Optum

D1625535

2023 coding guidelines included

Expert

ICD-10-CM Expert for Physicians

The complete official code set

Codes valid from October 1, 2022
through September 30, 2023

2023

optumcoding.com

Publisher's Notice

The *ICD-10-CM Expert for Physicians: The Complete Official Code Set* is designed to be an accurate and authoritative source regarding coding and every reasonable effort has been made to ensure accuracy and completeness of the content. However, Optum makes no guarantee, warranty, or representation that this publication is accurate, complete or without errors. It is understood that Optum is not rendering any legal or other professional services or advice in this publication and that Optum bears no liability for any results or consequences that may arise from the use of this book.

Acknowledgments

Karen Randall, CPC, *Product Manager*
Anita Schmidt, BS, RHIA, AHIMA-approved ICD-10-CM/PCS Trainer, *Subject Matter Expert*
Leanne Patterson, CPC, *Subject Matter Expert*
LaJuana Green, RHIA, CCS, *Subject Matter Expert*
Jacqueline R. Petersen, BS, RHIA, CHDA, CPC, *Subject Matter Expert*
Stacy Perry, *Manager, Desktop Publishing*
Tracy Betzler, *Senior Desktop Publishing Specialist*
Hope M. Dunn, *Senior Desktop Publishing Specialist*
Kate Russell, *Desktop Publishing Specialist*
Kate Holden, *Editor*

Our Commitment to Accuracy

Optum is committed to producing accurate and reliable materials.

To report corrections, please email customerassistance@optum.com. You can also reach customer service by calling 1.800.464.3649, option 1.

Leanne Patterson, CPC

Ms. Patterson has more than 15 years of experience in the healthcare profession. She has an extensive background in professional component coding, with expertise in E/M coding and auditing, and HIPAA compliance. Her experience includes general surgery coding, serving as Director of Compliance, conducting chart-to-claim audits, and physician education. She has been responsible for coding and denial management in large multi-specialty physician practices, and most recently has been part of a team developing content for educational products related to ICD-10-CM. Ms. Patterson is credentialed by the American Academy of Professional Coders (AAPC) as a Certified Professional Coder (CPC).

LaJuana Green, RHIA, CCS

Ms. Green is a Registered Health Information Administrator with over 35 years of experience in multiple areas of information management. She has proven expertise in the analysis of medical record documentation, assignment of ICD-10-CM and PCS codes, DRG validation, and CPT code assignment in ambulatory surgery units and the hospital outpatient setting. Her experience includes serving as a director of a health information management department, clinical technical editing, new technology research and writing, medical record management, utilization review activities, quality assurance, tumor registry, medical library services, and chargemaster maintenance. Ms. Green is an active member of the American Health Information Management Association (AHIMA).

2023 ICD-10-CM Official Guidelines for Coding and Reporting

Optum is pleased to provide you with this 2023 ICD-10-CM code book that INCLUDES the 2023 Official Guidelines for Coding and Reporting.

Product Updates

Significant updates to this manual will also be provided on our product updates page at Optumcoding.com, which can be accessed at the following:
https://www.optumcoding.com/ProductUpdates/
Password: Provider23

At our core, we're about coding

Essential medical code sets are just that — essential to your revenue cycle. In our ICD-10-CM/PCS, CPT®, HCPCS and DRG coding tools, we apply our collective coding expertise to present these code set resources in a way that is comprehensive, as well as easy to use and apply. Optum publications (print and eBook) are budget-friendly and easily referenced, created with intuitive features and formats, such as visual alerts, color-coding and symbols to identify important coding notes and instructions — plus, great coding tips.

Find the same content, tips and features of our code books in a variety of formats. Choose from print and eBook publications, online coding tools, data files or web services.

Your coding, billing and reimbursement product team,

Ryan Nichole Greg LaJuana Karen
Anita Ken Denise Leanne
Jacqui Marianne Elizabeth Nann Debbie

Put Optum medical coding, billing and reimbursement content at your fingertips today. Choose what works for you.

- Publications (print and eBook)
- Online coding tools
- Data files
- Web services

Visit us at **optumcoding.com** to browse our products, or call us at 1-800-464-3649, option 1, for more information.

Contents

How to Use ICD-10-CM Expert for Physicians 2023

Introduction

ICD-10-CM Expert for Physicians: The Complete Official Code Set is your definitive coding resource, combining the work of the National Center for Health Statistics (NCHS), Centers for Medicare and Medicaid Services (CMS), American Hospital Association (AHA), and Optum experts to provide the information you need for coding accuracy.

The International Classification of Diseases, 10th Revision, Clinical Modification (ICD-10-CM), is an adaptation of ICD-10, copyrighted by the World Health Organization (WHO). The development and maintenance of this clinical modification (CM) is the responsibility of the NCHS as authorized by WHO. Any new concepts added to ICD-10-CM are based on an established update process through the collaboration of WHO's Update and Revision Committee and the ICD-10-CM Coordination and Maintenance Committee.

In addition to the ICD-10-CM classification, other official government source information has been included in this manual. Depending on the source, updates to information may be annual or quarterly. This manual provides the most current information that was available at the time of publication. For updates to the source documents that may have occurred after this manual was published, please refer to the following:

- **NCHS, International Classification of Diseases, Tenth Revision, Clinical Modification (ICD-10-CM)**

  https://www.cms.gov/medicare/icd-10/2023-icd-10-cm

- **CMS Integrated Outpatient Code Editor (IOCE), version 23.2**

  https://www.cms.gov/Medicare/Coding/OutpatientCodeEdit/OCEQtrReleaseSpecs.html

- **CMS-HCC Risk Adjustment Model, version 24**

- **CMS ESRD-HCC Risk Adjustment Model, version 24**

- **CMS RxHCC Risk Adjustment Model, version 08**

  https://www.cms.gov/Medicare/Health-Plans/MedicareAdvtgSpecRateStats/Risk-Adjustors.html

- **HHS-HCC Commercial Risk Adjustment Model, version 07**

  https://www.cms.gov/CCIIO/Resources/Regulations-and-Guidance

- **CMS Quality Payment Program (QPP)**

  https://qpp.cms.gov/mips/explore-measures/quality-measures?tab=qualityMeasures&py=2022

- **AHA Coding Clinics**

  https://www.codingclinicadvisor.com/

The official NCHS ICD-10-CM classification includes three main sections: the guidelines, the indexes, and the tabular list, all of which make up the bulk of this coding manual. To complement the classification, Optum's coding experts have incorporated Medicare-related coding edits and proprietary features, such as supplementary notations, coding tools, and appendixes, into a comprehensive and easy-to-use reference. This publication is organized as follows:

What's New for 2023

This section provides a high-level overview of the code changes made for fiscal 2023. The list of codes provided identifies new, revised, and deleted codes. Asterisked codes identify prior midyear changes that were made to the classification, effective April 1, 2022. All changes are based on official addenda, provided by the National Center for Health Statistics (NCHS), the agency charged with maintaining and updating ICD-10-CM. NCHS is part of the Centers for Disease Control and Prevention (CDC).

Conversion Table

The conversion table was developed by National Center for Healthcare Statistics (NCHS) to help facilitate data retrieval as new codes are added to the ICD-10-CM classification. This table provides a crosswalk from each fiscal 2023 new code to the equivalent code(s) assigned, prior to October 1, 2022, for that diagnosis or condition. Asterisked codes identify prior midyear additions, effective April 1, 2022. For the full conversion table, refer to the Conversion Table zip file at https://www.cms.gov/medicare/icd-10/2023-icd-10-cm.

10 Steps to Correct Coding

This step-by-step tutorial walks the coder through the process of finding the correct code — from locating the code in the official indexes to verifying the code in the tabular section — while following applicable conventions, guidelines, and instructional notes. Specific examples are provided with detailed explanations of each coding step along with advice for proper sequencing.

Official ICD-10-CM Guidelines for Coding and Reporting

This section provides the full official conventions and guidelines regulating the appropriate assignment and reporting of ICD-10-CM codes. These conventions and guidelines are published by the U.S. Department of Health and Human Services (DHHS) and approved by the cooperating parties (American Health Information Management Association [AHIMA], National Center for Health Statistics [NCHS], Centers for Disease Control and Prevention [CDC], and the American Hospital Association [AHA]).

Indexes

Index to Diseases and Injuries

The Index to Diseases and Injuries is arranged in alphabetic order by terms specific to a disease, condition, illness, injury, eponym, or abbreviation as well as terms that describe circumstances other than a disease or injury that may require attention from a health care professional.

Neoplasm Table

The Neoplasm Table is arranged in alphabetic order by anatomical site. Codes are then listed in individual columns based upon the histological behavior (malignant, in situ, benign, uncertain, or unspecified) of the neoplasm.

Table of Drugs and Chemicals

The Table of Drugs and Chemicals is arranged in alphabetic order by the specific drug or chemical name. Codes are listed in individual columns based upon the associated intent (poisoning, adverse effect, or underdosing). Drugs with an asterisk identify substances added to the table by Optum subject matter experts.

External Causes Index

The External Causes Index is arranged in alphabetic order by main terms that describe the cause, the intent, the place of occurrence, the activity, and the status of the patient at the time the injury occurred or health condition arose.

Index Notations

With

The word "with" or "in" should be interpreted to mean "associated with" or "due to." The classification presumes a causal relationship between the two conditions linked by these terms in the index. These conditions should be coded as related even in the absence of provider documentation explicitly linking them unless the documentation clearly states the conditions are unrelated or when another guideline specifically requires a documented linkage between two conditions (e.g., the sepsis guideline for "acute organ dysfunction that is not clearly associated with the sepsis"). For conditions not specifically linked by these relational terms in the classification or when a guideline requires explicit documentation of a linkage between two conditions, provider documentation must link the conditions to code them as related.

The word "with" in the index is sequenced immediately following the main term, not in alphabetical order.

> **Dermatopolymyositis** M33.90
>   with
>   myopathy M33.92
>   respiratory involvement M33.91
>   specified organ involvement NEC M33.99
>   amyopathic M33.93

See

When the instruction "see" follows a term in the index, it indicates that another term must be referenced to locate the correct code.

> **Hematoperitoneum** — *see* Hemoperitoneum

See Also

The instructional note "see also" simply provides alternative terms the coder may reference that may be useful in determining the correct code but are not necessary to follow if the main term supplies the appropriate code.

> **Hematinuria** — *see also* Hemaglobinuria
>   malarial B50.8

Default Codes

In the index, the default code is the code listed next to the main term and represents the condition most commonly associated with that main term. This code may be assigned when documentation does not support reporting a more specific code. Alternatively, it may provide an unspecified code for the condition.

> **Hemiatrophy** R68.89
>   cerebellar G31.9
>   face, facial, progressive (Romberg) G51.8
>   tongue K14.8

Parentheses

Parentheses in the indexes enclose nonessential modifiers, supplementary words that may be present or absent in the statement of a disease without affecting the code.

> **Pseudomeningocele** (cerebral) (infective) (post-traumatic) G96.198
>   postprocedural (spinal) G97.82

Brackets

ICD-10-CM has a coding convention addressing code assignment for manifestations that occur as a result of an underlying condition. This convention requires the underlying condition to be sequenced first, followed by the code or codes for the associated manifestation. In the index, italicized codes in brackets identify manifestation codes.

> **Polyneuropathy** (peripheral) G62.9
>   alcoholic G62.1
>   amyloid (Portuguese) E85.1 *[G63]*
>   transthyretin-related (ATTR) familial E85.1*[G63]*

Shaded Guides

Exclusive vertical shaded guides in the Index to Diseases and Injuries and External Causes Index help the user easily follow the indent levels for the subentries under a main term. Sequencing rules may apply depending on the level of indent for separate subentries.

> **Hemicrania**
>   congenital malformation Q00.0
>   continua G44.51
>   meaning migraine — *see also* Migraine G43.909
>   paroxysmal G44.039
>   chronic G44.049
>   intractable G44.041
>   not intractable G44.049
>   episodic G44.039
>   intractable G44.031
>   not intractable G44.039
>   intractable G44.031
>   not intractable G44.039

Following References

The Index to Diseases and Injuries includes "following" references to assist in locating out-of-sequence codes in the tabular list. Out-of-sequence codes contain an alphabetic character (letter) in the third- or fourth-character position. These codes are placed according to the classification rules — according to condition — not according to alphabetic or numeric sequencing rules.

> **Carcinoma** (malignant) — *see also* Neoplasm, by site, malignant
>   neuroendocrine — *see also* Tumor, neuroendocrine
>   high grade, any site C7A.1- (*following* C75)
>   poorly differentiated, any site C7A.1 (*following* C75)

Additional Character Required

The Index to Diseases and Injuries, Neoplasm Table, and External Causes Index provide an icon after certain codes to signify to the user that additional characters are required to make the code valid. The tabular list should be consulted for appropriate character selection.

> **Fall, falling** (accidental) W19 ☑
>   building W20.1 ☑

Tabular List of Diseases

ICD-10-CM codes and descriptions are arranged numerically within the tabular list of diseases with 19 separate chapters providing codes associated with a particular body system or nature of injury or disease. There is also a chapter providing codes for external causes of an injury or health conditions, a chapter for codes that address encounters with healthcare facilities for circumstances other than a disease or injury, and finally, a chapter for codes that capture special circumstances such as new diseases of uncertain etiology or emergency use codes.

Code and Code Descriptions

ICD-10-CM is an alphanumeric classification system that contains categories, subcategories, and valid codes. The first character is always a letter with any additional characters represented by either a letter or number. A three-character category without further subclassification is equivalent to a valid three-character code. Valid codes may be three, four, five, six, or seven characters in length, with each level of subdivision after a three-character category representing a subcategory. The final level of subdivision is a valid code.

Boldface

Boldface type is used for all codes and descriptions in the tabular list.

Italics

Italicized type is used to identify manifestation codes, those codes that should not be reported as first-listed diagnoses.

Deleted Text

~~Strikethrough~~ on a code and code description indicates a deletion from the classification for the current year.

Key Word

Green font is used throughout the Tabular List of Diseases to differentiate the key words that appear in similar code descriptions in a given category or subcategory. The key word convention is used only in those categories in which there are multiple codes with very similar descriptions with only a few words that differentiate them.

For example, refer to the list of codes below from category H55:

✓4th **H55**	**Nystagmus and other irregular eye movements**	
✓5th	**H55.0 Nystagmus**	
	H55.00	**Unspecified nystagmus**
	H55.01	**Congenital nystagmus**
	H55.02	**Latent nystagmus**
	H55.03	**Visual deprivation nystagmus**
	H55.04	**Dissociated nystagmus**
	H55.09	**Other forms of nystagmus**

The portion of the code description that appears in green font in the tabular list helps the coder quickly identify the key terms and the correct code. This convention is especially useful when the codes describe laterality, such as the following codes from subcategory H40.22:

✓6th **H40.22**	**Chronic angle-closure glaucoma**	
	Chronic primary angle closure glaucoma	
✓7th	**H40.221**	**Chronic angle-closure glaucoma, right eye**
✓7th	**H40.222**	**Chronic angle-closure glaucoma, left eye**
✓7th	**H40.223**	**Chronic angle-closure glaucoma, bilateral**
✓7th	**H40.229**	**Chronic angle-closure glaucoma, unspecified eye**

Tabular Notations

Official parenthetical notes as well as Optum's supplementary notations are provided at the chapter, code block, category, subcategory, and individual code level to help the user assign proper codes. The information in the notation can apply to one or more codes depending on where the citation is placed.

Official Notations

Includes Notes

The word INCLUDES appears immediately under certain categories to further define, clarify, or give examples of the content of a code category.

Inclusion Terms

Lists of inclusion terms are included under certain codes. These terms indicate some of the conditions for which that code number may be used. Inclusion terms may be synonyms with the code title, or, in the case of "other specified" codes, the terms may also provide a list of various conditions included within a classification code. The inclusion terms are not exhaustive. The index may provide additional terms that may also be assigned to a given code.

Excludes Notes

ICD-10-CM has two types of excludes notes. Each note has a different definition for use. However, they are similar in that they both indicate that codes excluded from each other are independent of each other.

Excludes 1

An EXCLUDES 1 note is a "pure" excludes. It means "NOT CODED HERE!" An Excludes 1 note indicates mutually exclusive codes: two conditions that cannot be reported together. An Excludes1 note indicates that the code excluded should never be used at the same time as the code above the Excludes1 note. An Excludes1 is used when two conditions cannot occur together, such as a congenital form versus an acquired form of the same condition.

An exception to the Excludes 1 definition is when the two conditions are unrelated to each other. If it is not clear whether the two conditions involving an Excludes 1 note are related or not, query the provider. For example, code F45.8 Other somatoform disorders, has an Excludes 1 note for "sleep related teeth grinding (G47.63)" because "teeth grinding" is an inclusion term under F45.8. Only one of these two codes should be assigned for teeth grinding. However psychogenic dysmenorrhea is also an inclusion term under F45.8, and a patient could have both this condition and sleep-related teeth grinding. In this case, the two conditions are clearly unrelated to each other, so it would be appropriate to report F45.8 and G47.63 together.

Excludes 2

An EXCLUDES 2 note means "NOT INCLUDED HERE." An Excludes 2 note indicates that although the excluded condition is not part of the condition it is excluded from, a patient may have both conditions at the same time. Therefore, when an Excludes 2 note appears under a code, it may be acceptable to use both the code and the excluded code together if supported by the medical documentation.

Note

The term "NOTE" appears as an icon and precedes the instructional information. These notes function as alerts to highlight coding instructions within the text.

Code First/Use additional code

These instructional notes provide sequencing instruction. They may appear independently of each other or to designate certain etiology/manifestation paired codes. These instructions signal the coder that an additional code should be reported to provide a more complete picture of that diagnosis.

In etiology/manifestation coding, ICD-10-CM requires the underlying condition to be sequenced first, followed by the manifestation. In these situations, codes with "In diseases classified elsewhere" in the code description are never permitted as a first-listed or principal diagnosis code and must be sequenced following the underlying condition code.

Code Also

A "code also" note alerts the coder that more than one code may be required to fully describe the condition. The sequencing depends on the circumstances of the encounter. Factors that may determine sequencing include severity and reason for the encounter.

Revised Text

The revised text ▶◀ "bow ties" alert the user to changes in official notations for the current year. Revised text may include the following:

- A change in a current parenthetical description

- A change in the code(s) associated with a current parenthetical note

- A change in how a current parenthetical note is classified (e.g., an Excludes 1 note that changed to an Excludes 2 note)

- Addition of a new parenthetical note(s) to a code

Deleted Text

~~Strikethrough~~ on official notations indicate a deletion from the classification for the current year.

Optum Notations

AHA Coding Clinic Citations

Coding Clinics are official American Hospital Association (AHA) publications that provide coding advice specific to ICD-10-CM and ICD-10-PCS.

Coding Clinic citations included in this manual are current up to the second quarter of 2022.

These citations identify the year, quarter, and page number of one or more *Coding Clinic* publications that may have coding advice relevant to a particular code or group of codes. With the most current citation listed first, these notations are preceded by the symbol **AHA:** and appear in purple type.

I15.1	**Hypertension secondary to other renal disorders**
	AHA: 2016, 3Q, 22

Definitions

Definitions explain a specific term, condition, or disease process in layman's terms. These notations are preceded by the symbol **DEF:** and appear in purple type.

✓5ᵗʰ **M51.4**	**Schmorl's nodes**
	DEF: Irregular bone defect in the margin of the vertebral body that causes herniation into the end plate of the vertebral body.

Coding Tips

The tips in the tabular list offer coding advice that is not readily available within the ICD-10-CM classification. It may relate official coding guidelines, indexing nuances, or advice from *AHA's Coding Clinic for ICD-10-CM/PCS*. These notations are preceded by the symbol **TIP:** and appear in brown type.

✓5ᵗʰ **B97.2**	**Coronavirus as the cause of diseases classified elsewhere**
	TIP: Do not report a code from this subcategory for COVID-19, refer to U07.1.

Icons

Note: The following icons are placed to the left of the code.

Changes to ICD-10-CM codes, since the last published edition of this manual, are highlighted in two ways:

The following green icons identify new or revised codes effective April 1, 2022:

● **New Code – Midyear**

▲ **Revised Code – Midyear**

The following black icons identify new or revised codes effective October 1, 2022:

● **New Code**

▲ **Revised Code**

☑ **Additional Characters Required**

✓4ᵗʰ This symbol indicates that the code requires a 4th character.

✓5ᵗʰ This symbol indicates that the code requires a 5th character.

✓6ᵗʰ This symbol indicates that the code requires a 6th character.

✓7ᵗʰ This symbol indicates that the code requires a 7th character.

✓5ᵗʰ **H60.3**	**Other** infective **otitis externa**	
✓6ᵗʰ **H60.31**	Diffuse **otitis externa**	
H60.311	Diffuse otitis externa, right ear	
H60.312	Diffuse otitis externa, left ear	
H60.313	Diffuse otitis externa, bilateral	
H60.319	Diffuse otitis externa, unspecified ear	

✓x7ᵗʰ **Placeholder Alert**

This symbol indicates that the code requires a 7th character following the placeholder "X". Codes with fewer than six characters that require a 7th character must contain placeholder "X" to fill in the empty character(s).

✓x7ᵗʰ **T16.1**	**Foreign body in** right **ear**

This manual provides the most current information that was available at the time of publication. Except where otherwise noted, the icons and/or color bars reflect edits provided in the Integrated Outpatient Code Editor (IOCE) quarterly files utilized under the outpatient prospective payment system (OPPS). Because the October 2022 quarterly files were not available at the time this book was printed, the edits in this manual are based on the July 2022 quarterly files.

Note: In an effort to provide the most current edit information, Optum has provided a searchable data file that includes the final edit designations for all ICD-10-CM codes based on the IOCE October 2022 quarterly files. The edits included in the data file are as follows:

- Age

- Sex

- Manifestation

- Unacceptable principal diagnosis

This data file can be accessed at the following:

https://www.optumcoding.com/ProductUpdates/

Title: "2023 ICD-10-CM Outpatient Edits Data File"

Password: Provider23

Note: The following icons are placed at the end of the code description.

Age Edits

Ⓝ **Newborn Age: 0**
These diagnoses are intended for newborns and neonates and the patient's age must be 0 years.

> **N47.Ø** **Adherent prepuce, newborn**   Ⓝ ♂

Ⓟ **Pediatric Age: 0-17**
These diagnoses are intended for children and the patient's age must be between 0 and 17 years.

> **L21.1** **Seborrheic** infantile dermatitis   Ⓟ

Ⓜ **Maternity Age: 9-64**
These diagnoses are intended for childbearing patients between the age of 9 and 64 years.

> **OØ2.9** **Abnormal product of conception, unspecified**   Ⓜ ♀

Ⓐ **Adult Age: 15-124**
These diagnoses are intended for patients between the age of 15 and 124 years.

> **R54** **Age-related physical debility**   Ⓐ
>   Frailty
>   Old age
>   Senescence
>   Senile asthenia
>   Senile debility
>   **EXCLUDES 1** *age-related cognitive decline (R41.81)*
>   *sarcopenia (M62.84)*
>   *senile psychosis (FØ3)*
>   *senility NOS (R41.81)*

Sex Edits

♂ **Male diagnosis only**

> **Q98.Ø** **Klinefelter syndrome karyotype 47, XXY**   ♂

♀ **Female diagnosis only**

> **N35.12** **Postinfective urethral stricture, not elsewhere classified,** female   ♀

UPD **Unacceptable Principal Diagnosis**
This icon identifies codes that are not appropriate as a first-listed code for *outpatient* encounters. These codes describe circumstances that influence an individual's health status but are not a current illness or injury, or that are not specifically manifestations but may be due to an underlying cause.

> ✓7ᵗʰ **T48.5X5** **Adverse effect** of other anti-common-cold drugs **UPD**

HCC **CMS-HCC Condition**
This icon identifies codes that are considered a CMS-HCC (hierarchical condition category) diagnosis.

The HCC codes represented in this manual have been updated to reflect the 2023 Initial ICD-10-CM Mappings for CMS-HCC Model v24.

> **Y62.2** **Failure of sterile precautions during** kidney dialysis and other perfusion   **HCC**

Rx **Rx-HCC Condition**
This icon identifies codes that are included in the Rx-HCC risk-adjustment model, which covers the Part D (prescription drug) benefit.

The Rx-HCC codes represented in this manual have been updated to reflect the 2023 Initial ICD-10-CM Mappings for CMS Rx-HCC Model v08.

> **Z21** **Asymptomatic human immunodeficiency virus [HIV] infection status**   **HCC** **Rx** **ESR** **COM**

ESR **ESRD HCC Condition**
This icon identifies codes that are included in the end-stage renal disease (ESRD) HCC risk-adjustment model.

The ESRD HCC codes represented in this manual have been updated to reflect the 2023 Initial ICD-10-CM Mappings for CMS ESRD HCC Model v24.

> **Z21** **Asymptomatic human immunodeficiency virus [HIV] infection status**   **HCC** **Rx** **ESR** **COM**

COM **Commercial HCC Condition**
This icon identifies codes that are included in the commercial HHS-HCC risk-adjustment model.

The commercial HCC codes represented in this manual are based on the commercial HCC Model v07.

> **Z21** **Asymptomatic human immunodeficiency virus [HIV] infection status**   **HCC** **Rx** **ESR** **COM**

Note: Finalized ICD-10-CM to HCC mappings for CMS-HCC, Rx-HCC, ESRD HCC, and Commercial HCC have been provided in an easily searchable data file that can be accessed at the following:

https://www.optumcoding.com/ProductUpdates/

Title: "2023 Final ICD-10-CM to HCC Mappings Data File"

Password: Provider23

Q **QPP Condition**
This icon identifies codes recognized as a quality measure for claims-based reporting under CMS's Merit-based Incentive Payment System (MIPS) Claims Single Source v6.0.

> **G44.52** New daily persistent headache (NDPH)   **Q**

PDx **Z-code as First-Listed Diagnosis**
Section IV of the official guidelines states that the term "first-listed diagnosis" is used instead of principal diagnosis in the outpatient setting and represents the diagnosis that is chiefly responsible for the services provided during the encounter. This icon identifies Z codes that, in general, may be reported only as a first-listed diagnosis. According to guideline I.C.21.c.16, these are the only Z codes that are specifically meant to be utilized as a first-listed diagnosis; all other Z codes may be either first-listed or secondary diagnoses, depending upon the circumstances of the encounter, coding instructions, and guidelines.

Note: The codes identified with this icon may be used as a secondary diagnosis if the patient has multiple encounters on the same day and those medical records are combined.

A comprehensive list of all Z codes primarily used as first-listed diagnoses appears in appendix D of this book.

> **Z51.12** **Encounter for antineoplastic** immunotherapy   **PDx**

How to Use ICD-10-CM Expert for Physicians 2023

Color Bars

Manifestation Code

Codes defined as manifestation codes appear in italic type, with a blue color bar over the code description. A manifestation cannot be reported as a first-listed code; it is sequenced as a secondary diagnosis with the underlying disease code listed first.

> **G32.89** *Other specified degenerative disorders of nervous system in diseases classified elsewhere*
> Degenerative encephalopathy in diseases classified elsewhere

Unspecified Diagnosis

Codes that appear with a gray color bar over the alphanumeric code identify unspecified diagnoses. These codes should be used in limited circumstances, when neither the diagnostic statement nor the documentation provides enough information to assign a more specific diagnosis code. The abbreviation NOS, "not otherwise specified," in the tabular list may be interpreted as "unspecified."

> **G03.9** **Meningitis, unspecified**
> Arachnoiditis (spinal) NOS

Footnotes

Certain codes in the tabular section have a numerical superscript located to the upper left of the code. This numerical superscript corresponds to a specific footnote description.

For example:

> [1] ✓7ᵗʰ **M48.51** **Collapsed vertebra, not elsewhere classified, occipito-atlanto-axial region** HCC

For convenience, the footnote descriptions are provided on the front cover.

The following list also provides the footnote descriptions of all numerical superscripts found in the Tabular List of Diseases:

1 These codes are considered an HCC when reported as an initial encounter (7th character A, B, or C).

2 These codes are considered an HCC when reported as an initial encounter (7th character A or B) OR sequela (7th character S).

3 These codes are considered an HCC when reported as a sequela (7th character S).

Chapter-Level Notations

Chapter-specific Guidelines with Coding Examples

Each chapter begins with the Official Guidelines for Coding and Reporting specific to that chapter, where provided. Coding examples specific to outpatient care settings have been provided to illustrate the coding and/or sequencing guidance in these guidelines.

Muscle and Tendon Table

ICD-10-CM categorizes certain muscles and tendons in the upper and lower extremities by their action (e.g., extension or flexion) as well as their anatomical location. The Muscle/Tendon table is provided at the beginning of chapter 13 and chapter 19 to help users when code selection depends on the action of the muscle and/or tendon.

Note: This table is not all-inclusive, and proper code assignment should be based on the provider's documentation.

Appendixes

The additional resources described below have been included as appendixes for this book. These resources further instruct the professional coder on the appropriate application of the ICD-10-CM code set.

Appendix A: Valid 3-character ICD-10-CM Codes

The user may consult this table to confirm that no further specificity, such as the use of 4th, 5th, 6th, or 7th characters or placeholders (X), is necessary. All ICD-10-CM codes that are valid at the three-character level are listed.

Appendix B: Pharmacology List 2023

This reference is a comprehensive but not all-inclusive list of pharmacological agents used to treat acute and/or chronic conditions. Drugs are listed in alphabetical order by their brand and/or generic names along with their drug action and indications for which they may commonly be prescribed. Some drugs have also been mapped to their appropriate Z code for long-term drug use.

Appendix C: Z Codes for Long-Term Drug Use with Associated Drugs

This resource correlates Z codes that are used to identify current long-term drug use with a list of drugs that are typically categorized to that class of drug.

Note: These tables are not all-inclusive but list some of the more commonly used drugs.

Appendix D: Z Codes Only as Principal/First-Listed Diagnosis

This resource provides a comprehensive list of Z codes that are primarily used as first-listed diagnoses for outpatient encounters.

Appendix E: Centers for Medicare & Medicaid Services Hierarchical Condition Categories (CMS-HCC)

This resource provides the framework behind the Centers for Medicare and Medicaid Services' (CMS) Medicare Advantage (MA) program, a risk-adjustment model developed as a means of compensating health care plans with large numbers of Medicare Part C beneficiaries. It includes a brief synopsis of the evolution of the program from its inception; insight into the various elements needed to predict risk, including the principles used to develop the hierarchical condition categories (HCCs), which make up one of the fundamental components of the risk-adjustment model. This appendix also outlines the audit process used to ensure the accuracy of payments made to MA plans.

Appendix F: Centers for Medicare & Medicaid Services Quality Payment Program

This resource provides an overview of the Medicare Access and CHIP Reauthorization Act (MACRA), which replaced Medicare's sustainable growth rate (SGR) methodology with the Quality Payment Program (QPP). It summarizes the Merit-based Incentive Payment System (MIPS) track used by those who opt to participate in traditional Medicare and not an advanced alternative payment model (APM). This includes eligibility requirements and an overview of the four performance categories that combine to make up the MIPS.

Illustrations

This section includes illustrations of normal anatomy with ICD-10-CM-specific terminology.

What's New for 2023

Official Updates

A summary of changes to the official ICD-10-CM code set is provided below, identifying changes made for fiscal 2023, effective October 1, 2022, to September 30, 2023. Asterisked codes identify prior midyear changes that were made to the classification, effective April 1, 2022. All code changes were made by the agency charged with maintaining and updating the ICD-10-CM code set, the National Center for Health Statistics (NCHS), a section of the Centers for Disease Control and Prevention (CDC).

1179 New Codes

B37.31	B37.32	D59.30	D59.31	D59.32
D59.39	D68.00	D68.01	D68.020	D68.021
D68.022	D68.023	D68.029	D68.03	D68.04
D68.09	D75.821	D75.822	D75.828	D75.829
D75.84	D81.82	E34.30	E34.31	E34.321
E34.322	E34.328	E34.329	E34.39	E87.20
E87.21	E87.22	E87.29	F01.511	F01.518
F01.52	F01.53	F01.54	F01.A0	F01.A11
F01.A18	F01.A2	F01.A3	F01.A4	F01.B0
F01.B11	F01.B18	F01.B2	F01.B3	F01.B4
F01.C0	F01.C11	F01.C18	F01.C2	F01.C3
F01.C4	F02.811	F02.818	F02.82	F02.83
F02.84	F02.A0	F02.A11	F02.A18	F02.A2
F02.A3	F02.A4	F02.B0	F02.B11	F02.B18
F02.B2	F02.B3	F02.B4	F02.C0	F02.C11
F02.C18	F02.C2	F02.C3	F02.C4	F03.911
F03.918	F03.92	F03.93	F03.94	F03.A0
F03.A11	F03.A18	F03.A2	F03.A3	F03.A4
F03.B0	F03.B11	F03.B18	F03.B2	F03.B3
F03.B4	F03.C0	F03.C11	F03.C18	F03.C2
F03.C3	F03.C4	F06.70	F06.71	F10.90
F10.91	F11.91	F12.91	F13.91	F14.91
F15.91	F16.91	F18.91	F19.91	F43.81
F43.89	G71.031	G71.032	G71.033	G71.0340
G71.0341	G71.0342	G71.0349	G71.035	G71.038
G71.039	G90.A	G93.31	G93.32	G93.39
I20.2	I25.112	I25.702	I25.712	I25.722
I25.732	I25.752	I25.762	I25.792	I31.31
I31.39	I34.81	I34.89	I47.20	I47.21
I47.29	I71.010	I71.011	I71.012	I71.019
I71.10	I71.11	I71.12	I71.13	I71.20
I71.21	I71.22	I71.23	I71.30	I71.31
I71.32	I71.33	I71.40	I71.41	I71.42
I71.43	I71.50	I71.51	I71.52	I71.60
I71.61	I71.62	I77.82	J95.87	K76.82
M51.A0	M51.A1	M51.A2	M51.A3	M51.A4
M51.A5	M62.5A0	M62.5A1	M62.5A2	M62.5A9
M93.004	M93.014	M93.024	M93.034	M93.041
M93.042	M93.043	M93.044	M93.051	M93.052
M93.053	M93.054	M93.061	M93.062	M93.063
M93.064	M93.071	M93.072	M93.073	M93.074
M96.A1	M96.A2	M96.A3	M96.A4	M96.A9
N14.11	N14.19	N76.82	N80.00	N80.01
N80.02	N80.03	N80.101	N80.102	N80.103
N80.109	N80.111	N80.112	N80.113	N80.119
N80.121	N80.122	N80.123	N80.129	N80.201
N80.202	N80.203	N80.209	N80.211	N80.212
N80.213	N80.219	N80.221	N80.222	N80.223
N80.229	N80.30	N80.311	N80.312	N80.319
N80.321	N80.322	N80.329	N80.331	N80.332
N80.333	N80.339	N80.341	N80.342	N80.343
N80.349	N80.351	N80.352	N80.353	N80.359
N80.361	N80.362	N80.363	N80.369	N80.371
N80.372	N80.373	N80.379	N80.381	N80.382
N80.383	N80.389	N80.391	N80.392	N80.399
N80.3A1	N80.3A2	N80.3A3	N80.3A9	N80.3B1
N80.3B2	N80.3B3	N80.3B9	N80.3C1	N80.3C2
N80.3C3	N80.3C9	N80.40	N80.41	N80.42
N80.50	N80.511	N80.512	N80.519	N80.521
N80.522	N80.529	N80.531	N80.532	N80.539
N80.541	N80.542	N80.549	N80.551	N80.552
N80.559	N80.561	N80.562	N80.569	N80.A0
N80.A1	N80.A2	N80.A41	N80.A42	N80.A43
N80.A49	N80.A51	N80.A52	N80.A53	N80.A59
N80.A61	N80.A62	N80.A63	N80.A69	N80.B1
N80.B2	N80.B31	N80.B32	N80.B39	N80.B4
N80.B5	N80.B6	N80.C0	N80.C10	N80.C11
N80.C19	N80.C2	N80.C3	N80.C4	N80.C9
N80.D0	N80.D1	N80.D2	N80.D3	N80.D4
N80.D5	N80.D6	N80.D9	N85.A	O35.00X0
O35.00X1	O35.00X2	O35.00X3	O35.00X4	O35.00X5
O35.00X9	O35.01X0	O35.01X1	O35.01X2	O35.01X3
O35.01X4	O35.01X5	O35.01X9	O35.02X0	O35.02X1
O35.02X2	O35.02X3	O35.02X4	O35.02X5	O35.02X9
O35.03X0	O35.03X1	O35.03X2	O35.03X3	O35.03X4
O35.03X5	O35.03X9	O35.04X0	O35.04X1	O35.04X2
O35.04X3	O35.04X4	O35.04X5	O35.04X9	O35.05X0
O35.05X1	O35.05X2	O35.05X3	O35.05X4	O35.05X5
O35.05X9	O35.06X0	O35.06X1	O35.06X2	O35.06X3
O35.06X4	O35.06X5	O35.06X9	O35.07X0	O35.07X1
O35.07X2	O35.07X3	O35.07X4	O35.07X5	O35.07X9
O35.08X0	O35.08X1	O35.08X2	O35.08X3	O35.08X4
O35.08X5	O35.08X9	O35.09X0	O35.09X1	O35.09X2
O35.09X3	O35.09X4	O35.09X5	O35.09X9	O35.10X0
O35.10X1	O35.10X2	O35.10X3	O35.10X4	O35.10X5
O35.10X9	O35.11X0	O35.11X1	O35.11X2	O35.11X3
O35.11X4	O35.11X5	O35.11X9	O35.12X0	O35.12X1
O35.12X2	O35.12X3	O35.12X4	O35.12X5	O35.12X9
O35.13X0	O35.13X1	O35.13X2	O35.13X3	O35.13X4
O35.13X5	O35.13X9	O35.14X0	O35.14X1	O35.14X2
O35.14X3	O35.14X4	O35.14X5	O35.14X9	O35.15X0
O35.15X1	O35.15X2	O35.15X3	O35.15X4	O35.15X5
O35.15X9	O35.19X0	O35.19X1	O35.19X2	O35.19X3
O35.19X4	O35.19X5	O35.19X9	O35.AXX0	O35.AXX1
O35.AXX2	O35.AXX3	O35.AXX4	O35.AXX5	O35.AXX9
O35.BXX0	O35.BXX1	O35.BXX2	O35.BXX3	O35.BXX4
O35.BXX5	O35.BXX9	O35.CXX0	O35.CXX1	O35.CXX2
O35.CXX3	O35.CXX4	O35.CXX5	O35.CXX9	O35.DXX0
O35.DXX1	O35.DXX2	O35.DXX3	O35.DXX4	O35.DXX5
O35.DXX9	O35.EXX0	O35.EXX1	O35.EXX2	O35.EXX3
O35.EXX4	O35.EXX5	O35.EXX9	O35.FXX0	O35.FXX1
O35.FXX2	O35.FXX3	O35.FXX4	O35.FXX5	O35.FXX9
O35.GXX0	O35.GXX1	O35.GXX2	O35.GXX3	O35.GXX4
O35.GXX5	O35.GXX9	O35.HXX0	O35.HXX1	O35.HXX2
O35.HXX3	O35.HXX4	O35.HXX5	O35.HXX9	P28.30
P28.31	P28.32	P28.33	P28.39	P28.40
P28.41	P28.42	P28.43	P28.49	Q21.10
Q21.11	Q21.12	Q21.13	Q21.14	Q21.15
Q21.16	Q21.19	Q21.20	Q21.21	Q21.22
Q21.23	Q85.81	Q85.82	Q85.83	Q85.89
S06.0XAA	S06.0XAD	S06.0XAS	S06.1XAA	S06.1XAD
S06.1XAS	S06.2XAA	S06.2XAD	S06.2XAS	S06.30AA
S06.30AD	S06.30AS	S06.31AA	S06.31AD	S06.31AS
S06.32AA	S06.32AD	S06.32AS	S06.33AA	S06.33AD
S06.33AS	S06.34AA	S06.34AD	S06.34AS	S06.35AA
S06.35AD	S06.35AS	S06.36AA	S06.36AD	S06.36AS
S06.37AA	S06.37AD	S06.37AS	S06.38AA	S06.38AD
S06.38AS	S06.4XAA	S06.4XAD	S06.4XAS	S06.5XAA

S06.5XAD	S06.5XAS	S06.6XAA	S06.6XAD	S06.6XAS
S06.81AA	S06.81AD	S06.81AS	S06.82AA	S06.82AD
S06.82AS	S06.89AA	S06.89AD	S06.89AS	S06.8A0A
S06.8A0D	S06.8A0S	S06.8A1A	S06.8A1D	S06.8A1S
S06.8A2A	S06.8A2D	S06.8A2S	S06.8A3A	S06.8A3D
S06.8A3S	S06.8A4A	S06.8A4D	S06.8A4S	S06.8A5A
S06.8A5D	S06.8A5S	S06.8A6A	S06.8A6D	S06.8A6S
S06.8A7A	S06.8A8A	S06.8A9A	S06.8A9D	S06.8A9S
S06.8AAA	S06.8AAD	S06.8AAS	S06.9XAA	S06.9XAD
S06.9XAS	T43.651A	T43.651D	T43.651S	T43.652A
T43.652D	T43.652S	T43.653A	T43.653D	T43.653S
T43.654A	T43.654D	T43.654S	T43.655A	T43.655D
T43.655S	T43.656A	T43.656D	T43.656S	V20.01XA
V20.01XD	V20.01XS	V20.09XA	V20.09XD	V20.09XS
V20.11XA	V20.11XD	V20.19XA	V20.19XS	V20.19XD
V20.19XS	V20.21XA	V20.21XD	V20.21XS	V20.29XA
V20.29XD	V20.29XS	V20.31XA	V20.31XD	V20.31XS
V20.39XA	V20.39XD	V20.39XS	V20.41XA	V20.41XD
V20.41XS	V20.49XA	V20.49XD	V20.49XS	V20.51XA
V20.51XD	V20.51XS	V20.59XA	V20.59XD	V20.59XS
V20.91XA	V20.91XD	V20.91XS	V20.99XA	V20.99XD
V20.99XS	V21.01XA	V21.01XD	V21.01XS	V21.09XA
V21.09XD	V21.09XS	V21.11XA	V21.11XD	V21.11XS
V21.19XA	V21.19XD	V21.19XS	V21.21XA	V21.21XD
V21.21XS	V21.29XA	V21.29XD	V21.29XS	V21.31XA
V21.31XD	V21.31XS	V21.39XA	V21.39XD	V21.39XS
V21.41XA	V21.41XD	V21.41XS	V21.49XA	V21.49XD
V21.49XS	V21.51XA	V21.51XD	V21.51XS	V21.59XA
V21.59XD	V21.59XS	V21.91XA	V21.91XD	V21.91XS
V21.99XA	V21.99XD	V21.99XS	V22.01XA	V22.01XD
V22.01XS	V22.09XA	V22.09XD	V22.09XS	V22.11XA
V22.11XD	V22.11XS	V22.19XA	V22.19XD	V22.19XS
V22.21XA	V22.21XD	V22.21XS	V22.29XA	V22.29XD
V22.29XS	V22.31XA	V22.31XD	V22.31XS	V22.39XA
V22.39XD	V22.39XS	V22.41XA	V22.41XD	V22.41XS
V22.49XA	V22.49XD	V22.49XS	V22.51XA	V22.51XD
V22.51XS	V22.59XA	V22.59XD	V22.59XS	V22.91XA
V22.91XD	V22.91XS	V22.99XA	V22.99XD	V22.99XS
V23.01XA	V23.01XD	V23.01XS	V23.09XA	V23.09XD
V23.09XS	V23.11XA	V23.11XD	V23.11XS	V23.19XA
V23.19XD	V23.19XS	V23.21XA	V23.21XD	V23.21XS
V23.29XA	V23.29XD	V23.29XS	V23.31XA	V23.31XD
V23.31XS	V23.39XA	V23.39XD	V23.39XS	V23.41XA
V23.41XD	V23.41XS	V23.49XA	V23.49XD	V23.49XS
V23.51XA	V23.51XD	V23.51XS	V23.59XA	V23.59XD
V23.59XS	V23.91XA	V23.91XD	V23.91XS	V23.99XA
V23.99XD	V23.99XS	V24.01XA	V24.01XD	V24.01XS
V24.09XA	V24.09XD	V24.09XS	V24.11XA	V24.11XD
V24.11XS	V24.19XA	V24.19XD	V24.19XS	V24.21XA
V24.21XD	V24.21XS	V24.29XA	V24.29XD	V24.29XS
V24.31XA	V24.31XD	V24.31XS	V24.39XA	V24.39XD
V24.39XS	V24.41XA	V24.41XD	V24.41XS	V24.49XA
V24.49XD	V24.49XS	V24.51XA	V24.51XD	V24.51XS
V24.59XA	V24.59XD	V24.59XS	V24.91XA	V24.91XD
V24.91XS	V24.99XA	V24.99XD	V24.99XS	V25.01XA
V25.01XD	V25.01XS	V25.09XA	V25.09XD	V25.09XS
V25.11XA	V25.11XD	V25.11XS	V25.19XA	V25.19XD
V25.19XS	V25.21XA	V25.21XD	V25.21XS	V25.29XA
V25.29XD	V25.29XS	V25.31XA	V25.31XD	V25.31XS
V25.39XA	V25.39XD	V25.39XS	V25.41XA	V25.41XD
V25.41XS	V25.49XA	V25.49XD	V25.49XS	V25.51XA
V25.51XD	V25.51XS	V25.59XA	V25.59XD	V25.59XS
V25.91XA	V25.91XD	V25.91XS	V25.99XA	V25.99XD
V25.99XS	V26.01XA	V26.01XD	V26.01XS	V26.09XA
V26.09XD	V26.09XS	V26.11XA	V26.11XD	V26.11XS
V26.19XA	V26.19XD	V26.19XS	V26.21XA	V26.21XD
V26.21XS	V26.29XA	V26.29XD	V26.29XS	V26.31XA

V26.31XD	V26.31XS	V26.39XA	V26.39XD	V26.39XS
V26.41XA	V26.41XD	V26.41XS	V26.49XA	V26.49XD
V26.49XS	V26.51XA	V26.51XD	V26.51XS	V26.59XA
V26.59XD	V26.59XS	V26.91XA	V26.91XD	V26.91XS
V26.99XA	V26.99XD	V26.99XS	V27.01XA	V27.01XD
V27.01XS	V27.09XA	V27.09XD	V27.09XS	V27.11XA
V27.11XD	V27.11XS	V27.19XA	V27.19XD	V27.19XS
V27.21XA	V27.21XD	V27.21XS	V27.29XA	V27.29XD
V27.29XS	V27.31XA	V27.31XD	V27.31XS	V27.39XA
V27.39XD	V27.39XS	V27.41XA	V27.41XD	V27.41XS
V27.49XA	V27.49XD	V27.49XS	V27.51XA	V27.51XA
V27.51XS	V27.59XA	V27.59XD	V27.59XS	V27.91XA
V27.91XD	V27.91XS	V27.99XA	V27.99XD	V27.99XS
V28.01XA	V28.01XD	V28.01XS	V28.09XA	V28.09XD
V28.09XS	V28.11XA	V28.11XD	V28.11XS	V28.19XA
V28.19XD	V28.19XS	V28.21XA	V28.21XD	V28.21XS
V28.29XA	V28.29XD	V28.29XS	V28.31XA	V28.31XD
V28.31XS	V28.39XA	V28.39XD	V28.39XS	V28.41XA
V28.41XD	V28.41XS	V28.49XA	V28.49XD	V28.49XS
V28.51XA	V28.51XD	V28.51XS	V28.59XA	V28.59XD
V28.59XS	V28.91XA	V28.91XD	V28.91XS	V28.99XA
V28.99XD	V28.99XS	V29.001A	V29.001D	V29.001S
V29.008A	V29.008D	V29.008S	V29.091A	V29.091D
V29.091S	V29.098A	V29.098D	V29.098S	V29.101A
V29.101D	V29.101S	V29.108A	V29.108D	V29.108S
V29.191A	V29.191D	V29.191S	V29.198A	V29.198D
V29.198S	V29.201A	V29.201D	V29.201S	V29.208A
V29.208D	V29.208S	V29.291A	V29.291D	V29.291S
V29.298A	V29.298D	V29.298S	V29.31A	V29.31XD
V29.31XS	V29.39XA	V29.39XD	V29.39XS	V29.401A
V29.401D	V29.401S	V29.408A	V29.408D	V29.408S
V29.491A	V29.491D	V29.491S	V29.498A	V29.498D
V29.498S	V29.501A	V29.501D	V29.501S	V29.508A
V29.508D	V29.508S	V29.591A	V29.591D	V29.591S
V29.598A	V29.598D	V29.598S	V29.601A	V29.601D
V29.601S	V29.608A	V29.608D	V29.608S	V29.691A
V29.691D	V29.691S	V29.698A	V29.698D	V29.698S
V29.811A	V29.811D	V29.811S	V29.818A	V29.818D
V29.818S	V29.881A	V29.881D	V29.881S	V29.888A
V29.888D	V29.888S	V29.91XA	V29.91XD	V29.91XS
V29.99XA	V29.99XD	V29.99XS	W23.2XXA	W23.2XXD
W23.2XXS	Z03.83	*Z28.310	*Z28.311	*Z28.39
Z59.82	Z59.86	Z59.87	Z71.87	Z71.88
Z72.823	Z79.60	Z79.61	Z79.620	Z79.621
Z79.622	Z79.623	Z79.624	Z79.630	Z79.631
Z79.632	Z79.633	Z79.634	Z79.64	Z79.69
Z79.85	Z87.61	Z87.68	Z87.731	Z87.732
Z87.760	Z87.761	Z87.762	Z87.763	Z87.768
Z91.110	Z91.118	Z91.119	Z91.190	Z91.198
Z91.199	Z91.A10	Z91.A18	Z91.A20	Z91.A28
Z91.A3	Z91.A4	Z91.A5	Z91.A9	

28 Revised Codes

Note: Each code is listed with its revised description only.

C84.40   Peripheral T-cell lymphoma, not elsewhere classified, unspecified site

C84.41   Peripheral T-cell lymphoma, not elsewhere classified, lymph nodes of head, face, and neck

C84.42   Peripheral T-cell lymphoma, not elsewhere classified, intrathoracic lymph nodes

C84.43   Peripheral T-cell lymphoma, not elsewhere classified, intra-abdominal lymph nodes

C84.44   Peripheral T-cell lymphoma, not elsewhere classified, lymph nodes of axilla and upper limb

C84.45   Peripheral T-cell lymphoma, not elsewhere classified, lymph nodes of inguinal region and lower limb

Code	Description
C84.46	Peripheral T-cell lymphoma, not elsewhere classified, intrapelvic lymph nodes
C84.47	Peripheral T-cell lymphoma, not elsewhere classified, spleen
C84.48	Peripheral T-cell lymphoma, not elsewhere classified, lymph nodes of multiple sites
C84.49	Peripheral T-cell lymphoma, not elsewhere classified, extranodal and solid organ sites
C94.6	Myelodysplastic disease, not elsewhere classified
F01.50	Vascular dementia, unspecified severity, without behavioral disturbance, psychotic disturbance, mood disturbance, and anxiety
F02.80	Dementia in other diseases classified elsewhere, unspecified severity, without behavioral disturbance, psychotic disturbance, mood disturbance, and anxiety
F03.90	Unspecified dementia, unspecified severity, without behavioral disturbance, psychotic disturbance, mood disturbance, and anxiety
G31.09	Other frontotemporal neurocognitive disorder
G31.83	Neurocognitive disorder with Lewy bodies
G31.84	Mild cognitive impairment of uncertain or unknown etiology
K35.32	Acute appendicitis with perforation, localized peritonitis, and gangrene, without abscess
K35.33	Acute appendicitis with perforation, localized peritonitis, and gangrene, with abscess
M93.011	Acute slipped upper femoral epiphysis, stable (nontraumatic), right hip
M93.012	Acute slipped upper femoral epiphysis, stable (nontraumatic), left hip
M93.013	Acute slipped upper femoral epiphysis, stable (nontraumatic), unspecified hip
M93.021	Chronic slipped upper femoral epiphysis, stable (nontraumatic), right hip
M93.022	Chronic slipped upper femoral epiphysis, stable (nontraumatic), left hip
M93.023	Chronic slipped upper femoral epiphysis, stable (nontraumatic), unspecified hip
M93.031	Acute on chronic slipped upper femoral epiphysis, stable (nontraumatic), right hip
M93.032	Acute on chronic slipped upper femoral epiphysis, stable (nontraumatic), left hip
M93.033	Acute on chronic slipped upper femoral epiphysis, stable (nontraumatic), unspecified hip

251 Deleted Codes

O35.0XX0	O35.0XX1	O35.0XX2	O35.0XX3	O35.0XX4
O35.0XX5	O35.0XX9	O35.1XX0	O35.1XX1	O35.1XX2
O35.1XX3	O35.1XX4	O35.1XX5	O35.1XX9	V20.0XXA
V20.0XXD	V20.0XXS	V20.1XXA	V20.1XXD	V20.1XXS
V20.2XXA	V20.2XXD	V20.2XXS	V20.3XXA	V20.3XXD
V20.3XXS	V20.4XXA	V20.4XXD	V20.4XXS	V20.5XXA

V20.5XXD	V20.5XXS	V20.9XXA	V20.9XXD	V20.9XXS
V21.0XXA	V21.0XXD	V21.0XXS	V21.1XXA	V21.1XXD
V21.1XXS	V21.2XXA	V21.2XXD	V21.2XXS	V21.3XXA
V21.3XXD	V21.3XXS	V21.4XXA	V21.4XXD	V21.4XXS
V21.5XXA	V21.5XXD	V21.5XXS	V21.9XXA	V21.9XXD
V21.9XXS	V22.0XXA	V22.0XXD	V22.0XXS	V22.1XXA
V22.1XXD	V22.1XXS	V22.2XXA	V22.2XXD	V22.2XXS
V22.3XXA	V22.3XXD	V22.3XXS	V22.4XXA	V22.4XXD
V22.4XXS	V22.5XXA	V22.5XXD	V22.5XXS	V22.9XXA
V22.9XXD	V22.9XXS	V23.0XXA	V23.0XXD	V23.0XXS
V23.1XXA	V23.1XXD	V23.1XXS	V23.2XXA	V23.2XXD
V23.2XXS	V23.3XXA	V23.3XXD	V23.3XXS	V23.4XXA
V23.4XXD	V23.4XXS	V23.5XXA	V23.5XXD	V23.5XXS
V23.9XXA	V23.9XXD	V23.9XXS	V24.0XXA	V24.0XXD
V24.0XXS	V24.1XXA	V24.1XXD	V24.1XXS	V24.2XXA
V24.2XXD	V24.2XXS	V24.3XXA	V24.3XXD	V24.3XXS
V24.4XXS	V24.4XXD	V24.4XXS	V24.5XXA	V24.5XXD
V24.5XXS	V24.9XXA	V24.9XXD	V24.9XXS	V25.0XXA
V25.0XXD	V25.0XXS	V25.1XXA	V25.1XXD	V25.1XXS
V25.2XXA	V25.2XXD	V25.2XXS	V25.3XXA	V25.3XXD
V25.3XXS	V25.4XXA	V25.4XXD	V25.4XXS	V25.5XXA
V25.5XXD	V25.5XXS	V26.0XXA	V26.0XXD	V26.0XXS
V26.1XXA	V26.1XXD	V26.1XXS	V26.2XXA	V26.2XXD
V26.2XXS	V26.3XXA	V26.3XXD	V26.3XXS	V26.4XXA
V26.4XXD	V26.4XXS	V26.5XXA	V26.5XXD	V26.5XXS
V26.9XXA	V26.9XXD	V26.9XXS	V27.0XXA	V27.0XXD
V27.0XXS	V27.1XXA	V27.1XXD	V27.1XXS	V27.2XXA
V27.2XXD	V27.2XXS	V27.3XXA	V27.3XXD	V27.3XXS
V27.4XXA	V27.4XXD	V27.4XXS	V27.5XXD	V27.5XXS
V27.9XXA	V27.9XXD	V27.9XXS	V28.0XXA	V28.0XXD
V28.0XXS	V28.1XXA	V28.1XXD	V28.1XXS	V28.2XXA
V28.2XXD	V28.2XXS	V28.3XXD	V28.3XXS	V28.4XXA
V28.4XXA	V28.4XXS	V28.5XXA	V28.5XXD	V28.5XXS
V28.9XXA	V28.9XXD	V28.9XXS	V29.00XA	V29.00XD
V29.00XS	V29.09XA	V29.09XD	V29.09XS	V29.10XA
V29.10XD	V29.10XS	V29.19XA	V29.19XD	V29.19XS
V29.20XA	V29.20XD	V29.20XS	V29.29XA	V29.29XD
V29.29XS	V29.3XXD	V29.3XXS	V29.40XA	V29.40XD
V29.40XD	V29.40XS	V29.49XA	V29.49XD	V29.49XS
V29.50XA	V29.50XD	V29.50XS	V29.59XA	V29.59XD
V29.59XS	V29.60XA	V29.60XD	V29.60XS	V29.69XA
V29.69XD	V29.69XS	V29.81XA	V29.81XD	V29.81XS
V29.88XA	V29.88XD	V29.88XS	V29.9XXA	V29.9XXD
V29.9XXS				

Proprietary Updates

The following proprietary features have also been added:

- New definitions that describe, in lay terms, a specific condition or disease process

- New coding tips that provide coding advice beyond the code classification

- Updated *AHA Coding Clinic* references through second quarter 2022

Conversion Table of ICD-10-CM Codes

The fiscal 2023 (October 1, 2022–September 30, 2023) Conversion Table for new ICD-10-CM codes is provided to assist users in data retrieval. For each new code the table shows its previously assigned code equivalent. Asterisks identify new codes added to the classification April 1, 2022.

Code Assignment Beginning 10/1/2022	Previous Code(s) Assignment
B37.31	B37.3
B37.32	B37.3
D59.30	D59.3
D59.31	D59.3
D59.32	D59.3
D59.39	D59.3
D68.00	D68.0
D68.01	D68.0
D68.020	D68.0
D68.021	D68.0
D68.022	D68.0
D68.023	D68.0
D68.029	D68.0
D68.03	D68.0
D68.04	D68.0
D68.09	D68.0
D75.821	D75.82
D75.822	D75.82
D75.828	D75.82
D75.829	D75.82
D75.84	D75.89
D81.82	D81.89
E34.30	E34.3
E34.31	E34.3
E34.321	E34.3
E34.322	E34.3
E34.328	E34.3
E34.329	E34.3
E34.39	E34.3
E87.20	E87.2
E87.21	E87.2
E87.22	E87.2
E87.29	E87.2
F01.511	F01.51
F01.518	F01.51
F01.52	F01.51
F01.53	F01.51
F01.54	F01.51
F01.A0	F01.50
F01.A11	F01.51
F01.A18	F01.51
F01.A2	F01.51
F01.A3	F01.51
F01.A4	F01.51
F01.B0	F01.50
F01.B11	F01.51
F01.B18	F01.51
F01.B2	F01.51
F01.B3	F01.51
F01.B4	F01.51
F01.C0	F01.50
F01.C11	F01.51
F01.C18	F01.51
F01.C2	F01.51
F01.C3	F01.51
F01.C4	F01.51
F02.811	F02.81
F02.818	F02.81
F02.82	F02.81
F02.83	F02.81
F02.84	F02.81
F02.A0	F02.80
F02.A11	F02.81
F02.A18	F02.81
F02.A2	F02.81
F02.A3	F02.81
F02.A4	F02.81
F02.B0	F02.80
F02.B11	F02.81
F02.B18	F02.81
F02.B2	F02.81
F02.B3	F02.81
F02.B4	F02.81
F02.C0	F02.80
F02.C11	F02.81
F02.C18	F02.81
F02.C2	F02.81
F02.C3	F02.81
F02.C4	F02.81
F03.911	F03.91
F03.918	F03.91
F03.92	F03.91
F03.93	F03.91
F03.94	F03.91
F03.A0	F03.90
F03.A11	F03.91
F03.A18	F03.91
F03.A2	F03.91
F03.A3	F03.91
F03.A4	F03.91
F03.B0	F03.90
F03.B11	F03.91
F03.B18	F03.91
F03.B2	F03.91
F03.B3	F03.91
F03.B4	F03.91
F03.C0	F03.90
F03.C11	F03.91
F03.C18	F03.91
F03.C2	F03.91
F03.C3	F03.91
F03.C4	F03.91
F06.70	G31.84
F06.71	G31.84
F10.90	Z72.89
F10.91	Z72.89
F11.91	F11.90
F12.91	F12.90
F13.91	F13.90
F14.91	F14.90
F15.91	F15.90
F16.91	F16.90
F18.91	F18.90
F19.91	F19.90
F43.81	F43.8
F43.89	F43.8
G71.031	G71.09
G71.032	G71.09
G71.033	G71.09
G71.0340	G71.09
G71.0341	G71.09
G71.0342	G71.09
G71.0349	G71.09
G71.035	G71.09
G71.038	G71.09
G71.039	G71.09
G90.A	I49.8
G93.31	G93.3
G93.32	G93.3; R53.82
G93.39	G93.3
I20.2	I20.0-I20.1; I20.8
I25.112	I25.110-I25.111; I25.118
I25.702	I25.700-I25.701; I25.708
I25.712	I25.710-I25.711; I25.718
I25.722	I25.720-I25.721; I25.728
I25.732	I25.730-I25.731; I25.738
I25.752	I25.750-I25.751; I25.758
I25.762	I25.760-I25.761; I25.768
I25.792	I25.790-I25.791; I25.798
I31.31	I31.3
I31.39	I31.3
I34.81	I34.8
I34.89	I34.8
I47.20	I47.2
I47.21	I47.2
I47.29	I47.2
I71.010	I71.01
I71.011	I71.01
I71.012	I71.01
I71.019	I71.01
I71.10	I71.1
I71.11	I71.1
I71.12	I71.1
I71.13	I71.1
I71.20	I71.2
I71.21	I71.2
I71.22	I71.2
I71.23	I71.2
I71.30	I71.3
I71.31	I71.3
I71.32	I71.3
I71.33	I71.3
I71.40	I71.4
I71.41	I71.4
I71.42	I71.4
I71.43	I71.4
I71.50	I71.5
I71.51	I71.5
I71.52	I71.5
I71.60	I71.6
I71.61	I71.6
I71.62	I71.6
I77.82	I77.89
J95.87	J95.89
K76.82	K72.90-K72.91
M51.A0	M51.86
M51.A1	M51.86
M51.A2	M51.86
M51.A3	M51.87
M51.A4	M51.87
M51.A5	M51.87
M62.5A0	M62.58
M62.5A1	M62.58
M62.5A2	M62.58
M62.5A9	M62.58
M93.004	M93.001 & M93.002
M93.014	M93.011 & M93.012
M93.024	M93.021 & M93.022
M93.034	M93.031 & M93.032
M93.041	M93.011
M93.042	M93.012
M93.043	M93.013
M93.044	M93.011 & M93.012
M93.051	M93.031
M93.052	M93.032
M93.053	M93.033
M93.054	M93.031 & M93.032
M93.061	M93.011
M93.062	M93.012
M93.063	M93.013
M93.064	M93.011 & M93.012
M93.071	M93.031
M93.072	M93.032
M93.073	M93.033
M93.074	M93.031 & M93.032
M96.A1	M96.89 & Y84.8
M96.A2	M96.89 & Y84.8
M96.A3	M96.89 & Y84.8
M96.A4	M96.89 & Y84.8
M96.A9	M96.89 & Y84.8
N14.11	N14.1
N14.19	N14.1
N76.82	N76.89
N80.00	N80.0
N80.01	N80.0
N80.02	N80.0
N80.03	N80.0
N80.101	N80.1
N80.102	N80.1
N80.103	N80.1
N80.109	N80.1
N80.111	N80.1
N80.112	N80.1
N80.113	N80.1
N80.119	N80.1
N80.121	N80.1
N80.122	N80.1
N80.123	N80.1
N80.129	N80.1
N80.201	N80.2
N80.202	N80.2
N80.203	N80.2
N80.209	N80.2
N80.211	N80.2
N80.212	N80.2
N80.213	N80.2
N80.219	N80.2
N80.221	N80.2
N80.222	N80.2
N80.223	N80.2
N80.229	N80.2
N80.30	N80.3
N80.311	N80.3
N80.312	N80.3
N80.319	N80.3
N80.321	N80.3
N80.322	N80.3
N80.329	N80.3
N80.331	N80.3
N80.332	N80.3
N80.333	N80.3
N80.339	N80.3
N80.341	N80.3
N80.342	N80.3
N80.343	N80.3
N80.349	N80.3
N80.351	N80.3
N80.352	N80.3
N80.353	N80.3
N80.359	N80.3
N80.361	N80.3
N80.362	N80.3
N80.363	N80.3
N80.369	N80.3
N80.371	N80.3
N80.372	N80.3
N80.373	N80.3
N80.379	N80.3
N80.381	N80.3
N80.382	N80.3
N80.383	N80.3
N80.389	N80.3
N80.3A1	N80.3
N80.3A2	N80.3
N80.3A3	N80.3
N80.3A9	N80.3
N80.3B1	N80.3
N80.3B2	N80.3
N80.3B3	N80.3
N80.3B9	N80.3
N80.3C1	N80.3
N80.3C2	N80.3
N80.3C3	N80.3
N80.3C9	N80.3
N80.391	N80.3
N80.392	N80.3
N80.399	N80.3
N80.40	N80.3
N80.41	N80.4
N80.42	N80.4
N80.50	N80.5
N80.511	N80.5
N80.512	N80.5
N80.519	N80.5
N80.521	N80.5
N80.522	N80.5
N80.529	N80.5
N80.531	N80.5
N80.532	N80.5
N80.539	N80.5

Code Assignment Beginning 10/1/2022	Previous Code(s) Assignment	Code Assignment Beginning 10/1/2022	Previous Code(s) Assignment	Code Assignment Beginning 10/1/2022	Previous Code(s) Assignment	Code Assignment Beginning 10/1/2022	Previous Code(s) Assignment	Code Assignment Beginning 10/1/2022	Previous Code(s) Assignment	Code Assignment Beginning 10/1/2022	Previous Code(s) Assignment
N80.541	N80.5	O35.01X3	O35.0XX3	O35.09X9	O35.0XX9	O35.BXX2	O35.8XX2	Q21.12	Q21.1	S06.81AA	S06.819A
N80.542	N80.5	O35.01X4	O35.0XX4	O35.10X0	O35.1XX0	O35.BXX3	O35.8XX3	Q21.13	Q21.1	S06.81AD	S06.819D
N80.549	N80.5	O35.01X5	O35.0XX5	O35.10X1	O35.1XX1	O35.BXX4	O35.8XX4	Q21.14	Q21.1	S06.81AS	S06.819S
N80.551	N80.5	O35.01X9	O35.0XX9	O35.10X2	O35.1XX2	O35.BXX5	O35.8XX5	Q21.15	Q21.1	S06.82AA	S06.829A
N80.552	N80.5	O35.02X0	O35.0XX0	O35.10X3	O35.1XX3	O35.BXX9	O35.8XX9	Q21.16	Q21.1	S06.82AD	S06.829D
N80.559	N80.5	O35.02X1	O35.0XX1	O35.10X4	O35.1XX4	O35.CXX0	O35.8XX0	Q21.19	Q21.1	S06.82AS	S06.829S
N80.561	N80.5	O35.02X2	O35.0XX2	O35.10X5	O35.1XX5	O35.CXX1	O35.8XX1	Q21.20	Q21.2	S06.8A0A	S06.0X0A
N80.562	N80.5	O35.02X3	O35.0XX3	O35.10X9	O35.1XX9	O35.CXX2	O35.8XX2	Q21.21	Q21.2	S06.8A0D	S06.0X0D
N80.569	N80.5	O35.02X4	O35.0XX4	O35.11X0	O35.1XX0	O35.CXX3	O35.8XX3	Q21.22	Q21.2	S06.8A0S	S06.0X0S
N80.A0	N80.8	O35.02X5	O35.0XX5	O35.11X1	O35.1XX1	O35.CXX4	O35.8XX4	Q21.23	Q21.2	S06.8A1A	S06.0X9A
N80.A1	N80.8	O35.02X9	O35.0XX9	O35.11X2	O35.1XX2	O35.CXX5	O35.8XX5	Q85.81	Q85.8	S06.8A1D	S06.0X9D
N80.A2	N80.8	O35.03X0	O35.0XX0	O35.11X3	O35.1XX3	O35.CXX9	O35.8XX9	Q85.82	Q85.8	S06.8A1S	S06.0X9S
N80.A41	N80.8	O35.03X1	O35.0XX1	O35.11X4	O35.1XX4	O35.DXX0	O35.8XX0	Q85.83	Q85.8	S06.8A2A	S06.0X9A
N80.A42	N80.8	O35.03X2	O35.0XX2	O35.11X5	O35.1XX5	O35.DXX1	O35.8XX1	Q85.89	Q85.8	S06.8A2D	S06.0X9D
N80.A43	N80.8	O35.03X3	O35.0XX3	O35.11X9	O35.1XX9	O35.DXX2	O35.8XX2	S06.0XAA	S06.0X9A	S06.8A2S	S06.0X9S
N80.A49	N80.8	O35.03X4	O35.0XX4	O35.12X0	O35.1XX0	O35.DXX3	O35.8XX3	S06.0XAD	S06.0X9D	S06.8A3A	S06.0X9A
N80.A51	N80.8	O35.03X5	O35.0XX5	O35.12X1	O35.1XX1	O35.DXX4	O35.8XX4	S06.0XAS	S06.0X9S	S06.8A3D	S06.0X9D
N80.A52	N80.8	O35.03X9	O35.0XX9	O35.12X2	O35.1XX2	O35.DXX5	O35.8XX5	S06.1XAA	S06.1X9A	S06.8A3S	S06.0X9S
N80.A53	N80.8	O35.04X0	O35.0XX0	O35.12X3	O35.1XX3	O35.DXX9	O35.8XX9	S06.1XAD	S06.1X9D	S06.8A4A	S06.0X9A
N80.A59	N80.8	O35.04X1	O35.0XX1	O35.12X4	O35.1XX4	O35.EXX0	O35.8XX0	S06.1XAS	S06.1X9S	S06.8A4D	S06.0X9D
N80.A61	N80.8	O35.04X2	O35.0XX2	O35.12X5	O35.1XX5	O35.EXX1	O35.8XX1	S06.2XAA	S06.2X9A	S06.8A4S	S06.0X9S
N80.A62	N80.8	O35.04X3	O35.0XX3	O35.12X9	O35.1XX9	O35.EXX2	O35.8XX2	S06.2XAD	S06.2X9D	S06.8A5A	S06.0X9A
N80.A63	N80.8	O35.04X4	O35.0XX4	O35.13X0	O35.1XX0	O35.EXX3	O35.8XX3	S06.2XAS	S06.2X9S	S06.8A5D	S06.0X9D
N80.A69	N80.8	O35.04X5	O35.0XX5	O35.13X1	O35.1XX1	O35.EXX4	O35.8XX4	S06.30AA	S06.309A	S06.8A5S	S06.0X9S
N80.B1	N80.8	O35.04X9	O35.0XX9	O35.13X2	O35.1XX2	O35.EXX5	O35.8XX5	S06.30AD	S06.309D	S06.8A6A	S06.0X9A
N80.B2	N80.8	O35.05X0	O35.0XX0	O35.13X3	O35.1XX3	O35.EXX9	O35.8XX9	S06.30AS	S06.309S	S06.8A6D	S06.0X9D
N80.B31	N80.8	O35.05X1	O35.0XX1	O35.13X4	O35.1XX4	O35.FXX0	O35.8XX0	S06.31AA	S06.319A	S06.8A6S	S06.0X9S
N80.B32	N80.8	O35.05X2	O35.0XX2	O35.13X5	O35.1XX5	O35.FXX1	O35.8XX1	S06.31AD	S06.319D	S06.8A7A	S06.0X9A
N80.B39	N80.8	O35.05X3	O35.0XX3	O35.13X9	O35.1XX9	O35.FXX2	O35.8XX2	S06.31AS	S06.319S	S06.8A8A	S06.0X9A
N80.B4	N80.8	O35.05X4	O35.0XX4	O35.14X0	O35.1XX0	O35.FXX3	O35.8XX3	S06.32AA	S06.329A	S06.8AAA	S06.0X9A
N80.B5	N80.8	O35.05X5	O35.0XX5	O35.14X1	O35.1XX1	O35.FXX4	O35.8XX4	S06.32AD	S06.329D	S06.8AAD	S06.0X9D
N80.B6	N80.8	O35.05X9	O35.0XX9	O35.14X2	O35.1XX2	O35.FXX5	O35.8XX5	S06.32AS	S06.329S	S06.8AAS	S06.0X9S
N80.C0	N80.8	O35.06X0	O35.0XX0	O35.14X3	O35.1XX3	O35.FXX9	O35.8XX9	S06.33AA	S06.339A	S06.8A9A	S06.0X9A
N80.C10	N80.8	O35.06X1	O35.0XX1	O35.14X4	O35.1XX4	O35.GXX0	O35.8XX0	S06.33AD	S06.339D	S06.8A9D	S06.0X9D
N80.C11	N80.8	O35.06X2	O35.0XX2	O35.14X5	O35.1XX5	O35.GXX1	O35.8XX1	S06.33AS	S06.339S	S06.8A9S	S06.0X9S
N80.C19	N80.8	O35.06X3	O35.0XX3	O35.14X9	O35.1XX9	O35.GXX2	O35.8XX2	S06.34AA	S06.349A	S06.89AA	S06.0X9A
N80.C2	N80.8	O35.06X4	O35.0XX4	O35.15X0	O35.1XX0	O35.GXX3	O35.8XX3	S06.34AD	S06.349D	S06.89AD	S06.0X9D
N80.C3	N80.8	O35.06X5	O35.0XX5	O35.15X1	O35.1XX1	O35.GXX4	O35.8XX4	S06.34AS	S06.349S	S06.89AS	S06.0X9S
N80.C4	N80.8	O35.06X9	O35.0XX9	O35.15X2	O35.1XX2	O35.GXX5	O35.8XX5	S06.35AA	S06.359A	S06.9XAA	S06.9X9A
N80.C9	N80.8	O35.07X0	O35.0XX0	O35.15X3	O35.1XX3	O35.GXX9	O35.8XX9	S06.35AD	S06.359D	S06.9XAD	S06.9X9D
N80.D0	N80.8	O35.07X1	O35.0XX1	O35.15X4	O35.1XX4	O35.HXX0	O35.8XX0	S06.35AS	S06.359S	S06.9XAS	S06.9X9S
N80.D1	N80.8	O35.07X2	O35.0XX2	O35.15X5	O35.1XX5	O35.HXX1	O35.8XX1	S06.36AA	S06.369A	T43.651A	T43.621A
N80.D2	N80.8	O35.07X3	O35.0XX3	O35.15X9	O35.1XX9	O35.HXX2	O35.8XX2	S06.36AD	S06.369D	T43.651D	T43.621D
N80.D3	N80.8	O35.07X4	O35.0XX4	O35.19X0	O35.1XX0	O35.HXX3	O35.8XX3	S06.36AS	S06.369S	T43.651S	T43.621S
N80.D4	N80.8	O35.07X5	O35.0XX5	O35.19X1	O35.1XX1	O35.HXX4	O35.8XX4	S06.37AA	S06.379A	T43.652A	T43.622A
N80.D5	N80.8	O35.07X9	O35.0XX9	O35.19X2	O35.1XX2	O35.HXX5	O35.8XX5	S06.37AD	S06.379D	T43.652D	T43.621D
N80.D6	N80.8	O35.08X0	O35.0XX0	O35.19X3	O35.1XX3	O35.HXX9	O35.8XX9	S06.37AS	S06.379S	T43.652S	T43.621S
N80.D9	N80.8	O35.08X1	O35.0XX1	O35.19X4	O35.1XX4	P28.30	P28.3	S06.38AA	S06.389A	T43.653A	T43.623A
N85.A	N85.8	O35.08X2	O35.0XX2	O35.19X5	O35.1XX5	P28.31	P28.3	S06.38AD	S06.389D	T43.653D	T43.623D
O35.00X0	O35.0XX0	O35.08X3	O35.0XX3	O35.19X9	O35.1XX9	P28.32	P28.3	S06.38AS	S06.389S	T43.653S	T43.623S
O35.00X1	O35.0XX1	O35.08X4	O35.0XX4	O35.AXX0	O35.8XX0	P28.33	P28.3	S06.4XAA	S06.4X9A	T43.654A	T43.624A
O35.00X2	O35.0XX2	O35.08X5	O35.0XX5	O35.AXX1	O35.8XX1	P28.39	P28.3	S06.4XAD	S06.4X9D	T43.654D	T43.624D
O35.00X3	O35.0XX3	O35.08X9	O35.0XX9	O35.AXX2	O35.8XX2	P28.40	P28.4	S06.4XAS	S06.4X9S	T43.654S	T43.624S
O35.00X4	O35.0XX4	O35.09X0	O35.0XX0	O35.AXX3	O35.8XX3	P28.41	P28.4	S06.5XAA	S06.5X9A	T43.655A	T43.625A
O35.00X5	O35.0XX5	O35.09X1	O35.0XX1	O35.AXX4	O35.8XX4	P28.42	P28.4	S06.5XAD	S06.5X9D	T43.655D	T43.625D
O35.00X9	O35.0XX9	O35.09X2	O35.0XX2	O35.AXX5	O35.8XX5	P28.43	P28.4	S06.5XAS	S06.5X9S	T43.655S	T43.625S
O35.01X0	O35.0XX0	O35.09X3	O35.0XX3	O35.AXX9	O35.8XX9	P28.49	P28.4	S06.6XAA	S06.6X9A	T43.656A	T43.626A
O35.01X1	O35.0XX1	O35.09X4	O35.0XX4	O35.BXX0	O35.8XX0	Q21.10	Q21.1	S06.6XAD	S06.6X9D	T43.656D	T43.626D
O35.01X2	O35.0XX2	O35.09X5	O35.0XX5	O35.BXX1	O35.8XX1	Q21.11	Q21.1	S06.6XAS	S06.6X9S	T43.656S	T43.626S

Conversion Table of ICD-10-CM Codes

Code Assignment Beginning 10/1/2022	Previous Code(s) Assignment	Code Assignment Beginning 10/1/2022	Previous Code(s) Assignment	Code Assignment Beginning 10/1/2022	Previous Code(s) Assignment	Code Assignment Beginning 10/1/2022	Previous Code(s) Assignment	Code Assignment Beginning 10/1/2022	Previous Code(s) Assignment	Code Assignment Beginning 10/1/2022	Previous Code(s) Assignment
V20.01XA	V20.0XXA	V21.29XS	V21.2XXS	V22.59XD	V22.5XXD	V24.19XA	V24.1XXA	V25.41XS	V25.4XXS	V27.01XD	V27.0XXD
V20.01XD	V20.0XXD	V21.31XA	V21.3XXA	V22.59XS	V22.5XXS	V24.19XD	V24.1XXD	V25.49XA	V25.4XXA	V27.01XS	V27.0XXS
V20.01XS	V20.0XXS	V21.31XD	V21.3XXD	V22.91XA	V22.9XXA	V24.19XS	V24.1XXS	V25.49XD	V25.4XXD	V27.09XA	V27.0XXA
V20.09XA	V20.0XXA	V21.31XS	V21.3XXS	V22.91XD	V22.9XXD	V24.21XA	V24.2XXA	V25.49XS	V25.4XXS	V27.09XD	V27.0XXD
V20.09XD	V20.0XXD	V21.39XA	V21.3XXA	V22.91XS	V22.9XXS	V24.21XD	V24.2XXD	V25.51XA	V25.5XXA	V27.09XS	V27.0XXS
V20.09XS	V20.0XXS	V21.39XD	V21.3XXD	V22.99XA	V22.9XXA	V24.21XS	V24.2XXS	V25.51XD	V25.5XXD	V27.11XA	V27.1XXA
V20.11XA	V20.1XXA	V21.39XS	V21.3XXS	V22.99XD	V22.9XXD	V24.29XA	V24.2XXA	V25.51XS	V25.5XXS	V27.11XD	V27.1XXD
V20.11XD	V20.1XXD	V21.41XA	V21.4XXA	V22.99XS	V22.9XXS	V24.29XD	V24.2XXD	V25.59XA	V25.5XXA	V27.11XS	V27.1XXS
V20.11XS	V20.1XXS	V21.41XD	V21.4XXD	V23.01XA	V23.0XXA	V24.29XS	V24.2XXS	V25.59XD	V25.5XXD	V27.19XA	V27.1XXA
V20.19XA	V20.1XXA	V21.41XS	V21.4XXS	V23.01XD	V23.0XXD	V24.31XA	V24.3XXA	V25.59XS	V25.5XXS	V27.19XD	V27.1XXD
V20.19XD	V20.1XXD	V21.49XA	V21.4XXA	V23.01XS	V23.0XXS	V24.31XD	V24.3XXD	V25.91XA	V25.9XXA	V27.19XS	V27.1XXS
V20.19XS	V20.1XXS	V21.49XD	V21.4XXD	V23.09XA	V23.0XXA	V24.31XS	V24.3XXS	V25.91XD	V25.9XXD	V27.21XA	V27.2XXA
V20.21XA	V20.2XXA	V21.49XS	V21.4XXS	V23.09XD	V23.0XXD	V24.39XA	V24.3XXA	V25.91XS	V25.9XXS	V27.21XD	V27.2XXD
V20.21XD	V20.2XXD	V21.51XA	V21.5XXA	V23.09XS	V23.0XXS	V24.39XD	V24.3XXD	V25.99XA	V25.9XXA	V27.21XS	V27.2XXS
V20.21XS	V20.2XXS	V21.51XD	V21.5XXD	V23.11XA	V23.1XXA	V24.39XS	V24.3XXS	V25.99XD	V25.9XXD	V27.29XA	V27.2XXA
V20.29XA	V20.2XXA	V21.51XS	V21.5XXS	V23.11XD	V23.1XXD	V24.41XA	V24.4XXA	V25.99XS	V25.9XXS	V27.29XD	V27.2XXD
V20.29XD	V20.2XXD	V21.59XA	V21.5XXA	V23.11XS	V23.1XXS	V24.41XD	V24.4XXD	V26.01XA	V26.0XXA	V27.29XS	V27.2XXS
V20.29XS	V20.2XXS	V21.59XD	V21.5XXD	V23.19XA	V23.1XXA	V24.41XS	V24.4XXS	V26.01XD	V26.0XXD	V27.31XA	V27.3XXA
V20.31XA	V20.3XXA	V21.59XS	V21.5XXS	V23.19XD	V23.1XXD	V24.49XA	V24.4XXA	V26.01XS	V26.0XXS	V27.31XD	V27.3XXD
V20.31XD	V20.3XXD	V21.91XA	V21.9XXA	V23.19XS	V23.1XXS	V24.49XD	V24.4XXD	V26.09XA	V26.0XXA	V27.31XS	V27.3XXS
V20.31XS	V20.3XXS	V21.91XD	V21.9XXD	V23.21XA	V23.2XXA	V24.49XS	V24.4XXS	V26.09XD	V26.0XXD	V27.39XA	V27.3XXA
V20.39XA	V20.3XXA	V21.91XS	V21.9XXS	V23.21XD	V23.2XXD	V24.51XA	V24.5XXA	V26.09XS	V26.0XXS	V27.39XD	V27.3XXD
V20.39XD	V20.3XXD	V21.99XA	V21.9XXA	V23.21XS	V23.2XXS	V24.51XD	V24.5XXD	V26.11XA	V26.1XXA	V27.39XS	V27.3XXS
V20.39XS	V20.3XXS	V21.99XD	V21.9XXD	V23.29XA	V23.2XXA	V24.51XS	V24.5XXS	V26.11XD	V26.1XXD	V27.41XA	V27.4XXA
V20.41XA	V20.4XXA	V21.99XS	V21.9XXS	V23.29XD	V23.2XXD	V24.59XA	V24.5XXA	V26.11XS	V26.1XXS	V27.41XD	V27.4XXD
V20.41XD	V20.4XXD	V22.01XA	V22.0XXA	V23.29XS	V23.2XXS	V24.59XD	V24.5XXD	V26.19XA	V26.1XXA	V27.41XS	V27.4XXS
V20.41XS	V20.4XXS	V22.01XD	V22.0XXD	V23.31XA	V23.3XXA	V24.59XS	V24.5XXS	V26.19XD	V26.1XXD	V27.49XA	V27.4XXA
V20.49XA	V20.4XXA	V22.01XS	V22.0XXS	V23.31XD	V23.3XXD	V24.91XA	V24.9XXA	V26.19XS	V26.1XXS	V27.49XD	V27.4XXD
V20.49XD	V20.4XXD	V22.09XA	V22.0XXA	V23.31XS	V23.3XXS	V24.91XD	V24.9XXD	V26.21XA	V26.2XXA	V27.49XS	V27.4XXS
V20.49XS	V20.4XXS	V22.09XD	V22.0XXD	V23.39XA	V23.3XXA	V24.91XS	V24.9XXS	V26.21XD	V26.2XXD	V27.51XA	V27.5XXA
V20.51XA	V20.5XXA	V22.09XS	V22.0XXS	V23.39XD	V23.3XXD	V24.99XA	V24.9XXA	V26.21XS	V26.2XXS	V27.51XD	V27.5XXD
V20.51XD	V20.5XXD	V22.11XA	V22.1XXA	V23.39XS	V23.3XXS	V24.99XD	V24.9XXD	V26.29XA	V26.2XXA	V27.51XS	V27.5XXS
V20.51XS	V20.5XXS	V22.11XD	V22.1XXD	V23.41XA	V23.4XXA	V24.99XS	V24.9XXS	V26.29XD	V26.2XXD	V27.59XA	V27.5XXA
V20.59XA	V20.5XXA	V22.11XS	V22.1XXS	V23.41XD	V23.4XXD	V25.01XA	V25.0XXA	V26.29XS	V26.2XXS	V27.59XD	V27.5XXD
V20.59XD	V20.5XXD	V22.19XA	V22.1XXA	V23.41XS	V23.4XXS	V25.01XD	V25.0XXD	V26.31XA	V26.3XXA	V27.59XS	V27.5XXS
V20.59XS	V20.5XXS	V22.19XD	V22.1XXD	V23.49XA	V23.4XXA	V25.01XS	V25.0XXS	V26.31XD	V26.3XXD	V27.91XA	V27.9XXA
V20.91XA	V20.9XXA	V22.19XS	V22.1XXS	V23.49XD	V23.4XXD	V25.09XA	V25.0XXA	V26.31XS	V26.3XXS	V27.91XD	V27.9XXD
V20.91XD	V20.9XXD	V22.21XA	V22.2XXA	V23.49XS	V23.4XXS	V25.09XD	V25.0XXD	V26.39XA	V26.3XXA	V27.91XS	V27.9XXS
V20.91XS	V20.9XXS	V22.21XD	V22.2XXD	V23.51XD	V23.5XXA	V25.09XS	V25.0XXS	V26.39XD	V26.3XXD	V27.99XA	V27.9XXA
V20.99XA	V20.9XXA	V22.21XS	V22.2XXS	V23.51XD	V23.5XXD	V25.11XA	V25.1XXA	V26.39XS	V26.3XXS	V27.99XD	V27.9XXD
V20.99XD	V20.9XXD	V22.29XA	V22.2XXA	V23.51XS	V23.5XXS	V25.11XD	V25.1XXD	V26.41XA	V26.4XXA	V27.99XS	V27.9XXS
V20.99XS	V20.9XXS	V22.29XD	V22.2XXD	V23.59XA	V23.5XXA	V25.11XS	V25.1XXS	V26.41XD	V26.4XXD	V28.01XA	V28.0XXA
V21.01XA	V21.0XXA	V22.29XS	V22.2XXS	V23.59XD	V23.5XXD	V25.19XA	V25.1XXA	V26.41XS	V26.4XXS	V28.01XD	V28.0XXD
V21.01XD	V21.0XXD	V22.31XA	V22.3XXA	V23.59XS	V23.5XXS	V25.19XD	V25.1XXD	V26.49XA	V26.4XXA	V28.01XS	V28.0XXS
V21.01XS	V21.0XXS	V22.31XD	V22.3XXD	V23.91XA	V23.9XXA	V25.19XS	V25.1XXS	V26.49XD	V26.4XXD	V28.09XA	V28.0XXA
V21.09XA	V21.0XXA	V22.31XS	V22.3XXS	V23.91XD	V23.9XXD	V25.21XA	V25.2XXA	V26.49XS	V26.4XXS	V28.09XD	V28.0XXD
V21.09XD	V21.0XXD	V22.39XA	V22.3XXA	V23.91XS	V23.9XXS	V25.21XD	V25.2XXD	V26.51XA	V26.5XXA	V28.09XS	V28.0XXS
V21.09XS	V21.0XXS	V22.39XD	V22.3XXD	V23.99XA	V23.9XXA	V25.21XS	V25.2XXS	V26.51XD	V26.5XXD	V28.11XA	V28.1XXA
V21.11XA	V21.1XXA	V22.39XS	V22.3XXS	V23.99XD	V23.9XXD	V25.29XA	V25.2XXA	V26.51XS	V26.5XXS	V28.11XD	V28.1XXD
V21.11XD	V21.1XXD	V22.41XA	V22.4XXA	V23.99XS	V23.9XXS	V25.29XD	V25.2XXD	V26.59XA	V26.5XXA	V28.11XS	V28.1XXS
V21.11XS	V21.1XXS	V22.41XD	V22.4XXD	V24.01XA	V24.0XXA	V25.29XS	V25.2XXS	V26.59XD	V26.5XXD	V28.19XA	V28.1XXA
V21.19XA	V21.1XXA	V22.41XS	V22.4XXS	V24.01XD	V24.0XXD	V25.31XA	V25.3XXA	V26.59XS	V26.5XXS	V28.19XD	V28.1XXD
V21.19XD	V21.1XXD	V22.49XA	V22.4XXA	V24.01XS	V24.0XXS	V25.31XD	V25.3XXD	V26.91XA	V26.9XXA	V28.19XS	V28.1XXS
V21.19XS	V21.1XXS	V22.49XD	V22.4XXD	V24.09XA	V24.0XXA	V25.31XS	V25.3XXS	V26.91XD	V26.9XXD	V28.21XA	V28.2XXA
V21.21XA	V21.2XXA	V22.49XS	V22.4XXS	V24.09XD	V24.0XXD	V25.39XA	V25.3XXA	V26.91XS	V26.9XXS	V28.21XD	V28.2XXD
V21.21XD	V21.2XXD	V22.51XA	V22.5XXA	V24.09XS	V24.0XXS	V25.39XD	V25.3XXD	V26.99XA	V26.9XXA	V28.21XS	V28.2XXS
V21.21XS	V21.2XXS	V22.51XD	V22.5XXD	V24.11XA	V24.1XXA	V25.39XS	V25.3XXS	V26.99XD	V26.9XXD	V28.29XA	V28.2XXA
V21.29XA	V21.2XXA	V22.51XS	V22.5XXS	V24.11XD	V24.1XXD	V25.41XA	V25.4XXA	V26.99XS	V26.9XXS	V28.29XD	V28.2XXD
V21.29XD	V21.2XXD	V22.59XA	V22.5XXA	V24.11XS	V24.1XXS	V25.41XD	V25.4XXD	V27.01XA	V27.0XXA	V28.29XS	V28.2XXS

Conversion Table of ICD-10-CM Codes

Code Assignment Beginning 10/1/2022	Previous Code(s) Assignment
V28.31XA	V28.3XXA
V28.31XD	V28.3XXD
V28.31XS	V28.3XXS
V28.39XA	V28.3XXA
V28.39XD	V28.3XXD
V28.39XS	V28.3XXS
V28.41XA	V28.4XXA
V28.41XD	V28.4XXD
V28.41XS	V28.4XXS
V28.49XA	V28.4XXA
V28.49XD	V28.4XXD
V28.49XS	V28.4XXS
V28.51XA	V28.5XXA
V28.51XD	V28.5XXD
V28.51XS	V28.5XXS
V28.59XA	V28.5XXA
V28.59XD	V28.5XXD
V28.59XS	V28.5XXS
V28.91XA	V28.9XXA
V28.91XD	V28.9XXD
V28.91XS	V28.9XXS
V28.99XA	V28.9XXA
V28.99XD	V28.9XXD
V28.99XS	V28.9XXS
V29.001A	V29.00XA
V29.001D	V29.00XD
V29.001S	V29.00XS
V29.008A	V29.00XA
V29.008D	V29.00XD
V29.008S	V29.00XS

Code Assignment Beginning 10/1/2022	Previous Code(s) Assignment
V29.091A	V29.09XA
V29.091D	V29.09XD
V29.091S	V29.09XS
V29.098A	V29.09XA
V29.098D	V29.09XD
V29.098S	V29.09XS
V29.101A	V29.10XA
V29.101D	V29.10XD
V29.101S	V29.10XS
V29.108A	V29.10XA
V29.108D	V29.10XD
V29.108S	V29.10XS
V29.191A	V29.19XA
V29.191D	V29.19XD
V29.191S	V29.19XS
V29.198A	V29.19XA
V29.198D	V29.19XD
V29.198S	V29.19XS
V29.201A	V29.20XA
V29.201D	V29.20XD
V29.201S	V29.20XS
V29.208A	V29.20XA
V29.208D	V29.20XD
V29.208S	V29.20XS
V29.291A	V29.29XA
V29.291D	V29.29XD
V29.291S	V29.29XS
V29.298A	V29.29XA
V29.298D	V29.29XD
V29.298S	V29.29XS

Code Assignment Beginning 10/1/2022	Previous Code(s) Assignment
V29.31XA	V29.3XXA
V29.31XD	V29.3XXD
V29.31XS	V29.3XXS
V29.39XA	V29.3XXA
V29.39XD	V29.3XXD
V29.39XS	V29.3XXS
V29.401A	V29.40XA
V29.401D	V29.40XD
V29.401S	V29.40XS
V29.408A	V29.40XA
V29.408D	V29.40XD
V29.408S	V29.40XS
V29.491A	V29.49XA
V29.491D	V29.49XD
V29.491S	V29.49XS
V29.498A	V29.49XA
V29.498D	V29.49XD
V29.498S	V29.49XS
V29.501A	V29.50XA
V29.501D	V29.50XD
V29.501S	V29.50XS
V29.508A	V29.50XA
V29.508D	V29.50XD
V29.508S	V29.50XS
V29.591A	V29.59XA
V29.591D	V29.59XD
V29.591S	V29.59XS
V29.598A	V29.59XA
V29.598D	V29.59XD
V29.598S	V29.59XS

Code Assignment Beginning 10/1/2022	Previous Code(s) Assignment
V29.601A	V29.60XA
V29.601D	V29.60XD
V29.601S	V29.60XS
V29.608A	V29.60XA
V29.608D	V29.60XD
V29.608S	V29.60XS
V29.691A	V29.69XA
V29.691D	V29.69XD
V29.691S	V29.69XS
V29.698A	V29.69XA
V29.698D	V29.69XD
V29.698S	V29.69XS
V29.811A	V29.80XA
V29.811D	V29.80XD
V29.811S	V29.80XS
V29.818A	V29.80XA
V29.818D	V29.80XD
V29.818S	V29.80XS
V29.881A	V29.89XA
V29.881D	V29.89XD
V29.881S	V29.89XS
V29.888A	V29.89XA
V29.888D	V29.89XD
V29.888S	V29.89XS
V29.91XA	V29.9XXA
V29.91XD	V29.9XXD
V29.91XS	V29.9XXS
V29.99XA	V29.9XXA
V29.99XD	V29.9XXD
V29.99XS	V29.9XXS

Code Assignment Beginning 10/1/2022	Previous Code(s) Assignment
W23.2XXA	W23.0XXA & W23.1XXA
W23.2XXD	W23.0XXD & W23.1XXD
W23.2XXS	W23.0XXS & W23.1XXS
Z03.83	Z03.89
*Z28.310	Z28.3
*Z28.311	Z28.3
*Z28.39	Z28.3
Z59.82	Z59.89
Z59.86	Z59.89
Z59.87	Z59.89
Z71.87	Z71.89
Z71.88	Z71.89
Z72.823	Z72.89
Z79.60	Z79.899
Z79.61	Z79.899
Z79.620	Z79.899
Z79.621	Z79.899
Z79.622	Z79.899
Z79.623	Z79.899
Z79.624	Z79.899
Z79.630	Z79.899
Z79.631	Z79.899
Z79.632	Z79.899
Z79.633	Z79.899
Z79.634	Z79.899

Code Assignment Beginning 10/1/2022	Previous Code(s) Assignment
Z79.64	Z79.899
Z79.69	Z79.899
Z79.85	Z79.899
Z87.61	Z87.898
Z87.68	Z87.898
Z87.731	Z87.738
Z87.732	Z87.738
Z87.760	Z87.76
Z87.761	Z87.76
Z87.762	Z87.76
Z87.763	Z87.76
Z87.768	Z87.76
Z91.110	Z91.11
Z91.118	Z91.11
Z91.119	Z91.11
Z91.190	Z91.19
Z91.198	Z91.19
Z91.199	Z91.19
Z91.A10	Z91.19
Z91.A18	Z91.19
Z91.A20	Z91.19
Z91.A28	Z91.19
Z91.A3	Z91.19
Z91.A4	Z91.19
Z91.A5	Z91.19
Z91.A9	Z91.19

10 Steps to Correct Coding

Follow the 10 steps below to correctly code encounters for health care services.

Step 1: Identify the reason for the visit or encounter (i.e., a sign, symptom, diagnosis and/or condition).

The medical record documentation should accurately reflect the patient's condition, using terminology that includes specific diagnoses and symptoms or clearly states the reasons for the encounter.

Choosing the main term that best describes the reason chiefly responsible for the service provided is the most important step in coding. If symptoms are present and documented but a definitive diagnosis has not yet been determined, code the symptoms. *For outpatient cases, do not code conditions that are referred to as "rule out," "suspected," "probable," or "questionable."* Diagnoses often are not established at the time of the initial encounter/visit and may require two or more visits to be established. Code only what is documented in the available outpatient records and only to the highest degree of certainty known at the time of the patient's visit. For inpatient medical records, uncertain diagnoses may be reported if documented at the time of discharge.

Step 2: After selecting the reason for the encounter, consult the alphabetic index.

The most critical rule is to begin code selection in the alphabetic index. Never turn first to the tabular list. The index provides cross-references, essential and nonessential modifiers, and other instructional notations that may not be found in the tabular list.

Step 3: Locate the main term entry.

The alphabetic index lists conditions, which may be expressed as nouns or eponyms, with critical use of adjectives. Some conditions known by several names have multiple main entries. Reasons for encounters may be located under general terms such as admission, encounter, and examination. Other general terms such as history, status (post), or presence (of) can be used to locate other factors influencing health.

Step 4: Scan subterm entries.

Scan the subterm entries, as appropriate, being sure to review continued lines and additional subterms that may appear in the next column or on the next page. Shaded vertical guidelines in the index indicate the indentation level for each subterm in relation to the main terms.

Step 5: Pay close attention to index instructions.

- Parentheses ( ) enclose nonessential modifiers, terms that are supplementary words or explanatory information that may or may not appear in the diagnostic statement and do not affect code selection.

- Brackets [ ] enclose manifestation codes that can be used only as secondary codes to the underlying condition code immediately preceding it. If used, manifestation codes must be reported with the appropriate etiology codes.

- Default codes are listed next to the main term and represent the condition most commonly associated with the main term or the unspecified code for the main term.

- "*See*" cross-references, identified by italicized type and "code by" cross-references indicate that another term *must be referenced* to locate the correct code.

- "*See also*" cross-references, identified by italicized type, provide alternative terms that may be useful to look up but *are not mandatory*.

- "Omit code" cross-references identify instances when a code is not applicable depending on the condition being coded.

- "With" subterms are listed out of alphabetic order and identify a presumed causal relationship between the two conditions they link.

- "Due to" subterms identify a relationship between the two conditions they link.

- "NEC," abbreviation for "not elsewhere classified," follows some main terms or subterms and indicates that there is no specific code for the condition even though the medical documentation may be very specific.

- "NOS," abbreviation for "not otherwise specified," follows some main terms or subterms and is the equivalent of unspecified; NOS signifies that the information in the medical record is insufficient for assigning a more specific code.

- *Following* references help coders locate alphanumeric codes that are out of sequence in the tabular section.

- Check-additional-character symbols flag codes that require additional characters to make the code valid; the characters available to complete the code should be verified in the tabular section.

Step 6: Choose a potential code and locate it in the tabular list.

To prevent coding errors, always use both the alphabetic index (to identify a code) and the tabular list (to verify a code), as the index does not include the important instructional notes found in the tabular list. An added benefit of using the tabular list, which groups like things together, is that while looking at one code in the list, a coder might see a more specific one that would have been missed had the coder relied solely on the alphabetic index. Additionally, many of the codes require a fourth, fifth, sixth, or seventh character to be valid, and many of these characters can be found only in the tabular list.

Step 7: Read all instructional material in the tabular section.

The coder must follow any Includes, Excludes 1 and Excludes 2 notes, and other instructional notes, such as "Code first" and "Use additional code," listed in the tabular list for the chapter, category, subcategory, and subclassification levels of code selection that direct the coder to use a different or additional code. Any codes in the tabular range A00.0- through T88.9- may be used to identify the diagnostic reason for the encounter. The tabular list encompasses many codes describing disease and injury classifications (e.g., infectious and parasitic diseases, neoplasms, symptoms, nervous and circulatory system, etc.).

Codes that describe symptoms and signs, as opposed to definitive diagnoses, should be reported when an established diagnosis has not been made (confirmed) by the physician. Chapter 18 of the ICD-10-CM code book, "Symptoms, Signs, and Abnormal Clinical and Laboratory Findings, Not Elsewhere Classified" (codes R00–R99), contains many, but not all, codes for symptoms.

ICD-10-CM classifies encounters with health care providers for circumstances other than a disease or injury in chapter 21, "Factors Influencing Health Status and Contact with Health Services" (codes Z00–Z99). Circumstances other than a disease or injury often are recorded as chiefly responsible for the encounter.

A code is invalid if it does not include the full number of characters (greatest level of specificity) required. Codes in ICD-10-CM can contain from three to seven alphanumeric characters. A three-character code is to be used only if the category is not further subdivided into four-, five-, six-, or seven-character codes. Placeholder character X is used as part of an alphanumeric code to allow for future expansion and as a placeholder for empty characters in a code that requires a seventh character but has no fourth, fifth, or sixth character. Note that certain categories require seventh characters that apply to all codes in that category. Always check the category level for applicable seventh characters for that category.

Step 8: Consult the official ICD-10-CM conventions and guidelines.

The *ICD-10-CM Official Guidelines for Coding and Reporting* govern the use of certain codes. These guidelines provide both general and chapter-specific coding guidance.

Step 9: Confirm and assign the code.

Having reviewed all relevant information concerning the possible code choices, assign the code that most completely describes the condition.

Repeat steps 1 through 9 for all additional documented conditions that meet the following criteria:

- They exist at the time of the visit *AND*

- They require or affect patient care, treatment, or management

Step 10: Sequence codes correctly.

Sequencing is the order in which the codes are listed on the claim. List first the ICD-10-CM code for the diagnosis, condition, problem, or other reason for the encounter/visit that is shown in the medical record to be chiefly responsible for the services provided. List additional codes that describe any coexisting conditions. Follow the official coding guidelines (see the guidelines, section II, "Selection of Principal Diagnosis"; section III, "Reporting Additional Diagnoses"; and section IV, "Diagnostic Coding and Reporting Guidelines for Outpatient Services") on proper sequencing of codes.

Coding Examples

Diagnosis: Anorexia

Step 1: The reason for the encounter was the condition, anorexia.

Step 2: Consult the alphabetic index.

Step 3: Locate the main term "Anorexia."

Step 4: Two possible subterms are available, "hysterical" and "nervosa." Neither is documented in this instance, however, so they cannot be used in code selection.

Step 5: The code listed next to the main term is called the default code selection. Because the two subentries (essential modifiers) do not apply in this instance, the default code (R63.0) should be used.

Step 6: Turn to code R63.0 in the tabular list and read all instructional notes.

Step 7: The Excludes 1 note at code R63.0 indicates that anorexia nervosa and loss of appetite determined to be of nonorganic origin should be reported with a code from chapter 5. The diagnostic statement does not describe the condition as anorexia nervosa, however, and does not indicate that the anorexia is of a nonorganic origin. There is no further division of the category past the fourth-character subcategory. Therefore, code R63.0 is at the highest level of specificity.

Step 8: Review of official guideline I.C.18 indicates that a symptom code is appropriate when a more definitive diagnosis is not documented.

Step 9: The default code, R63.0 Anorexia, is the correct code selection.

Repeat steps 1 through 9 for any concomitant diagnoses.

Step 10: Since anorexia is listed as the chief reason for the health care encounter, the first-listed, or principal, diagnosis is R63.0. Note that this is a chapter 18 symptom code but can be assigned for both inpatient and outpatient records since the provider did not establish a more definitive diagnosis, according to sections II.A and IV.D.

Diagnosis: Acute bronchitis

Step 1: The reason for the encounter was the condition, acute bronchitis.

Step 2: Consult the alphabetic index.

Step 3: Locate the main term "Bronchitis."

Step 4: There is a subterm for "acute or subacute." Additional subterms are not included in the diagnostic statement.

Step 5: Nonessential modifiers (with bronchospasm or obstruction) are terms that do not affect code assignment. Since no other subterms indented under "acute" apply here, the code listed next to this subentry—in this case J20.9—should be chosen.

Step 6: Turn to code J20.9 in the tabular list and read all instructional notes.

Step 7: The Includes note under category J20 lists alternative terms for acute bronchitis. Note that the list is not exhaustive but is only a representative selection of diagnoses that are included in the subcategory. The Excludes 1 note refers to category J40 for bronchitis and tracheobronchitis NOS. There are several conditions in the Excludes 2 notes that, if applicable, can be coded in addition to this code.

Note that the codes included in J20 represent acute bronchitis due to various infectious organisms that could be selected if identified in the documentation. In this case, the organism was not identified and there is no further division of the category past the fourth character subcategory. Therefore, code J20.9 is at the highest level of specificity.

Step 8: Review of official guideline I.C.10 provides no additional information affecting the code selected.

Step 9: Assign code J20.9 Acute bronchitis, unspecified.

Repeat steps 1 through 9 for any concomitant diagnoses.

Step 10: In the absence of additional diagnoses that may affect sequencing, code J20.9 should be sequenced as the first-listed, or principal, diagnosis.

Diagnosis: Cerebellar ataxia in myxedema

Step 1: The reason for the encounter was the condition, cerebellar ataxia.

Step 2: Consult the alphabetic index.

Step 3: Locate the main term "Ataxia."

Step 4: Available subterms include "cerebellar (hereditary)," with additional indented subterms for "in" and "myxedema," all essential modifiers that are included in the diagnostic statement. Two codes are provided, E03.9 and G13.2, the latter of which is in brackets.

Step 5: Note the nonessential modifier (in parentheses) after the subterm cerebellar includes the term "hereditary." Because it is in parentheses, this term is not required in the diagnostic statement for this subentry to apply. The brackets around G13.2 identify this code as a manifestation of the condition described by code E03.9 and indicate that the two must be reported together and sequencing rules apply.

Step 6: Locate codes E03.9 and G13.2 in the tabular list, and read all instructional notes.

Step 7: For code E03.9, there are no instructional notes in the tabular list at the category E03 or code level that indicate that this condition should be coded elsewhere in the classification or that additional codes are required. Without further information from the diagnostic statement, myxedema, not otherwise specified (NOS), is appropriately reported with code E03.9 Hypothyroidism, unspecified, according to the inclusion term at this code.

Code G13.2 in the tabular list has an instructional note to "Code first underlying disease," which includes conditions found in category E03.-. Based on this note, codes E03.9 and G13.2 are to be coded together, with G13.2 listed only as a secondary diagnosis. This correlates with what the alphabetic index indicated. As there is no further division of codes in category G13 beyond the fourth character, G13.2 is at the highest level of specificity.

Step 8: Although there are some general conventions, such as how to interpret brackets in the alphabetic index, no chapter-specific guidelines apply to this coding scenario.

Step 9: Assign codes EØ3.9 Hypothyroidism, unspecified, and G13.2 Systemic atrophy primarily affecting the central nervous system in myxedema.

Repeat steps 1 through 9 for any concomitant diagnoses.

Step 10: Based on the alphabetic index and tabular instructional notations, code EØ3.9 should be sequenced as the first-listed, or principal, diagnosis followed by G13.2 as a secondary diagnosis.

Diagnosis: Decubitus ulcer of right elbow with skin loss and necrosis of subcutaneous tissue

Step 1: The reason for the encounter was the condition, decubitus ulcer.

Step 2: Consult the alphabetic index.

Step 3: Locate the main term "Ulcer."

Step 4: For the subterm "decubitus," there is no code provided or additional subterms indented, but a cross-reference is listed.

Step 5: The italicized cross-reference instructs the coder to "*see* Ulcer, pressure, by site."

Repeat steps 3 through 5 for the cross-reference:

Step 3: Locate the main term "Ulcer."

Step 4: Review the subentries for the subterm "pressure." The next level of indent lists either the site of the ulcer or the specific stage of the ulcer (stage 1–4, unstageable, and unspecified stages). The diagnostic statement provides the site, right elbow, and the extent of tissue damage (skin loss and necrosis of subcutaneous tissue) but does not specifically state that the ulcer is stage 1, stage 2, etc. Nonessential modifiers (in parentheses) at each stage include a description of the typical extent of damage at each stage. For example, stage 1 describes "pre-ulcer skin changes limited to persistent focal edema." Based on the documentation in the record, the coder can correlate the documentation to the nonessential modifiers and choose the specific stage from the index. The coder can also go directly to the body site, choosing the stage of the ulcer after reviewing the code options and instructional notations in the tabular list.

The diagnostic statement indicates that the extent of the damage to the elbow includes skin loss and necrosis of subcutaneous tissue, coinciding with the nonessential modifier next to the subentry "stage 3." The body site of elbow (L89.Ø-) is listed as another level of indent with other body sites.

Step 5: Note that code L89.Ø is followed by a dash and an additional-character-required icon, which indicate that more characters are needed to complete the code. From here, the tabular listing for L89.Ø- can be consulted.

Step 6: Locate code L89.Ø- in the tabular list and read all instructional notes.

Step 7: The tabular listing at category L89 has an Includes note for "decubitus ulcer," which confirms that category L89 is the appropriate category to represent what is documented in the diagnostic statement.

Several Excludes 2 notes are also listed at the category level. Excludes 2 notes represent conditions that can occur concomitantly with the decubitus ulcer and can be coded in addition to code L89, if supported by the documentation.

The subcategory codes under L89.Ø indicate that the fifth character describes laterality. Locate the right elbow at subcategory L89.Ø1. See that an additional sixth character to specify the stage of the ulcer is now needed to complete the code. The stage can be determined either by the specific documentation of the stage (e.g., stage 1, stage 2) or, in this case, a description that matches one of the inclusion terms that follow each stage code. For example, the diagnostic description in this case of "skin loss and necrosis of the subcutaneous tissue" matches the inclusion term under L89.Ø13 Pressure ulcer of right elbow, stage 3. No additional characters are required because code L89.Ø13 is at its highest level of specificity.

Step 8: The official guidelines contain quite a bit of information relating to pressure ulcers in chapter-specific guideline I.C.12 as well as information in general guideline I.B.14. These and any other pertinent guidelines should be reviewed to ensure appropriate code assignment.

Step 9: Assign code L89.Ø13 Pressure ulcer of right elbow, stage 3.

Repeat steps 1 through 9 for any concomitant diagnoses.

Step 10: Since the decubitus ulcer is listed as the chief reason for the health care encounter, the first-listed, or principal, diagnosis is L89.Ø13. However, according to the code first instructional note at the L89 category level, gangrene (I96) would be sequenced before the pressure ulcer if it were documented.

Diagnosis: Emergency department visit for bimalleolar fracture of the right ankle due to trauma

Step 1: The reason for the encounter was the condition, bimalleolar fracture.

Step 2: Consult the alphabetic index.

Step 3: Locate the main term "Fracture." Note that many main terms represent fractures: "Fracture, burst," "Fracture, chronic," "Fracture, insufficiency," "Fracture, nontraumatic NEC," "Fracture, pathological," and "Fracture, traumatic." Since the diagnostic statement specifically states that this fracture was the result of trauma, the main term "Fracture, traumatic" should be used.

Step 4: Subterms that should be referenced are "ankle" and "bimalleolar (displaced)," which lists code S82.84-.

Step 5: A nonessential modifier (in parentheses) next to the term bimalleolar for "displaced" indicates that S82.84- is the default category unless the fracture is specifically identified as "nondisplaced."

Note that code S82.84- is followed by a dash and an additional-character icon, both of which indicate that more characters are required. From here, the tabular list can be consulted.

Step 6: Locate code S82.84- in the tabular list and read all instructional notes.

Step: 7: The instructional notes at category S82 indicate that fractures not specified as displaced or nondisplaced default to displaced and that fractures not designated as open or closed default to closed. Additional instructional notes can be found at the category level but none pertain to the current scenario.

Read through the subcategory codes under S82.84, and note that the sixth character specifies displaced or nondisplaced and laterality. Based on the index nonessential modifier (displaced) and the code note at category S82, code selection should identify a displaced fracture of the right side. A displaced bimalleolar fracture of the right lower leg is coded to S82.841.

To complete the code, a seventh character must be assigned to identify the type of encounter (initial, subsequent, or sequela) and whether the fracture is open or closed. Most of the codes in category S82 require a seventh character represented in the list at the category level. However, it is important to note that some subcategories have their own specific set of seventh characters. In this instance, subcategory S82.84- does not have a unique set of seventh characters and the list provided at the category level should be used. Without documentation of the fracture being open, the tabular notation indicates that the default is closed. Character A, representing "initial encounter for closed fracture," listed in the box at the category level is the most appropriate option.

Step 8: Assign code S82.841A Displaced bimalleolar fracture of right lower leg, initial encounter for closed fracture.

Repeat steps 1 through 9 for any concomitant diagnoses.

Step 9: Review chapter-specific guideline I.C.19. and any other official conventions or guidelines to ensure appropriate code assignment.

Step 10: Additional codes can be applied to relate the specific cause of the injury, the place of occurrence, the activity of the patient at the time of the injury, and the patient's status, when this information is available in the record. However, coding this information is voluntary and reporting requirements depend on state mandates and/or facility-specific reporting requirements. If assigned, the external cause codes should be reported as secondary diagnoses only with the injury (fracture) sequenced first. Most codes in chapter 20, "External Causes of

Morbidity," require a seventh character to identify the type of encounter. The seventh character assigned to an external cause code should match the seventh character of the code assigned for the associated injury or condition for the encounter.

2023 ICD-10-CM Official Guidelines for Coding and Reporting

Narrative changes effective October 1, 2022 appear in **bold** text

Narrative changes effective April 1, 2022 appear in shaded text

Items underlined have been moved within the guidelines since the FY 2022 version

Italics are used to indicate revisions to heading changes

The Centers for Medicare and Medicaid Services (CMS) and the National Center for Health Statistics (NCHS), two departments within the U.S. Federal Government's Department of Health and Human Services (DHHS) provide the following guidelines for coding and reporting using the International Classification of Diseases, 10th Revision, Clinical Modification (ICD-10-CM). These guidelines should be used as a companion document to the official version of the ICD-10-CM as published on the NCHS website. The ICD-10-CM is a morbidity classification published by the United States for classifying diagnoses and reason for visits in all health care settings. The ICD-10-CM is based on the ICD-10, the statistical classification of disease published by the World Health Organization (WHO).

These guidelines have been approved by the four organizations that make up the Cooperating Parties for the ICD-10-CM: the American Hospital Association (AHA), the American Health Information Management Association (AHIMA), CMS, and NCHS.

These guidelines are a set of rules that have been developed to accompany and complement the official conventions and instructions provided within the ICD-10-CM itself. The instructions and conventions of the classification take precedence over guidelines. These guidelines are based on the coding and sequencing instructions in the Tabular List and Alphabetic Index of ICD-10-CM, but provide additional instruction. Adherence to these guidelines when assigning ICD-10-CM diagnosis codes is required under the Health Insurance Portability and Accountability Act (HIPAA). The diagnosis codes (Tabular List and Alphabetic Index) have been adopted under HIPAA for all healthcare settings. A joint effort between the healthcare provider and the coder is essential to achieve complete and accurate documentation, code assignment, and reporting of diagnoses and procedures. These guidelines have been developed to assist both the healthcare provider and the coder in identifying those diagnoses that are to be reported. The importance of consistent, complete documentation in the medical record cannot be overemphasized. Without such documentation accurate coding cannot be achieved. The entire record should be reviewed to determine the specific reason for the encounter and the conditions treated.

The term encounter is used for all settings, including hospital admissions. In the context of these guidelines, the term provider is used throughout the guidelines to mean physician or any qualified health care practitioner who is legally accountable for establishing the patient's diagnosis. Only this set of guidelines, approved by the Cooperating Parties, is official.

The guidelines are organized into sections. Section I includes the structure and conventions of the classification and general guidelines that apply to the entire classification, and chapter-specific guidelines that correspond to the chapters as they are arranged in the classification. Section II includes guidelines for selection of principal diagnosis for non-outpatient settings. Section III includes guidelines for reporting additional diagnoses in non-outpatient settings. Section IV is for outpatient coding and reporting. It is necessary to review all sections of the guidelines to fully understand all of the rules and instructions needed to code properly.

Section I. Conventions, general coding guidelines and chapter specific guidelines

The conventions, general guidelines and chapter-specific guidelines are applicable to all health care settings unless otherwise indicated. The conventions and instructions of the classification take precedence over guidelines.

A. Conventions for the ICD-10-CM

The conventions for the ICD-10-CM are the general rules for use of the classification independent of the guidelines. These conventions are incorporated within the Alphabetic Index and Tabular List of the ICD-10-CM as instructional notes.

1. **The Alphabetic Index and Tabular List**
   The ICD-10-CM is divided into the Alphabetic Index, an alphabetical list of terms and their corresponding code, and the Tabular List, a structured list of codes divided into chapters based on body system or condition. The Alphabetic Index consists of the following parts: the Index of Diseases and Injury, the Index of External Causes of Injury, the Table of Neoplasms and the Table of Drugs and Chemicals.
   See Section I.C.2. Neoplasms
   See Section I.C.19. Adverse effects, poisoning, underdosing and toxic effects

2. **Format and Structure:**
   The ICD-10-CM Tabular List contains categories, subcategories and codes. Characters for categories, subcategories and codes may be either a letter or a number. All categories are 3 characters. A three-character category that has no further subdivision is equivalent to a code. Subcategories are either 4 or 5 characters. Codes may be 3, 4, 5, 6 or 7 characters. That is, each level of subdivision after a category is a subcategory. The final level of subdivision is a code. Codes that have applicable 7th characters are still referred to as codes, not subcategories. A code that has an applicable 7th character is considered invalid without the 7th character.
   The ICD-10-CM uses an indented format for ease in reference.

3. **Use of codes for reporting purposes**
   For reporting purposes only codes are permissible, not categories or subcategories, and any applicable 7th character is required.

4. **Placeholder character**
   The ICD-10-CM utilizes a placeholder character "X". The "X" is used as a placeholder at certain codes to allow for future expansion. An example of this is at the poisoning, adverse effect and underdosing codes, categories T36-T50. Where a placeholder exists, the X must be used in order for the code to be considered a valid code.

5. **7th Characters**
   Certain ICD-10-CM categories have applicable 7th characters. The applicable 7th character is required for all codes within the category, or as the notes in the Tabular List instruct. The 7th character must always be the 7th character in the data field. If a code that requires a 7th character is not 6 characters, a placeholder X must be used to fill in the empty characters.

6. **Abbreviations**
   a. **Alphabetic Index abbreviations**
      NEC "Not elsewhere classifiable"
      This abbreviation in the Alphabetic Index represents "other specified." When a specific code is not available for a condition, the Alphabetic Index directs the coder to the "other specified" code in the Tabular List.
      NOS "Not otherwise specified"
      This abbreviation is the equivalent of unspecified.
   b. **Tabular List abbreviations**
      NEC "Not elsewhere classifiable"
      This abbreviation in the Tabular List represents "other specified". When a specific code is not available for a condition, the Tabular List includes an NEC entry under a code to identify the code as the "other specified" code.
      NOS "Not otherwise specified"
      This abbreviation is the equivalent of unspecified.

7. **Punctuation**
   [ ] Brackets are used in the Tabular List to enclose synonyms, alternative wording or explanatory phrases. Brackets are used in the Alphabetic Index to identify manifestation codes.
   ( ) Parentheses are used in both the Alphabetic Index and Tabular List to enclose supplementary words that may be present or absent in the statement of a disease or procedure without affecting the code number to which it is assigned. The terms within the parentheses are referred to as nonessential modifiers. The nonessential modifiers in the Alphabetic Index to Diseases apply to subterms following a main term except when a nonessential modifier and a subentry are

mutually exclusive, the subentry takes precedence. For example, in the ICD-10-CM Alphabetic Index under the main term Enteritis, "acute" is a nonessential modifier and "chronic" is a subentry. In this case, the nonessential modifier "acute" does not apply to the subentry "chronic".
   : Colons are used in the Tabular List after an incomplete term which needs one or more of the modifiers following the colon to make it assignable to a given category.

8. **Use of "and".**
   See Section I.A.14. Use of the term "And"

9. **Other and Unspecified codes**
   a. **"Other" codes**
      Codes titled "other" or "other specified" are for use when the information in the medical record provides detail for which a specific code does not exist. Alphabetic Index entries with NEC in the line designate "other" codes in the Tabular List. These Alphabetic Index entries represent specific disease entities for which no specific code exists, so the term is included within an "other" code.
   b. **"Unspecified" codes**
      Codes titled "unspecified" are for use when the information in the medical record is insufficient to assign a more specific code. For those categories for which an unspecified code is not provided, the "other specified" code may represent both other and unspecified.
      See Section I.B.18. Use of Signs/Symptom/Unspecified Codes

10. **Includes Notes**
    This note appears immediately under a three-character code title to further define, or give examples of, the content of the category.

11. **Inclusion terms**
    List of terms is included under some codes. These terms are the conditions for which that code is to be used. The terms may be synonyms of the code title, or, in the case of "other specified" codes, the terms are a list of the various conditions assigned to that code. The inclusion terms are not necessarily exhaustive. Additional terms found only in the Alphabetic Index may also be assigned to a code.

12. **Excludes Notes**
    The ICD-10-CM has two types of excludes notes. Each type of note has a different definition for use, but they are all similar in that they indicate that codes excluded from each other are independent of each other.
    a. **Excludes1**
       A type 1 Excludes note is a pure excludes note. It means "NOT CODED HERE!" An Excludes1 note indicates that the code excluded should never be used at the same time as the code above the Excludes1 note. An Excludes1 is used when two conditions cannot occur together, such as a congenital form versus an acquired form of the same condition.
       An exception to the Excludes1 definition is the circumstance when the two conditions are unrelated to each other. If it is not clear whether the two conditions involving an Excludes1 note are related or not, query the provider. For example, code F45.8, Other somatoform disorders, has an Excludes1 note for "sleep related teeth grinding (G47.63)," because "teeth grinding" is an inclusion term under F45.8. Only one of these two codes should be assigned for teeth grinding. However psychogenic dysmenorrhea is also an inclusion term under F45.8, and a patient could have both this condition and sleep related teeth grinding. In this case, the two conditions are clearly unrelated to each other, and so it would be appropriate to report F45.8 and G47.63 together.
    b. **Excludes2**
       A type 2 Excludes note represents "Not included here." An excludes2 note indicates that the condition excluded is not part of the condition represented by the code, but a patient may have both conditions at the same time. When an Excludes2 note appears under a code, it is acceptable to use both the code and the excluded code together, when appropriate.

13. **Etiology/manifestation convention ("code first", "use additional code" and "in diseases classified elsewhere" notes)**
    Certain conditions have both an underlying etiology and multiple body system manifestations due to the underlying etiology. For such conditions, the ICD-10-CM has a coding convention that requires the underlying condition be sequenced first, if applicable, followed by the manifestation. Wherever such a combination exists, there is a "use additional code" note at the etiology code, and a "code first" note at the manifestation code. These instructional notes indicate the proper sequencing order of the codes, etiology followed by manifestation.
    In most cases the manifestation codes will have in the code title, "in diseases classified elsewhere." Codes with this title are a component of the

etiology/ manifestation convention. The code title indicates that it is a manifestation code. "In diseases classified elsewhere" codes are never permitted to be used as first listed or principal diagnosis codes. They must be used in conjunction with an underlying condition code and they must be listed following the underlying condition. See category F02, Dementia in other diseases classified elsewhere, for an example of this convention.

There are manifestation codes that do not have "in diseases classified elsewhere" in the title. For such codes, there is a "use additional code" note at the etiology code and a "code first" note at the manifestation code, and the rules for sequencing apply.

In addition to the notes in the Tabular List, these conditions also have a specific Alphabetic Index entry structure. In the Alphabetic Index both conditions are listed together with the etiology code first followed by the manifestation codes in brackets. The code in brackets is always to be sequenced second.

An example of the etiology/manifestation convention is dementia **with** Parkinson's disease. In the Alphabetic Index, code G20 is listed first, followed by code F02.80 or F02.81- in brackets. Code G20 represents the underlying etiology, Parkinson's disease, and must be sequenced first, whereas code**s** F02.80 and F02.81- represent the manifestation of dementia in diseases classified elsewhere, with or without behavioral disturbance.

"Code first" and "Use additional code" notes are also used as sequencing rules in the classification for certain codes that are not part of an etiology/ manifestation combination.

See Section I.B.7. Multiple coding for a single condition.

14. "And"
The word "and" should be interpreted to mean either "and" or "or" when it appears in a title.

For example, cases of "tuberculosis of bones", "tuberculosis of joints" and "tuberculosis of bones and joints" are classified to subcategory A18.0, Tuberculosis of bones and joints.

15. "With"
The word "with" or "in" should be interpreted to mean "associated with" or "due to" when it appears in a code title, the Alphabetic Index (either under a main term or subterm), or an instructional note in the Tabular List. The classification presumes a causal relationship between the two conditions linked by these terms in the Alphabetic Index or Tabular List. These conditions should be coded as related even in the absence of provider documentation explicitly linking them, unless the documentation clearly states the conditions are unrelated or when another guideline exists that specifically requires a documented linkage between two conditions (e.g., sepsis guideline for "acute organ dysfunction that is not clearly associated with the sepsis").

For conditions not specifically linked by these relational terms in the classification or when a guideline requires that a linkage between two conditions be explicitly documented, provider documentation must link the conditions in order to code them as related.

The word "with" in the Alphabetic Index is sequenced immediately following the main term or subterm, not in alphabetical order.

16. "See" and "See Also"
The "see" instruction following a main term in the Alphabetic Index indicates that another term should be referenced. It is necessary to go to the main term referenced with the "see" note to locate the correct code.

A "see also" instruction following a main term in the Alphabetic Index instructs that there is another main term that may also be referenced that may provide additional Alphabetic Index entries that may be useful. It is not necessary to follow the "see also" note when the original main term provides the necessary code.

17. "Code also" note
A "code also" note instructs that two codes may be required to fully describe a condition, but this note does not provide sequencing direction. The sequencing depends on the circumstances of the encounter.

18. Default codes
A code listed next to a main term in the ICD-10-CM Alphabetic Index is referred to as a default code. The default code represents that condition that is most commonly associated with the main term or is the unspecified code for the condition. If a condition is documented in a medical record (for example, appendicitis) without any additional information, such as acute or chronic, the default code should be assigned.

19. Code assignment and Clinical Criteria
The assignment of a diagnosis code is based on the provider's diagnostic statement that the condition exists. The provider's statement that the patient has a particular condition is sufficient. Code assignment is not based on clinical criteria used by the provider to establish the diagnosis. **If**

there is conflicting medical record documentation, query the **provider.**

B. General Coding Guidelines

1. Locating a code in the ICD-10-CM
To select a code in the classification that corresponds to a diagnosis or reason for visit documented in a medical record, first locate the term in the Alphabetic Index, and then verify the code in the Tabular List. Read and be guided by instructional notations that appear in both the Alphabetic Index and the Tabular List.

It is essential to use both the Alphabetic Index and Tabular List when locating and assigning a code. The Alphabetic Index does not always provide the full code. Selection of the full code, including laterality and any applicable 7th character can only be done in the Tabular List. A dash (-) at the end of an Alphabetic Index entry indicates that additional characters are required. Even if a dash is not included at the Alphabetic Index entry, it is necessary to refer to the Tabular List to verify that no 7th character is required.

2. Level of Detail in Coding
Diagnosis codes are to be used and reported at their highest number of characters available and to the highest level of specificity documented in the medical record.

ICD-10-CM diagnosis codes are composed of codes with 3, 4, 5, 6 or 7 characters. Codes with three characters are included in ICD-10-CM as the heading of a category of codes that may be further subdivided by the use of fourth and/or fifth characters and/or sixth characters, which provide greater detail.

A three-character code is to be used only if it is not further subdivided. A code is invalid if it has not been coded to the full number of characters required for that code, including the 7th character, if applicable.

3. Code or codes from A00.0 through T88.9, Z00-Z99.8, U00-U85
The appropriate code or codes from A00.0 through T88.9, Z00-Z99.8, and U00-U85 must be used to identify diagnoses, symptoms, conditions, problems, complaints or other reason(s) for the encounter/visit.

4. Signs and symptoms
Codes that describe symptoms and signs, as opposed to diagnoses, are acceptable for reporting purposes when a related definitive diagnosis has not been established (confirmed) by the provider. Chapter 18 of ICD-10-CM, Symptoms, Signs, and Abnormal Clinical and Laboratory Findings, Not Elsewhere Classified (codes R00.0-R99) contains many, but not all, codes for symptoms.

See Section I.B.18. Use of Signs/Symptom/Unspecified Codes

5. Conditions that are an integral part of a disease process
Signs and symptoms that are associated routinely with a disease process should not be assigned as additional codes, unless otherwise instructed by the classification.

6. Conditions that are not an integral part of a disease process
Additional signs and symptoms that may not be associated routinely with a disease process should be coded when present.

7. Multiple coding for a single condition
In addition to the etiology/manifestation convention that requires two codes to fully describe a single condition that affects multiple body systems, there are other single conditions that also require more than one code. "Use additional code" notes are found in the Tabular List at codes that are not part of an etiology/manifestation pair where a secondary code is useful to fully describe a condition. The sequencing rule is the same as the etiology/manifestation pair, "use additional code" indicates that a secondary code should be added, if known.

For example, for bacterial infections that are not included in chapter 1, a secondary code from category B95, Streptococcus, Staphylococcus, and Enterococcus, as the cause of diseases classified elsewhere, or B96, Other bacterial agents as the cause of diseases classified elsewhere, may be required to identify the bacterial organism causing the infection. A "use additional code" note will normally be found at the infectious disease code, indicating a need for the organism code to be added as a secondary code.

"Code first" notes are also under certain codes that are not specifically manifestation codes but may be due to an underlying cause. When there is a "code first" note and an underlying condition is present, the underlying condition should be sequenced first, if known.

"Code, if applicable, any causal condition first" notes indicate that this code may be assigned as a principal diagnosis when the causal condition is unknown or not applicable. If a causal condition is known, then the code for that condition should be sequenced as the principal or first-listed diagnosis.

Multiple codes may be needed for sequela, complication codes and obstetric codes to more fully describe a condition. See the specific guidelines for these conditions for further instruction.

8. **Acute and Chronic Conditions**

If the same condition is described as both acute (subacute) and chronic, and separate subentries exist in the Alphabetic Index at the same indentation level, code both and sequence the acute (subacute) code first.

9. **Combination Code**

A combination code is a single code used to classify:

> Two diagnoses, or
>
> A diagnosis with an associated secondary process (manifestation)
>
> A diagnosis with an associated complication

Combination codes are identified by referring to subterm entries in the Alphabetic Index and by reading the inclusion and exclusion notes in the Tabular List.

Assign only the combination code when that code fully identifies the diagnostic conditions involved or when the Alphabetic Index so directs. Multiple coding should not be used when the classification provides a combination code that clearly identifies all of the elements documented in the diagnosis. When the combination code lacks necessary specificity in describing the manifestation or complication, an additional code should be used as a secondary code.

10. **Sequela (Late Effects)**

A sequela is the residual effect (condition produced) after the acute phase of an illness or injury has terminated. There is no time limit on when a sequela code can be used. The residual may be apparent early, such as in cerebral infarction, or it may occur months or years later, such as that due to a previous injury. Examples of sequela include: scar formation resulting from a burn, deviated septum due to a nasal fracture, and infertility due to tubal occlusion from old tuberculosis. Coding of sequela generally requires two codes sequenced in the following order: the condition or nature of the sequela is sequenced first. The sequela code is sequenced second.

An exception to the above guidelines are those instances where the code for the sequela is followed by a manifestation code identified in the Tabular List and title, or the sequela code has been expanded (at the fourth, fifth or sixth character levels) to include the manifestation(s). The code for the acute phase of an illness or injury that led to the sequela is never used with a code for the late effect.

See Section I.C.9. Sequelae of cerebrovascular disease

See Section I.C.15. Sequelae of complication of pregnancy, childbirth and the puerperium

See Section I.C.19. Application of 7th characters for Chapter 19

11. **Impending or Threatened Condition**

Code any condition described at the time of discharge as "impending" or "threatened" as follows:

> If it did occur, code as confirmed diagnosis.
>
> If it did not occur, reference the Alphabetic Index to determine if the condition has a subentry term for "impending" or "threatened" and also reference main term entries for "Impending" and for "Threatened."
>
> If the subterms are listed, assign the given code.
>
> If the subterms are not listed, code the existing underlying condition(s) and not the condition described as impending or threatened.

12. **Reporting Same Diagnosis Code More than Once**

Each unique ICD-10-CM diagnosis code may be reported only once for an encounter. This applies to bilateral conditions when there are no distinct codes identifying laterality or two different conditions classified to the same ICD-10-CM diagnosis code.

13. **Laterality**

Some ICD-10-CM codes indicate laterality, specifying whether the condition occurs on the left, right or is bilateral. If no bilateral code is provided and the condition is bilateral, assign separate codes for both the left and right side. If the side is not identified in the medical record, assign the code for the unspecified side.

When a patient has a bilateral condition and each side is treated during separate encounters, assign the "bilateral" code (as the condition still exists on both sides), including for the encounter to treat the first side. For the second encounter for treatment after one side has previously been treated and the condition no longer exists on that side, assign the appropriate unilateral code for the side where the condition still exists (e.g., cataract surgery performed on each eye in separate encounters). The bilateral code would not be assigned for the subsequent encounter, as the patient no longer has the condition in the previously-treated site. If the

treatment on the first side did not completely resolve the condition, then the bilateral code would still be appropriate.

When laterality is not documented by the patient's provider, code assignment for the affected side may be based on medical record documentation from other clinicians. If there is conflicting medical record documentation regarding the affected side, the patient's attending provider should be queried for clarification. Codes for "unspecified" side should rarely be used, such as when the documentation in the record is insufficient to determine the affected side and it is not possible to obtain clarification.

14. **Documentation by Clinicians Other than the Patient's Provider**

Code assignment is based on the documentation by the patient's provider (i.e., physician or other qualified healthcare practitioner legally accountable for establishing the patient's diagnosis). There are a few exceptions when code assignment may be based on medical record documentation from clinicians who are not the patient's provider (i.e., physician or other qualified healthcare practitioner legally accountable for establishing the patient's diagnosis). In this context, "clinicians" other than the patient's provider refer to healthcare professionals permitted, based on regulatory or accreditation requirements or internal hospital policies, to document in a patient's official medical record.

These exceptions include codes for:

- Body Mass Index (BMI)
- Depth of non-pressure chronic ulcers
- Pressure ulcer stage
- Coma scale
- NIH stroke scale (NIHSS)
- Social determinants of health (SDOH)
- Laterality
- Blood alcohol level
- **Underimmunization status**

This information is typically, or may be, documented by other clinicians involved in the care of the patient (e.g., a dietitian often documents the BMI, a nurse often documents the pressure ulcer stages, and an emergency medical technician often documents the coma scale). However, the associated diagnosis (such as overweight, obesity, acute stroke, pressure ulcer, or a condition classifiable to category F10, Alcohol related disorders) must be documented by the patient's provider. If there is conflicting medical record documentation, either from the same clinician or different clinicians, the patient's attending provider should be queried for clarification.

The BMI, coma scale, NIHSS, blood alcohol level codes, codes for social determinants of health **and underimmunization status** should only be reported as secondary diagnoses.

See Section I.C.21.c.17. for additional information regarding coding social determinants of health.

15. **Syndromes**

Follow the Alphabetic Index guidance when coding syndromes. In the absence of Alphabetic Index guidance, assign codes for the documented manifestations of the syndrome. Additional codes for manifestations that are not an integral part of the disease process may also be assigned when the condition does not have a unique code.

16. **Documentation of Complications of Care**

Code assignment is based on the provider's documentation of the relationship between the condition and the care or procedure, unless otherwise instructed by the classification. The guideline extends to any complications of care, regardless of the chapter the code is located in. It is important to note that not all conditions that occur during or following medical care or surgery are classified as complications. There must be a cause-and-effect relationship between the care provided and the condition, and **the documentation must support that the condition is clinically significant. It is not necessary for the provider to explicitly document the term "complication." For example, if the condition alters the course of the surgery as documented in the operative report, then it would be appropriate to report a complication code.** Query the provider for clarification **if the documentation is not clear as to the relationship between the condition and the care or procedure.**

17. **Borderline Diagnosis**

If the provider documents a "borderline" diagnosis at the time of discharge, the diagnosis is coded as confirmed, unless the classification provides a specific entry (e.g., borderline diabetes). If a borderline condition has a specific index entry in ICD-10-CM, it should be coded as such. Since borderline conditions are not uncertain diagnoses, no distinction is made between the care setting (inpatient versus outpatient). Whenever the documentation is unclear regarding a borderline condition, coders are encouraged to query for clarification.

18. Use of Sign/Symptom/Unspecified Codes

Sign/symptom and "unspecified" codes have acceptable, even necessary, uses. While specific diagnosis codes should be reported when they are supported by the available medical record documentation and clinical knowledge of the patient's health condition, there are instances when signs/symptoms or unspecified codes are the best choices for accurately reflecting the healthcare encounter. Each healthcare encounter should be coded to the level of certainty known for that encounter.

As stated in the introductory section of these official coding guidelines, a joint effort between the healthcare provider and the coder is essential to achieve complete and accurate documentation, code assignment, and reporting of diagnoses and procedures. The importance of consistent, complete documentation in the medical record cannot be overemphasized. Without such documentation accurate coding cannot be achieved. The entire record should be reviewed to determine the specific reason for the encounter and the conditions treated.

If a definitive diagnosis has not been established by the end of the encounter, it is appropriate to report codes for sign(s) and/or symptom(s) in lieu of a definitive diagnosis. When sufficient clinical information isn't known or available about a particular health condition to assign a more specific code, it is acceptable to report the appropriate "unspecified" code (e.g., a diagnosis of pneumonia has been determined, but not the specific type). Unspecified codes should be reported when they are the codes that most accurately reflect what is known about the patient's condition at the time of that particular encounter. It would be inappropriate to select a specific code that is not supported by the medical record documentation or conduct medically unnecessary diagnostic testing in order to determine a more specific code.

19. Coding for Healthcare Encounters in Hurricane Aftermath

a. Use of External Cause of Morbidity Codes

An external cause of morbidity code should be assigned to identify the cause of the injury(ies) incurred as a result of the hurricane. The use of external cause of morbidity codes is supplemental to the application of ICD-10-CM codes. External cause of morbidity codes are never to be recorded as a principal diagnosis (first-listed in non-inpatient settings). The appropriate injury code should be sequenced before any external cause codes. The external cause of morbidity codes capture how the injury or health condition happened (cause), the intent (unintentional or accidental; or intentional, such as suicide or assault), the place where the event occurred, the activity of the patient at the time of the event, and the person's status (e.g., civilian, military). They should not be assigned for encounters to treat hurricane victims' medical conditions when no injury, adverse effect or poisoning is involved. External cause of morbidity codes should be assigned for each encounter for care and treatment of the injury. External cause of morbidity codes may be assigned in all health care settings. For the purpose of capturing complete and accurate ICD-10-CM data in the aftermath of the hurricane, a healthcare setting should be considered as any location where medical care is provided by licensed healthcare professionals.

b. Sequencing of External Causes of Morbidity Codes

Codes for cataclysmic events, such as a hurricane, take priority over all other external cause codes except child and adult abuse and terrorism and should be sequenced before other external cause of injury codes. Assign as many external cause of morbidity codes as necessary to fully explain each cause. For example, if an injury occurs as a result of a building collapse during the hurricane, external cause codes for both the hurricane and the building collapse should be assigned, with the external causes code for hurricane being sequenced as the first external cause code. For injuries incurred as a direct result of the hurricane, assign the appropriate code(s) for the injuries, followed by the code X37.0-, Hurricane (with the appropriate 7th character), and any other applicable external cause of injury codes. Code X37.0- also should be assigned when an injury is incurred as a result of flooding caused by a levee breaking related to the hurricane. Code X38.-, Flood (with the appropriate 7th character), should be assigned when an injury is from flooding resulting directly from the storm. Code X36.0.-, Collapse of dam or man-made structure, should not be assigned when the cause of the collapse is due to the hurricane. Use of code X36.0- is limited to collapses of man-made structures due to earth surface movements, not due to storm surges directly from a hurricane.

c. Other External Causes of Morbidity Code Issues

For injuries that are not a direct result of the hurricane, such as an evacuee that has incurred an injury as a result of a motor vehicle accident, assign the appropriate external cause of morbidity code(s) to describe the cause of the injury, but do not assign code X37.0-, Hurricane. If it is not clear whether the injury was a direct result of the hurricane, assume the injury is due to the hurricane and assign code

X37.0-, Hurricane, as well as any other applicable external cause of morbidity codes. In addition to code X37.0-, Hurricane, other possible applicable external cause of morbidity codes include:

- X30-, Exposure to excessive natural heat
- X31-, Exposure to excessive natural cold
- X38-, Flood

d. Use of Z codes

Z codes (other reasons for healthcare encounters) may be assigned as appropriate to further explain the reasons for presenting for healthcare services, including transfers between healthcare facilities, or provide additional information relevant to a patient encounter. The ICD-10-CM Official Guidelines for Coding and Reporting identify which codes maybe assigned as principal or first-listed diagnosis only, secondary diagnosis only, or principal/first-listed or secondary (depending on the circumstances). Possible applicable Z codes include:

- Z59.0-, Homelessness
- Z59.1, Inadequate housing
- Z59.5, Extreme poverty
- Z75.1, Person awaiting admission to adequate facility elsewhere
- Z75.3, Unavailability and inaccessibility of health-care facilities
- Z75.4, Unavailability and inaccessibility of other helping agencies
- Z76.2, Encounter for health supervision and care of other healthy infant and child
- Z99.12, Encounter for respirator [ventilator] dependence during power failure

The external cause of morbidity codes and the Z codes listed above are not an all-inclusive list. Other codes may be applicable to the encounter based upon the documentation. Assign as many codes as necessary to fully explain each healthcare encounter. Since patient history information may be very limited, use any available documentation to assign the appropriate external cause of morbidity and Z codes.

C. Chapter-Specific Coding Guidelines

In addition to general coding guidelines, there are guidelines for specific diagnoses and/or conditions in the classification. Unless otherwise indicated, these guidelines apply to all health care settings. Please refer to Section II for guidelines on the selection of principal diagnosis.

1. Chapter 1: Certain Infectious and Parasitic Diseases (A00-B99), U07.1, U09.9

a. Human Immunodeficiency Virus (HIV) Infections

1) Code only confirmed cases

Code only confirmed cases of HIV infection/illness. This is an exception to the hospital inpatient guideline Section II, H.

In this context, "confirmation" does not require documentation of positive serology or culture for HIV; the provider's diagnostic statement that the patient is HIV positive or has an HIV-related illness is sufficient.

2) Selection and sequencing of HIV codes

(a) Patient admitted for HIV-related condition

If a patient is admitted for an HIV-related condition, the principal diagnosis should be B20, Human immunodeficiency virus [HIV] disease followed by additional diagnosis codes for all reported HIV-related conditions.

An exception to this guideline is if the reason for admission is hemolytic-uremic syndrome associated with HIV disease. Assign code D59.31, Infection-associated hemolytic-uremic syndrome, followed by code B20, Human immunodeficiency virus [HIV] disease.

(b) Patient with HIV disease admitted for unrelated condition

If a patient with HIV disease is admitted for an unrelated condition (such as a traumatic injury), the code for the unrelated condition (e.g., the nature of injury code) should be the principal diagnosis. Other diagnoses would be B20 followed by additional diagnosis codes for all reported HIV-related conditions.

(c) Whether the patient is newly diagnosed

Whether the patient is newly diagnosed or has had previous admissions/encounters for HIV conditions is irrelevant to the sequencing decision.

(d) Asymptomatic human immunodeficiency virus

Z21, Asymptomatic human immunodeficiency virus [HIV] infection status, is to be applied when the patient without any documentation of symptoms is listed as being "HIV positive," "known HIV," "HIV test positive," or similar terminology. Do not use this code if the term "AIDS" or "HIV disease" is used or if the patient is treated for any HIV-related illness or is described as having any condition(s) resulting from his/her HIV positive status; use B20 in these cases.

(e) Patients with inconclusive HIV serology
Patients with inconclusive HIV serology, but no definitive diagnosis or manifestations of the illness, may be assigned code R75, Inconclusive laboratory evidence of human immunodeficiency virus [HIV].

(f) Previously diagnosed HIV-related illness
Patients with any known prior diagnosis of an HIV-related illness should be coded to B20. Once a patient has developed an HIV-related illness, the patient should always be assigned code B20 on every subsequent admission/encounter. Patients previously diagnosed with any HIV illness (B20) should never be assigned to R75 or Z21, Asymptomatic human immunodeficiency virus [HIV] infection status.

(g) HIV Infection in Pregnancy, Childbirth and the Puerperium
During pregnancy, childbirth or the puerperium, a patient admitted (or presenting for a health care encounter) because of an HIV-related illness should receive a principal diagnosis code of O98.7-, Human immunodeficiency [HIV] disease complicating pregnancy, childbirth and the puerperium, followed by B20 and the code(s) for the HIV-related illness(es). Codes from Chapter 15 always take sequencing priority.

Patients with asymptomatic HIV infection status admitted (or presenting for a health care encounter) during pregnancy, childbirth, or the puerperium should receive codes of O98.7- and Z21.

(h) Encounters for testing for HIV
If a patient is being seen to determine his/her HIV status, use code Z11.4, Encounter for screening for human immunodeficiency virus [HIV]. Use additional codes for any associated high-risk behavior, if applicable.

If a patient with signs or symptoms is being seen for HIV testing, code the signs and symptoms. An additional counseling code Z71.7, Human immunodeficiency virus [HIV] counseling, may be used if counseling is provided during the encounter for the test.

When a patient returns to be informed of his/her HIV test results and the test result is negative, use code Z71.7, Human immunodeficiency virus [HIV] counseling.

If the results are positive, see previous guidelines and assign codes as appropriate.

(i) HIV managed by antiretroviral medication
If a patient with documented HIV disease, **HIV-related illness or AIDS** is currently managed on antiretroviral medications, assign code B20, Human immunodeficiency virus [HIV] disease. Code Z79.899, Other long term (current) drug therapy, may be assigned as an additional code to identify the long-term (current) use of antiretroviral medications.

b. Infectious agents as the cause of diseases classified to other chapters
Certain infections are classified in chapters other than Chapter 1 and no organism is identified as part of the infection code. In these instances, it is necessary to use an additional code from Chapter 1 to identify the organism. A code from category B95, Streptococcus, Staphylococcus, and Enterococcus as the cause of diseases classified to other chapters, B96, Other bacterial agents as the cause of diseases classified to other chapters, or B97, Viral agents as the cause of diseases classified to other chapters, is to be used as an additional code to identify the organism. An instructional note will be found at the infection code advising that an additional organism code is required.

c. Infections resistant to antibiotics
Many bacterial infections are resistant to current antibiotics. It is necessary to identify all infections documented as antibiotic resistant. Assign a code from category Z16, Resistance to antimicrobial drugs, following the infection code only if the infection code does not identify drug resistance.

d. Sepsis, Severe Sepsis, and Septic Shock Infections resistant to antibiotics

1) Coding of Sepsis and Severe Sepsis

(a) Sepsis
For a diagnosis of sepsis, assign the appropriate code for the underlying systemic infection. If the type of infection or causal organism is not further specified, assign code A41.9, Sepsis, unspecified organism.

A code from subcategory R65.2, Severe sepsis, should not be assigned unless severe sepsis or an associated acute organ dysfunction is documented.

(i) Negative or inconclusive blood cultures and sepsis
Negative or inconclusive blood cultures do not preclude a diagnosis of sepsis in patients with clinical evidence of the condition; however, the provider should be queried.

(ii) Urosepsis
The term urosepsis is a nonspecific term. It is not to be considered synonymous with sepsis. It has no default code in the Alphabetic Index. Should a provider use this term, he/she must be queried for clarification.

(iii) Sepsis with organ dysfunction
If a patient has sepsis and associated acute organ dysfunction or multiple organ dysfunction (MOD), follow the instructions for coding severe sepsis.

(iv) Acute organ dysfunction that is not clearly associated with the sepsis
If a patient has sepsis and an acute organ dysfunction, but the medical record documentation indicates that the acute organ dysfunction is related to a medical condition other than the sepsis, do not assign a code from subcategory R65.2, Severe sepsis. An acute organ dysfunction must be associated with the sepsis in order to assign the severe sepsis code. If the documentation is not clear as to whether an acute organ dysfunction is related to the sepsis or another medical condition, query the provider.

(b) Severe sepsis
The coding of severe sepsis requires a minimum of 2 codes: first a code for the underlying systemic infection, followed by a code from subcategory R65.2, Severe sepsis. If the causal organism is not documented, assign code A41.9, Sepsis, unspecified organism, for the infection. Additional code(s) for the associated acute organ dysfunction are also required.

Due to the complex nature of severe sepsis, some cases may require querying the provider prior to assignment of the codes.

2) Septic shock
Septic shock generally refers to circulatory failure associated with severe sepsis, and therefore, it represents a type of acute organ dysfunction.

For cases of septic shock, the code for the systemic infection should be sequenced first, followed by code R65.21, Severe sepsis with septic shock or code T81.12, Postprocedural septic shock.

Any additional codes for the other acute organ dysfunctions should also be assigned. As noted in the sequencing instructions in the Tabular List, the code for septic shock cannot be assigned as a principal diagnosis.

3) Sequencing of severe sepsis
If severe sepsis is present on admission, and meets the definition of principal diagnosis, the underlying systemic infection should be assigned as principal diagnosis followed by the appropriate code from subcategory R65.2 as required by the sequencing rules in the Tabular List. A code from subcategory R65.2 can never be assigned as a principal diagnosis.

When severe sepsis develops during an encounter (it was not present on admission), the underlying systemic infection and the appropriate code from subcategory R65.2 should be assigned as secondary diagnoses.

Severe sepsis may be present on admission, but the diagnosis may not be confirmed until sometime after admission. If the documentation is not clear whether severe sepsis was present on admission, the provider should be queried.

For infection-associated hemolytic-uremic syndrome with severe sepsis, see guideline I.C.1.d.9.

4) Sepsis or severe sepsis with a localized infection

If the reason for admission is sepsis or severe sepsis and a localized infection, such as pneumonia or cellulitis, a code(s) for the underlying systemic infection should be assigned first and the code for the localized infection should be assigned as a secondary diagnosis. If the patient has severe sepsis, a code from subcategory R65.2 should also be assigned as a secondary diagnosis. If the patient is admitted with a localized infection, such as pneumonia, and sepsis/severe sepsis doesn't develop until after admission, the localized infection should be assigned first, followed by the appropriate sepsis/severe sepsis codes.

For hemolytic-uremic syndrome associated with sepsis, see guideline I.C.1.d.9.

5) Sepsis due to a postprocedural infection

(a) Documentation of causal relationship

As with all postprocedural complications, code assignment is based on the provider's documentation of the relationship between the infection and the procedure.

(b) Sepsis due to a postprocedural infection

For infections following a procedure, a code from T81.40, to T81.43 Infection following a procedure, or a code from O86.00 to O86.03, Infection of obstetric surgical wound, that identifies the site of the infection should be coded first, if known. Assign an additional code for sepsis following a procedure (T81.44) or sepsis following an obstetrical procedure (O86.04). Use an additional code to identify the infectious agent. If the patient has severe sepsis, the appropriate code from subcategory R65.2 should also be assigned with the additional code(s) for any acute organ dysfunction.

For infections following infusion, transfusion, therapeutic injection, or immunization, a code from subcategory T80.2, Infections following infusion, transfusion, and therapeutic injection, or code T88.0-, Infection following immunization, should be coded first, followed by the code for the specific infection. If the patient has severe sepsis, the appropriate code from subcategory R65.2 should also be assigned, with the additional codes(s) for any acute organ dysfunction.

(c) Postprocedural infection and postprocedural septic shock

If a postprocedural infection has resulted in postprocedural septic shock, assign the codes indicated above for sepsis due to a postprocedural infection, followed by code T81.12-, Postprocedural septic shock. Do not assign code R65.21, Severe sepsis with septic shock. Additional code(s) should be assigned for any acute organ dysfunction.

6) Sepsis and severe sepsis associated with a noninfectious process (condition)

In some cases, a noninfectious process (condition) such as trauma, may lead to an infection which can result in sepsis or severe sepsis. If sepsis or severe sepsis is documented as associated with a noninfectious condition, such as a burn or serious injury, and this condition meets the definition for principal diagnosis, the code for the noninfectious condition should be sequenced first, followed by the code for the resulting infection. If severe sepsis is present, a code from subcategory R65.2 should also be assigned with any associated organ dysfunction(s) codes. It is not necessary to assign a code from subcategory R65.1, Systemic inflammatory response syndrome (SIRS) of non-infectious origin, for these cases.

If the infection meets the definition of principal diagnosis, it should be sequenced before the non-infectious condition. When both the associated non-infectious condition and the infection meet the definition of principal diagnosis, either may be assigned as principal diagnosis.

Only one code from category R65, Symptoms and signs specifically associated with systemic inflammation and infection, should be assigned. Therefore, when a non-infectious condition leads to an infection resulting in severe sepsis, assign the appropriate code from subcategory R65.2, Severe sepsis. Do not additionally assign a code from subcategory R65.1, Systemic inflammatory response syndrome (SIRS) of non-infectious origin.

See Section I.C.18. SIRS due to non-infectious process

7) Sepsis and septic shock complicating abortion, pregnancy, childbirth, and the puerperium

See Section I.C.15. Sepsis and septic shock complicating abortion, pregnancy, childbirth and the puerperium

8) Newborn sepsis

See Section I.C.16. f. Bacterial sepsis of Newborn

9) Hemolytic-uremic syndrome associated with sepsis

If the reason for admission is hemolytic-uremic syndrome that is associated with sepsis, assign code D59.31, Infection-associated hemolytic-uremic syndrome, as the principal diagnosis. Codes for the underlying systemic infection and any other conditions (such as severe sepsis) should be assigned as secondary diagnoses.

e. Methicillin Resistant Staphylococcus aureus (MRSA) Conditions

1) Selection and sequencing of MRSA codes

(a) Combination codes for MRSA infection

When a patient is diagnosed with an infection that is due to methicillin resistant *Staphylococcus aureus* (MRSA), and that infection has a combination code that includes the causal organism (e.g., sepsis, pneumonia) assign the appropriate combination code for the condition (e.g., code A41.02, Sepsis due to Methicillin resistant Staphylococcus aureus or code J15.212, Pneumonia due to Methicillin resistant Staphylococcus aureus). Do not assign code B95.62, Methicillin resistant Staphylococcus aureus infection as the cause of diseases classified elsewhere, as an additional code, because the combination code includes the type of infection and the MRSA organism. Do not assign a code from subcategory Z16.11, Resistance to penicillins, as an additional diagnosis.

See Section C.1. for instructions on coding and sequencing of sepsis and severe sepsis.

(b) Other codes for MRSA infection

When there is documentation of a current infection (e.g., wound infection, stitch abscess, urinary tract infection) due to MRSA, and that infection does not have a combination code that includes the causal organism, assign the appropriate code to identify the condition along with code B95.62, Methicillin resistant Staphylococcus aureus infection as the cause of diseases classified elsewhere for the MRSA infection. Do not assign a code from subcategory Z16.11, Resistance to penicillins.

(c) Methicillin susceptible Staphylococcus aureus (MSSA) and MRSA colonization

The condition or state of being colonized or carrying MSSA or MRSA is called colonization or carriage, while an individual person is described as being colonized or being a carrier.

Colonization means that MSSA or MSRA is present on or in the body without necessarily causing illness. A positive MRSA colonization test might be documented by the provider as "MRSA screen positive" or "MRSA nasal swab positive".

Assign code Z22.322, Carrier or suspected carrier of Methicillin resistant Staphylococcus aureus, for patients documented as having MRSA colonization. Assign code Z22.321, Carrier or suspected carrier of Methicillin susceptible Staphylococcus aureus, for patients documented as having MSSA colonization. Colonization is not necessarily indicative of a disease process or as the cause of a specific condition the patient may have unless documented as such by the provider.

(d) MRSA colonization and infection

If a patient is documented as having both MRSA colonization and infection during a hospital admission, code Z22.322, Carrier or suspected carrier of Methicillin resistant Staphylococcus aureus, and a code for the MRSA infection may both be assigned.

f. Zika virus infections

1) Code only confirmed cases

Code only a confirmed diagnosis of Zika virus (A92.5, Zika virus disease) as documented by the provider. This is an exception to the hospital inpatient guideline Section II, H. In this context, "confirmation" does not require documentation of the type of test performed; the provider's diagnostic statement that the condition is confirmed is sufficient. This code should be assigned regardless of the stated mode of transmission.

If the provider documents "suspected", "possible" or "probable" Zika, do not assign code A92.5. Assign a code(s) explaining the reason for encounter (such as fever, rash, or joint pain) or Z20.821, Contact with and (suspected) exposure to Zika virus.

g. **Coronavirus infections**
1) **COVID-19 infection (infection due to SARS-CoV-2)**
   (a) **Code only confirmed cases**
   Code only a confirmed diagnosis of the 2019 novel coronavirus disease (COVID-19) as documented by the provider, or documentation of a positive COVID-19 test result. For a confirmed diagnosis, assign code U07.1, COVID-19. This is an exception to the hospital inpatient guideline Section II, H. In this context, "confirmation" does not require documentation of a positive test result for COVID-19; the provider's documentation that the individual has COVID-19 is sufficient.

   If the provider documents "suspected," "possible," "probable," or "inconclusive" COVID-19, do not assign code U07.1. Instead, code the signs and symptoms reported. See guideline I.C.1.g.1.g.

   (b) **Sequencing of codes**
   When COVID-19 meets the definition of principal diagnosis, code U07.1, COVID-19, should be sequenced first, followed by the appropriate codes for associated manifestations, except when another guideline requires that certain codes be sequenced first, such as obstetrics, sepsis, or transplant complications.

   For a COVID-19 infection that progresses to sepsis, see Section I.C.1.d. Sepsis, Severe Sepsis, and Septic Shock

   See Section I.C.15.s. for COVID-19 infection in pregnancy, childbirth, and the puerperium

   See Section I.C.16.h. for COVID-19 infection in newborn

   For a COVID-19 infection in a lung transplant patient, see Section I.C.19.g.3.a. Transplant complications other than kidney.

   (c) **Acute respiratory manifestations of COVID-19**
   When the reason for the encounter/admission is a respiratory manifestation of COVID-19, assign code U07.1, COVID-19, as the principal/first-listed diagnosis and assign code(s) for the respiratory manifestation(s) as additional diagnoses.

   The following conditions are examples of common respiratory manifestations of COVID-19.

   (i) **Pneumonia**
   For a patient with pneumonia confirmed as due to COVID-19, assign codes U07.1, COVID-19, and J12.82, Pneumonia due to coronavirus disease 2019.

   (ii) **Acute bronchitis**
   For a patient with acute bronchitis confirmed as due to COVID-19, assign codes U07.1, and J20.8, Acute bronchitis due to other specified organisms.

   Bronchitis not otherwise specified (NOS) due to COVID-19 should be coded using code U07.1 and J40, Bronchitis, not specified as acute or chronic.

   (iii) **Lower respiratory infection**
   If the COVID-19 is documented as being associated with a lower respiratory infection, not otherwise specified (NOS), or an acute respiratory infection, NOS, codes U07.1 and J22, Unspecified acute lower respiratory infection, should be assigned.

   If the COVID-19 is documented as being associated with a respiratory infection, NOS, codes U07.1 and J98.8, Other specified respiratory disorders, should be assigned.

   (iv) **Acute respiratory distress syndrome**
   For acute respiratory distress syndrome (ARDS) due to COVID-19, assign codes U07.1, and J80, Acute respiratory distress syndrome.

   (v) **Acute respiratory failure**
   For acute respiratory failure due to COVID-19, assign code U07.1, and code J96.0-, Acute respiratory failure.

   (d) **Non-respiratory manifestations of COVID-19**
   When the reason for the encounter/admission is a non-respiratory manifestation (e.g., viral enteritis) of COVID-19, assign code U07.1, COVID-19, as the principal/first-listed diagnosis and assign code(s) for the manifestation(s) as additional diagnoses.

   (e) **Exposure to COVID-19**
   For asymptomatic individuals with actual or suspected exposure to COVID-19, assign code Z20.822, Contact with and (suspected) exposure to COVID-19.

   For symptomatic individuals with actual or suspected exposure to COVID-19 and the infection has been ruled out, or test results are inconclusive or unknown, assign code Z20.822, Contact with and (suspected) exposure to COVID-19. See guideline I.C.21.c.1, Contact/Exposure, for additional guidance regarding the use of category Z20 codes.

   If COVID-19 is confirmed, see guideline I.C.1.g.1.a.

   (f) **Screening for COVID-19**
   During the COVID-19 pandemic, a screening code is generally not appropriate. Do not assign code Z11.52, Encounter for screening for COVID-19. For encounters for COVID-19 testing, including preoperative testing, code as exposure to COVID-19 (guideline I.C.1.g.1.e).

   Coding guidance will be updated as new information concerning any changes in the pandemic status becomes available.

   (g) **Signs and symptoms without definitive diagnosis of COVID-19**
   For patients presenting with any signs/symptoms associated with COVID-19 (such as fever, etc.) but a definitive diagnosis has not been established, assign the appropriate code(s) for each of the presenting signs and symptoms such as:
   - R05.1, Acute cough, or R05.9, Cough, unspecified
   - R06.02 Shortness of breath
   - R50.9 Fever, unspecified

   If a patient with signs/symptoms associated with COVID-19 also has an actual or suspected contact with or exposure to COVID-19, assign Z20.822, Contact with and (suspected) exposure to COVID-19, as an additional code.

   (h) **Asymptomatic individuals who test positive for COVID-19**
   For asymptomatic individuals who test positive for COVID-19, see guideline I.C.1.g.1.a. Although the individual is asymptomatic, the individual has tested positive and is considered to have the COVID-19 infection.

   (i) **Personal history of COVID-19**
   For patients with a history of COVID-19, assign code Z86.16, Personal history of COVID-19.

   (j) **Follow-up visits after COVID-19 infection has resolved**
   For individuals who previously had COVID-19, without residual symptom(s) or condition(s), and are being seen for follow-up evaluation, and COVID-19 test results are negative, assign codes Z09, Encounter for follow-up examination after completed treatment for conditions other than malignant neoplasm, and Z86.16, Personal history of COVID-19.

   For follow-up visits for individuals with symptom(s) or condition(s) related to a previous COVID-19 infection, see guideline I.C.1.g.1.m.

   See Section I.C.21.c.8, Factors influencing health states and contact with health services, Follow-up

   (k) **Encounter for antibody testing**
   For an encounter for antibody testing that is not being performed to confirm a current COVID-19 infection, nor is a follow-up test after resolution of COVID-19, assign Z01.84, Encounter for antibody response examination.

   Follow the applicable guidelines above if the individual is being tested to confirm a current COVID-19 infection.

   For follow-up testing after a COVID-19 infection, see guideline I.C.1.g.1.j.

   (l) **Multisystem Inflammatory Syndrome**
   For individuals with multisystem inflammatory syndrome (MIS) and COVID-19, assign code U07.1, COVID-19, as the principal/first-listed diagnosis and assign code M35.81, Multisystem inflammatory syndrome, as an additional diagnosis.

   If an individual with a history of COVID-19 develops MIS, assign codes M35.81, Multisystem inflammatory syndrome, and U09.9, Post COVID-19 condition, unspecified.

   If an individual with a known or suspected exposure to COVID-19, and no current COVID-19 infection or history of

COVID-19, develops MIS, assign codes M35.81, Multisystem inflammatory syndrome, and Z20.822, Contact with and (suspected) exposure to COVID-19.

Additional codes should be assigned for any associated complications of MIS.

(m) Post COVID-19 Condition

For sequela of COVID-19, or associated symptoms or conditions that develop following a previous COVID-19 infection, assign a code(s) for the specific symptom(s) or condition(s) related to the previous COVID-19 infection, if known, and code U09.9, Post COVID-19 condition, unspecified.

Code U09.9 should not be assigned for manifestations of an active (current) COVID-19 infection.

If a patient has a condition(s) associated with a previous COVID-19 infection and develops a new active (current) COVID-19 infection, code U09.9 may be assigned in conjunction with code U07.1, COVID-19, to identify that the patient also has a condition(s) associated with a previous COVID-19 infection. Code(s) for the specific condition(s) associated with the previous COVID-19 infection and code(s) for manifestation(s) of the new active (current) COVID-19 infection should also be assigned.

(n) Underimmunization for COVID-19 Status

Code Z28.310, Unvaccinated for COVID-19, may be assigned when the patient has not received a COVID-19 vaccine of any type. Code Z28.311, Partially vaccinated for COVID-19, may be assigned when the patient has **been partially vaccinated for COVID-19 as per the recommendations of** the Centers for Disease Control and Prevention (CDC) in place at the time of the encounter. For information, visit the CDC's website https://www.cdc.gov/coronavirus/2019-ncov/vaccines/.

See Section I.B.14. for underimmunization documentation by clinicians other than patient's provider.

2. Chapter 2: Neoplasms (C00-D49)

General Guidelines

Chapter 2 of the ICD-10-CM contains the codes for most benign and all malignant neoplasms. Certain benign neoplasms, such as prostatic adenomas, may be found in the specific body system chapters. To properly code a neoplasm, it is necessary to determine from the record if the neoplasm is benign, in-situ, malignant, or of uncertain histologic behavior. If malignant, any secondary (metastatic) sites should also be determined.

Primary malignant neoplasms overlapping site boundaries

A primary malignant neoplasm that overlaps two or more contiguous (next to each other) sites should be classified to the subcategory/code .8 ('overlapping lesion'), unless the combination is specifically indexed elsewhere. For multiple neoplasms of the same site that are not contiguous such as tumors in different quadrants of the same breast, codes for each site should be assigned.

Malignant neoplasm of ectopic tissue

Malignant neoplasms of ectopic tissue are to be coded to the site of origin mentioned, e.g., ectopic pancreatic malignant neoplasms involving the stomach are coded to malignant neoplasm of pancreas, unspecified (C25.9).

The neoplasm table in the Alphabetic Index should be referenced first. However, if the histological term is documented, that term should be referenced first, rather than going immediately to the Neoplasm Table, in order to determine which column in the Neoplasm Table is appropriate. For example, if the documentation indicates "adenoma," refer to the term in the Alphabetic Index to review the entries under this term and the instructional note to "see also neoplasm, by site, benign." The table provides the proper code based on the type of neoplasm and the site. It is important to select the proper column in the table that corresponds to the type of neoplasm. The Tabular List should then be referenced to verify that the correct code has been selected from the table and that a more specific site code does not exist.

See Section I.C.21. Factors influencing health status and contact with health services, Status, for information regarding Z15.0, codes for genetic susceptibility to cancer.

a. Admission/Encounter for treatment of primary site

If the malignancy **is chiefly responsible for occasioning the patient admission/encounter and treatment is directed at the primary site**, designate the **primary** malignancy as the principal/**first-listed** diagnosis.

The only exception to this guideline is if the administration of chemotherapy, immunotherapy or external beam radiation therapy **is chiefly responsible for occasioning the admission/encounter. In that case**, assign the appropriate Z51.-- code as the first-listed or principal diagnosis, and the **underlying** diagnosis or problem for which the service is being performed as a secondary diagnosis.

b. Admission/Encounter for treatment of secondary site

When a patient is admitted because of a primary neoplasm with metastasis and treatment is directed toward the secondary site only, the secondary neoplasm is designated as the principal diagnosis even though the primary malignancy is still present.

c. Coding and sequencing of complications

Coding and sequencing of complications associated with the malignancies or with the therapy thereof are subject to the following guidelines:

1) Anemia associated with malignancy

When admission/encounter is for management of an anemia associated with the malignancy, and the treatment is only for anemia, the appropriate code for the malignancy is sequenced as the principal or first-listed diagnosis followed by the appropriate code for the anemia (such as code D63.0, Anemia in neoplastic disease).

2) Anemia associated with chemotherapy, immunotherapy and radiation therapy

When the admission/encounter is for management of an anemia associated with an adverse effect of the administration of chemotherapy or immunotherapy and the only treatment is for the anemia, the anemia code is sequenced first followed by the appropriate codes for the neoplasm and the adverse effect (T45.1X5-, Adverse effect of antineoplastic and immunosuppressive drugs).

When the admission/encounter is for management of an anemia associated with an adverse effect of radiotherapy, the anemia code should be sequenced first, followed by the appropriate neoplasm code and code Y84.2, Radiological procedure and radiotherapy as the cause of abnormal reaction of the patient, or of later complication, without mention of misadventure at the time of the procedure.

3) Management of dehydration due to the malignancy

When the admission/encounter is for management of dehydration due to the malignancy and only the dehydration is being treated (intravenous rehydration), the dehydration is sequenced first, followed by the code(s) for the malignancy.

4) Treatment of a complication resulting from a surgical procedure

When the admission/encounter is for treatment of a complication resulting from a surgical procedure, designate the complication as the principal or first-listed diagnosis if treatment is directed at resolving the complication.

d. Primary malignancy previously excised

When a primary malignancy has been previously excised or eradicated from its site and there is no further treatment directed to that site and there is no evidence of any existing primary malignancy at that site, a code from category Z85, Personal history of malignant neoplasm, should be used to indicate the former site of the malignancy. Any mention of extension, invasion, or metastasis to another site is coded as a secondary malignant neoplasm to that site. The secondary site may be the principal or first-listed diagnosis with the Z85 code used as a secondary code.

See section I.C.2.t. Secondary malignant neoplasm of lymphoid tissue.

e. Admissions/Encounters involving chemotherapy, immunotherapy and radiation therapy

1) Episode of care involves surgical removal of neoplasm

When an episode of care involves the surgical removal of a neoplasm, primary or secondary site, followed by adjunct chemotherapy or radiation treatment during the same episode of care, the code for the neoplasm should be assigned as principal or first-listed diagnosis.

2) Patient admission/encounter solely for administration of chemotherapy, immunotherapy and radiation therapy

If a patient admission/encounter is solely for the administration of chemotherapy, immunotherapy or external beam radiation therapy assign code Z51.0, Encounter for antineoplastic radiation therapy, or Z51.11, Encounter for antineoplastic chemotherapy, or Z51.12, Encounter for antineoplastic immunotherapy as the first-listed or principal diagnosis. If a patient receives more than one of these therapies during the same admission more than one of these codes may be assigned, in any sequence.

The malignancy for which the therapy is being administered should be assigned as a secondary diagnosis.

If a patient admission/encounter is for the insertion or implantation of radioactive elements (e.g., brachytherapy) the appropriate code for the malignancy is sequenced as the principal or first-listed diagnosis. Code Z51.0 should not be assigned.

3) Patient admitted for radiation therapy, chemotherapy or immunotherapy and develops complications
When a patient is admitted for the purpose of external beam radiotherapy, immunotherapy or chemotherapy and develops complications such as uncontrolled nausea and vomiting or dehydration, the principal or first-listed diagnosis is Z51.0, Encounter for antineoplastic radiation therapy, or Z51.11, Encounter for antineoplastic chemotherapy, or Z51.12, Encounter for antineoplastic immunotherapy followed by any codes for the complications.

When a patient is admitted for the purpose of insertion or implantation of radioactive elements (e.g., brachytherapy) and develops complications such as uncontrolled nausea and vomiting or dehydration, the principal or first-listed diagnosis is the appropriate code for the malignancy followed by any codes for the complications.

f. Admission/encounter to determine extent of malignancy
When the reason for admission/encounter is to determine the extent of the malignancy, or for a procedure such as paracentesis or thoracentesis, the primary malignancy or appropriate metastatic site is designated as the principal or first-listed diagnosis, even though chemotherapy or radiotherapy is administered.

g. Symptoms, signs, and abnormal findings listed in Chapter 18 associated with neoplasms
Symptoms, signs, and ill-defined conditions listed in Chapter 18 characteristic of, or associated with, an existing primary or secondary site malignancy cannot be used to replace the malignancy as principal or first-listed diagnosis, regardless of the number of admissions or encounters for treatment and care of the neoplasm.

See section I.C.21. Factors influencing health status and contact with health services, Encounter for prophylactic organ removal.

h. Admission/encounter for pain control/management
See Section I.C.6. for information on coding admission/encounter for pain control/management.

i. Malignancy in two or more noncontiguous sites
A patient may have more than one malignant tumor in the same organ. These tumors may represent different primaries or metastatic disease, depending on the site. Should the documentation be unclear, the provider should be queried as to the status of each tumor so that the correct codes can be assigned.

j. Disseminated malignant neoplasm, unspecified
Code C80.0, Disseminated malignant neoplasm, unspecified, is for use only in those cases where the patient has advanced metastatic disease and no known primary or secondary sites are specified. It should not be used in place of assigning codes for the primary site and all known secondary sites.

k. Malignant neoplasm without specification of site
Code C80.1, Malignant (primary) neoplasm, unspecified, equates to Cancer, unspecified. This code should only be used when no determination can be made as to the primary site of a malignancy. This code should rarely be used in the inpatient setting.

l. Sequencing of neoplasm codes
1) Encounter for treatment of primary malignancy
If the reason for the encounter is for treatment of a primary malignancy, assign the malignancy as the principal/first-listed diagnosis. The primary site is to be sequenced first, followed by any metastatic sites.

2) Encounter for treatment of secondary malignancy
When an encounter is for a primary malignancy with metastasis and treatment is directed toward the metastatic (secondary) site(s) only, the metastatic site(s) is designated as the principal/first-listed diagnosis. The primary malignancy is coded as an additional code.

3) Malignant neoplasm in a pregnant patient
When a pregnant patient has a malignant neoplasm, a code from subcategory O9A.1-, Malignant neoplasm complicating pregnancy, childbirth, and the puerperium, should be sequenced first, followed by the appropriate code from Chapter 2 to indicate the type of neoplasm.

4) Encounter for complication associated with a neoplasm
When an encounter is for management of a complication associated with a neoplasm, such as dehydration, and the treatment is only for the complication, the complication is coded first, followed by the appropriate code(s) for the neoplasm.

The exception to this guideline is anemia. When the admission/encounter is for management of an anemia associated with the malignancy, and the treatment is only for anemia, the appropriate code for the malignancy is sequenced as the principal or first-listed diagnosis followed by code D63.0, Anemia in neoplastic disease.

5) Complication from surgical procedure for treatment of a neoplasm
When an encounter is for treatment of a complication resulting from a surgical procedure performed for the treatment of the neoplasm, designate the complication as the principal/first-listed diagnosis. See the guideline regarding the coding of a current malignancy versus personal history to determine if the code for the neoplasm should also be assigned.

6) Pathologic fracture due to a neoplasm
When an encounter is for a pathological fracture due to a neoplasm, and the focus of treatment is the fracture, a code from subcategory M84.5, Pathological fracture in neoplastic disease, should be sequenced first, followed by the code for the neoplasm.

If the focus of treatment is the neoplasm with an associated pathological fracture, the neoplasm code should be sequenced first, followed by a code from M84.5 for the pathological fracture.

m. Current malignancy versus personal history of malignancy
When a primary malignancy has been excised but further treatment, such as an additional surgery for the malignancy, radiation therapy or chemotherapy is directed to that site, the primary malignancy code should be used until treatment is completed.

When a primary malignancy has been previously excised or eradicated from its site, there is no further treatment (of the malignancy) directed to that site, and there is no evidence of any existing primary malignancy at that site, a code from category Z85, Personal history of malignant neoplasm, should be used to indicate the former site of the malignancy.

Codes from subcategories Z85.0 – Z85.85 should only be assigned for the former site of a primary malignancy, not the site of a secondary malignancy. Code Z85.89 may be assigned for the former site(s) of either a primary or secondary malignancy.

See Section I.C.21. Factors influencing health status and contact with health services, History (of)

n. Leukemia, Multiple Myeloma, and Malignant Plasma Cell Neoplasms in remission versus personal history
The categories for leukemia, and category C90, Multiple myeloma and malignant plasma cell neoplasms, have codes indicating whether or not the leukemia has achieved remission. There are also codes Z85.6, Personal history of leukemia, and Z85.79, Personal history of other malignant neoplasms of lymphoid, hematopoietic and related tissues. If the documentation is unclear as to whether the leukemia has achieved remission, the provider should be queried.

See Section I.C.21. Factors influencing health status and contact with health services, History (of)

o. Aftercare following surgery for neoplasm
See Section I.C.21. Factors influencing health status and contact with health services, Aftercare

p. Follow-up care for completed treatment of a malignancy
See Section I.C.21. Factors influencing health status and contact with health services, Follow-up

q. Prophylactic organ removal for prevention of malignancy
See Section I.C. 21, Factors influencing health status and contact with health services, Prophylactic organ removal

r. Malignant neoplasm associated with transplanted organ
A malignant neoplasm of a transplanted organ should be coded as a transplant complication. Assign first the appropriate code from category T86.-, Complications of transplanted organs and tissue, followed by code C80.2, Malignant neoplasm associated with transplanted organ. Use an additional code for the specific malignancy.

s. **Breast Implant Associated Anaplastic Large Cell Lymphoma**
Breast implant associated anaplastic large cell lymphoma (BIA-ALCL) is a type of lymphoma that can develop around breast implants. Assign code C84.7A, Anaplastic large cell lymphoma, ALK-negative, breast, for BIA-ALCL. Do not assign a complication code from chapter 19.

t. **Secondary malignant neoplasm of lymphoid tissue**
When a malignant neoplasm of lymphoid tissue metastasizes beyond the lymph nodes, a code from categories C81-C85 with a final character "9" should be assigned identifying "extranodal and solid organ sites" rather than a code for the secondary neoplasm of the affected solid organ. For example, for metastasis of B-cell lymphoma to the lung, brain and left adrenal gland, assign code C83.39, Diffuse large B-cell lymphoma, extranodal and solid organ sites.

3. **Chapter 3: Disease of the blood and blood-forming organs and certain disorders involving the immune mechanism (D50-D89)**
Reserved for future guideline expansion

4. **Chapter 4: Endocrine, Nutritional, and Metabolic Diseases (E00-E89)**
a. **Diabetes mellitus**
The diabetes mellitus codes are combination codes that include the type of diabetes mellitus, the body system affected, and the complications affecting that body system. As many codes within a particular category as are necessary to describe all of the complications of the disease may be used. They should be sequenced based on the reason for a particular encounter. Assign as many codes from categories E08 – E13 as needed to identify all of the associated conditions that the patient has.

1) **Type of diabetes**
The age of a patient is not the sole determining factor, though most type 1 diabetics develop the condition before reaching puberty. For this reason, type 1 diabetes mellitus is also referred to as juvenile diabetes.

2) **Type of diabetes mellitus not documented**
If the type of diabetes mellitus is not documented in the medical record the default is E11.-, Type 2 diabetes mellitus.

3) **Diabetes mellitus and the use of insulin, oral hypoglycemics, and injectable non-insulin drugs**
If the documentation in a medical record does not indicate the type of diabetes but does indicate that the patient uses insulin, code E11.-, Type 2 diabetes mellitus, should be assigned. Additional code(s) should be assigned from category Z79 to identify the long-term (current) use of insulin, oral hypoglycemic drugs, or injectable non-insulin antidiabetic, as follows:

If the patient is treated with both oral **hypoglycemic drugs** and insulin, both code Z79.4, Long term (current) use of insulin, and code Z79.84, Long term (current) use of oral hypoglycemic drugs, should be assigned.

If the patient is treated with both insulin and an injectable non-insulin antidiabetic drug, assign codes Z79.4, Long term (current) use of insulin, and **Z79.85, Long-term (current) use of injectable non-insulin antidiabetic drugs.**

If the patient is treated with both oral hypoglycemic drugs and an injectable non-insulin antidiabetic drug, assign codes Z79.84, Long term (current) use of oral hypoglycemic drugs, and **Z79.85, Long-term (current) use of injectable non-insulin antidiabetic drugs.**

Code Z79.4 should not be assigned if insulin is given temporarily to bring a type 2 patient's blood sugar under control during an encounter.

4) **Diabetes mellitus in pregnancy and gestational diabetes**
See Section I.C.15. Diabetes mellitus in pregnancy.
See Section I.C.15. Gestational (pregnancy induced) diabetes

5) **Complications due to insulin pump malfunction**
(a) **Underdose of insulin due to insulin pump failure**
An underdose of insulin due to an insulin pump failure should be assigned to a code from subcategory T85.6, Mechanical complication of other specified internal and external prosthetic devices, implants and grafts, that specifies the type of pump malfunction, as the principal or first-listed code, followed by code T38.3X6-, Underdosing of insulin and oral hypoglycemic [antidiabetic] drugs. Additional codes for the type of diabetes mellitus and any associated complications due to the underdosing should also be assigned.

(b) **Overdose of insulin due to insulin pump failure**
The principal or first-listed code for an encounter due to an insulin pump malfunction resulting in an overdose of insulin, should also be T85.6-, Mechanical complication of other specified internal and external prosthetic devices, implants and grafts, followed by code T38.3X1-, Poisoning by insulin and oral hypoglycemic [antidiabetic] drugs, accidental (unintentional).

6) **Secondary diabetes mellitus**
Codes under categories E08, Diabetes mellitus due to underlying condition, E09, Drug or chemical induced diabetes mellitus, and E13, Other specified diabetes mellitus, identify complications/manifestations associated with secondary diabetes mellitus. Secondary diabetes is always caused by another condition or event (e.g., cystic fibrosis, malignant neoplasm of pancreas, pancreatectomy, adverse effect of drug, or poisoning).

(a) **Secondary diabetes mellitus and the use of insulin, oral hypoglycemic drugs, or injectable non-insulin drugs**
For patients with secondary diabetes mellitus who routinely use insulin, oral hypoglycemic drugs, or injectable non-insulin drugs, additional code(s) from category Z79 should be assigned to identify the long-term (current) use of insulin, oral hypoglycemic drugs, or non-injectable non-insulin drugs as follows:

If the patient is treated with both oral **hypoglycemic drugs** and insulin, both code Z79.4, Long term (current) use of insulin, and code Z79.84, Long term (current) use of oral hypoglycemic drugs, should be assigned.

If the patient is treated with both insulin and an injectable non-insulin antidiabetic drug, assign codes Z79.4, Long-term (current) use of insulin, and **Z79.85, Long-term (current) use of injectable non-insulin antidiabetic drugs**.

If the patient is treated with both oral hypoglycemic drugs and an injectable non-insulin antidiabetic drug, assign codes Z79.84, Long-term (current) use of oral hypoglycemic drugs, and **Z79.85, Long-term (current) use of injectable non-insulin antidiabetic drugs.**

Code Z79.4 should not be assigned if insulin is given temporarily to bring a secondary diabetic patient's blood sugar under control during an encounter.

(b) **Assigning and sequencing secondary diabetes codes and its causes**
The sequencing of the secondary diabetes codes in relationship to codes for the cause of the diabetes is based on the Tabular List instructions for categories E08, E09 and E13.

(i) **Secondary diabetes mellitus due to pancreatectomy**
For postpancreatectomy diabetes mellitus (lack of insulin due to the surgical removal of all or part of the pancreas), assign code E89.1, Postprocedural hypoinsulinemia.

Assign a code from category E13 and a code from subcategory Z90.41, Acquired absence of pancreas, as additional codes.

(ii) **Secondary diabetes due to drugs**
Secondary diabetes may be caused by an adverse effect of correctly administered medications, poisoning or sequela of poisoning.

See section I.C.19.e. for coding of adverse effects and poisoning, and section I.C.20 for external cause code reporting.

5. **Chapter 5: Mental, Behavioral and Neurodevelopmental disorders (F01-F99)**
a. **Pain disorders related to psychological factors**
Assign code F45.41, for pain that is exclusively related to psychological disorders. As indicated by the Excludes 1 note under category G89, a code from category G89 should not be assigned with code F45.41.

Code F45.42, Pain disorders with related psychological factors, should be used with a code from category G89, Pain, not elsewhere classified, if there is documentation of a psychological component for a patient with acute or chronic pain.

See Section I.C.6. Pain

b. Mental and behavioral disorders due to psychoactive substance use

1) In Remission

Selection of codes **describing** "in remission" for categories F10-F19, Mental and behavioral disorders due to psychoactive substance use (categories F10-F19 with -.11, -.21, **-.91**) requires the provider's clinical judgment **and** are assigned only on the basis of provider documentation (as defined in the Official Guidelines for Coding and Reporting), unless otherwise instructed by the classification.

Mild substance use disorders in early or sustained remission are classified to the appropriate codes for substance abuse in remission, and moderate or severe substance use disorders in early or sustained remission are classified to the appropriate codes for substance dependence in remission.

2) Psychoactive Substance Use, Abuse and Dependence

When the provider documentation refers to use, abuse and dependence of the same substance (e.g. alcohol, opioid, cannabis, etc.), only one code should be assigned to identify the pattern of use based on the following hierarchy:

- If both use and abuse are documented, assign only the code for abuse
- If both abuse and dependence are documented, assign only the code for dependence
- If use, abuse and dependence are all documented, assign only the code for dependence
- If both use and dependence are documented, assign only the code for dependence.

3) Psychoactive Substance Use, Unspecified

As with all other unspecified diagnoses, the codes for unspecified psychoactive substance use (F10.9-, F11.9-, F12.9-, F13.9-, F14.9-, F15.9-, F16.9-, F18.9-, F19.9-) should only be assigned based on provider documentation and when they meet the definition of a reportable diagnosis (see Section III, Reporting Additional Diagnoses). These codes are to be used only when the psychoactive substance use is associated with a substance related disorder (chapter 5 disorders such as sexual dysfunction, sleep disorder, or a mental or behavioral disorder) or medical condition, and such a relationship is documented by the provider.

4) Medical Conditions Due to Psychoactive Substance Use, Abuse and Dependence

Medical conditions due to substance use, abuse, and dependence are not classified as substance-induced disorders. Assign the diagnosis code for the medical condition as directed by the Alphabetical Index along with the appropriate psychoactive substance use, abuse or dependence code. For example, for alcoholic pancreatitis due to alcohol dependence, assign the appropriate code from subcategory K85.2, Alcohol induced acute pancreatitis, and the appropriate code from subcategory F10.2, such as code F10.20, Alcohol dependence, uncomplicated. It would not be appropriate to assign code F10.288, Alcohol dependence with other alcohol-induced disorder.

5) Blood Alcohol Level

A code from category Y90, Evidence of alcohol involvement determined by blood alcohol level, may be assigned when this information is documented and the patient's provider has documented a condition classifiable to category F10, Alcohol related disorders. The blood alcohol level does not need to be documented by the patient's provider in order for it to be coded.

See Section I.B.14. for blood alcohol level documentation by clinicians other than patient's provider.

c. Factitious Disorder

Factitious disorder imposed on self or Munchausen's syndrome is a disorder in which a person falsely reports or causes his or her own physical or psychological signs or symptoms. For patients with documented factitious disorder on self or Munchausen's syndrome, assign the appropriate code from subcategory F68.1-, Factitious disorder imposed on self.

Munchausen's syndrome by proxy (MSBP) is a disorder in which a caregiver (perpetrator) falsely reports or causes an illness or injury in another person (victim) under his or her care, such as a child, an elderly adult, or a person who has a disability. The condition is also referred to as "factitious disorder imposed on another" or "factitious disorder by proxy." The perpetrator, not the victim, receives this diagnosis. Assign code F68.A, Factitious disorder imposed on another,

to the perpetrator's record. For the victim of a patient suffering from MSBP, assign the appropriate code from categories T74, Adult and child abuse, neglect and other maltreatment, confirmed, or T76, Adult and child abuse, neglect and other maltreatment, suspected.

See Section I.C.19.f. Adult and child abuse, neglect and other maltreatment

d. Dementia

The ICD-10-CM classifies dementia (categories F01, F02, and F03) on the basis of the etiology and severity (unspecified, mild, moderate or severe). Selection of the appropriate severity level requires the provider's clinical judgment and codes should be assigned only on the basis of provider documentation (as defined in the *Official Guidelines for Coding and Reporting*), unless otherwise instructed by the classification. If the documentation does not provide information about the severity of the dementia, assign the appropriate code for unspecified severity.

If a patient is admitted to an inpatient acute care hospital or other inpatient facility setting with dementia at one severity level and it progresses to a higher severity level, assign one code for the highest severity level reported during the stay.

6. Chapter 6: Diseases of the Nervous System (G00-G99)

a. Dominant/nondominant side

Codes from category G81, Hemiplegia and hemiparesis, and subcategories G83.1, Monoplegia of lower limb, G83.2, Monoplegia of upper limb, and G83.3, Monoplegia, unspecified, identify whether the dominant or nondominant side is affected. Should the affected side be documented, but not specified as dominant or nondominant, and the classification system does not indicate a default, code selection is as follows:

- For ambidextrous patients, the default should be dominant.
- If the left side is affected, the default is non-dominant.
- If the right side is affected, the default is dominant.

b. Pain - Category G89

1) General coding information

Codes in category G89, Pain, not elsewhere classified, may be used in conjunction with codes from other categories and chapters to provide more detail about acute or chronic pain and neoplasm-related pain, unless otherwise indicated below.

If the pain is not specified as acute or chronic, post-thoracotomy, postprocedural, or neoplasm-related, do not assign codes from category G89.

A code from category G89 should not be assigned if the underlying (definitive) diagnosis is known, unless the reason for the encounter is pain control/ management and not management of the underlying condition.

When an admission or encounter is for a procedure aimed at treating the underlying condition (e.g., spinal fusion, kyphoplasty), a code for the underlying condition (e.g., vertebral fracture, spinal stenosis) should be assigned as the principal diagnosis. No code from category G89 should be assigned.

(a) Category G89 Codes as Principal or First-Listed Diagnosis

Category G89 codes are acceptable as principal diagnosis or the first-listed code:

- When pain control or pain management is the reason for the admission/encounter (e.g., a patient with displaced intervertebral disc, nerve impingement and severe back pain presents for injection of steroid into the spinal canal). The underlying cause of the pain should be reported as an additional diagnosis, if known.
- When a patient is admitted for the insertion of a neurostimulator for pain control, assign the appropriate pain code as the principal or first-listed diagnosis. When an admission or encounter is for a procedure aimed at treating the underlying condition and a neurostimulator is inserted for pain control during the same admission/encounter, a code for the underlying condition should be assigned as the principal diagnosis and the appropriate pain code should be assigned as a secondary diagnosis.

(b) Use of Category G89 Codes in Conjunction with Site Specific Pain Codes

(i) Assigning Category G89 and Site-Specific Pain Codes

Codes from category G89 may be used in conjunction with codes that identify the site of pain (including codes from chapter 18) if the category G89 code provides additional information. For example, if the code describes the site of the pain, but does not fully describe whether the pain is acute or chronic, then both codes should be assigned.

(ii) Sequencing of Category G89 Codes with Site-Specific Pain Codes

The sequencing of category G89 codes with site-specific pain codes (including chapter 18 codes), is dependent on the circumstances of the encounter/admission as follows:

- If the encounter is for pain control or pain management, assign the code from category G89 followed by the code identifying the specific site of pain (e.g., encounter for pain management for acute neck pain from trauma is assigned code G89.11, Acute pain due to trauma, followed by code M54.2, Cervicalgia, to identify the site of pain).

- If the encounter is for any other reason except pain control or pain management, and a related definitive diagnosis has not been established (confirmed) by the provider, assign the code for the specific site of pain first, followed by the appropriate code from category G89.

2) Pain due to devices, implants and grafts

See Section I.C.19. Pain due to medical devices

3) Postoperative Pain

The provider's documentation should be used to guide the coding of postoperative pain, as well as *Section III. Reporting Additional Diagnoses* and *Section IV. Diagnostic Coding and Reporting in the Outpatient Setting*.

The default for post-thoracotomy and other postoperative pain not specified as acute or chronic is the code for the acute form.

Routine or expected postoperative pain immediately after surgery should not be coded.

(a) Postoperative pain not associated with specific postoperative complication

Postoperative pain not associated with a specific postoperative complication is assigned to the appropriate postoperative pain code in category G89.

(b) Postoperative pain associated with specific postoperative complication

Postoperative pain associated with a specific postoperative complication (such as painful wire sutures) is assigned to the appropriate code(s) found in Chapter 19, Injury, poisoning, and certain other consequences of external causes. If appropriate, use additional code(s) from category G89 to identify acute or chronic pain (G89.18 or G89.28).

4) Chronic pain

Chronic pain is classified to subcategory G89.2. There is no time frame defining when pain becomes chronic pain. The provider's documentation should be used to guide use of these codes.

5) Neoplasm Related Pain

Code G89.3 is assigned to pain documented as being related, associated or due to cancer, primary or secondary malignancy, or tumor. This code is assigned regardless of whether the pain is acute or chronic.

This code may be assigned as the principal or first-listed code when the stated reason for the admission/encounter is documented as pain control/pain management. The underlying neoplasm should be reported as an additional diagnosis.

When the reason for the admission/encounter is management of the neoplasm and the pain associated with the neoplasm is also documented, code G89.3 may be assigned as an additional diagnosis. It is not necessary to assign an additional code for the site of the pain.

See Section I.C.2. for instructions on the sequencing of neoplasms for all other stated reasons for the admission/encounter (except for pain control/pain management).

6) Chronic pain syndrome

Central pain syndrome (G89.0) and chronic pain syndrome (G89.4) are different than the term "chronic pain," and therefore codes should only be used when the provider has specifically documented this condition.

See Section I.C.5. Pain disorders related to psychological factors

7. Chapter 7: Diseases of the Eye and Adnexa (H00-H59)

a. Glaucoma

1) Assigning Glaucoma Codes

Assign as many codes from category H40, Glaucoma, as needed to identify the type of glaucoma, the affected eye, and the glaucoma stage.

2) Bilateral glaucoma with same type and stage

When a patient has bilateral glaucoma and both eyes are documented as being the same type and stage, and there is a code for bilateral glaucoma, report only the code for the type of glaucoma, bilateral, with the seventh character for the stage.

When a patient has bilateral glaucoma and both eyes are documented as being the same type and stage, and the classification does not provide a code for bilateral glaucoma (i.e. subcategories H40.10, and H40.20) report only one code for the type of glaucoma with the appropriate seventh character for the stage.

3) Bilateral glaucoma stage with different types or stages

When a patient has bilateral glaucoma and each eye is documented as having a different type or stage, and the classification distinguishes laterality, assign the appropriate code for each eye rather than the code for bilateral glaucoma.

When a patient has bilateral glaucoma and each eye is documented as having a different type, and the classification does not distinguish laterality (i.e., subcategories H40.10, and H40.20), assign one code for each type of glaucoma with the appropriate seventh character for the stage.

When a patient has bilateral glaucoma and each eye is documented as having the same type, but different stage, and the classification does not distinguish laterality (i.e., subcategories H40.10 and H40.20), assign a code for the type of glaucoma for each eye with the seventh character for the specific glaucoma stage documented for each eye.

4) Patient admitted with glaucoma and stage evolves during the admission

If a patient is admitted with glaucoma and the stage progresses during the admission, assign the code for highest stage documented.

5) Indeterminate stage glaucoma

Assignment of the seventh character "4" for "indeterminate stage" should be based on the clinical documentation. The seventh character "4" is used for glaucomas whose stage cannot be clinically determined. This seventh character should not be confused with the seventh character "0", unspecified, which should be assigned when there is no documentation regarding the stage of the glaucoma.

b. Blindness

If "blindness" or "low vision" of both eyes is documented but the visual impairment category is not documented, assign code H54.3, Unqualified visual loss, both eyes. If "blindness" or "low vision" in one eye is documented but the visual impairment category is not documented, assign a code from H54.6-, Unqualified visual loss, one eye. If "blindness" or "visual loss" is documented without any information about whether one or both eyes are affected, assign code H54.7, Unspecified visual loss.

8. Chapter 8: Diseases of the Ear and Mastoid Process (H60-H95)

Reserved for future guideline expansion

9. Chapter 9: Diseases of the Circulatory System (I00-I99)

a. Hypertension

The classification presumes a causal relationship between hypertension and heart involvement and between hypertension and kidney involvement, as the two conditions are linked by the term "with" in the Alphabetic Index. These conditions should be coded as related even in the absence of provider documentation explicitly linking them, unless the documentation clearly states the conditions are unrelated.

For hypertension and conditions not specifically linked by relational terms such as "with," "associated with" or "due to" in the classification, provider documentation must link the conditions in order to code them as related.

1) **Hypertension with Heart Disease**

Hypertension with heart conditions classified to I50.- or I51.4-I51.7, I51.89, I51.9, are assigned to a code from category I11, Hypertensive heart disease. Use additional code(s) from category I50, Heart failure, to identify the type(s) of heart failure in those patients with heart failure.

The same heart conditions (I50.-, I51.4-I51.7, I51.89, I51.9) with hypertension are coded separately if the provider has documented they are unrelated to the hypertension. Sequence according to the circumstances of the admission/encounter.

2) **Hypertensive Chronic Kidney Disease**

Assign codes from category I12, Hypertensive chronic kidney disease, when both hypertension and a condition classifiable to category N18, Chronic kidney disease (CKD), are present. CKD should not be coded as hypertensive if the provider indicates the CKD is not related to the hypertension.

The appropriate code from category N18 should be used as a secondary code with a code from category I12 to identify the stage of chronic kidney disease.

See Section I.C.14. Chronic kidney disease.

If a patient has hypertensive chronic kidney disease and acute renal failure, the acute renal failure should also be coded. Sequence according to the circumstances of the admission/encounter.

3) **Hypertensive Heart and Chronic Kidney Disease**

Assign codes from combination category I13, Hypertensive heart and chronic kidney disease, when there is hypertension with both heart and kidney involvement. If heart failure is present, assign an additional code from category I50 to identify the type of heart failure.

The appropriate code from category N18, Chronic kidney disease, should be used as a secondary code with a code from category I13 to identify the stage of chronic kidney disease.

See Section I.C.14. Chronic kidney disease.

The codes in category I13, Hypertensive heart and chronic kidney disease, are combination codes that include hypertension, heart disease and chronic kidney disease. The Includes note at I13 specifies that the conditions included at I11 and I12 are included together in I13. If a patient has hypertension, heart disease and chronic kidney disease, then a code from I13 should be used, not individual codes for hypertension, heart disease and chronic kidney disease, or codes from I11 or I12.

For patients with both acute renal failure and chronic kidney disease, the acute renal failure should also be coded. Sequence according to the circumstances of the admission/encounter.

4) **Hypertensive Cerebrovascular Disease**

For hypertensive cerebrovascular disease, first assign the appropriate code from categories I60-I69, followed by the appropriate hypertension code.

5) **Hypertensive Retinopathy**

Subcategory H35.0, Background retinopathy and retinal vascular changes, should be used along with a code from categories I10-I15, in the Hypertensive diseases section, to include the systemic hypertension. The sequencing is based on the reason for the encounter.

6) **Hypertension, Secondary**

Secondary hypertension is due to an underlying condition. Two codes are required: one to identify the underlying etiology and one from category I15 to identify the hypertension. Sequencing of codes is determined by the reason for admission/encounter.

7) **Hypertension, Transient**

Assign code R03.0, Elevated blood pressure reading without diagnosis of hypertension, unless patient has an established diagnosis of hypertension. Assign code O13.-, Gestational [pregnancy-induced] hypertension without significant proteinuria, or O14.-, Pre-eclampsia, for transient hypertension of pregnancy.

8) **Hypertension, Controlled**

This diagnostic statement usually refers to an existing state of hypertension under control by therapy. Assign the appropriate code from categories I10-I15, Hypertensive diseases.

9) **Hypertension, Uncontrolled**

Uncontrolled hypertension may refer to untreated hypertension or hypertension not responding to current therapeutic regimen.

In either case, assign the appropriate code from categories I10-I15, Hypertensive diseases.

10) **Hypertensive Crisis**

Assign a code from category I16, Hypertensive crisis, for documented hypertensive urgency, hypertensive emergency or unspecified hypertensive crisis. Code also any identified hypertensive disease (I10-I15). The sequencing is based on the reason for the encounter.

11) **Pulmonary Hypertension**

Pulmonary hypertension is classified to category I27, Other pulmonary heart diseases. For secondary pulmonary hypertension (I27.1, I27.2-), code also any associated conditions or adverse effects of drugs or toxins. The sequencing is based on the reason for the encounter, except for adverse effects of drugs (See Section I.C.19.e.).

b. **Atherosclerotic Coronary Artery Disease and Angina**

ICD-10-CM has combination codes for atherosclerotic heart disease with angina pectoris. The subcategories for these codes are I25.11, Atherosclerotic heart disease of native coronary artery with angina pectoris and I25.7, Atherosclerosis of coronary artery bypass graft(s) and coronary artery of transplanted heart with angina pectoris.

When using one of these combination codes it is not necessary to use an additional code for angina pectoris. A causal relationship can be assumed in a patient with both atherosclerosis and angina pectoris, unless the documentation indicates the angina is due to something other than the atherosclerosis.

If a patient with coronary artery disease is admitted due to an acute myocardial infarction (AMI), the AMI should be sequenced before the coronary artery disease.

See Section I.C.9. Acute myocardial infarction (AMI)

c. **Intraoperative and Postprocedural Cerebrovascular Accident**

Medical record documentation should clearly specify the cause-and-effect relationship between the medical intervention and the cerebrovascular accident in order to assign a code for intraoperative or postprocedural cerebrovascular accident.

Proper code assignment depends on whether it was an infarction or hemorrhage and whether it occurred intraoperatively or postoperatively. If it was a cerebral hemorrhage, code assignment depends on the type of procedure performed.

d. **Sequelae of Cerebrovascular Disease**

1) **Category I69, Sequelae of Cerebrovascular disease**

Category I69 is used to indicate conditions classifiable to categories I60-I67 as the causes of sequela (neurologic deficits), themselves classified elsewhere. These "late effects" include neurologic deficits that persist after initial onset of conditions classifiable to categories I60-I67. The neurologic deficits caused by cerebrovascular disease may be present from the onset or may arise at any time after the onset of the condition classifiable to categories I60-I67.

Codes from category I69, Sequelae of cerebrovascular disease, that specify hemiplegia, hemiparesis and monoplegia identify whether the dominant or nondominant side is affected. Should the affected side be documented, but not specified as dominant or nondominant, and the classification system does not indicate a default, code selection is as follows:

- For ambidextrous patients, the default should be dominant.
- If the left side is affected, the default is non-dominant.
- If the right side is affected, the default is dominant.

2) **Codes from category I69 with codes from I60-I67**

Codes from category I69 may be assigned on a health care record with codes from I60-I67, if the patient has a current cerebrovascular disease and deficits from an old cerebrovascular disease.

3) **Codes from category I69 and Personal history of transient ischemic attack (TIA) and cerebral infarction (Z86.73)**

Codes from category I69 should not be assigned if the patient does not have neurologic deficits.

See Section I.C.21.4. History (of) for use of personal history codes

e. **Acute myocardial infarction (AMI)**

1) **Type 1 ST elevation myocardial infarction (STEMI) and non-ST elevation myocardial infarction (NSTEMI)**

The ICD-10-CM codes for type 1 acute myocardial infarction (AMI) identify the site, such as anterolateral wall or true posterior wall. Subcategories I21.0-I21.2 and code I21.3 are used for type 1 ST elevation myocardial infarction (STEMI). Code I21.4, Non-ST elevation (NSTEMI) myocardial infarction, is used for type 1 non-ST elevation myocardial infarction (NSTEMI) and nontransmural MIs.

If a type 1 NSTEMI evolves to STEMI, assign the STEMI code. If a type 1 STEMI converts to NSTEMI due to thrombolytic therapy, it is still coded as STEMI.

For encounters occurring while the myocardial infarction is equal to, or less than, four weeks old, including transfers to another acute setting or a postacute setting, and the myocardial infarction meets the definition for "other diagnoses" (see Section III, Reporting Additional Diagnoses), codes from category I21 may continue to be reported. For encounters after the 4-week time frame and the patient is still receiving care related to the myocardial infarction, the appropriate aftercare code should be assigned, rather than a code from category I21. For old or healed myocardial infarctions not requiring further care, code I25.2, Old myocardial infarction, may be assigned.

2) Acute myocardial infarction, unspecified
Code I21.9, Acute myocardial infarction, unspecified, is the default for unspecified acute myocardial infarction or unspecified type. If only type 1 STEMI or transmural MI without the site is documented, assign code I21.3, ST elevation (STEMI) myocardial infarction of unspecified site.

3) AMI documented as nontransmural or subendocardial but site provided
If an AMI is documented as nontransmural or subendocardial, but the site is provided, it is still coded as a subendocardial AMI.

See Section I.C.21.3. for information on coding status post administration of tPA in a different facility within the last 24 hours.

4) Subsequent acute myocardial infarction
A code from category I22, Subsequent ST elevation (STEMI) and non-ST elevation (NSTEMI) myocardial infarction, is to be used when a patient who has suffered a type 1 or unspecified AMI has a new AMI within the 4 week time frame of the initial AMI. A code from category I22 must be used in conjunction with a code from category I21. The sequencing of the I22 and I21 codes depends on the circumstances of the encounter.

Do not assign code I22 for subsequent myocardial infarctions other than type 1 or unspecified. For subsequent type 2 AMI assign only code I21.A1. For subsequent type 4 or type 5 AMI, assign only code I21.A9.

If a subsequent myocardial infarction of one type occurs within 4 weeks of a myocardial infarction of a different type, assign the appropriate codes from category I21 to identify each type. Do not assign a code from I22. Codes from category I22 should only be assigned if both the initial and subsequent myocardial infarctions are type 1 or unspecified.

5) Other Types of Myocardial Infarction
The ICD-10-CM provides codes for different types of myocardial infarction. Type 1 myocardial infarctions are assigned to codes I21.0-I21.4.

Type 2 myocardial infarction (myocardial infarction due to demand ischemia or secondary to ischemic imbalance) is assigned to code I21.A1, Myocardial infarction type 2 with the underlying cause coded first. Do not assign code I24.8, Other forms of acute ischemic heart disease, for the demand ischemia. If a type 2 AMI is described as NSTEMI or STEMI, only assign code I21.A1. Codes I21.01-I21.4 should only be assigned for type 1 AMIs.

Acute myocardial infarctions type 3, 4a, 4b, 4c and 5 are assigned to code I21.A9, Other myocardial infarction type.

The "Code also" and "Code first" notes should be followed related to complications, and for coding of postprocedural myocardial infarctions during or following cardiac surgery.

10. Chapter 10: Diseases of the Respiratory System (J00-J99), U07.0
a. Chronic Obstructive Pulmonary Disease [COPD] and Asthma
1) Acute exacerbation of chronic obstructive bronchitis and asthma
The codes in categories J44 and J45 distinguish between uncomplicated cases and those in acute exacerbation. An acute exacerbation is a worsening or a decompensation of a chronic condition. An acute exacerbation is not equivalent to an infection superimposed on a chronic condition, though an exacerbation may be triggered by an infection.

b. Acute Respiratory Failure
1) Acute respiratory failure as principal diagnosis
A code from subcategory J96.0, Acute respiratory failure, or subcategory J96.2, Acute and chronic respiratory failure, may be assigned as a principal diagnosis when it is the condition established after study to be chiefly responsible for occasioning the admission to the hospital, and the selection is supported by the Alphabetic Index and Tabular List. However, chapter-specific coding guidelines (such as obstetrics, poisoning, HIV, newborn) that provide sequencing direction take precedence.

2) Acute respiratory failure as secondary diagnosis
Respiratory failure may be listed as a secondary diagnosis if it occurs after admission, or if it is present on admission, but does not meet the definition of principal diagnosis.

3) Sequencing of acute respiratory failure and another acute condition
When a patient is admitted with respiratory failure and another acute condition, (e.g., myocardial infarction, cerebrovascular accident, aspiration pneumonia), the principal diagnosis will not be the same in every situation. This applies whether the other acute condition is a respiratory or nonrespiratory condition. Selection of the principal diagnosis will be dependent on the circumstances of admission. If both the respiratory failure and the other acute condition are equally responsible for occasioning the admission to the hospital, and there are no chapter-specific sequencing rules, the guideline regarding two or more diagnoses that equally meet the definition for principal diagnosis (Section II, C.) may be applied in these situations.

If the documentation is not clear as to whether acute respiratory failure and another condition are equally responsible for occasioning the admission, query the provider for clarification.

c. Influenza due to certain identified influenza viruses
Code only confirmed cases of influenza due to certain identified influenza viruses (category J09), and due to other identified influenza virus (category J10). This is an exception to the hospital inpatient guideline Section II, H. (Uncertain Diagnosis).

In this context, "confirmation" does not require documentation of positive laboratory testing specific for avian or other novel influenza A or other identified influenza virus. However, coding should be based on the provider's diagnostic statement that the patient has avian influenza, or other novel influenza A, for category J09, or has another particular identified strain of influenza, such as H1N1 or H3N2, but not identified as novel or variant, for category J10.

If the provider records "suspected" or "possible" or "probable" avian influenza, or novel influenza, or other identified influenza, then the appropriate influenza code from category J11, Influenza due to unidentified influenza virus, should be assigned. A code from category J09, Influenza due to certain identified influenza viruses, should not be assigned nor should a code from category J10, Influenza due to other identified influenza virus.

d. Ventilator associated Pneumonia
1) Documentation of Ventilator associated Pneumonia
As with all procedural or postprocedural complications, code assignment is based on the provider's documentation of the relationship between the condition and the procedure.

Code J95.851, Ventilator associated pneumonia, should be assigned only when the provider has documented ventilator associated pneumonia (VAP). An additional code to identify the organism (e.g., Pseudomonas aeruginosa, code B96.5) should also be assigned. Do not assign an additional code from categories J12-J18 to identify the type of pneumonia.

Code J95.851 should not be assigned for cases where the patient has pneumonia and is on a mechanical ventilator and the provider has not specifically stated that the pneumonia is ventilator-associated pneumonia. If the documentation is unclear as to whether the patient has a pneumonia that is a complication attributable to the mechanical ventilator, query the provider.

2) Ventilator associated Pneumonia Develops after Admission
A patient may be admitted with one type of pneumonia (e.g., code J13, Pneumonia due to Streptococcus pneumonia) and subsequently develop VAP. In this instance, the principal diagnosis would be the appropriate code from categories J12-J18 for the pneumonia diagnosed at the time of admission. Code J95.851, Ventilator associated pneumonia, would be assigned as an additional diagnosis when the provider has also documented the presence of ventilator associated pneumonia.

e. Vaping-related disorders

For patients presenting with condition(s) related to vaping, assign code U07.0, Vaping-related disorder, as the principal diagnosis. For lung injury due to vaping, assign only code U07.0. Assign additional codes for other manifestations, such as acute respiratory failure (subcategory J96.0-) or pneumonitis (code J68.0).

Associated respiratory signs and symptoms due to vaping, such as cough, shortness of breath, etc., are not coded separately, when a definitive diagnosis has been established. However, it would be appropriate to code separately any gastrointestinal symptoms, such as diarrhea and abdominal pain.

See Section I.C.1.g.1.c.i. for Pneumonia confirmed as due to COVID-19

11. Chapter 11: Diseases of the Digestive System (K00-K95)

Reserved for future guideline expansion

12. Chapter 12: Diseases of the Skin and Subcutaneous Tissue (L00-L99)

a. Pressure ulcer stage codes

1) Pressure ulcer stages

Codes in category L89, Pressure ulcer, identify the site and stage of the pressure ulcer.

The ICD-10-CM classifies pressure ulcer stages based on severity, which is designated by stages 1-4, deep tissue pressure injury, unspecified stage, and unstageable.

Assign as many codes from category L89 as needed to identify all the pressure ulcers the patient has, if applicable.

See Section I.B.14. for pressure ulcer stage documentation by clinicians other than patient's provider.

2) Unstageable pressure ulcers

Assignment of the code for unstageable pressure ulcer (L89.--0) should be based on the clinical documentation. These codes are used for pressure ulcers whose stage cannot be clinically determined (e.g., the ulcer is covered by eschar or has been treated with a skin or muscle graft). This code should not be confused with the codes for unspecified stage (L89.--9). When there is no documentation regarding the stage of the pressure ulcer, assign the appropriate code for unspecified stage (L89.-- 9).

If during an encounter, the stage of an unstageable pressure ulcer is revealed after debridement, assign only the code for the stage revealed following debridement.

3) Documented pressure ulcer stage

Assignment of the pressure ulcer stage code should be guided by clinical documentation of the stage or documentation of the terms found in the Alphabetic Index. For clinical terms describing the stage that are not found in the Alphabetic Index, and there is no documentation of the stage, the provider should be queried.

4) Patients admitted with pressure ulcers documented as healed

No code is assigned if the documentation states that the pressure ulcer is completely healed at the time of admission.

5) Pressure ulcers documented as healing

Pressure ulcers described as healing should be assigned the appropriate pressure ulcer stage code based on the documentation in the medical record. If the documentation does not provide information about the stage of the healing pressure ulcer, assign the appropriate code for unspecified stage.

If the documentation is unclear as to whether the patient has a current (new) pressure ulcer or if the patient is being treated for a healing pressure ulcer, query the provider.

For ulcers that were present on admission but healed at the time of discharge, assign the code for the site and stage of the pressure ulcer at the time of admission.

6) Patient admitted with pressure ulcer evolving into another stage during the admission

If a patient is admitted to an inpatient hospital with a pressure ulcer at one stage and it progresses to a higher stage, two separate codes should be assigned: one code for the site and stage of the ulcer on admission and a second code for the same ulcer site and the highest stage reported during the stay.

7) Pressure-induced deep tissue damage

For pressure-induced deep tissue damage or deep tissue pressure injury, assign only the appropriate code for pressure-induced deep tissue damage (L89.--6).

b. Non-Pressure Chronic Ulcers

1) Patients admitted with non-pressure ulcers documented as healed

No code is assigned if the documentation states that the non-pressure ulcer is completely healed at the time of admission.

2) Non-pressure ulcers documented as healing

Non-pressure ulcers described as healing should be assigned the appropriate non-pressure ulcer code based on the documentation in the medical record. If the documentation does not provide information about the severity of the healing non-pressure ulcer, assign the appropriate code for unspecified severity.

If the documentation is unclear as to whether the patient has a current (new) non-pressure ulcer or if the patient is being treated for a healing non-pressure ulcer, query the provider.

For ulcers that were present on admission but healed at the time of discharge, assign the code for the site and severity of the non-pressure ulcer at the time of admission.

3) Patient admitted with non-pressure ulcer that progresses to another severity level during the admission

If a patient is admitted to an inpatient hospital with a non-pressure ulcer at one severity level and it progresses to a higher severity level, two separate codes should be assigned: one code for the site and severity level of the ulcer on admission and a second code for the same ulcer site and the highest severity level reported during the stay.

See Section I.B.14. for pressure ulcer stage documentation by clinicians other than patient's provider

13. Chapter 13: Diseases of the Musculoskeletal System and Connective Tissue (M00-M99)

a. Site and laterality

Most of the codes within Chapter 13 have site and laterality designations. The site represents the bone, joint or the muscle involved. For some conditions where more than one bone, joint or muscle is usually involved, such as osteoarthritis, there is a "multiple sites" code available. For categories where no multiple site code is provided and more than one bone, joint or muscle is involved, multiple codes should be used to indicate the different sites involved.

1) Bone versus joint

For certain conditions, the bone may be affected at the upper or lower end, (e.g., avascular necrosis of bone, M87, Osteoporosis, M80, M81). Though the portion of the bone affected may be at the joint, the site designation will be the bone, not the joint.

b. Acute traumatic versus chronic or recurrent musculoskeletal conditions

Many musculoskeletal conditions are a result of previous injury or trauma to a site, or are recurrent conditions. Bone, joint or muscle conditions that are the result of a healed injury are usually found in chapter 13. Recurrent bone, joint or muscle conditions are also usually found in chapter 13. Any current, acute injury should be coded to the appropriate injury code from chapter 19. Chronic or recurrent conditions should generally be coded with a code from chapter 13. If it is difficult to determine from the documentation in the record which code is best to describe a condition, query the provider.

c. Coding of Pathologic Fractures

7th character A is for use as long as the patient is receiving active treatment for the fracture. While the patient may be seen by a new or different provider over the course of treatment for a pathological fracture, assignment of the 7th character is based on whether the patient is undergoing active treatment and not whether the provider is seeing the patient for the first time.

7th character D is to be used for encounters after the patient has completed active treatment for the fracture and is receiving routine care for the fracture during the healing or recovery phase. The other 7th characters, listed under each subcategory in the Tabular List, are to be used for subsequent encounters for treatment of problems associated with the healing, such as malunions, nonunions, and sequelae.

Care for complications of surgical treatment for fracture repairs during the healing or recovery phase should be coded with the appropriate complication codes.

See Section I.C.19. Coding of traumatic fractures.

d. Osteoporosis

Osteoporosis is a systemic condition, meaning that all bones of the musculoskeletal system are affected. Therefore, site is not a component of the codes under category M81, Osteoporosis without current pathological fracture. The site codes under category M80, Osteoporosis with current pathological fracture, identify the site of the fracture, not the osteoporosis.

1) Osteoporosis without pathological fracture

Category M81, Osteoporosis without current pathological fracture, is for use for patients with osteoporosis who do not currently have a pathologic fracture due to the osteoporosis, even if they have had a fracture in the past. For patients with a history of osteoporosis fractures, status code Z87.310, Personal history of (healed) osteoporosis fracture, should follow the code from M81.

2) Osteoporosis with current pathological fracture

Category M80, Osteoporosis with current pathological fracture, is for patients who have a current pathologic fracture at the time of an encounter. The codes under M80 identify the site of the fracture. A code from category M80, not a traumatic fracture code, should be used for any patient with known osteoporosis who suffers a fracture, even if the patient had a minor fall or trauma, if that fall or trauma would not usually break a normal, healthy bone.

e. Multisystem Inflammatory Syndrome

See Section I.C.1.g.1.l. for Multisystem Inflammatory Syndrome

14. Chapter 14: Diseases of Genitourinary System (N00-N99)

a. Chronic kidney disease

1) Stages of chronic kidney disease (CKD)

The ICD-10-CM classifies CKD based on severity. The severity of CKD is designated by stages 1-5. Stage 2, code N18.2, equates to mild CKD; stage 3, codes N18.30-N18.32, equate to moderate CKD; and stage 4, code N18.4, equates to severe CKD. Code N18.6, End stage renal disease (ESRD), is assigned when the provider has documented end-stage renal disease (ESRD).

If both a stage of CKD and ESRD are documented, assign code N18.6 only.

2) Chronic kidney disease and kidney transplant status

Patients who have undergone kidney transplant may still have some form of chronic kidney disease (CKD) because the kidney transplant may not fully restore kidney function. Therefore, the presence of CKD alone does not constitute a transplant complication. Assign the appropriate N18 code for the patient's stage of CKD and code Z94.0, Kidney transplant status. If a transplant complication such as failure or rejection or other transplant complication is documented, see section I.C.19.g for information on coding complications of a kidney transplant. If the documentation is unclear as to whether the patient has a complication of the transplant, query the provider.

3) Chronic kidney disease with other conditions

Patients with CKD may also suffer from other serious conditions, most commonly diabetes mellitus and hypertension. The sequencing of the CKD code in relationship to codes for other contributing conditions is based on the conventions in the Tabular List.

See I.C.9. Hypertensive chronic kidney disease.

See I.C.19. Chronic kidney disease and kidney transplant complications.

15. Chapter 15: Pregnancy, Childbirth, and the Puerperium (O00-O9A)

a. General Rules for Obstetric Cases

1) Codes from chapter 15 and sequencing priority

Obstetric cases require codes from chapter 15, codes in the range O00-O9A, Pregnancy, Childbirth, and the Puerperium. Chapter 15 codes have sequencing priority over codes from other chapters. Additional codes from other chapters may be used in conjunction with chapter 15 codes to further specify conditions. Should the provider document that the pregnancy is incidental to the encounter, then code Z33.1, Pregnant state, incidental, should be used in place of any chapter 15 codes. It is the provider's responsibility to state that the condition being treated is not affecting the pregnancy.

2) Chapter 15 codes used only on the maternal record

Chapter 15 codes are to be used only on the maternal record, never on the record of the newborn.

3) Final character for trimester

The majority of codes in Chapter 15 have a final character indicating the trimester of pregnancy. The timeframes for the trimesters are indicated at the beginning of the chapter. If trimester is not a component of a code, it is because the condition always occurs in a specific trimester, or the concept of trimester of

pregnancy is not applicable. Certain codes have characters for only certain trimesters because the condition does not occur in all trimesters, but it may occur in more than just one.

Assignment of the final character for trimester should be based on the provider's documentation of the trimester (or number of weeks) for the current admission/encounter. This applies to the assignment of trimester for pre-existing conditions as well as those that develop during or are due to the pregnancy. The provider's documentation of the number of weeks may be used to assign the appropriate code identifying the trimester.

Whenever delivery occurs during the current admission, and there is an "in childbirth" option for the obstetric complication being coded, the "in childbirth" code should be assigned. When the classification does not provide an obstetric code with an "in childbirth" option, it is appropriate to assign a code describing the current trimester.

4) Selection of trimester for inpatient admissions that encompass more than one trimester

In instances when a patient is admitted to a hospital for complications of pregnancy during one trimester and remains in the hospital into a subsequent trimester, the trimester character for the antepartum complication code should be assigned on the basis of the trimester when the complication developed, not the trimester of the discharge. If the condition developed prior to the current admission/encounter or represents a pre-existing condition, the trimester character for the trimester at the time of the admission/encounter should be assigned.

5) Unspecified trimester

Each category that includes codes for trimester has a code for "unspecified trimester." The "unspecified trimester" code should rarely be used, such as when the documentation in the record is insufficient to determine the trimester and it is not possible to obtain clarification.

6) 7th character for fetus identification

Where applicable, a 7th character is to be assigned for certain categories (O31, O32, O33.3-O33.6, O35, O36, O40, O41, O60.1, O60.2, O64, and O69) to identify the fetus for which the complication code applies.

Assign 7th character "0":

- For single gestations
- When the documentation in the record is insufficient to determine the fetus affected and it is not possible to obtain clarification.
- When it is not possible to clinically determine which fetus is affected.

7) Completed weeks of gestation

In ICD-10-CM, "completed" weeks of gestation refers to full weeks. For example, if the provider documents gestation at 39 weeks and 6 days, the code for 39 weeks of gestation should be assigned, as the patient has not yet reached 40 completed weeks.

b. Selection of OB Principal or First-listed Diagnosis

1) Routine outpatient prenatal visits

For routine outpatient prenatal visits when no complications are present, a code from category Z34, Encounter for supervision of normal pregnancy, should be used as the first-listed diagnosis. These codes should not be used in conjunction with chapter 15 codes.

2) Supervision of High-Risk Pregnancy

Codes from category O09, Supervision of high-risk pregnancy, are intended for use only during the prenatal period. For complications during the labor or delivery episode as a result of a high-risk pregnancy, assign the applicable complication codes from Chapter 15. If there are no complications during the labor or delivery episode, assign code O80, Encounter for full-term uncomplicated delivery.

For routine prenatal outpatient visits for patients with high-risk pregnancies, a code from category O09, Supervision of high-risk pregnancy, should be used as the first-listed diagnosis. Secondary chapter 15 codes may be used in conjunction with these codes if appropriate.

3) Episodes when no delivery occurs

In episodes when no delivery occurs, the principal diagnosis should correspond to the principal complication of the pregnancy which necessitated the encounter. Should more than one complication exist, all of which are treated or monitored, any of the complication codes may be sequenced first.

4) When a delivery occurs
When an obstetric patient is admitted and delivers during that admission, the condition that prompted the admission should be sequenced as the principal diagnosis. If multiple conditions prompted the admission, sequence the one most related to the delivery as the principal diagnosis. A code for any complication of the delivery should be assigned as an additional diagnosis. In cases of cesarean delivery, if the patient was admitted with a condition that resulted in the performance of a cesarean procedure, that condition should be selected as the principal diagnosis. If the reason for the admission was unrelated to the condition resulting in the cesarean delivery, the condition related to the reason for the admission should be selected as the principal diagnosis.

5) Outcome of delivery
A code from category Z37, Outcome of delivery, should be included on every maternal record when a delivery has occurred. These codes are not to be used on subsequent records or on the newborn record.

c. Pre-existing conditions versus conditions due to the pregnancy
Certain categories in Chapter 15 distinguish between conditions of the mother that existed prior to pregnancy (pre-existing) and those that are a direct result of pregnancy. When assigning codes from Chapter 15, it is important to assess if a condition was pre-existing prior to pregnancy or developed during or due to the pregnancy in order to assign the correct code.

Categories that do not distinguish between pre-existing and pregnancy-related conditions may be used for either. It is acceptable to use codes specifically for the puerperium with codes complicating pregnancy and childbirth if a condition arises postpartum during the delivery encounter.

d. Pre-existing hypertension in pregnancy
Category O10, Pre-existing hypertension complicating pregnancy, childbirth and the puerperium, includes codes for hypertensive heart and hypertensive chronic kidney disease. When assigning one of the O10 codes that includes hypertensive heart disease or hypertensive chronic kidney disease, it is necessary to add a secondary code from the appropriate hypertension category to specify the type of heart failure or chronic kidney disease.
See Section I.C.9. Hypertension.

e. Fetal Conditions Affecting the Management of the Mother
1) Codes from categories O35 and O36
Codes from categories O35, Maternal care for known or suspected fetal abnormality and damage, and O36, Maternal care for other fetal problems, are assigned only when the fetal condition is actually responsible for modifying the management of the mother, i.e., by requiring diagnostic studies, additional observation, special care, or termination of pregnancy. The fact that the fetal condition exists does not justify assigning a code from this series to the mother's record.

2) In utero surgery
In cases when surgery is performed on the fetus, a diagnosis code from category O35, Maternal care for known or suspected fetal abnormality and damage, should be assigned identifying the fetal condition. Assign the appropriate procedure code for the procedure performed.

No code from Chapter 16, the perinatal codes, should be used on the mother's record to identify fetal conditions. Surgery performed in utero on a fetus is still to be coded as an obstetric encounter.

f. HIV Infection in Pregnancy, Childbirth and the Puerperium
During pregnancy, childbirth or the puerperium, a patient admitted because of an HIV-related illness should receive a principal diagnosis from subcategory O98.7-, Human immunodeficiency [HIV] disease complicating pregnancy, childbirth and the puerperium, followed by the code(s) for the HIV-related illness(es).

Patients with asymptomatic HIV infection status admitted during pregnancy, childbirth, or the puerperium should receive codes of O98.7- and Z21, Asymptomatic human immunodeficiency virus [HIV] infection status.

g. Diabetes mellitus in pregnancy
Diabetes mellitus is a significant complicating factor in pregnancy. Pregnant patients who are diabetic should be assigned a code from category O24, Diabetes mellitus in pregnancy, childbirth, and the

puerperium, first, followed by the appropriate diabetes code(s) (E08-E13) from Chapter 4.

h. Long term use of insulin and oral hypoglycemics
See section I.C.4.a.3 for information on the long-term use of insulin and oral hypoglycemics.

i. Gestational (pregnancy induced) diabetes
Gestational (pregnancy induced) diabetes can occur during the second and third trimester of pregnancy in patients who were not diabetic prior to pregnancy. Gestational diabetes can cause complications in the pregnancy similar to those of pre-existing diabetes mellitus. It also puts the patient at greater risk of developing diabetes after the pregnancy.

Codes for gestational diabetes are in subcategory O24.4, Gestational diabetes mellitus. No other code from category O24, Diabetes mellitus in pregnancy, childbirth, and the puerperium, should be used with a code from O24.4.

The codes under subcategory O24.4 include diet controlled, insulin controlled, and controlled by oral hypoglycemic drugs. If a patient with gestational diabetes is treated with both diet and insulin, only the code for insulin-controlled is required. If a patient with gestational diabetes is treated with both diet and oral hypoglycemic medications, only the code for "controlled by oral hypoglycemic drugs" is required. Codes Z79.4, Long-term (current) use of insulin, Z79.84, Long-term (current) use of oral hypoglycemic drugs, **and Z79.85, Long-term (current) use of injectable non-insulin antidiabetic drugs,** should not be assigned with codes from subcategory O24.4.

An abnormal glucose tolerance in pregnancy is assigned a code from subcategory O99.81, Abnormal glucose complicating pregnancy, childbirth, and the puerperium.

j. Sepsis and septic shock complicating abortion, pregnancy, childbirth and the puerperium
When assigning a chapter 15 code for sepsis complicating abortion, pregnancy, childbirth, and the puerperium, a code for the specific type of infection should be assigned as an additional diagnosis. If severe sepsis is present, a code from subcategory R65.2, Severe sepsis, and code(s) for associated organ dysfunction(s) should also be assigned as additional diagnoses.

k. Puerperal sepsis
Code O85, Puerperal sepsis, should be assigned with a secondary code to identify the causal organism (e.g., for a bacterial infection, assign a code from category B95-B96, Bacterial infections in conditions classified elsewhere). A code from category A40, Streptococcal sepsis, or A41, Other sepsis, should not be used for puerperal sepsis. If applicable, use additional codes to identify severe sepsis (R65.2-) and any associated acute organ dysfunction.

Code O85 should not be assigned for sepsis following an obstetrical procedure (See Section I.C.1.d.5.b., Sepsis due to a postprocedural infection).

l. Alcohol, tobacco and drug use during pregnancy, childbirth and the puerperium
1) Alcohol use during pregnancy, childbirth and the puerperium
Codes under subcategory O99.31, Alcohol use complicating pregnancy, childbirth, and the puerperium, should be assigned for any pregnancy case when a patient uses alcohol during the pregnancy or postpartum. A secondary code from category F10, Alcohol related disorders, should also be assigned to identify manifestations of the alcohol use.

2) Tobacco use during pregnancy, childbirth and the puerperium
Codes under subcategory O99.33, Smoking (tobacco) complicating pregnancy, childbirth, and the puerperium, should be assigned for any pregnancy case when a patient uses any type of tobacco product during the pregnancy or postpartum.

A secondary code from category F17, Nicotine dependence, should also be assigned to identify the type of nicotine dependence.

3) Drug use during pregnancy, childbirth and the puerperium
Codes under subcategory O99.32, Drug use complicating pregnancy, childbirth, and the puerperium, should be assigned for any pregnancy case when a patient uses drugs during the pregnancy or postpartum. This can involve illegal drugs, or inappropriate use or abuse of prescription drugs. Secondary code(s) from categories F11-F16 and F18-F19 should also be assigned to identify manifestations of the drug use.

m. Poisoning, toxic effects, adverse effects and underdosing in a pregnant patient

A code from subcategory O9A.2, Injury, poisoning and certain other consequences of external causes complicating pregnancy, childbirth, and the puerperium, should be sequenced first, followed by the appropriate injury, poisoning, toxic effect, adverse effect or underdosing code, and then the additional code(s) that specifies the condition caused by the poisoning, toxic effect, adverse effect or underdosing.

See Section I.C.19. Adverse effects, poisoning, underdosing and toxic effects.

n. Normal Delivery, Code O80

1) Encounter for full term uncomplicated delivery

Code O80 should be assigned when a patient is admitted for a full-term normal delivery and delivers a single, healthy infant without any complications antepartum, during the delivery, or postpartum during the delivery episode. Code O80 is always a principal diagnosis. It is not to be used if any other code from chapter 15 is needed to describe a current complication of the antenatal, delivery, or postnatal period. Additional codes from other chapters may be used with code O80 if they are not related to or are in any way complicating the pregnancy.

2) Uncomplicated delivery with resolved antepartum complication

Code O80 may be used if the patient had a complication at some point during the pregnancy, but the complication is not present at the time of the admission for delivery.

3) Outcome of delivery for O80

Z37.0, Single live birth, is the only outcome of delivery code appropriate for use with O80.

o. The Peripartum and Postpartum Periods

1) Peripartum and Postpartum periods

The postpartum period begins immediately after delivery and continues for six weeks following delivery. The peripartum period is defined as the last month of pregnancy to five months postpartum.

2) Peripartum and postpartum complication

A postpartum complication is any complication occurring within the six-week period.

3) Pregnancy-related complications after 6-week period

Chapter 15 codes may also be used to describe pregnancy-related complications after the peripartum or postpartum period if the provider documents that a condition is pregnancy related.

4) Admission for routine postpartum care following delivery outside hospital

When the mother delivers outside the hospital prior to admission and is admitted for routine postpartum care and no complications are noted, code Z39.0, Encounter for care and examination of mother immediately after delivery, should be assigned as the principal diagnosis.

5) Pregnancy associated cardiomyopathy

Pregnancy associated cardiomyopathy, code O90.3, is unique in that it may be diagnosed in the third trimester of pregnancy but may continue to progress months after delivery. For this reason, it is referred to as peripartum cardiomyopathy. Code O90.3 is only for use when the cardiomyopathy develops as a result of pregnancy in a patient who did not have pre-existing heart disease.

p. Code O94, Sequelae of complication of pregnancy, childbirth, and the puerperium

1) Code O94

Code O94, Sequelae of complication of pregnancy, childbirth, and the puerperium, is for use in those cases when an initial complication of a pregnancy develops a sequela or sequelae requiring care or treatment at a future date.

2) After the initial postpartum period

This code may be used at any time after the initial postpartum period.

3) Sequencing of Code O94

This code, like all sequela codes, is to be sequenced following the code describing the sequelae of the complication.

q. Termination of Pregnancy and Spontaneous abortions

1) Abortion with Liveborn Fetus

When an attempted termination of pregnancy results in a liveborn fetus, assign code Z33.2, Encounter for elective termination of pregnancy and a code from category Z37, Outcome of Delivery.

2) Retained Products of Conception following an abortion

Subsequent encounters for retained products of conception following a spontaneous abortion or elective termination of pregnancy, without complications are assigned O03.4, Incomplete spontaneous abortion without complication, or code O07.4, Failed attempted termination of pregnancy without complication. This advice is appropriate even when the patient was discharged previously with a discharge diagnosis of complete abortion. If the patient has a specific complication associated with the spontaneous abortion or elective termination of pregnancy in addition to retained products of conception, assign the appropriate complication code (e.g., O03.-, O04.-, O07.-) instead of code O03.4 or O07.4.

3) Complications leading to abortion

Codes from Chapter 15 may be used as additional codes to identify any documented complications of the pregnancy in conjunction with codes in categories in O04, O07 and O08.

4) Hemorrhage following elective abortion

For hemorrhage post elective abortion, assign code O04.6, Delayed or excessive hemorrhage following (induced) termination of pregnancy. Do not assign code O72.1, Other immediate postpartum hemorrhage, as this code should not be assigned for post abortion conditions. Do not assign code Z33.2, Encounter for elective termination of pregnancy, when the patient experiences a complication post elective abortion.

r. Abuse in a pregnant patient

For suspected or confirmed cases of abuse of a pregnant patient, a code(s) from subcategories O9A.3, Physical abuse complicating pregnancy, childbirth, and the puerperium, O9A.4, Sexual abuse complicating pregnancy, childbirth, and the puerperium, and O9A.5, Psychological abuse complicating pregnancy, childbirth, and the puerperium, should be sequenced first, followed by the appropriate codes (if applicable) to identify any associated current injury due to physical abuse, sexual abuse, and the perpetrator of abuse.

See Section I.C.19. Adult and child abuse, neglect and other maltreatment.

s. COVID-19 infection in pregnancy, childbirth, and the puerperium

During pregnancy, childbirth or the puerperium, when COVID-19 is the reason for admission/encounter , code O98.5-, Other viral diseases complicating pregnancy, childbirth and the puerperium, should be sequenced as the principal/first-listed diagnosis, and code U07.1, COVID-19, and the appropriate codes for associated manifestation(s) should be assigned as additional diagnoses. Codes from Chapter 15 always take sequencing priority.

If the reason for admission/encounter is unrelated to COVID-19 but the patient tests positive for COVID-19 during the admission/encounter, the appropriate code for the reason for admission/encounter should be sequenced as the principal/first-listed diagnosis, and codes O98.5- and U07.1, as well as the appropriate codes for associated COVID-19 manifestations, should be assigned as additional diagnoses.

16. Chapter 16: Certain Conditions Originating in the Perinatal Period (P00-P96)

For coding and reporting purposes the perinatal period is defined as before birth through the 28th day following birth. The following guidelines are provided for reporting purposes.

a. General Perinatal Rules

1) Use of Chapter 16 Codes

Codes in this chapter are <u>never</u> for use on the maternal record. Codes from Chapter 15, the obstetric chapter, are never permitted on the newborn record. Chapter 16 codes may be used throughout the life of the patient if the condition is still present.

2) Principal Diagnosis for Birth Record

When coding the birth episode in a newborn record, assign a code from category Z38, Liveborn infants according to place of birth and type of delivery, as the principal diagnosis. A code from category Z38 is assigned only once, to a newborn at the time of birth. If a newborn is transferred to another institution, a code from category Z38 should not be used at the receiving hospital.

A code from category Z38 is used only on the newborn record, not on the mother's record.

3) Use of Codes from other Chapters with Codes from Chapter 16

Codes from other chapters may be used with codes from chapter 16 if the codes from the other chapters provide more specific detail. Codes for signs and symptoms may be assigned when a definitive diagnosis has not been established. If the reason for the encounter is a perinatal condition, the code from chapter 16 should be sequenced first.

4) Use of Chapter 16 Codes after the Perinatal Period

Should a condition originate in the perinatal period, and continue throughout the life of the patient, the perinatal code should continue to be used regardless of the patient's age.

5) Birth process or community acquired conditions

If a newborn has a condition that may be either due to the birth process or community acquired and the documentation does not indicate which it is, the default is due to the birth process and the code from Chapter 16 should be used. If the condition is community-acquired, a code from Chapter 16 should not be assigned.

For COVID-19 infection in a newborn, see guideline I.C.16.h.

6) Code all clinically significant conditions

All clinically significant conditions noted on routine newborn examination should be coded. A condition is clinically significant if it requires:

- clinical evaluation; or
- therapeutic treatment; or
- diagnostic procedures; or
- extended length of hospital stay; or
- increased nursing care and/or monitoring; or
- has implications for future health care needs

Note: The perinatal guidelines listed above are the same as the general coding guidelines for "additional diagnoses," except for the final point regarding implications for future health care needs. Codes should be assigned for conditions that have been specified by the provider as having implications for future health care needs.

b. Observation and Evaluation of Newborns for Suspected Conditions not Found

1) Use of Z05 codes

Assign a code from category Z05, Observation and evaluation of newborn for suspected **diseases and** conditions ruled out, to identify those instances when a healthy newborn is evaluated for a suspected condition/**disease** that is determined after study not to be present. Do not use a code from category Z05 when the patient **is documented to have** signs or symptoms of a suspected problem; in such cases code the sign or symptom.

2) Z05 on other than the birth record

A code from category Z05 may also be assigned as a principal or first-listed code for readmissions or encounters when the code from category Z38 code no longer applies. Codes from category Z05 are for use only for healthy newborns and infants for which no condition after study is found to be present.

3) Z05 on a birth record

A code from category Z05 is to be used as a secondary code after the code from category Z38, Liveborn infants according to place of birth and type of delivery.

c. Coding Additional Perinatal Diagnoses

1) Assigning codes for conditions that require treatment

Assign codes for conditions that require treatment or further investigation, prolong the length of stay, or require resource utilization.

2) Codes for conditions specified as having implications for future health care needs

Assign codes for conditions that have been specified by the provider as having implications for future health care needs.

Note: This guideline should not be used for adult patients.

d. Prematurity and Fetal Growth Retardation

Providers utilize different criteria in determining prematurity. A code for prematurity should not be assigned unless it is documented. Assignment of codes in categories P05, Disorders of newborn related to slow fetal growth and fetal malnutrition, and P07, Disorders of newborn related to short gestation and low birth weight, not elsewhere classified, should be based on the recorded birth weight and estimated gestational age.

When both birth weight and gestational age are available, two codes from category P07 should be assigned, with the code for birth weight sequenced before the code for gestational age.

e. Low birth weight and immaturity status

Codes from category P07, Disorders of newborn related to short gestation and low birth weight, not elsewhere classified, are for use for a child or adult who was premature or had a low birth weight as a newborn and this is affecting the patient's current health status.

See Section I.C.21. Factors influencing health status and contact with health services, Status.

f. Bacterial Sepsis of Newborn

Category P36, Bacterial sepsis of newborn, includes congenital sepsis. If a perinate is documented as having sepsis without documentation of congenital or community acquired, the default is congenital and a code from category P36 should be assigned. If the P36 code includes the causal organism, an additional code from category B95, Streptococcus, Staphylococcus, and Enterococcus as the cause of diseases classified elsewhere, or B96, Other bacterial agents as the cause of diseases classified elsewhere, should not be assigned. If the P36 code does not include the causal organism, assign an additional code from category B96. If applicable, use additional codes to identify severe sepsis (R65.2-) and any associated acute organ dysfunction.

g. Stillbirth

Code P95, Stillbirth, is only for use in institutions that maintain separate records for stillbirths. No other code should be used with P95. Code P95 should not be used on the mother's record.

h. COVID-19 Infection in Newborn

For a newborn that tests positive for COVID-19, assign code U07.1, COVID-19, and the appropriate codes for associated manifestation(s) in neonates/newborns in the absence of documentation indicating a specific type of transmission. For a newborn that tests positive for COVID-19 and the provider documents the condition was contracted in utero or during the birth process, assign codes P35.8, Other congenital viral diseases, and U07.1, COVID-19. When coding the birth episode in a newborn record, the appropriate code from category Z38, Liveborn infants according to place of birth and type of delivery, should be assigned as the principal diagnosis.

17. Chapter 17: Congenital malformations, deformations, and chromosomal abnormalities (Q00-Q99)

Assign an appropriate code(s) from categories Q00-Q99, Congenital malformations, deformations, and chromosomal abnormalities when a malformation/deformation or chromosomal abnormality is documented. A malformation/deformation or chromosomal abnormality may be the principal/first-listed diagnosis on a record or a secondary diagnosis.

When a malformation/deformation or chromosomal abnormality does not have a unique code assignment, assign additional code(s) for any manifestations that may be present.

When the code assignment specifically identifies the malformation/deformation or chromosomal abnormality, manifestations that are an inherent component of the anomaly should not be coded separately. Additional codes should be assigned for manifestations that are not an inherent component.

Codes from Chapter 17 may be used throughout the life of the patient. If a congenital malformation or deformity has been corrected, a personal history code should be used to identify the history of the malformation or deformity. Although present at birth, a malformation/deformation/or chromosomal abnormality may not be identified until later in life. Whenever the condition is diagnosed by the provider, it is appropriate to assign a code from codes Q00-Q99. For the birth admission, the appropriate code from category Z38, Liveborn infants, according to place of birth and type of delivery, should be sequenced as the principal diagnosis, followed by any congenital anomaly codes, Q00-Q99.

18. Chapter 18: Symptoms, signs, and abnormal clinical and laboratory findings, not elsewhere classified (R00-R99)

Chapter 18 includes symptoms, signs, abnormal results of clinical or other investigative procedures, and ill-defined conditions regarding which no diagnosis classifiable elsewhere is recorded. Signs and symptoms that point to a specific diagnosis have been assigned to a category in other chapters of the classification.

a. Use of symptom codes

Codes that describe symptoms and signs are acceptable for reporting purposes when a related definitive diagnosis has not been established (confirmed) by the provider.

b. Use of a symptom code with a definitive diagnosis code

Codes for signs and symptoms may be reported in addition to a related definitive diagnosis when the sign or symptom is not routinely associated with that diagnosis, such as the various signs and symptoms associated with complex syndromes. The definitive diagnosis code should be sequenced before the symptom code.

Signs or symptoms that are associated routinely with a disease process should not be assigned as additional codes, unless otherwise instructed by the classification.

c. Combination codes that include symptoms
ICD-10-CM contains a number of combination codes that identify both the definitive diagnosis and common symptoms of that diagnosis. When using one of these combination codes, an additional code should not be assigned for the symptom.

d. Repeated falls
Code R29.6, Repeated falls, is for use for encounters when a patient has recently fallen and the reason for the fall is being investigated.

Code Z91.81, History of falling, is for use when a patient has fallen in the past and is at risk for future falls. When appropriate, both codes R29.6 and Z91.81 may be assigned together.

e. Coma
Code R40.20, Unspecified coma, may be assigned in conjunction with codes for any medical condition.

Do not report codes for unspecified coma, individual or total Glasgow coma scale scores for a patient with a medically induced coma or a sedated patient.

1) Coma Scale
The coma scale codes (R40.21- to R40.24-) can be used in conjunction with traumatic brain injury codes. These codes are primarily for use by trauma registries, but they may be used in any setting where this information is collected. The coma scale codes should be sequenced after the diagnosis code(s).

These codes, one from each subcategory, are needed to complete the scale. The 7th character indicates when the scale was recorded. The 7th character should match for all three codes.

At a minimum, report the initial score documented on presentation at your facility. This may be a score from the emergency medicine technician (EMT) or in the emergency department. If desired, a facility may choose to capture multiple coma scale scores.

Assign code R40.24-, Glasgow coma scale, total score, when only the total score is documented in the medical record and not the individual score(s).

If multiple coma scores are captured within the first 24 hours after hospital admission, assign only the code for the score at the time of admission. ICD-10-CM does not classify coma scores that are reported after admission but less than 24 hours later.

See Section I.B.14. for coma scale documentation by clinicians other than patient's provider

f. Functional quadriplegia
GUIDELINE HAS BEEN DELETED EFFECTIVE OCTOBER 1, 2017

g. SIRS due to Non-Infectious Process
The systemic inflammatory response syndrome (SIRS) can develop as a result of certain non-infectious disease processes, such as trauma, malignant neoplasm, or pancreatitis. When SIRS is documented with a noninfectious condition, and no subsequent infection is documented, the code for the underlying condition, such as an injury, should be assigned, followed by code R65.10, Systemic inflammatory response syndrome (SIRS) of non-infectious origin without acute organ dysfunction, or code R65.11, Systemic inflammatory response syndrome (SIRS) of non-infectious origin with acute organ dysfunction. If an associated acute organ dysfunction is documented, the appropriate code(s) for the specific type of organ dysfunction(s) should be assigned in addition to code R65.11. If acute organ dysfunction is documented, but it cannot be determined if the acute organ dysfunction is associated with SIRS or due to another condition (e.g., directly due to the trauma), the provider should be queried.

h. Death NOS
Code R99, Ill-defined and unknown cause of mortality, is only for use in the very limited circumstance when a patient who has already died is brought into an emergency department or other healthcare facility and is pronounced dead upon arrival. It does not represent the discharge disposition of death.

i. NIHSS Stroke Scale
The NIH stroke scale (NIHSS) codes (R29.7- -) can be used in conjunction with acute stroke codes (I63) to identify the patient's neurological status and the severity of the stroke. The stroke scale codes should be sequenced after the acute stroke diagnosis code(s).

At a minimum, report the initial score documented. If desired, a facility may choose to capture multiple stroke scale scores.

See Section I.B.14. for NIHSS stroke scale documentation by clinicians other than patient's provider

19. Chapter 19: Injury, poisoning, and certain other consequences of external causes (S00-T88)

a. Application of 7th Characters in Chapter 19
Most categories in chapter 19 have a 7th character requirement for each applicable code. Most categories in this chapter have three 7th character values (with the exception of fractures): A, initial encounter, D, subsequent encounter and S, sequela. Categories for traumatic fractures have additional 7th character values. While the patient may be seen by a new or different provider over the course of treatment for an injury, assignment of the 7th character is based on whether the patient is undergoing active treatment and not whether the provider is seeing the patient for the first time.

For complication codes, active treatment refers to treatment for the condition described by the code, even though it may be related to an earlier precipitating problem. For example, code T84.50XA, Infection and inflammatory reaction due to unspecified internal joint prosthesis, initial encounter, is used when active treatment is provided for the infection, even though the condition relates to the prosthetic device, implant or graft that was placed at a previous encounter.

7th character "A", initial encounter is used for each encounter where the patient is receiving active treatment for the condition.

7th character "D" subsequent encounter is used for encounters after the patient has completed active treatment of the condition and is receiving routine care for the condition during the healing or recovery phase.

The aftercare Z codes should not be used for aftercare for conditions such as injuries or poisonings, where 7th characters are provided to identify subsequent care. For example, for aftercare of an injury, assign the acute injury code with the 7th character "D" (subsequent encounter).

7th character "S", sequela, is for use for complications or conditions that arise as a direct result of a condition, such as scar formation after a burn. The scars are sequelae of the burn. When using 7th character "S", it is necessary to use both the injury code that precipitated the sequela and the code for the sequela itself. The "S" is added only to the injury code, not the sequela code. The 7th character "S" identifies the injury responsible for the sequela. The specific type of sequela (e.g. scar) is sequenced first, followed by the injury code.

See Section I.B.10. Sequelae, (Late Effects)

b. Coding of Injuries
When coding injuries, assign separate codes for each injury unless a combination code is provided, in which case the combination code is assigned. Codes from category T07, Unspecified multiple injuries should not be assigned in the inpatient setting unless information for a more specific code is not available. Traumatic injury codes (S00-T14.9) are not to be used for normal, healing surgical wounds or to identify complications of surgical wounds.

The code for the most serious injury, as determined by the provider and the focus of treatment, is sequenced first.

1) Superficial injuries
Superficial injuries such as abrasions or contusions are not coded when associated with more severe injuries of the same site.

2) Primary injury with damage to nerves/blood vessels
When a primary injury results in minor damage to peripheral nerves or blood vessels, the primary injury is sequenced first with additional code(s) for injuries to nerves and spinal cord (such as category S04), and/or injury to blood vessels (such as category S15). When the primary injury is to the blood vessels or nerves, that injury should be sequenced first.

3) Iatrogenic injuries
Injury codes from Chapter 19 should not be assigned for injuries that occur during, or as a result of, a medical intervention. Assign the appropriate complication code(s).

c. Coding of Traumatic Fractures
The principles of multiple coding of injuries should be followed in coding fractures. Fractures of specified sites are coded individually by site in accordance with both the provisions within categories S02, S12, S22, S32, S42, S49, S52, S59, S62, S72, S79, S82, S89, S92 and the level of detail furnished by medical record content.

A fracture not indicated as open or closed should be coded to closed. A fracture not indicated whether displaced or not displaced should be coded to displaced.

More specific guidelines are as follows:

1) Initial vs. subsequent encounter for fractures

Traumatic fractures are coded using the appropriate 7th character for initial encounter (A, B, C) for each encounter where the patient is receiving active treatment for the fracture. The appropriate 7th character for initial encounter should also be assigned for a patient who delayed seeking treatment for the fracture or nonunion.

Fractures are coded using the appropriate 7th character for subsequent care for encounters after the patient has completed active treatment of the fracture and is receiving routine care for the fracture during the healing or recovery phase.

Care for complications of surgical treatment for fracture repairs during the healing or recovery phase should be coded with the appropriate complication codes.

Care of complications of fractures, such as malunion and nonunion, should be reported with the appropriate 7th character for subsequent care with nonunion (K, M, N,) or subsequent care with malunion (P, Q, R).

Malunion/nonunion: The appropriate 7th character for initial encounter should also be assigned for a patient who delayed seeking treatment for the fracture or nonunion.

The open fracture designations in the assignment of the 7th character for fractures of the forearm, femur and lower leg, including ankle are based on the Gustilo open fracture classification. When the Gustilo classification type is not specified for an open fracture, the 7th character for open fracture type I or II should be assigned (B, E, H, M, Q).

A code from category M80, not a traumatic fracture code, should be used for any patient with known osteoporosis who suffers a fracture, even if the patient had a minor fall or trauma, if that fall or trauma would not usually break a normal, healthy bone.

See Section I.C.13. Osteoporosis.

The aftercare Z codes should not be used for aftercare for traumatic fractures. For aftercare of a traumatic fracture, assign the acute fracture code with the appropriate 7th character.

2) Multiple fractures sequencing

Multiple fractures are sequenced in accordance with the severity of the fracture.

3) Physeal fractures

For physeal fractures, assign only the code identifying the type of physeal fracture. Do not assign a separate code to identify the specific bone that is fractured.

d. Coding of Burns and Corrosions

The ICD-10-CM makes a distinction between burns and corrosions. The burn codes are for thermal burns, except sunburns, that come from a heat source, such as a fire or hot appliance. The burn codes are also for burns resulting from electricity and radiation. Corrosions are burns due to chemicals. The guidelines are the same for burns and corrosions.

Current burns (T20-T25) are classified by depth, extent and by agent (X code). Burns are classified by depth as first degree (erythema), second degree (blistering), and third degree (full-thickness involvement). Burns of the eye and internal organs (T26-T28) are classified by site, but not by degree.

1) Sequencing of burn and related condition codes

Sequence first the code that reflects the highest degree of burn when more than one burn is present.

a. When the reason for the admission or encounter is for treatment of external multiple burns, sequence first the code that reflects the burn of the highest degree.

b. When a patient has both internal and external burns, the circumstances of admission govern the selection of the principal diagnosis or first-listed diagnosis.

c. When a patient is admitted for burn injuries and other related conditions such as smoke inhalation and/or respiratory failure, the circumstances of admission govern the selection of the principal or first-listed diagnosis.

2) Burns of the same anatomic site

Classify burns of the same anatomic site and on the same side but of different degrees to the subcategory identifying the highest

degree recorded in the diagnosis (e.g., for second and third degree burns of right thigh, assign only code T24.311-).

3) Non-healing burns

Non-healing burns are coded as acute burns.

Necrosis of burned skin should be coded as a non-healed burn.

4) Infected burn

For any documented infected burn site, use an additional code for the infection.

5) Assign separate codes for each burn site

When coding burns, assign separate codes for each burn site. Category T30, Burn and corrosion, body region unspecified is extremely vague and should rarely be used.

Codes for burns of "multiple sites" should only be assigned when the medical record documentation does not specify the individual sites.

6) Burns and corrosions classified according to extent of body surface involved

Assign codes from category T31, Burns classified according to extent of body surface involved, or T32, Corrosions classified according to extent of body surface involved, for acute burns or corrosions when the site of the burn or corrosion is not specified or when there is a need for additional data. It is advisable to use category T31 as additional coding when needed to provide data for evaluating burn mortality, such as that needed by burn units. It is also advisable to use category T31 as an additional code for reporting purposes when there is mention of a third-degree burn involving 20 percent or more of the body surface. Codes from categories T31 and T32 should not be used for sequelae of burns or corrosions.

Categories T31 and T32 are based on the classic "rule of nines" in estimating body surface involved: head and neck are assigned nine percent, each arm nine percent, each leg 18 percent, the anterior trunk 18 percent, posterior trunk 18 percent, and genitalia one percent. Providers may change these percentage assignments where necessary to accommodate infants and children who have proportionately larger heads than adults, and patients who have large buttocks, thighs, or abdomen that involve burns.

7) Encounters for treatment of sequela of burns

Encounters for the treatment of the late effects of burns or corrosions (i.e., scars or joint contractures) should be coded with a burn or corrosion code with the 7th character "S" for sequela.

8) Sequelae with a late effect code and current burn

When appropriate, both a code for a current burn or corrosion with 7th character "A" or "D" and a burn or corrosion code with 7th character "S" may be assigned on the same record (when both a current burn and sequelae of an old burn exist). Burns and corrosions do not heal at the same rate and a current healing wound may still exist with sequela of a healed burn or corrosion.

See Section I.B.10. Sequela (Late Effects)

9) Use of an external cause code with burns and corrosions

An external cause code should be used with burns and corrosions to identify the source and intent of the burn, as well as the place where it occurred.

e. Adverse Effects, Poisoning, Underdosing and Toxic Effects

Codes in categories T36-T65 are combination codes that include the substance that was taken as well as the intent. No additional external cause code is required for poisonings, toxic effects, adverse effects and underdosing codes.

1) Do not code directly from the Table of Drugs

Do not code directly from the Table of Drugs and Chemicals. Always refer back to the Tabular List.

2) Use as many codes as necessary to describe

Use as many codes as necessary to describe completely all drugs, medicinal or biological substances.

3) If the same code would describe the causative agent

If the same code would describe the causative agent for more than one adverse reaction, poisoning, toxic effect or underdosing, assign the code only once.

4) If two or more drugs, medicinal or biological substances

If two or more drugs, medicinal or biological substances are taken, code each individually unless a combination code is listed in the Table of Drugs and Chemicals.

If multiple unspecified drugs, medicinal or biological substances were taken, assign the appropriate code from subcategory

T50.91, Poisoning by, adverse effect of and underdosing of multiple unspecified drugs, medicaments and biological substances.

5) **The occurrence of drug toxicity is classified in ICD-10-CM as follows:**

(a) **Adverse Effect**
When coding an adverse effect of a drug that has been correctly prescribed and properly administered, assign the appropriate code for the nature of the adverse effect followed by the appropriate code for the adverse effect of the drug (T36-T50). The code for the drug should have a 5th or 6th character "5" (for example T36.0X5-) Examples of the nature of an adverse effect are tachycardia, delirium, gastrointestinal hemorrhaging, vomiting, hypokalemia, hepatitis, renal failure, or respiratory failure.

(b) **Poisoning**
When coding a poisoning or reaction to the improper use of a medication (e.g., overdose, wrong substance given or taken in error, wrong route of administration), first assign the appropriate code from categories T36-T50. The poisoning codes have an associated intent as their 5th or 6th character (accidental, intentional self-harm, assault and undetermined). If the intent of the poisoning is unknown or unspecified, code the intent as accidental intent. The undetermined intent is only for use if the documentation in the record specifies that the intent cannot be determined. Use additional code(s) for all manifestations of poisonings.

If there is also a diagnosis of abuse or dependence of the substance, the abuse or dependence is assigned as an additional code.

Examples of poisoning include:

(i) Error was made in drug prescription
Errors made in drug prescription or in the administration of the drug by provider, nurse, patient, or other person.

(ii) Overdose of a drug intentionally taken
If an overdose of a drug was intentionally taken or administered and resulted in drug toxicity, it would be coded as a poisoning.

(iii) Nonprescribed drug taken with correctly prescribed and properly administered drug
If a nonprescribed drug or medicinal agent was taken in combination with a correctly prescribed and properly administered drug, any drug toxicity or other reaction resulting from the interaction of the two drugs would be classified as a poisoning.

(iv) Interaction of drug(s) and alcohol
When a reaction results from the interaction of a drug(s) and alcohol, this would be classified as poisoning.

See Section I.C.4. if poisoning is the result of insulin pump malfunctions.

(c) **Underdosing**
Underdosing refers to taking less of a medication than is prescribed by a provider or a manufacturer's instruction. Discontinuing the use of a prescribed medication on the patient's own initiative (not directed by the patient's provider) is also classified as an underdosing. For underdosing, assign the code from categories T36-T50 (fifth or sixth character "6"). **Documentation of a change in the patient's condition is not required in order to assign an underdosing code. Documentation that the patient is taking less of a medication than is prescribed or discontinued the prescribed medication is sufficient for code assignment.**

Codes for underdosing should never be assigned as principal or first-listed codes. If a patient has a relapse or exacerbation of the medical condition for which the drug is prescribed because of the reduction in dose, then the medical condition itself should be coded.

Noncompliance (Z91.12-, Z91.13- and Z91.14-) or complication of care (Y63.6-Y63.9) codes are to be used with an underdosing code to indicate intent, if known.

(d) **Toxic Effects**
When a harmful substance is ingested or comes in contact with a person, this is classified as a toxic effect. The toxic effect codes are in categories T51-T65.

Toxic effect codes have an associated intent: accidental, intentional self-harm, assault and undetermined.

f. **Adult and child abuse, neglect and other maltreatment**
Sequence first the appropriate code from categories T74, Adult and child abuse, neglect and other maltreatment, confirmed, or T76, Adult and child abuse, neglect and other maltreatment, suspected, for abuse, neglect and other maltreatment, followed by any accompanying mental health or injury code(s).

If the documentation in the medical record states abuse or neglect, it is coded as confirmed (T74.-). It is coded as suspected if it is documented as suspected (T76.-).

For cases of confirmed abuse or neglect an external cause code from the assault section (X92-Y09) should be added to identify the cause of any physical injuries. A perpetrator code (Y07) should be added when the perpetrator of the abuse is known. For suspected cases of abuse or neglect, do not report external cause or perpetrator code.

If a suspected case of abuse, neglect or mistreatment is ruled out during an encounter code Z04.71, Encounter for examination and observation following alleged physical adult abuse, ruled out, or code Z04.72, Encounter for examination and observation following alleged child physical abuse, ruled out, should be used, not a code from T76.

If a suspected case of alleged rape or sexual abuse is ruled out during an encounter code Z04.41, Encounter for examination and observation following alleged adult rape or code Z04.42, Encounter for examination and observation following alleged child rape, should be used, not a code from T76.

If a suspected case of forced sexual exploitation or forced labor exploitation is ruled out during an encounter, code Z04.81, Encounter for examination and observation of victim following forced sexual exploitation, or code Z04.82, Encounter for examination and observation of victim following forced labor exploitation, should be used, not a code from T76.

See Section I.C.15. Abuse in a pregnant patient.

g. **Complications of care**

1) **General guidelines for complications of care**
(a) **Documentation of complications of care**
See Section I.B.16. for information on documentation of complications of care.

2) **Pain due to medical devices**
Pain associated with devices, implants or grafts left in a surgical site (for example painful hip prosthesis) is assigned to the appropriate code(s) found in Chapter 19, Injury, poisoning, and certain other consequences of external causes. Specific codes for pain due to medical devices are found in the T code section of the ICD-10-CM. Use additional code(s) from category G89 to identify acute or chronic pain due to presence of the device, implant or graft (G89.18 or G89.28).

3) **Transplant complications**
(a) **Transplant complications other than kidney**
Codes under category T86, Complications of transplanted organs and tissues, are for use for both complications and rejection of transplanted organs. A transplant complication code is only assigned if the complication affects the function of the transplanted organ. Two codes are required to fully describe a transplant complication: the appropriate code from category T86 and a secondary code that identifies the complication.

Pre-existing conditions or conditions that develop after the transplant are not coded as complications unless they affect the function of the transplanted organs.

See I.C.21. for transplant organ removal status

See I.C.2. for malignant neoplasm associated with transplanted organ.

(b) **Kidney transplant complications**
Patients who have undergone kidney transplant may still have some form of chronic kidney disease (CKD) because the kidney transplant may not fully restore kidney function. Code T86.1- should be assigned for documented complications of a kidney transplant, such as transplant failure or rejection or other transplant complication. Code T86.1- should not be assigned for post kidney transplant patients who have chronic kidney (CKD) unless a transplant complication such as transplant failure or rejection is documented. If the documentation is unclear as to whether the patient has a complication of the transplant, query the provider.

Conditions that affect the function of the transplanted kidney, other than CKD, should be assigned a code from subcategory T86.1, Complications of transplanted organ, Kidney, and a secondary code that identifies the complication.

For patients with CKD following a kidney transplant, but who do not have a complication such as failure or rejection, *see section I.C.14. Chronic kidney disease and kidney transplant status.*

4) Complication codes that include the external cause

As with certain other T codes, some of the complications of care codes have the external cause included in the code. The code includes the nature of the complication as well as the type of procedure that caused the complication. No external cause code indicating the type of procedure is necessary for these codes.

5) Complications of care codes within the body system chapters

Intraoperative and postprocedural complication codes are found within the body system chapters with codes specific to the organs and structures of that body system. These codes should be sequenced first, followed by a code(s) for the specific complication, if applicable.

Complication codes from the body system chapters should be assigned for intraoperative and postprocedural complications (e.g., the appropriate complication code from chapter 9 would be assigned for a vascular intraoperative or postprocedural complication) unless the complication is specifically indexed to a T code in chapter 19.

20. Chapter 20: External Causes of Morbidity (V00-Y99)

The external causes of morbidity codes should never be sequenced as the first-listed or principal diagnosis.

External cause codes are intended to provide data for injury research and evaluation of injury prevention strategies. These codes capture how the injury or health condition happened (cause), the intent (unintentional or accidental; or intentional, such as suicide or assault), the place where the event occurred the activity of the patient at the time of the event, and the person's status (e.g., civilian, military).

There is no national requirement for mandatory ICD-10-CM external cause code reporting. Unless a provider is subject to a state-based external cause code reporting mandate or these codes are required by a particular payer, reporting of ICD-10-CM codes in Chapter 20, External Causes of Morbidity, is not required. In the absence of a mandatory reporting requirement, providers are encouraged to voluntarily report external cause codes, as they provide valuable data for injury research and evaluation of injury prevention strategies.

a. General External Cause Coding Guidelines

1) Used with any code in the range of A00.0-T88.9, Z00-Z99

An external cause code may be used with any code in the range of A00.0-T88.9, Z00-Z99, classification that represents a health condition due to an external cause. Though they are most applicable to injuries, they are also valid for use with such things as infections or diseases due to an external source, and other health conditions, such as a heart attack that occurs during strenuous physical activity.

2) External cause code used for length of treatment

Assign the external cause code, with the appropriate 7th character (initial encounter, subsequent encounter or sequela) for each encounter for which the injury or condition is being treated.

Most categories in chapter 20 have a 7th character requirement for each applicable code. Most categories in this chapter have three 7th character values: A, initial encounter, D, subsequent encounter and S, sequela. While the patient may be seen by a new or different provider over the course of treatment for an injury or condition, assignment of the 7th character for external cause should match the 7th character of the code assigned for the associated injury or condition for the encounter.

3) Use the full range of external cause codes

Use the full range of external cause codes to completely describe the cause, the intent, the place of occurrence, and if applicable, the activity of the patient at the time of the event, and the patient's status, for all injuries, and other health conditions due to an external cause.

4) Assign as many external cause codes as necessary

Assign as many external cause codes as necessary to fully explain each cause. If only one external code can be recorded, assign the code most related to the principal diagnosis.

5) The selection of the appropriate external cause code

The selection of the appropriate external cause code is guided by the Alphabetic Index of External Causes and by Inclusion and Exclusion notes in the Tabular List.

6) External cause code can never be a principal diagnosis

An external cause code can never be a principal (first-listed) diagnosis.

7) Combination external cause codes

Certain of the external cause codes are combination codes that identify sequential events that result in an injury, such as a fall which results in striking against an object. The injury may be due to either event or both. The combination external cause code used should correspond to the sequence of events regardless of which caused the most serious injury.

8) No external cause code needed in certain circumstances

No external cause code from Chapter 20 is needed if the external cause and intent are included in a code from another chapter (e.g., T36.0X1-, Poisoning by penicillins, accidental (unintentional)).

b. Place of Occurrence Guideline

Codes from category Y92, Place of occurrence of the external cause, are secondary codes for use after other external cause codes to identify the location of the patient at the time of injury or other condition.

Generally, a place of occurrence code is assigned only once, at the initial encounter for treatment. However, in the rare instance that a new injury occurs during hospitalization, an additional place of occurrence code may be assigned. No 7th characters are used for Y92.

Do not use place of occurrence code Y92.9 if the place is not stated or is not applicable.

c. Activity Code

Assign a code from category Y93, Activity code, to describe the activity of the patient at the time the injury or other health condition occurred.

An activity code is used only once, at the initial encounter for treatment. Only one code from Y93 should be recorded on a medical record.

The activity codes are not applicable to poisonings, adverse effects, misadventures or sequela.

Do not assign Y93.9, Unspecified activity, if the activity is not stated.

A code from category Y93 is appropriate for use with external cause and intent codes if identifying the activity provides additional information about the event.

d. Place of Occurrence, Activity, and Status Codes Used with other External Cause Code

When applicable, place of occurrence, activity, and external cause status codes are sequenced after the main external cause code(s). Regardless of the number of external cause codes assigned, generally there should be only one place of occurrence code, one activity code, and one external cause status code assigned to an encounter. However, in the rare instance that a new injury occurs during hospitalization, an additional place of occurrence code may be assigned.

e. If the Reporting Format Limits the Number of External Cause Codes

If the reporting format limits the number of external cause codes that can be used in reporting clinical data, report the code for the cause/intent most related to the principal diagnosis. If the format permits capture of additional external cause codes, the cause/intent, including medical misadventures, of the additional events should be reported rather than the codes for place, activity, or external status.

f. Multiple External Cause Coding Guidelines

More than one external cause code is required to fully describe the external cause of an illness or injury. The assignment of external cause codes should be sequenced in the following priority:

If two or more events cause separate injuries, an external cause code should be assigned for each cause. The first-listed external cause code will be selected in the following order:

External codes for child and adult abuse take priority over all other external cause codes.

See Section I.C.19., Child and Adult abuse guidelines.

External cause codes for terrorism events take priority over all other external cause codes except child and adult abuse.

External cause codes for cataclysmic events take priority over all other external cause codes except child and adult abuse and terrorism.

External cause codes for transport accidents take priority over all other external cause codes except cataclysmic events, child and adult abuse and terrorism.

Activity and external cause status codes are assigned following all causal (intent) external cause codes.

The first-listed external cause code should correspond to the cause of the most serious diagnosis due to an assault, accident, or self-harm, following the order of hierarchy listed above.

g. Child and Adult Abuse Guideline

Adult and child abuse, neglect and maltreatment are classified as assault. Any of the assault codes may be used to indicate the external cause of any injury resulting from the confirmed abuse.

For confirmed cases of abuse, neglect and maltreatment, when the perpetrator is known, a code from Y07, Perpetrator of maltreatment and neglect, should accompany any other assault codes.

See Section I.C.19. Adult and child abuse, neglect and other maltreatment

h. Unknown or Undetermined Intent Guideline

If the intent (accident, self-harm, assault) of the cause of an injury or other condition is unknown or unspecified, code the intent as accidental intent. All transport accident categories assume accidental intent.

1) Use of undetermined intent

External cause codes for events of undetermined intent are only for use if the documentation in the record specifies that the intent cannot be determined.

i. Sequelae (Late Effects) of External Cause Guidelines

1) Sequelae external cause codes

Sequela are reported using the external cause code with the 7th character "S" for sequela. These codes should be used with any report of a late effect or sequela resulting from a previous injury.

See Section I.B.10. Sequela (Late Effects)

2) Sequela external cause code with a related current injury

A sequela external cause code should never be used with a related current nature of injury code.

3) Use of sequela external cause codes for subsequent visits

Use a late effect external cause code for subsequent visits when a late effect of the initial injury is being treated. Do not use a late effect external cause code for subsequent visits for follow-up care (e.g., to assess healing, to receive rehabilitative therapy) of the injury when no late effect of the injury has been documented.

j. Terrorism Guidelines

1) Cause of injury identified by the Federal Government (FBI) as terrorism

When the cause of an injury is identified by the Federal Government (FBI) as terrorism, the first-listed external cause code should be a code from category Y38, Terrorism. The definition of terrorism employed by the FBI is found at the inclusion note at the beginning of category Y38. Use additional code for place of occurrence (Y92.-). More than one Y38 code may be assigned if the injury is the result of more than one mechanism of terrorism.

2) Cause of an injury is suspected to be the result of terrorism

When the cause of an injury is suspected to be the result of terrorism a code from category Y38 should not be assigned. Suspected cases should be classified as assault.

3) Code Y38.9, Terrorism, secondary effects

Assign code Y38.9, Terrorism, secondary effects, for conditions occurring subsequent to the terrorist event. This code should not be assigned for conditions that are due to the initial terrorist act.

It is acceptable to assign code Y38.9 with another code from Y38 if there is an injury due to the initial terrorist event and an injury that is a subsequent result of the terrorist event.

k. External Cause Status

A code from category Y99, External cause status, should be assigned whenever any other external cause code is assigned for an encounter, including an Activity code, except for the events noted below. Assign a code from category Y99, External cause status, to indicate the work status of the person at the time the event occurred. The status code indicates whether the event occurred during military activity, whether a non-military person was at work, whether an individual including a student or volunteer was involved in a non-work activity at the time of the causal event.

A code from Y99, External cause status, should be assigned, when applicable, with other external cause codes, such as transport accidents and falls. The external cause status codes are not applicable to poisonings, adverse effects, misadventures or late effects.

Do not assign a code from category Y99 if no other external cause codes (cause, activity) are applicable for the encounter.

An external cause status code is used only once, at the initial encounter for treatment. Only one code from Y99 should be recorded on a medical record.

Do not assign code Y99.9, Unspecified external cause status, if the status is not stated.

21. Chapter 21: Factors influencing health status and contact with health services (Z00-Z99)

Note: The chapter specific guidelines provide additional information about the use of Z codes for specified encounters.

a. Use of Z Codes in Any Healthcare Setting

Z codes are for use in any healthcare setting. Z codes may be used as either a first-listed (principal diagnosis code in the inpatient setting) or secondary code, depending on the circumstances of the encounter. Certain Z codes may only be used as first-listed or principal diagnosis.

b. Z Codes Indicate a Reason for an Encounter or Provide Additional Information about a Patient Encounter

Z codes are not procedure codes. A corresponding procedure code must accompany a Z code to describe any procedure performed.

c. Categories of Z Codes

1) Contact/Exposure

Category Z20 indicates contact with, and suspected exposure to, communicable diseases. These codes are for patients who are suspected to have been exposed to a disease by close personal contact with an infected individual or are in an area where a disease is epidemic.

Category Z77, Other contact with and (suspected) exposures hazardous to health, indicates contact with and suspected exposures hazardous to health.

Contact/exposure codes may be used as a first-listed code to explain an encounter for testing, or, more commonly, as a secondary code to identify a potential risk.

2) Inoculations and vaccinations

Code Z23 is for encounters for inoculations and vaccinations. It indicates that a patient is being seen to receive a prophylactic inoculation against a disease. Procedure codes are required to identify the actual administration of the injection and the type(s) of immunizations given. Code Z23 may be used as a secondary code if the inoculation is given as a routine part of preventive health care, such as a well-baby visit.

3) Status

Status codes indicate that a patient is either a carrier of a disease or has the sequelae or residual of a past disease or condition. This includes such things as the presence of prosthetic or mechanical devices resulting from past treatment. A status code is informative, because the status may affect the course of treatment and its outcome. A status code is distinct from a history code. The history code indicates that the patient no longer has the condition.

A status code should not be used with a diagnosis code from one of the body system chapters, if the diagnosis code includes the information provided by the status code. For example, code Z94.1, Heart transplant status, should not be used with a code from subcategory T86.2, Complications of heart transplant. The status code does not provide additional information. The complication code indicates that the patient is a heart transplant patient.

For encounters for weaning from a mechanical ventilator, assign a code from subcategory J96.1, Chronic respiratory failure, followed by code Z99.11, Dependence on respirator [ventilator] status.

The status Z codes/categories are:

Z14   Genetic carrier
       Genetic carrier status indicates that a person carries a gene, associated with a particular disease, which may be passed to offspring who may develop that disease. The person does not have the disease and is not at risk of developing the disease.

Z15   Genetic susceptibility to disease
       Genetic susceptibility indicates that a person has a gene that increases the risk of that person developing the disease.

       Codes from category Z15 should not be used as principal or first-listed codes. If the patient has the condition to which he/she is susceptible, and that condition is the reason for the encounter, the code for the current condition should be sequenced first. If the patient is being seen for follow-up after completed treatment for this condition, and the condition no longer exists, a follow-up code should be sequenced first, followed by the appropriate personal history and genetic susceptibility codes. If the purpose of the encounter is genetic counseling associated with procreative management, code Z31.5, Encounter for genetic counseling, should be assigned as the first-listed code, followed by a code from category Z15. Additional codes should be assigned for any applicable family or personal history.

Z16   Resistance to antimicrobial drugs
This code indicates that a patient has a condition that is resistant to antimicrobial drug treatment. Sequence the infection code first.

Z17   Estrogen receptor status

Z18   Retained foreign body fragments

Z19   Hormone sensitivity malignancy status

Z21   Asymptomatic HIV infection status
This code indicates that a patient has tested positive for HIV but has manifested no signs or symptoms of the disease.

Z22   Carrier of infectious disease
Carrier status indicates that a person harbors the specific organisms of a disease without manifest symptoms and is capable of transmitting the infection.

Z28.3   Underimmunization status
See Section I.B.14. for underimmunization documentation by clinicians other than the patient's provider.

Z33.1   Pregnant state, incidental
This code is a secondary code only for use when the pregnancy is in no way complicating the reason for visit. Otherwise, a code from the obstetric chapter is required.

Z66   Do not resuscitate
This code may be used when it is documented by the provider that a patient is on do not resuscitate status at any time during the stay.

Z67   Blood type

Z68   Body mass index (BMI)
BMI codes should only be assigned when there is an associated, reportable diagnosis (such as obesity). Do not assign BMI codes during pregnancy.
See Section I.B.14. for BMI documentation by clinicians other than the patient's provider.

Z74.01   Bed confinement status

Z76.82   Awaiting organ transplant status

Z78   Other specified health status
Code Z78.1, Physical restraint status, may be used when it is documented by the provider that a patient has been put in restraints during the current encounter. Please note that this code should not be reported when it is documented by the provider that a patient is temporarily restrained during a procedure.

Z79   Long-term (current) drug therapy
Codes from this category indicate a patient's continuous use of a prescribed drug (including such things as aspirin therapy) for the long-term treatment of a condition or for prophylactic use. It is not for use for patients who have addictions to drugs. This subcategory is not for use of medications for detoxification or maintenance programs to prevent withdrawal symptoms (e.g., methadone maintenance for opiate dependence). Assign the appropriate code for the drug use, abuse, or dependence instead.
Assign a code from Z79 if the patient is receiving a medication for an extended period as a prophylactic measure (such as for the prevention of deep vein thrombosis) or as treatment of a chronic condition (such as arthritis) or a disease requiring a lengthy course of treatment (such as cancer). Do not assign a code from category Z79 for medication being administered for a brief period of time to treat an acute illness or injury (such as a course of antibiotics to treat acute bronchitis).

Z88   Allergy status to drugs, medicaments and biological substances
Except: Z88.9, Allergy status to unspecified drugs, medicaments and biological substances status

Z89   Acquired absence of limb

Z90   Acquired absence of organs, not elsewhere classified

Z91.0-   Allergy status, other than to drugs and biological substances

Z92.82   Status post administration of tPA (rtPA) in a different facility within the last 24 hours prior to admission to a current facility
Assign code Z92.82, Status post administration of tPA (rtPA) in a different facility within the last 24 hours prior to admission to current facility, as a secondary diagnosis when a patient is received by transfer into a facility and documentation indicates they were administered tissue plasminogen activator (tPA) within the last 24 hours prior to admission to the current facility.
This guideline applies even if the patient is still receiving the tPA at the time they are received into the current facility.
The appropriate code for the condition for which the tPA was administered (such as cerebrovascular disease or myocardial infarction) should be assigned first.
Code Z92.82 is only applicable to the receiving facility record and not to the transferring facility record.

Z93   Artificial opening status

Z94   Transplanted organ and tissue status

Z95   Presence of cardiac and vascular implants and grafts

Z96   Presence of other functional implants

Z97   Presence of other devices

Z98   Other postprocedural states
Assign code Z98.85, Transplanted organ removal status, to indicate that a transplanted organ has been previously removed. This code should not be assigned for the encounter in which the transplanted organ is removed. The complication necessitating removal of the transplant organ should be assigned for that encounter.
See section I.C.19. for information on the coding of organ transplant complications.

Z99   Dependence on enabling machines and devices, not elsewhere classified
Note: Categories Z89-Z90 and Z93-Z99 are for use only if there are no complications or malfunctions of the organ or tissue replaced, the amputation site or the equipment on which the patient is dependent.

4) History (of)

There are two types of history Z codes, personal and family. Personal history codes explain a patient's past medical condition that no longer exists and is not receiving any treatment, but that has the potential for recurrence, and therefore may require continued monitoring.

Family history codes are for use when a patient has a family member(s) who has had a particular disease that causes the patient to be at higher risk of also contracting the disease.

Personal history codes may be used in conjunction with follow-up codes and family history codes may be used in conjunction with screening codes to explain the need for a test or procedure. History codes are also acceptable on any medical record regardless of the reason for visit. A history of an illness, even if no longer present, is important information that may alter the type of treatment ordered.

The reason for the encounter (for example, screening or counseling) should be sequenced first and the appropriate personal and/or family history code(s) should be assigned as additional diagnos(es).

The history Z code categories are:

Z80   Family history of primary malignant neoplasm

Z81   Family history of mental and behavioral disorders

Z82   Family history of certain disabilities and chronic diseases (leading to disablement)

Z83   Family history of other specific disorders

Z84   Family history of other conditions

Z85   Personal history of malignant neoplasm

Z86   Personal history of certain other diseases

Z87	Personal history of other diseases and conditions
Z91.4-	Personal history of psychological trauma, not elsewhere classified
Z91.5-	Personal history of self-harm
Z91.81	History of falling
Z91.82	Personal history of military deployment
Z92	Personal history of medical treatment

Except: Z92.0, Personal history of contraception

Except: Z92.82, Status post administration of tPA (rtPA) in a different facility within the last 24 hours prior to admission to a current facility

5) Screening

Screening is the testing for disease or disease precursors in seemingly well individuals so that early detection and treatment can be provided for those who test positive for the disease (e.g., screening mammogram).

The testing of a person to rule out or confirm a suspected diagnosis because the patient has some sign or symptom is a diagnostic examination, not a screening. In these cases, the sign or symptom is used to explain the reason for the test.

A screening code may be a first-listed code if the reason for the visit is specifically the screening exam. It may also be used as an additional code if the screening is done during an office visit for other health problems. A screening code is not necessary if the screening is inherent to a routine examination, such as a pap smear done during a routine pelvic examination.

Should a condition be discovered during the screening then the code for the condition may be assigned as an additional diagnosis.

The Z code indicates that a screening exam is planned. A procedure code is required to confirm that the screening was performed.

The screening Z codes/categories:

Z11	Encounter for screening for infectious and parasitic diseases
Z12	Encounter for screening for malignant neoplasms
Z13	Encounter for screening for other diseases and disorders Except: Z13.9, Encounter for screening, unspecified
Z36	Encounter for antenatal screening for mother

6) Observation

There are three observation Z code categories. They are for use in very limited circumstances when a person is being observed for a suspected condition that is ruled out. The observation codes are not for use if an injury or illness or any signs or symptoms related to the suspected condition are present. In such cases the diagnosis/symptom code is used with the corresponding external cause code.

The observation codes are primarily to be used as a principal/first-listed diagnosis. An observation code may be assigned as a secondary diagnosis code when the patient is being observed for a condition that is ruled out and is unrelated to the principal/first-listed diagnosis. Also, when the principal diagnosis is required to be a code from category Z38, Liveborn infants according to place of birth and type of delivery, then a code from category Z05, Encounter for observation and evaluation of newborn for suspected diseases and conditions ruled out, is sequenced after the Z38 code. Additional codes may be used in addition to the observation code, but only if they are unrelated to the suspected condition being observed.

Codes from subcategory Z03.7, Encounter for suspected maternal and fetal conditions ruled out, may either be used as a first-listed or as an additional code assignment depending on the case. They are for use in very limited circumstances on a maternal record when an encounter is for a suspected maternal or fetal condition that is ruled out during that encounter (for example, a maternal or fetal condition may be suspected due to an abnormal test result). These codes should not be used when the condition is confirmed. In those cases, the confirmed condition should be coded. In addition, these codes are not for use if an illness or any signs or symptoms related to the suspected condition or problem are present. In such cases the diagnosis/symptom code is used.

Additional codes may be used in addition to the code from subcategory Z03.7, but only if they are unrelated to the suspected condition being evaluated.

Codes from subcategory Z03.7 may not be used for encounters for antenatal screening of mother. *See Section I.C.21. Screening.*

For encounters for suspected fetal condition that are inconclusive following testing and evaluation, assign the appropriate code from category O35, O36, O40 or O41.

The observation Z code categories:

Z03	Encounter for medical observation for suspected diseases and conditions ruled out
Z04	Encounter for examination and observation for other reasons Except: Z04.9, Encounter for examination and observation for unspecified reason
Z05	Encounter for observation and evaluation of newborn for suspected diseases and conditions ruled out

7) Aftercare

Aftercare visit codes cover situations when the initial treatment of a disease has been performed and the patient requires continued care during the healing or recovery phase, or for the long-term consequences of the disease. The aftercare Z code should not be used if treatment is directed at a current, acute disease. The diagnosis code is to be used in these cases. Exceptions to this rule are codes Z51.0, Encounter for antineoplastic radiation therapy, and codes from subcategory Z51.1, Encounter for antineoplastic chemotherapy and immunotherapy. These codes are to be first listed, followed by the diagnosis code when a patient's encounter is solely to receive radiation therapy, chemotherapy, or immunotherapy for the treatment of a neoplasm. If the reason for the encounter is more than one type of antineoplastic therapy, code Z51.0 and a code from subcategory Z51.1 may be assigned together, in which case one of these codes would be reported as a secondary diagnosis.

The aftercare Z codes should also not be used for aftercare for injuries. For aftercare of an injury, assign the acute injury code with the appropriate 7th character (for subsequent encounter).

The aftercare codes are generally first listed to explain the specific reason for the encounter. An aftercare code may be used as an additional code when some type of aftercare is provided in addition to the reason for admission and no diagnosis code is applicable. An example of this would be the closure of a colostomy during an encounter for treatment of another condition.

Aftercare codes should be used in conjunction with other aftercare codes or diagnosis codes to provide better detail on the specifics of an aftercare encounter visit, unless otherwise directed by the classification. The sequencing of multiple aftercare codes depends on the circumstances of the encounter.

Certain aftercare Z code categories need a secondary diagnosis code to describe the resolving condition or sequelae. For others, the condition is included in the code title.

Additional Z code aftercare category terms include fitting and adjustment, and attention to artificial openings.

Status Z codes may be used with aftercare Z codes to indicate the nature of the aftercare. For example, code Z95.1, Presence of aortocoronary bypass graft, may be used with code Z48.812, Encounter for surgical aftercare following surgery on the circulatory system, to indicate the surgery for which the aftercare is being performed. A status code should not be used when the aftercare code indicates the type of status, such as using Z43.0, Encounter for attention to tracheostomy, with Z93.0, Tracheostomy status.

The aftercare Z category/codes:

Z42	Encounter for plastic and reconstructive surgery following medical procedure or healed injury
Z43	Encounter for attention to artificial openings
Z44	Encounter for fitting and adjustment of external prosthetic device
Z45	Encounter for adjustment and management of implanted device
Z46	Encounter for fitting and adjustment of other devices
Z47	Orthopedic aftercare
Z48	Encounter for other postprocedural aftercare
Z49	Encounter for care involving renal dialysis
Z51	Encounter for other aftercare and medical care

8) Follow-up

The follow-up codes are used to explain continuing surveillance following completed treatment of a disease, condition, or injury. They imply that the condition has been fully treated and no longer exists. They should not be confused with aftercare codes, or injury codes with a 7th character for subsequent encounter, that explain ongoing care of a healing condition or its sequelae. Follow-up codes may be used in conjunction with history codes to provide the full picture of the healed condition and its treatment. The follow-up code is sequenced first, followed by the history code.

A follow-up code may be used to explain multiple visits. Should a condition be found to have recurred on the follow-up visit, then the diagnosis code for the condition should be assigned in place of the follow-up code.

The follow-up Z code categories:

Z08   Encounter for follow-up examination after completed treatment for malignant neoplasm

Z09   Encounter for follow-up examination after completed treatment for conditions other than malignant neoplasm

Z39   Encounter for maternal postpartum care and examination

9) Donor
Codes in category Z52, Donors of organs and tissues, are used for living individuals who are donating blood or other body tissue. These codes are for individuals donating for others, as well as for self-donations. They are not used to identify cadaveric donations.

10) Counseling
Counseling Z codes are used when a patient or family member receives assistance in the aftermath of an illness or injury, or when support is required in coping with family or social problems.

The counseling Z codes/categories:

Z30.0-   Encounter for general counseling and advice on contraception

Z31.5   Encounter for procreative genetic counseling

Z31.6-   Encounter for general counseling and advice on procreation

Z32.2   Encounter for childbirth instruction

Z32.3   Encounter for childcare instruction

Z69   Encounter for mental health services for victim and perpetrator of abuse

Z70   Counseling related to sexual attitude, behavior and orientation

Z71   Persons encountering health services for other counseling and medical advice, not elsewhere classified
Note: Code Z71.84, Encounter for health counseling related to travel, is to be used for health risk and safety counseling for future travel purposes.
Code Z71.85, Encounter for immunization safety counseling, is to be used for counseling of the patient or caregiver regarding the safety of a vaccine. This code should not be used for the provision of general information regarding risks and potential side effects during routine encounters for the administration of vaccines.
Code Z71.87, Encounter for pediatric-to-adult transition counseling, should be assigned when pediatric-to-adult transition counseling is the sole reason for the encounter or when this counseling is provided in addition to other services, such as treatment of a chronic condition. If both transition counseling and treatment of a medical condition are provided during the same encounter, the code(s) for the medical condition(s) treated and code Z71.87 should be assigned, with sequencing depending on the circumstances of the encounter.

Z76.81   Expectant mother prebirth pediatrician visit

11) Encounters for Obstetrical and Reproductive Services
See Section I.C.15. Pregnancy, Childbirth, and the Puerperium, for further instruction on the use of these codes.

Z codes for pregnancy are for use in those circumstances when none of the problems or complications included in the codes from the Obstetrics chapter exist (a routine prenatal visit or postpartum care). Codes in category Z34, Encounter for supervision of normal pregnancy, are always first listed and are not to be used with any other code from the OB chapter.

Codes in category Z3A, Weeks of gestation, may be assigned to provide additional information about the pregnancy. Category Z3A codes should not be assigned for pregnancies with abortive outcomes (categories O00-O08), elective termination of pregnancy (code Z33.2), nor for postpartum conditions, as

category Z3A is not applicable to these conditions. The date of the admission should be used to determine weeks of gestation for inpatient admissions that encompass more than one gestational week.

The outcome of delivery, category Z37, should be included on all maternal delivery records. It is always a secondary code.

Codes in category Z37 should not be used on the newborn record.

Z codes for family planning (contraceptive) or procreative management and counseling should be included on an obstetric record either during the pregnancy or the postpartum stage, if applicable.

Z codes/categories for obstetrical and reproductive services:

Z30   Encounter for contraceptive management

Z31   Encounter for procreative management

Z32.2   Encounter for childbirth instruction

Z32.3   Encounter for childcare instruction

Z33   Pregnant state

Z34   Encounter for supervision of normal pregnancy

Z36   Encounter for antenatal screening of mother

Z3A   Weeks of gestation

Z37   Outcome of delivery

Z39   Encounter for maternal postpartum care and examination

Z76.81   Expectant mother prebirth pediatrician visit

12) Newborns and Infants
See Section I.C.16. Newborn (Perinatal) Guidelines, for further instruction on the use of these codes.

Newborn Z codes/categories:

Z76.1   Encounter for health supervision and care of foundling

Z00.1-   Encounter for routine child health examination

Z38   Liveborn infants according to place of birth and type of delivery

13) Routine and Administrative Examinations
The Z codes allow for the description of encounters for routine examinations, such as, a general check-up, or, examinations for administrative purposes, such as, a pre-employment physical. The codes are not to be used if the examination is for diagnosis of a suspected condition or for treatment purposes. In such cases the diagnosis code is used. During a routine exam, should a diagnosis or condition be discovered, it should be coded as an additional code. Pre-existing and chronic conditions and history codes may also be included as additional codes as long as the examination is for administrative purposes and not focused on any particular condition.

Some of the codes for routine health examinations distinguish between "with" and "without" abnormal findings. Code assignment depends on the information that is known at the time the encounter is being coded. For example, if no abnormal findings were found during the examination, but the encounter is being coded before test results are back, it is acceptable to assign the code for "without abnormal findings." When assigning a code for "with abnormal findings," additional code(s) should be assigned to identify the specific abnormal finding(s).

Pre-operative examination and pre-procedural laboratory examination Z codes are for use only in those situations when a patient is being cleared for a procedure or surgery and no treatment is given.

The Z codes/categories for routine and administrative examinations:

Z00   Encounter for general examination without complaint, suspected or reported diagnosis

Z01   Encounter for other special examination without complaint, suspected or reported diagnosis

Z02   Encounter for administrative examination
Except: Z02.9, Encounter for administrative examinations, unspecified

Z32.0-   Encounter for pregnancy test

14) Miscellaneous Z Codes
The miscellaneous Z codes capture a number of other health care encounters that do not fall into one of the other categories. Some of these codes identify the reason for the encounter; others are for use as additional codes that provide useful information on circumstances that may affect a patient's care and treatment.

Prophylactic Organ Removal

For encounters specifically for prophylactic removal of an organ (such as prophylactic removal of breasts due to a genetic susceptibility to cancer or a family history of cancer), the principal or first-listed code should be a code from category Z40, Encounter for prophylactic surgery, followed by the appropriate codes to identify the associated risk factor (such as genetic susceptibility or family history).

If the patient has a malignancy of one site and is having prophylactic removal at another site to prevent either a new primary malignancy or metastatic disease, a code for the malignancy should also be assigned in addition to a code from subcategory Z40.0, Encounter for prophylactic surgery for risk factors related to malignant neoplasms. A Z40.0 code should not be assigned if the patient is having organ removal for treatment of a malignancy, such as the removal of the testes for the treatment of prostate cancer.

Miscellaneous Z codes/categories:

Z28   Immunization not carried out
        Except: Z28.3-, Underimmunization status

Z29   Encounter for other prophylactic measures

Z40   Encounter for prophylactic surgery

Z41   Encounter for procedures for purposes other than remedying health state
        Except: Z41.9, Encounter for procedure for purposes other than remedying health state, unspecified

Z53   Persons encountering health services for specific procedures and treatment, not carried out

Z72   Problems related to lifestyle
        Note: These codes should be assigned only when the documentation specifies that the patient has an associated problem

Z73   Problems related to life management difficulty
        Note: These codes should be assigned only when the documentation specifies that the patient has an associated problem.

Z74   Problems related to care provider dependency
        Except: Z74.01, Bed confinement status

Z75   Problems related to medical facilities and other health care

Z76.0   Encounter for issue of repeat prescription

Z76.3   Healthy person accompanying sick person

Z76.4   Other boarder to healthcare facility

Z76.5   Malingerer [conscious simulation]

Z91.1- Patient's noncompliance with medical treatment and regimen

Z91.83 Wandering in diseases classified elsewhere

Z91.84- Oral health risk factors

Z91.89 Other specified personal risk factors, not elsewhere classified

See Section I.B.14. for Z55-Z65 Persons with potential health hazards related to socioeconomic and psychosocial circumstances, documentation by clinicians other than the patient's provider

15) Nonspecific Z Codes

Certain Z codes are so non-specific, or potentially redundant with other codes in the classification, that there can be little justification for their use in the inpatient setting. Their use in the outpatient setting should be limited to those instances when there is no further documentation to permit more precise coding. Otherwise, any sign or symptom or any other reason for visit that is captured in another code should be used.

Nonspecific Z codes/categories:

Z02.9   Encounter for administrative examinations, unspecified

Z04.9   Encounter for examination and observation for unspecified reason

Z13.9   Encounter for screening, unspecified

Z41.9   Encounter for procedure for purposes other than remedying health state, unspecified

Z52.9   Donor of unspecified organ or tissue

Z86.59 Personal history of other mental and behavioral disorders

Z88.9   Allergy status to unspecified drugs, medicaments and biological substances status

Z92.0   Personal history of contraception

16) Z Codes That May Only be Principal/First-Listed Diagnosis

The following Z codes/categories may only be reported as the principal/first-listed diagnosis, except when there are multiple encounters on the same day and the medical records for the encounters are combined:

Z00   Encounter for general examination without complaint, suspected or reported diagnosis
        Except: Z00.6

Z01   Encounter for other special examination without complaint, suspected or reported diagnosis

Z02   Encounter for administrative examination

Z04   Encounter for examination and observation for other reasons

Z33.2   Encounter for elective termination of pregnancy

Z31.81 Encounter for male factor infertility in female patient

Z31.83 Encounter for assisted reproductive fertility procedure cycle

Z31.84 Encounter for fertility preservation procedure

Z34   Encounter for supervision of normal pregnancy

Z39   Encounter for maternal postpartum care and examination

Z38   Liveborn infants according to place of birth and type of delivery

Z40   Encounter for prophylactic surgery

Z42   Encounter for plastic and reconstructive surgery following medical procedure or healed injury

Z51.0   Encounter for antineoplastic radiation therapy

Z51.1- Encounter for antineoplastic chemotherapy and immunotherapy

Z52   Donors of organs and tissues
        Except: Z52.9, Donor of unspecified organ or tissue

Z76.1   Encounter for health supervision and care of foundling

Z76.2   Encounter for health supervision and care of other healthy infant and child

Z99.12 Encounter for respirator [ventilator] dependence during power failure

17) Social Determinants of Health

Codes describing **problems or risk factors related to** social determinants of health (SDOH) should be assigned when this information is documented. **Assign as many SDOH codes as are necessary to describe all of the problems or risk factors. These codes should be assigned only when the documentation specifies that the patient has an associated problem or risk factor. For example, not every individual living alone would be assigned code Z60.2, Problems related to living alone.**

For social determinants of health, such as information found in categories Z55-Z65, Persons with potential health hazards related to socioeconomic and psychosocial circumstances, code assignment may be based on medical record documentation from clinicians involved in the care of the patient who are not the patient's provider since this information represents social information, rather than medical diagnoses.

For example, coding professionals may utilize documentation of social information from social workers, community health workers, case managers, or nurses, if their documentation is included in the official medical record.

Patient self-reported documentation may be used to assign codes for social determinants of health, as long as the patient self-reported information is signed-off by and incorporated into the medical record by either a clinician or provider.

Social determinants of health codes are located primarily in these Z code categories:

Z55   Problems related to education and literacy

Z56   Problems related to employment and unemployment

Z57   Occupational exposure to risk factors

Z58   Problems related to physical environment

Z59   Problems related to housing and economic circumstances

Z60   Problems related to social environment

Z62   Problems related to upbringing

Z63   Other problems related to primary support group, including family circumstances

Z64   Problems related to certain psychosocial circumstances

Z65   Problems related to other psychosocial circumstances

See Section I.B.14. Documentation by Clinicians Other than the Patient's Provider.

22. Chapter 22: Codes for Special Purposes (U00-U85)
   U07.0   Vaping-related disorder (see Section I.C.10.e., Vaping-related disorders)
   U07.1   COVID-19 (see Section I.C.1.g.1., COVID-19 infection)
   U09.9   Post COVID-19 condition, unspecified (see Section I.C.1.g.1.m.)

Section II. Selection of Principal Diagnosis

The circumstances of inpatient admission always govern the selection of principal diagnosis. The principal diagnosis is defined in the Uniform Hospital Discharge Data Set (UHDDS) as "that condition established after study to be chiefly responsible for occasioning the admission of the patient to the hospital for care."

The UHDDS definitions are used by hospitals to report inpatient data elements in a standardized manner. These data elements and their definitions can be found in the July 31, 1985, Federal Register (Vol. 50, No, 147), pp. 31038-40.

Since that time, the application of the UHDDS definitions has been expanded to include all non-outpatient settings (acute care, short term, long term care and psychiatric hospitals; home health agencies; rehab facilities; nursing homes, etc.). The UHDDS definitions also apply to hospice services (all levels of care).

In determining principal diagnosis, coding conventions in the ICD-10-CM, the Tabular List and Alphabetic Index take precedence over these official coding guidelines.

(See Section I.A., Conventions for the ICD-10-CM)

The importance of consistent, complete documentation in the medical record cannot be overemphasized. Without such documentation the application of all coding guidelines is a difficult, if not impossible, task.

A. Codes for symptoms, signs, and ill-defined conditions
Codes for symptoms, signs, and ill-defined conditions from Chapter 18 are not to be used as principal diagnosis when a related definitive diagnosis has been established.

B. Two or more interrelated conditions, each potentially meeting the definition for principal diagnosis.
When there are two or more interrelated conditions (such as diseases in the same ICD-10-CM chapter or manifestations characteristically associated with a certain disease) potentially meeting the definition of principal diagnosis, either condition may be sequenced first, unless the circumstances of the admission, the therapy provided, the Tabular List, or the Alphabetic Index indicate otherwise.

C. Two or more diagnoses that equally meet the definition for principal diagnosis
In the unusual instance when two or more diagnoses equally meet the criteria for principal diagnosis as determined by the circumstances of admission, diagnostic workup and/or therapy provided, and the Alphabetic Index, Tabular List, or another coding guidelines does not provide sequencing direction, any one of the diagnoses may be sequenced first.

D. Two or more comparative or contrasting conditions
In those rare instances when two or more contrasting or comparative diagnoses are documented as "either/or" (or similar terminology), they are coded as if the diagnoses were confirmed and the diagnoses are sequenced according to the circumstances of the admission. If no further determination can be made as to which diagnosis should be principal, either diagnosis may be sequenced first.

E. A symptom(s) followed by contrasting/comparative diagnoses
GUIDELINE HAS BEEN DELETED EFFECTIVE OCTOBER 1, 2014

F. Original treatment plan not carried out
Sequence as the principal diagnosis the condition, which after study occasioned the admission to the hospital, even though treatment may not have been carried out due to unforeseen circumstances.

G. Complications of surgery and other medical care
When the admission is for treatment of a complication resulting from surgery or other medical care, the complication code is sequenced as the principal diagnosis. If the complication is classified to the T80-T88 series and the code lacks the necessary specificity in describing the complication, an additional code for the specific complication should be assigned.

H. Uncertain Diagnosis
If the diagnosis documented at the time of discharge is qualified as "probable," "suspected," "likely," "questionable," "possible," or "still to be ruled out," "compatible with," "consistent with," or other similar terms indicating uncertainty, code the condition as if it existed or was established. The bases for these guidelines are the diagnostic workup, arrangements for further workup or observation, and initial therapeutic approach that correspond most closely with the established diagnosis.

Note: This guideline is applicable only to inpatient admissions to short-term, acute, long-term care and psychiatric hospitals.

I. Admission from Observation Unit
   1. Admission Following Medical Observation
   When a patient is admitted to an observation unit for a medical condition, which either worsens or does not improve, and is subsequently admitted as an inpatient of the same hospital for this same medical condition, the principal diagnosis would be the medical condition which led to the hospital admission.

   2. Admission Following Post-Operative Observation
   When a patient is admitted to an observation unit to monitor a condition (or complication) that develops following outpatient surgery, and then is subsequently admitted as an inpatient of the same hospital, hospitals should apply the Uniform Hospital Discharge Data Set (UHDDS) definition of principal diagnosis as "that condition established after study to be chiefly responsible for occasioning the admission of the patient to the hospital for care."

J. Admission from Outpatient Surgery
When a patient receives surgery in the hospital's outpatient surgery department and is subsequently admitted for continuing inpatient care at the same hospital, the following guidelines should be followed in selecting the principal diagnosis for the inpatient admission:

   • If the reason for the inpatient admission is a complication, assign the complication as the principal diagnosis.

   • If no complication, or other condition, is documented as the reason for the inpatient admission, assign the reason for the outpatient surgery as the principal diagnosis.

   • If the reason for the inpatient admission is another condition unrelated to the surgery, assign the unrelated condition as the principal diagnosis.

K. Admissions/Encounters for Rehabilitation
When the purpose for the admission/encounter is rehabilitation, sequence first the code for the condition for which the service is being performed. For example, for an admission/encounter for rehabilitation for right-sided dominant hemiplegia following a cerebrovascular infarction, report code I69.351, Hemiplegia and hemiparesis following cerebral infarction affecting right dominant side, as the first-listed or principal diagnosis.

If the condition for which the rehabilitation service is being provided is no longer present, report the appropriate aftercare code as the first-listed or principal diagnosis, unless the rehabilitation service is being provided following an injury. For rehabilitation services following active treatment of an injury, assign the injury code with the appropriate seventh character for subsequent encounter as the first-listed or principal diagnosis. For example, if a patient with severe degenerative osteoarthritis of the hip, underwent hip replacement and the current encounter/admission is for rehabilitation, report code Z47.1, Aftercare following joint replacement surgery, as the first-listed or principal diagnosis. If the patient requires rehabilitation post hip replacement for right intertrochanteric femur fracture, report code S72.141D, Displaced intertrochanteric fracture of right femur, subsequent encounter for closed fracture with routine healing, as the first-listed or principal diagnosis.

See Section I.C.21.c.7., Factors influencing health states and contact with health services, Aftercare.

See Section I.C.19.a., for additional information about the use of 7th characters for injury codes.

Section III. Reporting Additional Diagnoses

GENERAL RULES FOR OTHER (ADDITIONAL) DIAGNOSES

For reporting purposes, the definition for "other diagnoses" is interpreted as additional conditions that affect patient care in terms of requiring:

   clinical evaluation; or

   therapeutic treatment; or

   diagnostic procedures; or

   extended length of hospital stay; or

   increased nursing care and/or monitoring.

The UHDDS item #11-b defines Other Diagnoses as "all conditions that coexist at the time of admission, that develop subsequently, or that affect the treatment received and/or the length of stay. Diagnoses that relate to an earlier episode which have no bearing on the current hospital stay are to be excluded." UHDDS definitions apply to inpatients in acute care, short-term, long term care and psychiatric hospital setting. The UHDDS definitions are used by acute care short-term hospitals to report inpatient data elements in a standardized manner. These data elements and their definitions can be found in the July 31, 1985, Federal Register (Vol. 50, No, 147), pp. 31038-40.

Since that time, the application of the UHDDS definitions has been expanded to include all non-outpatient settings (acute care, short term, long term care and psychiatric hospitals; home health agencies; rehab facilities; nursing homes, etc.). The UHDDS definitions also apply to hospice services (all levels of care).

The following guidelines are to be applied in designating "other diagnoses" when neither the Alphabetic Index nor the Tabular List in ICD-10-CM provide direction. The listing of the diagnoses in the patient record is the responsibility of the attending provider.

A. Previous conditions

If the provider has included a diagnosis in the final diagnostic statement, such as the discharge summary or the face sheet, it should ordinarily be coded. Some providers include in the diagnostic statement resolved conditions or diagnoses and status-post procedures from previous admissions that have no bearing on the current stay. Such conditions are not to be reported and are coded only if required by hospital policy.

However, history codes (categories Z80-Z87) may be used as secondary codes if the historical condition or family history has an impact on current care or influences treatment.

B. Abnormal findings

Abnormal findings (laboratory, x-ray, pathologic, and other diagnostic results) are not coded and reported unless the provider indicates their clinical significance. If the findings are outside the normal range and the attending provider has ordered other tests to evaluate the condition or prescribed treatment, it is appropriate to ask the provider whether the abnormal finding should be added.

Please note: This differs from the coding practices in the outpatient setting for coding encounters for diagnostic tests that have been interpreted by a provider.

C. Uncertain Diagnosis

If the diagnosis documented at the time of discharge is qualified as "probable," "suspected," "likely," "questionable," "possible," or "still to be ruled out," "compatible with," "consistent with," or other similar terms indicating uncertainty, code the condition as if it existed or was established. The bases for these guidelines are the diagnostic workup, arrangements for further workup or observation, and initial therapeutic approach that correspond most closely with the established diagnosis.

Note: This guideline is applicable only to inpatient admissions to short-term, acute, long-term care and psychiatric hospitals.

Section IV. Diagnostic Coding and Reporting Guidelines for Outpatient Services

These coding guidelines for outpatient diagnoses have been approved for use by hospitals/ providers in coding and reporting hospital-based outpatient services and provider-based office visits. Guidelines in Section I, Conventions, general coding guidelines and chapter-specific guidelines, should also be applied for outpatient services and office visits.

Information about the use of certain abbreviations, punctuation, symbols, and other conventions used in the ICD-10-CM Tabular List (code numbers and titles), can be found in Section IA of these guidelines, under "Conventions Used in the Tabular List." Section I.B. contains general guidelines that apply to the entire classification. Section I.C. contains chapter-specific guidelines that correspond to the chapters as they are arranged in the classification. Information about the correct sequence to use in finding a code is also described in Section I.

The terms encounter and visit are often used interchangeably in describing outpatient service contacts and, therefore, appear together in these guidelines without distinguishing one from the other.

Though the conventions and general guidelines apply to all settings, coding guidelines for outpatient and provider reporting of diagnoses will vary in a number of instances from those for inpatient diagnoses, recognizing that:

The Uniform Hospital Discharge Data Set (UHDDS) definition of principal diagnosis does not apply to hospital-based outpatient services and provider-based office visits.

Coding guidelines for inconclusive diagnoses (probable, suspected, rule out, etc.) were developed for inpatient reporting and do not apply to outpatients.

A. Selection of first-listed condition

In the outpatient setting, the term first-listed diagnosis is used in lieu of principal diagnosis.

In determining the first-listed diagnosis the coding conventions of ICD-10-CM, as well as the general and disease specific guidelines take precedence over the outpatient guidelines.

Diagnoses often are not established at the time of the initial encounter/visit. It may take two or more visits before the diagnosis is confirmed.

The most critical rule involves beginning the search for the correct code assignment through the Alphabetic Index. Never begin searching initially in the Tabular List as this will lead to coding errors.

1. Outpatient Surgery

When a patient presents for outpatient surgery (same day surgery), code the reason for the surgery as the first-listed diagnosis (reason for the encounter), even if the surgery is not performed due to a contraindication.

2. Observation Stay

When a patient is admitted for observation for a medical condition, assign a code for the medical condition as the first-listed diagnosis.

When a patient presents for outpatient surgery and develops complications requiring admission to observation, code the reason for the surgery as the first reported diagnosis (reason for the encounter), followed by codes for the complications as secondary diagnoses.

B. Codes from A00.0 through T88.9, Z00-Z99, U00-U85

The appropriate code(s) from A00.0 through T88.9, Z00-Z99 and U00-U85 must be used to identify diagnoses, symptoms, conditions, problems, complaints, or other reason(s) for the encounter/visit.

C. Accurate reporting of ICD-10-CM diagnosis codes

For accurate reporting of ICD-10-CM diagnosis codes, the documentation should describe the patient's condition, using terminology which includes specific diagnoses as well as symptoms, problems, or reasons for the encounter. There are ICD-10-CM codes to describe all of these.

D. Codes that describe symptoms and signs

Codes that describe symptoms and signs, as opposed to diagnoses, are acceptable for reporting purposes when a diagnosis has not been established (confirmed) by the provider. Chapter 18 of ICD-10-CM, Symptoms, Signs, and Abnormal Clinical and Laboratory Findings Not Elsewhere Classified (codes R00-R99) contain many, but not all codes for symptoms.

E. Encounters for circumstances other than a disease or injury

ICD-10-CM provides codes to deal with encounters for circumstances other than a disease or injury. The Factors Influencing Health Status and Contact with Health Services codes (Z00-Z99) are provided to deal with occasions when circumstances other than a disease or injury are recorded as diagnosis or problems.

See Section I.C.21. Factors influencing health status and contact with health services.

F. Level of Detail in Coding

1. ICD-10-CM codes with 3, 4, 5, 6 or 7 characters

ICD-10-CM is composed of codes with 3, 4, 5, 6 or 7 characters. Codes with three characters are included in ICD-10-CM as the heading of a category of codes that may be further subdivided by the use of fourth, fifth, sixth or seventh characters to provide greater specificity.

2. Use of full number of characters required for a code

A three-character code is to be used only if it is not further subdivided. A code is invalid if it has not been coded to the full number of characters required for that code, including the 7th character, if applicable.

3. Highest level of specificity

Code to the highest level of specificity when supported by the medical record documentation.

G. ICD-10-CM code for the diagnosis, condition, problem, or other reason for encounter/visit

List first the ICD-10-CM code for the diagnosis, condition, problem, or other reason for encounter/visit shown in the medical record to be chiefly responsible for the services provided. List additional codes that describe any coexisting conditions. In some cases, the first-listed diagnosis may be a symptom when a diagnosis has not been established (confirmed) by the provider.

H. Uncertain diagnosis

Do not code diagnoses documented as "probable", "suspected," "questionable," "rule out," "compatible with," "consistent with," or "working diagnosis" or other similar terms indicating uncertainty. Rather, code the condition(s) to the highest degree of certainty for that encounter/visit, such as symptoms, signs, abnormal test results, or other reason for the visit.

Please note: This differs from the coding practices used by short-term, acute care, long-term care and psychiatric hospitals.

I. Chronic diseases

Chronic diseases treated on an ongoing basis may be coded and reported as many times as the patient receives treatment and care for the condition(s)

J. Code all documented conditions that coexist

Code all documented conditions that coexist at the time of the encounter/visit and that require or affect patient care, treatment or management. Do not code conditions that were previously treated and no longer exist. However, history codes (categories Z80-Z87) may be used as secondary codes if the historical condition or family history has an impact on current care or influences treatment.

K. Patients receiving diagnostic services only

For patients receiving diagnostic services only during an encounter/visit, sequence first the diagnosis, condition, problem, or other reason for encounter/visit shown in the medical record to be chiefly responsible for the outpatient services provided during the encounter/visit. Codes for other diagnoses (e.g., chronic conditions) may be sequenced as additional diagnoses.

For encounters for routine laboratory/radiology testing in the absence of any signs, symptoms, or associated diagnosis, assign Z01.89, Encounter for other specified special examinations. If routine testing is performed during the same encounter as a test to evaluate a sign, symptom, or diagnosis, it is appropriate to assign both the Z code and the code describing the reason for the non-routine test.

For outpatient encounters for diagnostic tests that have been interpreted by a physician, and the final report is available at the time of coding, code any confirmed or definitive diagnosis(es) documented in the interpretation. Do not code related signs and symptoms as additional diagnoses.

Please note: This differs from the coding practice in the hospital inpatient setting regarding abnormal findings on test results.

L. Patients receiving therapeutic services only

For patients receiving therapeutic services only during an encounter/visit, sequence first the diagnosis, condition, problem, or other reason for encounter/visit shown in the medical record to be chiefly responsible for the outpatient services provided during the encounter/visit. Codes for other diagnoses (e.g., chronic conditions) may be sequenced as additional diagnoses.

The only exception to this rule is that when the primary reason for the admission/encounter is chemotherapy or radiation therapy, the appropriate Z code for the service is listed first, and the diagnosis or problem for which the service is being performed listed second.

M. Patients receiving preoperative evaluations only

For patients receiving preoperative evaluations only, sequence first a code from subcategory Z01.81, Encounter for pre-procedural examinations, to describe the pre-op consultations. Assign a code for the condition to describe the reason for the surgery as an additional diagnosis. Code also any findings related to the pre-op evaluation.

N. Ambulatory surgery

For ambulatory surgery, code the diagnosis for which the surgery was performed. If the postoperative diagnosis is known to be different from the preoperative diagnosis at the time the diagnosis is confirmed, select the postoperative diagnosis for coding, since it is the most definitive.

O. Routine outpatient prenatal visits

See Section I.C.15. Routine outpatient prenatal visits.

P. Encounters for general medical examinations with abnormal findings

The subcategories for encounters for general medical examinations, Z00.0- and encounter for routine child health examination, Z00.12-, provide codes for with and without abnormal findings. Should a general medical examination result in an abnormal finding, the code for general medical examination with abnormal finding should be assigned as the first-listed diagnosis. An examination with abnormal findings refers to a condition/diagnosis that is newly identified or a change in severity of a chronic condition (such as uncontrolled hypertension, or an acute exacerbation of chronic obstructive pulmonary disease) during a routine physical examination. A secondary code for the abnormal finding should also be coded.

Q. Encounters for routine health screenings

See Section I.C.21. Factors influencing health status and contact with health services, Screening

Appendix I. Present on Admission Reporting Guidelines

Introduction

These guidelines are to be used as a supplement to the *ICD-10-CM Official Guidelines for Coding and Reporting* to facilitate the assignment of the Present on Admission (POA) indicator for each diagnosis and external cause of injury code reported on claim forms (UB-04 and 837 Institutional).

These guidelines are not intended to replace any guidelines in the main body of the *ICD-10-CM Official Guidelines for Coding and Reporting*. The POA guidelines are not intended to provide guidance on when a condition should be coded, but rather, how to apply the POA indicator to the final set of diagnosis codes that have been assigned in accordance with Sections I, II, and III of the official coding guidelines. Subsequent to the assignment of the ICD-10-CM codes, the POA indicator should then be assigned to those conditions that have been coded.

As stated in the Introduction to the *ICD-10-CM Official Guidelines for Coding and Reporting*, a joint effort between the healthcare provider and the coder is essential to achieve complete and accurate documentation, code assignment, and reporting of diagnoses and procedures. The importance of consistent, complete documentation in the medical record cannot be overemphasized. Medical record documentation from any provider involved in the care and treatment of the patient may be used to support the determination of whether a condition was present on admission or not. In the context of the official coding guidelines, the term "provider" means a physician or any qualified healthcare practitioner who is legally accountable for establishing the patient's diagnosis.

These guidelines are not a substitute for the provider's clinical judgment as to the determination of whether a condition was/was not present on admission. The provider should be queried regarding issues related to the linking of signs/symptoms, timing of test results, and the timing of findings.

Please see the CDC website for the detailed list of ICD-10-CM codes that do not require the use of a POA indicator (https://www.cdc.gov/nchs/icd/icd10cm.htm). The codes and categories on this exempt list are for circumstances regarding the healthcare encounter or factors influencing health status that do not represent a current disease or injury or that describe conditions that are always present on admission.

General Reporting Requirements

All claims involving inpatient admissions to general acute care hospitals or other facilities that are subject to a law or regulation mandating collection of present on admission information.

Present on admission is defined as present at the time the order for inpatient admission occurs -- conditions that develop during an outpatient encounter, including emergency department, observation, or outpatient surgery, are considered as present on admission.

POA indicator is assigned to principal and secondary diagnoses (as defined in Section II of the Official Guidelines for Coding and Reporting) and the external cause of injury codes.

Issues related to inconsistent, missing, conflicting or unclear documentation must still be resolved by the provider.

If a condition would not be coded and reported based on UHDDS definitions and current official coding guidelines, then the POA indicator would not be reported.

Reporting Options

Y – Yes

N – No

U – Unknown

W – Clinically undetermined

Unreported/Not used – (Exempt from POA reporting)

Reporting Definitions

Y = present at the time of inpatient admission

N = not present at the time of inpatient admission

U = documentation is insufficient to determine if condition is present on admission

W = provider is unable to clinically determine whether condition was present on admission or not

Timeframe for POA Identification and Documentation

There is no required timeframe as to when a provider (per the definition of "provider" used in these guidelines) must identify or document a condition to be present on admission. In some clinical situations, it may not be possible for a provider to make a definitive diagnosis (or a condition may not be recognized or reported by the patient) for a period of time after admission. In some cases, it may be several days before the provider arrives at a definitive diagnosis. This does not mean that the condition was not present on admission. Determination of whether the condition was present on admission or not will be based on the applicable POA guideline as identified in this document, or on the provider's best clinical judgment.

If at the time of code assignment the documentation is unclear as to whether a condition was present on admission or not, it is appropriate to query the provider for clarification.

Assigning the POA Indicator

Condition is on the "Exempt from Reporting" list

Leave the "present on admission" field blank if the condition is on the list of ICD-10-CM codes for which this field is not applicable. This is the only circumstance in which the field may be left blank.

POA Explicitly Documented

Assign Y for any condition the provider explicitly documents as being present on admission.

Assign N for any condition the provider explicitly documents as not present at the time of admission.

Conditions diagnosed prior to inpatient admission

Assign "Y" for conditions that were diagnosed prior to admission (example: hypertension, diabetes mellitus, asthma)

Conditions diagnosed during the admission but clearly present before admission

Assign "Y" for conditions diagnosed during the admission that were clearly present but not diagnosed until after admission occurred.

Diagnoses subsequently confirmed after admission are considered present on admission if at the time of admission they are documented as suspected, possible, rule out, differential diagnosis, or constitute an underlying cause of a symptom that is present at the time of admission.

Condition develops during outpatient encounter prior to inpatient admission

Assign Y for any condition that develops during an outpatient encounter prior to a written order for inpatient admission.

Documentation does not indicate whether condition was present on admission

Assign "U" when the medical record documentation is unclear as to whether the condition was present on admission. "U" should not be routinely assigned and used only in very limited circumstances. Coders are encouraged to query the providers when the documentation is unclear.

Documentation states that it cannot be determined whether the condition was or was not present on admission

Assign "W" when the medical record documentation indicates that it cannot be clinically determined whether or not the condition was present on admission.

Chronic condition with acute exacerbation during the admission

If a single code identifies both the chronic condition and the acute exacerbation, see POA guidelines pertaining to codes that contain multiple clinical concepts.

If a single code only identifies the chronic condition and not the acute exacerbation (e.g., acute exacerbation of chronic leukemia), assign "Y."

Conditions documented as possible, probable, suspected, or rule out at the time of discharge

If the final diagnosis contains a possible, probable, suspected, or rule out diagnosis, and this diagnosis was based on signs, symptoms or clinical findings suspected at the time of inpatient admission, assign "Y."

If the final diagnosis contains a possible, probable, suspected, or rule out diagnosis, and this diagnosis was based on signs, symptoms or clinical findings that were not present on admission, assign "N".

Conditions documented as impending or threatened at the time of discharge

If the final diagnosis contains an impending or threatened diagnosis, and this diagnosis is based on symptoms or clinical findings that were present on admission, assign "Y".

If the final diagnosis contains an impending or threatened diagnosis, and this diagnosis is based on symptoms or clinical findings that were not present on admission, assign "N".

Acute and Chronic Conditions

Assign "Y" for acute conditions that are present at time of admission and N for acute conditions that are not present at time of admission.

Assign "Y" for chronic conditions, even though the condition may not be diagnosed until after admission.

If a single code identifies both an acute and chronic condition, see the POA guidelines for codes that contain multiple clinical concepts.

Codes That Contain Multiple Clinical Concepts

Assign "N" if at least one of the clinical concepts included in the code was not present on admission (e.g., COPD with acute exacerbation and the exacerbation was not present on admission; gastric ulcer that does not

start bleeding until after admission; asthma patient develops status asthmaticus after admission).

Assign "Y" if all of the clinical concepts included in the code were present on admission (e.g., duodenal ulcer that perforates prior to admission).

For infection codes that include the causal organism, assign "Y" if the infection (or signs of the infection) were present on admission, even though the culture results may not be known until after admission (e.g., patient is admitted with pneumonia and the provider documents Pseudomonas as the causal organism a few days later).

Same Diagnosis Code for Two or More Conditions

When the same ICD-10-CM diagnosis code applies to two or more conditions during the same encounter (e.g. two separate conditions classified to the same ICD-10-CM diagnosis code):

Assign "Y" if all conditions represented by the single ICD-10-CM code were present on admission (e.g. bilateral unspecified age-related cataracts).

Assign "N" if any of the conditions represented by the single ICD-10-CM code was not present on admission (e.g. traumatic secondary and recurrent hemorrhage and seroma is assigned to a single code T79.2, but only one of the conditions was present on admission).

Obstetrical conditions

Whether or not the patient delivers during the current hospitalization does not affect assignment of the POA indicator. The determining factor for POA assignment is whether the pregnancy complication or obstetrical condition described by the code was present at the time of admission or not.

If the pregnancy complication or obstetrical condition was present on admission (e.g., patient admitted in preterm labor), assign "Y".

If the pregnancy complication or obstetrical condition was not present on admission (e.g., 2nd degree laceration during delivery, postpartum hemorrhage that occurred during current hospitalization, fetal distress develops after admission), assign "N".

If the obstetrical code includes more than one diagnosis and any of the diagnoses identified by the code were not present on admission assign "N". (e.g., Category O11, Pre-existing hypertension with pre-eclampsia)

Perinatal conditions

Newborns are not considered to be admitted until after birth. Therefore, any condition present at birth or that developed in utero is considered present at admission and should be assigned "Y". This includes conditions that occur during delivery (e.g., injury during delivery, meconium aspiration, exposure to streptococcus B in the vaginal canal).

Congenital conditions and anomalies

Assign "Y" for congenital conditions and anomalies except for categories Q00-Q99, Congenital anomalies, which are on the exempt list. Congenital conditions are always considered present on admission.

External cause of injury codes

Assign "Y" for any external cause code representing an external cause of morbidity that occurred prior to inpatient admission (e.g., patient fell out of bed at home, patient fell out of bed in emergency room prior to admission)

Assign "N" for any external cause code representing an external cause of morbidity that occurred during inpatient hospitalization (e.g., patient fell out of hospital bed during hospital stay, patient experienced an adverse reaction to a medication administered after inpatient admission).

ICD-10-CM Index to Diseases and Injuries

A

Aarskog's syndrome Q87.19
Abandonment — *see* Maltreatment
Abasia (-astasia) (hysterical) F44.4
Abderhalden-Kaufmann-Lignac syndrome (cystinosis) E72.04
Abdomen, abdominal — *see also* condition
  muscle deficiency syndrome Q79.4
  angina K55.1
    acute R10.0
Abdominalgia — *see* Pain, abdominal
Abduction contracture, hip or other joint — *see* Contraction, joint
Aberrant (congenital) — *see also* Malposition, congenital
  adrenal gland Q89.1
  artery (peripheral) Q27.8
    basilar NEC Q28.1
    cerebral Q28.3
    coronary Q24.5
    digestive system Q27.8
    eye Q15.8
    lower limb Q27.8
    precerebral Q28.1
    pulmonary Q25.79
    renal Q27.2
    retina Q14.1
    specified site NEC Q27.8
    subclavian Q27.8
    upper limb Q27.8
    vertebral Q28.1
  breast Q83.8
  endocrine gland NEC Q89.2
  hepatic duct Q44.5
  pancreas Q45.3
  parathyroid gland Q89.2
  pituitary gland Q89.2
  sebaceous glands, mucous membrane, mouth, congenital Q38.6
  spleen Q89.09
  subclavian artery Q27.8
  thymus (gland) Q89.2
  thyroid gland Q89.2
  vein (peripheral) NEC Q27.8
    cerebral Q28.3
    digestive system Q27.8
    lower limb Q27.8
    precerebral Q28.1
    specified site NEC Q27.8
    upper limb Q27.8
Aberration
  distantial — *see* Disturbance, visual
  mental F99
Abetalipoproteinemia E78.6
Abiotrophy R68.89
Ablatio, ablation
  retinae — *see* Detachment, retina
Ablepharia, ablepharon Q10.3
Abnormal, abnormality, abnormalities — *see also* Anomaly
  acid-base balance (mixed) E87.4
  albumin R77.0
  alphafetoprotein R77.2
  alveolar ridge K08.9
  anatomical relationship Q89.9
  apertures, congenital, diaphragm Q79.1
  atrial septal, specified NEC Q21.19
  auditory perception H93.29- ☑
    diplacusis — *see* Diplacusis
    hyperacusis — *see* Hyperacusis
    recruitment — *see* Recruitment, auditory
    threshold shift — *see* Shift, auditory threshold
  autosomes Q99.9
    fragile site Q95.5
  basal metabolic rate R94.8
  biosynthesis, testicular androgen E29.1
  bleeding time R79.1
  blood amino-acid level R79.83
  blood level (of)
    cobalt R79.0
    copper R79.0
    iron R79.0

Abnormal, abnormality, abnormalities — *continued*
  blood level — *continued*
    lithium R78.89
    magnesium R79.0
    mineral NEC R79.0
    zinc R79.0
  blood pressure
    elevated R03.0
    low reading (nonspecific) R03.1
  blood sugar R73.09
  blood-gas level R79.81
  bowel sounds R19.15
    absent R19.11
    hyperactive R19.12
  brain scan R94.02
  breathing R06.9
  caloric test R94.138
  cerebrospinal fluid R83.9
    cytology R83.6
    drug level R83.2
    enzyme level R83.0
    hormones R83.1
    immunology R83.4
    microbiology R83.5
    nonmedicinal level R83.3
    specified type NEC R83.8
  chemistry, blood R79.9
    C-reactive protein R79.82
    drugs — *see* Findings, abnormal, in blood
    gas level R79.81
    minerals R79.0
    pancytopenia D61.818
    PTT R79.1
    specified NEC R79.89
    toxins — *see* Findings, abnormal, in blood
  chest sounds (friction) (rales) R09.89
  chromosome, chromosomal Q99.9
    with more than three X chromosomes, female Q97.1
    analysis result R89.8
      bronchial washings R84.8
      cerebrospinal fluid R83.8
      cervix uteri NEC R87.89
      nasal secretions R84.8
      nipple discharge R89.8
      peritoneal fluid R85.89
      pleural fluid R84.8
      prostatic secretions R86.8
      saliva R85.89
      seminal fluid R86.8
      sputum R84.8
      synovial fluid R89.8
      throat scrapings R84.8
      vagina R87.89
      vulva R87.89
      wound secretions R89.8
    dicentric replacement Q93.2
    ring replacement Q93.2
    sex Q99.8
      female phenotype Q97.9
        specified NEC Q97.8
      male phenotype Q98.9
        specified NEC Q98.8
      structural male Q98.6
    specified NEC Q99.8
  clinical findings NEC R68.89
  coagulation D68.9
    newborn, transient P61.6
    profile R79.1
    time R79.1
  communication — *see* Fistula
  conjunctiva, vascular H11.41- ☑
  coronary artery Q24.5
  cortisol-binding globulin E27.8
  course, eustachian tube Q17.8
  creatinine clearance R94.4
  cytology
    anus R85.619
      atypical squamous cells cannot exclude high grade squamous intraepithelial lesion (ASC-H) R85.611
      atypical squamous cells of undetermined significance (ASC-US) R85.610

Abnormal, abnormality, abnormalities — *continued*
  cytology — *continued*
    anus — *continued*
      cytologic evidence of malignancy R85.614
      high grade squamous intraepithelial lesion (HGSIL) R85.613
      human papillomavirus (HPV) DNA test
        high risk positive R85.81
        low risk postive R85.82
      inadequate smear R85.615
      low grade squamous intraepithelial lesion (LGSIL) R85.612
      satisfactory anal smear but lacking transformation zone R85.616
      specified NEC R85.618
      unsatisfactory smear R85.615
    female genital organs — *see* Abnormal, Papanicolaou (smear)
  dark adaptation curve H53.61
  dentofacial NEC — *see* Anomaly, dentofacial
  development, developmental Q89.9
    central nervous system Q07.9
  diagnostic imaging
    abdomen, abdominal region NEC R93.5
    biliary tract R93.2
    bladder R93.41
    breast R92.8
    central nervous system NEC R90.89
    cerebrovascular NEC R90.89
    coronary circulation R93.1
    digestive tract NEC R93.3
    gastrointestinal (tract) R93.3
    genitourinary organs R93.89
    head R93.0
    heart R93.1
    intrathoracic organ NEC R93.89
    kidney R93.42- ☑
    limbs R93.6
    liver R93.2
    lung (field) R91.8
    musculoskeletal system NEC R93.7
    renal pelvis R93.41
    retroperitoneum R93.5
    site specified NEC R93.89
    skin and subcutaneous tissue R93.89
    skull R93.0
    testis R93.81- ☑
    ureter R93.41
    urinary organs specified NEC R93.49
  direction, teeth, fully erupted M26.30
  ear ossicles, acquired NEC H74.39- ☑
    ankylosis — *see* Ankylosis, ear ossicles
    discontinuity — *see* Discontinuity, ossicles, ear
    partial loss — *see* Loss, ossicles, ear (partial)
  Ebstein Q22.5
  echocardiogram R93.1
  echoencephalogram R90.81
  echogram — *see* Abnormal, diagnostic imaging
  electrocardiogram [ECG] [EKG] R94.31
  electroencephalogram [EEG] R94.01
  electrolyte — *see* Imbalance, electrolyte
  electromyogram [EMG] R94.131
  electro-oculogram [EOG] R94.110
  electrophysiological intracardiac studies R94.39
  electroretinogram [ERG] R94.111
  erythrocytes
    congenital, with perinatal jaundice D58.9
  feces (color) (contents) (mucus) R19.5
  finding — *see* Findings, abnormal, without diagnosis
  fluid
    amniotic — *see* Abnormal, specimen, specified
    cerebrospinal — *see* Abnormal, cerebrospinal fluid
    peritoneal — *see* Abnormal, specimen, digestive organs
    pleural — *see* Abnormal, specimen, respiratory organs
    synovial — *see* Abnormal, specimen, specified
    thorax (bronchial washings) (pleural fluid) — *see* Abnormal, specimen, respiratory organs
    vaginal — *see* Abnormal, specimen, female genital organs

Abnormal, abnormality, abnormalities —
continued
form
teeth K00.2
uterus — *see* Anomaly, uterus
function studies
auditory R94.120
bladder R94.8
brain R94.09
cardiovascular R94.30
ear R94.128
endocrine NEC R94.7
eye NEC R94.118
kidney R94.4
liver R94.5
nervous system
central NEC R94.09
peripheral NEC R94.138
pancreas R94.8
placenta R94.8
pulmonary R94.2
special senses NEC R94.128
spleen R94.8
thyroid R94.6
vestibular R94.121
gait — *see* Gait
hysterical F44.4
gastrin secretion E16.4
globulin R77.1
cortisol-binding E27.8
thyroid-binding E07.89
glomerular, minor — *see also* N00-N07 with fourth
character .0 N05.0
glucagon secretion E16.3
glucose tolerance (test) (non-fasting) R73.09
gravitational (G) forces or states (effect of) T75.81 ☑
hair (color) (shaft) L67.9
specified NEC L67.8
hard tissue formation in pulp (dental) K04.3
head movement R25.0
heart
rate R00.9
specified NEC R00.8
shadow R93.1
sounds NEC R01.2
hemoglobin (disease) — *see also* Disease, hemoglobin
D58.2
trait — *see* Trait, hemoglobin, abnormal
histology NEC R89.7
immunological findings R89.4
in serum R76.9
specified NEC R76.8
increase in appetite R63.2
involuntary movement — *see* Abnormal, movement,
involuntary
jaw closure M26.51
karyotype R89.8
kidney function test R94.4
knee jerk R29.2
leukocyte (cell) (differential) NEC D72.9
liver function test — *see also* Elevated, liver function,
test R79.89
loss of
height R29.890
weight R63.4
mammogram NEC R92.8
calcification (calculus) R92.1
microcalcification R92.0
Mantoux test R76.11
movement (disorder) — *see also* Disorder, movement
head R25.0
involuntary R25.9
fasciculation R25.3
of head R25.0
spasm R25.2
specified type NEC R25.8
tremor R25.1
myoglobin (Aberdeen) (Annapolis) R89.7
neonatal screening P09.9
for
congenital adrenal hyperplasia P09.2
congenital endocrine disease P09.2
congenital hematologic disorders P09.3
critical congenital heart disease P09.5
cystic fibrosis P09.4
hemoglobinothies P09.3
hypothyroidism P09.2
inborn errors of metabolism P09.1

Abnormal, abnormality, abnormalities —
continued
neonatal screening — *continued*
for — *continued*
neonatal hearing loss P09.6
red cell membrane defects P09.3
sickle cell P09.3
specified NEC P09.8
oculomotor study R94.113
palmar creases Q82.8
Papanicolaou (smear)
anus R85.619
atypical squamous cells cannot exclude high
grade squamous intraepithelial lesion
(ASC-H) R85.611
atypical squamous cells of undetermined significance (ASC-US) R85.610
cytologic evidence of malignancy R85.614
high grade squamous intraepithelial lesion
(HGSIL) R85.613
human papillomavirus (HPV) DNA test
high risk positive R85.81
low risk postive R85.82
inadequate smear R85.615
low grade squamous intraepithelial lesion (LGSIL)
R85.612
satisfactory anal smear but lacking transformation zone R85.616
specified NEC R85.618
unsatisfactory smear R85.615
bronchial washings R84.6
cerebrospinal fluid R83.6
cervix R87.619
atypical squamous cells cannot exclude high
grade squamous intraepithelial lesion
(ASC-H) R87.611
atypical squamous cells of undetermined significance (ASC-US) R87.610
cytologic evidence of malignancy R87.614
high grade squamous intraepithelial lesion
(HGSIL) R87.613
inadequate smear R87.615
low grade squamous intraepithelial lesion (LGSIL)
R87.612
non-atypical endometrial cells R87.618
satisfactory cervical smear but lacking transformation zone R87.616
specified NEC R87.618
thin preparaton R87.619
unsatisfactory smear R87.615
nasal secretions R84.6
nipple discharge R89.6
peritoneal fluid R85.69
pleural fluid R84.6
prostatic secretions R86.6
saliva R85.69
seminal fluid R86.6
sites NEC R89.6
sputum R84.6
synovial fluid R89.6
throat scrapings R84.6
vagina R87.629
atypical squamous cells cannot exclude high
grade squamous intraepithelial lesion
(ASC-H) R87.621
atypical squamous cells of undetermined significance (ASC-US) R87.620
cytologic evidence of malignancy R87.624
high grade squamous intraepithelial lesion
(HGSIL) R87.623
inadequate smear R87.625
low grade squamous intraepithelial lesion (LGSIL)
R87.622
specified NEC R87.628
thin preparation R87.629
unsatisfactory smear R87.625
vulva R87.69
wound secretions R89.6
partial thromboplastin time (PTT) R79.1
pelvis (bony) — *see* Deformity, pelvis
percussion, chest (tympany) R09.89
periods (grossly) — *see* Menstruation
phonocardiogram R94.39
plantar reflex R29.2
plasma
protein R77.9
specified NEC R77.8
viscosity R70.1
pleural (folds) Q34.0

Abnormal, abnormality, abnormalities —
continued
posture R29.3
product of conception O02.9
specified type NEC O02.89
prothrombin time (PT) R79.1
pulmonary
artery, congenital Q25.79
function, newborn P28.89
test results R94.2
pulsations in neck R00.2
pupillary H21.56- ☑
function (reaction) (reflex) — *see* Anomaly, pupil,
function
radiological examination — *see* Abnormal, diagnostic
imaging
red blood cell(s) (morphology) (volume) R71.8
reflex — *see* Reflex
renal function test R94.4
response to nerve stimulation R94.130
retinal correspondence H53.31
retinal function study R94.111
rhythm, heart — *see also* Arrhythmia
saliva — *see* Abnormal, specimen, digestive organs
scan
kidney R94.4
liver R93.2
thyroid R94.6
secretion
gastrin E16.4
glucagon E16.3
semen, seminal fluid — *see* Abnormal, specimen, male
genital organs
serum level (of)
acid phosphatase R74.8
alkaline phosphatase R74.8
amylase R74.8
enzymes R74.9
specified NEC R74.8
lipase R74.8
triacylglycerol lipase R74.8
shape
gravid uterus — *see* Anomaly, uterus
sinus venosus Q21.16
size, tooth, teeth K00.2
spacing, tooth, teeth, fully erupted M26.30
specimen
digestive organs (peritoneal fluid) (saliva) R85.9
cytology R85.69
drug level R85.2
enzyme level R85.0
histology R85.7
hormones R85.1
immunology R85.4
microbiology R85.5
nonmedicinal level R85.3
specified type NEC R85.89
female genital organs (secretions) (smears) R87.9
cytology R87.69
cervix R87.619
human papillomavirus (HPV) DNA test
high risk positive R87.810
low risk positive R87.820
inadequate (unsatisfactory) smear
R87.615
non-atypical endometrial cells R87.618
specified NEC R87.618
vagina R87.629
human papillomavirus (HPV) DNA test
high risk positive R87.811
low risk positive R87.821
inadequate (unsatisfactory) smear
R87.625
vulva R87.69
drug level R87.2
enzyme level R87.0
histological R87.7
hormones R87.1
immunology R87.4
microbiology R87.5
nonmedicinal level R87.3
specified type NEC R87.89
male genital organs (prostatic secretions) (semen)
R86.9
cytology R86.6
drug level R86.2
enzyme level R86.0
histological R86.7

Abnormal, abnormality, abnormalities — *continued*
   specimen — *continued*
      male genital organs — *continued*
         hormones R86.1
         immunology R86.4
         microbiology R86.5
         nonmedicinal level R86.3
         specified type NEC R86.8
      nipple discharge — *see* Abnormal, specimen, specified
      respiratory organs (bronchial washings) (nasal secretions) (pleural fluid) (sputum) R84.9
         cytology R84.6
         drug level R84.2
         enzyme level R84.0
         histology R84.7
         hormones R84.1
         immunology R84.4
         microbiology R84.5
         nonmedicinal level R84.3
         specified type NEC R84.8
      specified organ, system and tissue NOS R89.9
         cytology R89.6
         drug level R89.2
         enzyme level R89.0
         histology R89.7
         hormones R89.1
         immunology R89.4
         microbiology R89.5
         nonmedicinal level R89.3
         specified type NEC R89.8
      synovial fluid — *see* Abnormal, specimen, specified
      thorax (bronchial washings) (pleural fluids) — *see* Abnormal, specimen, respiratory organs
      vagina (secretion) (smear) R87.629
      vulva (secretion) (smear) R87.69
      wound secretion — *see* Abnormal, specimen, specified
   spermatozoa — *see* Abnormal, specimen, male genital organs
   sputum (amount) (color) (odor) R09.3
   stool (color) (contents) (mucus) R19.5
      bloody K92.1
      guaiac positive R19.5
   synchondrosis Q78.8
   thermography — *see also* Abnormal, diagnostic imaging R93.89
   thyroid-binding globulin E07.89
   tooth, teeth (form) (size) K00.2
   toxicology (findings) R78.9
   transport protein E88.09
   tumor marker NEC R97.8
   ultrasound results — *see* Abnormal, diagnostic imaging
   umbilical cord complicating delivery O69.9 ☑
   urination NEC R39.198
   urine (constituents) R82.90
      bile R82.2
      cytological examination R82.89
      drugs R82.5
      fat R82.0
      glucose R81
      heavy metals R82.6
      hemoglobin R82.3
      histological examination R82.89
      ketones R82.4
      microbiological examination (culture) R82.79
      myoglobin R82.1
      positive culture R82.79
      protein — *see* Proteinuria
      specified substance NEC R82.998
         chromoabnormality NEC R82.91
      substances nonmedical R82.6
   uterine hemorrhage — *see* Hemorrhage, uterus
   vectorcardiogram R94.39
   visually evoked potential (VEP) R94.112
   white blood cells D72.9
      specified NEC D72.89
   X-ray examination — *see* Abnormal, diagnostic imaging
Abnormity (any organ or part) — *see* Anomaly
Abocclusion M26.29
   hemolytic disease (newborn) P55.1
   incompatibility reaction ABO — *see* Complication(s), transfusion, incompatibility reaction, ABO
Abolition, language R48.8
Aborter, habitual or recurrent — *see* Loss (of), pregnancy, recurrent
Abortion (complete) (spontaneous) O03.9

Abortion — *continued*
   with
      retained products of conception — *see* Abortion, incomplete
   attempted (elective) (failed) O07.4
      complicated by O07.30
         afibrinogenemia O07.1
         cardiac arrest O07.36
         chemical damage of pelvic organ(s) O07.34
         circulatory collapse O07.31
         cystitis O07.38
         defibrination syndrome O07.1
         electrolyte imbalance O07.33
         embolism (air) (amniotic fluid) (blood clot) (fat) (pulmonary) (septic) (soap) O07.2
         endometritis O07.0
         genital tract and pelvic infection O07.0
         hemolysis O07.1
         hemorrhage (delayed) (excessive) O07.1
         infection
            genital tract or pelvic O07.0
            urinary tract tract O07.38
         intravascular coagulation O07.1
         laceration of pelvic organ(s) O07.34
         metabolic disorder O07.33
         oliguria O07.32
         oophoritis O07.0
         parametritis O07.0
         pelvic peritonitis O07.0
         perforation of pelvic organ(s) O07.34
         renal failure or shutdown O07.32
         salpingitis or salpingo-oophoritis O07.0
         sepsis O07.37
         shock O07.31
         specified condition NEC O07.39
         tubular necrosis (renal) O07.32
         uremia O07.32
         urinary tract infection O07.38
         venous complication NEC O07.35
            embolism (air) (amniotic fluid) (blood clot) (fat) (pulmonary) (septic) (soap) O07.2
   complicated (by) (following) O03.80
      afibrinogenemia O03.6
      cardiac arrest O03.86
      chemical damage of pelvic organ(s) O03.84
      circulatory collapse O03.81
      cystitis O03.88
      defibrination syndrome O03.6
      electrolyte imbalance O03.83
      embolism (air) (amniotic fluid) (blood clot) (fat) (pulmonary) (septic) (soap) O03.7
      endometritis O03.5
      genital tract and pelvic infection O03.5
      hemolysis O03.6
      hemorrhage (delayed) (excessive) O03.6
      infection
         genital tract or pelvic O03.5
         urinary tract O03.88
      intravascular coagulation O03.6
      laceration of pelvic organ(s) O03.84
      metabolic disorder O03.83
      oliguria O03.82
      oophoritis O03.5
      parametritis O03.5
      pelvic peritonitis O03.5
      perforation of pelvic organ(s) O03.84
      renal failure or shutdown O03.82
      salpingitis or salpingo-oophoritis O03.5
      sepsis O03.87
      shock O03.81
      specified condition NEC O03.89
      tubular necrosis (renal) O03.82
      uremia O03.82
      urinary tract infection O03.88
      venous complication NEC O03.85
         embolism (air) (amniotic fluid) (blood clot) (fat) (pulmonary) (septic) (soap) O03.7
   failed — *see* Abortion, attempted
   habitual or recurrent N96
      with current abortion — *see* categories O03-O04
      without current pregnancy N96
      care in current pregnancy O26.2- ☑
   incomplete (spontaneous) O03.4
      complicated (by) (following) O03.30
         afibrinogenemia O03.1
         cardiac arrest O03.36
         chemical damage of pelvic organ(s) O03.34
         circulatory collapse O03.31
         cystitis O03.38

Abortion — *continued*
   incomplete — *continued*
      complicated — *continued*
         defibrination syndrome O03.1
         electrolyte imbalance O03.33
         embolism (air) (amniotic fluid) (blood clot) (fat) (pulmonary) (septic) (soap) O03.2
         endometritis O03.0
         genital tract and pelvic infection O03.0
         hemolysis O03.1
         hemorrhage (delayed) (excessive) O03.1
         infection
            genital tract or pelvic O03.0
            urinary tract O03.38
         intravascular coagulation O03.1
         laceration of pelvic organ(s) O03.34
         metabolic disorder O03.33
         oliguria O03.32
         oophoritis O03.0
         parametritis O03.0
         pelvic peritonitis O03.0
         perforation of pelvic organ(s) O03.34
         renal failure or shutdown O03.32
         salpingitis or salpingo-oophoritis O03.0
         sepsis O03.37
         shock O03.31
         specified condition NEC O03.39
         tubular necrosis (renal) O03.32
         uremia O03.32
         urinary infection O03.38
         venous complication NEC O03.35
            embolism (air) (amniotic fluid) (blood clot) (fat) (pulmonary) (septic) (soap) O03.2
   induced (encounter for) Z33.2
      complicated by O04.80
         afibrinogenemia O04.6
         cardiac arrest O04.86
         chemical damage of pelvic organ(s) O04.84
         circulatory collapse O04.81
         cystitis O04.88
         defibrination syndrome O04.6
         electrolyte imbalance O04.83
         embolism (air) (amniotic fluid) (blood clot) (fat) (pulmonary) (septic) (soap) O04.7
         endometritis O04.5
         genital tract and pelvic infection O04.5
         hemolysis O04.6
         hemorrhage (delayed) (excessive) O04.6
         infection
            genital tract or pelvic O04.5
            urinary tract O04.88
         intravascular coagulation O04.6
         laceration of pelvic organ(s) O04.84
         metabolic disorder O04.83
         oliguria O04.82
         oophoritis O04.5
         parametritis O04.5
         pelvic peritonitis O04.5
         perforation of pelvic organ(s) O04.84
         renal failure or shutdown O04.82
         salpingitis or salpingo-oophoritis O04.5
         sepsis O04.87
         shock O04.81
         specified condition NEC O04.89
         tubular necrosis (renal) O04.82
         uremia O04.82
         urinary tract infection O04.88
         venous complication NEC O04.85
            embolism (air) (amniotic fluid) (blood clot) (fat) (pulmonary) (septic) (soap) O04.7
   inevitable O03.4
   missed O02.1
   spontaneous — *see* Abortion (complete) (spontaneous)
      threatened O20.0
   threatened (spontaneous) O20.0
   tubal O00.10- ☑
      with intrauterine pregnancy O00.11- ☑
Abortus fever A23.1
Aboulomania F60.7
Abrami's disease D59.8
Abramov-Fiedler myocarditis (acute isolated myocarditis) I40.1
Abrasion T14.8 ☑
   abdomen, abdominal (wall) S30.811 ☑
   alveolar process S00.512 ☑
   ankle S90.51- ☑
   antecubital space — *see* Abrasion, elbow
   anus S30.817 ☑

Abscess — *continued*
cartilage — *see* Disorder, cartilage, specified type NEC
cecum K35.33
cerebellum, cerebellar G06.0
  sequelae G09
cerebral (embolic) G06.0
  sequelae G09
cervical (meaning neck) L02.11
  lymph gland or node L04.0
cervix (stump) (uteri) — *see* Cervicitis
cheek (external) L02.01
  inner K12.2
chest J86.9
  with fistula J86.0
  wall L02.213
chin L02.01
choroid — *see* Inflammation, chorioretinal
circumtonsillar J36
cold (lung) (tuberculous) — *see also* Tuberculosis, abscess, lung
  articular — *see* Tuberculosis, joint
colon (wall) K63.0
colostomy K94.02
conjunctiva — *see* Conjunctivitis, acute
cornea H16.31- ☑
corpus
  cavernosum N48.21
  luteum — *see* Oophoritis
Cowper's gland N34.0
cranium G06.0
cul-de-sac (Douglas') (posterior) — *see* Peritonitis, pelvic, female
cutaneous — *see* Abscess, by site
dental K04.7
  with sinus (alveolar) K04.6
dentoalveolar K04.7
  with sinus K04.6
diaphragm, diaphragmatic K65.1
Douglas' cul-de-sac or pouch — *see* Peritonitis, pelvic, female
Dubois A50.59
ear (middle) — *see also* Otitis, media, suppurative
  acute — *see* Otitis, media, suppurative, acute
  external H60.0- ☑
entamebic — *see* Abscess, amebic
enterostomy K94.12
epididymis N45.4
epidural G06.2
  brain G06.0
  spinal cord G06.1
epiglottis J38.7
epiploon, epiploic K65.1
erysipelatous — *see* Erysipelas
esophagus K20.80
ethmoid (bone) (chronic) (sinus) J32.2
external auditory canal — *see* Abscess, ear, external
extradural G06.2
  brain G06.0
    sequelae G09
  spinal cord G06.1
extraperitoneal K68.19
eye — *see* Endophthalmitis, purulent
eyelid H00.03- ☑
face (any part, except ear, eye and nose) L02.01
fallopian tube — *see* Salpingitis
fascia M72.8
fauces J39.1
fecal K63.0
femoral (region) — *see* Abscess, lower limb
filaria, filarial — *see* Infestation, filarial
finger (any) — *see also* Abscess, hand
  nail — *see* Cellulitis, finger
foot L02.61- ☑
forehead L02.01
frontal sinus (chronic) J32.1
gallbladder K81.0
genital organ or tract
  female (external) N76.4
  male N49.9
    multiple sites N49.8
    specified NEC N49.8
gestational mammary O91.11- ☑
gestational subareolar O91.11- ☑
gingival
  aggressive K05.20
    generalized K05.229
      moderate K05.222
      severe K05.223

Abscess — *continued*
gingival — *continued*
  aggressive — *continued*
    generalized — *continued*
      slight K05.221
    localized K05.219
      moderate K05.212
      severe K05.213
      slight K05.211
gland, glandular (lymph) (acute) — *see* Lymphadenitis, acute
gluteal (region) L02.31
gonorrheal — *see* Gonococcus
groin L02.214
gum
  aggressive K05.20
    generalized K05.229
      moderate K05.222
      severe K05.223
      slight K05.221
    localized K05.219
      moderate K05.212
      severe K05.213
      slight K05.211
hand L02.51- ☑
head NEC L02.811
  face (any part, except ear, eye and nose) L02.01
heart — *see* Carditis
heel — *see* Abscess, foot
helminthic — *see* Infestation, helminth
hepatic (cholangitic) (hematogenic) (lymphogenic) (pylephlebitic) K75.0
  amebic A06.4
hip (region) — *see* Abscess, lower limb
horseshoe K61.31
ileocecal K35.33
ileostomy (bud) K94.12
iliac (region) L02.214
  fossa K35.33
infraclavicular (fossa) — *see* Abscess, upper limb
inguinal (region) L02.214
  lymph gland or node L04.1
intersphincteric K61.4
intestine, intestinal NEC K63.0
  rectal K61.1
intra-abdominal — *see also* Abscess, peritoneum K65.1
  following procedure T81.43 ☑
    obstetrical O86.03
  postprocedural T81.43 ☑
    retroperitoneal K68.11
intracranial G06.0
intramammary — *see* Abscess, breast
intramuscular, following procedure T81.42 ☑
  obstetrical O86.02
intraorbital — *see* Abscess, orbit
intraperitoneal K65.1
intrasphincteric (anus) K61.4
intraspinal G06.1
intratonsillar J36
ischiorectal (fossa) (specified NEC) K61.39
jaw (bone) (lower) (upper) M27.2
joint — *see* Arthritis, pyogenic or pyemic
  spine (tuberculous) A18.01
    nontuberculous — *see* Spondylopathy, infective
kidney N15.1
  with calculus N20.0
    with hydronephrosis N13.6
  puerperal (postpartum) O86.21
knee — *see also* Abscess, lower limb
  joint M00.9
labium (majus) (minus) N76.4
lacrimal
  caruncle — *see* Inflammation, lacrimal, passages, acute
  gland — *see* Dacryoadenitis
  passages (duct) (sac) — *see* Inflammation, lacrimal, passages, acute
lacunar N34.0
larynx J38.7
lateral (alveolar) K04.7
  with sinus K04.6
leg (any part) — *see* Abscess, lower limb
lens H27.8
lingual K14.0
  tonsil J36
lip K13.0
Littre's gland N34.0

Abscess — *continued*
liver (cholangitic) (hematogenic) (lymphogenic) (pyle-phlebitic) (pyogenic) K75.0
  amebic (due to Entamoeba histolytica) (dysenteric) (tropical) A06.4
    with
      brain abscess (and liver or lung abscess) A06.6
      lung abscess A06.5
loin (region) L02.211
lower limb L02.41- ☑
lumbar (tuberculous) A18.01
  nontuberculous L02.212
lung (miliary) (putrid) J85.2
  with pneumonia J85.1
    due to specified organism (see Pneumonia, in (due to))
  amebic (with liver abscess) A06.5
    with
      brain abscess A06.6
      pneumonia A06.5
lymph, lymphatic, gland or node (acute) — *see also* Lymphadenitis, acute
  mesentery I88.0
malar M27.2
mammary gland — *see* Abscess, breast
marginal, anus K61.0
mastoid — *see* Mastoiditis, acute
maxilla, maxillary M27.2
  molar (tooth) K04.7
    with sinus K04.6
  premolar K04.7
  sinus (chronic) J32.0
mediastinum J85.3
meibomian gland — *see* Hordeolum
meninges G06.2
mesentery, mesenteric K65.1
mesosalpinx — *see* Salpingitis
mons pubis L02.215
mouth (floor) K12.2
muscle — *see* Myositis, infective
myocardium I40.0
nabothian (follicle) — *see* Cervicitis
nasal J32.9
nasopharyngeal J39.1
navel L02.216
  newborn P38.9
    with mild hemorrhage P38.1
    without hemorrhage P38.9
neck (region) L02.11
  lymph gland or node L04.0
nephritic — *see* Abscess, kidney
nipple N61.1
  associated with
    lactation — *see* Pregnancy, complicated by
    pregnancy — *see* Pregnancy, complicated by
nose (external) (fossa) (septum) J34.0
  sinus (chronic) — *see* Sinusitis
omentum K65.1
operative wound T81.49 ☑
orbit, orbital — *see* Cellulitis, orbit
otogenic G06.0
ovary, ovarian (corpus luteum) — *see* Oophoritis
oviduct — *see* Oophoritis
palate (soft) K12.2
  hard M27.2
palmar (space) — *see* Abscess, hand
pancreas (duct) — *see* Pancreatitis, acute
parafrenal N48.21
parametric, parametrium N73.2
  acute N73.0
  chronic N73.1
paranephric N15.1
parapancreatic — *see* Pancreatitis, acute
parapharyngeal J39.0
pararectal K61.1
parasinus — *see* Sinusitis
parauterine — *see also* Disease, pelvis, inflammatory N73.2
paravaginal — *see* Vaginitis
parietal region (scalp) L02.811
parodontal — *see* Periodontitis, aggressive, localized
parotid (duct) (gland) K11.3
  region K12.2
pectoral (region) L02.213
pelvis, pelvic
  female — *see* Disease, pelvis, inflammatory
  male, peritoneal K65.1
penis N48.21

Abscess — *continued*
penis — *continued*
gonococcal (accessory gland) (periurethral) A54.1
perianal K61.0
periapical K04.7
with sinus (alveolar) K04.6
periappendicular K35.33
pericardial I30.1
pericecal K35.33
pericemental — *see* Periodontitis, aggressive, localized
pericholecystic — *see* Cholecystitis, acute
pericoronal — *see* Periodontitis, aggressive, localized
peridental — *see* Periodontitis, aggressive, localized
perimetric — *see also* Disease, pelvis, inflammatory
N73.2
perinephric, perinephritic — *see* Abscess, kidney
perineum, perineal (superficial) L02.215
urethra N34.0
periodontal (parietal) — *see* Periodontitis, aggressive,
localized
apical K04.7
periosteum, periosteal — *see also* Osteomyelitis,
specified type NEC
with osteomyelitis — *see also* Osteomyelitis, specified type NEC
acute — *see* Osteomyelitis, acute
chronic — *see* Osteomyelitis, chronic
peripharyngeal J39.0
peripleuritic J86.9
with fistula J86.0
periprostatic N41.2
perirectal K61.1
perirenal (tissue) — *see* Abscess, kidney
perisinuous (nose) — *see* Sinusitis
peritoneum, peritoneal (perforated) (ruptured) K65.1
with appendicitis — *see also* Appendicitis K35.33
pelvic
female — *see* Peritonitis, pelvic, female
male K65.1
postoperative T81.43 ☑
puerperal, postpartum, childbirth O85
tuberculous A18.31
peritonsillar J36
perityphlic K35.33
periureteral N28.89
periurethral N34.0
gonococcal (accessory gland) (periurethral) A54.1
periuterine — *see also* Disease, pelvis, inflammatory
N73.2
perivesical — *see* Cystitis, specified type NEC
petrous bone — *see* Petrositis
phagedenic NOS L02.91
chancroid A57
pharynx, pharyngeal (lateral) J39.1
pilonidal L05.01
pituitary (gland) E23.6
pleura J86.9
with fistula J86.0
popliteal — *see* Abscess, lower limb
postcecal K35.33
postlaryngeal J38.7
postnasal J34.0
postoperative (any site) — *see also* Infection, postoperative wound T81.49 ☑
retroperitoneal K68.11
postpharyngeal J39.0
posttonsillar J36
post-typhoid A01.09
pouch of Douglas — *see* Peritonitis, pelvic, female
premammary — *see* Abscess, breast
prepatellar — *see* Abscess, lower limb
presacral K68.19
prostate N41.2
gonococcal (acute) (chronic) A54.22
psoas muscle K68.12
puerperal — *code by* site under Puerperal, abscess
pulmonary — *see* Abscess, lung
pulp, pulpal (dental) K04.01
irreversible K04.02
reversible K04.01
rectovaginal septum K63.0
rectovesical — *see* Cystitis, specified type NEC
rectum K61.1
renal — *see* Abscess, kidney
retina — *see* Inflammation, chorioretinal
retrobulbar — *see* Abscess, orbit
retrocecal K65.1
retrolaryngeal J38.7

Abscess — *continued*
retromammary — *see* Abscess, breast
retroperitoneal NEC K68.19
postprocedural K68.11
retropharyngeal J39.0
retrouterine — *see* Peritonitis, pelvic, female
retrovesical — *see* Cystitis, specified type NEC
root, tooth K04.7
with sinus (alveolar) K04.6
round ligament — *see also* Disease, pelvis, inflammatory N73.2
rupture (spontaneous) NOS L02.91
sacrum (tuberculous) A18.01
nontuberculous M46.28
salivary (duct) (gland) K11.3
scalp (any part) L02.811
scapular — *see* Osteomyelitis, specified type NEC
sclera — *see* Scleritis
scrofulous (tuberculous) A18.2
scrotum N49.2
seminal vesicle N49.0
septal, dental K04.7
with sinus (alveolar) K04.6
serous — *see* Periostitis
shoulder (region) — *see* Abscess, upper limb
sigmoid K63.0
sinus (accessory) (chronic) (nasal) — *see also* Sinusitis
intracranial venous (any) G06.0
Skene's duct or gland N34.0
skin — *see* Abscess, by site
specified site NEC L02.818
spermatic cord N49.1
sphenoidal (sinus) (chronic) J32.3
spinal cord (any part) (staphylococcal) G06.1
tuberculous A17.81
spine (column) (tuberculous) A18.01
epidural G06.1
nontuberculous — *see* Osteomyelitis, vertebra
spleen D73.3
amebic A06.89
stitch T81.41
following an obstetrical procedure O86.01
subarachnoid G06.2
brain G06.0
spinal cord G06.1
subareolar — *see* Abscess, breast
subcecal K35.33
subcutaneous — *see also* Abscess, by site
following procedure T81.41 ☑
obstetrical O86.01
pheomycotic (chromomycotic) B43.2
subdiaphragmatic K65.1
subdural G06.2
brain G06.0
sequelae G09
spinal cord G06.1
sub-fascial, following an obstetrical procedure O86.02
subgaleal L02.811
subhepatic K65.1
sublingual K12.2
gland K11.3
submammary — *see* Abscess, breast
submandibular (region) (space) (triangle) K12.2
gland K11.3
submaxillary (region) L02.01
gland K11.3
submental L02.01
gland K11.3
subperiosteal — *see* Osteomyelitis, specified type NEC
subphrenic K65.1
following an obstetrical procedure O86.03
postoperative T81.43 ☑
suburethral N34.0
sudoriparous L75.8
supraclavicular (fossa) — *see* Abscess, upper limb
supralevator K61.5
suprapelvic, acute N73.0
suprarenal (capsule) (gland) E27.8
sweat gland L74.8
tear duct — *see* Inflammation, lacrimal, passages, acute
temple L02.01
temporal region L02.01
temporosphenoidal G06.0
tendon (sheath) M65.00
ankle M65.07- ☑
foot M65.07- ☑
forearm M65.03- ☑
hand M65.04- ☑

Abscess — *continued*
tendon — *continued*
lower leg M65.06- ☑
pelvic region M65.05- ☑
shoulder region M65.01- ☑
specified site NEC M65.08
thigh M65.05- ☑
upper arm M65.02- ☑
testis N45.4
thigh — *see* Abscess, lower limb
thorax J86.9
with fistula J86.0
throat J39.1
thumb — *see also* Abscess, hand
nail — *see* Cellulitis, finger
thymus (gland) E32.1
thyroid (gland) E06.0
toe (any) — *see also* Abscess, foot
nail — *see* Cellulitis, toe
tongue (staphylococcal) K14.0
tonsil(s) (lingual) J36
tonsillopharyngeal J36
tooth, teeth (root) K04.7
with sinus (alveolar) K04.6
supporting structures NEC — *see* Periodontitis, aggressive, localized
trachea J39.8
trunk L02.219
abdominal wall L02.211
back L02.212
chest wall L02.213
groin L02.214
perineum L02.215
umbilicus L02.216
tubal — *see* Salpingitis
tuberculous — *see* Tuberculosis, abscess
tubo-ovarian — *see* Salpingo-oophoritis
tunica vaginalis N49.1
umbilicus L02.216
upper
limb L02.41- ☑
respiratory J39.8
urethral (gland) N34.0
urinary N34.0
uterus, uterine (wall) — *see also* Endometritis
ligament — *see also* Disease, pelvis, inflammatory
N73.2
neck — *see* Cervicitis
uvula K12.2
vagina (wall) — *see* Vaginitis
vaginorectal — *see* Vaginitis
vas deferens N49.1
vermiform appendix K35.33
vertebra (column) (tuberculous) A18.01
nontuberculous — *see* Osteomyelitis, vertebra
vesical — *see* Cystitis, specified type NEC
vesico-uterine pouch — *see* Peritonitis, pelvic, female
vitreous (humor) — *see* Endophthalmitis, purulent
vocal cord J38.3
von Bezold's — *see* Mastoiditis, acute
vulva N76.4
vulvovaginal gland N75.1
web space — *see* Abscess, hand
wound T81.49 ☑
wrist — *see* Abscess, upper limb
Absence (of) (organ or part) (complete or partial)
adrenal (gland) (congenital) Q89.1
acquired E89.6
albumin in blood E88.09
alimentary tract (congenital) Q45.8
upper Q40.8
alveolar process (acquired) — *see* Anomaly, alveolar
ankle (acquired) Z89.44- ☑
anus (congenital) Q42.3
with fistula Q42.2
aorta (congenital) Q25.41
appendix, congenital Q42.8
arm (acquired) Z89.20- ☑
above elbow Z89.22- ☑
congenital (with hand present) — *see* Agenesis,
arm, with hand present
and hand — *see* Agenesis, forearm, and hand
below elbow Z89.21- ☑
congenital (with hand present) — *see* Agenesis,
arm, with hand present
and hand — *see* Agenesis, forearm, and hand
congenital — *see* Defect, reduction, upper limb

Absence — *continued*
  arm — *continued*
    shoulder (following explanatation of shoulder joint prosthesis) (joint) (with or without presence of antibiotic-impregnated cement spacer) Z89.23- ☑
      congenital (with hand present) — *see* Agenesis, arm, with hand present
  artery (congenital) (peripheral) Q27.8
    brain Q28.3
    coronary Q24.5
    pulmonary Q25.79
    specified NEC Q27.8
    umbilical Q27.0
  atrial septum (congenital) Q21.19
  auditory canal (congenital) (external) Q16.1
  auricle (ear), congenital Q16.0
  bile, biliary duct, congenital Q44.5
  bladder (acquired) Z90.6
    congenital Q64.5
  bowel sounds R19.11
  brain Q00.0
    part of Q04.3
  breast(s) (and nipple(s)) (acquired) Z90.1- ☑
    congenital Q83.8
  broad ligament Q50.6
  bronchus (congenital) Q32.4
  canaliculus lacrimalis, congenital Q10.4
  cerebellum (vermis), congenital Q04.3
  cervix (acquired) (with uterus) Z90.710
    with remaining uterus Z90.712
    congenital Q51.5
  chin, congenital Q18.8
  cilia (congenital) Q10.3
    acquired — *see* Madarosis
  clitoris (congenital) Q52.6
  coccyx, congenital Q76.49
  cold sense R20.8
  congenital
    lumen — *see* Atresia
    organ or site NEC — *see* Agenesis
    septum — *see* Imperfect, closure
  corpus callosum Q04.0
  cricoid cartilage, congenital Q31.8
  diaphragm (with hernia), congenital Q79.1
  digestive organ(s) or tract, congenital Q45.8
    acquired NEC Z90.49
    upper Q40.8
  ductus arteriosus Q28.8
  duodenum (acquired) Z90.49
    congenital Q41.0
  ear, congenital Q16.9
    acquired H93.8- ☑
    auricle Q16.0
    external Q16.0
    inner Q16.5
    lobe, lobule Q17.8
    middle, except ossicles Q16.4
      ossicles Q16.3
    ossicles Q16.3
  ejaculatory duct (congenital) Q55.4
  endocrine gland (congenital) NEC Q89.2
    acquired E89.89
  epididymis (congenital) Q55.4
    acquired Z90.79
  epiglottis, congenital Q31.8
  esophagus (congenital) Q39.8
    acquired (partial) Z90.49
  eustachian tube (congenital) Q16.2
  extremity (acquired) Z89.9
    congenital Q73.8
    knee (following explantation of knee joint prosthesis) (joint) (with or without presence of antibiotic-impregnated cement spacer) Z89.52- ☑
    lower (above knee) Z89.619
      below knee Z89.51- ☑
    upper — *see* Absence, arm
  eye (acquired) Z90.01
    congenital Q11.1
    muscle (congenital) Q10.3
  eyeball (acquired) Z90.01
  eyelid (fold) (congenital) Q10.3
    acquired Z90.01
  face, specified part NEC Q18.8
  fallopian tube(s) (acquired) Z90.79
    congenital Q50.6
  family member (causing problem in home) NEC — *see also* Disruption, family Z63.32

Absence — *continued*
  femur, congenital — *see* Defect, reduction, lower limb, longitudinal, femur
  fibrinogen (congenital) D68.2
    acquired D65
  finger(s) (acquired) Z89.02- ☑
    congenital — *see* Agenesis, hand
  foot (acquired) Z89.43- ☑
    congenital — *see* Agenesis, foot
  forearm (acquired) — *see* Absence, arm, below elbow
  gallbladder (acquired) Z90.49
    congenital Q44.0
  gamma globulin in blood D80.1
    hereditary D80.0
  genital organs
    acquired (female) (male) Z90.79
    female, congenital Q52.8
      external Q52.71
      internal NEC Q52.8
    male, congenital Q55.8
  genitourinary organs, congenital NEC
    female Q52.8
    male Q55.8
  globe (acquired) Z90.01
    congenital Q11.1
  glottis, congenital Q31.8
  hand and wrist (acquired) Z89.11- ☑
    congenital — *see* Agenesis, hand
  head, part (acquired) NEC Z90.09
  heat sense R20.8
  hip (following explanation of hip joint prosthesis) (joint) (with or without presence of antibiotic-impregnated cement spacer) Z89.62- ☑
  hymen (congenital) Q52.4
  ileum (acquired) Z90.49
    congenital Q41.2
  immunoglobulin, isolated NEC D80.3
    IgA D80.2
    IgG D80.3
    IgM D80.4
  incus (acquired) — *see* Loss, ossicles, ear
    congenital Q16.3
  inner ear, congenital Q16.5
  intestine (acquired) (small) Z90.49
    congenital Q41.9
      specified NEC Q41.8
    large Z90.49
      congenital Q42.9
        specified NEC Q42.8
  iris, congenital Q13.1
  jejunum (acquired) Z90.49
    congenital Q41.1
  joint
    acquired
      hip (following explantation of hip joint prosthesis) (with or without presence of antibiotic-impregnated cement spacer) Z89.62- ☑
      knee (following explantation of knee joint prosthesis) (with or without presence of antibiotic-impregnated cement spacer) Z89.52- ☑
      shoulder (following explantation of shoulder joint prosthesis) (with or without presence of antibiotic-impregnated cement spacer) Z89.23- ☑
    congenital NEC Q74.8
  kidney(s) (acquired) Z90.5
    congenital Q60.2
      bilateral Q60.1
      unilateral Q60.0
  knee (following explantation of knee joint prosthesis) (joint) (with or without presence of antibiotic-impregnated cement spacer) Z89.52- ☑
  labyrinth, membranous Q16.5
  larynx (congenital) Q31.8
    acquired Z90.02
  leg (acquired) (above knee) Z89.61- ☑
    below knee (acquired) Z89.51- ☑
    congenital — *see* Defect, reduction, lower limb
  lens (acquired) — *see also* Aphakia
    congenital Q12.3
    post cataract extraction Z98.4- ☑
  limb (acquired) — *see* Absence, extremity
  lip Q38.6
  liver (congenital) Q44.7
  lung (fissure) (lobe) (bilateral) (unilateral) (congenital) Q33.3
    acquired (any part) Z90.2

Absence — *continued*
  menstruation — *see* Amenorrhea
  muscle (congenital) (pectoral) Q79.8
    ocular Q10.3
  neck, part Q18.8
  neutrophil — *see* Agranulocytosis
  nipple(s) (with breast(s)) (acquired) Z90.1- ☑
    congenital Q83.2
  nose (congenital) Q30.1
    acquired Z90.09
  organ
    of Corti, congenital Q16.5
    or site, congenital NEC Q89.8
      acquired NEC Z90.89
  osseous meatus (ear) Q16.4
  ovary
    bilateral Z90.722
    congenital
      bilateral Q50.02
      unilateral Q50.01
    unilateral Z90.721
  oviduct (acquired)
    bilateral Z90.722
    congenital Q50.6
    unilateral Z90.721
  pancreas (congenital) Q45.0
    acquired Z90.410
      complete Z90.410
      partial Z90.411
      total Z90.410
  parathyroid gland (acquired) E89.2
    congenital Q89.2
  patella, congenital Q74.1
  penis (congenital) Q55.5
    acquired Z90.79
  pericardium (congenital) Q24.8
  pituitary gland (congenital) Q89.2
    acquired E89.3
  prostate (acquired) Z90.79
    congenital Q55.4
  pulmonary valve Q22.0
  punctum lacrimale (congenital) Q10.4
  radius, congenital — *see* Defect, reduction, upper limb, longitudinal, radius
  rectum (congenital) Q42.1
    with fistula Q42.0
    acquired Z90.49
  respiratory organ NOS Q34.9
  rib (acquired) Z90.89
    congenital Q76.6
  sacrum, congenital Q76.49
  salivary gland(s), congenital Q38.4
  scrotum, congenital Q55.29
  seminal vesicles (congenital) Q55.4
    acquired Z90.79
  septum
    atrial (congenital) Q21.19
    between aorta and pulmonary artery Q21.4
    ventricular (congenital) Q20.4
  sex chromosome
    female phenotype Q97.8
    male phenotype Q98.8
  skull bone (congenital) Q75.8
    with
      anencephaly Q00.0
      encephalocele — *see* Encephalocele
      hydrocephalus Q03.9
        with spina bifida — *see* Spina bifida, by site, with hydrocephalus
      microcephaly Q02
  spermatic cord, congenital Q55.4
  spine, congenital Q76.49
  spleen (congenital) Q89.01
    acquired Z90.81
  sternum, congenital Q76.7
  stomach (acquired) (partial) Z90.3
    congenital Q40.2
  superior vena cava, congenital Q26.8
  teeth, tooth (congenital) K00.0
    acquired (complete) K08.109
      class I K08.101
      class II K08.102
      class III K08.103
      class IV K08.104
      due to
        caries K08.139
          class I K08.131
          class II K08.132
          class III K08.133

Index

Absence — Abuse

Absence — *continued*
  teeth, tooth — *continued*
    acquired — *continued*
      due to — *continued*
        caries — *continued*
          class IV K08.134
          periodontal disease K08.129
            class I K08.121
            class II K08.122
            class III K08.123
            class IV K08.124
          specified NEC K08.199
            class I K08.191
            class II K08.192
            class III K08.193
            class IV K08.194
          trauma K08.119
            class I K08.111
            class II K08.112
            class III K08.113
            class IV K08.114
      partial K08.409
        class I K08.401
        class II K08.402
        class III K08.403
        class IV K08.404
        due to
          caries K08.439
            class I K08.431
            class II K08.432
            class III K08.433
            class IV K08.434
          periodontal disease K08.429
            class I K08.421
            class II K08.422
            class III K08.423
            class IV K08.424
          specified NEC K08.499
            class I K08.491
            class II K08.492
            class III K08.493
            class IV K08.494
          trauma K08.419
            class I K08.411
            class II K08.412
            class III K08.413
            class IV K08.414
  tendon (congenital) Q79.8
  testis (congenital) Q55.0
    acquired Z90.79
  thumb (acquired) Z89.01- ☑
    congenital — *see* Agenesis, hand
  thymus gland Q89.2
  thyroid (gland) (acquired) E89.0
    cartilage, congenital Q31.8
    congenital E03.1
  toe(s) (acquired) Z89.42- ☑
    with foot — *see* Absence, foot and ankle
    congenital — *see* Agenesis, foot
    great Z89.41- ☑
  tongue, congenital Q38.3
  trachea (cartilage), congenital Q32.1
  transverse aortic arch, congenital Q25.49
  tricuspid valve Q22.4
  umbilical artery, congenital Q27.0
  upper arm and forearm with hand present, congenital
    — *see* Agenesis, arm, with hand present
  ureter (congenital) Q62.4
    acquired Z90.6
  urethra, congenital Q64.5
  uterus (acquired) Z90.710
    with cervix Z90.710
    with remaining cervical stump Z90.711
    congenital Q51.0
  uvula, congenital Q38.5
  vagina, congenital Q52.0
  vas deferens (congenital) Q55.4
    acquired Z90.79
  vein (peripheral) congenital NEC Q27.8
    cerebral Q28.3
    digestive system Q27.8
    great Q26.8
    lower limb Q27.8
    portal Q26.5
    precerebral Q28.1
    specified site NEC Q27.8
    upper limb Q27.8
  vena cava (inferior) (superior), congenital Q26.8

Absence — *continued*
  ventricular septum Q20.4
  vertebra, congenital Q76.49
  von Willebrand factor, complete (near) — *see also*
    Disease, von Willebrand D68.03
  vulva, congenital Q52.71
  wrist (acquired) Z89.12- ☑
Absorbent system disease I87.8
Absorption
  carbohydrate, disturbance K90.49
  chemical — *see* Table of Drugs and Chemicals
    through placenta (newborn) P04.9
      environmental substance P04.6
      nutritional substance P04.5
      obstetric anesthetic or analgesic drug P04.0
  drug NEC — *see* Table of Drugs and Chemicals
    addictive
      through placenta (newborn) — *see also* New-
        born, affected by, maternal, use of P04.40
        cocaine P04.41
        hallucinogens P04.42
        specified drug NEC P04.49
    medicinal
      through placenta (newborn) P04.19
    through placenta (newborn) P04.19
      obstetric anesthetic or analgesic drug P04.0
  fat, disturbance K90.49
    pancreatic K90.3
  noxious substance — *see* Table of Drugs and Chemicals
  protein, disturbance K90.49
  starch, disturbance K90.49
  toxic substance — *see* Table of Drugs and Chemicals
  uremic — *see* Uremia
Abstinence symptoms, syndrome
  alcohol F10.239
    with delirium F10.231
  cocaine F14.23
  neonatal P96.1
  nicotine — *see* Dependence, drug, nicotine, with,
    withdrawal
  opioid F11.93
    with dependence F11.23
  psychoactive NEC F19.939
    with
      delirium F19.931
      dependence F19.239
        with
          delirium F19.231
          perceptual disturbance F19.232
          uncomplicated F19.230
      perceptual disturbance F19.932
    uncomplicated F19.930
  sedative F13.939
    with
      delirium F13.931
      dependence F13.239
        with
          delirium F13.231
          perceptual disturbance F13.232
          uncomplicated F13.230
      perceptual disturbance F13.932
    uncomplicated F13.930
  stimulant NEC F15.93
    with dependence F15.23
Abulia R68.89
Abulomania F60.7
Abuse
  adult — *see* Maltreatment, adult
    as reason for
      couple seeking advice (including offender) Z63.0
  alcohol (non-dependent) F10.10
    with
      anxiety disorder F10.180
      intoxication F10.129
        with delirium F10.121
        uncomplicated F10.120
      mood disorder F10.14
      other specified disorder F10.188
      psychosis F10.159
        delusions F10.150
        hallucinations F10.151
      sexual dysfunction F10.181
      sleep disorder F10.182
      unspecified disorder F10.19
      withdrawal F10.139
        with
          perceptual disturbance F10.132
          delirium F10.131

Abuse — *continued*
  alcohol — *continued*
    with — *continued*
      withdrawal — *continued*
        uncomplicated F10.130
    counseling and surveillance Z71.41
    in remission (early) (sustained) F10.11
  amphetamine (or related substance) — *see also* Abuse,
    drug, stimulant NEC
    stimulant NEC F15.10
      with
        anxiety disorder F15.180
        intoxication F15.129
          with
            delirium F15.121
            perceptual disturbance F15.122
        withdrawal F15.13
  analgesics (non-prescribed) (over the counter) F55.8
  antacids F55.0
  antidepressants — *see* Abuse, drug, psychoactive NEC
  anxiolytic — *see* Abuse, drug, sedative
  barbiturates — *see* Abuse, drug, sedative
  caffeine — *see* Abuse, drug, stimulant NEC
  cannabis, cannabinoids — *see* Abuse, drug, cannabis
  child — *see* Maltreatment, child
  cocaine — *see* Abuse, drug, cocaine
  drug NEC (non-dependent) F19.10
    with sleep disorder F19.182
    amphetamine type — *see* Abuse, drug, stimulant
      NEC
    analgesics (non-prescribed) (over the counter) F55.8
    antacids F55.0
    antidepressants — *see* Abuse, drug, psychoactive
      NEC
    anxiolytics — *see* Abuse, drug, sedative
    barbiturates — *see* Abuse, drug, sedative
    caffeine — *see* Abuse, drug, stimulant NEC
    cannabis F12.10
      with
        anxiety disorder F12.180
        intoxication F12.129
          with
            delirium F12.121
            perceptual disturbance F12.122
          uncomplicated F12.120
        other specified disorder F12.188
        psychosis F12.159
          delusions F12.150
          hallucinations F12.151
        unspecified disorder F12.19
        withdrawal F12.13
      in remission (early) (sustained) F12.11
    cocaine F14.10
      with
        anxiety disorder F14.180
        intoxication F14.129
          with
            delirium F14.121
            perceptual disturbance F14.122
          uncomplicated F14.120
        mood disorder F14.14
        other specified disorder F14.188
        psychosis F14.159
          delusions F14.150
          hallucinations F14.151
        sexual dysfunction F14.181
        sleep disorder F14.182
        unspecified disorder F14.19
        withdrawal F14.13
      in remission (early) (sustained) F14.11
    counseling and surveillance Z71.51
    hallucinogen F16.10
      with
        anxiety disorder F16.180
        flashbacks F16.183
        intoxication F16.129
          with
            delirium F16.121
            perceptual disturbance F16.122
          uncomplicated F16.120
        mood disorder F16.14
        other specified disorder F16.188
        perception disorder, persisting F16.183
        psychosis F16.159
          delusions F16.150
          hallucinations F16.151
        unspecified disorder F16.19
      in remission (early) (sustained) F16.11

☑ **Additional Character Required** — **Refer to the Tabular List for Character Selection**

Abuse — *continued*
  drug — *continued*
    hashish — *see* Abuse, drug, cannabis
    herbal or folk remedies F55.1
    hormones F55.3
    hypnotics — *see* Abuse, drug, sedative
    in remission (early) (sustained) F19.11
    inhalant F18.10
      with
        anxiety disorder F18.180
        dementia, persisting F18.17
        intoxication F18.129
          with delirium F18.121
          uncomplicated F18.120
        mood disorder F18.14
        other specified disorder F18.188
        psychosis F18.159
          delusions F18.150
          hallucinations F18.151
        unspecified disorder F18.19
      in remission (early) (sustained) F18.11
    laxatives F55.2
    LSD — *see* Abuse, drug, hallucinogen
    marihuana — *see* Abuse, drug, cannabis
    morphine type (opioids) — *see* Abuse, drug, opioid
    opioid F11.10
      with
        intoxication F11.129
          with
            delirium F11.121
            perceptual disturbance F11.122
          uncomplicated F11.120
        mood disorder F11.14
        other specified disorder F11.188
        psychosis F11.159
          delusions F11.150
          hallucinations F11.151
        sexual dysfunction F11.181
        sleep disorder F11.182
        unspecified disorder F11.19
        withdrawal F11.13
      in remission (early) (sustained) F11.11
    PCP (phencyclidine) (or related substance) — *see*
      Abuse, drug, hallucinogen
    psychoactive NEC F19.10
      with
        amnestic disorder F19.16
        anxiety disorder F19.180
        dementia F19.17
        intoxication F19.129
          with
            delirium F19.121
            perceptual disturbance F19.122
          uncomplicated F19.120
        mood disorder F19.14
        other specified disorder F19.188
        psychosis F19.159
          delusions F19.150
          hallucinations F19.151
        sexual dysfunction F19.181
        sleep disorder F19.182
        unspecified disorder F19.19
        withdrawal F19.139
          with
            perceptual disturbance F19.132
          delirium F19.131
          uncomplicated F19.130
    sedative, hypnotic or anxiolytic F13.10
      with
        anxiety disorder F13.180
        intoxication F13.129
          with delirium F13.121
          uncomplicated F13.120
        mood disorder F13.14
        other specified disorder F13.188
        psychosis F13.159
          delusions F13.150
          hallucinations F13.151
        sexual dysfunction F13.181
        sleep disorder F13.182
        unspecified disorder F13.19
        withdrawal F13.139
          with
            perceptual disturbance F13.132
          delirium F13.131
          uncomplicated F13.130
      in remission (early) (sustained) F13.11
    solvent — *see* Abuse, drug, inhalant

Abuse — *continued*
  drug — *continued*
    steroids F55.3
    stimulant NEC F15.10
      with
        anxiety disorder F15.180
        intoxication F15.129
          with
            delirium F15.121
            perceptual disturbance F15.122
          uncomplicated F15.120
        mood disorder F15.14
        other specified disorder F15.188
        psychosis F15.159
          delusions F15.150
          hallucinations F15.151
        sexual dysfunction F15.181
        sleep disorder F15.182
        unspecified disorder F15.19
        withdrawal F15.13
      in remission (early) (sustained) F15.11
    tranquilizers — *see* Abuse, drug, sedative
    vitamins F55.4
  hallucinogens — *see* Abuse, drug, hallucinogen
  hashish — *see* Abuse, drug, cannabis
  herbal or folk remedies F55.1
  hormones F55.3
  hypnotic — *see* Abuse, drug, sedative
  inhalant — *see* Abuse, drug, inhalant
  laxatives F55.2
  LSD — *see* Abuse, drug, hallucinogen
  marihuana — *see* Abuse, drug, cannabis
  morphine type (opioids) — *see* Abuse, drug, opioid
  non-psychoactive substance NEC F55.8
    antacids F55.0
    folk remedies F55.1
    herbal remedies F55.1
    hormones F55.3
    laxatives F55.2
    steroids F55.3
    vitamins F55.4
  opioids — *see* Abuse, drug, opioid
  PCP (phencyclidine) (or related substance) — *see*
    Abuse, drug, hallucinogen
  physical (adult) (child) — *see* Maltreatment
  psychoactive substance — *see* Abuse, drug, psychoac-
    tive NEC
  psychological (adult) (child) — *see* Maltreatment
  sedative — *see* Abuse, drug, sedative
  sexual — *see* Maltreatment
  solvent — *see* Abuse, drug, inhalant
  steroids F55.3
  vitamins F55.4
Acalculia R48.8
  developmental F81.2
Acanthamebiasis (with) B60.10
  conjunctiva B60.12
  keratoconjunctivitis B60.13
  meningoencephalitis B60.11
  other specified B60.19
Acanthocephaliasis B83.8
Acanthocheilonemiasis B74.4
Acanthocytosis E78.6
Acantholysis L11.9
Acanthosis (acquired) (nigricans) L83
  benign Q82.8
  congenital Q82.8
  seborrheic L82.1
    inflamed L82.0
  tongue K14.3
Acapnia E87.3
Acarbia E87.29
Acardia, acardius Q89.8
Acardiacus amorphus Q89.8
Acardiotrophia I51.4
Acariasis B88.0
  scabies B86
Acarodermatitis (urticarioides) B88.0
Acarophobia F40.218
Acatalasemia, acatalasia E80.3
Acathisia (drug induced) G25.71
Accelerated atrioventricular conduction I45.6
Accentuation of personality traits (type A) Z73.1
Accessory (congenital)
  adrenal gland Q89.1
  anus Q43.4
  appendix Q43.4
  atrioventricular conduction I45.6

Accessory — *continued*
  auditory ossicles Q16.3
  auricle (ear) Q17.0
  biliary duct or passage Q44.5
  bladder Q64.79
  blood vessels NEC Q27.9
    coronary Q24.5
  bone NEC Q79.8
  breast tissue, axilla Q83.1
  carpal bones Q74.0
  cecum Q43.4
  chromosome(s) NEC (nonsex) Q92.9
    with complex rearrangements NEC Q92.5
      seen only at prometaphase Q92.8
    13 — *see* Trisomy, 13
    18 — *see* Trisomy, 18
    21 — *see* Trisomy, 21
    partial Q92.9
    sex
      female phenotype Q97.8
  coronary artery Q24.5
  cusp(s), heart valve NEC Q24.8
    pulmonary Q22.3
  cystic duct Q44.5
  digit(s) Q69.9
  ear (auricle) (lobe) Q17.0
  endocrine gland NEC Q89.2
  eye muscle Q10.3
  eyelid Q10.3
  face bone(s) Q75.8
  fallopian tube (fimbria) (ostium) Q50.6
  finger(s) Q69.0
  foreskin N47.8
  frontonasal process Q75.8
  gallbladder Q44.1
  genital organ(s)
    female Q52.8
      external Q52.79
      internal NEC Q52.8
    male Q55.8
  genitourinary organs NEC Q89.8
    female Q52.8
    male Q55.8
  hallux Q69.2
  heart Q24.8
    valve NEC Q24.8
      pulmonary Q22.3
  hepatic ducts Q44.5
  hymen Q52.4
  intestine (large) (small) Q43.4
  kidney Q63.0
  lacrimal canal Q10.6
  leaflet, heart valve NEC Q24.8
  ligament, broad Q50.6
  liver Q44.7
    duct Q44.5
  lobule (ear) Q17.0
  lung (lobe) Q33.1
  muscle Q79.8
  navicular of carpus Q74.0
  nervous system, part NEC Q07.8
  nipple Q83.3
  nose Q30.8
  organ or site not listed — *see* Anomaly, by site
  ovary Q50.31
  oviduct Q50.6
  pancreas Q45.3
  parathyroid gland Q89.2
  parotid gland (and duct) Q38.4
  pituitary gland Q89.2
  preauricular appendage Q17.0
  prepuce N47.8
  renal arteries (multiple) Q27.2
  rib Q76.6
    cervical Q76.5
  roots (teeth) K00.2
  salivary gland Q38.4
  sesamoid bones Q74.8
    foot Q74.2
    hand Q74.0
  skin tags Q82.8
  spleen Q89.09
  sternum Q76.7
  submaxillary gland Q38.4
  tarsal bones Q74.2
  teeth, tooth K00.1
  tendon Q79.8
  thumb Q69.1
  thymus gland Q89.2

Accessory — *continued*
　thyroid gland Q89.2
　toes Q69.2
　tongue Q38.3
　tooth, teeth K00.1
　tragus Q17.0
　ureter Q62.5
　urethra Q64.79
　urinary organ or tract NEC Q64.8
　uterus Q51.28
　vagina Q52.10
　valve, heart NEC Q24.8
　　pulmonary Q22.3
　vertebra Q76.49
　vocal cords Q31.8
　vulva Q52.79
Accident
　birth — *see* Birth, injury
　cardiac — *see* Infarct, myocardium
　cerebral I63.9
　cerebrovascular (embolic) (ischemic) (thrombotic) I63.9
　　aborted I63.9
　　hemorrhagic — *see* Hemorrhage, intracranial, intrac-
　　　erebral
　　old (without sequelae) Z86.73
　　　with sequelae (of) — *see* Sequelae, infarction,
　　　　cerebral
　coronary — *see* Infarct, myocardium
　craniovascular I63.9
　vascular, brain I63.9
Accidental — *see* condition
Accommodation (disorder) — *see also* condition
　hysterical paralysis of F44.89
　insufficiency of H52.4
　paresis — *see* Paresis, of accommodation
　spasm — *see* Spasm, of accommodation
Accouchement — *see* Delivery
Accreta placenta O43.21- ☑
Accretio cordis (nonrheumatic) I31.0
Accretions, tooth, teeth K03.6
Acculturation difficulty Z60.3
Accumulation secretion, prostate N42.89
Acephalia, acephalism, acephalus, acephaly Q00.0
Acephalobrachia monster Q89.8
Acephalochirus monster Q89.8
Acephalogaster Q89.8
Acephalostomus monster Q89.8
Acephalothorax Q89.8
Acerophobia F40.298
Acetonemia R79.89
　in Type 1 diabetes E10.10
　　with coma E10.11
Acetonuria R82.4
Achalasia (cardia) (esophagus) K22.0
　congenital Q39.5
　pylorus Q40.0
　sphincteral NEC K59.89
Ache(s) — *see* Pain
Acheilia Q38.6
Achillobursitis — *see* Tendinitis, Achilles
Achillodynia — *see* Tendinitis, Achilles
Achlorhydria, achlorhydric (neurogenic) K31.83
　anemia D50.8
　diarrhea K31.83
　psychogenic F45.8
　secondary to vagotomy K91.1
Achluophobia F40.228
Acholia K82.8
Acholuric jaundice (familial) (splenomegalic) — *see also*
　Spherocytosis
　acquired D59.8
Achondrogenesis Q77.0
Achondroplasia (osteosclerosis congenita) Q77.4
Achroma, cutis L80
Achromat (ism), achromatopsia (acquired) (congenital)
　H53.51
Achromia, congenital — *see* Albinism
Achromia parasitica B36.0
Achylia gastrica K31.89
　psychogenic F45.8
Acid
　burn — *see* Corrosion
　deficiency
　　amide nicotinic E52
　　ascorbic E54
　　folic E53.8
　　nicotinic E52

Acid — *continued*
　deficiency — *continued*
　　pantothenic E53.8
　intoxication — *see also* Acidosis E87.29
　peptic disease K30
　phosphatase deficiency E83.39
　stomach K30
　　psychogenic F45.8
Acidemia — *see also* Acidosis E87.20
　argininosuccinic E72.22
　isovaleric E71.110
　metabolic (newborn) P19.9
　　first noted before onset of labor P19.0
　　first noted during labor P19.1
　　noted at birth P19.2
　methylmalonic E71.120
　pipecolic E72.3
　propionic E71.121
Acidity, gastric (high) K30
　psychogenic F45.8
Acidocytopenia — *see* Agranulocytosis
Acidocytosis D72.10
Acidopenia — *see* Agranulocytosis
Acidosis (lactic) E87.20
　in Type 1 diabetes E10.10
　　with coma E10.11
　kidney, tubular N25.89
　lactic E87.20
　　acute E87.21
　　chronic E87.22
　metabolic NEC E87.20
　　with respiratory acidosis E87.4
　　acute E87.21
　　chronic E87.22
　　hyperchloremic, of newborn P74.421
　　late, of newborn P74.0
　mixed metabolic and respiratory, newborn P84
　newborn P84
　renal (hyperchloremic) (tubular) N25.89
　respiratory E87.29
　　acute J96.02
　　chronic J96.12
　　complicated by
　　　metabolic
　　　　acidosis E87.4
　　　　alkalosis E87.4
　specified NEC E87.29
Aciduria
　4-hydroxybutyric E72.81
　argininosuccinic E72.22
　gamma-hydroxybutyric E72.81
　glutaric (type I) E72.3
　　type II E71.313
　　type III E71.5- ☑
　orotic (congenital) (hereditary) (pyrimidine deficiency)
　　E79.8
　　anemia D53.0
Acladiosis (skin) B36.0
Aclasis, diaphyseal Q78.6
Acleistocardia Q21.19
Aclusion — *see* Anomaly, dentofacial, malocclusion
Acne L70.9
　artificialis L70.8
　atrophica L70.2
　cachecticorum (Hebra) L70.8
　conglobata L70.1
　cystic L70.0
　decalvans L66.2
　excoriée (des jeunes filles) L70.5
　frontalis L70.2
　indurata L70.0
　infantile L70.4
　keloid L73.0
　lupoid L70.2
　necrotic, necrotica (miliaris) L70.2
　neonatal L70.4
　nodular L70.0
　occupational L70.8
　picker's L70.5
　pustular L70.0
　rodens L70.2
　rosacea L71.9
　specified NEC L70.8
　tropica L70.3
　varioliformis L70.2
　vulgaris L70.0
Acnitis (primary) A18.4
Acosta's disease T70.29 ☑

Acoustic — *see* condition
Acousticophobia F40.298
ACPO (acute colonic pseudo-obstruction) K59.81
Acquired — *see also* condition
　immunodeficiency syndrome (AIDS) B20
Acrania Q00.0
Acroangiodermatitis I78.9
Acroasphyxia, chronic I73.89
Acrobystitis N47.7
Acrocephalopolysyndactyly Q87.0
Acrocephalosyndactyly Q87.0
Acrocephaly Q75.0
Acrochondrohyperplasia — *see* Syndrome, Marfan's
Acrocyanosis I73.89
　newborn P28.2
　　meaning transient blue hands and feet — *omit code*
Acrodermatitis L30.8
　atrophicans (chronica) L90.4
　continua (Hallopeau) L40.2
　enteropathica (hereditary) E83.2
　Hallopeau's L40.2
　infantile papular L44.4
　perstans L40.2
　pustulosa continua L40.2
　recalcitrant pustular L40.2
Acrodynia — *see* Poisoning, mercury
Acromegaly, acromegalia E22.0
Acromelalgia I73.81
Acromicria, acromikria Q79.8
Acronyx L60.0
Acropachy, thyroid — *see* Thyrotoxicosis
Acroparesthesia (simple) (vasomotor) I73.89
Acropathy, thyroid — *see* Thyrotoxicosis
Acrophobia F40.241
Acroposthitis N47.7
Acroscleriasis, acroscleroderma, acrosclerosis — *see*
　Sclerosis, systemic
Acrosphacelus I96
Acrospiroma, eccrine — *see* Neoplasm, skin, benign
Acrostealgia — *see* Osteochondropathy
Acrotrophodynia — *see* Immersion
ACTH ectopic syndrome E24.3
Actinic — *see* condition
Actinobacillosis, actinobacillus A28.8
　mallei A24.0
　muris A25.1
Actinomyces israelii (infection) — *see* Actinomycosis
Actinomycetoma (foot) B47.1
Actinomycosis, actinomycotic A42.9
　with pneumonia A42.0
　abdominal A42.1
　cervicofacial A42.2
　cutaneous A42.89
　gastrointestinal A42.1
　pulmonary A42.0
　sepsis A42.7
　specified site NEC A42.89
Actinoneuritis G62.82
Action, heart
　disorder I49.9
　irregular I49.9
　　psychogenic F45.8
Activated protein C resistance D68.51
Activation
　mast cell (disorder) (syndrome) D89.40
　　idiopathic D89.42
　　monoclonal D89.41
　　secondary D89.43
　　specified type NEC D89.49
Active — *see* condition
Acute — *see also* condition
　abdomen R10.0
　gallbladder — *see* Cholecystitis, acute
Acyanotic heart disease (congenital) Q24.9
Acystia Q64.5
Adair-Dighton syndrome (brittle bones and blue sclera,
　deafness) Q78.0
Adamantinoblastoma — *see* Ameloblastoma
Adamantinoma — *see also* Cyst, calcifying odontogenic
　long bones C40.90
　　lower limb C40.2- ☑
　　upper limb C40.0- ☑
　malignant C41.1
　　jaw (bone) (lower) C41.1
　　　upper C41.0
　tibial C40.2- ☑
Adamantoblastoma — *see* Ameloblastoma

Adams-Stokes (-Morgagni) disease or syndrome I45.9
Adaption reaction — *see* Disorder, adjustment
Addiction — *see also* Dependence F19.20
  alcohol, alcoholic (ethyl) (methyl) (wood) (without remission) F10.20
    with remission F10.21
  drug — *see* Dependence, drug
  ethyl alcohol (without remission) F10.20
    with remission F10.21
  heroin — *see* Dependence, drug, opioid
  methyl alcohol (without remission) F10.20
    with remission F10.21
  methylated spirit (without remission) F10.20
    with remission F10.21
  morphine (-like substances) — *see* Dependence, drug, opioid
  nicotine — *see* Dependence, drug, nicotine
  opium and opioids — *see* Dependence, drug, opioid
  tobacco — *see* Dependence, drug, nicotine
Addison-Biermer anemia (pernicious) D51.0
Addisonian crisis E27.2
Addison's
  anemia (pernicious) D51.0
  disease (bronze) or syndrome E27.1
    tuberculous A18.7
  keloid L94.0
Addison-Schilder complex E71.528
Additional — *see also* Accessory
  chromosome(s) Q99.8
    21 — *see* Trisomy, 21
    sex — *see* Abnormal, chromosome, sex
Adduction contracture, hip or other joint — *see* Contraction, joint
Adenitis — *see also* Lymphadenitis
  acute, unspecified site L04.9
  axillary I88.9
    acute L04.2
    chronic or subacute I88.1
  Bartholin's gland N75.8
  bulbourethral gland — *see* Urethritis
  cervical I88.9
    acute L04.0
    chronic or subacute I88.1
  chancroid (Hemophilus ducreyi) A57
  chronic, unspecified site I88.1
  Cowper's gland — *see* Urethritis
  due to Pasteurella multocida (P. septica) A28.0
  epidemic, acute B27.09
  gangrenous L04.9
  gonorrheal NEC A54.89
  groin I88.9
    acute L04.1
    chronic or subacute I88.1
  infectious (acute) (epidemic) B27.09
  inguinal I88.9
    acute L04.1
    chronic or subacute I88.1
  lymph gland or node, except mesenteric I88.9
    acute — *see* Lymphadenitis, acute
    chronic or subacute I88.1
  mesenteric (acute) (chronic) (nonspecific) (subacute) I88.0
  parotid gland (suppurative) — *see* Sialoadenitis
  salivary gland (any) (suppurative) — *see* Sialoadenitis
  scrofulous (tuberculous) A18.2
  Skene's duct or gland — *see* Urethritis
  strumous, tuberculous A18.2
  subacute, unspecified site I88.1
  sublingual gland (suppurative) — *see* Sialoadenitis
  submandibular gland (suppurative) — *see* Sialoadenitis
  submaxillary gland (suppurative) — *see* Sialoadenitis
  tuberculous — *see* Tuberculosis, lymph gland
  urethral gland — *see* Urethritis
  Wharton's duct (suppurative) — *see* Sialoadenitis
Adenoacanthoma — *see* Neoplasm, malignant, by site
Adenoameloblastoma — *see* Cyst, calcifying odontogenic
Adenocarcinoid (tumor) — *see* Neoplasm, malignant, by site
Adenocarcinoma — *see also* Neoplasm, malignant, by site
  acidophil
    specified site — *see* Neoplasm, malignant, by site
    unspecified site C75.1
  adrenal cortical C74.0- ☑
  alveolar — *see* Neoplasm, lung, malignant
  apocrine
    breast — *see* Neoplasm, breast, malignant

Adenocarcinoma — *continued*
  apocrine — *continued*
    in situ
      breast D05.8- ☑
      specified site NEC — *see* Neoplasm, skin, in situ
      unspecified site D04.9
    specified site NEC — *see* Neoplasm, skin, malignant
    unspecified site C44.99
  basal cell
    specified site — *see* Neoplasm, skin, malignant
    unspecified site C08.9
  basophil
    specified site — *see* Neoplasm, malignant, by site
    unspecified site C75.1
  bile duct type C22.1
    liver C22.1
    specified site NEC — *see* Neoplasm, malignant, by site
    unspecified site C22.1
  bronchiolar — *see* Neoplasm, lung, malignant
  bronchioloalveolar — *see* Neoplasm, lung, malignant
  ceruminous C44.29- ☑
  cervix, in situ — *see also* Carcinoma, cervix uteri, in situ D06.9
  chromophobe
    specified site — *see* Neoplasm, malignant, by site
    unspecified site C75.1
  diffuse type
    specified site — *see* Neoplasm, malignant, by site
    unspecified site C16.9
  duct
    infiltrating
      with Paget's disease — *see* Neoplasm, breast, malignant
      specified site — *see* Neoplasm, malignant, by site
      unspecified site (female) C50.91- ☑
        male C50.92- ☑
    specified site — *see* Neoplasm, malignant, by site
    unspecified site
      female C56.9
      male C61
  eosinophil
    specified site — *see* Neoplasm, malignant, by site
    unspecified site C75.1
  follicular
    with papillary C73
    moderately differentiated C73
    specified site — *see* Neoplasm, malignant, by site
    trabecular C73
    unspecified site C73
    well differentiated C73
  Hurthle cell C73
  in
    adenomatous
      polyposis coli C18.9
  infiltrating duct
    with Paget's disease — *see* Neoplasm, breast, malignant
    specified site — *see* Neoplasm, by site, malignant
    unspecified site (female) C50.91- ☑
      male C50.92- ☑
  inflammatory
    specified site — *see* Neoplasm, by site, malignant
    unspecified site (female) C50.91- ☑
      male C50.92- ☑
  intestinal type
    specified site — *see* Neoplasm, by site, malignant
    unspecified site C16.9
  intracystic papillary
  intraductal
    breast D05.1- ☑
    noninfiltrating
      breast D05.1- ☑
      papillary
        with invasion
          specified site — *see* Neoplasm, by site, malignant
          unspecified site (female) C50.91- ☑
            male C50.92- ☑
        breast D05.1- ☑
        specified site NEC — *see* Neoplasm, in situ, by site
        unspecified site D05.1- ☑
      specified site NEC — *see* Neoplasm, in situ, by site
      unspecified site D05.1- ☑

Adenocarcinoma — *continued*
  intraductal — *continued*
    papillary
      with invasion
        specified site — *see* Neoplasm, malignant, by site
        unspecified site (female) C50.91- ☑
          male C50.92- ☑
      breast D05.1- ☑
      specified site — *see* Neoplasm, in situ, by site
      unspecified site D05.1- ☑
    specified site NEC — *see* Neoplasm, in situ, by site
    unspecified site D05.1- ☑
  islet cell
    with exocrine, mixed
      specified site — *see* Neoplasm, malignant, by site
      unspecified site C25.9
    pancreas C25.4
    specified site NEC — *see* Neoplasm, malignant, by site
    unspecified site C25.4
  lobular
    in situ
      breast D05.0- ☑
      specified site NEC — *see* Neoplasm, in situ, by site
      unspecified site D05.0- ☑
    specified site — *see* Neoplasm, malignant, by site
    unspecified site (female) C50.91- ☑
      male C50.92- ☑
  mucoid — *see also* Neoplasm, malignant, by site
    cell
      specified site — *see* Neoplasm, malignant, by site
      unspecified site C75.1
  nonencapsulated sclerosing C73
  papillary
    with follicular C73
    follicular variant C73
    intraductal (noninfiltrating)
      with invasion
        specified site — *see* Neoplasm, malignant, by site
        unspecified site (female) C50.91- ☑
          male C50.92- ☑
      breast D05.1- ☑
      specified site NEC — *see* Neoplasm, in situ, by site
      unspecified site D05.1- ☑
    serous
      specified site — *see* Neoplasm, malignant, by site
      unspecified site C56.9
  papillocystic
    specified site — *see* Neoplasm, malignant, by site
    unspecified site C56.9
  pseudomucinous
    specified site — *see* Neoplasm, malignant, by site
    unspecified site C56.9
  renal cell C64- ☑
  sebaceous — *see* Neoplasm, skin, malignant
  serous — *see also* Neoplasm, malignant, by site
    papillary
      specified site — *see* Neoplasm, malignant, by site
      unspecified site C56.9
  sweat gland — *see* Neoplasm, skin, malignant
  water-clear cell C75.0
Adenocarcinoma-in-situ — *see also* Neoplasm, in situ, by site
  breast D05.9- ☑
Adenofibroma
  clear cell — *see* Neoplasm, benign, by site
  endometrioid D27.9
    borderline malignancy D39.10
    malignant C56- ☑
  mucinous
    specified site — *see* Neoplasm, benign, by site
    unspecified site D27.9
  papillary
    specified site — *see* Neoplasm, benign, by site
    unspecified site D27.9
  prostate — *see* Enlargement, enlarged, prostate
  serous
    specified site — *see* Neoplasm, benign, by site
    unspecified site D27.9

Adenofibroma — *continued*
specified site — *see* Neoplasm, benign, by site
unspecified site D27.9
Adenofibrosis
breast — *see* Fibroadenosis, breast
endometrioid N80.00
Adenoiditis (chronic) J35.02
with tonsillitis J35.03
acute J03.90
recurrent J03.91
specified organism NEC J03.80
recurrent J03.81
staphylococcal J03.80
recurrent J03.81
streptococcal J03.00
recurrent J03.01
Adenoids — *see* condition
Adenolipoma — *see* Neoplasm, benign, by site
Adenolipomatosis, Launois-Bensaude E88.89
Adenolymphoma
specified site — *see* Neoplasm, benign, by site
unspecified site D11.9
Adenoma — *see also* Neoplasm, benign, by site
acidophil
specified site — *see* Neoplasm, benign, by site
unspecified site D35.2
acidophil-basophil, mixed
specified site — *see* Neoplasm, benign, by site
unspecified site D35.2
adrenal (cortical) D35.00
clear cell D35.00
compact cell D35.00
glomerulosa cell D35.00
heavily pigmented variant D35.00
mixed cell D35.00
alpha-cell
pancreas D13.7
specified site NEC — *see* Neoplasm, benign, by site
unspecified site D13.7
alveolar D14.30
apocrine
breast D24- ☑
specified site NEC — *see* Neoplasm, skin, benign, by site
unspecified site D23.9
basal cell D11.9
basophil
specified site — *see* Neoplasm, benign, by site
unspecified site D35.2
basophil-acidophil, mixed
specified site — *see* Neoplasm, benign, by site
unspecified site D35.2
beta-cell
pancreas D13.7
specified site NEC — *see* Neoplasm, benign, by site
unspecified site D13.7
bile duct D13.4
common D13.5
extrahepatic D13.5
intrahepatic D13.4
specified site NEC — *see* Neoplasm, benign, by site
unspecified site D13.4
black D35.00
bronchial D38.1
cylindroid type — *see* Neoplasm, lung, malignant
ceruminous D23.2- ☑
chief cell D35.1
chromophobe
specified site — *see* Neoplasm, benign, by site
unspecified site D35.2
colloid
specified site — *see* Neoplasm, benign, by site
unspecified site D34
eccrine, papillary — *see* Neoplasm, skin, benign
endocrine, multiple
single specified site — *see* Neoplasm, uncertain behavior, by site
two or more specified sites D44- ☑
unspecified site D44.9
endometrioid — *see also* Neoplasm, benign
borderline malignancy — *see* Neoplasm, uncertain behavior, by site
eosinophil
specified site — *see* Neoplasm, benign, by site
unspecified site D35.2
fetal
specified site — *see* Neoplasm, benign, by site
unspecified site D34

Adenoma — *continued*
follicular
specified site — *see* Neoplasm, benign, by site
unspecified site D34
hepatocellular D13.4
Hurthle cell D34
islet cell
pancreas D13.7
specified site NEC — *see* Neoplasm, benign, by site
unspecified site D13.7
liver cell D13.4
macrofollicular
specified site — *see* Neoplasm, benign, by site
unspecified site D34
malignant, malignum — *see* Neoplasm, malignant, by site
microcystic
pancreas D13.6
specified site NEC — *see* Neoplasm, benign, by site
unspecified site D13.6
microfollicular
specified site — *see* Neoplasm, benign, by site
unspecified site D34
mucoid cell
specified site — *see* Neoplasm, benign, by site
unspecified site D35.2
multiple endocrine
single specified site — *see* Neoplasm, uncertain behavior, by site
two or more specified sites D44- ☑
unspecified site D44.9
nipple D24- ☑
papillary — *see also* Neoplasm, benign, by site
eccrine — *see* Neoplasm, skin, benign, by site
Pick's tubular
specified site — *see* Neoplasm, benign, by site
unspecified site
female D27.9
male D29.20
pleomorphic
carcinoma in — *see* Neoplasm, salivary gland, malignant
specified site — *see* Neoplasm, malignant, by site
unspecified site C08.9
polypoid — *see also* Neoplasm, benign
adenocarcinoma in — *see* Neoplasm, malignant, by site
adenocarcinoma in situ — *see* Neoplasm, in situ, by site
prostate — *see* Neoplasm, benign, prostate
rete cell D29.20
sebaceous — *see* Neoplasm, skin, benign
Sertoli cell
specified site — *see* Neoplasm, benign, by site
unspecified site
female D27.9
male D29.20
skin appendage — *see* Neoplasm, skin, benign
sudoriferous gland — *see* Neoplasm, skin, benign
sweat gland — *see* Neoplasm, skin, benign
testicular
specified site — *see* Neoplasm, benign, by site
unspecified site
female D27.9
male D29.20
tubular — *see also* Neoplasm, benign, by site
adenocarcinoma in — *see* Neoplasm, malignant, by site
adenocarcinoma in situ — *see* Neoplasm, in situ, by site
Pick's
specified site — *see* Neoplasm, benign, by site
unspecified site
female D27.9
male D29.20
tubulovillous — *see also* Neoplasm, benign, by site
adenocarcinoma in — *see* Neoplasm, malignant, by site
adenocarcinoma in situ — *see* Neoplasm, in situ, by site
villous — *see* Neoplasm, uncertain behavior, by site
adenocarcinoma in — *see* Neoplasm, malignant, by site
adenocarcinoma in situ — *see* Neoplasm, in situ, by site
water-clear cell D35.1

Adenomatosis
endocrine (multiple) E31.20
single specified site — *see* Neoplasm, uncertain behavior, by site
erosive of nipple D24- ☑
pluriendocrine — *see* Adenomatosis, endocrine
pulmonary D38.1
malignant — *see* Neoplasm, lung, malignant
specified site — *see* Neoplasm, benign, by site
unspecified site D12.6
Adenomatous
goiter (nontoxic) E04.9
with hyperthyroidism — *see* Hyperthyroidism, with, goiter, nodular
toxic — *see* Hyperthyroidism, with, goiter, nodular
Adenomyoma — *see also* Neoplasm, benign, by site
prostate — *see* Enlarged, prostate
Adenomyometritis N80.00
Adenomyosis (uterus) N80.03
Adenopathy (lymph gland) R59.9
generalized R59.1
inguinal R59.0
localized R59.0
mediastinal R59.0
mesentery R59.0
syphilitic (secondary) A51.49
tracheobronchial R59.0
tuberculous A15.4
primary (progressive) A15.7
tuberculous — *see also* Tuberculosis, lymph gland
tracheobronchial A15.4
primary (progressive) A15.7
Adenosalpingitis — *see* Salpingitis
Adenosarcoma — *see* Neoplasm, malignant, by site
Adenosclerosis I88.8
Adenosis (sclerosing) breast — *see* Fibroadenosis, breast
Adenovirus, as cause of disease classified elsewhere B97.0
Adentia (complete) (partial) — *see* Absence, teeth
Adherent — *see also* Adhesions
labia (minora) N90.89
pericardium (nonrheumatic) I31.0
rheumatic I09.2
placenta (with hemorrhage) O72.0
without hemorrhage O73.0
prepuce, newborn N47.0
scar (skin) L90.5
tendon in scar L90.5
Adhesions, adhesive (postinfective) K66.0
with intestinal obstruction K56.50
complete K56.52
incomplete K56.51
partial K56.51
abdominal (wall) — *see* Adhesions, peritoneum
appendix K38.8
bile duct (common) (hepatic) K83.8
bladder (sphincter) N32.89
bowel — *see* Adhesions, peritoneum
cardiac I31.0
rheumatic I09.2
cecum — *see* Adhesions, peritoneum
cervicovaginal N88.1
congenital Q52.8
postpartal O90.89
old N88.1
cervix N88.1
ciliary body NEC — *see* Adhesions, iris
clitoris N90.89
colon — *see* Adhesions, peritoneum
common duct K83.8
congenital — *see also* Anomaly, by site
fingers — *see* Syndactylism, complex, fingers
omental, anomalous Q43.3
peritoneal Q43.3
tongue (to gum or roof of mouth) Q38.3
conjunctiva (acquired) H11.21- ☑
congenital Q15.8
cystic duct K82.8
diaphragm — *see* Adhesions, peritoneum
due to foreign body — *see* Foreign body
duodenum — *see* Adhesions, peritoneum
ear
middle H74.1- ☑
epididymis N50.89
epidural — *see* Adhesions, meninges
epiglottis J38.7
eyelid H02.59
female pelvis N73.6

Adhesions, adhesive — *continued*
  gallbladder K82.8
  globe H44.89
  heart I31.Ø
    rheumatic I09.2
  ileocecal (coil) — *see* Adhesions, peritoneum
  ileum — *see* Adhesions, peritoneum
  intestine — *see also* Adhesions, peritoneum
    with obstruction K56.5Ø
      complete K56.52
      incomplete K56.51
      partial K56.51
  intra-abdominal — *see* Adhesions, peritoneum
  iris H21.5Ø- ✓
    anterior H21.51- ✓
    goniosynechiae H21.52- ✓
    posterior H21.54- ✓
    to corneal graft T85.898 ✓
  joint — *see* Ankylosis
    knee M23.8X ✓
    temporomandibular M26.61- ✓
  labium (majus) (minus), congenital Q52.5
  liver — *see* Adhesions, peritoneum
  lung J98.4
  mediastinum J98.59
  meninges (cerebral) (spinal) G96.12
    congenital Q07.8
    tuberculous (cerebral) (spinal) A17.Ø
  mesenteric — *see* Adhesions, peritoneum
  nasal (septum) (to turbinates) J34.89
  ocular muscle — *see* Strabismus, mechanical
  omentum — *see* Adhesions, peritoneum
  ovary N73.6
    congenital (to cecum, kidney or omentum) Q50.39
  paraovarian N73.6
  pelvic (peritoneal)
    female N73.6
      postprocedural N99.4
    male — *see* Adhesions, peritoneum
    postpartal (old) N73.6
    tuberculous A18.17
  penis to scrotum (congenital) Q55.8
  periappendiceal — *see also* Adhesions, peritoneum
  pericardium (nonrheumatic) I31.Ø
    focal I31.8
    rheumatic I09.2
    tuberculous A18.84
  pericholecystic K82.8
  perigastric — *see* Adhesions, peritoneum
  periovarian N73.6
  periprostatic N42.89
  perirectal — *see* Adhesions, peritoneum
  perirenal N28.89
  peritoneum, peritoneal (postinfective) K66.Ø
    with obstruction (intestinal) K56.5Ø
      complete K56.52
      incomplete K56.51
      partial K56.51
    congenital Q43.3
    pelvic, female N73.6
      postprocedural N99.4
    postpartal, pelvic N73.6
    postprocedural K66.Ø
    to uterus N73.6
  peritubal N73.6
  periureteral N28.89
  periuterine N73.6
  perivesical N32.89
  perivesicular (seminal vesicle) N50.89
  pleura, pleuritic J94.8
    tuberculous NEC A15.6
  pleuropericardial J94.8
  postoperative (gastrointestinal tract) K66.Ø
    with obstruction — *see also* Obstruction, intestine, postoperative K91.3Ø
    due to foreign body accidentally left in wound — *see* Foreign body, accidentally left during a procedure
    pelvic peritoneal N99.4
    urethra — *see* Stricture, urethra, postprocedural
    vagina N99.2
  postpartal, old (vulva or perineum) N90.89
  preputial, prepuce N47.5
  pulmonary J98.4
  pylorus — *see* Adhesions, peritoneum
  sciatic nerve — *see* Lesion, nerve, sciatic
  seminal vesicle N50.89
  shoulder (joint) — *see* Capsulitis, adhesive

Adhesions, adhesive — *continued*
  sigmoid flexure — *see* Adhesions, peritoneum
  spermatic cord (acquired) N50.89
    congenital Q55.4
  spinal canal G96.12
  stomach — *see* Adhesions, peritoneum
  subscapular — *see* Capsulitis, adhesive
  temporomandibular M26.61- ✓
  tendinitis (*see also* Tenosynovitis, specified type NEC)
    shoulder — *see* Capsulitis, adhesive
  testis N44.8
  tongue, congenital (to gum or roof of mouth) Q38.3
    acquired K14.8
  trachea J39.8
  tubo-ovarian N73.6
  tunica vaginalis N44.8
  uterus N73.6
    internal N85.6
    to abdominal wall N73.6
  vagina (chronic) N89.5
    postoperative N99.2
  vitreomacular H43.82- ✓
  vitreous H43.89
  vulva N90.89
Adiaspiromycosis B48.8
Adie (-Holmes) **pupil or syndrome** — *see* Anomaly, pupil, function, tonic pupil
Adiponecrosis neonatorum P83.88
Adiposis — *see also* Obesity
  cerebralis E23.6
  dolorosa E88.2
Adiposity — *see also* Obesity
  heart — *see* Degeneration, myocardial
  localized E65
Adiposogenital dystrophy E23.6
Adjustment
  disorder — *see* Disorder, adjustment
  implanted device — *see* Encounter (for), adjustment (of)
  prosthesis, external — *see* Fitting
  reaction — *see* Disorder, adjustment
Administration of tPA (rtPA) in a different facility within the last 24 hours prior to admission to current facility Z92.82
Admission (for) — *see also* Encounter (for)
  adjustment (of)
    artificial
      arm Z44.ØØ- ✓
        complete Z44.Ø1- ✓
        partial Z44.Ø2- ✓
      eye Z44.2 ✓
      leg Z44.1Ø- ✓
        complete Z44.11- ✓
        partial Z44.12- ✓
    brain neuropacemaker Z46.2
      implanted Z45.42
    breast
      implant Z45.81 ✓
      prosthesis (external) Z44.3 ✓
    colostomy belt Z46.89
    contact lenses Z46.Ø
    cystostomy device Z46.6
    dental prosthesis Z46.3
    device NEC
      abdominal Z46.89
      implanted Z45.89
        cardiac Z45.Ø9
          defibrillator (with synchronous cardiac pacemaker) Z45.Ø2
          pacemaker (cardiac resynchronization therapy (CRT-P)) Z45.Ø18
            pulse generator Z45.Ø1Ø
          resynchronization therapy defibrillator (CRT-D) Z45.Ø2
        hearing device Z45.328
          bone conduction Z45.32Ø
          cochlear Z45.321
        infusion pump Z45.1
        nervous system Z45.49
          CSF drainage Z45.41
          hearing device — *see* Admission, adjustment, device, implanted, hearing device
          neuropacemaker Z45.42
          visual substitution Z45.31
        specified NEC Z45.89
        vascular access Z45.2
        visual substitution Z45.31

Admission — *continued*
  adjustment — *continued*
    device — *continued*
      nervous system Z46.2
        implanted — *see* Admission, adjustment, device, implanted, nervous system
      orthodontic Z46.4
      prosthetic Z44.9
        arm — *see* Admission, adjustment, artificial, arm
        breast Z44.3 ✓
        dental Z46.3
        eye Z44.2 ✓
        leg — *see* Admission, adjustment, artificial, leg
        specified type NEC Z44.8
      substitution
        auditory Z46.2
          implanted — *see* Admission, adjustment, device, implanted, hearing device
        nervous system Z46.2
          implanted — *see* Admission, adjustment, device, implanted, nervous system
        visual Z46.2
          implanted Z45.31
      urinary Z46.6
    hearing aid Z46.1
      implanted — *see* Admission, adjustment, device, implanted, hearing device
    ileostomy device Z46.89
    intestinal appliance or device NEC Z46.89
    neuropacemaker (brain) (peripheral nerve) (spinal cord) Z46.2
      implanted Z45.42
    orthodontic device Z46.4
    orthopedic (brace) (cast) (device) (shoes) Z46.89
    pacemaker (cardiac resynchronization therapy (CRT-P))
      cardiac Z45.Ø18
        pulse generator Z45.Ø1Ø
      nervous system Z46.2
        implanted Z45.42
    portacath (port-a-cath) Z45.2
    prosthesis Z44.9
      arm — *see* Admission, adjustment, artificial, arm
      breast Z44.3 ✓
      dental Z46.3
      eye Z44.2 ✓
      leg — *see* Admission, adjustment, artificial, leg
      specified NEC Z44.8
    spectacles Z46.Ø
  aftercare — *see also* Aftercare Z51.89
    postpartum
      immediately after delivery Z39.Ø
      routine follow-up Z39.2
    radiation therapy (antineoplastic) Z51.Ø
  attention to artificial opening (of) Z43.9
    artificial vagina Z43.7
    colostomy Z43.3
    cystostomy Z43.5
    enterostomy Z43.4
    gastrostomy Z43.1
    ileostomy Z43.2
    jejunostomy Z43.4
    nephrostomy Z43.6
    specified site NEC Z43.8
      intestinal tract Z43.4
      urinary tract Z43.6
    tracheostomy Z43.Ø
    ureterostomy Z43.6
    urethrostomy Z43.6
  breast augmentation or reduction Z41.1
  breast reconstruction following mastectomy Z42.1
  change of
    dressing (nonsurgical) Z48.ØØ
    neuropacemaker device (brain) (peripheral nerve) (spinal cord) Z46.2
      implanted Z45.42
    surgical dressing Z48.Ø1
  circumcision, ritual or routine (in absence of diagnosis) Z41.2
  clinical research investigation (control) (normal comparison) (participant) Z00.6
  contraceptive management Z30.9
  cosmetic surgery NEC Z41.1
  counseling — *see also* Counseling
    dietary Z71.3
    gestational carrier Z31.7

Admission — *continued*
  counseling — *see also* Counseling — *continued*
    HIV Z71.7
    human immunodeficiency virus Z71.7
    nonattending third party Z71.0
    procreative management NEC Z31.69
  delivery, full-term, uncomplicated O80
    cesarean, without indication O82
  desensitization to allergens Z51.6
  dietary surveillance and counseling Z71.3
  ear piercing Z41.3
  examination at health care facility (adult) — *see also*
      Examination Z00.00
    with abnormal findings Z00.01
    clinical research investigation (control) (normal
        comparison) (participant) Z00.6
    dental Z01.20
      with abnormal findings Z01.21
    donor (potential) Z00.5
    ear Z01.10
      with abnormal findings NEC Z01.118
    eye Z01.00
      with abnormal findings Z01.01
      following failed vision screening Z01.020
        with abnormal findings Z01.021
    general, specified reason NEC Z00.8
    hearing Z01.10
      with abnormal findings NEC Z01.118
      infant or child (over 28 days old) Z00.129
        with abnormal findings Z00.121
    postpartum checkup Z39.2
    psychiatric (general) Z00.8
      requested by authority Z04.6
    vision Z01.00
      with abnormal findings Z01.01
      following failed vision screening Z01.020
        with abnormal findings Z01.021
      infant or child (over 28 days old) Z00.129
        with abnormal findings Z00.121
  fitting (of)
    artificial
      arm — *see* Admission, adjustment, artificial, arm
      eye Z44.2 ☑
      leg — *see* Admission, adjustment, artificial, leg
    brain neuropacemaker Z46.2
      implanted Z45.42
    breast prosthesis (external) Z44.3 ☑
    colostomy belt Z46.89
    contact lenses Z46.0
    cystostomy device Z46.6
    dental prosthesis Z46.3
    dentures Z46.3
    device NEC
      abdominal Z46.89
      nervous system Z46.2
        implanted — *see* Admission, adjustment,
            device, implanted, nervous system
      orthodontic Z46.4
      prosthetic Z44.9
        breast Z44.3 ☑
        dental Z46.3
        eye Z44.2 ☑
      substitution
        auditory Z46.2
          implanted — *see* Admission, adjustment,
              device, implanted, hearing device
        nervous system Z46.2
          implanted — *see* Admission, adjustment,
              device, implanted, nervous system
        visual Z46.2
          implanted Z45.31
    hearing aid Z46.1
    ileostomy device Z46.89
    intestinal appliance or device NEC Z46.89
    neuropacemaker (brain) (peripheral nerve) (spinal
        cord) Z46.2
      implanted Z45.42
    orthodontic device Z46.4
    orthopedic device (brace) (cast) (shoes) Z46.89
    prosthesis Z44.9
      arm — *see* Admission, adjustment, artificial, arm
      breast Z44.3 ☑
      dental Z46.3
      eye Z44.2 ☑
      leg — *see* Admission, adjustment, artificial, leg
      specified type NEC Z44.8
    spectacles Z46.0
  follow-up examination Z09

Admission — *continued*
  intrauterine device management Z30.431
    initial prescription Z30.014
  mental health evaluation Z00.8
    requested by authority Z04.6
  observation — *see* Observation
  Papanicolaou smear, cervix Z12.4
    for suspected malignant neoplasm Z12.4
  plastic and reconstructive surgery following medical
      procedure or healed injury NEC Z42.8
  plastic surgery, cosmetic NEC Z41.1
  postpartum observation
    immediately after delivery Z39.0
    routine follow-up Z39.2
  poststerilization (for restoration) Z31.0
    aftercare Z31.42
  procreative management Z31.9
  prophylactic (measure) — *see also* Encounter, prophy-
      lactic measures
    organ removal Z40.00
      breast Z40.01
      fallopian tube(s) Z40.03
        with ovary(s) Z40.02
      ovary(s) Z40.02
      specified organ NEC Z40.09
      testes Z40.09
    vaccination Z23
  psychiatric examination (general) Z00.8
    requested by authority Z04.6
  radiation therapy (antineoplastic) Z51.0
  reconstructive surgery following medical procedure or
      healed injury NEC Z42.8
  removal of
    cystostomy catheter Z43.5
    drains Z48.03
    dressing (nonsurgical) Z48.00
    implantable subdermal contraceptive Z30.46
    intrauterine contraceptive device Z30.432
    neuropacemaker (brain) (peripheral nerve) (spinal
        cord) Z46.2
      implanted Z45.42
    staples Z48.02
    surgical dressing Z48.01
    sutures Z48.02
    ureteral stent Z46.6
  respirator [ventilator] use during power failure Z99.12
  restoration of organ continuity (poststerilization) Z31.0
    aftercare Z31.42
  sensitivity test — *see also* Test, skin
    allergy NEC Z01.82
    Mantoux Z11.1
  tuboplasty following previous sterilization Z31.0
    aftercare Z31.42
  vasoplasty following previous sterilization Z31.0
    aftercare Z31.42
  vision examination Z01.00
    with abnormal findings Z01.01
    following failed vision screening Z01.020
      with abnormal findings Z01.021
    infant or child (over 28 days old) Z00.129
      with abnormal findings Z00.121
  waiting period for admission to other facility Z75.1
Adnexitis (suppurative) — *see* Salpingo-oophoritis
Adolescent X-linked adrenoleukodystrophy E71.521
Adrenal (gland) — *see* condition
Adrenalism, tuberculous A18.7
Adrenalitis, adrenitis E27.8
  autoimmune E27.1
  meningococcal, hemorrhagic A39.1
Adrenarche, premature E27.0
Adrenocortical syndrome — *see* Cushing's, syndrome
Adrenogenital syndrome E25.9
  acquired E25.8
  congenital E25.0
  salt loss E25.0
Adrenogenitalism, congenital E25.0
Adrenoleukodystrophy E71.529
  neonatal E71.511
  X-linked E71.529
    Addison only phenotype E71.528
    Addison-Schilder E71.528
    adolescent E71.521
    adrenomyeloneuropathy E71.522
    childhood cerebral E71.520
    other specified E71.528
Adrenomyeloneuropathy E71.522
Adventitious bursa — *see* Bursopathy, specified type
  NEC

Adverse effect — *see* Table of Drugs and Chemicals,
    categories T36-T50, with 6th character 5
Advice — *see* Counseling
Adynamia (episodica) (hereditary) (periodic) G72.3
Aeration lung imperfect, newborn — *see* Atelectasis
Aerobullosis T70.3 ☑
Aerocele — *see* Embolism, air
Aerodermectasia
  subcutaneous (traumatic) T79.7 ☑
Aerodontalgia T70.29 ☑
Aeroembolism T70.3 ☑
Aerogenes capsulatus infection A48.0
Aero-otitis media T70.0 ☑
Aerophagy, aerophagia (psychogenic) F45.8
Aerophobia F40.228
Aerosinusitis T70.1 ☑
Aerotitis T70.0 ☑
Affection — *see* Disease
Afibrinogenemia — *see also* Defect, coagulation D68.8
  acquired D65
  congenital D68.2
  following ectopic or molar pregnancy O08.1
  in abortion — *see* Abortion, by type, complicated by,
      afibrinogenemia
  puerperal O72.3
African
  sleeping sickness B56.9
  tick fever A68.1
  trypanosomiasis B56.9
    gambian B56.0
    rhodesian B56.1
Aftercare — *see also* Care Z51.89
  following surgery (for) (on)
    amputation Z47.81
    attention to
      drains Z48.03
      dressings (nonsurgical) Z48.00
        surgical Z48.01
      sutures Z48.02
    circulatory system Z48.812
    delayed (planned) wound closure Z48.1
    digestive system Z48.815
    explantation of joint prosthesis (staged procedure)
      hip Z47.32
      knee Z47.33
      shoulder Z47.31
    genitourinary system Z48.816
    joint replacement Z47.1
    neoplasm Z48.3
    nervous system Z48.811
    oral cavity Z48.814
    organ transplant
      bone marrow Z48.290
      heart Z48.21
      heart-lung Z48.280
      kidney Z48.22
      liver Z48.23
      lung Z48.24
      multiple organs NEC Z48.288
      specified NEC Z48.298
    orthopedic NEC Z47.89
    planned wound closure Z48.1
    removal of internal fixation device Z47.2
    respiratory system Z48.813
    scoliosis Z47.82
    sense organs Z48.810
    skin and subcutaneous tissue Z48.817
    specified body system
      circulatory Z48.812
      digestive Z48.815
      genitourinary Z48.816
      nervous Z48.811
      oral cavity Z48.814
      respiratory Z48.813
      sense organs Z48.810
      skin and subcutaneous tissue Z48.817
      teeth Z48.814
    specified NEC Z48.89
    spinal Z47.89
    teeth Z48.814
  fracture — *code to* fracture with seventh character D
  involving
    removal of
      drains Z48.03
      dressings (nonsurgical) Z48.00
      staples Z48.02
      surgical dressings Z48.01
      sutures Z48.02

☑ **Additional Character Required** — **Refer to the Tabular List for Character Selection**

Aftercare — *continued*
   neuropacemaker (brain) (peripheral nerve) (spinal cord)
       Z46.2
       implanted Z45.42
   orthopedic NEC Z47.89
   postprocedural — *see* Aftercare, following surgery
After-cataract — *see* Cataract, secondary
Agalactia (primary) O92.3
   elective, secondary or therapeutic O92.5
Agammaglobulinemia (acquired (secondary) (nonfamil-
       ial) D80.1
   with
       immunoglobulin-bearing B-lymphocytes D80.1
       lymphopenia D81.9
   autosomal recessive (Swiss type) D80.0
   Bruton's X-linked D80.0
   common variable (CVAgamma) D80.1
   congenital sex-linked D80.0
   hereditary D80.0
   lymphopenic D81.9
   Swiss type (autosomal recessive) D80.0
   X-linked (with growth hormone deficiency) (Bruton)
       D80.0
Aganglionosis (bowel) (colon) Q43.1
Age (old) — *see* Senility
Agenesis
   adrenal (gland) Q89.1
   alimentary tract (complete) (partial) NEC Q45.8
       upper Q40.8
   anus, anal (canal) Q42.3
       with fistula Q42.2
   aorta Q25.41
   appendix Q42.8
   arm (complete) Q71.0- ☑
       with hand present Q71.1- ☑
   artery (peripheral) Q27.9
       brain Q28.3
       coronary Q24.5
       pulmonary Q25.79
       specified NEC Q27.8
       umbilical Q27.0
   auditory (canal) (external) Q16.1
   auricle (ear) Q16.0
   bile duct or passage Q44.5
   bladder Q64.5
   bone Q79.9
   brain Q00.0
       part of Q04.3
   breast (with nipple present) Q83.8
       with absent nipple Q83.0
   bronchus Q32.4
   canaliculus lacrimalis Q10.4
   carpus — *see* Agenesis, hand
   cartilage Q79.9
   cecum Q42.8
   cerebellum Q04.3
   cervix Q51.5
   chin Q18.8
   cilia Q10.3
   circulatory system, part NOS Q28.9
   clavicle Q74.0
   clitoris Q52.6
   coccyx Q76.49
   colon Q42.9
       specified NEC Q42.8
   corpus callosum Q04.0
   cricoid cartilage Q31.8
   diaphragm (with hernia) Q79.1
   digestive organ(s) or tract (complete) (partial) NEC
       Q45.8
       upper Q40.8
   ductus arteriosus Q28.8
   duodenum Q41.0
   ear Q16.9
       auricle Q16.0
       lobe Q17.8
   ejaculatory duct Q55.4
   endocrine (gland) NEC Q89.2
   epiglottis Q31.8
   esophagus Q39.8
   eustachian tube Q16.2
   eye Q11.1
       adnexa Q15.8
   eyelid (fold) Q10.3
   face
       bones NEC Q75.8
       specified part NEC Q18.8
   fallopian tube Q50.6

Agenesis — *continued*
   femur — *see* Defect, reduction, lower limb, longitudi-
       nal, femur
   fibula — *see* Defect, reduction, lower limb, longitudinal,
       fibula
   finger (complete) (partial) — *see* Agenesis, hand
   foot (and toes) (complete) (partial) Q72.3- ☑
   forearm (with hand present) — *see* Agenesis, arm, with
       hand present
       and hand Q71.2- ☑
   gallbladder Q44.0
   gastric Q40.2
   genitalia, genital (organ(s))
       female Q52.8
           external Q52.71
           internal NEC Q52.8
       male Q55.8
   glottis Q31.8
   hair Q84.0
   hand (and fingers) (complete) (partial) Q71.3- ☑
   heart Q24.8
       valve NEC Q24.8
           pulmonary Q22.0
   hepatic Q44.7
   humerus — *see* Defect, reduction, upper limb
   hymen Q52.4
   ileum Q41.2
   incus Q16.3
   intestine (small) Q41.9
       large Q42.9
           specified NEC Q42.8
   iris (dilator fibers) Q13.1
   jaw M26.09
   jejunum Q41.1
   kidney(s) (partial) Q60.2
       bilateral Q60.1
       unilateral Q60.0
   labium (majus) (minus) Q52.71
   labyrinth, membranous Q16.5
   lacrimal apparatus Q10.4
   larynx Q31.8
   leg (complete) Q72.0- ☑
       with foot present Q72.1- ☑
       lower leg (with foot present) — *see* Agenesis, leg,
           with foot present
       and foot Q72.2- ☑
   lens Q12.3
   limb (complete) Q73.0
       lower — *see* Agenesis, leg
       upper — *see* Agenesis, arm
   lip Q38.0
   liver Q44.7
   lung (fissure) (lobe) (bilateral) (unilateral) Q33.3
   mandible, maxilla M26.09
   metacarpus — *see* Agenesis, hand
   metatarsus — *see* Agenesis, foot
   muscle Q79.8
       eyelid Q10.3
       ocular Q15.8
   musculoskeletal system NEC Q79.8
   nail(s) Q84.3
   neck, part Q18.8
   nerve Q07.8
   nervous system, part NEC Q07.8
   nipple Q83.2
   nose Q30.1
   nuclear Q07.8
   organ
       of Corti Q16.5
       or site not listed — *see* Anomaly, by site
   osseous meatus (ear) Q16.1
   ovary
       bilateral Q50.02
       unilateral Q50.01
   oviduct Q50.6
   pancreas Q45.0
   parathyroid (gland) Q89.2
   parotid gland(s) Q38.4
   patella Q74.1
   pelvic girdle (complete) (partial) Q74.2
   penis Q55.5
   pericardium Q24.8
   pituitary (gland) Q89.2
   prostate Q55.4
   punctum lacrimale Q10.4
   radioulnar — *see* Defect, reduction, upper limb
   radius — *see* Defect, reduction, upper limb, longitudi-
       nal, radius

Agenesis — *continued*
   rectum Q42.1
       with fistula Q42.0
   renal Q60.2
       bilateral Q60.1
       unilateral Q60.0
   respiratory organ NEC Q34.8
   rib Q76.6
   roof of orbit Q75.8
   round ligament Q52.8
   sacrum Q76.49
   salivary gland Q38.4
   scapula Q74.0
   scrotum Q55.29
   seminal vesicles Q55.4
   septum
       atrial Q21.19
       between aorta and pulmonary artery Q21.4
       ventricular Q20.4
   shoulder girdle (complete) (partial) Q74.0
   skull (bone) Q75.8
       with
           anencephaly Q00.0
           encephalocele — *see* Encephalocele
           hydrocephalus Q03.9
               with spina bifida — *see* Spina bifida, by site,
                   with hydrocephalus
           microcephaly Q02
   spermatic cord Q55.4
   spinal cord Q06.0
   spine Q76.49
   spleen Q89.01
   sternum Q76.7
   stomach Q40.2
   submaxillary gland(s) (congenital) Q38.4
   tarsus — *see* Agenesis, foot
   tendon Q79.8
   testicle Q55.0
   thymus (gland) Q89.2
   thyroid (gland) E03.1
       cartilage Q31.8
   tibia — *see* Defect, reduction, lower limb, longitudinal,
       tibia
   tibiofibular — *see* Defect, reduction, lower limb, speci-
       fied type NEC
   toe (and foot) (complete) (partial) — *see* Agenesis, foot
   tongue Q38.3
   trachea (cartilage) Q32.1
   ulna — *see* Defect, reduction, upper limb, longitudinal,
       ulna
   upper limb — *see* Agenesis, arm
   ureter Q62.4
   urethra Q64.5
   urinary tract NEC Q64.8
   uterus Q51.0
   uvula Q38.5
   vagina Q52.0
   vas deferens Q55.4
   vein(s) (peripheral) Q27.9
       brain Q28.3
       great NEC Q26.8
       portal Q26.5
   vena cava (inferior) (superior) Q26.8
   vermis of cerebellum Q04.3
   vertebra Q76.49
   vulva Q52.71
Ageusia R43.2
Agitated — *see* condition
Agitation R45.1
Aglossia (congenital) Q38.3
Aglossia-adactylia syndrome Q87.0
Aglycogenosis E74.00
Agnosia (body image) (other senses) (tactile) R48.1
   developmental F88
   verbal R48.1
       auditory R48.1
           developmental F80.2
       developmental F80.2
   visual (object) R48.3
Agoraphobia F40.00
   with panic disorder F40.01
   without panic disorder F40.02
Agrammatism R48.8
Agranulocytopenia — *see* Agranulocytosis
Agranulocytosis (chronic) (cyclical) (genetic) (infantile)
       (periodic) (pernicious) — *see also* Neutropenia
       D70.9
   congenital D70.0

Index

Agranulocytosis — Allergy, allergic

Agranulocytosis — *continued*
cytoreductive cancer chemotherapy sequela D70.1
drug-induced D70.2
due to cytoreductive cancer chemotherapy D70.1
due to infection D70.3
secondary D70.4
drug-induced D70.2
due to cytoreductive cancer chemotherapy D70.1
Agraphia (absolute) R48.8
with alexia R48.0
developmental F81.81
Ague (dumb) — *see* Malaria
Agyria Q04.3
Ahumada-del Castillo syndrome E23.0
Aichomophobia F40.298
AIDS (related complex) B20
Ailment heart — *see* Disease, heart
Ailurophobia F40.218
AIN — *see* Neoplasia, intraepithelial, anal
Ainhum (disease) L94.6
AIPHI (acute idiopathic pulmonary hemorrhage in infants
(over 28 days old)) R04.81
Air
anterior mediastinum J98.2
compressed, disease T70.3 ☑
conditioner lung or pneumonitis J67.7
embolism (artery) (cerebral) (any site) T79.0 ☑
with ectopic or molar pregnancy O08.2
due to implanted device NEC — *see* Complications,
by site and type, specified NEC
following
abortion — *see* Abortion by type, complicated
by, embolism
ectopic or molar pregnancy O08.2
infusion, therapeutic injection or transfusion
T80.0 ☑
in pregnancy, childbirth or puerperium — *see* Embolism, obstetric
traumatic T79.0 ☑
hunger, psychogenic F45.8
rarefied, effects of — *see* Effect, adverse, high altitude
sickness T75.3 ☑
Airplane sickness T75.3 ☑
Akathisia (drug-induced) (treatment-induced) G25.71
neuroleptic induced (acute) G25.71
tardive G25.71
Akinesia R29.898
Akinetic mutism R41.89
Akureyri's disease G93.39
Alactasia, congenital E73.0
Alagille's syndrome Q44.7
Alastrim B03
Albers-Schönberg syndrome Q78.2
Albert's syndrome — *see* Tendinitis, Achilles
Albinism, albino E70.30
with hematologic abnormality E70.339
Chédiak-Higashi syndrome E70.330
Hermansky-Pudlak syndrome E70.331
other specified E70.338
I E70.320
II E70.321
ocular E70.319
autosomal recessive E70.311
other specified E70.318
X-linked E70.310
oculocutaneous E70.329
other specified E70.328
tyrosinase (ty) negative E70.320
tyrosinase (ty) positive E70.321
other specified E70.39
Albinismus E70.30
Albright (-McCune)(-Sternberg) syndrome Q78.1
Albuminous — *see* condition
Albuminuria, albuminuric (acute) (chronic) (subacute)
— *see also* Proteinuria R80.9
complicating pregnancy — *see* Proteinuria, gestational
with
gestational hypertension — *see* Pre-eclampsia
pre-existing hypertension — *see* Hypertension,
complicating pregnancy, pre-existing,
with, pre-eclampsia
gestational — *see* Proteinuria, gestational
with
gestational hypertension — *see* Pre-eclampsia
pre-existing hypertension — *see* Hypertension,
complicating pregnancy, pre-existing,
with, pre-eclampsia

Albuminuria, albuminuric — *continued*
orthostatic R80.2
postural R80.2
pre-eclamptic — *see* Pre-eclampsia
scarlatinal A38.8
Albuminurophobia F40.298
Alcaptonuria E70.29
Alcohol, alcoholic, alcohol-induced
addiction (without remission) F10.20
with remission F10.21
amnestic disorder, persisting F10.96
with dependence F10.26
anxiety disorder F10.980
bipolar and related disorder F10.94
brain syndrome, chronic F10.97
with dependence F10.27
cardiopathy I42.6
counseling and surveillance Z71.41
family member Z71.42
delirium (acute) (tremens) (withdrawal) F10.921
with intoxication F10.921
in
abuse F10.121
dependence F10.221
dependence (acute) (tremens) (withdrawal) F10.231
dementia F10.97
with dependence F10.27
depressive disorder F10.94
deterioration F10.97
with dependence F10.27
hallucinosis (acute) F10.951
in
abuse F10.151
dependence F10.251
insanity F10.959
intoxication (acute) (without dependence) F10.129
with
delirium F10.121
dependence F10.229
with delirium F10.221
uncomplicated F10.220
uncomplicated F10.120
jealousy F10.988
Korsakoff's, Korsakov's, Korsakow's F10.26
liver K70.9
acute — *see* Disease, liver, alcoholic, hepatitis
major neurocognitive disorder, amnestic-confabulatory
type F10.96
major neurocognitive disorder, nonamnestic-confabulatory type F10.97
mania (acute) (chronic) F10.959
mild neurocognitive disorder F10.988
paranoia, paranoid (type) psychosis F10.950
pellagra E52
poisoning, accidental (acute) NEC — *see* Table of Drugs
and Chemicals, alcohol, poisoning
psychosis — *see* Psychosis, alcoholic
psychotic disorder F10.959
sexual dysfunction F10.981
sleep disorder F10.982
withdrawal (without convulsions) F10.239
with delirium F10.231
Alcoholism (chronic) (without remission) F10.20
with
psychosis — *see* Psychosis, alcoholic
remission F10.21
Korsakov's F10.96
with dependence F10.26
Alder (-Reilly) **anomaly or syndrome** (leukocyte granulation) D72.0
Aldosteronism E26.9
familial (type I) E26.02
glucocorticoid-remediable E26.02
primary (due to (bilateral) adrenal hyperplasia) E26.09
primary NEC E26.09
secondary E26.1
specified NEC E26.89
Aldosteronoma D44.10
Aldrich (-Wiskott) **syndrome** (eczema-thrombocytopenia) D82.0
Alektorophobia F40.218
Aleppo boil B55.1
Aleukemic — *see* condition
Aleukia
congenital D70.0
hemorrhagica D61.9
congenital D61.09
splenica D73.1

Alexia R48.0
developmental F81.0
secondary to organic lesion R48.0
Algoneurodystrophy M89.00
ankle M89.07- ☑
foot M89.07- ☑
forearm M89.03- ☑
hand M89.04- ☑
lower leg M89.06- ☑
multiple sites M89.0- ☑
shoulder M89.01- ☑
specified site NEC M89.08
thigh M89.05- ☑
upper arm M89.02- ☑
Algophobia F40.298
Alienation, mental — *see* Psychosis
Alkalemia E87.3
Alkalosis E87.3
metabolic E87.3
with respiratory acidosis E87.4
of newborn P74.41
respiratory E87.3
Alkaptonuria E70.29
Allen-Masters syndrome N83.8
Allergy, allergic (reaction) (to) T78.40 ☑
air-borne substance NEC (rhinitis) J30.89
alveolitis (extrinsic) J67.9
due to
Aspergillus clavatus J67.4
Cryptostroma corticale J67.6
organisms (fungal, thermophilic actinomycete)
growing in ventilation (air conditioning)
systems J67.7
specified type NEC J67.8
anaphylactic reaction or shock T78.2 ☑
angioneurotic edema T78.3 ☑
animal (dander) (epidermal) (hair) (rhinitis) J30.81
bee sting (anaphylactic shock) — *see* Toxicity, venom,
arthropod, bee
biological — *see* Allergy, drug
colitis — *see also* Colitis, allergic K52.29
dander (animal) (rhinitis) J30.81
dandruff (rhinitis) J30.81
dental restorative material (existing) K08.55
dermatitis — *see* Dermatitis, contact, allergic
diathesis — *see* History, allergy
drug, medicament & biological (any) (external) (internal) T78.40 ☑
correct substance properly administered — *see* Table of Drugs and Chemicals, by drug, adverse
effect
wrong substance given or taken NEC (by accident)
— *see* Table of Drugs and Chemicals, by drug,
poisoning
due to pollen J30.1
dust (house) (stock) (rhinitis) J30.89
with asthma — *see* Asthma, allergic extrinsic
eczema — *see* Dermatitis, contact, allergic
epidermal (animal) (rhinitis) J30.81
feathers (rhinitis) J30.89
food (any) (ingested) NEC T78.1 ☑
anaphylactic shock — *see* Shock, anaphylactic, due
to food
dermatitis — *see* Dermatitis, due to, food
dietary counseling and surveillance Z71.3
in contact with skin L23.6
rhinitis J30.5
status (without reaction) Z91.018
beef Z91.014
eggs Z91.012
lamb Z91.014
mammalian meats Z91.014
milk products Z91.011
peanuts Z91.010
pork Z91.014
red meats Z91.014
seafood Z91.013
specified NEC Z91.018
gastrointestinal — *see also* specific type of allergic reaction
meaning colitis — *see also* Colitis, allergic K52.29
meaning gastroenteritis — *see also* Gastroenteritis,
allergic K52.29
meaning other adverse food reaction not elsewhere
classified T78.1 ☑
grain J30.1
grass (hay fever) (pollen) J30.1

Allergy, allergic — *continued*
  grass — *continued*
    asthma — *see* Asthma, allergic extrinsic
  hair (animal) (rhinitis) J30.81
  history (of) — *see* History, allergy
  horse serum — *see* Allergy, serum
  inhalant (rhinitis) J30.89
    pollen J30.1
  kapok (rhinitis) J30.89
  medicine — *see* Allergy, drug
  milk protein — *see also* Allergy, food Z91.011
    anaphylactic reaction T78.07 ☑
    dermatitis L27.2
    enterocolitis syndrome K52.21
    enteropathy K52.22
    gastroenteritis K52.29
    gastroesophageal reflux — *see also* Reaction, adverse, food K21.9
      with esophagitis (without bleeding) K21.00
        with bleeding K21.01
    proctocolitis K52.29
  nasal, seasonal due to pollen J30.1
  pneumonia J82.89
  pollen (any) (hay fever) J30.1
    asthma — *see* Asthma, allergic extrinsic
  primrose J30.1
  primula J30.1
  proctocolitis K52.29
  purpura D69.0
  ragweed (hay fever) (pollen) J30.1
    asthma — *see* Asthma, allergic extrinsic
  rose (pollen) J30.1
  seasonal NEC J30.2
  Senecio jacobae (pollen) J30.1
  serum — *see also* Reaction, serum T80.69 ☑
    anaphylactic shock T80.59 ☑
  shock (anaphylactic) T78.2 ☑
    due to
      administration of blood and blood products T80.51 ☑
      adverse effect of correct medicinal substance properly administered T88.6 ☑
      immunization T80.52 ☑
      serum NEC T80.59 ☑
      vaccination T80.52 ☑
  specific NEC T78.49 ☑
  tree (any) (hay fever) (pollen) J30.1
    asthma — *see* Asthma, allergic extrinsic
  upper respiratory J30.9
  urticaria L50.0
  vaccine — *see* Allergy, serum
  wheat — *see* Allergy, food
Allescheriasis B48.2
Alligator skin disease Q80.9
Allocheiria, allochiria R20.8
Almeida's disease — *see* Paracoccidioidomycosis
Alopecia (hereditaria) (seborrheica) L65.9
  androgenic L64.9
    drug-induced L64.0
    specified NEC L64.8
  areata L63.9
    ophiasis L63.2
    specified NEC L63.8
    totalis L63.0
    universalis L63.1
  cicatricial L66.9
    specified NEC L66.8
  circumscripta L63.9
  congenital, congenitalis Q84.0
  due to cytotoxic drugs NEC L65.8
  mucinosa L65.2
  postinfective NEC L65.8
  postpartum L65.0
  premature L64.8
  specific (syphilitic) A51.32
  specified NEC L65.8
  syphilitic (secondary) A51.32
  totalis (capitis) L63.0
  universalis (entire body) L63.1
  X-ray L58.1
Alpers' disease G31.81
Alpine sickness T70.29 ☑
Alport syndrome Q87.81
ALTE (apparent life threatening event) **in newborn and infant** R68.13
Alteration (of), **Altered**
  awareness
    transient R40.4

Alteration (of), **Altered** — *continued*
  awareness — *continued*
    unintended under general anesthesia, during procedure T88.53 ☑
  mental status R41.82
  pattern of family relationships affecting child Z62.898
  sensation
    following
      cerebrovascular disease I69.998
        cerebral infarction I69.398
        intracerebral hemorrhage I69.198
        nontraumatic intracranial hemorrhage NEC I69.298
        specified disease NEC I69.898
        subarachnoid hemorrhage I69.098
Alternating — *see* condition
Altitude, high (effects) — *see* Effect, adverse, high altitude
Aluminosis (of lung) J63.0
Alveolitis
  allergic (extrinsic) — *see* Pneumonitis, hypersensitivity
  due to
    Aspergillus clavatus J67.4
    Cryptostroma corticale J67.6
  fibrosing (cryptogenic) (idiopathic) J84.112
  jaw M27.3
  sicca dolorosa M27.3
Alveolus, alveolar — *see* condition
Alymphocytosis D72.810
  thymic (with immunodeficiency) D82.1
Alymphoplasia, thymic D82.1
Alzheimer's disease or sclerosis — *see* Disease, Alzheimer's
Amastia (with nipple present) Q83.8
  with absent nipple Q83.0
Amathophobia F40.228
Amaurosis (acquired) (congenital) — *see also* Blindness
  fugax G45.3
  hysterical F44.6
  Leber's congenital H35.50
  uremic — *see* Uremia
Amaurotic idiocy (infantile) (juvenile) (late) E75.4
Amaxophobia F40.248
Ambiguous genitalia Q56.4
Amblyopia (congenital) (ex anopsia) (partial) (suppression) H53.00- ☑
  anisometropic — *see* Amblyopia, refractive
  deprivation H53.01- ☑
  hysterical F44.6
  nocturnal — *see also* Blindness, night
    vitamin A deficiency E50.5
  refractive H53.02- ☑
  strabismic H53.03- ☑
  suspect H53.04- ☑
  tobacco H53.8
  toxic NEC H53.8
  uremic — *see* Uremia
Ameba, amebic (histolytica) — *see also* Amebiasis
  abscess (liver) A06.4
Amebiasis A06.9
  with abscess — *see* Abscess, amebic
  acute A06.0
  chronic (intestine) A06.1
    with abscess — *see* Abscess, amebic
  cutaneous A06.7
  cutis A06.7
  cystitis A06.81
  genitourinary tract NEC A06.82
  hepatic — *see* Abscess, liver, amebic
  intestine A06.0
  nondysenteric colitis A06.2
  skin A06.7
  specified site NEC A06.89
Ameboma (of intestine) A06.3
Amelia Q73.0
  lower limb — *see* Agenesis, leg
  upper limb — *see* Agenesis, arm
Ameloblastoma — *see also* Cyst, calcifying odontogenic
  long bones C40.9- ☑
    lower limb C40.2- ☑
    upper limb C40.0- ☑
  malignant C41.1
    jaw (bone) (lower) C41.1
      upper C41.0
  tibial C40.2- ☑
Amelogenesis imperfecta K00.5
  nonhereditaria (segmentalis) K00.4

Amenorrhea N91.2
  hyperhormonal E28.8
  primary N91.0
  secondary N91.1
Amentia — *see* Disability, intellectual
  Meynert's (nonalcoholic) F04
American
  leishmaniasis B55.2
  mountain tick fever A93.2
Ametropia — *see* Disorder, refraction
AMH (asymptomatic microscopic hematuria) R31.21
Amianthosis J61
Amimia R48.8
Amino-acid disorder E72.9
  anemia D53.0
Aminoacidopathy E72.9
Aminoaciduria E72.9
Amnesia R41.3
  anterograde R41.1
  auditory R48.8
  dissociative F44.0
    with dissociative fugue F44.1
  hysterical F44.0
  postictal in epilepsy — *see* Epilepsy
  psychogenic F44.0
  retrograde R41.2
  transient global G45.4
Amnes(t)ic syndrome (post-traumatic) F04
  induced by
    alcohol F10.96
      with dependence F10.26
    psychoactive NEC F19.96
      with
        abuse F19.16
        dependence F19.26
    sedative F13.96
      with dependence F13.26
Amnion, amniotic — *see* condition
Amnionitis — *see* Pregnancy, complicated by
Amok F68.8
Amoral traits F60.89
Amphetamine (or other stimulant) **-induced**
  anxiety disorder F15.980
  bipolar and related disorder F15.94
  delirium F15.921
  depressive disorder F15.94
  obsessive-compulsive and related disorder F15.988
  psychotic disorder F15.959
  sexual dysfunction F15.981
  sleep disorder F15.982
  stimulant withdrawal F15.23
Ampulla
  lower esophagus K22.89
  phrenic K22.89
Amputation — *see also* Absence, by site, acquired
  neuroma (postoperative) (traumatic) — *see* Complications, amputation stump, neuroma
  stump (surgical)
    abnormal, painful, or with complication (late) — *see* Complications, amputation stump
    healed or old NOS Z89.9
  traumatic (complete) (partial)
    arm (upper) (complete) S48.91- ☑
      at
        elbow S58.01- ☑
          partial S58.02- ☑
        shoulder joint (complete) S48.01- ☑
          partial S48.02- ☑
      between
        elbow and wrist (complete) S58.11- ☑
          partial S58.12- ☑
        shoulder and elbow (complete) S48.11- ☑
          partial S48.12- ☑
      partial S48.92- ☑
    breast (complete) S28.21- ☑
      partial S28.22- ☑
    clitoris (complete) S38.211 ☑
      partial S38.212 ☑
    ear (complete) S08.11- ☑
      partial S08.12- ☑
    finger (complete) (metacarpophalangeal) S68.11- ☑
      index S68.11- ☑
      little S68.11- ☑
      middle S68.11- ☑
      partial S68.12- ☑
        index S68.12- ☑
        little S68.12- ☑

Amputation — continued
traumatic — continued
finger — continued
partial — continued
middle S68.12- ☑
ring S68.12- ☑
ring S68.11- ☑
thumb — see Amputation, traumatic, thumb
transphalangeal (complete) S68.61- ☑
index S68.61- ☑
little S68.61- ☑
middle S68.61- ☑
partial S68.62- ☑
index S68.62- ☑
little S68.62- ☑
middle S68.62- ☑
ring S68.62- ☑
ring S68.61- ☑
foot (complete) S98.91- ☑
at ankle level S98.01- ☑
partial S98.02- ☑
midfoot S98.31- ☑
partial S98.32- ☑
partial S98.92- ☑
forearm (complete) S58.91- ☑
at elbow level (complete) S58.01- ☑
partial S58.02- ☑
between elbow and wrist (complete) S58.11- ☑
partial S58.12- ☑
partial S58.92- ☑
genital organ(s) (external)
female (complete) S38.211 ☑
partial S38.212 ☑
male
penis (complete) S38.221 ☑
partial S38.222 ☑
scrotum (complete) S38.231 ☑
partial S38.232 ☑
testes (complete) S38.231 ☑
partial S38.232 ☑
hand (complete) (wrist level) S68.41- ☑
finger(s) alone — see Amputation, traumatic, finger
partial S68.42- ☑
thumb alone — see Amputation, traumatic, thumb
transmetacarpal (complete) S68.71- ☑
partial S68.72- ☑
head
ear — see Amputation, traumatic, ear
nose (partial) S08.812 ☑
complete S08.811 ☑
part S08.89 ☑
scalp S08.0 ☑
hip (and thigh) (complete) S78.91- ☑
at hip joint (complete) S78.01- ☑
partial S78.02- ☑
between hip and knee (complete) S78.11- ☑
partial S78.12- ☑
partial S78.92- ☑
labium (majus) (minus) (complete) S38.21- ☑
partial S38.21- ☑
leg (lower) S88.91- ☑
at knee level S88.01- ☑
partial S88.02- ☑
between knee and ankle S88.11- ☑
partial S88.12- ☑
partial S88.92- ☑
nose (partial) S08.812 ☑
complete S08.811 ☑
penis (complete) S38.221 ☑
partial S38.222 ☑
scrotum (complete) S38.231 ☑
partial S38.232 ☑
shoulder — see Amputation, traumatic, arm
at shoulder joint — see Amputation, traumatic, arm, at shoulder joint
testes (complete) S38.231 ☑
partial S38.232 ☑
thigh — see Amputation, traumatic, hip
thorax, part of S28.1 ☑
breast — see Amputation, traumatic, breast
thumb (complete) (metacarpophalangeal) S68.01- ☑
partial S68.02- ☑
transphalangeal (complete) S68.51- ☑

Amputation — continued
traumatic — continued
thumb — continued
transphalangeal — continued
partial S68.52- ☑
toe (lesser) S98.13- ☑
great S98.11- ☑
partial S98.12- ☑
more than one S98.21- ☑
partial S98.22- ☑
partial S98.14- ☑
vulva (complete) S38.211 ☑
partial S38.212 ☑
Amputee (bilateral) (old) Z89.9
Amsterdam dwarfism Q87.19
Amusia R48.8
developmental F80.89
Amyelencephalus, amyelencephaly Q00.0
Amyelia Q06.0
Amygdalitis — see Tonsillitis
Amygdalolith J35.8
Amyloid heart (disease) E85.4 [I43]
Amyloidosis (generalized) (primary) E85.9
with lung involvement E85.4 [J99]
familial E85.2
genetic E85.2
heart E85.4 [I43]
hemodialysis-associated E85.3
light chain (AL) E85.81
liver E85.4 [K77]
localized E85.4
neuropathic heredofamilial E85.1
non-neuropathic heredofamilial E85.0
organ limited E85.4
Portuguese E85.1
pulmonary E85.4 [J99]
secondary systemic E85.3
senile systemic (SSA) E85.82
skin (lichen) (macular) E85.4 [L99]
specified NEC E85.89
subglottic E85.4 [J99]
wild-type transthyretin-related (ATTR) E85.82
Amylopectinosis (brancher enzyme deficiency) E74.03
Amylophagia — see Pica
Amyoplasia congenita Q79.8
Amyotonia M62.89
congenita G70.2
Amyotrophia, amyotrophy, amyotrophic G71.8
congenita Q79.8
diabetic — see Diabetes, amyotrophy
lateral sclerosis G12.21
neuralgic G54.5
spinal progressive G12.25
Anacidity, gastric K31.83
psychogenic F45.8
Anaerosis of newborn P28.89
Analbuminemia E88.09
Analgesia — see Anesthesia
Analphalipoproteinemia E78.6
Anaphylactic
purpura D69.0
shock or reaction — see Shock, anaphylactic
Anaphylactoid shock or reaction — see Shock, anaphylactic
Anaphylactoid syndrome of pregnancy O88.01- ☑
Anaphylaxis — see Shock, anaphylactic
Anaplasia cervix — see also Dysplasia, cervix N87.9
Anaplasmosis [A. phagocytophilum] (transfusion transmitted) A79.82
human A77.49
Anarthria R47.1
Anasarca R60.1
cardiac — see Failure, heart, congestive
lung J18.2
newborn P83.2
nutritional E43
pulmonary J18.2
renal N04.9
Anastomosis
aneurysmal — see Aneurysm
arteriovenous ruptured brain I60.8
intracerebral I61.8
intraparenchymal I61.8
intraventricular I61.5
subarachnoid I60.8
intestinal K63.89
complicated NEC K91.89

Anastomosis — continued
intestinal — continued
complicated — continued
involving urinary tract N99.89
retinal and choroidal vessels (congenital) Q14.8
Anatomical narrow angle H40.03- ☑
Ancylostoma, ancylostomiasis (braziliense) (caninum) (ceylanicum) (duodenale) B76.0
Necator americanus B76.1
Andersen's disease (glycogen storage) E74.09
Anderson-Fabry disease E75.21
Andes disease T70.29 ☑
Andrews' disease (bacterid) L08.89
Androblastoma
benign
specified site — see Neoplasm, benign, by site
unspecified site
female D27.9
male D29.20
malignant
specified site — see Neoplasm, malignant, by site
unspecified site
female C56.9
male C62.90
specified site — see Neoplasm, uncertain behavior, by site
tubular
with lipid storage
specified site — see Neoplasm, benign, by site
unspecified site
female D27.9
male D29.20
specified site — see Neoplasm, benign, by site
unspecified site
female D27.9
male D29.20
unspecified site
female D39.10
male D40.10
Androgen insensitivity syndrome — see also Syndrome, androgen insensitivity E34.50
Androgen resistance syndrome — see also Syndrome, androgen insensitivity E34.50
Android pelvis Q74.2
with disproportion (fetopelvic) O33.3 ☑
causing obstructed labor O65.3
Androphobia F40.290
Anectasis, pulmonary (newborn) — see Atelectasis
Anemia (essential) (general) (hemoglobin deficiency) (infantile) (primary) (profound) D64.9
with (due to) (in)
disorder of
anaerobic glycolysis D55.29
pentose phosphate pathway D55.1
koilonychia D50.9
achlorhydric D50.8
achrestic D53.1
Addison (-Biermer) (pernicious) D51.0
agranulocytic — see Agranulocytosis
amino-acid-deficiency D53.0
aplastic D61.9
congenital D61.09
drug-induced D61.1
due to
drugs D61.1
external agents NEC D61.2
infection D61.2
radiation D61.2
idiopathic D61.3
red cell (pure) D60.9
chronic D60.0
congenital D60.01
specified type NEC D60.8
transient D60.1
specified type NEC D61.89
toxic D61.2
aregenerative
congenital D61.09
asiderotic D50.9
atypical (primary) D64.9
Baghdad spring D55.0
Balantidium coli A07.0
Biermer's (pernicious) D51.0
blood loss (chronic) D50.0
acute D62
bothriocephalus B70.0 [D63.8]
brickmaker's B76.9 [D63.8]
cerebral I67.89

Amputation — Anemia

Anemia — *continued*
childhood D58.9
chlorotic D50.8
chronic
  blood loss D50.0
  hemolytic D58.9
    idiopathic D59.9
  simple D53.9
chronica congenita aregenerativa D61.09
combined system disease NEC D51.0 [G32.0]
  due to dietary vitamin B12 deficiency D51.3 [G32.0]
complicating pregnancy, childbirth or puerperium —
  see Pregnancy, complicated by (management
  affected by), anemia
congenital P61.4
  aplastic D61.09
  due to isoimmunization NOS P55.9
  dyserythropoietic, dyshematopoietic D64.4
  following fetal blood loss P61.3
  Heinz body D58.2
  hereditary hemolytic NOS D58.9
  pernicious D51.0
  spherocytic D58.0
Cooley's (erythroblastic) D56.1
cytogenic D51.0
deficiency D53.9
  2, 3 diphosphoglycurate mutase D55.29
  2, 3 PG D55.29
  6 phosphogluconate dehydrogenase D55.1
  6-PGD D55.1
  amino-acid D53.0
  combined B12 and folate D53.1
  enzyme D55.9
    drug-induced (hemolytic) D59.2
    glucose-6-phosphate dehydrogenase (G6PD)
      D55.0
    glycolytic D55.29
    nucleotide metabolism D55.3
    related to hexose monophosphate (HMP) shunt
      pathway NEC D55.1
    specified type NEC D55.8
  erythrocytic glutathione D55.1
  folate D52.9
    dietary D52.0
    drug-induced D52.1
  folic acid D52.9
    dietary D52.0
    drug-induced D52.1
  G SH D55.1
  G6PD D55.0
  GGS-R D55.1
  glucose-6-phosphate dehydrogenase D55.0
  glutathione reductase D55.1
  glyceraldehyde phosphate dehydrogenase D55.29
  hexokinase D55.29
  iron D50.9
    secondary to blood loss (chronic) D50.0
  nutritional D53.9
    with
      poor iron absorption D50.8
      specified deficiency NEC D53.8
  phosphofructo-aldolase D55.29
  phosphoglycerate kinase D55.29
  PK D55.21
  protein D53.0
  pyruvate kinase D55.21
  transcobalamin II D51.2
  triose-phosphate isomerase D55.29
  vitamin B12 NOS D51.9
    dietary D51.3
    due to
      intrinsic factor deficiency D51.0
      selective vitamin B12 malabsorption with
        proteinuria D51.1
    pernicious D51.0
    specified type NEC D51.8
Diamond-Blackfan (congenital hypoplastic) D61.01
dibothriocephalus B70.0 [D63.8]
dimorphic D53.1
diphasic D53.1
Diphyllobothrium (Dibothriocephalus) B70.0 [D63.8]
due to (in) (with)
  antineoplastic chemotherapy D64.81
  blood loss (chronic) D50.0
    acute D62
  chemotherapy, antineoplastic D64.81
  chronic disease classified elsewhere NEC D63.8
  chronic kidney disease D63.1

Anemia — *continued*
due to — *continued*
  deficiency
    amino-acid D53.0
    copper D53.8
    folate (folic acid) D52.9
      dietary D52.0
      drug-induced D52.1
    molybdenum D53.8
    protein D53.0
    zinc D53.8
  dietary vitamin B12 deficiency D51.3
  disorder of
    glutathione metabolism D55.1
    nucleotide metabolism D55.3
  drug — *see* Anemia, by type — *see also* Table of
    Drugs and Chemicals
  end stage renal disease D63.1
  enzyme disorder D55.9
  fetal blood loss P61.3
  fish tapeworm (D.latum) infestation B70.0 [D63.8]
  hemorrhage (chronic) D50.0
    acute D62
  impaired absorption D50.9
  loss of blood (chronic) D50.0
    acute D62
  myxedema E03.9 [D63.8]
  Necator americanus B76.1 [D63.8]
  prematurity P61.2
  selective vitamin B12 malabsorption with protein-
    uria D51.1
  transcobalamin II deficiency D51.2
Dyke-Young type (secondary) (symptomatic) D59.19
dyserythropoietic (congenital) D64.4
dyshematopoietic (congenital) D64.4
Egyptian B76.9 [D63.8]
elliptocytosis — *see* Elliptocytosis
enzyme-deficiency, drug-induced D59.2
epidemic — *see also* Ancylostomiasis B76.9 [D63.8]
erythroblastic
  familial D56.1
  newborn — *see also* Disease, hemolytic P55.9
  of childhood D56.1
erythrocytic glutathione deficiency D55.1
erythropoietin-resistant anemia (EPO resistant anemia)
  D63.1
Faber's (achlorhydric anemia) D50.9
factitious (self-induced blood letting) D50.0
familial erythroblastic D56.1
Fanconi's (congenital pancytopenia) D61.09
favism D55.0
fish tapeworm (D. latum) infestation B70.0 [D63.8]
folate (folic acid) deficiency D52.9
glucose-6-phosphate dehydrogenase (G6PD) deficiency
  D55.0
glutathione-reductase deficiency D55.1
goat's milk D52.0
granulocytic — *see* Agranulocytosis
Heinz body, congenital D58.2
hemolytic D58.9
  acquired D59.9
    with hemoglobinuria NEC D59.6
    autoimmune NEC D59.19
    infectious D59.4
    specified type NEC D59.8
    toxic D59.4
  acute D59.9
    due to enzyme deficiency specified type NEC
      D55.8
    Lederer's D59.19
  autoimmune D59.10
    cold D59.12
    drug-induced D59.0
    mixed D59.13
    warm D59.11
  chronic D58.9
    idiopathic D59.9
  cold type (primary) (secondary) (symptomatic)
    D59.12
  congenital (spherocytic) — *see* Spherocytosis
  due to
    cardiac conditions D59.4
    drugs (nonautoimmune) D59.2
      autoimmune D59.0
    enzyme disorder D55.9
      drug-induced D59.2
    presence of shunt or other internal prosthetic
      device D59.4

Anemia — *continued*
hemolytic — *continued*
  familial D58.9
  hereditary D58.9
    due to enzyme disorder D55.9
      specified type NEC D55.8
    specified type NEC D58.8
  idiopathic (chronic) D59.9
  mechanical D59.4
  microangiopathic D59.4
  mixed type (primary) (secondary) (symptomatic)
    D59.13
  nonautoimmune D59.4
    drug-induced D59.2
  nonspherocytic
    congenital or hereditary NEC D55.8
      glucose-6-phosphate dehydrogenase deficien-
        cy D55.0
      pyruvate kinase deficiency D55.21
      type
        I D55.1
        II D55.29
    type
      I D55.1
      II D55.29
  primary
    autoimmune
      cold type D59.12
      mixed type D59.13
      warm type D59.11
  secondary D59.4
    autoimmune
      cold type D59.12
      mixed type D59.13
      warm type D59.11
  specified (hereditary) type NEC D58.8
  Stransky-Regala type — *see also* Hemoglobinopathy
    D58.8
  symptomatic D59.4
    autoimmune
      cold type D59.12
      mixed type D59.13
      warm type D59.11
  toxic D59.4
  warm type (primary) (secondary) (symptomatic)
    D59.11
hemorrhagic (chronic) D50.0
  acute D62
Herrick's D57.1
hexokinase deficiency D55.29
hookworm B76.9 [D63.8]
hypochromic (idiopathic) (microcytic) (normoblastic)
  D50.9
  due to blood loss (chronic) D50.0
    acute D62
  familial sex-linked D64.0
  pyridoxine-responsive D64.3
  sideroblastic, sex-linked D64.0
hypoplasia, red blood cells D61.9
  congenital or familial D61.01
hypoplastic (idiopathic) D61.9
  congenital or familial (of childhood) D61.01
hypoproliferative (refractive) D61.9
idiopathic D64.9
  aplastic D61.3
  hemolytic, chronic D59.9
in (due to) (with)
  chronic kidney disease D63.1
  end stage renal disease D63.1
  failure, kidney (renal) D63.1
  neoplastic disease — *see also* Neoplasm D63.0
intertropical — *see also* Ancylostomiasis D63.8
iron deficiency D50.9
  secondary to blood loss (chronic) D50.0
    acute D62
  specified type NEC D50.8
Joseph-Diamond-Blackfan (congenital hypoplastic)
  D61.01
Lederer's (hemolytic) D59.19
leukoerythroblastic D61.82
macrocytic D53.9
  nutritional D52.0
  tropical D52.8
malarial — *see also* Malaria B54 [D63.8]
malignant (progressive) D51.0
malnutrition D53.9
marsh — *see also* Malaria B54 [D63.8]
Mediterranean (with other hemoglobinopathy) D56.9
megaloblastic D53.1

Anemia — *continued*
  megaloblastic — *continued*
    combined B12 and folate deficiency D53.1
    hereditary D51.1
    nutritional D52.0
    orotic aciduria D53.0
    refractory D53.1
    specified type NEC D53.1
  megalocytic D53.1
  microcytic (hypochromic) D50.9
    due to blood loss (chronic) D50.0
      acute D62
    familial D56.8
  microdrepanocytosis D57.40
  microelliptopoikilocytic (Rietti-Greppi- Micheli) D56.9
  miner's B76.9 *[D63.8]*
  myelodysplastic D46.9
  myelofibrosis D75.81
  myelogenous D64.89
  myelopathic D64.89
  myelophthisic D61.82
  myeloproliferative D47.Z9 (*following D47.4*)
  newborn P61.4
    due to
      ABO (antibodies, isoimmunization, maternal/fetal incompatibility) P55.1
      Rh (antibodies, isoimmunization, maternal/fetal incompatibility) P55.0
    following fetal blood loss P61.3
    posthemorrhagic (fetal) P61.3
  nonspherocytic hemolytic — *see* Anemia, hemolytic, nonspherocytic
  normocytic (infectional) D64.9
    due to blood loss (chronic) D50.0
      acute D62
    myelophthisic D61.82
  nutritional (deficiency) D53.9
    with
      poor iron absorption D50.8
      specified deficiency NEC D53.8
    megaloblastic D52.0
  of prematurity P61.2
  orotaciduric (congenital) (hereditary) D53.0
  osteosclerotic D64.89
  ovalocytosis (hereditary) — *see* Elliptocytosis
  paludal — *see also* Malaria B54 *[D63.8]*
  pernicious (congenital) (malignant) (progressive) D51.0
  pleochromic D64.89
    of sprue D52.8
  posthemorrhagic (chronic) D50.0
    acute D62
    newborn P61.3
  postoperative (postprocedural)
    due to (acute) blood loss D62
      chronic blood loss D50.0
    specified NEC D64.89
  postpartum O90.81
  pressure D64.89
  progressive D64.9
    malignant D51.0
    pernicious D51.0
  protein-deficiency D53.0
  pseudoleukemica infantum D64.89
  pure red cell D60.9
    congenital D61.01
  pyridoxine-responsive D64.3
  pyruvate kinase deficiency D55.21
  refractory D46.4
    with
      excess of blasts D46.20
        1 (RAEB 1) D46.21
        2 (RAEB 2) D46.22
        in transformation (RAEB T) — *see* Leukemia, acute myeloblastic
      hemochromatosis D46.1
      sideroblasts (ring) (RARS) D46.1
    megaloblastic D53.1
    sideroblastic D46.1
    sideropenic D50.9
    without ring sideroblasts, so stated D46.0
    without sideroblasts without excess of blasts D46.0
  Rietti-Greppi-Micheli D56.9
  scorbutic D53.2
  secondary to
    blood loss (chronic) D50.0
      acute D62
    hemorrhage (chronic) D50.0
      acute D62
  semiplastic D61.89

Anemia — *continued*
  sickle-cell — *see* Disease, sickle-cell
  sideroblastic D64.3
    hereditary D64.0
    hypochromic, sex-linked D64.0
    pyridoxine-responsive NEC D64.3
    refractory D46.1
    secondary (due to)
      disease D64.1
      drugs and toxins D64.2
    specified type NEC D64.3
  sideropenic (refractory) D50.9
    due to blood loss (chronic) D50.0
      acute D62
  simple chronic D53.9
  specified type NEC D64.89
  spherocytic (hereditary) — *see* Spherocytosis
  splenic D64.89
  splenomegalic D64.89
  stomatocytosis D58.8
  syphilitic (acquired) (late) A52.79 *[D63.8]*
  target cell D64.89
  thalassemia D56.9
  thrombocytopenic — *see* Thrombocytopenia
  toxic D61.2
  tropical B76.9 *[D63.8]*
    macrocytic D52.8
  tuberculous A18.89 *[D63.8]*
  vegan D51.3
  vitamin
    B12 deficiency (dietary) pernicious D51.0
    B6-responsive D64.3
  von Jaksch's D64.89
  Witts' (achlorhydric anemia) D50.8
Anemophobia F40.228
Anencephalus, anencephaly Q00.0
Anergasia — *see* Psychosis, organic
Anesthesia, anesthetic R20.0
  complication or reaction NEC — *see also* Complications, anesthesia T88.59 ☑
    due to
      correct substance properly administered — *see* Table of Drugs and Chemicals, by drug, adverse effect
      overdose or wrong substance given — *see* Table of Drugs and Chemicals, by drug, poisoning
    unintended awareness under general anesthesia during procedure T88.53 ☑
      personal history of Z92.84
  cornea H18.81- ☑
  dissociative F44.6
  functional (hysterical) F44.6
  hyperesthetic, thalamic G89.0
  hysterical F44.6
  local skin lesion R20.0
  sexual (psychogenic) F52.1
  shock (due to) T88.2 ☑
  skin R20.0
  testicular N50.9
Anetoderma (maculosum) (of) L90.8
  Jadassohn-Pellizzari L90.2
  Schweniger-Buzzi L90.1
Aneurin deficiency E51.9
Aneurysm (anastomotic) (artery) (cirsoid) (diffuse) (false) (fusiform) (multiple) (saccular) I72.9
  abdominal (aorta) I71.40
    infrarenal I71.43
      ruptured I71.33
    juxtarenal I71.42
      ruptured I71.32
    pararenal I71.41
      ruptured I71.31
    ruptured I71.30
    syphilitic A52.01
  aorta, aortic (nonsyphilitic) I71.9
    abdominal I71.40
      dissecting — *see* Dissection, aorta, abdominal
      ruptured I71.30
    arch I71.22
      ruptured I71.12
    arteriosclerotic I71.9
      ruptured I71.8
    ascending I71.21
      ruptured I71.11
    congenital Q25.43
    descending I71.9
      abdominal I71.40

Aneurysm — *continued*
  aorta, aortic — *continued*
    descending — *continued*
      abdominal — *continued*
        ruptured I71.30
      ruptured I71.8
      thoracic I71.23
        ruptured I71.13
    dissecting — *see* Dissection, aorta
    root Q25.43
    ruptured I71.8
    sinus, congenital Q25.43
    syphilitic A52.01
    thoracic I71.20
      ruptured I71.10
    thoracoabdominal I71.60
      paravisceral I71.62
        ruptured I71.52
      ruptured I71.50
      supraceliac I71.61
        ruptured I71.51
    thorax, thoracic I71.20
      arch I71.22
        ruptured I71.12
      ascending I71.21
        ruptured I71.11
      descending I71.23
        ruptured I71.13
      ruptured I71.10
        arch I71.12
        ascending I71.11
        descending I71.13
    transverse I71.22
      ruptured I71.12
    valve (heart) — *see also* Endocarditis, aortic I35.8
  arteriosclerotic I72.9
    cerebral I67.1
      ruptured — *see* Hemorrhage, intracranial, subarachnoid
  arteriovenous (congenital) — *see also* Malformation, arteriovenous
    acquired I77.0
      brain I67.1
        ruptured — *see* Aneurysm, arteriovenous, brain, ruptured
      coronary I25.41
      pulmonary I28.0
    brain Q28.2
      ruptured I60.8
        intracerebral I61.8
        intraparenchymal I61.8
        intraventricular I61.5
        subarachnoid I60.8
    peripheral — *see* Malformation, arteriovenous, peripheral
    precerebral vessels Q28.0
    specified site NEC — *see also* Malformation, arteriovenous
      acquired I77.0
  basal — *see* Aneurysm, brain
  basilar (trunk) I72.5
  berry (congenital) (nonruptured) I67.1
    ruptured I60.7
  brain I67.1
    arteriosclerotic I67.1
      ruptured — *see* Hemorrhage, intracranial, subarachnoid
    arteriovenous (congenital) (nonruptured) Q28.2
      acquired I67.1
        ruptured — *see* Aneurysm, arteriovenous, brain, ruptured I60.8-
      ruptured — *see* Aneurysm, arteriovenous, brain, ruptured I60.8-
    berry (congenital) (nonruptured) I67.1
      ruptured — *see also* Hemorrhage, intracranial, subarachnoid I60.7
    congenital Q28.3
      ruptured I60.7
    meninges I67.1
      ruptured I60.8
    miliary (congenital) (nonruptured) I67.1
      ruptured — *see also* Hemorrhage, intracranial, subarachnoid I60.7
    mycotic I33.0
    ruptured — *see* Aneurysm, arteriovenous, brain, ruptured I60.8
    syphilitic (hemorrhage) A52.05
  cardiac (false) — *see also* Aneurysm, heart I25.3

Aneurysm — *continued*
  carotid artery (common) (external) I72.Ø
    internal (intracranial) I67.1
      extracranial portion I72.Ø
      ruptured into brain I6Ø.Ø- ☑
    syphilitic A52.Ø9
    intracranial A52.Ø5
  cavernous sinus I67.1
    arteriovenous (congenital) (nonruptured) Q28.3
      ruptured I6Ø.8
  celiac I72.8
  central nervous system, syphilitic A52.Ø5
  cerebral — *see* Aneurysm, brain
  chest — *see* Aneurysm, thorax
  circle of Willis I67.1
    congenital Q28.3
      ruptured I6Ø.6
    ruptured I6Ø.6
  common iliac artery I72.3
  congenital (peripheral) Q27.8
    aorta (root) (sinus) Q25.43
    brain Q28.3
      ruptured I6Ø.7
    coronary Q24.5
    digestive system Q27.8
    lower limb Q27.8
    pulmonary Q25.79
    retina Q14.1
    specified site NEC Q27.8
    upper limb Q27.8
  conjunctiva — *see* Abnormality, conjunctiva, vascular
  conus arteriosus — *see* Aneurysm, heart
  coronary (arteriosclerotic) (artery) I25.41
    arteriovenous, congenital Q24.5
    congenital Q24.5
    ruptured — *see* Infarct, myocardium
    syphilitic A52.Ø6
    vein I25.89
  cylindroid (aorta) I71.9
    ruptured I71.8
    syphilitic A52.Ø1
  ductus arteriosus Q25.Ø
  endocardial, infective (any valve) I33.Ø
  femoral (artery) (ruptured) I72.4
  gastroduodenal I72.8
  gastroepiploic I72.8
  heart (wall) (chronic or with a stated duration of over 4 weeks) I25.3
    valve — *see* Endocarditis
  hepatic I72.8
  iliac (common) (artery) (ruptured) I72.3
  infective I72.9
    endocardial (any valve) I33.Ø
  innominate (nonsyphilitic) I72.8
    syphilitic A52.Ø9
  interauricular septum — *see* Aneurysm, heart
  interventricular septum — *see* Aneurysm, heart
  intrathoracic (nonsyphilitic) — *see also* Aneurysm, aorta, thorax I71.2Ø
    ruptured — *see also* Aneurysm, aorta, thorax, ruptured I71.1Ø
    syphilitic A52.Ø1
  lower limb I72.4
  lung (pulmonary artery) I28.1
  mediastinal (nonsyphilitic) I72.8
    syphilitic A52.Ø9
  miliary (congenital) I67.1
    ruptured — *see* Hemorrhage, intracerebral, subarachnoid, intracranial
  mitral (heart) (valve) I34.89
  mural — *see* Aneurysm, heart
  mycotic I72.9
    endocardial (any valve) I33.Ø
    ruptured, brain — *see* Hemorrhage, intracerebral, subarachnoid
  myocardium — *see* Aneurysm, heart
  neck I72.Ø
  pancreaticoduodenal I72.8
  patent ductus arteriosus Q25.Ø
  peripheral NEC I72.8
    congenital Q27.8
      digestive system Q27.8
      lower limb Q27.8
      specified site NEC Q27.8
      upper limb Q27.8
  popliteal (artery) (ruptured) I72.4
  precerebral
    congenital (nonruptured) Q28.1

Aneurysm — *continued*
  precerebral — *continued*
    specified site, NEC I72.5
  pulmonary I28.1
    arteriovenous Q25.72
      acquired I28.Ø
    syphilitic A52.Ø9
    valve (heart) — *see* Endocarditis, pulmonary
  racemose (peripheral) I72.9
    congenital — *see* Aneurysm, congenital
  radial I72.1
  Rasmussen NEC A15.Ø
  renal (artery) I72.2
  retina — *see also* Disorder, retina, microaneurysms
    congenital Q14.1
    diabetic — *see* EØ8-E13 with .3-
  sinus of Valsalva Q25.49
  specified NEC I72.8
  spinal (cord) I72.8
    syphilitic (hemorrhage) A52.Ø9
  splenic I72.8
  subclavian (artery) (ruptured) I72.8
    syphilitic A52.Ø9
  superior mesenteric I72.8
  syphilitic (aorta) A52.Ø1
    central nervous system A52.Ø5
    congenital (late) A5Ø.54 *[I79.Ø]*
    spine, spinal A52.Ø9
  thoracoabdominal (aorta) I71.6Ø
    ruptured I71.5Ø
    syphilitic A52.Ø1
  thorax, thoracic (aorta) (arch) (nonsyphilitic) — *see* Aneurysm, aorta, thorax
    ruptured — *see* Aneurysm, aorta, thorax, ruptured
    syphilitic A52.Ø1
  traumatic (complication) (early), specified site — *see* Injury, blood vessel
  tricuspid (heart) (valve) IØ7.8
  ulnar I72.1
  upper limb (ruptured) I72.1
  valve, valvular — *see* Endocarditis
  venous — *see also* Varix I86.8
    congenital Q27.8
      digestive system Q27.8
      lower limb Q27.8
      specified site NEC Q27.8
      upper limb Q27.8
  ventricle — *see* Aneurysm, heart
  vertebral artery I72.6
  visceral NEC I72.8
Angelman syndrome Q93.51
Anger R45.4
Angiectasis, angiectopia I99.8
Angiitis I77.6
  allergic granulomatous M3Ø.1
  hypersensitivity M31.Ø
  necrotizing M31.9
    specified NEC M31.8
  nervous system, granulomatous I67.7
Angina (attack) (cardiac) (chest) (heart) (pectoris) (syndrome) (vasomotor) I2Ø.9
  with
    atherosclerotic heart disease — *see* Arteriosclerosis, coronary (artery),
    documented spasm I2Ø.1
  abdominal K55.1
  accelerated — *see* Angina, unstable
  agranulocytic — *see* Agranulocytosis
  angiospastic — *see* Angina, with documented spasm
  aphthous BØ8.5
  crescendo — *see* Angina, unstable
  croupous JØ5.Ø
  cruris I73.9
  de novo effort — *see* Angina, unstable
  diphtheritic, membranous A36.Ø
  equivalent I2Ø.8
  exudative, chronic J37.Ø
  following acute myocardial infarction I23.7
  gangrenous diphtheritic A36.Ø
  intestinal K55.1
  Ludovici K12.2
  Ludwig's K12.2
  malignant diphtheritic A36.Ø
  membranous JØ5.Ø
    diphtheritic A36.Ø
    Vincent's A69.1
  mesenteric K55.1
  monocytic — *see* Mononucleosis, infectious

Angina — *continued*
  of effort — *see* Angina, specified NEC
  phlegmonous J36
    diphtheritic A36.Ø
  post-infarctional I23.7
  pre-infarctional — *see* Angina, unstable
  Prinzmetal — *see* Angina, with documented spasm
  progressive — *see* Angina, unstable
  pseudomembranous A69.1
  pultaceous, diphtheritic A36.Ø
  refractory I2Ø.2
  spasm-induced — *see* Angina, with documented spasm
  specified NEC I2Ø.8
  stable I2Ø.8
  stenocardia — *see* Angina, specified NEC
  stridulous, diphtheritic A36.2
  tonsil J36
  trachealis JØ5.Ø
  unstable I2Ø.Ø
  variant — *see* Angina, with documented spasm
  Vincent's A69.1
  worsening effort — *see* Angina, unstable
Angioblastoma — *see* Neoplasm, connective tissue, uncertain behavior
Angiocholecystitis — *see* Cholecystitis, acute
Angiocholitis — *see also* Cholecystitis, acute K83.Ø9
Angiodysgenesis spinalis G95.19
Angiodysplasia (cecum) (colon) K55.2Ø
  with bleeding K55.21
  duodenum (and stomach) K31.819
    with bleeding K31.811
  stomach (and duodenum) K31.819
    with bleeding K31.811
Angioedema (allergic) (any site) (with urticaria) T78.3 ☑
  episodic, with eosinophilia D72.118
  hereditary D84.1
Angioendothelioma — *see* Neoplasm, uncertain behavior, by site
  benign D18.ØØ
    intra-abdominal D18.Ø3
    intracranial D18.Ø2
    skin D18.Ø1
    specified site NEC D18.Ø9
  bone — *see* Neoplasm, bone, malignant
  Ewing's — *see* Neoplasm, bone, malignant
Angioendotheliomatosis C85.8- ☑
Angiofibroma — *see also* Neoplasm, benign, by site
  juvenile
    specified site — *see* Neoplasm, benign, by site
    unspecified site D1Ø.6
Angiohemophilia (A) (B) — *see* Disease, von Willebrand
Angioid streaks (choroid) (macula) (retina) H35.33
Angiokeratoma — *see* Neoplasm, skin, benign
  corporis diffusum E75.21
Angioleiomyoma — *see* Neoplasm, connective tissue, benign
Angiolipoma — *see also* Lipoma
  infiltrating — *see* Lipoma
Angioma — *see also* Hemangioma, by site
  capillary I78.1
  hemorrhagicum hereditaria I78.Ø
  intra-abdominal D18.Ø3
  intracranial D18.Ø2
  malignant — *see* Neoplasm, connective tissue, malignant
  plexiform D18.ØØ
    intra-abdominal D18.Ø3
    intracranial D18.Ø2
    skin D18.Ø1
    specified site NEC D18.Ø9
  senile I78.1
  serpiginosum L81.7
  skin D18.Ø1
  specified site NEC D18.Ø9
  spider I78.1
  stellate I78.1
  venous Q28.3
Angiomatosis Q82.8
  bacillary A79.89
  encephalotrigeminal Q85.89
  hemorrhagic familial I78.Ø
  hereditary familial I78.Ø
  liver K76.4
Angiomyolipoma — *see* Lipoma
Angiomyoliposarcoma — *see* Neoplasm, connective tissue, malignant
Angiomyoma — *see* Neoplasm, connective tissue, benign

Angiomyosarcoma — *see* Neoplasm, connective tissue, malignant
Angiomyxoma — *see* Neoplasm, connective tissue, uncertain behavior
Angioneurosis F45.8
Angioneurotic edema (allergic) (any site) (with urticaria) T78.3 ☑
   hereditary D84.1
Angiopathia, angiopathy I99.9
   cerebral I67.9
      amyloid E85.4 *[I68.0]*
   diabetic (peripheral) — *see* Diabetes, angiopathy
   peripheral I73.9
      diabetic — *see* Diabetes, angiopathy
      specified type NEC I73.89
   retinae syphilitica A52.05
   retinalis (juvenilis)
      diabetic — *see* Diabetes, retinopathy
      proliferative — *see* Retinopathy, proliferative
Angiosarcoma — *see also* Neoplasm, connective tissue, malignant
   liver C22.3
Angiosclerosis — *see* Arteriosclerosis
Angiospasm (peripheral) (traumatic) (vessel) I73.9
   brachial plexus G54.0
   cerebral G45.9
   cervical plexus G54.2
   nerve
      arm — *see* Mononeuropathy, upper limb
         axillary G54.0
         median — *see* Lesion, nerve, median
         ulnar — *see* Lesion, nerve, ulnar
      axillary G54.0
      leg — *see* Mononeuropathy, lower limb
      median — *see* Lesion, nerve, median
      plantar — *see* Lesion, nerve, plantar
      ulnar — *see* Lesion, nerve, ulnar
Angiospastic disease or edema I73.9
Angiostrongyliasis
   due to
      Parastrongylus
         cantonensis B83.2
         costaricensis B81.3
   intestinal B81.3
Anguillulosis — *see* Strongyloidiasis
Angulation
   cecum — *see* Obstruction, intestine
   coccyx (acquired) — *see also* subcategory M43.8 ☑
      congenital NEC Q76.49
   femur (acquired) — *see also* Deformity, limb, specified type NEC, thigh
      congenital Q74.2
   intestine (large) (small) — *see* Obstruction, intestine
   sacrum (acquired) — *see also* subcategory M43.8 ☑
      congenital NEC Q76.49
   sigmoid (flexure) — *see* Obstruction, intestine
   spine — *see* Dorsopathy, deforming, specified NEC
   tibia (acquired) — *see also* Deformity, limb, specified type NEC, lower leg
      congenital Q74.2
   ureter N13.5
      with infection N13.6
   wrist (acquired) — *see also* Deformity, limb, specified type NEC, forearm
      congenital Q74.0
Angulus infectiosus (lips) K13.0
Anhedonia R45.84
   sexual F52.0
Anhidrosis L74.4
Anhydration E86.0
Anhydremia E86.0
Anidrosis L74.4
Aniridia (congenital) Q13.1
Anisakiasis (infection) (infestation) B81.0
Anisakis larvae infestation B81.0
Aniseikonia H52.32
Anisocoria (pupil) H57.02
   congenital Q13.2
Anisocytosis R71.8
Anisometropia (congenital) H52.31
Ankle — *see* condition
Ankyloblepharon (eyelid) (acquired) — *see also* Blepharophimosis
   filiforme (adnatum) (congenital) Q10.3
   total Q10.3
Ankyloglossia Q38.1
Ankylosis (fibrous) (osseous) (joint) M24.60

Ankylosis — *continued*
   ankle M24.67- ☑
   arthrodesis status Z98.1
   cricoarytenoid (cartilage) (joint) (larynx) J38.7
   dental K03.5
   ear ossicles H74.31- ☑
   elbow M24.62- ☑
   foot M24.67- ☑
   hand M24.64- ☑
   hip M24.65- ☑
   incostapedial joint (infectional) — *see* Ankylosis, ear ossicles
   jaw (temporomandibular) M26.61- ☑
   knee M24.66- ☑
   lumbosacral (joint) M43.27
   postoperative (status) Z98.1
   produced by surgical fusion, status Z98.1
   sacro-iliac (joint) M43.28
   shoulder M24.61- ☑
   specified site NEC M24.69
   spine (joint) — *see also* Fusion, spine
      spondylitic — *see* Spondylitis, ankylosing
   surgical Z98.1
   temporomandibular M26.61- ☑
   tooth, teeth (hard tissues) K03.5
   wrist M24.63- ☑
Ankylostoma — *see* Ancylostoma
Ankylostomiasis — *see* Ancylostomiasis
Ankylurethria — *see* Stricture, urethra
Annular — *see also* condition
   detachment, cervix N88.8
   organ or site, congenital NEC — *see* Distortion
   pancreas (congenital) Q45.1
Anoctaminopathy G71.035
Anodontia (complete) (partial) (vera) K00.0
   acquired K08.10 ☑
Anomaly, anomalous (congenital) (unspecified type) Q89.9
   abdominal wall NEC Q79.59
   acoustic nerve Q07.8
   adrenal (gland) Q89.1
   Alder (-Reilly) (leukocyte granulation) D72.0
   alimentary tract Q45.9
      upper Q40.9
   alveolar M26.70
      hyperplasia M26.79
         mandibular M26.72
         maxillary M26.71
      hypoplasia M26.79
         mandibular M26.74
         maxillary M26.73
      ridge (process) M26.79
      specified NEC M26.79
   ankle (joint) Q74.2
   anus Q43.9
   aorta (arch) NEC Q25.40
      coarctation (preductal) (postductal) Q25.1
   aortic cusp or valve Q23.9
   appendix Q43.8
   apple peel syndrome Q41.1
   aqueduct of Sylvius Q03.0
      with spina bifida — *see* Spina bifida, with hydrocephalus
   arm Q74.0
   arteriovenous NEC
      coronary Q24.5
      gastrointestinal Q27.33
         acquired — *see* Angiodysplasia
   artery (peripheral) Q27.9
      basilar NEC Q28.1
      cerebral Q28.3
      coronary Q24.5
      digestive system Q27.8
      eye Q15.8
      great Q25.9
         specified NEC Q25.8
      lower limb Q27.8
      peripheral Q27.9
         specified NEC Q27.8
      pulmonary NEC Q25.79
      renal Q27.2
      retina Q14.1
      specified site NEC Q27.8
      subclavian Q27.8
         origin Q25.48
      umbilical Q27.0
      upper limb Q27.8
      vertebral NEC Q28.1

Anomaly, anomalous — *continued*
   aryteno-epiglottic folds Q31.8
   atrial
      bands or folds Q20.8
      septa Q21.10
   atrioventricular
      excitation I45.6
      septum Q21.0
   auditory canal Q17.8
   auricle
      ear Q17.8
         causing impairment of hearing Q16.9
      heart Q20.8
   Axenfeld's Q15.0
   back Q89.9
   band
      atrial Q20.8
      heart Q24.8
      ventricular Q24.8
   Bartholin's duct Q38.4
   biliary duct or passage Q44.5
   bladder Q64.70
      absence Q64.5
      diverticulum Q64.6
      exstrophy Q64.10
         cloacal Q64.12
         extroversion Q64.19
         specified type NEC Q64.19
         supravesical fissure Q64.11
      neck obstruction Q64.31
      specified type NEC Q64.79
   bone Q79.9
      arm Q74.0
      face Q75.9
      leg Q74.2
      pelvic girdle Q74.2
      shoulder girdle Q74.0
      skull Q75.9
        with
            anencephaly Q00.0
            encephalocele — *see* Encephalocele
            hydrocephalus Q03.9
               with spina bifida — *see* Spina bifida, by site, with hydrocephalus
            microcephaly Q02
   brain (multiple) Q04.9
      vessel Q28.3
   breast Q83.9
   broad ligament Q50.6
   bronchus Q32.4
   bulbus cordis Q21.9
   bursa Q79.9
   canal of Nuck Q52.4
   canthus Q10.3
   capillary Q27.9
   cardiac Q24.9
      chambers Q20.9
         specified NEC Q20.8
      septal closure Q21.9
         specified NEC Q21.8
      valve NEC Q24.8
         pulmonary Q22.3
   cardiovascular system Q28.8
   carpus Q74.0
   caruncle, lacrimal Q10.6
   cascade stomach Q40.2
   cauda equina Q06.3
   cecum Q43.9
   cerebral Q04.9
      vessels Q28.3
   cervix Q51.9
   Chédiak-Higashi (-Steinbrinck) (congenital gigantism of peroxidase granules) E70.330
   cheek Q18.9
   chest wall Q67.8
      bones Q76.9
   chin Q18.9
   chordae tendineae Q24.8
   choroid Q14.3
      plexus Q07.8
   chromosomes, chromosomal Q99.9
      D (1) — *see* condition, chromosome 13
      E (3) — *see* condition, chromosome 18
      G — *see* condition, chromosome 21
      sex
         female phenotype Q97.8
         gonadal dysgenesis (pure) Q99.1
         Klinefelter's Q98.4
         male phenotype Q98.9

☑ **Additional Character Required — Refer to the Tabular List for Character Selection**

Anomaly, anomalous — *continued*
  chromosomes, chromosomal — *continued*
    sex — *continued*
      Turner's Q96.9
      specified NEC Q99.8
  cilia Q10.3
  circulatory system Q28.9
  clavicle Q74.0
  clitoris Q52.6
  coccyx Q76.49
  colon Q43.9
  common duct Q44.5
  communication
    coronary artery Q24.5
    left ventricle with right atrium Q21.0
  concha (ear) Q17.3
  connection
    portal vein Q26.5
    pulmonary venous Q26.4
      partial Q26.3
      total Q26.2
    renal artery with kidney Q27.2
  cornea (shape) Q13.4
  coronary artery or vein Q24.5
  cranium — *see* Anomaly, skull
  cricoid cartilage Q31.8
  cystic duct Q44.5
  dental
    alveolar — *see* Anomaly, alveolar
    arch relationship M26.20
      specified NEC M26.29
  dentofacial M26.9
    alveolar — *see* Anomaly, alveolar
    dental arch relationship M26.20
      specified NEC M26.29
    functional M26.50
      specified NEC M26.59
    jaw size M26.00
      macrogenia M26.05
      mandibular
        hyperplasia M26.03
        hypoplasia M26.04
      maxillary
        hyperplasia M26.01
        hypoplasia M26.02
      microgenia M26.06
      specified type NEC M26.09
    jaw-cranial base relationship M26.10
      asymmetry M26.12
        maxillary M26.11
      specified type NEC M26.19
    malocclusion M26.4
      dental arch relationship NEC M26.29
      jaw size — *see* Anomaly, dentofacial, jaw size
      jaw-cranial base relationship — *see* Anomaly,
        dentofacial, jaw-cranial base relationship
    specified type NEC M26.89
    temporomandibular joint M26.60- ☑
      adhesions M26.61- ☑
      ankylosis M26.61- ☑
      arthralgia M26.62- ☑
      articular disc M26.63- ☑
      specified type NEC M26.69
    tooth position, fully erupted M26.30
      specified NEC M26.39
  dermatoglyphic Q82.8
  diaphragm (apertures) NEC Q79.1
  digestive organ(s) or tract Q45.9
    lower Q43.9
    upper Q40.9
  distance, interarch (excessive) (inadequate) M26.25
  distribution, coronary artery Q24.5
  ductus
    arteriosus Q25.0
    botalli Q25.0
  duodenum Q43.9
  dura (brain) Q04.9
    spinal cord Q06.9
  ear (external) Q17.9
    causing impairment of hearing Q16.9
    inner Q16.5
    middle (causing impairment of hearing) Q16.4
      ossicles Q16.3
  Ebstein's (heart) (tricuspid valve) Q22.5
  ectodermal Q82.9
  Eisenmenger's (ventricular septal defect) Q21.8
  ejaculatory duct Q55.4
  elbow Q74.0

Anomaly, anomalous — *continued*
  endocrine gland NEC Q89.2
  epididymis Q55.4
  epiglottis Q31.8
  esophagus Q39.9
  eustachian tube Q17.8
  eye Q15.9
    anterior segment Q13.9
      specified NEC Q13.89
    posterior segment Q14.9
      specified NEC Q14.8
    ptosis (eyelid) Q10.0
    specified NEC Q15.8
  eyebrow Q18.8
  eyelid Q10.3
    ptosis Q10.0
  face Q18.9
    bone(s) Q75.9
  fallopian tube Q50.6
  fascia Q79.9
  femur NEC Q74.2
  fibula NEC Q74.2
  finger Q74.0
  fixation, intestine Q43.3
  flexion (joint) NOS Q74.9
    hip or thigh Q65.89
  foot NEC Q74.2
    varus (congenital) Q66.3- ☑
  foramen
    Botalli Q21.12
    ovale Q21.12
  forearm Q74.0
  forehead Q75.8
  form, teeth K00.2
  fovea centralis Q14.1
  frontal bone — *see* Anomaly, skull
  gallbladder (position) (shape) (size) Q44.1
  Gartner's duct Q52.4
  gastrointestinal tract Q45.9
  genitalia, genital organ(s) or system
    female Q52.9
      external Q52.70
      internal NOS Q52.9
    male Q55.9
      hydrocele P83.5
      specified NEC Q55.8
  genitourinary NEC
    female Q52.9
    male Q55.9
  Gerbode Q21.0
  glottis Q31.8
  granulation or granulocyte, genetic (constitutional)
    (leukocyte) D72.0
  gum Q38.6
  gyri Q07.9
  hair Q84.2
  hand Q74.0
  hard tissue formation in pulp K04.3
  head — *see* Anomaly, skull
  heart Q24.9
    auricle Q20.8
    bands or folds Q24.8
    fibroelastosis cordis I42.4
    obstructive NEC Q22.6
    patent ductus arteriosus (Botalli) Q25.0
    septum Q21.9
      auricular Q21.19
      interatrial Q21.19
      interventricular Q21.0
        with pulmonary stenosis or atresia, dextrapo-
          sition of aorta and hypertrophy of right
          ventricle Q21.3
      specified NEC Q21.8
      ventricular Q21.0
        with pulmonary stenosis or atresia, dextrapo-
          sition of aorta and hypertrophy of right
          ventricle Q21.3
    tetralogy of Fallot Q21.3
    valve NEC Q24.8
      aortic
        bicuspid valve Q23.1
        insufficiency Q23.1
        stenosis Q23.0
          subaortic Q24.4
      mitral
        insufficiency Q23.3
        stenosis Q23.2
      pulmonary Q22.3
        atresia Q22.0

Anomaly, anomalous — *continued*
  heart — *continued*
    valve — *continued*
      pulmonary — *continued*
        insufficiency Q22.2
        stenosis Q22.1
          infundibular Q24.3
          subvalvular Q24.3
      tricuspid
        atresia Q22.4
        stenosis Q22.4
    ventricle Q20.8
  heel NEC Q74.2
  Hegglin's D72.0
  hemianencephaly Q00.0
  hemicephaly Q00.0
  hemicrania Q00.0
  hepatic duct Q44.5
  hip NEC Q74.2
  hourglass stomach Q40.2
  humerus Q74.0
  hydatid of Morgagni
    female Q50.5
    male (epididymal) Q55.4
      testicular Q55.29
  hymen Q52.4
  hypersegmentation of neutrophils, hereditary D72.0
  hypophyseal Q89.2
  ileocecal (coil) (valve) Q43.9
  ileum Q43.9
  ilium NEC Q74.2
  integument Q84.9
    specified NEC Q84.8
  interarch distance (excessive) (inadequate) M26.25
  intervertebral cartilage or disc Q76.49
  intestine (large) (small) Q43.9
    with anomalous adhesions, fixation or malrotation
      Q43.3
  iris Q13.2
  ischium NEC Q74.2
  jaw — *see* Anomaly, dentofacial
    alveolar — *see* Anomaly, alveolar
  jaw-cranial base relationship — *see* Anomaly, dentofa-
    cial, jaw-cranial base relationship
  jejunum Q43.8
  joint Q74.9
    specified NEC Q74.8
  Jordan's D72.0
  kidney(s) (calyx) (pelvis) Q63.9
    artery Q27.2
    specified NEC Q63.8
  Klippel-Feil (brevicollis) Q76.1
  knee Q74.1
  labium (majus) (minus) Q52.70
  labyrinth, membranous Q16.5
  lacrimal apparatus or duct Q10.6
  larynx, laryngeal (muscle) Q31.9
    web (bed) Q31.0
  lens Q12.9
  leukocytes, genetic D72.0
    granulation (constitutional) D72.0
  lid (fold) Q10.3
  ligament Q79.9
    broad Q50.6
    round Q52.8
  limb Q74.9
    lower NEC Q74.2
      reduction deformity — *see* Defect, reduction,
        lower limb
    upper Q74.0
  lip Q38.0
  liver Q44.7
    duct Q44.5
  lower limb NEC Q74.2
  lumbosacral (joint) (region) Q76.49
    kyphosis — *see* Kyphosis, congenital
    lordosis — *see* Lordosis, congenital
  lung (fissure) (lobe) Q33.9
  mandible — *see* Anomaly, dentofacial
  maxilla — *see* Anomaly, dentofacial
  May (-Hegglin) D72.0
  meatus urinarius NEC Q64.79
  meningeal bands or folds Q07.9
    constriction Q07.8
    spinal Q06.9
  meninges Q07.9
    cerebral Q04.8
    spinal Q06.9

Anomaly, anomalous — *continued*
meningocele Q05.9
mesentery Q45.9
metacarpus Q74.0
metatarsus NEC Q74.2
middle ear Q16.4
  ossicles Q16.3
mitral (leaflets) (valve) Q23.9
  insufficiency Q23.3
  specified NEC Q23.8
  stenosis Q23.2
mouth Q38.6
Müllerian — *see also* Anomaly, by site
  uterus NEC Q51.818
multiple NEC Q89.7
muscle Q79.9
  eyelid Q10.3
musculoskeletal system, except limbs Q79.9
myocardium Q24.8
nail Q84.6
narrowness, eyelid Q10.3
nasal sinus (wall) Q30.8
neck (any part) Q18.9
nerve Q07.9
  acoustic Q07.8
  optic Q07.8
nervous system (central) Q07.9
nipple Q83.9
nose, nasal (bones) (cartilage) (septum) (sinus) Q30.9
  specified NEC Q30.8
ocular muscle Q15.8
omphalomesenteric duct Q43.0
opening, pulmonary veins Q26.4
optic
  disc Q14.2
  nerve Q07.8
opticociliary vessels Q13.2
orbit (eye) Q10.7
organ Q89.9
  of Corti Q16.5
origin
  artery
    innominate Q25.8
    pulmonary Q25.79
    renal Q27.2
    subclavian Q25.48
osseous meatus (ear) Q16.1
ovary Q50.39
oviduct Q50.6
palate (hard) (soft) NEC Q38.5
pancreas or pancreatic duct Q45.3
papillary muscles Q24.8
parathyroid gland Q89.2
paraurethral ducts Q64.79
parotid (gland) Q38.4
patella Q74.1
Pelger-Huët (hereditary hyposegmentation) D72.0
pelvic girdle NEC Q74.2
pelvis (bony) NEC Q74.2
  rachitic E64.3
penis (glans) Q55.69
pericardium Q24.8
peripheral vascular system Q27.9
Peter's Q13.4
pharynx Q38.8
pigmentation L81.9
  congenital Q82.8
pituitary (gland) Q89.2
pleural (folds) Q34.0
portal vein Q26.5
  connection Q26.5
position, tooth, teeth, fully erupted M26.30
  specified NEC M26.39
precerebral vessel Q28.1
prepuce Q55.69
prostate Q55.4
pulmonary Q33.9
  artery NEC Q25.79
  valve Q22.3
    atresia Q22.0
    insufficiency Q22.2
    specified type NEC Q22.3
    stenosis Q22.1
      infundibular Q24.3
      subvalvular Q24.3
  venous connection Q26.4
    partial Q26.3
    total Q26.2
pupil Q13.2

Anomaly, anomalous — *continued*
pupil — *continued*
  function H57.00
    anisocoria H57.02
    Argyll Robertson pupil H57.01
    miosis H57.03
    mydriasis H57.04
    specified type NEC H57.09
    tonic pupil H57.05- ☑
pylorus Q40.3
radius Q74.0
rectum Q43.9
reduction (extremity) (limb)
  femur (longitudinal) — *see* Defect, reduction, lower limb, longitudinal, femur
  fibula (longitudinal) — *see* Defect, reduction, lower limb, longitudinal, fibula
  lower limb — *see* Defect, reduction, lower limb
  radius (longitudinal) — *see* Defect, reduction, upper limb, longitudinal, radius
  tibia (longitudinal) — *see* Defect, reduction, lower limb, longitudinal, tibia
  ulna (longitudinal) — *see* Defect, reduction, upper limb, longitudinal, ulna
  upper limb — *see* Defect, reduction, upper limb
refraction — *see* Disorder, refraction
renal Q63.9
  artery Q27.2
  pelvis Q63.9
    specified NEC Q63.8
respiratory system Q34.9
  specified NEC Q34.8
retina Q14.1
rib Q76.6
  cervical Q76.5
Rieger's Q13.81
rotation — *see* Malrotation
  hip or thigh Q65.89
round ligament Q52.8
sacroiliac (joint) NEC Q74.2
sacrum NEC Q76.49
  kyphosis — *see* Kyphosis, congenital
  lordosis — *see* Lordosis, congenital
saddle nose, syphilitic A50.57
salivary duct or gland Q38.4
scapula Q74.0
scrotum — *see* Malformation, testis and scrotum
sebaceous gland Q82.9
seminal vesicles Q55.4
sense organs NEC Q07.8
sex chromosomes NEC — *see also* Anomaly, chromosomes
  female phenotype Q97.8
  male phenotype Q98.9
shoulder (girdle) (joint) Q74.0
sigmoid (flexure) Q43.9
simian crease Q82.8
sinus of Valsalva Q25.49
skeleton generalized Q78.9
skin (appendage) Q82.9
skull Q75.9
  with
    anencephaly Q00.0
    encephalocele — *see* Encephalocele
    hydrocephalus Q03.9
      with spina bifida — *see* Spina bifida, by site, with hydrocephalus
    microcephaly Q02
specified organ or site NEC Q89.8
spermatic cord Q55.4
spine, spinal NEC Q76.49
  column NEC Q76.49
    kyphosis — *see* Kyphosis, congenital
    lordosis — *see* Lordosis, congenital
  cord Q06.9
  nerve root Q07.8
spleen Q89.09
  agenesis Q89.01
stenonian duct Q38.4
sternum NEC Q76.7
stomach Q40.3
submaxillary gland Q38.4
tarsus NEC Q74.2
tendon Q79.9
testis — *see* Malformation, testis and scrotum
thigh NEC Q74.2
thorax (wall) Q67.8
  bony Q76.9

Anomaly, anomalous — *continued*
throat Q38.8
thumb Q74.0
thymus gland Q89.2
thyroid (gland) Q89.2
  cartilage Q31.8
tibia NEC Q74.2
  saber A50.56
toe Q74.2
tongue Q38.3
tooth, teeth K00.9
  eruption K00.6
  position, fully erupted M26.30
  spacing, fully erupted M26.30
trachea (cartilage) Q32.1
tragus Q17.9
tricuspid (leaflet) (valve) Q22.9
  atresia or stenosis Q22.4
  Ebstein's Q22.5
Uhl's (hypoplasia of myocardium, right ventricle) Q24.8
ulna Q74.0
umbilical artery Q27.0
union
  cricoid cartilage and thyroid cartilage Q31.8
  thyroid cartilage and hyoid bone Q31.8
  trachea with larynx Q31.8
upper limb Q74.0
urachus Q64.4
ureter Q62.8
  obstructive NEC Q62.39
    cecoureterocele Q62.32
    orthotopic ureterocele Q62.31
urethra Q64.70
  absence Q64.5
  double Q64.74
  fistula to rectum Q64.73
  obstructive Q64.39
    stricture Q64.32
  prolapse Q64.71
  specified type NEC Q64.79
urinary tract Q64.9
uterus Q51.9
  with only one functioning horn Q51.4
uvula Q38.5
vagina Q52.4
valleculae Q31.8
valve (heart) NEC Q24.8
  coronary sinus Q24.5
  inferior vena cava Q24.8
  pulmonary Q22.3
  sinus coronario Q24.5
  venae cavae inferioris Q24.8
vas deferens Q55.4
vascular Q27.9
  brain Q28.3
  ring Q25.45
vein(s) (peripheral) Q27.9
  brain Q28.3
  cerebral Q28.3
  coronary Q24.5
  developmental Q28.3
  great Q26.9
    specified NEC Q26.8
vena cava (inferior) (superior) Q26.9
venous — *see* Anomaly, vein(s)
venous return Q26.8
ventricular
  bands or folds Q24.8
  septa Q21.0
vertebra Q76.49
  kyphosis — *see* Kyphosis, congenital
  lordosis — *see* Lordosis, congenital
vesicourethral orifice Q64.79
vessel(s) Q27.9
  optic papilla Q14.2
  precerebral Q28.1
vitelline duct Q43.0
vitreous body or humor Q14.0
vulva Q52.70
wrist (joint) Q74.0
Anomia R48.8
Anonychia (congenital) Q84.3
  acquired L60.8
Anophthalmos, anophthalmus (congenital) (globe) Q11.1
  acquired Z90.01
Anopia, anopsia H53.46- ☑
  quadrant H53.46- ☑

Anorchia, anorchism, anorchidism Q55.0
Anorexia R63.0
hysterical F44.89
nervosa F50.00
atypical F50.9
binge-eating type F50.2
with purging F50.02
restricting type F50.01
Anorgasmy, psychogenic (female) F52.31
male F52.32
Anosmia R43.0
hysterical F44.6
postinfectional J39.8
Anosognosia R41.89
Anosteoplasia Q78.9
Anovulatory cycle N97.0
Anoxemia R09.02
newborn P84
Anoxia (pathological) R09.02
altitude T70.29 ☑
cerebral G93.1
complicating
anesthesia (general) (local) or other sedation T88.59 ☑
in labor and delivery O74.3
in pregnancy O29.21- ☑
postpartum, puerperal O89.2
delivery (cesarean) (instrumental) O75.4
during a procedure G97.81
newborn P84
resulting from a procedure G97.82
due to
drowning T75.1 ☑
high altitude T70.29 ☑
heart — see Insufficiency, coronary
intrauterine P84
myocardial — see Insufficiency, coronary
newborn P84
spinal cord G95.11
systemic (by suffocation) (low content in atmosphere) — see Asphyxia, traumatic
Anteflexion — see Anteversion
Antenatal
care (normal pregnancy) Z34.90
screening (encounter for) of mother — see also Encounter, antenatal screening Z36.9
Antepartum — see condition
Anterior — see condition
Antero-occlusion M26.220
Anteversion
cervix — see Anteversion, uterus
femur (neck), congenital Q65.89
uterus, uterine (cervix) (postinfectional) (postpartal, old) N85.4
congenital Q51.818
in pregnancy or childbirth — see Pregnancy, complicated by
Anthophobia F40.228
Anthracosilicosis J60
Anthracosis (lung) (occupational) J60
lingua K14.3
Anthrax A22.9
with pneumonia A22.1
cerebral A22.8
colitis A22.2
cutaneous A22.0
gastrointestinal A22.2
inhalation A22.1
intestinal A22.2
meningitis A22.8
pulmonary A22.1
respiratory A22.1
sepsis A22.7
specified manifestation NEC A22.8
Anthropoid pelvis Q74.2
with disproportion (fetopelvic) O33.0
Anthropophobia F40.10
generalized F40.11
Antibodies, maternal (blood group) — see Isoimmunization, affecting management of pregnancy
anti-D — see Isoimmunization, affecting management of pregnancy, Rh
newborn P55.0
Antibody
anticardiolipin R76.0
with
hemorrhagic disorder D68.312
hypercoagulable state D68.61

Antibody — continued
antiphosphatidylglycerol R76.0
with
hemorrhagic disorder D68.312
hypercoagulable state D68.61
antiphosphatidylinositol R76.0
with
hemorrhagic disorder D68.312
hypercoagulable state D68.61
antiphosphatidylserine R76.0
with
hemorrhagic disorder D68.312
hypercoagulable state D68.61
antiphospholipid R76.0
with
hemorrhagic disorder D68.312
hypercoagulable state D68.61
Anticardiolipin syndrome D68.61
Anticoagulant, circulating (intrinsic) — see also Disorder, hemorrhagic D68.318
drug-induced (extrinsic) — see also Disorder, hemorrhagic D68.32
iatrogenic D68.32
Antidiuretic hormone syndrome E22.2
Antimonial cholera — see Poisoning, antimony
Antiphospholipid
antibody
with hemorrhagic disorder D68.312
syndrome D68.61
Antisocial personality F60.2
Antithrombinemia — see Circulating anticoagulants
Antithromboplastinemia D68.318
Antithromboplastinogenemia D68.318
Antitoxin complication or reaction — see Complications, vaccination
Antlophobia F40.228
Antritis J32.0
maxilla J32.0
acute J01.00
recurrent J01.01
stomach K29.50
with bleeding K29.51
Antrum, antral — see condition
Anuria R34
calculous (impacted) (recurrent) — see also Calculus, urinary N20.9
following
abortion — see Abortion by type complicated by, renal failure
ectopic or molar pregnancy O08.4
newborn P96.0
postprocedural N99.0
postrenal N13.8
traumatic (following crushing) T79.5 ☑
Anus, anal — see condition
Anusitis K62.89
Anxiety F41.9
depression F41.8
episodic paroxysmal F41.0
generalized F41.1
hysteria F41.8
neurosis F41.1
panic type F41.0
reaction F41.1
separation, abnormal (of childhood) F93.0
specified NEC F41.8
state F41.1
Aorta, aortic — see condition
Aortectasia — see Ectasia, aorta
with aneurysm — see Aneurysm, aorta
Aortitis (nonsyphilitic) (calcific) I77.6
arteriosclerotic I70.0
Doehle-Heller A52.02
luetic A52.02
rheumatic — see Endocarditis, acute, rheumatic
specific (syphilitic) A52.02
syphilitic A52.02
congenital A50.54 [I79.1]
Apathetic thyroid storm — see Thyrotoxicosis
Apathy R45.3
Apeirophobia F40.228
Apepsia K30
psychogenic F45.8
Aperistalsis, esophagus K22.0
Apertognathia M26.29
Apert's syndrome Q87.0
Aphagia R13.0
psychogenic F50.9

Aphakia (acquired) (postoperative) H27.0- ☑
congenital Q12.3
Aphasia (amnestic) (global) (nominal) (semantic) (syntactic) R47.01
acquired, with epilepsy (Landau-Kleffner syndrome) — see Epilepsy, specified NEC
auditory (developmental) F80.2
developmental (receptive type) F80.2
expressive type F80.1
Wernicke's F80.2
following
cerebrovascular disease I69.920
cerebral infarction I69.320
intracerebral hemorrhage I69.120
nontraumatic intracranial hemorrhage NEC I69.220
specified disease NEC I69.820
subarachnoid hemorrhage I69.020
primary progressive — see also Dementia, in, diseases specified elsewhere G31.01 [F02.80]
with behavioral disturbance — see also Dementia, in, diseases specified elsewhere G31.01 [F02.81-] ☑
progressive isolated — see also Dementia, in, diseases specified elsewhere G31.01 [F02.80]
with behavioral disturbance — see also Dementia, in, diseases specified elsewhere G31.01 [F02.81-] ☑
sensory F80.2
syphilis, tertiary A52.19
Wernicke's (developmental) F80.2
Aphonia (organic) R49.1
hysterical F44.4
psychogenic F44.4
Aphthae, aphthous — see also condition
Bednar's K12.0
cachectic K14.0
epizootic B08.8
fever B08.8
oral (recurrent) K12.0
stomatitis (major) (minor) K12.0
thrush B37.0
ulcer (oral) (recurrent) K12.0
genital organ(s) NEC
female N76.6
male N50.89
larynx J38.7
Apical — see condition
Apiphobia F40.218
Aplasia — see also Agenesis
abdominal muscle syndrome Q79.4
alveolar process (acquired) — see Anomaly, alveolar
congenital Q38.6
aorta (congenital) Q25.41
axialis extracorticalis (congenita) E75.29
bone marrow (myeloid) D61.9
congenital D61.01
brain Q00.0
part of Q04.3
bronchus Q32.4
cementum K00.4
cerebellum Q04.3
cervix (congenital) Q51.5
congenital pure red cell D61.01
corpus callosum Q04.0
cutis congenita Q84.8
erythrocyte congenital D61.01
extracortical axial E75.29
eye Q11.1
fovea centralis (congenital) Q14.1
gallbladder, congenital Q44.0
iris Q13.1
labyrinth, membranous Q16.5
limb (congenital) Q73.8
lower — see Defect, reduction, lower limb
upper — see Agenesis, arm
lung, congenital (bilateral) (unilateral) Q33.3
pancreas Q45.0
parathyroid-thymic D82.1
Pelizaeus-Merzbacher E75.29
penis Q55.5
prostate Q55.4
red cell (with thymoma) D60.9
acquired D60.9
due to drugs D60.9
adult D60.9
chronic D60.0
congenital D61.01

Aplasia — *continued*
  red cell — *continued*
    constitutional D61.01
    due to drugs D60.9
    hereditary D61.01
    of infants D61.01
    primary D61.01
    pure D61.01
      due to drugs D60.9
    specified type NEC D60.8
    transient D60.1
  round ligament Q52.8
  skin Q84.8
  spermatic cord Q55.4
  spleen Q89.01
  testicle Q55.0
  thymic, with immunodeficiency D82.1
  thyroid (congenital) (with myxedema) E03.1
  uterus Q51.0
  ventral horn cell Q06.1
Apnea, apneic (of) (spells) R06.81
  newborn P28.40
    central P28.41
    mixed P28.43
    obstructive P28.42
    sleep
      primary P28.30
        central P28.31
        mixed P28.33
        obstructive P28.32
        specified NEC P28.39
    specified NEC P28.49
  prematurity P28.49
  sleep G47.30
    central (primary) G47.31
      idiopathic G47.31
      in conditions classified elsewhere G47.37
    obstructive (adult) (pediatric) G47.33
      hypopnea G47.33
    primary central G47.31
    specified NEC G47.39
Apneumatosis, newborn P28.0
Apocrine metaplasia (breast) — *see* Dysplasia, mammary, specified type NEC
Apophysitis (bone) — *see also* Osteochondropathy
  calcaneus M92.8
  juvenile M92.9
Apoplectiform convulsions (cerebral ischemia) I67.82
Apoplexia, apoplexy, apoplectic
  adrenal A39.1
  heart (auricle) (ventricle) — *see* Infarct, myocardium
  heat T67.01 ☑
  hemorrhagic (stroke) — *see* Hemorrhage, intracranial
  meninges, hemorrhagic — *see* Hemorrhage, intracranial, subarachnoid
  uremic N18.9 *[I68.8]*
Appearance
  bizarre R46.1
  specified NEC R46.89
  very low level of personal hygiene R46.0
Appendage
  epididymal (organ of Morgagni) Q55.4
  intestine (epiploic) Q43.8
  preauricular Q17.0
  testicular (organ of Morgagni) Q55.29
Appendicitis (pneumococcal) (retrocecal) K37
  with
    gangrene K35.891
      with localized peritonitis K35.31
    perforation NOS K35.32
    peritoneal abscess K35.33
    peritonitis NEC K35.33
      generalized (with perforation or rupture) K35.20
        with abscess K35.21
      localized K35.30
        with
          gangrene K35.31
          perforation K35.32
          and abscess K35.33
    rupture (with localized peritonitis) K35.32
  acute (catarrhal) (fulminating) (obstructive) (retrocecal) (suppurative) K35.80
    with
      gangrene K35.891
      peritoneal abscess K35.33
      peritonitis NEC K35.33
        generalized (with perforation or rupture) K35.20

Appendicitis — *continued*
  acute — *continued*
    with — *continued*
      peritonitis — *continued*
        generalized — *continued*
          with abscess K35.21
        localized K35.30
          with
            gangrene K35.31
            perforation K35.32
            and abscess K35.33
      specified NEC K35.890
        with gangrene K35.891
          with localized peritonitis K35.31
  amebic A06.89
  chronic (recurrent) K36
  exacerbation — *see* Appendicitis, with, gangrene
  gangrenous — *see* Appendicitis, acute
  healed (obliterative) K36
  interval K36
  neurogenic K36
  obstructive K36
  recurrent K36
  relapsing K36
  ruptured NOS (with localized peritonitis) K35.32
  subacute (adhesive) K36
  subsiding K36
  suppurative — *see* Appendicitis, acute
  tuberculous A18.32
Appendicopathia oxyurica B80
Appendix, appendicular — *see also* condition
  epididymis Q55.4
  Morgagni
    female Q50.5
    male (epididymal) Q55.4
      testicular Q55.29
  testis Q55.29
Appetite
  depraved — *see* Pica
  excessive R63.2
  lack or loss — *see also* Anorexia R63.0
    nonorganic origin F50.89
    psychogenic F50.89
  perverted (hysterical) — *see* Pica
Apple peel syndrome Q41.1
Apprehension state F41.1
Apprehensiveness, abnormal F41.9
Approximal wear K03.0
Apraxia (classic) (ideational) (ideokinetic) (ideomotor) (motor) (verbal) R48.2
  following
    cerebrovascular disease I69.990
      cerebral infarction I69.390
      intracerebral hemorrhage I69.190
      nontraumatic intracranial hemorrhage NEC I69.290
      specified disease NEC I69.890
      subarachnoid hemorrhage I69.090
  oculomotor, congenital H51.8
Aptyalism K11.7
Apudoma — *see* Neoplasm, uncertain behavior, by site
Aqueous misdirection H40.83- ☑
Arabicum elephantiasis — *see* Infestation, filarial
Arachnitis — *see* Meningitis
Arachnodactyly — *see* Syndrome, Marfan's
Arachnoiditis (acute) (adhesive) (basal) (brain) (cerebrospinal) — *see* Meningitis
Arachnophobia F40.210
Arboencephalitis, Australian A83.4
Arborization block (heart) I45.5
ARC (AIDS-related complex) B20
Arch
  aortic Q25.49
  bovine Q25.49
Arches — *see* condition
Arcuate uterus Q51.810
Arcuatus uterus Q51.810
Arcus (cornea) senilis — *see* Degeneration, cornea, senile
Arc-welder's lung J63.4
Areflexia R29.2
Areola — *see* condition
Argentaffinoma — *see also* Neoplasm, uncertain behavior, by site
  malignant — *see* Neoplasm, malignant, by site
  syndrome E34.0
Argininemia E72.21
Arginosuccinic aciduria E72.22

Argyll Robertson phenomenon, pupil or syndrome (syphilitic) A52.19
  atypical H57.09
  nonsyphilitic H57.09
Argyria, argyriasis
  conjunctival H11.13- ☑
  from drug or medicament — *see* Table of Drugs and Chemicals, by substance
Argyrosis, conjunctival H11.13- ☑
Arhinencephaly Q04.1
Ariboflavinosis E53.0
Arm — *see* condition
Arnold-Chiari disease, obstruction or syndrome (type II) Q07.00
  with
    hydrocephalus Q07.02
      with spina bifida Q07.03
    spina bifida Q07.01
      with hydrocephalus Q07.03
  type III — *see* Encephalocele
  type IV Q04.8
Aromatic amino-acid metabolism disorder E70.9
  specified NEC E70.89
Arousals, confusional G47.51
Arrest, arrested
  cardiac I46.9
    complicating
      abortion — *see* Abortion, by type, complicated by, cardiac arrest
      anesthesia (general) (local) or other sedation — *see* Table of Drugs and Chemicals, by drug
        in labor and delivery O74.2
        in pregnancy O29.11- ☑
        postpartum, puerperal O89.1
      delivery (cesarean) (instrumental) O75.4
    due to
      cardiac condition I46.2
      specified condition NEC I46.8
    intraoperative I97.71- ☑
    newborn P29.81
    personal history, successfully resuscitated Z86.74
    postprocedural I97.12- ☑
      obstetric procedure O75.4
  cardiorespiratory — *see* Arrest, cardiac
  circulatory — *see* Arrest, cardiac
  deep transverse O64.0 ☑
  development or growth
    bone — *see* Disorder, bone, development or growth
    child R62.50
    tracheal rings Q32.1
  epiphyseal
    complete
      femur M89.15- ☑
      humerus M89.12- ☑
      tibia M89.16- ☑
      ulna M89.13- ☑
      forearm M89.13- ☑
        specified NEC M89.13- ☑
      ulna — *see* Arrest, epiphyseal, by type, ulna
      lower leg M89.16- ☑
        specified NEC M89.168
        tibia — *see* Arrest, epiphyseal, by type, tibia
    partial
      femur M89.15- ☑
      humerus M89.12- ☑
      tibia M89.16- ☑
      ulna M89.13- ☑
    specified NEC M89.18
  granulopoiesis — *see* Agranulocytosis
  growth plate — *see* Arrest, epiphyseal
  heart — *see* Arrest, cardiac
  legal, anxiety concerning Z65.3
  physeal — *see* Arrest, epiphyseal
  respiratory R09.2
    newborn P28.81
  sinus I45.5
  spermatogenesis (complete) — *see* Azoospermia
    incomplete — *see* Oligospermia
  transverse (deep) O64.0 ☑
Arrhenoblastoma
  benign
    specified site — *see* Neoplasm, benign, by site
    unspecified site
      female D27.9
      male D29.20
  malignant
    specified site — *see* Neoplasm, malignant, by site

Arrhenoblastoma — *continued*
  malignant — *continued*
    unspecified site
      female C56.9
      male C62.90
    specified site — *see* Neoplasm, uncertain behavior, by
        site
    unspecified site
      female D39.10
      male D40.10
Arrhythmia (auricle) (cardiac) (juvenile) (nodal) (reflex)
    (supraventricular) (transitory) (ventricle) I49.9
  block I45.9
  extrasystolic I49.49
  newborn
    bradycardia P29.12
    occurring before birth P03.819
      before onset of labor P03.810
      during labor P03.811
    tachycardia P29.11
  psychogenic F45.8
  sinus I49.8
  specified NEC I49.8
  vagal R55
  ventricular re-entry I47.0
Arrillaga-Ayerza syndrome (pulmonary sclerosis with
    pulmonary hypertension) I27.0
Arsenical pigmentation L81.8
  from drug or medicament — *see* Table of Drugs and
      Chemicals
Arsenism — *see* Poisoning, arsenic
Arterial — *see* condition
Arteriofibrosis — *see* Arteriosclerosis
Arteriolar sclerosis — *see* Arteriosclerosis
Arteriolith — *see* Arteriosclerosis
Arteriolitis I77.6
  necrotizing, kidney I77.5
  renal — *see* Hypertension, kidney
Arteriolosclerosis — *see* Arteriosclerosis
Arterionephrosclerosis — *see* Hypertension, kidney
Arteriopathy I77.9
  cerebral autosomal dominant, with subcortical infarcts
      and leukoencephalopathy (CADASIL) I67.850
Arteriosclerosis, arteriosclerotic (diffuse) (obliterans)
    (of) (senile) (with calcification) I70.90
  with
    chronic limb-threatening ischemia — *see* Arteriosclerosis, with critical limb ischemia
    critical limb ischemia
      bypass graft I70.329
        autologous vein graft I70.429
          leg I70.429
            with
              gangrene (and intermittent claudication, rest pain, and ulcer) I70.469
              rest pain (and intermittent claudication) I70.429
            bilateral I70.423
              with
                gangrene (and intermittent claudication, rest pain, and ulcer) I70.463
                rest pain (and intermittent claudication) I70.423
            left I70.422
              with
                gangrene (and intermittent claudication, rest pain, and ulcer) I70.462
                rest pain (and intermittent claudication) I70.422
                ulceration (and intermittent claudication and rest pain) I70.449
                  ankle I70.443
                  calf I70.442
                  foot site NEC I70.445
                  heel I70.444
                  lower leg NEC I70.448
                  mid foot I70.444
                  thigh I70.441
            right I70.421
              with
                gangrene (and intermittent claudication, rest pain, and ulcer) I70.461

Arteriosclerosis, arteriosclerotic — *continued*
  with — *continued*
    critical limb ischemia — *continued*
      bypass graft — *continued*
        autologous vein graft — *continued*
          leg — *continued*
            right — *continued*
              with — *continued*
                rest pain (and intermittent claudication) I70.421
                ulceration (and intermittent claudication and rest pain) I70.439
                  ankle I70.433
                  calf I70.432
                  foot site NEC I70.435
                  heel I70.434
                  lower leg NEC I70.438
                  midfoot I70.434
                  thigh I70.431
          leg I70.329
            with
              gangrene (and intermittent claudication, rest pain, and ulcer) I70.369
              rest pain (and intermittent claudication) I70.329
            bilateral I70.323
              with
                gangrene (and intermittent claudication, rest pain, and ulcer) I70.363
                rest pain (and intermittent claudication) I70.323
            left I70.322
              with
                gangrene (and intermittent claudication, rest pain, and ulcer) I70.362
                rest pain (and intermittent claudication) I70.322
                ulceration (and intermittent claudication and rest pain) I70.349
                  ankle I70.343
                  calf I70.342
                  foot site NEC I70.345
                  heel I70.344
                  lower leg NEC I70.348
                  midfoot I70.344
                  thigh I70.341
            right I70.321
              with
                gangrene (and intermittent claudication, rest pain, and ulcer) I70.361
                rest pain (and intermittent claudication) I70.321
                ulceration (and intermittent claudication and rest pain) I70.339
                  ankle I70.333
                  calf I70.332
                  foot site NEC I70.335
                  heel I70.334
                  lower leg NEC I70.338
                  midfoot I70.334
                  thigh I70.331
        nonautologous biological graft I70.529
          leg I70.529
            with
              gangrene (and intermittent claudication, rest pain, and ulcer) I70.569
              rest pain (and intermittent claudication) I70.529
            bilateral I70.523
              with
                gangrene (and intermittent claudication, rest pain, and ulcer) I70.563
                rest pain (and intermittent claudication) I70.523
            left I70.522
              with
                gangrene (and intermittent claudication, rest pain, and ulcer) I70.562
                rest pain (and intermittent claudication) I70.522

Arteriosclerosis, arteriosclerotic — *continued*
  with — *continued*
    critical limb ischemia — *continued*
      bypass graft — *continued*
        nonautologous biological graft — *continued*
          leg — *continued*
            left — *continued*
              with — *continued*
                ulceration (and intermittent claudication and rest pain) I70.549
                  ankle I70.543
                  calf I70.542
                  foot site NEC I70.545
                  heel I70.544
                  lower leg NEC I70.548
                  midfoot I70.544
                  thigh I70.541
            right I70.521
              with
                gangrene (and intermittent claudication, rest pain, and ulcer) I70.561
                rest pain (and intermittent claudication) I70.521
                ulceration (and intermittent claudication and rest pain) I70.539
                  ankle I70.533
                  calf I70.532
                  foot site NEC I70.535
                  heel I70.534
                  lower leg NEC I70.538
                  midfoot I70.534
                  thigh I70.531
        nonbiological graft I70.629
          leg I70.629
            with
              gangrene (and intermittent claudication, rest pain, and ulcer) I70.669
              rest pain (and intermittent claudication) I70.629
            bilateral I70.623
              with
                gangrene (and intermittent claudication, rest pain, and ulcer) I70.663
                rest pain (intermittent claudication) I70.623
            left I70.622
              with
                gangrene (and intermittent claudication, rest pain, and ulcer) I70.662
                rest pain (and intermittent claudication) I70.622
                ulceration (and intermittent claudication and rest pain) I70.649
                  ankle I70.643
                  calf I70.642
                  foot site NEC I70.645
                  heel I70.644
                  lower leg NEC I70.648
                  midfoot I70.644
                  thigh I70.641
            right I70.621
              with
                gangrene (and intermittent claudication, rest pain, and ulcer) I70.661
                rest pain (and intermittent claudication) I70.621
                ulceration (and intermittent claudication and rest pain) I70.639
                  ankle I70.633
                  calf I70.632
                  foot site NEC I70.635
                  heel I70.634
                  lower leg NEC I70.638
                  midfoot I70.634
                  thigh I70.631
        specified graft NEC I70.729
          leg I70.729

Arteriosclerosis, arteriosclerotic — *continued*
  with — *continued*
    critical limb ischemia — *continued*
      bypass graft — *continued*
        specified graft — *continued*
          leg — *continued*
            with
              gangrene (and intermittent claudication, rest pain, and ulcer) I70.769
              rest pain (and intermittent claudication) I70.729
            bilateral I70.723
              with
                gangrene (and intermittent claudication, rest pain, and ulcer) I70.763
                rest pain (and intermittent claudication) I70.723
            left I70.722
              with
                gangrene (and intermittent claudication, rest pain, and ulcer) I70.762
                rest pain (and intermittent claudication) I70.722
                ulceration (and intermittent claudication and rest pain) I70.749
                  ankle I70.743
                  calf I70.742
                  foot site NEC I70.745
                  heel I70.744
                  lower leg NEC I70.748
                  midfoot I70.744
                  thigh I70.741
            right I70.721
              with
                gangrene (and intermittent claudication, rest pain, and ulcer) I70.761
                rest pain (and intermittent claudication) I70.721
                ulceration (and intermittent claudication and rest pain) I70.739
                  ankle I70.733
                  calf I70.732
                  foot site NEC I70.735
                  heel I70.734
                  lower leg NEC I70.738
                  midfoot I70.734
                  thigh I70.731
      leg I70.229
        with
          gangrene (and intermittent claudication, rest pain, and ulcer) I70.269
          rest pain (and intermittent claudication) I70.229
        bilateral I70.223
          with
           gangrene (and intermittent claudication, rest pain, and ulcer) I70.263
           rest pain (and intermittent claudication) I70.223
        left I70.222
          with
           gangrene (and intermittent claudication, rest pain, and ulcer) I70.262
           rest pain (and intermittent claudication) I70.222
           ulceration (and intermittent claudication and rest pain) I70.249
             ankle I70.243
             calf I70.242
             foot site NEC I70.245
             heel I70.244
             lower leg NEC I70.248
             midfoot I70.244
             thigh I70.241
        right I70.221
          with
           gangrene (and intermittent claudication, rest pain, and ulcer) I70.261
           rest pain (and intermittent claudication) I70.221

Arteriosclerosis, arteriosclerotic — *continued*
  with — *continued*
    critical limb ischemia — *continued*
      leg — *continued*
        right — *continued*
          with — *continued*
           ulceration (and intermittent claudication and rest pain) I70.239
             ankle I70.233
             calf I70.232
             foot site NEC I70.235
             heel I70.234
             lower leg NEC I70.238
             midfoot I70.234
             thigh I70.231
  aorta I70.0
  arteries of extremities — *see* Arteriosclerosis, extremities
    with
      chronic limb-threatening ischemia — *see* Arteriosclerosis, with critical limb ischemia
      critical limb ischemia — *see* Arteriosclerosis, with critical limb ischemia
  brain I67.2
  bypass graft
    with
      chronic limb-threatening ischemia — *see* Arteriosclerosis, with critical limb ischemia
      critical limb ischemia — *see* Arteriosclerosis, with critical limb ischemia
      coronary — *see* Arteriosclerosis, coronary, bypass graft
      extremities — *see* Arteriosclerosis, extremities, bypass graft
  cardiac — *see* Disease, heart, ischemic, atherosclerotic
  cardiopathy — *see* Disease, heart, ischemic, atherosclerotic
  cardiorenal — *see* Hypertension, cardiorenal
  cardiovascular — *see* Disease, heart, ischemic, atherosclerotic
  carotid — *see also* Occlusion, artery, carotid I65.2- ☑
  central nervous system I67.2
  cerebral I67.2
  cerebrovascular I67.2
  coronary (artery) I25.10
    due to
      calcified coronary lesion (severely) I25.84
      lipid rich plaque I25.83
      bypass graft I25.810
        with
          angina pectoris I25.709
            with documented spasm I25.701
            refractory I25.702
            specified type NEC I25.708
            unstable I25.700
          ischemic chest pain I25.709
        autologous artery I25.810
          with
           angina pectoris I25.729
             with documented spasm I25.721
             refractory I25.722
             specified type I25.728
             unstable I25.720
           ischemic chest pain I25.729
        autologous vein I25.810
          with
           angina pectoris I25.719
             with documented spasm I25.711
             refractory I25.712
             specified type I25.718
             unstable I25.710
           ischemic chest pain I25.719
        nonautologous biological I25.810
          with
           angina pectoris I25.739
             with documented spasm I25.731
             refractory I25.732
             specified type I25.738
             unstable I25.730
           ischemic chest pain I25.739
        specified type NEC I25.810
          with
           angina pectoris I25.799
             with documented spasm I25.791
             refractory I25.792
             specified type I25.798
             unstable I25.790
           ischemic chest pain I25.799

Arteriosclerosis, arteriosclerotic — *continued*
  coronary — *continued*
    native vessel
      with
        angina pectoris I25.119
          with documented spasm I25.111
          refractory I25.112
          specified type NEC I25.118
          unstable I25.110
        ischemic chest pain I25.119
    transplanted heart I25.811
      bypass graft I25.812
        with
          angina pectoris I25.769
           with documented spasm I25.761
           refractory I25.762
           specified type I25.768
           unstable I25.760
          ischemic chest pain I25.769
      native coronary artery I25.811
        with
          angina pectoris I25.759
           with documented spasm I25.751
           refractory I25.752
           specified type I25.758
           unstable I25.750
          ischemic chest pain I25.759
  extremities (native arteries) I70.209
    with
      chronic limb-threatening ischemia — *see* Arteriosclerosis, with critical limb ischemia
      critical limb ischemia — *see* Arteriosclerosis, with critical limb ischemia
    bypass graft I70.309
      with
        chronic limb-threatening ischemia — *see* Arteriosclerosis, with critical limb ischemia
        critical limb ischemia — *see* Arteriosclerosis, with critical limb ischemia
      autologous vein graft I70.409
        leg I70.409
          with
           gangrene (and intermittent claudication, rest pain and ulcer) I70.469
           intermittent claudication I70.419
           rest pain (and intermittent claudication) I70.429
          bilateral I70.403
           with
             gangrene (and intermittent claudication, rest pain and ulcer) I70.463
            intermittent claudication I70.463
            rest pain (and intermittent claudication) I70.423
           specified type NEC I70.493
          left I70.402
           with
             gangrene (and intermittent claudication, rest pain and ulcer) I70.462
            intermittent claudication I70.412
            rest pain (and intermittent claudication) I70.422
            ulceration (and intermittent claudication and rest pain) I70.449
             ankle I70.443
             calf I70.442
             foot site NEC I70.445
             heel I70.444
             lower leg NEC I70.448
             midfoot I70.444
             thigh I70.441
           specified type NEC I70.492
          right I70.401
           with
             gangrene (and intermittent claudication, rest pain and ulcer) I70.461
            intermittent claudication I70.411
            rest pain (and intermittent claudication) I70.421
            ulceration (and intermittent claudication and rest pain) I70.439
             ankle I70.433
             calf I70.432
             foot site NEC I70.435
             heel I70.434
             lower leg NEC I70.438

Arteriosclerosis, arteriosclerotic — *continued*
  extremities — *continued*
    bypass graft — *continued*
      autologous vein graft — *continued*
        leg — *continued*
          right — *continued*
            with — *continued*
              ulceration — *continued*
                midfoot I70.434
                thigh I70.431
              specified type NEC I70.491
            specified type NEC I70.499
        specified NEC I70.408
          with
            gangrene (and intermittent claudication, rest pain and ulcer) I70.468
            intermittent claudication I70.418
            rest pain (and intermittent claudication) I70.428
            ulceration (and intermittent claudication and rest pain) I70.45
            specified type NEC I70.498
      leg I70.309
        with
          gangrene (and intermittent claudication, rest pain and ulcer) I70.369
          intermittent claudication I70.319
          rest pain (and intermittent claudication) I70.329
        bilateral I70.303
          with
            gangrene (and intermittent claudication, rest pain and ulcer) I70.363
            intermittent claudication I70.313
            rest pain (and intermittent claudication) I70.323
            specified type NEC I70.393
        left I70.302
          with
            gangrene (and intermittent claudication, rest pain and ulcer) I70.362
            intermittent claudication I70.312
            rest pain (and intermittent claudication) I70.322
            ulceration (and intermittent claudication and rest pain) I70.349
              ankle I70.343
              calf I70.342
              foot site NEC I70.345
              heel I70.344
              lower leg NEC I70.348
              midfoot I70.344
              thigh I70.341
            specified type NEC I70.392
        right I70.301
          with
            gangrene (and intermittent claudication, rest pain and ulcer) I70.361
            intermittent claudication I70.311
            rest pain (and intermittent claudication) I70.321
            ulceration (and intermittent claudication and rest pain I70.339
              ankle I70.333
              calf I70.332
              foot site NEC I70.335
              heel I70.334
              lower leg NEC I70.338
              midfoot I70.334
              thigh I70.331
            specified type NEC I70.391
        specified type NEC I70.399
      nonautologous biological graft I70.509
        leg I70.509
          with
            gangrene (and intermittent claudication, rest pain and ulcer) I70.569
            intermittent claudication I70.519
            rest pain (and intermittent claudication) I70.529
        bilateral I70.503
          with
            gangrene (and intermittent claudication, rest pain and ulcer) I70.563
            intermittent claudication I70.513
            rest pain (and intermittent claudication) I70.523
            specified type NEC I70.593

Arteriosclerosis, arteriosclerotic — *continued*
  extremities — *continued*
    bypass graft — *continued*
      nonautologous biological graft — *continued*
        leg — *continued*
          left I70.502
            with
              gangrene (and intermittent claudication, rest pain and ulcer) I70.562
              intermittent claudication I70.512
              rest pain (and intermittent claudication) I70.522
              ulceration (and intermittent claudication and rest pain) I70.549
                ankle I70.543
                calf I70.542
                foot site NEC I70.545
                heel I70.544
                lower leg NEC I70.548
                midfoot I70.544
                thigh I70.541
            specified type NEC I70.592
          right I70.501
            with
              gangrene (and intermittent claudication, rest pain and ulcer) I70.561
              intermittent claudication I70.511
              rest pain (and intermittent claudication) I70.521
              ulceration (and intermittent claudication and rest pain) I70.539
                ankle I70.533
                calf I70.532
                foot site NEC I70.535
                heel I70.534
                lower leg NEC I70.538
                midfoot I70.534
                thigh I70.531
            specified type NEC I70.591
         specified type NEC I70.599
        specified NEC I70.508
          with
            gangrene (and intermittent claudication, rest pain and ulcer) I70.568
            intermittent claudication I70.518
            rest pain (and intermittent claudication) I70.528
            ulceration (and intermittent claudication and rest pain) I70.55
            specified type NEC I70.598
      nonbiological graft I70.609
        leg I70.609
          with
            gangrene (and intermittent claudication, rest pain and ulcer) I70.669
            intermittent claudication I70.619
            rest pain (and intermittent claudication) I70.629
        bilateral I70.603
          with
            gangrene (and intermittent claudication, rest pain and ulcer) I70.663
            intermittent claudication I70.613
            rest pain (and intermittent claudication) I70.623
            specified type NEC I70.693
        left I70.602
          with
            gangrene (and intermittent claudication, rest pain and ulcer) I70.662
            intermittent claudication I70.612
            rest pain (and intermittent claudication) I70.622
            ulceration (and intermittent claudication and rest pain) I70.649
              ankle I70.643
              calf I70.642
              foot site NEC I70.645
              heel I70.644
              lower leg NEC I70.648
              midfoot I70.644
              thigh I70.641
            specified type NEC I70.692
        right I70.601

Arteriosclerosis, arteriosclerotic — *continued*
  extremities — *continued*
    bypass graft — *continued*
      nonbiological graft — *continued*
        leg — *continued*
          right — *continued*
            with
              gangrene (and intermittent claudication, rest pain and ulcer) I70.661
              intermittent claudication I70.611
              rest pain (and intermittent claudication) I70.621
              ulceration (and intermittent claudication and rest pain) I70.639
                ankle I70.633
                calf I70.632
                foot site NEC I70.635
                heel I70.634
                lower leg NEC I70.638
                midfoot I70.634
                thigh I70.631
            specified type NEC I70.691
         specified type NEC I70.699
        specified NEC I70.608
          with
            gangrene (and intermittent claudication, rest pain and ulcer) I70.668
            intermittent claudication I70.618
            rest pain (and intermittent claudication) I70.628
            ulceration (and intermittent claudication and rest pain) I70.65
            specified type NEC I70.698
      specified graft NEC I70.709
        leg I70.709
          with
            gangrene (and intermittent claudication, rest pain and ulcer) I70.769
            intermittent claudication I70.719
            rest pain (and intermittent claudication) I70.729
        bilateral I70.703
          with
            gangrene (and intermittent claudication, rest pain and ulcer) I70.763
            intermittent claudication I70.713
            rest pain (and intermittent claudication) I70.723
            specified type NEC I70.793
        left I70.702
          with
            gangrene (and intermittent claudication, rest pain and ulcer) I70.762
            intermittent claudication I70.712
            rest pain (and intermittent claudication) I70.722
            ulceration (and intermittent claudication and rest pain) I70.749
              ankle I70.743
              calf I70.742
              foot site NEC I70.745
              heel I70.744
              lower leg NEC I70.748
              midfoot I70.744
              thigh I70.741
            specified type NEC I70.792
        right I70.701
          with
            gangrene (and intermittent claudication, rest pain and ulcer) I70.761
            intermittent claudication I70.711
            rest pain (and intermittent claudication) I70.721
            ulceration (and intermittent claudication and rest pain) I70.739
              ankle I70.733
              calf I70.732
              foot site NEC I70.735
              heel I70.734
              lower leg NEC I70.738
              midfoot I70.734
              thigh I70.731
            specified type NEC I70.791
        specified type NEC I70.799
        specified NEC I70.708

Arteriosclerosis, arteriosclerotic — *continued*
- extremities — *continued*
  - bypass graft — *continued*
    - specified graft — *continued*
      - specified — *continued*
        - with
          - gangrene (and intermittent claudication, rest pain and ulcer) I70.768
          - intermittent claudication I70.718
          - rest pain (and intermittent claudication) I70.728
          - ulceration (and intermittent claudication and rest pain) I70.75
          - specified type NEC I70.798
    - specified NEC I70.308
      - with
        - gangrene (and intermittent claudication, rest pain and ulcer) I70.368
        - intermittent claudication I70.318
        - rest pain (and intermittent claudication) I70.328
        - ulceration (and intermittent claudication and rest pain) I70.35
        - specifiec type NEC I70.398
  - leg I70.209
    - with
      - gangrene (and intermittent claudication, rest pain and ulcer) I70.269
      - intermittent claudication I70.219
      - rest pain (and intermittent claudication) I70.229
    - bilateral I70.203
      - with
        - gangrene (and intermittent claudication, rest pain and ulcer) I70.263
        - intermittent claudication I70.213
        - rest pain (and intermittent claudication) I70.223
        - specified type NEC I70.293
    - left I70.202
      - with
        - gangrene (and intermittent claudication, rest pain and ulcer) I70.262
        - intermittent claudication I70.212
        - rest pain (and intermittent claudication) I70.222
        - ulceration (and intermittent claudication and rest pain) I70.249
          - ankle I70.243
          - calf I70.242
          - foot site NEC I70.245
          - heel I70.244
          - lower leg NEC I70.248
          - midfoot I70.244
          - thigh I70.241
        - specified type NEC I70.292
    - right I70.201
      - with
        - gangrene (and intermittent claudication, rest pain and ulcer) I70.261
        - intermittent claudication I70.211
        - rest pain (and intermittent claudication) I70.221
        - ulceration (and intermittent claudication and rest pain) I70.239
          - ankle I70.233
          - calf I70.232
          - foot site NEC I70.235
          - heel I70.234
          - lower leg NEC I70.238
          - midfoot I70.234
          - thigh I70.231
        - specified type NEC I70.291
      - specified type NEC I70.299
  - specified site NEC I70.208
    - with
      - gangrene (and intermittent claudication, rest pain and ulcer) I70.268
      - intermittent claudication I70.218
      - rest pain (and intermittent claudication) I70.228
      - ulceration (and intermittent claudication and rest pain) I70.25
    - specified type NEC I70.298
- generalized I70.91
- heart (disease) — *see* Arteriosclerosis, coronary (artery),
- kidney — *see* Hypertension, kidney
- medial — *see* Arteriosclerosis, extremities
- mesenteric (artery) K55.1

Arteriosclerosis, arteriosclerotic — *continued*
- Mönckeberg's — *see* Arteriosclerosis, extremities
- myocarditis I51.4
- peripheral (of extremities) — *see* Arteriosclerosis, extremities
- pulmonary (idiopathic) I27.0
- renal (arterioles) — *see also* Hypertension, kidney
  - artery I70.1
- retina (vascular) I70.8 [H35.0-] ☑
- specified artery NEC I70.8
- spinal (cord) G95.19
- vertebral (artery) I67.2

Arteriospasm I73.9
Arteriovenous — *see* condition
Arteritis I77.6
- allergic M31.0
- aorta (nonsyphilitic) I77.6
  - syphilitic A52.02
- aortic arch M31.4
- brachiocephalic M31.4
- brain I67.7
  - syphilitic A52.04
- cerebral I67.7
  - in systemic lupus erythematosus M32.19
  - listerial A32.89
  - syphilitic A52.04
  - tuberculous A18.89
- coronary (artery) I25.89
  - rheumatic I01.8
    - chronic I09.89
  - syphilitic A52.06
- cranial (left) (right), giant cell M31.6
- deformans — *see* Arteriosclerosis
- giant cell NEC M31.6
  - with polymyalgia rheumatica M31.5
- necrosing or necrotizing M31.9
  - specified NEC M31.8
- nodosa M30.0
- obliterans — *see* Arteriosclerosis
- pulmonary I28.8
- rheumatic — *see* Fever, rheumatic
- senile — *see* Arteriosclerosis
- suppurative I77.2
- syphilitic (general) A52.09
  - brain A52.04
  - coronary A52.06
  - spinal A52.09
- temporal, giant cell M31.6
- young female aortic arch syndrome M31.4
Artery, arterial — *see also* condition
- abscess I77.89
- single umbilical Q27.0
Arthralgia (allergic) — *see also* Pain, joint
- in caisson disease T70.3 ☑
- temporomandibular M26.62- ☑
Arthritis, arthritic (acute) (chronic) (nonpyogenic) (subacute) M19.90
- allergic — *see* Arthritis, specified form NEC
- ankylosing (crippling) (spine) — *see also* Spondylitis, ankylosing
  - sites other than spine — *see* Arthritis, specified form NEC
- atrophic — *see* Osteoarthritis
  - spine — *see* Spondylitis, ankylosing
- back — *see* Spondylopathy, inflammatory
- blennorrhagic (gonococcal) A54.42
- Charcot's — *see* Arthropathy, neuropathic
  - diabetic — *see* Diabetes, arthropathy, neuropathic
  - syringomyelic G95.0
- chylous (filarial) — *see also* category M01 B74.9
- climacteric (any site) NEC — *see* Arthritis, specified form NEC
- crystal (-induced) — *see* Arthritis, in, crystals
- deformans — *see* Osteoarthritis
- degenerative — *see* Osteoarthritis
- due to or associated with
  - acromegaly E22.0
  - brucellosis — *see* Brucellosis
  - caisson disease T70.3 ☑
  - diabetes — *see* Diabetes, arthropathy
  - dracontiasis — *see also* category M01 B72
  - enteritis NEC
    - regional — *see* Enteritis, regional
  - erysipelas — *see also* category M01 A46
  - erythema
    - epidemic A25.1
    - nodosum L52
  - filariasis NOS B74.9

Arthritis, arthritic — *continued*
- due to or associated with — *continued*
  - glanders A24.0
  - helminthiasis — *see also* category M01 B83.9
  - hemophilia D66 [M36.2]
  - Henoch- (Schönlein) purpura D69.0 [M36.4]
  - human parvovirus — *see also* category M01 B97.6
  - infectious disease NEC M01 ☑
  - leprosy (see also category M01) — *see also* Leprosy A30.9
  - Lyme disease A69.23
  - mycobacteria — *see also* category M01 A31.8
  - parasitic disease NEC — *see also* category M01 B89
  - paratyphoid fever (see also category M01) — *see also* Fever, paratyphoid A01.4
  - rat bite fever — *see also* category M01 A25.1
  - regional enteritis — *see* Enteritis, regional
  - respiratory disorder NOS J98.9
  - serum sickness — *see also* Reaction, serum T80.69 ☑
  - syringomyelia G95.0
  - typhoid fever A01.04
- epidemic erythema A25.1
- facet joint — *see also* Spondylosis M47.819
- febrile — *see* Fever, rheumatic
- gonococcal A54.42
- gouty (acute) — *see* Gout
- in (due to)
  - acromegaly — *see also* subcategory M14.8- E22.0
  - amyloidosis — *see also* subcategory M14.8- E85.4
  - bacterial disease — *see also* subcategory M01 A49.9
  - Behçet's syndrome M35.2
  - caisson disease — *see also* subcategory M14.8- T70.3 ☑
  - coliform bacilli (Escherichia coli) — *see* Arthritis, in, pyogenic organism NEC
  - crystals M11.9
    - dicalcium phosphate — *see* Arthritis, in, crystals, specified type NEC
    - hydroxyapatite M11.0- ☑
    - pyrophosphate — *see* Arthritis, in, crystals, specified type NEC
    - specified type NEC M11.80
      - ankle M11.87- ☑
      - elbow M11.82- ☑
      - foot joint M11.87- ☑
      - hand joint M11.84- ☑
      - hip M11.85- ☑
      - knee M11.86- ☑
      - multiple sites M11.8- ☑
      - shoulder M11.81- ☑
      - vertebrae M11.88
      - wrist M11.83- ☑
  - dermatoarthritis, lipoid E78.81
  - dracontiasis (dracunculiasis) — *see also* category M01 B72
  - endocrine disorder NEC — *see also* subcategory M14.8- E34.9
  - enteritis, infectious NEC — *see also* category M01 A09
    - specified organism NEC — *see also* category M01 A08.8
  - erythema
    - multiforme — *see also* subcategory M14.8- L51.9
    - nodosum — *see also* subcategory M14.8- L52
  - gout — *see* Gout
  - helminthiasis NEC — *see also* category M01 B83.9
  - hemochromatosis — *see also* subcategory M14.8- E83.118
  - hemoglobinopathy NEC D58.2 [M36.3]
  - hemophilia NEC D66 [M36.2]
  - Hemophilus influenzae M00.8- ☑ [B96.3]
  - Henoch (-Schönlein) purpura D69.0 [M36.4]
  - hyperparathyroidism NEC — *see also* subcategory M14.8- E21.3
  - hypersensitivity reaction NEC T78.49 ☑ [M36.4]
  - hypogammaglobulinemia — *see also* subcategory M14.8- D80.1
  - hypothyroidism NEC — *see also* subcategory M14.8- E03.9
  - infection — *see* Arthritis, pyogenic or pyemic
    - spine — *see* Spondylopathy, infective
  - infectious disease NEC M01 ☑
  - leprosy — *see also* category M01 A30.9
  - leukemia NEC C95.9- ☑ [M36.1]
  - lipoid dermatoarthritis E78.81
  - Lyme disease A69.23

Arthritis, arthritic — *continued*
  in — *continued*
    Mediterranean fever, familial — *see also* subcategory M14.8- M04.1
    Meningococcus A39.83
    metabolic disorder NEC — *see also* subcategory M14.8- E88.9
    multiple myelomatosis C90.0- ☑ *[M36.1]*
    mumps B26.85
    mycosis NEC — *see also* category M01 B49
    myelomatosis (multiple) C90.0- ☑ *[M36.1]*
    neurological disorder NEC G98.0
    ochronosis — *see also* subcategory M14.8- E70.29
    O'nyong-nyong — *see also* category M01 A92.1
    parasitic disease NEC — *see also* category M01 B89
    paratyphoid fever — *see also* category M01 A01.4
    Pseudomonas — *see* Arthritis, pyogenic, bacterial NEC
    psoriasis L40.50
    pyogenic organism NEC — *see* Arthritis, pyogenic, bacterial NEC
    Reiter's disease — *see* Reiter's disease
    respiratory disorder NEC — *see also* subcategory M14.8- J98.9
    reticulosis, malignant — *see also* subcategory M14.8- C86.0
    rubella B06.82
    Salmonella (arizonae) (cholerae-suis) (enteritidis) (typhimurium) A02.23
    sarcoidosis D86.86
    specified bacteria NEC — *see* Arthritis, pyogenic, bacterial NEC
    sporotrichosis B42.82
    syringomyelia G95.0
    thalassemia NEC D56.9 *[M36.3]*
    tuberculosis — *see* Tuberculosis, arthritis
    typhoid fever A01.04
    urethritis, Reiter's — *see* Reiter's disease
    viral disease NEC — *see also* category M01 B34.9
  infectious or infective — *see also* Arthritis, pyogenic or pyemic
    spine — *see* Spondylopathy, infective
  juvenile M08.90
    with systemic onset — *see* Still's disease
    ankle M08.97- ☑
    elbow M08.92- ☑
    foot joint M08.97- ☑
    hand joint M08.94- ☑
    hip M08.95- ☑
    knee M08.96- ☑
    multiple site M08.99
    pauciarticular M08.40
      ankle M08.47- ☑
      elbow M08.42- ☑
      foot joint M08.47- ☑
      hand joint M08.44- ☑
      hip M08.45- ☑
      knee M08.46- ☑
      shoulder M08.41- ☑
      specified site NEC M08.4A
      vertebrae M08.48
      wrist M08.43- ☑
    psoriatic L40.54
    rheumatoid — *see* Arthritis, rheumatoid, juvenile
    shoulder M08.91- ☑
    specified site NEC M08.9A
    specified type NEC M08.80
      ankle M08.87- ☑
      elbow M08.82- ☑
      foot joint M08.87- ☑
      hand joint M08.84- ☑
      hip M08.85- ☑
      knee M08.86- ☑
      multiple site M08.89
      shoulder M08.81- ☑
      specified joint NEC M08.88
      vertebrae M08.88
      wrist M08.83- ☑
    wrist M08.93- ☑
  meaning osteoarthritis — *see* Osteoarthritis
  meningococcal A39.83
  menopausal (any site) NEC — *see* Arthritis, specified form NEC
  mutilans (psoriatic) L40.52
  mycotic NEC — *see also* category M01 B49
  neuropathic (Charcot) — *see* Arthropathy, neuropathic
    diabetic — *see* Diabetes, arthropathy, neuropathic

Arthritis, arthritic — *continued*
  neuropathic — *see* Arthropathy, neuropathic — *continued*
    nonsyphilitic NEC G98.0
    syringomyelic G95.0
  ochronotic — *see also* subcategory M14.8- E70.29
  palindromic (any site) — *see* Rheumatism, palindromic
  pneumococcal M00.10
    ankle M00.17- ☑
    elbow M00.12- ☑
    foot joint — *see* Arthritis, pneumococcal, ankle
    hand joint M00.14- ☑
    hip M00.15- ☑
    knee M00.16- ☑
    multiple site M00.19
    shoulder M00.11- ☑
    vertebra M00.18
    wrist M00.13- ☑
  postdysenteric — *see* Arthropathy, postdysenteric
  postmeningococcal A39.84
  postrheumatic, chronic — *see* Arthropathy, postrheumatic, chronic
  primary progressive — *see also* Arthritis, specified form NEC
    spine — *see* Spondylitis, ankylosing
  psoriatic L40.50
  purulent (any site except spine) — *see* Arthritis, pyogenic or pyemic
    spine — *see* Spondylopathy, infective
  pyogenic or pyemic (any site except spine) M00.9
    bacterial NEC M00.80
      ankle M00.87- ☑
      elbow M00.82- ☑
      foot joint — *see* Arthritis, pyogenic, bacterial NEC, ankle
      hand joint M00.84- ☑
      hip M00.85- ☑
      knee M00.86- ☑
      multiple site M00.89
      shoulder M00.81- ☑
      vertebra M00.88
      wrist M00.83- ☑
    pneumococcal — *see* Arthritis, pneumococcal
    spine — *see* Spondylopathy, infective
    staphylococcal — *see* Arthritis, staphylococcal
    streptococcal — *see* Arthritis, streptococcal NEC
      pneumococcal — *see* Arthritis, pneumococcal
  reactive — *see* Reiter's disease
  rheumatic — *see also* Arthritis, rheumatoid
    acute or subacute — *see* Fever, rheumatic
  rheumatoid M06.9
    with
      carditis — *see* Rheumatoid, carditis
      endocarditis — *see* Rheumatoid, carditis
      heart involvement NEC — *see* Rheumatoid, carditis
      lung involvement — *see* Rheumatoid, lung
      myocarditis — *see* Rheumatoid, carditis
      myopathy — *see* Rheumatoid, myopathy
      pericarditis — *see* Rheumatoid, carditis
      polyneuropathy — *see* Rheumatoid, polyneuropathy
      rheumatoid factor — *see* Arthritis, rheumatoid, seropositive
      splenoadenomegaly and leukopenia — *see* Felty's syndrome
      vasculitis — *see* Rheumatoid, vasculitis
      visceral involvement NEC — *see* Rheumatoid, arthritis, with involvement of organs NEC
    juvenile (with or without rheumatoid factor) M08.00
      with systemic onset — *see* Still's disease
      ankle M08.07- ☑
      elbow M08.02- ☑
      foot joint M08.07- ☑
      hand joint M08.04- ☑
      hip M08.05- ☑
      knee M08.06- ☑
      multiple site M08.09
      shoulder M08.01- ☑
      specified site NEC M08.0A
      vertebra M08.08
      wrist M08.03- ☑
    seronegative M06.00
      ankle M06.07- ☑
      elbow M06.02- ☑
      foot joint M06.07- ☑
      hand joint M06.04- ☑

Arthritis, arthritic — *continued*
  rheumatoid — *continued*
    seronegative — *continued*
      hip M06.05- ☑
      knee M06.06- ☑
      multiple site M06.09
      shoulder M06.01- ☑
      specified site NEC M06.0A
      vertebra M06.08
      wrist M06.03- ☑
    seropositive M05.9
      specified NEC M05.80
        ankle M05.87- ☑
        elbow M05.82- ☑
        foot joint M05.87- ☑
        hand joint M05.84- ☑
        hip M05.85- ☑
        knee M05.86- ☑
        multiple sites M05.89
        shoulder M05.81- ☑
        specified site NEC M05.8A
        vertebra — *see* Spondylitis, ankylosing
        wrist M05.83- ☑
      without organ involvement M05.70
        ankle M05.77- ☑
        elbow M05.72- ☑
        foot joint M05.77- ☑
        hand joint M05.74- ☑
        hip M05.75- ☑
        knee M05.76- ☑
        multiple sites M05.79
        shoulder M05.71- ☑
        specified site NEC M05.7A
        vertebra — *see* Spondylitis, ankylosing
        wrist M05.73- ☑
    specified type NEC M06.80
      ankle M06.87- ☑
      elbow M06.82- ☑
      foot joint M06.87- ☑
      hand joint M06.84- ☑
      hip M06.85- ☑
      knee M06.86- ☑
      multiple site M06.89
      shoulder M06.81- ☑
      specified site NEC M06.8A
      vertebra M06.88
      wrist M06.83- ☑
    spine — *see* Spondylitis, ankylosing
  rubella B06.82
  scorbutic — *see also* subcategory M14.8- E54
  senile or senescent — *see* Osteoarthritis
  septic (any site except spine) — *see* Arthritis, pyogenic or pyemic
    spine — *see* Spondylopathy, infective
  serum (nontherapeutic) (therapeutic) — *see* Arthropathy, postimmunization
  specified form NEC M13.80
    ankle M13.87- ☑
    elbow M13.82- ☑
    foot joint M13.87- ☑
    hand joint M13.84- ☑
    hip M13.85- ☑
    knee M13.86- ☑
    multiple site M13.89
    shoulder M13.81- ☑
    specified joint NEC M13.88
    wrist M13.83- ☑
  spine — *see also* Spondylosis
    infectious or infective NEC — *see* Spondylopathy, infective
    Marie-Strümpell — *see* Spondylitis, ankylosing
    pyogenic — *see* Spondylopathy, infective
    rheumatoid — *see* Spondylitis, ankylosing
    traumatic (old) — *see* Spondylopathy, traumatic
    tuberculous A18.01
  staphylococcal M00.00
    ankle M00.07- ☑
    elbow M00.02- ☑
    foot joint — *see* Arthritis, staphylococcal, ankle
    hand joint M00.04- ☑
    hip M00.05- ☑
    knee M00.06- ☑
    multiple site M00.09
    shoulder M00.01- ☑
    vertebra M00.08
    wrist M00.03- ☑
  streptococcal NEC M00.20

Arthritis, arthritic — *continued*
  streptococcal — *continued*
    ankle M00.27- ☑
    elbow M00.22- ☑
    foot joint — *see* Arthritis, streptococcal, ankle
    hand joint M00.24- ☑
    hip M00.25- ☑
    knee M00.26- ☑
    multiple site M00.29
    shoulder M00.21- ☑
    vertebra M00.28
    wrist M00.23- ☑
  suppurative — *see* Arthritis, pyogenic or pyemic
  syphilitic (late) A52.16
    congenital A50.55 *[M12.80]*
  syphilitica deformans (Charcot) A52.16
  temporomandibular joint M26.64- ☑
  toxic of menopause (any site) — *see* Arthritis, specified form NEC
  transient — *see* Arthropathy, specified form NEC
  traumatic (chronic) — *see* Arthropathy, traumatic
  tuberculous A18.02
    spine A18.01
  uratic — *see* Gout
  urethritica (Reiter's) — *see* Reiter's disease
  vertebral — *see* Spondylopathy, inflammatory
  villous (any site) — *see* Arthropathy, specified form NEC

Arthrocele — *see* Effusion, joint
Arthrodesis status Z98.1
Arthrodynia — *see also* Pain, joint
Arthrodysplasia Q74.9
Arthrofibrosis, joint — *see* Ankylosis
Arthrogryposis (congenital) Q68.8
  multiplex congenita Q74.3
Arthrokatadysis M24.7
Arthropathy — *see also* Arthritis M12.9
  Charcot's — *see* Arthropathy, neuropathic
    diabetic — *see* Diabetes, arthropathy, neuropathic
    syringomyelic G95.0
  cricoarytenoid J38.7
  crystal (-induced) — *see* Arthritis, in, crystals
  diabetic NEC — *see* Diabetes, arthropathy
  distal interphalangeal, psoriatic L40.51
  enteropathic M07.60
    ankle M07.67- ☑
    elbow M07.62- ☑
    foot joint M07.67- ☑
    hand joint M07.64- ☑
    hip M07.65- ☑
    knee M07.66- ☑
    multiple site M07.69
    shoulder M07.61- ☑
    vertebra M07.68
    wrist M07.63- ☑
  facet joint — *see also* Spondylosis M47.819
  following intestinal bypass M02.00
    ankle M02.07- ☑
    elbow M02.02- ☑
    foot joint M02.07- ☑
    hand joint M02.04- ☑
    hip M02.05- ☑
    knee M02.06- ☑
    multiple site M02.09
    shoulder M02.01- ☑
    vertebra M02.08
    wrist M02.03- ☑
  gouty — *see also* Gout
    in (due to)
      Lesch-Nyhan syndrome E79.1 *[M14.8-]* ☑
      sickle-cell disorders D57- ☑ *[M14.8-]* ☑
  hemophilic NEC D66 *[M36.2]*
    in (due to)
      hyperparathyroidism NEC E21.3 *[M14.8-]* ☑
      metabolic disease NOS E88.9 *[M14.8-]* ☑
  in (due to)
    acromegaly E22.0 *[M14.8-]* ☑
    amyloidosis E85.4 *[M14.8-]* ☑
    blood disorder NOS D75.9 *[M36.3]*
    diabetes — *see* Diabetes, arthropathy
    endocrine disease NOS E34.9 *[M14.8-]* ☑
    erythema
      multiforme L51.9 *[M14.8-]* ☑
      nodosum L52 *[M14.8-]* ☑
    hemochromatosis E83.118 *[M14.8-]* ☑
    hemoglobinopathy NEC D58.2 *[M36.3]*

Arthropathy — *continued*
  in — *continued*
    hemophilia NEC D66 *[M36.2]*
    Henoch-Schönlein purpura D69.0 *[M36.4]*
    hyperthyroidism E05.90 *[M14.8-]* ☑
    hypothyroidism E03.9 *[M14.8-]* ☑
    infective endocarditis I33.0 *[M12.80]*
    leukemia NEC C95.9- *[M36.1]*
    malignant histiocytosis C96.A *[M36.1]*
    metabolic disease NOS E88.9 *[M14.8-]* ☑
    multiple myeloma C90.0- *[M36.1]*
    neoplastic disease NOS (*see also* Neoplasm) D49.9 *[M36.1]*
    nutritional deficiency — *see also* subcategory M14.8- E63.9
    psoriasis NOS L40.50
    sarcoidosis D86.86
    syphilis (late) A52.77
      congenital A50.55 *[M12.80]*
    thyrotoxicosis — *see also* subcategory M14.8- E05.90
    ulcerative colitis K51.90 *[M07.60]*
    viral hepatitis (postinfectious) NEC B19.9 *[M12.80]*
    Whipple's disease — *see also* subcategory M14.8- K90.81
  Jaccoud — *see* Arthropathy, postrheumatic, chronic
  juvenile — *see* Arthritis, juvenile
    psoriatic L40.54
  mutilans (psoriatic) L40.52
  neuropathic (Charcot) M14.60
    ankle M14.67- ☑
    diabetic — *see* Diabetes, arthropathy, neuropathic
    elbow M14.62- ☑
    foot joint M14.67- ☑
    hand joint M14.64- ☑
    hip M14.65- ☑
    knee M14.66- ☑
    multiple site M14.69
    nonsyphilitic NEC G98.0
    shoulder M14.61- ☑
    syringomyelic G95.0
    vertebra M14.68
    wrist M14.63- ☑
  osteopulmonary — *see* Osteoarthropathy, hypertrophic, specified NEC
  postdysenteric M02.10
    ankle M02.17- ☑
    elbow M02.12- ☑
    foot joint M02.17- ☑
    hand joint M02.14- ☑
    hip M02.15- ☑
    knee M02.16- ☑
    multiple site M02.19
    shoulder M02.11- ☑
    vertebra M02.18
    wrist M02.13- ☑
  postimmunization M02.20
    ankle M02.27- ☑
    elbow M02.22- ☑
    foot joint M02.27- ☑
    hand joint M02.24- ☑
    hip M02.25- ☑
    knee M02.26- ☑
    multiple site M02.29
    shoulder M02.21- ☑
    vertebra M02.28
    wrist M02.23- ☑
  postinfectious NEC B99 ☑ *[M12.80]*
    in (due to)
      enteritis due to Yersinia enterocolitica A04.6 *[M12.80]*
      syphilis A52.77
      viral hepatitis NEC B19.9 *[M12.80]*
  postrheumatic, chronic (Jaccoud) M12.00
    ankle M12.07- ☑
    elbow M12.02- ☑
    foot joint M12.07- ☑
    hand joint M12.04- ☑
    hip M12.05- ☑
    knee M12.06- ☑
    multiple site M12.09
    shoulder M12.01- ☑
    specified joint NEC M12.08
    vertebrae M12.08
    wrist M12.03- ☑
  psoriatic NEC L40.59
    interphalangeal, distal L40.51

Arthropathy — *continued*
  reactive M02.9
    in (due to)
      infective endocarditis I33.0 *[M02.9]*
    specified type NEC M02.80
      ankle M02.87- ☑
      elbow M02.82- ☑
      foot joint M02.87- ☑
      hand joint M02.84- ☑
      hip M02.85- ☑
      knee M02.86- ☑
      multiple site M02.89
      shoulder M02.81- ☑
      vertebra M02.88
      wrist M02.83- ☑
  specified form NEC M12.80
    ankle M12.87- ☑
    elbow M12.82- ☑
    foot joint M12.87- ☑
    hand joint M12.84- ☑
    hip M12.85- ☑
    knee M12.86- ☑
    multiple site M12.89
    shoulder M12.81- ☑
    specified joint NEC M12.88
    vertebrae M12.88
    wrist M12.83- ☑
  syringomyelic G95.0
  tabes dorsalis A52.16
  tabetic A52.16
  temporomandibular joint M26.65- ☑
  transient — *see* Arthropathy, specified form NEC
  traumatic M12.50
    ankle M12.57- ☑
    elbow M12.52- ☑
    foot joint M12.57- ☑
    hand joint M12.54- ☑
    hip M12.55- ☑
    knee M12.56- ☑
    multiple site M12.59
    shoulder M12.51- ☑
    specified joint NEC M12.58
    vertebrae M12.58
    wrist M12.53- ☑

Arthropyosis — *see* Arthritis, pyogenic or pyemic
Arthrosis (deformans) (degenerative) (localized) — *see also* Osteoarthritis M19.90
  spine — *see* Spondylosis
Arthus' phenomenon or reaction T78.41 ☑
  due to
    drug — *see* Table of Drugs and Chemicals, by drug
Articular — *see* condition
Articulation, reverse (teeth) M26.24
Artificial
  insemination complication — *see* Complications, artificial, fertilization
  opening status (functioning) (without complication) Z93.9
    anus (colostomy) Z93.3
    colostomy Z93.3
    cystostomy Z93.50
      appendico-vesicostomy Z93.52
      cutaneous Z93.51
      specified NEC Z93.59
    enterostomy Z93.4
    gastrostomy Z93.1
    ileostomy Z93.2
    intestinal tract NEC Z93.4
    jejunostomy Z93.4
    nephrostomy Z93.6
    specified site NEC Z93.8
    tracheostomy Z93.0
    ureterostomy Z93.6
    urethrostomy Z93.6
    urinary tract NEC Z93.6
    vagina Z93.8
    vagina status Z93.8
Arytenoid — *see* condition
Asbestosis (occupational) J61
Ascariasis B77.9
  with
    complications NEC B77.89
    intestinal complications B77.0
    pneumonia, pneumonitis B77.81
Ascaridosis, ascaridiasis — *see* Ascariasis
Ascaris (infection) (infestation) (lumbricoides) — *see* Ascariasis

Ascending — *see* condition
ASC-H (atypical squamous cells cannot exclude high grade squamous intraepithelial lesion on cytologic smear)
  anus R85.611
  cervix R87.611
  vagina R87.621
Aschoff's bodies — *see* Myocarditis, rheumatic
Ascites (abdominal) R18.8
  cardiac — *see also* Failure, heart, right I50.810
  chylous (nonfilarial) I89.8
    filarial — *see* Infestation, filarial
  due to
    cirrhosis, alcoholic K70.31
    hepatitis
      alcoholic K70.11
      chronic active K71.51
    S. japonicum B65.2
  heart — *see also* Failure, heart, right I50.810
  malignant R18.0
  pseudochylous R18.8
  syphilitic A52.74
  tuberculous A18.31
ASC-US (atypical squamous cells of undetermined significance on cytologic smear)
  anus R85.610
  cervix R87.610
  vagina R87.620
Aseptic — *see* condition
Asherman's syndrome N85.6
Asialia K11.7
Asiatic cholera — *see* Cholera
Asimultagnosia (simultanagnosia) R48.3
Askin's tumor — *see* Neoplasm, connective tissue, malignant
Asocial personality F60.2
Asomatognosia R41.4
Aspartylglucosaminuria E77.1
Asperger's disease or syndrome F84.5
Aspergilloma — *see* Aspergillosis
Aspergillosis (with pneumonia) B44.9
  bronchopulmonary, allergic B44.81
  disseminated B44.7
  generalized B44.7
  pulmonary NEC B44.1
    allergic B44.81
    invasive B44.0
  specified NEC B44.89
  tonsillar B44.2
Aspergillus (flavus) (fumigatus) (infection) (terreus) — *see* Aspergillosis
Aspermatogenesis — *see* Azoospermia
Aspermia (testis) — *see* Azoospermia
Asphyxia, asphyxiation (by) R09.01
  antenatal P84
  birth P84
  bunny bag — *see* Asphyxia, due to, mechanical threat to breathing, trapped in bed clothes
  crushing S28.0 ☑
  drowning T75.1 ☑
  gas, fumes, or vapor — *see* Table of Drugs and Chemicals
  inhalation — *see* Inhalation
  intrauterine P84
  local I73.00
    with gangrene I73.01
  mucus — *see also* Foreign body, respiratory tract, causing asphyxia
  newborn P84
  pathological R09.01
  postnatal P84
    mechanical — *see* Asphyxia, due to, mechanical threat to breathing
  prenatal P84
  reticularis R23.1
  strangulation — *see* Asphyxia, due to, mechanical threat to breathing
  submersion T75.1 ☑
  traumatic T71.9 ☑
    due to
      crushed chest S28.0 ☑
      foreign body (in) — *see* Foreign body, respiratory tract, causing asphyxia
      low oxygen content of ambient air T71.20 ☑
        due to
          being trapped in
            low oxygen environment T71.29 ☑
              in car trunk T71.221 ☑

Asphyxia, asphyxiation — *continued*
  traumatic — *continued*
    due to — *continued*
      low oxygen content of ambient air — *continued*
        due to — *continued*
          being trapped in — *continued*
            low oxygen environment — *continued*
              in car trunk — *continued*
                circumstances undetermined T71.224 ☑
                done with intent to harm by
                  another person T71.223 ☑
                  self T71.222 ☑
            in refrigerator T71.231 ☑
              circumstances undetermined T71.234 ☑
              done with intent to harm by
                another person T71.233 ☑
                self T71.232 ☑
      cave-in T71.21 ☑
    mechanical threat to breathing (accidental) T71.191 ☑
      circumstances undetermined T71.194 ☑
      done with intent to harm by
        another person T71.193 ☑
        self T71.192 ☑
      hanging T71.161 ☑
        circumstances undetermined T71.164 ☑
        done with intent to harm by
          another person T71.163 ☑
          self T71.162 ☑
      plastic bag T71.121 ☑
        circumstances undetermined T71.124 ☑
        done with intent to harm by
          another person T71.123 ☑
          self T71.122 ☑
      smothering
        in furniture T71.151 ☑
          circumstances undetermined T71.154 ☑
          done with intent to harm by
            another person T71.153 ☑
            self T71.152 ☑
        under
          another person's body T71.141 ☑
            circumstances undetermined T71.144 ☑
            done with intent to harm T71.143 ☑
          pillow T71.111 ☑
            circumstances undetermined T71.114 ☑
            done with intent to harm by
              another person T71.113 ☑
              self T71.112 ☑
      trapped in bed clothes T71.131 ☑
        circumstances undetermined T71.134 ☑
        done with intent to harm by
          another person T71.133 ☑
          self T71.132 ☑
  vomiting, vomitus — *see* Foreign body, respiratory tract, causing asphyxia
Aspiration
  amniotic (clear) fluid (newborn) P24.10
    with
      pneumonia (pneumonitis) P24.11
      respiratory symptoms P24.11
  blood
    newborn (without respiratory symptoms) P24.20
      with
        pneumonia (pneumonitis) P24.21
        respiratory symptoms P24.21
    specified age NEC — *see* Foreign body, respiratory tract
  bronchitis J69.0
  food or foreign body — *see* Foreign body, by site
  liquor (amnii) (newborn) P24.10
    with
      pneumonia (pneumonitis) P24.11
      respiratory symptoms P24.11
  meconium (newborn) (without respiratory symptoms) P24.00
    with
      pneumonitis (pneumonitis) P24.01
      respiratory symptoms P24.01
  milk (newborn) (without respiratory symptoms) P24.30

Aspiration — *continued*
  milk — *continued*
    with
      pneumonia (pneumonitis) P24.31
      respiratory symptoms P24.31
    specified age NEC — *see* Foreign body, respiratory tract
  mucus — *see also* Foreign body, by site, causing asphyxia
    newborn P24.10
      with
        pneumonia (pneumonitis) P24.11
        respiratory symptoms P24.11
    neonatal P24.9
      specific NEC (without respiratory symptoms) P24.80
        with
          pneumonia (pneumonitis) P24.81
          respiratory symptoms P24.81
    newborn P24.9
      specific NEC (without respiratory symptoms) P24.80
        with
          pneumonia (pneumonitis) P24.81
          respiratory symptoms P24.81
  pneumonia J69.0
  pneumonitis J69.0
  syndrome of newborn — *see* Aspiration, by substance, with pneumonia
  vernix caseosa (newborn) P24.80
    with
      pneumonia (pneumonitis) P24.81
      respiratory symptoms P24.81
  vomitus — *see also* Foreign body, respiratory tract
    newborn (without respiratory symptoms) P24.30
      with
        pneumonia (pneumonitis) P24.31
        respiratory symptoms P24.31
Asplenia (congenital) Q89.01
  postsurgical Z90.81
Assam fever B55.0
Assault, sexual — *see* Maltreatment
Assmann's focus NEC A15.0
Astasia (-abasia) (hysterical) F44.4
Asteatosis cutis L85.3
Astereognosia, astereognosis R48.1
Asterixis R27.8
  in liver disease K71.3
Asteroid hyalitis — *see* Deposit, crystalline
Asthenia, asthenic R53.1
  cardiac — *see also* Failure, heart I50.9
    psychogenic F45.8
  cardiovascular — *see also* Failure, heart I50.9
    psychogenic F45.8
  heart — *see also* Failure, heart I50.9
    psychogenic F45.8
  hysterical F44.4
  myocardial — *see also* Failure, heart I50.9
    psychogenic F45.8
  nervous F48.8
  neurocirculatory F45.8
  neurotic F48.8
  psychogenic F48.8
  psychoneurotic F48.8
  psychophysiologic F48.8
  reaction (psychophysiologic) F48.8
  senile R54
Asthenopia — *see also* Discomfort, visual
  hysterical F44.6
  psychogenic F44.6
Asthenospermia — *see* Abnormal, specimen, male genital organs
Asthma, asthmatic (bronchial) (catarrh) (spasmodic) J45.909
  with
    chronic obstructive bronchitis J44.9
      with
        acute lower respiratory infection J44.0
        exacerbation (acute) J44.1
    chronic obstructive pulmonary disease J44.9
      with
        acute lower respiratory infection J44.0
        exacerbation (acute) J44.1
    exacerbation (acute) J45.901
    hay fever — *see* Asthma, allergic extrinsic
    rhinitis, allergic — *see* Asthma, allergic extrinsic
    status asthmaticus J45.902
  allergic extrinsic J45.909
    with
      exacerbation (acute) J45.901

Asthma, asthmatic — *continued*
allergic extrinsic — *continued*
with — *continued*
status asthmaticus J45.902
atopic — *see* Asthma, allergic extrinsic
cardiac — *see* Failure, ventricular, left
cardiobronchial I50.1
childhood J45.909
with
exacerbation (acute) J45.901
status asthmaticus J45.902
chronic obstructive J44.9
with
acute lower respiratory infection J44.0
exacerbation (acute) J44.1
collier's J60
cough variant J45.991
detergent J69.8
due to
detergent J69.8
inhalation of fumes J68.3
eosinophilic J82.83
extrinsic, allergic — *see* Asthma, allergic extrinsic
grinder's J62.8
hay — *see* Asthma, allergic extrinsic
heart I50.1
idiosyncratic — *see* Asthma, nonallergic
intermittent (mild) J45.20
with
exacerbation (acute) J45.21
status asthmaticus J45.22
intrinsic, nonallergic — *see* Asthma, nonallergic
Kopp's E32.8
late-onset J45.909
with
exacerbation (acute) J45.901
status asthmaticus J45.902
mild intermittent J45.20
with
exacerbation (acute) J45.21
status asthmaticus J45.22
mild persistent J45.30
with
exacerbation (acute) J45.31
status asthmaticus J45.32
Millar's (laryngismus stridulus) J38.5
miner's J60
mixed J45.909
with
exacerbation (acute) J45.901
status asthmaticus J45.902
moderate persistent J45.40
with
exacerbation (acute) J45.41
status asthmaticus J45.42
nervous — *see* Asthma, nonallergic
nonallergic (intrinsic) J45.909
with
exacerbation (acute) J45.901
status asthmaticus J45.902
persistent
mild J45.30
with
exacerbation (acute) J45.31
status asthmaticus J45.32
moderate J45.40
with
exacerbation (acute) J45.41
status asthmaticus J45.42
severe J45.50
with
exacerbation (acute) J45.51
status asthmaticus J45.52
platinum J45.998
pneumoconiotic NEC J64
potter's J62.8
predominantly allergic J45.909
psychogenic F54
pulmonary eosinophilic J82.83
red cedar J67.8
Rostan's I50.1
sandblaster's J62.8
sequoiosis J67.8
severe persistent J45.50
with
exacerbation (acute) J45.51
status asthmaticus J45.52
specified NEC J45.998

Asthma, asthmatic — *continued*
stonemason's J62.8
thymic E32.8
tuberculous — *see* Tuberculosis, pulmonary
Wichmann's (laryngismus stridulus) J38.5
wood J67.8
Astigmatism (compound) (congenital) H52.20- ☑
irregular H52.21- ☑
regular H52.22- ☑
Astraphobia F40.220
Astroblastoma
specified site — *see* Neoplasm, malignant, by site
unspecified site C71.9
Astrocytoma (cystic)
anaplastic
specified site — *see* Neoplasm, malignant, by site
unspecified site C71.9
fibrillary
specified site — *see* Neoplasm, malignant, by site
unspecified site C71.9
fibrous
specified site — *see* Neoplasm, malignant, by site
unspecified site C71.9
gemistocytic
specified site — *see* Neoplasm, malignant, by site
unspecified site C71.9
juvenile
specified site — *see* Neoplasm, malignant, by site
unspecified site C71.9
pilocytic
specified site — *see* Neoplasm, malignant, by site
unspecified site C71.9
piloid
specified site — *see* Neoplasm, malignant, by site
unspecified site C71.9
protoplasmic
specified site — *see* Neoplasm, malignant, by site
unspecified site C71.9
specified site NEC — *see* Neoplasm, malignant, by site
subependymal D43.2
giant cell
specified site — *see* Neoplasm, uncertain behavior, by site
unspecified site D43.2
specified site — *see* Neoplasm, uncertain behavior, by site
unspecified site D43.2
unspecified site C71.9
Astroglioma
specified site — *see* Neoplasm, malignant, by site
unspecified site C71.9
Asymbolia R48.8
Asymmetry — *see also* Distortion
between native and reconstructed breast N65.1
face Q67.0
jaw (lower) — *see* Anomaly, dentofacial, jaw-cranial base relationship, asymmetry
Asynergia, asynergy R27.8
ventricular I51.89
Asystole (heart) — *see* Arrest, cardiac
At risk
for
dental caries Z91.849
high Z91.843
low Z91.841
moderate Z91.842
falling Z91.81
Ataxia, ataxy, ataxic R27.0
acute R27.8
autosomal recessive Friedreich G11.11
brain (hereditary) G11.9
cerebellar (hereditary) G11.9
with defective DNA repair G11.3
alcoholic G31.2
early-onset G11.10
with
essential tremor G11.19
myoclonus [Hunt's ataxia] G11.19
retained tendon reflexes G11.19
in
alcoholism G31.2
myxedema E03.9 *[G13.2]*
neoplastic disease — *see also* Neoplasm D49.9 *[G32.81]*
specified disease NEC G32.81
late-onset (Marie's) G11.2
cerebral (hereditary) G11.9
congenital nonprogressive G11.0

Ataxia, ataxy, ataxic — *continued*
family, familial — *see* Ataxia, hereditary
following
cerebrovascular disease I69.993
cerebral infarction I69.393
intracerebral hemorrhage I69.193
nontraumatic intracranial hemorrhage NEC I69.293
specified disease NEC I69.893
subarachnoid hemorrhage I69.093
Friedreich's (heredofamilial) (cerebellar) (spinal) (with retained reflexes) G11.11
gait R26.0
hysterical F44.4
general R27.8
gluten M35.9 *[G32.81]*
with celiac disease K90.0 *[G32.81]*
hereditary G11.9
with neuropathy G60.2
cerebellar — *see* Ataxia, cerebellar
spastic G11.4
specified NEC G11.8
spinal (Friedreich's) G11.11
heredofamilial — *see* Ataxia, hereditary
Hunt's G11.19
hysterical F44.4
locomotor (progressive) (syphilitic) (partial) (spastic) A52.11
diabetic — *see* Diabetes, ataxia
Marie's (cerebellar) (heredofamilial) (late-onset) G11.2
nonorganic origin F44.4
nonprogressive, congenital G11.0
psychogenic F44.4
Roussy-Lévy G60.0
Sanger-Brown's (hereditary) G11.2
spastic hereditary G11.4
spinal
hereditary (Friedreich's) G11.11
progressive (syphilitic) A52.11
spinocerebellar, X-linked recessive G11.19
telangiectasia (Louis-Bar) G11.3
Ataxia-telangiectasia (Louis-Bar) G11.3
Atelectasis (massive) (partial) (pressure) (pulmonary) J98.11
newborn P28.10
due to resorption P28.11
partial P28.19
primary P28.0
secondary P28.19
primary (newborn) P28.0
tuberculous — *see* Tuberculosis, pulmonary
Atelocardia Q24.9
Atelomyelia Q06.1
Atheroembolism
of
extremities
lower I75.02- ☑
upper I75.01- ☑
kidney I75.81
specified NEC I75.89
Atheroma, atheromatous — *see also* Arteriosclerosis I70.90
aorta, aortic I70.0
valve — *see also* Endocarditis, aortic I35.8
aorto-iliac I70.0
artery — *see* Arteriosclerosis
basilar (artery) I67.2
carotid (artery) (common) (internal) I67.2
cerebral (arteries) I67.2
coronary (artery) I25.10
with angina pectoris — *see* Arteriosclerosis, coronary (artery),
degeneration — *see* Arteriosclerosis
heart, cardiac — *see* Disease, heart, ischemic, atherosclerotic
mitral (valve) I34.89
myocardium, myocardial — *see* Disease, heart, ischemic, atherosclerotic
pulmonary valve (heart) — *see also* Endocarditis, pulmonary I37.8
tricuspid (heart) (valve) I36.8
valve, valvular — *see* Endocarditis
vertebral (artery) I67.2
Atheromatosis — *see* Arteriosclerosis
Atherosclerosis — *see also* Arteriosclerosis
coronary
artery I25.10

☑ **Additional Character Required — Refer to the Tabular List for Character Selection**

Atherosclerosis — *continued*
  coronary — *continued*
    artery — *continued*
      with angina pectoris — *see* Arteriosclerosis, coronary (artery),
      due to
        calcified coronary lesion (severely) I25.84
        lipid rich plaque I25.83
    transplanted heart I25.811
      bypass graft I25.812
        with angina pectoris — *see* Arteriosclerosis, coronary (artery),
      native coronary artery I25.811
        with angina pectoris — *see* Arteriosclerosis, coronary (artery),
Athetosis (acquired) R25.8
  bilateral (congenital) G80.3
  congenital (bilateral) (double) G80.3
  double (congenital) G80.3
  unilateral R25.8
Athlete's
  foot B35.3
  heart I51.7
Athrepsia E41
Athyrea (acquired) — *see also* Hypothyroidism
  congenital E03.1
Atonia, atony, atonic
  bladder (sphincter) (neurogenic) N31.2
  capillary I78.8
  cecum K59.89
    psychogenic F45.8
  colon — *see* Atony, intestine
  congenital P94.2
  esophagus K22.89
  intestine K59.89
    psychogenic F45.8
  stomach K31.89
    neurotic or psychogenic F45.8
  uterus (during labor) O62.2
    with hemorrhage (postpartum) O72.1
    postpartum (with hemorrhage) O72.1
      without hemorrhage O75.89
Atopy — *see* History, allergy
Atransferrinemia, congenital E88.09
Atresia, atretic
  alimentary organ or tract NEC Q45.8
    upper Q40.8
  ani, anus, anal (canal) Q42.3
    with fistula Q42.2
  aorta (ring) Q25.29
  aortic (orifice) (valve) Q23.0
    arch Q25.21
    congenital with hypoplasia of ascending aorta and defective development of left ventricle (with mitral stenosis) Q23.4
    in hypoplastic left heart syndrome Q23.4
  aqueduct of Sylvius Q03.0
    with spina bifida — *see* Spina bifida, with hydrocephalus
  artery NEC Q27.8
    cerebral Q28.3
    coronary Q24.5
    digestive system Q27.8
    eye Q15.8
    lower limb Q27.8
    pulmonary Q25.5
    specified site NEC Q27.8
    umbilical Q27.0
    upper limb Q27.8
  auditory canal (external) Q16.1
  bile duct (common) (congenital) (hepatic) Q44.2
    acquired — *see* Obstruction, bile duct
  bladder (neck) Q64.39
    obstruction Q64.31
  bronchus Q32.4
  cecum Q42.8
  cervix (acquired) N88.2
    congenital Q51.828
    in pregnancy or childbirth — *see* Anomaly, cervix, in pregnancy or childbirth
      causing obstructed labor O65.5
  choana Q30.0
  colon Q42.9
    specified NEC Q42.8
  common duct Q44.2
  cricoid cartilage Q31.8
  cystic duct Q44.2
    acquired K82.8

Atresia, atretic — *continued*
  cystic duct — *continued*
    acquired — *continued*
      with obstruction K82.0
  digestive organs NEC Q45.8
  duodenum Q41.0
  ear canal Q16.1
  ejaculatory duct Q55.4
  epiglottis Q31.8
  esophagus Q39.0
    with tracheoesophageal fistula Q39.1
  eustachian tube Q17.8
  fallopian tube (congenital) Q50.6
    acquired N97.1
  follicular cyst N83.0- ☑
  foramen of
    Luschka Q03.1
      with spina bifida — *see* Spina bifida, with hydrocephalus
    Magendie Q03.1
      with spina bifida — *see* Spina bifida, with hydrocephalus
  gallbladder Q44.1
  genital organ
    external
      female Q52.79
      male Q55.8
    internal
      female Q52.8
      male Q55.8
  glottis Q31.8
  gullet Q39.0
    with tracheoesophageal fistula Q39.1
  heart valve NEC Q24.8
    pulmonary Q22.0
    tricuspid Q22.4
  hymen Q52.3
    acquired (postinfective) N89.6
  ileum Q41.2
  intestine (small) Q41.9
    large Q42.9
      specified NEC Q42.8
  iris, filtration angle Q15.0
  jejunum Q41.1
  lacrimal apparatus Q10.4
  larynx Q31.8
  meatus urinarius Q64.33
  mitral valve Q23.2
    in hypoplastic left heart syndrome Q23.4
  nares (anterior) (posterior) Q30.0
  nasopharynx Q34.8
  nose, nostril Q30.0
    acquired J34.89
  organ or site NEC Q89.8
  osseous meatus (ear) Q16.1
  oviduct (congenital) Q50.6
    acquired N97.1
  parotid duct Q38.4
    acquired K11.8
  pulmonary (artery) Q25.5
    valve Q22.0
  pulmonic Q22.0
  pupil Q13.2
  rectum Q42.1
    with fistula Q42.0
  salivary duct Q38.4
    acquired K11.8
  sublingual duct Q38.4
    acquired K11.8
  submandibular duct Q38.4
    acquired K11.8
  submaxillary duct Q38.4
    acquired K11.8
  thyroid cartilage Q31.8
  trachea Q32.1
  tricuspid valve Q22.4
  ureter Q62.10
    pelvic junction Q62.11
    vesical orifice Q62.12
  ureteropelvic junction Q62.11
  ureterovesical orifice Q62.12
  urethra (valvular) Q64.39
    stricture Q64.32
  urinary tract NEC Q64.8
  uterus Q51.818
    acquired N85.8
  vagina (congenital) Q52.4
    acquired (postinfectional) (senile) N89.5
  vas deferens Q55.3

Atresia, atretic — *continued*
  vascular NEC Q27.8
    cerebral Q28.3
    digestive system Q27.8
    lower limb Q27.8
    specified site NEC Q27.8
    upper limb Q27.8
  vein NEC Q27.8
    digestive system Q27.8
    great Q26.8
    lower limb Q27.8
    portal Q26.5
    pulmonary Q26.4
      partial Q26.3
      total Q26.2
    specified site NEC Q27.8
    upper limb Q27.8
  vena cava (inferior) (superior) Q26.8
  vesicourethral orifice Q64.31
  vulva Q52.79
    acquired N90.5
Atrichia, atrichosis — *see* Alopecia
Atrophia — *see also* Atrophy
  cutis senilis L90.8
    due to radiation L57.8
  gyrata of choroid and retina H31.23
  senilis R54
    dermatological L90.8
      due to radiation (nonionizing) (solar) L57.8
  unguium L60.3
    congenita Q84.6
Atrophie blanche (en plaque) (de Milian) L95.0
Atrophoderma, atrophodermia (of) L90.9
  diffusum (idiopathic) L90.4
  maculatum L90.8
    et striatum L90.8
      due to syphilis A52.79
    syphilitic A51.39
  neuriticum L90.8
  Pasini and Pierini L90.3
  pigmentosum Q82.1
  reticulatum symmetricum faciei L66.4
  senile L90.8
    due to radiation (nonionizing) (solar) L57.8
  vermiculata (cheeks) L66.4
Atrophy, atrophic (of)
  adrenal (capsule) (gland) E27.49
    primary (autoimmune) E27.1
  alveolar process or ridge (edentulous) K08.20
  anal sphincter (disuse) N81.84
  appendix K38.8
  arteriosclerotic — *see* Arteriosclerosis
  bile duct (common) (hepatic) K83.8
  bladder N32.89
    neurogenic N31.8
  blanche (en plaque) (of Milian) L95.0
  bone (senile) NEC — *see also* Disorder, bone, specified type NEC
    due to
      tabes dorsalis (neurogenic) A52.11
  brain (cortex) (progressive) G31.9
    frontotemporal circumscribed — *see also* Dementia, in, diseases specified elsewhere G31.01 *[F02.80]*
      with behavioral disturbance — *see also* Dementia, in, diseases specified elsewhere G31.01 *[F02.81-]* ☑
    senile NEC G31.1
  breast N64.2
    obstetric — *see* Disorder, breast, specified type NEC
  buccal cavity K13.79
  cardiac — *see* Degeneration, myocardial
  cartilage (infectional) (joint) — *see* Disorder, cartilage, specified NEC
  cerebellar — *see* Atrophy, brain
  cerebral — *see* Atrophy, brain
  cervix (mucosa) (senile) (uteri) N88.8
    menopausal N95.8
  Charcot-Marie-Tooth G60.0
  choroid (central) (macular) (myopic) (retina) H31.10- ☑
    diffuse secondary H31.12- ☑
    gyrate H31.23
    senile H31.11- ☑
  ciliary body — *see* Atrophy, iris
  conjunctiva (senile) H11.89
  corpus cavernosum N48.89
  cortical — *see* Atrophy, brain
  cystic duct K82.8

Atrophy, atrophic — *continued*
- Déjérine-Thomas G23.8
- disuse NEC — *see* Atrophy, muscle
- Duchenne-Aran G12.21
- ear H93.8- ☑
- edentulous alveolar ridge K08.20
- endometrium (senile) N85.8
  - cervix N88.8
- enteric K63.89
- epididymis N50.89
- eyeball — *see* Disorder, globe, degenerated condition, atrophy
- eyelid (senile) — *see* Disorder, eyelid, degenerative
- facial (skin) L90.9
- fallopian tube (senile) N83.32- ☑
  - with ovary N83.33- ☑
- fascioscapulohumeral (Landouzy- Déjérine) G71.02
- fatty, thymus (gland) E32.8
- gallbladder K82.8
- gastric K29.40
  - with bleeding K29.41
- gastrointestinal K63.89
- glandular I89.8
- globe H44.52- ☑
- gum — *see* Recession, gingival
- hair L67.8
- heart (brown) — *see* Degeneration, myocardial
- hemifacial Q67.4
  - Romberg G51.8
- infantile E41
  - paralysis, acute — *see* Poliomyelitis, paralytic
- intestine K63.89
- iris (essential) (progressive) H21.26- ☑
  - specified NEC H21.29
- kidney (senile) (terminal) — *see also* Sclerosis, renal N26.1
  - congenital or infantile Q60.5
    - bilateral Q60.4
    - unilateral Q60.3
  - hydronephrotic — *see* Hydronephrosis
- lacrimal gland (primary) H04.14- ☑
  - secondary H04.15- ☑
- Landouzy-Déjérine G71.02
- laryngitis, infective J37.0
- larynx J38.7
- Leber's optic (hereditary) H47.22
- lip K13.0
- liver (yellow) K72.90
  - with coma K72.91
  - acute, subacute K72.00
    - with coma K72.01
  - chronic K72.10
    - with coma K72.11
- lung (senile) J98.4
- macular (dermatological) L90.8
  - syphilitic, skin A51.39
    - striated A52.79
- mandible (edentulous) K08.20
  - minimal K08.21
  - moderate K08.22
  - severe K08.23
- maxilla K08.20
  - minimal K08.24
  - moderate K08.25
  - severe K08.26
- muscle, muscular (diffuse) (general) (idiopathic) (primary) M62.50
  - ankle M62.57- ☑
  - back M62.5A9
    - cervical M62.5A0
    - lumbosacral M62.5A2
    - thoracic M62.5A1
  - Duchenne-Aran G12.21
  - foot M62.57- ☑
  - forearm M62.53- ☑
  - hand M62.54- ☑
  - infantile spinal G12.0
  - lower leg M62.56- ☑
  - multiple sites M62.59
  - myelopathic — *see* Atrophy, muscle, spinal
  - myotonic G71.11
  - neuritic G58.9
  - neuropathic (peroneal) (progressive) G60.0
  - pelvic (disuse) N81.84
  - peroneal G60.0
  - progressive (bulbar) G12.21
    - adult G12.1
    - infantile (spinal) G12.0

Atrophy, atrophic — *continued*
- muscle, muscular — *continued*
  - progressive — *continued*
    - spinal G12.25
      - adult G12.1
      - infantile G12.0
    - pseudohypertrophic G71.02
  - shoulder region M62.51- ☑
  - specified site NEC M62.58
  - spinal G12.9
    - adult form G12.1
    - Aran-Duchenne G12.21
    - childhood form, type II G12.1
    - distal G12.1
    - hereditary NEC G12.1
    - infantile, type I (Werdnig-Hoffmann) G12.0
    - juvenile form, type III (Kugelberg- Welander) G12.1
    - progressive G12.25
    - scapuloperoneal form G12.1
    - specified NEC G12.8
  - syphilitic A52.78
  - thigh M62.55- ☑
  - upper arm M62.52- ☑
- myocardium — *see* Degeneration, myocardial
- myometrium (senile) N85.8
  - cervix N88.8
- myopathic NEC — *see* Atrophy, muscle
- myotonia G71.11
- nail L60.3
- nasopharynx J31.1
- nerve — *see also* Disorder, nerve
  - abducens — *see* Strabismus, paralytic, sixth nerve
  - accessory G52.8
  - acoustic or auditory H93.3 ☑
  - cranial G52.9
    - eighth (auditory) H93.3 ☑
    - eleventh (accessory) G52.8
    - fifth (trigeminal) G50.8
    - first (olfactory) G52.0
    - fourth (trochlear) — *see* Strabismus, paralytic, fourth nerve
    - second (optic) H47.20
    - sixth (abducens) — *see* Strabismus, paralytic, sixth nerve
    - tenth (pneumogastric) (vagus) G52.2
    - third (oculomotor) — *see* Strabismus, paralytic, third nerve
    - twelfth (hypoglossal) G52.3
  - hypoglossal G52.3
  - oculomotor — *see* Strabismus, paralytic, third nerve
  - olfactory G52.0
  - optic (papillomacular bundle)
    - syphilitic (late) A52.15
      - congenital A50.44
  - pneumogastric G52.2
  - trigeminal G50.8
  - trochlear — *see* Strabismus, paralytic, fourth nerve
  - vagus (pneumogastric) G52.2
- neurogenic, bone, tabetic A52.11
- nutritional E43
  - with marasmus E41
- old age R54
- olivopontocerebellar G23.8
- optic (nerve) H47.20
  - glaucomatous H47.23- ☑
  - hereditary H47.22
  - primary H47.21- ☑
  - specified type NEC H47.29- ☑
  - syphilitic (late) A52.15
    - congenital A50.44
- orbit H05.31- ☑
- ovary (senile) N83.31- ☑
  - with fallopian tube N83.33- ☑
- oviduct (senile) — *see* Atrophy, fallopian tube
- palsy, diffuse (progressive) G12.22
- pancreas (duct) (senile) K86.89
- parotid gland K11.0
- pelvic muscle N81.84
- penis N48.89
- pharynx J39.2
- pluriglandular E31.8
  - autoimmune E31.0
- polyarthritis M15.9
- prostate N42.89
- pseudohypertrophic (muscle) G71.02
- renal — *see also* Sclerosis, renal N26.1
- retina, retinal (postinfectional) H35.89

Atrophy, atrophic — *continued*
- rhinitis J31.0
- salivary gland K11.0
- scar L90.5
- sclerosis, lobar (of brain) — *see also* Dementia, in, diseases specified elsewhere G31.09 *[F02.80]*
  - with behavioral disturbance — *see also* Dementia, in, diseases specified elsewhere G31.09 *[F02.81-]* ☑
- scrotum N50.89
- seminal vesicle N50.89
- senile R54
  - due to radiation (nonionizing) (solar) L57.8
- skin (patches) (spots) L90.9
  - degenerative (senile) L90.8
  - due to radiation (nonionizing) (solar) L57.8
  - senile L90.8
- spermatic cord N50.89
- spinal (acute) (cord) G95.89
  - muscular — *see* Atrophy, muscle, spinal
  - paralysis G12.20
    - acute — *see* Poliomyelitis, paralytic
    - meaning progressive muscular atrophy G12.25
- spine (column) — *see* Spondylopathy, specified NEC
- spleen (senile) D73.0
- stomach K29.40
  - with bleeding K29.41
- striate (skin) L90.6
  - syphilitic A52.79
- subcutaneous L90.9
- sublingual gland K11.0
- submandibular gland K11.0
- submaxillary gland K11.0
- Sudeck's — *see* Algoneurodystrophy
- suprarenal (capsule) (gland) E27.49
  - primary E27.1
- systemic affecting central nervous system in
    - myxedema E03.9 *[G13.2]*
    - neoplastic disease — *see also* Neoplasm D49.9 *[G13.1]*
    - specified disease NEC G13.8
- tarso-orbital fascia, congenital Q10.3
- testis N50.0
- thenar, partial — *see* Syndrome, carpal tunnel
- thymus (fatty) E32.8
- thyroid (gland) (acquired) E03.4
  - with cretinism E03.1
  - congenital (with myxedema) E03.1
- tongue (senile) K14.8
  - papillae K14.4
- trachea J39.8
- tunica vaginalis N50.89
- turbinate J34.89
- tympanic membrane (nonflaccid) H73.82- ☑
  - flaccid H73.81- ☑
- upper respiratory tract J39.8
- uterus, uterine (senile) N85.8
  - cervix N88.8
  - due to radiation (intended effect) N85.8
    - adverse effect or misadventure N99.89
- vagina (senile) N95.2
- vas deferens N50.89
- vascular I99.8
- vertebra (senile) — *see* Spondylopathy, specified NEC
- vulva (senile) N90.5
- Werdnig-Hoffmann G12.0
- yellow — *see* Failure, hepatic

Attack, attacks
- with alteration of consciousness (with automatisms) — *see* Epilepsy, localization-related, symptomatic, with complex partial seizures
- Adams-Stokes I45.9
- akinetic — *see* Epilepsy, generalized, specified NEC
- angina — *see* Angina
- atonic — *see* Epilepsy, generalized, specified NEC
- benign shuddering G25.83
- cataleptic — *see* Catalepsy
- coronary — *see* Infarct, myocardium
- cyanotic, newborn P28.2
- drop NEC R55
- epileptic — *see* Epilepsy
- heart — *see* infarct, myocardium
- hysterical F44.9
- jacksonian — *see* Epilepsy, localization-related, symptomatic, with simple partial seizures
- myocardium, myocardial — *see* Infarct, myocardium
- myoclonic — *see* Epilepsy, generalized, specified NEC

☑ **Additional Character Required** — **Refer to the Tabular List for Character Selection**

Attack, attacks — *continued*
  panic F41.0
  psychomotor — *see* Epilepsy, localization-related,
    symptomatic, with complex partial seizures
  salaam — *see* Epilepsy, spasms
  schizophreniform, brief F23
  shuddering, benign G25.83
  Stokes-Adams I45.9
  syncope R55
  transient ischemic (TIA) G45.9
    specified NEC G45.8
  unconsciousness R55
    hysterical F44.89
  vasomotor R55
  vasovagal (paroxysmal) (idiopathic) R55
  without alteration of consciousness — *see* Epilepsy,
    localization-related, symptomatic, with simple
    partial seizures
Attention (to)
  artificial
    opening (of) Z43.9
      digestive tract NEC Z43.4
        colon Z43.3
        ilium Z43.2
        stomach Z43.1
      specified NEC Z43.8
      trachea Z43.0
      urinary tract NEC Z43.6
        cystostomy Z43.5
        nephrostomy Z43.6
        ureterostomy Z43.6
        urethrostomy Z43.6
      vagina Z43.7
  colostomy Z43.3
  cystostomy Z43.5
  deficit disorder or syndrome F98.8
    with hyperactivity — *see* Disorder, attention-deficit
      hyperactivity
  gastrostomy Z43.1
  ileostomy Z43.2
  jejunostomy Z43.4
  nephrostomy Z43.6
  surgical dressings Z48.01
  sutures Z48.02
  tracheostomy Z43.0
  ureterostomy Z43.6
  urethrostomy Z43.6
Attrition
  gum — *see* Recession, gingival
  tooth, teeth (excessive) (hard tissues) K03.0
Atypical, atypism — *see also* condition
  cells (on cytolgocial smear) (endocervical) (endometrial)
    (glandular)
      cervix R87.619
      vagina R87.629
  cervical N87.9
  endometrium N85.9
    hyperplasia N85.00
  parenting situation Z62.9
Auditory — *see* condition
Aujeszky's disease B33.8
Aurantiasis, cutis E67.1
Auricle, auricular — *see also* condition
  cervical Q18.2
Auriculotemporal syndrome G50.8
Austin Flint murmur (aortic insufficiency) I35.1
Australian
  Q fever A78
  X disease A83.4
Autism, autistic (childhood) (infantile) F84.0
  atypical F84.9
  spectrum disorder F84.0
Autodigestion R68.89
Autoerythrocyte sensitization (syndrome) D69.2
Autographism L50.3
Autoimmune
  disease (systemic) M35.9
  inhibitors to clotting factors D68.311
  lymphoproliferative syndrome [ALPS] D89.82
  thyroiditis E06.3
Autointoxication R68.89
Automatism G93.89
  with temporal sclerosis G93.81
  epileptic — *see* Epilepsy, localization-related, symp-
    tomatic, with complex partial seizures
  paroxysmal, idiopathic — *see* Epilepsy, localization-
    related, symptomatic, with complex partial
    seizures

Autonomic, autonomous
  bladder (neurogenic) N31.2
  hysteria seizure F44.5
Autosensitivity, erythrocyte D69.2
Autosensitization, cutaneous L30.2
Autosome — *see* condition by chromosome involved
Autotopagnosia R48.1
Autotoxemia R68.89
Autumn — *see* condition
Avellis' syndrome G46.8
Aversion
  oral R63.39
    newborn P92.- ☑
    nonorganic origin F98.2 ☑
  sexual F52.1
Aviator's
  disease or sickness — *see* Effect, adverse, high altitude
  ear T70.0 ☑
Avitaminosis (multiple) — *see also* Deficiency, vitamin
  E56.9
  B E53.9
    with
      beriberi E51.11
      pellagra E52
  B2 E53.0
  B6 E53.1
  B12 E53.8
  D E55.9
    with rickets E55.0
  G E53.0
  K E56.1
  nicotinic acid E52
AVNRT (atrioventricular nodal re-entrant tachycardia)
  I47.1
AVRT (atrioventricular nodal re-entrant tachycardia) I47.1
Avulsion (traumatic)
  blood vessel — *see* Injury, blood vessel
  bone — *see* Fracture, by site
  cartilage — *see also* Dislocation, by site
    symphyseal (inner), complicating delivery O71.6
  external site other than limb — *see* Wound, open, by
    site
  eye S05.7- ☑
  head (intracranial)
    external site NEC S08.89 ☑
    scalp S08.0 ☑
  internal organ or site — *see* Injury, by site
  joint — *see also* Dislocation, by site
    capsule — *see* Sprain, by site
  kidney S37.06- ☑
  ligament — *see* Sprain, by site
  limb — *see also* Amputation, traumatic, by site
    skin and subcutaneous tissue — *see* Wound, open,
      by site
  muscle — *see* Injury, muscle
  nerve (root) — *see* Injury, nerve
  scalp S08.0 ☑
  skin and subcutaneous tissue — *see* Wound, open, by
    site
  spleen S36.032 ☑
  symphyseal cartilage (inner), complicating delivery
    O71.6
  tendon — *see* Injury, muscle
  tooth S03.2 ☑
Awareness of heart beat R00.2
Axenfeld's
  anomaly or syndrome Q15.0
  degeneration (calcareous) Q13.4
Axilla, axillary — *see also* condition
  breast Q83.1
Axonotmesis — *see* Injury, nerve
Ayerza's disease or syndrome (pulmonary artery sclerosis with pulmonary hypertension) I27.0
Azoospermia (organic) N46.01
  due to
    drug therapy N46.021
    efferent duct obstruction N46.023
    infection N46.022
    radiation N46.024
    specified cause NEC N46.029
    systemic disease N46.025
Azotemia R79.89
  meaning uremia N19
Aztec ear Q17.3
Azygos
  continuation inferior vena cava Q26.8
  lobe (lung) Q33.1

B

Baastrup's disease — *see* Kissing spine
Babesiosis B60.00
  due to
    Babesia
      divergens B60.03
      duncani B60.02
      KO-1 B60.09
      microti B60.01
      MO-1 B60.03
      species
        unspecified B60.00
      venatorum B60.09
    specified NEC B60.09
Babington's disease (familial hemorrhagic telangiecta-
  sia) I78.0
Babinski's syndrome A52.79
Baby
  crying constantly R68.11
  floppy (syndrome) P94.2
Bacillary — *see* condition
Bacilluria R82.71
Bacillus — *see also* Infection, bacillus
  abortus infection A23.1
  anthracis infection A22.9
  coli infection — *see also* Escherichia coli B96.20
  Flexner's A03.1
  mallei infection A24.0
  Shiga's A03.0
  suipestifer infection — *see* Infection, salmonella
Back — *see* condition
Backache (postural) M54.9
  sacroiliac M53.3
  specified NEC M54.89
Backflow — *see* Reflux
Backward reading (dyslexia) F81.0
Bacteremia R78.81
  with sepsis — *see* Sepsis
Bactericholia — *see* Cholecystitis, acute
Bacterid, bacteride (pustular) L40.3
Bacterium, bacteria, bacterial
  agent NEC, as cause of disease classified elsewhere
    B96.89
  in blood — *see* Bacteremia
  in urine — *see* Bacteriuria
Bacteriuria, bacteruria R82.71
  asymptomatic R82.71
Bacteroides
  fragilis, as cause of disease classified elsewhere B96.6
Bad
  heart — *see* Disease, heart
  trip
    due to drug abuse — *see* Abuse, drug, hallucinogen
    due to drug dependence — *see* Dependence, drug,
      hallucinogen
Baelz's disease (cheilitis glandularis apostematosa) K13.0
Baerensprung's disease (eczema marginatum) B35.6
Bagasse disease or pneumonitis J67.1
Bagassosis J67.1
Baker's cyst — *see* Cyst, Baker's
Bakwin-Krida syndrome (metaphyseal dysplasia) Q78.5
Balancing side interference M26.56
Balanitis (circinata) (erosiva) (gangrenosa) (phagedenic)
  (vulgaris) N48.1
  amebic A06.82
  candidal B37.42
  due to Haemophilus ducreyi A57
  gonococcal (acute) (chronic) A54.23
  xerotica obliterans N48.0
Balanoposthitis N47.6
  gonococcal (acute) (chronic) A54.23
  ulcerative (specific) A63.8
Balanorrhagia — *see* Balanitis
Balantidiasis, balantidiosis A07.0
Bald tongue K14.4
Baldness — *see also* Alopecia
  male-pattern — *see* Alopecia, androgenic
Balkan grippe A78
Balloon disease — *see* Effect, adverse, high altitude
Balo's disease (concentric sclerosis) G37.5
Bamberger-Marie disease — *see* Osteoarthropathy,
  hypertrophic, specified type NEC
Bancroft's filariasis B74.0
Band(s)
  adhesive — *see* Adhesions, peritoneum

Band(s) — *continued*
 anomalous or congenital — *see also* Anomaly, by site
  heart (atrial) (ventricular) Q24.8
   intestine Q43.3
   omentum Q43.3
  cervix N88.1
  constricting, congenital Q79.8
  gallbladder (congenital) Q44.1
  intestinal (adhesive) — *see* Adhesions, peritoneum
  obstructive
   intestine K56.50
    complete K56.52
    incomplete K56.51
    partial K56.51
   peritoneum K56.50
    complete K56.52
    incomplete K56.51
    partial K56.51
  periappendiceal, congenital Q43.3
  peritoneal (adhesive) — *see* Adhesions, peritoneum
  uterus N73.6
   internal N85.6
  vagina N89.5
Bandemia D72.825
Bandl's ring (contraction), complicating delivery O62.4
Bangkok hemorrhagic fever A91
Bang's disease (brucella abortus) A23.1
Bankruptcy (anxiety concerning) Z59.86
Bannister's disease T78.3 ☑
 hereditary D84.1
Banti's disease or syndrome (with cirrhosis) (with portal hypertension) K76.6
Bar, median, prostate — *see* Enlargement, enlarged, prostate
Barcoo disease or rot — *see* Ulcer, skin
Barlow's disease E54
Barodontalgia T70.29 ☑
Baron Münchausen syndrome — *see* Disorder, factitious
Barosinusitis T70.1 ☑
Barotitis T70.0 ☑
Barotrauma T70.29 ☑
 odontalgia T70.29 ☑
 otitic T70.0 ☑
 sinus T70.1 ☑
Barraquer (-Simons) **disease or syndrome** (progressive lipodystrophy) E88.1
Barré-Guillain disease or syndrome G61.0
Barrel chest M95.4
Barré-Liéou syndrome (posterior cervical sympathetic) M53.0
Barrett's
 disease — *see* Barrett's, esophagus
 esophagus K22.70
  with dysplasia K22.719
   high grade K22.711
   low grade K22.710
  without dysplasia K22.70
 syndrome — *see* Barrett's, esophagus
 ulcer K22.10
  with bleeding K22.11
  without bleeding K22.10
Bársony (-Polgár) (-Teschendorf) **syndrome** (corkscrew esophagus) K22.4
Barth syndrome E78.71
Bartholinitis (suppurating) N75.8
 gonococcal (acute) (chronic) (with abscess) A54.1
Bartonellosis A44.9
 cutaneous A44.1
 mucocutaneous A44.1
 specified NEC A44.8
 systemic A44.0
Barton's fracture S52.56- ☑
Bartter's syndrome E26.81
Basal — *see* condition
Basan's (hidrotic) ectodermal dysplasia Q82.4
Baseball finger — *see* Dislocation, finger
Basedow's disease (exophthalmic goiter) — *see* Hyperthyroidism, with, goiter
Basic — *see* condition
Basilar — *see* condition
Bason's (hidrotic) ectodermal dysplasia Q82.4
Basopenia — *see* Agranulocytosis
Basophilia D72.824
Basophilism (cortico-adrenal) (Cushing's) (pituitary) E24.0
Bassen-Kornzweig disease or syndrome E78.6
Bat ear Q17.5

Bateman's
 disease B08.1
 purpura (senile) D69.2
Bathing cramp T75.1 ☑
Bathophobia F40.248
Batten (-Mayou) **disease** E75.4
 retina E75.4 [*H36*]
Batten-Steinert syndrome G71.11
Battered — *see* Maltreatment
Battey Mycobacterium infection A31.0
Battle exhaustion F43.0
Battledore placenta O43.19- ☑
Baumgarten-Cruveilhier cirrhosis, disease or syndrome K74.69
Bauxite fibrosis (of lung) J63.1
Bayle's disease (general paresis) A52.17
Bazin's disease (primary) (tuberculous) A18.4
Beach ear — *see* Swimmer's, ear
Beaded hair (congenital) Q84.1
Béal conjunctivitis or syndrome B30.2
Beard's disease (neurasthenia) F48.8
Beat(s)
 atrial, premature I49.1
 ectopic I49.49
 elbow — *see* Bursitis, elbow
 escaped, heart I49.49
 hand — *see* Bursitis, hand
 knee — *see* Bursitis, knee
 premature I49.40
  atrial I49.1
  auricular I49.1
  supraventricular I49.1
Beau's
 disease or syndrome — *see* Degeneration, myocardial
 lines (transverse furrows on fingernails) L60.4
Bechterev's syndrome — *see* Spondylitis, ankylosing
Becker's
 cardiomyopathy I42.8
 disease
  idiopathic mural endomyocardial disease I42.3
  myotonia congenita, recessive form G71.12
 dystrophy G71.01
 pigmented hairy nevus D22.5
Beck's syndrome (anterior spinal artery occlusion) I65.8
Beckwith-Wiedemann syndrome Q87.3
Bed confinement status Z74.01
Bed sore — *see* Ulcer, pressure, by site
Bedbug bite(s) — *see* Bite(s), by site, superficial, insect
Bedclothes, asphyxiation or suffocation by — *see* Asphyxia, traumatic, due to, mechanical, trapped
Bednar's
 aphthae K12.0
 tumor — *see* Neoplasm, malignant, by site
Bedridden Z74.01
Bed-sharing, infant Z72.823
Bedsore — *see* Ulcer, pressure, by site
Bedwetting — *see* Enuresis
Bee sting (with allergic or anaphylactic shock) — *see* Toxicity, venom, arthropod, bee
Beer drinker's heart (disease) I42.6
Begbie's disease (exophthalmic goiter) — *see* Hyperthyroidism, with, goiter
Behavior
 antisocial
  adult Z72.811
  child or adolescent Z72.810
 disorder, disturbance — *see* Disorder, conduct
 disruptive — *see* Disorder, conduct
 drug seeking Z76.5
 inexplicable R46.2
 marked evasiveness R46.5
 obsessive-compulsive R46.81
 overactivity R46.3
 poor responsiveness R46.4
 self-damaging (life-style) Z72.89
 sleep-incompatible Z72.821
 slowness R46.4
 specified NEC R46.89
 strange (and inexplicable) R46.2
 suspiciousness R46.5
 type A pattern Z73.1
 undue concern or preoccupation with stressful events R46.6
 verbosity and circumstantial detail obscuring reason for contact R46.7
Behçet's disease or syndrome M35.2
Behr's disease — *see* Degeneration, macula

Beigel's disease or morbus (white piedra) B36.2
Bejel A65
Bekhterev's syndrome — *see* Spondylitis, ankylosing
Belching — *see* Eructation
Bell's
 mania F30.8
 palsy, paralysis G51.0
  infant or newborn P11.3
 spasm G51.3- ☑
Bence Jones albuminuria or proteinuria NEC R80.3
Bends T70.3 ☑
Benedikt's paralysis or syndrome G46.3
Benign — *see also* condition
 prostatic hyperplasia — *see* Hyperplasia, prostate
Bennett's fracture (displaced) S62.21- ☑
Benson's disease — *see* Deposit, crystalline
Bent
 back (hysterical) F44.4
 nose M95.0
  congenital Q67.4
Bereavement (uncomplicated) Z63.4
Bergeron's disease (hysterical chorea) F44.4
Berger's disease — *see* Nephropathy, IgA
Beriberi (dry) E51.11
 heart (disease) E51.12
 polyneuropathy E51.11
 wet E51.12
  involving circulatory system E51.11
Berlin's disease or edema (traumatic) S05.8X- ☑
Berlock (berloque) **dermatitis** L56.2
Bernard-Horner syndrome G90.2
Bernard-Soulier disease or thrombopathia D69.1
Bernhardt (-Roth) **disease** — *see* Mononeuropathy, lower limb, meralgia paresthetica
Bernheim's syndrome — *see* Failure, heart, right
Bertielliasis B71.8
Berylliosis (lung) J63.2
Besnier-Boeck (-Schaumann) **disease** — *see* Sarcoidosis
Besnier's
 lupus pernio D86.3
 prurigo L20.0
Bestiality F65.89
Best's disease H35.50
Betalipoproteinemia, broad or floating E78.2
Beta-mercaptolactate-cysteine disulfiduria E72.09
Betting and gambling Z72.6
 pathological (compulsive) F63.0
Bezoar T18.9 ☑
 intestine T18.3 ☑
 stomach T18.2 ☑
Bezold's abscess — *see* Mastoiditis, acute
Bianchi's syndrome R48.8
Bicornate or bicornis uterus Q51.3
 in pregnancy or childbirth O34.00
  causing obstructed labor O65.5
Bicuspid aortic valve Q23.1
Biedl-Bardet syndrome Q87.89
Bielschowsky (-Jansky) disease E75.4
Biermer's (pernicious) anemia or disease D51.0
Biett's disease L93.0
Bifid (congenital)
 apex, heart Q24.8
 clitoris Q52.6
 kidney Q63.8
 nose Q30.2
 patella Q74.1
 scrotum Q55.29
 toe NEC Q74.2
 tongue Q38.3
 ureter Q62.8
 uterus Q51.3
 uvula Q35.7
Biforis uterus (suprasimplex) Q51.3
Bifurcation (congenital)
 gallbladder Q44.1
 kidney pelvis Q63.8
 renal pelvis Q63.8
 rib Q76.6
 tongue, congenital Q38.3
 trachea Q32.1
 ureter Q62.8
 urethra Q64.74
 vertebra Q76.49
Big spleen syndrome D73.1
Bigeminal pulse R00.8
Bilateral — *see* condition

Bile
- duct — *see* condition
- pigments in urine R82.2

Bilharziasis — *see also* Schistosomiasis
- chyluria B65.0
- cutaneous B65.3
- galacturia B65.0
- hematochyluria B65.0
- intestinal B65.1
- lipemia B65.9
- lipuria B65.0
- oriental B65.2
- piarhemia B65.9
- pulmonary NOS B65.9 *[J99]*
  - pneumonia B65.9 *[J17]*
- tropical hematuria B65.0
- vesical B65.0

Biliary — *see* condition

Bilirubin metabolism disorder E80.7
- specified NEC E80.6

Bilirubinemia, familial nonhemolytic E80.4

Bilirubinuria R82.2

Biliuria R82.2

Bilocular stomach K31.2

Binswanger's disease I67.3

Biparta, bipartite
- carpal scaphoid Q74.0
- patella Q74.1
- vagina Q52.10

Bird
- face Q75.8
- fancier's disease or lung J67.2

Birth
- complications in mother — *see* Delivery, complicated
- compression during NOS P15.9
- defect — *see* Anomaly
- immature (less than 37 completed weeks) — *see* Preterm, newborn
  - extremely (less than 28 completed weeks) — *see* Immaturity, extreme
- inattention, at or after — *see* Maltreatment, child, neglect
- injury NOS P15.9
  - basal ganglia P11.1
  - brachial plexus NEC P14.3
  - brain (compression) (pressure) P11.2
  - central nervous system NOS P11.9
  - cerebellum P11.1
  - cerebral hemorrhage P10.1
  - external genitalia P15.5
  - eye P15.3
  - face P15.4
  - fracture
    - bone P13.9
      - specified NEC P13.8
    - clavicle P13.4
    - femur P13.2
    - humerus P13.3
    - long bone, except femur P13.3
    - radius and ulna P13.3
    - skull P13.0
    - spine P11.5
    - tibia and fibula P13.3
  - intracranial P11.2
    - laceration or hemorrhage P10.9
      - specified NEC P10.8
  - intraventricular hemorrhage P10.2
  - laceration
    - brain P10.1
    - by scalpel P15.8
    - peripheral nerve P14.9
  - liver P15.0
  - meninges
    - brain P11.1
    - spinal cord P11.5
  - nerve
    - brachial plexus P14.3
    - cranial NEC (except facial) P11.4
    - facial P11.3
    - peripheral P14.9
    - phrenic (paralysis) P14.2
  - paralysis
    - facial nerve P11.3
    - spinal P11.5
  - penis P15.5
  - rupture
    - spinal cord P11.5
  - scalp P12.9

Birth — *continued*
- injury — *continued*
  - scalpel wound P15.8
  - scrotum P15.5
  - skull NEC P13.1
    - fracture P13.0
  - specified type NEC P15.8
  - spinal cord P11.5
  - spine P11.5
  - spleen P15.1
  - sternomastoid (hematoma) P15.2
  - subarachnoid hemorrhage P10.3
  - subcutaneous fat necrosis P15.6
  - subdural hemorrhage P10.0
  - tentorial tear P10.4
  - testes P15.5
  - vulva P15.5
- lack of care, at or after — *see* Maltreatment, child, neglect
- neglect, at or after — *see* Maltreatment, child, neglect
- palsy or paralysis, newborn, NOS (birth injury) P14.9
- premature (infant) — *see* Preterm, newborn
- shock, newborn P96.89
- trauma — *see* Birth, injury
- weight
  - low (2499 grams or less) — *see* Low, birthweight
    - extremely (999 grams or less) — *see* Low, birthweight, extreme
  - 4000 grams to 4499 grams P08.1
  - 4500 grams or more P08.0

Birthmark Q82.5

Birt-Hogg-Dube syndrome Q87.89

Bisalbuminemia E88.09

Biskra's button B55.1

Bite(s) (animal) (human)
- abdomen, abdominal
  - wall S31.159 ☑
    - with penetration into peritoneal cavity S31.659 ☑
    - epigastric region S31.152 ☑
      - with penetration into peritoneal cavity S31.652 ☑
    - left
      - lower quadrant S31.154 ☑
        - with penetration into peritoneal cavity S31.654 ☑
      - upper quadrant S31.151 ☑
        - with penetration into peritoneal cavity S31.651 ☑
    - periumbilic region S31.155 ☑
      - with penetration into peritoneal cavity S31.655 ☑
    - right
      - lower quadrant S31.153 ☑
        - with penetration into peritoneal cavity S31.653 ☑
      - upper quadrant S31.150 ☑
        - with penetration into peritoneal cavity S31.650 ☑
    - superficial NEC S30.871 ☑
      - insect S30.861 ☑
  - alveolar (process) — *see* Bite, oral cavity
- amphibian (venomous) — *see* Venom, bite, amphibian
- animal — *see also* Bite, by site
  - venomous — *see* Venom
- ankle S91.05- ☑
  - superficial NEC S90.57- ☑
    - insect S90.56- ☑
- antecubital space — *see* Bite, elbow
- anus S31.835 ☑
  - superficial NEC S30.877 ☑
    - insect S30.867 ☑
- arm (upper) S41.15- ☑
  - lower — *see* Bite, forearm
  - superficial NEC S40.87- ☑
    - insect S40.86- ☑
- arthropod NEC — *see* Venom, bite, arthropod
- auditory canal (external) (meatus) — *see* Bite, ear
- auricle, ear — *see* Bite, ear
- axilla — *see* Bite, arm
- back — *see also* Bite, thorax, back
  - lower S31.050 ☑
    - with penetration into retroperitoneal space S31.051 ☑
  - superficial NEC S30.870 ☑
    - insect S30.860 ☑
- bedbug — *see* Bite(s), by site, superficial, insect

Bite(s) — *continued*
- breast S21.05- ☑
  - superficial NEC S20.17- ☑
    - insect S20.16- ☑
- brow — *see* Bite, head, specified site NEC
- buttock S31.805 ☑
  - left S31.825 ☑
  - right S31.815 ☑
  - superficial NEC S30.870 ☑
    - insect S30.860 ☑
- calf — *see* Bite, leg
- canaliculus lacrimalis — *see* Bite, eyelid
- canthus, eye — *see* Bite, eyelid
- centipede — *see* Toxicity, venom, arthropod, centipede
- cheek (external) S01.45- ☑
  - internal — *see* Bite, oral cavity
  - superficial NEC S00.87 ☑
    - insect S00.86 ☑
- chest wall — *see* Bite, thorax
- chigger B88.0
- chin — *see* Bite, head, specified site NEC
- clitoris — *see* Bite, vulva
- costal region — *see* Bite, thorax
- digit(s)
  - hand — *see* Bite, finger
  - toe — *see* Bite, toe
- ear (canal) (external) S01.35- ☑
  - superficial NEC S00.47- ☑
    - insect S00.46- ☑
- elbow S51.05- ☑
  - superficial NEC S50.37- ☑
    - insect S50.36- ☑
- epididymis — *see* Bite, testis
- epigastric region — *see* Bite, abdomen
- epiglottis — *see* Bite, neck, specified site NEC
- esophagus, cervical S11.25 ☑
  - superficial NEC S10.17 ☑
    - insect S10.16 ☑
- eyebrow — *see* Bite, eyelid
- eyelid S01.15- ☑
  - superficial NEC S00.27- ☑
    - insect S00.26- ☑
- face NEC — *see* Bite, head, specified site NEC
- finger(s) S61.259 ☑
  - with
    - damage to nail S61.359 ☑
  - index S61.258 ☑
    - with
      - damage to nail S61.358 ☑
    - left S61.251 ☑
      - with
        - damage to nail S61.351 ☑
    - right S61.250 ☑
      - with
        - damage to nail S61.350 ☑
    - superficial NEC S60.478 ☑
      - insect S60.46- ☑
  - little S61.25- ☑
    - with
      - damage to nail S61.35- ☑
    - superficial NEC S60.47- ☑
      - insect S60.46- ☑
  - middle S61.25- ☑
    - with
      - damage to nail S61.35- ☑
    - superficial NEC S60.47- ☑
      - insect S60.46- ☑
  - ring S61.25- ☑
    - with
      - damage to nail S61.35- ☑
    - superficial NEC S60.47- ☑
      - insect S60.46- ☑
  - superficial NEC S60.479 ☑
    - insect S60.469 ☑
  - thumb — *see* Bite, thumb
- flank — *see* Bite, abdomen, wall
- flea — *see* Bite, by site, superficial, insect
- foot (except toe(s) alone) S91.35- ☑
  - superficial NEC S90.87- ☑
    - insect S90.86- ☑
  - toe — *see* Bite, toe
- forearm S51.85- ☑
  - elbow only — *see* Bite, elbow
  - superficial NEC S50.87- ☑
    - insect S50.86- ☑
- forehead — *see* Bite, head, specified site NEC

Bite(s) — *continued*
genital organs, external
female S31.552 ☑
superficial NEC S30.876 ☑
insect S30.866 ☑
vagina and vulva — *see* Bite, vulva
male S31.551 ☑
penis — *see* Bite, penis
scrotum — *see* Bite, scrotum
superficial NEC S30.875 ☑
insect S30.865 ☑
testes — *see* Bite, testis
groin — *see* Bite, abdomen, wall
gum — *see* Bite, oral cavity
hand S61.45- ☑
finger — *see* Bite, finger
superficial NEC S60.57- ☑
insect S60.56- ☑
thumb — *see* Bite, thumb
head S01.95 ☑
cheek — *see* Bite, cheek
ear — *see* Bite, ear
eyelid — *see* Bite, eyelid
lip — *see* Bite, lip
nose — *see* Bite, nose
oral cavity — *see* Bite, oral cavity
scalp — *see* Bite, scalp
specified site NEC S01.85 ☑
superficial NEC S00.87 ☑
insect S00.86 ☑
superficial NEC S00.97 ☑
insect S00.96 ☑
temporomandibular area — *see* Bite, cheek
heel — *see* Bite, foot
hip S71.05- ☑
superficial NEC S70.27- ☑
insect S70.26- ☑
hymen S31.45 ☑
hypochondrium — *see* Bite, abdomen, wall
hypogastric region — *see* Bite, abdomen, wall
inguinal region — *see* Bite, abdomen, wall
insect — *see* Bite, by site, superficial, insect
instep — *see* Bite, foot
interscapular region — *see* Bite, thorax, back
jaw — *see* Bite, head, specified site NEC
knee S81.05- ☑
superficial NEC S80.27- ☑
insect S80.26- ☑
labium (majus) (minus) — *see* Bite, vulva
lacrimal duct — *see* Bite, eyelid
larynx S11.015 ☑
superficial NEC S10.17 ☑
insect S10.16 ☑
leg (lower) S81.85- ☑
ankle — *see* Bite, ankle
foot — *see* Bite, foot
knee — *see* Bite, knee
superficial NEC S80.87- ☑
insect S80.86- ☑
toe — *see* Bite, toe
upper — *see* Bite, thigh
lip S01.551 ☑
superficial NEC S00.571 ☑
insect S00.561 ☑
lizard (venomous) — *see* Venom, bite, reptile
loin — *see* Bite, abdomen, wall
lower back — *see* Bite, back, lower
lumbar region — *see* Bite, back, lower
malar region — *see* Bite, head, specified site NEC
mammary — *see* Bite, breast
marine animals (venomous) — *see* Toxicity, venom, marine animal
mastoid region — *see* Bite, head, specified site NEC
mouth — *see* Bite, oral cavity
nail
finger — *see* Bite, finger
toe — *see* Bite, toe
nape — *see* Bite, neck, specified site NEC
nasal (septum) (sinus) — *see* Bite, nose
nasopharynx — *see* Bite, head, specified site NEC
neck S11.95 ☑
involving
cervical esophagus — *see* Bite, esophagus, cervical
larynx — *see* Bite, larynx
pharynx — *see* Bite, pharynx

Bite(s) — *continued*
neck — *continued*
involving — *continued*
thyroid gland S11.15 ☑
trachea — *see* Bite, trachea
specified site NEC S11.85 ☑
superficial NEC S10.87 ☑
insect S10.86 ☑
superficial NEC S10.97 ☑
insect S10.96 ☑
throat S11.85 ☑
superficial NEC S10.17 ☑
insect S10.16 ☑
nose (septum) (sinus) S01.25 ☑
superficial NEC S00.37 ☑
insect S00.36 ☑
occipital region — *see* Bite, scalp
oral cavity S01.552 ☑
superficial NEC S00.572 ☑
insect S00.562 ☑
orbital region — *see* Bite, eyelid
palate — *see* Bite, oral cavity
palm — *see* Bite, hand
parietal region — *see* Bite, scalp
pelvis S31.050 ☑
with penetration into retroperitoneal space S31.051 ☑
superficial NEC S30.870 ☑
insect S30.860 ☑
penis S31.25 ☑
superficial NEC S30.872 ☑
insect S30.862 ☑
perineum
female — *see* Bite, vulva
male — *see* Bite, pelvis
periocular area (with or without lacrimal passages) — *see* Bite, eyelid
phalanges
finger — *see* Bite, finger
toe — *see* Bite, toe
pharynx S11.25 ☑
superficial NEC S10.17 ☑
insect S10.16 ☑
pinna — *see* Bite, ear
poisonous — *see* Venom
popliteal space — *see* Bite, knee
prepuce — *see* Bite, penis
pubic region — *see* Bite, abdomen, wall
rectovaginal septum — *see* Bite, vulva
red bug B88.0
reptile NEC — *see also* Venom, bite, reptile
nonvenomous — *see* Bite, by site
snake — *see* Venom, bite, snake
sacral region — *see* Bite, back, lower
sacroiliac region — *see* Bite, back, lower
salivary gland — *see* Bite, oral cavity
scalp S01.05 ☑
superficial NEC S00.07 ☑
insect S00.06 ☑
scapular region — *see* Bite, shoulder
scrotum S31.35 ☑
superficial NEC S30.873 ☑
insect S30.863 ☑
sea-snake (venomous) — *see* Toxicity, venom, snake, sea snake
shin — *see* Bite, leg
shoulder S41.05- ☑
superficial NEC S40.27- ☑
insect S40.26- ☑
snake — *see also* Venom, bite, snake
nonvenomous — *see* Bite, by site
spermatic cord — *see* Bite, testis
spider (venomous) — *see* Toxicity, venom, spider
nonvenomous — *see* Bite, by site, superficial, insect
sternal region — *see* Bite, thorax, front
submaxillary region — *see* Bite, head, specified site NEC
submental region — *see* Bite, head, specified site NEC
subungual
finger(s) — *see* Bite, finger
toe — *see* Bite, toe
superficial — *see* Bite, by site, superficial
supraclavicular fossa S11.85 ☑
supraorbital — *see* Bite, head, specified site NEC
temple, temporal region — *see* Bite, head, specified site NEC

Bite(s) — *continued*
temporomandibular area — *see* Bite, cheek
testis S31.35 ☑
superficial NEC S30.873 ☑
insect S30.863 ☑
thigh S71.15- ☑
superficial NEC S70.37- ☑
insect S70.36- ☑
thorax, thoracic (wall) S21.95 ☑
back S21.25- ☑
with penetration into thoracic cavity S21.45- ☑
breast — *see* Bite, breast
front S21.15- ☑
with penetration into thoracic cavity S21.35- ☑
superficial NEC S20.97 ☑
back S20.47- ☑
front S20.37- ☑
insect S20.96 ☑
back S20.46- ☑
front S20.36- ☑
throat — *see* Bite, neck, throat
thumb S61.05- ☑
with
damage to nail S61.15- ☑
superficial NEC S60.37- ☑
insect S60.36- ☑
thyroid S11.15 ☑
superficial NEC S10.87 ☑
insect S10.86 ☑
toe(s) S91.15- ☑
with
damage to nail S91.25- ☑
great S91.15- ☑
with
damage to nail S91.25- ☑
lesser S91.15- ☑
with
damage to nail S91.25- ☑
superficial NEC S90.47- ☑
great S90.47-
insect S90.46- ☑
great S90.46- ☑
tongue S01.552 ☑
trachea S11.025 ☑
superficial NEC S10.17 ☑
insect S10.16 ☑
tunica vaginalis — *see* Bite, testis
tympanum, tympanic membrane — *see* Bite, ear
umbilical region S31.155 ☑
uvula — *see* Bite, oral cavity
vagina — *see* Bite, vulva
venomous — *see* Venom
vocal cords S11.035 ☑
superficial NEC S10.17 ☑
insect S10.16 ☑
vulva S31.45 ☑
superficial NEC S30.874 ☑
insect S30.864 ☑
wrist S61.55- ☑
superficial NEC S60.87- ☑
insect S60.86- ☑
Biting, cheek or lip K13.1
Biventricular failure (heart) I50.82
Björck (-Thorson) **syndrome** (malignant carcinoid) E34.0
Black
death A20.9
eye S00.1- ☑
hairy tongue K14.3
heel (foot) S90.3- ☑
lung (disease) J60
palm (hand) S60.22- ☑
Blackfan-Diamond anemia or syndrome (congenital hypoplastic anemia) D61.01
Blackhead L70.0
Blackout R55
Bladder — *see* condition
Blast (air) (hydraulic) (immersion) (underwater)
blindness S05.8X- ☑
injury
abdomen or thorax — *see* Injury, by site
ear (acoustic nerve trauma) — *see* Injury, nerve, acoustic, specified type NEC
syndrome NEC T70.8 ☑
Blastoma — *see* Neoplasm, malignant, by site
pulmonary — *see* Neoplasm, lung, malignant
Blastomycosis, blastomycotic B40.9

Blastomycosis, blastomycotic — *continued*
　Brazilian — *see* Paracoccidioidomycosis
　cutaneous B40.3
　disseminated B40.7
　European — *see* Cryptococcosis
　generalized B40.7
　keloidal B48.0
　North American B40.9
　primary pulmonary B40.0
　pulmonary B40.2
　　acute B40.0
　　chronic B40.1
　skin B40.3
　South American — *see* Paracoccidioidomycosis
　specified NEC B40.89
Bleb(s) R23.8
　emphysematous (lung) (solitary) J43.9
　endophthalmitis H59.43
　filtering (vitreous), after glaucoma surgery Z98.83
　inflamed (infected), postprocedural H59.40
　　stage 1 H59.41
　　stage 2 H59.42
　　stage 3 H59.43
　lung (ruptured) J43.9
　　congenital — *see* Atelectasis
　　newborn P25.8
　subpleural (emphysematous) J43.9
Blebitis, postprocedural H59.40
　stage 1 H59.41
　stage 2 H59.42
　stage 3 H59.43
Bleeder (familial) (hereditary) — *see* Hemophilia
Bleeding — *see also* Hemorrhage
　anal K62.5
　anovulatory N97.0
　atonic, following delivery O72.1
　capillary I78.8
　　puerperal O72.2
　contact (postcoital) N93.0
　due to uterine subinvolution N85.3
　ear — *see* Otorrhagia
　excessive, associated with menopausal onset N92.4
　familial — *see* Defect, coagulation
　following intercourse N93.0
　gastrointestinal K92.2
　hemorrhoids — *see* Hemorrhoids
　intermenstrual (regular) N92.3
　　irregular N92.1
　intraoperative — *see* Complication, intraoperative, hemorrhage
　irregular N92.6
　menopausal N92.4
　newborn, intraventricular — *see* Newborn, affected by, hemorrhage, intraventricular
　nipple N64.59
　nose R04.0
　ovulation N92.3
　perimenopausal N92.4
　postclimacteric N95.0
　postcoital N93.0
　postmenopausal N95.0
　postoperative — *see* Complication, postprocedural, hemorrhage
　preclimacteric N92.4
　pre-pubertal vaginal N93.1
　puberty (excessive, with onset of menstrual periods) N92.2
　rectum, rectal K62.5
　　newborn P54.2
　tendencies — *see* Defect, coagulation
　throat R04.1
　tooth socket (post-extraction) K91.840
　umbilical stump P51.9
　uterus, uterine NEC N93.9
　　climacteric N92.4
　　dysfunctional or functional N93.8
　　menopausal N92.4
　　preclimacteric or premenopausal N92.4
　　unrelated to menstrual cycle N93.9
　vagina, vaginal (abnormal) N93.9
　　dysfunctional or functional N93.8
　　newborn P54.6
　　pre-pubertal N93.1
　vicarious N94.89
Blennorrhagia, blennorrhagic — *see* Gonorrhea
Blennorrhea (acute) (chronic) — *see also* Gonorrhea
　inclusion (neonatal) (newborn) P39.1
　lower genitourinary tract (gonococcal) A54.00

Blennorrhea — *continued*
　neonatorum (gonococcal ophthalmia) A54.31
Blepharelosis — *see* Entropion
Blepharitis (angularis) (ciliaris) (eyelid) (marginal) (nonulcerative) H01.009
　herpes zoster B02.39
　left H01.006
　　lower H01.005
　　upper H01.004
　　upper and lower H01.00B
　right H01.003
　　lower H01.002
　　upper H01.001
　　upper and lower H01.00A
　squamous H01.029
　　left H01.026
　　　lower H01.025
　　　upper H01.024
　　　upper and lower H01.02B
　　right H01.023
　　　lower H01.022
　　　upper H01.021
　　　upper and lower H01.02A
　ulcerative H01.019
　　left H01.016
　　　lower H01.015
　　　upper H01.014
　　　upper and lower H01.01B
　　right H01.013
　　　lower H01.012
　　　upper H01.011
　　　upper and lower H01.01A
Blepharochalasis H02.30
　congenital Q10.0
　left H02.36
　　lower H02.35
　　upper H02.34
　right H02.33
　　lower H02.32
　　upper H02.31
Blepharoclonus H02.59
Blepharoconjunctivitis H10.50- ☑
　angular H10.52- ☑
　contact H10.53- ☑
　ligneous H10.51- ☑
Blepharophimosis (eyelid) H02.529
　congenital Q10.3
　left H02.526
　　lower H02.525
　　upper H02.524
　right H02.523
　　lower H02.522
　　upper H02.521
Blepharoptosis H02.40- ☑
　congenital Q10.0
　mechanical H02.41- ☑
　myogenic H02.42- ☑
　neurogenic H02.43- ☑
　paralytic H02.43- ☑
Blepharopyorrhea, gonococcal A54.39
Blepharospasm G24.5
　drug induced G24.01
Blighted ovum O02.0
Blind — *see also* Blindness
　bronchus (congenital) Q32.4
　loop syndrome K90.2
　　congenital Q43.8
　sac, fallopian tube (congenital) Q50.6
　spot, enlarged — *see* Defect, visual field, localized, scotoma, blind spot area
　tract or tube, congenital NEC — *see* Atresia, by site
Blindness (acquired) (congenital) (both eyes) H54.0X- ☑
　blast S05.8X- ☑
　color — *see* Deficiency, color vision
　concussion S05.8X- ☑
　cortical H47.619
　　left brain H47.612
　　right brain H47.611
　day H53.11
　due to injury (current episode) S05.9- ☑
　　sequelae — *code to* injury with seventh character S
　eclipse (total) — *see* Retinopathy, solar
　emotional (hysterical) F44.6
　face H53.16
　hysterical F44.6
　legal (both eyes) (USA definition) H54.8
　mind R48.8

Blindness — *continued*
　night H53.60
　　abnormal dark adaptation curve H53.61
　　acquired H53.62
　　congenital H53.63
　　specified type NEC H53.69
　　vitamin A deficiency E50.5
　one eye (other eye normal) H54.40
　　left (normal vision on right) H54.42- ☑
　　　low vision on right H54.12- ☑
　　low vision, other eye H54.10
　　right (normal vision on left) H54.41- ☑
　　　low vision on left H54.11- ☑
　psychic R48.8
　river B73.01
　snow — *see* Photokeratitis
　sun, solar — *see* Retinopathy, solar
　transient — *see* Disturbance, vision, subjective, loss, transient
　traumatic (current episode) S05.9- ☑
　word (developmental) F81.0
　　acquired R48.0
　　secondary to organic lesion R48.0
Blister (nonthermal)
　abdominal wall S30.821 ☑
　alveolar process S00.522 ☑
　ankle S90.52- ☑
　antecubital space — *see* Blister, elbow
　anus S30.827 ☑
　arm (upper) S40.82- ☑
　auditory canal — *see* Blister, ear
　auricle — *see* Blister, ear
　axilla — *see* Blister, arm
　back, lower S30.820 ☑
　beetle dermatitis L24.89
　breast S20.12- ☑
　brow S00.82 ☑
　calf — *see* Blister, leg
　canthus — *see* Blister, eyelid
　cheek S00.82 ☑
　　internal S00.522 ☑
　chest wall — *see* Blister, thorax
　chin S00.82 ☑
　costal region — *see* Blister, thorax
　digit(s)
　　foot — *see* Blister, toe
　　hand — *see* Blister, finger
　due to burn — *see* Burn, by site, second degree
　ear S00.42- ☑
　elbow S50.32- ☑
　epiglottis S10.12 ☑
　esophagus, cervical S10.12 ☑
　eyebrow — *see* Blister, eyelid
　eyelid S00.22- ☑
　face S00.82 ☑
　fever B00.1
　finger(s) S60.429 ☑
　　index S60.42- ☑
　　little S60.42- ☑
　　middle S60.42- ☑
　　ring S60.42- ☑
　foot (except toe(s) alone) S90.82- ☑
　　toe — *see* Blister, toe
　forearm S50.82- ☑
　　elbow only — *see* Blister, elbow
　forehead S00.82 ☑
　fracture — *omit code*
　genital organ
　　female S30.826 ☑
　　male S30.825 ☑
　gum S00.522 ☑
　hand S60.52- ☑
　head S00.92 ☑
　　ear — *see* Blister, ear
　　eyelid — *see* Blister, eyelid
　　lip S00.521 ☑
　　nose S00.32 ☑
　　oral cavity S00.522 ☑
　　scalp S00.02 ☑
　　specified site NEC S00.82 ☑
　heel — *see* Blister, foot
　hip S70.22- ☑
　interscapular region S20.429 ☑
　jaw S00.82 ☑
　knee S80.22- ☑
　larynx S10.12 ☑

Blister — continued
- leg (lower) S80.82- ☑
  - knee — see Blister, knee
  - upper — see Blister, thigh
- lip S00.521 ☑
- malar region S00.82 ☑
- mammary — see Blister, breast
- mastoid region S00.82 ☑
- mouth S00.522 ☑
- multiple, skin, nontraumatic R23.8
- nail
  - finger — see Blister, finger
  - toe — see Blister, toe
- nasal S00.32 ☑
- neck S10.92 ☑
  - specified site NEC S10.82 ☑
  - throat S10.12 ☑
- nose S00.32 ☑
- occipital region S00.02 ☑
- oral cavity S00.522 ☑
- orbital region — see Blister, eyelid
- palate S00.522 ☑
- palm — see Blister, hand
- parietal region S00.02 ☑
- pelvis S30.820 ☑
- penis S30.822 ☑
- periocular area — see Blister, eyelid
- phalanges
  - finger — see Blister, finger
  - toe — see Blister, toe
- pharynx S10.12 ☑
- pinna — see Blister, ear
- popliteal space — see Blister, knee
- scalp S00.02 ☑
- scapular region — see Blister, shoulder
- scrotum S30.823 ☑
- shin — see Blister, leg
- shoulder S40.22- ☑
- sternal region S20.329 ☑
- submaxillary region S00.82 ☑
- submental region S00.82 ☑
- subungual
  - finger(s) — see Blister, finger
  - toe(s) — see Blister, toe
- supraclavicular fossa S10.82 ☑
- supraorbital S00.82 ☑
- temple S00.82 ☑
- temporal region S00.82 ☑
- testis S30.823 ☑
- thermal — see Burn, second degree, by site
- thigh S70.32- ☑
- thorax, thoracic (wall) S20.92 ☑
  - back S20.42- ☑
  - front S20.32- ☑
- throat S10.12 ☑
- thumb S60.32- ☑
- toe(s) S90.42- ☑
  - great S90.42- ☑
- tongue S00.522 ☑
- trachea S10.12 ☑
- tympanum, tympanic membrane — see Blister, ear
- upper arm — see Blister, arm (upper)
- uvula S00.522 ☑
- vagina S30.824 ☑
- vocal cords S10.12 ☑
- vulva S30.824 ☑
- wrist S60.82- ☑

Bloating R14.0
Bloch-Sulzberger disease or syndrome Q82.3
Block, blocked
- alveolocapillary J84.10
- arborization (heart) I45.5
- arrhythmic I45.9
- atrioventricular (incomplete) (partial) I44.30
  - with atrioventricular dissociation I44.2
  - complete I44.2
    - congenital Q24.6
  - congenital Q24.6
  - first degree I44.0
  - second degree (types I and II) I44.1
  - specified NEC I44.39
  - third degree I44.2
  - types I and II I44.1
- auriculoventricular — see Block, atrioventricular
- bifascicular (cardiac) I45.2
- bundle-branch (complete) (false) (incomplete) I45.4

Block, blocked — continued
- bundle-branch — continued
  - bilateral I45.2
  - left I44.7
    - with right bundle branch block I45.2
    - hemiblock I44.60
      - anterior I44.4
      - posterior I44.5
    - incomplete I44.7
      - with right bundle branch block I45.2
  - right I45.10
    - with
      - left bundle branch block I45.2
      - left fascicular block I45.2
    - specified NEC I45.19
  - Wilson's type I45.19
- cardiac I45.9
- conduction I45.9
  - complete I44.2
- fascicular (left) I44.60
  - anterior I44.4
  - posterior I44.5
  - right I44.5
  - specified NEC I44.69
- foramen Magendie (acquired) G91.1
  - congenital Q03.1
    - with spina bifida — see Spina bifida, by site, with hydrocephalus
- heart I45.9
  - bundle branch I45.4
    - bilateral I45.2
  - complete (atrioventricular) I44.2
  - congenital Q24.6
  - first degree (atrioventricular) I44.0
  - second degree (atrioventricular) I44.1
  - specified type NEC I45.5
  - third degree (atrioventricular) I44.2
- hepatic vein I82.0
- intraventricular (nonspecific) I45.4
  - bundle branch
    - bilateral I45.2
- kidney N28.9
  - postcystoscopic or postprocedural N99.0
- Mobitz (types I and II) I44.1
- myocardial — see Block, heart
- nodal I45.5
- organ or site, congenital NEC — see Atresia, by site
- portal (vein) I81
- second degree (types I and II) I44.1
- sinoatrial I45.5
- sinoauricular I45.5
- third degree I44.2
- trifascicular I45.3
- tubal N97.1
- vein NOS I82.90
- Wenckebach (types I and II) I44.1

Blockage — see Obstruction
Blocq's disease F44.4
Blood
- constituents, abnormal R78.9
- disease D75.9
- donor — see Donor, blood
- dyscrasia D75.9
  - with
    - abortion — see Abortion, by type, complicated by, hemorrhage
    - ectopic pregnancy O08.1
    - molar pregnancy O08.1
  - following ectopic or molar pregnancy O08.1
  - newborn P61.9
  - puerperal, postpartum O72.3
- flukes NEC — see Schistosomiasis
- in
  - feces K92.1
    - occult R19.5
  - urine — see Hematuria
- mole O02.0
- occult in feces R19.5
- pressure
  - decreased, due to shock following injury T79.4 ☑
  - examination only Z01.30
  - fluctuating I99.8
  - high — see Hypertension
    - borderline R03.0
    - incidental reading, without diagnosis of hypertension R03.0
  - low — see also Hypotension

Blood — continued
- pressure — continued
  - low — see also Hypotension — continued
    - incidental reading, without diagnosis of hypotension R03.1
- spitting — see Hemoptysis
- staining cornea — see Pigmentation, cornea, stromal
- transfusion
  - reaction or complication — see Complications, transfusion
- type
  - A (Rh positive) Z67.10
    - Rh negative Z67.11
  - AB (Rh positive) Z67.30
    - Rh negative Z67.31
  - B (Rh positive) Z67.20
    - Rh negative Z67.21
  - O (Rh positive) Z67.40
    - Rh negative Z67.41
  - Rh (positive) Z67.90
    - negative Z67.91
- vessel rupture — see Hemorrhage
- vomiting — see Hematemesis

Blood-forming organs, disease D75.9
Bloodgood's disease — see Mastopathy, cystic
Bloom (-Machacek)(-Torre) **syndrome** Q82.8
Blount disease or osteochondrosis M92.51- ☑
Blue
- baby Q24.9
- diaper syndrome E72.09
- dome cyst (breast) — see Cyst, breast
- dot cataract Q12.0
- nevus D22.9
- sclera Q13.5
  - with fragility of bone and deafness Q78.0
- toe syndrome I75.02- ☑

Blueness — see Cyanosis
Blues, postpartal O90.6
- baby O90.6
Blurring, visual H53.8
Blushing (abnormal) (excessive) R23.2
BMI — see Body, mass index
Boarder, hospital NEC Z76.4
- accompanying sick person Z76.3
- healthy infant or child Z76.2
- foundling Z76.1
Bockhart's impetigo L01.02
Bodechtel-Guttman disease (subacute sclerosing panencephalitis) A81.1
Boder-Sedgwick syndrome (ataxia-telangiectasia) G11.3
Body, bodies
- Aschoff's — see Myocarditis, rheumatic
- asteroid, vitreous — see Deposit, crystalline
- cytoid (retina) — see Occlusion, artery, retina
- drusen (degenerative) (macula) (retinal) — see also Degeneration, macula, drusen
  - optic disc — see Drusen, optic disc
- foreign — see Foreign body
- loose
  - joint, except knee — see Loose, body, joint
    - knee M23.4- ☑
  - sheath, tendon — see Disorder, tendon, specified type NEC
- mass index (BMI)
  - adult
    - 19.9 or less Z68.1
    - 20.0-20.9 Z68.20
    - 21.0-21.9 Z68.21
    - 22.0-22.9 Z68.22
    - 23.0-23.9 Z68.23
    - 24.0-24.9 Z68.24
    - 25.0-25.9 Z68.25
    - 26.0-26.9 Z68.26
    - 27.0-27.9 Z68.27
    - 28.0-28.9 Z68.28
    - 29.0-29.9 Z68.29
    - 30.0-30.9 Z68.30
    - 31.0-31.9 Z68.31
    - 32.0-32.9 Z68.32
    - 33.0-33.9 Z68.33
    - 34.0-34.9 Z68.34
    - 35.0-35.9 Z68.35
    - 36.0-36.9 Z68.36
    - 37.0-37.9 Z68.37
    - 38.0-38.9 Z68.38
    - 39.0-39.9 Z68.39
    - 40.0-44.9 Z68.41
    - 45.0-49.9 Z68.42

Body, bodies — *continued*
   mass index — *continued*
      adult — *continued*
         50.0-59.9 Z68.43
         60.0-69.9 Z68.44
         70 and over Z68.45
      pediatric
         5th percentile to less than 85th percentile for age Z68.52
         85th percentile to less than 95th percentile for age Z68.53
         greater than or equal to ninety-fifth percentile for age Z68.54
         less than fifth percentile for age Z68.51
   Mooser's A75.2
   rice — *see also* Loose, body, joint
      knee M23.4- ☑
   rocking F98.4
Boeck's
   disease or sarcoid — *see* Sarcoidosis
   lupoid (miliary) D86.3
Boerhaave's syndrome (spontaneous esophageal rupture) K22.3
Boggy
   cervix N88.8
   uterus N85.8
Boil — *see also* Furuncle, by site
   Aleppo B55.1
   Baghdad B55.1
   Delhi B55.1
   lacrimal
      gland — *see* Dacryoadenitis
      passages (duct) (sac) — *see* Inflammation, lacrimal, passages, acute
   Natal B55.1
   orbit, orbital — *see* Abscess, orbit
   tropical B55.1
Bold hives — *see* Urticaria
Bombé, iris — *see* Membrane, pupillary
Bone — *see* condition
Bonnevie-Ullrich syndrome — *see also* Turner's syndrome Q87.19
Bonnier's syndrome H81.8 ☑
Bonvale dam fever T73.3 ☑
Bony block of joint — *see* Ankylosis
BOOP (bronchiolitis obliterans organized pneumonia) J84.89
Borderline
   diabetes mellitus R73.03
   hypertension R03.0
   osteopenia M85.8- ☑
   pelvis, with obstruction during labor O65.1
   personality F60.3
Borna disease A83.9
Bornholm disease B33.0
Boston exanthem A88.0
Botalli, ductus (patent) (persistent) Q25.0
Bothriocephalus latus infestation B70.0
Botulism (foodborne intoxication) A05.1
   infant A48.51
   non-foodborne A48.52
   wound A48.52
Bouba — *see* Yaws
Bouchard's nodes (with arthropathy) M15.2
Bouffée délirante F23
Bouillaud's disease or syndrome (rheumatic heart disease) I01.9
Bourneville's disease Q85.1
Boutonniere deformity (finger) — *see* Deformity, finger, boutonniere
Bouveret (-Hoffmann) **syndrome** (paroxysmal tachycardia) I47.9
Bovine heart — *see* Hypertrophy, cardiac
Bowel — *see* condition
Bowen's
   dermatosis (precancerous) — *see* Neoplasm, skin, in situ
   disease — *see* Neoplasm, skin, in situ
   epithelioma — *see* Neoplasm, skin, in situ
   type
      epidermoid carcinoma-in-situ — *see* Neoplasm, skin, in situ
      intraepidermal squamous cell carcinoma — *see* Neoplasm, skin, in situ
Bowing
   femur — *see also* Deformity, limb, specified type NEC, thigh

Bowing — *continued*
   femur — *see also* Deformity, limb, specified type, thigh — *continued*
      congenital Q68.3
   fibula — *see also* Deformity, limb, specified type NEC, lower leg
      congenital Q68.4
   forearm — *see* Deformity, limb, specified type NEC, forearm
   leg(s), long bones, congenital Q68.5
   radius — *see* Deformity, limb, specified type NEC, forearm
   tibia — *see also* Deformity, limb, specified type NEC, lower leg
      congenital Q68.4
Bowleg(s) (acquired) M21.16-
   congenital Q68.5
   rachitic E64.3
Boyd's dysentery A03.2
Brachial — *see* condition
Brachycardia R00.1
Brachycephaly Q75.0
Bradley's disease A08.19
Bradyarrhythmia, cardiac I49.8
Bradycardia (sinoatrial) (sinus) (vagal) R00.1
   neonatal P29.12
   reflex G90.09
   tachycardia syndrome I49.5
Bradykinesia R25.8
Bradypnea R06.89
Bradytachycardia I49.5
Brailsford's disease or osteochondrosis — *see* Osteochondrosis, juvenile, radius
Brain — *see also* condition
   death G93.82
   syndrome — *see* Syndrome, brain
Branched-chain amino-acid disorder E71.2
Branchial — *see* condition
   cartilage, congenital Q18.2
Branchiogenic remnant (in neck) Q18.0
Brandt's syndrome (acrodermatitis enteropathica) E83.2
Brash (water) R12
Bravais-jacksonian epilepsy — *see* Epilepsy, localization-related, symptomatic, with simple partial seizures
Braxton Hicks contractions — *see* False, labor
Brazilian leishmaniasis B55.2
BRBPR K62.5
Break, retina (without detachment) H33.30- ☑
   with retinal detachment — *see* Detachment, retina
   horseshoe tear H33.31- ☑
   multiple H33.33- ☑
   round hole H33.32- ☑
Breakdown
   device, graft or implant — *see also* Complications, by site and type, mechanical T85.618 ☑
      arterial graft NEC — *see* Complication, cardiovascular device, mechanical, vascular
      breast (implant) T85.41 ☑
      catheter NEC T85.618 ☑
         cystostomy T83.010 ☑
         dialysis (renal) T82.41 ☑
            intraperitoneal T85.611 ☑
         Hopkins T83.018 ☑
         ileostomy T83.018 ☑
         infusion NEC T82.514 ☑
            cranial T85.610- ☑
            epidural T85.610 ☑
            intrathecal T85.610 ☑
            spinal T85.610 ☑
            subarachnoid T85.610 ☑
            subdural T85.610 ☑
         nephrostomy T83.012 ☑
         urethral indwelling T83.011 ☑
         urinary NEC T83.018 ☑
         urostomy T83.018 ☑
      electronic (electrode) (pulse generator) (stimulator)
         bone T84.310 ☑
         cardiac T82.119 ☑
            electrode T82.110 ☑
            pulse generator T82.111 ☑
            specified type NEC T82.118 ☑
         nervous system — *see* Complication, prosthetic device, mechanical, electronic nervous system stimulator
         urinary — *see* Complication, genitourinary, device, urinary, mechanical

Breakdown — *continued*
   device, graft or implant — *see also* Complications, by site and type, mechanical — *continued*
      fixation, internal (orthopedic) NEC — *see* Complication, fixation device, mechanical
      gastrointestinal — *see* Complications, prosthetic device, mechanical, gastrointestinal device
      genital NEC T83.418 ☑
         intrauterine contraceptive device T83.31 ☑
         penile prosthesis (cylinder) (implanted) (pump) (resevoir) T83.410 ☑
         testicular prosthesis T83.411 ☑
      heart NEC — *see* Complication, cardiovascular device, mechanical
      intrathecal infusion pump T85.615 ☑
      joint prosthesis — *see* Complications, joint prosthesis, internal, mechanical, by site
      nervous system, specified device NEC T85.615 ☑
      ocular NEC — *see* Complications, prosthetic device, mechanical, ocular device
      orthopedic NEC — *see* Complication, orthopedic, device, mechanical
      specified NEC T85.618 ☑
      subcutaneous device pocket
         nervous system prosthetic device, implant, or graft T85.890 ☑
         other internal prosthetic device, implant, or graft T85.898 ☑
      sutures, permanent T85.612 ☑
         used in bone repair — *see* Complications, fixation device, internal (orthopedic), mechanical
      urinary NEC T83.118 ☑
         graft T83.21 ☑
         sphincter, implanted T83.111 ☑
         stent (ileal conduit) (nephroureteral) T83.113 ☑
            ureteral indwelling T83.112 ☑
      vascular NEC — *see* Complication, cardiovascular device, mechanical
      ventricular intracranial shunt T85.01 ☑
   nervous F48.8
   perineum O90.1
   respirator J95.850
      specified NEC J95.859
   ventilator J95.850
      specified NEC J95.859
Breast — *see also* condition
   buds E30.1
      in newborn P96.89
   dense R92.2
   nodule — *see also* Lump, breast N63.0
Breath
   foul R19.6
   holder, child R06.89
   holding spell R06.89
   shortness R06.02
Breathing
   labored — *see* Hyperventilation
   mouth R06.5
      causing malocclusion M26.5 ☑
   periodic R06.3
      high altitude G47.32
Breathlessness R06.81
Breda's disease — *see* Yaws
Breech presentation (mother) O32.1 ☑
   causing obstructed labor O64.1 ☑
   footling O32.8 ☑
      causing obstructed labor O64.8 ☑
   incomplete O32.8 ☑
      causing obstructed labor O64.8 ☑
Breisky's disease N90.4
Brennemann's syndrome I88.0
Brenner
   tumor (benign) D27.9
      borderline malignancy D39.1- ☑
      malignant C56 ☑
      proliferating D39.1- ☑
Bretonneau's disease or angina A36.0
Breus' mole O02.0
Brevicollis Q76.49
Brickmakers' anemia B76.9 *[D63.8]*
Bridge, myocardial Q24.5
Bright red blood per rectum (BRBPR) K62.5
Bright's disease — *see also* Nephritis
   arteriosclerotic — *see* Hypertension, kidney
Brill (-Zinsser) **disease** (recrudescent typhus) A75.1
Brill-Symmers' disease C82.90
Brion-Kayser disease — *see* Fever, parathyroid

Briquet's disorder or syndrome F45.0
Brissaud's
 infantilism or dwarfism E23.0
 motor-verbal tic F95.2
Brittle
 bones disease Q78.0
 nails L60.3
  congenital Q84.6
Broad — see also condition
 beta disease E78.2
 ligament laceration syndrome N83.8
Broad- or floating-betalipoproteinemia E78.2
Brock's syndrome (atelectasis due to enlarged lymph
  nodes) J98.19
Brocq-Duhring disease (dermatitis herpetiformis) L13.0
Brodie's abscess or disease M86.8X- ☑
Broken
 arches — see also Deformity, limb, flat foot
 arm (meaning upper limb) — see Fracture, arm
 back — see Fracture, vertebra
 bone — see Fracture
 implant or internal device — see Complications, by site
  and type, mechanical
 leg (meaning lower limb) — see Fracture, leg
 nose S02.2 ☑
 tooth, teeth — see Fracture, tooth
Bromhidrosis, bromidrosis L75.0
Bromidism, bromism G92.8
 due to
  correct substance properly administered — see Table of Drugs and Chemicals, by drug, adverse
   effect
  overdose or wrong substance given or taken — see
   Table of Drugs and Chemicals, by drug, poisoning
 chronic (dependence) F13.20
Bromidrosiphobia F40.298
Bronchi, bronchial — see condition
Bronchiectasis (cylindrical) (diffuse) (fusiform) (localized)
  (saccular) J47.9
 with
  acute
   bronchitis J47.0
   lower respiratory infection J47.0
  exacerbation (acute) J47.1
 congenital Q33.4
 tuberculous NEC — see Tuberculosis, pulmonary
Bronchiolectasis — see Bronchiectasis
Bronchiolitis (acute) (infective) (subacute) J21.9
 with
  bronchospasm or obstruction J21.9
  influenza, flu or grippe — see Influenza, with, respiratory manifestations NEC
 chemical (chronic) J68.4
  acute J68.0
 chronic (fibrosing) (obliterative) J44.9
 due to
  external agent — see Bronchitis, acute, due to
  human metapneumovirus J21.1
  respiratory syncytial virus (RSV) J21.0
  specified organism NEC J21.8
 fibrosa obliterans J44.9
 influenzal — see Influenza, with, respiratory manifestations NEC
 obliterans J42
  with organizing pneumonia (BOOP) J84.89
 obliterative (chronic) (subacute) J44.9
  due to fumes or vapors J68.4
  due to chemicals, gases, fumes or vapors (inhalation)
   J68.4
 respiratory, interstitial lung disease J84.115
Bronchitis (diffuse) (fibrinous) (hypostatic) (infective)
  (membranous) J40
 with
  influenza, flu or grippe — see Influenza, with, respiratory manifestations NEC
  obstruction (airway) (lung) J44.9
  tracheitis (15 years of age and above) J40
   acute or subacute J20.9
   chronic J42
   under 15 years of age J20.9
 acute or subacute (with bronchospasm or obstruction)
  J20.9
  with
   bronchiectasis J47.0
   chronic obstructive pulmonary disease J44.0
  chemical (due to gases, fumes or vapors) J68.0

Bronchitis — continued
 acute or subacute — continued
  due to
   fumes or vapors J68.0
   Haemophilus influenzae J20.1
   Mycoplasma pneumoniae J20.0
   radiation J70.0
   specified organism NEC J20.8
   Streptococcus J20.2
   virus
    coxsackie J20.3
    echovirus J20.7
    parainfluenzae J20.4
    respiratory syncytial (RSV) J20.5
    rhinovirus J20.6
  viral NEC J20.8
 allergic (acute) J45.909
  with
   exacerbation (acute) J45.901
   status asthmaticus J45.902
 arachidic T17.528 ☑
 aspiration (due to food and vomit) J69.0
 asthmatic J45.9 ☑
  chronic J44.9
   with
    acute lower respiratory infection J44.0
    exacerbation (acute) J44.1
 capillary — see Pneumonia, broncho
 caseous (tuberculous) A15.5
 Castellani's A69.8
 catarrhal (15 years of age and above) J40
  acute — see Bronchitis, acute
  chronic J41.0
  under 15 years of age J20.9
 chemical (acute) (subacute) J68.0
  chronic J68.4
  due to fumes or vapors J68.0
   chronic J68.4
 chronic J42
  with
   airways obstruction J44.9
   tracheitis (chronic) J42
  asthmatic (obstructive) J44.9
  catarrhal J41.0
  chemical (due to fumes or vapors) J68.4
  due to
   chemicals, gases, fumes or vapors (inhalation)
    J68.4
   radiation J70.1
   tobacco smoking J41.0
  emphysematous J44.9
  mucopurulent J41.1
  non-obstructive J41.0
  obliterans J44.9
  obstructive J44.9
  purulent J41.1
  simple J41.0
 croupous — see Bronchitis, acute
 due to gases, fumes or vapors (chemical) J68.0
 emphysematous (obstructive) J44.9
 exudative — see Bronchitis, acute
 fetid J41.1
 grippal — see Influenza, with, respiratory manifestations NEC
 in those under 15 years age — see Bronchitis, acute
  chronic — see Bronchitis, chronic
 influenzal — see Influenza, with, respiratory manifestations NEC
 mixed simple and mucopurulent J41.8
 moulder's J62.8
 mucopurulent (chronic) (recurrent) J41.1
  acute or subacute J20.9
  simple (mixed) J41.8
 obliterans (chronic) J44.9
 obstructive (chronic) (diffuse) J44.9
 pituitous J41.1
 pneumococcal, acute or subacute J20.2
 pseudomembranous, acute or subacute — see Bronchitis, acute
 purulent (chronic) (recurrent) J41.1
  acute or subacute — see Bronchitis, acute
 putrid J41.1
 senile (chronic) J42
 simple and mucopurulent (mixed) J41.8
 smokers' J41.0
 spirochetal NEC A69.8
 subacute — see Bronchitis, acute
 suppurative (chronic) J41.1

Bronchitis — continued
 suppurative — continued
  acute or subacute — see Bronchitis, acute
 tuberculous A15.5
 under 15 years of age — see Bronchitis, acute
  chronic — see Bronchitis, chronic
 viral NEC, acute or subacute — see also Bronchitis,
  acute J20.8
Bronchoalveolitis J18.0
Bronchoaspergillosis B44.1
Bronchocele meaning goiter E04.0
Broncholithiasis J98.09
 tuberculous NEC A15.5
Bronchomalacia J98.09
 congenital Q32.2
Bronchomycosis NOS B49 [J99]
 candidal B37.1
Bronchopleuropneumonia — see Pneumonia, broncho
Bronchopneumonia — see Pneumonia, broncho
Bronchopneumonitis — see Pneumonia, broncho
Bronchopulmonary — see condition
Bronchopulmonitis — see Pneumonia, broncho
Bronchorrhagia (see Hemoptysis)
Bronchorrhea J98.09
 acute J20.9
 chronic (infective) (purulent) J42
Bronchospasm (acute) J98.01
 with
  bronchiolitis, acute J21.9
  bronchitis, acute (conditions in J20) — see Bronchi-
   tis, acute
 due to external agent — see condition, respiratory,
  acute, due to
 exercise induced J45.990
Bronchospirochetosis A69.8
 Castellani A69.8
Bronchostenosis J98.09
Bronchus — see condition
Brontophobia F40.220
Bronze baby syndrome P83.88
Brooke's tumor — see Neoplasm, skin, benign
Brown enamel of teeth (hereditary) K00.5
Brown's sheath syndrome H50.61- ☑
Brown-Séquard disease, paralysis or syndrome
 G83.81
Bruce sepsis A23.0
Brucellosis (infection) A23.9
 abortus A23.1
 canis A23.3
 dermatitis A23.9
 melitensis A23.0
 mixed A23.8
 sepsis A23.9
  melitensis A23.0
  specified NEC A23.8
 suis A23.2
Bruck-de Lange disease Q87.19
Bruck's disease — see Deformity, limb
BRUE (brief resolved unexplained event) R68.13
Brugsch's syndrome Q82.8
Bruise (skin surface intact) — see also Contusion
 with
  open wound — see Wound, open
 internal organ — see Injury, by site
 newborn P54.5
 scalp, due to birth injury, newborn P12.3
 umbilical cord O69.5 ☑
Bruit (arterial) R09.89
 cardiac R01.1
Brush burn — see Abrasion, by site
Bruton's X-linked agammaglobulinemia D80.0
Bruxism
 psychogenic F45.8
 sleep related G47.63
Bubbly lung syndrome P27.0
Bubo I88.8
 blennorrhagic (gonococcal) A54.89
 chancroidal A57
 climatic A55
 due to Haemophilus ducreyi A57
 gonococcal A54.89
 indolent (nonspecific) I88.8
 inguinal (nonspecific) I88.8
  chancroidal A57
  climatic A55
  due to H. ducreyi A57
  infective I88.8

Bubo — *continued*
- scrofulous (tuberculous) A18.2
- soft chancre A57
- suppurating — *see* Lymphadenitis, acute
- syphilitic (primary) A51.0
  - congenital A50.07
- tropical A55
- virulent (chancroidal) A57

Bubonic plague A20.0
Bubonocele — *see* Hernia, inguinal
Buccal — *see* condition
Buchanan's disease or osteochondrosis M91.0
Buchem's syndrome (hyperostosis corticalis) M85.2
Bucket-handle fracture or tear (semilunar cartilage) — *see* Tear, meniscus
Budd-Chiari syndrome (hepatic vein thrombosis) I82.0
Budgerigar fancier's disease or lung J67.2
Buds
- breast E30.1
  - in newborn P96.89

Buerger's disease (thromboangiitis obliterans) I73.1
Bulbar — *see* condition
Bulbus cordis (left ventricle) (persistent) Q21.8
Bulimia (nervosa) F50.2
- atypical F50.9
- normal weight F50.9

Bulky
- stools R19.5
- uterus N85.2

Bulla (e) R23.8
- lung (emphysematous) (solitary) J43.9
  - newborn P25.8

Bullet wound — *see also* Puncture
- fracture — *code as* Fracture, by site
- internal organ — *see* Injury, by site

Bundle
- branch block (complete) (false) (incomplete) — *see* Block, bundle-branch
- of His — *see* condition

Bunion M21.61- ☑
- tailor's M21.62- ☑

Bunionette M21.62- ☑
Buphthalmia, buphthalmos (congenital) Q15.0
Burdwan fever B55.0
Bürger-Grütz disease or syndrome E78.3
Buried
- penis (congenital) Q55.64
  - acquired N48.83
- roots K08.3

Burke's syndrome K86.89
Burkitt
- cell leukemia C91.0- ☑
- lymphoma (malignant) C83.7- ☑
  - small noncleaved, diffuse C83.7- ☑
  - spleen C83.77
  - undifferentiated C83.7- ☑
- tumor C83.7- ☑
- type
  - acute lymphoblastic leukemia C91.0- ☑
  - undifferentiated C83.7- ☑

Burn (electricity) (flame) (hot gas, liquid or hot object) (radiation) (steam) (thermal) T30.0
- abdomen, abdominal (muscle) (wall) T21.02 ☑
  - first degree T21.12 ☑
  - second degree T21.22 ☑
  - third degree T21.32 ☑
- above elbow T22.039 ☑
  - first degree T22.139 ☑
  - left T22.032 ☑
    - first degree T22.132 ☑
    - second degree T22.232 ☑
    - third degree T22.332 ☑
  - right T22.031 ☑
    - first degree T22.131 ☑
    - second degree T22.231 ☑
    - third degree T22.331 ☑
  - second degree T22.239 ☑
  - third degree T22.339 ☑
- acid (caustic) (external) (internal) — *see* Corrosion, by site
- alimentary tract NEC T28.2 ☑
  - esophagus T28.1 ☑
  - mouth T28.0 ☑
  - pharynx T28.0 ☑
- alkaline (caustic) (external) (internal) — *see* Corrosion, by site

Burn — *continued*
- ankle T25.019 ☑
  - first degree T25.119 ☑
  - left T25.012 ☑
    - first degree T25.112 ☑
    - second degree T25.212 ☑
    - third degree T25.312 ☑
  - multiple with foot — *see* Burn, lower, limb, multiple, ankle and foot
  - right T25.011 ☑
    - first degree T25.111 ☑
    - second degree T25.211 ☑
    - third degree T25.311 ☑
  - second degree T25.219 ☑
  - third degree T25.319 ☑
- anus — *see* Burn, buttock
- arm (lower) (upper) — *see* Burn, upper, limb
- axilla T22.049 ☑
  - first degree T22.149 ☑
  - left T22.042 ☑
    - first degree T22.142 ☑
    - second degree T22.242 ☑
    - third degree T22.342 ☑
  - right T22.041 ☑
    - first degree T22.141 ☑
    - second degree T22.241 ☑
    - third degree T22.341 ☑
  - second degree T22.249 ☑
  - third degree T22.349 ☑
- back (lower) T21.04 ☑
  - first degree T21.14 ☑
  - second degree T21.24 ☑
  - third degree T21.34 ☑
  - upper T21.03 ☑
    - first degree T21.13 ☑
    - second degree T21.23 ☑
    - third degree T21.33 ☑
- blisters — *code as* Burn, second degree, by site
- breast(s) — *see* Burn, chest wall
- buttock(s) T21.05 ☑
  - first degree T21.15 ☑
  - second degree T21.25 ☑
  - third degree T21.35 ☑
- calf T24.039 ☑
  - first degree T24.139 ☑
  - left T24.032 ☑
    - first degree T24.132 ☑
    - second degree T24.232 ☑
    - third degree T24.332 ☑
  - right T24.031 ☑
    - first degree T24.131 ☑
    - second degree T24.231 ☑
    - third degree T24.331 ☑
  - second degree T24.239 ☑
  - third degree T24.339 ☑
- canthus (eye) — *see* Burn, eyelid
- caustic acid or alkaline — *see* Corrosion, by site
- cervix T28.3 ☑
- cheek T20.06 ☑
  - first degree T20.16 ☑
  - second degree T20.26 ☑
  - third degree T20.36 ☑
- chemical (acids) (alkalines) (caustics) (external) (internal) — *see* Corrosion, by site
- chest wall T21.01 ☑
  - first degree T21.11 ☑
  - second degree T21.21 ☑
  - third degree T21.31 ☑
- chin T20.03 ☑
  - first degree T20.13 ☑
  - second degree T20.23 ☑
  - third degree T20.33 ☑
- colon T28.2 ☑
- conjunctiva (and cornea) — *see* Burn, cornea
- cornea (and conjunctiva) T26.1- ☑
  - chemical — *see* Corrosion, cornea
- corrosion (external) (internal) — *see* Corrosion, by site
- deep necrosis of underlying tissue — *code as* Burn, third degree, by site
- dorsum of hand T23.069 ☑
  - first degree T23.169 ☑
  - left T23.062 ☑
    - first degree T23.162 ☑
    - second degree T23.262 ☑
    - third degree T23.362 ☑
  - right T23.061 ☑

Burn — *continued*
- dorsum of hand — *continued*
  - right — *continued*
    - first degree T23.161 ☑
    - second degree T23.261 ☑
    - third degree T23.361 ☑
  - second degree T23.269 ☑
  - third degree T23.369 ☑
- due to ingested chemical agent — *see* Corrosion, by site
- ear (auricle) (external) (canal) T20.01 ☑
  - first degree T20.11 ☑
  - second degree T20.21 ☑
  - third degree T20.31 ☑
- elbow T22.029 ☑
  - first degree T22.129 ☑
  - left T22.022 ☑
    - first degree T22.122 ☑
    - second degree T22.222 ☑
    - third degree T22.322 ☑
  - right T22.021 ☑
    - first degree T22.121 ☑
    - second degree T22.221 ☑
    - third degree T22.321 ☑
  - second degree T22.229 ☑
  - third degree T22.329 ☑
- epidermal loss — *code as* Burn, second degree, by site
- erythema, erythematous — *code as* Burn, first degree, by site
- esophagus T28.1 ☑
- extent (percentage of body surface)
  - less than 10 percent T31.0
  - 10-19 percent T31.10
    - with 0-9 percent third degree burns T31.10
    - with 10-19 percent third degree burns T31.11
  - 20-29 percent T31.20
    - with 0-9 percent third degree burns T31.20
    - with 10-19 percent third degree burns T31.21
    - with 20-29 percent third degree burns T31.22
  - 30-39 percent T31.30
    - with 0-9 percent third degree burns T31.30
    - with 10-19 percent third degree burns T31.31
    - with 20-29 percent third degree burns T31.32
    - with 30-39 percent third degree burns T31.33
  - 40-49 percent T31.40
    - with 0-9 percent third degree burns T31.40
    - with 10-19 percent third degree burns T31.41
    - with 20-29 percent third degree burns T31.42
    - with 30-39 percent third degree burns T31.43
    - with 40-49 percent third degree burns T31.44
  - 50-59 percent T31.50
    - with 0-9 percent third degree burns T31.50
    - with 10-19 percent third degree burns T31.51
    - with 20-29 percent third degree burns T31.52
    - with 30-39 percent third degree burns T31.53
    - with 40-49 percent third degree burns T31.54
    - with 50-59 percent third degree burns T31.55
  - 60-69 percent T31.60
    - with 0-9 percent third degree burns T31.60
    - with 10-19 percent third degree burns T31.61
    - with 20-29 percent third degree burns T31.62
    - with 30-39 percent third degree burns T31.63
    - with 40-49 percent third degree burns T31.64
    - with 50-59 percent third degree burns T31.65
    - with 60-69 percent third degree burns T31.66
  - 70-79 percent T31.70
    - with 0-9 percent third degree burns T31.70
    - with 10-19 percent third degree burns T31.71
    - with 20-29 percent third degree burns T31.72
    - with 30-39 percent third degree burns T31.73
    - with 40-49 percent third degree burns T31.74
    - with 50-59 percent third degree burns T31.75
    - with 60-69 percent third degree burns T31.76
    - with 70-79 percent third degree burns T31.77
  - 80-89 percent T31.80
    - with 0-9 percent third degree burns T31.80
    - with 10-19 percent third degree burns T31.81
    - with 20-29 percent third degree burns T31.82
    - with 30-39 percent third degree burns T31.83
    - with 40-49 percent third degree burns T31.84
    - with 50-59 percent third degree burns T31.85
    - with 60-69 percent third degree burns T31.86
    - with 70-79 percent third degree burns T31.87
    - with 80-89 percent third degree burns T31.88
  - 90 percent or more T31.90
    - with 0-9 percent third degree burns T31.90
    - with 10-19 percent third degree burns T31.91
    - with 20-29 percent third degree burns T31.92

Burn — continued
  extent — continued
    90 percent or more — continued
      with 30-39 percent third degree burns T31.93
      with 40-49 percent third degree burns T31.94
      with 50-59 percent third degree burns T31.95
      with 60-69 percent third degree burns T31.96
      with 70-79 percent third degree burns T31.97
      with 80-89 percent third degree burns T31.98
      with 90 percent or more third degree burns T31.99
  extremity — see Burn, limb
  eye(s) and adnexa T26.4- ☑
    with resulting rupture and destruction of eyeball T26.2- ☑
    conjunctival sac — see Burn, cornea
    cornea — see Burn, cornea
    lid — see Burn, eyelid
    periocular area — see Burn, eyelid
    specified site NEC T26.3- ☑
  eyeball — see Burn, eye
  eyelid(s) T26.0- ☑
    chemical — see Corrosion, eyelid
  face — see Burn, head
  finger T23.029 ☑
    first degree T23.129 ☑
    left T23.022 ☑
      first degree T23.122 ☑
      second degree T23.222 ☑
      third degree T23.322 ☑
      multiple sites (without thumb) T23.039 ☑
        with thumb T23.049 ☑
          first degree T23.149 ☑
          left T23.042 ☑
            first degree T23.142 ☑
            second degree T23.242 ☑
            third degree T23.342 ☑
          right T23.041 ☑
            first degree T23.141 ☑
            second degree T23.241 ☑
            third degree T23.341 ☑
          second degree T23.249 ☑
          third degree T23.349 ☑
      first degree T23.139 ☑
      left T23.032 ☑
        first degree T23.132 ☑
        second degree T23.232 ☑
        third degree T23.332 ☑
      right T23.031 ☑
        first degree T23.131 ☑
        second degree T23.231 ☑
        third degree T23.331 ☑
      second degree T23.239 ☑
      third degree T23.339 ☑
    right T23.021 ☑
      first degree T23.121 ☑
      second degree T23.221 ☑
      third degree T23.321 ☑
    second degree T23.229 ☑
    third degree T23.329 ☑
  flank — see Burn, abdominal wall
  foot T25.029 ☑
    first degree T25.129 ☑
    left T25.022 ☑
      first degree T25.122 ☑
      second degree T25.222 ☑
      third degree T25.322 ☑
    multiple with ankle — see Burn, lower, limb, multiple, ankle and foot
    right T25.021 ☑
      first degree T25.121 ☑
      second degree T25.221 ☑
      third degree T25.321 ☑
    second degree T25.229 ☑
    third degree T25.329 ☑
  forearm T22.019 ☑
    first degree T22.119 ☑
    left T22.012 ☑
      first degree T22.112 ☑
      second degree T22.212 ☑
      third degree T22.312 ☑
    right T22.011 ☑
      first degree T22.111 ☑
      second degree T22.211 ☑
      third degree T22.311 ☑
    second degree T22.219 ☑

Burn — continued
  forearm — continued
    third degree T22.319 ☑
  forehead T20.06 ☑
    first degree T20.16 ☑
    second degree T20.26 ☑
    third degree T20.36 ☑
  fourth degree — code as Burn, third degree, by site
  friction — see Burn, by site
  from swallowing caustic or corrosive substance NEC — see Corrosion, by site
  full thickness skin loss — code as Burn, third degree, by site
  gastrointestinal tract NEC T28.2 ☑
    from swallowing caustic or corrosive substance T28.7 ☑
  genital organs
    external
      female T21.07 ☑
        first degree T21.17 ☑
        second degree T21.27 ☑
        third degree T21.37 ☑
      male T21.06 ☑
        first degree T21.16 ☑
        second degree T21.26 ☑
        third degree T21.36 ☑
    internal T28.3 ☑
      from caustic or corrosive substance T28.8 ☑
  groin — see Burn, abdominal wall
  hand(s) T23.009 ☑
    back — see Burn, dorsum of hand
    finger — see Burn, finger
    first degree T23.109 ☑
    left T23.002 ☑
      first degree T23.102 ☑
      second degree T23.202 ☑
      third degree T23.302 ☑
    multiple sites with wrist T23.099 ☑
      first degree T23.199 ☑
      left T23.092 ☑
        first degree T23.192 ☑
        second degree T23.292 ☑
        third degree T23.392 ☑
      right T23.091 ☑
        first degree T23.191 ☑
        second degree T23.291 ☑
        third degree T23.391 ☑
      second degree T23.299 ☑
      third degree T23.399 ☑
    palm — see Burn, palm
    right T23.001 ☑
      first degree T23.101 ☑
      second degree T23.201 ☑
      third degree T23.301 ☑
    second degree T23.209 ☑
    third degree T23.309 ☑
    thumb — see Burn, thumb
  head (and face) (and neck) T20.00 ☑
    cheek — see Burn, cheek
    chin — see Burn, chin
    ear — see Burn, ear
    eye(s) only — see Burn, eye
    first degree T20.10 ☑
    forehead — see Burn, forehead
    lip — see Burn, lip
    multiple sites T20.09 ☑
      first degree T20.19 ☑
      second degree T20.29 ☑
      third degree T20.39 ☑
    neck — see Burn, neck
    nose — see Burn, nose
    scalp — see Burn, scalp
    second degree T20.20 ☑
    third degree T20.30 ☑
  hip(s) — see Burn, thigh
  inhalation — see Burn, respiratory tract
    caustic or corrosive substance (fumes) — see Corrosion, respiratory tract
  internal organ(s) T28.40 ☑
    alimentary tract T28.2 ☑
      esophagus T28.1 ☑
    eardrum T28.41 ☑
    esophagus T28.1 ☑
      from caustic or corrosive substance (swallowing) NEC — see Corrosion, by site
    genitourinary T28.3 ☑

Burn — continued
  internal organ(s) — continued
    mouth T28.0 ☑
    pharynx T28.0 ☑
    respiratory tract — see Burn, respiratory tract
    specified organ NEC T28.49 ☑
  interscapular region — see Burn, back, upper
  intestine (large) (small) T28.2 ☑
  knee T24.029 ☑
    first degree T24.129 ☑
    left T24.022 ☑
      first degree T24.122 ☑
      second degree T24.222 ☑
      third degree T24.322 ☑
    right T24.021 ☑
      first degree T24.121 ☑
      second degree T24.221 ☑
      third degree T24.321 ☑
    second degree T24.229 ☑
    third degree T24.329 ☑
  labium (majus) (minus) — see Burn, genital organs, external, female
  lacrimal apparatus, duct, gland or sac — see Burn, eye, specified site NEC
  larynx T27.0 ☑
    with lung T27.1 ☑
  leg(s) (lower) (upper) — see Burn, lower, limb
  lightning — see Burn, by site
  limb(s)
    lower (except ankle or foot alone) — see Burn, lower, limb
    upper — see Burn, upper limb
  lip(s) T20.02 ☑
    first degree T20.12 ☑
    second degree T20.22 ☑
    third degree T20.32 ☑
  lower
    back — see Burn, back
    limb T24.009 ☑
      ankle — see Burn, ankle
      calf — see Burn, calf
      first degree T24.109 ☑
      foot — see Burn, foot
      hip — see Burn, thigh
      knee — see Burn, knee
      left T24.002 ☑
        first degree T24.102 ☑
        second degree T24.202 ☑
        third degree T24.302 ☑
      multiple sites, except ankle and foot T24.099 ☑
        ankle and foot T25.099 ☑
          first degree T25.199 ☑
          left T25.092 ☑
            first degree T25.192 ☑
            second degree T25.292 ☑
            third degree T25.392 ☑
          right T25.091 ☑
            first degree T25.191 ☑
            second degree T25.291 ☑
            third degree T25.391 ☑
          second degree T25.299 ☑
          third degree T25.399 ☑
        first degree T24.199 ☑
        left T24.092 ☑
          first degree T24.192 ☑
          second degree T24.292 ☑
          third degree T24.392 ☑
        right T24.091 ☑
          first degree T24.191 ☑
          second degree T24.291 ☑
          third degree T24.391 ☑
        second degree T24.299 ☑
        third degree T24.399 ☑
      right T24.001 ☑
        first degree T24.101 ☑
        second degree T24.201 ☑
        third degree T24.301 ☑
      second degree T24.209 ☑
      thigh — see Burn, thigh
      third degree T24.309 ☑
      toe — see Burn, toe
  lung (with larynx and trachea) T27.1 ☑
  mouth T28.0 ☑
  neck T20.07 ☑
    first degree T20.17 ☑
    second degree T20.27 ☑

Burn — *continued*
neck — *continued*
   third degree T20.37 ☑
nose (septum) T20.04 ☑
  first degree T20.14 ☑
  second degree T20.24 ☑
  third degree T20.34 ☑
ocular adnexa — *see* Burn, eye
orbit region — *see* Burn, eyelid
palm T23.059 ☑
  first degree T23.159 ☑
  left T23.052 ☑
   first degree T23.152 ☑
   second degree T23.252 ☑
   third degree T23.352 ☑
  right T23.051 ☑
   first degree T23.151 ☑
   second degree T23.251 ☑
   third degree T23.351 ☑
  second degree T23.259 ☑
  third degree T23.359 ☑
partial thickness — *code as* Burn, by site, second degree
pelvis — *see* Burn, trunk
penis — *see* Burn, genital organs, external, male
perineum
  female — *see* Burn, genital organs, external, female
  male — *see* Burn, genital organs, external, male
periocular area — *see* Burn, eyelid
pharynx T28.0 ☑
rectum T28.2 ☑
respiratory tract T27.3 ☑
  larynx — *see* Burn, larynx
  specified part NEC T27.2 ☑
  trachea — *see* Burn, trachea
sac, lacrimal — *see* Burn, eye, specified site NEC
scalp T20.05 ☑
  first degree T20.15 ☑
  second degree T20.25 ☑
  third degree T20.35 ☑
scapular region T22.069 ☑
  first degree T22.169 ☑
  left T22.062 ☑
   first degree T22.162 ☑
   second degree T22.262 ☑
   third degree T22.362 ☑
  right T22.061 ☑
   first degree T22.161 ☑
   second degree T22.261 ☑
   third degree T22.361 ☑
  second degree T22.269 ☑
  third degree T22.369 ☑
sclera — *see* Burn, eye, specified site NEC
scrotum — *see* Burn, genital organs, external, male
shoulder T22.059 ☑
  first degree T22.159 ☑
  left T22.052 ☑
   first degree T22.152 ☑
   second degree T22.252 ☑
   third degree T22.352 ☑
  right T22.051 ☑
   first degree T22.151 ☑
   second degree T22.251 ☑
   third degree T22.351 ☑
  second degree T22.259 ☑
  third degree T22.359 ☑
stomach T28.2 ☑
temple — *see* Burn, head
testis — *see* Burn, genital organs, external, male
thigh T24.019 ☑
  first degree T24.119 ☑
  left T24.012 ☑
   first degree T24.112 ☑
   second degree T24.212 ☑
   third degree T24.312 ☑
  right T24.011 ☑
   first degree T24.111 ☑
   second degree T24.211 ☑
   third degree T24.311 ☑
  second degree T24.219 ☑
  third degree T24.319 ☑
thorax (external) — *see* Burn, trunk
throat (meaning pharynx) T28.0 ☑
thumb(s) T23.019 ☑
  first degree T23.119 ☑
  left T23.012 ☑
   first degree T23.112 ☑

Burn — *continued*
thumb(s) — *continued*
  left — *continued*
   second degree T23.212 ☑
   third degree T23.312 ☑
  multiple sites with fingers T23.049 ☑
   first degree T23.149 ☑
   left T23.042 ☑
    first degree T23.142 ☑
    second degree T23.242 ☑
    third degree T23.342 ☑
   right T23.041 ☑
    first degree T23.141 ☑
    second degree T23.241 ☑
    third degree T23.341 ☑
   second degree T23.249 ☑
   third degree T23.349 ☑
  right T23.011 ☑
   first degree T23.111 ☑
   second degree T23.211 ☑
   third degree T23.311 ☑
  second degree T23.219 ☑
  third degree T23.319 ☑
toe T25.039 ☑
  first degree T25.139 ☑
  left T25.032 ☑
   first degree T25.132 ☑
   second degree T25.232 ☑
   third degree T25.332 ☑
  right T25.031 ☑
   first degree T25.131 ☑
   second degree T25.231 ☑
   third degree T25.331 ☑
  second degree T25.239 ☑
  third degree T25.339 ☑
tongue T28.0 ☑
tonsil(s) T28.0 ☑
trachea T27.0 ☑
  with lung T27.1 ☑
trunk T21.00 ☑
  abdominal wall — *see* Burn, abdominal wall
  anus — *see* Burn, buttock
  axilla — *see* Burn, upper limb
  back — *see* Burn, back
  breast — *see* Burn, chest wall
  buttock — *see* Burn, buttock
  chest wall — *see* Burn, chest wall
  first degree T21.10 ☑
  flank — *see* Burn, abdominal wall
  genital
   female — *see* Burn, genital organs, external, female
   male — *see* Burn, genital organs, external, male
  groin — *see* Burn, abdominal wall
  interscapular region — *see* Burn, back, upper
  labia — *see* Burn, genital organs, external, female
  lower back — *see* Burn, back
  penis — *see* Burn, genital organs, external, male
  perineum
   female — *see* Burn, genital organs, external, female
   male — *see* Burn, genital organs, external, male
  scapula region — *see* Burn, scapular region
  scrotum — *see* Burn, genital organs, external, male
  second degree T21.20 ☑
  specified site NEC T21.09 ☑
   first degree T21.19 ☑
   second degree T21.29 ☑
   third degree T21.39 ☑
  testes — *see* Burn, genital organs, external, male
  third degree T21.30 ☑
  upper back — *see* Burn, back, upper
  vulva — *see* Burn, genital organs, external, female
unspecified site with extent of body surface involved specified
  less than 10 percent T31.0
  10-19 percent (0-9 percent third degree) T31.10
   with 10-19 percent third degree T31.11
  20-29 percent (0-9 percent third degree) T31.20
   with
    10-19 percent third degree T31.21
    20-29 percent third degree T31.22
  30-39 percent (0-9 percent third degree) T31.30
   with
    10-19 percent third degree T31.31
    20-29 percent third degree T31.32

Burn — *continued*
unspecified site with extent of body surface involved specified — *continued*
  30-39 percent — *continued*
   with — *continued*
    30-39 percent third degree T31.33
  40-49 percent (0-9 percent third degree) T31.40
   with
    10-19 percent third degree T31.41
    20-29 percent third degree T31.42
    30-39 percent third degree T31.43
    40-49 percent third degree T31.44
  50-59 percent (0-9 percent third degree) T31.50
   with
    10-19 percent third degree T31.51
    20-29 percent third degree T31.52
    30-39 percent third degree T31.53
    40-49 percent third degree T31.54
    50-59 percent third degree T31.55
  60-69 percent (0-9 percent third degree) T31.60
   with
    10-19 percent third degree T31.61
    20-29 percent third degree T31.62
    30-39 percent third degree T31.63
    40-49 percent third degree T31.64
    50-59 percent third degree T31.65
    60-69 percent third degree T31.66
  70-79 percent (0-9 percent third degree) T31.70
   with
    10-19 percent third degree T31.71
    20-29 percent third degree T31.72
    30-39 percent third degree T31.73
    40-49 percent third degree T31.74
    50-59 percent third degree T31.75
    60-69 percent third degree T31.76
    70-79 percent third degree T31.77
  80-89 percent (0-9 percent third degree) T31.80
   with
    10-19 percent third degree T31.81
    20-29 percent third degree T31.82
    30-39 percent third degree T31.83
    40-49 percent third degree T31.84
    50-59 percent third degree T31.85
    60-69 percent third degree T31.86
    70-79 percent third degree T31.87
    80-89 percent third degree T31.88
  90 percent or more (0-9 percent third degree) T31.90
   with
    10-19 percent third degree T31.91
    20-29 percent third degree T31.92
    30-39 percent third degree T31.93
    40-49 percent third degree T31.94
    50-59 percent third degree T31.95
    60-69 percent third degree T31.96
    70-79 percent third degree T31.97
    80-89 percent third degree T31.98
    90-99 percent third degree T31.99
upper limb T22.00 ☑
  above elbow — *see* Burn, above elbow
  axilla — *see* Burn, axilla
  elbow — *see* Burn, elbow
  first degree T22.10 ☑
  forearm — *see* Burn, forearm
  hand — *see* Burn, hand
  interscapular region — *see* Burn, back, upper
  multiple sites T22.099 ☑
   first degree T22.199 ☑
   left T22.092 ☑
    first degree T22.192 ☑
    second degree T22.292 ☑
    third degree T22.392 ☑
   right T22.091 ☑
    first degree T22.191 ☑
    second degree T22.291 ☑
    third degree T22.391 ☑
   second degree T22.299 ☑
   third degree T22.399 ☑
  scapular region — *see* Burn, scapular region
  second degree T22.20 ☑
  shoulder — *see* Burn, shoulder
  third degree T22.30 ☑
  wrist — *see* Burn, wrist
uterus T28.3 ☑
vagina T28.3 ☑
vulva — *see* Burn, genital organs, external, female
wrist T23.079 ☑
  first degree T23.179 ☑
  left T23.072 ☑

Burn — *continued*
  wrist — *continued*
    left — *continued*
      first degree T23.172 ☑
      second degree T23.272 ☑
      third degree T23.372 ☑
      multiple sites with hand T23.099 ☑
        first degree T23.199 ☑
        left T23.092 ☑
          first degree T23.192 ☑
          second degree T23.292 ☑
          third degree T23.392 ☑
        right T23.091 ☑
          first degree T23.191 ☑
          second degree T23.291 ☑
          third degree T23.391 ☑
        second degree T23.299 ☑
        third degree T23.399 ☑
      right T23.071 ☑
        first degree T23.171 ☑
        second degree T23.271 ☑
        third degree T23.371 ☑
      second degree T23.279 ☑
      third degree T23.379 ☑
Burnett's syndrome E83.52
Burning
  feet syndrome E53.9
  sensation R20.8
  tongue K14.6
Burn-out (state) Z73.0
Burns' disease or osteochondrosis — *see* Osteochondrosis, juvenile, ulna
Bursa — *see* condition
Bursitis M71.9
  Achilles — *see* Tendinitis, Achilles
  adhesive — *see* Bursitis, specified NEC
  ankle — *see* Enthesopathy, lower limb, ankle, specified type NEC
  calcaneal — *see* Enthesopathy, foot, specified type NEC
  collateral ligament, tibial — *see* Bursitis, tibial collateral
  due to use, overuse, pressure — *see also* Disorder, soft tissue, due to use, specified type NEC
    specified NEC — *see* Disorder, soft tissue, due to use, specified NEC
  Duplay's M75.0 ☑
  elbow NEC M70.3- ☑
    olecranon M70.2- ☑
  finger — *see* Disorder, soft tissue, due to use, specified type NEC, hand
  foot — *see* Enthesopathy, foot, specified type NEC
  gonococcal A54.49
  gouty — *see* Gout
  hand M70.1- ☑
  hip NEC M70.7- ☑
    trochanteric M70.6- ☑
  infective NEC M71.10
    abscess — *see* Abscess, bursa
    ankle M71.17- ☑
    elbow M71.12- ☑
    foot M71.17- ☑
    hand M71.14- ☑
    hip M71.15- ☑
    knee M71.16- ☑
    multiple sites M71.19
    shoulder M71.11- ☑
    specified site NEC M71.18
    wrist M71.13- ☑
  ischial — *see* Bursitis, hip
  knee NEC M70.5- ☑
    prepatellar M70.4- ☑
  occupational NEC — *see also* Disorder, soft tissue, due to use
  olecranon — *see* Bursitis, elbow, olecranon
  pharyngeal J39.1
  popliteal — *see* Bursitis, knee
  prepatellar M70.4- ☑
  radiohumeral M70.3- ☑
  rheumatoid M06.20
    ankle M06.27- ☑
    elbow M06.22- ☑
    foot joint M06.27- ☑
    hand joint M06.24- ☑
    hip M06.25- ☑
    knee M06.26- ☑
    multiple site M06.29
    shoulder M06.21- ☑

Bursitis — *continued*
  rheumatoid — *continued*
    vertebra M06.28
    wrist M06.23- ☑
  scapulohumeral — *see* Bursitis, shoulder
  semimembranous muscle (knee) — *see* Bursitis, knee
  shoulder M75.5-
    adhesive — *see* Capsulitis, adhesive
  specified NEC M71.50
    ankle M71.57- ☑
    due to use, overuse or pressure — *see* Disorder, soft tissue, due to, use
    elbow M71.52- ☑
    foot M71.57- ☑
    hand M71.54- ☑
    hip M71.55- ☑
    knee M71.56- ☑
    shoulder — *see* Bursitis, shoulder
    specified site NEC M71.58
    tibial collateral M76.4- ☑
    wrist M71.53- ☑
  subacromial — *see* Bursitis, shoulder
  subcoracoid — *see* Bursitis, shoulder
  subdeltoid — *see* Bursitis, shoulder
  syphilitic A52.78
  Thornwaldt, Tornwaldt J39.2
  tibial collateral M76.4- ☑
  toe — *see* Enthesopathy, foot, specified type NEC
  trochanteric (area) — *see* Bursitis, hip, trochanteric
  wrist — *see* Bursitis, hand
Bursopathy M71.9
  specified type NEC M71.80
    ankle M71.87- ☑
    elbow M71.82- ☑
    foot M71.87- ☑
    hand M71.84- ☑
    hip M71.85- ☑
    knee M71.86- ☑
    multiple sites M71.89
    shoulder M71.81- ☑
    specified site NEC M71.88
    wrist M71.83- ☑
Burst stitches or sutures (complication of surgery) T81.31
  external operation wound T81.31 ☑
  internal operation wound T81.32 ☑
Buruli ulcer A31.1
Bury's disease L95.1
Buschke's
  disease — *see* Cryptococcosis by site
  scleredema — *see* Sclerosis, systemic
Busse-Buschke disease — *see* Cryptococcosis by site
Buttock — *see* condition
Button
  Biskra B55.1
  Delhi B55.1
  oriental B55.1
Buttonhole deformity (finger) — *see* Deformity, finger, boutonniere
Bwamba fever A92.8
Byssinosis J66.0
Bywaters' syndrome T79.5 ☑

C

Cachexia R64
  cancerous R64
  cardiac — *see* Disease, heart
  dehydration E86.0
  due to malnutrition R64
  exophthalmic — *see* Hyperthyroidism
  heart — *see* Disease, heart
  hypophyseal E23.0
  hypopituitary E23.0
  lead — *see* Poisoning, lead
  malignant R64
  marsh — *see* Malaria
  nervous F48.8
  old age R54
  paludal — *see* Malaria
  pituitary E23.0
  pulmonary R64
  renal N28.9
  saturnine — *see* Poisoning, lead
  senile R54
  Simmonds' E23.0
  splenica D73.0

Cachexia — *continued*
  strumipriva E03.4
  tuberculous NEC — *see* Tuberculosis
CADASIL (cerebral autosomal dominant arteriopathy with subcortical infarcts and leukoencephalopathy) I67.850
Café, au lait spots L81.3
Caffeine-induced
  anxiety disorder F15.980
  sleep disorder F15.982
Caffey's syndrome Q78.8
Caisson disease T70.3 ☑
Cake kidney Q63.1
Caked breast (puerperal, postpartum) O92.79
Calabar swelling B74.3
Calcaneal spur — *see* Spur, bone, calcaneal
Calcaneo-apophysitis M92.8
Calcareous — *see* condition
Calcicosis J62.8
Calciferol (vitamin D) deficiency E55.9
  with rickets E55.0
Calcification
  adrenal (capsule) (gland) E27.49
    tuberculous B90.8 *[E35]*
  aorta I70.0
  artery (annular) — *see* Arteriosclerosis
  auricle (ear) — *see* Disorder, pinna, specified type NEC
  basal ganglia G23.8
  bladder N32.89
    due to Schistosoma hematobium B65.0
  brain (cortex) — *see* Calcification, cerebral
  bronchus J98.09
  bursa M71.40
    ankle M71.47- ☑
    elbow M71.42- ☑
    foot M71.47- ☑
    hand M71.44- ☑
    hip M71.45- ☑
    knee M71.46- ☑
    multiple sites M71.49
    shoulder M75.3- ☑
    specified site NEC M71.48
    wrist M71.43- ☑
  cardiac — *see* Degeneration, myocardial
  cerebral (cortex) G93.89
    artery I67.2
  cervix (uteri) N88.8
  choroid plexus G93.89
  conjunctiva — *see* Concretion, conjunctiva
  corpora cavernosa (penis) N48.89
  cortex (brain) — *see* Calcification, cerebral
  dental pulp (nodular) K04.2
  dentinal papilla K00.4
  fallopian tube N83.8
  falx cerebri G96.198
  gallbladder K82.8
  general E83.59
  heart — *see also* Degeneration, myocardial
    valve — *see also* Endocarditis
      mitral — *see* Calcification, mitral
  idiopathic infantile arterial (IIAC) Q28.8
  intervertebral cartilage or disc (postinfective) — *see* Disorder, disc, specified NEC
  intracranial — *see* Calcification, cerebral
  joint — *see* Disorder, joint, specified type NEC
  kidney N28.89
    tuberculous N29 *[B90.1]*
  larynx (senile) J38.7
  lens — *see* Cataract, specified NEC
  lung (active) (postinfectional) J98.4
    tuberculous B90.9
  lymph gland or node (postinfectional) I89.8
    tuberculous — *see also* Tuberculosis, lymph gland B90.8
  mammographic R92.1
  massive (paraplegic) — *see* Myositis, ossificans, in, quadriplegia
  medial — *see* Arteriosclerosis, extremities
  meninges (cerebral) (spinal) G96.198
  metastatic E83.59
  mitral (valve) I34.81
    annular I34.81
      nonrheumatic I34.81
      rheumatic I05.8
    annulus I34.81
      nonrheumatic I34.81
      rheumatic I05.8

Calcification — *continued*
  Mönckeberg's — *see* Arteriosclerosis, extremities
  muscle M61.9
    due to burns — *see* Myositis, ossificans, in, burns
    paralytic — *see* Myositis, ossificans, in, quadriplegia
    specified type NEC M61.40
      ankle M61.47- ☑
      foot M61.47- ☑
      forearm M61.43- ☑
      hand M61.44- ☑
      lower leg M61.46- ☑
      multiple sites M61.49
      pelvic region M61.45- ☑
      shoulder region M61.41- ☑
      specified site NEC M61.48
      thigh M61.45- ☑
      upper arm M61.42- ☑
  myocardium, myocardial — *see* Degeneration, myocardial
  ovary N83.8
  pancreas K86.89
  penis N48.89
  periarticular — *see* Disorder, joint, specified type NEC
  pericardium — *see also* Pericarditis I31.1
  pineal gland E34.8
  pleura J94.8
    postinfectional J94.8
    tuberculous NEC B90.9
  pulpal (dental) (nodular) K04.2
  sclera H15.89
  spleen D73.89
  subcutaneous L94.2
  suprarenal (capsule) (gland) E27.49
  tendon (sheath) — *see also* Tenosynovitis, specified type NEC
    with bursitis, synovitis or tenosynovitis — *see* Tendinitis, calcific
  trachea J39.8
  ureter N28.89
  uterus N85.8
  vitreous — *see* Deposit, crystalline
Calcified — *see* Calcification
Calcinosis (interstitial) (tumoral) (universalis) E83.59
  with Raynaud's phenomenon, esophageal dysfunction, sclerodactyly, telangiectasia (CREST syndrome) M34.1
  circumscripta (skin) L94.2
  cutis L94.2
Calciphylaxis — *see also* Calcification, by site E83.59
Calcium
  deposits — *see* Calcification, by site
  metabolism disorder E83.50
  salts or soaps in vitreous — *see* Deposit, crystalline
Calciuria R82.994
Calculi — *see* Calculus
Calculosis, intrahepatic — *see* Calculus, bile duct
Calculus, calculi, calculous
  ampulla of Vater — *see* Calculus, bile duct
  anuria (impacted) (recurrent) — *see also* Calculus, urinary N20.9
  appendix K38.1
  bile duct (common) (hepatic) K80.50
    with
      calculus of gallbladder — *see* Calculus, gallbladder and bile duct
      cholangitis K80.30
        with
          cholecystitis — *see* Calculus, bile duct, with cholecystitis
          obstruction K80.31
        acute K80.32
          with
            chronic cholangitis K80.36
              with obstruction K80.37
            obstruction K80.33
        chronic K80.34
          with
            acute cholangitis K80.36
              with obstruction K80.37
            obstruction K80.35
      cholecystitis (with cholangitis) K80.40
        with obstruction K80.41
        acute K80.42
          with
            chronic cholecystitis K80.46
              with obstruction K80.47
            obstruction K80.43
        chronic K80.44

Calculus, calculi, calculous — *continued*
  bile duct — *continued*
    with — *continued*
      cholecystitis — *continued*
        chronic — *continued*
          with
            acute cholecystitis K80.46
              with obstruction K80.47
            obstruction K80.45
  biliary — *see also* Calculus, gallbladder
    specified NEC K80.80
      with obstruction K80.81
  bilirubin, multiple — *see* Calculus, gallbladder
  bladder (encysted) (impacted) (urinary) (diverticulum) N21.0
  bronchus J98.09
  calyx (kidney) (renal) — *see* Calculus, kidney
  cholesterol (pure) (solitary) — *see* Calculus, gallbladder
  common duct (bile) — *see* Calculus, bile duct
  conjunctiva — *see* Concretion, conjunctiva
  cystic N21.0
    duct — *see* Calculus, gallbladder
  dental (subgingival) (supragingival) K03.6
  diverticulum
    bladder N21.0
    kidney N20.0
  epididymis N50.89
  gallbladder K80.20
    with
      bile duct calculus — *see* Calculus, gallbladder and bile duct
      cholecystitis K80.10
        with obstruction K80.11
        acute K80.00
          with
            chronic cholecystitis K80.12
              with obstruction K80.13
            obstruction K80.01
        chronic K80.10
          with
            acute cholecystitis K80.12
              with obstruction K80.13
            obstruction K80.11
        specified NEC K80.18
          with obstruction K80.19
      obstruction K80.21
  gallbladder and bile duct K80.70
    with
      cholecystitis K80.60
        with obstruction K80.61
        acute K80.62
          with
            chronic cholecystitis K80.66
              with obstruction K80.67
            obstruction K80.63
        chronic K80.64
          with
            acute cholecystitis K80.66
              with obstruction K80.67
            obstruction K80.65
      obstruction K80.71
  hepatic (duct) — *see* Calculus, bile duct
  ileal conduit N21.8
  intestinal (impaction) (obstruction) K56.49
  kidney (impacted) (multiple) (pelvis) (recurrent) (staghorn) N20.0
    with calculus, ureter N20.2
    congenital Q63.8
  lacrimal passages — *see* Dacryolith
  liver (impacted) — *see* Calculus, bile duct
  lung J98.4
  mammographic R92.1
  nephritic (impacted) (recurrent) — *see* Calculus, kidney
  nose J34.89
  pancreas (duct) K86.89
  parotid duct or gland K11.5
  pelvis, encysted — *see* Calculus, kidney
  prostate N42.0
  pulmonary J98.4
  pyelitis (impacted) (recurrent) N20.0
    with hydronephrosis N13.6
  pyelonephritis (impacted) (recurrent) — *see* category N20 ☑
    with hydronephrosis N13.6
  renal (impacted) (recurrent) — *see* Calculus, kidney
  salivary (duct) (gland) K11.5
  seminal vesicle N50.89
  staghorn — *see* Calculus, kidney

Calculus, calculi, calculous — *continued*
  Stensen's duct K11.5
  stomach K31.89
  sublingual duct or gland K11.5
    congenital Q38.4
  submandibular duct, gland or region K11.5
  submaxillary duct, gland or region K11.5
  suburethral N21.8
  tonsil J35.8
  tooth, teeth (subgingival) (supragingival) K03.6
  tunica vaginalis N50.89
  ureter (impacted) (recurrent) N20.1
    with calculus, kidney N20.2
      with hydronephrosis N13.2
        with infection N13.6
  ureteropelvic junction N20.1
  urethra (impacted) N21.1
  urinary (duct) (impacted) (passage) (tract) N20.9
    with hydronephrosis N13.2
      with infection N13.6
    in (due to)
      lower N21.9
        specified NEC N21.8
  vagina N89.8
  vesical (impacted) N21.0
  Wharton's duct K11.5
  xanthine E79.8 *[N22]*
Calicectasis N28.89
Caliectasis N28.89
California
  disease B38.9
  encephalitis A83.5
Caligo cornea — *see* Opacity, cornea, central
Callositas, callosity (infected) L84
Callus (infected) L84
  bone — *see* Osteophyte
    excessive, following fracture — *code as* Sequelae of fracture
CALME (childhood asymmetric labium majus enlargement) N90.61
Calorie deficiency or malnutrition — *see also* Malnutrition E46
Calpainopathy (primary) G71.032
  autosomal dominant G71.031
  autosomal recessive G71.032
Calvé-Perthes disease — *see* Legg-Calvé-Perthes disease
Calvé's disease — *see* Osteochondrosis, juvenile, spine
Calvities — *see* Alopecia, androgenic
Cameroon fever — *see* Malaria
Camptocormia (hysterical) F44.4
Camurati-Engelmann syndrome Q78.3
Canal — *see also* condition
  atrioventricular Q21.20
    common Q21.23
    incomplete Q21.21
    intermediate Q21.22
    partial Q21.21
    transitional Q21.22
Canaliculitis (lacrimal) (acute) (subacute) H04.33- ☑
  Actinomyces A42.89
  chronic H04.42- ☑
Canavan's disease E75.29
Canceled procedure (surgical) Z53.9
  because of
    contraindication Z53.09
      smoking Z53.01
    left against medical advice (AMA) Z53.29
    patient's decision Z53.20
      for reasons of belief or group pressure Z53.1
      specified reason NEC Z53.29
    specified reason NEC Z53.8
Cancer — *see also* Neoplasm, by site, malignant
  bile duct type liver C22.1
  blood — *see* Leukemia
  breast — *see also* Neoplasm, breast, malignant C50.91- ☑
  hepatocellular C22.0
  lung — *see also* Neoplasm, lung, malignant C34.90
  ovarian — *see also* Neoplasm ovary, malignant C56.9
  unspecified site (primary) C80.1
Cancer (o) phobia F45.29
Cancerous — *see* Neoplasm, malignant, by site
Cancrum oris A69.0
Candidiasis, candidal B37.9
  balanitis B37.42
  bronchitis B37.1
  cheilitis B37.83

Candidiasis, candidal — *continued*
congenital P37.5
cystitis B37.41
disseminated B37.7
endocarditis B37.6
enteritis B37.82
esophagitis B37.81
intertrigo B37.2
lung B37.1
meningitis B37.5
mouth B37.0
nails B37.2
neonatal P37.5
onychia B37.2
oral B37.0
osteomyelitis B37.89
otitis externa B37.84
paronychia B37.2
perionyxis B37.2
pneumonia B37.1
proctitis B37.82
pulmonary B37.1
pyelonephritis B37.49
sepsis B37.7
skin B37.2
specified site NEC B37.89
stomatitis B37.0
systemic B37.7
urethritis B37.41
urogenital site NEC B37.49
vagina (acute) B37.31
chronic (recurrent) B37.32
vulva (acute) B37.31
chronic (recurrent) B37.32
vulvovaginitis (acute) B37.31
chronic (recurrent) B37.32
Candidid L30.2
Candidosis — *see* Candidiasis
Candiru infection or infestation B88.8
Canities (premature) L67.1
congenital Q84.2
Canker (mouth) (sore) K12.0
rash A38.9
Cannabinosis J66.2
Cannabis induced
anxiety disorder F12.980
psychotic disorder F12.959
sleep disorder F12.988
Canton fever A75.9
Cantrell's syndrome Q87.89
Capillariasis (intestinal) B81.1
hepatic B83.8
Capillary — *see* condition
Caplan's syndrome — *see* Rheumatoid, lung
Capsule — *see* condition
Capsulitis (joint) — *see also* Enthesopathy
adhesive (shoulder) M75.0- ☑
hepatic K65.8
labyrinthine — *see* Otosclerosis, specified NEC
thyroid E06.9
Caput
crepitus Q75.8
medusae I86.8
succedaneum P12.81
Car sickness T75.3 ☑
Carapata (disease) A68.0
Carate — *see* Pinta
Carbon lung J60
Carbuncle L02.93
abdominal wall L02.231
anus K61.0
auditory canal, external — *see* Abscess, ear, external
auricle ear — *see* Abscess, ear, external
axilla L02.43- ☑
back (any part) L02.232
breast N61.1
buttock L02.33
cheek (external) L02.03
chest wall L02.233
chin L02.03
corpus cavernosum N48.21
ear (any part) (external) (middle) — *see* Abscess, ear, external
external auditory canal — *see* Abscess, ear, external
eyelid — *see* Abscess, eyelid
face NEC L02.03
femoral (region) — *see* Carbuncle, lower limb
finger — *see* Carbuncle, hand

Carbuncle — *continued*
flank L02.231
foot L02.63- ☑
forehead L02.03
genital — *see* Abscess, genital
gluteal (region) L02.33
groin L02.234
hand L02.53- ☑
head NEC L02.831
heel — *see* Carbuncle, foot
hip — *see* Carbuncle, lower limb
kidney — *see* Abscess, kidney
knee — *see* Carbuncle, lower limb
labium (majus) (minus) N76.4
lacrimal
gland — *see* Dacryoadenitis
passages (duct) (sac) — *see* Inflammation, lacrimal, passages, acute
leg — *see* Carbuncle, lower limb
lower limb L02.43- ☑
malignant A22.0
navel L02.236
neck L02.13
nose (external) (septum) J34.0
orbit, orbital — *see* Abscess, orbit
palmar (space) — *see* Carbuncle, hand
partes posteriores L02.33
pectoral region L02.233
penis N48.21
perineum L02.235
pinna — *see* Abscess, ear, external
popliteal — *see* Carbuncle, lower limb
scalp L02.831
seminal vesicle N49.0
shoulder — *see* Carbuncle, upper limb
specified site NEC L02.838
temple (region) L02.03
thumb — *see* Carbuncle, hand
toe — *see* Carbuncle, foot
trunk L02.239
abdominal wall L02.231
back L02.232
chest wall L02.233
groin L02.234
perineum L02.235
umbilicus L02.236
umbilicus L02.236
upper limb L02.43- ☑
urethra N34.0
vulva N76.4
Carbunculus — *see* Carbuncle
Carcinoid (tumor) — *see* Tumor, carcinoid
Carcinoidosis E34.0
Carcinoma (malignant) — *see also* Neoplasm, by site, malignant
acidophil
specified site — *see* Neoplasm, malignant, by site
unspecified site C75.1
acidophil-basophil, mixed
specified site — *see* Neoplasm, malignant, by site
unspecified site C75.1
adnexal (skin) — *see* Neoplasm, skin, malignant
adrenal cortical C74.0- ☑
alveolar — *see* Neoplasm, lung, malignant
cell — *see* Neoplasm, lung, malignant
ameloblastic C41.1
upper jaw (bone) C41.0
apocrine
breast — *see* Neoplasm, breast, malignant
specified site NEC — *see* Neoplasm, skin, malignant
unspecified site C44.99
basal cell (pigmented) (*see also* Neoplasm, skin, malignant) C44.91
fibro-epithelial — *see* Neoplasm, skin, malignant
morphea — *see* Neoplasm, skin, malignant
multicentric — *see* Neoplasm, skin, malignant
basaloid
basal-squamous cell, mixed — *see* Neoplasm, skin, malignant
basophil
specified site — *see* Neoplasm, malignant, by site
unspecified site C75.1
basophil-acidophil, mixed
specified site — *see* Neoplasm, malignant, by site
unspecified site C75.1
basosquamous — *see* Neoplasm, skin, malignant

Carcinoma — *continued*
bile duct
with hepatocellular, mixed C22.0
liver C22.1
specified site NEC — *see* Neoplasm, malignant, by site
unspecified site C22.1
branchial or branchiogenic C10.4
bronchial or bronchogenic — *see* Neoplasm, lung, malignant
bronchiolar — *see* Neoplasm, lung, malignant
bronchioloalveolar — *see* Neoplasm, lung, malignant
C cell
specified site — *see* Neoplasm, malignant, by site
unspecified site C73
ceruminous C44.29- ☑
cervix uteri
in situ D06.9
endocervix D06.0
exocervix D06.1
specified site NEC D06.7
chorionic
specified site — *see* Neoplasm, malignant, by site
unspecified site
female C58
male C62.90
chromophobe
specified site — *see* Neoplasm, malignant, by site
unspecified site C75.1
cloacogenic
specified site — *see* Neoplasm, malignant, by site
unspecified site C21.2
diffuse type
specified site — *see* Neoplasm, malignant, by site
unspecified site C16.9
duct (cell)
with Paget's disease — *see* Neoplasm, breast, malignant
infiltrating
with lobular carcinoma (in situ)
specified site — *see* Neoplasm, malignant, by site
unspecified site (female) C50.91- ☑
male C50.92- ☑
specified site — *see* Neoplasm, malignant, by site
unspecified site (female) C50.91- ☑
male C50.92- ☑
ductal
with lobular
specified site — *see* Neoplasm, malignant, by site
unspecified site (female) C50.91- ☑
male C50.92- ☑
ductular, infiltrating
specified site — *see* Neoplasm, malignant, by site
unspecified site (female) C50.91- ☑
male C50.92- ☑
embryonal
liver C22.7
endometrioid
specified site — *see* Neoplasm, malignant, by site
unspecified site
female C56.9
male C61
eosinophil
specified site — *see* Neoplasm, malignant, by site
unspecified site C75.1
epidermoid — *see also* Neoplasm, skin, malignant
in situ, Bowen's type — *see* Neoplasm, skin, in situ
fibroepithelial, basal cell — *see* Neoplasm, skin, malignant
follicular
with papillary (mixed) C73
moderately differentiated C73
pure follicle C73
specified site — *see* Neoplasm, malignant, by site
trabecular C73
unspecified site C73
well differentiated C73
generalized, with unspecified primary site C80.0
glycogen-rich — *see* Neoplasm, breast, malignant
granulosa cell C56- ☑
hepatic cell C22.0
hepatocellular C22.0
with bile duct, mixed C22.0
fibrolamellar C22.0
hepatocholangiolitic C22.0

☑ Additional Character Required — Refer to the Tabular List for Character Selection

Carcinoma — continued
  Hurthle cell C73
  in
    adenomatous
      polyposis coli C18.9
    pleomorphic adenoma — see Neoplasm, salivary
      glands, malignant
    situ — see Carcinoma-in-situ
  infiltrating
    duct
      with lobular
        specified site — see Neoplasm, malignant, by
          site
        unspecified site (female) C50.91- ☑
          male C50.92- ☑
      with Paget's disease — see Neoplasm, breast,
        malignant
      specified site — see Neoplasm, malignant
      unspecified site (female) C50.91- ☑
        male C50.92- ☑
    ductular
      specified site — see Neoplasm, malignant
      unspecified site (female) C50.91- ☑
        male C50.92- ☑
    lobular
      specified site — see Neoplasm, malignant
      unspecified site (female) C50.91- ☑
        male C50.92- ☑
  inflammatory
    specified site — see Neoplasm, malignant
    unspecified site (female) C50.91- ☑
      male C50.92- ☑
  intestinal type
    specified site — see Neoplasm, malignant, by site
    unspecified site C16.9
  intracystic
    noninfiltrating — see Neoplasm, in situ, by site
  intraductal (noninfiltrating)
    with Paget's disease — see Neoplasm, breast, ma-
      lignant
    breast D05.1- ☑
    papillary
      with invasion
        specified site — see Neoplasm, malignant, by
          site
        unspecified site (female) C50.91- ☑
          male C50.92- ☑
      breast D05.1- ☑
      specified site NEC — see Neoplasm, in situ, by
        site
      unspecified site (female) D05.1- ☑
    specified site NEC — see Neoplasm, in situ, by site
    unspecified site (female) D05.1- ☑
  intraepidermal — see Neoplasm, in situ
    squamous cell, Bowen's type — see Neoplasm, skin,
      in situ
  intraepithelial — see Neoplasm, in situ, by site
    squamous cell — see Neoplasm, in situ, by site
  intraosseous C41.1
    upper jaw (bone) C41.0
  islet cell
    with exocrine, mixed
      specified site — see Neoplasm, malignant, by
        site
      unspecified site C25.9
    pancreas C25.4
    specified site NEC — see Neoplasm, malignant, by
      site
    unspecified site C25.4
  juvenile, breast — see Neoplasm, breast, malignant
  large cell
    small cell
      specified site — see Neoplasm, malignant, by
        site
      unspecified site C34.90
  Leydig cell (testis)
    specified site — see Neoplasm, malignant, by site
    unspecified site
      female C56.9
      male C62.90
  lipid-rich (female) C50.91- ☑
    male C50.92- ☑
  liver cell C22.0
  liver NEC C22.7

Carcinoma — continued
  lobular (infiltrating)
    with intraductal
      specified site — see Neoplasm, malignant, by
        site
      unspecified site (female) C50.91- ☑
        male C50.92- ☑
    noninfiltrating
      breast D05.0- ☑
      specified site NEC — see Neoplasm, in situ, by
        site
      unspecified site D05.0- ☑
    specified site — see Neoplasm, malignant, by site
    unspecified site (female) C50.91- ☑
      male C50.92- ☑
  medullary
    with
      amyloid stroma
        specified site — see Neoplasm, malignant, by
          site
        unspecified site C73
      lymphoid stroma
        specified site — see Neoplasm, malignant, by
          site
        unspecified site (female) C50.91- ☑
          male C50.92- ☑
  Merkel cell C4A.9 (following C43)
    anal margin C4A.51 (following C43)
    anal skin C4A.51 (following C43)
    canthus C4A.1- ☑ (following C43)
    ear and external auricular canal C4A.2- ☑ (following
      C43)
    external auricular canal C4A.2- ☑ (following C43)
    eyelid, including canthus C4A.1- ☑ (following C43)
    face C4A.30 (following C43)
      specified NEC C4A.39 (following C43)
    hip C4A.7- ☑ (following C43)
    lip C4A.0 (following C43)
    lower limb, including hip C4A.7- ☑ (following C43)
    neck C4A.4 (following C43)
    nodal presentation C7B.1 (following C75)
    nose C4A.31 (following C43)
    overlapping sites C4A.8 (following C43)
    perianal skin C4A.51 (following C43)
    scalp C4A.4 (following C43)
    secondary C7B.1 (following C75)
    shoulder C4A.6- ☑ (following C43)
    skin of breast C4A.52 (following C43)
    trunk NEC C4A.59 (following C43)
    upper limb, including shoulder C4A.6- ☑ (following
      C43)
    visceral metastatic C7B.1 (following C75)
  metastatic — see Neoplasm, secondary, by site
  metatypical — see Neoplasm, skin, malignant
  morphea, basal cell — see Neoplasm, skin, malignant
  mucoid
    cell
      specified site — see Neoplasm, malignant, by
        site
      unspecified site C75.1
  neuroendocrine — see also Tumor, neuroendocrine
    high grade, any site C7A.1 (following C75)
    poorly differentiated, any site C7A.1 (following C75)
  nonencapsulated sclerosing C73
  noninfiltrating
    intracystic — see Neoplasm, in situ, by site
    intraductal
      breast D05.1- ☑
      papillary
        breast D05.1- ☑
        specified site NEC — see Neoplasm, in situ,
          by site
        unspecified site D05.1- ☑
      specified site — see Neoplasm, in situ, by site
      unspecified site D05.1- ☑
    lobular
      breast D05.0- ☑
      specified site NEC — see Neoplasm, in situ, by
        site
      unspecified site (female) D05.0- ☑
  oat cell
    specified site — see Neoplasm, malignant, by site
    unspecified site C34.90
  odontogenic C41.1
    upper jaw (bone) C41.0
  papillary
    with follicular (mixed) C73

Carcinoma — continued
  papillary — continued
    follicular variant C73
    intraductal (noninfiltrating)
      with invasion
        specified site — see Neoplasm, malignant, by
          site
        unspecified site (female) C50.91- ☑
          male C50.92- ☑
      breast D05.1- ☑
      specified site NEC — see Neoplasm, in situ, by
        site
      unspecified site D05.1- ☑
    serous
      specified site — see Neoplasm, malignant, by
        site
      surface
        specified site — see Neoplasm, malignant, by
          site
        unspecified site C56.9
      unspecified site C56.9
  papillocystic
    specified site — see Neoplasm, malignant, by site
    unspecified site C56.9
  parafollicular cell
    specified site — see Neoplasm, malignant, by site
    unspecified site C73
  pilomatrix — see Neoplasm, skin, malignant
  pseudomucinous
    specified site — see Neoplasm, malignant, by site
    unspecified site C56.9
  renal cell C64- ☑
  Schmincke — see Neoplasm, nasopharynx, malignant
  Schneiderian
    specified site — see Neoplasm, malignant, by site
    unspecified site C30.0
  sebaceous — see Neoplasm, skin, malignant
  secondary — see also Neoplasm, secondary, by site
    Merkel cell C7B.1 (following C75)
  secretory, breast — see Neoplasm, breast, malignant
  serous
    papillary
      specified site — see Neoplasm, malignant, by
        site
      unspecified site C56.9
    surface, papillary
      specified site — see Neoplasm, malignant, by
        site
      unspecified site C56.9
  Sertoli cell
    specified site — see Neoplasm, malignant, by site
    unspecified site C62.90
      female C56.9
      male C62.90
  skin appendage — see Neoplasm, skin, malignant
  small cell
    fusiform cell
      specified site — see Neoplasm, malignant, by
        site
      unspecified site C34.90
    intermediate cell
      specified site — see Neoplasm, malignant, by
        site
      unspecified site C34.90
    large cell
      specified site — see Neoplasm, malignant, by
        site
      unspecified site C34.90
  solid
    with amyloid stroma
      specified site — see Neoplasm, malignant, by
        site
      unspecified site C73
    microinvasive
      specified site — see Neoplasm, malignant, by
        site
      unspecified site C53.9
  sweat gland — see Neoplasm, skin, malignant
  theca cell C56.- ☑
  thymic C37
  unspecified site (primary) C80.1
  water-clear cell C75.0
Carcinoma-in-situ — see also Neoplasm, in situ, by site
  breast NOS D05.9- ☑
    specified type NEC D05.8- ☑
  epidermoid — see also Neoplasm, in situ, by site
    with questionable stromal invasion
      cervix D06.9

Carcinoma-in-situ — *continued*
  epidermoid — *see also* Neoplasm, in situ, by site — *continued*
    with questionable stromal invasion — *continued*
      specified site NEC — *see* Neoplasm, in situ, by site
      unspecified site D06.9
    Bowen's type — *see* Neoplasm, skin, in situ
  intraductal
    breast D05.1- ☑
    specified site NEC — *see* Neoplasm, in situ, by site
    unspecified site D05.1- ☑
  lobular
    with
      infiltrating duct
        breast (female) C50.91- ☑
          male C50.92- ☑
        specified site NEC — *see* Neoplasm, malignant
        unspecified site (female) C50.91- ☑
          male C50.92- ☑
      intraductal
        breast D05.8- ☑
        specified site NEC — *see* Neoplasm, in situ, by site
        unspecified site (female) D05.8- ☑
    breast D05.0- ☑
    specified site NEC — *see* Neoplasm, in situ, by site
    unspecified site D05.0- ☑
  squamous cell — *see also* Neoplasm, in situ, by site
    with questionable stromal invasion
      cervix D06.9
      specified site NEC — *see* Neoplasm, in situ, by site
      unspecified site D06.9
Carcinomaphobia F45.29
Carcinomatosis C80.0
  peritonei C78.6
  unspecified site (primary) (secondary) C80.0
Carcinosarcoma — *see* Neoplasm, malignant, by site
  embryonal — *see* Neoplasm, malignant, by site
Cardia, cardial — *see* condition
Cardiac — *see also* condition
  death, sudden — *see* Arrest, cardiac
  pacemaker
    in situ Z95.0
    management or adjustment Z45.018
  tamponade I31.4
Cardialgia — *see* Pain, precordial
Cardiectasis — *see* Hypertrophy, cardiac
Cardiochalasia K21.9
Cardiomalacia I51.5
Cardiomegalia glycogenica diffusa E74.02 *[I43]*
Cardiomegaly — *see also* Hypertrophy, cardiac
  congenital Q24.8
  glycogen E74.02 *[I43]*
  idiopathic I51.7
Cardiomyoliposis I51.5
Cardiomyopathy (familial) (idiopathic) I42.9
  alcoholic I42.6
  amyloid E85.4 *[I43]*
    transthyretin-related (ATTR) familial E85.4 *[I43]*
  arteriosclerotic — *see* Disease, heart, ischemic, atherosclerotic
  beriberi E51.12
  cobalt-beer I42.6
  congenital I42.4
  congestive I42.0
  constrictive NOS I42.5
  dilated I42.0
  due to
    alcohol I42.6
    beriberi E51.12
    cardiac glycogenosis E74.02 *[I43]*
    drugs I42.7
    external agents NEC I42.7
    Friedreich's ataxia G11.11
    myotonia atrophica G71.11 *[I43]*
    progressive muscular dystrophy — *see also* Dystrophy, muscular, by type G71.09 *[I43]*
  glycogen storage E74.02 *[I43]*
  hypertensive — *see* Hypertension, heart
  hypertrophic (nonobstructive) I42.2
    obstructive I42.1
      congenital Q24.8
  in
    Chagas' disease (chronic) B57.2
      acute B57.0

Cardiomyopathy — *continued*
  in — *continued*
    sarcoidosis D86.85
  ischemic I25.5
  metabolic E88.9 *[I43]*
    thyrotoxic E05.90 *[I43]*
      with thyroid storm E05.91 *[I43]*
  newborn I42.8
    congenital I42.4
  non-ischemic — *see also* by cause I42.8
  nutritional E63.9 *[I43]*
    beriberi E51.12
  obscure of Africa I42.8
  peripartum O90.3
  postpartum O90.3
  restrictive NEC I42.5
  rheumatic I09.0
  secondary I42.9
  specified NEC I42.8
  stress induced I51.81
  takotsubo I51.81
  thyrotoxic E05.90 *[I43]*
    with thyroid storm E05.91 *[I43]*
  toxic NEC I42.7
  transthyretin-related (ATTR) familial amyloid E85.4
  tuberculous A18.84
  viral B33.24
Cardionephritis — *see* Hypertension, cardiorenal
Cardionephropathy — *see* Hypertension, cardiorenal
Cardionephrosis — *see* Hypertension, cardiorenal
Cardiopathia nigra I27.0
Cardiopathy — *see also* Disease, heart I51.9
  idiopathic I42.9
  mucopolysaccharidosis E76.3 *[I52]*
Cardiopericarditis — *see* Pericarditis
Cardiophobia F45.29
Cardiorenal — *see* condition
Cardiorrhexis — *see* Infarct, myocardium
Cardiosclerosis — *see* Disease, heart, ischemic, atherosclerotic
Cardiosis — *see* Disease, heart
Cardiospasm (esophagus) (reflex) (stomach) K22.0
  congenital Q39.5
    with megaesophagus Q39.5
Cardiostenosis — *see* Disease, heart
Cardiosymphysis I31.0
Cardiovascular — *see* condition
Carditis (acute) (bacterial) (chronic) (subacute) I51.89
  meningococcal A39.50
  rheumatic — *see* Disease, heart, rheumatic
  rheumatoid — *see* Rheumatoid, carditis
  viral B33.20
Care (of) (for) (following)
  child (routine) Z76.2
  family member (handicapped) (sick)
    creating problem for family Z63.6
    provided away from home for holiday relief Z75.5
    unavailable, due to
      absence (person rendering care) (sufferer) Z74.2
      inability (any reason) of person rendering care Z74.2
  foundling Z76.1
  holiday relief Z75.5
  improper — *see* Maltreatment
  lack of (at or after birth) (infant) — *see* Maltreatment, child, neglect
  lactating mother Z39.1
  palliative Z51.5
  postpartum
    immediately after delivery Z39.0
    routine follow-up Z39.2
  respite Z75.5
  unavailable, due to
    absence of person rendering care Z74.2
    inability (any reason) of person rendering care Z74.2
  well-baby Z76.2
Caries
  bone NEC A18.03
  dental (dentino enamel junction) (early childhood) (of dentine) (pre-eruptive) (recurrent) (to the pulp) K02.9
    arrested (coronal) (root) K02.3
    chewing surface
      limited to enamel K02.51
      penetrating into dentin K02.52
      penetrating into pulp K02.53

Caries — *continued*
  dental — *continued*
    coronal surface
      chewing surface
        limited to enamel K02.51
        penetrating into dentin K02.52
        penetrating into pulp K02.53
      pit and fissure surface
        limited to enamel K02.51
        penetrating into dentin K02.52
        penetrating into pulp K02.53
      smooth surface
        limited to enamel K02.61
        penetrating into dentin K02.62
        penetrating into pulp K02.63
    pit and fissure surface
      limited to enamel K02.51
      penetrating into dentin K02.52
      penetrating into pulp K02.53
    primary, cervical origin K02.52
    root K02.7
    smooth surface
      limited to enamel K02.61
      penetrating into dentin K02.62
      penetrating into pulp K02.63
  external meatus — *see* Disorder, ear, external, specified type NEC
  hip (tuberculous) A18.02
  initial (tooth)
    chewing surface K02.51
    pit and fissure surface K02.51
    smooth surface K02.61
  knee (tuberculous) A18.02
  labyrinth H83.8 ☑
  limb NEC (tuberculous) A18.03
  mastoid process (chronic) — *see* Mastoiditis, chronic
    tuberculous A18.03
  middle ear H74.8 ☑
  nose (tuberculous) A18.03
  orbit (tuberculous) A18.03
  ossicles, ear — *see* Abnormal, ear ossicles
  petrous bone — *see* Petrositis
  root (dental) (tooth) K02.7
  sacrum (tuberculous) A18.01
  spine, spinal (column) (tuberculous) A18.01
  syphilitic A52.77
    congenital (early) A50.02 *[M90.80]*
  tooth, teeth — *see* Caries, dental
  tuberculous A18.03
  vertebra (column) (tuberculous) A18.01
Carious teeth — *see* Caries, dental
Carneous mole O02.0
Carnitine insufficiency E71.40
Carotenemia (dietary) E67.1
Carotenosis (cutis) (skin) E67.1
Carotid body or sinus syndrome G90.01
Carotidynia G90.01
Carpal tunnel syndrome — *see* Syndrome, carpal tunnel
Carpenter's syndrome Q87.0
Carpopedal spasm — *see* Tetany
Carr-Barr-Plunkett syndrome Q97.1
Carrier (suspected) of
  amebiasis Z22.1
  bacterial disease NEC Z22.39
    diphtheria Z22.2
    intestinal infectious NEC Z22.1
      typhoid Z22.0
    meningococcal Z22.31
    sexually transmitted Z22.4
    specified NEC Z22.39
    staphylococcal (Methicillin susceptible) Z22.321
      Methicillin resistant Z22.322
    streptococcal Z22.338
      group B Z22.330
        complicating pregnancy or delivery O99.82- ☑
    typhoid Z22.0
  cholera Z22.1
  diphtheria Z22.2
  gastrointestinal pathogens NEC Z22.1
  genetic Z14.8
    cystic fibrosis Z14.1
    hemophilia A (asymptomatic) Z14.01
      symptomatic Z14.02
  gestational, pregnant Z33.1
  gonorrhea Z22.4
  HAA (hepatitis Australian-antigen) B18.8
  HB (c)(s)-AG B18.1

Carrier of — *continued*
  hepatitis (viral) B18.9
    Australia-antigen (HAA) B18.8
    B surface antigen (HBsAg) B18.1
      with acute delta- (super)infection B17.0
    C B18.2
    specified NEC B18.8
  human T-cell lymphotropic virus type-1 (HTLV-1) infection Z22.6
  infectious organism Z22.9
    specified NEC Z22.8
  meningococci Z22.31
  Salmonella typhosa Z22.0
  serum hepatitis — *see* Carrier, hepatitis
  staphylococci (Methicillin susceptible) Z22.321
    Methicillin resistant Z22.322
  streptococci Z22.338
    group B Z22.330
      complicating pregnancy or delivery O99.82- ☑
  syphilis Z22.4
  typhoid Z22.0
  venereal disease NEC Z22.4
Carrion's disease A44.0
Carter's relapsing fever (Asiatic) A68.1
Cartilage — *see* condition
Caruncle (inflamed)
  conjunctiva (acute) — *see* Conjunctivitis, acute
  labium (majus) (minus) N90.89
  lacrimal — *see* Inflammation, lacrimal, passages
  myrtiform N89.8
  urethral (benign) N36.2
Cascade stomach K31.2
Caseation lymphatic gland (tuberculous) A18.2
Cassidy (-Scholte) syndrome (malignant carcinoid) E34.0
Castellani's disease A69.8
Castration, traumatic, male S38.231 ☑
Casts in urine R82.998
Cat
  cry syndrome Q93.4
  ear Q17.3
  eye syndrome Q92.8
Catabolism, senile R54
Catalepsy (hysterical) F44.2
  schizophrenic F20.2
Cataplexy (idiopathic) — *see* Narcolepsy
Cataract (cortical) (immature) (incipient) H26.9
  with
    neovascularization — *see* Cataract, complicated
  age-related — *see* Cataract, senile
  anterior
    and posterior axial embryonal Q12.0
    pyramidal Q12.0
  associated with
    galactosemia E74.21 *[H28]*
    myotonic disorders G71.19 *[H28]*
  blue Q12.0
  central Q12.0
  cerulean Q12.0
  complicated H26.20
    with
      neovascularization H26.21- ☑
      ocular disorder H26.22- ☑
    glaucomatous flecks H26.23- ☑
  congenital Q12.0
  coraliform Q12.0
  coronary Q12.0
  crystalline Q12.0
  diabetic — *see* Diabetes, cataract
  drug-induced H26.3- ☑
  due to
    ocular disorder — *see* Cataract, complicated
    radiation H26.8
  electric H26.8
  extraction status Z98.4- ☑
  glass-blower's H26.8
  heat ray H26.8
  heterochromic — *see* Cataract, complicated
  hypermature — *see* Cataract, senile, morgagnian type
  in (due to)
    chronic iridocyclitis — *see* Cataract, complicated
    diabetes — *see* Diabetes, cataract
    endocrine disease E34.9 *[H28]*
    eye disease — *see* Cataract, complicated
    hypoparathyroidism E20.9 *[H28]*
    malnutrition-dehydration E46 *[H28]*
    metabolic disease E88.9 *[H28]*
    myotonic disorders G71.19 *[H28]*

Cataract — *continued*
  in — *continued*
    nutritional disease E63.9 *[H28]*
  infantile — *see* Cataract, presenile
  irradiational — *see* Cataract, specified NEC
  juvenile — *see* Cataract, presenile
  malnutrition-dehydration E46 *[H28]*
  morgagnian — *see* Cataract, senile, morgagnian type
  myotonic G71.19 *[H28]*
  myxedema E03.9 *[H28]*
  nuclear
    embryonal Q12.0
    sclerosis — *see* Cataract, senile, nuclear
  presenile H26.00- ☑
    combined forms H26.06- ☑
    cortical H26.01- ☑
    lamellar — *see* Cataract, presenile, cortical
    nuclear H26.03- ☑
    specified NEC H26.09
    subcapsular polar (anterior) H26.04- ☑
      posterior H26.05- ☑
    zonular — *see* Cataract, presenile, cortical
  secondary H26.40
    Soemmering's ring H26.41- ☑
    specified NEC H26.49- ☑
    to eye disease — *see* Cataract, complicated
  senile H25.9
    brunescens — *see* Cataract, senile, nuclear
    combined forms H25.81- ☑
    coronary — *see* Cataract, senile, incipient
    cortical H25.01- ☑
    hypermature — *see* Cataract, senile, morgagnian type
    incipient (mature) (total) H25.09- ☑
      cortical — *see* Cataract, senile, cortical
      subcapsular — *see* Cataract, senile, subcapsular
    morgagnian type (hypermature) H25.2- ☑
    nuclear (sclerosis) H25.1- ☑
    polar subcapsular (anterior) (posterior) — *see* Cataract, senile, incipient
    punctate — *see* Cataract, senile, incipient
    specified NEC H25.89
    subcapsular polar (anterior) H25.03- ☑
      posterior H25.04- ☑
  snowflake — *see* Diabetes, cataract
  specified NEC H26.8
  toxic — *see* Cataract, drug-induced
  traumatic H26.10- ☑
    localized H26.11- ☑
    partially resolved H26.12- ☑
    total H26.13- ☑
  zonular (perinuclear) Q12.0
Cataracta — *see also* Cataract
  brunescens — *see* Cataract, senile, nuclear
  centralis pulverulenta Q12.0
  cerulea Q12.0
  complicata — *see* Cataract, complicated
  congenita Q12.0
  coralliformis Q12.0
  coronaria Q12.0
  diabetic — *see* Diabetes, cataract
  membranacea
    accreta — *see* Cataract, secondary
    congenita Q12.0
  nigra — *see* Cataract, senile, nuclear
  sunflower — *see* Cataract, complicated
Catarrh, catarrhal (acute) (febrile) (infectious) (inflammation) — *see also* condition J00
  bronchial — *see* Bronchitis
  chest — *see* Bronchitis
  chronic J31.0
  due to congenital syphilis A50.03
  enteric — *see* Enteritis
  eustachian H68.009
  fauces — *see* Pharyngitis
  gastrointestinal — *see* Enteritis
  gingivitis K05.00
    nonplaque induced K05.01
    plaque induced K05.00
  hay — *see* Fever, hay
  intestinal — *see* Enteritis
  larynx, chronic J37.0
  liver B15.9
    with hepatic coma B15.0
  lung — *see* Bronchitis
  middle ear, chronic — *see* Otitis, media, nonsuppurative, chronic, serous

Catarrh, catarrhal — *continued*
  mouth K12.1
  nasal (chronic) — *see* Rhinitis
  nasobronchial J31.1
  nasopharyngeal (chronic) J31.1
    acute J00
  pulmonary — *see* Bronchitis
  spring (eye) (vernal) — *see* Conjunctivitis, acute, atopic
  summer (hay) — *see* Fever, hay
  throat J31.2
  tubotympanal — *see also* Otitis, media, nonsuppurative
    chronic — *see* Otitis, media, nonsuppurative, chronic, serous
Catatonia (schizophrenic) F20.2
Catatonic
  disorder due to known physiologic condition F06.1
  schizophrenia F20.2
  stupor R40.1
Cat-scratch — *see also* Abrasion
  disease or fever A28.1
Cauda equina — *see* condition
Cauliflower ear M95.1- ☑
Causalgia (upper limb) G56.4- ☑
  lower limb G57.7- ☑
Cause
  external, general effects T75.89 ☑
Caustic burn — *see* Corrosion, by site
Cavare's disease (familial periodic paralysis) G72.3
Cave-in, injury
  crushing (severe) — *see* Crush
  suffocation — *see* Asphyxia, traumatic, due to low oxygen, due to cave-in
Cavernitis (penis) N48.29
Cavernositis N48.29
Cavernous — *see* condition
Cavitation of lung — *see also* Tuberculosis, pulmonary
  nontuberculous J98.4
Cavities, dental — *see* Caries, dental
Cavity
  lung — *see* Cavitation of lung
  optic papilla Q14.2
  pulmonary — *see* Cavitation of lung
Cavovarus foot, congenital Q66.1- ☑
Cavus foot (congenital) Q66.7- ☑
  acquired — *see* Deformity, limb, foot, specified NEC
Cazenave's disease L10.2
CDKL5 (Cyclin-Dependent Kinase-Like 5 Deficiency Disorder) G40.42
Cecitis K52.9
  with perforation, peritonitis, or rupture K65.8
Cecoureterocele Q62.32
Cecum — *see* condition
Celiac
  artery compression syndrome I77.4
  disease (with steatorrhea) K90.0
  infantilism K90.0
Cell(s), **cellular** — *see also* condition
  in urine R82.998
Cellulitis (diffuse) (phlegmonous) (septic) (suppurative) L03.90
  abdominal wall L03.311
  anaerobic A48.0
  ankle — *see* Cellulitis, lower limb
  anus K61.0
  arm — *see* Cellulitis, upper limb
  auricle (ear) — *see* Cellulitis, ear
  axilla L03.11- ☑
  back (any part) L03.312
  breast (acute) (nonpuerperal) (subacute) N61.0
    nipple N61.0
  broad ligament
    acute N73.0
  buttock L03.317
  cervical (meaning neck) L03.221
  cervix (uteri) — *see* Cervicitis
  cheek (external) L03.211
    internal K12.2
  chest wall L03.313
  chronic L03.90
  clostridial A48.0
  corpus cavernosum N48.22
  digit
    finger — *see* Cellulitis, finger
    toe — *see* Cellulitis, toe
  Douglas' cul-de-sac or pouch
    acute N73.0
  drainage site (following operation) T81.49 ☑

Cellulitis — continued
  ear (external) H60.1- ☑
  eosinophilic (granulomatous) L98.3
  erysipelatous — see Erysipelas
  external auditory canal — see Cellulitis, ear
  eyelid — see Abscess, eyelid
  face NEC L03.211
  finger (intrathecal) (periosteal) (subcutaneous) (subcu-
    ticular) L03.01- ☑
  foot — see Cellulitis, lower limb
  gangrenous — see Gangrene
  genital organ NEC
    female (external) N76.4
    male N49.9
      multiple sites N49.8
      specified NEC N49.8
  gluteal (region) L03.317
  gonococcal A54.89
  groin L03.314
  hand — see Cellulitis, upper limb
  head NEC L03.811
    face (any part, except ear, eye and nose) L03.211
  heel — see Cellulitis, lower limb
  hip — see Cellulitis, lower limb
  jaw (region) L03.211
  knee — see Cellulitis, lower limb
  labium (majus) (minus) — see Vulvitis
  lacrimal passages — see Inflammation, lacrimal, pas-
    sages
  larynx J38.7
  leg — see Cellulitis, lower limb
  lip K13.0
  lower limb L03.11- ☑
    toe — see Cellulitis, toe
  mouth (floor) K12.2
  multiple sites, so stated L03.90
  nasopharynx J39.1
  navel L03.316
    newborn P38.9
      with mild hemorrhage P38.1
      without hemorrhage P38.9
  neck (region) L03.221
  nipple (acute) (nonpuerperal) (subacute) N61.0
  nose (septum) (external) J34.0
  orbit, orbital H05.01- ☑
  palate (soft) K12.2
  pectoral (region) L03.313
  pelvis, pelvic (chronic)
    female — see also Disease, pelvis, inflammatory
      N73.2
      acute N73.0
    following ectopic or molar pregnancy O08.0
    male K65.0
  penis N48.22
  perineal, perineum L03.315
  periorbital L03.213
  perirectal K61.1
  peritonsillar J36
  periurethral N34.0
  periuterine — see also Disease, pelvis, inflammatory
    N73.2
    acute N73.0
  pharynx J39.1
  preseptal L03.213
  rectum K61.1
  retroperitoneal K68.9
  round ligament
    acute N73.0
  scalp (any part) L03.811
  scrotum N49.2
  seminal vesicle N49.0
  shoulder — see Cellulitis, upper limb
  specified site NEC L03.818
  submandibular (region) (space) (triangle) K12.2
    gland K11.3
  submaxillary (region) K12.2
    gland K11.3
  thigh — see Cellulitis, lower limb
  thumb (intrathecal) (periosteal) (subcutaneous) (sub-
    cuticular) — see Cellulitis, finger
  toe (intrathecal) (periosteal) (subcutaneous) (subcutic-
    ular) L03.03- ☑
  tonsil J36
  trunk L03.319
    abdominal wall L03.311
    back (any part) L03.312
    buttock L03.317
    chest wall L03.313

Cellulitis — continued
  trunk — continued
    groin L03.314
    perineal, perineum L03.315
    umbilicus L03.316
  tuberculous (primary) A18.4
  umbilicus L03.316
  upper limb L03.11- ☑
    axilla — see Cellulitis, axilla
    finger — see Cellulitis, finger
    thumb — see Cellulitis, finger
  vaccinal T88.0 ☑
  vocal cord J38.3
  vulva — see Vulvitis
  wrist — see Cellulitis, upper limb
Cementoblastoma, benign — see Cyst, calcifying
  odontogenic
Cementoma — see Cyst, calcifying odontogenic
Cementoperiostitis — see Periodontitis
Cementosis K03.4
Central auditory processing disorder H93.25
Central pain syndrome G89.0
Cephalematocele, cephal (o)hematocele
  newborn P52.8
    birth injury P10.8
  traumatic — see Hematoma, brain
Cephalematoma, cephalhematoma (calcified)
  newborn (birth injury) P12.0
  traumatic — see Hematoma, brain
Cephalgia, cephalalgia — see also Headache
  histamine G44.009
    intractable G44.001
    not intractable G44.009
  trigeminal autonomic (TAC) NEC G44.099
    intractable G44.091
    not intractable G44.099
Cephalic — see condition
Cephalitis — see Encephalitis
Cephalocele — see Encephalocele
Cephalomenia N94.89
Cephalopelvic — see condition
Cerclage (with cervical incompetence) in pregnancy —
  see Incompetence, cervix, in pregnancy
Cerebellitis — see Encephalitis
Cerebellum, cerebellar — see condition
Cerebral — see condition
Cerebritis — see Encephalitis
Cerebro-hepato-renal syndrome Q87.89
Cerebromalacia — see Softening, brain
  sequelae of cerebrovascular disease I69.398
Cerebroside lipidosis E75.22
Cerebrospasticity (congenital) G80.1
Cerebrospinal — see condition
Cerebrum — see condition
Ceroid-lipofuscinosis, neuronal E75.4
Cerumen (accumulation) (impacted) H61.2- ☑
Cervical — see also condition
  auricle Q18.2
  dysplasia in pregnancy — see Abnormal, cervix, in
    pregnancy or childbirth
  erosion in pregnancy — see Abnormal, cervix, in
    pregnancy or childbirth
  fibrosis in pregnancy — see Abnormal, cervix, in preg-
    nancy or childbirth
  fusion syndrome Q76.1
  rib Q76.5
  shortening (complicating pregnancy) O26.87- ☑
Cervicalgia M54.2
Cervicitis (acute) (atrophic) (chronic) (nonvenereal) (senile) (subacute) (with ulceration) N72
  with
    abortion — see Abortion, by type complicated by
      genital tract and pelvic infection
    ectopic pregnancy O08.0
    molar pregnancy O08.0
  chlamydial A56.09
  gonococcal A54.03
  herpesviral A60.03
  puerperal (postpartum) O86.11
  syphilitic A52.76
  trichomonal A59.09
  tuberculous A18.16
Cervicocolpitis (emphysematosa) — see also Cervicitis
  N72
Cervix — see condition
Cesarean delivery, previous, affecting management
  of pregnancy O34.219

Cesarean delivery, previous, affecting management
  of pregnancy — continued
  classical (vertical) scar O34.212
  isthmocele (non-pregnant state) N85.A
    maternal care for O34.22
  low transverse scar O34.211
  mid-transverse T incision O34.218
  scar
    defect (non-pregnant state) N85.A
      maternal care for O34.22
    specified type NEC O34.218
Céstan (-Chenais) paralysis or syndrome G46.3
Céstan-Raymond syndrome I65.8
Cestode infestation B71.9
  specified type NEC B71.8
Cestodiasis B71.9
Chabert's disease A22.9
Chacaleh E53.8
Chafing L30.4
Chagas' (-Mazza) disease (chronic) B57.2
  with
    cardiovascular involvement NEC B57.2
    digestive system involvement B57.30
      megacolon B57.32
      megaesophagus B57.31
      other specified B57.39
    megacolon B57.32
    megaesophagus B57.31
    myocarditis B57.2
    nervous system involvement B57.40
      meningitis B57.41
      meningoencephalitis B57.42
      other specified B57.49
    specified organ involvement NEC B57.5
  acute (with) B57.1
    cardiovascular NEC B57.0
    myocarditis B57.0
Chagres fever B50.9
Chairridden Z74.09
Chalasia (cardiac sphincter) K21.9
Chalazion H00.19
  left H00.16
    lower H00.15
    upper H00.14
  right H00.13
    lower H00.12
    upper H00.11
Chalcosis — see also Disorder, globe, degenerative,
  chalcosis
  cornea — see Deposit, cornea
  crystalline lens — see Cataract, complicated
  retina H35.89
Chalicosis (pulmonum) J62.8
Chancre (any genital site) (hard) (hunterian) (mixed)
  (primary) (seronegative) (seropositive) (syphilitic)
  A51.0
  congenital A50.07
  conjunctiva NEC A51.2
  Ducrey's A57
  extragenital A51.2
  eyelid A51.2
  lip A51.2
  nipple A51.2
  Nisbet's A57
  of
    carate A67.0
    pinta A67.0
    yaws A66.0
  palate, soft A51.2
  phagedenic A57
  simple A57
  soft A57
    bubo A57
    palate A51.2
  urethra A51.0
  yaws A66.0
Chancroid (anus) (genital) (penis) (perineum) (rectum)
  (urethra) (vulva) A57
Chandler's disease (osteochondritis dissecans, hip) —
  see Osteochondritis, dissecans, hip
Change(s) (in) (of) — see also Removal
  arteriosclerotic — see Arteriosclerosis
  bone — see also Disorder, bone
    diabetic — see Diabetes, bone change
  bowel habit R19.4
  cardiorenal (vascular) — see Hypertension, cardiorenal
  cardiovascular — see Disease, cardiovascular
  circulatory I99.9

Change(s) — *continued*
  cognitive (mild) (organic) R41.89
  color, tooth, teeth
    during formation K00.8
    posteruptive K03.7
  contraceptive device Z30.433
  corneal membrane H18.30
    Bowman's membrane fold or rupture H18.31- ☑
    Descemet's membrane
      fold H18.32- ☑
      rupture H18.33- ☑
  coronary — *see* Disease, heart, ischemic
  degenerative, spine or vertebra — *see* Spondylosis
  dental pulp, regressive K04.2
  dressing (nonsurgical) Z48.00
    surgical Z48.01
  heart — *see* Disease, heart
  hip joint — *see* Derangement, joint, hip
  hyperplastic larynx J38.7
  hypertrophic
    nasal sinus J34.89
    turbinate, nasal J34.3
    upper respiratory tract J39.8
  indwelling catheter Z46.6
  inflammatory — *see also* Inflammation
    sacroiliac M46.1
  job, anxiety concerning Z56.1
  joint — *see* Derangement, joint
  life — *see* Menopause
  mental status R41.82
  minimal (glomerular) — *see also* N00-N07 with fourth character .0 N05.0
  myocardium, myocardial — *see* Degeneration, myocardial
  of life — *see* Menopause
  pacemaker Z45.018
    pulse generator Z45.010
  personality (enduring) F68.8
    due to (secondary to)
      general medical condition F07.0
      secondary (nonspecific) F60.89
  regressive, dental pulp K04.2
  renal — *see* Disease, renal
  retina H35.9
    myopic — *see also* Myopia, degenerative H44.2- ☑
  sacroiliac joint M53.3
  senile — *see also* condition R54
  sensory R20.8
  skin R23.9
    acute, due to ultraviolet radiation L56.9
      specified NEC L56.8
    chronic, due to nonionizing radiation L57.9
      specified NEC L57.8
    cyanosis R23.0
    flushing R23.2
    pallor R23.1
    petechiae R23.3
    specified change NEC R23.8
    swelling — *see* Mass, localized
    texture R23.4
  trophic
    arm — *see* Mononeuropathy, upper limb
    leg — *see* Mononeuropathy, lower limb
  vascular I99.9
  vasomotor I73.9
  voice R49.9
    psychogenic F44.4
    specified NEC R49.8
Changing sleep-work schedule, affecting sleep G47.26
Changuinola fever A93.1
Chapping skin T69.8 ☑
Charcot-Marie-Tooth disease, paralysis or syndrome G60.0
Charcot's
  arthropathy — *see* Arthropathy, neuropathic
  cirrhosis K74.3
  disease (tabetic arthropathy) A52.16
  joint (disease) (tabetic) A52.16
    diabetic — *see* Diabetes, with, arthropathy
    syringomyelic G95.0
  syndrome (intermittent claudication) I73.9
CHARGE association Q89.8
Charley-horse (quadriceps) M62.831
  traumatic (quadriceps) S76.11- ☑
Charlouis' disease — *see* Yaws
Cheadle's disease E54

Checking (of)
  cardiac pacemaker (battery) (electrode(s)) Z45.018
    pulse generator Z45.010
  implantable subdermal contraceptive Z30.46
  intrauterine contraceptive device Z30.431
  wound Z48.0- ☑
    due to injury — code to Injury, by site, using appropriate seventh character for subsequent encounter
Check-up — *see* Examination
Chédiak-Higashi (-Steinbrinck) **syndrome** (congenital gigantism of peroxidase granules) E70.330
Cheek — *see* condition
Cheese itch B88.0
Cheese-washer's lung J67.8
Cheese-worker's lung J67.8
Cheilitis (acute) (angular) (catarrhal) (chronic) (exfoliative) (gangrenous) (glandular) (infectional) (suppurative) (ulcerative) (vesicular) K13.0
  actinic (due to sun) L56.8
    other than from sun L59.8
  candidal B37.83
Cheilodynia K13.0
Cheiloschisis — *see* Cleft, lip
Cheilosis (angular) K13.0
  with pellagra E52
  due to
    vitamin B2 (riboflavin) deficiency E53.0
Cheiromegaly M79.89
Cheiropompholyx L30.1
Cheloid — *see* Keloid
Chemical burn — *see* Corrosion, by site
Chemodectoma — *see* Paraganglioma, nonchromaffin
Chemosis, conjunctiva — *see* Edema, conjunctiva
Chemotherapy (session) (for)
  cancer Z51.11
  neoplasm Z51.11
Cherubism M27.8
Chest — *see* condition
Cheyne-Stokes breathing (respiration) R06.3
Chiari's
  disease or syndrome (hepatic vein thrombosis) I82.0
  malformation
    type I G93.5
    type II — *see* Spina bifida
  net Q24.8
Chicago disease B40.9
Chickenpox — *see* Varicella
Chiclero ulcer or sore B55.1
Chigger (infestation) B88.0
Chignon (disease) B36.8
  newborn (from vacuum extraction) (birth injury) P12.1
Chilaiditi's syndrome (subphrenic displacement, colon) Q43.3
Chilblain(s) (lupus) T69.1 ☑
Child
  custody dispute Z65.3
Childbirth — *see* Delivery
Childhood
  cerebral X-linked adrenoleukodystrophy E71.520
  period of rapid growth Z00.2
Chill(s) R68.83
  with fever R50.9
  congestive in malarial regions B54
  without fever R68.83
Chilomastigiasis A07.8
Chimera 46,XX/46,XY Q99.0
Chin — *see* condition
Chinese dysentery A03.9
Chionophobia F40.228
Chitral fever A93.1
Chlamydia, chlamydial A74.9
  cervicitis A56.09
  conjunctivitis A74.0
  cystitis A56.01
  endometritis A56.11
  epididymitis A56.19
  female
    pelvic inflammatory disease A56.11
    pelviperitonitis A56.11
  orchitis A56.19
  peritonitis A74.81
  pharyngitis A56.4
  proctitis A56.3
  psittaci (infection) A70
  salpingitis A56.11
  sexually-transmitted infection NEC A56.8

Chlamydia, chlamydial — *continued*
  specified NEC A74.89
  urethritis A56.01
  vulvovaginitis A56.02
Chlamydiosis — *see* Chlamydia
Chloasma (skin) (idiopathic) (symptomatic) L81.1
  eyelid H02.719
    hyperthyroid E05.90 [*H02.719*]
      with thyroid storm E05.91 [*H02.719*]
    left H02.716
      lower H02.715
      upper H02.714
    right H02.713
      lower H02.712
      upper H02.711
Chloroma C92.3- ☑
Chlorosis D50.9
  Egyptian B76.9 [*D63.8*]
  miner's B76.9 [*D63.8*]
Chlorotic anemia D50.8
Chocolate cyst (ovary) N80.10- ☑
Choked
  disc or disk — *see* Papilledema
  on food, phlegm, or vomitus NOS — *see* Foreign body, by site
  while vomiting NOS — *see* Foreign body, by site
Chokes (resulting from bends) T70.3 ☑
Choking sensation R09.89
Cholangiectasis K83.8
Cholangiocarcinoma
  with hepatocellular carcinoma, combined C22.0
  liver C22.1
  specified site NEC — *see* Neoplasm, malignant, by site
  unspecified site C22.1
Cholangiohepatitis K83.8
  due to fluke infestation B66.1
Cholangiohepatoma C22.0
Cholangiolitis (acute) (chronic) (extrahepatic) (gangrenous) (intrahepatic) K83.09
  paratyphoidal — *see* Fever, paratyphoid
  typhoidal A01.09
Cholangioma D13.4
  malignant — *see* Cholangiocarcinoma
Cholangitis (ascending) (recurrent) (secondary) (stenosing) (suppurative) K83.09
  with calculus, bile duct — *see* Calculus, bile duct, with cholangitis
  chronic nonsuppurative destructive K74.3
  primary K83.09
    sclerosing K83.01
  sclerosing K83.09
Cholecystectasia K82.8
Cholecystitis K81.9
  with
    calculus, stones in
      bile duct (common) (hepatic) — *see* Calculus, bile duct, with cholecystitis
      cystic duct — *see* Calculus, gallbladder, with cholecystitis
      gallbladder — *see* Calculus, gallbladder, with cholecystitis
      choledocholithiasis — *see* Calculus, bile duct, with cholecystitis
      cholelithiasis — *see* Calculus, gallbladder, with cholecystitis
    gangrene of gallbladder K82.A1
    perforation of gallbladder K82.A2
  acute (emphysematous) (gangrenous) (suppurative) K81.0
    with
      calculus, stones in
        cystic duct — *see* Calculus, gallbladder, with cholecystitis, acute
        gallbladder — *see* Calculus, gallbladder, with cholecystitis, acute
      choledocholithiasis — *see* Calculus, bile duct, with cholecystitis, acute
      cholelithiasis — *see* Calculus, gallbladder, with cholecystitis, acute
      chronic cholecystitis K81.2
        with gallbladder calculus K80.12
          with obstruction K80.13
  chronic K81.1
    with acute cholecystitis K81.2
      with gallbladder calculus K80.12
        with obstruction K80.13
  emphysematous (acute) — *see* Cholecystitis, acute

Cholecystitis — continued
  gangrenous — see Cholecystitis, acute
  paratyphoidal, current A01.4
  suppurative — see Cholecystitis, acute
  typhoidal A01.09
Cholecystolithiasis — see Calculus, gallbladder
Choledochitis (suppurative) K83.09
Choledocholith — see Calculus, bile duct
Choledocholithiasis (common duct) (hepatic duct) —
    see Calculus, bile duct
  cystic — see Calculus, gallbladder
  typhoidal A01.09
Cholelithiasis (cystic duct) (gallbladder) (impacted)
    (multiple) — see Calculus, gallbladder
  bile duct (common) (hepatic) — see Calculus, bile duct
  hepatic duct — see Calculus, bile duct
  specified NEC K80.80
    with obstruction K80.81
Cholemia — see also Jaundice
  familial (simple) (congenital) E80.4
  Gilbert's E80.4
Choleperitoneum, choleperitonitis K65.3
Cholera (Asiatic) (epidemic) (malignant) A00.9
  antimonial — see Poisoning, antimony
  classical A00.0
  due to Vibrio cholerae 01 A00.9
    biovar cholerae A00.0
    biovar eltor A00.1
    el tor A00.1
  el tor A00.1
Cholerine — see Cholera
Cholestasis NEC K83.1
  with hepatocyte injury K71.0
  due to total parenteral nutrition (TPN) K76.89
  pure K71.0
Cholesteatoma (ear) (middle) (with reaction) H71.9- ☑
  attic H71.0- ☑
  external ear (canal) H60.4- ☑
  mastoid H71.2- ☑
  postmastoidectomy cavity (recurrent) — see Complica-
    tions, postmastoidectomy, recurrent
    cholesteatoma
  recurrent (postmastoidectomy) — see Complications,
    postmastoidectomy, recurrent cholesteatoma
  tympanum H71.1- ☑
Cholesteatosis, diffuse H71.3- ☑
Cholesteremia E78.00
Cholesterin in vitreous — see Deposit, crystalline
Cholesterol
  deposit
    retina H35.89
    vitreous — see Deposit, crystalline
  elevated (high) E78.00
    with elevated (high) triglycerides E78.2
    screening for Z13.220
  imbibition of gallbladder K82.4
Cholesterolemia (essential) (pure) E78.00
  familial E78.01
  hereditary E78.01
Cholesterolosis, cholesterosis (gallbladder) K82.4
  cerebrotendinous E75.5
Cholocolic fistula K82.3
Choluria R82.2
Chondritis M94.8X9
  auricular H61.03- ☑
  costal (Tietze's) M94.0
  external ear H61.03- ☑
  patella, posttraumatic — see Chondromalacia, patella
  pinna H61.03- ☑
  purulent M94.8X- ☑
  tuberculous NEC A18.02
    intervertebral A18.01
Chondroblastoma — see also Neoplasm, bone, benign
  malignant — see Neoplasm, bone, malignant
Chondrocalcinosis M11.20
  ankle M11.27- ☑
  elbow M11.22- ☑
  familial M11.10
    ankle M11.17- ☑
    elbow M11.12- ☑
    foot joint M11.17- ☑
    hand joint M11.14- ☑
    hip M11.15- ☑
    knee M11.16- ☑
    multiple site M11.19
    shoulder M11.11- ☑
    vertebrae M11.18

Chondrocalcinosis — continued
  familial — continued
    wrist M11.13- ☑
  foot joint M11.27- ☑
  hand joint M11.24- ☑
  hip M11.25- ☑
  knee M11.26- ☑
  multiple site M11.29
  shoulder M11.21- ☑
  specified type NEC M11.20
    ankle M11.27- ☑
    elbow M11.22- ☑
    foot joint M11.27- ☑
    hand joint M11.24- ☑
    hip M11.25- ☑
    knee M11.26- ☑
    multiple site M11.29
    shoulder M11.21- ☑
    vertebrae M11.28
    wrist M11.23- ☑
  vertebrae M11.28
  wrist M11.23- ☑
Chondrodermatitis nodularis helicis or anthelicis —
    see Perichondritis, ear
Chondrodysplasia Q78.9
  with hemangioma Q78.4
  calcificans congenita Q77.3
  fetalis Q77.4
  metaphyseal (Jansen's) (McKusick's) (Schmid's) Q78.8
  punctata Q77.3
Chondrodystrophy, chondrodystrophia (familial) (fe-
    talis) (hypoplastic) Q78.9
  calcificans congenita Q77.3
  myotonic (congenital) G71.13
  punctata Q77.3
Chondroectodermal dysplasia Q77.6
Chondrogenesis imperfecta Q77.4
Chondrolysis M94.35- ☑
Chondroma — see also Neoplasm, cartilage, benign
  juxtacortical — see Neoplasm, bone, benign
  periosteal — see Neoplasm, bone, benign
Chondromalacia (systemic) M94.20
  acromioclavicular joint M94.21- ☑
  ankle M94.27- ☑
  elbow M94.22- ☑
  foot joint M94.27- ☑
  glenohumeral joint M94.21- ☑
  hand joint M94.24- ☑
  hip M94.25- ☑
  knee M94.26- ☑
    patella M22.4- ☑
  multiple sites M94.29
  patella M22.4- ☑
  rib M94.28
  sacroiliac joint M94.259
  shoulder M94.21- ☑
  sternoclavicular joint M94.21- ☑
  vertebral joint M94.28
  wrist M94.23- ☑
Chondromatosis — see also Neoplasm, cartilage, uncer-
    tain behavior
  internal Q78.4
Chondromyxosarcoma — see Neoplasm, cartilage,
    malignant
Chondro-osteodysplasia (Morquio-Brailsford type)
    E76.219
Chondro-osteodystrophy E76.29
Chondro-osteoma — see Neoplasm, bone, benign
Chondropathia tuberosa M94.0
Chondrosarcoma — see Neoplasm, cartilage, malignant
  juxtacortical — see Neoplasm, bone, malignant
  mesenchymal — see Neoplasm, connective tissue,
    malignant
  myxoid — see Neoplasm, cartilage, malignant
Chordee (nonvenereal) N48.89
  congenital Q54.4
  gonococcal A54.09
Chorditis (fibrinous) (nodosa) (tuberosa) J38.2
Chordoma — see Neoplasm, vertebral (column), malig-
    nant
Chorea (chronic) (gravis) (posthemiplegic) (senile) (spas-
    modic) G25.5
  with
    heart involvement I02.0
      active or acute (conditions in I01-) I02.0
      rheumatic I02.9
        with valvular disorder I02.0

Chorea — continued
  with — continued
    rheumatic heart disease (chronic) (inactive) (quies-
      cent) — code to rheumatic heart condition
      involved
  drug-induced G25.4
  habit F95.8
  hereditary G10
  Huntington's G10
  hysterical F44.4
  minor I02.9
    with heart involvement I02.0
  progressive G25.5
    hereditary G10
  rheumatic (chronic) I02.9
    with heart involvement I02.0
  Sydenham's I02.9
    with heart involvement — see Chorea, with
      rheumatic heart disease
    nonrheumatic G25.5
Choreoathetosis (paroxysmal) G25.5
Chorioadenoma (destruens) D39.2
Chorioamnionitis O41.12- ☑
Chorioangioma D26.7
Choriocarcinoma — see Neoplasm, malignant, by site
  combined with
    embryonal carcinoma — see Neoplasm, malignant,
      by site
    other germ cell elements — see Neoplasm, malig-
      nant, by site
    teratoma — see Neoplasm, malignant, by site
  specified site — see Neoplasm, malignant, by site
  unspecified site
    female C58
    male C62.90
Chorioencephalitis (acute) (lymphocytic) (serous) A87.2
Chorioepithelioma — see Choriocarcinoma
Choriomeningitis (acute) (lymphocytic) (serous) A87.2
Chorionepithelioma — see Choriocarcinoma
Chorioretinitis — see also Inflammation, chorioretinal
  disseminated — see also Inflammation, chorioretinal,
    disseminated
    in neurosyphilis A52.19
  Egyptian B76.9 [D63.8]
  focal — see also Inflammation, chorioretinal, focal
  histoplasmic B39.9 [H32]
  in (due to)
    histoplasmosis B39.9 [H32]
    syphilis (secondary) A51.43
      late A52.71
    toxoplasmosis (acquired) B58.01
      congenital (active) P37.1 [H32]
    tuberculosis A18.53
  juxtapapillary, juxtapapillaris — see Inflammation,
    chorioretinal, focal, juxtapapillary
  leprous A30.9 [H32]
  miner's B76.9 [D63.8]
  progressive myopia (degeneration) — see also Myopia,
    degenerative H44.2- ☑
  syphilitic (secondary) A51.43
    congenital (early) A50.01 [H32]
      late A50.32
    late A52.71
  tuberculous A18.53
Chorioretinopathy, central serous H35.71- ☑
Choroid — see condition
Choroideremia H31.21
Choroiditis — see Chorioretinitis
Choroidopathy — see Disorder, choroid
Choroidoretinitis — see Chorioretinitis
Choroidoretinopathy, central serous — see Chori-
    oretinopathy, central serous
Christian-Weber disease M35.6
Christmas disease D67
Chromaffinoma — see also Neoplasm, benign, by site
  malignant — see Neoplasm, malignant, by site
Chromatopsia — see Deficiency, color vision
Chromhidrosis, chromidrosis L75.1
Chromoblastomycosis — see Chromomycosis
Chromoconversion R82.91
Chromomycosis B43.9
  brain abscess B43.1
  cerebral B43.1
  cutaneous B43.0
  skin B43.0
  specified NEC B43.8
  subcutaneous abscess or cyst B43.2

Chromophytosis B36.0
Chromosome — *see* Anomaly, by chromosome involved
  D (1) — *see* Anomaly, chromosome 13
  E (3) — *see* Anomaly, chromosome 18
  G — *see* Anomaly, chromosome 21
Chromotrichomycosis B36.8
Chronic — *see* condition
  fracture — *see* Fracture, pathological
Churg-Strauss syndrome M30.1
Chyle cyst, mesentery I89.8
Chylocele (nonfilarial) I89.8
  filarial — *see also* Infestation, filarial B74.9 *[N51]*
  tunica vaginalis N50.89
    filarial — *see also* Infestation, filarial B74.9 *[N51]*
Chylomicronemia (fasting) (with hyperprebetalipoproteinemia) E78.3
Chylopericardium I31.39
  acute I30.9
Chylothorax (nonfilarial) J94.0
  filarial — *see also* Infestation, filarial B74.9 *[J91.8]*
Chylous — *see* condition
Chyluria (nonfilarial) R82.0
  due to
    bilharziasis B65.0
    Brugia (malayi) B74.1
      timori B74.2
    schistosomiasis (bilharziasis) B65.0
    Wuchereria (bancrofti) B74.0
  filarial — *see* Infestation, filarial
Cicatricial (deformity) — *see* Cicatrix
Cicatrix (adherent) (contracted) (painful) (vicious) — *see also* Scar L90.5
  adenoid (and tonsil) J35.8
  alveolar process M26.79
  anus K62.89
  auricle — *see* Disorder, pinna, specified type NEC
  bile duct (common) (hepatic) K83.8
  bladder N32.89
  bone — *see* Disorder, bone, specified type NEC
  brain G93.89
  cervix (postoperative) (postpartal) N88.1
  common duct K83.8
  cornea H17.9
    tuberculous A18.59
  duodenum (bulb), obstructive K31.5
  esophagus K22.2
  eyelid — *see* Disorder, eyelid function
  hypopharynx J39.2
  lacrimal passages — *see* Obstruction, lacrimal
  larynx J38.7
  lung J98.4
  middle ear H74.8 ☑
  mouth K13.79
  muscle M62.89
    with contracture — *see* Contraction, muscle NEC
  nasopharynx J39.2
  palate (soft) K13.79
  penis N48.89
  pharynx J39.2
  prostate N42.89
  rectum K62.89
  retina — *see* Scar, chorioretinal
  semilunar cartilage — *see* Derangement, meniscus
  seminal vesicle N50.89
  skin L90.5
    infected L08.89
    postinfective L90.5
    tuberculous B90.8
  specified site NEC L90.5
  throat J39.2
  tongue K14.8
  tonsil (and adenoid) J35.8
  trachea J39.8
  tuberculous NEC B90.9
  urethra N36.8
  uterus N85.8
  vagina N89.8
    postoperative N99.2
  vocal cord J38.3
  wrist, constricting (annular) L90.5
CIDP (chronic inflammatory demyelinating polyneuropathy) G61.81
CIN — *see* Neoplasia, intraepithelial, cervix
CINCA (chronic infantile neurological, cutaneous and articular syndrome) M04.2
Cinchonism — *see* Deafness, ototoxic
  correct substance properly administered — *see* Table of Drugs and Chemicals, by drug, adverse effect

Cinchonism — *continued*
  overdose or wrong substance given or taken — *see* Table of Drugs and Chemicals, by drug, poisoning
Circle of Willis — *see* condition
Circular — *see* condition
Circulating anticoagulants — *see also* Disorder, hemorrhagic D68.318
  due to drugs — *see also* Disorder, hemorrhagic D68.32
  following childbirth O72.3
Circulation
  collateral, any site I99.8
  defective (lower extremity) I99.9
    congenital Q28.9
  embryonic Q28.9
  failure (peripheral) R57.9
    newborn P29.89
  fetal, persistent P29.38
  heart, incomplete Q28.9
Circulatory system — *see* condition
Circulus senilis (cornea) — *see* Degeneration, cornea, senile
Circumcision (in absence of medical indication) (ritual) (routine) Z41.2
Circumscribed — *see* condition
Circumvallate placenta O43.11- ☑
Cirrhosis, cirrhotic (hepatic) (liver) K74.60
  alcoholic K70.30
    with ascites K70.31
  atrophic — *see* Cirrhosis, liver
  Baumgarten-Cruveilhier K74.69
  biliary (cholangiolitic) (cholangitic) (hypertrophic) (obstructive) (pericholangiolitic) K74.5
    due to
      Clonorchiasis B66.1
      flukes B66.3
    primary K74.3
    secondary K74.4
  cardiac (of liver) K76.1
  Charcot's K74.3
  cholangiolitic, cholangitic, cholestatic (primary) K74.3
  congestive K76.1
  Cruveilhier-Baumgarten K74.69
  cryptogenic (liver) K74.69
  due to
    hepatolenticular degeneration E83.01
    Wilson's disease E83.01
    xanthomatosis E78.2
  fatty K76.0
    alcoholic K70.0
  Hanot's (hypertrophic) K74.3
  hepatic — *see* Cirrhosis, liver
  hypertrophic K74.3
  Indian childhood K74.69
  kidney — *see* Sclerosis, renal
  Laennec's K70.30
    with ascites K70.31
    alcoholic K70.30
      with ascites K70.31
    nonalcoholic K74.69
  liver K74.60
    alcoholic K70.30
      with ascites K70.31
    fatty K70.0
    congenital P78.81
    syphilitic A52.74
  lung (chronic) J84.10
  macronodular K74.69
    alcoholic K70.30
      with ascites K70.31
  micronodular K74.69
    alcoholic K70.30
      with ascites K70.31
  mixed type K74.69
  monolobular K74.3
  nephritis — *see* Sclerosis, renal
  nutritional K74.69
    alcoholic K70.30
      with ascites K70.31
  obstructive — *see* Cirrhosis, biliary
  ovarian N83.8
  pancreas (duct) K86.89
  pigmentary E83.110
  portal K74.69
    alcoholic K70.30
      with ascites K70.31
  postnecrotic K74.69
    alcoholic K70.30
      with ascites K70.31

Cirrhosis, cirrhotic — *continued*
  pulmonary J84.10
  renal — *see* Sclerosis, renal
  spleen D73.2
  stasis K76.1
  Todd's K74.3
  unilobar K74.3
  xanthomatous (biliary) K74.5
    due to xanthomatosis (familial) (metabolic) (primary) E78.2
Cistern, subarachnoid R93.0
Citrullinemia E72.23
Citrullinuria E72.23
Civatte's disease or poikiloderma L57.3
Clam digger's itch B65.3
Clammy skin R23.1
Clap — *see* Gonorrhea
Clarke-Hadfield syndrome (pancreatic infantilism) K86.89
Clark's paralysis G80.9
Clastothrix L67.8
Claude Bernard-Horner syndrome G90.2
  traumatic — *see* Injury, nerve, cervical sympathetic
Claude's disease or syndrome G46.3
Claudicatio venosa intermittens I87.8
Claudication (intermittent) I73.9
  cerebral (artery) G45.9
  spinal cord (arteriosclerotic) G95.19
    syphilitic A52.09
  venous (axillary) I87.8
Claustrophobia F40.240
Clavus (infected) L84
Clawfoot (congenital) Q66.89
  acquired — *see* Deformity, limb, clawfoot
Clawhand (acquired) — *see also* Deformity, limb, clawhand
  congenital Q68.1
Clawtoe (congenital) Q66.89
  acquired — *see* Deformity, toe, specified NEC
Clay eating — *see* Pica
Cleansing of artificial opening — *see* Attention to, artificial, opening
Cleft (congenital) — *see also* Imperfect, closure
  alveolar process M26.79
  branchial (persistent) Q18.2
    cyst Q18.0
      fistula Q18.0
      sinus Q18.0
  cricoid cartilage, posterior Q31.8
  cyst Q18.0
    fistula Q18.0
    sinus Q18.0
  foot Q72.7 ☑
  hand Q71.6 ☑
  lip (unilateral) Q36.9
    with cleft palate Q37.9
      hard Q37.1
        with soft Q37.5
      soft Q37.3
        with hard Q37.5
    bilateral Q36.0
      with cleft palate Q37.8
        hard Q37.0
          with soft Q37.4
        soft Q37.2
          with hard Q37.4
    median Q36.1
  nose Q30.2
  palate Q35.9
    with cleft lip (unilateral) Q37.9
      bilateral Q37.8
    hard Q35.1
      with
        cleft lip (unilateral) Q37.1
          bilateral Q37.0
        soft Q35.5
          with cleft lip (unilateral) Q37.5
            bilateral Q37.4
    medial Q35.5
    soft Q35.3
      with
        cleft lip (unilateral) Q37.3
          bilateral Q37.2
        hard Q35.5
          with cleft lip (unilateral) Q37.5
            bilateral Q37.4
  penis Q55.69
  scrotum Q55.29

Cleft — *continued*
  thyroid cartilage Q31.8
  uvula Q35.7
Cleidocranial dysostosis Q74.0
Cleptomania F63.2
Clicking hip (newborn) R29.4
Climacteric (female) — *see also* Menopause
  arthritis (any site) NEC — *see* Arthritis, specified form NEC
  depression (single episode) F32.89
    recurrent episode F33.8
  male (symptoms) (syndrome) NEC N50.89
  melancholia (single episode) F32.89
    recurrent episode F33.8
  paranoid state F22
  polyarthritis NEC — *see* Arthritis, specified form NEC
  symptoms (female) N95.1
Clinical research investigation (clinical trial) (control subject) (normal comparison) (participant) Z00.6
Clitoris — *see* condition
Cloaca (persistent) Q43.7
Clonorchiasis, clonorchis infection (liver) B66.1
Clonus R25.8
Closed bite M26.29
Clostridium (C.) **perfringens, as cause of disease classified elsewhere** B96.7
Closure
  congenital, nose Q30.0
  cranial sutures, premature Q75.0
  defective or imperfect NEC — *see* Imperfect, closure
  fistula, delayed — *see* Fistula
  foramen ovale, imperfect Q21.12
  hymen N89.6
  interauricular septum, defective Q21.19
  interventricular septum, defective Q21.0
  lacrimal duct — *see also* Stenosis, lacrimal, duct
    congenital Q10.5
  nose (congenital) Q30.0
    acquired M95.0
  of artificial opening — *see* Attention to, artificial, opening
  vagina N89.5
  valve — *see* Endocarditis
  vulva N90.5
Clot (blood) — *see also* Embolism
  artery (obstruction) (occlusion) — *see* Embolism
  bladder N32.89
  brain (intradural or extradural) — *see* Occlusion, artery, cerebral
  circulation I74.9
  heart — *see also* Infarct, myocardium
    not resulting in infarction I51.3
  vein — *see* Thrombosis
Clouded state R40.1
  epileptic — *see* Epilepsy, specified NEC
  paroxysmal — *see* Epilepsy, specified NEC
Cloudy antrum, antra J32.0
Clouston's (hidrotic) **ectodermal dysplasia** Q82.4
Clubbed nail pachydermoperiostosis M89.40 [L62]
Clubbing of finger(s) (nails) R68.3
Clubfinger R68.3
  congenital Q68.1
Clubfoot (congenital) Q66.89
  acquired — *see* Deformity, limb, clubfoot
  equinovarus Q66.0- ☑
  paralytic — *see* Deformity, limb, clubfoot
Clubhand (congenital) (radial) Q71.4- ☑
  acquired — *see* Deformity, limb, clubhand
Clubnail R68.3
  congenital Q84.6
Clump, kidney Q63.1
Clumsiness, clumsy child syndrome F82
Cluttering F80.81
Clutton's joints A50.51 [M12.80]
Coagulation, intravascular (diffuse) (disseminated) — *see also* Defibrination syndrome
  complicating abortion — *see* Abortion, by type, complicated by, intravascular coagulation
  following ectopic or molar pregnancy O08.1
Coagulopathy — *see also* Defect, coagulation
  consumption D65
  intravascular D65
    newborn P60
Coalition
  calcaneo-scaphoid Q66.89
  tarsal Q66.89

Coalminer's
  elbow — *see* Bursitis, elbow, olecranon
  lung or pneumoconiosis J60
Coalworker's lung or pneumoconiosis J60
Coarctation
  aorta (preductal) (postductal) Q25.1
  pulmonary artery Q25.71
Coated tongue K14.3
Coats' disease (exudative retinopathy) — *see* Retinopathy, exudative
Cocaine-induced
  anxiety disorder F14.980
  bipolar and related disorder F14.94
  depressive disorder F14.94
  obsessive-compulsive and related disorder F14.988
  psychotic disorder F14.959
  sexual dysfunction F14.981
  sleep disorder F14.982
Cocainism — *see* Disorder, cocaine use
Coccidioidomycosis B38.9
  cutaneous B38.3
  disseminated B38.7
  generalized B38.7
  meninges B38.4
  prostate B38.81
  pulmonary B38.2
    acute B38.0
    chronic B38.1
  skin B38.3
  specified NEC B38.89
Coccidioidosis — *see* Coccidioidomycosis
Coccidiosis (intestinal) A07.3
Coccydynia, coccygodynia M53.3
Coccyx — *see* condition
Cochin-China diarrhea K90.1
Cockayne's syndrome Q87.19
Cocked up toe — *see* Deformity, toe, specified NEC
Cock's peculiar tumor L72.3
Codman's tumor — *see* Neoplasm, bone, benign
Coenurosis B71.8
Coffee-worker's lung J67.8
Cogan's syndrome H16.32- ☑
  oculomotor apraxia H51.8
Coitus, painful (female) N94.10
  male N53.12
  psychogenic F52.6
Cold J00
  with influenza, flu, or grippe — *see* Influenza, with, respiratory manifestations NEC
  agglutinin disease or hemoglobinuria (chronic) D59.12
  bronchial — *see* Bronchitis
  chest — *see* Bronchitis
  common (head) J00
  effects of T69.9 ☑
    specified effect NEC T69.8 ☑
  excessive, effects of T69.9 ☑
    specified effect NEC T69.8 ☑
  exhaustion from T69.8 ☑
  exposure to T69.9 ☑
    specified effect NEC T69.8 ☑
  head J00
  injury syndrome (newborn) P80.0
  on lung — *see* Bronchitis
  rose J30.1
  sensitivity, auto-immune D59.12
  symptoms J00
  virus J00
Coldsore B00.1
Colibacillosis A49.8
  as the cause of other disease — *see also* Escherichia coli B96.20
  generalized A41.50
Colic (bilious) (infantile) (intestinal) (recurrent) (spasmodic) R10.83
  abdomen R10.83
    psychogenic F45.8
  appendix, appendicular K38.8
  bile duct — *see* Calculus, bile duct
  biliary — *see* Calculus, bile duct
  common duct — *see* Calculus, bile duct
  cystic duct — *see* Calculus, gallbladder
  Devonshire NEC — *see* Poisoning, lead
  gallbladder — *see* Calculus, gallbladder
  gallstone — *see* Calculus, gallbladder
    gallbladder or cystic duct — *see* Calculus, gallbladder
  hepatic (duct) — *see* Calculus, bile duct

Colic — *continued*
  hysterical F45.8
  kidney N23
  lead NEC — *see* Poisoning, lead
  mucous K58.9
    with diarrhea K58.0
    psychogenic F54
  nephritic N23
  painter's NEC — *see* Poisoning, lead
  pancreas K86.89
  psychogenic F45.8
  renal N23
  saturnine NEC — *see* Poisoning, lead
  ureter N23
  urethral N36.8
    due to calculus N21.1
  uterus NEC N94.89
    menstrual — *see* Dysmenorrhea
  worm NOS B83.9
Colicystitis — *see* Cystitis
Colitis (acute) (catarrhal) (chronic) (noninfective) (hemorrhagic) — *see also* Enteritis K52.9
  allergic K52.29
    with
      food protein-induced enterocolitis syndrome K52.21
      proctocolitis K52.29
  amebic (acute) — *see also* Amebiasis A06.0
    nondysenteric A06.2
  anthrax A22.2
  bacillary — *see* Infection, Shigella
  balantidial A07.0
  Clostridium difficile
    not specified as recurrent A04.72
    recurrent A04.71
  coccidial A07.3
  collagenous K52.831
  cystica superficialis K52.89
  dietary counseling and surveillance (for) Z71.3
  dietetic — *see also* Colitis, allergic K52.29
  drug-induced K52.1
  due to radiation K52.0
  eosinophilic K52.82
  food hypersensitivity — *see also* Colitis, allergic K52.29
  giardial A07.1
  granulomatous — *see* Enteritis, regional, large intestine
  indeterminate, so stated K52.3
  infectious — *see* Enteritis, infectious
  ischemic K55.9
    acute (subacute) — *see also* Ischemia, intestine, acute K55.039
    chronic K55.1
    due to mesenteric artery insufficiency K55.1
    fulminant (acute) — *see also* Ischemia, intestine, acute K55.039
  left sided K51.50
    with
      abscess K51.514
      complication K51.519
        specified NEC K51.518
      fistula K51.513
      obstruction K51.512
      rectal bleeding K51.511
  lymphocytic K52.832
  membranous
    psychogenic F54
  microscopic K52.839
    specified NEC K52.838
  mucous — *see* Syndrome, irritable, bowel
    psychogenic F54
  noninfective K52.9
    specified NEC K52.89
  polyposa — *see* Polyp, colon, inflammatory
  protozoal A07.9
  pseudomembranous
    not specified as recurrent A04.72
    recurrent A04.71
  pseudomucinous — *see* Syndrome, irritable, bowel
  regional — *see* Enteritis, regional, large intestine
    infectious A09
  segmental — *see* Enteritis, regional, large intestine
  septic — *see* Enteritis, infectious
  spastic K58.9
    with diarrhea K58.0
    psychogenic F54
  staphylococcal A04.8
    foodborne A05.0

Index

Colitis — continued
  subacute ischemic — see also Ischemia, intestine, acute
    K55.039
  thromboulcerative — see also Ischemia, intestine, acute
    K55.039
  toxic NEC K52.1
    due to Clostridium difficile
      not specified as recurrent A04.72
      recurrent A04.71
  transmural — see Enteritis, regional, large intestine
  trichomonal A07.8
  tuberculous (ulcerative) A18.32
  ulcerative (chronic) K51.90
    with
      complication K51.919
        abscess K51.914
        fistula K51.913
        obstruction K51.912
        rectal bleeding K51.911
        specified complication NEC K51.918
    enterocolitis — see Enterocolitis, ulcerative
    ileocolitis — see Ileocolitis, ulcerative
    mucosal proctocolitis — see Proctocolitis, mucosal
    proctitis — see Proctitis, ulcerative
    pseudopolyposis — see Polyp, colon, inflammatory
    psychogenic F54
    rectosigmoiditis — see Rectosigmoiditis, ulcerative
    specified type NEC K51.80
      with
        complication K51.819
          abscess K51.814
          fistula K51.813
          obstruction K51.812
          rectal bleeding K51.811
          specified complication NEC K51.818
Collagenosis, collagen disease (nonvascular) (vascular)
  M35.9
  cardiovascular I42.8
  reactive perforating L87.1
  specified NEC M35.89
Collapse R55
  adrenal E27.2
  cardiorespiratory R57.0
  cardiovascular R57.0
    newborn P29.89
  circulatory (peripheral) R57.9
    during or after labor and delivery O75.1
    following ectopic or molar pregnancy O08.3
    newborn P29.89
  during or
    after labor and delivery O75.1
    resulting from a procedure, not elsewhere classified
      T81.10 ☑
  external ear canal — see Stenosis, external ear canal
  general R55
  heart — see Disease, heart
  heat T67.1 ☑
  hysterical F44.89
  labyrinth, membranous (congenital) Q16.5
  lung (massive) — see also Atelectasis J98.19
    pressure due to anesthesia (general) (local) or other
      sedation T88.2 ☑
      during labor and delivery O74.1
      in pregnancy O29.02- ☑
      postpartum, puerperal O89.09
  myocardial — see Disease, heart
  nervous F48.8
  neurocirculatory F45.8
  nose M95.0
  postoperative T81.10 ☑
  pulmonary — see also Atelectasis J98.19
    newborn — see Atelectasis
  trachea J39.8
  tracheobronchial J98.09
  valvular — see Endocarditis
  vascular (peripheral) R57.9
    during or after labor and delivery O75.1
    following ectopic or molar pregnancy O08.3
    newborn P29.89
  vertebra M48.50- ☑
    cervical region M48.52- ☑
    cervicothoracic region M48.53- ☑
    in (due to)
      neoplasm (metastasis) M84.58- ☑
      osteoporosis — see also Osteoporosis M80.88 ☑
        cervical region M80.88 ☑
        cervicothoracic region M80.88 ☑
        lumbar region M80.88 ☑

Collapse — continued
  vertebra — continued
    in — continued
      osteoporosis — see also Osteoporosis — continued
        lumbosacral region M80.88 ☑
        multiple sites M80.88 ☑
        occipito-atlanto-axial region M80.88 ☑
        sacrococcygeal region M80.88 ☑
        thoracic region M80.88 ☑
        thoracolumbar region M80.88 ☑
      specified disease NEC M48.50- ☑
        cervical region M48.52- ☑
        cervicothoracic region M48.53- ☑
        lumbar region M48.56- ☑
        lumbosacral region M48.57- ☑
        occipito-atlanto-axial region M48.51- ☑
        sacrococcygeal region M48.58- ☑
        thoracic region M48.54- ☑
        thoracolumbar region M48.55- ☑
    lumbar region M48.56- ☑
    lumbosacral region M48.57- ☑
    occipito-atlanto-axial region M48.51- ☑
    sacrococcygeal region M48.58- ☑
    thoracic region M48.54- ☑
    thoracolumbar region M48.55- ☑
Collateral — see also condition
  circulation (venous) I87.8
  dilation, veins I87.8
Colles' fracture S52.53- ☑
Collet (-Sicard) syndrome G52.7
Collier's asthma or lung J60
Collodion baby Q80.2
Colloid nodule (of thyroid) (cystic) E04.1
Coloboma (iris) Q13.0
  eyelid Q10.3
  fundus Q14.8
  lens Q12.2
  optic disc (congenital) Q14.2
    acquired H47.31- ☑
Coloenteritis — see Enteritis
Colon — see condition
Colonization
  MRSA (Methicillin resistant Staphylococcus aureus)
    Z22.322
  MSSA (Methicillin susceptible Staphylococcus aureus)
    Z22.321
  status — see Carrier (suspected) of
Coloptosis K63.4
Color blindness — see Deficiency, color vision
Colostomy
  attention to Z43.3
  fitting or adjustment Z46.89
  malfunctioning K94.03
  status Z93.3
Colpitis (acute) — see Vaginitis
Colpocele N81.5
Colpocystitis — see Vaginitis
Colpospasm N94.2
Column, spinal, vertebral — see condition
Coma R40.20
  with
    motor response (none) R40.231 ☑
      abnormal extensor posturing to pain or noxious
        stimuli (< 2 years of age) R40.232 ☑
      abnormal flexure posturing to pain or noxious
        stimuli (0-5 years of age) R40.233 ☑
      extensor posturing to pain or noxious stimuli (2-
        5 years of age) R40.232 ☑
      flexion/decorticate posturing (< 2 years of age)
        R40.233 ☑
      localizes pain (2-5 years of age) R40.235 ☑
      normal or spontaneous movement (< 2 years of
        age) R40.236 ☑
      obeys commands (2-5 years of age) R40.236 ☑
      score of
        1 R40.231 ☑
        2 R40.232 ☑
        3 R40.233 ☑
        4 R40.234 ☑
        5 R40.235 ☑
        6 R40.236 ☑
      withdraws from pain or noxious stimuli (0-5 years
        of age) R40.234 ☑
      withdraws to touch (< 2 years of age) R40.235 ☑
    opening of eyes (never) R40.211 ☑

Coma — continued
  with — continued
    opening of eyes — continued
      in response to
        pain R40.212 ☑
        sound R40.213 ☑
      score of
        1 R40.211 ☑
        2 R40.212 ☑
        3 R40.213 ☑
        4 R40.214 ☑
      spontaneous R40.214 ☑
    verbal response (none) R40.221 ☑
      confused conversation R40.224 ☑
      cooing or babbling or crying appropriately (<2
        years of age) R40.225 ☑
      inappropriate crying or screaming (< 2 years of
        age) R40.223 ☑
      inappropriate words (2-5 years of age)
        R40.224 ☑
      inappropriate words R40.223 ☑
      incomprehensible sounds (2-5 years of age)
        R40.222 ☑
      incomprehensible words R40.222 ☑
      irritable cries (< 2 years of age) R40.224 ☑
      moans/grunts to pain; restless (< 2 years old)
        R40.222 ☑
      oriented R40.225 ☑
      score of
        1 R40.221 ☑
        2 R40.222 ☑
        3 R40.223 ☑
        4 R40.224 ☑
        5 R40.225 ☑
      screaming (2-5 years of age) R40.223 ☑
      uses appropriate words (2-5 years of age)
        R40.225 ☑
  eclamptic — see Eclampsia
  epileptic — see Epilepsy
  Glasgow, scale score — see Glasgow coma scale
  hepatic — see Failure, hepatic, by type, with coma
  hyperglycemic (diabetic) — see Diabetes, by type, with
    hyperosmolarity, with coma
  hyperosmolar (diabetic) — see Diabetes, by type, with
    hyperosmolarity, with coma
  hypoglycemic (diabetic) — see Diabetes, by type, with
    hypoglycemia, with coma
    nondiabetic E15
  in diabetes — see Diabetes, coma
  insulin-induced — see Coma, hypoglycemic
  ketoacidotic (diabetic) — see Diabetes, by type, with
    ketoacidosis, with coma
  myxedematous E03.5
  newborn P91.5
  persistent vegetative state R40.3
  specified NEC, without documented Glasgow coma
    scale score, or with partial Glasgow coma scale
    score reported R40.244 ☑
Comatose — see Coma
Combat fatigue F43.0
Combined — see condition
Comedo, comedones (giant) L70.0
Comedocarcinoma — see also Neoplasm, breast, malignant
  noninfiltrating
    breast D05.8- ☑
    specified site — see Neoplasm, in situ, by site
    unspecified site D05.8- ☑
Comedomastitis — see Ectasia, mammary duct
Comminuted fracture — code as Fracture, closed
Common
  arterial trunk Q20.0
  atrioventricular canal Q21.23
  atrium Q21.19
  cold (head) J00
  truncus (arteriosus) Q20.0
  variable immunodeficiency — see Immunodeficiency,
    common variable
  ventricle Q20.4
Commotio, commotion (current)
  brain — see Injury, intracranial, concussion
  cerebri — see Injury, intracranial, concussion
  retinae S05.8X- ☑
  spinal cord — see Injury, spinal cord, by region
  spinalis — see Injury, spinal cord, by region

Colitis — Commotio, commotion

Communication
between
base of aorta and pulmonary artery Q21.4
left ventricle and right atrium Q20.5
pericardial sac and pleural sac Q34.8
pulmonary artery and pulmonary vein, congenital Q25.72
congenital between uterus and digestive or urinary tract Q51.7
Compartment syndrome (deep) (posterior) (traumatic) T79.A0 ☑ (*following* T79.7)
abdomen T79.A3 ☑ (*following* T79.7)
lower extremity (hip, buttock, thigh, leg, foot, toes) T79.A2 ☑ (*following* T79.7)
nontraumatic
abdomen M79.A3 (*following* M79.7)
lower extremity (hip, buttock, thigh, leg, foot, toes) M79.A2- ☑ (*following* M79.7)
specified site NEC M79.A9 (*following* M79.7)
upper extremity (shoulder, arm, forearm, wrist, hand, fingers) M79.A1- ☑ (*following* M79.7)
specified site NEC T79.A9 ☑ (*following* T79.7)
upper extremity (shoulder, arm, forearm, wrist, hand, fingers) T79.A1- ☑ (*following* T79.7)
Compensation
failure — *see* Disease, heart
neurosis, psychoneurosis — *see* Disorder, factitious
Complaint — *see also* Disease
bowel, functional K59.9
psychogenic F45.8
intestine, functional K59.9
psychogenic F45.8
kidney — *see* Disease, renal
miners' J60
Complete — *see* condition
Complex
Addison-Schilder E71.528
cardiorenal — *see* Hypertension, cardiorenal
Costen's M26.69
disseminated mycobacterium avium- intracellulare (DMAC) A31.2
Eisenmenger's (ventricular septal defect) I27.83
hypersexual F52.8
jumped process, spine — *see* Dislocation, vertebra
primary, tuberculous A15.7
Schilder-Addison E71.528
subluxation (vertebral) M99.19
abdomen M99.19
acromioclavicular M99.17
cervical region M99.11
cervicothoracic M99.11
costochondral M99.18
costovertebral M99.18
head region M99.10
hip M99.15
lower extremity M99.16
lumbar region M99.13
lumbosacral M99.13
occipitocervical M99.10
pelvic region M99.15
pubic M99.15
rib cage M99.18
sacral region M99.14
sacrococcygeal M99.14
sacroiliac M99.14
specified NEC M99.19
sternochondral M99.18
sternoclavicular M99.17
thoracic region M99.12
thoracolumbar M99.12
upper extremity M99.17
Taussig-Bing (transposition, aorta and overriding pulmonary artery) Q20.1
Complication(s) (from) (of)
accidental puncture or laceration during a procedure (of) — *see* Complications, intraoperative (intraprocedural), puncture or laceration
amputation stump (surgical) (late) NEC T87.9
dehiscence T87.81
infection or inflammation T87.40
lower limb T87.4- ☑
upper limb T87.4- ☑
necrosis T87.50
lower limb T87.5- ☑
upper limb T87.5- ☑
neuroma T87.30
lower limb T87.3- ☑
upper limb T87.3- ☑

Complication(s) — *continued*
amputation stump — *continued*
specified type NEC T87.89
anastomosis (and bypass) — *see also* Complications, prosthetic device or implant
intestinal (internal) NEC K91.89
involving urinary tract N99.89
urinary tract (involving intestinal tract) N99.89
vascular — *see* Complications, cardiovascular device or implant
anesthesia, anesthetic — *see also* Anesthesia, complication T88.59 ☑
brain, postpartum, puerperal O89.2
cardiac
in
labor and delivery O74.2
pregnancy O29.19- ☑
postpartum, puerperal O89.1
central nervous system
in
labor and delivery O74.3
pregnancy O29.29- ☑
postpartum, puerperal O89.2
difficult or failed intubation T88.4 ☑
in pregnancy O29.6- ☑
failed sedation (conscious) (moderate) during procedure T88.52 ☑
general, unintended awareness during procedure T88.53 ☑
hyperthermia, malignant T88.3 ☑
hypothermia T88.51 ☑
intubation failure T88.4 ☑
malignant hyperthermia T88.3 ☑
pulmonary
in
labor and delivery O74.1
pregnancy NEC O29.09- ☑
postpartum, puerperal O89.09
shock T88.2 ☑
spinal and epidural
in
labor and delivery NEC O74.6
headache O74.5
pregnancy NEC O29.5X- ☑
postpartum, puerperal NEC O89.5
headache O89.4
unintended awareness under general anesthesia during procedure T88.53 ☑
anti-reflux device — *see* Complications, esophageal anti-reflux device
aortic (bifurcation) graft — *see* Complications, graft, vascular
aortocoronary (bypass) graft — *see* Complications, coronary artery (bypass) graft
aortofemoral (bypass) graft — *see* Complications, extremity artery (bypass) graft
arteriovenous
fistula, surgically created T82.9 ☑
embolism T82.818 ☑
fibrosis T82.828 ☑
hemorrhage T82.838 ☑
infection or inflammation T82.7 ☑
mechanical
breakdown T82.510 ☑
displacement T82.520 ☑
leakage T82.530 ☑
malposition T82.520 ☑
obstruction T82.590 ☑
perforation T82.590 ☑
protrusion T82.590 ☑
pain T82.848 ☑
specified type NEC T82.898 ☑
stenosis T82.858 ☑
thrombosis T82.868 ☑
shunt, surgically created T82.9 ☑
embolism T82.818 ☑
fibrosis T82.828 ☑
hemorrhage T82.838 ☑
infection or inflammation T82.7 ☑
mechanical
breakdown T82.511 ☑
displacement T82.521 ☑
leakage T82.531 ☑
malposition T82.521 ☑
obstruction T82.591 ☑
perforation T82.591 ☑
protrusion T82.591 ☑

Complication(s) — *continued*
arteriovenous — *continued*
shunt, surgically created — *continued*
pain T82.848 ☑
specified type NEC T82.898 ☑
stenosis T82.858 ☑
thrombosis T82.868 ☑
arthroplasty — *see* Complications, joint prosthesis
artificial
fertilization or insemination N98.9
attempted introduction (of)
embryo in embryo transfer N98.3
ovum following in vitro fertilization N98.2
hyperstimulation of ovaries N98.1
infection N98.0
specified NEC N98.8
heart T82.9 ☑
embolism T82.817 ☑
fibrosis T82.827 ☑
hemorrhage T82.837 ☑
infection or inflammation T82.7 ☑
mechanical
breakdown T82.512 ☑
displacement T82.522 ☑
leakage T82.532 ☑
malposition T82.522 ☑
obstruction T82.592 ☑
perforation T82.592 ☑
protrusion T82.592 ☑
pain T82.847 ☑
specified type NEC T82.897 ☑
stenosis T82.857 ☑
thrombosis T82.867 ☑
opening
cecostomy — *see* Complications, colostomy
colostomy — *see* Complications, colostomy
cystostomy — *see* Complications, cystostomy
enterostomy — *see* Complications, enterostomy
gastrostomy — *see* Complications, gastrostomy
ileostomy — *see* Complications, enterostomy
jejunostomy — *see* Complications, enterostomy
nephrostomy — *see* Complications, stoma, urinary tract
tracheostomy — *see* Complications, tracheostomy
ureterostomy — *see* Complications, stoma, urinary tract
urethrostomy — *see* Complications, stoma, urinary tract
balloon implant or device
gastrointestinal T85.9 ☑
embolism T85.818 ☑
fibrosis T85.828 ☑
hemorrhage T85.838 ☑
infection and inflammation T85.79 ☑
pain T85.848 ☑
specified type NEC T85.898 ☑
stenosis T85.858 ☑
thrombosis T85.868 ☑
vascular (counterpulsation) T82.9 ☑
embolism T82.818 ☑
fibrosis T82.828 ☑
hemorrhage T82.838 ☑
infection or inflammation T82.7 ☑
mechanical
breakdown T82.513 ☑
displacement T82.523 ☑
leakage T82.533 ☑
malposition T82.523 ☑
obstruction T82.593 ☑
perforation T82.593 ☑
protrusion T82.593 ☑
pain T82.848 ☑
specified type NEC T82.898 ☑
stenosis T82.858 ☑
thrombosis T82.868 ☑
bariatric procedure
gastric band procedure K95.09
infection K95.01
specified procedure NEC K95.89
infection K95.81
bile duct implant (prosthetic) T85.9 ☑
embolism T85.818 ☑
fibrosis T85.828 ☑
hemorrhage T85.838 ☑
infection and inflammation T85.79 ☑

Complication(s) — *continued*
  bile duct implant — *continued*
    mechanical
      breakdown T85.510 ☑
      displacement T85.520 ☑
      malfunction T85.510 ☑
      malposition T85.520 ☑
      obstruction T85.590 ☑
      perforation T85.590 ☑
      protrusion T85.590 ☑
      specified NEC T85.590 ☑
    pain T85.848 ☑
    specified type NEC T85.898 ☑
    stenosis T85.858 ☑
    thrombosis T85.868 ☑
  bladder device (auxiliary) — *see* Complications, genitourinary, device or implant, urinary system
  bleeding (postoperative) — *see* Complication, postoperative, hemorrhage
    intraoperative — *see* Complication, intraoperative, hemorrhage
  blood vessel graft — *see* Complications, graft, vascular
  bone
    device NEC T84.9 ☑
      embolism T84.81 ☑
      fibrosis T84.82 ☑
      hemorrhage T84.83 ☑
      infection or inflammation T84.7 ☑
      mechanical
        breakdown T84.318 ☑
        displacement T84.328 ☑
        malposition T84.328 ☑
        obstruction T84.398 ☑
        perforation T84.398 ☑
        protrusion T84.398 ☑
      pain T84.84 ☑
      specified type NEC T84.89 ☑
      stenosis T84.85 ☑
      thrombosis T84.86 ☑
    graft — *see* Complications, graft, bone
    growth stimulator (electrode) — *see* Complications, electronic stimulator device, bone
    marrow transplant — *see* Complications, transplant, bone, marrow
  brain neurostimulator (electrode) — *see* Complications, electronic stimulator device, brain
  breast implant (prosthetic) T85.9 ☑
    capsular contracture T85.44 ☑
    embolism T85.818 ☑
    fibrosis T85.828 ☑
    hemorrhage T85.838 ☑
    infection and inflammation T85.79 ☑
    mechanical
      breakdown T85.41 ☑
      displacement T85.42 ☑
      leakage T85.43 ☑
      malposition T85.42 ☑
      obstruction T85.49 ☑
      perforation T85.49 ☑
      protrusion T85.49 ☑
      specified NEC T85.49 ☑
    pain T85.848 ☑
    specified type NEC T85.898 ☑
    stenosis T85.858 ☑
    thrombosis T85.868 ☑
  bypass — *see also* Complications, prosthetic device or implant
    aortocoronary — *see* Complications, coronary artery (bypass) graft
    arterial — *see also* Complications, graft, vascular
      extremity — *see* Complications, extremity artery (bypass) graft
    cardiac — *see also* Disease, heart
      device, implant or graft T82.9 ☑
        embolism T82.817 ☑
        fibrosis T82.827 ☑
        hemorrhage T82.837 ☑
        infection or inflammation T82.7 ☑
          valve prosthesis T82.6 ☑
        mechanical
          breakdown T82.519 ☑
            specified device NEC T82.518 ☑
          displacement T82.529 ☑
            specified device NEC T82.528 ☑
          leakage T82.539 ☑
            specified device NEC T82.538 ☑

Complication(s) — *continued*
  cardiac — *see also* Disease, heart — *continued*
    device, implant or graft — *continued*
      mechanical — *continued*
        malposition T82.529 ☑
          specified device NEC T82.528 ☑
        obstruction T82.599 ☑
          specified device NEC T82.598 ☑
        perforation T82.599 ☑
          specified device NEC T82.598 ☑
        protrusion T82.599 ☑
          specified device NEC T82.598 ☑
      pain T82.847 ☑
      specified type NEC T82.897 ☑
      stenosis T82.857 ☑
      thrombosis T82.867 ☑
  cardiovascular device, graft or implant T82.9 ☑
    aortic graft — *see* Complications, graft, vascular
    arteriovenous
      fistula, artificial — *see* Complication, arteriovenous, fistula, surgically created
      shunt — *see* Complication, arteriovenous, shunt, surgically created
    artificial heart — *see* Complication, artificial, heart
    balloon (counterpulsation) device — *see* Complication, balloon implant, vascular
    carotid artery graft — *see* Complications, graft, vascular
    coronary bypass graft — *see* Complications, coronary artery (bypass) graft
    dialysis catheter (vascular) — *see* Complication, catheter, dialysis
    electronic T82.9 ☑
      electrode T82.9 ☑
        embolism T82.817 ☑
        fibrosis T82.827 ☑
        hemorrhage T82.837 ☑
        infection T82.7 ☑
        mechanical
          breakdown T82.110 ☑
          displacement T82.120 ☑
          leakage T82.190 ☑
          obstruction T82.190 ☑
          perforation T82.190 ☑
          protrusion T82.190 ☑
          specified type NEC T82.190 ☑
        pain T82.847 ☑
        specified NEC T82.897 ☑
        stenosis T82.857 ☑
        thrombosis T82.867 ☑
      embolism T82.817 ☑
      fibrosis T82.827 ☑
      hemorrhage T82.837 ☑
      infection T82.7 ☑
      mechanical
        breakdown T82.119 ☑
        displacement T82.129 ☑
        leakage T82.199 ☑
        obstruction T82.199 ☑
        perforation T82.199 ☑
        protrusion T82.199 ☑
        specified type NEC T82.199 ☑
      pain T82.847 ☑
      pulse generator T82.9 ☑
        embolism T82.817 ☑
        fibrosis T82.827 ☑
        hemorrhage T82.837 ☑
        infection T82.7 ☑
        mechanical
          breakdown T82.111 ☑
          displacement T82.121 ☑
          leakage T82.191 ☑
          obstruction T82.191 ☑
          perforation T82.191 ☑
          protrusion T82.191 ☑
          specified type NEC T82.191 ☑
        pain T82.847 ☑
        specified NEC T82.897 ☑
        stenosis T82.857 ☑
        thrombosis T82.867 ☑
      specified condition NEC T82.897 ☑
    specified device NEC T82.9 ☑
      embolism T82.817 ☑
      fibrosis T82.827 ☑
      hemorrhage T82.837 ☑
      infection T82.7 ☑

Complication(s) — *continued*
  cardiovascular device, graft or implant — *continued*
    electronic — *continued*
      specified device — *continued*
        mechanical
          breakdown T82.118 ☑
          displacement T82.128 ☑
          leakage T82.198 ☑
          obstruction T82.198 ☑
          perforation T82.198 ☑
          protrusion T82.198 ☑
          specified type NEC T82.198 ☑
        pain T82.847 ☑
        specified NEC T82.897 ☑
        stenosis T82.857 ☑
        thrombosis T82.867 ☑
      stenosis T82.857 ☑
      thrombosis T82.867 ☑
    extremity artery graft — *see* Complication, extremity artery (bypass) graft
    femoral artery graft — *see* Complication, extremity artery (bypass) graft
    heart
      transplant — *see* Complication, transplant, heart
      valve — *see* Complication, prosthetic device, heart valve
      graft — *see* Complication, heart, valve, graft
    heart-lung transplant — *see* Complication, transplant, heart, with lung
    infection or inflammation T82.7 ☑
    umbrella device — *see* Complication, umbrella device, vascular
    vascular graft (or anastomosis) — *see* Complication, graft, vascular
  carotid artery (bypass) graft — *see* Complications, graft, vascular
  catheter (device) NEC — *see also* Complications, prosthetic device or implant
    cranial infusion
      infection and inflammation T85.735 ☑
      mechanical
        breakdown T85.610 ☑
        displacement T85.620 ☑
        leakage T85.630 ☑
        malfunction T85.690 ☑
        malposition T85.620 ☑
        obstruction T85.690 ☑
        perforation T85.690 ☑
        protrusion T85.690 ☑
        specified NEC T85.690 ☑
    cystostomy T83.9 ☑
      embolism T83.81 ☑
      fibrosis T83.82 ☑
      hemorrhage T83.83 ☑
      infection and inflammation T83.510 ☑
      mechanical
        breakdown T83.010 ☑
        displacement T83.020 ☑
        leakage T83.030 ☑
        malposition T83.020 ☑
        obstruction T83.090 ☑
        perforation T83.090 ☑
        protrusion T83.090 ☑
        specified NEC T83.090 ☑
      pain T83.84 ☑
      specified type NEC T83.89 ☑
      stenosis T83.85 ☑
      thrombosis T83.86 ☑
    dialysis (vascular) T82.9 ☑
      embolism T82.818 ☑
      fibrosis T82.828 ☑
      hemorrhage T82.838 ☑
      infection and inflammation T82.7 ☑
      intraperitoneal — *see* Complications, catheter, intraperitoneal
      mechanical
        breakdown T82.41 ☑
        displacement T82.42 ☑
        leakage T82.43 ☑
        malposition T82.42 ☑
        obstruction T82.49 ☑
        perforation T82.49 ☑
        protrusion T82.49 ☑
      pain T82.848 ☑
      specified type NEC T82.898 ☑
      stenosis T82.858 ☑

Complication(s) — *continued*
  catheter — *see also* Complications, prosthetic device
    or implant — *continued*
    dialysis — *continued*
      thrombosis T82.868 ☑
    epidural infusion T85.9 ☑
      embolism T85.810 ☑
      fibrosis T85.820 ☑
      hemorrhage T85.830 ☑
      infection and inflammation T85.735 ☑
      mechanical
        breakdown T85.610 ☑
        displacement T85.620 ☑
        leakage T85.630 ☑
        malfunction T85.610 ☑
        malposition T85.620 ☑
        obstruction T85.690 ☑
        perforation T85.690 ☑
        protrusion T85.690 ☑
        specified NEC T85.690 ☑
      pain T85.840 ☑
      specified type NEC T85.890 ☑
      stenosis T85.850 ☑
      thrombosis T85.860 ☑
    intraperitoneal dialysis T85.9 ☑
      embolism T85.818 ☑
      fibrosis T85.828 ☑
      hemorrhage T85.838 ☑
      infection and inflammation T85.71 ☑
      mechanical
        breakdown T85.611 ☑
        displacement T85.621 ☑
        leakage T85.631 ☑
        malfunction T85.611 ☑
        malposition T85.621 ☑
        obstruction T85.691 ☑
        perforation T85.691 ☑
        protrusion T85.691 ☑
        specified NEC T85.691 ☑
      pain T85.848 ☑
      specified type NEC T85.898 ☑
      stenosis T85.858 ☑
      thrombosis T85.868 ☑
    intrathecal infusion
      infection and inflammation T85.735 ☑
      mechanical
        breakdown T85.610 ☑
        displacement T85.620 ☑
        leakage T85.630 ☑
        malfunction T85.690 ☑
        malposition T85.620 ☑
        obstruction T85.690 ☑
        perforation T85.690 ☑
        protrusion T85.690 ☑
        specified NEC T85.690 ☑
    intravenous infusion T82.9 ☑
      embolism T82.818 ☑
      fibrosis T82.828 ☑
      hemorrhage T82.838 ☑
      infection or inflammation T82.7 ☑
      mechanical
        breakdown T82.514 ☑
        displacement T82.524 ☑
        leakage T82.534 ☑
        malposition T82.524 ☑
        obstruction T82.594 ☑
        perforation T82.594 ☑
        protrusion T82.594 ☑
      pain T82.848 ☑
      specified type NEC T82.898 ☑
      stenosis T82.858 ☑
      thrombosis T82.868 ☑
    spinal infusion
      infection and inflammation T85.735 ☑
      mechanical
        breakdown T85.610 ☑
        displacement T85.620 ☑
        leakage T85.630 ☑
        malfunction T85.690 ☑
        malposition T85.620 ☑
        obstruction T85.690 ☑
        perforation T85.690 ☑
        protrusion T85.690 ☑
        specified NEC T85.690 ☑
    subarachnoid infusion
      infection and inflammation T85.735 ☑

Complication(s) — *continued*
  catheter — *see also* Complications, prosthetic device
    or implant — *continued*
    subarachnoid infusion — *continued*
      mechanical
        breakdown T85.610 ☑
        displacement T85.620 ☑
        leakage T85.630 ☑
        malfunction T85.690 ☑
        malposition T85.620 ☑
        obstruction T85.690 ☑
        perforation T85.690 ☑
        specified NEC T85.690 ☑
    subdural infusion T85.9 ☑
      embolism T85.810 ☑
      fibrosis T85.820 ☑
      hemorrhage T85.830 ☑
      infection and inflammation T85.735 ☑
      mechanical
        breakdown T85.610 ☑
        displacement T85.620 ☑
        leakage T85.630 ☑
        malfunction T85.610 ☑
        malposition T85.620 ☑
        obstruction T85.690 ☑
        perforation T85.690 ☑
        protrusion T85.690 ☑
        specified NEC T85.690 ☑
      pain T85.840 ☑
      specified type NEC T85.890 ☑
      stenosis T85.850 ☑
      thrombosis T85.860 ☑
    urethral T83.9 ☑
      displacement T83.028 ☑
      embolism T83.81 ☑
      fibrosis T83.82 ☑
      hemorrhage T83.83 ☑
      indwelling
        breakdown T83.011 ☑
        displacement T83.021 ☑
        infection and inflammation T83.511 ☑
        leakage T83.031 ☑
        specified complication NEC T83.091 ☑
      infection and inflammation T83.511 ☑
      leakage T83.038 ☑
      malposition T83.028 ☑
      mechanical
        breakdown T83.011 ☑
      obstruction (mechanical) T83.091 ☑
      pain T83.84 ☑
      perforation T83.091 ☑
      protrusion T83.091 ☑
      specified type NEC T83.091 ☑
      stenosis T83.85 ☑
      thrombosis T83.86 ☑
    urinary NEC
      breakdown T83.018 ☑
      displacement T83.028 ☑
      infection and inflammation T83.518 ☑
      leakage T83.038 ☑
      specified complication NEC T83.098 ☑
  cecostomy (stoma) — *see* Complications, colostomy
  cesarean delivery wound NEC O90.89
    disruption O90.0
    hematoma O90.2
    infection (following delivery) O86.00
  chemotherapy (antineoplastic) NEC T88.7 ☑
  chimeric antigen receptor (CAR-T) cell therapy
    T80.82 ☑
  chin implant (prosthetic) — *see* Complication, prosthet-
    ic device or implant, specified NEC
  circulatory system I99.8
    intraoperative I97.88
    postprocedural I97.89
      following cardiac surgery — *see also* Infarct,
        myocardium, associated with revascular-
        ization procedure I97.19- ☑
        postcardiotomy syndrome I97.0
      hypertension I97.3
      lymphedema after mastectomy I97.2
      postcardiotomy syndrome I97.0
      specified NEC I97.89
  colostomy (stoma) K94.00
    hemorrhage K94.01
    infection K94.02

Complication(s) — *continued*
  colostomy — *continued*
    malfunction K94.03
    mechanical K94.03
    specified complication NEC K94.09
  contraceptive device, intrauterine — *see* Complications,
    intrauterine, contraceptive device
  cord (umbilical) — *see* Complications, umbilical cord
  corneal graft — *see* Complications, graft, cornea
  coronary artery (bypass) graft T82.9 ☑
    atherosclerosis — *see* Arteriosclerosis, coronary
      (artery)
    embolism T82.817 ☑
    fibrosis T82.827 ☑
    hemorrhage T82.837 ☑
    infection and inflammation T82.7 ☑
    mechanical
      breakdown T82.211 ☑
      displacement T82.212 ☑
      leakage T82.213 ☑
      malposition T82.212 ☑
      obstruction T82.218 ☑
      perforation T82.218 ☑
      protrusion T82.218 ☑
      specified NEC T82.218 ☑
    pain T82.847 ☑
    specified type NEC T82.898 ☑
    stenosis T82.857 ☑
    thrombosis T82.867 ☑
  counterpulsation device (balloon), intra- aortic — *see*
    Complications, balloon implant, vascular
  cystostomy (stoma) N99.518
    catheter — *see* Complications, catheter, cystostomy
    hemorrhage N99.510
    infection N99.511
    malfunction N99.512
    specified type NEC N99.518
  delivery — *see also* Complications, obstetric O75.9
    procedure (instrumental) (manual) (surgical) O75.4
    specified NEC O75.89
  dialysis (peritoneal) (renal) — *see also* Complications,
    infusion
    catheter (vascular) — *see* Complication, catheter,
      dialysis
    peritoneal, intraperitoneal — *see* Complications,
      catheter, intraperitoneal
  dorsal column (spinal) neurostimulator — *see* Compli-
    cations, electronic stimulator device, spinal cord
  drug NEC T88.7 ☑
  ear procedure — *see also* Disorder, ear
    intraoperative H95.88
      hematoma — *see* Complications, intraoperative,
        hemorrhage (hematoma) (of), ear
      hemorrhage — *see* Complications, intraopera-
        tive, hemorrhage (hematoma) (of), ear
      laceration — *see* Complications, intraoperative,
        puncture or laceration, ear
      specified NEC H95.88
    postoperative H95.89
      external ear canal stenosis H95.81- ☑
      hematoma — *see* Complications, postprocedural,
        hematoma (of), ear
      hemorrhage — *see* Complications, postprocedu-
        ral, hemorrhage (of), ear
      postmastoidectomy — *see* Complications, post-
        mastoidectomy
      seroma — *see* Complications, postprocedural,
        seroma (of), mastoid process
      specified NEC H95.89
  ectopic pregnancy O08.9
    damage to pelvic organs O08.6
    embolism O08.2
    genital infection O08.0
    hemorrhage (delayed) (excessive) O08.1
    metabolic disorder O08.5
    renal failure O08.4
    shock O08.3
    specified type NEC O08.0
    venous complication NEC O08.7
  electronic stimulator device
    bladder (urinary) — *see* Complications, electronic
      stimulator device, urinary
    bone T84.9 ☑
      breakdown T84.310 ☑
      displacement T84.320 ☑
      embolism T84.81 ☑
      fibrosis T84.82 ☑

Complication(s) — continued

electronic stimulator device — continued

  bone — continued
- hemorrhage T84.83 ☑
- infection or inflammation T84.7 ☑
- malfunction T84.310 ☑
- malposition T84.320 ☑
- mechanical NEC T84.390 ☑
- obstruction T84.390 ☑
- pain T84.84 ☑
- perforation T84.390 ☑
- protrusion T84.390 ☑
- specified type NEC T84.89 ☑
- stenosis T84.85 ☑
- thrombosis T84.86 ☑

  brain T85.9 ☑
- embolism T85.810 ☑
- fibrosis T85.820 ☑
- hemorrhage T85.830 ☑
- infection and inflammation T85.731 ☑
- mechanical
  - breakdown T85.110 ☑
  - displacement T85.120 ☑
  - leakage T85.190 ☑
  - malposition T85.120 ☑
  - obstruction T85.190 ☑
  - perforation T85.190 ☑
  - protrusion T85.190 ☑
  - specified NEC T85.190 ☑
- pain T85.840 ☑
- specified type NEC T85.890 ☑
- stenosis T85.850 ☑
- thrombosis T85.860 ☑

  cardiac (defibrillator) (pacemaker) — see Complications, cardiovascular device or implant, electronic

  generator (brain) (gastric) (peripheral) (sacral) (spinal)
- breakdown T85.113 ☑
- displacement T85.123 ☑
- leakage T85.193 ☑
- malposition T85.123 ☑
- obstruction T85.193 ☑
- perforation T85.193 ☑
- protrusion T85.193 ☑
- specified type NEC T85.193 ☑

  muscle T84.9 ☑
- breakdown T84.418 ☑
- displacement T84.428 ☑
- embolism T84.81 ☑
- fibrosis T84.82 ☑
- hemorrhage T84.83 ☑
- infection or inflammation T84.7 ☑
- mechanical NEC T84.498 ☑
- pain T84.84 ☑
- specified type NEC T84.89 ☑
- stenosis T84.85 ☑
- thrombosis T84.86 ☑

  nervous system T85.9 ☑
- brain — see Complications, electronic stimulator device, brain
- cranial nerve — see Complications, electronic stimulator device, peripheral nerve
- embolism T85.810 ☑
- fibrosis T85.820 ☑
- gastric nerve — see Complications, electronic stimulator device, peripheral nerve
- hemorrhage T85.830 ☑
- infection and inflammation T85.738 ☑
- mechanical
  - breakdown T85.118 ☑
  - displacement T85.128 ☑
  - leakage T85.199 ☑
  - malposition T85.128 ☑
  - obstruction T85.199 ☑
  - perforation T85.199 ☑
  - protrusion T85.199 ☑
  - specified NEC T85.199 ☑
- pain T85.840 ☑
- peripheral nerve — see Complications, electronic stimulator device, peripheral nerve
- sacral nerve — see Complications, electronic stimulator device, peripheral nerve
- specified type NEC T85.890 ☑
- spinal cord — see Complications, electronic stimulator device, spinal cord

Complication(s) — continued

electronic stimulator device — continued

  nervous system — continued
- stenosis T85.850 ☑
- thrombosis T85.860 ☑
- vagal nerve — see Complications, electronic stimulator device, peripheral nerve

  peripheral nerve T85.9 ☑
- embolism T85.810 ☑
- fibrosis T85.820 ☑
- hemorrhage T85.830 ☑
- infection and inflammation T85.732 ☑
- mechanical
  - breakdown T85.111 ☑
  - displacement T85.121 ☑
  - leakage T85.191 ☑
  - malposition T85.121 ☑
  - obstruction T85.191 ☑
  - perforation T85.191 ☑
  - protrusion T85.191 ☑
  - specified NEC T85.191 ☑
- pain T85.840 ☑
- specified type NEC T85.890 ☑
- stenosis T85.850 ☑
- thrombosis T85.860 ☑

  spinal cord T85.9 ☑
- embolism T85.810 ☑
- fibrosis T85.820 ☑
- hemorrhage T85.830 ☑
- infection and inflammation T85.733 ☑
- mechanical
  - breakdown T85.112 ☑
  - displacement T85.122 ☑
  - leakage T85.192 ☑
  - malposition T85.122 ☑
  - obstruction T85.192 ☑
  - perforation T85.192 ☑
  - protrusion T85.192 ☑
  - specified NEC T85.192 ☑
- pain T85.840 ☑
- specified type NEC T85.890 ☑
- stenosis T85.850 ☑
- thrombosis T85.860 ☑

  urinary T83.9 ☑
- embolism T83.81 ☑
- fibrosis T83.82 ☑
- hemorrhage T83.83 ☑
- infection and inflammation T83.598 ☑
- mechanical
  - breakdown T83.110 ☑
  - displacement T83.120 ☑
  - malposition T83.120 ☑
  - perforation T83.190 ☑
  - protrusion T83.190 ☑
  - specified NEC T83.190 ☑
- pain T83.84 ☑
- specified type NEC T83.89 ☑
- stenosis T83.85 ☑
- thrombosis T83.86 ☑

electroshock therapy T88.9 ☑

specified NEC T88.8 ☑

endocrine E34.9
- postprocedural
  - adrenal hypofunction E89.6
  - hypoinsulinemia E89.1
  - hypoparathyroidism E89.2
  - hypopituitarism E89.3
  - hypothyroidism E89.0
  - ovarian failure E89.40
    - asymptomatic E89.40
    - symptomatic E89.41
  - specified NEC E89.89
  - testicular hypofunction E89.5

endodontic treatment NEC M27.59

enterostomy (stoma) K94.10
- hemorrhage K94.11
- infection K94.12
- malfunction K94.13
- mechanical K94.13
- specified complication NEC K94.19

episiotomy, disruption O90.1

esophageal anti-reflux device T85.9 ☑
- embolism T85.818 ☑
- fibrosis T85.828 ☑
- hemorrhage T85.838 ☑
- infection and inflammation T85.79 ☑

Complication(s) — continued

esophageal anti-reflux device — continued

  mechanical
- breakdown T85.511 ☑
- displacement T85.521 ☑
- malfunction T85.511 ☑
- malposition T85.521 ☑
- obstruction T85.591 ☑
- perforation T85.591 ☑
- protrusion T85.591 ☑
- specified NEC T85.591 ☑

  pain T85.848 ☑
  specified type NEC T85.898 ☑
  stenosis T85.858 ☑
  thrombosis T85.868 ☑

esophagostomy K94.30
- hemorrhage K94.31
- infection K94.32
- malfunction K94.33
- mechanical K94.33
- specified complication NEC K94.39

extracorporeal circulation T80.90 ☑

extremity artery (bypass) graft T82.9 ☑
- arteriosclerosis — see Arteriosclerosis, extremities, bypass graft
- embolism T82.818 ☑
- fibrosis T82.828 ☑
- hemorrhage T82.838 ☑
- infection and inflammation T82.7 ☑
- mechanical
  - breakdown T82.318 ☑
    - femoral artery T82.312 ☑
  - displacement T82.328 ☑
    - femoral artery T82.322 ☑
  - leakage T82.338 ☑
    - femoral artery T82.332 ☑
  - malposition T82.328 ☑
    - femoral artery T82.322 ☑
  - obstruction T82.398 ☑
    - femoral artery T82.392 ☑
  - perforation T82.398 ☑
    - femoral artery T82.392 ☑
  - protrusion T82.398 ☑
    - femoral artery T82.392 ☑
- pain T82.848 ☑
- specified type NEC T82.898 ☑
- stenosis T82.858 ☑
- thrombosis T82.868 ☑

eye H57.9
- corneal graft — see Complications, graft, cornea
- implant (prosthetic) T85.9 ☑
  - embolism T85.818 ☑
  - fibrosis T85.828 ☑
  - hemorrhage T85.838 ☑
  - infection and inflammation T85.79 ☑
  - mechanical
    - breakdown T85.318 ☑
    - displacement T85.328 ☑
    - leakage T85.398 ☑
    - malposition T85.328 ☑
    - obstruction T85.398 ☑
    - perforation T85.398 ☑
    - protrusion T85.398 ☑
    - specified NEC T85.398 ☑
  - pain T85.848 ☑
  - specified type NEC T85.898 ☑
  - stenosis T85.858 ☑
  - thrombosis T85.868 ☑
- intraocular lens — see Complications, intraocular lens
- orbital prosthesis — see Complications, orbital prosthesis

female genital N94.9
- device, implant or graft NEC — see Complications, genitourinary, device or implant, genital tract

femoral artery (bypass) graft — see Complication, extremity artery (bypass) graft

fixation device, internal (orthopedic) T84.9 ☑
- infection and inflammation T84.60 ☑
  - arm T84.61- ☑
    - humerus T84.61- ☑
    - radius T84.61- ☑
    - ulna T84.61- ☑
  - leg T84.629 ☑
    - femur T84.62- ☑
    - fibula T84.62- ☑

Complication(s) — *continued*
  graft — *see also* Complications, prosthetic device or
    implant — *continued*
    genital organ or tract — *see* Complications, geni-
      tourinary, device or implant, genital tract
    muscle T84.9 ☑
      breakdown T84.410 ☑
      displacement T84.420 ☑
      embolism T84.81 ☑
      fibrosis T84.82 ☑
      hemorrhage T84.83 ☑
      infection and inflammation T84.7 ☑
      mechanical NEC T84.490 ☑
      pain T84.84 ☑
      specified type NEC T84.89 ☑
      stenosis T84.85 ☑
      thrombosis T84.86 ☑
    nerve — *see* Complication, prosthetic device or im-
      plant, specified NEC
    skin — *see* Complications, prosthetic device or im-
      plant, skin graft
    tendon T84.9 ☑
      breakdown T84.410 ☑
      displacement T84.420 ☑
      embolism T84.81 ☑
      fibrosis T84.82 ☑
      hemorrhage T84.83 ☑
      infection and inflammation T84.7 ☑
      mechanical NEC T84.490 ☑
      pain T84.84 ☑
      specified type NEC T84.89 ☑
      stenosis T84.85 ☑
      thrombosis T84.86 ☑
    urinary organ T83.9 ☑
      embolism T83.81 ☑
      fibrosis T83.82 ☑
      hemorrhage T83.83 ☑
      infection and inflammation T83.598 ☑
        indwelling urethral catheter T83.511 ☑
      mechanical
        breakdown T83.21 ☑
        displacement T83.22 ☑
        erosion T83.24 ☑
        exposure T83.25 ☑
        leakage T83.23 ☑
        malposition T83.22 ☑
        obstruction T83.29 ☑
        perforation T83.29 ☑
        protrusion T83.29 ☑
        specified NEC T83.29 ☑
      pain T83.84 ☑
      specified type NEC T83.89 ☑
      stenosis T83.85 ☑
      thrombosis T83.86 ☑
    vascular T82.9 ☑
      embolism T82.818 ☑
      femoral artery — *see* Complication, extremity
        artery (bypass) graft
      fibrosis T82.828 ☑
      hemorrhage T82.838 ☑
      mechanical
        breakdown T82.319 ☑
          aorta (bifurcation) T82.310 ☑
          carotid artery T82.311 ☑
          specified vessel NEC T82.318 ☑
        displacement T82.329 ☑
          aorta (bifurcation) T82.320 ☑
          carotid artery T82.321 ☑
          specified vessel NEC T82.328 ☑
        leakage T82.339 ☑
          aorta (bifurcation) T82.330 ☑
          carotid artery T82.331 ☑
          specified vessel NEC T82.338 ☑
        malposition T82.329 ☑
          aorta (bifurcation) T82.320 ☑
          carotid artery T82.321 ☑
          specified vessel NEC T82.328 ☑
        obstruction T82.399 ☑
          aorta (bifurcation) T82.390 ☑
          carotid artery T82.391 ☑
          specified vessel NEC T82.398 ☑
        perforation T82.399 ☑
          aorta (bifurcation) T82.390 ☑
          carotid artery T82.391 ☑
          specified vessel NEC T82.398 ☑
        protrusion T82.399 ☑

Complication(s) — *continued*
  graft — *see also* Complications, prosthetic device or
    implant — *continued*
    vascular — *continued*
      mechanical — *continued*
        protrusion — *continued*
          aorta (bifurcation) T82.390 ☑
          carotid artery T82.391 ☑
          specified vessel NEC T82.398 ☑
      pain T82.848 ☑
      specified complication NEC T82.898 ☑
      stenosis T82.858 ☑
      thrombosis T82.868 ☑
  heart I51.9
    assist device
      infection and inflammation T82.7 ☑
    following acute myocardial infarction — *see* Com-
      plications, following, acute myocardial infarc-
      tion
    postoperative — *see* Complications, circulatory
      system
    transplant — *see* Complication, transplant, heart
      and lung(s) — *see* Complications, transplant,
      heart, with lung
    valve
      graft (biological) T82.9 ☑
        embolism T82.817 ☑
        fibrosis T82.827 ☑
        hemorrhage T82.837 ☑
        infection and inflammation T82.7 ☑
        mechanical T82.228 ☑
          breakdown T82.221 ☑
          displacement T82.222 ☑
          leakage T82.223 ☑
          malposition T82.222 ☑
          obstruction T82.228 ☑
          perforation T82.228 ☑
          protrusion T82.228 ☑
        pain T82.847 ☑
        specified type NEC T82.897 ☑
        stenosis T82.857 ☑
        thrombosis T82.867 ☑
      prosthesis T82.9 ☑
        embolism T82.817 ☑
        fibrosis T82.827 ☑
        hemorrhage T82.837 ☑
        infection or inflammation T82.6 ☑
        mechanical T82.09 ☑
          breakdown T82.01 ☑
          displacement T82.02 ☑
          leakage T82.03 ☑
          malposition T82.02 ☑
          obstruction T82.09 ☑
          perforation T82.09 ☑
          protrusion T82.09 ☑
        pain T82.847 ☑
        specified type NEC T82.897 ☑
          mechanical T82.09 ☑
        stenosis T82.857 ☑
        thrombosis T82.867 ☑
  hematoma
    intraoperative — *see* Complication, intraoperative,
      hemorrhage
    postprocedural — *see* Complication, postprocedu-
      ral, hematoma
  hemodialysis — *see* Complications, dialysis
  hemorrhage
    intraoperative — *see* Complication, intraoperative,
      hemorrhage
    postprocedural — *see* Complication, postprocedu-
      ral, hemorrhage
  IEC (immune effector cellular) therapy T80.82 ☑
  ileostomy (stoma) — *see* Complications, enterostomy
  immune effector cellular (IEC) therapy T80.82 ☑
  immunization (procedure) — *see* Complications, vacci-
    nation
  implant — *see also* Complications, by site and type
    urinary sphincter T83.9 ☑
      embolism T83.81 ☑
      fibrosis T83.82 ☑
      hemorrhage T83.83 ☑
      infection and inflammation T83.591 ☑
      mechanical
        breakdown T83.111 ☑
        displacement T83.121 ☑
        leakage T83.191 ☑

Complication(s) — *continued*
  implant — *see also* Complications, by site and type —
    continued
    urinary sphincter — *continued*
      mechanical — *continued*
        malposition T83.121 ☑
        obstruction T83.191 ☑
        perforation T83.191 ☑
        protrusion T83.191 ☑
        specified NEC T83.191 ☑
      pain T83.84 ☑
      specified type NEC T83.89 ☑
      stenosis T83.85 ☑
      thrombosis T83.86 ☑
  infusion (procedure) T80.90 ☑
    air embolism T80.0 ☑
    blood — *see* Complications, transfusion
    catheter — *see* Complications, catheter
    infection T80.29 ☑
    pump — *see* Complications, cardiovascular, device
      or implant
    sepsis T80.29 ☑
    serum reaction — *see also* Reaction, serum
      T80.69 ☑
      anaphylactic shock — *see also* Shock, anaphylac-
        tic T80.59 ☑
    specified type NEC T80.89 ☑
  inhalation therapy NEC T81.81 ☑
  injection (procedure) T80.90 ☑
    drug reaction — *see* Reaction, drug
    infection T80.29 ☑
    sepsis T80.29 ☑
    serum (prophylactic) (therapeutic) — *see* Complica-
      tions, vaccination
    specified type NEC T80.89 ☑
    vaccine (any) — *see* Complications, vaccination
  inoculation (any) — *see* Complications, vaccination
  insulin pump
    infection and inflammation T85.72 ☑
    mechanical
      breakdown T85.614 ☑
      displacement T85.624 ☑
      leakage T85.633 ☑
      malposition T85.624 ☑
      obstruction T85.694 ☑
      perforation T85.694 ☑
      protrusion T85.694 ☑
      specified NEC T85.694 ☑
  intestinal pouch NEC K91.858
  intraocular lens (prosthetic) T85.9 ☑
    embolism T85.818 ☑
    fibrosis T85.828 ☑
    hemorrhage T85.838 ☑
    infection and inflammation T85.79 ☑
    mechanical
      breakdown T85.21 ☑
      displacement T85.22 ☑
      malposition T85.22 ☑
      obstruction T85.29 ☑
      perforation T85.29 ☑
      protrusion T85.29 ☑
      specified NEC T85.29 ☑
    pain T85.848 ☑
    specified type NEC T85.898 ☑
    stenosis T85.858 ☑
    thrombosis T85.868 ☑
  intraoperative (intraprocedural)
    cardiac arrest — *see also* Infarct, myocardium, asso-
      ciated with revascularization procedure
      during cardiac surgery I97.710
      during other surgery I97.711
    cardiac functional disturbance NEC — *see also* In-
      farct, myocardium, associated with revascular-
      ization procedure
      during cardiac surgery I97.790
      during other surgery I97.791
    hemorrhage (hematoma) (of)
      circulatory system organ or structure
        during cardiac bypass I97.411
        during cardiac catheterization I97.410
        during other circulatory system procedure
          I97.418
        during other procedure I97.42
      digestive system organ
        during procedure on digestive system K91.61
        during procedure on other organ K91.62

Complication(s) — *continued*
intraoperative — *continued*
hemorrhage — *continued*
ear
during procedure on ear and mastoid process H95.21
during procedure on other organ H95.22
endocrine system organ or structure
during procedure on endocrine system organ or structure E36.01
during procedure on other organ E36.02
eye and adnexa
during ophthalmic procedure H59.11- ☑
during other procedure H59.12- ☑
genitourinary organ or structure
during procedure on genitourinary organ or structure N99.61
during procedure on other organ N99.62
mastoid process
during procedure on ear and mastoid process H95.21
during procedure on other organ H95.22
musculoskeletal structure
during musculoskeletal surgery M96.810
during non-orthopedic surgery M96.811
during orthopedic surgery M96.810
nervous system
during a nervous system procedure G97.31
during other procedure G97.32
respiratory system
during other procedure J95.62
during procedure on respiratory system organ or structure J95.61
skin and subcutaneous tissue
during a dermatologic procedure L76.01
during a procedure on other organ L76.02
spleen
during a procedure on other organ D78.02
during a procedure on the spleen D78.01
puncture or laceration (accidental) (unintentional) (of)
brain
during a nervous system procedure G97.48
during other procedure G97.49
circulatory system organ or structure
during circulatory system procedure I97.51
during other procedure I97.52
digestive system
during procedure on digestive system K91.71
during procedure on other organ K91.72
ear
during procedure on ear and mastoid process H95.31
during procedure on other organ H95.32
endocrine system organ or structure
during procedure on endocrine system organ or structure E36.11
during procedure on other organ E36.12
eye and adnexa
during ophthalmic procedure H59.21- ☑
during other procedure H59.22- ☑
genitourinary organ or structure
during procedure on genitourinary organ or structure N99.71
during procedure on other organ N99.72
mastoid process
during procedure on ear and mastoid process H95.31
during procedure on other organ H95.32
musculoskeletal structure
during musculoskeletal surgery M96.820
during non-orthopedic surgery M96.821
during orthopedic surgery M96.820
nervous system
during a nervous system procedure G97.48
during other procedure G97.49
respiratory system
during other procedure J95.72
during procedure on respiratory system organ or structure J95.71
skin and subcutaneous tissue
during a dermatologic procedure L76.11
during a procedure on other organ L76.12
spleen
during a procedure on other organ D78.12
during a procedure on the spleen D78.11
specified NEC
circulatory system I97.88
digestive system K91.81

intraoperative — *continued*
specified — *continued*
ear H95.88
endocrine system E36.8
eye and adnexa H59.88
genitourinary system N99.81
mastoid process H95.88
musculoskeletal structure M96.89
nervous system G97.81
respiratory system J95.88
skin and subcutaneous tissue L76.81
spleen D78.81
intraperitoneal catheter (dialysis) (infusion) — *see* Complication(s), catheter, intraperitoneal dialysis
intrathecal infusion pump
infection and inflammation T85.738 ☑
mechanical
breakdown T85.615 ☑
displacement T85.625 ☑
leakage T85.635 ☑
malfunction T85.695 ☑
malposition T85.625 ☑
obstruction T85.695 ☑
perforation T85.695 ☑
protrusion T85.695 ☑
specified NEC T85.695 ☑
intrauterine
contraceptive device
embolism T83.81 ☑
fibrosis T83.82 ☑
hemorrhage T83.83 ☑
infection and inflammation T83.69 ☑
mechanical
breakdown T83.31 ☑
displacement T83.32 ☑
malposition T83.32 ☑
obstruction T83.39 ☑
perforation T83.39 ☑
protrusion T83.39 ☑
specified NEC T83.39 ☑
pain T83.84 ☑
specified type NEC T83.89 ☑
stenosis T83.85 ☑
thrombosis T83.86 ☑
procedure (fetal), to newborn P96.5
jejunostomy (stoma) — *see* Complications, enterostomy
joint prosthesis, internal T84.9 ☑
breakage (fracture) T84.01- ☑
dislocation T84.02- ☑
fracture T84.01- ☑
infection or inflammation T84.50 ☑
hip T84.5- ☑
knee T84.5- ☑
specified joint NEC T84.59 ☑
instability T84.02- ☑
malposition — *see* Complications, joint prosthesis, mechanical, displacement
mechanical
breakage, broken T84.01- ☑
dislocation T84.02- ☑
fracture T84.01- ☑
instability T84.02- ☑
leakage — *see* Complications, joint prosthesis, mechanical, specified NEC
loosening T84.039 ☑
hip T84.03- ☑
knee T84.03- ☑
specified joint NEC T84.038 ☑
obstruction — *see* Complications, joint prosthesis, mechanical, specified NEC
perforation — *see* Complications, joint prosthesis, mechanical, specified NEC
osteolysis T84.059 ☑
hip T84.05- ☑
knee T84.05- ☑
other specified joint T84.058 ☑
periprosthetic osteolysis, by site T84.05- ☑
protrusion — *see* Complications, joint prosthesis, mechanical, specified NEC
specified complication NEC T84.099 ☑
hip T84.09- ☑
knee T84.09- ☑
other specified joint T84.098 ☑
subluxation T84.02- ☑

Complication(s) — *continued*
joint prosthesis, internal — *continued*
mechanical — *continued*
wear of articular bearing surface T84.069 ☑
hip T84.06- ☑
knee T84.06- ☑
other specified joint T84.068 ☑
specified joint NEC T84.89 ☑
embolism T84.81 ☑
fibrosis T84.82 ☑
hemorrhage T84.83 ☑
pain T84.84 ☑
specified complication NEC T84.89 ☑
stenosis T84.85 ☑
thrombosis T84.86 ☑
subluxation T84.02- ☑
kidney transplant — *see* Complications, transplant, kidney
labor O75.9
specified NEC O75.89
liver transplant (immune or nonimmune) — *see* Complications, transplant, liver
lumbar puncture G97.1
cerebrospinal fluid leak G97.0
headache or reaction G97.1
lung transplant — *see* Complications, transplant, lung
and heart — *see* Complications, transplant, lung, with heart
male genital N50.9
device, implant or graft — *see* Complications, genitourinary, device or implant, genital tract
postprocedural or postoperative — *see* Complications, genitourinary, postprocedural
specified NEC N99.89
mastoid (process) procedure
intraoperative H95.88
hematoma — *see* Complications, intraoperative, hemorrhage (hematoma) (of), mastoid process
hemorrhage — *see* Complications, intraoperative, hemorrhage (hematoma) (of), mastoid process
laceration — *see* Complications, intraoperative, puncture or laceration, mastoid process
specified NEC H95.88
postmastoidectomy — *see* Complications, postmastoidectomy
postoperative H95.89
external ear canal stenosis H95.81 ☑
hematoma — *see* Complications, postprocedural, hematoma (of), mastoid process
hemorrhage — *see* Complications, postprocedural, hemorrhage (of), mastoid process
postmastoidectomy — *see* Complications, postmastoidectomy
seroma — *see* Complications, postprocedural, seroma (of), mastoid process
specified NEC H95.89
mastoidectomy cavity — *see* Complications, postmastoidectomy
mechanical — *see* Complications, by site and type, mechanical
medical procedures — *see also* Complication(s), intraoperative T88.9 ☑
metabolic E88.9
postoperative E89.89
specified NEC E89.89
molar pregnancy NOS O08.9
damage to pelvic organs O08.6
embolism O08.2
genital infection O08.0
hemorrhage (delayed) (excessive) O08.1
metabolic disorder O08.5
renal failure O08.4
shock O08.3
specified type NEC O08.0
venous complication NEC O08.7
musculoskeletal system — *see also* Complication, intraoperative (intraprocedural), by site
device, implant or graft NEC — *see* Complications, orthopedic, device or implant
internal fixation (nail) (plate) (rod) — *see* Complications, fixation device, internal
joint prosthesis — *see* Complications, joint prosthesis
post radiation M96.89
kyphosis M96.2

Complication(s) — *continued*
- musculoskeletal system — *see also* Complication, intra-operative, by site — *continued*
  - post radiation — *continued*
    - scoliosis M96.5
    - specified complication NEC M96.89
  - postoperative (postprocedural) M96.89
    - with osteoporosis — *see* Osteoporosis
    - fracture following insertion of device — *see* Fracture, following insertion of orthopedic implant, joint prosthesis or bone plate
    - joint instability after prosthesis removal M96.89
    - lordosis M96.4
    - postlaminectomy syndrome NEC M96.1
      - kyphosis M96.3
    - pseudarthrosis M96.0
    - specified complication NEC M96.89
- nephrostomy (stoma) — *see* Complications, stoma, urinary tract, external NEC
- nervous system G98.8
  - central G96.9
    - device, implant or graft — *see also* Complication, prosthetic device or implant, specified NEC
      - electronic stimulator (electrode(s)) — *see* Complications, electronic stimulator device
      - specified NEC
        - infection and inflammation T85.738 ☑
        - mechanical T85.695 ☑
          - breakdown T85.615 ☑
          - displacement T85.625 ☑
          - leakage T85.635 ☑
          - malfunction T85.695 ☑
          - malposition T85.625 ☑
          - obstruction T85.695 ☑
          - perforation T85.695 ☑
          - protrusion T85.695 ☑
          - specified NEC T85.695 ☑
      - ventricular shunt — *see* Complications, ventricular shunt
    - electronic stimulator (electrode(s)) — *see* Complications, electronic stimulator device
    - postprocedural G97.82
      - intracranial hypotension G97.2
      - specified NEC G97.82
      - spinal fluid leak G97.0
- newborn, due to intrauterine (fetal) procedure P96.5
- nonabsorbable (permanent) sutures — *see* Complication, sutures, permanent
- obstetric O75.9
  - procedure (instrumental) (manual) (surgical) specified NEC O75.4
  - specified NEC O75.89
  - surgical wound NEC O90.89
    - hematoma O90.2
    - infection O86.00
- ocular lens implant — *see* Complications, intraocular lens
- ophthalmologic
  - postprocedural bleb — *see* Blebitis
- orbital prosthesis T85.9 ☑
  - embolism T85.818 ☑
  - fibrosis T85.828 ☑
  - hemorrhage T85.838 ☑
  - infection and inflammation T85.79 ☑
  - mechanical
    - breakdown T85.31- ☑
    - displacement T85.32- ☑
    - malposition T85.32- ☑
    - obstruction T85.39- ☑
    - perforation T85.39- ☑
    - protrusion T85.39- ☑
    - specified NEC T85.39- ☑
  - pain T85.848 ☑
  - specified type NEC T85.898 ☑
  - stenosis T85.858 ☑
  - thrombosis T85.868 ☑
- organ or tissue transplant (partial) (total) — *see* Complications, transplant
- orthopedic — *see also* Disorder, soft tissue
  - device or implant T84.9 ☑
    - bone
      - device or implant — *see* Complication, bone, device NEC
      - graft — *see* Complication, graft, bone
      - breakdown T84.418 ☑
      - displacement T84.428 ☑

Complication(s) — *continued*
- orthopedic — *see also* Disorder, soft tissue — *continued*
  - device or implant — *continued*
    - electronic bone stimulator — *see* Complications, electronic stimulator device, bone
    - embolism T84.81 ☑
    - fibrosis T84.82 ☑
    - fixation device — *see* Complication, fixation device, internal
    - hemorrhage T84.83 ☑
    - infection or inflammation T84.7 ☑
    - joint prosthesis — *see* Complication, joint prosthesis, internal
    - malfunction T84.418 ☑
    - malposition T84.428 ☑
    - mechanical NEC T84.498 ☑
    - muscle graft — *see* Complications, graft, muscle
    - obstruction T84.498 ☑
    - pain T84.84 ☑
    - perforation T84.498 ☑
    - protrusion T84.498 ☑
    - specified complication NEC T84.89 ☑
    - stenosis T84.85 ☑
    - tendon graft — *see* Complications, graft, tendon
    - thrombosis T84.86 ☑
    - fracture (following insertion of device) — *see* Fracture, following insertion of orthopedic implant, joint prosthesis or bone plate
  - postprocedural M96.89
    - fracture — *see* Fracture, following insertion of orthopedic implant, joint prosthesis or bone plate
    - postlaminectomy syndrome NEC M96.1
      - kyphosis M96.3
      - lordosis M96.4
    - postradiation
      - kyphosis M96.2
      - scoliosis M96.5
    - pseudarthrosis post-fusion M96.0
    - specified type NEC M96.89
- pacemaker (cardiac) — *see* Complications, cardiovascular device or implant, electronic
- pancreas transplant — *see* Complications, transplant, pancreas
- penile prosthesis (implant) — *see* Complications, prosthetic device, penile
- perfusion NEC T80.90 ☑
- perineal repair (obstetrical) NEC O90.89
  - disruption O90.1
  - hematoma O90.2
  - infection (following delivery) O86.09
- phototherapy T88.9 ☑
  - specified NEC T88.8 ☑
- postmastoidectomy NEC H95.19- ☑
  - cyst, mucosal H95.13- ☑
  - granulation H95.12- ☑
  - inflammation, chronic H95.11- ☑
  - recurrent cholesteatoma H95.0- ☑
- postoperative — *see* Complications, postprocedural
  - circulatory — *see* Complications, circulatory system
  - ear — *see* Complications, ear
  - endocrine — *see* Complications, endocrine
  - eye — *see* Complications, eye
  - lumbar puncture G97.1
    - cerebrospinal fluid leak G97.0
  - nervous system (central) (peripheral) — *see* Complications, nervous system
  - respiratory system — *see* Complications, respiratory system
- postprocedural — *see also* Complications, surgical procedure
  - cardiac arrest — *see also* Infarct, myocardium, associated with revascularization procedure
    - following cardiac surgery I97.120
    - following other surgery I97.121
  - cardiac functional disturbance NEC — *see also* Infarct, myocardium, associated with revascularization procedure
    - following cardiac surgery I97.190
    - following other surgery I97.191
  - cardiac insufficiency
    - following cardiac surgery I97.110
    - following other surgery I97.111
  - chorioretinal scars following retinal surgery H59.81- ☑

Complication(s) — *continued*
- postprocedural — *see also* Complications, surgical procedure — *continued*
  - following cataract surgery
    - cataract (lens) fragments H59.02- ☑
    - cystoid macular edema H59.03- ☑
    - specified NEC H59.09- ☑
    - vitreous (touch) syndrome H59.01- ☑
  - heart failure
    - following cardiac surgery I97.130
    - following other surgery I97.131
  - hematoma (of)
    - circulatory system organ or structure
      - following cardiac bypass I97.631
      - following cardiac catheterization I97.630
      - following other circulatory system procedure I97.638
      - following other procedure I97.621
    - digestive system
      - following procedure on digestive system K91.870
      - following procedure on other organ K91.871
    - ear
      - following other procedure H95.52
      - following procedure on ear and mastoid process H95.51
    - endocrine system
      - following endocrine system procedure E89.820
      - following other procedure E89.821
    - eye and adnexa
      - following ophthalmic procedure H59.33- ☑
      - following other procedure H59.34- ☑
    - genitourinary organ or structure
      - following procedure on genitourinary organ or structure N99.840
      - following procedure on other organ N99.841
    - mastoid process
      - following other procedure H95.52
      - following procedure on ear and mastoid process H95.51
    - musculoskeletal structure
      - following musculoskeletal surgery M96.840
      - following non-orthopedic surgery M96.841
      - following orthopedic surgery M96.840
    - nervous system
      - following nervous system procedure G97.61
      - following other procedure G97.62
    - respiratory system
      - following other procedure J95.861
      - following procedure on respiratory system organ or structure J95.860
    - skin and subcutaneous tissue
      - following dermatologic procedure L76.31
      - following procedure on other organ L76.32
    - spleen
      - following procedure on other organ D78.32
      - following procedure on the spleen D78.31
  - hemorrhage (of)
    - circulatory system organ or structure
      - following cardiac bypass I97.611
      - following cardiac catheterization I97.610
      - following other circulatory system procedure I97.618
      - following other procedure I97.620
    - digestive system
      - following procedure on digestive system K91.840
      - following procedure on other organ K91.841
    - ear
      - following other procedure H95.42
      - following procedure on ear and mastoid process H95.41
    - endocrine system
      - following endocrine system procedure E89.810
      - following other procedure E89.811
    - eye and adnexa
      - following ophthalmic procedure H59.31- ☑
      - following other procedure H59.32- ☑
    - genitourinary organ or structure
      - following procedure on genitourinary organ or structure N99.820
      - following procedure on other organ N99.821
    - mastoid process
      - following other procedure H95.42
      - following procedure on ear and mastoid process H95.41

Complication(s) — *continued*
  postprocedural — *see also* Complications, surgical procedure — *continued*
    hemorrhage — *continued*
      musculoskeletal structure
        following musculoskeletal surgery M96.830
        following non-orthopedic surgery M96.831
        following orthopedic surgery M96.830
      nervous system
        following nervous system procedure G97.51
        following other procedure G97.52
      respiratory system
        following a respiratory system procedure J95.830
        following other procedure J95.831
      skin and subcutaneous tissue
        following a procedure on other organ L76.22
        following dermatologic procedure L76.21
      spleen
        following procedure on other organ D78.22
        following procedure on the spleen D78.21
    seroma (of)
      circulatory system organ or structure
        following cardiac bypass I97.641
        following cardiac catheterization I97.640
        following other circulatory system procedure I97.648
        following other procedure I97.622
      digestive system
        following procedure on digestive system K91.872
        following procedure on other organ K91.873
      ear
        following other procedure H95.54
        following procedure on ear and mastoid process H95.53
      endocrine system
        following endocrine system procedure E89.822
        following other procedure E89.823
      eye and adnexa
        following ophthalmic procedure H59.35- ☑
        following other procedure H59.36- ☑
      genitourinary organ or structure
        following procedure on genitourinary organ or structure N99.842
        following procedure on other organ N99.843
      mastoid process
        following other procedure H95.54
        following procedure on ear and mastoid process H95.53
      musculoskeletal structure
        following musculoskeletal surgery M96.842
        following non-orthopedic surgery M96.843
        following orthopedic surgery M96.842
      nervous system
        following nervous system procedure G97.63
        following other procedure G97.64
      respiratory system
        following other procedure J95.863
        following procedure on respiratory system organ or structure J95.862
      skin and subcutaneous tissue
        following dermatologic procedure L76.33
        following procedure on other organ L76.34
      spleen
        following procedure on other organ D78.34
        following procedure on the spleen D78.33
  specified NEC
    circulatory system I97.89
    digestive K91.89
    ear H95.89
    endocrine E89.89
    eye and adnexa H59.89
    genitourinary N99.89
    mastoid process H95.89
    metabolic E89.89
    musculoskeletal structure M96.89
    nervous system G97.82
    respiratory system J95.89
    skin and subcutaneous tissue L76.82
    spleen D78.89
  pregnancy NEC — *see* Pregnancy, complicated by
  prosthetic device or implant T85.9 ☑
    bile duct — *see* Complications, bile duct implant
    breast — *see* Complications, breast implant

Complication(s) — *continued*
  prosthetic device or implant — *continued*
    bulking agent
      ureteral
        erosion T83.714 ☑
        exposure T83.724 ☑
      urethral
        erosion T83.713 ☑
        exposure T83.723 ☑
    cardiac and vascular NEC — *see* Complications, cardiovascular device or implant
    corneal transplant — *see* Complications, graft, cornea
    electronic nervous system stimulator — *see* Complications, electronic stimulator device
    epidural infusion catheter — *see* Complications, catheter, epidural
    esophageal anti-reflux device — *see* Complications, esophageal anti-reflux device
    genital organ or tract — *see* Complications, genitourinary, device or implant, genital tract
      specified NEC T83.79-
    heart valve — *see* Complications, heart, valve, prosthesis
    infection or inflammation T85.79 ☑
      intestine transplant T86.852
      liver transplant T86.43
      lung transplant T86.812
      pancreas transplant T86.892
      skin graft T86.822
    intraocular lens — *see* Complications, intraocular lens
    intraperitoneal (dialysis) catheter — *see* Complication(s), catheter, intraperitoneal dialysis
    joint — *see* Complications, joint prosthesis, internal
    mechanical NEC T85.698 ☑
      dialysis catheter (vascular) — *see also* Complication, catheter, dialysis, mechanical
        peritoneal — *see* Complication(s), catheter, intraperitoneal dialysis
      gastrointestinal device T85.598 ☑
      ocular device T85.398 ☑
      subdural (infusion) catheter T85.690 ☑
      suture, permanent T85.692 ☑
        that for bone repair — *see* Complications, fixation device, internal (orthopedic), mechanical
      ventricular shunt
        breakdown T85.01 ☑
        displacement T85.02 ☑
        leakage T85.03 ☑
        malposition T85.02 ☑
        obstruction T85.09 ☑
        perforation T85.09 ☑
        protrusion T85.09 ☑
        specified NEC T85.09 ☑
    mesh
      erosion (to surrounding organ or tissue) T83.718 ☑
        urethral (into pelvic floor muscles) T83.712 ☑
        vaginal (into pelvic floor muscles) T83.711 ☑
      exposure (into surrounding organ or tissue) T83.728 ☑
        urethral (through urethral wall) T83.722 ☑
        vaginal (into vagina) (through vaginal wall) T83.721 ☑
    orbital — *see* Complications, orbital prosthesis
    penile T83.9 ☑
      embolism T83.81 ☑
      fibrosis T83.82 ☑
      hemorrhage T83.83 ☑
      infection and inflammation T83.61 ☑
      mechanical
        breakdown T83.410 ☑
        displacement T83.420 ☑
        leakage T83.490 ☑
        malposition T83.420 ☑
        obstruction T83.490 ☑
        perforation T83.490 ☑
        protrusion T83.490 ☑
        specified NEC T83.490 ☑
      pain T83.84 ☑
      specified type NEC T83.89 ☑
      stenosis T83.85 ☑
      thrombosis T83.86 ☑

Complication(s) — *continued*
  prosthetic device or implant — *continued*
    prosthetic materials NEC
      erosion (to surrounding organ or tissue) T83.718 ☑
      exposure (into surrounding organ or tissue) T83.728 ☑
    skin graft T86.829
      artificial skin or decellularized allodermis
        embolism T85.818 ☑
        fibrosis T85.828 ☑
        hemorrhage T85.838 ☑
        infection and inflammation T85.79 ☑
        mechanical
          breakdown T85.613 ☑
          displacement T85.623 ☑
          malfunction T85.613 ☑
          malposition T85.623 ☑
          obstruction T85.693 ☑
          perforation T85.693 ☑
          protrusion T85.693 ☑
          specified NEC T85.693 ☑
        pain T85.848 ☑
        specified type NEC T85.898 ☑
        stenosis T85.858 ☑
        thrombosis T85.868 ☑
      failure T86.821
      infection T86.822
      rejection T86.820
      specified NEC T86.828
    sling
      urethral (female) (male)
        erosion T83.712 ☑
        exposure T83.722 ☑
    specified NEC T85.9 ☑
      embolism T85.818 ☑
      fibrosis T85.828 ☑
      hemorrhage T85.838 ☑
      infection and inflammation T85.79 ☑
      mechanical
        breakdown T85.618 ☑
        displacement T85.628 ☑
        leakage T85.638 ☑
        malfunction T85.618 ☑
        malposition T85.628 ☑
        obstruction T85.698 ☑
        perforation T85.698 ☑
        protrusion T85.698 ☑
        specified NEC T85.698 ☑
      pain T85.848 ☑
      specified type NEC T85.898 ☑
      stenosis T85.858 ☑
      thrombosis T85.868 ☑
    subdural infusion catheter — *see* Complications, catheter, subdural
    sutures — *see* Complications, sutures
    urinary organ or tract NEC — *see* Complications, genitourinary, device or implant, urinary system
    vascular — *see* Complications, cardiovascular device or implant
    ventricular shunt — *see* Complications, ventricular shunt (device)
  puerperium — *see* Puerperal
  puncture, spinal G97.1
    cerebrospinal fluid leak G97.0
    headache or reaction G97.1
  pyelogram N99.89
  radiation
    kyphosis M96.2
    scoliosis M96.5
  reattached
    extremity (infection) (rejection)
      lower T87.1X- ☑
      upper T87.0X- ☑
    specified body part NEC T87.2
  reconstructed breast
    asymmetry between native and reconstructed breast N65.1
    deformity N65.0
    disproportion between native and reconstructed breast N65.1
    excess tissue N65.0
    misshapen N65.0
  reimplant NEC — *see also* Complications, prosthetic device or implant

☑ **Additional Character Required — Refer to the Tabular List for Character Selection**

Complication(s) — *continued*
  reimplant — *see also* Complications, prosthetic device
    or implant — *continued*
    limb (infection) (rejection) — *see* Complications,
      reattached, extremity
    organ (partial) (total) — *see* Complications, trans-
      plant
    prosthetic device NEC — *see* Complications, pros-
      thetic device
  renal N28.9
    allograft — *see* Complications, transplant, kidney
    dialysis — *see* Complications, dialysis
  respirator
    mechanical J95.850
      specified NEC J95.859
  respiratory system J98.9
    device, implant or graft — *see* Complication, pros-
      thetic device or implant, specified NEC
    lung transplant — *see* Complications, prosthetic
      device or implant, lung transplant
    postoperative J95.89
      air leak J95.812
      Mendelson's syndrome (chemical pneumonitis)
        J95.4
      pneumothorax J95.811
      pulmonary insufficiency (acute) (after nontho-
        racic surgery) J95.2
        chronic J95.3
        following thoracic surgery J95.1
      respiratory failure (acute) J95.821
        acute and chronic J95.822
      specified NEC J95.89
      subglottic stenosis J95.5
      tracheostomy complication — *see* Complica-
        tions, tracheostomy
  therapy T81.89 ☑
  sedation during labor and delivery O74.9
    cardiac O74.2
    central nervous system O74.3
    pulmonary NEC O74.1
  shunt — *see also* Complications, prosthetic device or
    implant
    arteriovenous — *see* Complications, arteriovenous,
      shunt
    ventricular (communicating) — *see* Complications,
      ventricular shunt
  skin
    graft T86.829
      failure T86.821
      infection T86.822
      rejection T86.820
      specified type NEC T86.828
  spinal
    anesthesia — *see* Complications, anesthesia, spinal
    catheter (epidural) (subdural) — *see* Complications,
      catheter
    puncture or tap G97.1
      cerebrospinal fluid leak G97.0
      headache or reaction G97.1
  stent
    bile duct — *see* Complications, bile duct prosthesis
    ureteral indwelling
      breakdown T83.112 ☑
      displacement T83.122 ☑
      leakage T83.192 ☑
      malposition T83.122 ☑
      obstruction T83.192 ☑
      perforation T83.192 ☑
      protrusion T83.192 ☑
      specified NEC T83.192 ☑
    urinary NEC (ileal conduit) (nephroureteral)
      T83.193 ☑
      embolism T83.81 ☑
      fibrosis T83.82 ☑
      hemorrhage T83.83 ☑
      infection and inflammation T83.593 ☑
      mechanical
        breakdown T83.113 ☑
        displacement T83.123 ☑
        leakage T83.193 ☑
        malposition T83.123 ☑
        obstruction T83.193 ☑
        perforation T83.193 ☑
        protrusion T83.193 ☑
        specified NEC T83.193 ☑
      pain T83.84 ☑
      specified type NEC T83.89 ☑

Complication(s) — *continued*
  stent — *continued*
    urinary — *continued*
      stenosis T83.85 ☑
      thrombosis T83.86 ☑
    vascular
      end stent stenosis — *see* Restenosis, stent
      in stent stenosis — *see* Restenosis, stent
  stoma
    digestive tract
      colostomy — *see* Complications, colostomy
      enterostomy — *see* Complications, enterostomy
      esophagostomy — *see* Complications,
        esophagostomy
      gastrostomy — *see* Complications, gastrostomy
    urinary tract N99.528
      continent N99.538
        hemorrhage N99.530
        herniation N99.533
        infection N99.531
        malfunction N99.532
        specified type NEC N99.538
        stenosis N99.534
      cystostomy — *see* Complications, cystostomy
      external NOS N99.528
      hemorrhage N99.520
      herniation N99.523
      incontinent N99.528
        hemorrhage N99.520
        herniation N99.523
        infection N99.521
        malfunction N99.522
        specified type NEC N99.528
        stenosis N99.524
      infection N99.521
      malfunction N99.522
      specified type NEC N99.528
      stenosis N99.524
  stomach banding — *see* Complication(s), bariatric
    procedure
  stomach stapling — *see* Complication(s), bariatric
    procedure
  surgical material, nonabsorbable — *see* Complication,
    suture, permanent
  surgical procedure (on) T81.9 ☑
    amputation stump (late) — *see* Complications,
      amputation stump
    cardiac — *see* Complications, circulatory system
    cholesteatoma, recurrent — *see* Complications,
      postmastoidectomy, recurrent cholesteatoma
    circulatory (early) — *see* Complications, circulatory
      system
    digestive system — *see* Complications, gastrointesti-
      nal
    dumping syndrome (postgastrectomy) K91.1
    ear — *see* Complications, ear
    elephantiasis or lymphedema I97.89
      postmastectomy I97.2
    emphysema (surgical) T81.82 ☑
    endocrine — *see* Complications, endocrine
    eye — *see* Complications, eye
    fistula (persistent postoperative) T81.83 ☑
    foreign body inadvertently left in wound (sponge)
      (suture) (swab) — *see* Foreign body, acciden-
      tally left during a procedure
    gastrointestinal — *see* Complications, gastrointesti-
      nal
    genitourinary NEC N99.89
    hematoma
      intraoperative — *see* Complication, intraopera-
        tive, hemorrhage
      postprocedural — *see* Complication, postproce-
        dural, hematoma
    hemorrhage
      intraoperative — *see* Complication, intraopera-
        tive, hemorrhage
      postprocedural — *see* Complication, postproce-
        dural, hemorrhage
    hepatic failure K91.82
    hyperglycemia (postpancreatectomy) E89.1
    hypoinsulinemia (postpancreatectomy) E89.1
    hypoparathyroidism (postparathyroidectomy) E89.2
    hypopituitarism (posthypophysectomy) E89.3
    hypothyroidism (post-thyroidectomy) E89.0
    intestinal obstruction — *see also* Obstruction, intes-
      tine, postoperative K91.30
    intracranial hypotension following ventricular
      shunting (ventriculostomy) G97.2

Complication(s) — *continued*
  surgical procedure — *continued*
    lymphedema I97.89
      postmastectomy I97.2
    malabsorption (postsurgical) NEC K91.2
      osteoporosis — *see* Osteoporosis, postsurgical
        malabsorption
    mastoidectomy cavity NEC — *see* Complications,
      postmastoidectomy
    metabolic E89.89
      specified NEC E89.89
    musculoskeletal — *see* Complications, musculoskele-
      tal system
    nervous system (central) (peripheral) — *see* Compli-
      cations, nervous system
    ovarian failure E89.40
      asymptomatic E89.40
      symptomatic E89.41
    peripheral vascular — *see* Complications, surgical
      procedure, vascular
    postcardiotomy syndrome I97.0
    postcholecystectomy syndrome K91.5
    postcommissurotomy syndrome I97.0
    postgastrectomy dumping syndrome K91.1
    postlaminectomy syndrome NEC M96.1
      kyphosis M96.3
    postmastectomy lymphedema syndrome I97.2
    postmastoidectomy cholesteatoma — *see* Compli-
      cations, postmastoidectomy, recurrent
      cholesteatoma
    postvagotomy syndrome K91.1
    postvalvulotomy syndrome I97.0
    pulmonary insufficiency (acute) J95.2
      chronic J95.3
      following thoracic surgery J95.1
    reattached body part — *see* Complications, reat-
      tached
    respiratory — *see* Complications, respiratory system
    shock (hypovolemic) T81.19 ☑
    spleen (postoperative) D78.89
      intraoperative D78.81
    stitch abscess T81.41 ☑
    subglottic stenosis (postsurgical) J95.5
    testicular hypofunction E89.5
    transplant — *see* Complications, organ or tissue
      transplant
    urinary NEC N99.89
    vaginal vault prolapse (posthysterectomy) N99.3
    vascular (peripheral)
      artery T81.719 ☑
        mesenteric T81.710 ☑
        renal T81.711 ☑
        specified NEC T81.718 ☑
      vein T81.72 ☑
    wound infection T81.49 ☑
  suture, permanent (wire) NEC T85.9 ☑
    with repair of bone — *see* Complications, fixation
      device, internal
    embolism T85.818 ☑
    fibrosis T85.828 ☑
    hemorrhage T85.838 ☑
    infection and inflammation T85.79 ☑
    mechanical
      breakdown T85.612 ☑
      displacement T85.622 ☑
      malfunction T85.612 ☑
      malposition T85.622 ☑
      obstruction T85.692 ☑
      perforation T85.692 ☑
      protrusion T85.692 ☑
      specified NEC T85.692 ☑
    pain T85.848 ☑
    specified type NEC T85.898 ☑
    stenosis T85.858 ☑
    thrombosis T85.868 ☑
  tracheostomy J95.00
    granuloma J95.09
    hemorrhage J95.01
    infection J95.02
    malfunction J95.03
    mechanical J95.03
    obstruction J95.03
    specified type NEC J95.09
    tracheo-esophageal fistula J95.04
  transfusion (blood) (lymphocytes) (plasma) T80.92 ☑
    air embolism T80.0 ☑
    circulatory overload E87.71

Complication(s) — *continued*
  transfusion — *continued*
    febrile nonhemolytic transfusion reaction R50.84
    hemochromatosis E83.111
    hemolysis T80.89 ☑
    hemolytic reaction (antigen unspecified) T80.919 ☑
    incompatibility reaction (antigen unspecified) T80.919 ☑
      ABO T80.30 ☑
        delayed serologic (DSTR) T80.39 ☑
        hemolytic transfusion reaction (HTR) (unspecified time after transfusion) T80.319 ☑
          acute (AHTR) (less than 24 hours after transfusion) T80.310 ☑
          delayed (DHTR) (24 hours or more after transfusion) T80.311 ☑
        specified NEC T80.39 ☑
      acute (antigen unspecified) T80.910 ☑
      delayed (antigen unspecified) T80.911 ☑
      delayed serologic (DSTR) T80.89 ☑
      non-ABO (minor antigens (Duffy) (K) (Kell) (Kidd) (Lewis) (M) (N) (P) (S)) T80.A0 ☑ (*following* T80.4)
        delayed serologic (DSTR) T80.A9 ☑ (*following* T80.4)
        hemolytic transfusion reaction (HTR) (unspecified time after transfusion) T80.A19 ☑ (*following* T80.4)
          acute (AHTR) (less than 24 hours after transfusion) T80.A10 ☑ (*following* T80.4)
          delayed (DHTR) (24 hours or more after transfusion) T80.A11 ☑ (*following* T80.4)
        specified NEC T80.A9 ☑ (*following* T80.4)
      Rh (antigens (C) (c) (D) (E) (e)) (factor) T80.40 ☑
        delayed serologic (DSTR) T80.49 ☑
        hemolytic transfusion reaction (HTR) (unspecified time after transfusion) T80.419 ☑
          acute (AHTR) (less than 24 hours after transfusion) T80.410 ☑
          delayed (DHTR) (24 hours or more after transfusion) T80.411 ☑
        specified NEC T80.49 ☑
    infection T80.29 ☑
      acute T80.22- ☑
    reaction NEC T80.89 ☑
    sepsis T80.29 ☑
    shock T80.89 ☑
  transplant T86.90
    bone T86.839
      failure T86.831
      infection T86.832
      rejection T86.830
      specified type NEC T86.838
    bone marrow T86.00
      failure T86.02
      infection T86.03
      rejection T86.01
      specified type NEC T86.09
    cornea T86.849-
      failure T86.841- ☑
      infection T86.842- ☑
      rejection T86.840- ☑
      specified type NEC T86.848- ☑
    failure T86.92
    heart T86.20
      with lung T86.30
      cardiac allograft vasculopathy T86.290
        failure T86.32
        infection T86.33
        rejection T86.31
        specified type NEC T86.39
      failure T86.22
      infection T86.23
      rejection T86.21
      specified type NEC T86.298
    infection T86.93
    intestine T86.859
      failure T86.851
      infection T86.852
      rejection T86.850
      specified type NEC T86.858
    kidney T86.10
      failure T86.12
      infection T86.13
      rejection T86.11

Complication(s) — *continued*
  transplant — *continued*
    kidney — *continued*
      specified type NEC T86.19
    liver T86.40
      failure T86.42
      infection T86.43
      rejection T86.41
      specified type NEC T86.49
    lung T86.819
      with heart T86.30
        failure T86.32
        infection T86.33
        rejection T86.31
        specified type NEC T86.39
      failure T86.811
      infection T86.812
      rejection T86.810
      specified type NEC T86.818
    malignant neoplasm C80.2
    pancreas T86.899
      failure T86.891
      infection T86.892
      rejection T86.890
      specified type NEC T86.898
    peripheral blood stem cells T86.5
    post-transplant lymphoproliferative disorder (PTLD) D47.Z1 (*following* D47.4)
    rejection T86.91
    skin T86.829
      failure T86.821
      infection T86.822
      rejection T86.820
      specified type NEC T86.828
    specified
      tissue T86.899
        failure T86.891
        infection T86.892
        rejection T86.890
        specified type NEC T86.898
      type NEC T86.99
    stem cell (from peripheral blood) (from umbilical cord) T86.5
    umbilical cord stem cells T86.5
  trauma (early) T79.9 ☑
    specified NEC T79.8 ☑
  ultrasound therapy NEC T88.9 ☑
  umbilical cord NEC
    complicating delivery O69.9 ☑
    specified NEC O69.89 ☑
  umbrella device, vascular T82.9 ☑
    embolism T82.818 ☑
    fibrosis T82.828 ☑
    hemorrhage T82.838 ☑
    infection or inflammation T82.7 ☑
    mechanical
      breakdown T82.515 ☑
      displacement T82.525 ☑
      leakage T82.535 ☑
      malposition T82.525 ☑
      obstruction T82.595 ☑
      perforation T82.595 ☑
      protrusion T82.595 ☑
    pain T82.848 ☑
    specified type NEC T82.898 ☑
    stenosis T82.858 ☑
    thrombosis T82.868 ☑
  urethral catheter — *see* Complications, catheter, urethral, indwelling
  vaccination T88.1 ☑
    anaphylaxis NEC T80.52 ☑
    arthropathy — *see* Arthropathy, postimmunization
    cellulitis T88.0 ☑
    encephalitis or encephalomyelitis G04.02
    infection (general) (local) NEC T88.0 ☑
    meningitis G03.8
    myelitis G04.02
    protein sickness T80.62 ☑
    rash T88.1 ☑
    reaction (allergic) T88.1 ☑
      serum T80.62 ☑
    sepsis T88.0 ☑
    serum intoxication, sickness, rash, or other serum reaction NEC T80.62 ☑
      anaphylactic shock T80.52 ☑
  shock (allergic) (anaphylactic) T80.52 ☑
  vaccinia (generalized) (localized) T88.1 ☑

Complication(s) — *continued*
  vas deferens device or implant — *see* Complications, genitourinary, device or implant, genital tract
  vascular I99.9
    device or implant T82.9 ☑
      embolism T82.818 ☑
      fibrosis T82.828 ☑
      hemorrhage T82.838 ☑
      infection or inflammation T82.7 ☑
      mechanical
        breakdown T82.519 ☑
          specified device NEC T82.518 ☑
        displacement T82.529 ☑
          specified device NEC T82.528 ☑
        leakage T82.539 ☑
          specified device NEC T82.538 ☑
        malposition T82.529 ☑
          specified device NEC T82.528 ☑
        obstruction T82.599 ☑
          specified device NEC T82.598 ☑
        perforation T82.599 ☑
          specified device NEC T82.598 ☑
        protrusion T82.599 ☑
          specified device NEC T82.598 ☑
      pain T82.848 ☑
      specified type NEC T82.898 ☑
      stenosis T82.858 ☑
      thrombosis T82.868 ☑
    dialysis catheter — *see* Complication, catheter, dialysis
    following infusion, therapeutic injection or transfusion T80.1 ☑
    graft T82.9 ☑
      embolism T82.818 ☑
      fibrosis T82.828 ☑
      hemorrhage T82.838 ☑
      mechanical
        breakdown T82.319 ☑
          aorta (bifurcation) T82.310 ☑
          carotid artery T82.311 ☑
          specified vessel NEC T82.318 ☑
        displacement T82.329 ☑
          aorta (bifurcation) T82.320 ☑
          carotid artery T82.321 ☑
          specified vessel NEC T82.328 ☑
        leakage T82.339 ☑
          aorta (bifurcation) T82.330 ☑
          carotid artery T82.331 ☑
          femoral artery T82.332 ☑
          specified vessel NEC T82.338 ☑
        malposition T82.329 ☑
          aorta (bifurcation) T82.320 ☑
          carotid artery T82.321 ☑
          specified vessel NEC T82.328 ☑
        obstruction T82.399 ☑
          aorta (bifurcation) T82.390 ☑
          carotid artery T82.391 ☑
          specified vessel NEC T82.398 ☑
        perforation T82.399 ☑
          aorta (bifurcation) T82.390 ☑
          carotid artery T82.391 ☑
          specified vessel NEC T82.398 ☑
        protrusion T82.399 ☑
          aorta (bifurcation) T82.390 ☑
          carotid artery T82.391 ☑
          specified vessel NEC T82.398 ☑
      pain T82.848 ☑
      specified complication NEC T82.898 ☑
      stenosis T82.858 ☑
      thrombosis T82.868 ☑
    postoperative — *see* Complications, postoperative, circulatory
  vena cava device (filter) (sieve) (umbrella) — *see* Complications, umbrella device, vascular
  ventilation therapy NEC T81.81 ☑
  ventilator
    mechanical J95.850
      specified NEC J95.859
  ventricular (communicating) shunt (device) T85.9 ☑
    embolism T85.810 ☑
    fibrosis T85.820 ☑
    hemorrhage T85.830 ☑
    infection and inflammation T85.730 ☑
    mechanical
      breakdown T85.01 ☑
      displacement T85.02 ☑

☑ Additional Character Required — Refer to the Tabular List for Character Selection

Complication(s) — *continued*
ventricular shunt — *continued*
mechanical — *continued*
leakage T85.03 ☑
malposition T85.02 ☑
obstruction T85.09 ☑
perforation T85.09 ☑
protrusion T85.09 ☑
specified NEC T85.09 ☑
pain T85.840 ☑
specified type NEC T85.890 ☑
stenosis T85.850 ☑
thrombosis T85.860 ☑
wire suture, permanent (implanted) — *see* Complications, suture, permanent
Compressed air disease T70.3 ☑
Compression
with injury — *code by* Nature of injury
artery I77.1
celiac, syndrome I77.4
brachial plexus G54.0
brain (stem) G93.5
due to
contusion (diffuse) — *see also* Injury, intracranial, diffuse S06.A0 ☑
with herniation S06.A1 ☑
focal — *see also* Injury, intracranial, focal S06.A0 ☑
with herniation S06.A1 ☑
injury NEC — *see also* Injury, intracranial, diffuse S06.A0 ☑
nontraumatic G93.5
traumatic — *see also* Injury, intracranial, diffuse S06.A0 ☑
with herniation S06.A1 ☑
bronchus J98.09
cauda equina G83.4
celiac (artery) (axis) I77.4
cerebral — *see* Compression, brain
cervical plexus G54.2
cord
spinal — *see* Compression, spinal
umbilical — *see* Compression, umbilical cord
cranial nerve G52.9
eighth H93.3 ☑
eleventh G52.8
fifth G50.8
first G52.0
fourth — *see* Strabismus, paralytic, fourth nerve
ninth G52.1
second — *see* Disorder, nerve, optic
seventh G51.8
sixth — *see* Strabismus, paralytic, sixth nerve
tenth G52.2
third — *see* Strabismus, paralytic, third nerve
twelfth G52.3
diver's squeeze T70.3 ☑
during birth (newborn) P15.9
esophagus K22.2
eustachian tube — *see* Obstruction, eustachian tube, cartilaginous
facies Q67.1
fracture
nontraumatic NOS — *see* Collapse, vertebra
pathological — *see* Fracture, pathological
traumatic — *see* Fracture, traumatic
heart — *see* Disease, heart
intestine — *see* Obstruction, intestine
laryngeal nerve, recurrent G52.2
with paralysis of vocal cords and larynx J38.00
bilateral J38.02
unilateral J38.01
lumbosacral plexus G54.1
lung J98.4
lymphatic vessel I89.0
medulla — *see* Compression, brain
nerve — *see also* Disorder, nerve G58.9
arm NEC — *see* Mononeuropathy, upper limb
axillary G54.0
cranial — *see* Compression, cranial nerve
leg NEC — *see* Mononeuropathy, lower limb
median (in carpal tunnel) — *see* Syndrome, carpal tunnel
optic — *see* Disorder, nerve, optic
plantar — *see* Lesion, nerve, plantar
posterior tibial (in tarsal tunnel) — *see* Syndrome, tarsal tunnel

Compression — *continued*
nerve — *see also* Disorder, nerve — *continued*
root or plexus NOS (in) G54.9
intervertebral disc disorder NEC — *see* Disorder, disc, with, radiculopathy
with myelopathy — *see* Disorder, disc, with, myelopathy
neoplastic disease — *see also* Neoplasm D49.9 *[G55]*
spondylosis — *see* Spondylosis, with radiculopathy
sciatic (acute) — *see* Lesion, nerve, sciatic
sympathetic G90.8
traumatic — *see* Injury, nerve
ulnar — *see* Lesion, nerve, ulnar
upper extremity NEC — *see* Mononeuropathy, upper limb
spinal (cord) G95.20
by displacement of intervertebral disc NEC — *see also* Disorder, disc, with, myelopathy
nerve root NOS G54.9
due to displacement of intervertebral disc NEC — *see* Disorder, disc, with, radiculopathy
with myelopathy — *see* Disorder, disc, with, myelopathy
specified NEC G95.29
spondylogenic (cervical) (lumbar, lumbosacral) (thoracic) — *see* Spondylosis, with myelopathy NEC
anterior — *see* Syndrome, anterior, spinal artery, compression
traumatic — *see* Injury, spinal cord, by region
subcostal nerve (syndrome) — *see* Mononeuropathy, upper limb, specified NEC
sympathetic nerve NEC G90.8
syndrome T79.5 ☑
trachea J39.8
ulnar nerve (by scar tissue) — *see* Lesion, nerve, ulnar
umbilical cord
complicating delivery O69.2 ☑
cord around neck O69.1 ☑
prolapse O69.0 ☑
specified NEC O69.2 ☑
ureter N13.5
vein I87.5
vena cava (inferior) (superior) I87.1
Compulsion, compulsive
gambling F63.0
neurosis F42.8
personality F60.5
states F42.8
swearing F42.8
in Gilles de la Tourette's syndrome F95.2
tics and spasms F95.9
Concato's disease (pericardial polyserositis) A19.9
nontubercular I31.1
pleural — *see* Pleurisy, with effusion
Concavity chest wall M95.4
Concealed penis Q55.64
Concern (normal) **about sick person in family** Z63.6
Concrescence (teeth) K00.2
Concretio cordis I31.1
rheumatic I09.2
Concretion — *see also* Calculus
appendicular K38.1
canaliculus — *see* Dacryolith
clitoris N90.89
conjunctiva H11.12-
eyelid — *see* Disorder, eyelid, specified type NEC
lacrimal passages — *see* Dacryolith
prepuce (male) N47.8
salivary gland (any) K11.5
seminal vesicle N50.89
tonsil J35.8
Concussion (brain) (cerebral) (current) S06.0X9 ☑
with
loss of consciousness
30 minutes or less S06.0X1 ☑
brief S06.0X1 ☑
status unknown S06.0XA ☑
unspecified duration S06.0X9 ☑
no loss of consciousness S06.0X0 ☑
blast (air) (hydraulic) (immersion) (underwater)
abdomen or thorax — *see* Injury, blast, by site
ear with acoustic nerve injury — *see* Injury, nerve, acoustic, specified type NEC
cauda equina S34.3 ☑

Concussion — *continued*
conus medullaris S34.02 ☑
ocular S05.8X- ☑
spinal (cord)
cervical S14.0 ☑
lumbar S34.01 ☑
sacral S34.02 ☑
thoracic S24.0 ☑
syndrome F07.81
without loss of consciousness S06.0X0 ☑
Condition — *see also* Disease
post COVID-19 U09.9
Conditions arising in the perinatal period — *see* Newborn, affected by
Conduct disorder — *see* Disorder, conduct
Condyloma A63.0
acuminatum A63.0
gonorrheal A54.09
latum A51.31
syphilitic A51.31
congenital A50.07
venereal, syphilitic A51.31
Conflagration — *see also* Burn
asphyxia (by inhalation of gases, fumes or vapors) — *see also* Table of Drugs and Chemicals T59.9- ☑
Conflict (with) — *see also* Discord
family Z73.9
marital Z63.0
involving divorce or estrangement Z63.5
parent-child Z62.820
parent-adopted child Z62.821
parent-biological child Z62.820
parent-foster child Z62.822
social role NEC Z73.5
Confluent — *see* condition
Confusion, confused R41.0
epileptic F05
mental state (psychogenic) F44.89
psychogenic F44.89
reactive (from emotional stress, psychological trauma) F44.89
Confusional arousals G47.51
Congelation T69.9 ☑
Congenital — *see also* condition
aortic septum Q25.49
intrinsic factor deficiency D51.0
malformation — *see* Anomaly
Congestion, congestive
bladder N32.89
bowel K63.89
brain G93.89
breast N64.59
bronchial J98.09
catarrhal J31.0
chest R09.89
chill, malarial — *see* Malaria
circulatory NEC I99.8
duodenum K31.89
eye — *see* Hyperemia, conjunctiva
facial, due to birth injury P15.4
general R68.89
glottis J37.0
heart — *see* Failure, heart, congestive
hepatic K76.1
hypostatic (lung) — *see* Edema, lung
intestine K63.89
kidney N28.89
labyrinth H83.8 ☑
larynx J37.0
liver K76.1
lung R09.89
active or acute — *see* Pneumonia
malaria, malarial — *see* Malaria
nasal R09.81
nose R09.81
orbit, orbital — *see also* Exophthalmos
inflammatory (chronic) — *see* Inflammation, orbit
ovary N83.8
pancreas K86.89
pelvic, female N94.89
pleural J94.8
prostate (active) N42.1
pulmonary — *see* Congestion, lung
renal N28.89
retina H35.81
seminal vesicle N50.1
spinal cord G95.19
spleen (chronic) D73.2

Congestion, congestive — continued
- stomach K31.89
- trachea — see Tracheitis
- urethra N36.8
- uterus N85.8
  - with subinvolution N85.3
- venous (passive) I87.8
- viscera R68.89

Congestive — see Congestion

Conical
- cervix (hypertrophic elongation) N88.4
- cornea — see Keratoconus
- teeth K00.2

Conjoined twins Q89.4

Conjugal maladjustment Z63.0
- involving divorce or estrangement Z63.5

Conjunctiva — see condition

Conjunctivitis (staphylococcal) (streptococcal) NOS H10.9
- Acanthamoeba B60.12
- acute H10.3- ☑
  - atopic H10.1- ☑
  - chemical — see also Corrosion, cornea H10.21- ☑
  - mucopurulent H10.02- ☑
    - follicular H10.01- ☑
  - pseudomembranous H10.22- ☑
  - serous except viral H10.23- ☑
    - viral — see Conjunctivitis, viral
  - toxic H10.21- ☑
- adenoviral (acute) (follicular) B30.1
- allergic (acute) — see Conjunctivitis, acute, atopic
  - chronic H10.45
    - vernal H10.44
- anaphylactic — see Conjunctivitis, acute, atopic
- Apollo B30.3
- atopic (acute) — see Conjunctivitis, acute, atopic
- Béal's B30.2
- blennorrhagic (gonococcal) (neonatorum) A54.31
- chemical (acute) — see also Corrosion, cornea H10.21- ☑
- chlamydial A74.0
  - due to trachoma A71.1
  - neonatal P39.1
- chronic (nodosa) (petrificans) (phlyctenular) H10.40- ☑
  - allergic H10.45
    - vernal H10.44
  - follicular H10.43- ☑
  - giant papillary H10.41- ☑
  - simple H10.42- ☑
  - vernal H10.44
- coxsackievirus 24 B30.3
- diphtheritic A36.86
- due to
  - dust — see Conjunctivitis, acute, atopic
  - filariasis B74.9
  - mucocutaneous leishmaniasis B55.2
- enterovirus type 70 (hemorrhagic) B30.3
- epidemic (viral) B30.9
  - hemorrhagic B30.3
- gonococcal (neonatorum) A54.31
- granular (trachomatous) A71.1
  - sequelae (late effect) B94.0
- hemorrhagic (acute) (epidemic) B30.3
- herpes zoster B02.31
- in (due to)
  - Acanthamoeba B60.12
  - adenovirus (acute) (follicular) B30.1
  - Chlamydia A74.0
  - coxsackievirus 24 B30.3
  - diphtheria A36.86
  - enterovirus type 70 (hemorrhagic) B30.3
  - filariasis B74.9
  - gonococci A54.31
  - herpes (simplex) virus B00.53
    - zoster B02.31
  - infectious disease NEC B99 ☑
  - meningococci A39.89
  - mucocutaneous leishmaniasis B55.2
  - rosacea H10.82- ☑
  - syphilis (late) A52.71
  - zoster B02.31
- inclusion A74.0
- infantile P39.1
  - gonococcal A54.31
- Koch-Weeks' — see Conjunctivitis, acute, mucopurulent
- light — see Conjunctivitis, acute, atopic
- ligneous — see Blepharoconjunctivitis, ligneous
- meningococcal A39.89

Conjunctivitis — continued
- mucopurulent — see Conjunctivitis, acute, mucopurulent
- neonatal P39.1
  - gonococcal A54.31
- Newcastle B30.8
- of Béal B30.2
- parasitic
  - filariasis B74.9
  - mucocutaneous leishmaniasis B55.2
- Parinaud's H10.89
- petrificans H10.89
- rosacea H10.82- ☑
- specified NEC H10.89
- swimming-pool B30.1
- trachomatous A71.1
  - acute A71.0
  - sequelae (late effect) B94.0
- traumatic NEC H10.89
- tuberculous A18.59
- tularemic A21.1
- tularensis A21.1
- viral B30.9
  - due to
    - adenovirus B30.1
    - enterovirus B30.3
  - specified NEC B30.8

Conjunctivochalasis H11.82- ☑

Connective tissue — see condition

Conn's syndrome E26.01

Conradi (-Hunermann) **disease** Q77.3

Consanguinity Z84.3
- counseling Z71.89

Conscious simulation (of illness) Z76.5

Consecutive — see condition

Consolidation lung (base) — see Pneumonia, lobar

Constipation (atonic) (neurogenic) (simple) (spastic) K59.00
- chronic K59.09
  - idiopathic K59.04
- drug-induced K59.03
- functional K59.04
- outlet dysfunction K59.02
- psychogenic F45.8
- slow transit K59.01
- specified NEC K59.09

Constitutional — see also condition
- substandard F60.7

Constitutionally substandard F60.7

Constriction — see also Stricture
- auditory canal — see Stenosis, external ear canal
- bronchial J98.09
- duodenum K31.5
- esophagus K22.2
- external
  - abdomen, abdominal (wall) S30.841 ☑
  - alveolar process S00.542 ☑
  - ankle S90.54- ☑
  - antecubital space — see Constriction, external, forearm
  - arm (upper) S40.84- ☑
  - auricle — see Constriction, external, ear
  - axilla — see Constriction, external, arm
  - back, lower S30.840 ☑
  - breast S20.14- ☑
  - brow S00.84 ☑
  - buttock S30.840 ☑
  - calf — see Constriction, external, leg
  - canthus — see Constriction, external, eyelid
  - cheek S00.84 ☑
    - internal S00.542 ☑
  - chest wall — see Constriction, external, thorax
  - chin S00.84 ☑
  - clitoris S30.844 ☑
  - costal region — see Constriction, external, thorax
  - digit(s)
    - foot — see Constriction, external, toe
    - hand — see Constriction, external, finger
  - ear S00.44- ☑
  - elbow S50.34- ☑
  - epididymis S30.843 ☑
  - epigastric region S30.841 ☑
  - esophagus, cervical S10.14 ☑
  - eyebrow — see Constriction, external, eyelid
  - eyelid S00.24- ☑
  - face S00.84 ☑
  - finger(s) S60.44- ☑

Constriction — continued
- external — continued
  - finger(s) — continued
    - index S60.44- ☑
    - little S60.44- ☑
    - middle S60.44- ☑
    - ring S60.44- ☑
  - flank S30.841
  - foot (except toe(s) alone) S90.84- ☑
    - toe — see Constriction, external, toe
  - forearm S50.84- ☑
    - elbow only — see Constriction, external, elbow
  - forehead S00.84 ☑
  - genital organs, external
    - female S30.846 ☑
    - male S30.845 ☑
  - groin S30.841 ☑
  - gum S00.542 ☑
  - hand S60.54- ☑
  - head S00.94 ☑
    - ear — see Constriction, external, ear
    - eyelid — see Constriction, external, eyelid
    - lip S00.541 ☑
    - nose S00.34 ☑
    - oral cavity S00.542 ☑
    - scalp S00.04 ☑
    - specified site NEC S00.84 ☑
  - heel — see Constriction, external, foot
  - hip S70.24- ☑
  - inguinal region S30.841 ☑
  - interscapular region S20.449 ☑
  - jaw S00.84 ☑
  - knee S80.24- ☑
  - labium (majus) (minus) S30.844 ☑
  - larynx S10.14 ☑
  - leg (lower) S80.84- ☑
    - knee — see Constriction, external, knee
    - upper — see Constriction, external, thigh
  - lip S00.541 ☑
  - lower back S30.840 ☑
  - lumbar region S30.840 ☑
  - malar region S00.84 ☑
  - mammary — see Constriction, external, breast
  - mastoid region S00.84 ☑
  - mouth S00.542 ☑
  - nail
    - finger — see Constriction, external, finger
    - toe — see Constriction, external, toe
  - nasal S00.34 ☑
  - neck S10.94 ☑
    - specified site NEC S10.84 ☑
    - throat S10.14 ☑
  - nose S00.34 ☑
  - occipital region S00.04 ☑
  - oral cavity S00.542 ☑
  - orbital region — see Constriction, external, eyelid
  - palate S00.542 ☑
  - palm — see Constriction, external, hand
  - parietal region S00.04 ☑
  - pelvis S30.840 ☑
  - penis S30.842 ☑
  - perineum
    - female S30.844 ☑
    - male S30.840 ☑
  - periocular area — see Constriction, external, eyelid
  - phalanges
    - finger — see Constriction, external, finger
    - toe — see Constriction, external, toe
  - pharynx S10.14 ☑
  - pinna — see Constriction, external, ear
  - popliteal space — see Constriction, external, knee
  - prepuce S30.842 ☑
  - pubic region S30.840 ☑
  - pudendum
    - female S30.846 ☑
    - male S30.845 ☑
  - sacral region S30.840 ☑
  - scalp S00.04 ☑
  - scapular region — see Constriction, external, shoulder
  - scrotum S30.843 ☑
  - shin — see Constriction, external, leg
  - shoulder S40.24- ☑
  - sternal region S20.349 ☑
  - submaxillary region S00.84 ☑
  - submental region S00.84 ☑

☑ Additional Character Required — Refer to the Tabular List for Character Selection

Constriction — *continued*
　external — *continued*
　　subungual
　　　finger(s) — *see* Constriction, external, finger
　　　toe(s) — *see* Constriction, external, toe
　　supraclavicular fossa S10.84 ☑
　　supraorbital S00.84 ☑
　　temple S00.84 ☑
　　temporal region S00.84 ☑
　　testis S30.843 ☑
　　thigh S70.34- ☑
　　thorax, thoracic (wall) S20.94 ☑
　　　back S20.44- ☑
　　　front S20.34- ☑
　　throat S10.14 ☑
　　thumb S60.34- ☑
　　toe(s) (lesser) S90.44- ☑
　　　great S90.44- ☑
　　tongue S00.542 ☑
　　trachea S10.14 ☑
　　tunica vaginalis S30.843 ☑
　　uvula S00.542 ☑
　　vagina S30.844 ☑
　　vulva S30.844 ☑
　　wrist S60.84- ☑
　gallbladder — *see* Obstruction, gallbladder
　intestine — *see* Obstruction, intestine
　larynx J38.6
　　congenital Q31.8
　　　specified NEC Q31.8
　　　subglottic Q31.1
　organ or site, congenital NEC — *see* Atresia, by site
　prepuce (acquired) (congenital) N47.1
　pylorus (adult hypertrophic) K31.1
　　congenital or infantile Q40.0
　　newborn Q40.0
　ring dystocia (uterus) O62.4
　spastic — *see also* Spasm
　　ureter N13.5
　ureter N13.5
　　with infection N13.6
　urethra — *see* Stricture, urethra
　visual field (peripheral) (functional) — *see* Defect, visual field
Constrictive — *see* condition
Consultation
　medical — *see* Counseling, medical
　religious Z71.81
　specified reason NEC Z71.89
　spiritual Z71.81
　without complaint or sickness Z71.9
　　feared complaint unfounded Z71.1
　　specified reason NEC Z71.89
Consumption — *see* Tuberculosis
Contact (with) — *see also* Exposure (to)
　acariasis Z20.7
　AIDS virus Z20.6
　air pollution Z77.110
　algae and algae toxins Z77.121
　algae bloom Z77.121
　anthrax Z20.810
　aromatic amines Z77.020
　aromatic (hazardous) compounds NEC Z77.028
　aromatic dyes NOS Z77.028
　arsenic Z77.010
　asbestos Z77.090
　bacterial disease NEC Z20.818
　benzene Z77.021
　blue-green algae bloom Z77.121
　body fluids (potentially hazardous) Z77.21
　brown tide Z77.121
　chemicals (chiefly nonmedicinal) (hazardous) NEC Z77.098
　cholera Z20.09
　chromium compounds Z77.018
　communicable disease Z20.9
　　bacterial NEC Z20.818
　　specified NEC Z20.89
　　viral NEC Z20.828
　　Zika virus Z20.821
　coronavirus (disease) (novel) 2019 Z20.822
　COVID-19 Z20.822
　cyanobacteria bloom Z77.121
　dyes Z77.098
　Escherichia coli (E. coli) Z20.01
　fiberglass — *see* Table of Drugs and Chemicals, fiberglass
　German measles Z20.4

Contact — *continued*
　gonorrhea Z20.2
　hazardous metals NEC Z77.018
　hazardous substances NEC Z77.29
　hazards in the physical environment NEC Z77.128
　hazards to health NEC Z77.9
　HIV Z20.6
　HTLV-III/LAV Z20.6
　human immunodeficiency virus (HIV) Z20.6
　infection Z20.9
　　specified NEC Z20.89
　infestation (parasitic) NEC Z20.7
　intestinal infectious disease NEC Z20.09
　　Escherichia coli (E. coli) Z20.01
　lead Z77.011
　meningococcus Z20.811
　mold (toxic) Z77.120
　nickel dust Z77.018
　noise Z77.122
　parasitic disease Z20.7
　pediculosis Z20.7
　pfiesteria piscicida Z77.121
　poliomyelitis Z20.89
　pollution
　　air Z77.110
　　environmental NEC Z77.118
　　soil Z77.112
　　water Z77.111
　polycyclic aromatic hydrocarbons Z77.028
　positive maternal group B streptococcus P00.82
　rabies Z20.3
　radiation, naturally occurring NEC Z77.123
　radon Z77.123
　red tide (Florida) Z77.121
　rubella Z20.4
　SARS-CoV-2 Z20.822
　sexually-transmitted disease Z20.2
　smallpox (laboratory) Z20.89
　syphilis Z20.2
　tuberculosis Z20.1
　uranium Z77.012
　varicella Z20.820
　venereal disease Z20.2
　viral disease NEC Z20.828
　viral hepatitis Z20.5
　water pollution Z77.111
　Zika virus Z20.821
Contamination, food — *see* Intoxication, foodborne
Contraception, contraceptive
　advice Z30.09
　counseling Z30.09
　device (intrauterine) (in situ) Z97.5
　　causing menorrhagia T83.83 ☑
　　checking Z30.431
　　complications — *see* Complications, intrauterine, contraceptive device
　　in place Z97.5
　　initial prescription Z30.014
　　reinsertion Z30.433
　　removal Z30.432
　　replacement Z30.433
　emergency (postcoital) Z30.012
　initial prescription Z30.019
　　barrier Z30.018
　　diaphragm Z30.018
　　injectable Z30.013
　　intrauterine device Z30.014
　　pills Z30.011
　　postcoital (emergency) Z30.012
　　specified type NEC Z30.018
　　subdermal implantable Z30.017
　　transdermal patch hormonal Z30.016
　　vaginal ring hormonal Z30.015
　maintenance Z30.40
　　barrier Z30.49
　　diaphragm Z30.49
　　examination Z30.8
　　injectable Z30.42
　　intrauterine device Z30.431
　　pills Z30.41
　　specified type NEC Z30.49
　　subdermal implantable Z30.46
　　transdermal patch hormonal Z30.45
　　vaginal ring hormonal Z30.44
　management Z30.9
　　specified NEC Z30.8
　postcoital (emergency) Z30.012
　prescription Z30.019
　　repeat Z30.40

Contraception, contraceptive — *continued*
　sterilization Z30.2
　surveillance (drug) — *see* Contraception, maintenance
Contraction(s), contracture, contracted
　Achilles tendon — *see also* Short, tendon, Achilles
　　congenital Q66.89
　amputation stump (surgical) (flexion) (late) (next proximal joint) T87.89
　anus K59.89
　bile duct (common) (hepatic) K83.8
　bladder N32.89
　　neck or sphincter N32.0
　bowel, cecum, colon or intestine, any part — *see* Obstruction, intestine
　Braxton Hicks — *see* False, labor
　breast implant, capsular T85.44 ☑
　bronchial J98.09
　burn (old) — *see* Cicatrix
　cervix — *see* Stricture, cervix
　cicatricial — *see* Cicatrix
　conjunctiva, trachomatous, active A71.1
　　sequelae (late effect) B94.0
　Dupuytren's M72.0
　eyelid — *see* Disorder, eyelid function
　fascia (lata) (postural) M72.8
　　Dupuytren's M72.0
　　palmar M72.0
　　plantar M72.2
　finger NEC — *see also* Deformity, finger
　　congenital Q68.1
　　joint — *see* Contraction, joint, hand
　flaccid — *see* Contraction, paralytic
　gallbladder K82.0
　heart valve — *see* Endocarditis
　hip — *see* Contraction, joint, hip
　hourglass
　　bladder N32.89
　　　congenital Q64.79
　　gallbladder K82.0
　　　congenital Q44.1
　　stomach K31.89
　　　congenital Q40.2
　　　psychogenic F45.8
　　uterus (complicating delivery) O62.4
　hysterical F44.4
　internal os — *see* Stricture, cervix
　joint (abduction) (acquired) (adduction) (flexion) (rotation) M24.50
　　ankle M24.57- ☑
　　congenital NEC Q68.8
　　　hip Q65.89
　　elbow M24.52- ☑
　　foot joint M24.57- ☑
　　hand joint M24.54- ☑
　　hip M24.55- ☑
　　　congenital Q65.89
　　hysterical F44.4
　　knee M24.56- ☑
　　shoulder M24.51- ☑
　　specified site NEC M24.59
　　wrist M24.53- ☑
　kidney (granular) (secondary) N26.9
　　congenital Q63.8
　　hydronephritic — *see* Hydronephrosis
　　Page N26.2
　　pyelonephritic — *see* Pyelitis, chronic
　　tuberculous A18.11
　ligament — *see also* Disorder, ligament
　　congenital Q79.8
　muscle (postinfective) (postural) NEC M62.40
　　with contracture of joint — *see* Contraction, joint
　　ankle M62.47- ☑
　　congenital Q79.8
　　　sternocleidomastoid Q68.0
　　extraocular — *see* Strabismus
　　eye (extrinsic) — *see* Strabismus
　　foot M62.47- ☑
　　forearm M62.43- ☑
　　hand M62.44- ☑
　　hysterical F44.4
　　ischemic (Volkmann's) T79.6 ☑
　　lower leg M62.46- ☑
　　multiple sites M62.49
　　pelvic region M62.45- ☑
　　posttraumatic — *see* Strabismus, paralytic
　　psychogenic F45.8
　　　conversion reaction F44.4

☑ **Additional Character Required — Refer to the Tabular List for Character Selection**

Contusion — *continued*
- parietal
  - lobe (brain) — *see* Injury, intracranial, diffuse
    - focal — *see* Injury, intracranial, focal
  - region (scalp) S00.03 ☑
- pelvic organ S37.92 ☑
  - adrenal gland S37.812 ☑
  - bladder S37.22 ☑
  - fallopian tube — *see* Contusion, fallopian tube
  - kidney — *see* Contusion, kidney
  - ovary — *see* Contusion, ovary
  - prostate S37.822 ☑
  - specified organ NEC S37.892 ☑
  - ureter S37.12 ☑
  - urethra S37.32 ☑
  - uterus S37.62 ☑
- pelvis S30.0 ☑
- penis S30.21 ☑
- perineum
  - female S30.23 ☑
  - male S30.0 ☑
- periocular area S00.1- ☑
- peritoneum S36.81 ☑
- periurethral tissue — *see* Contusion, urethra
- pharynx S10.0 ☑
- pinna — *see* Contusion, ear
- popliteal space — *see* Contusion, knee
- prepuce S30.21 ☑
- prostate S37.822 ☑
- pubic region S30.1 ☑
- pudendum
  - female S30.202 ☑
  - male S30.201 ☑
- quadriceps femoris — *see* Contusion, thigh
- rectum S36.62 ☑
- retroperitoneum S36.892 ☑
- round ligament S37.892 ☑
- sacral region S30.0 ☑
- scalp S00.03 ☑
  - due to birth injury P12.3
- scapular region — *see* Contusion, shoulder
- sclera — *see* Contusion, eyeball
- scrotum S30.22 ☑
- seminal vesicle S37.892 ☑
- shoulder S40.01- ☑
- skin NEC T14.8 ☑
- small intestine — *see* Injury, intestine, small, contusion
- spermatic cord S30.22 ☑
- spinal cord — *see* Injury, spinal cord, by region
  - cauda equina S34.3 ☑
  - conus medullaris S34.139 ☑
- spleen S36.029 ☑
  - major S36.021 ☑
  - minor S36.020 ☑
- sternal region S20.219 ☑
- stomach S36.32 ☑
- subconjunctival S05.1- ☑
- subcutaneous NEC T14.8 ☑
- submaxillary region S00.83 ☑
- submental region S00.83 ☑
- subperiosteal NEC T14.8 ☑
- subungual
  - finger — *see* Contusion, finger, with damage to nail
  - toe — *see* Contusion, toe, with damage to nail
- supraclavicular fossa S10.83 ☑
- supraorbital S00.83 ☑
- suprarenal gland S37.812 ☑
- temple (region) S00.83 ☑
- temporal
  - lobe (brain) — *see* Injury, intracranial, diffuse
    - focal — *see* Injury, intracranial, focal
  - region S00.83 ☑
- testis S30.22 ☑
- thigh S70.1- ☑
- thorax (wall) S20.20 ☑
  - back S20.22- ☑
  - front S20.21- ☑
- throat S10.0 ☑
- thumb S60.01- ☑
  - with damage to nail S60.11- ☑
- toe(s) (lesser) S90.12- ☑
  - with damage to nail S90.22- ☑
  - great S90.11- ☑
    - with damage to nail S90.21- ☑
- tongue S00.532 ☑
- trachea (cervical) S10.0 ☑

Contusion — *continued*
- trachea — *continued*
  - thoracic S27.52 ☑
- tunica vaginalis S30.22 ☑
- tympanum, tympanic membrane — *see* Contusion, ear
- ureter S37.12 ☑
- urethra S37.32 ☑
- urinary organ NEC S37.892 ☑
- uterus S37.62 ☑
- uvula S00.532 ☑
- vagina S30.23 ☑
- vas deferens S37.892 ☑
- vesical S37.22 ☑
- vocal cord(s) S10.0 ☑
- vulva S30.23 ☑
- wrist S60.21- ☑

Conus (congenital) (any type) Q14.8
- cornea — *see* Keratoconus
- medullaris syndrome G95.81

Conversion hysteria, neurosis or reaction F44.9

Converter, tuberculosis (test reaction) R76.11

Conviction (legal), **anxiety concerning** Z65.0
- with imprisonment Z65.1

Convulsions (idiopathic) — *see also* Seizure(s) R56.9
- apoplectiform (cerebral ischemia) I67.82
- dissociative F44.5
- epileptic — *see* Epilepsy
- epileptiform, epileptoid — *see* Seizure, epileptiform
- ether (anesthetic) — *see* Table of Drugs and Chemicals, by drug
- febrile R56.00
  - with status epilepticus G40.901
  - complex R56.01
    - with status epilepticus G40.901
  - simple R56.00
- hysterical F44.5
- infantile P90
  - epilepsy — *see* Epilepsy
- jacksonian — *see* Epilepsy, localization-related, symptomatic, with simple partial seizures
- myoclonic G25.3
- newborn P90
- obstetrical (nephritic) (uremic) — *see* Eclampsia
- paretic A52.17
- post traumatic R56.1
- psychomotor — *see* Epilepsy, localization-related, symptomatic, with complex partial seizures
- recurrent R56.9
- reflex R25.8
- scarlatinal A38.8
- tetanus, tetanic — *see* Tetanus
- thymic E32.8

Convulsive — *see also* Convulsions

Cooley's anemia D56.1

Coolie itch B76.9

Cooper's
- disease — *see* Mastopathy, cystic
- hernia — *see* Hernia, abdomen, specified site NEC

Copra itch B88.0

Coprophagy F50.89

Coprophobia F40.298

Coproporphyria, hereditary E80.29

Cor
- biloculare Q20.8
- bovis, bovinum — *see* Hypertrophy, cardiac
- pulmonale (chronic) I27.81
  - acute I26.09
- triatriatum, triatrium Q24.2
- triloculare Q20.8
  - biatrium Q20.4
  - biventriculare Q21.19

Corbus' disease (gangrenous balanitis) N48.1

Cord — *see also* condition
- around neck
  - complicating delivery O69.81 ☑
    - with compression O69.1 ☑
  - bladder G95.89
    - tabetic A52.19

Cordis ectopia Q24.8

Corditis (spermatic) N49.1

Corectopia Q13.2

Cori's disease (glycogen storage) E74.03

Corkhandler's disease or lung J67.3

Corkscrew esophagus K22.4

Corkworker's disease or lung J67.3

Corn (infected) L84

Cornea — *see also* condition
- donor Z52.5
- plana Q13.4

Cornelia de Lange syndrome Q87.19

Cornu cutaneum L85.8

Cornual gestation or pregnancy O00.80
- with intrauterine pregnancy O00.81

Coronary (artery) — *see* condition

Coronavirus (infection)
- 2019 — *see also* COVID-19 U07.1
- as cause of diseases classified elsewhere B97.29
- coronavirus-19 — *see also* COVID-19 U07.1
- COVID-19 — *see also* COVID-19 U07.1
- SARS-associated B97.21

Corpora — *see also* condition
- amylacea, prostate N42.89
- cavernosa — *see* condition

Corpulence — *see* Obesity

Corpus — *see* condition

Corrected transposition Q20.5

Corrosion (injury) (acid) (caustic) (chemical) (lime) (external) (internal) T30.4
- abdomen, abdominal (muscle) (wall) T21.42 ☑
  - first degree T21.52 ☑
  - second degree T21.62 ☑
  - third degree T21.72 ☑
- above elbow T22.439 ☑
  - first degree T22.539 ☑
  - left T22.432 ☑
    - first degree T22.532 ☑
    - second degree T22.632 ☑
    - third degree T22.732 ☑
  - right T22.431 ☑
    - first degree T22.531 ☑
    - second degree T22.631 ☑
    - third degree T22.731 ☑
  - second degree T22.639 ☑
  - third degree T22.739 ☑
- alimentary tract NEC T28.7 ☑
- ankle T25.419 ☑
  - first degree T25.519 ☑
  - left T25.412 ☑
    - first degree T25.512 ☑
    - second degree T25.612 ☑
    - third degree T25.712 ☑
  - multiple with foot — *see* Corrosion, lower, limb, multiple, ankle and foot
  - right T25.411 ☑
    - first degree T25.511 ☑
    - second degree T25.611 ☑
    - third degree T25.711 ☑
  - second degree T25.619 ☑
  - third degree T25.719 ☑
- anus — *see* Corrosion, buttock
- arm(s) (meaning upper limb(s)) — *see* Corrosion, upper limb
- axilla T22.449 ☑
  - first degree T22.549 ☑
  - left T22.442 ☑
    - first degree T22.542 ☑
    - second degree T22.642 ☑
    - third degree T22.742 ☑
  - right T22.441 ☑
    - first degree T22.541 ☑
    - second degree T22.641 ☑
    - third degree T22.741 ☑
  - second degree T22.649 ☑
  - third degree T22.749 ☑
- back (lower) T21.44 ☑
  - first degree T21.54 ☑
  - second degree T21.64 ☑
  - third degree T21.74 ☑
  - upper T21.43 ☑
    - first degree T21.53 ☑
    - second degree T21.63 ☑
    - third degree T21.73 ☑
- blisters — *code as* Corrosion, second degree, by site
- breast(s) — *see* Corrosion, chest wall
- buttock(s) T21.45 ☑
  - first degree T21.55 ☑
  - second degree T21.65 ☑
  - third degree T21.75 ☑
- calf T24.439 ☑
  - first degree T24.539 ☑
  - left T24.432 ☑
    - first degree T24.532 ☑

Corrosion — *continued*
  calf — *continued*
    left — *continued*
      second degree T24.632 ☑
      third degree T24.732 ☑
    right T24.431 ☑
      first degree T24.531 ☑
      second degree T24.631 ☑
      third degree T24.731 ☑
    second degree T24.639 ☑
    third degree T24.739 ☑
  canthus (eye) — *see* Corrosion, eyelid
  cervix T28.8 ☑
  cheek T20.46 ☑
    first degree T20.56 ☑
    second degree T20.66 ☑
    third degree T20.76 ☑
  chest wall T21.41 ☑
    first degree T21.51 ☑
    second degree T21.61 ☑
    third degree T21.71 ☑
  chin T20.43 ☑
    first degree T20.53 ☑
    second degree T20.63 ☑
    third degree T20.73 ☑
  colon T28.7 ☑
  conjunctiva (and cornea) — *see* Corrosion, cornea
  cornea (and conjunctiva) T26.6- ☑
  deep necrosis of underlying tissue — *code as* Corrosion, third degree, by site
  dorsum of hand T23.469 ☑
    first degree T23.569 ☑
    left T23.462 ☑
      first degree T23.562 ☑
      second degree T23.662 ☑
      third degree T23.762 ☑
    right T23.461 ☑
      first degree T23.561 ☑
      second degree T23.661 ☑
      third degree T23.761 ☑
    second degree T23.669 ☑
    third degree T23.769 ☑
  ear (auricle) (external) (canal) T20.41 ☑
    drum T28.91 ☑
    first degree T20.51 ☑
    second degree T20.61 ☑
    third degree T20.71 ☑
  elbow T22.429 ☑
    first degree T22.529 ☑
    left T22.422 ☑
      first degree T22.522 ☑
      second degree T22.622 ☑
      third degree T22.722 ☑
    right T22.421 ☑
      first degree T22.521 ☑
      second degree T22.621 ☑
      third degree T22.721 ☑
    second degree T22.629 ☑
    third degree T22.729 ☑
  entire body — *see* Corrosion, multiple body regions
  epidermal loss — *code as* Corrosion, second degree, by site
  epiglottis T27.4 ☑
  erythema, erythematous — *code as* Corrosion, first degree, by site
  esophagus T28.6 ☑
  extent (percentage of body surface)
    less than 10 percent T32.0
    10-19 percent (0-9 percent third degree) T32.10
      with 10-19 percent third degree T32.11
    20-29 percent (0-9 percent third degree) T32.20
      with
        10-19 percent third degree T32.21
        20-29 percent third degree T32.22
    30-39 percent (0-9 percent third degree) T32.30
      with
        10-19 percent third degree T32.31
        20-29 percent third degree T32.32
        30-39 percent third degree T32.33
    40-49 percent (0-9 percent third degree) T32.40
      with
        10-19 percent third degree T32.41
        20-29 percent third degree T32.42
        30-39 percent third degree T32.43
        40-49 percent third degree T32.44
    50-59 percent (0-9 percent third degree) T32.50

Corrosion — *continued*
  extent — *continued*
    50-59 percent — *continued*
      with
        10-19 percent third degree T32.51
        20-29 percent third degree T32.52
        30-39 percent third degree T32.53
        40-49 percent third degree T32.54
        50-59 percent third degree T32.55
    60-69 percent (0-9 percent third degree) T32.60
      with
        10-19 percent third degree T32.61
        20-29 percent third degree T32.62
        30-39 percent third degree T32.63
        40-49 percent third degree T32.64
        50-59 percent third degree T32.65
        60-69 percent third degree T32.66
    70-79 percent (0-9 percent third degree) T32.70
      with
        10-19 percent third degree T32.71
        20-29 percent third degree T32.72
        30-39 percent third degree T32.73
        40-49 percent third degree T32.74
        50-59 percent third degree T32.75
        60-69 percent third degree T32.76
        70-79 percent third degree T32.77
    80-89 percent (0-9 percent third degree) T32.80
      with
        10-19 percent third degree T32.81
        20-29 percent third degree T32.82
        30-39 percent third degree T32.83
        40-49 percent third degree T32.84
        50-59 percent third degree T32.85
        60-69 percent third degree T32.86
        70-79 percent third degree T32.87
        80-89 percent third degree T32.88
    90 percent or more (0-9 percent third degree) T32.90
      with
        10-19 percent third degree T32.91
        20-29 percent third degree T32.92
        30-39 percent third degree T32.93
        40-49 percent third degree T32.94
        50-59 percent third degree T32.95
        60-69 percent third degree T32.96
        70-79 percent third degree T32.97
        80-89 percent third degree T32.98
        90-99 percent third degree T32.99
  extremity — *see* Corrosion, limb
  eye(s) and adnexa T26.9- ☑
    with resulting rupture and destruction of eyeball T26.7- ☑
    conjunctival sac — *see* Corrosion, cornea
    cornea — *see* Corrosion, cornea
    lid — *see* Corrosion, eyelid
    periocular area — *see* Corrosion eyelid
    specified site NEC T26.8- ☑
  eyeball — *see* Corrosion, eye
  eyelid(s) T26.5- ☑
  face — *see* Corrosion, head
  finger T23.429 ☑
    first degree T23.529 ☑
    left T23.422 ☑
      first degree T23.522 ☑
      second degree T23.622 ☑
      third degree T23.722 ☑
    multiple sites (without thumb) T23.439 ☑
      with thumb T23.449 ☑
        first degree T23.549 ☑
        left T23.442 ☑
          first degree T23.542 ☑
          second degree T23.642 ☑
          third degree T23.742 ☑
        right T23.441 ☑
          first degree T23.541 ☑
          second degree T23.641 ☑
          third degree T23.741 ☑
      second degree T23.649 ☑
      third degree T23.749 ☑
    first degree T23.539 ☑
    left T23.432 ☑
      first degree T23.532 ☑
      second degree T23.632 ☑
      third degree T23.732 ☑
    right T23.431 ☑
      first degree T23.531 ☑
      second degree T23.631 ☑
      third degree T23.731 ☑

Corrosion — *continued*
  finger — *continued*
    multiple sites — *continued*
      second degree T23.639 ☑
      third degree T23.739 ☑
    right T23.421 ☑
      first degree T23.521 ☑
      second degree T23.621 ☑
      third degree T23.721 ☑
    second degree T23.629 ☑
    third degree T23.729 ☑
  flank — *see* Corrosion, abdomen
  foot T25.429 ☑
    first degree T25.529 ☑
    left T25.422 ☑
      first degree T25.522 ☑
      second degree T25.622 ☑
      third degree T25.722 ☑
    multiple with ankle — *see* Corrosion, lower, limb, multiple, ankle and foot
    right T25.421 ☑
      first degree T25.521 ☑
      second degree T25.621 ☑
      third degree T25.721 ☑
    second degree T25.629 ☑
    third degree T25.729 ☑
  forearm T22.419 ☑
    first degree T22.519 ☑
    left T22.412 ☑
      first degree T22.512 ☑
      second degree T22.612 ☑
      third degree T22.712 ☑
    right T22.411 ☑
      first degree T22.511 ☑
      second degree T22.611 ☑
      third degree T22.711 ☑
    second degree T22.619 ☑
    third degree T22.719 ☑
  forehead T20.46 ☑
    first degree T20.56 ☑
    second degree T20.66 ☑
    third degree T20.76 ☑
  fourth degree — *code as* Corrosion, third degree, by site
  full thickness skin loss — *code as* Corrosion, third degree, by site
  gastrointestinal tract NEC T28.7 ☑
  genital organs
    external
      female T21.47 ☑
        first degree T21.57 ☑
        second degree T21.67 ☑
        third degree T21.77 ☑
      male T21.46 ☑
        first degree T21.56 ☑
        second degree T21.66 ☑
        third degree T21.76 ☑
    internal T28.8 ☑
  groin — *see* Corrosion, abdominal wall
  hand(s) T23.409 ☑
    back — *see* Corrosion, dorsum of hand
    finger — *see* Corrosion, finger
    first degree T23.509 ☑
    left T23.402 ☑
      first degree T23.502 ☑
      second degree T23.602 ☑
      third degree T23.702 ☑
    multiple sites with wrist T23.499 ☑
      first degree T23.599 ☑
      left T23.492 ☑
        first degree T23.592 ☑
        second degree T23.692 ☑
        third degree T23.792 ☑
      right T23.491 ☑
        first degree T23.591 ☑
        second degree T23.691 ☑
        third degree T23.791 ☑
      second degree T23.699 ☑
      third degree T23.799 ☑
    palm — *see* Corrosion, palm
    right T23.401 ☑
      first degree T23.501 ☑
      second degree T23.601 ☑
      third degree T23.701 ☑
    second degree T23.609 ☑
    third degree T23.709 ☑

☑ Additional Character Required — Refer to the Tabular List for Character Selection

Corrosion — *continued*
  hand(s) — *continued*
    thumb — *see* Corrosion, thumb
  head (and face) (and neck) T20.40 ☑
    cheek — *see* Corrosion, cheek
    chin — *see* Corrosion, chin
    ear — *see* Corrosion, ear
    eye(s) only — *see* Corrosion, eye
    first degree T20.50 ☑
    forehead — *see* Corrosion, forehead
    lip — *see* Corrosion, lip
    multiple sites T20.49 ☑
      first degree T20.59 ☑
      second degree T20.69 ☑
      third degree T20.79 ☑
    neck — *see* Corrosion, neck
    nose — *see* Corrosion, nose
    scalp — *see* Corrosion, scalp
    second degree T20.60 ☑
    third degree T20.70 ☑
  hip(s) — *see* Corrosion, lower, limb
  inhalation — *see* Corrosion, respiratory tract
  internal organ(s) — *see also* Corrosion, by site
    T28.90 ☑
    alimentary tract T28.7 ☑
      esophagus T28.6 ☑
    esophagus T28.6 ☑
    genitourinary T28.8 ☑
    mouth T28.5 ☑
    pharynx T28.5 ☑
    specified organ NEC T28.99 ☑
  interscapular region — *see* Corrosion, back, upper
  intestine (large) (small) T28.7 ☑
  knee T24.429 ☑
    first degree T24.529 ☑
    left T24.422 ☑
      first degree T24.522 ☑
      second degree T24.622 ☑
      third degree T24.722 ☑
    right T24.421 ☑
      first degree T24.521 ☑
      second degree T24.621 ☑
      third degree T24.721 ☑
    second degree T24.629 ☑
    third degree T24.729 ☑
  labium (majus) (minus) — *see* Corrosion, genital organs, external, female
  lacrimal apparatus, duct, gland or sac — *see* Corrosion, eye, specified site NEC
  larynx T27.4 ☑
    with lung T27.5 ☑
  leg(s) (meaning lower limb(s)) — *see* Corrosion, lower, limb
  limb(s)
    lower — *see* Corrosion, lower, limb
    upper — *see* Corrosion, upper limb
  lip(s) T20.42 ☑
    first degree T20.52 ☑
    second degree T20.62 ☑
    third degree T20.72 ☑
  lower
    back — *see* Corrosion, back
    limb T24.409 ☑
      ankle — *see* Corrosion, ankle
      calf — *see* Corrosion, calf
      first degree T24.509 ☑
      foot — *see* Corrosion, foot
      knee — *see* Corrosion, knee
      left T24.402 ☑
        first degree T24.502 ☑
        second degree T24.602 ☑
        third degree T24.702 ☑
      multiple sites, except ankle and foot T24.499 ☑
        ankle and foot T25.499 ☑
          first degree T25.599 ☑
          left T25.492 ☑
            first degree T25.592 ☑
            second degree T25.692 ☑
            third degree T25.792 ☑
          right T25.491 ☑
            first degree T25.591 ☑
            second degree T25.691 ☑
            third degree T25.791 ☑
          second degree T25.699 ☑
          third degree T25.799 ☑
        first degree T24.599 ☑

Corrosion — *continued*
  lower — *continued*
    limb — *continued*
      multiple sites, except ankle and foot — *continued*
        left T24.492 ☑
          first degree T24.592 ☑
          second degree T24.692 ☑
          third degree T24.792 ☑
        right T24.491 ☑
          first degree T24.591 ☑
          second degree T24.691 ☑
          third degree T24.791 ☑
        second degree T24.699 ☑
        third degree T24.799 ☑
      right T24.401 ☑
        first degree T24.501 ☑
        second degree T24.601 ☑
        third degree T24.701 ☑
      second degree T24.609 ☑
      thigh — *see* Corrosion, thigh
      third degree T24.709 ☑
  lung (with larynx and trachea) T27.5 ☑
  mouth T28.5 ☑
  neck T20.47 ☑
    first degree T20.57 ☑
    second degree T20.67 ☑
    third degree T20.77 ☑
  nose (septum) T20.44 ☑
    first degree T20.54 ☑
    second degree T20.64 ☑
    third degree T20.74 ☑
  ocular adnexa — *see* Corrosion, eye
  orbit region — *see* Corrosion, eyelid
  palm T23.459 ☑
    first degree T23.559 ☑
    left T23.452 ☑
      first degree T23.552 ☑
      second degree T23.652 ☑
      third degree T23.752 ☑
    right T23.451 ☑
      first degree T23.551 ☑
      second degree T23.651 ☑
      third degree T23.751 ☑
    second degree T23.659 ☑
    third degree T23.759 ☑
  partial thickness — *code as* Corrosion, unspecified degree, by site
  pelvis — *see* Corrosion, trunk
  penis — *see* Corrosion, genital organs, external, male
  perineum
    female — *see* Corrosion, genital organs, external, female
    male — *see* Corrosion, genital organs, external, male
  periocular area — *see* Corrosion, eyelid
  pharynx T28.5 ☑
  rectum T28.7 ☑
  respiratory tract T27.7 ☑
    larynx — *see* Corrosion, larynx
    specified part NEC T27.6 ☑
    trachea — *see* Corrosion, larynx
  sac, lacrimal — *see* Corrosion, eye, specified site NEC
  scalp T20.45 ☑
    first degree T20.55 ☑
    second degree T20.65 ☑
    third degree T20.75 ☑
  scapular region T22.469 ☑
    first degree T22.569 ☑
    left T22.462 ☑
      first degree T22.562 ☑
      second degree T22.662 ☑
      third degree T22.762 ☑
    right T22.461 ☑
      first degree T22.561 ☑
      second degree T22.661 ☑
      third degree T22.761 ☑
    second degree T22.669 ☑
    third degree T22.769 ☑
  sclera — *see* Corrosion, eye, specified site NEC
  scrotum — *see* Corrosion, genital organs, external, male
  shoulder T22.459 ☑
    first degree T22.559 ☑
    left T22.452 ☑
      first degree T22.552 ☑
      second degree T22.652 ☑

Corrosion — *continued*
  shoulder — *continued*
    left — *continued*
      third degree T22.752 ☑
    right T22.451 ☑
      first degree T22.551 ☑
      second degree T22.651 ☑
      third degree T22.751 ☑
    second degree T22.659 ☑
    third degree T22.759 ☑
  stomach T28.7 ☑
  temple — *see* Corrosion, head
  testis — *see* Corrosion, genital organs, external, male
  thigh T24.419 ☑
    first degree T24.519 ☑
    left T24.412 ☑
      first degree T24.512 ☑
      second degree T24.612 ☑
      third degree T24.712 ☑
    right T24.411 ☑
      first degree T24.511 ☑
      second degree T24.611 ☑
      third degree T24.711 ☑
    second degree T24.619 ☑
    third degree T24.719 ☑
  thorax (external) — *see* Corrosion, trunk
  throat (meaning pharynx) T28.5 ☑
  thumb(s) T23.419 ☑
    first degree T23.519 ☑
    left T23.412 ☑
      first degree T23.512 ☑
      second degree T23.612 ☑
      third degree T23.712 ☑
    multiple sites with fingers T23.449 ☑
      first degree T23.549 ☑
      left T23.442 ☑
        first degree T23.542 ☑
        second degree T23.642 ☑
        third degree T23.742 ☑
      right T23.441 ☑
        first degree T23.541 ☑
        second degree T23.641 ☑
        third degree T23.741 ☑
    second degree T23.649 ☑
    third degree T23.749 ☑
    right T23.411 ☑
      first degree T23.511 ☑
      second degree T23.611 ☑
      third degree T23.711 ☑
    second degree T23.619 ☑
    third degree T23.719 ☑
  toe T25.439 ☑
    first degree T25.539 ☑
    left T25.432 ☑
      first degree T25.532 ☑
      second degree T25.632 ☑
      third degree T25.732 ☑
    right T25.431 ☑
      first degree T25.531 ☑
      second degree T25.631 ☑
      third degree T25.731 ☑
    second degree T25.639 ☑
    third degree T25.739 ☑
  tongue T28.5 ☑
  tonsil(s) T28.5 ☑
  total body — *see* Corrosion, multiple body regions
  trachea T27.4 ☑
    with lung T27.5 ☑
  trunk T21.40 ☑
    abdominal wall — *see* Corrosion, abdominal wall
    anus — *see* Corrosion, buttock
    axilla — *see* Corrosion, upper limb
    back — *see* Corrosion, back
    breast — *see* Corrosion, chest wall
    buttock — *see* Corrosion, buttock
    chest wall — *see* Corrosion, chest wall
    first degree T21.50 ☑
    flank — *see* Corrosion, abdominal wall
    genital
      female — *see* Corrosion, genital organs, external, female
      male — *see* Corrosion, genital organs, external, male
    groin — *see* Corrosion, abdominal wall
    interscapular region — *see* Corrosion, back, upper

Corrosion — *continued*
  trunk — *continued*
    labia — *see* Corrosion, genital organs, external, female
    lower back — *see* Corrosion, back
    penis — *see* Corrosion, genital organs, external, male
    perineum
      female — *see* Corrosion, genital organs, external, female
      male — *see* Corrosion, genital organs, external, male
    scapular region — *see* Corrosion, upper limb
    scrotum — *see* Corrosion, genital organs, external, male
    second degree T21.6Ø ☑
    shoulder — *see* Corrosion, upper limb
    specified site NEC T21.49 ☑
      first degree T21.59 ☑
      second degree T21.69 ☑
      third degree T21.79 ☑
    testes — *see* Corrosion, genital organs, external, male
    third degree T21.7Ø ☑
    upper back — *see* Corrosion, back, upper
    vagina T28.8 ☑
    vulva — *see* Corrosion, genital organs, external, female
  unspecified site with extent of body surface involved
    specified
      less than 10 percent T32.Ø
      10-19 percent (Ø-9 percent third degree) T32.1Ø
        with 10-19 percent third degree T32.11
      2Ø-29 percent (Ø-9 percent third degree) T32.2Ø
        with
          10-19 percent third degree T32.21
          2Ø-29 percent third degree T32.22
      3Ø-39 percent (Ø-9 percent third degree) T32.3Ø
        with
          10-19 percent third degree T32.31
          2Ø-29 percent third degree T32.32
          3Ø-39 percent third degree T32.33
      4Ø-49 percent (Ø-9 percent third degree) T32.4Ø
        with
          10-19 percent third degree T32.41
          2Ø-29 percent third degree T32.42
          3Ø-39 percent third degree T32.43
          4Ø-49 percent third degree T32.44
      5Ø-59 percent (Ø-9 percent third degree) T32.5Ø
        with
          10-19 percent third degree T32.51
          2Ø-29 percent third degree T32.52
          3Ø-39 percent third degree T32.53
          4Ø-49 percent third degree T32.54
          5Ø-59 percent third degree T32.55
      6Ø-69 percent (Ø-9 percent third degree) T32.6Ø
        with
          10-19 percent third degree T32.61
          2Ø-29 percent third degree T32.62
          3Ø-39 percent third degree T32.63
          4Ø-49 percent third degree T32.64
          5Ø-59 percent third degree T32.65
          6Ø-69 percent third degree T32.66
      7Ø-79 percent (Ø-9 percent third degree) T32.7Ø
        with
          10-19 percent third degree T32.71
          2Ø-29 percent third degree T32.72
          3Ø-39 percent third degree T32.73
          4Ø-49 percent third degree T32.74
          5Ø-59 percent third degree T32.75
          6Ø-69 percent third degree T32.76
          7Ø-79 percent third degree T32.77
      8Ø-89 percent (Ø-9 percent third degree) T32.8Ø
        with
          10-19 percent third degree T32.81
          2Ø-29 percent third degree T32.82
          3Ø-39 percent third degree T32.83
          4Ø-49 percent third degree T32.84
          5Ø-59 percent third degree T32.85
          6Ø-69 percent third degree T32.86
          7Ø-79 percent third degree T32.87
          8Ø-89 percent third degree T32.88
      9Ø percent or more (Ø-9 percent third degree) T32.9Ø
        with
          10-19 percent third degree T32.91
          2Ø-29 percent third degree T32.92
          3Ø-39 percent third degree T32.93
          4Ø-49 percent third degree T32.94

Corrosion — *continued*
  unspecified site with extent of body surface involved
    specified — *continued*
      9Ø percent or more — *continued*
        with — *continued*
          5Ø-59 percent third degree T32.95
          6Ø-69 percent third degree T32.96
          7Ø-79 percent third degree T32.97
          8Ø-89 percent third degree T32.98
          9Ø-99 percent third degree T32.99
  upper limb (axilla) (scapular region) T22.4Ø ☑
    above elbow — *see* Corrosion, above elbow
    axilla — *see* Corrosion, axilla
    elbow — *see* Corrosion, elbow
    first degree T22.5Ø ☑
    forearm — *see* Corrosion, forearm
    hand — *see* Corrosion, hand
    interscapular region — *see* Corrosion, back, upper
    multiple sites T22.499 ☑
      first degree T22.599 ☑
      left T22.492 ☑
        first degree T22.592 ☑
        second degree T22.692 ☑
        third degree T22.792 ☑
      right T22.491 ☑
        first degree T22.591 ☑
        second degree T22.691 ☑
        third degree T22.791 ☑
      second degree T22.699 ☑
      third degree T22.799 ☑
    scapular region — *see* Corrosion, scapular region
    second degree T22.6Ø ☑
    shoulder — *see* Corrosion, shoulder
    third degree T22.7Ø ☑
    wrist — *see* Corrosion, hand
  uterus T28.8 ☑
  vagina T28.8 ☑
  vulva — *see* Corrosion, genital organs, external, female
  wrist T23.479 ☑
    first degree T23.579 ☑
    left T23.472 ☑
      first degree T23.572 ☑
      second degree T23.672 ☑
      third degree T23.772 ☑
    multiple sites with hand T23.499 ☑
      first degree T23.599 ☑
      left T23.492 ☑
        first degree T23.592 ☑
        second degree T23.692 ☑
        third degree T23.792 ☑
      right T23.491 ☑
        first degree T23.591 ☑
        second degree T23.691 ☑
        third degree T23.791 ☑
      second degree T23.699 ☑
      third degree T23.799 ☑
    right T23.471 ☑
      first degree T23.571 ☑
      second degree T23.671 ☑
      third degree T23.771 ☑
    second degree T23.679 ☑
    third degree T23.779 ☑

Corrosive burn — *see* Corrosion
Corsican fever — *see* Malaria
Cortical — *see* condition
Cortico-adrenal — *see* condition
Coryza (acute) JØØ
  with grippe or influenza — *see* Influenza, with, respiratory manifestations NEC
  syphilitic
    congenital (chronic) A5Ø.Ø5
Co-sleeping, child-caregiver Z72.823
Costen's syndrome or complex M26.69
Costiveness — *see* Constipation
Costochondritis M94.Ø
Cot death R99
Cotard's syndrome F22
Cotia virus BØ8.8
Cotton wool spots (retinal) H35.81
Cotungo's disease — *see* Sciatica
Cough (affected) (epidemic) (nervous) RØ5.9
  with hemorrhage — *see* Hemoptysis
  acute RØ5.1
  bronchial RØ5.8
    with grippe or influenza — *see* Influenza, with, respiratory manifestations NEC

Cough — *continued*
  chronic RØ5.3
  functional F45.8
  hysterical F45.8
  laryngeal, spasmodic RØ5.8
  paroxysmal, due to Bordetella pertussis (without pneumonia) A37.ØØ
    with pneumonia A37.Ø1
  persistent RØ5.3
  psychogenic F45.8
  refractory RØ5.3
  smokers' J41.Ø
  specified NEC RØ5.8
  subacute RØ5.2
  syncope RØ5.4
  tea taster's B49
  unexplained RØ5.3
Counseling (for) Z71.9
  abuse NEC
    perpetrator Z69.82
    victim Z69.81
  alcohol abuser Z71.41
    family Z71.42
  child abuse
    nonparental
      perpetrator Z69.Ø21
      victim Z69.Ø2Ø
    parental
      perpetrator Z69.Ø11
      victim Z69.Ø1Ø
  consanguinity Z71.89
  contraceptive Z3Ø.Ø9
  dietary Z71.3
  drug abuser Z71.51
    family member Z71.52
  exercise Z71.82
  family Z71.89
  fertility preservation (prior to cancer therapy) (prior to removal of gonads) Z31.62
  for non-attending third party Z71.Ø
    related to sexual behavior or orientation Z7Ø.2
  genetic
    nonprocreative Z71.83
    procreative NEC Z31.5
  gestational carrier Z31.7
  health (advice) (education) (instruction) — *see* Counseling, medical
    risk for travel (international) Z71.84
  human immunodeficiency virus (HIV) Z71.7
  immunization safety Z71.85
  impotence Z7Ø.1
  insulin pump use Z46.81
  medical (for) Z71.9
    boarding school resident Z59.3
    consanguinity Z71.89
    feared complaint and no disease found Z71.1
    human immunodeficiency virus (HIV) Z71.7
    institutional resident Z59.3
    on behalf of another Z71.Ø
      related to sexual behavior or orientation Z7Ø.2
    person living alone Z6Ø.2
    specified reason NEC Z71.89
  natural family planning
    procreative Z31.61
    to avoid pregnancy Z3Ø.Ø2
  pediatric-to-adult transition Z71.87
  perpetrator (of)
    abuse NEC Z69.82
    child abuse
      non-parental Z69.Ø21
      parental Z69.Ø11
    rape NEC Z69.82
    spousal abuse Z69.12
  procreative NEC Z31.69
    fertility preservation (prior to cancer therapy) (prior to removal of gonads) Z31.62
    using natural family planning Z31.61
  promiscuity Z7Ø.1
  rape victim Z69.81
  religious Z71.81
  safety for travel (international) Z71.84
  sex, sexual (related to) Z7Ø.9
    attitude(s) Z7Ø.Ø
    behavior or orientation Z7Ø.1
    combined concerns Z7Ø.3
    non-responsiveness Z7Ø.1
    on behalf of third party Z7Ø.2
    specified reason NEC Z7Ø.8
  socioeconomic factors Z71.88

☑ Additional Character Required — Refer to the Tabular List for Character Selection

Counseling — *continued*
  specified reason NEC Z71.89
  spiritual Z71.81
  spousal abuse (perpetrator) Z69.12
    victim Z69.11
  substance abuse Z71.89
    alcohol Z71.41
    drug Z71.51
    tobacco Z71.6
  tobacco use Z71.6
  travel (international) Z71.84
  use (of)
    insulin pump Z46.81
  vaccine product safety Z71.85
  victim (of)
    abuse Z69.81
    child abuse
      by parent Z69.010
      non-parental Z69.020
    rape NEC Z69.81
Coupled rhythm R00.8
Couvelaire syndrome or uterus (complicating delivery)
  O45.8X- ☑
COVID-19 U07.1
  condition post U09.9
  contact (with) Z20.822
  exposure (to) Z20.822
  history of (personal) Z86.16
  long (haul) U09.9
  partially vaccinated (for) Z28.311
  pneumonia J12.82
  screening Z11.52
  sequelae (post acute) U09.9
  unvaccinated (for) Z28.310
Cowperitis — *see* Urethritis
Cowper's gland — *see* condition
Cowpox B08.010
  due to vaccination T88.1 ☑
Coxa
  magna M91.4- ☑
  plana M91.2- ☑
  valga (acquired) — *see also* Deformity, limb, specified
    type NEC, thigh
    congenital Q65.81
    sequelae (late effect) of rickets E64.3
  vara (acquired) — *see also* Deformity, limb, specified
    type NEC, thigh
    congenital Q65.82
    sequelae (late effect) of rickets E64.3
Coxalgia, coxalgic (nontuberculous) — *see also* Pain,
  joint, hip
  tuberculous A18.02
Coxitis — *see* Monoarthritis, hip
Coxsackie (virus) (infection) B34.1
  as cause of disease classified elsewhere B97.11
  carditis B33.20
  central nervous system NEC A88.8
  endocarditis B33.21
  enteritis A08.39
  meningitis (aseptic) A87.0
  myocarditis B33.22
  pericarditis B33.23
  pharyngitis B08.5
  pleurodynia B33.0
  specific disease NEC B33.8
Crabs, meaning pubic lice B85.3
Crack baby P04.41
Cracked nipple N64.0
  associated with
    lactation O92.13
      pregnancy O92.11- ☑
      puerperium O92.12
Cracked tooth K03.81
Cradle cap L21.0
Craft neurosis F48.8
Cramp(s) R25.2
  abdominal — *see* Pain, abdominal
  bathing T75.1 ☑
  colic R10.83
    psychogenic F45.8
  due to immersion T75.1 ☑
  fireman T67.2 ☑
  heat T67.2 ☑
  immersion T75.1 ☑
  intestinal — *see* Pain, abdominal
    psychogenic F45.8
  leg, sleep related G47.62
  limb (lower) (upper) NEC R25.2

Cramp(s) — *continued*
  limb — *continued*
    sleep related G47.62
  linotypist's F48.8
    organic G25.89
  muscle (limb) (general) R25.2
    due to immersion T75.1 ☑
    psychogenic F45.8
  occupational (hand) F48.8
    organic G25.89
  salt-depletion E87.1
  sleep related, leg G47.62
  stoker's T67.2 ☑
  swimmer's T75.1 ☑
  telegrapher's F48.8
    organic G25.89
  typist's F48.8
    organic G25.89
  uterus N94.89
    menstrual — *see* Dysmenorrhea
  writer's F48.8
    organic G25.89
Cranial — *see* condition
Craniocleidodysostosis Q74.0
Craniofenestria (skull) Q75.8
Craniolacunia (skull) Q75.8
Craniopagus Q89.4
Craniopathy, metabolic M85.2
Craniopharyngeal — *see* condition
Craniopharyngioma D44.4
Craniorachischisis (totalis) Q00.1
Cranioschisis Q75.8
Craniostenosis Q75.0
Craniosynostosis Q75.0
Craniotabes (cause unknown) M83.8
  neonatal P96.3
  rachitic E64.3
  syphilitic A50.56
Cranium — *see* condition
Craw-craw — *see* Onchocerciasis
Creaking joint — *see* Derangement, joint, specified type
  NEC
Creeping
  eruption B76.9
  palsy or paralysis G12.22
Crenated tongue K14.8
Creotoxism A05.9
Crepitus
  caput Q75.8
  joint — *see* Derangement, joint, specified type NEC
Crescent or conus choroid, congenital Q14.3
CREST syndrome M34.1
Cretin, cretinism (congenital) (endemic) (nongoitrous)
  (sporadic) E00.9
  pelvis
    with disproportion (fetopelvic) O33.0
      causing obstructed labor O65.0
  type
    hypothyroid E00.1
    mixed E00.2
    myxedematous E00.1
    neurological E00.0
Creutzfeldt-Jakob disease or syndrome (with dementia) A81.00
  familial A81.09
  iatrogenic A81.09
  specified NEC A81.09
  sporadic A81.09
  variant (vCJD) A81.01
Crib death R99
Cribriform hymen Q52.3
Cri-du-chat syndrome Q93.4
Crigler-Najjar disease or syndrome E80.5
Crime, victim of Z65.4
Crimean hemorrhagic fever A98.0
Criminalism F60.2
Crisis
  abdomen R10.0
  acute reaction F43.0
  addisonian E27.2
  adrenal (cortical) E27.2
  celiac K90.0
  Dietl's N13.8
  emotional — *see also* Disorder, adjustment
    acute reaction to stress F43.0
    specific to childhood and adolescence F93.8

Crisis — *continued*
  glaucomatocyclitic — *see* Glaucoma, secondary, inflam-
    mation
  heart — *see* Failure, heart
  nitritoid I95.2
    correct substance properly administered — *see* Ta-
      ble of Drugs and Chemicals, by drug, adverse
      effect
    overdose or wrong substance given or taken — *see*
      Table of Drugs and Chemicals, by drug, poi-
      soning
  oculogyric H51.8
    psychogenic F45.8
  Pel's (tabetic) A52.11
  psychosexual identity F64.2
  renal N28.0
  sickle-cell — *see also* Disease, sickle-cell, by type, with
    crisis D57.00
    with
      acute chest syndrome D57.01
      cerebral vascular involvement D57.03
      complication specified NEC D57.09
      splenic sequestration D57.02
      vasoocclusive pain D57.00
  state (acute reaction) F43.0
  tabetic A52.11
  thyroid — *see* Thyrotoxicosis with thyroid storm
  thyrotoxic — *see* Thyrotoxicosis with thyroid storm
Crocq's disease (acrocyanosis) I73.89
Crohn's disease — *see* Enteritis, regional
Crooked septum, nasal J34.2
Cross syndrome E70.328
Crossbite (anterior) (posterior) M26.24
Cross-eye — *see* Strabismus, convergent concomitant
Croup, croupous (catarrhal) (infectious) (inflammatory)
  (nondiphtheritic) J05.0
  bronchial J20.9
  diphtheritic A36.2
  false J38.5
  spasmodic J38.5
    diphtheritic A36.2
  stridulous J38.5
    diphtheritic A36.2
Crouzon's disease Q75.1
Crowding, tooth, teeth, fully erupted M26.31
CRST syndrome M34.1
Cruchet's disease A85.8
Cruelty in children — *see also* Disorder, conduct
Crural ulcer — *see* Ulcer, lower limb
Crush, crushed, crushing T14.8 ☑
  abdomen S38.1 ☑
  ankle S97.0- ☑
  arm (upper) (and shoulder) S47.- ☑
  axilla — *see* Crush, arm
  back, lower S38.1 ☑
  buttock S38.1 ☑
  cheek S07.0 ☑
  chest S28.0 ☑
  cranium S07.1 ☑
  ear S07.0 ☑
  elbow S57.0- ☑
  extremity
    lower
      ankle — *see* Crush, ankle
      below knee — *see* Crush, leg
      foot — *see* Crush, foot
      hip — *see* Crush, hip
      knee — *see* Crush, knee
      thigh — *see* Crush, thigh
      toe — *see* Crush, toe
    upper
      below elbow S67.9- ☑
      elbow — *see* Crush, elbow
      finger — *see* Crush, finger
      forearm — *see* Crush, forearm
      hand — *see* Crush, hand
      thumb — *see* Crush, thumb
      upper arm — *see* Crush, arm
      wrist — *see* Crush, wrist
  face S07.0 ☑
  finger(s) S67.1- ☑
    with hand (and wrist) — *see* Crush, hand, specified
      site NEC
    index S67.19- ☑
    little S67.19- ☑
    middle S67.19- ☑
    ring S67.19- ☑

Crush, crushed, crushing — *continued*
  finger(s) — *continued*
    thumb — *see* Crush, thumb
  foot S97.8- ☑
    toe — *see* Crush, toe
  forearm S57.8- ☑
  genitalia, external
    female S38.002 ☑
      vagina S38.03 ☑
      vulva S38.03 ☑
    male S38.001 ☑
      penis S38.01 ☑
      scrotum S38.02 ☑
      testis S38.02 ☑
  hand (except fingers alone) S67.2- ☑
    with wrist S67.4- ☑
  head S07.9
    specified NEC S07.8 ☑
  heel — *see* Crush, foot
  hip S77.0- ☑
    with thigh S77.2- ☑
  internal organ (abdomen, chest, or pelvis) NEC T14.8 ☑
  knee S87.0- ☑
  labium (majus) (minus) S38.03 ☑
  larynx S17.0 ☑
  leg (lower) S87.8- ☑
    knee — *see* Crush, knee
  lip S07.0 ☑
  lower
    back S38.1 ☑
    leg — *see* Crush, leg
  neck S17.9 ☑
  nerve — *see* Injury, nerve
  nose S07.0 ☑
  pelvis S38.1 ☑
  penis S38.01 ☑
  scalp S07.8 ☑
  scapular region — *see* Crush, arm
  scrotum S38.02 ☑
  severe, unspecified site T14.8 ☑
  shoulder (and upper arm) — *see* Crush, arm
  skull S07.1 ☑
  syndrome (complication of trauma) T79.5 ☑
  testis S38.02 ☑
  thigh S77.1- ☑
    with hip S77.2- ☑
  throat S17.8 ☑
  thumb S67.0- ☑
    with hand (and wrist) — *see* Crush, hand, specified site NEC
  toe(s) S97.10- ☑
    great S97.11- ☑
    lesser S97.12- ☑
  trachea S17.0 ☑
  vagina S38.03 ☑
  vulva S38.03 ☑
  wrist S67.3- ☑
    with hand S67.4- ☑
Crusta lactea L21.0
Crusts R23.4
Crutch paralysis — *see* Injury, brachial plexus
Cruveilhier-Baumgarten cirrhosis, disease or syndrome K74.69
Cruveilhier's atrophy or disease G12.8
Crying (constant) (continuous) (excessive)
  child, adolescent, or adult R45.83
  infant (baby) (newborn) R68.11
Cryofibrinogenemia D89.2
Cryoglobulinemia (essential) (idiopathic) (mixed) (primary) (purpura) (secondary) (vasculitis) D89.1
  with lung involvement D89.1 *[J99]*
Cryptitis (anal) (rectal) K62.89
Cryptococcosis, cryptococcus (infection) (neoformans) B45.9
  bone B45.3
  cerebral B45.1
  cutaneous B45.2
  disseminated B45.7
  generalized B45.7
  meningitis B45.1
  meningocerebralis B45.1
  osseous B45.3
  pulmonary B45.0
  skin B45.2
  specified NEC B45.8
Cryptopapillitis (anus) K62.89

Cryptophthalmos Q11.2
  syndrome Q87.0
Cryptorchid, cryptorchism, cryptorchidism Q53.9
  bilateral Q53.20
    abdominal Q53.211
    perineal Q53.22
  unilateral Q53.10
    abdominal Q53.111
    perineal Q53.12
Cryptosporidiosis A07.2
  hepatobiliary B88.8
  respiratory B88.8
Cryptostromosis J67.6
Crystalluria R82.998
Cubitus
  congenital Q68.8
  valgus (acquired) M21.0- ☑
    congenital Q68.8
    sequelae (late effect) of rickets E64.3
  varus (acquired) M21.1- ☑
    congenital Q68.8
    sequelae (late effect) of rickets E64.3
Cultural deprivation or shock Z60.3
Curling esophagus K22.4
Curling's ulcer — *see* Ulcer, peptic, acute
Curschmann (-Batten) (-Steinert) **disease or syndrome** G71.11
Curse, Ondine's — *see* Apnea, sleep
Curvature
  organ or site, congenital NEC — *see* Distortion
  penis (lateral) Q55.61
  Pott's (spinal) A18.01
  radius, idiopathic, progressive (congenital) Q74.0
  spine (acquired) (angular) (idiopathic) (incorrect) (postural) — *see* Dorsopathy, deforming
    congenital Q67.5
    due to or associated with
      Charcot-Marie-Tooth disease — *see also* subcategory M49.8 G60.0
      osteitis
        deformans M88.88
        fibrosa cystica — *see also* subcategory M49.8 E21.0
      tuberculosis (Pott's curvature) A18.01
    sequelae (late effect) of rickets E64.3
    tuberculous A18.01
Cushingoid due to steroid therapy E24.2
  correct substance properly administered — *see* Table of Drugs and Chemicals, by drug, adverse effect
  overdose or wrong substance given or taken — *see* Table of Drugs and Chemicals, by drug, poisoning
Cushing's
  syndrome or disease E24.9
    drug-induced E24.2
    iatrogenic E24.2
    pituitary-dependent E24.0
    specified NEC E24.8
  ulcer — *see* Ulcer, peptic, acute
Cusp, Carabelli — *omit code*
Cut (external) — *see also* Laceration
  muscle — *see* Injury, muscle
Cutaneous — *see also* condition
  hemorrhage R23.3
  larva migrans B76.9
Cutis — *see also* condition
  hyperelastica Q82.8
    acquired L57.4
  laxa (hyperelastica) — *see* Dermatolysis
  marmorata R23.8
  osteosis L94.2
  pendula — *see* Dermatolysis
  rhomboidalis nuchae L57.2
  verticis gyrata Q82.8
    acquired L91.8
Cyanosis R23.0
  due to
    patent foramen botalli Q21.12
    persistent foramen ovale Q21.12
  enterogenous D74.8
  paroxysmal digital — *see* Raynaud's disease
    with gangrene I73.01
  retina, retinal H35.89
Cyanotic heart disease I24.9
  congenital Q24.9
Cycle
  anovulatory N97.0
  menstrual, irregular N92.6
Cyclencephaly Q04.9

Cyclical vomiting, in migraine — *see also* Vomiting, cyclical G43.A0 (*following* G43.7)
  psychogenic F50.89
Cyclitis — *see also* Iridocyclitis H20.9
  chronic — *see* Iridocyclitis, chronic
  Fuchs' heterochromic H20.81- ☑
  granulomatous — *see* Iridocyclitis, chronic
  lens-induced — *see* Iridocyclitis, lens-induced
  posterior H30.2- ☑
Cycloid personality F34.0
Cyclophoria H50.54
Cyclopia, cyclops Q87.0
Cyclopism Q87.0
Cyclosporiasis A07.4
Cyclothymia F34.0
Cyclothymic personality F34.0
Cyclotropia H50.41- ☑
Cylindroma — *see also* Neoplasm, malignant, by site
  eccrine dermal — *see* Neoplasm, skin, benign
  skin — *see* Neoplasm, skin, benign
Cylindruria R82.998
Cynanche
  diphtheritic A36.2
  tonsillaris J36
Cynophobia F40.218
Cynorexia R63.2
Cyphosis — *see* Kyphosis
Cyprus fever — *see* Brucellosis
Cyst (colloid) (mucous) (simple) (retention)
  adenoid (infected) J35.8
  adrenal gland E27.8
    congenital Q89.1
  air, lung J98.4
  allantoic Q64.4
  alveolar process (jaw bone) M27.40
  amnion, amniotic O41.8X- ☑
  aneurysmal M27.49
  anterior
    chamber (eye) — *see* Cyst, iris
    nasopalatine K09.1
  antrum J34.1
  anus K62.89
  apical (tooth) (periodontal) K04.8
  appendix K38.8
  arachnoid, brain (acquired) G93.0
    congenital Q04.6
  arytenoid J38.7
  Baker's M71.2- ☑
    ruptured M66.0
    tuberculous A18.02
  Bartholin's gland N75.0
  bile duct (common) (hepatic) K83.5
  bladder (multiple) (trigone) N32.89
  blue dome (breast) — *see* Cyst, breast
  bone (local) NEC M85.60
    aneurysmal M85.50
      ankle M85.57- ☑
      foot M85.57- ☑
      forearm M85.53- ☑
      hand M85.54- ☑
      jaw M27.49
      lower leg M85.56- ☑
      multiple site M85.59
      neck M85.58
      rib M85.58
      shoulder M85.51- ☑
      skull M85.58
      specified site NEC M85.58
      thigh M85.55- ☑
      toe M85.57- ☑
      upper arm M85.52- ☑
      vertebra M85.58
    solitary M85.40
      ankle M85.47- ☑
      fibula M85.46- ☑
      foot M85.47- ☑
      hand M85.44- ☑
      humerus M85.42- ☑
      jaw M27.49
      neck M85.48
      pelvis M85.45- ☑
      radius M85.43- ☑
      rib M85.48
      shoulder M85.41- ☑
      skull M85.48
      specified site NEC M85.48
      tibia M85.46- ☑

Cyst — *continued*
  bone — *continued*
    solitary — *continued*
      toe M85.47- ☑
      ulna M85.43- ☑
      vertebra M85.48
    specified type NEC M85.60
      ankle M85.67- ☑
      foot M85.67- ☑
      forearm M85.63- ☑
      hand M85.64- ☑
      jaw M27.40
        developmental (nonodontogenic) K09.1
          odontogenic K09.0
        latent M27.0
      lower leg M85.66- ☑
      multiple site M85.69
      neck M85.68
      rib M85.68
      shoulder M85.61- ☑
      skull M85.68
      specified site NEC M85.68
      thigh M85.65- ☑
      toe M85.67- ☑
      upper arm M85.62- ☑
      vertebra M85.68
  brain (acquired) G93.0
    congenital Q04.6
    hydatid B67.99 *[G94]*
    third ventricle (colloid), congenital Q04.6
  branchial (cleft) Q18.0
  branchiogenic Q18.0
  breast (benign) (blue dome) (pedunculated) (solitary)
    N60.0- ☑
    involution — *see* Dysplasia, mammary, specified
      type NEC
    sebaceous — *see* Dysplasia, mammary, specified
      type NEC
  broad ligament (benign) N83.8
  bronchogenic (mediastinal) (sequestration) J98.4
    congenital Q33.0
  buccal K09.8
  bulbourethral gland N36.8
  bursa, bursal NEC M71.30
    with rupture — *see* Rupture, synovium
    ankle M71.37- ☑
    elbow M71.32- ☑
    foot M71.37- ☑
    hand M71.34- ☑
    hip M71.35- ☑
    multiple sites M71.39
    pharyngeal J39.2
    popliteal space — *see* Cyst, Baker's
    shoulder M71.31- ☑
    specified site NEC M71.38
    wrist M71.33- ☑
  calcifying odontogenic D16.5
    upper jaw (bone) (maxilla) D16.4
  canal of Nuck (female) N94.89
    congenital Q52.4
  canthus — *see* Cyst, conjunctiva
  carcinomatous — *see* Neoplasm, malignant, by site
  cauda equina G95.89
  cavum septi pellucidi — *see* Cyst, brain
  celomic (pericardium) Q24.8
  cerebellopontine (angle) — *see* Cyst, brain
  cerebellum — *see* Cyst, brain
  cerebral — *see* Cyst, brain
  cervical lateral Q18.0
  cervix NEC N88.8
    embryonic Q51.6
    nabothian N88.8
  chiasmal optic NEC — *see* Disorder, optic, chiasm
  chocolate (ovary) N80.10- ☑
  choledochus, congenital Q44.4
  chorion O41.8X- ☑
  choroid plexus G93.0
    congenital Q04.6
  ciliary body — *see* Cyst, iris
  clitoris N90.7
  colon K63.89
  common (bile) duct K83.5
  congenital NEC Q89.8
    adrenal gland Q89.1
    epiglottis Q31.8
    esophagus Q39.8
    fallopian tube Q50.4

Cyst — *continued*
  congenital — *continued*
    kidney Q61.00
      more than one (multiple) Q61.02
        specified as polycystic Q61.3
          adult type Q61.2
          infantile type NEC Q61.19
            collecting duct dilation Q61.11
      solitary Q61.01
    larynx Q31.8
    liver Q44.6
    lung Q33.0
    mediastinum Q34.1
    ovary Q50.1
    oviduct Q50.4
    periurethral (tissue) Q64.79
    prepuce Q55.69
    salivary gland (any) Q38.4
    sublingual Q38.6
    submaxillary gland Q38.6
    thymus (gland) Q89.2
    tongue Q38.3
    ureterovesical orifice Q62.8
    vulva Q52.79
  conjunctiva H11.44- ☑
  cornea H18.89- ☑
  corpora quadrigemina G93.0
  corpus
    albicans N83.29- ☑
    luteum (hemorrhagic) (ruptured) N83.1- ☑
  Cowper's gland (benign) (infected) N36.8
  cranial meninges G93.0
  craniobuccal pouch E23.6
  craniopharyngeal pouch E23.6
  cystic duct K82.8
  Cysticercus — *see* Cysticercosis
  Dandy-Walker Q03.1
    with spina bifida — *see* Spina bifida
  dental (root) K04.8
    developmental K09.0
    eruption K09.0
    primordial K09.0
  dentigerous (mandible) (maxilla) K09.0
  dermoid — *see* Neoplasm, benign, by site
    with malignant transformation C56.- ☑
    implantation
      external area or site (skin) NEC L72.0
      iris — *see* Cyst, iris, implantation
      vagina N89.8
      vulva N90.7
    mouth K09.8
    oral soft tissue K09.8
    sacrococcygeal — *see* Cyst, pilonidal
  developmental K09.1
    odontogenic K09.0
    oral region (nonodontogenic) K09.1
    ovary, ovarian Q50.1
  dura (cerebral) G93.0
    spinal G96.198
  ear (external) Q18.1
  echinococcal — *see* Echinococcus
  embryonic
    cervix uteri Q51.6
    fallopian tube Q50.4
    vagina Q52.4
  endometrium, endometrial (uterus) N85.8
    ectopic — *see* Endometriosis
  enterogenous Q43.8
  epidermal, epidermoid (inclusion) (*see also* Cyst, skin)
    L72.0
    mouth K09.8
    oral soft tissue K09.8
  epididymis N50.3
  epiglottis J38.7
  epiphysis cerebri E34.8
  epithelial (inclusion) L72.0
  epoophoron Q50.5
  eruption K09.0
  esophagus K22.89
  ethmoid sinus J34.1
  external female genital organs NEC N90.7
  eyelid (sebaceous) H02.829
    infected — *see* Hordeolum
    left H02.826
      lower H02.825
      upper H02.824
    right H02.823
      lower H02.822

Cyst — *continued*
  eyelid — *continued*
    right — *continued*
      upper H02.821
  eye NEC H57.89
    congenital Q15.8
  fallopian tube N83.8
    congenital Q50.4
  fimbrial (twisted) Q50.4
  fissural (oral region) K09.1
  follicle (graafian) (hemorrhagic) N83.0- ☑
    nabothian N88.8
  follicular (atretic) (hemorrhagic) (ovarian) N83.0- ☑
    dentigerous K09.0
    odontogenic K09.0
    skin L72.9
      specified NEC L72.8
  frontal sinus J34.1
  gallbladder K82.8
  ganglion — *see* Ganglion
  Gartner's duct Q52.4
  gingiva K09.0
  gland of Moll — *see* Cyst, eyelid
  globulomaxillary K09.1
  graafian follicle (hemorrhagic) N83.0- ☑
  granulosal lutein (hemorrhagic) N83.1- ☑
  hemangiomatous D18.00
    intra-abdominal D18.03
    intracranial D18.02
    skin D18.01
    specified site NEC D18.09
  hemorrhagic M27.49
  hydatid — *see also* Echinococcus B67.90
    brain B67.99 *[G94]*
    liver — *see also* Cyst, liver, hydatid B67.8
    lung NEC B67.99 *[J99]*
    Morgagni
      female Q50.5
      male (epididymal) Q55.4
        testicular Q55.29
    specified site NEC B67.99
  hymen N89.8
    embryonic Q52.4
  hypopharynx J39.2
  hypophysis, hypophyseal (duct) (recurrent) E23.6
    cerebri E23.6
  implantation (dermoid)
    external area or site (skin) NEC L72.0
    iris — *see* Cyst, iris, implantation
    vagina N89.8
    vulva N90.7
  incisive canal K09.1
  inclusion (epidermal) (epithelial) (epidermoid) (squa-
    mous) L72.0
    not of skin — *code under* Cyst, by site
  intestine (large) (small) K63.89
  intracranial — *see* Cyst, brain
  intraligamentous — *see also* Disorder, ligament
    knee — *see* Derangement, knee
  intrasellar E23.6
  iris H21.309
    exudative H21.31- ☑
    idiopathic H21.30- ☑
    implantation H21.32- ☑
    parasitic H21.33- ☑
    pars plana (primary) H21.34- ☑
      exudative H21.35- ☑
  jaw (bone) M27.40
    aneurysmal M27.49
    developmental (odontogenic) K09.0
    fissural K09.1
    hemorrhagic M27.49
    traumatic M27.49
  joint NEC — *see* Disorder, joint, specified type NEC
  kidney N28.1
    acquired N28.1
    calyceal — *see* Hydronephrosis
    congenital Q61.00
    more than one (multiple) Q61.02
      specified as polycystic Q61.3
        adult type (autosomal dominant) Q61.2
        infantile type (autosomal recessive) NEC
          Q61.19
            collecting duct dilation Q61.11
    pyelogenic — *see* Hydronephrosis
    simple N28.1
    solitary (single) N28.1
      acquired N28.1

Cyst — *continued*
  kidney — *continued*
    solitary — *continued*
      congenital Q61.01
  labium (majus) (minus) N90.7
    sebaceous N90.7
  lacrimal — *see also* Disorder, lacrimal system, specified NEC
    gland H04.13- ☑
    passages or sac — *see* Disorder, lacrimal system, specified NEC
  larynx J38.7
  lateral periodontal K09.0
  lens H27.8
    congenital Q12.8
  lip (gland) K13.0
  liver (idiopathic) (simple) K76.89
    congenital Q44.6
    hydatid B67.8
      granulosus B67.0
      multilocularis B67.5
  lung J98.4
    congenital Q33.0
    giant bullous J43.9
  lutein N83.1- ☑
  lymphangiomatous D18.1
  lymphoepithelial, oral soft tissue K09.8
  macula — *see* Degeneration, macula, hole
  malignant — *see* Neoplasm, malignant, by site
  mammary gland — *see* Cyst, breast
  mandible M27.40
    dentigerous K09.0
    radicular K04.8
  maxilla M27.40
    dentigerous K09.0
    radicular K04.8
  medial, face and neck Q18.8
  median
    anterior maxillary K09.1
    palatal K09.1
  mediastinum, congenital Q34.1
  meibomian (gland) — *see* Chalazion
    infected — *see* Hordeolum
  membrane, brain G93.0
  meninges (cerebral) G93.0
    spinal G96.198
  meniscus, knee — *see* Derangement, knee, meniscus, cystic
  mesentery, mesenteric K66.8
    chyle I89.8
  mesonephric duct
    female Q50.5
    male Q55.4
  milk N64.89
  Morgagni (hydatid)
    female Q50.5
    male (epididymal) Q55.4
      testicular Q55.29
  mouth K09.8
  Müllerian duct Q50.4
    appendix testis Q55.29
    cervix Q51.6
    fallopian tube Q50.4
    female Q50.4
    male Q55.29
    prostatic utricle Q55.4
    vagina (embryonal) Q52.4
  multilocular (ovary) D39.10
    benign — *see* Neoplasm, benign, by site
  myometrium N85.8
  nabothian (follicle) (ruptured) N88.8
  nasoalveolar K09.1
  nasolabial K09.1
  nasopalatine (anterior) (duct) K09.1
  nasopharynx J39.2
  neoplastic — *see* Neoplasm, uncertain behavior, by site
    benign — *see* Neoplasm, benign, by site
  nerve root
    cervical G96.191
    lumbar G96.191
    sacral G96.191
    thoracic G96.191
  nervous system NEC G96.89
  neuroenteric (congenital) Q06.8
  nipple — *see* Cyst, breast
  nose (turbinates) J34.1
    sinus J34.1

Cyst — *continued*
  odontogenic, developmental K09.0
  omentum (lesser) K66.8
    congenital Q45.8
  ora serrata — *see* Cyst, retina, ora serrata
  oral
    region K09.9
      developmental (nonodontogenic) K09.1
      specified NEC K09.8
    soft tissue K09.9
      specified NEC K09.8
  orbit H05.81- ☑
  ovary, ovarian (twisted) N83.20- ☑
    adherent N83.20- ☑
    chocolate N80.10- ☑
    corpus
      albicans N83.29- ☑
      luteum (hemorrhagic) N83.1- ☑
    dermoid D27.9
    developmental Q50.1
    due to failure of involution NEC N83.20- ☑
    endometrial N80.10- ☑
    follicular (graafian) (hemorrhagic) N83.0- ☑
    hemorrhagic N83.20- ☑
    in pregnancy or childbirth O34.8- ☑
      with obstructed labor O65.5
    multilocular D39.10
    pseudomucinous D27.9
    retention N83.29- ☑
    serous N83.20- ☑
    specified NEC N83.29- ☑
    theca lutein (hemorrhagic) N83.1- ☑
    tuberculous A18.18
  oviduct N83.8
  palate (median) (fissural) K09.1
  palatine papilla (jaw) K09.1
  pancreas, pancreatic (hemorrhagic) (true) K86.2
    congenital Q45.2
    false K86.3
  paralabral
    hip M24.85- ☑
    shoulder S43.43- ☑
  paramesonephric duct Q50.4
    female Q50.4
    male Q55.29
  paranephric N28.1
  paraphysis, cerebri, congenital Q04.6
  parasitic B89
  parathyroid (gland) E21.4
  paratubal N83.8
  paraurethral duct N36.8
  paroophoron Q50.5
  parotid gland K11.6
  parovarian Q50.5
  pelvis, female N94.89
    in pregnancy or childbirth O34.8- ☑
      causing obstructed labor O65.5
  penis (sebaceous) N48.89
  periapical K04.8
  pericardial (congenital) Q24.8
    acquired (secondary) I31.8
  pericoronal K09.0
  perineural G96.191
  periodontal K04.8
    lateral K09.0
  peripelvic (lymphatic) N28.1
  peritoneum K66.8
    chylous I89.8
  periventricular, acquired, newborn P91.1
  pharynx (wall) J39.2
  pilar L72.11
  pilonidal (infected) (rectum) L05.91
    with abscess L05.01
    malignant C44.59- ☑
  pituitary (duct) (gland) E23.6
  placenta O43.19- ☑
  pleura J94.8
  popliteal — *see* Cyst, Baker's
  porencephalic Q04.6
    acquired G93.0
  postanal (infected) — *see* Cyst, pilonidal
  postmastoidectomy cavity (mucosal) — *see* Complications, postmastoidectomy, cyst
  preauricular Q18.1
  prepuce N47.4
    congenital Q55.69
  primordial (jaw) K09.0
  prostate N42.83

Cyst — *continued*
  pseudomucinous (ovary) D27.9
  pupillary, miotic H21.27- ☑
  radicular (residual) K04.8
  radiculodental K04.8
  ranular K11.8
  Rathke's pouch E23.6
  rectum (epithelium) (mucous) K62.89
  renal — *see* Cyst, kidney
  residual (radicular) K04.8
  retention (ovary) N83.29- ☑
    salivary gland K11.6
  retina H33.19- ☑
    ora serrata H33.11- ☑
    parasitic H33.12- ☑
  retroperitoneal K68.9
  sacrococcygeal (dermoid) — *see* Cyst, pilonidal
  salivary gland or duct (mucous extravasation or retention) K11.6
  Sampson's N80.10- ☑
  sclera H15.89
  scrotum L72.9
    sebaceous L72.3
  sebaceous (duct) (gland) L72.3
    breast — *see* Dysplasia, mammary, specified type NEC
    eyelid — *see* Cyst, eyelid
    genital organ NEC
      female N94.89
      male N50.89
    scrotum L72.3
  semilunar cartilage (knee) (multiple) — *see* Derangement, knee, meniscus, cystic
  seminal vesicle N50.89
  serous (ovary) N83.20- ☑
  sinus (accessory) (nasal) J34.1
  Skene's gland N36.8
  skin L72.9
    breast — *see* Dysplasia, mammary, specified type NEC
    epidermal, epidermoid L72.0
    epithelial L72.0
    eyelid — *see* Cyst, eyelid
    genital organ NEC
      female N90.7
      male N50.89
    inclusion L72.0
    scrotum L72.9
    sebaceous L72.3
    sweat gland or duct L74.8
  solitary
    bone — *see* Cyst, bone, solitary
    jaw M27.40
    kidney N28.1
  spermatic cord N50.89
  sphenoid sinus J34.1
  spinal meninges G96.198
  spleen NEC D73.4
    congenital Q89.09
    hydatid — *see also* Echinococcus B67.99 *[D77]*
  Stafne's M27.0
  subarachnoid intrasellar R93.0
  subcutaneous, pheomycotic (chromomycotic) B43.2
  subdural (cerebral) G93.0
    spinal cord G96.198
  sublingual gland K11.6
  submandibular gland K11.6
  submaxillary gland K11.6
  suburethral N36.8
  suprarenal gland E27.8
  suprasellar — *see* Cyst, brain
  sweat gland or duct L74.8
  synovial — *see also* Cyst, bursa
    ruptured — *see* Rupture, synovium
  Tarlov G96.191
  tarsal — *see* Chalazion
  tendon (sheath) — *see* Disorder, tendon, specified type NEC
  testis N44.2
    tunica albuginea N44.1
  theca lutein (ovary) N83.1- ☑
  Thornwaldt's J39.2
  thymus (gland) E32.8
  thyroglossal duct (infected) (persistent) Q89.2
  thyroid (gland) E04.1
  thyrolingual duct (infected) (persistent) Q89.2
  tongue K14.8
  tonsil J35.8

☑ **Additional Character Required** — **Refer to the Tabular List for Character Selection**

Cyst — *continued*
  tooth — *see* Cyst, dental
  Tornwaldt's J39.2
  trichilemmal (proliferating) L72.12
  trichodermal L72.12
  tubal (fallopian) N83.8
    inflammatory — *see* Salpingitis, chronic
  tubo-ovarian N83.8
    inflammatory N70.13
  tunica
    albuginea testis N44.1
    vaginalis N50.89
  turbinate (nose) J34.1
  Tyson's gland N48.89
  urachus, congenital Q64.4
  ureter N28.89
  ureterovesical orifice N28.89
  urethra, urethral (gland) N36.8
  uterine ligament N83.8
  uterus (body) (corpus) (recurrent) N85.8
    embryonic Q51.818
      cervix Q51.6
  vagina, vaginal (implantation) (inclusion) (squamous cell) (wall) N89.8
    embryonic Q52.4
  vallecula, vallecular (epiglottis) J38.7
  vesical (orifice) N32.89
  vitreous body H43.89
  vulva (implantation) (inclusion) N90.7
    congenital Q52.79
    sebaceous gland N90.7
  vulvovaginal gland N90.7
  wolffian
    female Q50.5
    male Q55.4
Cystadenocarcinoma — *see* Neoplasm, malignant, by site
  bile duct C22.1
  endometrioid — *see* Neoplasm, malignant, by site
    specified site — *see* Neoplasm, malignant, by site
    unspecified site
      female C56.9
      male C61
  mucinous
    papillary
      specified site — *see* Neoplasm, malignant, by site
      unspecified site C56.9
    specified site — *see* Neoplasm, malignant, by site
    unspecified site C56.9
  papillary
    mucinous
      specified site — *see* Neoplasm, malignant, by site
      unspecified site C56.9
    pseudomucinous
      specified site — *see* Neoplasm, malignant, by site
      unspecified site C56.9
    serous
      specified site — *see* Neoplasm, malignant, by site
      unspecified site C56.9
    specified site — *see* Neoplasm, malignant, by site
    unspecified site C56.9
  pseudomucinous
    papillary
      specified site — *see* Neoplasm, malignant, by site
      unspecified site C56.9
    specified site — *see* Neoplasm, malignant, by site
    unspecified site C56.9
  serous
    papillary
      specified site — *see* Neoplasm, malignant, by site
      unspecified site C56.9
    specified site — *see* Neoplasm, malignant, by site
    unspecified site C56.9
Cystadenofibroma
  clear cell — *see* Neoplasm, benign, by site
  endometrioid D27.9
    borderline malignancy D39.1- ☑
    malignant C56.- ☑
  mucinous
    specified site — *see* Neoplasm, benign, by site
    unspecified site D27.9

Cystadenofibroma — *continued*
  serous
    specified site — *see* Neoplasm, benign, by site
    unspecified site D27.9
  specified site — *see* Neoplasm, benign, by site
  unspecified site D27.9
Cystadenoma — *see also* Neoplasm, benign, by site
  bile duct D13.4
  endometrioid — *see* Neoplasm, benign, by site
    borderline malignancy — *see* Neoplasm, uncertain behavior, by site
  malignant — *see* Neoplasm, malignant, by site
  mucinous
    borderline malignancy
      ovary C56.- ☑
      specified site NEC — *see* Neoplasm, uncertain behavior, by site
      unspecified site C56.9
    papillary
      borderline malignancy
        ovary C56.- ☑
        specified site NEC — *see* Neoplasm, uncertain behavior, by site
        unspecified site C56.9
      specified site — *see* Neoplasm, benign, by site
      unspecified site D27.9
    specified site — *see* Neoplasm, benign, by site
    unspecified site D27.9
  papillary
    borderline malignancy
      ovary C56.- ☑
      specified site NEC — *see* Neoplasm, uncertain behavior, by site
      unspecified site C56.9
    lymphomatosum
      specified site — *see* Neoplasm, benign, by site
      unspecified site D11.9
    mucinous
      borderline malignancy
        ovary C56.- ☑
        specified site NEC — *see* Neoplasm, uncertain behavior, by site
        unspecified site C56.9
      specified site — *see* Neoplasm, benign, by site
      unspecified site D27.9
    pseudomucinous
      borderline malignancy
        ovary C56.- ☑
        specified site NEC — *see* Neoplasm, uncertain behavior, by site
        unspecified site C56.9
      specified site — *see* Neoplasm, benign, by site
      unspecified site D27.9
    serous
      borderline malignancy
        ovary C56.- ☑
        specified site NEC — *see* Neoplasm, uncertain behavior, by site
        unspecified site C56.9
      specified site — *see* Neoplasm, benign, by site
      unspecified site D27.9
    specified site — *see* Neoplasm, benign, by site
    unspecified site D27.9
  pseudomucinous
    borderline malignancy
      ovary C56.- ☑
      specified site NEC — *see* Neoplasm, uncertain behavior, by site
      unspecified site C56.9
    papillary
      borderline malignancy
        ovary C56.- ☑
        specified site NEC — *see* Neoplasm, uncertain behavior, by site
        unspecified site C56.9
      specified site — *see* Neoplasm, benign, by site
      unspecified site D27.9
    specified site — *see* Neoplasm, benign, by site
    unspecified site D27.9
  serous
    borderline malignancy
      ovary C56.- ☑
      specified site NEC — *see* Neoplasm, uncertain behavior, by site
      unspecified site C56.9
    papillary
      borderline malignancy
        ovary C56.- ☑

Cystadenoma — *continued*
  serous — *continued*
    papillary — *continued*
      borderline malignancy — *continued*
        specified site NEC — *see* Neoplasm, uncertain behavior, by site
        unspecified site C56.9
      specified site — *see* Neoplasm, benign, by site
      unspecified site D27.9
    specified site — *see* Neoplasm, benign, by site
    unspecified site D27.9
Cystathionine synthase deficiency E72.11
Cystathioninemia E72.19
Cystathioninuria E72.19
Cystic — *see also* condition
  breast (chronic) — *see* Mastopathy, cystic
  corpora lutea (hemorrhagic) N83.1- ☑
  duct — *see* condition
  eyeball (congenital) Q11.0
  fibrosis — *see* Fibrosis, cystic
  kidney (congenital) Q61.9
    adult type Q61.2
    infantile type NEC Q61.19
      collecting duct dilatation Q61.11
    medullary Q61.5
  liver, congenital Q44.6
  lung disease J98.4
    congenital Q33.0
  mastitis, chronic — *see* Mastopathy, cystic
  medullary, kidney Q61.5
  meniscus — *see* Derangement, knee, meniscus, cystic
  ovary N83.20- ☑
Cysticercosis, cysticerciasis B69.9
  with
    epileptiform fits B69.0
    myositis B69.81
  brain B69.0
  central nervous system B69.0
  cerebral B69.0
  ocular B69.1
  specified NEC B69.89
Cysticercus cellulose infestation — *see* Cysticercosis
Cystinosis (malignant) E72.04
Cystinuria E72.01
Cystitis (exudative) (hemorrhagic) (septic) (suppurative) N30.90
  with
    fibrosis — *see* Cystitis, chronic, interstitial
    hematuria N30.91
    leukoplakia — *see* Cystitis, chronic, interstitial
    malakoplakia — *see* Cystitis, chronic, interstitial
    metaplasia — *see* Cystitis, chronic, interstitial
    prostatitis N41.3
  acute N30.00
    with hematuria N30.01
    of trigone N30.30
      with hematuria N30.31
  allergic — *see* Cystitis, specified type NEC
  amebic A06.81
  bilharzial B65.9 *[N33]*
  blennorrhagic (gonococcal) A54.01
  bullous — *see* Cystitis, specified type NEC
  calculous N21.0
  chlamydial A56.01
  chronic N30.20
    with hematuria N30.21
    interstitial N30.10
      with hematuria N30.11
    of trigone N30.30
      with hematuria N30.31
    specified NEC N30.20
      with hematuria N30.21
  cystic (a) — *see* Cystitis, specified type NEC
  diphtheritic A36.85
  echinococcal
    granulosus B67.39
    multilocularis B67.69
  emphysematous — *see* Cystitis, specified type NEC
  encysted — *see* Cystitis, specified type NEC
  eosinophilic — *see* Cystitis, specified type NEC
  follicular — *see* Cystitis, of trigone
  gangrenous — *see* Cystitis, specified type NEC
  glandularis — *see* Cystitis, specified type NEC
  gonococcal A54.01
  incrusted — *see* Cystitis, specified type NEC
  interstitial (chronic) — *see* Cystitis, chronic, interstitial
  irradiation N30.40
    with hematuria N30.41

Cystitis — *continued*
    irritation — *see* Cystitis, specified type NEC
    malignant — *see* Cystitis, specified type NEC
    of trigone N30.30
        with hematuria N30.31
    panmural — *see* Cystitis, chronic, interstitial
    polyposa — *see* Cystitis, specified type NEC
    prostatic N41.3
    puerperal (postpartum) O86.22
    radiation — *see* Cystitis, irradiation
    specified type NEC N30.80
        with hematuria N30.81
    subacute — *see* Cystitis, chronic
    submucous — *see* Cystitis, chronic, interstitial
    syphilitic (late) A52.76
    trichomonal A59.03
    tuberculous A18.12
    ulcerative — *see* Cystitis, chronic, interstitial
Cystocele (-urethrocele)
    female N81.10
        with prolapse of uterus — *see* Prolapse, uterus
        lateral N81.12
        midline N81.11
        paravaginal N81.12

Cystocele — *continued*
    in pregnancy or childbirth O34.8- ☑
        causing obstructed labor O65.5
    male N32.89
Cystolithiasis N21.0
Cystoma — *see also* Neoplasm, benign, by site
    endometrial, ovary N80.10- ☑
    mucinous
        specified site — *see* Neoplasm, benign, by site
        unspecified site D27.9
    serous
        specified site — *see* Neoplasm, benign, by site
        unspecified site D27.9
    simple (ovary) N83.29- ☑
Cystoplegia N31.2
Cystoptosis N32.89
Cystopyelitis — *see* Pyelonephritis
Cystorrhagia N32.89
Cystosarcoma phyllodes D48.6- ☑
    benign D24- ☑
    malignant — *see* Neoplasm, breast, malignant
Cystostomy
    attention to Z43.5
    complication — *see* Complications, cystostomy

Cystostomy — *continued*
    status Z93.50
        appendico-vesicostomy Z93.52
        cutaneous Z93.51
        specified NEC Z93.59
Cystourethritis — *see* Urethritis
Cystourethrocele — *see also* Cystocele
    female N81.10
        with uterine prolapse — *see* Prolapse, uterus
        lateral N81.12
        midline N81.11
        paravaginal N81.12
    male N32.89
Cytomegalic inclusion disease
    congenital P35.1
Cytomegalovirus infection B25.9
Cytomycosis (reticuloendothelial) B39.4
Cytopenia D75.9
    refractory
        with multilineage dysplasia D46.A (*following* D46.2)
            and ring sideroblasts (RCMD RS) D46.B (*following* D46.2)
Czerny's disease (periodic hydrarthrosis of the knee) — *see* Effusion, joint, knee

D

Da Costa's syndrome F45.8
Daae (-Finsen) **disease** (epidemic pleurodynia) B33.0
Dabney's grip B33.0
Dacryoadenitis, dacryadenitis H04.00- ☑
  acute H04.01- ☑
  chronic H04.02- ☑
Dacryocystitis H04.30- ☑
  acute H04.32- ☑
  chronic H04.41- ☑
  neonatal P39.1
  phlegmonous H04.31- ☑
  syphilitic A52.71
    congenital (early) A50.01
  trachomatous, active A71.1
    sequelae (late effect) B94.0
Dacryocystoblenorrhea — *see* Inflammation, lacrimal,
  passages, chronic
Dacryocystocele — *see* Disorder, lacrimal system,
  changes
Dacryolith, dacryolithiasis H04.51- ☑
Dacryoma — *see* Disorder, lacrimal system, changes
Dacryopericystitis — *see* Dacryocystitis
Dacryops H04.11- ☑
Dacryostenosis — *see also* Stenosis, lacrimal
  congenital Q10.5
Dactylitis
  bone — *see* Osteomyelitis
  sickle-cell D57.00
    Hb C D57.219
    Hb SS D57.00
    specified NEC D57.819
  skin L08.9
  syphilitic A52.77
  tuberculous A18.03
Dactylolysis spontanea (ainhum) L94.6
Dactylosymphysis Q70.9
  fingers — *see* Syndactylism, complex, fingers
  toes — *see* Syndactylism, complex, toes
Damage
  arteriosclerotic — *see* Arteriosclerosis
  brain (nontraumatic) G93.9
    anoxic, hypoxic G93.1
      resulting from a procedure G97.82
    child NEC G80.9
    due to birth injury P11.2
  cardiorenal (vascular) — *see* Hypertension, cardiorenal
  cerebral NEC — *see* Damage, brain
  coccyx, complicating delivery O71.6
  coronary — *see* Disease, heart, ischemic
  deep tissue, pressure-induced — *see also* L89 with final
    character .6
  eye, birth injury P15.3
  liver (nontraumatic) K76.9
    alcoholic K70.9
    due to drugs — *see* Disease, liver, toxic
    toxic — *see* Disease, liver, toxic
  lung
    dabbing (related) U07.0
    electronic cigarette (related) U07.0
    vaping (associated) (device) (product) (use) U07.0
  medication T88.7 ☑
  organ
    dabbing (related) U07.0
    electronic cigarette (related) U07.0
    vaping (associated) (device) (product) (use) U07.0
  pelvic
    joint or ligament, during delivery O71.6
    organ NEC
      during delivery O71.5
      following ectopic or molar pregnancy O08.6
  renal — *see* Disease, renal
  subendocardium, subendocardial — *see* Degeneration,
    myocardial
  vascular I99.9
Dana-Putnam syndrome (subacute combined sclerosis
  with pernicious anemia) — *see* Degeneration,
  combined
Danbolt (-Cross) **syndrome** (acrodermatitis enteropathica) E83.2
Dandruff L21.0
Dandy-Walker syndrome Q03.1
  with spina bifida — *see* Spina bifida
Danlos' syndrome — *see also* Syndrome, Ehlers-Danlos
  Q79.60

Darier (-White) **disease** (congenital) Q82.8
  meaning erythema annulare centrifugum L53.1
Darier-Roussy sarcoid D86.3
Darling's disease or histoplasmosis B39.4
Darwin's tubercle Q17.8
Dawson's (inclusion body) **encephalitis** A81.1
De Beurmann (-Gougerot) **disease** B42.1
De la Tourette's syndrome F95.2
De Lange's syndrome Q87.19
De Morgan's spots (senile angiomas) I78.1
De Quervain's
  disease (tendon sheath) M65.4
  syndrome E34.51
  thyroiditis (subacute granulomatous thyroiditis) E06.1
De Toni-Fanconi (-Debré) **syndrome** E72.09
  with cystinosis E72.04
Dead
  fetus, retained (mother) O36.4 ☑
    early pregnancy O02.1
  labyrinth H83.2 ☑
  ovum, retained O02.0
Deaf nonspeaking NEC H91.3
Deafmutism (acquired) (congenital) NEC H91.3
  hysterical F44.6
  syphilitic, congenital — *see also* subcategory H94.8
    A50.09
Deafness (acquired) (complete) (hereditary) (partial)
  H91.9- ☑
  with blue sclera and fragility of bone Q78.0
  auditory fatigue — *see* Deafness, specified type NEC
  aviation T70.0
    nerve injury — *see* Injury, nerve, acoustic, specified
      type NEC
  boilermaker's H83.3 ☑
  central — *see* Deafness, sensorineural
  conductive H90.2
    and sensorineural
      mixed H90.8
        bilateral H90.6
    bilateral H90.0
    unilateral H90.1- ☑
      with restricted hearing on the contralateral side
        H90.A- ☑
  congenital H90.5
    with blue sclera and fragility of bone Q78.0
  due to toxic agents — *see* Deafness, ototoxic
  emotional (hysterical) F44.6
  functional (hysterical) F44.6
  high frequency H91.9- ☑
  hysterical F44.6
  low frequency H91.9- ☑
  mental R48.8
  mixed conductive and sensorineural H90.8
    bilateral H90.6
    unilateral H90.7- ☑
  nerve — *see* Deafness, sensorineural
  neural — *see* Deafness, sensorineural
  noise-induced — *see also* subcategory H83.3 ☑
    nerve injury — *see* Injury, nerve, acoustic, specified
      type NEC
  nonspeaking H91.3
  ototoxic H91.0 ☑
  perceptive — *see* Deafness, sensorineural
  psychogenic (hysterical) F44.6
  sensorineural H90.5
    and conductive
      bilateral H90.6
      mixed H90.8
        bilateral H90.6
    bilateral H90.3
    unilateral H90.4- ☑
      with restricted hearing on the contralateral side
        H90.A- ☑
  sensory — *see* Deafness, sensorineural
  specified type NEC H91.8 ☑
  sudden (idiopathic) H91.2- ☑
  syphilitic A52.15
  transient ischemic H93.01- ☑
  traumatic — *see* Injury, nerve, acoustic, specified type
    NEC
  word (developmental) H93.25
Death (cause unknown) (of) (unexplained) (unspecified
  cause) R99
  brain G93.82
  cardiac (sudden) (with successful resuscitation) — *see*
    Arrest, cardiac
    family history of Z82.41

Death — *continued*
  cardiac — *see* Arrest, cardiac — *continued*
    personal history of Z86.74
  family member (assumed) Z63.4
Debility (chronic) (general) (nervous) R53.81
  congenital or neonatal NOS P96.9
  nervous R53.81
  old age R54
  senile R54
Débove's disease (splenomegaly) R16.1
Debt, burdensome Z59.86
Decalcification
  bone — *see* Osteoporosis
  teeth K03.89
Decapsulation, kidney N28.89
Decay
  dental — *see* Caries, dental
  senile R54
  tooth, teeth — *see* Caries, dental
Deciduitis (acute)
  following ectopic or molar pregnancy O08.0
Decline (general) — *see* Debility
  cognitive, age-associated R41.81
Decompensation
  cardiac (acute) (chronic) — *see* Disease, heart
  cardiovascular — *see* Disease, cardiovascular
  heart — *see* Disease, heart
  hepatic — *see* Failure, hepatic
  myocardial (acute) (chronic) — *see* Disease, heart
  respiratory J98.8
Decompression sickness T70.3 ☑
Decrease (d)
  absolute neutrophile count — *see* Neutropenia
  blood
    platelets — *see* Thrombocytopenia
    pressure R03.1
      due to shock following
        injury T79.4 ☑
        operation T81.19 ☑
  estrogen E28.39
    postablative E89.40
      asymptomatic E89.40
      symptomatic E89.41
  fragility of erythrocytes D58.8
  function
    lipase (pancreatic) K90.3
    ovary in hypopituitarism E23.0
    parenchyma of pancreas K86.89
    pituitary (gland) (anterior) (lobe) E23.0
      posterior (lobe) E23.0
  functional activity R68.89
  glucose R73.09
  hematocrit R71.0
  hemoglobin R71.0
  leukocytes D72.819
    specified NEC D72.818
  libido R68.82
  lymphocytes D72.810
  platelets D69.6
  respiration, due to shock following injury T79.4 ☑
  sexual desire R68.82
  tear secretion NEC — *see* Syndrome, dry eye
  tolerance
    fat K90.49
    glucose R73.09
    pancreatic K90.3
    salt and water E87.8
  vision NEC H54.7
  white blood cell count D72.819
    specified NEC D72.818
Decubitus (ulcer) — *see* Ulcer, pressure, by site
  cervix N86
Deepening acetabulum — *see* Derangement, joint,
  specified type NEC, hip
Defect, defective Q89.9
  3-beta-hydroxysteroid dehydrogenase E25.0
  11-hydroxylase E25.0
  21-hydroxylase E25.0
  abdominal wall, congenital Q79.59
  antibody immunodeficiency D80.9
  aorticopulmonary septum Q21.4
  atrial septal Q21.10
    coronary sinus Q21.13
    following acute myocardial infarction (current
      complication) I23.1
    ostium primum type (type I) Q21.20

Defect, defective — *continued*
- atrial septal — *continued*
  - ostium primum type — *continued*
    - with
      - common atrioventricular valves and moderate or larger inlet VSD Q21.23
      - separate atrioventricular valves Q21.21
        - and small or restrictive inlet VSD Q21.22
  - ostium secundum type (patent persistent) (type II) Q21.11
  - sinus venosus Q21.16
    - inferior Q21.15
    - superior Q21.14
  - specified NEC Q21.19
  - vena cava type
    - inferior Q21.15
    - superior Q21.14
- atrioventricular
  - canal Q21.20
  - septal
    - common Q21.23
    - complete Q21.23
    - incomplete Q21.21
    - intermediate Q21.22
    - partial Q21.21
    - transitional Q21.22
    - unspecified as to partial or complete Q21.20
  - septum Q21.20
- auricular septal Q21.10
- bilirubin excretion NEC E80.6
- biosynthesis, androgen (testicular) E29.1
- bulbar septum Q21.0
- catalase E80.3
- cell membrane receptor complex (CR3) D71
- circulation I99.9
  - congenital Q28.9
  - newborn Q28.9
- coagulation (factor) — *see also* Deficiency, factor D68.9
  - with
    - ectopic pregnancy O08.1
    - molar pregnancy O08.1
  - acquired D68.4
  - antepartum with hemorrhage — *see* Hemorrhage, antepartum, with coagulation defect
  - due to
    - liver disease D68.4
    - vitamin K deficiency D68.4
  - hereditary NEC D68.2
  - intrapartum O67.0
  - newborn, transient P61.6
  - postpartum O99.13
    - with hemorrhage O72.3
  - specified type NEC D68.8
- complement system D84.1
- conduction (heart) I45.9
  - bone — *see* Deafness, conductive
- congenital, organ or site not listed — *see* Anomaly, by site
- coronary sinus Q21.13
- cushion, endocardial Q21.20
  - common Q21.23
  - incomplete Q21.21
  - intermediate Q21.22
  - transitional Q21.22
- degradation, glycoprotein E77.1
- dental bridge, crown, fillings — *see* Defect, dental restoration
- dental restoration K08.50
  - specified NEC K08.59
- dentin (hereditary) K00.5
- Descemet's membrane, congenital Q13.89
- developmental — *see also* Anomaly
  - cauda equina Q06.3
- diaphragm
  - with elevation, eventration or hernia — *see* Hernia, diaphragm
  - congenital Q79.1
    - with hernia Q79.0
    - gross (with hernia) Q79.0
- ectodermal, congenital Q82.9
- Eisenmenger's Q21.8
- enzyme
  - catalase E80.3
  - peroxidase E80.3
- esophagus, congenital Q39.9
- extensor retinaculum M62.89
- fibrin polymerization D68.2

Defect, defective — *continued*
- filling
  - bladder R93.41
  - kidney R93.42-☑
  - renal pelvis R93.41
  - stomach R93.3
  - ureter R93.41
  - urinary organs, specified NEC R93.49
- GABA (gamma aminobutyric acid) metabolic E72.81
- Gerbode Q21.0
- glucose transport, blood-brain barrier E74.810
- glycoprotein degradation E77.1
- Hageman (factor) D68.2
- hearing — *see* Deafness
- high grade F70
- interatrial septal Q21.19
- interauricular septal Q21.19
- interventricular septal Q21.0
  - with dextroposition of aorta, pulmonary stenosis and hypertrophy of right ventricle Q21.3
  - in tetralogy of Fallot Q21.3
- intervertebral annular fibrosis — *see also* Disease, intervertebral disc, by site M51.9
  - lumbar M51.A0
    - large M51.A2
    - small M51.A1
  - lumbosacral M51.A3
    - large M51.A5
    - small M51.A4
- learning (specific) — *see* Disorder, learning
- lymphocyte function antigen-1 (LFA-1) D84.0
- lysosomal enzyme, post-translational modification E77.0
- major osseous M89.70
  - ankle M89.77-☑
  - carpus M89.74-☑
  - clavicle M89.71-☑
  - femur M89.75-☑
  - fibula M89.76-☑
  - fingers M89.74-☑
  - foot M89.77-☑
  - forearm M89.73-☑
  - hand M89.74-☑
  - humerus M89.72-☑
  - lower leg M89.76-☑
  - metacarpus M89.74-☑
  - metatarsus M89.77-☑
  - multiple sites M89.79
  - pelvic region M89.75-☑
  - pelvis M89.75-☑
  - radius M89.73-☑
  - scapula M89.71-☑
  - shoulder region M89.71-☑
  - specified NEC M89.78
  - tarsus M89.77-☑
  - thigh M89.75-☑
  - tibia M89.76-☑
  - toes M89.77-☑
  - ulna M89.73-☑
- mental — *see* Disability, intellectual
- modification, lysosomal enzymes, post-translational E77.0
- obstructive, congenital
  - renal pelvis Q62.39
  - ureter Q62.39
    - atresia — *see* Atresia, ureter
    - cecoureterocele Q62.32
    - megaureter Q62.2
    - orthotopic ureterocele Q62.31
- osseous, major M89.70
  - ankle M89.77-☑
  - carpus M89.74-☑
  - clavicle M89.71-☑
  - femur M89.75-☑
  - fibula M89.76-☑
  - fingers M89.74-☑
  - foot M89.77-☑
  - forearm M89.73-☑
  - hand M89.74-☑
  - humerus M89.72-☑
  - lower leg M89.76-☑
  - metacarpus M89.74-☑
  - metatarsus M89.77-☑
  - multiple sites M89.9
  - pelvic region M89.75-☑
  - pelvis M89.75-☑
  - radius M89.73-☑

Defect, defective — *continued*
- osseous, major — *continued*
  - scapula M89.71-☑
  - shoulder region M89.71-☑
  - specified NEC M89.78
  - tarsus M89.77-☑
  - thigh M89.75-☑
  - tibia M89.76-☑
  - toes M89.77-☑
  - ulna M89.73-☑
- osteochondral NEC — *see also* Deformity M95.8
- ostium
  - primum Q21.20
  - secundum Q21.11
- peroxidase E80.3
- placental blood supply — *see* Insufficiency, placental
- platelets, qualitative D69.1
  - constitutional — *see* Disease, von Willebrand
- postural NEC, spine — *see* Dorsopathy, deforming
- qualitative, of von Willebrand factor
  - with
    - decreased platelet adhesion and selective deficiency of high-molecular-weight multimers — *see also* Disease, von Willebrand D68.020
    - defective platelet adhesion with a normal size distribution of von Willebrand factor multimers — *see also* Disease, von Willebrand D68.022
    - defective von Willebrand factor to factor VIII binding — *see also* Disease, von Willebrand D68.023
    - high-molecular-weight von Willebrand factor loss — *see also* Disease, von Willebrand D68.021
    - hyper-adhesive forms — *see also* Disease, von Willebrand D68.021
    - increased affinity for platelet glycoprotein Ib — *see also* Disease, von Willebrand D68.021
    - markedly decreased affinity for factor VIII — *see also* Disease, von Willebrand D68.023
  - in von Willebrand factor function, with no further subtyping — *see also* Disease, von Willebrand D68.029
- reduction
  - limb Q73.8
    - lower Q72.9-☑
      - absence — *see* Agenesis, leg
        - foot — *see* Agenesis, foot
      - longitudinal
        - femur Q72.4-☑
        - fibula Q72.6-☑
        - tibia Q72.5-☑
      - specified type NEC Q72.89-☑
      - split foot Q72.7-☑
    - specified type NEC Q73.8
    - upper Q71.9-☑
      - absence — *see* Agenesis, arm
        - forearm — *see* Agenesis, forearm
        - hand — *see* Agenesis, hand
      - lobster-claw hand Q71.6-☑
      - longitudinal
        - radius Q71.4-☑
        - ulna Q71.5-☑
      - specified type NEC Q71.89-☑
- renal pelvis Q63.8
  - obstructive Q62.39
- respiratory system, congenital Q34.9
- restoration, dental K08.50
  - specified NEC K08.59
- retinal nerve bundle fibers H35.89
- septal (heart) NOS Q21.9
  - acquired (atrial) (auricular) (ventricular) (old) I51.0
  - atrial — *see also* Defect, atrial septal Q21.10
    - concurrent with acute myocardial infarction — *see* Infarct, myocardium
    - following acute myocardial infarction (current complication) I23.1
  - ventricular — *see also* Defect, ventricular septal Q21.0
- sinus venosus — *see also* Defect, atrial septal, sinus venosus Q21.16
- speech — *see* Disorder, speech
  - developmental F80.9
  - specified NEC R47.89
- Taussig-Bing (aortic transposition and overriding pulmonary artery) Q20.1

Defect, defective — continued
  teeth, wedge KØ3.1
  vascular (local) I99.9
    congenital Q27.9
  ventricular septal Q21.Ø
    concurrent with acute myocardial infarction — see Infarct, myocardium
    following acute myocardial infarction (current complication) I23.2
    in tetralogy of Fallot Q21.3
  vision NEC H54.7
  visual field H53.4Ø
    bilateral
      heteronymous H53.47
      homonymous H53.46- ☑
    generalized contraction H53.48- ☑
    localized
      arcuate H53.43- ☑
      scotoma (central area) H53.41- ☑
        blind spot area H53.42- ☑
      sector H53.43- ☑
      specified type NEC H53.45- ☑
  voice R49.9
    specified NEC R49.8
  wedge, tooth, teeth (abrasion) KØ3.1
Deferentitis N49.1
  gonorrheal (acute) (chronic) A54.23
Defibrination (syndrome) D65
  antepartum — see Hemorrhage, antepartum, with coagulation defect, disseminated intravascular coagulation
  following ectopic or molar pregnancy OØ8.1
  intrapartum O67.Ø
  newborn P6Ø
  postpartum O72.3
Deficiency, deficient
  3-beta hydroxysteroid dehydrogenase E25.Ø
  5-alpha reductase (with male pseudohermaphroditism) E29.1
  11-hydroxylase E25.Ø
  21-hydroxylase E25.Ø
  AADC (aromatic L-amino acid decarboxylase) E7Ø.81
  abdominal muscle syndrome Q79.4
  AC globulin (congenital) (hereditary) D68.2
    acquired D68.4
  accelerator globulin (Ac G) (blood) D68.2
  acid phosphatase E83.39
  acid sphingomyelinase (ASMD) E75.249
    type
      A E75.24Ø
      A/B E75.244
      B E75.241
  activating factor (blood) D68.2
  ADA2 (adenosine deaminase 2) D81.32
  adenosine deaminase (ADA) D81.3Ø
    with severe combined immunodeficiency (SCID) D81.31
    partial (type 1) D81.39
    specified NEC D81.39
    type 1 (without SCID) (without severe combined immunodeficiency) D81.39
    type 2 D81.32
  aldolase (hereditary) E74.19
  alpha-1-antitrypsin E88.Ø1
  amino-acids E72.9
  anemia — see Anemia
  aneurin E51.9
  antibody with
    hyperimmunoglobulinemia D8Ø.6
    near-normal immunoglobins D8Ø.6
  antidiuretic hormone E23.2
  anti-hemophilic
    factor (A) D66
      B D67
      C D68.1
    globulin (AHG) NEC D66
  antithrombin (antithrombin III) D68.59
  aromatic L-amino acid decarboxylase (AADC) E7Ø.81
  ascorbic acid E54
  attention (disorder) (syndrome) F98.8
    with hyperactivity — see Disorder, attention-deficit hyperactivity
  autoprothrombin
    I D68.2
    II D67
    C D68.2
  beta-glucuronidase E76.29
  biotin E53.8

Deficiency, deficient — continued
  biotin-dependent carboxylase D81.819
  biotinidase D81.81Ø
  brancher enzyme (amylopectinosis) E74.Ø3
  C1 esterase inhibitor (C1-INH) D84.1
  calciferol E55.9
    with
      adult osteomalacia M83.8
      rickets — see Rickets
  calcium (dietary) E58
  calorie, severe E43
    with marasmus E41
      and kwashiorkor E42
  cardiac — see Insufficiency, myocardial
  carnitine E71.4Ø
    due to
      hemodialysis E71.43
      inborn errors of metabolism E71.42
      Valproic acid therapy E71.43
    iatrogenic E71.43
    muscle palmityltransferase E71.314
    primary E71.41
    secondary E71.448
  carotene E5Ø.9
  central nervous system G96.89
  ceruloplasmin (Wilson) E83.Ø1
  choline E53.8
  Christmas factor D67
  chromium E61.4
  chronic neurovisceral acid sphingomyelinase E75.244
  chronic visceral acid sphingomyelinase E75.241
  clotting (blood) — see also Deficiency, coagulation factor D68.9
  clotting factor NEC (hereditary) — see also Deficiency, factor D68.2
  coagulation NOS D68.9
    with
      ectopic pregnancy OØ8.1
      molar pregnancy OØ8.1
    acquired (any) D68.4
    antepartum hemorrhage — see Hemorrhage, antepartum, with coagulation defect
    clotting factor NEC — see also Deficiency, factor D68.2
    due to
      hyperprothrombinemia D68.4
      liver disease D68.4
      vitamin K deficiency D68.4
    newborn, transient P61.6
    postpartum O72.3
    specified NEC D68.8
  cognitive FØ9
  color vision H53.5Ø
    achromatopsia H53.51
    acquired H53.52
    deuteranomaly H53.53
    protanomaly H53.54
    specified type NEC H53.59
    tritanomaly H53.55
  combined glucocorticoid and mineralocorticoid E27.49
  contact factor D68.2
  copper (nutritional) E61.Ø
  corticoadrenal E27.4Ø
    primary E27.1
  craniofacial axis Q75.Ø
  cyanocobalamin E53.8
  debrancher enzyme (limit dextrinosis) E74.Ø3
  dehydrogenase
    long chain/very long chain acyl CoA E71.31Ø
    medium chain acyl CoA E71.311
    short chain acyl CoA E71.312
  diet E63.9
  dihydropyrimidine dehydrogenase (DPD) E88.89
  disaccharidase E73.9
  edema — see Malnutrition, severe
  endocrine E34.9
  energy-supply — see Malnutrition
  enzymes, circulating NEC E88.Ø9
  ergosterol E55.9
    with
      adult osteomalacia M83.8
      rickets — see Rickets
  essential fatty acid (EFA) E63.Ø
  eye movements
    saccadic H55.81
    smooth pursuit H55.82
  factor — see also Deficiency, coagulation
    Hageman D68.2

Deficiency, deficient — continued
  factor — see also Deficiency, coagulation — continued
    I (congenital) (hereditary) D68.2
    II (congenital) (hereditary) D68.2
    IX (congenital) (functional) (hereditary) (with functional defect) D67
    multiple (congenital) D68.8
      acquired D68.4
    V (congenital) (hereditary) D68.2
    VII (congenital) (hereditary) D68.2
    VIII (congenital) (functional) (hereditary) (with functional defect) D66
      with vascular defect — see Disease, von Willebrand
    X (congenital) (hereditary) D68.2
    XI (congenital) (hereditary) D68.1
    XII (congenital) (hereditary) D68.2
    XIII (congenital) (hereditary) D68.2
  femoral, proximal focal (congenital) — see Defect, reduction, lower limb, longitudinal, femur
  fibrinase D68.2
  fibrinogen (congenital) (hereditary) D68.2
    acquired D65
  fibrin-stabilizing factor (congenital) (hereditary) D68.2
    acquired D68.4
  folate E53.8
  folic acid E53.8
  foreskin N47.3
  fructokinase E74.11
  fructose 1,6-diphosphatase E74.19
  fructose-1-phosphate aldolase E74.19
  GABA (gamma aminobutyric acid) transaminase E72.81
  GABA-T (gamma aminobutyric acid transaminase) E72.81
  galactokinase E74.29
  galactose-1-phosphate uridyl transferase E74.29
  gammaglobulin in blood D8Ø.1
    hereditary D8Ø.Ø
  glass factor D68.2
  glucocorticoid E27.49
    mineralocorticoid E27.49
  glucose transporter protein type 1 E74.81Ø
  glucose-6-phosphatase E74.Ø1
  glucose-6-phosphate dehydrogenase
    anemia D55.Ø
    without anemia D75.A
  glucuronyl transferase E8Ø.5
  Glut1 E74.81Ø
  glycogen synthetase E74.Ø9
  gonadotropin (isolated) E23.Ø
  growth hormone (idiopathic) (isolated) E23.Ø
  Hageman factor D68.2
  hemoglobin D64.9
  hepatophosphorylase E74.Ø9
  homogentisate 1,2-dioxygenase E7Ø.29
  hormone
    anterior pituitary (partial) NEC E23.Ø
      growth E23.Ø
    growth (isolated) E23.Ø
    pituitary E23.Ø
    testicular E29.1
  hypoxanthine- (guanine)-phosphoribosyltransferase (HG- PRT) (total H-PRT) E79.1
  immunity D84.9
    cell-mediated D84.89
      with thrombocytopenia and eczema D82.Ø
    combined D81.9
    humoral D8Ø.9
    IgA (secretory) D8Ø.2
    IgG D8Ø.3
    IgM D8Ø.4
  immuno — see Immunodeficiency
  immunoglobulin, selective
    A (IgA) D8Ø.2
    G (IgG) (subclasses) D8Ø.3
    M (IgM) D8Ø.4
  infantile neurovisceral acid sphingomyelinase E75.24Ø
  inositol (B complex) E53.8
  intrinsic
    factor (congenital) D51.Ø
    sphincter N36.42
      with urethral hypermobility N36.43
  iodine E61.8
    congenital syndrome — see Syndrome, iodine-deficiency, congenital
  iron E61.1
    anemia D5Ø.9
  kalium E87.6

Deficiency, deficient — *continued*

kappa-light chain D80.8
labile factor (congenital) (hereditary) D68.2
  acquired D68.4
lacrimal fluid (acquired) — *see also* Syndrome, dry eye
  congenital Q10.6
lactase
  congenital E73.0
  secondary E73.1
Laki-Lorand factor D68.2
lecithin cholesterol acyltransferase E78.6
lipocaic K86.89
lipoprotein (familial) (high density) E78.6
liver phosphorylase E74.09
lysosomal alpha-1, 4 glucosidase E74.02
magnesium E61.2
major histocompatibility complex
  class I D81.6
  class II D81.7
manganese E61.3
menadione (vitamin K) E56.1
  newborn P53
mental (familial) (hereditary) — *see* Disability, intellectual
methylenetetrahydrofolate reductase (MTHFR) E72.12
mevalonate kinase M04.1
mineralocorticoid E27.49
  with glucocorticoid E27.49
mineral NEC E61.8
molybdenum (nutritional) E61.5
moral F60.2
multiple nutrient elements E61.7
multiple sulfatase (MSD) E75.26
muscle
  carnitine (palmityltransferase) E71.314
  phosphofructokinase E74.09
myoadenylate deaminase E79.2
myocardial — *see* Insufficiency, myocardial
myophosphorylase E74.04
NADH diaphorase or reductase (congenital) D74.0
NADH-methemoglobin reductase (congenital) D74.0
natrium E87.1
niacin (amide) (-tryptophan) E52
nicotinamide E52
nicotinic acid E52
number of teeth — *see* Anodontia
nutrient element E61.9
  multiple E61.7
  specified NEC E61.8
nutrition, nutritional — *see also* Nutrition deficient
  E63.9
  sequelae — *see* Sequelae, nutritional deficiency
  specified NEC E63.8
of interleukin 1 receptor antagonist [DIRA] M04.8
ornithine transcarbamylase E72.4
ovarian E28.39
oxygen — *see* Anoxia
pantothenic acid E53.8
parathyroid (gland) E20.9
perineum (female) N81.89
phenylalanine hydroxylase E70.1
phosphoenolpyruvate carboxykinase E74.4
phosphofructokinase E74.19
phosphomannomutase E74.818
phosphomannose isomerase E74.818
phosphomannosyl mutase E74.818
phosphorylase kinase, liver E74.09
pituitary hormone (isolated) E23.0
plasma thromboplastin
  antecedent (PTA) D68.1
  component (PTC) D67
plasminogen (type 1) (type 2) E88.02
platelet NEC D69.1
  constitutional — *see* Disease, von Willebrand
polyglandular E31.8
  autoimmune E31.0
potassium (K) E87.6
prepuce N47.3
proaccelerin (congenital) (hereditary) D68.2
  acquired D68.4
proconvertin factor (congenital) (hereditary) D68.2
  acquired D68.4
protein — *see also* Malnutrition E46
  anemia D53.0
  C D68.59
  S D68.59
prothrombin (congenital) (hereditary) D68.2
  acquired D68.4

Deficiency, deficient — *continued*

Prower factor D68.2
pseudocholinesterase E88.09
PTA (plasma thromboplastin antecedent) D68.1
PTC (plasma thromboplastin component) D67
purine nucleoside phosphorylase (PNP) D81.5
pyracin (alpha) (beta) E53.1
pyridoxal E53.1
pyridoxamine E53.1
pyridoxine (derivatives) E53.1
pyruvate
  carboxylase E74.4
  dehydrogenase E74.4
riboflavin (vitamin B2) E53.0
salt E87.1
secretion
  ovary E28.39
  salivary gland (any) K11.7
  urine R34
selenium (dietary) E59
serum antitrypsin, familial E88.01
short stature homeobox gene (SHOX)
  with
    dyschondrosteosis Q78.8
    short stature (idiopathic) E34.328
    Turner's syndrome Q96.9
sodium (Na) E87.1
SPCA (factor VII) D68.2
sphincter, intrinsic N36.42
  with urethral hypermobility N36.43
stable factor (congenital) (hereditary) D68.2
  acquired D68.4
Stuart-Prower (factor X) D68.2
succinic semialdehyde dehydrogenase E72.81
sucrase E74.39
sulfatase E75.26
sulfite oxidase E72.19
thiamin, thiaminic (chloride) E51.9
  beriberi (dry) E51.11
  wet E51.12
thrombokinase D68.2
  newborn P53
thyroid (gland) — *see* Hypothyroidism
tocopherol E56.0
tooth bud K00.0
transcobalamine II (anemia) D51.2
vanadium E61.6
vascular I99.9
vasopressin E23.2
vertical ridge K06.8
viosterol — *see* Deficiency, calciferol
vitamin (multiple) NOS E56.9
  A E50.9
    with
      Bitot's spot (corneal) E50.1
      follicular keratosis E50.8
      keratomalacia E50.4
      manifestations NEC E50.8
      night blindness E50.5
      scar of cornea, xerophthalmic E50.6
      xeroderma E50.8
      xerophthalmia E50.7
      xerosis
        conjunctival E50.0
          and Bitot's spot E50.1
        cornea E50.2
          and ulceration E50.3
    sequelae E64.1
  B (complex) NOS E53.9
    with
      beriberi (dry) E51.11
        wet E51.12
      pellagra E52
  B1 NOS E51.9
    beriberi (dry) E51.11
      with circulatory system manifestations E51.11
      wet E51.12
  B12 E53.8
  B2 (riboflavin) E53.0
  B6 E53.1
  C E54
    sequelae E64.2
  D E55.9
    with
      adult osteomalacia M83.8
      rickets — *see* Rickets
    25-hydroxylase E83.32
  E E56.0
  folic acid E53.8

Deficiency, deficient — *continued*

vitamin — *continued*
  G E53.0
  group B E53.9
    specified NEC E53.8
  H (biotin) E53.8
  K E56.1
    of newborn P53
  nicotinic E52
  P E56.8
  PP (pellagra-preventing) E52
  specified NEC E56.8
  thiamin E51.9
    beriberi — *see* Beriberi
von Willebrand factor
  partial quantitative — *see also* Disease, von Willebrand D68.01
  total quantitative — *see also* Disease, von Willebrand D68.03
zinc, dietary E60

Deficit — *see also* Deficiency

attention and concentration R41.840
  disorder — *see* Attention, deficit
  following
    cerebral infarction I69.310
    cerebrovascular disease I69.910
      specified disease NEC I69.810
    nontraumatic
      intracerebral hemorrhage I69.110
      specified intracranial hemorrhage NEC I69.210
      subarachnoid hemorrhage I69.010
cognitive
  communication R41.841
  emotional
    following
      cerebral infarction I69.315
      cerebrovascular disease I69.915
        specified disease NEC I69.815
      nontraumatic
        intracerebral hemorrhage I69.115
        specified intracranial hemorrhage NEC I69.215
        subarachnoid hemorrhage I69.015
  following
    cerebral infarction I69.319
    cerebrovascular disease I69.919
      specified disease NEC I69.819
    nontraumatic
      intracerebral hemorrhage I69.119
      specified intracranial hemorrhage NEC I69.219
      subarachnoid hemorrhage I69.019
  social
    following
      cerebral infarction I69.315
      cerebrovascular disease I69.915
        specified disease NEC I69.815
      nontraumatic
        intracerebral hemorrhage I69.115
        specified intracranial hemorrhage NEC I69.215
        subarachnoid hemorrhage I69.015
cognitive NEC R41.89
  following
    cerebral infarction I69.318
    cerebrovascular disease I69.918
      specified disease NEC I69.818
    nontraumatic
      intracerebral hemorrhage I69.118
      specified intracranial hemorrhage NEC I69.218
      subarachnoid hemorrhage I69.018
concentration R41.840
executive function R41.844
  following
    cerebral infarction I69.314
    cerebrovascular disease I69.914
      specified disease NEC I69.814
    nontraumatic
      intracerebral hemorrhage I69.114
      specified intracranial hemorrhage NEC I69.214
      subarachnoid hemorrhage I69.014
frontal lobe R41.844
  following
    cerebral infarction I69.314
    cerebrovascular disease I69.914
      specified disease NEC I69.814
    nontraumatic
      intracerebral hemorrhage I69.114
      specified intracranial hemorrhage NEC I69.214
      subarachnoid hemorrhage I69.014

Deficit — *continued*
  memory
    following
      cerebral infarction I69.311
      cerebrovascular disease I69.911
        specified disease NEC I69.811
      nontraumatic
        intracerebral hemorrhage I69.111
        specified intracranial hemorrhage NEC I69.211
        subarachnoid hemorrhage I69.011
  neurologic NEC R29.818
    ischemic
      reversible (RIND) I63.9
        prolonged (PRIND) I63.9
  oxygen R09.02
  prolonged reversible ischemic neurologic (PRIND) I63.9
  psychomotor R41.843
    following
      cerebral infarction I69.313
      cerebrovascular disease I69.913
        specified disease NEC I69.813
      nontraumatic
        intracerebral hemorrhage I69.113
        specified intracranial hemorrhage NEC I69.213
        subarachnoid hemorrhage I69.013
  visuospatial R41.842
    following
      cerebral infarction I69.312
      cerebrovascular disease I69.912
        specified disease NEC I69.812
      nontraumatic
        intracerebral hemorrhage I69.112
        specified intracranial hemorrhage NEC I69.212
        subarachnoid hemorrhage I69.012

Deflection
  radius — *see* Deformity, limb, specified type NEC, forearm
  septum (acquired) (nasal) (nose) J34.2
  spine — *see* Curvature, spine
  turbinate (nose) J34.2

Defluvium
  capillorum — *see* Alopecia
  ciliorum — *see* Madarosis
  unguium L60.8

Deformity Q89.9
  abdomen, congenital Q89.9
  abdominal wall
    acquired M95.8
    congenital Q79.59
  acquired (unspecified site) M95.9
  adrenal gland Q89.1
  alimentary tract, congenital Q45.9
    upper Q40.9
  ankle (joint) (acquired) — *see also* Deformity, limb, lower leg
    abduction — *see* Contraction, joint, ankle
    congenital Q68.8
    contraction — *see* Contraction, joint, ankle
    specified type NEC — *see* Deformity, limb, foot, specified NEC
  anus (acquired) K62.89
    congenital Q43.9
  aorta (arch) (congenital) Q25.40
    acquired I77.89
  aortic
    arch, acquired I77.89
    cusp or valve (congenital) Q23.8
      acquired — *see also* Endocarditis, aortic I35.8
  arm (acquired) (upper) — *see also* Deformity, limb, upper arm
    congenital Q68.8
    forearm — *see* Deformity, limb, forearm
  artery (congenital) (peripheral) NOS Q27.9
    acquired I77.89
    coronary (acquired) I25.9
      congenital Q24.5
    umbilical Q27.0
  atrial septal — *see also* Defect, atrial septal Q21.10
  auditory canal (external) (congenital) — *see also* Malformation, ear, external
    acquired — *see* Disorder, ear, external, specified type NEC
  auricle
    ear (congenital) — *see also* Malformation, ear, external
      acquired — *see* Disorder, pinna, deformity
  back — *see* Dorsopathy, deforming
  bile duct (common) (congenital) (hepatic) Q44.5

Deformity — *continued*
  bile duct — *continued*
    acquired K83.8
  biliary duct or passage (congenital) Q44.5
    acquired K83.8
  bladder (neck) (trigone) (sphincter) (acquired) N32.89
    congenital Q64.79
  bone (acquired) NOS M95.9
    congenital Q79.9
    turbinate M95.0
  brain (congenital) Q04.9
    acquired G93.89
    reduction Q04.3
  breast (acquired) N64.89
    congenital Q83.9
    reconstructed N65.0
  bronchus (congenital) Q32.4
    acquired NEC J98.09
  bursa, congenital Q79.9
  canaliculi (lacrimalis) (acquired) — *see also* Disorder, lacrimal system, changes
    congenital Q10.6
  canthus, acquired — *see* Disorder, eyelid, specified type NEC
  capillary (acquired) I78.8
  cardiovascular system, congenital Q28.9
  caruncle, lacrimal (acquired) — *see also* Disorder, lacrimal system, changes
    congenital Q10.6
  cascade, stomach K31.2
  cecum (congenital) Q43.9
    acquired K63.89
  cerebral, acquired G93.89
    congenital Q04.9
  cervix (uterus) (acquired) NEC N88.8
    congenital Q51.9
  cheek (acquired) M95.2
    congenital Q18.9
  chest (acquired) (wall) M95.4
    congenital Q67.8
    sequelae (late effect) of rickets E64.3
  chin (acquired) M95.2
    congenital Q18.9
  choroid (congenital) Q14.3
    acquired H31.8
    plexus Q07.8
      acquired G96.198
  cicatricial — *see* Cicatrix
  cilia, acquired — *see* Disorder, eyelid, specified type NEC
  clavicle (acquired) M95.8
    congenital Q68.8
  clitoris (congenital) Q52.6
    acquired N90.89
  clubfoot — *see* Clubfoot
  coccyx (acquired) — *see* subcategory M43.8 ☑
  colon (congenital) Q43.9
    acquired K63.89
  concha (ear), congenital — *see also* Malformation, ear, external
    acquired — *see* Disorder, pinna, deformity
  cornea (acquired) H18.70
    congenital Q13.4
    descemetocele — *see* Descemetocele
    ectasia — *see* Ectasia, cornea
    specified NEC H18.79- ☑
    staphyloma — *see* Staphyloma, cornea
  coronary artery (acquired) I25.9
    congenital Q24.5
  cranium (acquired) — *see* Deformity, skull
  cricoid cartilage (congenital) Q31.8
    acquired J38.7
  cystic duct (congenital) Q44.5
    acquired K82.8
  Dandy-Walker Q03.1
    with spina bifida — *see* Spina bifida
  diaphragm (congenital) Q79.1
    acquired J98.6
  digestive organ NOS Q45.9
  ductus arteriosus Q25.0
  duodenal bulb K31.89
  duodenum (congenital) Q43.9
    acquired K31.89
  dura — *see* Deformity, meninges
  ear (acquired) — *see also* Disorder, pinna, deformity
    congenital (external) Q17.9
      internal Q16.5
      middle Q16.4

Deformity — *continued*
  ear — *see also* Disorder, pinna, deformity — *continued*
    congenital — *continued*
      middle — *continued*
        ossicles Q16.3
      ossicles Q16.3
  ectodermal (congenital) NEC Q84.9
  ejaculatory duct (congenital) Q55.4
    acquired N50.89
  elbow (joint) (acquired) — *see also* Deformity, limb, upper arm
    congenital Q68.8
    contraction — *see* Contraction, joint, elbow
  endocrine gland NEC Q89.2
  epididymis (congenital) Q55.4
    acquired N50.89
  epiglottis (congenital) Q31.8
    acquired J38.7
  esophagus (congenital) Q39.9
    acquired K22.89
  eustachian tube (congenital) NEC Q17.8
  eye, congenital Q15.9
  eyebrow (congenital) Q18.8
  eyelid (acquired) — *see also* Disorder, eyelid, specified type NEC
    congenital Q10.3
  face (acquired) M95.2
    congenital Q18.9
  fallopian tube, acquired N83.8
  femur (acquired) — *see* Deformity, limb, specified type NEC, thigh
  fetal
    with fetopelvic disproportion O33.7 ☑
    causing obstructed labor O66.3
  finger (acquired) M20.00- ☑
    boutonniere M20.02- ☑
    congenital Q68.1
    flexion contracture — *see* Contraction, joint, hand
    mallet finger M20.01- ☑
    specified NEC M20.09- ☑
    swan-neck M20.03- ☑
  flexion (joint) (acquired) — *see also* Deformity, limb, flexion M21.20
    congenital NOS Q74.9
    hip Q65.89
  foot (acquired) — *see also* Deformity, limb, lower leg
    cavovarus (congenital) Q66.1- ☑
    congenital NOS Q66.9- ☑
      specified type NEC Q66.89
    specified type NEC — *see* Deformity, limb, foot, specified NEC
    valgus (congenital) Q66.6
      acquired — *see* Deformity, valgus, ankle
    varus (congenital) NEC Q66.3- ☑
      acquired — *see* Deformity, varus, ankle
  forearm (acquired) — *see also* Deformity, limb, forearm
    congenital Q68.8
  forehead (acquired) M95.2
    congenital Q75.8
  frontal bone (acquired) M95.2
    congenital Q75.8
  gallbladder (congenital) Q44.1
    acquired K82.8
  gastrointestinal tract (congenital) NOS Q45.9
    acquired K63.89
  genitalia, genital organ(s) or system NEC
    female (congenital) Q52.9
      acquired N94.89
      external Q52.70
    male (congenital) Q55.9
      acquired N50.89
  globe (eye) (congenital) Q15.8
    acquired H44.89
  gum, acquired NEC K06.8
  hand (acquired) — *see* Deformity, limb, hand
    congenital Q68.1
  head (acquired) M95.2
    congenital Q75.8
  heart (congenital) Q24.9
    septum Q21.9
      auricular — *see also* Defect, atrial septal Q21.10
      ventricular Q21.0
    valve (congenital) NEC Q24.8
      acquired — *see* Endocarditis
  heel (acquired) — *see* Deformity, foot
  hepatic duct (congenital) Q44.5
    acquired K83.8

Deformity — *continued*
- hip (joint) (acquired) (*see also* Deformity, limb, thigh)
  - congenital Q65.9
  - due to (previous) juvenile osteochondrosis — *see* Coxa, plana
  - flexion — *see* Contraction, joint, hip
- hourglass — *see* Contraction, hourglass
- humerus (acquired) M21.82- ☑
  - congenital Q74.0
- hypophyseal (congenital) Q89.2
- ileocecal (coil) (valve) (acquired) K63.89
  - congenital Q43.9
- ileum (congenital) Q43.9
  - acquired K63.89
- ilium (acquired) M95.5
  - congenital Q74.2
- integument (congenital) Q84.9
- intervertebral cartilage or disc (acquired) — *see* Disorder, disc, specified NEC
- intestine (large) (small) (congenital) NOS Q43.9
  - acquired K63.89
- intrinsic minus or plus (hand) — *see* Deformity, limb, specified type NEC, forearm
- iris (acquired) H21.89
  - congenital Q13.2
- ischium (acquired) M95.5
  - congenital Q74.2
- jaw (acquired) (congenital) M26.9
- joint (acquired) NEC M21.90
  - congenital Q68.8
  - elbow M21.92- ☑
  - hand M21.94- ☑
  - hip M21.95- ☑
  - knee M21.96- ☑
  - shoulder M21.92- ☑
  - wrist M21.93- ☑
- kidney(s) (calyx) (pelvis) (congenital) Q63.9
  - acquired N28.89
  - artery (congenital) Q27.2
    - acquired I77.89
- Klippel-Feil (brevicollis) Q76.1
- knee (acquired) NEC — *see also* Deformity, limb, lower leg
  - congenital Q68.2
- labium (majus) (minus) (congenital) Q52.79
  - acquired N90.89
- lacrimal passages or duct (congenital) NEC Q10.6
  - acquired — *see* Disorder, lacrimal system, changes
- larynx (muscle) (congenital) Q31.8
  - acquired J38.7
  - web (glottic) Q31.0
- leg (upper) (acquired) NEC — *see also* Deformity, limb, thigh
  - congenital Q68.8
  - lower leg — *see* Deformity, limb, lower leg
- lens (acquired) H27.8
  - congenital Q12.9
- lid (fold) (acquired) — *see also* Disorder, eyelid, specified type NEC
  - congenital Q10.3
- ligament (acquired) — *see* Disorder, ligament
  - congenital Q79.9
- limb (acquired) M21.90
  - clawfoot M21.53- ☑
  - clawhand M21.51- ☑
    - congenital Q68.1
  - clubfoot M21.54- ☑
  - clubhand M21.52- ☑
  - congenital, except reduction deformity Q74.9
  - flat foot M21.4- ☑
  - flexion M21.20
    - ankle M21.27- ☑
    - elbow M21.22- ☑
    - finger M21.24- ☑
    - hip M21.25- ☑
    - knee M21.26- ☑
    - shoulder M21.21- ☑
    - toe M21.27- ☑
    - wrist M21.23- ☑
  - foot
    - claw — *see* Deformity, limb, clawfoot
    - club — *see* Deformity, limb, clubfoot
    - drop M21.37- ☑
    - flat — *see* Deformity, limb, flat foot
    - specified NEC M21.6X- ☑
  - forearm M21.93- ☑
  - hand M21.94- ☑

Deformity — *continued*
- limb — *continued*
  - lower leg M21.96- ☑
  - specified type NEC M21.80
    - forearm M21.83- ☑
    - lower leg M21.86- ☑
    - thigh M21.85- ☑
    - upper arm M21.82- ☑
  - thigh M21.95- ☑
  - unequal length M21.70
    - short site is
      - femur M21.75- ☑
      - fibula M21.76- ☑
      - humerus M21.72- ☑
      - radius M21.73- ☑
      - tibia M21.76- ☑
      - ulna M21.73- ☑
  - upper arm M21.92- ☑
  - valgus — *see* Deformity, valgus
  - varus — *see* Deformity, varus
  - wrist drop M21.33- ☑
- lip (acquired) NEC K13.0
  - congenital Q38.0
- liver (congenital) Q44.7
  - acquired K76.89
- lumbosacral (congenital) (joint) (region) Q76.49
  - acquired — *see* subcategory M43.8 ☑
  - kyphosis — *see* Kyphosis, congenital
  - lordosis — *see* Lordosis, congenital
- lung (congenital) Q33.9
  - acquired J98.4
- lymphatic system, congenital Q89.9
- Madelung's (radius) Q74.0
- mandible (acquired) (congenital) M26.9
- maxilla (acquired) (congenital) M26.9
- meninges or membrane (congenital) Q07.9
  - cerebral Q04.8
    - acquired G96.198
  - spinal cord (congenital) Q06.- ☑
    - acquired G96.198
- metacarpus (acquired) — *see* Deformity, limb, forearm
  - congenital Q74.0
- metatarsus (acquired) — *see* Deformity, foot
  - congenital Q66.9- ☑
- middle ear (congenital) Q16.4
  - ossicles Q16.3
- mitral (leaflets) (valve) I05.8
  - parachute Q23.2
  - stenosis, congenital Q23.2
- mouth (acquired) K13.79
  - congenital Q38.6
- multiple, congenital NEC Q89.7
- muscle (acquired) M62.89
  - congenital Q79.9
    - sternocleidomastoid Q68.0
- musculoskeletal system (acquired) M95.9
  - congenital Q79.9
  - specified NEC M95.8
- nail (acquired) L60.8
  - congenital Q84.6
- nasal — *see* Deformity, nose
- neck (acquired) M95.3
  - congenital Q18.9
    - sternocleidomastoid Q68.0
- nervous system (congenital) Q07.9
- nipple (congenital) Q83.9
  - acquired N64.89
- nose (acquired) (cartilage) M95.0
  - bone (turbinate) M95.0
  - congenital Q30.9
    - bent or squashed Q67.4
  - saddle M95.0
    - syphilitic A50.57
  - septum (acquired) J34.2
    - congenital Q30.8
  - sinus (wall) (congenital) Q30.8
    - acquired M95.0
  - syphilitic (congenital) A50.57
    - late A52.73
- ocular muscle (congenital) Q10.3
  - acquired — *see* Strabismus, mechanical
- opticociliary vessels (congenital) Q13.2
- orbit (eye) (acquired) H05.30
  - atrophy — *see* Atrophy, orbit
  - congenital Q10.7
  - due to
    - bone disease NEC H05.32- ☑
    - trauma or surgery H05.33- ☑

Deformity — *continued*
- orbit — *continued*
  - enlargement — *see* Enlargement, orbit
  - exostosis — *see* Exostosis, orbit
- organ of Corti (congenital) Q16.5
- ovary (congenital) Q50.39
  - acquired N83.8
- oviduct, acquired N83.8
- palate (congenital) Q38.5
  - acquired M27.8
  - cleft (congenital) — *see* Cleft, palate
- pancreas (congenital) Q45.3
  - acquired K86.89
- parathyroid (gland) Q89.2
- parotid (gland) (congenital) Q38.4
  - acquired K11.8
- patella (acquired) — *see* Disorder, patella, specified NEC
- pelvis, pelvic (acquired) (bony) M95.5
  - with disproportion (fetopelvic) O33.0
    - causing obstructed labor O65.0
  - congenital Q74.2
  - rachitic sequelae (late effect) E64.3
- penis (glans) (congenital) Q55.69
  - acquired N48.89
- pericardium (congenital) Q24.8
  - acquired — *see* Pericarditis
- pharynx (congenital) Q38.8
  - acquired J39.2
- pinna, acquired — *see also* Disorder, pinna, deformity
  - congenital Q17.9
- pituitary (congenital) Q89.2
- posture — *see* Dorsopathy, deforming
- prepuce (congenital) Q55.69
  - acquired N47.8
- prostate (congenital) Q55.4
  - acquired N42.89
- pupil (congenital) Q13.2
  - acquired — *see* Abnormality, pupillary
- pylorus (congenital) Q40.3
  - acquired K31.89
- rachitic (acquired), old or healed E64.3
- radius (acquired) — *see also* Deformity, limb, forearm
  - congenital Q68.8
- rectum (congenital) Q43.9
  - acquired K62.89
- reduction (extremity) (limb), congenital — *see also* condition and site Q73.8
  - brain Q04.3
  - lower — *see* Defect, reduction, lower limb
  - upper — *see* Defect, reduction, upper limb
- renal — *see* Deformity, kidney
- respiratory system (congenital) Q34.9
- rib (acquired) M95.4
  - congenital Q76.6
  - cervical Q76.5
- rotation (joint) (acquired) — *see* Deformity, limb, specified site NEC
  - congenital Q74.9
  - hip — *see* Deformity, limb, specified type NEC, thigh
    - congenital Q65.89
- sacroiliac joint (congenital) — *see* subcategory Q74.2
  - acquired — *see* subcategory M43.8 ☑
- sacrum (acquired) — *see* subcategory M43.8 ☑
- saddle
  - back — *see* Lordosis
  - nose M95.0
    - syphilitic A50.57
- salivary gland or duct (congenital) Q38.4
  - acquired K11.8
- scapula (acquired) M95.8
  - congenital Q68.8
- scrotum (congenital) — *see also* Malformation, testis and scrotum
  - acquired N50.89
- seminal vesicles (congenital) Q55.4
  - acquired N50.89
- septum, nasal (acquired) J34.2
- shoulder (joint) (acquired) — *see* Deformity, limb, upper arm
  - congenital Q74.0
  - contraction — *see* Contraction, joint, shoulder
- sigmoid (flexure) (congenital) Q43.9
  - acquired K63.89
- skin (congenital) Q82.9
- skull (acquired) M95.2
  - congenital Q75.8

Deformity — continued
  skull — continued
    congenital — continued
      with
        anencephaly Q00.0
        encephalocele — see Encephalocele
        hydrocephalus Q03.9
          with spina bifida — see Spina bifida, by
            site, with hydrocephalus
        microcephaly Q02
  soft parts, organs or tissues (of pelvis)
    in pregnancy or childbirth NEC O34.8- ☑
      causing obstructed labor O65.5
  spermatic cord (congenital) Q55.4
    acquired N50.89
      torsion — see Torsion, spermatic cord
  spinal — see Dorsopathy, deforming
    column (acquired) — see Dorsopathy, deforming
    congenital Q67.5
    cord (congenital) Q06.9
      acquired G95.89
    nerve root (congenital) Q07.9
  spine (acquired) — see also Dorsopathy, deforming
    congenital Q67.5
    rachitic E64.3
    specified NEC — see Dorsopathy, deforming, speci-
      fied NEC
  spleen
    acquired D73.89
    congenital Q89.09
  Sprengel's (congenital) Q74.0
  sternocleidomastoid (muscle), congenital Q68.0
  sternum (acquired) M95.4
    congenital NEC Q76.7
  stomach (congenital) Q40.3
    acquired K31.89
  submandibular gland (congenital) Q38.4
  submaxillary gland (congenital) Q38.4
    acquired K11.8
  talipes — see Talipes
  testis (congenital) — see also Malformation, testis and
    scrotum
    acquired N44.8
      torsion — see Torsion, testis
  thigh (acquired) — see also Deformity, limb, thigh
    congenital NEC Q68.8
  thorax (acquired) (wall) M95.4
    congenital Q67.8
    sequelae of rickets E64.3
  thumb (acquired) — see also Deformity, finger
    congenital NEC Q68.1
  thymus (tissue) (congenital) Q89.2
  thyroid (gland) (congenital) Q89.2
    cartilage Q31.8
      acquired J38.7
  tibia (acquired) — see also Deformity, limb, specified
    type NEC, lower leg
    congenital NEC Q68.8
    saber (syphilitic) A50.56
  toe (acquired) M20.6- ☑
    congenital Q66.9- ☑
    hallux rigidus M20.2- ☑
    hallux valgus M20.1- ☑
    hallux varus M20.3- ☑
    hammer toe M20.4- ☑
    specified NEC M20.5X- ☑
  tongue (congenital) Q38.3
    acquired K14.8
  tooth, teeth K00.2
  trachea (rings) (congenital) Q32.1
    acquired J39.8
  transverse aortic arch (congenital) Q25.49
  tricuspid (leaflets) (valve) I07.8
    atresia or stenosis Q22.4
    Ebstein's Q22.5
  trunk (acquired) M95.8
    congenital Q89.9
  ulna (acquired) — see also Deformity, limb, forearm
    congenital NEC Q68.8
  urachus, congenital Q64.4
  ureter (opening) (congenital) Q62.8
    acquired N28.89
  urethra (congenital) Q64.79
    acquired N36.8
  urinary tract (congenital) Q64.9
    urachus Q64.4
  uterus (congenital) Q51.9
    acquired N85.8

Deformity — continued
  uvula (congenital) Q38.5
  vagina (acquired) N89.8
    congenital Q52.4
  valgus NEC M21.00
    ankle M21.07- ☑
    elbow M21.02- ☑
    hip M21.05- ☑
    knee M21.06- ☑
  valve, valvular (congenital) (heart) Q24.8
    acquired — see Endocarditis
  varus NEC M21.10
    ankle M21.17- ☑
    elbow M21.12- ☑
    hip M21.15 ☑
    knee M21.16- ☑
    tibia — see Osteochondrosis, juvenile, tibia
  vas deferens (congenital) Q55.4
    acquired N50.89
  vein (congenital) Q27.9
    great Q26.9
  vertebra — see Dorsopathy, deforming
  vertical talus (congenital) Q66.80
    left foot Q66.82
    right foot Q66.81
  vesicourethral orifice (acquired) N32.89
    congenital NEC Q64.79
  vessels of optic papilla (congenital) Q14.2
  visual field (contraction) — see Defect, visual field
  vitreous body, acquired H43.89
  vulva (congenital) Q52.79
    acquired N90.89
  wrist (joint) (acquired) — see also Deformity, limb,
    forearm
    congenital Q68.8
    contraction — see Contraction, joint, wrist

Degeneration, degenerative
  adrenal (capsule) (fatty) (gland) (hyaline) (infectional)
    E27.8
  amyloid — see also Amyloidosis E85.9
  anterior cornua, spinal cord G12.29
  anterior labral S43.49- ☑
  aorta, aortic I70.0
    fatty I77.89
  aortic valve (heart) — see Endocarditis, aortic
  arteriovascular — see Arteriosclerosis
  artery, arterial (atheromatous) (calcareous) — see also
    Arteriosclerosis
    cerebral, amyloid E85.4 [I68.0]
    medial — see Arteriosclerosis, extremities
  articular cartilage NEC — see Derangement, joint, artic-
    ular cartilage, by site
  atheromatous — see Arteriosclerosis
  basal nuclei or ganglia G23.9
    specified NEC G23.8
  bone NEC — see Disorder, bone, specified type NEC
  brachial plexus G54.0
  brain (cortical) (progressive) G31.9
    alcoholic G31.2
    arteriosclerotic I67.2
    childhood G31.9
      specified NEC G31.89
    cystic G31.89
      congenital Q04.6
    in
      alcoholism G31.2
      beriberi E51.2
      cerebrovascular disease I67.9
      congenital hydrocephalus Q03.9
        with spina bifida — see also Spina bifida
      Fabry-Anderson disease E75.21
      Gaucher's disease E75.22
      Hunter's syndrome E76.1
      lipidosis
        cerebral E75.4
        generalized E75.6
      mucopolysaccharidosis — see Mucopolysaccha-
        ridosis
      myxedema E03.9 [G32.89]
      neoplastic disease — see also Neoplasm
        D49.6 [G32.89]
      Niemann-Pick disease E75.249 [G32.89]
      sphingolipidosis E75.3 [G32.89]
      vitamin B12 deficiency E53.8 [G32.89]
    senile NEC G31.1
  breast N64.89
  Bruch's membrane — see Degeneration, choroid
  capillaries (fatty) I78.8

Degeneration, degenerative — continued
  capillaries — continued
    amyloid E85.89 [I79.8]
  cardiac — see also Degeneration, myocardial
    valve, valvular — see Endocarditis
  cardiorenal — see Hypertension, cardiorenal
  cardiovascular — see also Disease, cardiovascular
    renal — see Hypertension, cardiorenal
  cerebellar NOS G31.9
    alcoholic G31.2
    primary (hereditary) (sporadic) G11.9
  cerebral — see Degeneration, brain
  cerebrovascular I67.9
    due to hypertension I67.4
  cervical plexus G54.2
  cervix N88.8
    due to radiation (intended effect) N88.8
      adverse effect or misadventure N99.89
  chamber angle H21.21- ☑
  changes, spine or vertebra — see Spondylosis
  chorioretinal — see also Degeneration, choroid
    hereditary H31.20
  choroid (colloid) (drusen) H31.10- ☑
    atrophy — see Atrophy, choroidal
    hereditary — see Dystrophy, choroidal, hereditary
  ciliary body H21.22- ☑
  cochlear — see subcategory H83.8 ☑
  combined (spinal cord) (subacute) E53.8 [G32.0]
    with anemia (pernicious) D51.0 [G32.0]
      due to dietary vitamin B12 deficiency
        D51.3 [G32.0]
    in (due to)
      vitamin B12 deficiency E53.8 [G32.0]
        anemia D51.9 [G32.0]
  conjunctiva H11.10
    concretions — see Concretion, conjunctiva
    deposits — see Deposit, conjunctiva
    pigmentations — see Pigmentation, conjunctiva
    pinguecula — see Pinguecula
    xerosis — see Xerosis, conjunctiva
  cornea H18.40
    calcerous H18.43
      band keratopathy H18.42- ☑
    familial, hereditary — see Dystrophy, cornea
    hyaline (of old scars) H18.49
    keratomalacia — see Keratomalacia
    nodular H18.45- ☑
    peripheral H18.46- ☑
    senile H18.41- ☑
    specified type NEC H18.49
  cortical (cerebellar) (parenchymatous) G31.89
    alcoholic G31.2
    diffuse, due to arteriopathy I67.2
  corticobasal G31.85
  cutis L98.8
    amyloid E85.4 [L99]
  dental pulp K04.2
  disc disease — see Degeneration, intervertebral disc,
    by site
  dorsolateral (spinal cord) — see Degeneration, com-
    bined
  extrapyramidal G25.9
  eye, macular — see also Degeneration, macula
    congenital or hereditary — see Dystrophy, retina
  facet joints — see Spondylosis
  fatty
    liver NEC K76.0
      alcoholic K70.0
  grey matter (brain) (Alpers') G31.81
  heart — see also Degeneration, myocardial
    amyloid E85.4 [I43]
    atheromatous — see Disease, heart, ischemic,
      atherosclerotic
    ischemic — see Disease, heart, ischemic
  hepatolenticular (Wilson's) E83.01
  hepatorenal K76.7
  hyaline (diffuse) (generalized)
    localized — see Degeneration, by site
  infrapatellar fat pad M79.4
  intervertebral disc NOS
    with
      myelopathy — see Disorder, disc, with,
        myelopathy
      radiculitis or radiculopathy — see Disorder, disc,
        with, radiculopathy
      cervical, cervicothoracic — see Disorder, disc, cervi-
        cal, degeneration

Index

Degeneration, degenerative — Delay, delayed

Degeneration, degenerative — continued
  intervertebral disc — continued
    cervical, cervicothoracic — see Disorder, disc, cervical, degeneration — continued
      with
        myelopathy — see Disorder, disc, cervical, with myelopathy
        neuritis, radiculitis or radiculopathy — see Disorder, disc, cervical, with neuritis
    lumbar region M51.36
      with
        myelopathy M51.06
        neuritis, radiculitis, radiculopathy or sciatica M51.16
    lumbosacral region M51.37
      with
        neuritis, radiculitis, radiculopathy or sciatica M51.17
    sacrococcygeal region M53.3
    thoracic region M51.34
      with
        myelopathy M51.04
        neuritis, radiculitis, radiculopathy M51.14
    thoracolumbar region M51.35
      with
        myelopathy M51.05
        neuritis, radiculitis, radiculopathy M51.15
  intestine, amyloid E85.4
  iris (pigmentary) H21.23- ☑
  ischemic — see Ischemia
  joint disease — see Osteoarthritis
  kidney N28.89
    amyloid E85.4 [N29]
    cystic, congenital Q61.9
    fatty N28.89
    polycystic Q61.3
      adult type (autosomal dominant) Q61.2
      infantile type (autosomal recessive) NEC Q61.19
        collecting duct dilatation Q61.11
  Kuhnt-Junius — see also Degeneration, macula H35.32- ☑
  lens — see Cataract
  lenticular (familial) (progressive) (Wilson's) (with cirrhosis of liver) E83.01
  liver (diffuse) NEC K76.89
    amyloid E85.4 [K77]
    cystic K76.89
      congenital Q44.6
    fatty NEC K76.0
      alcoholic K70.0
    hypertrophic K76.89
    parenchymatous, acute or subacute K72.00
      with coma K72.01
    pigmentary K76.89
    toxic (acute) K71.9
  lung J98.4
  lymph gland I89.8
    hyaline I89.8
  macula, macular (acquired) (age-related) (senile) H35.30
    angioid streaks H35.33
    atrophic age-related H35.31- ☑
    congenital or hereditary — see Dystrophy, retina
    cystoid H35.35- ☑
    drusen H35.36- ☑
    dry age-related H35.31- ☑
    exudative H35.32- ☑
    hole H35.34- ☑
    nonexudative H35.31- ☑
    puckering H35.37- ☑
    toxic H35.38- ☑
    wet age-related H35.32- ☑
  membranous labyrinth, congenital (causing impairment of hearing) Q16.5
  meniscus — see Derangement, meniscus
  mitral — see Insufficiency, mitral
  Mönckeberg's — see Arteriosclerosis, extremities
  motor centers, senile G31.1
  multi-system G90.3
  mural — see Degeneration, myocardial
  muscle (fatty) (fibrous) (hyaline) (progressive) M62.89
    heart — see Degeneration, myocardial
  myelin, central nervous system G37.9
  myocardial, myocardium (fatty) (hyaline) (senile) I51.5
    with rheumatic fever (conditions in I00) I09.0
      active, acute or subacute I01.2
        with chorea I02.0
      inactive or quiescent (with chorea) I09.0

Degeneration, degenerative — continued
  myocardial, myocardium — continued
    hypertensive — see Hypertension, heart
    rheumatic — see Degeneration, myocardial, with rheumatic fever
    syphilitic A52.06
  nasal sinus (mucosa) J32.9
    frontal J32.1
    maxillary J32.0
  nerve — see Disorder, nerve
  nervous system G31.9
    alcoholic G31.2
    amyloid E85.4 [G99.8]
    autonomic G90.9
    fatty G31.89
    specified NEC G31.89
  nipple N64.89
  olivopontocerebellar (hereditary) (familial) G23.8
  osseous labyrinth — see subcategory H83.8 ☑
  ovary N83.8
    cystic N83.20- ☑
    microcystic N83.20- ☑
  pallidal pigmentary (progressive) G23.0
  pancreas K86.89
    tuberculous A18.83
  penis N48.89
  pigmentary (diffuse) (general)
    localized — see Degeneration, by site
    pallidal (progressive) G23.0
  pineal gland E34.8
  pituitary (gland) E23.6
  popliteal fat pad M79.4
  posterolateral (spinal cord) — see Degeneration, combined
  pulmonary valve (heart) I37.8
  pulp (tooth) K04.2
  pupillary margin H21.24- ☑
  renal — see Degeneration, kidney
  retina H35.9
    hereditary (cerebroretinal) (congenital) (juvenile) (macula) (peripheral) (pigmentary) — see Dystrophy, retina
    Kuhnt-Junius — see also Degeneration, macula H35.32- ☑
    macula (cystic) (exudative) (hole) (nonexudative) (pseudohole) (senile) (toxic) — see Degeneration, macula
    peripheral H35.40
      lattice H35.41- ☑
      microcystoid H35.42- ☑
      paving stone H35.43- ☑
      secondary
        pigmentary H35.45- ☑
        vitreoretinal H35.46- ☑
      senile reticular H35.44- ☑
    pigmentary (primary) — see also Dystrophy, retina
      secondary — see Degeneration, retina, peripheral, secondary
    posterior pole — see Degeneration, macula
  saccule, congenital (causing impairment of hearing) Q16.5
  senile R54
    brain G31.1
    cardiac, heart or myocardium — see Degeneration, myocardial
    motor centers G31.1
    vascular — see Arteriosclerosis
  sinus (cystic) — see also Sinusitis
    polypoid J33.1
  skin L98.8
    amyloid E85.4 [L99]
    colloid L98.8
  spinal (cord) N31.89
    amyloid E85.4 [G32.89]
    combined (subacute) — see Degeneration, combined
    dorsolateral — see Degeneration, combined
    familial NEC G31.89
    fatty G31.89
    funicular — see Degeneration, combined
    posterolateral — see Degeneration, combined
    subacute combined — see Degeneration, combined
    tuberculous A17.81
  spleen D73.0
    amyloid E85.4 [D77]
  stomach K31.89
  striatonigral G23.2
  suprarenal (capsule) (gland) E27.8

Degeneration, degenerative — continued
  synovial membrane (pulpy) — see Disorder, synovium, specified type NEC
  tapetoretinal — see Dystrophy, retina
  thymus (gland) E32.8
    fatty E32.8
  thyroid (gland) E07.89
  tricuspid (heart) (valve) I07.9
  tuberculous NEC — see Tuberculosis
  turbinate J34.89
  uterus (cystic) N85.8
  vascular (senile) — see Arteriosclerosis
    hypertensive — see Hypertension
  vitreoretinal, secondary — see Degeneration, retina, peripheral, secondary, vitreoretinal
  vitreous (body) H43.81- ☑
  Wallerian — see Disorder, nerve
  Wilson's hepatolenticular E83.01
Deglutition
  paralysis R13.0
    hysterical F44.4
  pneumonia J69.0
Degos' disease I77.89
Dehiscence (of)
  amputation stump T87.81
  cesarean wound O90.0
  closure of
    cornea T81.31 ☑
    craniotomy T81.32 ☑
    fascia (muscular) (superficial) T81.32 ☑
    internal organ or tissue T81.32 ☑
    laceration (external) (internal) T81.33 ☑
    ligament T81.32 ☑
    mucosa T81.31 ☑
    muscle or muscle flap T81.32 ☑
    ribs or rib cage T81.32 ☑
    skin and subcutaneous tissue (full-thickness) (superficial) T81.31 ☑
    skull T81.32 ☑
    sternum (sternotomy) T81.32 ☑
    tendon T81.32 ☑
    traumatic laceration (external) (internal) T81.33 ☑
  episiotomy O90.1
  operation wound NEC T81.31 ☑
    external operation wound (superficial) T81.31 ☑
    internal operation wound (deep) T81.32 ☑
  perineal wound (postpartum) O90.1
  traumatic injury wound repair T81.33 ☑
  wound T81.30 ☑
    traumatic repair T81.33 ☑
Dehydration E86.0
  newborn P74.1
Déjérine-Roussy syndrome G89.0
Déjérine-Sottas disease or neuropathy (hypertrophic) G60.0
Déjérine-Thomas atrophy G23.8
Delay, delayed
  any plane in pelvis
    complicating delivery O66.9
  birth or delivery NOS O63.9
  closure, ductus arteriosus (Botalli) P29.38
  coagulation — see Defect, coagulation
  conduction (cardiac) (ventricular) I45.9
  delivery, second twin, triplet, etc O63.2
  development R62.50
    global F88
    intellectual (specific) F81.9
    language F80.9
      due to hearing loss F80.4
    learning F81.9
    milestone R62.0
    pervasive F84.9
    physiological R62.50
      specified stage NEC R62.0
    reading F81.0
    sexual E30.0
    speech F80.9
      due to hearing loss F80.4
    spelling F81.81
  ejaculation F52.32
  gastric emptying K30
  menarche E30.0
  menstruation (cause unknown) N91.0
  milestone R62.0
  passage of meconium (newborn) P76.0
  primary respiration P28.9
  puberty (constitutional) E30.0

☑ Additional Character Required — Refer to the Tabular List for Character Selection

Delay, delayed — *continued*
  separation of umbilical cord P96.82
  sexual maturation, female E30.0
  sleep phase syndrome G47.21
  union, fracture — *see* Fracture, by site
  vaccination Z28.9
Deletion(s)
  autosome Q93.9
    identified by fluorescence in situ hybridization (FISH)
      Q93.89
    identified by in situ hybridization (ISH) Q93.89
  chromosome
    with complex rearrangements NEC Q93.7
    part of NEC Q93.59
    seen only at prometaphase Q93.89
    short arm
      22q11.2 Q93.81
      4 Q93.3
      5p Q93.4
      specified NEC Q93.89
    long arm chromosome 18 or 21 Q93.89
      with complex rearrangements NEC Q93.7
  microdeletions NEC Q93.88
Delhi boil or button B55.1
Delinquency (juvenile) (neurotic) F91.8
  group Z72.810
Delinquent immunization status Z28.39
  COVID-19 Z28.31- ☑
Delirium, delirious (acute or subacute) (not alcohol- or
  drug-induced) (with dementia) R41.0
  alcoholic (acute) (tremens) (withdrawal) F10.921
    with intoxication F10.921
      in
        abuse F10.121
        dependence F10.221
  due to (secondary to)
    alcohol
      intoxication F10.921
        in
          abuse F10.121
          dependence F10.221
      withdrawal F10.231
    amphetamine intoxication F15.921
      in
        abuse F15.121
        dependence F15.221
    anxiolytic
      intoxication F13.921
        in
          abuse F13.121
          dependence F13.221
      withdrawal F13.231
    cannabis intoxication (acute) F12.921
      in
        abuse F12.121
        dependence F12.221
    cocaine intoxication (acute) F14.921
      in
        abuse F14.121
        dependence F14.221
    general medical condition F05
    hallucinogen intoxication F16.921
      in
        abuse F16.121
        dependence F16.221
    hypnotic
      intoxication F13.921
        in
          abuse F13.121
          dependence F13.221
      withdrawal F13.231
    inhalant intoxication (acute) F18.921
      in
        abuse F18.121
        dependence F18.221
    multiple etiologies F05
    opioid intoxication (acute) F11.921
      in
        abuse F11.121
        dependence F11.221
    other (or unknown) substance F19.921
    phencyclidine intoxication (acute) F16.921
      in
        abuse F16.121
        dependence F16.221
    psychoactive substance NEC intoxication (acute)
      F19.921

Delirium, delirious — *continued*
  due to — *continued*
    psychoactive substance intoxication — *contin-*
      ued
      in
        abuse F19.121
        dependence F19.221
    sedative
      intoxication F13.921
        in
          abuse F13.121
          dependence F13.221
      withdrawal F13.231
    unknown etiology R41.0
  exhaustion F43.0
  hysterical F44.89
  postprocedural (postoperative) F05
  puerperal F05
  thyroid — *see* Thyrotoxicosis with thyroid storm
  traumatic — *see* Injury, intracranial
  tremens (alcohol-induced) F10.231
    sedative-induced F13.231
Delivery (childbirth) (labor)
  arrested active phase O62.1
  cesarean (for)
    abnormal
      pelvis (bony) (deformity) (major) NEC with dispro-
        portion (fetopelvic) O33.0
        with obstructed labor O65.0
      presentation or position O32.9 ☑
    abruptio placentae — *see also* Abruptio placentae
      O45.9- ☑
    acromion presentation O32.2 ☑
    atony, uterus O62.2
    breech presentation O32.1 ☑
      incomplete O32.8 ☑
    brow presentation O32.3 ☑
    cephalopelvic disproportion O33.9
    cerclage O34.3- ☑
    chin presentation O32.3 ☑
    cicatrix of cervix O34.4- ☑
    contracted pelvis (general)
      inlet O33.2
      outlet O33.3 ☑
    cord presentation or prolapse O69.0 ☑
    cystocele O34.8- ☑
    deformity (acquired) (congenital)
      pelvic organs or tissues NEC O34.8- ☑
      pelvis (bony) NEC O33.0
    disproportion NOS O33.9
    eclampsia — *see* Eclampsia
    face presentation O32.3 ☑
    failed
      forceps O66.5
      induction of labor O61.9
        instrumental O61.1
        mechanical O61.1
        medical O61.0
        specified NEC O61.8
        surgical O61.1
      trial of labor NOS O66.40
        following previous cesarean delivery O66.41
      vacuum extraction O66.5
      ventouse O66.5
    fetal-maternal hemorrhage O43.01- ☑
    hemorrhage (intrapartum) O67.9
      with coagulation defect O67.0
      specified cause NEC O67.8
    high head at term O32.4 ☑
    hydrocephalic fetus O33.6 ☑
    incarceration of uterus O34.51- ☑
    incoordinate uterine action O62.4
    increased size, fetus O33.5 ☑
    inertia, uterus O62.2
      primary O62.0
      secondary O62.1
    isthmocele O34.22
    lateroversion, uterus O34.59- ☑
    mal lie O32.9 ☑
    malposition
      fetus O32.9 ☑
      pelvic organs or tissues NEC O34.8- ☑
      uterus NEC O34.59- ☑
    malpresentation NOS O32.9 ☑
    oblique presentation O32.2 ☑
    occurring after 37 completed weeks of gestation
      but before 39 completed weeks gestation due
      to (spontaneous) onset of labor O75.82

Delivery — *continued*
  cesarean — *continued*
    oversize fetus O33.5 ☑
    pelvic tumor NEC O34.8- ☑
    placenta previa O44.0- ☑
      complete O44.0- ☑
        with hemorrhage O44.1- ☑
    placental insufficiency O36.51- ☑
    planned, occurring after 37 completed weeks of
      gestation but before 39 completed weeks
      gestation due to (spontaneous) onset of labor
      O75.82
    polyp, cervix O34.4- ☑
      causing obstructed labor O65.5
    poor dilatation, cervix O62.0
    pre-eclampsia O14.94
      mild O14.04
      moderate O14.04
      severe O14.14
        with hemolysis, elevated liver enzymes and
          low platelet count (HELLP) O14.24
    previous
      cesarean delivery O34.219
        classical (vertical) scar O34.212
        isthmocele O34.22
        low transverse scar O34.211
        mid-transverse T incision O34.218
        scar
          defect (isthmocele) O34.22
          specified type NEC O34.218
      surgery (to)
        cervix O34.4- ☑
        gynecological NEC O34.8- ☑
        rectum O34.7- ☑
        uterus O34.29
        vagina O34.6- ☑
    prolapse
      arm or hand O32.2 ☑
      uterus O34.52- ☑
    prolonged labor NOS O63.9
    rectocele O34.8- ☑
    retroversion
      uterus O34.53- ☑
    rigid
      cervix O34.4- ☑
      pelvic floor O34.8- ☑
      perineum O34.7- ☑
      vagina O34.6- ☑
      vulva O34.7- ☑
    sacculation, pregnant uterus O34.59- ☑
    scar(s)
      cervix O34.4- ☑
      cesarean delivery O34.219
        classical (vertical) O34.212
        isthmocele O34.22
        low transverse O34.211
        mid-transverse T incision O34.218
        scar
          defect (isthmocele) O34.22
          specified type NEC O34.218
        defect (isthmocele) O34.22
        transmural uterine O34.29
        uterus O34.29
    Shirodkar suture in situ O34.3- ☑
    shoulder presentation O32.2 ☑
    stenosis or stricture, cervix O34.4- ☑
    streptococcus group B (GBS) carrier state O99.824
    transmural uterine scar O34.29
    transverse presentation or lie O32.2 ☑
    tumor, pelvic organs or tissues NEC O34.8- ☑
      cervix O34.4- ☑
    umbilical cord presentation or prolapse O69.0 ☑
    without indication O82
  completely normal case O80
  complicated O75.9
    by
      abnormal, abnormality (of)
        forces of labor O62.9
          specified type NEC O62.8
        glucose O99.814
        uterine contractions NOS O62.9
      abruptio placentae — *see also* Abruptio placen-
        tae O45.9- ☑
      abuse
        physical O9A.32 (*following* O99)
        psychological O9A.52 (*following* O99)
        sexual O9A.42 (*following* O99)

Index

Delay, delayed — Delivery

Delivery — *continued*
  complicated — *continued*
    by — *continued*
      adherent placenta O72.0
        without hemorrhage O73.0
      alcohol use O99.314
      anemia (pre-existing) O99.02
      anesthetic death O74.8
      annular detachment of cervix O71.3
      atony, uterus O62.2
      attempted vacuum extraction and forceps O66.5
      Bandl's ring O62.4
      bariatric surgery status O99.844
      biliary tract disorder O26.62
      bleeding — *see* Delivery, complicated by, hemorrhage
      blood disorder NEC O99.12
      cervical dystocia (hypotonic) O62.2
        primary O62.0
        secondary O62.1
      circulatory system disorder O99.42
      compression of cord (umbilical) NEC O69.2 ☑
      condition NEC O99.892
      contraction, contracted ring O62.4
      cord (umbilical)
        around neck
          with compression O69.1 ☑
          without compression O69.81 ☑
        bruising O69.5 ☑
        complication O69.9 ☑
          specified NEC O69.89 ☑
        compression NEC O69.2 ☑
        entanglement O69.2 ☑
          without compression O69.82 ☑
        hematoma O69.5 ☑
        presentation O69.0 ☑
        prolapse O69.0 ☑
        short O69.3 ☑
        thrombosis (vessels) O69.5 ☑
        vascular lesion O69.5 ☑
      Couvelaire uterus O45.8X- ☑
      damage to (injury to) NEC
        perineum O71.82
        periurethral tissue O71.82
        vulva O71.82
      delay following rupture of membranes (spontaneous) — *see* Pregnancy, complicated by, premature rupture of membranes
      depressed fetal heart tones O76
      diabetes O24.92
        gestational O24.429
          diet controlled O24.420
          insulin controlled O24.424
          oral drug controlled (antidiabetic) (hypoglycemic) O24.425
        pre-existing O24.32
          specified NEC O24.82
          type 1 O24.02
          type 2 O24.12
      diastasis recti (abdominis) O71.89
      dilatation
        bladder O66.8
        cervix incomplete, poor or slow O62.0
      disease NEC O99.892
      disruptio uteri — *see* Delivery, complicated by, rupture, uterus
      drug use O99.324
      dysfunction, uterus NOS O62.9
        hypertonic O62.4
        hypotonic O62.2
          primary O62.0
          secondary O62.1
        incoordinate O62.4
      eclampsia O15.1
      embolism (pulmonary) — *see* Embolism, obstetric
      endocrine, nutritional or metabolic disease NEC O99.284
      failed
        attempted vaginal birth after previous cesarean delivery O66.41
        induction of labor O61.9
          instrumental O61.1
          mechanical O61.1
          medical O61.0
          specified NEC O61.8
          surgical O61.1
        trial of labor O66.40

      female genital mutilation O65.5
      fetal
        abnormal acid-base balance O68
        acidemia O68
        acidosis O68
        alkalosis O68
        death, early O02.1
        deformity O66.3
        heart rate or rhythm (abnormal) (non-reassuring) O76
        hypoxia O77.8
        stress O77.9
          due to drug administration O77.1
          electrocardiographic evidence of O77.8
          specified NEC O77.8
          ultrasound evidence of O77.8
      fever during labor O75.2
      gastric banding status O99.844
      gastric bypass status O99.844
      gastrointestinal disease NEC O99.62
      gestational
        diabetes O24.429
          diet controlled O24.420
          insulin (and diet) controlled O24.424
          oral drug controlled (antidiabetic) (hypoglycemic) O24.425
        edema O12.04
          with proteinuria O12.24
        proteinuria O12.14
      gonorrhea O98.22
      hematoma O71.7
        ischial spine O71.7
        pelvic O71.7
        vagina O71.7
        vulva or perineum O71.7
      hemorrhage (uterine) O67.9
        associated with
          afibrinogenemia O67.0
          coagulation defect O67.0
          hyperfibrinolysis O67.0
          hypofibrinogenemia O67.0
        due to
          low implantation of placenta O44.5- ☑
          low-lying placenta O44.5- ☑
          placenta previa O44.1- ☑
            marginal O44.3- ☑
            partial O44.3- ☑
          premature separation of placenta (normally implanted) — *see also* Abruptio placentae O45.9- ☑
          retained placenta O72.0
          uterine leiomyoma O67.8
        placenta NEC O67.8
        postpartum NEC (atonic) (immediate) O72.1
          with retained or trapped placenta O72.0
          delayed O72.2
          secondary O72.2
          third stage O72.0
      hourglass contraction, uterus O62.4
      hypertension, hypertensive (pre-existing) — *see* Hypertension, complicated by, childbirth (labor)
      hypotension O26.5- ☑
      incomplete dilatation (cervix) O62.0
      incoordinate uterus contractions O62.4
      inertia, uterus O62.2
        during latent phase of labor O62.0
        primary O62.0
        secondary O62.1
      infection (maternal) O98.92
        carrier state NEC O99.834
        gonorrhea O98.22
        human immunodeficiency virus (HIV) O98.72
        sexually transmitted NEC O98.32
        specified NEC O98.82
        syphilis O98.12
        tuberculosis O98.02
        viral hepatitis O98.42
        viral NEC O98.52
      injury (to mother) — *see also* Delivery, complicated, by, damage to O71.9
        nonobstetric O9A.22 (*following* O99)
          caused by abuse — *see* Delivery, complicated by, abuse
      intrauterine fetal death, early O02.1

      inversion, uterus O71.2
      laceration (perineal) O70.9
        anus (sphincter) O70.4
          with third degree laceration — *see also* Delivery, complicated, by, laceration, perineum, third degree O70.20
            with mucosa O70.3
          without third degree laceration O70.2 ☑
        bladder (urinary) O71.5
        bowel O71.5
        cervix (uteri) O71.3
        fourchette O70.0
        hymen O70.0
        labia O70.0
        pelvic
          floor O70.1
          organ NEC O71.5
        perineum, perineal O70.9
          first degree O70.0
          fourth degree O70.3
          muscles O70.1
          second degree O70.1
          skin O70.0
          slight O70.0
          third degree O70.20
            with
              both external anal sphincter (EAS) and internal anal sphincter (IAS) torn (IIIc) O70.23
              less than 50% of external anal sphincter (EAS) thickness torn (IIIa) O70.21
              more than 50% external anal sphincter (EAS) thickness torn (IIIb) O70.22
            IIIa O70.21
            IIIb O70.22
            IIIc O70.23
        peritoneum (pelvic) O71.5
        rectovaginal (septum) (without perineal laceration) O71.4
          with perineum — *see also* Delivery, complicated, by, laceration, perineum, third degree O70.20
          with anal or rectal mucosa O70.3
        specified NEC O71.89
        sphincter ani — *see* Delivery, complicated, by, laceration, anus (sphincter)
        urethra O71.5
        uterus O71.81
          before labor O71.81
        vagina, vaginal (deep) (high) (without perineal laceration) O71.4
          with perineum O70.0
          muscles, with perineum O70.1
        vulva O70.0
      liver disorder O26.62
      malignancy O9A.12 (*following* O99)
      malnutrition O25.2
      malposition, malpresentation
        uterus or cervix O65.5
        placenta O44.0- ☑
          with hemorrhage O44.1- ☑
        without obstruction — *see also* Delivery, complicated by, obstruction O32.9 ☑
          breech O32.1 ☑
          compound O32.6 ☑
          face (brow) (chin) O32.3 ☑
          footling O32.8 ☑
          high head O32.4 ☑
          oblique O32.2 ☑
          specified NEC O32.8 ☑
          transverse O32.2 ☑
          unstable lie O32.0 ☑
      meconium in amniotic fluid O77.0
      mental disorder NEC O99.344
      metrorrhexis — *see* Delivery, complicated by, rupture, uterus
      nervous system disorder O99.354
      obesity (pre-existing) O99.214
      obesity surgery status O99.844
      obstetric trauma O71.9
        specified NEC O71.89

Delivery — *continued*
  complicated — *continued*
    by — *continued*
      obstructed labor
        due to
          breech (complete) (frank) presentation O64.1 ☑
            incomplete O64.8 ☑
          brow presentation O64.3 ☑
          buttock presentation O64.1 ☑
          chin presentation O64.2 ☑
          compound presentation O64.5 ☑
          contracted pelvis O65.1
          deep transverse arrest O64.0 ☑
          deformed pelvis O65.0
          dystocia (fetal) O66.9
            due to
              conjoined twins O66.3
              fetal
                abnormality NEC O66.3
                ascites O66.3
                hydrops O66.3
                meningomyelocele O66.3
                sacral teratoma O66.3
                tumor O66.3
              hydrocephalic fetus O66.3
              shoulder O66.0
          face presentation O64.2 ☑
          fetopelvic disproportion O65.4
          footling presentation O64.8 ☑
          impacted shoulders O66.0
          incomplete rotation of fetal head O64.0 ☑
          large fetus O66.2
          locked twins O66.1
          malposition O64.9 ☑
            specified NEC O64.8 ☑
          malpresentation O64.9 ☑
            specified NEC O64.8 ☑
          multiple fetuses NEC O66.6
          pelvic
            abnormality (maternal) O65.9
              organ O65.5
              specified NEC O65.8
            contraction
              inlet O65.2
              mid-cavity O65.3
              outlet O65.3
          persistent (position)
            occipitoiliac O64.0 ☑
            occipitoposterior O64.0 ☑
            occipitosacral O64.0 ☑
            occipitotransverse O64.0 ☑
          prolapsed arm O64.4 ☑
          shoulder presentation O64.4 ☑
          specified NEC O66.8
      pathological retraction ring, uterus O62.4
      penetration, pregnant uterus by instrument O71.1
      perforation — *see* Delivery, complicated by, laceration
      placenta, placental
        ablatio — *see also* Abruptio placentae O45.9-
        abnormality O43.9- ☑
          specified NEC O43.89- ☑
        abruptio — *see also* Abruptio placentae O45.9-
        accreta O43.21-
        adherent (with hemorrhage) O72.0
          without hemorrhage O73.0
        detachment (premature) — *see also* Abruptio placentae O45.9- ☑
        disorder O43.9- ☑
          specified NEC O43.89- ☑
        hemorrhage NEC O67.8
        increta O43.22- ☑
        low (implantation) (lying) O44.4- ☑
          with hemorrhage O44.5- ☑
        malformation O43.10- ☑
        malposition O44.0- ☑
          without hemorrhage O44.1- ☑
        percreta O43.23- ☑
        previa (central) (complete) (lateral) (total) O44.0- ☑
          with hemorrhage O44.1- ☑
            marginal O44.2- ☑

Delivery — *continued*
  complicated — *continued*
    by — *continued*
      placenta, placental — *continued*
        previa — *continued*
          marginal — *continued*
            with hemorrhage O44.3- ☑
          partial O44.2- ☑
            with hemorrhage O44.3- ☑
        retained (with hemorrhage) O72.0
          without hemorrhage O73.0
        separation (premature) O45.9- ☑
          specified NEC O45.8X- ☑
        vicious insertion O44.1- ☑
      precipitate labor O62.3
      premature rupture, membranes — *see also* Pregnancy, complicated by, premature rupture of membranes O42.90
      prolapse
        arm or hand O32.2 ☑
        cord (umbilical) O69.0 ☑
        foot or leg O32.8 ☑
        uterus O34.52- ☑
      prolonged labor O63.9
        first stage O63.0
        second stage O63.1
      protozoal disease (maternal) O98.62
      respiratory disease NEC O99.52
      retained membranes or portions of placenta O72.2
        without hemorrhage O73.1
      retarded birth O63.9
      retention of secundines (with hemorrhage) O72.0
        without hemorrhage O73.0
        partial O72.2
          without hemorrhage O73.1
      rupture
        bladder (urinary) O71.5
        cervix O71.3
        pelvic organ NEC O71.5
        urethra O71.5
        uterus (during or after labor) O71.1
          before labor O71.0- ☑
      separation, pubic bone (symphysis pubis) O71.6
      shock O75.1
      shoulder presentation O64.4 ☑
      skin disorder O99.72
      spasm, cervix O62.4
      stenosis or stricture, cervix O65.5
      streptococcus group B (GBS) carrier state O99.824
      subluxation of symphysis (pubis) O26.72
      syphilis (maternal) O98.12
      tear — *see* Delivery, complicated by, laceration
      tetanic uterus O62.4
      trauma (obstetrical) — *see also* Delivery, complicated, by, damage to O71.9
        non-obstetric O9A.22 (*following* O99)
        periurethral O71.82
        specified NEC O71.89
      tuberculosis (maternal) O98.02
      tumor, pelvic organs or tissues NEC O65.5
      umbilical cord around neck
        with compression O69.1 ☑
        without compression O69.81 ☑
      uterine inertia O62.2
        during latent phase of labor O62.0
        primary O62.0
        secondary O62.1
      vasa previa O69.4 ☑
      velamentous insertion of cord O43.12- ☑
    specified complication NEC O75.89
  delayed NOS O63.9
    following rupture of membranes
      artificial O75.5
    second twin, triplet, etc. O63.2
  forceps, low following failed vacuum extraction O66.5
  missed (at or near term) O36.4 ☑
  normal O80
  obstructed — *see* Delivery, complicated by, obstructed labor
  precipitate O62.3
  preterm — *see also* Pregnancy, complicated by, preterm labor O60.10 ☑
  spontaneous O80
  term pregnancy NOS O80
  uncomplicated O80
  vaginal, following previous cesarean delivery O34.219
    classical (vertical) scar O34.212

Delivery — *continued*
  vaginal, following previous cesarean delivery — *continued*
    low transverse scar O34.211
    mid-transverse T incision O34.218
    scar
      defect (isthmocele) O34.22
      specified type NEC O34.218

Delusions (paranoid) — *see* Disorder, delusional

Dementia (degenerative (primary)) (old age) (persisting) (unspecified severity) (without behavioral disturbance, psychotic disturbance, mood disturbance, and anxiety) F03.90
  with
    aberrant motor behavior (exit-seeking) (pacing) (restlessness) (rocking) F03.911
    agitation F03.911
    anxiety F03.94
    behavioral disturbances (sexual disinhibition) (sleep disturbance) (social disinhibition) F03.918
      specified NEC F03.918
    Lewy bodies — *see also* Dementia, in, diseases specified elsewhere G31.83 *[F02.80]*
      with behavioral disturbance — *see also* Dementia, in, diseases specified elsewhere G31.83 *[F02.81-]* ☑
    mood disturbance (anhedonia) (apathy) (depression) F03.93
    Parkinsonism — *see also* Dementia, in, diseases specified elsewhere G20 *[F02.80]*
      with behavioral disturbance — *see also* Dementia, in, diseases specified elsewhere G20 *[F02.81-]* ☑
    Parkinson's disease — *see also* Dementia, in, diseases specified elsewhere G20 *[F02.80]*
      with behavioral disturbance — *see also* Dementia, in, diseases specified elsewhere G20 *[F02.81-]* ☑
    psychotic disturbance (delusional state) (hallucinations) (paranoia) (suspiciousness) F03.92
    verbal or physical behaviors (anger) (aggression) (combativeness) (profanity) (shouting) (threatening) (violence) F03.911
  alcoholic F10.97
    with dependence F10.27
  Alzheimer's type — *see* Disease, Alzheimer's
  arteriosclerotic — *see* Dementia, vascular
  atypical, Alzheimer's type — *see* Disease, Alzheimer's, specified NEC
  congenital — *see* Disability, intellectual
  frontal (lobe) — *see also* Dementia, in, diseases specified elsewhere G31.09 *[F02.80]*
    with behavioral disturbance — *see also* Dementia, in, diseases specified elsewhere G31.09 *[F02.81-]* ☑
  frontotemporal G31.09 *[F02.80]*
    with behavioral disturbance G31.09 *[F02.81]* ☑
    specified NEC — *see also* Dementia, in, diseases specified elsewhere G31.09 *[F02.80]*
      with behavioral disturbance — *see also* Dementia, in, diseases specified elsewhere G31.09 *[F02.81-]* ☑
  in (due to)
    alcohol F10.97
      with dependence F10.27
    Alzheimer's disease — *see* Disease, Alzheimer's
    arteriosclerotic brain disease — *see* Dementia, vascular
    cerebral lipidoses — *see also* Dementia, in, diseases specified elsewhere E75.- ☑ *[F02.80]*
      with behavioral disturbance — *see also* Dementia, in, diseases specified elsewhere E75.- ☑ *[F02.81-]* ☑
    Creutzfeldt-Jakob disease — *see also* Creutzfeldt-Jakob disease or syndrome (with dementia) A81.00
    diseases specified elsewhere (unspecified severity) (without behavioral disturbance, psychotic disturbance, mood disturbance, and anxiety) F02.80
      with
        aberrant motor behavior (exit-seeking) (pacing) (restlessness) (rocking) F02.811
        agitation F02.811
        anxiety F02.84

Dementia — *continued*
  in — *continued*
    diseases specified elsewhere — *continued*
      with — *continued*
        behavioral disturbances (sexual disinhibition) (sleep disturbance) (social disinhibition) F02.818
          specified NEC F02.818
        mood disturbance (anhedonia) (apathy) (depression) F02.83
        psychotic disturbance (delusional state) (hallucinations) (paranoia) (suspiciousness) F02.82
        verbal or physical behaviors (anger) (aggression) (combativeness) (profanity) (shouting) (threatening) (violence) F02.811
    mild F02.A0
      with
        aberrant motor behavior (exit-seeking) (pacing) (restlessness) (rocking) F02.A11
        agitation F02.A11
        anxiety F02.A4
        behavioral disturbances (sexual disinhibition) (sleep disturbance) (social disinhibition) F02.A18
          specified NEC F02.A18
        mood disturbance (anhedonia) (apathy) (depression) F02.A3
        psychotic disturbance (delusional state) (hallucinations) (paranoia) (suspiciousness) F02.A2
        verbal or physical behaviors (anger) (aggression) (combativeness) (profanity) (shouting) (threatening) (violence) F02.A11
    moderate F02.B0
      with
        aberrant motor behavior (exit-seeking) (pacing) (restlessness) (rocking) F02.B11
        agitation F02.B11
        anxiety F02.B4
        behavioral disturbances (sexual disinhibition) (sleep disturbance) (social disinhibition) F02.B18
          specified NEC F02.B18
        mood disturbance (anhedonia) (apathy) (depression) F02.B3
        psychotic disturbance (delusional state) (hallucinations) (paranoia) (suspiciousness) F02.B2
        verbal or physical behaviors (anger) (aggression) (combativeness) (profanity) (shouting) (threatening) (violence) F02.B11
    severe F02.C0
      with
        aberrant motor behavior (exit-seeking) (pacing) (restlessness) (rocking) F02.C11
        agitation F02.C11
        anxiety F02.C4
        behavioral disturbances (sexual disinhibition) (sleep disturbance) (social disinhibition) F02.C18
          specified NEC F02.C18
        mood disturbance (anhedonia) (apathy) (depression) F02.C3
        psychotic disturbance (delusional state) (hallucinations) (paranoia) (suspiciousness) F02.C2
        verbal or physical behaviors (anger) (aggression) (combativeness) (profanity) (shouting) (threatening) (violence) F02.C11
    epilepsy — *see also* Dementia, in, diseases specified elsewhere G40.- ☑ *[F02.80]*
      with behavioral disturbance — *see also* Dementia, in, diseases specified elsewhere G40.- ☑ *[F02.81-]* ☑
    hepatolenticular degeneration — *see also* Dementia, in, diseases specified elsewhere E83.01 *[F02.80]*
      with behavioral disturbance — *see also* Dementia, in, diseases specified elsewhere E83.01 *[F02.81-]* ☑

Dementia — *continued*
  in — *continued*
    human immunodeficiency virus (HIV) disease — *see also* Dementia, in, diseases specified elsewhere B20 *[F02.80]*
      with behavioral disturbance — *see also* Dementia, in, diseases specified elsewhere B20 *[F02.81-]* ☑
    Huntington's disease or chorea — *see also* Dementia, in, diseases specified elsewhere G10 *[F02.80]*
      with behavioral disturbance — *see also* Dementia, in, diseases specified elsewhere G10 *[F02.81-]* ☑
    hypercalcemia — *see also* Dementia, in, diseases specified elsewhere E83.52 *[F02.80]*
      with behavioral disturbance — *see also* Dementia, in, diseases specified elsewhere E83.52 *[F02.81-]* ☑
    hypothyroidism, acquired — *see also* Dementia, in, diseases specified elsewhere E03.9 *[F02.80]*
      with behavioral disturbance — *see also* Dementia, in, diseases specified elsewhere E03.9 *[F02.81-]* ☑
      due to iodine deficiency — *see also* Dementia, in, diseases specified elsewhere E01.8 *[F02.80]*
        with behavioral disturbance — *see also* Dementia, in, diseases specified elsewhere E01.8 *[F02.81-]* ☑
    inhalants F18.97
      with dependence F18.27
    multiple
      etiologies F03 ☑
      sclerosis — *see also* Dementia, in, diseases specified elsewhere G35 *[F02.80]*
        with behavioral disturbance — *see also* Dementia, in, diseases specified elsewhere G35 *[F02.81-]* ☑
    neurosyphilis — *see also* Dementia, in, diseases specified elsewhere A52.17 *[F02.80]*
      with behavioral disturbance — *see also* Dementia, in, diseases specified elsewhere A52.17 *[F02.81-]* ☑
      juvenile — *see also* Dementia, in, diseases specified elsewhere A50.49 *[F02.80]*
        with behavioral disturbance — *see also* Dementia, in, diseases specified elsewhere A50.49 *[F02.81-]* ☑
    niacin deficiency — *see also* Dementia, in, diseases specified elsewhere E52 *[F02.80]*
      with behavioral disturbance — *see also* Dementia, in, diseases specified elsewhere E52 *[F02.81-]* ☑
    paralysis agitans — *see also* Dementia, in, diseases specified elsewhere G20 *[F02.80]*
      with behavioral disturbance — *see also* Dementia, in, diseases specified elsewhere G20 *[F02.81-]* ☑
    Parkinson's disease — *see also* Dementia, in, diseases specified elsewhere G20 *[F02.80]*
    pellagra — *see also* Dementia, in, diseases specified elsewhere E52 *[F02.80]*
      with behavioral disturbance — *see also* Dementia, in, diseases specified elsewhere E52 *[F02.81-]* ☑
    Pick's — *see also* Dementia, in, diseases specified elsewhere G31.01 *[F02.80]*
      with behavioral disturbance — *see also* Dementia, in, diseases specified elsewhere G31.01 *[F02.81-]* ☑
    polyarteritis nodosa — *see also* Dementia, in, diseases specified elsewhere M30.0 *[F02.80]*
      with behavioral disturbance — *see also* Dementia, in, diseases specified elsewhere M30.0 *[F02.81-]* ☑
    psychoactive drug F19.97
      with dependence F19.27
      inhalants F18.97
        with dependence F18.27
      sedatives, hypnotics or anxiolytics F13.97
        with dependence F13.27
    sedatives, hypnotics or anxiolytics F13.97
      with dependence F13.27
    systemic lupus erythematosus — *see also* Dementia, in, diseases specified elsewhere M32.- ☑ *[F02.80]*

Dementia — *continued*
  in — *continued*
    systemic lupus erythematosus — *see also* Dementia, in, diseases specified elsewhere — *continued*
      with behavioral disturbance — *see also* Dementia, in, diseases specified elsewhere M32.- ☑ *[F02.81-]* ☑
    trypanosomiasis
      African — *see also* Dementia, in, diseases specified elsewhere B56.9 *[F02.80]*
        with behavioral disturbance — *see also* Dementia, in, diseases specified elsewhere B56.9 *[F02.81-]* ☑
    unknown etiology F03.- ☑
    vitamin B12 deficiency — *see also* Dementia, in, diseases specified elsewhere E53.8 *[F02.80]*
      with behavioral disturbance — *see also* Dementia, in, diseases specified elsewhere E53.8 *[F02.81-]* ☑
    volatile solvents F18.97
      with dependence F18.27
  infantile, infantilis F84.3
  Lewy body — *see also* Dementia, in, diseases specified elsewhere G31.83 *[F02.80]*
    with behavioral disturbance — *see also* Dementia, in, diseases specified elsewhere G31.83 *[F02.81-]* ☑
  mild F03.A0
    with
      aberrant motor behavior (exit-seeking) (pacing) (restlessness) (rocking) F03.A11
      agitation F03.A11
      anxiety F03.A4
      behavioral disturbances (sexual disinhibition) (sleep disturbance) (social disinhibition) F03.A18
        specified NEC F03.A18
      mood disturbance (anhedonia) (apathy) (depression) F03.A3
      psychotic disturbance (delusional state) (hallucinations) (paranoia) (suspiciousness) F03.A2
      verbal or physical behaviors (anger) (aggression) (combativeness) (profanity) (shouting) (threatening) (violence) F03.A11
  moderate F03.B0
    with
      aberrant motor behavior (exit-seeking) (pacing) (restlessness) (rocking) F03.B11
      agitation F03.B11
      anxiety F03.B4
      behavioral disturbances (sexual disinhibition) (sleep disturbance) (social disinhibition) F03.B18
        specified NEC F03.B18
      mood disturbance (anhedonia) (apathy) (depression) F03.B3
      psychotic disturbance (delusional state) (hallucinations) (paranoia) (suspiciousness) F03.B2
      verbal or physical behaviors (anger) (aggression) (combativeness) (profanity) (shouting) (threatening) (violence) F03.B11
  multi-infarct — *see* Dementia, vascular
  paralytica, paralytic (syphilitic) — *see also* Dementia, in, diseases specified elsewhere A52.17 *[F02.80]*
    with behavioral disturbance — *see also* Dementia, in, diseases specified elsewhere A52.17 *[F02.81-]* ☑
    juvenilis A50.45
  paretic A52.17
  praecox — *see* Schizophrenia
  presenile F03 ☑
    Alzheimer's type — *see* Disease, Alzheimer's, early onset
  primary degenerative F03 ☑
  progressive, syphilitic A52.17
  senile F03 ☑
    with acute confusional state F05
    Alzheimer's type — *see* Disease, Alzheimer's, late onset
    depressed or paranoid type F03 ☑
  severe F03.C0
    with
      aberrant motor behavior (exit-seeking) (pacing) (restlessness) (rocking) F03.C11
      agitation F03.C11
      anxiety F03.C4

☑ **Additional Character Required — Refer to the Tabular List for Character Selection**

Dementia — *continued*
  severe — *continued*
    with — *continued*
      behavioral disturbances (sexual disinhibition) (sleep disturbance) (social disinhibition) F03.C18
        specified NEC F03.C18
      mood disturbance (anhedonia) (apathy) (depression) F03.C3
      psychotic disturbance (delusional state) (hallucinations) (paranoia) (suspiciousness) F03.C2
      verbal or physical behaviors (anger) (aggression) (combativeness) (profanity) (shouting) (threatening) (violence) F03.C11
  vascular (acute onset) (mixed) (multi-infarct) (subcortical) (unspecified severity) (without behavioral disturbance, psychotic disturbance, mood disturbance, and anxiety) F01.50
    with
      aberrant motor behavior (exit-seeking) (pacing) (restlessness) (rocking) F01.511
      agitation F01.511
      anxiety F01.54
      behavioral disturbances (sleep disturbance) (sexual disinhibition) (social disinhibition) F01.518
        specified NEC F01.518
      mood disturbance (anhedonia) (apathy) (depression) F01.53
      psychotic disturbance (delusional state) (hallucinations) (paranoia) (suspiciousness) F01.52
      verbal or physical behaviors (anger) (aggression) (combativeness) (profanity) (shouting) (threatening) (violence) F01.511
    mild F01.A0
      with
        aberrant motor behavior (exit-seeking) (pacing) (restlessness) (rocking) F01.A11
        agitation F01.A11
        anxiety F01.A4
        behavioral disturbances (sleep disturbance) (sexual disinhibition) (social disinhibition) F01.A18
          specified NEC F01.A18
        mood disturbance (anhedonia) (apathy) (depression) F01.A3
        psychotic disturbance (delusional state) (hallucinations) (paranoia) (suspiciousness) F01.A2
        verbal or physical behaviors (anger) (aggression) (combativeness) (profanity) (shouting) (threatening) (violence) F01.A11
    moderate F01.B0
      with
        aberrant motor behavior (exit-seeking) (pacing) (restlessness) (rocking) F01.B11
        agitation F01.B11
        anxiety F01.B4
        behavioral disturbances (sleep disturbance) (sexual disinhibition) (social disinhibition) F01.B18
          specified NEC F01.B18
        mood disturbance (anhedonia) (apathy) (depression) F01.B3
        psychotic disturbance (delusional state) (hallucinations) (paranoia) (suspiciousness) F01.B2
        verbal or physical behaviors (anger) (aggression) (combativeness) (profanity) (shouting) (threatening) (violence) F01.B11
    severe F01.C0
      with
        aberrant motor behavior (exit-seeking) (pacing) (restlessness) (rocking) F01.C11
        agitation F01.C11
        anxiety F01.C4
        behavioral disturbances (sleep disturbance) (sexual disinhibition) (social disinhibition) F01.C18
          specified NEC F01.C18
        mood disturbance (anhedonia) (apathy) (depression) F01.C3
        psychotic disturbance (delusional state) (hallucinations) (paranoia) (suspiciousness) F01.C2

Dementia — *continued*
  vascular — *continued*
    severe — *continued*
      with — *continued*
        verbal or physical behaviors (anger) (aggression) (combativeness) (profanity) (shouting) (threatening) (violence) F01.C11
Demineralization, bone — *see* Osteoporosis
Demodex folliculorum (infestation) B88.0
Demophobia F40.248
Demoralization R45.3
Demyelination, demyelinization
  central nervous system G37.9
    specified NEC G37.8
  corpus callosum (central) G37.1
  disseminated, acute G36.9
    specified NEC G36.8
  global G35
  in optic neuritis G36.0
Dengue (classical) (fever) A90
  hemorrhagic A91
  sandfly A93.1
Dennie-Marfan syphilitic syndrome A50.45
Dens evaginatus, in dente or invaginatus K00.2
Dense breasts R92.2
Density
  increased, bone (disseminated) (generalized) (spotted) — *see* Disorder, bone, density and structure, specified type NEC
  lung (nodular) J98.4
Dental — *see also* condition
  examination Z01.20
    with abnormal findings Z01.21
  restoration
    aesthetically inadequate or displeasing K08.56
    defective K08.50
      specified NEC K08.59
    failure of marginal integrity K08.51
    failure of periodontal anatomical integrity K08.54
Dentia praecox K00.6
Denticles (pulp) K04.2
Dentigerous cyst K09.0
Dentin
  irregular (in pulp) K04.3
  opalescent K00.5
  secondary (in pulp) K04.3
  sensitive K03.89
Dentinogenesis imperfecta K00.5
Dentinoma — *see* Cyst, calcifying odontogenic
Dentition (syndrome) K00.7
  delayed K00.6
  difficult K00.7
  precocious K00.6
  premature K00.6
  retarded K00.6
Dependence (on) (syndrome) F19.20
  with remission F19.21
  alcohol (ethyl) (methyl) (without remission) F10.20
    with
      amnestic disorder, persisting F10.26
      anxiety disorder F10.280
      dementia, persisting F10.27
      intoxication F10.229
        with delirium F10.221
        uncomplicated F10.220
      mood disorder F10.24
      psychotic disorder F10.259
        with
          delusions F10.250
          hallucinations F10.251
      remission F10.21
      sexual dysfunction F10.281
      sleep disorder F10.282
      specified disorder NEC F10.288
      withdrawal F10.239
        with
          delirium F10.231
          perceptual disturbance F10.232
        uncomplicated F10.230
    counseling and surveillance Z71.41
    in remission F10.21
  amobarbital — *see* Dependence, drug, sedative
  amphetamine(s) (type) — *see* Dependence, drug, stimulant NEC
  amytal (sodium) — *see* Dependence, drug, sedative
  analgesic NEC F55.8

Dependence — *continued*
  anesthetic (agent) (gas) (general) (local) NEC — *see* Dependence, drug, psychoactive NEC
  anxiolytic NEC — *see* Dependence, drug, sedative
  barbital(s) — *see* Dependence, drug, sedative
  barbiturate(s) (compounds) (drugs classifiable to T42) — *see* Dependence, drug, sedative
  benzedrine — *see* Dependence, drug, stimulant NEC
  bhang — *see* Dependence, drug, cannabis
  bromide(s) NEC — *see* Dependence, drug, sedative
  caffeine — *see* Dependence, drug, stimulant NEC
  cannabis (sativa) (indica) (resin) (derivatives) (type) — *see* Dependence, drug, cannabis
  chloral (betaine) (hydrate) — *see* Dependence, drug, sedative
  chlordiazepoxide — *see* Dependence, drug, sedative
  coca (leaf) (derivatives) — *see* Dependence, drug, cocaine
  cocaine — *see* Dependence, drug, cocaine
  codeine — *see* Dependence, drug, opioid
  combinations of drugs F19.20
  dagga — *see* Dependence, drug, cannabis
  demerol — *see* Dependence, drug, opioid
  dexamphetamine — *see* Dependence, drug, stimulant NEC
  dexedrine — *see* Dependence, drug, stimulant NEC
  dextromethorphan — *see* Dependence, drug, opioid
  dextromoramide — *see* Dependence, drug, opioid
  dextro-nor-pseudo-ephedrine — *see* Dependence, drug, stimulant NEC
  dextrorphan — *see* Dependence, drug, opioid
  diazepam — *see* Dependence, drug, sedative
  dilaudid — *see* Dependence, drug, opioid
  D-lysergic acid diethylamide — *see* Dependence, drug, hallucinogen
  drug NEC F19.20
    with sleep disorder F19.282
    cannabis F12.20
      with
        anxiety disorder F12.280
        intoxication F12.229
          with
            delirium F12.221
            perceptual disturbance F12.222
          uncomplicated F12.220
        other specified disorder F12.288
        psychosis F12.259
          delusions F12.250
          hallucinations F12.251
        unspecified disorder F12.29
        withdrawal F12.23
      in remission F12.21
    cocaine F14.20
      with
        anxiety disorder F14.280
        intoxication F14.229
          with
            delirium F14.221
            perceptual disturbance F14.222
          uncomplicated F14.220
        mood disorder F14.24
        other specified disorder F14.288
        psychosis F14.259
          delusions F14.250
          hallucinations F14.251
        sexual dysfunction F14.281
        sleep disorder F14.282
        unspecified disorder F14.29
        withdrawal F14.23
      in remission F14.21
      withdrawal symptoms in newborn P96.1
    counseling and surveillance Z71.51
    hallucinogen F16.20
      with
        anxiety disorder F16.280
        flashbacks F16.283
        intoxication F16.229
          with delirium F16.221
          uncomplicated F16.220
        mood disorder F16.24
        other specified disorder F16.288
        perception disorder, persisting F16.283
        psychosis F16.259
          delusions F16.250
          hallucinations F16.251
        unspecified disorder F16.29
      in remission F16.21
    in remission F19.21

Dependence — *continued*
  drug — *continued*
    inhalant F18.20
      with
        anxiety disorder F18.280
        dementia, persisting F18.27
        intoxication F18.229
          with delirium F18.221
          uncomplicated F18.220
        mood disorder F18.24
        other specified disorder F18.288
        psychosis F18.259
          delusions F18.250
          hallucinations F18.251
        unspecified disorder F18.29
      in remission F18.21
    nicotine F17.200
      with disorder F17.209
        in remission F17.201
        specified disorder NEC F17.208
        withdrawal F17.203
      chewing tobacco F17.220
        with disorder F17.229
          in remission F17.221
          specified disorder NEC F17.228
          withdrawal F17.223
      cigarettes F17.210
        with disorder F17.219
          in remission F17.211
          specified disorder NEC F17.218
          withdrawal F17.213
      specified product NEC F17.290
        with disorder F17.299
          remission F17.291
          specified disorder NEC F17.298
          withdrawal F17.293
    opioid F11.20
      with
        intoxication F11.229
          with
            delirium F11.221
              perceptual disturbance F11.222
            uncomplicated F11.220
        mood disorder F11.24
        other specified disorder F11.288
        psychosis F11.259
          delusions F11.250
          hallucinations F11.251
        sexual dysfunction F11.281
        sleep disorder F11.282
        unspecified disorder F11.29
        withdrawal F11.23
      in remission F11.21
    psychoactive NEC F19.20
      with
        amnestic disorder F19.26
        anxiety disorder F19.280
        dementia F19.27
        intoxication F19.229
          with
            delirium F19.221
              perceptual disturbance F19.222
            uncomplicated F19.220
        mood disorder F19.24
        other specified disorder F19.288
        psychosis F19.259
          delusions F19.250
          hallucinations F19.251
        sexual dysfunction F19.281
        sleep disorder F19.282
        unspecified disorder F19.29
        withdrawal F19.239
          with
            delirium F19.231
              perceptual disturbance F19.232
            uncomplicated F19.230
    sedative, hypnotic or anxiolytic F13.20
      with
        amnestic disorder F13.26
        anxiety disorder F13.280
        dementia, persisting F13.27
        intoxication F13.229
          with delirium F13.221
          uncomplicated F13.220
        mood disorder F13.24
        other specified disorder F13.288
        psychosis F13.259
          delusions F13.250
          hallucinations F13.251

Dependence — *continued*
  drug — *continued*
    sedative, hypnotic or anxiolytic — *continued*
      with — *continued*
        sexual dysfunction F13.281
        sleep disorder F13.282
        unspecified disorder F13.29
        withdrawal F13.239
          with
            delirium F13.231
              perceptual disturbance F13.232
            uncomplicated F13.230
      in remission F13.21
    stimulant NEC F15.20
      with
        anxiety disorder F15.280
        intoxication F15.229
          with
            delirium F15.221
              perceptual disturbance F15.222
            uncomplicated F15.220
        mood disorder F15.24
        other specified disorder F15.288
        psychosis F15.259
          delusions F15.250
          hallucinations F15.251
        sexual dysfunction F15.281
        sleep disorder F15.282
        unspecified disorder F15.29
        withdrawal F15.23
      in remission F15.21
  ethyl
    alcohol (without remission) F10.20
      with remission F10.21
    bromide — *see* Dependence, drug, sedative
    carbamate F19.20
    chloride F19.20
    morphine — *see* Dependence, drug, opioid
  ganja — *see* Dependence, drug, cannabis
  glue (airplane) (sniffing) — *see* Dependence, drug, inhalant
  glutethimide — *see* Dependence, drug, sedative
  hallucinogenics — *see* Dependence, drug, hallucinogen
  hashish — *see* Dependence, drug, cannabis
  hemp — *see* Dependence, drug, cannabis
  heroin (salt) (any) — *see* Dependence, drug, opioid
  hypnotic NEC — *see* Dependence, drug, sedative
  Indian hemp — *see* Dependence, drug, cannabis
  inhalants — *see* Dependence, drug, inhalant
  khat — *see* Dependence, drug, stimulant NEC
  laudanum — *see* Dependence, drug, opioid
  LSD (-25) (derivatives) — *see* Dependence, drug, hallucinogen
  luminal — *see* Dependence, drug, sedative
  lysergic acid — *see* Dependence, drug, hallucinogen
  maconha — *see* Dependence, drug, cannabis
  marihuana — *see* Dependence, drug, cannabis
  meprobamate — *see* Dependence, drug, sedative
  mescaline — *see* Dependence, drug, hallucinogen
  methadone — *see* Dependence, drug, opioid
  methamphetamine(s) — *see* Dependence, drug, stimulant NEC
  methaqualone — *see* Dependence, drug, sedative
  methyl
    alcohol (without remission) F10.20
      with remission F10.21
    bromide — *see* Dependence, drug, sedative
    morphine — *see* Dependence, drug, opioid
    phenidate — *see* Dependence, drug, stimulant NEC
    sulfonal — *see* Dependence, drug, sedative
  morphine (sulfate) (sulfite) (type) — *see* Dependence, drug, opioid
  narcotic (drug) NEC — *see* Dependence, drug, opioid
  nembutal — *see* Dependence, drug, sedative
  neraval — *see* Dependence, drug, sedative
  neravan — *see* Dependence, drug, sedative
  neurobarb — *see* Dependence, drug, sedative
  nicotine — *see* Dependence, drug, nicotine
  nitrous oxide F19.20
  nonbarbiturate sedatives and tranquilizers with similar effect — *see* Dependence, drug, sedative
  on
    artificial heart (fully implantable) (mechanical) Z95.812
    aspirator Z99.0
    care provider (because of) Z74.9
      impaired mobility Z74.09

Dependence — *continued*
  on — *continued*
    care provider — *continued*
      need for
        assistance with personal care Z74.1
        continuous supervision Z74.3
        no other household member able to render care Z74.2
        specified reason NEC Z74.8
    machine Z99.89
      enabling NEC Z99.89
      specified type NEC Z99.89
    renal dialysis (hemodialysis) (peritoneal) Z99.2
    respirator Z99.11
    ventilator Z99.11
    wheelchair Z99.3
  opiate — *see* Dependence, drug, opioid
  opioids — *see* Dependence, drug, opioid
  opium (alkaloids) (derivatives) (tincture) — *see* Dependence, drug, opioid
  oxygen (long-term) (supplemental) Z99.81
  paraldehyde — *see* Dependence, drug, sedative
  paregoric — *see* Dependence, drug, opioid
  PCP (phencyclidine) (or related substance) — *see* Dependence, drug, hallucinogen
  pentobarbital — *see* Dependence, drug, sedative
  pentobarbitone (sodium) — *see* Dependence, drug, sedative
  pentothal — *see* Dependence, drug, sedative
  peyote — *see* Dependence, drug, hallucinogen
  phencyclidine (PCP) (or related substance) — *see* Dependence, drug, hallucinogen
  phenmetrazine — *see* Dependence, drug, stimulant NEC
  phenobarbital — *see* Dependence, drug, sedative
  polysubstance F19.20
  psilocibin, psilocyn, psilocyn, psilocyline — *see* Dependence, drug, hallucinogen
  psychostimulant NEC — *see* Dependence, drug, stimulant NEC
  secobarbital — *see* Dependence, drug, sedative
  seconal — *see* Dependence, drug, sedative
  sedative NEC — *see* Dependence, drug, sedative
  specified drug NEC — *see* Dependence, drug
  stimulant NEC — *see* Dependence, drug, stimulant NEC
  substance NEC — *see* Dependence, drug
  supplemental oxygen Z99.81
  tobacco — *see* Dependence, drug, nicotine
    counseling and surveillance Z71.6
  tranquilizer NEC — *see* Dependence, drug, sedative
  vitamin B6 E53.1
  volatile solvents — *see* Dependence, drug, inhalant
Dependency
  care-provider Z74.9
  passive F60.7
  reactions (persistent) F60.7
Depersonalization (in neurotic state) (neurotic) (syndrome) F48.1
Depletion
  extracellular fluid E86.9
  plasma E86.1
  potassium E87.6
    nephropathy N25.89
  salt or sodium E87.1
    causing heat exhaustion or prostration T67.4 ☑
    nephropathy N28.9
  volume NOS E86.9
Deployment (current) (military) status Z56.82
  in theater or in support of military war, peacekeeping and humanitarian operations Z56.82
  personal history of Z91.82
    military war, peacekeeping and humanitarian deployment (current or past conflict) Z91.82
  returned from Z91.82
Depolarization, premature I49.40
  atrial I49.1
  junctional I49.2
  specified NEC I49.49
  ventricular I49.3
Deposit
  bone in Boeck's sarcoid D86.89
  calcareous, calcium — *see* Calcification
  cholesterol
    retina H35.89
    vitreous (body) (humor) — *see* Deposit, crystalline
  conjunctiva H11.11- ☑
  cornea H18.00- ☑
    argentous H18.02- ☑

Deposit — *continued*
  cornea — *continued*
    due to metabolic disorder H18.Ø3- ☑
    Kayser-Fleischer ring H18.Ø4- ☑
    pigmentation — *see* Pigmentation, cornea
  crystalline, vitreous (body) (humor) H43.2- ☑
  hemosiderin in old scars of cornea — *see* Pigmentation,
    cornea, stromal
  metallic in lens — *see* Cataract, specified NEC
  skin R23.8
  tooth, teeth (betel) (black) (green) (materia alba) (or-
    ange) (tobacco) KØ3.6
  urate, kidney — *see* Calculus, kidney
Depraved appetite — *see* Pica
Depressed
  HDL cholesterol E78.6
Depression (acute) (mental) F32.A
  agitated (single episode) F32.2
  anaclitic — *see* Disorder, adjustment
  anxiety F41.8
    persistent F34.1
  arches — *see also* Deformity, limb, flat foot
  atypical (single episode) F32.89
    recurrent episode F33.8
  basal metabolic rate R94.8
  bone marrow D75.89
  central nervous system RØ9.2
  cerebral R29.818
    newborn P91.4
  cerebrovascular I67.9
  chest wall M95.4
  climacteric (single episode) F32.89
    recurrent episode F33.8
  endogenous (without psychotic symptoms) F33.2
    with psychotic symptoms F33.3
  functional activity R68.89
  hysterical F44.89
  involutional (single episode) F32.89
    recurrent episode F33.8
  major F32.9
    with psychotic symptoms F32.3
    recurrent — *see* Disorder, depressive, recurrent
  manic-depressive — *see* Disorder, depressive, recurrent
  masked (single episode) F32.89
  medullary G93.89
  menopausal (single episode) F32.89
    recurrent episode F33.8
  metatarsus — *see* Depression, arches
  monopolar F33.9
  nervous F34.1
  neurotic F34.1
  nose M95.Ø
  postnatal (NOS) F53.Ø
  postpartum (NOS) F53.Ø
  post-psychotic of schizophrenia F32.89
  post-schizophrenic F32.89
  psychogenic (reactive) (single episode) F32.9
  psychoneurotic F34.1
  psychotic (single episode) F32.3
    recurrent F33.3
  reactive (psychogenic) (single episode) F32.9
    psychotic (single episode) F32.3
  recurrent — *see* Disorder, depressive, recurrent
  respiratory center G93.89
  seasonal — *see* Disorder, depressive, recurrent
  senile FØ3 ☑
  severe, single episode F32.2
  situational F43.21
  skull Q67.4
  specified NEC (single episode) F32.89
  sternum M95.4
  visual field — *see* Defect, visual field
  vital (recurrent) (without psychotic symptoms) F33.2
    with psychotic symptoms F33.3
    single episode F32.2
Deprivation
  cultural Z6Ø.3
  effects NOS T73.9 ☑
    specified NEC T73.8 ☑
  emotional NEC Z65.8
    affecting infant or child — *see* Maltreatment, child,
      psychological
  food T73.Ø ☑
  material Z59.87
  protein — *see* Malnutrition
  sleep Z72.82Ø
  social Z6Ø.4

Deprivation — *continued*
  social — *continued*
    affecting infant or child — *see* Maltreatment, child,
      psychological
  specified NEC T73.8 ☑
  vitamins — *see* Deficiency, vitamin
  water T73.1 ☑
Derangement
  ankle (internal) — *see* Derangement, joint, articular
    cartilage, ankle
  cartilage (articular) NEC — *see* Derangement, joint,
    articular cartilage, by site
    recurrent — *see* Dislocation, recurrent
  cruciate ligament, anterior, current injury — *see* Sprain,
    knee, cruciate, anterior
  elbow (internal) — *see* Derangement, joint, articular
    cartilage, elbow
  hip (joint) (internal) (old) — *see* Derangement, joint,
    articular cartilage, hip
  joint (internal) M24.9
    ankylosis — *see* Ankylosis
    articular cartilage M24.1Ø
      ankle M24.17- ☑
      elbow M24.12- ☑
      foot M24.17- ☑
      hand M24.14- ☑
      hip M24.15- ☑
      knee NEC M23.9- ☑
      loose body — *see* Loose, body
      shoulder M24.11- ☑
      specified site NEC M24.19
      wrist M24.13- ☑
    contracture — *see* Contraction, joint
    current injury — *see also* Dislocation
      knee, meniscus or cartilage — *see* Tear, meniscus
    dislocation
      pathological — *see* Dislocation, pathological
      recurrent — *see* Dislocation, recurrent
    knee — *see* Derangement, knee
    ligament — *see* Disorder, ligament
    loose body — *see* Loose, body
    recurrent — *see* Dislocation, recurrent
    specified type NEC M24.8Ø
      ankle M24.87- ☑
      elbow M24.82- ☑
      foot joint M24.87- ☑
      hand joint M24.84- ☑
      hip M24.85- ☑
      shoulder M24.81- ☑
      specified site NEC M24.89
      wrist M24.83- ☑
    temporomandibular M26.69
  knee (recurrent) M23.9- ☑
    ligament disruption, spontaneous M23.6Ø- ☑
      anterior cruciate M23.61- ☑
      capsular M23.67- ☑
      instability, chronic M23.5- ☑
      lateral collateral M23.64- ☑
      medial collateral M23.63- ☑
      posterior cruciate M23.62- ☑
    loose body M23.4- ☑
    meniscus M23.3Ø- ☑
      cystic M23.ØØ- ☑
        lateral M23.ØØ2
          anterior horn M23.Ø4- ☑
          posterior horn M23.Ø5- ☑
          specified NEC M23.Ø6- ☑
        medial M23.ØØ5
          anterior horn M23.Ø1- ☑
          posterior horn M23.Ø2- ☑
          specified NEC M23.Ø3- ☑
      degenerate — *see* Derangement, knee, menis-
        cus, specified NEC
      detached — *see* Derangement, knee, meniscus,
        specified NEC
      due to old tear or injury M23.2Ø- ☑
        lateral M23.2Ø- ☑
          anterior horn M23.24- ☑
          posterior horn M23.25- ☑
          specified NEC M23.26- ☑
        medial M23.2Ø- ☑
          anterior horn M23.21- ☑
          posterior horn M23.22- ☑
          specified NEC M23.23- ☑
      retained — *see* Derangement, knee, meniscus,
        specified NEC

Derangement — *continued*
  knee — *continued*
    meniscus — *continued*
      specified NEC M23.3Ø- ☑
        lateral M23.3Ø- ☑
          anterior horn M23.34- ☑
          posterior horn M23.35- ☑
          specified NEC M23.36- ☑
        medial M23.3Ø- ☑
          anterior horn M23.31- ☑
          posterior horn M23.32- ☑
          specified NEC M23.33- ☑
    old M23.8X- ☑
    specified NEC — *see* subcategory M23.8 ☑
  low back NEC — *see* Dorsopathy, specified NEC
  meniscus — *see* Derangement, knee, meniscus
  mental — *see* Psychosis
  patella, specified NEC — *see* Disorder, patella, derange-
    ment NEC
  semilunar cartilage (knee) — *see* Derangement, knee,
    meniscus, specified NEC
  shoulder (internal) — *see* Derangement, joint, shoulder
Dercum's disease E88.2
Derealization (neurotic) F48.1
Dermal — *see* condition
Dermaphytid — *see* Dermatophytosis
Dermatitis (eczematous) L3Ø.9
  ab igne L59.Ø
  acarine B88.Ø
  actinic (due to sun) L57.8
    other than from sun L59.8
  allergic — *see* Dermatitis, contact, allergic
  ambustionis, due to burn or scald — *see* Burn
  amebic AØ6.7
  ammonia L22
  arsenical (ingested) L27.8
  artefacta L98.1
    psychogenic F54
  atopic L2Ø.9
    psychogenic F54
    specified NEC L2Ø.89
  autoimmune progesterone L3Ø.8
  berlock, berloque L56.2
  blastomycotic B4Ø.3
  blister beetle L24.89
  bullous, bullosa L13.9
    mucosynechial, atrophic L12.1
    seasonal L3Ø.8
    specified NEC L13.8
  calorica L59.Ø
    due to burn or scald — *see* Burn
  caterpillar L24.89
  cercarial B65.3
  combustionis L59.Ø
    due to burn or scald — *see* Burn
  congelationis T69.1 ☑
  contact (occupational) L25.9
    allergic L23.9
      due to
        adhesives L23.1
        cement L23.5
        chemical products NEC L23.5
        chromium L23.Ø
        cosmetics L23.2
        dander (cat) (dog) L23.81
        drugs in contact with skin L23.3
        dyes L23.4
        food in contact with skin L23.6
        hair (cat) (dog) L23.81
        insecticide L23.5
        metals L23.Ø
        nickel L23.Ø
        plants, non-food L23.7
        plastic L23.5
        rubber L23.5
        specified agent NEC L23.89
      due to
        cement L25.3
        chemical products NEC L25.3
        cosmetics L25.Ø
        dander (cat) (dog) L23.81
        drugs in contact with skin L25.1
        dyes L25.2
        food in contact with skin L25.4
        hair (cat) (dog) L23.81
        plants, non-food L25.5
        specified agent NEC L25.8
    irritant L24.9

Dermatitis — continued
  contact — continued
    irritant — continued
      due to
        body fluids L24.A0
          incontinence (dual) (fecal) (urinary) L24.A2
          saliva L24.A1
          specified NEC L24.A9
        cement L24.5
        chemical products NEC L24.5
        cosmetics L24.3
        detergents L24.0
        drugs in contact with skin L24.4
        food in contact with skin L24.6
        oils and greases L24.1
        plants, non-food L24.7
        solvents L24.2
        specified agent NEC L24.89
      related to
        colostomy L24.B3
        endotracheal tube L24.A9
        enterocutaneous fistula L24.B3
        gastrostomy L24.B1
        ileostomy L24.B3
        jejunostomy L24.B1
        saliva or spit fistula L24.B1
        stoma or fistula L24.B0
          digestive L24.B1
          fecal or urinary L24.B3
          respiratory L24.B2
        tracheostomy L24.B2
  contusiformis L52
  desquamative L30.8
  diabetic — see E08-E13 with .620
  diaper L22
  diphtheritica A36.3
  dry skin L85.3
  due to
    acetone (contact) (irritant) L24.2
    acids (contact) (irritant) L24.5
    adhesive(s) (allergic) (contact) (plaster) L23.1
      irritant L24.5
    alcohol (irritant) (skin contact) (substances in category T51) L24.2
      taken internally L27.8
    alkalis (contact) (irritant) L24.5
    arsenic (ingested) L27.8
    carbon disulfide (contact) (irritant) L24.2
    caustics (contact) (irritant) L24.5
    cement (contact) L25.3
    cereal (ingested) L27.2
    chemical(s) NEC L25.3
      taken internally L27.8
    chlorocompounds L24.2
    chromium (contact) (irritant) L24.81
    coffee (ingested) L27.2
    cold weather L30.8
    cosmetics (contact) L25.0
      allergic L23.2
      irritant L24.3
    cyclohexanes L24.2
    dander (cat) (dog) L23.81
    Demodex species B88.0
    Dermanyssus gallinae B88.0
    detergents (contact) (irritant) L24.0
    dichromate L24.81
    drugs and medicaments (generalized) (internal use) L27.0
      external — see Dermatitis, due to, drugs, in contact with skin
      in contact with skin L25.1
        allergic L23.3
        irritant L24.4
      localized skin eruption L27.1
      specified substance — see Table of Drugs and Chemicals
    dyes (contact) L25.2
      allergic L23.4
      irritant L24.89
    epidermophytosis — see Dermatophytosis
    esters L24.2
    external irritant NEC L24.9
    fish (ingested) L27.2
    flour (ingested) L27.2
    food (ingested) L27.2
      in contact with skin L25.4
    fruit (ingested) L27.2
    furs (allergic) (contact) L23.81

Dermatitis — continued
  due to — continued
    glues — see Dermatitis, due to, adhesives
    glycols L24.2
    greases NEC (contact) (irritant) L24.1
    hair (cat) (dog) L23.81
    hot
      objects and materials — see Burn
      weather or places L59.0
    hydrocarbons L24.2
    infrared rays L59.8
    ingestion, ingested substance L27.9
      chemical NEC L27.8
      drugs and medicaments — see Dermatitis, due to, drugs
      food L27.2
      specified NEC L27.8
    insecticide in contact with skin L24.5
    internal agent L27.9
      drugs and medicaments (generalized) — see Dermatitis, due to, drugs
      food L27.2
    irradiation — see Dermatitis, due to, radioactive substance
    ketones L24.2
    lacquer tree (allergic) (contact) L23.7
    light (sun) NEC L57.8
      acute L56.8
      other L59.8
    Liponyssoides sanguineus B88.0
    low temperature L30.8
    meat (ingested) L27.2
    metals, metal salts (contact) (irritant) L24.81
    milk (ingested) L27.2
    nickel (contact) (irritant) L24.81
    nylon (contact) (irritant) L24.5
    oils NEC (contact) (irritant) L24.1
    paint solvent (contact) (irritant) L24.2
    petroleum products (contact) (irritant) (substances in T52.0) L24.2
    plants NEC (contact) L25.5
      allergic L23.7
      irritant L24.7
    plasters (adhesive) (any) (allergic) (contact) L23.1
      irritant L24.5
    plastic (contact) L25.3
    preservatives (contact) — see Dermatitis, due to, chemical, in contact with skin
    primrose (allergic) (contact) L23.7
    primula (allergic) (contact) L23.7
    radiation L59.8
      nonionizing (chronic exposure) L57.8
      sun NEC L57.8
        acute L56.8
    radioactive substance L58.9
      acute L58.0
      chronic L58.1
    radium L58.9
      acute L58.0
      chronic L58.1
    ragweed (allergic) (contact) L23.7
    Rhus (allergic) (contact) (diversiloba) (radicans) (toxicodendron) (venenata) (verniciflua) L23.7
    rubber (contact) L24.5
    Senecio jacobaea (allergic) (contact) L23.7
    solvents (contact) (irritant) (substances in category T52) L24.2
    specified agent NEC (contact) L25.8
      allergic L23.89
      irritant L24.89
    sunshine NEC L57.8
      acute L56.8
    tetrachlorethylene (contact) (irritant) L24.2
    toluene (contact) (irritant) L24.2
    turpentine (contact) L24.2
    ultraviolet rays (sun NEC) (chronic exposure) L57.8
      acute L56.8
    vaccine or vaccination L27.0
      specified substance — see Table of Drugs and Chemicals
    varicose veins — see Varix, leg, with, inflammation
    X-rays L58.9
      acute L58.0
      chronic L58.1
  dyshydrotic L30.1
  dysmenorrheica N94.6
  escharotica — see Burn
  exfoliative, exfoliativa (generalized) L26

Dermatitis — continued
  exfoliative, exfoliativa — continued
    neonatorum L00
    eyelid — see also Dermatosis, eyelid H01.9
      allergic H01.119
        left H01.116
          lower H01.115
          upper H01.114
        right H01.113
          lower H01.112
          upper H01.111
      contact — see Dermatitis, eyelid, allergic
      due to
        Demodex species B88.0
        herpes (zoster) B02.39
          simplex B00.59
      eczematous H01.139
        left H01.136
          lower H01.135
          upper H01.134
        right H01.133
          lower H01.132
          upper H01.131
      specified NEC H01.8
    facta, factitia, factitial L98.1
      psychogenic F54
    flexural NEC L20.82
    friction L30.4
    fungus B36.9
      specified type NEC B36.8
    gangrenosa, gangrenous infantum L08.0
    harvest mite B88.0
    heat L59.0
    herpesviral, vesicular (ear) (lip) B00.1
    herpetiformis (bullous) (erythematous) (pustular) (vesicular) L13.0
      juvenile L12.2
      senile L12.0
    hiemalis L30.8
    hypostatic, hypostatica — see Varix, leg, with, inflammation
    infectious eczematoid L30.3
    infective L30.3
    irritant — see Dermatitis, contact, irritant
    Jacquet's (diaper dermatitis) L22
    Leptus B88.0
    lichenified NEC L28.0
    medicamentosa (generalized) (internal use) — see Dermatitis, due to drugs
    mite B88.0
    multiformis L13.0
      juvenile L12.2
    napkin L22
    neurotica L13.0
    nummular L30.0
    papillaris capillitii L73.0
    pellagrous E52
    perioral L71.0
    photocontact L56.2
    polymorpha dolorosa L13.0
    pruriginosa L13.0
    pruritic NEC L30.8
    psychogenic F54
    purulent L08.0
    pustular
      contagious B08.02
      subcorneal L13.1
    pyococcal L08.0
    pyogenica L08.0
    repens L40.2
    Ritter's (exfoliativa) L00
    Schamberg's L81.7
    schistosome B65.3
    seasonal bullous L30.8
    seborrheic L21.9
      infantile L21.1
      specified NEC L21.8
    sensitization NOS L23.9
    septic L08.0
    solare L57.8
    specified NEC L30.8
    stasis I87.2
      with
        varicose ulcer — see Varix, leg, with ulcer, with inflammation
        varicose veins — see Varix, leg, with, inflammation

Dermatitis — *continued*
　　stasis — *continued*
　　　due to postthrombotic syndrome — *see* Syndrome,
　　　　postthrombotic
　　suppurative L08.0
　　traumatic NEC L30.4
　　trophoneurotica L13.0
　　ultraviolet (sun) (chronic exposure) L57.8
　　　acute L56.8
　　varicose — *see* Varix, leg, with, inflammation
　　vegetans L10.1
　　verrucosa B43.0
　　vesicular, herpesviral B00.1
Dermatoarthritis, lipoid E78.81
Dermatochalasis, eyelid H02.839
　　left H02.836
　　　lower H02.835
　　　upper H02.834
　　right H02.833
　　　lower H02.832
　　　upper H02.831
Dermatofibroma (lenticulare) — *see* Neoplasm, skin,
　　benign
　　protuberans — *see* Neoplasm, skin, uncertain behavior
Dermatofibrosarcoma (pigmented) (protuberans) —
　　see Neoplasm, skin, malignant
Dermatographia L50.3
Dermatolysis (exfoliativa) (congenital) Q82.8
　　acquired L57.4
　　eyelids — *see* Blepharochalasis
　　palpebrarum — *see* Blepharochalasis
　　senile L57.4
Dermatomegaly NEC Q82.8
Dermatomucosomyositis — *see also* Dermatomyositis
　　M33.10
　　with
　　　myopathy M33.12
　　　respiratory involvement M33.11
　　　specified organ involvement NEC M33.19
Dermatomycosis B36.9
　　furfuracea B36.0
　　specified type NEC B36.8
Dermatomyositis (acute) (chronic) — *see also* Der-
　　matopolymyositis
　　adult — *see also* Dermatomyositis, specified NEC
　　　M33.10
　　in (due to) neoplastic disease — *see also* Neoplasm
　　　D49.9 [M36.0]
　　juvenile M33.00
　　　with
　　　　myopathy M33.02
　　　　respiratory involvement M33.01
　　　　specified organ involvement NEC M33.09
　　　amyopathic M33.03
　　　without myopathy M33.03
　　specified NEC M33.10
　　　with
　　　　myopathy M33.12
　　　　respiratory involvement M33.11
　　　　specified organ involvement NEC M33.19
　　　amyopathic M33.13
　　　without myopathy M33.13
Dermatoneuritis of children — *see* Poisoning, mercury
Dermatophilosis A48.8
Dermatophytid L30.2
Dermatophytide — *see* Dermatophytosis
Dermatophytosis (epidermophyton) (infection) (Mi-
　　crosporum) (tinea) (Trichophyton) B35.9
　　beard B35.0
　　body B35.4
　　capitis B35.0
　　corporis B35.4
　　deep-seated B35.8
　　disseminated B35.8
　　foot B35.3
　　granulomatous B35.8
　　groin B35.6
　　hand B35.2
　　nail B35.1
　　perianal (area) B35.6
　　scalp B35.0
　　specified NEC B35.8
Dermatopolymyositis M33.90
　　with
　　　myopathy M33.92
　　　respiratory involvement M33.91
　　　specified organ involvement NEC M33.99
　　amyopathic M33.93

Dermatopolymyositis — *continued*
　　in neoplastic disease — *see also* Neoplasm
　　　D49.9 [M36.0]
　　juvenile M33.00
　　　with
　　　　myopathy M33.02
　　　　respiratory involvement M33.01
　　　　specified organ involvement NEC M33.09
　　　amyopathic M33.03
　　　without myopathy M33.03
　　specified NEC M33.10
　　　amyopathic M33.13
　　　myopathy M33.12
　　　respiratory involvement M33.11
　　　specified organ involvement NEC M33.19
　　　without myopathy M33.13
　　without myopathy M33.93
Dermatopolyneuritis — *see* Poisoning, mercury
Dermatorrhexis — *see also* Syndrome, Ehlers-Danlos
　　Q79.60
　　acquired L57.4
Dermatosclerosis — *see also* Scleroderma
　　localized L94.0
Dermatosis L98.9
　　Andrews' L08.89
　　Bowen's — *see* Neoplasm, skin, in situ
　　bullous L13.9
　　　specified NEC L13.8
　　exfoliativa L26
　　eyelid (noninfectious) — *see also* Dermatitis, eyelid
　　　H01.9
　　　discoid lupus erythematosus — *see* Lupus, erythe-
　　　　matosus, eyelid
　　　xeroderma — *see* Xeroderma, acquired, eyelid
　　factitial L98.1
　　febrile neutrophilic L98.2
　　gonococcal A54.89
　　herpetiformis L13.0
　　　juvenile L12.2
　　linear IgA L13.8
　　menstrual NEC L98.8
　　neutrophilic, febrile L98.2
　　occupational — *see* Dermatitis, contact
　　papulosa nigra L82.1
　　pigmentary L81.9
　　　progressive L81.7
　　　Schamberg's L81.7
　　psychogenic F54
　　purpuric, pigmented L81.7
　　pustular, subcorneal L13.1
　　transient acantholytic L11.1
Dermographia, dermographism L50.3
Dermoid (cyst) — *see also* Neoplasm, benign, by site
　　with malignant transformation C56- ☑
　　due to radiation (nonionizing) L57.8
Dermopathy
　　infiltrative with thyrotoxicosis — *see* Thyrotoxicosis
　　nephrogenic fibrosing L90.8
Dermophytosis — *see* Dermatophytosis
Descemetocele H18.73- ☑
Descemet's membrane — *see* condition
Descending — *see* condition
Descensus uteri — *see* Prolapse, uterus
Desert
　　rheumatism B38.0
　　sore — *see* Ulcer, skin
Desertion (newborn) — *see* Maltreatment
Desmoid (extra-abdominal) (tumor) — *see* Neoplasm,
　　connective tissue, uncertain behavior
　　abdominal D48.1
Despondency F32.A
Desquamation, skin R23.4
Destruction, destructive — *see also* Damage
　　articular facet — *see also* Derangement, joint, specified
　　　type NEC
　　　knee M23.8X- ☑
　　　vertebra — *see* Spondylosis
　　bone — *see also* Disorder, bone, specified type NEC
　　　syphilitic A52.77
　　joint — *see also* Derangement, joint, specified type
　　　NEC
　　　sacroiliac M53.3
　　rectal sphincter K62.89
　　septum (nasal) J34.89
　　tuberculous NEC — *see* Tuberculosis
　　tympanum, tympanic membrane (nontraumatic) —
　　　see Disorder, tympanic membrane, specified NEC
　　vertebral disc — *see* Degeneration, intervertebral disc

Destructiveness — *see also* Disorder, conduct
　　adjustment reaction — *see* Disorder, adjustment
Desultory labor O62.2
Detachment
　　cartilage — *see* Sprain
　　cervix, annular N88.8
　　　complicating delivery O71.3
　　choroid (old) (postinfectional) (simple) (spontaneous)
　　　H31.40- ☑
　　　hemorrhagic H31.41- ☑
　　　serous H31.42- ☑
　　ligament — *see* Sprain
　　meniscus (knee) — *see also* Derangement, knee,
　　　meniscus, specified NEC
　　　current injury — *see* Tear, meniscus
　　　due to old tear or injury — *see* Derangement, knee,
　　　　meniscus, due to old tear
　　retina (without retinal break) (serous) H33.2- ☑
　　　with retinal:
　　　　break H33.00- ☑
　　　　　giant H33.03- ☑
　　　　　multiple H33.02- ☑
　　　　　single H33.01- ☑
　　　　dialysis H33.04- ☑
　　　pigment epithelium — *see* Degeneration, retina,
　　　　separation of layers, pigment epithelium de-
　　　　tachment
　　　rhegmatogenous — *see* Detachment, retina, with
　　　　retinal, break
　　　specified NEC H33.8
　　　total H33.05- ☑
　　　traction H33.4- ☑
　　vitreous (body) H43.81 ☑
Detergent asthma J69.8
Deterioration
　　epileptic F06.8
　　general physical R53.81
　　heart, cardiac — *see* Degeneration, myocardial
　　mental — *see* Psychosis
　　myocardial, myocardium — *see* Degeneration, myocar-
　　　dial
　　senile (simple) R54
Deuteranomaly (anomalous trichromat) H53.53
Deuteranopia (complete) (incomplete) H53.53
Development
　　abnormal, bone Q79.9
　　arrested R62.50
　　　bone — *see* Arrest, development or growth, bone
　　　child R62.50
　　　due to malnutrition E45
　　defective, congenital — *see also* Anomaly, by site
　　　cauda equina Q06.3
　　　left ventricle Q24.8
　　　　in hypoplastic left heart syndrome Q23.4
　　　valve Q24.8
　　　　pulmonary Q22.3
　　delayed — *see also* Delay, development R62.50
　　　arithmetical skills F81.2
　　　language (skills) (expressive) F80.1
　　　learning skill F81.9
　　　mixed skills F88
　　　motor coordination F82
　　　reading F81.0
　　　specified learning skill NEC F81.89
　　　speech F80.9
　　　spelling F81.81
　　　written expression F81.81
　　imperfect, congenital — *see also* Anomaly, by site
　　　heart Q24.9
　　　lungs Q33.6
　　incomplete
　　　bronchial tree Q32.4
　　　organ or site not listed — *see* Hypoplasia, by site
　　　respiratory system Q34.9
　　sexual, precocious NEC E30.1
　　tardy, mental — *see also* Disability, intellectual F79
Developmental — *see* condition
　　testing, infant or child — *see* Examination, child
Devergie's disease (pityriasis rubra pilaris) L44.0
Deviation (in)
　　conjugate palsy (eye) (spastic) H51.0
　　esophagus (acquired) K22.89
　　eye, skew H51.8
　　midline (jaw) (teeth) (dental arch) M26.29
　　　specified site NEC — *see* Malposition
　　nasal septum J34.2
　　　congenital Q67.4

Deviation — *continued*
- opening and closing of the mandible M26.53
- organ or site, congenital NEC — *see* Malposition, congenital
- septum (nasal) (acquired) J34.2
    - congenital Q67.4
- sexual F65.9
    - bestiality F65.89
    - erotomania F52.8
    - exhibitionism F65.2
    - fetishism, fetishistic F65.0
        - transvestism F65.1
    - frotteurism F65.81
    - masochism F65.51
    - multiple F65.89
    - necrophilia F65.89
    - nymphomania F52.8
    - pederosis F65.4
    - pedophilia F65.4
    - sadism, sadomasochism F65.52
    - satyriasis F52.8
    - specified type NEC F65.89
    - transvestism F64.1
    - voyeurism F65.3
- teeth, midline M26.29
- trachea J39.8
- ureter, congenital Q62.61

Device
- cerebral ventricle (communicating) in situ Z98.2
- contraceptive — *see* Contraceptive, device
- drainage, cerebrospinal fluid, in situ Z98.2

Devic's disease G36.0

Devil's
- grip B33.0
- pinches (purpura simplex) D69.2

Devitalized tooth K04.99

Devonshire colic — *see* Poisoning, lead

Dextraposition, aorta Q20.3
- in tetralogy of Fallot Q21.3

Dextrinosis, limit (debrancher enzyme deficiency) E74.03

Dextrocardia (true) Q24.0
- with
    - complete transposition of viscera Q89.3
    - situs inversus Q89.3

Dextrotransposition, aorta Q20.3

d-glycericacidemia E72.59

Dhat syndrome F48.8

Dhobi itch B35.6

Di George's syndrome D82.1

Di Guglielmo's disease C94.0- ☑

Diabetes, diabetic (mellitus) (sugar) E11.9
- with
    - amyotrophy E11.44
    - arthropathy NEC E11.618
    - autonomic (poly)neuropathy E11.43
    - cataract E11.36
    - Charcot's joints E11.610
    - chronic kidney disease E11.22
    - circulatory complication NEC E11.59
    - coma due to
        - hyperosmolarity E11.01
        - hypoglycemia E11.641
        - ketoacidosis E11.11
    - complication E11.8
        - specified NEC E11.69
    - dermatitis E11.620
    - foot ulcer E11.621
    - gangrene E11.52
    - gastroparalysis E11.43
    - gastroparesis E11.43
    - glomerulonephrosis, intracapillary E11.21
    - glomerulosclerosis, intercapillary E11.21
    - hyperglycemia E11.65
    - hyperosmolarity E11.00
        - with coma E11.01
    - hypoglycemia E11.649
        - with coma E11.641
    - ketoacidosis E11.10
        - with coma E11.11
    - kidney complications NEC E11.29
    - Kimmelstiel-Wilson disease E11.21
    - loss of protective sensation (LOPS) — *see* Diabetes, by type, with neuropathy
    - mononeuropathy E11.41
    - myasthenia E11.44
    - necrobiosis lipoidica E11.620
    - nephropathy E11.21
    - neuralgia E11.42

Diabetes, diabetic — *continued*
- with — *continued*
    - neurologic complication NEC E11.49
    - neuropathic arthropathy E11.610
    - neuropathy E11.40
    - ophthalmic complication NEC E11.39
    - oral complication NEC E11.638
    - osteomyelitis E11.69
    - periodontal disease E11.630
    - peripheral angiopathy E11.51
        - with gangrene E11.52
    - polyneuropathy E11.42
    - renal complication NEC E11.29
    - renal tubular degeneration E11.29
    - retinopathy E11.319
        - with macular edema E11.311
            - resolved following treatment E11.37- ☑
        - nonproliferative E11.329 ☑
            - with macular edema E11.321 ☑
                - mild E11.329 ☑
                    - with macular edema E11.321 ☑
                - moderate E11.339 ☑
                    - with macular edema E11.331 ☑
                - severe E11.349 ☑
                    - with macular edema E11.341 ☑
        - proliferative E11.359 ☑
            - with
                - combined traction retinal detachment and rhegmatogenous retinal detachment E11.354 ☑
                - macular edema E11.351 ☑
                - stable proliferative diabetic retinopathy E11.355 ☑
                - traction retinal detachment involving the macula E11.352 ☑
                - traction retinal detachment not involving the macula E11.353 ☑
    - skin complication NEC E11.628
    - skin ulcer NEC E11.622
- brittle — *see* Diabetes, type 1
- bronzed E83.110
- complicating pregnancy — *see* Pregnancy, complicated by, diabetes
- dietary counseling and surveillance Z71.3
- due to
    - autoimmune process — *see* Diabetes, type 1
    - immune mediated pancreatic islet beta-cell destruction — *see* Diabetes, type 1
- due to drug or chemical E09.9
    - with
        - amyotrophy E09.44
        - arthropathy NEC E09.618
        - autonomic (poly)neuropathy E09.43
        - cataract E09.36
        - Charcot's joints E09.610
        - chronic kidney disease E09.22
        - circulatory complication NEC E09.59
        - complication E09.8
            - specified NEC E09.69
        - dermatitis E09.620
        - foot ulcer E09.621
        - gangrene E09.52
        - gastroparalysis E09.43
        - gastroparesis E09.43
        - glomerulonephrosis, intracapillary E09.21
        - glomerulosclerosis, intercapillary E09.21
        - hyperglycemia E09.65
        - hyperosmolarity E09.00
            - with coma E09.01
        - hypoglycemia E09.649
            - with coma E09.641
        - ketoacidosis E09.10
            - with coma E09.11
        - kidney complications NEC E09.29
        - Kimmelstiel-Wilson disease E09.21
        - mononeuropathy E09.41
        - myasthenia E09.44
        - necrobiosis lipoidica E09.620
        - nephropathy E09.21
        - neuralgia E09.42
        - neurologic complication NEC E09.49
        - neuropathic arthropathy E09.610
        - neuropathy E09.40
        - ophthalmic complication NEC E09.39
        - oral complication NEC E09.638
        - periodontal disease E09.630
        - peripheral angiopathy E09.51
            - with gangrene E09.52

Diabetes, diabetic — *continued*
- due to drug or chemical — *continued*
    - with — *continued*
        - polyneuropathy E09.42
        - renal complication NEC E09.29
        - renal tubular degeneration E09.29
        - retinopathy E09.319
            - with macular edema E09.311
            - resolved following treatment E09.37 ☑
            - nonproliferative E09.329 ☑
                - with macular edema E09.321 ☑
                    - mild E09.329 ☑
                        - with macular edema E09.321 ☑
                    - moderate E09.339 ☑
                        - with macular edema E09.331 ☑
                    - severe E09.349 ☑
                        - with macular edema E09.341 ☑
            - proliferative E09.359 ☑
                - with
                    - combined traction retinal detachment and rhegmatogenous retinal detachment E09.354 ☑
                    - macular edema E09.351 ☑
                    - stable proliferative diabetic retinopathy E09.355 ☑
                    - traction retinal detachment involving the macula E09.352 ☑
                    - traction retinal detachment not involving the macula E09.353 ☑
        - skin complication NEC E09.628
        - skin ulcer NEC E09.622
- due to underlying condition E08.9
    - with
        - amyotrophy E08.44
        - arthropathy NEC E08.618
        - autonomic (poly)neuropathy E08.43
        - cataract E08.36
        - Charcot's joints E08.610
        - chronic kidney disease E08.22
        - circulatory complication NEC E08.59
        - complication E08.8
            - specified NEC E08.69
        - dermatitis E08.620
        - foot ulcer E08.621
        - gangrene E08.52
        - gastroparalysis E08.43
        - gastroparesis E08.43
        - glomerulonephrosis, intracapillary E08.21
        - glomerulosclerosis, intercapillary E08.21
        - hyperglycemia E08.65
        - hyperosmolarity E08.00
            - with coma E08.01
        - hypoglycemia E08.649
            - with coma E08.641
        - ketoacidosis E08.10
            - with coma E08.11
        - kidney complications NEC E08.29
        - Kimmelstiel-WIlson disease E08.21
        - mononeuropathy E08.41
        - myasthenia E08.44
        - necrobiosis lipoidica E08.620
        - nephropathy E08.21
        - neuralgia E08.42
        - neurologic complication NEC E08.49
        - neuropathic arthropathy E08.610
        - neuropathy E08.40
        - ophthalmic complication NEC E08.39
        - oral complication NEC E08.638
        - periodontal disease E08.630
        - peripheral angiopathy E08.51
            - with gangrene E08.52
        - polyneuropathy E08.42
        - renal complication NEC E08.29
        - renal tubular degeneration E08.29
        - retinopathy E08.319
            - with macular edema E08.311
            - resolved following treatment E08.37 ☑
            - nonproliferative E08.329 ☑
                - with macular edema E08.321 ☑
                    - mild E08.329 ☑
                        - with macular edema E08.321 ☑
                    - moderate E08.339 ☑
                        - with macular edema E08.331 ☑
                    - severe E08.349 ☑
                        - with macular edema E08.341 ☑
            - proliferative E08.359 ☑

Disorder — *continued*
  depressive — *continued*
    major — *continued*
      single episode — *continued*
        severe (without psychotic symptoms) F32.2
          with psychotic symptoms F32.3
    organic F06.31
    persistent F34.1
    recurrent F33.9
      current episode
        mild F33.0
        moderate F33.1
        severe (without psychotic symptoms) F33.2
          with psychotic symptoms F33.3
      in remission F33.40
        full F33.42
        partial F33.41
      specified NEC F33.8
    single episode — *see* Episode, depressive
    specified NEC F32.89
  developmental F89
    arithmetical skills F81.2
    coordination (motor) F82
    expressive writing F81.81
    language F80.9
      expressive F80.1
      mixed receptive and expressive F80.2
      receptive type F80.2
      specified NEC F80.89
    learning F81.9
      arithmetical F81.2
      reading F81.0
    mixed F88
    motor coordination or function F82
    pervasive F84.9
      specified NEC F84.8
    phonological F80.0
    reading F81.0
    scholastic skills — *see also* Disorder, learning
      mixed F81.89
    specified NEC F88
    speech F80.9
      articulation F80.0
      specified NEC F80.89
    written expression F81.81
  diaphragm J98.6
  digestive (system) K92.9
    newborn P78.9
      specified NEC P78.89
    postprocedural — *see* Complication, gastrointestinal
    psychogenic F45.8
  disc (intervertebral) M51.9
    with
      myelopathy
        cervical region M50.00
        cervicothoracic region M50.03
        high cervical region M50.01
        lumbar region M51.06
        mid-cervical region M50.020
        sacrococcygeal region M53.3
        thoracic region M51.04
        thoracolumbar region M51.05
      radiculopathy
        cervical region M50.10
        cervicothoracic region M50.13
        high cervical region M50.11
        lumbar region M51.16
        lumbosacral region M51.17
        mid-cervical region M50.120
        sacrococcygeal region M53.3
        thoracic region M51.14
        thoracolumbar region M51.15
    cervical M50.90
      with
        myelopathy M50.00
          C2-C3 M50.01
          C3-C4 M50.01
          C4-C5 M50.021
          C5-C6 M50.022
          C6-C7 M50.023
          C7-T1 M50.03
          cervicothoracic region M50.03
          high cervical region M50.01
          mid-cervical region M50.020
        neuritis, radiculitis or radiculopathy M50.10
          C2-C3 M50.11
          C3-C4 M50.11
          C4-C5 M50.121
          C5-C6 M50.122

Disorder — *continued*
  disc — *continued*
    cervical — *continued*
      with
        neuritis, radiculitis or radiculopathy — *continued*
          C6-C7 M50.123
          C7-T1 M50.13
          cervicothoracic region M50.13
          high cervical region M50.11
          mid-cervical region M50.120
      C2-C3 M50.91
      C3-C4 M50.91
      C4-C5 M50.921
      C5-C6 M50.922
      C6-C7 M50.923
      C7-T1 M50.93
      cervicothoracic region M50.93
      degeneration M50.30
        C2-C3 M50.31
        C3-C4 M50.31
        C4-C5 M50.321
        C5-C6 M50.322
        C6-C7 M50.323
        C7-T1 M50.33
        cervicothoracic region M50.33
        high cervical region M50.31
        mid-cervical region M50.320
      displacement M50.20
        C2-C3 M50.21
        C3-C4 M50.21
        C4-C5 M50.221
        C5-C6 M50.222
        C6-C7 M50.223
        C7-T1 M50.23
        cervicothoracic region M50.23
        high cervical region M50.21
        mid-cervical region M50.220
      high cervical region M50.91
      mid-cervical region M50.920
      specified type NEC M50.80
        C2-C3 M50.81
        C3-C4 M50.81
        C4-C5 M50.821
        C5-C6 M50.822
        C6-C7 M50.823
        C7-T1 M50.83
        cervicothoracic region M50.83
        high cervical region M50.81
        mid-cervical region M50.820
    specified NEC
      lumbar region M51.86
      lumbosacral region M51.87
      sacrococcygeal region M53.3
      thoracic region M51.84
      thoracolumbar region M51.85
  disinhibited attachment (childhood) F94.2
  disintegrative, childhood NEC F84.3
  disruptive F91.9
    mood dysregulation F34.81
    specified NEC F91.8
  disruptive behavior — *see* Disorder, conduct
  dissocial personality F60.2
  dissociative F44.9
    affecting
      motor function F44.4
        and sensation F44.7
      sensation F44.6
        and motor function F44.7
    brief reactive F43.0
    due to (secondary to) general medical condition F06.8
    mixed F44.7
    organic F06.8
    other specified NEC F44.89
  double heterozygous sickling — *see* Disease, sickle-cell
  dream anxiety F51.5
  drug induced hemorrhagic D68.32
  drug related F19.99
    abuse — *see* Abuse, drug
    dependence — *see* Dependence, drug
  dysmorphic body F45.22
  dysthymic F34.1
  ear H93.9- ☑
    bleeding — *see* Otorrhagia
    deafness — *see* Deafness
    degenerative H93.09- ☑
    discharge — *see* Otorrhea

Disorder — *continued*
  ear — *continued*
    external H61.9- ☑
      auditory canal stenosis — *see* Stenosis, external ear canal
      exostosis — *see* Exostosis, external ear canal
      impacted cerumen — *see* Impaction, cerumen
      otitis — *see* Otitis, externa
      perichondritis — *see* Perichondritis, ear
      pinna — *see* Disorder, pinna
      specified type NEC H61.89- ☑
    inner H83.9- ☑
      vestibular dysfunction — *see* Disorder, vestibular function
    middle H74.9- ☑
      adhesive H74.1- ☑
      ossicle — *see* Abnormal, ear ossicles
      polyp — *see* Polyp, ear (middle)
      specified NEC, in diseases classified elsewhere H75.8- ☑
    postprocedural — *see* Complications, ear, procedure
    specified NEC, in diseases classified elsewhere H94.8- ☑
  eating (adult) (psychogenic) F50.9
    anorexia — *see* Anorexia
    binge F50.81
    bulimia F50.2
    child F98.29
      pica F98.3
      rumination disorder F98.21
    pica F50.89
      childhood F98.3
  electrolyte (balance) NEC E87.8
    with
      abortion — *see* Abortion by type complicated by specified condition NEC
      ectopic pregnancy O08.5
      molar pregnancy O08.5
    acidosis (lactic) (metabolic) E87.20
      acute E87.21
      chronic E87.22
      respiratory E87.29
      specified NEC E87.29
    alkalosis (metabolic) (respiratory) E87.3
  elimination, transepidermal L87.9
    specified NEC L87.8
  emotional (persistent) F34.9
    of childhood F93.9
      specified NEC F93.8
  endocrine E34.9
    postprocedural E89.89
    specified NEC E89.89
  erectile (male) (organic) — *see also* Dysfunction, sexual, male, erectile N52.9
    nonorganic F52.21
  erythematous — *see* Erythema
  esophagus K22.9
    functional K22.4
    psychogenic F45.8
  eustachian tube H69.9- ☑
    infection — *see* Salpingitis, eustachian
    obstruction — *see* Obstruction, eustachian tube
    patulous — *see* Patulous, eustachian tube
    specified NEC H69.8- ☑
  exhibitionistic F65.2
  extrapyramidal G25.9
    in deseases classified elsewhere — *see* category G26
    specified type NEC G25.89
  eye H57.9
    postprocedural — *see* Complication, postprocedural, eye
  eyelid H02.9
    cyst — *see* Cyst, eyelid
    degenerative H02.70
      chloasma — *see* Chloasma, eyelid
      madarosis — *see* Madarosis
      specified type NEC H02.79
      vitiligo — *see* Vitiligo, eyelid
      xanthelasma — *see* Xanthelasma
    dermatochalasis — *see* Dermatochalasis
    edema — *see* Edema, eyelid
    elephantiasis — *see* Elephantiasis, eyelid
    foreign body, retained — *see* Foreign body, retained, eyelid
    function H02.59

Disorder — *continued*
 eyelid — *continued*
  function — *continued*
   abnormal innervation syndrome — *see* Syndrome, abnormal innervation
   blepharochalasis — *see* Blepharochalasis
   blepharoclonus — *see* Blepharoclonus
   blepharophimosis — *see* Blepharophimosis
   blepharoptosis — *see* Blepharoptosis
   lagophthalmos — *see* Lagophthalmos
   lid retraction — *see* Retraction, lid
  hypertrichosis — *see* Hypertrichosis, eyelid
  specified type NEC H02.89
  vascular H02.879
   left H02.876
    lower H02.875
    upper H02.874
   right H02.873
    lower H02.872
    upper H02.871
 factitious
  by proxy F68.A
  imposed on another F68.A
  imposed on self F68.10
   with predominantly
    psychological symptoms F68.11
     with physical symptoms F68.13
    physical symptoms F68.12
     with psychological symptoms F68.13
 factor, coagulation — *see* Defect, coagulation
 fatty acid
  metabolism E71.30
   specified NEC E71.39
  oxidation
   LCAD E71.310
   MCAD E71.311
   SCAD E71.312
   specified deficiency NEC E71.318
 feeding (infant or child) — *see also* Disorder, eating R63.30
  or eating disorder F50.9
  pediatric
   acute R63.31
   chronic R63.32
  specified NEC F50.9
 feigned (with obvious motivation) Z76.5
  without obvious motivation — *see* Disorder, factitious
 female
  hypoactive sexual desire F52.0
  orgasmic F52.31
  sexual interest/arousal F52.22
 fetishistic F65.0
 fibroblastic M72.9
  specified NEC M72.8
 fluency
  adult onset F98.5
  childhood onset F80.81
  following
   cerebral infarction I69.323
   cerebrovascular disease I69.923
    specified disease NEC I69.823
   intracerebral hemorrhage I69.123
   nontraumatic intracranial hemorrhage NEC I69.223
   subarachnoid hemorrhage I69.023
  in conditions classified elsewhere R47.82
 fluid balance E87.8
 follicular (skin) L73.9
  specified NEC L73.8
 frotteuristic F65.81
 fructose metabolism E74.10
  essential fructosuria E74.11
  fructokinase deficiency E74.11
  fructose-1, 6-diphosphatase deficiency E74.19
  hereditary fructose intolerance E74.12
  other specified E74.19
 functional polymorphonuclear neutrophils D71
 gallbladder, biliary tract and pancreas in diseases classified elsewhere K87
 gambling F63.0
 gamma aminobutyric acid (GABA) metabolism E72.81
 gamma-glutamyl cycle E72.89
 gastric (functional) K31.9
  motility K30
  psychogenic F45.8
  secretion K30
 gastrointestinal (functional) NOS K92.9

Disorder — *continued*
 gastrointestinal — *continued*
  newborn P78.9
  psychogenic F45.8
 gender-identity or -role F64.9
  childhood F64.2
  effect on relationship F66
  of adolescence or adulthood F64.0
   nontranssexual F64.8
  specified NEC F64.8
  uncertainty F66
 genito-pelvic pain penetration F52.6
 genitourinary system
  female N94.9
  male N50.9
  psychogenic F45.8
 globe H44.9
  degenerated condition H44.50
   absolute glaucoma H44.51- ✓
   atrophy H44.52- ✓
   leucocoria H44.53- ✓
  degenerative H44.30
   chalcosis H44.31- ✓
   myopia — *see also* Myopia, degenerative H44.2- ✓
   siderosis H44.32- ✓
   specified type NEC H44.39- ✓
  endophthalmitis — *see* Endophthalmitis
  foreign body, retained — *see* Foreign body, intraocular, old, retained
  hemophthalmos — *see* Hemophthalmos
  hypotony H44.40
   due to
    ocular fistula H44.42- ✓
    specified disorder NEC H44.43- ✓
   flat anterior chamber H44.41- ✓
   primary H44.44- ✓
  luxation — *see* Luxation, globe
  specified type NEC H44.89
 glomerular (in) N05.9
  amyloidosis E85.4 [N08]
  cryoglobulinemia D89.1 [N08]
  disseminated intravascular coagulation D65 [N08]
  Fabry's disease E75.21 [N08]
  familial lecithin cholesterol acyltransferase deficiency E78.6 [N08]
  Goodpasture's syndrome M31.0
  hemolytic-uremic syndrome — *see* Syndrome, hemolytic-uremic
  Henoch (-Schönlein) purpura D69.0 [N08]
  malariae malaria B52.0
  microscopic polyangiitis M31.7 [N08]
  multiple myeloma C90.0- ✓ [N08]
  mumps B26.83
  schistosomiasis B65.9 [N08]
  sepsis NEC A41.- ✓ [N08]
   streptococcal A40.- ✓ [N08]
  sickle-cell disorders D57.- ✓ [N08]
  strongyloidiasis B78.9 [N08]
  subacute bacterial endocarditis I33.0 [N08]
  syphilis A52.75
  systemic lupus erythematosus M32.14
  thrombotic thrombocytopenic purpura M31.19 [N08]
  Waldenström macroglobulinemia C88.0 [N08]
  Wegener's granulomatosis M31.31
 gluconeogenesis E74.4
 glucosaminoglycan metabolism — *see* Disorder, metabolism, glucosaminoglycan
 glucose transport E74.819
  specified NEC E74.818
 glycine metabolism E72.50
  d-glycericacidemia E72.59
  hyperhydroxyprolinemia E72.59
  hyperoxaluria R82.992
   primary E72.53
  hyperprolinemia E72.59
  non-ketotic hyperglycinemia E72.51
  oxalosis E72.53
  oxaluria E72.53
  sarcosinemia E72.59
  trimethylaminuria E72.52
 glycoprotein metabolism E77.9
  specified NEC E77.8
 grief
  complicated F43.81
  prolonged F43.81
 habit (and impulse) F63.9

Disorder — *continued*
 habit — *continued*
  involving sexual behavior NEC F65.9
  specified NEC F63.89
 hallucinogen use
  mild F16.10
   with
    hallucinogen intoxication delirium F16.121
    hallucinogen-induced
     anxiety disorder F16.180
     bipolar and related disorder F16.14
     depressive disorder F16.14
     psychotic disorder F16.159
    other hallucinogen intoxication F16.129
   in remission (early) (sustained) F16.11
  moderate or severe F16.20
   with
    hallucinogen intoxication delirium F16.221
    hallucinogen-induced
     anxiety disorder F16.280
     bipolar and related disorder F16.24
     depressive disorder F16.24
     psychotic disorder F16.259
    other hallucinogen intoxication F16.229
   in remission (early) (sustained) F16.21
 heart action I49.9
 hematological D75.9
  newborn (transient) P61.9
  specified NEC P61.8
 hematopoietic organs D75.9
 hemorrhagic NEC D69.9
  drug-induced D68.32
  due to
   extrinsic circulating anticoagulants D68.32
   increase in
    anti-IIa D68.32
    anti-Xa D68.32
   intrinsic
    circulating anticoagulants D68.318
    increase in
     anti-IXa D68.318
     antithrombin D68.318
     anti-VIIIa D68.318
     anti-XIa D68.318
  following childbirth O72.3
 hemostasis — *see* Defect, coagulation
 histidine metabolism E70.40
  histidinemia E70.41
  other specified E70.49
 hoarding F42.3
 hyperkinetic — *see* Disorder, attention-deficit hyperactivity
 hyperleucine-isoleucinemia E71.19
 hypervalinemia E71.19
 hypoactive sexual desire F52.0
 hypochondriacal F45.20
  body dysmorphic F45.22
  neurosis F45.21
  other specified F45.29
 identity
  dissociative F44.81
  illness anxiety F45.21
  of childhood F93.8
 immune mechanism (immunity) D89.9
  specified type NEC D89.89
 impaired renal tubular function N25.9
  specified NEC N25.89
 impulse (control) F63.9
 inflammatory
  pelvic, in diseases classified elsewhere — *see* category N74
  penis N48.29
   abscess N48.21
   cellulitis N48.22
 inhalant use
  mild F18.10
   with
    inhalant intoxication F18.129
    inhalant intoxication delirium F18.121
    inhalant-induced
     anxiety disorder F18.180
     depressive disorder F18.14
     major neurocognitive disorder F18.17
     mild neurocognitive disorder F18.188
     psychotic disorder F18.159
   in remission (early) (sustained) F18.11
  moderate or severe F18.20
   with
    inhalant intoxication F18.229

Disorder — *continued*
  inhalant use — *continued*
    moderate or severe — *continued*
      with — *continued*
        inhalant intoxication delirium F18.221
        inhalant-induced
          anxiety disorder F18.280
          depressive disorder F18.24
          major neurocognitive disorder F18.27
          mild neurocognitive disorder F18.288
          psychotic disorder F18.259
        in remission (early) (sustained) F18.21
  integument, newborn P83.9
    specified NEC P83.88
  intermittent explosive F63.81
  internal secretion pancreas — *see* Increased, secretion, pancreas, endocrine
  intestine, intestinal
    carbohydrate absorption NEC E74.39
      postoperative K91.2
    functional NEC K59.9
      postoperative K91.89
    psychogenic F45.8
    vascular K55.9
      chronic K55.1
      specified NEC K55.8
  intraoperative (intraprocedural) — *see* Complications, intraoperative
  involuntary emotional expression (IEED) F07.89
  iris H21.9
    adhesions — *see* Adhesions, iris
    atrophy — *see* Atrophy, iris
    chamber angle recession — *see* Recession, chamber angle
    cyst — *see* Cyst, iris
    degeneration — *see* Degeneration, iris
    in diseases classified elsewhere H22
    iridodialysis — *see* Iridodialysis
    iridoschisis — *see* Iridoschisis
    miotic pupillary cyst — *see* Cyst, pupillary
    pupillary
      abnormality — *see* Abnormality, pupillary
      membrane — *see* Membrane, pupillary
    specified type NEC H21.89
    vascular NEC H21.1X- ☑
  iron metabolism E83.10
    specified NEC E83.19
  isovaleric acidemia E71.110
  jaw, developmental M27.0
    temporomandibular — *see also* Anomaly, dentofacial, temporomandibular joint M26.60- ☑
  joint M25.9
    derangement — *see* Derangement, joint
    effusion — *see* Effusion, joint
    fistula — *see* Fistula, joint
    hemarthrosis — *see* Hemarthrosis
    instability — *see* Instability, joint
    osteophyte — *see* Osteophyte
    pain — *see* Pain, joint
    psychogenic F45.8
    specified type NEC M25.80
      ankle M25.87- ☑
      elbow M25.82- ☑
      foot joint M25.87- ☑
      hand joint M25.84- ☑
      hip M25.85- ☑
      knee M25.86- ☑
      shoulder M25.81- ☑
      wrist M25.83- ☑
    stiffness — *see* Stiffness, joint
  ketone metabolism E71.32
  kidney N28.9
    functional (tubular) N25.9
    in
      schistosomiasis B65.9 *[N29]*
    tubular function N25.9
      specified NEC N25.89
  lacrimal system H04.9
    changes H04.69
      fistula — *see* Fistula, lacrimal
    gland H04.19
      atrophy — *see* Atrophy, lacrimal gland
      cyst — *see* Cyst, lacrimal, gland
      dacryops — *see* Dacryops
      dislocation — *see* Dislocation, lacrimal gland
      dry eye syndrome — *see* Syndrome, dry eye
      infection — *see* Dacryoadenitis

Disorder — *continued*
  lacrimal system — *continued*
    granuloma — *see* Granuloma, lacrimal
    inflammation — *see* Inflammation, lacrimal
    obstruction — *see* Obstruction, lacrimal
    specified NEC H04.89
  lactation NEC O92.79
  language (developmental) F80.9
    expressive F80.1
    mixed receptive and expressive F80.2
    receptive F80.2
  late luteal phase dysphoric N94.89
  learning (specific) F81.9
    acalculia R48.8
    alexia R48.0
    mathematics F81.2
    reading F81.0
    specified
      with impairment in
        mathematics F81.2
        reading F81.0
        written expression F81.81
    specified NEC F81.89
    spelling F81.81
    written expression F81.81
  lens H27.9
    aphakia — *see* Aphakia
    cataract — *see* Cataract
    dislocation — *see* Dislocation, lens
    specified type NEC H27.8
  ligament M24.20
    ankle M24.27- ☑
    attachment, spine — *see* Enthesopathy, spinal
    elbow M24.22- ☑
    foot joint M24.27- ☑
    hand joint M24.24- ☑
    hip M24.25- ☑
    knee — *see* Derangement, knee, specified NEC
    shoulder M24.21- ☑
    specified site NEC M24.29
    vertebra M24.28
    wrist M24.23- ☑
  ligamentous attachments — *see also* Enthesopathy
    spine — *see* Enthesopathy, spinal
  lipid
    metabolism, congenital E78.9
    storage E75.6
      specified NEC E75.5
  lipoprotein
    deficiency (familial) E78.6
    metabolism E78.9
      specified NEC E78.89
  liver K76.9
    malarial B54 *[K77]*
  low back — *see also* Dorsopathy, specified NEC
  lumbosacral
    plexus G54.1
    root (nerve) NEC G54.4
  lung, interstitial, drug-induced J70.4
    acute J70.2
    chronic J70.3
    dabbing (related) U07.0
    e-cigarette (related) U07.0
    electronic cigarette (related) U07.0
    vaping (associated) (device) (product) (related) (use) U07.0
  lymphoproliferative, post-transplant (PTLD) D47.Z1
    (following D47.4)
  lysine and hydroxylysine metabolism E72.3
  major neurocognitive — *see also* Dementia, in (due to) F03- ☑
  male
    erectile (organic) — *see also* Dysfunction, sexual, male, erectile N52.9
      nonorganic F52.21
    hypoactive sexual desire F52.0
    orgasmic F52.32
  manic F30.9
    organic F06.33
  mast cell activation — *see* Activation, mast cell
  mastoid — *see also* Disorder, ear, middle
    postprocedural — *see* Complications, ear, procedure
  meninges, specified type NEC G96.198
  meniscus — *see* Derangement, knee, meniscus
  menopausal N95.9
    specified NEC N95.8
  menstrual N92.6
    psychogenic F45.8

Disorder — *continued*
  menstrual — *continued*
    specified NEC N92.5
  mental (or behavioral) (nonpsychotic) F99
    due to (secondary to)
      amphetamine
        due to drug abuse — *see* Abuse, drug, stimulant
        due to drug dependence — *see* Dependence, drug, stimulant
      brain disease, damage and dysfunction F09
      caffeine use
        due to drug abuse — *see* Abuse, drug, stimulant
        due to drug dependence — *see* Dependence, drug, stimulant
      cannabis use
        due to drug abuse — *see* Abuse, drug, cannabis
        due to drug dependence — *see* Dependence, drug, cannabis
      general medical condition F09
      sedative or hypnotic use
        due to drug abuse — *see* Abuse, drug, sedative
        due to drug dependence — *see* Dependence, drug, sedative
      tobacco (nicotine) use — *see* Dependence, drug, nicotine
    following organic brain damage F07.9
      frontal lobe syndrome F07.0
      personality change F07.0
      postconcussional syndrome F07.81
      specified NEC F07.89
    infancy, childhood or adolescence F98.9
    neurotic — *see* Neurosis
    organic or symptomatic F09
    presenile, psychotic F03 ☑
    problem NEC
    psychoneurotic — *see* Neurosis
    psychotic — *see* Psychosis
    puerperal F53.0
    senile, psychotic NEC F03 ☑
  metabolic, amino acid, transitory, newborn P74.8
  metabolism NOS E88.9
    amino-acid E72.9
      aromatic E70.9
        albinism — *see* Albinism
        histidine E70.40
          histidinemia E70.41
          other specified E70.49
        hyperphenylalaninemia E70.1
          classical phenylketonuria E70.0
        other specified E70.89
        tryptophan E70.5
        tyrosine E70.20
          hypertyrosinemia E70.21
          other specified E70.29
      branched chain E71.2
        3-methylglutaconic aciduria E71.111
        hyperleucine-isoleucinemia E71.19
        hypervalinemia E71.19
        isovaleric acidemia E71.110
        maple syrup urine disease E71.0
        methylmalonic acidemia E71.120
        organic aciduria NEC E71.118
        other specified E71.19
        propionate NEC E71.128
        propionic acidemia E71.121
      glycine E72.50
        d-glycericacidemia E72.59
        hyperhydroxyprolinemia E72.59
        hyperoxaluria R82.992
          primary E72.53
        hyperprolinemia E72.59
        non-ketotic hyperglycinemia E72.51
        other specified E72.59
        sarcosinemia E72.59
        trimethylaminuria E72.52
      hydroxylysine E72.3
      lysine E72.3
      ornithine E72.4
      other specified E72.89
        beta-amino acid E72.89
        gamma-glutamyl cycle E72.89
      straight-chain E72.89
      sulfur-bearing E72.10
        homocystinuria E72.11

Disorder — *continued*
  metabolism — *continued*
    amino-acid — *continued*
      sulfur-bearing — *continued*
        methylenetetrahydrofolate reductase deficiency E72.12
        other specified E72.19
    bile acid and cholesterol metabolism E78.70
    bilirubin E80.7
      specified NEC E80.6
    calcium E83.50
      hypercalcemia E83.52
      hypocalcemia E83.51
      other specified E83.59
    carbohydrate E74.9
      specified NEC E74.89
    cholesterol and bile acid metabolism E78.70
    congenital E88.9
    copper E83.00
      specified type NEC E83.09
      Wilson's disease E83.01
    cystinuria E72.01
    fructose E74.10
    galactose E74.20
    glucosaminoglycan E76.9
      mucopolysaccharidosis — *see* Mucopolysaccharidosis
      specified NEC E76.8
    glutamine E72.89
    glycine E72.50
    glycogen storage (hepatorenal) E74.09
    glycoprotein E77.9
      specified NEC E77.8
    glycosaminoglycan E76.9
      specified NEC E76.8
    in labor and delivery O75.89
    iron E83.10
    isoleucine E71.19
    leucine E71.19
    lipoid E78.9
    lipoprotein E78.9
      specified NEC E78.89
    magnesium E83.40
      hypermagnesemia E83.41
      hypomagnesemia E83.42
      other specified E83.49
    mineral E83.9
      specified NEC E83.89
    mitochondrial E88.40
      MELAS syndrome E88.41
      MERRF syndrome (myoclonic epilepsy associated with ragged-red fibers) E88.42
      other specified E88.49
    ornithine E72.4
    phosphatases E83.30
    phosphorus E83.30
      acid phosphatase deficiency E83.39
      hypophosphatasia E83.39
      hypophosphatemia E83.39
        familial E83.31
      other specified E83.39
      pseudovitamin D deficiency E83.32
    plasma protein NEC E88.09
    porphyrin — *see* Porphyria
    postprocedural E89.89
      specified NEC E89.89
    purine E79.9
      specified NEC E79.8
    pyrimidine E79.9
      specified NEC E79.8
    pyruvate E74.4
    serine E72.89
    sodium E87.8
    specified NEC E88.89
    threonine E72.89
    valine E71.19
    zinc E83.2
  methylmalonic acidemia E71.120
  micturition NEC — *see also* Difficulty, micturition R39.198
    feeling of incomplete emptying R39.14
    hesitancy R39.11
    poor stream R39.12
    psychogenic F45.8
    split stream R39.13
    straining R39.16
    urgency R39.15
  mild neurocognitive G31.84

Disorder — *continued*
  mild neurocognitive — *continued*
    due to known physiological condition (without behavioral disturbance) F06.70
      with behavioral disturbance F06.71
  mitochondrial metabolism E88.40
  mitral (valve) — *see* Endocarditis, mitral
  mixed
    anxiety and depressive F41.8
    of scholastic skills (developmental) F81.89
    receptive expressive language F80.2
  mood F39
    bipolar — *see* Disorder, bipolar
    depressive — *see* Disorder, depressive
    due to (secondary to)
      alcohol F10.94
      amphetamine F15.94
        in
          abuse F15.14
          dependence F15.24
      anxiolytic F13.94
        in
          abuse F13.14
          dependence F13.24
      cocaine F14.94
        in
          abuse F14.14
          dependence F14.24
      general medical condition F06.30
      hallucinogen F16.94
        in
          abuse F16.14
          dependence F16.24
      hypnotic F13.94
        in
          abuse F13.14
          dependence F13.24
      inhalant F18.94
        in
          abuse F18.14
          dependence F18.24
      opioid F11.94
        in
          abuse F11.14
          dependence F11.24
      phencyclidine (PCP) F16.94
        in
          abuse F16.14
          dependence F16.24
      physiological condition F06.30
        with
          depressive features F06.31
          major depressive-like episode F06.32
          manic features F06.33
          mixed features F06.34
      psychoactive substance NEC F19.94
        in
          abuse F19.14
          dependence F19.24
      sedative F13.94
        in
          abuse F13.14
          dependence F13.24
      volatile solvents F18.94
        in
          abuse F18.14
          dependence F18.24
    manic episode F30.9
      with psychotic symptoms F30.2
      in remission (full) F30.4
        partial F30.3
      specified type NEC F30.8
      without psychotic symptoms F30.10
        mild F30.11
        moderate F30.12
        severe F30.13
    organic F06.30
      right hemisphere F07.89
    persistent F34.9
      cyclothymia F34.0
      dysthymia F34.1
      specified type NEC F34.89
    recurrent F39
    right hemisphere organic F07.89
  movement G25.9
    drug-induced G25.70
      akathisia G25.71
      specified NEC G25.79
    hysterical F44.4 .

Disorder — *continued*
  movement — *continued*
    in diseases classified elsewhere — *see* category G26
    periodic limb G47.61
      sleep related G47.61
    sleep related NEC G47.69
    specified NEC G25.89
    stereotyped F98.4
    treatment-induced G25.9
  multiple personality F44.81
  muscle M62.9
    attachment, spine — *see* Enthesopathy, spinal
    in trichinellosis — *see* Trichinellosis, with muscle disorder
    psychogenic F45.8
    specified type NEC M62.89
    tone, newborn P94.9
      specified NEC P94.8
  muscular
    attachments — *see also* Enthesopathy
      spine — *see* Enthesopathy, spinal
    urethra N36.44
  musculoskeletal system, soft tissue — *see* Disorder, soft tissue
    postprocedural M96.89
    psychogenic F45.8
  myoneural G70.9
    due to lead G70.1
    specified NEC G70.89
    toxic G70.1
  myotonic NEC G71.19
  nail, in diseases classified elsewhere L62
  neck region NEC — *see* Dorsopathy, specified NEC
  neonatal onset multisystemic inflammatory (NOMID) M04.2
  nerve G58.9
    abducent NEC — *see* Strabismus, paralytic, sixth nerve
    accessory G52.8
    acoustic — *see* subcategory H93.3 ☑
    auditory — *see* subcategory H93.3 ☑
    auriculotemporal G50.8
    axillary G54.0
    cerebral — *see* Disorder, nerve, cranial
    cranial G52.9
      eighth — *see* subcategory H93.3 ☑
      eleventh G52.8
      fifth G50.9
      first G52.0
      fourth NEC — *see* Strabismus, paralytic, fourth nerve
      multiple G52.7
      ninth G52.1
      second NEC — *see* Disorder, nerve, optic
      seventh NEC G51.8
      sixth NEC — *see* Strabismus, paralytic, sixth nerve
      specified NEC G52.8
      tenth G52.2
      third NEC — *see* Strabismus, paralytic, third nerve
      twelfth G52.3
    entrapment — *see* Neuropathy, entrapment
    facial G51.9
      specified NEC G51.8
    femoral — *see* Lesion, nerve, femoral
    glossopharyngeal NEC G52.1
    hypoglossal G52.3
    intercostal G58.0
    lateral
      cutaneous of thigh — *see* Mononeuropathy, lower limb, meralgia paresthetica
      popliteal — *see* Lesion, nerve, popliteal
    lower limb — *see* Mononeuropathy, lower limb
    medial popliteal — *see* Lesion, nerve, popliteal, medial
    median NEC — *see* Lesion, nerve, median
    multiple G58.7
    oculomotor NEC — *see* Strabismus, paralytic, third nerve
    olfactory G52.0
    optic NEC H47.09- ☑
      hemorrhage into sheath — *see* Hemorrhage, optic nerve
      ischemic H47.01- ☑
    peroneal — *see* Lesion, nerve, popliteal
    phrenic G58.8
    plantar — *see* Lesion, nerve, plantar
    pneumogastric G52.2
    posterior tibial — *see* Syndrome, tarsal tunnel

Disorder — *continued*
- nerve — *continued*
  - radial — *see* Lesion, nerve, radial
  - recurrent laryngeal G52.2
  - root G54.9
    - cervical G54.2
    - lumbosacral G54.1
    - specified NEC G54.8
    - thoracic G54.3
  - sciatic NEC — *see* Lesion, nerve, sciatic
  - specified NEC G58.8
    - lower limb — *see* Mononeuropathy, lower limb, specified NEC
    - upper limb — *see* Mononeuropathy, upper limb, specified NEC
  - sympathetic G90.9
  - tibial — *see* Lesion, nerve, popliteal, medial
  - trigeminal G50.9
    - specified NEC G50.8
  - trochlear NEC — *see* Strabismus, paralytic, fourth nerve
  - ulnar — *see* Lesion, nerve, ulnar
  - upper limb — *see* Mononeuropathy, upper limb
  - vagus G52.2
- nervous system G98.8
  - autonomic (peripheral) G90.9
    - specified NEC G90.8
  - central G96.9
    - specified NEC G96.89
  - parasympathetic G90.9
  - specified NEC G98.8
  - sympathetic G90.9
  - vegetative G90.9
- neurocognitive R41.9
  - with Lewy bodies — *see also* Dementia, in, diseases specified elsewhere G31.83 *[F02.-]* ☑
  - frontotemporal, specified NEC — *see also* Dementia, in, diseases specified elsewhere G31.09 *[F02.-]* ☑
  - major — *see also* Dementia F03.- ☑
    - due to vascular disease — *see* Dementia, vascular
    - mild — *see* Dementia, vascular, mild
    - moderate — *see* Dementia, vascular, moderate
    - severe — *see* Dementia, vascular, severe
    - in (due to) (other diseases classified elsewhere) — *see also* Dementia, in (due to) F02.80
      - with
        - aggressive behavior — *see also* Dementia, in (due to) F02.81- ☑
        - combative behavior — *see also* Dementia, in (due to) F02.81- ☑
        - violent behavior — *see also* Dementia, in (due to) F02.81- ☑
  - mild (of uncertain or unknown etiology) — *see also* Disorder, mild neurocognitive G31.84
- neurodevelopmental F89
  - specified NEC F88
- neurohypophysis NEC E23.3
- neurological NEC R29.818
- neuromuscular G70.9
  - hereditary NEC G71.9
  - specified NEC G70.89
  - toxic G70.1
- neurotic F48.9
  - specified NEC F48.8
- neutrophil, polymorphonuclear D71
- nicotine use — *see* Dependence, drug, nicotine
- nightmare F51.5
- non-rapid eye movement sleep arousal
  - sleep terror type F51.4
  - sleepwalking type F51.3
- nose J34.9
  - specified NEC J34.89
- obsessive-compulsive F42.9
  - and related disorder due to a known physiological condition F06.8
- odontogenesis NOS K00.9
- opioid use
  - with
    - opioid-induced psychotic disorder F11.959
      - with
        - delusions F11.950
        - hallucinations F11.951
    - due to drug abuse — *see* Abuse, drug, opioid
    - due to drug dependence — *see* Dependence, drug, opioid
  - mild F11.10

Disorder — *continued*
- opioid use — *continued*
  - mild — *continued*
    - with
      - opioid-induced
        - anxiety disorder F11.188
        - depressive disorder F11.14
        - sexual dysfunction F11.181
      - opioid intoxication
        - with perceptual disturbances F11.122
        - delirium F11.121
        - without perceptual disturbances F11.129
    - in remission (early) (sustained) F11.11
  - moderate or severe F11.20
    - with
      - opioid-induced
        - anxiety disorder F11.288
        - anxiety disorder F11.988
        - depressive disorder F11.24
        - depressive disorder F11.94
        - sexual dysfunction F11.281
        - sexual dysfunction F11.981
      - opioid intoxication
        - with perceptual disturbances F11.222
        - delirium F11.221
        - without perceptual disturbances F11.229
    - in remission (early) (sustained) F11.21
- oppositional defiant F91.3
- optic
  - chiasm H47.49
    - due to
      - inflammatory disorder H47.41
      - neoplasm H47.42
      - vascular disorder H47.43
  - disc H47.39- ☑
    - coloboma — *see* Coloboma, optic disc
    - drusen — *see* Drusen, optic disc
    - pseudopapilledema — *see* Pseudopapilledema
  - radiations — *see* Disorder, visual, pathway
  - tracts — *see* Disorder, visual, pathway
- orbit H05.9
  - cyst — *see* Cyst, orbit
  - deformity — *see* Deformity, orbit
  - edema — *see* Edema, orbit
  - enophthalmos — *see* Enophthalmos
  - exophthalmos — *see* Exophthalmos
  - hemorrhage — *see* Hemorrhage, orbit
  - inflammation — *see* Inflammation, orbit
  - myopathy — *see* Myopathy, extraocular muscles
  - retained foreign body — *see* Foreign body, orbit, old
  - specified type NEC H05.89
- organic
  - anxiety F06.4
  - catatonic F06.1
  - delusional F06.2
  - dissociative F06.8
  - emotionally labile (asthenic) F06.8
  - mood (affective) F06.30
  - schizophrenia-like F06.2
- orgasmic (female) F52.31
  - male F52.32
- ornithine metabolism E72.4
- overanxious F41.1
  - of childhood F93.8
- pain
  - with related psychological factors F45.42
  - exclusively related to psychological factors F45.41
  - genito-pelvic penetration disorder F52.6
- pancreatic internal secretion E16.9
  - specified NEC E16.8
- panic F41.0
  - with agoraphobia F40.01
- papulosquamous L44.9
  - in diseases classified elsewhere L45
  - specified NEC L44.8
- paranoid F22
  - induced F24
  - shared F24
- paraphilic F65.9
  - specified NEC F65.89
- parathyroid (gland) E21.5
  - specified NEC E21.4
- parietoalveolar NEC J84.09
- paroxysmal, mixed R56.9
- patella M22.9- ☑
  - chondromalacia — *see* Chondromalacia, patella
  - derangement NEC M22.3X- ☑

Disorder — *continued*
- patella — *continued*
  - recurrent
    - dislocation — *see* Dislocation, patella, recurrent
    - subluxation — *see* Dislocation, patella, recurrent, incomplete
  - specified NEC M22.8X- ☑
- patellofemoral M22.2X- ☑
- pedophilic F65.4
- pentose phosphate pathway with anemia D55.1
- perception, due to hallucinogens F16.983
  - in
    - abuse F16.183
    - dependence F16.283
- peripheral nervous system NEC G64
- peroxisomal E71.50
  - biogenesis
    - neonatal adrenoleukodystrophy E71.511
    - specified disorder NEC E71.518
    - Zellweger syndrome E71.510
  - rhizomelic chondrodysplasia punctata E71.540
  - specified form NEC E71.548
    - group 1 E71.518
    - group 2 E71.53
    - group 3 E71.542
  - X-linked adrenoleukodystrophy E71.529
    - adolescent E71.521
    - adrenomyeloneuropathy E71.522
    - childhood E71.520
    - specified form NEC E71.528
  - Zellweger-like syndrome E71.541
- persistent
  - (somatoform) pain F45.41
  - affective (mood) F34.9
- personality — *see also* Personality F60.9
  - affective F34.0
  - aggressive F60.3
  - amoral F60.2
  - anankastic F60.5
  - antisocial F60.2
  - anxious F60.6
  - asocial F60.2
  - asthenic F60.7
  - avoidant F60.6
  - borderline F60.3
  - change (secondary) due to general medical condition F07.0
  - compulsive F60.5
  - cyclothymic F34.0
  - dependent (passive) F60.7
  - depressive F34.1
  - dissocial F60.2
  - emotional instability F60.3
  - expansive paranoid F60.0
  - explosive F60.3
  - following organic brain damage F07.9
  - histrionic F60.4
  - hyperthymic F34.0
  - hypothymic F34.1
  - hysterical F60.4
  - immature F60.89
  - inadequate F60.7
  - labile F60.3
  - mixed (nonspecific) F60.89
  - moral deficiency F60.2
  - narcissistic F60.81
  - negativistic F60.89
  - obsessional F60.5
  - obsessive (-compulsive) F60.5
  - organic F07.9
  - overconscientious F60.5
  - paranoid F60.0
  - passive (-dependent) F60.7
  - passive-aggressive F60.89
  - pathological NEC F60.9
  - pseudosocial F60.2
  - psychopathic F60.2
  - schizoid F60.1
  - schizotypal F21
  - self-defeating F60.7
  - specified NEC F60.89
  - type A F60.5
  - unstable (emotional) F60.3
- pervasive, developmental F84.9
- phencyclidine use
  - mild F16.10
    - with
      - phencyclidine intoxication F16.129
      - phencyclidine intoxication delirium F16.121

Disorder — *continued*
  phencyclidine use — *continued*
    mild — *continued*
      with — *continued*
        phencyclidine-induced
          anxiety disorder F16.180
          bipolar and related disorder F16.14
          depressive disorder F16.14
          psychotic disorder F16.159
      in remission (early) (sustained) F16.11
    moderate or severe F16.20
      with
        phencyclidine intoxication F16.229
        phencyclidine intoxication delirium F16.221
        phencyclidine-induced
          anxiety disorder F16.280
          bipolar and related disorder F16.14
          depressive disorder F16.24
          psychotic disorder F16.259
      in remission (early) (sustained) F16.21
  phobic anxiety, childhood F40.8
  phosphate-losing tubular N25.0
  pigmentation L81.9
    choroid, congenital Q14.3
    diminished melanin formation L81.6
    iron L81.8
    specified NEC L81.8
  pinna (noninfective) H61.10- ☑
    deformity, acquired H61.11- ☑
    hematoma H61.12- ☑
    perichondritis — *see* Perichondritis, ear
    specified type NEC H61.19- ☑
  pituitary gland E23.7
    iatrogenic (postprocedural) E89.3
    specified NEC E23.6
  platelet-activating anti-PF4, specified NEC D75.84
  platelets D69.1
  plexus G54.9
    specified NEC G54.8
  polymorphonuclear neutrophils D71
  porphyrin metabolism — *see* Porphyria
  postconcussional F07.81
  posthallucinogen perception F16.983
    in
      abuse F16.183
      dependence F16.283
  postmenopausal N95.9
    specified NEC N95.8
  postprocedural (postoperative) — *see* Complications, postprocedural
  post-transplant lymphoproliferative D47.Z1 (*following* D47.4)
  post-traumatic stress (PTSD) F43.10
    acute F43.11
    chronic F43.12
  premenstrual dysphoric (PMDD) F32.81
  prepuce N47.8
  propionic acidemia E71.121
  prostate N42.9
    specified NEC N42.89
  psychogenic NOS — *see also* condition F45.9
    anxiety F41.8
    appetite F50.9
    asthenic F48.8
    cardiovascular (system) F45.8
    compulsive F42.8
    cutaneous F54
    depressive F32.9
    digestive (system) F45.8
    dysmenorrheic F45.8
    dyspneic F45.8
    endocrine (system) F54
    eye NEC F45.8
    feeding — *see* Disorder, eating
    functional NEC F45.8
    gastric F45.8
    gastrointestinal (system) F45.8
    genitourinary (system) F45.8
    heart (function) (rhythm) F45.8
    hyperventilatory F45.8
    hypochondriacal — *see* Disorder, hypochondriacal
    intestinal F45.8
    joint F45.8
    learning F81.9
    limb F45.8
    lymphatic (system) F45.8
    menstrual F45.8
    micturition F45.8

Disorder — *continued*
  psychogenic — *see also* condition — *continued*
    monoplegic NEC F44.4
    motor F44.4
    muscle F45.8
    musculoskeletal F45.8
    neurocirculatory F45.8
    obsessive F42.8
    occupational F48.8
    organ or part of body NEC F45.8
    paralytic NEC F44.4
    phobic F40.9
    physical NEC F45.8
    rectal F45.8
    respiratory (system) F45.8
    rheumatic F45.8
    sexual (function) F52.9
    skin (allergic) (eczematous) F54
    sleep F51.9
    specified part of body NEC F45.8
    stomach F45.8
  psychological F99
    associated with
      disease classified elsewhere F54
      sexual
        development F66
        relationship F66
      uncertainty about gender identity F64.9
  psychomotor NEC F44.4
    hysterical F44.4
  psychoneurotic — *see also* Neurosis
    mixed NEC F48.8
  psychophysiologic — *see* Disorder, somatoform
  psychosexual F65.9
    development F66
    identity of childhood F64.2
  psychosomatic NOS — *see* Disorder, somatoform
    multiple F45.0
    undifferentiated F45.1
  psychotic — *see* Psychosis
    transient (acute) F23
  puberty E30.9
    specified NEC E30.8
  pulmonary (valve) — *see* Endocarditis, pulmonary
  purine metabolism E79.9
  pyrimidine metabolism E79.9
  pyruvate metabolism E74.4
  reactive attachment (childhood) F94.1
  reading R48.0
    developmental (specific) F81.0
  receptive language F80.2
  receptor, hormonal, peripheral — *see also* Syndrome, androgen insensitivity E34.50
  recurrent brief depressive F33.8
  reflex R29.2
  refraction H52.7
    aniseikonia H52.32
    anisometropia H52.31
    astigmatism — *see* Astigmatism
    hypermetropia — *see* Hypermetropia
    myopia — *see* Myopia
    presbyopia H52.4
    specified NEC H52.6
  relationship F68.8
    due to sexual orientation F66
  REM sleep behavior G47.52
  renal function, impaired (tubular) N25.9
  resonance R49.9
    specified NEC R49.8
  respiratory function, impaired — *see also* Failure, respiration
    postprocedural — *see* Complication, postoperative, respiratory system
    psychogenic F45.8
  retina H35.9
    angioid streaks H35.33
    changes in vascular appearance H35.01- ☑
    degeneration — *see* Degeneration, retina
    dystrophy (hereditary) — *see* Dystrophy, retina
    edema H35.81
    hemorrhage — *see* Hemorrhage, retina
    ischemia H35.82
    macular degeneration — *see* Degeneration, macula
    microaneurysms H35.04- ☑
    microvascular abnormality NEC H35.09
    neovascularization — *see* Neovascularization, retina
    retinopathy — *see* Retinopathy
    separation of layers H35.70

Disorder — *continued*
  retina — *continued*
    separation of layers — *continued*
      central serous chorioretinopathy H35.71- ☑
      pigment epithelium detachment (serous) H35.72- ☑
      hemorrhagic H35.73- ☑
      specified type NEC H35.89
    telangiectasis — *see* Telangiectasis, retina
    vasculitis — *see* Vasculitis, retina
  retroperitoneal K68.9
  right hemisphere organic affective F07.89
  rumination (infant or child) F98.21
  sacrum, sacrococcygeal NEC M53.3
  schizoaffective F25.9
    bipolar type F25.0
    depressive type F25.1
    manic type F25.0
    mixed type F25.0
    specified NEC F25.8
  schizoid of childhood F84.5
  schizophrenia spectrum and other psychotic disorder F29
    specified NEC F28
  schizophreniform F20.81
    brief F23
  schizotypal (personality) F21
  seasonal affective, recurrent episodes F33.- ☑
  secretion, thyrocalcitonin E07.0
  sedative, hypnotic, or anxiolytic use
    mild F13.10
      with
        sedative, hypnotic, or anxiolytic intoxication F13.129
        sedative, hypnotic, or anxiolytic intoxication delirium F13.121
        sedative, hypnotic, or anxiolytic-induced
          anxiety disorder F13.180
          bipolar and related disorder F13.14
          depressive disorder F13.14
          psychotic disorder F13.159
          sexual dysfunction F13.181
      in remission (early) (sustained) F13.11
    moderate or severe F13.20
      with
        sedative, hypnotic, or anxiolytic intoxication F13.229
        sedative, hypnotic, or anxiolytic intoxication delirium F13.221
        sedative, hypnotic, or anxiolytic-induced
          anxiety disorder F13.280
          bipolar and related disorder F13.24
          depressive disorder F13.24
          major neurocognitive disorder F13.27
          mild neurocognitive disorder F13.288
          psychotic disorder F13.259
          sexual dysfunction F13.281
      in remission (early) (sustained) F13.21
  seizure — *see also* Epilepsy G40.909
    intractable G40.919
      with status epilepticus G40.911
  semantic pragmatic F80.89
    with autism F84.0
  sense of smell R43.1
    psychogenic F45.8
  separation anxiety, of childhood F93.0
  sexual
    aversion F52.1
    function, psychogenic F52.9
    interest/arousal, female F52.22
    masochism F65.51
    maturation F66
    nonorganic F52.9
    preference — *see also* Deviation, sexual F65.9
      fetishistic transvestism F65.1
    relationship F66
    sadism F65.52
  shyness, of childhood and adolescence F40.10
  sibling rivalry F93.8
  sickle-cell (sickling) (homozygous) — *see* Disease, sickle-cell
    heterozygous D57.3
    specified type NEC D57.8- ☑
    trait D57.3
  sinus (nasal) J34.9
    specified NEC J34.89
  skin L98.9
    atrophic L90.9

Disorder — *continued*
  skin — *continued*
    atrophic — *continued*
      specified NEC L90.8
    granulomatous L92.9
      specified NEC L92.8
    hypertrophic L91.9
      specified NEC L91.8
    infiltrative NEC L98.6
    newborn P83.9
      specified NEC P83.88
    picking F42.4
    psychogenic (allergic) (eczematous) F54
  sleep G47.9
    breathing-related — *see* Apnea, sleep
    circadian rhythm G47.20
      advance sleep phase type G47.22
      delayed sleep phase type G47.21
      due to
        alcohol
          abuse F10.182
          dependence F10.282
          use F10.982
        amphetamines
          abuse F15.182
          dependence F15.282
          use F15.982
        caffeine
          abuse F15.182
          dependence F15.282
          use F15.982
        cocaine
          abuse F14.182
          dependence F14.282
          use F14.982
        drug NEC
          abuse F19.182
          dependence F19.282
          use F19.982
        opioid
          abuse F11.182
          dependence F11.282
          use F11.982
        psychoactive substance NEC
          abuse F19.182
          dependence F19.282
          use F19.982
        sedative, hypnotic, or anxiolytic
          abuse F13.182
          dependence F13.282
          use F13.982
        stimulant NEC
          abuse F15.182
          dependence F15.282
          use F15.982
      free running type G47.24
      in conditions classified elsewhere G47.27
      irregular sleep wake type G47.23
      jet lag type G47.25
      non-24-hour sleep-wake type G47.24
      shift work type G47.26
      specified NEC G47.29
    due to
      alcohol
        abuse F10.182
        dependence F10.282
        use F10.982
      amphetamine
        abuse F15.182
        dependence F15.282
        use F15.982
      anxiolytic
        abuse F13.182
        dependence F13.282
        use F13.982
      caffeine
        abuse F15.182
        dependence F15.282
        use F15.982
      cocaine
        abuse F14.182
        dependence F14.282
        use F14.982
      drug NEC
        abuse F19.182
        dependence F19.282
        use F19.982
      hypnotic
        abuse F13.182

Disorder — *continued*
  sleep — *continued*
    due to — *continued*
      hypnotic — *continued*
        dependence F13.282
        use F13.982
      opioid
        abuse F11.182
        dependence F11.282
        use F11.982
      psychoactive substance NEC
        abuse F19.182
        dependence F19.282
        use F19.982
      sedative
        abuse F13.182
        dependence F13.282
        use F13.982
      stimulant NEC
        abuse F15.182
        dependence F15.282
        use F15.982
    emotional F51.9
    excessive somnolence — *see* Hypersomnia
    hypersomnia type — *see* Hypersomnia
    initiating or maintaining — *see* Insomnia
    nightmares F51.5
    nonorganic F51.9
      specified NEC F51.8
    parasomnia type G47.50
    specified NEC G47.8
    terrors F51.4
    walking F51.3
  sleep-wake pattern or schedule — *see also* Disorder, sleep, circadian rhythm G47.9
    specified NEC G47.8
  social
    anxiety (of childhood) F40.10
      generalized F40.11
    functioning in childhood F94.9
      specified NEC F94.8
    pragmatic F80.82
  soft tissue M79.9
    ankle M79.9
    due to use, overuse and pressure M70.90
      ankle M70.97- ☑
      bursitis — *see* Bursitis
      foot M70.97- ☑
      forearm M70.93- ☑
      hand M70.94- ☑
      lower leg M70.96- ☑
      multiple sites M70.99
      pelvic region M70.95- ☑
      shoulder region M70.91- ☑
      specified site NEC M70.98
      specified type NEC M70.80
        ankle M70.87- ☑
        foot M70.87- ☑
        forearm M70.83- ☑
        hand M70.84- ☑
        lower leg M70.86- ☑
        multiple sites M70.89
        pelvic region M70.85- ☑
        shoulder region M70.81- ☑
        specified site NEC M70.88
        thigh M70.85- ☑
        upper arm M70.82- ☑
      thigh M70.95- ☑
      upper arm M70.92- ☑
    foot M79.9
    forearm M79.9
    hand M79.9
    lower leg M79.9
    multiple sites M79.9
    occupational — *see* Disorder, soft tissue, due to use, overuse and pressure
    pelvic region M79.9
    shoulder region M79.9
    specified type NEC M79.89
    thigh M79.9
    upper arm M79.9
  somatic symptom F45.1
  somatization F45.0
  somatoform F45.9
    pain (persistent) F45.41
    somatization (multiple) (long-lasting) F45.0
    specified NEC F45.8
    undifferentiated F45.1

Disorder — *continued*
  somnolence, excessive — *see* Hypersomnia
  specific
    arithmetical F81.2
    developmental, of motor F82
    reading F81.0
    speech and language F80.9
    spelling F81.81
    written expression F81.81
  speech R47.9
    articulation (functional) (specific) F80.0
    developmental F80.9
    specified NEC R47.89
  speech-sound F80.0
  spelling (specific) F81.81
  spine — *see also* Dorsopathy
    ligamentous or muscular attachments, peripheral
      — *see* Enthesopathy, spinal
    specified NEC — *see* Dorsopathy, specified NEC
  stereotyped, habit or movement F98.4
  stimulant use (other) (unspecified)
    mild F15.10
      in remission (early) (sustained) F15.11
    moderate or severe F15.20
      in remission (early) (sustained) F15.21
  stomach (functional) — *see* Disorder, gastric
  stress F43.9
    acute F43.0
    post-traumatic F43.10
      acute F43.11
      chronic F43.12
  substance use (other) (unknown)
    mild F19.10
      with substance-induced
        anxiety disorder F19.180
        bipolar and related disorder F19.14
        depressive disorder F19.14
        major neurocognitive disorder F19.17
        mild neurocognitive disorder F19.188
        obsessive-compulsive and related disorder F19.188
        sexual dysfunction F19.181
      substance intoxication F19.129
      substance intoxication delirium F19.121
    moderate or severe F19.20
      with substance-induced
        anxiety disorder F19.280
        bipolar and related disorder F19.24
        depressive disorder F19.24
        major neurocognitive disorder F19.27
        mild neurocognitive disorder F19.288
        obsessive-compulsive and related disorder F19.288
        sexual dysfunction F19.281
      in remission (early) (sustained) F19.21
      substance intoxication F19.229
      substance intoxication delirium F19.221
  sulfur-bearing amino-acid metabolism E72.10
  sweat gland (eccrine) L74.9
    apocrine L75.9
      specified NEC L75.8
    specified NEC L74.8
  synovium M67.90
    acromioclavicular M67.91- ☑
    ankle M67.97- ☑
    elbow M67.92- ☑
    foot M67.97- ☑
    forearm M67.93- ☑
    hand M67.94- ☑
    hip M67.95- ☑
    knee M67.96- ☑
    multiple sites M67.99
    rupture — *see* Rupture, synovium
    shoulder M67.91- ☑
    specified type NEC M67.80
      acromioclavicular M67.81- ☑
      ankle M67.87- ☑
      elbow M67.82- ☑
      foot M67.87- ☑
      hand M67.84- ☑
      hip M67.85- ☑
      knee M67.86- ☑
      multiple sites M67.89
      wrist M67.83- ☑
    synovitis — *see* Synovitis
    upper arm M67.92- ☑
    wrist M67.93- ☑
  temperature regulation, newborn P81.9

Disorder — *continued*
  temperature regulation, newborn — *continued*
    specified NEC P81.8
  temporomandibular joint M26.60- ☑
  tendon M67.90
    acromioclavicular M67.91- ☑
    ankle M67.97- ☑
    contracture — *see* Contracture, tendon
    elbow M67.92- ☑
    foot M67.97- ☑
    forearm M67.93- ☑
    hand M67.94- ☑
    hip M67.95- ☑
    knee M67.96- ☑
    multiple sites M67.99
    rupture — *see* Rupture, tendon
    shoulder M67.91- ☑
    specified type NEC M67.80
      acromioclavicular M67.81- ☑
      ankle M67.87- ☑
      elbow M67.82- ☑
      foot M67.87- ☑
      hand M67.84- ☑
      hip M67.85- ☑
      knee M67.86- ☑
      multiple sites M67.89
      trunk M67.88
      wrist M67.83- ☑
    synovitis — *see* Synovitis
    tendinitis — *see* Tendinitis
    tenosynovitis — *see* Tenosynovitis
    trunk M67.98
    upper arm M67.92- ☑
    wrist M67.93- ☑
  thoracic root (nerve) NEC G54.3
  thyrocalcitonin hypersecretion E07.0
  thyroid (gland) E07.9
    function NEC, neonatal, transitory P72.2
    iodine-deficiency related E01.8
    specified NEC E07.89
  tic — *see* Tic
  tobacco use
    chewing tobacco (mild) (moderate) (severe)
      F17.221
      in remission (early) (sustained) F17.221
    cigarettes (mild) (moderate) (severe)
      F17.211
      in remission (early) (sustained) F17.211
    mild F17.200
      in remission (early) (sustained) F17.201
    moderate F17.200
      in remission (early) (sustained) F17.201
    severe F17.200
      in remission (early) (sustained) F17.201
    specified product NEC (mild) (moderate) (severe)
      F17.291
      in remission (early) (sustained) F17.291
  tooth K08.9
    development K00.9
      specified NEC K00.8
    eruption K00.6
  Tourette's F95.2
  trance and possession F44.89
  transvestic F65.1
  trauma and stressor-related NOS F43.9
    other specified F43.89
    unspecified F43.9
  tricuspid (valve) — *see* Endocarditis, tricuspid
  tryptophan metabolism E70.5
  tubular, phosphate-losing N25.0
  tubulo-interstitial (in)
    brucellosis A23.9 *[N16]*
    cystinosis E72.04
    diphtheria A36.84
    glycogen storage disease E74.00 *[N16]*
    leukemia NEC C95.9- ☑ *[N16]*
    lymphoma NEC C85.9- ☑ *[N16]*
    mixed cryoglobulinemia D89.1 *[N16]*
    multiple myeloma C90.0- ☑ *[N16]*
    Salmonella infection A02.25
    sarcoidosis D86.84
    sepsis A41.9 *[N16]*
      streptococcal A40.9 *[N16]*
    systemic lupus erythematosus M32.15
    toxoplasmosis B58.83
    transplant rejection T86.91 *[N16]*
    Wilson's disease E83.01 *[N16]*
  tubulo-renal function, impaired N25.9
    specified NEC N25.89
  tympanic membrane H73.9- ☑

Disorder — *continued*
  tympanic membrane — *continued*
    atrophy — *see* Atrophy, tympanic membrane
    infection — *see* Myringitis
    perforation — *see* Perforation, tympanum
    specified NEC H73.89- ☑
  unsocialized aggressive F91.1
  urea cycle metabolism E72.20
    argininemia E72.21
    arginosuccinic aciduria E72.22
    citrullinemia E72.23
    ornithine transcarbamylase deficiency E72.4
    other specified E72.29
  ureter (in) N28.9
    schistosomiasis B65.0 *[N29]*
    tuberculosis A18.11
  urethra N36.9
    specified NEC N36.8
  urinary system N39.9
    specified NEC N39.8
  valve, heart
    aortic — *see* Endocarditis, aortic
    mitral — *see* Endocarditis, mitral
    pulmonary — *see* Endocarditis, pulmonary
    rheumatic
      aortic — *see* Endocarditis, aortic, rheumatic
      mitral — *see* Endocarditis, mitral
      pulmonary — *see* Endocarditis, pulmonary,
        rheumatic
      tricuspid — *see* Endocarditis, tricuspid
    tricuspid — *see* Endocarditis, tricuspid
  vestibular function H81.9- ☑
    specified NEC — *see* subcategory H81.8 ☑
      in diseases classified elsewhere H82.- ☑
    vertigo — *see* Vertigo
  vision, binocular H53.30
    abnormal retinal correspondence H53.31
    diplopia H53.2
    fusion with defective stereopsis H53.32
    simultaneous perception H53.33
    suppression H53.34
  visual
    cortex
      blindness H47.619
        left brain H47.612
        right brain H47.611
      due to
        inflammatory disorder H47.629
          left brain H47.622
          right brain H47.621
        neoplasm H47.639
          left brain H47.632
          right brain H47.631
        vascular disorder H47.649
          left brain H47.642
          right brain H47.641
    pathway H47.9
      due to
        inflammatory disorder H47.51- ☑
        neoplasm H47.52- ☑
        vascular disorder H47.53- ☑
      optic chiasm — *see* Disorder, optic, chiasm
  vitreous body H43.9
    crystalline deposits — *see* Deposit, crystalline
    degeneration — *see* Degeneration, vitreous
    hemorrhage — *see* Hemorrhage, vitreous
    opacities — *see* Opacity, vitreous
    prolapse — *see* Prolapse, vitreous
    specified type NEC H43.89
  voice R49.9
    specified type NEC R49.8
  volatile solvent use
    due to drug abuse — *see* Abuse, drug, inhalant
    due to drug dependence — *see* Dependence, drug,
      inhalant
  voyeuristic F65.3
  white blood cells D72.9
    specified NEC D72.89
  withdrawing, child or adolescent F40.10
Disorientation R41.0
Displacement, displaced
  acquired traumatic of bone, cartilage, joint, tendon
    NEC — *see* Dislocation
  adrenal gland (congenital) Q89.1
  appendix, retrocecal (congenital) Q43.8
  auricle (congenital) Q17.4
  bladder (acquired) N32.89
    congenital Q64.19

Displacement, displaced — *continued*
  brachial plexus (congenital) Q07.8
  brain stem, caudal (congenital) Q04.8
  canaliculus (lacrimalis), congenital Q10.6
  cardia through esophageal hiatus (congenital) Q40.1
  cerebellum, caudal (congenital) Q04.8
  cervix — *see* Malposition, uterus
  colon (congenital) Q43.3
  device, implant or graft — *see also* Complications, by
    site and type, mechanical T85.628 ☑
    arterial graft NEC — *see* Complication, cardiovascu-
      lar device, mechanical, vascular
    breast (implant) T85.42 ☑
    catheter NEC T85.628 ☑
      dialysis (renal) T82.42 ☑
        intraperitoneal T85.621 ☑
      infusion NEC T82.524 ☑
        spinal (epidural) (subdural) T85.620 ☑
      urinary
        cystostomy T83.020 ☑
        Hopkins T83.028 ☑
        ileostomy T83.028 ☑
        indwelling T83.021 ☑
        nephrostomy T83.022 ☑
        specified NEC T83.028 ☑
        urostomy T83.028 ☑
    electronic (electrode) (pulse generator) (stimulator)
      — *see* Complication, electronic stimulator
    fixation, internal (orthopedic) NEC — *see* Complica-
      tion, fixation device, mechanical
    gastrointestinal — *see* Complications, prosthetic
      device, mechanical, gastrointestinal device
    genital NEC T83.428 ☑
      intrauterine contraceptive device (string)
        T83.32 ☑
      penile prosthesis (cylinder) (implanted) (pump)
        (reservoir) T83.420 ☑
      testicular prosthesis T83.421 ☑
    heart NEC — *see* Complication, cardiovascular de-
      vice, mechanical
    joint prosthesis — *see* Complications, joint prosthe-
      sis, mechanical
    ocular — *see* Complications, prosthetic device,
      mechanical, ocular device
    orthopedic NEC — *see* Complication, orthopedic,
      device or graft, mechanical
    specified NEC T85.628 ☑
    urinary NEC T83.128 ☑
      graft T83.22 ☑
      sphincter, implanted T83.121 ☑
      stent (ileal conduit) (nephroureteral) T83.123 ☑
        ureteral indwelling T83.122 ☑
    vascular NEC — *see* Complication, cardiovascular
      device, mechanical
    ventricular intracranial shunt T85.02 ☑
  electronic stimulator
    bone T84.320 ☑
    cardiac — *see* Complications, cardiac device, elec-
      tronic
    nervous system — *see* Complication, prosthetic
      device, mechanical, electronic nervous system
      stimulator
    urinary — *see* Complications, electronic stimulator,
      urinary
  esophageal mucosa into cardia of stomach, congenital
    Q39.8
  esophagus (acquired) K22.89
    congenital Q39.8
  eyeball (acquired) (lateral) (old) — *see* Displacement,
    globe
    congenital Q15.8
    current — *see* Avulsion, eye
  fallopian tube (acquired) N83.4- ☑
    congenital Q50.6
    opening (congenital) Q50.6
  gallbladder (congenital) Q44.1
  gastric mucosa (congenital) Q40.2
  globe (acquired) (old) (lateral) H05.21- ☑
    current — *see* Avulsion, eye
  heart (congenital) Q24.8
    acquired I51.89
  hymen (upward) (congenital) Q52.4
  intervertebral disc NEC
    with myelopathy — *see* Disorder, disc, with,
      myelopathy
    cervical, cervicothoracic (with) M50.20

Displacement, displaced — *continued*
  intervertebral disc — *continued*
    cervical, cervicothoracic — *continued*
      myelopathy — *see* Disorder, disc, cervical, with
        myelopathy
      neuritis, radiculitis or radiculopathy — *see* Disor-
        der, disc, cervical, with neuritis
    due to trauma — *see* Dislocation, vertebra
    lumbar region M51.26
      with
        myelopathy M51.06
        neuritis, radiculitis, radiculopathy or sciatica
          M51.16
    lumbosacral region M51.27
      with
        neuritis, radiculitis, radiculopathy or sciatica
          M51.17
    sacrococcygeal region M53.3
    thoracic region M51.24
      with
        myelopathy M51.04
        neuritis, radiculitis, radiculopathy M51.14
    thoracolumbar region M51.25
      with
        myelopathy M51.05
        neuritis, radiculitis, radiculopathy M51.15
  intrauterine device (string) T83.32 ☑
  kidney (acquired) N28.83
    congenital Q63.2
  lachrymal, lacrimal apparatus or duct (congenital) Q10.6
  lens, congenital Q12.1
  macula (congenital) Q14.1
  Meckel's diverticulum Q43.0
    malignant — *see* Table of Neoplasms, small intes-
      tine, malignant
  nail (congenital) Q84.6
    acquired L60.8
  opening of Wharton's duct in mouth Q38.4
  organ or site, congenital NEC — *see* Malposition, con-
    genital
  ovary (acquired) N83.4- ☑
    congenital Q50.39
    free in peritoneal cavity (congenital) Q50.39
    into hernial sac N83.4- ☑
  oviduct (acquired) N83.4- ☑
    congenital Q50.6
  parathyroid (gland) E21.4
  parotid gland (congenital) Q38.4
  punctum lacrimale (congenital) Q10.6
  sacro-iliac (joint) (congenital) Q74.2
    current injury S33.2 ☑
    old — *see* subcategory M53.2 ☑
  salivary gland (any) (congenital) Q38.4
  spleen (congenital) Q89.09
  stomach, congenital Q40.2
  sublingual duct Q38.4
  tongue (downward) (congenital) Q38.3
  tooth, teeth, fully erupted M26.30
    horizontal M26.33
    vertical M26.34
  trachea (congenital) Q32.1
  ureter or ureteric opening or orifice (congenital) Q62.62
  uterine opening of oviducts or fallopian tubes Q50.6
  uterus, uterine — *see* Malposition, uterus
  ventricular septum Q21.0
    with rudimentary ventricle Q20.4

Disproportion
  between native and reconstructed breast N65.1
  fiber-type G71.20
    congenital G71.29

Disruptio uteri — *see* Rupture, uterus

Disruption (of)
  ciliary body NEC H21.89
  closure of
    cornea T81.31 ☑
    craniotomy T81.32 ☑
    fascia (muscular) (superficial) T81.32 ☑
    internal organ or tissue T81.32 ☑
    laceration (external) (internal) T81.33 ☑
    ligament T81.32 ☑
    mucosa T81.31 ☑
    muscle or muscle flap T81.32 ☑
    ribs or rib cage T81.32 ☑
    skin and subcutaneous tissue (full-thickness) (super-
      ficial) T81.31 ☑
    skull T81.32 ☑
    sternum (sternotomy) T81.32 ☑
    tendon T81.32 ☑

Disruption — *continued*
  closure of — *continued*
    traumatic laceration (external) (internal) T81.33 ☑
  family Z63.8
    due to
      absence of family member due to military deploy-
        ment Z63.31
      absence of family member NEC Z63.32
      alcoholism and drug addiction in family Z63.72
      bereavement Z63.4
      death (assumed) or disappearance of family
        member Z63.4
      divorce or separation Z63.5
      drug addiction in family Z63.72
      return of family member from military deploy-
        ment (current or past conflict) Z63.71
      stressful life events NEC Z63.79
  iris NEC H21.89
  ligament(s) — *see also* Sprain
    knee
      current injury — *see* Dislocation, knee
      old (chronic) — *see* Derangement, knee, instabil-
        ity
      spontaneous NEC — *see* Derangement, knee,
        disruption ligament
  ossicular chain — *see* Discontinuity, ossicles, ear
  pelvic ring (stable) S32.810 ☑
    unstable S32.811 ☑
  traumatic injury wound repair T81.33 ☑
  wound T81.30 ☑
    episiotomy O90.1
    operation T81.31 ☑
      cesarean O90.0
      external operation wound (superficial) T81.31 ☑
      internal operation wound (deep) T81.32 ☑
    perineal (obstetric) O90.1
    traumatic injury repair T81.33 ☑

Dissatisfaction with
  employment Z56.9
  school environment Z55.4

Dissecting — *see* condition

Dissection
  aorta I71.00
    abdominal I71.02
    thoracic I71.019
      aortic arch I71.011
      ascending aorta I71.010
      descending thoracic aorta I71.012
    thoracoabdominal I71.03
  artery I77.70
    basilar (trunk) I77.75
    carotid I77.71
    cerebral (nonruptured) I67.0
      ruptured — *see* Hemorrhage, intracranial, sub-
        arachnoid
    coronary I25.42
    extremity
      lower I77.77
      upper I77.76
    iliac I77.72
    precerebral
      congenital (nonruptured) Q28.1
      specified site NEC I77.75
    renal I77.73
    specified NEC I77.79
    vertebral I77.74
  precerebral artery, congenital (nonruptured) Q28.1
    Heartland A93.8
  traumatic — *see* Wound, open, by site
  vascular I99.8
  wound — *see* Wound, open

Disseminated — *see* condition

Dissociation
  auriculoventricular or atrioventricular (AV) (any degree)
    (isorhythmic) I45.89
    with heart block I44.2
  interference I45.89

Dissociative reaction, state F44.9

Dissolution, vertebra — *see* Osteoporosis

Distension, distention
  abdomen R14.0
  bladder N32.89
  cecum K63.89
  colon K63.89
  gallbladder K82.8
  intestine K63.89
  kidney N28.89
  liver K76.89

Distension, distention — *continued*
  seminal vesicle N50.89
  stomach K31.89
    acute K31.0
    psychogenic F45.8
  ureter — *see* Dilatation, ureter
  uterus N85.8

Distoma hepaticum infestation B66.3

Distomiasis B66.9
  bile passages B66.3
  hemic B65.9
  hepatic B66.3
    due to Clonorchis sinensis B66.1
  intestinal B66.5
  liver B66.3
    due to Clonorchis sinensis B66.1
  lung B66.4
  pulmonary B66.4

Distomolar (fourth molar) K00.1

Disto-occlusion (Division I) (Division II) M26.212

Distortion(s) (congenital)
  adrenal (gland) Q89.1
  arm NEC Q68.8
  bile duct or passage Q44.5
  bladder Q64.79
  brain Q04.9
  cervix (uteri) Q51.9
  chest (wall) Q67.8
    bones Q76.8
  clavicle Q74.0
  clitoris Q52.6
  coccyx Q76.49
  common duct Q44.5
  coronary Q24.5
  cystic duct Q44.5
  ear (auricle) (external) Q17.3
    inner Q16.5
    middle Q16.4
      ossicles Q16.3
  endocrine NEC Q89.2
  eustachian tube Q17.8
  eye (adnexa) Q15.8
  face bone(s) NEC Q75.8
  fallopian tube Q50.6
  femur NEC Q68.8
  fibula NEC Q68.8
  finger(s) Q68.1
  foot Q66.9- ☑
  genitalia, genital organ(s)
    female Q52.8
      external Q52.79
      internal NEC Q52.8
  gyri Q04.8
  hand bone(s) Q68.1
  heart (auricle) (ventricle) Q24.8
    valve (cusp) Q24.8
  hepatic duct Q44.5
  humerus NEC Q68.8
  hymen Q52.4
  intrafamilial communications Z63.8
  jaw NEC M26.89
  labium (majus) (minus) Q52.79
  leg NEC Q68.8
  lens Q12.8
  liver Q44.7
  lumbar spine Q76.49
    with disproportion O33.8
      causing obstructed labor O65.0
  lumbosacral (joint) (region) Q76.49
    kyphosis — *see* Kyphosis, congenital
    lordosis — *see* Lordosis, congenital
  nerve Q07.8
  nose Q30.8
  organ
    of Corti Q16.5
    or site not listed — *see* Anomaly, by site
  ossicles, ear Q16.3
  oviduct Q50.6
  pancreas Q45.3
  parathyroid (gland) Q89.2
  pituitary (gland) Q89.2
  radius NEC Q68.8
  sacroiliac joint Q74.2
  sacrum Q76.49
  scapula Q74.0
  shoulder girdle Q74.0
  skull bone(s) NEC Q75.8

Distortion(s) — continued
 skull bone(s) — continued
  with
   anencephalus Q00.0
   encephalocele — see Encephalocele
   hydrocephalus Q03.9
    with spina bifida — see Spina bifida, with hydrocephalus
   microcephaly Q02
 spinal cord Q06.8
 spine Q76.49
  kyphosis — see Kyphosis, congenital
  lordosis — see Lordosis, congenital
 spleen Q89.09
 sternum NEC Q76.7
 thorax (wall) Q67.8
  bony Q76.8
 thymus (gland) Q89.2
 thyroid (gland) Q89.2
 tibia NEC Q68.8
 toe(s) Q66.9- ☑
 tongue Q38.3
 trachea (cartilage) Q32.1
 ulna NEC Q68.8
 ureter Q62.8
 urethra Q64.79
  causing obstruction Q64.39
 uterus Q51.9
 vagina Q52.4
 vertebra Q76.49
  kyphosis — see Kyphosis, congenital
  lordosis — see Lordosis, congenital
 visual — see also Disturbance, vision
  shape and size H53.15
 vulva Q52.79
 wrist (bones) (joint) Q68.8
Distress
 abdomen — see Pain, abdominal
 acute respiratory R06.03
  syndrome (adult) (child) J80
 epigastric R10.13
 fetal P84
  complicating pregnancy — see Stress, fetal
 gastrointestinal (functional) K30
  psychogenic F45.8
 intestinal (functional) NOS K59.9
  psychogenic F45.8
 maternal, during labor and delivery O75.0
 relationship, with spouse or intimate partner Z63.0
 respiratory (adult) (child) R06.03
  newborn P22.9
   specified NEC P22.8
  orthopnea R06.01
  psychogenic F45.8
  shortness of breath R06.02
  specified type NEC R06.09
Distribution vessel, atypical Q27.9
 coronary artery Q24.5
 precerebral Q28.1
Districhiasis L68.8
Disturbance(s) — see also Disease
 absorption K90.9
  calcium E58
  carbohydrate K90.49
  fat K90.49
   pancreatic K90.3
  protein K90.49
  starch K90.49
  vitamin — see Deficiency, vitamin
 acid-base equilibrium E87.8
  mixed E87.4
 activity and attention (with hyperkinesis) — see Disorder, attention-deficit hyperactivity
 amino acid transport E72.00
 assimilation, food K90.9
 auditory nerve, except deafness — see subcategory H93.3 ☑
 behavior — see Disorder, conduct
 blood clotting (mechanism) — see also Defect, coagulation D68.9
 cerebral
  nerve — see Disorder, nerve, cranial
  status, newborn P91.9
   specified NEC P91.88
 circulatory I99.9
 conduct — see also Disorder, conduct F91.9
  adjustment reaction — see Disorder, adjustment
  compulsive F63.9

Disturbance(s) — continued
 conduct — see also Disorder, conduct — continued
  disruptive F91.9
  hyperkinetic — see Disorder, attention-deficit hyperactivity
  socialized F91.2
  specified NEC F91.8
  unsocialized F91.1
 coordination R27.8
 cranial nerve — see Disorder, nerve, cranial
 deep sensibility — see Disturbance, sensation
 digestive K30
  psychogenic F45.8
 electrolyte — see also Imbalance, electrolyte
  newborn, transitory P74.49
   hyperammonemia P74.6
   hyperchloremia P74.421
   hyperchloremic metabolic acidosis P74.421
   hypochloremia P74.422
   potassium balance
    hyperkalemia P74.31
    hypokalemia P74.32
   sodium balance
    hypernatremia P74.21
    hyponatremia P74.22
   specified type NEC P74.49
 emotions specific to childhood and adolescence F93.9
  with
   anxiety and fearfulness NEC F93.8
   elective mutism F94.0
   oppositional disorder F91.3
   sensitivity (withdrawal) F40.10
   shyness F40.10
   social withdrawal F40.10
  involving relationship problems F93.8
  mixed F93.8
  specified NEC F93.8
 endocrine (gland) E34.9
  neonatal, transitory P72.9
   specified NEC P72.8
 equilibrium R42
 fructose metabolism E74.10
 gait — see Gait
  hysterical F44.4
  psychogenic F44.4
 gastrointestinal (functional) K30
  psychogenic F45.8
 habit, child F98.9
 hearing, except deafness and tinnitus — see Abnormal, auditory perception
 heart, functional (conditions in I44-I50)
  due to presence of (cardiac) prosthesis I97.19- ☑
  postoperative I97.89
   cardiac surgery — see also Infarct, myocardium, associated with revascularization procedure I97.19- ☑
 hormones E34.9
 innervation uterus (parasympathetic) (sympathetic) N85.8
 keratinization NEC
  gingiva K05.10
   nonplaque induced K05.11
   plaque induced K05.10
  lip K13.0
  oral (mucosa) (soft tissue) K13.29
  tongue K13.29
 learning (specific) — see Disorder, learning
 memory — see Amnesia
  mild, following organic brain damage F06.8
 mental F99
  associated with diseases classified elsewhere F54
 metabolism E88.9
  with
   abortion — see Abortion, by type with other specified complication
   ectopic pregnancy O08.5
   molar pregnancy O08.5
  amino-acid E72.9
   aromatic E70.9
   branched-chain E71.2
   straight-chain E72.89
   sulfur-bearing E72.10
  ammonia E72.20
  arginine E72.21
  arginosuccinic acid E72.22
  carbohydrate E74.9
  cholesterol E78.9
  citrulline E72.23

Disturbance(s) — continued
 metabolism — continued
  cystathionine E72.19
  general E88.9
  glutamine E72.89
  histidine E70.40
  homocystine E72.19
  hydroxylysine E72.3
  in labor or delivery O75.89
  iron E83.10
  lipoid E78.9
  lysine E72.3
  methionine E72.19
  neonatal, transitory P74.9
   calcium and magnesium P71.9
    specified type NEC P71.8
   carbohydrate metabolism P70.9
    specified type NEC P70.8
   specified NEC P74.8
  ornithine E72.4
  phosphate E83.39
  sodium NEC E87.8
  threonine E72.89
  tryptophan E70.5
  tyrosine E70.20
  urea cycle E72.20
 motor R29.2
 nervous, functional R45.0
 neuromuscular mechanism (eye), due to syphilis A52.15
 nutritional E63.9
  nail L60.3
 ocular motion H51.9
  psychogenic F45.8
 oculogyric H51.8
  psychogenic F45.8
 oculomotor H51.9
  psychogenic F45.8
 olfactory nerve R43.1
 optic nerve NEC — see Disorder, nerve, optic
 oral epithelium, including tongue NEC K13.29
 perceptual due to
  alcohol withdrawal F10.232
  amphetamine intoxication F15.922
   in
    abuse F15.122
    dependence F15.222
  anxiolytic withdrawal F13.232
  cannabis intoxication (acute) F12.922
   in
    abuse F12.122
    dependence F12.222
  cocaine intoxication (acute) F14.922
   in
    abuse F14.122
    dependence F14.222
  hypnotic withdrawal F13.232
  opioid intoxication (acute) F11.922
   in
    abuse F11.122
    dependence F11.222
  phencyclidine intoxication (acute) F16.122
  sedative withdrawal F13.232
 personality (pattern) (trait) — see also Disorder, personality F60.9
  following organic brain damage F07.9
 polyglandular E31.9
  specified NEC E31.8
 potassium balance, newborn
  hyperkalemia P74.31
  hypokalemia P74.32
 psychogenic F45.9
 psychomotor F44.4
 psychophysical visual H53.16
 pupillary — see Anomaly, pupil, function
 reflex R29.2
 rhythm, heart I49.9
 salivary secretion K11.7
 sensation (cold) (heat) (localization) (tactile discrimination) (texture) (vibratory) NEC R20.9
  hysterical F44.6
  skin R20.9
   anesthesia R20.0
   hyperesthesia R20.3
   hypoesthesia R20.1
   paresthesia R20.2
   specified type NEC R20.8
  smell R43.9
   and taste (mixed) R43.8
   anosmia R43.0

Disturbance(s) — *continued*
　sensation — *continued*
　　smell — *continued*
　　　parosmia R43.1
　　　specified NEC R43.8
　　taste R43.9
　　　and smell (mixed) R43.8
　　　parageusia R43.2
　　　specified NEC R43.8
　sensory — *see* Disturbance, sensation
　situational (transient) — *see also* Disorder, adjustment
　　acute F43.0
　sleep G47.9
　　nonorganic origin F51.9
　smell — *see* Disturbance, sensation, smell
　sociopathic F60.2
　sodium balance, newborn
　　hypernatremia P74.21
　　hyponatremia P74.22
　speech R47.9
　　developmental F80.9
　　specified NEC R47.89
　stomach (functional) K31.9
　sympathetic (nerve) G90.9
　taste — *see* Disturbance, sensation, taste
　temperature
　　regulation, newborn P81.9
　　　specified NEC P81.8
　　sense R20.8
　　　hysterical F44.6
　tooth
　　eruption K00.6
　　formation K00.4
　　structure, hereditary NEC K00.5
　touch — *see* Disturbance, sensation
　vascular I99.9
　　arteriosclerotic — *see* Arteriosclerosis
　vasomotor I73.9
　vasospastic I73.9
　vision, visual H53.9
　　following
　　　cerebral infarction I69.398
　　　cerebrovascular disease I69.998
　　　　specified NEC I69.898
　　　intracerebral hemorrhage I69.198
　　　nontraumatic intracranial hemorrhage NEC
　　　　I69.298
　　　specified disease NEC I69.898
　　　subarachnoid hemorrhage I69.098
　　psychophysical H53.16
　　specified NEC H53.8
　　subjective H53.10
　　　day blindness H53.11
　　　discomfort H53.14- ☑
　　　distortions of shape and size H53.15
　　　loss
　　　　sudden H53.13- ☑
　　　　transient H53.12- ☑
　　　specified type NEC H53.19
　voice R49.9
　　psychogenic F44.4
　　specified NEC R49.8
Diuresis R35.89
Diver's palsy, paralysis or squeeze T70.3 ☑
Diverticulitis (acute) K57.92
　bladder — *see* Cystitis
　ileum — *see* Diverticulitis, intestine, small
　intestine K57.92
　　with
　　　abscess, perforation K57.80
　　　　with bleeding K57.81
　　　bleeding K57.93
　　congenital Q43.8
　　large K57.32
　　　with
　　　　abscess, perforation K57.20
　　　　　with bleeding K57.21
　　　　bleeding K57.33
　　　　small intestine K57.52
　　　　　with
　　　　　　abscess, perforation K57.40
　　　　　　　with bleeding K57.41
　　　　　　bleeding K57.53
　　small K57.12
　　　with
　　　　abscess, perforation K57.00
　　　　　with bleeding K57.01
　　　　bleeding K57.13

Diverticulitis — *continued*
　intestine — *continued*
　　small — *continued*
　　　with — *continued*
　　　　large intestine K57.52
　　　　　with
　　　　　　abscess, perforation K57.40
　　　　　　　with bleeding K57.41
　　　　　　bleeding K57.53
Diverticulosis K57.90
　with bleeding K57.91
　large intestine K57.30
　　with
　　　bleeding K57.31
　　　small intestine K57.50
　　　　with bleeding K57.51
　small intestine K57.10
　　with
　　　bleeding K57.11
　　　large intestine K57.50
　　　　with bleeding K57.51
Diverticulum, diverticula (multiple) K57.90
　appendix (noninflammatory) K38.2
　bladder (sphincter) N32.3
　　congenital Q64.6
　bronchus (congenital) Q32.4
　　acquired J98.09
　calyx, calyceal (kidney) N28.89
　cardia (stomach) K31.4
　cecum — *see* Diverticulosis, intestine, large
　　congenital Q43.8
　colon — *see* Diverticulosis, intestine, large
　　congenital Q43.8
　duodenum — *see* Diverticulosis, intestine, small
　　congenital Q43.8
　epiphrenic (esophagus) K22.5
　esophagus (congenital) Q39.6
　　acquired (epiphrenic) (pulsion) (traction) K22.5
　eustachian tube — *see* Disorder, eustachian tube,
　　specified NEC
　fallopian tube N83.8
　gastric K31.4
　heart (congenital) Q24.8
　ileum — *see* Diverticulosis, intestine, small
　jejunum — *see* Diverticulosis, intestine, small
　kidney (pelvis) (calyces) N28.89
　　with calculus — *see* Calculus, kidney
　Meckel's (displaced) (hypertrophic) Q43.0
　　malignant — *see* Table of Neoplasms, small intes-
　　　tine, malignant
　midthoracic K22.5
　organ or site, congenital NEC — *see* Distortion
　pericardium (congenital) (cyst) Q24.8
　　acquired I31.8
　pharyngoesophageal (congenital) Q39.6
　　acquired K22.5
　pharynx (congenital) Q38.7
　rectosigmoid — *see* Diverticulosis, intestine, large
　　congenital Q43.8
　rectum — *see* Diverticulosis, intestine, large
　Rokitansky's K22.5
　seminal vesicle N50.89
　sigmoid — *see* Diverticulosis, intestine, large
　　congenital Q43.8
　stomach (acquired) K31.4
　　congenital Q40.2
　trachea (acquired) J39.8
　ureter (acquired) N28.89
　　congenital Q62.8
　ureterovesical orifice N28.89
　urethra (acquired) N36.1
　　congenital Q64.79
　ventricle, left (congenital) Q24.8
　vesical N32.3
　　congenital Q64.6
　Zenker's (esophagus) K22.5
Division
　cervix uteri (acquired) N88.8
　glans penis Q55.69
　labia minora (congenital) Q52.79
　ligament (partial or complete) (current) — *see also*
　　Sprain
　　with open wound — *see* Wound, open
　muscle (partial or complete) (current) — *see also* Injury,
　　muscle
　　with open wound — *see* Wound, open
　nerve (traumatic) — *see* Injury, nerve
　spinal cord — *see* Injury, spinal cord, by region

Division — *continued*
　vein I87.8
Divorce, causing family disruption Z63.5
Dix-Hallpike neurolabyrinthitis — *see* Neuronitis,
　vestibular
Dizziness R42
　hysterical F44.89
　psychogenic F45.8
DMAC (disseminated mycobacterium avium-intracellulare
　complex) A31.2
DNR (do not resuscitate) Z66
Doan-Wiseman syndrome (primary splenic neutropenia)
　— *see* Agranulocytosis
Doehle-Heller aortitis A52.02
Dog bite — *see* Bite
Dohle body panmyelopathic syndrome D72.0
Dolichocephaly Q67.2
Dolichocolon Q43.8
Dolichostenomelia — *see* Syndrome, Marfan's
Donohue's syndrome E34.8
Donor (organ or tissue) Z52.9
　blood (whole) Z52.000
　　autologous Z52.010
　　specified component (lymphocytes) (platelets) NEC
　　　Z52.008
　　　autologous Z52.018
　　　specified donor NEC Z52.098
　　specified donor NEC Z52.090
　　stem cells Z52.001
　　　autologous Z52.011
　　　specified donor NEC Z52.091
　bone Z52.20
　　autologous Z52.21
　　marrow Z52.3
　　specified type NEC Z52.29
　cornea Z52.5
　egg (Oocyte) Z52.819
　　age 35 and over Z52.812
　　　anonymous recipient Z52.812
　　　designated recipient Z52.813
　　under age 35 Z52.810
　　　anonymous recipient Z52.810
　　　designated recipient Z52.811
　kidney Z52.4
　liver Z52.6
　lung Z52.89
　lymphocyte — *see* Donor, blood, specified components
　　NEC
　Oocyte — *see* Donor, egg
　platelets Z52.008
　potential, examination of Z00.5
　semen Z52.89
　skin Z52.10
　　autologous Z52.11
　　specified type NEC Z52.19
　specified organ or tissue NEC Z52.89
　sperm Z52.89
Donovanosis A58
Dorsalgia M54.9
　psychogenic F45.41
　specified NEC M54.89
Dorsopathy M53.9
　deforming M43.9
　　specified NEC — *see* subcategory M43.8 ☑
　specified NEC M53.80
　　cervical region M53.82
　　cervicothoracic region M53.83
　　lumbar region M53.86
　　lumbosacral region M53.87
　　occipito-atlanto-axial region M53.81
　　sacrococcygeal region M53.88
　　thoracic region M53.84
　　thoracolumbar region M53.85
Double
　albumin E88.09
　aortic arch Q25.45
　auditory canal Q17.8
　auricle (heart) Q20.8
　bladder Q64.79
　cervix Q51.820
　　with doubling of uterus (and vagina) Q51.10
　　　with obstruction Q51.11
　inlet ventricle Q20.4
　kidney with double pelvis (renal) Q63.0
　meatus urinarius Q64.75
　monster Q89.4
　outlet
　　left ventricle Q20.2

Double — *continued*
  outlet — *continued*
    right ventricle Q20.1
  pelvis (renal) with double ureter Q62.5
  tongue Q38.3
  ureter (one or both sides) Q62.5
    with double pelvis (renal) Q62.5
  urethra Q64.74
  urinary meatus Q64.75
  uterus Q51.28
    with
      doubling of cervix (and vagina) Q51.10
        with obstruction Q51.11
    complete Q51.21
    in pregnancy or childbirth O34.0- ☑
      causing obstructed labor O65.5
    partial Q51.22
    specified NEC Q51.28
  vagina Q52.10
    with doubling of uterus (and cervix) Q51.10
      with obstruction Q51.11
  vision H53.2
  vulva Q52.79
Doubled up Z59.01
Douglas' pouch, cul-de-sac — *see* condition
Down syndrome Q90.9
  meiotic nondisjunction Q90.0
  mitotic nondisjunction Q90.1
  mosaicism Q90.1
  translocation Q90.2
DPD (dihydropyrimidine dehydrogenase deficiency) E88.89
Dracontiasis B72
Dracunculiasis, dracunculosis B72
Dream state, hysterical F44.89
Drepanocytic anemia — *see* Disease, sickle-cell
Dresbach's syndrome (elliptocytosis) D58.1
Dreschlera (hawaiiensis) (infection) B43.8
Dressler's syndrome I24.1
Drift, ulnar — *see* Deformity, limb, specified type NEC, forearm
Drinking (alcohol)
  excessive, to excess NEC (without dependence) F10.10
    habitual (continual) (without remission) F10.20
      with remission F10.21
Drip, postnasal (chronic) R09.82
  due to
    allergic rhinitis — *see* Rhinitis, allergic
    common cold J00
    gastroesophageal reflux — *see* Reflux, gastroesophageal
    nasopharyngitis — *see* Nasopharyngitis
    other known condition — *code to* condition
    sinusitis — *see* Sinusitis
Droop
  facial R29.810
    cerebrovascular disease I69.992
      cerebral infarction I69.392
      intracerebral hemorrhage I69.192
      nontraumatic intracranial hemorrhage NEC I69.292
      specified disease NEC I69.892
      subarachnoid hemorrhage I69.092
Drop (in)
  attack NEC R55
  finger — *see* Deformity, finger
  foot — *see* Deformity, limb, foot, drop
  hematocrit (precipitous) R71.0
  hemoglobin R71.0
  toe — *see* Deformity, toe, specified NEC
  wrist — *see* Deformity, limb, wrist drop
Dropped heart beats I45.9
Dropsy, dropsical — *see also* Hydrops
  abdomen R18.8
  brain — *see* Hydrocephalus
  cardiac, heart — *see* Failure, heart, congestive
  gangrenous — *see* Gangrene
  heart — *see* Failure, heart, congestive
  kidney — *see* Nephrosis
  lung — *see* Edema, lung
  newborn due to isoimmunization P56.0
  pericardium — *see* Pericarditis
Drowned, drowning (near) T75.1 ☑
Drowsiness R40.0
Drug
  abuse counseling and surveillance Z71.51
  addiction — *see* Dependence

Drug — *continued*
  dependence — *see* Dependence
  habit — *see* Dependence
  harmful use — *see* Abuse, drug
  induced fever R50.2
  overdose — *see* Table of Drugs and Chemicals, by drug, poisoning
  poisoning — *see* Table of Drugs and Chemicals, by drug, poisoning
  resistant organism infection — *see also* Resistant, organism, to, drug Z16.30
  therapy
    long term (current) (prophylactic) — *see* Therapy, drug long-term (current) (prophylactic)
    short term — *omit code*
  wrong substance given or taken in error — *see* Table of Drugs and Chemicals, by drug, poisoning
Drunkenness (without dependence) F10.129
  acute in alcoholism F10.229
  chronic (without remission) F10.20
    with remission F10.21
  pathological (without dependence) F10.129
    with dependence F10.229
  sleep F51.9
Drusen
  macula (degenerative) (retina) — *see* Degeneration, macula, drusen
  optic disc H47.32- ☑
Dry, dryness — *see also* condition
  larynx J38.7
  mouth R68.2
    due to dehydration E86.0
  nose J34.89
  socket (teeth) M27.3
  throat J39.2
DSAP L56.5
Duane's syndrome H50.81- ☑
Dubin-Johnson disease or syndrome E80.6
Dubois' disease (thymus gland) A50.59 *[E35]*
Dubowitz' syndrome Q87.19
Duchenne-Aran muscular atrophy G12.21
Duchenne-Griesinger disease G71.01
Duchenne's
  disease or syndrome
    motor neuron disease G12.22
    muscular dystrophy G71.01
  locomotor ataxia (syphilitic) A52.11
  paralysis
    birth injury P14.0
    due to or associated with
      motor neuron disease G12.22
      muscular dystrophy G71.01
Ducrey's chancre A57
Duct, ductus — *see* condition
Duhring's disease (dermatitis herpetiformis) L13.0
Dullness, cardiac (decreased) (increased) R01.2
Dumb ague — *see* Malaria
Dumbness — *see* Aphasia
Dumdum fever B55.0
Dumping syndrome (postgastrectomy) K91.1
Duodenitis (nonspecific) (peptic) K29.80
  with bleeding K29.81
Duodenocholangitis — *see* Cholangitis
Duodenum, duodenal — *see* condition
Duplay's bursitis or periarthritis M75.0 ☑
Duplication, duplex — *see also* Accessory
  alimentary tract Q45.8
  anus Q43.4
  appendix (and cecum) Q43.4
  biliary duct (any) Q44.5
  bladder Q64.79
  cecum (and appendix) Q43.4
  cervix Q51.820
  chromosome NEC
    with complex rearrangements NEC Q92.5
    seen only at prometaphase Q92.8
  cystic duct Q44.5
  digestive organs Q45.8
  esophagus Q39.8
  frontonasal process Q75.8
  intestine (large) (small) Q43.4
  kidney Q63.0
  liver Q44.7
  pancreas Q45.3
  penis Q55.69
  respiratory organs NEC Q34.8
  salivary duct Q38.4
  spinal cord (incomplete) Q06.2

Duplication, duplex — *continued*
  stomach Q40.2
Dupré's disease (meningism) R29.1
Dupuytren's contraction or disease M72.0
Durand-Nicolas-Favre disease A55
Durotomy (inadvertent) (incidental) G97.41
Duroziez's disease (congenital mitral stenosis) Q23.2
Dutton's relapsing fever (West African) A68.1
Dwarfism — *see also* Stature, short E34.328
  achondroplastic Q77.4
  congenital — *see also* Stature, short E34.328
  constitutional E34.31
  hypochondroplastic Q77.4
  hypophyseal E23.0
  infantile — *see also* Stature, short E34.328
  Laron-type — *see also* Stature, short E34.321
  Lorain (-Levi) type E23.0
  metatropic Q77.8
  nephrotic-glycosuric (with hypophosphatemic rickets) E72.09
  nutritional E45
  pancreatic K86.89
  pituitary E23.0
  renal N25.0
  thanatophoric Q77.1
Dyke-Young anemia (secondary) (symptomatic) D59.19
Dysacusis — *see* Abnormal, auditory perception
Dysadrenocortism E27.9
  hyperfunction E27.0
Dysarthria R47.1
  following
    cerebral infarction I69.322
    cerebrovascular disease I69.922
      specified disease NEC I69.822
    intracerebral hemorrhage I69.122
    nontraumatic intracranial hemorrhage NEC I69.222
    subarachnoid hemorrhage I69.022
Dysautonomia (familial) G90.1
Dysbarism T70.3 ☑
Dysbasia R26.2
  angiosclerotica intermittens I73.9
  hysterical F44.4
  lordotica (progressiva) G24.1
  nonorganic origin F44.4
  psychogenic F44.4
Dysbetalipoproteinemia (familial) E78.2
Dyscalculia R48.8
  developmental F81.2
Dyschezia K59.00
Dyschondroplasia (with hemangiomata) Q78.4
Dyschromia (skin) L81.9
Dyscollagenosis M35.9
Dyscranio-pygo-phalangy Q87.0
Dyscrasia
  blood (with) D75.9
    antepartum hemorrhage — *see* Hemorrhage, antepartum, with coagulation defect
    intrapartum hemorrhage O67.0
    newborn P61.9
      specified type NEC P61.8
    puerperal, postpartum O72.3
  polyglandular, pluriglandular E31.9
Dysendocrinism E34.9
Dysentery, dysenteric (catarrhal) (diarrhea) (epidemic) (hemorrhagic) (infectious) (sporadic) (tropical) A09
  abscess, liver A06.4
  amebic — *see also* Amebiasis A06.0
    with abscess — *see* Abscess, amebic
    acute A06.0
    chronic A06.1
  arthritis — *see also* category M01 A09
    bacillary (*see also* category M01) A03.9
  bacillary A03.9
    arthritis — *see also* category M01 A03.9
    Boyd A03.2
    Flexner A03.1
    Schmitz (-Stutzer) A03.0
    Shiga (-Kruse) A03.0
    Shigella A03.9
      boydii A03.2
      dysenteriae A03.0
      flexneri A03.1
      group A A03.0
      group B A03.1
      group C A03.2
      group D A03.3
      sonnei A03.3
      specified type NEC A03.8

Dysentery, dysenteric — *continued*
  bacillary — *continued*
    Sonne A03.3
    specified type NEC A03.8
  balantidial A07.0
  Balantidium coli A07.0
  Boyd's A03.2
  candidal B37.82
  Chilomastix A07.8
  Chinese A03.9
  coccidial A07.3
  Dientamoeba (fragilis) A07.8
  Embadomonas A07.8
  Entamoeba, entamebic — *see* Dysentery, amebic
  Flexner-Boyd A03.2
  Flexner's A03.1
  Giardia lamblia A07.1
  Hiss-Russell A03.1
  Lamblia A07.1
  leishmanial B55.0
  malarial — *see* Malaria
  metazoal B82.0
  monilial B37.82
  protozoal A07.9
  Salmonella A02.0
  schistosomal B65.1
  Schmitz (-Stutzer) A03.0
  Shiga (-Kruse) A03.0
  Shigella NOS — *see* Dysentery, bacillary
  Sonne A03.3
  strongyloidiasis B78.0
  trichomonal A07.8
  viral — *see also* Enteritis, viral A08.4
Dysequilibrium R42
Dysesthesia R20.8
  hysterical F44.6
Dysferlinopathy G71.033
Dysfibrinogenemia (congenital) D68.2
Dysfunction
  adrenal E27.9
    hyperfunction E27.0
  autonomic
    due to alcohol G31.2
    somatoform F45.8
  bladder N31.9
    neurogenic NOS — *see* Dysfunction, bladder, neu-
      romuscular
    neuromuscular NOS N31.9
      atonic (motor) (sensory) N31.2
      autonomous N31.2
      flaccid N31.2
      nonreflex N31.2
      reflex N31.1
      specified NEC N31.8
      uninhibited N31.0
  bleeding, uterus N93.8
  cerebral G93.89
  colon K59.9
    psychogenic F45.8
  colostomy K94.03
  cystic duct K82.8
  cystostomy (stoma) — *see* Complications, cystostomy
  ejaculatory N53.19
    anejaculatory orgasm N53.13
    painful N53.12
    premature F52.4
    retarded N53.11
  endocrine NOS E34.9
  endometrium N85.8
  enterostomy K94.13
  erectile — *see* Dysfunction, sexual, male, erectile
  feeding, pediatric
    acute R63.31
    chronic R63.32
  gallbladder K82.8
  gastrostomy (stoma) K94.23
  gland, glandular NOS E34.9
    meibomian, of eyelid — *see* Dysfunction, meibomi-
      an gland
  heart I51.89
  hemoglobin D75.89
  hepatic K76.89
  hypophysis E23.7
  hypothalamic NEC E23.3
  ileostomy (stoma) K94.13
  jejunostomy (stoma) K94.13
  kidney — *see* Disease, renal
  labyrinthine — *see* subcategory H83.2 ☑

Dysfunction — *continued*
  left ventricular, following sudden emotional stress
    I51.81
  liver K76.89
  male — *see* Dysfunction, sexual, male
  meibomian gland, of eyelid H02.889
    left H02.886
      lower H02.885
      upper H02.884
      upper and lower eyelids H02.88B
    right H02.883
      lower H02.882
      upper H02.881
      upper and lower eyelids H02.88A
  orgasmic (female) F52.31
    male F52.32
  ovary E28.9
    specified NEC E28.8
  papillary muscle I51.89
  parathyroid E21.4
  physiological NEC R68.89
    psychogenic F59
  pineal gland E34.8
  pituitary (gland) E23.3
  platelets D69.1
  polyglandular E31.9
    specified NEC E31.8
  psychophysiologic F59
  psychosexual F52.9
    with
      dyspareunia F52.6
      premature ejaculation F52.4
      vaginismus F52.5
  pylorus K31.9
  rectum K59.9
    psychogenic F45.8
  reflex (sympathetic) — *see* Syndrome, pain, complex
    regional I
  segmental — *see* Dysfunction, somatic
  senile R54
  sexual (due to) R37
    alcohol F10.981
    amphetamine F15.981
      in
        abuse F15.181
        dependence F15.281
    anxiolytic F13.981
      in
        abuse F13.181
        dependence F13.281
    cocaine F14.981
      in
        abuse F14.181
        dependence F14.281
    excessive sexual drive F52.8
    failure of genital response (male) F52.21
      female F52.22
    female N94.9
      aversion F52.1
      dyspareunia N94.10
        psychogenic F52.6
      frigidity F52.22
      nymphomania F52.8
      orgasmic F52.31
      psychogenic F52.9
        aversion F52.1
        dyspareunia F52.6
        frigidity F52.22
        nymphomania F52.8
        orgasmic F52.31
        vaginismus F52.5
      vaginismus N94.2
        psychogenic F52.5
    hypnotic F13.981
      in
        abuse F13.181
        dependence F13.281
    inhibited orgasm (female) F52.31
      male F52.32
    lack
      of sexual enjoyment F52.1
      or loss of sexual desire F52.0
    male N53.9
      anejaculatory orgasm N53.13
      ejaculatory N53.19
        painful N53.12
        premature N53.4
        retarded N53.11
      erectile N52.9

Dysfunction — *continued*
  sexual — *continued*
    male — *continued*
      erectile — *continued*
        drug induced N52.2
        due to
          disease classified elsewhere N52.1
          drug N52.2
        postoperative (postprocedural) N52.39
          following
            cryotherapy N52.37
            interstitial seed therapy N52.36
            prostate ablative therapy N52.37
            prostatectomy N52.34
              radical N52.31
            radiation therapy N52.35
            radical cystectomy N52.32
            ultrasound ablative therapy N52.37
            urethral surgery N52.33
        psychogenic F52.21
        specified cause NEC N52.8
        vasculogenic
          arterial insufficiency N52.01
            with corporo-venous occlusive N52.03
          corporo-venous occlusive N52.02
            with arterial insufficiency N52.03
      impotence — *see* Dysfunction, sexual, male,
        erectile
      psychogenic F52.9
        aversion F52.1
        erectile F52.21
        orgasmic F52.32
        premature ejaculation F52.4
        satyriasis F52.8
        specified type NEC F52.8
      specified type NEC N53.8
    nonorganic F52.9
      specified NEC F52.8
    opioid F11.981
      in
        abuse F11.181
        dependence F11.281
    orgasmic dysfunction (female) F52.31
      male F52.32
    premature ejaculation F52.4
    psychoactive substances NEC F19.981
      in
        abuse F19.181
        dependence F19.281
    psychogenic F52.9
    sedative F13.981
      in
        abuse F13.181
        dependence F13.281
    sexual aversion F52.1
    vaginismus (nonorganic) (psychogenic) F52.5
  sinoatrial node I49.5
  somatic M99.09
    abdomen M99.09
    acromioclavicular M99.07
    cervical region M99.01
    cervicothoracic M99.01
    costochondral M99.08
    costovertebral M99.08
    head region M99.00
    hip M99.05
    lower extremity M99.06
    lumbar region M99.03
    lumbosacral M99.03
    occipitocervical M99.00
    pelvic region M99.05
    pubic M99.05
    rib cage M99.08
    sacral region M99.04
    sacrococcygeal M99.04
    sacroiliac M99.04
    specified NEC M99.09
    sternochondral M99.08
    sternoclavicular M99.07
    thoracic region M99.02
    thoracolumbar M99.02
    upper extremity M99.07
  somatoform autonomic F45.8
  stomach K31.89
    psychogenic F45.8
  suprarenal E27.9
    hyperfunction E27.0
  symbolic R48.9
    specified type NEC R48.8

Dysfunction — *continued*
 temporomandibular (joint) M26.69
  joint-pain syndrome M26.62- ☑
 testicular (endocrine) E29.9
  specified NEC E29.8
 thymus E32.9
 thyroid E07.9
 ureterostomy (stoma) — *see* Complications, stoma, urinary tract
 urethrostomy (stoma) — *see* Complications, stoma, urinary tract
 uterus, complicating delivery O62.9
  hypertonic O62.4
  hypotonic O62.2
   primary O62.0
   secondary O62.1
 ventricular I51.9
  with congestive heart failure — *see also* Failure, heart I50.9
  left, reversible, following sudden emotional stress I51.81
Dysgenesis
 gonadal (due to chromosomal anomaly) Q96.9
  pure Q99.1
 renal Q60.5
  bilateral Q60.4
  unilateral Q60.3
 reticular D72.0
 tidal platelet D69.3
Dysgerminoma
 specified site — *see* Neoplasm, malignant, by site
 unspecified site
  female C56.9
  male C62.90
Dysgeusia R43.2
Dysgraphia R27.8
Dyshidrosis, dysidrosis L30.1
Dyskaryotic cervical smear R87.619
Dyskeratosis L85.8
 cervix — *see* Dysplasia, cervix
 congenital Q82.8
 uterus NEC N85.8
Dyskinesia G24.9
 biliary (cystic duct or gallbladder) K82.8
 drug induced
  orofacial G24.01
 esophagus K22.4
 hysterical F44.4
 intestinal K59.89
 nonorganic origin F44.4
 orofacial (idiopathic) G24.4
  drug induced G24.01
 psychogenic F44.4
 subacute, drug induced G24.01
 tardive G24.01
  neuroleptic induced G24.01
 trachea J39.8
 tracheobronchial J98.09
Dyslalia (developmental) F80.0
Dyslexia R48.0
 developmental F81.0
Dyslipidemia E78.5
 depressed HDL cholesterol E78.6
 elevated fasting triglycerides E78.1
Dysmaturity — *see also* Light for dates
 pulmonary (newborn) (Wilson-Mikity) P27.0
Dysmenorrhea (essential) (exfoliative) N94.6
 congestive (syndrome) N94.6
 primary N94.4
 psychogenic F45.8
 secondary N94.5
Dysmetabolic syndrome X E88.81
Dysmetria R27.8
Dysmorphism (due to)
 alcohol Q86.0
 exogenous cause NEC Q86.8
 hydantoin Q86.1
 warfarin Q86.2
Dysmorphophobia (nondelusional) F45.22
 delusional F22
Dysnomia R47.01
Dysorexia R63.0
 psychogenic F50.89
Dysostosis
 cleidocranial, cleidocranialis Q74.0
 craniofacial Q75.1
 Fairbank's (idiopathic familial generalized osteophytosis) Q78.9

Dysostosis — *continued*
 mandibulofacial (incomplete) Q75.4
 multiplex E76.01
 oculomandibular Q75.5
Dyspareunia (female) N94.10
 deep N94.12
 male N53.12
 nonorganic F52.6
 psychogenic F52.6
 secondary N94.19
 specified NEC N94.19
 superficial (introital) N94.11
Dyspepsia R10.13
 atonic K30
 functional (allergic) (congenital) (gastrointestinal) (occupational) (reflex) K30
 intestinal K59.89
 nervous F45.8
 neurotic F45.8
 psychogenic F45.8
Dysphagia R13.10
 cervical R13.19
 following
  cerebral infarction I69.391
  cerebrovascular disease I69.991
   specified NEC I69.891
  intracerebral hemorrhage I69.191
  nontraumatic intracranial hemorrhage NEC I69.291
  specified disease NEC I69.891
  subarachnoid hemorrhage I69.091
 functional (hysterical) F45.8
 hysterical F45.8
 nervous (hysterical) F45.8
 neurogenic R13.19
 oral phase R13.11
 oropharyngeal phase R13.12
 pharyngeal phase R13.13
 pharyngoesophageal phase R13.14
 psychogenic F45.8
 sideropenic D50.1
 spastica K22.4
 specified NEC R13.19
Dysphagocytosis, congenital D71
Dysphasia R47.02
 developmental
  expressive type F80.1
  receptive type F80.2
 following
  cerebrovascular disease I69.921
   cerebral infarction I69.321
   intracerebral hemorrhage I69.121
   nontraumatic intracranial hemorrhage NEC I69.221
  specified disease NEC I69.821
  subarachnoid hemorrhage I69.021
Dysphonia R49.0
 functional F44.4
 hysterical F44.4
 psychogenic F44.4
 spastica J38.3
Dysphoria
 gender F64.9
  in
   adolescence and adulthood F64.0
   children F64.2
  specified NEC F64.8
 postpartal O90.6
Dyspituitarism E23.3
Dysplasia — *see also* Anomaly
 acetabular, congenital Q65.89
 alveolar capillary, with vein misalignment J84.843
 anus (histologically confirmed) (mild) (moderate) K62.82
  severe D01.3
 arrhythmogenic right ventricular I42.8
 arterial, fibromuscular I77.3
 asphyxiating thoracic (congenital) Q77.2
 brain Q07.9
 bronchopulmonary, perinatal P27.1
 cervix (uteri) N87.9
  mild N87.0
  moderate N87.1
  severe D06.9
 chondroectodermal Q77.6
 colon D12.6
 craniometaphyseal Q78.8
 dentinal K00.5
 diaphyseal, progressive Q78.3

Dysplasia — *continued*
 dystrophic Q77.5
 ectodermal (anhidrotic) (congenital) (hereditary) Q82.4
  hydrotic Q82.8
 epithelial, uterine cervix — *see* Dysplasia, cervix
 eye (congenital) Q11.2
 fibrous
  bone NEC (monostotic) M85.00
   ankle M85.07- ☑
   foot M85.07- ☑
   forearm M85.03- ☑
   hand M85.04- ☑
   lower leg M85.06- ☑
   multiple site M85.09
   neck M85.08
   rib M85.08
   shoulder M85.01- ☑
   skull M85.08
   specified site NEC M85.08
   thigh M85.05- ☑
   toe M85.07- ☑
   upper arm M85.02- ☑
   vertebra M85.08
  diaphyseal, progressive Q78.3
  jaw M27.8
  polyostotic Q78.1
 florid osseous — *see also* Cyst, calcifying odontogenic
 high grade, focal D12.6
 hip, congenital Q65.89
 joint, congenital Q74.8
 kidney Q61.4
  multicystic Q61.4
 leg Q74.2
 lung, congenital (not associated with short gestation) Q33.6
 mammary (gland) (benign) N60.9- ☑
  cyst (solitary) — *see* Cyst, breast
  cystic — *see* Mastopathy, cystic
  duct ectasia — *see* Ectasia, mammary duct
  fibroadenosis — *see* Fibroadenosis, breast
  fibrosclerosis — *see* Fibrosclerosis, breast
  specified type NEC N60.8- ☑
 metaphyseal Q78.5
 muscle Q79.8
 oculodentodigital Q87.0
 periapical (cemental) (cemento-osseous) — *see* Cyst, calcifying odontogenic
 periosteum — *see* Disorder, bone, specified type NEC
 polyostotic fibrous Q78.1
 prostate — *see also* Neoplasia, intraepithelial, prostate N42.30
  severe D07.5
  specified NEC N42.39
 renal Q61.4
  multicystic Q61.4
 retinal, congenital Q14.1
 right ventricular, arrhythmogenic I42.8
 septo-optic Q04.4
 skin L98.8
 spinal cord Q06.1
 spondyloepiphyseal Q77.7
 thymic, with immunodeficiency D82.1
 vagina N89.3
  mild N89.0
  moderate N89.1
  severe NEC D07.2
 vulva N90.3
  mild N90.0
  moderate N90.1
  severe NEC D07.1
Dysplasminogenemia E88.02
Dyspnea (nocturnal) (paroxysmal) R06.00
 asthmatic (bronchial) J45.909
  with
   bronchitis J45.909
    with
     exacerbation (acute) J45.901
     status asthmaticus J45.902
    chronic J44.9
   exacerbation (acute) J45.901
   status asthmaticus J45.902
  cardiac — *see* Failure, ventricular, left
 cardiac — *see* Failure, ventricular, left
 functional F45.8
 hyperventilation R06.4
 hysterical F45.8
 newborn P28.89
 orthopnea R06.01

☑ **Additional Character Required** — Refer to the Tabular List for Character Selection

Dyspnea — *continued*
  psychogenic F45.8
  shortness of breath R06.02
  specified type NEC R06.09
  transfusion-associated [TAD] J95.87
Dyspraxia R27.8
  developmental (syndrome) F82
Dysproteinemia E88.09
Dysreflexia, autonomic G90.4
Dysrhythmia
  cardiac I49.9
    newborn
      bradycardia P29.12
      occurring before birth P03.819
        before onset of labor P03.810
        during labor P03.811
      tachycardia P29.11
    postoperative I97.89
  cerebral or cortical — *see* Epilepsy
Dyssomnia — *see* Disorder, sleep
Dyssynergia
  biliary K83.8
  bladder sphincter N36.44
  cerebellaris myoclonica (Hunt's ataxia) G11.19
Dysthymia F34.1
Dysthyroidism E07.9
Dystocia O66.9
  affecting newborn P03.1
  cervical (hypotonic) O62.2
    affecting newborn P03.6
    primary O62.0
    secondary O62.1
  contraction ring O62.4
  fetal O66.9
    abnormality NEC O66.3
    conjoined twins O66.3
    oversize O66.2
  maternal O66.9
  positional O64.9 ☑
  shoulder (girdle) O66.0
    causing obstructed labor O66.0
  uterine NEC O62.4
Dystonia G24.9
  cervical G24.3
  deformans progressiva G24.1
  drug induced NEC G24.09
    acute G24.02
    specified NEC G24.09
  familial G24.1
  idiopathic G24.1
    familial G24.1
    nonfamilial G24.2
    orofacial G24.4
  lenticularis G24.8
  musculorum deformans G24.1
  neuroleptic induced (acute) G24.02
  orofacial (idiopathic) G24.4
  oromandibular G24.4
    due to drug G24.01
  specified NEC G24.8
  torsion (familial) (idiopathic) G24.1
    acquired G24.8
    genetic G24.1
    symptomatic (nonfamilial) G24.2
Dystonic movements R25.8
Dystrophy, dystrophia
  adiposogenital E23.6
  autosomal recessive, childhood type, muscular dystrophy resembling Duchenne or Becker G71.01
  Becker's type G71.01
  cervical sympathetic G90.2
  choroid (hereditary) H31.20
    central areolar H31.22
    choroideremia H31.21
    gyrate atrophy H31.23
    specified type NEC H31.29
  cornea (hereditary) H18.50- ☑
    endothelial H18.51- ☑
    epithelial H18.52- ☑
    granular H18.53- ☑
    lattice H18.54- ☑
    macular H18.55- ☑
    specified type NEC H18.59- ☑
  Duchenne's type G71.01
  due to malnutrition E45
  Erb's G71.02
  Fuchs' H18.51- ☑
  Gower's muscular G71.01

Dystrophy, dystrophia — *continued*
  hair L67.8
  infantile neuraxonal G31.89
  Landouzy-Déjérine G71.02
  Leyden-Möbius — *see also* Dystrophy, muscular, limb-girdle, by type G71.039
    meaning Limb girdle muscular dystrophy NOS G71.039
    meaning Limb girdle muscular dystrophy, other specified type — *see* by type
    meaning Limb girdle muscular dystrophy, specified type NEC G71.038
    meaning Limb girdle muscular dystrophy type 2A (autosomal recessive) G71.032
  muscular G71.00
    autosomal recessive, childhood type, muscular dystrophy resembling Duchenne or Becker G71.01
    benign (Becker type) G71.01
      scapuloperoneal with early contractures [Emery-Dreifuss] G71.09
    congenital (hereditary) (progressive) (with specific morphological abnormalities of the muscle fiber) G71.09
      myotonic G71.11
    distal G71.09
    Duchenne type G71.01
    Emery-Dreifuss G71.09
    Erb type G71.02
    facioscapulohumeral G71.02
    Gower's G71.01
    hereditary (progressive) — *see also* Dystrophy, muscular, by type G71.09
    Landouzy-Déjérine type G71.02
    limb-girdle G71.039
      alpha-sarcoglycan-relate G71.0341
      anoctamin-5-related autosomal recessive (R12) G71.035
      autosomal recessive NEC G71.038
      beta-sarcoglycan-related G71.0342
      calpain-3-related G71.032
        autosomal dominant G71.031
        autosomal recessive G71.032
      collagen VI related
        autosomal dominant G71.031
        autosomal recessive G71.038
      D1 (autosomal dominant) G71.031
      D2 (autosomal dominant) G71.031
      D3 (autosomal dominant) G71.031
      D4 (autosomal dominant) G71.031
      D5 (autosomal dominant) G71.031
      delta-sarcoglycan-related G71.0349
      due to
        alpha sarcoglycan dysfunction G71.0341
        anoctamin-5 dysfunction G71.035
        beta sarcoglycan dysfunction G71.0342
        fukutin related protein dysfunction G71.038
        sarcoglycan dysfunction, specified NEC G71.0349
      FKRP-related autosomal recessive G71.038
      gamma-sarcoglycan-related G71.0349
      R1 (autosomal recessive) G71.032
      R2 (autosomal recessive) G71.033
      R3 (autosomal recessive) G71.0341
      R4 (autosomal recessive) G71.0342
      R5 (autosomal recessive) G71.0349
      R6 (autosomal recessive) G71.0349
      R7 (autosomal recessive) G71.038
      R8 (autosomal recessive) G71.038
      R9 (autosomal recessive) G71.038
      R10 (autosomal recessive) G71.038
      R11 (autosomal recessive) G71.038
      R12 (autosomal recessive) G71.035
      R13 (autosomal recessive) G71.038
      R14 (autosomal recessive) G71.038
      R15 (autosomal recessive) G71.038
      R16 (autosomal recessive) G71.038
      R17 (autosomal recessive) G71.038
      R18 (autosomal recessive) G71.038
      R19 (autosomal recessive) G71.038
      R20 (autosomal recessive) G71.038
      R21 (autosomal recessive) G71.038
      R22 (autosomal recessive) G71.038
      R23 (autosomal recessive) G71.038
      R24 (autosomal recessive) G71.038
      type 1 (autosomal dominant) G71.031
      type 1A (autosomal dominant) G71.031
      type 1B (autosomal dominant) G71.031
      type 1C (autosomal dominant) G71.031

Dystrophy, dystrophia — *continued*
  muscular — *continued*
    limb-girdle — *continued*
      type 1E (autosomal dominant) G71.031
      type 1H (autosomal dominant) G71.031
      type 1I (autosomal dominant) G71.031
      type 2 (autosomal recessive) G71.038
        specified NEC G71.038
      type 2A (autosomal recessive) G71.032
      type 2B (autosomal recessive) G71.033
      type 2C (autosomal recessive) G71.0349
      type 2D (autosomal recessive) G71.0341
      type 2E (autosomal recessive) G71.0342
      type 2F (autosomal recessive) G71.0349
      type 2I (autosomal recessive) G71.038
      type 2L (autosomal recessive) G71.035
    myotonic G71.11
    progressive (hereditary) — *see also* Dystrophy, muscular, by type G71.09
      Charcot-Marie (-Tooth) type G60.0
    pseudohypertrophic (infantile) G71.01
    scapulohumeral G71.02
    scapuloperoneal G71.09
    severe (Duchenne type) G71.01
    specified type NEC G71.09
  myocardium, myocardial — *see* Degeneration, myocardial
  nail L60.3
    congenital Q84.6
  nutritional E45
  ocular G71.09
  oculocerebrorenal E72.03
  oculopharyngeal G71.09
  ovarian N83.8
  polyglandular E31.8
  reflex (neuromuscular) (sympathetic) — *see* Syndrome, pain, complex regional I
  retinal (hereditary) H35.50
    in
      lipid storage disorders E75.6 *[H36]*
      systemic lipidoses E75.6 *[H36]*
    involving
      pigment epithelium H35.54
      sensory area H35.53
    pigmentary H35.52
    vitreoretinal H35.51
  Salzmann's nodular — *see* Degeneration, cornea, nodular
  scapuloperoneal G71.09
  skin NEC L98.8
  sympathetic (reflex) — *see* Syndrome, pain, complex regional I
    cervical G90.2
  tapetoretinal H35.54
  thoracic, asphyxiating Q77.2
  unguium L60.3
    congenital Q84.6
  vitreoretinal H35.51
  vulva N90.4
  yellow (liver) — *see* Failure, hepatic
Dysuria R30.0
  psychogenic F45.8

E

Eales' disease H35.06- ☑
Ear — *see also* condition
  piercing Z41.3
  tropical NEC B36.9 *[H62.40]*
    in
      aspergillosis B44.89
      candidiasis B37.84
      moniliasis B37.84
  wax (impacted) H61.20
    left H61.22
      with right H61.23
    right H61.21
      with left H61.23
Earache — *see* subcategory H92.0 ☑
Early satiety R68.81
Eaton-Lambert syndrome — *see* Syndrome, Lambert-Eaton
Eberth's disease (typhoid fever) A01.00
Ebola virus disease A98.4
Ebstein's anomaly or syndrome (heart) Q22.5
Eccentro-osteochondrodysplasia E76.29
Ecchondroma — *see* Neoplasm, bone, benign
Ecchondrosis D48.0

Ecchymosis R58
  conjunctiva — see Hemorrhage, conjunctiva
  eye (traumatic) — see Contusion, eyeball
  eyelid (traumatic) — see Contusion, eyelid
  newborn P54.5
  spontaneous R23.3
  traumatic — see Contusion
Echinococciasis — see Echinococcus
Echinococcosis — see Echinococcus
Echinococcus (infection) B67.90
  granulosus B67.4
    bone B67.2
    liver B67.0
    lung B67.1
    multiple sites B67.32
    specified site NEC B67.39
    thyroid B67.31
  liver NOS B67.8
    granulosus B67.0
    multilocularis B67.5
  lung NEC B67.99
    granulosus B67.1
    multilocularis B67.69
  multilocularis B67.7
    liver B67.5
    multiple sites B67.61
    specified site NEC B67.69
  specified site NEC B67.99
    granulosus B67.39
    multilocularis B67.69
  thyroid NEC B67.99
    granulosus B67.31
    multilocularis B67.69 [E35]
Echinorhynchiasis B83.8
Echinostomiasis B66.8
Echolalia R48.8
Echovirus, as cause of disease classified elsewhere B97.12
Eclampsia, eclamptic (coma) (convulsions) (delirium) (with hypertension) NEC O15.9
  complicating
    labor and delivery O15.1
    postpartum O15.2
    pregnancy O15.0- ☑
    puerperium O15.2
Economic circumstances affecting care Z59.9
Economo's disease A85.8
Ectasia, ectasis
  annuloaortic I35.8
  aorta I77.819
    with aneurysm — see Aneurysm, aorta
    abdominal I77.811
    thoracic I77.810
    thoracoabdominal I77.812
  breast — see Ectasia, mammary duct
  capillary I78.8
  cornea H18.71- ☑
  gastric antral vascular (GAVE) K31.819
    with hemorrhage K31.811
    without hemorrhage K31.819
  mammary duct N60.4- ☑
  salivary gland (duct) K11.8
  sclera — see Sclerectasia
Ecthyma L08.0
  contagiosum B08.02
  gangrenosum L08.0
  infectiosum B08.02
Ectocardia Q24.8
Ectodermal dysplasia (anhidrotic) Q82.4
Ectodermosis erosiva pluriorificialis L51.1
Ectopic, ectopia (congenital)
  abdominal viscera Q45.8
    due to defect in anterior abdominal wall Q79.59
  ACTH syndrome E24.3
  adrenal gland Q89.1
  anus Q43.5
  atrial beats I49.1
  beats I49.49
    atrial I49.1
    ventricular I49.3
  bladder Q64.10
  bone and cartilage in lung Q33.5
  brain Q04.8
  breast tissue Q83.8
  cardiac Q24.8
  cerebral Q04.8
  cordis Q24.8
  endometrium — see Endometriosis

Ectopic, ectopia — continued
  gastric mucosa Q40.2
  gestation — see Pregnancy, by site
  heart Q24.8
  hormone secretion NEC E34.2
  kidney (crossed) (pelvis) Q63.2
  lens, lentis Q12.1
  mole — see Pregnancy, by site
  organ or site NEC — see Malposition, congenital
  pancreas Q45.3
  pregnancy — see Pregnancy, ectopic
  pupil — see Abnormality, pupillary
  renal Q63.2
  sebaceous glands of mouth Q38.6
  spleen Q89.09
  testis Q53.00
    bilateral Q53.02
    unilateral Q53.01
  thyroid Q89.2
  tissue in lung Q33.5
  ureter Q62.63
  ventricular beats I49.3
  vesicae Q64.10
Ectromelia Q73.8
  lower limb — see Defect, reduction, limb, lower, specified type NEC
  upper limb — see Defect, reduction, limb, upper, specified type NEC
Ectropion H02.109
  cervix N86
    with cervicitis N72
  congenital Q10.1
  eyelid H02.109
    cicatricial H02.119
      left H02.116
        lower H02.115
        upper H02.114
      right H02.113
        lower H02.112
        upper H02.111
    congenital Q10.1
    left H02.106
      lower H02.105
      upper H02.104
    mechanical H02.129
      left H02.126
        lower H02.125
        upper H02.124
      right H02.123
        lower H02.122
        upper H02.121
    paralytic H02.159
      left H02.156
        lower H02.155
        upper H02.154
      right H02.153
        lower H02.152
        upper H02.151
    right H02.103
      lower H02.102
      upper H02.101
    senile H02.139
      left H02.136
        lower H02.135
        upper H02.134
      right H02.133
        lower H02.132
        upper H02.131
    spastic H02.149
      left H02.146
        lower H02.145
        upper H02.144
      right H02.143
        lower H02.142
        upper H02.141
  iris H21.89
  lip (acquired) K13.0
    congenital Q38.0
  urethra N36.8
  uvea H21.89
Eczema (acute) (chronic) (erythematous) (fissum) (rubrum) (squamous) — see also Dermatitis L30.9
  contact — see Dermatitis, contact
  dyshydrotic L30.1
  external ear — see Otitis, externa, acute, eczematoid
  flexural L20.82
  herpeticum B00.0
  hypertrophicum L28.0

Eczema — continued
  hypostatic — see Varix, leg, with, inflammation
  impetiginous L01.1
  infantile (due to any substance) L20.83
    intertriginous L21.1
    seborrheic L21.1
  intertriginous NEC L30.4
    infantile L21.1
  intrinsic (allergic) L20.84
  lichenified NEC L28.0
  marginatum (hebrae) B35.6
  pustular L30.3
  stasis I87.2
    with varicose veins — see Varix, leg, with, inflammation
  vaccination, vaccinatum T88.1 ☑
  varicose — see Varix, leg, with, inflammation
Eczematid L30.2
Eddowes (-Spurway) **syndrome** Q78.0
Edema, edematous (infectious) (pitting) (toxic) R60.9
  with nephritis — see Nephrosis
  allergic T78.3 ☑
  amputation stump (surgical) (sequelae (late effect)) T87.89
  angioneurotic (allergic) (any site) (with urticaria) T78.3 ☑
    hereditary D84.1
  angiospastic I73.9
  Berlin's (traumatic) S05.8X- ☑
  brain (cytotoxic) (vasogenic) G93.6
    due to birth injury P11.0
    newborn (anoxia or hypoxia) P52.4
      birth injury P11.0
    traumatic — see Injury, intracranial, cerebral edema
  cardiac — see Failure, heart, congestive
  cardiovascular — see Failure, heart, congestive
  cerebral — see Edema, brain
  cerebrospinal — see Edema, brain
  cervix (uteri) (acute) N88.8
    puerperal, postpartum O90.89
  chronic hereditary Q82.0
  circumscribed, acute T78.3 ☑
    hereditary D84.1
  conjunctiva H11.42- ☑
  cornea H18.2- ☑
    idiopathic H18.22- ☑
    secondary H18.23- ☑
      due to contact lens H18.21- ☑
  due to
    lymphatic obstruction I89.0
    salt retention E87.0
  epiglottis — see Edema, glottis
  essential, acute T78.3 ☑
    hereditary D84.1
  extremities, lower — see Edema, legs
  eyelid NEC H02.849
    left H02.846
      lower H02.845
      upper H02.844
    right H02.843
      lower H02.842
      upper H02.841
  familial, hereditary Q82.0
  famine — see Malnutrition, severe
  generalized R60.1
  glottis, glottic, glottidis (obstructive) (passive) J38.4
    allergic T78.3 ☑
      hereditary D84.1
  heart — see Failure, heart, congestive
  heat T67.7 ☑
  hereditary Q82.0
  inanition — see Malnutrition, severe
  intracranial G93.6
  iris H21.89
  joint — see Effusion, joint
  larynx — see Edema, glottis
  legs R60.0
    due to venous obstruction I87.1
    hereditary Q82.0
  localized R60.0
    due to venous obstruction I87.1
  lower limbs — see Edema, legs
  lung J81.1
    with heart condition or failure — see Failure, ventricular, left
    acute J81.0
    chemical (acute) J68.1
      chronic J68.1

Edema, edematous — *continued*
  lung — *continued*
    chronic J81.1
      due to
        chemicals, gases, fumes or vapors (inhalation)
          J68.1
        external agent J70.9
          specified NEC J70.8
        radiation J70.1
    due to
      chemicals, fumes or vapors (inhalation) J68.1
      external agent J70.9
        specified NEC J70.8
    high altitude T70.29 ☑
    near drowning T75.1 ☑
    radiation J70.0
    meaning failure, left ventricle I50.1
  lymphatic I89.0
    due to mastectomy I97.2
  macula H35.81
    cystoid, following cataract surgery — *see* Complications, postprocedural, following cataract surgery
    diabetic — *see* Diabetes, by type, with, retinopathy, with macular edema
  malignant — *see* Gangrene, gas
  Milroy's Q82.0
  nasopharynx J39.2
  newborn P83.30
    hydrops fetalis — *see* Hydrops, fetalis
    specified NEC P83.39
  nutritional — *see also* Malnutrition, severe
    with dyspigmentation, skin and hair E40
  optic disc or nerve — *see* Papilledema
  orbit H05.22- ☑
  pancreas K86.89
  papilla, optic — *see* Papilledema
  penis N48.89
  periodic T78.3 ☑
    hereditary D84.1
  pharynx J39.2
  pulmonary — *see* Edema, lung
  Quincke's T78.3 ☑
    hereditary D84.1
  renal — *see* Nephrosis
  retina H35.81
    diabetic — *see* Diabetes, by type, with, retinopathy, with macular edema
  salt E87.0
  scrotum N50.89
  seminal vesicle N50.89
  spermatic cord N50.89
  spinal (cord) (vascular) (nontraumatic) G95.19
  starvation — *see* Malnutrition, severe
  stasis — *see* Hypertension, venous, (chronic)
  subglottic — *see* Edema, glottis
  supraglottic — *see* Edema, glottis
  testis N44.8
  tunica vaginalis N50.89
  vas deferens N50.89
  vulva (acute) N90.89
Edentulism — *see* Absence, teeth, acquired
Edsall's disease T67.2 ☑
Educational handicap Z55.9
  less than a high school diploma Z55.5
  no general equivalence degree (GED) Z55.5
  specified NEC Z55.8
Edward's syndrome — *see* Trisomy, 18
Effect(s) (of) (from) — *see* Effect, adverse NEC
Effect, adverse
  abnormal gravitational (G) forces or states T75.81 ☑
  abuse — *see* Maltreatment
  air pressure T70.9 ☑
    specified NEC T70.8 ☑
  altitude (high) — *see* Effect, adverse, high altitude
  anesthesia — *see also* Anesthesia T88.59 ☑
    in labor and delivery O74.9
    local, toxic
      in labor and delivery O74.4
      in pregnancy NEC O29.3- ☑
      postpartum, puerperal O89.3
    postpartum, puerperal O89.9
    specified NEC T88.59 ☑
      in labor and delivery O74.8
      postpartum, puerperal O89.8
    spinal and epidural T88.59 ☑
      headache T88.59 ☑

Effect, adverse — *continued*
  anesthesia — *see also* Anesthesia — *continued*
    spinal and epidural — *continued*
      headache — *continued*
        in labor and delivery O74.5
        postpartum, puerperal O89.4
      specified NEC
        in labor and delivery O74.6
        postpartum, puerperal O89.5
  antitoxin — *see* Complications, vaccination
  atmospheric pressure T70.9 ☑
    due to explosion T70.8 ☑
    high T70.3 ☑
    low — *see* Effect, adverse, high altitude
    specified effect NEC T70.8 ☑
  biological, correct substance properly administered — *see* Effect, adverse, drug
  blood (derivatives) (serum) (transfusion) — *see* Complications, transfusion
  chemical substance — *see* Table of Drugs and Chemicals
  cold (temperature) (weather) T69.9 ☑
    chilblains T69.1 ☑
    frostbite — *see* Frostbite
    specified effect NEC T69.8 ☑
  drugs and medicaments T88.7 ☑
    specified drug — *see* Table of Drugs and Chemicals, by drug, adverse effect
    specified effect — *code to* condition
  electric current, electricity (shock) T75.4 ☑
    burn — *see* Burn
  exertion (excessive) T73.3 ☑
  exposure — *see* Exposure
  external cause NEC T75.89 ☑
  foodstuffs T78.1 ☑
    allergic reaction — *see* Allergy, food
      causing anaphylaxis — *see* Shock, anaphylactic, due to food
    noxious — *see* Poisoning, food, noxious
  gases, fumes, or vapors T59.9- ☑
    specified agent — *see* Table of Drugs and Chemicals
  glue (airplane) sniffing
    due to drug abuse — *see* Abuse, drug, inhalant
    due to drug dependence — *see* Dependence, drug, inhalant
  heat — *see* Heat
  high altitude NEC T70.29 ☑
    anoxia T70.29 ☑
    on
      ears T70.0 ☑
      sinuses T70.1 ☑
    polycythemia D75.1
  high pressure fluids T70.4 ☑
  hot weather — *see* Heat
  hunger T73.0 ☑
  immersion, foot — *see* Immersion
  immunization — *see* Complications, vaccination
  immunological agents — *see* Complications, vaccination
  infrared (radiation) (rays) NOS T66 ☑
    dermatitis or eczema L59.8
  infusion — *see* Complications, infusion
  lack of care of infants — *see* Maltreatment, child
  lightning — *see* Lightning
  medical care T88.9 ☑
    specified NEC T88.8 ☑
  medicinal substance, correct, properly administered — *see* Effect, adverse, drug
  motion T75.3 ☑
  noise, on inner ear — *see* subcategory H83.3 ☑
  overheated places — *see* Heat
  psychosocial, of work environment Z56.5
  radiation (diagnostic) (infrared) (natural source) (therapeutic) (ultraviolet) (X-ray) NOS T66 ☑
    dermatitis or eczema — *see* Dermatitis, due to, radiation
    fibrosis of lung J70.1
    pneumonitis J70.0
    pulmonary manifestations
      acute J70.0
      chronic J70.1
    skin L59.9
  radioactive substance NOS
    dermatitis or eczema — *see* Radiodermatitis
  reduced temperature T69.9 ☑
    immersion foot or hand — *see* Immersion
    specified effect NEC T69.8 ☑

Effect, adverse — *continued*
  serum NEC — *see also* Reaction, serum T80.69 ☑
  specified NEC T78.8 ☑
    external cause NEC T75.89 ☑
  strangulation — *see* Asphyxia, traumatic
  submersion T75.1 ☑
  thirst T73.1 ☑
  toxic — *see* Toxicity
  transfusion — *see* Complications, transfusion
  ultraviolet (radiation) (rays) NOS T66 ☑
    burn — *see* Burn
    dermatitis or eczema — *see* Dermatitis, due to, ultraviolet rays
      acute L56.8
  vaccine (any) — *see* Complications, vaccination
  vibration — *see* Vibration, adverse effects
  water pressure NEC T70.9 ☑
    specified NEC T70.8 ☑
  weightlessness T75.82 ☑
  whole blood — *see* Complications, transfusion
  work environment Z56.5
Effects, late — *see* Sequelae
Effluvium
  anagen L65.1
  telogen L65.0
Effort syndrome (psychogenic) F45.8
Effusion
  amniotic fluid — *see* Pregnancy, complicated by, premature rupture of membranes
  brain (serous) G93.6
  bronchial — *see* Bronchitis
  cerebral G93.6
  cerebrospinal — *see also* Meningitis
    vessel G93.6
  chest — *see* Effusion, pleura
  chylous, chyliform (pleura) J94.0
  intracranial G93.6
  joint M25.40
    ankle M25.47- ☑
    elbow M25.42- ☑
    foot joint M25.47- ☑
    hand joint M25.44- ☑
    hip M25.45- ☑
    knee M25.46- ☑
    shoulder M25.41- ☑
    specified joint NEC M25.48
    wrist M25.43- ☑
  malignant pleural J91.0
  meninges — *see* Meningitis
  pericardium, pericardial (noninflammatory) I31.39
    acute — *see* Pericarditis, acute
    malignant, in disease classified elsewhere I31.31
    specified type, NEC I31.39
  peritoneal (chronic) R18.8
  pleura, pleurisy, pleuritic, pleuropericardial J90
    chylous, chyliform J94.0
    due to systemic lupus erythematosis M32.13
    in conditions classified elsewhere J91.8
    influenzal — *see* Influenza, with, respiratory manifestations NEC
    malignant J91.0
    newborn P28.89
    tuberculous NEC A15.6
      primary (progressive) A15.7
  spinal — *see* Meningitis
  thorax, thoracic — *see* Effusion, pleura
Egg shell nails L60.3
  congenital Q84.6
EGPA (eosinophilic granulomatosis with polyangiitis) M30.1
Egyptian splenomegaly B65.1
Ehlers-Danlos syndrome — *see also* Syndrome, Ehlers-Danlos Q79.60
Ehrlichiosis A77.40
  due to
    E. chafeensis A77.41
    E. ewingii A77.49
    E. muris euclairensis A77.49
    E. sennetsu A79.81
    specified organism NEC A77.49
Eichstedt's disease B36.0
Eisenmenger's
  complex or syndrome I27.83
  defect Q21.8
Ejaculation
  delayed F52.32
  painful N53.12

Ejaculation — *continued*
  premature F52.4
  retarded N53.11
  retrograde N53.14
  semen, painful N53.12
    psychogenic F52.6
Ekbom's syndrome (restless legs) G25.81
Ekman's syndrome (brittle bones and blue sclera) Q78.0
Elastic skin Q82.8
  acquired L57.4
Elastofibroma — *see* Neoplasm, connective tissue, benign
Elastoma (juvenile) Q82.8
  Miescher's L87.2
Elastomyofibrosis I42.4
Elastosis
  actinic, solar L57.8
  atrophicans (senile) L57.4
  perforans serpiginosa L87.2
  senilis L57.4
Elbow — *see* condition
Electric current, electricity, effects (concussion) (fatal) (nonfatal) (shock) T75.4 ☑
  burn — *see* Burn
Electric feet syndrome E53.8
Electrocution T75.4 ☑
  from electroshock gun (taser) T75.4 ☑
Electrolyte imbalance E87.8
  with
    abortion — *see* Abortion by type, complicated by, electrolyte imbalance
    ectopic pregnancy O08.5
    molar pregnancy O08.5
Elephantiasis (nonfilarial) I89.0
  arabicum — *see* Infestation, filarial
  bancroftian B74.0
  congenital (any site) (hereditary) Q82.0
  due to
    Brugia (malayi) B74.1
      timori B74.2
    mastectomy I97.2
    Wuchereria (bancrofti) B74.0
  eyelid H02.859
    left H02.856
      lower H02.855
      upper H02.854
    right H02.853
      lower H02.852
      upper H02.851
  filarial, filariensis — *see* Infestation, filarial
  glandular I89.0
  graecorum A30.9
  lymphangiectatic I89.0
  lymphatic vessel I89.0
    due to mastectomy I97.2
  scrotum (nonfilarial) I89.0
  streptococcal I89.0
  surgical I97.89
    postmastectomy I97.2
  telangiectodes I89.0
  vulva (nonfilarial) N90.89
Elevated, elevation
  alanine transaminase (ALT) R74.01
  ALT (alanine transaminase) R74.01
  antibody titer R76.0
  aspartate transaminase (AST) R74.01
  AST (aspartate transaminase) R74.01
  basal metabolic rate R94.8
  blood pressure — *see also* Hypertension
    reading (incidental) (isolated) (nonspecific), no diagnosis of hypertension R03.0
  blood sugar R73.9
  body temperature (of unknown origin) R50.9
  cancer antigen 125 [CA 125] R97.1
  carcinoembryonic antigen [CEA] R97.0
  cholesterol E78.00
    with high triglycerides E78.2
  conjugate, eye H51.0
  C-reactive protein (CRP) R79.82
  diaphragm, congenital Q79.1
  erythrocyte sedimentation rate R70.0
  fasting glucose R73.01
  fasting triglycerides E78.1
  finding on laboratory examination — *see* Findings, abnormal, inconclusive, without diagnosis, by type of exam

Elevated, elevation — *continued*
  GFR (glomerular filtration rate) — *see* Findings, abnormal, inconclusive, without diagnosis, by type of exam
  glucose tolerance (oral) R73.02
  immunoglobulin level R76.8
  indoleacetic acid R82.5
  lactic acid dehydrogenase (LDH) level R74.02
  leukocytes D72.829
  lipoprotein a (Lp(a)) level E78.41
  liver function
    study R94.5
    test R79.89
      alkaline phosphatase R74.8
      aminotransferase R74.01
      bilirubin R17
      hepatic enzyme R74.8
      lactate dehydrogenase R74.02
  Lp(a) (lipoprotein(a)) E78.41
  lymphocytes D72.820
  prostate specific antigen [PSA] R97.20
  Rh titer — *see* Complication(s), transfusion, incompatibility reaction, Rh (factor)
  scapula, congenital Q74.0
  sedimentation rate R70.0
  SGOT R74.01
  SGPT R74.01
  transaminase level R74.01
  triglycerides E78.1
    with high cholesterol E78.2
  troponin R77.8
  tumor associated antigens [TAA] NEC R97.8
  tumor specific antigens [TSA] NEC R97.8
  urine level of
    17-ketosteroids R82.5
    catecholamine R82.5
    indoleacetic acid R82.5
    steroids R82.5
    vanillylmandelic acid (VMA) R82.5
  venous pressure I87.8
  white blood cell count D72.829
    specified NEC D72.828
Elliptocytosis (congenital) (hereditary) D58.1
  Hb C (disease) D58.1
  hemoglobin disease D58.1
  sickle-cell (disease) D57.8- ☑
    trait D57.3
Ellison-Zollinger syndrome E16.4
Ellis-van Creveld syndrome (chondroectodermal dysplasia) Q77.6
Elongated, elongation (congenital) — *see also* Distortion
  bone Q79.9
  cervix (uteri) Q51.828
    acquired N88.4
    hypertrophic N88.4
  colon Q43.8
  common bile duct Q44.5
  cystic duct Q44.5
  frenulum, penis Q55.69
  labia minora (acquired) N90.69
  ligamentum patellae Q74.1
  petiolus (epiglottidis) Q31.8
  tooth, teeth K00.2
  uvula Q38.6
Eltor cholera A00.1
Emaciation R64
  due to malnutrition E43
Embadomoniasis A07.8
Embedded tooth, teeth K01.0
  root only K08.3
Embolic — *see* condition
Embolism (multiple) (paradoxical) I74.9
  air (any site) (traumatic) T79.0 ☑
    following
      abortion — *see* Abortion by type complicated by embolism
      ectopic pregnancy O08.2
      infusion, therapeutic injection or transfusion T80.0 ☑
      molar pregnancy O08.2
      procedure NEC
        artery T81.719 ☑
          mesenteric T81.710 ☑
          renal T81.711 ☑
          specified NEC T81.718 ☑
        vein T81.72 ☑

Embolism — *continued*
  air — *continued*
    in pregnancy, childbirth or puerperium — *see* Embolism, obstetric
  amniotic fluid (pulmonary) — *see also* Embolism, obstetric
    following
      abortion — *see* Abortion by type complicated by embolism
      ectopic pregnancy O08.2
      molar pregnancy O08.2
  aorta, aortic I74.10
    abdominal I74.09
      saddle I74.01
    bifurcation I74.09
    saddle I74.01
    thoracic I74.11
  artery I74.9
    auditory, internal I65.8
    basilar — *see* Occlusion, artery, basilar
    carotid (common) (internal) — *see* Occlusion, artery, carotid
    cerebellar (anterior inferior) (posterior inferior) (superior) I66.3
    cerebral — *see* Occlusion, artery, cerebral
    choroidal (anterior) I65.8
    communicating posterior I65.8
    coronary — *see also* Infarct, myocardium
      not resulting in infarction I24.0
    extremity I74.4
      lower I74.3
      upper I74.2
    hypophyseal I65.8
    iliac I74.5
    limb I74.4
      lower I74.3
      upper I74.2
    mesenteric (with gangrene) — *see also* Ischemia, intestine, acute K55.059
    ophthalmic — *see* Occlusion, artery, retina
    peripheral I74.4
    pontine I65.8
    precerebral — *see* Occlusion, artery, precerebral
    pulmonary — *see* Embolism, pulmonary
    renal N28.0
    retinal — *see* Occlusion, artery, retina
    septic I76
    specified NEC I74.8
    vertebral — *see* Occlusion, artery, vertebral
  basilar (artery) I65.1
  blood clot
    following
      abortion — *see* Abortion by type complicated by embolism
      ectopic or molar pregnancy O08.2
    in pregnancy, childbirth or puerperium — *see* Embolism, obstetric
  brain — *see also* Occlusion, artery, cerebral
    following
      abortion — *see* Abortion by type complicated by embolism
      ectopic or molar pregnancy O08.2
    puerperal, postpartum, childbirth — *see* Embolism, obstetric
  capillary I78.8
  cardiac — *see also* Infarct, myocardium
    not resulting in infarction I51.3
  carotid (artery) (common) (internal) — *see* Occlusion, artery, carotid
  cavernous sinus (venous) — *see* Embolism, intracranial venous sinus
  cerebral — *see* Occlusion, artery, cerebral
  cholesterol — *see* Atheroembolism
  coronary (artery or vein) (systemic) — *see* Occlusion, coronary
  due to device, implant or graft — *see also* Complications, by site and type, specified NEC
    arterial graft NEC T82.818 ☑
    breast (implant) T85.818 ☑
    catheter NEC T85.818 ☑
      dialysis (renal) T82.818 ☑
        intraperitoneal T85.818 ☑
      infusion NEC T82.818 ☑
        spinal (epidural) (subdural) T85.810 ☑
      urinary (indwelling) T83.81 ☑
    electronic (electrode) (pulse generator) (stimulator)
      bone T84.81 ☑
      cardiac T82.817 ☑

Embolism — *continued*
due to device, implant or graft — *see also* Complications, by site and type, specified — *continued*
  electronic — *continued*
    nervous system (brain) (peripheral nerve) (spinal) T85.810 ☑
    urinary T83.81 ☑
  fixation, internal (orthopedic) NEC T84.81 ☑
  gastrointestinal (bile duct) (esophagus) T85.818 ☑
  genital NEC T83.81 ☑
  heart (graft) (valve) T82.817 ☑
  joint prosthesis T84.81 ☑
  ocular (corneal graft) (orbital implant) T85.818 ☑
  orthopedic (bone graft) NEC T86.838
  specified NEC T85.818 ☑
  urinary (graft) NEC T83.81 ☑
  vascular NEC T82.818 ☑
  ventricular intracranial shunt T85.810 ☑
extremities
  lower — *see* Embolism, vein, lower extremity
    arterial I74.3
  upper I74.2
eye H34.9
fat (cerebral) (pulmonary) (systemic) T79.1 ☑
  complicating delivery — *see* Embolism, obstetric
  following
    abortion — *see* Abortion by type complicated by embolism
    ectopic or molar pregnancy O08.2
following
  abortion — *see* Abortion by type complicated by embolism
  ectopic or molar pregnancy O08.2
  infusion, therapeutic injection or transfusion
    air T80.0 ☑
heart (fatty) — *see also* Infarct, myocardium
  not resulting in infarction I51.3
hepatic (vein) I82.0
in pregnancy, childbirth or puerperium — *see* Embolism, obstetric
intestine (artery) (vein) (with gangrene) — *see also* Ischemia, intestine, acute K55.039
intracranial — *see also* Occlusion, artery, cerebral
  venous sinus (any) G08
    nonpyogenic I67.6
intraspinal venous sinuses or veins G08
  nonpyogenic G95.19
kidney (artery) N28.0
lateral sinus (venous) — *see* Embolism, intracranial, venous sinus
leg — *see* Embolism, vein, lower extremity
  arterial I74.3
longitudinal sinus (venous) — *see* Embolism, intracranial, venous sinus
lung (massive) — *see* Embolism, pulmonary
meninges I66.8
mesenteric (artery) (vein) (with gangrene) — *see also* Ischemia, intestine, acute K55.059
obstetric (in) (pulmonary)
  childbirth O88.22
    air O88.02
    amniotic fluid O88.12
    blood clot O88.22
    fat O88.82
    pyemic O88.32
    septic O88.32
    specified type NEC O88.82
  pregnancy O88.21- ☑
    air O88.01- ☑
    amniotic fluid O88.11- ☑
    blood clot O88.21- ☑
    fat O88.81- ☑
    pyemic O88.31- ☑
    septic O88.31- ☑
    specified type NEC O88.81- ☑
  puerperal O88.23
    air O88.03
    amniotic fluid O88.13
    blood clot O88.23
    fat O88.83
    pyemic O88.33
    septic O88.33
    specified type NEC O88.83
ophthalmic — *see* Occlusion, artery, retina
penis N48.81
peripheral artery NOS I74.4
pituitary E23.6

Embolism — *continued*
popliteal (artery) I74.3
portal (vein) I81
postoperative, postprocedural
  artery T81.719 ☑
    mesenteric T81.710 ☑
    renal T81.711 ☑
    specified NEC T81.718 ☑
  vein T81.72 ☑
precerebral artery — *see* Occlusion, artery, precerebral
puerperal — *see* Embolism, obstetric
pulmonary (acute) (artery) (vein) I26.99
  with acute cor pulmonale I26.09
  chronic I27.82
  following
    abortion — *see* Abortion by type complicated by embolism
    ectopic or molar pregnancy O08.2
  healed or old Z86.711
  in pregnancy, childbirth or puerperium — *see* Embolism, obstetric
  multiple subsegmental without acute cor pulmonale I26.94
  personal history of Z86.711
  saddle I26.92
    with acute cor pulmonale I26.02
  septic I26.90
    with acute cor pulmonale I26.01
  single subsegmental without acute cor pulmonale I26.93
  subsegmental NOS I26.93
pyemic (multiple) I76
  following
    abortion — *see* Abortion by type complicated by embolism
    ectopic or molar pregnancy O08.2
  Hemophilus influenzae A41.3
  pneumococcal A40.3
    with pneumonia J13
  puerperal, postpartum, childbirth (any organism) — *see* Embolism, obstetric
  specified organism NEC A41.89
  staphylococcal A41.2
  streptococcal A40.9
renal (artery) N28.0
  vein I82.3
retina, retinal — *see* Occlusion, artery, retina
saddle
  abdominal aorta I74.01
  pulmonary artery I26.92
    with acute cor pulmonale I26.02
septic (arterial) I76
  complicating abortion — *see* Abortion, by type, complicated by, embolism
sinus — *see* Embolism, intracranial, venous sinus
soap complicating abortion — *see* Abortion, by type, complicated by, embolism
spinal cord G95.19
  pyogenic origin G06.1
spleen, splenic (artery) I74.8
upper extremity I74.2
vein (acute) I82.90
  antecubital I82.61- ☑
    chronic I82.71- ☑
  axillary I82.A1- ☑ (*following* I82.7)
    chronic I82.A2- ☑ (*following* I82.7)
  basilic I82.61- ☑
    chronic I82.71- ☑
  brachial I82.62- ☑
    chronic I82.72- ☑
  brachiocephalic (innominate) I82.290
    chronic I82.291
  calf, muscle I82.46- ☑
    chronic I82.56- ☑
  cephalic I82.61- ☑
    chronic I82.71- ☑
  chronic I82.91
  deep (DVT) I82.40- ☑
    calf I82.4Z- ☑
      chronic I82.5Z- ☑
    lower leg I82.4Z- ☑
      chronic I82.5Z- ☑
    thigh I82.4Y- ☑
      chronic I82.5Y- ☑
    upper leg I82.4Y ☑
      chronic I82.5Y-
  femoral I82.41- ☑

Embolism — *continued*
vein — *continued*
  femoral — *continued*
    chronic I82.51- ☑
  gastrocnemial I82.46- ☑
    chronic I82.56- ☑
  iliac (iliofemoral) I82.42- ☑
    chronic I82.52- ☑
  innominate I82.290
    chronic I82.291
  internal jugular I82.C1- ☑ (*following* I82.7)
    chronic I82.C2- ☑ (*following* I82.7)
  lower extremity
    deep I82.40- ☑
      chronic I82.50- ☑
      specified NEC I82.49- ☑
        chronic NEC I82.59- ☑
    distal
      deep I82.4Z- ☑
    proximal
      deep I82.4Y- ☑
        chronic I82.5Y- ☑
    superficial I82.81- ☑
  peroneal I82.45- ☑
    chronic I82.55- ☑
  popliteal I82.43- ☑
    chronic I82.53- ☑
  radial I82.62- ☑
    chronic I82.72- ☑
  renal I82.3
  saphenous (greater) (lesser) I82.81- ☑
  soleal I82.46- ☑
    chronic I82.56- ☑
  specified NEC I82.890
    chronic NEC I82.891
  subclavian I82.B1- ☑ (*following* I82.7)
    chronic I82.B2- ☑ (*following* I82.7)
  thoracic NEC I82.290
    chronic I82.291
  tibial I82.44- ☑
    chronic I82.54- ☑
  ulnar I82.62- ☑
    chronic I82.72- ☑
  upper extremity I82.60- ☑
    chronic I82.70- ☑
    deep I82.62- ☑
      chronic I82.72- ☑
    superficial I82.61- ☑
      chronic I82.71- ☑
  vena cava
    inferior (acute) I82.220
      chronic I82.221
    superior (acute) I82.210
      chronic I82.211
  venous sinus G08
  vessels of brain — *see* Occlusion, artery, cerebral
Embolus — *see* Embolism
Embryoma — *see also* Neoplasm, uncertain behavior, by site
benign — *see* Neoplasm, benign, by site
kidney C64.- ☑
liver C22.0
malignant — *see also* Neoplasm, malignant, by site
  kidney C64.- ☑
  liver C22.0
  testis C62.9- ☑
    descended (scrotal) C62.1- ☑
    undescended C62.0- ☑
testis C62.9- ☑
  descended (scrotal) C62.1- ☑
  undescended C62.0- ☑
Embryonic
circulation Q28.9
heart Q28.9
vas deferens Q55.4
Embryopathia NOS Q89.9
Embryotoxon Q13.4
Emesis — *see* Vomiting
Emotional lability R45.86
Emotionality, pathological F60.3
Emotogenic disease — *see* Disorder, psychogenic
Emphysema (atrophic) (bullous) (chronic) (interlobular) (lung) (obstructive) (pulmonary) (senile) (vesicular) J43.9
cellular tissue (traumatic) T79.7 ☑
  surgical T81.82 ☑

Emphysema — *continued*
centrilobular J43.2
compensatory J98.3
congenital (interstitial) P25.0
conjunctiva H11.89
connective tissue (traumatic) T79.7 ☑
  surgical T81.82 ☑
due to chemicals, gases, fumes or vapors J68.4
eyelid(s) — *see* Disorder, eyelid, specified type NEC
  surgical T81.82 ☑
  traumatic T79.7 ☑
interstitial J98.2
  congenital P25.0
  perinatal period P25.0
laminated tissue T79.7 ☑
  surgical T81.82 ☑
mediastinal J98.2
  newborn P25.2
orbit, orbital — *see* Disorder, orbit, specified type NEC
panacinar J43.1
panlobular J43.1
specified NEC J43.8
subcutaneous (traumatic) T79.7 ☑
  nontraumatic J98.2
  postprocedural T81.82 ☑
  surgical T81.82 ☑
surgical T81.82 ☑
thymus (gland) (congenital) E32.8
traumatic (subcutaneous) T79.7 ☑
unilateral J43.0
Empty nest syndrome Z60.0
Empyema (acute) (chest) (double) (pleura) (supradiaphragmatic) (thorax) J86.9
with fistula J86.0
accessory sinus (chronic) — *see* Sinusitis
antrum (chronic) — *see* Sinusitis, maxillary
brain (any part) — *see* Abscess, brain
ethmoidal (chronic) (sinus) — *see* Sinusitis, ethmoidal
extradural — *see* Abscess, extradural
frontal (chronic) (sinus) — *see* Sinusitis, frontal
gallbladder K81.0
mastoid (process) (acute) — *see* Mastoiditis, acute
maxilla, maxillary M27.2
  sinus (chronic) — *see* Sinusitis, maxillary
nasal sinus (chronic) — *see* Sinusitis
sinus (accessory) (chronic) (nasal) — *see* Sinusitis
sphenoidal (sinus) (chronic) — *see* Sinusitis, sphenoidal
subarachnoid — *see* Abscess, extradural
subdural — *see* Abscess, subdural
tuberculous A15.6
ureter — *see* Ureteritis
ventricular — *see* Abscess, brain
En coup de sabre lesion L94.1
Enamel pearls K00.2
Enameloma K00.2
Enanthema, viral B09
Encephalitis (chronic) (hemorrhagic) (idiopathic) (nonepidemic) (spurious) (subacute) G04.90
acute — *see also* Encephalitis, viral A86
  disseminated G04.00
    infectious G04.01
    noninfectious G04.81
    postimmunization (postvaccination) G04.02
    postinfectious G04.01
  inclusion body A85.8
  necrotizing hemorrhagic G04.30
    postimmunization G04.32
    postinfectious G04.31
    specified NEC G04.39
arboviral, arbovirus NEC A85.2
arthropod-borne NEC (viral) A85.2
Australian A83.4
California (virus) A83.5
Central European (tick-borne) A84.1
Czechoslovakian A84.1
Dawson's (inclusion body) A81.1
diffuse sclerosing A81.1
disseminated, acute G04.00
due to
  cat scratch disease A28.1
  human immunodeficiency virus (HIV) disease B20 *[G05.3]*
  malaria — *see* Malaria
  rickettsiosis — *see* Rickettsiosis
  smallpox inoculation G04.02
  typhus — *see* Typhus
Eastern equine A83.2

Encephalitis — *continued*
endemic (viral) A86
epidemic NEC (viral) A86
equine (acute) (infectious) (viral) A83.9
  Eastern A83.2
  Venezuelan A92.2
  Western A83.1
Far Eastern (tick-borne) A84.0
following vaccination or other immunization procedure G04.02
herpes zoster B02.0
herpesviral B00.4
  due to herpesvirus 6 B10.01
  due to herpesvirus 7 B10.09
  specified NEC B10.09
Ilheus (virus) A83.8
in (due to)
  actinomycosis A42.82
  adenovirus A85.1
  African trypanosomiasis B56.9 *[G05.3]*
  Chagas' disease (chronic) B57.42
  cytomegalovirus B25.8
  enterovirus A85.0
  herpes (simplex) virus B00.4
    due to herpesvirus 6 B10.01
    due to herpesvirus 7 B10.09
    specified NEC B10.09
  infectious disease NEC B99 ☑ *[G05.3]*
  influenza — *see* Influenza, with, encephalopathy
  listeriosis A32.12
  measles B05.0
  mumps B26.2
  naegleriasis B60.2
  parasitic disease NEC B89 *[G05.3]*
  poliovirus A80.9 *[G05.3]*
  rubella B06.01
  syphilis
    congenital A50.42
    late A52.14
  systemic lupus erythematosus M32.19
  toxoplasmosis (acquired) B58.2
    congenital P37.1
  tuberculosis A17.82
  zoster B02.0
inclusion body A81.1
infectious (acute) (virus) NEC A86
Japanese (B type) A83.0
La Crosse A83.5
lead — *see* Poisoning, lead
lethargica (acute) (infectious) A85.8
louping ill A84.89
lupus erythematosus, systemic M32.19
lymphatica A87.2
Mengo A85.8
meningococcal A39.81
Murray Valley A83.4
otitic NEC H66.40 *[G05.3]*
parasitic NOS B71.9
periaxial G37.0
periaxialis (concentrica) (diffuse) G37.5
postchickenpox B01.11
postexanthematous NEC B09
postimmunization G04.02
postinfectious NEC G04.01
postmeasles B05.0
postvaccinal G04.02
postvaricella B01.11
postviral NEC A86
Powassan A84.81
Rasmussen G04.81
Rio Bravo A85.8
Russian
  autumnal A83.0
  spring-summer (taiga) A84.0
saturnine — *see* Poisoning, lead
specified NEC G04.81
St. Louis A83.3
subacute sclerosing A81.1
summer A83.0
suppurative G04.81
tick-borne A84.9
Torula, torular (cryptococcal) B45.1
toxic NEC G92.8
trichinosis B75 *[G05.3]*
type
  B A83.0
  C A83.3
van Bogaert's A81.1

Encephalitis — *continued*
Venezuelan equine A92.2
Vienna A85.8
viral, virus A86
  arthropod-borne NEC A85.2
    mosquito-borne A83.9
      Australian X disease A83.4
      California virus A83.5
      Eastern equine A83.2
      Japanese (B type) A83.0
      Murray Valley A83.4
      specified NEC A83.8
      St. Louis A83.3
      type B A83.0
      type C A83.3
      Western equine A83.1
    tick-borne A84.9
      biundulant A84.1
      central European A84.1
      Czechoslovakian A84.1
      diphasic meningoencephalitis A84.1
      Far Eastern A84.0
      Russian spring-summer (taiga) A84.0
      specified NEC A84.89
  specified type NEC A85.8
  tick-borne, specified NEC A84.89
Western equine A83.1
Encephalocele Q01.9
frontal Q01.0
nasofrontal Q01.1
occipital Q01.2
specified NEC Q01.8
Encephalocystocele — *see* Encephalocele
Encephaloduroarteriomyosynangiosis (EDAMS) I67.5
Encephalomalacia (brain) (cerebellar) (cerebral) — *see* Softening, brain
Encephalomeningitis — *see* Meningoencephalitis
Encephalomeningocele — *see* Encephalocele
Encephalomeningomyelitis — *see* Meningoencephalitis
Encephalomyelitis — *see also* Encephalitis G04.90
acute disseminated G04.00
  infectious G04.01
  noninfectious G04.81
  postimmunization G04.02
  postinfectious G04.01
acute necrotizing hemorrhagic G04.30
  postimmunization G04.32
  postinfectious G04.31
  specified NEC G04.39
equine A83.9
  Eastern A83.2
  Venezuelan A92.2
  Western A83.1
in diseases classified elsewhere G05.3
myalgic G93.32
  chronic fatigue syndrome [ME/CFS] G93.32
postchickenpox B01.11
postinfectious NEC G04.01
postmeasles B05.0
postvaccinal G04.02
postvaricella B01.11
rubella B06.01
specified NEC G04.81
Venezuelan equine A92.2
Encephalomyelocele — *see* Encephalocele
Encephalomyelomeningitis — *see* Meningoencephalitis
Encephalomyelopathy G96.9
Encephalomyeloradiculitis (acute) G61.0
Encephalomyeloradiculoneuritis (acute) (Guillain-Barré) G61.0
Encephalomyeloradiculopathy G96.9
Encephalopathia hyperbilirubinemica, newborn P57.9
due to isoimmunization (conditions in P55) P57.0
Encephalopathy (acute) G93.40
acute necrotizing hemorrhagic G04.30
  postimmunization G04.32
  postinfectious G04.31
  specified NEC G04.39
alcoholic G31.2
anoxic — *see* Damage, brain, anoxic
arteriosclerotic I67.2
centrolobar progressive (Schilder) G37.0
congenital Q07.9
degenerative, in specified disease NEC G32.89
demyelinating callosal G37.1

Encephalopathy — *continued*
- due to
  - drugs — *see also* Table of Drugs and Chemicals G92.8
  - hepatic (without coma) K76.82
  - hyperbilirubinemic, newborn P57.9
    - due to isoimmunization (conditions in P55) P57.0
  - hypertensive I67.4
  - hypoglycemic E16.2
  - hypoxic — *see* Damage, brain, anoxic
  - hypoxic ischemic P91.60
    - mild P91.61
    - moderate P91.62
    - severe P91.63
  - in (due to) (with)
    - birth injury P11.1
    - hyperinsulinism E16.1 *[G94]*
    - influenza — *see* Influenza, with, encephalopathy
    - lack of vitamin — *see also* Deficiency, vitamin E56.9 *[G32.89]*
    - neoplastic disease — *see also* Neoplasm D49.9 *[G13.1]*
    - serum — *see also* Reaction, serum T80.69 ☑
    - syphilis A52.17
    - trauma (postconcussional) F07.81
      - current injury — *see* Injury, intracranial
    - vaccination G04.02
  - lead — *see* Poisoning, lead
  - metabolic G93.41
    - drug induced G92.8
    - toxic G92.8
  - myoclonic, early, symptomatic — *see* Epilepsy, generalized, specified NEC
  - necrotizing, subacute (Leigh) G31.82
  - neonatal P91.819
    - in diseases classified elsewhere P91.811
  - pellagrous E52 *[G32.89]*
  - portal-systemic K76.82
  - postcontusional F07.81
    - current injury — *see* Injury, intracranial, diffuse
  - posthypoglycemic (coma) E16.1 *[G94]*
  - postradiation G93.89
  - saturnine — *see* Poisoning, lead
  - septic G93.41
  - specified NEC G93.49
  - spongiform, subacute (viral) A81.09
  - toxic G92.9
    - metabolic G92.8
  - traumatic (postconcussional) F07.81
    - current injury — *see* Injury, intracranial
  - vitamin B deficiency NEC E53.9 *[G32.89]*
    - vitamin B1 E51.2
  - Wernicke's E51.2

Encephalorrhagia — *see* Hemorrhage, intracranial, intracerebral

Encephalosis, posttraumatic F07.81

Enchondroma — *see also* Neoplasm, bone, benign

Enchondromatosis (cartilaginous) (multiple) Q78.4

Encopresis R15.9
- functional F98.1
- nonorganic origin F98.1
- psychogenic F98.1

Encounter (with health service) (for) Z76.89
- adjustment and management (of)
  - breast implant Z45.81 ☑
  - implanted device NEC Z45.89
  - myringotomy device (stent) (tube) Z45.82
  - neurostimulator (brain) (gastric) (peripheral nerve) (sacral nerve) (spinal cord) (vagus nerve) Z45.42
- administrative purpose only Z02.9
  - examination for
    - adoption Z02.82
    - armed forces Z02.3
    - disability determination Z02.71
    - driving license Z02.4
    - employment Z02.1
    - insurance Z02.6
    - medical certificate NEC Z02.79
    - paternity testing Z02.81
    - residential institution admission Z02.2
    - school admission Z02.0
    - sports Z02.5
  - specified reason NEC Z02.89
- aftercare — *see* Aftercare
- antenatal screening Z36.9
  - cervical length Z36.86
  - chromosomal anomalies Z36.0

Encounter — *continued*
- antenatal screening — *continued*
  - congenital cardiac abnormalities Z36.83
  - elevated maternal serum alphafetoprotein Z36.1
  - fetal growth retardation Z36.4
  - fetal lung maturity Z36.84
  - fetal macrosomia Z36.88
  - hydrops fetalis Z36.81
  - intrauterine growth restriction (IUGR) /small-for-dates Z36.4
  - isoimmunization Z36.5
  - large-for-dates Z36.88
  - malformations Z36.3
  - non-visualized anatomy on a previous scan Z36.2
  - nuchal translucency Z36.82
  - raised alphafetoprotein level Z36.1
  - risk of pre-term labor Z36.86
  - specified follow-up NEC Z36.2
  - specified genetic defects NEC Z36.8A
  - specified type NEC Z36.89
  - Streptococcus B Z36.85
  - suspected anomaly Z36.3
  - uncertain dates Z36.87
- assisted reproductive fertility procedure cycle Z31.83
- blood typing Z01.83
  - Rh typing Z01.83
- breast augmentation or reduction Z41.1
- breast implant exchange (different material) (different size) Z45.81 ☑
- breast reconstruction following mastectomy Z42.1
- check-up — *see* Examination
- chemotherapy for neoplasm Z51.11
- colonoscopy, screening Z12.11
- counseling — *see* Counseling
- delivery, full-term, uncomplicated O80
  - cesarean, without indication O82
- desensitization to allergens Z51.6
- ear piercing Z41.3
- examination — *see* Examination
- expectant parent(s) (adoptive) pre-birth pediatrician visit Z76.81
- fertility preservation procedure (prior to cancer therapy) (prior to removal of gonads) Z31.84
- fitting (of) — *see* Fitting (and adjustment) (of)
- genetic
  - counseling
    - nonprocreative Z71.83
    - procreative Z31.5
  - testing — *see* Test, genetic
- hearing conservation and treatment Z01.12
- immunotherapy for neoplasm Z51.12
- in vitro fertilization cycle Z31.83
- instruction (in)
  - child care (postpartal) (prenatal) Z32.3
  - childbirth Z32.2
  - natural family planning
    - procreative Z31.61
    - to avoid pregnancy Z30.02
- insulin pump titration Z46.81
- joint prosthesis insertion following prior explantation of joint prosthesis (staged procedure)
  - hip Z47.32
  - knee Z47.33
  - shoulder Z47.31
- laboratory (as part of a general medical examination) Z00.00
  - with abnormal findings Z00.01
- mental health services (for)
  - abuse NEC
    - perpetrator Z69.82
    - victim Z69.81
  - child abuse
    - nonparental
      - perpetrator Z69.021
      - victim Z69.020
    - parental
      - perpetrator Z69.011
      - victim Z69.010
  - child neglect
    - nonparental
      - perpetrator Z69.021
      - victim Z69.020
    - parental
      - perpetrator Z69.011
      - victim Z69.010
  - child psychological abuse
    - nonparental
      - perpetrator Z69.021
      - victim Z69.020

Encounter — *continued*
- mental health services — *continued*
  - child psychological abuse — *continued*
    - parental
      - perpetrator Z69.011
      - victim Z69.010
  - child sexual abuse
    - nonparental
      - perpetrator Z69.021
      - victim Z69.020
    - parental
      - perpetrator Z69.011
      - victim Z69.010
  - non-spousal adult abuse
    - perpetrator Z69.82
    - victim Z69.81
  - spousal or partner
    - abuse
      - perpetrator Z69.12
      - victim Z69.11
    - neglect
      - perpetrator Z69.12
      - victim Z69.11
    - psychological abuse
      - perpetrator Z69.12
      - victim Z69.11
    - violence
      - perpetrator (physical) (sexual) Z69.12
      - victim (physical) Z69.11
        - sexual Z69.81
- observation (for) (ruled out)
  - alarm, without findings
    - apnea Z03.83
    - bradycardia Z03.83
    - oximeter Z03.83
  - condition suspected related to home physiologic monitoring device Z03.83
  - exposure to (suspected)
    - anthrax Z03.810
    - biological agent NEC Z03.818
  - malfunction of home cardiorespiratory monitor Z03.83
  - non-specific findings home physiologic monitoring device Z03.83
- pediatrician visit, by expectant parent(s) (adoptive) Z76.81
- placental sample (taken vaginally) — *see also* Encounter, antenatal screening Z36.9
- plastic and reconstructive surgery following medical procedure or healed injury NEC Z42.8
- pregnancy
  - supervision of — *see* Pregnancy, supervision of
  - test Z32.00
    - result negative Z32.02
    - result positive Z32.01
- procreative management and counseling for gestational carrier Z31.7
- prophylactic measures Z29.9
  - antivenin Z29.12
  - fluoride administration Z29.3
  - immunotherapy for respiratory syncytial virus (RSV) Z29.11
  - rabies immune globin Z29.14
  - Rho (D) immune globulin Z29.13
  - specified NEC Z29.8
- radiation therapy (antineoplastic) Z51.0
- radiological (as part of a general medical examination) Z00.00
  - with abnormal findings Z00.01
- reconstructive surgery following medical procedure or healed injury NEC Z42.8
- removal (of) — *see also* Removal
  - artificial
    - arm Z44.00- ☑
      - complete Z44.01- ☑
      - partial Z44.02- ☑
    - eye Z44.2- ☑
    - leg Z44.10- ☑
      - complete Z44.11- ☑
      - partial Z44.12- ☑
  - breast implant Z45.81 ☑
    - tissue expander (with or without synchronous insertion of permanent implant) Z45.81 ☑
  - device Z46.9
    - specified NEC Z46.89

Encounter — *continued*
  removal — *see also* Removal — *continued*
    external
      fixation device — *code to* fracture with seventh character D
      prosthesis, prosthetic device Z44.9
        breast Z44.3- ☑
        specified NEC Z44.8
    implanted device NEC Z45.89
    insulin pump Z46.81
    internal fixation device Z47.2
    myringotomy device (stent) (tube) Z45.82
    nervous system device NEC Z46.2
      brain neuropacemaker Z46.2
      visual substitution device Z46.2
        implanted Z45.31
    non-vascular catheter Z46.82
    orthodontic device Z46.4
    stent
      ureteral Z46.6
    urinary device Z46.6
  repeat cervical smear to confirm findings of recent normal smear following initial abnormal smear Z01.42
  respirator [ventilator] use during power failure Z99.12
  Rh typing Z01.83
  screening — *see* Screening
  specified NEC Z76.89
  sterilization Z30.2
  suspected condition, ruled out
    amniotic cavity and membrane Z03.71
    cervical shortening Z03.75
    fetal anomaly Z03.73
    fetal growth Z03.74
    maternal and fetal conditions NEC Z03.79
    oligohydramnios Z03.71
    placental problem Z03.72
    polyhydramnios Z03.71
  suspected exposure (to), ruled out
    anthrax Z03.810
    biological agents NEC Z03.818
  termination of pregnancy, elective Z33.2
  testing — *see* Test
  therapeutic drug level monitoring Z51.81
  titration, insulin pump Z46.81
  to determine fetal viability of pregnancy O36.80 ☑
  training
    insulin pump Z46.81
  X-ray of chest (as part of a general medical examination) Z00.00
    with abnormal findings Z00.01
Encystment — *see* Cyst
Endarteritis (bacterial, subacute) (infective) I77.6
  brain I67.7
  cerebral or cerebrospinal I67.7
  deformans — *see* Arteriosclerosis
  embolic — *see* Embolism
  obliterans — *see also* Arteriosclerosis
    pulmonary I28.8
  pulmonary I28.8
  retina — *see* Vasculitis, retina
  senile — *see* Arteriosclerosis
  syphilitic A52.09
    brain or cerebral A52.04
    congenital A50.54 [I79.8]
  tuberculous A18.89
Endemic — *see* condition
Endocarditis (chronic) (marantic) (nonbacterial) (thrombotic) (valvular) I38
  with rheumatic fever (conditions in I00)
    active — *see* Endocarditis, acute, rheumatic
    inactive or quiescent (with chorea) I09.1
  acute or subacute I33.9
    infective I33.0
    rheumatic (aortic) (mitral) (pulmonary) (tricuspid) I01.1
      with chorea (acute) (rheumatic) (Sydenham's) I02.0
  aortic (heart) (nonrheumatic) (valve) I35.8
    with
      mitral disease I08.0
        with tricuspid (valve) disease I08.3
          active or acute I01.1
            with chorea (acute) (rheumatic) (Sydenham's) I02.0
      rheumatic fever (conditions in I00)
        active — *see* Endocarditis, acute, rheumatic
        inactive or quiescent (with chorea) I06.9

Endocarditis — *continued*
  aortic — *continued*
    with — *continued*
      tricuspid (valve) disease I08.2
        with mitral (valve) disease I08.3
    acute or subacute I33.9
    arteriosclerotic I35.8
    rheumatic I06.9
      with mitral disease I08.0
        with tricuspid (valve) disease I08.3
          active or acute I01.1
            with chorea (acute) (rheumatic) (Sydenham's) I02.0
      active or acute I01.1
        with chorea (acute) (rheumatic) (Sydenham's) I02.0
      specified NEC I06.8
    specified cause NEC I35.8
    syphilitic A52.03
  arteriosclerotic I38
  atypical verrucous (Libman-Sacks) M32.11
  bacterial (acute) (any valve) (subacute) I33.0
  candidal B37.6
  congenital Q24.8
  constrictive I33.0
  Coxiella burnetii A78 [I39]
  Coxsackie B33.21
  due to
    prosthetic cardiac valve T82.6 ☑
    Q fever A78 [I39]
    Serratia marcescens I33.0
    typhoid (fever) A01.02
  gonococcal A54.83
  infectious or infective (acute) (any valve) (subacute) I33.0
  lenta (acute) (any valve) (subacute) I33.0
  Libman-Sacks M32.11
  listerial A32.82
  Löffler's I42.3
  malignant (acute) (any valve) (subacute) I33.0
  meningococcal A39.51
  mitral (chronic) (double) (fibroid) (heart) (inactive) (valve) (with chorea) I05.9
    with
      aortic (valve) disease I08.0
        with tricuspid (valve) disease I08.3
          active or acute I01.1
            with chorea (acute) (rheumatic) (Sydenham's) I02.0
      rheumatic fever (conditions in I00)
        active — *see* Endocarditis, acute, rheumatic
        inactive or quiescent (with chorea) I05.9
      tricuspid (valve) disease I08.1
        with aortic (valve) disease I08.3
    active or acute I01.1
      with chorea (acute) (rheumatic) (Sydenham's) I02.0
    bacterial I33.0
    arteriosclerotic I34.89
    nonrheumatic I34.89
      acute or subacute I33.9
    specified NEC I05.8
  monilial B37.6
  multiple valves I08.9
    specified disorders I08.8
  mycotic (acute) (any valve) (subacute) I33.0
  pneumococcal (acute) (any valve) (subacute) I33.0
  pulmonary (chronic) (heart) (valve) I37.8
    with rheumatic fever (conditions in I00)
      active — *see* Endocarditis, acute, rheumatic
      inactive or quiescent (with chorea) I09.89
        with aortic, mitral or tricuspid disease I08.8
    acute or subacute I33.9
      rheumatic I01.1
        with chorea (acute) (rheumatic) (Sydenham's) I02.0
    arteriosclerotic I37.8
    congenital Q22.2
    rheumatic (chronic) (inactive) (with chorea) I09.89
      active or acute I01.1
        with chorea (acute) (rheumatic) (Sydenham's) I02.0
    syphilitic A52.03
  purulent (acute) (any valve) (subacute) I33.0
  Q fever A78 [I39]
  rheumatic (chronic) (inactive) (with chorea) I09.1
    active or acute (aortic) (mitral) (pulmonary) (tricuspid) I01.1

Endocarditis — *continued*
  rheumatic — *continued*
    active or acute — *continued*
      with chorea (acute) (rheumatic) (Sydenham's) I02.0
  rheumatoid — *see* Rheumatoid, carditis
  septic (acute) (any valve) (subacute) I33.0
  streptococcal (acute) (any valve) (subacute) I33.0
  subacute — *see* Endocarditis, acute
  suppurative (acute) (any valve) (subacute) I33.0
  syphilitic A52.03
  toxic I33.9
  tricuspid (chronic) (heart) (inactive) (rheumatic) (valve) (with chorea) I07.9
    with
      aortic (valve) disease I08.2
        mitral (valve) disease I08.3
      mitral (valve) disease I08.1
        aortic (valve) disease I08.3
      rheumatic fever (conditions in I00)
        active — *see* Endocarditis, acute, rheumatic
        inactive or quiescent (with chorea) I07.8
    active or acute I01.1
      with chorea (acute) (rheumatic) (Sydenham's) I02.0
    arteriosclerotic I36.8
    nonrheumatic I36.8
      acute or subacute I33.9
    specified cause, except rheumatic I36.8
  tuberculous — *see* Tuberculosis, endocarditis
  typhoid A01.02
  ulcerative (acute) (any valve) (subacute) I33.0
  vegetative (acute) (any valve) (subacute) I33.0
  verrucous (atypical) (nonbacterial) (nonrheumatic) M32.11
Endocardium, endocardial — *see also* condition
  cushion defect Q21.20
Endocervicitis — *see also* Cervicitis
  due to intrauterine (contraceptive) device T83.69 ☑
  hyperplastic N72
Endocrine — *see* condition
Endocrinopathy, pluriglandular E31.9
Endodontic
  overfill M27.52
  underfill M27.53
Endodontitis K04.01
  irreversible K04.02
  reversible K04.01
Endomastoiditis — *see* Mastoiditis
Endometrioma N80.12- ☑
Endometriosis N80.9
  abdomen, abdominal N80.C0
    specified site, NEC N80.C9
    wall N80.C19
      fascia and muscular layers N80.C11
      subcutaneous tissue N80.C10
      unspecified depth N80.C19
  appendix N80.549
    deep N80.542
    superficial N80.541
  bladder (unspecified depth) N80.A0
    deep N80.A2
    superficial N80.A1
  bowel N80.50
  broad ligament N80.3C ☑
  cardiothoracic space N80.B6
  cecum N80.539
    deep N80.532
    superficial N80.531
  cervix N80.0- ☑
  colon N80.559
    descending N80.559
      deep N80.552
      superficial N80.551
    sigmoid N80.529
      deep N80.522
      superficial N80.521
    transverse N80.559
      deep N80.552
      superficial N80.551
  cul-de-sac (Douglas')
    anterior (unspecified depth) N80.319
      deep N80.312
      superficial N80.311
    posterior (unspecified depth) N80.329
      deep N80.322
      superficial N80.321

Endometriosis — *continued*
- deep
  - involving muscular wall of fallopian tube N80.22 ☑
  - retrocervical N80.02
- diaphragm N80.B39
  - deep N80.B32
  - superficial N80.B31
  - unspecified depth N80.B39
- exocervix N80.01
- extra-pelvic abdominal peritoneum N80.C4
- fallopian tube (unspecified depth) N80.20- ☑
  - deep N80.22- ☑
  - superficial N80.21- ☑
- female genital organ NEC N80.8
- gallbladder N80.8
- in scar of skin N80.6
- inguinal canal N80.C3
- internal N80.02
- intestine N80.50
- lung N80.B2
- mediastinal space N80.B5
- myometrium N80.03
- nerve
  - femoral N80.D6
  - obturator N80.D3
  - pelvic N80.D0
    - splanchnic N80.D1
  - pudendal N80.D5
  - retroperitoneum, NEC N80.D9
  - sacral splanchnic N80.D1
  - sciatic N80.D4
  - specified, NEC N80.D9
- ovary (unspecified depth) N80.10- ☑
  - deep N80.12- ☑
  - superficial N80.11- ☑
- parametrium N80.399
- pelvic
  - brim N80.38- ☑
    - deep N80.37- ☑
    - superficial N80.36- ☑
  - peritoneum N80.30
    - specified sites, NEC N80.399
      - deep N80.392
      - superficial N80.391
  - sidewall N80.35- ☑
    - deep N80.34- ☑
    - superficial N80.33- ☑
- pericardial space N80.B4
- peritoneal (pelvic) N80.30
- pleura N80.B1
- rectovaginal septum N80.40
  - with involvement of vagina N80.42
  - without involvement of vagina N80.41
- rectum N80.519
  - deep (multifocal) N80.512
  - superficial N80.511
- retroperitoneum N80.30
- round ligament N80.3C9
- sacral nerve roots N80.D2
- skin (scar) N80.6
- small N80.569
  - deep (multifocal) N80.562
  - superficial N80.561
- specified site NEC N80.8
- stromal D39.0
- thorax N80.B- ☑
- umbilicus N80.C2
- ureter N80.A69
  - deep N80.A5- ☑
  - extrinsic N80.A4- ☑
  - intrinsic N80.A5- ☑
  - superficial N80.A4- ☑
  - unspecified depth N80.A6- ☑
- uterosacral ligament(s) N80.3C- ☑
  - deep N80.3B- ☑
  - superficial N80.3A- ☑
- uterus N80.00
  - deep N80.02
  - internal N80.02
  - superficial N80.01
- vagina N80.42
- vulva N80.8

Endometritis (decidual) (nonspecific) (purulent) (senile) (atrophic) (suppurative) N71.9
- with ectopic pregnancy O08.0
- acute N71.0
- blenorrhagic (gonococcal) (acute) (chronic) A54.24

Endometritis — *continued*
- cervix, cervical (with erosion or ectropion) — *see also* Cervicitis
  - hyperplastic N72
- chlamydial A56.11
- chronic N71.1
- following
  - abortion — *see* Abortion by type complicated by genital infection
  - ectopic or molar pregnancy O08.0
- gonococcal, gonorrheal (acute) (chronic) A54.24
- hyperplastic — *see also* Hyperplasia, endometrial N85.00
  - cervix N72
- puerperal, postpartum, childbirth O86.12
- subacute N71.0
- tuberculous A18.17
Endometrium — *see* condition
Endomyocardiopathy, South African I42.3
Endomyocarditis — *see* Endocarditis
Endomyofibrosis I42.3
Endomyometritis — *see* Endometritis
Endopericarditis — *see* Endocarditis
Endoperineuritis — *see* Disorder, nerve
Endophlebitis — *see* Phlebitis
Endophthalmia — *see* Endophthalmitis, purulent
Endophthalmitis (acute) (infective) (metastatic) (subacute) H44.009
- bleb associated — *see also* Bleb, inflamed (infected), postprocedural H59.4 ☑
- gonorrheal A54.39
- in (due to)
  - cysticercosis B69.1
  - onchocerciasis B73.01
  - toxocariasis B83.0
- panuveitis — *see* Panuveitis
- parasitic H44.12- ☑
- purulent H44.00- ☑
  - panophthalmitis — *see* Panophthalmitis
  - vitreous abscess H44.02- ☑
- specified NEC H44.19
- sympathetic — *see* Uveitis, sympathetic
Endosalpingioma D28.2
Endosalpingiosis N94.89
Endosteitis — *see* Osteomyelitis
Endothelioma, bone — *see* Neoplasm, bone, malignant
Endotheliosis (hemorrhagic infectional) D69.8
Endotoxemia — code to condition
Endotrachelitis — *see* Cervicitis
Engelmann (-Camurati) **syndrome** Q78.3
English disease — *see* Rickets
Engman's disease L30.3
Engorgement
- breast N64.59
  - newborn P83.4
  - puerperal, postpartum O92.79
- lung (passive) — *see* Edema, lung
- pulmonary (passive) — *see* Edema, lung
- stomach K31.89
- venous, retina — *see* Occlusion, retina, vein, engorgement
Enlargement, enlarged — *see also* Hypertrophy
- adenoids J35.2
  - with tonsils J35.3
- alveolar ridge K08.89
  - congenital — *see* Anomaly, alveolar
- apertures of diaphragm (congenital) Q79.1
- gingival K06.1
- heart, cardiac — *see* Hypertrophy, cardiac
- labium majus, childhood asymmetric (CALME) N90.61
- lacrimal gland, chronic H04.03- ☑
- liver — *see* Hypertrophy, liver
- lymph gland or node R59.9
  - generalized R59.1
  - localized R59.0
- orbit H05.34- ☑
- organ or site, congenital NEC — *see* Anomaly, by site
- parathyroid (gland) E21.0
- pituitary fossa R93.0
- prostate N40.0
  - with lower urinary tract symptoms (LUTS) N40.1
  - without lower urinary tract symtpoms (LUTS) N40.0
- sella turcica R93.0
- spleen — *see* Splenomegaly
- thymus (gland) (congenital) E32.0
- thyroid (gland) — *see* Goiter
- tongue K14.8

Enlargement, enlarged — *continued*
- tonsils J35.1
  - with adenoids J35.3
- uterus N85.2
- vestibular aqueduct Q16.5
Enophthalmos H05.40- ☑
- due to
  - orbital tissue atrophy H05.41- ☑
  - trauma or surgery H05.42- ☑
Enostosis M27.8
Entamebic, entamebiasis — *see* Amebiasis
Entanglement
- umbilical cord(s) O69.82 ☑
  - with compression O69.2 ☑
  - around neck (with compression) O69.81 ☑
    - with compression O69.1 ☑
    - without compression O69.81 ☑
  - of twins in monoamniotic sac O69.2 ☑
  - without compression O69.82 ☑
Enteralgia — *see* Pain, abdominal
Enteric — *see* condition
Enteritis (acute) (diarrheal) (hemorrhagic) (noninfective) K52.9
- adenovirus A08.2
- aertrycke infection A02.0
- allergic K52.29
  - with
    - eosinophilic gastritis or gastroenteritis K52.81
    - food protein-induced enterocolitis syndrome K52.21
    - food protein-induced enteropathy K52.22 FPIES K52.21
- amebic (acute) A06.0
  - with abscess — *see* Abscess, amebic
  - chronic A06.1
    - with abscess — *see* Abscess, amebic
    - nondysenteric A06.2
  - nondysenteric A06.2
- astrovirus A08.32
- bacillary NOS A03.9
- bacterial A04.9
  - specified NEC A04.8
- calicivirus A08.31
- candidal B37.82
- Chilomastix A07.8
- choleriformis A00.1
- chronic (noninfectious) K52.9
  - ulcerative — *see* Colitis, ulcerative
- cicatrizing (chronic) — *see* Enteritis, regional, small intestine
- Clostridium
  - botulinum (food poisoning) A05.1
  - difficile
    - not specified as recurrent A04.72
    - recurrent A04.71
- coccidial A07.3
- coxsackie virus A08.39
- dietetic — *see also* Enteritis, allergic K52.29
- drug-induced K52.1
- due to
  - astrovirus A08.32
  - calicivirus A08.31
  - coxsackie virus A08.39
  - drugs K52.1
  - echovirus A08.39
  - enterovirus NEC A08.39
  - food hypersensitivity — *see also* Enteritis, allergic K52.29
  - infectious organism (bacterial) (viral) — *see* Enteritis, infectious
  - torovirus A08.39
  - Yersinia enterocolitica A04.6
- echovirus A08.39
- eltor A00.1
- enterovirus NEC A08.39
- eosinophilic K52.81
- epidemic (infectious) A09
- fulminant — *see also* Ischemia, intestine, acute K55.019
- gangrenous — *see* Enteritis, infectious
- giardial A07.1
- infectious NOS A09
  - due to
    - adenovirus A08.2
    - Aerobacter aerogenes A04.8
    - Arizona (bacillus) A02.0
    - bacteria NOS A04.9
      - specified NEC A04.8
    - Campylobacter A04.5

Enteritis — continued
  infectious — continued
    due to — continued
      Clostridium difficile
        not specified as recurrent A04.72
        recurrent A04.71
      Clostridium perfringens A04.8
      Enterobacter aerogenes A04.8
      enterovirus A08.39
      Escherichia coli A04.4
        enteroaggregative A04.4
        enterohemorrhagic A04.3
        enteroinvasive A04.2
        enteropathogenic A04.0
        enterotoxigenic A04.1
        specified NEC A04.4
      specified
        bacteria NEC A04.8
        virus NEC A08.39
      Staphylococcus A04.8
      virus NEC A08.4
        specified type NEC A08.39
      Yersinia enterocolitica A04.6
    specified organism NEC A08.8
  influenzal — see Influenza, with, digestive manifestations
  ischemic K55.9
    acute — see also Ischemia, intestine, acute K55.019
    chronic K55.1
  microsporidial A07.8
  mucomembranous, myxomembranous — see Syndrome, irritable bowel
  mucous — see Syndrome, irritable bowel
  necroticans A05.2
  necrotizing of newborn — see Enterocolitis, necrotizing, in newborn
  neurogenic — see Syndrome, irritable bowel
  newborn necrotizing — see Enterocolitis, necrotizing, in newborn
  noninfectious K52.9
  norovirus A08.11
  parasitic NEC B82.9
  paratyphoid (fever) — see Fever, paratyphoid
  protozoal A07.9
    specified NEC A07.8
  radiation K52.0
  regional (of) K50.90
    with
      complication K50.919
        abscess K50.914
        fistula K50.913
        intestinal obstruction K50.912
        rectal bleeding K50.911
        specified complication NEC K50.918
    colon — see Enteritis, regional, large intestine
    duodenum — see Enteritis, regional, small intestine
    ileum — see Enteritis, regional, small intestine
    jejunum — see Enteritis, regional, small intestine
    large bowel — see Enteritis, regional, large intestine
    large intestine (colon) (rectum) K50.10
      with
        complication K50.119
          abscess K50.114
          fistula K50.113
          intestinal obstruction K50.112
          rectal bleeding K50.111
          small intestine (duodenum) (ileum) (jejunum) involvement K50.80
            with
              complication K50.819
                abscess K50.814
                fistula K50.813
                intestinal obstruction K50.812
                rectal bleeding K50.811
                specified complication NEC K50.818
          specified complication NEC K50.118
    rectum — see Enteritis, regional, large intestine
    small intestine (duodenum) (ileum) (jejunum) K50.00
      with
        complication K50.019
          abscess K50.014
          fistula K50.013
          intestinal obstruction K50.012
          large intestine (colon) (rectum) involvement K50.80

Enteritis — continued
  regional — continued
    small intestine — continued
      with — continued
        complication — continued
          large intestine involvement — continued
            with
              complication K50.819
                abscess K50.814
                fistula K50.813
                intestinal obstruction K50.812
                rectal bleeding K50.811
                specified complication NEC K50.818
          rectal bleeding K50.011
          specified complication NEC K50.018
    rotaviral A08.0
    Salmonella, salmonellosis (arizonae) (cholerae-suis) (enteritidis) (typhimurium) A02.0
    segmental — see Enteritis, regional
    septic A09
    Shigella — see Infection, Shigella
    small round structured NEC A08.19
    spasmodic, spastic — see Syndrome, irritable bowel
    staphylococcal A04.8
      due to food A05.0
    torovirus A08.39
    toxic NEC K52.1
      due to Clostridium difficile
        not specified as recurrent A04.72
        recurrent A04.71
    trichomonal A07.8
    tuberculous A18.32
    typhosa A01.00
    ulcerative (chronic) — see Colitis, ulcerative
    viral A08.4
      adenovirus A08.2
      enterovirus A08.39
      Rotavirus A08.0
      small round structured NEC A08.19
      specified NEC A08.39
      virus specified NEC A08.39
Enterobiasis B80
Enterobius vermicularis (infection) (infestation) B80
Enterocele — see also Hernia, abdomen
  pelvic, pelvis (acquired) (congenital) N81.5
  vagina, vaginal (acquired) (congenital) NEC N81.5
Enterocolitis — see also Enteritis K52.9
  due to Clostridium difficile
    not specified as recurrent A04.72
    recurrent A04.71
  fulminant ischemic — see also Ischemia, intestine, acute K55.059
  granulomatous — see Enteritis, regional
  hemorrhagic (acute) — see also Ischemia, intestine, acute K55.059
  chronic K55.1
  infectious NEC A09
  ischemic K55.9
  necrotizing K55.30
    with
      perforation K55.33
      pneumatosis K55.32
        and perforation K55.33
    due to Clostridium difficile
      not specified as recurrent A04.72
      recurrent A04.71
    in non-newborn K55.30
      stage 1 (without pneumatosis, without perforation) K55.31
      stage 2 (with pneumatosis, without perforation) K55.32
      stage 3 (with pneumatosis, with perforation) K55.33
    in newborn P77.9
      stage 1 (without pneumatosis, without perforation) P77.1
      stage 2 (with pneumatosis, without perforation) P77.2
      stage 3 (with pneumatosis, with perforation) P77.3
    without pneumatosis or perforation K55.31
  noninfectious K52.9
    newborn — see Enterocolitis, necrotizing, in newborn
  pseudomembranous (newborn)
    not specified as recurrent A04.72

Enterocolitis — continued
  pseudomembranous — continued
    recurrent A04.71
  radiation K52.0
    newborn — see Enterocolitis, necrotizing, in newborn
  ulcerative (chronic) — see Pancolitis, ulcerative (chronic)
Enterogastritis — see Enteritis
Enteropathy K63.9
  celiac-gluten-sensitive K90.0
    non-celiac K90.41
  food protein-induced K52.22
  hemorrhagic, terminal — see also Ischemia, intestine, acute K55.059
  protein-losing K90.49
Enteroperitonitis — see Peritonitis
Enteroptosis K63.4
Enterorrhagia K92.2
Enterospasm — see also Syndrome, irritable, bowel
  psychogenic F45.8
Enterostenosis — see also Obstruction, intestine, specified NEC K56.699
Enterostomy
  complication — see Complication, enterostomy
  status Z93.4
Enterovirus, as cause of disease classified elsewhere B97.10
  coxsackievirus B97.11
  echovirus B97.12
  other specified B97.19
Enthesopathy (peripheral) M77.9
  Achilles tendinitis — see Tendinitis, Achilles
  ankle and tarsus M77.5- ☑
    specified type NEC — see Enthesopathy, foot, specified type NEC
  anterior tibial syndrome M76.81- ☑
  calcaneal spur — see Spur, bone, calcaneal
  elbow region M77.8
    lateral epicondylitis — see Epicondylitis, lateral
    medial epicondylitis — see Epicondylitis, medial
  foot NEC M77.8
    metatarsalgia — see Metatarsalgia
    specified type NEC M77.5- ☑
  forearm M77.8
  gluteal tendinitis — see Tendinitis, gluteal
  hand M77.8
  hip — see Enthesopathy, lower limb, specified type NEC
  iliac crest spur — see Spur, bone, iliac crest
  iliotibial band syndrome — see Syndrome, iliotibial band
  knee — see Enthesopathy, lower limb, lower leg, specified type NEC
  lateral epicondylitis — see Epicondylitis, lateral
  lower limb (excluding foot) M76.9
    Achilles tendinitis — see Tendinitis, Achilles
    ankle and tarsus M77.5- ☑
      specified type NEC — see Enthesopathy, foot, specified type NEC
    anterior tibial syndrome M76.81- ☑
    gluteal tendinitis — see Tendinitis, gluteal
    iliac crest spur — see Spur, bone, iliac crest
    iliotibial band syndrome — see Syndrome, iliotibial band
    patellar tendinitis — see Tendinitis, patellar
    pelvic region — see Enthesopathy, lower limb, specified type NEC
    peroneal tendinitis — see Tendinitis, peroneal
    posterior tibial syndrome M76.82- ☑
    psoas tendinitis — see Tendinitis, psoas
    specified type NEC M76.89- ☑
    tibial collateral bursitis — see Bursitis, tibial collateral
  medial epicondylitis — see Epicondylitis, medial
  metatarsalgia — see Metatarsalgia
  multiple sites M77.8
  patellar tendinitis — see Tendinitis, patellar
  pelvis M77.8
  periarthritis of wrist — see Periarthritis, wrist
  peroneal tendinitis — see Tendinitis, peroneal
  posterior tibial syndrome M76.82- ☑
  psoas tendinitis — see Tendinitis, psoas
  shoulder M77.8
  shoulder region — see Lesion, shoulder
  specified type NEC M77.8
  spinal M46.00

Enthesopathy — continued
　spinal — continued
　　cervical region M46.02
　　cervicothoracic region M46.03
　　lumbar region M46.06
　　lumbosacral region M46.07
　　multiple sites M46.09
　　occipito-atlanto-axial region M46.01
　　sacrococcygeal region M46.08
　　thoracic region M46.04
　　thoracolumbar region M46.05
　　tibial collateral bursitis — see Bursitis, tibial collateral
　upper arm M77.8
　wrist and carpus NEC M77.8
　　calcaneal spur — see Spur, bone, calcaneal
　　periarthritis of wrist — see Periarthritis, wrist
Entomophobia F40.218
Entomophthoromycosis B46.8
Entrance, air into vein — see Embolism, air
Entrapment, nerve — see Neuropathy, entrapment
Entropion (eyelid) (paralytic) H02.009
　cicatricial H02.019
　　left H02.016
　　　lower H02.015
　　　upper H02.014
　　right H02.013
　　　lower H02.012
　　　upper H02.011
　congenital Q10.2
　left H02.006
　　lower H02.005
　　upper H02.004
　mechanical H02.029
　　left H02.026
　　　lower H02.025
　　　upper H02.024
　　right H02.023
　　　lower H02.022
　　　upper H02.021
　right H02.003
　　lower H02.002
　　upper H02.001
　senile H02.039
　　left H02.036
　　　lower H02.035
　　　upper H02.034
　　right H02.033
　　　lower H02.032
　　　upper H02.031
　spastic H02.049
　　left H02.046
　　　lower H02.045
　　　upper H02.044
　　right H02.043
　　　lower H02.042
　　　upper H02.041
Enucleated eye (traumatic, current) S05.7- ✓
Enuresis R32
　functional F98.0
　habit disturbance F98.0
　nocturnal N39.44
　　psychogenic F98.0
　nonorganic origin F98.0
　psychogenic F98.0
Eosinopenia — see Agranulocytosis
Eosinophilia (allergic) (idiopathic) (secondary) D72.10
　with
　　angiolymphoid hyperplasia (ALHE) D18.01
　familial D72.19
　hereditary D72.19
　in disease classified elsewhere D72.18
　infiltrative — see Eosinophilia, pulmonary
　Löffler's J82.89
　peritoneal — see Peritonitis, eosinophilic
　pulmonary NEC J82.89
　　acute J82.82
　　asthmatic J82.83
　　chronic J82.81
　specified NEC D72.19
　tropical (pulmonary) J82.89
Eosinophilia-myalgia syndrome M35.89
Ependymitis (acute) (cerebral) (chronic) (granular) —
　　see Encephalomyelitis
Ependymoblastoma
　specified site — see Neoplasm, malignant, by site
　unspecified site C71.9

Ependymoma (epithelial) (malignant)
　anaplastic
　　specified site — see Neoplasm, malignant, by site
　　unspecified site C71.9
　benign
　　specified site — see Neoplasm, benign, by site
　　unspecified site D33.2
　myxopapillary D43.2
　　specified site — see Neoplasm, uncertain behavior,
　　　by site
　　unspecified site D43.2
　papillary D43.2
　　specified site — see Neoplasm, uncertain behavior,
　　　by site
　　unspecified site D43.2
　specified site — see Neoplasm, malignant, by site
　unspecified site C71.9
Ependymopathy G93.89
Ephelis, ephelides L81.2
Epiblepharon (congenital) Q10.3
Epicanthus, epicanthic fold (eyelid) (congenital) Q10.3
Epicondylitis (elbow)
　lateral M77.1- ✓
　medial M77.0- ✓
Epicystitis — see Cystitis
Epidemic — see condition
Epidermidalization, cervix — see Dysplasia, cervix
Epidermis, epidermal — see condition
Epidermodysplasia verruciformis B07.8
Epidermolysis
　bullosa (congenital) Q81.9
　　acquired L12.30
　　　drug-induced L12.31
　　　specified cause NEC L12.35
　　dystrophica Q81.2
　　letalis Q81.1
　　simplex Q81.0
　　specified NEC Q81.8
　necroticans combustiformis L51.2
　　due to drug — see Table of Drugs and Chemicals,
　　　by drug
Epidermophytid — see Dermatophytosis
Epidermophytosis (infected) — see Dermatophytosis
Epididymis — see condition
Epididymitis (acute) (nonvenereal) (recurrent) (residual)
　　N45.1
　with orchitis N45.3
　blennorrhagic (gonococcal) A54.23
　caseous (tuberculous) A18.15
　chlamydial A56.19
　filarial — see also Infestation, filarial B74.9 [N51]
　gonococcal A54.23
　syphilitic A52.76
　tuberculous A18.15
Epididymo-orchitis — see also Epididymitis N45.3
Epidural — see condition
Epigastrium, epigastric — see condition
Epigastrocele — see Hernia, ventral
Epiglottis — see condition
Epiglottitis, epiglottiditis (acute) J05.10
　with obstruction J05.11
　chronic J37.0
Epignathus Q89.4
Epilepsia partialis continua — see also Kozhevnikof's
　　epilepsy G40.1- ✓
Epilepsy, epileptic, epilepsia (attack) (cerebral) (convul-
　　sion) (fit) (seizure) G40.909

Note: the following terms are to be considered
equivalent to intractable: pharmacoresistant
(pharmacologically resistant), treatment resistant,
refractory (medically) and poorly controlled

　with
　　complex partial seizures — see Epilepsy, localiza-
　　　tion-related, symptomatic, with complex
　　　partial seizures
　　grand mal seizures on awakening — see Epilepsy,
　　　generalized, specified NEC
　　myoclonic absences — see Epilepsy, generalized,
　　　specified NEC
　　myoclonic-astatic seizures — see Epilepsy, general-
　　　ized, specified NEC
　　simple partial seizures — see Epilepsy, localization-
　　　related, symptomatic, with simple partial
　　　seizures
　akinetic — see Epilepsy, generalized, specified NEC

Epilepsy, epileptic, epilepsia — continued
　benign childhood with centrotemporal EEG spikes —
　　see Epilepsy, localization-related, idiopathic
　benign myoclonic in infancy G40.80- ✓
　Bravais-jacksonian — see Epilepsy, localization-related,
　　symptomatic, with simple partial seizures
　childhood
　　with occipital EEG paroxysms — see Epilepsy, local-
　　　ization-related, idiopathic
　　absence G40.A09 (following G40.3)
　　　intractable G40.A19 (following G40.3)
　　　　with status epilepticus G40.A11 (following
　　　　　G40.3)
　　　　without status epilepticus G40.A19 (following
　　　　　G40.3)
　　　not intractable G40.A09 (following G40.3)
　　　　with status epilepticus G40.A01 (following
　　　　　G40.3)
　　　　without status epilepticus G40.A09 (following
　　　　　G40.3)
　climacteric — see Epilepsy, specified NEC
　cysticercosis B69.0
　deterioration (mental) F06.8
　due to syphilis A52.19
　focal — see Epilepsy, localization-related, symptomatic,
　　with simple partial seizures
　generalized
　　idiopathic G40.309
　　　intractable G40.319
　　　　with status epilepticus G40.311
　　　　without status epilepticus G40.319
　　　not intractable G40.309
　　　　with status epilepticus G40.301
　　　　without status epilepticus G40.309
　　specified NEC G40.409
　　　intractable G40.419
　　　　with status epilepticus G40.411
　　　　without status epilepticus G40.419
　　　not intractable G40.409
　　　　with status epilepticus G40.401
　　　　without status epilepticus G40.409
　impulsive petit mal — see Epilepsy, juvenile myoclonic
　intractable G40.919
　　with status epilepticus G40.911
　　without status epilepticus G40.919
　juvenile absence G40.A09 (following G40.3)
　　intractable G40.A19 (following G40.3)
　　　with status epilepticus G40.A11 (following G40.3)
　　　without status epilepticus G40.A19 (following
　　　　G40.3)
　　not intractable G40.A09 (following G40.3)
　　　with status epilepticus G40.A01 (following G40.3)
　　　without status epilepticus G40.A09 (following
　　　　G40.3)
　juvenile myoclonic G40.B09 (following G40.3)
　　intractable G40.B19 (following G40.3)
　　　with status epilepticus G40.B11 (following G40.3)
　　　without status epilepticus G40.B19 (following
　　　　G40.3)
　　not intractable G40.B09 (following G40.3)
　　　with status epilepticus G40.B01 (following G40.3)
　　　without status epilepticus G40.B09 (following
　　　　G40.3)
　localization-related (focal) (partial)
　　idiopathic G40.009
　　　with seizures of localized onset G40.009
　　　　intractable G40.019
　　　　　with status epilepticus G40.011
　　　　　without status epilepticus G40.019
　　　　not intractable G40.009
　　　　　with status epilepticus G40.001
　　　　　without status epilepticus G40.009
　　symptomatic
　　　with complex partial seizures G40.209
　　　　intractable G40.219
　　　　　with status epilepticus G40.211
　　　　　without status epilepticus G40.219
　　　　not intractable G40.209
　　　　　with status epilepticus G40.201
　　　　　without status epilepticus G40.209
　　　with simple partial seizures G40.109
　　　　intractable G40.119
　　　　　with status epilepticus G40.111
　　　　　without status epilepticus G40.119
　　　　not intractable G40.109
　　　　　with status epilepticus G40.101
　　　　　without status epilepticus G40.109

Epilepsy, epileptic, epilepsia — *continued*
  myoclonus, myoclonic — *see also* Epilepsy, generalized,
      specified NEC
    progressive — *see* Epilepsy, generalized, idiopathic
    severe, in infancy (SMEI) G40.83- ☑
    not intractable G40.909
      with status epilepticus G40.901
      without status epilepticus G40.909
    on awakening — *see* Epilepsy, generalized, specified
        NEC
  parasitic NOS B71.9 *[G94]*
  partialis continua — *see also* Kozhevnikof's epilepsy
      G40.1- ☑
  peripheral — *see* Epilepsy, specified NEC
  polymorphic, in infancy (PMEI) G40.83- ☑
  procursiva — *see* Epilepsy, localization-related, symp-
      tomatic, with simple partial seizures
  progressive (familial) myoclonic — *see* Epilepsy, gener-
      alized, idiopathic
  reflex — *see* Epilepsy, specified NEC
  related to
    alcohol G40.509
      not intractable G40.509
        with status epilepticus G40.501
        without status epilepticus G40.509
    drugs G40.509
      not intractable G40.509
        with status epilepticus G40.501
        without status epilepticus G40.509
    external causes G40.509
      not intractable G40.509
        with status epilepticus G40.501
        without status epilepticus G40.509
    hormonal changes G40.509
      not intractable G40.509
        with status epilepticus G40.501
        without status epilepticus G40.509
    sleep deprivation G40.509
      not intractable G40.509
        with status epilepticus G40.501
        without status epilepticus G40.509
    stress G40.509
      not intractable G40.509
        with status epilepticus G40.501
        without status epilepticus G40.509
  somatomotor — *see* Epilepsy, localization-related,
      symptomatic, with simple partial seizures
  somatosensory — *see* Epilepsy, localization-related,
      symptomatic, with simple partial seizures
  spasms G40.822
    intractable G40.824
      with status epilepticus G40.823
      without status epilepticus G40.824
    not intractable G40.822
      with status epilepticus G40.821
      without status epilepticus G40.822
    specified NEC G40.802
      intractable G40.804
        with status epilepticus G40.803
        without status epilepticus G40.804
      not intractable G40.802
        with status epilepticus G40.801
        without status epilepticus G40.802
  syndromes
    generalized
      idiopathic G40.309
        intractable G40.319
          with status epilepticus G40.311
          without status epilepticus G40.319
        not intractable G40.309
          with status epilepticus G40.301
          without status epilepticus G40.309
      specified NEC G40.409
        intractable G40.419
          with status epilepticus G40.411
          without status epilepticus G40.419
        not intractable G40.409
          with status epilepticus G40.401
          without status epilepticus G40.409
    localization-related (focal) (partial)
      idiopathic G40.009
        with seizures of localized onset G40.009
          intractable G40.019
            with status epilepticus G40.011
            without status epilepticus G40.019
          not intractable G40.009
            with status epilepticus G40.001
            without status epilepticus G40.009

Epilepsy, epileptic, epilepsia — *continued*
  syndromes — *continued*
    localization-related — *continued*
      symptomatic
        with complex partial seizures G40.209
          intractable G40.219
            with status epilepticus G40.211
            without status epilepticus G40.219
          not intractable G40.209
            with status epilepticus G40.201
            without status epilepticus G40.209
        with simple partial seizures G40.109
          intractable G40.119
            with status epilepticus G40.111
            without status epilepticus G40.119
          not intractable G40.109
            with status epilepticus G40.101
            without status epilepticus G40.109
        specified NEC G40.802
          intractable G40.804
            with status epilepticus G40.803
            without status epilepticus G40.804
          not intractable G40.802
            with status epilepticus G40.801
            without status epilepticus G40.802
    tonic (-clonic) — *see* Epilepsy, generalized, specified
        NEC
    twilight F05
    uncinate (gyrus) — *see* Epilepsy, localization-related,
        symptomatic, with complex partial seizures
    Unverricht (-Lundborg) (familial myoclonic) — *see*
        Epilepsy, generalized, idiopathic
    visceral — *see* Epilepsy, specified NEC
    visual — *see* Epilepsy, specified NEC
Epiloia Q85.1
Epimenorrhea N92.0
Epipharyngitis — *see* Nasopharyngitis
Epiphora H04.20- ☑
  due to
    excess lacrimation H04.21- ☑
    insufficient drainage H04.22- ☑
Epiphyseal arrest — *see* Arrest, epiphyseal
Epiphyseolysis, epiphysiolysis — *see* Osteochondropa-
    thy
Epiphysitis — *see also* Osteochondropathy
  juvenile M92.9
  syphilitic (congenital) A50.02
Epiplocele — *see* Hernia, abdomen
Epiploitis — *see* Peritonitis
Epiplosarcomphalocele — *see* Hernia, umbilicus
Episcleritis (suppurative) H15.10- ☑
  in (due to)
    syphilis A52.71
    tuberculosis A18.51
  nodular H15.12- ☑
  periodica fugax H15.11- ☑
    angioneurotic — *see* Edema, angioneurotic
  syphilitic (late) A52.71
  tuberculous A18.51
Episode
  affective, mixed F39
  depersonalization (in neurotic state) F48.1
  depressive F32.A
    major F32.9
      mild F32.0
      moderate F32.1
      severe (without psychotic symptoms) F32.2
        with psychotic symptoms F32.3
    recurrent F33.9
      brief F33.8
    specified NEC F32.89
  hypomanic F30.8
  manic F30.9
    with
      psychotic symptoms F30.2
      remission (full) F30.4
        partial F30.3
    other specified F30.8
    recurrent F31.89
    without psychotic symptoms F30.10
      mild F30.11
      moderate F30.12
      severe (without psychotic symptoms) F30.13
        with psychotic symptoms F30.2
  psychotic F23
    organic F06.8
  schizophrenic (acute) NEC, brief F23
Epispadias (female) (male) Q64.0

Episplenitis D73.89
Epistaxis (multiple) R04.0
  hereditary I78.0
  vicarious menstruation N94.89
Epithelioma (malignant) — *see also* Neoplasm, malig-
    nant, by site
  adenoides cysticum — *see* Neoplasm, skin, benign
  basal cell — *see* Neoplasm, skin, malignant
  benign — *see* Neoplasm, benign, by site
  Bowen's — *see* Neoplasm, skin, in situ
  calcifying, of Malherbe — *see* Neoplasm, skin, benign
  external site — *see* Neoplasm, skin, malignant
  intraepidermal, Jadassohn — *see* Neoplasm, skin, be-
      nign
  squamous cell — *see* Neoplasm, malignant, by site
Epitheliomatosis pigmented Q82.1
Epitheliopathy, multifocal placoid pigment
    H30.14- ☑
Epithelium, epithelial — *see* condition
Epituberculosis (with atelectasis) (allergic) A15.7
Eponychia Q84.6
Epstein's
  nephrosis or syndrome — *see* Nephrosis
  pearl K09.8
Epulis (gingiva) (fibrous) (giant cell) K06.8
Equinia A24.0
Equinovarus (congenital) (talipes) Q66.0- ☑
  acquired — *see* Deformity, limb, clubfoot
Equivalent
  convulsive (abdominal) — *see* Epilepsy, specified NEC
  epileptic (psychic) — *see* Epilepsy, localization-related,
      symptomatic, with complex partial seizures
Erb (-Duchenne) **paralysis** (birth injury) (newborn) P14.0
Erb-Goldflam disease or syndrome G70.00
  with exacerbation (acute) G70.01
  in crisis G70.01
Erb's
  disease G71.02
  palsy, paralysis (brachial) (birth) (newborn) P14.0
    spinal (spastic) syphilitic A52.17
  pseudohypertrophic muscular dystrophy G71.02
Erdheim's syndrome (acromegalic macrospondylitis)
    E22.0
Erection, painful (persistent) — *see* Priapism
Ergosterol deficiency (vitamin D) E55.9
  with
    adult osteomalacia M83.8
    rickets — *see* Rickets
Ergotism — *see also* Poisoning, food, noxious, plant
  from ergot used as drug (migraine therapy) — *see* Ta-
      ble of Drugs and Chemicals
Erosio interdigitalis blastomycetica B37.2
Erosion
  artery I77.2
    without rupture I77.89
  bone — *see* Disorder, bone, density and structure,
      specified NEC
  bronchus J98.09
  cartilage (joint) — *see* Disorder, cartilage, specified
      type NEC
  cervix (uteri) (acquired) (chronic) (congenital) N86
    with cervicitis N72
  cornea (nontraumatic) — *see* Ulcer, cornea
    recurrent H18.83- ☑
    traumatic — *see* Abrasion, cornea
  dental (idiopathic) (occupational) (due to diet, drugs
      or vomiting) K03.2
  duodenum, postpyloric — *see* Ulcer, duodenum
  esophagus K22.10
    with bleeding K22.11
  gastric — *see* Ulcer, stomach
  gastrojejunal — *see* Ulcer, gastrojejunal
  implanted mesh — *see* Complications, prosthetic de-
      vice or implant, mesh
  intestine K63.3
  lymphatic vessel I89.8
  pylorus, pyloric (ulcer) — *see* Ulcer, stomach
  spine, aneurysmal A52.09
  stomach — *see* Ulcer, stomach
  subcutaneous device pocket
    nervous system prosthetic device, implant, or graft
        T85.890 ☑
    other internal prosthetic device, implant, or graft
        T85.898 ☑
  teeth (idiopathic) (occupational) (due to diet, drugs or
      vomiting) K03.2
  urethra N36.8

Erosion — *continued*
  uterus N85.8
Erotomania F52.8
Error
  metabolism, inborn — *see* Disorder, metabolism
  refractive — *see* Disorder, refraction
Eructation R14.2
  nervous or psychogenic F45.8
Eruption
  creeping B76.9
  drug (generalized) (taken internally) L27.0
    fixed L27.1
    in contact with skin — *see* Dermatitis, due to drugs
    localized L27.1
  Hutchinson, summer L56.4
  Kaposi's varicelliform B00.0
  napkin L22
  polymorphous light (sun) L56.4
  recalcitrant pustular L13.8
  ringed R23.8
  skin (nonspecific) R21
    creeping (meaning hookworm) B76.9
    due to inoculation/vaccination (generalized) — *see also* Dermatitis, due to, vaccine L27.0
      localized L27.1
    erysipeloid A26.0
    feigned L98.1
    Kaposi's varicelliform B00.0
    lichenoid L28.0
    meaning dermatitis — *see* Dermatitis
    toxic NEC L53.0
  tooth, teeth, abnormal (incomplete) (late) (premature) (sequence) K00.6
  vesicular R23.8
Erysipelas (gangrenous) (infantile) (newborn) (phlegmonous) (suppurative) A46
  external ear A46 *[H62.40]*
  puerperal, postpartum O86.89
Erysipeloid A26.9
  cutaneous (Rosenbach's) A26.0
  disseminated A26.8
  sepsis A26.7
  specified NEC A26.8
Erythema, erythematous (infectional) (inflammation) L53.9
  ab igne L59.0
  annulare (centrifugum) (rheumaticum) L53.1
  arthriticum epidemicum A25.1
  brucellum — *see* Brucellosis
  chronic figurate NEC L53.3
  chronicum migrans (Borrelia burgdorferi) A69.20
  diaper L22
  due to
    chemical NEC L53.0
      in contact with skin L24.5
    drug (internal use) — *see* Dermatitis, due to, drugs
  elevatum diutinum L95.1
  endemic E52
  epidemic, arthritic A25.1
  figuratum perstans L53.3
  gluteal L22
  heat — *code by site under* Burn, first degree
  ichthyosiforme congenitum bullous Q80.3
  in diseases classified elsewhere L54
  induratum (nontuberculous) L52
    tuberculous A18.4
  infectiosum B08.3
  intertrigo L30.4
  iris L51.9
  marginatum L53.2
    in (due to) acute rheumatic fever I00
  medicamentosum — *see* Dermatitis, due to, drugs
  migrans A26.0
    chronicum A69.20
    tongue K14.1
  multiforme (major) (minor) L51.9
    bullous, bullosum L51.1
    conjunctiva L51.1
    nonbullous L51.0
    pemphigoides L12.0
    specified NEC L51.8
  napkin L22
  neonatorum P83.88
    toxic P83.1
  nodosum L52
    tuberculous A18.4
  palmar L53.8
  pernio T69.1 ☑

Erythema, erythematous — *continued*
  rash, newborn P83.88
  scarlatiniform (recurrent) (exfoliative) L53.8
  solare L55.0
  specified NEC L53.8
  toxic, toxicum NEC L53.0
    newborn P83.1
  tuberculous (primary) A18.4
Erythematous, erythematosus — *see* condition
Erythermalgia (primary) I73.81
Erythralgia I73.81
Erythrasma L08.1
Erythredema (polyneuropathy) — *see* Poisoning, mercury
Erythremia (acute) C94.0- ☑
  chronic D45
  secondary D75.1
Erythroblastopenia — *see also* Aplasia, red cell D60.9
  congenital D61.01
Erythroblastophthisis D61.09
Erythroblastosis (fetalis) (newborn) P55.9
  due to
    ABO (antibodies) (incompatibility) (isoimmunization) P55.1
    Rh (antibodies) (incompatibility) (isoimmunization) P55.0
Erythrocyanosis (crurum) I73.89
Erythrocythemia — *see* Erythremia
Erythrocytosis (megalosplenic) (secondary) D75.1
  familial D75.0
  oval, hereditary — *see* Elliptocytosis
  secondary D75.1
  stress D75.1
Erythroderma (secondary) — *see also* Erythema L53.9
  bullous ichthyosiform, congenital Q80.3
  desquamativum L21.1
  ichthyosiform, congenital (bullous) Q80.3
  neonatorum P83.88
  psoriaticum L40.8
Erythrodysesthesia, palmar plantar (PPE) L27.1
Erythrogenesis imperfecta D61.09
Erythroleukemia C94.0- ☑
Erythromelalgia I73.81
Erythrophagocytosis D75.89
Erythrophobia F40.298
Erythroplakia, oral epithelium, and tongue K13.29
Erythroplasia (Queyrat) D07.4
  specified site — *see* Neoplasm, skin, in situ
  unspecified site D07.4
Escherichia coli (E. coli), **as cause of disease classified elsewhere** B96.20
  non-O157 Shiga toxin-producing (with known O group) B96.22
  non-Shiga toxin-producing B96.29
  O157 B96.21
  O157 with confirmation of Shiga toxin when H antigen is unknown, or is not H7 B96.21
  O157:H- (nonmotile) with confirmation of Shiga toxin B96.21
  O157:H7 with or without confirmation of Shiga toxin-production B96.21
    specified NEC B96.22
  Shiga toxin-producing (with unspecified O group) (STEC) B96.23
  specified NEC B96.29
Esophagismus K22.4
Esophagitis (acute) (alkaline) (chemical) (chronic) (infectional) (necrotic) (peptic) (postoperative) (without bleeding) K20.90
  with bleeding K20.91
  candidal B37.81
  due to gastrointestinal reflux disease (without bleeding) K21.00
    with bleeding K21.01
  eosinophilic K20.0
  reflux K21.00
  specified NEC (without bleeding) K20.80
    with bleeding K20.81
  tuberculous A18.83
  ulcerative K22.10
    with bleeding K22.11
Esophagocele K22.5
Esophagomalacia K22.89
Esophagospasm K22.4
Esophagostenosis K22.2
Esophagostomiasis B81.8
Esophagotracheal — *see* condition
Esophagus — *see* condition

Esophoria H50.51
  convergence, excess H51.12
  divergence, insufficiency H51.8
Esotropia — *see* Strabismus, convergent concomitant
Espundia B55.2
Essential — *see* condition
Esthesioneuroblastoma C30.0
Esthesioneurocytoma C30.0
Esthesioneuroepithelioma C30.0
Esthiomene A55
Estivo-autumnal malaria (fever) B50.9
Estrangement (marital) Z63.5
  parent-child NEC Z62.890
Estriasis — *see* Myiasis
Ethanolism — *see* Alcoholism
Etherism — *see* Dependence, drug, inhalant
Ethmoid, ethmoidal — *see* condition
Ethmoiditis (chronic) (nonpurulent) (purulent) — *see also* Sinusitis, ethmoidal
  influenzal — *see* Influenza, with, respiratory manifestations NEC
  Woakes' J33.1
Ethylism — *see* Alcoholism
Eulenburg's disease (congenital paramyotonia) G71.19
Eumycetoma B47.0
Eunuchoidism E29.1
  hypogonadotropic E23.0
European blastomycosis — *see* Cryptococcosis
Eustachian — *see* condition
Evaluation (for) (of)
  development state
    adolescent Z00.3
    period of
      delayed growth in childhood Z00.70
        with abnormal findings Z00.71
      rapid growth in childhood Z00.2
      puberty Z00.3
  growth and developmental state (period of rapid growth) Z00.2
    delayed growth Z00.70
      with abnormal findings Z00.71
  mental health (status) Z00.8
    requested by authority Z04.6
  period of
    delayed growth in childhood Z00.70
      with abnormal findings Z00.71
    rapid growth in childhood Z00.2
  suspected condition — *see* Observation
Evans syndrome D69.41
Event
  apparent life threatening in newborn and infant (ALTE) R68.13
  brief resolved unexplained event (BRUE) R68.13
Eventration — *see also* Hernia, ventral
  colon into chest — *see* Hernia, diaphragm
  diaphragm (congenital) Q79.1
Eversion
  bladder N32.89
  cervix (uteri) N86
    with cervicitis N72
  foot NEC — *see also* Deformity, valgus, ankle
    congenital Q66.6
  punctum lacrimale (postinfectional) (senile) H04.52- ☑
  ureter (meatus) N28.89
  urethra (meatus) N36.8
  uterus N81.4
Evidence
  cytologic
    of malignancy on anal smear R85.614
    of malignancy on cervical smear R87.614
    of malignancy on vaginal smear R87.624
Evisceration
  birth injury P15.8
  traumatic NEC
    eye — *see* Enucleated eye
Evulsion — *see* Avulsion
Ewing's sarcoma or tumor — *see* Neoplasm, bone, malignant
Examination (for) (following) (general) (of) (routine) Z00.00
  with abnormal findings Z00.01
  abuse, physical (alleged), ruled out
    adult Z04.71
    child Z04.72
  adolescent (development state) Z00.3
  alleged rape or sexual assault (victim), ruled out
    adult Z04.41
    child Z04.42

Examination — *continued*
allergy Z01.82
annual (adult) (periodic) (physical) Z00.00
  with abnormal findings Z00.01
  gynecological Z01.419
    with abnormal findings Z01.411
antibody response Z01.84
blood — *see* Examination, laboratory
blood pressure Z01.30
  with abnormal findings Z01.31
cancer staging — *see* Neoplasm, malignant, by site
cervical Papanicolaou smear Z12.4
  as part of routine gynecological examination
    Z01.419
    with abnormal findings Z01.411
child (over 28 days old) Z00.129
  with abnormal findings Z00.121
  under 28 days old — *see* Newborn, examination
clinical research control or normal comparison (control)
  (participant) Z00.6
contraceptive (drug) maintenance (routine) Z30.8
  device (intrauterine) Z30.431
dental Z01.20
  with abnormal findings Z01.21
developmental — *see* Examination, child
donor (potential) Z00.5
ear Z01.10
  with abnormal findings NEC Z01.118
eye Z01.00
  with abnormal findings Z01.01
  following failed vision screening Z01.020
    with abnormal findings Z01.021
follow-up (routine) (following) Z09
  chemotherapy NEC Z09
    malignant neoplasm Z08
  fracture Z09
  malignant neoplasm Z08
  postpartum Z39.2
  psychotherapy Z09
  radiotherapy NEC Z09
    malignant neoplasm Z08
  surgery NEC Z09
    malignant neoplasm Z08
following
  accident NEC Z04.3
    transport Z04.1
    work Z04.2
  assault, alleged, ruled out
    adult Z04.71
    child Z04.72
  motor vehicle accident Z04.1
  treatment (for) Z09
    combined NEC Z09
      fracture Z09
      malignant neoplasm Z08
    malignant neoplasm Z08
    mental disorder Z09
    specified condition NEC Z09
forced sexual exploitation Z04.81
forced labor exploitation Z04.82
gynecological Z01.419
  with abnormal findings Z01.411
  for contraceptive maintenance Z30.8
health — *see* Examination, medical
hearing Z01.10
  with abnormal findings NEC Z01.118
  following failed hearing screening Z01.110
  infant or child (over 28 days old) Z00.129
    with abnormal findings Z00.121
immunity status testing Z01.84
laboratory (as part of a general medical examination)
  Z00.00
  with abnormal findings Z00.01
  preprocedural Z01.812
lactating mother Z39.1
medical (adult) (for) (of) Z00.00
  with abnormal findings Z00.01
  administrative purpose only Z02.9
    specified NEC Z02.89
  admission to
    armed forces Z02.3
    old age home Z02.2
    prison Z02.89
    residential institution Z02.2
    school Z02.0
      following illness or medical treatment Z02.0
    summer camp Z02.89
  adoption Z02.82
  blood alcohol or drug level Z02.83

Examination — *continued*
medical — *continued*
  camp (summer) Z02.89
  clinical research, normal subject (control) (partici-
    pant) Z00.6
  control subject in clinical research (normal compar-
    ison) (participant) Z00.6
  donor (potential) Z00.5
  driving license Z02.4
  general (adult) Z00.00
    with abnormal findings Z00.01
  immigration Z02.89
  insurance purposes Z02.6
  marriage Z02.89
  medicolegal reasons NEC Z04.89
  naturalization Z02.89
  participation in sport Z02.5
  paternity testing Z02.81
  population survey Z00.8
  pre-employment Z02.1
  pre-operative — *see* Examination, pre-procedural
  pre-procedural
    cardiovascular Z01.810
    respiratory Z01.811
    specified NEC Z01.818
  preschool children
    for admission to school Z02.0
  prisoners
    for entrance into prison Z02.89
  recruitment for armed forces Z02.3
  specified NEC Z00.8
  sport competition Z02.5
medicolegal reason NEC Z04.89
  following
    forced sexual exploitation Z04.81
    forced labor exploitation Z04.82
newborn — *see* Newborn, examination
pelvic (annual) (periodic) Z01.419
  with abnormal findings Z01.411
period of rapid growth in childhood Z00.2
periodic (adult) (annual) (routine) Z00.00
  with abnormal findings Z00.01
physical (adult) — *see also* Examination, medical Z00.00
  sports Z02.5
postpartum
  immediately after delivery Z39.0
  routine follow-up Z39.2
pre-chemotherapy (antineoplastic) Z01.818
prenatal (normal pregnancy) — *see also* Pregnancy,
  normal Z34.9- ☑
pre-procedural (pre-operative)
  cardiovascular Z01.810
  laboratory Z01.812
  respiratory Z01.811
  specified NEC Z01.818
prior to chemotherapy (antineoplastic) Z01.818
psychiatric NEC Z00.8
  follow-up not needing further care Z09
  requested by authority Z04.6
radiological (as part of a general medical examination)
  Z00.00
  with abnormal findings Z00.01
repeat cervical smear to confirm findings of recent
  normal smear following initial abnormal smear
  Z01.42
skin (hypersensitivity) Z01.82
special — *see also* Examination, by type Z01.89
  specified type NEC Z01.89
specified type or reason NEC Z04.89
teeth Z01.20
  with abnormal findings Z01.21
urine — *see* Examination, laboratory
vision Z01.00
  with abnormal findings Z01.01
  following failed vision screening Z01.020
    with abnormal findings Z01.021
  infant or child (over 28 days old) Z00.129
    with abnormal findings Z00.121

Exanthem, exanthema — *see also* Rash
with enteroviral vesicular stomatitis B08.4
Boston A88.0
epidemic with meningitis A88.0 *[G02]*
subitum B08.20
  due to human herpesvirus 6 B08.21
  due to human herpesvirus 7 B08.22
viral, virus B09
  specified type NEC B08.8

Excess, excessive, excessively
alcohol level in blood R78.0
androgen (ovarian) E28.1
attrition, tooth, teeth K03.0
carotene, carotin (dietary) E67.1
cold, effects of T69.9 ☑
  specified effect NEC T69.8 ☑
convergence H51.12
crying
  in child, adolescent, or adult R45.83
  in infant R68.11
development, breast N62
divergence H51.8
drinking (alcohol) NEC (without dependence) F10.10
  habitual (continual) (without remission) F10.20
eating R63.2
estrogen E28.0
fat — *see also* Obesity
  in heart — *see* Degeneration, myocardial
  localized E65
foreskin N47.8
gas R14.0
glucagon E16.3
heat — *see* Heat
intermaxillary vertical dimension of fully erupted teeth
  M26.37
interocclusal distance of fully erupted teeth M26.37
kalium E87.5
large
  colon K59.39
    congenital Q43.8
  infant P08.0
  organ or site, congenital NEC — *see* Anomaly, by
    site
long
  organ or site, congenital NEC — *see* Anomaly, by
    site
menstruation (with regular cycle) N92.0
  with irregular cycle N92.1
napping Z72.821
natrium E87.0
number of teeth K00.1
nutrient (dietary) NEC R63.2
potassium (K) E87.5
salivation K11.7
secretion — *see also* Hypersecretion
  milk O92.6
  sputum R09.3
  sweat R61
sexual drive F52.8
short
  organ or site, congenital NEC — *see* Anomaly, by
    site
  umbilical cord in labor or delivery O69.3 ☑
skin L98.7
  and subcutaneous tissue L98.7
  eyelid (acquired) — *see* Blepharochalasis
    congenital Q10.3
sodium (Na) E87.0
spacing of fully erupted teeth M26.32
sputum R09.3
sweating R61
thirst R63.1
  due to deprivation of water T73.1 ☑
transportation time Z59.82
tuberosity of jaw M26.07
vitamin
  A (dietary) E67.0
    administered as drug (prolonged intake) — *see*
      Table of Drugs and Chemicals, vitamins,
      adverse effect
    overdose or wrong substance given or taken —
      see Table of Drugs and Chemicals, vita-
      mins, poisoning
  D (dietary) E67.3
    administered as drug (prolonged intake) — *see*
      Table of Drugs and Chemicals, vitamins,
      adverse effect
    overdose or wrong substance given or taken —
      see Table of Drugs and Chemicals, vita-
      mins, poisoning
weight
  gain R63.5
  loss R63.4

Excitability, abnormal, under minor stress (personality disorder) F60.3

Excitation
anomalous atrioventricular I45.6

Excitation — *continued*
  psychogenic F30.8
  reactive (from emotional stress, psychological trauma)
     F30.8
Excitement
  hypomanic F30.8
  manic F30.9
  mental, reactive (from emotional stress, psychological
     trauma) F30.8
  state, reactive (from emotional stress, psychological
     trauma) F30.8
Excoriation (traumatic) — *see also* Abrasion
  neurotic L98.1
  skin picking disorder F42.4
Exfoliation
  due to erythematous conditions according to extent
     of body surface involved L49.0
     10-19 percent of body surface L49.1
     20-29 percent of body surface L49.2
     30-39 percent of body surface L49.3
     40-49 percent of body surface L49.4
     50-59 percent of body surface L49.5
     60-69 percent of body surface L49.6
     70-79 percent of body surface L49.7
     80-89 percent of body surface L49.8
     90-99 percent of body surface L49.9
     less than 10 percent of body surface L49.0
  teeth, due to systemic causes K08.0
Exfoliative — *see* condition
Exhaustion, exhaustive (physical NEC) R53.83
  battle F43.0
  cardiac — *see* Failure, heart
  delirium F43.0
  due to
     cold T69.8 ☑
     excessive exertion T73.3 ☑
     exposure T73.2 ☑
     neurasthenia F48.8
  heart — *see* Failure, heart
  heat — *see also* Heat, exhaustion T67.5 ☑
     due to
        salt depletion T67.4 ☑
        water depletion T67.3 ☑
  maternal, complicating delivery O75.81
  mental F48.8
  myocardium, myocardial — *see* Failure, heart
  nervous F48.8
  old age R54
  psychogenic F48.8
  psychosis F43.0
  senile R54
  vital NEC Z73.0
Exhibitionism F65.2
Exocervicitis — *see* Cervicitis
Exomphalos Q79.2
  meaning hernia — *see* Hernia, umbilicus
Exophoria H50.52
  convergence, insufficiency H51.11
  divergence, excess H51.8
Exophthalmos H05.2- ☑
  congenital Q15.8
  constant NEC H05.24- ☑
  displacement, globe — *see* Displacement, globe
  due to thyrotoxicosis (hyperthyroidism) — *see* Hyper-
     thyroidism, with, goiter (diffuse)
  dysthyroid — *see* Hyperthyroidism, with, goiter (dif-
     fuse)
  goiter — *see* Hyperthyroidism, with, goiter (diffuse)
  intermittent NEC H05.25- ☑
  malignant — *see* Hyperthyroidism, with, goiter (diffuse)
  orbital
     edema — *see* Edema, orbit
     hemorrhage — *see* Hemorrhage, orbit
  pulsating NEC H05.26- ☑
  thyrotoxic, thyrotropic — *see* Hyperthyroidism, with,
     goiter (diffuse)
Exostosis — *see also* Disorder, bone
  cartilaginous — *see* Neoplasm, bone, benign
  congenital (multiple) Q78.6
  external ear canal H61.81- ☑
  gonococcal A54.49
  jaw (bone) M27.8
  multiple, congenital Q78.6
  orbit H05.35- ☑
  osteocartilaginous — *see* Neoplasm, bone, benign
  syphilitic A52.77
Exotropia — *see* Strabismus, divergent concomitant

Explanation of
  investigation finding Z71.2
  medication Z71.89
Exploitation
  labor
     confirmed
        adult forced T74.61 ☑
        child forced T74.62 ☑
     suspected
        adult forced T76.61 ☑
        child forced T76.62 ☑
  sexual
     confirmed
        adult forced T74.51 ☑
        child T74.52 ☑
     suspected
        adult forced T76.51 ☑
        child T76.52 ☑
Exposure (to) — *see also* Contact, with T75.89 ☑
  acariasis Z20.7
  AIDS virus Z20.6
  air pollution Z77.110
  algae and algae toxins Z77.121
  algae bloom Z77.121
  anthrax Z20.810
  aromatic amines Z77.020
  aromatic (hazardous) compounds NEC Z77.028
  aromatic dyes NOS Z77.028
  arsenic Z77.010
  asbestos Z77.090
  bacterial disease NEC Z20.818
  benzene Z77.021
  blue-green algae bloom Z77.121
  body fluids (potentially hazardous) Z77.21
  brown tide Z77.121
  chemicals (chiefly nonmedicinal) (hazardous) NEC
     Z77.098
  cholera Z20.09
  chromium compounds Z77.018
  cold, effects of T69.9 ☑
     specified effect NEC T69.8 ☑
  communicable disease Z20.9
     bacterial NEC Z20.818
     specified NEC Z20.89
     viral NEC Z20.828
     Zika virus Z20.821
  coronavirus (disease) (novel) 2019 Z20.822
  COVID-19 Z20.822
  cyanobacteria bloom Z77.121
  disaster Z65.5
  discrimination Z60.5
  dyes Z77.098
  effects of T73.9 ☑
  environmental tobacco smoke (acute) (chronic) Z77.22
  Escherichia coli (E. coli) Z20.01
  exhaustion due to T73.2 ☑
  fiberglass — *see* Table of Drugs and Chemicals, fiber-
     glass
  German measles Z20.4
  gonorrhea Z20.2
  hazardous metals NEC Z77.018
  hazardous substances NEC Z77.29
  hazards in the physical environment NEC Z77.128
  hazards to health NEC Z77.9
  human immunodeficiency virus (HIV) Z20.6
  human T-lymphotropic virus type-1 (HTLV-1) Z20.89
  implanted
     mesh — *see* Complications, prosthetic device or
        implant, mesh
     prosthetic materials NEC — *see* Complications,
        prosthetic materials NEC
  infestation (parasitic) NEC Z20.7
  intestinal infectious disease NEC Z20.09
     Escherichia coli (E. coli) Z20.01
  lead Z77.011
  meningococcus Z20.811
  mold (toxic) Z77.120
  nickel dust Z77.018
  noise Z77.122
  occupational
     air contaminants NEC Z57.39
     dust Z57.2
     environmental tobacco smoke Z57.31
     extreme temperature Z57.6
     noise Z57.0
     radiation Z57.1
     risk factors Z57.9
        specified NEC Z57.8

Exposure — *continued*
  occupational — *continued*
     toxic agents (gases) (liquids) (solids) (vapors) in
        agriculture Z57.4
     toxic agents (gases) (liquids) (solids) (vapors) in in-
        dustry NEC Z57.5
     vibration Z57.7
  parasitic disease NEC Z20.7
  pediculosis Z20.7
  persecution Z60.5
  pfiesteria piscicida Z77.121
  poliomyelitis Z20.89
  pollution
     air Z77.110
     environmental NEC Z77.118
     soil Z77.112
     water Z77.111
  polycyclic aromatic hydrocarbons Z77.028
  prenatal (drugs) (toxic chemicals) — *see* Newborn, af-
     fected by, noxious substances transmitted via
     placenta or breast milk
  rabies Z20.3
  radiation, naturally occurring NEC Z77.123
  radon Z77.123
  red tide (Florida) Z77.121
  rubella Z20.4
  SARS-CoV-2 Z20.822
  second hand tobacco smoke (acute) (chronic) Z77.22
     in the perinatal period P96.81
  sexually-transmitted disease Z20.2
  smallpox (laboratory) Z20.89
  syphilis Z20.2
  terrorism Z65.4
  torture Z65.4
  tuberculosis Z20.1
  uranium Z77.012
  varicella Z20.820
  venereal disease Z20.2
  viral disease NEC Z20.828
  war Z65.5
  water pollution Z77.111
  Zika virus Z20.821
Exsanguination — *see* Hemorrhage
Exstrophy
  abdominal contents Q45.8
  bladder Q64.10
     cloacal Q64.12
     specified type NEC Q64.19
     supravesical fissure Q64.11
Extensive — *see* condition
Extra — *see also* Accessory
  marker chromosomes (normal individual) Q92.61
     in abnormal individual Q92.62
  rib Q76.6
     cervical Q76.5
Extrasystoles (supraventricular) I49.49
  atrial I49.1
  auricular I49.1
  junctional I49.2
  ventricular I49.3
Extrauterine gestation or pregnancy — *see* Pregnancy,
  by site
Extravasation
  blood R58
  chyle into mesentery I89.8
  pelvicalyceal N13.8
  pyelosinus N13.8
  urine (from ureter) R39.0
  vesicant agent
     antineoplastic chemotherapy T80.810 ☑
     other agent NEC T80.818 ☑
Extremity — *see* condition, limb
Extrophy — *see* Exstrophy
Extroversion
  bladder Q64.19
  uterus N81.4
     complicating delivery O71.2
     postpartal (old) N81.4
Extruded tooth (teeth) M26.34
Extrusion
  breast implant (prosthetic) T85.42 ☑
  eye implant (globe) (ball) T85.328 ☑
  intervertebral disc — *see* Displacement, intervertebral
     disc
  ocular lens implant (prosthetic) — *see* Complications,
     intraocular lens
  vitreous — *see* Prolapse, vitreous

Exudate
pleural — *see* Effusion, pleura
retina H35.89
wound fluids L24.A9
Exudative — *see* condition
Eye, eyeball, eyelid — *see* condition
Eyestrain — *see* Disturbance, vision, subjective
Eyeworm disease of Africa B74.3

F

Faber's syndrome (achlorhydric anemia) D50.9
Fabry (-Anderson) **disease** E75.21
Facet syndrome M47.89- ☑
Faciocephalalgia, autonomic — *see also* Neuropathy, peripheral, autonomic G90.09
Factor(s)
psychic, associated with diseases classified elsewhere F54
psychological
affecting physical conditions F54
or behavioral
affecting general medical condition F54
associated with disorders or diseases classified elsewhere F54
Fahr disease (of brain) G23.8
Fahr Volhard disease (of kidney) I12.- ☑
Failure, failed
abortion — *see* Abortion, attempted
aortic (valve) I35.8
rheumatic I06.8
attempted abortion — *see* Abortion, attempted
biventricular I50.82
due to left heart failure I50.814
bone marrow — *see* Anemia, aplastic
cardiac — *see* Failure, heart
cardiorenal (chronic) — *see also* Failure, renal, and Failure, heart I50.9
hypertensive I13.2
cardiorespiratory — *see also* Failure, heart R09.2
cardiovascular (chronic) — *see* Failure, heart
cerebrovascular I67.9
cervical dilatation in labor O62.0
circulation, circulatory (peripheral) R57.9
newborn P29.89
compensation — *see* Disease, heart
compliance with medical treatment or regimen — *see* Noncompliance
congestive — *see* Failure, heart, congestive
dental implant (endosseous) M27.69
due to
failure of dental prosthesis M27.63
lack of attached gingiva M27.62
occlusal trauma (poor prosthetic design) M27.62
parafunctional habits M27.62
periodontal infection (peri-implantitis) M27.62
poor oral hygiene M27.62
osseointegration M27.61
due to
complications of systemic disease M27.61
poor bone quality M27.61
iatrogenic M27.61
post-osseointegration
biological M27.62
due to complications of systemic disease M27.62
iatrogenic M27.62
mechanical M27.63
pre-integration M27.61
pre-osseointegration M27.61
specified NEC M27.69
descent of head (at term) of pregnancy (mother) O32.4 ☑
endosseous dental implant — *see* Failure, dental implant
engagement of head (term of pregnancy) (mother) O32.4 ☑
erection (penile) — *see also* Dysfunction, sexual, male, erectile N52.9
nonorganic F52.21
examination(s), anxiety concerning Z55.2
expansion terminal respiratory units (newborn) (primary) P28.0
forceps NOS (with subsequent cesarean delivery) O66.5
gain weight (child over 28 days old) R62.51
adult R62.7
newborn P92.6
genital response (male) F52.21
female F52.22

Failure, failed — *continued*
heart (acute) (senile) (sudden) I50.9
with
acute pulmonary edema — *see* Failure, ventricular, left
decompensation I50.9
with
normal ejection fraction I50.33
preserved ejection fraction I50.33
reduced ejection fraction I50.23
with diastolic dysfunction I50.43
combined systolic and diastolic I50.43
diastolic I50.33
right I50.813
systolic I50.23
dilatation — *see* Disease, heart
hypertension — *see* Hypertension, heart
normal ejection fraction — *see* Failure, heart, diastolic
preserved ejection fraction — *see* Failure, heart, diastolic
reduced ejection fraction — *see* Failure, heart, systolic
arteriosclerotic I70.90
biventricular I50.82
due to left heart failure I50.814
combined left-right sided I50.82
due to left heart failure I50.814
compensated — *see also* Failure, heart, by type as diastolic or systolic, chronic I50.9
complicating
anesthesia (general) (local) or other sedation in labor and delivery O74.2
in pregnancy O29.12- ☑
postpartum, puerperal O89.1
delivery (cesarean) (instrumental) O75.4
congestive I50.9
with rheumatic fever (conditions in I00)
active I01.8
inactive or quiescent (with chorea) I09.81
newborn P29.0
rheumatic (chronic) (inactive) (with chorea) I09.81
active or acute I01.8
with chorea I02.0
decompensated — *see also* Failure, heart, by type as diastolic or systolic, acute and chronic I50.9
degenerative — *see* Degeneration, myocardial
diastolic (congestive) (left ventricular) I50.30
acute (congestive) I50.31
and (on) chronic (congestive) I50.33
chronic (congestive) I50.32
and (on) acute (congestive) I50.33
combined with systolic (congestive) I50.40
acute (congestive) I50.41
and (on) chronic (congestive) I50.43
chronic (congestive) I50.42
and (on) acute (congestive) I50.43
due to presence of cardiac prosthesis I97.13- ☑
end stage — *see also* Failure, heart, by type as diastolic or systolic, chronic I50.84
following cardiac surgery I97.13- ☑
high output NOS I50.83
hypertensive — *see* Hypertension, heart
left (ventricular) — *see also* Failure, ventricular, left
combined diastolic and systolic — *see* Failure, heart, diastolic, combined with systolic
diastolic — *see* Failure, heart, diastolic
systolic — *see* Failure, heart, systolic
low output (syndrome) NOS I50.9
newborn P29.0
organic — *see* Disease, heart
peripartum O90.3
postprocedural I97.13- ☑
rheumatic (chronic) (inactive) I09.9
right (isolated) (ventricular) I50.810
acute I50.811
and (on) chronic I50.813
chronic I50.812
and acute I50.813
secondary to left heart failure I50.814
specified NEC I50.89

Note: heart failure stages A, B, C, and D are based on the American College of Cardiology and American Heart Association stages of heart failure, which complement and should not be confused with the New York Heart Association Classification of Heart Failure, into Class I, Class II, Class III, and Class IV

Failure, failed — *continued*
heart — *continued*
stage A Z91.89
stage B — *see also* Failure, heart, by type as diastolic or systolic I50.9
stage C — *see also* Failure, heart, by type as diastolic or systolic I50.9
stage D — *see also* Failure, heart, by type as diastolic or systolic, chronic I50.84
systolic (congestive) (left ventricular) I50.20
acute (congestive) I50.21
and (on) chronic (congestive) I50.23
chronic (congestive) I50.22
and (on) acute (congestive) I50.23
combined with diastolic (congestive) I50.40
acute (congestive) I50.41
and (on) chronic (congestive) I50.43
chronic (congestive) I50.42
and (on) acute (congestive) I50.43
thyrotoxic — *see also* Thyrotoxicosis E05.90 *[I43]*
with
high output — *see also* Thyrotoxicosis I50.83
thyroid storm E05.91 *[I43]*
high output — *see also* Thyrotoxicosis I50.83
valvular — *see* Endocarditis
hepatic K72.90
with coma K72.91
acute or subacute K72.00
with coma K72.01
due to drugs K71.10
with coma K71.11
alcoholic (acute) (chronic) (subacute) K70.40
with coma K70.41
chronic K72.10
with coma K72.11
due to drugs (acute) (subacute) (chronic) K71.10
with coma K71.11
due to drugs (acute) (subacute) (chronic) K71.10
with coma K71.11
postprocedural K91.82
hepatorenal K76.7
induction (of labor) O61.9
abortion — *see* Abortion, attempted
by
oxytocic drugs O61.0
prostaglandins O61.0
instrumental O61.1
mechanical O61.1
medical O61.0
specified NEC O61.8
surgical O61.1
intubation during anesthesia T88.4 ☑
in pregnancy O29.6- ☑
labor and delivery O74.7
postpartum, puerperal O89.6
involution, thymus (gland) E32.0
kidney — *see also* Disease, kidney, chronic N19
acute — *see also* Failure, renal, acute N17.9
lactation (complete) O92.3
partial O92.4
Leydig's cell, adult E29.1
liver — *see* Failure, hepatic
menstruation at puberty N91.0
mitral I05.8
myocardial, myocardium — *see also* Failure, heart I50.9
chronic — *see also* Failure, heart, congestive I50.9
congestive — *see also* Failure, heart, congestive I50.9
newborn screening — *see* Abnormal, neonatal screening
neonatal congenital heart disease P09.5
orgasm (female) (psychogenic) F52.31
male F52.32
ovarian (primary) E28.39
iatrogenic E89.40
asymptomatic E89.40
symptomatic E89.41
postprocedural (postablative) (postirradiation) (postsurgical) E89.40
asymptomatic E89.40
symptomatic E89.41
ovulation causing infertility N97.0
polyglandular, autoimmune E31.0
prosthetic joint implant — *see* Complications, joint prosthesis, mechanical, breakdown, by site
renal N19

Failure, failed — *continued*
  renal — *continued*
    with
      tubular necrosis (acute) N17.0
      acute N17.9
        with
          cortical necrosis N17.1
          medullary necrosis N17.2
          tubular necrosis N17.0
        specified NEC N17.8
    chronic N18.9
      hypertensive — *see* Hypertension, kidney
    congenital P96.0
    end stage (chronic) N18.6
      due to hypertension I12.0
    following
      abortion — *see* Abortion by type complicated
          by specified condition NEC
      crushing T79.5 ☑
      ectopic or molar pregnancy O08.4
      labor and delivery (acute) O90.4
    hypertensive — *see* Hypertension, kidney
    postprocedural N99.0
  respiration, respiratory J96.90
    with
      hypercapnia J96.92
      hypercarbia J96.92
      hypoxia J96.91
    acute J96.00
      with
        hypercapnia J96.02
        hypercarbia J96.02
        hypoxia J96.01
      center G93.89
    acute and (on) chronic J96.20
      with
        hypercapnia J96.22
        hypercarbia J96.22
        hypoxia J96.21
    chronic J96.10
      with
        hypercapnia J96.12
        hypercarbia J96.12
        hypoxia J96.11
    newborn P28.5
    postprocedural (acute) J95.821
      acute and chronic J95.822
  rotation
    cecum Q43.3
    colon Q43.3
    intestine Q43.3
    kidney Q63.2
  sedation (conscious) (moderate) during procedure
      T88.52 ☑
    history of Z92.83
  segmentation — *see also* Fusion
    fingers — *see* Syndactylism, complex, fingers
    vertebra Q76.49
      with scoliosis Q76.3
  seminiferous tubule, adult E29.1
  senile (general) R54
  sexual arousal (male) F52.21
    female F52.22
  testicular endocrine function E29.1
  to thrive (child over 28 days old) R62.51
    adult R62.7
    newborn P92.6
  transplant T86.92
    bone T86.831
      marrow T86.02
    cornea T86.841- ☑
    heart T86.22
      with lung(s) T86.32
    intestine T86.851
    kidney T86.12
    liver T86.42
    lung(s) T86.811
      with heart T86.32
    pancreas T86.891
    skin (allograft) (autograft) T86.821
    specified organ or tissue NEC T86.891
    stem cell (peripheral blood) (umbilical cord) T86.5
  trial of labor (with subsequent cesarean delivery)
      O66.40
    following previous cesarean delivery O66.41
  tubal ligation N99.89
  urinary — *see* Disease, kidney, chronic

Failure, failed — *continued*
  vacuum extraction NOS (with subsequent cesarean
      delivery) O66.5
  vasectomy N99.89
  ventouse NOS (with subsequent cesarean delivery)
      O66.5
  ventricular — *see also* Failure, heart I50.9
    left — *see also* Failure, heart, left I50.1
      with rheumatic fever (conditions in I00)
        active I01.8
          with chorea I02.0
        inactive or quiescent (with chorea) I09.81
        rheumatic (chronic) (inactive) (with chorea)
            I09.81
        active or acute I01.8
          with chorea I02.0
    right — *see* Failure, heart, right
  vital centers, newborn P91.88
Fainting (fit) R55
Fallen arches — *see* Deformity, limb, flat foot
Falling, falls (repeated) R29.6
  any organ or part — *see* Prolapse
Fallopian
  insufflation Z31.41
  tube — *see* condition
Fallot's
  pentalogy Q21.8
  tetrad or tetralogy Q21.3
  triad or trilogy Q22.3
False — *see also* condition
  croup J38.5
  joint — *see* Nonunion, fracture
  labor (pains) O47.9
    at or after 37 completed weeks of gestation O47.1
    before 37 completed weeks of gestation O47.0- ☑
  passage, urethra (prostatic) N36.5
  pregnancy F45.8
Family, familial — *see also* condition
  disruption Z63.8
    involving divorce or separation Z63.5
  Li-Fraumeni (syndrome) Z15.01
  planning advice Z30.09
  problem Z63.9
    specified NEC Z63.8
  retinoblastoma C69.2- ☑
Famine (effects of) T73.0 ☑
  edema — *see* Malnutrition, severe
Fanconi (-de Toni)(-Debré) **syndrome** E72.09
  with cystinosis E72.04
Fanconi's anemia (congenital pancytopenia) D61.09
Farber's disease or syndrome E75.29
Farcy A24.0
Farmer's
  lung J67.0
  skin L57.8
Farsightedness — *see* Hypermetropia
Fascia — *see* condition
Fasciculation R25.3
Fasciitis M72.9
  diffuse (eosinophilic) M35.4
  infective M72.8
    necrotizing M72.6
  necrotizing M72.6
  nodular M72.4
  perirenal (with ureteral obstruction) N13.5
    with infection N13.6
  plantar M72.2
  specified NEC M72.8
  traumatic (old) M72.8
    current — *code by* site under Sprain
Fascioliasis B66.3
Fasciolopsis, fasciolopsiasis (intestinal) B66.5
Fascioscapulohumeral myopathy G71.02
Fast pulse R00.0
Fat
  embolism — *see* Embolism, fat
  excessive — *see also* Obesity
    in heart — *see* Degeneration, myocardial
  in stool R19.5
  localized (pad) E65
    heart — *see* Degeneration, myocardial
    knee M79.4
    retropatellar M79.4
  necrosis
    breast N64.1
    mesentery K65.4
    omentum K65.4
  pad E65

Fat — *continued*
  pad — *continued*
    knee M79.4
Fatigue R53.83
  auditory deafness — *see* Deafness
  chronic R53.82
  combat F43.0
  general R53.83
    psychogenic F48.8
  heat (transient) T67.6 ☑
  muscle M62.89
  myocardium — *see* Failure, heart
  neoplasm-related R53.0
  nervous, neurosis F48.8
  operational F48.8
  psychogenic (general) F48.8
  senile R54
  voice R49.8
Fatness — *see* Obesity
Fatty — *see also* condition
  apron E65
  degeneration — *see* Degeneration, fatty
  heart (enlarged) — *see* Degeneration, myocardial
  liver NEC K76.0
    alcoholic K70.0
    nonalcoholic K76.0
  necrosis — *see* Degeneration, fatty
Fauces — *see* condition
Fauchard's disease (periodontitis) — *see* Periodontitis
Faucitis J02.9
Favism (anemia) D55.0
Favus — *see* Dermatophytosis
Fazio-Londe disease or syndrome G12.1
Fear complex or reaction F40.9
Fear of — *see* Phobia
Feared complaint unfounded Z71.1
Febris, febrile — *see also* Fever
  flava — *see also* Fever, yellow A95.9
  melitensis A23.0
  pestis — *see* Plague
  recurrens — *see* Fever, relapsing
  rubra A38.9
Fecal
  incontinence R15.9
  smearing R15.1
  soiling R15.1
  urgency R15.2
Fecalith (impaction) K56.41
  appendix K38.1
  congenital P76.8
Fede's disease K14.0
Feeble rapid pulse due to shock following injury
    T79.4 ☑
Feeble-minded F70
Feeding
  difficulties R63.30
  problem (elderly) (infant) R63.39
    newborn P92.9
      specified NEC P92.8
    nonorganic (adult) — *see* Disorder, eating
Feeling (of)
  foreign body in throat R09.89
Feer's disease — *see* Poisoning, mercury
Feet — *see* condition
Feigned illness Z76.5
Feil-Klippel syndrome (brevicollis) Q76.1
Feinmesser's (hidrotic) **ectodermal dysplasia** Q82.4
Felinophobia F40.218
Felon — *see also* Cellulitis, digit
  with lymphangitis — *see* Lymphangitis, acute, digit
Felty's syndrome M05.00
  ankle M05.07- ☑
  elbow M05.02- ☑
  foot joint M05.07- ☑
  hand joint M05.04- ☑
  hip M05.05- ☑
  knee M05.06- ☑
  multiple site M05.09
  shoulder M05.01- ☑
  vertebra — *see* Spondylitis, ankylosing
  wrist M05.03- ☑
Female genital cutting status — *see* Female genital
    mutilation status (FGM)
Female genital mutilation status (FGM) N90.810
  specified NEC N90.818
  type I (clitorectomy status) N90.811

Female genital mutilation status — continued
- type II (clitorectomy with excision of labia minora status) N90.812
- type III (infibulation status) N90.813
- type IV N90.818

Femur, femoral — see condition

Fenestration, fenestrated — see also Imperfect, closure
- aortico-pulmonary Q21.4
- atrial septum Q21.11
- cusps, heart valve NEC Q24.8
  - pulmonary Q22.3
- pulmonic cusps Q22.3

Fernell's disease (aortic aneurysm) I71.9

Fertile eunuch syndrome E23.0

Fetid
- breath R19.6
- sweat L75.0

Fetishism F65.0
- transvestic F65.1

Fetus, fetal — see also condition
- alcohol syndrome (dysmorphic) Q86.0
- compressus O31.0- ☑
- hydantoin syndrome Q86.1
- lung tissue P28.0
- papyraceous O31.0- ☑

Fever (inanition) (of unknown origin) (persistent) (with chills) (with rigor) R50.9
- abortus A23.1
- Aden (dengue) A90
- African tick bite A77.8
- African tick-borne A68.1
- American
  - mountain (tick) A93.2
  - spotted A77.0
- aphthous B08.8
- arbovirus, arboviral A94
  - hemorrhagic A94
  - specified NEC A93.8
- Argentinian hemorrhagic A96.0
- Assam B55.0
- Australian Q A78
- Bangkok hemorrhagic A91
- Barmah forest A92.8
- Bartonella A44.0
- bilious, hemoglobinuric B50.8
- blackwater B50.8
- blister B00.1
- Bolivian hemorrhagic A96.1
- Bonvale dam T73.3 ☑
- boutonneuse A77.1
- brain — see Encephalitis
- Brazilian purpuric A48.4
- breakbone A90
- Bullis A77.0
- Bunyamwera A92.8
- Burdwan B55.0
- Bwamba A92.8
- Cameroon — see Malaria
- Canton A75.9
- catarrhal (acute) J00
  - chronic J31.0
- cat-scratch A28.1
- Central Asian hemorrhagic A98.0
- cerebral — see Encephalitis
- cerebrospinal meningococcal A39.0
- Chagres B50.9
- Chandipura A92.8
- Changuinola A93.1
- Charcot's (biliary) (hepatic) (intermittent) — see Calculus, bile duct
- Chikungunya (viral) (hemorrhagic) A92.0
- Chitral A93.1
- Colombo — see Fever, paratyphoid
- Colorado tick (virus) A93.2
- congestive (remittent) — see Malaria
- Congo virus A98.0
- continued malarial B50.9
- Corsican — see Malaria
- Crimean-Congo hemorrhagic A98.0
- Cyprus — see Brucellosis
- dandy A90
- deer fly — see Tularemia
- dengue (virus) A90
  - hemorrhagic A91
  - sandfly A93.1
- desert B38.0
- drug induced R50.2

Fever — continued
- due to
  - conditions classified elsewhere R50.81
  - heat T67.01 ☑
- enteric A01.00
- enteroviral exanthematous (Boston exanthem) A88.0
- ephemeral (of unknown origin) R50.9
- epidemic hemorrhagic A98.5
- erysipelatous — see Erysipelas
- estivo-autumnal (malarial) B50.9
- famine A75.0
- five day A79.0
- following delivery O86.4
- Fort Bragg A27.89
- gastroenteric A01.00
- gastromalarial — see Malaria
- Gibraltar — see Brucellosis
- glandular — see Mononucleosis, infectious
- Guama (viral) A92.8
- Haverhill A25.1
- hay (allergic) J30.1
  - with asthma (bronchial) J45.909
    - with
      - exacerbation (acute) J45.901
      - status asthmaticus J45.902
  - due to
    - allergen other than pollen J30.89
    - pollen, any plant or tree J30.1
- heat (effects) T67.01 ☑
- hematuric, bilious B50.8
- hemoglobinuric (malarial) (bilious) B50.8
- hemorrhagic (arthropod-borne) NOS A94
  - with renal syndrome A98.5
  - arenaviral A96.9
    - specified NEC A96.8
  - Argentinian A96.0
  - Bangkok A91
  - Bolivian A96.1
  - Central Asian A98.0
  - Chikungunya A92.0
  - Crimean-Congo A98.0
  - dengue (virus) A91
  - epidemic A98.5
  - Junin (virus) A96.0
  - Korean A98.5
  - Kyasanur forest A98.2
  - Machupo (virus) A96.1
  - mite-borne A93.8
  - mosquito-borne A92.8
  - Omsk A98.1
  - Philippine A91
  - Russian A98.5
  - Singapore A91
  - Southeast Asia A91
  - Thailand A91
  - tick-borne NEC A93.8
  - viral A99
    - specified NEC A98.8
- hepatic — see Cholecystitis
- herpetic — see Herpes
- icterohemorrhagic A27.0
- Indiana A93.8
- infective B99.9
  - specified NEC B99.8
- intermittent (bilious) — see also Malaria
  - of unknown origin R50.9
  - pernicious B50.9
- iodide R50.2
- Japanese river A75.3
- jungle — see also Malaria
  - yellow A95.0
- Junin (virus) hemorrhagic A96.0
- Katayama B65.2
- kedani A75.3
- Kenya (tick) A77.1
- Kew Garden A79.1
- Korean hemorrhagic A98.5
- Lassa A96.2
- Lone Star A77.0
- Machupo (virus) hemorrhagic A96.1
- malaria, malarial — see Malaria
- Malta A23.9
- Marseilles A77.1
- marsh — see Malaria
- Mayaro (viral) A92.8
- Mediterranean — see also Brucellosis A23.9
  - familial M04.1
  - tick A77.1

Fever — continued
- meningeal — see Meningitis
- Meuse A79.0
- Mexican A75.2
- mianeh A68.1
- miasmatic — see Malaria
- mosquito-borne (viral) A92.9
  - hemorrhagic A92.8
- mountain — see also Brucellosis
  - meaning Rocky Mountain spotted fever A77.0
  - tick (American) (Colorado) (viral) A93.2
- Mucambo (viral) A92.8
- mud A27.9
- Neapolitan — see Brucellosis
- neutropenic D70.9
- newborn P81.9
  - environmental P81.0
- Nine-Mile A78
- non-exanthematous tick A93.2
- North Asian tick-borne A77.2
- Omsk hemorrhagic A98.1
- O'nyong-nyong (viral) A92.1
- Oropouche (viral) A93.0
- Oroya A44.0
- pacific coast tick A77.8
- paludal — see Malaria
- Panama (malarial) B50.9
- Pappataci A93.1
- paratyphoid A01.4
  - A A01.1
  - B A01.2
  - C A01.3
- parrot A70
- periodic (Mediterranean) M04.1
- persistent (of unknown origin) R50.9
- petechial A39.0
- pharyngoconjunctival B30.2
- Philippine hemorrhagic A91
- phlebotomus A93.1
- Piry (virus) A93.8
- Pixuna (viral) A92.8
- Plasmodium ovale B53.0
- polioviral (nonparalytic) A80.4
- Pontiac A48.2
- postimmunization R50.83
- postoperative R50.82
  - due to infection T81.40 ☑
- posttransfusion R50.84
- postvaccination R50.83
- presenting with conditions classified elsewhere R50.81
- pretibial A27.89
- puerperal O86.4
- Q A78
- quadrilateral A78
- quartan (malaria) B52.9
- Queensland (coastal) (tick) A77.3
- quintan A79.0
- rabbit — see Tularemia
- rat-bite A25.9
  - due to
    - Spirillum A25.0
    - Streptobacillus moniliformis A25.1
- recurrent — see Fever, relapsing
- relapsing (Borrelia) A68.9
  - Carter's (Asiatic) A68.1
  - Dutton's (West African) A68.1
  - Koch's A68.9
  - louse-borne A68.0
  - Novy's
    - louse-borne A68.0
    - tick-borne A68.1
  - Obermeyer's (European) A68.0
  - tick-borne A68.1
- remittent (bilious) (congestive) (gastric) — see Malaria
- rheumatic (active) (acute) (chronic) (subacute) I00
  - with central nervous system involvement I02.9
  - active with heart involvement — see category I01 ☑
  - inactive or quiescent with
    - cardiac hypertrophy I09.89
    - carditis I09.9
    - endocarditis I09.1
      - aortic (valve) I06.9
        - with mitral (valve) disease I08.0
      - mitral (valve) I05.9
        - with aortic (valve) disease I08.0
      - pulmonary (valve) I09.89
      - tricuspid (valve) I07.8
    - heart disease NEC I09.89

☑ Additional Character Required — Refer to the Tabular List for Character Selection

Fever — *continued*
  rheumatic — *continued*
    inactive or quiescent with — *continued*
      heart failure (congestive) (conditions in category I50.) I09.81
      left ventricular failure (conditions in I50.1-I50.4-) I09.81
      myocarditis, myocardial degeneration (conditions in I51.4) I09.0
      pancarditis I09.9
      pericarditis I09.2
  Rift Valley (viral) A92.4
  Rocky Mountain spotted A77.0
  rose J30.1
  Ross River B33.1
  Russian hemorrhagic A98.5
  San Joaquin (Valley) B38.0
  sandfly A93.1
  Sao Paulo A77.0
  scarlet A38.9
  seven day (leptospirosis) (autumnal) (Japanese) A27.89
    dengue A90
  shin-bone A79.0
  Singapore hemorrhagic A91
  solar A90
  Songo A98.5
  sore B00.1
  South African tick-bite A68.1
  Southeast Asia hemorrhagic A91
  spinal — *see* Meningitis
  spirillary A25.0
  splenic — *see* Anthrax
  spotted A77.9
    American A77.0
    Brazilian A77.0
    cerebrospinal meningitis A39.0
    Colombian A77.0
    due to Rickettsia
      africae (African tick bite fever) A77.8
      australis A77.3
      conorii A77.1
      parkeri A77.8
      rickettsii A77.0
      sibirica A77.2
      specified type NEC A77.8
    Ehrlichiosis A77.40
      due to
        E. chafeensis A77.41
        specified organism NEC A77.49
    Rocky Mountain A77.0
  steroid R50.2
  streptobacillary A25.1
  subtertian B50.9
  Sumatran mite A75.3
  sun A90
  swamp A27.9
  swine A02.8
  sylvatic, yellow A95.0
  Tahyna B33.8
  tertian — *see* Malaria, tertian
  Thailand hemorrhagic A91
  thermic T67.01 ☑
  three-day A93.1
  tick
    American mountain A93.2
    Colorado A93.2
    Kemerovo A93.8
    Mediterranean A77.1
    mountain A93.2
    nonexanthematous A93.2
    Quaranfil A93.8
  tick-bite NEC A93.8
  tick-borne (hemorrhagic) NEC A93.8
  trench A79.0
  tsutsugamushi A75.3
  typhogastric A01.00
  typhoid (abortive) (hemorrhagic) (intermittent) (malignant) A01.00
    complicated by
      arthritis A01.04
      heart involvement A01.02
      meningitis A01.01
      osteomyelitis A01.05
      pneumonia A01.03
      specified NEC A01.09
  typhomalarial — *see* Malaria
  typhus — *see* Typhus (fever)
  undulant — *see* Brucellosis

Fever — *continued*
  unknown origin R50.9
  uveoparotid D86.89
  valley B38.0
  Venezuelan equine A92.2
  vesicular stomatitis A93.8
  viral hemorrhagic — *see* Fever, hemorrhagic, by type of virus
  Volhynian A79.0
  Wesselsbron (viral) A92.8
  West
    African B50.8
    Nile (viral) A92.30
      with
        complications NEC A92.39
        cranial nerve disorders A92.32
        encephalitis A92.31
        encephalomyelitis A92.31
        neurologic manifestation NEC A92.32
        optic neuritis A92.32
        polyradiculitis A92.32
  Whitmore's — *see* Melioidosis
  Wolhynian A79.0
  worm B83.9
  yellow A95.9
    jungle A95.0
    sylvatic A95.0
    urban A95.1
  Zika virus A92.5
Fibrillation
  atrial or auricular (established) I48.91
    chronic I48.20
      persistent I48.19
    paroxysmal I48.0
    permanent I48.21
    persistent (chronic) (NOS) (other) I48.19
      longstanding I48.11
  cardiac I49.8
  heart I49.8
  muscular M62.89
  ventricular I49.01
Fibrin
  ball or bodies, pleural (sac) J94.1
  chamber, anterior (eye) (gelatinous exudate) — *see* Iridocyclitis, acute
Fibrinogenolysis — *see* Fibrinolysis
Fibrinogenopenia D68.8
  acquired D65
  congenital D68.2
Fibrinolysis (hemorrhagic) (acquired) D65
  antepartum hemorrhage — *see* Hemorrhage, antepartum, with coagulation defect
  following
    abortion — *see* Abortion by type complicated by hemorrhage
    ectopic or molar pregnancy O08.1
  intrapartum O67.0
  newborn, transient P60
  postpartum O72.3
Fibrinopenia (hereditary) D68.2
  acquired D68.4
Fibrinopurulent — *see* condition
Fibrinous — *see* condition
Fibroadenoma
  cellular intracanalicular D24- ☑
  giant D24- ☑
  intracanalicular
    cellular D24- ☑
    giant D24- ☑
    specified site — *see* Neoplasm, benign, by site
    unspecified site D24- ☑
  juvenile D24- ☑
  pericanalicular
    specified site — *see* Neoplasm, benign, by site
    unspecified site D24- ☑
  phyllodes D24- ☑
  prostate D29.1
  specified site NEC — *see* Neoplasm, benign, by site
  unspecified site D24- ☑
Fibroadenosis, breast (chronic) (cystic) (diffuse) (periodic) (segmental) N60.2- ☑
Fibroangioma — *see also* Neoplasm, benign, by site
  juvenile
    specified site — *see* Neoplasm, benign, by site
    unspecified site D10.6
Fibrochondrosarcoma — *see* Neoplasm, cartilage, malignant

Fibrocystic
  disease — *see also* Fibrosis, cystic
    breast — *see* Mastopathy, cystic
    jaw M27.49
    kidney (congenital) Q61.8
    liver Q44.6
    pancreas E84.9
  kidney (congenital) Q61.8
Fibrodysplasia ossificans progressiva — *see* Myositis, ossificans, progressiva
Fibroelastosis (cordis) (endocardial) (endomyocardial) I42.4
Fibroid (tumor) — *see also* Neoplasm, connective tissue, benign
  disease, lung (chronic) — *see* Fibrosis, lung
  heart (disease) — *see* Myocarditis
  in pregnancy or childbirth O34.1- ☑
    causing obstructed labor O65.5
  induration, lung (chronic) — *see* Fibrosis, lung
  lung — *see* Fibrosis, lung
  pneumonia (chronic) — *see* Fibrosis, lung
  uterus — *see also* Leiomyoma, uterus D25.9
Fibrolipoma — *see* Lipoma
Fibroliposarcoma — *see* Neoplasm, connective tissue, malignant
Fibroma — *see also* Neoplasm, connective tissue, benign
  ameloblastic — *see* Cyst, calcifying odontogenic
  bone (nonossifying) — *see* Disorder, bone, specified type NEC
    ossifying — *see* Neoplasm, bone, benign
  cementifying — *see* Neoplasm, bone, benign
  chondromyxoid — *see* Neoplasm, bone, benign
  desmoplastic — *see* Neoplasm, connective tissue, uncertain behavior
  durum — *see* Neoplasm, connective tissue, benign
  fascial — *see* Neoplasm, connective tissue, benign
  invasive — *see* Neoplasm, connective tissue, uncertain behavior
  molle — *see* Lipoma
  myxoid — *see* Neoplasm, connective tissue, benign
  nasopharynx, nasopharyngeal (juvenile) D10.6
  nonosteogenic (nonossifying) — *see* Dysplasia, fibrous
  odontogenic (central) — *see* Cyst, calcifying odontogenic
  ossifying — *see* Neoplasm, bone, benign
  periosteal — *see* Neoplasm, bone, benign
  soft — *see* Lipoma
Fibromatosis M72.9
  abdominal — *see* Neoplasm, connective tissue, uncertain behavior
  aggressive — *see* Neoplasm, connective tissue, uncertain behavior
  congenital generalized — *see* Neoplasm, connective tissue, uncertain behavior
  Dupuytren's M72.0
  gingival K06.1
  palmar (fascial) M72.0
  plantar (fascial) M72.2
  pseudosarcomatous (proliferative) (subcutaneous) M72.4
  retroperitoneal D48.3
  specified NEC M72.8
Fibromyalgia M79.7
Fibromyoma — *see also* Neoplasm, connective tissue, benign
  uterus (corpus) — *see also* Leiomyoma, uterus
    in pregnancy or childbirth — *see* Fibroid, in pregnancy or childbirth
    causing obstructed labor O65.5
Fibromyositis M79.7
Fibromyxolipoma D17.9
Fibromyxoma — *see* Neoplasm, connective tissue, benign
Fibromyxosarcoma — *see* Neoplasm, connective tissue, malignant
Fibro-odontoma, ameloblastic — *see* Cyst, calcifying odontogenic
Fibro-osteoma — *see* Neoplasm, bone, benign
Fibroplasia, retrolental H35.17- ☑
Fibropurulent — *see* condition
Fibrosarcoma — *see also* Neoplasm, connective tissue, malignant
  ameloblastic C41.1
    upper jaw (bone) C41.0
  congenital — *see* Neoplasm, connective tissue, malignant
  fascial — *see* Neoplasm, connective tissue, malignant

Fibrosarcoma — *continued*
    infantile — *see* Neoplasm, connective tissue, malignant
    odontogenic C41.1
        upper jaw (bone) C41.0
    periosteal — *see* Neoplasm, bone, malignant
Fibrosclerosis
    breast N60.3- ☑
    multifocal M35.5
    penis (corpora cavernosa) N48.6
Fibrosis, fibrotic
    adrenal (gland) E27.8
    amnion O41.8X- ☑
    anal papillae K62.89
    arteriocapillary — *see* Arteriosclerosis
    bladder N32.89
        interstitial — *see* Cystitis, chronic, interstitial
        localized submucosal — *see* Cystitis, chronic, interstitial
        panmural — *see* Cystitis, chronic, interstitial
    breast — *see* Fibrosclerosis, breast
    capillary — *see also* Arteriosclerosis I70.90
        lung (chronic) — *see* Fibrosis, lung
    cardiac — *see* Myocarditis
    cervix N88.8
    chorion O41.8X- ☑
    corpus cavernosum (sclerosing) N48.6
    cystic (of pancreas) E84.9
        with
            distal intestinal obstruction syndrome E84.19
            fecal impaction E84.19
            intestinal manifestations NEC E84.19
            pulmonary manifestations E84.0
            specified manifestations NEC E84.8
    due to device, implant or graft — *see also* Complications, by site and type, specified NEC T85.828 ☑
        arterial graft NEC T82.828 ☑
        breast (implant) T85.828 ☑
        catheter NEC T85.828 ☑
            dialysis (renal) T82.828 ☑
                intraperitoneal T85.828 ☑
            infusion NEC T82.828 ☑
                spinal (epidural) (subdural) T85.820 ☑
            urinary (indwelling) T83.82 ☑
        electronic (electrode) (pulse generator) (stimulator)
            bone T84.82 ☑
            cardiac T82.827 ☑
            nervous system (brain) (peripheral nerve) (spinal) T85.820 ☑
            urinary T83.82 ☑
        fixation, internal (orthopedic) NEC T84.82 ☑
        gastrointestinal (bile duct) (esophagus) T85.828 ☑
        genital NEC T83.82 ☑
        heart NEC T82.827 ☑
        joint prosthesis T84.82 ☑
        ocular (corneal graft) (orbital implant) NEC T85.828 ☑
        orthopedic NEC T84.82 ☑
        specified NEC T85.828 ☑
        urinary NEC T83.82 ☑
        vascular NEC T82.828 ☑
        ventricular intracranial shunt T85.820 ☑
    ejaculatory duct N50.89
    endocardium — *see* Endocarditis
    endomyocardial (tropical) I42.3
    epididymis N50.89
    eye muscle — *see* Strabismus, mechanical
    heart — *see* Myocarditis
    hepatic — *see* Fibrosis, liver
    hepatolienal (portal hypertension) K76.6
    hepatosplenic (portal hypertension) K76.6
    infrapatellar fat pad M79.4
    intrascrotal N50.89
    kidney N26.9
    liver K74.00
        with sclerosis K74.2
        advanced K74.02
        alcoholic K70.2
        early K74.01
        stage
            F1 or F2 K74.01
            F3 K74.02
    lung (atrophic) (chronic) (confluent) (massive) (perialveolar) (peribronchial) J84.10
        with
            anthracosilicosis J60
            anthracosis J60
            asbestosis J61

Fibrosis, fibrotic — *continued*
    lung — *continued*
        with — *continued*
            bagassosis J67.1
            bauxite J63.1
            berylliosis J63.2
            byssinosis J66.0
            calcicosis J62.8
            chalicosis J62.8
            dust reticulation J64
            farmer's lung J67.0
            ganister disease J62.8
            graphite J63.3
            pneumoconiosis NOS J64
            siderosis J63.4
            silicosis J62.8
        capillary J84.10
        congenital P27.8
        diffuse (idiopathic) J84.10
            chemicals, gases, fumes or vapors (inhalation) J68.4
            interstitial J84.10
                acute J84.114
            talc J62.0
        following radiation J70.1
        idiopathic J84.112
        postinflammatory J84.10
        silicotic J62.8
        tuberculous — *see* Tuberculosis, pulmonary
    lymphatic gland I89.8
    median bar — *see* Hyperplasia, prostate
    mediastinum (idiopathic) J98.59
    meninges G96.198
    myocardium, myocardial — *see* Myocarditis
    ovary N83.8
    oviduct N83.8
    pancreas K86.89
    penis NEC N48.6
    pericardium I31.0
    perineum, in pregnancy or childbirth O34.7- ☑
        causing obstructed labor O65.5
    pleura J94.1
    popliteal fat pad M79.4
    prostate (chronic) — *see* Hyperplasia, prostate
    pulmonary — *see also* Fibrosis, lung J84.10
        congenital P27.8
        idiopathic J84.112
    rectal sphincter K62.89
    retroperitoneal, idiopathic (with ureteral obstruction) N13.5
        with infection N13.6
    sclerosing mesenteric (idiopathic) K65.4
    scrotum N50.89
    seminal vesicle N50.89
    senile R54
    skin L90.5
    spermatic cord N50.89
    spleen D73.89
        in schistosomiasis (bilharziasis) B65.9 *[D77]*
    subepidermal nodular — *see* Neoplasm, skin, benign
    submucous (oral) (tongue) K13.5
    testis N44.8
        chronic, due to syphilis A52.76
    thymus (gland) E32.8
    tongue, submucous K13.5
    tunica vaginalis N50.89
    uterus (non-neoplastic) N85.8
    vagina N89.8
    valve, heart — *see* Endocarditis
    vas deferens N50.89
    vein I87.8
Fibrositis (periarticular) M79.7
    nodular, chronic (Jaccoud's) (rheumatoid) — *see* Arthropathy, postrheumatic, chronic
Fibrothorax J94.1
Fibrotic — *see* Fibrosis
Fibrous — *see* condition
Fibroxanthoma — *see also* Neoplasm, connective tissue, benign
    atypical — *see* Neoplasm, connective tissue, uncertain behavior
    malignant — *see* Neoplasm, connective tissue, malignant
Fibroxanthosarcoma — *see* Neoplasm, connective tissue, malignant
Fiedler's
    disease (icterohemorrhagic leptospirosis) A27.0
    myocarditis (acute) I40.1

Fifth disease B08.3
    venereal A55
Filaria, filarial, filariasis — *see* Infestation, filarial
Filatov's disease — *see* Mononucleosis, infectious
File-cutter's disease — *see* Poisoning, lead
Filling defect
    biliary tract R93.2
    bladder R93.41
    duodenum R93.3
    gallbladder R93.2
    gastrointestinal tract R93.3
    intestine R93.3
    kidney R93.42- ☑
    stomach R93.3
    ureter R93.41
    urinary organs, specified NEC R93.49
Fimbrial cyst Q50.4
Financial problem affecting care NOS Z59.9
    bankruptcy Z59.89
    foreclosure on loan Z59.89
        home loan Z59.81- ☑
    strain Z59.86
Findings, abnormal, inconclusive, without diagnosis
    — *see also* Abnormal
    17-ketosteroids, elevated R82.5
    acetonuria R82.4
    alcohol in blood R78.0
    anisocytosis R71.8
    antenatal screening of mother O28.9
        biochemical O28.1
        chromosomal O28.5
        cytological O28.2
        genetic O28.5
        hematological O28.0
        radiological O28.4
        specified NEC O28.8
        ultrasonic O28.3
    antibody titer, elevated R76.0
    anticardiolipin antibody R76.0
    antiphosphatidylglycerol antibody R76.0
    antiphosphatidylinositol antibody R76.0
    antiphosphatidylserine antibody R76.0
    antiphospholipid antibody R76.0
    bacteriuria R82.71
    bicarbonate E87.8
    bile in urine R82.2
    blood sugar R73.09
        high R73.9
        low (transient) E16.2
    body fluid or substance, specified NEC R88.8
    casts, urine R82.998
    catecholamines R82.5
    cells, urine R82.998
    chloride E87.8
    cholesterol E78.9
        high E78.00
            with high triglycerides E78.2
    chyluria R82.0
    cloudy
        dialysis effluent R88.0
        urine R82.90
    creatinine clearance R94.4
    crystals, urine R82.998
    culture
        blood R78.81
        positive — *see* Positive, culture
    echocardiogram R93.1
    electrolyte level, urinary R82.998
    function study NEC R94.8
        bladder R94.8
        endocrine NEC R94.7
            thyroid R94.6
        kidney R94.4
        liver R94.5
        pancreas R94.8
        placenta R94.8
        pulmonary R94.2
        spleen R94.8
    gallbladder, nonvisualization R93.2
    glucose (tolerance test) (non-fasting) R73.09
    glycosuria R81
    heart
        shadow R93.1
        sounds R01.2
    hematinuria R82.3
    hematocrit drop (precipitous) R71.0
    hemoglobinuria R82.3

Findings, abnormal, inconclusive, without diagnosis
— *continued*

human papillomavirus (HPV) DNA test positive
 cervix
  high risk R87.810
  low risk R87.820
 vagina
  high risk R87.811
  low risk R87.821
in blood (of substance not normally found in blood) R78.9
 addictive drug NEC R78.4
 alcohol (excessive level) R78.0
 cocaine R78.2
 hallucinogen R78.3
 heavy metals (abnormal level) R78.79
 lead R78.71
 lithium (abnormal level) R78.89
 opiate drug R78.1
 psychotropic drug R78.5
 specified substance NEC R78.89
 steroid agent R78.6
indoleacetic acid, elevated R82.5
ketonuria R82.4
lactic acid dehydrogenase (LDH) R74.02
liver function test — *see also* Elevated, liver function, test R79.89
mammogram NEC R92.8
 calcification (calculus) R92.1
 inconclusive result (due to dense breasts) R92.2
 microcalcification R92.0
mediastinal shift R93.89
melanin, urine R82.998
myoglobinuria R82.1
neonatal screening — *see* Abnormal, neonatal screening
newborn screens, state mandated — *see* Abnormal, neonatal screening
nonvisualization of gallbladder R93.2
odor of urine NOS R82.90
Papanicolaou cervix R87.619
 non-atypical endometrial cells R87.618
pneumoencephalogram R93.0
poikilocytosis R71.8
potassium (deficiency) E87.6
 excess E87.5
PPD R76.11
radiologic (X-ray) R93.89
 abdomen R93.5
 biliary tract R93.2
 breast R92.8
 gastrointestinal tract R93.3
 genitourinary organs R93.89
 head R93.0
 inconclusive due to excess body fat of patient R93.9
 intrathoracic organs NEC R93.1
 musculoskeletal
  limbs R93.6
  other than limb R93.7
 placenta R93.89
 retroperitoneum R93.5
 skin R93.89
 skull R93.0
 subcutaneous tissue R93.89
 testis R93.81- ☑
red blood cell (count) (morphology) (sickling) (volume) R71.8
scan NEC R94.8
 bladder R94.8
 bone R94.8
 kidney R94.4
 liver R93.2
 lung R94.2
 pancreas R94.8
 placental R94.8
 spleen R94.8
 thyroid R94.6
sedimentation rate, elevated R70.0
SGOT R74.01
SGPT R74.01
sodium (deficiency) E87.1
 excess E87.0
specified body fluid NEC R88.8
stress test R94.39
testis R93.81- ☑
thyroid (function) (metabolic rate) (scan) (uptake) R94.6
transaminase (level) R74.01
triglycerides E78.9
 high E78.1

Findings, abnormal, inconclusive, without diagnosis
— *continued*

triglycerides — *continued*
 high — *continued*
  with high cholesterol E78.2
tuberculin skin test (without active tuberculosis) R76.11
urine R82.90
 acetone R82.4
 bacteria R82.71
 bile R82.2
 casts or cells R82.998
 chyle R82.0
 culture positive R82.79
 glucose R81
 hemoglobin R82.3
 ketone R82.4
 sugar R81
vanillylmandelic acid (VMA), elevated R82.5
vectorcardiogram (VCG) R94.39
ventriculogram R93.0
white blood cell (count) (differential) (morphology) D72.9
xerography R92.8

Finger — *see* condition
Fire, Saint Anthony's — *see* Erysipelas
Fire-setting
 pathological (compulsive) F63.1
Fish hook stomach K31.89
Fishmeal-worker's lung J67.8
Fissure, fissured
anus, anal K60.2
 acute K60.0
 chronic K60.1
 congenital Q43.8
ear, lobule, congenital Q17.8
epiglottis (congenital) Q31.8
larynx J38.7
 congenital Q31.8
lip K13.0
 congenital — *see* Cleft, lip
nipple N64.0
 associated with
  lactation O92.13
  pregnancy O92.11- ☑
  puerperium O92.12
nose Q30.2
palate (congenital) — *see* Cleft, palate
skin R23.4
spine (congenital) — *see also* Spina bifida
 with hydrocephalus — *see* Spina bifida, by site, with hydrocephalus
tongue (acquired) K14.5
 congenital Q38.3

Fistula (cutaneous) L98.8
abdomen (wall) K63.2
 bladder N32.2
 intestine NEC K63.2
 ureter N28.89
 uterus N82.5
abdominorectal K63.2
abdominosigmoidal K63.2
abdominothoracic J86.0
abdominouterine N82.5
 congenital Q51.7
abdominovesical N32.2
accessory sinuses — *see* Sinusitis
actinomycotic — *see* Actinomycosis
alveolar antrum — *see* Sinusitis, maxillary
alveolar process K04.6
anorectal K60.5
antrobuccal — *see* Sinusitis, maxillary
antrum — *see* Sinusitis, maxillary
anus, anal (recurrent) (infectional) K60.3
 congenital Q43.6
  with absence, atresia and stenosis Q42.2
 tuberculous A18.32
aorta-duodenal I77.2
appendix, appendicular K38.3
arteriovenous (acquired) (nonruptured) I77.0
 brain I67.1
  congenital Q28.2
   ruptured — *see* Fistula, arteriovenous, brain, ruptured
  ruptured I60.8
   intracerebral I61.8
   intraparenchymal I61.8
   intraventricular I61.5
   subarachnoid I60.8

Fistula — *continued*
arteriovenous — *continued*
 cerebral — *see* Fistula, arteriovenous, brain
 congenital (peripheral) — *see also* Malformation, arteriovenous
  brain Q28.2
   ruptured — *see* Fistula, arteriovenous, brain, ruptured
  coronary Q24.5
  pulmonary Q25.72
 coronary I25.41
  congenital Q24.5
 pulmonary I28.0
  congenital Q25.72
 surgically created (for dialysis) Z99.2
  complication — *see* Complication, arteriovenous, fistula, surgically created
 traumatic — *see* Injury, blood vessel
artery I77.2
aural (mastoid) — *see* Mastoiditis, chronic
auricle — *see also* Disorder, pinna, specified type NEC
 congenital Q18.1
Bartholin's gland N82.8
bile duct (common) (hepatic) K83.3
 with calculus, stones — *see also* Calculus, bile duct K83.3
biliary (tract) — *see* Fistula, bile duct
bladder (sphincter) NEC — *see* Fistula, vesico- N32.2
 into seminal vesicle N32.2
bone — *see also* Disorder, bone, specified type NEC
 with osteomyelitis, chronic — *see* Osteomyelitis, chronic, with draining sinus
brain G93.89
 arteriovenous (acquired) — *see also* Fistula, arteriovenous, brain I67.1
 congenital Q28.2
branchial (cleft) Q18.0
branchiogenous Q18.0
breast N61.0
 puerperal, postpartum or gestational, due to mastitis (purulent) — *see* Mastitis, obstetric, purulent
bronchial J86.0
bronchocutaneous, bronchomediastinal, bronchopleural, bronchopleuromediastinal (infective) J86.0
 tuberculous NEC A15.5
bronchoesophageal J86.0
 congenital Q39.2
  with atresia of esophagus Q39.1
bronchovisceral J86.0
buccal cavity (infective) K12.2
cecosigmoidal K63.2
cecum K63.2
cerebrospinal (fluid) G96.08
cervical, lateral Q18.1
cervicoaural Q18.1
cervicosigmoidal N82.4
cervicovesical N82.1
cervix N82.8
chest (wall) J86.0
cholecystenteric — *see* Fistula, gallbladder
cholecystocolic — *see* Fistula, gallbladder
cholecystocolonic — *see* Fistula, gallbladder
cholecystoduodenal — *see* Fistula, gallbladder
cholecystogastric — *see* Fistula, gallbladder
cholecystointestinal — *see* Fistula, gallbladder
choledochoduodenal — *see* Fistula, bile duct
cholocolic K82.3
coccyx — *see* Sinus, pilonidal
colon K63.2
colostomy K94.09
colovesical N32.1
common duct — *see* Fistula, bile duct
congenital, site not listed — *see* Anomaly, by site
coronary, arteriovenous I25.41
 congenital Q24.5
costal region J86.0
cul-de-sac, Douglas' N82.8
cystic duct — *see also* Fistula, gallbladder
 congenital Q44.5
dental K04.6
diaphragm J86.0
duodenum K31.6
ear (external) (canal) — *see* Disorder, ear, external, specified type NEC
enterocolic K63.2
enterocutaneous K63.2
enterouterine N82.4

Fistula — *continued*
  enterouterine — *continued*
    congenital Q51.7
  enterovaginal N82.4
    congenital Q52.2
    large intestine N82.3
    small intestine N82.2
  enterovesical N32.1
  epididymis N50.89
    tuberculous A18.15
  esophagobronchial J86.0
    congenital Q39.2
      with atresia of esophagus Q39.1
  esophagocutaneous K22.89
  esophagopleural-cutaneous J86.0
  esophagotracheal J86.0
    congenital Q39.2
      with atresia of esophagus Q39.1
  esophagus K22.89
    congenital Q39.2
      with atresia of esophagus Q39.1
  ethmoid — *see* Sinusitis, ethmoidal
  eyeball (cornea) (sclera) — *see* Disorder, globe, hypotony
  eyelid H01.8
  fallopian tube, external N82.5
  fecal K63.2
    congenital Q43.6
  from periapical abscess K04.6
  frontal sinus — *see* Sinusitis, frontal
  gallbladder K82.3
    with calculus, cholelithiasis, stones — *see* Calculus, gallbladder
  gastric K31.6
  gastrocolic K31.6
    congenital Q40.2
    tuberculous A18.32
  gastroenterocolic K31.6
  gastroesophageal K31.6
  gastrojejunal K31.6
  gastrojejunocolic K31.6
  genital tract (female) N82.9
    specified NEC N82.8
    to intestine NEC N82.4
    to skin N82.5
  hepatic artery-portal vein, congenital Q26.6
  hepatopleural J86.0
  hepatopulmonary J86.0
  ileorectal or ileosigmoidal K63.2
  ileovaginal N82.2
  ileovesical N32.1
  ileum K63.2
  in ano K60.3
    tuberculous A18.32
  inner ear (labyrinth) — *see* subcategory H83.1 ☑
  intestine NEC K63.2
  intestinocolonic (abdominal) K63.2
  intestinoureteral N28.89
  intestinouterine N82.4
  intestinovaginal N82.4
    large intestine N82.3
    small intestine N82.2
  intestinovesical N32.1
  ischiorectal (fossa) K61.39
  jejunum K63.2
  joint M25.10
    ankle M25.17- ☑
    elbow M25.12- ☑
    foot joint M25.17- ☑
    hand joint M25.14- ☑
    hip M25.15- ☑
    knee M25.16- ☑
    shoulder M25.11- ☑
    specified joint NEC M25.18
    tuberculous — *see* Tuberculosis, joint
    vertebrae M25.18
    wrist M25.13- ☑
  kidney N28.89
  labium (majus) (minus) N82.8
  labyrinth — *see* subcategory H83.1 ☑
  lacrimal (gland) (sac) H04.61- ☑
  lacrimonasal duct — *see* Fistula, lacrimal
  laryngotracheal, congenital Q34.8
  larynx J38.7
  lip K13.0
    congenital Q38.0
  lumbar, tuberculous A18.01
  lung J86.0

Fistula — *continued*
  lymphatic I89.8
  mammary (gland) N61.0
  mastoid (process) (region) — *see* Mastoiditis, chronic
  maxillary J32.0
  medial, face and neck Q18.8
  mediastinal J86.0
  mediastinobronchial J86.0
  mediastinocutaneous J86.0
  middle ear — *see* subcategory H74.8 ☑
  mouth K12.2
  nasal J34.89
    sinus — *see* Sinusitis
  nasopharynx J39.2
  nipple N64.0
  nose J34.89
  oral (cutaneous) K12.2
    maxillary J32.0
    nasal (with cleft palate) — *see* Cleft, palate
  orbit, orbital — *see* Disorder, orbit, specified type NEC
  oroantral J32.0
  oviduct, external N82.5
  palate (hard) M27.8
  pancreatic K86.89
  pancreaticoduodenal K86.89
  parotid (gland) K11.4
    region K12.2
  penis N48.89
  perianal K60.3
  pericardium (pleura) (sac) — *see* Pericarditis
  pericecal K63.2
  perineorectal K60.4
  perineosigmoidal K63.2
  perineum, perineal (with urethral involvement) NEC N36.0
    tuberculous A18.13
    ureter N28.89
  perirectal K60.4
    tuberculous A18.32
  peritoneum K65.9
  pharyngoesophageal J39.2
  pharynx J39.2
    branchial cleft (congenital) Q18.0
  pilonidal (infected) (rectum) — *see* Sinus, pilonidal
  pleura, pleural, pleurocutaneous, pleuroperitoneal J86.0
    tuberculous NEC A15.6
  pleuropericardial I31.8
  portal vein-hepatic artery, congenital Q26.6
  postauricular H70.81- ☑
  postoperative, persistent T81.83 ☑
    specified site — *see* Fistula, by site
  preauricular (congenital) Q18.1
  prostate N42.89
  pulmonary J86.0
    arteriovenous I28.0
      congenital Q25.72
    tuberculous — *see* Tuberculosis, pulmonary
  pulmonoperitoneal J86.0
  rectolabial N82.4
  rectosigmoid (intercommunicating) K63.2
  rectoureteral N28.89
  rectourethral N36.0
    congenital Q64.73
  rectouterine N82.4
    congenital Q51.7
  rectovaginal N82.3
    congenital Q52.2
    tuberculous A18.18
  rectovesical N32.1
    congenital Q64.79
  rectovesicovaginal N82.3
  rectovulval N82.4
    congenital Q52.79
  rectum (to skin) K60.4
    congenital Q43.6
      with absence, atresia and stenosis Q42.0
    tuberculous A18.32
  renal N28.89
  retroauricular — *see* Fistula, postauricular
  salivary duct or gland (any) K11.4
    congenital Q38.4
  scrotum (urinary) N50.89
    tuberculous A18.15
  semicircular canals — *see* subcategory H83.1 ☑
  sigmoid K63.2
    to bladder N32.1
  sinus — *see* Sinusitis

Fistula — *continued*
  skin L98.8
    to genital tract (female) N82.5
  splenocolic D73.89
  stercoral K63.2
  stomach K31.6
  sublingual gland K11.4
  submandibular gland K11.4
  submaxillary (gland) K11.4
    region K12.2
  thoracic J86.0
    duct I89.8
  thoracoabdominal J86.0
  thoracogastric J86.0
  thoracointestinal J86.0
  thorax J86.0
  thyroglossal duct Q89.2
  thyroid E07.89
  trachea, congenital (external) (internal) Q32.1
  tracheoesophageal J86.0
    congenital Q39.2
      with atresia of esophagus Q39.1
    following tracheostomy J95.04
  traumatic arteriovenous — *see* Injury, blood vessel, by site
  tuberculous — *code by* site under Tuberculosis
  typhoid A01.09
  umbilicourinary Q64.8
  urachus, congenital Q64.4
  ureter (persistent) N28.89
  ureteroabdominal N28.89
  ureterorectal N28.89
  ureterosigmoido-abdominal N28.89
  ureterovaginal N82.1
  ureterovesical N32.2
  urethra N36.0
    congenital Q64.79
    tuberculous A18.13
  urethroperineal N36.0
  urethroperineovesical N32.2
  urethrorectal N36.0
    congenital Q64.73
  urethroscrotal N50.89
  urethrovaginal N82.1
  urethrovesical N32.2
  urinary (tract) (persistent) (recurrent) N36.0
  uteroabdominal N82.5
    congenital Q51.7
  uteroenteric, uterointestinal N82.4
    congenital Q51.7
  uterorectal N82.4
    congenital Q51.7
  uteroureteric N82.1
  uterourethral Q51.7
  uterovaginal N82.8
  uterovesical N82.1
    congenital Q51.7
  uterus N82.8
  vagina (postpartal) (wall) N82.8
  vaginocutaneous (postpartal) N82.5
  vaginointestinal NEC N82.4
    large intestine N82.3
    small intestine N82.2
  vaginoperineal N82.5
  vasocutaneous, congenital Q55.7
  vesical NEC N32.2
  vesicoabdominal N32.2
  vesicocervicovaginal N82.1
  vesicocolic N32.1
  vesicocutaneous N32.2
  vesicoenteric N32.1
  vesicointestinal N32.1
  vesicometrorectal N82.4
  vesicoperineal N32.2
  vesicorectal N32.1
    congenital Q64.79
  vesicosigmoidal N32.1
  vesicosigmoidovaginal N82.3
  vesicoureteral N32.2
  vesicoureterovaginal N82.1
  vesicourethral N32.2
  vesicourethrorectal N32.1
  vesicouterine N82.1
    congenital Q51.7
  vesicovaginal N82.0
  vulvorectal N82.4
    congenital Q52.79
Fit R56.9
  epileptic — *see* Epilepsy

☑ **Additional Character Required — Refer to the Tabular List for Character Selection**

Fit — *continued*
 fainting R55
 hysterical F44.5
 newborn P90
Fitting (and adjustment) (of)
 artificial
  arm — *see* Admission, adjustment, artificial, arm
  breast Z44.3 ☑
  eye Z44.2 ☑
  leg — *see* Admission, adjustment, artificial, leg
 automatic implantable cardiac defibrillator (with synchronous cardiac pacemaker) Z45.02
 brain neuropacemaker Z46.2
  implanted Z45.42
 cardiac defibrillator — *see* Fitting (and adjustment) (of), automatic implantable cardiac defibrillator
 catheter, non-vascular Z46.82
 colostomy belt Z46.89
 contact lenses Z46.0
 CRT-D (resynchronization therapy defibrillator) Z45.02
 CRT-P (cardiac resynchronization therapy pacemaker) Z45.018
  pulse generator Z45.010
 cystostomy device Z46.6
 defibrillator, cardiac — *see* Fitting (and adjustment) (of), automatic implantable cardiac defibrillator
 dentures Z46.3
 device NOS Z46.9
  abdominal Z46.89
  gastrointestinal NEC Z46.59
  implanted NEC Z45.89
  nervous system Z46.2
   implanted — *see* Admission, adjustment, device, implanted, nervous system
  orthodontic Z46.4
  orthoptic Z46.0
  orthotic Z46.89
  prosthetic (external) Z44.9
   breast Z44.3 ☑
   dental Z46.3
   eye Z44.2 ☑
   specified NEC Z44.8
  specified NEC Z46.89
  substitution
   auditory Z46.2
    implanted — *see* Admission, adjustment, device, implanted, hearing device
   nervous system Z46.2
    implanted — *see* Admission, adjustment, device, implanted, nervous system
   visual Z46.2
    implanted Z45.31
  urinary Z46.6
 gastric lap band Z46.51
 gastrointestinal appliance NEC Z46.59
 glasses (reading) Z46.0
 hearing aid Z46.1
 ileostomy device Z46.89
 insulin pump Z46.81
 intestinal appliance NEC Z46.89
 myringotomy device (stent) (tube) Z45.82
 neuropacemaker Z46.2
  implanted Z45.42
 non-vascular catheter Z46.82
 orthodontic device Z46.4
 orthopedic device (brace) (cast) (corset) (shoes) Z46.89
 pacemaker (cardiac) (cardiac resynchronization therapy (CRT-P)) Z45.018
  nervous system (brain) (peripheral nerve) (spinal cord) Z46.2
  implanted Z45.42
  pulse generator Z45.010
 portacath (port-a-cath) Z45.2
 prosthesis (external) Z44.9
  arm — *see* Admission, adjustment, artificial, arm
  breast Z44.3 ☑
  dental Z46.3
  eye Z44.2 ☑
  leg — *see* Admission, adjustment, artificial, leg
  specified NEC Z44.8
 spectacles Z46.0
 wheelchair Z46.89
Fitzhugh-Curtis syndrome
 due to
  Chlamydia trachomatis A74.81
  Neisseria gonorrhoea (gonococcal peritonitis) A54.85

Fitz's syndrome (acute hemorrhagic pancreatitis) — *see also* Pancreatitis, acute K85.80
Fixation
 joint — *see* Ankylosis
 larynx J38.7
 stapes — *see* Ankylosis, ear ossicles
  deafness — *see* Deafness, conductive
 uterus (acquired) — *see* Malposition, uterus
 vocal cord J38.3
Flabby ridge K06.8
Flaccid — *see also* condition
 palate, congenital Q38.5
Flail
 chest S22.5 ☑
  associated with chest compression and cardiopulmonary resuscitation M96.A4
  newborn (birth injury) P13.8
 joint (paralytic) M25.20
  ankle M25.27- ☑
  elbow M25.22- ☑
  foot joint M25.27- ☑
  hand joint M25.24- ☑
  hip M25.25- ☑
  knee M25.26- ☑
  shoulder M25.21- ☑
  specified joint NEC M25.28
  wrist M25.23- ☑
Flajani's disease — *see* Hyperthyroidism, with, goiter (diffuse)
Flap, liver K71.3
Flashbacks (residual to hallucinogen use) F16.283
Flat
 chamber (eye) — *see* Disorder, globe, hypotony, flat anterior chamber
 chest, congenital Q67.8
 foot (acquired) (fixed type) (painful) (postural) — *see also* Deformity, limb, flat foot
  congenital (rigid) (spastic (everted)) Q66.5- ☑
  rachitic sequelae (late effect) E64.3
 organ or site, congenital NEC — *see* Anomaly, by site
 pelvis M95.5
  with disproportion (fetopelvic) O33.0
   causing obstructed labor O65.0
  congenital Q74.2
Flatau-Schilder disease G37.0
Flatback syndrome M40.30
 lumbar region M40.36
 lumbosacral region M40.37
 thoracolumbar region M40.35
Flattening
 head, femur M89.8X5
 hip — *see* Coxa, plana
 lip (congenital) Q18.8
 nose (congenital) Q67.4
  acquired M95.0
Flatulence R14.3
 psychogenic F45.8
Flatus R14.3
 vaginalis N89.8
Flax-dresser's disease J66.1
Flea bite — *see* Injury, bite, by site, superficial, insect
Flecks, glaucomatous (subcapsular) — *see* Cataract, complicated
Fleischer (-Kayser) **ring** (cornea) H18.04- ☑
Fleshy mole O02.0
Flexibilitas cerea — *see* Catalepsy
Flexion
 amputation stump (surgical) T87.89
 cervix — *see* Malposition, uterus
 contracture, joint — *see* Contraction, joint
 deformity, joint — *see also* Deformity, limb, flexion M21.20
  hip, congenital Q65.89
 uterus — *see also* Malposition, uterus
  lateral — *see* Lateroversion, uterus
Flexner-Boyd dysentery A03.2
Flexner's dysentery A03.1
Flexure — *see* Flexion
Flint murmur (aortic insufficiency) I35.1
Floater, vitreous — *see* Opacity, vitreous
Floating
 cartilage (joint) — *see also* Loose, body, joint
  knee — *see* Derangement, knee, loose body
 gallbladder, congenital Q44.1
 kidney N28.89
  congenital Q63.8
 spleen D73.89

Flooding N92.0
Floor — *see* condition
Floppy
 baby syndrome (nonspecific) P94.2
 iris syndrome (intraoperative) (IFIS) H21.81
 nonrheumatic mitral valve syndrome I34.1
Flu — *see also* Influenza
 avian — *see also* Influenza, due to, identified novel influenza A virus J09.X2
 bird — *see also* Influenza, due to, identified novel influenza A virus J09.X2
 intestinal NEC A08.4
 swine (viruses that normally cause infections in pigs) — *see also* Influenza, due to, identified novel influenza A virus J09.X2
Fluctuating blood pressure I99.8
Fluid
 abdomen R18.8
 chest J94.8
 heart — *see* Failure, heart, congestive
 joint — *see* Effusion, joint
 loss (acute) E86.9
 lung — *see* Edema, lung
 overload E87.70
  specified NEC E87.79
 peritoneal cavity R18.8
 pleural cavity J94.8
 retention R60.9
Flukes NEC — *see also* Infestation, fluke
 blood NEC — *see* Schistosomiasis
 liver B66.3
Fluor (vaginalis) N89.8
 trichomonal or due to Trichomonas (vaginalis) A59.00
Fluorosis
 dental K00.3
 skeletal M85.10
  ankle M85.17- ☑
  foot M85.17- ☑
  forearm M85.13- ☑
  hand M85.14- ☑
  lower leg M85.16- ☑
  multiple site M85.19
  neck M85.18
  rib M85.18
  shoulder M85.11- ☑
  skull M85.18
  specified site NEC M85.18
  thigh M85.15- ☑
  toe M85.17- ☑
  upper arm M85.12- ☑
  vertebra M85.18
Flush syndrome E34.0
Flushing R23.2
 menopausal N95.1
Flutter
 atrial or auricular I48.92
  atypical I48.4
  type I I48.3
  type II I48.4
  typical I48.3
 heart I49.8
  atrial or auricular I48.92
   atypical I48.4
   type I I48.3
   type II I48.4
   typical I48.3
  ventricular I49.02
 ventricular I49.02
FNHTR (febrile nonhemolytic transfusion reaction) R50.84
Fochier's abscess — *code by* site under Abscess
Focus, Assmann's — *see* Tuberculosis, pulmonary
Fogo selvagem L10.3
Foix-Alajouanine syndrome G95.19
Fold, folds (anomalous) — *see also* Anomaly, by site
 Descemet's membrane — *see* Change, corneal membrane, Descemet's, fold
 epicanthic Q10.3
 heart Q24.8
Folie à deux F24
Follicle
 cervix (nabothian) (ruptured) N88.8
 graafian, ruptured, with hemorrhage N83.0- ☑
 nabothian N88.8
Follicular — *see* condition
Folliculitis (superficial) L73.9
 abscedens et suffodiens L66.3
 cyst N83.0- ☑

Folliculitis — *continued*
  decalvans L66.2
  deep — *see* Furuncle, by site
  gonococcal (acute) (chronic) A54.01
  keloid, keloidalis L73.0
  pustular L01.02
  ulerythematosa reticulata L66.4
Folliculome lipidique
  specified site — *see* Neoplasm, benign, by site
  unspecified site
    female D27.9
    male D29.20
Følling's disease E70.0
Follow-up — *see* Examination, follow-up
Fong's syndrome (hereditary osteo-onychodysplasia)
    Q87.2
Food
  allergy L27.2
  asphyxia (from aspiration or inhalation) — *see* Foreign
      body, by site
  choked on — *see* Foreign body, by site
  deprivation T73.0 ☑
    specified kind of food NEC E63.8
  insecurity Z59.41
  intoxication — *see* Poisoning, food
  lack of T73.0 ☑
  poisoning — *see* Poisoning, food
  rejection NEC — *see* Disorder, eating
  strangulation or suffocation — *see* Foreign body, by
      site
  toxemia — *see* Poisoning, food
Foot — *see* condition
Foramen ovale (nonclosure) (patent) (persistent) Q21.12
Forbes' glycogen storage disease E74.03
Fordyce-Fox disease L75.2
Fordyce's disease (mouth) Q38.6
Forearm — *see* condition
Foreclosure on loan Z59.89
Foreign body
  with
    laceration — *see* Laceration, by site, with foreign
        body
    puncture wound — *see* Puncture, by site, with for-
        eign body
  accidentally left following a procedure T81.509 ☑
    aspiration T81.506 ☑
      resulting in
        adhesions T81.516 ☑
        obstruction T81.526 ☑
        perforation T81.536 ☑
        specified complication NEC T81.596 ☑
    cardiac catheterization T81.505 ☑
      resulting in
        acute reaction T81.60 ☑
          aseptic peritonitis T81.61 ☑
          specified NEC T81.69 ☑
        adhesions T81.515 ☑
        obstruction T81.525 ☑
        perforation T81.535 ☑
        specified complication NEC T81.595 ☑
    causing
      acute reaction T81.60 ☑
        aseptic peritonitis T81.61 ☑
        specified complication NEC T81.69 ☑
      adhesions T81.519 ☑
      aseptic peritonitis T81.61 ☑
      obstruction T81.529 ☑
      perforation T81.539 ☑
      specified complication NEC T81.599 ☑
    endoscopy T81.504 ☑
      resulting in
        adhesions T81.514 ☑
        obstruction T81.524 ☑
        perforation T81.534 ☑
        specified complication NEC T81.594 ☑
    immunization T81.503 ☑
      resulting in
        adhesions T81.513 ☑
        obstruction T81.523 ☑
        perforation T81.533 ☑
        specified complication NEC T81.593 ☑
    infusion T81.501 ☑
      resulting in
        adhesions T81.511 ☑
        obstruction T81.521 ☑
        perforation T81.531 ☑

Foreign body — *continued*
  accidentally left following a procedure — *continued*
    infusion — *continued*
      resulting in — *continued*
        specified complication NEC T81.591 ☑
    injection T81.503 ☑
      resulting in
        adhesions T81.513 ☑
        obstruction T81.523 ☑
        perforation T81.533 ☑
        specified complication NEC T81.593 ☑
    kidney dialysis T81.502 ☑
      resulting in
        adhesions T81.512 ☑
        obstruction T81.522 ☑
        perforation T81.532 ☑
        specified complication NEC T81.592 ☑
    packing removal T81.507 ☑
      resulting in
        acute reaction T81.60 ☑
          aseptic peritonitis T81.61 ☑
          specified NEC T81.69 ☑
        adhesions T81.517 ☑
        obstruction T81.527 ☑
        perforation T81.537 ☑
        specified complication NEC T81.597 ☑
    puncture T81.506 ☑
      resulting in
        adhesions T81.516 ☑
        obstruction T81.526 ☑
        perforation T81.536 ☑
        specified complication NEC T81.596 ☑
    specified procedure NEC T81.508 ☑
      resulting in
        acute reaction T81.60 ☑
          aseptic peritonitis T81.61 ☑
          specified NEC T81.69 ☑
        adhesions T81.518 ☑
        obstruction T81.528 ☑
        perforation T81.538 ☑
        specified complication NEC T81.598 ☑
    surgical operation T81.500 ☑
      resulting in
        acute reaction T81.60 ☑
          aseptic peritonitis T81.61 ☑
          specified NEC T81.69 ☑
        adhesions T81.510 ☑
        obstruction T81.520 ☑
        perforation T81.530 ☑
        specified complication NEC T81.590 ☑
    transfusion T81.501 ☑
      resulting in
        adhesions T81.511 ☑
        obstruction T81.521 ☑
        perforation T81.531 ☑
        specified complication NEC T81.591 ☑
  alimentary tract T18.9 ☑
    anus T18.5 ☑
    colon T18.4 ☑
    esophagus — *see* Foreign body, esophagus
    mouth T18.0 ☑
    multiple sites T18.8 ☑
    rectosigmoid (junction) T18.5 ☑
    rectum T18.5 ☑
    small intestine T18.3 ☑
    specified site NEC T18.8 ☑
    stomach T18.2 ☑
  anterior chamber (eye) S05.5- ☑
  auditory canal — *see* Foreign body, entering through
      orifice, ear
  bronchus T17.508 ☑
    causing
      asphyxiation T17.500 ☑
        food (bone) (seed) T17.520 ☑
        gastric contents (vomitus) T17.510 ☑
        specified type NEC T17.590 ☑
      injury NEC T17.508 ☑
        food (bone) (seed) T17.528 ☑
        gastric contents (vomitus) T17.518 ☑
        specified type NEC T17.598 ☑
  canthus — *see* Foreign body, conjunctival sac
  ciliary body (eye) S05.5- ☑
  conjunctival sac T15.1- ☑
  cornea T15.0- ☑
  entering through orifice
    accessory sinus T17.0 ☑

Foreign body — *continued*
  entering through orifice — *continued*
    alimentary canal T18.9 ☑
      multiple parts T18.8 ☑
      specified part NEC T18.8 ☑
    alveolar process T18.0 ☑
    antrum (Highmore's) T17.0 ☑
    anus T18.5 ☑
    appendix T18.4 ☑
    auditory canal — *see* Foreign body, entering
        through orifice, ear
    auricle — *see* Foreign body, entering through ori-
        fice, ear
    bladder T19.1 ☑
    bronchioles — *see* Foreign body, respiratory tract,
        specified site NEC
    bronchus (main) — *see* Foreign body, bronchus
    buccal cavity T18.0 ☑
    canthus (inner) — *see* Foreign body, conjunctival
        sac
    cecum T18.4 ☑
    cervix (canal) (uteri) T19.3 ☑
    colon T18.4 ☑
    conjunctival sac — *see* Foreign body, conjunctival
        sac
    cornea — *see* Foreign body, cornea
    digestive organ or tract NOS T18.9 ☑
      multiple parts T18.8 ☑
      specified part NEC T18.8 ☑
    duodenum T18.3 ☑
    ear (external) T16.- ☑
    esophagus — *see* Foreign body, esophagus
    eye (external) NOS T15.9- ☑
      conjunctival sac — *see* Foreign body, conjuncti-
          val sac
      cornea — *see* Foreign body, cornea
      specified part NEC T15.8- ☑
    eyeball — *see also* Foreign body, entering through
        orifice, eye, specified part NEC
      with penetrating wound — *see* Puncture, eyeball
    eyelid — *see also* Foreign body, conjunctival sac
      with
        laceration — *see* Laceration, eyelid, with for-
            eign body
        puncture — *see* Puncture, eyelid, with foreign
            body
        superficial injury — *see* Foreign body, super-
            ficial, eyelid
    gastrointestinal tract T18.9 ☑
      multiple parts T18.8 ☑
      specified part NEC T18.8 ☑
    genitourinary tract T19.9 ☑
      multiple parts T19.8 ☑
      specified part NEC T19.8 ☑
    globe — *see* Foreign body, entering through orifice,
        eyeball
    gum T18.0 ☑
    Highmore's antrum T17.0 ☑
    hypopharynx — *see* Foreign body, pharynx
    ileum T18.3 ☑
    intestine (small) T18.3 ☑
      large T18.4 ☑
    lacrimal apparatus (punctum) — *see* Foreign body,
        entering through orifice, eye, specified part
        NEC
    large intestine T18.4 ☑
    larynx — *see* Foreign body, larynx
    lung — *see* Foreign body, respiratory tract, specified
        site NEC
    maxillary sinus T17.0 ☑
    mouth T18.0 ☑
    nasal sinus T17.0 ☑
    nasopharynx — *see* Foreign body, pharynx
    nose (passage) T17.1 ☑
    nostril T17.1 ☑
    oral cavity T18.0 ☑
    palate T18.0 ☑
    penis T19.4 ☑
    pharynx — *see* Foreign body, pharynx
    piriform sinus — *see* Foreign body, pharynx
    rectosigmoid (junction) T18.5 ☑
    rectum T18.5 ☑
    respiratory tract — *see* Foreign body, respiratory
        tract
    sinus (accessory) (frontal) (maxillary) (nasal) T17.0 ☑
      piriform — *see* Foreign body, pharynx

☑ Additional Character Required — Refer to the Tabular List for Character Selection

Foreign body — *continued*
  entering through orifice — *continued*
    small intestine T18.3 ☑
    stomach T18.2 ☑
    suffocation by — *see* Foreign body, by site
    tear ducts or glands — *see* Foreign body, entering
      through orifice, eye, specified part NEC
    throat — *see* Foreign body, pharynx
    tongue T18.0 ☑
    tonsil, tonsillar (fossa) — *see* Foreign body, pharynx
    trachea — *see* Foreign body, trachea
    ureter T19.8 ☑
    urethra T19.0 ☑
    uterus (any part) T19.3 ☑
    vagina T19.2 ☑
    vulva T19.2 ☑
  esophagus T18.108 ☑
    causing
      injury NEC T18.108 ☑
        food (bone) (seed) T18.128 ☑
        gastric contents (vomitus) T18.118 ☑
        specified type NEC T18.198 ☑
      tracheal compression T18.100 ☑
        food (bone) (seed) T18.120 ☑
        gastric contents (vomitus) T18.110 ☑
        specified type NEC T18.190 ☑
  feeling of, in throat R09.89
  fragment — *see* Retained, foreign body fragments
    (type of)
  genitourinary tract T19.9 ☑
    bladder T19.1 ☑
    multiple parts T19.8 ☑
    penis T19.4 ☑
    specified site NEC T19.8 ☑
    urethra T19.0 ☑
    uterus T19.3 ☑
      IUD Z97.5
    vagina T19.2 ☑
      contraceptive device Z97.5
    vulva T19.2 ☑
  granuloma (old) (soft tissue) — *see also* Granuloma,
    foreign body
    skin L92.3
  in
    laceration — *see* Laceration, by site, with foreign
      body
    puncture wound — *see* Puncture, by site, with for-
      eign body
    soft tissue (residual) M79.5
  inadvertently left in operation wound — *see* Foreign
    body, accidentally left during a procedure
  ingestion, ingested NOS T18.9 ☑
  inhalation or inspiration — *see* Foreign body, by site
  internal organ, not entering through a natural orifice
    — code as specific injury with foreign body
  intraocular S05.5- ☑
    old, retained (nonmagnetic) H44.70- ☑
      anterior chamber H44.71- ☑
      ciliary body H44.72- ☑
      iris H44.72- ☑
      lens H44.73- ☑
      magnetic H44.60- ☑
        anterior chamber H44.61- ☑
        ciliary body H44.62- ☑
        iris H44.62- ☑
        lens H44.63- ☑
        posterior wall H44.64- ☑
        specified site NEC H44.69- ☑
        vitreous body H44.65- ☑
      posterior wall H44.74- ☑
      specified site NEC H44.79- ☑
      vitreous body H44.75- ☑
    iris — *see* Foreign body, intraocular
  lacrimal punctum — *see* Foreign body, entering
    through orifice, eye, specified part NEC
  larynx T17.308 ☑
    causing
      asphyxiation T17.300 ☑
        food (bone) (seed) T17.320 ☑
        gastric contents (vomitus) T17.310 ☑
        specified type NEC T17.390 ☑
      injury NEC T17.308 ☑
        food (bone) (seed) T17.328 ☑
        gastric contents (vomitus) T17.318 ☑
        specified type NEC T17.398 ☑
  lens — *see* Foreign body, intraocular

Foreign body — *continued*
  ocular muscle S05.4- ☑
    old, retained — *see* Foreign body, orbit, old
  old or residual
    soft tissue (residual) M79.5
  operation wound, left accidentally — *see* Foreign body,
    accidentally left during a procedure
  orbit S05.4- ☑
    old, retained H05.5- ☑
  pharynx T17.208 ☑
    causing
      asphyxiation T17.200 ☑
        food (bone) (seed) T17.220 ☑
        gastric contents (vomitus) T17.210 ☑
        specified type NEC T17.290 ☑
      injury NEC T17.208 ☑
        food (bone) (seed) T17.228 ☑
        gastric contents (vomitus) T17.218 ☑
        specified type NEC T17.298 ☑
  respiratory tract T17.908 ☑
    bronchioles — *see* Foreign body, respiratory tract,
      specified site NEC
    bronchus — *see* Foreign body, bronchus
    causing
      asphyxiation T17.900 ☑
        food (bone) (seed) T17.920 ☑
        gastric contents (vomitus) T17.910 ☑
        specified type NEC T17.990 ☑
      injury NEC T17.908 ☑
        food (bone) (seed) T17.928 ☑
        gastric contents (vomitus) T17.918 ☑
        specified type NEC T17.998 ☑
    larynx — *see* Foreign body, larynx
    lung — *see* Foreign body, respiratory tract, specified
      site NEC
    multiple parts — *see* Foreign body, respiratory tract,
      specified site NEC
    nasal sinus T17.0 ☑
    nasopharynx — *see* Foreign body, pharynx
    nose T17.1 ☑
    nostril T17.1 ☑
    pharynx — *see* Foreign body, pharynx
    specified site NEC T17.808 ☑
      causing
        asphyxiation T17.800 ☑
          food (bone) (seed) T17.820 ☑
          gastric contents (vomitus) T17.810 ☑
          specified type NEC T17.890 ☑
        injury NEC T17.808 ☑
          food (bone) (seed) T17.828 ☑
          gastric contents (vomitus) T17.818 ☑
          specified type NEC T17.898 ☑
    throat — *see* Foreign body, pharynx
    trachea — *see* Foreign body, trachea
  retained (old) (nonmagnetic) (in)
    anterior chamber (eye) — *see* Foreign body, intraoc-
      ular, old, retained, anterior chamber
      magnetic — *see* Foreign body, intraocular, old,
        retained, magnetic, anterior chamber
    ciliary body — *see* Foreign body, intraocular, old,
      retained, ciliary body
      magnetic — *see* Foreign body, intraocular, old,
        retained, magnetic, ciliary body
    eyelid H02.819
      left H02.816
        lower H02.815
        upper H02.814
      right H02.813
        lower H02.812
        upper H02.811
    fragments — *see* Retained, foreign body fragments
      (type of)
    globe — *see* Foreign body, intraocular, old, retained
      magnetic — *see* Foreign body, intraocular, old,
        retained, magnetic
    intraocular — *see* Foreign body, intraocular, old,
      retained
      magnetic — *see* Foreign body, intraocular, old,
        retained, magnetic
    iris — *see* Foreign body, intraocular, old, retained,
      iris
      magnetic — *see* Foreign body, intraocular, old,
        retained, magnetic, iris
    lens — *see* Foreign body, intraocular, old, retained,
      lens
      magnetic — *see* Foreign body, intraocular, old,
        retained, magnetic, lens

Foreign body — *continued*
  retained — *continued*
    muscle — *see* Foreign body, retained, soft tissue
    orbit — *see* Foreign body, orbit, old
    posterior wall of globe — *see* Foreign body, intraoc-
      ular, old, retained, posterior wall
      magnetic — *see* Foreign body, intraocular, old,
        retained, magnetic, posterior wall
    retrobulbar — *see* Foreign body, orbit, old, retrob-
      ulbar
    soft tissue M79.5
    vitreous — *see* Foreign body, intraocular, old, re-
      tained, vitreous body
      magnetic — *see* Foreign body, intraocular, old,
        retained, magnetic, vitreous body
  retina S05.5- ☑
  superficial, without open wound
    abdomen, abdominal (wall) S30.851 ☑
    alveolar process S00.552 ☑
    ankle S90.55- ☑
    antecubital space — *see* Foreign body, superficial,
      forearm
    anus S30.857 ☑
    arm (upper) S40.85- ☑
    auditory canal — *see* Foreign body, superficial, ear
    auricle — *see* Foreign body, superficial, ear
    axilla — *see* Foreign body, superficial, arm
    back, lower S30.850 ☑
    breast S20.15- ☑
    brow S00.85 ☑
    buttock S30.850 ☑
    calf — *see* Foreign body, superficial, leg
    canthus — *see* Foreign body, superficial, eyelid
    cheek S00.85 ☑
      internal S00.552 ☑
    chest wall — *see* Foreign body, superficial, thorax
    chin S00.85 ☑
    clitoris S30.854 ☑
    costal region — *see* Foreign body, superficial, thorax
    digit(s)
      foot — *see* Foreign body, superficial, toe
      hand — *see* Foreign body, superficial, finger
    ear S00.45- ☑
    elbow S50.35- ☑
    epididymis S30.853 ☑
    epigastric region S30.851 ☑
    epiglottis S10.15 ☑
    esophagus, cervical S10.15 ☑
    eyebrow — *see* Foreign body, superficial, eyelid
    eyelid S00.25- ☑
    face S00.85 ☑
    finger(s) S60.459 ☑
      index S60.45- ☑
      little S60.45- ☑
      middle S60.45- ☑
      ring S60.45- ☑
    flank S30.851 ☑
    foot (except toe(s) alone) S90.85- ☑
      toe — *see* Foreign body, superficial, toe
    forearm S50.85- ☑
      elbow only — *see* Foreign body, superficial, el-
        bow
    forehead S00.85 ☑
    genital organs, external
      female S30.856 ☑
      male S30.855 ☑
    groin S30.851 ☑
    gum S00.552 ☑
    hand S60.55- ☑
    head S00.95 ☑
      ear — *see* Foreign body, superficial, ear
      eyelid — *see* Foreign body, superficial, eyelid
      lip S00.551 ☑
      nose S00.35 ☑
      oral cavity S00.552 ☑
      scalp S00.05 ☑
      specified site NEC S00.85 ☑
    heel — *see* Foreign body, superficial, foot
    hip S70.25- ☑
    inguinal region S30.851 ☑
    interscapular region S20.459 ☑
    jaw S00.85 ☑
    knee S80.25- ☑
    labium (majus) (minus) S30.854 ☑
    larynx S10.15 ☑
    leg (lower) S80.85- ☑

Foreign body — *continued*
superficial, without open wound — *continued*
- leg — *continued*
  - knee — *see* Foreign body, superficial, knee
  - upper — *see* Foreign body, superficial, thigh
- lip S00.551 ☑
- lower back S30.850 ☑
- lumbar region S30.850 ☑
- malar region S00.85 ☑
- mammary — *see* Foreign body, superficial, breast
- mastoid region S00.85 ☑
- mouth S00.552 ☑
- nail
  - finger — *see* Foreign body, superficial, finger
  - toe — *see* Foreign body, superficial, toe
- nape S10.85 ☑
- nasal S00.35 ☑
- neck S10.95 ☑
  - specified site NEC S10.85 ☑
  - throat S10.15 ☑
- nose S00.35 ☑
- occipital region S00.05 ☑
- oral cavity S00.552 ☑
- orbital region — *see* Foreign body, superficial, eyelid
- palate S00.552 ☑
- palm — *see* Foreign body, superficial, hand
- parietal region S00.05 ☑
- pelvis S30.850 ☑
- penis S30.852 ☑
- perineum
  - female S30.854 ☑
  - male S30.850 ☑
- periocular area — *see* Foreign body, superficial, eyelid
- phalanges
  - finger — *see* Foreign body, superficial, finger
  - toe — *see* Foreign body, superficial, toe
- pharynx S10.15 ☑
- pinna — *see* Foreign body, superficial, ear
- popliteal space — *see* Foreign body, superficial, knee
- prepuce S30.852 ☑
- pubic region S30.850 ☑
- pudendum
  - female S30.856 ☑
  - male S30.855 ☑
- sacral region S30.850 ☑
- scalp S00.05 ☑
- scapular region — *see* Foreign body, superficial, shoulder
- scrotum S30.853 ☑
- shin — *see* Foreign body, superficial, leg
- shoulder S40.25- ☑
- sternal region S20.359 ☑
- submaxillary region S00.85 ☑
- submental region S00.85 ☑
- subungual
  - finger(s) — *see* Foreign body, superficial, finger
  - toe(s) — *see* Foreign body, superficial, toe
- supraclavicular fossa S10.85 ☑
- supraorbital S00.85 ☑
- temple S00.85 ☑
- temporal region S00.85 ☑
- testis S30.853 ☑
- thigh S70.35- ☑
- thorax, thoracic (wall) S20.95 ☑
  - back S20.45- ☑
  - front S20.35- ☑
- throat S10.15 ☑
- thumb S60.35- ☑
- toe(s) (lesser) S90.456 ☑
  - great S90.45- ☑
- tongue S00.552 ☑
- trachea S10.15 ☑
- tunica vaginalis S30.853 ☑
- tympanum, tympanic membrane — *see* Foreign body, superficial, ear
- uvula S00.552 ☑
- vagina S30.854 ☑
- vocal cords S10.15 ☑
- vulva S30.854 ☑
- wrist S60.85- ☑
- swallowed T18.9 ☑
- trachea T17.408 ☑
  - causing
    - asphyxiation T17.400 ☑

Foreign body — *continued*
trachea — *continued*
- causing — *continued*
  - asphyxiation — *continued*
    - food (bone) (seed) T17.420 ☑
    - gastric contents (vomitus) T17.410 ☑
    - specified type NEC T17.490 ☑
  - injury NEC T17.408 ☑
    - food (bone) (seed) T17.428 ☑
    - gastric contents (vomitus) T17.418 ☑
    - specified type NEC T17.498 ☑
- type of fragment — *see* Retained, foreign body fragments (type of)
- vitreous (humor) S05.5- ☑

Forestier's disease (rhizomelic pseudopolyarthritis) M35.3
- meaning ankylosing hyperostosis — *see* Hyperostosis, ankylosing

Formation
- hyalin in cornea — *see* Degeneration, cornea
- sequestrum in bone (due to infection) — *see* Osteomyelitis, chronic
- valve
  - colon, congenital Q43.8
  - ureter (congenital) Q62.39

Formication R20.2
Fort Bragg fever A27.89
Fossa — *see also* condition
- pyriform — *see* condition
Foster-Kennedy syndrome H47.14- ☑
Fothergill's
- disease (trigeminal neuralgia) — *see also* Neuralgia, trigeminal
  - scarlatina anginosa A38.9
Foul breath R19.6
Foundling Z76.1
Fournier disease or gangrene N49.3
- female N76.82
- vagina and vulva N76.82
Fourth
- cranial nerve — *see* condition
- molar K00.1
Foville's (peduncular) **disease or syndrome** G46.3
Fox (-Fordyce) disease (apocrine miliaria) L75.2
FPIES (food protein-induced enterocolitis syndrome) K52.21
Fracture, burst — *see* Fracture, traumatic, by site
Fracture, chronic — *see* Fracture, pathological, by site
Fracture, insufficiency — *see* Fracture, pathological, by site
Fracture, nontraumatic, NEC
- atypical
  - femur M84.750- ☑
    - complete
      - oblique M84.759 ☑
        - left side M84.758 ☑
        - right side M84.757 ☑
      - transverse M84.756 ☑
        - left side M84.755 ☑
        - right side M84.754 ☑
    - incomplete M84.753 ☑
      - left side M84.752 ☑
      - right side M84.751 ☑
Fracture, pathological (pathologic) — *see also* Fracture, traumatic M84.40 ☑
- ankle M84.47- ☑
- carpus M84.44- ☑
- clavicle M84.41- ☑
- compression (not due to trauma) — *see also* Collapse, vertebra M48.50- ☑
- dental implant M27.63
- dental restorative material K08.539
  - with loss of material K08.531
  - without loss of material K08.530
- due to
  - neoplastic disease NEC — *see also* Neoplasm M84.50 ☑
    - ankle M84.57- ☑
    - carpus M84.54- ☑
    - clavicle M84.51- ☑
    - femur M84.55- ☑
    - fibula M84.56- ☑
    - finger M84.54- ☑
    - hip M84.559 ☑
    - humerus M84.52- ☑
    - ilium M84.550 ☑

Fracture, pathological — *continued*
due to — *continued*
- neoplastic disease — *see also* Neoplasm - *continued*
  - ischium M84.550 ☑
  - metacarpus M84.54- ☑
  - metatarsus M84.57- ☑
  - neck M84.58 ☑
  - pelvis M84.550 ☑
  - radius M84.53- ☑
  - rib M84.58 ☑
  - scapula M84.51- ☑
  - skull M84.58 ☑
  - specified site NEC M84.58 ☑
  - tarsus M84.57- ☑
  - tibia M84.56- ☑
  - toe M84.57- ☑
  - ulna M84.53- ☑
  - vertebra M84.58 ☑
- osteoporosis M80.00 ☑
  - disuse — *see* Osteoporosis, specified type NEC, with pathological fracture
  - drug-induced — *see* Osteoporosis, drug induced, with pathological fracture
  - idiopathic — *see* Osteoporosis, specified type NEC, with pathological fracture
  - postmenopausal — *see* Osteoporosis, postmenopausal, with pathological fracture
  - postoophorectomy — *see* Osteoporosis, postoophorectomy, with pathological fracture
  - postsurgical malabsorption — *see* Osteoporosis, specified type NEC, with pathological fracture
  - specified cause NEC — *see* Osteoporosis, specified type NEC, with pathological fracture
- specified disease NEC M84.60 ☑
  - ankle M84.67- ☑
  - carpus M84.64- ☑
  - clavicle M84.61- ☑
  - femur M84.65- ☑
  - fibula M84.66- ☑
  - finger M84.64- ☑
  - hip M84.65- ☑
  - humerus M84.62- ☑
  - ilium M84.650 ☑
  - ischium M84.650 ☑
  - metacarpus M84.64- ☑
  - metatarsus M84.67- ☑
  - neck M84.68 ☑
  - radius M84.63- ☑
  - rib M84.68 ☑
  - scapula M84.61- ☑
  - skull M84.68 ☑
  - tarsus M84.67- ☑
  - tibia M84.66- ☑
  - toe M84.67- ☑
  - ulna M84.63- ☑
  - vertebra M84.68 ☑
- femur M84.45- ☑
- fibula M84.46- ☑
- finger M84.44- ☑
- hip M84.459 ☑
- humerus M84.42- ☑
- ilium M84.454 ☑
- ischium M84.454 ☑
- joint prosthesis — *see* Complications, joint prosthesis, mechanical, breakdown, by site
  - periprosthetic — *see* Fracture, pathological, periprosthetic
- metacarpus M84.44- ☑
- metatarsus M84.47- ☑
- neck M84.48 ☑
- pelvis M84.454 ☑
- periprosthetic M97.9 ☑
  - ankle M97.2- ☑
  - elbow M97.4- ☑
  - finger M97.8 ☑
  - hip M97.0- ☑
  - knee M97.1- ☑
  - other specified joint M97.8 ☑
  - shoulder M97.3- ☑
  - spinal joint M97.8 ☑
  - toe joint M97.8 ☑
  - wrist joint M97.8 ☑
- radius M84.43- ☑
- restorative material (dental) K08.539

Fracture, pathological — *continued*
  restorative material — *continued*
    with loss of material K08.531
    without loss of material K08.530
  rib M84.48 ☑
  scapula M84.41- ☑
  skull M84.48 ☑
  tarsus M84.47- ☑
  tibia M84.46- ☑
  toe M84.47- ☑
  ulna M84.43- ☑
  vertebra M84.48 ☑
Fracture, traumatic (abduction) (adduction) (separation)
    — *see also* Fracture, pathological T14.8 ☑
  acetabulum S32.40- ☑
    column
      anterior (displaced) (iliopubic) S32.43- ☑
        nondisplaced S32.436 ☑
      posterior (displaced) (ilioischial) S32.443 ☑
        nondisplaced S32.44- ☑
    dome (displaced) S32.48- ☑
      nondisplaced S32.48 ☑
    specified NEC S32.49- ☑
    transverse (displaced) S32.45- ☑
      with associated posterior wall fracture (displaced)
        S32.46- ☑
        nondisplaced S32.46- ☑
      nondisplaced S32.45- ☑
    wall
      anterior (displaced) S32.41- ☑
        nondisplaced S32.41- ☑
      medial (displaced) S32.47- ☑
        nondisplaced S32.47- ☑
      posterior (displaced) S32.42- ☑
        with associated transverse fracture (displaced)
          S32.46- ☑
          nondisplaced S32.46- ☑
        nondisplaced S32.42- ☑
  acromion — *see* Fracture, scapula, acromial process
  ankle S82.899 ☑
    bimalleolar (displaced) S82.84- ☑
      nondisplaced S82.84- ☑
    lateral malleolus only (displaced) S82.6- ☑
      nondisplaced S82.6- ☑
    medial malleolus (displaced) S82.5- ☑
      associated with Maisonneuve's fracture — *see*
        Fracture, Maisonneuve's
      nondisplaced S82.5- ☑
    talus — *see* Fracture, tarsal, talus
    trimalleolar (displaced) S82.85- ☑
      nondisplaced S82.85- ☑
  arm (upper) — *see also* Fracture, humerus, shaft
    humerus — *see* Fracture, humerus
    radius — *see* Fracture, radius
    ulna — *see* Fracture, ulna
  associated with chest compression and cardiopul-
    monary resuscitation M96.A9
  astragalus — *see* Fracture, tarsal, talus
  atlas — *see* Fracture, neck, cervical vertebra, first
  axis — *see* Fracture, neck, cervical vertebra, second
  back — *see* Fracture, vertebra
  Barton's — *see* Barton's fracture
  base of skull — *see* Fracture, skull, base
  basicervical (basal) (femoral) S72.0 ☑
  Bennett's — *see* Bennett's fracture
  bimalleolar — *see* Fracture, ankle, bimalleolar
  blow-out S02.3- ☑
  bone NEC T14.8 ☑
    birth injury P13.9
    following insertion of orthopedic implant, joint
      prosthesis or bone plate — *see* Fracture, fol-
      lowing insertion of orthopedic implant, joint
      prosthesis or bone plate
    in (due to) neoplastic disease NEC — *see* Fracture,
      pathological, due to, neoplastic disease
    pathological (cause unknown) — *see* Fracture,
      pathological
  breast bone — *see* Fracture, sternum
  bucket handle (semilunar cartilage) — *see* Tear,
    meniscus
  buckle — *see* Fracture, by site, torus
  burst — *see* Fracture, traumatic, by site
  calcaneus — *see* Fracture, tarsal, calcaneus
  carpal bone(s) S62.10- ☑
    capitate (displaced) S62.13- ☑
      nondisplaced S62.13- ☑

Fracture, traumatic — *continued*
  carpal bone(s) — *continued*
    cuneiform — *see* Fracture, carpal bone, triquetrum
    hamate (body) (displaced) S62.143 ☑
      hook process (displaced) S62.15- ☑
        nondisplaced S62.15- ☑
      nondisplaced S62.14- ☑
    larger multangular — *see* Fracture, carpal bones,
      trapezium
    lunate (displaced) S62.12- ☑
      nondisplaced S62.12- ☑
    navicular S62.00- ☑
      distal pole (displaced) S62.01- ☑
        nondisplaced S62.01- ☑
      middle third (displaced) S62.02- ☑
        nondisplaced S62.02- ☑
      proximal third (displaced) S62.03- ☑
        nondisplaced S62.03- ☑
      volar tuberosity — *see* Fracture, carpal bones,
        navicular, distal pole
    os magnum — *see* Fracture, carpal bones, capitate
    pisiform (displaced) S62.16- ☑
      nondisplaced S62.16- ☑
    semilunar — *see* Fracture, carpal bones, lunate
    smaller multangular — *see* Fracture, carpal bones,
      trapezoid
    trapezium (displaced) S62.17- ☑
      nondisplaced S62.17- ☑
    trapezoid (displaced) S62.18- ☑
      nondisplaced S62.18- ☑
    triquetrum (displaced) S62.11- ☑
      nondisplaced S62.11- ☑
    unciform — *see* Fracture, carpal bones, hamate
  cervical — *see* Fracture, vertebra, cervical
  clavicle S42.00- ☑
    acromial end (displaced) S42.03- ☑
      nondisplaced S42.03- ☑
    birth injury P13.4
    lateral end — *see* Fracture, clavicle, acromial end
    shaft (displaced) S42.02- ☑
      nondisplaced S42.02- ☑
    sternal end (anterior) (displaced) S42.01- ☑
      nondisplaced S42.01- ☑
      posterior S42.01- ☑
  coccyx S32.2 ☑
  collapsed — *see* Collapse, vertebra
  collar bone — *see* Fracture, clavicle
  Colles' — *see* Colles' fracture
  coronoid process — *see* Fracture, ulna, upper end,
    coronoid process
  corpus cavernosum penis S39.840 ☑
  costochondral cartilage S23.41
  costochondral, costosternal junction — *see* Fracture,
    rib
  cranium — *see* Fracture, skull
  cricoid cartilage S12.8 ☑
  cuboid (ankle) — *see* Fracture, tarsal, cuboid
  cuneiform
    foot — *see* Fracture, tarsal, cuneiform
    wrist — *see* Fracture, carpal, triquetrum
  delayed union — *see* Delay, union, fracture
  dental restorative material K08.539
    with loss of material K08.531
    without loss of material K08.530
  due to
    birth injury — *see* Birth, injury, fracture
    osteoporosis — *see* Osteoporosis, with fracture
  Dupuytren's — *see* Fracture, ankle, lateral malleolus
  elbow S42.40- ☑
  ethmoid (bone) (sinus) — *see* Fracture, skull, base
  face bone S02.92 ☑
  fatigue — *see also* Fracture, stress
    vertebra M48.40 ☑
      cervical region M48.42 ☑
      cervicothoracic region M48.43 ☑
      lumbar region M48.46 ☑
      lumbosacral region M48.47 ☑
      occipito-atlanto-axial region M48.41 ☑
      sacrococcygeal region M48.48 ☑
      thoracic region M48.44 ☑
      thoracolumbar region M48.45 ☑
  femur, femoral S72.9- ☑
    basicervical (basal) S72.0 ☑
    birth injury P13.2
    capital epiphyseal S79.01- ☑

Fracture, traumatic — *continued*
  femur, femoral — *continued*
    condyles, epicondyles — *see* Fracture, femur, lower
      end
    distal end — *see* Fracture, femur, lower end
    epiphysis
      head — *see* Fracture, femur, upper end, epiphysis
      lower — *see* Fracture, femur, lower end, epiph-
        ysis
      upper — *see* Fracture, femur, upper end, epiph-
        ysis
    following insertion of implant, prosthesis or plate
      M96.66- ☑
    head — *see* Fracture, femur, upper end, head
    intertrochanteric — *see* Fracture, femur,
      trochanteric
    intratrochanteric — *see* Fracture, femur,
      trochanteric
    lower end S72.40- ☑
      condyle (displaced) S72.41- ☑
        lateral (displaced) S72.42- ☑
          nondisplaced S72.42- ☑
        medial (displaced) S72.43- ☑
          nondisplaced S72.43- ☑
        nondisplaced S72.41- ☑
      epiphysis (displaced) S72.44- ☑
        nondisplaced S72.44- ☑
      physeal S79.10- ☑
        Salter-Harris
          Type I S79.11- ☑
          Type II S79.12- ☑
          Type III S79.13- ☑
          Type IV S79.14- ☑
        specified NEC S79.19- ☑
      specified NEC S72.49- ☑
      supracondylar (displaced) S72.45- ☑
        with intracondylar extension (displaced)
          S72.46- ☑
          nondisplaced S72.46- ☑
        nondisplaced S72.45- ☑
      torus S72.47- ☑
    neck — *see* Fracture, femur, upper end, neck
    pertrochanteric — *see* Fracture, femur, trochanteric
    shaft (lower third) (middle third) (upper third)
      S72.30- ☑
      comminuted (displaced) S72.35- ☑
        nondisplaced S72.35- ☑
      oblique (displaced) S72.33- ☑
        nondisplaced S72.33- ☑
      segmental (displaced) S72.36- ☑
        nondisplaced S72.36- ☑
      specified NEC S72.39- ☑
      spiral (displaced) S72.34- ☑
        nondisplaced S72.34- ☑
      transverse (displaced) S72.32- ☑
        nondisplaced S72.32- ☑
    specified site NEC — *see* subcategory S72.8 ☑
    subcapital (displaced) S72.01- ☑
    subtrochanteric (region) (section) (displaced)
      S72.2- ☑
      nondisplaced S72.2- ☑
    transcervical — *see* Fracture, femur, midcervical
    transtrochanteric — *see* Fracture, femur,
      trochanteric
    trochanteric S72.10- ☑
      apophyseal (displaced) S72.13- ☑
        nondisplaced S72.13- ☑
      greater trochanter (displaced) S72.11- ☑
        nondisplaced S72.11- ☑
      intertrochanteric (displaced) S72.14- ☑
        nondisplaced S72.14- ☑
      lesser trochanter (displaced) S72.12- ☑
        nondisplaced S72.12- ☑
    upper end S72.00- ☑
      apophyseal (displaced) S72.13- ☑
        nondisplaced S72.13- ☑
      cervicotrochanteric — *see* Fracture, femur, upper
        end, neck, base
      epiphysis (displaced) S72.02- ☑
        nondisplaced S72.02- ☑
      head S72.05- ☑
        articular (displaced) S72.06- ☑
          nondisplaced S72.06- ☑
        specified NEC S72.09- ☑
      intertrochanteric (displaced) S72.14- ☑
        nondisplaced S72.14- ☑

Fracture, traumatic — *continued*
  femur, femoral — *continued*
    upper end — *continued*
      intracapsular S72.01- ☑
      midcervical (displaced) S72.03- ☑
        nondisplaced S72.03- ☑
      neck S72.00- ☑
        base (displaced) S72.04- ☑
          nondisplaced S72.04- ☑
        specified NEC S72.09- ☑
      pertrochanteric — *see* Fracture, femur, upper
        end, trochanteric
      physeal S79.00- ☑
        Salter-Harris type I S79.01- ☑
        specified NEC S79.09- ☑
      subcapital (displaced) S72.01- ☑
      subtrochanteric (displaced) S72.2- ☑
        nondisplaced S72.2- ☑
      transcervical — *see* Fracture, femur, upper end,
        midcervical
      trochanteric S72.10- ☑
        greater (displaced) S72.11- ☑
          nondisplaced S72.11- ☑
        lesser (displaced) S72.12- ☑
          nondisplaced S72.12- ☑
  fibula (shaft) (styloid) S82.40- ☑
    comminuted (displaced) S82.45- ☑
      nondisplaced S82.45- ☑
    following insertion of implant, prosthesis or plate
      M96.67- ☑
    involving ankle or malleolus — *see* Fracture, fibula,
      lateral malleolus
    lateral malleolus (displaced) S82.6- ☑
      nondisplaced S82.6- ☑
    lower end
      physeal S89.30- ☑
        Salter-Harris
          Type I S89.31- ☑
          Type II S89.32- ☑
        specified NEC S89.39- ☑
      specified NEC S82.83- ☑
      torus S82.82- ☑
    oblique (displaced) S82.43- ☑
      nondisplaced S82.43- ☑
    segmental (displaced) S82.46- ☑
      nondisplaced S82.46- ☑
    specified NEC S82.49- ☑
    spiral (displaced) S82.44- ☑
      nondisplaced S82.44- ☑
    transverse (displaced) S82.42- ☑
      nondisplaced S82.42- ☑
    upper end
      physeal S89.20- ☑
        Salter-Harris
          Type I S89.21- ☑
          Type II S89.22- ☑
        specified NEC S89.29- ☑
      specified NEC S82.83- ☑
      torus S82.81- ☑
  finger (except thumb) S62.60- ☑
    distal phalanx (displaced) S62.63- ☑
      nondisplaced S62.66- ☑
    index S62.60- ☑
      distal phalanx (displaced) S62.63- ☑
        nondisplaced S62.66- ☑
      middle phalanx (displaced) S62.62- ☑
        nondisplaced S62.65- ☑
      proximal phalanx (displaced) S62.61- ☑
        nondisplaced S62.64- ☑
    little S62.60- ☑
      distal phalanx (displaced) S62.63- ☑
        nondisplaced S62.66- ☑
      middle phalanx (displaced) S62.62- ☑
        nondisplaced S62.65- ☑
      proximal phalanx (displaced) S62.61- ☑
        nondisplaced S62.64- ☑
    middle S62.60- ☑
      distal phalanx (displaced) S62.63- ☑
        nondisplaced S62.66- ☑
      middle phalanx (displaced) S62.62- ☑
        nondisplaced S62.65- ☑
      proximal phalanx (displaced) S62.61- ☑
        nondisplaced S62.64- ☑
    middle phalanx (displaced) S62.62- ☑
      nondisplaced S62.65- ☑
    proximal phalanx (displaced) S62.61- ☑

Fracture, traumatic — *continued*
  finger — *continued*
    proximal phalanx — *continued*
      nondisplaced S62.64- ☑
    ring S62.60- ☑
      distal phalanx (displaced) S62.63- ☑
        nondisplaced S62.66- ☑
      middle phalanx (displaced) S62.62- ☑
        nondisplaced S62.65- ☑
      proximal phalanx (displaced) S62.61- ☑
        nondisplaced S62.64- ☑
    thumb — *see* Fracture, thumb
  following insertion (intraoperative) (postoperative) of
    orthopedic implant, joint prosthesis or bone
    plate M96.69
    femur M96.66- ☑
    fibula M96.67- ☑
    humerus M96.62- ☑
    pelvis M96.65
    radius M96.63- ☑
    specified bone NEC M96.69
    tibia M96.67- ☑
    ulna M96.63- ☑
  foot S92.90- ☑
    astragalus — *see* Fracture, tarsal, talus
    calcaneus — *see* Fracture, tarsal, calcaneus
    cuboid — *see* Fracture, tarsal, cuboid
    cuneiform — *see* Fracture, tarsal, cuneiform
    metatarsal — *see* Fracture, metatarsal
    navicular — *see* Fracture, tarsal, navicular
    sesamoid S92.81- ☑
    specified NEC S92.81- ☑
    talus — *see* Fracture, tarsal, talus
    tarsal — *see* Fracture, tarsal
    toe — *see* Fracture, toe
  forearm S52.9- ☑
    radius — *see* Fracture, radius
    ulna — *see* Fracture, ulna
  fossa (anterior) (middle) (posterior) S02.19 ☑
  fragility — *see* Fracture, pathological, due to osteoporo-
    sis
  frontal (bone) (skull) S02.0 ☑
    sinus S02.19 ☑
  glenoid (cavity) (scapula) — *see* Fracture, scapula,
    glenoid cavity
  greenstick — *see* Fracture, by site
  hallux — *see* Fracture, toe, great
  hand S62.9- ☑
    carpal — *see* Fracture, carpal bone
    finger (except thumb) — *see* Fracture, finger
    metacarpal — *see* Fracture, metacarpal
    navicular (scaphoid) (hand) — *see* Fracture, carpal
      bone, navicular
    thumb — *see* Fracture, thumb
  healed or old
    with complications — *code by* Nature of the compli-
      cation
  heel bone — *see* Fracture, tarsal, calcaneus
  Hill-Sachs S42.29- ☑
  hip — *see* Fracture, femur, neck
  humerus S42.30- ☑
    anatomical neck — *see* Fracture, humerus, upper
      end
    articular process — *see* Fracture, humerus, lower
      end
    capitellum — *see* Fracture, humerus, lower end,
      condyle, lateral
    distal end — *see* Fracture, humerus, lower end
    epiphysis
      lower — *see* Fracture, humerus, lower end, phy-
        seal
      upper — *see* Fracture, humerus, upper end,
        physeal
    external condyle — *see* Fracture, humerus, lower
      end, condyle, lateral
    following insertion of implant, prosthesis or plate
      M96.62- ☑
    great tuberosity — *see* Fracture, humerus, upper
      end, greater tuberosity
    intercondylar — *see* Fracture, humerus, lower end
    internal epicondyle — *see* Fracture, humerus, lower
      end, epicondyle, medial
    lesser tuberosity — *see* Fracture, humerus, upper
      end, lesser tuberosity
    lower end S42.40- ☑
      condyle
        lateral (displaced) S42.45- ☑

Fracture, traumatic — *continued*
  humerus — *continued*
    lower end — *continued*
      condyle — *continued*
        lateral — *continued*
          nondisplaced S42.45- ☑
        medial (displaced) S42.46- ☑
          nondisplaced S42.46- ☑
      epicondyle
        lateral (displaced) S42.43- ☑
          nondisplaced S42.43- ☑
        medial (displaced) S42.44- ☑
          incarcerated S42.44- ☑
          nondisplaced S42.44- ☑
      physeal S49.10- ☑
        Salter-Harris
          Type I S49.11- ☑
          Type II S49.12- ☑
          Type III S49.13- ☑
          Type IV S49.14- ☑
        specified NEC S49.19- ☑
      specified NEC (displaced) S42.49- ☑
        nondisplaced S42.49- ☑
      supracondylar (simple) (displaced) S42.41- ☑
        with intercondylar fracture — *see* Fracture,
          humerus, lower end
        comminuted (displaced) S42.42- ☑
          nondisplaced S42.42- ☑
        nondisplaced S42.41- ☑
      torus S42.48- ☑
      transcondylar (displaced) S42.47- ☑
        nondisplaced S42.47- ☑
    proximal end — *see* Fracture, humerus, upper end
    shaft S42.30- ☑
      comminuted (displaced) S42.35- ☑
        nondisplaced S42.35- ☑
      greenstick S42.31- ☑
      oblique (displaced) S42.33- ☑
        nondisplaced S42.33- ☑
      segmental (displaced) S42.36- ☑
        nondisplaced S42.36- ☑
      specified NEC S42.39- ☑
      spiral (displaced) S42.34- ☑
        nondisplaced S42.34- ☑
      transverse (displaced) S42.32- ☑
        nondisplaced S42.32- ☑
    supracondylar — *see* Fracture, humerus, lower end
    surgical neck — *see* Fracture, humerus, upper end,
      surgical neck
    trochlea — *see* Fracture, humerus, lower end,
      condyle, medial
    tuberosity — *see* Fracture, humerus, upper end
    upper end S42.20- ☑
      anatomical neck — *see* Fracture, humerus, upper
        end, specified NEC
      articular head — *see* Fracture, humerus, upper
        end, specified NEC
      epiphysis — *see* Fracture, humerus, upper end,
        physeal
      greater tuberosity (displaced) S42.25- ☑
        nondisplaced S42.25- ☑
      lesser tuberosity (displaced) S42.26- ☑
        nondisplaced S42.26- ☑
      physeal S49.00- ☑
        Salter-Harris
          Type I S49.01- ☑
          Type II S49.02- ☑
          Type III S49.03- ☑
          Type IV S49.04- ☑
        specified NEC S49.09- ☑
      specified NEC (displaced) S42.29- ☑
        nondisplaced S42.29- ☑
      surgical neck (displaced) S42.21- ☑
        four-part S42.24- ☑
        nondisplaced S42.21- ☑
        three-part S42.23- ☑
        two-part (displaced) S42.22- ☑
          nondisplaced S42.22- ☑
      torus S42.27- ☑
      transepiphyseal — *see* Fracture, humerus, upper
        end, physeal
  hyoid bone S12.8 ☑
  ilium S32.30- ☑
    with disruption of pelvic ring — *see* Disruption,
      pelvic ring
    avulsion (displaced) S32.31- ☑

Fracture, traumatic — *continued*
  ilium — *continued*
    avulsion — *continued*
      nondisplaced S32.31- ☑
    specified NEC S32.39- ☑
  impaction, impacted — *code as* Fracture, by site
  innominate bone — *see* Fracture, ilium
  instep — *see* Fracture, foot
  ischium S32.60- ☑
    with disruption of pelvic ring — *see* Disruption,
      pelvic ring
    avulsion (displaced) S32.61- ☑
      nondisplaced S32.61- ☑
    specified NEC S32.69- ☑
  jaw (bone) (lower) — *see* Fracture, mandible
    upper — *see* Fracture, maxilla
  joint prosthesis — *see* Complications, joint prosthesis,
    mechanical, breakdown, by site
    periprosthetic — *see* Fracture, traumatic, peripros-
      thetic
  knee cap — *see* Fracture, patella
  larynx S12.8 ☑
  late effects — *see* Sequelae, fracture
  leg (lower) S82.9- ☑
    ankle — *see* Fracture, ankle
    femur — *see* Fracture, femur
    fibula — *see* Fracture, fibula
    malleolus — *see* Fracture, ankle
    patella — *see* Fracture, patella
    specified site NEC S82.89- ☑
    tibia — *see* Fracture, tibia
  lumbar spine — *see* Fracture, vertebra, lumbar
  lumbosacral spine S32.9 ☑
  Maisonneuve's (displaced) S82.86- ☑
    nondisplaced S82.86- ☑
  malar bone — *see also* Fracture, maxilla S02.400 ☑
    left side S02.40B ☑
    right side S02.40A ☑
  malleolus — *see* Fracture, ankle
  malunion — *see* Fracture, by site
  mandible (lower jaw (bone)) S02.609 ☑
    alveolus S02.67- ☑
    angle (of jaw) S02.65- ☑
    body, unspecified S02.600 ☑
      left side S02.602 ☑
      right side S02.601 ☑
    condylar process S02.61- ☑
    coronoid process S02.63- ☑
    ramus, unspecified S02.64- ☑
    specified site NEC S02.69 ☑
    subcondylar process S02.62- ☑
    symphysis S02.66 ☑
  manubrium (sterni) S22.21 ☑
    dissociation from sternum S22.23 ☑
  march — *see* Fracture, traumatic, stress, by site
  maxilla, maxillary (bone) (sinus) (superior) (upper jaw)
    S02.401 ☑
    alveolus S02.42 ☑
    inferior — *see* Fracture, mandible
    LeFort I S02.411 ☑
    LeFort II S02.412 ☑
    LeFort III S02.413 ☑
    left side S02.40D ☑
    right side S02.40C ☑
  metacarpal S62.309 ☑
    base (displaced) S62.319 ☑
      nondisplaced S62.349 ☑
    fifth S62.30- ☑
      base (displaced) S62.31- ☑
        nondisplaced S62.34- ☑
      neck (displaced) S62.33- ☑
        nondisplaced S62.36- ☑
      shaft (displaced) S62.32- ☑
        nondisplaced S62.35- ☑
      specified NEC S62.398 ☑
    first S62.20- ☑
      base NEC (displaced) S62.23- ☑
        nondisplaced S62.23- ☑
      Bennett's — *see* Bennett's fracture
      neck (displaced) S62.25- ☑
        nondisplaced S62.25- ☑
      shaft (displaced) S62.24- ☑
        nondisplaced S62.24- ☑
      specified NEC S62.29- ☑
    fourth S62.30- ☑
      base (displaced) S62.31- ☑

Fracture, traumatic — *continued*
  metacarpal — *continued*
    fourth — *continued*
      base — *continued*
        nondisplaced S62.34- ☑
      neck (displaced) S62.33- ☑
        nondisplaced S62.36- ☑
      shaft (displaced) S62.32- ☑
        nondisplaced S62.35- ☑
      specified NEC S62.39- ☑
    neck (displaced) S62.33- ☑
      nondisplaced S62.36- ☑
    Rolando's — *see* Rolando's fracture
    second S62.30- ☑
      base (displaced) S62.31- ☑
        nondisplaced S62.34- ☑
      neck (displaced) S62.33- ☑
        nondisplaced S62.36- ☑
      shaft (displaced) S62.32- ☑
        nondisplaced S62.35- ☑
      specified NEC S62.39- ☑
    shaft (displaced) S62.32- ☑
      nondisplaced S62.35- ☑
    specified NEC S62.399 ☑
    third S62.30- ☑
      base (displaced) S62.31- ☑
        nondisplaced S62.34- ☑
      neck (displaced) S62.33- ☑
        nondisplaced S62.36- ☑
      shaft (displaced) S62.32- ☑
        nondisplaced S62.35- ☑
      specified NEC S62.39- ☑
  metaphyseal — *see* Fracture, traumatic, by site, shaft
  metastatic — *see* Fracture, pathological, due to, neo-
    plastic disease — *see also* Neoplasm
  metatarsal bone S92.30- ☑
    fifth (displaced) S92.35- ☑
      nondisplaced S92.35- ☑
    first (displaced) S92.31- ☑
      nondisplaced S92.31- ☑
    fourth (displaced) S92.34- ☑
      nondisplaced S92.34- ☑
    physeal S99.10- ☑
      Salter-Harris
        Type I S99.11- ☑
        Type II S99.12- ☑
        Type III S99.13- ☑
        Type IV S99.14- ☑
      specified NEC S99.19- ☑
    second (displaced) S92.32- ☑
      nondisplaced S92.32- ☑
    third (displaced) S92.33- ☑
      nondisplaced S92.33- ☑
  Monteggia's — *see* Monteggia's fracture
  multiple
    hand (and wrist) NEC — *see* Fracture, by site
    ribs — *see* Fracture, rib, multiple
  nasal (bone(s)) S02.2 ☑
  navicular (scaphoid) (foot) — *see also* Fracture, tarsal,
    navicular
    hand — *see* Fracture, carpal, navicular
  neck S12.9 ☑
    cervical vertebra S12.9 ☑
      fifth (displaced) S12.400 ☑
        nondisplaced S12.401 ☑
        specified type NEC (displaced) S12.490 ☑
          nondisplaced S12.491 ☑
      first (displaced) S12.000 ☑
        burst (stable) S12.01 ☑
          unstable S12.02 ☑
        lateral mass (displaced) S12.040 ☑
          nondisplaced S12.041 ☑
        nondisplaced S12.001 ☑
        posterior arch (displaced) S12.030 ☑
          nondisplaced S12.031 ☑
        specified type NEC (displaced) S12.090 ☑
          nondisplaced S12.091 ☑
      fourth (displaced) S12.300 ☑
        nondisplaced S12.301 ☑
        specified type NEC (displaced) S12.390 ☑
          nondisplaced S12.391 ☑
      second (displaced) S12.100 ☑
        dens (anterior) (displaced) (type II) S12.110 ☑
          nondisplaced S12.112 ☑
          posterior S12.111 ☑
          specified type NEC (displaced) S12.120 ☑

Fracture, traumatic — *continued*
  neck — *continued*
    cervical vertebra — *continued*
      second — *continued*
        dens — *continued*
          specified type — *continued*
            nondisplaced S12.121 ☑
        nondisplaced S12.101 ☑
        specified type NEC (displaced) S12.190 ☑
          nondisplaced S12.191 ☑
      seventh (displaced) S12.600 ☑
        nondisplaced S12.601 ☑
        specified type NEC (displaced) S12.690 ☑
          nondisplaced S12.691 ☑
      sixth (displaced) S12.500 ☑
        nondisplaced S12.501 ☑
        specified type NEC (displaced) S12.590 ☑
          nondisplaced S12.591 ☑
      third (displaced) S12.200 ☑
        nondisplaced S12.201 ☑
        specified type NEC (displaced) S12.290 ☑
          nondisplaced S12.291 ☑
    hyoid bone S12.8 ☑
    larynx S12.8 ☑
    specified site NEC S12.8 ☑
    thyroid cartilage S12.8 ☑
    trachea S12.8 ☑
  neoplastic NEC — *see* Fracture, pathological, due to,
    neoplastic disease
  neural arch — *see* Fracture, vertebra
  newborn — *see* Birth, injury, fracture
  nontraumatic — *see* Fracture, pathological
  nonunion — *see* Nonunion, fracture
  nose, nasal (bone) (septum) S02.2 ☑
  occiput — *see* Fracture, skull, base, occiput
  odontoid process — *see* Fracture, neck, cervical verte-
    bra, second
  olecranon (process) (ulna) — *see* Fracture, ulna, upper
    end, olecranon process
  orbit, orbital (bone) (region) S02.85 ☑
    floor (blow-out) S02.3- ☑
    roof S02.12- ☑
    wall S02.85 ☑
      lateral S02.84- ☑
      medial S02.83- ☑
  os
    calcis — *see* Fracture, tarsal, calcaneus
    magnum — *see* Fracture, carpal, capitate
    pubis — *see* Fracture, pubis
  palate S02.8- ☑
  parietal bone (skull) S02.0 ☑
  patella S82.00- ☑
    comminuted (displaced) S82.04- ☑
      nondisplaced S82.04- ☑
    longitudinal (displaced) S82.02- ☑
      nondisplaced S82.02- ☑
    osteochondral (displaced) S82.01- ☑
      nondisplaced S82.01- ☑
    specified NEC S82.09- ☑
    transverse (displaced) S82.03- ☑
      nondisplaced S82.03- ☑
  pedicle (of vertebral arch) — *see* Fracture, vertebra
  pelvis, pelvic (bone) S32.9 ☑
    acetabulum — *see* Fracture, acetabulum
    circle — *see* Disruption, pelvic ring
    following insertion of implant, prosthesis or plate
      M96.65
    ilium — *see* Fracture, ilium
    ischium — *see* Fracture, ischium
    multiple
      with disruption of pelvic ring (circle) — *see* Dis-
        ruption, pelvic ring
      without disruption of pelvic ring (circle)
        S32.82 ☑
    pubis — *see* Fracture, pubis
    sacrum — *see* Fracture, sacrum
    specified site NEC S32.89 ☑
  periprosthetic, around internal prosthetic joint
    M97.9 ☑
    ankle M97.2- ☑
    elbow M97.4- ☑
    finger M97.8 ☑
    hip M97.0- ☑
    knee M97.1- ☑
    shoulder M97.3- ☑
    specified joint NEC M97.8 ☑

Fracture, traumatic — *continued*
- periprosthetic, around internal prosthetic joint — *continued*
    - spine M97.8 ☑
    - toe M97.8 ☑
    - wrist M97.8 ☑
- phalanx
    - foot — *see* Fracture, toe
    - hand — *see* Fracture, finger
- pisiform — *see* Fracture, carpal, pisiform
- pond — *see* Fracture, skull
- prosthetic device, internal — *see* Complications, prosthetic device, by site, mechanical
- pubis S32.50- ☑
    - with disruption of pelvic ring — *see* Disruption, pelvic ring
    - specified site NEC S32.59- ☑
    - superior rim S32.51- ☑
- radius S52.9- ☑
    - distal end — *see* Fracture, radius, lower end
    - following insertion of implant, prosthesis or plate M96.63- ☑
    - head — *see* Fracture, radius, upper end, head
    - lower end S52.50- ☑
        - Barton's — *see* Barton's fracture
        - Colles' — *see* Colles' fracture
        - extraarticular NEC S52.55- ☑
        - intraarticular NEC S52.57- ☑
        - physeal S59.20- ☑
            - Salter-Harris
                - Type I S59.21- ☑
                - Type II S59.22- ☑
                - Type III S59.23- ☑
                - Type IV S59.24- ☑
            - specified NEC S59.29- ☑
        - Smith's — *see* Smith's fracture
        - specified NEC S52.59- ☑
        - styloid process (displaced) S52.51- ☑
            - nondisplaced S52.51- ☑
        - torus S52.52- ☑
    - neck — *see* Fracture, radius, upper end
    - proximal end — *see* Fracture, radius, upper end
    - shaft S52.30- ☑
        - bent bone S52.38- ☑
        - comminuted (displaced) S52.35- ☑
            - nondisplaced S52.35- ☑
        - Galeazzi's — *see* Galeazzi's fracture
        - greenstick S52.31- ☑
        - oblique (displaced) S52.33- ☑
            - nondisplaced S52.33- ☑
        - segmental (displaced) S52.36- ☑
            - nondisplaced S52.36- ☑
        - specified NEC S52.39- ☑
        - spiral (displaced) S52.34- ☑
            - nondisplaced S52.34- ☑
        - transverse (displaced) S52.32- ☑
            - nondisplaced S52.32- ☑
    - upper end S52.10- ☑
        - head (displaced) S52.12- ☑
            - nondisplaced S52.12- ☑
        - neck (displaced) S52.13- ☑
            - nondisplaced S52.13- ☑
        - physeal S59.10- ☑
            - Salter-Harris
                - Type I S59.11- ☑
                - Type II S59.12- ☑
                - Type III S59.13- ☑
                - Type IV S59.14- ☑
            - specified NEC S59.19- ☑
        - specified NEC S52.18- ☑
        - torus S52.11- ☑
- ramus
    - inferior or superior, pubis — *see* Fracture, pubis
    - mandible — *see* Fracture, mandible
- restorative material (dental) K08.539
    - with loss of material K08.531
    - without loss of material K08.530
- rib S22.3- ☑
    - with flail chest — *see* Flail, chest
    - associated with chest compression and cardiopulmonary resuscitation M96.A2
    - multiple S22.4- ☑
        - with flail chest — *see* Flail, chest
        - associated with chest compression and cardiopulmonary resuscitation M96.A3
- root, tooth — *see* Fracture, tooth

Fracture, traumatic — *continued*
- sacrum S32.10 ☑
    - specified NEC S32.19 ☑
    - Type
        - 1 S32.14 ☑
        - 2 S32.15 ☑
        - 3 S32.16 ☑
        - 4 S32.17 ☑
    - Zone
        - I S32.119 ☑
            - displaced (minimally) S32.111 ☑
                - severely S32.112 ☑
            - nondisplaced S32.110 ☑
        - II S32.129 ☑
            - displaced (minimally) S32.121 ☑
                - severely S32.122 ☑
            - nondisplaced S32.120 ☑
        - III S32.139 ☑
            - displaced (minimally) S32.131 ☑
                - severely S32.132 ☑
            - nondisplaced S32.130 ☑
- scaphoid (hand) — *see also* Fracture, carpal, navicular
    - foot — *see* Fracture, tarsal, navicular
- scapula S42.10- ☑
    - acromial process (displaced) S42.12- ☑
        - nondisplaced S42.12- ☑
    - body (displaced) S42.11- ☑
        - nondisplaced S42.11- ☑
    - coracoid process (displaced) S42.13- ☑
        - nondisplaced S42.13- ☑
    - glenoid cavity (displaced) S42.14- ☑
        - nondisplaced S42.14- ☑
    - neck (displaced) S42.15- ☑
        - nondisplaced S42.15- ☑
    - specified NEC S42.19- ☑
- semilunar bone, wrist — *see* Fracture, carpal, lunate
- sequelae — *see* Sequelae, fracture
- sesamoid bone
    - foot S92.81- ☑
    - hand — *see* Fracture, carpal
    - other — *see* Fracture, traumatic, by site
- shepherd's — *see* Fracture, tarsal, talus
- shoulder (girdle) S42.9- ☑
    - blade — *see* Fracture, scapula
- sinus (ethmoid) (frontal) S02.19 ☑
- skull S02.91 ☑
    - base S02.10- ☑
        - occiput S02.119 ☑
            - condyle S02.113 ☑
                - specified NEC S02.118 ☑
                    - left side S02.11H ☑
                    - right side S02.11G ☑
                - type I S02.110 ☑
                    - left side S02.11B ☑
                    - right side S02.11A ☑
                - type II S02.111 ☑
                    - left side S02.11D ☑
                    - right side S02.11C ☑
                - type III S02.112 ☑
                    - left side S02.11F ☑
                    - right side S02.11E ☑
        - specified NEC S02.19 ☑
    - birth injury P13.0
    - frontal bone S02.0 ☑
    - parietal bone S02.0 ☑
    - specified site NEC S02.8- ☑
    - temporal bone S02.19 ☑
    - vault S02.0 ☑
- Smith's — *see* Smith's fracture
- sphenoid (bone) (sinus) S02.19 ☑
- spine — *see* Fracture, vertebra
- spinous process — *see* Fracture, vertebra
- spontaneous (cause unknown) — *see* Fracture, pathological
- stave (of thumb) — *see* Fracture, metacarpal, first
- sternum S22.20 ☑
    - with flail chest — *see* Flail, chest
    - associated with chest compression and cardiopulmonary resuscitation M96.A1
    - body S22.22 ☑
    - manubrium S22.21 ☑
    - xiphoid (process) S22.24 ☑
        - associated with chest compression and cardiopulmonary resuscitation M96.A1
- stress M84.30 ☑
    - ankle M84.37- ☑

Fracture, traumatic — *continued*
- stress — *continued*
    - carpus M84.34- ☑
    - clavicle M84.31- ☑
    - femoral neck M84.359 ☑
    - femur M84.35- ☑
    - fibula M84.36- ☑
    - finger M84.34- ☑
    - hip M84.359 ☑
    - humerus M84.32- ☑
    - ilium M84.350 ☑
    - ischium M84.350 ☑
    - metacarpus M84.34- ☑
    - metatarsus M84.37- ☑
    - neck — *see* Fracture, fatigue, vertebra
    - pelvis M84.350 ☑
    - radius M84.33- ☑
    - rib M84.38 ☑
    - scapula M84.31- ☑
    - skull M84.38 ☑
    - tarsus M84.37- ☑
    - tibia M84.36- ☑
    - toe M84.37- ☑
    - ulna M84.33- ☑
    - vertebra — *see* Fracture, fatigue, vertebra
- supracondylar, elbow — *see* Fracture, humerus, lower end, supracondylar
- symphysis pubis — *see* Fracture, pubis
- talus (ankle bone) — *see* Fracture, tarsal, talus
- tarsal bone(s) S92.20- ☑
    - astragalus — *see* Fracture, tarsal, talus
    - calcaneus S92.00- ☑
        - anterior process (displaced) S92.02- ☑
            - nondisplaced S92.02- ☑
        - body (displaced) S92.01- ☑
            - nondisplaced S92.01- ☑
        - extraarticular NEC (displaced) S92.05- ☑
            - nondisplaced S92.05- ☑
        - intraarticular (displaced) S92.06- ☑
            - nondisplaced S92.06- ☑
        - physeal S99.00- ☑
            - Salter-Harris
                - Type I S99.01- ☑
                - Type II S99.02- ☑
                - Type III S99.03- ☑
                - Type IV S99.04- ☑
            - specified NEC S99.09- ☑
        - tuberosity (displaced) S92.04- ☑
            - avulsion (displaced) S92.03- ☑
                - nondisplaced S92.03- ☑
            - nondisplaced S92.04- ☑
    - cuboid (displaced) S92.21- ☑
        - nondisplaced S92.21- ☑
    - cuneiform
        - intermediate (displaced) S92.23- ☑
            - nondisplaced S92.23- ☑
        - lateral (displaced) S92.22- ☑
            - nondisplaced S92.22- ☑
        - medial (displaced) S92.24- ☑
            - nondisplaced S92.24- ☑
    - navicular (displaced) S92.25- ☑
        - nondisplaced S92.25- ☑
    - scaphoid — *see* Fracture, tarsal, navicular
    - talus S92.10- ☑
        - avulsion (displaced) S92.15- ☑
            - nondisplaced S92.15- ☑
        - body (displaced) S92.12- ☑
            - nondisplaced S92.12- ☑
        - dome (displaced) S92.14- ☑
            - nondisplaced S92.14- ☑
        - head (displaced) S92.12- ☑
            - nondisplaced S92.12- ☑
        - lateral process (displaced) S92.14- ☑
            - nondisplaced S92.14- ☑
        - neck (displaced) S92.11- ☑
            - nondisplaced S92.11- ☑
        - posterior process (displaced) S92.13- ☑
            - nondisplaced S92.13- ☑
        - specified NEC S92.19- ☑
- temporal bone (styloid) S02.19 ☑
- thorax (bony) S22.9 ☑
    - with flail chest — *see* Flail, chest
    - rib S22.3- ☑
        - multiple S22.4- ☑
            - with flail chest — *see* Flail, chest
    - sternum S22.20 ☑

Fracture, traumatic — *continued*
  thorax — *continued*
    sternum — *continued*
      body S22.22 ☑
      manubrium S22.21 ☑
      xiphoid process S22.24 ☑
        associated with chest compression and cardiopulmonary resuscitation M96.A1
    vertebra (displaced) S22.009 ☑
      burst (stable) S22.001 ☑
        unstable S22.002 ☑
      eighth S22.069 ☑
        burst (stable) S22.061 ☑
          unstable S22.062 ☑
        specified type NEC S22.068 ☑
        wedge compression S22.060 ☑
      eleventh S22.089 ☑
        burst (stable) S22.081 ☑
          unstable S22.082 ☑
        specified type NEC S22.088 ☑
        wedge compression S22.080 ☑
      fifth S22.059 ☑
        burst (stable) S22.051 ☑
          unstable S22.052 ☑
        specified type NEC S22.058 ☑
        wedge compression S22.050 ☑
      first S22.019 ☑
        burst (stable) S22.011 ☑
          unstable S22.012 ☑
        specified type NEC S22.018 ☑
        wedge compression S22.010 ☑
      fourth S22.049 ☑
        burst (stable) S22.041 ☑
          unstable S22.042 ☑
        specified type NEC S22.048 ☑
        wedge compression S22.040 ☑
      ninth S22.079 ☑
        burst (stable) S22.071 ☑
          unstable S22.072 ☑
        specified type NEC S22.078 ☑
        wedge compression S22.070 ☑
      nondisplaced S22.001 ☑
      second S22.029 ☑
        burst (stable) S22.021 ☑
          unstable S22.022 ☑
        specified type NEC S22.028 ☑
        wedge compression S22.020 ☑
      seventh S22.069 ☑
        burst (stable) S22.061 ☑
          unstable S22.062 ☑
        specified type NEC S22.068 ☑
        wedge compression S22.060 ☑
      sixth S22.059 ☑
        burst (stable) S22.051 ☑
          unstable S22.052 ☑
        specified type NEC S22.058 ☑
        wedge compression S22.050 ☑
      specified type NEC S22.008 ☑
      tenth S22.079 ☑
        burst (stable) S22.071 ☑
          unstable S22.072 ☑
        specified type NEC S22.078 ☑
        wedge compression S22.070 ☑
      third S22.039 ☑
        burst (stable) S22.031 ☑
          unstable S22.032 ☑
        specified type NEC S22.038 ☑
        wedge compression S22.030 ☑
      twelfth S22.089 ☑
        burst (stable) S22.081 ☑
          unstable S22.082 ☑
        specified type NEC S22.088 ☑
        wedge compression S22.080 ☑
      wedge compression S22.000 ☑
  thumb S62.50- ☑
    distal phalanx (displaced) S62.52- ☑
      nondisplaced S62.52- ☑
    proximal phalanx (displaced) S62.51- ☑
      nondisplaced S62.51- ☑
  thyroid cartilage S12.8 ☑
  tibia (shaft) S82.20- ☑
    comminuted (displaced) S82.25- ☑
      nondisplaced S82.25- ☑
    condyles — *see* Fracture, tibia, upper end
    distal end — *see* Fracture, tibia, lower end

Fracture, traumatic — *continued*
  tibia — *continued*
    epiphysis
      lower — *see* Fracture, tibia, lower end
      upper — *see* Fracture, tibia, upper end
    following insertion of implant, prosthesis or plate M96.67-
    head (involving knee joint) — *see* Fracture, tibia, upper end
    intercondyloid eminence — *see* Fracture, tibia, upper end
    involving ankle or malleolus — *see* Fracture, ankle, medial malleolus
    lower end S82.30- ☑
      physeal S89.10- ☑
        Salter-Harris
          Type I S89.11- ☑
          Type II S89.12- ☑
          Type III S89.13- ☑
          Type IV S89.14- ☑
        specified NEC S89.19- ☑
      pilon (displaced) S82.87- ☑
        nondisplaced S82.87- ☑
      specified NEC S82.39- ☑
      torus S82.31- ☑
    malleolus — *see* Fracture, ankle, medial malleolus
    oblique (displaced) S82.23- ☑
      nondisplaced S82.23- ☑
    pilon — *see* Fracture, tibia, lower end, pilon
    proximal end — *see* Fracture, tibia, upper end
    segmental (displaced) S82.26- ☑
      nondisplaced S82.26- ☑
    specified NEC S82.29- ☑
    spine — *see* Fracture, tibia, upper end, spine
    spiral (displaced) S82.24- ☑
      nondisplaced S82.24- ☑
    transverse (displaced) S82.22- ☑
      nondisplaced S82.22- ☑
    tuberosity — *see* Fracture, tibia, upper end, tuberosity
    upper end S82.10- ☑
      bicondylar (displaced) S82.14- ☑
        nondisplaced S82.14- ☑
      lateral condyle (displaced) S82.12- ☑
        nondisplaced S82.12- ☑
      medial condyle (displaced) S82.13- ☑
        nondisplaced S82.13- ☑
      physeal S89.00- ☑
        Salter-Harris
          Type I S89.01- ☑
          Type II S89.02- ☑
          Type III S89.03- ☑
          Type IV S89.04- ☑
        specified NEC S89.09- ☑
      plateau — *see* Fracture, tibia, upper end, bicondylar
      specified NEC S82.19- ☑
      spine (displaced) S82.11- ☑
        nondisplaced S82.11- ☑
      torus S82.16- ☑
      tuberosity (displaced) S82.15- ☑
        nondisplaced S82.15- ☑
  toe S92.91- ☑
    great (displaced) S92.40- ☑
      distal phalanx (displaced) S92.42- ☑
        nondisplaced S92.42- ☑
      nondisplaced S92.40- ☑
      proximal phalanx (displaced) S92.41- ☑
        nondisplaced S92.41- ☑
      specified NEC S92.49- ☑
    lesser (displaced) S92.50- ☑
      distal phalanx (displaced) S92.53- ☑
        nondisplaced S92.53- ☑
      middle phalanx (displaced) S92.52- ☑
        nondisplaced S92.52- ☑
      nondisplaced S92.50- ☑
      proximal phalanx (displaced) S92.51- ☑
        nondisplaced S92.51- ☑
      specified NEC S92.59- ☑
    physeal
      phalanx S99.20- ☑
        Salter-Harris
          Type I S99.21- ☑
          Type II S99.22- ☑
          Type III S99.23- ☑
          Type IV S99.24- ☑

Fracture, traumatic — *continued*
  toe — *continued*
    physeal — *continued*
      phalanx — *continued*
        specified NEC S99.29- ☑
  tooth (root) S02.5 ☑
  trachea (cartilage) S12.8 ☑
  transverse process — *see* Fracture, vertebra
  trapezium or trapezoid bone — *see* Fracture, carpal
  trimalleolar — *see* Fracture, ankle, trimalleolar
  triquetrum (cuneiform of carpus) — *see* Fracture, carpal, triquetrum
  trochanter — *see* Fracture, femur, trochanteric
  tuberosity (external) — *see* Fracture, traumatic, by site
  ulna (shaft) S52.20- ☑
    bent bone S52.28- ☑
    coronoid process — *see* Fracture, ulna, upper end, coronoid process
    distal end — *see* Fracture, ulna, lower end
    following insertion of implant, prosthesis or plate M96.63- ☑
    head S52.60- ☑
    lower end S52.60- ☑
      physeal S59.00- ☑
        Salter-Harris
          Type I S59.01- ☑
          Type II S59.02- ☑
          Type III S59.03- ☑
          Type IV S59.04- ☑
        specified NEC S59.09- ☑
      specified NEC S52.69- ☑
      styloid process (displaced) S52.61- ☑
        nondisplaced S52.61- ☑
      torus S52.62- ☑
    proximal end — *see* Fracture, ulna, upper end
    shaft S52.20- ☑
      comminuted (displaced) S52.25- ☑
        nondisplaced S52.25- ☑
      greenstick S52.21- ☑
      Monteggia's — *see* Monteggia's fracture
      oblique (displaced) S52.23- ☑
        nondisplaced S52.23- ☑
      segmental (displaced) S52.26- ☑
        nondisplaced S52.26- ☑
      specified NEC S52.29- ☑
      spiral (displaced) S52.24- ☑
        nondisplaced S52.24- ☑
      transverse (displaced) S52.22- ☑
        nondisplaced S52.22- ☑
    upper end S52.00- ☑
      coronoid process (displaced) S52.04- ☑
        nondisplaced S52.04- ☑
      olecranon process (displaced) S52.02- ☑
        with intraarticular extension S52.03- ☑
        nondisplaced S52.02- ☑
          with intraarticular extension S52.03- ☑
      specified NEC S52.09- ☑
      torus S52.01- ☑
  unciform — *see* Fracture, carpal, hamate
  vault of skull S02.0 ☑
  vertebra, vertebral (arch) (body) (column) (neural arch) (pedicle) (spinous process) (transverse process)
    atlas — *see* Fracture, neck, cervical vertebra, first
    axis — *see* Fracture, neck, cervical vertebra, second
    cervical (teardrop) S12.9 ☑
      axis — *see* Fracture, neck, cervical vertebra, second
      first (atlas) — *see* Fracture, neck, cervical vertebra, first
      second (axis) — *see* Fracture, neck, cervical vertebra, second
    chronic M84.48 ☑
    coccyx S32.2 ☑
    dorsal — *see* Fracture, thorax, vertebra
    lumbar S32.009 ☑
      burst (stable) S32.001 ☑
        unstable S32.002 ☑
      fifth S32.059 ☑
        burst (stable) S32.051 ☑
          unstable S32.052 ☑
        specified type NEC S32.058 ☑
        wedge compression S32.050 ☑
      first S32.019 ☑
        burst (stable) S32.011 ☑
          unstable S32.012 ☑
        specified type NEC S32.018 ☑

Fracture, traumatic — *continued*
　vertebra, vertebral — *continued*
　　lumbar — *continued*
　　　first — *continued*
　　　　wedge compression S32.010 ☑
　　　fourth S32.049 ☑
　　　　burst (stable) S32.041 ☑
　　　　　unstable S32.042 ☑
　　　　specified type NEC S32.048 ☑
　　　　wedge compression S32.040 ☑
　　　second S32.029 ☑
　　　　burst (stable) S32.021 ☑
　　　　　unstable S32.022 ☑
　　　　specified type NEC S32.028 ☑
　　　　wedge compression S32.020 ☑
　　　specified type NEC S32.008 ☑
　　　third S32.039 ☑
　　　　burst (stable) S32.031 ☑
　　　　　unstable S32.032 ☑
　　　　specified type NEC S32.038 ☑
　　　　wedge compression S32.030 ☑
　　　wedge compression S32.000 ☑
　　metastatic — *see* Collapse, vertebra, in, specified
　　　disease NEC — *see also* Neoplasm
　　newborn (birth injury) P11.5
　　sacrum S32.10 ☑
　　　specified NEC S32.19 ☑
　　　Type
　　　　1 S32.14 ☑
　　　　2 S32.15 ☑
　　　　3 S32.16 ☑
　　　　4 S32.17 ☑
　　　Zone
　　　　I S32.119 ☑
　　　　　displaced (minimally) S32.111 ☑
　　　　　　severely S32.112 ☑
　　　　　nondisplaced S32.110 ☑
　　　　II S32.129 ☑
　　　　　displaced (minimally) S32.121 ☑
　　　　　　severely S32.122 ☑
　　　　　nondisplaced S32.120 ☑
　　　　III S32.139 ☑
　　　　　displaced (minimally) S32.131 ☑
　　　　　　severely S32.132 ☑
　　　　　nondisplaced S32.130 ☑
　　thoracic — *see* Fracture, thorax, vertebra
　vertex S02.0 ☑
　vomer (bone) S02.2 ☑
　wrist S62.10- ☑
　　carpal — *see* Fracture, carpal bone
　　navicular (scaphoid) (hand) — *see* Fracture, carpal,
　　　navicular
　xiphisternum, xiphoid (process) S22.24 ☑
　　associated with chest compression and cardiopul-
　　　monary resuscitation M96.A1
　zygoma S02.402 ☑
　　left side S02.40F ☑
　　right side S02.40E ☑
Fragile, fragility
　autosomal site Q95.5
　bone, congenital (with blue sclera) Q78.0
　capillary (hereditary) D69.8
　hair L67.8
　nails L60.3
　non-sex chromosome site Q95.5
　X chromosome Q99.2
Fragilitas
　crinium L67.8
　ossium (with blue sclerae) (hereditary) Q78.0
　unguium L60.3
　　congenital Q84.6
Fragments, cataract (lens), **following cataract surgery**
　　H59.02- ☑
　retained foreign body — *see* Retained, foreign body
　　fragments (type of)
Frailty (frail) R54
　mental R41.81
Frambesia, frambesial (tropica) — *see also* Yaws
　initial lesion or ulcer A66.0
　primary A66.0
Frambeside
　gummatous A66.4
　of early yaws A66.2
Frambesioma A66.1
Franceschetti-Klein (-Wildervanck) **disease or syn-**
　　drome Q75.4
Francis' disease — *see* Tularemia

Franklin disease C88.2
Frank's essential thrombocytopenia D69.3
Fraser's syndrome Q87.0
Freckle(s) L81.2
　malignant melanoma in — *see* Melanoma
　melanotic (Hutchinson's) — *see* Melanoma, in situ
　retinal D49.81
Frederickson's hyperlipoproteinemia, type
　I and V E78.3
　IIA E78.00
　IIB and III E78.2
　IV E78.1
Freeman Sheldon syndrome Q87.0
Freezing — *see also* Effect, adverse, cold T69.9 ☑
Freiberg's disease (infraction of metatarsal head or os-
　　teochondrosis) — *see* Osteochondrosis, juvenile,
　　metatarsus
Frei's disease A55
Fremitus, friction, cardiac R01.2
Frenum, frenulum
　external os Q51.828
　tongue (shortening) (congenital) Q38.1
Frequency micturition (nocturnal) R35.0
　psychogenic F45.8
Frey's syndrome
　auriculotemporal G50.8
　hyperhidrosis L74.52
Friction
　burn — *see* Burn, by site
　fremitus, cardiac R01.2
　precordial R01.2
　sounds, chest R09.89
Friderichsen-Waterhouse syndrome or disease A39.1
Friedländer's B (bacillus) **NEC** — *see also* condition A49.8
Friedreich's
　ataxia G11.11
　combined systemic disease G11.11
　facial hemihypertrophy Q67.4
　sclerosis (cerebellum) (spinal cord) G11.11
Frigidity F52.22
Fröhlich's syndrome E23.6
Frontal — *see also* condition
　lobe syndrome F07.0
Frostbite (superficial) T33.90 ☑
　with
　　partial thickness skin loss — *see* Frostbite (superfi-
　　　cial), by site
　　tissue necrosis T34.90 ☑
　abdominal wall T33.3 ☑
　　with tissue necrosis T34.3 ☑
　ankle T33.81- ☑
　　with tissue necrosis T34.81- ☑
　arm T33.4- ☑
　　with tissue necrosis T34.4- ☑
　　finger(s) — *see* Frostbite, finger
　　hand — *see* Frostbite, hand
　　wrist — *see* Frostbite, wrist
　ear T33.01- ☑
　　with tissue necrosis T34.01- ☑
　face T33.09 ☑
　　with tissue necrosis T34.09 ☑
　finger T33.53- ☑
　　with tissue necrosis T34.53- ☑
　foot T33.82- ☑
　　with tissue necrosis T34.82- ☑
　hand T33.52- ☑
　　with tissue necrosis T34.52- ☑
　head T33.09 ☑
　　with tissue necrosis T34.09 ☑
　　ear — *see* Frostbite, ear
　　nose — *see* Frostbite, nose
　hip (and thigh) T33.6- ☑
　　with tissue necrosis T34.6- ☑
　knee T33.7- ☑
　　with tissue necrosis T34.7- ☑
　leg T33.9- ☑
　　with tissue necrosis T34.9- ☑
　　ankle — *see* Frostbite, ankle
　　foot — *see* Frostbite, foot
　　knee — *see* Frostbite, knee
　　lower T33.7- ☑
　　　with tissue necrosis T34.7- ☑
　　thigh — *see* Frostbite, hip
　　toe — *see* Frostbite, toe
　limb
　　lower T33.99 ☑

Frostbite — *continued*
　limb — *continued*
　　lower — *continued*
　　　with tissue necrosis T34.99 ☑
　　upper — *see* Frostbite, arm
　neck T33.1 ☑
　　with tissue necrosis T34.1 ☑
　nose T33.02 ☑
　　with tissue necrosis T34.02 ☑
　pelvis T33.3 ☑
　　with tissue necrosis T34.3 ☑
　specified site NEC T33.99 ☑
　　with tissue necrosis T34.99 ☑
　thigh — *see* Frostbite, hip
　thorax T33.2 ☑
　　with tissue necrosis T34.2 ☑
　toes T33.83- ☑
　　with tissue necrosis T34.83- ☑
　trunk T33.99 ☑
　　with tissue necrosis T34.99 ☑
　wrist T33.51- ☑
　　with tissue necrosis T34.51- ☑
Frotteurism F65.81
Frozen — *see also* Effect, adverse, cold T69.9 ☑
　pelvis (female) N94.89
　　male K66.8
　shoulder — *see* Capsulitis, adhesive
Fructokinase deficiency E74.11
Fructose 1,6 diphosphatase deficiency E74.19
Fructosemia (benign) (essential) E74.12
Fructosuria (benign) (essential) E74.11
Fuchs'
　black spot (myopic) — *see also* Myopia, degenerative
　　H44.2- ☑
　dystrophy (corneal endothelium) H18.51- ☑
　heterochromic cyclitis — *see* Cyclitis, Fuchs' hete-
　　rochromic
Fucosidosis E77.1
Fugue R68.89
　dissociative F44.1
　hysterical (dissociative) F44.1
　postictal in epilepsy — *see* Epilepsy
　reaction to exceptional stress (transient) F43.0
Fulminant, fulminating — *see* condition
Functional — *see also* condition
　bleeding (uterus) N93.8
Functioning, intellectual, borderline R41.83
Fundus — *see* condition
Fungemia NOS B49
Fungus, fungous
　cerebral G93.89
　disease NOS B49
　infection — *see* Infection, fungus
Funiculitis (acute) (chronic) (endemic) N49.1
　gonococcal (acute) (chronic) A54.23
　tuberculous A18.15
Funnel
　breast (acquired) M95.4
　　congenital Q67.6
　　sequelae (late effect) of rickets E64.3
　chest (acquired) M95.4
　　congenital Q67.6
　　sequelae (late effect) of rickets E64.3
　pelvis (acquired) M95.5
　　with disproportion (fetopelvic) O33.3 ☑
　　　causing obstructed labor O65.3
　　congenital Q74.2
FUO (fever of unknown origin) R50.9
Furfur L21.0
　microsporon B36.0
Furrier's lung J67.8
Furrowed K14.5
　nail(s) (transverse) L60.4
　　congenital Q84.6
　tongue K14.5
　　congenital Q38.3
Furuncle L02.92
　abdominal wall L02.221
　ankle — *see* Furuncle, lower limb
　antecubital space — *see* Furuncle, upper limb
　anus K61.0
　arm — *see* Furuncle, upper limb
　auditory canal, external — *see* Abscess, ear, external
　auricle (ear) — *see* Abscess, ear, external
　axilla (region) L02.42- ☑
　back (any part) L02.222
　breast N61.1

Furuncle — *continued*
buttock L02.32
cheek (external) L02.02
chest wall L02.223
chin L02.02
corpus cavernosum N48.21
ear, external — *see* Abscess, ear, external
external auditory canal — *see* Abscess, ear, external
eyelid — *see* Abscess, eyelid
face L02.02
femoral (region) — *see* Furuncle, lower limb
finger — *see* Furuncle, hand
flank L02.221
foot L02.62- ☑
forehead L02.02
gluteal (region) L02.32
groin L02.224
hand L02.52- ☑
head L02.821
   face L02.02
hip — *see* Furuncle, lower limb
kidney — *see* Abscess, kidney
knee — *see* Furuncle, lower limb
labium (majus) (minus) N76.4
lacrimal
   gland — *see* Dacryoadenitis
   passages (duct) (sac) — *see* Inflammation, lacrimal,
      passages, acute
leg (any part) — *see* Furuncle, lower limb
lower limb L02.42- ☑
malignant A22.0
mouth K12.2
navel L02.226
neck L02.12
nose J34.0
orbit, orbital — *see* Abscess, orbit
palmar (space) — *see* Furuncle, hand
partes posteriores L02.32
pectoral region L02.223
penis N48.21
perineum L02.225
pinna — *see* Abscess, ear, external
popliteal — *see* Furuncle, lower limb

Furuncle — *continued*
prepatellar — *see* Furuncle, lower limb
scalp L02.821
seminal vesicle N49.0
shoulder — *see* Furuncle, upper limb
specified site NEC L02.828
submandibular K12.2
temple (region) L02.02
thumb — *see* Furuncle, hand
toe — *see* Furuncle, foot
trunk L02.229
   abdominal wall L02.221
   back L02.222
   chest wall L02.223
   groin L02.224
   perineum L02.225
   umbilicus L02.226
umbilicus L02.226
upper limb L02.42- ☑
vulva N76.4
Furunculosis — *see* Furuncle
Fused — *see* Fusion, fused
Fusion, fused (congenital)
astragaloscaphoid Q74.2
atria Q21.19
auditory canal Q16.1
auricles, heart Q21.19
binocular with defective stereopsis H53.32
bone Q79.8
cervical spine M43.22
choanal Q30.0
commissure, mitral valve Q23.2
cusps, heart valve NEC Q24.8
   mitral Q23.2
   pulmonary Q22.1
   tricuspid Q22.4
ear ossicles Q16.3
fingers Q70.0 ☑
hymen Q52.3
joint (acquired) — *see also* Ankylosis
   congenital Q74.8
kidneys (incomplete) Q63.1
labium (majus) (minus) Q52.5
larynx and trachea Q34.8

Fusion, fused — *continued*
limb, congenital Q74.8
   lower Q74.2
   upper Q74.0
lobes, lung Q33.8
lumbosacral (acquired) M43.27
   arthrodesis status Z98.1
   congenital Q76.49
   postprocedural status Z98.1
nares, nose, nasal, nostril(s) Q30.0
organ or site not listed — *see* Anomaly, by site
ossicles Q79.9
   auditory Q16.3
pulmonic cusps Q22.1
ribs Q76.6
sacroiliac (joint) (acquired) M43.28
   arthrodesis status Z98.1
   congenital Q74.2
   postprocedural status Z98.1
spine (acquired) NEC M43.20
   arthrodesis status Z98.1
   cervical region M43.22
   cervicothoracic region M43.23
   congenital Q76.49
   lumbar M43.26
   lumbosacral region M43.27
   occipito-atlanto-axial region M43.21
   postoperative status Z98.1
   sacrococcygeal region M43.28
   thoracic region M43.24
   thoracolumbar region M43.25
sublingual duct with submaxillary duct at opening in
     mouth Q38.4
testes Q55.1
toes Q70.2- ☑
tooth, teeth K00.2
trachea and esophagus Q39.8
twins Q89.4
vagina Q52.4
ventricles, heart Q21.0
vertebra (arch) — *see* Fusion, spine
vulva Q52.5
Fusospirillosis (mouth) (tongue) (tonsil) A69.1
Fussy baby R68.12

G

Gain in weight (abnormal) (excessive) — *see also* Weight, gain
Gaisböck's disease (polycythemia hypertonica) D75.1
Gait abnormality R26.9
  ataxic R26.0
  falling R29.6
  hysterical (ataxic) (staggering) F44.4
  paralytic R26.1
  spastic R26.1
  specified type NEC R26.89
  staggering R26.0
  unsteadiness R26.81
  walking difficulty NEC R26.2
Galactocele (breast) N64.89
  puerperal, postpartum O92.79
Galactokinase deficiency E74.29
Galactophoritis N61.0
  gestational, puerperal, postpartum O91.2-
Galactorrhea O92.6
  not associated with childbirth N64.3
Galactosemia (classic) (congenital) E74.21
Galactosuria E74.29
Galacturia R82.0
  schistosomiasis (bilharziasis) B65.0
GALD (gestational alloimmune liver disease) P78.84
Galeazzi's fracture S52.37-
Galen's vein — *see* condition
Galeophobia F40.218
Gall duct — *see* condition
Gallbladder — *see also* condition
  acute K81.0
Gallop rhythm R00.8
Gallstone (colic) (cystic duct) (gallbladder) (impacted) (multiple) — *see also* Calculus, gallbladder
  with
    cholecystitis — *see* Calculus, gallbladder, with cholecystitis
    bile duct (common) (hepatic) — *see* Calculus, bile duct
  causing intestinal obstruction K56.3
  specified NEC K80.80
    with obstruction K80.81
Gambling Z72.6
  pathological (compulsive) F63.0
Gammopathy (of undetermined significance [MGUS]) D47.2
  associated with lymphoplasmacytic dyscrasia D47.2
  monoclonal D47.2
  polyclonal D89.0
Gamna's disease (siderotic splenomegaly) D73.1
Gamophobia F40.298
Gampsodactylia (congenital) Q66.7-
Gamstorp's disease (adynamia episodica hereditaria) G72.3
Gandy-Nanta disease (siderotic splenomegaly) D73.1
Gang
  membership offenses Z72.810
Gangliocytoma D36.10
Ganglioglioma — *see* Neoplasm, uncertain behavior, by site
Ganglion (compound) (diffuse) (joint) (tendon (sheath)) M67.40
  ankle M67.47-
  foot M67.47-
  forearm M67.43-
  hand M67.44-
  lower leg M67.46-
  multiple sites M67.49
  of yaws (early) (late) A66.6
  pelvic region M67.45-
  periosteal — *see* Periostitis
  shoulder region M67.41-
  specified site NEC M67.48
  thigh region M67.45-
  tuberculous A18.09
  upper arm M67.42-
  wrist M67.43-
Ganglioneuroblastoma — *see* Neoplasm, nerve, malignant
Ganglioneuroma D36.10
  malignant — *see* Neoplasm, nerve, malignant
Ganglioneuromatosis D36.10
Ganglionitis
  fifth nerve — *see* Neuralgia, trigeminal
  gasserian (postherpetic) (postzoster) B02.21

Ganglionitis — *continued*
  geniculate G51.1
    newborn (birth injury) P11.3
    postherpetic, postzoster B02.21
  herpes zoster B02.21
  postherpetic geniculate B02.21
Gangliosidosis E75.10
  GM1 E75.19
  GM2 E75.00
    other specified E75.09
    Sandhoff disease E75.01
    Tay-Sachs disease E75.02
  GM3 E75.19
  mucolipidosis IV E75.11
Gangosa A66.5
Gangrene, gangrenous (connective tissue) (dropsical) (dry) (moist) (skin) (ulcer) — *see also* Necrosis I96
  with diabetes (mellitus) — *see* Diabetes, with, gangrene
  abdomen (wall) I96
  alveolar M27.3
  appendix K35.80
    with
      peritonitis, localized — *see also* Appendicitis K35.31
  arteriosclerotic (general) (senile) — *see* Arteriosclerosis, extremities, with, gangrene
  auricle I96
  Bacillus welchii A48.0
  bladder (infectious) — *see* Cystitis, specified type NEC
  bowel, cecum, or colon — *see* Gangrene, intestine
  Clostridium perfringens or welchii A48.0
  cornea H18.89-
  corpora cavernosa N48.29
    noninfective N48.89
  cutaneous, spreading I96
  decubital — *see* Ulcer, pressure, by site
  diabetic (any site) — *see* Diabetes, with, gangrene
  emphysematous — *see* Gangrene, gas
  epidemic — *see* Poisoning, food, noxious, plant
  epididymis (infectional) N45.1
  erysipelas — *see* Erysipelas
  extremity (lower) (upper) I96
  Fournier N49.3
    female N76.82
    vagina and vulva N76.82
  fusospirochetal A69.0
  gallbladder — *see* Cholecystitis, acute
  gas (bacillus) A48.0
    following
      abortion — *see* Abortion by type complicated by infection
      ectopic or molar pregnancy O08.0
  glossitis K14.0
  hernia — *see* Hernia, by site, with gangrene
  intestine, intestinal (hemorrhagic) (massive) — *see also* Infarct, intestine K55.069
    with
      mesenteric embolism — *see also* Infarct, intestine K55.069
      obstruction — *see* Obstruction, intestine
  laryngitis J04.0
  limb (lower) (upper) I96
  lung J85.0
    spirochetal A69.8
  lymphangitis I89.1
  Meleney's (synergistic) — *see* Ulcer, skin
  mesentery — *see also* Infarct, intestine K55.069
    with
      embolism — *see also* Infarct, intestine K55.069
      intestinal obstruction — *see* Obstruction, intestine
  mouth A69.0
  ovary — *see* Oophoritis
  pancreas — *see* Pancreatitis, acute
  penis N48.29
    noninfective N48.89
  perineum I96
  pharynx — *see also* Pharyngitis
    Vincent's A69.1
  presenile I73.1
  progressive synergistic — *see* Ulcer, skin
  pulmonary J85.0
  pulpal (dental) K04.1
  quinsy J36
  Raynaud's (symmetric gangrene) I73.01
  retropharyngeal J39.2
  scrotum N49.3
    noninfective N50.89

Gangrene, gangrenous — *continued*
  senile (atherosclerotic) — *see* Arteriosclerosis, extremities, with, gangrene
  spermatic cord N49.1
    noninfective N50.89
  spine I96
  spirochetal NEC A69.8
  spreading cutaneous I96
  stomatitis A69.0
  symmetrical I73.01
  testis (infectional) N45.2
    noninfective N44.8
  throat — *see also* Pharyngitis
    diphtheritic A36.0
    Vincent's A69.1
  thyroid (gland) E07.89
  tooth (pulp) K04.1
  tuberculous NEC — *see* Tuberculosis
  tunica vaginalis N49.1
    noninfective N50.89
  umbilicus I96
  uterus — *see* Endometritis
  uvulitis K12.2
  vas deferens N49.1
    noninfective N50.89
  vulva N76.82
Ganister disease J62.8
Ganser's syndrome (hysterical) F44.89
Gardner-Diamond syndrome (autoerythrocyte sensitization) D69.2
Gargoylism E76.01
Garré's disease, osteitis (sclerosing), osteomyelitis — *see* Osteomyelitis, specified type NEC
Garrod's pad, knuckle M72.1
Gartner's duct
  cyst Q52.4
  persistent Q50.6
Gas R14.3
  asphyxiation, inhalation, poisoning, suffocation NEC — *see* Table of Drugs and Chemicals
  excessive R14.0
  gangrene A48.0
    following
      abortion — *see* Abortion by type complicated by infection
      ectopic or molar pregnancy O08.0
  on stomach R14.0
  pains R14.1
Gastralgia — *see also* Pain, abdominal
Gastrectasis K31.0
  psychogenic F45.8
Gastric — *see* condition
Gastrinoma
  malignant
    pancreas C25.4
    specified site NEC — *see* Neoplasm, malignant, by site
    unspecified site C25.4
  specified site — *see* Neoplasm, uncertain behavior
  unspecified site D37.9
Gastritis (simple) K29.70
  with bleeding K29.71
  acute (erosive) K29.00
    with bleeding K29.01
  alcoholic K29.20
    with bleeding K29.21
  allergic K29.60
    with bleeding K29.61
  atrophic (chronic) K29.40
    with bleeding K29.41
  chronic (antral) (fundal) K29.50
    with bleeding K29.51
    atrophic K29.40
      with bleeding K29.41
    superficial K29.30
      with bleeding K29.31
  dietary counseling and surveillance Z71.3
  due to diet deficiency E63.9
  eosinophilic K52.81
  giant hypertrophic K29.60
    with bleeding K29.61
  granulomatous K29.60
    with bleeding K29.61
  hypertrophic (mucosa) K29.60
    with bleeding K29.61
  nervous F54
  spastic K29.60
    with bleeding K29.61

Gastritis — *continued*
  specified NEC K29.60
    with bleeding K29.61
  superficial chronic K29.30
    with bleeding K29.31
  tuberculous A18.83
  viral NEC A08.4
Gastrocarcinoma — *see* Neoplasm, malignant, stomach
Gastrocolic — *see* condition
Gastrodisciasis, gastrodiscoidiasis B66.8
Gastroduodenitis K29.90
  with bleeding K29.91
  virus, viral A08.4
    specified type NEC A08.39
Gastrodynia — *see* Pain, abdominal
Gastroenteritis (acute) (chronic) (noninfectious) — *see also* Enteritis K52.9
  allergic K52.29
    with
      eosinophilic gastritis or gastroenteritis K52.81
      food protein-induced enterocolitis syndrome K52.21
      food protein-induced enteropathy K52.22
  dietetic — *see also* Gastroenteritis, allergic K52.29
  drug-induced K52.1
  due to
    Cryptosporidium A07.2
    drugs K52.1
    food poisoning — *see* Intoxication, foodborne
    radiation K52.0
  eosinophilic K52.81
  epidemic (infectious) A09
  food hypersensitivity — *see also* Gastroenteritis, allergic K52.29
  infectious — *see* Enteritis, infectious
  influenzal — *see* Influenza, with gastroenteritis
  noninfectious K52.9
    specified NEC K52.89
  rotaviral A08.0
  Salmonella A02.0
  toxic K52.1
  viral NEC A08.4
    acute infectious A08.39
      type Norwalk A08.11
    infantile (acute) A08.39
    Norwalk agent A08.11
    rotaviral A08.0
    severe of infants A08.39
    specified type NEC A08.39
Gastroenteropathy — *see also* Gastroenteritis K52.9
  acute, due to Norovirus A08.11
  acute, due to Norwalk agent A08.11
  infectious A09
Gastroenteroptosis K63.4
Gastroesophageal laceration- hemorrhage syndrome K22.6
Gastrointestinal — *see* condition
Gastrojejunal — *see* condition
Gastrojejunitis — *see also* Enteritis K52.9
Gastrojejunocolic — *see* condition
Gastroliths K31.89
Gastromalacia K31.89
Gastroparalysis K31.84
  diabetic — *see* Diabetes, gastroparalysis
Gastroparesis K31.84
  diabetic — *see* Diabetes, by type, with gastroparesis
Gastropathy K31.9
  congestive portal — *see also* Hypertension, portal K31.89
  erythematous K29.70
  exudative K90.89
  portal hypertensive — *see also* Hypertension, portal K31.89
Gastroptosis K31.89
Gastrorrhagia K92.2
  psychogenic F45.8
Gastroschisis (congenital) Q79.3
Gastrospasm (neurogenic) (reflex) K31.89
  neurotic F45.8
  psychogenic F45.8
Gastrostaxis — *see* Gastritis, with bleeding
Gastrostenosis K31.89
Gastrostomy
  attention to Z43.1
  status Z93.1
Gastrosuccorrhea (continuous) (intermittent) K31.89
  neurotic F45.8
  psychogenic F45.8

Gatophobia F40.218
Gaucher's disease or splenomegaly (adult) (infantile) E75.22
Gee (-Herter)(-Thaysen) **disease** (nontropical sprue) K90.0
Gélineau's syndrome G47.419
  with cataplexy G47.411
Gemination, tooth, teeth K00.2
Gemistocytoma
  specified site — *see* Neoplasm, malignant, by site
  unspecified site C71.9
General, generalized — *see* condition
Genetic
  carrier (status)
    cystic fibrosis Z14.1
    hemophilia A (asymptomatic) Z14.01
      symptomatic Z14.02
    specified NEC Z14.8
  susceptibility to disease NEC Z15.89
    malignant neoplasm Z15.09
      breast Z15.01
      endometrium Z15.04
      ovary Z15.02
      prostate Z15.03
      specified NEC Z15.09
    multiple endocrine neoplasia Z15.81
Genital — *see* condition
Genito-anorectal syndrome A55
Genitourinary system — *see* condition
Genu
  congenital Q74.1
  extrorsum (acquired) — *see also* Deformity, varus, knee
    congenital Q74.1
    sequelae (late effect) of rickets E64.3
  introrsum (acquired) — *see also* Deformity, valgus, knee
    congenital Q74.1
    sequelae (late effect) of rickets E64.3
  rachitic (old) E64.3
  recurvatum (acquired) — *see also* Deformity, limb, specified type NEC, lower leg
    congenital Q68.2
    sequelae (late effect) of rickets E64.3
  valgum (acquired) (knock-knee) M21.06- ☑
    congenital Q74.1
    sequelae (late effect) of rickets E64.3
  varum (acquired) (bowleg) M21.16- ☑
    congenital Q74.1
    sequelae (late effect) of rickets E64.3
Geographic tongue K14.1
Geophagia — *see* Pica
Geotrichosis B48.3
  stomatitis B48.3
Gephyrophobia F40.242
Gerbode defect Q21.0
GERD (gastroesophageal reflux disease) K21.9
Gerhardt's
  disease (erythromelalgia) I73.81
  syndrome (vocal cord paralysis) J38.00
    bilateral J38.02
    unilateral J38.01
German measles — *see also* Rubella
  exposure to Z20.4
Germinoblastoma (diffuse) C85.9- ☑
  follicular C82.9- ☑
Germinoma — *see* Neoplasm, malignant, by site
Gerontoxon — *see* Degeneration, cornea, senile
Gerstmann's syndrome R48.8
  developmental F81.2
Gerstmann-Sträussler-Scheinker syndrome (GSS) A81.82
Gestation (period) — *see also* Pregnancy
  ectopic — *see* Pregnancy, by site
  multiple O30.9- ☑
    greater than quadruplets — *see* Pregnancy, multiple (gestation), specified NEC
    specified NEC — *see* Pregnancy, multiple (gestation), specified NEC
Gestational
  mammary abscess O91.11- ☑
  purulent mastitis O91.11- ☑
  subareolar abscess O91.11- ☑
Ghon tubercle, primary infection A15.7
Ghost
  teeth K00.4
  vessels (cornea) H16.41- ☑
Ghoul hand A66.3
Gianotti-Crosti disease L44.4

Giant
  cell
    epulis K06.8
    peripheral granuloma K06.8
  esophagus, congenital Q39.5
  kidney, congenital Q63.3
  urticaria T78.3 ☑
    hereditary D84.1
Giardiasis A07.1
Gibert's disease or pityriasis L42
Giddiness R42
  hysterical F44.89
  psychogenic F45.8
Gierke's disease (glycogenosis I) E74.01
Gigantism (cerebral) (hypophyseal) (pituitary) E22.0
  constitutional E34.4
Gilbert's disease or syndrome E80.4
Gilchrist's disease B40.9
Gilford-Hutchinson disease E34.8
Gilles de la Tourette's disease or syndrome (motor-verbal tic) F95.2
Gingivitis K05.10
  acute (catarrhal) K05.00
    necrotizing A69.1
    nonplaque induced K05.01
    plaque induced K05.00
  chronic (desquamative) (hyperplastic) (simple marginal) (pregnancy associated) (ulcerative) K05.10
    nonplaque induced K05.11
    plaque induced K05.10
  expulsiva — *see* Periodontitis
  necrotizing ulcerative (acute) A69.1
  pellagrous E52
    acute necrotizing A69.1
  Vincent's A69.1
Gingivoglossitis K14.0
Gingivopericementitis — *see* Periodontitis
Gingivosis — *see* Gingivitis, chronic
Gingivostomatitis K05.10
  herpesviral B00.2
  necrotizing ulcerative (acute) A69.1
Gland, glandular — *see* condition
Glanders A24.0
Glanzmann (-Naegeli) **disease or thrombasthenia** D69.1
Glasgow coma scale
  total score
    3-8 R40.243 ☑
    9-12 R40.242 ☑
    13-15 R40.241 ☑
Glass-blower's disease (cataract) — *see* Cataract, specified NEC
Glaucoma H40.9
  with
    increased episcleral venous pressure H40.81- ☑
    pseudoexfoliation of lens — *see* Glaucoma, open angle, primary, capsular
  absolute H44.51- ☑
  angle-closure (primary) H40.20- ☑
    acute (attack) (crisis) H40.21- ☑
    chronic H40.22- ☑
    intermittent H40.23- ☑
    residual stage H40.24- ☑
  borderline H40.00- ☑
  capsular (with pseudoexfoliation of lens) — *see* Glaucoma, open angle, primary, capsular
  childhood Q15.0
  closed angle — *see* Glaucoma, angle-closure
  congenital Q15.0
  corticosteroid-induced — *see* Glaucoma, secondary, drugs
  hypersecretion H40.82- ☑
  in (due to)
    amyloidosis E85.4 *[H42]*
    aniridia Q13.1 *[H42]*
    concussion of globe — *see* Glaucoma, secondary, trauma
    dislocation of lens — *see* Glaucoma, secondary
    disorder of lens NEC — *see* Glaucoma, secondary
    drugs — *see* Glaucoma, secondary, drugs
    endocrine disease NOS E34.9 *[H42]*
    eye
      inflammation — *see* Glaucoma, secondary, inflammation
      trauma — *see* Glaucoma, secondary, trauma
    hypermature cataract — *see* Glaucoma, secondary

Glaucoma — *continued*
in — *continued*
  iridocyclitis — *see* Glaucoma, secondary, inflammation
  lens disorder — *see* Glaucoma, secondary
  Lowe's syndrome E72.03 *[H42]*
  metabolic disease NOS E88.9 *[H42]*
  ocular disorders NEC — *see* Glaucoma, secondary
  onchocerciasis B73.02
  pupillary block — *see* Glaucoma, secondary
  retinal vein occlusion — *see* Glaucoma, secondary
  Rieger's anomaly Q13.81 *[H42]*
  rubeosis of iris — *see* Glaucoma, secondary
  tumor of globe — *see* Glaucoma, secondary
  infantile Q15.0
  low tension — *see* Glaucoma, open angle, primary, low-tension
  malignant H40.83- ☑
  narrow angle — *see* Glaucoma, angle-closure
  newborn Q15.0
  noncongestive (chronic) — *see* Glaucoma, open angle
  nonobstructive — *see* Glaucoma, open angle
  obstructive — *see also* Glaucoma, angle-closure
    due to lens changes — *see* Glaucoma, secondary
  open angle H40.10- ☑
    primary H40.11- ☑
      capsular (with pseudoexfoliation of lens) H40.14- ☑
      low-tension H40.12- ☑
      pigmentary H40.13- ☑
      residual stage H40.15- ☑
  phacolytic — *see* Glaucoma, secondary
  pigmentary — *see* Glaucoma, open angle, primary, pigmentary
  postinfectious — *see* Glaucoma, secondary, inflammation
  secondary (to) H40.5- ☑
    drugs H40.6- ☑
    inflammation H40.4- ☑
    trauma H40.3- ☑
  simple (chronic) H40.11- ☑
  simplex H40.11- ☑
  specified type NEC H40.89
  suspect H40.00- ☑
  syphilitic A52.71
  traumatic — *see also* Glaucoma, secondary, trauma
    newborn (birth injury) P15.3
  tuberculous A18.59
Glaucomatous flecks (subcapsular) — *see* Cataract, complicated
Glazed tongue K14.4
Gleet (gonococcal) A54.01
Glénard's disease K63.4
Glioblastoma (multiforme)
  with sarcomatous component
    specified site — *see* Neoplasm, malignant, by site
    unspecified site C71.9
  giant cell
    specified site — *see* Neoplasm, malignant, by site
    unspecified site C71.9
  specified site — *see* Neoplasm, malignant, by site
  unspecified site C71.9
Glioma (malignant)
  astrocytic
    specified site — *see* Neoplasm, malignant, by site
    unspecified site C71.9
  mixed
    specified site — *see* Neoplasm, malignant, by site
    unspecified site C71.9
  nose Q30.8
  specified site NEC — *see* Neoplasm, malignant, by site
  subependymal D43.2
    specified site — *see* Neoplasm, uncertain behavior, by site
    unspecified site D43.2
  unspecified site C71.9
Gliomatosis cerebri C71.0
Glioneuroma — *see* Neoplasm, uncertain behavior, by site
Gliosarcoma
  specified site — *see* Neoplasm, malignant, by site
  unspecified site C71.9
Gliosis (cerebral) G93.89
  spinal G95.89
Glisson's disease — *see* Rickets
Globinuria R82.3
Globus (hystericus) F45.8

Glomangioma D18.00
  intra-abdominal D18.03
  intracranial D18.02
  skin D18.01
  specified site NEC D18.09
Glomangiomyoma D18.00
  intra-abdominal D18.03
  intracranial D18.02
  skin D18.01
  specified site NEC D18.09
Glomangiosarcoma — *see* Neoplasm, connective tissue, malignant
Glomerular
  disease in syphilis A52.75
  nephritis — *see* Glomerulonephritis
Glomerulitis — *see* Glomerulonephritis
Glomerulonephritis — *see also* Nephritis N05.9
  with
    C3
      glomerulonephritis N05.A
      glomerulopathy N05.A
        with dense deposit disease N05.6
    edema — *see* Nephrosis
    minimal change N05.0
    minor glomerular abnormality N05.0
  acute N00.9
  chronic N03.9
  crescentic (diffuse) NEC — *see also* N00-N07 with fourth character .7 N05.7
  dense deposit — *see also* N00-N07 with fourth character .6 N05.6
  diffuse
    crescentic — *see also* N00-N07 with fourth character .7 N05.7
    endocapillary proliferative — *see also* N00-N07 with fourth character .4 N05.4
    membranous — *see also* N00-N07 with fourth character .2 N05.2
    mesangial proliferative — *see also* N00-N07 with fourth character .3 N05.3
    mesangiocapillary — *see also* N00-N07 with fourth character .5 N05.5
    sclerosing N18.9
  endocapillary proliferative (diffuse) NEC — *see also* N00-N07 with fourth character .4 N05.4
  extracapillary NEC — *see also* N00-N07 with fourth character .7 N05.7
  focal (and segmental) — *see also* N00-N07 with fourth character .1 N05.1
  hypocomplementemic — *see* Glomerulonephritis, membranoproliferative
  IgA — *see* Nephropathy, IgA
  immune complex (circulating) NEC N05.8
  in (due to)
    amyloidosis E85.4 *[N08]*
    bilharziasis B65.9 *[N08]*
    cryoglobulinemia D89.1 *[N08]*
    defibrination syndrome D65 *[N08]*
    diabetes mellitus — *see* Diabetes, glomerulosclerosis
    disseminated intravascular coagulation D65 *[N08]*
    Fabry (-Anderson) disease E75.21 *[N08]*
    Goodpasture's syndrome M31.0
    hemolytic-uremic syndrome — *see* Syndrome, hemolytic-uremic
    Henoch (-Schönlein) purpura D69.0 *[N08]*
    lecithin cholesterol acyltransferase deficiency E78.6 *[N08]*
    microscopic polyangiitis M31.7 *[N08]*
    multiple myeloma C90.0- ☑ *[N08]*
    Plasmodium malariae B52.0
    schistosomiasis B65.9 *[N08]*
    sepsis A41.9 *[N08]*
      streptococcal A40- ☑ *[N08]*
    sickle-cell disorders D57.- ☑ *[N08]*
    strongyloidiasis B78.9 *[N08]*
    subacute bacterial endocarditis I33.0 *[N08]*
    syphilis (late) congenital A50.59 *[N08]*
    systemic lupus erythematosus M32.14
    thrombotic thrombocytopenic purpura M31.19 *[N08]*
    typhoid fever A01.09
    Waldenström macroglobulinemia C88.0 *[N08]*
    Wegener's granulomatosis M31.31
  latent or quiescent N03.9
  lobular, lobulonodular — *see* Glomerulonephritis, membranoproliferative

Glomerulonephritis — *continued*
  membranoproliferative (diffuse)(type 1 or 3) — *see also* N00-N07 with fourth character .5 N05.5
    dense deposit (type 2) NEC — *see also* N00-N07 with fourth character .6 N05.6
  membranous (diffuse) NEC — *see also* N00-N07 with fourth character .2 N05.2
  mesangial
    IgA/IgG — *see* Nephropathy, IgA
    proliferative (diffuse) NEC — *see also* N00-N07 with fourth character .3 N05.3
  mesangiocapillary (diffuse) NEC — *see also* N00-N07 with fourth character .5 N05.5
  necrotic, necrotizing NEC — *see also* N00- N07 with fourth character .8 N05.8
  nodular — *see* Glomerulonephritis, membranoproliferative
  poststreptococcal NEC N05.9
    acute N00.9
    chronic N03.9
    rapidly progressive N01.9
  proliferative NEC — *see also* N00-N07 with fourth character .8 N05.8
    diffuse (lupus) M32.14
    rapidly progressive N01.9
  sclerosing, diffuse N18.9
  specified pathology NEC — *see also* N00- N07 with fourth character .8 N05.8
  subacute N01.9
Glomerulopathy — *see* Glomerulonephritis
Glomerulosclerosis — *see also* Sclerosis, renal
  intercapillary (nodular) (with diabetes) — *see* Diabetes, glomerulosclerosis
  intracapillary — *see* Diabetes, glomerulosclerosis
Glossagra K14.6
Glossalgia K14.6
Glossitis (chronic superficial) (gangrenous) (Moeller's) K14.0
  areata exfoliativa K14.1
  atrophic K14.4
  benign migratory K14.1
  cortical superficial, sclerotic K14.0
  Hunter's D51.0
  interstitial, sclerous K14.0
  median rhomboid K14.2
  pellagrous E52
  superficial, chronic K14.0
Glossocele K14.8
Glossodynia K14.6
  exfoliativa K14.4
Glossoncus K14.8
Glossopathy K14.9
Glossophytia K14.3
Glossoplegia K14.8
Glossoptosis K14.8
Glossopyrosis K14.6
Glossotrichia K14.3
Glossy skin L90.8
Glottis — *see* condition
Glottitis — *see also* Laryngitis J04.0
Glucagonoma
  pancreas
    benign D13.7
    malignant C25.4
    uncertain behavior D37.8
  specified site NEC
    benign — *see* Neoplasm, benign, by site
    malignant — *see* Neoplasm, malignant, by site
    uncertain behavior — *see* Neoplasm, uncertain behavior, by site
  unspecified site
    benign D13.7
    malignant C25.4
    uncertain behavior D37.8
Glucoglycinuria E72.51
Glucose-galactose malabsorption E74.39
Glue
  ear — *see* Otitis, media, nonsuppurative, chronic, mucoid
  sniffing (airplane) — *see* Abuse, drug, inhalant
    dependence — *see* Dependence, drug, inhalant
GLUT1 deficiency syndrome 1, infantile onset E74.810
GLUT1 deficiency syndrome 2, childhood onset E74.810
Glutaric aciduria E72.3
Glycinemia E72.51
Glycinuria (renal) (with ketosis) E72.09

☑ Additional Character Required — Refer to the Tabular List for Character Selection

Glycogen
infiltration — *see* Disease, glycogen storage
storage disease — *see* Disease, glycogen storage
Glycogenosis (diffuse) (generalized) — *see also* Disease, glycogen storage
cardiac E74.02 *[I43]*
diabetic, secondary — *see* Diabetes, glycogenosis, secondary
pulmonary interstitial J84.842
Glycopenia E16.2
Glycosuria R81
renal E74.818
Gnathostoma spinigerum (infection) (infestation), **gnathostomiasis** (wandering swelling) B83.1
Goiter (plunging) (substernal) E04.9
with
hyperthyroidism (recurrent) — *see* Hyperthyroidism, with, goiter
thyrotoxicosis — *see* Hyperthyroidism, with, goiter
adenomatous — *see* Goiter, nodular
cancerous C73
congenital (nontoxic) E03.0
diffuse E03.0
parenchymatous E03.0
transitory, with normal functioning P72.0
cystic E04.2
due to iodine-deficiency E01.1
due to
enzyme defect in synthesis of thyroid hormone E07.1
iodine-deficiency (endemic) E01.2
dyshormonogenetic (familial) E07.1
endemic (iodine-deficiency) E01.2
diffuse E01.0
multinodular E01.1
exophthalmic — *see* Hyperthyroidism, with, goiter
iodine-deficiency (endemic) E01.2
diffuse E01.0
multinodular E01.1
nodular E01.1
lingual Q89.2
lymphadenoid E06.3
malignant C73
multinodular (cystic) (nontoxic) E04.2
toxic or with hyperthyroidism E05.20
with thyroid storm E05.21
neonatal NEC P72.0
nodular (nontoxic) (due to) E04.9
with
hyperthyroidism E05.20
with thyroid storm E05.21
thyrotoxicosis E05.20
with thyroid storm E05.21
endemic E01.1
iodine-deficiency E01.1
sporadic E04.9
toxic E05.20
with thyroid storm E05.21
nontoxic E04.9
diffuse (colloid) E04.0
multinodular E04.2
simple E04.0
specified NEC E04.8
uninodular E04.1
simple E04.0
toxic — *see* Hyperthyroidism, with, goiter
uninodular (nontoxic) E04.1
toxic or with hyperthyroidism E05.10
with thyroid storm E05.11
Goiter-deafness syndrome E07.1
Goldberg syndrome Q89.8
Goldberg-Maxwell syndrome E34.51
Goldblatt's hypertension or kidney I70.1
Goldenhar (-Gorlin) **syndrome** Q87.0
Goldflam-Erb disease or syndrome G70.00
with exacerbation (acute) G70.01
in crisis G70.01
Goldscheider's disease Q81.8
Goldstein's disease (familial hemorrhagic telangiectasia) I78.0
Golfer's elbow — *see* Epicondylitis, medial
Gonadoblastoma
specified site — *see* Neoplasm, uncertain behavior, by site
unspecified site
female D39.10
male D40.10
Gonecystitis — *see* Vesiculitis

Gongylonemiasis B83.8
Goniosynechiae — *see* Adhesions, iris, goniosynechiae
Goniosynechia A54.86
Gonococcus, gonococcal (disease) (infection) — *see also* condition A54.9
anus A54.6
bursa, bursitis A54.49
conjunctiva, conjunctivitis (neonatorum) A54.31
endocardium A54.83
eye A54.30
conjunctivitis A54.31
iridocyclitis A54.32
keratitis A54.33
newborn A54.31
other specified A54.39
fallopian tubes (acute) (chronic) A54.24
genitourinary (organ) (system) (tract) (acute)
lower A54.00
with abscess (accessory gland) (periurethral) A54.1
upper — *see also* condition A54.29
heart A54.83
iridocyclitis A54.32
joint A54.42
lymphatic (gland) (node) A54.89
meninges, meningitis A54.81
musculoskeletal A54.40
arthritis A54.42
osteomyelitis A54.43
other specified A54.49
spondylopathy A54.41
pelviperitonitis A54.24
pelvis (acute) (chronic) A54.24
pharynx A54.5
proctitis A54.6
pyosalpinx (acute) (chronic) A54.24
rectum A54.6
skin A54.89
specified site NEC A54.89
tendon sheath A54.49
throat A54.5
urethra (acute) (chronic) A54.01
with abscess (accessory gland) (periurethral) A54.1
vulva (acute) (chronic) A54.02
Gonocytoma
specified site — *see* Neoplasm, uncertain behavior, by site
unspecified site
female D39.10
male D40.10
Gonorrhea (acute) (chronic) A54.9
Bartholin's gland (acute) (chronic) (purulent) A54.02
with abscess (accessory gland) (periurethral) A54.1
bladder A54.01
cervix A54.03
conjunctiva, conjunctivitis (neonatorum) A54.31
contact Z20.2
Cowper's gland (with abscess) A54.1
exposure to Z20.2
fallopian tube (acute) (chronic) A54.24
kidney (acute) (chronic) A54.21
lower genitourinary tract A54.00
with abscess (accessory gland) (periurethral) A54.1
ovary (acute) (chronic) A54.24
pelvis (acute) (chronic) A54.24
female pelvic inflammatory disease A54.24
penis A54.09
prostate (acute) (chronic) A54.22
seminal vesicle (acute) (chronic) A54.23
specified site not listed — *see also* Gonococcus A54.89
spermatic cord (acute) (chronic) A54.23
urethra A54.01
with abscess (accessory gland) (periurethral) A54.1
vagina A54.02
vas deferens (acute) (chronic) A54.23
vulva A54.02
Goodall's disease A08.19
Goodpasture's syndrome M31.0
Gopalan's syndrome (burning feet) E53.0
Gorlin-Chaudry-Moss syndrome Q87.0
Gottron's papules L94.4
Gougerot-Blum syndrome (pigmented purpuric lichenoid dermatitis) L81.7
Gougerot-Carteaud disease or syndrome (confluent reticulate papillomatosis) L83
Gougerot's syndrome (trisymptomatic) L81.7
Gouley's syndrome (constrictive pericarditis) I31.1
Goundou A66.6

Gout, chronic — *see also* Gout, gouty M1A.9 ☑ (*following* M08)
drug-induced M1A.20 ☑ (*following* M08)
ankle M1A.27- ☑ (*following* M08)
elbow M1A.22- ☑ (*following* M08)
foot joint M1A.27- ☑ (*following* M08)
hand joint M1A.24- ☑ (*following* M08)
hip M1A.25- ☑ (*following* M08)
knee M1A.26- ☑ (*following* M08)
multiple site M1A.29- ☑ (*following* M08)
shoulder M1A.21- ☑ (*following* M08)
vertebrae M1A.28 ☑ (*following* M08)
wrist M1A.23- ☑ (*following* M08)
idiopathic M1A.00 ☑ (*following* M08)
ankle M1A.07- ☑ (*following* M08)
elbow M1A.02- ☑ (*following* M08)
foot joint M1A.07- ☑ (*following* M08)
hand joint M1A.04- ☑ (*following* M08)
hip M1A.05- ☑ (*following* M08)
knee M1A.06- ☑ (*following* M08)
multiple site M1A.09 ☑ (*following* M08)
shoulder M1A.01- ☑ (*following* M08)
vertebrae M1A.08 ☑ (*following* M08)
wrist M1A.03- ☑ (*following* M08)
in (due to) renal impairment M1A.30 ☑ (*following* M08)
ankle M1A.37- ☑ (*following* M08)
elbow M1A.32- ☑ (*following* M08)
foot joint M1A.37- ☑ (*following* M08)
hand joint M1A.34- ☑ (*following* M08)
hip M1A.35- ☑ (*following* M08)
knee M1A.36- ☑ (*following* M08)
multiple site M1A.39 ☑ (*following* M08)
shoulder M1A.31- ☑ (*following* M08)
vertebrae M1A.38 ☑ (*following* M08)
wrist M1A.33- ☑ (*following* M08)
lead-induced M1A.10 ☑ (*following* M08)
ankle M1A.17- ☑ (*following* M08)
elbow M1A.12- ☑ (*following* M08)
foot joint M1A.17- ☑ (*following* M08)
hand joint M1A.14- ☑ (*following* M08)
hip M1A.15- ☑ (*following* M08)
knee M1A.16- ☑ (*following* M08)
multiple site M1A.19 ☑ (*following* M08)
shoulder M1A.11- ☑ (*following* M08)
vertebrae M1A.18 ☑ (*following* M08)
wrist M1A.13- ☑ (*following* M08)
primary — *see* Gout, chronic, idiopathic
saturnine — *see* Gout, chronic, lead-induced
secondary NEC M1A.40 ☑ (*following* M08)
ankle M1A.47- ☑ (*following* M08)
elbow M1A.42- ☑ (*following* M08)
foot joint M1A.47- ☑ (*following* M08)
hand joint M1A.44- ☑ (*following* M08)
hip M1A.45- ☑ (*following* M08)
knee M1A.46- ☑ (*following* M08)
multiple site M1A.49 ☑ (*following* M08)
shoulder M1A.41- ☑ (*following* M08)
vertebrae M1A.48 ☑ (*following* M08)
wrist M1A.43- ☑ (*following* M08)
syphilitic — *see also* subcategory M14.8- A52.77
tophi M1A.9 ☑ (*following* M08)
Gout, gouty (acute) (attack) (flare) — *see also* Gout, chronic M10.9
drug-induced M10.20
ankle M10.27- ☑
elbow M10.22- ☑
foot joint M10.27- ☑
hand joint M10.24- ☑
hip M10.25- ☑
knee M10.26- ☑
multiple site M10.29
shoulder M10.21- ☑
vertebrae M10.28
wrist M10.23- ☑
idiopathic M10.00
ankle M10.07- ☑
elbow M10.02- ☑
foot joint M10.07- ☑
hand joint M10.04- ☑
hip M10.05- ☑
knee M10.06- ☑
multiple site M10.09
shoulder M10.01- ☑
vertebrae M10.08
wrist M10.03- ☑
in (due to) renal impairment M10.30

Gout, gouty — *continued*
  in renal impairment — *continued*
      ankle M10.37- ☑
      elbow M10.32- ☑
      foot joint M10.37- ☑
      hand joint M10.34- ☑
      hip M10.35- ☑
      knee M10.36- ☑
      multiple site M10.39
      shoulder M10.31- ☑
      vertebrae M10.38
      wrist M10.33- ☑
  lead-induced M10.10
      ankle M10.17- ☑
      elbow M10.12- ☑
      foot joint M10.17- ☑
      hand joint M10.14- ☑
      hip M10.15- ☑
      knee M10.16- ☑
      multiple site M10.19
      shoulder M10.11- ☑
      vertebrae M10.18
      wrist M10.13- ☑
  primary — *see* Gout, idiopathic
  saturnine — *see* Gout, lead-induced
  secondary NEC M10.40
      ankle M10.47- ☑
      elbow M10.42- ☑
      foot joint M10.47- ☑
      hand joint M10.44- ☑
      hip M10.45- ☑
      knee M10.46- ☑
      multiple site M10.49
      shoulder M10.41- ☑
      vertebrae M10.48
      wrist M10.43- ☑
  syphilitic — *see also* subcategory M14.8- A52.77
  tophi — *see* Gout, chronic

Gower's
  muscular dystrophy G71.01
  syndrome (vasovagal attack) R55

Gradenigo's syndrome — *see* Otitis, media, suppurative, acute

Graefe's disease — *see* Strabismus, paralytic, ophthalmoplegia, progressive

Graft-versus-host disease D89.813
  acute D89.810
  acute on chronic D89.812
  chronic D89.811

Grain mite (itch) B88.0

Grainhandler's disease or lung J67.8

Grand mal — *see* Epilepsy, generalized, specified NEC

Grand multipara status only (not pregnant) Z64.1
  pregnant — *see* Pregnancy, complicated by, grand multiparity

Granite worker's lung J62.8

Granular — *see also* condition
  inflammation, pharynx J31.2
  kidney (contracting) — *see* Sclerosis, renal
  liver K74.69

Granulation tissue (abnormal) (excessive) L92.9
  postmastoidectomy cavity — *see* Complications, postmastoidectomy, granulation

Granulocytopenia (primary) (malignant) — *see* Agranulocytosis

Granuloma L92.9
  abdomen K66.8
    from residual foreign body L92.3
    pyogenicum L98.0
  actinic L57.5
  annulare (perforating) L92.0
  apical K04.5
  aural — *see* Otitis, externa, specified NEC
  beryllium (skin) L92.3
  bone
    eosinophilic C96.6
    from residual foreign body — *see* Osteomyelitis, specified type NEC
    lung C96.6
  brain (any site) G06.0
    schistosomiasis B65.9 [G07]
  canaliculus lacrimalis — *see* Granuloma, lacrimal
  candidal (cutaneous) B37.2
  cerebral (any site) G06.0
  coccidioidal (primary) (progressive) B38.7
    lung B38.1
    meninges B38.4

Granuloma — *continued*
  colon K63.89
  conjunctiva H11.22- ☑
  dental K04.5
  ear, middle — *see* Cholesteatoma
  eosinophilic C96.6
    bone C96.6
    lung C96.6
    oral mucosa K13.4
    skin L92.2
  eyelid H01.8
  facial (e) L92.2
  foreign body (in soft tissue) NEC M60.20
    ankle M60.27- ☑
    foot M60.27- ☑
    forearm M60.23- ☑
    hand M60.24- ☑
    in operation wound — *see* Foreign body, accidentally left during a procedure
    lower leg M60.26- ☑
    pelvic region M60.25- ☑
    shoulder region M60.21- ☑
    skin L92.3
    specified site NEC M60.28
    subcutaneous tissue L92.3
    thigh M60.25- ☑
    upper arm M60.22- ☑
  gangraenescens M31.2
  genito-inguinale A58
  giant cell (central) (reparative) (jaw) M27.1
    gingiva (peripheral) K06.8
  gland (lymph) I88.8
  hepatic NEC K75.3
    in (due to)
      berylliosis J63.2 [K77]
      sarcoidosis D86.89
  Hodgkin C81.9 ☑
  ileum K63.89
  infectious B99.9
    specified NEC B99.8
  inguinale (Donovan) (venereal) A58
  intestine NEC K63.89
  intracranial (any site) G06.0
  intraspinal (any part) G06.1
  iridocyclitis — *see* Iridocyclitis, chronic
  jaw (bone) (central) M27.1
    reparative giant cell M27.1
  kidney — *see also* Infection, kidney N15.8
  lacrimal H04.81- ☑
  larynx J38.7
  lethal midline (faciale(e)) M31.2
  liver NEC — *see* Granuloma, hepatic
  lung (infectious) — *see also* Fibrosis, lung
    coccidioidal B38.1
    eosinophilic C96.6
  Majocchi's B35.8
  malignant (facial(e)) M31.2
  mandible (central) M27.1
  midline (lethal) M31.2
  monilial (cutaneous) B37.2
  nasal sinus — *see* Sinusitis
  operation wound T81.89 ☑
    foreign body — *see* Foreign body, accidentally left during a procedure
    stitch T81.89 ☑
    talc — *see* Foreign body, accidentally left during a procedure
  oral mucosa K13.4
  orbit, orbital H05.11- ☑
  paracoccidioidal B41.8
  penis, venereal A58
  periapical K04.5
  peritoneum K66.8
    due to ova of helminths NOS — *see also* Helminthiasis B83.9 [K67]
  postmastoidectomy cavity — *see* Complications, postmastoidectomy, recurrent cholesteatoma
  prostate N42.89
  pudendi (ulcerating) A58
  pulp, internal (tooth) K03.3
  pyogenic, pyogenicum (of) (skin) L98.0
    gingiva K06.8
    maxillary alveolar ridge K04.5
    oral mucosa K13.4
  rectum K62.89
  reticulohistiocytic D76.3
  rubrum nasi L74.8
  Schistosoma — *see* Schistosomiasis

Granuloma — *continued*
  septic (skin) L98.0
  silica (skin) L92.3
  sinus (accessory) (infective) (nasal) — *see* Sinusitis
  skin L92.9
    from residual foreign body L92.3
    pyogenicum L98.0
  spine
    syphilitic (epidural) A52.19
    tuberculous A18.01
  stitch (postoperative) T81.89 ☑
  suppurative (skin) L98.0
  swimming pool A31.1
  talc — *see also* Granuloma, foreign body
    in operation wound — *see* Foreign body, accidentally left during a procedure
  telangiectaticum (skin) L98.0
  tracheostomy J95.09
  trichophyticum B35.8
  tropicum A66.4
  umbilical P83.81
  umbilicus P83.81
  urethra N36.8
  uveitis — *see* Iridocyclitis, chronic
  vagina A58
  venereum A58
  vocal cord J38.3

Granulomatosis L92.9
  with polyangiitis M31.3- ☑
  eosinophilic, with polyangiitis [EGPA] M30.1
  lymphoid C83.8- ☑
  miliary (listerial) A32.89
  necrotizing, respiratory M31.30
  progressive septic D71
  specified NEC L92.8
  Wegener's M31.30
    with renal involvement M31.31

Granulomatous tissue (abnormal) (excessive) L92.9

Granulosis rubra nasi L74.8

Graphite fibrosis (of lung) J63.3

Graphospasm F48.8
  organic G25.89

Grating scapula M89.8X1

Gravel (urinary) — *see* Calculus, urinary

Graves' disease — *see* Hyperthyroidism, with, goiter

Gravis — *see* condition

Grawitz tumor C64.- ☑

Gray syndrome (newborn) P93.0

Grayness, hair (premature) L67.1
  congenital Q84.2

Green sickness D50.8

Greenfield's disease
  meaning
    concentric sclerosis (encephalitis periaxialis concentrica) G37.5
    metachromatic leukodystrophy E75.25

Greenstick fracture — *code as* Fracture, by site

Grey syndrome (newborn) P93.0

Grief F43.21
  complicated F34.81
  prolonged F43.29
  reaction — *see also* Disorder, adjustment F43.20

Griesinger's disease B76.0

Grinder's lung or pneumoconiosis J62.8

Grinding, teeth
  psychogenic F45.8
  sleep related G47.63

Grip
  Dabney's B33.0
  devil's B33.0

Grippe, grippal — *see also* Influenza
  Balkan A78
  summer, of Italy A93.1

Grisel's disease M43.6

Groin — *see* condition

Grooved tongue K14.5

Ground itch B76.9

Grover's disease or syndrome L11.1

Growing pains, children R29.898

Growth (fungoid) (neoplastic) (new) — *see also* Neoplasm
  adenoid (vegetative) J35.8
  benign — *see* Neoplasm, benign, by site
  malignant — *see* Neoplasm, malignant, by site
  rapid, childhood Z00.2
  secondary — *see* Neoplasm, secondary, by site

Gruby's disease B35.0

Gubler-Millard paralysis or syndrome G46.3

Guerin-Stern syndrome Q74.3
Guidance, insufficient anterior (occlusal) M26.54
Guillain-Barré disease or syndrome G61.0
    sequelae G65.0
Guinea worms (infection) (infestation) B72
Guinon's disease (motor-verbal tic) F95.2
Gull's disease E03.4
Gum — *see* condition
Gumboil K04.7
    with sinus K04.6
Gumma (syphilitic) A52.79
    artery A52.09
        cerebral A52.04
    bone A52.77
        of yaws (late) A66.6
    brain A52.19
    cauda equina A52.19
    central nervous system A52.3
    ciliary body A52.71
    congenital A50.59
    eyelid A52.71
    heart A52.06
    intracranial A52.19
    iris A52.71
    kidney A52.75
    larynx A52.73
    leptomeninges A52.19
    liver A52.74
    meninges A52.19
    myocardium A52.06
    nasopharynx A52.73
    neurosyphilitic A52.3
    nose A52.73
    orbit A52.71
    palate (soft) A52.79
    penis A52.76
    pericardium A52.06
    pharynx A52.73
    pituitary A52.79
    scrofulous (tuberculous) A18.4
    skin A52.79
    specified site NEC A52.79
    spinal cord A52.19
    tongue A52.79
    tonsil A52.73
    trachea A52.73
    tuberculous A18.4
    ulcerative due to yaws A66.4
    ureter A52.75
    yaws A66.4
        bone A66.6
Gunn's syndrome Q07.8
Gunshot wound — *see also* Puncture, open
    fracture — *code as* Fracture, by site
    internal organs — *see* Injury, by site
Gynandrism Q56.0
Gynandroblastoma
    specified site — *see* Neoplasm, uncertain behavior, by
        site
    unspecified site
        female D39.10
        male D40.10
Gynecological examination (periodic) (routine) Z01.419
    with abnormal findings Z01.411
Gynecomastia N62
Gynephobia F40.291
Gyrate scalp Q82.8

H

H (Hartnup's) **disease** E72.02
Haas' disease or osteochondrosis (juvenile) (head of
    humerus) — *see* Osteochondrosis, juvenile, humerus
Habit, habituation
    bad sleep Z72.821
    chorea F95.8
    disturbance, child F98.9
    drug — *see* Dependence, drug
    irregular sleep Z72.821
    laxative F55.2
    spasm — *see* Tic
    tic — *see* Tic
Haemophilus (H.) **influenzae, as cause of disease
    classified elsewhere** B96.3
Haff disease — *see* Poisoning, mercury
Hageman's factor defect, deficiency or disease D68.2

Haglund's disease or osteochondrosis (juvenile) (os
    tibiale externum) — *see* Osteochondrosis, juvenile,
    tarsus
Hailey-Hailey disease Q82.8
Hair — *see also* condition
    plucking F63.3
        in stereotyped movement disorder F98.4
    tourniquet syndrome — *see also* Constriction, external,
        by site
        finger S60.44- ☑
        penis S30.842 ☑
        thumb S60.34- ☑
        toe S90.44- ☑
Hairball in stomach T18.2 ☑
Hair-pulling, pathological (compulsive) F63.3
Hairy black tongue K14.3
Half vertebra Q76.49
Halitosis R19.6
Hallerman-Streiff syndrome Q87.0
Hallervorden-Spatz disease G23.0
Hallopeau's acrodermatitis or disease L40.2
Hallucination R44.3
    auditory R44.0
    gustatory R44.2
    olfactory R44.2
    specified NEC R44.2
    tactile R44.2
    visual R44.1
Hallucinosis (chronic) F28
    alcoholic (acute) F10.951
        in
            abuse F10.151
            dependence F10.251
    drug-induced F19.951
        cannabis F12.951
        cocaine F14.951
        hallucinogen F16.151
        in
            abuse F19.151
                cannabis F12.151
                cocaine F14.151
                hallucinogen F16.151
                inhalant F18.151
                opioid F11.151
                sedative, anxiolytic or hypnotic F13.151
                stimulant NEC F15.151
            dependence F19.251
                cannabis F12.251
                cocaine F14.251
                hallucinogen F16.251
                inhalant F18.251
                opioid F11.251
                sedative, anxiolytic or hypnotic F13.251
                stimulant NEC F15.251
        inhalant F18.951
        opioid F11.951
        sedative, anxiolytic or hypnotic F13.951
        stimulant NEC F15.951
    organic F06.0
Hallux
    deformity (acquired) NEC M20.5X- ☑
    limitus M20.5X- ☑
    malleus (acquired) NEC M20.3- ☑
    rigidus (acquired) M20.2- ☑
        congenital Q74.2
        sequelae (late effect) of rickets E64.3
    valgus (acquired) M20.1- ☑
        congenital Q66.6
    varus (acquired) M20.3- ☑
        congenital Q66.3- ☑
Halo, visual H53.19
Hamartoma, hamartoblastoma Q85.9
    epithelial (gingival), odontogenic, central or peripheral
        — *see* Cyst, calcifying odontogenic
Hamartosis Q85.9
Hamman-Rich syndrome J84.114
Hammer toe (acquired) NEC — *see also* Deformity, toe,
    hammer toe
    congenital Q66.89
    sequelae (late effect) of rickets E64.3
Hand — *see* condition
Hand-foot syndrome L27.1
Handicap, handicapped
    educational Z55.9
        specified NEC Z55.8
Hand-Schüller-Christian disease or syndrome C96.5

Hanging (asphyxia) (strangulation) (suffocation) — *see*
    Asphyxia, traumatic, due to mechanical threat
Hangnail — *see also* Cellulitis, digit
    with lymphangitis — *see* Lymphangitis, acute, digit
Hangover (alcohol) F10.129
Hanhart's syndrome Q87.0
Hanot-Chauffard (-Troisier) **syndrome** E83.19
Hanot's cirrhosis or disease K74.3
Hansen's disease — *see* Leprosy
Hantaan virus disease (Korean hemorrhagic fever) A98.5
Hantavirus disease (with renal manifestations) (Dobrava)
    (Puumala) (Seoul) A98.5
    with pulmonary manifestations (Andes) (Bayou)
        (Bermejo) (Black Creek Canal) (Choclo) (Juquitiba)
        (Laguna negra) (Lechiguanas) (New York) (Oran)
        (Sin nombre) B33.4
Happy puppet syndrome Q93.51
Harada's disease or syndrome H30.81- ☑
Hardening
    artery — *see* Arteriosclerosis
    brain G93.89
Hardship, material Z59.87
Harelip (complete) (incomplete) — *see* Cleft, lip
Harlequin (newborn) Q80.4
Harley's disease D59.6
Harmful use (of)
    alcohol F10.10
    anxiolytics — *see* Abuse, drug, sedative
    cannabinoids — *see* Abuse, drug, cannabis
    cocaine — *see* Abuse, drug, cocaine
    drug — *see* Abuse, drug
    hallucinogens — *see* Abuse, drug, hallucinogen
    hypnotics — *see* Abuse, drug, sedative
    opioids — *see* Abuse, drug, opioid
    PCP (phencyclidine) — *see* Abuse, drug, hallucinogen
    sedatives — *see* Abuse, drug, sedative
    stimulants NEC — *see* Abuse, drug, stimulant
Harris' lines — *see* Arrest, epiphyseal
Hartnup's disease E72.02
Harvester's lung J67.0
Harvesting ovum for in vitro fertilization Z31.83
Hashimoto's disease or thyroiditis E06.3
Hashitoxicosis (transient) E06.3
Hassal-Henle bodies or warts (cornea) H18.49
Haut mal — *see* Epilepsy, generalized, specified NEC
Haverhill fever A25.1
Hay fever — *see also* Fever, hay J30.1
Hayem-Widal syndrome D59.8
Haygarth's nodes M15.8
Haymaker's lung J67.0
Hb (abnormal)
    Bart's disease D56.0
    disease — *see* Disease, hemoglobin
    trait — *see* Trait
Head — *see* condition
Headache R51.9
    with
        orthostatic component NEC R51.0
        positional component NEC R51.0
    allergic NEC G44.89
    associated with sexual activity G44.82
    cervicogenic G44.86
    chronic daily R51.9
    cluster G44.009
        chronic G44.029
            intractable G44.021
            not intractable G44.029
        episodic G44.019
            intractable G44.011
            not intractable G44.019
        intractable G44.001
        not intractable G44.009
    cough (primary) G44.83
    daily chronic R51.9
    drug-induced NEC G44.40
        intractable G44.41
        not intractable G44.40
    exertional (primary) G44.84
    histamine G44.009
        intractable G44.001
        not intractable G44.009
    hypnic G44.81
    lumbar puncture G97.1
    medication overuse G44.40
        intractable G44.41
        not intractable G44.40
    menstrual — *see* Migraine, menstrual

Headache — *continued*
  migraine (type) — *see also* Migraine G43.909
  nasal septum R51.9
  neuralgiform, short lasting unilateral, with conjunctival
      injection and tearing (SUNCT) G44.059
    intractable G44.051
    not intractable G44.059
  new daily persistent (NDPH) G44.52
  orgasmic G44.82
  periodic syndromes in adults and children G43.C0 (*following* G43.7)
    with refractory migraine G43.C1 (*following* G43.7)
      intractable G43.C1 (*following* G43.7)
      not intractable G43.C0 (*following* G43.7)
    without refractory migraine G43.C0 (*following* G43.7)
  postspinal puncture G97.1
  post-traumatic G44.309
    acute G44.319
      intractable G44.311
      not intractable G44.319
    chronic G44.329
      intractable G44.321
      not intractable G44.329
    intractable G44.301
    not intractable G44.309
  pre-menstrual — *see* Migraine, menstrual
  preorgasmic G44.82
  primary
    cough G44.83
    exertional G44.84
    stabbing G44.85
    thunderclap G44.53
  rebound G44.40
    intractable G44.41
    not intractable G44.40
  short lasting unilateral neuralgiform, with conjunctival
      injection and tearing (SUNCT) G44.059
    intractable G44.051
    not intractable G44.059
  specified syndrome NEC G44.89
  spinal and epidural anesthesia - induced T88.59 ☑
    in labor and delivery O74.5
    in pregnancy O29.4- ☑
    postpartum, puerperal O89.4
  spinal fluid loss (from puncture) G97.1
  stabbing (primary) G44.85
  tension (-type) G44.209
    chronic G44.229
      intractable G44.221
      not intractable G44.229
    episodic G44.219
      intractable G44.211
      not intractable G44.219
    intractable G44.201
    not intractable G44.209
  thunderclap (primary) G44.53
  vascular NEC G44.1
Healthy
  infant
    accompanying sick mother Z76.3
    receiving care Z76.2
  person accompanying sick person Z76.3
Hearing examination Z01.10
  with abnormal findings NEC Z01.118
  following failed hearing screening Z01.110
  for hearing conservation and treatment Z01.12
  infant or child (over 28 days old) Z00.129
    with abnormal findings Z00.121
Heart — *see* condition
Heart beat
  abnormality R00.9
    specified NEC R00.8
  awareness R00.2
  rapid R00.0
  slow R00.1
Heartburn R12
  psychogenic F45.8
Heartland virus disease A93.8
Heat (effects) T67.9 ☑
  apoplexy T67.01 ☑
  burn — *see also* Burn L55.9
  collapse T67.1 ☑
  cramps T67.2 ☑
  dermatitis or eczema L59.0
  edema T67.7 ☑
  erythema — *code by site under* Burn, first degree
  excessive T67.9 ☑
    specified effect NEC T67.8 ☑

Heat — *continued*
  exhaustion T67.5 ☑
    anhydrotic T67.3 ☑
    due to
      salt (and water) depletion T67.4 ☑
      water depletion T67.3 ☑
        with salt depletion T67.4 ☑
  fatigue (transient) T67.6 ☑
  fever T67.01 ☑
  hyperpyrexia T67.01 ☑
  prickly L74.0
  prostration — *see* Heat, exhaustion
  pyrexia T67.01 ☑
  rash L74.0
  specified effect NEC T67.8 ☑
  stroke T67.01 ☑
    exertional T67.02 ☑
    specified NEC T67.09 ☑
  sunburn — *see* Sunburn
  syncope T67.1 ☑
Heavy-for-dates NEC (infant) (4000g to 4499g) P08.1
  exceptionally (4500g or more) P08.0
Hebephrenia, hebephrenic (schizophrenia) F20.1
Heberden's disease or nodes (with arthropathy) M15.1
Hebra's
  pityriasis L26
  prurigo L28.2
Heel — *see* condition
Heerfordt's disease D86.89
Hegglin's anomaly or syndrome D72.0
Heilmeyer-Schoner disease D45
Heine-Medin disease A80.9
Heinz body anemia, congenital D58.2
Heliophobia F40.228
Heller's disease or syndrome F84.3
HELLP syndrome (hemolysis, elevated liver enzymes and
    low platelet count) O14.2- ☑
  complicating
    childbirth O14.24
    puerperium O14.25
Helminthiasis — *see also* Infestation, helminth
  Ancylostoma B76.0
  intestinal B82.0
    mixed types (types classifiable to more than one of
      the titles B65.0-B81.3 and B81.8) B81.4
    specified type NEC B81.8
  mixed types (intestinal) (types classifiable to more than
      one of the titles B65.0-B81.3 and B81.8) B81.4
  Necator (americanus) B76.1
  specified type NEC B83.8
Heloma L84
Hemangioblastoma — *see* Neoplasm, connective tissue,
  uncertain behavior
  malignant — *see* Neoplasm, connective tissue, malig-
    nant
Hemangioendothelioma — *see also* Neoplasm, uncertain behavior, by site
  benign D18.00
    intra-abdominal D18.03
    intracranial D18.02
    skin D18.01
    specified site NEC D18.09
  bone (diffuse) — *see* Neoplasm, bone, malignant
  epithelioid — *see also* Neoplasm, uncertain behavior,
    by site
    malignant — *see* Neoplasm, malignant, by site
  malignant — *see* Neoplasm, connective tissue, malig-
    nant
Hemangiofibroma — *see* Neoplasm, benign, by site
Hemangiolipoma — *see* Lipoma
Hemangioma D18.00
  arteriovenous D18.00
    intra-abdominal D18.03
    intracranial D18.02
    skin D18.01
    specified site NEC D18.09
  capillary I78.1
    intra-abdominal D18.03
    intracranial D18.02
    skin D18.01
    specified site NEC D18.09
  cavernous D18.00
    intra-abdominal D18.03
    intracranial D18.02
    skin D18.01
    specified site NEC D18.09
  epithelioid D18.00

Hemangioma — *continued*
  epithelioid — *continued*
    intra-abdominal D18.03
    intracranial D18.02
    skin D18.01
    specified site NEC D18.09
  histiocytoid D18.00
    intra-abdominal D18.03
    intracranial D18.02
    skin D18.01
    specified site NEC D18.09
  infantile D18.00
    intra-abdominal D18.03
    intracranial D18.02
    skin D18.01
    specified site NEC D18.09
  intra-abdominal D18.03
  intracranial D18.02
  intramuscular D18.00
    intra-abdominal D18.03
    intracranial D18.02
    skin D18.01
    specified site NEC D18.09
  intrathoracic structures D18.09
  juvenile D18.00
  malignant — *see* Neoplasm,connective tissue, malig-
    nant
  plexiform D18.00
    intra-abdominal D18.03
    intracranial D18.02
    skin D18.01
    specified site NEC D18.09
  racemose D18.00
    intra-abdominal D18.03
    intracranial D18.02
    skin D18.01
    specified site NEC D18.09
  sclerosing — *see* Neoplasm, skin, benign
  simplex D18.00
    intra-abdominal D18.03
    intracranial D18.02
    skin D18.01
    specified site NEC D18.09
  skin D18.01
  specified site NEC D18.09
  venous D18.00
    intra-abdominal D18.03
    intracranial D18.02
    skin D18.01
    specified site NEC D18.09
  verrucous keratotic D18.00
    intra-abdominal D18.03
    intracranial D18.02
    skin D18.01
    specified site NEC D18.09
Hemangiomatosis (systemic) I78.8
  involving single site — *see* Hemangioma
Hemangiopericytoma — *see also* Neoplasm, connective
  tissue, uncertain behavior
  benign — *see* Neoplasm, connective tissue, benign
  malignant — *see* Neoplasm, connective tissue, malig-
    nant
Hemangiosarcoma — *see* Neoplasm, connective tissue,
  malignant
Hemarthrosis (nontraumatic) M25.00
  ankle M25.07- ☑
  elbow M25.02- ☑
  foot joint M25.07- ☑
  hand joint M25.04- ☑
  hip M25.05- ☑
  in hemophilic arthropathy — *see* Arthropathy,
    hemophilic
  knee M25.06- ☑
  shoulder M25.01- ☑
  specified joint NEC M25.08
  traumatic — *see* Sprain, by site
  vertebrae M25.08
  wrist M25.03- ☑
Hematemesis K92.0
  with ulcer — *code by site under* Ulcer, with hemorrhage
    K27.4
  newborn, neonatal P54.0
    due to swallowed maternal blood P78.2
Hematidrosis L74.8
Hematinuria — *see also* Hemoglobinuria
  malarial B50.8
Hematobilia K83.8

Hematocele
  female NEC N94.89
    with ectopic pregnancy O00.90
      with intrauterine pregnancy O00.91
    ovary N83.8
  male N50.1
Hematochezia — see also Melena K92.1
Hematochyluria — see also Infestation, filarial
  schistosomiasis (bilharziasis) B65.0
Hematocolpos (with hematometra or hematosalpinx)
  N89.7
Hematocornea — see Pigmentation, cornea, stromal
Hematogenous — see condition
Hematoma (traumatic) (skin surface intact) — see also
  Contusion
  with
    injury of internal organs — see Injury, by site
    open wound — see Wound, open
  amputation stump (surgical) (late) T87.89
  aorta, dissecting I71.00
    abdominal I71.02
    thoracic — see also Dissection, aorta, thoracic
      I71.019
    thoracoabdominal I71.03
  aortic intramural — see Dissection, aorta
  arterial (complicating trauma) — see Injury, blood
    vessel, by site
  auricle — see Contusion, ear
    nontraumatic — see Disorder, pinna, hematoma
  birth injury NEC P15.8
  brain (traumatic)
    with
      cerebral laceration or contusion (diffuse) — see
        Injury, intracranial, diffuse
        focal — see Injury, intracranial, focal
    cerebellar, traumatic S06.37- ☑
    intracerebral, traumatic — see Injury, intracranial,
      intracerebral hemorrhage
    newborn NEC P52.4
      birth injury P10.1
    nontraumatic — see Hemorrhage, intracranial
    subarachnoid, arachnoid, traumatic — see Injury,
      intracranial, subarachnoid hemorrhage
    subdural, traumatic — see Injury, intracranial, sub-
      dural hemorrhage
  breast (nontraumatic) N64.89
  broad ligament (nontraumatic) N83.7
    traumatic S37.892 ☑
  cerebellar, traumatic S06.37- ☑
  cerebral — see Hematoma, brain
  cerebrum S06.36- ☑
    left S06.35- ☑
    right S06.34- ☑
  cesarean delivery wound O90.2
  complicating delivery (perineal) (pelvic) (vagina) (vulva)
    O71.7
  corpus cavernosum (nontraumatic) N48.89
  epididymis (nontraumatic) N50.1
  epidural (traumatic) — see Injury, intracranial, epidural
    hemorrhage
    spinal — see Injury, spinal cord, by region
  episiotomy O90.2
  face, birth injury P15.4
  genital organ NEC (nontraumatic)
    female (nonobstetric) N94.89
      traumatic S30.202 ☑
    male N50.1
      traumatic S30.201 ☑
  internal organs — see Injury, by site
  intracerebral, traumatic — see Injury, intracranial, in-
    tracerebral hemorrhage
  intraoperative — see Complications, intraoperative,
    hemorrhage
  labia (nontraumatic) (nonobstetric) N90.89
  liver (subcapsular) (nontraumatic) K76.89
    birth injury P15.0
  mediastinum — see Injury, intrathoracic
  mesosalpinx (nontraumatic) N83.7
    traumatic S37.898 ☑
  muscle — code by site under Contusion
  nontraumatic
    muscle M79.81
    soft tissue M79.81
  obstetrical surgical wound O90.2
  orbit, orbital (nontraumatic) — see also Hemorrhage,
    orbit
    traumatic — see Contusion, orbit

Hematoma — continued
  pelvis (female) (nontraumatic) (nonobstetric) N94.89
    obstetric O71.7
    traumatic — see Injury, by site
  penis (nontraumatic) N48.89
    birth injury P15.5
  perianal (nontraumatic) K64.5
  perineal S30.23 ☑
    complicating delivery O71.7
  perirenal — see Injury, kidney
  pinna — see Contusion, ear
    nontraumatic — see Disorder, pinna, hematoma
  placenta O43.89- ☑
  postoperative (postprocedural) — see Complication,
    postprocedural, hematoma
  retroperitoneal (nontraumatic) K66.1
    traumatic S36.892 ☑
  scrotum, superficial S30.22 ☑
    birth injury P15.5
  seminal vesicle (nontraumatic) N50.1
    traumatic S37.892 ☑
  spermatic cord (traumatic) S37.892 ☑
    nontraumatic N50.1
  spinal (cord) (meninges) — see also Injury, spinal cord,
    by region
    newborn (birth injury) P11.5
  spleen D73.5
    intraoperative — see Complications, intraoperative,
      hemorrhage, spleen
    postprocedural (postoperative) — see Complica-
      tions, postprocedural, hemorrhage, spleen
  sternocleidomastoid, birth injury P15.2
  sternomastoid, birth injury P15.2
  subarachnoid (traumatic) — see Injury, intracranial,
    subarachnoid hemorrhage
    newborn (nontraumatic) P52.5
      due to birth injury P10.3
    nontraumatic — see Hemorrhage, intracranial,
      subarachnoid
  subdural (traumatic) — see Injury, intracranial, subdural
    hemorrhage
    newborn (localized) P52.8
      birth injury P10.0
    nontraumatic — see Hemorrhage, intracranial,
      subdural
  superficial, newborn P54.5
  testis (nontraumatic) N50.1
    birth injury P15.5
  tunica vaginalis (nontraumatic) N50.1
  umbilical cord, complicating delivery O69.5 ☑
  uterine ligament (broad) (nontraumatic) N83.7
    traumatic S37.892 ☑
  vagina (ruptured) (nontraumatic) N89.8
    complicating delivery O71.7
  vas deferens (nontraumatic) N50.1
    traumatic S37.892 ☑
  vitreous — see Hemorrhage, vitreous
  vulva (nontraumatic) (nonobstetric) N90.89
    complicating delivery O71.7
    newborn (birth injury) P15.5
Hematometra N85.7
  with hematocolpos N89.7
Hematomyelia (central) G95.19
  newborn (birth injury) P11.5
  traumatic T14.8 ☑
Hematomyelitis G04.90
Hematoperitoneum — see Hemoperitoneum
Hematophobia F40.230
Hematopneumothorax (see Hemothorax)
Hematopoiesis, cyclic D70.4
Hematoporphyria — see Porphyria
Hematorachis, hematorrhachis G95.19
  newborn (birth injury) P11.5
Hematosalpinx N83.6
  with
    hematocolpos N89.7
    hematometra N85.7
      with hematocolpos N89.7
  infectional — see Salpingitis
Hematospermia R36.1
Hematothorax (see Hemothorax)
Hematuria R31.9
  benign (familial) (of childhood) — see also Hematuria,
    idiopathic
    essential microscopic R31.1
  due to sulphonamide, sulfonamide — see Table of
    Drugs and Chemicals, by drug

Hematuria — continued
  endemic — see also Schistosomiasis B65.0
  gross R31.0
  idiopathic N02.9
    with glomerular lesion
      C3
        glomerulonephritis N02.A
        glomerulopathy N02.A
          with dense deposit disease N02.6
      crescentic (diffuse) glomerulonephritis N02.7
      dense deposit disease N02.6
      endocapillary proliferative glomerulonephritis
        N02.4
      focal and segmental hyalinosis or sclerosis N02.1
      membranoproliferative (diffuse) N02.5
      membranous (diffuse) N02.2
      mesangial proliferative (diffuse) N02.3
      mesangiocapillary (diffuse) N02.5
      minor abnormality N02.0
      proliferative NEC N02.8
      specified pathology NEC N02.8
  intermittent — see Hematuria, idiopathic
  malarial B50.8
  microscopic NEC (with symptoms) R31.29
    asymptomatic R31.21
    benign essential R31.1
  paroxysmal — see also Hematuria, idiopathic
    nocturnal D59.5
  persistent — see Hematuria, idiopathic
  recurrent — see Hematuria, idiopathic
  tropical — see also Schistosomiasis B65.0
  tuberculous A18.13
Hemeralopia (day blindness) H53.11
  vitamin A deficiency E50.5
Hemi-akinesia R41.4
Hemianalgesia R20.0
Hemianencephaly Q00.0
Hemianesthesia R20.0
Hemianopia, hemianopsia (heteronymous) H53.47
  homonymous H53.46- ☑
  syphilitic A52.71
Hemiathetosis R25.8
Hemiatrophy R68.89
  cerebellar G31.9
  face, facial, progressive (Romberg) G51.8
  tongue K14.8
Hemiballism (us) G25.5
Hemicardia Q24.8
Hemicephalus, hemicephaly Q00.0
Hemichorea G25.5
Hemicolitis, left — see Colitis, left sided
Hemicrania
  congenital malformation Q00.0
  continua G44.51
  meaning migraine — see also Migraine G43.909
  paroxysmal G44.039
    chronic G44.049
      intractable G44.041
      not intractable G44.049
    episodic G44.039
      intractable G44.031
      not intractable G44.039
    intractable G44.031
    not intractable G44.039
Hemidystrophy — see Hemiatrophy
Hemiectromelia Q73.8
Hemihypalgesia R20.8
Hemihypesthesia R20.1
Hemi-inattention R41.4
Hemimelia Q73.8
  lower limb — see Defect, reduction, lower limb, speci-
    fied type NEC
  upper limb — see Defect, reduction, upper limb, spec-
    ified type NEC
Hemiparalysis — see Hemiplegia
Hemiparesis — see Hemiplegia
Hemiparesthesia R20.2
Hemiparkinsonism G20
Hemiplegia G81.9- ☑
  alternans facialis G83.89
  ascending NEC G81.90
    spinal G95.89
  congenital (cerebral) G80.8
    spastic G80.2
  embolic (current episode) I63.4- ☑
  flaccid G81.0- ☑
  following
    cerebrovascular disease I69.959

Index

Hematocele — Hemiplegia

Hemiplegia — *continued*
following — *continued*
cerebrovascular disease — *continued*
cerebral infarction I69.35- ☑
intracerebral hemorrhage I69.15- ☑
nontraumatic intracranial hemorrhage NEC
I69.25- ☑
specified disease NEC I69.85- ☑
stroke NOS I69.35- ☑
subarachnoid hemorrhage I69.05- ☑
hysterical F44.4
newborn NEC P91.88
birth injury P11.9
spastic G81.1- ☑
congenital G80.2
thrombotic (current episode) I63.3- ☑
Hemisection, spinal cord — *see* Injury, spinal cord, by
region
Hemispasm (facial) R25.2
Hemisporosis B48.8
Hemitremor R25.1
Hemivertebra Q76.49
failure of segmentation with scoliosis Q76.3
fusion with scoliosis Q76.3
Hemochromatosis E83.119
with refractory anemia D46.1
due to repeated red blood cell transfusion E83.111
hereditary (primary) E83.110
neonatal P78.84
primary E83.110
specified NEC E83.118
Hemoglobin — *see also* condition
abnormal (disease) — *see* Disease, hemoglobin
AS genotype D57.3
Constant Spring D58.2
E-beta thalassemia D56.5
fetal, hereditary persistence (HPFH) D56.4
H Constant Spring D56.0
low NOS D64.9
S (Hb S), heterozygous D57.3
Hemoglobinemia D59.9
due to blood transfusion T80.89 ☑
paroxysmal D59.6
nocturnal D59.5
Hemoglobinopathy (mixed) D58.2
with thalassemia D56.8
sickle-cell D57.1
with thalassemia D57.40
with
acute chest syndrome D57.411
cerebral vascular involvement D57.413
crisis (painful) D57.419
with specified complication NEC D57.418
splenic sequestration D57.412
vasoocclusive pain D57.419
without crisis D57.40
Hemoglobinuria R82.3
with anemia, hemolytic, acquired (chronic) NEC D59.6
cold (paroxysmal) (with Raynaud's syndrome) D59.6
agglutinin D59.12
due to exertion or hemolysis NEC D59.6
intermittent D59.6
malarial B50.8
march D59.6
nocturnal (paroxysmal) D59.5
paroxysmal (cold) D59.6
nocturnal D59.5
Hemolymphangioma D18.1
Hemolysis
intravascular
with
abortion — *see* Abortion, by type, complicated
by, hemorrhage
ectopic or molar pregnancy O08.1
hemorrhage
antepartum — *see* Hemorrhage, antepartum,
with coagulation defect
intrapartum — *see also* Hemorrhage, complicating, delivery O67.0
postpartum O72.3
neonatal (excessive) P58.9
specified NEC P58.8
Hemolytic — *see* condition
Hemopericardium I31.2
following acute myocardial infarction (current complication) I23.0
newborn P54.8
traumatic — *see* Injury, heart, with hemopericardium

Hemoperitoneum K66.1
infectional K65.9
traumatic S36.899 ☑
with open wound — *see* Wound, open, with penetration into peritoneal cavity
Hemophilia (classical) (familial) (hereditary) D66
A D66
acquired D68.311
autoimmune D68.311
B D67
C D68.1
calcipriva — *see also* Defect, coagulation D68.4
nonfamilial — *see also* Defect, coagulation D68.4
secondary D68.311
vascular — *see* Disease, von Willebrand
Hemophthalmos H44.81- ☑
Hemopneumothorax — *see also* Hemothorax
traumatic S27.2 ☑
Hemoptysis R04.2
newborn P26.9
tuberculous — *see* Tuberculosis, pulmonary
Hemorrhage, hemorrhagic (concealed) R58
abdomen R58
accidental antepartum — *see* Hemorrhage, antepartum
acute idiopathic pulmonary, in infants R04.81
adenoid J35.8
adrenal (capsule) (gland) E27.49
medulla E27.8
newborn P54.4
after delivery — *see* Hemorrhage, postpartum
alveolar
lung, newborn P26.8
process K08.89
alveolus K08.89
amputation stump (surgical) T87.89
anemia (chronic) D50.0
acute D62
antepartum (with) O46.90
with coagulation defect O46.00- ☑
afibrinogenemia O46.01- ☑
disseminated intravascular coagulation
O46.02- ☑
hypofibrinogenemia O46.01- ☑
specified defect NEC O46.09- ☑
before 20 weeks gestation O20.9
specified type NEC O20.8
threatened abortion O20.0
due to
abruptio placenta — *see also* Abruptio placentae
O45.9- ☑
leiomyoma, uterus — *see* Hemorrhage, antepartum, specified cause NEC
placenta previa O44.1- ☑
specified cause NEC — *see* subcategory O46.8X- ☑
anus (sphincter) K62.5
apoplexy (stroke) — *see* Hemorrhage, intracranial, intracerebral
arachnoid — *see* Hemorrhage, intracranial, subarachnoid
artery R58
brain — *see* Hemorrhage, intracranial, intracerebral
basilar (ganglion) I61.0
bladder N32.89
bowel K92.2
newborn P54.3
brain (miliary) (nontraumatic) — *see* Hemorrhage, intracranial, intracerebral
due to
birth injury P10.1
syphilis A52.05
epidural or extradural (traumatic) — *see* Injury, intracranial, epidural hemorrhage
newborn P52.4
birth injury P10.1
subarachnoid — *see* Hemorrhage, intracranial,
subarachnoid
subdural — *see* Hemorrhage, intracranial, subdural
brainstem (nontraumatic) I61.3
traumatic S06.38- ☑
breast N64.59
bronchial tube — *see* Hemorrhage, lung
bronchopulmonary — *see* Hemorrhage, lung
bronchus — *see* Hemorrhage, lung
bulbar I61.5
capillary I78.8
primary D69.8
cecum K92.2

Hemorrhage, hemorrhagic — *continued*
cerebellar, cerebellum (nontraumatic) I61.4
newborn P52.6
traumatic S06.37- ☑
cerebral, cerebrum — *see also* Hemorrhage, intracranial, intracerebral
lobe I61.1
newborn (anoxic) P52.4
birth injury P10.1
cerebromeningeal I61.8
cerebrospinal — *see* Hemorrhage, intracranial, intracerebral
cervix (uteri) (stump) NEC N88.8
chamber, anterior (eye) — *see* Hyphema
childbirth — *see* Hemorrhage, complicating, delivery
choroid H31.30- ☑
expulsive H31.31- ☑
ciliary body — *see* Hyphema
cochlea — *see* subcategory H83.8 ☑
colon K92.2
complicating
abortion — *see* Abortion, by type, complicated by,
hemorrhage
delivery O67.9
associated with coagulation defect (afibrinogenemia) (DIC) (hyperfibrinolysis) O67.0
specified cause NEC O67.8
surgical procedure — *see* Hemorrhage, intraoperative
conjunctiva H11.3- ☑
newborn P54.8
cord, newborn (stump) P51.9
corpus luteum (ruptured) cyst N83.1- ☑
cortical (brain) I61.1
cranial — *see* Hemorrhage, intracranial
cutaneous R23.3
due to autosensitivity, erythrocyte D69.2
newborn P54.5
delayed
following ectopic or molar pregnancy O08.1
postpartum O72.2
diathesis (familial) D69.9
disease D69.9
newborn P53
specified type NEC D69.8
due to or associated with
afibrinogenemia or other coagulation defect (conditions in categories D65- D69)
antepartum — *see* Hemorrhage, antepartum,
with coagulation defect
intrapartum O67.0
dental implant M27.61
device, implant or graft — *see also* Complications,
by site and type, specified NEC T85.838 ☑
arterial graft NEC T82.838 ☑
breast T85.838 ☑
catheter NEC T85.838 ☑
dialysis (renal) T82.838 ☑
intraperitoneal T85.838 ☑
infusion NEC T82.838 ☑
spinal (epidural) (subdural) T85.830 ☑
urinary (indwelling) T83.83 ☑
electronic (electrode) (pulse generator) (stimulator)
bone T84.83 ☑
cardiac T82.837 ☑
nervous system (brain) (peripheral nerve)
(spinal) T85.830 ☑
urinary T83.83 ☑
fixation, internal (orthopedic) NEC T84.83 ☑
gastrointestinal (bile duct) (esophagus)
T85.838 ☑
genital NEC T83.83 ☑
heart NEC T82.837 ☑
joint prosthesis T84.83 ☑
ocular (corneal graft) (orbital implant) NEC
T85.838 ☑
orthopedic NEC T84.83 ☑
bone graft T86.838
specified NEC T85.838 ☑
urinary NEC T83.83 ☑
vascular NEC T82.838 ☑
ventricular intracranial shunt T85.830 ☑
duodenum, duodenal K92.2
ulcer — *see* Ulcer, duodenum, with hemorrhage
dura mater — *see* Hemorrhage, intracranial, subdural
endotracheal — *see* Hemorrhage, lung

Hemorrhage, hemorrhagic — *continued*
epicranial subaponeurotic (massive), birth injury P12.2
epidural (traumatic) — *see also* Injury, intracranial, epidural hemorrhage
   nontraumatic I62.1
esophagus K22.89
   varix I85.01
      secondary I85.11
excessive, following ectopic gestation (subsequent episode) O08.1
extradural (traumatic) — *see* Injury, intracranial, epidural hemorrhage
   birth injury P10.8
   newborn (anoxic) (nontraumatic) P52.8
   nontraumatic I62.1
eye NEC H57.89
   fundus — *see* Hemorrhage, retina
   lid — *see* Disorder, eyelid, specified type NEC
fallopian tube N83.6
fibrinogenolysis — *see* Fibrinolysis
fibrinolytic (acquired) — *see* Fibrinolysis
from
   ear (nontraumatic) — *see* Otorrhagia
   tracheostomy stoma J95.01
fundus, eye — *see* Hemorrhage, retina
funis — *see* Hemorrhage, umbilicus, cord
gastric — *see* Hemorrhage, stomach
gastroenteric K92.2
   newborn P54.3
gastrointestinal (tract) K92.2
   newborn P54.3
genital organ, male N50.1
genitourinary (tract) NOS R31.9
gingiva K06.8
globe (eye) — *see* Hemophthalmos
graafian follicle cyst (ruptured) N83.0- ☑
gum K06.8
heart I51.89
hypopharyngeal (throat) R04.1
intermenstrual (regular) N92.3
   irregular N92.1
internal (organs) NEC R58
   capsule I61.0
   ear — *see* subcategory H83.8 ☑
   newborn P54.8
intestine K92.2
   newborn P54.3
intra-abdominal R58
intra-alveolar (lung), newborn P26.8
intracerebral (nontraumatic) — *see* Hemorrhage, intracranial, intracerebral
intracranial (nontraumatic) I62.9
   birth injury P10.9
   epidural, nontraumatic I62.1
   extradural, nontraumatic I62.1
   intracerebral (nontraumatic) (in) I61.9
      brain stem I61.3
      cerebellum I61.4
      hemisphere I61.2
         cortical (superficial) I61.1
         subcortical (deep) I61.0
      intraoperative
         during a nervous system procedure G97.31
         during other procedure G97.32
      intraventricular I61.5
      multiple localized I61.6
      newborn P52.4
         birth injury P10.1
      postprocedural
         following a nervous system procedure G97.51
         following other procedure G97.52
      specified NEC I61.8
      superficial I61.1
      traumatic (diffuse) — *see* Injury, intracranial, diffuse
         focal — *see* Injury, intracranial, focal
   newborn P52.9
      specified NEC P52.8
   subarachnoid (nontraumatic) (from) I60.9
      intracranial (cerebral) artery I60.7
         anterior communicating I60.2
         basilar I60.4
         carotid siphon and bifurcation I60.0- ☑
         communicating I60.7
            anterior I60.2
            posterior I60.3- ☑
         middle cerebral I60.1- ☑
         posterior communicating I60.3- ☑

Hemorrhage, hemorrhagic — *continued*
intracranial — *continued*
   subarachnoid — *continued*
      intracranial artery — *continued*
         specified artery NEC I60.6
         vertebral I60.5- ☑
      newborn P52.5
         birth injury P10.3
      specified NEC I60.8
      traumatic S06.6X- ☑
   subdural (nontraumatic) I62.00
      acute I62.01
      birth injury P10.0
      chronic I62.03
      newborn (anoxic) (hypoxic) P52.8
         birth injury P10.0
      spinal G95.19
      subacute I62.02
      traumatic — *see* Injury, intracranial, subdural hemorrhage
   traumatic — *see* Injury, intracranial, focal brain injury
intramedullary NEC G95.19
intraocular — *see* Hemophthalmos
intraoperative, intraprocedural — *see* Complication, hemorrhage (hematoma), intraoperative (intraprocedural), by site
intrapartum — *see* Hemorrhage, complicating, delivery
intrapelvic
   female N94.89
   male K66.1
intraperitoneal K66.1
intrapontine I61.3
intraprocedural — *see* Complication, hemorrhage (hematoma), intraoperative (intraprocedural), by site
intrauterine N85.7
   complicating delivery — *see also* Hemorrhage, complicating, delivery O67.9
   postpartum — *see* Hemorrhage, postpartum
intraventricular I61.5
   newborn (nontraumatic) — *see also* Newborn, affected by, hemorrhage P52.3
      due to birth injury P10.2
      grade
         1 P52.0
         2 P52.1
         3 P52.21
         4 P52.22
intravesical N32.89
iris (postinfectional) (postinflammatory) (toxic) — *see* Hyphema
joint (nontraumatic) — *see* Hemarthrosis
kidney N28.89
knee (joint) (nontraumatic) — *see* Hemarthrosis, knee
labyrinth — *see* subcategory H83.8 ☑
lenticular striate artery I61.0
ligature, vessel — *see* Hemorrhage, postoperative
liver K76.89
lung R04.89
   newborn P26.9
      massive P26.1
      specified NEC P26.8
   tuberculous — *see* Tuberculosis, pulmonary
massive umbilical, newborn P51.0
mediastinum — *see* Hemorrhage, lung
medulla I61.3
membrane (brain) I60.8
   spinal cord — *see* Hemorrhage, spinal cord
meninges, meningeal (brain) (middle) I60.8
   spinal cord — *see* Hemorrhage, spinal cord
mesentery K66.1
metritis — *see* Endometritis
mouth K13.79
mucous membrane NEC R58
   newborn P54.8
muscle M62.89
nail (subungual) L60.8
nasal turbinate R04.0
   newborn P54.8
navel, newborn P51.9
newborn P54.9
   specified NEC P54.8
nipple N64.59
nose R04.0
   newborn P54.8
omentum K66.1
optic nerve (sheath) H47.02- ☑

Hemorrhage, hemorrhagic — *continued*
orbit, orbital H05.23- ☑
ovary NEC N83.8
oviduct N83.6
pancreas K86.89
parathyroid (gland) (spontaneous) E21.4
parturition — *see* Hemorrhage, complicating, delivery
penis N48.89
pericardium, pericarditis I31.2
peritoneum, peritoneal K66.1
peritonsillar tissue J35.8
   due to infection J36
petechial R23.3
   due to autosensitivity, erythrocyte D69.2
pituitary (gland) E23.6
pleura — *see* Hemorrhage, lung
polioencephalitis, superior E51.2
polymyositis — *see* Polymyositis
pons, pontine I61.3
posterior fossa (nontraumatic) I61.8
   newborn P52.6
postmenopausal N95.0
postnasal R04.0
postoperative — *see* Complications, postprocedural, hemorrhage, by site
postpartum NEC (following delivery of placenta) O72.1
   delayed or secondary O72.2
   retained placenta O72.0
   third stage O72.0
pregnancy — *see* Hemorrhage, antepartum
preretinal — *see* Hemorrhage, retina
prostate N42.1
puerperal — *see* Hemorrhage, postpartum
   delayed or secondary O72.2
pulmonary R04.89
   newborn P26.9
      massive P26.1
      specified NEC P26.8
   tuberculous — *see* Tuberculosis, pulmonary
purpura (primary) D69.3
rectum (sphincter) K62.5
   newborn P54.2
recurring, following initial hemorrhage at time of injury T79.2 ☑
renal N28.89
respiratory passage or tract R04.9
   specified NEC R04.89
retina, retinal (vessels) H35.6- ☑
   diabetic — *see* Microaneurysm, retinal, diabetic
retroperitoneal R58
scalp R58
scrotum N50.1
secondary (nontraumatic) R58
   following initial hemorrhage at time of injury T79.2 ☑
seminal vesicle N50.1
skin R23.3
   newborn P54.5
slipped umbilical ligature P51.8
spermatic cord N50.1
spinal (cord) G95.19
   newborn (birth injury) P11.5
spleen D73.5
   intraoperative — *see* Complications, intraoperative, hemorrhage, spleen
   postprocedural — *see* Complications, postprocedural, hemorrhage, spleen
stomach K92.2
   newborn P54.3
   ulcer — *see* Ulcer, stomach, with hemorrhage
subarachnoid (nontraumatic) — *see* Hemorrhage, intracranial, subarachnoid
subconjunctival — *see also* Hemorrhage, conjunctiva
   birth injury P15.3
subcortical (brain) I61.0
subcutaneous R23.3
subdiaphragmatic R58
subdural (acute) (nontraumatic) — *see* Hemorrhage, intracranial, subdural
subependymal
   newborn P52.0
      with intraventricular extension P52.1
      and intracerebral extension P52.22
subgaleal P12.2
subhyaloid — *see* Hemorrhage, retina
subperiosteal — *see* Disorder, bone, specified type NEC
subretinal — *see* Hemorrhage, retina
subtentorial — *see* Hemorrhage, intracranial, subdural

Hemorrhage, hemorrhagic — *continued*
  subungual L60.8
  suprarenal (capsule) (gland) E27.49
    newborn P54.4
  tentorium (traumatic) NEC — *see* Hemorrhage, brain
    newborn (birth injury) P10.4
  testis N50.1
  third stage (postpartum) O72.0
  thorax — *see* Hemorrhage, lung
  throat R04.1
  thymus (gland) E32.8
  thyroid (cyst) (gland) E07.89
  tongue K14.8
  tonsil J35.8
  trachea — *see* Hemorrhage, lung
  tracheobronchial R04.89
    newborn P26.0
  traumatic — *code to* specific injury
    cerebellar — *see* Hemorrhage, brain
    intracranial — *see* Hemorrhage, brain
    recurring or secondary (following initial hemorrhage
      at time of injury) T79.2 ☑
  tuberculous NEC — *see also* Tuberculosis, pulmonary
    A15.0
  tunica vaginalis N50.1
  ulcer — *code by* site under Ulcer, with hemorrhage
    K27.4
  umbilicus, umbilical
    cord
      after birth, newborn P51.9
      complicating delivery O69.5 ☑
    newborn P51.9
      massive P51.0
      slipped ligature P51.8
    stump P51.9
  urethra (idiopathic) N36.8
  uterus, uterine (abnormal) N93.9
    climacteric N92.4
    complicating delivery — *see* Hemorrhage, compli-
      cating, delivery
    dysfunctional or functional N93.8
    intermenstrual (regular) N92.3
      irregular N92.1
    postmenopausal N95.0
    postpartum — *see* Hemorrhage, postpartum
    preclimacteric or premenopausal N92.4
    prepubertal N93.8
    pubertal N92.2
  vagina (abnormal) N93.9
    newborn P54.6
  vas deferens N50.1
  vasa previa O69.4 ☑
  ventricular I61.5
  vesical N32.89
  viscera NEC R58
    newborn P54.8
  vitreous (humor) (intraocular) H43.1- ☑
  vulva N90.89
Hemorrhoids (bleeding) (without mention of degree)
    K64.9
  1st degree (grade/stage I) (without prolapse outside
    of anal canal) K64.0
  2nd degree (grade/stage II) (that prolapse with strain-
    ing but retract spontaneously) K64.1
  3rd degree (grade/stage III) (that prolapse with strain-
    ing and require manual replacement back inside
    anal canal) K64.2
  4th degree (grade/stage IV) (with prolapsed tissue that
    cannot be manually replaced) K64.3
  complicating
    pregnancy O22.4 ☑
    puerperium O87.2
  external K64.4
    with
      thrombosis K64.5
  internal (without mention of degree) K64.8
  prolapsed K64.8
  skin tags
    anus K64.4
    residual K64.4
  specified NEC K64.8
  strangulated — *see also* Hemorrhoids, by degree K64.8
  thrombosed — *see also* Hemorrhoids, by degree K64.5
  ulcerated — *see also* Hemorrhoids, by degree K64.8
Hemosalpinx N83.6
  with
    hematocolpos N89.7
    hematometra N85.7

Hemosalpinx — *continued*
  with — *continued*
    hematometra — *continued*
      with hematocolpos N89.7
Hemosiderosis (dietary) E83.19
  pulmonary, idiopathic E83.1- ☑ *[J84.03]*
  transfusion T80.89 ☑
Hemothorax (bacterial) (nontuberculous) J94.2
  newborn P54.8
  traumatic S27.1 ☑
    with pneumothorax S27.2 ☑
  tuberculous NEC A15.6
Henoch (-Schönlein) **disease or syndrome** (purpura)
    D69.0
Henpue, henpuye A66.6
Hepar lobatum (syphilitic) A52.74
Hepatalgia K76.89
Hepatitis K75.9
  acute B17.9
    with coma K72.01
    with hepatic failure — *see* Failure, hepatic
    alcoholic — *see* Hepatitis, alcoholic
    infectious B17.9
    non-viral K72.0 ☑
    viral B17.9
  alcoholic (acute) (chronic) K70.10
    with ascites K70.11
  amebic — *see* Abscess, liver, amebic
  anicteric, (viral) — *see* Hepatitis, viral
  antigen-associated (HAA) — *see* Hepatitis, B
  Australia-antigen (positive) — *see* Hepatitis, B
  autoimmune K75.4
  B B19.10
    with hepatic coma B19.11
    acute B16.9
      with
        delta-agent (coinfection) (without hepatic
          coma) B16.1
          with hepatic coma B16.0
        hepatic coma (without delta-agent coinfec-
          tion) B16.2
    chronic B18.1
      with delta-agent B18.0
  bacterial NEC K75.89
  C (viral) B19.20
    with hepatic coma B19.21
    acute B17.10
      with hepatic coma B17.11
    chronic B18.2
  catarrhal (acute) B15.9
    with hepatic coma B15.0
  cholangiolitic K75.89
  cholestatic K75.89
  chronic K73.9
    active NEC K73.2
    lobular NEC K73.1
    persistent NEC K73.0
    specified NEC K73.8
  cytomegaloviral B25.1
  due to ethanol (acute) (chronic) — *see* Hepatitis, alco-
    holic
  epidemic B15.9
    with hepatic coma B15.0
  fulminant NEC (viral) — *see* Hepatitis, viral
  granulomatous NEC K75.3
  herpesviral B00.81
  history of
    B Z86.19
    C Z86.19
  homologous serum — *see* Hepatitis, viral, type B
  in (due to)
    mumps B26.81
    toxoplasmosis (acquired) B58.1
      congenital (active) P37.1 *[K77]*
  infectious, infective B15.9
    acute (subacute) B17.9
    chronic B18.9
  inoculation — *see* Hepatitis, viral, type B
  interstitial (chronic) K74.69
  ischemia, ischemic K72.00
  lupoid NEC K75.4
  malignant NEC (with hepatic failure) K72.90
    with coma K72.91
  neonatal (idiopathic) (toxic) P59.29
  neonatal giant cell P59.29
  newborn P59.29
  non-viral K72.0 ☑
  postimmunization — *see* Hepatitis, viral, type B

Hepatitis — *continued*
  post-transfusion — *see* Hepatitis, viral, type B
  reactive, nonspecific K75.2
  serum — *see* Hepatitis, viral, type B
  shock K72.00
  specified type NEC
    with hepatic failure — *see* Failure, hepatic
  syphilitic (late) A52.74
    congenital (early) A50.08 *[K77]*
      late A50.59 *[K77]*
    secondary A51.45
  toxic — *see also* Disease, liver, toxic K71.6
  tuberculous A18.83
  viral, virus B19.9
    with hepatic coma B19.0
    acute B17.9
    chronic B18.9
      specified NEC B18.8
      type
        B B18.1
          with delta-agent B18.0
        C B18.2
    congenital P35.3
    coxsackie B33.8 *[K77]*
    cytomegalic inclusion B25.1
    in remission, any type — *code to* Hepatitis, chronic,
      by type
    non-A, non-B B17.8
    specified type NEC (with or without coma) B17.8
    type
      A B15.9
        with hepatic coma B15.0
      B B19.10
        with hepatic coma B19.11
        acute B16.9
          with
            delta-agent (coinfection) (without
              hepatic coma) B16.1
              with hepatic coma B16.0
            hepatic coma (without delta-agent
              coinfection) B16.2
        chronic B18.1
          with delta-agent B18.0
      C B19.20
        with hepatic coma B19.21
        acute B17.10
          with hepatic coma B17.11
        chronic B18.2
      E B17.2
    non-A, non-B B17.8
Hepatization lung (acute) — *see* Pneumonia, lobar
Hepatoblastoma C22.2
Hepatocarcinoma C22.0
Hepatocholangiocarcinoma C22.0
Hepatocholangioma, benign D13.4
Hepatocholangitis K75.89
Hepatolenticular degeneration E83.01
Hepatoma (malignant) C22.0
  benign D13.4
  embryonal C22.0
Hepatomegaly — *see also* Hypertrophy, liver
  with splenomegaly R16.2
  congenital Q44.7
  in mononucleosis
    gammaherpesviral B27.09
    infectious specified NEC B27.89
Hepatoptosis K76.89
Hepatorenal syndrome following labor and delivery
    O90.4
Hepatosis K76.89
Hepatosplenomegaly R16.2
  hyperlipemic (Bürger-Grütz type) E78.3 *[K77]*
Hereditary — *see* condition
Hereditary alpha tryptasemia (syndrome) D89.44
Heredodegeneration, macular — *see* Dystrophy, retina
Heredopathia atactica polyneuritiformis G60.1
Heredosyphilis — *see* Syphilis, congenital
Herlitz' syndrome Q81.1
Hermansky-Pudlak syndrome E70.331
Hermaphrodite, hermaphroditism (true) Q56.0
  46,XX with streak gonads Q99.1
  46,XX/46,XY Q99.0
  46,XY with streak gonads Q99.1
  chimera 46,XX/46,XY Q99.0
Hernia, hernial (acquired) (recurrent) K46.9
  with
    gangrene — *see* Hernia, by site, with, gangrene
    incarceration — *see* Hernia, by site, with, obstruction

☑ Additional Character Required — Refer to the Tabular List for Character Selection

Hernia, hernial — *continued*
with — *continued*
irreducible — *see* Hernia, by site, with, obstruction
obstruction — *see* Hernia, by site, with, obstruction
strangulation — *see* Hernia, by site, with, obstruction
abdomen, abdominal K46.9
with
gangrene (and obstruction) K46.1
obstruction K46.0
femoral — *see* Hernia, femoral
incisional — *see* Hernia, incisional
inguinal — *see* Hernia, inguinal
specified site NEC K45.8
with
gangrene (and obstruction) K45.1
obstruction K45.0
umbilical — *see* Hernia, umbilical
wall — *see* Hernia, ventral
appendix — *see* Hernia, abdomen
bladder (mucosa) (sphincter)
congenital (female) (male) Q79.51
female — *see* Cystocele
male N32.89
brain, congenital — *see* Encephalocele
cartilage, vertebra — *see* Displacement, intervertebral
disc
cerebral, congenital — *see also* Encephalocele
endaural Q01.8
ciliary body (traumatic) S05.2- ☑
colon — *see* Hernia, abdomen
Cooper's — *see* Hernia, abdomen, specified site NEC
crural — *see* Hernia, femoral
diaphragm, diaphragmatic K44.9
with
gangrene (and obstruction) K44.1
obstruction K44.0
congenital Q79.0
direct (inguinal) — *see* Hernia, inguinal
diverticulum, intestine — *see* Hernia, abdomen
double (inguinal) — *see* Hernia, inguinal, bilateral
due to adhesions (with obstruction) K56.50
epigastric — *see also* Hernia, ventral K43.9
esophageal hiatus — *see* Hernia, hiatal
external (inguinal) — *see* Hernia, inguinal
fallopian tube N83.4- ☑
fascia M62.89
femoral K41.90
with
gangrene (and obstruction) K41.40
not specified as recurrent K41.40
recurrent K41.41
obstruction K41.30
not specified as recurrent K41.30
recurrent K41.31
not specified as recurrent K41.90
recurrent K41.91
bilateral K41.20
with
gangrene (and obstruction) K41.10
not specified as recurrent K41.10
recurrent K41.11
obstruction K41.00
not specified as recurrent K41.00
recurrent K41.01
not specified as recurrent K41.20
recurrent K41.21
unilateral K41.90
with
gangrene (and obstruction) K41.40
not specified as recurrent K41.40
recurrent K41.41
obstruction K41.30
not specified as recurrent K41.30
recurrent K41.31
not specified as recurrent K41.90
recurrent K41.91
foramen magnum G93.5
congenital Q01.8
funicular (umbilical) — *see also* Hernia, umbilicus
spermatic (cord) — *see* Hernia, inguinal
gastrointestinal tract — *see* Hernia, abdomen
Hesselbach's — *see* Hernia, femoral, specified site NEC
hiatal (esophageal) (sliding) K44.9
with
gangrene (and obstruction) K44.1
obstruction K44.0
congenital Q40.1

Hernia, hernial — *continued*
hypogastric — *see* Hernia, ventral
incarcerated — *see also* Hernia, by site, with obstruction
with gangrene — *see* Hernia, by site, with gangrene
incisional K43.2
with
gangrene (and obstruction) K43.1
obstruction K43.0
indirect (inguinal) — *see* Hernia, inguinal
inguinal (direct) (external) (funicular) (indirect) (internal) (oblique) (scrotal) (sliding) K40.90
with
gangrene (and obstruction) K40.40
not specified as recurrent K40.40
recurrent K40.41
obstruction K40.30
not specified as recurrent K40.30
recurrent K40.31
not specified as recurrent K40.90
recurrent K40.91
bilateral K40.20
with
gangrene (and obstruction) K40.10
not specified as recurrent K40.10
recurrent K40.11
obstruction K40.00
not specified as recurrent K40.00
recurrent K40.01
not specified as recurrent K40.20
recurrent K40.21
unilateral K40.90
with
gangrene (and obstruction) K40.40
not specified as recurrent K40.40
recurrent K40.41
obstruction K40.30
not specified as recurrent K40.30
recurrent K40.31
not specified as recurrent K40.90
recurrent K40.91
internal — *see also* Hernia, abdomen
inguinal — *see* Hernia, inguinal
interstitial — *see* Hernia, abdomen
intervertebral cartilage or disc — *see* Displacement, intervertebral disc
intestine, intestinal — *see* Hernia, by site
intra-abdominal — *see* Hernia, abdomen
iris (traumatic) S05.2- ☑
irreducible — *see also* Hernia, by site, with obstruction
with gangrene — *see* Hernia, by site, with gangrene
ischiatic — *see* Hernia, abdomen, specified site NEC
ischiorectal — *see* Hernia, abdomen, specified site NEC
lens (traumatic) S05.2- ☑
linea (alba) (semilunaris) — *see* Hernia, ventral
Littre's — *see* Hernia, abdomen
lumbar — *see* Hernia, abdomen, specified site NEC
lung (subcutaneous) J98.4
mediastinum J98.59
mesenteric (internal) — *see* Hernia, abdomen
midline — *see* Hernia, ventral
muscle (sheath) M62.89
nucleus pulposus — *see* Displacement, intervertebral disc
oblique (inguinal) — *see* Hernia, inguinal
obstructive — *see also* Hernia, by site, with obstruction
with gangrene — *see* Hernia, by site, with gangrene
obturator — *see* Hernia, abdomen, specified site NEC
omental — *see* Hernia, abdomen
ovary N83.4- ☑
oviduct N83.4- ☑
paraesophageal — *see also* Hernia, diaphragm
congenital Q40.1
parastomal K43.5
with
gangrene (and obstruction) K43.4
obstruction K43.3
paraumbilical — *see* Hernia, umbilicus
perineal — *see* Hernia, abdomen, specified site NEC
Petit's — *see* Hernia, abdomen, specified site NEC
postoperative — *see* Hernia, incisional
pregnant uterus — *see* Abnormal, uterus in pregnancy or childbirth
prevesical N32.89
properitoneal — *see* Hernia, abdomen, specified site NEC
pudendal — *see* Hernia, abdomen, specified site NEC
rectovaginal N81.6

Hernia, hernial — *continued*
retroperitoneal — *see* Hernia, abdomen, specified site NEC
Richter's — *see* Hernia, abdomen, with obstruction
Rieux's, Riex's — *see* Hernia, abdomen, specified site NEC
sac condition (adhesion) (dropsy) (inflammation) (laceration) (suppuration) — *code by site under* Hernia
sciatic — *see* Hernia, abdomen, specified site NEC
scrotum, scrotal — *see* Hernia, inguinal
sliding (inguinal) — *see also* Hernia, inguinal
hiatus — *see* Hernia, hiatal
spigelian — *see* Hernia, ventral
spinal — *see* Spina bifida
strangulated — *see also* Hernia, by site, with obstruction
with gangrene — *see* Hernia, by site, with gangrene
subxiphoid — *see* Hernia, ventral
supra-umbilicus — *see* Hernia, ventral
tendon — *see* Disorder, tendon, specified type NEC
Treitz's (fossa) — *see* Hernia, abdomen, specified site NEC
tunica vaginalis Q55.29
umbilicus, umbilical K42.9
with
gangrene (and obstruction) K42.1
obstruction K42.0
ureter N28.89
urethra, congenital Q64.79
urinary meatus, congenital Q64.79
uterus N81.4
pregnant — *see* Abnormal, uterus in pregnancy or childbirth
vaginal (anterior) (wall) — *see* Cystocele
Velpeau's — *see* Hernia, femoral
ventral K43.9
with
gangrene (and obstruction) K43.7
obstruction K43.6
incisional K43.2
with
gangrene (and obstruction) K43.1
obstruction K43.0
recurrent — *see* Hernia, incisional
specified NEC K43.9
with
gangrene (and obstruction) K43.7
obstruction K43.6
vesical
congenital (female) (male) Q79.51
female — *see* Cystocele
male N32.89
vitreous (into wound) S05.2- ☑
into anterior chamber — *see* Prolapse, vitreous
Herniation — *see also* Hernia
brain (stem) G93.5
nontraumatic G93.5
traumatic S06.A1 ☑
cerebellar S06.A1 ☑
subfalcine (cingulate) S06.A1 ☑
tonsillar S06.A1 ☑
transtentorial (central) (upward cerebellar) S06.A1 ☑
uncal S06.A1 ☑
cerebral G93.5
nontraumatic G93.5
traumatic S06.A1 ☑
mediastinum J98.59
nucleus pulposus — *see* Displacement, intervertebral disc
Herpangina B08.5
Herpes, herpesvirus, herpetic B00.9
anogenital A60.9
perianal skin A60.1
rectum A60.1
urogenital tract A60.00
cervix A60.03
male genital organ NEC A60.02
penis A60.01
specified site NEC A60.09
vagina A60.04
vulva A60.04
blepharitis (zoster) B02.39
simplex B00.59
circinatus B35.4
bullosus L12.0
conjunctivitis (simplex) B00.53

Herpes, herpesvirus, herpetic — *continued*
  conjunctivitis — *continued*
    zoster B02.31
  cornea B02.33
  encephalitis B00.4
    due to herpesvirus 6 B10.01
    due to herpesvirus 7 B10.09
    specified NEC B10.09
  eye (zoster) B02.30
    simplex B00.50
  eyelid (zoster) B02.39
    simplex B00.59
  facialis B00.1
  febrilis B00.1
  geniculate ganglionitis B02.21
  genital, genitalis A60.00
    female A60.09
    male A60.02
  gestational, gestationis O26.4- ☑
  gingivostomatitis B00.2
  human B00.9
    1 — *see* Herpes, simplex
    2 — *see* Herpes, simplex
    3 — *see* Varicella
    4 — *see* Mononucleosis, Epstein-Barr (virus)
    5 — *see* Disease, cytomegalic inclusion (generalized)
    6
      encephalitis B10.01
      specified NEC B10.81
    7
      encephalitis B10.09
      specified NEC B10.82
    8 B10.89
  infection NEC B10.89
    Kaposi's sarcoma associated B10.89
  iridocyclitis (simplex) B00.51
    zoster B02.32
  iris (vesicular erythema multiforme) L51.9
  iritis (simplex) B00.51
  Kaposi's sarcoma associated B10.89
  keratitis (simplex) (dendritic) (disciform) (interstitial) B00.52
    zoster (interstitial) B02.33
  keratoconjunctivitis (simplex) B00.52
    zoster B02.33
  labialis B00.1
  lip B00.1
  meningitis (simplex) B00.3
    zoster B02.1
  ophthalmicus (zoster) NEC B02.30
    simplex B00.50
  penis A60.01
  perianal skin A60.1
  pharyngitis, pharyngotonsillitis B00.2
  rectum A60.1
  scrotum A60.02
  sepsis B00.7
  simplex B00.9
    complicated NEC B00.89
    congenital P35.2
    conjunctivitis B00.53
    external ear B00.1
    eyelid B00.59
    hepatitis B00.81
    keratitis (interstitial) B00.52
    myleitis B00.82
    specified complication NEC B00.89
    visceral B00.89
  stomatitis B00.2
  tonsurans B35.0
  visceral B00.89
  vulva A60.04
  whitlow B00.89
  zoster — *see also* condition B02.9
    auricularis B02.21
    complicated NEC B02.8
    conjunctivitis B02.31
    disseminated B02.7
    encephalitis B02.0
    eye (lid) B02.39
    geniculate ganglionitis B02.21
    keratitis (interstitial) B02.33
    meningitis B02.1
    myelitis B02.24
    neuritis, neuralgia B02.29
    ophthalmicus NEC B02.30
    oticus B02.21
    polyneuropathy B02.23

Herpes, herpesvirus, herpetic — *continued*
  zoster — *see also* condition — *continued*
    specified complication NEC B02.8
    trigeminal neuralgia B02.22
Herpesvirus (human) — *see* Herpes
Herpetophobia F40.218
Herrick's anemia — *see* Disease, sickle-cell
Hers' disease E74.09
Herter-Gee syndrome K90.0
Herxheimer's reaction R68.89
Hesitancy
  of micturition R39.11
  urinary R39.11
Hesselbach's hernia — *see* Hernia, femoral, specified site NEC
Heterochromia (congenital) Q13.2
  cataract — *see* Cataract, complicated
  cyclitis (Fuchs) — *see* Cyclitis, Fuchs' heterochromic
  hair L67.1
  iritis — *see* Cyclitis, Fuchs' heterochromic
  retained metallic foreign body (nonmagnetic) — *see* Foreign body, intraocular, old, retained
    magnetic — *see* Foreign body, intraocular, old, retained, magnetic
  uveitis — *see* Cyclitis, Fuchs' heterochromic
Heterophoria — *see* Strabismus, heterophoria
Heterophyes, heterophyiasis (small intestine) B66.8
Heterotopia, heterotopic — *see also* Malposition, congenital
  cerebralis Q04.8
Heterotropia — *see* Strabismus
Heubner-Herter disease K90.0
Hexadactylism Q69.9
HGSIL (cytology finding) (high grade squamous intraepithelial lesion on cytologic smear) (Pap smear finding)
  anus R85.613
  cervix R87.613
    biopsy (histology) finding — *see* Neoplasia, intraepithelial, cervix, grade II or grade III
  vagina R87.623
    biopsy (histology) finding — *see* Neoplasia, intraepithelial, cervix, grade II or grade III
Hibernoma — *see* Lipoma
Hiccup, hiccough R06.6
  epidemic B33.0
  psychogenic F45.8
Hidden penis (congenital) Q55.64
  acquired N48.83
Hidradenitis (axillaris) (suppurative) L73.2
Hidradenoma (nodular) — *see also* Neoplasm, skin, benign
  clear cell — *see* Neoplasm, skin, benign
  papillary — *see* Neoplasm, skin, benign
Hidrocystoma — *see* Neoplasm, skin, benign
High
  altitude effects T70.20 ☑
    anoxia T70.29 ☑
    on
      ears T70.0 ☑
      sinuses T70.1 ☑
    polycythemia D75.1
  arch
    foot Q66.7- ☑
    palate, congenital Q38.5
  arterial tension — *see* Hypertension
  basal metabolic rate R94.8
  blood pressure — *see also* Hypertension
    borderline R03.0
    reading (incidental) (isolated) (nonspecific), without diagnosis of hypertension R03.0
  cholesterol E78.00
    with high triglycerides E78.2
  diaphragm (congenital) Q79.1
  expressed emotional level within family Z63.8
  head at term O32.4 ☑
  palate, congenital Q38.5
  risk
    infant NEC Z76.2
    sexual behavior (heterosexual) Z72.51
      bisexual Z72.53
      homosexual Z72.52
  scrotal testis, testes
    bilateral Q53.23
    unilateral Q53.13
  temperature (of unknown origin) R50.9
  thoracic rib Q76.6

High — *continued*
  triglycerides E78.1
    with high cholesterol E78.2
Hildenbrand's disease A75.0
Hilum — *see* condition
Hip — *see* condition
Hippel's disease Q85.83
Hippophobia F40.218
Hippus H57.09
Hirschsprung's disease or megacolon Q43.1
Hirsutism, hirsuties L68.0
Hirudiniasis
  external B88.3
  internal B83.4
Hiss-Russell dysentery A03.1
Histidinemia, histidinuria E70.41
Histiocytoma — *see also* Neoplasm, skin, benign
  fibrous — *see also* Neoplasm, skin, benign
    atypical — *see* Neoplasm, connective tissue, uncertain behavior
    malignant — *see* Neoplasm, connective tissue, malignant
Histiocytosis D76.3
  acute differentiated progressive C96.0
  Langerhans' cell NEC C96.6
    multifocal X
      multisystemic (disseminated) C96.0
      unisystemic C96.5
    pulmonary, adult (adult PLCH) J84.82
    unifocal (X) C96.6
  lipid, lipoid D76.3
    essential E75.29
  malignant C96.A (*following* C96.6)
  mononuclear phagocytes NEC D76.1
    Langerhans' cells C96.6
  non-Langerhans cell D76.3
  polyostotic sclerosing D76.3
  sinus, with massive lymphadenopathy D76.3
  syndrome NEC D76.3
  X NEC C96.6
    acute (progressive) C96.0
    chronic C96.6
    multifocal C96.5
    multisystemic C96.0
    unifocal C96.6
Histoplasmosis B39.9
  with pneumonia NEC B39.2
  African B39.5
  American — *see* Histoplasmosis, capsulati
  capsulati B39.4
    disseminated B39.3
    generalized B39.3
    pulmonary B39.2
      acute B39.0
      chronic B39.1
  Darling's B39.4
  duboisii B39.5
  lung NEC B39.2
History
  family (of) — *see also* History, personal (of)
    alcohol abuse Z81.1
    allergy NEC Z84.89
    anemia Z83.2
    arthritis Z82.61
    asthma Z82.5
    blindness Z82.1
    cardiac death (sudden) Z82.41
    carrier of genetic disease Z84.81
    chromosomal anomaly Z82.79
    chronic
      disabling disease NEC Z82.8
      lower respiratory disease Z82.5
    colonic polyps Z83.71
    congenital malformations and deformations Z82.79
      polycystic kidney Z82.71
    consanguinity Z84.3
    deafness Z82.2
    diabetes mellitus Z83.3
    disability NEC Z82.8
    disease or disorder (of)
      allergic NEC Z84.89
      behavioral NEC Z81.8
      blood and blood-forming organs Z83.2
      cardiovascular NEC Z82.49
      chronic disabling NEC Z82.8
      digestive Z83.79
      ear NEC Z83.52
      elevated lipoprotein (a) (Lp(a)) Z83.430

Index

History — History

History — *continued*
  personal — *see also* History, family — *continued*
    dysplasia — *continued*
      cervical — *continued*
        severe (grade III) Z86.001
      prostatic Z87.430
      vaginal (mild) (moderate) Z87.411
        severe (grade III) Z86.002
      vulvar (mild) (moderate) Z87.412
        severe (grade III) Z86.002
    embolism (venous) Z86.718
      pulmonary Z86.711
    encephalitis Z86.61
    estrogen therapy Z92.23
    extracorporeal membrane oxygenation (ECMO)
        Z92.81
    failed conscious sedation Z92.83
    failed moderate sedation Z92.83
    fall, falling Z91.81
    forced labor or sexual exploitation Z91.42
      in childhood Z62.813
    fracture (healed)
      fatigue Z87.312
      fragility Z87.310
      osteoporosis Z87.310
      pathological NEC Z87.311
      stress Z87.312
      traumatic Z87.81
    gene therapy Z92.86
    gestational diabetes Z86.32
    hepatitis
      B Z86.19
      C Z86.19
    Hodgkin disease Z85.71
    hyperthermia, malignant Z88.4
    hypospadias (corrected) Z87.710
    hysterectomy Z90.710
    immunosuppression therapy Z92.25
    in situ neoplasm
      breast Z86.000
      cervix uteri Z86.001
      digestive organs, specified NEC Z86.004
      esophagus Z86.003
      genital organs, specified NEC Z86.002
      melanoma Z86.006
      middle ear Z86.005
      oral cavity Z86.003
      respiratory system Z86.005
      skin Z86.007
      specified NEC Z86.008
      stomach Z86.003
    in utero procedure during pregnancy Z98.870
    in utero procedure while a fetus Z98.871
    infection NEC Z86.19
      central nervous system Z86.61
      coronavirus (disease) (novel) 2019 Z86.16
      COVID-19 Z86.16
      latent tuberculosis Z86.15
      Methicillin resistant Staphylococcus aureus
          (MRSA) Z86.14
      SARS-CoV-2 Z86.16
      urinary (recurrent) (tract) Z87.440
    injury NEC Z87.828
    irradiation Z92.3
    kidney stones Z87.442
    latent tuberculosis infection Z86.15
    leukemia Z85.6
    lymphoma (non-Hodgkin) Z85.72
    malignant melanoma (skin) Z85.820
    malignant neoplasm (of) Z85.9
      accessory sinuses Z85.22
      anus NEC Z85.048
        carcinoid Z85.040
      bladder Z85.51
      bone Z85.830
      brain Z85.841
      breast Z85.3
      bronchus NEC Z85.118
        carcinoid Z85.110
      carcinoid — *see* History, personal (of), malignant
          neoplasm, by site, carcinioid
      cervix Z85.41
      colon NEC Z85.038
        carcinoid Z85.030
      digestive organ Z85.00
        specified NEC Z85.09
      endocrine gland NEC Z85.858
      epididymis Z85.48
      esophagus Z85.01

History — *continued*
  personal — *see also* History, family — *continued*
    malignant neoplasm — *continued*
      eye Z85.840
      gastrointestinal tract — *see* History, malignant
          neoplasm, digestive organ
      genital organ
        female Z85.40
          specified NEC Z85.44
        male Z85.45
          specified NEC Z85.49
      hematopoietic NEC Z85.79
      intrathoracic organ Z85.20
      kidney NEC Z85.528
        carcinoid Z85.520
      large intestine NEC Z85.038
        carcinoid Z85.030
      larynx Z85.21
      liver Z85.05
      lung NEC Z85.118
        carcinoid Z85.110
      mediastinum Z85.29
      Merkel cell Z85.821
      middle ear Z85.22
      nasal cavities Z85.22
      nervous system NEC Z85.848
      oral cavity Z85.819
        specified site NEC Z85.818
      ovary Z85.43
      pancreas Z85.07
      pelvis Z85.53
      pharynx Z85.819
        specified site NEC Z85.818
      pleura Z85.29
      prostate Z85.46
      rectosigmoid junction NEC Z85.048
        carcinoid Z85.040
      rectum NEC Z85.048
        carcinoid Z85.040
      respiratory organ Z85.20
      sinuses, accessory Z85.22
      skin NEC Z85.828
        melanoma Z85.820
        Merkel cell Z85.821
      small intestine NEC Z85.068
        carcinoid Z85.060
      soft tissue Z85.831
      specified site NEC Z85.89
      stomach NEC Z85.028
        carcinoid Z85.020
      testis Z85.47
      thymus NEC Z85.238
        carcinoid Z85.230
      thyroid Z85.850
      tongue Z85.810
      trachea Z85.12
      urinary organ or tract Z85.50
        specified NEC Z85.59
      uterus Z85.42
    maltreatment Z91.89
    medical treatment NEC Z92.89
    melanoma Z85.820
      in situ Z86.006
      malignant (skin) Z85.820
    meningitis Z86.61
    mental disorder Z86.59
    Merkel cell carcinoma (skin) Z85.821
    Methicillin resistant Staphylococcus aureus (MRSA)
        Z86.14
    military deployment Z91.82
    military war, peacekeeping and humanitarian de-
        ployment (current or past conflict) Z91.82
    myocardial infarction (old) I25.2
    necrotizing enterocolitis of newborn (corrected)
        Z87.61
    neglect (in)
      adult Z91.412
      childhood Z62.812
    neoplasia
      anal intraepithelial, III [AIN III] Z86.004
      high-grade prostatic intraepithelial, III [HGPIN
          III] Z86.002
      vaginal intraepithelial, III [VAIN III] Z86.002
      vulvar intraepithelial, III [VIN III] Z86.002
    neoplasm
      benign Z86.018
        brain Z86.011
        colon polyp Z86.010

History — *continued*
  personal — *see also* History, family — *continued*
    neoplasm — *continued*
      in situ
        breast Z86.000
        cervix uteri Z86.001
        digestive organs, specified NEC Z86.004
        esophagus Z86.003
        genital organs, specified NEC Z86.002
        melanoma Z86.006
        middle ear Z86.005
        oral cavity Z86.003
        respiratory system Z86.005
        skin Z86.007
        specified NEC Z86.008
        stomach Z86.003
      malignant — *see* History of, malignant neoplasm
      uncertain behavior Z86.03
    nephrotic syndrome Z87.441
    nicotine dependence Z87.891
    noncompliance with medical treatment or regimen
        — *see* Noncompliance
    nutritional deficiency Z86.39
    obstetric complications Z87.59
      childbirth Z87.59
      pregnancy Z87.59
      pre-term labor Z87.51
      puerperium Z87.59
    osteoporosis fractures Z87.31 ☑
    parasuicide (attempt) Z91.51
    physical trauma NEC Z87.828
      self-harm or suicide attempt Z91.51
    pneumonia (recurrent) Z87.01
    poisoning NEC Z91.89
      self-harm or suicide attempt Z91.51
    poor personal hygiene Z91.89
    preterm labor Z87.51
    procedure during pregnancy Z98.870
    procedure while a fetus Z98.871
    prolonged reversible ischemic neurologic deficit
        (PRIND) Z86.73
    prostatic dysplasia Z87.430
    psychological
      abuse
        adult Z91.411
        child Z62.811
      trauma, specified NEC Z91.49
    radiation therapy Z92.3
    removal
      implant
        breast Z98.86
    renal calculi Z87.442
    respiratory condition NEC Z87.09
    retained foreign body fully removed Z87.821
    risk factors NEC Z91.89
    SARS-CoV-2 infection Z86.16
    self-harm
      nonsuicidal Z91.52
      suicidal Z91.51
    self-inflicted injury without suicidal intent Z91.52
    self-injury
      nonsuicidal Z91.52
    self-mutilation Z91.52
    self-poisoning attempt Z91.51
    sex reassignment Z87.890
    sleep-wake cycle problem Z72.821
    specified NEC Z87.898
    steroid therapy (systemic) Z92.241
      inhaled Z92.240
    stroke without residual deficits Z86.73
    substance abuse NEC F10-F19
    sudden cardiac arrest Z86.74
    sudden cardiac death successfully resuscitated
        Z86.74
    suicidal behavior Z91.51
    suicide attempt Z91.51
    surgery NEC Z98.890
      with uterine scar Z98.891
      sex reassignment Z87.890
      transplant — *see* Transplant
    thrombophlebitis Z86.72
    thrombosis (venous) Z86.718
      pulmonary Z86.711
    tobacco dependence Z87.891
    tracheoesophageal
      atresia Z87.731
      fistula Z87.731
    transient ischemic attack (TIA) without residual
        deficits Z86.73

☑ **Additional Character Required — Refer to the Tabular List for Character Selection**

History — *continued*
  personal — *see also* History, family — *continued*
    trauma (physical) NEC Z87.828
      psychological NEC Z91.49
      self-harm Z91.51
    traumatic brain injury Z87.820
    tuberculosis, latent infection Z86.15
    unhealthy sleep-wake cycle Z72.821
    unintended awareness under general anesthesia
        Z92.84
    urinary calculi Z87.442
    urinary (recurrent) (tract) infection(s) Z87.440
    uterine scar from previous surgery Z98.891
    vaginal dysplasia Z87.411
    venous thrombosis or embolism Z86.718
      pulmonary Z86.711
    vulvar dysplasia Z87.412
His-Werner disease A79.0
HIV — *see also* Human, immunodeficiency virus B20
  laboratory evidence (nonconclusive) R75
  nonconclusive test (in infants) R75
  positive, seropositive Z21
Hives (bold) — *see* Urticaria
Hoarseness R49.0
Hobo Z59.00
Hodgkin disease — *see* Lymphoma, Hodgkin
Hodgson's — *see also* Aneurysm, aorta, thorax I71.20
  ruptured — *see also* Aneurysm, aorta, thorax, ruptured
      I71.10
Hoffa-Kastert disease E88.89
Hoffa's disease E88.89
Hoffmann-Bouveret syndrome I47.9
Hoffmann's syndrome E03.9 *[G73.7]*
Hole (round)
  macula H35.34- ☑
  retina (without detachment) — *see* Break, retina, round
      hole
    with detachment — *see* Detachment, retina, with
        retinal, break
Holiday relief care Z75.5
Hollenhorst's plaque — *see* Occlusion, artery, retina
Hollow foot (congenital) Q66.7- ☑
  acquired — *see* Deformity, limb, foot, specified NEC
Holoprosencephaly Q04.2
Holt-Oram syndrome Q87.2
Homelessness Z59.00
  sheltered Z59.01
  unsheltered Z59.02
Homesickness — *see* Disorder, adjustment
Homocysteinemia R79.83
Homocystinemia, homocystinuria E72.11
Homogentisate 1,2-dioxygenase deficiency E70.29
Homologous serum hepatitis (prophylactic) (therapeu-
    tic) — *see* Hepatitis, viral, type B
Honeycomb lung J98.4
  congenital Q33.0
Hooded
  clitoris Q52.6
  penis Q55.69
Hookworm (disease) (infection) (infestation) B76.9
  with anemia B76.9 *[D63.8]*
  specified NEC B76.8
Hordeolum (eyelid) (externum) (recurrent) H00.019
  internum H00.029
    left H00.026
      lower H00.025
      upper H00.024
    right H00.023
      lower H00.022
      upper H00.021
  left H00.016
    lower H00.015
    upper H00.014
  right H00.013
    lower H00.012
    upper H00.011
Horn
  cutaneous L85.8
  nail L60.2
    congenital Q84.6
Horner (-Claude Bernard) **syndrome** G90.2
  traumatic — *see* Injury, nerve, cervical sympathetic
Horseshoe kidney (congenital) Q63.1
Horton's headache or neuralgia G44.099
  intractable G44.091
  not intractable G44.099
Hospital hopper syndrome — *see* Disorder, factitious

Hospitalism in children — *see* Disorder, adjustment
Hostility R45.5
  towards child Z62.3
Hot flashes
  menopausal N95.1
Hourglass (contracture) — *see also* Contraction, hour-
    glass
  stomach K31.89
    congenital Q40.2
    stricture K31.2
Household, housing circumstance affecting care
    Z59.9
  specified NEC Z59.89
Housemaid's knee — *see* Bursitis, prepatellar
HSCT-TMA (hematopoietic stem cell transplantation-as-
    sociated thrombotic microangiopathy) M31.11
Hudson (-Stähli) **line** (cornea) — *see* Pigmentation,
    cornea, anterior
Human
  bite (open wound) — *see also* Bite
    intact skin surface — *see* Bite, superficial
  herpesvirus — *see* Herpes
  immunodeficiency virus (HIV) disease (infection) B20
    asymptomatic status Z21
    contact Z20.6
    counseling Z71.7
    dementia — *see also* Dementia, in, diseases speci-
        fied elsewhere B20 *[F02.80]*
      with behavioral disturbance — *see also* Demen-
          tia, in, diseases specified elsewhere
          B20 *[F02.81-]* ☑
    exposure to Z20.6
    laboratory evidence R75
    type-2 (HIV 2) as cause of disease classified else-
        where B97.35
  papillomavirus (HPV)
    DNA test positive
      high risk
        cervix R87.810
        vagina R87.811
      low risk
        cervix R87.820
        vagina R87.821
    screening for Z11.51
  T-cell lymphotropic virus
    type-1 (HTLV-I) infection B33.3
      as cause of disease classified elsewhere B97.33
      carrier Z22.6
    type-2 (HTLV-II) as cause of disease classified else-
        where B97.34
Humidifier lung or pneumonitis J67.7
Humiliation (experience) **in childhood** Z62.898
Humpback (acquired) — *see* Kyphosis
Hunchback (acquired) — *see* Kyphosis
Hunger T73.0 ☑
  air, psychogenic F45.8
Hungry bone syndrome E83.81
Hunner's ulcer — *see* Cystitis, chronic, interstitial
Hunter's
  glossitis D51.0
  syndrome E76.1
Huntington's disease or chorea G10
  with dementia — *see also* Dementia, in, diseases
      specified elsewhere G10 *[F02.80]*
    with behavioral disturbance — *see also* Dementia,
        in, diseases specified elsewhere
        G10 *[F02.81-]* ☑
Hunt's
  disease or syndrome (herpetic geniculate ganglionitis)
      B02.21
    dyssynergia cerebellaris myoclonica G11.19
  neuralgia B02.21
Hurler (-Scheie) **disease or syndrome** E76.02
Hurst's disease G36.1
Hurthle cell
  adenocarcinoma C73
  adenoma D34
  carcinoma C73
  tumor D34
Hutchinson-Boeck disease or syndrome — *see* Sar-
    coidosis
Hutchinson-Gilford disease or syndrome E34.8
Hutchinson's
  disease, meaning
    angioma serpiginosum L81.7
    pompholyx (cheiropompholyx) L30.1
    prurigo estivalis L56.4
    summer eruption or summer prurigo L56.4

Hutchinson's — *continued*
  melanotic freckle — *see* Melanoma, in situ
    malignant melanoma in — *see* Melanoma
  teeth or incisors (congenital syphilis) A50.52
  triad (congenital syphilis) A50.53
Hyalin plaque, sclera, senile H15.89
Hyaline membrane (disease) (lung) (pulmonary) (new-
    born) P22.0
Hyalinosis
  cutis (et mucosae) E78.89
  focal and segmental (glomerular) — *see also* N00-N07
    with fourth character .1 N05.1
Hyalitis, hyalosis, asteroid — *see also* Deposit, crys-
    talline
  syphilitic (late) A52.71
Hydatid
  cyst or tumor — *see* Echinococcus
  mole — *see* Hydatidiform mole
  Morgagni
    female Q50.5
    male (epididymal) Q55.4
    testicular Q55.29
Hydatidiform mole (benign) (complicating pregnancy)
    (delivered) (undelivered) O01.9
  classical O01.0
  complete O01.0
  incomplete O01.1
  invasive D39.2
  malignant D39.2
  partial O01.1
Hydatidosis — *see* Echinococcus
Hydradenitis (axillaris) (suppurative) L73.2
Hydradenoma — *see* Hidradenoma
Hydramnios O40.- ☑
Hydrancephaly, hydranencephaly Q04.3
  with spina bifida — *see* Spina bifida, with hydro-
      cephalus
Hydrargyrism NEC — *see* Poisoning, mercury
Hydrarthrosis — *see also* Effusion, joint
  gonococcal A54.42
  intermittent M12.40
    ankle M12.47- ☑
    elbow M12.42- ☑
    foot joint M12.47- ☑
    hand joint M12.44- ☑
    hip M12.45- ☑
    knee M12.46- ☑
    multiple site M12.49
    shoulder M12.41- ☑
    specified joint NEC M12.48
    wrist M12.43- ☑
  of yaws (early) (late) — *see also* subcategory M14.8-
      A66.6
  syphilitic (late) A52.77
    congenital A50.55 *[M12.80]*
Hydremia D64.89
Hydrencephalocele (congenital) — *see* Encephalocele
Hydrencephalomeningocele (congenital) — *see* En-
    cephalocele
Hydroa R23.8
  aestivale L56.4
  vacciniforme L56.4
Hydroadenitis (axillaris) (suppurative) L73.2
Hydrocalycosis — *see* Hydronephrosis
Hydrocele (spermatic cord) (testis) (tunica vaginalis)
    N43.3
  canal of Nuck N94.89
  communicating N43.2
    congenital P83.5
  congenital P83.5
  encysted N43.0
  female NEC N94.89
  infected N43.1
  newborn P83.5
  round ligament N94.89
  specified NEC N43.2
  spinalis — *see* Spina bifida
  vulva N90.89
Hydrocephalus (acquired) (external) (internal) (malig-
    nant) (recurrent) G91.9
  aqueduct Sylvius stricture Q03.0
  causing disproportion O33.6 ☑
    with obstructed labor O66.3
  communicating G91.0
  congenital (external) (internal) Q03.9
    with spina bifida Q05.4
      cervical Q05.0

Hydrocephalus — *continued*
  congenital — *continued*
    with spina bifida — *continued*
      dorsal Q05.1
      lumbar Q05.2
      lumbosacral Q05.2
      sacral Q05.3
      thoracic Q05.1
      thoracolumbar Q05.1
    specified NEC Q03.8
  due to toxoplasmosis (congenital) P37.1
  foramen Magendie block (acquired) G91.1
    congenital — *see also* Hydrocephalus, congenital Q03.1
  in (due to)
    infectious disease NEC B89 *[G91.4]*
    neoplastic disease NEC — *see also* Neoplasm G91.4
    parasitic disease B89 *[G91.4]*
  newborn Q03.9
    with spina bifida — *see* Spina bifida, with hydrocephalus
  noncommunicating G91.1
  normal pressure G91.2
    secondary G91.0
  obstructive G91.1
  otitic G93.2
  post-traumatic NEC G91.3
  secondary G91.4
    post-traumatic G91.3
  specified NEC G91.8
  syphilitic, congenital A50.49
Hydrocolpos (congenital) N89.8
Hydrocystoma — *see* Neoplasm, skin, benign
Hydroencephalocele (congenital) — *see* Encephalocele
Hydroencephalomeningocele (congenital) — *see* Encephalocele
Hydrohematopneumothorax — *see* Hemothorax
Hydromeningitis — *see* Meningitis
Hydromeningocele (spinal) — *see also* Spina bifida
  cranial — *see* Encephalocele
Hydrometra N85.8
Hydrometrocolpos N89.8
Hydromicrocephaly Q02
Hydromphalos (since birth) Q45.8
Hydromyelia Q06.4
Hydromyelocele — *see* Spina bifida
Hydronephrosis (atrophic) (early) (functionless) (intermittent) (primary) (secondary) NEC N13.30
  with
    infection N13.6
    obstruction (by) (of)
      renal calculus N13.2
        with infection N13.6
      ureteral NEC N13.1
        with infection N13.6
        calculus N13.2
          with infection N13.6
      ureteropelvic junction (congenital) Q62.11
        acquired N13.0
          with infection N13.6
      ureteral stricture NEC N13.1
        with infection N13.6
  congenital Q62.0
  due to acquired occlusion of ureteropelvic junction N13.0
  specified type NEC N13.39
  tuberculous A18.11
Hydropericarditis — *see* Pericarditis
Hydropericardium — *see* Pericarditis
Hydroperitoneum R18.8
Hydrophobia — *see* Rabies
Hydrophthalmos Q15.0
Hydropneumohemothorax — *see* Hemothorax
Hydropneumopericarditis — *see* Pericarditis
Hydropneumopericardium — *see* Pericarditis
Hydropneumothorax J94.8
  traumatic — *see* Injury, intrathoracic, lung
  tuberculous NEC A15.6
Hydrops R60.9
  abdominis R18.8
  articulorum intermittens — *see* Hydrarthrosis, intermittent
  cardiac — *see* Failure, heart, congestive
  causing obstructed labor (mother) O66.3
  endolymphatic H81.0- ☑
  fetal — *see* Pregnancy, complicated by, hydrops, fetalis
  fetalis P83.2

Hydrops — *continued*
  fetalis — *continued*
    due to
      ABO isoimmunization P56.0
      alpha thalassemia D56.0
      hemolytic disease P56.90
        specified NEC P56.99
      isoimmunization (ABO) (Rh) P56.0
      other specified nonhemolytic disease NEC P83.2
      Rh incompatibility P56.0
    during pregnancy — *see* Pregnancy, complicated by, hydrops, fetalis
  gallbladder K82.1
  joint — *see* Effusion, joint
  labyrinth H81.0- ☑
  newborn (idiopathic) P83.2
    due to
      ABO isoimmunization P56.0
      alpha thalassemia D56.0
      hemolytic disease P56.90
        specified NEC P56.99
      isoimmunization (ABO) (Rh) P56.0
      Rh incompatibility P56.0
  nutritional — *see* Malnutrition, severe
  pericardium — *see* Pericarditis
  pleura — *see* Hydrothorax
  spermatic cord — *see* Hydrocele
Hydropyonephrosis N13.6
Hydrorachis Q06.4
Hydrorrhea (nasal) J34.89
  pregnancy — *see* Rupture, membranes, premature
Hydrosadenitis (axillaris) (suppurative) L73.2
Hydrosalpinx (fallopian tube) (follicularis) N70.11
Hydrothorax (double) (pleura) J94.8
  chylous (nonfilarial) I89.8
    filarial — *see also* Infestation, filarial B74.9 *[J91.8]*
  traumatic — *see* Injury, intrathoracic
  tuberculous NEC (non primary) A15.6
Hydroureter — *see also* Hydronephrosis N13.4
  with infection N13.6
  congenital Q62.39
Hydroureteronephrosis — *see* Hydronephrosis
Hydrourethra N36.8
Hydroxykynureninuria E70.89
Hydroxylysinemia E72.3
Hydroxyprolinemia E72.59
Hygiene, sleep
  abuse Z72.821
  inadequate Z72.821
  poor Z72.821
Hygroma (congenital) (cystic) D18.1
  praepatellare, prepatellar — *see* Bursitis, prepatellar
Hymen — *see* condition
Hymenolepis, hymenolepiasis (diminuta) (infection) (infestation) (nana) B71.0
Hypalgesia R20.8
Hyperacidity (gastric) K31.89
  psychogenic F45.8
Hyperactive, hyperactivity F90.9
  basal cell, uterine cervix — *see* Dysplasia, cervix
  bowel sounds R19.12
  cervix epithelial (basal) — *see* Dysplasia, cervix
  child F90.9
    attention deficit — *see* Disorder, attention-deficit hyperactivity
  detrusor muscle N32.81
  gastrointestinal K31.89
    psychogenic F45.8
  nasal mucous membrane J34.3
  stomach K31.89
  thyroid (gland) — *see* Hyperthyroidism
Hyperacusis H93.23- ☑
Hyperadrenalism E27.5
Hyperadrenocorticism E24.9
  congenital E25.0
  iatrogenic E24.2
    correct substance properly administered — *see* Table of Drugs and Chemicals, by drug, adverse effect
    overdose or wrong substance given or taken — *see* Table of Drugs and Chemicals, by drug, poisoning
  not associated with Cushing's syndrome E27.0
  pituitary-dependent E24.0
Hyperaldosteronism E26.9
  familial (type I) E26.02
  glucocorticoid-remediable E26.02

Hyperaldosteronism — *continued*
  primary (due to (bilateral) adrenal hyperplasia) E26.09
  primary NEC E26.09
  secondary E26.1
  specified NEC E26.89
Hyperalgesia R20.8
Hyperalimentation R63.2
  carotene, carotin E67.1
  specified NEC E67.8
  vitamin
    A E67.0
    D E67.3
Hyperaminoaciduria
  arginine E72.21
  cystine E72.01
  lysine E72.3
  ornithine E72.4
Hyperammonemia (congenital) E72.20
Hyperazotemia — *see* Uremia
Hyperbetalipoproteinemia (familial) E78.00
  with prebetalipoproteinemia E78.2
Hyperbicarbonatemia P74.41
Hyperbilirubinemia
  constitutional E80.6
  familial conjugated E80.6
  neonatal (transient) — *see* Jaundice, newborn
Hypercalcemia, hypocalciuric, familial E83.52
Hypercalciuria, idiopathic R82.994
Hypercapnia R06.89
  newborn P84
Hypercarotenemia (dietary) E67.1
Hypercementosis K03.4
Hyperchloremia E87.8
Hyperchlorhydria K31.89
  neurotic F45.8
  psychogenic F45.8
Hypercholesterinemia — *see* Hypercholesterolemia
Hypercholesterolemia (essential) (primary) (pure) E78.00
  with hyperglyceridemia, endogenous E78.2
  dietary counseling and surveillance Z71.3
  familial E78.01
  hereditary E78.01
Hyperchylia gastrica, psychogenic F45.8
Hyperchylomicronemia (familial) (primary) E78.3
  with hyperbetalipoproteinemia E78.3
Hypercoagulable (state) D68.59
  activated protein C resistance D68.51
  antithrombin (III) deficiency D68.59
  factor V Leiden mutation D68.51
  primary NEC D68.59
  protein C deficiency D68.59
  protein S deficiency D68.59
  prothrombin gene mutation D68.52
  secondary D68.69
  specified NEC D68.69
Hypercoagulation (state) D68.59
Hypercorticalism, pituitary-dependent E24.0
Hypercorticosolism — *see* Cushing's, syndrome
Hypercorticosteronism E24.2
  correct substance properly administered — *see* Table of Drugs and Chemicals, by drug, adverse effect
  overdose or wrong substance given or taken — *see* Table of Drugs and Chemicals, by drug, poisoning
Hypercortisonism E24.2
  correct substance properly administered — *see* Table of Drugs and Chemicals, by drug, adverse effect
  overdose or wrong substance given or taken — *see* Table of Drugs and Chemicals, by drug, poisoning
Hyperekplexia Q89.8
Hyperelectrolytemia E87.8
Hyperemesis R11.10
  with nausea R11.2
  gravidarum (mild) O21.0
    with
      carbohydrate depletion O21.1
      dehydration O21.1
      electrolyte imbalance O21.1
      metabolic disturbance O21.1
      severe (with metabolic disturbance) O21.1
  projectile R11.12
  psychogenic F45.8
Hyperemia (acute) (passive) R68.89
  anal mucosa K62.89
  bladder N32.89
  cerebral I67.89
  conjunctiva H11.43- ☑
  ear internal, acute — *see* subcategory H83.0 ☑
  enteric K59.89

☑ **Additional Character Required — Refer to the Tabular List for Character Selection**

Hyperemia — *continued*
  eye — *see* Hyperemia, conjunctiva
  eyelid (active) (passive) — *see* Disorder, eyelid, specified type NEC
  intestine K59.89
  iris — *see* Disorder, iris, vascular
  kidney N28.89
  labyrinth — *see* subcategory H83.0 ☑
  liver (active) K76.89
  lung (passive) — *see* Edema, lung
  pulmonary (passive) — *see* Edema, lung
  renal N28.89
  retina H35.89
  stomach K31.89
Hyperesthesia (body surface) R20.3
  larynx (reflex) J38.7
    hysterical F44.89
  pharynx (reflex) J39.2
    hysterical F44.89
Hyperestrogenism (drug-induced) (iatrogenic) E28.0
Hyperexplexia Q89.8
Hyperfibrinolysis — *see* Fibrinolysis
Hyperfructosemia E74.19
Hyperfunction
  adrenal cortex, not associated with Cushing's syndrome E27.0
    medulla E27.5
      adrenomedullary E27.5
    virilism E25.9
      congenital E25.0
  ovarian E28.8
  pancreas K86.89
  parathyroid (gland) E21.3
  pituitary (gland) (anterior) E22.9
    specified NEC E22.8
  polyglandular E31.1
  testicular E29.0
Hypergammaglobulinemia D89.2
  polyclonal D89.0
  Waldenström D89.0
Hypergastrinemia E16.4
Hyperglobulinemia R77.1
Hyperglycemia, hyperglycemic (transient) R73.9
  coma — *see* Diabetes, by type, with coma
  postpancreatectomy E89.1
Hyperglyceridemia (endogenous) (essential) (familial) (hereditary) (pure) E78.1
  mixed E78.3
Hyperglycinemia (non-ketotic) E72.51
Hypergonadism
  ovarian E28.8
  testicular (primary) (infantile) E29.0
Hyperheparinemia D68.32
Hyperhidrosis, hyperidrosis R61
  focal
    primary L74.519
      axilla L74.510
      face L74.511
      palms L74.512
      soles L74.513
    secondary L74.52
  generalized R61
  localized
    primary L74.519
      axilla L74.510
      face L74.511
      palms L74.512
      soles L74.513
    secondary L74.52
  psychogenic F45.8
  secondary R61
    focal L74.52
Hyperhistidinemia E70.41
Hyperhomocysteinemia E72.11
Hyperhydroxyprolinemia E72.59
Hyperinsulinism (functional) E16.1
  with
    coma (hypoglycemic) E15
    encephalopathy E16.1 *[G94]*
  ectopic E16.1
  therapeutic misadventure (from administration of insulin) — *see* subcategory T38.3 ☑
Hyperkalemia E87.5
Hyperkeratosis — *see also* Keratosis L85.9
  cervix N88.0
  due to yaws (early) (late) (palmar or plantar) A66.3
  follicularis Q82.8
    penetrans (in cutem) L87.0

Hyperkeratosis — *continued*
  palmoplantaris climacterica L85.1
  pinta A67.1
  senile (with pruritus) L57.0
  universalis congenita Q80.8
  vocal cord J38.3
  vulva N90.4
Hyperkinesia, hyperkinetic (disease) (reaction) (syndrome) (childhood) (adolescence) — *see also* Disorder, attention-deficit hyperactivity
  heart I51.89
Hyperleucine-isoleucinemia E71.19
Hyperlipemia, hyperlipidemia E78.5
  combined E78.2
    familial E78.49
  group
    A E78.00
    B E78.1
    C E78.2
    D E78.3
  mixed E78.2
  specified NEC E78.49
Hyperlipidosis E75.6
  hereditary NEC E75.5
Hyperlipoproteinemia E78.5
  Fredrickson's type
    I E78.3
    IIa E78.00
    IIb E78.2
    III E78.2
    IV E78.1
    V E78.3
  low-density-lipoprotein-type (LDL) E78.00
  very-low-density-lipoprotein-type (VLDL) E78.1
Hyperlucent lung, unilateral J43.0
Hyperlysinemia E72.3
Hypermagnesemia E83.41
  neonatal P71.8
Hypermenorrhea N92.0
Hypermethioninemia E72.19
Hypermetropia (congenital) H52.0- ☑
Hypermobility, hypermotility
  cecum — *see* Syndrome, irritable bowel
  coccyx — *see* subcategory M53.2 ☑
  colon — *see* Syndrome, irritable bowel
    psychogenic F45.8
  ileum K58.9
  intestine — *see also* Syndrome, irritable bowel K58.9
    psychogenic F45.8
  meniscus (knee) — *see* Derangement, knee, meniscus
  scapula — *see* Instability, joint, shoulder
  stomach K31.89
    psychogenic F45.8
  syndrome M35.7
  urethra N36.41
    with intrinsic sphincter deficiency N36.43
Hypernasality R49.21
Hypernatremia E87.0
Hypernephroma C64.- ☑
Hyperopia — *see* Hypermetropia
Hyperorexia nervosa F50.2
Hyperornithinemia E72.4
Hyperosmia R43.1
Hyperosmolality E87.0
Hyperostosis (monomelic) — *see also* Disorder, bone, density and structure, specified NEC
  ankylosing (spine) M48.10
    cervical region M48.12
    cervicothoracic region M48.13
    lumbar region M48.16
    lumbosacral region M48.17
    multiple sites M48.19
    occipito-atlanto-axial region M48.11
    sacrococcygeal region M48.18
    thoracic region M48.14
    thoracolumbar region M48.15
  cortical (skull) M85.2
    infantile M89.8X- ☑
  frontal, internal of skull M85.2
  interna frontalis M85.2
  skeletal, diffuse idiopathic — *see* Hyperostosis, ankylosing
  skull M85.2
    congenital Q75.8
  vertebral, ankylosing — *see* Hyperostosis, ankylosing
Hyperovarism E28.8
Hyperoxaluria R82.992
  primary E72.53

Hyperparathyroidism E21.3
  primary E21.0
  secondary (renal) N25.81
    non-renal E21.1
  specified NEC E21.2
  tertiary E21.2
Hyperpathia R20.8
Hyperperistalsis R19.2
  psychogenic F45.8
Hyperpermeability, capillary I78.8
Hyperphagia R63.2
Hyperphenylalaninemia NEC E70.1
Hyperphoria (alternating) H50.53
Hyperphosphatemia E83.39
Hyperpiesis, hyperpiesia — *see* Hypertension
Hyperpigmentation — *see also* Pigmentation
  melanin NEC L81.4
  postinflammatory L81.0
Hyperpinealism E34.8
Hyperpituitarism E22.9
Hyperplasia, hyperplastic
  adenoids J35.2
  adrenal (capsule) (cortex) (gland) E27.8
    with
      sexual precocity (male) E25.9
        congenital E25.0
      virilism, adrenal E25.9
        congenital E25.0
      virilization (female) E25.9
        congenital E25.0
    congenital E25.0
      salt-losing E25.0
  adrenomedullary E27.5
  angiolymphoid, eosinophilia (ALHE) D18.01
  appendix (lymphoid) K38.0
  artery, fibromuscular I77.3
  bone — *see also* Hypertrophy, bone
    marrow D75.89
  breast — *see also* Hypertrophy, breast
    atypical, atypia N60.9- ☑
      ductal N60.9- ☑
      lobular N60.9- ☑
  C-cell, thyroid E07.0
  cementation (tooth) (teeth) K03.4
  cervical gland R59.0
  cervix (uteri) (basal cell) (endometrium) (polypoid) — *see also* Dysplasia, cervix
    congenital Q51.828
  clitoris, congenital Q52.6
  denture K06.2
  endocervicitis N72
  endometrium, endometrial (adenomatous) (cystic) (glandular) (glandular-cystic) (polypoid) N85.00
    with atypia N85.02
    benign N85.01
    cervix — *see* Dysplasia, cervix
    complex (without atypia) N85.01
    simple (without atypia) N85.01
  epithelial L85.9
    focal, oral, including tongue K13.29
    nipple N62
    skin L85.9
    tongue K13.29
    vaginal wall N89.3
  erythroid D75.89
  fibromuscular of artery (carotid) (renal) I77.3
  genital
    female NEC N94.89
    male N50.89
  gingiva K06.1
  glandularis cystica uteri (interstitialis) — *see also* Hyperplasia, endometrial N85.00
  gum K06.1
  hymen, congenital Q52.4
  irritative, edentulous (alveolar) K06.2
  jaw M26.09
    alveolar M26.79
      lower M26.03
        alveolar M26.72
      upper M26.01
        alveolar M26.71
  kidney (congenital) Q63.3
  labia N90.69
    epithelial N90.3
  liver (congenital) Q44.7
    nodular, focal K76.89
  lymph gland or node R59.9
  mandible, mandibular M26.03

Hyperplasia, hyperplastic — *continued*
 mandible, mandibular — *continued*
  alveolar M26.72
  unilateral condylar M27.8
 maxilla, maxillary M26.01
  alveolar M26.71
 myometrium, myometrial N85.2
 neuroendocrine cell, of infancy J84.841
 nose
  lymphoid J34.89
  polypoid J33.9
 oral mucosa (irritative) K13.6
 organ or site, congenital NEC — *see* Anomaly, by site
 ovary N83.8
 palate, papillary (irritative) K13.6
 pancreatic islet cells E16.9
  alpha E16.8
   with excess
    gastrin E16.4
    glucagon E16.3
  beta E16.1
 parathyroid (gland) E21.0
 pharynx (lymphoid) J39.2
 prostate (adenofibromatous) (nodular) N40.0
  with lower urinary tract symptoms (LUTS) N40.1
  without lower urinary tract symtpoms (LUTS) N40.0
 renal artery I77.89
 reticulo-endothelial (cell) D75.89
 salivary gland (any) K11.1
 Schimmelbusch's — *see* Mastopathy, cystic
 suprarenal capsule (gland) E27.8
 thymus (gland) (persistent) E32.0
 thyroid (gland) — *see* Goiter
 tonsils (faucial) (infective) (lingual) (lymphoid) J35.1
  with adenoids J35.3
 unilateral condylar M27.8
 uterus, uterine N85.2
  endometrium (glandular) — *see also* Hyperplasia, endometrial N85.00
 vulva N90.69
  epithelial N90.3
Hyperpnea — *see* Hyperventilation
Hyperpotassemia E87.5
Hyperprebetalipoproteinemia (familial) E78.1
Hyperprolactinemia E22.1
Hyperprolinemia (type I) (type II) E72.59
Hyperproteinemia E88.09
Hyperprothrombinemia, causing coagulation factor deficiency D68.4
Hyperpyrexia R50.9
 heat (effects) T67.01 ☑
 malignant, due to anesthetic T88.3 ☑
 rheumatic — *see* Fever, rheumatic
 unknown origin R50.9
Hyper-reflexia R29.2
Hypersalivation K11.7
Hypersecretion
 ACTH (not associated with Cushing's syndrome) E27.0
  pituitary E24.0
 adrenaline E27.5
 adrenomedullary E27.5
 androgen (testicular) E29.0
  ovarian (drug-induced) (iatrogenic) E28.1
 calcitonin E07.0
 catecholamine E27.5
 corticoadrenal E24.9
 cortisol E24.9
 epinephrine E27.5
 estrogen E28.0
 gastric K31.89
  psychogenic F45.8
 gastrin E16.4
 glucagon E16.3
 hormone(s)
  ACTH (not associated with Cushing's syndrome) E27.0
   pituitary E24.0
  antidiuretic E22.2
  growth E22.0
  intestinal NEC E34.1
  ovarian androgen E28.1
  pituitary E22.9
  testicular E29.0
  thyroid stimulating E05.80
   with thyroid storm E05.81
 insulin — *see* Hyperinsulinism
 lacrimal glands — *see* Epiphora
 medulloadrenal E27.5

Hypersecretion — *continued*
 milk O92.6
 ovarian androgens E28.1
 salivary gland (any) K11.7
 thyrocalcitonin E07.0
 upper respiratory J39.8
Hypersegmentation, leukocytic, hereditary D72.0
Hypersensitive, hypersensitiveness, hypersensitivity — *see also* Allergy
 carotid sinus G90.01
 colon — *see* Irritable, colon
 drug T88.7 ☑
 gastrointestinal K52.29
  immediate K52.29
  psychogenic F45.8
 labyrinth — *see* subcategory H83.2 ☑
 pain R20.8
 pneumonitis — *see* Pneumonitis, allergic
 reaction T78.40 ☑
  upper respiratory tract NEC J39.3
Hypersomnia (organic) G47.10
 due to
  alcohol
   abuse F10.182
   dependence F10.282
   use F10.982
  amphetamines
   abuse F15.182
   dependence F15.282
   use F15.982
  caffeine
   abuse F15.182
   dependence F15.282
   use F15.982
  cocaine
   abuse F14.182
   dependence F14.282
   use F14.982
  drug NEC
   abuse F19.182
   dependence F19.282
   use F19.982
  medical condition G47.14
  mental disorder F51.13
  opioid
   abuse F11.182
   dependence F11.282
   use F11.982
  psychoactive substance NEC
   abuse F19.182
   dependence F19.282
   use F19.982
  sedative, hypnotic, or anxiolytic
   abuse F13.182
   dependence F13.282
   use F13.982
  stimulant NEC
   abuse F15.182
   dependence F15.282
   use F15.982
 idiopathic G47.11
  with long sleep time G47.11
  without long sleep time G47.12
 menstrual related G47.13
 nonorganic origin F51.11
  specified NEC F51.19
 not due to a substance or known physiological condition F51.11
  specified NEC F51.19
 primary F51.11
 recurrent G47.13
 specified NEC G47.19
Hypersplenia, hypersplenism D73.1
Hyperstimulation, ovaries (associated with induced ovulation) N98.1
Hypersusceptibility — *see* Allergy
Hypertelorism (ocular) (orbital) Q75.2
Hypertension, hypertensive (accelerated) (benign) (essential) (idiopathic) (malignant) (systemic) I10
 with
  heart failure (congestive) I11.0
  heart involvement (conditions in I50.- or I51.4-I51.7, I51.89, I51.9, due to hypertension) — *see* Hypertension, heart
  kidney involvement — *see* Hypertension, kidney
 benign, intracranial G93.2
 borderline R03.0
 cardiorenal (disease) I13.10

Hypertension, hypertensive — *continued*
 cardiorenal — *continued*
  with heart failure I13.0
   with stage 1 through stage 4 chronic kidney disease I13.0
   with stage 5 or end stage renal disease I13.2
  without heart failure I13.10
   with stage 1 through stage 4 chronic kidney disease I13.10
   with stage 5 or end stage renal disease I13.11
 cardiovascular
  disease (arteriosclerotic) (sclerotic) — *see* Hypertension, heart
  renal (disease) — *see* Hypertension, cardiorenal
 chronic venous — *see* Hypertension, venous (chronic)
 complicating
  childbirth (labor) O16.4
  pre-existing O10.92
   with
    heart disease O10.12
     with renal disease O10.32
    pre-eclampsia O11.4
    renal disease O10.22
     with heart disease O10.32
    essential O10.02
   secondary O10.42
  pregnancy O16.- ☑
   with edema — *see also* Pre-eclampsia O14.9- ☑
   gestational (pregnancy induced) (without proteinuria) O13.- ☑
    with proteinuria O14.9- ☑
     mild pre-eclampsia O14.0- ☑
     moderate pre-eclampsia O14.0- ☑
     severe pre-eclampsia O14.1- ☑
      with hemolysis, elevated liver enzymes and low platelet count (HELLP) O14.2- ☑
   pre-existing O10.91- ☑
    with
     heart disease O10.11- ☑
      with renal disease O10.31- ☑
     pre-eclampsia — *see* category O11
     renal disease O10.21- ☑
      with heart disease O10.31- ☑
     essential O10.01- ☑
     secondary O10.41- ☑
   transient O13- ☑
  puerperium, pre-existing O16.5
   pre-existing
    with
     heart disease O10.13
      with renal disease O10.33
     pre-eclampsia O11.5
     renal disease O10.23
      with heart disease O10.33
     essential O10.03
   pregnancy-induced O13.9
   secondary O10.43
 crisis I16.9
 due to
  endocrine disorders I15.2
  pheochromocytoma I15.2
  renal disorders NEC I15.1
   arterial I15.0
  renovascular disorders I15.0
  specified disease NEC I15.8
 emergency I16.1
 encephalopathy I67.4
 gestational (without significant proteinuria) (pregnancy-induced) (transient) O13.- ☑
  with significant proteinuria — *see* Pre-eclampsia
  complicating
   delivery O13.4
   puerperium O13.5
 Goldblatt's I70.1
 heart (disease) (conditions in I51.4-I51.9 due to hypertension) I11.9
  with
   heart failure (congestive) I11.0
   kidney disease (chronic) — *see* Hypertension, cardiorenal
 intracranial, benign G93.2
 kidney I12.9
  with
   heart disease — *see* Hypertension, cardiorenal
   stage 1 through stage 4 chronic kidney disease I12.9

Hypertension, hypertensive — *continued*
  kidney — *continued*
    with — *continued*
      stage 5 chronic kidney disease (CKD) or end stage
        renal disease (ESRD) I12.0
    lesser circulation I27.0
    maternal O16- ☑
    newborn P29.2
      pulmonary (persistent) P29.30
    ocular H40.05- ☑
    pancreatic duct — *code to* underlying condition
      with chronic pancreatitis K86.1
    portal (due to chronic liver disease) (idiopathic) K76.6
      gastropathy K31.89
      in (due to) schistosomiasis (bilharziasis) B65.9 *[K77]*
    postoperative I97.3
    psychogenic F45.8
    pulmonary I27.20
      with
        cor pulmonale (chronic) I27.29
          acute I26.09
        right heart ventricular strain/failure I27.29
          acute I26.09
        right to left shunt related to congenital heart
          disease I27.83
        unclear multifactorial mechanisms I27.29
      arterial (associated) (drug-induced) (toxin-induced)
        I27.21
      chronic thromboembolic I27.24
      due to
        hematologic disorders I27.29
        kyphoscoliotic heart disease I27.1
        left heart disease I27.22
        lung diseases and hypoxia I27.23
        metabolic disorders I27.29
        specified systemic disorders I27.29
      group 1 (associated) (drug-induced) (toxin-induced)
        I27.21
      group 2 I27.22
      group 3 I27.23
      group 4 I27.24
      group 5 I27.29
      of newborn (persistent) P29.30
      primary (idiopathic) I27.0
      secondary
        arterial I27.21
        specified NEC I27.29
    renal — *see* Hypertension, kidney
    renovascular I15.0
    secondary NEC I15.9
      due to
        endocrine disorders I15.2
        pheochromocytoma I15.2
        renal disorders NEC I15.1
          arterial I15.0
        renovascular disorders I15.0
      specified NEC I15.8
    transient R03.0
      of pregnancy O13.- ☑
    urgency I16.0
    venous (chronic)
      due to
        deep vein thrombosis — *see* Syndrome, post-
          thrombotic
      idiopathic I87.309
        with
          inflammation I87.32- ☑
            with ulcer I87.33- ☑
          specified complication NEC I87.39- ☑
          ulcer I87.31- ☑
            with inflammation I87.33- ☑
        asymptomatic I87.30- ☑

Hypertensive urgency — *see* Hypertension
Hyperthecosis ovary E28.8
Hyperthermia (of unknown origin) — *see also* Hyperpyrexia
  malignant, due to anesthesia T88.3 ☑
  newborn P81.9
    environmental P81.0
Hyperthyroid (recurrent) — *see* Hyperthyroidism
Hyperthyroidism (latent) (pre-adult) (recurrent) E05.90
  with
    goiter (diffuse) E05.00
      with thyroid storm E05.01
      nodular (multinodular) E05.20
        with thyroid storm E05.21
        uninodular E05.10
          with thyroid storm E05.11

Hyperthyroidism — *continued*
  with — *continued*
    storm E05.91
  due to ectopic thyroid tissue E05.30
    with thyroid storm E05.31
  neonatal, transitory P72.1
  specified NEC E05.80
    with thyroid storm E05.81
Hypertony, hypertonia, hypertonicity
  bladder N31.8
  congenital P94.1
  stomach K31.89
    psychogenic F45.8
  uterus, uterine (contractions) (complicating delivery)
    O62.4
Hypertrichosis L68.9
  congenital Q84.2
  eyelid H02.869
    left H02.866
      lower H02.865
      upper H02.864
    right H02.863
      lower H02.862
      upper H02.861
  lanuginosa Q84.2
    acquired L68.1
  localized L68.2
  specified NEC L68.8
Hypertriglyceridemia, essential E78.1
Hypertrophy, hypertrophic
  adenofibromatous, prostate — *see* Enlargement, en-
    larged, prostate
  adenoids (infective) J35.2
    with tonsils J35.3
  adrenal cortex E27.8
  alveolar process or ridge — *see* Anomaly, alveolar
  anal papillae K62.89
  artery I77.89
    congenital NEC Q27.8
      digestive system Q27.8
      lower limb Q27.8
      specified site NEC Q27.8
      upper limb Q27.8
  auricular — *see* Hypertrophy, cardiac
  Bartholin's gland N75.8
  bile duct (common) (hepatic) K83.8
  bladder (sphincter) (trigone) N32.89
  bone M89.30
    carpus M89.34- ☑
    clavicle M89.31- ☑
    femur M89.35- ☑
    fibula M89.36- ☑
    finger M89.34- ☑
    humerus M89.32- ☑
    ilium M89.359
    ischium M89.359
    metacarpus M89.34- ☑
    metatarsus M89.37- ☑
    multiple sites M89.39
    neck M89.38
    radius M89.33- ☑
    rib M89.38
    scapula M89.31- ☑
    skull M89.38
    tarsus M89.37- ☑
    tibia M89.36- ☑
    toe M89.37- ☑
    ulna M89.33- ☑
    vertebra M89.38
  brain G93.89
  breast N62
    cystic — *see* Mastopathy, cystic
    newborn P83.4
    pubertal, massive N62
    puerperal, postpartum — *see* Disorder, breast,
      specified type NEC
    senile (parenchymatous) N62
  cardiac (chronic) (idiopathic) I51.7
    with rheumatic fever (conditions in I00)
      active I01.8
      inactive or quiescent (with chorea) I09.89
    congenital NEC Q24.8
    fatty — *see* Degeneration, myocardial
    hypertensive — *see* Hypertension, heart
    rheumatic (with chorea) I09.89
      active or acute I01.8
        with chorea I02.0
    valve — *see* Endocarditis

Hypertrophy, hypertrophic — *continued*
  cartilage — *see* Disorder, cartilage, specified type NEC
  cecum — *see* Megacolon
  cervix (uteri) N88.8
    congenital Q51.828
    elongation N88.4
  clitoris (cirrhotic) N90.89
    congenital Q52.6
  colon — *see also* Megacolon
    congenital Q43.2
  conjunctiva, lymphoid H11.89
  corpora cavernosa N48.89
  cystic duct K82.8
  duodenum K31.89
  endometrium (glandular) — *see also* Hyperplasia, en-
    dometrial N85.00
    cervix N88.8
  epididymis N50.89
  esophageal hiatus (congenital) Q79.1
    with hernia — *see* Hernia, hiatal
  eyelid — *see* Disorder, eyelid, specified type NEC
  facet joint — *see also* Spondylosis M47.819
  fat pad E65
    knee (infrapatellar) (popliteal) (prepatellar)
      (retropatellar) M79.4
  foot (congenital) Q74.2
  frenulum, frenum (tongue) K14.8
    lip K13.0
  gallbladder K82.8
  gastric mucosa K29.60
    with bleeding K29.61
  gland, glandular R59.9
    generalized R59.1
    localized R59.0
  gum (mucous membrane) K06.1
  heart (idiopathic) — *see also* Hypertrophy, cardiac
    valve — *see also* Endocarditis I38
  hemifacial Q67.4
  hepatic — *see* Hypertrophy, liver
  hiatus (esophageal) Q79.1
  hilus gland R59.0
  hymen, congenital Q52.4
  ileum K63.89
  intestine NEC K63.89
  jejunum K63.89
  kidney (compensatory) N28.81
    congenital Q63.3
  labium (majus) (minus) N90.60
  ligament — *see* Disorder, ligament
  lingual tonsil (infective) J35.1
    with adenoids J35.3
  lip K13.0
    congenital Q18.6
  liver R16.0
    acute K76.89
    cirrhotic — *see* Cirrhosis, liver
    congenital Q44.7
    fatty — *see* Fatty, liver
  lymph, lymphatic gland R59.9
    generalized R59.1
    localized R59.0
    tuberculous — *see* Tuberculosis, lymph gland
  mammary gland — *see* Hypertrophy, breast
  Meckel's diverticulum (congenital) Q43.0
    malignant — *see* Table of Neoplasms, small intes-
      tine, malignant
  median bar — *see* Hyperplasia, prostate
  meibomian gland — *see* Chalazion
  meniscus, knee, congenital Q74.1
  metatarsal head — *see* Hypertrophy, bone, metatarsus
  metatarsus — *see* Hypertrophy, bone, metatarsus
  mucous membrane
    alveolar ridge K06.2
    gum K06.1
    nose (turbinate) J34.3
  muscle M62.89
  muscular coat, artery I77.89
  myocardium — *see also* Hypertrophy, cardiac
    idiopathic I42.2
  myometrium N85.2
  nail L60.2
    congenital Q84.5
  nasal J34.89
    alae J34.89
    bone J34.89
    cartilage J34.89
    mucous membrane (septum) J34.3
    sinus J34.89

Hypertrophy, hypertrophic — *continued*
  nasal — *continued*
    turbinate J34.3
  nasopharynx, lymphoid (infectional) (tissue) (wall) J35.2
  nipple N62
  organ or site, congenital NEC — *see* Anomaly, by site
  ovary N83.8
  palate (hard) M27.8
    soft K13.79
  pancreas, congenital Q45.3
  parathyroid (gland) E21.0
  parotid gland K11.1
  penis N48.89
  pharyngeal tonsil J35.2
  pharynx J39.2
    lymphoid (infectional) (tissue) (wall) J35.2
  pituitary (anterior) (fossa) (gland) E23.6
  prepuce (congenital) N47.8
    female N90.89
  prostate — *see* Enlargement, enlarged, prostate
    congenital Q55.4
  pseudomuscular — *see also* Dystrophy, muscular, by
    type, if applicable G71.09
  pylorus (adult) (muscle) (sphincter) K31.1
    congenital or infantile Q40.0
  rectal, rectum (sphincter) K62.89
  rhinitis (turbinate) J31.0
  salivary gland (any) K11.1
    congenital Q38.4
  scaphoid (tarsal) — *see* Hypertrophy, bone, tarsus
  scar L91.0
  scrotum N50.89
  seminal vesicle N50.89
  sigmoid — *see* Megacolon
  skin L91.9
    specified NEC L91.8
  spermatic cord N50.89
  spleen — *see* Splenomegaly
  spondylitis — *see* Spondylosis
  stomach K31.89
  sublingual gland K11.1
  submandibular gland K11.1
  suprarenal cortex (gland) E27.8
  synovial NEC M67.20
    acromioclavicular M67.21- ☑
    ankle M67.27- ☑
    elbow M67.22- ☑
    foot M67.27- ☑
    hand M67.24- ☑
    hip M67.25- ☑
    knee M67.26- ☑
    multiple sites M67.29
    specified site NEC M67.28
    wrist M67.23- ☑
  tendon — *see* Disorder, tendon, specified type NEC
  testis N44.8
    congenital Q55.29
  thymic, thymus (gland) (congenital) E32.0
  thyroid (gland) — *see* Goiter
  toe (congenital) Q74.2
    acquired — *see also* Deformity, toe, specified NEC
  tongue K14.8
    congenital Q38.2
    papillae (foliate) K14.3
  tonsils (faucial) (infective) (lingual) (lymphoid) J35.1
    with adenoids J35.3
  tunica vaginalis N50.89
  ureter N28.89
  urethra N36.8
  uterus N85.2
    neck (with elongation) N88.4
    puerperal O90.89
  uvula K13.79
  vagina N89.8
  vas deferens N50.89
  vein I87.8
  ventricle, ventricular (heart) — *see also* Hypertrophy,
    cardiac
    congenital Q24.8
    in tetralogy of Fallot Q21.3
  verumontanum N36.8
  vocal cord J38.3
  vulva N90.60
    stasis (nonfilarial) N90.69
Hypertropia H50.2- ☑
Hypertyrosinemia E70.21
Hyperuricemia (asymptomatic) E79.0
Hyperuricosuria R82.993

Hypervalinemia E71.19
Hyperventilation (tetany) R06.4
  hysterical F45.8
  psychogenic F45.8
  syndrome F45.8
Hypervitaminosis (dietary) NEC E67.8
  A E67.0
    administered as drug (prolonged intake) — *see* Table of Drugs and Chemicals, vitamins, adverse effect
    overdose or wrong substance given or taken — *see* Table of Drugs and Chemicals, vitamins, poisoning
  B6 E67.2
  D E67.3
    administered as drug (prolonged intake) — *see* Table of Drugs and Chemicals, vitamins, adverse effect
    overdose or wrong substance given or taken — *see* Table of Drugs and Chemicals, vitamins, poisoning
  K E67.8
    administered as drug (prolonged intake) — *see* Table of Drugs and Chemicals, vitamins, adverse effect
    overdose or wrong substance given or taken — *see* Table of Drugs and Chemicals, vitamins, poisoning
Hypervolemia E87.70
  specified NEC E87.79
Hypesthesia R20.1
  cornea — *see* Anesthesia, cornea
Hyphema H21.0- ☑
  traumatic S05.1- ☑
Hypoacidity, gastric K31.89
  psychogenic F45.8
Hypoadrenalism, hypoadrenia E27.40
  primary E27.1
  tuberculous A18.7
Hypoadrenocorticism E27.40
  pituitary E23.0
  primary E27.1
Hypoalbuminemia E88.09
Hypoaldosteronism E27.40
Hypoalphalipoproteinemia E78.6
Hypobarism T70.29 ☑
Hypobaropathy T70.29 ☑
Hypobetalipoproteinemia (familial) E78.6
Hypocalcemia E83.51
  dietary E58
  neonatal P71.1
    due to cow's milk P71.0
  phosphate-loading (newborn) P71.1
Hypochloremia E87.8
Hypochlorhydria K31.89
  neurotic F45.8
  psychogenic F45.8
Hypochondria, hypochondriac, hypochondriasis (reaction) F45.21
  sleep F51.03
Hypochondrogenesis Q77.0
Hypochondroplasia Q77.4
Hypochromasia, blood cells D50.8
Hypocitraturia R82.991
Hypodontia — *see* Anodontia
Hypoeosinophilia D72.89
Hypoesthesia R20.1
Hypofibrinogenemia D68.8
  acquired D65
  congenital (hereditary) D68.2
Hypofunction
  adrenocortical E27.40
    drug-induced E27.3
    postprocedural E89.6
    primary E27.1
  adrenomedullary, postprocedural E89.6
  cerebral R29.818
  corticoadrenal NEC E27.40
  intestinal K59.89
  labyrinth — *see* subcategory H83.2 ☑
  ovary E28.39
  pituitary (gland) (anterior) E23.0
  testicular E29.1
    postprocedural (postsurgical) (postirradiation) (iatrogenic) E89.5
Hypogalactia O92.4

Hypogammaglobulinemia — *see also* Agammaglobulinemia D80.1
  hereditary D80.0
  nonfamilial D80.1
  transient, of infancy D80.7
Hypogenitalism (congenital) — *see* Hypogonadism
Hypoglossia Q38.3
Hypoglycemia (spontaneous) E16.2
  coma E15
    diabetic — *see* Diabetes, by type, with hypoglycemia, with coma
  diabetic — *see* Diabetes, hypoglycemia
  dietary counseling and surveillance Z71.3
  drug-induced E16.0
    with coma (nondiabetic) E15
  due to insulin E16.0
    with coma (nondiabetic) E15
    therapeutic misadventure — *see* subcategory T38.3 ☑
  functional, nonhyperinsulinemic E16.1
  iatrogenic E16.0
    with coma (nondiabetic) E15
  in infant of diabetic mother P70.1
    gestational diabetes P70.0
  infantile E16.1
  leucine-induced E71.19
  neonatal (transitory) P70.4
    iatrogenic P70.3
  reactive (not drug-induced) E16.1
  transitory neonatal P70.4
Hypogonadism
  female E28.39
  hypogonadotropic E23.0
  male E29.1
  ovarian (primary) E28.39
  pituitary E23.0
  testicular (primary) E29.1
Hypohidrosis, hypoidrosis L74.4
Hypoinsulinemia, postprocedural E89.1
Hypokalemia E87.6
Hypoleukocytosis — *see* Agranulocytosis
Hypolipoproteinemia (alpha) (beta) E78.6
Hypomagnesemia E83.42
  neonatal P71.2
Hypomania, hypomanic reaction F30.8
Hypomenorrhea — *see* Oligomenorrhea
Hypometabolism R63.8
Hypomotility
  gastrointestinal (tract) K31.89
    psychogenic F45.8
  intestine K59.89
    psychogenic F45.8
  stomach K31.89
    psychogenic F45.8
Hyponasality R49.22
Hyponatremia E87.1
Hypo-osmolality E87.1
Hypo-ovarianism, hypo-ovarism E28.39
Hypoparathyroidism E20.9
  familial E20.8
  idiopathic E20.0
  neonatal, transitory P71.4
  postprocedural E89.2
  specified NEC E20.8
Hypoperfusion (in)
  newborn P96.89
Hypopharyngitis — *see* Laryngopharyngitis
Hypophoria H50.53
Hypophosphatemia, hypophosphatasia (acquired) (congenital) (renal) E83.39
  familial E83.31
Hypophyseal, hypophysis — *see also* condition
  dwarfism E23.0
  gigantism E22.0
Hypopiesis — *see* Hypotension
Hypopinealism E34.8
Hypopituitarism (juvenile) E23.0
  drug-induced E23.1
  due to
    hypophysectomy E89.3
    radiotherapy E89.3
  iatrogenic NEC E23.1
  postirradiation E89.3
  postpartum O99.285
  postprocedural E89.3
Hypoplasia, hypoplastic
  adrenal (gland), congenital Q89.1
  alimentary tract, congenital Q45.8

Hypoplasia, hypoplastic — *continued*
  alimentary tract, congenital — *continued*
    upper Q40.8
  anus, anal (canal) Q42.3
    with fistula Q42.2
  aorta, aortic Q25.42
    ascending, in hypoplastic left heart syndrome Q23.4
    valve Q23.1
      in hypoplastic left heart syndrome Q23.4
  areola, congenital Q83.8
  arm (congenital) — *see* Defect, reduction, upper limb
  artery (peripheral) Q27.8
    brain (congenital) Q28.3
    coronary Q24.5
    digestive system Q27.8
    lower limb Q27.8
    pulmonary Q25.79
      functional, unilateral J43.0
    retinal (congenital) Q14.1
    specified site NEC Q27.8
    umbilical Q27.0
    upper limb Q27.8
  auditory canal Q17.8
    causing impairment of hearing Q16.9
  biliary duct or passage Q44.5
  bone NOS Q79.9
    face Q75.8
    marrow D61.9
      megakaryocytic D69.49
    skull — *see* Hypoplasia, skull
  brain Q02
    gyri Q04.3
    part of Q04.3
  breast (areola) N64.82
  bronchus Q32.4
  cardiac Q24.8
  carpus — *see* Defect, reduction, upper limb, specified type NEC
  cartilage hair Q78.8
  cecum Q42.8
  cementum K00.4
  cephalic Q02
  cerebellum Q04.3
  cervix (uteri), congenital Q51.821
  clavicle (congenital) Q74.0
  coccyx Q76.49
  colon Q42.9
    specified NEC Q42.8
  corpus callosum Q04.0
  cricoid cartilage Q31.2
  digestive organ(s) or tract NEC Q45.8
    upper (congenital) Q40.8
  ear (auricle) (lobe) Q17.2
    middle Q16.4
  enamel of teeth (neonatal) (postnatal) (prenatal) K00.4
  endocrine (gland) NEC Q89.2
  endometrium N85.8
  epididymis (congenital) Q55.4
  epiglottis Q31.2
  erythroid, congenital D61.01
  esophagus (congenital) Q39.8
  eustachian tube Q17.8
  eye Q11.2
  eyelid (congenital) Q10.3
  face Q18.8
    bone(s) Q75.8
  femur (congenital) — *see* Defect, reduction, lower limb, specified type NEC
  fibula (congenital) — *see* Defect, reduction, lower limb, specified type NEC
  finger (congenital) — *see* Defect, reduction, upper limb, specified type NEC
  focal dermal Q82.8
  foot — *see* Defect, reduction, lower limb, specified type NEC
  gallbladder Q44.0
  genitalia, genital organ(s)
    female, congenital Q52.8
      external Q52.79
      internal NEC Q52.8
    in adiposogenital dystrophy E23.6
  glottis Q31.2
  hair Q84.2
  hand (congenital) — *see* Defect, reduction, upper limb, specified type NEC
  heart Q24.8
  humerus (congenital) — *see* Defect, reduction, upper limb, specified type NEC

Hypoplasia, hypoplastic — *continued*
  intestine (small) Q41.9
    large Q42.9
      specified NEC Q42.8
  jaw M26.09
    alveolar M26.79
    lower M26.04
      alveolar M26.74
    upper M26.02
      alveolar M26.73
  kidney(s) Q60.5
    bilateral Q60.4
    unilateral Q60.3
  labium (majus) (minus), congenital Q52.79
  larynx Q31.2
  left heart syndrome Q23.4
  leg (congenital) — *see* Defect, reduction, lower limb
  limb Q73.8
    lower (congenital) — *see* Defect, reduction, lower limb
    upper (congenital) — *see* Defect, reduction, upper limb
  liver Q44.7
  lung (lobe) (not associated with short gestation) Q33.6
    associated with immaturity, low birth weight, prematurity, or short gestation P28.0
  mammary (areola), congenital Q83.8
  mandible, mandibular M26.04
    alveolar M26.74
    unilateral condylar M27.8
  maxillary M26.02
    alveolar M26.73
  medullary D61.9
  megakaryocytic D69.49
  metacarpus — *see* Defect, reduction, upper limb, specified type NEC
  metatarsus — *see* Defect, reduction, lower limb, specified type NEC
  muscle Q79.8
  nail(s) Q84.6
  nose, nasal Q30.1
  optic nerve H47.03- ☑
  osseous meatus (ear) Q17.8
  ovary, congenital Q50.39
  pancreas Q45.0
  parathyroid (gland) Q89.2
  parotid gland Q38.4
  patella Q74.1
  pelvis, pelvic girdle Q74.2
  penis (congenital) Q55.62
  peripheral vascular system Q27.8
    digestive system Q27.8
    lower limb Q27.8
    specified site NEC Q27.8
    upper limb Q27.8
  pituitary (gland) (congenital) Q89.2
  pulmonary (not associated with short gestation) Q33.6
    artery, functional J43.0
    associated with short gestation P28.0
  radioulnar — *see* Defect, reduction, upper limb, specified type NEC
  radius — *see* Defect, reduction, upper limb
  rectum Q42.1
    with fistula Q42.0
  respiratory system NEC Q34.8
  rib Q76.6
  right heart syndrome Q22.6
  sacrum Q76.49
  scapula Q74.0
  scrotum Q55.1
  shoulder girdle Q74.0
  skin Q82.8
  skull (bone) Q75.8
    with
      anencephaly Q00.0
      encephalocele — *see* Encephalocele
      hydrocephalus Q03.9
        with spina bifida — *see* Spina bifida, by site, with hydrocephalus
      microcephaly Q02
  spinal (cord) (ventral horn cell) Q06.1
  spine Q76.49
  sternum Q76.7
  tarsus — *see* Defect, reduction, lower limb, specified type NEC
  testis Q55.1
  thymic, with immunodeficiency D82.1
  thymus (gland) Q89.2

Hypoplasia, hypoplastic — *continued*
  thymus — *continued*
    with immunodeficiency D82.1
  thyroid (gland) E03.1
    cartilage Q31.2
  tibiofibular (congenital) — *see* Defect, reduction, lower limb, specified type NEC
  toe — *see* Defect, reduction, lower limb, specified type NEC
  tongue Q38.3
  Turner's K00.4
  ulna (congenital) — *see* Defect, reduction, upper limb
  umbilical artery Q27.0
  unilateral condylar M27.8
  ureter Q62.8
  uterus, congenital Q51.811
  vagina Q52.4
  vascular NEC peripheral Q27.8
    brain Q28.3
    digestive system Q27.8
    lower limb Q27.8
    specified site NEC Q27.8
    upper limb Q27.8
  vein(s) (peripheral) Q27.8
    brain Q28.3
    digestive system Q27.8
    great Q26.8
    lower limb Q27.8
    specified site NEC Q27.8
    upper limb Q27.8
  vena cava (inferior) (superior) Q26.8
  vertebra Q76.49
  vulva, congenital Q52.79
  zonule (ciliary) Q12.8
Hypoplasminogenemia E88.02
Hypopnea, obstructive sleep apnea G47.33
Hypopotassemia E87.6
Hypoproconvertinemia, congenital (hereditary) D68.2
Hypoproteinemia E77.8
Hypoprothrombinemia (congenital) (hereditary) (idiopathic) D68.2
  acquired D68.4
  newborn, transient P61.6
Hypoptyalism K11.7
Hypopyon (eye) (anterior chamber) — *see* Iridocyclitis, acute, hypopyon
Hypopyrexia R68.0
Hyporeflexia R29.2
Hyposecretion
  ACTH E23.0
  antidiuretic hormone E23.2
  ovary E28.39
  salivary gland (any) K11.7
  vasopressin E23.2
Hyposegmentation, leukocytic, hereditary D72.0
Hyposiderinemia D50.9
Hypospadias Q54.9
  balanic Q54.0
  coronal Q54.0
  glandular Q54.0
  penile Q54.1
  penoscrotal Q54.2
  perineal Q54.3
  specified NEC Q54.8
Hypospermatogenesis — *see* Oligospermia
Hyposplenism D73.0
Hypostasis pulmonary, passive — *see* Edema, lung
Hypostatic — *see* condition
Hyposthenuria N28.89
Hypotension (arterial) (constitutional) I95.9
  chronic I95.89
  due to (of) hemodialysis I95.3
  drug-induced I95.2
  iatrogenic I95.89
  idiopathic (permanent) I95.0
  intracranial G96.810
    following
      lumbar cerebrospinal fluid shunting G97.83
      specified procedure NEC G97.84
      ventricular shunting (ventriculostomy) G97.2
    specified NEC G96.819
    spontaneous G96.811
  intra-dialytic I95.3
  maternal, syndrome (following labor and delivery) O26.5- ☑
  neurogenic, orthostatic G90.3
  orthostatic (chronic) I95.1
    due to drugs I95.2

Hypotension — continued

Hypotension | ICD-10-CM 2023

Hypotension — *continued*
orthostatic — *continued*
neurogenic G90.3
postoperative I95.81
postural I95.1
specified NEC I95.89
Hypothermia (accidental) T68 ☑
due to anesthesia, anesthetic T88.51 ☑
low environmental temperature T68 ☑
neonatal P80.9
environmental (mild) NEC P80.8
mild P80.8
severe (chronic) (cold injury syndrome) P80.0
specified NEC P80.8
not associated with low environmental temperature
R68.0
Hypothyroidism (acquired) E03.9
autoimmune — *see* Thyroiditis, autoimmune
congenital (without goiter) E03.1
with goiter (diffuse) E03.0
due to
exogenous substance NEC E03.2
iodine-deficiency, acquired E01.8
subclinical E02
irradiation therapy E89.0
medicament NEC E03.2
P-aminosalicylic acid (PAS) E03.2
phenylbutazone E03.2
resorcinol E03.2
sulfonamide E03.2
surgery E89.0
thiourea group drugs E03.2
iatrogenic NEC E03.2
iodine-deficiency (acquired) E01.8
congenital — *see* Syndrome, iodine- deficiency,
congenital
subclinical E02
neonatal, transitory P72.2
postinfectious E03.3
postirradiation E89.0
postprocedural E89.0
postsurgical E89.0
specified NEC E03.8
subclinical, iodine-deficiency related E02
Hypotonia, hypotonicity, hypotony
bladder N31.2
congenital (benign) P94.2
eye — *see* Disorder, globe, hypotony
Hypotrichosis — *see* Alopecia
Hypotropia H50.2- ☑
Hypoventilation R06.89
congenital central alveolar G47.35
sleep related
idiopathic nonobstructive alveolar G47.34
in conditions classified elsewhere G47.36
Hypovitaminosis — *see* Deficiency, vitamin
Hypovolemia E86.1
surgical shock T81.19 ☑
traumatic (shock) T79.4 ☑
Hypoxemia R09.02
newborn P84
sleep related, in conditions classified elsewhere G47.36
Hypoxia — *see also* Anoxia R09.02
cerebral, during a procedure NEC G97.81
postprocedural NEC G97.82
intrauterine P84
myocardial — *see* Insufficiency, coronary
newborn P84
sleep-related G47.34
Hypsarrhythmia — *see* Epilepsy, generalized, specified
NEC
Hysteralgia, pregnant uterus O26.89- ☑
Hysteria, hysterical (conversion) (dissociative state)
F44.9
anxiety F41.8
convulsions F44.5
psychosis, acute F44.9
Hysteroepilepsy F44.5

IBDU (colonic inflammatory bowel disease unclassified)
K52.3
ICANS (immune effector cell-associated neurotoxicity
syndrome) — *see* Syndrome, immune effector cell-
associated neurotoxicity
Ichthyoparasitism due to Vandellia cirrhosa B88.8
Ichthyosis (congenital) Q80.9

Ichthyosis — *continued*
acquired L85.0
fetalis Q80.4
hystrix Q80.8
lamellar Q80.2
lingual K13.29
palmaris and plantaris Q82.8
simplex Q80.0
vera Q80.8
vulgaris Q80.0
X-linked Q80.1
Ichthyotoxism — *see* Poisoning, fish
bacterial — *see* Intoxication, foodborne
Icteroanemia, hemolytic (acquired) D59.9
congenital — *see* Spherocytosis
Icterus — *see also* Jaundice
conjunctiva R17
gravis, newborn P55.0
hematogenous (acquired) D59.9
hemolytic (acquired) D59.9
congenital — *see* Spherocytosis
hemorrhagic (acute) (leptospiral) (spirochetal) A27.0
newborn P53
infectious B15.9
with hepatic coma B15.0
leptospiral A27.0
spirochetal A27.0
neonatorum — *see* Jaundice, newborn
newborn P59.9
spirochetal A27.0
Ictus solaris, solis T67.01 ☑
Id reaction (due to bacteria) L30.2
Ideation
homicidal R45.850
suicidal R45.851
Identity disorder (child) F64.9
gender role F64.2
psychosexual F64.2
Idioglossia F80.0
Idiopathic — *see* condition
Idiot, idiocy (congenital) F73
amaurotic (Bielschowsky(-Jansky)) (family) (infantile
(late)) (juvenile (late)) (Vogt-Spielmeyer) E75.4
microcephalic Q02
IgE asthma J45.909
IIAC (idiopathic infantile arterial calcification) Q28.8
Ileitis (chronic) (noninfectious) — *see also* Enteritis K52.9
backwash — *see* Pancolitis, ulcerative (chronic)
infectious A09
regional (ulcerative) — *see* Enteritis, regional, small
intestine
segmental — *see* Enteritis, regional
terminal (ulcerative) — *see* Enteritis, regional, small
intestine
Ileocolitis — *see also* Enteritis K52.9
infectious A09
regional — *see* Enteritis, regional
ulcerative K51.0- ☑
Ileostomy
attention to Z43.2
malfunctioning K94.13
status Z93.2
with complication — *see* Complications, enterostomy
Ileotyphus — *see* Typhoid
Ileum — *see* condition
Ileus (bowel) (colon) (inhibitory) (intestine) K56.7
adynamic K56.0
due to gallstone (in intestine) K56.3
duodenal (chronic) K31.5
gallstone K56.3
mechanical NEC — *see also* Obstruction, intestine,
specified NEC K56.699
meconium P76.0
in cystic fibrosis E84.11
meaning meconium plug (without cystic fibrosis)
P76.0
myxedema K59.89
neurogenic K56.0
Hirschsprung's disease or megacolon Q43.1
newborn
due to meconium P76.0
in cystic fibrosis E84.11
meaning meconium plug (without cystic fibrosis)
P76.0
transitory P76.1
obstructive — *see also* Obstruction, intestine, specified
NEC K56.699

Ileus — *continued*
paralytic K56.0
postoperative K91.89
Iliac — *see* condition
Iliotibial band syndrome M76.3- ☑
Illiteracy Z55.0
Illness — *see also* Disease R69
manic-depressive — *see* Disorder, bipolar
Imbalance R26.89
autonomic G90.8
constituents of food intake E63.1
electrolyte E87.8
with
abortion — *see* Abortion by type, complicated
by, electrolyte imbalance
molar pregnancy O08.5
due to hyperemesis gravidarum O21.1
following ectopic or molar pregnancy O08.5
neonatal, transitory NEC P74.49
potassium
hyperkalemia P74.31
hypokalemia P74.32
sodium
hypernatremia P74.21
hyponatremia P74.22
endocrine E34.9
eye muscle NOS H50.9
hormone E34.9
hysterical F44.4
labyrinth — *see* subcategory H83.2 ☑
posture R29.3
protein-energy — *see* Malnutrition
sympathetic G90.8
Imbecile, imbecility (I.Q. 35-49) F71
Imbedding, intrauterine device T83.39 ☑
Imbibition, cholesterol (gallbladder) K82.4
Imbrication, teeth,, fully erupted M26.30
Imerslund (-Gräsbeck) **syndrome** D51.1
Immature — *see also* Immaturity
birth (less than 37 completed weeks) — *see* Preterm,
newborn
extremely (less than 28 completed weeks) — *see*
Immaturity, extreme
personality F60.89
Immaturity (less than 37 completed weeks) — *see also*
Preterm, newborn
extreme of newborn (less than 28 completed weeks of
gestation) (less than 196 completed days of
gestation) (unspecified weeks of gestation)
P07.20
gestational age
23 completed weeks (23 weeks, 0 days through
23 weeks, 6 days) P07.22
24 completed weeks (24 weeks, 0 days through
24 weeks, 6 days) P07.23
25 completed weeks (25 weeks, 0 days through
25 weeks, 6 days) P07.24
26 completed weeks (26 weeks, 0 days through
26 weeks, 6 days) P07.25
27 completed weeks (27 weeks, 0 days through
27 weeks, 6 days) P07.26
less than 23 completed weeks P07.21
fetus or infant light-for-dates — *see* Light-for-dates
lung, newborn P28.0
organ or site NEC — *see* Hypoplasia
pulmonary, newborn P28.0
reaction F60.89
sexual (female) (male), after puberty E30.0
Immersion T75.1 ☑
foot T69.02- ☑
hand T69.01- ☑
Immobile, immobility
complete, due to severe physical disability or frailty
R53.2
intestine K59.89
syndrome (paraplegic) M62.3
Immune reconstitution (inflammatory) syndrome [IRIS]
D89.3
Immunization — *see also* Vaccination
ABO — *see* Incompatibility, ABO
in newborn P55.1
appropriate for age
child (over 28 days old) Z00.129
with abnormal findings Z00.121
complication — *see* Complications, vaccination
encounter for Z23
not done (not carried out) — *see also* Underimmunization status Z28.9

Immunization — *continued*
not done — *see also* Underimmunization status — *continued*
because (of)
acute illness of patient Z28.Ø1
allergy to vaccine (or component) Z28.Ø4
caregiver refusal Z28.82
chronic illness of patient Z28.Ø2
contraindication NEC Z28.Ø9
delay in delivery of vaccine Z28.83
group pressure Z28.1
guardian refusal Z28.82
immune compromised state of patient Z28.Ø3
lack of availability of vaccine Z28.83
manufacturer delay of vaccine Z28.83
parent refusal Z28.82
patient had disease being vaccinated against Z28.81
patient refusal Z28.21
patient's belief Z28.1
religious beliefs of patient Z28.1
specified reason NEC Z28.89
of patient Z28.29
unavailability of vaccine Z28.83
unspecified patient reason Z28.2Ø
partial — *see also* Underimmunization status
for COVID-19 Z28.311
Rh factor
affecting management of pregnancy NEC O36.Ø9- ☑
anti-D antibody O36.Ø1- ☑
from transfusion — *see* Complication(s), transfusion, incompatibility reaction, Rh (factor)
Immunocompromised NOS D84.9
Immunocytoma C83.Ø- ☑
Immunodeficiency D84.9
with
adenosine-deaminase deficiency — *see also* Deficiency, adenosine deaminase D81.3Ø
antibody defects D8Ø.9
specified type NEC D8Ø.8
hyperimmunoglobulinemia D8Ø.6
increased immunoglobulin M (IgM) D8Ø.5
major defect D82.9
specified type NEC D82.8
partial albinism D82.8
short-limbed stature D82.2
thrombocytopenia and eczema D82.Ø
antibody with
hyperimmunoglobulinemia D8Ø.6
near-normal immunoglobulins D8Ø.6
autosomal recessive, Swiss type D8Ø.Ø
combined D81.9
biotin-dependent carboxylase D81.819
biotinidase D81.81Ø
holocarboxylase synthetase D81.818
specified type NEC D81.818
severe (SCID) D81.9
with
low or normal B-cell numbers D81.2
low T- and B-cell numbers D81.1
reticular dysgenesis D81.Ø
specified type NEC D81.89
common variable D83.9
with
abnormalities of B-cell numbers and function D83.Ø
autoantibodies to B- or T-cells D83.2
immunoregulatory T-cell disorders D83.1
specified type NEC D83.8
due to
conditions classified elsewhere D84.81
drugs D84.821
external causes D84.822
medication (current or past) D84.821
following hereditary defective response to Epstein-Barr virus (EBV) D82.3
selective, immunoglobulin
A (IgA) D8Ø.2
G (IgG) (subclasses) D8Ø.3
M (IgM) D8Ø.4
severe combined (SCID) D81.9
due to adenosine deaminase deficiency D81.31
specified type NEC D84.89
X-linked, with increased IgM D8Ø.5
Immunodeficient NOS D84.9
Immunosuppressed NOS D84.9
Immunotherapy (encounter for)
antineoplastic Z51.12

Impaction, impacted
bowel, colon, rectum — *see also* Impaction, fecal K56.49
by gallstone K56.3
calculus — *see* Calculus
cerumen (ear) (external) H61.2- ☑
cuspid — *see* Impaction, tooth
dental (same or adjacent tooth) KØ1.1
fecal, feces K56.41
fracture — *see* Fracture, by site
gallbladder — *see* Calculus, gallbladder
gallstone(s) — *see* Calculus, gallbladder
bile duct (common) (hepatic) — *see* Calculus, bile duct
cystic duct — *see* Calculus, gallbladder
in intestine, with obstruction (any part) K56.3
intestine (calculous) NEC — *see also* Impaction, fecal K56.49
gallstone, with ileus K56.3
intrauterine device (IUD) T83.39 ☑
molar — *see* Impaction, tooth
shoulder, causing obstructed labor O66.Ø
tooth, teeth KØ1.1
turbinate J34.89
Impaired, impairment (function)
auditory discrimination — *see* Abnormal, auditory perception
cognitive, mild, of uncertain or unknown etiology G31.84
dual sensory Z73.82
fasting glucose R73.Ø1
glucose tolerance (oral) R73.Ø2
hearing — *see* Deafness
heart — *see* Disease, heart
kidney N28.9
disorder resulting from N25.9
specified NEC N25.89
liver K72.9Ø
with coma K72.91
mastication KØ8.89
mild cognitive G31.84
of uncertain or unknown etiology G31.84
mild neurocognitive
due to known physiological condition (without behavioral disturbance) FØ6.7Ø
with behavioral disturbance FØ6.71
mobility
ear ossicles — *see* Ankylosis, ear ossicles
requiring care provider Z74.Ø9
myocardium, myocardial — *see* Insufficiency, myocardial
rectal sphincter R19.8
renal (acute) (chronic) N28.9
disorder resulting from N25.9
specified NEC N25.89
vision NEC H54.7
both eyes H54.3
Impediment, speech — *see also* Disorder, speech R47.9
psychogenic (childhood) F98.8
slurring R47.81
specified NEC R47.89
Impending
coronary syndrome I2Ø.Ø
delirium tremens F1Ø.239
myocardial infarction I2Ø.Ø
Imperception auditory (acquired) — *see also* Deafness
congenital H93.25
Imperfect
aeration, lung (newborn) NEC — *see* Atelectasis
closure (congenital)
alimentary tract NEC Q45.8
lower Q43.8
upper Q4Ø.8
atrioventricular ostium Q21.2Ø
atrium (secundum) Q21.11
branchial cleft NOS Q18.2
cyst Q18.Ø
fistula Q18.Ø
sinus Q18.Ø
choroid Q14.3
cricoid cartilage Q31.8
cusps, heart valve NEC Q24.8
pulmonary Q22.3
ductus
arteriosus Q25.Ø
Botalli Q25.Ø
ear drum (causing impairment of hearing) Q16.4

Imperfect — *continued*
closure — *continued*
esophagus with communication to bronchus or trachea Q39.1
eyelid Q1Ø.3
foramen
botalli Q21.12
ovale Q21.12
genitalia, genital organ(s) or system
female Q52.8
external Q52.79
internal NEC Q52.8
male Q55.8
glottis Q31.8
interatrial ostium or septum Q21.19
interauricular ostium or septum Q21.19
interventricular ostium or septum Q21.Ø
larynx Q31.8
lip — *see* Cleft, lip
nasal septum Q3Ø.3
nose Q3Ø.2
omphalomesenteric duct Q43.Ø
optic nerve entry Q14.2
organ or site not listed — *see* Anomaly, by site
ostium
interatrial Q21.19
interauricular Q21.19
interventricular Q21.Ø
palate — *see* Cleft, palate
preauricular sinus Q18.1
retina Q14.1
roof of orbit Q75.8
sclera Q13.5
septum
aorticopulmonary Q21.4
atrial (secundum) Q21.19
between aorta and pulmonary artery Q21.4
heart Q21.9
interatrial (secundum) Q21.19
interauricular (secundum) Q21.19
interventricular Q21.Ø
in tetralogy of Fallot Q21.3
nasal Q3Ø.3
ventricular Q21.Ø
with pulmonary stenosis or atresia, dextraposition of aorta, and hypertrophy of right ventricle Q21.3
in tetralogy of Fallot Q21.3
skull Q75.Ø
with
anencephaly QØØ.Ø
encephalocele — *see* Encephalocele
hydrocephalus QØ3.9
with spina bifida — *see* Spina bifida, by site, with hydrocephalus
microcephaly QØ2
spine (with meningocele) — *see* Spina bifida
trachea Q32.1
tympanic membrane (causing impairment of hearing) Q16.4
uterus Q51.818
vitelline duct Q43.Ø
erection — *see* Dysfunction, sexual, male, erectile
fusion — *see* Imperfect, closure
inflation, lung (newborn) — *see* Atelectasis
posture R29.3
rotation, intestine Q43.3
septum, ventricular Q21.Ø
Imperfectly descended testis — *see* Cryptorchid
Imperforate (congenital) — *see also* Atresia
anus Q42.3
with fistula Q42.2
cervix (uteri) Q51.828
esophagus Q39.Ø
with tracheoesophageal fistula Q39.1
hymen Q52.3
jejunum Q41.1
pharynx Q38.8
rectum Q42.1
with fistula Q42.Ø
urethra Q64.39
vagina Q52.4
Impervious (congenital) — *see also* Atresia
anus Q42.3
with fistula Q42.2
bile duct Q44.2
esophagus Q39.Ø
with tracheoesophageal fistula Q39.1

Impervious — continued
- intestine (small) Q41.9
  - large Q42.9
    - specified NEC Q42.8
  - rectum Q42.1
    - with fistula Q42.0
  - ureter — see Atresia, ureter
  - urethra Q64.39

Impetiginization of dermatoses L01.1

Impetigo (any organism) (any site) (circinate) (contagiosa) (simplex) (vulgaris) L01.00
- Bockhart's L01.02
- bullous, bullosa L01.03
- external ear L01.00 [H62.40]
- follicularis L01.02
- furfuracea L30.5
- herpetiformis L40.1
  - nonobstetrical L40.1
- neonatorum L01.03
- nonbullous L01.01
- specified type NEC L01.09
- ulcerative L01.09

Impingement (on teeth)
- joint — see Disorder, joint, specified type NEC
- soft tissue
  - anterior M26.81
  - posterior M26.82

Implant, endometrial N80.9

Implantation
- anomalous — see Anomaly, by site
  - ureter Q62.63
- cyst
  - external area or site (skin) NEC L72.0
  - iris — see Cyst, iris, implantation
  - vagina N89.8
  - vulva N90.7
- dermoid (cyst) — see Implantation, cyst

Impotence (sexual) N52.9
- counseling Z70.1
- organic origin — see also Dysfunction, sexual, male, erectile N52.9
- psychogenic F52.21

Impression, basilar Q75.8

Imprisonment, anxiety concerning Z65.1

Improper care (child) (newborn) — see Maltreatment

Improperly tied umbilical cord (causing hemorrhage) P51.8

Impulsiveness (impulsive) R45.87

Inability to swallow — see Aphagia
- comply with dietary regimen Z91.118
- swallow — see Aphagia

Inaccessible, inaccessibility
- health care NEC Z75.3
  - due to
    - waiting period Z75.2
      - for admission to facility elsewhere Z75.1
  - other helping agencies Z75.4
  - transportation Z59.82

Inactive — see condition

Inadequate, inadequacy
- aesthetics of dental restoration K08.56
- biologic, constitutional, functional, or social F60.7
- development
  - child R62.50
  - genitalia
    - after puberty NEC E30.0
    - congenital
      - female Q52.8
        - external Q52.79
        - internal Q52.8
      - male Q55.8
  - lungs Q33.6
    - associated with short gestation P28.0
  - organ or site not listed — see Anomaly, by site
- diet (causing nutritional deficiency) E63.9
- drinking-water supply Z58.6
- eating habits Z72.4
- environment, household Z59.1
- family support Z63.8
- food (supply) NEC Z59.48
  - hunger effects T73.0 ☑
- functional F60.7
- household care, due to
  - family member
    - handicapped or ill Z74.2
    - on vacation Z75.5
    - temporarily away from home Z74.2
  - technical defects in home Z59.1

Inadequate, inadequacy — continued
- household care, due to — continued
  - temporary absence from home of person rendering care Z74.2
- housing (heating) (space) Z59.1
- income (financial) Z59.6
- intrafamilial communication Z63.8
- material resources Z59.87
- mental — see Disability, intellectual
- parental supervision or control of child Z62.0
- personality F60.7
- pulmonary
  - function R06.89
    - newborn P28.5
  - ventilation, newborn P28.5
- sample of cytologic smear
  - anus R85.615
  - cervix R87.615
  - vagina R87.625
- social F60.7
  - insurance Z59.7
  - skills NEC Z73.4
- supervision of child by parent Z62.0
- teaching affecting education Z55.8
- transportation Z59.82
- welfare support Z59.7

Inanition R64
- with edema — see Malnutrition, severe
- due to
  - deprivation of food T73.0 ☑
  - malnutrition — see Malnutrition
- fever R50.9

Inappropriate
- change in quantitative human chorionic gonadotropin (hCG) in early pregnancy O02.81
- diet or eating habits Z72.4
- level of quantitative human chorionic gonadotropin (hCG) for gestational age in early pregnancy O02.81
- secretion
  - antidiuretic hormone (ADH) (excessive) E22.2
    - deficiency E23.2
  - pituitary (posterior) E22.2

Inattention at or after birth — see Neglect

Incarceration, incarcerated
- enterocele K46.0
  - gangrenous K46.1
- epiplocele K46.0
  - gangrenous K46.1
- exomphalos K42.0
  - gangrenous K42.1
- hernia — see also Hernia, by site, with obstruction
  - with gangrene — see Hernia, by site, with gangrene
- iris, in wound — see Injury, eye, laceration, with prolapse
- lens, in wound — see Injury, eye, laceration, with prolapse
- omphalocele K42.0
- prison, anxiety concerning Z65.1
- rupture — see Hernia, by site
- sarcoepiplocele K46.0
  - gangrenous K46.1
- sarcoepiplomphalocele K42.0
  - with gangrene K42.1
- uterus N85.8
  - gravid O34.51- ☑
    - causing obstructed labor O65.5

Incised wound
- external — see Laceration
- internal organs — see Injury, by site

Incision, incisional
- hernia K43.2
  - with
    - gangrene (and obstruction) K43.1
    - obstruction K43.0
  - surgical, complication — see Complications, surgical procedure
- traumatic
  - external — see Laceration
  - internal organs — see Injury, by site

Inclusion
- azurophilic leukocytic D72.0
- blennorrhea (neonatal) (newborn) P39.1
- gallbladder in liver (congenital) Q44.1

Incompatibility
- ABO
  - affecting management of pregnancy O36.11- ☑
    - anti-A sensitization O36.11- ☑

Incompatibility — continued
- ABO — continued
  - affecting management of pregnancy — continued
    - anti-B sensitization O36.19- ☑
    - specified NEC O36.19- ☑
  - infusion or transfusion reaction — see Complication(s), transfusion, incompatibility reaction, ABO
  - newborn P55.1
- blood (group) (Duffy) (K) (Kell) (Kidd) (Lewis) (M) (S) NEC
  - affecting management of pregnancy O36.11- ☑
    - anti-A sensitization O36.11- ☑
    - anti-B sensitization O36.19- ☑
  - infusion or transfusion reaction T80.89 ☑
  - newborn P55.8
- divorce or estrangement Z63.5
- Rh (blood group) (factor) Z31.82
  - affecting management of pregnancy NEC O36.09- ☑
    - anti-D antibody O36.01- ☑
  - infusion or transfusion reaction — see Complication(s), transfusion, incompatibility reaction, Rh (factor)
  - newborn P55.0
- rhesus — see Incompatibility, Rh

Incompetency, incompetent, incompetence
- annular
  - aortic (valve) — see Insufficiency, aortic
  - mitral (valve) I34.0
  - pulmonary valve (heart) I37.1
- aortic (valve) — see Insufficiency, aortic
- cardiac valve — see Endocarditis
- cervix, cervical (os) N88.3
  - in pregnancy O34.3- ☑
- chronotropic I45.89
  - with
    - autonomic dysfunction G90.8
    - ischemic heart disease I25.89
    - left ventricular dysfunction I51.89
    - sinus node dysfunction I49.8
- esophagogastric (junction) (sphincter) K22.0
- mitral (valve) — see Insufficiency, mitral
- pelvic fundus N81.89
- pubocervical tissue N81.82
- pulmonary valve (heart) I37.1
  - congenital Q22.3
- rectovaginal tissue N81.83
- tricuspid (annular) (valve) — see Insufficiency, tricuspid
- valvular — see Endocarditis
  - congenital Q24.8
- vein, venous (saphenous) (varicose) — see Varix, leg

Incomplete — see also condition
- atrioventricular
  - canal Q21.21
  - septal defect Q21.21
- bladder, emptying R33.9
- defecation R15.0
- endocardial cushion defect Q21.21
- expansion lungs (newborn) NEC — see Atelectasis
- rotation, intestine Q43.3

Inconclusive
- diagnostic imaging due to excess body fat of patient R93.9
- findings on diagnostic imaging of breast NEC R92.8
- mammogram (due to dense breasts) R92.2

Incontinence R32
- anal sphincter R15.9
- coital N39.491
- feces R15.9
  - nonorganic origin F98.1
- insensible (urinary) N39.42
- overflow N39.490
- postural (urinary) N39.492
- psychogenic F45.8
- rectal R15.9
- reflex N39.498
- stress (female) (male) N39.3
  - and urge N39.46
- urethral sphincter R32
- urge N39.41
  - and stress (female) (male) N39.46
- urine (urinary) R32
  - continuous N39.45
  - due to cognitive impairment, or severe physical disability or immobility R39.81
  - functional R39.81
  - insensible N39.42

Incontinence — continued
urine — continued
mixed (stress and urge) N39.46
nocturnal N39.44
nonorganic origin F98.0
overflow N39.490
post dribbling N39.43
postural N39.492
reflex N39.498
specified NEC N39.498
stress (female) (male) N39.3
and urge N39.46
total N39.498
unaware N39.42
urge N39.41
and stress (female) (male) N39.46

Incontinentia pigmenti Q82.3

Incoordinate, incoordination
esophageal-pharyngeal (newborn) — see Dysphagia
muscular R27.8
uterus (action) (contractions) (complicating delivery) O62.4

Increase, increased
abnormal, in development R63.8
androgens (ovarian) E28.1
anticoagulants (antithrombin) (anti-VIIIa) (anti-IXa) (anti-Xa) (anti-XIa) — see Circulating anticoagulants
cold sense R20.8
estrogen E28.0
function
adrenal
cortex — see Cushing's, syndrome
medulla E27.5
pituitary (gland) (anterior) (lobe) E22.9
posterior E22.2
heat sense R20.8
intracranial pressure (benign) G93.2
permeability, capillaries I78.8
pressure, intracranial G93.2
secretion
gastrin E16.4
glucagon E16.3
pancreas, endocrine E16.9
growth hormone-releasing hormone E16.8
pancreatic polypeptide E16.8
somatostatin E16.8
vasoactive-intestinal polypeptide E16.8
sphericity, lens Q12.4
splenic activity D73.1
venous pressure I87.8
portal K76.6

Increta placenta O43.22- ☑

Incrustation, cornea, foreign body (lead)(zinc) — see Foreign body, cornea

Incyclophoria H50.54

Incyclotropia — see Cyclotropia

Indeterminate sex Q56.4

India rubber skin Q82.8

Indigestion (acid) (bilious) (functional) K30
catarrhal K31.89
due to decomposed food NOS A05.9
nervous F45.8
psychogenic F45.8

Indirect — see condition

Induratio penis plastica N48.6

Induration, indurated
brain G93.89
breast (fibrous) N64.51
puerperal, postpartum O92.29
broad ligament N83.8
chancre
anus A51.1
congenital A50.07
extragenital NEC A51.2
corpora cavernosa (penis) (plastic) N48.6
liver (chronic) K76.89
lung (black) (chronic) (fibroid) — see also Fibrosis, lung J84.10
essential brown J84.03
penile (plastic) N48.6
phlebitic — see Phlebitis
skin R23.4

Inebriety (without dependence) — see Alcohol, intoxication

Inefficiency, kidney N28.9

Inelasticity, skin R23.4

Inequality, leg (length) (acquired) — see also Deformity, limb, unequal length
congenital — see Defect, reduction, lower limb
lower leg — see Deformity, limb, unequal length

Inertia
bladder (neurogenic) N31.2
stomach K31.89
psychogenic F45.8
uterus, uterine during labor O62.2
during latent phase of labor O62.0
primary O62.0
secondary O62.1
vesical (neurogenic) N31.2

Infancy, infantile, infantilism — see also condition
celiac K90.0
genitalia, genitals (after puberty) E30.0
Herter's (nontropical sprue) K90.0
intestinal K90.0
Lorain E23.0
pancreatic K86.89
pelvis M95.5
with disproportion (fetopelvic) O33.1
causing obstructed labor O65.1
pituitary E23.0
renal N25.0
uterus — see Infantile, genitalia

Infant(s) — see also Infancy
excessive crying R68.11
irritable child R68.12
lack of care — see Neglect
liveborn (singleton) Z38.2
born in hospital Z38.00
by cesarean Z38.01
born outside hospital Z38.1
multiple NEC Z38.8
born in hospital Z38.68
by cesarean Z38.69
born outside hospital Z38.7
quadruplet Z38.8
born in hospital Z38.63
by cesarean Z38.64
born outside hospital Z38.7
quintuplet Z38.8
born in hospital Z38.65
by cesarean Z38.66
born outside hospital Z38.7
triplet Z38.8
born in hospital Z38.61
by cesarean Z38.62
born outside hospital Z38.7
twin Z38.5
born in hospital Z38.30
by cesarean Z38.31
born outside hospital Z38.4
of diabetic mother (syndrome of) P70.1
gestational diabetes P70.0

Infantile — see also condition
genitalia, genitals E30.0
os, uterine E30.0
penis E30.0
testis E29.1
uterus E30.0

Infantilism — see Infancy

Infarct, infarction
adrenal (capsule) (gland) E27.49
appendices epiploicae — see also Infarct, intestine K55.069
bowel — see also Infarct, intestine K55.069
brain (stem) — see Infarct, cerebral
breast N64.89
brewer's (kidney) N28.0
cardiac — see Infarct, myocardium
cerebellar — see Infarct, cerebral
cerebral (acute) (chronic) — see also Occlusion, artery cerebral or precerebral, with infarction I63.9-
aborted I63.9
cortical I63.9
due to
cerebral venous thrombosis, nonpyogenic I63.6
embolism
cerebral arteries I63.4- ☑
precerebral arteries I63.1- ☑
occlusion NEC
cerebral arteries I63.5- ☑
precerebral arteries I63.2- ☑
small artery I63.81
stenosis NEC
cerebral arteries I63.5- ☑

Infarct, infarction — continued
cerebral — see also Occlusion, artery cerebral or precerebral, with infarction — continued
due to — continued
stenosis — continued
precerebral arteries I63.2- ☑
small artery I63.81
thrombosis
cerebral artery I63.3- ☑
precerebral artery I63.0- ☑
intraoperative
during cardiac surgery I97.810
during other surgery I97.811
neonatal P91.82- ☑
perinatal (arterial ischemic) P91.82- ☑
postprocedural
following cardiac surgery I97.820
following other surgery I97.821
specified NEC I63.89
colon (acute) (agnogenic) (embolic) (hemorrhagic) (nonocclusive) (nonthrombotic) (occlusive) (segmental) (thrombotic) (with gangrene) — see also Infarct, intestine K55.049
coronary artery — see Infarct, myocardium
embolic — see Embolism
fallopian tube N83.8
gallbladder K82.8
heart — see Infarct, myocardium
hepatic K76.3
hypophysis (anterior lobe) E23.6
impending (myocardium) I20.0
intestine (acute) (agnogenic) (embolic) (hemorrhagic) (nonocclusive) (nonthrombotic) (occlusive) (thrombotic) (with gangrene) K55.069
diffuse K55.062
focal K55.061
large K55.049
diffuse K55.042
focal K55.041
small K55.029
diffuse K55.022
focal K55.021
kidney N28.0
lacunar I63.81
liver K76.3
lung (embolic) (thrombotic) — see Embolism, pulmonary
lymph node I89.8
mesentery, mesenteric (embolic) (thrombotic) (with gangrene) — see also Infarct, intestine K55.069
muscle (ischemic) M62.20
ankle M62.27- ☑
foot M62.27- ☑
forearm M62.23- ☑
hand M62.24- ☑
lower leg M62.26- ☑
pelvic region M62.25- ☑
shoulder region M62.21- ☑
specified site NEC M62.28
thigh M62.25- ☑
upper arm M62.22- ☑
myocardium, myocardial (acute) (with stated duration of 4 weeks or less) I21.9
associated with revascularization procedure I21.A9
diagnosed on ECG, but presenting no symptoms I25.2
due to
demand ischemia I21.A1
ischemic imbalance I21.A1
healed or old I25.2
intraoperative — see also Infarct, myocardium, associated with revascularization procedure
during cardiac surgery I97.790
during other surgery I97.791
non-Q wave I21.4
non-ST elevation (NSTEMI) I21.4
subsequent I22.2
nontransmural I21.4
past (diagnosed on ECG or other investigation, but currently presenting no symptoms) I25.2
postprocedural — see also Infarct, myocardium, associated with revascularization procedure
following cardiac surgery — see also Infarct, myocardium, type 4 or type 5 I97.190
following other surgery I97.191
Q wave (see also Infarct, myocardium, by site) I21.3
secondary to
demand ischemia I21.A1

Infarct, infarction — continued
myocardium, myocardial — continued
  secondary to — continued
    ischemic imbalance I21.A1
  ST elevation (STEMI) I21.3
    anterior (anteroapical) (anterolateral) (anteroseptal) (Q wave) (wall) I21.09
      subsequent I22.0
    inferior (diaphragmatic) (inferolateral) (inferoposterior) (wall) NEC I21.19
      subsequent I22.1
    inferoposterior transmural (Q wave) I21.11
    involving
      coronary artery of anterior wall NEC I21.09
      coronary artery of inferior wall NEC I21.19
      diagonal coronary artery I21.02
      left anterior descending coronary artery I21.02
      left circumflex coronary artery I21.21
      left main coronary artery I21.01
      oblique marginal coronary artery I21.21
      right coronary artery I21.11
    lateral (apical-lateral) (basal-lateral) (high) I21.29
      subsequent I22.8
    posterior (posterobasal) (posterolateral) (posteroseptal) (true) I21.29
      subsequent I22.8
    septal I21.29
      subsequent I22.8
    specified NEC I21.29
      subsequent I22.8
  subsequent I22.9
  subsequent (recurrent) (reinfarction) I22.9
    anterior (anteroapical) (anterolateral) (anteroseptal) (wall) I22.0
    diaphragmatic (wall) I22.1
    inferior (diaphragmatic) (inferolateral) (inferoposterior) (wall) I22.1
    lateral (apical-lateral) (basal-lateral) (high) I22.8
    non-ST elevation (NSTEMI) I22.2
    posterior (posterobasal) (posterolateral) (posteroseptal) (true) I22.8
    septal I22.8
    specified NEC I22.8
    ST elevation I22.9
      anterior (anteroapical) (anterolateral) (anteroseptal) (wall) I22.0
      inferior (diaphragmatic) (inferolateral) (inferoposterior) (wall) I22.1
      specified NEC I22.8
    subendocardial I22.2
    transmural I22.9
      anterior (anteroapical) (anterolateral) (anteroseptal) (wall) I22.0
      diaphragmatic (wall) I22.1
      inferior (diaphragmatic) (inferolateral) (inferoposterior) (wall) I22.1
      lateral (apical-lateral) (basal-lateral) (high) I22.8
      posterior (posterobasal) (posterolateral) (posteroseptal) (true) I22.8
      specified NEC I22.8
    type 1 — see also Infarction, myocardial, subsequent, by site, or by ST elevation or non-ST elevation I22.9
    type 2 I21.A1
    type 3 I21.A9
    type 4 I21.A9
    type 5 I21.A9
  syphilitic A52.06
  transmural I21.9
    anterior (anteroapical) (anterolateral) (anteroseptal) (Q wave) (wall) NEC I21.09
    inferior (diaphragmatic) (inferolateral) (inferoposterior) (Q wave) (wall) NEC I21.19
    inferoposterior (Q wave) I21.11
    lateral (apical-lateral) (basal-lateral) (high) NEC I21.29
    posterior (posterobasal) (posterolateral) (posteroseptal) (true) NEC I21.29
    septal NEC I21.29
    specified NEC I21.29
    type 1 — see also Infarction, myocardial, by site, or by ST elevation or non-ST elevation I21.9
    type 2 I21.A1
    type 3 I21.A9
    type 4 (a) (b) (c) I21.A9
    type 5 I21.A9
nontransmural I21.4
omentum — see also Infarct, intestine K55.069

Infarct, infarction — continued
ovary N83.8
pancreas K86.89
papillary muscle — see Infarct, myocardium
parathyroid gland E21.4
pituitary (gland) E23.6
placenta O43.81- ☑
prostate N42.89
pulmonary (artery) (vein) (hemorrhagic) — see Embolism, pulmonary
renal (embolic) (thrombotic) N28.0
retina, retinal (artery) — see Occlusion, artery, retina
spinal (cord) (acute) (embolic) (nonembolic) G95.11
spleen D73.5
  embolic or thrombotic I74.8
subendocardial (acute) (nontransmural) I21.4
suprarenal (capsule) (gland) E27.49
testis N50.1
thrombotic — see also Thrombosis
  artery, arterial — see Embolism
thyroid (gland) E07.89
ventricle (heart) — see Infarct, myocardium
Infecting — see condition
Infection, infected, infective (opportunistic) B99.9
with
    drug resistant organism — see Resistance (to), drug — see also specific organism
    lymphangitis — see Lymphangitis
    organ dysfunction (acute) R65.20
      with septic shock R65.21
abscess (skin) — code by site under Abscess
Absidia — see Mucormycosis
Acanthamoeba — see Acanthamebiasis
Acanthocheilonema (perstans) (streptocerca) B74.4
accessory sinus (chronic) — see Sinusitis
achorion — see Dermatophytosis
Acremonium falciforme B47.0
acromioclavicular M00.9
Actinobacillus (actinomycetem-comitans) A28.8
  mallei A24.0
  muris A25.1
Actinomadura B47.1
Actinomyces (israelii) — see also Actinomycosis A42.9
Actinomycetales — see Actinomycosis
actinomycotic NOS — see Actinomycosis
adenoid (and tonsil) J03.90
  chronic J35.02
adenovirus NEC
  as cause of disease classified elsewhere B97.0
  unspecified nature or site B34.0
aerogenes capsulatus A48.0
aertrycke — see Infection, salmonella
alimentary canal NOS — see Enteritis, infectious
Allescheria boydii B48.2
Alternaria B48.8
alveolus, alveolar (process) K04.7
Ameba, amebic (histolytica) — see Amebiasis
amniotic fluid, sac or cavity O41.10- ☑
  chorioamnionitis O41.12- ☑
  placentitis O41.14- ☑
amputation stump (surgical) — see Complication, amputation stump, infection
Ancylostoma (duodenalis) B76.0
Anisakiasis, Anisakis larvae B81.0
anthrax — see Anthrax
antrum (chronic) — see Sinusitis, maxillary
anus, anal (papillae) (sphincter) K62.89
arbovirus (arbor virus) A94
  specified type NEC A93.8
artificial insemination N98.0
Ascaris lumbricoides — see Ascariasis
Ascomycetes B47.0
Aspergillus (flavus) (fumigatus) (terreus) — see Aspergillosis
atypical
  acid-fast (bacilli) — see Mycobacterium, atypical
  mycobacteria — see Mycobacterium, atypical
  virus A81.9
    specified type NEC A81.89
auditory meatus (external) — see Otitis, externa, infective
auricle (ear) — see Otitis, externa, infective
axillary gland (lymph) L04.2
Bacillus A49.9
  abortus A23.1
  anthracis — see Anthrax
  Ducrey's (any location) A57
  Flexner's A03.1

Infection, infected, infective — continued
Bacillus — continued
  Friedländer's NEC A49.8
  gas (gangrene) A48.0
  mallei A24.0
  melitensis A23.0
  paratyphoid, paratyphosus A01.4
    A A01.1
    B A01.2
    C A01.3
  Shiga (-Kruse) A03.0
  suipestifer — see Infection, salmonella
  swimming pool A31.1
  typhosa A01.00
  welchii — see Gangrene, gas
bacterial NOS A49.9
  as cause of disease classified elsewhere B96.89
    Bacteroides fragilis [B. fragilis] B96.6
    Clostridium perfringens [C. perfringens] B96.7
    Enterobacter sakazakii B96.89
    Enterococcus B95.2
    Escherichia coli [E. coli] — see also Escherichia coli B96.20
    Helicobacter pylori [H.pylori] B96.81
    Hemophilus influenzae [H. influenzae] B96.3
    Klebsiella pneumoniae [K. pneumoniae] B96.1
    Mycoplasma pneumoniae [M. pneumoniae] B96.0
    Proteus (mirabilis) (morganii) B96.4
    Pseudomonas (aeruginosa) (mallei) (pseudomallei) B96.5
    Staphylococcus B95.8
      aureus (methicillin susceptible) (MSSA) B95.61
        methicillin resistant (MRSA) B95.62
      specified NEC B95.7
    Streptococcus B95.5
      group A B95.0
      group B B95.1
      pneumoniae B95.3
      specified NEC B95.4
    Vibrio vulnificus B96.82
  specified NEC A48.8
Bacterium
  paratyphosum A01.4
    A A01.1
    B A01.2
    C A01.3
  typhosum A01.00
Bacteroides NEC A49.8
  fragilis, as cause of disease classified elsewhere B96.6
Balantidium coli A07.0
Bartholin's gland N75.8
Basidiobolus B46.8
bile duct (common) (hepatic) — see Cholangitis
bladder — see Cystitis
Blastomyces, blastomycotic — see also Blastomycosis
  brasiliensis — see Paracoccidioidomycosis
  dermatitidis — see Blastomycosis
  European — see Cryptococcosis
  Loboi B48.0
  North American B40.9
  South American — see Paracoccidioidomycosis
bleb, postprocedure — see Blebitis
bone — see Osteomyelitis
Bordetella — see Whooping cough
Borrelia bergdorfi A69.20
brain — see also Encephalitis G04.90
  membranes — see Meningitis
  septic G06.0
    meninges — see Meningitis, bacterial
branchial cyst Q18.0
breast — see Mastitis
bronchus — see Bronchitis
Brucella A23.9
  abortus A23.1
  canis A23.3
  melitensis A23.0
  mixed A23.8
  specified NEC A23.8
  suis A23.2
Brugia (malayi) B74.1
  timori B74.2
bursa — see Bursitis, infective
buttocks (skin) L08.9
Campylobacter, intestinal A04.5
  as cause of disease classified elsewhere B96.81
Candida (albicans) (tropicalis) — see Candidiasis

☑ Additional Character Required — Refer to the Tabular List for Character Selection

Infection, infected, infective — *continued*
candiru B88.8
Capillaria (intestinal) B81.1
   hepatica B83.8
   philippinensis B81.1
cartilage — *see* Disorder, cartilage, specified type NEC
cat liver fluke B66.0
catheter-related bloodstream (CRBSI) T80.211 ☑
cellulitis — *code by* site under Cellulitis
central line-associated T80.219 ☑
   bloodstream (CLABSI) T80.211 ☑
   specified NEC T80.218 ☑
Cephalosporium falciforme B47.0
cerebrospinal — *see* Meningitis
cervical gland (lymph) L04.0
cervix — *see* Cervicitis
cesarean delivery wound (puerperal) O86.00
cestodes — *see* Infestation, cestodes
chest J22
Chilomastix (intestinal) A07.8
Chlamydia, chlamydial A74.9
   anus A56.3
   genitourinary tract A56.2
      lower A56.00
      specified NEC A56.19
   lymphogranuloma A55
   pharynx A56.4
   psittaci A70
   rectum A56.3
   sexually transmitted NEC A56.8
cholera — *see* Cholera
Cladosporium
   bantianum (brain abscess) B43.1
   carrionii B43.0
   castellanii B36.1
   trichoides (brain abscess) B43.1
   werneckii B36.1
Clonorchis (sinensis) (liver) B66.1
Clostridium NEC
   bifermentans A48.0
   botulinum (food poisoning) A05.1
      infant A48.51
      wound A48.52
   difficile
      as cause of disease classified elsewhere B96.89
      foodborne (disease)
         not specified as recurrent A04.72
         recurrent A04.71
      gas gangrene A48.0
      necrotizing enterocolitis
         not specified as recurrent A04.72
         recurrent A04.71
      sepsis A41.4
   gas-forming NEC A48.0
   histolyticum A48.0
   novyi, causing gas gangrene A48.0
   oedematiens A48.0
   perfringens
      as cause of disease classified elsewhere B96.7
      due to food A05.2
      foodborne (disease) A05.2
      gas gangrene A48.0
      sepsis A41.4
   septicum, causing gas gangrene A48.0
   sordellii, causing gas gangrene A48.0
   welchii
      as cause of disease classified elsewhere B96.7
      foodborne (disease) A05.2
      gas gangrene A48.0
      necrotizing enteritis A05.2
      sepsis A41.4
Coccidioides (immitis) — *see* Coccidioidomycosis
colon — *see* Enteritis, infectious
colostomy K94.02
common duct — *see* Cholangitis
congenital P39.9
   Candida (albicans) P37.5
   cytomegalovirus P35.1
   hepatitis, viral P35.3
   herpes simplex P35.2
   infectious or parasitic disease P37.9
      specified NEC P37.8
   listeriosis (disseminated) P37.2
   malaria NEC P37.4
      falciparum P37.3
   Plasmodium falciparum P37.3
   poliomyelitis P35.8
   rubella P35.0

Infection, infected, infective — *continued*
congenital — *continued*
   skin P39.4
   toxoplasmosis (acute) (subacute) (chronic) P37.1
   tuberculosis P37.0
   urinary (tract) P39.3
   vaccinia P35.8
   virus P35.9
      specified type NEC P35.8
Conidiobolus B46.8
coronavirus-2019 U07.1
coronavirus NEC B34.2
   as cause of disease classified elsewhere B97.29
   severe acute respiratory syndrome (SARS associated) B97.21
corpus luteum — *see* Salpingo-oophoritis
Corynebacterium diphtheriae — *see* Diphtheria
cotia virus B08.8
COVID-19 — *see also* COVID-19 U07.1
Coxiella burnetii A78
coxsackie — *see* Coxsackie
Cryptococcus neoformans — *see* Cryptococcosis
Cryptosporidium A07.2
Cunninghamella — *see* Mucormycosis
cyst — *see* Cyst
cystic duct — *see also* Cholecystitis K81.9
Cysticercus cellulosae — *see* Cysticercosis
cytomegalovirus, cytomegaloviral B25.9
   congenital P35.1
   maternal, maternal care for (suspected) damage to fetus O35.3 ☑
   mononucleosis B27.10
      with
         complication NEC B27.19
         meningitis B27.12
         polyneuropathy B27.11
delta-agent (acute), in hepatitis B carrier B17.0
dental (pulpal origin) K04.7
Deuteromycetes B47.0
Dicrocoelium dendriticum B66.2
Dipetalonema (perstans) (streptocerca) B74.4
diphtherial — *see* Diphtheria
Diphyllobothrium (adult) (latum) (pacificum) B70.0
   larval B70.1
Diplogonoporus (grandis) B71.8
Dipylidium caninum B67.4
Dirofilaria B74.8
Dracunculus medinensis B72
Drechslera (hawaiiensis) B43.8
Ducrey Haemophilus (any location) A57
due to or resulting from
   artificial insemination N98.0
   Babesia
      divergens (-like) strain B60.03
      duncani (-type) species B60.02
      microti B60.01
      species
         specified NEC B60.09
   central venous catheter T80.219 ☑
      bloodstream T80.211 ☑
      exit or insertion site T80.212 ☑
      localized T80.212 ☑
      port or reservoir T80.212 ☑
      specified NEC T80.218 ☑
      tunnel T80.212 ☑
   device, implant or graft — *see also* Complications, by site and type, infection or inflammation T85.79 ☑
      arterial graft NEC T82.7 ☑
      breast (implant) T85.79 ☑
      catheter NEC T85.79 ☑
         dialysis (renal) T82.7 ☑
            central line T80.211 ☑
            intraperitoneal T85.71 ☑
         infusion NEC T82.7 ☑
            cranial T85.735 ☑
            intrathecal T85.735 ☑
            spinal (epidural) (subdural) T85.735 ☑
            subarachnoid T85.735 ☑
         urinary T83.518 ☑
            cystostomy T83.510 ☑
            Hopkins T83.518 ☑
            ileostomy T83.518 ☑
            nephrostomy T83.512 ☑
            specified NEC T83.518 ☑
            urethral indwelling T83.511 ☑
            urostomy T83.518 ☑

Infection, infected, infective — *continued*
due to or resulting from — *continued*
   device, implant or graft — *see also* Complications, by site and type, infection or inflammation — *continued*
      electronic (electrode) (pulse generator) (stimulator)
         bone T84.7 ☑
         cardiac T82.7 ☑
         nervous system T85.738 ☑
            brain T85.731 ☑
            cranial nerve T85.732 ☑
            gastric nerve T85.732 ☑
            generator pocket T85.734 ☑
            neurostimulator generator T85.734 ☑
            peripheral nerve T85.732 ☑
            sacral nerve T85.732 ☑
            spinal cord T85.733 ☑
            vagal nerve T85.732 ☑
         urinary (indwelling) T83.51 ☑
      fixation, internal (orthopedic) NEC — *see* Complication, fixation device, infection
      gastrointestinal (bile duct) (esophagus) T85.79 ☑
      neurostimulator electrode (lead) T85.732 ☑
      genital NEC T83.69 ☑
      heart NEC T82.7 ☑
         valve (prosthesis) T82.6 ☑
            graft T82.7 ☑
      joint prosthesis — *see* Complication, joint prosthesis, infection
      ocular (corneal graft) (orbital implant) NEC T85.79 ☑
      orthopedic NEC T84.7 ☑
      penile (cylinder) (pump) (resevoir) T83.61 ☑
      specified NEC T85.79 ☑
      testicular T83.62 ☑
      urinary NEC T83.598 ☑
         ileal conduit stent T83.593 ☑
         implanted neurostimulation T83.590 ☑
         implanted sphincter T83.591 ☑
         indwelling ureteral stent T83.592 ☑
         nephroureteral stent T83.593 ☑
         specified stent NEC T83.593 ☑
      vascular NEC T82.7 ☑
      ventricular intracranial (communicating) shunt T85.730 ☑
   Hickman catheter T80.219 ☑
      bloodstream T80.211 ☑
      localized T80.212 ☑
      specified NEC T80.218 ☑
   immunization or vaccination T88.0 ☑
   infusion, injection or transfusion NEC T80.29 ☑
   injury NEC — *code by* site under Wound, open
   peripherally inserted central catheter (PICC) T80.219 ☑
      bloodstream T80.211 ☑
      localized T80.212 ☑
      specified NEC T80.218 ☑
   portacath (port-a-cath) T80.219 ☑
      bloodstream T80.211 ☑
      localized T80.212 ☑
      specified NEC T80.218 ☑
   protozoa of the order Piroplasmida NEC B60.09
   pulmonary artery catheter — *see* Infection, due to or resulting from, central venous catheter
   surgery T81.40 ☑
   Swan Ganz catheter — *see* Infection, due to or resulting from, central venous catheter
   triple lumen catheter T80.219 ☑
      bloodstream T80.211 ☑
      localized T80.212 ☑
      specified NEC T80.218 ☑
   umbilical venous catheter T80.219 ☑
      bloodstream T80.211 ☑
      localized T80.212 ☑
      specified NEC T80.218 ☑
during labor NEC O75.3
ear (middle) — *see also* Otitis media
   external — *see* Otitis, externa, infective
   inner — *see* subcategory H83.0 ☑
Eberthella typhosa A01.00
Echinococcus — *see* Echinococcus
echovirus
   as cause of disease classified elsewhere B97.12
   unspecified nature or site B34.1
endocardium I33.0

Infection, infected, infective — *continued*
- endocervix — *see* Cervicitis
- Entamoeba — *see* Amebiasis
- enteric — *see* Enteritis, infectious
- Enterobacter sakazakii B96.89
- Enterobius vermicularis B80
- enterostomy K94.12
- enterovirus B34.1
    - as cause of disease classified elsewhere B97.10
        - coxsackievirus B97.11
        - echovirus B97.12
        - specified NEC B97.19
- Entomophthora B46.8
- Epidermophyton — *see* Dermatophytosis
- epididymis — *see* Epididymitis
- episiotomy (puerperal) O86.09
- Erysipelothrix (insidiosa) (rhusiopathiae) — *see* Erysipeloid
- erythema infectiosum B08.3
- Escherichia (E.) coli NEC A49.8
    - as cause of disease classified elsewhere — *see also* Escherichia coli B96.20
    - congenital P39.8
        - sepsis P36.4
    - generalized A41.51
    - intestinal — *see* Enteritis, infectious, due to, Escherichia coli
- ethmoidal (chronic) (sinus) — *see* Sinusitis, ethmoidal
- eustachian tube (ear) — *see* Salpingitis, eustachian
- external auditory canal (meatus) NEC — *see* Otitis, externa, infective
- eye (purulent) — *see* Endophthalmitis, purulent
- eyelid — *see* Inflammation, eyelid
- fallopian tube — *see* Salpingo-oophoritis
- Fasciola (gigantica) (hepatica) (indica) B66.3
- Fasciolopsis (buski) B66.5
- filarial — *see* Infestation, filarial
- finger (skin) L08.9
    - nail L03.01- ☑
        - fungus B35.1
- fish tapeworm B70.0
    - larval B70.1
- flagellate, intestinal A07.9
- fluke — *see* Infestation, fluke
- focal
    - teeth (pulpal origin) K04.7
    - tonsils J35.01
- Fonsecaea (compactum) (pedrosoi) B43.0
- food — *see* Intoxication, foodborne
- foot (skin) L08.9
    - dermatophytic fungus B35.3
- Francisella tularensis — *see* Tularemia
- frontal (sinus) (chronic) — *see* Sinusitis, frontal
- fungus NOS B49
    - beard B35.0
    - dermatophytic — *see* Dermatophytosis
    - foot B35.3
    - groin B35.6
    - hand B35.2
    - nail B35.1
    - pathogenic to compromised host only B48.8
    - perianal (area) B35.6
    - scalp B35.0
    - skin B36.9
        - foot B35.3
        - hand B35.2
        - toenails B35.1
- Fusarium B48.8
- gallbladder — *see* Cholecystitis
- gas bacillus — *see* Gangrene, gas
- gastrointestinal — *see* Enteritis, infectious
- generalized NEC — *see* Sepsis
- generator pocket, implanted electronic neurostimulator T85.734 ☑
- genital organ or tract
    - female — *see* Disease, pelvis, inflammatory
    - male N49.9
        - multiple sites N49.8
        - specified NEC N49.8
- Ghon tubercle, primary A15.7
- Giardia lamblia A07.1
- gingiva (chronic) K05.10
    - acute K05.00
        - nonplaque induced K05.01
        - plaque induced K05.00
    - nonplaque induced K05.11
    - plaque induced K05.10
- glanders A24.0

Infection, infected, infective — *continued*
- glenosporopsis B48.0
- Gnathostoma (spinigerum) B83.1
- Gongylonema B83.8
- gonococcal — *see* Gonococcus
- gram-negative bacilli NOS A49.9
- guinea worm B72
- gum (chronic) K05.10
    - acute K05.00
        - nonplaque induced K05.01
        - plaque induced K05.00
    - nonplaque induced K05.11
    - plaque induced K05.10
- Haemophilus — *see* Infection, Hemophilus
- heart — *see* Carditis
- Helicobacter pylori A04.8
    - as cause of disease classified elsewhere B96.81
- helminths B83.9
    - intestinal B82.0
        - mixed (types classifiable to more than one of the titles B65.0-B81.3 and B81.8) B81.4
        - specified type NEC B81.8
    - specified type NEC B83.8
- Hemophilus
    - aegyptius, systemic A48.4
    - ducrey (any location) A57
    - generalized A41.3
    - influenzae NEC A49.2
        - as cause of disease classified elsewhere B96.3
- herpes (simplex) — *see also* Herpes
    - congenital P35.2
    - disseminated B00.7
    - zoster B02.9
- herpesvirus, herpesviral — *see* Herpes
- Heterophyes (heterophyes) B66.8
- hip (joint) NEC M00.9
    - due to internal joint prosthesis
        - left T84.52 ☑
        - right T84.51 ☑
    - skin NEC L08.9
- Histoplasma — *see* Histoplasmosis
    - American B39.4
    - capsulatum B39.4
- hookworm B76.9
- human
    - papilloma virus A63.0
    - T-cell lymphotropic virus type-1 (HTLV-1) B33.3
- hydrocele N43.0
- Hymenolepis B71.0
- hypopharynx — *see* Pharyngitis
- inguinal (lymph) glands L04.1
    - due to soft chancre A57
- intervertebral disc, pyogenic M46.30
    - cervical region M46.32
    - cervicothoracic region M46.33
    - lumbar region M46.36
    - lumbosacral region M46.37
    - multiple sites M46.39
    - occipito-atlanto-axial region M46.31
    - sacrococcygeal region M46.38
    - thoracic region M46.34
    - thoracolumbar region M46.35
- intestine, intestinal — *see* Enteritis, infectious
    - specified NEC A08.8
- intra-amniotic affecting newborn NEC P39.2
- intrauterine inflammation O41.12- ☑
- Isospora belli or hominis A07.3
- Japanese B encephalitis A83.0
- jaw (bone) (lower) (upper) M27.2
- joint NEC M00.9
    - due to internal joint prosthesis T84.50 ☑
- kidney (cortex) (hematogenous) N15.9
    - with calculus N20.0
        - with hydronephrosis N13.6
    - following ectopic gestation O08.83
    - pelvis and ureter (cystic) N28.85
    - puerperal (postpartum) O86.21
    - specified NEC N15.8
- Klebsiella (K.) pneumoniae NEC A49.8
    - as cause of disease classified elsewhere B96.1
- knee (joint) NEC M00.9
    - joint M00.9
    - due to internal joint prosthesis
        - left T84.54 ☑
        - right T84.53 ☑
    - skin L08.9
- Koch's — *see* Tuberculosis
- labia (majora) (minora) (acute) — *see* Vulvitis

Infection, infected, infective — *continued*
- lacrimal
    - gland — *see* Dacryoadenitis
    - passages (duct) (sac) — *see* Inflammation, lacrimal, passages
- lancet fluke B66.2
- larynx NEC J38.7
- leg (skin) NOS L08.9
- Legionella pneumophila A48.1
    - nonpneumonic A48.2
- Leishmania — *see also* Leishmaniasis
    - aethiopica B55.1
    - braziliensis B55.2
    - chagasi B55.0
    - donovani B55.0
    - infantum B55.0
    - major B55.1
    - mexicana B55.1
    - tropica B55.1
- lentivirus, as cause of disease classified elsewhere B97.31
- Leptosphaeria senegalensis B47.0
- Leptospira interrogans A27.9
    - autumnalis A27.89
    - canicola A27.89
    - hebdomadis A27.89
    - icterohaemorrhagiae A27.0
    - pomona A27.89
    - specified type NEC A27.89
- leptospirochetal NEC — *see* Leptospirosis
- Listeria monocytogenes — *see also* Listeriosis
    - congenital P37.2
- Loa loa B74.3
    - with conjunctival infestation B74.3
    - eyelid B74.3
- Loboa loboi B48.0
- local, skin (staphylococcal) (streptococcal) L08.9
    - abscess — *code by* site under Abscess
    - cellulitis — *code by* site under Cellulitis
    - specified NEC L08.89
    - ulcer — *see* Ulcer, skin
- Loefflerella mallei A24.0
- lung — *see also* Pneumonia J18.9
    - atypical Mycobacterium A31.0
    - spirochetal A69.8
    - tuberculous — *see* Tuberculosis, pulmonary
    - virus — *see* Pneumonia, viral
- lymph gland — *see also* Lymphadenitis, acute
    - mesenteric I88.0
- lymphoid tissue, base of tongue or posterior pharynx, NEC (chronic) J35.03
- Madurella (grisea) (mycetomii) B47.0
- major
    - following ectopic or molar pregnancy O08.0
    - puerperal, postpartum, childbirth O85
- Malassezia furfur B36.0
- Malleomyces
    - mallei A24.0
    - pseudomallei (whitmori) — *see* Melioidosis
- mammary gland N61.0
- Mansonella (ozzardi) (perstans) (streptocerca) B74.4
- mastoid — *see* Mastoiditis
- maxilla, maxillary M27.2
    - sinus (chronic) — *see* Sinusitis, maxillary
- mediastinum J98.51
- Medina (worm) B72
- meibomian cyst or gland — *see* Hordeolum
- meninges — *see* Meningitis, bacterial
- meningococcal — *see also* condition A39.9
    - adrenals A39.1
    - brain A39.81
    - cerebrospinal A39.0
    - conjunctiva A39.89
    - endocardium A39.51
    - heart A39.50
        - endocardium A39.51
        - myocardium A39.52
        - pericardium A39.53
    - joint A39.83
    - meninges A39.0
    - meningococcemia A39.4
        - acute A39.2
        - chronic A39.3
    - myocardium A39.52
    - pericardium A39.53
    - retrobulbar neuritis A39.82
    - specified site NEC A39.89
- mesenteric lymph nodes or glands NEC I88.0

☑ **Additional Character Required — Refer to the Tabular List for Character Selection**

Infection, infected, infective — *continued*
- Metagonimus B66.8
- metatarsophalangeal M00.9
- methicillin
  - resistant Staphylococcus aureus (MRSA) A49.02
  - susceptible Staphylococcus aureus (MSSA) A49.01
- Microsporum, microsporic — *see* Dermatophytosis
- mixed flora (bacterial) NEC A49.8
- Monilia — *see* Candidiasis
- Monosporium apiospermum B48.2
- mouth, parasitic B37.0
- Mucor — *see* Mucormycosis
- muscle NEC — *see* Myositis, infective
- mycelium NOS B49
- mycetoma B47.9
  - actinomycotic NEC B47.1
  - mycotic NEC B47.0
- Mycobacterium, mycobacterial — *see* Mycobacterium
- Mycoplasma NEC A49.3
  - pneumoniae, as cause of disease classified elsewhere B96.0
- mycotic NOS B49
  - pathogenic to compromised host only B48.8
  - skin NOS B36.9
- myocardium NEC I40.0
- nail (chronic)
  - with lymphangitis — *see* Lymphangitis, acute, digit
  - finger L03.01- ☑
    - fungus B35.1
  - ingrowing L60.0
  - toe L03.03- ☑
    - fungus B35.1
- nasal sinus (chronic) — *see* Sinusitis
- nasopharynx — *see* Nasopharyngitis
- navel L08.82
- Necator americanus B76.1
- Neisseria — *see* Gonococcus
- Neotestudina rosatii B47.0
- newborn P39.9
  - intra-amniotic NEC P39.2
  - skin P39.4
  - specified type NEC P39.8
- nipple N61.0
  - associated with
    - lactation O91.03
    - pregnancy O91.01- ☑
    - puerperium O91.02
- Nocardia — *see* Nocardiosis
- obstetrical surgical wound (puerperal) O86.00
  - incisional site
    - deep O86.02
    - superficial O86.01
  - organ and space site O86.03
  - surgical site specified NEC O86.09
- Oesophagostomum (apiostomum) B81.8
- Oestrus ovis — *see* Myiasis
- Oidium albicans B37.9
- Onchocerca (volvulus) — *see* Onchocerciasis
- oncovirus, as cause of disease classified elsewhere B97.32
- operation wound T81.49 ☑
- Opisthorchis (felineus) (viverrini) B66.0
- orbit, orbital — *see* Inflammation, orbit
- orthopoxvirus NEC B08.09
- ovary — *see* Salpingo-oophoritis
- Oxyuris vermicularis B80
- pancreas (acute) — *see* Pancreatitis, acute
  - abscess — *see* Pancreatitis, acute
  - specified NEC — *see also* Pancreatitis, acute K85.80
- papillomavirus, as cause of disease classified elsewhere B97.7
- papovavirus NEC B34.4
- Paracoccidioides brasiliensis — *see* Paracoccidioidomycosis
- Paragonimus (westermani) B66.4
- parainfluenza virus B34.8
- parameningococcus NOS A39.9
- parapoxvirus B08.60
  - specified NEC B08.69
- parasitic B89
- Parastrongylus
  - cantonensis B83.2
  - costaricensis B81.3
  - paratyphoid A01.4
    - Type A A01.1
    - Type B A01.2
    - Type C A01.3
- paraurethral ducts N34.2

Infection, infected, infective — *continued*
- parotid gland — *see* Sialoadenitis
- parvovirus NEC B34.3
  - as cause of disease classified elsewhere B97.6
- Pasteurella NEC A28.0
  - multocida A28.0
  - pestis — *see* Plague
  - pseudotuberculosis A28.0
  - septica (cat bite) (dog bite) A28.0
  - tularensis — *see* Tularemia
- pelvic, female — *see* Disease, pelvis, inflammatory
- penis (glans) (retention) NEC N48.29
- periapical K04.5
- peridental, periodontal K05.20
  - generalized — *see* Periodontitis, aggressive, generalized
  - localized — *see* Periodontitis, aggressive, localized
- perinatal period P39.9
  - specified type NEC P39.8
- perineal repair (puerperal) O86.09
- periorbital — *see* Inflammation, orbit
- perirectal K62.89
- perirenal — *see* Infection, kidney
- peritoneal — *see* Peritonitis
- periureteral N28.89
- Petriellidium boydii B48.2
- pharynx — *see also* Pharyngitis
  - coxsackievirus B08.5
  - posterior, lymphoid (chronic) J35.03
- Phialophora
  - gougerotii (subcutaneous abscess or cyst) B43.2
  - jeanselmei (subcutaneous abscess or cyst) B43.2
  - verrucosa (skin) B43.0
- Piedraia hortae B36.3
- pinta A67.9
  - intermediate A67.1
  - late A67.2
  - mixed A67.3
  - primary A67.0
- pinworm B80
- pityrosporum furfur B36.0
- pleuro-pneumonia-like organism (PPLO) NEC A49.3
  - as cause of disease classified elsewhere B96.0
- pneumococcus, pneumococcal NEC A49.1
  - as cause of disease classified elsewhere B95.3
  - generalized (purulent) A40.3
    - with pneumonia J13
- Pneumocystis carinii (pneumonia) B59
- Pneumocystis jiroveci (pneumonia) B59
- port or reservoir T80.212 ☑
- postoperative T81.40 ☑
- postoperative wound T81.49 ☑
  - surgical site
    - deep incisional T81.42 ☑
    - organ and space T81.43 ☑
    - specified NEC T81.49 ☑
    - superficial incisional T81.41 ☑
- postprocedural T81.40 ☑
- postvaccinal T88.0 ☑
- prepuce NEC N47.7
  - with penile inflammation N47.6
- prion — *see* Disease, prion, central nervous system
- prostate (capsule) — *see* Prostatitis
- Proteus (mirabilis) (morganii) (vulgaris) NEC A49.8
  - as cause of disease classified elsewhere B96.4
- protozoal NEC B64
  - intestinal A07.9
    - specified NEC A07.8
  - specified NEC B60.8
- Pseudoallescheria boydii B48.2
- Pseudomonas NEC A49.8
  - as cause of disease classified elsewhere B96.5
  - mallei A24.0
  - pneumonia J15.1
  - pseudomallei — *see* Melioidosis
- puerperal O86.4
  - genitourinary tract NEC O86.89
  - major or generalized O85
  - minor O86.4
  - specified NEC O86.89
- pulmonary — *see* Infection, lung
- purulent — *see* Abscess
- Pyrenochaeta romeroi B47.0
- Q fever A78
- rectum (sphincter) K62.89
- renal — *see also* Infection, kidney
  - pelvis and ureter (cystic) N28.85

Infection, infected, infective — *continued*
- reovirus, as cause of disease classified elsewhere B97.5
- respiratory (tract) NEC J98.8
  - acute J22
  - chronic J98.8
  - influenzal (upper) (acute) — *see* Influenza, with, respiratory manifestations NEC
  - lower (acute) J22
    - chronic — *see* Bronchitis, chronic
  - rhinovirus J00
  - syncytial virus (RSV) — *see* Infection, virus, respiratory syncytial (RSV)
  - upper (acute) NOS J06.9
    - chronic J39.8
    - streptococcal J06.9
    - viral NOS J06.9
      - due to respiratory syncytial virus (RSV) J06.9 [B97.4]
- resulting from
  - presence of internal prosthesis, implant, graft — *see* Complications, by site and type, infection
- retortamoniasis A07.8
- retroperitoneal NEC K68.9
- retrovirus B33.3
  - as cause of disease classified elsewhere B97.30
    - human
      - immunodeficiency, type 2 (HIV 2) B97.35
      - T-cell lymphotropic
        - type I (HTLV-I) B97.33
        - type II (HTLV-II) B97.34
    - lentivirus B97.31
    - oncovirus B97.32
    - specified NEC B97.39
- Rhinosporidium (seeberi) B48.1
- rhinovirus
  - as cause of disease classified elsewhere B97.89
  - unspecified nature or site B34.8
- Rhizopus — *see* Mucormycosis
- rickettsial NOS A79.9
- roundworm (large) NEC B82.0
  - Ascariasis — *see also* Ascariasis B77.9
- rubella — *see* Rubella
- Saccharomyces — *see* Candidiasis
- salivary duct or gland (any) — *see* Sialoadenitis
- Salmonella (aertrycke) (arizonae) (callinarum) (choleraesuis) (enteritidis) (suipestifer) (typhimurium) A02.9
  - with
    - (gastro)enteritis A02.0
    - sepsis A02.1
    - specified manifestation NEC A02.8
  - due to food (poisoning) A02.9
  - hirschfeldii A01.3
  - localized A02.20
    - arthritis A02.23
    - meningitis A02.21
    - osteomyelitis A02.24
    - pneumonia A02.22
    - pyelonephritis A02.25
    - specified NEC A02.29
  - paratyphi A01.4
    - A A01.1
    - B A01.2
    - C A01.3
  - schottmuelleri A01.2
  - typhi, typhosa — *see* Typhoid
- Sarcocystis A07.8
- SARS-CoV-2 — *see* Infection, COVID-19
- scabies B86
- Schistosoma — *see* Infestation, Schistosoma
- scrotum (acute) NEC N49.2
- seminal vesicle — *see* Vesiculitis
- septic
  - localized, skin — *see* Abscess
- sheep liver fluke B66.3
- Shigella A03.9
  - boydii A03.2
  - dysenteriae A03.0
  - flexneri A03.1
  - group
    - A A03.0
    - B A03.1
    - C A03.2
    - D A03.3
  - Schmitz (-Stutzer) A03.0
  - schmitzii A03.0
  - shigae A03.0
  - sonnei A03.3

Infection, infected, infective — *continued*
  Shigella — *continued*
    specified NEC A03.8
  shoulder (joint) NEC M00.9
    due to internal joint prosthesis T84.59 ☑
    skin NEC L08.9
  sinus (accessory) (chronic) (nasal) — *see also* Sinusitis
    pilonidal — *see* Sinus, pilonidal
    skin NEC L08.89
  Skene's duct or gland — *see* Urethritis
  skin (local) (staphylococcal) (streptococcal) L08.9
    abscess — *code by* site under Abscess
    cellulitis — *code by* site under Cellulitis
    due to fungus B36.9
      specified type NEC B36.8
    mycotic B36.9
      specified type NEC B36.8
    newborn P39.4
    ulcer — *see* Ulcer, skin
  slow virus A81.9
    specified NEC A81.89
  Sparganum (mansoni) (proliferum) (baxteri) B70.1
  specific — *see also* Syphilis
    to perinatal period — *see* Infection, congenital
  specified NEC B99.8
  spermatic cord NEC N49.1
  sphenoidal (sinus) — *see* Sinusitis, sphenoidal
  spinal cord NOS — *see also* Myelitis G04.91
    abscess G06.1
    meninges — *see* Meningitis
    streptococcal G04.89
  Spirillum A25.0
  spirochetal NOS A69.9
    lung A69.8
    specified NEC A69.8
  Spirometra larvae B70.1
  spleen D73.89
  Sporotrichum, Sporothrix (schenckii) — *see* Sporotrichosis
  staphylococcal, unspecified site
    as cause of disease classified elsewhere B95.8
      aureus (methicillin susceptible) (MSSA) B95.61
        methicillin resistant (MRSA) B95.62
      specified NEC B95.7
    aureus (methicillin susceptible) (MSSA) A49.01
      methicillin resistant (MRSA) A49.02
    food poisoning A05.0
    generalized (purulent) A41.2
    pneumonia — *see* Pneumonia, staphylococcal
  Stellantchasmus falcatus B66.8
  streptobacillus moniliformis A25.1
  streptococcal NEC A49.1
    as cause of disease classified elsewhere B95.5
    B genitourinary complicating
      childbirth O98.82
      pregnancy O98.81- ☑
      puerperium O98.83
    congenital
      sepsis P36.10
        group B P36.0
        specified NEC P36.19
    generalized (purulent) A40.9
  Streptomyces B47.1
  Strongyloides (stercoralis) — *see* Strongyloidiasis
  stump (amputation) (surgical) — *see* Complication, amputation stump, infection
  subcutaneous tissue, local L08.9
  suipestifer — *see* Infection, salmonella
  swimming pool bacillus A31.1
  Taenia — *see* Infestation, Taenia
  Taeniarhynchus saginatus B68.1
  tapeworm — *see* Infestation, tapeworm
  tendon (sheath) — *see* Tenosynovitis, infective NEC
  testis — *see* Orchitis
  threadworm B80
  throat — *see* Pharyngitis
  thyroglossal duct K14.8
  toe (skin) L08.9
    cellulitis L03.03- ☑
      fungus B35.1
    nail L03.03- ☑
      fungus B35.1
  tongue NEC K14.0
    parasitic B37.0
  tonsil (and adenoid) (faucial) (lingual) (pharyngeal) — *see* Tonsillitis
  tooth, teeth K04.7

Infection, infected, infective — *continued*
  tooth, teeth — *continued*
    periapical K04.7
    peridental, periodontal K05.20
      generalized — *see* Periodontitis, aggressive, generalized
      localized — *see* Periodontitis, aggressive, localized
    pulp K04.01
      irreversible K04.02
      reversible K04.01
    socket M27.3
  TORCH — *see* Infection, congenital
    without active infection P00.2
  Torula histolytica — *see* Cryptococcosis
  Toxocara (canis) (cati) (felis) B83.0
  Toxoplasma gondii — *see* Toxoplasma
  trachea, chronic J42
  trematode NEC — *see* Infestation, fluke
  trench fever A79.0
  Treponema pallidum — *see* Syphilis
  Trichinella (spiralis) B75
  Trichomonas A59.9
    cervix A59.09
    intestine A07.8
    prostate A59.02
    specified site NEC A59.8
    urethra A59.03
    urogenitalis A59.00
    vagina A59.01
    vulva A59.01
  Trichophyton, trichophytic — *see* Dermatophytosis
  Trichosporon (beigelii) cutaneum B36.2
  Trichostrongylus B81.2
  Trichuris (trichiura) B79
  Trombicula (irritans) B88.0
  Trypanosoma
    brucei
      gambiense B56.0
      rhodesiense B56.1
    cruzi — *see* Chagas' disease
  tubal — *see* Salpingo-oophoritis
  tuberculous
    latent (LTBI) Z22.7
    NEC — *see* Tuberculosis
  tubo-ovarian — *see* Salpingo-oophoritis
  tunica vaginalis N49.1
  tunnel T80.212 ☑
  tympanic membrane NEC — *see* Myringitis
  typhoid (abortive) (ambulant) (bacillus) — *see* Typhoid
  typhus A75.9
    flea-borne A75.2
    mite-borne A75.3
    recrudescent A75.1
    tick-borne A77.9
      African A77.1
      North Asian A77.2
  umbilicus L08.82
  ureter — *see* Ureteritis
  urethra — *see* Urethritis
  urinary (tract) N39.0
    bladder — *see* Cystitis
    complicating
      pregnancy O23.4- ☑
        specified type NEC O23.3- ☑
    kidney — *see* Infection, kidney
    newborn P39.3
    puerperal (postpartum) O86.20
    tuberculous A18.13
    urethra — *see* Urethritis
  uterus, uterine — *see* Endometritis
  vaccination T88.0 ☑
  vaccinia not from vaccination B08.011
  vagina (acute) — *see* Vaginitis
  varicella B01.9
  varicose veins — *see* Varix
  vas deferens NEC N49.1
  vesical — *see* Cystitis
  Vibrio
    cholerae A00.0
      El Tor A00.1
    parahaemolyticus (food poisoning) A05.3
    vulnificus
      as cause of disease classified elsewhere B96.82
      foodborne intoxication A05.5
  Vincent's (gum) (mouth) (tonsil) A69.1
  virus, viral NOS B34.9

Infection, infected, infective — *continued*
  virus, viral — *continued*
    adenovirus
      as cause of disease classified elsewhere B97.0
      unspecified nature or site B34.0
    arborvirus, arbovirus arthropod-borne A94
    as cause of disease classified elsewhere B97.89
      adenovirus B97.0
      coronavirus B97.29
        SARS-associated B97.21
      coxsackievirus B97.11
      echovirus B97.12
      enterovirus B97.10
        coxsackievirus B97.11
        echovirus B97.12
        specified NEC B97.19
      human
        immunodeficiency, type 2 (HIV 2) B97.35
        metapneumovirus B97.81
        T-cell lymphotropic,
          type I (HTLV-I) B97.33
          type II (HTLV-II) B97.34
      papillomavirus B97.7
      parvovirus B97.6
      reovirus B97.5
      respiratory syncytial (RSV) — *see* Infection, virus, respiratory syncytial (RSV)
      retrovirus B97.30
        human
          immunodeficiency, type 2 (HIV 2) B97.35
          T-cell lymphotropic,
            type I (HTLV-I) B97.33
            type II (HTLV-II) B97.34
        lentivirus B97.31
        oncovirus B97.32
        specified NEC B97.39
      specified NEC B97.89
    central nervous system A89
      atypical A81.9
        specified NEC A81.89
      enterovirus NEC A88.8
        meningitis A87.0
      slow virus A81.9
        specified NEC A81.89
      specified NEC A88.8
    chest J98.8
    cotia B08.8
    COVID-19 U07.1
    coxsackie — *see also* Infection, coxsackie B34.1
      as cause of disease classified elsewhere B97.11
    ECHO
      as cause of disease classified elsewhere B97.12
      unspecified nature or site B34.1
    encephalitis, tick-borne A84.9
    enterovirus, as cause of disease classified elsewhere B97.10
      coxsackievirus B97.11
      echovirus B97.12
      specified NEC B97.19
    exanthem NOS B09
    human metapneumovirus as cause of disease classified elsewhere B97.81
    human papilloma as cause of disease classified elsewhere B97.7
    intestine — *see* Enteritis, viral
    respiratory syncytial (RSV)
      as cause of disease classified elsewhere B97.4
      bronchiolitis J21.0
      bronchitis J20.5
      bronchopneumonia J12.1
      otitis media H65- ☑ [B97.4]
      pneumonia J12.1
      upper respiratory infection J06.9 [B97.4]
    rhinovirus
      as cause of disease classified elsewhere B97.89
      unspecified nature or site B34.8
    slow A81.9
      specified NEC A81.89
    specified type NEC B33.8
      as cause of disease classified elsewhere B97.89
      unspecified nature or site B34.8
    unspecified nature or site B34.9
    West Nile — *see* Virus, West Nile
  vulva (acute) — *see* Vulvitis
  West Nile — *see* Virus, West Nile
  whipworm B79
  worms B83.9
    specified type NEC B83.8

☑ **Additional Character Required — Refer to the Tabular List for Character Selection**

Infection, infected, infective — *continued*
  Wuchereria (bancrofti) B74.0
    malayi B74.1
  yatapoxvirus B08.70
    specified NEC B08.79
  yeast — *see also* Candidiasis B37.9
  yellow fever — *see* Fever, yellow
  Yersinia
    enterocolitica (intestinal) A04.6
    pestis — *see* Plague
    pseudotuberculosis A28.2
  Zeis' gland — *see* Hordeolum
  Zika virus A92.5
    congenital P35.4
  zoonotic bacterial NOS A28.9
  Zopfia senegalensis B47.0
Infective, infectious — *see* condition
Infertility
  female N97.9
    age-related N97.8
    associated with
      anovulation N97.0
      cervical (mucus) disease or anomaly N88.3
      congenital anomaly
        cervix N88.3
        fallopian tube N97.1
        uterus N97.2
        vagina N97.8
      dysmucorrhea N88.3
      fallopian tube disease or anomaly N97.1
      pituitary-hypothalamic origin E23.0
      specified origin NEC N97.8
      Stein-Leventhal syndrome E28.2
      uterine disease or anomaly N97.2
      vaginal disease or anomaly N97.8
    due to
      cervical anomaly N88.3
      fallopian tube anomaly N97.1
      ovarian failure E28.39
      Stein-Leventhal syndrome E28.2
      uterine anomaly N97.2
      vaginal anomaly N97.8
    nonimplantation N97.2
    origin
      cervical N88.3
      tubal (block) (occlusion) (stenosis) N97.1
      uterine N97.2
      vaginal N97.8
  male N46.9
    azoospermia N46.01
      extratesticular cause N46.029
        drug therapy N46.021
        efferent duct obstruction N46.023
        infection N46.022
        radiation N46.024
        specified cause NEC N46.029
        systemic disease N46.025
    oligospermia N46.11
      extratesticular cause N46.129
        drug therapy N46.121
        efferent duct obstruction N46.123
        infection N46.122
        radiation N46.124
        specified cause NEC N46.129
        systemic disease N46.125
    specified type NEC N46.8
Infestation B88.9
  Acanthocheilonema (perstans) (streptocerca) B74.4
  Acariasis B88.0
    demodex folliculorum B88.0
    sarcoptes scabiei B86
    trombiculae B88.0
  Agamofilaria streptocerca B74.4
  Ancylostoma, ankylostoma (braziliense) (caninum) (ceylanicum) (duodenale) B76.0
    americanum B76.1
    new world B76.1
  Anisakis larvae, anisakiasis B81.0
  arthropod NEC B88.2
  Ascaris lumbricoides — *see* Ascariasis
  Balantidium coli A07.0
  beef tapeworm B68.1
  Bothriocephalus (latus) B70.0
    larval B70.1
  broad tapeworm B70.0
    larval B70.1
  Brugia (malayi) B74.1
    timori B74.2

Infestation — *continued*
  candiru B88.8
  Capillaria
    hepatica B83.8
    philippinensis B81.1
  cat liver fluke B66.0
  cestodes B71.9
    diphyllobothrium — *see* Infestation, diphyllobothrium
    dipylidiasis B71.1
    hymenolepiasis B71.0
    specified type NEC B71.8
  chigger B88.0
  chigo, chigoe B88.1
  Clonorchis (sinensis) (liver) B66.1
  coccidial A07.3
  crab-lice B85.3
  Cysticercus cellulosae — *see* Cysticercosis
  Demodex (folliculorum) B88.0
  Dermanyssus gallinae B88.0
  Dermatobia (hominis) — *see* Myiasis
  Dibothriocephalus (latus) B70.0
    larval B70.1
  Dicrocoelium dendriticum B66.2
  Diphyllobothrium (adult) (latum) (intestinal) (pacificum) B70.0
    larval B70.1
  Diplogonoporus (grandis) B71.8
  Dipylidium caninum B67.4
  Distoma hepaticum B66.3
  dog tapeworm B67.4
  Dracunculus medinensis B72
  dragon worm B72
  dwarf tapeworm B71.0
  Echinococcus — *see* Echinococcus
  Echinostomum ilocanum B66.8
  Entamoeba (histolytica) — *see* Infection, Ameba
  Enterobius vermicularis B80
  eyelid
    in (due to)
      leishmaniasis B55.1
      loiasis B74.3
      onchocerciasis B73.09
      phthiriasis B85.3
    parasitic NOS B89
  eyeworm B74.3
  Fasciola (gigantica) (hepatica) (indica) B66.3
  Fasciolopsis (buski) (intestine) B66.5
  filarial B74.9
    bancroftian B74.0
    conjunctiva B74.9
    due to
      Acanthocheilonema (perstans) (streptocerca) B74.4
      Brugia (malayi) B74.1
        timori B74.2
      Dracunculus medinensis B72
      guinea worm B72
      loa loa B74.3
      Mansonella (ozzardi) (perstans) (streptocerca) B74.4
      Onchocerca volvulus B73.00
        eye B73.00
        eyelid B73.09
      Wuchereria (bancrofti) B74.0
    Malayan B74.1
    ozzardi B74.4
    specified type NEC B74.8
  fish tapeworm B70.0
    larval B70.1
  fluke B66.9
    blood NOS — *see* Schistosomiasis
    cat liver B66.0
    intestinal B66.5
    lancet B66.2
    liver (sheep) B66.3
      cat B66.0
      Chinese B66.1
      due to clonorchiasis B66.1
      oriental B66.1
    lung (oriental) B66.4
    sheep liver B66.3
    specified type NEC B66.8
  fly larvae — *see* Myiasis
  Gasterophilus (intestinalis) — *see* Myiasis
  Gastrodiscoides hominis B66.8
  Giardia lamblia A07.1
  Gnathostoma (spinigerum) B83.1

Infestation — *continued*
  Gongylonema B83.8
  guinea worm B72
  helminth B83.9
    angiostrongyliasis B83.2
      intestinal B81.3
    gnathostomiasis B83.1
    hirudiniasis, internal B83.4
    intestinal B82.0
      angiostrongyliasis B81.3
      anisakiasis B81.0
      ascariasis — *see* Ascariasis
      capillariasis B81.1
      cysticercosis — *see* Cysticercosis
      diphyllobothriasis — *see* Infestation, diphyllobothriasis
      dracunculiasis B72
      echinococcus — *see* Echinococcosis
      enterobiasis B80
      filariasis — *see* Infestation, filarial
      fluke — *see* Infestation, fluke
      hookworm — *see* Infestation, hookworm
      mixed (types classifiable to more than one of the titles B65.0-B81.3 and B81.8) B81.4
      onchocerciasis — *see* Onchocerciasis
      schistosomiasis — *see* Infestation, schistosoma
      specified
        cestode NEC — *see* Infestation, cestode type NEC B81.8
      strongyloidiasis — *see* Strongyloidiasis
      taenia — *see* Infestation, taenia
      trichinellosis B75
      trichostrongyliasis B81.2
      trichuriasis B79
    specified type NEC B83.8
    syngamiasis B83.3
    visceral larva migrans B83.0
  Heterophyes (heterophyes) B66.8
  hookworm B76.9
    ancylostomiasis B76.0
    necatoriasis B76.1
    specified type NEC B76.8
  Hymenolepis (diminuta) (nana) B71.0
  intestinal NEC B82.9
  leeches (aquatic) (land) — *see* Hirudiniasis
  Leishmania — *see* Leishmaniasis
  lice, louse — *see* Infestation, Pediculus
  Linguatula B88.8
  Liponyssoides sanguineus B88.0
  Loa loa B74.3
    conjunctival B74.3
    eyelid B74.3
  louse — *see* Infestation, Pediculus
  maggots — *see* Myiasis
  Mansonella (ozzardi) (perstans) (streptocerca) B74.4
  Medina (worm) B72
  Metagonimus (yokogawai) B66.8
  microfilaria streptocerca — *see* Onchocerciasis
    eye B73.00
    eyelid B73.09
  mites B88.9
    scabic B86
  Monilia (albicans) — *see* Candidiasis
  mouth B37.0
  Necator americanus B76.1
  nematode NEC (intestinal) B82.0
    Ancylostoma B76.0
    conjunctiva NEC B83.9
    Enterobius vermicularis B80
    Gnathostoma spinigerum B83.1
    physaloptera B80
    specified NEC B81.8
    trichostrongylus B81.2
    trichuris (trichuria) B79
  Oesophagostomum (apiostomum) B81.8
  Oestrus ovis — *see also* Myiasis B87.9
  Onchocerca (volvulus) — *see* Onchocerciasis
  Opisthorchis (felineus) (viverrini) B66.0
  orbit, parasitic NOS B89
  Oxyuris vermicularis B80
  Paragonimus (westermani) B66.4
  parasite, parasitic B89
    eyelid B89
    intestinal NOS B82.9
    mouth B37.0
    skin B88.9
    tongue B37.0

Infestation — *continued*
- Parastrongylus
  - cantonensis B83.2
  - costaricensis B81.3
- Pediculus B85.2
  - body B85.1
  - capitis (humanus) (any site) B85.0
  - corporis (humanus) (any site) B85.1
  - head B85.0
  - mixed (classifiable to more than one of the titles B85.0 - B85.3) B85.4
  - pubis (any site) B85.3
- Pentastoma B88.8
- Phthirus (pubis) (any site) B85.3
  - with any infestation classifiable to B85.0 - B85.2 B85.4
- pinworm B80
- pork tapeworm (adult) B68.0
- protozoal NEC B64
  - intestinal A07.9
    - specified NEC A07.8
  - specified NEC B60.8
- pubic, louse B85.3
- rat tapeworm B71.0
- red bug B88.0
- roundworm (large) NEC B82.0
  - Ascariasis — *see also* Ascariasis B77.9
- sandflea B88.1
- Sarcoptes scabiei B86
- scabies B86
- Schistosoma B65.9
  - bovis B65.8
  - cercariae B65.3
  - haematobium B65.0
  - intercalatum B65.8
  - japonicum B65.2
  - mansoni B65.1
  - mattheei B65.8
  - mekongi B65.8
  - specified type NEC B65.8
  - spindale B65.8
- screw worms — *see* Myiasis
- skin NOS B88.9
- Sparganum (mansoni) (proliferum) (baxteri) B70.1
  - larval B70.1
- specified type NEC B88.8
- Spirometra larvae B70.1
- Stellantchasmus falcatus B66.8
- Strongyloides stercoralis — *see* Strongyloidiasis
- Taenia B68.9
  - diminuta B71.0
  - echinococcus — *see* Echinococcus
  - mediocanellata B68.1
  - nana B71.0
  - saginata B68.1
  - solium (intestinal form) B68.0
    - larval form — *see* Cysticercosis
- Taeniarhynchus saginatus B68.1
- tapeworm B71.9
  - beef B68.1
  - broad B70.0
    - larval B70.1
  - dog B67.4
  - dwarf B71.0
  - fish B70.0
    - larval B70.1
  - pork B68.0
  - rat B71.0
- Ternidens diminutus B81.8
- Tetranychus molestissimus B88.0
- threadworm B80
- tongue B37.0
- Toxocara (canis) (cati) (felis) B83.0
- trematode(s) NEC — *see* Infestation, fluke
- Trichinella (spiralis) B75
- Trichocephalus B79
- Trichomonas — *see* Trichomoniasis
- Trichostrongylus B81.2
- Trichuris (trichiura) B79
- Trombicula (irritans) B88.0
- Tunga penetrans B88.1
- Uncinaria americana B76.1
- Vandellia cirrhosa B88.8
- whipworm B79
- worms B83.9
  - intestinal B82.0
- Wuchereria (bancrofti) B74.0

Infiltrate, infiltration
- amyloid (generalized) (localized) — *see* Amyloidosis
- calcareous NEC R89.7
  - localized — *see* Degeneration, by site
- calcium salt R89.7
- cardiac
  - fatty — *see* Degeneration, myocardial
  - glycogenic E74.02 *[I43]*
- corneal — *see* Edema, cornea
- eyelid — *see* Inflammation, eyelid
- glycogen, glycogenic — *see* Disease, glycogen storage
- heart, cardiac
  - fatty — *see* Degeneration, myocardial
  - glycogenic E74.02 *[I43]*
- inflammatory in vitreous H43.89
- kidney N28.89
- leukemic — *see* Leukemia
- liver K76.89
  - fatty — *see* Fatty, liver NEC
  - glycogen — *see also* Disease, glycogen storage E74.03 *[K77]*
- lung R91.8
  - eosinophilic — *see* Eosinophilia, pulmonary
- lymphatic — *see also* Leukemia, lymphatic C91.9- ☑
  - gland I88.9
- muscle, fatty M62.89
- myocardium, myocardial
  - fatty — *see* Degeneration, myocardial
  - glycogenic E74.02 *[I43]*
- on chest x-ray R91.8
- pulmonary R91.8
  - with eosinophilia — *see* Eosinophilia, pulmonary
- skin (lymphocytic) L98.6
- thymus (gland) (fatty) E32.8
- urine R39.0
- vesicant agent
  - antineoplastic chemotherapy T80.810 ☑
  - other agent NEC T80.818 ☑
- vitreous body H43.89

Infirmity R68.89
- senile R54

Inflammation, inflamed, inflammatory (with exudation)
- abducent (nerve) — *see* Strabismus, paralytic, sixth nerve
- accessory sinus (chronic) — *see* Sinusitis
- adrenal (gland) E27.8
- alveoli, teeth M27.3
  - scorbutic E54
- anal canal, anus K62.89
- antrum (chronic) — *see* Sinusitis, maxillary
- appendix — *see* Appendicitis
- arachnoid — *see* Meningitis
- areola N61.0
  - puerperal, postpartum or gestational — *see* Infection, nipple
- areolar tissue NOS L08.9
- artery — *see* Arteritis
- auditory meatus (external) — *see* Otitis, externa
- Bartholin's gland N75.8
- bile duct (common) (hepatic) or passage — *see* Cholangitis
- bladder — *see* Cystitis
- bone — *see* Osteomyelitis
- brain — *see also* Encephalitis
  - membrane — *see* Meningitis
- breast N61.0
  - puerperal, postpartum, gestational — *see* Mastitis, obstetric
- broad ligament — *see* Disease, pelvis, inflammatory
- bronchi — *see* Bronchitis
- catarrhal J00
- cecum — *see* Appendicitis
- cerebral — *see also* Encephalitis
  - membrane — *see* Meningitis
- cerebrospinal
  - meningococcal A39.0
- cervix (uteri) — *see* Cervicitis
- chest J98.8
- chorioretinal H30.9- ☑
  - cyclitis — *see* Cyclitis
  - disseminated H30.10- ☑
    - generalized H30.13- ☑
    - peripheral H30.12- ☑
    - posterior pole H30.11- ☑
  - epitheliopathy — *see* Epitheliopathy
  - focal H30.00- ☑

Inflammation, inflamed, inflammatory — *continued*
- chorioretinal — *continued*
  - focal — *continued*
    - juxtapapillary H30.01- ☑
    - macular H30.04- ☑
    - paramacular — *see* Inflammation, chorioretinal, focal, macular
    - peripheral H30.03- ☑
    - posterior pole H30.02- ☑
    - specified type NEC H30.89- ☑
- choroid — *see* Inflammation, chorioretinal
- chronic, postmastoidectomy cavity — *see* Complications, postmastoidectomy, inflammation
- colon — *see* Enteritis
- connective tissue (diffuse) NEC — *see* Disorder, soft tissue, specified type NEC
- cornea — *see* Keratitis
- corpora cavernosa N48.29
- cranial nerve — *see* Disorder, nerve, cranial
- Douglas' cul-de-sac or pouch (chronic) N73.0
- due to device, implant or graft — *see also* Complications, by site and type, infection or inflammation
  - arterial graft T82.7 ☑
  - breast (implant) T85.79 ☑
  - catheter T85.79 ☑
    - dialysis (renal) T82.7 ☑
      - intraperitoneal T85.71 ☑
    - infusion T82.7 ☑
      - cranial T85.735 ☑
      - intrathecal T85.735 ☑
      - spinal (epidural) (subdural) T85.735 ☑
      - subarachnoid T85.735 ☑
    - urinary T83.518 ☑
      - cystostomy T83.510 ☑
      - Hopkins T83.518 ☑
      - ileostomy T83.518 ☑
      - nephrostomy T83.512 ☑
      - specified NEC T83.518 ☑
      - urethral indwelling T83.511 ☑
      - urostomy T83.518 ☑
  - electronic (electrode) (pulse generator) (stimulator)
    - bone T84.7 ☑
    - cardiac T82.7 ☑
    - nervous system T85.738 ☑
      - brain T85.731 ☑
      - cranial nerve T85.732 ☑
      - gastric nerve T85.732 ☑
      - neurostimulator generator T85.734 ☑
      - peripheral nerve T85.732 ☑
      - sacral nerve T85.732 ☑
      - spinal cord T85.733 ☑
      - vagal nerve T85.732 ☑
    - urinary T83.590 ☑
  - fixation, internal (orthopedic) NEC — *see* Complication, fixation device, infection
  - gastrointestinal (bile duct) (esophagus) T85.79 ☑
    - neurostimulator electrode (lead) T85.732 ☑
  - genital NEC T83.69 ☑
  - heart NEC T82.7 ☑
    - valve (prosthesis) T82.6 ☑
      - graft T82.7 ☑
  - joint prosthesis — *see* Complication, joint prosthesis, infection
  - ocular (corneal graft) (orbital implant) NEC T85.79 ☑
  - orthopedic NEC T84.7 ☑
  - penile (cylinder) (pump) (reservoir) T83.61 ☑
  - specified NEC T85.79 ☑
  - testicular T83.62 ☑
  - urinary NEC T83.598 ☑
    - ileal conduit stent T83.593 ☑
    - implanted neurostimulation T83.590 ☑
    - implanted sphincter T83.591 ☑
    - indwelling ureteral stent T83.592 ☑
    - nephroureteral stent T83.593 ☑
    - specified stent NEC T83.593 ☑
  - vascular NEC T82.7 ☑
  - ventricular intracranial (communicating) shunt T85.730 ☑
- duodenum K29.80
  - with bleeding K29.81
- dura mater — *see* Meningitis
- ear (middle) — *see also* Otitis, media
  - external — *see* Otitis, externa
  - inner — *see* subcategory H83.0 ☑
- epididymis — *see* Epididymitis

Inflammation, inflamed, inflammatory —
  continued
  esophagus — *see* Esophagitis
  ethmoidal (sinus) (chronic) — *see* Sinusitis, ethmoidal
  eustachian tube (catarrhal) — *see* Salpingitis, eustachi-
     an
  eyelid H01.9
    abscess — *see* Abscess, eyelid
    blepharitis — *see* Blepharitis
    chalazion — *see* Chalazion
    dermatosis (noninfectious) — *see* Dermatosis, eyelid
    hordeolum — *see* Hordeolum
    specified NEC H01.8
  fallopian tube — *see* Salpingo-oophoritis
  fascia — *see* Myositis
  follicular, pharynx J31.2
  frontal (sinus) (chronic) — *see* Sinusitis, frontal
  gallbladder — *see* Cholecystitis
  gastric — *see* Gastritis
  gastrointestinal — *see* Enteritis
  genital organ (internal) (diffuse)
    female — *see* Disease, pelvis, inflammatory
    male N49.9
      multiple sites N49.8
      specified NEC N49.8
  gland (lymph) — *see* Lymphadenitis
  glottis — *see* Laryngitis
  granular, pharynx J31.2
  gum K05.10
    nonplaque induced K05.11
    plaque induced K05.10
  heart — *see* Carditis
  hepatic duct — *see* Cholangitis
  ileoanal (internal) pouch K91.850
  ileum — *see also* Enteritis
    regional or terminal — *see* Enteritis, regional
  intestinal pouch K91.850
  intestine (any part) — *see* Enteritis
  jaw (acute) (bone) (chronic) (lower) (suppurative) (up-
     per) M27.2
  joint NEC — *see* Arthritis
    sacroiliac M46.1
  kidney — *see* Nephritis
  knee (joint) M13.169
    tuberculous A18.02
  labium (majus) (minus) — *see* Vulvitis
  lacrimal
    gland — *see* Dacryoadenitis
    passages (duct) (sac) — *see also* Dacryocystitis
      canaliculitis — *see* Canaliculitis, lacrimal
  larynx — *see* Laryngitis
  leg NOS L08.9
  lip K13.0
  liver (capsule) — *see also* Hepatitis
    chronic K73.9
    suppurative K75.0
  lung (acute) — *see also* Pneumonia
    chronic J98.4
  lymph gland or node — *see* Lymphadenitis
  lymphatic vessel — *see* Lymphangitis
  maxilla, maxillary M27.2
    sinus (chronic) — *see* Sinusitis, maxillary
  membranes of brain or spinal cord — *see* Meningitis
  meninges — *see* Meningitis
  mouth K12.1
  muscle — *see* Myositis
  myocardium — *see* Myocarditis
  nasal sinus (chronic) — *see* Sinusitis
  nasopharynx — *see* Nasopharyngitis
  navel L08.82
  nerve NEC — *see* Neuritis
  nipple N61.0
    puerperal, postpartum or gestational — *see* Infec-
      tion, nipple
  nose — *see* Rhinitis
  oculomotor (nerve) — *see* Strabismus, paralytic, third
    nerve
  optic nerve — *see* Neuritis, optic
  orbit (chronic) H05.10
    acute H05.00
      abscess — *see* Abscess, orbit
      cellulitis — *see* Cellulitis, orbit
      osteomyelitis — *see* Osteomyelitis, orbit
      periostitis — *see* Periostitis, orbital
      tenonitis — *see* Tenonitis, eye
    granuloma — *see* Granuloma, orbit
    myositis — *see* Myositis, orbital

Inflammation, inflamed, inflammatory —
  continued
  ovary — *see* Salpingo-oophoritis
  oviduct — *see* Salpingo-oophoritis
  pancreas (acute) — *see* Pancreatitis
  parametrium N73.0
  parotid region L08.9
  pelvis, female — *see* Disease, pelvis, inflammatory
  penis (corpora cavernosa) N48.29
  perianal K62.89
  pericardium — *see* Pericarditis
  perineum (female) (male) L08.9
  perirectal K62.89
  peritoneum — *see* Peritonitis
  periuterine — *see* Disease, pelvis, inflammatory
  perivesical — *see* Cystitis
  petrous bone (acute) (chronic) — *see* Petrositis
  pharynx (acute) — *see* Pharyngitis
  pia mater — *see* Meningitis
  pleura — *see* Pleurisy
  polyp, colon — *see also* Polyp, colon, inflammatory
    K51.40
  prostate — *see also* Prostatitis
    specified type NEC N41.8
  rectosigmoid — *see* Rectosigmoiditis
  rectum — *see also* Proctitis K62.89
  respiratory, upper — *see also* Infection, respiratory,
    upper J06.9
    acute, due to radiation J70.0
    chronic, due to external agent — *see* condition,
      respiratory, chronic, due to
    due to
      chemicals, gases, fumes or vapors (inhalation)
        J68.2
      radiation J70.1
  retina — *see* Chorioretinitis
  retrocecal — *see* Appendicitis
  retroperitoneal — *see* Peritonitis
  salivary duct or gland (any) (suppurative) — *see*
    Sialoadenitis
  scorbutic, alveoli, teeth E54
  scrotum N49.2
  seminal vesicle — *see* Vesiculitis
  sigmoid — *see* Enteritis
  sinus — *see* Sinusitis
  Skene's duct or gland — *see* Urethritis
  skin L08.9
  spermatic cord N49.1
  sphenoidal (sinus) — *see* Sinusitis, sphenoidal
  spinal
    cord — *see* Encephalitis
    membrane — *see* Meningitis
    nerve — *see* Disorder, nerve
  spine — *see* Spondylopathy, inflammatory
  spleen (capsule) D73.89
  stomach — *see* Gastritis
  subcutaneous tissue L08.9
  suprarenal (gland) E27.8
  synovial — *see* Tenosynovitis
  tendon (sheath) NEC — *see* Tenosynovitis
  testis — *see* Orchitis
  throat (acute) — *see* Pharyngitis
  thymus (gland) E32.8
  thyroid (gland) — *see* Thyroiditis
  tongue K14.0
  tonsil — *see* Tonsillitis
  trachea — *see* Tracheitis
  trochlear (nerve) — *see* Strabismus, paralytic, fourth
    nerve
  tubal — *see* Salpingo-oophoritis
  tuberculous NEC — *see* Tuberculosis
  tubo-ovarian — *see* Salpingo-oophoritis
  tunica vaginalis N49.1
  tympanic membrane — *see* Tympanitis
  umbilicus, umbilical L08.82
  uterine ligament — *see* Disease, pelvis, inflammatory
  uterus (catarrhal) — *see* Endometritis
  uveal tract (anterior) NOS — *see also* Iridocyclitis
    posterior — *see* Chorioretinitis
  vagina — *see* Vaginitis
  vas deferens N49.1
  vein — *see also* Phlebitis
    intracranial or intraspinal (septic) G08
    thrombotic I80.9
      leg — *see* Phlebitis, leg
      lower extremity — *see* Phlebitis, leg
  vocal cord J38.3

Inflammation, inflamed, inflammatory —
  continued
  vulva — *see* Vulvitis
  Wharton's duct (suppurative) — *see* Sialoadenitis
Inflation, lung, imperfect (newborn) — *see* Atelectasis
Influenza (bronchial) (epidemic) (respiratory (upper))
  (unidentified influenza virus) J11.1
  with
    digestive manifestations J11.2
    encephalopathy J11.81
    enteritis J11.2
    gastroenteritis J11.2
    gastrointestinal manifestations J11.2
    laryngitis J11.1
    myocarditis J11.82
    otitis media J11.83
    pharyngitis J11.1
    pneumonia J11.00
      specified type J11.08
    respiratory manifestations NEC J11.1
    specified manifestation NEC J11.89
  A (non-novel) J10- ☑
  A/H5N1 — *see also* Influenza, due to, identified novel
    influenza A virus J09.X2
  avian — *see also* Influenza, due to, identified novel in-
    fluenza A virus J09.X2
  B J10- ☑
  bird — *see also* Influenza, due to, identified novel in-
    fluenza A virus J09.X2
  C J10- ☑
  due to
    avian — *see also* Influenza, due to, identified novel
      influenza A virus J09.X2
    identified influenza virus NEC J10.1
      with
        digestive manifestations J10.2
        encephalopathy J10.81
        enteritis J10.2
        gastroenteritis J10.2
        gastrointestinal manifestations J10.2
        laryngitis J10.1
        myocarditis J10.82
        otitis media J10.83
        pharyngitis J10.1
        pneumonia (unspecified type) J10.00
          with same identified influenza virus
            J10.01
          specified type NEC J10.08
        respiratory manifestations NEC J10.1
        specified manifestation NEC J10.89
    identified novel influenza A virus J09.X2
      with
        digestive manifestations J09.X3
        encephalopathy J09.X9
        enteritis J09.X3
        gastroenteritis J09.X3
        gastrointestinal manifestations J09.X3
        laryngitis J09.X2
        myocarditis J09.X9
        otitis media J09.X9
        pharyngitis J09.X2
        pneumonia J09.X1
        respiratory manifestations NEC J09.X2
        specified manifestation NEC J09.X9
        upper respiratory symptoms J09.X2
    novel (2009) H1N1 influenza — *see also* Influenza, due
      to, identified influenza virus NEC J10.1
    novel influenza A/H1N1 — *see also* Influenza, due to,
      identified influenza virus NEC J10.1
    of other animal origin, not bird or swine — *see also*
      Influenza, due to, identified novel influenza A
      virus J09.X2
    swine (viruses that normally cause infections in pigs)
      — *see also* Influenza, due to, identified novel
      influenza A virus J09.X2
Influenzal — *see* Influenza
Influenza-like disease — *see* Influenza
Infraction, Freiberg's (metatarsal head) — *see* Osteo-
  chondrosis, juvenile, metatarsus
Infraeruption of tooth (teeth) M26.34
Infusion complication, misadventure, or reaction —
  see Complications, infusion
Ingestion
  chemical — *see* Table of Drugs and Chemicals, by
    substance, poisoning

Index

Inflammation, inflamed, inflammatory — Ingestion

Ingestion — continued
drug or medicament
correct substance properly administered — see Table of Drugs and Chemicals, by drug, adverse effect
overdose or wrong substance given or taken — see Table of Drugs and Chemicals, by drug, poisoning
foreign body — see Foreign body, alimentary tract
multiple drug — see Table of Drugs and Chemicals, multiple
tularemia A21.3
Ingrowing
hair (beard) L73.1
nail (finger) (toe) L60.0
Inguinal — see also condition
testicle Q53.9
bilateral Q53.212
unilateral Q53.112
Inhalant-induced
anxiety disorder F18.980
depressive disorder F18.94
major neurocognitive disorder F18.97
mild neurocognitive disorder F18.988
psychotic disorder F18.959
Inhalation
anthrax A22.1
flame T27.3
food or foreign body — see Foreign body, by site
gases, fumes, or vapors T59.9- ☑
specified agent NEC — see Table of Drugs and Chemicals, by substance T59.89- ☑
liquid or vomitus — see Asphyxia
meconium (newborn) P24.00
with
with respiratory symptoms P24.01
pneumonia (pneumonitis) P24.01
mucus — see Asphyxia, mucus
oil or gasoline (causing suffocation) — see Foreign body, by site
smoke T59.81- ☑
with respiratory conditions J70.5
due to chemicals, gases, fumes and vapors J68.9
steam — see also Burn, respiratory tract T59.9- ☑
stomach contents or secretions — see Foreign body, by site
due to anesthesia (general) (local) or other sedation T88.59 ☑
in labor and delivery O74.0
in pregnancy O29.01- ☑
postpartum, puerperal O89.01
Inhibition, orgasm
female F52.31
male F52.32
Inhibitor, systemic lupus erythematosus (presence of) D68.62
Iniencephalus, iniencephaly Q00.2
Injection, traumatic jet (air) (industrial) (water) (paint or dye) T70.4 ☑
Injury — see also specified injury type T14.90 ☑
abdomen, abdominal S39.91 ☑
blood vessel — see Injury, blood vessel, abdomen
cavity — see Injury, intra-abdominal
contusion S30.1 ☑
internal — see Injury, intra-abdominal
intra-abdominal organ — see Injury, intra-abdominal
nerve — see Injury, nerve, abdomen
open — see Wound, open, abdomen
specified NEC S39.81 ☑
superficial — see Injury, superficial, abdomen
Achilles tendon S86.00- ☑
laceration S86.02- ☑
specified type NEC S86.09- ☑
strain S86.01- ☑
acoustic, resulting in deafness — see Injury, nerve, acoustic
adrenal (gland) S37.819 ☑
contusion S37.812 ☑
laceration S37.813 ☑
specified type NEC S37.818 ☑
alveolar (process) S09.93 ☑
ankle S99.91- ☑
contusion — see Contusion, ankle
dislocation — see Dislocation, ankle
fracture — see Fracture, ankle
nerve — see Injury, nerve, ankle

Injury — continued
ankle — continued
open — see Wound, open, ankle
specified type NEC S99.81- ☑
sprain — see Sprain, ankle
superficial — see Injury, superficial, ankle
anterior chamber, eye — see Injury, eye, specified site NEC
anus — see Injury, abdomen
aorta (thoracic) S25.00 ☑
abdominal S35.00 ☑
laceration (minor) (superficial) S35.01 ☑
major S35.02 ☑
specified type NEC S35.09 ☑
laceration (minor) (superficial) S25.01 ☑
major S25.02 ☑
specified type NEC S25.09 ☑
arm (upper) S49.9- ☑
blood vessel — see Injury, blood vessel, arm
contusion — see Contusion, arm, upper
fracture — see Fracture, humerus
lower — see Injury, forearm
muscle — see Injury, muscle, shoulder
nerve — see Injury, nerve, arm
open — see Wound, open, arm
specified type NEC S49.8- ☑
superficial — see Injury, superficial, arm
artery (complicating trauma) — see also Injury, blood vessel, by site
cerebral or meningeal — see Injury, intracranial
auditory canal (external) (meatus) S09.91
auricle, auris, ear S09.91
axilla — see Injury, shoulder
back — see Injury, back, lower
bile duct S36.13
birth — see also Birth, injury P15.9
bladder (sphincter) S37.20 ☑
at delivery O71.5
contusion S37.22 ☑
laceration S37.23 ☑
obstetrical trauma O71.5
specified type NEC S37.29 ☑
blast (air) (hydraulic) (immersion) (underwater) NEC T14.8 ☑
acoustic nerve trauma — see Injury, nerve, acoustic
bladder — see Injury, bladder
brain — see Concussion
primary, specified NEC S06.8A- ☑
colon — see Injury, intestine, large
ear (primary) S09.31- ☑
secondary S09.39- ☑
generalized T70.8 ☑
lung — see Injury, intrathoracic, lung
multiple body organs T70.8 ☑
peritoneum S36.81 ☑
rectum S36.61 ☑
retroperitoneum S36.898 ☑
small intestine S36.419 ☑
duodenum S36.410 ☑
specified site NEC S36.418 ☑
specified
intra-abdominal organ NEC S36.898 ☑
pelvic organ NEC S37.899 ☑
blood vessel NEC T14.8 ☑
abdomen S35.9 ☑
aorta — see Injury, aorta, abdominal
celiac artery — see Injury, blood vessel, celiac artery
iliac vessel — see Injury, blood vessel, iliac
laceration S35.91 ☑
mesenteric vessel — see Injury, mesenteric
portal vein — see Injury, blood vessel, portal vein
renal vessel — see Injury, blood vessel, renal
specified vessel NEC S35.8X- ☑
splenic vessel — see Injury, blood vessel, splenic
vena cava — see Injury, vena cava, inferior
ankle — see Injury, blood vessel, foot
aorta (abdominal) (thoracic) — see Injury, aorta
arm (upper) NEC S45.90- ☑
forearm — see Injury, blood vessel, forearm
laceration S45.91- ☑
specified
site NEC S45.80- ☑
laceration S45.81- ☑
specified type NEC S45.89- ☑
type NEC S45.99- ☑

Injury — continued
blood vessel — continued
arm — continued
superficial vein S45.30- ☑
laceration S45.31- ☑
specified type NEC S45.39- ☑
axillary
artery S45.00- ☑
laceration S45.01- ☑
specified type NEC S45.09- ☑
vein S45.20- ☑
laceration S45.21- ☑
specified type NEC S45.29- ☑
azygos vein — see Injury, blood vessel, thoracic, specified site NEC
brachial
artery S45.10- ☑
laceration S45.11- ☑
specified type NEC S45.19- ☑
vein S45.20- ☑
laceration S45.219 ☑
specified type NEC S45.29- ☑
carotid artery (common) (external) (internal, extracranial) S15.00- ☑
internal, intracranial S06.8- ☑
laceration (minor) (superficial) S15.01- ☑
major S15.02- ☑
specified type NEC S15.09- ☑
celiac artery S35.219 ☑
branch S35.299 ☑
laceration (minor) (superficial) S35.291 ☑
major S35.292 ☑
specified NEC S35.298 ☑
laceration (minor) (superficial) S35.211 ☑
major S35.212 ☑
specified type NEC S35.218 ☑
cerebral — see Injury, intracranial
deep plantar — see Injury, blood vessel, plantar artery
digital (hand) — see Injury, blood vessel, finger
dorsal
artery (foot) S95.00- ☑
laceration S95.01- ☑
specified type NEC S95.09- ☑
vein (foot) S95.20- ☑
laceration S95.21- ☑
specified type NEC S95.29- ☑
due to accidental laceration during procedure — see Laceration, accidental complicating surgery
extremity — see Injury, blood vessel, limb
femoral
artery (common) (superficial) S75.00- ☑
laceration (minor) (superficial) S75.01- ☑
major S75.02- ☑
specified type NEC S75.09- ☑
vein (hip level) (thigh level) S75.10- ☑
laceration (minor) (superficial) S75.11- ☑
major S75.12- ☑
specified type NEC S75.19- ☑
finger S65.50- ☑
index S65.50- ☑
laceration S65.51- ☑
specified type NEC S65.59- ☑
laceration S65.51- ☑
little S65.50- ☑
laceration S65.51- ☑
specified type NEC S65.59- ☑
middle S65.50- ☑
laceration S65.51- ☑
specified type NEC S65.59- ☑
specified type NEC S65.59- ☑
thumb — see Injury, blood vessel, thumb
foot S95.90- ☑
dorsal
artery — see Injury, blood vessel, dorsal, artery
vein — see Injury, blood vessel, dorsal, vein
laceration S95.91- ☑
plantar artery — see Injury, blood vessel, plantar artery
specified
site NEC S95.80- ☑
laceration S95.81- ☑
specified type NEC S95.89- ☑
specified type NEC S95.99- ☑

Injury — *continued*
  blood vessel — *continued*
    forearm S55.90- ☑
      laceration S55.91- ☑
      radial artery — *see* Injury, blood vessel, radial artery
      specified
        site NEC S55.80- ☑
          laceration S55.81- ☑
          specified type NEC S55.89- ☑
        type NEC S55.99- ☑
      ulnar artery — *see* Injury, blood vessel, ulnar artery
      vein S55.20- ☑
        laceration S55.21- ☑
        specified type NEC S55.29- ☑
    gastric
      artery — *see* Injury, mesenteric, artery, branch
      vein — *see* Injury, blood vessel, abdomen
    gastroduodenal artery — *see* Injury, mesenteric, artery, branch
    greater saphenous vein (lower leg level) S85.30- ☑
      hip (and thigh) level S75.20- ☑
        laceration (minor) (superficial) S75.21- ☑
          major S75.22- ☑
        specified type NEC S75.29- ☑
      laceration S85.31- ☑
      specified type NEC S85.39- ☑
    hand (level) S65.90- ☑
      finger — *see* Injury, blood vessel, finger
      laceration S65.91- ☑
      palmar arch — *see* Injury, blood vessel, palmar arch
      radial artery — *see* Injury, blood vessel, radial artery, hand
      specified
        site NEC S65.80- ☑
          laceration S65.81- ☑
          specified type NEC S65.89- ☑
        type NEC S65.99- ☑
      thumb — *see* Injury, blood vessel, thumb
      ulnar artery — *see* Injury, blood vessel, ulnar artery, hand
    head S09.0 ☑
      intracranial — *see* Injury, intracranial
      multiple S09.0 ☑
    hepatic
      artery — *see* Injury, mesenteric, artery
      vein — *see* Injury, vena cava, inferior
    hip S75.90- ☑
      femoral artery — *see* Injury, blood vessel, femoral, artery
      femoral vein — *see* Injury, blood vessel, femoral, vein
      greater saphenous vein — *see* Injury, blood vessel, greater saphenous, hip level
      laceration S75.91- ☑
      specified
        site NEC S75.80- ☑
          laceration S75.81- ☑
          specified type NEC S75.89- ☑
        type NEC S75.99- ☑
    hypogastric (artery) (vein) — *see* Injury, blood vessel, iliac
    iliac S35.5- ☑
      artery S35.51- ☑
      specified vessel NEC S35.5- ☑
      uterine vessel — *see* Injury, blood vessel, uterine
      vein S35.51- ☑
    innominate — *see* Injury, blood vessel, thoracic, innominate
    intercostal (artery) (vein) — *see* Injury, blood vessel, thoracic, intercostal
    jugular vein (external) S15.20- ☑
      internal S15.30- ☑
        laceration (minor) (superficial) S15.31- ☑
          major S15.32- ☑
        specified type NEC S15.39- ☑
      laceration (minor) (superficial) S15.21- ☑
        major S15.22- ☑
      specified type NEC S15.29- ☑
    leg (level) (lower) S85.90- ☑
      greater saphenous — *see* Injury, blood vessel, greater saphenous
      laceration S85.91- ☑

Injury — *continued*
  blood vessel — *continued*
    leg — *continued*
      lesser saphenous — *see* Injury, blood vessel, lesser saphenous
      peroneal artery — *see* Injury, blood vessel, peroneal artery
      popliteal
        artery — *see* Injury, blood vessel, popliteal, artery
        vein — *see* Injury, blood vessel, popliteal, vein
      specified
        site NEC S85.80- ☑
          laceration S85.81- ☑
          specified type NEC S85.89- ☑
        type NEC S85.99- ☑
      thigh — *see* Injury, blood vessel, hip
      tibial artery — *see* Injury, blood vessel, tibial artery
    lesser saphenous vein (lower leg level) S85.40- ☑
      laceration S85.41- ☑
      specified type NEC S85.49- ☑
    limb
      lower — *see* Injury, blood vessel, leg
      upper — *see* Injury, blood vessel, arm
    lower back — *see* Injury, blood vessel, abdomen
      specified NEC — *see* Injury, blood vessel, abdomen, specified, site NEC
    mammary (artery) (vein) — *see* Injury, blood vessel, thoracic, specified site NEC
    mesenteric (inferior) (superior)
      artery — *see* Injury, mesenteric, artery
      vein — *see* Injury, blood vessel, mesenteric, vein
    neck S15.9 ☑
      specified site NEC S15.8 ☑
    ovarian (artery) (vein) — *see* subcategory S35.8 ☑
    palmar arch (superficial) S65.20- ☑
      deep S65.30- ☑
        laceration S65.31- ☑
        specified type NEC S65.39- ☑
      laceration S65.21- ☑
      specified type NEC S65.29- ☑
    pelvis — *see* Injury, blood vessel, abdomen
      specified NEC — *see* Injury, blood vessel, abdomen, specified, site NEC
    peroneal artery S85.20- ☑
      laceration S85.21- ☑
      specified type NEC S85.29- ☑
    plantar artery (deep) (foot) S95.10- ☑
      laceration S95.11- ☑
      specified type NEC S95.19- ☑
    popliteal
      artery S85.00- ☑
        laceration S85.01- ☑
        specified type NEC S85.09- ☑
      vein S85.50- ☑
        laceration S85.51- ☑
        specified type NEC S85.59- ☑
    portal vein S35.319 ☑
      laceration S35.311 ☑
      specified type NEC S35.318 ☑
    precerebral — *see* Injury, blood vessel, neck
    pulmonary — *see* Injury, blood vessel, thoracic, pulmonary
    radial artery (forearm level) S55.10- ☑
      hand and wrist (level) S65.10- ☑
        laceration S65.11- ☑
        specified type NEC S65.19- ☑
      laceration S55.11- ☑
      specified type NEC S55.19- ☑
    renal
      artery S35.40- ☑
        laceration S35.41- ☑
        specified NEC S35.49- ☑
      vein S35.40- ☑
        laceration S35.41- ☑
        specified NEC S35.49- ☑
    saphenous vein (greater) (lower leg level) — *see* Injury, blood vessel, greater saphenous
      hip and thigh level — *see* Injury, blood vessel, greater saphenous, hip level
      lesser — *see* Injury, blood vessel, lesser saphenous
    shoulder
      specified NEC — *see* Injury, blood vessel, arm, specified site NEC

Injury — *continued*
  blood vessel — *continued*
    shoulder — *continued*
      superficial vein — *see* Injury, blood vessel, arm, superficial vein
    specified NEC T14.8 ☑
    splenic
      artery — *see* Injury, blood vessel, celiac artery, branch
      vein S35.329 ☑
        laceration S35.321 ☑
        specified NEC S35.328 ☑
    subclavian — *see* Injury, blood vessel, thoracic, innominate
    thigh — *see* Injury, blood vessel, hip
    thoracic S25.90 ☑
      aorta S25.00 ☑
        laceration (minor) (superficial) S25.01 ☑
          major S25.02 ☑
        specified type NEC S25.09 ☑
      azygos vein — *see* Injury, blood vessel, thoracic, specified, site NEC
      innominate
        artery S25.10- ☑
          laceration (minor) (superficial) S25.11- ☑
            major S25.12- ☑
          specified type NEC S25.19- ☑
        vein S25.30- ☑
          laceration (minor) (superficial) S25.31- ☑
            major S25.32- ☑
          specified type NEC S25.39- ☑
      intercostal S25.50- ☑
        laceration S25.51- ☑
        specified type NEC S25.59- ☑
      laceration S25.91 ☑
      mammary vessel — *see* Injury, blood vessel, thoracic, specified, site NEC
      pulmonary S25.40- ☑
        laceration (minor) (superficial) S25.41- ☑
          major S25.42- ☑
        specified type NEC S25.49- ☑
      specified
        site NEC S25.80- ☑
          laceration S25.81 ☑
          specified type NEC S25.89 ☑
        type NEC S25.99 ☑
      subclavian — *see* Injury, blood vessel, thoracic, innominate
      vena cava (superior) S25.20 ☑
        laceration (minor) (superficial) S25.21 ☑
          major S25.22 ☑
        specified type NEC S25.29 ☑
    thumb S65.40- ☑
      laceration S65.41- ☑
      specified type NEC S65.49- ☑
    tibial artery S85.10- ☑
      anterior S85.13- ☑
        laceration S85.14- ☑
        specified injury NEC S85.15- ☑
      laceration S85.11- ☑
      posterior S85.16- ☑
        laceration S85.17- ☑
        specified injury NEC S85.18- ☑
      specified injury NEC S85.12- ☑
    ulnar artery (forearm level) S55.00- ☑
      hand and wrist (level) S65.00- ☑
        laceration S65.01- ☑
        specified type NEC S65.09- ☑
      laceration S55.01- ☑
      specified type NEC S55.09- ☑
    upper arm (level) — *see* Injury, blood vessel, arm
      superficial vein — *see* Injury, blood vessel, arm, superficial vein
    uterine S35.5- ☑
      artery S35.53- ☑
      vein S35.53- ☑
    vena cava — *see* Injury, vena cava
    vertebral artery S15.10- ☑
      laceration (minor) (superficial) S15.11- ☑
        major S15.12- ☑
      specified type NEC S15.19- ☑
    wrist (level) — *see* Injury, blood vessel, hand
  brachial plexus S14.3 ☑
    newborn P14.3
  brain (traumatic) S06.9- ☑
    diffuse (axonal) S06.2X- ☑

Injury — *continued*
  brain — *continued*
    focal S06.30- ☑
  brainstem S06.38- ☑
  breast NOS S29.9 ☑
  broad ligament — *see* Injury, pelvic organ, specified site NEC
  bronchus, bronchi — *see* Injury, intrathoracic, bronchus
  brow S09.90 ☑
  buttock S39.92 ☑
  canthus, eye S05.90 ☑
  cardiac plexus — *see* Injury, nerve, thorax, sympathetic
  cauda equina S34.3 ☑
  cavernous sinus — *see* Injury, intracranial
  cecum — *see* Injury, colon
  celiac ganglion or plexus — *see* Injury, nerve, lumbosacral, sympathetic
  cerebellum — *see* Injury, intracranial
  cerebral — *see* Injury, intracranial
  cervix (uteri) — *see* Injury, uterus
  cheek (wall) S09.93 ☑
  chest — *see* Injury, thorax
  childbirth (newborn) — *see also* Birth, injury
    maternal NEC O71.9
  chin S09.93 ☑
  choroid (eye) — *see* Injury, eye, specified site NEC
  clitoris S39.94 ☑
  coccyx — *see also* Injury, back, lower
    complicating delivery O71.6
  colon — *see* Injury, intestine, large
  common bile duct — *see* Injury, liver
  conjunctiva (superficial) — *see* Injury, eye, conjunctiva
  conus medullaris — *see* Injury, spinal, sacral
  cord
    spermatic (pelvic region) S37.898 ☑
      scrotal region S39.848 ☑
    spinal — *see* Injury, spinal cord, by region
  cornea — *see* Injury, eye, specified site NEC
    abrasion — *see* Injury, eye, cornea, abrasion
  cortex (cerebral) — *see also* Injury, intracranial
    visual — *see* Injury, nerve, optic
  costal region NEC S29.9 ☑
  costochondral NEC S29.9 ☑
  cranial
    cavity — *see* Injury, intracranial
    nerve — *see* Injury, nerve, cranial
  crushing — *see* Crush
  cutaneous sensory nerve
  cystic duct — *see* Injury, liver
  deep tissue — *see* Contusion, by site
    meaning pressure ulcer — *see* Ulcer, pressure L89 with final character .6
  delivery (newborn) P15.9
    maternal NEC O71.9
  Descemet's membrane — *see* Injury, eyeball, penetrating
  diaphragm — *see* Injury, intrathoracic, diaphragm
  duodenum — *see* Injury, intestine, small, duodenum
  ear (auricle) (external) (canal) S09.91 ☑
    abrasion — *see* Abrasion, ear
    bite — *see* Bite, ear
    blister — *see* Blister, ear
    bruise — *see* Contusion, ear
    contusion — *see* Contusion, ear
    external constriction — *see* Constriction, external, ear
    hematoma — *see* Hematoma, ear
    inner — *see* Injury, ear, middle
    laceration — *see* Laceration, ear
    middle S09.30- ☑
      blast — *see* Injury, blast, ear
      specified NEC S09.39- ☑
    puncture — *see* Puncture, ear
    superficial — *see* Injury, superficial, ear
  eighth cranial nerve (acoustic or auditory) — *see* Injury, nerve, acoustic
  elbow S59.90- ☑
    contusion — *see* Contusion, elbow
    dislocation — *see* Dislocation, elbow
    fracture — *see* Fracture, ulna, upper end
    open — *see* Wound, open, elbow
    specified NEC S59.80- ☑
    sprain — *see* Sprain, elbow
    superficial — *see* Injury, superficial, elbow
  eleventh cranial nerve (accessory) — *see* Injury, nerve, accessory

Injury — *continued*
  epididymis S39.94 ☑
  epigastric region S39.91 ☑
  epiglottis NEC S19.89 ☑
  esophageal plexus — *see* Injury, nerve, thorax, sympathetic
  esophagus (thoracic part) — *see also* Injury, intrathoracic, esophagus
    cervical NEC S19.85 ☑
  eustachian tube S09.30 ☑
  eye S05.9- ☑
    avulsion S05.7- ☑
    ball — *see* Injury, eyeball
    conjunctiva S05.0- ☑
    cornea
      abrasion S05.0- ☑
      laceration S05.3- ☑
        with prolapse S05.2- ☑
    lacrimal apparatus S05.8X- ☑
    orbit penetration S05.4- ☑
    specified site NEC S05.8X- ☑
  eyeball S05.8X- ☑
    contusion S05.1- ☑
    penetrating S05.6- ☑
      with
        foreign body S05.5- ☑
        prolapse or loss of intraocular tissue S05.2- ☑
      without prolapse or loss of intraocular tissue S05.3- ☑
    specified type NEC S05.8- ☑
  eyebrow S09.93 ☑
  eyelid S09.93 ☑
    abrasion — *see* Abrasion, eyelid
    contusion — *see* Contusion, eyelid
    open — *see* Wound, open, eyelid
  face S09.93 ☑
  fallopian tube S37.509 ☑
    bilateral S37.502 ☑
      blast injury S37.512 ☑
      contusion S37.522 ☑
      laceration S37.532 ☑
      specified type NEC S37.592 ☑
    blast injury (primary) S37.519 ☑
      bilateral S37.512 ☑
      secondary — *see* Injury, fallopian tube, specified type NEC
      unilateral S37.511 ☑
    contusion S37.529 ☑
      bilateral S37.522 ☑
      unilateral S37.521 ☑
    laceration S37.539 ☑
      bilateral S37.532 ☑
      unilateral S37.531 ☑
    specified type NEC S37.599 ☑
      bilateral S37.592 ☑
      unilateral S37.591 ☑
    unilateral S37.501 ☑
      blast injury S37.511 ☑
      contusion S37.521 ☑
      laceration S37.531 ☑
      specified type NEC S37.591 ☑
  fascia — *see* Injury, muscle
  fifth cranial nerve (trigeminal) — *see* Injury, nerve, trigeminal
  finger (nail) S69.9- ☑
    blood vessel — *see* Injury, blood vessel, finger
    contusion — *see* Contusion, finger
    dislocation — *see* Dislocation, finger
    fracture — *see* Fracture, finger
    muscle — *see* Injury, muscle, finger
    nerve — *see* Injury, nerve, digital, finger
    open — *see* Wound, open, finger
    specified NEC S69.8- ☑
    sprain — *see* Sprain, finger
    superficial — *see* Injury, superficial, finger
  first cranial nerve (olfactory) — *see* Injury, nerve, olfactory
  flank — *see* Injury, abdomen
  foot S99.92- ☑
    blood vessel — *see* Injury, blood vessel, foot
    contusion — *see* Contusion, foot
    dislocation — *see* Dislocation, foot
    fracture — *see* Fracture, foot
    muscle — *see* Injury, muscle, foot
    open — *see* Wound, open, foot
    specified type NEC S99.82- ☑

Injury — *continued*
  foot — *continued*
    sprain — *see* Sprain, foot
    superficial — *see* Injury, superficial, foot
  forceps NOS P15.9
  forearm S59.91- ☑
    blood vessel — *see* Injury, blood vessel, forearm
    contusion — *see* Contusion, forearm
    fracture — *see* Fracture, forearm
    muscle — *see* Injury, muscle, forearm
    nerve — *see* Injury, nerve, forearm
    open — *see* Wound, open, forearm
    specified NEC S59.81- ☑
    superficial — *see* Injury, superficial, forearm
  forehead S09.90 ☑
  fourth cranial nerve (trochlear) — *see* Injury, nerve, trochlear
  gallbladder S36.129 ☑
    contusion S36.122 ☑
    laceration S36.123 ☑
    specified NEC S36.128 ☑
  ganglion
    celiac, coeliac — *see* Injury, nerve, lumbosacral, sympathetic
    gasserian — *see* Injury, nerve, trigeminal
    stellate — *see* Injury, nerve, thorax, sympathetic
    thoracic sympathetic — *see* Injury, nerve, thorax, sympathetic
  gasserian ganglion — *see* Injury, nerve, trigeminal
  gastric artery — *see* Injury, blood vessel, celiac artery, branch
  gastroduodenal artery — *see* Injury, blood vessel, celiac artery, branch
  gastrointestinal tract — *see* Injury, intra-abdominal
    with open wound into abdominal cavity — *see* Wound, open, with penetration into peritoneal cavity
    colon — *see* Injury, intestine, large
    rectum — *see* Injury, intestine, large, rectum
      with open wound into abdominal cavity S36.61 ☑
    small intestine — *see* Injury, intestine, small
    specified site NEC — *see* Injury, intra-abdominal, specified, site NEC
    stomach — *see* Injury, stomach
  genital organ(s)
    external S39.94 ☑
      specified NEC S39.848 ☑
    internal S37.90 ☑
      fallopian tube — *see* Injury, fallopian tube
      ovary — *see* Injury, ovary
      prostate — *see* Injury, prostate
      seminal vesicle — *see* Injury, pelvis, organ, specified site NEC
      uterus — *see* Injury, uterus
      vas deferens — *see* Injury, pelvis, organ, specified site NEC
    obstetrical trauma O71.9
  gland
    lacrimal laceration — *see* Injury, eye, specified site NEC
    salivary S09.93 ☑
    thyroid NEC S19.84 ☑
  globe (eye) S05.90 ☑
    specified NEC S05.8X- ☑
  groin — *see* Injury, abdomen
  gum S09.90 ☑
  hand S69.9- ☑
    blood vessel — *see* Injury, blood vessel, hand
    contusion — *see* Contusion, hand
    fracture — *see* Fracture, hand
    muscle — *see* Injury, muscle, hand
    nerve — *see* Injury, nerve, hand
    open — *see* Wound, open, hand
    specified NEC S69.8- ☑
    sprain — *see* Sprain, hand
    superficial — *see* Injury, superficial, hand
  head S09.90 ☑
    with loss of consciousness S06.9- ☑
    specified NEC S09.8 ☑
  heart (traumatic) S26.90 ☑
    with hemopericardium S26.00 ☑
      contusion S26.01 ☑
      laceration (mild) S26.020 ☑
        major S26.022 ☑
        moderate S26.021 ☑

Injury — *continued*
  heart — *continued*
    with hemopericardium — *continued*
      specified type NEC S26.09 ☑
    contusion S26.91 ☑
    laceration S26.92 ☑
    non-traumatic (acute) (chronic) (non-ischemic) I5A
    specified type NEC S26.99 ☑
    without hemopericardium S26.10 ☑
      contusion S26.11 ☑
      laceration S26.12 ☑
      specified type NEC S26.19 ☑
  heel — *see* Injury, foot
  hepatic
    artery — *see* Injury, blood vessel, celiac artery, branch
    duct — *see* Injury, liver
    vein — *see* Injury, vena cava, inferior
  hip S79.91- ☑
    blood vessel — *see* Injury, blood vessel, hip
    contusion — *see* Contusion, hip
    dislocation — *see* Dislocation, hip
    fracture — *see* Fracture, femur, neck
    muscle — *see* Injury, muscle, hip
    nerve — *see* Injury, nerve, hip
    open — *see* Wound, open, hip
    specified NEC S79.81- ☑
    sprain — *see* Sprain, hip
    superficial — *see* Injury, superficial, hip
  hymen S39.94 ☑
  hypogastric
    blood vessel — *see* Injury, blood vessel, iliac
    plexus — *see* Injury, nerve, lumbosacral, sympathetic
  ileum — *see* Injury, intestine, small
  iliac region S39.91 ☑
  instrumental (during surgery) — *see* Laceration, accidental complicating surgery
    birth injury — *see* Birth, injury
    nonsurgical — *see* Injury, by site
    obstetrical O71.9
      bladder O71.5
      cervix O71.3
      high vaginal O71.4
      perineal NOS O70.9
      urethra O71.5
      uterus O71.5
        with rupture or perforation O71.1
  internal T14.8 ☑
    aorta — *see* Injury, aorta
    bladder (sphincter) — *see* Injury, bladder
      with
        ectopic or molar pregnancy O08.6
        following ectopic or molar pregnancy O08.6
        obstetrical trauma O71.5
    bronchus, bronchi — *see* Injury, intrathoracic, bronchus
    cecum — *see* Injury, intestine, large
    cervix (uteri) — *see also* Injury, uterus
      with ectopic or molar pregnancy O08.6
      following ectopic or molar pregnancy O08.6
      obstetrical trauma O71.3
    chest — *see* Injury, intrathoracic
    gastrointestinal tract — *see* Injury, intra-abdominal
    heart — *see* Injury, heart
    intestine NEC — *see* Injury, intestine
    intrauterine — *see* Injury, uterus
    mesentery — *see* Injury, intra-abdominal, specified, site NEC
    pelvis, pelvic (organ) S37.90 ☑
      following ectopic or molar pregnancy (subsequent episode) O08.6
      obstetrical trauma NEC O71.5
        rupture or perforation O71.1
      specified NEC S39.83 ☑
    rectum — *see* Injury, intestine, large, rectum
    stomach — *see* Injury, stomach
    ureter — *see* Injury, ureter
    urethra (sphincter) following ectopic or molar pregnancy O08.6
    uterus — *see* Injury, uterus
  interscapular area — *see* Injury, thorax
  intestine
    large S36.509 ☑
      ascending (right) S36.500 ☑
        blast injury (primary) S36.510 ☑
          secondary S36.590 ☑

Injury — *continued*
  intestine — *continued*
    large — *continued*
      ascending — *continued*
        contusion S36.520 ☑
        laceration S36.530 ☑
        specified type NEC S36.590 ☑
      blast injury (primary) S36.519 ☑
        ascending (right) S36.510 ☑
        descending (left) S36.512 ☑
        rectum S36.61 ☑
        sigmoid S36.513 ☑
        specified site NEC S36.518 ☑
        transverse S36.511 ☑
      contusion S36.529 ☑
        ascending (right) S36.520 ☑
        descending (left) S36.522 ☑
        rectum S36.62 ☑
        sigmoid S36.523 ☑
        specified site NEC S36.528 ☑
        transverse S36.521 ☑
      descending (left) S36.502 ☑
        blast injury (primary) S36.512 ☑
          secondary S36.592 ☑
        contusion S36.522 ☑
        laceration S36.532 ☑
        specified type NEC S36.592 ☑
      laceration S36.539 ☑
        ascending (right) S36.530 ☑
        descending (left) S36.532 ☑
        rectum S36.63 ☑
        sigmoid S36.533 ☑
        specified site NEC S36.538 ☑
        transverse S36.531 ☑
      rectum S36.60 ☑
        blast injury (primary) S36.61 ☑
          secondary S36.69 ☑
        contusion S36.62 ☑
        laceration S36.63 ☑
        specified type NEC S36.69 ☑
      sigmoid S36.503 ☑
        blast injury (primary) S36.513 ☑
          secondary S36.593 ☑
        contusion S36.523 ☑
        laceration S36.533 ☑
        specified type NEC S36.593 ☑
      specified
        site NEC S36.508 ☑
          blast injury (primary) S36.518 ☑
            secondary S36.598 ☑
          contusion S36.528 ☑
          laceration S36.538 ☑
          specified type NEC S36.598 ☑
        type NEC S36.599 ☑
          ascending (right) S36.590 ☑
          descending (left) S36.592 ☑
          rectum S36.69 ☑
          sigmoid S36.593 ☑
          specified site NEC S36.598 ☑
          transverse S36.591 ☑
      transverse S36.501 ☑
        blast injury (primary) S36.511 ☑
          secondary S36.591 ☑
        contusion S36.521 ☑
        laceration S36.531 ☑
        specified type NEC S36.591 ☑
    small S36.409 ☑
      blast injury (primary) S36.419 ☑
        duodenum S36.410 ☑
          secondary S36.499 ☑
            duodenum S36.490 ☑
            specified site NEC S36.498 ☑
          specified site NEC S36.418 ☑
      contusion S36.429 ☑
        duodenum S36.420 ☑
        specified site NEC S36.428 ☑
      duodenum S36.400 ☑
        blast injury (primary) S36.410 ☑
          secondary S36.490 ☑
        contusion S36.420 ☑
        laceration S36.430 ☑
        specified NEC S36.490 ☑
      laceration S36.439 ☑
        duodenum S36.430 ☑
        specified site NEC S36.438 ☑

Injury — *continued*
  intestine — *continued*
    small — *continued*
      specified
        site NEC S36.408 ☑
        type NEC S36.499 ☑
          duodenum S36.490 ☑
          specified site NEC S36.498 ☑
  intra-abdominal S36.90 ☑
    adrenal gland — *see* Injury, adrenal gland
    bladder — *see* Injury, bladder
    colon — *see* Injury, intestine, large
    contusion S36.92 ☑
    fallopian tube — *see* Injury, fallopian tube
    gallbladder — *see* Injury, gallbladder
    intestine — *see* Injury, intestine
    kidney — *see* Injury, kidney
    laceration S36.93 ☑
    liver — *see* Injury, liver
    ovary — *see* Injury, ovary
    pancreas — *see* Injury, pancreas
    pelvic NOS S37.90 ☑
    peritoneum — *see* Injury, intra-abdominal, specified, site NEC
    prostate — *see* Injury, prostate
    rectum — *see* Injury, intestine, large, rectum
    retroperitoneum — *see* Injury, intra-abdominal, specified, site NEC
    seminal vesicle — *see* Injury, pelvis, organ, specified site NEC
    small intestine — *see* Injury, intestine, small
    specified
      pelvic S37.90 ☑
        specified
          site NEC S37.899 ☑
            specified type NEC S37.898 ☑
          type NEC S37.99 ☑
      site NEC S36.899 ☑
        contusion S36.892 ☑
        laceration S36.893 ☑
        specified type NEC S36.898 ☑
      type NEC S36.99 ☑
    spleen — *see* Injury, spleen
    stomach — *see* Injury, stomach
    ureter — *see* Injury, ureter
    urethra — *see* Injury, urethra
    uterus — *see* Injury, uterus
    vas deferens — *see* Injury, pelvis, organ, specified site NEC
  intracranial (traumatic) — *see also* if applicable, Compression, brain, traumatic S06.9- ☑
    cerebellar hemorrhage, traumatic — *see* Injury, intracranial, focal
    cerebral edema, traumatic S06.1X- ☑
      diffuse S06.1X- ☑
      focal S06.1X- ☑
    diffuse (axonal) S06.2X- ☑
    epidural hemorrhage (traumatic) S06.4X- ☑
    focal brain injury S06.30- ☑
      contusion — *see* Contusion, cerebral
      laceration — *see* Laceration, cerebral
      intracerebral hemorrhage, traumatic S06.36- ☑
        left side S06.35- ☑
        right side S06.34- ☑
      specified NEC S06.89- ☑
    subarachnoid hemorrhage, traumatic S06.6X- ☑
    subdural hemorrhage, traumatic S06.5X- ☑
  intraocular — *see* Injury, eyeball, penetrating
  intrathoracic S27.9 ☑
    bronchus S27.409 ☑
      bilateral S27.402 ☑
      blast injury (primary) S27.419 ☑
        bilateral S27.412 ☑
          secondary — *see* Injury, intrathoracic, bronchus, specified type NEC
        unilateral S27.411 ☑
      contusion S27.429 ☑
        bilateral S27.422 ☑
        unilateral S27.421 ☑
      laceration S27.439 ☑
        bilateral S27.432 ☑
        unilateral S27.431 ☑
      specified type NEC S27.499 ☑
        bilateral S27.492 ☑
        unilateral S27.491 ☑
      unilateral S27.401 ☑

Injury — *continued*
  intrathoracic — *continued*
    diaphragm S27.809 ☑
      contusion S27.802 ☑
      laceration S27.803 ☑
      specified type NEC S27.808 ☑
    esophagus (thoracic) S27.819 ☑
      contusion S27.812 ☑
      laceration S27.813 ☑
      specified type NEC S27.818 ☑
    heart — *see* Injury, heart
    hemopneumothorax S27.2
    hemothorax S27.1 ☑
    lung S27.309 ☑
      aspiration J69.0
      bilateral S27.302 ☑
      blast injury (primary) S27.319 ☑
        bilateral S27.312 ☑
        secondary — *see* Injury, intrathoracic, lung, specified type NEC
        unilateral S27.311 ☑
      contusion S27.329 ☑
        bilateral S27.322 ☑
        unilateral S27.321 ☑
      laceration S27.339 ☑
        bilateral S27.332 ☑
        unilateral S27.331 ☑
      specified type NEC S27.399 ☑
        bilateral S27.392 ☑
        unilateral S27.391 ☑
      unilateral S27.301 ☑
    pleura S27.60 ☑
      laceration S27.63 ☑
      specified type NEC S27.69 ☑
    pneumothorax S27.0 ☑
    specified organ NEC S27.899 ☑
      contusion S27.892 ☑
      laceration S27.893 ☑
      specified type NEC S27.898 ☑
    thoracic duct — *see* Injury, intrathoracic, specified organ NEC
    thymus gland — *see* Injury, intrathoracic, specified organ NEC
    trachea, thoracic S27.50 ☑
      blast (primary) S27.51 ☑
      contusion S27.52 ☑
      laceration S27.53 ☑
      specified type NEC S27.59 ☑
  iris — *see* Injury, eye, specified site NEC
    penetrating — *see* Injury, eyeball, penetrating
  jaw S09.93 ☑
  jejunum — *see* Injury, intestine, small
  joint NOS T14.8 ☑
    old or residual — *see* Disorder, joint, specified type NEC
  kidney S37.00- ☑
    acute (nontraumatic) N17.9
    contusion — *see* Contusion, kidney
    laceration — *see* Laceration, kidney
    specified NEC S37.09- ☑
  knee S89.9- ☑
    contusion — *see* Contusion, knee
    dislocation — *see* Dislocation, knee
    meniscus (lateral) (medial) — *see* Sprain, knee, specified site NEC
      old injury or tear — *see* Derangement, knee, meniscus, due to old injury
    open — *see* Wound, open, knee
    specified NEC S89.8- ☑
    sprain — *see* Sprain, knee
    superficial — *see* Injury, superficial, knee
  labium (majus) (minus) S39.94 ☑
  labyrinth, ear S09.30- ☑
  lacrimal apparatus, duct, gland, or sac — *see* Injury, eye, specified site NEC
  larynx NEC S19.81 ☑
  leg (lower) S89.9- ☑
    blood vessel — *see* Injury, blood vessel, leg
    contusion — *see* Contusion, leg
    fracture — *see* Fracture, leg
    muscle — *see* Injury, muscle, leg
    nerve — *see* Injury, nerve, leg
    open — *see* Wound, open, leg
    specified NEC S89.8- ☑
    superficial — *see* Injury, superficial, leg
  lens, eye — *see* Injury, eye, specified site NEC

Injury — *continued*
  lens, eye — *see* Injury, eye, specified site — *continued*
    penetrating — *see* Injury, eyeball, penetrating
  limb NEC T14.8 ☑
  lip S09.93 ☑
  liver S36.119 ☑
    contusion S36.112 ☑
    laceration S36.113 ☑
      major (stellate) S36.116 ☑
      minor S36.114 ☑
      moderate S36.115 ☑
    specified NEC S36.118 ☑
  lower back S39.92 ☑
    specified NEC S39.82 ☑
  lumbar, lumbosacral (region) S39.92 ☑
    plexus — *see* Injury, lumbosacral plexus
  lumbosacral plexus S34.4 ☑
  lung — *see also* Injury, intrathoracic, lung
    aspiration J69.0
    dabbing (related) U07.0
    electronic cigarette (related) U07.0
    EVALI - [e-cigarette, or vaping, product use associated] U07.0
    transfusion-related (TRALI) J95.84
    vaping (associated) (device) (product) (use) U07.0
  lymphatic thoracic duct — *see* Injury, intrathoracic, specified organ NEC
  malar region S09.93 ☑
  mastoid region S09.90 ☑
  maxilla S09.93 ☑
  mediastinum — *see* Injury, intrathoracic, specified organ NEC
  membrane, brain — *see* Injury, intracranial
  meningeal artery — *see* Injury, intracranial, subdural hemorrhage
  meninges (cerebral) — *see* Injury, intracranial
  mesenteric
    artery
      branch S35.299 ☑
        laceration (minor) (superficial) S35.291 ☑
          major S35.292 ☑
        specified NEC S35.298 ☑
      inferior S35.239 ☑
        laceration (minor) (superficial) S35.231 ☑
          major S35.232 ☑
        specified NEC S35.238 ☑
      superior S35.229 ☑
        laceration (minor) (superficial) S35.221 ☑
          major S35.222 ☑
        specified NEC S35.228 ☑
      plexus (inferior) (superior) — *see* Injury, nerve, lumbosacral, sympathetic
    vein
      inferior S35.349 ☑
        laceration S35.341 ☑
        specified NEC S35.348 ☑
      superior S35.339 ☑
        laceration S35.331 ☑
        specified NEC S35.338 ☑
  mesentery — *see* Injury, intra-abdominal, specified site NEC
  mesosalpinx — *see* Injury, pelvic organ, specified site NEC
  middle ear S09.30- ☑
  midthoracic region NOS S29.9 ☑
  mouth S09.93 ☑
  multiple NOS T07 ☑
  muscle (and fascia) (and tendon)
    abdomen S39.001 ☑
      laceration S39.021 ☑
      specified type NEC S39.091 ☑
      strain S39.011 ☑
    abductor
      thumb, forearm level — *see* Injury, muscle, thumb, abductor
    adductor
      thigh S76.20- ☑
        laceration S76.22- ☑
        specified type NEC S76.29- ☑
        strain S76.21- ☑
    ankle — *see* Injury, muscle, foot
    anterior muscle group, at leg level (lower) S86.20- ☑
      laceration S86.22- ☑
      specified type NEC S86.29- ☑
      strain S86.21- ☑

Injury — *continued*
  muscle — *continued*
    arm (upper) — *see* Injury, muscle, shoulder
    biceps (parts NEC) S46.20- ☑
      laceration S46.22- ☑
      long head S46.10- ☑
        laceration S46.12- ☑
        specified type NEC S46.19- ☑
        strain S46.11- ☑
      specified type NEC S46.29- ☑
      strain S46.21- ☑
    extensor
      finger(s) (other than thumb) — *see* Injury, muscle, finger by site, extensor
      forearm level, specified NEC — *see* Injury, muscle, forearm, extensor
      thumb — *see* Injury, muscle, thumb, extensor
      toe (large) (ankle level) (foot level) — *see* Injury, muscle, toe, extensor
    finger
      extensor (forearm level) S56.40- ☑
        hand level S66.309 ☑
          laceration S66.329 ☑
          specified type NEC S66.399 ☑
          strain S66.319 ☑
        laceration S56.429 ☑
        specified type NEC S56.499 ☑
        strain S56.419 ☑
      flexor (forearm level) S56.10- ☑
        hand level S66.109 ☑
          laceration S66.129 ☑
          specified type NEC S66.199 ☑
          strain S66.119 ☑
        laceration S56.129 ☑
        specified type NEC S56.199 ☑
        strain S56.119 ☑
      index
        extensor (forearm level)
          hand level S66.308 ☑
            laceration S66.32- ☑
            specified type NEC S66.39- ☑
            strain S66.31- ☑
          specified type NEC S56.492 ☑
        flexor (forearm level)
          hand level S66.108 ☑
            laceration S66.12- ☑
            specified type NEC S66.19- ☑
            strain S66.11- ☑
          specified type NEC S56.19- ☑
          strain S56.11- ☑
        intrinsic S66.50- ☑
          laceration S66.52- ☑
          specified type NEC S66.59- ☑
          strain S66.51- ☑
      intrinsic S66.509 ☑
        laceration S66.529 ☑
        specified type NEC S66.599 ☑
        strain S66.519 ☑
      little
        extensor (forearm level)
          hand level S66.30- ☑
            laceration S66.32- ☑
            specified type NEC S66.39- ☑
            strain S66.31- ☑
          laceration S56.42- ☑
          specified type NEC S56.49- ☑
          strain S56.41- ☑
        flexor (forearm level)
          hand level S66.10- ☑
            laceration S66.12- ☑
            specified type NEC S66.19- ☑
            strain S66.11- ☑
          laceration S56.12- ☑
          specified type NEC S56.19- ☑
          strain S56.11- ☑
        intrinsic S66.50- ☑
          laceration S66.52- ☑
          specified type NEC S66.59- ☑
          strain S66.51- ☑
      middle
        extensor (forearm level)
          hand level S66.30- ☑
            laceration S66.32- ☑
            specified type NEC S66.39- ☑
            strain S66.31- ☑
          laceration S56.42- ☑

☑ **Additional Character Required — Refer to the Tabular List for Character Selection**

Injury — *continued*
  muscle — *continued*
    finger — *continued*
      middle — *continued*
        extensor — *continued*
          specified type NEC S56.49- ☑
          strain S56.41- ☑
        flexor (forearm level)
          hand level S66.10- ☑
            laceration S66.12- ☑
            specified type NEC S66.19- ☑
            strain S66.11- ☑
          laceration S56.12- ☑
          specified type NEC S56.19- ☑
          strain S56.11- ☑
        intrinsic S66.50- ☑
          laceration S66.52- ☑
          specified type NEC S66.59- ☑
          strain S66.51- ☑
      ring
        extensor (forearm level)
          hand level S66.30- ☑
            laceration S66.32- ☑
            specified type NEC S66.39- ☑
            strain S66.31- ☑
          laceration S56.42- ☑
          specified type NEC S56.49- ☑
          strain S56.41- ☑
        flexor (forearm level)
          hand level S66.10- ☑
            laceration S66.12- ☑
            specified type NEC S66.19- ☑
            strain S66.11- ☑
          laceration S56.12- ☑
          specified type NEC S56.19- ☑
          strain S56.11- ☑
        intrinsic S66.50- ☑
          laceration S66.52- ☑
          specified type NEC S66.59- ☑
          strain S66.51- ☑
    flexor
      finger(s) (other than thumb) — *see* Injury, muscle, finger
      forearm level, specified NEC — *see* Injury, muscle, forearm, flexor
      thumb — *see* Injury, muscle, thumb, flexor
      toe (long) (ankle level) (foot level) — *see* Injury, muscle, toe, flexor
    foot S96.90- ☑
      intrinsic S96.20- ☑
        laceration S96.22- ☑
        specified type NEC S96.29- ☑
        strain S96.21- ☑
      laceration S96.92- ☑
      long extensor, toe — *see* Injury, muscle, toe, extensor
      long flexor, toe — *see* Injury, muscle, toe, flexor
      specified
        site NEC S96.80- ☑
          laceration S96.82- ☑
          specified type NEC S96.89- ☑
          strain S96.81- ☑
        type S96.99- ☑
      strain S96.91- ☑
    forearm (level) S56.90- ☑
      extensor S56.50- ☑
        laceration S56.52- ☑
        specified type NEC S56.59- ☑
        strain S56.51- ☑
      flexor S56.20- ☑
        laceration S56.22- ☑
        specified type NEC S56.29- ☑
        strain S56.21- ☑
      laceration S56.92- ☑
      specified S56.99- ☑
        site NEC S56.80- ☑
          laceration S56.82- ☑
          strain S56.81- ☑
          type NEC S56.89- ☑
      strain S56.91- ☑
    hand (level) S66.90- ☑
      laceration S66.92- ☑
      specified
        site NEC S66.80- ☑
          laceration S66.82- ☑
          specified type NEC S66.89- ☑

Injury — *continued*
  muscle — *continued*
    hand — *continued*
      specified — *continued*
        site — *continued*
          strain S66.81- ☑
          type NEC S66.99- ☑
      strain S66.91- ☑
    head S09.10 ☑
      laceration S09.12 ☑
      specified type NEC S09.19 ☑
      strain S09.11 ☑
    hip NEC S76.00- ☑
      laceration S76.02- ☑
      specified type NEC S76.09- ☑
      strain S76.01- ☑
    intrinsic
      ankle and foot level — *see* Injury, muscle, foot, intrinsic
      finger (other than thumb) — *see* Injury, muscle, finger by site, intrinsic
      foot (level) — *see* Injury, muscle, foot, intrinsic
      thumb — *see* Injury, muscle, thumb, intrinsic
    leg (level) (lower) S86.90- ☑
      Achilles tendon — *see* Injury, Achilles tendon
      anterior muscle group — *see* Injury, muscle, anterior muscle group
      laceration S86.92- ☑
      peroneal muscle group — *see* Injury, muscle, peroneal muscle group
      posterior muscle group — *see* Injury, muscle, posterior muscle group, leg level
      specified
        site NEC S86.80- ☑
          laceration S86.82- ☑
          specified type NEC S86.89- ☑
          strain S86.81- ☑
        type NEC S86.99- ☑
      strain S86.91- ☑
    long
      extensor toe, at ankle and foot level — *see* Injury, muscle, toe, extensor
      flexor, toe, at ankle and foot level — *see* Injury, muscle, toe, flexor
      head, biceps — *see* Injury, muscle, biceps, long head
    lower back S39.002 ☑
      laceration S39.022 ☑
      specified type NEC S39.092 ☑
      strain S39.012 ☑
    neck (level) S16.9 ☑
      laceration S16.2 ☑
      specified type NEC S16.8 ☑
      strain S16.1 ☑
    pelvis S39.003 ☑
      laceration S39.023 ☑
      specified type NEC S39.093 ☑
      strain S39.013 ☑
    peroneal muscle group, at leg level (lower) S86.30- ☑
      laceration S86.32- ☑
      specified type NEC S86.39- ☑
      strain S86.31- ☑
    posterior muscle (group)
      leg level (lower) S86.10- ☑
        laceration S86.12- ☑
        specified type NEC S86.19- ☑
        strain S86.11- ☑
      thigh level S76.30- ☑
        laceration S76.32- ☑
        specified type NEC S76.39- ☑
        strain S76.31- ☑
    quadriceps (thigh) S76.10- ☑
      laceration S76.12- ☑
      specified type NEC S76.19- ☑
      strain S76.11- ☑
    shoulder S46.90- ☑
      laceration S46.92- ☑
      rotator cuff — *see* Injury, rotator cuff
      specified site NEC S46.80- ☑
        laceration S46.82- ☑
        specified type NEC S46.89- ☑
        strain S46.81- ☑
      specified type NEC S46.99- ☑
      strain S46.91- ☑
    thigh NEC (level) S76.90- ☑

Injury — *continued*
  muscle — *continued*
    thigh — *continued*
      adductor — *see* Injury, muscle, adductor, thigh
      laceration S76.92- ☑
      posterior muscle (group) — *see* Injury, muscle, posterior muscle, thigh level
      quadriceps — *see* Injury, muscle, quadriceps
      specified
        site NEC S76.80- ☑
          laceration S76.82- ☑
          specified type NEC S76.89- ☑
          strain S76.81- ☑
        type NEC S76.99- ☑
      strain S76.91- ☑
    thorax (level) S29.009 ☑
      back wall S29.002 ☑
      front wall S29.001 ☑
      laceration S29.029 ☑
        back wall S29.022 ☑
        front wall S29.021 ☑
      specified type NEC S29.099 ☑
        back wall S29.092 ☑
        front wall S29.091 ☑
      strain S29.019 ☑
        back wall S29.012 ☑
        front wall S29.011 ☑
    thumb
      abductor (forearm level) S56.30- ☑
        laceration S56.32- ☑
        specified type NEC S56.39- ☑
        strain S56.31- ☑
      extensor (forearm level) S56.30- ☑
        hand level S66.20- ☑
          laceration S66.22- ☑
          specified type NEC S66.29- ☑
          strain S66.21- ☑
        laceration S56.32- ☑
        specified type NEC S56.39- ☑
        strain S56.31- ☑
      flexor (forearm level) S56.00- ☑
        hand level S66.00- ☑
          laceration S66.02- ☑
          specified type NEC S66.09- ☑
          strain S66.01- ☑
        laceration S56.02- ☑
        specified type NEC S56.09- ☑
        strain S56.01- ☑
        wrist level — *see* Injury, muscle, thumb, flexor, hand level
      intrinsic S66.40- ☑
        laceration S66.42- ☑
        specified type NEC S66.49- ☑
        strain S66.41- ☑
    toe — *see also* Injury, muscle, foot
      extensor, long S96.10- ☑
        laceration S96.12- ☑
        specified type NEC S96.19- ☑
        strain S96.11- ☑
      flexor, long S96.00- ☑
        laceration S96.02- ☑
        specified type NEC S96.09- ☑
        strain S96.01- ☑
    triceps S46.30- ☑
      laceration S46.32- ☑
      specified type NEC S46.39- ☑
      strain S46.31- ☑
    wrist (and hand) level — *see* Injury, muscle, hand
  musculocutaneous nerve — *see* Injury, nerve, musculocutaneous
  myocardial (acute) (chronic) (non-ischemic) (non-traumatic) I5A
    traumatic — *see* Injury, heart
  myocardium — *see also* Injury, heart
    non-traumatic — *see* Injury, myocardial
  nape — *see* Injury, neck
  nasal (septum) (sinus) S09.92 ☑
  nasopharynx S09.92 ☑
  neck S19.9 ☑
    specified NEC S19.80 ☑
      specified site NEC S19.89 ☑
  nerve NEC T14.8 ☑
    abdomen S34.9 ☑
      peripheral S34.6 ☑
      specified site NEC S34.8 ☑
    abducens S04.4- ☑

Injury — *continued*
  nerve — *continued*
    abducens — *continued*
      contusion S04.4- ☑
      laceration S04.4- ☑
      specified type NEC S04.4- ☑
    abducent — *see* Injury, nerve, abducens
    accessory S04.7- ☑
      contusion S04.7- ☑
      laceration S04.7- ☑
      specified type NEC S04.7- ☑
    acoustic S04.6- ☑
      contusion S04.6- ☑
      laceration S04.6- ☑
      specified type NEC S04.6- ☑
    ankle S94.9- ☑
      cutaneous sensory S94.3- ☑
      specified site NEC — *see* subcategory S94.8 ☑
    anterior crural, femoral — *see* Injury, nerve, femoral
    arm (upper) S44.9- ☑
      axillary — *see* Injury, nerve, axillary
      cutaneous — *see* Injury, nerve, cutaneous, arm
      median — *see* Injury, nerve, median, upper arm
      musculocutaneous — *see* Injury, nerve, musculocutaneous
      radial — *see* Injury, nerve, radial, upper arm
      specified site NEC — *see* subcategory S44.8 ☑
      ulnar — *see* Injury, nerve, ulnar, arm
    auditory — *see* Injury, nerve, acoustic
    axillary S44.3- ☑
    brachial plexus — *see* Injury, brachial plexus
    cervical sympathetic S14.5 ☑
    cranial S04.9 ☑
      contusion S04.9 ☑
      eighth (acoustic or auditory) — *see* Injury, nerve, acoustic
      eleventh (accessory) — *see* Injury, nerve, accessory
      fifth (trigeminal) — *see* Injury, nerve, trigeminal
      first (olfactory) — *see* Injury, nerve, olfactory
      fourth (trochlear) — *see* Injury, nerve, trochlear
      laceration S04.9 ☑
      ninth (glossopharyngeal) — *see* Injury, nerve, glossopharyngeal
      second (optic) — *see* Injury, nerve, optic
      seventh (facial) — *see* Injury, nerve, facial
      sixth (abducent) — *see* Injury, nerve, abducens
      specified
        nerve NEC S04.89- ☑
          contusion S04.89- ☑
          laceration S04.89- ☑
          specified type NEC S04.89- ☑
        type NEC S04.9
      tenth (pneumogastric or vagus) — *see* Injury, nerve, vagus
      third (oculomotor) — *see* Injury, nerve, oculomotor
      twelfth (hypoglossal) — *see* Injury, nerve, hypoglossal
    cutaneous sensory
      ankle (level) S94.3- ☑
      arm (upper) (level) S44.5- ☑
      foot (level) — *see* Injury, nerve, cutaneous sensory, ankle
      forearm (level) S54.3- ☑
      hip (level) S74.2- ☑
      leg (lower level) S84.2- ☑
      shoulder (level) — *see* Injury, nerve, cutaneous sensory, arm
      thigh (level) — *see* Injury, nerve, cutaneous sensory, hip
    deep peroneal — *see* Injury, nerve, peroneal, foot
    digital
      finger S64.4- ☑
        index S64.49- ☑
        little S64.49- ☑
        middle S64.49- ☑
        ring S64.49- ☑
        thumb S64.3- ☑
      toe — *see* Injury, nerve, ankle, specified site NEC
    eighth cranial (acoustic or auditory) — *see* Injury, nerve, acoustic
    eleventh cranial (accessory) — *see* Injury, nerve, accessory
    facial S04.5- ☑
      contusion S04.5- ☑

Injury — *continued*
  nerve — *continued*
    facial — *continued*
      laceration S04.5- ☑
      newborn P11.3
      specified type NEC S04.5- ☑
    femoral (hip level) (thigh level) S74.1- ☑
    fifth cranial (trigeminal) — *see* Injury, nerve, trigeminal
    finger (digital) — *see* Injury, nerve, digital, finger
    first cranial (olfactory) — *see* Injury, nerve, olfactory
    foot S94.9- ☑
      cutaneous sensory S94.3- ☑
      deep peroneal S94.2- ☑
      lateral plantar S94.0- ☑
      medial plantar S94.1- ☑
      specified site NEC — *see* subcategory S94.8 ☑
    forearm (level) S54.9- ☑
      cutaneous sensory — *see* Injury, nerve, cutaneous, forearm
      median — *see* Injury, nerve, median
      radial — *see* Injury, nerve, radial
      specified site NEC — *see* subcategory S54.8 ☑
      ulnar — *see* Injury, nerve, ulnar
    fourth cranial (trochlear) — *see* Injury, nerve, trochlear
    glossopharyngeal S04.89- ☑
      specified type NEC S04.89- ☑
    hand S64.9- ☑
      median — *see* Injury, nerve, median, hand
      radial — *see* Injury, nerve, radial, hand
      specified NEC — *see* subcategory S64.8 ☑
      ulnar — *see* Injury, nerve, ulnar, hand
    hip (level) S74.9- ☑
      cutaneous sensory — *see* Injury, nerve, cutaneous sensory, hip
      femoral — *see* Injury, nerve, femoral
      sciatic — *see* Injury, nerve, sciatic
      specified site NEC — *see* subcategory S74.8 ☑
    hypoglossal S04.89- ☑
      specified type NEC S04.89- ☑
    lateral plantar S94.0- ☑
    leg (lower) S84.9- ☑
      cutaneous sensory — *see* Injury, nerve, cutaneous sensory, leg
      peroneal — *see* Injury, nerve, peroneal
      specified site NEC — *see* subcategory S84.8 ☑
      tibial — *see* Injury, nerve, tibial
      upper — *see* Injury, nerve, thigh
    lower
      back — *see* Injury, nerve, abdomen, specified site NEC
        peripheral — *see* Injury, nerve, abdomen, peripheral
      limb — *see* Injury, nerve, leg
    lumbar plexus — *see* Injury, nerve, lumbosacral, sympathetic
    lumbar spinal — *see* Injury, spinal, lumbar
      peripheral S34.6 ☑
      root S34.21 ☑
      sympathetic S34.5 ☑
    lumbosacral
      plexus — *see* Injury, nerve, lumbosacral, sympathetic
      sympathetic S34.5 ☑
    medial plantar S94.1- ☑
    median (forearm level) S54.1- ☑
      hand (level) S64.1- ☑
      upper arm (level) S44.1- ☑
      wrist (level) — *see* Injury, nerve, median, hand
    musculocutaneous S44.4- ☑
    musculospiral (upper arm level) — *see* Injury, nerve, radial, upper arm
    neck S14.9 ☑
      peripheral S14.4 ☑
      specified site NEC S14.8 ☑
      sympathetic S14.5 ☑
    ninth cranial (glossopharyngeal) — *see* Injury, nerve, glossopharyngeal
    oculomotor S04.1- ☑
      contusion S04.1- ☑
      laceration S04.1- ☑
      specified type NEC S04.1- ☑
    olfactory S04.81- ☑
      specified type NEC S04.81- ☑
    optic S04.01- ☑

Injury — *continued*
  nerve — *continued*
    optic — *continued*
      contusion S04.01- ☑
      laceration S04.01- ☑
      specified type NEC S04.01- ☑
    pelvic girdle — *see* Injury, nerve, hip
    pelvis — *see* Injury, nerve, abdomen, specified site NEC
      peripheral — *see* Injury, nerve, abdomen, peripheral
    peripheral NEC T14.8 ☑
      abdomen — *see* Injury, nerve, abdomen, peripheral
      lower back — *see* Injury, nerve, abdomen, peripheral
      neck — *see* Injury, nerve, neck, peripheral
      pelvis — *see* Injury, nerve, abdomen, peripheral
      specified NEC T14.8 ☑
    peroneal (lower leg level) S84.1- ☑
      foot S94.2- ☑
    plexus
      brachial — *see* Injury, brachial plexus
      celiac, coeliac — *see* Injury, nerve, lumbosacral, sympathetic
      mesenteric, inferior — *see* Injury, nerve, lumbosacral, sympathetic
      sacral — *see* Injury, lumbosacral plexus
      spinal
        brachial — *see* Injury, brachial plexus
        lumbosacral — *see* Injury, lumbosacral plexus
    pneumogastric — *see* Injury, nerve, vagus
    radial (forearm level) S54.2- ☑
      hand (level) S64.2- ☑
      upper arm (level) S44.2- ☑
      wrist (level) — *see* Injury, nerve, radial, hand
    root — *see* Injury, nerve, spinal, root
    sacral plexus — *see* Injury, lumbosacral plexus
    sacral spinal — *see* Injury, spinal, sacral
      peripheral S34.6 ☑
      root S34.22 ☑
      sympathetic S34.5 ☑
    sciatic (hip level) (thigh level) S74.0- ☑
    second cranial (optic) — *see* Injury, nerve, optic
    seventh cranial (facial) — *see* Injury, nerve, facial
    shoulder — *see* Injury, nerve, arm
    sixth cranial (abducent) — *see* Injury, nerve, abducens
    spinal
      plexus — *see* Injury, nerve, plexus, spinal
      root
        cervical S14.2 ☑
        dorsal S24.2 ☑
        lumbar S34.21 ☑
        sacral S34.22 ☑
        thoracic — *see* Injury, nerve, spinal, root, dorsal
    splanchnic — *see* Injury, nerve, lumbosacral, sympathetic
    sympathetic NEC — *see* Injury, nerve, lumbosacral, sympathetic
      cervical — *see* Injury, nerve, cervical sympathetic
    tenth cranial (pneumogastric or vagus) — *see* Injury, nerve, vagus
    thigh (level) — *see* Injury, nerve, hip
      cutaneous sensory — *see* Injury, nerve, cutaneous sensory, hip
      femoral — *see* Injury, nerve, femoral
      sciatic — *see* Injury, nerve, sciatic
      specified NEC — *see* Injury, nerve, hip
    third cranial (oculomotor) — *see* Injury, nerve, oculomotor
    thorax S24.9 ☑
      peripheral S24.3 ☑
      specified site NEC S24.8 ☑
      sympathetic S24.4 ☑
    thumb, digital — *see* Injury, nerve, digital, thumb
    tibial (lower leg level) (posterior) S84.0- ☑
    toe — *see* Injury, nerve, ankle
    trigeminal S04.3- ☑
      contusion S04.3- ☑
      laceration S04.3- ☑
      specified type NEC S04.3- ☑
    trochlear S04.2- ☑
      contusion S04.2- ☑
      laceration S04.2- ☑

Injury — *continued*
　nerve — *continued*
　　trochlear — *continued*
　　　specified type NEC S04.2- ☑
　　twelfth cranial (hypoglossal) — *see* Injury, nerve, hypoglossal
　　ulnar (forearm level) S54.0- ☑
　　　arm (upper) (level) S44.0- ☑
　　　hand (level) S64.0- ☑
　　　wrist (level) — *see* Injury, nerve, ulnar, hand
　　vagus S04.89- ☑
　　　specified type NEC S04.89- ☑
　　wrist (level) — *see* Injury, nerve, hand
　　ninth cranial nerve (glossopharyngeal) — *see* Injury, nerve, glossopharyngeal
　nose (septum) S09.92 ☑
　obstetrical O71.9
　　specified NEC O71.89
　occipital (region) (scalp) S09.90 ☑
　　lobe — *see* Injury, intracranial
　optic chiasm S04.02 ☑
　optic radiation S04.03- ☑
　optic tract and pathways S04.03- ☑
　orbit, orbital (region) — *see* Injury, eye
　　penetrating (with foreign body) — *see* Injury, eye, orbit, penetrating
　　specified NEC — *see* Injury, eye, specified site NEC
　ovary, ovarian S37.409 ☑
　　bilateral S37.402 ☑
　　　contusion S37.422 ☑
　　　laceration S37.432 ☑
　　　specified type NEC S37.492 ☑
　　blood vessel — *see* Injury, blood vessel, ovarian
　　contusion S37.429 ☑
　　　bilateral S37.422 ☑
　　　unilateral S37.421 ☑
　　laceration S37.439 ☑
　　　bilateral S37.432 ☑
　　　unilateral S37.431 ☑
　　specified type NEC S37.499 ☑
　　　bilateral S37.492 ☑
　　　unilateral S37.491 ☑
　　unilateral S37.401 ☑
　　　contusion S37.421 ☑
　　　laceration S37.431 ☑
　　　specified type NEC S37.491 ☑
　palate (hard) (soft) S09.93 ☑
　pancreas S36.209 ☑
　　body S36.201 ☑
　　　contusion S36.221 ☑
　　　laceration S36.231 ☑
　　　　major S36.261 ☑
　　　　minor S36.241 ☑
　　　　moderate S36.251 ☑
　　　specified type NEC S36.291 ☑
　　contusion S36.229 ☑
　　head S36.200 ☑
　　　contusion S36.220 ☑
　　　laceration S36.230 ☑
　　　　major S36.260 ☑
　　　　minor S36.240 ☑
　　　　moderate S36.250 ☑
　　　specified type NEC S36.290 ☑
　　laceration S36.239 ☑
　　　major S36.269 ☑
　　　minor S36.249 ☑
　　　moderate S36.259 ☑
　　specified type NEC S36.299 ☑
　　tail S36.202 ☑
　　　contusion S36.222 ☑
　　　laceration S36.232 ☑
　　　　major S36.262 ☑
　　　　minor S36.242 ☑
　　　　moderate S36.252 ☑
　　　specified type NEC S36.292 ☑
　parietal (region) (scalp) S09.90 ☑
　　lobe — *see* Injury, intracranial
　patellar ligament (tendon) S76.10- ☑
　　laceration S76.12- ☑
　　specified NEC S76.19- ☑
　　strain S76.11- ☑
　pelvis, pelvic (floor) S39.93 ☑
　　complicating delivery O70.1
　　joint or ligament, complicating delivery O71.6
　　organ S37.90 ☑
　　　with ectopic or molar pregnancy O08.6

Injury — *continued*
　pelvis, pelvic — *continued*
　　organ — *continued*
　　　complication of abortion — *see* Abortion
　　　contusion S37.92 ☑
　　　following ectopic or molar pregnancy O08.6
　　　laceration S37.93 ☑
　　　obstetrical trauma NEC O71.5
　　　specified
　　　　site NEC S37.899 ☑
　　　　　contusion S37.892 ☑
　　　　　laceration S37.893 ☑
　　　　　specified type NEC S37.898 ☑
　　　　type NEC S37.99 ☑
　　　specified NEC S39.83 ☑
　penis S39.94 ☑
　perineum S39.94 ☑
　peritoneum S36.81 ☑
　　laceration S36.893 ☑
　periurethral tissue — *see* Injury, urethra
　　complicating delivery O71.82
　phalanges
　　foot — *see* Injury, foot
　　hand — *see* Injury, hand
　pharynx NEC S19.85 ☑
　pleura — *see* Injury, intrathoracic, pleura
　plexus
　　brachial — *see* Injury, brachial plexus
　　cardiac — *see* Injury, nerve, thorax, sympathetic
　　celiac, coeliac — *see* Injury, nerve, lumbosacral, sympathetic
　　esophageal — *see* Injury, nerve, thorax, sympathetic
　　hypogastric — *see* Injury, nerve, lumbosacral, sympathetic
　　lumbar, lumbosacral — *see* Injury, lumbosacral plexus
　　mesenteric — *see* Injury, nerve, lumbosacral, sympathetic
　　pulmonary — *see* Injury, nerve, thorax, sympathetic
　postcardiac surgery (syndrome) I97.0
　prepuce S39.94 ☑
　pressure
　　injury — *see* Ulcer, pressure, by site
　prostate S37.829 ☑
　　contusion S37.822 ☑
　　laceration S37.823 ☑
　　specified type NEC S37.828 ☑
　pubic region S39.94 ☑
　pudendum S39.94 ☑
　pulmonary plexus — *see* Injury, nerve, thorax, sympathetic
　rectovaginal septum NEC S39.83 ☑
　rectum — *see* Injury, intestine, large, rectum
　retina — *see* Injury, eye, specified site NEC
　　penetrating — *see* Injury, eyeball, penetrating
　retroperitoneal — *see* Injury, intra-abdominal, specified site NEC
　rotator cuff (muscle(s)) (tendon(s)) S46.00- ☑
　　laceration S46.02- ☑
　　specified type NEC S46.09- ☑
　　strain S46.01- ☑
　round ligament — *see* Injury, pelvic organ, specified site NEC
　sacral plexus — *see* Injury, lumbosacral plexus
　salivary duct or gland S09.93 ☑
　scalp S09.90 ☑
　　newborn (birth injury) P12.9
　　　due to monitoring (electrode) (sampling incision) P12.4
　　　specified NEC P12.89
　　　　caput succedaneum P12.81
　scapular region — *see* Injury, shoulder
　sclera — *see* Injury, eye, specified site NEC
　　penetrating — *see* Injury, eyeball, penetrating
　scrotum S39.94 ☑
　second cranial nerve (optic) — *see* Injury, nerve, optic
　self-inflicted, without suicidal intent R45.88
　seminal vesicle — *see* Injury, pelvic organ, specified site NEC
　seventh cranial nerve (facial) — *see* Injury, nerve, facial
　shoulder S49.9- ☑
　　blood vessel — *see* Injury, blood vessel, arm
　　contusion — *see* Contusion, shoulder
　　dislocation — *see* Dislocation, shoulder
　　fracture — *see* Fracture, shoulder
　　muscle — *see* Injury, muscle, shoulder
　　nerve — *see* Injury, nerve, shoulder

Injury — *continued*
　shoulder — *continued*
　　open — *see* Wound, open, shoulder
　　specified type NEC S49.8- ☑
　　sprain — *see* Sprain, shoulder girdle
　　superficial — *see* Injury, superficial, shoulder
　sinus
　　cavernous — *see* Injury, intracranial
　　nasal S09.92 ☑
　sixth cranial nerve (abducent) — *see* Injury, nerve, abducens
　skeleton, birth injury P13.9
　　specified part NEC P13.8
　skin NEC T14.8 ☑
　　surface intact — *see* Injury, superficial
　skull NEC S09.90 ☑
　specified NEC T14.8 ☑
　spermatic cord (pelvic region) S37.898 ☑
　　scrotal region S39.848 ☑
　spinal (cord) S14.109 ☑
　　cervical (neck) S14.109 ☑
　　　anterior cord syndrome S14.139 ☑
　　　　C1 level S14.131 ☑
　　　　C2 level S14.132 ☑
　　　　C3 level S14.133 ☑
　　　　C4 level S14.134 ☑
　　　　C5 level S14.135 ☑
　　　　C6 level S14.136 ☑
　　　　C7 level S14.137 ☑
　　　　C8 level S14.138 ☑
　　　Brown-Séquard syndrome S14.149 ☑
　　　　C1 level S14.141 ☑
　　　　C2 level S14.142 ☑
　　　　C3 level S14.143 ☑
　　　　C4 level S14.144 ☑
　　　　C5 level S14.145 ☑
　　　　C6 level S14.146 ☑
　　　　C7 level S14.147 ☑
　　　　C8 level S14.148 ☑
　　　C1 level S14.101 ☑
　　　C2 level S14.102 ☑
　　　C3 level S14.103 ☑
　　　C4 level S14.104 ☑
　　　C5 level S14.105 ☑
　　　C6 level S14.106 ☑
　　　C7 level S14.107 ☑
　　　C8 level S14.108 ☑
　　　central cord syndrome S14.129 ☑
　　　　C1 level S14.121 ☑
　　　　C2 level S14.122 ☑
　　　　C3 level S14.123 ☑
　　　　C4 level S14.124 ☑
　　　　C5 level S14.125 ☑
　　　　C6 level S14.126 ☑
　　　　C7 level S14.127 ☑
　　　　C8 level S14.128 ☑
　　　complete lesion S14.119 ☑
　　　　C1 level S14.111 ☑
　　　　C2 level S14.112 ☑
　　　　C3 level S14.113 ☑
　　　　C4 level S14.114 ☑
　　　　C5 level S14.115 ☑
　　　　C6 level S14.116 ☑
　　　　C7 level S14.117 ☑
　　　　C8 level S14.118 ☑
　　　concussion S14.0 ☑
　　　edema S14.0 ☑
　　　incomplete lesion specified NEC S14.159 ☑
　　　　C1 level S14.151 ☑
　　　　C2 level S14.152 ☑
　　　　C3 level S14.153 ☑
　　　　C4 level S14.154 ☑
　　　　C5 level S14.155 ☑
　　　　C6 level S14.156 ☑
　　　　C7 level S14.157 ☑
　　　　C8 level S14.158 ☑
　　　posterior cord syndrome S14.159 ☑
　　　　C1 level S14.151 ☑
　　　　C2 level S14.152 ☑
　　　　C3 level S14.153 ☑
　　　　C4 level S14.154 ☑
　　　　C5 level S14.155 ☑
　　　　C6 level S14.156 ☑
　　　　C7 level S14.157 ☑
　　　　C8 level S14.158 ☑
　　dorsal — *see* Injury, spinal, thoracic

Injury — *continued*
  spinal — *continued*
    lumbar S34.109 ☑
      complete lesion S34.119 ☑
        L1 level S34.111 ☑
        L2 level S34.112 ☑
        L3 level S34.113 ☑
        L4 level S34.114 ☑
        L5 level S34.115 ☑
      concussion S34.01 ☑
      edema S34.01 ☑
      incomplete lesion S34.129 ☑
        L1 level S34.121 ☑
        L2 level S34.122 ☑
        L3 level S34.123 ☑
        L4 level S34.124 ☑
        L5 level S34.125 ☑
      L1 level S34.101 ☑
      L2 level S34.102 ☑
      L3 level S34.103 ☑
      L4 level S34.104 ☑
      L5 level S34.105 ☑
    nerve root NEC
      cervical — *see* Injury, nerve, spinal, root, cervical
      dorsal — *see* Injury, nerve, spinal, root, dorsal
      lumbar S34.21 ☑
      sacral S34.22 ☑
      thoracic — *see* Injury, nerve, spinal, root, dorsal
    plexus
      brachial — *see* Injury, brachial plexus
      lumbosacral — *see* Injury, lumbosacral plexus
    sacral S34.139 ☑
      complete lesion S34.131 ☑
      incomplete lesion S34.132 ☑
    thoracic S24.109 ☑
      anterior cord syndrome S24.139 ☑
        T1 level S24.131 ☑
        T2-T6 level S24.132 ☑
        T7-T10 level S24.133 ☑
        T11-T12 level S24.134 ☑
      Brown-Séquard syndrome S24.149 ☑
        T1 level S24.141 ☑
        T2-T6 level S24.142 ☑
        T7-T10 level S24.143 ☑
        T11-T12 level S24.144 ☑
      complete lesion S24.119 ☑
        T1 level S24.111 ☑
        T2-T6 level S24.112 ☑
        T7-T10 level S24.113 ☑
        T11-T12 level S24.114 ☑
      concussion S24.0 ☑
      edema S24.0 ☑
      incomplete lesion specified NEC S24.159 ☑
        T1 level S24.151 ☑
        T2-T6 level S24.152 ☑
        T7-T10 level S24.153 ☑
        T11-T12 level S24.154 ☑
      posterior cord syndrome S24.159 ☑
        T1 level S24.151 ☑
        T2-T6 level S24.152 ☑
        T7-T10 level S24.153 ☑
        T11-T12 level S24.154 ☑
      T1 level S24.101 ☑
      T2-T6 level S24.102 ☑
      T7-T10 level S24.103 ☑
      T11-T12 level S24.104 ☑
  splanchnic nerve — *see* Injury, nerve, lumbosacral, sympathetic
  spleen S36.00 ☑
    contusion S36.029 ☑
      major S36.021 ☑
      minor S36.020 ☑
    laceration S36.039 ☑
      major (massive) (stellate) S36.032 ☑
      moderate S36.031 ☑
      superficial (capsular) (minor) S36.030 ☑
    specified type NEC S36.09 ☑
  splenic artery — *see* Injury, blood vessel, celiac artery, branch
  stellate ganglion — *see* Injury, nerve, thorax, sympathetic
  sternal region S29.9 ☑
  stomach S36.30 ☑
    contusion S36.32 ☑
    laceration S36.33 ☑
    specified type NEC S36.39 ☑

Injury — *continued*
  subconjunctival — *see* Injury, eye, conjunctiva
  subcutaneous NEC T14.8 ☑
  submaxillary region S09.93 ☑
  submental region S09.93 ☑
  subungual
    fingers — *see* Injury, hand
    toes — *see* Injury, foot
  superficial NEC T14.8 ☑
    abdomen, abdominal (wall) S30.92 ☑
      abrasion S30.811 ☑
      bite S30.871 ☑
        insect S30.861 ☑
      contusion S30.1 ☑
      external constriction S30.841 ☑
      foreign body S30.851 ☑
    abrasion — *see* Abrasion, by site
    adnexa, eye NEC — *see* Injury, eye, specified site NEC
    alveolar process — *see* Injury, superficial, oral cavity
    ankle S90.91- ☑
      abrasion — *see* Abrasion, ankle
      bite — *see* Bite, ankle
      blister — *see* Blister, ankle
      contusion — *see* Contusion, ankle
      external constriction — *see* Constriction, external, ankle
      foreign body — *see* Foreign body, superficial, ankle
    anus S30.98 ☑
    arm (upper) S40.92- ☑
      abrasion — *see* Abrasion, arm
      bite — *see* Bite, superficial, arm
      blister — *see* Blister, arm (upper)
      contusion — *see* Contusion, arm
      external constriction — *see* Constriction, external, arm
      foreign body — *see* Foreign body, superficial, arm
    auditory canal (external) (meatus) — *see* Injury, superficial, ear
    auricle — *see* Injury, superficial, ear
    axilla — *see* Injury, superficial, arm
    back — *see also* Injury, superficial, thorax, back
      lower S30.91 ☑
        abrasion S30.810 ☑
        contusion S30.0 ☑
        external constriction S30.840 ☑
        superficial
          bite NEC S30.870 ☑
            insect S30.860 ☑
          foreign body S30.850 ☑
    bite NEC — *see* Bite, superficial NEC, by site
    blister — *see* Blister, by site
    breast S20.10- ☑
      abrasion — *see* Abrasion, breast
      bite — *see* Bite, superficial, breast
      contusion — *see* Contusion, breast
      external constriction — *see* Constriction, external, breast
      foreign body — *see* Foreign body, superficial, breast
    brow — *see* Injury, superficial, head, specified NEC
    buttock S30.91 ☑
    calf — *see* Injury, superficial, leg
    canthus, eye — *see* Injury, superficial, periocular area
    cheek (external) — *see* Injury, superficial, head, specified NEC
      internal — *see* Injury, superficial, oral cavity
    chest wall — *see* Injury, superficial, thorax
    chin — *see* Injury, superficial, head NEC
    clitoris S30.95 ☑
    conjunctiva — *see* Injury, eye, conjunctiva
      with foreign body (in conjunctival sac) — *see* Foreign body, conjunctival sac
    contusion — *see* Contusion, by site
    costal region — *see* Injury, superficial, thorax
    digit(s)
      hand — *see* Injury, superficial, finger
    ear (auricle) (canal) (external) S00.40- ☑
      abrasion — *see* Abrasion, ear
      bite — *see* Bite, superficial, ear
      contusion — *see* Contusion, ear
      external constriction — *see* Constriction, external, ear

Injury — *continued*
  superficial — *continued*
    ear — *continued*
      foreign body — *see* Foreign body, superficial, ear
    elbow S50.90- ☑
      abrasion — *see* Abrasion, elbow
      bite — *see* Bite, superficial, elbow
      blister — *see* Blister, elbow
      contusion — *see* Contusion, elbow
      external constriction — *see* Constriction, external, elbow
      foreign body — *see* Foreign body, superficial, elbow
    epididymis S30.94 ☑
    epigastric region S30.92 ☑
    epiglottis — *see* Injury, superficial, throat
    esophagus
      cervical — *see* Injury, superficial, throat
    external constriction — *see* Constriction, external, by site
    extremity NEC T14.8 ☑
    eyeball NEC — *see* Injury, eye, specified site NEC
    eyebrow — *see* Injury, superficial, periocular area
    eyelid S00.20- ☑
      abrasion — *see* Abrasion, eyelid
      bite — *see* Bite, superficial, eyelid
      contusion — *see* Contusion, eyelid
      external constriction — *see* Constriction, external, eyelid
      foreign body — *see* Foreign body, superficial, eyelid
    face NEC — *see* Injury, superficial, head, specified NEC
    finger(s) S60.949 ☑
      abrasion — *see* Abrasion, finger
      bite — *see* Bite, superficial, finger
      blister — *see* Blister, finger
      contusion — *see* Contusion, finger
      external constriction — *see* Constriction, external, finger
      foreign body — *see* Foreign body, superficial, finger
      index S60.94- ☑
      insect bite — *see* Bite, by site, superficial, insect
      little S60.94- ☑
      middle S60.94- ☑
      ring S60.94- ☑
    flank S30.92 ☑
    foot S90.92- ☑
      abrasion — *see* Abrasion, foot
      bite — *see* Bite, foot
      blister — *see* Blister, foot
      contusion — *see* Contusion, foot
      external constriction — *see* Constriction, external, foot
      foreign body — *see* Foreign body, superficial, foot
    forearm S50.91- ☑
      abrasion — *see* Abrasion, forearm
      bite — *see* Bite, forearm, superficial
      blister — *see* Blister, forearm
      contusion — *see* Contusion, forearm
      elbow only — *see* Injury, superficial, elbow
      external constriction — *see* Constriction, external, forearm
      foreign body — *see* Foreign body, superficial, forearm
    forehead — *see* Injury, superficial, head NEC
    foreign body — *see* Foreign body, superficial
    genital organs, external
      female S30.97 ☑
      male S30.96 ☑
    globe (eye) — *see* Injury, eye, specified site NEC
    groin S30.92 ☑
    gum — *see* Injury, superficial, oral cavity
    hand S60.92- ☑
      abrasion — *see* Abrasion, hand
      bite — *see* Bite, superficial, hand
      contusion — *see* Contusion, hand
      external constriction — *see* Constriction, external, hand
      foreign body — *see* Foreign body, superficial, hand
    head S00.90 ☑
      ear — *see* Injury, superficial, ear

Injury — continued
  superficial — continued
    head — continued
      eyelid — see Injury, superficial, eyelid
      nose S00.30 ☑
      oral cavity S00.502 ☑
      scalp S00.00 ☑
      specified site NEC S00.80 ☑
    heel — see Injury, superficial, foot
    hip S70.91- ☑
      abrasion — see Abrasion, hip
      bite — see Bite, superficial, hip
      blister — see Blister, hip
      contusion — see Contusion, hip
      external constriction — see Constriction, external, hip
      foreign body — see Foreign body, superficial, hip
    iliac region — see Injury, superficial, abdomen
    inguinal region — see Injury, superficial, abdomen
    insect bite — see Bite, by site, superficial, insect
    interscapular region — see Injury, superficial, thorax, back
    jaw — see Injury, superficial, head, specified NEC
    knee S80.91- ☑
      abrasion — see Abrasion, knee
      bite — see Bite, superficial, knee
      blister — see Blister, knee
      contusion — see Contusion, knee
      external constriction — see Constriction, external, knee
      foreign body — see Foreign body, superficial, knee
    labium (majus) (minus) S30.95 ☑
    lacrimal (apparatus) (gland) (sac) — see Injury, eye, specified site NEC
    larynx — see Injury, superficial, throat
    leg (lower) S80.92- ☑
      abrasion — see Abrasion, leg
      bite — see Bite, superficial, leg
      contusion — see Contusion, leg
      external constriction — see Constriction, external, leg
      foreign body — see Foreign body, superficial, leg
      knee — see Injury, superficial, knee
    limb NEC T14.8 ☑
    lip S00.501 ☑
    lower back S30.91 ☑
    lumbar region S30.91 ☑
    malar region — see Injury, superficial, head, specified NEC
    mammary — see Injury, superficial, breast
    mastoid region — see Injury, superficial, head, specified NEC
    mouth — see Injury, superficial, oral cavity
    muscle NEC T14.8 ☑
    nail NEC T14.8 ☑
      finger — see Injury, superficial, finger
      toe — see Injury, superficial, toe
    nasal (septum) — see Injury, superficial, nose
    neck S10.90 ☑
      specified site NEC S10.80 ☑
    nose (septum) S00.30 ☑
    occipital region — see Injury, superficial, scalp
    oral cavity S00.502 ☑
    orbital region — see Injury, superficial, periocular area
    palate — see Injury, superficial, oral cavity
    palm — see Injury, superficial, hand
    parietal region — see Injury, superficial, scalp
    pelvis S30.91 ☑
      girdle — see Injury, superficial, hip
    penis S30.93 ☑
    perineum
      female S30.95 ☑
      male S30.91 ☑
    periocular area S00.20- ☑
      abrasion — see Abrasion, eyelid
      bite — see Bite, superficial, eyelid
      contusion — see Contusion, eyelid
      external constriction — see Constriction, external, eyelid
      foreign body — see Foreign body, superficial, eyelid

Injury — continued
  superficial — continued
    phalanges
      finger — see Injury, superficial, finger
      toe — see Injury, superficial, toe
    pharynx — see Injury, superficial, throat
    pinna — see Injury, superficial, ear
    popliteal space — see Injury, superficial, knee
    prepuce S30.93 ☑
    pubic region S30.91 ☑
    pudendum
      female S30.97 ☑
      male S30.96 ☑
    sacral region S30.91 ☑
    scalp S00.00 ☑
    scapular region — see Injury, superficial, shoulder
    sclera — see Injury, eye, specified site NEC
    scrotum S30.94 ☑
    shin — see Injury, superficial, leg
    shoulder S40.91- ☑
      abrasion — see Abrasion, shoulder
      bite — see Bite, superficial, shoulder
      blister — see Blister, shoulder
      contusion — see Contusion, shoulder
      external constriction — see Constriction, external, shoulder
      foreign body — see Foreign body, superficial, shoulder
    skin NEC T14.8 ☑
    sternal region — see Injury, superficial, thorax, front
    subconjunctival — see Injury, eye, specified site NEC
    subcutaneous NEC T14.8 ☑
    submaxillary region — see Injury, superficial, head, specified NEC
    submental region — see Injury, superficial, head, specified NEC
    subungual
      finger(s) — see Injury, superficial, finger
      toe(s) — see Injury, superficial, toe
    supraclavicular fossa — see Injury, superficial, neck
    supraorbital — see Injury, superficial, head, specified NEC
    temple — see Injury, superficial, head, specified NEC
    temporal region — see Injury, superficial, head, specified NEC
    testis S30.94 ☑
    thigh S70.92- ☑
      abrasion — see Abrasion, thigh
      bite — see Bite, superficial, thigh
      blister — see Blister, thigh
      contusion — see Contusion, thigh
      external constriction — see Constriction, external, thigh
      foreign body — see Foreign body, superficial, thigh
    thorax, thoracic (wall) S20.90 ☑
      abrasion — see Abrasion, thorax
      back S20.40- ☑
      bite — see Bite, thorax, superficial
      blister — see Blister, thorax
      contusion — see Contusion, thorax
      external constriction — see Constriction, external, thorax
      foreign body — see Foreign body, superficial, thorax
      front S20.30- ☑
    throat S10.10 ☑
      abrasion S10.11 ☑
      bite S10.17 ☑
        insect S10.16 ☑
      blister S10.12 ☑
      contusion S10.0 ☑
      external constriction S10.14 ☑
      foreign body S10.15 ☑
    thumb S60.93- ☑
      abrasion — see Abrasion, thumb
      bite — see Bite, superficial, thumb
      blister — see Blister, thumb
      contusion — see Contusion, thumb
      external constriction — see Constriction, external, thumb
      foreign body — see Foreign body, superficial, thumb
      insect bite — see Bite, by site, superficial, insect
      specified type NEC S60.39 ☑
    toe(s) S90.93- ☑

Injury — continued
  superficial — continued
    toe(s) — continued
      abrasion — see Abrasion, toe
      bite — see Bite, toe
      blister — see Blister, toe
      contusion — see Contusion, toe
      external constriction — see Constriction, external, toe
      foreign body — see Foreign body, superficial, toe
      great S90.93- ☑
    tongue — see Injury, superficial, oral cavity
    tooth, teeth — see Injury, superficial, oral cavity
    trachea S10.10 ☑
    tunica vaginalis S30.94 ☑
    tympanum, tympanic membrane — see Injury, superficial, ear
    uvula — see Injury, superficial, oral cavity
    vagina S30.95 ☑
    vocal cords — see Injury, superficial, throat
    vulva S30.95 ☑
    wrist S60.91- ☑
  supraclavicular region — see Injury, neck
  supraorbital S09.93 ☑
  suprarenal gland (multiple) — see Injury, adrenal
  surgical complication (external or internal site) — see Laceration, accidental complicating surgery
  temple S09.90 ☑
  temporal region S09.90 ☑
  tendon — see also Injury, muscle, by site
    abdomen — see Injury, muscle, abdomen
    Achilles — see Injury, Achilles tendon
    lower back — see Injury, muscle, lower back
    pelvic organs — see Injury, muscle, pelvis
  tenth cranial nerve (pneumogastric or vagus) — see Injury, nerve, vagus
  testis S39.94 ☑
  thigh S79.92- ☑
    blood vessel — see Injury, blood vessel, hip
    contusion — see Contusion, thigh
    fracture — see Fracture, femur
    muscle — see Injury, muscle, thigh
    nerve — see Injury, nerve, thigh
    open — see Wound, open, thigh
    specified NEC S79.82- ☑
    superficial — see Injury, superficial, thigh
  third cranial nerve (oculomotor) — see Injury, nerve, oculomotor
  thorax, thoracic S29.9 ☑
    blood vessel — see Injury, blood vessel, thorax
    cavity — see Injury, intrathoracic
    dislocation — see Dislocation, thorax
    external (wall) S29.9 ☑
      contusion — see Contusion, thorax
      nerve — see Injury, nerve, thorax
      open — see Wound, open, thorax
      specified NEC S29.8 ☑
      sprain — see Sprain, thorax
      superficial — see Injury, superficial, thorax
    fracture — see Fracture, thorax
    internal — see Injury, intrathoracic
    intrathoracic organ — see Injury, intrathoracic
    sympathetic ganglion — see Injury, nerve, thorax, sympathetic
  throat — see also Injury, neck S19.9 ☑
  thumb S69.9- ☑
    blood vessel — see Injury, blood vessel, thumb
    contusion — see Contusion, thumb
    dislocation — see Dislocation, thumb
    fracture — see Fracture, thumb
    muscle — see Injury, muscle, thumb
    nerve — see Injury, nerve, digital, thumb
    open — see Wound, open, thumb
    specified NEC S69.8- ☑
    sprain — see Sprain, thumb
    superficial — see Injury, superficial, thumb
  thymus (gland) — see Injury, intrathoracic, specified organ NEC
  thyroid (gland) NEC S19.84 ☑
  toe S99.92- ☑
    contusion — see Contusion, toe
    dislocation — see Dislocation, toe
    fracture — see Fracture, toe
    muscle — see Injury, muscle, toe
    open — see Wound, open, toe

Injury — *continued*
  toe — *continued*
    specified type NEC S99.82- ☑
    sprain — *see* Sprain, toe
    superficial — *see* Injury, superficial, toe
  tongue S09.93 ☑
  tonsil S09.93 ☑
  tooth S09.93 ☑
  trachea (cervical) NEC S19.82 ☑
    thoracic — *see* Injury, intrathoracic, trachea, thoracic
  transfusion-related acute lung (TRALI) J95.84
  tunica vaginalis S39.94 ☑
  twelfth cranial nerve (hypoglossal) — *see* Injury, nerve, hypoglossal
  ureter S37.10 ☑
    contusion S37.12 ☑
    laceration S37.13 ☑
    specified type NEC S37.19 ☑
  urethra (sphincter) S37.30 ☑
    at delivery O71.5
    contusion S37.32 ☑
    laceration S37.33 ☑
    specified type NEC S37.39 ☑
  urinary organ S37.90 ☑
    contusion S37.92 ☑
    laceration S37.93 ☑
    specified
      site NEC S37.899 ☑
        contusion S37.892 ☑
        laceration S37.893 ☑
        specified type NEC S37.898 ☑
      type NEC S37.99 ☑
  uterus, uterine S37.60 ☑
    with ectopic or molar pregnancy O08.6
    blood vessel — *see* Injury, blood vessel, iliac
    contusion S37.62 ☑
    laceration S37.63 ☑
      cervix at delivery O71.3
    rupture associated with obstetrics — *see* Rupture, uterus
    specified type NEC S37.69 ☑
  uvula S09.93 ☑
  vagina S39.93 ☑
    abrasion S30.814 ☑
    bite S31.45 ☑
      insect S30.864 ☑
      superficial NEC S30.874 ☑
    contusion S30.23 ☑
    crush S38.03 ☑
    during delivery — *see* Laceration, vagina, during delivery
    external constriction S30.844 ☑
    insect bite S30.864 ☑
    laceration S31.41 ☑
      with foreign body S31.42 ☑
    open wound S31.40 ☑
    puncture S31.43 ☑
      with foreign body S31.44 ☑
    superficial S30.95 ☑
      foreign body S30.854 ☑
  vas deferens — *see* Injury, pelvic organ, specified site NEC
  vascular NEC T14.8 ☑
  vein — *see* Injury, blood vessel
  vena cava (superior) S25.20 ☑
    inferior S35.10 ☑
      laceration (minor) (superficial) S35.11 ☑
        major S35.12 ☑
      specified type NEC S35.19 ☑
    laceration (minor) (superficial) S25.21 ☑
      major S25.22 ☑
    specified type NEC S25.29 ☑
  vesical (sphincter) — *see* Injury, bladder
  visual cortex S04.04- ☑
  vitreous (humor) S05.90 ☑
    specified NEC S05.8X- ☑
  vocal cord NEC S19.83 ☑
  vulva S39.94 ☑
    abrasion S30.814 ☑
    bite S31.45 ☑
      insect S30.864 ☑
      superficial NEC S30.874 ☑
    contusion S30.23 ☑
    crush S38.03 ☑
    during delivery — *see* Laceration, perineum, female, during delivery

Injury — *continued*
  vulva — *continued*
    external constriction S30.844 ☑
    insect bite S30.864 ☑
    laceration S31.41 ☑
      with foreign body S31.42 ☑
    open wound S31.40 ☑
    puncture S31.43 ☑
      with foreign body S31.44 ☑
    superficial S30.95 ☑
      foreign body S30.854 ☑
  whiplash (cervical spine) S13.4 ☑
  wrist S69.9- ☑
    blood vessel — *see* Injury, blood vessel, hand
    contusion — *see* Contusion, wrist
    dislocation — *see* Dislocation, wrist
    fracture — *see* Fracture, wrist
    muscle — *see* Injury, muscle, hand
    nerve — *see* Injury, nerve, hand
    open — *see* Wound, open, wrist
    specified NEC S69.8- ☑
    sprain — *see* Sprain, wrist
    superficial — *see* Injury, superficial, wrist
Inoculation — *see also* Vaccination
  complication or reaction — *see* Complications, vaccination
Insanity, insane — *see also* Psychosis
  adolescent — *see* Schizophrenia
  confusional F28
    acute or subacute F05
  delusional F22
  senile F03 ☑
Insect
  bite — *see* Bite, by site, superficial, insect
  venomous, poisoning NEC (by) — *see* Venom, arthropod
Insecurity
  financial Z59.86
  food Z59.41
  transportation Z59.82
Insensitivity
  adrenocorticotropin hormone (ACTH) E27.49
  androgen E34.50
    complete E34.51
    partial E34.52
Insertion
  cord (umbilical) lateral or velamentous O43.12- ☑
  intrauterine contraceptive device (encounter for) — *see* Intrauterine contraceptive device
Insolation (sunstroke) T67.01 ☑
Insomnia (organic) G47.00
  adjustment F51.02
  adjustment disorder F51.02
  behavioral, of childhood Z73.819
    combined type Z73.812
    limit setting type Z73.811
    sleep-onset association type Z73.810
  childhood Z73.819
  chronic F51.04
    somatized tension F51.04
  conditioned F51.04
  due to
    alcohol
      abuse F10.182
      dependence F10.282
      use F10.982
    amphetamines
      abuse F15.182
      dependence F15.282
      use F15.982
    anxiety disorder F51.05
    caffeine
      abuse F15.182
      dependence F15.282
      use F15.982
    cocaine
      abuse F14.182
      dependence F14.282
      use F14.982
    depression F51.05
    drug NEC
      abuse F19.182
      dependence F19.282
      use F19.982
    medical condition G47.01
    mental disorder NEC F51.05

Insomnia — *continued*
  due to — *continued*
    opioid
      abuse F11.182
      dependence F11.282
      use F11.982
    psychoactive substance NEC
      abuse F19.182
      dependence F19.182
      use F19.982
    sedative, hypnotic, or anxiolytic
      abuse F13.182
      dependence F13.282
      use F13.982
    stimulant NEC
      abuse F15.182
      dependence F15.282
      use F15.982
  fatal familial (FFI) A81.83
  idiopathic F51.01
  learned F51.3
  nonorganic origin F51.01
  not due to a substance or known physiological condition F51.01
    specified NEC F51.09
  paradoxical F51.03
  primary F51.01
  psychiatric F51.05
  psychophysiologic F51.04
  related to psychopathology F51.05
  short-term F51.02
  specified NEC G47.09
  stress-related F51.02
  transient F51.02
  without objective findings F51.02
Inspiration
  food or foreign body — *see* Foreign body, by site
  mucus — *see* Asphyxia, mucus
Inspissated bile syndrome (newborn) P59.1
Instability
  emotional (excessive) F60.3
  housing
    housed Z59.819
      with risk of homelessness Z59.811
      homelessness in past 12 months Z59.812
  joint (post-traumatic) M25.30
    ankle M25.37- ☑
    due to old ligament injury — *see* Disorder, ligament
    elbow M25.32- ☑
    flail — *see* Flail, joint
    foot M25.37- ☑
    hand M25.34- ☑
    hip M25.35- ☑
    knee M25.36- ☑
    lumbosacral — *see* subcategory M53.2 ☑
    prosthesis — *see* Complications, joint prosthesis, mechanical, displacement, by site
    sacroiliac — *see* subcategory M53.2 ☑
    secondary to
      old ligament injury — *see* Disorder, ligament
      removal of joint prosthesis M96.89
    shoulder (region) M25.31- ☑
    specified site NEC M25.39
    spine — *see* subcategory M53.2 ☑
    wrist M25.33- ☑
  knee (chronic) M23.5- ☑
  lumbosacral — *see* subcategory M53.2 ☑
  nervous F48.8
  personality (emotional) F60.3
  spine — *see* Instability, joint, spine
  vasomotor R55
Institutional syndrome (childhood) F94.2
Institutionalization, affecting child Z62.22
  disinhibited attachment F94.2
Insufficiency, insufficient
  accommodation, old age H52.4
  adrenal (gland) E27.40
    primary E27.1
  adrenocortical E27.40
    drug-induced E27.3
    iatrogenic E27.3
    primary E27.1
  anatomic crown height K08.89
  anterior (occlusal) guidance M26.54
  anus K62.89
  aortic (valve) I35.1
    with
      mitral (valve) disease I08.0

☑ **Additional Character Required** — Refer to the Tabular List for Character Selection

Insufficiency, insufficient — *continued*
 aortic — *continued*
  with — *continued*
   mitral disease — *continued*
    with tricuspid (valve) disease I08.3
    stenosis I35.2
    tricuspid (valve) disease I08.2
     with mitral (valve) disease I08.3
   congenital Q23.1
   rheumatic I06.1
    with
     mitral (valve) disease I08.0
      with tricuspid (valve) disease I08.3
     stenosis I06.2
      with mitral (valve) disease I08.0
       with tricuspid (valve) disease I08.3
     tricuspid (valve) disease I08.2
      with mitral (valve) disease I08.3
   specified cause NEC I35.1
   syphilitic A52.03
 arterial I77.1
  basilar G45.0
  carotid (hemispheric) G45.1
  cerebral I67.81
  coronary (acute or subacute) I24.8
  mesenteric K55.1
  peripheral I73.9
  precerebral (multiple) (bilateral) G45.2
  vertebral G45.0
 arteriovenous I99.8
 biliary K83.8
 cardiac — *see also* Insufficiency, myocardial
  due to presence of (cardiac) prosthesis I97.11- ☑
  postprocedural I97.11- ☑
 cardiorenal, hypertensive I13.2
 cardiovascular — *see* Disease, cardiovascular
 cerebrovascular (acute) I67.81
  with transient focal neurological signs and symptoms G45.8
 circulatory NEC I99.8
  newborn P29.89
 clinical crown length K08.89
 convergence H51.11
 coronary (acute or subacute) I24.8
  chronic or with a stated duration of over 4 weeks I25.89
 corticoadrenal E27.40
  primary E27.1
 dietary E63.9
 divergence H51.8
 food T73.0 ☑
 gastroesophageal K22.89
 gonadal
  ovary E28.39
  testis E29.1
 heart — *see also* Insufficiency, myocardial
  newborn P29.0
  valve — *see* Endocarditis
 hepatic — *see* Failure, hepatic
 idiopathic autonomic G90.09
 interocclusal distance of fully erupted teeth (ridge) M26.36
 kidney N28.9
  acute N28.9
  chronic N18.9
 lacrimal (secretion) H04.12- ☑
  passages — *see* Stenosis, lacrimal
 liver — *see* Failure, hepatic
 lung — *see* Insufficiency, pulmonary
 mental (congenital) — *see* Disability, intellectual
 mesenteric K55.1
 mitral (valve) I34.0
  with
   aortic valve disease I08.0
    with tricuspid (valve) disease I08.3
   obstruction or stenosis I05.2
    with aortic valve disease I08.0
   tricuspid (valve) disease I08.1
    with aortic (valve) disease I08.3
  congenital Q23.3
  rheumatic I05.1
   with
    aortic valve disease I08.0
     with tricuspid (valve) disease I08.3
    obstruction or stenosis I05.2
     with aortic valve disease I08.0
      with tricuspid (valve) disease I08.3
     tricuspid (valve) disease I08.1

Insufficiency, insufficient — *continued*
 mitral — *continued*
  rheumatic — *continued*
   with — *continued*
    tricuspid disease — *continued*
     with aortic (valve) disease I08.3
    active or acute I01.1
     with chorea, rheumatic (Sydenham's) I02.0
   specified cause, except rheumatic I34.0
 muscle — *see also* Disease, muscle
  heart — *see* Insufficiency, myocardial
  ocular NEC H50.9
 myocardial, myocardium (with arteriosclerosis) — *see also* Failure, heart I50.9
  with
   rheumatic fever (conditions in I00) I09.0
    active, acute or subacute I01.2
     with chorea I02.0
    inactive or quiescent (with chorea) I09.0
  congenital Q24.8
  hypertensive — *see* Hypertension, heart
  newborn P29.0
  rheumatic I09.0
   active, acute, or subacute I01.2
  syphilitic A52.06
 nourishment — *see also* Nutrition deficient T73.0 ☑
 pancreatic K86.89
  exocrine K86.81
 parathyroid (gland) E20.9
 peripheral vascular (arterial) I73.9
 pituitary E23.0
 placental (mother) O36.51- ☑
 platelets D69.6
 prenatal care affecting management of pregnancy O09.3- ☑
 progressive pluriglandular E31.0
 pulmonary J98.4
  acute, following surgery (nonthoracic) J95.2
   thoracic J95.1
  chronic, following surgery J95.3
  following
   shock J98.4
   trauma J98.4
  newborn P28.89
  valve I37.1
   with stenosis I37.2
   congenital Q22.2
   rheumatic I09.89
    with aortic, mitral or tricuspid (valve) disease I08.8
 pyloric K31.89
 renal (acute) N28.9
  chronic N18.9
 respiratory R06.89
  newborn P28.5
 rotation — *see* Malrotation
 sleep syndrome F51.12
 social insurance Z59.7
 suprarenal E27.40
  primary E27.1
 tarso-orbital fascia, congenital Q10.3
 testis E29.1
 thyroid (gland) (acquired) E03.9
  congenital E03.1
 tricuspid (valve) (rheumatic) I07.1
  with
   aortic (valve) disease I08.2
    with mitral (valve) disease I08.3
   mitral (valve) disease I08.1
    with aortic (valve) disease I08.3
   obstruction or stenosis I07.2
    with aortic (valve) disease I08.2
     with mitral (valve) disease I08.3
  congenital Q22.8
  nonrheumatic I36.1
   with stenosis I36.2
 urethral sphincter R32
 valve, valvular (heart) I38
  aortic — *see* Insufficiency, aortic (valve)
  congenital Q24.8
  mitral — *see* Insufficiency, mitral (valve)
  pulmonary — *see* Insufficiency, pulmonary, valve
  tricuspid — *see* Insufficiency, tricuspid (valve)
 vascular I99.8
  intestine K55.9
   acute — *see also* Ischemia, intestine, acute K55.059
   mesenteric K55.1

Insufficiency, insufficient — *continued*
 vascular — *continued*
  peripheral I73.9
  renal — *see* Hypertension, kidney
 velopharyngeal
  acquired K13.79
  congenital Q38.8
 venous (chronic) (peripheral) I87.2
 ventricular — *see* Insufficiency, myocardial
 welfare support Z59.7
Insufflation, fallopian Z31.41
Insular — *see* condition
Insulinoma
 pancreas
  benign D13.7
  malignant C25.4
  uncertain behavior D37.8
 specified site
  benign — *see* Neoplasm, by site, benign
  malignant — *see* Neoplasm, by site, malignant
  uncertain behavior — *see* Neoplasm, by site, uncertain behavior
 unspecified site
  benign D13.7
  malignant C25.4
  uncertain behavior D37.8
Insuloma — *see* Insulinoma
Interference
 balancing side M26.56
 non-working side M26.56
Intermenstrual — *see* condition
Intermittent — *see* condition
Internal — *see* condition
Interrogation
 cardiac defibrillator (automatic) (implantable) Z45.02
 cardiac pacemaker Z45.018
 cardiac (event) (loop) recorder Z45.09
 infusion pump (implanted) (intrathecal) Z45.1
 neurostimulator Z46.2
Interruption
 aortic arch Q25.21
 bundle of His I44.30
 phase-shift, sleep cycle — *see* Disorder, sleep, circadian rhythm
 sleep phase-shift, or 24 hour sleep-wake cycle — *see* Disorder, sleep, circadian rhythm
Interstitial — *see* condition
Intertrigo L30.4
 labialis K13.0
Intervertebral disc — *see* condition
Intestine, intestinal — *see* condition
Intolerance
 carbohydrate K90.49
 disaccharide, hereditary E73.0
 fat NEC K90.49
  pancreatic K90.3
 food K90.49
  dietary counseling and surveillance Z71.3
 fructose E74.10
  hereditary E74.12
 glucose (-galactose) E74.39
 gluten K90.41
 lactose E73.9
  specified NEC E73.8
 lysine E72.3
 milk NEC K90.49
  lactose E73.9
  orthostatic, chronic G90.A
 protein K90.49
 starch NEC K90.49
 sucrose (-isomaltose) E74.31
Intoxicated NEC (without dependence) — *see* Alcohol, intoxication
Intoxication
 acid — *see also* Acidosis E87.29
 alcoholic (acute) (without dependence) — *see* Alcohol, intoxication
 alimentary canal K52.1
 amphetamine (without dependence) — *see also* Abuse, drug, stimulant, with intoxication
  with dependence — *see* Dependence, drug, stimulant, with intoxication
  stimulant NEC F15.10
   with
    anxiety disorder F15.180
    intoxication F15.129
     with
      delirium F15.121

Intoxication — *continued*
  amphetamine — *see also* Abuse, drug, stimulant, with intoxication — *continued*
    stimulant — *continued*
      with — *continued*
        intoxication — *continued*
          with — *continued*
            perceptual disturbance F15.122
  anxiolytic (acute) (without dependence) — *see* Abuse, drug, sedative, with intoxication
    with dependence — *see* Dependence, drug, sedative, with intoxication
  caffeine F15.929
    with dependence — *see* Dependence, drug, stimulant, with intoxication
  cannabinoids (acute) (without dependence) — *see* Use, cannabis, with intoxication
    with
      abuse — *see* Abuse, drug, cannabis, with intoxication
      dependence — *see* Dependence, drug, cannabis, with intoxication
  chemical — *see* Table of Drugs and Chemicals
    via placenta or breast milk — *see* - Absorption, chemical, through placenta
  cocaine (acute) (without dependence) — *see* Abuse, drug, cocaine, with intoxication
    with dependence — *see* Dependence, drug, cocaine, with intoxication
  drug
    acute (without dependence) — *see* Abuse, drug, by type with intoxication
      with dependence — *see* Dependence, drug, by type with intoxication
    addictive
      via placenta or breast milk — *see* Absorption, drug, addictive, through placenta
    newborn P93.8
      gray baby syndrome P93.0
    overdose or wrong substance given or taken — *see* Table of Drugs and Chemicals, by drug, poisoning
  enteric K52.1
  foodborne A05.9
    bacterial A05.9
    classical (Clostridium botulinum) A05.1
    due to
      Bacillus cereus A05.4
      bacterium A05.9
        specified NEC A05.8
      Clostridium
        botulinum A05.1
        perfringens A05.2
        welchii A05.2
      Salmonella A02.9
        with
          (gastro)enteritis A02.0
          localized infection(s) A02.20
            arthritis A02.23
            meningitis A02.21
            osteomyelitis A02.24
            pneumonia A02.22
            pyelonephritis A02.25
            specified NEC A02.29
          sepsis A02.1
          specified manifestation NEC A02.8
      Staphylococcus A05.0
      Vibrio
        parahaemolyticus A05.3
        vulnificus A05.5
    enterotoxin, staphylococcal A05.0
    noxious — *see* Poisoning, food, noxious
  gastrointestinal K52.1
  hallucinogenic (without dependence) — *see* Abuse, drug, hallucinogen, with intoxication
    with dependence — *see* Dependence, drug, hallucinogen, with intoxication
  hepatocerebral intoxication K76.82
  hypnotic (acute) (without dependence) — *see* Abuse, drug, sedative, with intoxication
    with dependence — *see* Dependence, drug, sedative, with intoxication
  inhalant (acute) (without dependence) — *see* Abuse, drug, inhalant, with intoxication
    with dependence — *see* Dependence, drug, inhalant, with intoxication
  meaning
    inebriation — *see* category F10 ☑

Intoxication — *continued*
  meaning — *continued*
    poisoning — *see* Table of Drugs and Chemicals
  methyl alcohol (acute) (without dependence) — *see* Alcohol, intoxication
  opioid (acute) (without dependence) — *see* Abuse, drug, opioid, with intoxication
    with dependence — *see* Dependence, drug, opioid, with intoxication
  pathologic NEC (without dependence) — *see* Alcohol, intoxication
  phencyclidine (without dependence) — *see* Abuse, drug, hallucinogen, with intoxication
    with dependence — *see* Dependence, drug, hallucinogen, with intoxication
  potassium (K) E87.5
  psychoactive substance NEC (without dependence) — *see* Abuse, drug, psychoactive NEC, with intoxication
    with dependence — *see* Dependence, drug, psychoactive NEC, with intoxication
  sedative (acute) (without dependence) — *see* Abuse, drug, sedative, with intoxication
    with dependence — *see* Dependence, drug, sedative, with intoxication
  serum — *see also* Reaction, serum T80.69 ☑
  uremic — *see* Uremia
  volatile solvents (acute) (without dependence) — *see* Abuse, drug, inhalant, with intoxication
    with dependence — *see* Dependence, drug, inhalant, with intoxication
  water E87.79

Intraabdominal testis, testes
  bilateral Q53.211
  unilateral Q53.111
Intracranial — *see* condition
Intrahepatic gallbladder Q44.1
Intraligamentous — *see* condition
Intrathoracic — *see also* condition
  kidney Q63.2
Intrauterine contraceptive device
  checking Z30.431
  in situ Z97.5
  insertion Z30.430
    immediately following removal Z30.433
  management Z30.431
  reinsertion Z30.433
  removal Z30.432
  replacement Z30.433
  retention in pregnancy O26.3- ☑
Intraventricular — *see* condition
Intrinsic deformity — *see* Deformity
Intubation, difficult or failed T88.4 ☑
Intumescence, lens (eye) (cataract) — *see* Cataract
Intussusception (bowel) (colon) (enteric) (ileocecal) (ileocolic) (intestine) (rectum) K56.1
  appendix K38.8
  congenital Q43.8
  ureter (with obstruction) N13.5
Invagination (bowel, colon, intestine or rectum) K56.1
Inversion
  albumin-globulin (A-G) ratio E88.09
  bladder N32.89
  cecum — *see* Intussusception
  cervix N88.8
  chromosome in normal individual Q95.1
  circadian rhythm — *see* Disorder, sleep, circadian rhythm
  nipple N64.59
    congenital Q83.8
    gestational — *see* Retraction, nipple
    puerperal, postpartum — *see* Retraction, nipple
  nyctohemeral rhythm — *see* Disorder, sleep, circadian rhythm
  optic papilla Q14.2
  organ or site, congenital NEC — *see* Anomaly, by site
  sleep rhythm — *see* Disorder, sleep, circadian rhythm
  testis (congenital) Q55.29
  uterus (chronic) (postinfectional) (postpartal, old) N85.5
    postpartum O71.2
  vagina (posthysterectomy) N99.3
  ventricular Q20.5
Investigation — *see also* Examination Z04.9
  clinical research subject (control) (normal comparison) (participant) Z00.6
Involuntary movement, abnormal R25.9
Involution, involutional — *see also* condition

Involution, involutional — *continued*
  breast, cystic — *see* Dysplasia, mammary, specified type NEC
  depression (single episode) F32.89
    recurrent episode F33.9
  melancholia (single episode) F32.89
    recurrent episode F33.8
  ovary, senile — *see* Atrophy, ovary
  thymus failure E32.8
I.Q.
  20-34 F72
  35-49 F71
  50-69 F70
  under 20 F73
IRDS (type I) P22.0
  type II P22.1
Irideremia Q13.1
Iridis rubeosis — *see* Disorder, iris, vascular
Iridochoroiditis (panuveitis) — *see* Panuveitis
Iridocyclitis H20.9
  acute H20.0- ☑
    hypopyon H20.05- ☑
    primary H20.01- ☑
    recurrent H20.02- ☑
    secondary (noninfectious) H20.04- ☑
      infectious H20.03- ☑
  chronic H20.1- ☑
  due to allergy — *see* Iridocyclitis, acute, secondary
  endogenous — *see* Iridocyclitis, acute, primary
  Fuchs' — *see* Cyclitis, Fuchs' heterochromic
  gonococcal A54.32
  granulomatous — *see* Iridocyclitis, chronic
  herpes, herpetic (simplex) B00.51
    zoster B02.32
  hypopyon — *see* Iridocyclitis, acute, hypopyon
  in (due to)
    ankylosing spondylitis M45.9
    gonococcal infection A54.32
    herpes (simplex) virus B00.51
      zoster B02.32
    infectious disease NOS B99 ☑
    parasitic disease NOS B89 *[H22]*
    sarcoidosis D86.83
    syphilis A51.43
    tuberculosis A18.54
    zoster B02.32
  lens-induced H20.2- ☑
  nongranulomatous — *see* Iridocyclitis, acute
  recurrent — *see* Iridocyclitis, acute, recurrent
  rheumatic — *see* Iridocyclitis, chronic
  subacute — *see* Iridocyclitis, acute
  sympathetic — *see* Uveitis, sympathetic
  syphilitic (secondary) A51.43
  tuberculous (chronic) A18.54
  Vogt-Koyanagi H20.82- ☑
Iridocyclochoroiditis (panuveitis) — *see* Panuveitis
Iridodialysis H21.53- ☑
Iridodonesis H21.89
Iridoplegia (complete) (partial) (reflex) H57.09
Iridoschisis H21.25- ☑
Iris — *see also* condition
  bombé — *see* Membrane, pupillary
Iritis — *see also* Iridocyclitis
  chronic — *see* Iridocyclitis, chronic
  diabetic — *see* E08-E13 with .39
  due to
    herpes simplex B00.51
    leprosy A30.9 *[H22]*
  gonococcal A54.32
  gouty — *see also* Gout, by type M10.9 *[H22]*
  granulomatous — *see* Iridocyclitis, chronic
  lens induced — *see* Iridocyclitis, lens-induced
  papulosa (syphilitic) A52.71
  rheumatic — *see* Iridocyclitis, chronic
  syphilitic (secondary) A51.43
    congenital (early) A50.01
    late A52.71
  tuberculous A18.54
Iron — *see* condition
Iron-miner's lung J63.4
Irradiated enamel (tooth, teeth) K03.89
Irradiation effects, adverse T66 ☑
Irreducible, irreducibility — *see* condition
Irregular, irregularity
  action, heart I49.9
  alveolar process K08.89
  bleeding N92.6

Irregular, irregularity — *continued*
- breathing R06.89
- contour of cornea (acquired) — *see* Deformity, cornea
  - congenital Q13.4
- contour, reconstructed breast N65.0
- dentin (in pulp) K04.3
- eye movements H55.89
  - deficient
    - saccadic H55.81
    - smooth H55.82
  - nystagmus — *see* Nystagmus
- labor O62.2
- menstruation (cause unknown) N92.6
- periods N92.6
- prostate N42.9
- pupil — *see* Abnormality, pupillary
- reconstructed breast N65.0
- respiratory R06.89
- septum (nasal) J34.2
- shape, organ or site, congenital NEC — *see* Distortion
- sleep-wake pattern (rhythm) G47.23

Irritable, irritability R45.4
- bladder N32.89
- bowel (syndrome) K58.9
  - with
    - constipation K58.1
    - diarrhea K58.0
  - mixed K58.2
  - psychogenic F45.8
  - specified NEC K58.8
- bronchial — *see* Bronchitis
- cerebral, in newborn P91.3
- colon — *see also* Irritable, bowel K58.9
  - with diarrhea K58.0
  - psychogenic F45.8
- duodenum K59.89
- heart (psychogenic) F45.8
- hip — *see* Derangement, joint, specified type NEC, hip
- ileum K59.89
- infant R68.12
- jejunum K59.89
- rectum K59.89
- stomach K31.89
  - psychogenic F45.8
- sympathetic G90.8
- urethra N36.8

Irritation
- anus K62.89
- axillary nerve G54.0
- bladder N32.89
- brachial plexus G54.0
- bronchial — *see* Bronchitis
- cervical plexus G54.2
- cervix — *see* Cervicitis
- choroid, sympathetic — *see* Endophthalmitis
- cranial nerve — *see* Disorder, nerve, cranial
- gastric K31.89
  - psychogenic F45.8
- globe, sympathetic — *see* Uveitis, sympathetic
- labyrinth — *see* subcategory H83.2 ☑
- lumbosacral plexus G54.1
- meninges (traumatic) — *see* Injury, intracranial
  - nontraumatic — *see* Meningismus
- nerve — *see* Disorder, nerve
- nervous R45.0
- penis N48.89
- perineum NEC L29.3
- peripheral autonomic nervous system G90.8
- peritoneum — *see* Peritonitis
- pharynx J39.2
- plantar nerve — *see* Lesion, nerve, plantar
- spinal (cord) (traumatic) — *see also* Injury, spinal cord, by region
  - nerve G58.9
    - root NEC — *see* Radiculopathy
  - nontraumatic — *see* Myelopathy
- stomach K31.89
  - psychogenic F45.8
- sympathetic nerve NEC G90.8
- ulnar nerve — *see* Lesion, nerve, ulnar
- vagina N89.8

Ischemia, ischemic I99.8
- bowel (transient)
  - acute — *see also* Ischemia, intestine, acute K55.059
  - chronic K55.1
    - due to mesenteric artery insufficiency K55.1
- brain — *see* Ischemia, cerebral
- cardiac (see Disease, heart, ischemic)

Ischemia, ischemic — *continued*
- cardiomyopathy I25.5
- cerebral (chronic) (generalized) I67.82
  - arteriosclerotic I67.2
  - intermittent G45.9
  - newborn P91.0
  - recurrent focal G45.8
  - transient G45.9
- colon chronic (due to mesenteric artery insufficiency) K55.1
- coronary — *see* Disease, heart, ischemic
- demand (coronary) — *see also* Angina I24.8
  - with myocardial infarction I21.A1
  - resulting in myocardial infarction I21.A1
- heart (chronic or with a stated duration of over 4 weeks) I25.9
  - acute or with a stated duration of 4 weeks or less I24.9
  - subacute I24.9
- infarction, muscle — *see* Infarct, muscle
- intestine (large) (small) (transient) K55.9
  - acute K55.059
    - diffuse K55.052
    - focal K55.051
    - large K55.039
      - diffuse K55.032
      - focal K55.031
    - small K55.019
      - diffuse K55.012
      - focal K55.011
  - chronic K55.1
  - due to mesenteric artery insufficiency K55.1
- kidney N28.0
- limb, critical — *see* Arteriosclerosis, with critical limb ischemia
- limb-threatening, chronic — *see* Arteriosclerosis, with critical limb ischemia
- mesenteric, acute — *see also* Ischemia, intestine, acute K55.059
- muscle, traumatic T79.6 ☑
- myocardium, myocardial (chronic or with a stated duration of over 4 weeks) I25.9
  - acute, without myocardial infarction I51.3
  - silent (asymptomatic) I25.6
  - transient of newborn P29.4
- renal N28.0
- retina, retinal — *see* Occlusion, artery, retina
- small bowel
  - acute K55.019
    - diffuse K55.012
    - focal K55.011
  - chronic K55.1
  - due to mesenteric artery insufficiency K55.1
- spinal cord G95.11
- subendocardial — *see* Insufficiency, coronary
- supply (coronary) — *see also* Angina I25.9
  - due to vasospasm I20.1

Ischial spine — *see* condition
Ischialgia — *see* Sciatica
Ischiopagus Q89.4
Ischium, ischial — *see* condition
Ischuria R34
Iselin's disease or osteochondrosis — *see* Osteochondrosis, juvenile, metatarsus
Islands of
- parotid tissue in
  - lymph nodes Q38.6
  - neck structures Q38.6
- submaxillary glands in
  - fascia Q38.6
  - lymph nodes Q38.6
  - neck muscles Q38.6

Islet cell tumor, pancreas D13.7
Isoimmunization NEC — *see also* Incompatibility
- affecting management of pregnancy (ABO) (with hydrops fetalis) O36.11- ☑
  - anti-A sensitization O36.11- ☑
  - anti-B sensitization O36.19- ☑
  - anti-c sensitization O36.09- ☑
  - anti-C sensitization O36.09- ☑
  - anti-e sensitization O36.09- ☑
  - anti-E sensitization O36.09- ☑
  - Rh NEC O36.09- ☑
    - anti-D antibody O36.01- ☑
  - specified NEC O36.19- ☑
- newborn P55.9
  - with
    - hydrops fetalis P56.0

Isoimmunization — *continued*
- newborn — *continued*
  - with — *continued*
    - kernicterus P57.0
    - ABO (blood groups) P55.1
    - Rhesus (Rh) factor P55.0
    - specified type NEC P55.8

Isolation, isolated
- dwelling Z59.89
- family Z63.79
- social Z60.4

Isoleucinosis E71.19
Isomerism atrial appendages (with asplenia or polysplenia) Q20.6
Isosporiasis, isosporosis A07.3
Isovaleric acidemia E71.110
Issue of
- medical certificate Z02.79
  - for disability determination Z02.71
- repeat prescription (appliance) (glasses) (medicinal substance, medicament, medicine) Z76.0
  - contraception — *see* Contraception

Itch, itching — *see also* Pruritus
- baker's L23.6
- barber's B35.0
- bricklayer's L24.5
- cheese B88.0
- clam digger's B65.3
- coolie B76.9
- copra B88.0
- dew B76.9
- dhobi B35.6
- filarial — *see* Infestation, filarial
- grain B88.0
- grocer's B88.0
- ground B76.9
- harvest B88.0
- jock B35.6
- Malabar B35.5
  - beard B35.0
  - foot B35.3
  - scalp B35.0
- meaning scabies B86
- Norwegian B86
- perianal L29.0
- poultrymen's B88.0
- sarcoptic B86
- scabies B86
- scrub B88.0
- straw B88.0
- swimmer's B65.3
- water B76.9
- winter L29.8

Ivemark's syndrome (asplenia with congenital heart disease) Q89.01
Ivory bones Q78.2
Ixodiasis NEC B88.8

J

Jaccoud's syndrome — *see* Arthropathy, postrheumatic, chronic
Jackson's
- membrane Q43.3
- paralysis or syndrome G83.89
- veil Q43.3

Jacquet's dermatitis (diaper dermatitis) L22
Jadassohn-Pellizari's disease or anetoderma L90.2
Jadassohn's
- blue nevus — *see* Nevus
- intraepidermal epithelioma — *see* Neoplasm, skin, benign

Jaffe-Lichtenstein (-Uehlinger) **syndrome** — *see* Dysplasia, fibrous, bone NEC
Jakob-Creutzfeldt disease or syndrome — *see* Creutzfeldt-Jakob disease or syndrome
Jaksch-Luzet disease D64.89
Jamaican
- neuropathy G92.8
- paraplegic tropical ataxic-spastic syndrome G92.8

Janet's disease F48.8
Janiceps Q89.4
Jansky-Bielschowsky amaurotic idiocy E75.4
Japanese
- B-type encephalitis A83.0
- river fever A75.3

Jaundice (yellow) R17

Jaundice — *continued*
acholuric (familial) (splenomegalic) — *see also* Spherocytosis
acquired D59.8
breast-milk (inhibitor) P59.3
catarrhal (acute) B15.9
with hepatic coma B15.0
cholestatic (benign) R17
due to or associated with
delayed conjugation P59.8
associated with (due to) preterm delivery P59.0
preterm delivery P59.0
epidemic (catarrhal) B15.9
with hepatic coma B15.0
leptospiral A27.0
spirochetal A27.0
familial nonhemolytic (congenital) (Gilbert) E80.4
Crigler-Najjar E80.5
febrile (acute) B15.9
with hepatic coma B15.0
leptospiral A27.0
spirochetal A27.0
hematogenous D59.9
hemolytic (acquired) D59.9
congenital — *see* Spherocytosis
hemorrhagic (acute) (leptospiral) (spirochetal) A27.0
infectious (acute) (subacute) B15.9
with hepatic coma B15.0
leptospiral A27.0
spirochetal A27.0
leptospiral (hemorrhagic) A27.0
malignant (without coma) K72.90
with coma K72.91
neonatal — *see* Jaundice, newborn
newborn P59.9
due to or associated with
ABO
antibodies P55.1
incompatibility, maternal/fetal P55.1
isoimmunization P55.1
absence or deficiency of enzyme system for
bilirubin conjugation (congenital) P59.8
bleeding P58.1
breast milk inhibitors to conjugation P59.3
associated with preterm delivery P59.0
bruising P58.0
Crigler-Najjar syndrome E80.5
delayed conjugation P59.8
associated with preterm delivery P59.0
drugs or toxins
given to newborn P58.42
transmitted from mother P58.41
excessive hemolysis P58.9
due to
bleeding P58.1
bruising P58.0
drugs or toxins
given to newborn P58.42
transmitted from mother P58.41
infection P58.2
polycythemia P58.3
swallowed maternal blood P58.5
specified type NEC P58.8
galactosemia E74.21
Gilbert syndrome E80.4
hemolytic disease P55.9
ABO isoimmunization P55.1
Rh isoimmunization P55.0
specified NEC P55.8
hepatocellular damage P59.20
specified NEC P59.29
hereditary hemolytic anemia P58.8
hypothyroidism, congenital E03.1
incompatibility, maternal/fetal NOS P55.9
infection P58.2
inspissated bile syndrome P59.1
isoimmunization NOS P55.9
mucoviscidosis E84.9
polycythemia P58.3
preterm delivery P59.0
Rh
antibodies P55.0
incompatibility, maternal/fetal P55.0
isoimmunization P55.0
specified cause NEC P59.8
swallowed maternal blood P58.5
spherocytosis (congenital) D58.0
nonhemolytic congenital familial (Gilbert) E80.4

Jaundice — *continued*
nuclear, newborn — *see also* Kernicterus of newborn
P57.9
obstructive — *see also* Obstruction, bile duct K83.1
post-immunization — *see* Hepatitis, viral, type, B
post-transfusion — *see* Hepatitis, viral, type, B
regurgitation — *see also* Obstruction, bile duct K83.1
serum (homologous) (prophylactic) (therapeutic) —
see Hepatitis, viral, type, B
spirochetal (hemorrhagic) A27.0
symptomatic R17
newborn P59.9
Jaw — *see* condition
Jaw-winking phenomenon or syndrome Q07.8
Jealousy
alcoholic F10.988
childhood F93.8
sibling F93.8
Jejunitis — *see* Enteritis
Jejunostomy status Z93.4
Jejunum, jejunal — *see* condition
Jensen's disease — *see* Inflammation, chorioretinal, fo-
cal, juxtapapillary
Jerks, myoclonic G25.3
Jervell-Lange-Nielsen syndrome I45.81
Jeune's disease Q77.2
Jigger disease B88.1
Job's syndrome (chronic granulomatous disease) D71
Joint — *see also* condition
mice — *see* Loose, body, joint
knee M23.4- ☑
Jordan's anomaly or syndrome D72.0
Joseph-Diamond-Blackfan anemia (congenital hy-
poplastic) D61.01
Jungle yellow fever A95.0
Jüngling's disease — *see* Sarcoidosis
Juvenile — *see* condition

K

Kahler's disease C90.0- ☑
Kakke E51.11
Kala-azar B55.0
Kallmann's syndrome E23.0
Kanner's syndrome (autism) — *see* Psychosis, childhood
Kaposi's
dermatosis (xeroderma pigmentosum) Q82.1
lichen ruber L44.0
acuminatus L44.0
sarcoma
colon C46.4
connective tissue C46.1
gastrointestinal organ C46.4
lung C46.5- ☑
lymph node (multiple) C46.3
palate (hard) (soft) C46.2
rectum C46.4
skin (multiple sites) C46.0
specified site NEC C46.7
stomach C46.4
unspecified site C46.9
varicelliform eruption B00.0
vaccinia T88.1 ☑
Kartagener's syndrome or triad (sinusitis, bronchiectasis, situs inversus) Q89.3
Karyotype
with abnormality except iso (Xq) Q96.2
45,X Q96.0
46,X
iso (Xq) Q96.1
46,XX Q98.3
with streak gonads Q50.32
hermaphrodite (true) Q99.1
male Q98.3
46,XY
with streak gonads Q56.1
female Q97.3
hermaphrodite (true) Q99.1
47,XXX Q97.0
47,XXY Q98.0
47,XYY Q98.5
Kaschin-Beck disease — *see* Disease, Kaschin-Beck
Katayama's disease or fever B65.2
Kawasaki's syndrome M30.3
Kayser-Fleischer ring (cornea) (pseudosclerosis)
H18.04- ☑

Kaznelson's syndrome (congenital hypoplastic anemia)
D61.01
Kearns-Sayre syndrome H49.81- ☑
Kedani fever A75.3
Kelis L91.0
Kelly (-Patterson) **syndrome** (sideropenic dysphagia)
D50.1
Keloid, cheloid L91.0
acne L73.0
Addison's L94.0
cornea — *see* Opacity, cornea
Hawkin's L91.0
scar L91.0
Keloma L91.0
Kenya fever A77.1
Keratectasia — *see also* Ectasia, cornea
congenital Q13.4
Keratinization of alveolar ridge mucosa
excessive K13.23
minimal K13.22
Keratinized residual ridge mucosa
excessive K13.23
minimal K13.22
Keratitis (nodular) (nonulcerative) (simple) (zonular)
H16.9
with ulceration (central) (marginal) (perforated) (ring)
— *see* Ulcer, cornea
actinic — *see* Photokeratitis
arborescens (herpes simplex) B00.52
areolar H16.11- ☑
bullosa H16.8
deep H16.309
specified type NEC H16.399
dendritic (a) (herpes simplex) B00.52
disciform (is) (herpes simplex) B00.52
varicella B01.81
filamentary H16.12- ☑
gonococcal (congenital or prenatal) A54.33
herpes, herpetic (simplex) B00.52
zoster B02.33
in (due to)
acanthamebiasis B60.13
adenovirus B30.0
exanthema — *see also* Exanthem B09
herpes (simplex) virus B00.52
measles B05.81
syphilis A50.31
tuberculosis A18.52
zoster B02.33
interstitial (nonsyphilitic) H16.30- ☑
diffuse H16.32- ☑
herpes, herpetic (simplex) B00.52
zoster B02.33
sclerosing H16.33- ☑
specified type NEC H16.39- ☑
syphilitic (congenital) (late) A50.31
tuberculous A18.52
macular H16.11- ☑
nummular H16.11- ☑
oyster shuckers' H16.8
parenchymatous — *see* Keratitis, interstitial
petrificans H16.8
postmeasles B05.81
punctata
leprosa A30.9 *[H16.14-]* ☑
syphilitic (profunda) A50.31
punctate H16.14- ☑
purulent H16.8
rosacea L71.8
sclerosing H16.33- ☑
specified type NEC H16.8
stellate H16.11- ☑
striate H16.11- ☑
superficial H16.10- ☑
with conjunctivitis — *see* Keratoconjunctivitis
due to light — *see* Photokeratitis
suppurative H16.8
syphilitic (congenital) (prenatal) A50.31
trachomatous A71.1
sequelae B94.0
tuberculous A18.52
vesicular H16.8
xerotic — *see also* Keratomalacia H16.8
vitamin A deficiency E50.4
Keratoacanthoma L85.8
Keratocele — *see* Descemetocele
Keratoconjunctivitis H16.20- ☑

Keratoconjunctivitis — *continued*
  Acanthamoeba B60.13
  adenoviral B30.0
  epidemic B30.0
  exposure H16.21- ☑
  herpes, herpetic (simplex) B00.52
    zoster B02.33
  in exanthema — *see also* Exanthem B09
  infectious B30.0
  lagophthalmic — *see* Keratoconjunctivitis, specified
    type NEC
  neurotrophic H16.23- ☑
  phlyctenular H16.25- ☑
  postmeasles B05.81
  shipyard B30.0
  sicca (Sjogren's) M35.0- ☑
    not Sjogren's H16.22- ☑
  specified type NEC H16.29- ☑
  tuberculous (phlyctenular) A18.52
  vernal H16.26- ☑
Keratoconus H18.60- ☑
  congenital Q13.4
  stable H18.61- ☑
  unstable H18.62- ☑
Keratocyst (dental) (odontogenic) — *see* Cyst, calcifying odontogenic
Keratoderma, keratodermia (congenital) (palmaris et plantaris) (symmetrical) Q82.8
  acquired L85.1
    in diseases classified elsewhere L86
  climactericum L85.1
  gonococcal A54.89
  gonorrheal A54.89
  punctata L85.2
  Reiter's — *see* Reiter's disease
Keratodermatocele — *see* Descemetocele
Keratoglobus H18.79 ☑
  congenital Q15.8
    with glaucoma Q15.0
Keratohemia — *see* Pigmentation, cornea, stromal
Keratoiritis — *see also* Iridocyclitis
  syphilitic A50.39
  tuberculous A18.54
Keratoma L57.0
  palmaris and plantaris hereditarium Q82.8
  senile L57.0
Keratomalacia H18.44- ☑
  vitamin A deficiency E50.4
Keratomegaly Q13.4
Keratomycosis B49
  nigrans, nigricans (palmaris) B36.1
Keratopathy H18.9
  band H18.42- ☑
  bullous (aphakic), following cataract surgery H59.01- ☑
  bullous H18.1- ☑
Keratoscleritis, tuberculous A18.52
Keratosis L57.0
  actinic L57.0
  arsenical L85.8
  congenital, specified NEC Q80.8
  female genital NEC N94.89
  follicularis Q82.8
    acquired L11.0
    congenita Q82.8
    et parafollicularis in cutem penetrans L87.0
    spinulosa (decalvans) Q82.8
    vitamin A deficiency E50.8
  gonococcal A54.89
  male genital (external) N50.89
  nigricans L83
  obturans, external ear (canal) — *see* Cholesteatoma, external ear
  palmaris et plantaris (inherited) (symmetrical) Q82.8
    acquired L85.1
  penile N48.89
  pharynx J39.2
  pilaris, acquired L85.8
  punctata (palmaris et plantaris) L85.2
  scrotal N50.89
  seborrheic L82.1
    inflamed L82.0
  senile L57.0
  solar L57.0
  tonsillaris J35.8
  vagina N89.4
  vegetans Q82.8
  vitamin A deficiency E50.8
  vocal cord J38.3

Kerato-uveitis — *see* Iridocyclitis
Kerion (celsi) B35.0
Kernicterus of newborn (not due to isoimmunization) P57.9
  due to isoimmunization (conditions in P55.0-P55.9) P57.0
  specified type NEC P57.8
Kerunoparalysis T75.09 ☑
Keshan disease E59
Ketoacidosis E87.29
  diabetic — *see* Diabetes, by type, with ketoacidosis
Ketonuria R82.4
Ketosis NEC E88.89
  diabetic — *see* Diabetes, by type, with ketoacidosis
Kew Garden fever A79.1
Kidney — *see* condition
Kienböck's disease — *see also* Osteochondrosis, juvenile, hand, carpal lunate
  adult M93.1
Kimmelstiel (-Wilson) **disease** — *see* Diabetes, Kimmelstiel (-Wilson) disease
Kink, kinking
  artery I77.1
  hair (acquired) L67.8
  ileum or intestine — *see* Obstruction, intestine
  Lane's — *see* Obstruction, intestine
  organ or site, congenital NEC — *see* Anomaly, by site
  ureter (pelvic junction) N13.5
    with
      hydronephrosis N13.1
        with infection N13.6
      pyelonephritis (chronic) N11.1
    congenital Q62.39
  vein(s) I87.8
    caval I87.1
    peripheral I87.1
Kinnier Wilson's disease (hepatolenticular degeneration) E83.01
Kissing spine M48.20
  cervical region M48.22
  cervicothoracic region M48.23
  lumbar region M48.26
  lumbosacral region M48.27
  occipito-atlanto-axial region M48.21
  thoracic region M48.24
  thoracolumbar region M48.25
Klatskin's tumor C22.1
Klauder's disease A26.8
Klebs' disease — *see also* Glomerulonephritis N05- ☑
Klebsiella (K.) **pneumoniae, as cause of disease classified elsewhere** B96.1
Klein (e)-**Levin syndrome** G47.13
Kleptomania F63.2
Klinefelter's syndrome Q98.4
  karyotype 47,XXY Q98.0
  male with more than two X chromosomes Q98.1
Klippel-Feil deficiency, disease, or syndrome (brevicollis) Q76.1
Klippel's disease I67.2
Klippel-Trenaunay (-Weber) **syndrome** Q87.2
Klumpke (-Déjerine) **palsy, paralysis** (birth) (newborn) P14.1
Knee — *see* condition
Knock knee (acquired) M21.06- ☑
  congenital Q74.1
Knot(s)
  intestinal, syndrome (volvulus) K56.2
  surfer S89.8- ☑
  umbilical cord (true) O69.2 ☑
Knotting (of)
  hair L67.8
  intestine K56.2
Knuckle pad (Garrod's) M72.1
Koch's
  infection — *see* Tuberculosis
  relapsing fever A68.9
Koch-Weeks' conjunctivitis — *see* Conjunctivitis, acute, mucopurulent
Köebner's syndrome Q81.8
Köenig's disease (osteochondritis dissecans) — *see* Osteochondritis, dissecans
Köhler-Pellegrini-Steida disease or syndrome (calcification, knee joint) — *see* Bursitis, tibial collateral
Köhler's disease
  patellar — *see* Osteochondrosis, juvenile, patella
  tarsal navicular — *see* Osteochondrosis, juvenile, tarsus
Koilonychia L60.3

Koilonychia — *continued*
  congenital Q84.6
Kojevnikov's, epilepsy — *see* Kozhevnikof's epilepsy
Koplik's spots B05.9
Kopp's asthma E32.8
Korsakoff's (Wernicke) **disease, psychosis or syndrome** (alcoholic) F10.96
  with dependence F10.26
  drug-induced
    due to drug abuse — *see* Abuse, drug, by type, with amnestic disorder
    due to drug dependence — *see* Dependence, drug, by type, with amnestic disorder
  nonalcoholic F04
Korsakov's disease, psychosis or syndrome — *see* Korsakoff's disease
Korsakow's disease, psychosis or syndrome — *see* Korsakoff's disease
Kostmann's disease or syndrome (infantile genetic agranulocytosis) — *see* Agranulocytosis
Kozhevnikof's epilepsy G40.109
  intractable G40.119
    with status epilepticus G40.111
    without status epilepticus G40.119
  not intractable G40.109
    with status epilepticus G40.101
    without status epilepticus G40.109
Krabbe's
  disease E75.23
  syndrome, congenital muscle hypoplasia Q79.8
Kraepelin-Morel disease — *see* Schizophrenia
Kraft-Weber-Dimitri disease Q85.89
Kraurosis
  ani K62.89
  penis N48.0
  vagina N89.8
  vulva N90.4
Kreotoxism A05.9
Krukenberg's
  spindle — *see* Pigmentation, cornea, posterior
  tumor C79.6- ☑
Kufs' disease E75.4
Kugelberg-Welander disease G12.1
Kuhnt-Junius degeneration — *see also* Degeneration, macula H35.32- ☑
Kümmell's disease or spondylitis — *see* Spondylopathy, traumatic
Kupffer cell sarcoma C22.3
Kuru A81.81
Kussmaul's
  disease M30.0
  respiration E87.29
    in diabetic acidosis — *see* Diabetes, by type, with ketoacidosis
Kwashiorkor E40
  marasmic, marasmus type E42
Kyasanur Forest disease A98.2
Kyphoscoliosis, kyphoscoliotic (acquired) — *see also* Scoliosis M41.9
  congenital Q67.5
  heart (disease) I27.1
  sequelae of rickets E64.3
  tuberculous A18.01
Kyphosis, kyphotic (acquired) M40.209
  cervical region M40.202
  cervicothoracic region M40.203
  congenital Q76.419
    cervical region Q76.412
    cervicothoracic region Q76.413
    occipito-atlanto-axial region Q76.411
    thoracic region Q76.414
    thoracolumbar region Q76.415
  Morquio-Brailsford type (spinal) — *see also* subcategory M49.8 E76.219
  postlaminectomy M96.3
  postradiation therapy M96.2
  postural (adolescent) M40.00
    cervicothoracic region M40.03
    thoracic region M40.04
    thoracolumbar region M40.05
  secondary NEC M40.10
    cervical region M40.12
    cervicothoracic region M40.13
    thoracic region M40.14
    thoracolumbar region M40.15
  sequelae of rickets E64.3
  specified type NEC M40.299
    cervical region M40.292

Kyphosis, kyphotic — *continued*
　specified type — *continued*
　　cervicothoracic region M40.293
　　thoracic region M40.294
　　thoracolumbar region M40.295
　syphilitic, congenital A50.56
　thoracic region M40.204
　thoracolumbar region M40.205
　tuberculous A18.01
Kyrle disease L87.0

L

Labia, labium — *see* condition
Labile
　blood pressure R09.89
　vasomotor system I73.9
Labioglossal paralysis G12.29
Labium leporinum — *see* Cleft, lip
Labor — *see* Delivery
Labored breathing — *see* Hyperventilation
Labyrinthitis (circumscribed) (destructive) (diffuse) (inner ear) (latent) (purulent) (suppurative) — *see also* subcategory H83.0 ☑
　syphilitic A52.79
Laceration
　with abortion — *see* Abortion, by type, complicated by laceration of pelvic organs
　abdomen, abdominal
　　wall S31.119 ☑
　　　with
　　　　foreign body S31.129 ☑
　　　　penetration into peritoneal cavity S31.619 ☑
　　　　　with foreign body S31.629 ☑
　　　　epigastric region S31.112 ☑
　　　　　with
　　　　　　foreign body S31.122 ☑
　　　　　　penetration into peritoneal cavity S31.612 ☑
　　　　　　　with foreign body S31.622 ☑
　　　　left
　　　　　lower quadrant S31.114 ☑
　　　　　　with
　　　　　　　foreign body S31.124 ☑
　　　　　　　penetration into peritoneal cavity S31.614 ☑
　　　　　　　　with foreign body S31.624 ☑
　　　　　upper quadrant S31.111 ☑
　　　　　　with
　　　　　　　foreign body S31.121 ☑
　　　　　　　penetration into peritoneal cavity S31.611 ☑
　　　　　　　　with foreign body S31.621 ☑
　　　　periumbilic region S31.115 ☑
　　　　　with
　　　　　　foreign body S31.125 ☑
　　　　　　penetration into peritoneal cavity S31.615 ☑
　　　　　　　with foreign body S31.625 ☑
　　　　right
　　　　　lower quadrant S31.113 ☑
　　　　　　with
　　　　　　　foreign body S31.123 ☑
　　　　　　　penetration into peritoneal cavity S31.613 ☑
　　　　　　　　with foreign body S31.623 ☑
　　　　　upper quadrant S31.110 ☑
　　　　　　with
　　　　　　　foreign body S31.120 ☑
　　　　　　　penetration into peritoneal cavity S31.610 ☑
　　　　　　　　with foreign body S31.620 ☑
　accidental, complicating surgery — *see* Complications, surgical, accidental puncture or laceration
　Achilles tendon S86.02- ☑
　adrenal gland S37.813 ☑
　alveolar (process) — *see* Laceration, oral cavity
　ankle S91.01- ☑
　　with
　　　foreign body S91.02- ☑
　antecubital space — *see* Laceration, elbow
　anus (sphincter) S31.831 ☑
　　with
　　　ectopic or molar pregnancy O08.6
　　　foreign body S31.832 ☑
　　complicating delivery — *see* Delivery, complicated, by, laceration, anus (sphincter)

Laceration — *continued*
　anus — *continued*
　　following ectopic or molar pregnancy O08.6
　　nontraumatic, nonpuerperal — *see* Fissure, anus
　arm (upper) S41.11- ☑
　　with foreign body S41.12- ☑
　　lower — *see* Laceration, forearm
　auditory canal (external) (meatus) — *see* Laceration, ear
　auricle, ear — *see* Laceration, ear
　axilla — *see* Laceration, arm
　back — *see also* Laceration, thorax, back
　　lower S31.010 ☑
　　　with
　　　　foreign body S31.020 ☑
　　　　　with penetration into retroperitoneal space S31.021 ☑
　　　　penetration into retroperitoneal space S31.011 ☑
　bile duct S36.13 ☑
　bladder S37.23 ☑
　　with ectopic or molar pregnancy O08.6
　　following ectopic or molar pregnancy O08.6
　　obstetrical trauma O71.5
　blood vessel — *see* Injury, blood vessel
　bowel — *see also* Laceration, intestine
　　with ectopic or molar pregnancy O08.6
　　complicating abortion — *see* Abortion, by type, complicated by, specified condition NEC
　　following ectopic or molar pregnancy O08.6
　　obstetrical trauma O71.5
　brain (any part) (cortex) (diffuse) (membrane) — *see also* Injury, intracranial, diffuse
　　during birth P10.8
　　　with hemorrhage P10.1
　　focal — *see* Injury, intracranial, focal brain injury
　brainstem S06.38- ☑
　breast S21.01- ☑
　　with foreign body S21.02- ☑
　broad ligament S37.893 ☑
　　with ectopic or molar pregnancy O08.6
　　following ectopic or molar pregnancy O08.6
　　laceration syndrome N83.8
　　obstetrical trauma O71.6
　　syndrome (laceration) N83.8
　buttock S31.801 ☑
　　with foreign body S31.802 ☑
　　left S31.821 ☑
　　　with foreign body S31.822 ☑
　　right S31.811 ☑
　　　with foreign body S31.812 ☑
　calf — *see* Laceration, leg
　canaliculus lacrimalis — *see* Laceration, eyelid
　canthus, eye — *see* Laceration, eyelid
　capsule, joint — *see* Sprain
　causing eversion of cervix uteri (old) N86
　central (perineal), complicating delivery O70.9
　cerebellum, traumatic S06.37- ☑
　cerebral S06.33- ☑
　　during birth P10.8
　　　with hemorrhage P10.1
　　left side S06.32- ☑
　　right side S06.31- ☑
　cervix (uteri)
　　with ectopic or molar pregnancy O08.6
　　following ectopic or molar pregnancy O08.6
　　nonpuerperal, nontraumatic N88.1
　　obstetrical trauma (current) O71.3
　　old (postpartal) N88.1
　　traumatic S37.63 ☑
　cheek (external) S01.41- ☑
　　with foreign body S01.42- ☑
　　internal — *see* Laceration, oral cavity
　chest wall — *see* Laceration, thorax
　chin — *see* Laceration, head, specified site NEC
　chordae tendinae NEC I51.1
　　concurrent with acute myocardial infarction — *see* Infarct, myocardium
　　following acute myocardial infarction (current complication) I23.4
　clitoris — *see* Laceration, vulva
　colon — *see* Laceration, intestine, large, colon
　common bile duct S36.13 ☑
　cortex (cerebral) — *see* Injury, intracranial, diffuse
　costal region — *see* Laceration, thorax
　cystic duct S36.13 ☑
　diaphragm S27.803 ☑

Laceration — *continued*
　digit(s)
　　foot — *see* Laceration, toe
　　hand — *see* Laceration, finger
　duodenum S36.430 ☑
　ear (canal) (external) S01.31- ☑
　　with foreign body S01.32- ☑
　　drum S09.2- ☑
　elbow S51.01- ☑
　　with
　　　foreign body S51.02- ☑
　epididymis — *see* Laceration, testis
　epigastric region — *see* Laceration, abdomen, wall, epigastric region
　esophagus K22.89
　　traumatic
　　　cervical S11.21 ☑
　　　　with foreign body S11.22 ☑
　　　thoracic S27.813 ☑
　eye (ball) S05.3- ☑
　　with prolapse or loss of intraocular tissue S05.2- ☑
　　penetrating S05.6- ☑
　eyebrow — *see* Laceration, eyelid
　eyelid S01.11- ☑
　　with foreign body S01.12- ☑
　face NEC — *see* Laceration, head, specified site NEC
　fallopian tube S37.539 ☑
　　bilateral S37.532 ☑
　　unilateral S37.531 ☑
　finger(s) S61.219 ☑
　　with
　　　damage to nail S61.319 ☑
　　　　with
　　　　　foreign body S61.329 ☑
　　　foreign body S61.229 ☑
　　index S61.218 ☑
　　　with
　　　　damage to nail S61.318 ☑
　　　　　with
　　　　　　foreign body S61.328 ☑
　　　　foreign body S61.228 ☑
　　　left S61.211 ☑
　　　　with
　　　　　damage to nail S61.311 ☑
　　　　　　with
　　　　　　　foreign body S61.321 ☑
　　　　　foreign body S61.221 ☑
　　　right S61.210 ☑
　　　　with
　　　　　damage to nail S61.310 ☑
　　　　　　with
　　　　　　　foreign body S61.320 ☑
　　　　　foreign body S61.220 ☑
　　little S61.218 ☑
　　　with
　　　　damage to nail S61.318 ☑
　　　　　with
　　　　　　foreign body S61.328 ☑
　　　　foreign body S61.228 ☑
　　　left S61.217 ☑
　　　　with
　　　　　damage to nail S61.317 ☑
　　　　　　with
　　　　　　　foreign body S61.327 ☑
　　　　　foreign body S61.227 ☑
　　　right S61.216 ☑
　　　　with
　　　　　damage to nail S61.316 ☑
　　　　　　with
　　　　　　　foreign body S61.326 ☑
　　　　　foreign body S61.226 ☑
　　middle S61.218 ☑
　　　with
　　　　damage to nail S61.318 ☑
　　　　　with
　　　　　　foreign body S61.328 ☑
　　　　foreign body S61.228 ☑
　　　left S61.213 ☑
　　　　with
　　　　　damage to nail S61.313 ☑
　　　　　　with
　　　　　　　foreign body S61.323 ☑
　　　　　foreign body S61.223 ☑
　　　right S61.212 ☑
　　　　with
　　　　　damage to nail S61.312 ☑

Laceration — *continued*
  finger(s) — *continued*
    middle — *continued*
      right — *continued*
        with — *continued*
          damage to nail — *continued*
            with
              foreign body S61.322 ☑
            foreign body S61.222 ☑
      ring S61.218 ☑
        with
          damage to nail S61.318 ☑
            with
              foreign body S61.328 ☑
          foreign body S61.228 ☑
        left S61.215 ☑
          with
            damage to nail S61.315 ☑
              with
                foreign body S61.325 ☑
            foreign body S61.225 ☑
        right S61.214 ☑
          with
            damage to nail S61.314 ☑
              with
                foreign body S61.324 ☑
            foreign body S61.224 ☑
  flank S31.119 ☑
    with foreign body S31.129 ☑
  foot (except toe(s) alone) S91.319 ☑
    with foreign body S91.329 ☑
    left S91.312 ☑
      with foreign body S91.322 ☑
    right S91.311 ☑
      with foreign body S91.321 ☑
    toe — *see* Laceration, toe
  forearm S51.819 ☑
    with
      foreign body S51.829 ☑
    elbow only — *see* Laceration, elbow
    left S51.812 ☑
      with
        foreign body S51.822 ☑
    right S51.811 ☑
      with
        foreign body S51.821 ☑
  forehead S01.81 ☑
    with foreign body S01.82 ☑
  fourchette O70.0
    with ectopic or molar pregnancy O08.6
    complicating delivery O70.0
    following ectopic or molar pregnancy O08.6
  gallbladder S36.123 ☑
  genital organs, external
    female S31.512 ☑
      with foreign body S31.522 ☑
      vagina — *see* Laceration, vagina
      vulva — *see* Laceration, vulva
    male S31.511 ☑
      with foreign body S31.521 ☑
      penis — *see* Laceration, penis
      scrotum — *see* Laceration, scrotum
      testis — *see* Laceration, testis
  groin — *see* Laceration, abdomen, wall
  gum — *see* Laceration, oral cavity
  hand S61.419 ☑
    with
      foreign body S61.429 ☑
    finger — *see* Laceration, finger
    left S61.412 ☑
      with
        foreign body S61.422 ☑
    right S61.411 ☑
      with
        foreign body S61.421 ☑
    thumb — *see* Laceration, thumb
  head S01.91 ☑
    with foreign body S01.92 ☑
    cheek — *see* Laceration, cheek
    ear — *see* Laceration, ear
    eyelid — *see* Laceration, eyelid
    lip — *see* Laceration, lip
    nose — *see* Laceration, nose
    oral cavity — *see* Laceration, oral cavity
    scalp S01.01 ☑
      with foreign body S01.02 ☑

Laceration — *continued*
  head — *continued*
    specified site NEC S01.81 ☑
      with foreign body S01.82 ☑
    temporomandibular area — *see* Laceration, cheek
  heart — *see* Injury, heart, laceration
  heel — *see* Laceration, foot
  hepatic duct S36.13 ☑
  hip S71.019 ☑
    with foreign body S71.029 ☑
    left S71.012 ☑
      with foreign body S71.022 ☑
    right S71.011 ☑
      with foreign body S71.021 ☑
  hymen — *see* Laceration, vagina
  hypochondrium — *see* Laceration, abdomen, wall
  hypogastric region — *see* Laceration, abdomen, wall
  ileum S36.438 ☑
  inguinal region — *see* Laceration, abdomen, wall
  instep — *see* Laceration, foot
  internal organ — *see* Injury, by site
  interscapular region — *see* Laceration, thorax, back
  intestine
    large
      colon S36.539 ☑
        ascending S36.530 ☑
        descending S36.532 ☑
        sigmoid S36.533 ☑
        specified site NEC S36.538 ☑
      rectum S36.63 ☑
        transverse S36.531 ☑
    small S36.439 ☑
      duodenum S36.430 ☑
      specified site NEC S36.438 ☑
  intra-abdominal organ S36.93 ☑
    intestine — *see* Laceration, intestine
    liver — *see* Laceration, liver
    pancreas — *see* Laceration, pancreas
    peritoneum S36.81 ☑
    specified site NEC S36.893 ☑
    spleen — *see* Laceration, spleen
    stomach — *see* Laceration, stomach
  intracranial NEC — *see also* Injury, intracranial, diffuse
    birth injury P10.9
  jaw — *see* Laceration, head, specified site NEC
  jejunum S36.438 ☑
  joint capsule — *see* Sprain, by site
  kidney S37.03- ☑
    major (greater than 3 cm) (massive) (stellate) S37.06- ☑
    minor (less than 1 cm) S37.04- ☑
    moderate (1 to 3 cm) S37.05- ☑
      multiple S37.06- ☑
  knee S81.01- ☑
    with foreign body S81.02- ☑
  labium (majus) (minus) — *see* Laceration, vulva
  lacrimal duct — *see* Laceration, eyelid
  large intestine — *see* Laceration, intestine, large
  larynx S11.011 ☑
    with foreign body S11.012 ☑
  leg (lower) S81.819 ☑
    with foreign body S81.829 ☑
    foot — *see* Laceration, foot
    knee — *see* Laceration, knee
    left S81.812 ☑
      with foreign body S81.822 ☑
    right S81.811 ☑
      with foreign body S81.821 ☑
    upper — *see* Laceration, thigh
  ligament — *see* Sprain
  lip S01.511 ☑
    with foreign body S01.521 ☑
  liver S36.113 ☑
    major (stellate) S36.116 ☑
    minor S36.114 ☑
    moderate S36.115 ☑
  loin — *see* Laceration, abdomen, wall
  lower back — *see* Laceration, back, lower
  lumbar region — *see* Laceration, back, lower
  lung S27.339 ☑
    bilateral S27.332 ☑
    unilateral S27.331 ☑
  malar region — *see* Laceration, head, specified site NEC
  mammary — *see* Laceration, breast
  mastoid region — *see* Laceration, head, specified site NEC

Laceration — *continued*
  meninges — *see* Injury, intracranial, diffuse
  meniscus — *see* Tear, meniscus
  mesentery S36.893 ☑
  mesosalpinx S37.893 ☑
  mouth — *see* Laceration, oral cavity
  muscle — *see* Injury, muscle, by site, laceration
  nail
    finger — *see* Laceration, finger, with damage to nail
    toe — *see* Laceration, toe, with damage to nail
  nasal (septum) (sinus) — *see* Laceration, nose
  nasopharynx — *see* Laceration, head, specified site NEC
  neck S11.91 ☑
    with foreign body S11.92 ☑
    involving
      cervical esophagus S11.21 ☑
        with foreign body S11.22 ☑
      larynx — *see* Laceration, larynx
      pharynx — *see* Laceration, pharynx
      thyroid gland — *see* Laceration, thyroid gland
      trachea — *see* Laceration, trachea
    specified site NEC S11.81 ☑
      with foreign body S11.82 ☑
  nerve — *see* Injury, nerve
  nose (septum) (sinus) S01.21 ☑
    with foreign body S01.22 ☑
  ocular NOS S05.3- ☑
    adnexa NOS S01.11- ☑
  oral cavity S01.512 ☑
    with foreign body S01.522 ☑
  orbit (eye) — *see* Wound, open, ocular, orbit
  ovary S37.439 ☑
    bilateral S37.432 ☑
    unilateral S37.431 ☑
  palate — *see* Laceration, oral cavity
  palm — *see* Laceration, hand
  pancreas S36.239 ☑
  pelvic S31.010 ☑
    with
      foreign body S31.020 ☑
        penetration into retroperitoneal cavity S31.021 ☑
      penetration into retroperitoneal cavity S31.011 ☑
    floor — *see also* Laceration, back, lower
      with ectopic or molar pregnancy O08.6
      complicating delivery O70.1
      following ectopic or molar pregnancy O08.6
      old (postpartal) N81.89
    organ S37.93 ☑
  penis S31.21 ☑
    with foreign body S31.22 ☑
  perineum
    female S31.41 ☑
      with
        ectopic or molar pregnancy O08.6
        foreign body S31.42 ☑
      during delivery O70.9
        first degree O70.0
        fourth degree O70.3
        second degree O70.1
        third degree — *see also* Delivery, complicated, by, laceration, perineum, third degree O70.20
      old (postpartal) N81.89
      postpartal N81.89
      secondary (postpartal) O90.1
    male S31.119 ☑
      with foreign body S31.129 ☑
  periocular area (with or without lacrimal passages) — *see* Laceration, eyelid
  peritoneum S36.893 ☑
  periumbilic region — *see* Laceration, abdomen, wall, periumbilic
  periurethral tissue — *see* Laceration, urethra
  phalanges
    finger — *see* Laceration, finger
    toe — *see* Laceration, toe
  pharynx S11.21 ☑
    with foreign body S11.22 ☑
  pinna — *see* Laceration, ear
  popliteal space — *see* Laceration, knee
  prepuce — *see* Laceration, penis
  prostate S37.823 ☑
  pubic region S31.119 ☑
    with foreign body S31.129 ☑

☑ **Additional Character Required** — Refer to the Tabular List for Character Selection

Laceration — *continued*
 pudendum — *see* Laceration, genital organs, external
 rectovaginal septum — *see* Laceration, vagina
 rectum S36.63 ☑
 retroperitoneum S36.893 ☑
 round ligament S37.893 ☑
 sacral region — *see* Laceration, back, lower
 sacroiliac region — *see* Laceration, back, lower
 salivary gland — *see* Laceration, oral cavity
 scalp S01.01 ☑
  with foreign body S01.02 ☑
 scapular region — *see* Laceration, shoulder
 scrotum S31.31 ☑
  with foreign body S31.32 ☑
 seminal vesicle S37.893 ☑
 shin — *see* Laceration, leg
 shoulder S41.019 ☑
  with foreign body S41.029 ☑
  left S41.012 ☑
   with foreign body S41.022 ☑
  right S41.011 ☑
   with foreign body S41.021 ☑
 small intestine — *see* Laceration, intestine, small
 spermatic cord — *see* Laceration, testis
 spinal cord (meninges) — *see also* Injury, spinal cord, by region
  due to injury at birth P11.5
  newborn (birth injury) P11.5
 spleen S36.039 ☑
  major (massive) (stellate) S36.032 ☑
  moderate S36.031 ☑
  superficial (minor) S36.030 ☑
 sternal region — *see* Laceration, thorax, front
 stomach S36.33 ☑
 submaxillary region — *see* Laceration, head, specified site NEC
 submental region — *see* Laceration, head, specified site NEC
 subungual
  finger(s) — *see* Laceration, finger, with damage to nail
  toe(s) — *see* Laceration, toe, with damage to nail
 suprarenal gland — *see* Laceration, adrenal gland
 temple, temporal region — *see* Laceration, head, specified site NEC
 temporomandibular area — *see* Laceration, cheek
 tendon — *see* Injury, muscle, by site, laceration
  Achilles S86.02- ☑
 tentorium cerebelli — *see* Injury, intracranial, diffuse
 testis S31.31 ☑
  with foreign body S31.32 ☑
 thigh S71.11- ☑
  with foreign body S71.12- ☑
 thorax, thoracic (wall) S21.91 ☑
  with foreign body S21.92 ☑
  back S21.22- ☑
   with penetration into thoracic cavity S21.42- ☑
  front S21.12- ☑
   with penetration into thoracic cavity S21.32- ☑
  back S21.21- ☑
   with
    foreign body S21.22- ☑
     with penetration into thoracic cavity S21.42- ☑
    penetration into thoracic cavity S21.41- ☑
  breast — *see* Laceration, breast
  front S21.11- ☑
   with
    foreign body S21.12- ☑
     with penetration into thoracic cavity S21.32- ☑
    penetration into thoracic cavity S21.31- ☑
 thumb S61.019 ☑
  with
   damage to nail S61.119 ☑
    with
     foreign body S61.129 ☑
   foreign body S61.029 ☑
  left S61.012 ☑
   with
    damage to nail S61.112 ☑
     with
      foreign body S61.122 ☑
    foreign body S61.022 ☑

Laceration — *continued*
 thumb — *continued*
  right S61.011 ☑
   with
    damage to nail S61.111 ☑
     with
      foreign body S61.121 ☑
    foreign body S61.021 ☑
 thyroid gland S11.11 ☑
  with foreign body S11.12 ☑
 toe(s) S91.119 ☑
  with
   damage to nail S91.219 ☑
    with
     foreign body S91.229 ☑
   foreign body S91.129 ☑
  great S91.113 ☑
   with
    damage to nail S91.213 ☑
     with
      foreign body S91.223 ☑
    foreign body S91.123 ☑
   left S91.112 ☑
    with
     damage to nail S91.212 ☑
      with
       foreign body S91.222 ☑
     foreign body S91.122 ☑
   right S91.111 ☑
    with
     damage to nail S91.211 ☑
      with
       foreign body S91.221 ☑
     foreign body S91.121 ☑
  lesser S91.116 ☑
   with
    damage to nail S91.216 ☑
     with
      foreign body S91.226 ☑
    foreign body S91.126 ☑
   left S91.115 ☑
    with
     damage to nail S91.215 ☑
      with
       foreign body S91.225 ☑
     foreign body S91.125 ☑
   right S91.114 ☑
    with
     damage to nail S91.214 ☑
      with
       foreign body S91.224 ☑
     foreign body S91.124 ☑
 tongue — *see* Laceration, oral cavity
 trachea S11.021 ☑
  with foreign body S11.022 ☑
 tunica vaginalis — *see* Laceration, testis
 tympanum, tympanic membrane — *see* Laceration, ear, drum
 umbilical region S31.115 ☑
  with foreign body S31.125 ☑
 ureter S37.13 ☑
 urethra S37.33 ☑
  with or following ectopic or molar pregnancy O08.6
  obstetrical trauma O71.5
 urinary organ NEC S37.893 ☑
 uterus S37.63 ☑
  with ectopic or molar pregnancy O08.6
  following ectopic or molar pregnancy O08.6
  nonpuerperal, nontraumatic N85.8
  obstetrical trauma NEC O71.81
  old (postpartal) N85.8
 uvula — *see* Laceration, oral cavity
 vagina S31.41 ☑
  with
   ectopic or molar pregnancy O08.6
   foreign body S31.42 ☑
  during delivery O71.4
   with perineal laceration — *see* Laceration, perineum, female, during delivery
  following ectopic or molar pregnancy O08.6
  nonpuerperal, nontraumatic N89.8
  old (postpartal) N89.8
 vas deferens S37.893 ☑
 vesical — *see* Laceration, bladder
 vocal cords S11.031 ☑
  with foreign body S11.032 ☑
 vulva S31.41 ☑

Laceration — *continued*
 vulva — *continued*
  with
   ectopic or molar pregnancy O08.6
   foreign body S31.42 ☑
  complicating delivery O70.0
  following ectopic or molar pregnancy O08.6
  nonpuerperal, nontraumatic N90.89
  old (postpartal) N90.89
 wrist S61.519 ☑
  with
   foreign body S61.529 ☑
  left S61.512 ☑
   with
    foreign body S61.522 ☑
  right S61.511 ☑
   with
    foreign body S61.521 ☑

Lack of
 achievement in school Z55.3
 adequate
  food Z59.48
  intermaxillary vertical dimension of fully erupted teeth M26.36
  sleep Z72.820
 appetite (see Anorexia) R63.0
 awareness R41.9
 care
  in home Z74.2
  of infant (at or after birth) T76.02 ☑
   confirmed T74.02 ☑
 cognitive functions R41.9
 coordination R27.9
  ataxia R27.0
  specified type NEC R27.8
 development (physiological) R62.50
  failure to thrive (child over 28 days old) R62.51
   adult R62.7
   newborn P92.6
  short stature R62.52
  specified type NEC R62.59
 energy R53.83
 financial resources Z59.6
 food Z59.48
 growth R62.52
 heating Z59.1
 housing (permanent) (temporary) Z59.00
  adequate Z59.1
 learning experiences in childhood Z62.898
 leisure time (affecting life-style) Z73.2
 material resources Z59.87
 memory — *see also* Amnesia
  mild, following organic brain damage F06.8
 ovulation N97.0
 parental supervision or control of child Z62.0
 person able to render necessary care Z74.2
 physical exercise Z72.3
 play experience in childhood Z62.898
 posterior occlusal support M26.57
 relaxation (affecting life-style) Z73.2
 safe drinking water Z58.6
 sexual
  desire F52.0
  enjoyment F52.1
 shelter Z59.02
 sleep (adequate) Z72.820
 supervision of child by parent Z62.0
 support, posterior occlusal M26.57
 transportation Z59.82
 water T73.1
  safe drinking Z58.6
Lacrimal — *see* condition
Lacrimation, abnormal — *see* Epiphora
Lacrimonasal duct — *see* condition
Lactation, lactating (breast) (puerperal, postpartum)
 associated
  cracked nipple O92.13
  retracted nipple O92.03
 defective O92.4
 disorder NEC O92.79
 excessive O92.6
 failed (complete) O92.3
  partial O92.4
 mastitis NEC — *see* Mastitis, obstetric
 mother (care and/or examination) Z39.1
 nonpuerperal N64.3
Lacticemia, excessive — *see also* Acidosis E87.20
Lacunar skull Q75.8

Laennec's cirrhosis K70.30
  with ascites K70.31
  nonalcoholic K74.69
Lafora's disease — *see* Epilepsy, generalized, idiopathic
Lag, lid (nervous) — *see* Retraction, lid
Lagophthalmos (eyelid) (nervous) H02.209
  bilateral, upper and lower eyelids H02.20C
  cicatricial H02.219
    bilateral, upper and lower eyelids H02.21C
    left H02.216
      lower H02.215
      upper H02.214
      upper and lower eyelids H02.21B
    right H02.213
      lower H02.212
      upper H02.211
      upper and lower eyelids H02.21A
  keratoconjunctivitis — *see* Keratoconjunctivitis
  left H02.206
    lower H02.205
    upper H02.204
    upper and lower eyelids H02.20B
  mechanical H02.229
    bilateral, upper and lower eyelids H02.22C
    left H02.226
      lower H02.225
      upper H02.224
      upper and lower eyelids H02.22B
    right H02.223
      lower H02.222
      upper H02.221
      upper and lower eyelids H02.22A
  paralytic H02.239
    bilateral, upper and lower eyelids H02.23C
    left H02.236
      lower H02.235
      upper H02.234
      upper and lower eyelids H02.23B
    right H02.233
      lower H02.232
      upper H02.231
      upper and lower eyelids H02.23A
  right H02.203
    lower H02.202
    upper H02.201
    upper and lower eyelids H02.20A
Laki-Lorand factor deficiency — *see* Defect, coagulation, specified type NEC
Lalling F80.0
Lambert-Eaton syndrome — *see* Syndrome, Lambert-Eaton
Lambliasis, lambliosis A07.1
Landau-Kleffner syndrome — *see* Epilepsy, specified NEC
Landouzy-Déjérine dystrophy or facioscapulohumeral atrophy G71.02
Landouzy's disease (icterohemorrhagic leptospirosis) A27.0
Landry-Guillain-Barré, syndrome or paralysis G61.0
Landry's disease or paralysis G61.0
Lane's
  band Q43.3
  kink — *see* Obstruction, intestine
  syndrome K90.2
Langdon Down syndrome — *see* Trisomy, 21
Lapsed immunization schedule status Z28.39
Large
  baby (regardless of gestational age) (4000g to 4499g) P08.1
  ear, congenital Q17.1
  physiological cup Q14.2
  stature R68.89
Large-for-dates NEC (infant) (4000g to 4499g) P08.1
  affecting management of pregnancy O36.6- ☑
  exceptionally (4500g or more) P08.0
Larsen-Johansson disease orosteochondrosis — *see* Osteochondrosis, juvenile, patella
Larsen's syndrome (flattened facies and multiple congenital dislocations) Q74.8
Larva migrans
  cutaneous B76.9
    Ancylostoma B76.0
  visceral B83.0
Laryngeal — *see* condition
Laryngismus (stridulus) J38.5
  congenital P28.89
  diphtheritic A36.2

Laryngitis (acute) (edematous) (fibrinous) (infective) (infiltrative) (malignant) (membranous) (phlegmonous) (pneumococcal) (pseudomembranous) (septic) (subglottic) (suppurative) (ulcerative) J04.0
  with
    influenza, flu, or grippe — *see* Influenza, with, laryngitis
    tracheitis (acute) — *see* Laryngotracheitis
  atrophic J37.0
  catarrhal J37.0
  chronic J37.0
    with tracheitis (chronic) J37.1
  diphtheritic A36.2
  due to external agent — *see* Inflammation, respiratory, upper, due to
  H. influenzae J04.0
  Hemophilus influenzae J04.0
  hypertrophic J37.0
  influenzal — *see* Influenza, with, respiratory manifestations NEC
  obstructive J05.0
  sicca J37.0
  spasmodic J05.0
    acute J04.0
  streptococcal J04.0
  stridulous J05.0
  syphilitic (late) A52.73
    congenital A50.59 [J99]
      early A50.03 [J99]
  tuberculous A15.5
  Vincent's A69.1
Laryngocele (congenital) (ventricular) Q31.3
Laryngofissure J38.7
  congenital Q31.8
Laryngomalacia (congenital) Q31.5
Laryngopharyngitis (acute) J06.0
  chronic J37.0
  due to external agent — *see* Inflammation, respiratory, upper, due to
Laryngoplegia J38.00
  bilateral J38.02
  unilateral J38.01
Laryngoptosis J38.7
Laryngospasm J38.5
Laryngostenosis J38.6
Laryngotracheitis (acute) (Infectional) (infective) (viral) J04.2
  atrophic J37.1
  catarrhal J37.1
  chronic J37.1
  diphtheritic A36.2
  due to external agent — *see* Inflammation, respiratory, upper, due to
  Hemophilus influenzae J04.2
  hypertrophic J37.1
  influenzal — *see* Influenza, with, respiratory manifestations NEC
  pachydermic J38.7
  sicca J37.1
  spasmodic J38.5
    acute J05.0
  streptococcal J04.2
  stridulous J38.5
  syphilitic (late) A52.73
    congenital A50.59 [J99]
      early A50.03 [J99]
  tuberculous A15.5
  Vincent's A69.1
Laryngotracheobronchitis — *see* Bronchitis
Larynx, laryngeal — *see* condition
Lassa fever A96.2
Lassitude — *see* Weakness
Late
  talker R62.0
  walker R62.0
Late effect(s) — *see* Sequelae
Latent — *see* condition
Laterocession — *see* Lateroversion
Lateroflexion — *see* Lateroversion
Lateroversion
  cervix — *see* Lateroversion, uterus
  uterus, uterine (cervix) (postinfectional) (postpartal, old) N85.4
    congenital Q51.818
    in pregnancy or childbirth O34.59- ☑
Lathyrism — *see* Poisoning, food, noxious, plant
Launois' syndrome (pituitary gigantism) E22.0
Launois-Bensaude adenolipomatosis E88.89

Laurence-Moon (-Bardet)-**Biedl syndrome** Q87.89
Lax, laxity — *see also* Relaxation
  ligament (ous) — *see also* Disorder, ligament
    familial M35.7
    knee — *see* Derangement, knee
  skin (acquired) L57.4
    congenital Q82.8
Laxative habit F55.2
Lazy leukocyte syndrome D70.8
Lead miner's lung J63.6
Leak, leakage
  air NEC J93.82
    postprocedural J95.812
  amniotic fluid — *see* Rupture, membranes, premature
  blood (microscopic), fetal, into maternal circulation affecting management of pregnancy — *see* Pregnancy, complicated by
  cerebrospinal fluid G96.00
    cranial
      postoperative G96.08
      specified NEC G96.08
      spontaneous G96.01
      traumatic G96.08
    from spinal (lumbar) puncture G97.0
    spinal
      postoperative G96.09
      post-traumatic G96.09
      specified NEC G96.09
      spontaneous G96.02
    spontaneous
      from
        skull base G96.01
        spine G96.02
  CSF — *see* Leak, cerebrospinal fluid
  device, implant or graft — *see also* Complications, by site and type, mechanical
    arterial graft NEC — *see* Complication vascular, graft, mechanical, leakage T82.838 ☑
    breast (implant) T85.43 ☑
    catheter NEC T85.638 ☑
      dialysis (renal) T82.43 ☑
        intraperitoneal T85.631 ☑
      infusion NEC T82.534 ☑
        spinal (epidural) (subdural) T85.630 ☑
      urinary T83.038 ☑
        cystostomy T83.030 ☑
        Hopkins T83.038 ☑
        ileostomy T83.038 ☑
        indwelling T83.031 ☑
        nephrostomy T83.032 ☑
        specified T83.038 ☑
        urostomy T83.038 ☑
    gastrointestinal — *see* Complications, prosthetic device, mechanical, gastrointestinal device
    genital NEC T83.498 ☑
      penile prosthesis (cylinder) (implanted) (pump) (reservoir) T83.490 ☑
      testicular prosthesis T83.491 ☑
    heart NEC — *see* Complication, cardiovascular device, mechanical
    joint prosthesis — *see* Complications, joint prosthesis, mechanical, specified NEC, by site
    ocular NEC — *see* Complications, prosthetic device, mechanical, ocular device
    orthopedic NEC — *see* Complication, orthopedic, device, mechanical
    persistent air J93.82
    specified NEC T85.638 ☑
    urinary NEC — *see also* Complication, genitourinary, device, urinary, mechanical
      graft T83.23 ☑
    vascular NEC — *see* Complication, cardiovascular device, mechanical
    ventricular intracranial shunt T85.03 ☑
  urine — *see* Incontinence
Leaky heart — *see* Endocarditis
Learning defect (specific) F81.9
Leather bottle stomach C16.9
Leber's
  congenital amaurosis H35.50
  optic atrophy (hereditary) H47.22
Lederer's anemia D59.19
Leeches (external) — *see* Hirudiniasis
Leg — *see* condition
Legg (-Calvé)-**Perthes disease, syndrome or osteochondrosis** M91.1- ☑
Legionellosis A48.1

Legionellosis — continued

Legionellosis — *continued*
  nonpneumonic A48.2
Legionnaires'
  disease A48.1
    nonpneumonic A48.2
  pneumonia A48.1
Leigh's disease G31.82
Leiner's disease L21.1
Leiofibromyoma — *see* Leiomyoma
Leiomyoblastoma — *see* Neoplasm, connective tissue, benign
Leiomyofibroma — *see also* Neoplasm, connective tissue, benign
  uterus (cervix) (corpus) D25.9
Leiomyoma — *see also* Neoplasm, connective tissue, benign
  bizarre — *see* Neoplasm, connective tissue, benign
  cellular — *see* Neoplasm, connective tissue, benign
  epithelioid — *see* Neoplasm, connective tissue, benign
  uterus (cervix) (corpus) D25.9
    intramural D25.1
    submucous D25.0
    subserosal D25.2
  vascular — *see* Neoplasm, connective tissue, benign
Leiomyoma, leiomyomatosis (intravascular) — *see* Neoplasm, connective tissue, uncertain behavior
Leiomyosarcoma — *see also* Neoplasm, connective tissue, malignant
  epithelioid — *see* Neoplasm, connective tissue, malignant
  myxoid — *see* Neoplasm, connective tissue, malignant
Leishmaniasis B55.9
  American (mucocutaneous) B55.2
    cutaneous B55.1
  Asian Desert B55.1
  Brazilian B55.2
  cutaneous (any type) B55.1
  dermal — *see also* Leishmaniasis, cutaneous
    post-kala-azar B55.0
  eyelid B55.1
  infantile B55.0
  Mediterranean B55.0
  mucocutaneous (American) (New World) B55.2
  naso-oral B55.2
  nasopharyngeal B55.2
  old world B55.1
  tegumentaria diffusa B55.1
  visceral B55.0
Leishmanoid, dermal — *see also* Leishmaniasis, cutaneous
    post-kala-azar B55.0
Lenegre's disease I44.2
Lengthening, leg — *see* Deformity, limb, unequal length
Lennert's lymphoma — *see* Lymphoma, Lennert's
Lennox-Gastaut syndrome G40.812
  intractable G40.814
    with status epilepticus G40.813
    without status epilepticus G40.814
  not intractable G40.812
    with status epilepticus G40.811
    without status epilepticus G40.812
Lens — *see* condition
Lenticonus (anterior) (posterior) (congenital) Q12.8
Lenticular degeneration, progressive E83.01
Lentiglobus (posterior) (congenital) Q12.8
Lentigo (congenital) L81.4
  maligna — *see also* Melanoma, in situ
    melanoma — *see* Melanoma
Lentivirus, as cause of disease classified elsewhere B97.31
Leontiasis
  ossium M85.2
  syphilitic (late) A52.78
    congenital A50.59
Lepothrix A48.8
Lepra — *see* Leprosy
Leprechaunism E34.8
Leprosy A30.- ☑
  with muscle disorder A30.9 [M63.80]
    ankle A30.9 [M63.87-] ☑
    foot A30.9 [M63.87-] ☑
    forearm A30.9 [M63.83-] ☑
    hand A30.9 [M63.84-] ☑
    lower leg A30.9 [M63.86-] ☑
    multiple sites A30.9 [M63.89]
    pelvic region A30.9 [M63.85-] ☑
    shoulder region A30.9 [M63.81-] ☑

Leprosy — *continued*
  with muscle disorder — *continued*
    specified site NEC A30.9 [M63.88]
    thigh A30.9 [M63.85-] ☑
    upper arm A30.9 [M63.82-] ☑
  anesthetic A30.9
  BB A30.3
  BL A30.4
  borderline (infiltrated) (neuritic) A30.3
    lepromatous A30.4
    tuberculoid A30.2
  BT A30.2
  dimorphous (infiltrated) (neuritic) A30.3
  I A30.0
  indeterminate (macular) (neuritic) A30.0
  lepromatous (diffuse) (infiltrated) (macular) (neuritic) (nodular) A30.5
  LL A30.5
  macular (early) (neuritic) (simple) A30.9
  maculoanesthetic A30.9
  mixed A30.3
  neural A30.9
  nodular A30.5
  primary neuritic A30.3
  specified type NEC A30.8
  TT A30.1
  tuberculoid (major) (minor) A30.1
Leptocytosis, hereditary D56.9
Leptomeningitis (chronic) (circumscribed) (hemorrhagic) (nonsuppurative) — *see* Meningitis
Leptomeningopathy G96.198
Leptospiral — *see* condition
Leptospirochetal — *see* condition
Leptospirosis A27.9
  canicola A27.89
  due to Leptospira interrogans serovar icterohaemorrhagiae A27.0
  icterohemorrhagica A27.0
  pomona A27.89
  Weil's disease A27.0
Leptus dermatitis B88.0
Leriche's syndrome (aortic bifurcation occlusion) I74.09
Leri's pleonosteosis Q78.8
Leri-Weill syndrome Q77.8
Lermoyez' syndrome — *see* Vertigo, peripheral NEC
Lesch-Nyhan syndrome E79.1
Leser-Trélat disease L82.1
  inflamed L82.0
Lesion(s) (nontraumatic)
  abducens nerve — *see* Strabismus, paralytic, sixth nerve
  alveolar process K08.9
  angiocentric immunoproliferative D47.Z9 (*following* D47.4)
  anorectal K62.9
  aortic (valve) I35.9
  auditory nerve — *see* subcategory H93.3 ☑
  basal ganglion G25.9
  bile duct — *see* Disease, bile duct
  biomechanical M99.9
    specified type NEC M99.89
      abdomen M99.89
      acromioclavicular M99.87
      cervical region M99.81
      cervicothoracic M99.81
      costochondral M99.88
      costovertebral M99.88
      head region M99.80
      hip M99.85
      lower extremity M99.86
      lumbar region M99.83
      lumbosacral M99.83
      occipitocervical M99.80
      pelvic region M99.85
      pubic M99.85
      rib cage M99.88
      sacral region M99.84
      sacrococcygeal M99.84
      sacroiliac M99.84
      specified NEC M99.89
      sternochondral M99.88
      sternoclavicular M99.87
      thoracic region M99.82
      thoracolumbar M99.82
      upper extremity M99.87
  bladder N32.9
  bone — *see* Disorder, bone
  brachial plexus G54.0
  brain G93.9

Lesion(s) — *continued*
  brain — *continued*
    congenital Q04.9
    vascular I67.9
      degenerative I67.9
      hypertensive I67.4
  buccal cavity K13.79
  calcified — *see* Calcification
  canthus — *see* Disorder, eyelid
  carate — *see* Pinta, lesions
  cardia K31.9
  cardiac — *see also* Disease, heart I51.9
    congenital Q24.9
    valvular — *see* Endocarditis
  cauda equina G83.4
  cecum K63.9
  cerebral — *see* Lesion, brain
  cerebrovascular I67.9
    degenerative I67.9
    hypertensive I67.4
  cervical (nerve) root NEC G54.2
  chiasmal — *see* Disorder, optic, chiasm
  chorda tympani G51.8
  coin, lung R91.1
  colon K63.9
  combined periodontic - endodontic K05.5
  congenital — *see* Anomaly, by site
  conjunctiva H11.9
  conus medullaris — *see* Injury, conus medullaris
  coronary artery — *see* Ischemia, heart
  cranial nerve G52.9
    eighth — *see* Disorder, ear
    eleventh G52.9
    fifth G50.9
    first G52.0
    fourth — *see* Strabismus, paralytic, fourth nerve
    seventh G51.9
    sixth — *see* Strabismus, paralytic, sixth nerve
    tenth G52.2
    twelfth G52.3
  cystic — *see* Cyst
  degenerative — *see* Degeneration
  duodenum K31.9
  edentulous (alveolar) ridge, associated with trauma, due to traumatic occlusion K06.2
  en coup de sabre L94.1
  eyelid — *see* Disorder, eyelid
  gasserian ganglion G50.8
  gastric K31.9
  gastroduodenal K31.9
  gastrointestinal K63.9
  gingiva, associated with trauma K06.2
  glomerular
    focal and segmental — *see also* N00-N07 with fourth character .1 N05.1
    minimal change — *see also* N00-N07 with fourth character .0 N05.0
  heart (organic) — *see* Disease, heart
  hyperchromic, due to pinta (carate) A67.1
  hyperkeratotic — *see* Hyperkeratosis
  hypothalamic E23.7
  ileocecal K63.9
  ileum K63.9
  iliohypogastric nerve G57.8- ☑
  inflammatory — *see* Inflammation
  intestine K63.9
  intracerebral — *see* Lesion, brain
  intrachiasmal (optic) — *see* Disorder, optic, chiasm
  intracranial, space-occupying R90.0
  joint — *see* Disorder, joint
    sacroiliac (old) M53.3
  keratotic — *see* Keratosis
  kidney — *see* Disease, renal
  laryngeal nerve (recurrent) G52.2
  lip K13.0
  liver K76.9
  lumbosacral
    plexus G54.1
    root (nerve) NEC G54.4
  lung (coin) R91.1
  maxillary sinus J32.0
  mitral I05.9
  Morel-Lavallée — *see* Hematoma, by site
  motor cortex NEC G93.89
  mouth K13.79
  nerve G58.9
    femoral G57.2- ☑
    median G56.1- ☑

Lesion(s) — *continued*
  nerve — *continued*
    median — *continued*
      carpal tunnel syndrome — *see* Syndrome, carpal tunnel
    plantar G57.6- ☑
    popliteal (lateral) G57.3- ☑
      medial G57.4- ☑
    radial G56.3- ☑
    sciatic G57.0- ☑
    spinal — *see* Injury, nerve, spinal
    ulnar G56.2- ☑
  nervous system, congenital Q07.9
  nonallopathic — *see* Lesion, biomechanical
  nose (internal) J34.89
  obstructive — *see* Obstruction
  obturator nerve G57.8- ☑
  oral mucosa K13.70
  organ or site NEC — *see* Disease, by site
  osteolytic — *see* Osteolysis
  peptic K27.9
  periodontal, due to traumatic occlusion K05.5
  pharynx J39.2
  pigment, pigmented (skin) L81.9
  pinta — *see* Pinta, lesions
  polypoid — *see* Polyp
  prechiasmal (optic) — *see* Disorder, optic, chiasm
  primary — *see also* Syphilis, primary A51.0
    carate A67.0
    pinta A67.0
    yaws A66.0
  pulmonary J98.4
    valve I37.9
  pylorus K31.9
  rectosigmoid K63.9
  retina, retinal H35.9
  sacroiliac (joint) (old) M53.3
  salivary gland K11.9
    benign lymphoepithelial K11.8
  saphenous nerve G57.8- ☑
  sciatic nerve G57.0- ☑
  secondary — *see* Syphilis, secondary
  shoulder (region) M75.9- ☑
    specified NEC M75.8- ☑
  sigmoid K63.9
  sinus (accessory) (nasal) J34.89
  skin L98.9
    suppurative L08.0
  SLAP S43.43- ☑
  spinal cord G95.9
    congenital Q06.9
  spleen D73.89
  stomach K31.9
  superior glenoid labrum S43.43- ☑
  syphilitic — *see* Syphilis
  tertiary — *see* Syphilis, tertiary
  thoracic root (nerve) NEC G54.3
  tonsillar fossa J35.9
  tooth, teeth K08.9
    white spot
      chewing surface K02.51
      pit and fissure surface K02.51
      smooth surface K02.61
  traumatic — *see* specific type of injury by site
  tricuspid (valve) I07.9
    nonrheumatic I36.9
  trigeminal nerve G50.9
  ulcerated or ulcerative — *see* Ulcer, skin
  uterus N85.9
  vagina N89.8
  vagus nerve G52.2
  valvular — *see* Endocarditis
  vascular I99.9
    affecting central nervous system I67.9
    following trauma NEC T14.8 ☑
    umbilical cord, complicating delivery O69.5 ☑
  vulva N90.89
  warty — *see* Verruca
  white spot (tooth)
    chewing surface K02.51
    pit and fissure surface K02.51
    smooth surface K02.61
Less than a high school diploma Z55.5
Lethargic — *see* condition
Lethargy R53.83
Letterer-Siwe's disease C96.0
Leukemia, leukemic C95.9- ☑

Leukemia, leukemic — *continued*
  acute basophilic C94.8- ☑
  acute bilineal C95.0- ☑
  acute erythroid C94.0- ☑
  acute lymphoblastic C91.0- ☑
  acute megakaryoblastic C94.2- ☑
  acute megakaryocytic C94.2- ☑
  acute mixed lineage C95.0- ☑
  acute monoblastic (monoblastic/monocytic) C93.0- ☑
  acute monocytic (monoblastic/monocytic) C93.0- ☑
  acute myeloblastic (minimal differentiation) (with maturation) C92.0- ☑
  acute myeloid, NOS C92.0- ☑
    with
      11q23-abnormality C92.6- ☑
      dysplasia of remaining hematopoesis and/or myelodysplastic disease in its history C92.A- ☑ (*following* C92.6)
      multilineage dysplasia C92.A- ☑ (*following* C92.6)
      variation of MLL-gene C92.6- ☑
    M6 (a)(b) C94.0- ☑
    M7 C94.2- ☑
  acute myelomonocytic C92.5- ☑
  acute promyelocytic C92.4- ☑
  adult T-cell (HTLV-1-associated) (acute variant) (chronic variant) (lymphomatoid variant) (smouldering variant) C91.5- ☑
  aggressive NK-cell C94.8- ☑
  AML (1/ETO) (M0) (M1) (M2) (without a FAB classification) C92.0- ☑
  AML M3 C92.4- ☑
  AML M4 (Eo with inv(16) or t(16;16)) C92.5- ☑
  AML M5 C93.0- ☑
  AML M5a C93.0- ☑
  AML M5b C93.0- ☑
  AML Me with t (15;17) and variants C92.4- ☑
  atypical chronic myeloid, BCR/ABL-negative C92.2- ☑
  biphenotypic acute C95.0- ☑
  blast cell C95.0- ☑
  Burkitt-type, mature B-cell C91.A- ☑ (*following* C91.6)
  chronic eosinophilic — *see also* Syndrome, hypereosinophilic, myeloid C94.8- ☑
  chronic lymphocytic, of B-cell type C91.1- ☑
  chronic monocytic C93.1- ☑
  chronic myelogenous (Philadelphia chromosome (Ph1) positive) (t(9;22)) (q34;q11) (with crisis of blast cells) C92.1- ☑
  chronic myeloid, BCR/ABL-positive C92.1- ☑
    atypical, BCR/ABL-negative C92.2- ☑
  chronic myelomonocytic C93.1- ☑
  chronic neutrophilic D47.1
  CMML (-1) (-2) (with eosinophilia) C93.1- ☑
  granulocytic — *see also* Category C92 C92.9- ☑
  hairy cell C91.4- ☑
  juvenile myelomonocytic C93.3- ☑
  lymphoid C91.9- ☑
    specified NEC C91.Z- ☑ (*following* C91.6)
  mast cell C94.3- ☑
  mature B-cell, Burkitt-type C91.A- ☑ (*following* C91.6)
  monocytic (subacute) C93.9- ☑
    specified NEC C93.Z- ☑ (*following* C93.3)
  myelogenous — *see also* Category C92 C92.9- ☑
  myeloid C92.9- ☑
    specified NEC C92.Z- ☑ (*following* C92.6)
  plasma cell C90.1- ☑
  plasmacytic C90.1- ☑
  prolymphocytic
    of B-cell type C91.3- ☑
    of T-cell type C91.6- ☑
  specified NEC C94.8- ☑
  stem cell, of unclear lineage C95.0- ☑
  subacute lymphocytic C91.9- ☑
  T-cell large granular lymphocytic C91.Z- ☑ (*following* C91.6)
  unspecified cell type C95.9- ☑
    acute C95.0- ☑
    chronic C95.1- ☑
Leukemoid reaction — *see also* Reaction, leukemoid D72.823
Leukoaraiosis (hypertensive) I67.81
Leukoariosis — *see* Leukoaraiosis
Leukocoria — *see* Disorder, globe, degenerated condition, leucocoria
Leukocytopenia D72.819
Leukocytosis D72.829

Leukocytosis — *continued*
  eosinophilic D72.19
Leukoderma, leukodermia NEC L81.5
  syphilitic A51.39
    late A52.79
Leukodystrophy E75.29
Leukoedema, oral epithelium K13.29
Leukoencephalitis G04.81
  acute (subacute) hemorrhagic G36.1
    postimmunization or postvaccinal G04.02
  postinfectious G04.01
  subacute sclerosing A81.1
  van Bogaert's (sclerosing) A81.1
Leukoencephalopathy — *see also* Encephalopathy G93.49
  Binswanger's I67.3
  heroin vapor G92.8
  metachromatic E75.25
  multifocal (progressive) A81.2
  postimmunization and postvaccinal G04.02
  progressive multifocal A81.2
  reversible, posterior G93.6
  van Bogaert's (sclerosing) A81.1
  vascular, progressive I67.3
Leukoerythroblastosis D75.9
Leukokeratosis — *see also* Leukoplakia
  mouth K13.21
  nicotina palati K13.24
  oral mucosa K13.21
  tongue K13.21
  vocal cord J38.3
Leukokraurosis vulva (e) N90.4
Leukoma (cornea) — *see also* Opacity, cornea
  adherent H17.0- ☑
  interfering with central vision — *see* Opacity, cornea, central
Leukomalacia, cerebral, newborn P91.2
  periventricular P91.2
Leukomelanopathy, hereditary D72.0
Leukonychia (punctata) (striata) L60.8
  congenital Q84.4
Leukopathia unguium L60.8
  congenital Q84.4
Leukopenia D72.819
  basophilic D72.818
  chemotherapy (cancer) induced D70.1
  congenital D70.0
  cyclic D70.0
  drug induced NEC D70.2
    due to cytoreductive cancer chemotherapy D70.1
  eosinophilic D72.818
  familial D70.0
  infantile genetic D70.0
  malignant D70.9
  periodic D70.0
  transitory neonatal P61.5
Leukopenic — *see* condition
Leukoplakia
  anus K62.89
  bladder (postinfectional) N32.89
  buccal K13.21
  cervix (uteri) N88.0
  esophagus K22.89
  gingiva K13.21
  hairy (oral mucosa) (tongue) K13.3
  kidney (pelvis) N28.89
  larynx J38.7
  lip K13.21
  mouth K13.21
  oral epithelium, including tongue (mucosa) K13.21
  palate K13.21
  pelvis (kidney) N28.89
  penis (infectional) N48.0
  rectum K62.89
  syphilitic (late) A52.79
  tongue K13.21
  ureter (postinfectional) N28.89
  urethra (postinfectional) N36.8
  uterus N85.8
  vagina N89.4
  vocal cord J38.3
  vulva N90.4
Leukorrhea N89.8
  due to Trichomonas (vaginalis) A59.00
  trichomonal A59.00
Leukosarcoma C85.9- ☑
Levocardia (isolated) Q24.1
  with situs inversus Q89.3

Levotransposition Q20.5
Lev's disease or syndrome (acquired complete heart block) I44.2
Levulosuria — *see* Fructosuria
Levurid L30.2
Lewy body (ies) (disease) G31.83
Leyden-Möbius dystrophy — *see* Dystrophy, Leyden-Möbius
Leydig cell
carcinoma
specified site — *see* Neoplasm, malignant, by site
unspecified site
female C56.9
male C62.9- ☑
tumor
benign
specified site — *see* Neoplasm, benign, by site
unspecified site
female D27.- ☑
male D29.2- ☑
malignant
specified site — *see* Neoplasm, malignant, by site
unspecified site
female C56.- ☑
male C62.9- ☑
specified site — *see* Neoplasm, uncertain behavior, by site
unspecified site
female D39.1- ☑
male D40.1- ☑
Leydig-Sertoli cell tumor
specified site — *see* Neoplasm, benign, by site
unspecified site
female D27.- ☑
male D29.2- ☑
LGMD — *see* Dystrophy, muscular, limb-girdle
LGSIL (Low grade squamous intraepithelial lesion on cytologic smear of)
anus R85.612
cervix R87.612
vagina R87.622
Liar, pathologic F60.2
Libido
decreased R68.82
Libman-Sacks disease M32.11
Lice (infestation) B85.2
body (Pediculus corporis) B85.1
crab B85.3
head (Pediculus capitis) B85.0
mixed (classifiable to more than one of the titles B85.0-B85.3) B85.4
pubic (Phthirus pubis) B85.3
Lichen L28.0
albus L90.0
penis N48.0
vulva N90.4
amyloidosis E85.4 [L99]
atrophicus L90.0
penis N48.0
vulva N90.4
congenital Q82.8
myxedematosus L98.5
nitidus L44.1
pilaris Q82.8
acquired L85.8
planopilaris L66.1
planus (chronicus) L43.9
annularis L43.8
bullous L43.1
follicular L66.1
hypertrophic L43.0
moniliformis L44.3
of Wilson L43.9
specified NEC L43.8
subacute (active) L43.3
tropicus L43.3
ruber
acuminatus L44.0
moniliformis L44.3
planus L43.9
sclerosus (et atrophicus) L90.0
penis N48.0
vulva N90.4
scrofulosus (primary) (tuberculous) A18.4
simplex (chronicus) (circumscriptus) L28.0
striatus L44.2
urticatus L28.2

Lichenification L28.0
Lichenoides tuberculosis (primary) A18.4
Lichtheim's disease or syndrome D51.0
Lien migrans D73.89
Ligament — *see* condition
Light
for gestational age — *see* Light for dates
headedness R42
Light-for-dates (infant) P05.00
with weight of
499 grams or less P05.01
500-749 grams P05.02
750-999 grams P05.03
1000-1249 grams P05.04
1250-1499 grams P05.05
1500-1749 grams P05.06
1750-1999 grams P05.07
2000-2499 grams P05.08
2500 grams and over P05.09
affecting management of pregnancy O36.59- ☑
and small-for-dates — *see* Small for dates
specified NEC P05.09
Lightning (effects) (stroke) (struck by) T75.00 ☑
burn — *see* Burn
foot E53.8
shock T75.01 ☑
specified effect NEC T75.09 ☑
Lightwood-Albright syndrome N25.89
Lightwood's disease or syndrome (renal tubular acidosis) N25.89
Lignac (-de Toni) (-Fanconi) (-Debré) **disease or syndrome** E72.09
with cystinosis E72.04
Ligneous thyroiditis E06.5
Likoff's syndrome I20.8
Limb — *see* condition
Limbic epilepsy personality syndrome F07.0
Limitation, limited
activities due to disability Z73.6
cardiac reserve — *see* Disease, heart
eye muscle duction, traumatic — *see* Strabismus, mechanical
mandibular range of motion M26.52
Lindau (-von Hippel) **disease** Q85.83
Line(s)
Beau's L60.4
Harris' — *see* Arrest, epiphyseal
Hudson's (cornea) — *see* Pigmentation, cornea, anterior
Stähli's (cornea) — *see* Pigmentation, cornea, anterior
Linea corneae senilis — *see* Change, cornea, senile
Lingua
geographica K14.1
nigra (villosa) K14.3
plicata K14.5
tylosis K13.29
Lingual — *see* condition
Linguatulosis B88.8
Linitis (gastric) **plastica** C16.9
Lip — *see* condition
Lipedema — *see* Edema
Lipemia — *see also* Hyperlipidemia
retina, retinalis E78.3
Lipidosis E75.6
cerebral (infantile) (juvenile) (late) E75.4
cerebroretinal E75.4
cerebroside E75.22
cholesterol (cerebral) E75.5
glycolipid E75.21
hepatosplenomegalic E78.3
sphingomyelin — *see* Niemann-Pick disease or syndrome
sulfatide E75.29
Lipoadenoma — *see* Neoplasm, benign, by site
Lipoblastoma — *see* Lipoma
Lipoblastomatosis — *see* Lipoma
Lipochondrodystrophy E76.01
Lipochrome histiocytosis (familial) D71
Lipodermatosclerosis — *see* Varix, leg, with, inflammation
ulcerated — *see* Varix, leg, with, ulcer, with inflammation by site
Lipodystrophia progressiva E88.1
Lipodystrophy (progressive) E88.1
insulin E88.1
intestinal K90.81
mesenteric K65.4
Lipofibroma — *see* Lipoma

Lipofuscinosis, neuronal (with ceroidosis) E75.4
Lipogranuloma, sclerosing L92.8
Lipogranulomatosis E78.89
Lipoid — *see also* condition
histiocytosis D76.3
essential E75.29
nephrosis N04.9
proteinosis of Urbach E78.89
Lipoidemia — *see* Hyperlipidemia
Lipoidosis — *see* Lipidosis
Lipoma D17.9
fetal D17.9
fat cell D17.9
infiltrating D17.9
intramuscular D17.9
pleomorphic D17.9
site classification
arms (skin) (subcutaneous) D17.2- ☑
connective tissue D17.30
intra-abdominal D17.5
intrathoracic D17.4
peritoneum D17.79
retroperitoneum D17.79
specified site NEC D17.39
spermatic cord D17.6
face (skin) (subcutaneous) D17.0
genitourinary organ NEC D17.72
head (skin) (subcutaneous) D17.0
intra-abdominal D17.5
intrathoracic D17.4
kidney D17.71
legs (skin) (subcutaneous) D17.2- ☑
neck (skin) (subcutaneous) D17.0
peritoneum D17.79
retroperitoneum D17.79
skin D17.30
specified site NEC D17.39
specified site NEC D17.79
spermatic cord D17.6
subcutaneous D17.30
specified site NEC D17.39
trunk (skin) (subcutaneous) D17.1
unspecified D17.9
spindle cell D17.9
Lipomatosis E88.2
dolorosa (Dercum) E88.2
fetal — *see* Lipoma
Launois-Bensaude E88.89
Lipomyoma — *see* Lipoma
Lipomyxoma — *see* Lipoma
Lipomyxosarcoma — *see* Neoplasm, connective tissue, malignant
Lipoprotein metabolism disorder E78.9
Lipoproteinemia E78.5
broad-beta E78.2
floating-beta E78.2
hyper-pre-beta E78.1
Liposarcoma — *see also* Neoplasm, connective tissue, malignant
dedifferentiated — *see* Neoplasm, connective tissue, malignant
differentiated type — *see* Neoplasm, connective tissue, malignant
embryonal — *see* Neoplasm, connective tissue, malignant
mixed type — *see* Neoplasm, connective tissue, malignant
myxoid — *see* Neoplasm, connective tissue, malignant
pleomorphic — *see* Neoplasm, connective tissue, malignant
round cell — *see* Neoplasm, connective tissue, malignant
well differentiated type — *see* Neoplasm, connective tissue, malignant
Liposynovitis prepatellaris E88.89
Lipping, cervix N86
Lipschütz disease or ulcer N76.6
Lipuria R82.0
schistosomiasis (bilharziasis) B65.0
Lisping F80.0
Lissauer's paralysis A52.17
Lissencephalia, lissencephaly Q04.3
Listeriosis, listerellosis A32.9
congenital (disseminated) P37.2
cutaneous A32.0
neonatal, newborn (disseminated) P37.2
oculoglandular A32.81
specified NEC A32.89

Lithemia E79.0
Lithiasis — *see* Calculus
Lithosis J62.8
Lithuria R82.998
Litigation, anxiety concerning Z65.3
Little leaguer's elbow — *see* Epicondylitis, medial
Little's disease G80.9
Littre's
  gland — *see* condition
  hernia — *see* Hernia, abdomen
Littritis — *see* Urethritis
Livedo (annularis) (racemosa) (reticularis) R23.1
Liver — *see* condition
Living alone (problems with) Z60.2
  with handicapped person Z74.2
Living in a shelter (motel) (scattered site housing)
  (temporary or transitional living situation) Z59.01
Lloyd's syndrome — *see* Adenomatosis, endocrine
Loa loa, loaiasis, loasis B74.3
Lobar — *see* condition
Lobomycosis B48.0
Lobo's disease B48.0
Lobotomy syndrome F07.0
Lobstein (-Ekman) **disease or syndrome** Q78.0
Lobster-claw hand Q71.6- ☑
Lobulation (congenital) — *see also* Anomaly, by site
  kidney, Q63.1
  liver, abnormal Q44.7
  spleen Q89.09
Lobule, lobular — *see* condition
Local, localized — *see* condition
Locked twins causing obstructed labor O66.1
Locked-in state G83.5
Locking
  joint — *see* Derangement, joint, specified type NEC
  knee — *see* Derangement, knee
Lockjaw — *see* Tetanus
Löffler's
  endocarditis I42.3
  eosinophilia J82.89
  pneumonia J82.89
  syndrome (eosinophilic pneumonitis) J82.89
Loiasis (with conjunctival infestation) (eyelid) B74.3
Lone Star fever A77.0
Long
  COVID (-19) — *see also* COVID-19 U09.9
  labor O63.9
    first stage O63.0
    second stage O63.1
  QT syndrome I45.81
Longitudinal stripes or grooves, nails L60.8
  congenital Q84.6
Long-term (current) (prophylactic) **drug therapy** (use
  of)
  5-fluorouracil Z79.631
  6-mercaptopurine Z79.631
  adalimumab Z79.620
  agents affecting estrogen receptors and estrogen levels
    NEC Z79.818
  alkylating agent Z79.630
  anastrozole (Arimidex) Z79.811
  antibiotics Z79.2
    short-term use — *omit code*
  anticoagulants Z79.01
  antidiabetic drugs, injectable, non-insulin Z79.85
  anti-inflammatory, non-steroidal (NSAID) Z79.1
  antimetabolite agent Z79.631
  antiplatelet Z79.02
  antithrombotics Z79.02
  antitumor antibiotic Z79.632
  apremilast Z79.61
  aromatase inhibitors Z79.811
  aspirin Z79.82
  azathioprine Z79.624
  birth control pill or patch Z79.3
  bisphosphonates Z79.83
  bleomycin Z79.632
  calcineurin inhibitor Z79.621
  chlorambucil Z79.630
  cisplatin Z79.630
  contraceptive, oral Z79.3
  cyclophosphamide Z79.630
  cyclosporine Z79.621
  cytarabine Z79.631
  doxorubicin Z79.632
  drug, specified NEC Z79.899
  estrogen receptor downregulators Z79.818

Long-term (current) (prophylactic) **drug therapy** —
  continued
  etanercept Z79.620
  etoposide Z79.634
  Evista Z79.810
  exemestane (Aromasin) Z79.811
  Fareston Z79.810
  fulvestrant (Faslodex) Z79.818
  gonadotropin-releasing hormone (GnRH) agonist
    Z79.818
  goserelin acetate (Zoladex) Z79.818
  hormone replacement Z79.890
  hydroxyurea Z79.64
  immunomodulators, unspecified Z79.60
    specified NEC Z79.69
  immunomodulatory imide drug Z79.61
  immunosuppressants, unspecified Z79.60
    specified NEC Z79.69
  immunosuppressive biologic Z79.620
  infliximab Z79.620
  inhibitors of nucleotide synthesis Z79.624
  insulin Z79.4
  irinotecan Z79.634
  Janus kinase inhibitor Z79.622
  lenalidomide Z79.61
  letrozole (Femara) Z79.811
  leuprolide acetate (leuprorelin) (Lupron) Z79.818
  mammalian target of rapamycin (mTOR) inhibitor
    Z79.623
  megestrol acetate (Megace) Z79.818
  methadone for pain management Z79.891
  mitomycin C Z79.632
  mitotic inhibitor Z79.633
  monoclonal antibodies Z79.620
  myelosuppressive agent Z79.64
  Nolvadex Z79.810
  non-insulin antidiabetic drug, injectable Z79.899
  non-steroidal anti-inflammatories (NSAID) Z79.1
  omycophenolate Z79.624
  opiate analgesic Z79.891
  oral
    antidiabetic Z79.84
    contraceptive Z79.3
    hypoglycemic Z79.84
  paclitaxel Z79.633
  plant alkaloids Z79.633
  pomalidomide Z79.61
  purine synthesis (IMDH) inhibitors Z79.624
  raloxifene (Evista) Z79.810
  selective estrogen receptor modulators (SERMs)
    Z79.810
  sirolimus Z79.623
  steroids
    inhaled Z79.51
    systemic Z79.52
  tacrolimus Z79.621
  tamoxifen (Nolvadex) Z79.810
  tofacitinib Z79.622
  topoisomerase inhibitor Z79.634
  topotecan Z79.634
  toremifene (Fareston) Z79.810
  vinblastine Z79.633
  vincristine Z79.633
Loop
  intestine — *see* Volvulus
  vascular on papilla (optic) Q14.2
Loose — *see also* condition
  body
    joint M24.00
      ankle M24.07- ☑
      elbow M24.02- ☑
      hand M24.04- ☑
      hip M24.05- ☑
      knee M23.4- ☑
      shoulder (region) M24.01- ☑
      specified site NEC M24.08
      toe M24.07- ☑
      vertebra M24.08
      wrist M24.03- ☑
    knee M23.4- ☑
    sheath, tendon — *see* Disorder, tendon, specified
      type NEC
  cartilage — *see* Loose, body, joint
  skin and subcutaneous tissue (following bariatric
    surgery weight loss) (following dietary weight
    loss) L98.7
  tooth, teeth K08.89

Loosening
  aseptic
    joint prosthesis — *see* Complications, joint prosthe-
      sis, mechanical, loosening, by site
    epiphysis — *see* Osteochondropathy
  mechanical
    joint prosthesis — *see* Complications, joint prosthe-
      sis, mechanical, loosening, by site
Looser-Milkman (-Debray) **syndrome** M83.8
Lop ear (deformity) Q17.3
Lorain (-Levi) **short stature syndrome** E23.0
Lordosis M40.50
  acquired — *see* Lordosis, specified type NEC
  congenital Q76.429
    lumbar region Q76.426
    lumbosacral region Q76.427
    sacral region Q76.428
    sacrococcygeal region Q76.428
    thoracolumbar region Q76.425
  lumbar region M40.56
  lumbosacral region M40.57
  postsurgical M96.4
  postural — *see* Lordosis, specified type NEC
  rachitic (late effect) (sequelae) E64.3
  sequelae of rickets E64.3
  specified type NEC M40.40
    lumbar region M40.46
    lumbosacral region M40.47
    thoracolumbar region M40.45
  thoracolumbar region M40.55
  tuberculous A18.01
Loss (of)
  appetite — *see also* Anorexia R63.0
    hysterical F50.89
    nonorganic origin F50.89
    psychogenic F50.89
  blood — *see* Hemorrhage
  bone —*see* Loss, substance of, bone
  consciousness, transient R55
    traumatic — *see* Injury, intracranial
  control, sphincter, rectum R15.9
    nonorganic origin F98.1
  elasticity, skin R23.4
  family (member) in childhood Z62.898
  fluid (acute) E86.9
  function of labyrinth — *see* subcategory H83.2 ☑
  hair, nonscarring — *see* Alopecia
  hearing — *see also* Deafness
    central NOS H90.5
    conductive H90.2
      bilateral H90.0
      unilateral
        with
          restricted hearing on the contralateral
            side H90.A1- ☑
          unrestricted hearing on the contralateral
            side H90.1- ☑
    mixed conductive and sensorineural hearing loss
      H90.8
      bilateral H90.6
      unilateral
        with
          restricted hearing on the contralateral
            side H90.A3- ☑
          unrestricted hearing on the contralateral
            side H90.7- ☑
    neural NOS H90.5
    perceptive NOS H90.5
    sensorineural NOS H90.5
      bilateral H90.3
      unilateral
        with
          restricted hearing onthe contralateral
            side H90.A2- ☑
          unrestricted hearing on the contralateral
            side H90.4- ☑
    sensory NOS H90.5
  height R29.890
  limb or member, traumatic, current — *see* Amputation,
    traumatic
  love relationship in childhood Z62.898
  memory — *see also* Amnesia
    mild, following organic brain damage F06.8
  mind — *see* Psychosis
  occlusal vertical dimension of fully erupted teeth
    M26.37
  organ or part — *see* Absence, by site, acquired
  ossicles, ear (partial) H74.32- ☑

Loss — *continued*
  parent in childhood Z63.4
  pregnancy, recurrent N96
    care in current pregnancy O26.2- ☑
    without current pregnancy N96
  recurrent pregnancy — *see* Loss, pregnancy, recurrent
  self-esteem, in childhood Z62.898
  sense of
    smell — *see* Disturbance, sensation, smell
    taste — *see* Disturbance, sensation, taste
    touch R20.8
  sensory R44.9
    dissociative F44.6
  sexual desire F52.0
  sight (acquired) (complete) (congenital) — *see* Blindness
  substance of
    bone — *see* Disorder, bone, density and structure, specified NEC
      horizontal alveolar K06.3
    cartilage — *see* Disorder, cartilage, specified type NEC
      auricle (ear) — *see* Disorder, pinna, specified type NEC
    vitreous (humor) H15.89
  tooth, teeth — *see* Absence, teeth, acquired
  vision, visual H54.7
    both eyes H54.3
    one eye H54.60
      left (normal vision on right) H54.62
      right (normal vision on left) H54.61
    specified as blindness — *see* Blindness
    subjective
      sudden H53.13- ☑
      transient H53.12- ☑
  vitreous — *see* Prolapse, vitreous
  voice — *see* Aphonia
  weight (abnormal) (cause unknown) R63.4
Louis-Bar syndrome (ataxia-telangiectasia) G11.3
Louping ill (encephalitis) A84.89
Louse, lousiness — *see* Lice
Low
  achiever, school Z55.3
  back syndrome M54.50
  basal metabolic rate R94.8
  birthweight (2499 grams or less) P07.10
    with weight of
      1000-1249 grams P07.14
      1250-1499 grams P07.15
      1500-1749 grams P07.16
      1750-1999 grams P07.17
      2000-2499 grams P07.18
    extreme (999 grams or less) P07.00
      with weight of
        499 grams or less P07.01
        500-749 grams P07.02
        750-999 grams P07.03
    for gestational age — *see* Light for dates
  blood pressure — *see also* Hypotension
    reading (incidental) (isolated) (nonspecific) R03.1
  cardiac reserve — *see* Disease, heart
  function — *see also* Hypofunction
    kidney N28.9
  hematocrit D64.9
  hemoglobin D64.9
  income Z59.6
  level of literacy Z55.0
  lying
    kidney N28.89
    organ or site, congenital — *see* Malposition, congenital
  output syndrome (cardiac) — *see* Failure, heart
  platelets (blood) — *see* Thrombocytopenia
  reserve, kidney N28.89
  salt syndrome E87.1
  self esteem R45.81
  set ears Q17.4
  vision H54.2X- ☑
    one eye (other eye normal) H54.50
      left (normal vision on right) H54.52A- ☑
      other eye blind — *see* Blindness
      right (normal vision on left) H54.511- ☑
  von Willebrand factor R79.1
Low-density-lipoprotein-type (LDL) **hyperlipoproteinemia** E78.00
Lowe's syndrome E72.03
Lown-Ganong-Levine syndrome I45.6
LSD reaction (acute) (without dependence) F16.90

LSD reaction — *continued*
  with dependence F16.20
L-shaped kidney Q63.8
LTBI (latent tuberculosis infection) Z22.7
Ludwig's angina or disease K12.2
Lues (venerea), **luetic** — *see* Syphilis
Luetscher's syndrome (dehydration) E86.0
Lumbago, lumbalgia M54.50
  with sciatica M54.4- ☑
    due to intervertebral disc disorder M51.17
  due to displacement, intervertebral disc M51.27
    with sciatica M51.17
Lumbar — *see* condition
Lumbarization, vertebra, congenital Q76.49
Lumbermen's itch B88.0
Lump — *see also* Mass
  breast N63.0
    axillary tail
      left N63.32
      right N63.31
    left
      lower inner quadrant N63.24
      lower outer quadrant N63.23
      overlapping quadrants N63.25
      unspecified quadrant N63.20
      upper inner quadrant N63.22
      upper outer quadrant N63.21
    right
      lower inner quadrant N63.14
      lower outer quadrant N63.13
      overlapping quadrants N63.15
      unspecified quadrant N63.10
      upper inner quadrant N63.12
      upper outer quadrant N63.11
    subareolar
      left N63.42
      right N63.41
Lunacy — *see* Psychosis
Lung — *see* condition
Lupoid (miliary) **of Boeck** D86.3
Lupus
  anticoagulant D68.62
    with
      hemorrhagic disorder D68.312
      hypercoagulable state D68.62
    finding without diagnosis R76.0
  discoid (local) L93.0
  erythematosus (discoid) (local) L93.0
    disseminated — *see* Lupus, erythematosus, systemic
    eyelid H01.129
      left H01.126
        lower H01.125
        upper H01.124
      right H01.123
        lower H01.122
        upper H01.121
    profundus L93.2
    specified NEC L93.2
    subacute cutaneous L93.1
    systemic M32.9
      with organ or system involvement M32.10
        endocarditis M32.11
        lung M32.13
        pericarditis M32.12
        renal (glomerular) M32.14
          tubulo-interstitial M32.15
        specified organ or system NEC M32.19
      drug-induced M32.0
      inhibitor (presence of) D68.62
        with
          hemorrhagic disorder D68.312
          hypercoagulable state D68.62
        finding without diagnosis R76.0
      specified NEC M32.8
  exedens A18.4
  hydralazine M32.0
    correct substance properly administered — *see* Table of Drugs and Chemicals, by drug, adverse effect
    overdose or wrong substance given or taken — *see* Table of Drugs and Chemicals, by drug, poisoning
  nephritis (chronic) M32.14
  nontuberculous, not disseminated L93.0
  panniculitis L93.2
  pernio (Besnier) D86.3
  systemic — *see* Lupus, erythematosus, systemic
  tuberculous A18.4

Lupus — *continued*
  tuberculous — *continued*
    eyelid A18.4
    vulgaris A18.4
      eyelid A18.4
Luteinoma D27.- ☑
Lutembacher's disease or syndrome (atrial septal defect with mitral stenosis) Q21.19
Luteoma D27.- ☑
Lutz (-Splendore-de Almeida) **disease** — *see* Paracoccidioidomycosis
Luxation — *see also* Dislocation
  eyeball (nontraumatic) — *see* Luxation, globe
    birth injury P15.3
  globe, nontraumatic H44.82- ☑
  lacrimal gland — *see* Dislocation, lacrimal gland
  lens (old) (partial) (spontaneous)
    congenital Q12.1
    syphilitic A50.39
Lycanthropy F22
Lyell's syndrome L51.2
  due to drug L51.2
    correct substance properly administered — *see* Table of Drugs and Chemicals, by drug, adverse effect
    overdose or wrong substance given or taken — *see* Table of Drugs and Chemicals, by drug, poisoning
Lyme disease A69.20
Lymph
  gland or node — *see* condition
  scrotum — *see* Infestation, filarial
Lymphadenitis I88.9
  with ectopic or molar pregnancy O08.0
  acute L04.9
    axilla L04.2
    face L04.0
    head L04.0
    hip L04.3
    limb
      lower L04.3
      upper L04.2
    neck L04.0
    shoulder L04.2
    specified site NEC L04.8
    trunk L04.1
  anthracosis (occupational) J60
  any site, except mesenteric I88.9
    chronic I88.1
    subacute I88.1
  breast
    gestational — *see* Mastitis, obstetric
    puerperal, postpartum (nonpurulent) O91.22
  chancroidal (congenital) A57
  chronic I88.1
    mesenteric I88.0
  due to
    Brugia (malayi) B74.1
      timori B74.2
    chlamydial lymphogranuloma A55
    diphtheria (toxin) A36.89
    lymphogranuloma venereum A55
    Wuchereria bancrofti B74.0
  following ectopic or molar pregnancy O08.0
  gonorrheal A54.89
  infective — *see* Lymphadenitis, acute
  mesenteric (acute) (chronic) (nonspecific) (subacute) I88.0
    due to Salmonella typhi A01.09
    tuberculous A18.39
  mycobacterial A31.8
  purulent — *see* Lymphadenitis, acute
  pyogenic — *see* Lymphadenitis, acute
  regional, nonbacterial I88.8
  septic — *see* Lymphadenitis, acute
  subacute, unspecified site I88.1
  suppurative — *see* Lymphadenitis, acute
  syphilitic (early) (secondary) A51.49
    late A52.79
  tuberculous — *see* Tuberculosis, lymph gland
  venereal (chlamydial) A55
Lymphadenoid goiter E06.3
Lymphadenopathy (generalized) R59.1
  angioimmunoblastic, with dysproteinemia (AILD) C86.5
  due to toxoplasmosis (acquired) B58.89
    congenital (acute) (subacute) (chronic) P37.1
  localized R59.0
  syphilitic (early) (secondary) A51.49

☑ **Additional Character Required** — **Refer to the Tabular List for Character Selection**

Lymphadenosis R59.1
Lymphangiectasis I89.0
　conjunctiva H11.89
　postinfectional I89.0
　scrotum I89.0
Lymphangiectatic elephantiasis, nonfilarial I89.0
Lymphangioendothelioma D18.1
　malignant — *see* Neoplasm, connective tissue, malignant
Lymphangioleiomyomatosis J84.81
Lymphangioma D18.1
　capillary D18.1
　cavernous D18.1
　cystic D18.1
　malignant — *see* Neoplasm, connective tissue, malignant
Lymphangiomyoma D18.1
Lymphangiomyomatosis J84.81
Lymphangiosarcoma — *see* Neoplasm, connective tissue, malignant
Lymphangitis I89.1
　with
　　abscess — *code by* site under Abscess
　　cellulitis — *code by* site under Cellulitis
　　ectopic or molar pregnancy O08.0
　acute L03.91
　　abdominal wall L03.321
　　ankle — *see* Lymphangitis, acute, lower limb
　　arm — *see* Lymphangitis, acute, upper limb
　　auricle (ear) — *see* Lymphangitis, acute, ear
　　axilla L03.12- ☑
　　back (any part) L03.322
　　buttock L03.327
　　cervical (meaning neck) L03.222
　　cheek (external) L03.212
　　chest wall L03.323
　　digit
　　　finger — *see* Lymphangitis, acute, finger
　　　toe — *see* Lymphangitis, acute, toe
　　ear (external) H60.1- ☑
　　external auditory canal — *see* Lymphangitis, acute, ear
　　eyelid — *see* Abscess, eyelid
　　face NEC L03.212
　　finger (intrathecal) (periosteal) (subcutaneous) (subcuticular) L03.02- ☑
　　foot — *see* Lymphangitis, acute, lower limb
　　gluteal (region) L03.327
　　groin L03.324
　　hand — *see* Lymphangitis, acute, upper limb
　　head NEC L03.891
　　　face (any part, except ear, eye and nose) L03.212
　　heel — *see* Lymphangitis, acute, lower limb
　　hip — *see* Lymphangitis, acute, lower limb
　　jaw (region) L03.212
　　knee — *see* Lymphangitis, acute, lower limb
　　leg — *see* Lymphangitis, acute, lower limb
　　lower limb L03.12- ☑
　　　toe — *see* Lymphangitis, acute, toe
　　navel L03.326
　　neck (region) L03.222
　　orbit, orbital — *see* Cellulitis, orbit
　　pectoral (region) L03.323
　　perineal, perineum L03.325
　　scalp (any part) L03.891
　　shoulder — *see* Lymphangitis, acute, upper limb
　　specified site NEC L03.898
　　thigh — *see* Lymphangitis, acute, lower limb
　　thumb (intrathecal) (periosteal) (subcutaneous) (subcuticular) — *see* Lymphangitis, acute, finger
　　toe (intrathecal) (periosteal) (subcutaneous) (subcuticular) L03.04- ☑
　　trunk L03.329
　　　abdominal wall L03.321
　　　back (any part) L03.322
　　　buttock L03.327
　　　chest wall L03.323
　　　groin L03.324
　　　perineal, perineum L03.325
　　　umbilicus L03.326
　　umbilicus L03.326
　　upper limb L03.12- ☑
　　　axilla — *see* Lymphangitis, acute, axilla
　　　finger — *see* Lymphangitis, acute, finger
　　　thumb — *see* Lymphangitis, acute, finger
　　wrist — *see* Lymphangitis, acute, upper limb

Lymphangitis — *continued*
　breast
　　gestational — *see* Mastitis, obstetric
　chancroidal A57
　chronic (any site) I89.1
　due to
　　Brugia (malayi) B74.1
　　　timori B74.2
　　Wuchereria bancrofti B74.0
　following ectopic or molar pregnancy O08.89
　penis
　　acute N48.29
　　gonococcal (acute) (chronic) A54.09
　puerperal, postpartum, childbirth O86.89
　strumous, tuberculous A18.2
　subacute (any site) I89.1
　tuberculous — *see* Tuberculosis, lymph gland
Lymphatic (vessel) — *see* condition
Lymphatism E32.8
Lymphectasia I89.0
Lymphedema (acquired) — *see also* Elephantiasis
　congenital Q82.0
　hereditary (chronic) (idiopathic) Q82.0
　postmastectomy I97.2
　praecox I89.0
　secondary I89.0
　surgical NEC I97.89
　　postmastectomy (syndrome) I97.2
Lymphoblastic — *see* condition
Lymphoblastoma (diffuse) — *see* Lymphoma, lymphoblastic (diffuse)
　giant follicular — *see* Lymphoma, lymphoblastic (diffuse)
　macrofollicular — *see* Lymphoma, lymphoblastic (diffuse)
Lymphocele I89.8
Lymphocytic
　chorioencephalitis (acute) (serous) A87.2
　choriomeningitis (acute) (serous) A87.2
　meningoencephalitis A87.2
Lymphocytoma, benign cutis L98.8
Lymphocytopenia D72.810
Lymphocytosis (symptomatic) D72.820
　infectious (acute) B33.8
Lymphoepithelioma — *see* Neoplasm, malignant, by site
Lymphogranuloma (malignant) — *see also* Lymphoma, Hodgkin
　chlamydial A55
　inguinale A55
　venereum (any site) (chlamydial) (with stricture of rectum) A55
Lymphogranulomatosis (malignant) — *see also* Lymphoma, Hodgkin
　benign (Boeck's sarcoid) (Schaumann's) D86.1
Lymphohistiocytosis, hemophagocytic (familial) D76.1
Lymphoid — *see* condition
Lymphoma (of) (malignant) C85.90
　adult T-cell (HTLV-1-associated) (acute variant) (chronic variant) (lymphomatoid variant) (smouldering variant) C91.5- ☑
　anaplastic large cell
　　ALK-negative C84.7- ☑
　　ALK-positive C84.6- ☑
　　breast implant associated (BIA-ALCL) C84.7A
　　CD30-positive C84.6- ☑
　　primary cutaneous C86.6
　angioimmunoblastic T-cell C86.5
　BALT C88.4
　B-cell C85.1- ☑
　blastic NK-cell C86.4
　blastic plasmacytoid dendritic cell neoplasm (BPDCN) C86.4
　B-precursor C83.5- ☑
　bronchial-associated lymphoid tissue [BALT-lymphoma] C88.4
　Burkitt (atypical) C83.7- ☑
　Burkitt-like C83.7- ☑
　centrocytic C83.1- ☑
　cutaneous follicle center C82.6- ☑
　cutaneous T-cell C84.A- ☑ (*following* C84.7)
　diffuse follicle center C82.5- ☑
　diffuse large cell C83.3- ☑
　　anaplastic C83.3- ☑
　　B-cell C83.3- ☑
　　CD30-positive C83.3- ☑
　　centroblastic C83.3- ☑

Lymphoma — *continued*
　diffuse large cell — *continued*
　　immunoblastic C83.3- ☑
　　plasmablastic C83.3- ☑
　　subtype not specified C83.3- ☑
　　T-cell rich C83.3- ☑
　enteropathy-type (associated) (intestinal) T-cell C86.2
　extranodal marginal zone B-cell lymphoma of mucosa-associated lymphoid tissue [MALT-lymphoma] C88.4
　extranodal NK/T-cell, nasal type C86.0
　follicular C82.9- ☑
　　grade
　　　I C82.0- ☑
　　　II C82.1- ☑
　　　III C82.2- ☑
　　　IIIa C82.3- ☑
　　　IIIb C82.4- ☑
　　specified NEC C82.8- ☑
　hepatosplenic T-cell (alpha-beta) (gamma-delta) C86.1
　histiocytic C85.9- ☑
　　true C96.A (*following* C96.6)
　Hodgkin C81.9 ☑
　　lymphocyte depleted (classical) C81.3- ☑
　　lymphocyte-rich (classical) C81.4- ☑
　　mixed cellularity (classical) C81.2- ☑
　　nodular
　　　lymphocyte predominant C81.0- ☑
　　　sclerosis (classical) C81.1- ☑
　　nodular sclerosis (classical) C81.1- ☑
　　specified NEC (classical) C81.7- ☑
　intravascular large B-cell C83.8- ☑
　Lennert's C84.4- ☑
　lymphoblastic (diffuse) C83.5- ☑
　lymphoblastic B-cell C83.5- ☑
　lymphoblastic T-cell C83.5- ☑
　lymphoepithelioid C84.4- ☑
　lymphoplasmacytic C83.0- ☑
　　with IgM-production C88.0
　MALT C88.4
　mantle cell C83.1- ☑
　mature T-cell NEC C84.4- ☑
　mature T/NK-cell C84.9- ☑
　　specified NEC C84.Z- ☑ (*following* C84.7)
　mediastinal (thymic) large B-cell C85.2- ☑
　Mediterranean C88.3
　mucosa-associated lymphoid tissue [MALT-lymphoma] C88.4
　NK/T cell C84.9- ☑
　nodal marginal zone C83.0- ☑
　non-follicular (diffuse) C83.9- ☑
　　specified NEC C83.8- ☑
　non-Hodgkin — *see also* Lymphoma, by type C85.9- ☑
　　specified NEC C85.8- ☑
　non-leukemic variant of B-CLL C83.0- ☑
　peripheral T-cell NEC C84.4- ☑
　primary cutaneous
　　anaplastic large cell C86.6
　　CD30-positive large T-cell C86.6
　primary effusion B-cell C83.8- ☑
　SALT C88.4
　skin-associated lymphoid tissue [SALT-lymphoma] C88.4
　small cell B-cell C83.0- ☑
　splenic marginal zone C83.0- ☑
　subcutaneous panniculitis-like T-cell C86.3
　T-precursor C83.5- ☑
　true histiocytic C96.A (*following* C96.6)
Lymphomatosis — *see* Lymphoma
Lymphopathia venereum, veneris A55
Lymphopenia D72.810
Lymphoplasmacytic leukemia — *see* Leukemia, chronic lymphocytic, B-cell type
Lymphoproliferation, X-linked disease D82.3
Lymphoreticulosis, benign (of inoculation) A28.1
Lymphorrhea I89.8
Lymphosarcoma (diffuse) — *see also* Lymphoma C85.9- ☑
Lymphostasis I89.8
Lypemania — *see* Melancholia
Lysine and hydroxylysine metabolism disorder E72.3
Lyssa — *see* Rabies

M

Macacus ear Q17.3

Maceration, wet feet, tropical (syndrome) T69.02- ☑
MacLeod's syndrome J43.0
Macrocephalia, macrocephaly Q75.3
Macrocheilia, macrochilia (congenital) Q18.6
Macrocolon — *see also* Megacolon Q43.1
Macrocornea Q15.8
  with glaucoma Q15.0
Macrocytic — *see* condition
Macrocytosis D75.89
Macrodactylia, macrodactylism (fingers) (thumbs) Q74.0
  toes Q74.2
Macrodontia K00.2
Macrogenia M26.05
Macrogenitosomia (adrenal) (male) (praecox) E25.9
  congenital E25.0
Macroglobulinemia (idiopathic) (primary) C88.0
  monoclonal (essential) D47.2
  Waldenström C88.0
Macroglossia (congenital) Q38.2
  acquired K14.8
Macrognathia, macrognathism (congenital) (mandibular) (maxillary) M26.09
Macrogyria (congenital) Q04.8
Macrohydrocephalus — *see* Hydrocephalus
Macromastia — *see* Hypertrophy, breast
Macrophthalmos Q11.3
  in congenital glaucoma Q15.0
Macropsia H53.15
Macrosigmoid K59.39
  congenital Q43.2
Macrospondylitis , acromegalic E22.0
Macrostomia (congenital) Q18.4
Macrotia (external ear) (congenital) Q17.1
Macula
  cornea, corneal — *see* Opacity, cornea
  degeneration (atrophic) (exudative) (senile) — *see also* Degeneration, macula
  hereditary — *see* Dystrophy, retina
Maculae ceruleae B85.1
Maculopathy, toxic — *see* Degeneration, macula, toxic
Madarosis (eyelid) H02.729
  left H02.726
    lower H02.725
    upper H02.724
  right H02.723
    lower H02.722
    upper H02.721
Madelung's
  deformity (radius) Q74.0
  disease
    radial deformity Q74.0
    symmetrical lipomas, neck E88.89
Madness — *see* Psychosis
Madura
  foot B47.9
    actinomycotic B47.1
    mycotic B47.0
Maduromycosis B47.0
Maffucci's syndrome Q78.4
Magnesium metabolism disorder — *see* Disorder, metabolism, magnesium
Main en griffe (acquired) — *see also* Deformity, limb, clawhand
  congenital Q68.1
Maintenance (encounter for)
  antineoplastic chemotherapy Z51.11
  antineoplastic radiation therapy Z51.0
  methadone F11.20
Majocchi's
  disease L81.7
  granuloma B35.8
Major — *see* condition
Mal de los pintos — *see* Pinta
Mal de mer T75.3 ☑
Malabar itch (any site) B35.5
Malabsorption K90.9
  calcium K90.89
  carbohydrate K90.49
  disaccharide E73.9
  fat K90.49
  galactose E74.20
  glucose (-galactose) E74.39
  intestinal K90.9
    specified NEC K90.89
  isomaltose E74.31
  lactose E73.9

Malabsorption — *continued*
  methionine E72.19
  monosaccharide E74.39
  postgastrectomy K91.2
  postsurgical K91.2
  protein K90.49
  starch K90.49
  sucrose E74.39
  syndrome K90.9
    postsurgical K91.2
Malacia, bone (adult) M83.9
  juvenile — *see* Rickets
Malacoplakia
  bladder N32.89
  pelvis (kidney) N28.89
  ureter N28.89
  urethra N36.8
Malacosteon, juvenile — *see* Rickets
Maladaptation — *see* Maladjustment
Maladie de Roger Q21.0
Maladjustment
  conjugal Z63.0
    involving divorce or estrangement Z63.5
  educational Z55.4
  family Z63.9
  marital Z63.0
    involving divorce or estrangement Z63.5
  occupational NEC Z56.89
  simple, adult — *see* Disorder, adjustment
  situational — *see* Disorder, adjustment
  social Z60.9
    due to
      acculturation difficulty Z60.3
      discrimination and persecution (perceived) Z60.5
      exclusion and isolation Z60.4
      life-cycle (phase of life) transition Z60.0
      rejection Z60.4
      specified reason NEC Z60.8
Malaise R53.81
Malakoplakia — *see* Malacoplakia
Malaria, malarial (fever) B54
  with
    blackwater fever B50.8
      hemoglobinuric (bilious) B50.8
    hemoglobinuria B50.8
  accidentally induced (therapeutically) — *code by* type under Malaria
  algid B50.9
  cerebral B50.0 *[G94]*
  clinically diagnosed (without parasitological confirmation) B54
  congenital NEC P37.4
    falciparum P37.3
  congestion, congestive B54
  continued (fever) B50.9
  estivo-autumnal B50.9
  falciparum B50.9
    with complications NEC B50.8
      cerebral B50.0 *[G94]*
    severe B50.8
  hemorrhagic B54
  malariae B52.9
    with
      complications NEC B52.8
      glomerular disorder B52.0
  malignant (tertian) — *see* Malaria, falciparum
  mixed infections — *code to* first listed type in B50-B53
  ovale B53.0
  parasitologically confirmed NEC B53.8
  pernicious, acute — *see* Malaria, falciparum
  Plasmodium (P.)
    falciparum NEC — *see* Malaria, falciparum
    malariae NEC B52.9
      with Plasmodium
        falciparum (and or vivax) — *see* Malaria, falciparum
        vivax — *see also* Malaria, vivax
          and falciparum — *see* Malaria, falciparum
      ovale B53.0
        with Plasmodium malariae — *see also* Malaria, malariae
          and vivax — *see also* Malaria, vivax
            and falciparum — *see* Malaria, falciparum
      simian B53.1
        with Plasmodium malariae — *see also* Malaria, malariae
          and vivax — *see also* Malaria, vivax
            and falciparum — *see* Malaria, falciparum

Malaria, malarial — *continued*
  Plasmodium — *continued*
    vivax NEC B51.9
      with Plasmodium falciparum — *see* Malaria, falciparum
    quartan — *see* Malaria, malariae
    quotidian — *see* Malaria, falciparum
    recurrent B54
    remittent B54
    specified type NEC (parasitologically confirmed) B53.8
    spleen B54
    subtertian (fever) — *see* Malaria, falciparum
    tertian (benign) — *see also* Malaria, vivax
      malignant B50.9
    tropical B50.9
    typhoid B54
    vivax B51.9
      with
        complications NEC B51.8
        ruptured spleen B51.0
Malassez's disease (cystic) N50.89
Malassimilation K90.9
Maldescent, testis Q53.9
  bilateral Q53.20
    abdominal Q53.211
    perineal Q53.22
  unilateral Q53.10
    abdominal Q53.111
    perineal Q53.12
Maldevelopment — *see also* Anomaly
  brain Q07.9
  colon Q43.9
  hip Q74.2
    congenital dislocation Q65.2
      bilateral Q65.1
      unilateral Q65.0- ☑
  mastoid process Q75.8
  middle ear Q16.4
    except ossicles Q16.4
    ossicles Q16.3
  ossicles Q16.3
  spine Q76.49
  toe Q74.2
Male type pelvis Q74.2
  with disproportion (fetopelvic) O33.3 ☑
    causing obstructed labor O65.3
Malformation (congenital) — *see also* Anomaly
  adrenal gland Q89.1
  affecting multiple systems with skeletal changes NEC Q87.5
  alimentary tract Q45.9
    specified type NEC Q45.8
    upper Q40.9
      specified type NEC Q40.8
  aorta Q25.40
    absence Q25.41
    aneurysm, congenital Q25.43
    aplasia Q25.41
    atresia Q25.29
      aortic arch Q25.21
    coarctation (preductal) (postductal) Q25.1
    dilatation, congenital Q25.44
    hypoplasia Q25.42
    patent ductus arteriosus Q25.0
    specified type NEC Q25.49
    stenosis Q25.1
      supravalvular Q25.3
  aortic valve Q23.9
    specified NEC Q23.8
  arteriovenous, aneurysmatic (congenital) Q27.30
    brain Q28.2
      ruptured I60.8
        intracerebral I61.8
        intraparenchymal I61.8
        intraventricular I61.5
        subarachnoid I60.8
      cerebral — *see also* Malformation, arteriovenous, brain Q28.2
    peripheral Q27.30
      digestive system — *see* Angiodysplasia
        congenital Q27.33
      lower limb Q27.32
      other specified site Q27.39
      renal vessel Q27.34
      upper limb Q27.31
    precerebral vessels (nonruptured) Q28.0
  auricle
    ear (congenital) Q17.3

Malfunction — continued
urinary device NEC — see Complication, genitourinary, device, urinary, mechanical
valve
  colostomy K94.03
  heart T82.09 ☑
  ileostomy K94.13
vascular graft or shunt NEC — see Complication, cardiovascular device, mechanical, vascular
ventricular (communicating shunt) T85.01 ☑
Malherbe's tumor — see Neoplasm, skin, benign
Malibu disease L98.8
Malignancy — see also Neoplasm, malignant, by site
unspecified site (primary) C80.1
Malignant — see condition
Malingerer, malingering Z76.5
Mallet finger (acquired) — see Deformity, finger, mallet
finger
  congenital Q74.0
  sequelae of rickets E64.3
Malleus A24.0
Mallory's bodies R89.7
Mallory-Weiss syndrome K22.6
Malnutrition E46
degree
  first E44.1
  mild (protein) E44.1
  moderate (protein) E44.0
  second E44.0
  severe (protein-energy) E43
    intermediate form E42
      with
        kwashiorkor E42
        marasmus E41
  third E43
following gastrointestinal surgery K91.2
intrauterine
  light-for-dates — see Light for dates
  small-for-dates — see Small for dates
lack of care, or neglect (child) (infant) T76.02 ☑
  confirmed T74.02 ☑
malignant E40
protein E46
  calorie E46
    mild E44.1
    moderate E44.0
    severe E43
      intermediate form E42
        with
          kwashiorkor (and marasmus) E42
          marasmus E41
  energy E46
    mild E44.1
    moderate E44.0
    severe E43
      intermediate form E42
        with
          kwashiorkor (and marasmus) E42
          marasmus E41
severe (protein-energy) E43
  with
    kwashiorkor (and marasmus) E42
    marasmus E41
Malocclusion (teeth) M26.4
Angle's M26.219
  class I M26.211
  class II M26.212
  class III M26.213
due to
  abnormal swallowing M26.59
  mouth breathing M26.59
  tongue, lip or finger habits M26.59
temporomandibular (joint) M26.69
Malposition
cervix — see Malposition, uterus
congenital
  adrenal (gland) Q89.1
  alimentary tract Q45.8
    lower Q43.8
    upper Q40.8
  aorta Q25.49
  appendix Q43.8
  arterial trunk Q20.0
  artery (peripheral) Q27.8
    coronary Q24.5
    digestive system Q27.8
    lower limb Q27.8
    pulmonary Q25.79

Malposition — continued
congenital — continued
  artery — continued
    specified site NEC Q27.8
    upper limb Q27.8
  auditory canal Q17.8
    causing impairment of hearing Q16.9
  auricle (ear) Q17.4
    causing impairment of hearing Q16.9
    cervical Q18.2
  biliary duct or passage Q44.5
  bladder (mucosa) — see Exstrophy, bladder
  brachial plexus Q07.8
  brain tissue Q04.8
  breast Q83.8
  bronchus Q32.4
  cecum Q43.8
  clavicle Q74.0
  colon Q43.8
  digestive organ or tract NEC Q45.8
    lower Q43.8
    upper Q40.8
  ear (auricle) (external) Q17.4
    ossicles Q16.3
  endocrine (gland) NEC Q89.2
  epiglottis Q31.8
  eustachian tube Q17.8
  eye Q15.8
  facial features Q18.8
  fallopian tube Q50.6
  finger(s) Q68.1
    supernumerary Q69.0
  foot Q66.9-
  gallbladder Q44.1
  gastrointestinal tract Q45.8
  genitalia, genital organ(s) or tract
    female Q52.8
      external Q52.79
      internal NEC Q52.8
    male Q55.8
  glottis Q31.8
  hand Q68.1
  heart Q24.8
    dextrocardia Q24.0
      with complete transposition of viscera Q89.3
  hepatic duct Q44.5
  hip (joint) Q65.89
  intestine (large) (small) Q43.8
    with anomalous adhesions, fixation or malrotation Q43.3
  joint NEC Q68.8
  kidney Q63.2
  larynx Q31.8
  limb Q68.8
    lower Q68.8
    upper Q68.8
  liver Q44.7
  lung (lobe) Q33.8
  nail(s) Q84.6
  nerve Q07.8
  nervous system NEC Q07.8
  nose, nasal (septum) Q30.8
  organ or site not listed — see Anomaly, by site
  ovary Q50.39
  pancreas Q45.3
  parathyroid (gland) Q89.2
  patella Q74.1
  peripheral vascular system Q27.8
  pituitary (gland) Q89.2
  respiratory organ or system NEC Q34.8
  rib (cage) Q76.6
    supernumerary in cervical region Q76.5
  scapula Q74.0
  shoulder Q74.0
  spinal cord Q06.8
  spleen Q89.09
  sternum NEC Q76.7
  stomach Q40.2
  symphysis pubis Q74.2
  thymus (gland) Q89.2
  thyroid (gland) (tissue) Q89.2
    cartilage Q31.8
  toe(s) Q66.9- ☑
    supernumerary Q69.2
  tongue Q38.3
  trachea Q32.1
  ureter Q62.60
    deviation Q62.61
    displacement Q62.62

Malposition — continued
congenital — continued
  ureter — continued
    ectopia Q62.63
    specified type NEC Q62.69
  uterus Q51.818
  vein(s) (peripheral) Q27.8
    great Q26.8
  vena cava (inferior) (superior) Q26.8
device, implant or graft — see also Complications, by site and type, mechanical T85.628 ☑
  arterial graft NEC — see Complication, cardiovascular device, mechanical, vascular
  breast (implant) T85.42 ☑
  catheter NEC T85.628 ☑
    cystostomy T83.020 ☑
    dialysis (renal) T82.42 ☑
      intraperitoneal T85.621 ☑
    infusion NEC T82.524 ☑
      spinal (epidural) (subdural) T85.620 ☑
    urinary — see also Displacement, device, catheter, urinary T83.028 ☑
  electronic (electrode) (pulse generator) (stimulator)
    bone T84.320 ☑
    cardiac T82.129 ☑
      electrode T82.120 ☑
      pulse generator T82.121 ☑
      specified type NEC T82.128 ☑
    nervous system — see Complication, prosthetic device, mechanical, electronic nervous system stimulator
    urinary — see Complication, genitourinary, device, urinary, mechanical
  fixation, internal (orthopedic) NEC — see Complication, fixation device, mechanical
  gastrointestinal — see Complications, prosthetic device, mechanical, gastrointestinal device
  genital NEC T83.428 ☑
    intrauterine contraceptive device (string) T83.32 ☑
    penile prosthesis (cylinder) (implanted) (pump) (reservoir) T83.420 ☑
    testicular prosthesis T83.421 ☑
  heart NEC — see Complication, cardiovascular device, mechanical
  joint prosthesis — see Complication, joint prosthesis, mechanical
  ocular NEC — see Complications, prosthetic device, mechanical, ocular device
  orthopedic NEC — see Complication, orthopedic, device, mechanical
  specified NEC T85.628 ☑
  urinary NEC — see also Complication, genitourinary, device, urinary, mechanical
    graft T83.22 ☑
  vascular NEC — see Complication, cardiovascular device, mechanical
  ventricular intracranial shunt T85.02 ☑
fetus — see Pregnancy, complicated by (management affected by), presentation, fetal
gallbladder K82.8
gastrointestinal tract, congenital Q45.8
heart, congenital NEC Q24.8
joint prosthesis — see Complications, joint prosthesis, mechanical, displacement, by site
stomach K31.89
  congenital Q40.2
tooth, teeth, fully erupted M26.30
uterus (acute) (acquired) (adherent) (asymptomatic) (postinfectional) (postpartal) (old) N85.4
  anteflexion or anteversion N85.4
    congenital Q51.818
  flexion N85.4
    lateral — see Lateroversion, uterus
  inversion N85.5
  lateral (flexion) (version) — see Lateroversion, uterus
    in pregnancy or childbirth — see subcategory O34.5 ☑
  retroflexion or retroversion — see Retroversion, uterus
Malposture R29.3
Malrotation
cecum Q43.3
colon Q43.3
intestine Q43.3
kidney Q63.2
Malta fever — see Brucellosis

Maltreatment
  adult
    abandonment
      confirmed T74.01 ☑
      suspected T76.01 ☑
    bullying
      confirmed T74.31 ☑
      suspected T76.31 ☑
    confirmed T74.91 ☑
    history of Z91.419
    intimidation (through social media)
      confirmed T74.31 ☑
      suspected T76.31 ☑
    neglect
      confirmed T74.01 ☑
      suspected T76.01 ☑
    physical abuse
      confirmed T74.11 ☑
      suspected T76.11 ☑
    psychological abuse
      confirmed T74.31 ☑
      history of Z91.411
      suspected T76.31 ☑
    sexual abuse
      confirmed T74.21 ☑
      suspected T76.21 ☑
    suspected T76.91 ☑
  child
    abandonment
      confirmed T74.02 ☑
      suspected T76.02 ☑
    bullying
      confirmed T74.32 ☑
      suspected T76.32 ☑
    confirmed T74.92 ☑
    history of — *see* History, personal (of), abuse
    intimidation (through social media)
      confirmed T74.32 ☑
      suspected T76.32 ☑
    neglect
      confirmed T74.02 ☑
      history of — *see* History, personal (of), abuse
      suspected T76.02 ☑
    physical abuse
      confirmed T74.12 ☑
      history of — *see* History, personal (of), abuse
      suspected T76.12 ☑
    psychological abuse
      confirmed T74.32 ☑
      history of — *see* History, personal (of), abuse
      suspected T76.32 ☑
    sexual abuse
      confirmed T74.22 ☑
      history of — *see* History, personal (of), abuse
      suspected T76.22 ☑
    suspected T76.92 ☑
  personal history of Z91.89
Maltworker's lung J67.4
Malunion, fracture — *see* Fracture, by site
Mammillitis N61.0
  puerperal, postpartum O91.02
Mammitis — *see* Mastitis
Mammogram (examination) Z12.39
  routine Z12.31
Mammoplasia N62
Management (of)
  bone conduction hearing device (implanted) Z45.320
  cardiac pacemaker NEC Z45.018
  cerebrospinal fluid drainage device Z45.41
  cochlear device (implanted) Z45.321
  contraceptive Z30.9
    specified NEC Z30.8
  implanted device Z45.9
    specified NEC Z45.89
  infusion pump Z45.1
  procreative Z31.9
    male factor infertility in female Z31.81
    specified NEC Z31.89
  prosthesis (external) — *see also* Fitting Z44.9
    implanted Z45.9
      specified NEC Z45.89
  renal dialysis catheter Z49.01
  vascular access device Z45.2
Mangled — *see* specified injury by site
Mania (monopolar) — *see also* Disorder, mood, manic
  episode
    with psychotic symptoms F30.2

Mania — *continued*
  without psychotic symptoms F30.10
    mild F30.11
    moderate F30.12
    severe F30.13
  Bell's F30.8
  chronic (recurrent) F31.89
  hysterical F44.89
  puerperal F30.8
  recurrent F31.89
Manic depression F31.9
Manic-depressive insanity, psychosis, or syndrome
  — *see* Disorder, bipolar
Mannosidosis E77.1
Mansonelliasis, mansonellosis B74.4
Manson's
  disease B65.1
  schistosomiasis B65.1
Manual — *see* condition
Maple-bark-stripper's lung (disease) J67.6
Maple-syrup-urine disease E71.0
Marable's syndrome (celiac artery compression) I77.4
Marasmus E41
  due to malnutrition E41
  intestinal E41
  nutritional E41
  senile R54
  tuberculous NEC — *see* Tuberculosis
Marble
  bones Q78.2
  skin R23.8
Marburg virus disease A98.3
March
  fracture — *see* Fracture, traumatic, stress, by site
  hemoglobinuria D59.6
Marchesani (-Weill) **syndrome** Q87.0
Marchiafava (-Bignami) **syndrome or disease** G37.1
Marchiafava-Micheli syndrome D59.5
Marcus Gunn's syndrome Q07.8
Marfan's syndrome — *see* Syndrome, Marfan's
Marie-Bamberger disease — *see* Osteoarthropathy,
  hypertrophic, specified NEC
Marie-Charcot-Tooth neuropathic muscular atrophy
  G60.0
Marie's
  cerebellar ataxia (late-onset) G11.2
  disease or syndrome (acromegaly) E22.0
Marie-Strümpell arthritis, disease or spondylitis —
  see Spondylitis, ankylosing
Marion's disease (bladder neck obstruction) N32.0
Marital conflict Z63.0
Mark
  port wine Q82.5
  raspberry Q82.5
  strawberry Q82.5
  stretch L90.6
  tattoo L81.8
Marker heterochromatin — *see* Extra, marker chromo-
  somes
Maroteaux-Lamy syndrome (mild) (severe) E76.29
Marrow (bone)
  arrest D61.9
  poor function D75.89
Marseilles fever A77.1
Marsh fever — *see* Malaria
Marshall's (hidrotic) **ectodermal dysplasia** Q82.4
Marsh's disease (exophthalmic goiter) E05.00
  with storm E05.01
Masculinization (female) **with adrenal hyperplasia**
  E25.9
  congenital E25.0
Masculinovoblastoma D27.- ☑
Masochism (sexual) F65.51
Mason's lung J62.8
Mass
  abdominal R19.00
    epigastric R19.06
    generalized R19.07
    left lower quadrant R19.04
    left upper quadrant R19.02
    periumbilic R19.05
    right lower quadrant R19.03
    right upper quadrant R19.01
    specified site NEC R19.09
  breast — *see also* Lump, breast N63.0
  chest R22.2
  cystic — *see* Cyst

Mass — *continued*
  ear H93.8- ☑
  head R22.0
  intra-abdominal (diffuse) (generalized) — *see* Mass,
    abdominal
  kidney N28.89
  liver R16.0
  localized (skin) R22.9
    chest R22.2
    head R22.0
    limb
      lower R22.4- ☑
      upper R22.3- ☑
    neck R22.1
    trunk R22.2
  lung R91.8
  malignant — *see* Neoplasm, malignant, by site
  neck R22.1
  pelvic (diffuse) (generalized) — *see* Mass, abdominal
  specified organ NEC — *see* Disease, by site
  splenic R16.1
  substernal thyroid — *see* Goiter
  superficial (localized) R22.9
  umbilical (diffuse) (generalized) R19.09
Massive — *see* condition
Mast cell
  disease, systemic tissue D47.02
  leukemia C94.3- ☑
  neoplasm
    malignant C96.20
      specified type NEC C96.29
    of uncertain behavior NEC D47.09
  sarcoma C96.22
  tumor D47.09
Mastalgia N64.4
Masters-Allen syndrome N83.8
Mastitis (acute) (diffuse) (nonpuerperal) (subacute) N61.0
  with abscess N61.1
  chronic (cystic) — *see* Mastopathy, cystic
  cystic (Schimmelbusch's type) — *see* Mastopathy, cystic
  fibrocystic — *see* Mastopathy, cystic
  granulomatous N61.2- ☑
  infective N61.0
    newborn P39.0
  interstitial, gestational or puerperal — *see* Mastitis,
    obstetric
  neonatal (noninfective) P83.4
    infective P39.0
  obstetric (interstitial) (nonpurulent)
    associated with
      lactation O91.23
      pregnancy O91.21- ☑
      puerperium O91.22
    purulent
      associated with
        lactation O91.13
        pregnancy O91.11- ☑
        puerperium O91.12
  periductal — *see* Ectasia, mammary duct
  phlegmonous — *see* Mastopathy, cystic
  plasma cell — *see* Ectasia, mammary duct
  without abscess N61.0
Mastocytoma (extracutaneous) D47.09
  malignant C96.29
  solitary D47.01
Mastocytosis D47.09
  aggressive systemic C96.21
  cutaneous (diffuse) (maculopapular) D47.01
    congenital Q82.2
    of neonatal onset Q82.2
    of newborn onset Q82.2
  indolent systemic D47.02
  isolated bone marrow D47.02
  malignant C96.29
  systemic (indolent) (smoldering)
    with an associated hematological non-mast cell
      lineage disease (SM-AHNMD) D47.02
Mastodynia N64.4
Mastoid — *see* condition
Mastoidalgia — *see* subcategory H92.0 ☑
Mastoiditis (coalescent) (hemorrhagic) (suppurative)
  H70.9- ☑
  acute, subacute H70.00- ☑
    complicated NEC H70.09- ☑
    subperiosteal H70.01- ☑
  chronic (necrotic) (recurrent) H70.1- ☑

Mastoiditis — *continued*
in (due to)
infectious disease NEC B99 ☑ *[H75.0-]* ☑
parasitic disease NEC B89 *[H75.0-]* ☑
tuberculosis A18.03
petrositis — *see* Petrositis
postauricular fistula — *see* Fistula, postauricular
specified NEC H70.89- ☑
tuberculous A18.03
Mastopathy, mastopathia N64.9
chronica cystica — *see* Mastopathy, cystic
cystic (chronic) (diffuse) N60.1- ☑
with epithelial proliferation N60.3- ☑
diffuse cystic — *see* Mastopathy, cystic
estrogenic, oestrogenica N64.89
ovarian origin N64.89
Mastoplasia, mastoplastia N62
Masturbation (excessive) F98.8
Maternal care (for) — *see* Pregnancy (complicated by) (management affected by)
Matheiu's disease (leptospiral jaundice) A27.0
Mauclaire's disease or osteochondrosis — *see* Osteochondrosis, juvenile, hand, metacarpal
Maxcy's disease A75.2
Maxilla, maxillary — *see* condition
May (-Hegglin) **anomaly or syndrome** D72.0
McArdle (-Schmid)(-Pearson) **disease** (glycogen storage) E74.04
McCune-Albright syndrome Q78.1
McQuarrie's syndrome (idiopathic familial hypoglycemia) E16.2
Meadow's syndrome Q86.1
Measles (black) (hemorrhagic) (suppressed) B05.9
with
complications NEC B05.89
encephalitis B05.0
intestinal complications B05.4
keratitis (keratoconjunctivitis) B05.81
meningitis B05.1
otitis media B05.3
pneumonia B05.2
French — *see* Rubella
German — *see* Rubella
Liberty — *see* Rubella
Meatitis, urethral — *see* Urethritis
Meatus, meatal — *see* condition
Meat-wrappers' asthma J68.9
ME/CFS (myalgic encephalomyelitis/chronic fatigue syndrome) G93.32
Meckel-Gruber syndrome Q61.9
Meckel's diverticulitis, diverticulum (displaced) (hypertrophic) Q43.0
malignant — *see* Table of Neoplasms, small intestine, malignant
Meconium
ileus, newborn P76.0
in cystic fibrosis E84.11
meaning meconium plug (without cystic fibrosis) P76.0
obstruction, newborn P76.0
due to fecaliths P76.0
in mucoviscidosis E84.11
peritonitis P78.0
plug syndrome (newborn) NEC P76.0
Median — *see also* condition
arcuate ligament syndrome I77.4
bar (prostate) (vesical orifice) — *see* Hyperplasia, prostate
rhomboid glossitis K14.2
Mediastinal shift R93.89
Mediastinitis (acute) (chronic) J98.51
syphilitic A52.73
tuberculous A15.8
Mediastinopericarditis — *see also* Pericarditis
acute I30.9
adhesive I31.0
chronic I31.8
rheumatic I09.2
Mediastinum, mediastinal — *see* condition
Medicine poisoning — *see* Table of Drugs and Chemicals, by drug, poisoning
Mediterranean
fever — *see* Brucellosis
familial M04.1
tick A77.1
kala-azar B55.0
leishmaniasis B55.0

Mediterranean — *continued*
tick fever A77.1
Medulla — *see* condition
Medullary cystic kidney Q61.5
Medullated fibers
optic (nerve) Q14.8
retina Q14.1
Medulloblastoma
desmoplastic C71.6
specified site — *see* Neoplasm, malignant, by site
unspecified site C71.6
Medulloepithelioma — *see also* Neoplasm, malignant, by site
teratoid — *see* Neoplasm, malignant, by site
Medullomyoblastoma
specified site — *see* Neoplasm, malignant, by site
unspecified site C71.6
Meekeren-Ehlers-Danlos syndrome — *see also* Syndrome, Ehlers-Danlos Q79.69
Megacolon (acquired) (functional) (not Hirschsprung's disease) (in) K59.39
Chagas' disease B57.32
congenital, congenitum (aganglionic) Q43.1
Hirschsprung's (disease) Q43.1
toxic NEC K59.31
due to Clostridium difficile
not specified as recurrent A04.72
recurrent A04.71
Megaesophagus (functional) K22.0
congenital Q39.5
in (due to) Chagas' disease B57.31
Megalencephaly Q04.5
Megalerythema (epidemic) B08.3
Megaloappendix Q43.8
Megalocephalus, megalocephaly NEC Q75.3
Megalocornea Q15.8
with glaucoma Q15.0
Megalocytic anemia D53.1
Megalodactylia (fingers) (thumbs) (congenital) Q74.0
toes Q74.2
Megaloduodenum Q43.8
Megaloesophagus (functional) K22.0
congenital Q39.5
Megalogastria (acquired) K31.89
congenital Q40.2
Megalophthalmos Q11.3
Megalopia H53.15
Megalopsia H53.15
Megalosplenia — *see* Splenomegaly
Megaloureter N28.82
congenital Q62.2
Megarectum K62.89
Megasigmoid K59.39
congenital Q43.2
Megaureter N28.82
congenital Q62.2
Megavitamin-B6 syndrome E67.2
Megrim — *see* Migraine
Meibomian
cyst, infected — *see* Hordeolum
gland — *see* condition
sty, stye — *see* Hordeolum
Meibomitis — *see* Hordeolum
Meige-Milroy disease (chronic hereditary edema) Q82.0
Meige's syndrome Q82.0
Melalgia, nutritional E53.8
Melancholia F32.A
climacteric (single episode) F32.89
recurrent episode F33.8
hypochondriac F45.29
intermittent (single episode) F32.89
recurrent episode F33.8
involutional (single episode) F32.89
recurrent episode F33.8
menopausal (single episode) F32.89
recurrent episode F33.8
puerperal F32.89
reactive (emotional stress or trauma) F32.3
recurrent F33.9
senile F03 ☑
stuporous (single episode) F32.89
recurrent episode F33.8
Melanemia R79.89
Melanoameloblastoma — *see* Neoplasm, bone, benign
Melanoblastoma — *see* Melanoma
Melanocarcinoma — *see* Melanoma
Melanocytoma, eyeball D31.9- ☑
Melanocytosis, neurocutaneous Q82.8

Melanoderma, melanodermia L81.4
Melanodontia, infantile K03.89
Melanodontoclasia K03.89
Melanoepithelioma — *see* Melanoma
Melanoma (malignant) C43.9
acral lentiginous, malignant — *see* Melanoma, skin, by site
amelanotic — *see* Melanoma, skin, by site
balloon cell — *see* Melanoma, skin, by site
benign — *see* Nevus
desmoplastic, malignant — *see* Melanoma, skin, by site
epithelioid cell — *see* Melanoma, skin, by site
with spindle cell, mixed — *see* Melanoma, skin, by site
in
giant pigmented nevus — *see* Melanoma, skin, by site
Hutchinson's melanotic freckle — *see* Melanoma, skin, by site
junctional nevus — *see* Melanoma, skin, by site
precancerous melanosis — *see* Melanoma, skin, by site
in situ D03.9
abdominal wall D03.59
ala nasi D03.39
ankle D03.7- ☑
anus, anal (margin) (skin) D03.51
arm D03.6- ☑
auditory canal D03.2- ☑
auricle (ear) D03.2- ☑
auricular canal (external) D03.2- ☑
axilla, axillary fold D03.59
back D03.59
breast D03.52
brow D03.39
buttock D03.59
canthus (eye) D03.1- ☑
cheek (external) D03.39
chest wall D03.59
chin D03.39
choroid D03.8
conjunctiva D03.8
ear (external) D03.2- ☑
external meatus (ear) D03.2- ☑
eye D03.8
eyebrow D03.39
eyelid (lower) (upper) D03.1- ☑
face D03.30
specified NEC D03.39
female genital organ (external) NEC D03.8
finger D03.6- ☑
flank D03.59
foot D03.7- ☑
forearm D03.6- ☑
forehead D03.39
foreskin D03.8
gluteal region D03.59
groin D03.59
hand D03.6- ☑
heel D03.7- ☑
helix D03.2- ☑
hip D03.7- ☑
interscapular region D03.59
iris D03.8
jaw D03.39
knee D03.7- ☑
labium (majus) (minus) D03.8
lacrimal gland D03.8
leg D03.7- ☑
lip (lower) (upper) D03.0
lower limb NEC D03.7- ☑
male genital organ (external) NEC D03.8
nail D03.9
finger D03.6- ☑
toe D03.7- ☑
neck D03.4
nose (external) D03.39
orbit D03.8
penis D03.8
perianal skin D03.51
perineum D03.51
pinna D03.2- ☑
popliteal fossa or space D03.7- ☑
prepuce D03.8
pudendum D03.8
retina D03.8

☑ **Additional Character Required — Refer to the Tabular List for Character Selection**

Melanoma — *continued*
  in situ — *continued*
    retrobulbar D03.8
    scalp D03.4
    scrotum D03.8
    shoulder D03.6- ☑
    specified site NEC D03.8
    submammary fold D03.52
    temple D03.39
    thigh D03.7- ☑
    toe D03.7- ☑
    trunk NEC D03.59
    umbilicus D03.59
    upper limb NEC D03.6- ☑
    vulva D03.8
  juvenile — *see* Nevus
  malignant, of soft parts except skin — *see* Neoplasm,
      connective tissue, malignant
  metastatic
    breast C79.81
    genital organ C79.82
    specified site NEC C79.89
  neurotropic, malignant — *see* Melanoma, skin, by site
  nodular — *see* Melanoma, skin, by site
  regressing, malignant — *see* Melanoma, skin, by site
  skin C43.9
    abdominal wall C43.59
    ala nasi C43.31
    ankle C43.7- ☑
    anus, anal (skin) C43.51
    arm C43.6- ☑
    auditory canal (external) C43.2- ☑
    auricle (ear) C43.2- ☑
    auricular canal (external) C43.2- ☑
    axilla, axillary fold C43.59
    back C43.59
    breast (female) (male) C43.52
    brow C43.39
    buttock C43.59
    canthus (eye) C43.1- ☑
    cheek (external) C43.39
    chest wall C43.59
    chin C43.39
    ear (external) C43.2- ☑
    elbow C43.6- ☑
    external meatus (ear) C43.2- ☑
    eyebrow C43.39
    eyelid (lower) (upper) C43.1- ☑
    face C43.30
      specified NEC C43.39
    female genital organ (external) NEC C51.9
    finger C43.6- ☑
    flank C43.59
    foot C43.7- ☑
    forearm C43.6- ☑
    forehead C43.39
    foreskin C60.0
    glabella C43.39
    gluteal region C43.59
    groin C43.59
    hand C43.6- ☑
    heel C43.7- ☑
    helix C43.2- ☑
    hip C43.7- ☑
    interscapular region C43.59
    jaw (external) C43.39
    knee C43.7- ☑
    labium C51.9
      majus C51.0
      minus C51.1
    leg C43.7- ☑
    lip (lower) (upper) C43.0
    lower limb NEC C43.7- ☑
    male genital organ (external) NEC C63.9
    nail
      finger C43.6- ☑
      toe C43.7- ☑
    nasolabial groove C43.39
    nates C43.59
    neck C43.4
    nose (external) C43.31
    overlapping site C43.8
    palpebra C43.1- ☑
    penis C60.9
    perianal skin C43.51
    perineum C43.51
    pinna C43.2- ☑

Melanoma — *continued*
  skin — *continued*
    popliteal fossa or space C43.7- ☑
    prepuce C51.9
    pudendum C51.9
    scalp C43.4
    scrotum C63.2
    shoulder C43.6- ☑
    skin NEC C43.9
    submammary fold C43.52
    temple C43.39
    thigh C43.7- ☑
    toe C43.7- ☑
    trunk NEC C43.59
    umbilicus C43.59
    upper limb NEC C43.6- ☑
    vulva C51.9
      overlapping sites C51.8
  spindle cell
    with epithelioid, mixed — *see* Melanoma, skin, by
        site
    type A C69.4- ☑
    type B C69.4- ☑
  superficial spreading — *see* Melanoma, skin, by site
Melanosarcoma — *see also* Melanoma
  epithelioid cell — *see* Melanoma
Melanosis L81.4
  addisonian E27.1
    tuberculous A18.7
  adrenal E27.1
  colon K63.89
  conjunctiva — *see* Pigmentation, conjunctiva
    congenital Q13.89
  cornea (presenile) (senile) — *see also* Pigmentation,
      cornea
    congenital Q13.4
  eye NEC H57.89
    congenital Q15.8
  lenticularis progressiva Q82.1
  liver K76.89
  precancerous — *see also* Melanoma, in situ
    malignant melanoma in — *see* Melanoma
  Riehl's L81.4
  sclera H15.89
    congenital Q13.89
  suprarenal E27.1
  tar L81.4
  toxic L81.4
Melanuria R82.998
MELAS syndrome E88.41
Melasma L81.1
  adrenal (gland) E27.1
  suprarenal (gland) E27.1
Melena K92.1
  with ulcer — *code by* site under Ulcer, with hemorrhage
      K27.4
  due to swallowed maternal blood P78.2
  newborn, neonatal P54.1
    due to swallowed maternal blood P78.2
Meleney's
  gangrene (cutaneous) — *see* Ulcer, skin
  ulcer (chronic undermining) — *see* Ulcer, skin
Melioidosis A24.9
  acute A24.1
  chronic A24.2
  fulminating A24.1
  pneumonia A24.1
  pulmonary (chronic) A24.2
    acute A24.1
    subacute A24.2
  sepsis A24.1
  specified NEC A24.3
  subacute A24.2
Melitensis, febris A23.0
Melkersson (-Rosenthal) **syndrome** G51.2
Mellitus, diabetes — *see* Diabetes
Melorheostosis (bone) — *see* Disorder, bone, density
      and structure, specified NEC
Meloschisis Q18.4
Melotia Q17.4
Membrana
  capsularis lentis posterior Q13.89
  epipapillaris Q14.2
Membranacea placenta O43.19- ☑
Membranaceous uterus N85.8
Membrane(s), membranous — *see also* condition
  cyclitic — *see* Membrane, pupillary

Membrane(s), membranous — *continued*
  folds, congenital — *see* Web
  Jackson's Q43.3
  over face of newborn P28.9
  premature rupture — *see* Rupture, membranes, prema-
      ture
  pupillary H21.4- ☑
    persistent Q13.89
  retained (with hemorrhage) (complicating delivery)
      O72.2
    without hemorrhage O73.1
  secondary cataract — *see* Cataract, secondary
  unruptured (causing asphyxia) — *see* Asphyxia, new-
      born
  vitreous — *see* Opacity, vitreous, membranes and
      strands
Membranitis — *see* Chorioamnionitis
Memory disturbance, lack or loss — *see also* Amnesia
  mild, following organic brain damage F06.8
Menadione deficiency E56.1
Menarche
  delayed E30.0
  precocious E30.1
Mendacity, pathologic F60.2
Mendelson's syndrome (due to anesthesia) J95.4
  in labor and delivery O74.0
  in pregnancy O29.01- ☑
  obstetric O74.0
  postpartum, puerperal O89.01
Ménétrier's disease or syndrome K29.60
  with bleeding K29.61
Ménière's disease, syndrome or vertigo H81.0- ☑
Meninges, meningeal — *see* condition
Meningioma — *see also* Neoplasm, meninges, benign
  angioblastic — *see* Neoplasm, meninges, benign
  angiomatous — *see* Neoplasm, meninges, benign
  atypical — *see* Neoplasm, meninges, uncertain behav-
      ior
  endotheliomatous — *see* Neoplasm, meninges, benign
  fibroblastic — *see* Neoplasm, meninges, benign
  fibrous — *see* Neoplasm, meninges, benign
  hemangioblastic — *see* Neoplasm, meninges, benign
  hemangiopericytic — *see* Neoplasm, meninges, benign
  malignant — *see* Neoplasm, meninges, malignant
  meningothelial — *see* Neoplasm, meninges, benign
  meningotheliomatous — *see* Neoplasm, meninges,
      benign
  mixed — *see* Neoplasm, meninges, benign
  multiple — *see* Neoplasm, meninges, uncertain behav-
      ior
  papillary — *see* Neoplasm, meninges, uncertain behav-
      ior
  psammomatous — *see* Neoplasm, meninges, benign
  syncytial — *see* Neoplasm, meninges, benign
  transitional — *see* Neoplasm, meninges, benign
Meningiomatosis (diffuse) — *see* Neoplasm, meninges,
      uncertain behavior
Meningism — *see* Meningismus
Meningismus (infectional) (pneumococcal) R29.1
  due to serum or vaccine R29.1
  influenzal — *see* Influenza, with, manifestations NEC
Meningitis (basal) (basic) (brain) (cerebral) (cervical)
      (congestive) (diffuse) (hemorrhagic) (infantile)
      (membranous) (metastatic) (nonspecific) (pontine)
      (progressive) (simple) (spinal) (subacute) (sympa-
      thetic) (toxic) G03.9
  abacterial G03.0
  actinomycotic A42.81
  adenoviral A87.1
  arbovirus A87.8
  aseptic (acute) G03.0
  bacterial G00.9
    Escherichia coli (E. coli) G00.8
    Friedländer (bacillus) G00.8
    gram-negative G00.9
    H. influenzae G00.0
    Klebsiella G00.8
    pneumococcal G00.1
    specified organism NEC G00.8
    staphylococcal G00.3
    streptococcal (acute) G00.2
  benign recurrent (Mollaret) G03.2
  candidal B37.5
  caseous (tuberculous) A17.0
  cerebrospinal A39.0
  chronic NEC G03.1
  clear cerebrospinal fluid NEC G03.0

Meningitis — *continued*
- coxsackievirus A87.0
- cryptococcal B45.1
- diplococcal (gram positive) A39.0
- echovirus A87.0
- enteroviral A87.0
- eosinophilic B83.2
- epidemic NEC A39.0
- Escherichia coli (E. coli) G00.8
- fibrinopurulent G00.9
  - specified organism NEC G00.8
- Friedländer (bacillus) G00.8
- gonococcal A54.81
- gram-negative cocci G00.9
- gram-positive cocci G00.9
- H. influenzae G00.0
- Haemophilus (influenzae) G00.0
- in (due to)
  - adenovirus A87.1
  - African trypanosomiasis B56.9 *[G02]*
  - anthrax A22.8
  - bacterial disease NEC A48.8 *[G01]*
  - Chagas' disease (chronic) B57.41
  - chickenpox B01.0
  - coccidioidomycosis B38.4
  - Diplococcus pneumoniae G00.1
  - enterovirus A87.0
  - herpes (simplex) virus B00.3
    - zoster B02.1
  - infectious mononucleosis B27.92
  - leptospirosis A27.81
  - Listeria monocytogenes A32.11
  - Lyme disease A69.21
  - measles B05.1
  - mumps (virus) B26.1
  - neurosyphilis (late) A52.13
  - parasitic disease NEC B89 *[G02]*
  - poliovirus A80.9 *[G02]*
  - preventive immunization, inoculation or vaccination G03.8
  - rubella B06.02
  - Salmonella infection A02.21
  - specified cause NEC G03.8
  - Streptococcal pneumoniae G00.1
  - typhoid fever A01.01
  - varicella B01.0
  - viral disease NEC A87.8
  - whooping cough A37.90
  - zoster B02.1
- infectious G00.9
- influenzal (H. influenzae) G00.0
- Klebsiella G00.8
- leptospiral (aseptic) A27.81
- lymphocytic (acute) (benign) (serous) A87.2
- meningococcal A39.0
- Mima polymorpha G00.8
- Mollaret (benign recurrent) G03.2
- monilial B37.5
- mycotic NEC B49 *[G02]*
- Neisseria A39.0
- nonbacterial G03.0
- nonpyogenic NEC G03.0
- ossificans G96.198
- pneumococcal streptococcus pneumoniae G00.1
- poliovirus A80.9 *[G02]*
- postmeasles B05.1
- purulent G00.9
  - specified organism NEC G00.8
- pyogenic G00.9
  - specified organism NEC G00.8
- Salmonella (arizonae) (Cholerae-Suis) (enteritidis) (typhimurium) A02.21
- septic G00.9
  - specified organism NEC G00.8
- serosa circumscripta NEC G03.0
- serous NEC G93.2
- specified organism NEC G00.8
- sporotrichosis B42.81
- staphylococcal G00.3
- sterile G03.0
- Streptococcal (acute) G00.2
  - pneumoniae G00.1
- suppurative G00.9
  - specified organism NEC G00.8
- syphilitic (late) (tertiary) A52.13
  - acute A51.41
  - congenital A50.41
  - secondary A51.41
- Torula histolytica (cryptococcal) B45.1

Meningitis — *continued*
- traumatic (complication of injury) T79.8 ☑
- tuberculous A17.0
- typhoid A01.01
- viral NEC A87.9
- Yersinia pestis A20.3

Meningocele (spinal) — *see also* Spina bifida
- with hydrocephalus — *see* Spina bifida, by site, with hydrocephalus
- acquired (traumatic) G96.198
- cerebral — *see* Encephalocele

Meningocerebritis — *see* Meningoencephalitis

Meningococcemia A39.4
- acute A39.2
- chronic A39.3

Meningococcus, meningococcal — *see also* condition A39.9
- adrenalitis, hemorrhagic A39.1
- carrier (suspected) of Z22.31
- meningitis (cerebrospinal) A39.0

Meningoencephalitis — *see also* Encephalitis G04.90
- acute NEC — *see also* Encephalitis, viral A86
- bacterial NEC G04.2
- California A83.5
- diphasic A84.1
- eosinophilic B83.2
- epidemic A39.81
- herpesviral, herpetic B00.4
  - due to herpesvirus 6 B10.01
  - due to herpesvirus 7 B10.09
  - specified NEC B10.09
- in (due to)
  - blastomycosis NEC B40.81
  - diseases classified elsewhere G05.3
  - free-living amebae B60.2
  - H. influenzae G00.0
  - Hemophilus influenzae (H .influenzae) G00.0
  - herpes B00.4
    - due to herpesvirus 6 B10.01
    - due to herpesvirus 7 B10.09
    - specified NEC B10.09
  - Lyme disease A69.22
  - mercury — *see* subcategory T56.1 ☑
  - mumps B26.2
  - Naegleria (amebae) (organisms) (fowleri) B60.2
  - Parastrongylus cantonensis B83.2
  - toxoplasmosis (acquired) B58.2
    - congenital P37.1
- infectious (acute) (viral) A86
- influenzal (H. influenzae) G00.0
- Listeria monocytogenes A32.12
- lymphocytic (serous) A87.2
- mumps B26.2
- parasitic NEC B89 *[G05.3]*
- pneumococcal G04.2
- primary amebic B60.2
- specific (syphilitic) A52.14
- specified organism NEC G04.81
- staphylococcal G04.2
- streptococcal G04.2
- syphilitic A52.14
- toxic NEC G92.8
  - due to mercury — *see* subcategory T56.1 ☑
- tuberculous A17.82
- virus NEC A86

Meningoencephalocele — *see also* Encephalocele
- syphilitic A52.19
  - congenital A50.49

Meningoencephalomyelitis — *see also* Meningoencephalitis
- acute NEC (viral) A86
  - disseminated G04.00
    - postimmunization or postvaccination G04.02
    - postinfectious G04.01
  - due to
    - actinomycosis A42.82
    - Torula B45.1
    - Toxoplasma or toxoplasmosis (acquired) B58.2
      - congenital P37.1
  - postimmunization or postvaccination G04.02

Meningoencephalomyelopathy G96.9

Meningoencephalopathy G96.9

Meningomyelitis — *see also* Meningoencephalitis
- bacterial NEC G04.2
- blastomycotic NEC B40.81
- cryptococcal B45.1
- in diseases classified elsewhere G05.4
- meningococcal A39.81

Meningomyelitis — *continued*
- syphilitic A52.14
- tuberculous A17.82

Meningomyelocele — *see also* Spina bifida
- syphilitic A52.19

Meningomyeloneuritis — *see* Meningoencephalitis

Meningoradiculitis — *see* Meningitis

Meningovascular — *see* condition

Menkes' disease or syndrome E83.09
- meaning maple-syrup-urine disease E71.0

Menometrorrhagia N92.1

Menopause, menopausal (asymptomatic) (state) Z78.0
- arthritis (any site) NEC — *see* Arthritis, specified form NEC
- bleeding N92.4
- depression (single episode) F32.89
  - agitated (single episode) F32.2
    - recurrent episode F33.9
  - psychotic (single episode) F32.89
    - recurrent episode F33.9
  - recurrent episode F33.8
- melancholia (single episode) F32.89
  - recurrent episode F33.8
- paranoid state F22
- postirradiation (postprocedural)
  - asymptomatic E89.40
  - symptomatic E89.41
- premature E28.319
  - asymptomatic E28.319
    - postirradiation E89.40
    - postsurgical E89.40
  - symptomatic E28.310
    - postirradiation E89.41
    - postsurgical E89.41
- psychosis NEC F28
- symptomatic N95.1
- toxic polyarthritis NEC — *see* Arthritis, specified form NEC

Menorrhagia (primary) N92.0
- climacteric N92.4
  - menopausal N92.4
- menopausal N92.4
- perimenopausal N92.4
- postclimacteric N95.0
- postmenopausal N95.0
- preclimacteric or premenopausal N92.4
- pubertal (menses retained) N92.2

Menostaxis N92.0

Menses, retention N94.89

Menstrual — *see* Menstruation

Menstruation
- absent — *see* Amenorrhea
- anovulatory N97.0
- cycle, irregular N92.6
- delayed N91.0
- disorder N93.9
  - psychogenic F45.8
- during pregnancy O20.8
- excessive (with regular cycle) N92.0
  - with irregular cycle N92.1
    - at puberty N92.2
- frequent N92.0
- infrequent — *see* Oligomenorrhea
- irregular N92.6
  - specified NEC N92.5
- latent N92.5
- membranous N92.5
- painful — *see also* Dysmenorrhea N94.6
  - primary N94.4
  - psychogenic F45.8
  - secondary N94.5
- passage of clots N92.0
- precocious E30.1
- protracted N92.5
- rare — *see* Oligomenorrhea
- retained N94.89
- retrograde N92.5
- scanty — *see* Oligomenorrhea
- suppression N94.89
- vicarious (nasal) N94.89

Mental — *see also* condition
- deficiency — *see* Disability, intellectual
- deterioration — *see* Psychosis
- disorder — *see* Disorder, mental
- exhaustion F48.8
- insufficiency (congenital) — *see* Disability, intellectual
- observation without need for further medical care Z03.89

Mental — *continued*
  retardation — *see* Disability, intellectual
  subnormality — *see* Disability, intellectuall
  upset — *see* Disorder, mental
Meralgia paresthetica G57.1- ☑
Mercurial — *see* condition
Mercurialism — *see* subcategory T56.1 ☑
Merkel cell tumor — *see* Carcinoma, Merkel cell
Merocele — *see* Hernia, femoral
Meromelia
  lower limb — *see* Defect, reduction, lower limb
    intercalary
      femur — *see* Defect, reduction, lower limb,
        specified type NEC
        tibiofibular (complete) (incomplete) — *see*
          Defect, reduction, lower limb
  upper limb — *see* Defect, reduction, upper limb
    intercalary, humeral, radioulnar — *see* Agenesis,
      arm, with hand present
MERRF syndrome (myoclonic epilepsy associated with
  ragged-red fiber) E88.42
Merzbacher-Pelizaeus disease E75.29
Mesaortitis — *see* Aortitis
Mesarteritis — *see* Arteritis
Mesencephalitis — *see* Encephalitis
Mesenchymoma — *see also* Neoplasm, connective tis-
  sue, uncertain behavior
  benign — *see* Neoplasm, connective tissue, benign
  malignant — *see* Neoplasm, connective tissue, malig-
    nant
Mesenteritis
  retractile K65.4
  sclerosing K65.4
Mesentery, mesenteric — *see* condition
Mesiodens, mesiodentes K00.1
Mesio-occlusion M26.213
Mesocolon — *see* condition
Mesonephroma (malignant) — *see* Neoplasm, malig-
  nant, by site
  benign — *see* Neoplasm, benign, by site
Mesophlebitis — *see* Phlebitis
Mesostromal dysgenesia Q13.89
Mesothelioma (malignant) C45.9
  benign
    mesentery D19.1
    mesocolon D19.1
    omentum D19.1
    peritoneum D19.1
    pleura D19.0
    specified site NEC D19.7
    unspecified site D19.9
  biphasic C45.9
    benign
      mesentery D19.1
      mesocolon D19.1
      omentum D19.1
      peritoneum D19.1
      pleura D19.0
      specified site NEC D19.7
      unspecified site D19.9
  cystic D48.4
  epithelioid C45.9
    benign
      mesentery D19.1
      mesocolon D19.1
      omentum D19.1
      peritoneum D19.1
      pleura D19.0
      specified site NEC D19.7
      unspecified site D19.9
  fibrous C45.9
    benign
      mesentery D19.1
      mesocolon D19.1
      omentum D19.1
      peritoneum D19.1
      pleura D19.0
      specified site NEC D19.7
      unspecified site D19.9
  site classification
    liver C45.7
    lung C45.7
    mediastinum C45.7
    mesentery C45.1
    mesocolon C45.1
    omentum C45.1
    pericardium C45.2
    peritoneum C45.1

Mesothelioma — *continued*
  site classification — *continued*
    pleura C45.0
      parietal C45.0
    retroperitoneum C45.7
    specified site NEC C45.7
    unspecified C45.9
Metabolic syndrome E88.81
Metagonimiasis B66.8
Metagonimus infestation (intestine) B66.8
Metal
  pigmentation L81.8
  polisher's disease J62.8
Metamorphopsia H53.15
Metaplasia
  apocrine (breast) — *see* Dysplasia, mammary, specified
    type NEC
  cervix (squamous) — *see* Dysplasia, cervix
  endometrium (squamous) (uterus) N85.8
  esophagus K22.7- ☑
  gastric intestinal K31.A0
    with dysplasia K31.A29
      high grade K31.A22
      low grade K31.A21
    indefinite for dysplasia K31.A0
    without dysplasia K31.A19
      involving
        antrum K31.A11
        body (corpus) K31.A12
        cardia K31.A14
        fundus K31.A13
        multiple sites K31.A15
  kidney (pelvis) (squamous) N28.89
  myelogenous D73.1
  myeloid (agnogenic) (megakaryocytic) D73.1
  spleen D73.1
  squamous cell, bladder N32.89
Metastasis, metastatic
  abscess — *see* Abscess
  calcification E83.59
  cancer
    from specified site — *see* Neoplasm, malignant, by
      site
    to specified site — *see* Neoplasm, secondary, by site
  deposits (in) — *see* Neoplasm, secondary, by site
  disease — *see also* Neoplasm, secondary, by site C79.9
  spread (to) — *see* Neoplasm, secondary, by site
Metastrongyliasis B83.8
Metatarsalgia M77.4- ☑
  anterior G57.6- ☑
  Morton's G57.6- ☑
Metatarsus, metatarsal — *see also* condition
  adductus, congenital Q66.22- ☑
  valgus (abductus), congenital Q66.6
  varus (congenital) Q66.22- ☑
  primus Q66.21- ☑
Methadone use — *see* Use, opioid
Methemoglobinemia D74.9
  acquired (with sulfhemoglobinemia) D74.8
  congenital D74.0
  enzymatic (congenital) D74.0
  Hb M disease D74.0
  hereditary D74.0
  toxic D74.8
Methemoglobinuria — *see* Hemoglobinuria
Methioninemia E72.19
Methylmalonic acidemia E71.120
Metritis (catarrhal) (hemorrhagic) (septic) (suppurative)
  — *see also* Endometritis
  cervical — *see* Cervicitis
Metropathia hemorrhagica N93.8
Metroperitonitis — *see* Peritonitis, pelvic, female
Metrorrhagia N92.1
  climacteric N92.4
  menopausal N92.4
  perimenopausal N92.4
  postpartum NEC (atonic) (following delivery of placen-
    ta) O72.1
    delayed or secondary O72.2
  preclimacteric or premenopausal N92.4
  psychogenic F45.8
Metrorrhexis — *see* Rupture, uterus
Metrosalpingitis N70.91
Metrostaxis N93.8
Metrovaginitis — *see* Endometritis
Meyer-Schwickerath and Weyers syndrome Q87.0
Meynert's amentia (nonalcoholic) F04

Meynert's amentia — *continued*
  alcoholic F10.96
    with dependence F10.26
Mibelli's disease (porokeratosis) Q82.8
Mice, joint — *see* Loose, body, joint
  knee M23.4- ☑
Micrencephalon, micrencephaly Q02
Microalbuminuria R80.9
Microaneurysm, retinal — *see also* Disorder, retina,
  microaneurysms
  diabetic — *see* E08-E13 with .31
Microangiopathy (peripheral) I73.9
  thrombotic M31.10
    hematopoietic stem cell transplantation-associated
      [HSCT-TMA] M31.10
Microcalcifications, breast R92.0
Microcephalus, microcephalic, microcephaly Q02
  due to toxoplasmosis (congenital) P37.1
Microcheilia Q18.7
Microcolon (congenital) Q43.8
Microcornea (congenital) Q13.4
Microcytic — *see* condition
Microdeletions NEC Q93.88
Microdontia K00.2
Microdrepanocytosis D57.40
  with
    acute chest syndrome D57.411
    cerebral vascular involvement D57.413
    crisis (painful) D57.419
      with specified complication NEC D57.418
    splenic sequestration D57.412
    vasoocclusive pain D57.419
Microembolism
  atherothrombotic — *see* Atheroembolism
  retinal — *see* Occlusion, artery, retina
Microencephalon Q02
Microfilaria streptocerca infestation — *see* Onchocer-
  ciasis
Microgastria (congenital) Q40.2
Microgenia M26.06
Microgenitalia, congenital
  female Q52.8
  male Q55.8
Microglioma — *see* Lymphoma, non-Hodgkin, specified
  NEC
Microglossia (congenital) Q38.3
Micrognathia, micrognathism (congenital) (mandibu-
  lar) (maxillary) M26.09
Microgyria (congenital) Q04.3
Microinfarct of heart — *see* Insufficiency, coronary
Microlentia (congenital) Q12.8
Microlithiasis, alveolar, pulmonary J84.02
Micromastia N64.82
Micromyelia (congenital) Q06.8
Micropenis Q55.62
Microphakia (congenital) Q12.8
Microphthalmos, microphthalmia (congenital) Q11.2
  due to toxoplasmosis P37.1
Micropsia H53.15
Microscopic polyangiitis (polyarteritis) M31.7
Microsporidiosis B60.8
  intestinal A07.8
Microsporon furfur infestation B36.0
Microsporosis — *see also* Dermatophytosis
  nigra B36.1
Microstomia (congenital) Q18.5
Microtia (congenital) (external ear) Q17.2
Microtropia H50.40
Microvillus inclusion disease (MVD) (MVID) Q43.8
Micturition
  disorder NEC — *see also* Difficulty, micturition R39.198
    psychogenic F45.8
  frequency R35.0
    psychogenic F45.8
  hesitancy R39.11
  incomplete emptying R39.14
  nocturnal R35.1
  painful R30.9
    dysuria R30.0
    psychogenic F45.8
    tenesmus R30.1
  poor stream R39.12
  position dependent R39.192
  split stream R39.13
  straining R39.16
  urgency R39.15
Mid plane — *see* condition

Middle
  ear — *see* condition
  lobe (right) syndrome J98.19
Miescher's elastoma L87.2
Mietens' syndrome Q87.2
Migraine (idiopathic) G43.909
  with refractory migraine G43.919
    with status migrainosus G43.911
    without status migrainosus G43.919
  with aura (acute-onset) (prolonged) (typical) (without
      headache) G43.109
    with refractory migraine G43.119
      with status migrainosus G43.111
      without status migrainosus G43.119
    intractable G43.119
      with status migrainosus G43.111
      without status migrainosus G43.119
    not intractable G43.109
      with status migrainosus G43.101
      without status migrainosus G43.109
    persistent G43.509
      with cerebral infarction G43.609
        with refractory migraine G43.619
          with status migrainosus G43.611
          without status migrainosus G43.619
        intractable G43.619
          with status migrainosus G43.611
          without status migrainosus G43.619
        not intractable G43.609
          with status migrainosus G43.601
          without status migrainosus G43.609
        without refractory migraine G43.609
          with status migrainosus G43.601
          without status migrainosus G43.609
      without cerebral infarction G43.509
        with refractory migraine G43.519
          with status migrainosus G43.511
          without status migrainosus G43.519
        intractable G43.519
          with status migrainosus G43.511
          without status migrainosus G43.519
        not intractable G43.509
          with status migrainosus G43.501
          without status migrainosus G43.509
        without refractory migraine G43.509
          with status migrainosus G43.501
          without status migrainosus G43.509
    without mention of refractory migraine G43.109
      with status migrainosus G43.101
      without status migrainosus G43.109
  abdominal G43.D0 (*following* G43.7)
    with refractory migraine G43.D1 (*following* G43.7)
    intractable G43.D1 (*following* G43.7)
    not intractable G43.D0 (*following* G43.7)
    without refractory migraine G43.D0 (*following* G43.7)
  basilar — *see* Migraine, with aura
  classical — *see* Migraine, with aura
  common — *see* Migraine, without aura
  complicated G43.109
  equivalents — *see* Migraine, with aura
  familiar — *see* Migraine, hemiplegic
  hemiplegic G43.409
    with refractory migraine G43.419
      with status migrainosus G43.411
      without status migrainosus G43.419
    intractable G43.419
      with status migrainosus G43.411
      without status migrainosus G43.419
    not intractable G43.409
      with status migrainosus G43.401
      without status migrainosus G43.409
    without refractory migraine G43.409
      with status migrainosus G43.401
      without status migrainosus G43.409
  intractable G43.919
    with status migrainosus G43.911
    without status migrainosus G43.919
  menstrual G43.829
    with refractory migraine G43.839
      with status migrainosus G43.831
      without status migrainosus G43.839
    intractable G43.839
      with status migrainosus G43.831
      without status migrainosus G43.839
    not intractable G43.829
      with status migrainosus G43.821
      without status migrainosus G43.829
    without refractory migraine G43.829

Migraine — *continued*
  menstrual — *continued*
    without refractory migraine — *continued*
      with status migrainosus G43.821
      without status migrainosus G43.829
  menstrually related — *see* Migraine, menstrual
  not intractable G43.909
    with status migrainosus G43.901
    without status migrainosus G43.919
  ophthalmoplegic G43.B0 (*following* G43.7)
    with refractory migraine G43.B1 (*following* G43.7)
    intractable G43.B1 (*following* G43.7)
    not intractable G43.B0 (*following* G43.7)
    without refractory migraine G43.B0 (*following* G43.7)
  persistent aura (with, without) cerebral infarction —
      see Migraine, with aura, persistent
  preceded or accompanied by transient focal neurolog-
      ical phenomena — *see* Migraine, with aura
  pre-menstrual — *see* Migraine, menstrual
  pure menstrual — *see* Migraine, menstrual
  retinal — *see* Migraine, with aura
  specified NEC G43.809
    intractable G43.819
      with status migrainosus G43.811
      without status migrainosus G43.819
    not intractable G43.809
      with status migrainosus G43.801
      without status migrainosus G43.809
  sporadic — *see* Migraine, hemiplegic
  transformed — *see* Migraine, without aura, chronic
  triggered seizures — *see* Migraine, with aura
  without aura G43.009
    with refractory migraine G43.019
      with status migrainosus G43.011
      without status migrainosus G43.019
    chronic G43.709
      with refractory migraine G43.719
        with status migrainosus G43.711
        without status migrainosus G43.719
      intractable
        with status migrainosus G43.711
        without status migrainosus G43.719
      not intractable
        with status migrainosus G43.701
        without status migrainosus G43.709
      without refractory migraine G43.709
        with status migrainosus G43.701
        without status migrainosus G43.709
    intractable
      with status migrainosus G43.011
      without status migrainosus G43.019
    not intractable
      with status migrainosus G43.001
      without status migrainosus G43.009
    without mention of refractory migraine G43.009
      with status migrainosus G43.001
      without status migrainosus G43.009
  without refractory migraine G43.909
    with status migrainosus G43.901
    without status migrainosus G43.909
Migrant, social Z59.00
Migration, anxiety concerning Z60.3
Migratory, migrating — *see also* condition
  person Z59.00
  testis Q55.29
Mikity-Wilson disease or syndrome P27.0
Mikulicz' disease or syndrome K11.8
Miliaria L74.3
  alba L74.1
  apocrine L75.2
  crystallina L74.1
  profunda L74.2
  rubra L74.0
  tropicalis L74.2
Miliary — *see* condition
Milium L72.0
  colloid L57.8
Milk
  crust L21.0
  excessive secretion O92.6
  poisoning — *see* Poisoning, food, noxious
  retention O92.79
  sickness — *see* Poisoning, food, noxious
  spots I31.0
Milk-alkali disease or syndrome E83.52
Milk-leg (deep vessels) (nonpuerperal) — *see* Embolism,
    vein, lower extremity
  complicating pregnancy O22.3- ☑

Milk-leg — *continued*
  puerperal, postpartum, childbirth O87.1
Milkman's disease or syndrome M83.8
Milky urine — *see* Chyluria
Millard-Gubler (-Foville) **paralysis or syndrome** G46.3
Millar's asthma J38.5
Miller Fisher syndrome G61.0
Mills' disease — *see* Hemiplegia
Millstone maker's pneumoconiosis J62.8
Milroy's disease (chronic hereditary edema) Q82.0
Minamata disease T56.1 ☑
Miners' asthma or lung J60
Minkowski-Chauffard syndrome — *see* Spherocytosis
Minor — *see* condition
Minor's disease (hematomyelia) G95.19
Minot's disease (hemorrhagic disease), newborn P53
Minot-von Willebrand-Jurgens disease or syndrome
    (angiohemophilia) — *see* Disease, von Willebrand
Minus (and plus) **hand** (intrinsic) — *see* Deformity, limb,
    specified type NEC, forearm
Miosis (pupil) H57.03
Mirizzi's syndrome (hepatic duct stenosis) K83.1
Mirror writing F81.0
MIS-A M35.81
Misadventure (of) (prophylactic) (therapeutic) — *see
    also* Complications T88.9 ☑
  administration of insulin (by accident) — *see* subcate-
      gory T38.3 ☑
  infusion — *see* Complications, infusion
  local applications (of fomentations, plasters, etc.)
      T88.9 ☑
    burn or scald — *see* Burn
    specified NEC T88.8 ☑
  medical care (early) (late) T88.9 ☑
    adverse effect of drugs or chemicals — *see* Table of
        Drugs and Chemicals
    burn or scald — *see* Burn
    specified NEC T88.8 ☑
  specified NEC T88.8 ☑
  surgical procedure (early) (late) — *see* Complications,
      surgical procedure
  transfusion — *see* Complications, transfusion
  vaccination or other immunological procedure — *see*
      Complications, vaccination
MIS-C M35.81
Miscarriage O03.9
Misdirection, aqueous H40.83- ☑
Misperception, sleep state F51.02
Misplaced, misplacement
  ear Q17.4
  kidney (acquired) N28.89
    congenital Q63.2
  organ or site, congenital NEC — *see* Malposition, con-
      genital
Missed
  abortion O02.1
  delivery O36.4 ☑
Missing — *see also* Absence
  string of intrauterine contraceptive device T83.32- ☑
Misuse of drugs F19.99
Mitchell's disease (erythromelalgia) I73.81
Mite(s) (infestation) B88.9
  diarrhea B88.0
  grain (itch) B88.0
  hair follicle (itch) B88.0
  in sputum B88.0
Mitral — *see* condition
Mittelschmerz N94.0
Mixed — *see* condition
MMN (multifocal motor neuropathy) G61.82
MNGIE (Mitochondrial Neurogastrointestinal Encephalopa-
    thy) **syndrome** E88.49
Mobile, mobility
  cecum Q43.3
  excessive — *see* Hypermobility
  gallbladder, congenital Q44.1
  kidney N28.89
  organ or site, congenital NEC — *see* Malposition, con-
      genital
Mobitz heart block (atrioventricular) I44.1
Moebius, Möbius
  disease (ophthalmoplegic migraine) — *see* Migraine,
      ophthalmoplegic
  syndrome Q87.0
    congenital oculofacial paralysis (with other anoma-
        lies) Q87.0

☑ Additional Character Required — Refer to the Tabular List for Character Selection

Moebius, Möbius — *continued*
  syndrome — *continued*
    ophthalmoplegic migraine — *see* Migraine, ophthal-
      moplegic
Moeller's glossitis K14.0
Mohr's syndrome (Types I and II) Q87.0
Mola destruens D39.2
Molar pregnancy O02.0
Molarization of premolars K00.2
Molding, head (during birth) — *omit code*
Mole (pigmented) — *see also* Nevus
  blood O02.0
  Breus' O02.0
  cancerous — *see* Melanoma
  carneous O02.0
  destructive D39.2
  fleshy O02.0
  hydatid, hydatidiform (benign) (complicating pregnan-
    cy) (delivered) (undelivered) O01.9
    classical O01.0
    complete O01.0
    incomplete O01.1
    invasive D39.2
    malignant D39.2
    partial O01.1
  intrauterine O02.0
  invasive (hydatidiform) D39.2
  malignant
    meaning
      malignant hydatidiform mole D39.2
      melanoma — *see* Melanoma
  nonhydatidiform O02.0
  nonpigmented — *see* Nevus
  pregnancy NEC O02.0
  skin — *see* Nevus
  tubal O00.10- ☑
    with intrauterine pregnancy O00.11- ☑
  vesicular — *see* Mole, hydatidiform
Molimen, molimina (menstrual) N94.3
Molluscum contagiosum (epitheliale) B08.1
Mönckeberg's arteriosclerosis, disease, or sclerosis
    — *see* Arteriosclerosis, extremities
Mondini's malformation (cochlea) Q16.5
Mondor's disease I80.8
Monge's disease T70.29 ☑
Monilethrix (congenital) Q84.1
Moniliasis — *see also* Candidiasis B37.9
  neonatal P37.5
Monitoring (encounter for)
  therapeutic drug level Z51.81
Monkey malaria B53.1
Monkeypox B04
Monoarthritis M13.10
  ankle M13.17- ☑
  elbow M13.12- ☑
  foot joint M13.17- ☑
  hand joint M13.14- ☑
  hip M13.15- ☑
  knee M13.16- ☑
  shoulder M13.11- ☑
  wrist M13.13- ☑
Monoblastic — *see* condition
Monochromat (ism), monochromatopsia (acquired)
  (congenital) H53.51
Monocytic — *see* condition
Monocytopenia D72.818
Monocytosis (symptomatic) D72.821
Monomania — *see* Psychosis
Mononeuritis G58.9
  cranial nerve — *see* Disorder, nerve, cranial
  femoral nerve G57.2- ☑
  lateral
    cutaneous nerve of thigh G57.1- ☑
    popliteal nerve G57.3- ☑
  lower limb G57.9- ☑
    specified nerve NEC G57.8- ☑
  medial popliteal nerve G57.4- ☑
  median nerve G56.1- ☑
  multiplex G58.7
  plantar nerve G57.6- ☑
  posterior tibial nerve G57.5- ☑
  radial nerve G56.3- ☑
  sciatic nerve G57.0- ☑
  specified NEC G58.8
  tibial nerve G57.4- ☑
  ulnar nerve G56.2- ☑
  upper limb G56.9- ☑

Mononeuritis — *continued*
  upper limb — *continued*
    specified nerve NEC G56.8- ☑
  vestibular — *see* subcategory H93.3 ☑
Mononeuropathy G58.9
  carpal tunnel syndrome — *see* Syndrome, carpal tunnel
  diabetic NEC — *see* E08-E13 with .41
  femoral nerve — *see* Lesion, nerve, femoral
  ilioinguinal nerve G57.8- ☑
  in diseases classified elsewhere — *see* category G59
  intercostal G58.0
  lower limb G57.9-
    causalgia — *see* Causalgia, lower limb
    femoral nerve — *see* Lesion, nerve, femoral
    meralgia paresthetica G57.1- ☑
    plantar nerve — *see* Lesion, nerve, plantar
    popliteal nerve — *see* Lesion, nerve, popliteal
    sciatic nerve — *see* Lesion, nerve, sciatic
    specified NEC G57.8- ☑
    tarsal tunnel syndrome — *see* Syndrome, tarsal
      tunnel
  median nerve — *see* Lesion, nerve, median
  multiplex G58.7
  obturator nerve G57.8- ☑
  popliteal nerve — *see* Lesion, nerve, popliteal
  radial nerve — *see* Lesion, nerve, radial
  saphenous nerve G57.8- ☑
  specified NEC G58.8
  tarsal tunnel syndrome — *see* Syndrome, tarsal tunnel
  tuberculous A17.83
  ulnar nerve — *see* Lesion, nerve, ulnar
  upper limb G56.9- ☑
    carpal tunnel syndrome — *see* Syndrome, carpal
      tunnel
    causalgia — *see* Causalgia
    median nerve — *see* Lesion, nerve, median
    radial nerve — *see* Lesion, nerve, radial
    specified site NEC G56.8- ☑
    ulnar nerve — *see* Lesion, nerve, ulnar
Mononucleosis, infectious B27.90
  with
    complication NEC B27.99
    meningitis B27.92
    polyneuropathy B27.91
  cytomegaloviral B27.10
    with
      complication NEC B27.19
      meningitis B27.12
      polyneuropathy B27.11
  Epstein-Barr (virus) B27.00
    with
      complication NEC B27.09
      meningitis B27.02
      polyneuropathy B27.01
  gammaherpesviral B27.00
    with
      complication NEC B27.09
      meningitis B27.02
      polyneuropathy B27.01
  specified NEC B27.80
    with
      complication NEC B27.89
      meningitis B27.82
      polyneuropathy B27.81
Monoplegia G83.3- ☑
  congenital (cerebral) G80.8
    spastic G80.1
  embolic (current episode) I63.4- ☑
  following
    cerebrovascular disease
      cerebral infarction
        lower limb I69.34- ☑
        upper limb I69.33- ☑
      intracerebral hemorrhage
        lower limb I69.14- ☑
        upper limb I69.13- ☑
      lower limb I69.94- ☑
      nontraumatic intracranial hemorrhage NEC
        lower limb I69.24- ☑
        upper limb I69.23- ☑
      specified disease NEC
        lower limb I69.84- ☑
        upper limb I69.83- ☑
      stroke NOS
        lower limb I69.34- ☑
        upper limb I69.33- ☑

Monoplegia — *continued*
  following — *continued*
    cerebrovascular disease — *continued*
      subarachnoid hemorrhage
        lower limb I69.04- ☑
        upper limb I69.03- ☑
      upper limb I69.93- ☑
  hysterical (transient) F44.4
  lower limb G83.1- ☑
  psychogenic (conversion reaction) F44.4
  thrombotic (current episode) I63.3- ☑
  transient R29.818
  upper limb G83.2- ☑
Monorchism, monorchidism Q55.0
Monosomy — *see also* Deletion, chromosome Q93.9
  specified NEC Q93.89
  whole chromosome
    meiotic nondisjunction Q93.0
    mitotic nondisjunction Q93.1
    mosaicism Q93.1
  X Q96.9
Monster, monstrosity (single) Q89.7
  acephalic Q00.0
  twin Q89.4
Monteggia's fracture (-dislocation) S52.27- ☑
Mooren's ulcer (cornea) — *see* Ulcer, cornea, Mooren's
Moore's syndrome — *see* Epilepsy, specified NEC
Mooser-Neill reaction A75.2
Mooser's bodies A75.2
Morbidity not stated or unknown R69
Morbilli — *see* Measles
Morbus — *see also* Disease
  angelicus, anglorum E55.0
  Beigel B36.2
  caducus — *see* Epilepsy
  celiacus K90.0
  comitialis — *see* Epilepsy
  cordis — *see also* Disease, heart I51.9
    valvulorum — *see* Endocarditis
  coxae senilis M16.9
    tuberculous A18.02
  hemorrhagicus neonatorum P53
  maculosus neonatorum P54.5
Morel (-Stewart)(-Morgagni) **syndrome** M85.2
Morel-Kraepelin disease — *see* Schizophrenia
Morel-Moore syndrome M85.2
Morgagni's
  cyst, organ, hydatid, or appendage
    female Q50.5
    male (epididymal) Q55.4
      testicular Q55.29
  syndrome M85.2
Morgagni-Stewart-Morel syndrome M85.2
Morgagni-Stokes-Adams syndrome I45.9
Morgagni-Turner (-Albright) **syndrome** Q96.9
Moria F07.0
Moron (I.Q. 50-69) F70
Morphea L94.0
Morphinism (without remission) F11.20
  with remission F11.21
Morphinomania (without remission) F11.20
  with remission F11.21
Morquio (-Ullrich)(-Brailsford) **disease or syndrome** —
    see Mucopolysaccharidosis
Mortification (dry) (moist) — *see* Gangrene
Morton's metatarsalgia (neuralgia) (neuroma) (syn-
  drome) G57.6- ☑
Morvan's disease or syndrome G60.8
Mosaicism, mosaic (autosomal) (chromosomal)
  45,X/46,XX Q96.3
  45,X/other cell lines NEC with abnormal sex chromo-
    some Q96.4
  sex chromosome
    female Q97.8
    lines with various numbers of X chromosomes Q97.2
    male Q98.7
  XY Q96.3
Moschowitz' disease M31.19
Mother yaw A66.0
Motion sickness (from travel, any vehicle) (from round-
  abouts or swings) T75.3 ☑
Mottled, mottling, teeth (enamel) (endemic) (nonen-
  demic) K00.3
Mounier-Kuhn syndrome Q32.4
  with bronchiectasis J47.9
    exacerbation (acute) J47.1
    lower respiratory infection J47.0

Mounier-Kuhn syndrome — *continued*
  acquired J98.09
    with bronchiectasis J47.9
      with
        exacerbation (acute) J47.1
        lower respiratory infection J47.0
Mountain
  sickness T70.29 ☑
    with polycythemia , acquired (acute) D75.1
  tick fever A93.2
Mouse, joint — *see* Loose, body, joint
  knee M23.4- ☑
Mouth — *see* condition
Movable
  coccyx — *see* subcategory M53.2 ☑
  kidney N28.89
    congenital Q63.8
  spleen D73.89
Movements, dystonic R25.8
Moyamoya disease I67.5
MRSA (Methicillin resistant Staphylococcus aureus)
  infection A49.02
    as the cause of diseases classified elsewhere B95.62
  sepsis A41.02
MSD (multiple sulfatase deficiency) E75.26
MSSA (Methicillin susceptible Staphylococcus aureus)
  infection A49.01
    as the cause of diseases classified elsewhere B95.61
  sepsis A41.01
Mucha-Habermann disease L41.0
Mucinosis (cutaneous) (focal) (papular) (skin) L98.5
  oral K13.79
Mucocele
  appendix K38.8
  buccal cavity K13.79
  gallbladder K82.1
  lacrimal sac, chronic H04.43- ☑
  nasal sinus J34.1
  nose J34.1
  salivary gland (any) K11.6
  sinus (accessory) (nasal) J34.1
  turbinate (bone) (middle) (nasal) J34.1
  uterus N85.8
Mucolipidosis
  I E77.1
  II, III E77.0
  IV E75.11
Mucopolysaccharidosis E76.3
  beta-gluduronidase deficiency E76.29
  cardiopathy E76.3 *[I52]*
  Hunter's syndrome E76.1
  Hurler's syndrome E76.01
  Hurler-Scheie syndrome E76.02
  Maroteaux-Lamy syndrome E76.29
  Morquio syndrome E76.219
    A E76.210
    B E76.211
    classic E76.210
  Sanfilippo syndrome E76.22
  Scheie's syndrome E76.03
  specified NEC E76.29
  type
    I
        Hurler's syndrome E76.01
        Hurler-Scheie syndrome E76.02
        Scheie's syndrome E76.03
    II E76.1
    III E76.22
    IV E76.219
    IVA E76.210
    IVB E76.211
    VI E76.29
    VII E76.29
Mucormycosis B46.5
  cutaneous B46.3
  disseminated B46.4
  gastrointestinal B46.2
  generalized B46.4
  pulmonary B46.0
  rhinocerebral B46.1
  skin B46.3
  subcutaneous B46.3
Mucositis (ulcerative) K12.30
  due to drugs NEC K12.32
  gastrointestinal K92.81
  mouth (oral) (oropharyngeal) K12.30
    due to antineoplastic therapy K12.31
    due to drugs NEC K12.32

Mucositis — *continued*
  mouth — *continued*
    due to radiation K12.33
    specified NEC K12.39
    viral K12.39
  nasal J34.81
  oral cavity — *see* Mucositis, mouth
  oral soft tissues — *see* Mucositis, mouth
  vagina and vulva N76.81
Mucositis necroticans agranulocytica — *see* Agranulocytosis
Mucous — *see also* condition
  patches (syphilitic) A51.39
    congenital A50.07
Mucoviscidosis E84.9
  with meconium obstruction E84.11
Mucus
  asphyxia or suffocation — *see* Asphyxia, mucus
  in stool R19.5
  plug — *see* Asphyxia, mucus
Muguet B37.0
Mulberry molars (congenital syphilis) A50.52
Müllerian mixed tumor
  specified site — *see* Neoplasm, malignant, by site
  unspecified site C54.9
Multicystic kidney (development) Q61.4
Multiparity (grand) Z64.1
  affecting management of pregnancy, labor and delivery (supervision only) O09.4- ☑
  requiring contraceptive management — *see* Contraception
Multipartita placenta O43.19- ☑
Multiple, multiplex — *see also* condition
  digits (congenital) Q69.9
  endocrine neoplasia — *see* Neoplasia, endocrine, multiple (MEN)
  personality F44.81
Multisystem inflammatory syndrome (in adult) (in children) M35.81
Mumps B26.9
  arthritis B26.85
  complication NEC B26.89
  encephalitis B26.2
  hepatitis B26.81
  meningitis (aseptic) B26.1
  meningoencephalitis B26.2
  myocarditis B26.82
  oophoritis B26.89
  orchitis B26.0
  pancreatitis B26.3
  polyneuropathy B26.84
Mumu — *see also* Infestation, filarial B74.9 *[N51]*
Münchhausen's syndrome — *see* Disorder, factitious
Münchmeyer's syndrome — *see* Myositis, ossificans, progressiva
Mural — *see* condition
Murmur (cardiac) (heart) (organic) R01.1
  abdominal R19.15
  aortic (valve) — *see* Endocarditis, aortic
  benign R01.0
  diastolic — *see* Endocarditis
  Flint I35.1
  functional R01.0
  Graham Steell I37.1
  innocent R01.0
  mitral (valve) — *see* Insufficiency, mitral
  nonorganic R01.0
  presystolic, mitral — *see* Insufficiency, mitral
  pulmonic (valve) I37.8
  systolic R01.1
  tricuspid (valve) I07.9
  valvular — *see* Endocarditis
Murri's disease (intermittent hemoglobinuria) D59.6
Muscle, muscular — *see also* condition
  carnitine (palmityltransferase) deficiency E71.314
Musculoneuralgia — *see* Neuralgia
Mushrooming hip — *see* Derangement, joint, specified NEC, hip
Mushroom-workers' (pickers') **disease or lung** J67.5
Mutation(s)
  factor V Leiden D68.51
  prothrombin gene D68.52
  surfactant, of lung J84.83
Mutism — *see also* Aphasia
  deaf (acquired) (congenital) NEC H91.3
  elective (adjustment reaction) (childhood) F94.0
  hysterical F44.4

Mutism — *continued*
  selective (childhood) F94.0
MVD (microvillus inclusion disease) Q43.8
MVID (microvillus inclusion disease) Q43.8
Myalgia M79.10
  auxiliary muscles, head and neck M79.12
  epidemic (cervical) B33.0
  mastication muscle M79.11
  site specified NEC M79.18
  traumatic NEC T14.8 ☑
Myasthenia G70.9
  congenital G70.2
  cordis — *see* Failure, heart
  developmental G70.2
  gravis G70.00
    with exacerbation (acute) G70.01
    in crisis G70.01
    neonatal, transient P94.0
    pseudoparalytica G70.00
      with exacerbation (acute) G70.01
      in crisis G70.01
  stomach, psychogenic F45.8
  syndrome
    in
        diabetes mellitus — *see* E08-E13 with .44
        neoplastic disease — *see also* Neoplasm D49.9 *[G73.3]*
        pernicious anemia D51.0 *[G73.3]*
        thyrotoxicosis E05.90 *[G73.3]*
          with thyroid storm E05.91 *[G73.3]*
Myasthenic M62.81
Mycelium infection B49
Mycetismus — *see* Poisoning, food, noxious, mushroom
Mycetoma B47.9
  actinomycotic B47.1
  bone (mycotic) B47.9 *[M90.80]*
  eumycotic B47.0
  foot B47.9
    actinomycotic B47.1
    mycotic B47.0
  madurae NEC B47.9
    mycotic B47.0
  maduromycotic B47.0
  mycotic B47.0
  nocardial B47.1
Mycobacteriosis — *see* Mycobacterium
Mycobacterium, mycobacterial (infection) A31.9
  anonymous A31.9
  atypical A31.9
    cutaneous A31.1
    pulmonary A31.0
      tuberculous — *see* Tuberculosis, pulmonary
    specified site NEC A31.8
  avium (intracellulare complex) A31.0
  balnei A31.1
  Battey A31.0
  chelonei A31.8
  cutaneous A31.1
  extrapulmonary systemic A31.8
  fortuitum A31.8
  intracellulare (Battey bacillus) A31.0
  kakaferifu A31.8
  kansasii (yellow bacillus) A31.0
  kasongo A31.8
  leprae — *see also* Leprosy A30.9
  luciflavum A31.1
  marinum (M. balnei) A31.1
  nonspecific — *see* Mycobacterium, atypical
  pulmonary (atypical) A31.0
    tuberculous — *see* Tuberculosis, pulmonary
  scrofulaceum A31.8
  simiae A31.8
  systemic, extrapulmonary A31.8
  szulgai A31.8
  terrae A31.8
  triviale A31.8
  tuberculosis (human, bovine) — *see* Tuberculosis
  ulcerans A31.1
  xenopi A31.8
Mycoplasma (M.) **pneumoniae, as cause of disease classified elsewhere** B96.0
Mycosis, mycotic B49
  cutaneous NEC B36.9
  ear B36.9
    in
        aspergillosis B44.89
        candidiasis B37.84
        moniliasis B37.84

☑ **Additional Character Required — Refer to the Tabular List for Character Selection**

Mycosis, mycotic — *continued*
  fungoides (extranodal) (solid organ) C84.0- ☑
  mouth B37.0
  nails B35.1
  opportunistic B48.8
  skin NEC B36.9
  specified NEC B48.8
  stomatitis B37.0
  vagina, vaginitis (candidal) (acute) B37.31
    chronic (recurrent) B37.32
Mydriasis (pupil) H57.04
Myelatelia Q06.1
Myelinolysis, pontine, central G37.2
Myelitis (acute) (ascending) (childhood) (chronic) (descending) (diffuse) (disseminated) (idiopathic) (pressure) (progressive) (spinal cord) (subacute) — *see also* Encephalitis G04.91
  flaccid G04.82
  herpes simplex B00.82
  herpes zoster B02.24
  in diseases classified elsewhere G05.4
  necrotizing, subacute G37.4
  optic neuritis in G36.0
  postchickenpox B01.12
  postherpetic B02.24
  postimmunization G04.02
  postinfectious NEC G04.89
  postvaccinal G04.02
  specified NEC G04.89
  syphilitic (transverse) A52.14
  toxic G92.9
  transverse (in demyelinating diseases of central nervous system) G37.3
  tuberculous A17.82
  varicella B01.12
Myeloblastic — *see* condition
Myeloblastoma
  granular cell — *see also* Neoplasm, connective tissue
    malignant — *see* Neoplasm, connective tissue, malignant
    tongue D10.1
Myelocele — *see* Spina bifida
Myelocystocele — *see* Spina bifida
Myelocytic — *see* condition
Myelodysplasia D46.9
  specified NEC D46.Z (*following* D46.4)
  spinal cord (congenital) Q06.1
Myelodysplastic syndrome — *see also* Syndrome, myelodysplastic D46.9
  with
    5q deletion D46.C (*following* D46.2)
    isolated del (5q) chromosomal abnormality D46.C (*following* D46.2)
  specified NEC D46.Z (*following* D46.4)
Myeloencephalitis — *see* Encephalitis
Myelofibrosis D75.81
  with myeloid metaplasia D47.4
  acute C94.4- ☑
  idiopathic (chronic) D47.4
  primary D47.1
  secondary D75.81
    in myeloproliferative disease D47.4
Myelogenous — *see* condition
Myeloid — *see* condition
Myelokathexis D70.9
Myeloleukodystrophy E75.29
Myelolipoma — *see* Lipoma
Myeloma (multiple) C90.0- ☑
  monostotic C90.3 ☑
    plasma cell C90.0- ☑
  plasma cell C90.0- ☑
  solitary — *see also* Plasmacytoma, solitary C90.3- ☑
Myelomalacia G95.89
Myelomatosis C90.0- ☑
Myelomeningitis — *see* Meningoencephalitis
Myelomeningocele (spinal cord) — *see* Spina bifida
Myelo-osteo-musculodysplasia hereditaria Q79.8
Myelopathic
  anemia D64.89
  muscle atrophy — *see* Atrophy, muscle, spinal
  pain syndrome G89.0
Myelopathy (spinal cord) G95.9
  drug-induced G95.89
  in (due to)
    degeneration or displacement, intervertebral disc NEC — *see* Disorder, disc, with, myelopathy
    infection — *see* Encephalitis

Myelopathy — *continued*
  in — *continued*
    intervertebral disc disorder — *see also* Disorder, disc, with, myelopathy
    mercury — *see* subcategory T56.1 ☑
    neoplastic disease — *see also* Neoplasm D49.9 *[G99.2]*
    pernicious anemia D51.0 *[G99.2]*
    spondylosis — *see* Spondylosis, with myelopathy NEC
  necrotic (subacute) (vascular) G95.19
  radiation-induced G95.89
  spondylogenic NEC — *see* Spondylosis, with myelopathy NEC
  toxic G95.89
  transverse, acute G37.3
  vascular G95.19
  vitamin B12 E53.8 *[G32.0]*
Myelophthisis D61.82
Myeloradiculitis G04.91
Myeloradiculodysplasia (spinal) Q06.1
Myelosarcoma C92.3- ☑
Myelosclerosis D75.89
  with myeloid metaplasia D47.4
  disseminated, of nervous system G35
  megakaryocytic D47.4
    with myeloid metaplasia D47.4
Myelosis
  acute C92.0- ☑
  aleukemic C92.9- ☑
  chronic D47.1
  erythremic (acute) C94.0- ☑
  megakaryocytic C94.2- ☑
  nonleukemic D72.828
  subacute C92.9- ☑
Myiasis (cavernous) B87.9
  aural B87.4
  creeping B87.0
  cutaneous B87.0
  dermal B87.0
  ear (external) (middle) B87.4
  eye B87.2
  genitourinary B87.81
  intestinal B87.82
  laryngeal B87.3
  nasopharyngeal B87.3
  ocular B87.2
  orbit B87.2
  skin B87.0
  specified site NEC B87.89
  traumatic B87.1
  wound B87.1
Myoadenoma, prostate — *see* Hyperplasia, prostate
Myoblastoma
  granular cell — *see also* Neoplasm, connective tissue, benign
    malignant — *see* Neoplasm, connective tissue, malignant
    tongue D10.1
Myocardial — *see* condition
Myocardiopathy (congestive) (constrictive) (familial) (hypertrophic nonobstructive) (idiopathic) (infiltrative) (obstructive) (primary) (restrictive) (sporadic) — *see also* Cardiomyopathy I42.9
  alcoholic I42.6
  cobalt-beer I42.6
  glycogen storage E74.02 *[I43]*
  hypertrophic obstructive I42.1
  in (due to)
    beriberi E51.12
    cardiac glycogenosis E74.02 *[I43]*
    Friedreich's ataxia G11.11 *[I43]*
    myotonia atrophica G71.11 *[I43]*
    progressive muscular dystrophy — *see also* Dystrophy, muscular, by type G71.09 *[I43]*
  obscure (African) I42.8
  secondary I42.9
  thyrotoxic E05.90 *[I43]*
    with storm E05.91 *[I43]*
  toxic NEC I42.7
Myocarditis (with arteriosclerosis) (chronic) (fibroid) (interstitial) (old) (progressive) (senile) I51.4
  with
    rheumatic fever (conditions in I00) I09.0
      active — *see* Myocarditis, acute, rheumatic
      inactive or quiescent (with chorea) I09.0
  active I40.9

Myocarditis — *continued*
  active — *continued*
    rheumatic I01.2
      with chorea (acute) (rheumatic) (Sydenham's) I02.0
  acute or subacute (interstitial) I40.9
    due to
      streptococcus (beta-hemolytic) I01.2
    idiopathic I40.1
    rheumatic I01.2
      with chorea (acute) (rheumatic) (Sydenham's) I02.0
    specified NEC I40.8
  aseptic of newborn B33.22
  bacterial (acute) I40.0
  Coxsackie (virus) B33.22
  diphtheritic A36.81
  eosinophilic I40.1
  epidemic of newborn (Coxsackie) B33.22
  Fiedler's (acute) (isolated) I40.1
  giant cell (acute) (subacute) I40.1
  gonococcal A54.83
  granulomatous (idiopathic) (isolated) (nonspecific) I40.1
  hypertensive — *see* Hypertension, heart
  idiopathic (granulomatous) I40.1
  in (due to)
    diphtheria A36.81
    epidemic louse-borne typhus A75.0 *[I41]*
    Lyme disease A69.29
    sarcoidosis D86.85
    scarlet fever A38.1
    toxoplasmosis (acquired) B58.81
    typhoid A01.02
    typhus NEC A75.9 *[I41]*
  infective I40.0
  influenzal — *see* Influenza, with, myocarditis
  isolated (acute) I40.1
  meningococcal A39.52
  mumps B26.82
  nonrheumatic, active I40.9
  parenchymatous I40.9
  pneumococcal I40.0
  rheumatic (chronic) (inactive) (with chorea) I09.0
    active or acute I01.2
      with chorea (acute) (rheumatic) (Sydenham's) I02.0
  rheumatoid — *see* Rheumatoid, carditis
  septic I40.0
  staphylococcal I40.0
  suppurative I40.0
  syphilitic (chronic) A52.06
  toxic I40.8
    rheumatic — *see* Myocarditis, acute, rheumatic
  tuberculous A18.84
  typhoid A01.02
  valvular — *see* Endocarditis
  virus, viral I40.0
    of newborn (Coxsackie) B33.22
Myocardium, myocardial — *see* condition
Myocardosis — *see* Cardiomyopathy
Myoclonus, myoclonic, myoclonia (familial) (essential) (multifocal) (simplex) G25.3
  drug-induced G25.3
  epilepsy — *see also* Epilepsy, generalized, specified NEC G40.4- ☑
    familial (progressive) G25.3
  epileptica G40.409
    with status epilepticus G40.401
  facial G51.3- ☑
  familial progressive G25.3
  Friedreich's G25.3
  jerks G25.3
  massive G25.3
  palatal G25.3
  pharyngeal G25.3
Myocytolysis I51.5
Myodiastasis — *see* Diastasis, muscle
Myoendocarditis — *see* Endocarditis
Myoepithelioma — *see* Neoplasm, benign, by site
Myofasciitis (acute) — *see* Myositis
Myofibroma — *see also* Neoplasm, connective tissue, benign
  uterus (cervix) (corpus) — *see* Leiomyoma
Myofibromatosis D48.1
  infantile Q89.8
Myofibrosis M62.89
  heart — *see* Myocarditis
  scapulohumeral — *see* Lesion, shoulder, specified NEC

Myofibrositis M79.7
  scapulohumeral — *see* Lesion, shoulder, specified NEC
Myoglobulinuria, myoglobinuria (primary) R82.1
Myokymia, facial G51.4
Myolipoma — *see* Lipoma
Myoma — *see also* Neoplasm, connective tissue, benign
  malignant — *see* Neoplasm, connective tissue, malignant
  prostate D29.1
  uterus (cervix) (corpus) — *see* Leiomyoma
Myomalacia M62.89
Myometritis — *see* Endometritis
Myometrium — *see* condition
Myonecrosis, clostridial A48.0
Myopathy G72.9
  acute
    necrotizing G72.81
    quadriplegic G72.81
  alcoholic G72.1
  benign congenital G71.20
  central core G71.29
  centronuclear G71.228
    autosomal (dominant) (recessive) G71.228
    other specified NEC G71.228
  congenital (benign) G71.20
  critical illness G72.81
  distal G71.09
  drug-induced G72.0
  endocrine NEC E34.9 *[G73.7]*
  extraocular muscles H05.82-
  facioscapulohumeral G71.02
  hereditary G71.9
    specified NEC G71.8
  hyaline body G71.29
  immune NEC G72.49
  in (due to)
    Addison's disease E27.1 *[G73.7]*
    alcohol G72.1
    amyloidosis E85.0 *[G73.7]*
    cretinism E00.9 *[G73.7]*
    Cushing's syndrome E24.9 *[G73.7]*
    drugs G72.0
    endocrine disease NEC E34.9 *[G73.7]*
    giant cell arteritis M31.6 *[G73.7]*
    glycogen storage disease E74.00 *[G73.7]*
    hyperadrenocorticism E24.9 *[G73.7]*
    hyperparathyroidism NEC E21.3 *[G73.7]*
    hypoparathyroidism E20.9 *[G73.7]*
    hypopituitarism E23.0 *[G73.7]*
    hypothyroidism E03.9 *[G73.7]*
    infectious disease NEC B99 ☑ *[G73.7]*
    lipid storage disease E75.6 *[G73.7]*
    metabolic disease NEC E88.9 *[G73.7]*
    myxedema E03.9 *[G73.7]*
    parasitic disease NEC B89 *[G73.7]*
    polyarteritis nodosa M30.0 *[G73.7]*
    rheumatoid arthritis — *see* Rheumatoid, myopathy
    sarcoidosis D86.87
    scleroderma M34.82
    sicca syndrome M35.03
    Sjögren's syndrome M35.03
    systemic lupus erythematosus M32.19
    thyrotoxicosis (hyperthyroidism) E05.90 *[G73.7]*
      with thyroid storm E05.91 *[G73.7]*
    toxic agent NEC G72.2
  inflammatory NEC G72.49
  intensive care (ICU) G72.81
  limb-girdle — *see* Dystrophy, muscular, limb-girdle
  mitochondrial NEC
  Miyoshi, type 3 G71.035
  myosin storage G71.29
  myotubular (centronuclear) G71.220
    X-linked G71.220
  mytonic, proximal (PROMM) G71.11
  nemaline G71.21
  ocular G71.09
  oculopharyngeal G71.09
  of critical illness G72.81
  primary G71.9
    specified NEC G71.8
  progressive NEC G72.89
  proximal myotonic (PROMM) G71.11
  rod (body) G71.21
  scapulohumeral G71.02
  specified NEC G72.89
  toxic G72.2
Myopericarditis — *see also* Pericarditis
  chronic rheumatic I09.2

Myopia (axial) (congenital) H52.1- ☑
  degenerative (malignant) H44.20
    with
      choroidal neovascularization H44.2A- ☑
      foveoschisis H44.2D- ☑
      macular hole H44.2B- ☑
      retinal detachment H44.2C- ☑
      specified maculopathy NEC H44.2E- ☑
    bilateral H44.23
    left eye H44.22
    right eye H44.21
  malignant — *see also* Myopia, degenerative H44.2- ☑
  pernicious — *see also* Myopia, degenerative H44.2- ☑
  progressive high (degenerative) — *see also* Myopia, degenerative H44.2- ☑
Myosarcoma — *see* Neoplasm, connective tissue, malignant
Myosis (pupil) H57.03
  stromal (endolymphatic) D39.0
Myositis M60.9
  clostridial A48.0
  due to posture — *see* Myositis, specified type NEC
  epidemic B33.0
  fibrosa or fibrous (chronic), Volkmann's T79.6 ☑
  foreign body granuloma — *see* Granuloma, foreign body
  in (due to)
    bilharziasis B65.9 *[M63.8-]* ☑
    cysticercosis B69.81
    leprosy A30.9 *[M63.8-]* ☑
    mycosis B49 *[M63.8-]* ☑
    sarcoidosis D86.87
    schistosomiasis B65.9 *[M63.8-]* ☑
    syphilis
      late A52.78
      secondary A51.49
    toxoplasmosis (acquired) B58.82
    trichinellosis B75 *[M63.8-]* ☑
    tuberculosis A18.09
  inclusion body [IBM] G72.41
  infective M60.009
    arm M60.002
      left M60.001
      right M60.000
    leg M60.005
      left M60.004
      right M60.003
    lower limb M60.005
      ankle M60.07- ☑
      foot M60.07- ☑
      lower leg M60.06- ☑
      thigh M60.05- ☑
      toe M60.07- ☑
    multiple sites M60.09
    specified site NEC M60.08
    upper limb M60.002
      finger M60.04- ☑
      forearm M60.03- ☑
      hand M60.04- ☑
      shoulder region M60.01- ☑
      upper arm M60.02- ☑
  interstitial M60.10
    ankle M60.17- ☑
    foot M60.17- ☑
    forearm M60.13- ☑
    hand M60.14- ☑
    lower leg M60.16- ☑
    multiple sites M60.19
    shoulder region M60.11- ☑
    specified site NEC M60.18
    thigh M60.15- ☑
    upper arm M60.12- ☑
  mycotic B49 *[M63.8-]* ☑
  orbital, chronic H05.12- ☑
  ossificans or ossifying (circumscripta) — *see also* Ossification, muscle, specified NEC
    in (due to)
      burns M61.30
        ankle M61.37- ☑
        foot M61.37- ☑
        forearm M61.33- ☑
        hand M61.34- ☑
        lower leg M61.36- ☑
        multiple sites M61.39
        pelvic region M61.35- ☑
        shoulder region M61.31- ☑
        specified site NEC M61.38

Myositis — *continued*
  ossificans or ossifying — *see also* Ossification, muscle, specified — *continued*
    in — *continued*
      burns — *continued*
        thigh M61.35- ☑
        upper arm M61.32- ☑
      quadriplegia or paraplegia M61.20
        ankle M61.27- ☑
        foot M61.27- ☑
        forearm M61.23- ☑
        hand M61.24- ☑
        lower leg M61.26- ☑
        multiple sites M61.29
        pelvic region M61.25- ☑
        shoulder region M61.21- ☑
        specified site NEC M61.28
        thigh M61.25- ☑
        upper arm M61.22- ☑
    progressiva M61.10
      ankle M61.17- ☑
      finger M61.14- ☑
      foot M61.17- ☑
      forearm M61.13- ☑
      hand M61.14- ☑
      lower leg M61.16- ☑
      multiple sites M61.19
      pelvic region M61.15- ☑
      shoulder region M61.11- ☑
      specified site NEC M61.18
      thigh M61.15- ☑
      toe M61.17- ☑
      upper arm M61.12- ☑
    traumatica M61.00
      ankle M61.07- ☑
      foot M61.07- ☑
      forearm M61.03- ☑
      hand M61.04- ☑
      lower leg M61.06- ☑
      multiple sites M61.09
      pelvic region M61.05- ☑
      shoulder region M61.01- ☑
      specified site NEC M61.08
      thigh M61.05- ☑
      upper arm M61.02- ☑
  purulent — *see* Myositis, infective
  specified type NEC M60.80
    ankle M60.87- ☑
    foot M60.87- ☑
    forearm M60.83- ☑
    hand M60.84- ☑
    lower leg M60.86- ☑
    multiple sites M60.89
    pelvic region M60.85- ☑
    shoulder region M60.81- ☑
    specified site NEC M60.88
    thigh M60.85- ☑
    upper arm M60.82- ☑
  suppurative — *see* Myositis, infective
  traumatic (old) — *see* Myositis, specified type NEC
Myospasia impulsiva F95.2
Myotonia (acquisita) (intermittens) M62.89
  atrophica G71.11
  chondrodystrophic G71.13
  congenita (acetazolamide responsive) (dominant) (recessive) G71.12
  drug-induced G71.14
  dystrophica G71.11
  fluctuans G71.19
  levior G71.12
  permanens G71.19
  symptomatic G71.19
Myotonic pupil — *see* Anomaly, pupil, function, tonic pupil
Myriapodiasis B88.2
Myringitis H73.2- ☑
  with otitis media — *see* Otitis, media
  acute H73.00- ☑
    bullous H73.01- ☑
    specified NEC H73.09- ☑
  bullous — *see* Myringitis, acute, bullous
  chronic H73.1- ☑
Mysophobia F40.228
Mytilotoxism — *see* Poisoning, fish
Myxadenitis labialis K13.0

☑ **Additional Character Required — Refer to the Tabular List for Character Selection**

Myxedema (adult) (idiocy) (infantile) (juvenile) — *see also* Hypothyroidism E03.9
  circumscribed E05.90
    with storm E05.91
  coma E03.5
  congenital E00.1
  cutis L98.5
  localized (pretibial) E05.90
    with storm E05.91

Myxedema — *continued*
  papular L98.5
Myxochondrosarcoma — *see* Neoplasm, cartilage, malignant
Myxofibroma — *see* Neoplasm, connective tissue, benign
  odontogenic — *see* Cyst, calcifying odontogenic
Myxofibrosarcoma — *see* Neoplasm, connective tissue, malignant

Myxolipoma D17.9
Myxoliposarcoma — *see* Neoplasm, connective tissue, malignant
Myxoma — *see also* Neoplasm, connective tissue, benign
  nerve sheath — *see* Neoplasm, nerve, benign
  odontogenic — *see* Cyst, calcifying odontogenic
Myxosarcoma — *see* Neoplasm, connective tissue, malignant

N

Naegeli's
  disease Q82.8
  leukemia, monocytic C93.1- ☑
Naegleriasis (with meningoencephalitis) B60.2
Naffziger's syndrome G54.0
Naga sore — see Ulcer, skin
Nägele's pelvis M95.5
  with disproportion (fetopelvic) O33.0
    causing obstructed labor O65.0
Nail — see also condition
  biting F98.8
  patella syndrome Q87.2
Nanism, nanosomia — see Dwarfism
Nanophyetiasis B66.8
Nanukayami A27.89
Napkin rash L22
Narcolepsy G47.419
  with cataplexy G47.411
  in conditions classified elsewhere G47.429
    with cataplexy G47.421
Narcosis R06.89
Narcotism — see Dependence
NARP (Neuropathy, Ataxia and Retinitis pigmentosa)
    syndrome E88.49
Narrow
  anterior chamber angle H40.03- ☑
  gingival width (of periodontal soft tissue) K05.5
  pelvis — see Contraction, pelvis
Narrowing — see also Stenosis
  artery I77.1
    auditory, internal I65.8
    basilar — see Occlusion, artery, basilar
    carotid — see Occlusion, artery, carotid
    cerebellar — see Occlusion, artery, cerebellar
    cerebral — see Occlusion artery, cerebral
    choroidal — see Occlusion, artery, precerebral,
      specified NEC
    communicating posterior — see Occlusion, artery,
      precerebral, specified NEC
    coronary — see also Disease, heart, ischemic,
      atherosclerotic
      congenital Q24.5
      syphilitic A50.54 [I52]
      due to syphilis NEC A52.06
    hypophyseal — see Occlusion, artery, precerebral,
      specified NEC
    pontine — see Occlusion, artery, precerebral, spec-
      ified NEC
    precerebral — see Occlusion, artery, precerebral
    vertebral — see Occlusion, artery, vertebral
  auditory canal (external) — see Stenosis, external ear
    canal
  eustachian tube — see Obstruction, eustachian tube
  eyelid — see Disorder, eyelid function
  larynx J38.6
  mesenteric artery — see also Ischemia, intestine, acute
    K55.059
  palate M26.89
  palpebral fissure — see Disorder, eyelid function
  ureter N13.5
    with infection N13.6
  urethra — see Stricture, urethra
Narrowness, abnormal, eyelid Q10.3
Nasal — see condition
Nasolachrymal, nasolacrimal — see condition
Nasopharyngeal — see also condition
  pituitary gland Q89.2
  torticollis M43.6
Nasopharyngitis (acute) (infective) (streptococcal)
    (subacute) J00
  chronic (suppurative) (ulcerative) J31.1
Nasopharynx, nasopharyngeal — see condition
Natal tooth, teeth K00.6
Nausea (without vomiting) R11.0
  with vomiting R11.2
  gravidarum — see Hyperemesis, gravidarum
  marina T75.3 ☑
  navalis T75.3 ☑
Navel — see condition
Neapolitan fever — see Brucellosis
Near drowning T75.1 ☑
Nearsightedness — see Myopia
Near-syncope R55
Nebula, cornea — see Opacity, cornea

Necator americanus infestation B76.1
Necatoriasis B76.1
Neck — see condition
Necrobiosis R68.89
  lipoidica NEC L92.1
    with diabetes — see E08-E13 with .620
Necrolysis, toxic epidermal L51.2
  due to drug
    correct substance properly administered — see Ta-
      ble of Drugs and Chemicals, by drug, adverse
      effect
    overdose or wrong substance given or taken — see
      Table of Drugs and Chemicals, by drug, poi-
      soning
Necrophilia F65.89
Necrosis, necrotic (ischemic) — see also Gangrene
  adrenal (capsule) (gland) E27.49
  amputation stump (surgical) (late) T87.50
    arm T87.5- ☑
    leg T87.5- ☑
  antrum J32.0
  aorta (hyaline) — see also Aneurysm, aorta
    cystic medial — see Dissection, aorta
  artery I77.5
  bladder (aseptic) (sphincter) N32.89
  bone — see also Osteonecrosis M87.9
    aseptic or avascular — see Osteonecrosis
      idiopathic M87.00
    ethmoid J32.2
    jaw M27.2
    tuberculous — see Tuberculosis, bone
  brain I67.89
  breast (aseptic) (fat) (segmental) N64.1
  bronchus J98.09
  central nervous system NEC I67.89
  cerebellar I67.89
  cerebral I67.89
  colon — see also Infarct, intestine K55.049
  cornea H18.89- ☑
  cortical (acute) (renal) N17.1
  cystic medial (aorta) — see Dissection, aorta
  dental pulp K04.1
  esophagus K22.89
  ethmoid (bone) J32.2
  eyelid — see Disorder, eyelid, degenerative
  fat, fatty (generalized) — see also Disorder, soft tissue,
      specified type NEC
    abdominal wall K65.4
    breast (aseptic) (segmental) N64.1
    localized — see Degeneration, by site, fatty
    mesentery K65.4
    omentum K65.4
    pancreas K86.89
    peritoneum K65.4
    skin (subcutaneous), newborn P83.0
    subcutaneous, due to birth injury P15.6
  gallbladder — see Cholecystitis, acute
  heart — see Infarct, myocardium
  hip, aseptic or avascular — see Osteonecrosis, by type,
    femur
  intestine (acute) (hemorrhagic) (massive) — see also
    Infarct, intestine K55.069
  jaw M27.2
  kidney (bilateral) N28.0
    acute N17.9
    cortical (acute) (bilateral) N17.1
      with ectopic or molar pregnancy O08.4
    medullary (bilateral) (in acute renal failure) (papil-
      lary) N17.2
    papillary (bilateral) (in acute renal failure) N17.2
    tubular N17.0
      with ectopic or molar pregnancy O08.4
      complicating
        abortion — see Abortion, by type, complicat-
          ed by, tubular necrosis
        ectopic or molar pregnancy O08.4
        pregnancy — see Pregnancy, complicated by,
          diseases of, specified type or system
          NEC
      following ectopic or molar pregnancy O08.4
      traumatic T79.5 ☑
  larynx J38.7
  liver (with hepatic failure) (cell) — see Failure, hepatic
    hemorrhagic, central K76.2
  lung J85.0
  lymphatic gland — see Lymphadenitis, acute
  mammary gland (fat) (segmental) N64.1
  mastoid (chronic) — see Mastoiditis, chronic

Necrosis, necrotic — continued
  medullary (acute) (renal) N17.2
  mesentery — see also Infarct, intestine K55.069
    fat K65.4
  mitral valve — see Insufficiency, mitral
  myocardium, myocardial — see Infarct, myocardium
  nose J34.0
  omentum (with mesenteric infarction) — see also In-
    farct, intestine K55.069
    fat K65.4
  orbit, orbital — see Osteomyelitis, orbit
  ossicles, ear — see Abnormal, ear ossicles
  ovary N70.92
  pancreas (aseptic) (duct) (fat) K86.89
    acute (infective) — see Pancreatitis, acute
    infective — see Pancreatitis, acute
  papillary (acute) (renal) N17.2
  perineum N90.89
  peritoneum (with mesenteric infarction) — see also
    Infarct, intestine K55.069
    fat K65.4
  pharynx J02.9
    in granulocytopenia — see Neutropenia
    Vincent's A69.1
  phosphorus — see subcategory T54.2 ☑
  pituitary (gland) E23.0
    postpartum O99.285
    Sheehan O99.285
  pressure — see Ulcer, pressure, by site
  pulmonary J85.0
  pulp (dental) K04.1
  radiation — see Necrosis, by site
  radium — see Necrosis, by site
  renal — see Necrosis, kidney
  sclera H15.89
  scrotum N50.89
  skin or subcutaneous tissue NEC I96
  spine, spinal (column) — see also Osteonecrosis, by
    type, vertebra
    cord G95.19
  spleen D73.5
  stomach K31.89
  stomatitis (ulcerative) A69.0
  subcutaneous fat, newborn P83.88
  subendocardial (acute) I21.4
    chronic I25.89
  suprarenal (capsule) (gland) E27.49
  testis N50.89
  thymus (gland) E32.8
  tonsil J35.8
  trachea J39.8
  tuberculous NEC — see Tuberculosis
  tubular (acute) (anoxic) (renal) (toxic) N17.0
    postprocedural N99.0
  vagina N89.8
  vertebra — see also Osteonecrosis, by type, vertebra
    tuberculous A18.01
  vulva N90.89
  X-ray — see Necrosis, by site
Necrospermia — see Infertility, male
Need (for)
  care provider because (of)
    assistance with personal care Z74.1
    continuous supervision required Z74.3
    impaired mobility Z74.09
    no other household member able to render care
      Z74.2
    specified reason NEC Z74.8
  immunization — see Vaccination
  vaccination — see Vaccination
Neglect
  adult
    confirmed T74.01 ☑
    history of Z91.412
    suspected T76.01 ☑
  child (childhood)
    confirmed T74.02 ☑
    history of Z62.812
    suspected T76.02 ☑
  emotional, in childhood Z62.898
  hemispatial R41.4
  left-sided R41.4
  sensory R41.4
  visuospatial R41.4
Neisserian infection NEC — see Gonococcus
Nelaton's syndrome G60.8
Nelson's syndrome E24.1
Nematodiasis (intestinal) B82.0

☑ Additional Character Required — Refer to the Tabular List for Character Selection

Nematodiasis — *continued*
  Ancylostoma B76.0
Neonatal — *see also* Newborn
  acne L70.4
  bradycardia P29.12
  screening, abnormal findings on — *see* Abnormal,
    neonatal screening
  tachycardia P29.11
  tooth, teeth K00.6
Neonatorum — *see* condition
Neoplasia
  endocrine, multiple (MEN) E31.20
    type I E31.21
    type IIA E31.22
    type IIB E31.23
  intraepithelial (histologically confirmed)
    anal (AIN) (histologically confirmed) K62.82
      grade I K62.82
      grade II K62.82
      severe D01.3
    cervical glandular (histologically confirmed) D06.9
    cervix (uteri) (CIN) (histologically confirmed) N87.9
      glandular D06.9
      grade I N87.0
      grade II N87.1
      grade III (severe dysplasia) — *see also* Carcinoma,
        cervix uteri, in situ D06.9
    prostate (histologically confirmed) (PIN) N42.31
      grade I N42.31
      grade II N42.31
      grade III (severe dysplasia) D07.5
    vagina (histologically confirmed) (VAIN) N89.3
      grade I N89.0
      grade II N89.1
      grade III (severe dysplasia) D07.2
    vulva (histologically confirmed) (VIN) N90.3
      grade I N90.0
      grade II N90.1
      grade III (severe dysplasia) D07.1
Neoplasm, neoplastic — *see also* Table of Neoplasms
  lipomatous, benign — *see* Lipoma
  malignant mast cell C96.20
    specified type NEC C96.29
  mast cell, of uncertain behavior NEC D47.09
  myelodysplastic/myeloproliferative, unclassifiable
    C94.6
Neovascularization
  ciliary body — *see* Disorder, iris, vascular
  cornea H16.40- ☑
    deep H16.44- ☑
    ghost vessels — *see* Ghost, vessels
    localized H16.43- ☑
    pannus — *see* Pannus
  iris — *see* Disorder, iris, vascular
  retina H35.05- ☑
Nephralgia N23
Nephritis, nephritic (albuminuric) (azotemic) (congenital) (disseminated) (epithelial) (familial) (focal) (granulomatous) (hemorrhagic) (infantile) (nonsuppurative, excretory) (uremic) N05.9
  with
    C3
      glomerulonephritis N05.A
      glomerulopathy N05.A
        with dense deposit disease N05.6
      dense deposit disease N05.6
      diffuse
        crescentic glomerulonephritis N05.7
        endocapillary proliferative glomerulonephritis
          N05.4
        membranous glomerulonephritis N05.2
        mesangial proliferative glomerulonephritis N05.3
        mesangiocapillary glomerulonephritis N05.5
    edema — *see* Nephrosis
    focal and segmental glomerular lesions N05.1
    foot process disease N04.9
    glomerular lesion
      diffuse sclerosing N05.8
      hypocomplementemic — *see* Nephritis, membranoproliferative
      IgA — *see* Nephropathy, IgA
      lobular, lobulonodular — *see* Nephritis, membranoproliferative
      nodular — *see* Nephritis, membranoproliferative
    lesion of
      glomerulonephritis, proliferative N05.8
      renal necrosis N05.9
    minor glomerular abnormality N05.0

Nephritis, nephritic — *continued*
  with — *continued*
    specified morphological changes NEC N05.8
  acute N00.9
    with
      C3
        glomerulonephritis N00.A
        glomerulopathy N00.A
          with dense deposit disease N00.6
        dense deposit disease N00.6
        diffuse
          crescentic glomerulonephritis N00.7
          endocapillary proliferative glomerulonephritis
            N00.4
          membranous glomerulonephritis N00.2
          mesangial proliferative glomerulonephritis
            N00.3
          mesangiocapillary glomerulonephritis N00.5
        focal and segmental glomerular lesions N00.1
        minor glomerular abnormality N00.0
        specified morphological changes NEC N00.8
  amyloid E85.4 *[N08]*
  antiglomerular basement membrane (anti-GBM) antibody NEC
    in Goodpasture's syndrome M31.0
  antitubular basement membrane (tubulo-interstitial)
    NEC N12
    toxic — *see* Nephropathy, toxic
  arteriolar — *see* Hypertension, kidney
  arteriosclerotic — *see* Hypertension, kidney
  ascending — *see* Nephritis, tubulo-interstitial
  atrophic N03.9
  Balkan (endemic) N15.0
  calculous, calculus — *see* Calculus, kidney
  cardiac — *see* Hypertension, kidney
  cardiovascular — *see* Hypertension, kidney
  chronic N03.9
    with
      C3
        glomerulonephritis N03.A
        glomerulopathy N03.A
          with dense deposit disease N03.6
        dense deposit disease N03.6
        diffuse
          crescentic glomerulonephritis N03.7
          endocapillary proliferative glomerulonephritis
            N03.4
          membranous glomerulonephritis N03.2
          mesangial proliferative glomerulonephritis
            N03.3
          mesangiocapillary glomerulonephritis N03.5
        focal and segmental glomerular lesions N03.1
        minor glomerular abnormality N03.0
        specified morphological changes NEC N03.8
    arteriosclerotic — *see* Hypertension, kidney
  cirrhotic N26.9
  complicating pregnancy O26.83- ☑
  croupous N00.9
  degenerative — *see* Nephrosis
  diffuse sclerosing N05.8
  due to
    diabetes mellitus — *see* E08-E13 with .21
    subacute bacterial endocarditis I33.0
    systemic lupus erythematosus (chronic) M32.14
    typhoid fever A01.09
  gonococcal (acute) (chronic) A54.21
  hypocomplementemic — *see* Nephritis, membranoproliferative
  IgA — *see* Nephropathy, IgA
  immune complex (circulating) NEC N05.8
  infective — *see* Nephritis, tubulo-interstitial
  interstitial — *see* Nephritis, tubulo-interstitial
  lead N14.3
  membranoproliferative (diffuse) (type 1 or 3) — *see
    also* N00-N07 with fourth character .5 N05.5
    type 2 — *see also* N00-N07 with fourth character .6
      N05.6
  minimal change N05.0
  necrotic, necrotizing NEC — *see also* N00-N07 with
    fourth character .8 N05.8
  nephrotic — *see* Nephrosis
  nodular — *see* Nephritis, membranoproliferative
  polycystic Q61.3
    adult type Q61.2
    autosomal
      dominant Q61.2
      recessive NEC Q61.19
    childhood type NEC Q61.19

Nephritis, nephritic — *continued*
  polycystic — *continued*
    infantile type NEC Q61.19
  poststreptococcal N05.9
    acute N00.9
    chronic N03.9
    rapidly progressive N01.9
  proliferative NEC — *see also* N00-N07 with fourth
    character .8 N05.8
  purulent — *see* Nephritis, tubulo-interstitial
  rapidly progressive N01.9
    with
      C3
        glomerulonephritis N01.A
        glomerulopathy N01.A
          with dense deposit disease N01.6
        dense deposit disease N01.6
        diffuse
          crescentic glomerulonephritis N01.7
          endocapillary proliferative glomerulonephritis
            N01.4
          membranous glomerulonephritis N01.2
          mesangial proliferative glomerulonephritis
            N01.3
          mesangiocapillary glomerulonephritis N01.5
        focal and segmental glomerular lesions N01.1
        minor glomerular abnormality N01.0
        specified morphological changes NEC N01.8
  salt losing or wasting NEC N28.89
  saturnine N14.3
  sclerosing, diffuse N05.8
  septic — *see* Nephritis, tubulo-interstitial
  specified pathology NEC — *see also* N00-N07 with
    fourth character .8 N05.8
  subacute N01.9
  suppurative — *see* Nephritis, tubulo-interstitial
  syphilitic (late) A52.75
    congenital A50.59 *[N08]*
    early (secondary) A51.44
  toxic — *see* Nephropathy, toxic
  tubal, tubular — *see* Nephritis, tubulo-interstitial
  tuberculous A18.11
  tubulo-interstitial (in) N12
    acute (infectious) N10
    chronic (infectious) N11.9
      nonobstructive N11.8
        reflux-associated N11.0
      obstructive N11.1
      specified NEC N11.8
    due to
      brucellosis A23.9 *[N16]*
      cryoglobulinemia D89.1 *[N16]*
      glycogen storage disease E74.00 *[N16]*
      Sjögren's syndrome M35.04
  vascular — *see* Hypertension, kidney
  war N00.9
Nephroblastoma (epithelial) (mesenchymal) C64- ☑
Nephrocalcinosis E83.59 *[N29]*
Nephrocystitis, pustular — *see* Nephritis, tubulo-interstitial
Nephrolithiasis (congenital) (pelvis) (recurrent) — *see
  also* Calculus, kidney
Nephroma C64- ☑
  mesoblastic D41.0- ☑
Nephronephritis — *see* Nephrosis
Nephronophthisis Q61.5
Nephropathia epidemica A98.5
Nephropathy — *see also* Nephritis N28.9
  with
    edema — *see* Nephrosis
    glomerular lesion — *see* Glomerulonephritis
  amyloid, hereditary E85.0
  analgesic N14.0
    with medullary necrosis, acute N17.2
  Balkan (endemic) N15.0
  chemical — *see* Nephropathy, toxic
  contrast medium, radiography N14.11
  contrast-induced N14.11
  diabetic — *see* E08-E13 with .21
  drug-induced N14.2
    contrast-induced N14.11
    specified NEC N14.19
  focal and segmental hyalinosis or sclerosis N02.1
  heavy metal-induced N14.3
  hereditary NEC N07.9
    with
      C3
        glomerulonephritis N07.A

Nephropathy — *continued*
hereditary — *continued*
with — *continued*
C3 — *continued*
glomerulopathy N07.A
with dense deposit disease N07.6
dense deposit disease N07.6
diffuse
crescentic glomerulonephritis N07.7
endocapillary proliferative glomerulonephritis N07.4
membranous glomerulonephritis N07.2
mesangial proliferative glomerulonephritis N07.3
mesangiocapillary glomerulonephritis N07.5
focal and segmental glomerular lesions N07.1
minor glomerular abnormality N07.0
specified morphological changes NEC N07.8
hypercalcemic N25.89
hypertensive — *see* Hypertension, kidney
hypokalemic (vacuolar) N25.89
IgA N02.8
with glomerular lesion N02.9
focal and segmental hyalinosis or sclerosis N02.1
membranoproliferative (diffuse) N02.5
membranous (diffuse) N02.2
mesangial proliferative (diffuse) N02.3
mesangiocapillary (diffuse) N02.5
proliferative NEC N02.8
specified pathology NEC N02.8
lead N14.3
membranoproliferative (diffuse) N02.5
membranous (diffuse) N02.2
mesangial (IgA/IgG) — *see* Nephropathy, IgA
proliferative (diffuse) N02.3
mesangiocapillary (diffuse) N02.5
obstructive N13.8
phenacetin N17.2
phosphate-losing N25.0
potassium depletion N25.89
pregnancy-related O26.83- ☑
proliferative NEC — *see also* N00-N07 with fourth character .8 N05.8
protein-losing N25.89
saturnine N14.3
sickle-cell D57.- ☑ *[N08]*
toxic NEC N14.4
due to
drugs N14.2
analgesic N14.0
specified NEC N14.19
heavy metals N14.3
vasomotor N17.0
water-losing N25.89
Nephroptosis N28.83
Nephropyosis — *see* Abscess, kidney
Nephrorrhagia N28.89
Nephrosclerosis (arteriolar) (arteriosclerotic) (chronic) (hyaline) — *see also* Hypertension, kidney
hyperplastic — *see* Hypertension, kidney
senile N26.9
Nephrosis, nephrotic (Epstein's) (syndrome) (congenital) N04.9
with
foot process disease N04.9
glomerular lesion N04.1
hypocomplementemic N04.5
acute N04.9
anoxic — *see* Nephrosis, tubular
chemical — *see* Nephrosis, tubular
cholemic K76.7
diabetic — *see* E08-E13 with .21
Finnish type (congenital) Q89.8
hemoglobin N10
hemoglobinuric — *see* Nephrosis, tubular
in
amyloidosis E85.4 *[N08]*
diabetes mellitus — *see* E08-E13 with .21
epidemic hemorrhagic fever A98.5
malaria (malariae) B52.0
ischemic — *see* Nephrosis, tubular
lipoid N04.9
lower nephron — *see* Nephrosis, tubular
malarial (malariae) B52.0
minimal change N04.0
myoglobin N10
necrotizing — *see* Nephrosis, tubular
osmotic (sucrose) N25.89

Nephrosis, nephrotic — *continued*
radiation N04.9
syphilitic (late) A52.75
toxic — *see* Nephrosis, tubular
tubular (acute) N17.0
postprocedural N99.0
radiation N04.9
Nephrosonephritis, hemorrhagic (endemic) A98.5
Nephrostomy
attention to Z43.6
status Z93.6
Nerve — *see also* condition
injury — *see* Injury, nerve, by body site
Nerves R45.0
Nervous — *see also* condition R45.0
heart F45.8
stomach F45.8
tension R45.0
Nervousness R45.0
Nesidioblastoma
pancreas D13.7
specified site NEC — *see* Neoplasm, benign, by site
unspecified site D13.7
Nettleship's syndrome — *see* Urticaria pigmentosa
Neumann's disease or syndrome L10.1
Neuralgia, neuralgic (acute) M79.2
accessory (nerve) G52.8
acoustic (nerve) — *see* subcategory H93.3 ☑
auditory (nerve) — *see* subcategory H93.3 ☑
ciliary G44.009
intractable G44.001
not intractable G44.009
cranial
nerve — *see also* Disorder, nerve, cranial
fifth or trigeminal — *see* Neuralgia, trigeminal
postherpetic, postzoster B02.29
ear — *see* subcategory H92.0 ☑
facialis vera G51.1
Fothergill's — *see* Neuralgia, trigeminal
glossopharyngeal (nerve) G52.1
Horton's G44.099
intractable G44.091
not intractable G44.099
Hunt's B02.21
hypoglossal (nerve) G52.3
infraorbital — *see* Neuralgia, trigeminal
malarial — *see* Malaria
migrainous G44.009
intractable G44.001
not intractable G44.009
Morton's G57.6- ☑
nerve, cranial — *see* Disorder, nerve, cranial
nose G52.0
occipital M54.81
olfactory G52.0
penis N48.9
perineum R10.2
postherpetic NEC B02.29
trigeminal B02.22
pubic region R10.2
scrotum R10.2
Sluder's G44.89
specified nerve NEC G58.8
spermatic cord R10.2
sphenopalatine (ganglion) G90.09
trifacial — *see* Neuralgia, trigeminal
trigeminal G50.0
postherpetic, postzoster B02.22
vagus (nerve) G52.2
writer's F48.8
organic G25.89
Neurapraxia — *see* Injury, nerve
Neurasthenia F48.8
cardiac F45.8
gastric F45.8
heart F45.8
Neurilemmoma — *see also* Neoplasm, nerve, benign
acoustic (nerve) D33.3
malignant — *see also* Neoplasm, nerve, malignant
acoustic (nerve) C72.4- ☑
Neurilemmosarcoma — *see* Neoplasm, nerve, malignant
Neurinoma — *see* Neoplasm, nerve, benign
Neurinomatosis — *see* Neoplasm, nerve, uncertain behavior
Neuritis (rheumatoid) M79.2
abducens (nerve) — *see* Strabismus, paralytic, sixth nerve
accessory (nerve) G52.8

Neuritis — *continued*
acoustic (nerve) — *see also* subcategory H93.3 ☑
in (due to)
infectious disease NEC B99 ☑ *[H94.0-]* ☑
parasitic disease NEC B89 *[H94.0-]* ☑
syphilitic A52.15
alcoholic G62.1
with psychosis — *see* Psychosis, alcoholic
amyloid, any site E85.4 *[G63]*
auditory (nerve) — *see* subcategory H93.3 ☑
brachial — *see* Radiculopathy
due to displacement, intervertebral disc — *see* Disorder, disc, cervical, with neuritis
cranial nerve
due to Lyme disease A69.22
eighth or acoustic or auditory — *see* subcategory H93.3 ☑
eleventh or accessory G52.8
fifth or trigeminal G50.- ☑
first or olfactory G52.0
fourth or trochlear — *see* Strabismus, paralytic, fourth nerve
second or optic — *see* Neuritis, optic
seventh or facial G51.8
newborn (birth injury) P11.3
sixth or abducent — *see* Strabismus, paralytic, sixth nerve
tenth or vagus G52.2
third or oculomotor — *see* Strabismus, paralytic, third nerve
twelfth or hypoglossal G52.3
Déjérine-Sottas G60.0
diabetic (mononeuropathy) — *see* E08-E13 with .41
polyneuropathy — *see* E08-E13 with .42
due to
beriberi E51.11
displacement, prolapse or rupture, intervertebral disc — *see* Disorder, disc, with, radiculopathy
herniation, nucleus pulposus M51.9 *[G55]*
endemic E51.11
facial G51.8
newborn (birth injury) P11.3
general — *see* Polyneuropathy
geniculate ganglion G51.1
due to herpes (zoster) B02.21
gouty — *see also* Gout, by type M10.9 *[G63]*
hypoglossal (nerve) G52.3
ilioinguinal (nerve) G57.9- ☑
infectious (multiple) NEC G61.0
interstitial hypertrophic progressive G60.0
lumbar M54.16
lumbosacral M54.17
multiple — *see also* Polyneuropathy
endemic E51.11
infective, acute G61.0
multiplex endemica E51.11
nerve root — *see* Radiculopathy
oculomotor (nerve) — *see* Strabismus, paralytic, third nerve
olfactory nerve G52.0
optic (nerve) (hereditary) (sympathetic) H46.9
with demyelination G36.0
in myelitis G36.0
nutritional H46.2
papillitis — *see* Papillitis, optic
retrobulbar H46.1- ☑
specified type NEC H46.8
toxic H46.3
peripheral (nerve) G62.9
multiple — *see* Polyneuropathy
single — *see* Mononeuritis
pneumogastric (nerve) G52.2
postherpetic, postzoster B02.29
progressive hypertrophic interstitial G60.0
retrobulbar — *see also* Neuritis, optic, retrobulbar
in (due to)
late syphilis A52.15
meningococcal infection A39.82
meningococcal A39.82
syphilitic A52.15
sciatic (nerve) — *see also* Sciatica
due to displacement of intervertebral disc — *see* Disorder, disc, with, radiculopathy
serum — *see also* Reaction, serum T80.69 ☑
shoulder-girdle G54.5
specified nerve NEC G58.8
spinal (nerve) root — *see* Radiculopathy
syphilitic A52.15

☑ Additional Character Required — Refer to the Tabular List for Character Selection

Neuritis — *continued*
  thenar (median) G56.1- ☑
  thoracic M54.14
  toxic NEC G62.2
  trochlear (nerve) — *see* Strabismus, paralytic, fourth
      nerve
  vagus (nerve) G52.2
Neuroastrocytoma — *see* Neoplasm, uncertain behavior,
      by site
Neuroavitaminosis E56.9 *[G99.8]*
Neuroblastoma
  olfactory C30.0
  specified site — *see* Neoplasm, malignant, by site
  unspecified site C74.90
Neurochorioretinitis — *see* Chorioretinitis
Neurocirculatory asthenia F45.8
Neurocysticercosis B69.0
Neurocytoma — *see* Neoplasm, benign, by site
Neurodermatitis (circumscribed) (circumscripta) (local)
      L28.0
  atopic L20.81
  diffuse (Brocq) L20.81
  disseminated L20.81
Neuroencephalomyelopathy, optic G36.0
Neuroepithelioma — *see also* Neoplasm, malignant, by
      site
  olfactory C30.0
Neurofibroma — *see also* Neoplasm, nerve, benign
  melanotic — *see* Neoplasm, nerve, benign
  multiple — *see* Neurofibromatosis
  plexiform — *see* Neoplasm, nerve, benign
Neurofibromatosis (multiple) (nonmalignant) Q85.00
  acoustic Q85.02
  malignant — *see* Neoplasm, nerve, malignant
  specified NEC Q85.09
  type 1 (von Recklinghausen) Q85.01
  type 2 Q85.02
Neurofibrosarcoma — *see* Neoplasm, nerve, malignant
Neurogenic — *see also* condition
  bladder — *see also* Dysfunction, bladder, neuromuscu-
      lar N31.9
    cauda equina syndrome G83.4
  bowel NEC K59.2
  heart F45.8
Neuroglioma — *see* Neoplasm, uncertain behavior, by
      site
Neurolabyrinthitis (of Dix and Hallpike) — *see* Neuroni-
      tis, vestibular
Neurolathyrism — *see* Poisoning, food, noxious, plant
Neuroleprosy A30.9
Neuroma — *see also* Neoplasm, nerve, benign
  acoustic (nerve) D33.3
  amputation (stump) (traumatic) (surgical complication)
      (late) T87.3- ☑
    arm T87.3- ☑
    leg T87.3- ☑
  digital (toe) G57.6- ☑
  interdigital G58.8
    lower limb (toe) G57.8- ☑
    upper limb G56.8- ☑
  intermetatarsal G57.8- ☑
  Morton's G57.6- ☑
  nonneoplastic
    arm G56.9- ☑
    leg G57.9- ☑
    lower extremity G57.9- ☑
    upper extremity G56.9- ☑
  optic (nerve) D33.3
  plantar G57.6- ☑
  plexiform — *see* Neoplasm, nerve, benign
  surgical (nonneoplastic)
    arm G56.9- ☑
    leg G57.9- ☑
    lower extremity G57.9- ☑
    upper extremity G56.9- ☑
Neuromyalgia — *see* Neuralgia
Neuromyasthenia (epidemic) (postinfectious) G93.39
Neuromyelitis G36.9
  ascending G61.0
  optica G36.0
Neuromyopathy G70.9
  paraneoplastic D49.9 *[G13.0]*
Neuromyotonia (Isaacs) G71.19
Neuronevus — *see* Nevus
Neuronitis G58.9
  ascending (acute) G57.2- ☑
  vestibular H81.2- ☑

Neuroparalytic — *see* condition
Neuropathy, neuropathic G62.9
  acute motor G62.81
  alcoholic G62.1
    with psychosis — *see* Psychosis, alcoholic
  arm G56.9- ☑
  autonomic, peripheral — *see* Neuropathy, peripheral,
      autonomic
  axillary G56.9- ☑
  bladder N31.9
    atonic (motor) (sensory) N31.2
    autonomous N31.2
    flaccid N31.2
    nonreflex N31.2
    reflex N31.1
    uninhibited N31.0
  brachial plexus G54.0
  cervical plexus G54.2
  chronic
    progressive segmentally demyelinating G62.89
    relapsing demyelinating G62.89
  Déjérine-Sottas G60.0
  diabetic — *see* E08-E13 with .40
    mononeuropathy — *see* E08-E13 with .41
    polyneuropathy — *see* E08-E13 with .42
  entrapment G58.9
    iliohypogastric nerve G57.8- ☑
    ilioinguinal nerve G57.8- ☑
    lateral cutaneous nerve of thigh G57.1- ☑
    median nerve G56.0- ☑
    obturator nerve G57.8- ☑
    peroneal nerve G57.3- ☑
    posterior tibial nerve G57.5- ☑
    saphenous nerve G57.8- ☑
    ulnar nerve G56.2- ☑
  facial nerve G51.9
  hereditary G60.9
    motor and sensory (types I-IV) G60.0
    sensory G60.8
    specified NEC G60.8
  hypertrophic G60.0
    Charcot-Marie-Tooth G60.0
    Déjérine-Sottas G60.0
    interstitial progressive G60.0
    of infancy G60.0
    Refsum G60.1
  idiopathic G60.9
    progressive G60.3
    specified NEC G60.8
  in association with hereditary ataxia G60.2
  intercostal G58.0
  ischemic — *see* Disorder, nerve
  Jamaica (ginger) G62.2
  leg NEC G57.9- ☑
  lower extremity G57.9- ☑
  lumbar plexus G54.1
  median nerve G56.1- ☑
  motor and sensory — *see also* Polyneuropathy
    hereditary (types I-IV) G60.0
  multifocal motor (MMN) G61.82
  multiple (acute) (chronic) — *see* Polyneuropathy
  optic (nerve) — *see also* Neuritis, optic
    ischemic H47.01- ☑
  paraneoplastic (sensorial) (Denny Brown) D49.9 *[G13.0]*
  peripheral (nerve) — *see also* Polyneuropathy G62.9
    autonomic G90.9
      idiopathic G90.09
      in (due to)
        amyloidosis E85.4 *[G99.0]*
        diabetes mellitus — *see* E08-E13 with .43
        endocrine disease NEC E34.9 *[G99.0]*
        gout M10.00 *[G99.0]*
        hyperthyroidism E05.90 *[G99.0]*
          with thyroid storm E05.91 *[G99.0]*
        metabolic disease NEC E88.9 *[G99.0]*
    idiopathic G60.9
      progressive G60.3
    in (due to)
      antitetanus serum G62.0
      arsenic G62.2
      drugs NEC G62.0
      lead G62.2
      organophosphate compounds G62.2
      toxic agent NEC G62.2
  plantar nerves G57.6- ☑
  progressive
    hypertrophic interstitial G60.0

Neuropathy, neuropathic — *continued*
  progressive — *continued*
    inflammatory G62.81
  radicular NEC — *see* Radiculopathy
  sacral plexus G54.1
  sciatic G57.0- ☑
  serum G61.1
  toxic NEC G62.2
  trigeminal sensory G50.8
  ulnar nerve G56.2- ☑
  uremic N18.9 *[G63]*
  vitamin B12 E53.8 *[G63]*
    with anemia (pernicious) D51.0 *[G63]*
      due to dietary deficiency D51.3 *[G63]*
Neurophthisis — *see also* Disorder, nerve
  peripheral, diabetic — *see* E08-E13 with .42
Neuroretinitis — *see* Chorioretinitis
Neuroretinopathy, hereditary optic H47.22
Neurosarcoma — *see* Neoplasm, nerve, malignant
Neurosclerosis — *see* Disorder, nerve
Neurosis, neurotic F48.9
  anankastic F42.8
  anxiety (state) F41.1
    panic type F41.0
  asthenic F48.8
  bladder F45.8
  cardiac (reflex) F45.8
  cardiovascular F45.8
  character F60.9
  colon F45.8
  compensation F68.10
  compulsive, compulsion F42.8
  conversion F44.9
  craft F48.8
  cutaneous F45.8
  depersonalization F48.1
  depressive (reaction) (type) F34.1
  environmental F48.8
  excoriation L98.1
  fatigue F48.8
  functional — *see* Disorder, somatoform
  gastric F45.8
  gastrointestinal F45.8
  heart F45.8
  hypochondriacal F45.21
  hysterical F44.9
  incoordination F45.8
    larynx F45.8
    vocal cord F45.8
  intestine F45.8
  larynx (sensory) F45.8
    hysterical F44.4
  mixed NEC F48.8
  musculoskeletal F45.8
  obsessional F42.8
  obsessive-compulsive F42.8
  occupational F48.8
  ocular NEC F45.8
  organ — *see* Disorder, somatoform
  pharynx F45.8
  phobic F40.9
  posttraumatic (situational) F43.10
    acute F43.11
    chronic F43.12
  psychasthenic (type) F48.8
  railroad F48.8
  rectum F45.8
  respiratory F45.8
  rumination F45.8
  sexual F65.9
  situational F48.8
  social F40.10
    generalized F40.11
  specified type NEC F48.8
  state F48.9
    with depersonalization episode F48.1
  stomach F45.8
  traumatic F43.10
    acute F43.11
    chronic F43.12
  vasomotor F45.8
  visceral F45.8
  war F48.8
Neurospongioblastosis diffusa Q85.1
Neurosyphilis (arrested) (early) (gumma) (late) (latent)
      (recurrent) (relapse) A52.3
  with ataxia (cerebellar) (locomotor) (spastic) (spinal)
      A52.19

Neurosyphilis — *continued*
 aneurysm (cerebral) A52.05
 arachnoid (adhesive) A52.13
 arteritis (any artery) (cerebral) A52.04
 asymptomatic A52.2
 congenital A50.40
 dura (mater) A52.13
 general paresis A52.17
 hemorrhagic A52.05
 juvenile (asymptomatic) (meningeal) A50.40
 leptomeninges (aseptic) A52.13
 meningeal, meninges (adhesive) A52.13
 meningitis A52.13
 meningovascular (diffuse) A52.13
 optic atrophy A52.15
 parenchymatous (degenerative) A52.19
 paresis, paretic A52.17
  juvenile A50.45
 remission in (sustained) A52.3
 serological (without symptoms) A52.2
 specified nature or site NEC A52.19
 tabes, tabetic (dorsalis) A52.11
  juvenile A50.45
 taboparesis A52.17
  juvenile A50.45
 thrombosis (cerebral) A52.05
 vascular (cerebral) NEC A52.05
Neurothekeoma — *see* Neoplasm, nerve, benign
Neurotic — *see* Neurosis
Neurotoxemia — *see* Toxemia
Neutroclusion M26.211
Neutropenia, neutropenic (chronic) (genetic) (idiopathic) (immune) (infantile) (malignant) (pernicious) (splenic) D70.9
 congenital (primary) D70.0
 cyclic D70.4
 cytoreductive cancer chemotherapy sequela D70.1
 drug-induced D70.2
  due to cytoreductive cancer chemotherapy D70.1
 due to infection D70.3
 fever D70.9
 neonatal, transitory (isoimmune) (maternal transfer) P61.5
 periodic D70.4
 secondary (cyclic) (periodic) (splenic) D70.4
  drug-induced D70.2
   due to cytoreductive cancer chemotherapy D70.1
 toxic D70.8
Neutrophilia, hereditary giant D72.0
Nevocarcinoma — *see* Melanoma
Nevus D22.9
 achromic — *see* Neoplasm, skin, benign
 amelanotic — *see* Neoplasm, skin, benign
 angiomatous D18.00
  intra-abdominal D18.03
  intracranial D18.02
  skin D18.01
  specified site NEC D18.09
 araneus I78.1
 balloon cell — *see* Neoplasm, skin, benign
 bathing trunk D48.5
 blue — *see* Neoplasm, skin, benign
  cellular — *see* Neoplasm, skin, benign
  giant — *see* Neoplasm, skin, benign
  Jadassohn's — *see* Neoplasm, skin, benign
  malignant — *see* Melanoma
 capillary D18.00
  intra-abdominal D18.03
  intracranial D18.02
  skin D18.01
  specified site NEC D18.09
 cavernous D18.00
  intra-abdominal D18.03
  intracranial D18.02
  skin D18.01
  specified site NEC D18.09
 cellular — *see* Neoplasm, skin, benign
  blue — *see* Neoplasm, skin, benign
 choroid D31.3- ☑
 comedonicus Q82.5
 conjunctiva D31.0- ☑
 dermal — *see* Neoplasm, skin, benign
  with epidermal nevus — *see* Neoplasm, skin, benign
 dysplastic — *see* Neoplasm, skin, benign
 eye D31.9- ☑
 flammeus Q82.5
 hemangiomatous D18.00
  intra-abdominal D18.03

Nevus — *continued*
 hemangiomatous — *continued*
  intracranial D18.02
  skin D18.01
  specified site NEC D18.09
 iris D31.4- ☑
 lacrimal gland D31.5- ☑
 lymphatic D18.1
 magnocellular
  specified site — *see* Neoplasm, benign, by site
  unspecified site D31.40
 malignant — *see* Melanoma
 meaning hemangioma D18.00
  intra-abdominal D18.03
  intracranial D18.02
  skin D18.01
  specified site NEC D18.09
 mouth (mucosa) D10.30
  specified site NEC D10.39
  white sponge Q38.6
 multiplex Q85.1
 non-neoplastic I78.1
 oral mucosa D10.30
  specified site NEC D10.39
  white sponge Q38.6
 orbit D31.6- ☑
 pigmented
  giant — *see also* Neoplasm, skin, uncertain behavior D48.5
   malignant melanoma in — *see* Melanoma
 portwine Q82.5
 retina D31.2- ☑
 retrobulbar D31.6- ☑
 sanguineous Q82.5
 senile I78.1
 skin D22.9
  abdominal wall D22.5
  ala nasi D22.39
  ankle D22.7- ☑
  anus, anal D22.5
  arm D22.6- ☑
  auditory canal (external) D22.2- ☑
  auricle (ear) D22.2- ☑
  auricular canal (external) D22.2- ☑
  axilla, axillary fold D22.5
  back D22.5
  breast D22.5
  brow D22.39
  buttock D22.5
  canthus (eye) D22.1- ☑
  cheek (external) D22.39
  chest wall D22.5
  chin D22.39
  ear (external) D22.2- ☑
  external meatus (ear) D22.2- ☑
  eyebrow D22.39
  eyelid (lower) (upper) D22.1- ☑
  face D22.30
   specified NEC D22.39
  female genital organ (external) NEC D28.0
  finger D22.6- ☑
  flank D22.5
  foot D22.7- ☑
  forearm D22.6- ☑
  forehead D22.39
  foreskin D29.0
  genital organ (external) NEC
   female D28.0
   male D29.9
  gluteal region D22.5
  groin D22.5
  hand D22.6- ☑
  heel D22.7- ☑
  helix D22.2- ☑
  hip D22.7- ☑
  interscapular region D22.5
  jaw D22.39
  knee D22.7- ☑
  labium (majus) (minus) D28.0
  leg D22.7- ☑
  lip (lower) (upper) D22.0
  lower limb D22.7- ☑
  male genital organ (external) D29.9
  nail D22.9
   finger D22.6- ☑
   toe D22.7- ☑
  nasolabial groove D22.39
  nates D22.5

Nevus — *continued*
 skin — *continued*
  neck D22.4
  nose (external) D22.39
  palpebra D22.1- ☑
  penis D29.0
  perianal skin D22.5
  perineum D22.5
  pinna D22.2- ☑
  popliteal fossa or space D22.7- ☑
  prepuce D29.0
  pudendum D28.0
  scalp D22.4
  scrotum D29.4
  shoulder D22.6- ☑
  submammary fold D22.5
  temple D22.39
  thigh D22.7- ☑
  toe D22.7- ☑
  trunk NEC D22.5
  umbilicus D22.5
  upper limb D22.6- ☑
  vulva D28.0
 specified site NEC — *see* Neoplasm, by site, benign
 spider I78.1
 stellar I78.1
 strawberry Q82.5
 Sutton's benign D22.9
 temporal site NEC — *see* Neoplasm, by site, benign
 unius lateris Q82.5
 Unna's Q82.5
 vascular Q82.5
 verrucous Q82.5
Newborn (infant) (liveborn) (singleton) Z38.2
 abstinence syndrome P96.1
 acne L70.4
 affected by
  abnormalities of membranes P02.9
   specified NEC P02.8
  abruptio placenta P02.1
  amino-acid metabolic disorder, transitory P74.8
  amniocentesis (while in utero) P00.6
  amnionitis P02.78
  apparent life threatening event (ALTE) R68.13
  bleeding (into)
   cerebral cortex P52.22
   germinal matrix P52.0
   ventricles P52.1
  breech delivery P03.0
  cardiac arrest P29.81
  cardiomyopathy I42.8
   congenital I42.4
  cerebral ischemia P91.0
  Cesarean delivery P03.4
  chemotherapy agents P04.11
  chorioamnionitis P02.78
  cocaine (crack) P04.41
  complications of labor and delivery P03.9
   specified NEC P03.89
  compression of umbilical cord NEC P02.5
  contracted pelvis P03.1
  cyanosis P28.2
  delivery P03.9
   Cesarean P03.4
   forceps P03.2
   vacuum extractor P03.3
  drugs of addiction P04.40
   cocaine P04.41
   hallucinogens P04.42
   specified drug NEC P04.49
  entanglement (knot) in umbilical cord P02.5
  environmental chemicals P04.6
  fetal (intrauterine)
   growth retardation P05.9
   inflammatory response syndrome (FIRS) P02.70
   malnutrition not light or small for gestational age P05.2
  FIRS (fetal inflammatory response syndrome) P02.70
  forceps delivery P03.2
  heart rate abnormalities
   bradycardia P29.12
   intrauterine P03.819
    before onset of labor P03.810
    during labor P03.811
   tachycardia P29.11
  hemorrhage (antepartum) P02.1
   cerebellar (nontraumatic) P52.6
   intracerebral (nontraumatic) P52.4
   intracranial (nontraumatic) P52.9

Newborn — *continued*
  affected by — *continued*
    hemorrhage — *continued*
      intracranial — *continued*
        specified NEC P52.8
        intraventricular (nontraumatic) P52.3
          grade 1 P52.0
          grade 2 P52.1
          grade 3 P52.21
          grade 4 P52.22
        posterior fossa (nontraumatic) P52.6
        subarachnoid (nontraumatic) P52.5
        subependymal P52.0
          with intracerebral extension P52.22
          with intraventricular extension P52.1
            with enlargment of ventricles P52.21
          without intraventricular extension P52.0
    hypoxic ischemic encephalopathy [HIE] P91.60
      mild P91.61
      moderate P91.62
      severe P91.63
    induction of labor P03.89
    intestinal perforation P78.0
    intrauterine (fetal) blood loss P50.9
      due to (from)
        cut end of co-twin cord P50.5
        hemorrhage into
          co-twin P50.3
            maternal circulation P50.4
        placenta P50.2
        ruptured cord blood P50.1
        vasa previa P50.0
      specified NEC P50.8
    intrauterine (fetal) hemorrhage P50.9
    intrauterine (in utero) procedure P96.5
    malpresentation (malposition) NEC P03.1
    maternal (complication of) (use of)
      alcohol P04.3
      amphetamines P04.16
      analgesia (maternal) P04.0
      anesthesia (maternal) P04.0
      anticonvulsants P04.13
      antidepressants P04.15
      antineoplastic chemotherapy P04.11
      anxiolytics P04.1A
      blood loss P02.1
      cannabis P04.81
      circulatory disease P00.3
      condition P00.9
        specified NEC P00.89
      cytotoxic drugs P04.12
      delivery P03.9
        Cesarean P03.4
        forceps P03.2
        vacuum extractor P03.3
      diabetes mellitus (pre-existing) P70.1
      disorder P00.9
        specified NEC P00.89
      drugs (addictive) (illegal) NEC P04.49
      ectopic pregnancy P01.4
      gestational diabetes P70.0
      group B streptococcus (GBS) colonization (positive) P00.82
      hemorrhage P02.1
      hypertensive disorder P00.0
      incompetent cervix P01.0
      infectious disease P00.2
      injury P00.5
      labor and delivery P03.9
      malpresentation before labor P01.7
      maternal death P01.6
      medical procedure P00.7
      medication P04.19
        specified type NEC P04.18
      multiple pregnancy P01.5
      nutritional disorder P00.4
      oligohydramnios P01.2
      opiates P04.14
        administered for procedures during pregnancy or labor and delivery P04.0
      parasitic disease P00.2
      periodontal disease P00.81
      placenta previa P02.0
      polyhydramnios P01.3
      precipitate delivery P03.5
      pregnancy P01.9
        specified P01.8
      premature rupture of membranes P01.1
      renal disease P00.1

Newborn — *continued*
  affected by — *continued*
    maternal — *continued*
      respiratory disease P00.3
      sedative-hypnotics P04.17
      surgical procedure P00.6
      tranquilizers administered for procedures during pregnancy or labor and delivery P04.0
      urinary tract disease P00.1
      uterine contraction (abnormal) P03.6
    meconium peritonitis P78.0
    medication (legal) (maternal use) (prescribed) P04.19
    membrane abnormalities P02.9
      specified NEC P02.8
    membranitis P02.78
    methamphetamine(s) P04.49
    mixed metabolic and respiratory acidosis P84
    neonatal abstinence syndrome P96.1
    noxious substances transmitted via placenta or breast milk P04.9
      cannabis P04.81
      specified NEC P04.89
    nutritional supplements P04.5
    placenta previa P02.0
    placental
      abnormality (functional) (morphological) P02.20
        specified NEC P02.29
      dysfunction P02.29
      infarction P02.29
      insufficiency P02.29
      separation NEC P02.1
      transfusion syndromes P02.3
    placentitis P02.78
    precipitate delivery P03.5
    prolapsed cord P02.4
    respiratory arrest P28.81
    slow intrauterine growth P05.9
    tobacco P04.2
    twin to twin transplacental transfusion P02.3
    umbilical cord (tightly) around neck P02.5
    umbilical cord condition P02.60
      short cord P02.69
      specified NEC P02.69
    uterine contractions (abnormal) P03.6
    vasa previa P02.69
      from intrauterine blood loss P50.0
  apnea — *see also* Apnea, newborn P28.40
    obstructive P28.42
    primary — *see also* Apnea, newborn, sleep, primary P28.30
    sleep (central) (obstructive) (primary) — *see also* Apnea, newborn, sleep, primary P28.30
  born in hospital Z38.00
    by cesarean Z38.01
  born outside hospital Z38.1
  breast buds P96.89
  breast engorgement P83.4
  check-up — *see* Newborn, examination
  convulsion P90
  dehydration P74.1
  examination
    8 to 28 days old Z00.111
    under 8 days old Z00.110
  fever P81.9
    environmentally-induced P81.0
  hyperbilirubinemia P59.9
    of prematurity P59.0
  hypernatremia P74.21
  hyponatremia P74.22
  infection P39.9
    candidal P37.5
    specified NEC P39.8
    urinary tract P39.3
  jaundice P59.9
    due to
      breast milk inhibitor P59.3
      hepatocellular damage P59.20
        specified NEC P59.29
      preterm delivery P59.0
    of prematurity P59.0
    specified NEC P59.8
  late metabolic acidosis P74.0
  mastitis P39.0
    infective P39.0
    noninfective P83.4
  multiple born NEC Z38.8
    born in hospital Z38.68
      by cesarean Z38.69

Newborn — *continued*
  multiple born — *continued*
    born outside hospital Z38.7
  omphalitis P38.9
    with mild hemorrhage P38.1
    without hemorrhage P38.9
  post-term P08.21
  prolonged gestation (over 42 completed weeks) P08.22
  quadruplet Z38.8
    born in hospital Z38.63
      by cesarean Z38.64
    born outside hospital Z38.7
  quintuplet Z38.8
    born in hospital Z38.65
      by cesarean Z38.66
    born outside hospital Z38.7
  seizure P90
  sepsis (congenital) P36.9
    due to
      anaerobes NEC P36.5
      Escherichia coli P36.4
      Staphylococcus P36.30
        aureus P36.2
        specified NEC P36.39
      Streptococcus P36.10
        group B P36.0
        specified NEC P36.19
    specified NEC P36.8
  triplet Z38.8
    born in hospital Z38.61
      by cesarean Z38.62
    born outside hospital Z38.7
  twin Z38.5
    born in hospital Z38.30
      by cesarean Z38.31
    born outside hospital Z38.4
  vomiting P92.09
    bilious P92.01
  weight check Z00.111
Newcastle conjunctivitis or disease B30.8
Nezelof's syndrome (pure alymphocytosis) D81.4
Niacin (amide) **deficiency** E52
Nicolas (-Durand)-**Favre disease** A55
Nicotine — *see* Tobacco
Nicotinic acid deficiency E52
Niemann-Pick disease or syndrome E75.249
  specified NEC E75.248
  type
    A E75.240
    A/B E75.244
    B E75.241
    C E75.242
    D E75.243
Night
  blindness — *see* Blindness, night
  sweats R61
  terrors (child) F51.4
Nightmares (REM sleep type) F51.5
NIHSS (National Institutes of Health Stroke Scale) **score** R29.7- ☑
Nipple — *see* condition
Nisbet's chancre A57
Nishimoto (-Takeuchi) **disease** I67.5
Nitritoid crisis or reaction — *see* Crisis, nitritoid
Nitrosohemoglobinemia D74.8
Njovera A65
No general equivalence degree (GED) Z55.5
Nocardiosis, nocardiasis A43.9
  cutaneous A43.1
  lung A43.0
  pneumonia A43.0
  pulmonary A43.0
  specified site NEC A43.8
Nocturia R35.1
  psychogenic F45.8
Nocturnal — *see* condition
Nodal rhythm I49.8
Node(s) — *see also* Nodule
  Bouchard's (with arthropathy) M15.2
  Haygarth's M15.8
  Heberden's (with arthropathy) M15.1
  larynx J38.7
  lymph — *see* condition
  milker's B08.03
  Osler's I33.0
  Schmorl's — *see* Schmorl's disease
  singer's J38.2
  teacher's J38.2

Node(s) — *continued*
  tuberculous — *see* Tuberculosis, lymph gland
  vocal cord J38.2
Nodule(s), nodular
  actinomycotic — *see* Actinomycosis
  breast NEC — *see also* Lump, breast N63.Ø
  colloid (cystic), thyroid EØ4.1
  cutaneous — *see* Swelling, localized
  endometrial (stromal) D26.1
  Haygarth's M15.8
  inflammatory — *see* Inflammation
  juxta-articular
    syphilitic A52.77
    yaws A66.7
  larynx J38.7
  lung, solitary (subsegmental branch of the bronchial
    tree) R91.1
    multiple R91.8
  milker's BØ8.Ø3
  prostate N4Ø.2
    with lower urinary tract symptoms (LUTS) N4Ø.3
    without lower urinary tract symtpoms (LUTS) N4Ø.2
  pulmonary, solitary (subsegmental branch of the
    bronchial tree) R91.1
  retrocardiac RØ9.89
  rheumatoid MØ6.3Ø
    ankle MØ6.37- ☑
    elbow MØ6.32- ☑
    foot joint MØ6.37- ☑
    hand joint MØ6.34- ☑
    hip MØ6.35- ☑
    knee MØ6.36- ☑
    multiple site MØ6.39
    shoulder MØ6.31- ☑
    vertebra MØ6.38
    wrist MØ6.33- ☑
  scrotum (inflammatory) N49.2
  singer's J38.2
  solitary, lung (subsegmental branch of the bronchial
    tree) R91.1
    multiple R91.8
  subcutaneous — *see* Swelling, localized
  teacher's J38.2
  thyroid (cold) (gland) (nontoxic) EØ4.1
    with thyrotoxicosis EØ5.2Ø
      with thyroid storm EØ5.21
    toxic or with hyperthyroidism EØ5.2Ø
      with thyroid storm EØ5.21
  vocal cord J38.2
Noma (gangrenous) (hospital) (infective) A69.Ø
  auricle I96
  mouth A69.Ø
  pudendi N76.89
  vulvae N76.89
Nomad, nomadism Z59.ØØ
NOMID (neonatal onset multisystemic inflammatory disorder) MØ4.2
Nonadherence to medical treatment, specified NEC
  Z91.199
  due to
    financial hardship Z91.19Ø
    specified reason NEC Z91.198
Nonautoimmune hemolytic anemia D59.4
  drug-induced D59.2
Nonclosure — *see also* Imperfect, closure
  ductus arteriosus (Botallo's) Q25.Ø
  foramen
    botalli Q21.12
    ovale Q21.12
Noncompliance Z91.199
  with
    dialysis Z91.15
    dietary regimen Z91.119
      due to
        financial hardship Z91.11Ø
        specified reason NEC Z91.118
    medical treatment, specified NEC Z91.199
      due to
        financial hardship Z91.19Ø
        specified reason NEC Z91.198
    medication regimen NEC Z91.14
      underdosing — *see also* Table of Drugs and
        Chemicals, categories T36-T5Ø, with final
        character 6 Z91.14
        intentional NEC Z91.128
          by caregiver Z91.A4
            due to
              financial hardship Z91.A2Ø

Noncompliance — *continued*
  with — *continued*
    medication regimen — *continued*
      underdosing — *see also* Table of Drugs and
        Chemicals, categories T36-T5Ø, with final
        character 6 — *continued*
        intentional — *continued*
          by caregiver — *continued*
            due to — *continued*
              specified reason NEC Z91.A28
            due to financial hardship of patient
              Z91.12Ø
        unintentional NEC Z91.138
          by caregiver Z91.A3
          due to patient's age related debility
            Z91.13Ø
    renal dialysis Z91.15
  caregiver
    with patient's
      dietary regimen
        due to
          financial hardship Z91.A1Ø
          specified reason NEC Z91.A18
      medical treatment and regimen Z91.A9
      medication regimen, specified NEC Z91.A4
      renal dialysis Z91.A5
Nondescent (congenital) — *see also* Malposition, congenital
  cecum Q43.3
  colon Q43.3
  testicle Q53.9
    bilateral Q53.2Ø
      abdominal Q53.211
      perineal Q53.22
    unilateral Q53.1Ø
      abdominal Q53.111
      perineal Q53.12
Nondevelopment
  brain QØ2
    part of QØ4.3
  heart Q24.8
  organ or site, congenital NEC — *see* Hypoplasia
Nonengagement
  head NEC O32.4 ☑
    in labor, causing obstructed labor O64.8 ☑
Nonexanthematous tick fever A93.2
Nonexpansion, lung (newborn) P28.Ø
Nonfunctioning
  cystic duct — *see also* Disease, gallbladder K82.8
  gallbladder — *see also* Disease, gallbladder K82.8
  kidney N28.9
  labyrinth — *see* subcategory H83.2 ☑
Non-Hodgkin lymphoma NEC — *see* Lymphoma, non-Hodgkin
Nonimplantation, ovum N97.2
Noninsufflation, fallopian tube N97.1
Non-ketotic hyperglycinemia E72.51
Nonne-Milroy syndrome Q82.Ø
Nonovulation N97.Ø
Non-palpable testicle(s)
  bilateral R39.84
  unilateral R39.83
Nonpatent fallopian tube N97.1
Nonpneumatization, lung NEC P28.Ø
Nonrotation — *see* Malrotation
Nonsecretion, urine — *see* Anuria
Nonunion
  fracture — *see* Fracture, by site
  joint, following fusion or arthrodesis M96.Ø
  organ or site, congenital NEC — *see* Imperfect, closure
  symphysis pubis, congenital Q74.2
Nonvisualization, gallbladder R93.2
Nonvital, nonvitalized tooth KØ4.99
Non-working side interference M26.56
Noonan's syndrome Q87.19
Normocytic anemia (infectional) due to blood loss
  (chronic) D5Ø.Ø
  acute D62
Norrie's disease (congenital) Q15.8
North American blastomycosis B4Ø.9
Norwegian itch B86
Nose, nasal — *see* condition
Nosebleed RØ4.Ø
Nose-picking F98.8
Nosomania F45.21
Nosophobia F45.22
Nostalgia F43.2Ø

Notch of iris Q13.2
Notching nose, congenital (tip) Q3Ø.2
Nothnagel's
  syndrome — *see* Strabismus, paralytic, third nerve
  vasomotor acroparesthesia I73.89
Novy's relapsing fever A68.9
  louse-borne A68.Ø
  tick-borne A68.1
Noxious
  foodstuffs, poisoning by — *see* Poisoning, food, noxious, plant
  substances transmitted through placenta or breast milk
    PØ4.9
Nucleus pulposus — *see* condition
Numbness R2Ø.Ø
Nuns' knee — *see* Bursitis, prepatellar
Nursemaid's elbow S53.Ø3- ☑
Nutcracker esophagus K22.4
Nutmeg liver K76.1
Nutrient element deficiency E61.9
  specified NEC E61.8
Nutrition deficient or insufficient — *see also* Malnutrition E63.9
  due to
    insufficient food T73.Ø ☑
    lack of
      care (child) T76.Ø2 ☑
        adult T76.Ø1 ☑
      food T73.Ø ☑
    specific element deficiency — *see* Nutrient element
      deficiency, or by element
  sequelae — *see* Sequalae, nutritional deficiency
  specified NEC E63.8
Nutritional stunting E45
Nyctalopia (night blindness) — *see* Blindness, night
Nycturia R35.1
  psychogenic F45.8
Nymphomania F52.8
Nystagmus H55.ØØ
  benign paroxysmal — *see* Vertigo, benign paroxysmal
  central positional H81.4
  congenital H55.Ø1
  dissociated H55.Ø4
  latent H55.Ø2
  miners' H55.Ø9
  positional
    benign paroxysmal H81.4
    central H81.4
  specified form NEC H55.Ø9
  visual deprivation H55.Ø3

O

Obermeyer's relapsing fever (European) A68.Ø
Obesity E66.9
  with alveolar hypoventilation E66.2
  adrenal E27.8
  complicating
    childbirth O99.214
    pregnancy O99.21- ☑
    puerperium O99.215
  constitutional E66.8
  dietary counseling and surveillance Z71.3
  drug-induced E66.1
  due to
    drug E66.1
    excess calories E66.Ø9
      morbid E66.Ø1
      severe E66.Ø1
  endocrine E66.8
  endogenous E66.8
  exogenous E66.Ø9
  familial E66.8
  glandular E66.8
  hypothyroid — *see* Hypothyroidism
  hypoventilation syndrome (OHS) E66.2
  morbid E66.Ø1
    with
      alveolar hypoventilation E66.2
      obesity hypoventilation syndrome (OHS) E66.2
    due to excess calories E66.Ø1
  nutritional E66.Ø9
  pituitary E23.6
  severe E66.Ø1
  specified type NEC E66.8
Oblique — *see* condition

Obliteration

appendix (lumen) K38.8
artery I77.1
bile duct (noncalculous) K83.1
common duct (noncalculous) K83.1
cystic duct — *see* Obstruction, gallbladder
disease, arteriolar I77.1
endometrium N85.8
eye, anterior chamber — *see* Disorder, globe, hypotony
fallopian tube N97.1
lymphatic vessel I89.0
  due to mastectomy I97.2
organ or site, congenital NEC — *see* Atresia, by site
ureter N13.5
  with infection N13.6
urethra — *see* Stricture, urethra
vein I87.8
vestibule (oral) K08.89

Observation (following) (for) (without need for further medical care) Z04.9

accident NEC Z04.3
  at work Z04.2
  transport Z04.1
adverse effect of drug Z03.6
alleged rape or sexual assault (victim), ruled out
  adult Z04.41
  child Z04.42
criminal assault Z04.89
development state
  adolescent Z00.3
  period of rapid growth in childhood Z00.2
  puberty Z00.3
disease, specified NEC Z03.89
following work accident Z04.2
forced sexual exploitation Z04.81
forced labor exploitation Z04.82
growth and development state — *see* Observation, development state
injuries (accidental) NEC — *see also* Observation, accident
newborn (for)
  suspected condition, related to exposure from the mother or birth process — *see* Newborn, affected by, maternal
  ruled out Z05.9
    cardiac Z05.0
    connective tissue Z05.73
    gastrointestinal Z05.5
    genetic Z05.41
    genitourinary Z05.6
    immunologic Z05.43
    infectious Z05.1
    metabolic Z05.42
    musculoskeletal Z05.72
    neurological Z05.2
    respiratory Z05.3
    skin and subcutaneous tissue Z05.71
    specified condition NEC Z05.8
postpartum
  immediately after delivery Z39.0
  routine follow-up Z39.2
pregnancy (normal) (without complication) Z34.9- ☑
  high risk O09.9- ☑
suicide attempt, alleged NEC Z03.89
  self-poisoning Z03.6
suspected, ruled out — *see also* Suspected condition, ruled out
  abuse, physical
    adult Z04.71
    child Z04.72
  accident at work Z04.2
  adult battering victim Z04.71
  child battering victim Z04.72
  condition NEC Z03.89
    newborn — *see also* Observation, newborn (for), suspected condition, ruled out Z05.9
  drug poisoning or adverse effect Z03.6
  exposure (to)
    anthrax Z03.810
    biological agent NEC Z03.818
  foreign body
    aspirated (inhaled) Z03.822
    ingested Z03.821
    inserted (injected), in (eye) (orifice) (skin) Z03.823
  inflicted injury NEC Z04.89
  suicide attempt, alleged Z03.89
    self-poisoning Z03.6

Observation — *continued*

suspected, ruled out — *see also* Suspected condition, ruled out — *continued*
  toxic effects from ingested substance (drug) (poison) Z03.6
  toxic effects from ingested substance (drug) (poison) Z03.6

Obsession, obsessional state F42.8

mixed thoughts and acts F42.2

Obsessive-compulsive neurosis or reaction F42.8

Obstetric embolism, septic — *see* Embolism, obstetric, septic

Obstetrical trauma (complicating delivery) O71.9
with or following ectopic or molar pregnancy O08.6
specified type NEC O71.89

Obstipation — *see* Constipation

Obstruction, obstructed, obstructive

airway J98.8
  with
    allergic alveolitis J67.9
    asthma J45.909
      with
        exacerbation (acute) J45.901
        status asthmaticus J45.902
    bronchiectasis J47.9
      with
        exacerbation (acute) J47.1
        lower respiratory infection J47.0
    bronchitis (chronic) J44.9
    emphysema J43.9
  chronic J44.9
    with
      allergic alveolitis — *see* Pneumonitis, hypersensitivity
      bronchiectasis J47.9
        with
          exacerbation (acute) J47.1
          lower respiratory infection J47.0
  due to
    foreign body — *see* Foreign body, by site, causing asphyxia
    inhalation of fumes or vapors J68.9
    laryngospasm J38.5
ampulla of Vater K83.1
aortic (heart) (valve) — *see* Stenosis, aortic
aortoiliac I74.09
aqueduct of Sylvius G91.1
  congenital Q03.0
    with spina bifida — *see* Spina bifida, by site, with hydrocephalus
Arnold-Chiari — *see* Arnold-Chiari disease
artery — *see also* Atherosclerosis, artery I70.9 ☑
  basilar (complete) (partial) — *see* Occlusion, artery, basilar
  carotid (complete) (partial) — *see* Occlusion, artery, carotid
  cerebellar — *see* Occlusion, artery, cerebellar
  cerebral (anterior) (middle) (posterior) — *see* Occlusion, artery, cerebral
  precerebral — *see* Occlusion, artery, precerebral
  renal N28.0
  retinal NEC — *see* Occlusion, artery, retina
  stent — *see* Restenosis, stent
  vertebral (complete) (partial) — *see* Occlusion, artery, vertebral
band (intestinal) — *see also* Obstruction, intestine, specified NEC K56.699
bile duct or passage (common) (hepatic) (noncalculous) K83.1
  with calculus K80.51
  congenital (causing jaundice) Q44.3
biliary (duct) (tract) K83.1
  gallbladder K82.0
bladder-neck (acquired) N32.0
  congenital Q64.31
  due to hyperplasia (hypertrophy) of prostate — *see* Hyperplasia, prostate
bowel — *see* Obstruction, intestine
bronchus J98.09
canal, ear — *see* Stenosis, external ear canal
cardia K22.2
caval veins (inferior) (superior) I87.1
cecum — *see* Obstruction, intestine
circulatory I99.8
colon — *see* Obstruction, intestine
common duct (noncalculous) K83.1
coronary (artery) — *see* Occlusion, coronary
cystic duct — *see also* Obstruction, gallbladder

Obstruction, obstructed, obstructive — *continued*

cystic duct — *see also* Obstruction, gallbladder — *continued*
  with calculus K80.21
device, implant or graft — *see also* Complications, by site and type, mechanical T85.698 ☑
  arterial graft NEC — *see* Complication, cardiovascular device, mechanical, vascular
  catheter NEC T85.628 ☑
    cystostomy T83.090 ☑
    dialysis (renal) T82.49 ☑
      intraperitoneal T85.691 ☑
    Hopkins T83.098 ☑
    ileostomy T83.098 ☑
    infusion NEC T82.594 ☑
      spinal (epidural) (subdural) T85.690 ☑
    nephrostomy T83.092 ☑
    urethral indwelling T83.091 ☑
    urinary T83.098 ☑
    urostomy T83.098 ☑
  due to infection T85.79 ☑
  gastrointestinal — *see* Complications, prosthetic device, mechanical, gastrointestinal device
  genital NEC T83.498 ☑
    intrauterine contraceptive device T83.39 ☑
    penile prosthesis (cylinder) (implanted) (pump) (resevoir) T83.490 ☑
    testicular prosthesis T83.491 ☑
  heart NEC — *see* Complication, cardiovascular device, mechanical
  joint prosthesis — *see* Complications, joint prosthesis, mechanical, specified NEC, by site
  orthopedic NEC — *see* Complication, orthopedic, device, mechanical
  specified NEC T85.628 ☑
  urinary NEC — *see also* Complication, genitourinary, device, urinary, mechanical
    graft T83.29 ☑
  vascular NEC — *see* Complication, cardiovascular device, mechanical
  ventricular intracranial shunt T85.09 ☑
due to foreign body accidentally left in operative wound T81.529 ☑
duodenum K31.5
ejaculatory duct N50.89
esophagus K22.2
eustachian tube (complete) (partial) H68.10- ☑
  cartilagenous (extrinsic) H68.13- ☑
    intrinsic H68.12- ☑
  osseous H68.11- ☑
fallopian tube (bilateral) N97.1
fecal K56.41
  with hernia — *see* Hernia, by site, with obstruction
foramen of Monro (congenital) Q03.8
  with spina bifida — *see* Spina bifida, by site, with hydrocephalus
foreign body — *see* Foreign body
gallbladder K82.0
  with calculus, stones K80.21
  congenital Q44.1
gastric outlet K31.1
gastrointestinal — *see* Obstruction, intestine
hepatic K76.89
  duct (noncalculous) K83.1
ileum — *see* Obstruction, intestine
iliofemoral (artery) I74.5
intestine K56.609
  with
    adhesions (intestinal) (peritoneal) K56.50
      complete K56.52
      incomplete K56.51
      partial K56.51
  adynamic K56.0
  by gallstone K56.3
  complete K56.601
  congenital (small) Q41.9
    large Q42.9
      specified part NEC Q42.8
  incomplete K56.600
  neurogenic K56.0
    Hirschsprung's disease or megacolon Q43.1
  newborn P76.9
    due to
      fecaliths P76.8
      inspissated milk P76.2
      meconium (plug) P76.0
        in mucoviscidosis E84.11

Obstruction, obstructed, obstructive — *continued*
  intestine — *continued*
    newborn — *continued*
      specified NEC P76.8
    partial K56.600
    postoperative K91.30
      complete K91.32
      incomplete K91.31
      partial K91.31
    reflex K56.0
    specified NEC K56.699
      complete K56.691
      incomplete K56.690
      partial K56.690
    volvulus K56.2
  intracardiac ball valve prosthesis T82.09 ☑
  jejunum — *see* Obstruction, intestine
  joint prosthesis — *see* Complications, joint prosthesis, mechanical, specified NEC, by site
  kidney (calices) — *see also* Hydronephrosis N28.89
  labor — *see* Delivery
  lacrimal (passages) (duct)
    by
      dacryolith — *see* Dacryolith
      stenosis — *see* Stenosis, lacrimal
    congenital Q10.5
    neonatal H04.53- ☑
  lacrimonasal duct — *see* Obstruction, lacrimal
  lacteal, with steatorrhea K90.2
  laryngitis — *see* Laryngitis
  larynx NEC J38.6
    congenital Q31.8
  lung J98.4
    disease, chronic J44.9
  lymphatic I89.0
  meconium (plug)
    newborn P76.0
      due to fecaliths P76.0
      in mucoviscidosis E84.11
  mitral — *see* Stenosis, mitral
  nasal J34.89
  nasolacrimal duct — *see also* Obstruction, lacrimal
    congenital Q10.5
  nasopharynx J39.2
  nose J34.89
  organ or site, congenital NEC — *see* Atresia, by site
  pancreatic duct K86.89
  parotid duct or gland K11.8
  pelviureteral junction N13.5
    with hydronephrosis N13.0
    congenital Q62.39
  pharynx J39.2
  portal (circulation) (vein) I81
  prostate — *see also* Hyperplasia, prostate
    valve (urinary) N32.0
  pulmonary valve (heart) I37.0
  pyelonephritis (chronic) N11.1
  pylorus
    adult K31.1
    congenital or infantile Q40.0
  rectosigmoid — *see* Obstruction, intestine
  rectum K62.4
  renal — *see also* Hydronephrosis N28.89
    outflow N13.8
    pelvis, congenital Q62.39
  respiratory J98.8
    chronic J44.9
  retinal (vessels) H34.9
  salivary duct (any) K11.8
    with calculus K11.5
  sigmoid — *see* Obstruction, intestine
  sinus (accessory) (nasal) J34.89
  Stensen's duct K11.8
  stomach NEC K31.89
    acute K31.0
    congenital Q40.2
    due to pylorospasm K31.3
  submandibular duct K11.8
  submaxillary gland K11.8
    with calculus K11.5
  thoracic duct I89.0
  thrombotic — *see* Thrombosis
  trachea J39.8
  tracheostomy airway J95.03
  tricuspid (valve) — *see* Stenosis, tricuspid
  upper respiratory, congenital Q34.8
  ureter (functional) (pelvic junction) NEC N13.5

Obstruction, obstructed, obstructive — *continued*
  ureter — *continued*
    with
      hydronephrosis N13.1
        with infection N13.6
        congenital Q62.39
      pyelonephritis (chronic) N11.1
    congenital Q62.39
    due to calculus — *see* Calculus, ureter
  urethra NEC N36.8
    congenital Q64.39
  urinary (moderate) N13.9
    due to hyperplasia (hypertrophy) of prostate — *see* Hyperplasia, prostate
    organ or tract (lower) N13.9
    prostatic valve N32.0
    specified NEC N13.8
  uropathy N13.9
  uterus N85.8
  vagina N89.5
  valvular — *see* Endocarditis
  vein, venous I87.1
    caval (inferior) (superior) I87.1
    thrombotic — *see* Thrombosis
  vena cava (inferior) (superior) I87.1
  vesical NEC N32.0
  vesicourethral orifice N32.0
    congenital Q64.31
  vessel NEC I99.8
    stent — *see* Restenosis, stent
Obturator — *see* condition
Occlusal wear, teeth K03.0
Occlusio pupillae — *see* Membrane, pupillary
Occlusion, occluded
  anus K62.4
    congenital Q42.3
      with fistula Q42.2
  aortoiliac (chronic) I74.09
  aqueduct of Sylvius G91.1
    congenital Q03.0
      with spina bifida — *see* Spina bifida, by site, with hydrocephalus
  artery — *see also* Atherosclerosis, artery I70.9 ☑
    auditory, internal I65.8
    basilar I65.1
      with
        infarction I63.22
          due to
            embolism I63.12
            thrombosis I63.02
    brain or cerebral I66.9
      with infarction (due to) I63.5- ☑
        embolism I63.4- ☑
        thrombosis I63.3- ☑
    carotid I65.2- ☑
      with
        infarction I63.23- ☑
          due to
            embolism I63.13- ☑
            thrombosis I63.03- ☑
    cerebellar (anterior inferior) (posterior inferior) (superior) I66.3
      with infarction I63.54- ☑
        due to
          embolism I63.44- ☑
          thrombosis I63.34- ☑
    cerebral I66.9
      with infarction I63.50
        due to
          embolism I63.40
            specified NEC I63.49
          thrombosis I63.30
            specified NEC I63.39
      anterior I66.1- ☑
        with infarction I63.52- ☑
          due to
            embolism I63.42- ☑
            thrombosis I63.32- ☑
      middle I66.0- ☑
        with infarction I63.51- ☑
          due to
            embolism I63.41- ☑
            thrombosis I63.31- ☑
      posterior I66.2- ☑
        with infarction I63.53- ☑
          due to
            embolism I63.43- ☑

Occlusion, occluded — *continued*
  artery — *see also* Atherosclerosis, artery — *continued*
    cerebral — *continued*
      posterior — *continued*
        with infarction — *continued*
          due to — *continued*
            thrombosis I63.33- ☑
        specified NEC I66.8
          with infarction I63.59
            due to
              embolism I63.4- ☑
              thrombosis I63.3- ☑
    choroidal (anterior) — *see* Occlusion, artery, precerebral, specified NEC
    communicating posterior — *see* Occlusion, artery, precerebral, specified NEC
    complete
      coronary I25.82
      extremities I70.92
    coronary (acute) (thrombotic) (without myocardial infarction) I24.0
      with myocardial infarction — *see* Infarction, myocardium
      chronic total I25.82
      complete I25.82
      healed or old I25.2
      total (chronic) I25.82
    hypophyseal — *see* Occlusion, artery, precerebral, specified NEC
    iliac I74.5
    lower extremities due to stenosis or stricture I77.1
    mesenteric (embolic) (thrombotic) — *see also* Infarct, intestine K55.069
    perforating — *see* Occlusion, artery, cerebral, specified NEC
    peripheral I77.9
      thrombotic or embolic I74.4
    pontine — *see* Occlusion, artery, precerebral, specified NEC
    precerebral I65.9
      with infarction I63.20
        specified NEC I63.29
        due to
          embolism I63.10
            specified NEC I63.19
          thrombosis I63.00
            specified NEC I63.09
      basilar — *see* Occlusion, artery, basilar
      carotid — *see* Occlusion, artery, carotid
      puerperal O88.23
      specified NEC I65.8
        with infarction I63.29
          due to
            embolism I63.19
            thrombosis I63.09
      vertebral — *see* Occlusion, artery, vertebral
    renal N28.0
    retinal
      branch H34.23- ☑
      central H34.1- ☑
      partial H34.21- ☑
      transient H34.0- ☑
    spinal — *see* Occlusion, artery, precerebral, vertebral
    total (chronic)
      coronary I25.82
      extremities I70.92
    vertebral I65.0- ☑
      with
        infarction I63.21- ☑
          due to
            embolism I63.11- ☑
            thrombosis I63.01- ☑
  basilar artery — *see* Occlusion, artery, basilar
  bile duct (common) (hepatic) (noncalculous) K83.1
  bowel — *see* Obstruction, intestine
  carotid (artery) (common) (internal) — *see* Occlusion, artery, carotid
  centric (of teeth) M26.59
    maximum intercuspation discrepancy M26.55
  cerebellar (artery) — *see* Occlusion, artery, cerebellar
  cerebral (artery) — *see* Occlusion, artery, cerebral
  cerebrovascular — *see also* Occlusion, artery, cerebral
    with infarction I63.5- ☑
  cervical canal — *see* Stricture, cervix
  cervix (uteri) — *see* Stricture, cervix
  choanal Q30.0

Occlusion, occluded — *continued*
  choroidal (artery) — *see* Occlusion, artery, precerebral, specified NEC
  colon — *see* Obstruction, intestine
  communicating posterior artery — *see* Occlusion, artery, precerebral, specified NEC
  coronary (artery) (vein) (thrombotic) — *see also* Infarct, myocardium
    chronic total I25.82
    healed or old I25.2
    not resulting in infarction I24.0
    total (chronic) I25.82
  cystic duct — *see* Obstruction, gallbladder
  embolic — *see* Embolism
  fallopian tube N97.1
    congenital Q50.6
  gallbladder — *see also* Obstruction, gallbladder
    congenital (causing jaundice) Q44.1
  gingiva, traumatic K06.2
  hymen N89.6
    congenital Q52.3
  hypophyseal (artery) — *see* Occlusion, artery, precerebral, specified NEC
  iliac artery I74.5
  intestine — *see* Obstruction, intestine
  lacrimal passages — *see* Obstruction, lacrimal
  lung J98.4
  lymph or lymphatic channel I89.0
  mammary duct N64.89
  mesenteric artery (embolic) (thrombotic) — *see also* Infarct, intestine K55.069
  nose J34.89
    congenital Q30.0
  organ or site, congenital NEC — *see* Atresia, by site
  oviduct N97.1
    congenital Q50.6
  peripheral arteries
    due to stricture or stenosis I77.1
    upper extremity I74.2
  pontine (artery) — *see* Occlusion, artery, precerebral, specified NEC
  posterior lingual, of mandibular teeth M26.29
  precerebral artery — *see* Occlusion, artery, precerebral
  punctum lacrimale — *see* Obstruction, lacrimal
  pupil — *see* Membrane, pupillary
  pylorus, adult — *see also* Stricture, pylorus K31.1
  renal artery N28.0
  retina, retinal
    artery — *see* Occlusion, artery, retinal
    vein (central) H34.81- ☑
      engorgement H34.82- ☑
      tributary H34.83- ☑
      vessels H34.9
  spinal artery — *see* Occlusion, artery, precerebral, vertebral
  teeth (mandibular) (posterior lingual) M26.29
  thoracic duct I89.0
  thrombotic — *see* Thrombosis, artery
  traumatic
    edentulous (alveolar) ridge K06.2
    gingiva K06.2
    periodontal K05.5
  tubal N97.1
  ureter (complete) (partial) N13.5
    congenital Q62.10
  ureteropelvic junction N13.5
    congenital Q62.11
  ureterovesical orifice N13.5
    congenital Q62.12
  urethra — *see* Stricture, urethra
  uterus N85.8
  vagina N89.5
  vascular NEC I99.8
  vein — *see* Thrombosis
    retinal — *see* Occlusion, retinal, vein
  vena cava (inferior) (superior) — *see* Embolism, vena cava
  ventricle (brain) NEC G91.1
  vertebral (artery) — *see* Occlusion, artery, vertebral
  vessel (blood) I99.8
  vulva N90.5
Occult
  blood in feces (stools) R19.5
Occupational
  problems NEC Z56.89
Ochlophobia — *see* Agoraphobia
Ochronosis (endogenous) E70.29
Ocular muscle — *see* condition

Oculogyric crisis or disturbance H51.8
  psychogenic F45.8
Oculomotor syndrome H51.9
Oculopathy
  syphilitic NEC A52.71
    congenital
      early A50.01
      late A50.30
    early (secondary) A51.43
    late A52.71
Oddi's sphincter spasm K83.4
Odontalgia K08.89
Odontoameloblastoma — *see* Cyst, calcifying odontogenic
Odontoclasia K03.89
Odontodysplasia, regional K00.4
Odontogenesis imperfecta K00.5
Odontoma (ameloblastic) (complex) (compound) (fibroameloblastic) — *see* Cyst, calcifying odontogenic
Odontomyelitis (closed) (open) K04.01
  irreversible K04.02
  reversible K04.01
Odontorrhagia K08.89
Odontosarcoma, ameloblastic C41.1
  upper jaw (bone) C41.0
Oestriasis — *see* Myiasis
Oguchi's disease H53.63
Ohara's disease — *see* Tularemia
OHS (obesity hypoventilation syndrome) E66.2
Oidiomycosis — *see* Candidiasis
Oidium albicans infection — *see* Candidiasis
Old age (without mention of debility) R54
  dementia F03 ☑
Old (previous) **myocardial infarction** I25.2
Olfactory — *see* condition
Oligemia — *see* Anemia
Oligoastrocytoma
  specified site — *see* Neoplasm, malignant, by site
  unspecified site C71.9
Oligocythemia D64.9
Oligodendroblastoma
  specified site — *see* Neoplasm, malignant
  unspecified site C71.9
Oligodendroglioma
  anaplastic type
    specified site — *see* Neoplasm, malignant, by site
    unspecified site C71.9
  specified site — *see* Neoplasm, malignant, by site
  unspecified site C71.9
Oligodontia — *see* Anodontia
Oligoencephalon Q02
Oligohidrosis L74.4
Oligohydramnios O41.0- ☑
Oligohydrosis L74.4
Oligomenorrhea N91.5
  primary N91.3
  secondary N91.4
Oligophrenia — *see also* Disability, intellectual
  phenylpyruvic E70.0
Oligospermia N46.11
  due to
    drug therapy N46.121
    efferent duct obstruction N46.123
    infection N46.122
    radiation N46.124
    specified cause NEC N46.129
    systemic disease N46.125
Oligotrichia — *see* Alopecia
Oliguria R34
  with, complicating or following ectopic or molar pregnancy O08.4
  postprocedural N99.0
Ollier's disease Q78.4
Omenotocele — *see* Hernia, abdomen, specified site NEC
Omentitis — *see* Peritonitis
Omentum, omental — *see* condition
Omphalitis (congenital) (newborn) P38.9
  with mild hemorrhage P38.1
  without hemorrhage P38.9
  not of newborn L08.82
  tetanus A33
Omphalocele Q79.2
Omphalomesenteric duct, persistent Q43.0
Omphalorrhagia, newborn P51.9
Omsk hemorrhagic fever A98.1
Onanism (excessive) F98.8
Onchocerciasis, onchocercosis B73.1

Onchocerciasis, onchocercosis — *continued*
  with
    eye disease B73.00
      endophthalmitis B73.01
      eyelid B73.09
      glaucoma B73.02
      specified NEC B73.09
    eyelid B73.09
    eye NEC B73.00
Oncocytoma — *see* Neoplasm, benign, by site
Oncovirus, as cause of disease classified elsewhere B97.32
Ondine's curse — *see* Apnea, sleep
Oneirophrenia F23
Onychauxis L60.2
  congenital Q84.5
Onychia — *see also* Cellulitis, digit
  with lymphangitis — *see* Lymphangitis, acute, digit
  candidal B37.2
  dermatophytic B35.1
Onychitis — *see also* Cellulitis, digit
  with lymphangitis — *see* Lymphangitis, acute, digit
Onychocryptosis L60.0
Onychodystrophy L60.3
  congenital Q84.6
Onychogryphosis, onychogryposis L60.2
Onycholysis L60.1
Onychomadesis L60.8
Onychomalacia L60.3
Onychomycosis (finger) (toe) B35.1
Onycho-osteodysplasia Q87.2
Onychophagia F98.8
Onychophosis L60.8
Onychoptosis L60.8
Onychorrhexis L60.3
  congenital Q84.6
Onychoschizia L60.3
Onyxis (finger) (toe) L60.0
Onyxitis — *see also* Cellulitis, digit
  with lymphangitis — *see* Lymphangitis, acute, digit
Oophoritis (cystic) (infectional) (interstitial) N70.92
  with salpingitis N70.93
  acute N70.02
    with salpingitis N70.03
  chronic N70.12
    with salpingitis N70.13
  complicating abortion — *see* Abortion, by type, complicated by, oophoritis
Oophorocele N83.4- ☑
Opacity, opacities
  cornea H17.- ☑
    central H17.1- ☑
    congenital Q13.3
    degenerative — *see* Degeneration, cornea
    hereditary — *see* Dystrophy, cornea
    inflammatory — *see* Keratitis
    minor H17.81- ☑
    peripheral H17.82- ☑
    sequelae of trachoma (healed) B94.0
    specified NEC H17.89
  enamel (teeth) (fluoride) (nonfluoride) K00.3
  lens — *see* Cataract
  snowball — *see* Deposit, crystalline
  vitreous (humor) NEC H43.39- ☑
    congenital Q14.0
    membranes and strands H43.31- ☑
Opalescent dentin (hereditary) K00.5
Open, opening
  abnormal, organ or site, congenital — *see* Imperfect, closure
  angle with
    borderline
      findings
        high risk H40.02- ☑
        low risk H40.01- ☑
      intraocular pressure H40.00- ☑
    cupping of discs H40.01- ☑
    glaucoma (primary) — *see* Glaucoma, open angle
  bite
    anterior M26.220
    posterior M26.221
  false — *see* Imperfect, closure
  margin on tooth restoration K08.51
  restoration margins of tooth K08.51
  wound — *see* Wound, open
Operational fatigue F48.8
Operative — *see* condition

Operculitis — see Periodontitis
Operculum — see Break, retina
Ophiasis L63.2
Ophthalmia — see also Conjunctivitis H10.9
   actinic rays — see Photokeratitis
   allergic (acute) — see Conjunctivitis, acute, atopic
   blennorrhagic (gonococcal) (neonatorum) A54.31
   diphtheritic A36.86
   Egyptian A71.1
   electrica — see Photokeratitis
   gonococcal (neonatorum) A54.31
   metastatic — see Endophthalmitis, purulent
   migraine — see Migraine, ophthalmoplegic
   neonatorum, newborn P39.1
      gonococcal A54.31
   nodosa H16.24- ☑
   purulent — see Conjunctivitis, acute, mucopurulent
   spring — see Conjunctivitis, acute, atopic
   sympathetic — see Uveitis, sympathetic
Ophthalmitis — see Ophthalmia
Ophthalmocele (congenital) Q15.8
Ophthalmoneuromyelitis G36.0
Ophthalmoplegia — see also Strabismus, paralytic
   anterior internuclear — see Ophthalmoplegia, internuclear
   ataxia-areflexia G61.0
   diabetic — see E08-E13 with .39
   exophthalmic E05.00
      with thyroid storm E05.01
   external H49.88- ☑
      progressive H49.4- ☑
         with pigmentary retinopathy — see Kearns-Sayre syndrome
      total H49.3- ☑
   internal (complete) (total) H52.51- ☑
   internuclear H51.2- ☑
   migraine — see Migraine, ophthalmoplegic
   Parinaud's H49.88- ☑
   progressive external — see Ophthalmoplegia, external, progressive
   supranuclear, progressive G23.1
   total (external) — see Ophthalmoplegia, external, total
Opioid(s)
   abuse — see Abuse, drug, opioids
   dependence — see Dependence, drug, opioids
   induced, without use disorder
      anxiety disorder F11.988
      delirium F11.921
      depressive disorder F11.94
      sexual dysfunction F11.981
      sleep disorder F11.982
Opisthognathism M26.09
Opisthorchiasis (felineus) (viverrini) B66.0
Opitz' disease D73.2
Opiumism — see Dependence, drug, opioid
Oppenheim's disease G70.2
Oppenheim-Urbach disease (necrobiosis lipoidica diabeticorum) — see E08-E13 with .620
Optic nerve — see condition
Orbit — see condition
Orchioblastoma C62.9- ☑
Orchitis (gangrenous) (nonspecific) (septic) (suppurative) N45.2
   blennorrhagic (gonococcal) (acute) (chronic) A54.23
   chlamydial A56.19
   filarial — see also Infestation, filarial B74.9 [N51]
   gonococcal (acute) (chronic) A54.23
   mumps B26.0
   syphilitic A52.76
   tuberculous A18.15
Orf (virus disease) B08.02
Organic — see also condition
   brain syndrome F09
   heart — see Disease, heart
   mental disorder F09
   psychosis F09
Orgasm
   anejaculatory N53.13
Oriental
   bilharziasis B65.2
   schistosomiasis B65.2
Orifice — see condition
Origin of both great vessels from right ventricle Q20.1
Ormond's disease (with ureteral obstruction) N13.5
   with infection N13.6
Ornithine metabolism disorder E72.4

Ornithinemia (Type I) (Type II) E72.4
Ornithosis A70
Orotaciduria, oroticaciduria (congenital) (hereditary) (pyrimidine deficiency) E79.8
   anemia D53.0
Orthodontics
   adjustment Z46.4
   fitting Z46.4
Orthopnea R06.01
Orthopoxvirus B08.09
Os, uterus — see condition
Osgood-Schlatter disease or osteochondrosis M92.52- ☑
Osler (-Weber)-Rendu disease I78.0
Osler's nodes I33.0
Osmidrosis L75.0
Osseous — see condition
Ossification
   artery — see Arteriosclerosis
   auricle (ear) — see Disorder, pinna, specified type NEC
   bronchial J98.09
   cardiac — see Degeneration, myocardial
   cartilage (senile) — see Disorder, cartilage, specified type NEC
   coronary (artery) — see Disease, heart, ischemic, atherosclerotic
   diaphragm J98.6
   ear, middle — see Otosclerosis
   falx cerebri G96.198
   fontanel, premature Q75.0
   heart — see also Degeneration, myocardial
      valve — see Endocarditis
   larynx J38.7
   ligament — see Disorder, tendon, specified type NEC
      posterior longitudinal — see Spondylopathy, specified NEC
   meninges (cerebral) (spinal) G96.198
   multiple, eccentric centers — see Disorder, bone, development or growth
   muscle — see also Calcification, muscle
      due to burns — see Myositis, ossificans, in, burns
      paralytic — see Myositis, ossificans, in, quadriplegia
      progressive — see Myositis, ossificans, progressiva
      specified NEC M61.50
         ankle M61.57- ☑
         foot M61.57- ☑
         forearm M61.53- ☑
         hand M61.54- ☑
         lower leg M61.56- ☑
         multiple sites M61.59
         pelvic region M61.55- ☑
         shoulder region M61.51- ☑
         specified site NEC M61.58
         thigh M61.55- ☑
         upper arm M61.52- ☑
      traumatic — see Myositis, ossificans, traumatica
   myocardium, myocardial — see Degeneration, myocardial
   penis N48.89
   periarticular — see Disorder, joint, specified type NEC
   pinna — see Disorder, pinna, specified type NEC
   rider's bone — see Ossification, muscle, specified NEC
   sclera H15.89
   subperiosteal, post-traumatic M89.8X- ☑
   tendon — see Disorder, tendon, specified type NEC
   trachea J39.8
   tympanic membrane — see Disorder, tympanic membrane, specified NEC
   vitreous (humor) — see Deposit, crystalline
Osteitis — see also Osteomyelitis
   alveolar M27.3
   condensans M85.30
      ankle M85.37- ☑
      foot M85.37- ☑
      forearm M85.33- ☑
      hand M85.34- ☑
      lower leg M85.36- ☑
      multiple site M85.39
      neck M85.38
      rib M85.38
      shoulder M85.31- ☑
      skull M85.38
      specified site NEC M85.38
      thigh M85.35- ☑
      toe M85.37- ☑
      upper arm M85.32- ☑
      vertebra M85.38

Osteitis — continued
   deformans M88.9
      in (due to)
         malignant neoplasm of bone C41.9 [M90.60]
         neoplastic disease — see also Neoplasm D49.9 [M90.60]
            carpus D49.9 [M90.64-] ☑
            clavicle D49.9 [M90.61-] ☑
            femur D49.9 [M90.65-] ☑
            fibula D49.9 [M90.66-] ☑
            finger D49.9 [M90.64-] ☑
            humerus D49.9 [M90.62-] ☑
            ilium D49.9 [M90.65-] ☑
            ischium D49.9 [M90.65-] ☑
            metacarpus D49.9 [M90.64-] ☑
            metatarsus D49.9 [M90.67-] ☑
            multiple sites D49.9 [M90.69]
            neck D49.9 [M90.68]
            radius D49.9 [M90.63-] ☑
            rib D49.9 [M90.68]
            scapula D49.9 [M90.61-] ☑
            skull D49.9 [M90.68]
            tarsus D49.9 [M90.67-] ☑
            tibia D49.9 [M90.66-] ☑
            toe D49.9 [M90.67-] ☑
            ulna D49.9 [M90.63-] ☑
            vertebra D49.9 [M90.68]
      skull M88.0
      specified NEC — see Paget's disease, bone, by site
      vertebra M88.1
   due to yaws A66.6
   fibrosa NEC — see Cyst, bone, by site
      circumscripta — see Dysplasia, fibrous, bone NEC
      cystica (generalisata) E21.0
      disseminata Q78.1
      osteoplastica E21.0
   fragilitans Q78.0
   Garr's (sclerosing) — see Osteomyelitis, specified type NEC
   jaw (acute) (chronic) (lower) (suppurative) (upper) M27.2
   parathyroid E21.0
   petrous bone (acute) (chronic) — see Petrositis
   sclerotic, nonsuppurative — see Osteomyelitis, specified type NEC
   tuberculosa A18.09
      cystica D86.89
      multiplex cystoides D86.89
Osteoarthritis M19.90
   ankle M19.07- ☑
      post-traumatic M19.17- ☑
      primary M19.07- ☑
      secondary M19.27- ☑
   elbow M19.02- ☑
      post-traumatic M19.12- ☑
      primary M19.02- ☑
      secondary M19.22- ☑
   foot joint M19.07- ☑
      post-traumatic M19.17- ☑
      primary M19.07- ☑
      secondary M19.27- ☑
   generalized (multiple joints) M15.9
      erosive M15.4
      primary M15.0
      specified NEC M15.8
   hand joint M19.04- ☑
      first carpometacarpal joint M18.9
         post-traumatic — see Osteoarthritis, post-traumatic NEC, hand joint, first carpometacarpal joint
         primary — see Osteoarthritis, primary, hand joint, first carpometacarpal joint
         secondary — see Osteoarthritis, secondary, hand joint, first carpometacarpal joint
      post-traumatic M19.14- ☑
      primary M19.04- ☑
      secondary M19.24- ☑
   hip M16.9
      bilateral M16.0
         due to hip dysplasia M16.2
         post-traumatic M16.4
         secondary M16.6
      due to hip dysplasia (unilateral) M16.3- ☑
         bilateral M16.2
      post-traumatic — see Osteoarthritis, post-traumatic, hip
      primary M16.1- ☑

☑ **Additional Character Required** — Refer to the Tabular List for Character Selection

Osteoarthritis — *continued*
hip — *continued*
secondary — *see* Osteoarthritis, secondary, hip
unilateral M16.1- ☑
due to hip dysplasia M16.3- ☑
post-traumatic M16.5- ☑
primary M16.1- ☑
secondary NEC M16.7
interphalangeal
distal (Heberden) M15.1
proximal (Bouchard) M15.2
knee M17.9
bilateral M17.0
post-traumatic M17.2
secondary M17.4
post-traumatic — *see* Osteoarthritis, post-traumatic, knee
primary M17.1- ☑
bilateral M17.0
secondary — *see* Osteoarthritis, secondary, knee
unilateral M17.1- ☑
post-traumatic M17.3- ☑
primary M17.1- ☑
secondary NEC M17.5
post-traumatic NEC M19.92
ankle M19.17- ☑
elbow M19.12- ☑
foot joint M19.17- ☑
hand joint M19.14- ☑
first carpometacarpal joint M18.3- ☑
bilateral M18.2
hip M16.5- ☑
bilateral M16.4
knee M17.3- ☑
bilateral M17.2
shoulder M19.11- ☑
specified site NEC M19.19
wrist M19.13- ☑
primary M19.91
ankle M19.07- ☑
elbow M19.02- ☑
foot joint M19.07- ☑
hand joint M19.04- ☑
first carpometacarpal joint M18.1- ☑
bilateral M18.0
hip M16.1- ☑
bilateral M16.0
knee M17.1- ☑
bilateral M17.0
multiple sites M15.9
shoulder M19.01- ☑
specified site NEC M19.09
spine — *see* Spondylosis
wrist M19.03- ☑
secondary M19.93
ankle M19.27- ☑
elbow M19.22- ☑
foot joint M19.27- ☑
hand joint M19.24- ☑
first carpometacarpal joint M18.5- ☑
bilateral M18.4
hip M16.7- ☑
bilateral M16.6
knee M17.5- ☑
bilateral M17.4
multiple M15.3
shoulder M19.21- ☑
specified site NEC M19.29
spine — *see* Spondylosis
wrist M19.23- ☑
shoulder M19.01- ☑
post-traumatic M19.11- ☑
primary M19.01- ☑
secondary M19.21- ☑
specified site NEC M19.09
spine — *see* Spondylosis
wrist M19.03- ☑
first carpometacarpal joint — *see* Osteoarthritis, hand joint, first carpometacarpal joint
post-traumatic M19.13- ☑
primary M19.03- ☑
secondary M19.23 ☑

Osteoarthropathy (hypertrophic) M19.90
ankle — *see* Osteoarthritis, primary, ankle
elbow — *see* Osteoarthritis, primary, elbow
foot joint — *see* Osteoarthritis, primary, foot
hand joint — *see* Osteoarthritis, primary, hand joint

Osteoarthropathy — *continued*
knee joint — *see* Osteoarthritis, primary, knee
multiple site — *see* Osteoarthritis, primary, multiple joint
pulmonary — *see also* Osteoarthropathy, specified type NEC
hypertrophic — *see* Osteoarthropathy, hypertrophic, specified type NEC
secondary — *see* Osteoarthropathy, specified type NEC
secondary hypertrophic — *see* Osteoarthropathy, specified type NEC
shoulder — *see* Osteoarthritis, primary, shoulder
specified joint NEC — *see* Osteoarthritis, primary, specified joint NEC
specified type NEC M89.40
carpus M89.44- ☑
clavicle M89.41- ☑
femur M89.45- ☑
fibula M89.46- ☑
finger M89.44- ☑
humerus M89.42- ☑
ilium M89.459
ischium M89.459
metacarpus M89.44- ☑
metatarsus M89.47- ☑
multiple sites M89.49
neck M89.48
radius M89.43- ☑
rib M89.48
scapula M89.41- ☑
skull M89.48
tarsus M89.47- ☑
tibia M89.46- ☑
toe M89.47- ☑
ulna M89.43- ☑
vertebra M89.48
spine — *see* Spondylosis
wrist — *see* Osteoarthritis, primary, wrist

Osteoarthrosis (degenerative) (hypertrophic) (joint) — *see also* Osteoarthritis
deformans alkaptonurica E70.29 *[M36.8]*
erosive M15.4
generalized M15.9
primary M15.0
polyarticular M15.9
spine — *see* Spondylosis

Osteoblastoma — *see* Neoplasm, bone, benign
aggressive — *see* Neoplasm, bone, uncertain behavior

Osteochondritis — *see also* Osteochondropathy, by site
Brailsford's — *see* Osteochondrosis, juvenile, radius
dissecans M93.20
ankle M93.27- ☑
elbow M93.22- ☑
foot M93.27- ☑
hand M93.24- ☑
hip M93.25- ☑
knee M93.26- ☑
multiple sites M93.29
shoulder joint M93.21- ☑
specified site NEC M93.28
wrist M93.23- ☑
juvenile M92.9
patellar — *see* Osteochondrosis, juvenile, patella
syphilitic (congenital) (early) A50.02 *[M90.80]*
ankle A50.02 *[M90.87-]* ☑
elbow A50.02 *[M90.82-]* ☑
foot A50.02 *[M90.87-]* ☑
forearm A50.02 *[M90.83-]* ☑
hand A50.02 *[M90.84-]* ☑
hip A50.02 *[M90.85-]* ☑
knee A50.02 *[M90.86-]* ☑
multiple sites A50.02 *[M90.89]*
shoulder joint A50.02 *[M90.81-]* ☑
specified site NEC A50.02 *[M90.88]*

Osteochondroarthrosis deformans endemica — *see* Disease, Kaschin-Beck

Osteochondrodysplasia Q78.9
with defects of growth of tubular bones and spine Q77.9
specified NEC Q77.8
specified NEC Q78.8

Osteochondrodystrophy E78.9

Osteochondrolysis — *see* Osteochondritis, dissecans

Osteochondroma — *see* Neoplasm, bone, benign

Osteochondromatosis D16.9
syndrome Q78.4

Osteochondromyxosarcoma — *see* Neoplasm, bone, malignant

Osteochondropathy M93.90
ankle M93.97- ☑
elbow M93.92- ☑
foot M93.97- ☑
hand M93.94- ☑
hip M93.95- ☑
Kienböck's disease of adults M93.1
knee M93.96- ☑
multiple joints M93.99
osteochondritis dissecans — *see* Osteochondritis, dissecans
osteochondrosis — *see* Osteochondrosis
shoulder region M93.91- ☑
slipped upper femoral epiphysis — *see* Slipped, epiphysis, upper femoral
specified joint NEC M93.98
specified type NEC M93.80
ankle M93.87- ☑
elbow M93.82- ☑
foot M93.87- ☑
hand M93.84- ☑
hip M93.85- ☑
knee M93.86- ☑
multiple joints M93.89
shoulder region M93.81- ☑
specified joint NEC M93.88
wrist M93.83- ☑
syphilitic, congenital
early A50.02 *[M90.80]*
late A50.56 *[M90.80]*
wrist M93.93- ☑

Osteochondrosarcoma — *see* Neoplasm, bone, malignant

Osteochondrosis — *see also* Osteochondropathy, by site
acetabulum (juvenile) M91.0
adult — *see* Osteochondropathy, specified type NEC, by site
astragalus (juvenile) — *see* Osteochondrosis, juvenile, tarsus
Blount M92.51- ☑
Buchanan's M91.0
Burns' — *see* Osteochondrosis, juvenile, ulna
calcaneus (juvenile) — *see* Osteochondrosis, juvenile, tarsus
capitular epiphysis (femur) (juvenile) — *see* Legg-Calvé-Perthes disease
carpal (juvenile) (lunate) (scaphoid) — *see* Osteochondrosis, juvenile, hand, carpal lunate
adult M93.1
coxae juvenilis — *see* Legg-Calvé-Perthes disease
deformans juvenilis, coxae — *see* Legg-Calvé-Perthes disease
Diaz's — *see* Osteochondrosis, juvenile, tarsus
dissecans (knee) (shoulder) — *see* Osteochondritis, dissecans
femoral capital epiphysis (juvenile) — *see* Legg-Calvé-Perthes disease
femur (head), juvenile — *see* Legg-Calvé-Perthes disease
fibula (juvenile) — *see* Osteochondrosis, juvenile, fibula
foot NEC (juvenile) M92.8
Freiberg's — *see* Osteochondrosis, juvenile, metatarsus
Haas' (juvenile) — *see* Osteochondrosis, juvenile, humerus
Haglund's — *see* Osteochondrosis, juvenile, tarsus
hip (juvenile) — *see* Legg-Calvé-Perthes disease
humerus (capitulum) (head) (juvenile) — *see* Osteochondrosis, juvenile, humerus
ilium, iliac crest (juvenile) M91.0
ischiopubic synchondrosis M91.0
Iselin's — *see* Osteochondrosis, juvenile, metatarsus
juvenile, juvenilis M92.9
after congenital dislocation of hip reduction — *see* Osteochondrosis, juvenile, hip, specified NEC
arm — *see* Osteochondrosis, juvenile, upper limb NEC
capitular epiphysis (femur) — *see* Legg-Calvé-Perthes disease
clavicle, sternal epiphysis — *see* Osteochondrosis, juvenile, upper limb NEC
coxae — *see* Legg-Calvé-Perthes disease
deformans M92.9
fibula M92.50- ☑

Osteochondrosis — *continued*
  juvenile, juvenilis — *continued*
    foot NEC M92.8
    hand M92.20- ☑
      carpal lunate M92.21- ☑
      metacarpal head M92.22- ☑
      specified site NEC M92.29- ☑
    head of femur — *see* Legg-Calvé-Perthes disease
    hip and pelvis M91.9- ☑
      coxa plana — *see* Coxa, plana
      femoral head — *see* Legg-Calvé-Perthes disease
      pelvis M91.0
      pseudocoxalgia — *see* Pseudocoxalgia
      specified NEC M91.8- ☑
    humerus M92.0- ☑
    limb
      lower NEC M92.8
      upper NEC — *see* Osteochondrosis, juvenile,
        upper limb NEC
    medial cuneiform bone — *see* Osteochondrosis,
      juvenile, tarsus
    metatarsus M92.7- ☑
    patella M92.4- ☑
    radius M92.1- ☑
    specified
      site NEC M92.8
      type NEC M92.8
        tibia and fibula M92.59- ☑
    spine M42.00
      cervical region M42.02
      cervicothoracic region M42.03
      lumbar region M42.06
      lumbosacral region M42.07
      multiple sites M42.09
      occipito-atlanto-axial region M42.01
      sacrococcygeal region M42.08
      thoracic region M42.04
      thoracolumbar region M42.05
    tarsus M92.6- ☑
    tibia M92.50- ☑
      proximal M92.51- ☑
      tubercle M92.52- ☑
    ulna M92.1- ☑
    upper limb NEC M92.3- ☑
    vertebra (body) (epiphyseal plates) (Calvé's)
      (Scheuermann's) — *see* Osteochondrosis, ju-
      venile, spine
  Kienböck's — *see* Osteochondrosis, juvenile, hand,
    carpal lunate
    adult M93.1
  Köhler's
    patellar — *see* Osteochondrosis, juvenile, patella
    tarsal navicular — *see* Osteochondrosis, juvenile,
      tarsus
  Legg-Perthes (-Calvé) (-Waldenström) — *see* Legg-
    Calvé-Perthes disease
  limb
    lower NEC (juvenile) M92.8
      tibia and fibula M92.59- ☑
    upper NEC (juvenile) — *see* Osteochondrosis, juve-
      nile, upper limb NEC
  lunate bone (carpal) (juvenile) — *see also* Osteochon-
    drosis, juvenile, hand, carpal lunate
    adult M93.1
  Mauclaire's — *see* Osteochondrosis, juvenile, hand,
    metacarpal
  metacarpal (head) (juvenile) — *see* Osteochondrosis,
    juvenile, hand, metacarpal
  metatarsus (fifth) (head) (juvenile) (second) — *see* Os-
    teochondrosis, juvenile, metatarsus
  navicular (juvenile) — *see* Osteochondrosis, juvenile,
    tarsus
  os
    calcis (juvenile) — *see* Osteochondrosis, juvenile,
      tarsus
    tibiale externum (juvenile) — *see* Osteochondrosis,
      juvenile, tarsus
  Osgood-Schlatter M92.52- ☑
  Panner's — *see* Osteochondrosis, juvenile, humerus
  patellar center (juvenile) (primary) (secondary) — *see*
    Osteochondrosis, juvenile, patella
  pelvis (juvenile) M91.0
  Pierson's M91.0
  radius (head) (juvenile) — *see* Osteochondrosis, juve-
    nile, radius
  Scheuermann's — *see* Osteochondrosis, juvenile, spine
  Sever's — *see* Osteochondrosis, juvenile, tarsus

Osteochondrosis — *continued*
  Sinding-Larsen — *see* Osteochondrosis, juvenile,
    patella
  spine M42.9
    adult M42.10
      cervical region M42.12
      cervicothoracic region M42.13
      lumbar region M42.16
      lumbosacral region M42.17
      multiple sites M42.19
      occipito-atlanto-axial region M42.11
      sacrococcygeal region M42.18
      thoracic region M42.14
      thoracolumbar region M42.15
    juvenile — *see* Osteochondrosis, juvenile, spine
  symphysis pubis (juvenile) M91.0
  syphilitic (congenital) A50.02
  talus (juvenile) — *see* Osteochondrosis, juvenile, tarsus
  tarsus (navicular) (juvenile) — *see* Osteochondrosis,
    juvenile, tarsus
  tibia (proximal) (tubercle) (juvenile) — *see* Osteochon-
    drosis, juvenile, tibia
  tuberculous — *see* Tuberculosis, bone
  ulna (lower) (juvenile) — *see* Osteochondrosis, juvenile,
    ulna
  van Neck's M91.0
  vertebral — *see* Osteochondrosis, spine
Osteoclastoma D48.0
  malignant — *see* Neoplasm, bone, malignant
Osteodynia — *see* Disorder, bone, specified type NEC
Osteodystrophy Q78.9
  azotemic N25.0
  congenital Q78.9
  parathyroid, secondary E21.1
  renal N25.0
Osteofibroma — *see* Neoplasm, bone, benign
Osteofibrosarcoma — *see* Neoplasm, bone, malignant
Osteogenesis imperfecta Q78.0
Osteogenic — *see* condition
Osteolysis M89.50
  carpus M89.54- ☑
  clavicle M89.51- ☑
  femur M89.55- ☑
  fibula M89.56- ☑
  finger M89.54- ☑
  humerus M89.52- ☑
  ilium M89.559
  ischium M89.559
  joint prosthesis (periprosthetic) — *see* Complications,
    joint prosthesis, mechanical, periprosthetic, oste-
    olysis, by site
  metacarpus M89.54- ☑
  metatarsus M89.57- ☑
  multiple sites M89.59
  neck M89.58
  periprosthetic — *see* Complications, joint prosthesis,
    mechanical, periprosthetic, osteolysis, by site
  radius M89.53- ☑
  rib M89.58
  scapula M89.51- ☑
  skull M89.58
  tarsus M89.57- ☑
  tibia M89.56- ☑
  toe M89.57- ☑
  ulna M89.53- ☑
  vertebra M89.58
Osteoma — *see also* Neoplasm, bone, benign
  osteoid — *see also* Neoplasm, bone, benign
    giant — *see* Neoplasm, bone, benign
Osteomalacia M83.9
  adult M83.9
    drug-induced NEC M83.5
    due to
      malabsorption (postsurgical) M83.2
      malnutrition M83.3
    specified NEC M83.8
  aluminium-induced M83.4
  infantile — *see* Rickets
  juvenile — *see* Rickets
  oncogenic E83.89
  pelvis M83.8
  puerperal M83.0
  senile M83.1
  vitamin-D-resistant in adults E83.31 *[M90.8-]* ☑
    carpus E83.31 *[M90.84-]* ☑
    clavicle E83.31 *[M90.81-]* ☑
    femur E83.31 *[M90.85-]* ☑

Osteomalacia — *continued*
  vitamin-D-resistant in adults — *continued*
    fibula E83.31 *[M90.86-]* ☑
    finger E83.31 *[M90.84-]* ☑
    humerus E83.31 *[M90.82-]* ☑
    ilium E83.31 *[M90.859]*
    ischium E83.31 *[M90.859]*
    metacarpus E83.31 *[M90.84-]* ☑
    metatarsus E83.31 *[M90.87-]* ☑
    multiple sites E83.31 *[M90.89]*
    neck E83.31 *[M90.88]*
    radius E83.31 *[M90.83-]* ☑
    rib E83.31 *[M90.88]*
    scapula E83.31 *[M90.819]*
    skull E83.31 *[M90.88]*
    tarsus E83.31 *[M90.879]*
    tibia E83.31 *[M90.869]*
    toe E83.31 *[M90.879]*
    ulna E83.31 *[M90.839]*
    vertebra E83.31 *[M90.88]*
Osteomyelitis (general) (infective) (localized) (neonatal)
  (purulent) (septic) (staphylococcal) (streptococcal)
  (suppurative) (with periostitis) M86.9
  acute M86.10
    carpus M86.14- ☑
    clavicle M86.11- ☑
    femur M86.15- ☑
    fibula M86.16- ☑
    finger M86.14- ☑
    hematogenous M86.00
      carpus M86.04- ☑
      clavicle M86.01- ☑
      femur M86.05- ☑
      fibula M86.06- ☑
      finger M86.04- ☑
      humerus M86.02- ☑
      ilium M86.08
      ischium M86.08
      mandible M27.2
      metacarpus M86.04- ☑
      metatarsus M86.07- ☑
      multiple sites M86.09
      neck M86.08
      orbit H05.02- ☑
      petrous bone — *see* Petrositis
      radius M86.03- ☑
      rib M86.08
      scapula M86.01- ☑
      skull M86.08
      tarsus M86.07- ☑
      tibia M86.06- ☑
      toe M86.07- ☑
      ulna M86.03- ☑
      vertebra — *see* Osteomyelitis, vertebra
    humerus M86.12- ☑
    ilium M86.18
    ischium M86.18
    mandible M27.2
    metacarpus M86.14- ☑
    metatarsus M86.17- ☑
    multiple sites M86.19
    neck M86.18
    orbit H05.02- ☑
    petrous bone — *see* Petrositis
    radius M86.13- ☑
    rib M86.18
    scapula M86.11- ☑
    skull M86.18
    tarsus M86.17- ☑
    tibia M86.16- ☑
    toe M86.17- ☑
    ulna M86.13- ☑
    vertebra — *see* Osteomyelitis, vertebra
  chronic (or old) M86.60
    with draining sinus M86.40
      carpus M86.44- ☑
      clavicle M86.41- ☑
      femur M86.45- ☑
      fibula M86.46- ☑
      finger M86.44- ☑
      humerus M86.42- ☑
      ilium M86.459
      ischium M86.459
      mandible M27.2
      metacarpus M86.44- ☑
      metatarsus M86.47- ☑

Osteomyelitis — *continued*
  chronic — *continued*
    with draining sinus — *continued*
      multiple sites M86.49
      neck M86.48
      orbit H05.02- ☑
      petrous bone — *see* Petrositis
      radius M86.43- ☑
      rib M86.48
      scapula M86.41- ☑
      skull M86.48
      tarsus M86.47- ☑
      tibia M86.46- ☑
      toe M86.47- ☑
      ulna M86.43- ☑
      vertebra — *see* Osteomyelitis, vertebra
    carpus M86.64- ☑
    clavicle M86.61- ☑
    femur M86.65- ☑
    fibula M86.66- ☑
    finger M86.64- ☑
    hematogenous NEC M86.50
      carpus M86.54- ☑
      clavicle M86.51- ☑
      femur M86.55- ☑
      fibula M86.56- ☑
      finger M86.54- ☑
      humerus M86.52- ☑
      ilium M86.559
      ischium M86.559
      mandible M27.2
      metacarpus M86.54- ☑
      metatarsus M86.57- ☑
      multifocal M86.30
        carpus M86.34- ☑
        clavicle M86.31- ☑
        femur M86.35- ☑
        fibula M86.36- ☑
        finger M86.34- ☑
        humerus M86.32- ☑
        ilium M86.359
        ischium M86.359
        metacarpus M86.34- ☑
        metatarsus M86.37- ☑
        multiple sites M86.39
        neck M86.38
        radius M86.33- ☑
        rib M86.38
        scapula M86.31- ☑
        skull M86.38
        tarsus M86.37- ☑
        tibia M86.36- ☑
        toe M86.37- ☑
        ulna M86.33- ☑
        vertebra — *see* Osteomyelitis, vertebra
      multiple sites M86.59
      neck M86.58
      orbit H05.02- ☑
      petrous bone — *see* Petrositis
      radius M86.53- ☑
      rib M86.58
      scapula M86.51- ☑
      skull M86.58
      tarsus M86.57- ☑
      tibia M86.56- ☑
      toe M86.57- ☑
      ulna M86.53- ☑
      vertebra — *see* Osteomyelitis, vertebra
    humerus M86.62- ☑
    ilium M86.659
    ischium M86.659
    mandible M27.2
    metacarpus M86.64- ☑
    metatarsus M86.67- ☑
    multifocal — *see* Osteomyelitis, chronic,
        hematogenous, multifocal
    multiple sites M86.69
    neck M86.68
    orbit H05.02- ☑
    petrous bone — *see* Petrositis
    radius M86.63- ☑
    rib M86.68
    scapula M86.61- ☑
    skull M86.68
    tarsus M86.67- ☑
    tibia M86.66- ☑
    toe M86.67- ☑

Osteomyelitis — *continued*
  chronic — *continued*
    ulna M86.63- ☑
    vertebra — *see* Osteomyelitis, vertebra
  echinococcal B67.2
  Garr's — *see* Osteomyelitis, specified type NEC
  in diabetes mellitus — *see* E08-E13 with .69
  jaw (acute) (chronic) (lower) (neonatal) (suppurative)
      (upper) M27.2
  nonsuppurating — *see* Osteomyelitis, specified type
      NEC
  orbit H05.02- ☑
  petrous bone — *see* Petrositis
  Salmonella (arizonae) (cholerae-suis) (enteritidis) (ty-
      phimurium) A02.24
  sclerosing, nonsuppurative — *see* Osteomyelitis,
      specified type NEC
  specified type NEC — *see also* subcategory M86.8X- ☑
    mandible M27.2
    orbit H05.02- ☑
    petrous bone — *see* Petrositis
    vertebra — *see* Osteomyelitis, vertebra
  subacute M86.20
    carpus M86.24- ☑
    clavicle M86.21- ☑
    femur M86.25- ☑
    fibula M86.26- ☑
    finger M86.24- ☑
    humerus M86.22- ☑
    mandible M27.2
    metacarpus M86.24- ☑
    metatarsus M86.27- ☑
    multiple sites M86.29
    neck M86.28
    orbit H05.02- ☑
    petrous bone — *see* Petrositis
    radius M86.23- ☑
    rib M86.28
    scapula M86.21- ☑
    skull M86.28
    tarsus M86.27- ☑
    tibia M86.26- ☑
    toe M86.27- ☑
    ulna M86.23- ☑
    vertebra — *see* Osteomyelitis, vertebra
  syphilitic A52.77
    congenital (early) A50.02 *[M90.80]*
  tuberculous — *see* Tuberculosis, bone
  typhoid A01.05
  vertebra M46.20
    cervical region M46.22
    cervicothoracic region M46.23
    lumbar region M46.26
    lumbosacral region M46.27
    occipito-atlanto-axial region M46.21
    sacrococcygeal region M46.28
    thoracic region M46.24
    thoracolumbar region M46.25

Osteomyelofibrosis D47.4
Osteomyelosclerosis D75.89
Osteonecrosis M87.9
  due to
    drugs — *see* Osteonecrosis, secondary, due to, drugs
    trauma — *see* Osteonecrosis, secondary, due to,
        trauma
  idiopathic aseptic M87.00
    ankle M87.07- ☑
    carpus M87.03- ☑
    clavicle M87.01- ☑
    femur M87.05- ☑
    fibula M87.06- ☑
    finger M87.04- ☑
    humerus M87.02- ☑
    ilium M87.050
    ischium M87.050
    metacarpus M87.04- ☑
    metatarsus M87.07- ☑
    multiple sites M87.09
    neck M87.08
    pelvis M87.050
    radius M87.03- ☑
    rib M87.08
    scapula M87.01- ☑
    skull M87.08
    tarsus M87.07- ☑
    tibia M87.06- ☑
    toe M87.07- ☑

Osteonecrosis — *continued*
  idiopathic aseptic — *continued*
    ulna M87.03- ☑
    vertebra M87.08
  secondary NEC M87.30
    carpus M87.33- ☑
    clavicle M87.31- ☑
    due to
      drugs M87.10
        carpus M87.13- ☑
        clavicle M87.11- ☑
        femur M87.15- ☑
        fibula M87.16- ☑
        finger M87.14- ☑
        humerus M87.12- ☑
        ilium M87.159
        ischium M87.159
        jaw M87.180
        metacarpus M87.14- ☑
        metatarsus M87.17- ☑
        multiple sites M87.19
        neck M87.18
        radius M87.13- ☑
        rib M87.18
        scapula M87.11- ☑
        skull M87.18
        tarsus M87.17- ☑
        tibia M87.16- ☑
        toe M87.17- ☑
        ulna M87.13- ☑
        vertebra M87.18
      hemoglobinopathy NEC D58.2 *[M90.50]*
        carpus D58.2 *[M90.54-]* ☑
        clavicle D58.2 *[M90.51-]* ☑
        femur D58.2 *[M90.55-]* ☑
        fibula D58.2 *[M90.56-]* ☑
        finger D58.2 *[M90.54-]* ☑
        humerus D58.2 *[M90.52-]* ☑
        ilium D58.2 *[M90.55-]* ☑
        ischium D58.2 *[M90.55-]* ☑
        metacarpus D58.2 *[M90.54-]* ☑
        metatarsus D58.2 *[M90.57-]* ☑
        multiple sites D58.2 *[M90.58]*
        neck D58.2 *[M90.58]*
        radius D58.2 *[M90.53-]* ☑
        rib D58.2 *[M90.58]*
        scapula D58.2 *[M90.51-]* ☑
        skull D58.2 *[M90.58]*
        tarsus D58.2 *[M90.57-]* ☑
        tibia D58.2 *[M90.56-]* ☑
        toe D58.2 *[M90.57-]* ☑
        ulna D58.2 *[M90.53-]* ☑
        vertebra D58.2 *[M90.58]*
      trauma (previous) M87.20
        carpus M87.23- ☑
        clavicle M87.21- ☑
        femur M87.25- ☑
        fibula M87.26- ☑
        finger M87.24- ☑
        humerus M87.22- ☑
        ilium M87.25- ☑
        ischium M87.25- ☑
        metacarpus M87.24- ☑
        metatarsus M87.27- ☑
        multiple sites M87.29
        neck M87.28
        radius M87.23- ☑
        rib M87.28
        scapula M87.21- ☑
        skull M87.28
        tarsus M87.27- ☑
        tibia M87.26- ☑
        toe M87.27- ☑
        ulna M87.23- ☑
        vertebra M87.28
    femur M87.35- ☑
    fibula M87.36- ☑
    finger M87.34- ☑
    humerus M87.32- ☑
    ilium M87.350
    in
      caisson disease T70.3 ☑ *[M90.50]*
        carpus T70.3 ☑ *[M90.54-]* ☑
        clavicle T70.3 ☑ *[M90.51-]* ☑
        femur T70.3 ☑ *[M90.55-]* ☑
        fibula T70.3 ☑ *[M90.56-]* ☑

Osteonecrosis — continued
secondary — continued
in — continued
caisson disease — continued
finger T70.3 ☑ [M90.54-] ☑
humerus T70.3 ☑ [M90.52-] ☑
ilium T70.3 ☑ [M90.55-] ☑
ischium T70.3 ☑ [M90.55-] ☑
metacarpus T70.3 ☑ [M90.54-] ☑
metatarsus T70.3 ☑ [M90.57-] ☑
multiple sites T70.3 ☑ [M90.59]
neck T70.3 [M90.58]
radius T70.3 ☑ [M90.53-] ☑
rib T70.3 ☑ [M90.58]
scapula T70.3 ☑ [M90.51-] ☑
skull T70.3 ☑ [M90.58]
tarsus T70.3 ☑ [M90.57-] ☑
tibia T70.3 ☑ [M90.56-] ☑
toe T70.3 ☑ [M90.57-] ☑
ulna T70.3 ☑ [M90.53-] ☑
vertebra T70.3 ☑ [M90.58]
ischium M87.350
metacarpus M87.34- ☑
metatarsus M87.37- ☑
multiple site M87.39
neck M87.38
radius M87.33- ☑
rib M87.38
scapula M87.319
skull M87.38
tarsus M87.379
tibia M87.366
toe M87.379
ulna M87.33- ☑
vertebra M87.38
specified type NEC M87.80
carpus M87.83- ☑
clavicle M87.81- ☑
femur M87.85- ☑
fibula M87.86- ☑
finger M87.84- ☑
humerus M87.82- ☑
ilium M87.85- ☑
ischium M87.85- ☑
metacarpus M87.84- ☑
metatarsus M87.87- ☑
multiple sites M87.89
neck M87.88
radius M87.83- ☑
rib M87.88
scapula M87.81- ☑
skull M87.88
tarsus M87.87- ☑
tibia M87.86- ☑
toe M87.87- ☑
ulna M87.83- ☑
vertebra M87.88
Osteo-onycho-arthro-dysplasia Q87.2
Osteo-onychodysplasia, hereditary Q87.2
Osteopathia condensans disseminata Q78.8
Osteopathy — see also Osteomyelitis, Osteonecrosis, Osteoporosis
after poliomyelitis M89.60
carpus M89.64- ☑
clavicle M89.61- ☑
femur M89.65- ☑
fibula M89.66- ☑
finger M89.64- ☑
humerus M89.62- ☑
ilium M89.659
ischium M89.659
metacarpus M89.64- ☑
metatarsus M89.67- ☑
multiple sites M89.69
neck M89.68
radius M89.63- ☑
rib M89.68
scapula M89.61- ☑
skull M89.68
tarsus M89.67- ☑
tibia M89.66- ☑
toe M89.67- ☑
ulna M89.63- ☑
vertebra M89.68
in (due to)
renal osteodystrophy N25.0

Osteopathy — continued
in — continued
specified diseases classified elsewhere — see subcategory M90.8 ☑
Osteopenia M85.8- ☑
borderline M85.8- ☑
Osteoperiostitis — see Osteomyelitis, specified type NEC
Osteopetrosis (familial) Q78.2
Osteophyte M25.70
ankle M25.77- ☑
elbow M25.72- ☑
foot joint M25.77- ☑
hand joint M25.74- ☑
hip M25.75- ☑
knee M25.76- ☑
shoulder M25.71- ☑
spine M25.78
vertebrae M25.78
wrist M25.73- ☑
Osteopoikilosis Q78.8
Osteoporosis (female) (male) M81.0
with current pathological fracture M80.00 ☑
age-related M81.0
with current pathologic fracture M80.00 ☑
carpus M80.04- ☑
clavicle M80.01- ☑
fibula M80.06- ☑
finger M80.04- ☑
humerus M80.02- ☑
ilium M80.05- ☑
ischium M80.05- ☑
metacarpus M80.04- ☑
metatarsus M80.07- ☑
pelvis M80.05- ☑
radius M80.03- ☑
rib(s) — see Osteoporosis, specified site NEC
scapula M80.01- ☑
site specified NEC M80.0A ☑
specified site NEC M80.0A ☑
tarsus M80.07- ☑
tibia M80.06- ☑
toe M80.07- ☑
ulna M80.03- ☑
vertebra M80.08 ☑
disuse M81.8
with current pathological fracture M80.80 ☑
carpus M80.84- ☑
clavicle M80.81- ☑
fibula M80.86- ☑
finger M80.84- ☑
humerus M80.82- ☑
ilium M80.85- ☑
ischium M80.85- ☑
metacarpus M80.84- ☑
metatarsus M80.87- ☑
pelvis M80.85- ☑
radius M80.83- ☑
scapula M80.81- ☑
site specified NEC M80.8A ☑
tarsus M80.87- ☑
tibia M80.86- ☑
toe M80.87- ☑
ulna M80.83- ☑
vertebra M80.88 ☑
drug-induced — see Osteoporosis, specified type NEC
idiopathic — see Osteoporosis, specified type NEC
involutional — see Osteoporosis, age-related
Lequesne M81.6
localized M81.6
postmenopausal M81.0
with pathological fracture M80.00 ☑
carpus M80.04- ☑
clavicle M80.01- ☑
fibula M80.06- ☑
finger M80.04- ☑
humerus M80.02- ☑
ilium M80.05- ☑
ischium M80.05- ☑
metacarpus M80.04- ☑
metatarsus M80.07- ☑
pelvis M80.05- ☑
radius M80.03- ☑
scapula M80.01- ☑
site specified NEC M80.0A ☑
tarsus M80.07- ☑

Osteoporosis — continued
postmenopausal — continued
with pathological fracture — continued
tibia M80.06- ☑
toe M80.07- ☑
ulna M80.03- ☑
vertebra M80.08 ☑
postoophorectomy — see Osteoporosis, specified type NEC
postsurgical malabsorption — see Osteoporosis, specified type NEC
post-traumatic — see Osteoporosis, specified type NEC
senile — see Osteoporosis, age-related
specified type NEC M81.8
with pathological fracture M80.80 ☑
carpus M80.84- ☑
clavicle M80.81- ☑
fibula M80.86- ☑
finger M80.84- ☑
humerus M80.82- ☑
ilium M80.85- ☑
ischium M80.85- ☑
metacarpus M80.84- ☑
metatarsus M80.87- ☑
pelvis M80.85- ☑
radius M80.83- ☑
scapula M80.81- ☑
site specified NEC M80.8A ☑
tarsus M80.87- ☑
tibia M80.86- ☑
toe M80.87- ☑
ulna M80.83- ☑
vertebra M80.88 ☑
Osteopsathyrosis (idiopathica) Q78.0
Osteoradionecrosis, jaw (acute) (chronic) (lower) (suppurative) (upper) M27.2
Osteosarcoma (any form) — see Neoplasm, bone, malignant
Osteosclerosis Q78.2
acquired M85.8- ☑
congenita Q77.4
fragilitas (generalisata) Q78.2
myelofibrosis D75.81
Osteosclerotic anemia D64.89
Osteosis
cutis L94.2
renal fibrocystic N25.0
Österreicher-Turner syndrome Q87.2
Ostium
atrioventriculare commune Q21.23
primum (arteriosum) (defect) (persistent) Q21.20
secundum (arteriosum) (defect) (patent) (persistent) Q21.11
Ostrum-Furst syndrome Q75.8
Otalgia H92.0 ☑
Otitis (acute) H66.90
with effusion — see also Otitis, media, nonsuppurative
purulent — see Otitis, media, suppurative
adhesive — see subcategory H74.1 ☑
chronic — see also Otitis, media, chronic
with effusion — see also Otitis, media, nonsuppurative, chronic
externa H60.9- ☑
abscess — see Abscess, ear, external
acute (noninfective) H60.50- ☑
actinic H60.51- ☑
chemical H60.52- ☑
contact H60.53- ☑
eczematoid H60.54- ☑
infective — see Otitis, externa, infective
reactive H60.55- ☑
specified NEC H60.59- ☑
cellulitis — see Cellulitis, ear
chronic H60.6- ☑
diffuse — see Otitis, externa, infective, diffuse
hemorrhagic — see Otitis, externa, infective, hemorrhagic
in (due to)
aspergillosis B44.89
candidiasis B37.84
erysipelas A46 [H62.40]
herpes (simplex) virus infection B00.1
zoster B02.8
impetigo L01.00 [H62.40]
infectious disease NEC B99 ☑ [H62.4-] ☑
mycosis NEC B36.9 [H62.40]

Otitis — *continued*
  externa — *continued*
    in — *continued*
      parasitic disease NEC B89 *[H62.40]*
      viral disease NEC B34.9 *[H62.40]*
      zoster B02.8
    infective NEC H60.39- ☑
      abscess — *see* Abscess, ear, external
      cellulitis — *see* Cellulitis, ear
      diffuse H60.31- ☑
      hemorrhagic H60.32- ☑
      swimmer's ear — *see* Swimmer's, ear
    malignant H60.2- ☑
    mycotic NEC B36.9 *[H62.40]*
      in
        aspergillosis B44.89
        candidiasis B37.84
        moniliasis B37.84
    necrotizing — *see* Otitis, externa, malignant
    Pseudomonas aeruginosa — *see* Otitis, externa, malignant
    reactive — *see* Otitis, externa, acute, reactive
    specified NEC — *see* subcategory H60.8 ☑
    tropical NEC B36.9 *[H62.40]*
      in
        aspergillosis B44.89
        candidiasis B37.84
        moniliasis B37.84
  insidiosa — *see* Otosclerosis
  interna H83.0 ☑
  media (hemorrhagic) (staphylococcal) (streptococcal) H66.9- ☑
    with effusion (nonpurulent) — *see* Otitis, media, nonsuppurative
    acute, subacute H66.90
      allergic — *see* Otitis, media, nonsuppurative, acute, allergic
      exudative — *see* Otitis, media, suppurative, acute
      mucoid — *see* Otitis, media, nonsuppurative, acute
      necrotizing — *see also* Otitis, media, suppurative, acute
        in
          measles B05.3
          scarlet fever A38.0
      nonsuppurative NEC — *see* Otitis, media, nonsuppurative, acute
      purulent — *see* Otitis, media, suppurative, acute
      sanguinous — *see* Otitis, media, nonsuppurative, acute
      secretory — *see* Otitis, media, nonsuppurative, acute, serous
      seromucinous — *see* Otitis, media, nonsuppurative, acute
      serous — *see* Otitis, media, nonsuppurative, acute, serous
      suppurative — *see* Otitis, media, suppurative, acute
    allergic — *see* Otitis, media, nonsuppurative
    catarrhal — *see* Otitis, media, nonsuppurative
    chronic H66.90
      with effusion (nonpurulent) — *see* Otitis, media, nonsuppurative, chronic
      allergic — *see* Otitis, media, nonsuppurative, chronic, allergic
      benign suppurative — *see* Otitis, media, suppurative, chronic, tubotympanic
      catarrhal — *see* Otitis, media, nonsuppurative, chronic, serous
      exudative — *see* Otitis, media, nonsuppurative, chronic
      mucinous — *see* Otitis, media, nonsuppurative, chronic, mucoid
      mucoid — *see* Otitis, media, nonsuppurative, chronic, mucoid
      nonsuppurative NEC — *see* Otitis, media, nonsuppurative, chronic
      purulent — *see* Otitis, media, suppurative, chronic
      secretory — *see* Otitis, media, nonsuppurative, chronic, mucoid
      seromucinous — *see* Otitis, media, nonsuppurative, chronic
      serous — *see* Otitis, media, nonsuppurative, chronic, serous
      suppurative — *see* Otitis, media, suppurative, chronic

Otitis — *continued*
  media — *continued*
    chronic — *continued*
      transudative — *see* Otitis, media, nonsuppurative, chronic, mucoid
    exudative — *see* Otitis, media, suppurative
    in (due to) (with)
      influenza — *see* Influenza, with, otitis media
      measles B05.3
      scarlet fever A38.0
      tuberculosis A18.6
      viral disease NEC B34.- ☑ *[H67.-]* ☑
    mucoid — *see* Otitis, media, nonsuppurative
    nonsuppurative H65.9- ☑
      acute or subacute NEC H65.19- ☑
        allergic H65.11- ☑
          recurrent H65.11- ☑
        recurrent H65.19- ☑
        secretory — *see* Otitis, media, nonsuppurative, serous
        serous H65.0- ☑
          recurrent H65.0- ☑
      chronic H65.49- ☑
        allergic H65.41- ☑
        mucoid H65.3- ☑
        serous H65.2- ☑
    postmeasles B05.3
    purulent — *see* Otitis, media, suppurative
    secretory — *see* Otitis, media, nonsuppurative
    seromucinous — *see* Otitis, media, nonsuppurative
    serous — *see* Otitis, media, nonsuppurative
    suppurative H66.4- ☑
      acute H66.00- ☑
        with rupture of ear drum H66.01- ☑
        recurrent H66.00- ☑
          with rupture of ear drum H66.01- ☑
      chronic — *see also* subcategory H66.3 ☑
        atticoantral H66.2- ☑
        benign — *see* Otitis, media, suppurative, chronic, tubotympanic
        tubotympanic H66.1- ☑
    transudative — *see* Otitis, media, nonsuppurative
    tuberculous A18.6
Otocephaly Q18.2
Otolith syndrome — *see* subcategory H81.8 ☑
Otomycosis (diffuse) **NEC** B36.9 *[H62.40]*
  in
    aspergillosis B44.89
    candidiasis B37.84
    moniliasis B37.84
Otoporosis — *see* Otosclerosis
Otorrhagia (nontraumatic) H92.2- ☑
  traumatic — *code by* Type of injury
Otorrhea H92.1- ☑
  cerebrospinal (fluid) G96.01
    postoperative G96.08
    specified NEC G96.08
    spontaneous G96.01
    traumatic G96.08
Otosclerosis (general) H80.9- ☑
  cochlear (endosteal) H80.2- ☑
  involving
    otic capsule — *see* Otosclerosis, cochlear
    oval window
      nonobliterative H80.0- ☑
      obliterative H80.1- ☑
    round window — *see* Otosclerosis, cochlear
  nonobliterative — *see* Otosclerosis, involving, oval window, nonobliterative
  obliterative — *see* Otosclerosis, involving, oval window, obliterative
  specified NEC H80.8- ☑
Otospongiosis — *see* Otosclerosis
Otto's disease or pelvis M24.7
Outcome of delivery Z37.9
  multiple births Z37.9
    all liveborn Z37.50
      quadruplets Z37.52
      quintuplets Z37.53
      sextuplets Z37.54
      specified number NEC Z37.59
      triplets Z37.51
    all stillborn Z37.7
    some liveborn Z37.60
      quadruplets Z37.62
      quintuplets Z37.63
      sextuplets Z37.64

Outcome of delivery — *continued*
  multiple births — *continued*
    some liveborn — *continued*
      specified number NEC Z37.69
      triplets Z37.61
  single NEC Z37.9
    liveborn Z37.0
    stillborn Z37.1
  twins NEC Z37.9
    both liveborn Z37.2
    both stillborn Z37.4
    one liveborn, one stillborn Z37.3
Outlet — *see* condition
Ovalocytosis (congenital) (hereditary) — *see* Elliptocytosis
Ovarian — *see* Condition
Ovariocele N83.4- ☑
Ovaritis (cystic) — *see* Oophoritis
Ovary, ovarian — *see also* condition
  resistant syndrome E28.39
  vein syndrome N13.8
Overactive — *see also* Hyperfunction
  adrenal cortex NEC E27.0
  bladder N32.81
  hypothalamus E23.3
  thyroid — *see* Hyperthyroidism
Overactivity R46.3
  child — *see* Disorder, attention-deficit hyperactivity
Overbite (deep) (excessive) (horizontal) (vertical) M26.29
Overbreathing — *see* Hyperventilation
Overconscientious personality F60.5
Overdevelopment — *see* Hypertrophy
Overdistension — *see* Distension
Overdose, overdosage (drug) — *see* Table of Drugs and Chemicals, by drug, poisoning
Overeating R63.2
  nonorganic origin F50.89
  psychogenic F50.89
Overexertion (effects) (exhaustion) T73.3 ☑
Overexposure (effects) T73.9 ☑
  exhaustion T73.2 ☑
Overfeeding — *see* Overeating
  newborn P92.4
Overfill, endodontic M27.52
Overgrowth, bone — *see* Hypertrophy, bone
Overhanging of dental restorative material (unrepairable) K08.52
Overheated (places) (effects) — *see* Heat
Overjet (excessive horizontal) M26.23
Overlaid, overlying (suffocation) — *see* Asphyxia, traumatic, due to mechanical threat
Overlap, excessive horizontal (teeth) M26.23
Overlapping toe (acquired) — *see also* Deformity, toe, specified NEC
  congenital (fifth toe) Q66.89
Overload
  circulatory, due to transfusion (blood) (blood components) (TACO) E87.71
  fluid E87.70
    due to transfusion (blood) (blood components) E87.71
    specified NEC E87.79
  iron, due to repeated red blood cell transfusions E83.111
  potassium (K) E87.5
  sodium (Na) E87.0
Overnutrition — *see* Hyperalimentation
Overproduction — *see also* Hypersecretion
  ACTH E27.0
  catecholamine E27.5
  growth hormone E22.0
Overprotection, child by parent Z62.1
Overriding
  aorta Q25.49
  finger (acquired) — *see* Deformity, finger
    congenital Q68.1
  toe (acquired) — *see also* Deformity, toe, specified NEC
    congenital Q66.89
Overstrained R53.83
  heart — *see* Hypertrophy, cardiac
Overuse, muscle NEC M70.8- ☑
Overweight E66.3
Overworked R53.83
Oviduct — *see* condition
Ovotestis Q56.0
Ovulation (cycle)
  failure or lack of N97.0

Ovulation — *continued*
pain N94.0
Ovum — *see* condition
Owren's disease or syndrome (parahemophilia) D68.2
Ox heart — *see* Hypertrophy, cardiac
Oxalosis E72.53
Oxaluria E72.53
Oxycephaly, oxycephalic Q75.0
syphilitic, congenital A50.02
Oxyuriasis B80
Oxyuris vermicularis (infestation) B80
Ozena J31.0

P

Pachyderma, pachydermia L85.9
larynx (verrucosa) J38.7
Pachydermatocele (congenital) Q82.8
Pachydermoperiostosis — *see also* Osteoarthropathy, hypertrophic, specified type NEC
clubbed nail M89.40 [L62]
Pachygyria Q04.3
Pachymeningitis (adhesive) (basal) (brain) (cervical) (chronic) (circumscribed) (external) (fibrous) (hemorrhagic) (hypertrophic) (internal) (purulent) (spinal) (suppurative) — *see* Meningitis
Pachyonychia (congenital) Q84.5
Pacinian tumor — *see* Neoplasm, skin, benign
Pad, knuckle or Garrod's M72.1
Paget's disease
with infiltrating duct carcinoma — *see* Neoplasm, breast, malignant
bone M88.9
carpus M88.84- ☑
clavicle M88.81- ☑
femur M88.85- ☑
fibula M88.86- ☑
finger M88.84- ☑
humerus M88.82- ☑
ilium M88.85- ☑
in neoplastic disease — *see* Osteitis, deformans, in neoplastic disease
ischium M88.85- ☑
metacarpus M88.84- ☑
metatarsus M88.87- ☑
multiple sites M88.89
neck M88.88
radius M88.83- ☑
rib M88.88
scapula M88.81- ☑
skull M88.0
specified NEC M88.88
tarsus M88.87- ☑
tibia M88.86- ☑
toe M88.87- ☑
ulna M88.83- ☑
vertebra M88.1
breast (female) C50.01- ☑
male C50.02- ☑
extramammary — *see also* Neoplasm, skin, malignant
anus C21.0
margin C44.590
skin C44.590
intraductal carcinoma — *see* Neoplasm, breast, malignant
malignant — *see* Neoplasm, skin, malignant
breast (female) C50.01- ☑
male C50.02- ☑
unspecified site (female) C50.01- ☑
male C50.02- ☑
mammary — *see* Paget's disease, breast
nipple — *see* Paget's disease, breast
osteitis deformans — *see* Paget's disease, bone
Paget-Schroetter syndrome I82.890
Pain(s) — *see also* Painful R52
abdominal R10.9
colic R10.83
generalized R10.84
with acute abdomen R10.0
lower R10.30
left quadrant R10.32
pelvic or perineal R10.2
periumbilical R10.33
right quadrant R10.31
rebound — *see* Tenderness, abdominal, rebound
severe with abdominal rigidity R10.0
tenderness — *see* Tenderness, abdominal

Pain(s) — *continued*
abdominal — *continued*
upper R10.10
epigastric R10.13
left quadrant R10.12
right quadrant R10.11
acute R52
due to trauma G89.11
neoplasm related G89.3
postprocedural NEC G89.18
post-thoracotomy G89.12
specified by site — *code to* Pain, by site
adnexa (uteri) R10.2
anginoid — *see* Pain, precordial
anus K62.89
arm — *see* Pain, limb, upper
axillary (axilla) M79.62- ☑
back (postural) M54.9
bladder R39.89
associated with micturition — *see* Micturition, painful
chronic R39.82
bone — *see* Disorder, bone, specified type NEC
breast N64.4
broad ligament R10.2
cancer associated (acute) (chronic) G89.3
cecum — *see* Pain, abdominal
cervicobrachial M53.1
chest (central) R07.9
anterior wall R07.89
atypical R07.89
ischemic I20.9
musculoskeletal R07.89
non-cardiac R07.89
on breathing R07.1
pleurodynia R07.81
precordial R07.2
wall (anterior) R07.89
chronic G89.29
associated with significant psychosocial dysfunction G89.4
due to trauma G89.21
neoplasm related G89.3
postoperative NEC G89.28
postprocedural NEC G89.28
post-thoracotomy G89.22
specified NEC G89.29
coccyx M53.3
colon — *see* Pain, abdominal
coronary — *see* Angina
costochondral R07.1
diaphragm R07.1
due to cancer G89.3
due to device, implant or graft — *see also* Complications, by site and type, specified NEC T85.848 ☑
arterial graft NEC T82.848 ☑
breast (implant) T85.848 ☑
catheter NEC T85.848 ☑
dialysis (renal) T82.848 ☑
intraperitoneal T85.848 ☑
infusion NEC T82.848 ☑
spinal (epidural) (subdural) T85.840 ☑
urinary (indwelling) T83.84 ☑
electronic (electrode) (pulse generator) (stimulator)
bone T85.840 ☑
cardiac T82.847 ☑
nervous system (brain) (peripheral nerve) (spinal) T85.84 ☑
urinary T83.84 ☑
fixation, internal (orthopedic) NEC T84.84 ☑
gastrointestinal (bile duct) (esophagus) T85.848 ☑
genital NEC T83.84 ☑
heart NEC T82.847 ☑
infusion NEC T85.848 ☑
joint prosthesis T84.84 ☑
ocular (corneal graft) (orbital implant) NEC T85.848 ☑
orthopedic NEC T84.84 ☑
specified NEC T85.848 ☑
urinary NEC T83.84 ☑
vascular NEC T82.848 ☑
ventricular intracranial shunt T85.840 ☑
due to malignancy (primary) (secondary) G89.3
ear — *see* subcategory H92.0 ☑
epigastric, epigastrium R10.13
eye — *see* Pain, ocular
face, facial R51.9

Pain(s) — *continued*
face, facial — *continued*
atypical G50.1
female genital organs NEC N94.89
finger — *see* Pain, limb, upper
flank — *see* Pain, abdominal
foot — *see* Pain, limb, lower
gallbladder K82.9
gas (intestinal) R14.1
gastric — *see* Pain, abdominal
generalized NOS R52
genital organ
female N94.89
male N50.89
groin — *see* Pain, abdominal, lower
hand — *see* Pain, limb, upper
head — *see* Headache
heart — *see* Pain, precordial
infra-orbital — *see* Neuralgia, trigeminal
intercostal R07.82
intermenstrual N94.0
jaw R68.84
joint M25.50
ankle M25.57- ☑
elbow M25.52- ☑
finger M25.54- ☑
foot M25.57- ☑
hand M25.54- ☑
hip M25.55- ☑
knee M25.56- ☑
shoulder M25.51- ☑
specified site NEC M25.59
toe M25.57- ☑
wrist M25.53- ☑
kidney N23
laryngeal R07.0
leg — *see* Pain, limb, lower
limb M79.609
lower M79.60- ☑
foot M79.67- ☑
lower leg M79.66- ☑
thigh M79.65- ☑
toe M79.67- ☑
upper M79.60- ☑
axilla M79.62- ☑
finger M79.64- ☑
forearm M79.63- ☑
hand M79.64- ☑
upper arm M79.62- ☑
loin M54.50
low back M54.50
specified NEC M54.59
vertebral end plate M54.51
vertebrogenic M54.51
lumbar region M54.50
vertebral end plate M54.51
vertebrogenic M54.51
mandibular R68.84
mastoid — *see* subcategory H92.0 ☑
maxilla R68.84
menstrual — *see also* Dysmenorrhea N94.6
metacarpophalangeal (joint) — *see* Pain, joint, hand
metatarsophalangeal (joint) — *see* Pain, joint, foot
mouth K13.79
muscle — *see* Myalgia
musculoskeletal — *see also* Pain, by site M79.18
myofascial M79.18
nasal J34.89
nasopharynx J39.2
neck NEC M54.2
nerve NEC — *see* Neuralgia
neuromuscular — *see* Neuralgia
nose J34.89
ocular H57.1- ☑
ophthalmic — *see* Pain, ocular
orbital region — *see* Pain, ocular
ovary N94.89
over heart — *see* Pain, precordial
ovulation N94.0
pelvic (female) R10.2
penis N48.89
pericardial — *see* Pain, precordial
perineal, perineum R10.2
pharynx J39.2
pleura, pleural, pleuritic R07.81
postoperative NOS G89.18
postprocedural NOS G89.18

Pain(s) — *continued*
post-thoracotomy G89.12
precordial (region) R07.2
premenstrual N94.3
psychogenic (persistent) (any site) F45.41
radicular (spinal) — *see* Radiculopathy
rectum K62.89
respiration R07.1
retrosternal R07.2
rheumatoid, muscular — *see* Myalgia
rib R07.81
root (spinal) — *see* Radiculopathy
round ligament (stretch) R10.2
sacroiliac M53.3
sciatic — *see* Sciatica
scrotum N50.82
seminal vesicle N50.89
shoulder M25.51- ☑
spermatic cord N50.89
spinal root — *see* Radiculopathy
spine M54.9
cervical M54.2
low back M54.50
with sciatica M54.4- ☑
thoracic M54.6
stomach — *see* Pain, abdominal
substernal R07.2
temporomandibular (joint) M26.62- ☑
testis N50.81- ☑
thoracic spine M54.6
with radicular and visceral pain M54.14
throat R07.0
tibia — *see* Pain, limb, lower
toe — *see* Pain, limb, lower
tongue K14.6
tooth K08.89
trigeminal — *see* Neuralgia, trigeminal
tumor associated G89.3
ureter N23
urinary (organ) (system) N23
uterus NEC N94.89
vagina R10.2
vertebral end plate — *see* Pain, vertebrogenic
vertebrogenic M54.89
low back M54.51
lumbar M54.51
syndrome M54.89
vesical R39.89
associated with micturition — *see* Micturition, painful
vulva R10.2
Painful — *see also* Pain
coitus
female N94.10
male N53.12
psychogenic F52.6
ejaculation (semen) N53.12
psychogenic F52.6
erection — *see* Priapism
feet syndrome E53.8
joint replacement (hip) (knee) T84.84 ☑
menstruation — *see* Dysmenorrhea
psychogenic F45.8
micturition — *see* Micturition, painful
respiration R07.1
scar NEC L90.5
wire sutures T81.89 ☑
Painter's colic — *see* subcategory T56.0 ☑
Palate — *see* condition
Palatoplegia K13.79
Palatoschisis — *see* Cleft, palate
Palilalia R48.8
Palliative care Z51.5
Pallor R23.1
optic disc, temporal — *see* Atrophy, optic
Palmar — *see also* condition
fascia — *see* condition
Palpable
cecum K63.89
kidney N28.89
ovary N83.8
prostate N42.9
spleen — *see* Splenomegaly
Palpitations (heart) R00.2
psychogenic F45.8
Palsy — *see also* Paralysis G83.9
atrophic diffuse (progressive) G12.22
Bell's — *see also* Palsy, facial

Palsy — *continued*
Bell's — *see also* Palsy, facial — *continued*
newborn P11.3
brachial plexus NEC G54.0
newborn (birth injury) P14.3
brain — *see* Palsy, cerebral
bulbar (progressive) (chronic) G12.22
of childhood (Fazio-Londe) G12.1
pseudo NEC G12.29
supranuclear (progressive) G23.1
cerebral (congenital) G80.9
ataxic G80.4
athetoid G80.3
choreathetoid G80.3
diplegic G80.8
spastic G80.1
dyskinetic G80.3
athetoid G80.3
choreathetoid G80.3
distonic G80.3
dystonic G80.3
hemiplegic G80.8
spastic G80.2
mixed G80.8
monoplegic G80.8
spastic G80.1
paraplegic G80.8
spastic G80.1
quadriplegic G80.8
spastic G80.0
spastic G80.1
diplegic G80.1
hemiplegic G80.2
monoplegic G80.1
quadriplegic G80.0
specified NEC G80.1
tetraplegic G80.0
specified NEC G80.8
syphilitic A52.12
congenital A50.49
tetraplegic G80.8
spastic G80.0
cranial nerve — *see also* Disorder, nerve, cranial
multiple G52.7
in
infectious disease B99 ☑ *[G53]*
neoplastic disease — *see also* Neoplasm D49.9 *[G53]*
parasitic disease B89 *[G53]*
sarcoidosis D86.82
creeping G12.22
diver's T70.3 ☑
Erb's P14.0
facial G51.0
newborn (birth injury) P11.3
glossopharyngeal G52.1
Klumpke (-Déjérine) P14.1
lead — *see* subcategory T56.0 ☑
median nerve (tardy) G56.1- ☑
nerve G58.9
specified NEC G58.8
peroneal nerve (acute) (tardy) G57.3- ☑
progressive supranuclear G23.1
pseudobulbar NEC G12.29
radial nerve (acute) G56.3- ☑
seventh nerve — *see also* Palsy, facial
newborn P11.3
shaking — *see* Parkinsonism
spastic (cerebral) (spinal) G80.1
ulnar nerve (tardy) G56.2- ☑
wasting G12.29
Paludism — *see* Malaria
Panangiitis M30.0
Panaris, panaritium — *see also* Cellulitis, digit
with lymphangitis — *see* Lymphangitis, acute, digit
Panarteritis nodosa M30.0
brain or cerebral I67.7
Pancake heart R93.1
with cor pulmonale (chronic) I27.81
Pancarditis (acute) (chronic) I51.89
rheumatic I09.89
active or acute I01.8
Pancoast's syndrome or tumor C34.1- ☑
Pancolitis, ulcerative (chronic) K51.00
with
abscess K51.014
complication K51.019
fistula K51.013

Pancolitis, ulcerative — *continued*
with — *continued*
obstruction K51.012
rectal bleeding K51.011
specified complication NEC K51.018
Pancreas, pancreatic — *see* condition
Pancreatitis (annular) (apoplectic) (calcareous) (edematous) (hemorrhagic) (malignant) (subacute) (suppurative) K85.90
with necrosis (uninfected) K85.91
infected K85.92
acute (without necrosis or infection) K85.90
with necrosis (uninfected) K85.91
infected K85.92
alcohol induced (without necrosis or infection) K85.20
with necrosis (uninfected) K85.21
infected K85.22
biliary (without necrosis or infection) K85.10
with necrosis (uninfected) K85.11
infected K85.12
drug induced (without necrosis or infection) K85.30
with necrosis (uninfected) K85.31
infected K85.32
gallstone (without necrosis or infection) K85.10
with necrosis (uninfected) K85.11
infected K85.12
idiopathic (without necrosis or infection) K85.00
with necrosis (uninfected) K85.01
infected K85.02
specified NEC (without necrosis or infection) K85.80
with necrosis (uninfected) K85.81
infected K85.82
chronic (infectious) K86.1
alcohol-induced K86.0
recurrent K86.1
relapsing K86.1
cystic (chronic) K86.1
cytomegaloviral B25.2
fibrous (chronic) K86.1
gallstone (without necrosis or infection) K85.10
with necrosis (uninfected) K85.11
infected K85.12
gangrenous — *see* Pancreatitis, acute
interstitial (chronic) K86.1
acute — *see also* Pancreatitis, acute K85.80
mumps B26.3
recurrent
acute — *see* Pancreatitis, acute by type
chronic K86.1
relapsing, chronic K86.1
syphilitic A52.74
Pancreatoblastoma — *see* Neoplasm, pancreas, malignant
Pancreolithiasis K86.89
Pancytolysis D75.89
Pancytopenia (acquired) D61.818
with
malformations D61.09
myelodysplastic syndrome — *see* Syndrome, myelodysplastic
antineoplastic chemotherapy induced D61.810
congenital D61.09
drug-induced NEC D61.811
PANDAS (pediatric autoimmune neuropsychiatric disorders associated with streptococcal infections syndrome) D89.89
Panencephalitis, subacute, sclerosing A81.1
Panhematopenia D61.9
congenital D61.09
constitutional D61.09
splenic, primary D73.1
Panhemocytopenia D61.9
congenital D61.09
constitutional D61.09
Panhypogonadism E29.1
Panhypopituitarism E23.0
prepubertal E23.0
Panic (attack) (state) F41.0
reaction to exceptional stress (transient) F43.0
Panmyelopathy, familial, constitutional D61.09
Panmyelophthisis D61.82
congenital D61.09
Panmyelosis (acute) (with myelofibrosis) C94.4- ☑
Panner's disease — *see* Osteochondrosis, juvenile, humerus
Panneuritis endemica E51.11
Panniculitis (nodular) (nonsuppurative) M79.3

Pain — Panniculitis

Panniculitis — continued
- back M54.00
  - cervical region M54.02
  - cervicothoracic region M54.03
  - lumbar region M54.06
  - lumbosacral region M54.07
  - multiple sites M54.09
  - occipito-atlanto-axial region M54.01
  - sacrococcygeal region M54.08
  - thoracic region M54.04
  - thoracolumbar region M54.05
- lupus L93.2
- mesenteric K65.4
- neck M54.02
  - cervicothoracic region M54.03
  - occipito-atlanto-axial region M54.01
- relapsing M35.6

Panniculus adiposus (abdominal) E65

Pannus (allergic) (cornea) (degenerativus) (keratic) H16.42- ☑
- abdominal (symptomatic) E65
- trachomatosus, trachomatous (active) A71.1

Panophthalmitis H44.01- ☑

Pansinusitis (chronic) (hyperplastic) (nonpurulent) (purulent) J32.4
- acute J01.40
  - recurrent J01.41
- tuberculous A15.8

Panuveitis (sympathetic) H44.11- ☑

Panvalvular disease I08.9
- specified NEC I08.8

PAPA (pyogenic arthritis, pyoderma gangrenosum, and acne syndrome) M04.8

Papanicolaou smear, cervix Z12.4
- as part of routine gynecological examination Z01.419
  - with abnormal findings Z01.411
- for suspected neoplasm Z12.4
- nonspecific abnormal finding R87.619
- routine Z01.419
  - with abnormal findings Z01.411

Papilledema (choked disc) H47.10
- associated with
  - decreased ocular pressure H47.12
  - increased intracranial pressure H47.11
  - retinal disorder H47.13
- Foster-Kennedy syndrome H47.14- ☑

Papillitis H46.00
- anus K62.89
- chronic lingual K14.4
- necrotizing, kidney N17.2
- optic H46.0- ☑
- rectum K62.89
- renal, necrotizing N17.2
- tongue K14.0

Papilloma — see also Neoplasm, benign, by site
- acuminatum (female) (male) (anogenital) A63.0
- basal cell L82.1
  - inflamed L82.0
- benign pinta (primary) A67.0
- bladder (urinary) (transitional cell) D41.4
- choroid plexus (lateral ventricle) (third ventricle) D33.0
  - anaplastic C71.5
  - fourth ventricle D33.1
  - malignant C71.5
- renal pelvis (transitional cell) D41.1- ☑
  - benign D30.1- ☑
- Schneiderian
  - specified site — see Neoplasm, benign, by site
  - unspecified site D14.0
- serous surface
  - borderline malignancy
    - specified site — see Neoplasm, uncertain behavior, by site
    - unspecified site D39.10
  - specified site — see Neoplasm, benign, by site
  - unspecified site D27.9
- transitional (cell)
  - bladder (urinary) D41.4
  - inverted type — see Neoplasm, uncertain behavior, by site
  - renal pelvis D41.1- ☑
  - ureter D41.2- ☑
- ureter (transitional cell) D41.2- ☑
  - benign D30.2- ☑
- urothelial — see Neoplasm, uncertain behavior, by site
- villous — see Neoplasm, uncertain behavior, by site
  - adenocarcinoma in — see Neoplasm, malignant, by site

Papilloma — continued
- villous — see Neoplasm, uncertain behavior, by site — continued
  - adenocarcinoma in — see Neoplasm, malignant, by site — continued
    - in situ — see Neoplasm, in situ
- yaws, plantar or palmar A66.1

Papillomata, multiple, of yaws A66.1

Papillomatosis — see also Neoplasm, benign, by site
- confluent and reticulated L83
- cystic, breast — see Mastopathy, cystic
- ductal, breast — see Mastopathy, cystic
- intraductal (diffuse) — see Neoplasm, benign, by site
- subareolar duct D24- ☑

Papillomavirus, as cause of disease classified elsewhere B97.7

Papillon-Léage and Psaume syndrome Q87.0

Papule(s) R23.8
- carate (primary) A67.0
- fibrous, of nose D22.39
- Gottron's L94.4
- pinta (primary) A67.0

Papulosis
- lymphomatoid C86.6
- malignant I77.89

Papyraceous fetus O31.0- ☑

Para-albuminemia E88.09

Paracephalus Q89.7

Parachute mitral valve Q23.2

Paracoccidioidomycosis B41.9
- disseminated B41.7
- generalized B41.7
- mucocutaneous-lymphangitic B41.8
- pulmonary B41.0
- specified NEC B41.8
- visceral B41.8

Paradentosis K05.4

Paraffinoma T88.8 ☑

Paraganglioma D44.7
- adrenal D35.0- ☑
  - malignant C74.1- ☑
- aortic body D44.7
  - malignant C75.5
- carotid body D44.6
  - malignant C75.4
- chromaffin — see also Neoplasm, benign, by site
  - malignant — see Neoplasm, malignant, by site
- extra-adrenal D44.7
  - malignant C75.5
    - specified site — see Neoplasm, malignant, by site
    - unspecified site C75.5
  - specified site — see Neoplasm, uncertain behavior, by site
  - unspecified site D44.7
- gangliocytic D13.2
  - specified site — see Neoplasm, benign, by site
  - unspecified site D13.2
- glomus jugulare D44.7
  - malignant C75.5
- jugular D44.7
- malignant C75.5
  - specified site — see Neoplasm, malignant, by site
  - unspecified site C75.5
- nonchromaffin D44.7
  - malignant C75.5
    - specified site — see Neoplasm, malignant, by site
    - unspecified site C75.5
  - specified site — see Neoplasm, uncertain behavior, by site
  - unspecified site D44.7
- parasympathetic D44.7
  - specified site — see Neoplasm, uncertain behavior, by site
  - unspecified site D44.7
- specified site — see Neoplasm, uncertain behavior, by site
- sympathetic D44.7
  - specified site — see Neoplasm, uncertain behavior, by site
  - unspecified site D44.7
- unspecified site D44.7

Parageusia R43.2
- psychogenic F45.8

Paragonimiasis B66.4

Paragranuloma, Hodgkin — see Lymphoma, Hodgkin, specified NEC

Parahemophilia — see also Defect, coagulation D68.2

Parakeratosis R23.4
- variegata L41.0

Paralysis, paralytic (complete) (incomplete) G83.9
- with
  - syphilis A52.17
- abducens, abducent (nerve) — see Strabismus, paralytic, sixth nerve
- abductor, lower extremity G57.9- ☑
- accessory nerve G52.8
- accommodation — see also Paresis, of accommodation
  - hysterical F44.89
- acoustic nerve (except Deafness) H93.3 ☑
- agitans — see also Parkinsonism G20
  - arteriosclerotic G21.4
- alternating (oculomotor) G83.89
- amyotrophic G12.21
- ankle G57.9- ☑
- anus (sphincter) K62.89
- arm — see Monoplegia, upper limb
- ascending (spinal), acute G61.0
- association G12.29
- asthenic bulbar G70.00
  - with exacerbation (acute) G70.01
  - in crisis G70.01
- ataxic (hereditary) G11.9
  - general (syphilitic) A52.17
- atrophic G58.9
  - infantile, acute — see Poliomyelitis, paralytic
  - progressive G12.22
  - spinal (acute) — see Poliomyelitis, paralytic
- axillary G54.0
- Babinski-Nageotte's G83.89
- Bell's G51.0
  - newborn P11.3
- Benedikt's G46.3
- birth injury P14.9
  - spinal cord P11.5
- bladder (neurogenic) (sphincter) N31.2
- bowel, colon or intestine K56.0
- brachial plexus G54.0
  - birth injury P14.3
  - newborn (birth injury) P14.3
- brain G83.9
  - diplegia G83.0
  - triplegia G83.89
- bronchial J98.09
- Brown-Séquard G83.81
- bulbar (chronic) (progressive) G12.22
  - infantile — see Poliomyelitis, paralytic
  - poliomyelitic — see Poliomyelitis, paralytic
  - pseudo G12.29
- bulbospinal G70.00
  - with exacerbation (acute) G70.01
  - in crisis G70.01
- cardiac — see also Failure, heart I50.9
- cerebrocerebellar, diplegic G80.1
- cervical
  - plexus G54.2
  - sympathetic G90.09
- Céstan-Chenais G46.3
- Charcot-Marie-Tooth type G60.0
- Clark's G80.9
- colon K56.0
- compressed air T70.3 ☑
- compression
  - arm G56.9- ☑
  - leg G57.9- ☑
  - lower extremity G57.9- ☑
  - upper extremity G56.9- ☑
- congenital (cerebral) — see Palsy, cerebral
- conjugate movement (gaze) (of eye) H51.0
  - cortical (nuclear) (supranuclear) H51.0
- cordis — see Failure, heart
- cranial or cerebral nerve G52.9
- creeping G12.22
- crossed leg G83.89
- crutch — see Injury, brachial plexus
- deglutition R13.0
  - hysterical F44.4
- dementia A52.17
- descending (spinal) NEC G12.29
- diaphragm (flaccid) J98.6
  - due to accidental dissection of phrenic nerve during procedure — see Puncture, accidental complicating surgery

Paralysis, paralytic — *continued*
- digestive organs NEC K59.89
- diplegic — *see* Diplegia
- divergence (nuclear) H51.8
- diver's T70.3 ☑
- Duchenne's
  - birth injury P14.0
  - due to or associated with
    - motor neuron disease G12.22
    - muscular dystrophy G71.01
  - due to intracranial or spinal birth injury — *see* Palsy, cerebral
- embolic (current episode) I63.4- ☑
- Erb (-Duchenne) (birth) (newborn) P14.0
- Erb's syphilitic spastic spinal A52.17
- esophagus K22.89
- eye muscle (extrinsic) H49.9
  - intrinsic — *see also* Paresis, of accommodation
- facial (nerve) G51.0
  - birth injury P11.3
  - congenital P11.3
  - following operation NEC — *see* Puncture, accidental complicating surgery
  - newborn (birth injury) P11.3
- familial (recurrent) (periodic) G72.3
  - spastic G11.4
- fauces J39.2
- finger G56.9- ☑
- gait R26.1
- gastric nerve (nondiabetic) G52.2
- gaze, conjugate H51.0
- general (progressive) (syphilitic) A52.17
  - juvenile A50.45
- glottis J38.00
  - bilateral J38.02
  - unilateral J38.01
- gluteal G54.1
- Gubler (-Millard) G46.3
- hand — *see* Monoplegia, upper limb
- heart — *see* Arrest, cardiac
- hemiplegic — *see* Hemiplegia
- hyperkalemic periodic (familial) G72.3
- hypoglossal (nerve) G52.3
- hypokalemic periodic G72.3
- hysterical F44.4
- ileus K56.0
- infantile — *see also* Poliomyelitis, paralytic A80.30
  - bulbar — *see* Poliomyelitis, paralytic
  - cerebral — *see* Palsy, cerebral
  - spastic — *see* Palsy, cerebral, spastic
- infective — *see* Poliomyelitis, paralytic
- inferior nuclear G83.9
- internuclear — *see* Ophthalmoplegia, internuclear
- intestine K56.0
- iris H57.09
  - due to diphtheria (toxin) A36.89
- ischemic, Volkmann's (complicating trauma) T79.6 ☑
- Jackson's G83.89
- jake — *see* Poisoning, food, noxious, plant
- Jamaica ginger (jake) G62.2
- juvenile general A50.45
- Klumpke (-Déjérine) (birth) (newborn) P14.1
- labioglossal (laryngeal) (pharyngeal) G12.29
- Landry's G61.0
- laryngeal nerve (recurrent) (superior) (unilateral) J38.00
  - bilateral J38.02
  - unilateral J38.01
- larynx J38.00
  - bilateral J38.02
  - due to diphtheria (toxin) A36.2
  - unilateral J38.01
- lateral G12.23
- lead T56.0 ☑
- left side — *see* Hemiplegia
- leg G83.1- ☑
  - both — *see* Paraplegia
  - crossed G83.89
  - hysterical F44.4
  - psychogenic F44.4
  - transient or transitory R29.818
    - traumatic NEC — *see* Injury, nerve, leg
- levator palpebrae superioris — *see* Blepharoptosis, paralytic
- limb — *see* Monoplegia
- lip K13.0
- Lissauer's A52.17
- lower limb — *see* Monoplegia, lower limb
  - both — *see* Paraplegia

Paralysis, paralytic — *continued*
- lung J98.4
- median nerve G56.1- ☑
- medullary (tegmental) G83.89
- mesencephalic NEC G83.89
  - tegmental G83.89
- middle alternating G83.89
- Millard-Gubler-Foville G46.3
- monoplegic — *see* Monoplegia
- motor G83.9
- muscle, muscular NEC G72.89
  - due to nerve lesion G58.9
  - eye (extrinsic) H49.9
    - intrinsic — *see* Paresis, of accommodation
    - oblique — *see* Strabismus, paralytic, fourth nerve
  - iris sphincter H21.9
  - ischemic (Volkmann's) (complicating trauma) T79.6 ☑
  - progressive G12.21
  - progressive, spinal G12.25
  - pseudohypertrophic G71.02
  - spinal progressive G12.25
- musculocutaneous nerve G56.9- ☑
- musculospiral G56.9- ☑
- nerve — *see also* Disorder, nerve
  - abducent — *see* Strabismus, paralytic, sixth nerve
  - accessory G52.8
  - auditory (except Deafness) H93.3 ☑
  - birth injury P14.9
  - cranial or cerebral G52.9
  - facial G51.0
    - birth injury P11.3
    - congenital P11.3
    - newborn (birth injury) P11.3
  - fourth or trochlear — *see* Strabismus, paralytic, fourth nerve
  - newborn (birth injury) P14.9
  - oculomotor — *see* Strabismus, paralytic, third nerve
  - phrenic (birth injury) P14.2
  - radial G56.3- ☑
  - seventh or facial G51.0
    - newborn (birth injury) P11.3
  - sixth or abducent — *see* Strabismus, paralytic, sixth nerve
  - syphilitic A52.15
  - third or oculomotor — *see* Strabismus, paralytic, third nerve
  - trigeminal G50.9
  - trochlear — *see* Strabismus, paralytic, fourth nerve
  - ulnar G56.2- ☑
- normokalemic periodic G72.3
- ocular H49.9
  - alternating G83.89
- oculofacial, congenital (Moebius) Q87.0
- oculomotor (external bilateral) (nerve) — *see* Strabismus, paralytic, third nerve
- palate (soft) K13.79
- paratrigeminal G50.9
- periodic (familial) (hyperkalemic) (hypokalemic) (myotonic) (normokalemic) (potassium sensitive) (secondary) G72.3
- peripheral autonomic nervous system — *see* Neuropathy, peripheral, autonomic
- peroneal (nerve) G57.3- ☑
- pharynx J39.2
- phrenic nerve G56.8- ☑
- plantar nerve(s) G57.6- ☑
- pneumogastric nerve G52.2
- poliomyelitis (current) — *see* Poliomyelitis, paralytic
- popliteal nerve G57.3- ☑
- postepileptic transitory G83.84
- progressive (atrophic) (bulbar) (spinal) G12.22
  - general A52.17
  - infantile acute — *see* Poliomyelitis, paralytic
  - supranuclear G23.1
- pseudobulbar G12.29
- pseudohypertrophic (muscle) — *see also* Dystrophy, muscular, by type, if applicable G71.09
- psychogenic F44.4
- quadriceps G57.9- ☑
- quadriplegic — *see* Tetraplegia
- radial nerve G56.3- ☑
- rectus muscle (eye) H49.9
- recurrent isolated sleep G47.53
- respiratory (muscle) (system) (tract) R06.81
  - center NEC G93.89
  - congenital P28.89
  - newborn P28.89

Paralysis, paralytic — *continued*
- right side — *see* Hemiplegia
- saturnine T56.0 ☑
- sciatic nerve G57.0- ☑
- senile G83.9
- shaking — *see* Parkinsonism
- shoulder G56.9- ☑
- sleep, recurrent isolated G47.53
- spastic G83.9
  - cerebral — *see* Palsy, cerebral, spastic
  - congenital (cerebral) — *see* Palsy, cerebral, spastic
  - familial G11.4
  - hereditary G11.4
  - quadriplegic G80.0
  - syphilitic (spinal) A52.17
- sphincter, bladder — *see* Paralysis, bladder
- spinal (cord) G83.9
  - accessory nerve G52.8
  - acute — *see* Poliomyelitis, paralytic
  - ascending acute G61.0
  - atrophic (acute) — *see also* Poliomyelitis, paralytic spastic, syphilitic A52.17
  - congenital NEC — *see* Palsy, cerebral
  - hereditary G95.89
  - infantile — *see* Poliomyelitis, paralytic
  - progressive G12.21
    - muscle G12.25
  - sequelae NEC G83.89
- sternomastoid G52.8
- stomach K31.84
  - diabetic — *see* Diabetes, by type, with gastroparesis
  - nerve G52.2
    - diabetic — *see* Diabetes, by type, with gastroparesis
- stroke — *see* Infarct, brain
- subcapsularis G56.8- ☑
- supranuclear (progressive) G23.1
- sympathetic G90.8
  - cervical G90.09
  - nervous system — *see* Neuropathy, peripheral, autonomic
- syndrome G83.9
  - specified NEC G83.89
- syphilitic spastic spinal (Erb's) A52.17
- thigh G57.9- ☑
- throat J39.2
  - diphtheritic A36.0
  - muscle J39.2
- thrombotic (current episode) I63.3- ☑
- thumb G56.9- ☑
- tick — *see* Toxicity, venom, arthropod, specified NEC
- Todd's (postepileptic transitory paralysis) G83.84
- toe G57.6- ☑
- tongue K14.8
- transient R29.5
  - arm or leg NEC R29.818
  - traumatic NEC — *see* Injury, nerve
- trapezius G52.8
- traumatic, transient NEC — *see* Injury, nerve
- trembling — *see* Parkinsonism
- triceps brachii G56.9- ☑
- trigeminal nerve G50.9
- trochlear (nerve) — *see* Strabismus, paralytic, fourth nerve
- ulnar nerve G56.2- ☑
- upper limb — *see* Monoplegia, upper limb
- uremic N18.9 *[G99.8]*
- uveoparotitic D86.89
- uvula K13.79
  - postdiphtheritic A36.0
- vagus nerve G52.2
- vasomotor NEC G90.8
- velum palati K13.79
- vesical — *see* Paralysis, bladder
- vestibular nerve (except Vertigo) H93.3 ☑
- vocal cords J38.00
  - bilateral J38.02
  - unilateral J38.01
- Volkmann's (complicating trauma) T79.6 ☑
- wasting G12.29
- Weber's G46.3
- wrist G56.9- ☑

Paramedial urethrovesical orifice Q64.79

Paramenia N92.6

Parametritis — *see also* Disease, pelvis, inflammatory N73.2
- acute N73.0

Parametritis — *continued*
   complicating abortion — *see* Abortion, by type, complicated by, parametritis
Parametrium, parametric — *see* condition
Paramnesia — *see* Amnesia
Paramolar K00.1
Paramyloidosis E85.89
Paramyoclonus multiplex G25.3
Paramyotonia (congenita) G71.19
Parangi — *see* Yaws
Paranoia (querulans) F22
   senile F03 ☑
Paranoid
   dementia (senile) F03 ☑
      praecox — *see* Schizophrenia
   personality F60.0
   psychosis (climacteric) (involutional) (menopausal) F22
      psychogenic (acute) F23
      senile F03 ☑
   reaction (acute) F23
      chronic F22
   schizophrenia F20.0
   state (climacteric) (involutional) (menopausal) (simple) F22
      senile F03 ☑
   tendencies F60.0
   traits F60.0
   trends F60.0
   type, psychopathic personality F60.0
Paraparesis — *see* Paraplegia
Paraphasia R47.02
Paraphilia F65.9
Paraphimosis (congenital) N47.2
   chancroidal A57
Paraphrenia, paraphrenic (late) F22
   schizophrenia F20.0
Paraplegia (lower) G82.20
   ataxic — *see* Degeneration, combined, spinal cord
   complete G82.21
   congenital (cerebral) G80.8
      spastic G80.1
   familial spastic G11.4
   functional (hysterical) F44.4
   hereditary, spastic G11.4
   hysterical F44.4
   incomplete G82.22
   Pott's A18.01
   psychogenic F44.4
   spastic
      Erb's spinal, syphilitic A52.17
      hereditary G11.4
      tropical G04.1
   syphilitic (spastic) A52.17
   traumatic
      current injury — code to injury with seventh character A
      sequela of previous injury — code to injury with seventh character S
   tropical spastic G04.1
Parapoxvirus B08.60
   specified NEC B08.69
Paraproteinemia D89.2
   benign (familial) D89.2
   monoclonal D47.2
   secondary to malignant disease D47.2
Parapsoriasis L41.9
   en plaques L41.4
   guttata L41.1
   large plaque L41.4
   retiform, retiformis L41.5
   small plaque L41.3
   specified NEC L41.8
   varioliformis (acuta) L41.0
Parasitic — *see also* condition
   disease NEC B89
   stomatitis B37.0
   sycosis (beard) (scalp) B35.0
   twin Q89.4
Parasitism B89
   intestinal B82.9
   skin B88.9
   specified — *see* Infestation
Parasitophobia F40.218
Parasomnia G47.50
   due to
      alcohol
         abuse F10.182
         dependence F10.282

Parasomnia — *continued*
   due to — *continued*
      alcohol — *continued*
         use F10.982
      amphetamines
         abuse F15.182
         dependence F15.282
         use F15.982
      caffeine
         abuse F15.182
         dependence F15.282
         use F15.982
      cocaine
         abuse F14.182
         dependence F14.282
         use F14.982
      drug NEC
         abuse F19.182
         dependence F19.282
         use F19.982
      opioid
         abuse F11.182
         dependence F11.282
         use F11.982
      psychoactive substance NEC
         abuse F19.182
         dependence F19.282
         use F19.982
      sedative, hypnotic, or anxiolytic
         abuse F13.182
         dependence F13.282
         use F13.982
      stimulant NEC
         abuse F15.182
         dependence F15.282
         use F15.982
   in conditions classified elsewhere G47.54
   nonorganic origin F51.8
   organic G47.50
   specified NEC G47.59
Paraspadias Q54.9
Paraspasmus facialis G51.8
Parasuicide (attempt)
   history of (personal) Z91.51
      in family Z81.8
Parathyroid gland — *see* condition
Parathyroid tetany E20.9
Paratrachoma A74.0
Paratyphilitis — *see* Appendicitis
Paratyphoid (fever) — *see* Fever, paratyphoid
Paratyphus — *see* Fever, paratyphoid
Paraurethral duct Q64.79
Paraurethritis — *see also* Urethritis
   gonococcal (acute) (chronic) (with abscess) A54.1
Paravaccinia NEC B08.04
Paravaginitis — *see* Vaginitis
Parencephalitis — *see also* Encephalitis
   sequelae G09
Parent-child conflict — *see* Conflict, parent-child
   estrangement NEC Z62.890
Paresis — *see also* Paralysis
   accommodation — *see* Paresis, of accommodation
   Bernhardt's G57.1- ☑
   bladder (sphincter) — *see also* Paralysis, bladder
      tabetic A52.17
   bowel, colon or intestine K56.0
   extrinsic muscle, eye H49.9
   general (progressive) (syphilitic) A52.17
      juvenile A50.45
   heart — *see* Failure, heart
   insane (syphilitic) A52.17
   juvenile (general) A50.45
   of accommodation H52.52- ☑
   peripheral progressive (idiopathic) G60.3
   pseudohypertrophic — *see also* Dystrophy, muscular, by type, if applicable G71.09
   senile G83.9
   syphilitic (general) A52.17
      congenital A50.45
   vesical NEC N31.2
Paresthesia — *see also* Disturbance, sensation, skin R20.2
   Bernhardt G57.1- ☑
Paretic — *see* condition
Parinaud's
   conjunctivitis H10.89
   oculoglandular syndrome H10.89
   ophthalmoplegia H49.88- ☑
Parkinsonism (idiopathic) (primary) G20

Parkinsonism — *continued*
   with neurogenic orthostatic hypotension (symptomatic) G90.3
   arteriosclerotic G21.4
   dementia — *see also* Dementia, in, diseases specified elsewhere G20 *[F02.80]*
      with behavioral disturbance — *see also* Dementia, in, diseases specified elsewhere G20 *[F02.81-]* ☑
   due to
      drugs NEC G21.19
         neuroleptic G21.11
   medication-induced NEC G21.19
   neuroleptic induced G21.11
   postencephalitic G21.3
   secondary G21.9
      due to
         arteriosclerosis G21.4
         drugs NEC G21.19
            neuroleptic G21.11
         encephalitis G21.3
         external agents NEC G21.2
         syphilis A52.19
      specified NEC G21.8
   syphilitic A52.19
   treatment-induced NEC G21.19
   vascular G21.4
Parkinson's disease, syndrome or tremor — *see* Parkinsonism
Parodontitis — *see* Periodontitis
Parodontosis K05.4
Paronychia — *see also* Cellulitis, digit
   with lymphangitis — *see* Lymphangitis, acute, digit
   candidal (chronic) B37.2
   tuberculous (primary) A18.4
Parorexia (psychogenic) F50.89
Parosmia R43.1
   psychogenic F45.8
Parotid gland — *see* condition
Parotitis, parotiditis (allergic) (nonspecific toxic) (purulent) (septic) (suppurative) — *see also* Sialoadenitis
   epidemic — *see* Mumps
   infectious — *see* Mumps
   postoperative K91.89
   surgical K91.89
Parrot fever A70
Parrot's disease (early congenital syphilitic pseudoparalysis) A50.02
Parry-Romberg syndrome G51.8
Parry's disease or syndrome E05.00
   with thyroid storm E05.01
Pars planitis — *see* Cyclitis
Parsonage (-Aldren)-**Turner syndrome** G54.5
Parson's disease (exophthalmic goiter) E05.00
   with thyroid storm E05.01
Particolored infant Q82.8
Parturition — *see* Delivery
Parulis K04.7
   with sinus K04.6
Parvovirus, as cause of disease classified elsewhere B97.6
Pasini and Pierini's atrophoderma L90.3
Passage
   false, urethra N36.5
   meconium (newborn) during delivery P03.82
   of sounds or bougies — *see* Attention to, artificial, opening
Passive — *see* condition
   smoking Z77.22
Past due on rent or mortgage Z59.81- ☑
Pasteurella septica A28.0
Pasteurellosis — *see* Infection, Pasteurella
PAT (paroxysmal atrial tachycardia) I47.1
Patau's syndrome — *see* Trisomy, 13
Patches
   mucous (syphilitic) A51.39
      congenital A50.07
   smokers' (mouth) K13.24
Patellar — *see* condition
Patent — *see also* Imperfect, closure
   canal of Nuck Q52.4
   cervix N88.3
   ductus arteriosus or Botallo's Q25.0
   foramen
      botalli Q21.12
      ovale Q21.12
   interauricular septum Q21.19

☑ **Additional Character Required** — **Refer to the Tabular List for Character Selection**

Patent — *continued*
- interventricular septum Q21.0
- omphalomesenteric duct Q43.0
- os (uteri) — *see* Patent, cervix
- ostium secundum (type II) Q21.11
- urachus Q64.4
- vitelline duct Q43.0

Paterson (-Brown) (-Kelly) **syndrome or web** D50.1
Pathologic, pathological — *see also* condition
- asphyxia R09.01
- fire-setting F63.1
- gambling F63.0
- ovum O02.0
- resorption, tooth K03.3
- stealing F63.2

Pathology (of) — *see* Disease
- periradicular, associated with previous endodontic treatment NEC M27.59

Pattern, sleep-wake, irregular G47.23
Patulous — *see also* Imperfect, closure (congenital)
- alimentary tract Q45.8
  - lower Q43.8
  - upper Q40.8
- eustachian tube H69.0- ☑

Pause, sinoatrial I49.5
Paxton's disease B36.2
Pearl(s)
- enamel K00.2
- Epstein's K09.8

Pearl-worker's disease — *see* Osteomyelitis, specified type NEC
Pectenosis K62.4
Pectoral — *see* condition
Pectus
- carinatum (congenital) Q67.7
  - acquired M95.4
  - rachitic sequelae (late effect) E64.3
- excavatum (congenital) Q67.6
  - acquired M95.4
  - rachitic sequelae (late effect) E64.3
- recurvatum (congenital) Q67.6

Pedatrophia E41
Pederosis F65.4
Pediatric inflammatory multisystem syndrome M35.81
Pediculosis (infestation) B85.2
- capitis (head-louse) (any site) B85.0
- corporis (body-louse) (any site) B85.1
- eyelid B85.0
- mixed (classifiable to more than one of the titles B85.0-B85.3) B85.4
- pubis (pubic louse) (any site) B85.3
- vestimenti B85.1
- vulvae B85.3

Pediculus (infestation) — *see* Pediculosis
Pedophilia F65.4
Peg-shaped teeth K00.2
Pelade — *see* Alopecia, areata
Pelger-Huët anomaly or syndrome D72.0
Peliosis (rheumatica) D69.0
- hepatis K76.4
  - with toxic liver disease K71.8

Pelizaeus-Merzbacher disease E75.29
Pellagra (alcoholic) (with polyneuropathy) E52
Pellagra-cerebellar-ataxia-renal aminoaciduria syndrome E72.02
Pellegrini (-Stieda) **disease or syndrome** — *see* Bursitis, tibial collateral
Pellizzi's syndrome E34.8
Pel's crisis A52.11
Pelvic — *see also* condition
- examination (periodic) (routine) Z01.419
  - with abnormal findings Z01.411
- kidney, congenital Q63.2

Pelviolithiasis — *see* Calculus, kidney
Pelviperitonitis — *see also* Peritonitis, pelvic
- gonococcal A54.24
- puerperal O85

Pelvis — *see* condition or type
Pemphigoid L12.9
- benign, mucous membrane L12.1
- bullous L12.0
- cicatricial L12.1
- juvenile L12.2
- ocular L12.1
- specified NEC L12.8

Pemphigus L10.9
- benign familial (chronic) Q82.8

Pemphigus — *continued*
- Brazilian L10.3
- circinatus L13.0
- conjunctiva L12.1
- drug-induced L10.5
- erythematosus L10.4
- foliaceous L10.2
- gangrenous — *see* Gangrene
- neonatorum L01.03
- ocular L12.1
- paraneoplastic L10.81
- specified NEC L10.89
- syphilitic (congenital) A50.06
- vegetans L10.1
- vulgaris L10.0
- wildfire L10.3

Pendred's syndrome E07.1
Pendulous
- abdomen, in pregnancy — *see* Pregnancy, complicated by, abnormal, pelvic organs or tissues NEC
- breast N64.89

Penetrating wound — *see also* Puncture
- with internal injury — *see* Injury, by site
- eyeball — *see* Puncture, eyeball
- orbit (with or without foreign body) — *see* Puncture, orbit
- uterus by instrument with or following ectopic or molar pregnancy O08.6

Penicillosis B48.4
Penis — *see* condition
Penitis N48.29
Pentalogy of Fallot Q21.8
Pentasomy X syndrome Q97.1
Pentosuria (essential) E74.89
Percreta placenta - O43.23 ☑
Peregrinating patient — *see* Disorder, factitious
Perforation, perforated (nontraumatic) (of)
- accidental during procedure (blood vessel) (nerve) (organ) — *see* Complication, accidental puncture or laceration
- antrum — *see* Sinusitis, maxillary
- appendix K35.32
  - with localized peritonitis K35.32
- atrial septum, multiple Q21.19
- attic, ear — *see* Perforation, tympanum, attic
- bile duct (common) (hepatic) K83.2
  - cystic K82.2
- bladder (urinary)
  - with or following ectopic or molar pregnancy O08.6
  - obstetrical trauma O71.5
  - traumatic S37.29 ☑
    - at delivery O71.5
- bowel K63.1
  - with or following ectopic or molar pregnancy O08.6
  - newborn P78.0
  - obstetrical trauma O71.5
  - traumatic — *see* Laceration, intestine
- broad ligament N83.8
  - with or following ectopic or molar pregnancy O08.6
  - obstetrical trauma O71.6
- by
  - device, implant or graft — *see also* Complications, by site and type, mechanical T85.628 ☑
    - arterial graft NEC — *see* Complication, cardiovascular device, mechanical, vascular
    - breast (implant) T85.49 ☑
    - catheter NEC T85.698 ☑
      - cystostomy T83.090 ☑
      - dialysis (renal) T82.49 ☑
        - intraperitoneal T85.691 ☑
      - infusion NEC T82.594 ☑
        - spinal (epidural) (subdural) T85.690 ☑
      - urinary — *see also* Complications, catheter, urinary T83.098 ☑
    - electronic (electrode) (pulse generator) (stimulator)
      - bone T84.390 ☑
      - cardiac T82.199 ☑
        - electrode T82.190 ☑
        - pulse generator T82.191 ☑
        - specified type NEC T82.198 ☑
      - nervous system — *see* Complication, prosthetic device, mechanical, electronic nervous system stimulator
      - urinary — *see* Complication, genitourinary, device, urinary, mechanical

Perforation, perforated — *continued*
- by — *continued*
  - device, implant or graft — *see also* Complications, by site and type, mechanical — *continued*
    - fixation, internal (orthopedic) NEC — *see* Complication, fixation device, mechanical
    - gastrointestinal — *see* Complications, prosthetic device, mechanical, gastrointestinal device
    - genital NEC T83.498 ☑
      - intrauterine contraceptive device T83.39 ☑
      - penile prosthesis T83.490 ☑
    - heart NEC — *see* Complication, cardiovascular device, mechanical
    - joint prosthesis — *see* Complications, joint prosthesis, mechanical, specified NEC, by site
    - ocular NEC — *see* Complications, prosthetic device, mechanical, ocular device
    - orthopedic NEC — *see* Complication, orthopedic, device, mechanical
    - specified NEC T85.628 ☑
    - urinary NEC — *see also* Complication, genitourinary, device, urinary, mechanical
      - graft T83.29 ☑
    - vascular NEC — *see* Complication, cardiovascular device, mechanical
    - ventricular intracranial shunt T85.09 ☑
  - foreign body left accidentally in operative wound T81.539 ☑
  - instrument (any) during a procedure, accidental — *see* Puncture, accidental complicating surgery
- cecum K35.32
  - with localized peritonitis K35.32
- cervix (uteri) N88.8
  - with or following ectopic or molar pregnancy O08.6
  - obstetrical trauma O71.3
- colon K63.1
  - newborn P78.0
  - obstetrical trauma O71.5
  - traumatic — *see* Laceration, intestine, large
- common duct (bile) K83.2
- cornea (due to ulceration) — *see* Ulcer, cornea, perforated
- cystic duct K82.2
- diverticulum (intestine) K57.80
  - with bleeding K57.81
  - large intestine K57.20
    - with
      - bleeding K57.21
      - small intestine K57.40
        - with bleeding K57.41
  - small intestine K57.00
    - with
      - bleeding K57.01
      - large intestine K57.40
        - with bleeding K57.41
- ear drum — *see* Perforation, tympanum
- esophagus K22.3
- ethmoidal sinus — *see* Sinusitis, ethmoidal
- frontal sinus — *see* Sinusitis, frontal
- gallbladder K82.2
- heart valve — *see* Endocarditis
- ileum K63.1
  - newborn P78.0
  - obstetrical trauma O71.5
  - traumatic — *see* Laceration, intestine, small
- instrumental, surgical (accidental) (blood vessel) (nerve) (organ) — *see* Puncture, accidental complicating surgery
- intestine NEC K63.1
  - with ectopic or molar pregnancy O08.6
  - newborn P78.0
  - obstetrical trauma O71.5
  - traumatic — *see* Laceration, intestine
  - ulcerative NEC K63.1
    - newborn P78.0
- jejunum, jejunal K63.1
  - obstetrical trauma O71.5
  - traumatic — *see* Laceration, intestine, small
  - ulcer — *see* Ulcer, gastrojejunal, with perforation
- joint prosthesis — *see* Complications, joint prosthesis, mechanical, specified NEC, by site
- mastoid (antrum) (cell) — *see* Disorder, mastoid, specified NEC
- maxillary sinus — *see* Sinusitis, maxillary
- membrana tympani — *see* Perforation, tympanum
- nasal
  - septum J34.89

Perforation, perforated — continued
- nasal — continued
  - septum — continued
    - congenital Q30.3
    - syphilitic A52.73
  - sinus J34.89
    - congenital Q30.8
    - due to sinusitis — see Sinusitis
- palate — see also Cleft, palate Q35.9
  - syphilitic A52.79
- palatine vault — see also Cleft, palate, hard Q35.1
  - syphilitic A52.79
    - congenital A50.59
- pars flaccida (ear drum) — see Perforation, tympanum, attic
- pelvic
  - floor S31.030 ☑
    - with
      - ectopic or molar pregnancy O08.6
      - penetration into retroperitoneal space S31.031
      - retained foreign body S31.040 ☑
        - with penetration into retroperitoneal space S31.041 ☑
    - following ectopic or molar pregnancy O08.6
    - obstetrical trauma O70.1
  - organ S37.99 ☑
    - adrenal gland S37.818 ☑
    - bladder — see Perforation, bladder
    - fallopian tube S37.599 ☑
      - bilateral S37.592 ☑
      - unilateral S37.591 ☑
    - kidney S37.09- ☑
    - obstetrical trauma O71.5
    - ovary S37.499 ☑
      - bilateral S37.492 ☑
      - unilateral S37.491 ☑
    - prostate S37.828 ☑
    - specified organ NEC S37.898 ☑
    - ureter — see Perforation, ureter
    - urethra — see Perforation, urethra
    - uterus — see Perforation, uterus
- perineum — see Laceration, perineum
- pharynx J39.2
- rectum K63.1
  - newborn P78.0
  - obstetrical trauma O71.5
  - traumatic S36.63 ☑
- root canal space due to endodontic treatment M27.51
- sigmoid K63.1
  - newborn P78.0
  - obstetrical trauma O71.5
  - traumatic S36.533 ☑
- sinus (accessory) (chronic) (nasal) J34.89
- sphenoidal sinus — see Sinusitis, sphenoidal
- surgical (accidental) (by instrument) (blood vessel) (nerve) (organ) — see Puncture, accidental complicating surgery
- traumatic
  - external — see Puncture
  - eye — see Puncture, eyeball
  - internal organ — see Injury, by site
- tympanum, tympanic (membrane) (persistent post-traumatic) (postinflammatory) H72.9- ☑
  - attic H72.1- ☑
    - multiple — see Perforation, tympanum, multiple
    - total — see Perforation, tympanum, total
  - central H72.0- ☑
    - multiple — see Perforation, tympanum, multiple
    - total — see Perforation, tympanum, total
  - marginal NEC — see subcategory H72.2 ☑
  - multiple H72.81- ☑
  - pars flaccida — see Perforation, tympanum, attic
  - total H72.82- ☑
  - traumatic, current episode S09.2- ☑
- typhoid, gastrointestinal — see Typhoid
- ulcer — see Ulcer, by site, with perforation
- ureter N28.89
  - traumatic S37.19 ☑
- urethra N36.8
  - with ectopic or molar pregnancy O08.6
  - following ectopic or molar pregnancy O08.6
  - obstetrical trauma O71.5
  - traumatic S37.39 ☑
    - at delivery O71.5
- uterus
  - with ectopic or molar pregnancy O08.6

Perforation, perforated — continued
- uterus — continued
  - by intrauterine contraceptive device T83.39 ☑
  - following ectopic or molar pregnancy O08.6
  - obstetrical trauma O71.1
  - traumatic S37.69 ☑
    - obstetric O71.1
- uvula K13.79
  - syphilitic A52.79
- vagina O71.4
  - obstetrical trauma O71.4
  - other trauma — see Puncture, vagina
Periadenitis mucosa necrotica recurrens K12.0
Periappendicitis (acute) — see Appendicitis
Periarteritis nodosa (disseminated) (infectious) (necrotizing) M30.0
Periarthritis (joint) — see also Enthesopathy
- Duplay's M75.0- ☑
- gonococcal A54.42
- humeroscapularis — see Capsulitis, adhesive
- scapulohumeral — see Capsulitis, adhesive
- shoulder — see Capsulitis, adhesive
- wrist M77.2- ☑
Periarthrosis (angioneural) — see Enthesopathy
Pericapsulitis, adhesive (shoulder) — see Capsulitis, adhesive
Pericarditis (with decompensation) (with effusion) I31.9
- with rheumatic fever (conditions in I00)
  - active — see Pericarditis, rheumatic
  - inactive or quiescent I09.2
- acute (hemorrhagic) (nonrheumatic) (Sicca) I30.9
  - with chorea (acute) (rheumatic) (Sydenham's) I02.0
  - benign I30.8
  - nonspecific I30.0
  - rheumatic I01.0
    - with chorea (acute) (Sydenham's) I02.0
- adhesive or adherent (chronic) (external) (internal) I31.0
  - acute — see Pericarditis, acute
  - rheumatic I09.2
- bacterial (acute) (subacute) (with serous or seropurulent effusion) I30.1
- calcareous I31.1
- cholesterol (chronic) I31.8
  - acute I30.9
- chronic (nonrheumatic) I31.9
  - rheumatic I09.2
- constrictive (chronic) I31.1
- coxsackie B33.23
- fibrinocaseous (tuberculous) A18.84
- fibrinopurulent I30.1
- fibrinous I30.8
- fibrous I31.0
- gonococcal A54.83
- idiopathic I30.0
- in systemic lupus erythematosus M32.12
- infective I30.1
- meningococcal A39.53
- neoplastic (chronic) I31.8
  - acute I30.9
- obliterans, obliterating I31.0
- plastic I31.0
- pneumococcal I30.1
- postinfarction I24.1
- purulent I30.1
- rheumatic (active) (acute) (with effusion) (with pneumonia) I01.0
  - with chorea (acute) (rheumatic) (Sydenham's) I02.0
  - chronic or inactive (with chorea) I09.2
- rheumatoid — see Rheumatoid, carditis
- septic I30.1
- serofibrinous I30.8
- staphylococcal I30.1
- streptococcal I30.1
- suppurative I30.1
- syphilitic A52.06
- tuberculous A18.84
- uremic N18.9 [I32]
- viral I30.1
Pericardium, pericardial — see condition
Pericellulitis — see Cellulitis
Pericementitis (chronic) (suppurative) — see also Periodontitis
- acute K05.20
  - generalized — see Periodontitis, aggressive, generalized
  - localized — see Periodontitis, aggressive, localized
Perichondritis
- auricle — see Perichondritis, ear

Perichondritis — continued
- bronchus J98.09
- ear (external) H61.00- ☑
  - acute H61.01- ☑
  - chronic H61.02- ☑
- external auditory canal — see Perichondritis, ear
- larynx J38.7
  - syphilitic A52.73
  - typhoid A01.09
- nose J34.89
- pinna — see Perichondritis, ear
- trachea J39.8
Periclasia K05.4
Pericoronitis — see Periodontitis
Pericystitis N30.90
- with hematuria N30.91
Peridiverticulitis (intestine) K57.92
- cecum — see Diverticulitis, intestine, large
- colon — see Diverticulitis, intestine, large
- duodenum — see Diverticulitis, intestine, small
- intestine — see Diverticulitis, intestine
- jejunum — see Diverticulitis, intestine, small
- rectosigmoid — see Diverticulitis, intestine, large
- rectum — see Diverticulitis, intestine, large
- sigmoid — see Diverticulitis, intestine, large
Periendocarditis — see Endocarditis
Periepididymitis N45.1
Perifolliculitis L01.02
- abscedens, caput, scalp L66.3
- capitis, abscedens (et suffodiens) L66.3
- superficial pustular L01.02
Perihepatitis K65.8
Perilabyrinthitis (acute) — see subcategory H83.0 ☑
Perimeningitis — see Meningitis
Perimetritis — see Endometritis
Perimetrosalpingitis — see Salpingo-oophoritis
Perineocele N81.81
Perinephric, perinephritic — see condition
Perinephritis — see also Infection, kidney
- purulent — see Abscess, kidney
Perineum, perineal — see condition
Perineuritis NEC — see Neuralgia
Periodic — see condition
Periodontitis (chronic) (complex) (compound) (local) (simplex) K05.30
- acute K05.20
  - generalized K05.229
    - moderate K05.222
    - severe K05.223
    - slight K05.221
  - localized K05.219
    - moderate K05.212
    - severe K05.213
    - slight K05.211
- aggressive K05.20
  - generalized K05.229
    - moderate K05.222
    - severe K05.223
    - slight K05.221
  - localized K05.219
    - moderate K05.212
    - severe K05.213
    - slight K05.211
- apical K04.5
  - acute (pulpal origin) K04.4
- generalized K05.329
  - moderate K05.322
  - severe K05.323
  - slight K05.321
- localized K05.319
  - moderate K05.312
  - severe K05.313
  - slight K05.311
Periodontoclasia K05.4
Periodontosis (juvenile) K05.4
Periods — see also Menstruation
- heavy N92.0
- irregular N92.6
- shortened intervals (irregular) N92.1
Perionychia — see also Cellulitis, digit
- with lymphangitis — see Lymphangitis, acute, digit
Periophoritis — see Salpingo-oophoritis
Periorchitis N45.2
Periosteum, periosteal — see condition
Periostitis (albuminosa) (circumscribed) (diffuse) (infective) (monomelic) — see also Osteomyelitis
- alveolar M27.3

Periostitis — *continued*
  alveolodental M27.3
  dental M27.3
  gonorrheal A54.43
  jaw (lower) (upper) M27.2
  orbit H05.03- ☑
  syphilitic A52.77
    congenital (early) A50.02 *[M90.80]*
    secondary A51.46
  tuberculous — *see* Tuberculosis, bone
  yaws (hypertrophic) (early) (late) A66.6 *[M90.80]*
Periostosis (hyperplastic) — *see also* Disorder, bone, specified type NEC
  with osteomyelitis — *see* Osteomyelitis, specified type NEC
Peripartum
  cardiomyopathy O90.3
Periphlebitis — *see* Phlebitis
Periproctitis K62.89
Periprostatitis — *see* Prostatitis
Perirectal — *see* condition
Perirenal — *see* condition
Perisalpingitis — *see* Salpingo-oophoritis
Perisplenitis (infectional) D73.89
Peristalsis, visible or reversed R19.2
Peritendinitis — *see* Enthesopathy
Peritoneum, peritoneal — *see* condition
Peritonitis (adhesive) (bacterial) (fibrinous) (hemorrhagic) (idiopathic) (localized) (perforative) (primary) (with adhesions) (with effusion) K65.9
  with or following
    abscess K65.1
    appendicitis
      with perforation or rupture K35.32
      generalized — *see also* Appendicitis K35.20
      localized — *see also* Appendicitis K35.30
    diverticular disease (intestine) K57.80
      with bleeding K57.81
    ectopic or molar pregnancy O08.0
    large intestine K57.20
      with
        bleeding K57.21
        small intestine K57.40
          with bleeding K57.41
    small intestine K57.00
      with
        bleeding K57.01
        large intestine K57.40
          with bleeding K57.41
  acute (generalized) K65.0
  aseptic T81.61 ☑
  bile, biliary K65.3
  chemical T81.61 ☑
  chlamydial A74.81
  chronic proliferative K65.8
  complicating abortion — *see* Abortion, by type, complicated by, pelvic peritonitis
  congenital P78.1
  diaphragmatic K65.0
  diffuse K65.0
  diphtheritic A36.89
  disseminated K65.0
  due to
    bile K65.3
    foreign
      body or object accidentally left during a procedure (instrument) (sponge) (swab) T81.599 ☑
      substance accidentally left during a procedure (chemical) (powder) (talc) T81.61 ☑
    talc T81.61 ☑
    urine K65.8
  eosinophilic K65.8
    acute K65.0
  fibrocaseous (tuberculous) A18.31
  fibropurulent K65.0
  following ectopic or molar pregnancy O08.0
  general (ized) K65.0
  gonococcal A54.85
  meconium (newborn) P78.0
  neonatal P78.1
    meconium P78.0
  pancreatic K65.0
  paroxysmal, familial E85.0
    benign E85.0
  pelvic
    female N73.5
      acute N73.3

Peritonitis — *continued*
  pelvic — *continued*
    female — *continued*
      chronic N73.4
        with adhesions N73.6
    male K65.0
  periodic, familial E85.0
  proliferative, chronic K65.8
  puerperal, postpartum, childbirth O85
  purulent K65.0
  septic K65.0
  specified NEC K65.8
  spontaneous bacterial K65.2
  subdiaphragmatic K65.0
  subphrenic K65.0
  suppurative K65.0
  syphilitic A52.74
    congenital (early) A50.08 *[K67]*
  talc T81.61 ☑
  tuberculous A18.31
  urine K65.8
Peritonsillar — *see* condition
Peritonsillitis J36
Perityphlitis — *see also* Cecitis K37
Periureteritis N28.89
Periurethral — *see* condition
Periurethritis (gangrenous) — *see* Urethritis
Periuterine — *see* condition
Perivaginitis — *see* Vaginitis
Perivasculitis, retinal H35.06- ☑
Perivasitis (chronic) N49.1
Perivesiculitis (seminal) — *see* Vesiculitis
Perlèche NEC K13.0
  due to
    candidiasis B37.83
    moniliasis B37.83
    riboflavin deficiency E53.0
    vitamin B2 (riboflavin) deficiency E53.0
Pernicious — *see* condition
Pernio, perniosis T69.1 ☑
Perpetrator (of abuse) — *see* Index to External Causes of Injury, Perpetrator
Persecution
  delusion F22
  social Z60.5
Perseveration (tonic) R48.8
Persistence, persistent (congenital)
  anal membrane Q42.3
    with fistula Q42.2
  arteria stapedia Q16.3
  atrioventricular canal Q21.20
  branchial cleft NOS Q18.2
    cyst Q18.0
    fistula Q18.0
    sinus Q18.0
  bulbus cordis in left ventricle Q21.8
  canal of Cloquet Q14.0
  capsule (opaque) Q12.8
  cilioretinal artery or vein Q14.8
  cloaca Q43.7
  communication — *see* Fistula, congenital
  convolutions
    aortic arch Q25.46
    fallopian tube Q50.6
    oviduct Q50.6
    uterine tube Q50.6
  double aortic arch Q25.45
  ductus arteriosus (Botalli) Q25.0
  fetal
    circulation P29.38
    form of cervix (uteri) Q51.828
    hemoglobin, hereditary (HPFH) D56.4
  foramen
    Botalli Q21.12
    ovale Q21.12
  Gartner's duct Q52.4
  hemoglobin, fetal (hereditary) (HPFH) D56.4
  hyaloid
    artery (generally incomplete) Q14.0
    system Q14.8
  hymen, in pregnancy or childbirth — *see* Pregnancy, complicated by, abnormal, vulva
  lanugo Q84.2
  left
    posterior cardinal vein Q26.8
    root with right arch of aorta Q25.49
    superior vena cava Q26.1
  Meckel's diverticulum Q43.0

Persistence, persistent — *continued*
  Meckel's diverticulum — *continued*
    malignant — *see* Table of Neoplasms, small intestine, malignant
  mucosal disease (middle ear) — *see* Otitis, media, suppurative, chronic, tubotympanic
  nail(s), anomalous Q84.6
  omphalomesenteric duct Q43.0
  organ or site not listed — *see* Anomaly, by site
  ostium
    atrioventriculare commune Q21.23
    primum Q21.20
    secundum Q21.11
  ovarian rests in fallopian tube Q50.6
  pancreatic tissue in intestinal tract Q43.8
  primary (deciduous)
    teeth K00.6
    vitreous hyperplasia Q14.0
  pupillary membrane Q13.89
  rhesus (Rh) titer — *see* Complication(s), transfusion, incompatibility reaction, Rh (factor)
  right aortic arch Q25.47
  sinus
    urogenitalis
      female Q52.8
      male Q55.8
    venosus with imperfect incorporation in right auricle Q26.8
  thymus (gland) (hyperplasia) E32.0
  thyroglossal duct Q89.2
  thyrolingual duct Q89.2
  truncus arteriosus or communis Q20.0
  tunica vasculosa lentis Q12.2
  umbilical sinus Q64.4
  urachus Q64.4
  vitelline duct Q43.0
Person (with)
  admitted for clinical research, as a control subject (normal comparison) (participant) Z00.6
  awaiting admission to adequate facility elsewhere Z75.1
  concern (normal) about sick person in family Z63.6
  consulting on behalf of another Z71.0
  feigning illness Z76.5
  living (in)
    alone Z60.2
    boarding school Z59.3
    residential institution Z59.3
    without
      adequate housing (heating) (space) Z59.1
      housing (permanent) (temporary) Z59.00
      person able to render necessary care Z74.2
      shelter Z59.02
  on waiting list Z75.1
  sick or handicapped in family Z63.6
Personality (disorder) F60.9
  accentuation of traits (type A pattern) Z73.1
  affective F34.0
  aggressive F60.3
  amoral F60.2
  anacastic, anankastic F60.5
  antisocial F60.2
  anxious F60.6
  asocial F60.2
  asthenic F60.7
  avoidant F60.6
  borderline F60.3
  change due to organic condition (enduring) F07.0
  compulsive F60.5
  cycloid F34.0
  cyclothymic F34.0
  dependent F60.7
  depressive F34.1
  dissocial F60.2
  dual F44.81
  eccentric F60.89
  emotionally unstable F60.3
  expansive paranoid F60.0
  explosive F60.3
  fanatic F60.0
  haltose type F60.89
  histrionic F60.4
  hyperthymic F34.0
  hypothymic F34.1
  hysterical F60.4
  immature F60.89
  inadequate F60.7
  labile (emotional) F60.3
  mixed (nonspecific) F60.89

Personality — *continued*
  morally defective F60.2
  multiple F44.81
  narcissistic F60.81
  obsessional F60.5
  obsessive (-compulsive) F60.5
  organic F07.0
  overconscientious F60.5
  paranoid F60.0
  passive (-dependent) F60.7
  passive-aggressive F60.89
  pathologic F60.9
  pattern defect or disturbance F60.9
  pseudopsychopathic (organic) F07.0
  pseudoretarded (organic) F07.0
  psychoinfantile F60.4
  psychoneurotic NEC F60.89
  psychopathic F60.2
  querulant F60.0
  sadistic F60.89
  schizoid F60.1
  self-defeating F60.89
  sensitive paranoid F60.0
  sociopathic (amoral) (antisocial) (asocial) (dissocial)
    F60.2
  specified NEC F60.89
  type A Z73.1
  unstable (emotional) F60.3
Perthes' disease — *see* Legg-Calvé-Perthes disease
Pertussis — *see also* Whooping cough A37.90
Perversion, perverted
  appetite F50.89
    psychogenic F50.89
  function
    pituitary gland E23.2
      posterior lobe E22.2
  sense of smell and taste R43.8
    psychogenic F45.8
  sexual — *see* Deviation, sexual
Pervious, congenital — *see also* Imperfect, closure
  ductus arteriosus Q25.0
Pes (congenital) — *see also* Talipes
  acquired — *see also* Deformity, limb, foot, specified
    NEC
    planus — *see* Deformity, limb, flat foot
  adductus Q66.89
  cavus Q66.7- ☑
  deformity NEC, acquired — *see* Deformity, limb, foot,
    specified NEC
  planus (acquired) (any degree) — *see also* Deformity,
    limb, flat foot
    rachitic sequelae (late effect) E64.3
  valgus Q66.6
Pest, pestis — *see* Plague
Petechia, petechiae R23.3
  newborn P54.5
Petechial typhus A75.9
Peter's anomaly Q13.4
Petit mal seizure — *see* Epilepsy, childhood, absence
Petit's hernia — *see* Hernia, abdomen, specified site NEC
Petrellidosis B48.2
Petrositis H70.20- ☑
  acute H70.21- ☑
  chronic H70.22- ☑
Peutz-Jeghers disease or syndrome Q85.89
Peyronie's disease N48.6
PFAPA (periodic fever, aphthous stomatitis, pharyngitis,
    and adenopathy syndrome) M04.8
Pfeiffer's disease — *see* Mononucleosis, infectious
Phagedena (dry) (moist) (sloughing) — *see also* Gan-
    grene
  geometric L88
  penis N48.29
  tropical — *see* Ulcer, skin
  vulva N76.6
Phagedenic — *see* condition
Phakoma H35.89
Phakomatosis — *see also* specific eponymous syndromes
    Q85.9
  Bourneville's Q85.1
  specified NEC Q85.89
Phantom limb syndrome (without pain) G54.7
  with pain G54.6
Pharyngeal pouch syndrome D82.1
Pharyngitis (acute) (catarrhal) (gangrenous) (infective)
    (malignant) (membranous) (phlegmonous) (pseu-
    domembranous) (simple) (subacute) (suppurative)
    (ulcerative) (viral) J02.9

Pharyngitis — *continued*
  with influenza, flu, or grippe — *see* Influenza, with,
    pharyngitis
  aphthous B08.5
  atrophic J31.2
  chlamydial A56.4
  chronic (atrophic) (granular) (hypertrophic) J31.2
  coxsackievirus B08.5
  diphtheritic A36.0
  enteroviral vesicular B08.5
  follicular (chronic) J31.2
  fusospirochetal A69.1
  gonococcal A54.5
  granular (chronic) J31.2
  herpesviral B00.2
  hypertrophic J31.2
  infectional, chronic J31.2
  influenzal — *see* Influenza, with, respiratory manifesta-
    tions NEC
  lymphonodular, acute (enteroviral) B08.8
  pneumococcal J02.8
  purulent J02.9
  putrid J02.9
  septic J02.0
  sicca J31.2
  specified organism NEC J02.8
  staphylococcal J02.8
  streptococcal J02.0
  syphilitic, congenital (early) A50.03
  tuberculous A15.8
  vesicular, enteroviral B08.5
  viral NEC J02.8
Pharyngoconjunctivitis, viral B30.2
Pharyngolaryngitis (acute) J06.0
  chronic J37.0
Pharyngoplegia J39.2
Pharyngotonsillitis, herpesviral B00.2
Pharyngotracheitis, chronic J42
Pharynx, pharyngeal — *see* condition
Phencyclidine-induced
  anxiety disorder F16.980
  bipolar and related disorder F16.94
  depressive disorder F16.94
  psychotic disorder F16.959
Phenomenon
  Arthus' — *see* Arthus' phenomenon
  jaw-winking Q07.8
  lupus erythematosus (LE) cell M32.9
  Raynaud's (secondary) I73.00
    with gangrene I73.01
  vasomotor R55
  vasospastic I73.9
  vasovagal R55
  Wenckebach's I44.1
Phenylketonuria E70.1
  classical E70.0
  maternal E70.1
Pheochromoblastoma
  specified site — *see* Neoplasm, malignant, by site
  unspecified site C74.10
Pheochromocytoma
  malignant
    specified site — *see* Neoplasm, malignant, by site
    unspecified site C74.10
  specified site — *see* Neoplasm, benign, by site
  unspecified site D35.00
Pheohyphomycosis — *see* Chromomycosis
Pheomycosis — *see* Chromomycosis
Phimosis (congenital) (due to infection) N47.1
  chancroidal A57
Phlebectasia — *see also* Varix
  congenital Q27.4
Phlebitis (infective) (pyemic) (septic) (suppurative) I80.9
  antepartum — *see* Thrombophlebitis, antepartum
  blue — *see* Phlebitis, leg, deep
  breast, superficial I80.8
  calf muscular vein (NOS) I80.25- ☑
  cavernous (venous) sinus — *see* Phlebitis, intracranial
    (venous) sinus
  cerebral (venous) sinus — *see* Phlebitis, intracranial
    (venous) sinus
  chest wall, superficial I80.8
  cranial (venous) sinus — *see* Phlebitis, intracranial
    (venous) sinus
  deep (vessels) — *see* Phlebitis, leg, deep
  due to implanted device — *see* Complications, by site
    and type, specified NEC
  during or resulting from a procedure T81.72 ☑

Phlebitis — *continued*
  femoral vein (superficial) I80.1- ☑
  femoropopliteal vein I80.0- ☑
  gastrocnemial vein I80.25- ☑
  gestational — *see* Phlebopathy, gestational
  hepatic veins I80.8
  iliac vein (common) (external) (internal) I80.21- ☑
  iliofemoral — *see* Phlebitis, femoral vein
  intracranial (venous) sinus (any) G08
    nonpyogenic I67.6
  intraspinal venous sinuses and veins G08
    nonpyogenic G95.19
  lateral (venous) sinus — *see* Phlebitis, intracranial (ve-
    nous) sinus
  leg I80.3
    antepartum — *see* Thrombophlebitis, antepartum
    deep (vessels) NEC I80.20- ☑
      iliac I80.21- ☑
      popliteal vein I80.22- ☑
      specified vessel NEC I80.29- ☑
      tibial vein (anterior) (posterior) I80.23- ☑
    femoral vein (superficial) I80.1- ☑
    superficial (vessels) I80.0- ☑
  longitudinal sinus — *see* Phlebitis, intracranial (venous)
    sinus
  lower limb — *see* Phlebitis, leg
  migrans, migrating (superficial) I82.1
  pelvic
    with ectopic or molar pregnancy O08.0
    following ectopic or molar pregnancy O08.0
    puerperal, postpartum O87.1
  peroneal vein I80.24- ☑
  popliteal vein — *see* Phlebitis, leg, deep, popliteal
  portal (vein) K75.1
  postoperative T81.72 ☑
  pregnancy — *see* Thrombophlebitis, antepartum
  puerperal, postpartum, childbirth O87.0
    deep O87.1
    pelvic O87.1
    superficial O87.0
  retina — *see* Vasculitis, retina
  saphenous (accessory) (great) (long) (small) — *see*
    Phlebitis, leg, superficial
  sinus (meninges) — *see* Phlebitis, intracranial (venous)
    sinus
  soleal vein I80.25- ☑
  specified site NEC I80.8
  syphilitic A52.09
  tibial vein — *see* Phlebitis, leg, deep, tibial
  ulcerative I80.9
    leg — *see* Phlebitis, leg
  umbilicus I80.8
  uterus (septic) — *see* Endometritis
  varicose (leg) (lower limb) — *see* Varix, leg, with, inflam-
    mation
Phlebofibrosis I87.8
Phleboliths I87.8
Phlebopathy,
  gestational O22.9- ☑
  puerperal O87.9
Phlebosclerosis I87.8
Phlebothrombosis — *see also* Thrombosis
  antepartum — *see* Thrombophlebitis, antepartum
  pregnancy — *see* Thrombophlebitis, antepartum
  puerperal — *see* Thrombophlebitis, puerperal
Phlebotomus fever A93.1
Phlegmasia
  alba dolens O87.1
    nonpuerperal — *see* Phlebitis, femoral vein
  cerulea dolens — *see* Phlebitis, leg, deep
Phlegmon — *see* Abscess
Phlegmonous — *see* condition
Phlyctenulosis (allergic) (keratoconjunctivitis) (nontuber-
    culous) — *see also* Keratoconjunctivitis
  cornea — *see* Keratoconjunctivitis
  tuberculous A18.52
Phobia, phobic F40.9
  animal F40.218
    spiders F40.210
  examination F40.298
  reaction F40.9
  simple F40.298
  social F40.10
    generalized F40.11
  specific (isolated) F40.298
    animal F40.218
      spiders F40.210

Phobia, phobic — *continued*
  specific — *continued*
    blood F40.230
    injection F40.231
    injury F40.233
    men F40.290
    natural environment F40.228
      thunderstorms F40.220
    situational F40.248
      bridges F40.242
      closed in spaces F40.240
      flying F40.243
      heights F40.241
    specified focus NEC F40.298
    transfusion F40.231
    women F40.291
  specified NEC F40.8
    medical care NEC F40.232
  state F40.9
Phocas' disease — *see* Mastopathy, cystic
Phocomelia Q73.1
  lower limb — *see* Agenesis, leg, with foot present
  upper limb — *see* Agenesis, arm, with hand present
Phoria H50.50
Phosphate-losing tubular disorder N25.0
Phosphatemia E83.39
Phosphaturia E83.39
Photodermatitis (sun) L56.8
  chronic L57.8
  due to drug L56.8
  light other than sun L59.8
Photokeratitis H16.13- ☑
Photophobia H53.14- ☑
Photophthalmia — *see* Photokeratitis
Photopsia H53.19
Photoretinitis — *see* Retinopathy, solar
Photosensitivity, photosensitization (sun) skin L56.8
  light other than sun L59.8
Phrenitis — *see* Encephalitis
Phrynoderma (vitamin A deficiency) E50.8
Phthiriasis (pubis) B85.3
  with any infestation classifiable to B85.0-B85.2 B85.4
Phthirus infestation — *see* Phthiriasis
Phthisis — *see also* Tuberculosis
  bulbi (infectional) — *see* Disorder, globe, degenerated
    condition, atrophy
  eyeball (due to infection) — *see* Disorder, globe, degen-
    erated condition, atrophy
PHTS Q85.81
Phycomycosis — *see* Zygomycosis
Physalopteriasis B81.8
Physical restraint status Z78.1
Phytobezoar T18.9 ☑
  intestine T18.3 ☑
  stomach T18.2 ☑
Pian — *see* Yaws
Pianoma A66.1
Pica F50.89
  in adults F50.89
  infant or child F98.3
Picking, nose F98.8
Pick-Niemann disease — *see* Niemann-Pick disease or
  syndrome
Pick's
  cerebral atrophy — *see also* Dementia, in, diseases
    specified elsewhere G31.01 *[F02.80]*
    with behavioral disturbance — *see also* Dementia,
      in, diseases specified elsewhere
      G31.01 *[F02.81-]* ☑
  disease or syndrome (brain) — *see also* Dementia, in,
    diseases specified elsewhere G31.01 *[F02.80]*
    with behavioral disturbance — *see also* Dementia,
      in, diseases specified elsewhere
      G31.01 *[F02.81-]* ☑
    brain — *see also* Dementia, in, diseases specified
      elsewhere G31.01 *[F02.80]*
      with behavioral disturbance — *see also* Demen-
        tia, in, diseases specified elsewhere
        G31.01 *[F02.81-]* ☑
  pericardium (pericardial pseudocirrhosis of liver)
    I31.1
  syndrome
    brain — *see also* Dementia, in, diseases specified
      elsewhere G31.01 *[F02.80]*
      with behavioral disturbance — *see also* Demen-
        tia, in, diseases specified elsewhere
        G31.01 *[F02.81-]* ☑

Pick's — *continued*
  syndrome — *continued*
    of heart (pericardial pseudocirrhosis of liver) I31.1
Pickwickian syndrome E66.2
Piebaldism E70.39
Piedra (beard) (scalp) B36.8
  black B36.3
  white B36.2
Pierre Robin deformity or syndrome Q87.0
Pierson's disease or osteochondrosis M91.0
Pig-bel A05.2
Pigeon
  breast or chest (acquired) M95.4
    congenital Q67.7
      rachitic sequelae (late effect) E64.3
  breeder's disease or lung J67.2
  fancier's disease or lung J67.2
  toe — *see* Deformity, toe, specified NEC
Pigmentation (abnormal) (anomaly) L81.9
  conjunctiva H11.13- ☑
  cornea (anterior) H18.01- ☑
    posterior H18.05- ☑
    stromal H18.06- ☑
  diminished melanin formation NEC L81.6
  iron L81.8
  lids, congenital Q82.8
  limbus corneae — *see* Pigmentation, cornea
  metals L81.8
  optic papilla, congenital Q14.2
  retina, congenital (grouped) (nevoid) Q14.1
  scrotum, congenital Q82.8
  tattoo L81.8
Piles — *see also* Hemorrhoids K64.9
Pili
  annulati or torti (congenital) Q84.1
  incarnati L73.1
Pill roller hand (intrinsic) — *see* Parkinsonism
Pilomatrixoma — *see* Neoplasm, skin, benign
  malignant — *see* Neoplasm, skin, malignant
Pilonidal — *see* condition
Pimple R23.8
PIMS M35.81
PIN — *see* Neoplasia, intraepithelial, prostate
Pinched nerve — *see* Neuropathy, entrapment
Pindborg tumor — *see* Cyst, calcifying odontogenic
Pineal body or gland — *see* condition
Pinealoblastoma C75.3
Pinealoma D44.5
  malignant C75.3
Pineoblastoma C75.3
Pineocytoma D44.5
Pinguecula H11.15- ☑
Pingueculitis H10.81- ☑
Pinhole meatus — *see also* Stricture, urethra N35.919
Pink
  disease — *see* subcategory T56.1 ☑
  eye — *see* Conjunctivitis, acute, mucopurulent
Pinkus' disease (lichen nitidus) L44.1
Pinpoint
  meatus — *see* Stricture, urethra
  os (uteri) — *see* Stricture, cervix
Pins and needles R20.2
Pinta A67.9
  cardiovascular lesions A67.2
  chancre (primary) A67.0
  erythematous plaques A67.1
  hyperchromic lesions A67.1
  hyperkeratosis A67.1
  lesions A67.9
    cardiovascular A67.2
    hyperchromic A67.1
    intermediate A67.1
    late A67.2
    mixed A67.3
    primary A67.0
    skin (achromic) (cicatricial) (dyschromic) A67.2
      hyperchromic A67.1
      mixed (achromic and hyperchromic) A67.3
  papule (primary) A67.0
  skin lesions (achromic) (cicatricial) (dyschromic) A67.2
    hyperchromic A67.1
    mixed (achromic and hyperchromic) A67.3
  vitiligo A67.2
Pintids A67.1
Pinworm (disease) (infection) (infestation) B80
Piroplasmosis — *see also* Babesiosis B60.00
  specified NEC B60.09

Pistol wound — *see* Gunshot wound
Pitchers' elbow — *see* Derangement, joint, specified
  type NEC, elbow
Pithecoid pelvis Q74.2
  with disproportion (fetopelvic) O33.0
    causing obstructed labor O65.0
Pithiatism F48.8
Pitted — *see* Pitting
Pitting — *see also* Edema R60.9
  lip R60.0
  nail L60.8
  teeth K00.4
Pituitary gland — *see* condition
Pituitary-snuff-taker's disease J67.8
Pityriasis (capitis) L21.0
  alba L30.5
  circinata (et maculata) L42
  furfuracea L21.0
  Hebra's L26
  lichenoides L41.0
    chronica L41.1
    et varioliformis (acuta) L41.0
  maculata (et circinata) L30.5
  nigra B36.1
  pilaris, Hebra's L44.0
  rosea L42
  rotunda L44.8
  rubra (Hebra) pilaris L44.0
  simplex L30.5
  specified type NEC L30.5
  streptogenes L30.5
  versicolor (scrotal) B36.0
Placenta, placental — *see* Pregnancy, complicated by
  (care of) (management affected by), specified condition
Placentitis O41.14- ☑
Plagiocephaly Q67.3
Plague A20.9
  abortive A20.8
  ambulatory A20.8
  asymptomatic A20.8
  bubonic A20.0
  cellulocutaneous A20.1
  cutaneobubonic A20.1
  lymphatic gland A20.0
  meningitis A20.3
  pharyngeal A20.8
  pneumonic (primary) (secondary) A20.2
  pulmonary, pulmonic A20.2
  septicemic A20.7
  tonsillar A20.8
    septicemic A20.7
Planning, family
  contraception Z30.9
  procreation Z31.69
Plaque(s)
  artery, arterial — *see* Arteriosclerosis
  calcareous — *see* Calcification
  coronary, lipid rich I25.83
  epicardial I31.8
  erythematous, of pinta A67.1
  Hollenhorst's — *see* Occlusion, artery, retina
  lipid rich, coronary I25.83
  pleural (without asbestos) J92.9
    with asbestos J92.0
  tongue K13.29
Plasmacytoma C90.3- ☑
  extramedullary C90.2- ☑
  medullary C90.0- ☑
  solitary C90.3- ☑
Plasmacytopenia D72.818
Plasmacytosis D72.822
Plaster ulcer — *see* Ulcer, pressure, by site
Plateau iris syndrome (post-iridectomy) (postprocedural) (without glaucoma) H21.82
  with glaucoma H40.22- ☑
Platybasia Q75.8
Platyonychia (congenital) Q84.6
  acquired L60.8
Platypelloid pelvis M95.5
  with disproportion (fetopelvic) O33.0
    causing obstructed labor O65.0
  congenital Q74.2
Platyspondylisis Q76.49
Plaut (-Vincent) **disease** — *see also* Vincent's A69.1
Plethora R23.2
  newborn P61.1
Pleura, pleural — *see* condition

Pleuralgia R07.81
Pleurisy (acute) (adhesive) (chronic) (costal) (diaphragmatic) (double) (dry) (fibrinous) (fibrous) (interlobar) (latent) (plastic) (primary) (residual) (sicca) (sterile) (subacute) (unresolved) R09.1
  with
    adherent pleura J86.0
    effusion J90
      chylous, chyliform J94.0
      tuberculous (non primary) A15.6
        primary (progressive) A15.7
    tuberculosis — *see* Pleurisy, tuberculous (non primary)
  encysted — *see* Pleurisy, with effusion
  exudative — *see* Pleurisy, with effusion
  fibrinopurulent, fibripurulent — *see* Pyothorax
  hemorrhagic — *see* Hemothorax
  pneumococcal J90
  purulent — *see* Pyothorax
  septic — *see* Pyothorax
  serofibrinous — *see* Pleurisy, with effusion
  seropurulent — *see* Pyothorax
  serous — *see* Pleurisy, with effusion
  staphylococcal J86.9
  streptococcal J90
  suppurative — *see* Pyothorax
  traumatic (post) (current) — *see* Injury, intrathoracic, pleura
  tuberculous (with effusion) (non primary) A15.6
    primary (progressive) A15.7
Pleuritis sicca — *see* Pleurisy
Pleurobronchopneumonia — *see* Pneumonia, broncho-
Pleurodynia R07.81
  epidemic B33.0
  viral B33.0
Pleuropericarditis — *see also* Pericarditis
  acute I30.9
Pleuropneumonia (acute) (bilateral) (double) (septic) — *see also* Pneumonia J18.8
  chronic — *see* Fibrosis, lung
Pleuro-pneumonia-like-organism (PPLO), as cause of disease classified elsewhere B96.0
Pleurorrhea — *see* Pleurisy, with effusion
Plexitis, brachial G54.0
Plica
  polonica B85.0
  syndrome, knee M67.5- ☑
  tonsil J35.8
Plicated tongue K14.5
Plug
  bronchus NEC J98.09
  meconium (newborn) NEC syndrome P76.0
  mucus — *see* Asphyxia, mucus
Plumbism — *see* subcategory T56.0 ☑
Plummer's disease E05.20
  with thyroid storm E05.21
Plummer-Vinson syndrome D50.1
Pluricarential syndrome of infancy E40
Plus (and minus) **hand** (intrinsic) — *see* Deformity, limb, specified type NEC, forearm
PMEI (polymorphic epilepsy in infancy) G40.83- ☑
Pneumathemia — *see* Air, embolism
Pneumatic hammer (drill) syndrome T75.21 ☑
Pneumatocele (lung) J98.4
  intracranial G93.89
  tension J44.9
Pneumatosis
  cystoides intestinalis K63.89
  intestinalis K63.89
  peritonei K66.8
Pneumaturia R39.89
Pneumoblastoma — *see* Neoplasm, lung, malignant
Pneumocephalus G93.89
Pneumococcemia A40.3
Pneumococcus, pneumococcal — *see* condition
Pneumoconiosis (due to) (inhalation of) J64
  with tuberculosis (any type in A15) J65
  aluminum J63.0
  asbestos J61
  bagasse, bagassosis J67.1
  bauxite J63.1
  beryllium J63.2
  coal miners' (simple) J60
  coalworkers' (simple) J60
  collier's J60
  cotton dust J66.0
  diatomite (diatomaceous earth) J62.8

Pneumoconiosis — *continued*
  dust
    inorganic NEC J63.6
    lime J62.8
    marble J62.8
    organic NEC J66.8
  fumes or vapors (from silo) J68.9
  graphite J63.3
  grinder's J62.8
  kaolin J62.8
  mica J62.8
  millstone maker's J62.8
  mineral fibers NEC J61
  miner's J60
  moldy hay J67.0
  potter's J62.8
  rheumatoid — *see* Rheumatoid, lung
  sandblaster's J62.8
  silica, silicate NEC J62.8
    with carbon J60
  stonemason's J62.8
  talc (dust) J62.0
Pneumocystis carinii pneumonia B59
Pneumocystis jiroveci (pneumonia) B59
Pneumocystosis (with pneumonia) B59
Pneumohemopericardium I31.2
Pneumohemothorax J94.2
  traumatic S27.2 ☑
Pneumohydropericardium — *see* Pericarditis
Pneumohydrothorax — *see* Hydrothorax
Pneumomediastinum J98.2
  congenital or perinatal P25.2
Pneumomycosis B49 [*J99*]
Pneumonia (acute) (double) (migratory) (purulent) (septic) (unresolved) J18.9
  with
    influenza — *see* Influenza, with, pneumonia
    lung abscess J85.1
      due to specified organism — *see* Pneumonia, in (due to)
  2019 (novel) coronavirus J12.82
  adenoviral J12.0
  adynamic J18.2
  alba A50.04
  allergic — *see also* Pneumonitis, hypersensitivity J82.89
  alveolar — *see* Pneumonia, lobar
  anaerobes J15.8
  anthrax A22.1
  apex, apical — *see* Pneumonia, lobar
  Ascaris B77.81
  aspiration J69.0
    due to
      aspiration of microorganisms
        bacterial J15.9
        viral J12.9
      food (regurgitated) J69.0
      gastric secretions J69.0
      milk (regurgitated) J69.0
      oils, essences J69.1
      solids, liquids NEC J69.8
      vomitus J69.0
    newborn P24.81
      amniotic fluid (clear) P24.11
      blood P24.21
      food (regurgitated) P24.31
      liquor (amnii) P24.11
      meconium P24.01
      milk P24.31
      mucus P24.11
      specified NEC P24.81
      stomach contents P24.31
    postprocedural J95.4
  atypical NEC J18.9
  bacillus J15.9
    specified NEC J15.8
  bacterial J15.9
    specified NEC J15.8
  Bacteroides (fragilis) (oralis) (melaninogenicus) J15.8
  basal, basic, basilar — *see* Pneumonia, by type
  bronchiolitis obliterans organized (BOOP) J84.89
  broncho-, bronchial (confluent) (croupous) (diffuse) (disseminated) (hemorrhagic) (involving lobes) (lobar) (terminal) J18.0
    allergic — *see also* Pneumonitis, hypersensitivity J82.89
    aspiration — *see* Pneumonia, aspiration
    bacterial J15.9
      specified NEC J15.8

Pneumonia — *continued*
  broncho-, bronchial — *continued*
    chronic — *see* Fibrosis, lung
    diplococcal J13
    Eaton's agent J15.7
    Escherichia coli (E. coli) J15.5
    Friedländer's bacillus J15.0
    Hemophilus influenzae J14
    hypostatic J18.2
    inhalation — *see also* Pneumonia, aspiration
      due to fumes or vapors (chemical) J68.0
      of oils or essences J69.1
    Klebsiella (pneumoniae) J15.0
    lipid, lipoid J69.1
      endogenous J84.89
    Mycoplasma (pneumoniae) J15.7
    pleuro-pneumonia-like-organisms (PPLO) J15.7
    pneumococcal J13
    Proteus J15.6
    Pseudomonas J15.1
    Serratia marcescens J15.6
    specified organism NEC J16.8
    staphylococcal — *see* Pneumonia, staphylococcal
    streptococcal NEC J15.4
      group B J15.3
      pneumoniae J13
    viral, virus — *see* Pneumonia, viral
  Butyrivibrio (fibriosolvens) J15.8
  Candida B37.1
  caseous — *see* Tuberculosis, pulmonary
  catarrhal — *see* Pneumonia, broncho
  chlamydial J16.0
    congenital P23.1
  cholesterol J84.89
  cirrhotic (chronic) — *see* Fibrosis, lung
  Clostridium (haemolyticum) (novyi) J15.8
  confluent — *see* Pneumonia, broncho
  congenital (infective) P23.9
    due to
      bacterium NEC P23.6
      Chlamydia P23.1
      Escherichia coli P23.4
      Haemophilus influenzae P23.6
      infective organism NEC P23.8
      Klebsiella pneumoniae P23.6
      Mycoplasma P23.6
      Pseudomonas P23.5
      Staphylococcus P23.2
      Streptococcus (except group B) P23.6
        group B P23.3
      viral agent P23.0
    specified NEC P23.8
  coronavirus (novel) (disease) 2019 J12.82
  COVID-19 J12.82
  croupous — *see* Pneumonia, lobar
  cryptogenic organizing J84.116
  cytomegalic inclusion B25.0
  cytomegaloviral B25.0
  deglutition — *see* Pneumonia, aspiration
  desquamative interstitial J84.117
  diffuse — *see* Pneumonia, broncho
  diplococcal, diplococcus (broncho-) (lobar) J13
  disseminated (focal) — *see* Pneumonia, broncho
  Eaton's agent J15.7
  embolic, embolism — *see* Embolism, pulmonary
  Enterobacter J15.6
  eosinophilic J82.81
    acute J82.82
    chronic J82.81
  Escherichia coli (E. coli) J15.5
  Eubacterium J15.8
  fibrinous — *see* Pneumonia, lobar
  fibroid, fibrous (chronic) — *see* Fibrosis, lung
  Friedländer's bacillus J15.0
  Fusobacterium (nucleatum) J15.8
  gangrenous J85.0
  giant cell (measles) B05.2
  gonococcal A54.84
  gram-negative bacteria NEC J15.6
    anaerobic J15.8
  Hemophilus influenzae (broncho) (lobar) J14
  human metapneumovirus J12.3
  hypostatic (broncho) (lobar) J18.2
  in (due to)
    actinomycosis A42.0
    adenovirus J12.0
    anthrax A22.1
    ascariasis B77.81

Pneumonia — *continued*
- in — *continued*
  - aspergillosis B44.9
  - Bacillus anthracis A22.1
  - Bacterium anitratum J15.6
  - candidiasis B37.1
  - chickenpox B01.2
  - Chlamydia J16.0
    - neonatal P23.1
  - coccidioidomycosis B38.2
    - acute B38.0
    - chronic B38.1
  - cytomegalovirus disease B25.0
  - Diplococcus (pneumoniae) J13
  - Eaton's agent J15.7
  - Enterobacter J15.6
  - Escherichia coli (E. coli) J15.5
  - Friedländer's bacillus J15.0
  - fumes and vapors (chemical) (inhalation) J68.0
  - gonorrhea A54.84
  - Hemophilus influenzae (H. influenzae) J14
  - Herellea J15.6
  - histoplasmosis B39.2
    - acute B39.0
    - chronic B39.1
  - human metapneumovirus J12.3
  - Klebsiella (pneumoniae) J15.0
  - measles B05.2
  - Mycoplasma (pneumoniae) J15.7
  - nocardiosis, nocardiasis A43.0
  - ornithosis A70
  - parainfluenza virus J12.2
  - pleuro-pneumonia-like-organism (PPLO) J15.7
  - pneumococcus J13
  - pneumocystosis (Pneumocystis carinii) (Pneumocystis jiroveci) B59
  - Proteus J15.6
  - Pseudomonas NEC J15.1
    - pseudomallei A24.1
  - psittacosis A70
  - Q fever A78
  - respiratory syncytial virus (RSV) J12.1
  - rheumatic fever I00 *[J17]*
  - rubella B06.81
  - Salmonella (infection) A02.22
    - typhi A01.03
  - schistosomiasis B65.9 *[J17]*
  - Serratia marcescens J15.6
  - specified
    - bacterium NEC J15.8
    - organism NEC J16.8
  - spirochetal NEC A69.8
  - Staphylococcus J15.20
    - aureus (methicillin susceptible) (MSSA) J15.211
      - methicillin resistant (MRSA) J15.212
    - specified NEC J15.29
  - Streptococcus J15.4
    - group B J15.3
    - pneumoniae J13
    - specified NEC J15.4
  - toxoplasmosis B58.3
  - tularemia A21.2
  - typhoid (fever) A01.03
  - varicella B01.2
  - virus — *see* Pneumonia, viral
  - whooping cough A37.91
    - due to
      - Bordetella parapertussis A37.11
      - Bordetella pertussis A37.01
      - specified NEC A37.81
  - Yersinia pestis A20.2
- inhalation of food or vomit — *see* Pneumonia, aspiration
- interstitial J84.9
  - chronic J84.111
  - desquamative J84.117
  - due to
    - collagen vascular disease J84.178
    - known underlying cause J84.178
  - idiopathic NOS J84.111
  - in disease classified elsewhere J84.178
  - lymphocytic (due to collagen vascular disease) (in diseases classified elsewhere) J84.178
  - lymphoid J84.2
  - non-specific J84.89
    - due to
      - collagen vascular disease J84.178
      - known underlying cause J84.178
    - idiopathic J84.113

Pneumonia — *continued*
- interstitial — *continued*
  - non-specific — *continued*
    - in diseases classified elsewhere J84.178
  - plasma cell B59
  - pseudomonas J15.1
  - usual J84.112
    - due to collagen vascular disease J84.178
    - idiopathic J84.112
    - in diseases classified elsewhere J84.178
- Klebsiella (pneumoniae) J15.0
- lipid, lipoid (exogenous) J69.1
  - endogenous J84.89
- lobar (disseminated) (double) (interstitial) J18.1
  - bacterial J15.9
    - specified NEC J15.8
  - chronic — *see* Fibrosis, lung
  - Escherichia coli (E. coli) J15.5
  - Friedländer's bacillus J15.0
  - Hemophilus influenzae J14
  - hypostatic J18.2
  - Klebsiella (pneumoniae) J15.0
  - pneumococcal J13
  - Proteus J15.6
  - Pseudomonas J15.1
  - specified organism NEC J16.8
  - staphylococcal — *see* Pneumonia, staphylococcal
  - streptococcal NEC J15.4
  - Streptococcus pneumoniae J13
  - viral, virus — *see* Pneumonia, viral
- lobular — *see* Pneumonia, broncho
- Löffler's J82.89
- lymphoid interstitial J84.2
- massive — *see* Pneumonia, lobar
- meconium P24.01
- MRSA (methicillin resistant Staphylococcus aureus) J15.212
- MSSA (methicillin susceptible Staphylococcus aureus) J15.211
- multilobar — *see* Pneumonia, by type
- Mycoplasma (pneumoniae) J15.7
- necrotic J85.0
- neonatal P23.9
  - aspiration — *see* Aspiration, by substance, with pneumonia
- nitrogen dioxide J68.0
- organizing J84.89
  - due to
    - collagen vascular disease J84.178
    - known underlying cause J84.178
  - in diseases classified elsewhere J84.178
- orthostatic J18.2
- parainfluenza virus J12.2
- parenchymatous — *see* Fibrosis, lung
- passive J18.2
- patchy — *see* Pneumonia, broncho
- Peptococcus J15.8
- Peptostreptococcus J15.8
- plasma cell (of infants) B59
- pleurolobar — *see* Pneumonia, lobar
- pleuro-pneumonia-like organism (PPLO) J15.7
- pneumococcal (broncho) (lobar) J13
- Pneumocystis (carinii) (jiroveci) B59
- postinfectional NEC B99 ☑ *[J17]*
- postmeasles B05.2
- Proteus J15.6
- Pseudomonas J15.1
- psittacosis A70
- radiation J70.0
- respiratory syncytial virus (RSV) J12.1
- resulting from a procedure J95.89
- rheumatic I00 *[J17]*
- Salmonella (arizonae) (cholerae-suis) (enteritidis) (typhimurium) A02.22
  - typhi A01.03
  - typhoid fever A01.03
- SARS-associated coronavirus J12.81
- SARS-CoV-2 J12.82
- segmented, segmental — *see* Pneumonia, broncho-
- Serratia marcescens J15.6
- specified NEC J18.8
  - bacterium NEC J15.8
  - organism NEC J16.8
  - virus NEC J12.89
- spirochetal NEC A69.8
- staphylococcal (broncho) (lobar) J15.20
  - aureus (methicillin susceptible) (MSSA) J15.211
    - methicillin resistant (MRSA) J15.212

Pneumonia — *continued*
- staphylococcal — *continued*
  - specified NEC J15.29
- static, stasis J18.2
- streptococcal NEC (broncho) (lobar) J15.4
  - group
    - A J15.4
    - B J15.3
    - specified NEC J15.4
- Streptococcus pneumoniae J13
- syphilitic, congenital (early) A50.04
- traumatic (complication) (early) (secondary) T79.8 ☑
- tuberculous (any) — *see* Tuberculosis, pulmonary
- tularemic A21.2
- varicella B01.2
- Veillonella J15.8
- ventilator associated J95.851
- viral, virus (broncho) (interstitial) (lobar) J12.9
  - adenoviral J12.0
  - congenital P23.0
  - human metapneumovirus J12.3
  - parainfluenza J12.2
  - respiratory syncytial (RSV) J12.1
  - SARS-associated coronavirus J12.81
  - specified NEC J12.89
- white (congenital) A50.04

Pneumonic — *see* condition

Pneumonitis (acute) (primary) — *see also* Pneumonia
- air-conditioner J67.7
- allergic (due to) J67.9
  - organic dust NEC J67.8
  - red cedar dust J67.8
  - sequoiosis J67.8
  - wood dust J67.8
- aspiration J69.0
  - due to
    - anesthesia J95.4
      - during
        - labor and delivery O74.0
        - pregnancy O29.01- ☑
        - puerperium O89.01
    - fumes or gases J68.0
    - obstetric O74.0
- chemical (due to gases, fumes or vapors) (inhalation) J68.0
  - due to anesthesia J95.4
- cholesterol J84.89
- chronic — *see* Fibrosis, lung
- congenital rubella P35.0
- crack (cocaine) J68.0
- due to
  - beryllium J68.0
  - cadmium J68.0
  - crack (cocaine) J68.0
  - detergent J69.8
  - fluorocarbon-polymer J68.0
  - food, vomit (aspiration) J69.0
  - fumes or vapors J68.0
  - gases, fumes or vapors (inhalation) J68.0
  - inhalation
    - blood J69.8
    - essences J69.1
    - food (regurgitated), milk, vomit J69.0
    - oils, essences J69.1
    - saliva J69.0
    - solids, liquids NEC J69.8
  - manganese J68.0
  - nitrogen dioxide J68.0
  - oils, essences J69.1
  - solids, liquids NEC J69.8
  - toxoplasmosis (acquired) B58.3
    - congenital P37.1
  - vanadium J68.0
  - ventilator J95.851
- eosinophilic J82.81
  - acute J82.82
  - chronic J82.81
- hypersensitivity J67.9
  - air conditioner lung J67.7
  - bagassosis J67.1
  - bird fancier's lung J67.2
  - farmer's lung J67.0
  - maltworker's lung J67.4
  - maple bark-stripper's lung J67.6
  - mushroom worker's lung J67.5
  - specified organic dust NEC J67.8
  - suberosis J67.3
- interstitial (chronic) J84.89

Pneumonitis — continued
  interstitial — continued
    acute J84.114
    lymphoid J84.2
    non-specific J84.89
      idiopathic J84.113
  lymphoid, interstitial J84.2
  meconium P24.01
  postanesthetic J95.4
    correct substance properly administered — see Table of Drugs and Chemicals, by drug, adverse effect
    in labor and delivery O74.0
    in pregnancy O29.01- ☑
    obstetric O74.0
    overdose or wrong substance given or taken (by accident) — see Table of Drugs and Chemicals, by drug, poisoning
  postpartum, puerperal O89.01
  postoperative J95.4
    obstetric O74.0
  radiation J70.0
  rubella, congenital P35.0
  ventilation (air-conditioning) J67.7
  ventilator associated J95.851
  wood-dust J67.8
Pneumonoconiosis — see Pneumoconiosis
Pneumoparotid K11.8
Pneumopathy NEC J98.4
  alveolar J84.09
  due to organic dust NEC J66.8
  parietoalveolar J84.09
Pneumopericarditis — see also Pericarditis
  acute I30.9
Pneumopericardium — see also Pericarditis
  congenital P25.3
  newborn P25.3
  traumatic (post) — see Injury, heart
Pneumophagia (psychogenic) F45.8
Pneumopleurisy, pneumopleuritis — see also Pneumonia J18.8
Pneumopyopericardium I30.1
Pneumopyothorax — see Pyopneumothorax
  with fistula J86.0
Pneumorrhagia — see also Hemorrhage, lung
  tuberculous — see Tuberculosis, pulmonary
Pneumothorax NOS J93.9
  acute J93.83
  chronic J93.81
  congenital P25.1
  perinatal period P25.1
  postprocedural J95.811
  specified NEC J93.83
  spontaneous NOS J93.83
    newborn P25.1
    primary J93.11
    secondary J93.12
    tension J93.0
  tense valvular, infectional J93.0
  tension (spontaneous) J93.0
  traumatic S27.0 ☑
    with hemothorax S27.2 ☑
  tuberculous — see Tuberculosis, pulmonary
Podagra — see also Gout M10.9
Podencephalus Q01.9
Poikilocytosis R71.8
Poikiloderma L81.6
  Civatte's L57.3
  congenital Q82.8
  vasculare atrophicans L94.5
Poikilodermatomyositis M33.10
  with
    myopathy M33.12
    respiratory involvement M33.11
    specified organ involvement NEC M33.19
  amyopathic M33.13
  without myopathy M33.13
Pointed ear (congenital) Q17.3
Poison ivy, oak, sumac or other plant dermatitis (allergic) (contact) L23.7
Poisoning (acute) — see also Table of Drugs and Chemicals
  algae and toxins T65.82- ☑
  Bacillus B (aertrycke) (cholerae (suis)) (paratyphosus) (suipestifer) A02.9
    botulinus A05.1
  bacterial toxins A05.9
  berries, noxious — see Poisoning, food, noxious, berries

Poisoning — continued
  botulism A05.1
  ciguatera fish T61.0- ☑
  Clostridium botulinum A05.1
  death-cap (Amanita phalloides) (Amanita verna) — see Poisoning, food, noxious, mushrooms
  drug — see Table of Drugs and Chemicals, by drug, poisoning
  epidemic, fish (noxious) — see Poisoning, seafood
    bacterial A05.9
  fava bean D55.0
  fish (noxious) T61.9- ☑
    bacterial — see Intoxication, foodborne, by agent
    ciguatera fish — see Poisoning, ciguatera fish
    scombroid fish — see Poisoning, scombroid fish
    specified type NEC T61.77- ☑
  food NEC A05.9
    bacterial — see Intoxication, foodborne, by agent
    due to
      Bacillus (aertrycke) (choleraesuis) (suipestifer) A02.9
        botulinus A05.1
      Clostridium (perfringens) (Welchii) A05.2
      salmonella (aertrycke) (callinarum) (choleraesuis) (enteritidis) (paratyphi) (suipestifer) A02.9
        with
          gastroenteritis A02.0
          sepsis A02.1
      staphylococcus A05.0
      Vibrio
        parahaemolyticus A05.3
        vulnificus A05.5
    noxious or naturally toxic T62.9- ☑
      berries — see subcategory T62.1 ☑
      fish — see Poisoning, seafood
      mushrooms — see subcategory T62.0X ☑
      plants NEC — see subcategory T62.2X ☑
      seafood — see Poisoning, seafood
      specified NEC — see subcategory T62.8X ☑
  ichthyotoxism — see Poisoning, seafood
  kreotoxism, food A05.9
  latex T65.81- ☑
  lead T56.0- ☑
  mushroom — see Poisoning, food, noxious, mushroom
  mussels — see also Poisoning, shellfish
    bacterial — see Intoxication, foodborne, by agent
  nicotine (tobacco) T65.2- ☑
  noxious foodstuffs — see Poisoning, food, noxious
  plants, noxious — see Poisoning, food, noxious, plants NEC
  ptomaine — see Poisoning, food
  radiation J70.0
  Salmonella (arizonae) (cholerae-suis) (enteritidis) (typhimurium) A02.9
  scombroid fish T61.1- ☑
  seafood (noxious) T61.9- ☑
    bacterial — see Intoxication, foodborne, by agent
    fish — see Poisoning, fish
    shellfish — see Poisoning, shellfish
    specified NEC — see subcategory T61.8X ☑
  shellfish (amnesic) (azaspiracid) (diarrheic) (neurotoxic) (noxious) (paralytic) T61.78- ☑
    bacterial — see Intoxication, foodborne, by agent
    ciguatera mollusk — see Poisoning, ciguatera fish
  specified substance NEC T65.891 ☑
  Staphylococcus, food A05.0
  tobacco (nicotine) T65.2- ☑
  water E87.79
Poker spine — see Spondylitis, ankylosing
Poland syndrome Q79.8
Polioencephalitis (acute) (bulbar) A80.9
  inferior G12.22
  influenzal — see Influenza, with, encephalopathy
  superior hemorrhagic (acute) (Wernicke's) E51.2
  Wernicke's E51.2
Polioencephalomyelitis (acute) (anterior) A80.9
  with beriberi E51.2
Polioencephalopathy, superior hemorrhagic E51.2
  with
    beriberi E51.11
    pellagra E52
Poliomeningoencephalitis — see Meningoencephalitis
Poliomyelitis (acute) (anterior) (epidemic) A80.9
  with paralysis (bulbar) — Poliomyelitis, paralytic
  abortive A80.4
  ascending (progressive) — see Poliomyelitis, paralytic
  bulbar (paralytic) — see Poliomyelitis, paralytic

Poliomyelitis — continued
  congenital P35.8
  nonepidemic A80.9
  nonparalytic A80.4
  paralytic A80.30
    specified NEC A80.39
    vaccine-associated A80.0
    wild virus
      imported A80.1
      indigenous A80.2
  spinal, acute A80.9
Poliosis (eyebrow) (eyelashes) L67.1
  circumscripta, acquired L67.1
Pollakiuria R35.0
  psychogenic F45.8
Pollinosis J30.1
Pollitzer's disease L73.2
Polyadenitis — see also Lymphadenitis
  malignant A20.0
Polyalgia M79.89
Polyangiitis M30.0
  microscopic M31.7
  overlap syndrome M30.8
Polyarteritis
  microscopic M31.7
  nodosa M30.0
    with lung involvement M30.1
    juvenile M30.2
    related condition NEC M30.8
Polyarthralgia — see Pain, joint
Polyarthritis, polyarthropathy — see also Arthritis M13.0
  due to or associated with other specified conditions — see Arthritis
  epidemic (Australian) (with exanthema) B33.1
  infective — see Arthritis, pyogenic or pyemic
  inflammatory M06.4
  juvenile (chronic) (seronegative) M08.3
  migratory M13.8- ☑
  rheumatic, acute — see Fever, rheumatic
Polyarthrosis M15.9
  post-traumatic M15.3
  primary M15.0
  specified NEC M15.8
Polycarential syndrome of infancy E40
Polychondritis (atrophic) (chronic) — see also Disorder, cartilage, specified type NEC
  relapsing M94.1
Polycoria Q13.2
Polycystic (disease)
  degeneration, kidney Q61.3
    autosomal dominant (adult type) Q61.2
    autosomal recessive (infantile type) NEC Q61.19
  kidney Q61.3
    autosomal
      dominant Q61.2
      recessive NEC Q61.19
    autosomal dominant (adult type) Q61.2
    autosomal recessive (childhood type) NEC Q61.19
    infantile type NEC Q61.19
  liver Q44.6
  lung J98.4
    congenital Q33.0
  ovary, ovaries E28.2
  spleen Q89.09
Polycythemia (secondary) D75.1
  acquired D75.1
  benign (familial) D75.0
  due to
    donor twin P61.1
    erythropoietin D75.1
    fall in plasma volume D75.1
    high altitude D75.1
    maternal-fetal transfusion P61.1
    stress D75.1
  emotional D75.1
  erythropoietin D75.1
  familial (benign) D75.0
  Gaisböck's (hypertonica) D75.1
  high altitude D75.1
  hypertonica D75.1
  hypoxemic D75.1
  neonatorum P61.1
  nephrogenous D75.1
  relative D75.1
  secondary D75.1
  spurious D75.1
  stress D75.1

Polycythemia — *continued*
  vera D45
Polycytosis cryptogenica D75.1
Polydactylism, polydactyly Q69.9
  toes Q69.2
Polydipsia R63.1
Polydystrophy, pseudo-Hurler E77.0
Polyembryoma — *see* Neoplasm, malignant, by site
Polyglandular
  deficiency E31.0
  dyscrasia E31.9
  dysfunction E31.9
  syndrome E31.8
Polyhydramnios O40.- ☑
Polymastia Q83.1
Polymenorrhea N92.0
Polymyalgia M35.3
  arteritica, giant cell M31.5
  rheumatica M35.3
    with giant cell arteritis M31.5
Polymyositis (acute) (chronic) (hemorrhagic) M33.20
  with
    myopathy M33.22
    respiratory involvement M33.21
    skin involvement — *see* Dermatopolymyositis
    specified organ involvement NEC M33.29
  ossificans (generalisata) (progressiva) — *see* Myositis,
    ossificans, progressiva
Polyneuritis, polyneuritic — *see also* Polyneuropathy
  acute (post-)infective G61.0
  alcoholic G62.1
  cranialis G52.7
  demyelinating, chronic inflammatory (CIDP) G61.81
  diabetic — *see* Diabetes, polyneuropathy
  diphtheritic A36.83
  due to lack of vitamin NEC E56.9 *[G63]*
  endemic E51.11
  erythredema — *see* subcategory T56.1 ☑
  febrile, acute G61.0
  hereditary ataxic G60.1
  idiopathic, acute G61.0
  infective (acute) G61.0
  inflammatory, chronic demyelinating (CIDP) G61.81
  nutritional E63.9 *[G63]*
  postinfective (acute) G61.0
  specified NEC G62.89
Polyneuropathy (peripheral) G62.9
  alcoholic G62.1
  amyloid (Portuguese) E85.1 *[G63]*
    transthyretin-related (ATTR) familial E85.1 *[G63]*
  arsenical G62.2
  critical illness G62.81
  demyelinating, chronic inflammatory (CIDP) G61.81
  diabetic — *see* Diabetes, polyneuropathy
  drug-induced G62.0
  hereditary G60.9
    specified NEC G60.8
  idiopathic G60.9
    progressive G60.3
  in (due to)
    alcohol G62.1
      sequelae G65.2
    amyloidosis, familial (Portuguese) E85.1 *[G63]*
    antitetanus serum G61.1
    arsenic G62.2
      sequelae G65.2
    avitaminosis NEC E56.9 *[G63]*
    beriberi E51.11
    collagen vascular disease NEC M35.9 *[G63]*
    deficiency (of)
      B (-complex) vitamins E53.9 *[G63]*
      vitamin B6 E53.1 *[G63]*
    diabetes — *see* Diabetes, polyneuropathy
    diphtheria A36.83
    drug or medicament G62.0
      correct substance properly administered — *see*
        Table of Drugs and Chemicals, by drug,
        adverse effect
      overdose or wrong substance given or taken —
        see Table of Drugs and Chemicals, by drug,
        poisoning
    endocrine disease NEC E34.9 *[G63]*
    herpes zoster B02.23
    hypoglycemia E16.2 *[G63]*
    infectious
      disease NEC B99 ☑ *[G63]*
      mononucleosis B27.91
    lack of vitamin NEC E56.9 *[G63]*

Polyneuropathy — *continued*
  in — *continued*
    lead G62.2
      sequelae G65.2
    leprosy A30.9 *[G63]*
    Lyme disease A69.22
    metabolic disease NEC E88.9 *[G63]*
    microscopic polyangiitis M31.7 *[G63]*
    mumps B26.84
    neoplastic disease — *see also* Neoplasm D49.9 *[G63]*
    nutritional deficiency NEC E63.9 *[G63]*
    organophosphate compounds G62.2
      sequelae G65.2
    parasitic disease NEC B89 *[G63]*
    pellagra E52 *[G63]*
    polyarteritis nodosa M30.0
    porphyria E80.20 *[G63]*
    radiation G62.82
    rheumatoid arthritis — *see* Rheumatoid, polyneu-
      ropathy
    sarcoidosis D86.89
    serum G61.1
    syphilis (late) A52.15
      congenital A50.43
    systemic
      connective tissue disorder M35.9 *[G63]*
      lupus erythematosus M32.19
    toxic agent NEC G62.2
      sequelae G65.2
    transthyretin-related (ATTR) familial amyloid E85.1
    triorthocresyl phosphate G62.2
      sequelae G65.2
    tuberculosis A17.89
    uremia N18.9 *[G63]*
    vitamin B12 deficiency E53.8 *[G63]*
      with anemia (pernicious) D51.0 *[G63]*
        due to dietary deficiency D51.3, G63
    zoster B02.23
  inflammatory G61.9
    chronic demyelinating (CIDP) G61.81
    sequelae G65.1
    specified NEC G61.89
  lead G62.2
    sequelae G65.2
  nutritional NEC E63.9 *[G63]*
  postherpetic (zoster) B02.23
  progressive G60.3
  radiation-induced G62.82
  sensory (hereditary) (idiopathic) G60.8
  specified NEC G62.89
  syphilitic (late) A52.15
    congenital A50.43
Polyopia H53.8
Polyorchism, polyorchidism Q55.21
Polyosteoarthritis — *see also* Osteoarthritis, generalized
    M15.9
  post-traumatic M15.3
  specified NEC M15.8
Polyostotic fibrous dysplasia Q78.1
Polyotia Q17.0
Polyp, polypus
  accessory sinus J33.8
  adenocarcinoma in — *see* Neoplasm, malignant, by
    site
  adenocarcinoma in situ in — *see* Neoplasm, in situ, by
    site
  adenoid tissue J33.0
  adenomatous — *see also* Neoplasm, benign, by site
    adenocarcinoma in — *see* Neoplasm, malignant, by
      site
    adenocarcinoma in situ in — *see* Neoplasm, in situ,
      by site
    carcinoma in — *see* Neoplasm, malignant, by site
    carcinoma in situ in — *see* Neoplasm, in situ, by site
    multiple — *see* Neoplasm, benign
      adenocarcinoma in — *see* Neoplasm, malignant,
        by site
      adenocarcinoma in situ in — *see* Neoplasm, in
        situ, by site
  antrum J33.8
  anus, anal (canal) K62.0
  Bartholin's gland N84.3
  bladder D41.4
  carcinoma in — *see* Neoplasm, malignant, by site
  carcinoma in situ in — *see* Neoplasm, in situ, by site
  cecum D12.0
  cervix (uteri) N84.1

Polyp, polypus — *continued*
  cervix — *continued*
    in pregnancy or childbirth — *see* Pregnancy, com-
      plicated by, abnormal, cervix
    mucous N84.1
    nonneoplastic N84.1
  choanal J33.0
  cholesterol K82.4
  clitoris N84.3
  colon K63.5
    adenomatous D12.6
      ascending D12.2
      cecum D12.0
      descending D12.4
      sigmoid D12.5
      transverse D12.3
    ascending K63.5
    cecum K63.5
    descending K63.5
    hyperplastic, (any site) K63.5
    inflammatory K51.40
      with
        abscess K51.414
        complication K51.419
          specified NEC K51.418
        fistula K51.413
        intestinal obstruction K51.412
        rectal bleeding K51.411
    sigmoid K63.5
    transverse K63.5
  corpus uteri N84.0
  dental K04.01
    irreversible K04.02
    reversible K04.01
  duodenum K31.7
  ear (middle) H74.4- ☑
  endometrium N84.0
  esophageal K22.81
  esophagogastric junction K22.82
  ethmoidal (sinus) J33.8
  fallopian tube N84.8
  female genital tract N84.9
    specified NEC N84.8
  frontal (sinus) J33.8
  gallbladder K82.4
  gingiva, gum K06.8
  labia, labium (majus) (minus) N84.3
  larynx (mucous) J38.1
    adenomatous D14.1
  malignant — *see* Neoplasm, malignant, by site
  maxillary (sinus) J33.8
  middle ear — *see* Polyp, ear (middle)
  myometrium N84.0
  nares
    anterior J33.9
    posterior J33.0
  nasal (mucous) J33.9
    cavity J33.0
    septum J33.0
  nasopharyngeal J33.0
  nose (mucous) J33.9
  oviduct N84.8
  pharynx J39.2
  placenta O90.89
  prostate — *see* Enlargement, enlarged, prostate
  pudenda, pudendum N84.3
  pulpal (dental) K04.01
    irreversible K04.02
    reversible K04.01
  rectum (nonadenomatous) K62.1
    adenomatous — *see* Polyp, adenomatous
  septum (nasal) J33.0
  sinus (accessory) (ethmoidal) (frontal) (maxillary)
    (sphenoidal) J33.8
  sphenoidal (sinus) J33.8
  stomach K31.7
    adenomatous D13.1
  tube, fallopian N84.8
  turbinate, mucous membrane J33.8
  umbilical, newborn P83.6
  ureter N28.89
  urethra N36.2
  uterus (body) (corpus) (mucous) N84.0
    cervix N84.1
    in pregnancy or childbirth — *see* Pregnancy, com-
      plicated by, tumor, uterus
  vagina N84.2
  vocal cord (mucous) J38.1

Polyp, polypus — *continued*
  vulva N84.3
Polyphagia R63.2
Polyploidy Q92.7
Polypoid — *see* condition
Polyposis — *see also* Polyp
  coli (adenomatous) D12.6
    adenocarcinoma in C18.9
    adenocarcinoma in situ in — *see* Neoplasm, in situ, by site
    carcinoma in C18.9
  colon (adenomatous) D12.6
  familial D12.6
    adenocarcinoma in situ in — *see* Neoplasm, in situ, by site
  intestinal (adenomatous) D12.6
  malignant lymphomatous C83.1- ☑
  multiple, adenomatous — *see also* Neoplasm, benign D36.9
Polyradiculitis — *see* Polyneuropathy
Polyradiculoneuropathy (acute) (postinfective) (segmentally demyelinating) G61.0
Polyserositis
  due to pericarditis I31.1
  pericardial I31.1
  periodic, familial E85.0
  tuberculous A19.9
    acute A19.1
    chronic A19.8
Polysplenia syndrome Q89.09
Polysyndactyly — *see also* Syndactylism, syndactyly Q70.4
Polytrichia L68.3
Polyunguia Q84.6
Polyuria R35.89
  nocturnal R35.81
  psychogenic F45.8
  specified NEC R35.89
Pompe's disease (glycogen storage) E74.02
Pompholyx L30.1
Poncet's disease (tuberculous rheumatism) A18.09
Pond fracture — *see* Fracture, skull
Ponos B55.0
Pons, pontine — *see* condition
Poor
  aesthetic of existing restoration of tooth K08.56
  contractions, labor O62.2
  gingival margin to tooth restoration K08.51
  personal hygiene R46.0
  prenatal care, affecting management of pregnancy — *see* Pregnancy, complicated by, insufficient, prenatal care
  sucking reflex (newborn) R29.2
  urinary stream R39.12
  vision NEC H54.7
Poradenitis, nostras inguinalis or venerea A55
Porencephaly (congenital) (developmental) (true) Q04.6
  acquired G93.0
  nondevelopmental G93.0
  traumatic (post) F07.89
Porocephaliasis B88.8
Porokeratosis Q82.8
Poroma, eccrine — *see* Neoplasm, skin, benign
Porphyria (South African) E80.20
  acquired E80.20
  acute intermittent (hepatic) (Swedish) E80.21
  cutanea tarda (hereditary) (symptomatic) E80.1
  due to drugs E80.20
    correct substance properly administered — *see* Table of Drugs and Chemicals, by drug, adverse effect
    overdose or wrong substance given or taken — *see* Table of Drugs and Chemicals, by drug, poisoning
  erythropoietic (congenital) (hereditary) E80.0
  hepatocutaneous type E80.1
  secondary E80.20
  toxic NEC E80.20
  variegata E80.20
Porphyrinuria — *see* Porphyria
Porphyruria — *see* Porphyria
Port wine nevus, mark, or stain Q82.5
Portal — *see* condition
Posadas-Wernicke disease B38.9
Positive
  culture (nonspecific)
    blood R78.81
    bronchial washings R84.5

Positive — *continued*
  culture — *continued*
    cerebrospinal fluid R83.5
    cervix uteri R87.5
    nasal secretions R84.5
    nipple discharge R89.5
    nose R84.5
      staphylococcus (Methicillin susceptible) Z22.321
        Methicillin resistant Z22.322
    peritoneal fluid R85.5
    pleural fluid R84.5
    prostatic secretions R86.5
    saliva R85.5
    seminal fluid R86.5
    sputum R84.5
    synovial fluid R89.5
    throat scrapings R84.5
    urine R82.79
    vagina R87.5
    vulva R87.5
    wound secretions R89.5
  PPD (skin test) R76.11
  serology for syphilis A53.0
    false R76.8
    with signs or symptoms — *code as* Syphilis, by site and stage
  skin test, tuberculin (without active tuberculosis) R76.11
  test, human immunodeficiency virus (HIV) R75
  VDRL A53.0
    with signs or symptoms — *code by* site and stage under Syphilis A53.9
  Wassermann reaction A53.0
Post COVID-19 condition, unspecified U09.9
Postcardiotomy syndrome I97.0
Postcaval ureter Q62.62
Postcholecystectomy syndrome K91.5
Postclimacteric bleeding N95.0
Postcommissurotomy syndrome I97.0
Postconcussional syndrome F07.81
Postcontusional syndrome F07.81
Postcricoid region — *see* condition
Post-dates (40-42 weeks) (pregnancy) (mother) O48.0
  more than 42 weeks gestation O48.1
Postencephalitic syndrome F07.89
Posterior — *see* condition
Posterolateral sclerosis (spinal cord) — *see* Degeneration, combined
Postexanthematous — *see* condition
Postfebrile — *see* condition
Postgastrectomy dumping syndrome K91.1
Posthemiplegic chorea — *see* Monoplegia
Posthemorrhagic anemia (chronic) D50.0
  acute D62
  newborn P61.3
Postherpetic neuralgia (zoster) B02.29
  trigeminal B02.22
Posthitis N47.7
Postimmunization complication or reaction — *see* Complications, vaccination
Postinfectious — *see* condition
Postlaminectomy syndrome NEC M96.1
Postleukotomy syndrome F07.0
Postmastectomy lymphedema (syndrome) I97.2
Postmaturity, postmature (over 42 weeks)
  maternal (over 42 weeks gestation) O48.1
  newborn P08.22
Postmeasles complication NEC — *see also* condition B05.89
Postmenopausal
  endometrium (atrophic) N95.8
    suppurative — *see also* Endometritis N71.9
  osteoporosis — *see* Osteoporosis, postmenopausal
Postnasal drip R09.82
  due to
    allergic rhinitis — *see* Rhinitis, allergic
    common cold J00
    gastroesophageal reflux — *see* Reflux, gastroesophageal
    nasopharyngitis — *see* Nasopharyngitis
    other known condition — *code to* condition
    sinusitis — *see* Sinusitis
Postnatal — *see* condition
Postoperative (postprocedural) — *see* Complication, postoperative
  pneumothorax, therapeutic Z98.3
  state NEC Z98.890
Postpancreatectomy hyperglycemia E89.1

Postpartum — *see* Puerperal
Postphlebitic syndrome — *see* Syndrome, postthrombotic
Postpolio (myelitic) **syndrome** G14
Postpoliomyelitic — *see also* condition
  osteopathy — *see* Osteopathy, after poliomyelitis
Postprocedural — *see also* Postoperative
  hypoinsulinemia E89.1
Postschizophrenic depression F32.89
Postsurgery status — *see also* Status (post)
  pneumothorax, therapeutic Z98.3
Post-term (40-42 weeks) (pregnancy) (mother) O48.0
  infant P08.21
  more than 42 weeks gestation (mother) O48.1
Post-traumatic brain syndrome, nonpsychotic F07.81
Post-typhoid abscess A01.09
Postures, hysterical F44.2
Postvaccinal reaction or complication — *see* Complications, vaccination
Postvalvulotomy syndrome I97.0
Potain's
  disease (pulmonary edema) — *see* Edema, lung
  syndrome (gastrectasis with dyspepsia) K31.0
POTS (postural orthostatic tachycardia syndrome) G90.A
Potter's
  asthma J62.8
  facies Q60.6
  lung J62.8
  syndrome (with renal agenesis) Q60.6
Pott's
  curvature (spinal) A18.01
  disease or paraplegia A18.01
  spinal curvature A18.01
  tumor, puffy — *see* Osteomyelitis, specified type NEC
Pouch
  bronchus Q32.4
  Douglas' — *see* condition
  esophagus, esophageal, congenital Q39.6
    acquired K22.5
  gastric K31.4
  Hartmann's K82.8
  pharynx, pharyngeal (congenital) Q38.7
Pouchitis K91.850
Poultrymen's itch B88.0
Poverty NEC Z59.6
  extreme Z59.5
Poxvirus NEC B08.8
Prader-Willi syndrome Q87.11
Prader-Willi-like syndrome Q87.19
Preauricular appendage or tag Q17.0
Prebetalipoproteinemia (acquired) (essential) (familial) (hereditary) (primary) (secondary) E78.1
  with chylomicronemia E78.3
Precipitate labor or delivery O62.3
Preclimacteric bleeding (menorrhagia) N92.4
Precocious
  adrenarche E30.1
  menarche E30.1
  menstruation E30.1
  pubarche E30.1
  puberty E30.1
    central E22.8
  sexual development NEC E30.1
  thelarche E30.8
Precocity, sexual (constitutional) (cryptogenic) (female) (idiopathic) (male) E30.1
  with adrenal hyperplasia E25.9
    congenital E25.0
Precordial pain R07.2
Predeciduous teeth K00.2
Prediabetes, prediabetic R73.03
  complicating
    pregnancy — *see* Pregnancy, complicated by, diseases of, specified type or system NEC
    puerperium O99.893
Predislocation status of hip at birth Q65.6
Pre-eclampsia O14.9- ☑
  with pre-existing hypertension — *see* Hypertension, complicating pregnancy, pre-existing, with, pre-eclampsia
  complicating
    childbirth O14.94
    puerperium O14.95
  mild O14.0- ☑
    complicating
      childbirth O14.04
      puerperium O14.05

Pre-eclampsia — *continued*
- moderate O14.0- ☑
  - complicating
    - childbirth O14.04
    - puerperium O14.05
- severe O14.1- ☑
  - with hemolysis, elevated liver enzymes and low platelet count (HELLP) O14.2- ☑
  - complicating
    - childbirth O14.24
    - puerperium O14.25
- complicating
  - childbirth O14.14
  - puerperium O14.15

Pre-eruptive color change, teeth, tooth K00.8
Pre-excitation atrioventricular conduction I45.6
Preglaucoma H40.00- ☑
Pregnancy (single) (uterine) — *see also* Delivery and Puerperal Z33.1

> Note: The Tabular must be reviewed for assignment of appropriate seventh character for multiple gestation codes in Chapter 15

> Note: The Tabular must be reviewed for assignment of the appropriate character indicating the trimester of the pregnancy

- abdominal (ectopic) O00.00
  - with intrauterine pregnancy O00.01
  - with viable fetus O36.7- ☑
- ampullar O00.10- ☑
  - with intrauterine pregnancy O00.11- ☑
- biochemical O02.81
- broad ligament O00.80
  - with intrauterine pregnancy O00.81
- cervical O00.8
  - with intrauterine pregnancy O00.81
- chemical O02.81
- complicated by (care of) (management affected by)
  - abnormal, abnormality
    - cervix O34.4- ☑
      - causing obstructed labor O65.5
    - cord (umbilical) O69.9
    - fetal heart rate or rhythm O36.83- ☑
    - findings on antenatal screening of mother O28.9
      - biochemical O28.1
      - chromosomal O28.5
      - cytological O28.2
      - genetic O28.5
      - hematological O28.0
      - radiological O28.4
      - specified NEC O28.8
      - ultrasonic O28.3
    - glucose (tolerance) NEC O99.810
    - pelvic organs O34.9- ☑
      - specified NEC O34.8- ☑
        - causing obstructed labor O65.5
    - pelvis (bony) (major) NEC O33.0
    - perineum O34.7- ☑
    - position
      - placenta O44.0- ☑
        - with hemorrhage O44.1- ☑
      - uterus O34.59- ☑
    - uterus O34.59- ☑
      - causing obstructed labor O65.5
      - congenital O34.0- ☑
    - vagina O34.6- ☑
      - causing obstructed labor O65.5
    - vulva O34.7- ☑
      - causing obstructed labor O65.5
  - abruptio placentae — *see* Abruptio placentae
  - abscess or cellulitis
    - bladder O23.1- ☑
    - breast O91.11- ☑
    - genital organ or tract O23.9- ☑
  - abuse
    - physical O9A.31 ☑ (*following* O99)
    - psychological O9A.51 ☑ (*following* O99)
    - sexual O9A.41 ☑ (*following* O99)
  - adverse effect anesthesia O29.9- ☑
    - aspiration pneumonitis O29.01- ☑
    - cardiac arrest O29.11- ☑
    - cardiac complication NEC O29.19- ☑
    - cardiac failure O29.12- ☑
    - central nervous system complication NEC O29.29- ☑
    - cerebral anoxia O29.21- ☑

Pregnancy — *continued*
- complicated by — *continued*
  - adverse effect anesthesia — *continued*
    - failed or difficult intubation O29.6- ☑
    - inhalation of stomach contents or secretions NOS O29.01- ☑
    - local, toxic reaction O29.3X ☑
    - Mendelson's syndrome O29.01- ☑
    - pressure collapse of lung O29.02- ☑
    - pulmonary complications NEC O29.09- ☑
    - specified NEC O29.8X- ☑
    - spinal and epidural type NEC O29.5X ☑
      - induced headache O29.4- ☑
  - albuminuria — *see also* Proteinuria, gestational O12.1- ☑
  - alcohol use O99.31- ☑
  - amnionitis O41.12- ☑
  - anaphylactoid syndrome of pregnancy O88.01- ☑
  - anemia (conditions in D50-D64) (pre-existing) O99.01- ☑
    - complicating the puerperium O99.03
  - antepartum hemorrhage O46.9- ☑
    - with coagulation defect — *see* Hemorrhage, antepartum, with coagulation defect
    - specified NEC O46.8X- ☑
  - appendicitis O99.61- ☑
  - atrophy (yellow) (acute) liver (subacute) O26.61- ☑
  - bariatric surgery status O99.84- ☑
  - bicornis or bicornuate uterus O34.0- ☑
  - biliary tract problems O26.61- ☑
  - breech presentation O32.1 ☑
  - cardiovascular diseases (conditions in I00-I09, I20-I52, I70-I99) O99.41- ☑
  - cerebrovascular disorders (conditions in I60-I69) O99.41- ☑
  - cervical shortening O26.87- ☑
  - cervicitis O23.51- ☑
  - cesarean scar defect (isthmocele) O34.22
  - chloasma (gravidarum) O26.89- ☑
  - cholecystitis O99.61- ☑
  - cholestasis (intrahepatic) O26.61- ☑
  - chorioamnionitis O41.12- ☑
  - circulatory system disorder (conditions in I00-I09, I20-I99, O99.41-)
  - compound presentation O32.6 ☑
  - conjoined twins O30.02- ☑
  - connective system disorders (conditions in M00-M99) O99.891
  - contracted pelvis (general) O33.1
    - inlet O33.2
    - outlet O33.3 ☑
  - convulsions (eclamptic) (uremic) — *see also* Eclampsia O15.9
  - cracked nipple O92.11- ☑
  - cystitis O23.1- ☑
  - cystocele O34.8- ☑
  - death of fetus (near term) O36.4 ☑
    - early pregnancy O02.1
    - of one fetus or more in multiple gestation O31.2- ☑
  - deciduitis O41.14- ☑
  - decreased fetal movement O36.81- ☑
  - dental problems O99.61- ☑
  - diabetes (mellitus) O24.91- ☑
    - gestational (pregnancy induced) — *see* Diabetes, gestational
    - pre-existing O24.31- ☑
      - specified NEC O24.81- ☑
      - type 1 O24.01- ☑
      - type 2 O24.11- ☑
  - digestive system disorders (conditions in K00-K93) O99.61- ☑
  - diseases of — *see* Pregnancy, complicated by, specified body system disease
    - biliary tract O26.61- ☑
    - blood NEC (conditions in D65-D77) O99.11- ☑
    - liver O26.61- ☑
    - specified NEC O99.891
  - disorders of — *see* Pregnancy, complicated by, specified body system disorder
    - amniotic fluid and membranes O41.9- ☑
      - specified NEC O41.8X- ☑
    - biliary tract O26.61- ☑
    - ear and mastoid process (conditions in H60-H95) O99.891
    - eye and adnexa (conditions in H00-H59) O99.891

Pregnancy — *continued*
- complicated by — *continued*
  - disorders of — *see* Pregnancy, complicated by, specified body system disorder — *continued*
    - liver O26.61- ☑
    - skin (conditions in L00-L99) O99.71- ☑
    - specified NEC O99.891
  - displacement, uterus NEC O34.59- ☑
    - causing obstructed labor O65.5
  - disproportion (due to) O33.9
    - fetal (ascites) (hydrops) (meningomyelocele) (sacral teratoma) (tumor) deformities NEC O33.7
    - generally contracted pelvis O33.1
    - hydrocephalic fetus O33.6
    - inlet contraction of pelvis O33.2
    - mixed maternal and fetal origin O33.4 ☑
    - specified NEC O33.8
  - double uterus O34.0- ☑
    - causing obstructed labor O65.5
  - drug use (conditions in F11-F19) O99.32- ☑
  - eclampsia, eclamptic (coma) (convulsions) (delirium) (nephritis) (uremia) — *see also* Eclampsia O15.- ☑
  - ectopic pregnancy — *see* Pregnancy, ectopic
  - edema O12.0- ☑
    - with
      - gestational hypertension, mild — *see also* Pre-eclampsia O14.0- ☑
      - proteinuria O12.2- ☑
  - effusion, amniotic fluid — *see* Pregnancy, complicated by, premature rupture of membranes
  - elderly
    - multigravida O09.52- ☑
    - primigravida O09.51- ☑
  - embolism — *see also* Embolism, obstetric, pregnancy O88.- ☑
  - endocrine diseases NEC O99.28- ☑
  - endometritis O86.12
  - excessive weight gain O26.0- ☑
  - exhaustion O26.81- ☑
    - during labor and delivery O75.81
  - face presentation O32.3 ☑
  - failed induction of labor O61.9
    - instrumental O61.1
    - mechanical O61.1
    - medical O61.0
    - specified NEC O61.8
    - surgical O61.1
  - failed or difficult intubation for anesthesia O29.6- ☑
  - false labor (pains) O47.9
    - at or after 37 completed weeks of pregnancy O47.1
    - before 37 completed weeks of pregnancy O47.0-
  - fatigue O26.81- ☑
    - during labor and delivery O75.81
  - fatty metamorphosis of liver O26.61- ☑
  - female genital mutilation O34.8- ☑ *[N90.81-]* ☑
  - fetal (maternal care for)
    - abnormality or damage O35.9 ☑
      - acid-base balance O68
      - specified type NEC O35.8 ☑
    - acidemia O68
    - acidosis O68
    - agenesis of corpus callosum O35.01 ☑
    - alkalosis O68
    - anemia and thrombocytopenia O36.82- ☑
    - anencephaly O35.02 ☑
    - bradycardia O36.83- ☑
    - cardiac anomalies O35.B ☑
    - central nervous system malformation or damage O35.00 ☑
      - specified type NEC O35.09 ☑
    - choroid plexus cysts O35.03 ☑
    - chromosomal abnormality (conditions in Q90-Q99) O35.10 ☑
      - sex chromosome O35.15 ☑
      - specified NEC O35.19 ☑
      - Trisomy 13 O35.11 ☑
      - Trisomy 18 O35.12 ☑
      - Trisomy 21 O35.13 ☑
      - Turner Syndrome O35.14 ☑
    - conjoined twins O30.02- ☑
    - damage from
      - amniocentesis O35.7 ☑

Pregnancy — *continued*
  complicated by — *continued*
    fetal — *continued*
      damage from — *continued*
        biopsy procedures O35.7 ☑
        drug addiction O35.5 ☑
        hematological investigation O35.7 ☑
        intrauterine contraceptive device O35.7 ☑
        maternal
          alcohol addiction O35.4 ☑
          cytomegalovirus infection O35.3 ☑
          disease NEC O35.8 ☑
          drug addiction O35.5 ☑
          listeriosis O35.8 ☑
          rubella O35.3 ☑
          toxoplasmosis O35.8 ☑
          viral infection O35.3 ☑
        medical procedure NEC O35.7 ☑
        radiation O35.6 ☑
      death (near term) O36.4 ☑
        early pregnancy O02.1
      decreased movement O36.81- ☑
      depressed heart rate tones O36.83- ☑
      disproportion due to deformity (fetal) O33.7 ☑
      encephalocele O35.04 ☑
      excessive growth (large for dates) O36.6- ☑
      facial anomalies O35.A ☑
      gastrointestinal anomalies O35.D ☑
      genitourinary anomalies O35.E ☑
      growth retardation O36.59- ☑
        light for dates O36.59- ☑
        small for dates O36.59- ☑
      heart rate irregularity (abnormal variability)
        (bradycardia) (decelerations) (tachycardia)
        O36.83- ☑
      hereditary disease O35.2 ☑
      holoprosencephaly O35.05 ☑
      hydrocephalus O35.06 ☑
      hydrocephaly O35.06 ☑
      intrauterine death O36.4 ☑
      microcephaly O35.07 ☑
      musculoskeletal anomalies
        lower extremities O35.H ☑
        trunk O35.F ☑
        upper extremities O35.G ☑
      non-reassuring heart rate or rhythm O36.83- ☑
      poor growth O36.59- ☑
        light for dates O36.59- ☑
        small for dates O36.59- ☑
      problem O36.9- ☑
        specified NEC O36.89- ☑
      pulmonary anomalies O35.C ☑
      reduction (elective) O31.3- ☑
      selective termination O31.3- ☑
      spina bifida O35.08 ☑
      thrombocytopenia O36.82- ☑
    fibroid (tumor) (uterus) O34.1- ☑
    fissure of nipple O92.11- ☑
    gallstones O99.61- ☑
    gastric banding status O99.84- ☑
    gastric bypass status O99.84- ☑
    genital herpes (asymptomatic) (history of) (inactive)
      O98.3- ☑
    genital tract infection O23.9- ☑
    glomerular diseases (conditions in N00-N07)
      O26.83- ☑
      with hypertension, pre-existing — *see* Hyperten-
        sion, complicating, pregnancy, pre-exist-
        ing, with, renal disease
    gonorrhea O98.21- ☑
    grand multiparity O09.4 ☑
    habitual aborter — *see* Pregnancy, complicated by,
      recurrent pregnancy loss
    HELLP syndrome (hemolysis, elevated liver enzymes
      and low platelet count) O14.2- ☑
    hemorrhage
      antepartum — *see* Hemorrhage, antepartum
      before 20 completed weeks gestation O20.9
        specified NEC O20.8
      due to premature separation, placenta — *see*
        also Abruptio placentae O45.9- ☑
      early O20.9
        specified NEC O20.8
        threatened abortion O20.0
    hemorrhoids O22.4- ☑
    hepatitis (viral) O98.41- ☑

Pregnancy — *continued*
  complicated by — *continued*
    herniation of uterus O34.59- ☑
    high
      head at term O32.4 ☑
      risk — *see* Supervision (of) (for), high-risk
    history of in utero procedure during previous preg-
      nancy O09.82- ☑
    HIV O98.71- ☑
    human immunodeficiency virus (HIV) disease
      O98.71- ☑
    hydatidiform mole — *see also* Mole, hydatidiform
      O01.9
    hydramnios O40.- ☑
    hydrocephalic fetus (disproportion) O33.6 ☑
    hydrops
      amnii O40.- ☑
      fetalis O36.2- ☑
        associated with isoimmunization — *see also*
          Pregnancy, complicated by, isoimmu-
          nization O36.11- ☑
    hydrorrhea O42.90
    hyperemesis (gravidarum) (mild) — *see also* Hyper-
      emesis, gravidarum O21.0
    hypertension — *see* Hypertension, complicating
      pregnancy
    hypertensive
      heart and renal disease, pre-existing — *see* Hy-
        pertension, complicating, pregnancy, pre-
        existing, with, heart disease, with renal
        disease
      heart disease, pre-existing — *see* Hypertension,
        complicating, pregnancy, pre-existing,
        with, heart disease
      renal disease, pre-existing — *see* Hypertension,
        complicating, pregnancy, pre-existing,
        with, renal disease
    hypotension O26.5- ☑
    immune disorders NEC (conditions in D80-D89)
      O99.11- ☑
    incarceration, uterus O34.51- ☑
    incompetent cervix O34.3- ☑
    inconclusive fetal viability O36.80 ☑
    infection(s) O98.91- ☑
      amniotic fluid or sac O41.10- ☑
      bladder O23.1- ☑
      carrier state NEC O99.830
        streptococcus B O99.820
      genital organ or tract O23.9- ☑
        specified NEC O23.59- ☑
      genitourinary tract O23.9- ☑
      gonorrhea O98.21- ☑
      hepatitis (viral) O98.41- ☑
      HIV O98.71- ☑
      human immunodeficiency virus (HIV) O98.71- ☑
      intrauterine O41.12 ☑
      kidney O23.0- ☑
      nipple O91.01- ☑
      parasitic disease O98.91- ☑
        specified NEC O98.81- ☑
      protozoal disease O98.61- ☑
      sexually transmitted NEC O98.31- ☑
      specified type NEC O98.81- ☑
      syphilis O98.11- ☑
      tuberculosis O98.01- ☑
      urethra O23.2- ☑
      urinary (tract) O23.4- ☑
        specified NEC O23.3- ☑
      viral disease O98.51- ☑
    inflammation
      intrauterine O41.12 ☑
    injury or poisoning (conditions in S00-T88)
      O9A.21- ☑ (*following* O99)
      due to abuse
        physical O9A.31- ☑ (*following* O99)
        psychological O9A.51- ☑ (*following* O99)
        sexual O9A.41- ☑ (*following* O99)
    insufficient
      prenatal care O09.3- ☑
      weight gain O26.1- ☑
    insulin resistance O26.89 ☑
    intrauterine fetal death (near term) O36.4 ☑
      early pregnancy O02.1
      multiple gestation (one fetus or more) O31.2- ☑
    isoimmunization O36.11- ☑
      anti-A sensitization O36.11- ☑

Pregnancy — *continued*
  complicated by — *continued*
    isoimmunization — *continued*
      anti-B sensitization O36.19- ☑
      Rh O36.09- ☑
        anti-D antibody O36.01- ☑
      specified NEC O36.19- ☑
    laceration of uterus NEC O71.81
    malformation
      central nervous system O35.00 ☑
        specified type NEC O35.09 ☑
      placenta, placental (vessel) O43.10- ☑
        specified NEC O43.19- ☑
      uterus (congenital) O34.0- ☑
    malnutrition (conditions in E40-E46) O25.1- ☑
    maternal hypotension syndrome O26.5- ☑
    mental disorders (conditions in F01-F09, F20-F52
      and F54-F99) O99.34- ☑
      alcohol use O99.31- ☑
      drug use O99.32- ☑
      smoking O99.33- ☑
    mentum presentation O32.3 ☑
    metabolic disorders O99.28- ☑
    missed
      abortion O02.1
      delivery O36.4
    multiple gestations O30.9- ☑
      conjoined twins O30.02- ☑
      quadruplet — *see* Pregnancy, quadruplet
      specified complication NEC O31.8X- ☑
      specified number of multiples NEC — *see* Preg-
        nancy, multiple (gestation), specified NEC
      triplet — *see* Pregnancy, triplet
      twin — *see* Pregnancy, twin
    musculoskeletal condition (conditions is M00-M99)
      O99.891
    necrosis, liver (conditions in K72) O26.61- ☑
    neoplasm
      benign
        cervix O34.4- ☑
        corpus uteri O34.1- ☑
        uterus O34.1- ☑
      malignant O9A.11- ☑ (*following* O99)
    nephropathy NEC O26.83- ☑
    nervous system condition (conditions in G00-G99)
      O99.35- ☑
    nutritional diseases NEC O99.28- ☑
    obesity (pre-existing) O99.21- ☑
    obesity surgery status O99.84- ☑
    oblique lie or presentation O32.2 ☑
    older mother — *see* Pregnancy, complicated by,
      elderly
    oligohydramnios O41.0- ☑
      with premature rupture of membranes — *see*
        also Pregnancy, complicated by, prema-
        ture rupture of membranes O42.- ☑
    onset (spontaneous) of labor after 37 completed
      weeks of gestation but before 39 completed
      weeks gestation, with delivery by (planned)
      cesarean section O75.82
    oophoritis O23.52- ☑
    overdose, drug — *see also* Table of Drugs and
      Chemicals, by drug, poisoning O9A.21- ☑
      (*following* O99)
    oversize fetus O33.5 ☑
    papyraceous fetus O31.0- ☑
    pelvic inflammatory disease O99.891
    periodontal disease O99.61- ☑
    peripheral neuritis O26.82- ☑
    peritoneal (pelvic) adhesions O99.891
    phlebitis O22.9- ☑
    phlebopathy O22.9- ☑
    phlebothrombosis (superficial) O22.2- ☑
      deep O22.3- ☑
    placenta accreta O43.21- ☑
    placenta increta O43.22- ☑
    placenta percreta O43.23- ☑
    placenta previa O44.0- ☑
      complete O44.0- ☑
        with hemorrhage O44.1- ☑
      marginal O44.2- ☑
        with hemorrhage O44.3- ☑
      partial O44.2- ☑
        with hemorrhage O44.3- ☑
    placental disorder O43.9- ☑
      specified NEC O43.89- ☑

☑ **Additional Character Required — Refer to the Tabular List for Character Selection**

Pregnancy — *continued*
  isthmian O00.10- ☑
    with intrauterine pregnancy O00.11- ☑
  mesometric (mural) O00.80
    with intrauterine pregnancy O00.81
  molar NEC O02.0
    complicated (by) O08.9
      afibrinogenemia O08.1
      cardiac arrest O08.81
      chemical damage of pelvic organ(s) O08.6
      circulatory collapse O08.3
      defibrination syndrome O08.1
      electrolyte imbalance O08.5
      embolism (amniotic fluid) (blood clot) (pulmonary) (septic) O08.2
      endometritis O08.0
      genital tract and pelvic infection O08.0
      hemorrhage (delayed) (excessive) O08.1
      infection
        genital tract or pelvic O08.0
        kidney O08.83
        urinary tract O08.83
      intravascular coagulation O08.1
      laceration of pelvic organ(s) O08.6
      metabolic disorder O08.5
      oliguria O08.4
      oophoritis O08.0
      parametritis O08.0
      pelvic peritonitis O08.0
      perforation of pelvic organ(s) O08.6
      renal failure or shutdown O08.4
      salpingitis or salpingo-oophoritis O08.0
      sepsis O08.82
      shock O08.3
        septic O08.82
      specified condition NEC O08.89
      tubular necrosis (renal) O08.4
      uremia O08.4
      urinary infection O08.83
      venous complication NEC O08.7
        embolism O08.2
    hydatidiform — *see also* Mole, hydatidiform O01.9
  multiple (gestation) O30.9- ☑
    greater than quadruplets — *see* Pregnancy, multiple (gestation), specified NEC
    specified NEC O30.80- ☑
      with
        two or more monoamniotic fetuses O30.82- ☑
        two or more monochorionic fetuses O30.81- ☑
        number of chorions and amnions are both equal to the number of fetuses O30.83- ☑
        two or more monoamniotic fetuses O30.82- ☑
        two or more monochorionic fetuses O30.81- ☑
        unable to determine number of placenta and number of amniotic sacs O30.89- ☑
        unspecified number of placenta and unspecified number of amniotic sacs O30.80- ☑
  mural O00.80
    with intrauterine pregnancy O00.81
  normal (supervision of) Z34.9- ☑
    first Z34.0- ☑
    high-risk — *see* Pregnancy, supervision of, high-risk
    specified Z34.8- ☑
  ovarian O00.20- ☑
    with intrauterine pregnancy O00.21- ☑
  pentachorionic, penta-amniotic (quintuplets) O30.83- ☑
  postmature (40 to 42 weeks) O48.0
    more than 42 weeks gestation O48.1
  post-term (40 to 42 weeks) O48.0
  prenatal care only Z34.9- ☑
    first Z34.0- ☑
    high-risk — *see* Pregnancy, supervision of, high-risk
    specified Z34.8- ☑
  prolonged (more than 42 weeks gestation) O48.1
  quadruplet O30.20- ☑
    with
      two or more monoamniotic fetuses O30.22- ☑
      two or more monochorionic fetuses O30.21- ☑
      quadrachorionic/quadra-amniotic O30.23- ☑
      two or more monoamniotic fetuses O30.22- ☑
      two or more monochorionic fetuses O30.21- ☑
      unable to determine number of placenta and number of amniotic sacs O30.29- ☑
      unspecified number of placenta and unspecified number of amniotic sacs O30.20- ☑

Pregnancy — *continued*
  quintuplet — *see* Pregnancy, multiple (gestation), specified NEC
  sextuplet — *see* Pregnancy, multiple (gestation), specified NEC
  supervision of
    concealed pregnancy O09.3- ☑
    elderly mother
      multigravida O09.52- ☑
      primigravida O09.51- ☑
    hidden pregnancy O09.3- ☑
    high-risk O09.9- ☑
      due to (history of)
        ectopic pregnancy O09.1- ☑
        elderly — *see* Pregnancy, supervision, elderly mother
        grand multiparity O09.4 ☑
        in utero procedure during previous pregnancy O09.82- ☑
        in vitro fertilization O09.81- ☑
        infertility O09.0- ☑
        insufficient prenatal care O09.3- ☑
        molar pregnancy O09.A- ☑
        multiple previous pregnancies O09.4- ☑
        older mother — *see* Pregnancy, supervision of, elderly mother
        poor reproductive or obstetric history NEC O09.29- ☑
        pre-term labor O09.21- ☑
        previous
          neonatal death O09.29- ☑
        social problems O09.7- ☑
        specified NEC O09.89- ☑
        very young mother — *see* Pregnancy, supervision, young mother
    resulting from in vitro fertilization O09.81- ☑
    normal Z34.9- ☑
      first Z34.0- ☑
      specified NEC Z34.8- ☑
    young mother
      multigravida O09.62- ☑
      primigravida O09.61- ☑
  triplet O30.10- ☑
    with
      two or more monoamniotic fetuses O30.12- ☑
      two or more monochorionic fetuses O30.11- ☑
    trichorionic/triamniotic O30.13- ☑
    two or more monoamniotic fetuses O30.12- ☑
    two or more monochorionic fetuses O30.11- ☑
    unable to determine number of placenta and number of amniotic sacs O30.19- ☑
    unspecified number of placenta and unspecified number of amniotic sacs O30.10- ☑
  tubal (with abortion) (with rupture) O00.10- ☑
    with intrauterine pregnancy O00.11- ☑
  twin O30.00- ☑
    conjoined O30.02- ☑
    dichorionic/diamniotic (two placenta, two amniotic sacs) O30.04- ☑
    monochorionic/diamniotic (one placenta, two amniotic sacs) O30.03- ☑
    monochorionic/monoamniotic (one placenta, one amniotic sac) O30.01- ☑
    unable to determine number of placenta and number of amniotic sacs O30.09- ☑
    unspecified number of placenta and unspecified number of amniotic sacs O30.00- ☑
  unwanted Z64.0
  weeks of gestation
    8 weeks Z3A.08 (*following* Z36)
    9 weeks Z3A.09 (*following* Z36)
    10 weeks Z3A.10 (*following* Z36)
    11 weeks Z3A.11 (*following* Z36)
    12 weeks Z3A.12 (*following* Z36)
    13 weeks Z3A.13 (*following* Z36)
    14 weeks Z3A.14 (*following* Z36)
    15 weeks Z3A.15 (*following* Z36)
    16 weeks Z3A.16 (*following* Z36)
    17 weeks Z3A.17 (*following* Z36)
    18 weeks Z3A.18 (*following* Z36)
    19 weeks Z3A.19 (*following* Z36)
    20 weeks Z3A.20 (*following* Z36)
    21 weeks Z3A.21 (*following* Z36)
    22 weeks Z3A.22 (*following* Z36)
    23 weeks Z3A.23 (*following* Z36)
    24 weeks Z3A.24 (*following* Z36)
    25 weeks Z3A.25 (*following* Z36)

Pregnancy — *continued*
  weeks of gestation — *continued*
    26 weeks Z3A.26 (*following* Z36)
    27 weeks Z3A.27 (*following* Z36)
    28 weeks Z3A.28 (*following* Z36)
    29 weeks Z3A.29 (*following* Z36)
    30 weeks Z3A.30 (*following* Z36)
    31 weeks Z3A.31 (*following* Z36)
    32 weeks Z3A.32 (*following* Z36)
    33 weeks Z3A.33 (*following* Z36)
    34 weeks Z3A.34 (*following* Z36)
    35 weeks Z3A.35 (*following* Z36)
    36 weeks Z3A.36 (*following* Z36)
    37 weeks Z3A.37 (*following* Z36)
    38 weeks Z3A.38 (*following* Z36)
    39 weeks Z3A.39 (*following* Z36)
    40 weeks Z3A.40 (*following* Z36)
    41 weeks Z3A.41 (*following* Z36)
    42 weeks Z3A.42 (*following* Z36)
    greater than 42 weeks Z3A.49 (*following* Z36)
    less than 8 weeks Z3A.01 (*following* Z36)
    not specified Z3A.00 (*following* Z36)
Preiser's disease — *see* Osteonecrosis, secondary, due to, trauma, metacarpus
Pre-kwashiorkor — *see* Malnutrition, severe
Preleukemia (syndrome) D46.9
Preluxation, hip, congenital Q65.6
Premature — *see also* condition
  adrenarche E27.0
  aging E34.8
  beats I49.40
    atrial I49.1
    auricular I49.1
    supraventricular I49.1
  birth NEC — *see* Preterm, newborn
  closure, foramen ovale Q21.8
  contraction
    atrial I49.1
    atrioventricular I49.2
    auricular I49.1
    auriculoventricular I49.49
    heart (extrasystole) I49.49
    junctional I49.2
    ventricular I49.3
  delivery — *see also* Pregnancy, complicated by, preterm labor O60.10 ☑
  ejaculation F52.4
  infant NEC — *see* Preterm, newborn
    light-for-dates — *see* Light for dates
  labor — *see* Pregnancy, complicated by, preterm labor
  lungs P28.0
  menopause E28.319
    asymptomatic E28.319
    symptomatic E28.310
  newborn
    extreme (less than 28 completed weeks) — *see* Immaturity, extreme
    less than 37 completed weeks — *see* Preterm, newborn
  puberty E30.1
  rupture membranes or amnion — *see* Pregnancy, complicated by, premature rupture of membranes
  senility E34.8
  thelarche E30.8
  ventricular systole I49.3
Prematurity NEC (less than 37 completed weeks) — *see* Preterm, newborn
  extreme (less than 28 completed weeks) — *see* Immaturity, extreme
Premenstrual
  dysphoric disorder (PMDD) F32.81
  tension (syndrome) N94.3
Premolarization, cuspids K00.2
Prenatal
  care, normal pregnancy — *see* Pregnancy, normal
  screening of mother — *see also* Encounter, antenatal screening Z36.9
  teeth K00.6
Preparatory care for subsequent treatment NEC
  for dialysis Z49.01
    peritoneal Z49.02
Prepartum — *see* condition
Preponderance, left or right ventricular I51.7
Prepuce — *see* condition
PRES (posterior reversible encephalopathy syndrome) I67.83
Presbycardia R54

Presbycusis, presbyacusia H91.1- ☑
Presbyesophagus K22.89
Presbyophrenia F03 ☑
Presbyopia H52.4
Prescription of contraceptives (initial) Z30.019
  barrier Z30.018
  diaphragm Z30.018
  emergency (postcoital) Z30.012
  implantable subdermal Z30.017
  injectable Z30.013
  intrauterine contraceptive device Z30.014
  pills Z30.011
  postcoital (emergency) Z30.012
  repeat Z30.40
    barrier Z30.49
    diaphragm Z30.49
    implantable subdermal Z30.46
    injectable Z30.42
    pills Z30.41
    specified type NEC Z30.49
    transdermal patch hormonal Z30.45
    vaginal ring hormonal Z30.44
  specified type NEC Z30.018
    transdermal patch hormonal Z30.016
    vaginal ring hormonal Z30.015
Presence (of)
  ankle-joint implant (functional) (prosthesis) Z96.66- ☑
  aortocoronary (bypass) graft Z95.1
  arterial-venous shunt (dialysis) Z99.2
  artificial
    eye (globe) Z97.0
    heart (fully implantable) (mechanical) Z95.812
      valve Z95.2
    larynx Z96.3
    lens (intraocular) Z96.1
    limb (complete) (partial) Z97.1- ☑
      arm Z97.1- ☑
        bilateral Z97.15
      leg Z97.1- ☑
        bilateral Z97.16
  audiological implant (functional) Z96.29
  bladder implant (functional) Z96.0
  bone
    conduction hearing device Z96.29
    implant (functional) NEC Z96.7
    joint (prosthesis) — see Presence, joint implant
  cardiac
    defibrillator (functional) (with synchronous cardiac
      pacemaker) Z95.810
    implant or graft Z95.9
      specified type NEC Z95.818
    pacemaker Z95.0
    resynchronization therapy
      defibrillator Z95.810
      pacemaker Z95.0
  cardioverter-defibrillator (ICD) Z95.810
  cerebrospinal fluid drainage device Z98.2
  cochlear implant (functional) Z96.21
  contact lens (es) Z97.3
  coronary artery graft or prosthesis Z95.5
  CRT-D (cardiac resynchronization therapy defibrillator)
    Z95.810
  CRT-P (cardiac resynchronization therapy pacemaker)
    Z95.0
  CSF shunt Z98.2
  dental prosthesis device Z97.2
  dentures Z97.2
  device (external) NEC Z97.8
    cardiac NEC Z95.818
    heart assist Z95.811
    implanted (functional) Z96.9
      specified NEC Z96.89
    prosthetic Z97.8
  ear implant Z96.20
    cochlear implant Z96.21
    myringotomy tube Z96.22
    specified type NEC Z96.29
  elbow-joint implant (functional) (prosthesis) Z96.62- ☑
  endocrine implant (functional) NEC Z96.49
  eustachian tube stent or device (functional) Z96.29
  external hearing-aid or device Z97.4
  finger-joint implant (functional) (prosthetic) Z96.69- ☑
  functional implant Z96.9
    specified NEC Z96.89
  graft
    cardiac NEC Z95.818
    vascular NEC Z95.828
  hearing-aid or device (external) Z97.4

Presence — continued
  hearing-aid or device — continued
    implant (bone) (cochlear) (functional) Z96.21
  heart assist device Z95.811
  heart valve implant (functional) Z95.2
    prosthetic Z95.2
    specified type NEC Z95.4
    xenogenic Z95.3
  hip-joint implant (functional) (prosthesis) Z96.64- ☑
  ICD (cardioverter-defibrillator) Z95.810
  implanted device (artificial) (functional) (prosthetic)
    Z96.9
    automatic cardiac defibrillator (with synchronous
      cardiac pacemaker) Z95.810
    cardiac pacemaker Z95.0
    cochlear Z96.21
    dental Z96.5
    heart Z95.812
    heart valve Z95.2
      prosthetic Z95.2
      specified NEC Z95.4
      xenogenic Z95.3
    insulin pump Z96.41
    intraocular lens Z96.1
    joint Z96.60
      ankle Z96.66- ☑
      elbow Z96.62- ☑
      finger Z96.69- ☑
      hip Z96.64- ☑
      knee Z96.65- ☑
      shoulder Z96.61- ☑
      specified NEC Z96.698
      wrist Z96.63- ☑
    larynx Z96.3
    myringotomy tube Z96.22
    otological Z96.20
      cochlear Z96.21
      eustachian stent Z96.29
      myringotomy Z96.22
      specified NEC Z96.29
      stapes Z96.29
    skin Z96.81
    skull plate Z96.7
    specified NEC Z96.89
    urogenital Z96.0
  insulin pump (functional) Z96.41
  intestinal bypass or anastomosis Z98.0
  intraocular lens (functional) Z96.1
  intrauterine contraceptive device (IUD) Z97.5
  intravascular implant (functional) (prosthetic) NEC
    Z95.9
    coronary artery Z95.5
    defibrillator (with synchronous cardiac pacemaker)
      Z95.810
    peripheral vessel (with angioplasty) Z95.820
  joint implant (prosthetic) (any) Z96.60
    ankle — see Presence, ankle joint implant
    elbow — see Presence, elbow joint implant
    finger — see Presence, finger joint implant
    hip — see Presence, hip joint implant
    knee — see Presence, knee joint implant
    shoulder — see Presence, shoulder joint implant
    specified joint NEC Z96.698
    wrist — see Presence, wrist joint implant
  knee-joint implant (functional) (prosthesis) Z96.65- ☑
  laryngeal implant (functional) Z96.3
  mandibular implant (dental) Z96.5
  myringotomy tube(s) Z96.22
  neurostimulator (brain) (gastric) (peripheral nerve)
    (sacral nerve) (spinal cord) (vagus nerve) Z96.82
  orthopedic-joint implant (prosthetic) (any) — see
    Presence, joint implant
  otological implant (functional) Z96.29
  shoulder-joint implant (functional) (prosthesis)
    Z96.61- ☑
  skull-plate implant Z96.7
  spectacles Z97.3
  stapes implant (functional) Z96.29
  systemic lupus erythematosus [SLE] inhibitor D68.62
  tendon implant (functional) (graft) Z96.7
  tooth root(s) implant Z96.5
  ureteral stent Z96.0
  urethral stent Z96.0
  urogenital implant (functional) Z96.0
  vascular implant or device Z95.9
    access port device Z95.828
    specified type NEC Z95.828
  wrist-joint implant (functional) (prosthesis) Z96.63- ☑

Presenile — see also condition
  dementia F03 ☑
  premature aging E34.8
Presentation, fetal — see Delivery, complicated by,
  malposition
Prespondylolisthesis (congenital) Q76.2
Pressure
  area, skin — see Ulcer, pressure, by site
  brachial plexus G54.0
  brain G93.5
    injury at birth NEC P11.1
  cerebral — see Pressure, brain
  chest R07.89
  cone, tentorial G93.5
  hyposystolic — see also Hypotension
    incidental reading, without diagnosis of hypoten-
      sion R03.1
  increased
    intracranial benign G93.2
      injury at birth P11.0
    intraocular H40.05- ☑
  injury — see Ulcer, pressure, by site
  lumbosacral plexus G54.1
  mediastinum J98.59
  necrosis (chronic) — see Ulcer, pressure, by site
  parental, inappropriate (excessive) Z62.6
  sore (chronic) — see Ulcer, pressure, by site
  spinal cord G95.20
  ulcer (chronic) — see Ulcer, pressure, by site
  venous, increased I87.8
Pre-syncope R55
Preterm
  delivery — see also Pregnancy, complicated by,
    preterm labor O60.10 ☑
  labor — see Pregnancy, complicated by, preterm labor
  newborn (infant) P07.30
    gestational age
      28 completed weeks (28 weeks, 0 days through
        28 weeks, 6 days) P07.31
      29 completed weeks (29 weeks, 0 days through
        29 weeks, 6 days) P07.32
      30 completed weeks (30 weeks, 0 days through
        30 weeks, 6 days) P07.33
      31 completed weeks (31 weeks, 0 days through
        31 weeks, 6 days) P07.34
      32 completed weeks (32 weeks, 0 days through
        32 weeks, 6 days) P07.35
      33 completed weeks (33 weeks, 0 days through
        33 weeks, 6 days) P07.36
      34 completed weeks (34 weeks, 0 days through
        34 weeks, 6 days) P07.37
      35 completed weeks (35 weeks, 0 days through
        35 weeks, 6 days) P07.38
      36 completed weeks (36 weeks, 0 days through
        36 weeks, 6 days) P07.39
Previa
  placenta (total) (without hemorrhage) O44.0- ☑
    with hemorrhage O44.1- ☑
    complete O44.0- ☑
      with hemorrhage O44.1- ☑
    low — see also Delivery, complicated, by, placenta,
      low O44.4- ☑
    with hemorrhage O44.5- ☑
    marginal O44.2- ☑
      with hemorrhage O44.3- ☑
    partial O44.2- ☑
      with hemorrhage O44.3- ☑
  vasa O69.4 ☑
Priapism N48.30
  due to
    disease classified elsewhere N48.32
    drug N48.33
    specified cause NEC N48.39
    trauma N48.31
Prickling sensation (skin) R20.2
Prickly heat L74.0
Primary — see condition
Primigravida
  elderly, affecting management of pregnancy, labor and
    delivery (supervision only) — see Pregnancy,
    complicated by, elderly, primigravida
  older, affecting management of pregnancy, labor and
    delivery (supervision only) — see Pregnancy,
    complicated by, elderly, primigravida
  very young, affecting management of pregnancy, labor
    and delivery (supervision only) — see Pregnancy,
    complicated by, young mother, primigravida

Primipara
- elderly, affecting management of pregnancy, labor and delivery (supervision only) — *see* Pregnancy, complicated by, elderly, primigravida
- older, affecting management of pregnancy, labor and delivery (supervision only) — *see* Pregnancy, complicated by, elderly, primigravida
- very young, affecting management of pregnancy, labor and delivery (supervision only) — *see* Pregnancy, complicated by, young mother, primigravida

Primus varus Q66.21- ☑

PRIND (Prolonged reversible ischemic neurologic deficit) I63.9

Pringle's disease (tuberous sclerosis) Q85.1

Prinzmetal angina I20.1

Prizefighter ear — *see* Cauliflower ear

Problem (with) (related to)
- academic Z55.8
- acculturation Z60.3
- adjustment (to)
  - change of job Z56.1
  - life-cycle transition Z60.0
  - pension Z60.0
  - retirement Z60.0
- adopted child Z62.821
- alcoholism in family Z63.72
- atypical parenting situation Z62.9
- bankruptcy Z59.89
- behavioral (adult) F69
  - drug seeking Z76.5
- birth of sibling affecting child Z62.898
- care (of)
  - provider dependency Z74.9
    - specified NEC Z74.8
  - sick or handicapped person in family or household Z63.6
- child
  - abuse (affecting the child) — *see* Maltreatment, child
  - custody or support proceedings Z65.3
  - in care of non-parental family member Z62.21
  - in foster care Z62.21
  - in welfare custody Z62.21
  - living in orphanage or group home Z62.22
- child-rearing Z62.9
  - specified NEC Z62.898
- communication (developmental) F80.9
- conflict or discord (with)
  - boss Z56.4
  - classmates Z55.4
  - counselor Z64.4
  - employer Z56.4
  - family Z63.9
    - specified NEC Z63.8
  - probation officer Z64.4
  - social worker Z64.4
  - teachers Z55.4
  - workmates Z56.4
- conviction in legal proceedings Z65.0
  - with imprisonment Z65.1
- counselor Z64.4
- creditors Z59.89
- digestive K92.9
- drug addict in family Z63.72
- ear — *see* Disorder, ear
- economic Z59.9
  - affecting care Z59.9
  - specified NEC Z59.89
  - strain Z59.86
- education Z55.9
  - specified NEC Z55.8
- employment Z56.9
  - change of job Z56.1
  - discord Z56.4
  - environment Z56.5
  - sexual harassment Z56.81
  - specified NEC Z56.89
  - stressful schedule Z56.3
  - stress NEC Z56.6
  - threat of job loss Z56.2
  - unemployment Z56.0
- enuresis, child F98.0
- eye H57.9
- failed examinations (school) Z55.2
- falling Z91.81
- family — *see also* Disruption, family Z63.9
  - specified NEC Z63.8
- feeding (elderly) (infant) R63.39

Problem — *continued*
- feeding — *continued*
  - newborn P92.9
    - breast P92.5
    - overfeeding P92.4
    - slow P92.2
    - specified NEC P92.8
    - underfeeding P92.3
  - nonorganic F50.89
- finance Z59.9
  - specified NEC Z59.89
  - foreclosure on loan Z59.89
- foster child Z62.822
- frightening experience(s) in childhood Z62.898
- genital NEC
  - female N94.9
  - male N50.9
- health care Z75.9
  - specified NEC Z75.8
- hearing — *see* Deafness
- homelessness Z59.00
- housing Z59.9
  - inadequate Z59.1
  - isolated Z59.89
  - specified NEC Z59.89
- identity (of childhood) F93.8
- illegitimate pregnancy (unwanted) Z64.0
- illiteracy Z55.0
- impaired mobility Z74.09
- imprisonment or incarceration Z65.1
- inadequate teaching affecting education Z55.8
- inappropriate (excessive) parental pressure Z62.6
- influencing health status NEC Z78.9
- in-law Z63.1
- institutionalization, affecting child Z62.22
- intrafamilial communication Z63.8
- jealousy, child F93.8
- landlord Z59.2
- language (developmental) F80.9
- learning (developmental) F81.9
- legal Z65.3
  - conviction without imprisonment Z65.0
  - imprisonment Z65.1
  - release from prison Z65.2
- life-management Z73.9
  - specified NEC Z73.89
- life-style Z72.9
  - gambling Z72.6
  - high-risk sexual behavior (heterosexual) Z72.51
    - bisexual Z72.53
    - homosexual Z72.52
  - inappropriate eating habits Z72.4
  - self-damaging behavior NEC Z72.89
  - specified NEC Z72.89
  - tobacco use Z72.0
- literacy Z55.9
  - low level Z55.0
  - specified NEC Z55.8
- living alone Z60.2
- lodgers Z59.2
- loss of love relationship in childhood Z62.898
- marital Z63.0
  - involving
    - divorce Z63.5
    - estrangement Z63.5
    - gender identity F66
- mastication K08.89
- medical
  - care, within family Z63.6
  - facilities Z75.9
    - specified NEC Z75.8
- mental F48.9
- money Z59.86
- multiparity Z64.1
- negative life events in childhood Z62.9
  - altered pattern of family relationships Z62.898
  - frightening experience Z62.898
  - loss of
    - love relationship Z62.898
    - self-esteem Z62.898
  - physical abuse (alleged) — *see* Maltreatment, child
  - removal from home Z62.29
  - specified event NEC Z62.898
- neighbor Z59.2
- neurological NEC R29.818
- new step-parent affecting child Z62.898
- none (feared complaint unfounded) Z71.1
- occupational NEC Z56.89
- parent-child — *see* Conflict, parent-child

Problem — *continued*
- personal hygiene Z91.89
- personality F69
- phase-of-life transition, adjustment Z60.0
- presence of sick or disabled person in family or household Z63.79
  - needing care Z63.6
- primary support group (family) Z63.9
  - specified NEC Z63.8
- probation officer Z64.4
- psychiatric F99
- psychosexual (development) F66
- psychosocial Z65.9
  - religious or spiritual Z65.8
  - specified NEC Z65.8
- relationship Z63.9
  - childhood F93.8
- release from prison Z65.2
  - religious or spiritual Z65.8
- removal from home affecting child Z62.29
- seeking and accepting known hazardous and harmful
  - behavioral or psychological interventions Z65.8
  - chemical, nutritional or physical interventions Z65.8
- sexual function (nonorganic) F52.9
- sight H54.7
- sleep disorder, child F51.9
- smell — *see* Disturbance, sensation, smell
- social
  - environment Z60.9
    - specified NEC Z60.8
  - exclusion and rejection Z60.4
  - worker Z64.4
- speech R47.9
  - developmental F80.9
  - specified NEC R47.89
- swallowing — *see* Dysphagia
- taste — *see* Disturbance, sensation, taste
- tic, child F95.0
- underachievement in school Z55.3
- unemployment Z56.0
  - threatened Z56.2
- unwanted pregnancy Z64.0
- upbringing Z62.9
  - specified NEC Z62.898
- urinary N39.9
- voice production R47.89
- work schedule (stressful) Z56.3

Procedure (surgical)
- converted
  - arthroscopic to open Z53.33
  - laparoscopic to open Z53.31
  - specified procedure NEC to open Z53.39
  - thoracoscopic to open Z53.32
- for purpose other than remedying health state Z41.9
  - specified NEC Z41.8
- not done Z53.9
  - because of
    - administrative reasons Z53.8
    - contraindication Z53.09
      - smoking Z53.01
    - patient's decision Z53.20
      - for reasons of belief or group pressure Z53.1
      - left against medical advice (AMA) Z53.29
      - left without being seen Z53.21
      - specified reason NEC Z53.29
    - specified reason NEC Z53.8

Procidentia (uteri) N81.3

Proctalgia K62.89
- fugax K59.4
- spasmodic K59.4

Proctitis K62.89
- amebic (acute) A06.0
- chlamydial A56.3
- gonococcal A54.6
- granulomatous — *see* Enteritis, regional, large intestine
- herpetic A60.1
- radiation K62.7
- tuberculous A18.32
- ulcerative (chronic) K51.20
  - with
    - complication K51.219
      - abscess K51.214
      - fistula K51.213
      - obstruction K51.212
      - rectal bleeding K51.211
      - specified NEC K51.218

Proctocele
- female (without uterine prolapse) N81.6

Proctocele — *continued*
female — *continued*
with uterine prolapse N81.2
complete N81.3
male K62.3
Proctocolitis
allergic K52.29
food protein-induced K52.29
food-induced eosinophilic K52.29
milk protein-induced K52.29
mucosal — *see* Rectosigmoiditis, ulcerative
Proctoptosis K62.3
Proctorrhagia K62.5
Proctosigmoiditis K63.89
ulcerative (chronic) — *see* Rectosigmoiditis, ulcerative
Proctospasm K59.4
psychogenic F45.8
Profichet's disease — *see* Disorder, soft tissue, specified type NEC
Progeria E34.8
Prognathism (mandibular) (maxillary) M26.19
Progonoma (melanotic) — *see* Neoplasm, benign, by site
Progressive — *see* condition
Prolactinoma
specified site — *see* Neoplasm, benign, by site
unspecified site D35.2
Prolapse, prolapsed
anus, anal (canal) (sphincter) K62.2
arm or hand O32.2 ☑
causing obstructed labor O64.4 ☑
bladder (mucosa) (sphincter) (acquired)
congenital Q79.4
female — *see* Cystocele
male N32.89
breast implant (prosthetic) T85.49 ☑
cecostomy K94.09
cecum K63.4
cervix, cervical (hypertrophied) N81.2
anterior lip, obstructing labor O65.5
congenital Q51.828
postpartal, old N81.2
stump N81.85
ciliary body (traumatic) — *see* Laceration, eye(ball), with prolapse or loss of interocular tissue
colon (pedunculated) K63.4
colostomy K94.09
disc (intervertebral) — *see* Displacement, intervertebral disc
eye implant (orbital) T85.398 ☑
lens (ocular) — *see* Complications, intraocular lens
fallopian tube N83.4- ☑
gastric (mucosa) K31.89
genital, female N81.9
specified NEC N81.89
globe, nontraumatic — *see* Luxation, globe
ileostomy bud K94.19
intervertebral disc — *see* Displacement, intervertebral disc
intestine (small) K63.4
iris (traumatic) — *see* Laceration, eye(ball), with prolapse or loss of interocular tissue
nontraumatic H21.89
kidney N28.83
congenital Q63.2
laryngeal muscles or ventricle J38.7
liver K76.89
meatus urinarius N36.8
mitral (valve) I34.1
ocular lens implant — *see* Complications, intraocular lens
organ or site, congenital NEC — *see* Malposition, congenital
ovary N83.4- ☑
pelvic floor, female N81.89
perineum, female N81.89
rectum (mucosa) (sphincter) K62.3
due to trichuris trichuria B79
spleen D73.89
stomach K31.89
umbilical cord
complicating delivery O69.0 ☑
urachus, congenital Q64.4
ureter N28.89
with obstruction N13.5
with infection N13.6
ureterovesical orifice N28.89
urethra (acquired) (infected) (mucosa) N36.8

Prolapse, prolapsed — *continued*
urethra — *continued*
congenital Q64.71
urinary meatus N36.8
congenital Q64.72
uterovaginal N81.4
complete N81.3
incomplete N81.2
uterus (with prolapse of vagina) N81.4
complete N81.3
congenital Q51.818
first degree N81.2
in pregnancy or childbirth — *see* Pregnancy, complicated by, abnormal, uterus
incomplete N81.2
postpartal (old) N81.4
second degree N81.2
third degree N81.3
uveal (traumatic) — *see* Laceration, eye(ball), with prolapse or loss of interocular tissue
vagina (anterior) (wall) — *see* Cystocele
with prolapse of uterus N81.4
complete N81.3
incomplete N81.2
posterior wall N81.6
posthysterectomy N99.3
vitreous (humor) H43.0- ☑
in wound — *see* Laceration, eye(ball), with prolapse or loss of interocular tissue
womb — *see* Prolapse, uterus
Prolapsus, female N81.9
specified NEC N81.89
Proliferation(s)
primary cutaneous CD30-positive large T-cell C86.6
prostate, atypical small acinar N42.32
Proliferative — *see* condition
Prolonged, prolongation (of)
bleeding (time) (idiopathic) R79.1
coagulation (time) R79.1
gestation (over 42 completed weeks)
mother O48.1
newborn P08.22
interval I44.0
labor O63.9
first stage O63.0
second stage O63.1
partial thromboplastin time (PTT) R79.1
pregnancy (more than 42 weeks gestation) O48.1
prothrombin time R79.1
QT interval R94.31
uterine contractions in labor O62.4
Prominence, prominent
auricle (congenital) (ear) Q17.5
ischial spine or sacral promontory with disproportion (fetopelvic) O33.0
causing obstructed labor O65.0
nose (congenital) acquired M95.0
Promiscuity — *see* High, risk, sexual behavior
Pronation
ankle — *see* Deformity, limb, foot, specified NEC
foot — *see also* Deformity, limb, foot, specified NEC
congenital Q74.2
Prophylactic
administration of
antibiotics, long-term Z79.2
short-term use — *omit code*
drug — *see also* Long-term (current) drug therapy (use of) Z79.899
medication Z79.899
organ removal (for neoplasia management) Z40.00
breast Z40.01
fallopian tube(s) Z40.03
with ovary(s) Z40.02
ovary(s) Z40.02
specified site NEC Z40.09
surgery Z40.9
for risk factors related to malignant neoplasm — *see* Prophylactic, organ removal
specified NEC Z40.8
vaccination Z23
Propionic acidemia E71.121
Proptosis (ocular) — *see also* Exophthalmos
thyroid — *see* Hyperthyroidism, with goiter
Prosecution, anxiety concerning Z65.3
Prosopagnosia R48.3
Prostadynia N42.81
Prostate, prostatic — *see* condition
Prostatism — *see* Hyperplasia, prostate

Prostatitis (congestive) (suppurative) (with cystiti
acute N41.0
cavitary N41.8
chronic N41.1
diverticular N41.8
due to Trichomonas (vaginalis) A59.02
fibrous N41.1
gonococcal (acute) (chronic) A54.22
granulomatous N41.4
hypertrophic N41.1
subacute N41.1
trichomonal A59.02
tuberculous A18.14
Prostatocystitis N41.3
Prostatorrhea N42.89
Prostatosis N42.82
Prostration R53.83
heat — *see also* Heat, exhaustion
anhydrotic T67.3 ☑
due to
salt (and water) depletion T67.4 ☑
water depletion T67.3 ☑
nervous F48.8
senile R54
Protanomaly (anomalous trichromat) H53.54
Protanopia (complete) (incomplete) H53.54
Protection (against) (from) — *see* Prophylactic
Protein
deficiency NEC — *see* Malnutrition
malnutrition — *see* Malnutrition
sickness — *see also* Reaction, serum T80.69 ☑
Proteinemia R77.9
Proteinosis
alveolar (pulmonary) J84.01
lipid or lipoid (of Urbach) E78.89
Proteinuria R80.9
Bence Jones R80.3
complicating pregnancy — *see* Proteinuria, gestational
gestational
complicating
childbirth O12.14
pregnancy O12.1- ☑
with edema O12.2- ☑
puerperium O12.15
idiopathic R80.0
isolated R80.0
with glomerular lesion N06.9
C3
glomerulonephritis N06.A
glomerulopathy N06.A
with dense deposit disease N06.6
dense deposit disease N06.6
diffuse
crescentic glomerulonephritis N06.7
endocapillary proliferative glomerulonephritis N06.4
mesangiocapillary glomerulonephritis N06.5
focal and segmental hyalinosis or sclerosis N06.1
membranous (diffuse) N06.2
mesangial proliferative (diffuse) N06.3
minimal change N06.0
specified pathology NEC N06.8
orthostatic R80.2
with glomerular lesion — *see* Proteinuria, isolated, with glomerular lesion
persistent R80.1
with glomerular lesion — *see* Proteinuria, isolated, with glomerular lesion
postural R80.2
with glomerular lesion — *see* Proteinuria, isolated, with glomerular lesion
pre-eclamptic — *see* Pre-eclampsia
puerperal O12.15
specified type NEC R80.8
Proteolysis, pathologic D65
Proteus (mirabilis) (morganii), **as cause of disease classified elsewhere** B96.4
Prothrombin gene mutation D68.52
Protoporphyria, erythropoietic E80.0
Protozoal — *see also* condition
disease B64
specified NEC B60.8
Protrusion, protrusio
acetabuli M24.7
acetabulum (into pelvis) M24.7
device, implant or graft — *see also* Complications, by site and type, mechanical T85.698 ☑

Protrusion, protrusio — *continued*
    device, implant or graft — *see also* Complications, by
      site and type, mechanical — *continued*
      arterial graft NEC — *see* Complication, cardiovascular device, mechanical, vascular
      breast (implant) T85.49 ☑
      catheter NEC T85.698 ☑
        cystostomy T83.090 ☑
        dialysis (renal) T82.49 ☑
          intraperitoneal T85.691 ☑
        infusion NEC T82.594 ☑
          spinal (epidural) (subdural) T85.690 ☑
        urinary — *see also* Complications, catheter, urinary T83.098 ☑
      electronic (electrode) (pulse generator) (stimulator)
        bone T84.390 ☑
        nervous system — *see* Complication, prosthetic device, mechanical, electronic nervous system stimulator
      fixation, internal (orthopedic) NEC — *see* Complication, fixation device, mechanical
      gastrointestinal — *see* Complications, prosthetic device, mechanical, gastrointestinal device
      genital NEC T83.498 ☑
        intrauterine contraceptive device T83.39 ☑
        penile prosthesis (cylinder) (implanted) (pump) (resevoir) T83.490 ☑
        testicular prosthesis T83.491 ☑
      heart NEC — *see* Complication, cardiovascular device, mechanical
      joint prosthesis — *see* Complications, joint prosthesis, mechanical, specified NEC, by site
      ocular NEC — *see* Complications, prosthetic device, mechanical, ocular device
      orthopedic NEC — *see* Complication, orthopedic, device, mechanical
      specified NEC T85.628 ☑
      urinary NEC — *see also* Complication, genitourinary, device, urinary, mechanical
        graft T83.29 ☑
      vascular NEC — *see* Complication, cardiovascular device, mechanical
      ventricular intracranial shunt T85.09 ☑
    intervertebral disc — *see* Displacement, intervertebral disc
    joint prosthesis — *see* Complications, joint prosthesis, mechanical, specified NEC, by site
    nucleus pulposus — *see* Displacement, intervertebral disc
Prune belly (syndrome) Q79.4
Prurigo (ferox) (gravis) (Hebrae) (Hebra's) (mitis) (simplex) L28.2
    Besnier's L20.0
    estivalis L56.4
    nodularis L28.1
    psychogenic F45.8
Pruritus, pruritic (essential) L29.9
    ani, anus L29.0
      psychogenic F45.8
    anogenital L29.3
      psychogenic F45.8
    due to onchocerca volvulus B73.1
    gravidarum — *see* Pregnancy, complicated by, specified pregnancy-related condition NEC
    hiemalis L29.8
    neurogenic (any site) F45.8
    perianal L29.0
    psychogenic (any site) F45.8
    scroti, scrotum L29.1
      psychogenic F45.8
    senile, senilis L29.8
    specified NEC L29.8
      psychogenic F45.8
    Trichomonas A59.9
    vulva, vulvae L29.2
      psychogenic F45.8
Pseudarthrosis, pseudoarthrosis (bone) — *see* Nonunion, fracture
    clavicle, congenital Q74.0
    joint, following fusion or arthrodesis M96.0
Pseudoaneurysm — *see* Aneurysm
Pseudoangina (pectoris) — *see* Angina
Pseudoangioma I81
Pseudoarteriosus Q28.8
Pseudoarthrosis — *see* Pseudarthrosis
Pseudobulbar affect (PBA) F48.2
Pseudochromhidrosis L67.8

Pseudocirrhosis, liver, pericardial I31.1
Pseudocowpox B08.03
Pseudocoxalgia M91.3- ☑
Pseudocroup J38.5
Pseudo-Cushing's syndrome, alcohol-induced E24.4
Pseudocyesis F45.8
Pseudocyst
    lung J98.4
    pancreas K86.3
    retina — *see* Cyst, retina
Pseudoelephantiasis neuroarthritica Q82.0
Pseudoexfoliation, capsule (lens) — *see* Cataract, specified NEC
Pseudofolliculitis barbae L73.1
Pseudoglioma H44.89
Pseudohemophilia (Bernuth's) (hereditary) (type B) — *see* Disease, von Willebrand
    Type A D69.8
    vascular D69.8
Pseudohermaphroditism Q56.3
    adrenal E25.8
    female — *see also* Disorder, adrenogenital Q56.2
      with adrenocortical disorder E25.8
      without adrenocortical disorder Q56.2
      adrenal (congenital) E25.0
    male — *see also* Disorder, adrenogenital Q56.1
      with
        5-alpha-reductase deficiency E29.1
        adrenocortical disorder E25.8
        androgen resistance E34.51
        cleft scrotum Q56.1
        feminizing testis E34.51
      without gonadal disorder Q56.1
      adrenal E25.8
Pseudo-Hurler's polydystrophy E77.0
Pseudohydrocephalus G93.2
Pseudohypertrophic muscular dystrophy (Erb's) G71.02
Pseudohypertrophy, muscle — *see also* Dystrophy, muscular, by type, if applicable G71.09
Pseudohypoparathyroidism E20.1
Pseudoinsomnia F51.03
Pseudoleukemia, infantile D64.89
Pseudomembranous — *see* condition
Pseudomeningocele (cerebral) (infective) (post-traumatic) G96.198
    postprocedural (spinal) G97.82
Pseudomenses (newborn) P54.6
Pseudomenstruation (newborn) P54.6
Pseudomonas
    aeruginosa, as cause of disease classified elsewhere B96.5
    mallei infection A24.0
      as cause of disease classified elsewhere B96.5
    pseudomallei, as cause of disease classified elsewhere B96.5
Pseudomyotonia G71.19
Pseudomyxoma peritonei C78.6
Pseudoneuritis, optic (nerve) (disc) (papilla), **congenital** Q14.2
Pseudo-obstruction intestine (acute) (chronic) (idiopathic) (intermittent secondary) (primary) K59.89
    colonic K59.81
Pseudopapilledema H47.33- ☑
    congenital Q14.2
Pseudoparalysis
    arm or leg R29.818
    atonic, congenital P94.2
Pseudopelade L66.0
Pseudophakia Z96.1
Pseudopolyarthritis, rhizomelic M35.3
Pseudopolycythemia D75.1
Pseudopseudohypoparathyroidism E20.1
Pseudopterygium H11.81- ☑
Pseudoptosis (eyelid) — *see* Blepharochalasis
Pseudopuberty, precocious
    female heterosexual E25.8
    male isosexual E25.8
Pseudorickets (renal) N25.0
Pseudorubella B08.20
Pseudosclerema, newborn P83.88
Pseudosclerosis (brain)
    Jakob's — *see* Creutzfeldt-Jakob disease or syndrome of Westphal (Strümpell) E83.01
    spastic — *see* Creutzfeldt-Jakob disease or syndrome
Pseudotetanus — *see* Convulsions
Pseudotetany R29.0

Pseudotetany — *continued*
    hysterical F44.5
Pseudotruncus arteriosus Q25.49
Pseudotuberculosis A28.2
    enterocolitis A04.8
    pasteurella (infection) A28.0
Pseudotumor G93.2
    cerebri G93.2
    orbital H05.11 ☑
Pseudoxanthoma elasticum Q82.8
Psilosis (sprue) (tropical) K90.1
    nontropical K90.0
Psittacosis A70
Psoitis M60.88
Psoriasis L40.9
    arthropathic L40.50
      arthritis mutilans L40.52
      distal interphalangeal L40.51
      juvenile L40.54
      other specified L40.59
      spondylitis L40.53
    buccal K13.29
    flexural L40.8
    guttate L40.4
    mouth K13.29
    nummular L40.0
    plaque L40.0
    psychogenic F54
    pustular (generalized) L40.1
      palmaris et plantaris L40.3
    specified NEC L40.8
    vulgaris L40.0
Psychasthenia F48.8
Psychiatric disorder or problem F99
Psychogenic — *see also* condition
    factors associated with physical conditions F54
Psychological and behavioral factors affecting medical condition F59
Psychoneurosis, psychoneurotic — *see also* Neurosis
    anxiety (state) F41.1
    depersonalization F48.1
    hypochondriacal F45.21
    hysteria F44.9
    neurasthenic F48.8
    personality NEC F60.89
Psychopathy, psychopathic
    affectionless F94.2
    autistic F84.5
    constitution, post-traumatic F07.81
    personality — *see* Disorder, personality
    sexual — *see* Deviation, sexual
    state F60.2
Psychosexual identity disorder of childhood F64.2
Psychosis, psychotic F29
    acute (transient) F23
      hysterical F44.9
    affective — *see* Disorder, mood
    alcoholic F10.959
      with
        abuse F10.159
        anxiety disorder F10.980
          with
            abuse F10.180
            dependence F10.280
        delirium tremens F10.231
        delusions F10.950
          with
            abuse F10.150
            dependence F10.250
        dementia F10.97
          with dependence F10.27
        dependence F10.259
        hallucinosis F10.951
          with
            abuse F10.151
            dependence F10.251
        mood disorder F10.94
          with
            abuse F10.14
            dependence F10.24
        paranoia F10.950
          with
            abuse F10.150
            dependence F10.250
        persisting amnesia F10.96
          with dependence F10.26
      amnestic confabulatory F10.96
        with dependence F10.26

Psychosis, psychotic — *continued*
  alcoholic — *continued*
    delirium tremens F10.231
    Korsakoff's, Korsakov's, Korsakow's F10.26
    paranoid type F10.950
      with
        abuse F10.150
        dependence F10.250
  anergastic — *see* Psychosis, organic
  arteriosclerotic (simple type) (uncomplicated) — *see also* Dementia, vascular F01.50
    with behavioral disturbance — *see* Dementia, vascular
  childhood F84.0
    atypical F84.8
  climacteric — *see* Psychosis, involutional
  confusional F29
    acute or subacute F05
    reactive F23
  cycloid F23
  depressive — *see* Disorder, depressive
  disintegrative (childhood) F84.3
  drug-induced — *see* F11-F19 with .X59
    paranoid and hallucinatory states — *see* F11-F19 with .X50 or .X51
  due to or associated with
    addiction, drug — *see* F11-F19 with .X59
    dependence
      alcohol F10.259
      drug — *see* F11-F19 with .X59
    epilepsy F06.8
    Huntington's chorea F06.8
    ischemia, cerebrovascular (generalized) F06.8
    multiple sclerosis F06.8
    physical disease F06.8
    presenile dementia F03 ☑
    senile dementia F03 ☑
    vascular disease (arteriosclerotic) (cerebral) — *see also* Dementia, vascular F01.50
      with behavioral disturbance — *see* Dementia, vascular
  epileptic F06.8
  episode F23
    due to or associated with physical condition F06.8
  exhaustive F43.0
  hallucinatory, chronic F28
  hypomanic F30.8
  hysterical (acute) F44.9
  induced F24
  infantile F84.0
    atypical F84.8
  infective (acute) (subacute) F05
  involutional F28
    depressive — *see* Disorder, depressive
    melancholic — *see* Disorder, depressive
    paranoid (state) F22
  Korsakoff's, Korsakov's, Korsakow's (nonalcoholic) F04
    alcoholic F10.96
      in dependence F10.26
    induced by other psychoactive substance — *see* categories F11-F19 with .X5X
  mania, manic (single episode) F30.2
    recurrent type F31.89
  manic-depressive — *see* Disorder, bipolar
  menopausal — *see* Psychosis, involutional
  mixed schizophrenic and affective F25.8
  multi-infarct (cerebrovascular) — *see also* Dementia, vascular F01.50
    with behavioral disturbance — *see* Dementia, vascular
  nonorganic F29
    specified NEC F28
  organic F09
    due to or associated with
      arteriosclerosis (cerebral) — *see* Psychosis, arteriosclerotic
      cerebrovascular disease, arteriosclerotic — *see* Psychosis, arteriosclerotic
      childbirth — *see* Psychosis, puerperal
      Creutzfeldt-Jakob disease or syndrome — *see* Creutzfeldt-Jakob disease or syndrome
      dependence, alcohol F10.259
      disease
        alcoholic liver F10.259
        brain, arteriosclerotic — *see* Psychosis, arteriosclerotic
        cerebrovascular — *see also* Dementia, vascular F01.50

Psychosis, psychotic — *continued*
  organic — *continued*
    due to or associated with — *continued*
      disease — *continued*
        cerebrovascular — *see also* Dementia, vascular — *continued*
          with behavioral disturbance — *see* Dementia, vascular
        Creutzfeldt-Jakob — *see* Creutzfeldt-Jakob disease or syndrome
        endocrine or metabolic F06.8
          acute or subacute F05
        liver, alcoholic F10.259
      epilepsy transient (acute) F05
      infection
        brain (intracranial) F06.8
          acute or subacute F05
      intoxication
        alcoholic (acute) F10.259
        drug F11-F19 with .x59
      ischemia, cerebrovascular (generalized) — *see* Psychosis, arteriosclerotic
      puerperium — *see* Psychosis, puerperal
      trauma, brain (birth) (from electric current) (surgical) F06.8
        acute or subacute F05
    infective F06.8
      acute or subacute F05
    post-traumatic F06.8
      acute or subacute F05
  paranoiac F22
  paranoid (climacteric) (involutional) (menopausal) F22
    psychogenic (acute) F23
    schizophrenic F20.0
    senile F03 ☑
  postpartum (NOS) F53.1
  presbyophrenic (type) F03 ☑
  presenile F03 ☑
  psychogenic (paranoid) F23
    depressive F32.3
  puerperal (NOS) F53.1
    specified type — *see* Psychosis, by type
  reactive (brief) (transient) (emotional stress) (psychological trauma) F23
    depressive F32.3
      recurrent F33.3
    excitative type F30.8
  schizoaffective F25.9
    depressive type F25.1
    manic type F25.0
  schizophrenia, schizophrenic — *see* Schizophrenia
  schizophrenia-like, in epilepsy F06.2
  schizophreniform F20.81
    affective type F25.9
    brief F23
    confusional type F23
    mixed type F25.0
  senile NEC F03 ☑
    depressed or paranoid type F03 ☑
    simple deterioration F03 ☑
    specified type — *code to* condition
  shared F24
  situational (reactive) F23
  symbiotic (childhood) F84.3
  symptomatic F09
Psychosomatic — *see* Disorder, psychosomatic
Psychosyndrome, organic F07.9
Psychotic episode due to or associated with physical condition F06.8
Pterygium (eye) H11.00- ☑
  amyloid H11.01- ☑
  central H11.02- ☑
  colli Q18.3
  double H11.03- ☑
  peripheral
    progressive H11.05- ☑
    stationary H11.04- ☑
  recurrent H11.06- ☑
Ptilosis (eyelid) — *see* Madarosis
Ptomaine (poisoning) — *see* Poisoning, food
Ptosis — *see also* Blepharoptosis
  adiposa (false) — *see* Blepharoptosis
  breast N64.81-
  brow H57.81- ☑
  cecum K63.4
  colon K63.4
  congenital (eyelid) Q10.0
    specified site NEC — *see* Anomaly, by site

Ptosis — *continued*
  eyebrow H57.81- ☑
  eyelid — *see* Blepharoptosis
    congenital Q10.0
  gastric K31.89
  intestine K63.4
  kidney N28.83
  liver K76.89
  renal N28.83
  splanchnic K63.4
  spleen D73.89
  stomach K31.89
  viscera K63.4
PTP D69.51
Ptyalism (periodic) K11.7
  hysterical F45.8
  pregnancy — *see* Pregnancy, complicated by, specified pregnancy-related condition NEC
  psychogenic F45.8
Ptyalolithiasis K11.5
Pubarche, precocious E30.1
Pubertas praecox E30.1
Puberty (development state) Z00.3
  bleeding (excessive) N92.2
  delayed E30.0
  precocious (constitutional) (cryptogenic) (idiopathic) E30.1
    central E22.8
    due to
      ovarian hyperfunction E28.1
        estrogen E28.0
      testicular hyperfunction E29.0
  premature E30.1
    due to
      adrenal cortical hyperfunction E25.8
      pineal tumor E34.8
      pituitary (anterior) hyperfunction E22.8
Puckering, macula — *see* Degeneration, macula, puckering
Pudenda, pudendum — *see* condition
Puente's disease (simple glandular cheilitis) K13.0
Puerperal, puerperium (complicated by, complications)
  abnormal glucose (tolerance test) O99.815
  abscess
    areola O91.02
      associated with lactation O91.03
    Bartholin's gland O86.19
    breast O91.12
      associated with lactation O91.13
    cervix (uteri) O86.11
    genital organ NEC O86.19
    kidney O86.21
    mammary O91.12
      associated with lactation O91.13
    nipple O91.02
      associated with lactation O91.03
    peritoneum O85
    subareolar O91.12
      associated with lactation O91.13
    urinary tract — *see* Puerperal, infection, urinary
    uterus O86.12
    vagina (wall) O86.13
    vaginorectal O86.13
    vulvovaginal gland O86.13
  adnexitis O86.19
  afibrinogenemia, or other coagulation defect O72.3
  albuminuria (acute) (subacute) — *see* Proteinuria, gestational
  alcohol use O99.315
  anemia O90.81
    pre-existing (pre-pregnancy) O99.03
  anesthetic death O89.8
  apoplexy O99.43
  bariatric surgery status O99.845
  blood disorder NEC O99.13
  blood dyscrasia O72.3
  cardiomyopathy O90.3
  cerebrovascular disorder (conditions in I60-I69) O99.43
  cervicitis O86.11
  circulatory system disorder O99.43
  coagulopathy (any) O99.13
    with hemorrhage O72.3
  complications O90.9
    specified NEC O90.89
  convulsions — *see* Eclampsia
  cystitis O86.22
  cystopyelitis O86.29
  delirium NEC F05

Puerperal, puerperium — *continued*
- diabetes O24.93
  - gestational — *see* Puerperal, gestational diabetes
  - pre-existing O24.33
    - specified NEC O24.83
      - type 1 O24.03
      - type 2 O24.13
- digestive system disorder O99.63
- disease O90.9
  - breast NEC O92.29
  - cerebrovascular (acute) O99.43
  - nonobstetric NEC O99.893
  - tubo-ovarian O86.19
  - Valsuani's O99.03
- disorder O90.9
  - biliary tract O26.63
  - lactation O92.70
  - liver O26.63
  - nonobstetric NEC O99.893
- disruption
  - cesarean wound O90.0
  - episiotomy wound O90.1
  - perineal laceration wound O90.1
- drug use O99.325
- eclampsia (with pre-existing hypertension) O15.2
- embolism (pulmonary) (blood clot) — *see* Embolism, obstetric, puerperal
- endocrine, nutritional or metabolic disease NEC O99.285
- endophlebitis — *see* Puerperal, phlebitis
- endotrachelitis O86.11
- failure
  - lactation (complete) O92.3
    - partial O92.4
  - renal, acute O90.4
- fever (of unknown origin) O86.4
  - septic O85
- fissure, nipple O92.12
  - associated with lactation O92.13
- fistula
  - breast (due to mastitis) O91.12
    - associated with lactation O91.13
  - nipple O91.02
    - associated with lactation O91.03
- galactophoritis O91.22
  - associated with lactation O91.23
- galactorrhea O92.6
- gastric banding status O99.845
- gastric bypass status O99.845
- gastrointestinal disease NEC O99.63
- gestational
  - diabetes O24.439
    - diet controlled O24.430
    - insulin (and diet) controlled O24.434
    - oral drug controlled (antidiabetic) (hypoglycemic) O24.435
  - edema O12.05
    - with proteinuria O12.25
  - proteinuria O12.15
- gonorrhea O98.23
- hematoma, subdural O99.43
- hemiplegia, cerebral O99.355
  - due to cerbrovascular disorder O99.43
- hemorrhage O72.1
  - brain O99.43
  - bulbar O99.43
  - cerebellar O99.43
  - cerebral O99.43
  - cortical O99.43
  - delayed or secondary O72.2
  - extradural O99.43
  - internal capsule O99.43
  - intracranial O99.43
  - intrapontine O99.43
  - meningeal O99.43
  - pontine O99.43
  - retained placenta O72.0
  - subarachnoid O99.43
  - subcortical O99.43
  - subdural O99.43
  - third stage O72.0
  - uterine, delayed O72.2
  - ventricular O99.43
- hemorrhoids O87.2
- hepatorenal syndrome O90.4
- hypertension — *see* Hypertension, complicating, puerperium
- hypertrophy, breast O92.29
- induration breast (fibrous) O92.29

Puerperal, puerperium — *continued*
- infection O86.4
  - cervix O86.11
  - generalized O85
  - genital tract NEC O86.19
    - obstetric surgical wound O86.09
  - kidney (bacillus coli) O86.21
  - maternal O98.93
    - carrier state NEC O99.835
    - gonorrhea O98.23
    - human immunodeficiency virus (HIV) O98.73
    - protozoal O98.63
    - sexually transmitted NEC O98.33
    - specified NEC O98.83
    - streptococcus group B (GBS) carrier state O99.825
    - syphilis O98.13
    - tuberculosis O98.03
    - viral hepatitis O98.43
    - viral NEC O98.53
  - nipple O91.02
    - associated with lactation O91.03
  - peritoneum O85
  - renal O86.21
  - specified NEC O86.89
  - urinary (asymptomatic) (tract) NEC O86.20
    - bladder O86.22
    - kidney O86.21
    - specified site NEC O86.29
    - urethra O86.22
  - vagina O86.13
  - vein — *see* Puerperal, phlebitis
- ischemia, cerebral O99.43
- lymphangitis O86.89
  - breast O91.22
    - associated with lactation O91.23
- malignancy O9A.13 (*following* O99)
- malnutrition O25.3
- mammillitis O91.02
  - associated with lactation O91.03
- mammitis O91.22
  - associated with lactation O91.23
- mania F30.8
- mastitis O91.22
  - associated with lactation O91.23
  - purulent O91.12
    - associated with lactation O91.13
- melancholia — *see* Disorder, depressive
- mental disorder NEC O99.345
- metroperitonitis O85
- metrorrhagia — *see* Hemorrhage, postpartum
- metrosalpingitis O86.19
- metrovaginitis O86.13
- milk leg O87.1
- monoplegia, cerebral O99.43
- mood disturbance O90.6
- necrosis, liver (acute) (subacute) (conditions in subcategory K72.0) O26.63
  - with renal failure O90.4
- nervous system disorder O99.355
- obesity (pre-existing prior to pregnancy) O99.215
- obesity surgery status O99.845
- occlusion, precerebral artery O99.43
- paralysis
  - bladder (sphincter) O90.89
  - cerebral O99.43
- paralytic stroke O99.43
- parametritis O85
- paravaginitis O86.13
- pelviperitonitis O85
- perimetritis O86.12
- perimetrosalpingitis O86.19
- perinephritis O86.21
- periphlebitis — *see* Puerperal phlebitis
- peritoneal infection O85
- peritonitis (pelvic) O85
- perivaginitis O86.13
- phlebitis O87.0
  - deep O87.1
  - pelvic O87.1
  - superficial O87.0
- phlebothrombosis, deep O87.1
- phlegmasia alba dolens O87.1
- placental polyp O90.89
- pneumonia, embolic — *see* Embolism, obstetric, puerperal
- pre-eclampsia — *see* Pre-eclampsia
- psychosis (NOS) F53.1
- pyelitis O86.21
- pyelocystitis O86.29

Puerperal, puerperium — *continued*
- pyelonephritis O86.21
- pyelonephrosis O86.21
- pyemia O85
- pyocystitis O86.29
- pyohemia O85
- pyometra O86.12
- pyonephritis O86.21
- pyosalpingitis O86.19
- pyrexia (of unknown origin) O86.4
- renal
  - disease NEC O90.89
  - failure O90.4
- respiratory disease NEC O99.53
- retention
  - decidua — *see* Retention, decidua
  - placenta O72.0
  - secundines — *see* Retention, secundines
- retracted nipple O92.02
- salpingo-ovaritis O86.19
- salpingoperitonitis O85
- secondary perineal tear O90.1
- sepsis (pelvic) O85
- sepsis O85
- septic thrombophlebitis O86.81
- skin disorder NEC O99.73
- specified condition NEC O99.893
- stroke O99.43
- subinvolution (uterus) O90.89
- subluxation of symphysis (pubis) O26.73
- suppuration — *see* Puerperal, abscess
- tetanus A34
- thelitis O91.02
  - associated with lactation O91.03
- thrombocytopenia O72.3
- thrombophlebitis (superficial) O87.0
  - deep O87.1
  - pelvic O87.1
  - septic O86.81
- thrombosis (venous) — *see* Thrombosis, puerperal
- thyroiditis O90.5
- toxemia (eclamptic) (pre-eclamptic) (with convulsions) O15.2
- trauma, non-obstetric O9A.23 (*following* O99)
  - caused by abuse (physical) (suspected) O9A.33 (*following* O99)
    - confirmed O9A.33 (*following* O99)
    - psychological (suspected) O9A.53 (*following* O99)
      - confirmed O9A.53 (*following* O99)
    - sexual (suspected) O9A.43 (*following* O99)
      - confirmed O9A.43 (*following* O99)
- uremia (due to renal failure) O90.4
- urethritis O86.22
- vaginitis O86.13
- varicose veins (legs) O87.4
  - vulva or perineum O87.8
- venous O87.9
- vulvitis O86.19
- vulvovaginitis O86.13
- white leg O87.1

Puerperium — *see* Puerperal
Pulmolithiasis J98.4
Pulmonary — *see* condition
Pulpitis (acute) (anachoretic) (chronic) (hyperplastic) (putrescent) (suppurative) (ulcerative) K04.01
- irreversible K04.02
- reversible K04.01
Pulpless tooth K04.99
Pulse
- alternating R00.8
- bigeminal R00.8
- fast R00.0
- feeble, rapid due to shock following injury T79.4 ☑
- rapid R00.0
- weak R09.89
Pulsus alternans or trigeminus R00.8
Punch drunk F07.81
Punctum lacrimale occlusion — *see* Obstruction, lacrimal
Puncture
- abdomen, abdominal
  - wall S31.139 ☑
    - with
      - foreign body S31.149 ☑
      - penetration into peritoneal cavity S31.639 ☑
        - with foreign body S31.649 ☑
  - epigastric region S31.132 ☑

Puncture — *continued*
  abdomen, abdominal — *continued*
    wall — *continued*
      epigastric region — *continued*
        with
          foreign body S31.142 ☑
          penetration into peritoneal cavity
            S31.632 ☑
            with foreign body S31.642 ☑
      left
        lower quadrant S31.134 ☑
          with
            foreign body S31.144 ☑
            penetration into peritoneal cavity
              S31.634 ☑
              with foreign body S31.644 ☑
        upper quadrant S31.131 ☑
          with
            foreign body S31.141 ☑
            penetration into peritoneal cavity
              S31.631 ☑
              with foreign body S31.641 ☑
      periumbilic region S31.135 ☑
        with
          foreign body S31.145 ☑
          penetration into peritoneal cavity
            S31.635 ☑
            with foreign body S31.645 ☑
      right
        lower quadrant S31.133 ☑
          with
            foreign body S31.143 ☑
            penetration into peritoneal cavity
              S31.633 ☑
              with foreign body S31.643 ☑
        upper quadrant S31.130 ☑
          with
            foreign body S31.140 ☑
            penetration into peritoneal cavity
              S31.630 ☑
              with foreign body S31.640 ☑
  accidental, complicating surgery — *see* Complication, accidental puncture or laceration
  alveolar (process) — *see* Puncture, oral cavity
  ankle S91.039 ☑
    with
      foreign body S91.049 ☑
    left S91.032 ☑
      with
        foreign body S91.042 ☑
    right S91.031 ☑
      with
        foreign body S91.041 ☑
  anus S31.833 ☑
    with foreign body S31.834 ☑
  arm (upper) S41.139 ☑
    with foreign body S41.149 ☑
    left S41.132 ☑
      with foreign body S41.142 ☑
    lower — *see* Puncture, forearm
    right S41.131 ☑
      with foreign body S41.141 ☑
  auditory canal (external) (meatus) — *see* Puncture, ear
  auricle, ear — *see* Puncture, ear
  axilla — *see* Puncture, arm
  back — *see also* Puncture, thorax, back
    lower S31.030 ☑
      with
        foreign body S31.040 ☑
          with penetration into retroperitoneal space S31.041 ☑
        penetration into retroperitoneal space
          S31.031 ☑
  bladder (traumatic) S37.29 ☑
    nontraumatic N32.89
  breast S21.039 ☑
    with foreign body S21.049 ☑
    left S21.032 ☑
      with foreign body S21.042 ☑
    right S21.031 ☑
      with foreign body S21.041 ☑
  buttock S31.803 ☑
    with foreign body S31.804 ☑
    left S31.823 ☑
      with foreign body S31.824 ☑
    right S31.813 ☑

Puncture — *continued*
  buttock — *continued*
    right — *continued*
      with foreign body S31.814 ☑
  by
    device, implant or graft — *see* Complications, by site and type, mechanical
    foreign body left accidentally in operative wound T81.539 ☑
    instrument (any) during a procedure, accidental — *see* Puncture, accidental complicating surgery
  calf — *see* Puncture, leg
  canaliculus lacrimalis — *see* Puncture, eyelid
  canthus, eye — *see* Puncture, eyelid
  cervical esophagus S11.23 ☑
    with foreign body S11.24 ☑
  cheek (external) S01.439 ☑
    with foreign body S01.449 ☑
    internal — *see* Puncture, oral cavity
    left S01.432 ☑
      with foreign body S01.442 ☑
    right S01.431 ☑
      with foreign body S01.441 ☑
  chest wall — *see* Puncture, thorax
  chin — *see* Puncture, head, specified site NEC
  clitoris — *see* Puncture, vulva
  costal region — *see* Puncture, thorax
  digit(s)
    foot — *see* Puncture, toe
    hand — *see* Puncture, finger
  ear (canal) (external) S01.339 ☑
    with foreign body S01.349 ☑
    drum S09.2- ☑
    left S01.332 ☑
      with foreign body S01.342 ☑
    right S01.331 ☑
      with foreign body S01.341 ☑
  elbow S51.039 ☑
    with
      foreign body S51.049 ☑
    left S51.032 ☑
      with
        foreign body S51.042 ☑
    right S51.031 ☑
      with
        foreign body S51.041 ☑
  epididymis — *see* Puncture, testis
  epigastric region — *see* Puncture, abdomen, wall, epigastric
  epiglottis S11.83 ☑
    with foreign body S11.84 ☑
  esophagus
    cervical S11.23 ☑
      with foreign body S11.24 ☑
    thoracic S27.818 ☑
  eyeball S05.6- ☑
    with foreign body S05.5- ☑
  eyebrow — *see* Puncture, eyelid
  eyelid S01.13- ☑
    with foreign body S01.14- ☑
    left S01.132 ☑
      with foreign body S01.142 ☑
    right S01.131 ☑
      with foreign body S01.141 ☑
  face NEC — *see* Puncture, head, specified site NEC
  finger(s) S61.239 ☑
    with
      damage to nail S61.339 ☑
        with
          foreign body S61.349 ☑
      foreign body S61.249 ☑
    index S61.238 ☑
      with
        damage to nail S61.338 ☑
          with
            foreign body S61.348 ☑
        foreign body S61.248 ☑
      left S61.231 ☑
        with
          damage to nail S61.331 ☑
            with
              foreign body S61.341 ☑
          foreign body S61.241 ☑
      right S61.230 ☑
        with
          damage to nail S61.330 ☑

Puncture — *continued*
  finger(s) — *continued*
    index — *continued*
      right — *continued*
        with — *continued*
          damage to nail — *continued*
            with
              foreign body S61.340 ☑
          foreign body S61.240 ☑
    little S61.238 ☑
      with
        damage to nail S61.338 ☑
          with
            foreign body S61.348 ☑
        foreign body S61.248 ☑
      left S61.237 ☑
        with
          damage to nail S61.337 ☑
            with
              foreign body S61.347 ☑
          foreign body S61.247 ☑
      right S61.236 ☑
        with
          damage to nail S61.336 ☑
            with
              foreign body S61.346 ☑
          foreign body S61.246 ☑
    middle S61.238 ☑
      with
        damage to nail S61.338 ☑
          with
            foreign body S61.348 ☑
        foreign body S61.248 ☑
      left S61.233 ☑
        with
          damage to nail S61.333 ☑
            with
              foreign body S61.343 ☑
          foreign body S61.243 ☑
      right S61.232 ☑
        with
          damage to nail S61.332 ☑
            with
              foreign body S61.342 ☑
          foreign body S61.242 ☑
    ring S61.238 ☑
      with
        damage to nail S61.338 ☑
          with
            foreign body S61.348 ☑
        foreign body S61.248 ☑
      left S61.235 ☑
        with
          damage to nail S61.335 ☑
            with
              foreign body S61.345 ☑
          foreign body S61.245 ☑
      right S61.234 ☑
        with
          damage to nail S61.334 ☑
            with
              foreign body S61.344 ☑
          foreign body S61.244 ☑
  flank S31.139 ☑
    with foreign body S31.149 ☑
  foot (except toe(s) alone) S91.339 ☑
    with foreign body S91.349 ☑
    left S91.332 ☑
      with foreign body S91.342 ☑
    right S91.331 ☑
      with foreign body S91.341 ☑
    toe — *see* Puncture, toe
  forearm S51.839 ☑
    with
      foreign body S51.849 ☑
    elbow only — *see* Puncture, elbow
    left S51.832 ☑
      with
        foreign body S51.842 ☑
    right S51.831 ☑
      with
        foreign body S51.841 ☑
  forehead — *see* Puncture, head, specified site NEC
  genital organs, external
    female S31.532 ☑
      with foreign body S31.542 ☑

☑ **Additional Character Required** — **Refer to the Tabular List for Character Selection**

Puncture — *continued*
  toe(s) — *continued*
    lesser — *continued*
      with — *continued*
        foreign body S91.146 ☑
      left S91.135 ☑
        with
          damage to nail S91.235 ☑
            with
              foreign body S91.245 ☑
          foreign body S91.145 ☑
      right S91.134 ☑
        with
          damage to nail S91.234 ☑
            with
              foreign body S91.244 ☑
          foreign body S91.144 ☑
  tongue — *see* Puncture, oral cavity
  trachea S11.023 ☑
    with foreign body S11.024 ☑
  tunica vaginalis — *see* Puncture, testis
  tympanum, tympanic membrane S09.2- ☑
  umbilical region S31.135 ☑
    with foreign body S31.145 ☑
  uvula — *see* Puncture, oral cavity
  vagina S31.43 ☑
    with foreign body S31.44 ☑
  vocal cords S11.033 ☑
    with foreign body S11.034 ☑
  vulva S31.43 ☑
    with foreign body S31.44 ☑
  wrist S61.539 ☑
    with
      foreign body S61.549 ☑
    left S61.532 ☑
      with
        foreign body S61.542 ☑
    right S61.531 ☑
      with
        foreign body S61.541 ☑
PUO (pyrexia of unknown origin) R50.9
Pupillary membrane (persistent) Q13.89
Pupillotonia — *see* Anomaly, pupil, function, tonic pupil
Purpura D69.2
  abdominal D69.0
  allergic D69.0
  anaphylactoid D69.0
  annularis telangiectodes L81.7
  arthritic D69.0
  autoerythrocyte sensitization D69.2
  autoimmune D69.0
  bacterial D69.0
  Bateman's (senile) D69.2
  capillary fragility (hereditary) (idiopathic) D69.8
  cryoglobulinemic D89.1
  Devil's pinches D69.2
  fibrinolytic — *see* Fibrinolysis
  fulminans, fulminous D65
  gangrenous D65
  hemorrhagic, hemorrhagica D69.3
    not due to thrombocytopenia D69.0
  Henoch (-Schönlein) (allergic) D69.0
  hypergammaglobulinemic (benign) (Waldenström)
    D89.0
  idiopathic (thrombocytopenic) D69.3
    nonthrombocytopenic D69.0
  immune thrombocytopenic D69.3
  infectious D69.0
  malignant D69.0
  neonatorum P54.5
  nervosa D69.0
  newborn P54.5
  nonthrombocytopenic D69.2
    hemorrhagic D69.0
    idiopathic D69.0
  nonthrombopenic D69.2
  peliosis rheumatica D69.0
  posttransfusion (post-transfusion) (from (fresh) whole
    blood or blood products) D69.51
  primary D69.49
  red cell membrane sensitivity D69.2
  rheumatica D69.0
  Schönlein (-Henoch) (allergic) D69.0
  scorbutic E54 *[D77]*
  senile D69.2
  simplex D69.2
  symptomatica D69.0

Purpura — *continued*
  telangiectasia annularis L81.7
  thrombocytopenic D69.49
    congenital D69.42
    hemorrhagic D69.3
    hereditary D69.42
    idiopathic D69.3
    immune D69.3
    neonatal, transitory P61.0
    thrombotic M31.19
  thrombohemolytic — *see* Fibrinolysis
  thrombolytic — *see* Fibrinolysis
  thrombopenic D69.49
  thrombotic, thrombocytopenic M31.19
  toxic D69.0
  vascular D69.0
  visceral symptoms D69.0
Purpuric spots R23.3
Purulent — *see* condition
Pus
  in
    stool R19.5
    urine N39.0
  tube (rupture) — *see* Salpingo-oophoritis
Pustular rash L08.0
Pustule (nonmalignant) L08.9
  malignant A22.0
Pustulosis palmaris et plantaris L40.3
Putnam (-Dana) **disease or syndrome** — *see* Degeneration, combined
Putrescent pulp (dental) K04.1
Pyarthritis, pyarthrosis — *see* Arthritis, pyogenic or pyemic
  tuberculous — *see* Tuberculosis, joint
Pyelectasis — *see* Hydronephrosis
Pyelitis (congenital) (uremic) — *see also* Pyelonephritis
  with
    calculus — *see* category N20 ☑
      with hydronephrosis N13.6
    contracted kidney N11.9
  acute N10
  chronic N11.9
    with calculus — *see* category N20 ☑
      with hydronephrosis N13.6
  cystica N28.84
  puerperal (postpartum) O86.21
  tuberculous A18.11
Pyelocystitis — *see* Pyelonephritis
Pyelonephritis — *see also* Nephritis, tubulo-interstitial
  with
    calculus — *see* category N20 ☑
      with hydronephrosis N13.6
    contracted kidney N11.9
  acute N10
  calculous — *see* category N20 ☑
    with hydronephrosis N13.6
  chronic N11.9
    with calculus — *see* category N20 ☑
      with hydronephrosis N13.6
    associated with ureteral obstruction or stricture
      N11.1
    nonobstructive N11.8
      with reflux (vesicoureteral) N11.0
    obstructive N11.1
    specified NEC N11.8
  in (due to)
    brucellosis A23.9 *[N16]*
    cryoglobulinemia (mixed) D89.1 *[N16]*
    cystinosis E72.04
    diphtheria A36.84
    glycogen storage disease E74.09 *[N16]*
    leukemia NEC C95.9- ☑ *[N16]*
    lymphoma NEC C85.90 *[N16]*
    multiple myeloma C90.0- ☑ *[N16]*
    obstruction N11.1
    Salmonella infection A02.25
    sarcoidosis D86.84
    sepsis A41.9 *[N16]*
    Sjögren's disease M35.04
    toxoplasmosis B58.83
    transplant rejection T86.91 *[N16]*
    Wilson's disease E83.01 *[N16]*
  nonobstructive N12
    with reflux (vesicoureteral) N11.0
    chronic N11.8
  syphilitic A52.75
Pyelonephrosis (obstructive) N11.1
  chronic N11.9

Pyelophlebitis I80.8
Pyeloureteritis cystica N28.85
Pyemia, pyemic (fever) (infection) (purulent) — *see also* Sepsis
  joint — *see* Arthritis, pyogenic or pyemic
  liver K75.1
  pneumococcal A40.3
  portal K75.1
  postvaccinal T88.0 ☑
  puerperal, postpartum, childbirth O85
  specified organism NEC A41.89
  tuberculous — *see* Tuberculosis, miliary
Pygopagus Q89.4
Pyknoepilepsy (idiopathic) — *see* Pyknolepsy
Pyknolepsy G40.A09 (*following* G40.3)
  intractable G40.A19 (*following* G40.3)
    with status epilepticus G40.A11 (*following* G40.3)
    without status epilepticus G40.A19 (*following* G40.3)
  not intractable G40.A09 (*following* G40.3)
    with status epilepticus G40.A01 (*following* G40.3)
    without status epilepticus G40.A09 (*following* G40.3)
Pylephlebitis K75.1
Pyle's syndrome Q78.5
Pylethrombophlebitis K75.1
Pylethrombosis K75.1
Pyloritis K29.90
  with bleeding K29.91
Pylorospasm (reflex) **NEC** K31.3
  congenital or infantile Q40.0
  neurotic F45.8
  newborn Q40.0
  psychogenic F45.8
Pylorus, pyloric — *see* condition
Pyoarthrosis — *see* Arthritis, pyogenic or pyemic
Pyocele
  mastoid — *see* Mastoiditis, acute
  sinus (accessory) — *see* Sinusitis
  turbinate (bone) J32.9
  urethra — *see also* Urethritis N34.0
Pyocolpos — *see* Vaginitis
Pyocystitis N30.80
  with hematuria N30.81
Pyoderma, pyodermia L08.0
  gangrenosum L88
  newborn P39.4
  phagedenic L88
  vegetans L08.81
Pyodermatitis L08.0
  vegetans L08.81
Pyogenic — *see* condition
Pyohydronephrosis N13.6
Pyometra, pyometrium, pyometritis — *see* Endometritis
Pyomyositis (tropical) — *see* Myositis, infective
Pyonephritis N12
Pyonephrosis N13.6
  tuberculous A18.11
Pyo-oophoritis — *see* Salpingo-oophoritis
Pyo-ovarium — *see* Salpingo-oophoritis
Pyopericarditis, pyopericardium I30.1
Pyophlebitis — *see* Phlebitis
Pyopneumopericardium I30.1
Pyopneumothorax (infective) J86.9
  with fistula J86.0
  tuberculous NEC A15.6
Pyosalpinx, pyosalpingitis — *see also* Salpingo-oophoritis
Pyothorax J86.9
  with fistula J86.0
  tuberculous NEC A15.6
Pyoureter N28.89
  tuberculous A18.11
Pyramidopallidonigral syndrome G20
Pyrexia (of unknown origin) R50.9
  atmospheric T67.01 ☑
  during labor NEC O75.2
  heat T67.01 ☑
  newborn P81.9
    environmentally-induced P81.0
  persistent R50.9
  puerperal O86.4
Pyroglobulinemia NEC E88.09
Pyromania F63.1
Pyrosis R12
Pyuria (bacterial) (sterile) R82.81

Q

Q fever A78
 with pneumonia A78
Quadricuspid aortic valve Q23.8
Quadrilateral fever A78
Quadriparesis — see Quadriplegia
 meaning muscle weakness M62.81
Quadriplegia G82.50
 complete
  C1-C4 level G82.51
  C5-C7 level G82.53
 congenital (cerebral) (spinal) G80.8
  spastic G80.0
 embolic (current episode) I63.4- ☑
 functional R53.2
 incomplete
  C1-C4 level G82.52
  C5-C7 level G82.54
 thrombotic (current episode) I63.3- ☑
 traumatic — code to injury with seventh character S
  current episode — see Injury, spinal (cord), cervical
Quadruplet, pregnancy — see Pregnancy, quadruplet
Quarrelsomeness F60.3
Queensland fever A77.3
Quervain's disease M65.4
 thyroid E06.1
Queyrat's erythroplasia D07.4
 penis D07.4
 specified site — see Neoplasm, skin, in situ
 unspecified site D07.4
Quincke's disease or edema T78.3 ☑
 hereditary D84.1
Quinsy (gangrenous) J36
Quintan fever A79.0
Quintuplet, pregnancy — see Pregnancy, quintuplet

R

Rabbit fever — see Tularemia
Rabies A82.9
 contact Z20.3
 exposure to Z20.3
 inoculation reaction — see Complications, vaccination
 sylvatic A82.0
 urban A82.1
Rachischisis — see Spina bifida
Rachitic — see also condition
 deformities of spine (late effect) (sequelae) E64.3
 pelvis (late effect) (sequelae) E64.3
  with disproportion (fetopelvic) O33.0
   causing obstructed labor O65.0
Rachitis, rachitism (acute) (tarda) — see also Rickets
 renalis N25.0
 sequelae E64.3
Radial nerve — see condition
Radiation
 burn — see Burn
 effects NOS T66 ☑
 sickness NOS T66 ☑
 therapy, encounter for Z51.0
Radiculitis (pressure) (vertebrogenic) — see Radiculopathy
Radiculomyelitis — see also Encephalitis
 toxic, due to
  Clostridium tetani A35
  Corynebacterium diphtheriae A36.82
Radiculopathy M54.10
 cervical region M54.12
 cervicothoracic region M54.13
 due to
  disc disorder
   C3 M50.11
   C4 M50.11
   C5 M50.121
   C6 M50.122
   C7 M50.123
  displacement of intervertebral disc — see Disorder, disc, with, radiculopathy
 leg M54.1- ☑
 lumbar region M54.16
 lumbosacral region M54.17
 occipito-atlanto-axial region M54.11
 postherpetic B02.29
 sacrococcygeal region M54.18
 syphilitic A52.11

Radiculopathy — continued
 thoracic region (with visceral pain) M54.14
 thoracolumbar region M54.15
Radiodermal burns (acute, chronic, or occupational) — see Burn
Radiodermatitis L58.9
 acute L58.0
 chronic L58.1
Radiotherapy session Z51.0
RAEB (refractory anemia with excess blasts) D46.2- ☑
Rage, meaning rabies — see Rabies
Ragpicker's disease A22.1
Ragsorter's disease A22.1
Raillietiniasis B71.8
Railroad neurosis F48.8
Railway spine F48.8
Raised — see also Elevated
 antibody titer R76.0
Rake teeth, tooth M26.39
Rales R09.89
Ramifying renal pelvis Q63.8
Ramsay-Hunt disease or syndrome — see also Hunt's disease B02.21
 meaning dyssynergia cerebellaris myoclonica G11.19
Ranula K11.6
 congenital Q38.4
Rape
 adult
  confirmed T74.21 ☑
  suspected T76.21 ☑
 alleged, observation or examination, ruled out
  adult Z04.41
  child Z04.42
 child
  confirmed T74.22 ☑
  suspected T76.22 ☑
Rapid
 feeble pulse, due to shock, following injury T79.4 ☑
 heart (beat) R00.0
  psychogenic F45.8
 second stage (delivery) O62.3
 time-zone change syndrome G47.25
Rarefaction, bone — see Disorder, bone, density and structure, specified NEC
Rash (toxic) R21
 canker A38.9
 diaper R21
 drug (internal use) L27.0
  contact — see also Dermatitis, due to, drugs, external L25.1
 following immunization T88.1 ☑
 food — see Dermatitis, due to, food
 heat L74.0
 napkin (psoriasiform) L22
 nettle — see Urticaria
 pustular L08.0
 rose R21
  epidemic B06.9
 scarlet A38.9
 serum — see also Reaction, serum T80.69 ☑
 wandering tongue K14.1
Rasmussen aneurysm — see Tuberculosis, pulmonary
Rasmussen encephalitis G04.81
Rat-bite fever A25.9
 due to Streptobacillus moniliformis A25.1
 spirochetal (morsus muris) A25.0
Rathke's pouch tumor D44.3
Raymond (-Céstan) **syndrome** I65.8
Raynaud's disease, phenomenon or syndrome (secondary) I73.00
 with gangrene (symmetric) I73.01
RDS (newborn) (type I) P22.0
 type II P22.1
Reaction — see also Disorder
 withdrawing, child or adolescent F93.8
 adaptation — see Disorder, adjustment
 adjustment (anxiety) (conduct disorder) (depressiveness) (distress) — see Disorder, adjustment
  with
   mutism, elective (child) (adolescent) F94.0
 adverse
  food (any) (ingested) NEC T78.1 ☑
   anaphylactic — see Shock, anaphylactic, due to food
 affective — see Disorder, mood
 allergic — see Allergy
 anaphylactic — see Shock, anaphylactic

Reaction — continued
 anaphylactoid — see Shock, anaphylactic
 anesthesia — see Anesthesia, complication
 antitoxin (prophylactic) (therapeutic) — see Complications, vaccination
 anxiety F41.1
 Arthus — see Arthus' phenomenon
 asthenic F48.8
 combat and operational stress F43.0
 compulsive F42.8
 conversion F44.9
 crisis, acute F43.0
 deoxyribonuclease (DNA) (DNase) hypersensitivity D69.2
 depressive (single episode) F32.9
  affective (single episode) F31.4
   recurrent episode F33.9
  neurotic F34.1
  psychoneurotic F34.1
  psychotic F32.3
  recurrent — see Disorder, depressive, recurrent
 dissociative F44.9
 drug NEC T88.7 ☑
  addictive — see Dependence, drug
   transmitted via placenta or breast milk — see Absorption, drug, addictive, through placenta
  allergic — see Allergy, drug
  lichenoid L43.2
  newborn P93.8
   gray baby syndrome P93.0
  overdose or poisoning (by accident) — see Table of Drugs and Chemicals, by drug, poisoning
  photoallergic L56.1
  phototoxic L56.0
  withdrawal — see Dependence, by drug, with, withdrawal
   infant of dependent mother P96.1
   newborn P96.1
  wrong substance given or taken (by accident) — see Table of Drugs and Chemicals, by drug, poisoning
 fear F40.9
  child (abnormal) F93.8
 febrile nonhemolytic transfusion (FNHTR) R50.84
 fluid loss, cerebrospinal G97.1
 foreign
  body NEC — see Granuloma, foreign body
   in operative wound (inadvertently left) — see Foreign body, accidentally left during a procedure
  substance accidentally left during a procedure (chemical) (powder) (talc) T81.60 ☑
   aseptic peritonitis T81.61 ☑
   body or object (instrument) (sponge) (swab) — see Foreign body, accidentally left during a procedure
   specified reaction NEC T81.69 ☑
 grief — see Disorder, adjustment
 Herxheimer's R68.89
 hyperkinetic — see Hyperkinesia
 hypochondriacal F45.20
 hypoglycemic, due to insulin E16.0
  with coma (diabetic) — see Diabetes, coma nondiabetic E15
  therapeutic misadventure — see subcategory T38.3 ☑
 hypomanic F30.8
 hysterical F44.9
 immunization — see Complications, vaccination
 incompatibility
  ABO blood group (infusion) (transfusion) — see Complication(s), transfusion, incompatibility reaction, ABO
   delayed serologic T80.39 ☑
  minor blood group (Duffy) (E) (K) (Kell) (Kidd) (Lewis) (M) (N) (P) (S) T80.89 ☑
  Rh (factor) (infusion) (transfusion) — see Complication(s), transfusion, incompatibility reaction, Rh (factor)
 inflammatory — see Infection
 infusion — see Complications, infusion
 inoculation (immune serum) — see Complications, vaccination
 insulin T38.3- ☑
 involutional psychotic — see Disorder, depressive
 leukemoid D72.823
  basophilic D72.823

Reaction — *continued*
  leukemoid — *continued*
    lymphocytic D72.823
    monocytic D72.823
    myelocytic D72.823
    neutrophilic D72.823
  LSD (acute)
    due to drug abuse — *see* Abuse, drug, hallucinogen
    due to drug dependence — *see* Dependence, drug,
      hallucinogen
  lumbar puncture G97.1
  manic-depressive — *see* Disorder, bipolar
  neurasthenic F48.8
  neurogenic — *see* Neurosis
  neurotic F48.9
  neurotic-depressive F34.1
  nitritoid — *see* Crisis, nitritoid
  nonspecific
    to
      cell mediated immunity measurement of gamma
        interferon antigen response without active
        tuberculosis R76.12
      QuantiFERON-TB test (QFT) without active tuber-
        culosis R76.12
      tuberculin test — *see also* Reaction, tuberculin
        skin test R76.11
  obsessive-compulsive F42.8
  organic, acute or subacute — *see* Delirium
  paranoid (acute) F23
    chronic F22
    senile F03 ☑
  passive dependency F60.7
  phobic F40.9
  post-traumatic stress, uncomplicated Z73.3
  psychogenic F99
  psychoneurotic — *see also* Neurosis
    compulsive F42.8
    depersonalization F48.1
    depressive F34.1
    hypochondriacal F45.20
    neurasthenic F48.8
    obsessive F42.8
  psychophysiologic — *see* Disorder, somatoform
  psychosomatic — *see* Disorder, somatoform
  psychotic — *see* Psychosis
  scarlet fever toxin — *see* Complications, vaccination
  schizophrenic F23
    acute (brief) (undifferentiated) F23
    latent F21
    undifferentiated (acute) (brief) F23
  serological for syphilis — *see* Serology for syphilis
  serum T80.69 ☑
    anaphylactic (immediate) — *see also* Shock, anaphy-
      lactic T80.59 ☑
    specified reaction NEC
      due to
        administration of blood and blood products
          T80.61 ☑
        immunization T80.62 ☑
        serum specified NEC T80.69 ☑
        vaccination T80.62 ☑
  situational — *see* Disorder, adjustment
  somatization — *see* Disorder, somatoform
  spinal puncture G97.1
    dural G97.1
  stress (severe) F43.9
    acute (agitation) ("daze") (disorientation) (distur-
      bance of consciousness) (flight reaction)
      (fugue) F43.0
    specified NEC F43.89
  surgical procedure — *see* Complications, surgical pro-
    cedure
  tetanus antitoxin — *see* Complications, vaccination
  toxic, to local anesthesia T88.59 ☑
    in labor and delivery O74.4
    in pregnancy O29.3X- ☑
    postpartum, puerperal O89.3
  toxin-antitoxin — *see* Complications, vaccination
  transfusion (blood) (bone marrow) (lymphocytes) (al-
    lergic) — *see* Complications, transfusion
  tuberculin skin test, abnormal R76.11
  vaccination (any) — *see* Complications, vaccination
Reactive airway disease — *see* Asthma
Reactive depression — *see* Reaction, depressive
Rearrangement
  chromosomal
    balanced (in) Q95.9
      abnormal individual (autosomal) Q95.2

Rearrangement — *continued*
  chromosomal — *continued*
    balanced — *continued*
      abnormal individual — *continued*
        non-sex (autosomal) chromosomes Q95.2
        sex/non-sex chromosomes Q95.3
        specified NEC Q95.8
Recalcitrant patient — *see* Noncompliance
Recanalization, thrombus — *see* Thrombosis
Recession, receding
  chamber angle (eye) H21.55- ☑
  chin M26.09
  gingival (postinfective) (postoperative)
    generalized K06.020
      minimal K06.021
      moderate K06.022
      severe K06.023
    localized K06.010
      minimal K06.011
      moderate K06.012
      severe K06.013
Recklinghausen disease Q85.01
  bones E21.0
Reclus' disease (cystic) — *see* Mastopathy, cystic
Recrudescent typhus (fever) A75.1
Recruitment, auditory H93.21- ☑
Rectalgia K62.89
Rectitis K62.89
Rectocele
  female (without uterine prolapse) N81.6
    with uterine prolapse N81.4
      incomplete N81.2
  in pregnancy — *see* Pregnancy, complicated by, abnor-
    mal, pelvic organs or tissues NEC
  male K62.3
Rectosigmoid junction — *see* condition
Rectosigmoiditis K63.89
  ulcerative (chronic) K51.30
    with
      complication K51.319
        abscess K51.314
        fistula K51.313
        obstruction K51.312
        rectal bleeding K51.311
        specified NEC K51.318
Rectourethral — *see* condition
Rectovaginal — *see* condition
Rectovesical — *see* condition
Rectum, rectal — *see* condition
Recurrent — *see* condition
  pregnancy loss — *see* Loss (of), pregnancy, recurrent
Red bugs B88.0
Red tide — *see also* Table of Drugs and Chemicals
  T65.82- ☑
Red-cedar lung or pneumonitis J67.8
Reduced
  mobility Z74.09
  ventilatory or vital capacity R94.2
Redundant, redundancy
  anus (congenital) Q43.8
  clitoris N90.89
  colon (congenital) Q43.8
  foreskin (congenital) N47.8
  intestine (congenital) Q43.8
  labia N90.89
  organ or site, congenital NEC — *see* Accessory
  panniculus (abdominal) E65
  prepuce (congenital) N47.8
  pylorus K31.89
  rectum (congenital) Q43.8
  scrotum N50.89
  sigmoid (congenital) Q43.8
  skin L98.7
    and subcutaneous tissue L98.7
    of face L57.4
      eyelids — *see* Blepharochalasis
  stomach K31.89
Reduplication — *see* Duplication
Reflex R29.2
  hyperactive gag J39.2
  pupillary, abnormal — *see* Anomaly, pupil, function
  vasoconstriction I73.9
  vasovagal R55
Reflux K21.9
  acid K21.9
  esophageal K21.9
    with esophagitis (without bleeding) K21.00
      with bleeding K21.01

Reflux — *continued*
  esophageal — *continued*
    newborn P78.83
  gastroesophageal K21.9
    with esophagitis (without bleeding) K21.00
      with bleeding K21.01
  mitral — *see* Insufficiency, mitral
  ureteral — *see* Reflux, vesicoureteral
  vesicoureteral (with scarring) N13.70
    with
      nephropathy N13.729
        with hydroureter N13.739
          bilateral N13.732
          unilateral N13.731
        bilateral N13.722
        unilateral N13.721
        without hydroureter N13.729
          bilateral N13.722
          unilateral N13.721
      pyelonephritis (chronic) N11.0
    congenital Q62.7
    without nephropathy N13.71
Reforming, artificial openings — *see* Attention to, artificial, opening
Refractive error — *see* Disorder, refraction
Refsum's disease or syndrome G60.1
Refusal of
  food, psychogenic F50.89
  treatment (because of) Z53.20
    left against medical advice (AMA) Z53.29
    left without being seen Z53.21
    patient's decision NEC Z53.29
    reasons of belief or group pressure Z53.1
Regional — *see* condition
Regurgitation R11.10
  aortic (valve) — *see* Insufficiency, aortic
  food — *see also* Vomiting
    with reswallowing — *see* Rumination
    newborn P92.1
  gastric contents — *see* Vomiting
  heart — *see* Endocarditis
  mitral (valve) — *see* Insufficiency, mitral
    congenital Q23.3
  myocardial — *see* Endocarditis
  pulmonary (valve) (heart) I37.1
    congenital Q22.2
    syphilitic A52.03
  tricuspid — *see* Insufficiency, tricuspid
  valve, valvular — *see* Endocarditis
    congenital Q24.8
  vesicoureteral — *see* Reflux, vesicoureteral
Reichmann's disease or syndrome K31.89
Reifenstein syndrome E34.52
Reinsertion
  implantable subdermal contraceptive Z30.46
  intrauterine contraceptive device Z30.433
Reiter's disease, syndrome, or urethritis M02.30
  ankle M02.37- ☑
  elbow M02.32- ☑
  foot joint M02.37- ☑
  hand joint M02.34- ☑
  hip M02.35- ☑
  knee M02.36- ☑
  multiple site M02.39
  shoulder M02.31- ☑
  vertebra M02.38
  wrist M02.33- ☑
Rejection
  food, psychogenic F50.89
  transplant T86.91
    bone T86.830
      marrow T86.01
    cornea T86.840- ☑
    heart T86.21
      with lung(s) T86.31
    intestine T86.850
    kidney T86.11
    liver T86.41
    lung(s) T86.810
      with heart T86.31
    organ (immune or nonimmune cause) T86.91
    pancreas T86.890
    skin (allograft) (autograft) T86.820
    specified NEC T86.890
    stem cell (peripheral blood) (umbilical cord) T86.5
Relapsing fever A68.9
  Carter's (Asiatic) A68.1
  Dutton's (West African) A68.1

Relapsing fever — *continued*
  Koch's A68.9
  louse-borne (epidemic) A68.0
  Novy's (American) A68.1
  Obermeyers's (European) A68.0
  Spirillum A68.9
  tick-borne (endemic) A68.1
Relationship
  occlusal
    open anterior M26.220
    open posterior M26.221
Relaxation
  anus (sphincter) K62.89
    psychogenic F45.8
  arch (foot) — *see also* Deformity, limb, flat foot
  back ligaments — *see* Instability, joint, spine
  bladder (sphincter) N31.2
  cardioesophageal K21.9
  cervix — *see* Incompetency, cervix
  diaphragm J98.6
  joint (capsule) (ligament) (paralytic) — *see* Flail, joint
    congenital NEC Q74.8
  lumbosacral (joint) — *see* subcategory M53.2 ☑
  pelvic floor N81.89
  perineum N81.89
  posture R29.3
  rectum (sphincter) K62.89
  sacroiliac (joint) — *see* subcategory M53.2 ☑
  scrotum N50.89
  urethra (sphincter) N36.44
  vesical N31.2
Release from prison, anxiety concerning Z65.2
Remains
  canal of Cloquet Q14.0
  capsule (opaque) Q14.8
Remittent fever (malarial) B54
Remnant
  canal of Cloquet Q14.0
  capsule (opaque) Q14.8
  cervix, cervical stump (acquired) (postoperative) N88.8
  cystic duct, postcholecystectomy K91.5
  fingernail L60.8
    congenital Q84.6
  meniscus, knee — *see* Derangement, knee, meniscus,
    specified NEC
  thyroglossal duct Q89.2
  tonsil J35.8
    infected (chronic) J35.01
  urachus Q64.4
Removal (from) (of)
  artificial
    arm Z44.00- ☑
      complete Z44.01- ☑
      partial Z44.02- ☑
    eye Z44.2- ☑
    leg Z44.10- ☑
      complete Z44.11- ☑
      partial Z44.12- ☑
  breast implant Z45.81 ☑
  cardiac pulse generator (battery) (end-of-life) Z45.010
  catheter (urinary) (indwelling) Z46.6
    from artificial opening — *see* Attention to, artificial,
      opening
    non-vascular Z46.82
    vascular NEC Z45.2
  device Z46.9
    contraceptive Z30.432
      implantable subdermal Z30.46
    implanted NEC Z45.89
    specified NEC Z46.89
  drains Z48.03
  dressing (nonsurgical) Z48.00
    surgical Z48.01
  external
    fixation device — *code to* fracture with seventh
      character D
    prosthesis, prosthetic device Z44.9
      breast Z44.3- ☑
      specified NEC Z44.8
  home in childhood (to foster home or institution)
    Z62.29
  ileostomy Z43.2
  insulin pump Z46.81
  myringotomy device (stent) (tube) Z45.82
  nervous system device NEC Z46.2
    brain neuropacemaker Z46.2
    visual substitution device Z46.2
      implanted Z45.31

Removal — *continued*
  non-vascular catheter Z46.82
  organ, prophylactic (for neoplasia management) —
    see Prophylactic, organ removal
  orthodontic device Z46.4
  staples Z48.02
  stent
    ureteral Z46.6
  suture Z48.02
  urinary device Z46.6
  vascular access device or catheter Z45.2
Ren
  arcuatus Q63.1
  mobile, mobilis N28.89
    congenital Q63.8
  unguliformis Q63.1
Renal — *see* condition
Rendu-Osler-Weber disease or syndrome I78.0
Reninoma D41.0- ☑
Renon-Delille syndrome E23.3
Reovirus, as cause of disease classified elsewhere
  B97.5
Repeated falls NEC R29.6
Replaced chromosome by dicentric ring Q93.2
Replacement by artificial or mechanical device or
  prosthesis of
  bladder Z96.0
  blood vessel NEC Z95.828
  bone NEC Z96.7
  cochlea Z96.21
  coronary artery Z95.5
  eustachian tube Z96.29
  eye globe Z97.0
  heart Z95.812
    valve Z95.2
      prosthetic Z95.2
      specified NEC Z95.4
      xenogenic Z95.3
  intestine Z96.89
  joint Z96.60
    hip — *see* Presence, hip joint implant
    knee — *see* Presence, knee joint implant
    specified site NEC Z96.698
  larynx Z96.3
  lens Z96.1
  limb(s) — *see* Presence, artificial, limb
  mandible NEC (for tooth root implant(s)) Z96.5
  organ NEC Z96.89
  peripheral vessel NEC Z95.828
  stapes Z96.29
  teeth Z97.2
  tendon Z96.7
  tissue NEC Z96.89
  tooth root(s) Z96.5
  vessel NEC Z95.828
    coronary (artery) Z95.5
Request for expert evidence Z04.89
Reserve, decreased or low
  cardiac — *see* Disease, heart
  kidney N28.89
Residing
  in place not meant for human habitation (abandoned
    building) (car) (park) (sidewalk) Z59.02
  on the street Z59.02
Residual — *see also* condition
  ovary syndrome N99.83
  state, schizophrenic F20.5
  urine R39.198
Resistance, resistant (to)
  activated protein C D68.51
  complicating pregnancy O26.89 ☑
  insulin E88.81
  organism(s)
    to
      drug Z16.30
        aminoglycosides Z16.29
        amoxicillin Z16.11
        ampicillin Z16.11
        antibiotic(s) Z16.20
          multiple Z16.24
          specified NEC Z16.29
        antifungal Z16.32
        antimicrobial (single) Z16.30
          multiple Z16.35
          specified NEC Z16.39
        antimycobacterial (single) Z16.341
          multiple Z16.342
        antiparasitic Z16.31

Resistance, resistant — *continued*
  organism(s) — *continued*
    to — *continued*
      drug — *continued*
        antiviral Z16.33
        beta lactam antibiotics Z16.10
          specified NEC Z16.19
        cephalosporins Z16.19
        extended beta lactamase (ESBL) Z16.12
        fluoroquinolones Z16.23
        macrolides Z16.29
        methicillin — *see* MRSA
        multiple drugs (MDRO)
          antibiotics Z16.24
          antimicrobial Z16.35
          antimycobacterials Z16.342
        penicillins Z16.11
        quinine (and related compounds) Z16.31
        quinolones Z16.23
        sulfonamides Z16.29
        tetracyclines Z16.29
        tuberculostatics (single) Z16.341
          multiple Z16.342
        vancomycin Z16.21
          related antibiotics Z16.22
  thyroid hormone E07.89
Resorption
  dental (roots) K03.3
    alveoli M26.79
  teeth (external) (internal) (pathological) (roots) K03.3
Respiration
  Cheyne-Stokes R06.3
  decreased due to shock, following injury T79.4 ☑
  disorder of, psychogenic F45.8
  insufficient, or poor R06.89
    newborn P28.5
  painful R07.1
  sighing, psychogenic F45.8
Respiratory — *see also* condition
  distress syndrome (newborn) (type I) P22.0
    type II P22.1
  syncytial virus, as cause of disease classified elsewhere
    — *see also* Virus, respiratory syncytial (RSV) B97.4
Respite care Z75.5
Response (drug)
  photoallergic L56.1
  phototoxic L56.0
Restenosis
  stent
    vascular
      end stent
        adjacent to stent — *see* Arteriosclerosis
        within the stent
          coronary T82.855 ☑
          peripheral T82.856 ☑
      in stent
        coronary vessel T82.855 ☑
        peripheral vessel T82.856 ☑
Restless legs (syndrome) G25.81
Restlessness R45.1
Restoration (of)
  dental
    aesthetically inadequate or displeasing K08.56
    defective K08.50
      specified NEC K08.59
    failure of marginal integrity K08.51
    failure of periodontal anatomical intergrity K08.54
  organ continuity from previous sterilization (tuboplas-
    ty) (vasoplasty) Z31.0
    aftercare Z31.42
  tooth (existing)
    contours biologically incompatible with oral health
      K08.54
    open margins K08.51
    overhanging K08.52
    poor aesthetic K08.56
    poor gingival margins K08.51
  unsatisfactory, of tooth K08.50
    specified NEC K08.59
Restorative material (dental)
  allergy to K08.55
  fractured K08.539
    with loss of material K08.531
    without loss of material K08.530
  unrepairable overhanging of K08.52
Restriction of housing space Z59.1
Rests, ovarian, in fallopian tube Q50.6
Restzustand (schizophrenic) F20.5

Retained — *see also* Retention
  cholelithiasis following cholecystectomy K91.86
  foreign body fragments (type of) Z18.9
    acrylics Z18.2
    animal quill(s) or spines Z18.31
    cement Z18.83
    concrete Z18.83
    crystalline Z18.83
    depleted isotope Z18.09
    depleted uranium Z18.01
    diethylhexyl phthalates Z18.2
    glass Z18.81
    isocyanate Z18.2
    magnetic metal Z18.11
    metal Z18.10
    nonmagnectic metal Z18.12
    nontherapeutic radioactive Z18.09
    organic NEC Z18.39
    plastic Z18.2
    quill(s) (animal) Z18.31
    radioactive (nontherapeutic) NEC Z18.09
    specified NEC Z18.89
    spine(s) (animal) Z18.31
    stone Z18.83
    tooth (teeth) Z18.32
    wood Z18.33
  fragments (type of) Z18.9
    acrylics Z18.2
    animal quill(s) or spines Z18.31
    cement Z18.83
    concrete Z18.83
    crystalline Z18.83
    depleted isotope Z18.09
    depleted uranium Z18.01
    diethylhexyl phthalates Z18.2
    glass Z18.81
    isocyanate Z18.2
    magnetic metal Z18.11
    metal Z18.10
    nonmagnectic metal Z18.12
    nontherapeutic radioactive Z18.09
    organic NEC Z18.39
    plastic Z18.2
    quill(s) (animal) Z18.31
    radioactive (nontherapeutic) NEC Z18.09
    specified NEC Z18.89
    spine(s) (animal) Z18.31
    stone Z18.83
    tooth (teeth) Z18.32
    wood Z18.33
  gallstones, following cholecystectomy K91.86
Retardation
  development, developmental, specific — *see* Disorder, developmental
  endochondral bone growth — *see* Disorder, bone, development or growth
  growth R62.50
    due to malnutrition E45
  mental — *see* Disability, intellectual
  motor function, specific F82
  physical (child) R62.52
    due to malnutrition E45
  reading (specific) F81.0
  spelling (specific) (without reading disorder) F81.81
Retching — *see* Vomiting
Retention — *see also* Retained
  bladder — *see* Retention, urine
  carbon dioxide E87.29
  cholelithiasis following cholecystectomy K91.86
  cyst — *see* Cyst
  dead
    fetus (at or near term) (mother) O36.4 ☑
      early fetal death O02.1
    ovum O02.0
  decidua (fragments) (following delivery) (with hemorrhage) O72.2
    without hemorrhage O73.1
  deciduous tooth K00.6
  dental root K08.3
  fecal — *see* Constipation
  fetus
    dead O36.4 ☑
      early O02.1
  fluid R60.9
  foreign body — *see also* Foreign body, retained
    current trauma — *code as* Foreign body, by site or type
  gallstones, following cholecystectomy K91.86

Retention — *continued*
  gastric K31.89
  intrauterine contraceptive device, in pregnancy — *see* Pregnancy, complicated by, retention, intrauterine device
  membranes (complicating delivery) (with hemorrhage) O72.2
    with abortion — *see* Abortion, by type
    without hemorrhage O73.1
  meniscus — *see* Derangement, meniscus
  menses N94.89
  milk (puerperal, postpartum) O92.79
  nitrogen, extrarenal R39.2
  ovary syndrome N99.83
  placenta (total) (with hemorrhage) O72.0
    without hemorrhage O73.0
    portions or fragments (with hemorrhage) O72.2
      without hemorrhage O73.1
  products of conception
    early pregnancy (dead fetus) O02.1
    following
      delivery (with hemorrhage) O72.2
        without hemorrhage O73.1
  secundines (following delivery) (with hemorrhage) O72.0
    without hemorrhage O73.0
    complicating puerperium (delayed hemorrhage) O72.2
    partial O72.2
      without hemorrhage O73.1
  smegma, clitoris N90.89
  urine R33.9
    due to hyperplasia (hypertrophy) of prostate — *see* Hyperplasia, prostate
    drug-induced R33.0
    organic R33.8
      drug-induced R33.0
    psychogenic F45.8
    specified NEC R33.8
  water (in tissues) — *see* Edema
Reticulation, dust — *see* Pneumoconiosis
Reticulocytosis R70.1
Reticuloendotheliosis
  acute infantile C96.0
  leukemic C91.4- ☑
  nonlipid C96.0
Reticulohistiocytoma (giant-cell) D76.3
Reticuloid, actinic L57.1
Reticulosis (skin)
  acute of infancy C96.0
  hemophagocytic, familial D76.1
  histiocytic medullary C96.A (*following* C96.6)
  lipomelanotic I89.8
  malignant (midline) C86.0
  polymorphic C83.8- ☑
  Sézary — *see* Sézary disease
Retina, retinal — *see also* condition
  dark area D49.81
Retinitis — *see also* Inflammation, chorioretinal
  albuminurica N18.9 *[H32]*
  diabetic — *see* Diabetes, retinitis
  disciformis — *see* Degeneration, macula
  focal — *see* Inflammation, chorioretinal, focal
  gravidarum — *see* Pregnancy, complicated by, specified pregnancy-related condition NEC
  juxtapapillaris — *see* Inflammation, chorioretinal, focal, juxtapapillary
  luetic — *see* Retinitis, syphilitic
  pigmentosa H35.52
  proliferans — *see* Disorder, globe, degenerative, specified type NEC
  proliferating — *see* Disorder, globe, degenerative, specified type NEC
  renal N18.9 *[H32]*
  syphilitic (early) (secondary) A51.43
    central, recurrent A52.71
    congenital (early) A50.01 *[H32]*
    late A52.71
  tuberculous A18.53
Retinoblastoma C69.2- ☑
  differentiated C69.2- ☑
  undifferentiated C69.2- ☑
Retinochoroiditis — *see also* Inflammation, chorioretinal
  disseminated — *see* Inflammation, chorioretinal, disseminated
  syphilitic A52.71
  focal — *see* Inflammation, chorioretinal

Retinochoroiditis — *continued*
  juxtapapillaris — *see* Inflammation, chorioretinal, focal, juxtapapillary
Retinopathy (background) H35.00
  arteriosclerotic I70.8 *[H35.0-]* ☑
  atherosclerotic I70.8 *[H35.0-]* ☑
  central serous — *see* Chorioretinopathy, central serous
  Coats H35.02- ☑
  diabetic — *see* Diabetes, retinopathy
  exudative H35.02- ☑
  hypertensive H35.03- ☑
  in (due to)
    diabetes — *see* Diabetes, retinopathy
    sickle-cell disorders D57.- ☑ *[H36]*
  of prematurity H35.10- ☑
    stage 0 H35.11- ☑
    stage 1 H35.12- ☑
    stage 2 H35.13- ☑
    stage 3 H35.14- ☑
    stage 4 H35.15- ☑
    stage 5 H35.16- ☑
  pigmentary, congenital — *see* Dystrophy, retina
  proliferative NEC H35.2- ☑
    diabetic — *see* Diabetes, retinopathy, proliferative
    sickle-cell D57.- ☑ *[H36]*
  solar H31.02- ☑
Retinoschisis H33.10- ☑
  congenital Q14.1
  specified type NEC H33.19- ☑
Retortamoniasis A07.8
Retractile testis Q55.22
Retraction
  cervix — *see* Retroversion, uterus
  drum (membrane) — *see* Disorder, tympanic membrane, specified NEC
  finger — *see* Deformity, finger
  lid H02.539
    left H02.536
      lower H02.535
      upper H02.534
    right H02.533
      lower H02.532
      upper H02.531
  lung J98.4
  mediastinum J98.59
  nipple N64.53
    associated with
      lactation O92.03
      pregnancy O92.01- ☑
      puerperium O92.02
    congenital Q83.8
  palmar fascia M72.0
  pleura — *see* Pleurisy
  ring, uterus (Bandl's) (pathological) O62.4
  sternum (congenital) Q76.7
    acquired M95.4
  uterus — *see* Retroversion, uterus
  valve (heart) — *see* Endocarditis
Retrobulbar — *see* condition
Retrocecal — *see* condition
Retrocession — *see* Retroversion
Retrodisplacement — *see* Retroversion
Retroflection, retroflexion — *see* Retroversion
Retrognathia, retrognathism (mandibular) (maxillary) M26.19
Retrograde menstruation N92.5
Retroperineal — *see* condition
Retroperitoneal — *see* condition
Retroperitonitis K68.9
Retropharyngeal — *see* condition
Retroplacental — *see* condition
Retroposition — *see* Retroversion
Retroprosthetic membrane T85.398 ☑
Retrosternal thyroid (congenital) Q89.2
Retroversion, retroverted
  cervix — *see* Retroversion, uterus
  female NEC — *see* Retroversion, uterus
  iris H21.89
  testis (congenital) Q55.29
  uterus (acquired) (acute) (any degree) (asymptomatic) (cervix) (postinfectional) (postpartal, old) N85.4
    congenital Q51.818
    in pregnancy O34.53- ☑
Retrovirus, as cause of disease classified elsewhere B97.30
  human
    immunodeficiency, type 2 (HIV 2) B97.35

Retrovirus, as cause of disease classified elsewhere
— *continued*
  human — *continued*
    T-cell lymphotropic
      type I (HTLV-I) B97.33
      type II (HTLV-II) B97.34
    lentivirus B97.31
    oncovirus B97.32
    specified NEC B97.39
Retrusion, premaxilla (developmental) M26.09
Rett's disease or syndrome F84.2
Reverse peristalsis R19.2
Reye's syndrome G93.7
Rh (factor)
  hemolytic disease (newborn) P55.0
  incompatibility, immunization or sensitization
    affecting management of pregnancy NEC O36.09- ☑
      anti-D antibody O36.01- ☑
    newborn P55.0
    transfusion reaction — *see* Complication(s), transfusion, incompatibility reaction, Rh (factor)
  negative mother affecting newborn P55.0
  titer elevated — *see* Complication(s), transfusion, incompatibility reaction, Rh (factor)
  transfusion reaction — *see* Complication(s), transfusion, incompatibility reaction, Rh (factor)
Rhabdomyolysis (idiopathic) NEC M62.82
  traumatic T79.6 ☑
Rhabdomyoma — *see also* Neoplasm, connective tissue, benign
  adult — *see* Neoplasm, connective tissue, benign
  fetal — *see* Neoplasm, connective tissue, benign
  glycogenic — *see* Neoplasm, connective tissue, benign
Rhabdomyosarcoma (any type) — *see* Neoplasm, connective tissue, malignant
Rhabdosarcoma — *see* Rhabdomyosarcoma
Rhesus (factor) **incompatibility** — *see* Rh, incompatibility
Rheumatic (acute) (subacute)
  adherent pericardium I09.2
  chronic I09.89
  coronary arteritis I01.8
  degeneration, myocardium I09.0
  fever (acute) — *see* Fever, rheumatic
  heart — *see* Disease, heart, rheumatic
  myocardial degeneration — *see* Degeneration, myocardium
  myocarditis (chronic) (inactive) (with chorea) I09.0
    active or acute I01.2
    with chorea (acute) (rheumatic) (Sydenham's) I02.0
  pancarditis, acute I01.8
    with chorea, acute I01.8
  pericarditis (active) (acute) (with effusion) (with pneumonia) I01.0
    with chorea (acute) (rheumatic) (Sydenham's) I02.0
    chronic or inactive I09.2
  pneumonia I00 [*J17*]
  torticollis M43.6
  typhoid fever A01.09
Rheumatism (articular) (neuralgic) (nonarticular) M79.0
  gout — *see* Arthritis, rheumatoid
  intercostal, meaning Tietze's disease M94.0
  palindromic (any site) M12.30
    ankle M12.37- ☑
    elbow M12.32- ☑
    foot joint M12.37- ☑
    hand joint M12.34- ☑
    hip M12.35- ☑
    knee M12.36- ☑
    multiple site M12.39
    shoulder M12.31- ☑
    specified joint NEC M12.38
    vertebrae M12.38
    wrist M12.33- ☑
  sciatic M54.4- ☑
Rheumatoid — *see also* condition
  arthritis — *see also* Arthritis, rheumatoid
    with involvement of organs NEC M05.60
      ankle M05.67- ☑
      elbow M05.62- ☑
      foot joint M05.67- ☑
      hand joint M05.64- ☑
      hip M05.65- ☑
      knee M05.66- ☑
      multiple site M05.69
      shoulder M05.61- ☑
      vertebra — *see* Spondylitis, ankylosing

Rheumatoid — *continued*
  arthritis — *see also* Arthritis, rheumatoid — *continued*
    with involvement of organs — *continued*
      wrist M05.63- ☑
    seronegative — *see* Arthritis, rheumatoid, seronegative
    seropositive — *see* Arthritis, rheumatoid, seropositive
  carditis M05.30
    ankle M05.37- ☑
    elbow M05.32- ☑
    foot joint M05.37- ☑
    hand joint M05.34- ☑
    hip M05.35- ☑
    knee M05.36- ☑
    multiple site M05.39
    shoulder M05.31- ☑
    vertebra — *see* Spondylitis, ankylosing
    wrist M05.33- ☑
  endocarditis — *see* Rheumatoid, carditis
  lung (disease) M05.10
    ankle M05.17- ☑
    elbow M05.12- ☑
    foot joint M05.17- ☑
    hand joint M05.14- ☑
    hip M05.15- ☑
    knee M05.16- ☑
    multiple site M05.19
    shoulder M05.11- ☑
    vertebra — *see* Spondylitis, ankylosing
    wrist M05.13- ☑
  myocarditis — *see* Rheumatoid, carditis
  myopathy M05.40
    ankle M05.47- ☑
    elbow M05.42- ☑
    foot joint M05.47- ☑
    hand joint M05.44- ☑
    hip M05.45- ☑
    knee M05.46- ☑
    multiple site M05.49
    shoulder M05.41- ☑
    vertebra — *see* Spondylitis, ankylosing
    wrist M05.43- ☑
  pericarditis — *see* Rheumatoid, carditis
  polyarthritis — *see* Arthritis, rheumatoid
  polyneuropathy M05.50
    ankle M05.57- ☑
    elbow M05.52- ☑
    foot joint M05.57- ☑
    hand joint M05.54- ☑
    hip M05.55- ☑
    knee M05.56- ☑
    multiple site M05.59
    shoulder M05.51- ☑
    vertebra — *see* Spondylitis, ankylosing
    wrist M05.53- ☑
  vasculitis M05.20
    ankle M05.27- ☑
    elbow M05.22- ☑
    foot joint M05.27- ☑
    hand joint M05.24- ☑
    hip M05.25- ☑
    knee M05.26- ☑
    multiple site M05.29
    shoulder M05.21- ☑
    vertebra — *see* Spondylitis, ankylosing
    wrist M05.23- ☑
Rhinitis (atrophic) (catarrhal) (chronic) (croupous) (fibrinous) (granulomatous) (hyperplastic) (hypertrophic) (membranous) (obstructive) (purulent) (suppurative) (ulcerative) J31.0
  with
    sore throat — *see* Nasopharyngitis
  acute J00
  allergic J30.9
    with asthma J45.909
      with
        exacerbation (acute) J45.901
        status asthmaticus J45.902
      due to
        food J30.5
        pollen J30.1
    nonseasonal J30.89
    perennial J30.89
    seasonal NEC J30.2
    specified NEC J30.89

Rhinitis — *continued*
  infective J00
  pneumococcal J00
  syphilitic A52.73
    congenital A50.05 [*J99*]
  tuberculous A15.8
  vasomotor J30.0
Rhinoantritis (chronic) — *see* Sinusitis, maxillary
Rhinodacryolith — *see* Dacryolith
Rhinolith (nasal sinus) J34.89
Rhinomegaly J34.89
Rhinopharyngitis (acute) (subacute) — *see also* Nasopharyngitis
  chronic J31.1
  destructive ulcerating A66.5
  mutilans A66.5
Rhinophyma L71.1
Rhinorrhea J34.89
  cerebrospinal (fluid) G96.01
    postoperative G96.08
    specified NEC G96.08
    spontaneous G96.01
    traumatic G96.08
  paroxysmal — *see* Rhinitis, allergic
  spasmodic — *see* Rhinitis, allergic
Rhinosalpingitis — *see* Salpingitis, eustachian
Rhinoscleroma A48.8
Rhinosporidiosis B48.1
Rhinovirus infection NEC B34.8
Rhizomelic chondrodysplasia punctata E71.540
Rhythm
  atrioventricular nodal I49.8
  disorder I49.9
    coronary sinus I49.8
    ectopic I49.8
    nodal I49.8
  escape I49.9
  heart, abnormal I49.9
  idioventricular I44.2
  nodal I49.8
  sleep, inversion G47.2- ☑
    nonorganic origin — *see* Disorder, sleep, circadian rhythm, psychogenic
Rhytidosis facialis L98.8
Rib — *see also* condition
  cervical Q76.5
Riboflavin deficiency E53.0
Rice bodies — *see also* Loose, body, joint
  knee M23.4- ☑
Richter syndrome — *see* Leukemia, chronic lymphocytic, B-cell type
Richter's hernia — *see* Hernia, abdomen, with obstruction
Ricinism — *see* Poisoning, food, noxious, plant
Rickets (active) (acute) (adolescent) (chest wall) (congenital) (current) (infantile) (intestinal) E55.0
  adult — *see* Osteomalacia
  celiac K90.0
  hypophosphatemic with nephrotic-glycosuric dwarfism E72.09
  inactive E64.3
  kidney N25.0
  renal N25.0
  sequelae, any E64.3
  vitamin-D-resistant E83.31 [*M90.80*]
Rickettsia 364D/R. philipii (Pacific Coast tick fever) A77.8
Rickettsial disease A79.9
  specified type NEC A79.89
Rickettsialpox (Rickettsia akari) A79.1
Rickettsiosis A79.9
  due to
    Ehrlichia sennetsu A79.81
    Neorickettsia sennetsu A79.81
    Rickettsia akari (rickettsialpox) A79.1
  specified type NEC A79.89
  tick-borne A77.9
  vesicular A79.1
Rider's bone — *see* Ossification, muscle, specified NEC
Ridge, alveolus — *see also* condition
  flabby K06.8
Ridged ear, congenital Q17.3
Riedel's
  lobe, liver Q44.7
  struma, thyroiditis or disease E06.5
Rieger's anomaly or syndrome Q13.81
Riehl's melanosis L81.4

Rietti-Greppi-Micheli anemia D56.9
Rieux's hernia — see Hernia, abdomen, specified site NEC
Riga (-Fede) disease K14.0
Riggs' disease — see Periodontitis
Right aortic arch Q25.47
Right middle lobe syndrome J98.11
Rigid, rigidity — see also condition
  abdominal R19.30
    with severe abdominal pain R10.0
    epigastric R19.36
    generalized R19.37
    left lower quadrant R19.34
    left upper quadrant R19.32
    periumbilic R19.35
    right lower quadrant R19.33
    right upper quadrant R19.31
  articular, multiple, congenital Q68.8
  cervix (uteri) in pregnancy — see Pregnancy, complicated by, abnormal, cervix
  hymen (acquired) (congenital) N89.6
  nuchal R29.1
  pelvic floor in pregnancy — see Pregnancy, complicated by, abnormal, pelvic organs or tissues NEC
  perineum or vulva in pregnancy — see Pregnancy, complicated by, abnormal, vulva
  spine — see Dorsopathy, specified NEC
  vagina in pregnancy — see Pregnancy, complicated by, abnormal, vagina
Rigors R68.89
  with fever R50.9
Riley-Day syndrome G90.1
RIND (reversible ischemic neurologic deficit) I63.9
Ring(s)
  aorta (vascular) Q25.45
  Bandl's O62.4
  contraction, complicating delivery O62.4
  esophageal, lower (muscular) K22.2
  Fleischer's (cornea) H18.04- ☑
  hymenal, tight (acquired) (congenital) N89.6
  Kayser-Fleischer (cornea) H18.04- ☑
  retraction, uterus, pathological O62.4
  Schatzki's (esophagus) (lower) K22.2
    congenital Q39.3
  Soemmerring's — see Cataract, secondary
  vascular (congenital) Q25.8
    aorta Q25.45
Ringed hair (congenital) Q84.1
Ringworm B35.9
  beard B35.0
  black dot B35.0
  body B35.4
  Burmese B35.5
  corporeal B35.4
  foot B35.3
  groin B35.6
  hand B35.2
  honeycomb B35.0
  nails B35.1
  perianal (area) B35.6
  scalp B35.0
  specified NEC B35.8
  Tokelau B35.5
Rise, venous pressure I87.8
Rising, PSA following treatment for malignant neoplasm of prostate R97.21
Risk
  for
    dental caries Z91.849
      high Z91.843
      low Z91.841
      moderate Z91.842
    homelessness, imminent Z59.811
    suffocation (smothering) under another while sleeping Z72.823
  suicidal
    meaning personal history of attempted suicide Z91.51
    meaning suicidal ideation — see Ideation, suicidal
Ritter's disease L00
Rivalry, sibling Z62.891
Rivalta's disease A42.2
River blindness B73.01
Robert's pelvis Q74.2
  with disproportion (fetopelvic) O33.0
    causing obstructed labor O65.0
Robin (-Pierre) syndrome Q87.0
Robinow-Silvermann-Smith syndrome Q87.19

Robinson's (hidrotic) ectodermal dysplasia or syndrome Q82.4
Robles' disease B73.01
Rocky Mountain (spotted) fever A77.0
Roetheln — see Rubella
Roger's disease Q21.0
Rokitansky-Aschoff sinuses (gallbladder) K82.8
Rolando's fracture (displaced) S62.22- ☑
  nondisplaced S62.22- ☑
Romano-Ward (prolonged QT interval) syndrome I45.81
Romberg's disease or syndrome G51.8
Roof, mouth — see condition
Rosacea L71.9
  acne L71.9
  keratitis L71.8
  specified NEC L71.8
Rosary, rachitic E55.0
Rose
  cold J30.1
  fever J30.1
  rash R21
    epidemic B06.9
Rosenbach's erysipeloid A26.0
Rosenthal's disease or syndrome D68.1
Roseola B09
  infantum B08.20
    due to human herpesvirus 6 B08.21
    due to human herpesvirus 7 B08.22
Ross River disease or fever B33.1
Rossbach's disease K31.89
  psychogenic F45.8
Rostan's asthma (cardiac) — see Failure, ventricular, left
Rotation
  anomalous, incomplete or insufficient, intestine Q43.3
  cecum (congenital) Q43.3
  colon (congenital) Q43.3
  spine, incomplete or insufficient — see Dorsopathy, deforming, specified NEC
  tooth, teeth, fully erupted M26.35
  vertebra, incomplete or insufficient — see Dorsopathy, deforming, specified NEC
Rotes Quérol disease or syndrome — see Hyperostosis, ankylosing
Roth (-Bernhardt) disease or syndrome — see Meralgia paraesthetica
Rothmund (-Thomson) syndrome Q82.8
Rotor's disease or syndrome E80.6
Round
  back (with wedging of vertebrae) — see Kyphosis
    sequelae (late effect) of rickets E64.3
  worms (large) (infestation) NEC B82.0
    Ascariasis — see also Ascariasis B77.9
Roussy-Lévy syndrome G60.0
Rubella (German measles) B06.9
  complication NEC B06.09
    neurological B06.00
  congenital P35.0
  contact Z20.4
  exposure to Z20.4
  maternal
    care for (suspected) damage to fetus O35.3 ☑
    manifest rubella in infant P35.0
    suspected damage to fetus affecting management of pregnancy O35.3 ☑
  specified complications NEC B06.89
Rubeola (meaning measles) — see Measles
  meaning rubella — see Rubella
Rubeosis, iris — see Disorder, iris, vascular
Rubinstein-Taybi syndrome Q87.2
Rudimentary (congenital) — see also Agenesis
  arm — see Defect, reduction, upper limb
  bone Q79.9
  cervix uteri Q51.828
  eye Q11.2
  lobule of ear Q17.3
  patella Q74.1
  respiratory organs in thoracopagus Q89.4
  tracheal bronchus Q32.4
  uterus Q51.818
    in male Q56.1
  vagina Q52.0
Ruled out condition — see Observation, suspected
Rumination R11.10
  with nausea R11.2
  disorder of infancy F98.21
  neurotic F42.8
  newborn P92.1

Rumination — continued
  obsessional F42.8
  psychogenic F42.8
Runeberg's disease D51.0
Running out of money Z59.86
Runny nose R09.89
Rupia (syphilitic) A51.39
  congenital A50.06
  tertiary A52.79
Rupture, ruptured
  abscess (spontaneous) — code by site under Abscess
  aneurysm — see Aneurysm
  anus (sphincter) — see Laceration, anus
  aorta, aortic I71.8
    abdominal I71.30
      infrarenal I71.33
      juxtarenal I71.32
      pararenal I71.31
    arch I71.12
    ascending I71.11
    descending I71.8
      abdominal I71.30
      thoracic I71.13
    syphilitic A52.01
    thoracoabdominal I71.50
      paravisceral I71.52
      supraceliac I71.51
    thorax, thoracic I71.10
    transverse I71.12
    traumatic — see Injury, aorta, laceration, major
    valve or cusp — see also Endocarditis, aortic I35.8
  appendix (with peritonitis) — see also Appendicitis K35.32
    with localized peritonitis — see also Appendicitis K35.32
  arteriovenous fistula, brain — see Fistula, arteriovenous, brain, ruptured
  artery I77.2
    brain — see Hemorrhage, intracranial, intracerebral
    coronary — see Infarct, myocardium
    heart — see Infarct, myocardium
    pulmonary I28.8
    traumatic (complication) — see Injury, blood vessel
  bile duct (common) (hepatic) K83.2
    cystic K82.2
  bladder (sphincter) (nontraumatic) (spontaneous) N32.89
    following ectopic or molar pregnancy O08.6
    obstetrical trauma O71.5
    traumatic S37.29 ☑
  blood vessel — see also Hemorrhage
    brain — see Hemorrhage, intracranial, intracerebral
    heart — see Infarct, myocardium
    traumatic (complication) — see Injury, blood vessel, laceration, major, by site
  bone — see Fracture
  bowel (nontraumatic) K63.1
  brain
    aneurysm (congenital) — see also Hemorrhage, intracranial, subarachnoid
      syphilitic A52.05
    hemorrhagic — see Hemorrhage, intracranial, intracerebral
  capillaries I78.8
  cardiac (auricle) (ventricle) (wall) I23.3
    with hemopericardium I23.0
    infectional I40.9
    traumatic — see Injury, heart
  cartilage (articular) (current) — see also Sprain
    knee S83.3- ☑
    semilunar — see Tear, meniscus
  cecum (with peritonitis) K65.0
    with peritoneal abscess K35.33
    traumatic S36.598 ☑
  celiac artery, traumatic — see Injury, blood vessel, celiac artery, laceration, major
  cerebral aneurysm (congenital) (see Hemorrhage, intracranial, subarachnoid)
  cervix (uteri)
    with ectopic or molar pregnancy O08.6
    following ectopic or molar pregnancy O08.6
    obstetrical trauma O71.3
    traumatic S37.69 ☑
  chordae tendineae NEC I51.1
    concurrent with acute myocardial infarction — see Infarct, myocardium
    following acute myocardial infarction (current complication) I23.4

Rupture, ruptured — *continued*
- choroid (direct) (indirect) (traumatic) H31.32- ☑
- circle of Willis I60.6
- colon (nontraumatic) K63.1
  - traumatic — *see* Injury, intestine, large
- cornea (traumatic) — *see* Injury, eye, laceration
- coronary (artery) (thrombotic) — *see* Infarct, myocardium
- corpus luteum (infected) (ovary) N83.1- ☑
- cyst — *see* Cyst
- cystic duct K82.2
- Descemet's membrane — *see* Change, corneal membrane, Descemet's, rupture
  - traumatic — *see* Injury, eye, laceration
- diaphragm, traumatic — *see* Injury, intrathoracic, diaphragm
- disc — *see* Rupture, intervertebral disc
- diverticulum (intestine) K57.80
  - with bleeding K57.81
  - bladder N32.3
  - large intestine K57.20
    - with
      - bleeding K57.21
      - small intestine K57.40
        - with bleeding K57.41
  - small intestine K57.00
    - with
      - bleeding K57.01
      - large intestine K57.40
        - with bleeding K57.41
- duodenal stump K31.89
- ear drum (nontraumatic) — *see also* Perforation, tympanum
  - traumatic S09.2- ☑
    - due to blast injury — *see* Injury, blast, ear
- esophagus K22.3
- eye (without prolapse or loss of intraocular tissue) — *see* Injury, eye, laceration
- fallopian tube NEC (nonobstetric) (nontraumatic) N83.8
  - due to pregnancy O00.10- ☑
    - with intrauterine pregnancy O00.11- ☑
- fontanel P13.1
- gallbladder K82.2
  - traumatic S36.128 ☑
- gastric — *see also* Rupture, stomach
  - vessel K92.2
- globe (eye) (traumatic) — *see* Injury, eye, laceration
- graafian follicle (hematoma) N83.0- ☑
- heart — *see* Rupture, cardiac
- hymen (nontraumatic) (nonintentional) N89.8
- internal organ, traumatic — *see* Injury, by site
- intervertebral disc — *see* Displacement, intervertebral disc
  - traumatic — *see* Rupture, traumatic, intervertebral disc
- intestine NEC (nontraumatic) K63.1
  - traumatic — *see* Injury, intestine
- iris — *see also* Abnormality, pupillary
  - traumatic — *see* Injury, eye, laceration
- joint capsule, traumatic — *see* Sprain
- kidney (traumatic) S37.06- ☑
  - birth injury P15.8
  - nontraumatic N28.89
- lacrimal duct (traumatic) — *see* Injury, eye, specified site NEC
- lens (cataract) (traumatic) — *see* Cataract, traumatic
- ligament, traumatic — *see* Rupture, traumatic, ligament, by site
- liver S36.116 ☑
  - birth injury P15.0
- lymphatic vessel I89.8
- marginal sinus (placental) (with hemorrhage) — *see* Hemorrhage, antepartum, specified cause NEC
- membrana tympani (nontraumatic) — *see* Perforation, tympanum
- membranes (spontaneous)
  - artificial
    - delayed delivery following O75.5
  - delayed delivery following — *see* Pregnancy, complicated by, premature rupture of membranes
- meningeal artery I60.8
- meniscus (knee) — *see also* Tear, meniscus
  - old — *see* Derangement, meniscus
  - site other than knee — *code as* Sprain
- mesenteric artery, traumatic — *see* Injury, mesenteric, artery, laceration, major
- mesentery (nontraumatic) K66.8

Rupture, ruptured — *continued*
- mesentery — *continued*
  - traumatic — *see* Injury, intra-abdominal, specified, site NEC
- mitral (valve) I34.89
- muscle (traumatic) — *see also* Strain
  - diastasis — *see* Diastasis, muscle
  - nontraumatic M62.10
    - ankle M62.17- ☑
    - foot M62.17- ☑
    - forearm M62.13- ☑
    - hand M62.14- ☑
    - lower leg M62.16- ☑
    - pelvic region M62.15- ☑
    - shoulder region M62.11- ☑
    - specified site NEC M62.18
    - thigh M62.15- ☑
    - upper arm M62.12- ☑
  - traumatic — *see* Strain, by site
- musculotendinous junction NEC, nontraumatic — *see* Rupture, tendon, spontaneous
- mycotic aneurysm causing cerebral hemorrhage — *see* Hemorrhage, intracranial, subarachnoid
- myocardium, myocardial — *see* Rupture, cardiac
  - traumatic — *see* Injury, heart
- nontraumatic, meaning hernia — *see* Hernia
- obstructed — *see* Hernia, by site, obstructed
- operation wound — *see* Disruption, wound, operation
- ovary, ovarian N83.8
  - corpus luteum cyst N83.1- ☑
  - follicle (graafian) N83.0- ☑
- oviduct (nonobstetric) (nontraumatic) N83.8
  - due to pregnancy O00.10- ☑
    - with intrauterine pregnancy O00.11- ☑
- pancreas (nontraumatic) K86.89
  - traumatic S36.299 ☑
- papillary muscle NEC I51.2
  - following acute myocardial infarction (current complication) I23.5
- pelvic
  - floor, complicating delivery O70.1
  - organ NEC, obstetrical trauma O71.5
- perineum (nonobstetric) (nontraumatic) N90.89
  - complicating delivery — *see* Delivery, complicated, by, laceration, anus (sphincter)
- postoperative wound — *see* Disruption, wound, operation
- prostate (traumatic) S37.828 ☑
- pulmonary
  - artery I28.8
  - valve (heart) I37.8
  - vein I28.8
  - vessel I28.8
- pus tube — *see* Salpingitis
- pyosalpinx — *see* Salpingitis
- rectum (nontraumatic) K63.1
  - traumatic S36.69 ☑
- retina, retinal (traumatic) (without detachment) — *see also* Break, retina
  - with detachment — *see* Detachment, retina, with retinal, break
- rotator cuff (nontraumatic) M75.10- ☑
  - complete M75.12- ☑
  - incomplete M75.11- ☑
- sclera — *see* Injury, eye, laceration
- sigmoid (nontraumatic) K63.1
  - traumatic S36.593 ☑
- spinal cord — *see also* Injury, spinal cord, by region
  - due to injury at birth P11.5
  - newborn (birth injury) P11.5
- spleen (traumatic) S36.09 ☑
  - birth injury P15.1
  - congenital (birth injury) P15.1
  - due to P. vivax malaria B51.0
  - nontraumatic D73.5
  - spontaneous D73.5
- splenic vein R58
  - traumatic — *see* Injury, blood vessel, splenic vein
- stomach (nontraumatic) (spontaneous) K31.89
  - traumatic S36.39 ☑
- supraspinatus (complete) (incomplete) (nontraumatic) — *see* Tear, rotator cuff
- symphysis pubis
  - obstetric O71.6
  - traumatic S33.4 ☑
- synovium (cyst) M66.10
  - ankle M66.17- ☑

Rupture, ruptured — *continued*
- synovium — *continued*
  - elbow M66.12- ☑
  - finger M66.14- ☑
  - foot M66.17- ☑
  - forearm M66.13- ☑
  - hand M66.14- ☑
  - pelvic region M66.15- ☑
  - shoulder region M66.11- ☑
  - specified site NEC M66.18
  - thigh M66.15- ☑
  - toe M66.17- ☑
  - upper arm M66.12- ☑
  - wrist M66.13- ☑
- tendon (traumatic) — *see* Strain
  - nontraumatic (spontaneous) M66.9
    - ankle M66.87- ☑
    - extensor M66.20
      - ankle M66.27- ☑
      - foot M66.27- ☑
      - forearm M66.23- ☑
      - hand M66.24- ☑
      - lower leg M66.26- ☑
      - multiple sites M66.29
      - pelvic region M66.25- ☑
      - shoulder region M66.21- ☑
      - specified site NEC M66.28
      - thigh M66.25- ☑
      - upper arm M66.22- ☑
    - flexor M66.30
      - ankle M66.37- ☑
      - foot M66.37- ☑
      - forearm M66.33- ☑
      - hand M66.34- ☑
      - lower leg M66.36- ☑
      - multiple sites M66.39
      - pelvic region M66.35- ☑
      - shoulder region M66.31- ☑
      - specified site NEC M66.38
      - thigh M66.35- ☑
      - upper arm M66.32- ☑
    - foot M66.87- ☑
    - forearm M66.83- ☑
    - hand M66.84- ☑
    - lower leg M66.86- ☑
    - multiple sites M66.89
    - pelvic region M66.85- ☑
    - shoulder region M66.81- ☑
    - specified
      - site NEC M66.88
      - tendon M66.80
    - thigh M66.85- ☑
    - upper arm M66.82- ☑
- thoracic duct I89.8
- tonsil J35.8
- traumatic
  - aorta — *see* Injury, aorta, laceration, major
  - diaphragm — *see* Injury, intrathoracic, diaphragm
  - external site — *see* Wound, open, by site
  - eye — *see* Injury, eye, laceration
  - internal organ — *see* Injury, by site
  - intervertebral disc
    - cervical S13.0 ☑
    - lumbar S33.0 ☑
    - thoracic S23.0 ☑
  - kidney S37.06- ☑
  - ligament — *see also* Sprain
    - ankle — *see* Sprain, ankle
    - carpus — *see* Rupture, traumatic, ligament, wrist
    - collateral (hand) — *see* Rupture, traumatic, ligament, finger, collateral
    - finger (metacarpophalangeal) (interphalangeal) S63.40- ☑
      - collateral S63.41- ☑
        - index S63.41- ☑
        - little S63.41- ☑
        - middle S63.41- ☑
        - ring S63.41- ☑
      - index S63.40- ☑
      - little S63.40- ☑
      - middle S63.40- ☑
      - palmar S63.42- ☑
        - index S63.42- ☑
        - little S63.42- ☑
        - middle S63.42- ☑
        - ring S63.42- ☑

☑ Additional Character Required — Refer to the Tabular List for Character Selection

Rupture, ruptured — *continued*
  traumatic — *continued*
    ligament — *see also* Sprain — *continued*
      finger — *continued*
        ring S63.40- ☑
        specified site NEC S63.499 ☑
          index S63.49- ☑
          little S63.49- ☑
          middle S63.49- ☑
          ring S63.49- ☑
        volar plate S63.43- ☑
          index S63.43- ☑
          little S63.43- ☑
          middle S63.43- ☑
          ring S63.43- ☑
      foot — *see* Sprain, foot
      radial collateral S53.2- ☑
      radiocarpal — *see* Rupture, traumatic, ligament, wrist, radiocarpal
      ulnar collateral S53.3- ☑
      ulnocarpal — *see* Rupture, traumatic, ligament, wrist, ulnocarpal
      wrist S63.30- ☑
        collateral S63.31- ☑
        radiocarpal S63.32- ☑
        specified site NEC S63.39- ☑
        ulnocarpal (palmar) S63.33- ☑
    liver S36.116 ☑
    membrana tympani — *see* Rupture, ear drum, traumatic
    muscle or tendon — *see* Strain
    myocardium — *see* Injury, heart
    pancreas S36.299 ☑
    rectum S36.69 ☑
    sigmoid S36.593 ☑
    spleen S36.09 ☑
    stomach S36.39 ☑
    symphysis pubis S33.4 ☑
    tympanum, tympanic (membrane) — *see* Rupture, ear drum, traumatic
    ureter S37.19 ☑
    uterus S37.69 ☑
    vagina — *see* Injury, vagina
    vena cava — *see* Injury, vena cava, laceration, major
  tricuspid (heart) (valve) I07.8
  tube, tubal (nonobstetric) (nontraumatic) N83.8
    abscess — *see* Salpingitis
    due to pregnancy O00.10- ☑
      with intrauterine pregnancy O00.11- ☑
  tympanum, tympanic (membrane) (nontraumatic) — *see also* Perforation, tympanic membrane H72.9- ☑
    traumatic — *see* Rupture, ear drum, traumatic
  umbilical cord, complicating delivery O69.89 ☑
  ureter (traumatic) S37.19 ☑
    nontraumatic N28.89
  urethra (nontraumatic) N36.8
    with ectopic or molar pregnancy O08.6
    following ectopic or molar pregnancy O08.6
    obstetrical trauma O71.5
    traumatic S37.39 ☑
  uterosacral ligament (nonobstetric) (nontraumatic) N83.8
  uterus (traumatic) S37.69 ☑
    before labor O71.0- ☑
    during or after labor O71.1
    nonpuerperal, nontraumatic N85.8
    pregnant (during labor) O71.1
      before labor O71.0- ☑
  vagina — *see* Injury, vagina
  valve, valvular (heart) — *see* Endocarditis
  varicose vein — *see* Varix
  varix — *see* Varix
  vena cava R58
    traumatic — *see* Injury, vena cava, laceration, major
  vesical (urinary) N32.89
  vessel (blood) R58
    pulmonary I28.8
    traumatic — *see* Injury, blood vessel
  viscus R19.8
  vulva complicating delivery O70.0
Russell-Silver syndrome Q87.19
Russian spring-summer type encephalitis A84.0
Rust's disease (tuberculous cervical spondylitis) A18.01
Ruvalcaba-Myhre-Smith syndrome E71.440
Rytand-Lipsitch syndrome I44.2

S

Saber, sabre shin or tibia (syphilitic) A50.56 *[M90.8-]* ☑
Sac lacrimal — *see* condition
Saccharomyces infection B37.9
Saccharopinuria E72.3
Saccular — *see* condition
Sacculation
  aorta (nonsyphilitic) — *see* Aneurysm, aorta
  bladder N32.3
  intralaryngeal (congenital) (ventricular) Q31.3
  larynx (congenital) (ventricular) Q31.3
  organ or site, congenital — *see* Distortion
  pregnant uterus — *see* Pregnancy, complicated by, abnormal, uterus
  ureter N28.89
  urethra N36.1
  vesical N32.3
Sachs' amaurotic familial idiocy or disease E75.02
Sachs-Tay disease E75.02
Sacks-Libman disease M32.11
Sacralgia M53.3
Sacralization Q76.49
Sacrodynia M53.3
Sacroiliac joint — *see* condition
Sacroiliitis NEC M46.1
Sacrum — *see* condition
Saddle
  back — *see* Lordosis
  embolus
    abdominal aorta I74.01
    pulmonary artery I26.92
      with acute cor pulmonale I26.02
  injury — *code to* condition
  nose M95.0
    due to syphilis A50.57
Sadism (sexual) F65.52
Sadness, postpartal O90.6
Sadomasochism F65.50
Saemisch's ulcer (cornea) — *see* Ulcer, cornea, central
Sagging
  skin and subcutaneous tissue (following bariatric surgery weight loss) (following dietary weight loss) L98.7
Sahib disease B55.0
Sailors' skin L57.8
Saint
  Anthony's fire — *see* Erysipelas
  triad — *see* Hernia, diaphragm
  Vitus' dance — *see* Chorea, Sydenham's
Salaam
  attack(s) — *see* Epilepsy, spasms
  tic R25.8
Salicylism
  abuse F55.8
  overdose or wrong substance given — *see* Table of Drugs and Chemicals, by drug, poisoning
Salivary duct or gland — *see* condition
Salivation, excessive K11.7
Salmonella — *see* Infection, Salmonella
Salmonellosis A02.0
Salpingitis (catarrhal) (fallopian tube) (nodular) (pseudofollicular) (purulent) (septic) N70.91
  with oophoritis N70.93
  acute N70.01
    with oophoritis N70.03
  chlamydial A56.11
  chronic N70.11
    with oophoritis N70.13
  complicating abortion — *see* Abortion, by type, complicated by, salpingitis
  ear — *see* Salpingitis, eustachian
  eustachian (tube) H68.00- ☑
    acute H68.01- ☑
    chronic H68.02- ☑
  follicularis N70.11
    with oophoritis N70.13
  gonococcal (acute) (chronic) A54.24
  interstitial, chronic N70.11
    with oophoritis N70.13
  isthmica nodosa N70.11
    with oophoritis N70.13
  specific (gonococcal) (acute) (chronic) A54.24
  tuberculous (acute) (chronic) A18.17
  venereal (gonococcal) (acute) (chronic) A54.24
Salpingocele N83.4- ☑

Salpingo-oophoritis (catarrhal) (purulent) (ruptured) (septic) (suppurative) N70.93
  acute N70.03
    with ectopic or molar pregnancy O08.0
    following ectopic or molar pregnancy O08.0
    gonococcal A54.24
  chronic N70.13
  following ectopic or molar pregnancy O08.0
  gonococcal (acute) (chronic) A54.24
  puerperal O86.19
  specific (gonococcal) (acute) (chronic) A54.24
  subacute N70.03
  tuberculous (acute) (chronic) A18.17
  venereal (gonococcal) (acute) (chronic) A54.24
Salpingo-ovaritis — *see* Salpingo-oophoritis
Salpingoperitonitis — *see* Salpingo-oophoritis
Salzmann's nodular dystrophy — *see* Degeneration, cornea, nodular
Sampson's cyst or tumor N80.10- ☑
San Joaquin (Valley) **fever** B38.0
Sandblaster's asthma, lung or pneumoconiosis J62.8
Sander's disease (paranoia) F22
Sandfly fever A93.1
Sandhoff's disease E75.01
Sanfilippo (Type B) (Type C) (Type D) **syndrome** E76.22
Sanger-Brown ataxia G11.2
Sao Paulo fever or typhus A77.0
Saponification, mesenteric K65.8
Sarcocele (benign)
  syphilitic A52.76
    congenital A50.59
Sarcocystosis A07.8
Sarcoepiplocele — *see* Hernia
Sarcoepiplomphalocele Q79.2
Sarcoglycanopathy G71.0340
  alpha G71.0341
  beta G71.0342
  delta G71.0349
  gamma G71.0349
Sarcoid — *see also* Sarcoidosis
  arthropathy D86.86
  Boeck's D86.9
  Darier-Roussy D86.3
  iridocyclitis D86.83
  meningitis D86.81
  myocarditis D86.85
  myositis D86.87
  pyelonephritis D86.84
  Spiegler-Fendt L08.89
Sarcoidosis D86.9
  with
    cranial nerve palsies D86.82
    hepatic granuloma D86.89
    polyarthritis D86.86
    tubulo-interstitial nephropathy D86.84
  combined sites NEC D86.89
  lung D86.0
    and lymph nodes D86.2
  lymph nodes D86.1
    and lung D86.2
  meninges D86.81
  skin D86.3
  specified type NEC D86.89
Sarcoma (of) — *see also* Neoplasm, connective tissue, malignant
  alveolar soft part — *see* Neoplasm, connective tissue, malignant
  ameloblastic C41.1
    upper jaw (bone) C41.0
  botryoid — *see* Neoplasm, connective tissue, malignant
  botryoides — *see* Neoplasm, connective tissue, malignant
  cerebellar C71.6
    circumscribed (arachnoidal) C71.6
  circumscribed (arachnoidal) cerebellar C71.6
  clear cell — *see also* Neoplasm, connective tissue, malignant
    kidney C64.- ☑
  dendritic cells (accessory cells) C96.4
  embryonal — *see* Neoplasm, connective tissue, malignant
  endometrial (stromal) C54.1
    isthmus C54.0
  epithelioid (cell) — *see* Neoplasm, connective tissue, malignant
  Ewing's — *see* Neoplasm, bone, malignant
  follicular dendritic cell C96.4

Sarcoma — *continued*
  germinoblastic (diffuse) — *see* Lymphoma, diffuse large cell
    follicular — *see* Lymphoma, follicular, specified NEC
  giant cell (except of bone) — *see also* Neoplasm, connective tissue, malignant
    bone — *see* Neoplasm, bone, malignant
  glomoid — *see* Neoplasm, connective tissue, malignant
  granulocytic C92.3- ☑
  hemangioendothelial — *see* Neoplasm, connective tissue, malignant
  hemorrhagic, multiple — *see* Sarcoma, Kaposi's
  histiocytic C96.A (*following* C96.6)
  Hodgkin — *see* Lymphoma, Hodgkin
  immunoblastic (diffuse) — *see* Lymphoma, diffuse large cell
  interdigitating dendritic cell C96.4
  Kaposi's
    colon C46.4
    connective tissue C46.1
    gastrointestinal organ C46.4
    lung C46.5- ☑
    lymph node(s) C46.3
    palate (hard) (soft) C46.2
    rectum C46.4
    skin C46.0
    specified site NEC C46.7
    stomach C46.4
    unspecified site C46.9
  Kupffer cell C22.3
  Langerhans cell C96.4
  leptomeningeal — *see* Neoplasm, meninges, malignant
  liver NEC C22.4
  lymphangioendothelial — *see* Neoplasm, connective tissue, malignant
  lymphoblastic — *see* Lymphoma, lymphoblastic (diffuse)
  lymphocytic — *see* Lymphoma, small cell B-cell
  mast cell C96.22
  melanotic — *see* Melanoma
  meningeal — *see* Neoplasm, meninges, malignant
  meningothelial — *see* Neoplasm, meninges, malignant
  mesenchymal — *see also* Neoplasm, connective tissue, malignant
    mixed — *see* Neoplasm, connective tissue, malignant
  mesothelial — *see* Mesothelioma
  monstrocellular
    specified site — *see* Neoplasm, malignant, by site
    unspecified site C71.9
  myeloid C92.3- ☑
  neurogenic — *see* Neoplasm, nerve, malignant
  odontogenic C41.1
    upper jaw (bone) C41.0
  osteoblastic — *see* Neoplasm, bone, malignant
  osteogenic — *see also* Neoplasm, bone, malignant
    juxtacortical — *see* Neoplasm, bone, malignant
    periosteal — *see* Neoplasm, bone, malignant
  periosteal — *see also* Neoplasm, bone, malignant
    osteogenic — *see* Neoplasm, bone, malignant
  pleomorphic cell — *see* Neoplasm, connective tissue, malignant
  reticulum cell (diffuse) — *see* Lymphoma, diffuse large cell
    nodular — *see* Lymphoma, follicular
    pleomorphic cell type — *see* Lymphoma, diffuse large cell
  rhabdoid — *see* Neoplasm, malignant, by site
  round cell — *see* Neoplasm, connective tissue, malignant
  small cell — *see* Neoplasm, connective tissue, malignant
  soft tissue — *see* Neoplasm, connective tissue, malignant
  spindle cell — *see* Neoplasm, connective tissue, malignant
  stromal (endometrial) C54.1
    isthmus C54.0
  synovial — *see also* Neoplasm, connective tissue, malignant
    biphasic — *see* Neoplasm, connective tissue, malignant
    epithelioid cell — *see* Neoplasm, connective tissue, malignant
    spindle cell — *see* Neoplasm, connective tissue, malignant

Sarcomatosis
  meningeal — *see* Neoplasm, meninges, malignant
  specified site NEC — *see* Neoplasm, connective tissue, malignant
  unspecified site C80.1
Sarcopenia (age-related) M62.84
Sarcosinemia E72.59
Sarcosporidiosis (intestinal) A07.8
SARS-CoV-2 — *see also* COVID-19
  sequelae (post acute) U09.9
Satiety, early R68.81
Saturnine — *see* condition
Saturnism
  overdose or wrong substance given or taken — *see* Table of Drugs and Chemicals, by drug, poisoning
Satyriasis F52.8
Sauriasis — *see* Ichthyosis
SBE (subacute bacterial endocarditis) I33.0
Scabies (any site) B86
Scabs R23.4
Scaglietti-Dagnini syndrome E22.0
Scald — *see* Burn
Scalenus anticus (anterior) **syndrome** G54.0
Scales R23.4
Scaling, skin R23.4
Scalp — *see* condition
Scapegoating affecting child Z62.3
Scaphocephaly Q75.0
Scapulalgia M89.8X1
Scapulohumeral myopathy G71.02
Scar, scarring — *see also* Cicatrix L90.5
  adherent L90.5
  atrophic L90.5
  cervix
    in pregnancy or childbirth — *see* Pregnancy, complicated by, abnormal cervix
  cheloid L91.0
  chorioretinal H31.00- ☑
    posterior pole macula H31.01- ☑
    postsurgical H59.81- ☑
    solar retinopathy H31.02- ☑
    specified type NEC H31.09- ☑
  choroid — *see* Scar, chorioretinal
  conjunctiva H11.24- ☑
  cornea H17.9
    xerophthalmic — *see also* Opacity, cornea
      vitamin A deficiency E50.6
  defect (isthmocele) O34.22
  duodenum, obstructive K31.5
  hypertrophic L91.0
  keloid L91.0
  labia N90.89
  lung (base) J98.4
  macula — *see* Scar, chorioretinal, posterior pole
  muscle M62.89
  myocardium, myocardial I25.2
  painful L90.5
  posterior pole (eye) — *see* Scar, chorioretinal, posterior pole
  retina — *see* Scar, chorioretinal
  trachea J39.8
  transmural uterine, in pregnancy O34.29
  uterus N85.8
    in pregnancy O34.29
  vagina N89.8
    postoperative N99.2
  vulva N90.89
Scarabiasis B88.2
Scarlatina (anginosa) (maligna) A38.9
  myocarditis (acute) A38.1
    old — *see* Myocarditis
  otitis media A38.0
  ulcerosa A38.8
Scarlet fever (albuminuria) (angina) A38.9
Schamberg's disease (progressive pigmentary dermatosis) L81.7
Schatzki's ring (acquired) (esophagus) (lower) K22.2
  congenital Q39.3
Schaufenster krankheit I20.8
Schaumann's
  benign lymphogranulomatosis D86.1
  disease or syndrome — *see* Sarcoidosis
Scheie's syndrome E76.03
Schenck's disease B42.1
Scheuermann's disease or osteochondrosis — *see* Osteochondrosis, juvenile, spine
Schilder (-Flatau) **disease** G37.0

Schilling-type monocytic leukemia C93.0- ☑
Schimmelbusch's disease, cystic mastitis, or hyperplasia — *see* Mastopathy, cystic
Schistosoma infestation — *see* Infestation, Schistosoma
Schistosomiasis B65.9
  with muscle disorder B65.9 *[M63.80]*
    ankle B65.9 *[M63.87-]* ☑
    foot B65.9 *[M63.87-]* ☑
    forearm B65.9 *[M63.83-]* ☑
    hand B65.9 *[M63.84-]* ☑
    lower leg B65.9 *[M63.86-]* ☑
    multiple sites B65.9 *[M63.89]*
    pelvic region B65.9 *[M63.85-]* ☑
    shoulder region B65.9 *[M63.81-]* ☑
    specified site NEC B65.9 *[M63.88]*
    thigh B65.9 *[M63.85-]* ☑
    upper arm B65.9 *[M63.82-]* ☑
  Asiatic B65.2
  bladder B65.0
  chestermani B65.8
  colon B65.1
  cutaneous B65.3
  due to
    S. haematobium B65.0
    S. japonicum B65.2
    S. mansoni B65.1
    S. mattheii B65.8
  Eastern B65.2
  genitourinary tract B65.0
  intestinal B65.1
  lung NEC B65.9 *[J99]*
    pneumonia B65.9 *[J17]*
  Manson's (intestinal) B65.1
  oriental B65.2
  pulmonary NEC B65.9 *[J99]*
    pneumonia B65.9
  Schistosoma
    haematobium B65.0
    japonicum B65.2
    mansoni B65.1
  specified type NEC B65.8
  urinary B65.0
  vesical B65.0
Schizencephaly Q04.6
Schizoaffective psychosis F25.9
Schizodontia K00.2
Schizoid personality F60.1
Schizophrenia, schizophrenic F20.9
  acute (brief) (undifferentiated) F23
  atypical (form) F20.3
  borderline F21
  catalepsy F20.2
  catatonic (type) (excited) (withdrawn) F20.2
  cenesthopathic, cenesthesiopathic F20.89
  childhood type F84.5
  chronic undifferentiated F20.9
  cyclic F25.0
  disorganized (type) F20.1
  flexibilitas cerea F20.2
  hebephrenic (type) F20.1
  incipient F21
  latent F21
  negative type F20.5
  paranoid (type) F20.0
  paraphrenic F20.0
  post-psychotic depression F32.89
  prepsychotic F21
  prodromal F21
  pseudoneurotic F21
  pseudopsychopathic F21
  reaction F23
  residual (state) (type) F20.5
  restzustand F20.5
  schizoaffective (type) — *see* Psychosis, schizoaffective
  simple (type) F20.89
  simplex F20.89
  specified type NEC F20.89
  spectrum and other psychotic disorder F29
    specified NEC F28
  stupor F20.2
  syndrome of childhood F84.5
  undifferentiated (type) F20.3
    chronic F20.9
Schizothymia (persistent) F60.1
Schlatter-Osgood disease or osteochondrosis M92.52- ☑
Schlatter's tibia — *see* Osteochondrosis, juvenile, tibia
Schmidt's syndrome (polyglandular, autoimmune) E31.0

☑ Additional Character Required — Refer to the Tabular List for Character Selection

Schmincke's carcinoma or tumor — *see* Neoplasm, nasopharynx, malignant
Schmitz (-Stutzer) **dysentery** A03.0
Schmorl's disease or nodes
    lumbar region M51.46
    lumbosacral region M51.47
    sacrococcygeal region M53.3
    thoracic region M51.44
    thoracolumbar region M51.45
Schneiderian
    papilloma — *see* Neoplasm, nasopharynx, benign
        specified site — *see* Neoplasm, benign, by site
        unspecified site D14.0
        specified site — *see* Neoplasm, malignant, by site
        unspecified site C30.0
Scholte's syndrome (malignant carcinoid) E34.0
Scholz (-Bielchowsky-Henneberg) **disease or syndrome** E75.25
Schönlein (-Henoch) disease or purpura (primary) (rheumatic) D69.0
Schottmuller's disease A01.4
Schroeder's syndrome (endocrine hypertensive) E27.0
Schüller-Christian disease or syndrome C96.5
Schultze's type acroparesthesia, simple I73.89
Schultz's disease or syndrome — *see* Agranulocytosis
Schwalbe-Ziehen-Oppenheim disease G24.1
Schwannoma — *see also* Neoplasm, nerve, benign
    malignant — *see also* Neoplasm, nerve, malignant
        with rhabdomyoblastic differentiation — *see* Neoplasm, nerve, malignant
    melanocytic — *see* Neoplasm, nerve, benign
    pigmented — *see* Neoplasm, nerve, benign
Schwannomatosis Q85.03
Schwartz (-Jampel) **syndrome** G71.13
Schwartz-Bartter syndrome E22.2
Schweniger-Buzzi anetoderma L90.1
Sciatic — *see* condition
Sciatica (infective) M54.3 ☑
    with lumbago M54.4- ☑
        due to intervertebral disc disorder — *see* Disorder, disc, with, radiculopathy
    due to displacement of intervertebral disc (with lumbago) — *see* Disorder, disc, with, radiculopathy
    wallet M54.3- ☑
Scimitar syndrome Q26.8
Sclera — *see* condition
Sclerectasia H15.84- ☑
Scleredema
    adultorum — *see* Sclerosis, systemic
    Buschke's — *see* Sclerosis, systemic
    newborn P83.0
Sclerema (adiposum) (edematosum) (neonatorum) (newborn) P83.0
    adultorum — *see* Sclerosis, systemic
Scleriasis — *see* Scleroderma
Scleritis H15.00- ☑
    with corneal involvement H15.04- ☑
    anterior H15.01- ☑
    brawny H15.02- ☑
    in (due to) zoster B02.34
    posterior H15.03- ☑
    specified type NEC H15.09- ☑
    syphilitic A52.71
    tuberculous (nodular) A18.51
Sclerochoroiditis H31.8
Scleroconjunctivitis — *see* Scleritis
Sclerocystic ovary syndrome E28.2
Sclerodactyly, sclerodactylia L94.3
Scleroderma, sclerodermia (acrosclerotic) (diffuse) (generalized) (progressive) (pulmonary) — *see also* Sclerosis, systemic M34.9
    circumscribed L94.0
    linear L94.1
    localized L94.0
    newborn P83.88
    systemic M34.9
Sclerokeratitis H16.8
    tuberculous A18.52
Scleroma nasi A48.8
Scleromalacia (perforans) H15.05- ☑
Scleromyxedema L98.5
Sclérose en plaques G35
Sclerosis, sclerotic
    adrenal (gland) E27.8
    Alzheimer's — *see* Disease, Alzheimer's
    amyotrophic (lateral) G12.21
    aorta, aortic I70.0

Sclerosis, sclerotic — *continued*
    aorta, aortic — *continued*
        valve — *see* Endocarditis, aortic
    artery, arterial, arteriolar, arteriovascular — *see* Arteriosclerosis
    ascending multiple G35
    brain (generalized) (lobular) G37.9
        artery, arterial I67.2
        diffuse G37.0
        disseminated G35
        insular G35
        Krabbe's E75.23
        miliary G35
        multiple G35
        presenile (Alzheimer's) — *see* Disease, Alzheimer's, early onset
        senile (arteriosclerotic) I67.2
        stem, multiple G35
        tuberous Q85.1
    bulbar, multiple G35
    bundle of His I44.39
    cardiac — *see* Disease, heart, ischemic, atherosclerotic
    cardiorenal — *see* Hypertension, cardiorenal
    cardiovascular — *see also* Disease, cardiovascular
        renal — *see* Hypertension, cardiorenal
    cerebellar — *see* Sclerosis, brain
    cerebral — *see* Sclerosis, brain
    cerebrospinal (disseminated) (multiple) G35
    cerebrovascular I67.2
    choroid — *see* Degeneration, choroid
    combined (spinal cord) — *see also* Degeneration, combined
        multiple G35
    concentric (Balo) G37.5
    cornea — *see* Opacity, cornea
    coronary (artery) I25.10
        with angina pectoris — *see* Arteriosclerosis, coronary (artery),
    corpus cavernosum
        female N90.89
        male N48.6
    diffuse (brain) (spinal cord) G37.0
    disseminated G35
    dorsal G35
    dorsolateral (spinal cord) — *see* Degeneration, combined
    endometrium N85.5
    extrapyramidal G25.9
    eye, nuclear (senile) — *see* Cataract, senile, nuclear
    focal and segmental (glomerular) — *see also* N00-N07
        with fourth character .1 N05.1
    Friedreich's (spinal cord) G11.11
    funicular (spermatic cord) N50.89
    general (vascular) — *see* Arteriosclerosis
    gland (lymphatic) I89.8
    hepatic K74.1
        alcoholic K70.2
    hereditary
        cerebellar G11.9
        spinal (Friedreich's ataxia) G11.11
    hippocampal G93.81
    insular G35
    kidney — *see* Sclerosis, renal
    larynx J38.7
    lateral (amyotrophic) (descending) (spinal) G12.21
        primary G12.23
    lens, senile nuclear — *see* Cataract, senile, nuclear
    liver K74.1
        with fibrosis K74.2
            alcoholic K70.2
        alcoholic K70.2
        cardiac K76.1
    lung — *see* Fibrosis, lung
    mastoid — *see* Mastoiditis, chronic
    mesial temporal G93.81
    mitral I05.8
    Mönckeberg's (medial) — *see* Arteriosclerosis, extremities
    multiple (brain stem) (cerebral) (generalized) (spinal cord) G35
    myocardium, myocardial — *see* Disease, heart, ischemic, atherosclerotic
    nuclear (senile), eye — *see* Cataract, senile, nuclear
    ovary N83.8
    pancreas K86.89
    penis N48.6
    peripheral arteries — *see* Arteriosclerosis, extremities
    plaques G35

Sclerosis, sclerotic — *continued*
    pluriglandular E31.8
    polyglandular E31.8
    posterolateral (spinal cord) — *see* Degeneration, combined
    presenile (Alzheimer's) — *see* Disease, Alzheimer's, early onset
    primary, lateral G12.23
    progressive, systemic M34.0
    pulmonary — *see* Fibrosis, lung
        artery I27.0
        valve (heart) — *see* Endocarditis, pulmonary
    renal N26.9
        with
            cystine storage disease E72.09
            hypertensive heart disease (conditions in I11) — *see* Hypertension, cardiorenal
            arteriolar (hyaline) (hyperplastic) — *see* Hypertension, kidney
    retina (senile) (vascular) H35.00
    senile (vascular) — *see* Arteriosclerosis
    spinal (cord) (progressive) G95.89
        ascending G61.0
        combined — *see also* Degeneration, combined
            multiple G35
            syphilitic A52.11
        disseminated G35
        dorsolateral — *see* Degeneration, combined
        hereditary (Friedreich's) (mixed form) G11.11
        lateral (amyotrophic) G12.21
            progressive G12.23
        multiple G35
        posterior (syphilitic) A52.11
    stomach K31.89
    subendocardial, congenital I42.4
    systemic M34.9
        with
            lung involvement M34.81
            myopathy M34.82
            polyneuropathy M34.83
        drug-induced M34.2
        due to chemicals NEC M34.2
        progressive M34.0
        specified NEC M34.89
    temporal (mesial) G93.81
    tricuspid (heart) (valve) I07.8
    tuberous (brain) Q85.1
    tympanic membrane — *see* Disorder, tympanic membrane, specified NEC
    valve, valvular (heart) — *see* Endocarditis
    vascular — *see* Arteriosclerosis
    vein I87.8
Scoliosis (acquired) (postural) M41.9
    adolescent (idiopathic) — *see* Scoliosis, idiopathic, adolescent
    congenital Q67.5
        due to bony malformation Q76.3
        failure of segmentation (hemivertebra) Q76.3
        hemivertebra fusion Q76.3
        postural Q67.5
    degenerative M41.5- ☑
    idiopathic M41.20
        adolescent M41.129
            cervical region M41.122
            cervicothoracic region M41.123
            lumbar region M41.126
            lumbosacral region M41.127
            thoracic region M41.124
            thoracolumbar region M41.125
        cervical region M41.22
        cervicothoracic region M41.23
        infantile M41.00
            cervical region M41.02
            cervicothoracic region M41.03
            lumbar region M41.06
            lumbosacral region M41.07
            sacrococcygeal region M41.08
            thoracic region M41.04
            thoracolumbar region M41.05
        juvenile M41.119
            cervical region M41.112
            cervicothoracic region M41.113
            lumbar region M41.116
            lumbosacral region M41.117
            thoracic region M41.114
            thoracolumbar region M41.115
        lumbar region M41.26
        lumbosacral region M41.27

Scoliosis — continued
  idiopathic — continued
    thoracic region M41.24
    thoracolumbar region M41.25
  infantile — see Scoliosis, idiopathic, infantile
  neuromuscular M41.40
    cervical region M41.42
    cervicothoracic region M41.43
    lumbar region M41.46
    lumbosacral region M41.47
    occipito-atlanto-axial region M41.41
    thoracic region M41.44
    thoracolumbar region M41.45
  paralytic — see Scoliosis, neuromuscular
  postradiation therapy M96.5
  rachitic (late effect or sequelae) E64.3 [M49.80]
    cervical region E64.3 [M49.82]
    cervicothoracic region E64.3 [M49.83]
    lumbar region E64.3 [M49.86]
    lumbosacral region E64.3 [M49.87]
    multiple sites E64.3 [M49.89]
    occipito-atlanto-axial region E64.3 [M49.81]
    sacrococcygeal region E64.3 [M49.88]
    thoracic region E64.3 [M49.84]
    thoracolumbar region E64.3 [M49.85]
  sciatic M54.4- ☑
  secondary (to) NEC M41.50
    cerebral palsy, Friedreich's ataxia, poliomyelitis, neuromuscular disorders — see Scoliosis, neuromuscular
    cervical region M41.52
    cervicothoracic region M41.53
    lumbar region M41.56
    lumbosacral region M41.57
    thoracic region M41.54
    thoracolumbar region M41.55
  specified form NEC M41.80
    cervical region M41.82
    cervicothoracic region M41.83
    lumbar region M41.86
    lumbosacral region M41.87
    thoracic region M41.84
    thoracolumbar region M41.85
  thoracogenic M41.30
    thoracic region M41.34
    thoracolumbar region M41.35
  tuberculous A18.01
Scoliotic pelvis
  with disproportion (fetopelvic) O33.0
    causing obstructed labor O65.0
Scorbutus, scorbutic — see also Scurvy
  anemia D53.2
Score, NIHSS (National Institutes of Health Stroke Scale) R29.7- ☑
Scotoma (arcuate) (Bjerrum) (central) (ring) — see also Defect, visual field, localized, scotoma
  scintillating H53.12- ☑
Scratch — see Abrasion
Scratchy throat R09.89
Screening (for) Z13.9
  alcoholism Z13.39
  anemia Z13.0
  anomaly, congenital Z13.89
  antenatal, of mother — see also Encounter, antenatal screening Z36.9
  arterial hypertension Z13.6
  arthropod-borne viral disease NEC Z11.59
  autism Z13.41
  bacteriuria, asymptomatic Z13.89
  behavioral disorder Z13.30
    specified NEC Z13.39
  brain injury, traumatic Z13.850
  bronchitis, chronic Z13.83
  brucellosis Z11.2
  cardiovascular disorder Z13.6
  cataract Z13.5
  chlamydial diseases Z11.8
  cholera Z11.0
  chromosomal abnormalities (nonprocreative) NEC Z13.79
  colonoscopy Z12.11
  congenital
    dislocation of hip Z13.89
    eye disorder Z13.5
    malformation or deformation Z13.89
  contamination NEC Z13.88
  coronavirus (disease) (novel) 2019 Z11.52
  COVID-19 Z11.52

Screening — continued
  cystic fibrosis Z13.228
  dengue fever Z11.59
  dental disorder Z13.84
  depression (adult) (adolescent) (child) Z13.31
    maternal Z13.32
    perinatal Z13.32
  developmental
    delays Z13.40
      global (milestones) Z13.42
      specified NEC Z13.49
    handicap Z13.42
      in early childhood Z13.42
  diabetes mellitus Z13.1
  diphtheria Z11.2
  disability, intellectual Z13.39
  disease or disorder Z13.9
    bacterial NEC Z11.2
      intestinal infectious Z11.0
      respiratory tuberculosis Z11.1
    behavioral Z13.30
      specified NEC Z13.39
    blood or blood-forming organ Z13.0
    cardiovascular Z13.6
    Chagas' Z11.6
    chlamydial Z11.8
    coronavirus (novel) 2019 Z11.52
    COVID-19 Z11.52
    dental Z13.89
    developmental delays Z13.40
      global (milestones) Z13.42
      specified NEC Z13.49
    digestive tract NEC Z13.818
      lower GI Z13.811
      upper GI Z13.810
    ear Z13.5
    endocrine Z13.29
    eye Z13.5
    genitourinary Z13.89
    heart Z13.6
    human immunodeficiency virus (HIV) infection Z11.4
    immunity Z13.0
    infection
      intestinal Z11.0
        specified NEC Z11.6
    infectious Z11.9
    mental health and behavioral Z13.30
      specified NEC Z13.39
    metabolic Z13.228
    neurological Z13.89
    nutritional Z13.21
      metabolic Z13.228
        lipoid disorders Z13.220
    protozoal Z11.6
      intestinal Z11.0
    respiratory Z13.83
    rheumatic Z13.828
    rickettsial Z11.8
    sexually-transmitted NEC Z11.3
      human immunodeficiency virus (HIV) Z11.4
    sickle-cell (trait) Z13.0
    skin Z13.89
    specified NEC Z13.89
    spirochetal Z11.8
    thyroid Z13.29
    vascular Z13.6
    venereal Z11.3
    viral NEC Z11.59
      coronavirus (novel) 2019 Z11.52
      COVID-19 Z11.52
      human immunodeficiency virus (HIV) Z11.4
      intestinal Z11.0
      SARS-CoV-2 Z11.52
  elevated titer Z13.89
  emphysema Z13.83
  encephalitis, viral (mosquito- or tick-borne) Z11.59
  exposure to contaminants (toxic) Z13.88
  fever
    dengue Z11.59
    hemorrhagic Z11.59
    yellow Z11.59
  filariasis Z11.6
  galactosemia Z13.228
  gastrointestinal condition Z13.818
  genetic (nonprocreative) - for procreative management — see Testing, genetic, for procreative management
    disease carrier status (nonprocreative) Z13.71
    specified NEC (nonprocreative) Z13.79

Screening — continued
  genitourinary condition Z13.89
  glaucoma Z13.5
  gonorrhea Z11.3
  gout Z13.89
  helminthiasis (intestinal) Z11.6
  hematopoietic malignancy Z12.89
  hemoglobinopathies NEC Z13.0
  hemorrhagic fever Z11.59
  Hodgkin disease Z12.89
  human immunodeficiency virus (HIV) Z11.4
  human papillomavirus Z11.51
  hypertension Z13.6
  immunity disorders Z13.0
  infant or child (over 28 days old) Z00.129
    with abnormal findings Z00.121
  infection
    mycotic Z11.8
    parasitic Z11.8
  ingestion of radioactive substance Z13.88
  intellectual disability Z13.39
  intestinal
    helminthiasis Z11.6
    infectious disease Z11.0
  leishmaniasis Z11.6
  leprosy Z11.2
  leptospirosis Z11.8
  leukemia Z12.89
  lymphoma Z12.89
  malaria Z11.6
  malnutrition Z13.29
    metabolic Z13.228
    nutritional Z13.21
  measles Z11.59
  mental health disorder Z13.30
    specified NEC Z13.39
  metabolic errors, inborn Z13.228
  multiphasic Z13.89
  musculoskeletal disorder Z13.828
    osteoporosis Z13.820
  mycoses Z11.8
  myocardial infarction (acute) Z13.6
  neoplasm (malignant) (of) Z12.9
    bladder Z12.6
    blood Z12.89
    breast Z12.39
      routine mammogram Z12.31
    cervix Z12.4
    colon Z12.11
    genitourinary organs NEC Z12.79
      bladder Z12.6
      cervix Z12.4
      ovary Z12.73
      prostate Z12.5
      testis Z12.71
      vagina Z12.72
    hematopoietic system Z12.89
    intestinal tract Z12.10
      colon Z12.11
      rectum Z12.12
      small intestine Z12.13
    lung Z12.2
    lymph (glands) Z12.89
    nervous system Z12.82
    oral cavity Z12.81
    prostate Z12.5
    rectum Z12.12
    respiratory organs Z12.2
    skin Z12.83
    small intestine Z12.13
    specified site NEC Z12.89
    stomach Z12.0
  nephropathy Z13.89
  nervous system disorders NEC Z13.858
  neurological condition Z13.89
  osteoporosis Z13.820
  parasitic infestation Z11.9
    specified NEC Z11.8
  phenylketonuria Z13.228
  plague Z11.2
  poisoning (chemical) (heavy metal) Z13.88
  poliomyelitis Z11.59
  postnatal, chromosomal abnormalities Z13.89
  prenatal, of mother — see also Encounter, antenatal screening Z36.9
  protozoal disease Z11.6
    intestinal Z11.0
  pulmonary tuberculosis Z11.1
  radiation exposure Z13.88

Screening — *continued*
  respiratory condition Z13.83
  respiratory tuberculosis Z11.1
  rheumatoid arthritis Z13.828
  rubella Z11.59
  SARS-CoV-2 Z11.52
  schistosomiasis Z11.6
  sexually-transmitted disease NEC Z11.3
    human immunodeficiency virus (HIV) Z11.4
  sickle-cell disease or trait Z13.0
  skin condition Z13.89
  sleeping sickness Z11.6
  special Z13.9
    specified NEC Z13.89
  syphilis Z11.3
  tetanus Z11.2
  trachoma Z11.8
  traumatic brain injury Z13.850
  trypanosomiasis Z11.6
  tuberculosis, respiratory Z11.1
    active Z11.1
    latent Z11.7
  venereal disease Z11.3
  viral encephalitis (mosquito- or tick-borne) Z11.59
  whooping cough Z11.2
  worms, intestinal Z11.6
  yaws Z11.8
  yellow fever Z11.59
Scrofula, scrofulosis (tuberculosis of cervical lymph glands) A18.2
Scrofulide (primary) (tuberculous) A18.4
Scrofuloderma, scrofulodermia (any site) (primary) A18.4
Scrofulosus lichen (primary) (tuberculous) A18.4
Scrofulous — *see* condition
Scrotal tongue K14.5
Scrotum — *see* condition
Scurvy, scorbutic E54
  anemia D53.2
  gum E54
  infantile E54
  rickets E55.0 [M90.80]
Sealpox B08.62
Seasickness T75.3 ☑
Seatworm (infection) (infestation) B80
Sebaceous — *see also* condition
  cyst — *see* Cyst, sebaceous
Seborrhea, seborrheic L21.9
  capillitii R23.8
  capitis L21.0
  dermatitis L21.9
    infantile L21.1
  eczema L21.9
    infantile L21.1
  sicca L21.0
Seckel's syndrome Q87.19
Seclusion, pupil — *see* Membrane, pupillary
Second hand tobacco smoke exposure (acute) (chronic) Z77.22
  in the perinatal period P96.81
Secondary
  dentin (in pulp) K04.3
  neoplasm, secondaries — *see* Table of Neoplasms, secondary
Secretion
  antidiuretic hormone, inappropriate E22.2
  catecholamine, by pheochromocytoma E27.5
  hormone
    antidiuretic, inappropriate (syndrome) E22.2
    by
      carcinoid tumor E34.0
      pheochromocytoma E27.5
    ectopic NEC E34.2
  urinary
    excessive R35.89
    suppression R34
Section
  nerve, traumatic — *see* Injury, nerve
Sedative, hypnotic, or anxiolytic-induced
  anxiety disorder F13.980
  bipolar and related disorder F13.94
  delirium F13.921
  depressive disorder F13.94
  major neurocognitive disorder F13.97
  mild neurocognitive disorder F13.988
  psychotic disorder F13.959
  sexual dysfunction F13.981
  sleep disorder F13.982

Segmentation, incomplete (congenital) — *see also* Fusion
  bone NEC Q78.8
  lumbosacral (joint) (vertebra) Q76.49
SEID (systemic exertion intolerance disease) G93.32
Seitelberger's syndrome (infantile neuraxonal dystrophy) G31.89
Seizure(s) — *see also* Convulsions R56.9
  absence G40.A- ☑ (*following* G40.3)
  akinetic — *see* Epilepsy, generalized, specified NEC
  atonic — *see* Epilepsy, generalized, specified NEC
  autonomic (hysterical) F44.5
  convulsive — *see* Convulsions
  cortical (focal) (motor) — *see* Epilepsy, localization-related, symptomatic, with simple partial seizures
  disorder — *see also* Epilepsy G40.909
  due to stroke — *see* Sequelae (of), disease, cerebrovascular, by type, specified NEC
  epileptic — *see* Epilepsy
  febrile (simple) R56.00
    with status epilepticus G40.901
    complex (atypical) (complicated) R56.01
      with status epilepticus G40.901
  grand mal G40.409
    intractable G40.419
      with status epilepticus G40.411
      without status epilepticus G40.419
    not intractable G40.409
      with status epilepticus G40.401
      without status epilepticus G40.409
  heart — *see* Disease, heart
  hysterical F44.5
  intractable G40.919
    with status epilepticus G40.911
  Jacksonian (focal) (motor type) (sensory type) — *see* Epilepsy, localization-related, symptomatic, with simple partial seizures
  newborn P90
  nonspecific epileptic
    atonic — *see* Epilepsy, generalized, specified NEC
    clonic — *see* Epilepsy, generalized, specified NEC
    myoclonic — *see* Epilepsy, generalized, specified NEC
    tonic — *see* Epilepsy, generalized, specified NEC
    tonic-clonic — *see* Epilepsy, generalized, specified NEC
  partial, developing into secondarily generalized seizures
    complex — *see* Epilepsy, localization-related, symptomatic, with complex partial seizures
    simple — *see* Epilepsy, localization-related, symptomatic, with simple partial seizures
  petit mal G40.A- ☑ (*following* G40.3)
    intractable G40.A1- ☑ (*following* G40.3)
      with status epilepticus G40.A11 (*following* G40.3)
      without status epilepticus G40.A19 (*following* G40.3)
    not intractable G40.A0- ☑ (*following* G40.3)
      with status epilepticus G40.A01 (*following* G40.3)
      without status epilepticus G40.A09 (*following* G40.3)
  post traumatic R56.1
  recurrent G40.909
  specified NEC G40.89
  uncinate — *see* Epilepsy, localization-related, symptomatic, with complex partial seizures
Selenium deficiency, dietary E59
Self-damaging behavior (life-style) Z72.89
Self-harm (attempted)
  history (personal)
    in family Z81.8
    nonsuicidal Z91.52
    suicidal Z91.51
  nonsuicidal R45.88
Self-injury, nonsuicidal R45.88
  personal history Z91.52
Self-mutilation (attempted)
  history (personal)
    in family Z81.8
    nonsuicidal Z91.52
    suicidal Z91.51
  nonsuicidal R45.88
Self-poisoning
  history (personal) Z91.51
    in family Z81.8
  observation following (alleged) attempt Z03.6
Semicoma R40.1
Seminal vesiculitis N49.0

Seminoma C62.9- ☑
  specified site — *see* Neoplasm, malignant, by site
Senear-Usher disease or syndrome L10.4
Senectus R54
Senescence (without mention of psychosis) R54
Senile, senility — *see also* condition R41.81
  with
    acute confusional state F05
    mental changes NOS F03 ☑
    psychosis NEC — *see* Psychosis, senile
  asthenia R54
  cervix (atrophic) N88.8
  debility R54
  endometrium (atrophic) N85.8
  fallopian tube (atrophic) — *see* Atrophy, fallopian tube
  heart (failure) R54
  ovary (atrophic) — *see* Atrophy, ovary
  premature E34.8
  vagina, vaginitis (atrophic) N95.2
  wart L82.1
Sensation
  burning (skin) R20.8
    tongue K14.6
  loss of R20.8
  prickling (skin) R20.2
  tingling (skin) R20.2
Sense loss
  smell — *see* Disturbance, sensation, smell
  taste — *see* Disturbance, sensation, taste
  touch R20.8
Sensibility disturbance (cortical) (deep) (vibratory) R20.9
Sensitive, sensitivity — *see also* Allergy
  carotid sinus G90.01
  child (excessive) F93.8
  cold, autoimmune D59.12
  dentin K03.89
  gluten (non-celiac) K90.41
  latex Z91.040
  methemoglobin D74.8
  tuberculin, without clinical or radiological symptoms R76.11
  visual
    glare H53.71
    impaired contrast H53.72
Sensitiver Beziehungswahn F22
Sensitization, auto-erythrocytic D69.2
Separation
  anxiety, abnormal (of childhood) F93.0
  apophysis, traumatic — *code as* Fracture, by site
  choroid — *see* Detachment, choroid
  epiphysis, epiphyseal
    nontraumatic — *see also* Osteochondropathy, specified type NEC
      upper femoral — *see* Slipped, epiphysis, upper femoral
    traumatic — *code as* Fracture, by site
  fracture — *see* Fracture
  infundibulum cardiac from right ventricle by a partition Q24.3
  joint (traumatic) (current) — *code by* site under Dislocation
  muscle (nontraumatic) — *see* Diastasis, muscle
  pubic bone, obstetrical trauma O71.6
  retina, retinal — *see* Detachment, retina
  symphysis pubis, obstetrical trauma O71.6
  tracheal ring, incomplete, congenital Q32.1
Sepsis (generalized) (unspecified organism) A41.9
  with
    organ dysfunction (acute) (multiple) R65.20
      with septic shock R65.21
  actinomycotic A42.7
  adrenal hemorrhage syndrome (meningococcal) A39.1
  anaerobic A41.4
  Bacillus anthracis A22.7
  Brucella — *see also* Brucellosis A23.9
  candidal B37.7
  cryptogenic A41.9
  due to device, implant or graft T85.79 ☑
    arterial graft NEC T82.7 ☑
    breast (implant) T85.79 ☑
    catheter NEC T85.79 ☑
      dialysis (renal) T82.7 ☑
        intraperitoneal T85.71 ☑
      infusion NEC T82.7 ☑
        spinal (cranial) (epidural) (intrathecal) (spinal) (subarachnoid) (subdural) T85.735 ☑
      urethral indwelling T83.511 ☑

Sepsis — *continued*
- due to device, implant or graft — *continued*
  - catheter — *continued*
    - urinary T83.518 ☑
  - ectopic or molar pregnancy O08.82
  - electronic (electrode) (pulse generator) (stimulator)
    - bone T84.7 ☑
    - cardiac T82.7 ☑
    - nervous system T85.738 ☑
      - brain T85.731 ☑
      - neurostimulator generator T85.734 ☑
      - peripheral nerve T85.732 ☑
      - spinal cord T85.733 ☑
    - urinary T83.590 ☑
  - fixation, internal (orthopedic) — *see* Complication, fixation device, infection
  - gastrointestinal (bile duct) (esophagus) T85.79 ☑
    - neurostimulator electrode (lead) T85.732 ☑
  - genital T83.69 ☑
  - heart NEC T82.7 ☑
    - valve (prosthesis) T82.6 ☑
      - graft T82.7 ☑
  - joint prosthesis — *see* Complication, joint prosthesis, infection
  - ocular (corneal graft) (orbital implant) T85.79 ☑
  - orthopedic NEC T84.7 ☑
    - fixation device, internal — *see* Complication, fixation device, infection
  - specified NEC T85.79 ☑
  - vascular T82.7 ☑
  - ventricular intracranial (communicating) shunt T85.730 ☑
- during labor O75.3
- Enterococcus A41.81
- Erysipelothrix (rhusiopathiae) (erysipeloid) A26.7
- Escherichia coli (E. coli) A41.5 ☑
- extraintestinal yersiniosis A28.2
- following
  - abortion (subsequent episode) O08.0
    - current episode — *see* Abortion
  - ectopic or molar pregnancy O08.82
  - immunization T88.0 ☑
  - infusion, therapeutic injection or transfusion NEC T80.29 ☑
  - obstetrical procedure O86.04
- gangrenous A41.9
- gonococcal A54.86
- Gram-negative (organism) A41.5 ☑
  - anaerobic A41.4
- Haemophilus influenzae A41.3
- herpesviral B00.7
- intra-abdominal K65.1
- intraocular — *see* Endophthalmitis, purulent
- Listeria monocytogenes A32.7
- localized — *code to* specific localized infection
  - in operation wound T81.49 ☑
  - skin — *see* Abscess
- malleus A24.0
- melioidosis A24.1
- meningeal — *see* Meningitis
- meningococcal A39.4
  - acute A39.2
  - chronic A39.3
- MSSA (Methicillin susceptible Staphylococcus aureus) A41.01
- newborn P36.9
  - due to
    - anaerobes NEC P36.5
    - Escherichia coli P36.4
    - Staphylococcus P36.30
      - aureus P36.2
      - specified NEC P36.39
    - Streptococcus P36.10
      - group B P36.0
      - specified NEC P36.19
    - specified NEC P36.8
- Pasteurella multocida A28.0
- pelvic, puerperal, postpartum, childbirth O85
- pneumococcal A40.3
- postprocedural T81.44 ☑
- puerperal, postpartum, childbirth (pelvic) O85
- Salmonella (arizonae) (cholerae-suis) (enteritidis) (typhimurium) A02.1
- severe R65.20
  - with septic shock R65.21
- Shigella — *see also* Dysentery, bacillary A03.9
- skin, localized — *see* Abscess

Sepsis — *continued*
- specified organism NEC A41.89
- Staphylococcus, staphylococcal A41.2
  - aureus (methicillin susceptible) (MSSA) A41.01
    - methicillin resistant (MRSA) A41.02
  - coagulase-negative A41.1
  - specified NEC A41.1
- Streptococcus, streptococcal A40.9
  - agalactiae A40.1
  - group
    - A A40.0
    - B A40.1
    - D A41.81
  - neonatal P36.10
    - group B P36.0
    - specified NEC P36.19
  - pneumoniae A40.3
  - pyogenes A40.0
  - specified NEC A40.8
- tracheostomy stoma J95.02
- tularemic A21.7
- umbilical, umbilical cord (newborn) — *see* Sepsis, newborn
- Yersinia pestis A20.7

Septate — *see* Septum

Septic — *see* condition
- arm — *see* Cellulitis, upper limb
  - with lymphangitis — *see* Lymphangitis, acute, upper limb
- embolus — *see* Embolism
- finger — *see* Cellulitis, digit
  - with lymphangitis — *see* Lymphangitis, acute, digit
- foot — *see* Cellulitis, lower limb
  - with lymphangitis — *see* Lymphangitis, acute, lower limb
- gallbladder (acute) K81.0
- hand — *see* Cellulitis, upper limb
  - with lymphangitis — *see* Lymphangitis, acute, upper limb
- joint — *see* Arthritis, pyogenic or pyemic
- leg — *see* Cellulitis, lower limb
  - with lymphangitis — *see* Lymphangitis, acute, lower limb
- nail — *see also* Cellulitis, digit
  - with lymphangitis — *see* Lymphangitis, acute, digit
- sore — *see also* Abscess
  - throat J02.0
    - streptococcal J02.0
- spleen (acute) D73.89
- teeth, tooth (pulpal origin) K04.4
- throat — *see* Pharyngitis
- thrombus — *see* Thrombosis
- toe — *see* Cellulitis, digit
  - with lymphangitis — *see* Lymphangitis, acute, digit
- tonsils, chronic J35.01
  - with adenoiditis J35.03
- uterus — *see* Endometritis

Septicemia A41.9
- meaning sepsis — *see* Sepsis

Septum, septate (congenital) — *see also* Anomaly, by site
- anal Q42.3
  - with fistula Q42.2
- aqueduct of Sylvius Q03.0
  - with spina bifida — *see* Spina bifida, by site, with hydrocephalus
- uterus Q51.28
  - complete Q51.21
  - partial Q51.22
  - specified NEC Q51.28
- vagina Q52.10
  - in pregnancy — *see* Pregnancy, complicated by, abnormal vagina
    - causing obstructed labor O65.5
  - longitudinal Q52.129
    - microperforate
      - left side Q52.124
      - right side Q52.123
    - nonobstruction Q52.120
    - obstructing Q52.129
      - left side Q52.122
      - right side Q52.121
  - transverse Q52.11

Sequelae (of) — *see also* condition
- abscess, intracranial or intraspinal (conditions in G06) G09

Sequelae — *continued*
- amputation — *code to* injury with seventh character S
- burn and corrosion — *code to* injury with seventh character S
- calcium deficiency E64.8
- cerebrovascular disease — *see* Sequelae, disease, cerebrovascular
- childbirth O94
- contusion — *code to* injury with seventh character S
- corrosion — *see* Sequelae, burn and corrosion
- COVID-19 (post acute) U09.9
- crushing injury — *code to* injury with seventh character S
- disease
  - cerebrovascular I69.90
    - alteration of sensation I69.998
    - aphasia I69.920
    - apraxia I69.990
    - ataxia I69.993
    - cognitive deficits I69.91 ☑
    - disturbance of vision I69.998
    - dysarthria I69.922
    - dysphagia I69.991
    - dysphasia I69.921
    - facial droop I69.992
    - facial weakness I69.992
    - fluency disorder I69.923
    - hemiplegia I69.95- ☑
    - hemorrhage
      - intracerebral — *see* Sequelae, hemorrhage, intracerebral
      - intracranial, nontraumatic NEC — *see* Sequelae, hemorrhage, intracranial, nontraumatic
      - subarachnoid — *see* Sequelae, hemorrhage, subarachnoid
    - language deficit I69.928
    - monoplegia
      - lower limb I69.94- ☑
      - upper limb I69.93- ☑
    - paralytic syndrome I69.96- ☑
    - specified effect NEC I69.998
    - specified type NEC I69.80
      - alteration of sensation I69.898
      - aphasia I69.820
      - apraxia I69.890
      - ataxia I69.893
      - cognitive deficits I69.81 ☑
      - disturbance of vision I69.898
      - dysarthria I69.822
      - dysphagia I69.891
      - dysphasia I69.821
      - facial droop I69.892
      - facial weakness I69.892
      - fluency disorder I69.823
      - hemiplegia I69.85- ☑
      - language deficit I69.828
      - monoplegia
        - lower limb I69.84- ☑
        - upper limb I69.83- ☑
      - paralytic syndrome I69.86- ☑
      - specified effect NEC I69.898
    - speech deficit I69.928
      - speech deficit I69.828
    - stroke NOS — *see* Sequelae, stroke NOS
- dislocation — *code to* injury with seventh character S
- encephalitis or encephalomyelitis (conditions in G04) G09
  - in infectious disease NEC B94.8
  - viral B94.1
- external cause — *code to* injury with seventh character S
- foreign body entering natural orifice — *code to* injury with seventh character S
- fracture — *code to* injury with seventh character S
- frostbite — *code to* injury with seventh character S
- Hansen's disease B92
- hemorrhage
  - intracerebral I69.10
    - alteration of sensation I69.198
    - aphasia I69.120
    - apraxia I69.190
    - ataxia I69.193
    - cognitive deficits I69.11 ☑
    - disturbance of vision I69.198
    - dysarthria I69.122
    - dysphagia I69.191

Sequelae — *continued*
- hemorrhage — *continued*
  - intracerebral — *continued*
    - dysphasia I69.121
    - facial droop I69.192
    - facial weakness I69.192
    - fluency disorder I69.123
    - hemiplegia I69.15- ☑
    - language deficit NEC I69.128
    - monoplegia
      - lower limb I69.14- ☑
      - upper limb I69.13- ☑
    - paralytic syndrome I69.16- ☑
    - specified effect NEC I69.198
    - speech deficit NEC I69.128
  - intracranial, nontraumatic NEC I69.20
    - alteration of sensation I69.298
    - aphasia I69.220
    - apraxia I69.290
    - ataxia I69.293
    - cognitive deficits I69.21 ☑
    - disturbance of vision I69.298
    - dysarthria I69.222
    - dysphagia I69.291
    - dysphasia I69.221
    - facial droop I69.292
    - facial weakness I69.292
    - fluency disorder I69.223
    - hemiplegia I69.25- ☑
    - language deficit NEC I69.228
    - monoplegia
      - lower limb I69.24- ☑
      - upper limb I69.23- ☑
    - paralytic syndrome I69.26- ☑
    - specified effect NEC I69.298
    - speech deficit NEC I69.228
  - subarachnoid I69.00
    - alteration of sensation I69.098
    - aphasia I69.020
    - apraxia I69.090
    - ataxia I69.093
    - cognitive deficits — *see* subcategory I69.01- ☑
    - disturbance of vision I69.098
    - dysarthria I69.022
    - dysphagia I69.091
    - dysphasia I69.021
    - facial droop I69.092
    - facial weakness I69.092
    - fluency disorder I69.023
    - hemiplegia I69.05- ☑
    - language deficit NEC I69.028
    - monoplegia
      - lower limb I69.04- ☑
      - upper limb I69.03- ☑
    - paralytic syndrome I69.06- ☑
    - specified effect NEC I69.098
    - speech deficit NEC I69.028
- hepatitis, viral B94.2
- hyperalimentation E68
- infarction
  - cerebral I69.30
    - alteration of sensation I69.398
    - aphasia I69.320
    - apraxia I69.390
    - ataxia I69.393
    - cognitive deficits I69.31 ☑
    - disturbance of vision I69.398
    - dysarthria I69.322
    - dysphagia I69.391
    - dysphasia I69.321
    - facial droop I69.392
    - facial weakness I69.392
    - fluency disorder I69.323
    - hemiplegia I69.35- ☑
    - language deficit NEC I69.328
    - monoplegia
      - lower limb I69.34- ☑
      - upper limb I69.33- ☑
    - paralytic syndrome I69.36- ☑
    - specified effect NEC I69.398
    - speech deficit NEC I69.328
- infection, pyogenic, intracranial or intraspinal G09
- infectious disease B94.9
  - specified NEC B94.8
- injury — *code to* injury with seventh character S
- leprosy B92
- meningitis
  - bacterial (conditions in G00) G09

Sequelae — *continued*
- meningitis — *continued*
  - other or unspecified cause (conditions in G03) G09
- muscle (and tendon) injury — *code to* injury with seventh character S
- myelitis — *see* Sequelae, encephalitis
- niacin deficiency E64.8
- nutritional deficiency E64.9
  - specified NEC E64.8
- obstetrical condition O94
- parasitic disease B94.9
- phlebitis or thrombophlebitis of intracranial or intraspinal venous sinuses and veins (conditions in G08) G09
- poisoning — *code to* poisoning with seventh character S
  - nonmedicinal substance — *see* Sequelae, toxic effect, nonmedicinal substance
- poliomyelitis (acute) B91
- pregnancy O94
- protein-energy malnutrition E64.0
- puerperium O94
- rickets E64.3
- SARS-CoV-2 (post acute) U09.9
- selenium deficiency E64.8
- sprain and strain — *code to* injury with seventh character S
- stroke NOS I69.30
  - alteration in sensation I69.398
  - aphasia I69.320
  - apraxia I69.390
  - ataxia I69.393
  - cognitive deficits I69.31 ☑
  - disturbance of vision I69.398
  - dysarthria I69.322
  - dysphagia I69.391
  - dysphasia I69.321
  - facial droop I69.392
  - facial weakness I69.392
  - hemiplegia I69.35- ☑
  - language deficit NEC I69.328
  - monoplegia
    - lower limb I69.34- ☑
    - upper limb I69.33- ☑
  - paralytic syndrome I69.36- ☑
  - specified effect NEC I69.398
  - speech deficit NEC I69.328
- tendon and muscle injury — *code to* injury with seventh character S
- thiamine deficiency E64.8
- trachoma B94.0
- tuberculosis B90.9
  - bones and joints B90.2
  - central nervous system B90.0
  - genitourinary B90.1
  - pulmonary (respiratory) B90.9
  - specified organs NEC B90.8
- viral
  - encephalitis B94.1
  - hepatitis B94.2
- vitamin deficiency NEC E64.8
  - A E64.1
  - B E64.8
  - C E64.2
- wound, open — *code to* injury with seventh character S

Sequestration — *see also* Sequestrum
- disc — *see* Displacement, intervertebral disc
- lung, congenital Q33.2

Sequestrum
- bone — *see* Osteomyelitis, chronic
- dental M27.2
- jaw bone M27.2
- orbit — *see* Osteomyelitis, orbit
- sinus (accessory) (nasal) — *see* Sinusitis

Sequoiosis lung or pneumonitis J67.8

Serology for syphilis
- doubtful
  - with signs or symptoms — *code by* site and stage under Syphilis
  - follow-up of latent syphilis — *see* Syphilis, latent
- negative, with signs or symptoms — *code by* site and stage under Syphilis
- positive A53.0
  - with signs or symptoms — *code by* site and stage under Syphilis
- reactivated A53.0

Seroma — *see also* Hematoma

Seroma — *continued*
- postprocedural — *see* Complication, postprocedural, seroma
- traumatic, secondary and recurrent T79.2 ☑

Seropurulent — *see* condition

Serositis, multiple K65.8
- pericardial I31.1
- peritoneal K65.8

Serous — *see* condition

Sertoli cell
- adenoma
  - specified site — *see* Neoplasm, benign, by site
  - unspecified site
    - female D27.9
    - male D29.20
- carcinoma
  - specified site — *see* Neoplasm, malignant, by site
  - unspecified site (male) C62.9- ☑
    - female C56.9
- tumor
  - with lipid storage
    - specified site — *see* Neoplasm, benign, by site
    - unspecified site
      - female D27.9
      - male D29.20
  - specified site — *see* Neoplasm, benign, by site
  - unspecified site
    - female D27.9
    - male D29.20

Sertoli-Leydig cell tumor — *see* Neoplasm, benign, by site
- specified site — *see* Neoplasm, benign, by site
- unspecified site
  - female D27.9
  - male D29.20

Serum
- allergy, allergic reaction — *see also* Reaction, serum T80.69 ☑
  - shock — *see also* Shock, anaphylactic T80.59 ☑
- arthritis — *see also* Reaction, serum T80.69 ☑
- complication or reaction NEC — *see also* Reaction, serum T80.69 ☑
- disease NEC — *see also* Reaction, serum T80.69 ☑
- hepatitis — *see also* Hepatitis, viral, type B carrier (suspected) of B18.1
- intoxication — *see also* Reaction, serum T80.69 ☑
- neuritis — *see also* Reaction, serum T80.69 ☑
- neuropathy G61.1
- poisoning NEC — *see also* Reaction, serum T80.69 ☑
- rash NEC — *see also* Reaction, serum T80.69 ☑
- reaction NEC — *see also* Reaction, serum T80.69 ☑
- sickness NEC — *see also* Reaction, serum T80.69 ☑
- urticaria — *see also* Reaction, serum T80.69 ☑

Sesamoiditis M25.8- ☑

Severe sepsis R65.20
- with septic shock R65.21

Sever's disease or osteochondrosis — *see* Osteochondrosis, juvenile, tarsus

Sex
- chromosome mosaics Q97.8
  - lines with various numbers of X chromosomes Q97.2
- education Z70.8
- reassignment surgery status Z87.890

Sextuplet pregnancy — *see* Pregnancy, sextuplet

Sexual
- function, disorder of (psychogenic) F52.9
- immaturity (female) (male) E30.0
- impotence (psychogenic) organic origin NEC — *see* Dysfunction, sexual, male
- precocity (constitutional) (cryptogenic) (female) (idiopathic) (male) E30.1

Sexuality, pathologic — *see* Deviation, sexual

Sézary disease C84.1- ☑

Shadow, lung R91.8

Shaking palsy or paralysis — *see* Parkinsonism

Shallowness, acetabulum — *see* Derangement, joint, specified type NEC, hip

Shaver's disease J63.1

Sheath (tendon) — *see* condition

Sheathing, retinal vessels H35.01- ☑

Shedding
- nail L60.8
- premature, primary (deciduous) teeth K00.6

Sheehan's disease or syndrome E23.0

Shelf, rectal K62.89

Shell teeth K00.5

Shellshock (current) F43.0

Shellshock — continued
lasting state — see Disorder, post-traumatic stress
Shield kidney Q63.1
Shift
auditory threshold (temporary) H93.24- ☑
mediastinal R93.89
Shifting sleep-work schedule (affecting sleep) G47.26
Shiga (-Kruse) **dysentery** A03.0
Shiga's bacillus A03.0
Shigella (dysentery) — see Dysentery, bacillary
Shigellosis A03.9
Group A A03.0
Group B A03.1
Group C A03.2
Group D A03.3
Shin splints S86.89- ☑
Shingles — see Herpes, zoster
Shipyard disease or eye B30.0
Shirodkar suture, in pregnancy — see Pregnancy, complicated by, incompetent cervix
Shock R57.9
with ectopic or molar pregnancy O08.3
adrenal (cortical) (Addisonian) E27.2
adverse food reaction (anaphylactic) — see Shock, anaphylactic, due to food
allergic — see Shock, anaphylactic
anaphylactic T78.2 ☑
chemical — see Table of Drugs and Chemicals
due to drug or medicinal substance
correct substance properly administered T88.6 ☑
overdose or wrong substance given or taken (by accident) — see Table of Drugs and Chemicals, by drug, poisoning
due to food (nonpoisonous) T78.00 ☑
additives T78.06 ☑
dairy products T78.07 ☑
eggs T78.08 ☑
fish T78.03 ☑
shellfish T78.02 ☑
fruit T78.04 ☑
milk T78.07 ☑
nuts T78.05 ☑
multiple types T78.05 ☑
peanuts T78.01 ☑
peanuts T78.01 ☑
seeds T78.05 ☑
specified type NEC T78.09 ☑
vegetable T78.04 ☑
following sting(s) — see Venom
immunization T80.52 ☑
serum T80.59 ☑
blood and blood products T80.51 ☑
immunization T80.52 ☑
specified NEC T80.59 ☑
vaccination T80.52 ☑
anaphylactoid — see Shock, anaphylactic
anesthetic
correct substance properly administered T88.2 ☑
overdose or wrong substance given or taken — see Table of Drugs and Chemicals, by drug, poisoning
specified anesthetic — see Table of Drugs and Chemicals, by drug, poisoning
cardiogenic R57.0
chemical substance — see Table of Drugs and Chemicals
complicating ectopic or molar pregnancy O08.3
culture — see Disorder, adjustment
drug
due to correct substance properly administered T88.6 ☑
overdose or wrong substance given or taken (by accident) — see Table of Drugs and Chemicals, by drug, poisoning
during or after labor and delivery O75.1
electric T75.4 ☑
(taser) T75.4 ☑
endotoxic R65.21
postprocedural (resulting from a procedure, not elsewhere classified) T81.12 ☑
following
ectopic or molar pregnancy O08.3
injury (immediate) (delayed) T79.4 ☑
labor and delivery O75.1
food (anaphylactic) — see Shock, anaphylactic, due to food
from electroshock gun (taser) T75.4 ☑

Shock — continued
gram-negative R65.21
postprocedural (resulting from a procedure, not elsewhere classified) T81.12 ☑
hematologic R57.8
hemorrhagic R57.8
surgery (intraoperative) (postoperative) T81.19 ☑
trauma T79.4 ☑
hypovolemic R57.1
surgical T81.19 ☑
traumatic T79.4 ☑
insulin E15
therapeutic misadventure — see subcategory T38.3 ☑
kidney N17.0
traumatic (following crushing) T79.5 ☑
lightning T75.01 ☑
liver K72.00
lung J80
obstetric O75.1
with ectopic or molar pregnancy O08.3
following ectopic or molar pregnancy O08.3
pleural (surgical) T81.19 ☑
due to trauma T79.4 ☑
postprocedural (postoperative) T81.10 ☑
with ectopic or molar pregnancy O08.3
cardiogenic T81.11 ☑
endotoxic T81.12 ☑
following ectopic or molar pregnancy O08.3
gram-negative T81.12 ☑
hypovolemic T81.19 ☑
septic T81.12 ☑
specified type NEC T81.19 ☑
psychic F43.0
septic (due to severe sepsis) R65.21
specified NEC R57.8
surgical T81.10 ☑
taser gun (taser) T75.4 ☑
therapeutic misadventure NEC T81.10 ☑
thyroxin
overdose or wrong substance given or taken — see Table of Drugs and Chemicals, by drug, poisoning
toxic, syndrome A48.3
transfusion — see Complications, transfusion
traumatic (immediate) (delayed) T79.4 ☑
Shoemaker's chest M95.4
Short, shortening, shortness
arm (acquired) — see also Deformity, limb, unequal length
congenital Q71.81- ☑
forearm — see Deformity, limb, unequal length
bowel syndrome K91.2
breath R06.02
cervical (complicating pregnancy) O26.87- ☑
non-gravid uterus N88.3
common bile duct, congenital Q44.5
cord (umbilical), complicating delivery O69.3 ☑
cystic duct, congenital Q44.5
esophagus (congenital) Q39.8
femur (acquired) — see Deformity, limb, unequal length, femur
congenital — see Defect, reduction, lower limb, longitudinal, femur
frenum, frenulum, linguae (congenital) Q38.1
hip (acquired) — see also Deformity, limb, unequal length
congenital Q65.89
leg (acquired) — see also Deformity, limb, unequal length
congenital Q72.81- ☑
lower leg — see also Deformity, limb, unequal length
limbed stature, with immunodeficiency D82.2
lower limb (acquired) — see also Deformity, limb, unequal length
congenital Q72.81- ☑
organ or site, congenital NEC — see Distortion
palate, congenital Q38.5
radius (acquired) — see also Deformity, limb, unequal length
congenital — see Defect, reduction, upper limb, longitudinal, radius
rib syndrome Q77.2
stature (child) (hereditary) (idiopathic) NEC R62.52
constitutional E34.31

Short, shortening, shortness — continued
stature — continued
due to
endocrine disorder E34.30
specified type NEC, due to endocrine dosorder E34.39
genetic causes E34.329
ACAN gene variant E34.328
acid-labile subunit gene (IGFALS) defect E34.321
aggrecan deficiency E34.328
genetic syndrome with resistance to insulin-like growth factor-1 E34.322
growth hormone gene 1 (GH1) defect with growth hormone neutralizing antibodies E34.321
growth hormone insensitivity syndrome (GHIS) E34.321
insulin-like growth factor 1 gene (IGF1) defect E34.321
insulin-like growth factor-1 receptor (IGF-1R) defect E34.322
insulin-like growth factor-1 (IGF-1) resistance E34.322
NPR-2 gene variant E34.328
post-insulin-like growth factor-1 receptor signaling defect E34.322
primary insulin-like growth factor-1 (IGF-1) deficiency E34.321
severe primary insulin-like growth factor-1 deficiency (SPIGFD) E34.321
signal transducer and activator of transcription 5B gene (STAT5b) defect E34.321
specified genetic cause NEC E34.328
Laron-type E34.321
tendon — see also Contraction, tendon
with contracture of joint — see Contraction, joint
Achilles (acquired) M67.0- ☑
congenital Q66.89
congenital Q79.8
thigh (acquired) — see also Deformity, limb, unequal length, femur
congenital — see Defect, reduction, lower limb, longitudinal, femur
tibialis anterior (tendon) — see Contraction, tendon
umbilical cord
complicating delivery O69.3 ☑
upper limb, congenital — see Defect, reduction, upper limb, specified type NEC
urethra N36.8
uvula, congenital Q38.5
vagina (congenital) Q52.4
Shortsightedness — see Myopia
Shoshin (acute fulminating beriberi) E51.11
Shoulder — see condition
Shovel-shaped incisors K00.2
Shower, thromboembolic — see Embolism
Shunt
arterial-venous (dialysis) Z99.2
arteriovenous, pulmonary (acquired) I28.0
congenital Q25.72
cerebral ventricle (communicating) in situ Z98.2
surgical, prosthetic, with complications — see Complications, cardiovascular, device or implant
Shutdown, renal N28.9
Shy-Drager syndrome G90.3
Sialadenitis, sialadenosis (any gland) (chronic) (periodic) (suppurative) — see Sialoadenitis
Sialectasia K11.8
Sialidosis E77.1
Sialitis, silitis (any gland) (chronic) (suppurative) — see Sialoadenitis
Sialoadenitis (any gland) (periodic) (suppurative) K11.20
acute K11.21
recurrent K11.22
chronic K11.23
Sialoadenopathy K11.9
Sialoangitis — see Sialoadenitis
Sialodochitis (fibrinosa) — see Sialoadenitis
Sialodocholithiasis K11.5
Sialolithiasis K11.5
Sialometaplasia, necrotizing K11.8
Sialorrhea — see also Ptyalism
periodic — see Sialoadenitis
Sialosis K11.7
Siamese twin Q89.4
Sibling rivalry Z62.891
Sicard's syndrome G52.7

☑ Additional Character Required — Refer to the Tabular List for Character Selection

Sicca syndrome — *see* Syndrome, Sjögren
Sick R69
or handicapped person in family Z63.79
needing care at home Z63.6
sinus (syndrome) I49.5
Sick-euthyroid syndrome E07.81
Sickle-cell
anemia — *see* Disease, sickle-cell
beta plus — *see* Disease, sickle-cell, thalassemia, beta
plus
beta zero — *see* Disease, sickle-cell, thalassemia, beta
zero
trait D57.3
Sicklemia — *see also* Disease, sickle-cell
trait D57.3
Sickness
air (travel) T75.3 ☑
airplane T75.3 ☑
alpine T70.29 ☑
altitude T70.20 ☑
Andes T70.29 ☑
aviator's T70.29 ☑
balloon T70.29 ☑
car T75.3 ☑
compressed air T70.3 ☑
decompression T70.3 ☑
green D50.8
milk — *see* Poisoning, food, noxious
motion T75.3 ☑
mountain T70.29 ☑
acute D75.1
protein — *see also* Reaction, serum T80.69 ☑
radiation T66 ☑
roundabout (motion) T75.3 ☑
sea T75.3 ☑
serum NEC — *see also* Reaction, serum T80.69 ☑
sleeping (African) B56.9
by Trypanosoma B56.9
brucei
gambiense B56.0
rhodesiense B56.1
East African B56.1
Gambian B56.0
Rhodesian B56.1
West African B56.0
swing (motion) T75.3 ☑
train (railway) (travel) T75.3 ☑
travel (any vehicle) T75.3 ☑
Sideropenia — *see* Anemia, iron deficiency
Siderosilicosis J62.8
Siderosis (lung) J63.4
brain G93.89
eye (globe) — *see* Disorder, globe, degenerative,
siderosis
Siemens' syndrome (ectodermal dysplasia) Q82.8
Sighing R06.89
psychogenic F45.8
Sigmoid — *see also* condition
flexure — *see* condition
kidney Q63.1
Sigmoiditis — *see also* Enteritis K52.9
infectious A09
noninfectious K52.9
Silfverskiöld's syndrome Q78.9
Silicosiderosis J62.8
Silicosis, silicotic (simple) (complicated) J62.8
with tuberculosis J65
Silicotuberculosis J65
Silo-fillers' disease J68.8
bronchitis J68.0
pneumonitis J68.0
pulmonary edema J68.1
Silver's syndrome Q87.19
Simian malaria B53.1
Simmonds' cachexia or disease E23.0
Simons' disease or syndrome (progressive lipodystrophy) E88.1
Simple, simplex — *see* condition
Simulation, conscious (of illness) Z76.5
Simultanagnosia (asimultagnosia) R48.3
Sin Nombre virus disease (Hantavirus) (cardio)-pulmonary syndrome) B33.4
Sinding-Larsen disease or osteochondrosis — *see*
Osteochondrosis, juvenile, patella
Singapore hemorrhagic fever A91
Singer's node or nodule J38.2

Single
atrium Q21.20
coronary artery Q24.5
umbilical artery Q27.0
ventricle Q20.4
Singultus R06.6
epidemicus B33.0
Sinus — *see also* Fistula
abdominal K63.89
arrest I45.5
arrhythmia I49.8
bradycardia R00.1
branchial cleft (internal) (external) Q18.0
coccygeal — *see* Sinus, pilonidal
dental K04.6
dermal (congenital) Q06.8
with abscess Q06.8
coccygeal, pilonidal — *see* Sinus, coccygeal
infected, skin NEC L08.89
marginal, ruptured or bleeding — *see* Hemorrhage,
antepartum, specified cause NEC
medial, face and neck Q18.8
pause I45.5
pericranii Q01.9
pilonidal (infected) (rectum) L05.92
with abscess L05.02
preauricular Q18.1
rectovaginal N82.3
Rokitansky-Aschoff (gallbladder) K82.8
sacrococcygeal (dermoid) (infected) — *see* Sinus, pilonidal
tachycardia R00.0
paroxysmal I47.1
tarsi syndrome M25.57- ☑
testis N50.89
tract (postinfective) — *see* Fistula
urachus Q64.4
Sinusitis (accessory) (chronic) (hyperplastic) (nasal)
(nonpurulent) (purulent) J32.9
acute J01.90
ethmoidal J01.20
recurrent J01.21
frontal J01.10
recurrent J01.11
involving more than one sinus, other than pansinusitis J01.80
recurrent J01.81
maxillary J01.00
recurrent J01.01
pansinusitis J01.40
recurrent J01.41
recurrent J01.91
specified NEC J01.80
recurrent J01.81
sphenoidal J01.30
recurrent J01.31
allergic — *see* Rhinitis, allergic
due to high altitude T70.1 ☑
ethmoidal J32.2
acute J01.20
recurrent J01.21
frontal J32.1
acute J01.10
recurrent J01.11
influenzal — *see* Influenza, with, respiratory manifestations NEC
involving more than one sinus but not pansinusitis
J32.8
acute J01.80
recurrent J01.81
maxillary J32.0
acute J01.00
recurrent J01.01
sphenoidal J32.3
acute J01.30
recurrent J01.31
tuberculous, any sinus A15.8
Sinusitis-bronchiectasis-situs inversus (syndrome)
(triad) Q89.3
Sipple's syndrome E31.22
Sirenomelia (syndrome) Q87.2
Siriasis T67.01 ☑
Sirkari's disease B55.0
Siti A65
Situation, psychiatric F99
Situational
disturbance (transient) — *see* Disorder, adjustment
acute F43.0

Situational — *continued*
maladjustment — *see* Disorder, adjustment
reaction — *see* Disorder, adjustment
acute F43.0
Situs inversus or transversus (abdominalis) (thoracis)
Q89.3
Sixth disease B08.20
due to human herpesvirus 6 B08.21
due to human herpesvirus 7 B08.22
Sjögren-Larsson syndrome Q87.19
Sjögren's syndrome or disease — *see* Syndrome, Sjögren
Skeletal — *see* condition
Skene's gland — *see* condition
Skenitis — *see* Urethritis
Skerljevo A65
Skevas-Zerfus disease — *see* Toxicity, venom, marine
animal, sea anemone
Skin — *see also* condition
clammy R23.1
donor — *see* Donor, skin
dry L85.3
hidebound M35.9
Slate-dressers' or slate-miners' lung J62.8
Sleep
apnea — *see* Apnea, sleep
deprivation Z72.820
disorder or disturbance G47.9
child F51.9
nonorganic origin F51.9
specified NEC G47.8
disturbance G47.9
nonorganic origin F51.9
drunkenness F51.9
rhythm inversion G47.2- ☑
terrors F51.4
walking F51.3
hysterical F44.89
Sleep hygiene
abuse Z72.821
inadequate Z72.821
poor Z72.821
Sleeping sickness — *see* Sickness, sleeping
Sleeplessness — *see* Insomnia
menopausal N95.1
Sleep-wake schedule disorder G47.20
Slim disease (in HIV infection) B20
Slipped, slipping
epiphysis (traumatic) — *see also* Osteochondropathy,
specified type NEC
capital femoral (traumatic) [SCFE]
acute (on chronic) S79.01- ☑
nontraumatic M93.00- ☑
current traumatic — *code as* Fracture, by site
upper femoral (nontraumatic) [SUFE] M93.00- ☑
acute M93.01- ☑
on chronic M93.03- ☑
chronic M93.02- ☑
intervertebral disc — *see* Displacement, intervertebral
disc
ligature, umbilical P51.8
patella — *see* Disorder, patella, derangement NEC
rib M89.8X8
sacroiliac joint — *see* subcategory M53.2 ☑
tendon — *see* Disorder, tendon
ulnar nerve, nontraumatic — *see* Lesion, nerve, ulnar
vertebra NEC — *see* Spondylolisthesis
Slocumb's syndrome E27.0
Sloughing (multiple) (phagedena) (skin) — *see also*
Gangrene
abscess — *see* Abscess
appendix K38.8
fascia — *see* Disorder, soft tissue, specified type NEC
scrotum N50.89
tendon — *see* Disorder, tendon
transplanted organ — *see* Rejection, transplant
ulcer — *see* Ulcer, skin
Slow
feeding, newborn P92.2
flow syndrome, coronary I20.8
heart (beat) R00.1
Slowing, urinary stream R39.198
Sluder's neuralgia (syndrome) G44.89
Slurred, slurring speech R47.81
Small (ness)
for gestational age — *see* Small for dates
introitus, vagina N89.6

Small — *continued*
kidney (unknown cause) N27.9
  bilateral N27.1
  unilateral N27.0
ovary (congenital) Q50.39
pelvis
  with disproportion (fetopelvic) O33.1
    causing obstructed labor O65.1
uterus N85.8
white kidney N03.9
Small-and-light-for-dates — *see* Small for dates
Small-for-dates (infant) P05.10
with weight of
  499 grams or less P05.11
  500-749 grams P05.12
  750-999 grams P05.13
  1000-1249 grams P05.14
  1250-1499 grams P05.15
  1500-1749 grams P05.16
  1750-1999 grams P05.17
  2000-2499 grams P05.18
  2500 grams and over P05.19
specified NEC P05.19
Smallpox B03
Smearing, fecal R15.1
SMEI (severe myoclonic epilepsy in infancy) G40.83-
Smith-Lemli-Opitz syndrome E78.72
Smith's fracture S52.54- ☑
Smoker — *see* Dependence, drug, nicotine
Smoker's
bronchitis J41.0
cough J41.0
palate K13.24
throat J31.2
tongue K13.24
Smoking
passive Z77.22
Smothering spells R06.81
Snaggle teeth, tooth M26.39
Snapping
finger — *see* Trigger finger
hip — *see* Derangement, joint, specified type NEC, hip
  involving the iliotiblial band M76.3- ☑
knee — *see* Derangement, knee
  involving the iliotiblial band M76.3- ☑
Sneddon-Wilkinson disease or syndrome (sub-corneal
  pustular dermatosis) L13.1
Sneezing (intractable) R06.7
Sniffing
cocaine
  abuse — *see* Abuse, drug, cocaine
  dependence — *see* Dependence, drug, cocaine
gasoline
  abuse — *see* Abuse, drug, inhalant
  dependence — *see* Dependence, drug, inhalant
glue (airplane)
  abuse — *see* Abuse, drug, inhalant
  drug dependence — *see* Dependence, drug, in-
    halant
Sniffles
newborn P28.89
Snoring R06.83
Snow blindness — *see* Photokeratitis
Snuffles (non-syphilitic) R06.5
newborn P28.89
syphilitic (infant) A50.05 *[J99]*
Social
exclusion Z60.4
  due to discrimination or persecution (perceived)
    Z60.5
migrant Z59.00
  acculturation difficulty Z60.3
rejection Z60.4
  due to discrimination or persecution Z60.5
role conflict NEC Z73.5
skills inadequacy NEC Z73.4
transplantation Z60.3
Sodoku A25.0
Soemmerring's ring — *see* Cataract, secondary
Soft — *see also* condition
nails L60.3
Softening
bone — *see* Osteomalacia
brain (necrotic) (progressive) G93.89
  congenital Q04.8
  embolic I63.4- ☑

Softening — *continued*
brain — *continued*
  hemorrhagic — *see* Hemorrhage, intracranial, intrac-
    erebral
  occlusive I63.5- ☑
  thrombotic I63.3- ☑
cartilage M94.2- ☑
  patella M22.4- ☑
cerebellar — *see* Softening, brain
cerebral — *see* Softening, brain
cerebrospinal — *see* Softening, brain
myocardial, heart — *see* Degeneration, myocardial
spinal cord G95.89
stomach K31.89
Soldier's
heart F45.8
patches I31.0
Solitary
cyst, kidney N28.1
kidney, congenital Q60.0
Solvent abuse — *see* Abuse, drug, inhalant
dependence — *see* Dependence, drug, inhalant
Somatization reaction, somatic reaction — *see* Disorder, somatoform
Somnambulism F51.3
hysterical F44.89
Somnolence R40.0
nonorganic origin F51.11
Sonne dysentery A03.3
Soor B37.0
Sore
bed — *see* Ulcer, pressure, by site
chiclero B55.1
Delhi B55.1
desert — *see* Ulcer, skin
eye H57.1- ☑
Lahore B55.1
mouth K13.79
  canker K12.0
muscle M79.10
Naga — *see* Ulcer, skin
of skin — *see* Ulcer, skin
oriental B55.1
pressure — *see* Ulcer, pressure, by site
skin L98.9
soft A57
throat (acute) — *see also* Pharyngitis
  with influenza, flu, or grippe — *see* Influenza, with,
    respiratory manifestations NEC
  chronic J31.2
  coxsackie (virus) B08.5
  diphtheritic A36.0
  herpesviral B00.2
  influenzal — *see* Influenza, with, respiratory mani-
    festations NEC
  septic J02.0
  streptococcal (ulcerative) J02.0
  viral NEC J02.8
    coxsackie B08.5
tropical — *see* Ulcer, skin
veldt — *see* Ulcer, skin
Soto's syndrome (cerebral gigantism) Q87.3
South African cardiomyopathy syndrome I42.8
Southeast Asian hemorrhagic fever A91
Spacing
abnormal, tooth, teeth, fully erupted M26.30
excessive, tooth, fully erupted M26.32
Spade-like hand (congenital) Q68.1
Spading nail L60.8
congenital Q84.6
Spanish collar N47.1
Sparganosis B70.1
Spasm(s), **spastic, spasticity** — *see also* condition R25.2
accommodation — *see* Spasm, of accommodation
ampulla of Vater K83.4
anus, ani (sphincter) (reflex) K59.4
  psychogenic F45.8
artery I73.9
  cerebral G45.9
Bell's G51.3- ☑
bladder (sphincter, external or internal) N32.89
  psychogenic F45.8
bronchus, bronchiole J98.01
cardia K22.0
cardiac I20.1
carpopedal — *see* Tetany
cerebral (arteries) (vascular) G45.9

Spasm(s), **spastic, spasticity** — *continued*
cervix, complicating delivery O62.4
ciliary body (of accommodation) — *see* Spasm, of accommodation
colon — *see also* Irritable, bowel K58.9
  with diarrhea K58.0
  psychogenic F45.8
common duct K83.8
compulsive — *see* Tic
conjugate H51.8
coronary (artery) I20.1
diaphragm (reflex) R06.6
  epidemic B33.0
  psychogenic F45.8
duodenum K59.89
epidemic diaphragmatic (transient) B33.0
esophagus (diffuse) K22.4
  psychogenic F45.8
facial G51.3- ☑
fallopian tube N83.8
gastrointestinal (tract) K31.89
  psychogenic F45.8
glottis J38.5
  hysterical F44.4
  psychogenic F45.8
    conversion reaction F44.4
  reflex through recurrent laryngeal nerve J38.5
habit — *see* Tic
heart I20.1
hemifacial (clonic) G51.3- ☑
hourglass — *see* Contraction, hourglass
hysterical F44.4
infantile — *see* Epilepsy, spasms
inferior oblique, eye H51.8
intestinal — *see also* Syndrome, irritable bowel K58.9
  psychogenic F45.8
larynx, laryngeal J38.5
  hysterical F44.4
  psychogenic F45.8
    conversion reaction F44.4
levator palpebrae superioris — *see* Disorder, eyelid
  function
muscle NEC M62.838
  back M62.830
nerve, trigeminal G51.0
nervous F45.8
nodding F98.4
occupational F48.8
oculogyric H51.8
  psychogenic F45.8
of accommodation H52.53- ☑
ophthalmic artery — *see* Occlusion, artery, retina
perineal, female N94.89
peroneo-extensor — *see also* Deformity, limb, flat foot
pharynx (reflex) J39.2
  hysterical F45.8
  psychogenic F45.8
psychogenic F45.8
pylorus NEC K31.3
  adult hypertrophic K31.89
  congenital or infantile Q40.0
  psychogenic F45.8
rectum (sphincter) K59.4
  psychogenic F45.8
retinal (artery) — *see* Occlusion, artery, retina
sigmoid — *see also* Syndrome, irritable bowel K58.9
  psychogenic F45.8
sphincter of Oddi K83.4
stomach K31.89
  neurotic F45.8
throat J39.2
  hysterical F45.8
  psychogenic F45.8
tic F95.9
  chronic F95.1
  transient of childhood F95.0
tongue K14.8
torsion (progressive) G24.1
trigeminal nerve — *see* Neuralgia, trigeminal
ureter N13.5
urethra (sphincter) N35.919
uterus N85.8
  complicating labor O62.4
vagina N94.2
  psychogenic F52.5
vascular I73.9
vasomotor I73.9
vein NEC I87.8

Spasm(s), spastic, spasticity — *continued*
  viscera — *see* Pain, abdominal
Spasmodic — *see* condition
Spasmophilia — *see* Tetany
Spasmus nutans F98.4
Spastic, spasticity — *see also* Spasm
  child (cerebral) (congenital) (paralysis) G80.1
Speaker's throat R49.8
Specific, specified — *see* condition
Speech
  defect, disorder, disturbance, impediment — *see* Disorder, speech R47.9
  psychogenic, in childhood and adolescence F98.8
  slurring R47.81
  specified NEC R47.89
Spells, transient oxygen desaturation of newborn
  — *see also* Apnea, newborn P28.40
  during sleep — *see also* Apnea, newborn, sleep, primary P28.30
Spencer's disease A08.19
Spens' syndrome (syncope with heart block) I45.9
Sperm counts (fertility testing) Z31.41
  postvasectomy Z30.8
    reversal Z31.42
Spermatic cord — *see* condition
Spermatocele N43.40
  congenital Q55.4
  multiple N43.42
  single N43.41
Spermatocystitis N49.0
Spermatocytoma C62.9- ☑
  specified site — *see* Neoplasm, malignant, by site
Spermatorrhea N50.89
Sphacelus — *see* Gangrene
Sphenoidal — *see* condition
Sphenoiditis (chronic) — *see* Sinusitis, sphenoidal
Sphenopalatine ganglion neuralgia G90.09
Sphericity, increased, lens (congenital) Q12.4
Spherocytosis (congenital) (familial) (hereditary) D58.0
  hemoglobin disease D58.0
  sickle-cell (disease) D57.8- ☑
Spherophakia Q12.4
Sphincter — *see* condition
Sphincteritis, sphincter of Oddi — *see* Cholangitis
Sphingolipidosis E75.3
  specified NEC E75.29
Sphingomyelinosis E75.3
Spicule tooth K00.2
Spider
  bite — *see* Toxicity, venom, spider
    nonvenomous — *see* Bite, by site, superficial, insect
  fingers — *see* Syndrome, Marfan's
  nevus I78.1
  toes — *see* Syndrome, Marfan's
  vascular I78.1
Spiegler-Fendt
  benign lymphocytoma L98.8
  sarcoid L08.89
Spielmeyer-Vogt disease E75.4
Spina bifida (aperta) Q05.9
  with hydrocephalus NEC Q05.4
  cervical Q05.5
    with hydrocephalus Q05.0
  dorsal Q05.6
  lumbar Q05.7
    with hydrocephalus Q05.2
  lumbosacral Q05.7
    with hydrocephalus Q05.2
  occulta Q76.0
  sacral Q05.8
    with hydrocephalus Q05.3
  thoracic Q05.6
    with hydrocephalus Q05.1
  thoracolumbar Q05.6
    with hydrocephalus Q05.1
Spindle, Krukenberg's — *see* Pigmentation, cornea, posterior
Spine, spinal — *see* condition
Spiradenoma (eccrine) — *see* Neoplasm, skin, benign
Spirillosis A25.0
Spirillum
  minus A25.0
  obermeieri infection A68.0
Spirochetal — *see* condition
Spirochetosis A69.9
  arthritic, arthritica A69.9

Spirochetosis — *continued*
  bronchopulmonary A69.8
  icterohemorrhagic A27.0
  lung A69.8
Spirometrosis B70.1
Spitting blood — *see* Hemoptysis
Splanchnoptosis K63.4
Spleen, splenic — *see* condition
Splenectasis — *see* Splenomegaly
Splenitis (interstitial) (malignant) (nonspecific) D73.89
  malarial — *see also* Malaria B54 *[D77]*
  tuberculous A18.85
Splenocele D73.89
Splenomegaly, splenomegalia (Bengal) (cryptogenic) (idiopathic) (tropical) R16.1
  with hepatomegaly R16.2
  cirrhotic D73.2
  congenital Q89.09
  congestive, chronic D73.2
  Egyptian B65.1
  Gaucher's E75.22
  malarial — *see also* Malaria B54 *[D77]*
  neutropenic D73.81
  Niemann-Pick — *see* Niemann-Pick disease or syndrome
  siderotic D73.2
  syphilitic A52.79
    congenital (early) A50.08 *[D77]*
Splenopathy D73.9
Splenoptosis D73.89
Splenosis D73.89
Splinter — *see* Foreign body, superficial, by site
Split, splitting
  foot Q72.7- ☑
  hand Q71.6 ☑
  heart sounds R01.2
  lip, congenital — *see* Cleft, lip
  nails L60.3
  urinary stream R39.13
Spondylarthrosis — *see* Spondylosis
Spondylitis (chronic) — *see also* Spondylopathy, inflammatory
  ankylopoietica — *see* Spondylitis, ankylosing
  ankylosing (chronic) M45.9
    with lung involvement M45.9 *[J99]*
    cervical region M45.2
    cervicothoracic region M45.3
    juvenile M08.1
    lumbar region M45.6
    lumbosacral region M45.7
    multiple sites M45.0
    occipito-atlanto-axial region M45.1
    sacrococcygeal region M45.8
    thoracic region M45.4
    thoracolumbar region M45.5
  atrophic (ligamentous) — *see* Spondylitis, ankylosing
  deformans (chronic) — *see* Spondylosis
  gonococcal A54.41
  gouty — *see also* Gout, by type, vertebrae M10.08
  in (due to)
    brucellosis A23.9 *[M49.80]*
      cervical region A23.9 *[M49.82]*
      cervicothoracic region A23.9 *[M49.83]*
      lumbar region A23.9 *[M49.86]*
      lumbosacral region A23.9 *[M49.87]*
      multiple sites A23.9 *[M49.89]*
      occipito-atlanto-axial region A23.9 *[M49.81]*
      sacrococcygeal region A23.9 *[M49.88]*
      thoracic region A23.9 *[M49.84]*
      thoracolumbar region A23.9 *[M49.85]*
    enterobacteria — *see also* subcategory M49.8 A04.9
    tuberculosis A18.01
  infectious NEC — *see* Spondylopathy, infective
  juvenile ankylosing (chronic) M08.1
  Kümmell's — *see* Spondylopathy, traumatic
  Marie-Strümpell — *see* Spondylitis, ankylosing
  muscularis — *see* Spondylopathy, specified NEC
  psoriatic L40.53
  rheumatoid — *see* Spondylitis, ankylosing
  rhizomelica — *see* Spondylitis, ankylosing
  sacroiliac NEC M46.1
  senescent, senile — *see* Spondylosis
  traumatic (chronic) or post-traumatic — *see* Spondylopathy, traumatic
  tuberculous A18.01
  typhosa A01.05

Spondyloarthritis
  axial — *see also* Spondlyitis, ankylosing
    non-radiographic M45.A0
      cervical M45.A2
      cervicothoracic M45.A3
      lumbar M45.A6
      lumbosacral M45.A7
      multiple sites M45.AB
      occipito-atlanto-axial region M45.A1
      sacral and sacrococcygeal M45.A8
      thoracic M45.A4
      thoracolumbar M45.A5
Spondylolisthesis (acquired) (degenerative) M43.10
  with disproportion (fetopelvic) O33.0
    causing obstructed labor O65.0
  cervical region M43.12
  cervicothoracic region M43.13
  congenital Q76.2
  lumbar region M43.16
  lumbosacral region M43.17
  multiple sites M43.19
  occipito-atlanto-axial region M43.11
  sacrococcygeal region M43.18
  thoracic region M43.14
  thoracolumbar region M43.15
  traumatic (old) M43.10
    acute
      fifth cervical (displaced) S12.430 ☑
        nondisplaced S12.431 ☑
        specified type NEC (displaced) S12.450 ☑
          nondisplaced S12.451 ☑
        type III S12.44 ☑
      fourth cervical (displaced) S12.330 ☑
        nondisplaced S12.331 ☑
        specified type NEC (displaced) S12.350 ☑
          nondisplaced S12.351 ☑
        type III S12.34 ☑
      second cervical (displaced) S12.130 ☑
        nondisplaced S12.131 ☑
        specified type NEC (displaced) S12.150 ☑
          nondisplaced S12.151 ☑
        type III S12.14 ☑
      seventh cervical (displaced) S12.630 ☑
        nondisplaced S12.631 ☑
        specified type NEC (displaced) S12.650 ☑
          nondisplaced S12.651 ☑
        type III S12.64 ☑
      sixth cervical (displaced) S12.530 ☑
        nondisplaced S12.531 ☑
        specified type NEC (displaced) S12.550 ☑
          nondisplaced S12.551 ☑
        type III S12.54 ☑
      third cervical (displaced) S12.230 ☑
        nondisplaced S12.231 ☑
        specified type NEC (displaced) S12.250 ☑
          nondisplaced S12.251 ☑
        type III S12.24 ☑
Spondylolysis (acquired) M43.00
  cervical region M43.02
  cervicothoracic region M43.03
  congenital Q76.2
  lumbar region M43.06
  lumbosacral region M43.07
    with disproportion (fetopelvic) O33.0
      causing obstructed labor O65.8
  multiple sites M43.09
  occipito-atlanto-axial region M43.01
  sacrococcygeal region M43.08
  thoracic region M43.04
  thoracolumbar region M43.05
Spondylopathy M48.9
  infective NEC M46.50
    cervical region M46.52
    cervicothoracic region M46.53
    lumbar region M46.56
    lumbosacral region M46.57
    multiple sites M46.59
    occipito-atlanto-axial region M46.51
    sacrococcygeal region M46.58
    thoracic region M46.54
    thoracolumbar region M46.55
  inflammatory M46.90
    cervical region M46.92
    cervicothoracic region M46.93
    lumbar region M46.96
    lumbosacral region M46.97
    multiple sites M46.99

Spondylopathy — continued
- inflammatory — continued
  - occipito-atlanto-axial region M46.91
  - sacrococcygeal region M46.98
  - specified type NEC M46.80
    - cervical region M46.82
    - cervicothoracic region M46.83
    - lumbar region M46.86
    - lumbosacral region M46.87
    - multiple sites M46.89
    - occipito-atlanto-axial region M46.81
    - sacrococcygeal region M46.88
    - thoracic region M46.84
    - thoracolumbar region M46.85
  - thoracic region M46.94
  - thoracolumbar region M46.95
- neuropathic, in
  - syringomyelia and syringobulbia G95.0
  - tabes dorsalis A52.11
- specified NEC — see subcategory M48.8 ☑
- traumatic M48.30
  - cervical region M48.32
  - cervicothoracic region M48.33
  - lumbar region M48.36
  - lumbosacral region M48.37
  - occipito-atlanto-axial region M48.31
  - sacrococcygeal region M48.38
  - thoracic region M48.34
  - thoracolumbar region M48.35

Spondylosis M47.9
- with
  - disproportion (fetopelvic) O33.0
    - causing obstructed labor O65.0
  - myelopathy NEC M47.10
    - cervical region M47.12
    - cervicothoracic region M47.13
    - lumbar region M47.16
    - occipito-atlanto-axial region M47.11
    - thoracic region M47.14
    - thoracolumbar region M47.15
  - radiculopathy M47.20
    - cervical region M47.22
    - cervicothoracic region M47.23
    - lumbar region M47.26
    - lumbosacral region M47.27
    - occipito-atlanto-axial region M47.21
    - sacrococcygeal region M47.28
    - thoracic region M47.24
    - thoracolumbar region M47.25
- specified NEC M47.899
  - cervical region M47.892
  - cervicothoracic region M47.893
  - facet joint — see also Spondylosis M47.819
  - lumbar region M47.896
  - lumbosacral region M47.897
  - occipito-atlanto-axial region M47.891
  - sacrococcygeal region M47.898
  - thoracic region M47.894
  - thoracolumbar region M47.895
- traumatic — see Spondylopathy, traumatic
- without myelopathy or radiculopathy M47.819
  - cervical region M47.812
  - cervicothoracic region M47.813
  - lumbar region M47.816
  - lumbosacral region M47.817
  - occipito-atlanto-axial region M47.811
  - sacrococcygeal region M47.818
  - thoracic region M47.814
  - thoracolumbar region M47.815

Sponge
- inadvertently left in operation wound — see Foreign body, accidentally left during a procedure
- kidney (medullary) Q61.5

Sponge-diver's disease — see Toxicity, venom, marine animal, sea anemone

Spongioblastoma (any type) — see Neoplasm, malignant, by site
- specified site — see Neoplasm, malignant, by site
- unspecified site C71.9

Spongioneuroblastoma — see Neoplasm, malignant, by site

Spontaneous — see also condition
- fracture (cause unknown) — see Fracture, pathological

Spoon nail L60.3
- congenital Q84.6

Sporadic — see condition

Sporothrix schenckii infection — see Sporotrichosis

Sporotrichosis B42.9

Sporotrichosis — continued
- arthritis B42.82
- disseminated B42.7
- generalized B42.7
- lymphocutaneous (fixed) (progressive) B42.1
- pulmonary B42.0
- specified NEC B42.89

Spots, spotting (in) (of)
- Bitot's — see also Pigmentation, conjunctiva
  - in the young child E50.1
    - vitamin A deficiency E50.1
- café, au lait L81.3
- Cayenne pepper I78.1
- cotton wool, retina — see Occlusion, artery, retina
- de Morgan's (senile angiomas) I78.1
- Fuchs' black (myopic) — see also Myopia, degenerative H44.2-
- intermenstrual (regular) N92.0
  - irregular N92.1
- Koplik's B05.9
- liver L81.4
- pregnancy O26.85- ☑
- purpuric R23.3
- ruby I78.1

Spotted fever — see Fever, spotted A77.9

Sprain (joint) (ligament)
- acromioclavicular joint or ligament S43.5- ☑
- ankle S93.40- ☑
  - calcaneofibular ligament S93.41- ☑
  - deltoid ligament S93.42- ☑
  - internal collateral ligament — see Sprain, ankle, specified ligament NEC
  - specified ligament NEC S93.49- ☑
  - talofibular ligament — see Sprain, ankle, specified ligament NEC
  - tibiofibular ligament S93.43- ☑
- anterior longitudinal, cervical S13.4 ☑
- atlas, atlanto-axial, atlanto-occipital S13.4 ☑
- breast bone — see Sprain, sternum
- calcaneofibular — see Sprain, ankle
- carpal — see Sprain, wrist
- carpometacarpal — see Sprain, hand, specified site NEC
- cartilage
  - costal S23.41 ☑
  - semilunar (knee) — see Sprain, knee, specified site NEC
    - with current tear — see Tear, meniscus
  - thyroid region S13.5 ☑
  - xiphoid — see Sprain, sternum
- cervical, cervicodorsal, cervicothoracic S13.4 ☑
- chondrosternal S23.421 ☑
- coracoclavicular S43.8- ☑
- coracohumeral S43.41- ☑
- coronary, knee — see Sprain, knee, specified site NEC
- costal cartilage S23.41 ☑
- cricoarytenoid articulation or ligament S13.5 ☑
- cricothyroid articulation S13.5 ☑
- cruciate, knee — see Sprain, knee, cruciate
- deltoid, ankle — see Sprain, ankle
- dorsal (spine) S23.3 ☑
- elbow S53.40- ☑
  - radial collateral ligament S53.43- ☑
  - radiohumeral S53.41- ☑
  - rupture
    - radial collateral ligament — see Rupture, traumatic, ligament, radial collateral
    - ulnar collateral ligament — see Rupture, traumatic, ligament, ulnar collateral
  - specified type NEC S53.49- ☑
  - ulnar collateral ligament S53.44- ☑
  - ulnohumeral S53.42- ☑
- femur, head — see Sprain, hip
- fibular collateral, knee — see Sprain, knee, collateral
- fibulocalcaneal — see Sprain, ankle
- finger(s) S63.61- ☑
  - index S63.61- ☑
  - interphalangeal (joint) S63.63- ☑
    - index S63.63- ☑
    - little S63.63- ☑
    - middle S63.63- ☑
    - ring S63.63- ☑
  - little S63.61- ☑
  - metacarpophalangeal (joint) S63.65- ☑
  - middle S63.61- ☑
  - ring S63.61- ☑

Sprain — continued
- finger(s) — continued
  - specified site NEC S63.69- ☑
    - index S63.69- ☑
    - little S63.69- ☑
    - middle S63.69- ☑
    - ring S63.69- ☑
- foot S93.60- ☑
  - specified ligament NEC S93.69- ☑
  - tarsal ligament S93.61- ☑
  - tarsometatarsal ligament S93.62- ☑
  - toe — see Sprain, toe
- hand S63.9- ☑
  - finger — see Sprain, finger
  - specified site NEC — see subcategory S63.8 ☑
  - thumb — see Sprain, thumb
- head S03.9 ☑
- hip S73.10- ☑
  - iliofemoral ligament S73.11- ☑
  - ischiocapsular (ligament) S73.12- ☑
  - specified NEC S73.19- ☑
- iliofemoral — see Sprain, hip
- innominate
  - acetabulum — see Sprain, hip
  - sacral junction S33.6 ☑
- internal
  - collateral, ankle — see Sprain, ankle
  - semilunar cartilage — see Sprain, knee, specified site NEC
- interphalangeal
  - finger — see Sprain, finger, interphalangeal (joint)
  - toe — see Sprain, toe, interphalangeal joint
- ischiocapsular — see Sprain, hip
- ischiofemoral — see Sprain, hip
- jaw (articular disc) (cartilage) (meniscus) S03.4- ☑
  - old M26.69
- knee S83.9- ☑
  - collateral ligament S83.40- ☑
    - lateral (fibular) S83.42- ☑
    - medial (tibial) S83.41- ☑
  - cruciate ligament S83.50- ☑
    - anterior S83.51- ☑
    - posterior S83.52- ☑
  - lateral (fibular) collateral ligament S83.42- ☑
  - medial (tibial) collateral ligament S83.41- ☑
  - patellar ligament S76.11- ☑
  - specified site NEC S83.8X- ☑
  - superior tibiofibular joint (ligament) S83.6- ☑
- lateral collateral, knee — see Sprain, knee, collateral
- lumbar (spine) S33.5 ☑
- lumbosacral S33.9 ☑
- mandible (articular disc) S03.4- ☑
  - old M26.69
- medial collateral, knee — see Sprain, knee, collateral
- meniscus
  - jaw S03.4- ☑
    - old M26.69
  - knee — see Sprain, knee, specified site NEC
    - with current tear — see Tear, meniscus
      - old — see Derangement, knee, meniscus, due to old tear
  - mandible S03.4- ☑
    - old M26.69
- metacarpal (distal) (proximal) — see Sprain, hand, specified site NEC
- metacarpophalangeal — see Sprain, finger, metacarpophalangeal (joint)
- metatarsophalangeal — see Sprain, toe, metatarsophalangeal joint
- midcarpal — see Sprain, hand, specified site NEC
- midtarsal — see Sprain, foot, specified site NEC
- neck S13.9 ☑
  - anterior longitudinal cervical ligament S13.4 ☑
  - atlanto-axial joint S13.4 ☑
  - atlanto-occipital joint S13.4 ☑
  - cervical spine S13.4 ☑
  - cricoarytenoid ligament S13.5 ☑
  - cricothyroid ligament S13.5 ☑
  - specified site NEC S13.8 ☑
  - thyroid region (cartilage) S13.5 ☑
- nose S03.8 ☑
- orbicular, hip — see Sprain, hip
- patella — see Sprain, knee, specified site NEC
- patellar ligament S76.11- ☑
- pelvis NEC S33.8 ☑

☑ Additional Character Required — Refer to the Tabular List for Character Selection

Sprain — *continued*
  phalanx
    finger — *see* Sprain, finger
    toe — *see* Sprain, toe
  pubofemoral — *see* Sprain, hip
  radiocarpal — *see* Sprain, wrist
  radiohumeral — *see* Sprain, elbow
  radius, collateral — *see* Rupture, traumatic, ligament, radial collateral
  rib (cage) S23.41 ☑
  rotator cuff (capsule) S43.42- ☑
  sacroiliac (region)
    chronic or old — *see* subcategory M53.2 ☑
    joint S33.6 ☑
  scaphoid (hand) — *see* Sprain, hand, specified site NEC
  scapula (r) — *see* Sprain, shoulder girdle, specified site NEC
  semilunar cartilage (knee) — *see* Sprain, knee, specified site NEC
    with current tear — *see* Tear, meniscus
      old — *see* Derangement, knee, meniscus, due to old tear
  shoulder joint S43.40- ☑
    acromioclavicular joint (ligament) — *see* Sprain, acromioclavicular joint
    blade — *see* Sprain, shoulder, girdle, specified site NEC
    coracoclavicular joint (ligament) — *see* Sprain, coracoclavicular joint
    coracohumeral ligament — *see* Sprain, coracohumeral joint
    girdle S43.9- ☑
      specified site NEC S43.8- ☑
    rotator cuff — *see* Sprain, rotator cuff
    specified site NEC S43.49- ☑
    sternoclavicular joint (ligament) — *see* Sprain, sternoclavicular joint
  spine
    cervical S13.4 ☑
    lumbar S33.5 ☑
    thoracic S23.3 ☑
  sternoclavicular joint S43.6- ☑
  sternum S23.429
    chondrosternal joint S23.421 ☑
    specified site NEC S23.428 ☑
    sternoclavicular (joint) (ligament) S23.420 ☑
  symphysis
    jaw S03.4- ☑
      old M26.69
    mandibular S03.4- ☑
      old M26.69
  talofibular — *see* Sprain, ankle
  tarsal — *see* Sprain, foot, specified site NEC
  tarsometatarsal — *see* Sprain, foot, specified site NEC
  temporomandibular S03.4- ☑
    old M26.69
  thorax S23.9 ☑
    ribs S23.41 ☑
    specified site NEC S23.8 ☑
    spine S23.3 ☑
    sternum — *see* Sprain, sternum
  thumb S63.60- ☑
    interphalangeal (joint) S63.62- ☑
    metacarpophalangeal (joint) S63.64- ☑
    specified site NEC S63.68- ☑
  thyroid cartilage or region S13.5 ☑
  tibia (proximal end) — *see* Sprain, knee, specified site NEC
  tibial collateral, knee — *see* Sprain, knee, collateral
  tibiofibular
    distal — *see* Sprain, ankle
    superior — *see* Sprain, knee, specified site NEC
  toe(s) S93.50- ☑
    great S93.50- ☑
    interphalangeal joint S93.51- ☑
      great S93.51- ☑
      lesser S93.51- ☑
    lesser S93.50- ☑
    metatarsophalangeal joint S93.52- ☑
      great S93.52- ☑
      lesser S93.52- ☑
  ulna, collateral — *see* Rupture, traumatic, ligament, ulnar collateral
  ulnohumeral — *see* Sprain, elbow
  wrist S63.50- ☑
    carpal S63.51- ☑

Sprain — *continued*
  wrist — *continued*
    radiocarpal S63.52- ☑
    specified site NEC S63.59- ☑
  xiphoid cartilage — *see* Sprain, sternum
Sprengel's deformity (congenital) Q74.0
Sprue (tropical) K90.1
  celiac K90.0
  idiopathic K90.49
  meaning thrush B37.0
  nontropical K90.0
Spur, bone — *see also* Enthesopathy
  calcaneal M77.3-
  iliac crest M76.2- ☑
  nose (septum) J34.89
Spurway's syndrome Q78.0
Sputum
  abnormal (amount) (color) (odor) (purulent) R09.3
  blood-stained R04.2
  excessive (cause unknown) R09.3
Squamous — *see also* condition
  epithelium in
    cervical canal (congenital) Q51.828
    uterine mucosa (congenital) Q51.818
Squashed nose M95.0
  congenital Q67.4
Squeeze, diver's T70.3 ☑
Squint — *see also* Strabismus
  accommodative — *see* Strabismus, convergent concomitant
SSADHD (succinic semialdehyde dehydrogenase deficiency) E72.81
St. Hubert's disease A82.9
Stab — *see also* Laceration
  internal organs — *see* Injury, by site
Stafne's cyst or cavity M27.0
Staggering gait R26.0
  hysterical F44.4
Staghorn calculus — *see* Calculus, kidney
Stähli's line (cornea) (pigment) — *see* Pigmentation, cornea, anterior
Stain, staining
  meconium (newborn) P96.83
  port wine Q82.5
  tooth, teeth (hard tissues) (extrinsic) K03.6
    due to
      accretions K03.6
      deposits (betel) (black) (green) (materia alba) (orange) (soft) (tobacco) K03.6
      metals (copper) (silver) K03.7
      nicotine K03.6
      pulpal bleeding K03.7
      tobacco K03.6
    intrinsic K00.8
Stammering — *see also* Disorder, fluency F80.81
Standstill
  auricular I45.5
  cardiac — *see* Arrest, cardiac
  sinoatrial I45.5
  ventricular — *see* Arrest, cardiac
Stannosis J63.5
Stanton's disease — *see* Melioidosis
Staphylitis (acute) (catarrhal) (chronic) (gangrenous) (membranous) (suppurative) (ulcerative) K12.2
Staphylococcal scalded skin syndrome L00
Staphylococcemia A41.2
Staphylococcus, staphylococcal — *see also* condition
  as cause of disease classified elsewhere B95.8
    aureus (methicillin susceptible) (MSSA) B95.61
      methicillin resistant (MRSA) B95.62
    specified NEC, as cause of disease classified elsewhere B95.7
Staphyloma (sclera)
  cornea H18.72- ☑
  equatorial H15.81- ☑
  localized (anterior) H15.82- ☑
  posticum H15.83- ☑
  ring H15.85- ☑
Stargardt's disease — *see* Dystrophy, retina
Starvation (inanition) (due to lack of food) T73.0 ☑
  edema — *see* Malnutrition, severe
Stasis
  bile (noncalculous) K83.1
  bronchus J98.09
    with infection — *see* Bronchitis
  cardiac — *see* Failure, heart, congestive
  cecum K59.89

Stasis — *continued*
  colon K59.89
  dermatitis I87.2
    with
      varicose ulcer — *see* Varix, leg, with ulcer, with inflammation
      varicose veins — *see* Varix, leg, with, inflammation
    due to postthrombotic syndrome — *see* Syndrome, postthrombotic
  duodenal K31.5
  eczema — *see* Varix, leg, with, inflammation
  edema — *see* Hypertension, venous (chronic), idiopathic
  foot T69.0- ☑
  ileocecal coil K59.89
  ileum K59.89
  intestinal K59.89
  jejunum K59.89
  kidney N19
  liver (cirrhotic) K76.1
  lymphatic I89.8
  pneumonia J18.2
  pulmonary — *see* Edema, lung
  rectal K59.89
  renal N19
    tubular N17.0
  ulcer — *see* Varix, leg, with, ulcer
    without varicose veins I87.2
  urine — *see* Retention, urine
  venous I87.8
State (of)
  affective and paranoid, mixed, organic psychotic F06.8
  agitated R45.1
    acute reaction to stress F43.0
  anxiety (neurotic) F41.1
  apprehension F41.1
  burn-out Z73.0
  climacteric, female Z78.0
    symptomatic N95.1
  compulsive F42.8
    mixed with obsessional thoughts F42.2
  confusional (psychogenic) F44.89
    acute — *see also* Delirium
      with
        arteriosclerotic dementia — *see also* Dementia, vascular F01.50
          with behavioral disturbance — *see* Dementia, vascular
        senility or dementia F05
      alcoholic F10.231
      epileptic F05
      reactive (from emotional stress, psychological trauma) F44.89
    subacute — *see* Delirium
  convulsive — *see* Convulsions
  crisis F43.0
  depressive F32.A
    neurotic F34.1
  dissociative F44.9
  emotional shock (stress) R45.7
  hypercoagulation — *see* Hypercoagulable
  locked-in G83.5
  menopausal Z78.0
    symptomatic N95.1
  neurotic F48.9
    with depersonalization F48.1
  obsessional F42.8
  oneiroid (schizophrenia-like) F23
  organic
    hallucinatory (nonalcoholic) F06.0
    paranoid (-hallucinatory) F06.2
  panic F41.0
  paranoid F22
    climacteric F22
    involutional F22
    menopausal F22
    organic F06.2
    senile F03 ☑
    simple F22
  persistent vegetative R40.3
  phobic F40.9
  postleukotomy F07.0
  pregnant
    gestational carrier Z33.3
    incidental Z33.1
  psychogenic, twilight F44.89
  psychopathic (constitutional) F60.2

State — *continued*
psychotic, organic — *see also* Psychosis, organic
  mixed paranoid and affective F06.8
  senile or presenile F03 ☑
  transient NEC F06.8
    with
      depression F06.31
      hallucinations F06.0
residual schizophrenic F20.5
restlessness R45.1
stress (emotional) R45.7
tension (mental) F48.9
  specified NEC F48.8
transient organic psychotic NEC F06.8
  depressive type F06.31
  hallucinatory type F06.0
twilight
  epileptic F05
  psychogenic F44.89
vegetative, persistent R40.3
vital exhaustion Z73.0
withdrawal, — *see* Withdrawal, state
Status (post) — *see also* Presence (of)
absence, epileptic — *see* Epilepsy, by type, with status epilepticus
administration of tPA (rtPA) in a different facility within the last 24 hours prior to admission to current facility Z92.82
adrenalectomy (unilateral) (bilateral) E89.6
anastomosis Z98.0
anginosus I20.9
angioplasty (peripheral) Z98.62
  with implant Z95.820
  coronary artery Z98.61
    with implant Z95.5
aortocoronary bypass Z95.1
arthrodesis Z98.1
artificial opening (of) Z93.9
  gastrointestinal tract Z93.4
  specified NEC Z93.8
  urinary tract Z93.6
  vagina Z93.8
asthmaticus — *see* Asthma, by type, with status asthmaticus
awaiting organ transplant Z76.82
bariatric surgery Z98.84
bed confinement Z74.01
bleb, filtering (vitreous), after glaucoma surgery Z98.83
breast implant Z98.82
  removal Z98.86
cataract extraction Z98.4- ☑
cholecystectomy Z90.49
clitorectomy N90.811
  with excision of labia minora N90.812
colectomy (complete) (partial) Z90.49
colonization — *see* Carrier (suspected) of
colostomy Z93.3
convulsivus idiopathicus — *see* Epilepsy, by type, with status epilepticus
coronary artery angioplasty — *see* Status, angioplasty, coronary artery
coronary artery bypass graft Z95.1
cystectomy (urinary bladder) Z90.6
cystostomy Z93.50
  appendico-vesicostomy Z93.52
  cutaneous Z93.51
  specified NEC Z93.59
delinquent immunization Z28.39
  COVID-19 Z28.31- ☑
dental Z98.818
  crown Z98.811
  fillings Z98.811
  restoration Z98.811
  sealant Z98.810
  specified NEC Z98.818
deployment (current) (military) Z56.82
dialysis (hemodialysis) (peritoneal) Z99.2
do not resuscitate (DNR) Z66
donor — *see* Donor
embedded fragments — *see* Retained, foreign body fragments (type of)
embedded splinter — *see* Retained, foreign body fragments (type of)
enterostomy Z93.4
epileptic, epilepticus — *see also* Epilepsy, by type, with status epilepticus G40.901
estrogen receptor
  negative Z17.1

Status — *continued*
estrogen receptor — *continued*
  positive Z17.0
female genital cutting — *see* Female genital mutilation status
female genital mutilation — *see* Female genital mutilation status
filtering (vitreous) bleb after glaucoma surgery Z98.83
gastrectomy (complete) (partial) Z90.3
gastric banding Z98.84
gastric bypass for obesity Z98.84
gastrostomy Z93.1
human immunodeficiency virus (HIV) infection, asymptomatic Z21
hysterectomy (complete) (total) Z90.710
  partial (with remaining cervial stump) Z90.711
ileostomy Z93.2
implant
  breast Z98.82
infibulation N90.813
intestinal bypass Z98.0
jejunostomy Z93.4
lapsed immunization schedule Z28.39
laryngectomy Z90.02
lymphaticus E32.8
malignancy
  castrate resistant prostate Z19.2
  hormone resistant Z19.2
  hormone sensitive Z19.1
marmoratus G80.3
mastectomy (unilateral) (bilateral) Z90.1- ☑
military deployment status (current) Z56.82
  in theater or in support of military war, peacekeeping and humanitarian operations Z56.82
nephrectomy (unilateral) (bilateral) Z90.5
nephrostomy Z93.6
obesity surgery Z98.84
oophorectomy
  bilateral Z90.722
  unilateral Z90.721
organ replacement
  by artificial or mechanical device or prosthesis of
    artery Z95.828
    bladder Z96.0
    blood vessel Z95.828
    breast Z97.8
    eye globe Z97.0
    heart Z95.812
      valve Z95.2
    intestine Z97.8
    joint Z96.60
      hip — *see* Presence, hip joint implant
      knee — *see* Presence, knee joint implant
      specified site NEC Z96.698
    kidney Z97.8
    larynx Z96.3
    lens Z96.1
    limbs — *see* Presence, artificial, limb
    liver Z97.8
    lung Z97.8
    pancreas Z97.8
  by organ transplant (heterologous) (homologous) — *see* Transplant
pacemaker
  brain Z96.89
  cardiac Z95.0
  specified NEC Z96.89
pancreatectomy Z90.410
  complete Z90.410
  partial Z90.411
  total Z90.410
physical restraint Z78.1
pneumonectomy (complete) (partial) Z90.2
pneumothorax, therapeutic Z98.3
postcommotio cerebri F07.81
postoperative (postprocedural) NEC Z98.890
  breast implant Z98.82
  dental Z98.818
    crown Z98.811
    fillings Z98.811
    restoration Z98.811
    sealant Z98.810
    specified NEC Z98.818
  pneumothorax, therapeutic Z98.3
  uterine scar Z98.891
postpartum (routine follow-up) Z39.2
  care immediately after delivery Z39.0
postsurgical (postprocedural) NEC Z98.890
  pneumothorax, therapeutic Z98.3

Status — *continued*
pregnancy, incidental Z33.1
prosthesis coronary angioplasty Z95.5
pseudophakia Z96.1
renal dialysis (hemodialysis) (peritoneal) Z99.2
retained foreign body — *see* Retained, foreign body fragments (type of)
reversed jejunal transposition (for bypass) Z98.0
salpingo-oophorectomy
  bilateral Z90.722
  unilateral Z90.721
sex reassignment surgery status Z87.890
shunt
  arteriovenous (for dialysis) Z99.2
  cerebrospinal fluid Z98.2
  ventricular (communicating) (for drainage) Z98.2
splenectomy Z90.81
thymicolymphaticus E32.8
thymicus E32.8
thymolymphaticus E32.8
thyroidectomy (hypothyroidism) E89.0
tooth (teeth) extraction — *see also* Absence, teeth, acquired K08.409
tPA (rtPA) administration in a different facility within the last 24 hours prior to admission to current facility Z92.82
tracheostomy Z93.0
transplant — *see* Transplant
  organ removed Z98.85
tubal ligation Z98.51
underimmunization Z28.39
  COVID-19 Z28.31- ☑
    partially vaccinated (for) Z28.311
    unvaccinated (for) Z28.310
ureterostomy Z93.6
urethrostomy Z93.6
vagina, artificial Z93.8
vasectomy Z98.52
wheelchair confinement Z99.3
Stealing
child problem F91.8
  in company with others Z72.810
pathological (compulsive) F63.2
Steam burn — *see* Burn
Steatocystoma multiplex L72.2
Steatohepatitis (nonalcoholic) (NASH) K75.81
Steatoma L72.3
eyelid (cystic) — *see* Dermatosis, eyelid
  infected — *see* Hordeolum
Steatorrhea (chronic) K90.9
with lacteal obstruction K90.2
idiopathic (adult) (infantile) K90.9
pancreatic K90.3
primary K90.0
tropical K90.1
Steatosis E88.89
heart — *see* Degeneration, myocardial
kidney N28.89
liver NEC K76.0
Steele-Richardson-Olszewski disease or syndrome G23.1
Steinbrocker's syndrome G90.8
Steinert's disease G71.11
Stein-Leventhal syndrome E28.2
Stein's syndrome E28.2
STEMI — *see also* Infarct, myocardium, ST elevation I21.3
Stenocardia I20.8
Stenocephaly Q75.8
Stenosis, stenotic (cicatricial) — *see also* Stricture
ampulla of Vater K83.1
anus, anal (canal) (sphincter) K62.4
  and rectum K62.4
  congenital Q42.3
    with fistula Q42.2
aorta (ascending) (supraventricular) (congenital) Q25.1
  arteriosclerotic I70.0
  calcified I70.0
  supravalvular Q25.3
aortic (valve) I35.0
  with insufficiency I35.2
  congenital Q23.0
  rheumatic I06.0
    with
      incompetency, insufficiency or regurgitation I06.2
        with mitral (valve) disease I08.0
          with tricuspid (valve) disease I08.3
      mitral (valve) disease I08.0

Stenosis, stenotic — continued
- aortic — continued
  - rheumatic — continued
    - with — continued
      - mitral disease — continued
        - with tricuspid (valve) disease I08.3
        - tricuspid (valve) disease I08.2
          - with mitral (valve) disease I08.3
  - specified cause NEC I35.0
  - syphilitic A52.03
- aqueduct of Sylvius (congenital) Q03.0
  - with spina bifida — see Spina bifida, by site, with hydrocephalus
  - acquired G91.1
- artery NEC — see also Arteriosclerosis I77.1
  - celiac I77.4
  - cerebral — see Occlusion, artery, cerebral
  - extremities — see Arteriosclerosis, extremities
  - precerebral — see Occlusion, artery, precerebral
  - pulmonary (congenital) Q25.6
    - acquired I28.8
  - renal I70.1
  - stent
    - coronary T82.855 ☑
    - peripheral T82.856 ☑
- bile duct (common) (hepatic) K83.1
  - congenital Q44.3
- bladder-neck (acquired) N32.0
  - congenital Q64.31
- brain G93.89
- bronchus J98.09
  - congenital Q32.3
  - syphilitic A52.72
- cardia (stomach) K22.2
  - congenital Q39.3
- cardiovascular — see Disease, cardiovascular
- caudal M48.08
- cervix, cervical (canal) N88.2
  - congenital Q51.828
  - in pregnancy or childbirth — see Pregnancy, complicated by, abnormal cervix
- colon — see also Obstruction, intestine
  - congenital Q42.9
    - specified NEC Q42.8
- colostomy K94.03
- common (bile) duct K83.1
  - congenital Q44.3
- coronary (artery) — see Disease, heart, ischemic, atherosclerotic
- cystic duct — see Obstruction, gallbladder
- due to presence of device, implant or graft — see also Complications, by site and type, specified NEC T85.858 ☑
  - arterial graft NEC T82.858 ☑
  - breast (implant) T85.858 ☑
  - catheter T85.858 ☑
    - dialysis (renal) T82.858 ☑
      - intraperitoneal T85.858 ☑
    - infusion NEC T82.858 ☑
      - spinal (epidural) (subdural) T85.850 ☑
    - urinary (indwelling) T83.85 ☑
  - fixation, internal (orthopedic) NEC T84.85 ☑
  - gastrointestinal (bile duct) (esophagus) T85.858 ☑
  - genital NEC T83.85 ☑
  - heart NEC T82.857 ☑
  - joint prosthesis T84.85 ☑
  - ocular (corneal graft) (orbital implant) NEC T85.858 ☑
  - orthopedic NEC T84.85 ☑
  - specified NEC T85.858 ☑
  - urinary NEC T83.85 ☑
  - vascular NEC T82.858 ☑
  - ventricular intracranial shunt T85.850 ☑
- duodenum K31.5
  - congenital Q41.0
- ejaculatory duct NEC N50.89
  - stent
    - vascular
      - end stent
        - adjacent to stent — see Arteriosclerosis
        - within the stent
          - coronary T82.855 ☑
          - peripheral T82.856 ☑
      - in stent
        - coronary vessel T82.855 ☑
        - peripheral vessel T82.856 ☑
- endocervical os — see Stenosis, cervix

Stenosis, stenotic — continued
- enterostomy K94.13
- esophagus K22.2
  - congenital Q39.3
  - syphilitic A52.79
    - congenital A50.59 [K23]
- eustachian tube — see Obstruction, eustachian tube
- external ear canal (acquired) H61.30- ☑
  - congenital Q16.1
  - due to
    - inflammation H61.32- ☑
    - trauma H61.31- ☑
  - postprocedural H95.81- ☑
  - specified cause NEC H61.39- ☑
- gallbladder — see Obstruction, gallbladder
- glottis J38.6
- heart valve — see also Endocarditis I38
  - aortic — see Stenosis, aortic
  - congenital Q24.8
  - mitral — see Stenosis, mitral
  - pulmonary — see Stenosis, pulmonary valve
  - tricuspid — see Stenosis, tricuspid
- hepatic duct K83.1
- hymen N89.6
- hypertrophic subaortic (idiopathic) I42.1
- ileum — see also Obstruction, intestine, specified NEC K56.699
  - congenital Q41.2
- infundibulum cardia Q24.3
- intervertebral foramina — see also Lesion, biomechanical, specified NEC
  - connective tissue M99.79
    - abdomen M99.79
    - cervical region M99.71
    - cervicothoracic M99.71
    - head region M99.70
    - lumbar region M99.73
    - lumbosacral M99.73
    - occipitocervical M99.70
    - sacral region M99.74
    - sacrococcygeal M99.74
    - sacroiliac M99.74
    - specified NEC M99.79
    - thoracic region M99.72
    - thoracolumbar M99.72
  - disc M99.79
    - abdomen M99.79
    - cervical region M99.71
    - cervicothoracic M99.71
    - head region M99.70
    - lower extremity M99.76
    - lumbar region M99.73
    - lumbosacral M99.73
    - occipitocervical M99.70
    - pelvic M99.75
    - rib cage M99.78
    - sacral region M99.74
    - sacrococcygeal M99.74
    - sacroiliac M99.74
    - specified NEC M99.79
    - thoracic region M99.72
    - thoracolumbar M99.72
    - upper extremity M99.77
  - osseous M99.69
    - abdomen M99.69
    - cervical region M99.61
    - cervicothoracic M99.61
    - head region M99.60
    - lower extremity M99.66
    - lumbar region M99.63
    - lumbosacral M99.63
    - occipitocervical M99.60
    - pelvic M99.65
    - rib cage M99.68
    - sacral region M99.64
    - sacrococcygeal M99.64
    - sacroiliac M99.64
    - specified NEC M99.69
    - thoracic region M99.62
    - thoracolumbar M99.62
    - upper extremity M99.67
  - subluxation — see Stenosis, intervertebral foramina, osseous
- intestine — see also Obstruction, intestine
  - congenital (small) Q41.9
    - large Q42.9
      - specified NEC Q42.8
    - specified NEC Q41.8

Stenosis, stenotic — continued
- jejunum — see also Obstruction, intestine, specified NEC K56.699
  - congenital Q41.1
- lacrimal (passage)
  - canaliculi H04.54- ☑
  - congenital Q10.5
  - duct H04.55- ☑
  - punctum H04.56- ☑
  - sac H04.57- ☑
- lacrimonasal duct — see Stenosis, lacrimal, duct
  - congenital Q10.5
- larynx J38.6
  - congenital NEC Q31.8
    - subglottic Q31.1
  - syphilitic A52.73
    - congenital A50.59 [J99]
- mitral (chronic) (inactive) (valve) I05.0
  - with
    - aortic valve disease I08.0
    - incompetency, insufficiency or regurgitation I05.2
  - active or acute I01.1
    - with rheumatic or Sydenham's chorea I02.0
  - congenital Q23.2
  - specified cause, except rheumatic I34.2
  - syphilitic A52.03
- myocardium, myocardial — see also Degeneration, myocardial
  - hypertrophic subaortic (idiopathic) I42.1
- nares (anterior) (posterior) J34.89
  - congenital Q30.0
- nasal duct — see also Stenosis, lacrimal, duct
  - congenital Q10.5
- nasolacrimal duct — see also Stenosis, lacrimal, duct
  - congenital Q10.5
- neural canal — see also Lesion, biomechanical, specified NEC
  - connective tissue M99.49
    - abdomen M99.49
    - cervical region M99.41
    - cervicothoracic M99.41
    - head region M99.40
    - lower extremity M99.46
    - lumbar region M99.43
    - lumbosacral M99.43
    - occipitocervical M99.40
    - pelvic M99.45
    - rib cage M99.48
    - sacral region M99.44
    - sacrococcygeal M99.44
    - sacroiliac M99.44
    - specified NEC M99.49
    - thoracic region M99.42
    - thoracolumbar M99.42
    - upper extremity M99.47
  - intervertebral disc M99.59
    - abdomen M99.59
    - cervical region M99.51
    - cervicothoracic M99.51
    - head region M99.50
    - lower extremity M99.56
    - lumbar region M99.53
    - lumbosacral M99.53
    - occipitocervical M99.50
    - pelvic M99.55
    - rib cage M99.58
    - sacral region M99.54
    - sacrococcygeal M99.54
    - sacroiliac M99.54
    - specified NEC M99.59
    - thoracic region M99.52
    - thoracolumbar M99.52
    - upper extremity M99.57
  - osseous M99.39
    - abdomen M99.39
    - cervical region M99.31
    - cervicothoracic M99.31
    - head region M99.30
    - lower extremity M99.36
    - lumbar region M99.33
    - lumbosacral M99.33
    - occipitocervical M99.30
    - pelvic M99.35
    - rib cage M99.38
    - sacral region M99.34
    - sacrococcygeal M99.34
    - sacroiliac M99.34

Stenosis, stenotic — *continued*
  neural canal — *see also* Lesion, biomechanical, specified — *continued*
    osseous — *continued*
      specified NEC M99.39
      thoracic region M99.32
      thoracolumbar M99.32
      upper extremity M99.37
    subluxation M99.29
      cervical region M99.21
      cervicothoracic M99.21
      head region M99.20
      lower extremity M99.26
      lumbar region M99.23
      lumbosacral M99.23
      occipitocervical M99.20
      pelvic M99.25
      rib cage M99.28
      sacral region M99.24
      sacrococcygeal M99.24
      sacroiliac M99.24
      specified NEC M99.29
      thoracic region M99.22
      thoracolumbar M99.22
      upper extremity M99.27
  organ or site, congenital NEC — *see* Atresia, by site
  papilla of Vater K83.1
  pulmonary (artery) (congenital) Q25.6
    with ventricular septal defect, transposition of aorta, and hypertrophy of right ventricle Q21.3
    acquired I28.8
    in tetralogy of Fallot Q21.3
    infundibular Q24.3
    subvalvular Q24.3
    supravalvular Q25.6
    valve I37.0
      with insufficiency I37.2
      congenital Q22.1
      rheumatic I09.89
        with aortic, mitral or tricuspid (valve) disease I08.8
    vein, acquired I28.8
    vessel NEC I28.8
  pulmonic (congenital) Q22.1
    infundibular Q24.3
    subvalvular Q24.3
  pylorus (hypertrophic) (acquired) K31.1
    adult K31.1
    congenital Q40.0
    infantile Q40.0
  rectum (sphincter) — *see* Stricture, rectum
  renal artery I70.1
    congenital Q27.1
  salivary duct (any) K11.8
  sphincter of Oddi K83.1
  spinal M48.00
    cervical region M48.02
    cervicothoracic region M48.03
    lumbar region (NOS) (without neurogenic claudication) M48.061
      with neurogenic claudication M48.062
    lumbosacral region M48.07
    occipito-atlanto-axial region M48.01
    sacrococcygeal region M48.08
    thoracic region M48.04
    thoracolumbar region M48.05
  stomach, hourglass K31.2
  subaortic (congenital) Q24.4
    hypertrophic (idiopathic) I42.1
  subglottic J38.6
    congenital Q31.1
    postprocedural J95.5
  trachea J39.8
    congenital Q32.1
    syphilitic A52.73
    tuberculous NEC A15.5
  tracheostomy J95.03
  tricuspid (valve) I07.0
    with
      aortic (valve) disease I08.2
      incompetency, insufficiency or regurgitation I07.2
        with aortic (valve) disease I08.2
          with mitral (valve) disease I08.3
      mitral (valve) disease I08.1
        with aortic (valve) disease I08.3
    congenital Q22.4
    nonrheumatic I36.0
      with insufficiency I36.2

Stenosis, stenotic — *continued*
  tubal N97.1
  ureter — *see* Atresia, ureter
  ureteropelvic junction, congenital Q62.11
  ureterovesical orifice, congenital Q62.12
  urethra (valve) *see also* Stricture, urethra
    congenital Q64.32
  urinary meatus, congenital Q64.33
  vagina N89.5
    congenital Q52.4
    in pregnancy — *see* Pregnancy, complicated by, abnormal vagina
    causing obstructed labor O65.5
  valve (cardiac) (heart) — *see also* Endocarditis I38
    congenital Q24.8
      aortic Q23.0
      mitral Q23.2
      pulmonary Q22.1
      tricuspid Q22.4
  vena cava (inferior) (superior) I87.1
    congenital Q26.0
  vesicourethral orifice Q64.31
  vulva N90.5
Stent jail T82.897 ☑
Stercolith (impaction) K56.41
  appendix K38.1
Stercoraceous, stercoral ulcer K63.3
  anus or rectum K62.6
Stereotypies NEC F98.4
Sterility — *see* Infertility
Sterilization — *see* Encounter (for), sterilization
Sternalgia — *see* Angina
Sternopagus Q89.4
Sternum bifidum Q76.7
Steroid
  effects (adverse) (adrenocortical) (iatrogenic)
    cushingoid E24.2
      correct substance properly administered — *see* Table of Drugs and Chemicals, by drug, adverse effect
      overdose or wrong substance given or taken — *see* Table of Drugs and Chemicals, by drug, poisoning
    diabetes — *see* subcategory E09 ☑
      correct substance properly administered — *see* Table of Drugs and Chemicals, by drug, adverse effect
      overdose or wrong substance given or taken — *see* Table of Drugs and Chemicals, by drug, poisoning
    fever R50.2
    insufficiency E27.3
      correct substance properly administered — *see* Table of Drugs and Chemicals, by drug, adverse effect
      overdose or wrong substance given or taken — *see* Table of Drugs and Chemicals, by drug, poisoning
    responder H40.04- ☑
Stevens-Johnson disease or syndrome L51.1
  toxic epidermal necrolysis overlap L51.3
Stewart-Morel syndrome M85.2
Sticker's disease B08.3
Sticky eye — *see* Conjunctivitis, acute, mucopurulent
Stieda's disease — *see* Bursitis, tibial collateral
Stiff neck — *see* Torticollis
Stiff-man syndrome G25.82
Stiffness, joint NEC M25.60
  ankle M25.67- ☑
  ankylosis — *see* Ankylosis, joint
  contracture — *see* Contraction, joint
  elbow M25.62- ☑
  foot M25.67- ☑
  hand M25.64- ☑
  hip M25.65- ☑
  knee M25.66- ☑
  shoulder M25.61- ☑
  specified site NEC M25.69
  wrist M25.63- ☑
Stigmata congenital syphilis A50.59
Stillbirth P95
Still-Felty syndrome — *see* Felty's syndrome
Still's disease or syndrome (juvenile) M08.20
  adult-onset M06.1
  ankle M08.27- ☑
  elbow M08.22- ☑
  foot joint M08.27- ☑

Still's disease or syndrome — *continued*
  hand joint M08.24- ☑
  hip M08.25- ☑
  knee M08.26- ☑
  multiple site M08.29
  shoulder M08.21- ☑
  specified site NEC M08.2A
  vertebra M08.28
  wrist M08.23- ☑
Stimulation, ovary E28.1
Sting (venomous) (with allergic or anaphylactic shock) — *see* Table of Drugs and Chemicals, by animal or substance, poisoning
Stippled epiphyses Q78.8
Stitch
  abscess T81.41 ☑
  burst (in operation wound) — *see* Disruption, wound, operation
Stokes' disease E05.00
  with thyroid storm E05.01
Stokes-Adams disease or syndrome I45.9
Stokvis (-Talma) **disease** D74.8
Stoma malfunction
  colostomy K94.03
  enterostomy K94.13
  gastrostomy K94.23
  ileostomy K94.13
  tracheostomy J95.03
Stomach — *see* condition
Stomatitis (denture) (ulcerative) K12.1
  angular K13.0
    due to dietary or vitamin deficiency E53.0
  aphthous K12.0
  bovine B08.61
  candidal B37.0
  catarrhal K12.1
  diphtheritic A36.89
  due to
    dietary deficiency E53.0
    thrush B37.0
    vitamin deficiency
      B group NEC E53.9
      B2 (riboflavin) E53.0
  epidemic B08.8
  epizootic B08.8
  follicular K12.1
  gangrenous A69.0
  Geotrichum B48.3
  herpesviral, herpetic B00.2
  herpetiformis K12.0
  malignant K12.1
  membranous acute K12.1
  monilial B37.0
  mycotic B37.0
  necrotizing ulcerative A69.0
  parasitic B37.0
  septic K12.1
  spirochetal A69.1
  suppurative (acute) K12.2
  ulceromembranous A69.1
  vesicular K12.1
    with exanthem (enteroviral) B08.4
    virus disease A93.8
  Vincent's A69.1
Stomatocytosis D58.8
Stomatomycosis B37.0
Stomatorrhagia K13.79
Stone(s) — *see also* Calculus
  bladder (diverticulum) N21.0
  cystine E72.09
  heart syndrome I50.1
  kidney N20.0
  prostate N42.0
  pulpal (dental) K04.2
  renal N20.0
  salivary gland or duct (any) K11.5
  urethra (impacted) N21.1
  urinary (duct) (impacted) (passage) N20.9
    bladder (diverticulum) N21.0
    lower tract N21.9
    specified NEC N21.8
  xanthine E79.8 *[N22]*
Stonecutter's lung J62.8
Stonemason's asthma, disease, lung or pneumoconiosis J62.8
Stoppage
  heart — *see* Arrest, cardiac
  urine — *see* Retention, urine

Storm, thyroid — *see* Thyrotoxicosis
Strabismus (congenital) (nonparalytic) H50.9
  concomitant H50.40
    convergent — *see* Strabismus, convergent concomitant
    divergent — *see* Strabismus, divergent concomitant
  convergent concomitant H50.00
    accommodative component H50.43
    alternating H50.05
      with
        A pattern H50.06
        specified nonconcomitances NEC H50.08
        V pattern H50.07
    monocular H50.01- ☑
      with
        A pattern H50.02-
        specified nonconcomitances NEC H50.04- ☑
        V pattern H50.03- ☑
      intermittent H50.31- ☑
        alternating H50.32
  cyclotropia H50.41 ☑
  divergent concomitant H50.10
    alternating H50.15
      with
        A pattern H50.16
        specified noncomitances NEC H50.18
        V pattern H50.17
    monocular H50.11- ☑
      with
        A pattern H50.12- ☑
        specified noncomitances NEC H50.14- ☑
        V pattern H50.13- ☑
      intermittent H50.33 ☑
        alternating H50.34
  Duane's syndrome H50.81- ☑
  due to adhesions, scars H50.69
  heterophoria H50.50
    alternating H50.55
    cyclophoria H50.54
    esophoria H50.51
    exophoria H50.52
    vertical H50.53
  heterotropia H50.40
    intermittent H50.30
  hypertropia H50.2- ☑
  hypotropia — *see* Hypertropia
  latent H50.50
  mechanical H50.60
    Brown's sheath syndrome H50.61- ☑
    specified type NEC H50.69
  monofixation syndrome H50.42
  paralytic H49.9
    abducens nerve H49.2- ☑
    fourth nerve H49.1- ☑
    Kearns-Sayre syndrome H49.81- ☑
    ophthalmoplegia (external)
      progressive H49.4- ☑
        with pigmentary retinopathy H49.81- ☑
      total H49.3- ☑
    sixth nerve H49.2- ☑
    specified type NEC H49.88- ☑
    third nerve H49.0- ☑
    trochlear nerve H49.1- ☑
  specified type NEC H50.89
  vertical H50.2- ☑
Strain
  back S39.012 ☑
  cervical S16.1 ☑
  eye NEC — *see* Disturbance, vision, subjective
  heart — *see* Disease, heart
  low back S39.012 ☑
  mental NOS Z73.3
    work-related Z56.6
  muscle (tendon) — *see* Injury, muscle, by site, strain
  neck S16.1 ☑
  physical NOS Z73.3
    work-related Z56.6
  postural — *see also* Disorder, soft tissue, due to use
  psychological NEC Z73.3
  tendon — *see* Injury, muscle, by site, strain
Straining, on urination R39.16
Strand, vitreous — *see* Opacity, vitreous, membranes and strands
Strangulation, strangulated — *see also* Asphyxia, traumatic
  appendix K38.8
  bladder-neck N32.0

Strangulation, strangulated — *continued*
  bowel or colon K56.2
  food or foreign body — *see* Foreign body, by site
  hemorrhoids — *see* Hemorrhoids, with complication
  hernia — *see also* Hernia, by site, with obstruction
    with gangrene — *see* Hernia, by site, with gangrene
  intestine (large) (small) K56.2
    with hernia — *see also* Hernia, by site, with obstruction
      with gangrene — *see* Hernia, by site, with gangrene
  mesentery K56.2
  mucus — *see* Asphyxia, mucus
  omentum K56.2
  organ or site, congenital NEC — *see* Atresia, by site
  ovary — *see* Torsion, ovary
  penis N48.89
    foreign body T19.4 ☑
  rupture — *see* Hernia, by site, with obstruction
  stomach due to hernia — *see also* Hernia, by site, with obstruction
    with gangrene — *see* Hernia, by site, with gangrene
  vesicourethral orifice N32.0
Strangury R30.0
Straw itch B88.0
Strawberry
  gallbladder K82.4
  mark Q82.5
  tongue (red) (white) K14.3
Streak(s)
  macula, angioid H35.33
  ovarian Q50.32
Strephosymbolia F81.0
  secondary to organic lesion R48.8
Streptobacillary fever A25.1
Streptobacillosis A25.1
Streptobacillus moniliformis A25.1
Streptococcus, streptococcal — *see also* condition
  as cause of disease classified elsewhere B95.5
  group
    A, as cause of disease classified elsewhere B95.0
    B, as cause of disease classified elsewhere B95.1
    D, as cause of disease classified elsewhere B95.2
    pneumoniae, as cause of disease classified elsewhere B95.3
    specified NEC, as cause of disease classified elsewhere B95.4
Streptomycosis B47.1
Streptotrichosis A48.8
Stress F43.9
  family — *see* Disruption, family
  fetal P84
    complicating pregnancy O77.9
      due to drug administration O77.1
  mental NEC Z73.3
    work-related Z56.6
  physical NEC Z73.3
    work-related Z56.6
  polycythemia D75.1
  reaction — *see also* Reaction, stress F43.9
  work schedule Z56.3
Stretching, nerve — *see* Injury, nerve
Striae albicantes, atrophicae or distensae (cutis) L90.6
Stricture — *see also* Stenosis
  ampulla of Vater K83.1
  anus (sphincter) K62.4
    congenital Q42.3
      with fistula Q42.2
    infantile Q42.3
      with fistula Q42.2
  aorta (ascending) (congenital) Q25.1
    arteriosclerotic I70.0
    calcified I70.0
    supravalvular, congenital Q25.3
  aortic (valve) — *see* Stenosis, aortic
  aqueduct of Sylvius (congenital) Q03.0
    with spina bifida — *see* Spina bifida, by site, with hydrocephalus
    acquired G91.1
  artery I77.1
    basilar — *see* Occlusion, artery, basilar
    carotid — *see* Occlusion, artery, carotid
    celiac I77.4
    congenital (peripheral) Q27.8
      cerebral Q28.3
      coronary Q24.5
      digestive system Q27.8
      lower limb Q27.8

Stricture — *continued*
  artery — *continued*
    congenital — *continued*
      retinal Q14.1
      specified site NEC Q27.8
      umbilical Q27.0
      upper limb Q27.8
    coronary — *see* Disease, heart, ischemic, atherosclerotic
      congenital Q24.5
    precerebral — *see* Occlusion, artery, precerebral
    pulmonary (congenital) Q25.6
      acquired I28.8
    renal I70.1
    vertebral — *see* Occlusion, artery, vertebral
  auditory canal (external) (congenital)
    acquired — *see* Stenosis, external ear canal
  bile duct (common) (hepatic) K83.1
    congenital Q44.3
    postoperative K91.89
  bladder N32.89
    neck N32.0
  bowel — *see* Obstruction, intestine
  brain G93.89
  bronchus J98.09
    congenital Q32.3
    syphilitic A52.72
  cardia (stomach) K22.2
    congenital Q39.3
  cardiac — *see also* Disease, heart
    orifice (stomach) K22.2
  cecum — *see* Obstruction, intestine
  cervix, cervical (canal) N88.2
    congenital Q51.828
    in pregnancy — *see* Pregnancy, complicated by, abnormal cervix
    causing obstructed labor O65.5
  colon — *see also* Obstruction, intestine
    congenital Q42.9
    specified NEC Q42.8
  colostomy K94.03
  common (bile) duct K83.1
  coronary (artery) — *see* Disease, heart, ischemic, atherosclerotic
  cystic duct — *see* Obstruction, gallbladder
  digestive organs NEC, congenital Q45.8
  duodenum K31.5
    congenital Q41.0
  ear canal (external) (congenital) Q16.1
    acquired — *see* Stricture, auditory canal, acquired
  ejaculatory duct N50.89
  enterostomy K94.13
  esophagus K22.2
    congenital Q39.3
    syphilitic A52.79
      congenital A50.59 *[K23]*
  eustachian tube — *see also* Obstruction, eustachian tube
    congenital Q17.8
  fallopian tube N97.1
    gonococcal A54.24
    tuberculous A18.17
  gallbladder — *see* Obstruction, gallbladder
  glottis J38.6
  heart — *see also* Disease, heart
    valve — *see also* Endocarditis I38
      aortic Q23.0
      mitral Q23.2
      pulmonary Q22.1
      tricuspid Q22.4
  hepatic duct K83.1
  hourglass, of stomach K31.2
  hymen N89.6
  hypopharynx J39.2
  ileum — *see also* Obstruction, intestine, specified NEC K56.699
    congenital Q41.2
  intestine — *see also* Obstruction, intestine
    congenital (small) Q41.9
      large Q42.9
        specified NEC Q42.8
      specified NEC Q41.8
    ischemic K55.1
  jejunum — *see also* Obstruction, intestine, specified NEC K56.699
    congenital Q41.1
  lacrimal passages — *see also* Stenosis, lacrimal
    congenital Q10.5

Stricture — *continued*
- larynx J38.6
  - congenital NEC Q31.8
    - subglottic Q31.1
  - syphilitic A52.73
    - congenital A50.59 *[J99]*
- meatus
  - ear (congenital) Q16.1
    - acquired — *see* Stricture, auditory canal, acquired
  - osseous (ear) (congenital) Q16.1
    - acquired — *see* Stricture, auditory canal, acquired
  - urinarius — *see also* Stricture, urethra
    - congenital Q64.33
- mitral (valve) — *see* Stenosis, mitral
- myocardium, myocardial I51.5
  - hypertrophic subaortic (idiopathic) I42.1
- nares (anterior) (posterior) J34.89
  - congenital Q30.0
- nasal duct — *see also* Stenosis, lacrimal, duct
  - congenital Q10.5
- nasolacrimal duct — *see also* Stenosis, lacrimal, duct
  - congenital Q10.5
- nasopharynx J39.2
  - syphilitic A52.73
- nose J34.89
  - congenital Q30.0
- nostril (anterior) (posterior) J34.89
  - congenital Q30.0
  - syphilitic A52.73
    - congenital A50.59 *[J99]*
- organ or site, congenital NEC — *see* Atresia, by site
- os uteri — *see* Stricture, cervix
- osseous meatus (ear) (congenital) Q16.1
  - acquired — *see* Stricture, auditory canal, acquired
- oviduct — *see* Stricture, fallopian tube
- pelviureteric junction (congenital) Q62.11
  - acquired, with hydronephrosis N13.0
- penis, by foreign body T19.4 ☑
- pharynx J39.2
- prostate N42.89
- pulmonary, pulmonic
  - artery (congenital) Q25.6
    - acquired I28.8
    - noncongenital I28.8
  - infundibulum (congenital) Q24.3
  - valve I37.0
    - congenital Q22.1
  - vein, acquired I28.8
  - vessel NEC I28.8
- punctum lacrimale — *see also* Stenosis, lacrimal, punctum
  - congenital Q10.5
- pylorus (hypertrophic) K31.1
  - adult K31.1
  - congenital Q40.0
  - infantile Q40.0
- rectosigmoid — *see also* Obstruction, intestine, specified NEC K56.699
- rectum (sphincter) K62.4
  - congenital Q42.1
    - with fistula Q42.0
  - due to
    - chlamydial lymphogranuloma A55
    - irradiation K91.89
    - lymphogranuloma venereum A55
  - gonococcal A54.6
  - inflammatory (chlamydial) A55
  - syphilitic A52.74
  - tuberculous A18.32
- renal artery I70.1
  - congenital Q27.1
- salivary duct or gland (any) K11.8
- sigmoid (flexure) — *see* Obstruction, intestine
- spermatic cord N50.89
- stoma (following) (of)
  - colostomy K94.03
  - enterostomy K94.13
  - gastrostomy K94.23
  - ileostomy K94.13
  - tracheostomy J95.03
- stomach K31.89
  - congenital Q40.2
  - hourglass K31.2
- subaortic Q24.4
  - hypertrophic (acquired) (idiopathic) I42.1
- subglottic J38.6

Stricture — *continued*
- syphilitic NEC A52.79
- trachea J39.8
  - congenital Q32.1
  - syphilitic A52.73
  - tuberculous NEC A15.5
- tracheostomy J95.03
- tricuspid (valve) — *see* Stenosis, tricuspid
- tunica vaginalis N50.89
- ureter (postoperative) N13.5
  - with
    - hydronephrosis N13.1
      - with infection N13.6
    - pyelonephritis (chronic) N11.1
  - congenital — *see* Atresia, ureter
  - tuberculous A18.11
- ureteropelvic junction (congenital) Q62.11
  - acquired, with hydronephrosis N13.0
- ureterovesical orifice N13.5
  - with infection N13.6
- urethra (organic) (spasmodic) — *see also* Stricture, urethra, male N35.919
  - associated with schistosomiasis B65.0 *[N37]*
  - congenital Q64.39
    - valvular (posterior) Q64.2
  - due to
    - infection — *see* Stricture, urethra, postinfective
    - trauma — *see* Stricture, urethra, post-traumatic
  - female N35.92
  - gonococcal, gonorrheal A54.01
  - infective NEC — *see* Stricture, urethra, postinfective
  - late effect (sequelae) of injury — *see* Stricture, urethra, post-traumatic
  - male N35.919
    - anterior urethra N35.914
    - bulbous urethra N35.912
    - meatal N35.911
    - membranous urethra N35.913
    - overlapping sites N35.916
  - postcatheterization — *see* Stricture, urethra, postprocedural
  - postinfective NEC
    - female N35.12
    - male N35.119
      - anterior urethra N35.114
      - bulbous urethra N35.112
      - meatal N35.111
      - membranous urethra N35.113
      - overlapping sites N35.116
  - postobstetric N35.021
  - postoperative — *see* Stricture, urethra, postprocedural
  - postprocedural
    - female N99.12
    - male N99.114
      - anterior bulbous urethra N99.113
      - bulbous urethra N99.111
      - fossa navicularis N99.115
      - meatal N99.110
      - membranous urethra N99.112
      - overlapping sites N99.116
  - post-traumatic
    - female N35.028
      - due to childbirth N35.021
    - male N35.014
      - anterior urethra N35.013
      - bulbous urethra N35.011
      - meatal N35.010
      - membranous urethra N35.012
      - overlapping sites N35.016
  - sequela (late effect) of
    - childbirth N35.021
    - injury — *see* Stricture, urethra, post-traumatic
  - specified cause NEC
    - female N35.82
    - male N35.819
      - anterior urethra N35.814
      - bulbous urethra N35.812
      - meatal N35.811
      - membranous urethra N35.813
      - overlapping sites N35.816
  - syphilitic A52.76
  - traumatic — *see* Stricture, urethra, post-traumatic
  - valvular (posterior), congenital Q64.2
- urinary meatus — *see* Stricture, urethra
- uterus, uterine (synechiae) N85.6
  - os (external) (internal) — *see* Stricture, cervix
- vagina (outlet) — *see* Stenosis, vagina

Stricture — *continued*
- valve (cardiac) (heart) — *see also* Endocarditis
  - congenital
    - aortic Q23.0
    - mitral Q23.2
    - pulmonary Q22.1
    - tricuspid Q22.4
- vas deferens N50.89
  - congenital Q55.4
- vein I87.1
- vena cava (inferior) (superior) NEC I87.1
  - congenital Q26.0
- vesicourethral orifice N32.0
  - congenital Q64.31
- vulva (acquired) N90.5

Stridor R06.1
- congenital (larynx) P28.89

Stridulous — *see* condition

Stroke (apoplectic) (brain) (embolic) (ischemic) (paralytic) (thrombotic) I63.9
- cerebral, perinatal P91.82- ☑
- cryptogenic — *see also* infarction, cerebral I63.9
- epileptic — *see* Epilepsy
- heat T67.01 ☑
  - exertional T67.02 ☑
  - specified NEC T67.09 ☑
- in evolution I63.9
- intraoperative
  - during cardiac surgery I97.810
  - during other surgery I97.811
- ischemic, perinatal arterial P91.82- ☑
- lightning — *see* Lightning
- meaning
  - cerebral hemorrhage — *code to* Hemorrhage, intracranial
  - cerebral infarction — *code to* Infarction, cerebral
- neonatal P91.82- ☑
- postprocedural
  - following cardiac surgery I97.820
  - following other surgery I97.821
- sun T67.01 ☑
  - specified NEC T67.09 ☑
- unspecified (NOS) I63.9

Stromatosis, endometrial D39.0

Strongyloidiasis, strongyloidosis B78.9
- cutaneous B78.1
- disseminated B78.7
- intestinal B78.0

Strophulus pruriginosus L28.2

Struck by lightning — *see* Lightning

Struma — *see also* Goiter
- Hashimoto E06.3
- lymphomatosa E06.3
- nodosa (simplex) E04.9
  - endemic E01.2
    - multinodular E01.1
  - multinodular E04.2
    - iodine-deficiency related E01.1
  - toxic or with hyperthyroidism E05.20
    - with thyroid storm E05.21
    - multinodular E05.20
      - with thyroid storm E05.21
    - uninodular E05.10
      - with thyroid storm E05.11
  - toxicosa E05.20
    - with thyroid storm E05.21
    - multinodular E05.20
      - with thyroid storm E05.21
    - uninodular E05.10
      - with thyroid storm E05.11
  - uninodular E04.1
- ovarii D27.- ☑
- Riedel's E06.5

Strumipriva cachexia E03.4

Strümpell-Marie spine — *see* Spondylitis, ankylosing

Strümpell-Westphal pseudosclerosis E83.01

Stuart deficiency disease (factor X) D68.2

Stuart-Prower factor deficiency (factor X) D68.2

Student's elbow — *see* Bursitis, elbow, olecranon

Stump — *see* Amputation

Stunting, nutritional E45

Stupor (catatonic) R40.1
- depressive (single episode) F32.89
  - recurrent episode F33.8
- dissociative F44.2
- manic F30.2
- manic-depressive F31.89
- psychogenic (aergic) F44.2

Stupor — *continued*
   reaction to exceptional stress (transient) F43.Ø
Sturge (-Weber) (-Dimitri) (-Kalischer) **disease or syndrome** Q85.89
Stuttering F8Ø.81
   adult onset F98.5
   childhood onset F8Ø.81
   following cerebrovascular disease — *see* Disorder, fluency. following cerebrovascular disease
   in conditions classified elsewhere R47.82
Sty, stye (external) (internal) (meibomian) (zeisian) — *see* Hordeolum
Subacidity, gastric K31.89
   psychogenic F45.8
Subacute — *see* condition
Subarachnoid — *see* condition
Subcortical — *see* condition
Subcostal syndrome, nerve compression — *see* Mononeuropathy, upper limb, specified site NEC
Subcutaneous, subcuticular — *see* condition
Subdural — *see* condition
Subendocardium — *see* condition
Subependymoma
   specified site — *see* Neoplasm, uncertain behavior, by site
   unspecified site D43.2
Suberosis J67.3
Subglossitis — *see* Glossitis
Subhemophilia D66
Subinvolution
   breast (postlactational) (postpuerperal) N64.89
   puerperal O9Ø.89
   uterus (chronic) (nonpuerperal) N85.3
     puerperal O9Ø.89
Sublingual — *see* condition
Sublinguitis — *see* Sialoadenitis
Subluxatable hip Q65.6
Subluxation — *see also* Dislocation
   acromioclavicular S43.11- ☑
   ankle S93.Ø- ☑
   atlantoaxial, recurrent M43.4
     with myelopathy M43.3
   carpometacarpal (joint) NEC S63.Ø5- ☑
     thumb S63.Ø4- ☑
   complex, vertebral — *see* Complex, subluxation
   congenital — *see also* Malposition, congenital
     hip — *see* Dislocation, hip, congenital, partial
     joint (excluding hip)
       lower limb Q68.8
       shoulder Q68.8
       upper limb Q68.8
   elbow (traumatic) S53.1Ø- ☑
     anterior S53.11- ☑
     lateral S53.14- ☑
     medial S53.13- ☑
     posterior S53.12- ☑
     specified type NEC S53.19- ☑
   finger S63.2Ø- ☑
     index S63.2Ø- ☑
     interphalangeal S63.22- ☑
       distal S63.24- ☑
         index S63.24- ☑
         little S63.24- ☑
         middle S63.24- ☑
         ring S63.24- ☑
       index S63.22- ☑
       little S63.22- ☑
       middle S63.22- ☑
       proximal S63.23- ☑
         index S63.23- ☑
         little S63.23- ☑
         middle S63.23- ☑
         ring S63.23- ☑
       ring S63.22- ☑
     little S63.2Ø- ☑
     metacarpophalangeal S63.21- ☑
       index S63.21- ☑
       little S63.21- ☑
       middle S63.21- ☑
       ring S63.21- ☑
     middle S63.2Ø- ☑
     ring S63.2Ø- ☑
   foot S93.3Ø- ☑
     specified site NEC S93.33- ☑
     tarsal joint S93.31- ☑
     tarsometatarsal joint S93.32- ☑

Subluxation — *continued*
   foot — *continued*
     toe — *see* Subluxation, toe
   hip S73.ØØ- ☑
     anterior S73.Ø3- ☑
       obturator S73.Ø2- ☑
     central S73.Ø4- ☑
     posterior S73.Ø1- ☑
   interphalangeal (joint)
     finger S63.22- ☑
       distal joint S63.24- ☑
         index S63.24- ☑
         little S63.24- ☑
         middle S63.24- ☑
         ring S63.24- ☑
       index S63.22- ☑
       little S63.22- ☑
       middle S63.22- ☑
       proximal joint S63.23- ☑
         index S63.23- ☑
         little S63.23- ☑
         middle S63.23- ☑
         ring S63.23- ☑
       ring S63.22- ☑
     thumb S63.12- ☑
     toe S93.13- ☑
       great S93.13- ☑
       lesser S93.13- ☑
   joint prosthesis — *see* Complications, joint prosthesis, mechanical, displacement, by site
   knee S83.1Ø- ☑
     cap — *see* Subluxation, patella
     patella — *see* Subluxation, patella
     proximal tibia
       anteriorly S83.11- ☑
       laterally S83.14- ☑
       medially S83.13- ☑
       posteriorly S83.12- ☑
     specified type NEC S83.19- ☑
   lens — *see* Dislocation, lens, partial
   ligament, traumatic — *see* Sprain, by site
   metacarpal (bone)
     proximal end S63.Ø6- ☑
   metacarpophalangeal (joint)
     finger S63.21- ☑
       index S63.21- ☑
       little S63.21- ☑
       middle S63.21- ☑
       ring S63.21- ☑
     thumb S63.11- ☑
   metatarsophalangeal joint S93.14- ☑
     great toe S93.14- ☑
     lesser toe S93.14- ☑
   midcarpal (joint) S63.Ø3- ☑
   patella S83.ØØ- ☑
     lateral S83.Ø1- ☑
     recurrent (nontraumatic) — *see* Dislocation, patella, recurrent, incomplete
     specified type NEC S83.Ø9- ☑
   pathological — *see* Dislocation, pathological
   radial head S53.ØØ- ☑
     anterior S53.Ø1- ☑
     nursemaid's elbow S53.Ø3- ☑
     posterior S53.Ø2- ☑
     specified type NEC S53.Ø9- ☑
   radiocarpal (joint) S63.Ø2- ☑
   radioulnar (joint)
     distal S63.Ø1- ☑
     proximal — *see* Subluxation, elbow
   shoulder
     congenital Q68.8
     girdle S43.3Ø- ☑
       scapula S43.31- ☑
       specified site NEC S43.39- ☑
     traumatic S43.ØØ- ☑
       anterior S43.Ø1- ☑
       inferior S43.Ø3- ☑
       posterior S43.Ø2- ☑
       specified type NEC S43.Ø8- ☑
   sternoclavicular (joint) S43.2Ø- ☑
     anterior S43.21- ☑
     posterior S43.22- ☑
   symphysis (pubis) — *see also* Dislocation, symphysis pubis
   thumb S63.1Ø3 ☑

Subluxation — *continued*
   thumb — *continued*
     interphalangeal joint — *see* Subluxation, interphalangeal (joint), thumb
     metacarpophalangeal joint — *see* Subluxation, metacarpophalangeal (joint), thumb
   toe(s) S93.1Ø- ☑
     great S93.1Ø- ☑
       interphalangeal joint S93.13- ☑
       metatarsophalangeal joint S93.14- ☑
     interphalangeal joint S93.13- ☑
     lesser S93.1Ø- ☑
       interphalangeal joint S93.13- ☑
       metatarsophalangeal joint S93.14- ☑
     metatarsophalangeal joint S93.149 ☑
   ulna
     distal end S63.Ø7- ☑
     proximal end — *see* Subluxation, elbow
   ulnohumeral joint — *see* Subluxation, elbow
   vertebral
     recurrent NEC — *see* subcategory M43.5 ☑
     traumatic
       cervical S13.1ØØ ☑
         atlantoaxial joint S13.12Ø ☑
         atlantooccipital joint S13.11Ø ☑
         atloidoccipital joint S13.11Ø ☑
         joint between
           CØ and C1 S13.11Ø ☑
           C1 and C2 S13.12Ø ☑
           C2 and C3 S13.13Ø ☑
           C3 and C4 S13.14Ø ☑
           C4 and C5 S13.15Ø ☑
           C5 and C6 S13.16Ø ☑
           C6 and C7 S13.17Ø ☑
           C7 and T1 S13.18Ø ☑
         occipitoatloid joint S13.11Ø ☑
       lumbar S33.1ØØ ☑
         joint between
           L1 and L2 S33.11Ø ☑
           L2 and L3 S33.12Ø ☑
           L3 and L4 S33.13Ø ☑
           L4 and L5 S33.14Ø ☑
       thoracic S23.1ØØ ☑
         joint between
           T1 and T2 S23.11Ø ☑
           T2 and T3 S23.12Ø ☑
           T3 and T4 S23.122 ☑
           T4 and T5 S23.13Ø ☑
           T5 and T6 S23.132 ☑
           T6 and T7 S23.14Ø ☑
           T7 and T8 S23.142 ☑
           T8 and T9 S23.15Ø ☑
           T9 and T1Ø S23.152 ☑
           T1Ø and T11 S23.16Ø ☑
           T11 and T12 S23.162 ☑
           T12 and L1 S23.17Ø ☑
   wrist (carpal bone) S63.ØØ- ☑
     carpometacarpal joint — *see* Subluxation, carpometacarpal (joint)
     distal radioulnar joint — *see* Subluxation, radioulnar (joint), distal
     metacarpal bone, proximal — *see* Subluxation, metacarpal (bone), proximal end
     midcarpal — *see* Subluxation, midcarpal (joint)
     radiocarpal joint — *see* Subluxation, radiocarpal (joint)
     recurrent — *see* Dislocation, recurrent, wrist
     specified site NEC S63.Ø9- ☑
     ulna — *see* Subluxation, ulna, distal end
Submaxillary — *see* condition
Submersion (fatal) (nonfatal) T75.1 ☑
Submucous — *see* condition
Subnormal, subnormality
   accommodation (old age) H52.4
   mental — *see* Disability, intellectual
   temperature (accidental) T68 ☑
Subphrenic — *see* condition
Subscapular nerve — *see* condition
Subseptus uterus Q51.28
Subsiding appendicitis K36
Substance (other psychoactive) **-induced**
   anxiety disorder F19.98Ø
   bipolar and related disorder F19.94
   delirium F19.921
   depressive disorder F19.94
   major neurocognitive disorder F19.97

Substance (other psychoactive) **-induced** — *continued*
  mild neurocognitive disorder F19.988
  obsessive-compulsive and related disorder F19.988
  psychotic disorder F19.959
  sexual dysfunction F19.981
  sleep disorder F19.982
Substernal thyroid E04.9
  congenital Q89.2
Substitution disorder F44.9
Subtentorial — *see* condition
Subthyroidism (acquired) — *see also* Hypothyroidism
  congenital E03.1
Succenturiate placenta O43.19- ☑
Sucking thumb, child (excessive) F98.8
Sudamen, sudamina L74.1
Sudanese kala-azar B55.0
Sudden
  hearing loss — *see* Deafness, sudden
  heart failure — *see* Failure, heart
Sudeck's atrophy, disease, or syndrome — *see* Algoneurodystrophy
Suffocation — *see* Asphyxia, traumatic
Sugar
  blood
    high (transient) R73.9
    low (transient) E16.2
  in urine R81
Suicide, suicidal (attempted) T14.91 ☑
  by poisoning — *see* Table of Drugs and Chemicals
  history of (personal) Z91.51
    in family Z81.8
  ideation — *see* Ideation, suicidal
  risk
    meaning personal history of attempted suicide
      Z91.51
    meaning suicidal ideation — *see* Ideation, suicidal
  tendencies
    meaning personal history of attempted suicide
      Z91.51
    meaning suicidal ideation — *see* Ideation, suicidal
  trauma — *see* nature of injury by site
Suipestifer infection — *see* Infection, salmonella
Sulfhemoglobinemia, sulphemoglobinemia (acquired) (with methemoglobinemia) D74.8
Sumatran mite fever A75.3
Summer — *see* condition
Sunburn L55.9
  due to
    tanning bed (acute) L56.8
      chronic L57.8
    ultraviolet radiation (acute) L56.8
      chronic L57.8
  first degree L55.0
  second degree L55.1
  third degree L55.2
SUNCT (short lasting unilateral neuralgiform headache
  with conjunctival injection and tearing) G44.059
  intractable G44.051
  not intractable G44.059
Sundowning F05
Sunken acetabulum — *see* Derangement, joint, specified type NEC, hip
Sunstroke T67.01 ☑
  specified NEC T67.09 ☑
Superfecundation — *see* Pregnancy, multiple
Superfetation — *see* Pregnancy, multiple
Superinvolution (uterus) N85.8
Supernumerary (congenital)
  aortic cusps Q23.8
  auditory ossicles Q16.3
  bone Q79.8
  breast Q83.1
  carpal bones Q74.0
  cusps, heart valve NEC Q24.8
    aortic Q23.8
    mitral Q23.2
    pulmonary Q22.3
  digit(s) Q69.9
  ear (lobule) Q17.0
  fallopian tube Q50.6
  finger Q69.0
  hymen Q52.4
  kidney Q63.0
  lacrimonasal duct Q10.6
  lobule (ear) Q17.0
  mitral cusps Q23.2
  muscle Q79.8

Supernumerary — *continued*
  nipple(s) Q83.3
  organ or site not listed — *see* Accessory
  ossicles, auditory Q16.3
  ovary Q50.31
  oviduct Q50.6
  pulmonary, pulmonic cusps Q22.3
  rib Q76.6
    cervical or first (syndrome) Q76.5
  roots (of teeth) K00.2
  spleen Q89.09
  tarsal bones Q74.2
  teeth K00.1
  testis Q55.29
  thumb Q69.1
  toe Q69.2
  uterus Q51.28
  vagina Q52.1 ☑
  vertebra Q76.49
Supervision (of)
  contraceptive — *see* Prescription, contraceptives
  dietary (for) Z71.3
    allergy (food) Z71.3
    colitis Z71.3
    diabetes mellitus Z71.3
    food allergy or intolerance Z71.3
    gastritis Z71.3
    hypercholesterolemia Z71.3
    hypoglycemia Z71.3
    intolerance (food) Z71.3
    obesity Z71.3
    specified NEC Z71.3
  healthy infant or child Z76.2
    foundling Z76.1
  high-risk pregnancy — *see* Pregnancy, supervision of,
    high-risk
  lactation Z39.1
  pregnancy — *see* Pregnancy, supervision of
Supplemental teeth K00.1
Suppression
  binocular vision H53.34
  lactation O92.5
  menstruation N94.89
  ovarian secretion E28.39
  renal N28.9
  urine, urinary secretion R34
Suppuration, suppurative — *see also* condition
  accessory sinus (chronic) — *see* Sinusitis
  adrenal gland
  antrum (chronic) — *see* Sinusitis, maxillary
  bladder — *see* Cystitis
  brain G06.0
    sequelae G09
  breast N61.1
    puerperal, postpartum or gestational — *see* Mastitis,
      obstetric, purulent
  dental periosteum M27.3
  ear (middle) — *see* Otitis, media
    external NEC — *see* Otitis, externa, infective
    internal — *see* subcategory H83.0 ☑
  ethmoidal (chronic) (sinus) — *see* Sinusitis, ethmoidal
  fallopian tube — *see* Salpingo-oophoritis
  frontal (chronic) (sinus) — *see* Sinusitis, frontal
  gallbladder (acute) K81.0
  gum K05.20
    generalized — *see* Periodontitis, aggressive, gener-
      alized
    localized — *see* Periodontitis, aggressive, localized
  intracranial G06.0
  joint — *see* Arthritis, pyogenic or pyemic
  labyrinthine — *see* subcategory H83.0 ☑
  lung — *see* Abscess, lung
  mammary gland N61.1
    puerperal, postpartum O91.12
      associated with lactation O91.13
  maxilla, maxillary M27.2
    sinus (chronic) — *see* Sinusitis, maxillary
  muscle — *see* Myositis, infective
  nasal sinus (chronic) — *see* Sinusitis
  pancreas, acute — *see also* Pancreatitis, acute K85.80
  parotid gland — *see* Sialoadenitis
  pelvis, pelvic
    female — *see* Disease, pelvis, inflammatory
    male K65.0
  pericranial — *see* Osteomyelitis
  salivary duct or gland (any) — *see* Sialoadenitis
  sinus (accessory) (chronic) (nasal) — *see* Sinusitis
  sphenoidal sinus (chronic) — *see* Sinusitis, sphenoidal

Suppuration, suppurative — *continued*
  thymus (gland) E32.1
  thyroid (gland) E06.0
  tonsil — *see* Tonsillitis
  uterus — *see* Endometritis
Supraeruption of tooth (teeth) M26.34
Supraglottitis J04.30
  with obstruction J04.31
Suprarenal (gland) — *see* condition
Suprascapular nerve — *see* condition
Suprasellar — *see* condition
Surfer's knots or nodules S89.8- ☑
Surgical
  emphysema T81.82 ☑
  procedures, complication or misadventure — *see*
    Complications, surgical procedures
  shock T81.10 ☑
Surveillance (of) (for) — *see also* Observation
  alcohol abuse Z71.41
  contraceptive — *see* Prescription, contraceptives
  dietary Z71.3
  drug abuse Z71.51
Susceptibility to disease, genetic Z15.89
  malignant neoplasm Z15.09
    breast Z15.01
    endometrium Z15.04
    ovary Z15.02
    prostate Z15.03
    specified NEC Z15.09
  multiple endocrine neoplasia Z15.81
Suspected condition, ruled out — *see also* Observation,
  suspected
  amniotic cavity and membrane Z03.71
  cervical shortening Z03.75
  fetal anomaly Z03.73
  fetal growth Z03.74
  maternal and fetal conditions NEC Z03.79
  newborn — *see also* Observation, newborn, suspected
    condition ruled out Z05.9
  oligohydramnios Z03.71
  placental problem Z03.72
  polyhydramnios Z03.71
Suspended uterus
  in pregnancy or childbirth — *see* Pregnancy, compli-
    cated by, abnormal uterus
Sutton's nevus D22.9
Suture
  burst (in operation wound) T81.31 ☑
    external operation wound T81.31 ☑
    internal operation wound T81.32 ☑
  inadvertently left in operation wound — *see* Foreign
    body, accidentally left during a procedure
  removal Z48.02
Swab inadvertently left in operation wound — *see*
  Foreign body, accidentally left during a procedure
Swallowed, swallowing
  difficulty — *see* Dysphagia
  foreign body — *see* Foreign body, alimentary tract
Swan-neck deformity (finger) — *see* Deformity, finger,
  swan-neck
Swearing, compulsive F42.8
  in Gilles de la Tourette's syndrome F95.2
Sweat, sweats
  fetid L75.0
  night R61
Sweating, excessive R61
Sweeley-Klionsky disease E75.21
Sweet's disease or dermatosis L98.2
Swelling (of) R60.9
  abdomen, abdominal (not referable to any particular
    organ) — *see* Mass, abdominal
  ankle — *see* Effusion, joint, ankle
  arm M79.89
    forearm M79.89
  breast — *see also* Lump, breast N63.0
  Calabar B74.3
  cervical gland R59.0
  chest, localized R22.2
  ear H93.8- ☑
  extremity (lower) (upper) — *see* Disorder, soft tissue,
    specified type NEC
  finger M79.89
  foot M79.89
  glands R59.9
    generalized R59.1
    localized R59.0
  hand M79.89

Swelling — continued
head (localized) R22.0
inflammatory — see Inflammation
intra-abdominal — see Mass, abdominal
joint — see Effusion, joint
leg M79.89
lower M79.89
limb — see Disorder, soft tissue, specified type NEC
localized (skin) R22.9
chest R22.2
head R22.0
limb
lower — see Mass, localized, limb, lower
upper — see Mass, localized, limb, upper
neck R22.1
trunk R22.2
neck (localized) R22.1
pelvic — see Mass, abdominal
scrotum N50.89
splenic — see Splenomegaly
testis N50.89
toe M79.89
umbilical R19.09
wandering, due to Gnathostoma (spinigerum) B83.1
white — see Tuberculosis, arthritis
Swift (-Feer) disease
overdose or wrong substance given or taken — see
Table of Drugs and Chemicals, by drug, poisoning
Swimmer's
cramp T75.1 ☑
ear H60.33- ☑
itch B65.3
Swimming in the head R42
Swollen — see Swelling
Swyer syndrome Q99.1
Sycosis L73.8
barbae (not parasitic) L73.8
contagiosa (mycotic) B35.0
lupoides L73.8
mycotic B35.0
parasitic B35.0
vulgaris L73.8
Sydenham's chorea — see Chorea, Sydenham's
Sylvatic yellow fever A95.0
Sylvest's disease B33.0
Symblepharon H11.23- ☑
congenital Q10.3
Symond's syndrome G93.2
Sympathetic — see condition
Sympatheticotonia G90.8
Sympathicoblastoma
specified site — see Neoplasm, malignant, by site
unspecified site C74.90
Sympathogonioma — see Sympathicoblastoma
Symphalangy (fingers) (toes) Q70.9
Symptoms NEC R68.89
breast NEC N64.59
cold J00
development NEC R63.8
factitious, self-induced — see Disorder, factitious
genital organs, female R10.2
involving
abdomen NEC R19.8
appearance NEC R46.89
awareness R41.9
altered mental status R41.82
amnesia — see Amnesia
borderline intellectual functioning R41.83
coma — see Coma
disorientation R41.0
neurologic neglect syndrome R41.4
senile cognitive decline R41.81
specified symptom NEC R41.89
behavior NEC R46.89
cardiovascular system NEC R09.89
chest NEC R09.89
circulatory system NEC R09.89
cognitive functions R41.9
altered mental status R41.82
amnesia — see Amnesia
borderline intellectual functioning R41.83
coma — see Coma
disorientation R41.0
neurologic neglect syndrome R41.4
senile cognitive decline R41.81
specified symptom NEC R41.89
development NEC R62.50
digestive system NEC R19.8

Symptoms — continued
involving — continued
emotional state NEC R45.89
emotional lability R45.86
food and fluid intake R63.8
general perceptions and sensations R44.9
specified NEC R44.8
musculoskeletal system R29.91
specified NEC R29.898
nervous system R29.90
specified NEC R29.818
pelvis NEC R19.8
respiratory system NEC R09.89
skin and integument R23.9
urinary system R39.9
menopausal N95.1
metabolism NEC R63.8
neurotic F48.8
of infancy R68.19
pelvis NEC, female R10.2
skin and integument NEC R23.9
subcutaneous tissue NEC R23.9
viral cold J00
Sympus Q74.2
Syncephalus Q89.4
Synchondrosis
abnormal (congenital) Q78.8
ischiopubic M91.0
Synchysis (scintillans) (senile) (vitreous body) H43.89
Syncope (near) (pre-) R55
anginosa I20.8
bradycardia R00.1
cardiac R55
carotid sinus G90.01
due to spinal (lumbar) puncture G97.1
heart R55
heat T67.1 ☑
laryngeal R05.4
psychogenic F48.8
tussive R05.8
vasoconstriction R55
vasodepressor R55
vasomotor R55
vasovagal R55
Syndactylism, syndactyly Q70.9
complex (with synostosis)
fingers Q70.0- ☑
toes Q70.2- ☑
simple (without synostosis)
fingers Q70.1- ☑
toes Q70.3- ☑
Syndrome — see also Disease
5q minus NOS D46.C (following D46.2)
48,XXXX Q97.1
49,XXXXX Q97.1
abdominal
acute R10.0
muscle deficiency Q79.4
abnormal innervation H02.519
left H02.516
lower H02.515
upper H02.514
right H02.513
lower H02.512
upper H02.511
abstinence, neonatal P96.1
acid pulmonary aspiration, obstetric O74.0
acquired immunodeficiency — see Human, immunodeficiency virus (HIV) disease
activated phosphoinositide 3-kinase delta syndrome
[APDS] D81.82
acute abdominal R10.0
acute respiratory distress (adult) (child) J80
idiopathic J84.114
Adair-Dighton Q78.0
Adams-Stokes (-Morgagni) I45.9
adiposogenital E23.6
adrenal
hemorrhage (meningococcal) A39.1
meningococcic A39.1
adrenocortical — see Cushing's, syndrome
adrenogenital E25.9
congenital, associated with enzyme deficiency E25.0
afferent loop NEC K91.89
Alagille's Q44.7
alcohol withdrawal (without convulsions) — see Dependence, alcohol, with, withdrawal
Alder's D72.0

Syndrome — continued
Aldrich (-Wiskott) D82.0
alien hand R41.4
Alport Q87.81
alveolar hypoventilation E66.2
alveolocapillary block J84.10
amnesic, amnestic (confabulatory) (due to) — see Disorder, amnesic
amyostatic (Wilson's disease) E83.01
androgen insensitivity E34.50
complete E34.51
partial E34.52
androgen resistance — see also Syndrome, androgen
insensitivity E34.50
Angelman Q93.51
anginal — see Angina
ankyloglossia superior Q38.1
anterior
chest wall R07.89
cord G83.82
spinal artery G95.19
compression M47.019
cervical region M47.012
cervicothoracic region M47.013
lumbar region M47.016
occipito-atlanto-axial region M47.011
thoracic region M47.014
thoracolumbar region M47.015
tibial M76.81- ☑
antibody deficiency D80.9
agammaglobulinemic D80.1
hereditary D80.0
congenital D80.0
hypogammaglobulinemic D80.1
hereditary D80.0
anticardiolipin (-antibody) D68.61
antidepressant discontinuation T43.205 ☑
antiphospholipid (-antibody) D68.61
aortic
arch M31.4
bifurcation I74.09
aortomesenteric duodenum occlusion K31.5
apical ballooning (transient left ventricular) I51.81
arcuate ligament I77.4
argentaffin, argintaffinoma E34.0
Arnold-Chiari — see Arnold-Chiari disease
Arrillaga-Ayerza I27.0
arterial tortuosity Q87.82
arteriovenous steal T82.898- ☑
Asherman's N85.6
aspiration, of newborn — see Aspiration, by substance,
with pneumonia
meconium P24.01
ataxia-telangiectasia G11.3
auriculotemporal G50.8
autoerythrocyte sensitization (Gardner-Diamond) D69.2
autoimmune lymphoproliferative [ALPS] D89.82
autoimmune polyglandular E31.0
autoinflammatory M04.9
specified type NEC M04.8
autosomal — see Abnormal, autosomes
Avellis' G46.8
Ayerza (-Arrillaga) I27.0
Babinski-Nageotte G83.89
Bakwin-Krida Q78.5
bare lymphocyte D81.6
Barré-Guillain G61.0
Barré-Liéou M53.0
Barrett's — see Barrett's, esophagus
Barsony-Polgar K22.4
Bársony-Teschendorf K22.4
Barth E78.71
Bartter's E26.81
basal cell nevus Q87.89
Basedow's E05.00
with thyroid storm E05.01
basilar artery G45.0
Batten-Steinert G71.11
battered
baby or child — see Maltreatment, child, physical
abuse
spouse — see Maltreatment, adult, physical abuse
Beals Q87.40
Beau's I51.5
Beck's I65.8
Benedikt's G46.3
Béquez César (-Steinbrinck-Chédiak-Higashi) E70.330
Bernhardt-Roth — see Meralgia paresthetica

Syndrome — *continued*
Bernheim's — *see* Failure, heart, right
big spleen D73.1
bilateral polycystic ovarian E28.2
Bing-Horton's — *see* Horton's headache
Birt-Hogg-Dube syndrome Q87.89
Björck (-Thorsen) E34.0
black
lung J60
widow spider bite — *see* Toxicity, venom, spider, black widow
Blackfan-Diamond D61.01
Blau M04.8
blind loop K90.2
congenital Q43.8
postsurgical K91.2
blue sclera Q78.0
blue toe I75.02- ☑
Boder-Sedgewick G11.3
Boerhaave's K22.3
Borjeson Forssman Lehmann Q89.8
Bouillaud's I01.9
Bourneville (-Pringle) Q85.1
Bouveret (-Hoffman) I47.9
brachial plexus G54.0
bradycardia-tachycardia I49.5
brain (nonpsychotic) F09
with psychosis, psychotic reaction F09
acute or subacute — *see* Delirium
congenital — *see* Disability, intellectual
organic F09
post-traumatic (nonpsychotic) F07.81
psychotic F09
personality change F07.0
postcontusional F07.81
post-traumatic, nonpsychotic F07.81
psycho-organic F09
psychotic F06.8
brain stem stroke G46.3
Brandt's (acrodermatitis enteropathica) E83.2
broad ligament laceration N83.8
Brock's J98.11
bronze baby P83.88
Brown-Sequard G83.81
Brugada I49.8
bubbly lung P27.0
Buchem's M85.2
Budd-Chiari I82.0
bulbar (progressive) G12.22
Bürger-Grütz E78.3
Burke's K86.89
Burnett's (milk-alkali) E83.52
burning feet E53.9
Bywaters' T79.5 ☑
Call-Fleming I67.841
carbohydrate-deficient glycoprotein (CDGS) E77.8
carcinogenic thrombophlebitis I82.1
carcinoid E34.0
cardiac asthma I50.1
cardiacos negros I27.0
cardiofaciocutaneous Q87.89
cardiopulmonary-obesity E66.2
cardiorenal — *see* Hypertension, cardiorenal
cardiorespiratory distress (idiopathic), newborn P22.0
cardiovascular renal — *see* Hypertension, cardiorenal
carotid
artery (hemispheric) (internal) G45.1
body G90.01
sinus G90.01
carpal tunnel G56.0- ☑
Cassidy (-Scholte) E34.0
cat cry Q93.4
cat eye Q92.8
cauda equina G83.4
causalgia — *see* Causalgia
celiac K90.0
artery compression I77.4
axis I77.4
central pain G89.0
cerebellar
hereditary G11.9
stroke G46.4
cerebellomedullary malformation — *see* Spina bifida
cerebral
artery
anterior G46.1
middle G46.0
posterior G46.2

Syndrome — *continued*
cerebral — *continued*
gigantism E22.0
cervical (root) M53.1
disc — *see* Disorder, disc, cervical, with neuritis
fusion Q76.1
posterior, sympathicus M53.0
rib Q76.5
sympathetic paralysis G90.2
cervicobrachial (diffuse) M53.1
cervicocranial M53.0
cervicodorsal outlet G54.2
cervicothoracic outlet G54.0
Céstan (-Raymond) I65.8
Charcot's (angina cruris) (intermittent claudication) I73.9
Charcot-Weiss-Baker G90.09
CHARGE Q89.8
Chédiak-Higashi (-Steinbrinck) E70.330
chest wall R07.1
Chiari's (hepatic vein thrombosis) I82.0
Chilaiditi's Q43.3
child maltreatment — *see* Maltreatment, child
chondrocostal junction M94.0
chondroectodermal dysplasia Q77.6
chromosome 4 short arm deletion Q93.3
chromosome 5 short arm deletion Q93.4
chronic
infantile neurological, cutaneous and articular (CINCA) M04.2
pain G89.4
personality F68.8
Churg-Strauss M30.1
Clarke-Hadfield K86.89
Clerambault's automatism G93.89
Clouston's (hidrotic ectodermal dysplasia) Q82.4
clumsiness, clumsy child F82
cluster headache G44.009
intractable G44.001
not intractable G44.009
Coffin-Lowry Q89.8
cold injury (newborn) P80.0
combined immunity deficiency D81.9
compartment (deep) (posterior) (traumatic) T79.A0 ☑
(*following* T79.7)
abdomen T79.A3 ☑ (*following* T79.7)
lower extremity (hip, buttock, thigh, leg, foot, toes) T79.A2 ☑ (*following* T79.7)
nontraumatic
abdomen M79.A3 (*following* M79.7)
lower extremity (hip, buttock, thigh, leg, foot, toes) M79.A2- ☑ (*following* M79.7)
specified site NEC M79.A9 (*following* M79.7)
upper extremity (shoulder, arm, forearm, wrist, hand, fingers) M79.A1- ☑ (*following* M79.7)
postprocedural — *see* Syndrome, compartment, nontraumatic
specified site NEC T79.A9 ☑ (*following* T79.7)
upper extremity (shoulder, arm, forearm, wrist, hand, fingers) T79.A1 ☑ (*following* T79.7)
complex regional pain — *see* Syndrome, pain, complex regional
compression T79.5 ☑
anterior spinal — *see* Syndrome, anterior, spinal artery, compression
cauda equina G83.4
celiac artery I77.4
vertebral artery M47.029
cervical region M47.022
occipito-atlanto-axial region M47.021
concussion F07.81
congenital
affecting multiple systems NEC Q87.89
central alveolar hypoventilation G47.35
facial diplegia Q87.0
muscular hypertrophy-cerebral Q87.89
oculo-auriculovertebral Q87.0
oculofacial diplegia (Moebius) Q87.0
rubella (manifest) P35.0
congestion-fibrosis (pelvic), female N94.89
congestive dysmenorrhea N94.6
connective tissue M35.9
overlap NEC M35.1
Conn's E26.01
conus medullaris G95.81
cord
anterior G83.82

Syndrome — *continued*
cord — *continued*
posterior G83.83
coronary
acute NEC I24.9
insufficiency or intermediate I20.0
slow flow I20.8
Costen's (complex) M26.69
costochondral junction M94.0
costoclavicular G54.0
costovertebral E22.0
Cowden
PTEN related Q85.81
specified NEC Q85.82
craniovertebral M53.0
Creutzfeldt-Jakob — *see* Creutzfeldt-Jakob disease or syndrome
crib death R99
cricopharyngeal — *see* Dysphagia
cri-du-chat Q93.4
croup J05.0
CRPS I — *see* Syndrome, pain, complex regional I
crush T79.5 ☑
cryopyrin-associated perodic M04.2
cryptophthalmos Q87.0
cubital tunnel — *see* Lesion, nerve, ulnar
Curschmann (-Batten) (-Steinert) G71.11
Cushing's E24.9
alcohol-induced E24.4
due to
alcohol
drugs E24.2
ectopic ACTH E24.3
overproduction of pituitary ACTH E24.0
drug-induced E24.2
overdose or wrong substance given or taken — *see* Table of Drugs and Chemicals, by drug, poisoning
pituitary-dependent E24.0
specified type NEC E24.8
cystic duct stump K91.5
cytokine release D89.839
grade 1 D89.831
grade 2 D89.832
grade 3 D89.833
grade 4 D89.834
grade 5 D89.835
Dana-Putnam D51.0
Danbolt (-Cross) (acrodermatitis enteropathica) E83.2
Dandy-Walker Q03.1
with spina bifida Q07.01
Danlos' — *see also* Syndrome, Ehlers-Danlos Q79.60
De Quervain E34.51
de Toni-Fanconi (-Debré) E72.09
with cystinosis E72.04
de Vivo syndrome E74.810
defibrination — *see also* Fibrinolysis
with
antepartum hemorrhage — *see* Hemorrhage, antepartum, with coagulation defect
intrapartum hemorrhage — *see* Hemorrhage, complicating, delivery
newborn P60
postpartum O72.3
Degos' I77.89
Déjérine-Roussy G89.0
delayed sleep phase G47.21
demyelinating G37.9
dependence — *see* F10-F19 with fourth character .2
depersonalization (-derealization) F48.1
di George's D82.1
diabetes mellitus in newborn infant P70.2
diabetes mellitus-hypertension-nephrosis — *see* Diabetes, nephrosis
diabetes-nephrosis — *see* Diabetes, nephrosis
diabetic amyotrophy — *see* Diabetes, amyotrophy
dialysis associated steal T82.898- ☑
Diamond-Blackfan D61.01
Diamond-Gardener D69.2
DIC (diffuse or disseminated intravascular coagulopathy) D65
Dighton's Q78.0
disequilibrium E87.8
Döhle body-panmyelopathic D72.0
dorsolateral medullary G46.4
double athetosis G80.3
Down — *see also* Down syndrome Q90.9
Dravet (intractable) G40.834

Syndrome — *continued*
  Dravet — *continued*
    with status epilepticus G40.833
    without status epilepticus G40.834
  Dresbach's (elliptocytosis) D58.1
  DRESS (drug rash with eosinophilia and systemic symptoms) D72.12
  Dressler's (postmyocardial infarction) I24.1
    postcardiotomy I97.0
  drug rash with eosinophilia and systemic symptoms (DRESS) D72.12
  drug withdrawal, infant of dependent mother P96.1
  dry eye H04.12- ☑
  due to abnormality
    chromosomal Q99.9
      sex
        female phenotype Q97.9
        male phenotype Q98.9
      specified NEC Q99.8
  dumping (postgastrectomy) K91.1
    nonsurgical K31.89
  Dupré's (meningism) R29.1
  dysmetabolic X E88.81
  dyspraxia, developmental F82
  Eagle-Barrett Q79.4
  Eaton-Lambert — *see* Syndrome, Lambert-Eaton
  Ebstein's Q22.5
  ectopic ACTH E24.3
  eczema-thrombocytopenia D82.0
  Eddowes' Q78.0
  effort (psychogenic) F45.8
  Ehlers-Danlos Q79.60
    classical (cEDS) (classical EDS) Q79.61
    hypermobile (hEDS) (hypermobile EDS) Q79.62
    specified NEC Q79.69
    vascular (vascular EDS) (vEDS) Q79.63
  Eisenmenger's I27.83
  Ekman's Q78.0
  electric feet E53.8
  Ellis-van Creveld Q77.6
  empty nest Z60.0
  endocrine-hypertensive E27.0
  entrapment — *see* Neuropathy, entrapment
  eosinophilia-myalgia M35.89
  epileptic — *see also* Epilepsy, by type
    absence G40.A09 (*following G40.3*)
      intractable G40.A19 (*following G40.3*)
        with status epilepticus G40.A11 (*following G40.3*)
        without status epilepticus G40.A19 (*following G40.3*)
      not intractable G40.A09 (*following G40.3*)
        with status epilepticus G40.A01 (*following G40.3*)
        without status epilepticus G40.A09 (*following G40.3*)
  Erdheim-Chester (ECD) E88.89
  Erdheim's E22.0
  erythrocyte fragmentation D59.4
  Evans D69.41
  exhaustion F48.8
  extrapyramidal G25.9
    specified NEC G25.89
  eye retraction — *see* Strabismus
  eyelid-malar-mandible Q87.0
  Faber's D50.9
  facet M47.89- ☑
  facet joint — *see also* Spondylosis M47.819
  facial pain, paroxysmal G50.0
  Fallot's Q21.3
  familial cold autoinflammatory M04.2
  familial eczema-thrombocytopenia (Wiskott-Aldrich) D82.0
  Fanconi (-de Toni) (-Debré) E72.09
    with cystinosis E72.04
  Fanconi's (anemia) (congenital pancytopenia) D61.09
  fatigue
    chronic G93.32
    postviral G93.31
    psychogenic F48.8
  faulty bowel habit K59.39
  Feil-Klippel (brevicollis) Q76.1
  Felty's — *see* Felty's syndrome
  fertile eunuch E23.0
  fetal
    alcohol (dysmorphic) Q86.0
    hydantoin Q86.1
  Fiedler's I40.1

Syndrome — *continued*
  first arch Q87.0
  fish odor E72.89
  Fisher's G61.0
  Fitzhugh-Curtis
    due to
      Chlamydia trachomatis A74.81
      Neisseria gonorrhorea (gonococcal peritonitis) A54.85
  Fitz's — *see also* Pancreatitis, acute K85.80
  Flajani (-Basedow) E05.00
    with thyroid storm E05.01
  flatback — *see* Flatback syndrome
  floppy
    baby P94.2
    iris (intraoeprative) (IFIS) H21.81
    mitral valve I34.1
  flush E34.0
  Foix-Alajouanine G95.19
  Fong's Q87.2
  food protein-induced enterocolitis (FPIES) K52.21
  foramen magnum G93.5
  Foster-Kennedy H47.14- ☑
  Foville's (peduncular) G46.3
  fragile X Q99.2
  Franceschetti Q75.4
  Frey's
    auriculotemporal G50.8
    hyperhidrosis L74.52
  Friderichsen-Waterhouse A39.1
  Froin's G95.89
  frontal lobe F07.0
  Fukuhara E88.49
  functional
    bowel K59.9
    prepubertal castrate E29.1
  Gaisböck's D75.1
  ganglion (basal ganglia brain) G25.9
    geniculi G51.1
  Gardner-Diamond D69.2
  gastroesophageal
    junction K22.0
    laceration-hemorrhage K22.6
  gastrojejunal loop obstruction K91.89
  Gee-Herter-Heubner K90.0
  Gelineau's G47.419
    with cataplexy G47.411
  genito-anorectal A55
  Gerstmann-Sträussler-Scheinker (GSS) A81.82
  Gianotti-Crosti L44.4
  giant platelet (Bernard-Soulier) D69.1
  Gilles de la Tourette's F95.2
  Glass Q87.89
  Gleich's D72.118
  goiter-deafness E07.1
  Goldberg Q89.8
  Goldberg-Maxwell E34.51
  Good's D83.8
  Gopalan' (burning feet) E53.8
  Gorlin's Q87.89
  Gougerot-Blum L81.7
  Gouley's I31.1
  Gower's R55
  gray or grey (newborn) P93.0
    platelet D69.1
  Gubler-Millard G46.3
  Guillain-Barré (-Strohl) G61.0
  gustatory sweating G50.8
  Hadfield-Clarke K86.89
  hair tourniquet — *see* Constriction, external, by site
  Hamman's J98.19
  hand-foot L27.1
  hand-shoulder G90.8
  hantavirus (cardio)-pulmonary (HPS) (HCPS) B33.4
  happy puppet Q93.51
  Harada's H30.81- ☑
  Hayem-Faber D50.9
  headache NEC G44.89
    complicated NEC G44.59
  Heberden's I20.8
  Hedinger's E34.0
  Hegglin's D72.0
  HELLP (hemolysis, elevated liver enzymes and low platelet count) O14.2- ☑
    complicating
      childbirth O14.24
      puerperium O14.25
  hemolytic-uremic D59.30
    atypical D59.39

Syndrome — *continued*
  hemolytic-uremic — *continued*
    atypical — *continued*
      genetic D59.32
      hereditary D59.32
      infection-associated D59.31
      secondary D59.39
      specified NEC D59.39
    due to genetic disorder D59.32
    familial D59.32
    hereditary D59.32
    infection-associated D59.31
    secondary D59.39
    Shiga toxin-producing E. coli [STEC] related D59.31
    specified NEC D59.39
    typical D59.31
  hemophagocytic, infection-associated D76.2
  Henoch-Schönlein D69.0
  hepatic flexure K59.89
  hepatopulmonary K76.81
  hepatorenal K76.7
    following delivery O90.4
    postoperative or postprocedural K91.83
    postpartum, puerperal O90.4
  hepatourologic K76.7
  hereditary alpha tryptasemia D89.44
  Herter (-Gee) (nontropical sprue) K90.0
  Heubner-Herter K90.0
  Heyd's K76.7
  Hilger's G90.09
  histamine-like (fish poisoning) — *see* Poisoning, fish
  histiocytic D76.3
  histiocytosis NEC D76.3
  HIV infection, acute B20
  Hoffmann-Werdnig G12.0
  Hollander-Simons E88.1
  Hoppe-Goldflam G70.00
    with exacerbation (acute) G70.01
    in crisis G70.01
  Horner's G90.2
  hungry bone E83.81
  hunterian glossitis D51.0
  Hutchinson's triad A50.53
  hyperabduction G54.0
  hyperammonemia-hyperornithinemia-homocitrulline-mia E72.4
  hypereosinophilic (HES) D72.119
    idiopathic (IHES) D72.110
    lymphocytic variant (LHES) D72.111
    myeloid D72.118
    specified NEC D72.118
  hyperimmunoglobulin D M04.1
  hyperimmunoglobulin E (IgE) D82.4
  hyperkalemic E87.5
  hyperkinetic — *see* Hyperkinesia
  hypermobility M35.7
  hypernatremia E87.0
  hyperosmolarity E87.0
  hyperperfusion G97.82
  hypersplenic D73.1
  hypertransfusion, newborn P61.1
  hyperventilation F45.8
  hyperviscosity (of serum)
    polycythemic D75.1
    sclerothymic D58.8
  hypoglycemic (familial) (neonatal) E16.2
  hypokalemic E87.6
  hyponatremic E87.1
  hypopituitarism E23.0
  hypoplastic left-heart Q23.4
  hypopotassemia E87.6
  hyposmolality E87.1
  hypotension, maternal O26.5- ☑
  hypothenar hammer I73.89
  hypoventilation, obesity (OHS) E66.2
  ICF (intravascular coagulation-fibrinolysis) D65
  idiopathic
    cardiorespiratory distress, newborn P22.0
    nephrotic (infantile) N04.9
  iliotibial band M76.3- ☑
  immobility, immobilization (paraplegic) M62.3
  immune effector cell-associated neurotoxicity (ICANS) G92.00
    grade
      1 G92.01
      2 G92.02
      3 G92.03
      4 G92.04
      5 G92.05

Syndrome — *continued*
  immune effector cell-associated neurotoxicity — *continued*
    grade — *continued*
      unspecified G92.00
  immune reconstitution D89.3
  immune reconstitution inflammatory [IRIS] D89.3
  immunity deficiency, combined D81.9
  immunodeficiency
    acquired — *see* Human, immunodeficiency virus (HIV) disease
    combined D81.9
  impending coronary I20.0
  impingement, shoulder M75.4- ☑
  inappropriate secretion of antidiuretic hormone E22.2
  infant
    gestational diabetes P70.0
    of diabetic mother P70.1
  infantilism (pituitary) E23.0
  inferior vena cava I87.1
  inspissated bile (newborn) P59.1
  institutional (childhood) F94.2
  insufficient sleep F51.12
  intermediate coronary (artery) I20.0
  interspinous ligament — *see* Spondylopathy, specified NEC
  intestinal
    carcinoid E34.0
    knot K56.2
  intravascular coagulation-fibrinolysis (ICF) D65
  iodine-deficiency, congenital E00.9
    type
      mixed E00.2
      myxedematous E00.1
      neurological E00.0
  IRDS (idiopathic respiratory distress, newborn) P22.0
  irritable
    bowel K58.9
      with
        constipation K58.1
        diarrhea K58.0
      mixed K58.2
      psychogenic F45.8
      specified NEC K58.8
    heart (psychogenic) F45.8
    weakness F48.8
  ischemic
    bowel (transient) K55.9
      chronic K55.1
      due to mesenteric artery insufficiency K55.1
    steal T82.898 ☑
  IVC (intravascular coagulopathy) D65
  Ivemark's Q89.01
  Jaccoud's — *see* Arthropathy, postrheumatic, chronic
  Jackson's G83.89
  Jakob-Creutzfeldt — *see* Creutzfeldt-Jakob disease or syndrome
  jaw-winking Q07.8
  Jervell-Lange-Nielsen I45.81
  jet lag G47.25
  Job's D71
  Joseph-Diamond-Blackfan D61.01
  jugular foramen G52.7
  Kabuki Q89.8
  Kanner's (autism) F84.0
  Kartagener's Q89.3
  Kelly's D50.1
  Kimmelsteil-Wilson — *see* Diabetes, specified type, with Kimmelsteil-Wilson disease
  Klein (e)-Levine G47.13
  Klippel-Feil (brevicollis) Q76.1
  Köhler-Pellegrini-Steida — *see* Bursitis, tibial collateral
  König's K59.89
  Korsakoff (-Wernicke) (nonalcoholic) F04
    alcoholic F10.26
  Kostmann's D70.0
  Krabbe's congenital muscle hypoplasia Q79.8
  labyrinthine — *see* subcategory H83.2 ☑
  lacunar NEC G46.7
  Lambert-Eaton G70.80
    in
      neoplastic disease G73.1
      specified disease NEC G70.81
  Landau-Kleffner — *see* Epilepsy, specified NEC
  Larsen's Q74.8
  lateral
    cutaneous nerve of thigh G57.1- ☑
    medullary G46.4

Syndrome — *continued*
  Launois' E22.0
  lazy
    leukocyte D70.8
    posture M62.3
  Lemiere I80.8
  Lennox-Gastaut G40.812
    intractable G40.814
      with status epilepticus G40.813
      without status epilepticus G40.814
    not intractable G40.812
      with status epilepticus G40.811
      without status epilepticus G40.812
  lenticular, progressive E83.01
  Leopold-Levi's E05.90
  Lev's I44.2
  Lichtheim's D51.0
  Li-Fraumeni Z15.01
  Lightwood's N25.89
  Lignac (de Toni) (-Fanconi) (-Debré) E72.09
    with cystinosis E72.04
  Likoff's I20.8
  limbic epilepsy personality F07.0
  liver-kidney K76.7
  lobotomy F07.0
  Löffler's J82.89
  long arm 18 or 21 deletion Q93.89
  long QT I45.81
  Louis-Barré G11.3
  low
    atmospheric pressure T70.29 ☑
    back M54.50
    output (cardiac) I50.9
  lower radicular, newborn (birth injury) P14.8
  Luetscher's (dehydration) E86.0
  Lupus anticoagulant D68.62
  Lutembacher's Q21.19
  macrophage activation D76.1
    due to infection D76.2
  magnesium-deficiency R29.0
  Majeed M04.8
  Mal de Debarquement R42
  malabsorption K90.9
    postsurgical K91.2
  malformation, congenital, due to
    alcohol Q86.0
    exogenous cause NEC Q86.8
    hydantoin Q86.1
    warfarin Q86.2
  malignant
    carcinoid E34.0
    neuroleptic G21.0
  Mallory-Weiss K22.6
  mandibulofacial dysostosis Q75.4
  manic-depressive — *see* Disorder, bipolar
  maple-syrup-urine E71.0
  Marable's I77.4
  Marfan's Q87.40
    with
      cardiovascular manifestations Q87.418
        aortic dilation Q87.410
      ocular manifestations Q87.42
      skeletal manifestations Q87.43
  Marie's (acromegaly) E22.0
  mast cell activation — *see* Activation, mast cell
  maternal hypotension — *see* Syndrome, hypotension, maternal
  May (-Hegglin) D72.0
  McArdle (-Schmidt) (-Pearson) E74.04
  McQuarrie's E16.2
  meconium plug (newborn) P76.0
  median arcuate ligament I77.4
  Meekeren-Ehlers-Danlos Q79.6 ☑
  megavitamin-B6 E67.2
  Meige G24.4
  MELAS E88.41
  Mendelson's O74.0
  MERRF (myoclonic epilepsy associated with ragged-red fibers) E88.42
  mesenteric
    artery (superior) K55.1
    vascular insufficiency K55.1
  metabolic E88.81
  metastatic carcinoid E34.0
  micrognathia-glossoptosis Q87.0
  midbrain NEC G93.89
  middle lobe (lung) J98.19
  middle radicular G54.0
  migraine — *see also* Migraine G43.909

Syndrome — *continued*
  Mikulicz' K11.8
  milk-alkali E83.52
  Millard-Gubler G46.3
  Miller-Dieker Q93.88
  Miller-Fisher G61.0
  Minkowski-Chauffard D58.0
  Mirizzi's K83.1
  MNGIE (Mitochondrial Neurogastrointestinal Encephalopathy) E88.49
  Möbius, ophthalmoplegic migraine — *see* Migraine, ophthalmoplegic
  monofixation H50.42
  Morel-Moore M85.2
  Morel-Morgagni M85.2
  Morgagni (-Morel) (-Stewart) M85.2
  Morgagni-Adams-Stokes I45.9
  Mounier-Kuhn Q32.4
    with bronchiectasis J47.9
      with
        exacerbation (acute) J47.1
        lower respiratory infection J47.0
    acquired J98.09
      with bronchiectasis J47.9
        with
          exacerbation (acute) J47.1
          lower respiratory infection J47.0
  Muckle-Wells M04.2
  mucocutaneous lymph node (acute febrile) (MCLS) M30.3
  multiple endocrine neoplasia (MEN) — *see* Neoplasia, endocrine, multiple (MEN)
  multiple operations — *see* Disorder, factitious
  multisystem inflammatory (in adults) (in children) M35.81
  myasthenic G70.9
    in
      diabetes mellitus — *see* Diabetes, amyotrophy
      endocrine disease NEC E34.9 *[G73.3]*
      neoplastic disease — *see also* Neoplasm D49.9 *[G73.3]*
      thyrotoxicosis (hyperthyroidism) E05.90 *[G73.3]*
        with thyroid storm E05.91 *[G73.3]*
  myelodysplastic D46.9
    with
      5q deletion D46.C (*following* D46.2)
      isolated del (5q) chromosomal abnormality D46.C (*following* D46.2)
      multilineage dysplasia D46.A (*following* D46.2)
        with ringed sideroblasts D46.B (*following* D46.2)
      lesions, low grade D46.20
      specified NEC D46.Z (*following* D46.4)
  myeloid hypereosinophilic D72.118
  myelopathic pain G89.0
  myeloproliferative (chronic) D47.1
  myofascial pain M79.18
  Naffziger's G54.0
  nail patella Q87.2
  NARP (Neuropathy, Ataxia and Retinitis pigmentosa) E88.49
  neonatal abstinence P96.1
  nephritic — *see also* Nephritis
    with edema — *see* Nephrosis
    acute N00.9
    chronic N03.9
    rapidly progressive N01.9
  nephrotic (congenital) — *see also* Nephrosis N04.9
    with
      C3
        glomerulonephritis N04.A
        glomerulopathy N04.A
          with dense deposit disease N04.6
      dense deposit disease N04.6
      diffuse
        crescentic glomerulonephritis N04.7
        endocapillary proliferative glomerulonephritis N04.4
        membranous glomerulonephritis N04.2
        mesangial proliferative glomerulonephritis N04.3
        mesangiocapillary glomerulonephritis N04.5
      focal and segmental glomerular lesions N04.1
      minor glomerular abnormality N04.0
      specified morphological changes NEC N04.8
    diabetic — *see* Diabetes, nephrosis
  neurologic neglect R41.4
  Nezelof's D81.4

Syndrome — Syndrome

Syndrome — continued

Nonne-Milroy-Meige Q82.0
Nothnagel's vasomotor acroparesthesia I73.89
obesity hypoventilation (OHS) E66.2
oculomotor H51.9
Ogilvie K59.81
ophthalmoplegia-cerebellar ataxia — see Strabismus, paralytic, third nerve
oral allergy T78.1 ☑
oral-facial-digital Q87.0
organic
  affective F06.30
  amnesic (not alcohol- or drug-induced) F04
  brain F09
  depressive F06.31
  hallucinosis F06.0
  personality F07.0
Ormond's N13.5
oro-facial-digital Q87.0
os trigonum Q68.8
Osler-Weber-Rendu I78.0
osteoporosis-osteomalacia M83.8
Osterreicher-Turner Q87.2
otolith — see subcategory H81.8 ☑
oto-palatal-digital Q87.0
outlet (thoracic) G54.0
ovary
  polycystic E28.2
  resistant E28.39
  sclerocystic E28.2
Owren's D68.2
Paget-Schroetter I82.890
pain — see also Pain
  complex regional I G90.50
    lower limb G90.52- ☑
    specified site NEC G90.59
    upper limb G90.51- ☑
  complex regional II — see Causalgia
painful
  bruising D69.2
  feet E53.8
  prostate N42.81
paralysis agitans — see Parkinsonism
paralytic G83.9
  specified NEC G83.89
Parinaud's H51.0
parkinsonian — see Parkinsonism
Parkinson's — see Parkinsonism
paroxysmal facial pain G50.0
Parry's E05.00
  with thyroid storm E05.01
Parsonage (-Aldren)-Turner G54.5
patella clunk M25.86- ☑
Paterson (-Brown) (-Kelly) D50.1
pectoral girdle I77.89
pectoralis minor I77.89
pediatric autoimmune neuropsychiatric disorders associated with streptococcal infections (PANDAS) D89.89
pediatric inflammatory multisystem M35.81
Pelger-Huet D72.0
pellagra-cerebellar ataxia-renal aminoaciduria E72.02
pellagroid E52
Pellegrini-Stieda — see Bursitis, tibial collateral
pelvic congestion-fibrosis, female N94.89
penta X Q97.1
peptic ulcer — see Ulcer, peptic
perabduction I77.89
periodic fever M04.1
periodic fever, aphthous stomatitis, pharyngitis, and adenopathy [PFAPA] M04.8
periodic headache, in adults and children — see Headache, periodic syndromes in adults and children
periurethral fibrosis N13.5
Peutz-Jeghers Q85.89
phantom limb (without pain) G54.7
  with pain G54.6
pharyngeal pouch D82.1
Pick's — see Disease, Pick's
Pickwickian E66.2
PIE (pulmonary infiltration with eosinophilia) — see also Eosinophilia, pulmonary J82.89
pigmentary pallidal degeneration (progressive) G23.0
pineal E34.8
pituitary E22.0
placental transfusion — see Pregnancy, complicated by, placental transfusion syndromes

Syndrome — continued

plantar fascia M72.2
plateau iris (post-iridectomy) (postprocedural) H21.82
Plummer-Vinson D50.1
pluricarential of infancy E40
plurideficiency E40
pluriglandular (compensatory) E31.8
  autoimmune E31.0
pneumatic hammer T75.21 ☑
polyangiitis overlap M30.8
polycarential of infancy E40
polyglandular E31.8
  autoimmune E31.0
polysplenia Q89.09
pontine NEC G93.89
popliteal
  artery entrapment I77.89
  web Q87.89
post chemoembolization — code to associated conditions
post endometrial ablation N99.85
postbacterial fatigue G93.39
postcardiac injury
  postcardiotomy I97.0
  postmyocardial infarction I24.1
postcardiotomy I97.0
postcholecystectomy K91.5
postcommissurotomy I97.0
postconcussional F07.81
postcontusional F07.81
post-COVID (-19) U09.9
postencephalitic F07.89
posterior
  cervical sympathetic M53.0
  cord G83.83
  fossa compression G93.5
  reversible encephalopathy (PRES) I67.83
postgastrectomy (dumping) K91.1
postgastric surgery K91.1
postinfarction I24.1
postinfectious fatigue G93.39
postlaminectomy NEC M96.1
postleukotomy F07.0
postmastectomy lymphedema I97.2
postmyocardial infarction I24.1
postoperative NEC T81.9 ☑
  blind loop K90.2
postpartum panhypopituitary (Sheehan) E23.0
postpolio (myelitic) G14
postthrombotic I87.009
  with
    inflammation I87.02- ☑
      with ulcer I87.03- ☑
    specified complication NEC I87.09- ☑
    ulcer I87.01- ☑
      with inflammation I87.03- ☑
  asymptomatic I87.00- ☑
postural
  orthostatic tachycardia [POTS] G90.A
  tachycardia G90.A
postvagotomy K91.1
postvalvulotomy I97.0
postviral NEC G93.31
  fatigue G93.31
Potain's K31.0
potassium intoxication E87.5
Prader-Willi Q87.11
Prader-Willi-like Q87.19
precerebral artery (multiple) (bilateral) G45.2
preinfarction I20.0
preleukemic D46.9
premature senility E34.8
premenstrual dysphoric F32.81
premenstrual tension N94.3
Prinzmetal-Massumi R07.1
prune belly Q79.4
pseudo -Turner's Q87.19
pseudocarpal tunnel (sublimis) — see Syndrome, carpal tunnel
pseudoparalytica G70.00
  with exacerbation (acute) G70.01
  in crisis G70.01
psycho-organic (nonpsychotic severity) F07.9
  acute or subacute F05
  depressive type F06.31
  hallucinatory type F06.0
  nonpsychotic severity F07.0
  specified NEC F07.89

Syndrome — continued

PTEN (hamartoma) tumor Q85.81
pulmonary
  arteriosclerosis I27.0
  dysmaturity (Wilson-Mikity) P27.0
  hypoperfusion (idiopathic) P22.0
  renal (hemorrhagic) (Goodpasture's) M31.0
pure
  motor lacunar G46.5
  sensory lacunar G46.6
Putnam-Dana D51.0
pyogenic arthritis, pyoderma gangrenosum, and acne [PAPA] M04.8
pyramidopallidonigral G20
pyriformis — see Lesion, nerve, sciatic
QT interval prolongation I45.81
radicular NEC — see Radiculopathy
  upper limbs, newborn (birth injury) P14.3
rapid time-zone change G47.25
Rasmussen G04.81
Raymond (-Céstan) I65.8
Raynaud's I73.00
  with gangrene I73.01
RDS (respiratory distress syndrome, newborn) P22.0
reactive airways dysfunction J68.3
Refsum's G60.1
Reifenstein E34.52
renal glomerulohyalinosis-diabetic — see Diabetes, nephrosis
Rendu-Osler-Weber I78.0
residual ovary N99.83
resistant ovary E28.39
respiratory
  distress
    acute J80
      adult J80
      child J80
      idiopathic J84.114
      newborn (idiopathic) (type I) P22.0
      type II P22.1
restless legs G25.81
retinoblastoma (familial) C69.2 ☑
retroperitoneal fibrosis N13.5
Reye's G93.7
Richter — see Leukemia, chronic lymphocytic, B-cell type
Ridley's I50.1
right
  heart, hypoplastic Q22.6
  ventricular obstruction — see Failure, heart, right
Romano-Ward (prolonged QT interval) I45.81
rotator cuff, shoulder — see also Tear, rotator cuff M75.10- ☑
Rotes Quérol — see Hyperostosis, ankylosing
Roth — see Meralgia paresthetica
rubella (congenital) P35.0
Ruvalcaba-Myhre-Smith E71.440
Rytand-Lipsitch I44.2
salt
  depletion E87.1
    due to heat NEC T67.8 ☑
      causing heat exhaustion or prostration T67.4 ☑
  low E87.1
salt-losing N28.89
SATB2-associated Q87.89
Scaglietti-Dagnini E22.0
scalenus anticus (anterior) G54.0
scapulocostal — see Mononeuropathy, upper limb, specified site NEC
scapuloperoneal G71.09
schizophrenic, of childhood NEC F84.5
Schnitzler D47.2
Scholte's E34.0
Schroeder's E27.0
Schüller-Christian C96.5
Schwachman's — see Syndrome, Shwachman's
Schwartz (-Jampel) G71.13
Schwartz-Bartter E22.2
scimitar Q26.8
sclerocystic ovary E28.2
Seitelberger's G31.89
septicemic adrenal hemorrhage A39.1
seroconversion, retroviral (acute) Z21
serous meningitis G93.2
severe acute respiratory (SARS) J12.81
  coronavirus 2 (see also COVID-19) U07.1

Syndrome — *continued*

severe acute respiratory — *continued*
 coronavirus 2 (*see also* COVID-19) — *continued*
  pneumonia J12.82
shaken infant T74.4 ☑
shock (traumatic) T79.4 ☑
 kidney N17.0
  following crush injury T79.5 ☑
 toxic A48.3
shock-lung J80
Shone's — *code to* specific anomalies
short
 bowel K91.2
 rib Q77.2
shoulder-hand — *see* Algoneurodystrophy
Shwachman's D70.4
sicca — *see* Syndrome, Sjögren
sick
 cell E87.1
 sinus I49.5
sick-euthyroid E07.81
sideropenic D50.1
Siemens' ectodermal dysplasia Q82.4
Silfverskjöld's Q78.9
Simons' E88.1
sinus tarsi M25.57- ☑
sinusitis-bronchiectasis-situs inversus Q89.3
Sipple's E31.22
sirenomelia Q87.2
Sjögren M35.00
 with
  central nervous system involvement M35.07
  dental involvement M35.0C
  gastrointestinal involvement M35.08
  glomerular disease M35.0A
  inflammatory arthritis M35.05
  keratoconjunctivitis M35.01
  lung involvement M35.02
  myopathy M35.03
  peripheral nervous system involvement M35.06
  renal tubular acidosis M35.04
  specified organ involvement, NEC M35.09
  tubulo-interstitial nephropathy M35.04
  vasculitis M35.0B
Slocumb's E27.0
slow flow, coronary I20.8
Sluder's G44.89
Smith-Magenis Q93.88
Sneddon-Wilkinson L13.1
Sotos' Q87.3
South African cardiomyopathy I42.8
spasmodic
 upward movement, eyes H51.8
 winking F95.8
Spen's I45.9
splenic
 agenesis Q89.01
 flexure K59.89
 neutropenia D73.81
Spurway's Q78.0
staphylococcal scalded skin L00
steal
 arteriovenous T82.898- ☑
 ischemic T82.898- ☑
 subclavian G45.8
Stein-Leventhal E28.2
Stein's E28.2
Stevens-Johnson syndrome L51.1
 toxic epidermal necrolysis overlap L51.3
Stewart-Morel M85.2
Stickler Q89.8
stiff baby Q89.8
stiff man G25.82
Still-Felty — *see* Felty's syndrome
Stokes (-Adams) I45.9
stone heart I50.1
straight back, congenital Q76.49
Sturge-Weber (-Dimitri) Q85.89
subclavian steal G45.8
subcoracoid-pectoralis minor G54.0
subcostal nerve compression I77.89
subphrenic interposition Q43.3
superior
 cerebellar artery I63.89
 mesenteric artery K55.1
 semi-circular canal dehiscence H83.8X- ☑
 vena cava I87.1

Syndrome — *continued*

supine hypotensive (maternal) — *see* Syndrome, hypotension, maternal
suprarenal cortical E27.0
supraspinatus — *see also* Tear, rotator cuff M75.10- ☑
Susac G93.49
swallowed blood P78.2
sweat retention L74.0
Swyer Q99.1
Symond's G93.2
sympathetic
 cervical paralysis G90.2
 pelvic, female N94.89
systemic inflammatory response (SIRS), of non-infectious origin (without organ dysfunction) R65.10
 with acute organ dysfunction R65.11
tachycardia-bradycardia I49.5
takotsubo I51.81
TAR (thrombocytopenia with absent radius) Q87.2
tarsal tunnel G57.5- ☑
teething K00.7
tegmental G93.89
telangiectasic-pigmentation-cataract Q82.8
temporal pyramidal apex — *see* Otitis, media, suppurative, acute
temporomandibular joint-pain-dysfunction M26.62- ☑
Terry's — *see also* Myopia, degenerative H44.2- ☑
testicular feminization — *see also* Syndrome, androgen insensitivity E34.51
thalamic pain (hyperesthetic) G89.0
thoracic outlet (compression) G54.0
Thorson-Björck E34.0
thrombocytopenia with absent radius (TAR) Q87.2
thrombosis with thrombocytopenia D75.84
thyroid-adrenocortical insufficiency E31.0
tibial
 anterior M76.81- ☑
 posterior M76.82- ☑
Tietze's M94.0
time-zone (rapid) G47.25
Toni-Fanconi E72.09
 with cystinosis E72.04
Touraine's Q79.8
tourniquet — *see* Constriction, external, by site
toxic shock A48.3
transient left ventricular apical balderning I51.81
traumatic vasospastic T75.22 ☑
Treacher Collins Q75.4
triple X, female Q97.0
trisomy Q92.9
 13 Q91.7
  meiotic nondisjunction Q91.4
  mitotic nondisjunction Q91.5
  mosaicism Q91.5
  translocation Q91.6
 18 Q91.3
  meiotic nondisjunction Q91.0
  mitotic nondisjunction Q91.1
  mosaicism Q91.1
  translocation Q91.2
 20 (q)(p) Q92.8
 21 Q90.9
  meiotic nondisjunction Q90.0
  mitotic nondisjunction Q90.1
  mosaicism Q90.1
  translocation Q90.2
 22 Q92.8
tropical wet feet T69.0- ☑
Trousseau's I82.1
tumor lysis (following antineoplastic chemotherapy) (spontaneous) NEC E88.3
tumor necrosis factor receptor associated periodic (TRAPS) M04.1
Twiddler's (due to)
 automatic implantable defibrillator T82.198 ☑
 cardiac pacemaker T82.198 ☑
Unverricht (-Lundborg) — *see* Epilepsy, generalized, idiopathic
upward gaze H51.8
uremia, chronic — *see also* Disease, kidney, chronic N18.9
urethral N34.3
urethro-oculo-articular — *see* Reiter's disease
urohepatic K76.7
vago-hypoglossal G52.7
van Buchem's M85.2
van der Hoeve's Q78.0
vascular NEC in cerebrovascular disease G46.8

Syndrome — *continued*

vasoconstriction, reversible cerebrovascular I67.841
vasomotor I73.9
vasospastic (traumatic) T75.22 ☑
vasovagal R55
VATER Q87.2
velo-cardio-facial Q93.81
vena cava (inferior) (superior) (obstruction) I87.1
vertebral
 artery G45.0
  compression — *see* Syndrome, anterior, spinal artery, compression
 steal G45.0
vertebro-basilar artery G45.0
vertebrogenic (pain) — *see also* Pain, vertebrogenic M54.89
vertiginous — *see* Disorder, vestibular function
Vinson-Plummer D50.1
virus B34.9
visceral larva migrans B83.0
visual disorientation H53.8
vitamin B6 deficiency E53.1
vitreal corneal H59.01- ☑
vitreous (touch) H59.01- ☑
Vogt-Koyanagi H20.82- ☑
Volkmann's T79.6 ☑
von Hippel-Lindau Q85.83
von Schroetter's I82.890
von Willebrand (-Jürgen) — *see* Disease, von Willebrand
 acquired — *see also* Disease, von Willebrand D68.04
Waldenström-Kjellberg D50.1
Wallenberg's G46.3
water retention E87.79
Waterhouse (-Friderichsen) A39.1
Weber-Gubler G46.3
Weber-Leyden G46.3
Weber's G46.3
Wegener's M31.30
 with
  kidney involvement M31.31
  lung involvement M31.30
   with kidney involvement M31.31
Weingarten's (tropical eosinophilia) J82.89
Weiss-Baker G90.09
Werdnig-Hoffman G12.0
Wermer's E31.21
Werner's E34.8
Wernicke-Korsakoff (nonalcoholic) F04
 alcoholic F10.26
Westphal-Strümpell E83.01
West's — *see* Epilepsy, spasms
wet
 feet (maceration) (tropical) T69.0- ☑
 lung, newborn P22.1
whiplash S13.4 ☑
whistling face Q87.0
Wilkie's K55.1
Wilkinson-Sneddon L13.1
Willebrand (-Jürgens) — *see* Disease, von Willebrand
Williams Q93.82
Wilson's (hepatolenticular degeneration) E83.01
Wiskott-Aldrich D82.0
withdrawal — *see* Withdrawal, state
 drug
  infant of dependent mother P96.1
  therapeutic use, newborn P96.2
Woakes' (ethmoiditis) J33.1
Wright's (hyperabduction) G54.0
X I20.9
XXXX Q97.1
XXXXX Q97.1
XXXXY Q98.1
XXY Q98.0
Yao M04.8
yellow nail L60.5
Zahorsky's B08.5
Zellweger syndrome E71.510
Zellweger-like syndrome E71.541

Synechia (anterior) (iris) (posterior) (pupil) — *see also* Adhesions, iris
 intra-uterine (traumatic) N85.6

Synesthesia R20.8

Syngamiasis, syngamosis B83.3

Synodontia K00.2

Synorchidism, synorchism Q55.1

Synostosis (congenital) Q78.8
 astragalo-scaphoid Q74.2

Synostosis — *continued*
  radioulnar Q74.0
Synovial sarcoma — *see* Neoplasm, connective tissue, malignant
Synovioma (malignant) — *see also* Neoplasm, connective tissue, malignant
  benign — *see* Neoplasm, connective tissue, benign
Synoviosarcoma — *see* Neoplasm, connective tissue, malignant
Synovitis — *see also* Tenosynovitis M65.9
  crepitant
    hand M70.0- ☑
    wrist M70.03- ☑
  gonococcal A54.49
  gouty — *see* Gout
  in (due to)
    crystals M65.8- ☑
    gonorrhea A54.49
    syphilis (late) A52.78
    use, overuse, pressure — *see* Disorder, soft tissue, due to use
  infective NEC — *see* Tenosynovitis, infective NEC
  specified NEC — *see* Tenosynovitis, specified type NEC
  syphilitic A52.78
    congenital (early) A50.02
  toxic — *see* Synovitis, transient
  transient M67.3- ☑
    ankle M67.37- ☑
    elbow M67.32- ☑
    foot joint M67.37- ☑
    hand joint M67.34- ☑
    hip M67.35- ☑
    knee M67.36- ☑
    multiple site M67.39
    pelvic region M67.35- ☑
    shoulder M67.31- ☑
    specified joint NEC M67.38
    wrist M67.33- ☑
  traumatic, current — *see* Sprain
  tuberculous — *see* Tuberculosis, synovitis
  villonodular (pigmented) M12.2- ☑
    ankle M12.27- ☑
    elbow M12.22- ☑
    foot joint M12.27- ☑
    hand joint M12.24- ☑
    hip M12.25- ☑
    knee M12.26- ☑
    multiple site M12.29
    pelvic region M12.25- ☑
    shoulder M12.21- ☑
    specified joint NEC M12.28
    vertebrae M12.28
    wrist M12.23- ☑
Syphilid A51.39
  congenital A50.06
  newborn A50.06
  tubercular (late) A52.79
Syphilis, syphilitic (acquired) A53.9
  abdomen (late) A52.79
  acoustic nerve A52.15
  adenopathy (secondary) A51.49
  adrenal (gland) (with cortical hypofunction) A52.79
  age under 2 years NOS — *see also* Syphilis, congenital, early
    acquired A51.9
  alopecia (secondary) A51.32
  anemia (late) A52.79 *[D63.8]*
  aneurysm (aorta) (ruptured) A52.01
    central nervous system A52.05
    congenital A50.54 *[I79.0]*
  anus (late) A52.74
    primary A51.1
    secondary A51.39
  aorta (arch) (abdominal) (thoracic) A52.02
    aneurysm A52.01
  aortic (insufficiency) (regurgitation) (stenosis) A52.03
    aneurysm A52.01
  arachnoid (adhesive) (cerebral) (spinal) A52.13
  asymptomatic — *see* Syphilis, latent
  ataxia (locomotor) A52.11
  atrophoderma maculatum A51.39
  auricular fibrillation A52.06
  bladder (late) A52.76
  bone A52.77
    secondary A51.46
  brain A52.17
  breast (late) A52.79

Syphilis, syphilitic — *continued*
  bronchus (late) A52.72
  bubo (primary) A51.0
  bulbar palsy A52.19
  bursa (late) A52.78
  cardiac decompensation A52.06
  cardiovascular A52.00
  central nervous system (late) (recurrent) (relapse) (tertiary) A52.3
    with
      ataxia A52.11
      general paralysis A52.17
        juvenile A50.45
      paresis (general) A52.17
        juvenile A50.45
      tabes (dorsalis) A52.11
        juvenile A50.45
      taboparesis A52.17
        juvenile A50.45
    aneurysm A52.05
    congenital A50.40
    juvenile A50.40
    remission in (sustained) A52.3
    serology doubtful, negative, or positive A52.3
    specified nature or site NEC A52.19
    vascular A52.05
  cerebral A52.17
    meningovascular A52.13
    nerves (multiple palsies) A52.15
    sclerosis A52.17
    thrombosis A52.05
  cerebrospinal (tabetic type) A52.12
  cerebrovascular A52.05
  cervix (late) A52.76
  chancre (multiple) A51.0
    extragenital A51.2
    Rollet's A51.0
  Charcot's joint A52.16
  chorioretinitis A51.43
    congenital A50.01
    late A52.71
    prenatal A50.01
  choroiditis — *see* Syphilitic chorioretinitis
  choroidoretinitis — *see* Syphilitic chorioretinitis
  ciliary body (secondary) A51.43
    late A52.71
  colon (late) A52.74
  combined spinal sclerosis A52.11
  condyloma (latum) A51.31
  congenital A50.9
    with
      paresis (general) A50.45
      tabes (dorsalis) A50.45
      taboparesis A50.45
    chorioretinitis, choroiditis A50.01 *[H32]*
    early, or less than 2 years after birth NEC A50.2
      with manifestations — *see* Syphilis, congenital, early, symptomatic
      latent (without manifestations) A50.1
        negative spinal fluid test A50.1
        serology positive A50.1
      symptomatic A50.09
        cutaneous A50.06
        mucocutaneous A50.07
        oculopathy A50.01
        osteochondropathy A50.02
        pharyngitis A50.03
        pneumonia A50.04
        rhinitis A50.05
        visceral A50.08
    interstitial keratitis A50.31
    juvenile neurosyphilis A50.45
    late, or 2 years or more after birth NEC A50.7
      chorioretinitis, choroiditis A50.32
      interstitial keratitis A50.31
      juvenile neurosyphilis A50.45
      latent (without manifestations) A50.6
        negative spinal fluid test A50.6
        serology positive A50.6
      symptomatic or with manifestations NEC A50.59
        arthropathy A50.55
        cardiovascular A50.54
        Clutton's joints A50.51
        Hutchinson's teeth A50.52
        Hutchinson's triad A50.53
        osteochondropathy A50.56
        saddle nose A50.57
  conjugal A53.9
    tabes A52.11

Syphilis, syphilitic — *continued*
  conjunctiva (late) A52.71
  contact Z20.2
  cord bladder A52.19
  cornea, late A52.71
  coronary (artery) (sclerosis) A52.06
  coryza, congenital A50.05
  cranial nerve A52.15
    multiple palsies A52.15
  cutaneous — *see* Syphilis, skin
  dacryocystitis (late) A52.71
  degeneration, spinal cord A52.12
  dementia paralytica A52.17
    juvenilis A50.45
  destruction of bone A52.77
  dilatation, aorta A52.01
  due to blood transfusion A53.9
  dura mater A52.13
  ear A52.79
    inner A52.79
      nerve (eighth) A52.15
      neurorecurrence A52.15
  early A51.9
    cardiovascular A52.00
    central nervous system A52.3
    latent (without manifestations) (less than 2 years after infection) A51.5
      negative spinal fluid test A51.5
      serological relapse after treatment A51.5
      serology positive A51.5
    relapse (treated, untreated) A51.9
    skin A51.39
    symptomatic A51.9
      extragenital chancre A51.2
      primary, except extragenital chancre A51.0
      secondary — *see also* Syphilis, secondary A51.39
        relapse (treated, untreated) A51.49
    ulcer A51.39
  eighth nerve (neuritis) A52.15
  endemic A65
  endocarditis A52.03
    aortic A52.03
    pulmonary A52.03
  epididymis (late) A52.76
  epiglottis (late) A52.73
  epiphysitis (congenital) (early) A50.02
  episcleritis (late) A52.71
  esophagus A52.79
  eustachian tube A52.73
  exposure to Z20.2
  eye A52.71
  eyelid (late) (with gumma) A52.71
  fallopian tube (late) A52.76
  fracture A52.77
  gallbladder (late) A52.74
  gastric (polyposis) (late) A52.74
  general A53.9
    paralysis A52.17
      juvenile A50.45
  genital (primary) A51.0
  glaucoma A52.71
  gumma NEC A52.79
    cardiovascular system A52.00
    central nervous system A52.3
    congenital A50.59
  heart (block) (decompensation) (disease) (failure) A52.06 *[I52]*
    valve NEC A52.03
  hemianesthesia A52.19
  hemianopsia A52.71
  hemiparesis A52.17
  hemiplegia A52.17
  hepatic artery A52.09
  hepatis A52.74
  hepatomegaly, congenital A50.08
  hereditaria tarda — *see* Syphilis, congenital, late
  hereditary — *see* Syphilis, congenital
  Hutchinson's teeth A50.52
  hyalitis A52.71
  inactive — *see* Syphilis, latent
  infantum — *see* Syphilis, congenital
  inherited — *see* Syphilis, congenital
  internal ear A52.79
  intestine (late) A52.74
  iris, iritis (secondary) A51.43
    late A52.71
  joint (late) A52.77
  keratitis (congenital) (interstitial) (late) A50.31

Syphilis, syphilitic — *continued*
  kidney (late) A52.75
  lacrimal passages (late) A52.71
  larynx (late) A52.73
  late A52.9
    cardiovascular A52.00
    central nervous system A52.3
    kidney A52.75
    latent or 2 years or more after infection (without
      manifestations) A52.8
      negative spinal fluid test A52.8
      serology positive A52.8
    paresis A52.17
    specified site NEC A52.79
    symptomatic or with manifestations A52.79
    tabes A52.11
  latent A53.0
    with signs or symptoms — *code by* site and stage
      under Syphilis
    central nervous system A52.2
    date of infection unspecified A53.0
    early, or less than 2 years after infection A51.5
    follow-up of latent syphilis A53.0
      date of infection unspecified A53.0
      late, or 2 years or more after infection A52.8
    late, or 2 years or more after infection A52.8
    positive serology (only finding) A53.0
      date of infection unspecified A53.0
      early, or less than 2 years after infection A51.5
      late, or 2 years or more after infection A52.8
  lens (late) A52.71
  leukoderma A51.39
    late A52.79
  lienitis A52.79
  lip A51.39
    chancre (primary) A51.2
    late A52.79
  Lissauer's paralysis A52.17
  liver A52.74
  locomotor ataxia A52.11
  lung A52.72
  lymph gland (early) (secondary) A51.49
    late A52.79
  lymphadenitis (secondary) A51.49
  macular atrophy of skin A51.39
    striated A52.79
  mediastinum (late) A52.73
  meninges (adhesive) (brain) (spinal cord) A52.13
  meningitis A52.13
    acute (secondary) A51.41
    congenital A50.41
  meningoencephalitis A52.14
  meningovascular A52.13
    congenital A50.41
  mesarteritis A52.09
    brain A52.04
  middle ear A52.77
  mitral stenosis A52.03
  monoplegia A52.17
  mouth (secondary) A51.39
    late A52.79
  mucocutaneous (secondary) A51.39
    late A52.79
  mucous
    membrane (secondary) A51.39
      late A52.79
    patches A51.39
      congenital A50.07
  mulberry molars A50.52
  muscle A52.78
  myocardium A52.06
  nasal sinus (late) A52.73
  neonatorum — *see* Syphilis, congenital
  nephrotic syndrome (secondary) A51.44
  nerve palsy (any cranial nerve) A52.15
    multiple A52.15
  nervous system, central A52.3
  neuritis A52.15
    acoustic A52.15
  neurorecidive of retina A52.19
  neuroretinitis A52.19
  newborn — *see* Syphilis, congenital
  nodular superficial (late) A52.79
  nonvenereal A65
  nose (late) A52.73
    saddle back deformity A50.57
  occlusive arterial disease A52.09
  oculopathy A52.71
  ophthalmic (late) A52.71

Syphilis, syphilitic — *continued*
  optic nerve (atrophy) (neuritis) (papilla) A52.15
  orbit (late) A52.71
  organic A53.9
  osseous (late) A52.77
  osteochondritis (congenital) (early) A50.02 [M90.80]
  osteoporosis A52.77
  ovary (late) A52.76
  oviduct (late) A52.76
  palate (late) A52.79
  pancreas A52.74
  paralysis A52.17
    general A52.17
      juvenile A50.45
  paresis (general) A52.17
    juvenile A50.45
  paresthesia A52.19
  Parkinson's disease or syndrome A52.19
  paroxysmal tachycardia A52.06
  pemphigus (congenital) A50.06
  penis (chancre) A51.0
    late A52.76
  pericardium A52.06
  perichondritis, larynx (late) A52.73
  periosteum (late) A52.77
    congenital (early) A50.02 [M90.80]
    early (secondary) A51.46
  peripheral nerve A52.79
  petrous bone (late) A52.77
  pharynx (late) A52.73
    secondary A51.39
  pituitary (gland) A52.79
  pleura (late) A52.73
  pneumonia, white A50.04
  pontine lesion A52.17
  portal vein A52.09
  primary A51.0
    anal A51.1
    and secondary — *see* Syphilis, secondary
    central nervous system A52.3
    extragenital chancre NEC A51.2
    fingers A51.2
    genital A51.0
    lip A51.2
    specified site NEC A51.2
    tonsils A51.2
  prostate (late) A52.76
  ptosis (eyelid) A52.71
  pulmonary (late) A52.72
    artery A52.09
  pyelonephritis (late) A52.75
  recently acquired, symptomatic A51.9
  rectum (late) A52.74
  respiratory tract (late) A52.73
  retina, late A52.71
  retrobulbar neuritis A52.15
  salpingitis A52.76
  sclera (late) A52.71
  sclerosis
    cerebral A52.17
    coronary A52.06
    multiple A52.11
  scotoma (central) A52.71
  scrotum (late) A52.76
  secondary (and primary) A51.49
    adenopathy A51.49
    anus A51.39
    bone A51.46
    chorioretinitis, choroiditis A51.43
    hepatitis A51.45
    liver A51.45
    lymphadenitis A51.49
    meningitis (acute) A51.41
    mouth A51.39
    mucous membranes A51.39
    periosteum, periostitis A51.46
    pharynx A51.39
    relapse (treated, untreated) A51.49
    skin A51.39
    specified form NEC A51.49
    tonsil A51.39
    ulcer A51.39
    viscera NEC A51.49
    vulva A51.39
  seminal vesicle (late) A52.76

Syphilis, syphilitic — *continued*
  seronegative with signs or symptoms — *code by* site
    and stage under Syphilis
  seropositive
    with signs or symptoms — *code by* site and stage
      under Syphilis
    follow-up of latent syphilis — *see* Syphilis, latent
    only finding — *see* Syphilis, latent
  seventh nerve (paralysis) A52.15
  sinus, sinusitis (late) A52.73
  skeletal system A52.77
  skin (with ulceration) (early) (secondary) A51.39
    late or tertiary A52.79
  small intestine A52.74
  spastic spinal paralysis A52.17
  spermatic cord (late) A52.76
  spinal (cord) A52.12
  spleen A52.79
  splenomegaly A52.79
  spondylitis A52.77
  staphyloma A52.71
  stigmata (congenital) A50.59
  stomach A52.74
  synovium A52.78
  tabes dorsalis (late) A52.11
    juvenile A50.45
  tabetic type A52.11
    juvenile A50.45
  taboparesis A52.17
    juvenile A50.45
  tachycardia A52.06
  tendon (late) A52.78
  testis A52.76
  thorax A52.73
  throat A52.73
  thymus (gland) (late) A52.79
  thyroid (late) A52.79
  tongue (late) A52.79
  tonsil (lingual) (late) A52.73
    primary A51.2
    secondary A51.39
  trachea (late) A52.73
  tunica vaginalis (late) A52.76
  ulcer (any site) (early) (secondary) A51.39
    late A52.79
    perforating A52.79
      foot A52.11
  urethra (late) A52.76
  urogenital (late) A52.76
  uterus (late) A52.76
  uveal tract (secondary) A51.43
    late A52.71
  uveitis (secondary) A51.43
    late A52.71
  uvula (late) (perforated) A52.79
  vagina A51.0
    late A52.76
  valvulitis NEC A52.03
  vascular A52.00
    brain (cerebral) A52.05
  ventriculi A52.74
  vesicae urinariae (late) A52.76
  viscera (abdominal) (late) A52.74
    secondary A51.49
  vitreous (opacities) (late) A52.71
    hemorrhage A52.71
  vulva A51.0
    late A52.76
    secondary A51.39
Syphiloma A52.79
  cardiovascular system A52.00
  central nervous system A52.3
  circulatory system A52.00
  congenital A50.59
Syphilophobia F45.29
Syringadenoma — *see also* Neoplasm, skin, benign
  papillary — *see* Neoplasm, skin, benign
Syringobulbia G95.0
Syringocystadenoma — *see* Neoplasm, skin, benign
  papillary — *see* Neoplasm, skin, benign
Syringoma — *see also* Neoplasm, skin, benign
  chondroid — *see* Neoplasm, skin, benign

Syringomyelia G95.0
Syringomyelitis — *see* Encephalitis
Syringomyelocele — *see* Spina bifida
Syringopontia G95.0

System, systemic — *see also* condition
  disease, combined — *see* Degeneration, combined
  inflammatory response syndrome (SIRS) of non-infec-
    tious origin (without organ dysfunction) R65.10
    with acute organ dysfunction R65.11

System, systemic — *continued*
  lupus erythematosus M32.9
    inhibitor present D68.62
Systemic exertion intolerance disease [SEID] G93.32

T

Tabacism, tabacosis, tabagism — *see also* Poisoning, tobacco
  meaning dependence (without remission) F17.200
    with
      disorder F17.299
        in remission F17.211
        specified disorder NEC F17.298
        withdrawal F17.203
Tabardillo A75.9
  flea-borne A75.2
  louse-borne A75.0
Tabes, tabetic A52.10
  with
    central nervous system syphilis A52.10
    Charcot's joint A52.16
    cord bladder A52.19
    crisis, viscera (any) A52.19
    paralysis, general A52.17
    paresis (general) A52.17
    perforating ulcer (foot) A52.19
  arthropathy (Charcot) A52.16
  bladder A52.19
  bone A52.11
  cerebrospinal A52.12
  congenital A50.45
  conjugal A52.10
  dorsalis A52.11
    juvenile A50.49
  juvenile A50.49
  latent A52.19
  mesenterica A18.39
  paralysis, insane, general A52.17
  spasmodic A52.17
  syphilis (cerebrospinal) A52.12
Taboparalysis A52.17
Taboparesis (remission) A52.17
  juvenile A50.45
TAC (trigeminal autonomic cephalgia) **NEC** G44.099
  intractable G44.091
  not intractable G44.099
Tache noir S60.22- ☑
Tachyalimentation K91.2
Tachyarrhythmia, tachyrhythmia — *see* Tachycardia
Tachycardia R00.0
  atrial (paroxysmal) I47.1
  auricular I47.1
  AV nodal re-entry (re-entrant) I47.1
  junctional (paroxysmal) I47.1
  newborn P29.11
  nodal (paroxysmal) I47.1
  non-paroxysmal AV nodal I45.89
  paroxysmal (sustained) (nonsustained) I47.9
    with sinus bradycardia I49.5
    atrial (PAT) I47.1
    atrioventricular (AV) (re-entrant) I47.1
      psychogenic F54
    junctional I47.1
      ectopic I47.1
    nodal I47.1
    psychogenic (atrial) (supraventricular) (ventricular) F54
    supraventricular (sustained) I47.1
      psychogenic F54
    ventricular I47.20
      psychogenic F54
      specified type NEC I47.29
  psychogenic F45.8
  sick sinus I49.5
  sinoauricular NOS R00.0
    paroxysmal I47.1
  sinus [sinusal] NOS R00.0
    paroxysmal I47.1
  supraventricular I47.1
  ventricular (paroxysmal) (sustained) I47.20
    psychogenic F54
    specified NEC I47.29
Tachygastria K31.89
Tachypnea R06.82
  hysterical F45.8
  newborn (idiopathic) (transitory) P22.1
  psychogenic F45.8
  transitory, of newborn P22.1
TACO (transfusion associated circulatory overload) E87.71
TAD (transfusion-associated dyspnea) J95.87
Taenia (infection) (infestation) B68.9

Taenia — *continued*
  diminuta B71.0
  echinococcal infestation B67.90
  mediocanellata B68.1
  nana B71.0
  saginata B68.1
  solium (intestinal form) B68.0
    larval form — *see* Cysticercosis
Taeniasis (intestine) — *see* Taenia
Tag (hypertrophied skin) (infected) L91.8
  adenoid J35.8
  anus K64.4
  hemorrhoidal K64.4
  hymen N89.8
  perineal N90.89
  preauricular Q17.0
  sentinel K64.4
  skin L91.8
    accessory (congenital) Q82.8
    anus K64.4
    congenital Q82.8
    preauricular Q17.0
  tonsil J35.8
  urethra, urethral N36.8
  vulva N90.89
Tahyna fever B33.8
Takahara's disease E80.3
Takayasu's disease or syndrome M31.4
Talaromycosis B48.4
Talcosis (pulmonary) J62.0
Talipes (congenital) Q66.89
  acquired, planus — *see* Deformity, limb, flat foot
  asymmetric Q66.89
  calcaneovalgus Q66.4- ☑
  calcaneovarus Q66.1- ☑
  calcaneus Q66.89
  cavus Q66.7- ☑
  equinovalgus Q66.6
  equinovarus Q66.0- ☑
  equinus Q66.89
  percavus Q66.7- ☑
  planovalgus Q66.6
  planus (acquired) (any degree) — *see also* Deformity, limb, flat foot
    congenital Q66.5- ☑
    due to rickets (sequelae) E64.3
  valgus Q66.6
  varus Q66.3- ☑
Tall stature, constitutional E34.4
Talma's disease M62.89
Talon noir S90.3- ☑
  hand S60.22- ☑
  heel S90.3- ☑
  toe S90.1- ☑
Tamponade, heart I31.4
Tanapox (virus disease) B08.71
Tangier disease E78.6
Tantrum, child problem F91.8
Tapeworm (infection) (infestation) — *see* Infestation, tapeworm
Tapia's syndrome G52.7
TAR (thrombocytopenia with absent radius) **syndrome** Q87.2
Tarral-Besnier disease L44.0
Tarsal tunnel syndrome — *see* Syndrome, tarsal tunnel
Tarsalgia — *see* Pain, limb, lower
Tarsitis (eyelid) H01.8
  syphilitic A52.71
  tuberculous A18.4
Tartar (teeth) (dental calculus) K03.6
Tattoo (mark) L81.8
Tauri's disease E74.09
Taurodontism K00.2
Taussig-Bing syndrome Q20.1
Taybi's syndrome Q87.2
Tay-Sachs amaurotic familial idiocy or disease E75.02
TBI (traumatic brain injury) S06.9 ☑
Teacher's node or nodule J38.2
Tear, torn (traumatic) — *see also* Laceration
  with abortion — *see* Abortion
  annular fibrosis M51.35
  anus, anal (sphincter) S31.831 ☑
    complicating delivery
      with third degree perineal laceration — *see also* Delivery, complicated, by, laceration, perineum, third degree O70.20
        with mucosa O70.3

Tear, torn — *continued*
  anus, anal — *continued*
    complicating delivery — *continued*
      without third degree perineal laceration O70.4
    nontraumatic (healed) (old) K62.81
  articular cartilage, old — *see* Derangement, joint, articular cartilage, by site
  bladder
    with ectopic or molar pregnancy O08.6
    following ectopic or molar pregnancy O08.6
    obstetrical O71.5
    traumatic — *see* Injury, bladder
  bowel
    with ectopic or molar pregnancy O08.6
    following ectopic or molar pregnancy O08.6
    obstetrical trauma O71.5
  broad ligament
    with ectopic or molar pregnancy O08.6
    following ectopic or molar pregnancy O08.6
    obstetrical trauma O71.6
  bucket handle (knee) (meniscus) — *see* Tear, meniscus
  capsule, joint — *see* Sprain
  cartilage — *see also* Sprain
    articular, old — *see* Derangement, joint, articular cartilage, by site
  cervix
    with ectopic or molar pregnancy O08.6
    following ectopic or molar pregnancy O08.6
    obstetrical trauma (current) O71.3
    old N88.1
    traumatic — *see* Injury, uterus
  dural G97.41
    nontraumatic G96.11
  internal organ — *see* Injury, by site
  knee cartilage
    articular (current) S83.3- ☑
    old — *see* Derangement, knee, meniscus, due to old tear
  ligament — *see* Sprain
  meniscus (knee) (current injury) S83.209 ☑
    bucket-handle S83.20- ☑
    lateral
      bucket-handle S83.25- ☑
      complex S83.27- ☑
      peripheral S83.26- ☑
      specified type NEC S83.28- ☑
    medial
      bucket-handle S83.21- ☑
      complex S83.23- ☑
      peripheral S83.22- ☑
      specified type NEC S83.24- ☑
    old — *see* Derangement, knee, meniscus, due to old tear
    site other than knee — *code as* Sprain
    specified type NEC S83.20- ☑
  muscle — *see* Strain
  pelvic
    floor, complicating delivery O70.1
    organ NEC, obstetrical trauma O71.5
      with ectopic or molar pregnancy O08.6
      following ectopic or molar pregnancy O08.6
  perineal, secondary O90.1
  periurethral tissue, obstetrical trauma O71.82
    with ectopic or molar pregnancy O08.6
    following ectopic or molar pregnancy O08.6
  rectovaginal septum — *see* Laceration, vagina
  retina, retinal (without detachment) (horseshoe) — *see also* Break, retina, horseshoe
    with detachment — *see* Detachment, retina, with retinal, break
  rotator cuff (nontraumatic) M75.10- ☑
    complete M75.12- ☑
    incomplete M75.11- ☑
    traumatic S46.01- ☑
      capsule S43.42- ☑
  semilunar cartilage, knee — *see* Tear, meniscus
  supraspinatus (complete) (incomplete) (nontraumatic) — *see also* Tear, rotator cuff M75.10- ☑
  tendon — *see* Strain
  tentorial, at birth P10.4
  umbilical cord
    complicating delivery O69.89 ☑
  urethra
    with ectopic or molar pregnancy O08.6
    following ectopic or molar pregnancy O08.6
    obstetrical trauma O71.5
  uterus — *see* Injury, uterus

Tear, torn — *continued*
  vagina — *see* Laceration, vagina
  vessel, from catheter — *see* Puncture, accidental
      complicating surgery
  vulva, complicating delivery O70.0
Tear-stone — *see* Dacryolith
Teeth — *see also* condition
  grinding
      psychogenic F45.8
      sleep related G47.63
Teething (syndrome) K00.7
Telangiectasia, telangiectasis (verrucous) I78.1
  ataxic (cerebellar) (Louis-Bar) G11.3
  familial I78.0
  hemorrhagic, hereditary (congenital) (senile) I78.0
  hereditary, hemorrhagic (congenital) (senile) I78.0
  juxtafoveal H35.07- ☑
  macular H35.07- ☑
  macularis eruptiva perstans D47.01
  parafoveal H35.07- ☑
  retinal (idiopathic) (juxtafoveal) (macular) (parafoveal)
      H35.07- ☑
  spider I78.1
Telephone scatologia F65.89
Telescoped bowel or intestine K56.1
  congenital Q43.8
Temperature
  body, high (of unknown origin) R50.9
  cold, trauma from T69.9 ☑
      newborn P80.0
      specified effect NEC T69.8 ☑
Temple — *see* condition
Temporal — *see* condition
Temporomandibular joint pain-dysfunction syn-
    drome M26.62- ☑
Temporosphenoidal — *see* condition
Tendency
  bleeding — *see* Defect, coagulation
  suicide
      meaning personal history of attempted suicide
          Z91.51
      meaning suicidal ideation — *see* Ideation, suicidal
  to fall R29.6
Tenderness, abdominal R10.819
  epigastric R10.816
  generalized R10.817
  left lower quadrant R10.814
  left upper quadrant R10.812
  periumbilic R10.815
  rebound R10.829
      epigastric R10.826
      generalized R10.827
      left lower quadrant R10.824
      left upper quadrant R10.822
      periumbilic R10.825
      right lower quadrant R10.823
      right upper quadrant R10.821
  right lower quadrant R10.813
  right upper quadrant R10.811
Tendinitis, tendonitis — *see also* Enthesopathy
  Achilles M76.6- ☑
  adhesive — *see* Tenosynovitis, specified type NEC
      shoulder — *see* Capsulitis, adhesive
  bicipital M75.2- ☑
  calcific M65.2- ☑
      ankle M65.27- ☑
      foot M65.27- ☑
      forearm M65.23- ☑
      hand M65.24- ☑
      lower leg M65.26- ☑
      multiple sites M65.29
      pelvic region M65.25- ☑
      shoulder M75.3- ☑
      specified site NEC M65.28
      thigh M65.25- ☑
      upper arm M65.22- ☑
  due to use, overuse, pressure — *see also* Disorder, soft
      tissue, due to use
      specified NEC — *see* Disorder, soft tissue, due to
          use, specified NEC
  gluteal M76.0- ☑
  patellar M76.5- ☑
  peroneal M76.7- ☑
  psoas M76.1- ☑
  tibial (posterior) M76.82- ☑
      anterior M76.81- ☑
  trochanteric — *see* Bursitis, hip, trochanteric

Tendon — *see* condition
Tendosynovitis — *see* Tenosynovitis
Tenesmus (rectal) R19.8
  vesical R30.1
Tennis elbow — *see* Epicondylitis, lateral
Tenonitis — *see also* Tenosynovitis
  eye (capsule) H05.04- ☑
Tenontosynovitis — *see* Tenosynovitis
Tenontothecitis — *see* Tenosynovitis
Tenophyte — *see* Disorder, synovium, specified type NEC
Tenosynovitis — *see also* Synovitis M65.9
  adhesive — *see* Tenosynovitis, specified type NEC
      shoulder — *see* Capsulitis, adhesive
  bicipital (calcifying) — *see* Tendinitis, bicipital
  gonococcal A54.49
  in (due to)
      crystals M65.8- ☑
      gonorrhea A54.49
      syphilis (late) A52.78
      use, overuse, pressure — *see also* Disorder, soft tis-
          sue, due to use
          specified NEC — *see* Disorder, soft tissue, due to
              use, specified NEC
  infective NEC M65.1- ☑
      ankle M65.17- ☑
      foot M65.17- ☑
      forearm M65.13- ☑
      hand M65.14- ☑
      lower leg M65.16- ☑
      multiple sites M65.19
      pelvic region M65.15- ☑
      shoulder region M65.11- ☑
      specified site NEC M65.18
      thigh M65.15- ☑
      upper arm M65.12- ☑
  radial styloid M65.4
  shoulder region M65.81- ☑
      adhesive — *see* Capsulitis, adhesive
  specified type NEC M65.88
      ankle M65.87- ☑
      foot M65.87- ☑
      forearm M65.83- ☑
      hand M65.84- ☑
      lower leg M65.86- ☑
      multiple sites M65.89
      pelvic region M65.85- ☑
      shoulder region M65.81- ☑
      specified site NEC M65.88
      thigh M65.85- ☑
      upper arm M65.82- ☑
  tuberculous — *see* Tuberculosis, tenosynovitis
Tenovaginitis — *see* Tenosynovitis
Tension
  arterial, high — *see also* Hypertension
      without diagnosis of hypertension R03.0
  headache G44.209
      intractable G44.201
      not intractable G44.209
  nervous R45.0
  pneumothorax J93.0
  premenstrual N94.3
  state (mental) F48.9
Tentorium — *see* condition
Teratencephalus Q89.8
Teratism Q89.7
Teratoblastoma (malignant) — *see* Neoplasm, malig-
    nant, by site
Teratocarcinoma — *see also* Neoplasm, malignant, by
    site
  liver C22.7
Teratoma (solid) — *see also* Neoplasm, uncertain behav-
    ior, by site
  with embryonal carcinoma, mixed — *see* Neoplasm,
      malignant, by site
  with malignant transformation — *see* Neoplasm, ma-
      lignant, by site
  adult (cystic) — *see* Neoplasm, benign, by site
  benign — *see* Neoplasm, benign, by site
  combined with choriocarcinoma — *see* Neoplasm,
      malignant, by site
  cystic (adult) — *see* Neoplasm, benign, by site
  differentiated — *see* Neoplasm, benign, by site
  embryonal — *see also* Neoplasm, malignant, by site
      liver C22.7
  immature — *see* Neoplasm, malignant, by site
  liver C22.7

Teratoma — *continued*
  liver — *continued*
      adult, benign, cystic, differentiated type or mature
          D13.4
  malignant — *see also* Neoplasm, malignant, by site
      anaplastic — *see* Neoplasm, malignant, by site
      intermediate — *see* Neoplasm, malignant, by site
          specified site — *see* Neoplasm, malignant, by
              site
          unspecified site C62.90
      undifferentiated — *see* Neoplasm, malignant, by
          site
  mature — *see* Neoplasm, uncertain behavior, by site
      malignant — *see* Neoplasm, by site, malignant, by
          site
  ovary D27.- ☑
      embryonal, immature or malignant C56- ☑
  solid — *see* Neoplasm, uncertain behavior, by site
  testis C62.9- ☑
      adult, benign, cystic, differentiated type or mature
          D29.2- ☑
      scrotal C62.1- ☑
      undescended C62.0- ☑
Termination
  anomalous — *see also* Malposition, congenital
      right pulmonary vein Q26.3
  pregnancy, elective Z33.2
Ternidens diminutus infestation B81.8
Ternidensiasis B81.8
Terror(s) night (child) F51.4
Terrorism, victim of Z65.4
Terry's syndrome — *see also* Myopia, degenerative
    H44.2- ☑
Tertiary — *see* condition
Test, tests, testing (for)
  adequacy (for dialysis)
      hemodialysis Z49.31
      peritoneal Z49.32
  blood pressure Z01.30
      abnormal reading — *see* Blood, pressure
  blood typing Z01.83
      Rh typing Z01.83
  blood-alcohol Z02.83
      positive — *see* Findings, abnormal, in blood
  blood-drug Z02.83
      positive — *see* Findings, abnormal, in blood
  cardiac pulse generator (battery) Z45.010
  fertility Z31.41
  genetic
      disease carrier status for procreative management
          female Z31.430
          male Z31.440
      male partner of patient with recurrent pregnancy
          loss Z31.441
      procreative management NEC
          female Z31.438
          male Z31.448
  hearing Z01.10
      with abnormal findings NEC Z01.118
      infant or child (over 28 days old) Z00.129
          with abnormal findings Z00.121
  HIV (human immunodeficiency virus)
      nonconclusive (in infants) R75
      positive Z21
      seropositive Z21
  immunity status Z01.84
  intelligence NEC Z01.89
  laboratory (as part of a general medical examination)
      Z00.00
      with abnormal finding Z00.01
      for medicolegal reason NEC Z04.89
  male partner of patient with recurrent pregnancy loss
      Z31.441
  Mantoux (for tuberculosis) Z11.1
      abnormal result R76.11
  pregnancy, positive first pregnancy — *see* Pregnancy,
      normal, first
  procreative Z31.49
      fertility Z31.41
  skin, diagnostic
      allergy Z01.82
          special screening examination — *see* Screening,
              by name of disease
      Mantoux Z11.1
      tuberculin Z11.1
  specified NEC Z01.89
  tuberculin Z11.1
      abnormal result R76.11

Test, tests, testing — *continued*
  vision Z01.00
    with abnormal findings Z01.01
    following failed vision screening Z01.020
      with abnormal findings Z01.021
    infant or child (over 28 days old) Z00.129
      with abnormal findings Z00.121
  Wassermann Z11.3
    positive — *see* Serology for syphilis, positive
Testicle, testicular, testis — *see also* condition
  feminization syndrome — *see also* Syndrome, androgen insensitivity E34.51
  migrans Q55.29
Tetanus, tetanic (cephalic) (convulsions) A35
  with
    abortion A34
    ectopic or molar pregnancy O08.0
  following ectopic or molar pregnancy O08.0
  inoculation reaction (due to serum) — *see* Complications, vaccination
  neonatorum A33
  obstetrical A34
  puerperal, postpartum, childbirth A34
Tetany (due to) R29.0
  alkalosis E87.3
  associated with rickets E55.0
  convulsions R29.0
    hysterical F44.5
  functional (hysterical) F44.5
  hyperkinetic R29.0
    hysterical F44.5
  hyperpnea R06.4
    hysterical F44.5
    psychogenic F45.8
  hyperventilation — *see also* Hyperventilation R06.4
    hysterical F44.5
  neonatal (without calcium or magnesium deficiency) P71.3
  parathyroid (gland) E20.9
  parathyroprival E89.2
  post- (para)thyroidectomy E89.2
  postoperative E89.2
  pseudotetany R29.0
  psychogenic (conversion reaction) F44.5
Tetralogy of Fallot Q21.3
Tetraplegia (chronic) — *see also* Quadriplegia G82.50
Thailand hemorrhagic fever A91
Thalassanemia — *see* Thalassemia
Thalassemia (anemia) (disease) D56.9
  with other hemoglobinopathy D56.8
  alpha (major) (severe) (triple gene defect) D56.0
    minor D56.3
    silent carrier D56.3
    trait D56.3
  beta (severe) D56.1
    homozygous D56.1
    major D56.1
    minor D56.3
    trait D56.3
  delta-beta (homozygous) D56.2
    minor D56.3
    trait D56.3
  dominant D56.8
  hemoglobin
    C D56.8
    E-beta D56.5
  intermedia D56.1
  major D56.1
  minor D56.3
  mixed D56.8
  sickle-cell — *see* Disease, sickle-cell, thalassemia
  specified type NEC D56.8
  trait D56.3
  variants D56.8
Thanatophoric dwarfism or short stature Q77.1
Thaysen-Gee disease (nontropical sprue) K90.0
Thaysen's disease K90.0
Thecoma D27- ☑
  luteinized D27- ☑
  malignant C56- ☑
Thelarche, premature E30.8
Thelaziasis B83.8
Thelitis N61.0
  puerperal, postpartum or gestational — *see* Infection, nipple
Therapeutic — *see* condition

Therapy
  drug, long-term (current) (prophylactic)
    agents affecting estrogen receptors and estrogen levels NEC Z79.818
    anastrozole (Arimidex) Z79.811
    antibiotics Z79.2
      short-term use — *omit code*
    anticoagulants Z79.01
    anti-inflammatory Z79.1
    antiplatelet Z79.02
    antithrombotics Z79.02
    aromatase inhibitors Z79.811
    aspirin Z79.82
    birth control pill or patch Z79.3
    bisphosphonates Z79.83
    contraceptive, oral Z79.3
    drug, specified NEC Z79.899
    estrogen receptor downregulators Z79.818
    Evista Z79.810
    exemestane (Aromasin) Z79.811
    Fareston Z79.810
    fulvestrant (Faslodex) Z79.818
    gonadotropin-releasing hormone (GnRH) agonist Z79.818
    goserelin acetate (Zoladex) Z79.818
    hormone replacement Z79.890
    insulin Z79.4
    letrozole (Femara) Z79.811
    leuprolide acetate (leuprorelin) (Lupron) Z79.818
    megestrol acetate (Megace) Z79.818
    methadone
      for pain management Z79.891
      maintenance therapy F11.20
    Nolvadex Z79.810
    opiate analgesic Z79.891
    oral contraceptive Z79.3
    raloxifene (Evista) Z79.810
    selective estrogen receptor modulators (SERMs) Z79.810
    short term — *omit code*
    steroids
      inhaled Z79.51
      systemic Z79.52
    tamoxifen (Nolvadex) Z79.810
    toremifene (Fareston) Z79.810
Thermic — *see* condition
Thermography (abnormal) — *see also* Abnormal, diagnostic imaging R93.89
  breast R92.8
Thermoplegia T67.01 ☑
Thesaurismosis, glycogen — *see* Disease, glycogen storage
Thiamin deficiency E51.9
  specified NEC E51.8
Thiaminic deficiency with beriberi E51.11
Thibierge-Weissenbach syndrome — *see* Sclerosis, systemic
Thickening
  bone — *see* Hypertrophy, bone
  breast N64.59
  endometrium R93.89
  epidermal L85.9
    specified NEC L85.8
  hymen N89.6
  larynx J38.7
  nail L60.2
    congenital Q84.5
  periosteal — *see* Hypertrophy, bone
  pleura J92.9
    with asbestos J92.0
  skin R23.4
  subepiglottic J38.7
  tongue K14.8
  valve, heart — *see* Endocarditis
Thigh — *see* condition
Thinning vertebra — *see* Spondylopathy, specified NEC
Thirst, excessive R63.1
  due to deprivation of water T73.1 ☑
Thomsen disease G71.12
Thoracic — *see also* condition
  kidney Q63.2
  outlet syndrome G54.0
Thoracogastroschisis (congenital) Q79.8
Thoracopagus Q89.4
Thorax — *see* condition
Thorn's syndrome N28.89
Thorson-Björck syndrome E34.0
Threadworm (infection) (infestation) B80

Threatened
  abortion O20.0
    with subsequent abortion O03.9
  job loss, anxiety concerning Z56.2
  labor (without delivery) O47.9
    at or after 37 completed weeks of gestation O47.1
    before 37 completed weeks of gestation O47.0- ☑
  loss of job, anxiety concerning Z56.2
  miscarriage O20.0
  unemployment, anxiety concerning Z56.2
Three-day fever A93.1
Threshers' lung J67.0
Thrix annulata (congenital) Q84.1
Throat — *see* condition
Thrombasthenia (Glanzmann) (hemorrhagic) (hereditary) D69.1
Thromboangiitis I73.1
  obliterans (general) I73.1
    cerebral I67.89
    vessels
      brain I67.89
      spinal cord I67.89
Thromboarteritis — *see* Arteritis
Thromboasthenia (Glanzmann) (hemorrhagic) (hereditary) D69.1
Thrombocytasthenia (Glanzmann) D69.1
Thrombocythemia (hemorrhagic) *see also* Thrombocytosis D75.839
  essential D47.3
  idiopathic D47.3
  primary D47.3
Thrombocytopathy (dystrophic) (granulopenic) D69.1
Thrombocytopenia, thrombocytopenic D69.6
  with absent radius (TAR) Q87.2
  congenital D69.42
  dilutional D69.59
  due to
    (massive) blood transfusion D69.59
    drugs D69.59
    extracorporeal circulation of blood D69.59
    platelet alloimmunization D69.59
  essential D69.3
  heparin induced (HIT) D75.829
    delayed-onset D75.828
    immune-mediated D75.822
    non-immune D75.821
    persisting D75.828
    syndrome
      autoimmune D75.828
      specified NEC D75.828
      spontaneous (without heparin exposure) D75.84
    type 1 D75.821
    type 2 D75.822
  heparin-associated D75.821
  hereditary D69.42
  idiopathic D69.3
  neonatal, transitory P61.0
    due to
      exchange transfusion P61.0
      idiopathic maternal thrombocytopenia P61.0
      isoimmunization P61.0
  primary NEC D69.49
    idiopathic D69.3
  puerperal, postpartum O72.3
  secondary D69.59
  transient neonatal P61.0
  vaccine-induced thrombotic D75.84
Thrombocytosis D75.839
  essential D47.3
  idiopathic D47.3
  primary D47.3
  reactive D75.838
  secondary D75.838
  specified NEC D75.838
Thromboembolism — *see* Embolism
Thrombopathy (Bernard-Soulier) D69.1
  constitutional — *see* Disease, von Willebrand
  Willebrand-Jurgens — *see* Disease, von Willebrand
Thrombopenia — *see* Thrombocytopenia
Thrombophilia D68.59
  primary NEC D68.59
  secondary NEC D68.69
  specified NEC D68.69
Thrombophlebitis I80.9
  antepartum O22.2- ☑
    deep O22.3- ☑
    superficial O22.2- ☑
  calf muscular vein (NOS) I80.25- ☑

☑ **Additional Character Required — Refer to the Tabular List for Character Selection**

Thrombophlebitis — *continued*
- cavernous (venous) sinus G08
  - complicating pregnancy O22.5- ☑
  - nonpyogenic I67.6
- cerebral (sinus) (vein) G08
  - nonpyogenic I67.6
  - sequelae G09
- due to implanted device — *see* Complications, by site and type, specified NEC
- during or resulting from a procedure NEC T81.72 ☑
- femoral vein (superficial) I80.1- ☑
- femoropopliteal vein I80.0- ☑
- gastrocnemial vein I80.25- ☑
- hepatic (vein) I80.8
- idiopathic, recurrent I82.1
- iliac vein (common) (external) (internal) I80.21- ☑
- iliofemoral I80.1- ☑
- intracranial venous sinus (any) G08
  - nonpyogenic I67.6
  - sequelae G09
- intraspinal venous sinuses and veins G08
  - nonpyogenic G95.19
- lateral (venous) sinus G08
  - nonpyogenic I67.6
- leg I80.3
  - superficial I80.0- ☑
- longitudinal (venous) sinus G08
  - nonpyogenic I67.6
- lower extremity I80.299
- migrans, migrating I82.1
- pelvic
  - with ectopic or molar pregnancy O08.0
  - following ectopic or molar pregnancy O08.0
  - puerperal O87.1
- peroneal vein I80.24- ☑
- popliteal vein — *see* Phlebitis, leg, deep, popliteal
- portal (vein) K75.1
- postoperative T81.72 ☑
- pregnancy — *see* Thrombophlebitis, antepartum
- puerperal, postpartum, childbirth O87.0
  - deep O87.1
  - pelvic O87.1
  - septic O86.81
  - superficial O87.0
- saphenous (greater) (lesser) I80.0- ☑
- sinus (intracranial) G08
  - nonpyogenic I67.6
- soleal vein I80.25- ☑
- specified site NEC I80.8
- tibial vein (anterior) (posterior) I80.23- ☑

Thrombosis, thrombotic (bland) (multiple) (progressive) (silent) (vessel) I82.90
- anal K64.5
- antepartum — *see* Thrombophlebitis, antepartum
- aorta, aortic I74.10
  - abdominal I74.09
    - saddle I74.01
  - bifurcation I74.09
  - saddle I74.01
  - specified site NEC I74.19
  - terminal I74.09
  - thoracic I74.11
  - valve — *see* Endocarditis, aortic
- apoplexy I63.3- ☑
- artery, arteries (postinfectional) I74.9
  - auditory, internal — *see* Occlusion, artery, precerebral, specified NEC
  - basilar — *see* Occlusion, artery, basilar
  - carotid (common) (internal) — *see* Occlusion, artery, carotid
  - cerebellar (anterior inferior) (posterior inferior) (superior) — *see* Occlusion, artery, cerebellar
  - cerebral — *see* Occlusion, artery, cerebral
  - choroidal (anterior) — *see* Occlusion, artery, precerebral, specified NEC
  - communicating, posterior — *see* Occlusion, artery, precerebral, specified NEC
  - coronary — *see also* Infarct, myocardium
    - not resulting in infarction I24.0
  - hepatic I74.8
  - hypophyseal — *see* Occlusion, artery, precerebral, specified NEC
  - iliac I74.5
  - limb I74.4
    - lower I74.3
    - upper I74.2
  - meningeal, anterior or posterior — *see* Occlusion, artery, cerebral, specified NEC

Thrombosis, thrombotic — *continued*
- artery, arteries — *continued*
  - mesenteric (with gangrene) — *see also* Infarct, intestine K55.069
  - ophthalmic — *see* Occlusion, artery, retina
  - pontine — *see* Occlusion, artery, precerebral, specified NEC
  - precerebral — *see* Occlusion, artery, precerebral
  - pulmonary (iatrogenic) — *see* Embolism, pulmonary
  - renal N28.0
  - retinal — *see* Occlusion, artery, retina
  - spinal, anterior or posterior G95.11
  - traumatic NEC T14.8 ☑
  - vertebral — *see* Occlusion, artery, vertebral
- atrium, auricular — *see also* Infarct, myocardium
  - following acute myocardial infarction (current complication) I23.6
  - not resulting in infarction I51.3
  - old I51.3
- basilar (artery) — *see* Occlusion, artery, basilar
- brain (artery) (stem) — *see also* Occlusion, artery, cerebral
  - due to syphilis A52.05
  - puerperal O99.43
  - sinus — *see* Thrombosis, intracranial venous sinus
- capillary I78.8
- cardiac — *see also* Infarct, myocardium
  - not resulting in infarction I51.3
  - old I51.3
  - valve — *see* Endocarditis
- carotid (artery) (common) (internal) — *see* Occlusion, artery, carotid
- cavernous (venous) sinus — *see* Thrombosis, intracranial venous sinus
- cerebellar artery (anterior inferior) (posterior inferior) (superior) I66.3
- cerebral (artery) — *see* Occlusion, artery, cerebral
- cerebrovenous sinus — *see also* Thrombosis, intracranial venous sinus
  - puerperium O87.3
- chronic I82.91
- coronary (artery) (vein) — *see also* Infarct, myocardium
  - not resulting in infarction I24.0
- corpus cavernosum N48.89
- cortical I66.9
- deep — *see* Embolism, vein, lower extremity
- due to device, implant or graft — *see also* Complications, by site and type, specified NEC T85.868 ☑
  - arterial graft NEC T82.868 ☑
  - breast (implant) T85.868 ☑
  - catheter NEC T85.868 ☑
    - dialysis (renal) T82.868 ☑
      - intraperitoneal T85.868 ☑
    - infusion NEC T82.868 ☑
      - spinal (epidural) (subdural) T85.860 ☑
    - urinary (indwelling) T83.86 ☑
  - electronic (electrode) (pulse generator) (stimulator)
    - bone T84.86 ☑
    - cardiac T82.867 ☑
    - nervous system (brain) (peripheral nerve) (spinal) T85.860 ☑
    - urinary T83.86 ☑
  - fixation, internal (orthopedic) NEC T84.86 ☑
  - gastrointestinal (bile duct) (esophagus) T85.868 ☑
  - genital NEC T83.86 ☑
  - heart T82.867 ☑
  - joint prosthesis T84.86 ☑
  - ocular (corneal graft) (orbital implant) NEC T85.868 ☑
  - orthopedic NEC T84.86 ☑
  - specified NEC T85.868 ☑
  - urinary NEC T83.86 ☑
  - vascular NEC T82.868 ☑
  - ventricular intracranial shunt T85.860 ☑
- during the puerperium — *see* Thrombosis, puerperal
- endocardial — *see also* Infarct, myocardium
  - not resulting in infarction I51.3
- eye — *see* Occlusion, retina
- genital organ
  - female NEC N94.89
    - pregnancy — *see* Thrombophlebitis, antepartum
  - male N50.1
- gestational — *see* Phlebopathy, gestational
- heart (chamber) — *see also* Infarct, myocardium
  - not resulting in infarction I51.3
  - old I51.3
- hepatic (vein) I82.0

Thrombosis, thrombotic — *continued*
- hepatic — *continued*
  - artery I74.8
- history (of) Z86.718
- intestine (with gangrene) — *see also* Infarct, intestine K55.069
- intracardiac NEC (apical) (atrial) (auricular) (ventricular) (old) I51.3
- intracranial (arterial) I66.9
  - venous sinus (any) G08
    - nonpyogenic origin I67.6
    - puerperium O87.3
- intramural — *see also* Infarct, myocardium
  - not resulting in infarction I51.3
  - old I51.3
- intraspinal venous sinuses and veins G08
  - nonpyogenic G95.19
- kidney (artery) N28.0
- lateral (venous) sinus — *see* Thrombosis, intracranial venous sinus
- leg — *see* Thrombosis, vein, lower extremity
  - arterial I74.3
- liver (venous) I82.0
  - artery I74.8
  - portal vein I81
- longitudinal (venous) sinus — *see* Thrombosis, intracranial venous sinus
- lower limb — *see* Thrombosis, vein, lower extremity
- lung (iatrogenic) (postoperative) — *see* Embolism, pulmonary
- meninges (brain) (arterial) I66.8
- mesenteric (artery) (with gangrene) — *see also* Infarct, intestine K55.069
  - vein (inferior) (superior) K55.0- ☑
- mitral I34.89
- mural — *see also* Infarct, myocardium
  - due to syphilis A52.06
  - not resulting in infarction I51.3
  - old I51.3
- omentum (with gangrene) — *see also* Infarct, intestine K55.069
- ophthalmic — *see* Occlusion, retina
- pampiniform plexus (male) N50.1
- parietal — *see also* Infarct, myocardium
  - not resulting in infarction I24.0
- penis, superficial vein N48.81
- perianal venous K64.5
- peripheral arteries I74.4
  - upper I74.2
- personal history (of) Z86.718
- portal I81
  - due to syphilis A52.09
- precerebral artery — *see* Occlusion, artery, precerebral
- puerperal, postpartum O87.0
  - brain (artery) O99.43
    - venous (sinus) O87.3
  - cardiac O99.43
  - cerebral (artery) O99.43
    - venous (sinus) O87.3
  - superficial O87.0
- pulmonary (artery) (iatrogenic) (postoperative) (vein) — *see* Embolism, pulmonary
- renal (artery) N28.0
  - vein I82.3
- resulting from presence of device, implant or graft — *see* Complications, by site and type, specified NEC
- retina, retinal — *see* Occlusion, retina
- scrotum N50.1
- seminal vesicle N50.1
- sigmoid (venous) sinus — *see* Thrombosis, intracranial venous sinus
- sinus, intracranial (any) — *see* Thrombosis, intracranial venous sinus
- specified site NEC I82.890
  - chronic I82.891
- spermatic cord N50.1
- spinal cord (arterial) G95.11
  - due to syphilis A52.09
  - pyogenic origin G06.1
- spleen, splenic D73.5
  - artery I74.8
- testis N50.1
- traumatic NEC T14.8 ☑
- tricuspid I07.8
- tumor — *see* Neoplasm, unspecified behavior, by site
- tunica vaginalis N50.1
- umbilical cord (vessels), complicating delivery O69.5 ☑

Thrombosis, thrombotic — *continued*
  vas deferens N50.1
  vein (acute) I82.90
    antecubital I82.61- ☑
      chronic I82.71- ☑
    axillary I82.A1- ☑ (*following* I82.7)
      chronic I82.A2- ☑ (*following* I82.7)
    basilic I82.61- ☑
      chronic I82.71- ☑
    brachial I82.62- ☑
      chronic I82.72- ☑
    brachiocephalic (innominate) I82.290
      chronic I82.291
    cephalic I82.61- ☑
      chronic I82.71- ☑
    cerebral, nonpyogenic I67.6
    chronic I82.91
    deep (DVT) I82.40- ☑
      calf I82.4Z- ☑
        chronic I82.5Z- ☑
      lower leg I82.4Z- ☑
        chronic I82.5Z- ☑
      thigh I82.4Y- ☑
        chronic I82.5Y- ☑
      upper leg I82.4Y- ☑
        chronic I82.5Y- ☑
    femoral I82.41- ☑
      chronic I82.51- ☑
    iliac (iliofemoral) I82.42- ☑
      chronic I82.52- ☑
    innominate I82.290
      chronic I82.291
    internal jugular I82.C1- ☑ (*following* I82.7)
      chronic I82.C2- ☑ (*following* I82.7)
    lower extremity
      deep I82.40- ☑
        chronic I82.50- ☑
        specified NEC I82.49- ☑
          chronic NEC I82.59- ☑
      distal
        deep I82.4Z- ☑
      proximal
        deep I82.4Y- ☑
          chronic I82.5Y- ☑
      superficial I82.81- ☑
    perianal K64.5
    popliteal I82.43- ☑
      chronic I82.53- ☑
    radial I82.62- ☑
      chronic I82.72- ☑
    renal I82.3
    saphenous (greater) (lesser) I82.81- ☑
    specified NEC I82.890
      chronic NEC I82.891
    subclavian I82.B1- ☑ (*following* I82.7)
      chronic I82.B2- ☑ (*following* I82.7)
    thoracic NEC I82.290
      chronic I82.291
    tibial I82.44- ☑
      chronic I82.54- ☑
    ulnar I82.62- ☑
      chronic I82.72- ☑
    upper extremity I82.60- ☑
      chronic I82.70- ☑
      deep I82.62- ☑
        chronic I82.72- ☑
      superficial I82.61- ☑
        chronic I82.71- ☑
  vena cava
    inferior I82.220
      chronic I82.221
    superior I82.210
      chronic I82.211
  venous, perianal K64.5
  ventricle — *see also* Infarct, myocardium
    following acute myocardial infarction (current complication) I23.6
    not resulting in infarction I24.0
    old I51.3
Thrombus — *see* Thrombosis
Thrush — *see also* Candidiasis
  newborn P37.5
  oral B37.0
  vaginal (acute) B37.31
    chronic (recurrent) B37.32
Thumb — *see also* condition
  sucking (child problem) F98.8

Thymitis E32.8
Thymoma — *see also* Neoplasm, thymus, by type
  malignant C37
  metaplastic C37
  microscopic D15.0
  sclerosing C37
  type A C37
  type AB C37
  type B1 C37
  type B2 C37
  type B3 C37
Thymus, thymic (gland) — *see* condition
Thyrocele — *see* Goiter
Thyroglossal — *see also* condition
  cyst Q89.2
  duct, persistent Q89.2
Thyroid (gland) (body) — *see also* condition
  hormone resistance E07.89
  lingual Q89.2
  nodule (cystic) (nontoxic) (single) E04.1
Thyroiditis E06.9
  acute (nonsuppurative) (pyogenic) (suppurative) E06.0
  autoimmune E06.3
  chronic (nonspecific) (sclerosing) E06.5
    with thyrotoxicosis, transient E06.2
    fibrous E06.5
    lymphadenoid E06.3
    lymphocytic E06.3
    lymphoid E06.3
  de Quervain's E06.1
  drug-induced E06.4
  fibrous (chronic) E06.5
  giant-cell (follicular) E06.1
  granulomatous (de Quervain) (subacute) E06.1
  Hashimoto's (struma lymphomatosa) E06.3
  iatrogenic E06.4
  ligneous E06.5
  lymphocytic (chronic) E06.3
  lymphoid E06.3
  lymphomatous E06.3
  nonsuppurative E06.1
  postpartum, puerperal O90.5
  pseudotuberculous E06.1
  pyogenic E06.0
  radiation E06.4
  Riedel's E06.5
  subacute (granulomatous) E06.1
  suppurative E06.0
  tuberculous A18.81
  viral E06.1
  woody E06.5
Thyrolingual duct, persistent Q89.2
Thyromegaly E01.0
Thyrotoxic
  crisis — *see* Thyrotoxicosis
  heart disease or failure — *see also* Thyrotoxicosis E05.90 [I43]
    with thyroid storm E05.91 [I43]
  storm — *see* Thyrotoxicosis
Thyrotoxicosis (recurrent) E05.90
  with
    goiter (diffuse) E05.00
      with thyroid storm E05.01
      adenomatous uninodular E05.10
        with thyroid storm E05.11
      multinodular E05.20
        with thyroid storm E05.21
      nodular E05.20
        with thyroid storm E05.21
      uninodular E05.10
        with thyroid storm E05.11
    infiltrative
      dermopathy E05.00
        with thyroid storm E05.01
      ophthalmopathy E05.00
        with thyroid storm E05.01
    single thyroid nodule E05.10
      with thyroid storm E05.11
    thyroid storm E05.91
  due to
    ectopic thyroid nodule or tissue E05.30
      with thyroid storm E05.31
    ingestion of (excessive) thyroid material E05.40
      with thyroid storm E05.41
    overproduction of thyroid-stimulating hormone E05.80
      with thyroid storm E05.81
    specified cause NEC E05.80

Thyrotoxicosis — *continued*
  due to — *continued*
    specified cause — *continued*
      with thyroid storm E05.81
    factitia E05.40
      with thyroid storm E05.41
    heart — *see also* Failure, heart, high-output E05.90 [I43]
      with thyroid storm — *see also* Failure, heart, high-output E05.91 [I43]
      failure — *see also* Failure, heart, high-output E05.90 [I43]
    neonatal (transient) P72.1
    transient with chronic thyroiditis E06.2
Tibia vara M92.51- ☑
Tic (disorder) F95.9
  breathing F95.8
  child problem F95.0
  compulsive F95.1
  de la Tourette F95.2
  degenerative (generalized) (localized) G25.69
    facial G25.69
  disorder
    chronic
      motor F95.1
      vocal F95.1
    combined vocal and multiple motor F95.2
    transient F95.0
  douloureux G50.0
    atypical G50.1
    postherpetic, postzoster B02.22
  drug-induced G25.61
  eyelid F95.8
  habit F95.9
    chronic F95.1
    transient of childhood F95.0
  lid, transient of childhood F95.0
  motor-verbal F95.2
  occupational F48.8
  orbicularis F95.8
    transient of childhood F95.0
  organic origin G25.69
  postchoreic G25.69
  provisional F95.0
  psychogenic, compulsive F95.1
  salaam R25.8
  spasm (motor or vocal) F95.9
    chronic F95.1
    transient of childhood F95.0
  specified NEC F95.8
Tick-borne — *see* condition
Tietze's disease or syndrome M94.0
Tight, tightness
  anus K62.89
  chest R07.89
  fascia (lata) M62.89
  foreskin (congenital) N47.1
  hymen, hymenal ring N89.6
  introitus (acquired) (congenital) N89.6
  rectal sphincter K62.89
  tendon — *see* Short, tendon
  urethral sphincter N35.919
Tilting vertebra — *see* Dorsopathy, deforming, specified NEC
Timidity, child F93.8
Tinea (intersecta) (tarsi) B35.9
  amiantacea L44.8
  asbestina B35.0
  barbae B35.0
  beard B35.0
  black dot B35.0
  blanca B36.2
  capitis B35.0
  corporis B35.4
  cruris B35.6
  flava B36.0
  foot B35.3
  furfuracea B36.0
  imbricata (Tokelau) B35.5
  kerion B35.0
  manuum B35.2
  microsporic — *see* Dermatophytosis
  nigra B36.1
  nodosa — *see* Piedra
  pedis B35.3
  scalp B35.0
  specified NEC B35.8
  sycosis B35.0
  tonsurans B35.0

Tinea — *continued*
  trichophytic — *see* Dermatophytosis
  unguium B35.1
  versicolor B36.0
Tingling sensation (skin) R20.2
Tin-miner's lung J63.5
Tinnitus NOS H93.1- ☑
  audible H93.1- ☑
  aurium H93.1- ☑
  pulsatile H93.A- ☑
  subjective H93.1- ☑
Tipped tooth (teeth) M26.33
Tipping
  pelvis M95.5
    with disproportion (fetopelvic) O33.0
      causing obstructed labor O65.0
  tooth (teeth), fully erupted M26.33
Tiredness R53.83
Tissue — *see* condition
Tobacco (nicotine)
  abuse — *see* Tobacco, use
  dependence — *see* Dependence, drug, nicotine
  harmful use Z72.0
  heart — *see* Tobacco, toxic effect
  maternal use, affecting newborn P04.2
  toxic effect — *see* Table of Drugs and Chemicals, by
      substance, poisoning
    chewing tobacco — *see* Table of Drugs and Chemi-
        cals, by substance, poisoning
    cigarettes — *see* Table of Drugs and Chemicals, by
        substance, poisoning
  use Z72.0
    complicating
      childbirth O99.334
      pregnancy O99.33- ☑
      puerperium O99.335
    counseling and surveillance Z71.6
    history Z87.891
  withdrawal state — *see also* Dependence, drug, nico-
      tine F17.203
Tocopherol deficiency E56.0
Todd's
  cirrhosis K74.3
  paralysis (postepileptic) (transitory) G83.84
Toe — *see* condition
Toilet, artificial opening — *see* Attention to, artificial,
    opening
Tokelau (ringworm) B35.5
Tollwut — *see* Rabies
Tommaselli's disease R31.9
  correct substance properly administered — *see* Table
      of Drugs and Chemicals, by drug, adverse effect
  overdose or wrong substance given or taken — *see*
      Table of Drugs and Chemicals, by drug, poisoning
Tongue — *see also* condition
  tie Q38.1
Tonic pupil — *see* Anomaly, pupil, function, tonic pupil
Toni-Fanconi syndrome (cystinosis) E72.09
  with cystinosis E72.04
Tonsil — *see* condition
Tonsillitis (acute) (catarrhal) (croupous) (follicular) (gan-
    grenous) (infective) (lacunar) (lingual) (malignant)
    (membranous) (parenchymatous) (phlegmonous)
    (pseudomembranous) (purulent) (septic) (subacute)
    (suppurative) (toxic) (ulcerative) (vesicular) (viral)
    J03.90
  chronic J35.01
    with adenoiditis J35.03
  diphtheritic A36.0
  hypertrophic J35.01
    with adenoiditis J35.03
  recurrent J03.91
  specified organism NEC J03.80
    recurrent J03.81
  staphylococcal J03.80
    recurrent J03.81
  streptococcal J03.00
    recurrent J03.01
  tuberculous A15.8
  Vincent's A69.1
Tooth, teeth — *see* condition
Toothache K08.89
Topagnosis R20.8
Tophi — *see* Gout, chronic
TORCH infection — *see* Infection, congenital
  without active infection P00.2
Torn — *see* Tear

Tornwaldt's cyst or disease J39.2
Torsades de pointes I47.21
Torsion
  accessory tube — *see* Torsion, fallopian tube
  adnexa (female) — *see* Torsion, fallopian tube
  aorta, acquired I77.1
  appendix epididymis N44.04
  appendix testis N44.03
  bile duct (common) (hepatic) K83.8
    congenital Q44.5
  bowel, colon or intestine K56.2
  cervix — *see* Malposition, uterus
  cystic duct K82.8
  dystonia — *see* Dystonia, torsion
  epididymis (appendix) N44.04
  fallopian tube N83.52- ☑
    with ovary N83.53
  gallbladder K82.8
    congenital Q44.1
  hydatid of Morgagni
    female N83.52- ☑
    male N44.03
  kidney (pedicle) (leading to infarction) N28.0
  Meckel's diverticulum (congenital) Q43.0
    malignant — *see* Table of Neoplasms, small intes-
        tine, malignant
  mesentery K56.2
  omentum K56.2
  organ or site, congenital NEC — *see* Anomaly, by site
  ovary (pedicle) N83.51- ☑
    with fallopian tube N83.53
    congenital Q50.2
  oviduct — *see* Torsion, fallopian tube
  penis (acquired) N48.82
    congenital Q55.63
  spasm — *see* Dystonia, torsion
  spermatic cord N44.02
    extravaginal N44.01
    intravaginal N44.02
  spleen D73.5
  testis, testicle N44.00
    appendix N44.03
  tibia — *see* Deformity, limb, specified type NEC, lower
      leg
  uterus — *see* Malposition, uterus
Torticollis (intermittent) (spastic) M43.6
  congenital (sternomastoid) Q68.0
  due to birth injury P15.8
  hysterical F44.4
  ocular R29.891
  psychogenic F45.8
    conversion reaction F44.4
  rheumatic M43.6
  rheumatoid M06.88
  spasmodic G24.3
  traumatic, current S13.4 ☑
Tortipelvis G24.1
Tortuous
  aortic arch Q25.46
  artery I77.1
  organ or site, congenital NEC — *see* Distortion
  retinal vessel, congenital Q14.1
  ureter N13.8
  urethra N36.8
  vein — *see* Varix
Torture, victim of Z65.4
Torula, torular (histolytica) (infection) — *see* Cryptococ-
    cosis
Torulosis — *see* Cryptococcosis
Torus (mandibularis) (palatinus) M27.0
  fracture — *see* Fracture, by site, torus
Touraine's syndrome Q79.8
Tourette's syndrome F95.2
Tourniquet syndrome — *see* Constriction, external, by
    site
Tower skull Q75.0
  with exophthalmos Q87.0
Toxemia R68.89
  bacterial — *see* Sepsis
  burn — *see* Burn
  eclamptic (with pre-existing hypertension) — *see*
      Eclampsia
  erysipelatous — *see* Erysipelas
  fatigue R68.89
  food — *see* Poisoning, food
  gastrointestinal K52.1
  intestinal K52.1
  kidney — *see* Uremia

Toxemia — *continued*
  malarial — *see* Malaria
  myocardial — *see* Myocarditis, toxic
  of pregnancy — *see* Pre-eclampsia
  pre-eclamptic — *see* Pre-eclampsia
  small intestine K52.1
  staphylococcal, due to food A05.0
  stasis R68.89
  uremic — *see* Uremia
  urinary — *see* Uremia
Toxemica cerebropathia psychica (nonalcoholic) F04
  alcoholic — *see* Alcohol, amnestic disorder
Toxic (poisoning) — *see also* condition T65.91 ☑
  effect — *see* Table of Drugs and Chemicals, by sub-
      stance, poisoning
  shock syndrome A48.3
  thyroid (gland) — *see* Thyrotoxicosis
Toxicemia — *see* Toxemia
Toxicity — *see* Table of Drugs and Chemicals, by sub-
    stance, poisoning
  fava bean D55.0
  food, noxious — *see* Poisoning, food
  from drug or nonmedicinal substance — *see* Table of
      Drugs and Chemicals, by drug
Toxicosis — *see also* Toxemia
  capillary, hemorrhagic D69.0
Toxinfection, gastrointestinal K52.1
Toxocariasis B83.0
Toxoplasma, toxoplasmosis (acquired) B58.9
  with
    hepatitis B58.1
    meningoencephalitis B58.2
    ocular involvement B58.00
    other organ involvement B58.89
    pneumonia, pneumonitis B58.3
  congenital (acute) (subacute) (chronic) P37.1
  maternal, manifest toxoplasmosis in infant (acute)
      (subacute) (chronic) P37.1
**tPA (rtPA) administration in a different facility within
    the last 24 hours prior to admission to current
    facility** Z92.82
Trabeculation, bladder N32.89
Trachea — *see* condition
Tracheitis (catarrhal) (infantile) (membranous) (plastic)
    (septal) (suppurative) (viral) J04.10
  with
    bronchitis (15 years of age and above) J40
      acute or subacute — *see* Bronchitis, acute
      chronic J42
      tuberculous NEC A15.5
      under 15 years of age J20.9
    laryngitis (acute) J04.2
      chronic J37.1
      tuberculous NEC A15.5
  acute J04.10
    with obstruction J04.11
  chronic J42
    with
      bronchitis (chronic) J42
      laryngitis (chronic) J37.1
  diphtheritic (membranous) A36.89
  due to external agent — *see* Inflammation, respiratory,
      upper, due to
  syphilitic A52.73
  tuberculous A15.5
Trachelitis (nonvenereal) — *see* Cervicitis
Tracheobronchial — *see* condition
Tracheobronchitis (15 years of age and above) — *see
    also* Bronchitis
  due to
    Bordetella bronchiseptica A37.80
      with pneumonia A37.81
    Francisella tularensis A21.8
Tracheobronchomegaly Q32.4
  with bronchiectasis J47.9
    with
      exacerbation (acute) J47.1
      lower respiratory infection J47.0
  acquired J98.09
    with bronchiectasis J47.9
      with
        exacerbation (acute) J47.1
        lower respiratory infection J47.0
Tracheobronchopneumonitis — *see* Pneumonia,
    broncho-
Tracheocele (external) (internal) J39.8
  congenital Q32.1
Tracheomalacia J39.8

ICD-10-CM 2023

Index

Tracheomalacia — Trichomoniasis

Tracheomalacia — *continued*
  congenital Q32.0
Tracheopharyngitis (acute) J06.9
  chronic J42
  due to external agent — *see* Inflammation, respiratory, upper, due to
Tracheostenosis J39.8
Tracheostomy
  complication — *see* Complication, tracheostomy
  status Z93.0
    attention to Z43.0
    malfunctioning J95.03
Trachoma, trachomatous A71.9
  active (stage) A71.1
  contraction of conjunctiva A71.1
  dubium A71.0
  healed or sequelae B94.0
  initial (stage) A71.0
  pannus A71.1
  Türck's J37.0
Traction, vitreomacular H43.82- ☑
Train sickness T75.3 ☑
Trait(s)
  Hb-S D57.3
  hemoglobin
    abnormal NEC D58.2
      with thalassemia D56.3
    C — *see* Disease, hemoglobin C
    S (Hb-S) D57.3
  Lepore D56.3
  personality, accentuated Z73.1
  sickle-cell D57.3
    with elliptocytosis or spherocytosis D57.3
  type A personality Z73.1
Tramp Z59.00
Trance R41.89
  hysterical F44.89
Transaminasemia R74.01
Transection
  abdomen (partial) S38.3 ☑
  aorta (incomplete) — *see also* Injury, aorta
    complete — *see* Injury, aorta, laceration, major
  carotid artery (incomplete) — *see also* Injury, blood vessel, carotid, laceration
    complete — *see* Injury, blood vessel, carotid, laceration, major
  celiac artery (incomplete) S35.211 ☑
    branch (incomplete) S35.291 ☑
      complete S35.292 ☑
    complete S35.212 ☑
  innominate
    artery (incomplete) — *see also* Injury, blood vessel, thoracic, innominate, artery, laceration
      complete — *see* Injury, blood vessel, thoracic, innominate, artery, laceration, major
    vein (incomplete) — *see also* Injury, blood vessel, thoracic, innominate, vein, laceration
      complete — *see* Injury, blood vessel, thoracic, innominate, vein, laceration, major
  jugular vein (external) (incomplete) — *see also* Injury, blood vessel, jugular vein, laceration
    complete — *see* Injury, blood vessel, jugular vein, laceration, major
    internal (incomplete) — *see also* Injury, blood vessel, jugular vein, internal, laceration
      complete — *see* Injury, blood vessel, jugular vein, internal, laceration, major
  mesenteric artery (incomplete) — *see also* Injury, mesenteric artery, laceration
    complete — *see* Injury, mesenteric artery, laceration, major
  pulmonary vessel (incomplete) — *see also* Injury, blood vessel, thoracic, pulmonary, laceration
    complete — *see* Injury, blood vessel, thoracic, pulmonary, laceration, major
  subclavian — *see* Transection, innominate
  vena cava (incomplete) — *see also* Injury, vena cava
    complete — *see* Injury, vena cava, laceration, major
  vertebral artery (incomplete) — *see also* Injury, blood vessel, vertebral, laceration
    complete — *see* Injury, blood vessel, vertebral, laceration, major
Transfusion
  associated (red blood cell) hemochromatosis E83.111
  blood
    ABO incompatible — *see* Complication(s), transfusion, incompatibility reaction, ABO

Transfusion — *continued*
  blood — *continued*
    minor blood group (Duffy) (E) (K) (Kell) (Kidd) (Lewis) (M) (N) (P) (S) T80.89 ☑
    reaction or complication — *see* Complications, transfusion
  fetomaternal (mother) — *see* Pregnancy, complicated by, placenta, transfusion syndrome
  maternofetal (mother) — *see* Pregnancy, complicated by, placenta, transfusion syndrome
  placental (syndrome) (mother) — *see* Pregnancy, complicated by, placenta, transfusion syndrome
  reaction (adverse) — *see* Complications, transfusion
  related acute lung injury (TRALI) J95.84
  twin-to-twin — *see* Pregnancy, complicated by, placenta, transfusion syndrome, fetus to fetus
Transient (meaning homeless) — *see also* condition Z59.00
Translocation
  balanced autosomal Q95.9
    in normal individual Q95.0
  chromosomes NEC Q99.8
    balanced and insertion in normal individual Q95.0
  Down syndrome Q90.2
  trisomy
    13 Q91.6
    18 Q91.2
    21 Q90.2
Translucency, iris — *see* Degeneration, iris
Transmission of chemical substances through the placenta — *see* Absorption, chemical, through placenta
Transparency, lung, unilateral J43.0
Transplant (ed) (status) Z94.9
  awaiting organ Z76.82
  bone Z94.6
    marrow Z94.81
  candidate Z76.82
  complication — *see* Complication, transplant
  cornea Z94.7
  heart Z94.1
    and lung(s) Z94.3
    valve Z95.2
      prosthetic Z95.2
      specified NEC Z95.4
      xenogenic Z95.3
  intestine Z94.82
  kidney Z94.0
  liver Z94.4
  lung(s) Z94.2
    and heart Z94.3
  organ (failure) (infection) (rejection) Z94.9
    removal status Z98.85
  pancreas Z94.83
  skin Z94.5
  social Z60.3
  specified organ or tissue NEC Z94.89
  stem cells Z94.84
  tissue Z94.9
Transplants, ovarian, endometrial N80.10- ☑
Transposed — *see* Transposition
Transposition (congenital) — *see also* Malposition, congenital
  abdominal viscera Q89.3
  aorta (dextra) Q20.3
  appendix Q43.8
  colon Q43.8
  corrected Q20.5
  great vessels (complete) (partial) Q20.3
  heart Q24.0
    with complete transposition of viscera Q89.3
  intestine (large) (small) Q43.8
  reversed jejunal (for bypass) (status) Z98.0
  scrotum Q55.23
  stomach Q40.2
    with general transposition of viscera Q89.3
  tooth, teeth, fully erupted M26.30
  vessels, great (complete) (partial) Q20.3
  viscera (abdominal) (thoracic) Q89.3
Transsexualism F64.0
Transverse — *see also* condition
  arrest (deep), in labor O64.0 ☑
  lie (mother) O32.2 ☑
    causing obstructed labor O64.8 ☑
Transvestism, transvestitism (dual-role) F64.1
  fetishistic F65.1
Trapped placenta (with hemorrhage) O72.0
  without hemorrhage O73.0

TRAPS (tumor necrosis factor receptor associated periodic syndrome) M04.1
Trauma, traumatism — *see also* Injury
  acoustic — *see* subcategory H83.3 ☑
  birth — *see* Birth, injury
  complicating ectopic or molar pregnancy O08.6
  during delivery O71.9
  following ectopic or molar pregnancy O08.6
  obstetric O71.9
    specified NEC O71.89
  occlusal
    primary K08.81
    secondary K08.82
Traumatic — *see also* condition
  brain injury S06.9 ☑
Treacher Collins syndrome Q75.4
Treitz's hernia — *see* Hernia, abdomen, specified site NEC
Trematode infestation — *see* Infestation, fluke
Trematodiasis — *see* Infestation, fluke
Trembling paralysis — *see* Parkinsonism
Tremor(s) R25.1
  drug induced G25.1
  essential (benign) G25.0
  familial G25.0
  hereditary G25.0
  hysterical F44.4
  intention G25.2
  medication induced postural G25.1
  mercurial — *see* subcategory T56.1 ☑
  Parkinson's — *see* Parkinsonism
  psychogenic (conversion reaction) F44.4
  senilis R54
  specified type NEC G25.2
Trench
  fever A79.0
  foot — *see* Immersion, foot
  mouth A69.1
Treponema pallidum infection — *see* Syphilis
Treponematosis
  due to
    T. pallidum — *see* Syphilis
    T. pertenue — *see* Yaws
Triad
  Hutchinson's (congenital syphilis) A50.53
  Kartagener's Q89.3
  Saint's — *see* Hernia, diaphragm
Trichiasis (eyelid) H02.059
  with entropion — *see* Entropion
  left H02.056
    lower H02.055
    upper H02.054
  right H02.053
    lower H02.052
    upper H02.051
Trichinella spiralis (infection) (infestation) B75
Trichinellosis, trichiniasis, trichinelliasis, trichinosis B75
  with muscle disorder B75 *[M63.80]*
    ankle B75 *[M63.87-]* ☑
    foot B75 *[M63.87-]* ☑
    forearm B75 *[M63.83-]* ☑
    hand B75 *[M63.84-]* ☑
    lower leg B75 *[M63.86-]* ☑
    multiple sites B75 *[M63.89]*
    pelvic region B75 *[M63.85-]* ☑
    shoulder region B75 *[M63.81-]* ☑
    specified site NEC B75 *[M63.88]*
    thigh B75 *[M63.85-]* ☑
    upper arm B75 *[M63.82-]* ☑
Trichobezoar T18.9 ☑
  intestine T18.3 ☑
  stomach T18.2 ☑
Trichocephaliasis, trichocephalosis B79
Trichocephalus infestation B79
Trichoclasis L67.8
Trichoepithelioma — *see also* Neoplasm, skin, benign
  malignant — *see* Neoplasm, skin, malignant
Trichofolliculoma — *see* Neoplasm, skin, benign
Tricholemmoma — *see* Neoplasm, skin, benign
Trichomoniasis A59.9
  bladder A59.03
  cervix A59.09
  intestinal A07.8
  prostate A59.02
  seminal vesicles A59.09
  specified site NEC A59.8

☑ **Additional Character Required** — Refer to the Tabular List for Character Selection

Trichomoniasis — *continued*
  urethra A59.03
  urogenitalis A59.00
  vagina A59.01
  vulva A59.01
Trichomycosis
  axillaris A48.8
  nodosa, nodularis B36.8
Trichonodosis L67.8
Trichophytid, trichophyton infection — *see* Dermatophytosis
Trichophytobezoar T18.9 ☑
  intestine T18.3 ☑
  stomach T18.2 ☑
Trichophytosis — *see* Dermatophytosis
Trichoptilosis L67.8
Trichorrhexis (nodosa) (invaginata) L67.0
Trichosis axillaris A48.8
Trichosporosis nodosa B36.2
Trichostasis spinulosa (congenital) Q84.1
Trichostrongyliasis, trichostrongylosis (small intestine) B81.2
Trichostrongylus infection B81.2
Trichotillomania F63.3
Trichromat, trichromatopsia, anomalous (congenital) H53.55
Trichuriasis B79
Trichuris trichiura (infection) (infestation) (any site) B79
Tricuspid (valve) — *see* condition
Trifid — *see also* Accessory
  kidney (pelvis) Q63.8
  tongue Q38.3
Trigeminal neuralgia — *see* Neuralgia, trigeminal
Trigeminy R00.8
Trigger finger (acquired) M65.30
  congenital Q74.0
  index finger M65.32- ☑
  little finger M65.35- ☑
  middle finger M65.33- ☑
  ring finger M65.34- ☑
  thumb M65.31- ☑
Trigonitis (bladder) (chronic) (pseudomembranous) N30.30
  with hematuria N30.31
Trigonocephaly Q75.0
Trilocular heart — *see* Cor triloculare
Trimethylaminuria E72.52
Tripartite placenta O43.19- ☑
Triphalangeal thumb Q74.0
Triple — *see also* Accessory
  kidneys Q63.0
  uteri Q51.818
  X, female Q97.0
Triple I O41.12- ☑
Triplegia G83.89
  congenital G80.8
Triplet (newborn) — *see also* Newborn, triplet
  complicating pregnancy — *see* Pregnancy, triplet
Triplication — *see* Accessory
Triploidy Q92.7
Trismus R25.2
  neonatorum A33
  newborn A33
Trisomy (syndrome) Q92.9
  13 (partial) Q91.7
    meiotic nondisjunction Q91.4
    mitotic nondisjunction Q91.5
    mosaicism Q91.5
    translocation Q91.6
  18 (partial) Q91.3
    meiotic nondisjunction Q91.0
    mitotic nondisjunction Q91.1
    mosaicism Q91.1
    translocation Q91.2
  20 Q92.8
  21 (partial) Q90.9
    meiotic nondisjunction Q90.0
    mitotic nondisjunction Q90.1
    mosaicism Q90.1
    translocation Q90.2
  22 Q92.8
  autosomes Q92.9
  chromosome specified NEC Q92.8
    partial Q92.2
      due to unbalanced translocation Q92.5
    specified NEC Q92.8

Trisomy — *continued*
  chromosome specified — *continued*
    whole (nonsex chromosome)
      meiotic nondisjunction Q92.0
      mitotic nondisjunction Q92.1
      mosaicism Q92.1
  due to
    dicentrics — *see* Extra, marker chromosomes
    extra rings — *see* Extra, marker chromosomes
    isochromosomes — *see* Extra, marker chromosomes
  specified NEC Q92.8
  whole chromosome Q92.9
    meiotic nondisjunction Q92.0
    mitotic nondisjunction Q92.1
    mosaicism Q92.1
    partial Q92.9
    specified NEC Q92.8
Tritanomaly, tritanopia H53.55
Trombiculosis, trombiculiasis, trombidiosis B88.0
Trophedema (congenital) (hereditary) Q82.0
Trophoblastic disease — *see also* Mole, hydatidiform O01.9
Tropholymphedema Q82.0
Trophoneurosis NEC G96.89
  disseminated M34.9
Tropical — *see* condition
Trouble — *see also* Disease
  heart — *see* Disease, heart
  kidney — *see* Disease, renal
  nervous R45.0
  sinus — *see* Sinusitis
Trousseau's syndrome (thrombophlebitis migrans) I82.1
Truancy, childhood
  from school Z72.810
Truncus
  arteriosus (persistent) Q20.0
  communis Q20.0
Trunk — *see* condition
Trypanosomiasis
  African B56.9
    by Trypanosoma brucei
      gambiense B56.0
      rhodesiense B56.1
  American — *see* Chagas' disease
  Brazilian — *see* Chagas' disease
  by Trypanosoma
    brucei gambiense B56.0
    brucei rhodesiense B56.1
    cruzi — *see* Chagas' disease
  gambiensis, Gambian B56.0
  rhodesiensis, Rhodesian B56.1
  South American — *see* Chagas' disease
  where
    African trypanosomiasis is prevalent B56.9
    Chagas' disease is prevalent B57.2
Tryptasemia, hereditary alpha D89.44
T-shaped incisors K00.2
Tsutsugamushi (disease) (fever) A75.3
Tube, tubal, tubular — *see* condition
Tubercle — *see also* Tuberculosis
  brain, solitary A17.81
  Darwin's Q17.8
  Ghon, primary infection A15.7
Tuberculid, tuberculide (indurating, subcutaneous) (lichenoid) (miliary) (papulonecrotic) (primary) (skin) A18.4
Tuberculoma — *see also* Tuberculosis
  brain A17.81
  meninges (cerebral) (spinal) A17.1
  spinal cord A17.81
Tuberculosis, tubercular, tuberculous (calcification) (calcified) (caseous) (chromogenic acid-fast bacilli) (degeneration) (fibrocaseous) (fistula) (interstitial) (isolated circumscribed lesions) (necrosis) (parenchymatous) (ulcerative) A15.9
  with pneumoconiosis (any condition in J60-J64) J65
  abdomen (lymph gland) A18.39
  abscess (respiratory) A15.9
    bone A18.03
      hip A18.02
      knee A18.02
      sacrum A18.01
      specified site NEC A18.03
      spinal A18.01
      vertebra A18.01
    brain A17.81
    breast A18.89
    Cowper's gland A18.15

Tuberculosis, tubercular, tuberculous — *continued*
  abscess — *continued*
    dura (mater) (cerebral) (spinal) A17.81
    epidural (cerebral) (spinal) A17.81
    female pelvis A18.17
    frontal sinus A15.8
    genital organs NEC A18.10
    genitourinary A18.10
    gland (lymphatic) — *see* Tuberculosis, lymph gland
    hip A18.02
    intestine A18.32
    ischiorectal A18.32
    joint NEC A18.02
      hip A18.02
      knee A18.02
      specified NEC A18.02
      vertebral A18.01
    kidney A18.11
    knee A18.02
    latent Z22.7
    lumbar (spine) A18.01
    lung — *see* Tuberculosis, pulmonary
    meninges (cerebral) (spinal) A17.0
    muscle A18.09
    perianal (fistula) A18.32
    perinephritic A18.11
    perirectal A18.32
    rectum A18.32
    retropharyngeal A15.8
    sacrum A18.01
    scrofulous A18.2
    scrotum A18.15
    skin (primary) A18.4
    spinal cord A17.81
    spine or vertebra (column) A18.01
    subdiaphragmatic A18.31
    testis A18.15
    urinary A18.13
    uterus A18.17
  accessory sinus — *see* Tuberculosis, sinus
  Addison's disease A18.7
  adenitis — *see* Tuberculosis, lymph gland
  adenoids A15.8
  adenopathy — *see* Tuberculosis, lymph gland
  adherent pericardium A18.84
  adnexa (uteri) A18.17
  adrenal (capsule) (gland) A18.7
  alimentary canal A18.32
  anemia A18.89
  ankle (joint) (bone) A18.02
  anus A18.32
  apex, apical — *see* Tuberculosis, pulmonary
  appendicitis, appendix A18.32
  arachnoid A17.0
  artery, arteritis A18.89
    cerebral A18.89
  arthritis (chronic) (synovial) A18.02
    spine or vertebra (column) A18.01
  articular — *see* Tuberculosis, joint
  ascites A18.31
  asthma — *see* Tuberculosis, pulmonary
  axilla, axillary (gland) A18.2
  bladder A18.12
  bone A18.03
    hip A18.02
    knee A18.02
    limb NEC A18.03
    sacrum A18.01
    spine or vertebral column A18.01
  bowel (miliary) A18.32
  brain A17.81
  breast A18.89
  broad ligament A18.17
  bronchi, bronchial, bronchus A15.5
    ectasia, ectasis (bronchiectasis) — *see* Tuberculosis, pulmonary
    fistula A15.5
      primary (progressive) A15.7
    gland or node A15.4
      primary (progressive) A15.7
    lymph gland or node A15.4
      primary (progressive) A15.7
  bronchiectasis — *see* Tuberculosis, pulmonary
  bronchitis A15.5
  bronchopleural A15.6
  bronchopneumonia, bronchopneumonic — *see* Tuberculosis, pulmonary
  bronchorrhagia A15.5

Tuberculosis, tubercular, tuberculous — *continued*
bronchotracheal A15.5
bronze disease A18.7
buccal cavity A18.83
bulbourethral gland A18.15
bursa A18.09
cachexia A15.9
cardiomyopathy A18.84
caries — *see* Tuberculosis, bone
cartilage A18.02
    intervertebral A18.01
catarrhal — *see* Tuberculosis, respiratory
cecum A18.32
cellulitis (primary) A18.4
cerebellum A17.81
cerebral, cerebrum A17.81
cerebrospinal A17.81
    meninges A17.0
cervical (lymph gland or node) A18.2
cervicitis, cervix (uteri) A18.16
chest — *see* Tuberculosis, respiratory
chorioretinitis A18.53
choroid, choroiditis A18.53
ciliary body A18.54
colitis A18.32
collier's J65
colliquativa (primary) A18.4
colon A18.32
complex, primary A15.7
congenital P37.0
conjunctiva A18.59
connective tissue (systemic) A18.89
contact Z20.1
cornea (ulcer) A18.52
Cowper's gland A18.15
coxae A18.02
coxalgia A18.02
cul-de-sac of Douglas A18.17
curvature, spine A18.01
cutis (colliquativa) (primary) A18.4
cyst, ovary A18.18
cystitis A18.12
dactylitis A18.03
diarrhea A18.32
diffuse — *see* Tuberculosis, miliary
digestive tract A18.32
disseminated — *see* Tuberculosis, miliary
duodenum A18.32
dura (mater) (cerebral) (spinal) A17.0
    abscess (cerebral) (spinal) A17.81
dysentery A18.32
ear (inner) (middle) A18.6
    bone A18.03
    external (primary) A18.4
    skin (primary) A18.4
elbow A18.02
emphysema — *see* Tuberculosis, pulmonary
empyema A15.6
encephalitis A17.82
endarteritis A18.89
endocarditis A18.84
    aortic A18.84
    mitral A18.84
    pulmonary A18.84
    tricuspid A18.84
endocrine glands NEC A18.82
endometrium A18.17
enteric, enterica, enteritis A18.32
enterocolitis A18.32
epididymis, epididymitis A18.15
epidural abscess (cerebral) (spinal) A17.81
epiglottis A15.5
episcleritis A18.51
erythema (induratum) (nodosum) (primary) A18.4
esophagus A18.83
eustachian tube A18.6
exposure (to) Z20.1
exudative — *see* Tuberculosis, pulmonary
eye A18.50
eyelid (primary) (lupus) A18.4
fallopian tube (acute) (chronic) A18.17
fascia A18.09
fauces A15.8
female pelvic inflammatory disease A18.17
finger A18.03
first infection A15.7
gallbladder A18.83
ganglion A18.09

Tuberculosis, tubercular, tuberculous — *continued*
gastritis A18.83
gastrocolic fistula A18.32
gastroenteritis A18.32
gastrointestinal tract A18.32
general, generalized — *see* Tuberculosis, miliary
genital organs A18.10
genitourinary A18.10
genu A18.02
glandula suprarenalis A18.7
glandular, general A18.2
glottis A15.5
grinder's J65
gum A18.83
hand A18.03
heart A18.84
hematogenous — *see* Tuberculosis, miliary
hemoptysis — *see* Tuberculosis, pulmonary
hemorrhage NEC — *see* Tuberculosis, pulmonary
hemothorax A15.6
hepatitis A18.83
hilar lymph nodes A15.4
    primary (progressive) A15.7
hip (joint) (disease) (bone) A18.02
hydropneumothorax A15.6
hydrothorax A15.6
hypoadrenalism A18.7
hypopharynx A15.8
ileocecal (hyperplastic) A18.32
ileocolitis A18.32
ileum A18.32
iliac spine (superior) A18.03
immunological findings only A15.7
indurativa (primary) A18.4
infantile A15.7
infection A15.9
    without clinical manifestations A15.7
infraclavicular gland A18.2
inguinal gland A18.2
inguinalis A18.2
intestine (any part) A18.32
iridocyclitis A18.54
iris, iritis A18.54
ischiorectal A18.32
jaw A18.03
jejunum A18.32
joint A18.02
    vertebral A18.01
keratitis (interstitial) A18.52
keratoconjunctivitis A18.52
kidney A18.11
knee (joint) A18.02
kyphosis, kyphoscoliosis A18.01
laryngitis A15.5
larynx A15.5
latent Z22.7
leptomeninges, leptomeningitis (cerebral) (spinal) A17.0
lichenoides (primary) A18.4
linguae A18.83
lip A18.83
liver A18.83
lordosis A18.01
lung — *see* Tuberculosis, pulmonary
lupus vulgaris A18.4
lymph gland or node (peripheral) A18.2
    abdomen A18.39
    bronchial A15.4
        primary (progressive) A15.7
    cervical A18.2
    hilar A15.4
        primary (progressive) A15.7
    intrathoracic A15.4
        primary (progressive) A15.7
    mediastinal A15.4
        primary (progressive) A15.7
    mesenteric A18.39
    retroperitoneal A18.39
    tracheobronchial A15.4
        primary (progressive) A15.7
lymphadenitis — *see* Tuberculosis, lymph gland
lymphangitis — *see* Tuberculosis, lymph gland
lymphatic (gland) (vessel) — *see* Tuberculosis, lymph gland
mammary gland A18.89
marasmus A15.9
mastoiditis A18.03
mediastinal lymph gland or node A15.4

Tuberculosis, tubercular, tuberculous — *continued*
mediastinal lymph gland or node — *continued*
    primary (progressive) A15.7
mediastinitis A15.8
    primary (progressive) A15.7
mediastinum A15.8
    primary (progressive) A15.7
medulla A17.81
melanosis, Addisonian A18.7
meninges, meningitis (basilar) (cerebral) (cerebrospinal) (spinal) A17.0
meningoencephalitis A17.82
mesentery, mesenteric (gland or node) A18.39
miliary A19.9
    acute A19.2
        multiple sites A19.1
        single specified site A19.0
    chronic A19.8
    specified NEC A19.8
millstone makers' J65
miner's J65
molder's J65
mouth A18.83
multiple A19.9
    acute A19.1
    chronic A19.8
muscle A18.09
myelitis A17.82
myocardium, myocarditis A18.84
nasal (passage) (sinus) A15.8
nasopharynx A15.8
neck gland A18.2
nephritis A18.11
nerve (mononeuropathy) A17.83
nervous system A17.9
nose (septum) A15.8
ocular A18.50
omentum A18.31
oophoritis (acute) (chronic) A18.17
optic (nerve trunk) (papilla) A18.59
orbit A18.59
orchitis A18.15
organ, specified NEC A18.89
osseous — *see* Tuberculosis, bone
osteitis — *see* Tuberculosis, bone
osteomyelitis — *see* Tuberculosis, bone
otitis media A18.6
ovary, ovaritis (acute) (chronic) A18.17
oviduct (acute) (chronic) A18.17
pachymeningitis A17.0
palate (soft) A18.83
pancreas A18.83
papulonecrotic (a) (primary) A18.4
parathyroid glands A18.82
paronychia (primary) A18.4
parotid gland or region A18.83
pelvis (bony) A18.03
penis A18.15
peribronchitis A15.5
pericardium, pericarditis A18.84
perichondritis, larynx A15.5
periostitis — *see* Tuberculosis, bone
perirectal fistula A18.32
peritoneum NEC A18.31
peritonitis A18.31
pharynx, pharyngitis A15.8
phlyctenulosis (keratoconjunctivitis) A18.52
phthisis NEC — *see* Tuberculosis, pulmonary
pituitary gland A18.82
pleura, pleural, pleurisy, pleuritis (fibrinous) (obliterative) (purulent) (simple plastic) (with effusion) A15.6
    primary (progressive) A15.7
pneumonia, pneumonic — *see* Tuberculosis, pulmonary
pneumothorax (spontaneous) (tense valvular) — *see* Tuberculosis, pulmonary
polyneuropathy A17.89
polyserositis A19.9
    acute A19.1
    chronic A19.8
potter's J65
prepuce A18.15
primary (complex) A15.7
proctitis A18.32
prostate, prostatitis A18.14
pulmonalis — *see* Tuberculosis, pulmonary

☑ **Additional Character Required — Refer to the Tabular List for Character Selection**

Tuberculosis, tubercular, tuberculous — *continued*
  pulmonary (cavitated) (fibrotic) (infiltrative) (nodular) A15.0
    childhood type or first infection A15.7
      primary (complex) A15.7
  pyelitis A18.11
  pyelonephritis A18.11
  pyemia — *see* Tuberculosis, miliary
  pyonephrosis A18.11
  pyopneumothorax A15.6
  pyothorax A15.6
  rectum (fistula) (with abscess) A18.32
  reinfection stage — *see* Tuberculosis, pulmonary
  renal A18.11
  renis A18.11
  respiratory A15.9
    primary A15.7
    specified site NEC A15.8
  retina, retinitis A18.53
  retroperitoneal (lymph gland or node) A18.39
  rheumatism NEC A18.09
  rhinitis A15.8
  sacroiliac (joint) A18.01
  sacrum A18.01
  salivary gland A18.83
  salpingitis (acute) (chronic) A18.17
  sandblaster's J65
  sclera A18.51
  scoliosis A18.01
  scrofulous A18.2
  scrotum A18.15
  seminal tract or vesicle A18.15
  senile A15.9
  septic — *see* Tuberculosis, miliary
  shoulder (joint) A18.02
    blade A18.03
  sigmoid A18.32
  sinus (any nasal) A15.8
    bone A18.03
    epididymis A18.15
  skeletal NEC A18.03
  skin (any site) (primary) A18.4
  small intestine A18.32
  soft palate A18.83
  spermatic cord A18.15
  spine, spinal (column) A18.01
    cord A17.81
    medulla A17.81
    membrane A17.0
    meninges A17.0
  spleen, splenitis A18.85
  spondylitis A18.01
  sternoclavicular joint A18.02
  stomach A18.83
  stonemason's J65
  subcutaneous tissue (cellular) (primary) A18.4
  subcutis (primary) A18.4
  subdeltoid bursa A18.83
  submaxillary (region) A18.83
  supraclavicular gland A18.2
  suprarenal (capsule) (gland) A18.7
  swelling, joint (*see also* category M01) — *see also* Tuberculosis, joint A18.02
  symphysis pubis A18.02
  synovitis A18.09
    articular A18.02
    spine or vertebra A18.01
  systemic — *see* Tuberculosis, miliary
  tarsitis A18.4
  tendon (sheath) — *see* Tuberculosis, tenosynovitis
  tenosynovitis A18.09
    spine or vertebra A18.01
  testis A18.15
  throat A15.8
  thymus gland A18.82
  thyroid gland A18.81
  tongue A18.83
  tonsil, tonsillitis A15.8
  trachea, tracheal A15.5
    lymph gland or node A15.4
      primary (progressive) A15.7
  tracheobronchial A15.5
    lymph gland or node A15.4
      primary (progressive) A15.7
  tubal (acute) (chronic) A18.17
  tunica vaginalis A18.15
  ulcer (skin) (primary) A18.4
    bowel or intestine A18.32

Tuberculosis, tubercular, tuberculous — *continued*
  ulcer — *continued*
    specified NEC — *see* Tuberculosis, by site
  unspecified site A15.9
  ureter A18.11
  urethra, urethral (gland) A18.13
  urinary organ or tract A18.13
  uterus A18.17
  uveal tract A18.54
  uvula A18.83
  vagina A18.18
  vas deferens A18.15
  verruca, verrucosa (cutis) (primary) A18.4
  vertebra (column) A18.01
  vesiculitis A18.15
  vulva A18.18
  wrist (joint) A18.02
Tuberculum
  Carabelli — *see* Excludes Note at K00.2
  occlusal — *see* Excludes Note at K00.2
  paramolare K00.2
Tuberosity, enitre maxillary M26.07
Tuberous sclerosis (brain) Q85.1
Tubo-ovarian — *see* condition
Tuboplasty, after previous sterilization Z31.0
  aftercare Z31.42
Tubotympanitis, catarrhal (chronic) — *see* Otitis, media, nonsuppurative, chronic, serous
Tularemia A21.9
  with
    conjunctivitis A21.1
    pneumonia A21.2
  abdominal A21.3
  bronchopneumonic A21.2
  conjunctivitis A21.1
  cryptogenic A21.3
  enteric A21.3
  gastrointestinal A21.3
  generalized A21.7
  ingestion A21.3
  intestinal A21.3
  oculoglandular A21.1
  ophthalmic A21.1
  pneumonia (any), pneumonic A21.2
  pulmonary A21.2
  sepsis A21.7
  specified NEC A21.8
  typhoidal A21.7
  ulceroglandular A21.0
Tularensis conjunctivitis A21.1
Tumefaction — *see also* Swelling
  liver — *see* Hypertrophy, liver
Tumor — *see also* Neoplasm, unspecified behavior, by site
  acinar cell — *see* Neoplasm, uncertain behavior, by site
  acinic cell — *see* Neoplasm, uncertain behavior, by site
  adenocarcinoid — *see* Neoplasm, malignant, by site
  adenomatoid — *see also* Neoplasm, benign, by site
    odontogenic — *see* Cyst, calcifying odontogenic
  adnexal (skin) — *see* Neoplasm, skin, benign, by site
  adrenal
    cortical (benign) D35.0- ☑
      malignant C74.0- ☑
    rest — *see* Neoplasm, benign, by site
  alpha-cell
    malignant
      pancreas C25.4
      specified site NEC — *see* Neoplasm, malignant, by site
      unspecified site C25.4
    pancreas D13.7
    specified site NEC — *see* Neoplasm, benign, by site
    unspecified site D13.7
  aneurysmal — *see* Aneurysm
  aortic body D44.7
    malignant C75.5
  Askin's — *see* Neoplasm, connective tissue, malignant
  basal cell — *see also* Neoplasm, skin, uncertain behavior D48.5
  Bednar — *see* Neoplasm, skin, malignant
  benign (unclassified) — *see* Neoplasm, benign, by site
  beta-cell
    malignant
      pancreas C25.4
      specified site NEC — *see* Neoplasm, malignant, by site
      unspecified site C25.4
    pancreas D13.7

Tumor — *continued*
  beta-cell — *continued*
    specified site NEC — *see* Neoplasm, benign, by site
    unspecified site D13.7
  Brenner D27.9
    borderline malignancy D39.1- ☑
    malignant C56- ☑
    proliferating D39.1- ☑
  bronchial alveolar, intravascular D38.1
  Brooke's — *see* Neoplasm, skin, benign
  brown fat — *see* Lipoma
  Burkitt — *see* Lymphoma, Burkitt
  calcifying epithelial odontogenic — *see* Cyst, calcifying odontogenic
  carcinoid D3A.00 (*following* D36)
    benign D3A.00 (*following* D36)
      appendix D3A.020 (*following* D36)
      ascending colon D3A.022 (*following* D36)
      bronchus (lung) D3A.090 (*following* D36)
      cecum D3A.021 (*following* D36)
      colon D3A.029 (*following* D36)
      descending colon D3A.024 (*following* D36)
      duodenum D3A.010 (*following* D36)
      foregut NOS D3A.094 (*following* D36)
      hindgut NOS D3A.096 (*following* D36)
      ileum D3A.012 (*following* D36)
      jejunum D3A.011 (*following* D36)
      kidney D3A.093 (*following* D36)
      large intestine D3A.029 (*following* D36)
      lung (bronchus) D3A.090 (*following* D36)
      midgut NOS D3A.095 (*following* D36)
      rectum D3A.026 (*following* D36)
      sigmoid colon D3A.025 (*following* D36)
      small intestine D3A.019 (*following* D36)
      specified NEC D3A.098 (*following* D36)
      stomach D3A.092 (*following* D36)
      thymus D3A.091 (*following* D36)
      transverse colon D3A.023 (*following* D36)
    malignant C7A.00 (*following* C75)
      appendix C7A.020 (*following* C75)
      ascending colon C7A.022 (*following* C75)
      bronchus (lung) C7A.090 (*following* C75)
      cecum C7A.021 (*following* C75)
      colon C7A.029 (*following* C75)
      descending colon C7A.024 (*following* C75)
      duodenum C7A.010 (*following* C75)
      foregut NOS C7A.094 (*following* C75)
      hindgut NOS C7A.096 (*following* C75)
      ileum C7A.012 (*following* C75)
      jejunum C7A.011 (*following* C75)
      kidney C7A.093 (*following* C75)
      large intestine C7A.029 (*following* C75)
      lung (bronchus) C7A.090 (*following* C75)
      midgut NOS C7A.095 (*following* C75)
      rectum C7A.026 (*following* C75)
      sigmoid colon C7A.025 (*following* C75)
      small intestine C7A.019 (*following* C75)
      specified NEC C7A.098 (*following* C75)
      stomach C7A.092 (*following* C75)
      thymus C7A.091 (*following* C75)
      transverse colon C7A.023 (*following* C75)
    mesentary metastasis C7B.04 (*following* C75)
    secondary C7B.00 (*following* C75)
      bone C7B.03 (*following* C75)
      distant lymph nodes C7B.01 (*following* C75)
      liver C7B.02 (*following* C75)
      peritoneum C7B.04 (*following* C75)
      specified NEC C7B.09 (*following* C75)
  carotid body D44.6
    malignant C75.4
  cells — *see also* Neoplasm, unspecified behavior, by site
    benign — *see* Neoplasm, benign, by site
    malignant — *see* Neoplasm, malignant, by site
    uncertain whether benign or malignant — *see* Neoplasm, uncertain behavior, by site
  cervix, in pregnancy or childbirth — *see* Pregnancy, complicated by, tumor, cervix
  chondromatous giant cell — *see* Neoplasm, bone, benign
  chromaffin — *see also* Neoplasm, benign, by site
    malignant — *see* Neoplasm, malignant, by site
  Cock's peculiar L72.3
  Codman's — *see* Neoplasm, bone, benign
  dentigerous, mixed — *see* Cyst, calcifying odontogenic
  dermoid — *see* Neoplasm, benign, by site
    with malignant transformation C56- ☑

Tumor — *continued*

desmoid (extra-abdominal) — *see also* Neoplasm,
    connective tissue, uncertain behavior
    abdominal — *see* Neoplasm, connective tissue, un-
        certain behavior
embolus — *see* Neoplasm, secondary, by site
embryonal (mixed) — *see also* Neoplasm, uncertain
    behavior, by site
    liver C22.7
endodermal sinus
    specified site — *see* Neoplasm, malignant, by site
    unspecified site
        female C56.- ☑
        male C62.90
epithelial
    benign — *see* Neoplasm, benign, by site
    malignant — *see* Neoplasm, malignant, by site
Ewing's — *see* Neoplasm, bone, malignant, by site
fatty — *see* Lipoma
fibroid — *see* Leiomyoma
G cell
    malignant
        pancreas C25.4
        specified site NEC — *see* Neoplasm, malignant,
            by site
        unspecified site C25.4
    specified site — *see* Neoplasm, uncertain behavior,
        by site
    unspecified site D37.8
germ cell — *see also* Neoplasm, malignant, by site
    mixed — *see* Neoplasm, malignant, by site
ghost cell, odontogenic — *see* Cyst, calcifying odonto-
    genic
giant cell — *see also* Neoplasm, uncertain behavior,
    by site
    bone D48.0
        malignant — *see* Neoplasm, bone, malignant
        chondromatous — *see* Neoplasm, bone, benign
        malignant — *see* Neoplasm, malignant, by site
    soft parts — *see* Neoplasm, connective tissue, un-
        certain behavior
        malignant — *see* Neoplasm, connective tissue,
            malignant
glomus D18.00
    intra-abdominal D18.03
    intracranial D18.02
    jugulare D44.7
        malignant C75.5
    skin D18.01
    specified site NEC D18.09
gonadal stromal — *see* Neoplasm, uncertain behavior,
    by site
granular cell — *see also* Neoplasm, connective tissue,
    benign
    malignant — *see* Neoplasm, connective tissue, ma-
        lignant
granulosa cell D39.1- ☑
    juvenile D39.1- ☑
    malignant C56- ☑
granulosa cell-theca cell D39.1- ☑
    malignant C56- ☑
Grawitz's C64- ☑
hemorrhoidal — *see* Hemorrhoids
hilar cell D27- ☑
hilus cell D27- ☑
Hurthle cell (benign) D34
    malignant C73
hydatid — *see* Echinococcus
hypernephroid — *see also* Neoplasm, uncertain behav-
    ior, by site
interstitial cell — *see also* Neoplasm, uncertain behav-
    ior, by site
    benign — *see* Neoplasm, benign, by site
    malignant — *see* Neoplasm, malignant, by site
intravascular bronchial alveolar D38.1
islet cell — *see* Neoplasm, benign, by site
    malignant — *see* Neoplasm, malignant, by site
        pancreas C25.4
        specified site NEC — *see* Neoplasm, malignant,
            by site
        unspecified site C25.4
    pancreas D13.7
    specified site NEC — *see* Neoplasm, benign, by site
    unspecified site D13.7
juxtaglomerular D41.0- ☑
Klatskin's C22.1
Krukenberg's C79.6- ☑

Tumor — *continued*

Leydig cell — *see* Neoplasm, uncertain behavior, by
    site
    benign — *see* Neoplasm, benign, by site
        specified site — *see* Neoplasm, benign, by site
        unspecified site
            female D27.9
            male D29.20
    malignant — *see* Neoplasm, malignant, by site
        specified site — *see* Neoplasm, malignant, by
            site
        unspecified site
            female C56.9
            male C62.90
    specified site — *see* Neoplasm, uncertain behavior,
        by site
    unspecified site
        female D39.10
        male D40.10
lipid cell, ovary D27- ☑
lipoid cell, ovary D27- ☑
malignant — *see also* Neoplasm, malignant, by site
    C80.1
    fusiform cell (type) C80.1
    giant cell (type) C80.1
    localized, plasma cell — *see* Plasmacytoma, solitary
    mixed NEC C80.1
    small cell (type) C80.1
    spindle cell (type) C80.1
    unclassified C80.1
mast cell D47.09
melanotic, neuroectodermal — *see* Neoplasm, benign,
    by site
Merkel cell — *see* Carcinoma, Merkel cell
mesenchymal
    malignant — *see* Neoplasm, connective tissue, ma-
        lignant
    mixed — *see* Neoplasm, connective tissue, uncertain
        behavior
mesodermal, mixed — *see also* Neoplasm, malignant,
    by site
    liver C22.4
mesonephric — *see also* Neoplasm, uncertain behavior,
    by site
    malignant — *see* Neoplasm, malignant, by site
metastatic
    from specified site — *see* Neoplasm, malignant, by
        site
    of specified site — *see* Neoplasm, malignant, by site
    to specified site — *see* Neoplasm, secondary, by site
mixed NEC — *see also* Neoplasm, benign, by site
    malignant — *see* Neoplasm, malignant, by site
mucinous of low malignant potential
    specified site — *see* Neoplasm, malignant, by site
    unspecified site C56.9
mucocarcinoid
    specified site — *see* Neoplasm, malignant, by site
    unspecified site C18.1
mucoepidermoid — *see* Neoplasm, uncertain behavior,
    by site
Müllerian, mixed
    specified site — *see* Neoplasm, malignant, by site
    unspecified site C54.9
myoepithelial — *see* Neoplasm, benign, by site
neuroectodermal (peripheral) — *see* Neoplasm, malig-
    nant, by site
    primitive
        specified site — *see* Neoplasm, malignant, by
            site
        unspecified site C71.9
neuroendocrine D3A.8 (*following* D36)
    malignant poorly differentiated C7A.1 (*following*
        C75)
    secondary NEC C7B.8 (*following* C75)
    specified NEC C7A.8 (*following* C75)
neurogenic olfactory C30.0
nonencapsulated sclerosing C73
odontogenic (adenomatoid) (benign) (calcifying epithe-
    lial) (keratocystic) (squamous) — *see* Cyst, calci-
    fying odontogenic
    malignant C41.1
        upper jaw (bone) C41.0
ovarian stromal D39.1- ☑
ovary, in pregnancy — *see* Pregnancy, complicated by
pacinian — *see* Neoplasm, skin, benign
Pancoast's — *see* Pancoast's syndrome
papillary — *see also* Papilloma
    cystic D37.9

Tumor — *continued*

papillary — *see also* Papilloma — *continued*
    mucinous of low malignant potential C56- ☑
        specified site — *see* Neoplasm, malignant, by
            site
        unspecified site C56.9
    serous of low malignant potential
        specified site — *see* Neoplasm, malignant, by
            site
        unspecified site C56.9
pelvic, in pregnancy or childbirth — *see* Pregnancy,
    complicated by
phantom F45.8
phyllodes D48.6- ☑
    benign D24- ☑
    malignant — *see* Neoplasm, breast, malignant
Pindborg — *see* Cyst, calcifying odontogenic
placental site trophoblastic D39.2
plasma cell (malignant) (localized) — *see* Plasmacy-
    toma, solitary
polyvesicular vitelline
    specified site — *see* Neoplasm, malignant, by site
    unspecified site
        female C56.9
        male C62.90
Pott's puffy — *see* Osteomyelitis, specified NEC
Rathke's pouch D44.3
retinal anlage — *see* Neoplasm, benign, by site
salivary gland type, mixed — *see* Neoplasm, salivary
    gland, benign
    malignant — *see* Neoplasm, salivary gland, malig-
        nant
Sampson's N80.10- ☑
Schmincke's — *see* Neoplasm, nasopharynx, malignant
sclerosing stromal D27- ☑
sebaceous — *see* Cyst, sebaceous
secondary — *see* Neoplasm, secondary, by site
    carcinoid C7B.00 (*following* C75)
        bone C7B.03 (*following* C75)
        distant lymph nodes C7B.01 (*following* C75)
        liver C7B.02 (*following* C75)
        peritoneum C7B.04 (*following* C75)
        specified NEC C7B.09 (*following* C75)
    neuroendocrine NEC C7B.8 (*following* C75)
serous of low malignant potential
    specified site — *see* Neoplasm, malignant, by site
    unspecified site C56.9
Sertoli cell — *see* Neoplasm, benign, by site
    with lipid storage
        specified site — *see* Neoplasm, benign, by site
        unspecified site
            female D27.9
            male D29.20
    specified site — *see* Neoplasm, benign, by site
    unspecified site
        female D27.9
        male D29.20
Sertoli-Leydig cell — *see* Neoplasm, benign, by site
    specified site — *see* Neoplasm, benign, by site
    unspecified site
        female D27.9
        male D29.20
sex cord (-stromal) — *see* Neoplasm, uncertain behav-
    ior, by site
    with annular tubules D39.1- ☑
skin appendage — *see* Neoplasm, skin, benign
smooth muscle — *see* Neoplasm, connective tissue,
    uncertain behavior
soft tissue
    benign — *see* Neoplasm, connective tissue, benign
    malignant — *see* Neoplasm, connective tissue, ma-
        lignant
sternomastoid (congenital) Q68.0
stromal
    endometrial D39.0
    gastric D48.1
        benign D21.4
        malignant C16.9
        uncertain behavior D48.1
    gastrointestinal C49.A- ☑
        benign D21.4
        esophagus C49.A1
        malignant C49.A0
            colon C49.A4
            duodenum C49.A3
            esophagus C49.A1
            ileum C49.A3
            jejunum C49.A3

☑ **Additional Character Required** — **Refer to the Tabular List for Character Selection**

Tumor — *continued*
  stromal — *continued*
    gastrointestinal — *continued*
      malignant — *continued*
        large intestine C49.A4
        Meckel diverticulum C49.A3
        omentum C49.A9
        peritoneum C49.A9
        rectum C49.A5
        small intestine C49.A3
        specified site NEC C49.A9
        stomach C49.A2
      rectum C49.A5
      small intestine C49.A3
      specified site NEC C49.A9
      stomach C49.A2
      uncertain behavior D48.1
    intestine
      benign D21.4
      malignant
        large C49.A4
        small C49.A3
      uncertain behavior D48.1
    ovarian D39.1- ☑
    stomach C49.A2
      benign D21.4
      malignant C49.A2
      uncertain behavior D48.1
  sweat gland — *see also* Neoplasm, skin, uncertain behavior
    benign — *see* Neoplasm, skin, benign
    malignant — *see* Neoplasm, skin, malignant
  syphilitic, brain A52.17
  testicular D40.10
  testicular stromal D40.1- ☑
  theca cell D27.- ☑
  theca cell-granulosa cell D39.1- ☑
  Triton, malignant — *see* Neoplasm, nerve, malignant
  trophoblastic, placental site D39.2
  turban D23.4
  uterus (body), in pregnancy or childbirth — *see* Pregnancy, complicated by, tumor, uterus
  vagina, in pregnancy or childbirth — *see* Pregnancy, complicated by
  varicose — *see* Varix
  von Recklinghausen's — *see* Neurofibromatosis
  vulva or perineum, in pregnancy or childbirth — *see* Pregnancy, complicated by
    causing obstructed labor O65.5
  Warthin's — *see* Neoplasm, salivary gland, benign
  Wilms' C64- ☑
  yolk sac — *see* Neoplasm, malignant, by site
    specified site — *see* Neoplasm, malignant, by site
    unspecified site
      female C56.9
      male C62.90
Tumor lysis syndrome (following antineoplastic chemotherapy) (spontaneous) NEC E88.3
Tumorlet — *see* Neoplasm, uncertain behavior, by site
Tungiasis B88.1
Tunica vasculosa lentis Q12.2
Turban tumor D23.4
Türck's trachoma J37.0
Turner-Kieser syndrome Q87.2
Turner-like syndrome Q87.19
Turner's
  hypoplasia (tooth) K00.4
  syndrome Q96.9
    specified NEC Q96.8
  tooth K00.4
Turner-Ullrich syndrome Q96.9
Tussis convulsiva — *see* Whooping cough
Twiddler's syndrome (due to)
  automatic implantable defibrillator T82.198
  cardiac pacemaker T82.198 ☑
Twilight state
  epileptic F05
  psychogenic F44.89
Twin (newborn) — *see also* Newborn, twin
  conjoined Q89.4
  pregnancy — *see* Pregnancy, twin
Twinning, teeth K00.2
Twist, twisted
  bowel, colon or intestine K56.2
  hair (congenital) Q84.1
  mesentery K56.2
  omentum K56.2
  organ or site, congenital NEC — *see* Anomaly, by site

Twist, twisted — *continued*
  ovarian pedicle — *see* Torsion, ovary
Twitching R25.3
Tylosis (acquired) L84
  buccalis K13.29
  linguae K13.29
  palmaris et plantaris (congenital) (inherited) Q82.8
    acquired L85.1
Tympanism R14.0
Tympanites (abdominal) (intestinal) R14.0
Tympanitis — *see* Myringitis
Tympanosclerosis H74.0 ☑
Tympanum — *see* condition
Tympany
  abdomen R14.0
  chest R09.89
Type A behavior pattern Z73.1
Typhlitis — *see* Cecitis
Typhoenteritis — *see* Typhoid
Typhoid (abortive) (ambulant) (any site) (clinical) (fever) (hemorrhagic) (infection) (intermittent) (malignant) (rheumatic) (Widal negative) A01.00
  with pneumonia A01.03
  abdominal A01.09
  arthritis A01.04
  carrier (suspected) of Z22.0
  cholecystitis (current) A01.09
  endocarditis A01.02
  heart involvement A01.02
  inoculation reaction — *see* Complications, vaccination
  meningitis A01.01
  mesenteric lymph nodes A01.09
  myocarditis A01.02
  osteomyelitis A01.05
  perichondritis, larynx A01.09
  pneumonia A01.03
  specified NEC A01.09
  spine A01.05
  ulcer (perforating) A01.09
Typhomalaria (fever) — *see* Malaria
Typhomania A01.00
Typhoperitonitis A01.09
Typhus (fever) A75.9
  abdominal, abdominalis — *see* Typhoid
  African tick A77.1
  amarillic A95.9
  brain A75.9 *[G94]*
  cerebral A75.9 *[G94]*
  classical A75.0
  due to Rickettsia
    prowazekii A75.0
      recrudescent A75.1
    tsutsugamushi A75.3
    typhi A75.2
  endemic (flea-borne) A75.2
  epidemic (louse-borne) A75.0
  exanthematicus SAI A75.0
    brillii SAI A75.1
    mexicanus SAI A75.2
    typhus murinus A75.2
  exanthematic NEC A75.0
  flea-borne A75.2
  India tick A77.1
  Kenya (tick) A77.1
  louse-borne A75.0
  Mexican A75.2
  mite-borne A75.3
  murine A75.2
  North Asian tick-borne A77.2
  Orientia Tsutsugamushi (scrub typhus) A75.3
  petechial A75.9
  Queensland tick A77.3
  rat A75.2
  recrudescent A75.1
  recurrens — *see* Fever, relapsing
  Sao Paulo A77.0
  scrub (China) (India) (Malaysia) (New Guinea) A75.3
  shop (of Malaysia) A75.2
  Siberian tick A77.2
  tick-borne A77.9
  tropical (mite-borne) A75.3
Tyrosinemia E70.21
  newborn, transitory P74.5
Tyrosinosis E70.21
Tyrosinuria E70.29

U

Uhl's anomaly or disease Q24.8
Ulcer, ulcerated, ulcerating, ulceration, ulcerative
  alveolar process M27.3
  amebic (intestine) A06.1
    skin A06.7
  anastomotic — *see* Ulcer, gastrojejunal
  anorectal K62.6
  antral — *see* Ulcer, stomach
  anus (sphincter) (solitary) K62.6
  aorta — *see* Aneurysm
  aphthous (oral) (recurrent) K12.0
    genital organ(s)
      female N76.6
      male N50.89
  artery I77.2
  atrophic — *see* Ulcer, skin
    decubitus — *see* Ulcer, pressure, by site
  back L98.429
    with
      bone involvement without evidence of necrosis L98.426
      bone necrosis L98.424
      exposed fat layer L98.422
      muscle involvement without evidence of necrosis L98.425
      muscle necrosis L98.423
      skin breakdown only L98.421
      specified severity NEC L98.428
  Barrett's (esophagus) K22.10
    with bleeding K22.11
  bile duct (common) (hepatic) K83.8
  bladder (solitary) (sphincter) NEC N32.89
    bilharzial B65.9 *[N33]*
    in schistosomiasis (bilharzial) B65.9 *[N33]*
    submucosal — *see* Cystitis, interstitial
    tuberculous A18.12
  bleeding K27.4
  bone — *see* Osteomyelitis, specified type NEC
  bowel — *see* Ulcer, intestine
  breast N61.1
  bronchus J98.09
  buccal (cavity) (traumatic) K12.1
  Buruli A31.1
  buttock L98.419
    with
      bone involvement without evidence of necrosis L98.416
      bone necrosis L98.414
      exposed fat layer L98.412
      muscle involvement without evidence of necrosis L98.415
      muscle necrosis L98.413
      skin breakdown only L98.411
      specified severity NEC L98.418
  cancerous — *see* Neoplasm, malignant, by site
  cardia K22.10
    with bleeding K22.11
  cardioesophageal (peptic) K22.10
    with bleeding K22.11
  cecum — *see* Ulcer, intestine
  cervix (uteri) (decubitus) (trophic) N86
    with cervicitis N72
  chancroidal A57
  chiclero B55.1
  chronic (cause unknown) — *see* Ulcer, skin
  Cochin-China B55.1
  colon — *see* Ulcer, intestine
  conjunctiva H10.89
  cornea H16.00- ☑
    with hypopyon H16.03- ☑
    central H16.01- ☑
    dendritic (herpes simplex) B00.52
    marginal H16.04- ☑
    Mooren's H16.05- ☑
    mycotic H16.06- ☑
    perforated H16.07- ☑
    ring H16.02- ☑
    tuberculous (phlyctenular) A18.52
  corpus cavernosum (chronic) N48.5
  crural — *see* Ulcer, lower limb
  Curling's — *see* Ulcer, peptic, acute
  Cushing's — *see* Ulcer, peptic, acute
  cystic duct K82.8
  cystitis (interstitial) — *see* Cystitis, interstitial
  decubitus — *see* Ulcer, pressure, by site

Ulcer, ulcerated, ulcerating, ulceration, ulcerative
— *continued*
dendritic, cornea (herpes simplex) B00.52
diabetes, diabetic — *see* Diabetes, ulcer
Dieulafoy's K25.0
due to
infection NEC — *see* Ulcer, skin
radiation NEC L59.8
trophic disturbance (any region) — *see* Ulcer, skin
X-ray L58.1
duodenum, duodenal (eroded) (peptic) K26.9
with
hemorrhage K26.4
and perforation K26.6
perforation K26.5
acute K26.3
with
hemorrhage K26.0
and perforation K26.2
perforation K26.1
chronic K26.7
with
hemorrhage K26.4
and perforation K26.6
perforation K26.5
dysenteric A09
elusive — *see* Cystitis, interstitial
endocarditis (acute) (chronic) (subacute) I28.8
epiglottis J38.7
esophagus (peptic) K22.10
with bleeding K22.11
due to
aspirin K22.10
with bleeding K22.11
gastrointestinal reflux disease (without bleeding)
K21.00
with bleeding K21.01
ingestion of chemical or medicament K22.10
with bleeding K22.11
fungal K22.10
with bleeding K22.11
infective K22.10
with bleeding K22.11
varicose — *see* Varix, esophagus
eyelid (region) H01.8
fauces J39.2
Fenwick (-Hunner) (solitary) — *see* Cystitis, interstitial
fistulous — *see* Ulcer, skin
foot (indolent) (trophic) — *see* Ulcer, lower limb
frambesial, initial A66.0
frenum (tongue) K14.0
gallbladder or duct K82.8
gangrenous — *see* Gangrene
gastric — *see* Ulcer, stomach
gastrocolic — *see* Ulcer, gastrojejunal
gastroduodenal — *see* Ulcer, peptic
gastroesophageal — *see* Ulcer, stomach
gastrointestinal — *see* Ulcer, gastrojejunal
gastrojejunal (peptic) K28.9
with
hemorrhage K28.4
and perforation K28.6
perforation K28.5
acute K28.3
with
hemorrhage K28.0
and perforation K28.2
perforation K28.1
chronic K28.7
with
hemorrhage K28.4
and perforation K28.6
perforation K28.5
gastrojejunocolic — *see* Ulcer, gastrojejunal
gingiva K06.8
gingivitis K05.10
nonplaque induced K05.11
plaque induced K05.10
glottis J38.7
granuloma of pudenda A58
gum K06.8
gumma, due to yaws A66.4
heel — *see* Ulcer, lower limb
hemorrhoid — *see also* Hemorrhoids, by degree K64.8
Hunner's — *see* Cystitis, interstitial
hypopharynx J39.2
hypopyon (chronic) (subacute) — *see* Ulcer, cornea,
with hypopyon

Ulcer, ulcerated, ulcerating, ulceration, ulcerative
— *continued*
hypostaticum — *see* Ulcer, varicose
ileum — *see* Ulcer, intestine
intestine, intestinal K63.3
with perforation K63.1
amebic A06.1
duodenal — *see* Ulcer, duodenum
granulocytopenic (with hemorrhage) — *see* Neutropenia
marginal — *see* Ulcer, gastrojejunal
perforating K63.1
newborn P78.0
primary, small intestine K63.3
rectum K62.6
stercoraceous, stercoral K63.3
tuberculous A18.32
typhoid (fever) — *see* Typhoid
varicose I86.8
jejunum, jejunal — *see* Ulcer, gastrojejunal
keratitis — *see* Ulcer, cornea
knee — *see* Ulcer, lower limb
labium (majus) (minus) N76.6
laryngitis — *see* Laryngitis
larynx (aphthous) (contact) J38.7
diphtheritic A36.2
leg — *see* Ulcer, lower limb
lip K13.0
Lipschütz's N76.6
lower limb (atrophic) (chronic) (neurogenic) (perforating) (pyogenic) (trophic) (tropical) L97.909
with
bone involvement without evidence of necrosis
L97.906
bone necrosis L97.904
exposed fat layer L97.902
muscle involvement without evidence of necrosis
L97.905
muscle necrosis L97.903
skin breakdown only L97.901
specified severity NEC L97.908
ankle L97.309
with
bone involvement without evidence of
necrosis L97.306
bone necrosis L97.304
exposed fat layer L97.302
muscle involvement without evidence of
necrosis L97.305
muscle necrosis L97.303
skin breakdown only L97.301
specified severity NEC L97.308
left L97.329
with
bone involvement without evidence of
necrosis L97.326
bone necrosis L97.324
exposed fat layer L97.322
muscle involvement without evidence of
necrosis L97.325
muscle necrosis L97.323
skin breakdown only L97.321
specified severity NEC L97.328
right L97.319
with
bone involvement without evidence of
necrosis L97.316
bone necrosis L97.314
exposed fat layer L97.312
muscle involvement without evidence of
necrosis L97.315
muscle necrosis L97.313
skin breakdown only L97.311
specified severity NEC L97.318
calf L97.209
with
bone involvement without evidence of
necrosis L97.206
bone necrosis L97.204
exposed fat layer L97.202
muscle involvement without evidence of
necrosis L97.205
muscle necrosis L97.203
skin breakdown only L97.201
specified severity NEC L97.208
left L97.229

Ulcer, ulcerated, ulcerating, ulceration, ulcerative
— *continued*
lower limb — *continued*
calf — *continued*
left — *continued*
with
bone involvement without evidence of
necrosis L97.226
bone necrosis L97.224
exposed fat layer L97.222
muscle involvement without evidence of
necrosis L97.225
muscle necrosis L97.223
skin breakdown only L97.221
specified severity NEC L97.228
right L97.219
with
bone involvement without evidence of
necrosis L97.216
bone necrosis L97.214
exposed fat layer L97.212
muscle involvement without evidence of
necrosis L97.215
muscle necrosis L97.213
skin breakdown only L97.211
specified severity NEC L97.218
decubitus — *see* Ulcer, pressure, by site
foot specified NEC L97.509
with
bone involvement without evidence of
necrosis L97.506
bone necrosis L97.504
exposed fat layer L97.502
muscle involvement without evidence of
necrosis L97.505
muscle necrosis L97.503
skin breakdown only L97.501
specified severity NEC L97.508
left L97.529
with
bone involvement without evidence of
necrosis L97.526
bone necrosis L97.524
exposed fat layer L97.522
muscle involvement without evidence of
necrosis L97.525
muscle necrosis L97.523
skin breakdown only L97.521
specified severity NEC L97.528
right L97.519
with
bone involvement without evidence of
necrosis L97.516
bone necrosis L97.514
exposed fat layer L97.512
muscle involvement without evidence of
necrosis L97.515
muscle necrosis L97.513
skin breakdown only L97.511
specified severity NEC L97.518
heel L97.409
with
bone involvement without evidence of
necrosis L97.406
bone necrosis L97.404
exposed fat layer L97.402
muscle involvement without evidence of
necrosis L97.405
muscle necrosis L97.403
skin breakdown only L97.401
specified severity NEC L97.408
left L97.429
with
bone involvement without evidence of
necrosis L97.426
bone necrosis L97.424
exposed fat layer L97.422
muscle involvement without evidence of
necrosis L97.425
muscle necrosis L97.423
skin breakdown only L97.421
specified severity NEC L97.428
right L97.419
with
bone involvement without evidence of
necrosis L97.416
bone necrosis L97.414
exposed fat layer L97.412

☑ **Additional Character Required** — Refer to the Tabular List for Character Selection

Ulcer, ulcerated, ulcerating, ulceration, ulcerative
— *continued*
  lower limb — *continued*
    heel — *continued*
      right — *continued*
        with — *continued*
          muscle involvement without evidence of
            necrosis L97.415
          muscle necrosis L97.413
          skin breakdown only L97.411
          specified severity NEC L97.418
      left L97.929
        with
          bone involvement without evidence of
            necrosis L97.926
          bone necrosis L97.924
          exposed fat layer L97.922
          muscle involvement without evidence of
            necrosis L97.925
          muscle necrosis L97.923
          skin breakdown only L97.921
          specified severity NEC L97.928
    leprous A30.1
    lower leg NOS L97.909
      with
        bone involvement without evidence of
          necrosis L97.906
        bone necrosis L97.904
        exposed fat layer L97.902
        muscle involvement without evidence of
          necrosis L97.905
        muscle necrosis L97.903
        skin breakdown only L97.901
        specified severity NEC L97.908
      left L97.929
        with
          bone involvement without evidence of
            necrosis L97.926
          bone necrosis L97.924
          exposed fat layer L97.922
          muscle involvement without evidence of
            necrosis L97.925
          muscle necrosis L97.923
          skin breakdown only L97.921
          specified severity NEC L97.928
      right L97.919
        with
          bone involvement without evidence of
            necrosis L97.916
          bone necrosis L97.914
          exposed fat layer L97.912
          muscle involvement without evidence of
            necrosis L97.915
          muscle necrosis L97.913
          skin breakdown only L97.911
          specified severity NEC L97.918
    specified site NEC L97.809
      with
        bone involvement without evidence of
          necrosis L97.806
        bone necrosis L97.804
        exposed fat layer L97.802
        muscle involvement without evidence of
          necrosis L97.805
        muscle necrosis L97.803
        skin breakdown only L97.801
        specified severity NEC L97.808
      left L97.829
        with
          bone involvement without evidence
            of necrosis L97.826
          bone necrosis L97.824
          exposed fat layer L97.822
          muscle involvement without evidence
            of necrosis L97.825
          muscle necrosis L97.823
          skin breakdown only L97.821
          specified severity NEC L97.828
      right L97.819
        with
          bone involvement without evidence
            of necrosis L97.816
          bone necrosis L97.814
          exposed fat layer L97.812
          muscle involvement without evidence
            of necrosis L97.815
          muscle necrosis L97.813
          skin breakdown only L97.811
          specified severity NEC L97.818

Ulcer, ulcerated, ulcerating, ulceration, ulcerative
— *continued*
  lower limb — *continued*
    midfoot L97.409
      with
        bone involvement without evidence of
          necrosis L97.406
        bone necrosis L97.404
        exposed fat layer L97.402
        muscle involvement without evidence of
          necrosis L97.405
        muscle necrosis L97.403
        skin breakdown only L97.401
        specified severity NEC L97.408
      left L97.429
        with
          bone involvement without evidence of
            necrosis L97.426
          bone necrosis L97.424
          exposed fat layer L97.422
          muscle involvement without evidence of
            necrosis L97.425
          muscle necrosis L97.423
          skin breakdown only L97.421
          specified severity NEC L97.428
      right L97.419
        with
          bone involvement without evidence of
            necrosis L97.416
          bone necrosis L97.414
          exposed fat layer L97.412
          muscle involvement without evidence of
            necrosis L97.415
          muscle necrosis L97.413
          skin breakdown only L97.411
          specified severity NEC L97.418
    right L97.919
      with
        bone involvement without evidence of
          necrosis L97.916
        bone necrosis L97.914
        exposed fat layer L97.912
        muscle involvement without evidence of
          necrosis L97.915
        muscle necrosis L97.913
        skin breakdown only L97.911
        specified severity NEC L97.918
    syphilitic A52.19
    thigh L97.109
      with
        bone involvement without evidence of
          necrosis L97.106
        bone necrosis L97.104
        exposed fat layer L97.102
        muscle involvement without evidence of
          necrosis L97.105
        muscle necrosis L97.103
        skin breakdown only L97.101
        specified severity NEC L97.108
      left L97.129
        with
          bone involvement without evidence of
            necrosis L97.126
          bone necrosis L97.124
          exposed fat layer L97.122
          muscle involvement without evidence of
            necrosis L97.125
          muscle necrosis L97.123
          skin breakdown only L97.121
          specified severity NEC L97.128
      right L97.119
        with
          bone involvement without evidence of
            necrosis L97.116
          bone necrosis L97.114
          exposed fat layer L97.112
          muscle involvement without evidence of
            necrosis L97.115
          muscle necrosis L97.113
          skin breakdown only L97.111
          specified severity NEC L97.118
    toe L97.509
      with
        bone involvement without evidence of
          necrosis L97.506
        bone necrosis L97.504
        exposed fat layer L97.502
        muscle involvement without evidence of
          necrosis L97.505

Ulcer, ulcerated, ulcerating, ulceration, ulcerative
— *continued*
  lower limb — *continued*
    toe — *continued*
      with — *continued*
        muscle necrosis L97.503
        skin breakdown only L97.501
        specified severity NEC L97.508
      left L97.529
        with
          bone involvement without evidence of
            necrosis L97.526
          bone necrosis L97.524
          exposed fat layer L97.522
          muscle involvement without evidence of
            necrosis L97.525
          muscle necrosis L97.523
          skin breakdown only L97.521
          specified severity NEC L97.528
      right L97.519
        with
          bone involvement without evidence of
            necrosis L97.516
          bone necrosis L97.514
          exposed fat layer L97.512
          muscle involvement without evidence of
            necrosis L97.515
          muscle necrosis L97.513
          skin breakdown only L97.511
          specified severity NEC L97.518
    varicose — *see* Varix, leg, with, ulcer
    luetic — *see* Ulcer, syphilitic
  lung J98.4
    tuberculous — *see* Tuberculosis, pulmonary
  malignant — *see* Neoplasm, malignant, by site
  marginal NEC — *see* Ulcer, gastrojejunal
  meatus (urinarius) N34.2
  Meckel's diverticulum Q43.0
    malignant — *see* Table of Neoplasms, small intestine, malignant
  Meleney's (chronic undermining) — *see* Ulcer, skin
  Mooren's (cornea) — *see* Ulcer, cornea, Mooren's
  mycobacterial (skin) A31.1
  nasopharynx J39.2
  neck, uterus N86
  neurogenic NEC — *see* Ulcer, skin
  nose, nasal (passage) (infective) (septum) J34.0
    skin — *see* Ulcer, skin
    spirochetal A69.8
    varicose (bleeding) I86.8
  oral mucosa (traumatic) K12.1
  palate (soft) K12.1
  penis (chronic) N48.5
  peptic (site unspecified) K27.9
    with
      hemorrhage K27.4
        and perforation K27.6
      perforation K27.5
    acute K27.3
      with
        hemorrhage K27.0
          and perforation K27.2
        perforation K27.1
    chronic K27.7
      with
        hemorrhage K27.4
          and perforation K27.6
        perforation K27.5
    esophagus K22.10
      with bleeding K22.11
    newborn P78.82
  perforating K27.5
    skin — *see* Ulcer, skin
  peritonsillar J35.8
  phagedenic (tropical) — *see* Ulcer, skin
  pharynx J39.2
  phlebitis — *see* Phlebitis
  plaster — *see* Ulcer, pressure, by site
  popliteal space — *see* Ulcer, lower limb
  postpyloric — *see* Ulcer, duodenum
  prepuce N47.7
  prepyloric — *see* Ulcer, stomach
  pressure (pressure area) L89.9- ☑
    ankle L89.5- ☑
    back L89.1- ☑
    buttock L89.3- ☑
    coccyx L89.15- ☑
    contiguous site of back, buttock, hip L89.4- ☑

Ulcer, ulcerated, ulcerating, ulceration, ulcerative
— continued
pressure *— continued*
  elbow L89.0- ☑
  face L89.81- ☑
  head L89.81- ☑
  heel L89.6- ☑
  hip L89.2- ☑
  sacral region (tailbone) L89.15- ☑
  specified site NEC L89.89- ☑
  stage 1 (healing) (pre-ulcer skin changes limited to persistent focal edema)
    ankle L89.5- ☑
    back L89.1- ☑
    buttock L89.3- ☑
    coccyx L89.15- ☑
    contiguous site of back, buttock, hip L89.4- ☑
    elbow L89.0- ☑
    face L89.81- ☑
    head L89.81- ☑
    heel L89.6- ☑
    hip L89.2- ☑
    sacral region (tailbone) L89.15- ☑
    specified site NEC L89.89- ☑
  stage 2 (healing) (abrasion, blister, partial thickness skin loss involving epidermis and/or dermis)
    ankle L89.5- ☑
    back L89.1- ☑
    buttock L89.3- ☑
    coccyx L89.15- ☑
    contiguous site of back, buttock, hip L89.4- ☑
    elbow L89.0- ☑
    face L89.81- ☑
    head L89.81- ☑
    heel L89.6- ☑
    hip L89.2- ☑
    sacral region (tailbone) L89.15- ☑
    specified site NEC L89.89- ☑
  stage 3 (healing) (full thickness skin loss involving damage or necrosis of subcutaneous tissue)
    ankle L89.5- ☑
    back L89.1- ☑
    buttock L89.3- ☑
    coccyx L89.15- ☑
    contiguous site of back, buttock, hip L89.4- ☑
    elbow L89.0- ☑
    face L89.81- ☑
    head L89.81- ☑
    heel L89.6- ☑
    hip L89.2- ☑
    sacral region (tailbone) L89.15- ☑
    specified site NEC L89.89- ☑
  stage 4 (healing) (necrosis of soft tissues through to underlying muscle, tendon, or bone)
    ankle L89.5- ☑
    back L89.1- ☑
    buttock L89.3- ☑
    coccyx L89.15- ☑
    contiguous site of back, buttock, hip L89.4- ☑
    elbow L89.0- ☑
    face L89.81- ☑
    head L89.81- ☑
    heel L89.6- ☑
    hip L89.2- ☑
    sacral region (tailbone) L89.15- ☑
    specified site NEC L89.89- ☑
  unspecified stage
    ankle L89.5- ☑
    back L89.1- ☑
    buttock L89.3- ☑
    coccyx L89.15- ☑
    contiguous site of back, buttock, hip L89.4- ☑
    elbow L89.0- ☑
    face L89.81- ☑
    head L89.81- ☑
    heel L89.6- ☑
    hip L89.2- ☑
    sacral region (tailbone) L89.15- ☑
    specified site NEC L89.89- ☑
  unstageable
    ankle L89.5- ☑
    back L89.1- ☑
    buttock L89.3- ☑
    coccyx L89.15- ☑
    contiguous site of back, buttock, hip L89.4- ☑
    elbow L89.0- ☑

Ulcer, ulcerated, ulcerating, ulceration, ulcerative
— continued
pressure *— continued*
  unstageable *— continued*
    face L89.81- ☑
    head L89.81- ☑
    heel L89.6- ☑
    hip L89.2- ☑
    sacral region (tailbone) L89.15- ☑
    specified site NEC L89.89- ☑
primary of intestine K63.3
  with perforation K63.1
prostate N41.9
pyloric *— see* Ulcer, stomach
rectosigmoid K63.3
  with perforation K63.1
rectum (sphincter) (solitary) K62.6
  stercoraceous, stercoral K62.6
retina *— see* Inflammation, chorioretinal
rodent *— see also* Neoplasm, skin, malignant
sclera *— see* Scleritis
scrofulous (tuberculous) A18.2
scrotum N50.89
  tuberculous A18.15
  varicose I86.1
seminal vesicle N50.89
sigmoid *— see* Ulcer, intestine
skin (atrophic) (chronic) (neurogenic) (non-healing) (perforating) (pyogenic) (trophic) (tropical) L98.499
  with gangrene *— see* Gangrene
  amebic A06.7
  back *— see* Ulcer, back
  buttock *— see* Ulcer, buttock
  decubitus *— see* Ulcer, pressure
  lower limb *— see* Ulcer, lower limb
  mycobacterial A31.1
  specified site NEC L98.499
    with
      bone involvement without evidence of necrosis L98.496
      bone necrosis L98.494
      exposed fat layer L98.492
      muscle involvement without evidence of necrosis L98.495
      muscle necrosis L98.493
      skin breakdown only L98.491
      specified severity NEC L98.498
  tuberculous (primary) A18.4
  varicose *— see* Ulcer, varicose
sloughing *— see* Ulcer, skin
solitary, anus or rectum (sphincter) K62.6
sore throat J02.9
  streptococcal J02.0
spermatic cord N50.89
spine (tuberculous) A18.01
stasis (venous) *— see* Varix, leg, with, ulcer
  without varicose veins I87.2
stercoraceous, stercoral K63.3
  with perforation K63.1
  anus or rectum K62.6
stoma, stomal *— see* Ulcer, gastrojejunal
stomach (eroded) (peptic) (round) K25.9
  with
    hemorrhage K25.4
      and perforation K25.6
    perforation K25.5
  acute K25.3
    with
      hemorrhage K25.0
        and perforation K25.2
      perforation K25.1
  chronic K25.7
    with
      hemorrhage K25.4
        and perforation K25.6
      perforation K25.5
stomal *— see* Ulcer, gastrojejunal
stomatitis K12.1
stress *— see* Ulcer, peptic
strumous (tuberculous) A18.2
submucosal, bladder *— see* Cystitis, interstitial
syphilitic (any site) (early) (secondary) A51.39
  late A52.79
  perforating A52.79
    foot A52.11
testis N50.89
thigh *— see* Ulcer, lower limb

Ulcer, ulcerated, ulcerating, ulceration, ulcerative
— continued
throat J39.2
  diphtheritic A36.0
toe *— see* Ulcer, lower limb
tongue (traumatic) K14.0
tonsil J35.8
  diphtheritic A36.0
trachea J39.8
trophic *— see* Ulcer, skin
tropical *— see* Ulcer, skin
tuberculous *— see* Tuberculosis, ulcer
tunica vaginalis N50.89
turbinate J34.89
typhoid (perforating) *— see* Typhoid
unspecified site *— see* Ulcer, skin
urethra (meatus) *— see* Urethritis
uterus N85.8
  cervix N86
    with cervicitis N72
  neck N86
    with cervicitis N72
vagina N76.5
  in Behçet's disease M35.2 *[N77.0]*
  pessary N89.8
valve, heart I33.0
varicose (lower limb, any part) *— see also* Varix, leg, with, ulcer
  broad ligament I86.2
  esophagus *— see* Varix, esophagus
  inflamed or infected *— see* Varix, leg, with ulcer, with inflammation
  nasal septum I86.8
  perineum I86.3
  scrotum I86.1
  specified site NEC I86.8
  sublingual I86.0
  vulva I86.3
vas deferens N50.89
vulva (acute) (infectional) N76.6
  in (due to)
    Behçet's disease M35.2 *[N77.0]*
    herpesviral (herpes simplex) infection A60.04
    tuberculosis A18.18
vulvobuccal, recurring N76.6
X-ray L58.1
yaws A66.4
Ulcerosa scarlatina A38.8
Ulcus *— see also* Ulcer
  cutis tuberculosum A18.4
  duodeni *— see* Ulcer, duodenum
  durum (syphilitic) A51.0
    extragenital A51.2
  gastrojejunale *— see* Ulcer, gastrojejunal
  hypostaticum *— see* Ulcer, varicose
  molle (cutis) (skin) A57
  serpens corneae *— see* Ulcer, cornea, central
  ventriculi *— see* Ulcer, stomach
Ulegyria Q04.8
Ulerythema
  ophryogenes, congenital Q84.2
  sycosiforme L73.8
Ullrich (-Bonnevie) (-Turner) syndrome *— see also* Turner's syndrome Q87.19
Ullrich-Feichtiger syndrome Q87.0
Ulnar *— see* condition
Ulorrhagia, ulorrhea K06.8
Umbilicus, umbilical *— see* condition
Unable to
  make ends meet Z59.86
  obtain
    adequate
      childcare Z59.87
      clothing Z59.87
      utilities Z59.87
    basic needs Z59.87
Unacceptable
  contours of tooth K08.54
  morphology of tooth K08.54
Unaffordable transportation Z59.82
Unavailability (of)
  bed at medical facility Z75.1
  health service-related agencies Z75.4
  medical facilities (at) Z75.3
    due to
      investigation by social service agency Z75.2
      lack of services at home Z75.0
      remoteness from facility Z75.3

☑ **Additional Character Required — Refer to the Tabular List for Character Selection**

Unavailability — *continued*
　medical facilities — *continued*
　　due to — *continued*
　　　waiting list Z75.1
　　home Z75.Ø
　　outpatient clinic Z75.3
　schooling Z55.1
　social service agencies Z75.4
Uncinaria americana infestation B76.1
Uncinariasis B76.9
Uncongenial work Z56.5
Unconscious (ness) — *see* Coma
Under observation — *see* Observation
Underachievement in school Z55.3
Underdevelopment — *see also* Undeveloped
　nose Q3Ø.1
　sexual E3Ø.Ø
Underdosing — *see also* Table of Drugs and Chemicals,
　　categories T36-T5Ø, with final character 6 Z91.14
　intentional NEC Z91.128
　　due to financial hardship of patient Z91.12Ø
　unintentional NEC Z91.138
　　due to patient's age related debility Z91.13Ø
Underfeeding, newborn P92.3
Underfill, endodontic M27.53
Underimmunization status Z28.39
　COVID-19 Z28.31- ☑
　　partially vaccinated (for) Z28.311
　　unvaccinated (for) Z28.31Ø
Undernourishment — *see* Malnutrition
Undernutrition — *see* Malnutrition
Underweight R63.6
　for gestational age — *see* Light for dates
Underwood's disease P83.Ø
Undescended — *see also* Malposition, congenital
　cecum Q43.3
　colon Q43.3
　testicle — *see* Cryptorchid
Undeveloped, undevelopment — *see also* Hypoplasia
　brain (congenital) QØ2
　cerebral (congenital) QØ2
　heart Q24.8
　lung Q33.6
　testis E29.1
　uterus E3Ø.Ø
Undiagnosed (disease) R69
Undulant fever — *see* Brucellosis
Unemployment, anxiety concerning Z56.Ø
　threatened Z56.2
Unequal length (acquired) (limb) — *see also* Deformity,
　　limb, unequal length
　leg — *see also* Deformity, limb, unequal length
　　congenital Q72.9- ☑
Unextracted dental root KØ8.3
Unguis incarnatus L6Ø.Ø
Unhappiness R45.2
Unicornate uterus Q51.4
　in pregnancy or childbirth O34.ØØ
Unilateral — *see also* condition
　development, breast N64.89
　organ or site, congenital NEC — *see* Agenesis, by site
Unilocular heart Q2Ø.8
Unimmunized — *see also* Underimmunization status
　for COVID-19 Z28.31Ø
Union, abnormal — *see also* Fusion
　larynx and trachea Q34.8
Universal mesentery Q43.3
Unreliable transportation Z59.82
Unrepairable overhanging of dental restorative
　　materials KØ8.52
Unroofed coronary sinus Q21.13
Unsafe transportation Z59.82
Unsatisfactory
　restoration of tooth KØ8.5Ø
　　specified NEC KØ8.59
　sample of cytologic smear
　　anus R85.615
　　cervix R87.615
　　vagina R87.625
　surroundings Z59.1
　work Z56.5
Unsoundness of mind — *see* Psychosis
Unstable
　back NEC — *see* Instability, joint, spine
　hip (congenital) Q65.6
　　acquired — *see* Derangement, joint, specified type
　　　NEC, hip

Unstable — *continued*
　joint — *see* Instability, joint
　　secondary to removal of joint prosthesis M96.89
　lie (mother) O32.Ø ☑
　lumbosacral joint (congenital) — *see* subcategory
　　M53.2
　sacroiliac — *see* subcategory M53.2 ☑
　spine NEC — *see* Instability, joint, spine
Unsteadiness on feet R26.81
Untruthfulness, child problem F91.8
Unvaccinated — *see also* Underimmunization status
　for COVID-19 Z28.31Ø
Unverricht (-Lundborg) **disease or epilepsy** — *see*
　　Epilepsy, generalized, idiopathic
Unwanted
　multiple moves in the last 12 months Z59.81- ☑
　pregnancy Z64.Ø
Upbringing, institutional Z62.22
　away from parents NEC Z62.29
　in care of non-parental family member Z62.21
　in foster care Z62.21
　in orphanage or group home Z62.22
　in welfare custody Z62.21
Upper respiratory — *see* condition
Upset
　gastric K3Ø
　gastrointestinal K3Ø
　　psychogenic F45.8
　intestinal (large) (small) K59.9
　　psychogenic F45.8
　menstruation N93.9
　mental F48.9
　stomach K3Ø
　　psychogenic F45.8
Urachus — *see also* condition
　patent or persistent Q64.4
Urbach-Oppenheim disease (necrobiosis lipoidica dia-
　　beticorum) — *see* EØ8-E13 with .62Ø
Urbach's lipoid proteinosis E78.89
Urbach-Wiethe disease E78.89
Urban yellow fever A95.1
Urea
　blood, high — *see* Uremia
　cycle metabolism disorder — *see* Disorder, urea cycle
　　metabolism
Uremia, uremic N19
　with
　　ectopic or molar pregnancy OØ8.4
　　polyneuropathy N18.9 *[G63]*
　chronic NOS — *see also* Disease, kidney, chronic N18.9
　　due to hypertension — *see* Hypertensive, kidney
　complicating
　　ectopic or molar pregnancy OØ8.4
　congenital P96.Ø
　extrarenal R39.2
　following ectopic or molar pregnancy OØ8.4
　newborn P96.Ø
　prerenal R39.2
Ureter, ureteral — *see* condition
Ureteralgia N23
Ureterectasis — *see* Hydroureter
Ureteritis N28.89
　cystica N28.86
　due to calculus N2Ø.1
　　with calculus, kidney N2Ø.2
　　　with hydronephrosis N13.2
　gonococcal (acute) (chronic) A54.21
　nonspecific N28.89
Ureterocele N28.89
　congenital (orthotopic) Q62.31
　　ectopic Q62.32
Ureterolith, ureterolithiasis — *see* Calculus, ureter
Ureterostomy
　attention to Z43.6
　status Z93.6
Urethra, urethral — *see* condition
Urethralgia R39.89
Urethritis (anterior) (posterior) N34.2
　calculous N21.1
　candidal B37.41
　chlamydial A56.Ø1
　diplococcal (gonococcal) A54.Ø1
　　with abscess (accessory gland) (periurethral) A54.1
　gonococcal A54.Ø1
　　with abscess (accessory gland) (periurethral) A54.1
　nongonococcal N34.1
　　Reiter's — *see* Reiter's disease

Urethritis — *continued*
　nonspecific N34.1
　nonvenereal N34.1
　postmenopausal N34.2
　puerperal O86.22
　Reiter's — *see* Reiter's disease
　specified NEC N34.2
　trichomonal or due to Trichomonas (vaginalis) A59.Ø3
Urethrocele N81.Ø
　with
　　cystocele — *see* Cystocele
　　prolapse of uterus — *see* Prolapse, uterus
Urethrolithiasis (with colic or infection) N21.1
Urethrorectal — *see* condition
Urethrorrhagia N36.8
Urethrorrhea R36.9
Urethrostomy
　attention to Z43.6
　status Z93.6
Urethrotrigonitis — *see* Trigonitis
Urethrovaginal — *see* condition
Urgency
　fecal R15.2
　hypertensive — *see* Hypertension
　urinary R39.15
Urhidrosis, uridrosis L74.8
Uric acid in blood (increased) E79.Ø
Uricacidemia (asymptomatic) E79.Ø
Uricemia (asymptomatic) E79.Ø
Uricosuria R82.998
Urinary — *see* condition
Urination
　frequent R35.Ø
　painful R3Ø.9
Urine
　blood in — *see* Hematuria
　discharge, excessive R35.89
　enuresis, nonorganic origin F98.Ø
　extravasation R39.Ø
　frequency R35.Ø
　incontinence R32
　　nonorganic origin F98.Ø
　intermittent stream R39.198
　pus in N39.Ø
　retention or stasis R33.9
　　organic R33.8
　　　drug-induced R33.Ø
　　psychogenic F45.8
　secretion
　　deficient R34
　　excessive R35.89
　　frequency R35.Ø
　stream
　　intermittent R39.198
　　slowing R39.198
　　splitting R39.13
　　weak R39.12
Urinemia — *see* Uremia
Urinoma, urethra N36.8
Uroarthritis, infectious (Reiter's) — *see* Reiter's disease
Urodialysis R34
Urolithiasis — *see* Calculus, urinary
Uronephrosis — *see* Hydronephrosis
Uropathy N39.9
　obstructive N13.9
　　specified NEC N13.8
　reflux N13.9
　　specified NEC N13.8
　vesicoureteral reflux-associated — *see* Reflux, vesi-
　　coureteral
Urosepsis — *code to* condition
Urticaria L5Ø.9
　with angioneurotic edema T78.3 ☑
　　hereditary D84.1
　allergic L5Ø.Ø
　cholinergic L5Ø.5
　chronic L5Ø.8
　cold, familial L5Ø.2
　contact L5Ø.6
　dermatographic L5Ø.3
　due to
　　cold or heat L5Ø.2
　　drugs L5Ø.Ø
　　food L5Ø.Ø
　　inhalants L5Ø.Ø
　　plants L5Ø.6
　　serum — *see also* Reaction, serum T8Ø.69 ☑
　factitial L5Ø.3

Urticaria — *continued*
  familial cold M04.2
  giant T78.3 ☑
    hereditary D84.1
  gigantea T78.3 ☑
  idiopathic L50.1
  larynx T78.3 ☑
    hereditary D84.1
  neonatorum P83.88
  nonallergic L50.1
  papulosa (Hebra) L28.2
  pigmentosa D47.01
    congenital Q82.2
    of neonatal onset Q82.2
    of newborn onset Q82.2
  recurrent periodic L50.8
  serum — *see also* Reaction, serum T80.69 ☑
  solar L56.3
  specified type NEC L50.8
  thermal (cold) (heat) L50.2
  vibratory L50.4
  xanthelasmoidea — *see* Urticaria pigmentosa
Use (of)
  alcohol F10.90
    with
      intoxication F10.929
      sleep disorder F10.982
      withdrawal F10.939
        with
          perceptual disturbance F10.932
        delirium F10.931
        uncomplicated F10.930
    harmful — *see* Abuse, alcohol
    in remission F10.91
  amphetamines — *see* Use, stimulant NEC
  caffeine — *see* Use, stimulant NEC
  cannabis F12.90
    with
      anxiety disorder F12.980
      intoxication F12.929
        with
          delirium F12.921
          perceptual disturbance F12.922
        uncomplicated F12.920
      other specified disorder F12.988
      psychosis F12.959
        delusions F12.950
        hallucinations F12.951
      unspecified disorder F12.99
      withdrawal F12.93
    in remission F12.91
  cocaine F14.90
    with
      anxiety disorder F14.980
      intoxication F14.929
        with
          delirium F14.921
          perceptual disturbance F14.922
        uncomplicated F14.920
      other specified disorder F14.988
      psychosis F14.959
        delusions F14.950
        hallucinations F14.951
      sexual dysfunction F14.981
      sleep disorder F14.982
      unspecified disorder F14.99
      withdrawal F14.93
    harmful — *see* Abuse, drug, cocaine
    in remission F14.91
  drug(s) NEC F19.90
    with sleep disorder F19.982
    harmful — *see* Abuse, drug, by type
  hallucinogen NEC F16.90
    with
      anxiety disorder F16.980
      intoxication F16.929
        with
          delirium F16.921
        uncomplicated F16.920
      mood disorder F16.94
      other specified disorder F16.988
      perception disorder (flashbacks) F16.983
      psychosis F16.959
        delusions F16.950
        hallucinations F16.951
      unspecified disorder F16.99
    harmful — *see* Abuse, drug, hallucinogen NEC
    in remission F16.91

Use — *continued*
  inhalants F18.90
    with
      anxiety disorder F18.980
      intoxication F18.929
        with delirium F18.921
        uncomplicated F18.920
      mood disorder F18.94
      other specified disorder F18.988
      persisting dementia F18.97
      psychosis F18.959
        delusions F18.950
        hallucinations F18.951
      unspecified disorder F18.99
    harmful — *see* Abuse, drug, inhalant
    in remission F18.91
  methadone — *see* Use, opioid
  nonprescribed drugs F19.90
    harmful — *see* Abuse, non-psychoactive substance
  opioid F11.90
    with
      disorder F11.99
        mood F11.94
        sleep F11.982
        specified type NEC F11.988
      intoxication F11.929
        with
          delirium F11.921
          perceptual disturbance F11.922
        uncomplicated F11.920
      withdrawal F11.93
    harmful — *see* Abuse, drug, opioid
    in remission F11.91
  patent medicines F19.90
    harmful — *see* Abuse, non-psychoactive substance
  psychoactive drug NEC F19.90
    with
      anxiety disorder F19.980
      intoxication F19.929
        with
          delirium F19.921
          perceptual disturbance F19.922
        uncomplicated F19.920
      mood disorder F19.94
      other specified disorder F19.988
      persisting
        amnestic disorder F19.96
        dementia F19.97
      psychosis F19.959
        delusions F19.950
        hallucinations F19.951
      sexual dysfunction F19.981
      sleep disorder F19.982
      unspecified disorder F19.99
      withdrawal F19.939
        with
          delirium F19.931
          perceptual disturbance F19.932
        uncomplicated F19.930
    harmful — *see* Abuse, drug NEC, psychoactive NEC
    in remission F19.91
  sedative, hypnotic, or anxiolytic F13.90
    with
      anxiety disorder F13.980
      intoxication F13.929
        with
          delirium F13.921
        uncomplicated F13.920
      other specified disorder F13.988
      persisting
        amnestic disorder F13.96
        dementia F13.97
      psychosis F13.959
        delusions F13.950
        hallucinations F13.951
      sexual dysfunction F13.981
      sleep disorder F13.982
      unspecified disorder F13.99
    harmful — *see* Abuse, drug, sedative, hypnotic, or anxiolytic
    in remission F13.91
  stimulant NEC F15.90
    with
      anxiety disorder F15.980
      intoxication F15.929
        with
          delirium F15.921
          perceptual disturbance F15.922

Use — *continued*
  stimulant — *continued*
    with — *continued*
      intoxication — *continued*
        uncomplicated F15.920
      mood disorder F15.94
      other specified disorder F15.988
      psychosis F15.959
        delusions F15.950
        hallucinations F15.951
      sexual dysfunction F15.981
      sleep disorder F15.982
      unspecified disorder F15.99
      withdrawal F15.93
    harmful — *see* Abuse, drug, stimulant NEC
    in remission F15.91
  tobacco Z72.0
    with dependence — *see* Dependence, drug, nicotine
  volatile solvents — *see also* Use, inhalant F18.90
    harmful — *see* Abuse, drug, inhalant
Usher-Senear disease or syndrome L10.4
Uta B55.1
Uteromegaly N85.2
Uterovaginal — *see* condition
Uterovesical — *see* condition
Uveal — *see* condition
Uveitis (anterior) — *see also* Iridocyclitis
  acute — *see* Iridocyclitis, acute
  chronic — *see* Iridocyclitis, chronic
  due to toxoplasmosis (acquired) B58.09
    congenital P37.1
  granulomatous — *see* Iridocyclitis, chronic
  heterochromic — *see* Cyclitis, Fuchs' heterochromic
  lens-induced — *see* Iridocyclitis, lens-induced
  posterior — *see* Chorioretinitis
  sympathetic H44.13- ☑
  syphilitic (secondary) A51.43
    congenital (early) A50.01
    late A52.71
  tuberculous A18.54
Uveoencephalitis — *see* Inflammation, chorioretinal
Uveokeratitis — *see* Iridocyclitis
Uveoparotitis D86.89
Uvula — *see* condition
Uvulitis (acute) (catarrhal) (chronic) (membranous) (suppurative) (ulcerative) K12.2

V

Vaccination (prophylactic)
  complication or reaction — *see* Complications, vaccination
  delayed Z28.9
  encounter for Z23
  not done — *see* Immunization, not done
  partial — *see also* Underimmunization status
    for COVID-19 Z28.311
Vaccinia (generalized) (localized) T88.1 ☑
  congenital P35.8
  without vaccination B08.011
Vacuum, in sinus (accessory) (nasal) J34.89
Vagabond, vagabondage Z59.00
Vagabond's disease B85.1
Vagina, vaginal — *see* condition
Vaginalitis (tunica) (testis) N49.1
Vaginismus (reflex) N94.2
  functional F52.5
  nonorganic F52.5
  psychogenic F52.5
  secondary N94.2
Vaginitis (acute) (circumscribed) (diffuse) (emphysematous) (nonvenereal) (ulcerative) N76.0
  with ectopic or molar pregnancy O08.0
  amebic A06.82
  atrophic, postmenopausal N95.2
  bacterial N76.0
  blennorrhagic (gonococcal) A54.02
  candidal (acute) B37.31
    chronic (recurrent) B37.32
  chlamydial A56.02
  chronic N76.1
  due to Trichomonas (vaginalis) A59.01
  following ectopic or molar pregnancy O08.0
  gonococcal A54.02
    with abscess (accessory gland) (periurethral) A54.1
  granuloma A58

Vaginitis — *continued*
  in (due to)
    candidiasis (acute) B37.31
      chronic (recurrent) B37.32
    herpesviral (herpes simplex) infection A60.04
    pinworm infection B80 *[N77.1]*
    monilial (acute) B37.31
      chronic (recurrent) B37.32
    mycotic (candidal) (acute) B37.31
      chronic (recurrent) B37.32
  postmenopausal atrophic N95.2
  puerperal (postpartum) O86.13
  senile (atrophic) N95.2
  subacute or chronic N76.1
  syphilitic (early) A51.0
    late A52.76
  trichomonal A59.01
  tuberculous A18.18
Vaginosis — *see* Vaginitis
Vagotonia G52.2
Vagrancy Z59.00
VAIN — *see* Neoplasia, intraepithelial, vagina
Vallecula — *see* condition
Valley fever B38.0
Valsuani's disease — *see* Anemia, obstetric
Valve, valvular (formation) — *see also* condition
  cerebral ventricle (communicating) in situ Z98.2
  cervix, internal os Q51.828
  congenital NEC — *see* Atresia, by site
  ureter (pelvic junction) (vesical orifice) Q62.39
  urethra (congenital) (posterior) Q64.2
Valvulitis (chronic) — *see* Endocarditis
Valvulopathy — *see* Endocarditis
Van Bogaert's leukoencephalopathy (sclerosing) (subacute) A81.1
Van Bogaert-Scherer-Epstein disease or syndrome E75.5
Van Buchem's syndrome M85.2
Van Creveld-von Gierke disease E74.01
Van der Hoeve (-de Kleyn) **syndrome** Q78.0
Van der Woude's syndrome Q38.0
Van Neck's disease or osteochondrosis M91.0
Vanishing lung J44.9
Vapor asphyxia or suffocation T59.9 ☑
  specified agent — *see* Table of Drugs and Chemicals
Variance, lethal ball, prosthetic heart valve T82.09 ☑
Variants, thalassemic D56.8
Variations in hair color L67.1
Varicella B01.9
  with
    complications NEC B01.89
    encephalitis B01.11
    encephalomyelitis B01.11
    meningitis B01.0
    myelitis B01.12
    pneumonia B01.2
  congenital P35.8
Varices — *see* Varix
Varicocele (scrotum) (thrombosed) I86.1
  ovary I86.2
  perineum I86.3
  spermatic cord (ulcerated) I86.1
Varicose
  aneurysm (ruptured) I77.0
  dermatitis — *see* Varix, leg, with, inflammation
  eczema — *see* Varix, leg, with, inflammation
  phlebitis — *see* Varix, with, inflammation
  tumor — *see* Varix
  ulcer (lower limb, any part) — *see also* Varix, leg, with, ulcer
    anus — *see also* Hemorrhoids K64.8
    esophagus — *see* Varix, esophagus
    inflamed or infected — *see* Varix, leg, with ulcer, with inflammation
    nasal septum I86.8
    perineum I86.3
    scrotum I86.1
    specified site NEC I86.8
  vein — *see* Varix
  vessel — *see* Varix, leg
Varicosis, varicosities, varicosity — *see* Varix
Variola (major) (minor) B03
Varioloid B03
Varix (lower limb) I83.90
  with
    bleeding I83.899
    edema I83.899

Varix — *continued*
  with — *continued*
    inflammation I83.10
      with ulcer (venous) I83.209
    pain I83.819
    rupture I83.899
    specified complication NEC I83.899
    stasis dermatitis I83.10
      with ulcer (venous) I83.209
    swelling I83.899
    ulcer I83.009
      with inflammation I83.209
  aneurysmal I77.0
  asymptomatic I83.9- ☑
  bladder I86.2
  broad ligament I86.2
  complicating
    childbirth (lower extremity) O87.4
      anus or rectum O87.2
      genital (vagina, vulva or perineum) O87.8
    pregnancy (lower extremity) O22.0- ☑
      anus or rectum O22.4- ☑
      genital (vagina, vulva or perineum) O22.1- ☑
    puerperium (lower extremity) O87.4
      anus or rectum O87.2
      genital (vagina, vulva, perineum) O87.8
  congenital (any site) Q27.8
  esophagus (idiopathic) (primary) (ulcerated) I85.00
    bleeding I85.01
    congenital Q27.8
    in (due to)
      alcoholic liver disease I85.10
        bleeding I85.11
      cirrhosis of liver I85.10
        bleeding I85.11
      portal hypertension I85.10
        bleeding I85.11
      schistosomiasis I85.10
        bleeding I85.11
      toxic liver disease I85.10
        bleeding I85.11
    secondary I85.10
      bleeding I85.11
  gastric I86.4
  inflamed or infected I83.10
    ulcerated I83.209
  labia (majora) I86.3
  leg (asymptomatic) I83.9- ☑
    with
      edema I83.899
      inflammation I83.10
        with ulcer — *see* Varix, leg, with, ulcer, with inflammation by site
      pain I83.819
      specified complication NEC I83.899
      swelling I83.899
      ulcer I83.0- ☑
        with inflammation I83.2- ☑
        ankle I83.003
          with inflammation I83.203
        calf I83.002
          with inflammation I83.202
        foot NEC I83.005
          with inflammation I83.205
        heel I83.004
          with inflammation I83.204
        lower leg NEC I83.008
          with inflammation I83.208
        midfoot I83.004
          with inflammation I83.204
        thigh I83.001
          with inflammation I83.201
    bilateral (asymptomatic) I83.93
      with
        edema I83.893
        pain I83.813
        specified complication NEC I83.893
        swelling I83.893
        ulcer I83.0- ☑
          with inflammation I83.209
    left (asymptomatic) I83.92
      with
        edema I83.892
        inflammation I83.12
          with ulcer — *see* Varix, leg, with, ulcer, with inflammation by site
        pain I83.812
        specified complication NEC I83.892

Varix — *continued*
  leg — *continued*
    left — *continued*
      with — *continued*
        swelling I83.892
        ulcer I83.029
          with inflammation I83.229
          ankle I83.023
            with inflammation I83.223
          calf I83.022
            with inflammation I83.222
          foot NEC I83.025
            with inflammation I83.225
          heel I83.024
            with inflammation I83.224
          lower leg NEC I83.028
            with inflammation I83.228
          midfoot I83.024
            with inflammation I83.224
          thigh I83.021
            with inflammation I83.221
    right (asymptomatic) I83.91
      with
        edema I83.891
        inflammation I83.11
          with ulcer — *see* Varix, leg, with, ulcer, with inflammation by site
        pain I83.811
        specified complication NEC I83.891
        swelling I83.891
        ulcer I83.019
          with inflammation I83.219
          ankle I83.013
            with inflammation I83.213
          calf I83.012
            with inflammation I83.212
          foot NEC I83.015
            with inflammation I83.215
          heel I83.014
            with inflammation I83.214
          lower leg NEC I83.018
            with inflammation I83.218
          midfoot I83.014
            with inflammation I83.214
          thigh I83.011
            with inflammation I83.211
  nasal septum I86.8
  orbit I86.8
    congenital Q27.8
  ovary I86.2
  papillary I78.1
  pelvis I86.2
  perineum I86.3
  pharynx I86.8
  placenta O43.89- ☑
  renal papilla I86.8
  retina H35.09
  scrotum (ulcerated) I86.1
  sigmoid colon I86.8
  specified site NEC I86.8
  spinal (cord) (vessels) I86.8
  spleen, splenic (vein) (with phlebolith) I86.8
  stomach I86.4
  sublingual I86.0
  ulcerated I83.009
    inflamed or infected I83.209
  uterine ligament I86.2
  vagina I86.8
  vocal cord I86.8
  vulva I86.3
Vas deferens — *see* condition
Vas deferentitis N49.1
Vasa previa O69.4 ☑
  hemorrhage from, affecting newborn P50.0
Vascular — *see also* condition
  loop on optic papilla Q14.2
  spasm I73.9
  spider I78.1
Vascularization, cornea — *see* Neovascularization, cornea
Vasculitis I77.6
  allergic D69.0
  ANCA (antineutrophilic cytoplasmic antibody) associated I77.82
  ANCA (antineutrophilic cytoplasmic antibody) positive I77.82
  antineutrophilic cytoplasmic antibody [ANCA] I77.82
  cryoglobulinemic D89.1

Volvulus — *continued*
  with perforation K56.2
  congenital Q43.8
  duodenum K31.5
  fallopian tube — *see* Torsion, fallopian tube
  oviduct — *see* Torsion, fallopian tube
  stomach (due to absence of gastrocolic ligament)
    K31.89
Vomiting R11.10
  with nausea R11.2
  asphyxia — *see* Foreign body, by site, causing asphyxia,
    gastric contents
  bilious (cause unknown) R11.14
    following gastro-intestinal surgery K91.0
    in newborn P92.01
  blood — *see* Hematemesis
  causing asphyxia, choking, or suffocation — *see* Foreign body, by site
  cyclical, in migraine G43.A0 (*following* G43.7)
    with refractory migraine G43.A1 (*following* G43.7)
    intractable G43.A1 (*following* G43.7)
    not intractable G43.A0 (*following* G43.7)
    psychogenic F50.89
    without refractory migraine G43.A0 (*following* G43.7)
  cyclical syndrome NOS (unrelated to migraine) R11.15
  fecal mater R11.13
  following gastrointestinal surgery K91.0
    psychogenic F50.89
  functional K31.89
  hysterical F50.89
  nervous F50.89
  neurotic F50.89
  newborn NEC P92.09
    bilious P92.01
  periodic R11.10
    psychogenic F50.89
  persistent R11.15
  projectile R11.12
  psychogenic F50.89
  uremic — *see* Uremia
  without nausea R11.11
Vomito negro — *see* Fever, yellow
Von Bezold's abscess — *see* Mastoiditis, acute
Von Economo-Cruchet disease A85.8
Von Eulenburg's disease G71.19
Von Gierke's disease E74.01
Von Hippel (-Lindau) **disease or syndrome** Q85.83
Von Jaksch's anemia or disease D64.89
Von Recklinghausen
  disease (neurofibromatosis) Q85.01
    bones E21.0
Von Schroetter's syndrome I82.890
Von Willebrand (-Jurgens) (-Minot) **disease or syndrome** — *see* Disease, von Willebrand
Von Zumbusch's disease L40.1
Voyeurism F65.3
Vrolik's disease Q78.0
Vulva — *see* condition
Vulvismus N94.2
Vulvitis (acute) (allergic) (atrophic) (hypertrophic) (intertriginous) (senile) N76.2
  with ectopic or molar pregnancy O08.0
  adhesive, congenital Q52.79
  blennorrhagic (gonococcal) A54.02
  candidal (acute) B37.31
    chronic (recurrent) B37.32
  chlamydial A56.02
  due to Haemophilus ducreyi A57
  following ectopic or molar pregnancy O08.0
  gonococcal A54.02
    with abscess (accessory gland) (periurethral) A54.1
  herpesviral A60.04
  leukoplakic N90.4
  monilial (acute) B37.31
    chronic (recurrent) B37.32
  puerperal (postpartum) O86.19
  subacute or chronic N76.3
  syphilitic (early) A51.0
    late A52.76
  trichomonal A59.01
  tuberculous A18.18
Vulvodynia N94.819
  specified NEC N94.818
Vulvorectal — *see* condition
Vulvovaginitis (acute) — *see* Vaginitis

W

Waiting list, person on Z75.1
  for organ transplant Z76.82
  undergoing social agency investigation Z75.2
Waldenström
  hypergammaglobulinemia D89.0
  syndrome or macroglobulinemia C88.0
Waldenström-Kjellberg syndrome D50.1
Walking
  difficulty R26.2
    psychogenic F44.4
  sleep F51.3
    hysterical F44.89
Wall, abdominal — *see* condition
Wallenberg's disease or syndrome G46.3
Wallgren's disease I87.8
Wandering
  gallbladder, congenital Q44.1
  in diseases classified elsewhere Z91.83
  kidney, congenital Q63.8
  organ or site, congenital NEC — *see* Malposition, congenital, by site
  pacemaker (heart) I49.8
  spleen D73.89
War neurosis F48.8
Wart (due to HPV) (filiform) (infectious) (viral) B07.9
  anogenital region (venereal) A63.0
  common B07.8
  external genital organs (venereal) A63.0
  flat B07.8
  Hassal-Henle's (of cornea) H18.49
  Peruvian A44.1
  plantar B07.0
  prosector (tuberculous) A18.4
  seborrheic L82.1
    inflamed L82.0
  senile (seborrheic) L82.1
    inflamed L82.0
  tuberculous A18.4
  venereal A63.0
Warthin's tumor — *see* Neoplasm, salivary gland, benign
Wassilieff's disease A27.0
Wasting
  disease R64
    due to malnutrition E43
      with marasmus E41
  extreme (due to malnutrition) E43
    with marasmus E41
  muscle NEC — *see* Atrophy, muscle
Water
  clefts (senile cataract) — *see* Cataract, senile, incipient
  deprivation of T73.1 ☑
  intoxication E87.79
  itch B76.9
  lack of T73.1 ☑
    safe drinking Z58.6
  loading E87.70
  on
    brain — *see* Hydrocephalus
    chest J94.8
  poisoning E87.79
Waterbrash R12
Waterhouse (-Friderichsen) **syndrome or disease** (meningococcal) A39.1
Water-losing nephritis N25.89
Watermelon stomach K31.819
  with hemorrhage K31.811
  without hemorrhage K31.819
Watsoniasis B66.8
Wax in ear — *see* Impaction, cerumen
Weak, weakening, weakness (generalized) R53.1
  arches (acquired) — *see also* Deformity, limb, flat foot
  bladder (sphincter) R32
  facial R29.810
    following
      cerebrovascular disease I69.992
        cerebral infarction I69.392
        intracerebral hemorrhage I69.192
        nontraumatic intracranial hemorrhage NEC I69.292
        specified disease NEC I69.892
        stroke I69.392
        subarachnoid hemorrhage I69.092
  foot (double) — *see also* Weak, arches
  heart, cardiac — *see* Failure, heart
  mind F70

Weak, weakening, weakness — *continued*
  muscle M62.81
  myocardium — *see* Failure, heart
  newborn P96.89
  pelvic fundus N81.89
  pubocervical tissue N81.82
  rectovaginal tissue N81.83
  senile R54
  urinary stream R39.12
  valvular — *see* Endocarditis
Wear, worn (with normal or routine use)
  articular bearing surface of internal joint prosthesis — *see* Complications, joint prosthesis, mechanical, wear of articular bearing surfaces, by site
  device, implant or graft — *see* Complications, by site, mechanical complication
  tooth, teeth (approximal) (hard tissues) (interproximal) (occlusal) K03.0
Weather, weathered
  effects of
    cold T69.9 ☑
      specified effect NEC T69.8 ☑
    hot — *see* Heat
  skin L57.8
Weaver's syndrome Q87.3
Web, webbed (congenital)
  duodenal Q43.8
  esophagus Q39.4
  fingers Q70.1- ☑
  larynx (glottic) (subglottic) Q31.0
  neck (pterygium colli) Q18.3
  Paterson-Kelly D50.1
  popliteal syndrome Q87.89
  toes Q70.3- ☑
Weber-Christian disease M35.6
Weber-Cockayne syndrome (epidermolysis bullosa) Q81.8
Weber-Gubler syndrome G46.3
Weber-Leyden syndrome G46.3
Weber-Osler syndrome I78.0
Weber's paralysis or syndrome G46.3
Wedge-shaped or wedging vertebra — *see* Collapse, vertebra NEC
Wegener's granulomatosis or syndrome M31.30
  with
    kidney involvement M31.31
    lung involvement M31.30
      with kidney involvement M31.31
Wegner's disease A50.02
Weight
  1000-2499 grams at birth (low) — *see* Low, birthweight
  999 grams or less at birth (extremely low) — *see* Low, birthweight, extreme
  and length below 10th percentile for gestational age P05.1- ☑
  below but length above 10th percentile for gestational age P05.0- ☑
  gain (abnormal) (excessive) R63.5
    in pregnancy — *see* Pregnancy, complicated by, excessive weight gain
    low — *see* Pregnancy, complicated by, insufficient, weight gain
  loss (abnormal) (cause unknown) R63.4
Weightlessness (effect of) T75.82 ☑
Weil (I)-**Marchesani syndrome** Q87.19
Weil's disease A27.0
Weingarten's syndrome J82.89
Weir Mitchell's disease I73.81
Weiss-Baker syndrome G90.09
Wells' disease L98.3
Wen — *see* Cyst, sebaceous
Wenckebach's block or phenomenon I44.1
Werdnig-Hoffmann syndrome (muscular atrophy) G12.0
Werlhof's disease D69.3
Wermer's disease or syndrome E31.21
Werner-His disease A79.0
Werner's disease or syndrome E34.8
Wernicke-Korsakoff's syndrome or psychosis (alcoholic) F10.96
  with dependence F10.26
  drug-induced
    due to drug abuse — *see* Abuse, drug, by type, with amnestic disorder
    due to drug dependence — *see* Dependence, drug, by type, with amnestic disorder
  nonalcoholic F04

Wernicke-Posadas disease B38.9
Wernicke's
  developmental aphasia F80.2
  disease or syndrome E51.2
  encephalopathy E51.2
  polioencephalitis, superior E51.2
West African fever B50.8
Westphal-Strümpell syndrome E83.01
West's syndrome — *see* Epilepsy, spasms
Wet
  feet, tropical (maceration) (syndrome) — *see* Immersion, foot
  lung (syndrome), newborn P22.1
Wharton's duct — *see* condition
Wheal — *see* Urticaria
Wheezing R06.2
Whiplash injury S13.4 ☑
Whipple's disease — *see also* subcategory M14.8- K90.81
Whipworm (disease) (infection) (infestation) B79
Whistling face Q87.0
White — *see also* condition
  kidney, small N03.9
  leg, puerperal, postpartum, childbirth O87.1
  mouth B37.0
  patches of mouth K13.29
  spot lesions, teeth
    chewing surface K02.51
    pit and fissure surface K02.51
    smooth surface K02.61
Whitehead L70.0
Whitlow — *see also* Cellulitis, digit
  with lymphangitis — *see* Lymphangitis, acute, digit
  herpesviral B00.89
Whitmore's disease or fever — *see* Melioidosis
Whooping cough A37.90
  with pneumonia A37.91
    due to Bordetella
      bronchiseptica A37.81
      parapertussis A37.11
      pertussis A37.01
      specified organism NEC A37.81
  due to
    Bordetella
      bronchiseptica A37.80
        with pneumonia A37.81
      parapertussis A37.10
        with pneumonia A37.11
      pertussis A37.00
        with pneumonia A37.01
      specified NEC A37.80
        with pneumonia A37.81
Wichman's asthma J38.5
Wide cranial sutures, newborn P96.3
Widening aorta — *see* Ectasia, aorta
  with aneurysm — *see* Aneurysm, aorta
Wilkie's disease or syndrome K55.1
Wilkinson-Sneddon disease or syndrome L13.1
Willebrand (-Jürgens) **thrombopathy** — *see* Disease, von Willebrand
Williams syndrome Q93.82
Willige-Hunt disease or syndrome G23.1
Wilms' tumor C64- ☑
Wilson-Mikity syndrome P27.0
Wilson's
  disease or syndrome E83.01
  hepatolenticular degeneration E83.01
  lichen ruber L43.9
Window — *see also* Imperfect, closure
  aorticopulmonary Q21.4
Winter — *see* condition
Wiskott-Aldrich syndrome D82.0
Withdrawal state — *see also* Dependence, drug by type, with withdrawal
  alcohol
    with perceptual disturbances F10.232
      due to alcohol abuse F10.132
      due to alcohol use F10.932
    abuse — *see* Abuse, alcohol, with, withdrawal
    dependence — *see* Dependence, alcohol, with, withdrawal
    use — *see* Use, alcohol, with, withdrawal
    without perceptual disturbances F10.239
      due to alcohol abuse F10.139
      due to alcohol use F10.939
  caffeine F15.93
  cannabis F12.23

Withdrawal state — *continued*
  newborn
    correct therapeutic substance properly administered P96.2
    infant of dependent mother P96.1
  therapeutic substance, neonatal P96.2
Witts' anemia D50.8
Witzelsucht F07.0
Woakes' ethmoiditis or syndrome J33.1
Wolff-Hirschorn syndrome Q93.3
Wolff-Parkinson-White syndrome I45.6
Wolhynian fever A79.0
Wolman's disease E75.5
Wood lung or pneumonitis J67.8
Woolly, wooly hair (congenital) (nevus) Q84.1
Woolsorter's disease A22.1
Word
  blindness (congenital) (developmental) F81.0
  deafness (congenital) (developmental) H93.25
Worm(s) (infection) (infestation) — *see also* Infestation, helminth
  guinea B72
  in intestine NEC B82.0
Worm-eaten soles A66.3
Worn out — *see* Exhaustion
  cardiac
    defibrillator (with synchronous cardiac pacemaker) Z45.02
    pacemaker
      battery Z45.010
      lead Z45.018
  device, implant or graft — *see* Complications, by site, mechanical
Worried well Z71.1
Worries R45.82
Wound check Z48.0- ☑
  due to injury — *code to* Injury, by site, using appropriate seventh character for subsequent encounter
Wound, open T14.8-
  abdomen, abdominal
    wall S31.109 ☑
      with penetration into peritoneal cavity S31.609 ☑
      bite — *see* Bite, abdomen, wall
      epigastric region S31.102 ☑
        with penetration into peritoneal cavity S31.602 ☑
        bite — *see* Bite, abdomen, wall, epigastric region
        laceration — *see* Laceration, abdomen, wall, epigastric region
        puncture — *see* Puncture, abdomen, wall, epigastric region
      laceration — *see* Laceration, abdomen, wall
      left
        lower quadrant S31.104 ☑
          with penetration into peritoneal cavity S31.604 ☑
          bite — *see* Bite, abdomen, wall, left, lower quadrant
          laceration — *see* Laceration, abdomen, wall, left, lower quadrant
          puncture — *see* Puncture, abdomen, wall, left, lower quadrant
        upper quadrant S31.101 ☑
          with penetration into peritoneal cavity S31.601 ☑
          bite — *see* Bite, abdomen, wall, left, upper quadrant
          laceration — *see* Laceration, abdomen, wall, left, upper quadrant
          puncture — *see* Puncture, abdomen, wall, left, upper quadrant
      periumbilic region S31.105 ☑
        with penetration into peritoneal cavity S31.605 ☑
        bite — *see* Bite, abdomen, wall, periumbilic region
        laceration — *see* Laceration, abdomen, wall, periumbilic region
        puncture — *see* Puncture, abdomen, wall, periumbilic region
      puncture — *see* Puncture, abdomen, wall
      right
        lower quadrant S31.103 ☑
          with penetration into peritoneal cavity S31.603 ☑

Wound, open — *continued*
  abdomen, abdominal — *continued*
    wall — *continued*
      right — *continued*
        lower quadrant — *continued*
          bite — *see* Bite, abdomen, wall, right, lower quadrant
          laceration — *see* Laceration, abdomen, wall, right, lower quadrant
          puncture — *see* Puncture, abdomen, wall, right, lower quadrant
        upper quadrant S31.100 ☑
          with penetration into peritoneal cavity S31.600 ☑
          bite — *see* Bite, abdomen, wall, right, upper quadrant
          laceration — *see* Laceration, abdomen, wall, right, upper quadrant
          puncture — *see* Puncture, abdomen, wall, right, upper quadrant
  alveolar (process) — *see* Wound, open, oral cavity
  ankle S91.00- ☑
    bite — *see* Bite, ankle
    laceration — *see* Laceration, ankle
    puncture — *see* Puncture, ankle
  antecubital space — *see* Wound, open, elbow
  anterior chamber, eye — *see* Wound, open, ocular
  anus S31.839 ☑
    bite S31.835 ☑
    laceration — *see* Laceration, anus
    puncture — *see* Puncture, anus
  arm (upper) S41.10- ☑
    with amputation — *see* Amputation, traumatic, arm
    bite — *see* Bite, arm
    forearm — *see* Wound, open, forearm
    laceration — *see* Laceration, arm
    puncture — *see* Puncture, arm
  auditory canal (external) (meatus) — *see* Wound, open, ear
  auricle, ear — *see* Wound, open, ear
  axilla — *see* Wound, open, arm
  back — *see also* Wound, open, thorax, back
    lower S31.000 ☑
      with penetration into retroperitoneal space S31.001 ☑
      bite — *see* Bite, back, lower
      laceration — *see* Laceration, back, lower
      puncture — *see* Puncture, back, lower
  bite — *see* Bite
  blood vessel — *see* Injury, blood vessel
  breast S21.00- ☑
    with amputation — *see* Amputation, traumatic, breast
    bite — *see* Bite, breast
    laceration — *see* Laceration, breast
    puncture — *see* Puncture, breast
  buttock S31.809 ☑
    bite — *see* Bite, buttock
    laceration — *see* Laceration, buttock
    left S31.829 ☑
    puncture — *see* Puncture, buttock
    right S31.819 ☑
  calf — *see* Wound, open, leg
  canaliculus lacrimalis — *see* Wound, open, eyelid
  canthus, eye — *see* Wound, open, eyelid
  cervical esophagus S11.20 ☑
    bite S11.25 ☑
    laceration — *see* Laceration, esophagus, traumatic, cervical
    puncture — *see* Puncture, cervical esophagus
  cheek (external) S01.40- ☑
    bite — *see* Bite, cheek
    internal — *see* Wound, open, oral cavity
    laceration — *see* Laceration, cheek
    puncture — *see* Puncture, cheek
  chest wall — *see* Wound, open, thorax
  chin — *see* Wound, open, head, specified site NEC
  choroid — *see* Wound, open, ocular
  ciliary body (eye) — *see* Wound, open, ocular
  clitoris S31.40 ☑
    with amputation — *see* Amputation, traumatic, clitoris
    bite S31.45 ☑
    laceration — *see* Laceration, vulva
    puncture — *see* Puncture, vulva
  conjunctiva — *see* Wound, open, ocular

Wound, open — *continued*

cornea — *see* Wound, open, ocular
costal region — *see* Wound, open, thorax
Descemet's membrane — *see* Wound, open, ocular
digit(s)
  foot — *see* Wound, open, toe
  hand — *see* Wound, open, finger
ear (canal) (external) S01.30- ☑
  with amputation — *see* Amputation, traumatic, ear
  bite — *see* Bite, ear
  drum S09.2- ☑
  laceration — *see* Laceration, ear
  puncture — *see* Puncture, ear
elbow S51.00- ☑
  bite — *see* Bite, elbow
  laceration — *see* Laceration, elbow
  puncture — *see* Puncture, elbow
epididymis — *see* Wound, open, testis
epigastric region S31.102 ☑
  with penetration into peritoneal cavity S31.602 ☑
  bite — *see* Bite, abdomen, wall, epigastric region
  laceration — *see* Laceration, abdomen, wall, epigastric region
  puncture — *see* Puncture, abdomen, wall, epigastric region
epiglottis — *see* Wound, open, neck, specified site NEC
esophagus (thoracic) S27.819 ☑
  cervical — *see* Wound, open, cervical esophagus
  laceration S27.813 ☑
  specified type NEC S27.818 ☑
eye — *see* Wound, open, ocular
eyeball — *see* Wound, open, ocular
eyebrow — *see* Wound, open, eyelid
eyelid S01.10- ☑
  bite — *see* Bite, eyelid
  laceration — *see* Laceration, eyelid
  puncture — *see* Puncture, eyelid
face NEC — *see* Wound, open, head, specified site NEC
finger(s) S61.209 ☑
  with
    amputation — *see* Amputation, traumatic, finger
    damage to nail S61.309 ☑
  bite — *see* Bite, finger
  index S61.208 ☑
    with
      damage to nail S61.308 ☑
    left S61.201 ☑
      with
        damage to nail S61.301 ☑
    right S61.200 ☑
      with
        damage to nail S61.300 ☑
  laceration — *see* Laceration, finger
  little S61.208 ☑
    with
      damage to nail S61.308 ☑
    left S61.207 ☑
      with damage to nail S61.307 ☑
    right S61.206 ☑
      with damage to nail S61.306 ☑
  middle S61.208 ☑
    with
      damage to nail S61.308 ☑
    left S61.203 ☑
      with damage to nail S61.303 ☑
    right S61.202 ☑
      with damage to nail S61.302 ☑
  puncture — *see* Puncture, finger
  ring S61.208 ☑
    with
      damage to nail S61.308 ☑
    left S61.205 ☑
      with damage to nail S61.305 ☑
    right S61.204 ☑
      with damage to nail S61.304 ☑
flank — *see* Wound, open, abdomen, wall
foot (except toe(s) alone) S91.30- ☑
  with amputation — *see* Amputation, traumatic, foot
  bite — *see* Bite, foot
  laceration — *see* Laceration, foot
  puncture — *see* Puncture, foot
  toe — *see* Wound, open, toe
forearm S51.80- ☑
  with
    amputation — *see* Amputation, traumatic, forearm

Wound, open — *continued*

forearm — *continued*
  bite — *see* Bite, forearm
  elbow only — *see* Wound, open, elbow
  laceration — *see* Laceration, forearm
  puncture — *see* Puncture, forearm
forehead — *see* Wound, open, head, specified site NEC
genital organs, external
  with amputation — *see* Amputation, traumatic, genital organs
  bite — *see* Bite, genital organ
  female S31.502 ☑
    vagina S31.40 ☑
    vulva S31.40 ☑
  laceration — *see* Laceration, genital organ
  male S31.501 ☑
    penis S31.20 ☑
    scrotum S31.30 ☑
    testes S31.30 ☑
  puncture — *see* Puncture, genital organ
globe (eye) — *see* Wound, open, ocular
groin — *see* Wound, open, abdomen, wall
gum — *see* Wound, open, oral cavity
hand S61.40- ☑
  with
    amputation — *see* Amputation, traumatic, hand
  bite — *see* Bite, hand
  finger(s) — *see* Wound, open, finger
  laceration — *see* Laceration, hand
  puncture — *see* Puncture, hand
  thumb — *see* Wound, open, thumb
head S01.90 ☑
  bite — *see* Bite, head
  cheek — *see* Wound, open, cheek
  ear — *see* Wound, open, ear
  eyelid — *see* Wound, open, eyelid
  laceration — *see* Laceration, head
  lip — *see* Wound, open, lip
  nose S01.20 ☑
  oral cavity — *see* Wound, open, oral cavity
  puncture — *see* Puncture, head
  scalp — *see* Wound, open, scalp
  specified site NEC S01.80 ☑
  temporomandibular area — *see* Wound, open, cheek
heel — *see* Wound, open, foot
hip S71.00- ☑
  with amputation — *see* Amputation, traumatic, hip
  bite — *see* Bite, hip
  laceration — *see* Laceration, hip
  puncture — *see* Puncture, hip
hymen S31.40 ☑
  bite — *see* Bite, vulva
  laceration — *see* Laceration, vagina
  puncture — *see* Puncture, vagina
hypochondrium S31.109 ☑
  bite — *see* Bite, hypochondrium
  laceration — *see* Laceration, hypochondrium
  puncture — *see* Puncture, hypochondrium
hypogastric region S31.109 ☑
  bite — *see* Bite, hypogastric region
  laceration — *see* Laceration, hypogastric region
  puncture — *see* Puncture, hypogastric region
iliac (region) — *see* Wound, open, inguinal region
inguinal region S31.109 ☑
  bite — *see* Bite, abdomen, wall, lower quadrant
  laceration — *see* Laceration, inguinal region
  puncture — *see* Puncture, inguinal region
instep — *see* Wound, open, foot
interscapular region — *see* Wound, open, thorax, back
intraocular — *see* Wound, open, ocular
iris — *see* Wound, open, ocular
jaw — *see* Wound, open, head, specified site NEC
knee S81.00- ☑
  bite — *see* Bite, knee
  laceration — *see* Laceration, knee
  puncture — *see* Puncture, knee
labium (majus) (minus) — *see* Wound, open, vulva
laceration — *see* Laceration, by site
lacrimal duct — *see* Wound, open, eyelid
larynx S11.019 ☑
  bite — *see* Bite, larynx
  laceration — *see* Laceration, larynx
  puncture — *see* Puncture, larynx
left
  lower quadrant S31.104 ☑

Wound, open — *continued*

left — *continued*
  lower quadrant — *continued*
    with penetration into peritoneal cavity S31.604 ☑
    bite — *see* Bite, abdomen, wall, left, lower quadrant
    laceration — *see* Laceration, abdomen, wall, left, lower quadrant
    puncture — *see* Puncture, abdomen, wall, left, lower quadrant
  upper quadrant S31.101 ☑
    with penetration into peritoneal cavity S31.601 ☑
    bite — *see* Bite, abdomen, wall, left, upper quadrant
    laceration — *see* Laceration, abdomen, wall, left, upper quadrant
    puncture — *see* Puncture, abdomen, wall, left, upper quadrant
leg (lower) S81.80- ☑
  with amputation — *see* Amputation, traumatic, leg
  ankle — *see* Wound, open, ankle
  bite — *see* Bite, leg
  foot — *see* Wound, open, foot
  knee — *see* Wound, open, knee
  laceration — *see* Laceration, leg
  puncture — *see* Puncture, leg
  toe — *see* Wound, open, toe
  upper — *see* Wound, open, thigh
lip S01.501 ☑
  bite — *see* Bite, lip
  laceration — *see* Laceration, lip
  puncture — *see* Puncture, lip
loin S31.109 ☑
  bite — *see* Bite, abdomen, wall
  laceration — *see* Laceration, loin
  puncture — *see* Puncture, loin
lower back — *see* Wound, open, back, lower
lumbar region — *see* Wound, open, back, lower
malar region — *see* Wound, open, head, specified site NEC
mammary — *see* Wound, open, breast
mastoid region — *see* Wound, open, head, specified site NEC
mouth — *see* Wound, open, oral cavity
nail
  finger — *see* Wound, open, finger, with damage to nail
  toe — *see* Wound, open, toe, with damage to nail
nape (neck) — *see* Wound, open, neck
nasal (septum) (sinus) — *see* Wound, open, nose
nasopharynx — *see* Wound, open, head, specified site NEC
neck S11.90 ☑
  bite — *see* Bite, neck
  involving
    cervical esophagus S11.20 ☑
    larynx — *see* Wound, open, larynx
    pharynx S11.20 ☑
    thyroid S11.10 ☑
    trachea (cervical) S11.029 ☑
      bite — *see* Bite, trachea
      laceration S11.021 ☑
        with foreign body S11.022 ☑
      puncture S11.023 ☑
        with foreign body S11.024 ☑
  laceration — *see* Laceration, neck
  puncture — *see* Puncture, neck
  specified site NEC S11.80 ☑
    specified type NEC S11.89 ☑
nose (septum) (sinus) S01.20 ☑
  with amputation — *see* Amputation, traumatic, nose
  bite — *see* Bite, nose
  laceration — *see* Laceration, nose
  puncture — *see* Puncture, nose
ocular S05.90 ☑
  avulsion (traumatic enucleation) S05.7- ☑
  eyeball S05.6- ☑
    with foreign body S05.5- ☑
  eyelid — *see* Wound, open, eyelid
  laceration and rupture S05.3- ☑
    with prolapse or loss of intraocular tissue S05.2- ☑

Wound, open — *continued*

ocular — *continued*
  orbit (penetrating) (with or without foreign body) S05.4- ☑
  periocular area — *see* Wound, open, eyelid
  specified NEC S05.8X- ☑
oral cavity S01.502 ☑
  bite S01.552 ☑
  laceration — *see* Laceration, oral cavity
  puncture — *see* Puncture, oral cavity
orbit — *see* Wound, open, ocular, orbit
palate — *see* Wound, open, oral cavity
palm — *see* Wound, open, hand
pelvis, pelvic — *see also* Wound, open, back, lower
  girdle — *see* Wound, open, hip
penetrating — *see* Puncture, by site
penis S31.20 ☑
  with amputation — *see* Amputation, traumatic, penis
  bite S31.25 ☑
  laceration — *see* Laceration, penis
  puncture — *see* Puncture, penis
perineum
  bite — *see* Bite, perineum
  female S31.502 ☑
  laceration — *see* Laceration, perineum
  male S31.501 ☑
  puncture — *see* Puncture, perineum
periocular area (with or without lacrimal passages) — *see* Wound, open, eyelid
periumbilic region S31.105 ☑
  with penetration into peritoneal cavity S31.605 ☑
  bite — *see* Bite, abdomen, wall, periumbilic region
  laceration — *see* Laceration, abdomen, wall, periumbilic region
  puncture — *see* Puncture, abdomen, wall, periumbilic region
phalanges
  finger — *see* Wound, open, finger
  toe — *see* Wound, open, toe
pharynx S11.20 ☑
pinna — *see* Wound, open, ear
popliteal space — *see* Wound, open, knee
prepuce — *see* Wound, open, penis
pubic region — *see* Wound, open, back, lower
pudendum — *see* Wound, open, genital organs, external
puncture wound — *see* Puncture
rectovaginal septum — *see* Wound, open, vagina
right
  lower quadrant S31.103 ☑
   with penetration into peritoneal cavity S31.603 ☑
   bite — *see* Bite, abdomen, wall, right, lower quadrant
   laceration — *see* Laceration, abdomen, wall, right, lower quadrant
   puncture — *see* Puncture, abdomen, wall, right, lower quadrant
  upper quadrant S31.100 ☑
   with penetration into peritoneal cavity S31.600 ☑
   bite — *see* Bite, abdomen, wall, right, upper quadrant
   laceration — *see* Laceration, abdomen, wall, right, upper quadrant
   puncture — *see* Puncture, abdomen, wall, right, upper quadrant
sacral region — *see* Wound, open, back, lower
sacroiliac region — *see* Wound, open, back, lower
salivary gland — *see* Wound, open, oral cavity
scalp S01.00 ☑
  bite S01.05 ☑
  laceration — *see* Laceration, scalp
  puncture — *see* Puncture, scalp
scalpel, newborn (birth injury) P15.8
scapular region — *see* Wound, open, shoulder
sclera — *see* Wound, open, ocular
scrotum S31.30 ☑
  with amputation — *see* Amputation, traumatic, scrotum
  bite S31.35 ☑
  laceration — *see* Laceration, scrotum
  puncture — *see* Puncture, scrotum
shin — *see* Wound, open, leg
shoulder S41.00- ☑

Wound, open — *continued*

shoulder — *continued*
  with amputation — *see* Amputation, traumatic, arm
  bite — *see* Bite, shoulder
  laceration — *see* Laceration, shoulder
  puncture — *see* Puncture, shoulder
skin NOS T14.8 ☑
spermatic cord — *see* Wound, open, testis
sternal region — *see* Wound, open, thorax, front wall
submaxillary region — *see* Wound, open, head, specified site NEC
submental region — *see* Wound, open, head, specified site NEC
subungual
  finger(s) — *see* Wound, open, finger
  toe(s) — *see* Wound, open, toe
supraclavicular region — *see* Wound, open, neck, specified site NEC
temple, temporal region — *see* Wound, open, head, specified site NEC
temporomandibular area — *see* Wound, open, cheek
testis S31.30 ☑
  with amputation — *see* Amputation, traumatic, testes
  bite S31.35 ☑
  laceration — *see* Laceration, testis
  puncture — *see* Puncture, testis
thigh S71.10- ☑
  with amputation — *see* Amputation, traumatic, hip
  bite — *see* Bite, thigh
  laceration — *see* Laceration, thigh
  puncture — *see* Puncture, thigh
thorax, thoracic (wall) S21.90 ☑
  back S21.20- ☑
   with penetration S21.40 ☑
  bite — *see* Bite, thorax
  breast — *see* Wound, open, breast
  front S21.10- ☑
   with penetration S21.30 ☑
  laceration — *see* Laceration, thorax
  puncture — *see* Puncture, thorax
throat — *see* Wound, open, neck
thumb S61.009 ☑
  with
   amputation — *see* Amputation, traumatic, thumb
   damage to nail S61.109 ☑
  bite — *see* Bite, thumb
  laceration — *see* Laceration, thumb
  left S61.002 ☑
   with
    damage to nail S61.102 ☑
   puncture — *see* Puncture, thumb
  right S61.001 ☑
   with
    damage to nail S61.101 ☑
thyroid (gland) — *see* Wound, open, neck, thyroid
toe(s) S91.109 ☑
  with
   amputation — *see* Amputation, traumatic, toe
   damage to nail S91.209 ☑
  bite — *see* Bite, toe
  great S91.103 ☑
   with
    damage to nail S91.203 ☑
   left S91.102 ☑
    with
     damage to nail S91.202 ☑
   right S91.101 ☑
    with
     damage to nail S91.201 ☑
  laceration — *see* Laceration, toe
  lesser S91.106 ☑
   with
    damage to nail S91.206 ☑
   left S91.105 ☑
    with
     damage to nail S91.205 ☑
   right S91.104 ☑
    with
     damage to nail S91.204 ☑
  puncture — *see* Puncture, toe
tongue — *see* Wound, open, oral cavity
trachea (cervical region) — *see* Wound, open, neck, trachea
tunica vaginalis — *see* Wound, open, testis

Wound, open — *continued*

tympanum, tympanic membrane S09.2- ☑
  laceration — *see* Laceration, ear, drum
  puncture — *see* Puncture, tympanum
umbilical region — *see* Wound, open, abdomen, wall, periumbilic region
uvula — *see* Wound, open, oral cavity
vagina S31.40 ☑
  bite S31.45 ☑
  laceration — *see* Laceration, vagina
  puncture — *see* Puncture, vagina
vitreous (humor) — *see* Wound, open, ocular
vocal cord S11.039 ☑
  bite — *see* Bite, vocal cord
  laceration S11.031 ☑
   with foreign body S11.032 ☑
  puncture S11.033 ☑
   with foreign body S11.034 ☑
vulva S31.40 ☑
  with amputation — *see* Amputation, traumatic, vulva
  bite S31.45 ☑
  laceration — *see* Laceration, vulva
  puncture — *see* Puncture, vulva
wrist S61.50- ☑
  bite — *see* Bite, wrist
  laceration — *see* Laceration, wrist
  puncture — *see* Puncture, wrist
Wound, superficial — *see* Injury — *see also* specified injury type
Wright's syndrome G54.0
Wrist — *see* condition
Wrong drug (by accident) (given in error) — *see* Table of Drugs and Chemicals, by drug, poisoning
Wry neck — *see* Torticollis
Wuchereria (bancrofti) **infestation** B74.0
Wuchereriasis B74.0
Wuchernde Struma Langhans C73

X

Xanthelasma (eyelid) (palpebrarum) H02.60
  left H02.66
   lower H02.65
   upper H02.64
  right H02.63
   lower H02.62
   upper H02.61
Xanthelasmatosis (essential) E78.2
Xanthinuria, hereditary E79.8
Xanthoastrocytoma
  specified site — *see* Neoplasm, malignant, by site
  unspecified site C71.9
Xanthofibroma — *see* Neoplasm, connective tissue, benign
Xanthogranuloma D76.3
Xanthoma(s), xanthomatosis (primary) (familial) (hereditary) E75.5
  with
   hyperlipoproteinemia
    Type I E78.3
    Type III E78.2
    Type IV E78.1
    Type V E78.3
  bone (generalisata) C96.5
  cerebrotendinous E75.5
  cutaneotendinous E75.5
  disseminatum (skin) E78.2
  eruptive E78.2
  hypercholesterinemic E78.00
  hypercholesterolemic E78.00
  hyperlipidemic E78.5
  joint E75.5
  multiple (skin) E78.2
  tendon (sheath) E75.5
  tuberosum E78.2
  tuberous E78.2
  tubo-eruptive E78.2
  verrucous, oral mucosa K13.4
Xanthosis R23.8
Xenophobia F40.10
Xeroderma — *see also* Ichthyosis
  acquired L85.0
  eyelid H01.149
   left H01.146
    lower H01.145
    upper H01.144

Xeroderma — *continued*
  acquired — *continued*
    eyelid — *continued*
      right H01.143
        lower H01.142
        upper H01.141
  pigmentosum Q82.1
  vitamin A deficiency E50.8
Xerophthalmia (vitamin A deficiency) E50.7
  unrelated to vitamin A deficiency — *see* Keratoconjunctivitis
Xerosis
  conjunctiva H11.14- ☑
    with Bitot's spots — *see also* Pigmentation, conjunctiva
      vitamin A deficiency E50.1
      vitamin A deficiency E50.0
  cornea H18.89- ☑
    with ulceration — *see* Ulcer, cornea
      vitamin A deficiency E50.3
      vitamin A deficiency E50.2
  cutis (dry skin) L85.3
  skin L85.3
Xerostomia K11.7
Xiphopagus Q89.4
XO syndrome Q96.9
X-ray (of)
  abnormal findings — *see* Abnormal, diagnostic imaging
  breast (mammogram) (routine) Z12.31
  chest
    routine (as part of a general medical examination) Z00.00
      with abnormal findings Z00.01
  routine (as part of a general medical examination) Z00.00
    with abnormal findings Z00.01
XXXXY syndrome Q98.1
XXY syndrome Q98.0

Y

Yaba pox (virus disease) B08.72
Yatapoxvirus B08.70
  specified NEC B08.79
Yawning R06.89
  psychogenic F45.8
Yaws A66.9
  bone lesions A66.6
  butter A66.1
  chancre A66.0
  cutaneous, less than five years after infection A66.2
  early (cutaneous) (macular) (maculopapular) (micropapular) (papular) A66.2
    frambeside A66.2
    skin lesions NEC A66.2
  eyelid A66.2
  ganglion A66.6
  gangosis, gangosa A66.5
  gumma, gummata A66.4
    bone A66.6
  gummatous
    frambeside A66.4
    osteitis A66.6
    periostitis A66.6
  hydrarthrosis — *see also* subcategory M14.8- A66.6
  hyperkeratosis (early) (late) A66.3
  initial lesions A66.0
  joint lesions — *see also* subcategory M14.8- A66.6
  juxta-articular nodules A66.7
  late nodular (ulcerated) A66.4
  latent (without clinical manifestations) (with positive serology) A66.8
  mother A66.0
  mucosal A66.7
  multiple papillomata A66.1
  nodular, late (ulcerated) A66.4

Yaws — *continued*
  osteitis A66.6
  papilloma, plantar or palmar A66.1
  periostitis (hypertrophic) A66.6
  specified NEC A66.7
  ulcers A66.4
  wet crab A66.1
Yeast infection — *see also* Candidiasis B37.9
Yellow
  atrophy (liver) — *see* Failure, hepatic
  fever — *see* Fever, yellow
  jack — *see* Fever, yellow
  jaundice — *see* Jaundice
  nail syndrome L60.5
Yersiniosis — *see also* Infection, Yersinia
  extraintestinal A28.2
  intestinal A04.6

Z

Zahorsky's syndrome (herpangina) B08.5
Zellweger's syndrome E71.510
Zenker's diverticulum (esophagus) K22.5
Ziehen-Oppenheim disease G24.1
Zieve's syndrome K70.0
Zika NOS A92.5
  congenital P35.4
Zinc
  deficiency, dietary E60
  metabolism disorder E83.2
Zollinger-Ellison syndrome E16.4
Zona — *see* Herpes, zoster
Zoophobia F40.218
Zoster (herpes) — *see* Herpes, zoster
Zygomycosis B46.9
  specified NEC B46.8
Zymotic — *see* condition

Neoplasm Table

Neoplasm, abdomen, abdominal — Neoplasm, abdominal — Neoplasm, bile or biliary

> **Note:** The list below gives the code number for neoplasms by anatomical site. For each site there are six possible code numbers according to whether the neoplasm in question is malignant, benign, in situ, of uncertain behavior, or of unspecified nature. The description of the neoplasm will often indicate which of the six columns is appropriate; e.g., malignant melanoma of skin, benign fibroadenoma of breast, carcinoma in situ of cervix uteri. Where such descriptors are not present, the remainder of the Index should be consulted where guidance is given to the appropriate column for each morphological (histological) variety listed; e.g., Mesonephroma – see Neoplasm, malignant; Embryoma — see also Neoplasm, uncertain behavior; Disease, Bowen's – see Neoplasm, skin, in situ. However, the guidance in the Index can be overridden if one of the descriptors mentioned above is present; e.g., malignant adenoma of colon is coded to C18.9 and not to D12.6 as the adjective "malignant" overrides the Index entry "Adenoma — see also Neoplasm, benign, by site." Codes listed with a dash -, following the code have a required additional character for laterality. The tabular list must be reviewed for the complete code.

	Malignant Primary	Malignant Secondary	Ca in situ	Benign	Uncertain Behavior	Unspecified Behavior
Neoplasm, neoplastic	C80.1	C79.9	D09.9	D36.9	D48.9	D49.9
abdomen, abdominal	C76.2	C79.8-☑	D09.8	D36.7	D48.7	D49.89
cavity	C76.2	C79.8-☑	D09.8	D36.7	D48.7	D49.89
organ	C76.2	C79.8-☑	D09.8	D36.7	D48.7	D49.89
viscera	C76.2	C79.8-☑	D09.8	D36.7	D48.7	D49.89
wall — *see also* Neoplasm, abdomen, wall, skin	C44.509	C79.2	D04.5	D23.5	D48.5	D49.2
connective tissue	C49.4	C79.8-☑	—	D21.4	D48.1	D49.2
skin	C44.509	—	—	—	—	—
basal cell carcinoma	C44.519	—	—	—	—	—
specified type NEC	C44.599	—	—	—	—	—
squamous cell carcinoma	C44.529	—	—	—	—	—
abdominopelvic	C76.8	C79.8-☑		D36.7	D48.7	D49.89
accessory sinus — *see* Neoplasm, sinus						
acoustic nerve	C72.4-☑	C79.49		D33.3	D43.3	D49.7
adenoid (pharynx) (tissue)	C11.1	C79.89	D00.08	D10.6	D37.05	D49.0
adipose tissue — *see also* Neoplasm, connective tissue	C49.4	C79.89	—	D21.9	D48.1	D49.2
adnexa (uterine)	C57.4	C79.89	D07.39	D28.7	D39.8	D49.59
adrenal	C74.9-☑	C79.7-☑	D09.3	D35.0-☑	D44.1-☑	D49.7
capsule	C74.9-☑	C79.7-☑	D09.3	D35.0-☑	D44.1-☑	D49.7
cortex	C74.0-☑	C79.7-☑	D09.3	D35.0-☑	D44.1-☑	D49.7
gland	C74.9-☑	C79.7-☑	D09.3	D35.0-☑	D44.1-☑	D49.7
medulla	C74.1-☑	C79.7-☑	D09.3	D35.0-☑	D44.1-☑	D49.7
ala nasi (external) — *see also* Neoplasm, skin, nose	C44.301	C79.2	D04.39	D23.39	D48.5	D49.2
alimentary canal or tract NEC	C26.9	C78.80	D01.9	D13.9	D37.9	D49.0
alveolar	C03.9	C79.89	D00.03	D10.39	D37.09	D49.0
mucosa	C03.9	C79.89	D00.03	D10.39	D37.09	D49.0
lower	C03.1	C79.89	D00.03	D10.39	D37.09	D49.0
upper	C03.0	C79.89	D00.03	D10.39	D37.09	D49.0
ridge or process	C41.1	C79.51	—	D16.5	D48.0	D49.2
carcinoma	C03.9	C79.8-☑	—	—	—	—
lower	C03.1	C79.8-☑	—	—	—	—
upper	C03.0	C79.8-☑	—	—	—	—
lower	C41.1	C79.51	—	D16.5	D48.0	D49.2
mucosa	C03.9	C79.89	D00.03	D10.39	D37.09	D49.0
lower	C03.1	C79.89	D00.03	D10.39	D37.09	D49.0
upper	C03.0	C79.89	D00.03	D10.39	D37.09	D49.0
upper	C41.0	C79.51	—	D16.4	D48.0	D49.2
sulcus	C06.1	C79.89	D00.02	D10.39	D37.09	D49.0
alveolus	C03.9	C79.89	D00.03	D10.39	D37.09	D49.0
lower	C03.1	C79.89	D00.03	D10.39	D37.09	D49.0
upper	C03.0	C79.89	D00.03	D10.39	D37.09	D49.0
ampulla of Vater	C24.1	C78.89	D01.5	D13.5	D37.6	D49.0
ankle NEC	C76.5-☑	C79.89	D04.7-☑	D36.7	D48.7	D49.89
anorectum, anorectal (junction)	C21.8	C78.5	D01.3	D12.9	D37.8	D49.0
antecubital fossa or space	C76.4-☑	C79.89	D04.6-☑	D36.7	D48.7	D49.89

	Malignant Primary	Malignant Secondary	Ca in situ	Benign	Uncertain Behavior	Unspecified Behavior
Neoplasm, neoplastic — *continued*						
antrum (Highmore) (maxillary)	C31.0	C78.39	D02.3	D14.0	D38.5	D49.1
pyloric	C16.3	C78.89	D00.2	D13.1	D37.1	D49.0
tympanicum	C30.1	C78.39	D02.3	D14.0	D38.5	D49.1
anus, anal	C21.0	C78.5	D01.3	D12.9	D37.8	D49.0
canal	C21.1	C78.5	D01.3	D12.9	D37.8	D49.0
cloacogenic zone	C21.2	C78.5	D01.3	D12.9	D37.8	D49.0
margin — *see also* Neoplasm, anus, skin	C44.500	C79.2	D04.5	D23.5	D48.5	D49.2
overlapping lesion with rectosigmoid junction or rectum	C21.8	—				
skin	C44.500	C79.2	D04.5	D23.5	D48.5	D49.2
basal cell carcinoma	C44.510					
specified type NEC	C44.590					
squamous cell carcinoma	C44.520					
sphincter	C21.1	C78.5	D01.3	D12.9	D37.8	D49.0
aorta (thoracic)	C49.3	C79.89	—	D21.3	D48.1	D49.2
abdominal	C49.4	C79.89	—	D21.4	D48.1	D49.2
aortic body	C75.5	C79.89	—	D35.6	D44.7	D49.7
aponeurosis	C49.9	C79.89	—	D21.9	D48.1	D49.2
palmar	C49.1-☑	C79.89	—	D21.1-☑	D48.1	D49.2
plantar	C49.2-☑	C79.89	—	D21.2-☑	D48.1	D49.2
appendix	C18.1	C78.5	D01.0	D12.1	D37.3	D49.0
arachnoid	C70.9	C79.49	—	D32.9	D42.9	D49.7
cerebral	C70.0	C79.32	—	D32.0	D42.0	D49.7
spinal	C70.1	C79.49	—	D32.1	D42.1	D49.7
areola	C50.0-☑	C79.81	D05-☑	D24-☑	D48.6-☑	D49.3
arm NEC	C76.4-☑	C79.89	D04.6-☑	D36.7	D48.7	D49.89
artery — *see* Neoplasm, connective tissue						
aryepiglottic fold	C13.1	C79.89	D00.08	D10.7	D37.05	D49.0
hypopharyngeal aspect	C13.1	C79.89	D00.08	D10.7	D37.05	D49.0
laryngeal aspect	C32.1	C78.39	D02.0	D14.1	D38.0	D49.1
marginal zone	C13.1	C79.89	D00.08	D10.7	D37.05	D49.0
arytenoid (cartilage)	C32.3	C78.39	D02.0	D14.1	D38.0	D49.1
fold — *see* Neoplasm, aryepiglottic						
associated with transplanted organ	C80.2	—		—		—
atlas	C41.2	C79.51	—	D16.6	D48.0	D49.2
atrium, cardiac	C38.0	C79.89	—	D15.1	D48.7	D49.89
auditory						
canal (external) (skin)	C44.20-☑	C79.2	D04.2-☑	D23.2-☑	D48.5	D49.2
internal	C30.1	C78.39	D02.3	D14.0	D38.5	D49.1
nerve	C72.4-☑	C79.49	—	D33.3	D43.3	D49.7
tube	C30.1	C78.39	D02.3	D14.0	D38.5	D49.1
opening	C11.2	C79.89	D00.08	D10.6	D37.05	D49.0
auricle, ear — *see also* Neoplasm, skin, ear	C44.20-☑	C79.2	D04.2-☑	D23.2-☑	D48.5	D49.2
auricular canal (external) — *see also* Neoplasm, skin, ear	C44.20-☑	C79.2	D04.2-☑	D23.2-☑	D48.5	D49.2
internal	C30.1	C78.39	D02.3	D14.0	D38.5	D49.2
autonomic nerve or nervous system NEC (see Neoplasm, nerve, peripheral)						
axilla, axillary	C76.1	C79.89	D09.8	D36.7	D48.7	D49.89
fold — *see also* Neoplasm, skin, trunk	C44.509	C79.2	D04.5	D23.5	D48.5	D49.2
back NEC	C76.8	C79.89	D04.5	D36.7	D48.7	D49.89
Bartholin's gland	C51.0	C79.82	D07.1	D28.0	D39.8	D49.59
basal ganglia	C71.0	C79.31	—	D33.0	D43.0	D49.6
basis pedunculi	C71.7	C79.31	—	D33.1	D43.1	D49.6
bile or biliary (tract)	C24.9	C78.89	D01.5	D13.5	D37.6	D49.0

☑ **Additional Character Required — Refer to the Tabular List for Character Selection**

Neoplasm, neoplastic	Malignant Primary	Malignant Secondary	Ca in situ	Benign	Uncertain Behavior	Unspecified Behavior
— *continued*						
bile or biliary — *continued*						
canaliculi (biliferi) (intrahepatic)	C22.1	C78.7	D01.5	D13.4	D37.6	D49.0
canals, interlobular	C22.1	C78.89	D01.5	D13.4	D37.6	D49.0
duct or passage (common) (cystic) (extrahepatic)	C24.0	C78.89	D01.5	D13.5	D37.6	D49.0
interlobular	C22.1	C78.89	D01.5	D13.4	D37.6	D49.0
intrahepatic and	C22.1	C78.7	D01.5	D13.4	D37.6	D49.0
extrahepatic	C24.8	C78.89	D01.5	D13.5	D37.6	D49.0
bladder (urinary)	C67.9	C79.11	D09.0	D30.3	D41.4	D49.4
dome	C67.1	C79.11	D09.0	D30.3	D41.4	D49.4
neck	C67.5	C79.11	D09.0	D30.3	D41.4	D49.4
orifice	C67.9	C79.11	D09.0	D30.3	D41.4	D49.4
ureteric	C67.6	C79.11	D09.0	D30.3	D41.4	D49.4
urethral	C67.5	C79.11	D09.0	D30.3	D41.4	D49.4
overlapping lesion	C67.8	—	—	—	—	—
sphincter	C67.8	C79.11	D09.0	D30.3	D41.4	D49.4
trigone	C67.0	C79.11	D09.0	D30.3	D41.4	D49.4
urachus	C67.7	C79.11	D09.0	D30.3	D41.4	D49.4
wall	C67.9	C79.11	D09.0	D30.3	D41.4	D49.4
anterior	C67.3	C79.11	D09.0	D30.3	D41.4	D49.4
lateral	C67.2	C79.11	D09.0	D30.3	D41.4	D49.4
posterior	C67.4	C79.11	D09.0	D30.3	D41.4	D49.4
blood vessel — *see* Neoplasm, connective tissue						
bone (periosteum)	C41.9	C79.51	—	D16.9-	D48.0	D49.2
acetabulum						
ankle	C40.3-☑	C79.51	—	D16.3-☑	—	—
arm NEC	C40.0-☑	C79.51	—	D16.0-☑	—	—
astragalus	C40.3-☑	C79.51	—	D16.3-☑	—	—
atlas	C41.2	C79.51	—	D16.6	D48.0	D49.2
axis	C41.2	C79.51	—	D16.6	D48.0	D49.2
back NEC	C41.2	C79.51	—	D16.6	D48.0	D49.2
calcaneus	C40.3-☑	C79.51	—	D16.3-☑	—	—
calvarium	C41.0	C79.51	—	D16.4	D48.0	D49.2
carpus (any)	C40.1-☑	C79.51	—	D16.1-☑	—	—
cartilage NEC	C41.9	C79.51	—	D16.9	D48.0	D49.2
clavicle	C41.3	C79.51	—	D16.7	D48.0	D49.2
clivus	C41.0	C79.51	—	D16.4	D48.0	D49.2
coccygeal vertebra	C41.4	C79.51	—	D16.8	D48.0	D49.2
coccyx	C41.4	C79.51	—	D16.8	D48.0	D49.2
costal cartilage	C41.3	C79.51	—	D16.7	D48.0	D49.2
costovertebral joint	C41.3	C79.51	—	D16.7	D48.0	D49.2
cranial	C41.0	C79.51	—	D16.4	D48.0	D49.2
cuboid	C40.3-☑	C79.51	—	D16.3-☑	—	—
cuneiform	C41.9	C79.51	—	D16.9	D48.0	D49.2
elbow	C40.0-☑	C79.51	—	D16.0-☑	—	—
ethmoid (labyrinth)	C41.0	C79.51	—	D16.4	D48.0	D49.2
face	C41.0	C79.51	—	D16.4	D48.0	D49.2
femur (any part)	C40.2-☑	C79.51	—	D16.2-☑	—	—
fibula (any part)	C40.2-☑	C79.51	—	D16.2-☑	—	—
finger (any)	C40.1-☑	C79.51	—	D16.1-☑	—	—
foot	C40.3-☑	C79.51	—	D16.3-☑	—	—
forearm	C40.0-☑	C79.51	—	D16.0-☑	—	—
frontal	C41.0	C79.51	—	D16.4	D48.0	D49.2
hand	C40.1-☑	C79.51	—	D16.1-☑	—	—
heel	C40.3-☑	C79.51	—	D16.3-☑	—	—
hip	C41.4	C79.51	—	D16.8	D48.0	D49.2
humerus (any part)	C40.0-☑	C79.51	—	D16.0-☑	—	—
hyoid	C41.0	C79.51	—	D16.4	D48.0	D49.2
ilium	C41.4	C79.51	—	D16.8	D48.0	D49.2
innominate	C41.4	C79.51	—	D16.8	D48.0	D49.2
intervertebral cartilage or disc	C41.2	C79.51	—	D16.6	D48.0	D49.2
ischium	C41.4	C79.51	—	D16.8	D48.0	D49.2
jaw (lower)	C41.1	C79.51	—	D16.5	D48.0	D49.2
knee	C40.2-☑	C79.51	—	D16.2-☑	—	—
leg NEC	C40.2-☑	C79.51	—	D16.2-☑	—	—
limb NEC	C40.9-☑	C79.51	—	D16.9	—	—

Neoplasm, neoplastic	Malignant Primary	Malignant Secondary	Ca in situ	Benign	Uncertain Behavior	Unspecified Behavior
— *continued*						
bone — *continued*						
limb — *continued*						
lower (long bones)	C40.2-☑	C79.51	—	D16.2-☑	—	—
short bones	C40.3-☑	C79.51	—	D16.3-☑	—	—
upper (long bones)	C40.0-☑	C79.51	—	D16.0-☑	—	—
short bones	C40.1-☑	C79.51	—	D16.1-☑	—	—
malar	C41.0	C79.51	—	D16.4	D48.0	D49.2
mandible	C41.1	C79.51	—	D16.5	D48.0	D49.2
marrow NEC (any bone)	C96.9	C79.52	—	—	D47.9	D49.89
mastoid	C41.0	C79.51	—	D16.4	D48.0	D49.2
maxilla, maxillary (superior)	C41.0	C79.51	—	D16.4	D48.0	D49.2
inferior	C41.1	C79.51	—	D16.5	D48.0	D49.2
metacarpus (any)	C40.1-☑	C79.51	—	D16.1-☑	—	—
metatarsus (any)	C40.3-☑	C79.51	—	D16.3-☑	—	—
navicular						
ankle	C40.3-☑	C79.51	—	—	—	—
hand	C40.1-☑	C79.51	—	—	—	—
nose, nasal	C41.0	C79.51	—	D16.4	D48.0	D49.2
occipital	C41.0	C79.51	—	D16.4	D48.0	D49.2
orbit	C41.0	C79.51	—	D16.4	D48.0	D49.2
overlapping sites	C40.8-☑	—	—	—	—	—
parietal	C41.0	C79.51	—	D16.4	D48.0	D49.2
patella	C40.2-☑	C79.51	—	—	—	—
pelvic	C41.4	C79.51	—	D16.8	D48.0	D49.2
phalanges						
foot	C40.3-☑	C79.51	—	—	—	—
hand	C40.1-☑	C79.51	—	—	—	—
pubic	C41.4	C79.51	—	D16.8	D48.0	D49.2
radius (any part)	C40.0-☑	C79.51	—	D16.0-☑	—	—
rib	C41.3	C79.51	—	D16.7	D48.0	D49.2
sacral vertebra	C41.4	C79.51	—	D16.8	D48.0	D49.2
sacrum	C41.4	C79.51	—	D16.8	D48.0	D49.2
scaphoid						
of ankle	C40.3-☑	C79.51	—	—	—	—
of hand	C40.1-☑	C79.51	—	—	—	—
scapula (any part)	C40.0-☑	C79.51	—	D16.0-☑	—	—
sella turcica	C41.0	C79.51	—	D16.4	D48.0	D49.2
shoulder	C40.0-☑	C79.51	—	D16.0-☑	—	—
skull	C41.0	C79.51	—	D16.4	D48.0	D49.2
sphenoid	C41.0	C79.51	—	D16.4	D48.0	D49.2
spine, spinal (column)	C41.2	C79.51	—	D16.6	D48.0	D49.2
coccyx	C41.4	C79.51	—	D16.8	D48.0	D49.2
sacrum	C41.4	C79.51	—	D16.8	D48.0	D49.2
sternum	C41.3	C79.51	—	D16.7	D48.0	D49.2
tarsus (any)	C40.3-☑	C79.51	—	—	—	—
temporal	C41.0	C79.51	—	D16.4	D48.0	D49.2
thumb	C40.1-☑	C79.51	—	—	—	—
tibia (any part)	C40.2-☑	C79.51	—	—	—	—
toe (any)	C40.3-☑	C79.51	—	—	—	—
trapezium	C40.1-☑	C79.51	—	—	—	—
trapezoid	C40.1-☑	C79.51	—	—	—	—
turbinate	C41.0	C79.51	—	D16.4	D48.0	D49.2
ulna (any part)	C40.0-☑	C79.51	—	D16.0-☑	—	—
unciform	C40.1-☑	C79.51	—	—	—	—
vertebra (column)	C41.2	C79.51	—	D16.6	D48.0	D49.2
coccyx	C41.4	C79.51	—	D16.8	D48.0	D49.2
sacrum	C41.4	C79.51	—	D16.8	D48.0	D49.2
vomer	C41.0	C79.51	—	D16.4	D48.0	D49.2
wrist	C40.1-☑	C79.51	—	—	—	—
xiphoid process	C41.3	C79.51	—	D16.7	D48.0	D49.2
zygomatic	C41.0	C79.51	—	D16.4	D48.0	D49.2
book-leaf (mouth) — *ventral surface of tongue and floor of mouth*	C06.89	C79.89	D00.00	D10.39	D37.09	D49.0
bowel — *see* Neoplasm, intestine						
brachial plexus	C47.1-☑	C79.89	—	D36.12	D48.2	D49.2
brain NEC	C71.9	C79.31	—	D33.2	D43.2	D49.6

☑ **Additional Character Required — Refer to the Tabular List for Character Selection**

Neoplasm Table

Neoplasm, brain NEC — Neoplasm, cartilage

Neoplasm, neoplastic	Malignant Primary	Malignant Secondary	Ca in situ	Benign	Uncertain Behavior	Unspecified Behavior
— continued						
brain — continued						
basal ganglia	C71.0	C79.31	—	D33.0	D43.0	D49.6
cerebellopontine angle	C71.6	C79.31	—	D33.1	D43.1	D49.6
cerebellum NOS	C71.6	C79.31	—	D33.1	D43.1	D49.6
cerebrum	C71.0	C79.31	—	D33.0	D43.0	D49.6
choroid plexus	C71.7	C79.31	—	D33.1	D43.1	D49.6
corpus callosum	C71.8	C79.31	—	D33.2	D43.2	D49.6
corpus striatum	C71.0	C79.31	—	D33.0	D43.0	D49.6
cortex (cerebral)	C71.0	C79.31	—	D33.0	D43.0	D49.6
frontal lobe	C71.1	C79.31	—	D33.0	D43.0	D49.6
globus pallidus	C71.0	C79.31	—	D33.0	D43.0	D49.6
hippocampus	C71.2	C79.31	—	D33.0	D43.0	D49.6
hypothalamus	C71.0	C79.31	—	D33.0	D43.0	D49.6
internal capsule	C71.0	C79.31	—	D33.0	D43.0	D49.6
medulla oblongata	C71.7	C79.31	—	D33.1	D43.1	D49.6
meninges	C70.0	C79.32	—	D32.0	D42.0	D49.7
midbrain	C71.7	C79.31	—	D33.1	D43.1	D49.6
occipital lobe	C71.4	C79.31	—	D33.0	D43.0	D49.6
overlapping lesion	C71.8	C79.31	—	—	—	—
parietal lobe	C71.3	C79.31	—	D33.0	D43.0	D49.6
peduncle	C71.7	C79.31	—	D33.1	D43.1	D49.6
pons	C71.7	C79.31	—	D33.1	D43.1	D49.6
stem	C71.7	C79.31	—	D33.1	D43.1	D49.6
tapetum	C71.8	C79.31	—	D33.2	D43.2	D49.6
temporal lobe	C71.2	C79.31	—	D33.0	D43.0	D49.6
thalamus	C71.0	C79.31	—	D33.0	D43.0	D49.6
uncus	C71.2	C79.31	—	D33.0	D43.0	D49.6
ventricle (floor)	C71.5	C79.31	—	D33.0	D43.0	D49.6
fourth	C71.7	C79.31	—	D33.1	D43.1	D49.6
branchial (cleft) (cyst) (vestiges)	C10.4	C79.89	D00.08	D10.5	D37.05	D49.0
breast (connective tissue) (glandular tissue) (soft parts)	C50.9-✓	C79.81	D05.-✓	D24.-✓	D48.6-✓	D49.3
areola	C50.0-✓	C79.81	D05.-✓	D24.-✓	D48.6-✓	D49.3
axillary tail	C50.6-✓	C79.81	D05.-✓	D24.-✓	D48.6-✓	D49.3
central portion	C50.1-✓	C79.81	D05.-✓	D24.-✓	D48.6-✓	D49.3
inner	C50.8-✓	C79.81	D05.-✓	D24.-✓	D48.6-✓	D49.3
lower	C50.8-✓	C79.81	D05.-✓	D24.-✓	D48.6-✓	D49.3
lower-inner quadrant	C50.3-✓	C79.81	D05.-✓	D24.-✓	D48.6-✓	D49.3
lower-outer quadrant	C50.5-✓	C79.81	D05.-✓	D24.-✓	D48.6-✓	D49.3
mastectomy site (skin) — see also Neoplasm, breast, skin	C44.501	C79.2	—	—	—	—
specified as breast tissue	C50.8-✓	C79.81	—	—	—	—
midline	C50.8-✓	C79.81	D05.-✓	D24.-✓	D48.6-✓	D49.3
nipple	C50.0-✓	C79.81	D05.-✓	D24.-✓	D48.6-✓	D49.3
outer	C50.8-✓	C79.81	D05.-✓	D24.-✓	D48.6-✓	D49.3
overlapping lesion	C50.8-✓	—	—	—	—	—
skin	C44.501	C79.2	D04.5	D23.5	D48.5	D49.2
basal cell carcinoma	C44.511	—	—	—	—	—
specified type NEC	C44.591	—	—	—	—	—
squamous cell carcinoma	C44.521	—	—	—	—	—
tail (axillary)	C50.6-✓	C79.81	D05.-✓	D24.-✓	D48.6-✓	D49.3
upper	C50.8-✓	C79.81	D05.-✓	D24.-✓	D48.6-✓	D49.3
upper-inner quadrant	C50.2-✓	C79.81	D05.-✓	D24.-✓	D48.6-✓	D49.3
upper-outer quadrant	C50.4-✓	C79.81	D05.-✓	D24.-✓	D48.6-✓	D49.3
broad ligament	C57.1-✓	C79.82	D07.39	D28.2	D39.8	D49.59
bronchiogenic, bronchogenic (lung)	C34.9-✓	C78.0-✓	D02.2-✓	D14.3-✓	D38.1	D49.1
bronchiole	C34.9-✓	C78.0-✓	D02.2-✓	D14.3-✓	D38.1	D49.1
bronchus	C34.9-✓	C78.0-✓	D02.2-✓	D14.3-✓	D38.1	D49.1
carina	C34.0-✓	C78.0-✓	D02.2-✓	D14.3-✓	D38.1	D49.1
lower lobe of lung	C34.3-✓	C78.0-✓	D02.2-✓	D14.3-✓	D38.1	D49.1

Neoplasm, neoplastic	Malignant Primary	Malignant Secondary	Ca in situ	Benign	Uncertain Behavior	Unspecified Behavior
— continued						
bronchus — continued						
main	C34.0-✓	C78.0-✓	D02.2-✓	D14.3-✓	D38.1	D49.1
middle lobe of lung	C34.2	C78.0-✓	D02.21	D14.31	D38.1	D49.1
overlapping lesion	C34.8-✓	—	—	—	—	—
upper lobe of lung	C34.1-✓	C78.0-✓	D02.2-✓	D14.3-✓	D38.1	D49.1
brow	C44.309	C79.2	D04.39	D23.39	D48.5	D49.2
basal cell carcinoma	C44.319	—	—	—	—	—
specified type NEC	C44.399	—	—	—	—	—
squamous cell carcinoma	C44.329	—	—	—	—	—
buccal (cavity)	C06.9	C79.89	D00.00	D10.39	D37.09	D49.0
commissure	C06.0	C79.89	D00.02	D10.39	D37.09	D49.0
groove (lower) (upper)	C06.1	C79.89	D00.02	D10.39	D37.09	D49.0
mucosa	C06.0	C79.89	D00.02	D10.39	D37.09	D49.0
sulcus (lower) (upper)	C06.1	C79.89	D00.02	D10.39	D37.09	D49.0
bulbourethral gland	C68.0	C79.19	D09.19	D30.4	D41.3	D49.59
bursa — see Neoplasm, connective tissue						
buttock NEC	C76.3	C79.89	D04.5	D36.7	D48.7	D49.89
calf	C76.5-✓	C79.89	D04.7-✓	D36.7	D48.7	D49.89
calvarium	C41.0	C79.51	—	D16.4	D48.0	D49.2
calyx, renal	C65.-✓	C79.0-✓	D09.19	D30.1-✓	D41.1-✓	D49.51-✓
canal						
anal	C21.1	C78.5	D01.3	D12.9	D37.8	D49.0
auditory (external) — see also Neoplasm, skin, ear	C44.20-✓	C79.2	D04.2-✓	D23.2-✓	D48.5	D49.2
auricular (external) — see also Neoplasm, skin, ear	C44.20-✓	C79.2	D04.2-✓	D23.2-✓	D48.5	D49.2
canaliculi, biliary (biliferi) (intrahepatic)	C22.1	C78.7	D01.5	D13.4	D37.6	D49.0
canthus (eye) (inner) (outer)	C44.10-✓	C79.2	D04.1-✓	D23.1-✓	D48.5	D49.2
basal cell carcinoma	C44.11-✓	—	—	—	—	—
sebaceous cell	C44.13-✓	—	—	—	—	—
specified type NEC	C44.19-✓	—	—	—	—	—
squamous cell carcinoma	C44.12-✓	—	—	—	—	—
capillary — see Neoplasm, connective tissue						
caput coli	C18.0	C78.5	D01.0	D12.0	D37.4	D49.0
carcinoid — see Tumor, carcinoid						
cardia (gastric)	C16.0	C78.89	D00.2	D13.1	D37.1	D49.0
cardiac orifice (stomach)	C16.0	C78.89	D00.2	D13.1	D37.1	D49.0
cardio-esophageal junction	C16.0	C78.89	D00.2	D13.1	D37.1	D49.0
cardio-esophagus	C16.0	C78.89	D00.2	D13.1	D37.1	D49.0
carina (bronchus)	C34.0-✓	C78.0-✓	D02.2-✓	D14.3-✓	D38.1	D49.1
carotid (artery)	C49.0	C79.89	—	D21.0	D48.1	D49.2
body	C75.4	C79.89	—	D35.5	D44.6	D49.7
carpus (any bone)	C40.1-✓	C79.51	—	D16.1-✓	—	—
cartilage (articular) (joint) NEC — see also Neoplasm, bone	C41.9	C79.51	—	D16.9	D48.0	D49.2
arytenoid	C32.3	C78.39	D02.0	D14.1	D38.0	D49.1
auricular	C49.0	C79.89	—	D21.0	D48.1	D49.2
bronchi	C34.0-✓	C78.39	—	D14.3-✓	D38.1	D49.2
costal	C41.3	C79.51	—	D16.7	D48.0	D49.2
cricoid	C32.3	C78.39	D02.0	D14.1	D38.0	D49.1
cuneiform	C32.3	C78.39	D02.0	D14.1	D38.0	D49.1
ear (external)	C49.0	C79.89	—	D21.0	D48.1	D49.2
ensiform	C41.3	C79.51	—	D16.7	D48.0	D49.2
epiglottis	C32.1	C78.39	D02.0	D14.1	D38.0	D49.1

✓ Additional Character Required — Refer to the Tabular List for Character Selection

Neoplasm, neoplastic	Malignant Primary	Malignant Secondary	Ca in situ	Benign	Uncertain Behavior	Unspecified Behavior
— continued						
cartilage — see also						
Neoplasm, bone —						
continued						
epiglottis —						
continued						
anterior						
surface	C10.1	C79.89	D00.08	D10.5	D37.05	D49.0
eyelid	C49.0	C79.89	—	D21.0	D48.1	D49.2
intervertebral	C41.2	C79.51	—	D16.6	D48.0	D49.2
larynx, laryngeal	C32.3	C78.39	D02.0	D14.1	D38.0	D49.1
nose, nasal	C30.0	C78.39	D02.3	D14.0	D38.5	D49.1
pinna	C49.0	C79.89	—	D21.0	D48.1	D49.2
rib	C41.3	C79.51	—	D16.7	D48.0	D49.2
semilunar						
(knee)	C40.2-☑	C79.51	—	D16.2-☑	D48.0	D49.2
thyroid	C32.3	C78.39	D02.0	D14.1	D38.0	D49.1
trachea	C33	C78.39	D02.1	D14.2	D38.1	D49.1
cauda equina	C72.1	C79.49	—	D33.4	D43.4	D49.7
cavity						
buccal	C06.9	C79.89	D00.00	D10.30	D37.09	D49.0
nasal	C30.0	C78.39	D02.3	D14.0	D38.5	D49.1
oral	C06.9	C79.89	D00.00	D10.30	D37.09	D49.0
peritoneal	C48.2	C78.6	—	D20.1	D48.4	D49.0
tympanic	C30.1	C78.39	D02.3	D14.0	D38.5	D49.1
cecum	C18.0	C78.5	D01.0	D12.0	D37.4	D49.0
central nervous						
system	C72.9	C79.40	—	—	—	—
cerebellopontine						
(angle)	C71.6	C79.31		D33.1	D43.1	D49.6
cerebellum,						
cerebellar	C71.6	C79.31		D33.1	D43.1	D49.6
cerebrum, cerebra						
(cortex)						
(hemisphere)						
(white matter)	C71.0	C79.31	—	D33.0	D43.0	D49.6
meninges	C70.0	C79.32	—	D32.0	D42.0	D49.7
peduncle	C71.7	C79.31	—	D33.1	D43.1	D49.6
ventricle	C71.5	C79.31	—	D33.0	D43.0	D49.6
fourth	C71.7	C79.31	—	D33.1	D43.1	D49.6
cervical region	C76.0	C79.89	D09.8	D36.7	D48.7	D49.89
cervix (cervical) (uteri)						
(uterus)	C53.9	C79.82	D06.9	D26.0	D39.0	D49.59
canal	C53.0	C79.82	D06.0	D26.0	D39.0	D49.59
endocervix (canal)						
(gland)	C53.0	C79.82	D06.0	D26.0	D39.0	D49.59
exocervix	C53.1	C79.82	D06.1	D26.0	D39.0	D49.59
external os	C53.1	C79.82	D06.1	D26.0	D39.0	D49.59
internal os	C53.0	C79.82	D06.0	D26.0	D39.0	D49.59
nabothian gland	C53.0	C79.82	D06.0	D26.0	D39.0	D49.59
overlapping						
lesion	C53.8	—	—	—	—	—
squamocolumnar						
junction	C53.8	C79.82	D06.7	D26.0	D39.0	D49.59
stump	C53.8	C79.82	D06.7	D26.0	D39.0	D49.59
cheek	C76.0	C79.89	D09.8	D36.7	D48.7	D49.89
external	C44.309	C79.2	D04.39	D23.39	D48.5	D49.2
basal cell						
carcinoma	C44.319	—	—	—	—	—
specified type						
NEC	C44.399	—	—	—	—	—
squamous cell						
carcinoma	C44.329	—	—	—	—	—
inner aspect	C06.0	C79.89	D00.02	D10.39	D37.09	D49.0
internal	C06.0	C79.89	D00.02	D10.39	D37.09	D49.0
mucosa	C06.0	C79.89	D00.02	D10.39	D37.09	D49.0
chest (wall) NEC	C76.1	C79.89	D09.8	D36.7	D48.7	D49.89
chiasma opticum	C72.3-☑	C79.49	—	D33.3	D43.3	D49.7
chin	C44.309	C79.2	D04.39	D23.39	D48.5	D49.2
basal cell						
carcinoma	C44.319	—	—	—	—	—
specified type						
NEC	C44.399	—	—	—	—	—
squamous cell						
carcinoma	C44.329	—	—	—	—	—
choana	C11.3	C79.89	D00.08	D10.6	D37.05	D49.0
cholangiole	C22.1	C78.89	D01.5	D13.4	D37.6	D49.0
choledochal duct	C24.0	C78.89	D01.5	D13.5	D37.6	D49.0
choroid	C69.3-☑	C79.49	D09.2-☑	D31.3-☑	D48.7	D49.81
plexus	C71.5	C79.31	—	D33.0	D43.0	D49.6
ciliary body	C69.4-☑	C79.49	D09.2-☑	D31.4-☑	D48.7	D49.89
clavicle	C41.3	C79.51	—	D16.7	D48.0	D49.2

Right table

Neoplasm, neoplastic	Malignant Primary	Malignant Secondary	Ca in situ	Benign	Uncertain Behavior	Unspecified Behavior
— continued						
clitoris	C51.2	C79.82	D07.1	D28.0	D39.8	D49.59
clivus	C41.0	C79.51	—	D16.4	D48.0	D49.2
cloacogenic zone	C21.2	C78.5	D01.3	D12.9	D37.8	D49.0
coccygeal						
body or glomus	C49.5	C79.89	—	D21.5	D48.1	D49.2
vertebra	C41.4	C79.51	—	D16.8	D48.0	D49.2
coccyx	C41.4	C79.51	—	D16.8	D48.0	D49.2
colon — see also						
Neoplasm,						
intestine,						
large	C18.9	C78.5	—	—	—	—
with rectum	C19	C78.5	D01.1	D12.7	D37.5	D49.0
columnella — see also						
Neoplasm, skin,						
face	C44.390	C79.2	D04.39	D23.39	D48.5	D49.2
column, spinal — see						
Neoplasm, spine						
commissure						
labial, lip	C00.6	C79.89	D00.01	D10.39	D37.01	D49.0
laryngeal	C32.0	C78.39	D02.0	D14.1	D38.0	D49.1
common (bile)						
duct	C24.0	C78.89	D01.5	D13.5	D37.6	D49.0
concha — see also						
Neoplasm, skin,						
ear	C44.20-☑	C79.2	D04.2-☑	D23.2-☑	D48.5	D49.2
nose	C30.0	C78.39	D02.3	D14.0	D38.5	D49.1
conjunctiva	C69.0-☑	C79.49	D09.2-☑	D31.0-☑	D48.7	D49.89
connective tissue						
NEC	C49.9	C79.89	—	D21.9	D48.1	D49.2

Note: For neoplasms of connective tissue (blood vessel, bursa, fascia, ligament, muscle, peripheral nerves, sympathetic and parasympathetic nerves and ganglia, synovia, tendon, etc.) or of morphological types that indicate connective tissue, code according to the list under "Neoplasm, connective tissue". For sites that do not appear in this list, code to neoplasm of that site; e.g., fibrosarcoma, pancreas (C25.9)

Note: Morphological types that indicate connective tissue appear in their proper place in the alphabetic index with the instruction "see Neoplasm, connective tissue …."

	Malignant Primary	Malignant Secondary	Ca in situ	Benign	Uncertain Behavior	Unspecified Behavior
abdomen	C49.4	C79.89	—	D21.4	D48.1	D49.2
abdominal wall	C49.4	C79.89	—	D21.4	D48.1	D49.2
ankle	C49.2-☑	C79.89	—	D21.2-☑	D48.1	D49.2
antecubital fossa or						
space	C49.1-☑	C79.89	—	D21.1-☑	D48.1	D49.2
arm	C49.1-☑	C79.89	—	D21.1-☑	D48.1	D49.2
auricle (ear)	C49.0	C79.89	—	D21.0	D48.1	D49.2
axilla	C49.3	C79.89	—	D21.3	D48.1	D49.2
back	C49.6	C79.89	—	D21.6	D48.1	D49.2
breast — see						
Neoplasm,						
breast						
buttock	C49.5	C79.89	—	D21.5	D48.1	D49.2
calf	C49.2-☑	C79.89	—	D21.2-☑	D48.1	D49.2
cervical region	C49.0	C79.89	—	D21.0	D48.1	D49.2
cheek	C49.0	C79.89	—	D21.0	D48.1	D49.2
chest (wall)	C49.3	C79.89	—	D21.3	D48.1	D49.2
chin	C49.0	C79.89	—	D21.0	D48.1	D49.2
diaphragm	C49.3	C79.89	—	D21.3	D48.1	D49.2
ear (external)	C49.0	C79.89	—	D21.0	D48.1	D49.2
elbow	C49.1-☑	C79.89	—	D21.1-☑	D48.1	D49.2
extrarectal	C49.5	C79.89	—	D21.5	D48.1	D49.2
extremity	C49.9	C79.89	—	D21.9	D48.1	D49.2
lower	C49.2-☑	C79.89	—	D21.2-☑	D48.1	D49.2
upper	C49.1-☑	C79.89	—	D21.1-☑	D48.1	D49.2
eyelid	C49.0	C79.89	—	D21.0	D48.1	D49.2
face	C49.0	C79.89	—	D21.0	D48.1	D49.2
finger	C49.1-☑	C79.89	—	D21.1-☑	D48.1	D49.2
flank	C49.6	C79.89	—	D21.6	D48.1	D49.2
foot	C49.2-☑	C79.89	—	D21.2-☑	D48.1	D49.2
forearm	C49.1-☑	C79.89	—	D21.1-☑	D48.1	D49.2
forehead	C49.0	C79.89	—	D21.0	D48.1	D49.2
gastric	C49.4	C79.89	—	D21.4	D48.1	D49.2
gastrointestinal	C49.4	C79.89	—	D21.4	D48.1	D49.2
gluteal region	C49.5	C79.89	—	D21.5	D48.1	D49.2
great vessels						
NEC	C49.3	C79.89	—	D21.3	D48.1	D49.2
groin	C49.5	C79.89	—	D21.5	D48.1	D49.2
hand	C49.1-☑	C79.89	—	D21.1-☑	D48.1	D49.2
head	C49.0	C79.89	—	D21.0	D48.1	D49.2

	Malignant Primary	Malignant Secondary	Ca in situ	Benign	Uncertain Behavior	Unspecified Behavior
Neoplasm, neoplastic						
— *continued*						
connective tissue —						
continued						
heel	C49.2-☑	C79.89	—	D21.2-☑	D48.1	D49.2
hip	C49.2-☑	C79.89	—	D21.2-☑	D48.1	D49.2
hypochondrium	C49.4	C79.89	—	D21.4	D48.1	D49.2
iliopsoas muscle	C49.5	C79.89	—	D21.5	D48.1	D49.2
infraclavicular						
region	C49.3	C79.89	—	D21.3	D48.1	D49.2
inguinal (canal)						
(region)	C49.5	C79.89	—	D21.5	D48.1	D49.2
intestinal	C49.4	C79.89	—	D21.4	D48.1	D49.2
intrathoracic	C49.3	C79.89	—	D21.3	D48.1	D49.2
ischiorectal						
fossa	C49.5	C79.89	—	D21.5	D48.1	D49.2
jaw	C03.9	C79.89	D00.03	D10.39	D48.1	D49.0
knee	C49.2-☑	C79.89	—	D21.2-☑	D48.1	D49.2
leg	C49.2-☑	C79.89	—	D21.2-☑	D48.1	D49.2
limb NEC	C49.9	C79.89	—	D21.9	D48.1	D49.2
lower	C49.2-☑	C79.89	—	D21.2-☑	D48.1	D49.2
upper	C49.1-☑	C79.89	—	D21.1-☑	D48.1	D49.2
nates	C49.5	C79.89	—	D21.5	D48.1	D49.2
neck	C49.0	C79.89	—	D21.0	D48.1	D49.2
orbit	C69.6-☑	C79.49	D09.2-☑	D31.6-☑	D48.1	D49.89
overlapping						
lesion	C49.8	—	—	—	—	—
pararectal	C49.5	C79.89	—	D21.5	D48.1	D49.2
para-urethral	C49.5	C79.89	—	D21.5	D48.1	D49.2
paravaginal	C49.5	C79.89	—	D21.5	D48.1	D49.2
pelvis (floor)	C49.5	C79.89	—	D21.5	D48.1	D49.2
pelvo-abdominal	C49.8	C79.89	—	D21.6	D48.1	D49.2
perineum	C49.5	C79.89	—	D21.5	D48.1	D49.2
perirectal						
(tissue)	C49.5	C79.89	—	D21.5	D48.1	D49.2
periurethral						
(tissue)	C49.5	C79.89	—	D21.5	D48.1	D49.2
popliteal fossa or						
space	C49.2-☑	C79.89	—	D21.2-☑	D48.1	D49.2
presacral	C49.5	C79.89	—	D21.5	D48.1	D49.2
psoas muscle	C49.4	C79.89	—	D21.4	D48.1	D49.2
pterygoid fossa	C49.0	C79.89	—	D21.0	D48.1	D49.2
rectovaginal septum						
or wall	C49.5	C79.89	—	D21.5	D48.1	D49.2
rectovesical	C49.5	C79.89	—	D21.5	D48.1	D49.2
retroperitoneum	C48.0	C78.6	—	D20.0	D48.3	D49.0
sacrococcygeal						
region	C49.5	C79.89	—	D21.5	D48.1	D49.2
scalp	C49.0	C79.89	—	D21.0	D48.1	D49.2
scapular region	C49.3	C79.89	—	D21.3	D48.1	D49.2
shoulder	C49.1-☑	C79.89	—	D21.1-☑	D48.1	D49.2
skin (dermis) NEC —						
see also						
Neoplasm, skin,						
by site	C44.90	C79.2	D04.9	D23.9	D48.5	D49.2
stomach	C49.4	C79.89	—	D21.4	D48.1	D49.2
submental	C49.0	C79.89	—	D21.0	D48.1	D49.2
supraclavicular						
region	C49.0	C79.89	—	D21.0	D48.1	D49.2
temple	C49.0	C79.89	—	D21.0	D48.1	D49.2
temporal region	C49.0	C79.89	—	D21.0	D48.1	D49.2
thigh	C49.2-☑	C79.89	—	D21.2-☑	D48.1	D49.2
thoracic (duct)						
(wall)	C49.3	C79.89	—	D21.3	D48.1	D49.2
thorax	C49.3	C79.89	—	D21.3	D48.1	D49.2
thumb	C49.1-☑	C79.89	—	D21.1-☑	D48.1	D49.2
toe	C49.2-☑	C79.89	—	D21.2-☑	D48.1	D49.2
trunk	C49.6	C79.89	—	D21.6	D48.1	D49.2
umbilicus	C49.4	C79.89	—	D21.4	D48.1	D49.2
vesicorectal	C49.5	C79.89	—	D21.5	D48.1	D49.2
wrist	C49.1-☑	C79.89	—	D21.1-☑	D48.1	D49.2
conus medullaris	C72.0	C79.49	—	D33.4	D43.4	D49.7
cord (true) (vocal)	C32.0	C78.39	D02.0	D14.1	D38.0	D49.1
false	C32.1	C78.39	D02.0	D14.1	D38.0	D49.1
spermatic	C63.1-☑	C79.82	D07.69	D29.8	D40.8	D49.59
spinal (cervical)						
(lumbar)						
(thoracic)	C72.0	C79.49	—	D33.4	D43.4	D49.7
cornea (limbus)	C69.1-☑	C79.49	D09.2-☑	D31.1-☑	D48.7	D49.89
corpus						
albicans	C56.-☑	C79.6-☑	D07.39	D27.-☑	D39.1-☑	D49.59
callosum, brain	C71.0	C79.31	—	D33.2	D43.2	D49.6

	Malignant Primary	Malignant Secondary	Ca in situ	Benign	Uncertain Behavior	Unspecified Behavior
Neoplasm, neoplastic						
— *continued*						
corpus — *continued*						
cavernosum	C60.2	C79.82	D07.4	D29.0	D40.8	D49.59
gastric	C16.2	C78.89	D00.2	D13.1	D37.1	D49.0
overlapping						
sites	C54.8	—	—	—	—	—
penis	C60.2	C79.82	D07.4	D29.0	D40.8	D49.59
striatum,						
cerebrum	C71.0	C79.31	—	D33.0	D43.0	D49.6
uteri	C54.9	C79.82	D07.0	D26.1	D39.0	D49.59
isthmus	C54.0	C79.82	D07.0	D26.1	D39.0	D49.59
cortex						
adrenal	C74.0-☑	C79.7-☑	D09.3	D35.0-☑	D44.1-☑	D49.7
cerebral	C71.0	C79.31	—	D33.0	D43.0	D49.6
costal cartilage	C41.3	C79.51	—	D16.7	D48.0	D49.2
costovertebral						
joint	C41.3	C79.51	—	D16.7	D48.0	D49.2
Cowper's gland	C68.0	C79.19	D09.19	D30.4	D41.3	D49.59
cranial (fossa, any)	C71.9	C79.31	—	D33.2	D43.2	D49.6
meninges	C70.0	C79.32	—	D32.0	D42.0	D49.7
nerve	C72.50	C79.49	—	D33.3	D43.3	D49.7
specified NEC	C72.59	C79.49	—	D33.3	D43.3	D49.7
craniobuccal						
pouch	C75.2	C79.89	D09.3	D35.2	D44.3	D49.7
craniopharyngeal (duct)						
(pouch)	C75.2	C79.89	D09.3	D35.3	D44.4	D49.7
cricoid	C13.0	C79.89	D00.08	D10.7	D37.05	D49.0
cartilage	C32.3	C78.39	D02.0	D14.1	D38.0	D49.1
cricopharynx	C13.0	C79.89	D00.08	D10.7	D37.05	D49.0
crypt of Morgagni	C21.8	C78.5	D01.3	D12.9	D37.8	D49.0
crystalline lens	C69.4-☑	C79.49	D09.2-☑	D31.4-☑	D48.7	D49.89
cul-de-sac						
(Douglas')	C48.1	C78.6	—	D20.1	D48.4	D49.0
cuneiform						
cartilage	C32.3	C78.39	D02.0	D14.1	D38.0	D49.1
cutaneous — *see*						
Neoplasm, skin						
cutis — *see* Neoplasm,						
skin						
cystic (bile) duct						
(common)	C24.0	C78.89	D01.5	D13.5	D37.6	D49.0
dermis — *see*						
Neoplasm, skin						
diaphragm	C49.3	C79.89	—	D21.3	D48.1	D49.2
digestive organs,						
system, tube, or						
tract NEC	C26.9	C78.89	D01.9	D13.9	D37.9	D49.0
disc,						
intervertebral	C41.2	C79.51	—	D16.6	D48.0	D49.2
disease,						
generalized	C80.0	—	—	—	—	—
disseminated	C80.0	—	—	—	—	—
Douglas' cul-de-sac or						
pouch	C48.1	C78.6	—	D20.1	D48.4	D49.0
duodenojejunal						
junction	C17.0	C78.4	D01.49	D13.39	D37.2	D49.0
duodenum	C17.0	C78.4	D01.49	D13.2	D37.2	D49.0
dura (cranial)						
(mater)	C70.9	C79.49	—	D32.9	D42.9	D49.7
cerebral	C70.0	C79.32	—	D32.0	D42.0	D49.7
spinal	C70.1	C79.49	—	D32.1	D42.1	D49.7
ear (external) — *see*						
also Neoplasm, skin,						
ear	C44.20-☑	C79.2	D04.2-☑	D23.2-☑	D48.5	D49.2
auricle or auris — *see*						
also Neoplasm,						
skin, ear	C44.20-☑	C79.2	D04.2-☑	D23.2-☑	D48.5	D49.2
canal, external — *see*						
also Neoplasm,						
skin, ear	C44.20-☑	C79.2	D04.2-☑	D23.2-☑	D48.5	D49.2
cartilage	C49.0	C79.89	—	D21.0	D48.1	D49.2
external meatus —						
see also						
Neoplasm, skin,						
ear	C44.20-☑	C79.2	D04.2-☑	D23.2-☑	D48.5	D49.2
inner	C30.1	C78.39	D02.3	D14.0	D38.5	D49.1
lobule — *see also*						
Neoplasm, skin,						
ear	C44.20-☑	C79.2	D04.2-☑	D23.2-☑	D48.5	D49.2
middle	C30.1	C78.39	D02.3	D14.0	D38.5	D49.1
overlapping lesion						
with accessory						
sinuses	C31.8	—	—	—	—	—

Neoplasm, neoplastic	Malignant Primary	Malignant Secondary	Ca in situ	Benign	Uncertain Behavior	Unspecified Behavior
— continued						
ear — see also						
Neoplasm, skin, ear						
— continued						
skin	C44.20-☑	C79.2	D04.2-☑	D23.2-☑	D48.5	D49.2
basal cell						
carcinoma	C44.21-☑	—	—	—	—	—
specified type						
NEC	C44.29-☑	—	—	—	—	—
squamous cell						
carcinoma	C44.22-☑	—	—	—	—	—
earlobe	C44.20-☑	C79.2	D04.2-☑	D23.2-☑	D48.5	D49.2
basal cell						
carcinoma	C44.21-☑	—	—	—	—	—
specified type						
NEC	C44.29-☑	—	—	—	—	—
squamous cell						
carcinoma	C44.22-☑	—	—	—	—	—
ejaculatory duct	C63.7	C79.82	D07.69	D29.8	D40.8	D49.59
elbow NEC	C76.4-☑	C79.89	D04.6-☑	D36.7	D48.7	D49.89
endocardium	C38.0	C79.89	—	D15.1	D48.7	D49.89
endocervix (canal)						
(gland)	C53.0	C79.82	D06.0	D26.0	D39.0	D49.59
endocrine gland						
NEC	C75.9	C79.89	D09.3	D35.9	D44.9	D49.7
pluriglandular	C75.8	C79.89	D09.3	D35.7	D44.9	D49.7
endometrium (gland)						
(stroma)	C54.1	C79.82	D07.0	D26.1	D39.0	D49.59
ensiform cartilage	C41.3	C79.51	—	D16.7	D48.0	D49.2
enteric — see						
Neoplasm,						
intestine						
ependyma (brain)	C71.5	C79.31	—	D33.0	D43.0	D49.6
fourth ventricle	C71.7	C79.31	—	D33.1	D43.1	D49.6
epicardium	C38.0	C79.89	—	D15.1	D48.7	D49.89
epididymis	C63.0-☑	C79.82	D07.69	D29.3-☑	D40.8	D49.59
epidural	C72.9	C79.49	—	D33.9	D43.9	D49.7
epiglottis	C32.1	C78.39	D02.0	D14.1	D38.0	D49.1
anterior aspect or						
surface	C10.1	C79.89	D00.08	D10.5	D37.05	D49.0
cartilage	C32.3	C78.39	D02.0	D14.1	D38.0	D49.1
free border						
(margin)	C10.1	C79.89	D00.08	D10.5	D37.05	D49.0
junctional						
region	C10.8	C79.89	D00.08	D10.5	D37.05	D49.0
posterior (laryngeal)						
surface	C32.1	C78.39	D02.0	D14.1	D38.0	D49.1
suprahyoid						
portion	C32.1	C78.39	D02.0	D14.1	D38.0	D49.1
esophagogastric						
junction	C16.0	C78.89	D00.2	D13.1	D37.1	D49.0
esophagus	C15.9	C78.89	D00.1	D13.0	D37.8	D49.0
abdominal	C15.5	C78.89	D00.1	D13.0	D37.8	D49.0
cervical	C15.3	C78.89	D00.1	D13.0	D37.8	D49.0
distal (third)	C15.5	C78.89	D00.1	D13.0	D37.8	D49.0
lower (third)	C15.5	C78.89	D00.1	D13.0	D37.8	D49.0
middle (third)	C15.4	C78.89	D00.1	D13.0	D37.8	D49.0
overlapping						
lesion	C15.8	—	—	—	—	—
proximal (third)	C15.3	C78.89	D00.1	D13.0	D37.8	D49.0
thoracic	C15.4	C78.89	D00.1	D13.0	D37.8	D49.0
upper (third)	C15.3	C78.89	D00.1	D13.0	D37.8	D49.0
ethmoid (sinus)	C31.1	C78.39	D02.3	D14.0	D38.5	D49.1
bone or						
labyrinth	C41.0	C79.51	—	D16.4	D48.0	D49.2
eustachian tube	C30.1	C78.39	D02.3	D14.0	D38.5	D49.1
exocervix	C53.1	C79.82	D06.1	D26.0	D39.0	D49.59
external						
meatus (ear) — see						
also Neoplasm,						
skin, ear	C44.20-☑	C79.2	D04.2-☑	D23.2-☑	D48.5	D49.2
os, cervix uteri	C53.1	C79.82	D06.1	D26.0	D39.0	D49.59
extradural	C72.9	C79.49	—	D33.9	D43.9	D49.7
extrahepatic (bile)						
duct	C24.0	C78.89	D01.5	D13.5	D37.6	D49.0
overlapping lesion						
with						
gallbladder	C24.8	—	—	—	—	—
extraocular						
muscle	C69.6-☑	C79.49	D09.2-☑	D31.6-☑	D48.7	D49.89
extrarectal	C76.3	C79.89	D09.8	D36.7	D48.7	D49.89
extremity	C76.8	C79.89	D04.8	D36.7	D48.7	D49.89

Neoplasm, neoplastic	Malignant Primary	Malignant Secondary	Ca in situ	Benign	Uncertain Behavior	Unspecified Behavior
— continued						
extremity — continued						
lower	C76.5-☑	C79.89	D04.7-☑	D36.7	D48.7	D49.89
upper	C76.4-☑	C79.89	D04.6-☑	D36.7	D48.7	D49.89
eyeball	C69.9-☑	C79.49	D09.2-☑	D31.9-☑	D48.7	D49.89
eyebrow	C44.309	C79.2	D04.39	D23.39	D48.5	D49.2
basal cell						
carcinoma	C44.319	—	—	—	—	—
specified type						
NEC	C44.399	—	—	—	—	—
squamous cell						
carcinoma	C44.329	—	—	—	—	—
eyelid (lower) (skin)						
(upper)	C44.10-☑	—	—	—	—	—
basal cell						
carcinoma	C44.11-☑	—	—	—	—	—
cartilage	C49.0	C79.89	—	D21.0	D48.1	D49.2
sebaceous cell	C44.13-☑	—	—	—	—	—
specified type						
NEC	C44.19-☑	—	—	—	—	—
squamous cell						
carcinoma	C44.12-☑	—	—	—	—	—
eye NEC	C69.9-☑	C79.49	D09.2-☑	D31.9-☑	D48.7	D49.89
overlapping						
sites	C69.8-☑	—	—	—	—	—
face NEC	C76.0	C79.89	D04.39	D36.7	D48.7	D49.89
fallopian tube						
(accessory)	C57.0-☑	C79.82	D07.39	D28.2	D39.8	D49.59
falx (cerebella)						
(cerebri)	C70.0	C79.32	—	D32.0	D42.0	D49.7
fascia — see also						
Neoplasm,						
connective tissue						
palmar	C49.1-☑	C79.89	—	D21.1-☑	D48.1	D49.2
plantar	C49.2-☑	C79.89	—	D21.2-☑	D48.1	D49.2
fatty tissue — see						
Neoplasm,						
connective tissue						
fauces, faucial NEC	C10.9	C79.89	D00.08	D10.5	D37.05	D49.0
pillars	C09.1	C79.89	D00.08	D10.5	D37.05	D49.0
tonsil	C09.9	C79.89	D00.08	D10.4	D37.05	D49.0
femur (any part)	C40.2-☑	—	—	D16.2-☑	—	—
fetal membrane	C58	C79.82	D07.0	D26.7	D39.2	D49.59
fibrous tissue — see						
Neoplasm,						
connective tissue						
fibula (any part)	C40.2-☑	C79.51	—	D16.2-☑	—	—
filum terminale	C72.0	C79.49	—	D33.4	D43.4	D49.7
finger NEC	C76.4-☑	C79.89	D04.6-☑	D36.7	D48.7	D49.89
flank NEC	C76.8	C79.89	D04.5	D36.7	D48.7	D49.89
follicle, nabothian	C53.0	C79.82	D06.0	D26.0	D39.0	D49.59
foot NEC	C76.5-☑	C79.89	D04.7-☑	D36.7	D48.7	D49.89
forearm NEC	C76.4-☑	C79.89	D04.6-☑	D36.7	D48.7	D49.89
forehead (skin)	C44.309	C79.2	D04.39	D23.39	D48.5	D49.2
basal cell						
carcinoma	C44.319	—	—	—	—	—
specified type						
NEC	C44.399	—	—	—	—	—
squamous cell						
carcinoma	C44.329	—	—	—	—	—
foreskin	C60.0	C79.82	D07.4	D29.0	D40.8	D49.59
fornix						
pharyngeal	C11.3	C79.89	D00.08	D10.6	D37.05	D49.0
vagina	C52	C79.82	D07.2	D28.1	D39.8	D49.59
fossa (of)						
anterior (cranial)	C71.9	C79.31	—	D33.2	D43.2	D49.6
cranial	C71.9	C79.31	—	D33.2	D43.2	D49.6
ischiorectal	C76.3	C79.89	D09.8	D36.7	D48.7	D49.89
middle (cranial)	C71.9	C79.31	—	D33.2	D43.2	D49.6
piriform	C12	C79.89	D00.08	D10.7	D37.05	D49.0
pituitary	C75.1	C79.89	D09.3	D35.2	D44.3	D49.7
posterior						
(cranial)	C71.9	C79.31	—	D33.2	D43.2	D49.6
pterygoid	C49.0	C79.89	—	D21.0	D48.1	D49.2
pyriform	C12	C79.89	D00.08	D10.7	D37.05	D49.0
Rosenmuller	C11.2	C79.89	D00.08	D10.6	D37.05	D49.0
tonsillar	C09.0	C79.89	D00.08	D10.5	D37.05	D49.0
fourchette	C51.9	C79.82	D07.1	D28.0	D39.8	D49.59
frenulum						
labii — see						
Neoplasm, lip,						
internal						

Neoplasm Table

Neoplasm, ear — Neoplasm, frenulum

	Malignant Primary	Malignant Secondary	Ca in situ	Benign	Uncertain Behavior	Unspecified Behavior
Neoplasm, neoplastic						
— *continued*						
frenulum — *continued*						
linguae	C02.2	C79.89	D00.07	D10.1	D37.02	D49.0
frontal						
bone	C41.0	C79.51	—	D16.4	D48.0	D49.2
lobe, brain	C71.1	C79.31	—	D33.0	D43.0	D49.6
pole	C71.1	C79.31	—	D33.0	D43.0	D49.6
sinus	C31.2	C78.39	D02.3	D14.0	D38.5	D49.1
fundus						
stomach	C16.1	C78.89	D00.2	D13.1	D37.1	D49.0
uterus	C54.3	C79.82	D07.0	D26.1	D39.0	D49.59
gallbladder	C23	C78.89	D01.5	D13.5	D37.6	D49.0
overlapping lesion with extrahepatic bile ducts	C24.8	—	—	—	—	—
gall duct (extrahepatic)	C24.0	C78.89	D01.5	D13.5	D37.6	D49.0
intrahepatic	C22.1	C78.7	D01.5	D13.4	D37.6	D49.0
ganglia — *see also* Neoplasm, nerve, peripheral	C47.9	C79.89	—	D36.10	D48.2	D49.2
basal	C71.0	C79.31	—	D33.0	D43.0	D49.6
cranial nerve	C72.50	C79.49	—	D33.3	D43.3	D49.7
Gartner's duct	C52	C79.82	D07.2	D28.1	D39.8	D49.59
gastric — *see* Neoplasm, stomach						
gastrocolic	C26.9	C78.89	D01.9	D13.9	D37.9	D49.0
gastroesophageal junction	C16.0	C78.89	D00.2	D13.1	D37.1	D49.0
gastrointestinal (tract) NEC	C26.9	C78.89	D01.9	D13.9	D37.9	D49.0
generalized	C80.0	—	—	—	—	—
genital organ or tract						
female NEC	C57.9	C79.82	D07.30	D28.9	D39.9	D49.59
overlapping lesion	C57.8	—	—	—	—	—
specified site NEC	C57.7	C79.82	D07.39	D28.7	D39.8	D49.59
male NEC	C63.9	C79.82	D07.60	D29.9	D40.9	D49.59
overlapping lesion	C63.8	—	—	—	—	—
specified site NEC	C63.7	C79.82	D07.69	D29.8	D40.8	D49.59
genitourinary tract						
female	C57.9	C79.82	D07.30	D28.9	D39.9	D49.59
male	C63.9	C79.82	D07.60	D29.9	D40.9	D49.59
gingiva (alveolar) (marginal)	C03.9	C79.89	D00.03	D10.39	D37.09	D49.0
lower	C03.1	C79.89	D00.03	D10.39	D37.09	D49.0
mandibular	C03.1	C79.89	D00.03	D10.39	D37.09	D49.0
maxillary	C03.0	C79.89	D00.03	D10.39	D37.09	D49.0
upper	C03.0	C79.89	D00.03	D10.39	D37.09	D49.0
gland, glandular (lymphatic) (system) — *see also* Neoplasm, lymph gland						
endocrine NEC	C75.9	C79.89	D09.3	D35.9	D44.9	D49.7
salivary — *see* Neoplasm, salivary gland						
glans penis	C60.1	C79.82	D07.4	D29.0	D40.8	D49.59
globus pallidus	C71.0	C79.31	—	D33.0	D43.0	D49.6
glomus						
coccygeal	C49.5	C79.89	—	D21.5	D48.1	D49.2
jugularis	C75.5	C79.89	—	D35.6	D44.7	D49.7
glosso-epiglottic fold(s)	C10.1	C79.89	D00.08	D10.5	D37.05	D49.0
glossopalatine fold	C09.1	C79.89	D00.08	D10.5	D37.05	D49.0
glossopharyngeal sulcus	C09.0	C79.89	D00.08	D10.5	D37.05	D49.0
glottis	C32.0	C78.39	D02.0	D14.1	D38.0	D49.1
gluteal region	C76.3	C79.89	D04.5	D36.7	D48.7	D49.89
great vessels NEC	C49.3	C79.89	—	D21.3	D48.1	D49.2
groin NEC	C76.3	C79.89	D04.5	D36.7	D48.7	D49.89
gum	C03.9	C79.89	D00.03	D10.39	D37.09	D49.0
lower	C03.1	C79.89	D00.03	D10.39	D37.09	D49.0
upper	C03.0	C79.89	D00.03	D10.39	D37.09	D49.0
hand NEC	C76.4-✓	C79.89	D04.6-✓	D36.7	D48.7	D49.89
head NEC	C76.0	C79.89	D04.4	D36.7	D48.7	D49.89
heart	C38.0	C79.89	—	D15.1	D48.7	D49.89

	Malignant Primary	Malignant Secondary	Ca in situ	Benign	Uncertain Behavior	Unspecified Behavior
Neoplasm, neoplastic						
— *continued*						
heel NEC	C76.5-✓	C79.89	D04.7-✓	D36.7	D48.7	D49.89
helix — *see also* Neoplasm, skin, ear	C44.20-✓	C79.2	D04.2-✓	D23.2-✓	D48.5	D49.2
hematopoietic, hemopoietic tissue NEC	C96.9	—	—	—	—	—
specified NEC	C96.Z	—	—	—	—	—
hemisphere, cerebral	C71.0	C79.31	—	D33.0	D43.0	D49.6
hemorrhoidal zone	C21.1	C78.5	D01.3	D12.9	D37.8	D49.0
hepatic — *see also* Index to disease, by histology	C22.9	C78.7	D01.5	D13.4	D37.6	D49.0
duct (bile)	C24.0	C78.89	D01.5	D13.5	D37.6	D49.0
flexure (colon)	C18.3	C78.5	D01.0	D12.3	D37.4	D49.0
primary	C22.8	C78.7	D01.5	D13.4	D37.6	D49.0
hepatobiliary	C24.9	C78.89	D01.5	D13.5	D37.6	D49.0
hepatoblastoma	C22.2	C78.7	D01.5	D13.4	D37.6	D49.0
hepatoma	C22.0	C78.7	D01.5	D13.4	D37.6	D49.0
hilus of lung	C34.0-✓	C78.0-✓	D02.2-✓	D14.3-✓	D38.1	D49.1
hippocampus, brain	C71.2	C79.31	—	D33.0	D43.0	D49.6
hip NEC	C76.5-✓	C79.89	D04.7-✓	D36.7	D48.7	D49.89
humerus (any part)	C40.0-✓	C79.51	—	D16.0-✓	—	—
hymen	C52	C79.82	D07.2	D28.1	D39.8	D49.59
hypopharynx, hypopharyngeal NEC	C13.9	C79.89	D00.08	D10.7	D37.05	D49.0
overlapping lesion	C13.8	—	—	—	—	—
postcricoid region	C13.0	C79.89	D00.08	D10.7	D37.05	D49.0
posterior wall	C13.2	C79.89	D00.08	D10.7	D37.05	D49.0
pyriform fossa (sinus)	C12	C79.89	D00.08	D10.7	D37.05	D49.0
hypophysis	C75.1	C79.89	D09.3	D35.2	D44.3	D49.7
hypothalamus	C71.0	C79.31	—	D33.0	D43.0	D49.6
ileocecum, ileocecal (coil) (junction) (valve)	C18.0	C78.5	D01.0	D12.0	D37.4	D49.0
ileum	C17.2	C78.4	D01.49	D13.39	D37.2	D49.0
ilium	C41.4	C79.51	—	D16.8	D48.0	D49.2
immunoproliferative NEC	C88.9	—	—	—	—	—
infraclavicular (region)	C76.1	C79.89	D04.5	D36.7	D48.7	D49.89
inguinal (region)	C76.3	C79.89	D04.5	D36.7	D48.7	D49.89
insula	C71.0	C79.31	—	D33.0	D43.0	D49.6
insular tissue (pancreas)	C25.4	C78.89	D01.7	D13.7	D37.8	D49.0
brain	C71.0	C79.31	—	D33.0	D43.0	D49.6
interarytenoid fold	C13.1	C78.39	D00.08	D10.7	D37.05	D49.0
hypopharyngeal aspect	C13.1	C79.89	D00.08	D10.7	D37.05	D49.0
laryngeal aspect	C32.1	C78.39	D02.0	D14.1	D38.0	D49.1
marginal zone	C13.1	C79.89	D00.08	D10.7	D37.05	D49.0
interdental papillae	C03.9	C79.89	D00.03	D10.39	D37.09	D49.0
lower	C03.1	C79.89	D00.03	D10.39	D37.09	D49.0
upper	C03.0	C79.89	D00.03	D10.39	D37.09	D49.0
internal						
capsule	C71.0	C79.31	—	D33.0	D43.0	D49.6
os (cervix)	C53.0	C79.82	D06.0	D26.0	D39.0	D49.59
intervertebral cartilage or disc	C41.2	C79.51	—	D16.6	D48.0	D49.2
intestine, intestinal	C26.0	C78.80	D01.40	D13.9	D37.8	D49.0
large	C18.9	C78.5	D01.0	D12.6	D37.4	D49.0
appendix	C18.1	C78.5	D01.0	D12.1	D37.3	D49.0
caput coli	C18.0	C78.5	D01.0	D12.0	D37.4	D49.0
cecum	C18.0	C78.5	D01.0	D12.0	D37.4	D49.0
colon	C18.9	C78.5	D01.0	D12.6	D37.4	D49.0
and rectum	C19	C78.5	D01.1	D12.7	D37.5	D49.0
ascending	C18.2	C78.5	D01.0	D12.2	D37.4	D49.0
caput	C18.0	C78.5	D01.0	D12.0	D37.4	D49.0
descending	C18.6	C78.5	D01.0	D12.4	D37.4	D49.0
distal	C18.6	C78.5	D01.0	D12.4	D37.4	D49.0

✓ **Additional Character Required — Refer to the Tabular List for Character Selection**

Neoplasm Table

Neoplasm, frenulum — Neoplasm, intestine, intestinal

Neoplasm, neoplastic — continued	Malignant Primary	Malignant Secondary	Ca in situ	Benign	Uncertain Behavior	Unspecified Behavior
intestine, intestinal — continued						
large — continued						
colon — continued						
left	C18.6	C78.5	D01.0	D12.4	D37.4	D49.0
overlapping lesion	C18.8	—	—	—	—	—
pelvic	C18.7	C78.5	D01.0	D12.5	D37.4	D49.0
right	C18.2	C78.5	D01.0	D12.2	D37.4	D49.0
sigmoid (flexure)	C18.7	C78.5	D01.0	D12.5	D37.4	D49.0
transverse	C18.4	C78.5	D01.0	D12.3	D37.4	D49.0
hepatic flexure	C18.3	C78.5	D01.0	D12.3	D37.4	D49.0
ileocecum, ileocecal (coil) (valve)	C18.0	C78.5	D01.0	D12.0	D37.4	D49.0
overlapping lesion	C18.8	—	—	—	—	—
sigmoid flexure (lower) (upper)	C18.7	C78.5	D01.0	D12.5	D37.4	D49.0
splenic flexure	C18.5	C78.5	D01.0	D12.3	D37.4	D49.0
small	C17.9	C78.4	D01.40	D13.30	D37.2	D49.0
duodenum	C17.0	C78.4	D01.49	D13.2	D37.2	D49.0
ileum	C17.2	C78.4	D01.49	D13.39	D37.2	D49.0
jejunum	C17.1	C78.4	D01.49	D13.39	D37.2	D49.0
overlapping lesion	C17.8	—	—	—	—	—
tract NEC	C26.0	C78.89	D01.40	D13.9	D37.8	D49.0
intra-abdominal	C76.2	C79.89	D09.8	D36.7	D48.7	D49.89
intracranial NEC	C71.9	C79.31	—	D33.2	D43.2	D49.6
intrahepatic (bile) duct	C22.1	C78.7	D01.5	D13.4	D37.6	D49.0
intraocular	C69.9-☑	C79.49	D09.2-☑	D31.9-☑	D48.7	D49.89
intraorbital	C69.6-☑	C79.49	D09.2-☑	D31.6-☑	D48.7	D49.89
intrasellar	C75.1	C79.89	D09.3	D35.2	D44.3	D49.7
intrathoracic (cavity) (organs)	C76.1	C79.89	D09.8	D15.9	D48.7	D49.89
specified NEC	C76.1	C79.89	D09.8	D15.7	—	—
iris	C69.4-☑	C79.49	D09.2-☑	D31.4-☑	D48.7	D49.89
ischiorectal (fossa)	C76.3	C79.89	D09.8	D36.7	D48.7	D49.89
ischium	C41.4	C79.51	—	D16.8	D48.0	D49.2
island of Reil	C71.0	C79.31	—	D33.0	D43.0	D49.6
islands or islets of Langerhans	C25.4	C78.89	D01.7	D13.7	D37.8	D49.0
isthmus uteri	C54.0	C79.82	D07.0	D26.1	D39.0	D49.59
jaw	C76.0	C79.89	D09.8	D36.7	D48.7	D49.89
bone	C41.1	C79.51	—	D16.5	D48.0	D49.2
lower	C41.1	C79.51	—	D16.5	—	—
upper	C41.0	C79.51	—	D16.4	—	—
carcinoma (any type) (lower) (upper)	C76.0	C79.89	—	—	—	—
skin — see also Neoplasm, skin, face	C44.309	C79.2	D04.39	D23.39	D48.5	D49.2
soft tissues	C03.9	C79.89	D00.03	D10.39	D37.09	D49.0
lower	C03.1	C79.89	D00.03	D10.39	D37.09	D49.0
upper	C03.0	C79.89	D00.03	D10.39	D37.09	D49.0
jejunum	C17.1	C78.4	D01.49	D13.39	D37.2	D49.0
joint NEC — see also Neoplasm, bone	C41.9	C79.51	—	D16.9	D48.0	D49.2
acromioclavicular	C40.0-☑	C79.51	—	D16.0-☑	—	—
bursa or synovial membrane — see Neoplasm, connective tissue						
costovertebral	C41.3	C79.51	—	D16.7	D48.0	D49.2
sternocostal	C41.3	C79.51	—	D16.7	D48.0	D49.2
temporomandibular	C41.1	C79.51	—	D16.5	D48.0	D49.2
junction						
anorectal	C21.8	C78.5	D01.3	D12.9	D37.8	D49.0
cardioesophageal	C16.0	C78.89	D00.2	D13.1	D37.1	D49.0
esophagogastric	C16.0	C78.89	D00.2	D13.1	D37.1	D49.0
gastroesophageal	C16.0	C78.89	D00.2	D13.1	D37.1	D49.0
hard and soft palate	C05.9	C79.89	D00.00	D10.39	D37.09	D49.0
ileocecal	C18.0	C78.5	D01.0	D12.0	D37.4	D49.0

Neoplasm, neoplastic — continued	Malignant Primary	Malignant Secondary	Ca in situ	Benign	Uncertain Behavior	Unspecified Behavior
junction — continued						
pelvirectal	C19	C78.5	D01.1	D12.7	D37.5	D49.0
pelviureteric	C65.-☑	C79.0-☑	D09.19	D30.1-☑	D41.1-☑	D49.59
rectosigmoid	C19	C78.5	D01.1	D12.7	D37.5	D49.0
squamocolumnar, of cervix	C53.8	C79.82	D06.7	D26.0	D39.0	D49.59
Kaposi's sarcoma — see Kaposi's, sarcoma						
kidney (parenchymal)	C64.-☑	C79.0-☑	D09.19	D30.0-☑	D41.0-☑	D49.51-☑
calyx	C65.-☑	C79.0-☑	D09.19	D30.1-☑	D41.1-☑	D49.51-☑
hilus	C65.-☑	C79.0-☑	D09.19	D30.1-☑	D41.1-☑	D49.51-☑
pelvis	C65.-☑	C79.0-☑	D09.19	D30.1-☑	D41.1-☑	D49.51-☑
knee NEC	C76.5-☑	C79.89	D04.7-☑	D36.7	D48.7	D49.89
labia (skin)	C51.9	C79.82	D07.1	D28.0	D39.8	D49.59
majora	C51.0	C79.82	D07.1	D28.0	D39.8	D49.59
minora	C51.1	C79.82	D07.1	D28.0	D39.8	D49.59
labial — see also Neoplasm, lip	C00.9	C79.89	D00.01	D10.0	D37.01	D49.0
sulcus (lower) (upper)	C06.1	C79.89	D00.02	D10.39	D37.09	D49.0
labium (skin)	C51.9	C79.82	D07.1	D28.0	D39.8	D49.59
majus	C51.0	C79.82	D07.1	D28.0	D39.8	D49.59
minus	C51.1	C79.82	D07.1	D28.0	D39.8	D49.59
lacrimal						
canaliculi	C69.5-☑	C79.49	D09.2-☑	D31.5-☑	D48.7	D49.89
duct (nasal)	C69.5-☑	C79.49	D09.2-☑	D31.5-☑	D48.7	D49.89
gland	C69.5-☑	C79.49	D09.2-☑	D31.5-☑	D48.7	D49.89
punctum	C69.5-☑	C79.49	D09.2-☑	D31.5-☑	D48.7	D49.89
sac	C69.5-☑	C79.49	D09.2-☑	D31.5-☑	D48.7	D49.89
Langerhans, islands or islets	C25.4	C78.89	D01.7	D13.7	D37.8	D49.0
laryngopharynx	C13.9	C79.89	D00.08	D10.7	D37.05	D49.0
larynx, laryngeal NEC	C32.9	C78.39	D02.0	D14.1	D38.0	D49.1
aryepiglottic fold	C32.1	C78.39	D02.0	D14.1	D38.0	D49.1
cartilage (arytenoid) (cricoid) (cuneiform) (thyroid)	C32.3	C78.39	D02.0	D14.1	D38.0	D49.1
commissure (anterior) (posterior)	C32.0	C78.39	D02.0	D14.1	D38.0	D49.1
extrinsic NEC	C32.1	C78.39	D02.0	D14.1	D38.0	D49.1
meaning hypopharynx	C13.9	C79.89	D00.08	D10.7	D37.05	D49.0
interarytenoid fold	C32.1	C78.39	D02.0	D14.1	D38.0	D49.1
intrinsic	C32.0	C78.39	D02.0	D14.1	D38.0	D49.1
overlapping lesion	C32.8	—	—	—	—	—
ventricular band	C32.1	C78.39	D02.0	D14.1	D38.0	D49.1
leg NEC	C76.5-☑	C79.89	D04.7-☑	D36.7	D48.7	D49.89
lens, crystalline	C69.4-☑	C79.49	D09.2-☑	D31.4-☑	D48.7	D49.89
lid (lower) (upper)	C44.10-☑	C79.2	D04.1-☑	D23.1-☑	D48.5	D49.2
basal cell carcinoma	C44.11-☑	—	—	—	—	—
sebaceous cell	C44.13-☑	—	—	—	—	—
specified type NEC	C44.19-☑	—	—	—	—	—
squamous cell carcinoma	C44.12-☑	—	—	—	—	—
ligament — see also Neoplasm, connective tissue						
broad	C57.1-☑	C79.82	D07.39	D28.2	D39.8	D49.59
Mackenrodt's	C57.7	C79.82	D07.39	D28.7	D39.8	D49.59
non-uterine — see Neoplasm, connective tissue						
round	C57.2-☑	C79.82	—	D28.2	D39.8	D49.59
sacro-uterine	C57.3	C79.82	—	D28.2	D39.8	D49.59
uterine	C57.3	C79.82	—	D28.2	D39.8	D49.59
utero-ovarian	C57.7	C79.82	D07.39	D28.2	D39.8	D49.59
uterosacral	C57.3	C79.82	—	D28.2	D39.8	D49.59
limb	C76.8	C79.89	D04.8	D36.7	D48.7	D49.89
lower	C76.5-☑	C79.89	D04.7-☑	D36.7	D48.7	D49.89
upper	C76.4-☑	C79.89	D04.6-☑	D36.7	D48.7	D49.89
limbus of cornea	C69.1-☑	C79.49	D09.2-☑	D31.1-☑	D48.7	D49.89

☑ Additional Character Required — Refer to the Tabular List for Character Selection

Neoplasm, neoplastic	Malignant Primary	Malignant Secondary	Ca in situ	Benign	Uncertain Behavior	Unspecified Behavior
— continued						
lingual NEC — see also Neoplasm, tongue	C02.9	C79.89	D00.07	D10.1	D37.02	D49.0
lingula, lung	C34.1-☑	C78.0-☑	D02.2-☑	D14.3-☑	D38.1	D49.1
lip	C00.9	C79.89	D00.01	D10.0	D37.01	D49.0
buccal aspect — see Neoplasm, lip, internal						
commissure	C00.6	C79.89	D00.01	D10.0	D37.01	D49.0
external	C00.2	C79.89	D00.01	D10.0	D37.01	D49.0
lower	C00.1	C79.89	D00.01	D10.0	D37.01	D49.0
upper	C00.0	C79.89	D00.01	D10.0	D37.01	D49.0
frenulum — see Neoplasm, lip, internal						
inner aspect — see Neoplasm, lip, internal						
internal	C00.5	C79.89	D00.01	D10.0	D37.01	D49.0
lower	C00.4	C79.89	D00.01	D10.0	D37.01	D49.0
upper	C00.3	C79.89	D00.01	D10.0	D37.01	D49.0
lipstick area	C00.2	C79.89	D00.01	D10.0	D37.01	D49.0
lower	C00.1	C79.89	D00.01	D10.0	D37.01	D49.0
upper	C00.0	C79.89	D00.01	D10.0	D37.01	D49.0
lower	C00.1	C79.89	D00.01	D10.0	D37.01	D49.0
internal	C00.4	C79.89	D00.01	D10.0	D37.01	D49.0
mucosa — see Neoplasm, lip, internal						
oral aspect — see Neoplasm, lip, internal						
overlapping lesion	C00.8	—	—	—	—	—
with oral cavity or pharynx	C14.8	—	—	—	—	—
skin (commissure) (lower) (upper)	C44.00	C79.2	D04.0	D23.0	D48.5	D49.2
basal cell carcinoma	C44.01	—	—	—	—	—
specified type NEC	C44.09	—	—	—	—	—
squamous cell carcinoma	C44.02	—	—	—	—	—
upper	C00.0	C79.89	D00.01	D10.0	D37.01	D49.0
internal	C00.3	C79.89	D00.01	D10.0	D37.01	D49.0
vermilion border	C00.2	C79.89	D00.01	D10.0	D37.01	D49.0
lower	C00.1	C79.89	D00.01	D10.0	D37.01	D49.0
upper	C00.0	C79.89	D00.01	D10.0	D37.01	D49.0
lipomatous — see Lipoma, by site						
liver — see also Index to disease, by histology	C22.9	C78.7	D01.5	D13.4	D37.6	D49.0
primary	C22.8	C78.7	D01.5	D13.4	D37.6	D49.0
lumbosacral plexus	C47.5	C79.89	—	D36.16	D48.2	D49.2
lung	C34.9-☑	C78.0-☑	D02.2-☑	D14.3-☑	D38.1	D49.1
azygos lobe	C34.1-☑	C78.0-☑	D02.2-☑	D14.3-☑	D38.1	D49.1
carina	C34.0-☑	C78.0-☑	D02.2-☑	D14.3-☑	D38.1	D49.1
hilus	C34.0-☑	C78.0-☑	D02.2-☑	D14.3-☑	D38.1	D49.1
linqula	C34.1-☑	C78.0-☑	D02.2-☑	D14.3-☑	D38.1	D49.1
lobe NEC	C34.9-☑	C78.0-☑	D02.2-☑	D14.3-☑	D38.1	D49.1
lower lobe	C34.3-☑	C78.0-☑	D02.2-☑	D14.3-☑	D38.1	D49.1
main bronchus	C34.0-☑	C78.0-☑	D02.2-☑	D14.3-☑	D38.1	D49.1
mesothelioma — see Mesothelioma						
middle lobe	C34.2	C78.0-☑	D02.21	D14.31	D38.1	D49.1
overlapping lesion	C34.8-☑	—	—	—	—	—
upper lobe	C34.1-☑	C78.0-☑	D02.2-☑	D14.3-☑	D38.1	D49.1
lymph, lymphatic channel NEC	C49.9	C79.89	—	D21.9	D48.1	D49.2
gland (secondary)	—	C77.9	—	D36.0	D48.7	D49.89
abdominal	—	C77.2	—	D36.0	D48.7	D49.89
aortic	—	C77.2	—	D36.0	D48.7	D49.89
arm	—	C77.3	—	D36.0	D48.7	D49.89

Neoplasm, neoplastic	Malignant Primary	Malignant Secondary	Ca in situ	Benign	Uncertain Behavior	Unspecified Behavior
— continued						
lymph, lymphatic channel — continued						
gland — continued						
auricular (anterior) (posterior)	—	C77.0	—	D36.0	D48.7	D49.89
axilla, axillary	—	C77.3	—	D36.0	D48.7	D49.89
brachial	—	C77.3	—	D36.0	D48.7	D49.89
bronchial	—	C77.1	—	D36.0	D48.7	D49.89
bronchopulmonary	—	C77.1	—	D36.0	D48.7	D49.89
celiac	—	C77.2	—	D36.0	D48.7	D49.89
cervical	—	C77.0	—	D36.0	D48.7	D49.89
cervicofacial	—	C77.0	—	D36.0	D48.7	D49.89
Cloquet	—	C77.4	—	D36.0	D48.7	D49.89
colic	—	C77.2	—	D36.0	D48.7	D49.89
common duct	—	C77.2	—	D36.0	D48.7	D49.89
cubital	—	C77.3	—	D36.0	D48.7	D49.89
diaphragmatic	—	C77.1	—	D36.0	D48.7	D49.89
epigastric, inferior	—	C77.1	—	D36.0	D48.7	D49.89
epitrochlear	—	C77.3	—	D36.0	D48.7	D49.89
esophageal	—	C77.1	—	D36.0	D48.7	D49.89
face	—	C77.0	—	D36.0	D48.7	D49.89
femoral	—	C77.4	—	D36.0	D48.7	D49.89
gastric	—	C77.2	—	D36.0	D48.7	D49.89
groin	—	C77.4	—	D36.0	D48.7	D49.89
head	—	C77.0	—	D36.0	D48.7	D49.89
hepatic	—	C77.2	—	D36.0	D48.7	D49.89
hilar (pulmonary)	—	C77.1	—	D36.0	D48.7	D49.89
splenic	—	C77.2	—	D36.0	D48.7	D49.89
hypogastric	—	C77.5	—	D36.0	D48.7	D49.89
ileocolic	—	C77.2	—	D36.0	D48.7	D49.89
iliac	—	C77.5	—	D36.0	D48.7	D49.89
infraclavicular	—	C77.3	—	D36.0	D48.7	D49.89
inguina, inguinal	—	C77.4	—	D36.0	D48.7	D49.89
innominate	—	C77.1	—	D36.0	D48.7	D49.89
intercostal	—	C77.1	—	D36.0	D48.7	D49.89
intestinal	—	C77.2	—	D36.0	D48.7	D49.89
intrabdominal	—	C77.2	—	D36.0	D48.7	D49.89
intrapelvic	—	C77.5	—	D36.0	D48.7	D49.89
intrathoracic	—	C77.1	—	D36.0	D48.7	D49.89
jugular	—	C77.0	—	D36.0	D48.7	D49.89
leg	—	C77.4	—	D36.0	D48.7	D49.89
limb						
lower	—	C77.4	—	D36.0	D48.7	D49.89
upper	—	C77.3	—	D36.0	D48.7	D49.89
lower limb	—	C77.4	—	D36.0	D48.7	D49.89
lumbar	—	C77.2	—	D36.0	D48.7	D49.89
mandibular	—	C77.0	—	D36.0	D48.7	D49.89
mediastinal	—	C77.1	—	D36.0	D48.7	D49.89
mesenteric (inferior) (superior)	—	C77.2	—	D36.0	D48.7	D49.89
midcolic	—	C77.2	—	D36.0	D48.7	D49.89
multiple sites in categories C77.0 - C77.5	—	C77.8	—	D36.0	D48.7	D49.89
neck	—	C77.0	—	D36.0	D48.7	D49.89
obturator	—	C77.5	—	D36.0	D48.7	D49.89
occipital	—	C77.0	—	D36.0	D48.7	D49.89
pancreatic	—	C77.2	—	D36.0	D48.7	D49.89
para-aortic	—	C77.2	—	D36.0	D48.7	D49.89
paracervical	—	C77.5	—	D36.0	D48.7	D49.89
parametrial	—	C77.5	—	D36.0	D48.7	D49.89
parasternal	—	C77.1	—	D36.0	D48.7	D49.89
parotid	—	C77.0	—	D36.0	D48.7	D49.89
pectoral	—	C77.3	—	D36.0	D48.7	D49.89
pelvic	—	C77.5	—	D36.0	D48.7	D49.89
peri-aortic	—	C77.2	—	D36.0	D48.7	D49.89
peripancreatic	—	C77.2	—	D36.0	D48.7	D49.89
popliteal	—	C77.4	—	D36.0	D48.7	D49.89
porta hepatis	—	C77.2	—	D36.0	D48.7	D49.89
portal	—	C77.2	—	D36.0	D48.7	D49.89
preauricular	—	C77.0	—	D36.0	D48.7	D49.89
prelaryngeal	—	C77.0	—	D36.0	D48.7	D49.89
presymphysial	—	C77.5	—	D36.0	D48.7	D49.89
pretracheal	—	C77.0	—	D36.0	D48.7	D49.89
primary (any site) NEC	C96.9	—	—	—	—	—

☑ Additional Character Required — Refer to the Tabular List for Character Selection

Neoplasm, neoplastic — continued	Malignant Primary	Malignant Secondary	Ca in situ	Benign	Uncertain Behavior	Unspecified Behavior
lymph, lymphatic channel — continued						
gland — continued						
pulmonary (hiler)	—	C77.1	—	D36.0	D48.7	D49.89
pyloric	—	C77.2	—	D36.0	D48.7	D49.89
retroperitoneal	—	C77.2	—	D36.0	D48.7	D49.89
retropharyngeal	—	C77.0	—	D36.0	D48.7	D49.89
Rosenmuller's	—	C77.4	—	D36.0	D48.7	D49.89
sacral	—	C77.5	—	D36.0	D48.7	D49.89
scalene	—	C77.0	—	D36.0	D48.7	D49.89
site NEC	—	C77.9	—	D36.0	D48.7	D49.89
splenic (hilar)	—	C77.2	—	D36.0	D48.7	D49.89
subclavicular	—	C77.3	—	D36.0	D48.7	D49.89
subinguinal	—	C77.4	—	D36.0	D48.7	D49.89
sublingual	—	C77.0	—	D36.0	D48.7	D49.89
submandibular	—	C77.0	—	D36.0	D48.7	D49.89
submaxillary	—	C77.0	—	D36.0	D48.7	D49.89
submental	—	C77.0	—	D36.0	D48.7	D49.89
subscapular	—	C77.3	—	D36.0	D48.7	D49.89
supraclavicular	—	C77.0	—	D36.0	D48.7	D49.89
thoracic	—	C77.1	—	D36.0	D48.7	D49.89
tibial	—	C77.4	—	D36.0	D48.7	D49.89
tracheal	—	C77.1	—	D36.0	D48.7	D49.89
tracheobronchial	—	C77.1	—	D36.0	D48.7	D49.89
upper limb	—	C77.3	—	D36.0	D48.7	D49.89
Virchow's	—	C77.0	—	D36.0	D48.7	D49.89
node — see also Neoplasm, lymph gland						
primary NEC	C96.9	—	—	—	—	—
vessel — see also Neoplasm, connective tissue	C49.9	C79.89	—	D21.9	D48.1	D49.2
Mackenrodt's ligament	C57.7	C79.82	D07.39	D28.7	D39.8	D49.59
malar	C41.0	C79.51	—	D16.4	D48.0	D49.2
region — see Neoplasm, cheek						
mammary gland — see Neoplasm, breast						
mandible	C41.1	C79.51	—	D16.5	D48.0	D49.2
alveolar						
mucosa (carcinoma)	C03.1	C79.89	D00.03	D10.39	D37.09	D49.0
ridge or process	C41.1	C79.51	—	D16.5	D48.0	D49.2
marrow (bone) NEC	C96.9	C79.52	—	—	D47.9	D49.89
mastectomy site (skin) — see also Neoplasm, breast, skin	C44.501	C79.2	—	—	—	—
specified as breast tissue	C50.8-☑	C79.81	—	—	—	—
mastoid (air cells) (antrum) (cavity)	C30.1	C78.39	D02.3	D14.0	D38.5	D49.1
bone or process	C41.0	C79.51	—	D16.4	D48.0	D49.2
maxilla, maxillary (superior)	C41.0	C79.51	—	D16.4	D48.0	D49.2
alveolar						
mucosa	C03.0	C79.89	D00.03	D10.39	D37.09	D49.0
ridge or process (carcinoma)	C41.0	C79.51	—	D16.4	D48.0	D49.2
antrum	C31.0	C78.39	D02.3	D14.0	D38.5	D49.1
carcinoma	C03.0	C79.51	—	—	—	—
inferior — see Neoplasm, mandible						
sinus	C31.0	C78.39	D02.3	D14.0	D38.5	D49.1
meatus external (ear) — see also Neoplasm, skin, ear	C44.20-☑	C79.2	D04.2-☑	D23.2-☑	D48.5	D49.2
Meckel diverticulum, malignant	C17.3	C78.4	D01.49	D13.39	D37.2	D49.0
mediastinum, mediastinal	C38.3	C78.1	—	D15.2	D38.3	D49.89
anterior	C38.1	C78.1	—	D15.2	D38.3	D49.89

Neoplasm, neoplastic — continued	Malignant Primary	Malignant Secondary	Ca in situ	Benign	Uncertain Behavior	Unspecified Behavior
mediastinum, mediastinal — continued						
posterior	C38.2	C78.1	—	D15.2	D38.3	D49.89
medulla						
adrenal	C74.1-☑	C79.7-☑	D09.3	D35.0-☑	D44.1-☑	D49.7
oblongata	C71.7	C79.31	—	D33.1	D43.1	D49.6
meibomian gland	C44.10-☑	C79.2	D04.1-☑	D23.1-☑	D48.5	D49.2
basal cell carcinoma	C44.11-☑	—	—	—	—	—
sebaceous cell	C44.13-☑	—	—	—	—	—
specified type NEC	C44.19-☑	—	—	—	—	—
squamous cell carcinoma	C44.12-☑	—	—	—	—	—
melanoma — see Melanoma						
meninges	C70.9	C79.49	—	D32.9	D42.9	D49.7
brain	C70.0	C79.32	—	D32.0	D42.0	D49.7
cerebral	C70.0	C79.32	—	D32.0	D42.0	D49.7
crainial	C70.0	C79.32	—	D32.0	D42.0	D49.7
intracranial	C70.0	C79.32	—	D32.0	D42.0	D49.7
spinal (cord)	C70.1	C79.49	—	D32.1	D42.1	D49.7
meniscus, knee joint (lateral)						
(medial)	C40.2-☑	C79.51	—	D16.2-☑	D48.0	D49.2
Merkel cell — see Carcinoma, Merkel cell						
mesentery, mesenteric	C48.1	C78.6	—	D20.1	D48.4	D49.0
mesoappendix	C48.1	C78.6	—	D20.1	D48.4	D49.0
mesocolon	C48.1	C78.6	—	D20.1	D48.4	D49.0
mesopharynx — see Neoplasm, oropharynx						
mesosalpinx	C57.1-☑	C79.82	D07.39	D28.2	D39.8	D49.59
mesothelial tissue — see Mesothelioma						
mesothelioma — see Mesothelioma						
mesovarium	C57.1-☑	C79.82	D07.39	D28.2	D39.8	D49.59
metacarpus (any bone)	C40.1-☑	C79.51	—	D16.1-☑	—	—
metastatic NEC — see also Neoplasm, by site, secondary	—	C79.9	—	—	—	—
metatarsus (any bone)	C40.3-☑	C79.51	—	D16.3-☑	—	—
midbrain	C71.7	C79.31	—	D33.1	D43.1	D49.6
milk duct — see Neoplasm, breast						
mons						
pubis	C51.9	C79.82	D07.1	D28.0	D39.8	D49.59
veneris	C51.9	C79.82	D07.1	D28.0	D39.8	D49.59
motor tract	C72.9	C79.49	—	D33.9	D43.9	D49.7
brain	C71.9	C79.31	—	D33.2	D43.2	D49.6
cauda equina	C72.1	C79.49	—	D33.4	D43.4	D49.7
spinal	C72.0	C79.49	—	D33.4	D43.4	D49.7
mouth	C06.9	C79.89	D00.00	D10.30	D37.09	D49.0
book-leaf	C06.89	C79.89	—	—	—	—
floor	C04.9	C79.89	D00.06	D10.2	D37.09	D49.0
anterior portion	C04.0	C79.89	D00.06	D10.2	D37.09	D49.0
lateral portion	C04.1	C79.89	D00.06	D10.2	D37.09	D49.0
overlapping lesion	C04.8	—	—	—	—	—
overlapping NEC	C06.80	—	—	—	—	—
roof	C05.9	C79.89	D00.00	D10.39	D37.09	D49.0
specified part NEC	C06.89	C79.89	D00.00	D10.39	D37.09	D49.0
vestibule	C06.1	C79.89	D00.00	D10.39	D37.09	D49.0
mucosa						
alveolar (ridge or process)	C03.9	C79.89	D00.03	D10.39	D37.09	D49.0
lower	C03.1	C79.89	D00.03	D10.39	D37.09	D49.0
upper	C03.0	C79.89	D00.03	D10.39	D37.09	D49.0
buccal	C06.0	C79.89	D00.02	D10.39	D37.09	D49.0
cheek	C06.0	C79.89	D00.02	D10.39	D37.09	D49.0

☑ **Additional Character Required — Refer to the Tabular List for Character Selection**

	Malignant Primary	Malignant Secondary	Ca in situ	Benign	Uncertain Behavior	Unspecified Behavior
Neoplasm, neoplastic						
— *continued*						
mucosa — *continued*						
lip — *see* Neoplasm, lip, internal						
nasal	C30.0	C78.39	D02.3	D14.0	D38.5	D49.1
oral	C06.0	C79.89	D00.02	D10.39	D37.09	D49.0
Mullerian duct						
female	C57.7	C79.82	D07.39	D28.7	D39.8	D49.59
male	C63.7	C79.82	D07.69	D29.8	D40.8	D49.59
muscle — *see also* Neoplasm, connective tissue						
extraocular	C69.6-☑	C79.49	D09.2-☑	D31.6-☑	D48.7	D49.89
myocardium	C38.0	C79.89	—	D15.1	D48.7	D49.89
myometrium	C54.2	C79.82	D07.0	D26.1	D39.0	D49.59
myopericardium	C38.0	C79.89	—	D15.1	D48.7	D49.89
nabothian gland (follicle)	C53.0	C79.82	D06.0	D26.0	D39.0	D49.59
nail — *see also* Neoplasm, skin, limb						
	C44.90	C79.2	D04.9	D23.9	D48.5	D49.2
finger — *see also* Neoplasm, skin, limb, upper						
	C44.60-☑	C79.2	D04.6-☑	D23.6-☑	D48.5	D49.2
toe — *see also* Neoplasm, skin, limb, lower						
	C44.70-☑	C79.2	D04.7-☑	D23.7-☑	D48.5	D49.2
nares, naris (anterior) (posterior)	C30.0	C78.39	D02.3	D14.0	D38.5	D49.1
nasal — *see* Neoplasm, nose						
nasolabial groove — *see also* Neoplasm, skin, face	C44.309	C79.2	D04.39	D23.39	D48.5	D49.2
nasolacrimal duct	C69.5-☑	C79.49	D09.2-☑	D31.5-☑	D48.7	D49.89
nasopharynx, nasopharyngeal	C11.9	C79.89	D00.08	D10.6	D37.05	D49.0
floor	C11.3	C79.89	D00.08	D10.6	D37.05	D49.0
overlapping lesion	C11.8	—	—	—	—	—
roof	C11.0	C79.89	D00.08	D10.6	D37.05	D49.0
wall	C11.9	C79.89	D00.08	D10.6	D37.05	D49.0
anterior	C11.3	C79.89	D00.08	D10.6	D37.05	D49.0
lateral	C11.2	C79.89	D00.08	D10.6	D37.05	D49.0
posterior	C11.1	C79.89	D00.08	D10.6	D37.05	D49.0
superior	C11.0	C79.89	D00.08	D10.6	D37.05	D49.0
nates — *see also* Neoplasm, skin, trunk	C44.509	C79.2	D04.5	D23.5	D48.5	D49.2
neck NEC	C76.0	C79.89	D09.8	D36.7	D48.7	D49.89
skin	C44.40	—	—	—	—	—
basal cell carcinoma	C44.41	—	—	—	—	—
specified type NEC	C44.49	—	—	—	—	—
squamous cell carcinoma	C44.42	—	—	—	—	—
nerve (ganglion)	C47.9	C79.89	—	D36.10	D48.2	D49.2
abducens	C72.59	C79.49	—	D33.3	D43.3	D49.7
accessory (spinal)	C72.59	C79.49	—	D33.3	D43.3	D49.7
acoustic	C72.4-☑	C79.49	—	D33.3	D43.3	D49.7
auditory	C72.4-☑	C79.49	—	D33.3	D43.3	D49.7
autonomic NEC — *see also* Neoplasm, nerve, peripheral	C47.9	C79.89	—	D36.10	D48.2	D49.2
brachial	C47.1-☑	C79.89	—	D36.12	D48.2	D49.2
cranial	C72.50	C79.49	—	D33.3	D43.3	D49.7
specified NEC	C72.59	C79.49	—	D33.3	D43.3	D49.7
facial	C72.59	C79.49	—	D33.3	D43.3	D49.7
femoral	C47.2-☑	C79.89	—	D36.13	D48.2	D49.2
ganglion NEC — *see also* Neoplasm, nerve, peripheral	C47.9	C79.89	—	D36.10	D48.2	D49.2
glossopharyngeal	C72.59	C79.49	—	D33.3	D43.3	D49.7
hypoglossal	C72.59	C79.49	—	D33.3	D43.3	D49.7
intercostal	C47.3	C79.89	—	D36.14	D48.2	D49.2
lumbar	C47.6	C79.89	—	D36.17	D48.2	D49.2
median	C47.1-☑	C79.89	—	D36.12	D48.2	D49.2
obturator	C47.2-☑	C79.89	—	D36.13	D48.2	D49.2

	Malignant Primary	Malignant Secondary	Ca in situ	Benign	Uncertain Behavior	Unspecified Behavior
Neoplasm, neoplastic						
— *continued*						
nerve — *continued*						
oculomotor	C72.59	C79.49	—	D33.3	D43.3	D49.7
olfactory	C47.2-☑	C79.49	—	D33.3	D43.3	D49.7
optic	C72.3-☑	C79.49	—	D33.3	D43.3	D49.7
parasympathetic NEC	C47.9	C79.89	—	D36.10	D48.2	D49.2
peripheral NEC	C47.9	C79.89	—	D36.10	D48.2	D49.2
abdomen	C47.4	C79.89	—	D36.15	D48.2	D49.2
abdominal wall	C47.4	C79.89	—	D36.15	D48.2	D49.2
ankle	C47.2-☑	C79.89	—	D36.13	D48.2	D49.2
antecubital fossa or space	C47.1-☑	C79.89	—	D36.12	D48.2	D49.2
arm	C47.1-☑	C79.89	—	D36.12	D48.2	D49.2
auricle (ear)	C47.0	C79.89	—	D36.11	D48.2	D49.2
axilla	C47.3	C79.89	—	D36.12	D48.2	D49.2
back	C47.6	C79.89	—	D36.17	D48.2	D49.2
buttock	C47.5	C79.89	—	D36.16	D48.2	D49.2
calf	C47.2-☑	C79.89	—	D36.13	D48.2	D49.2
cervical region	C47.0	C79.89	—	D36.11	D48.2	D49.2
cheek	C47.0	C79.89	—	D36.11	D48.2	D49.2
chest (wall)	C47.3	C79.89	—	D36.14	D48.2	D49.2
chin	C47.0	C79.89	—	D36.11	D48.2	D49.2
ear (external)	C47.0	C79.89	—	D36.11	D48.2	D49.2
elbow	C47.1-☑	C79.89	—	D36.12	D48.2	D49.2
extrarectal	C47.5	C79.89	—	D36.16	D48.2	D49.2
extremity	C47.9	C79.89	—	D36.10	D48.2	D49.2
lower	C47.2-☑	C79.89	—	D36.13	D48.2	D49.2
upper	C47.1-☑	C79.89	—	D36.12	D48.2	D49.2
eyelid	C47.0	C79.89	—	D36.11	D48.2	D49.2
face	C47.0	C79.89	—	D36.11	D48.2	D49.2
finger	C47.1-☑	C79.89	—	D36.12	D48.2	D49.2
flank	C47.6	C79.89	—	D36.17	D48.2	D49.2
foot	C47.2-☑	C79.89	—	D36.13	D48.2	D49.2
forearm	C47.1-☑	C79.89	—	D36.12	D48.2	D49.2
forehead	C47.0	C79.89	—	D36.11	D48.2	D49.2
gluteal region	C47.5	C79.89	—	D36.16	D48.2	D49.2
groin	C47.5	C79.89	—	D36.16	D48.2	D49.2
hand	C47.1-☑	C79.89	—	D36.12	D48.2	D49.2
head	C47.0	C79.89	—	D36.11	D48.2	D49.2
heel	C47.2-☑	C79.89	—	D36.13	D48.2	D49.2
hip	C47.2-☑	C79.89	—	D36.13	D48.2	D49.2
infraclavicular region	C47.3	C79.89	—	D36.14	D48.2	D49.2
inguinal (canal) (region)	C47.5	C79.89	—	D36.16	D48.2	D49.2
intrathoracic	C47.3	C79.89	—	D36.14	D48.2	D49.2
ischiorectal fossa	C47.5	C79.89	—	D36.16	D48.2	D49.2
knee	C47.2-☑	C79.89	—	D36.13	D48.2	D49.2
leg	C47.2-☑	C79.89	—	D36.13	D48.2	D49.2
limb NEC	C47.9	C79.89	—	D36.10	D48.2	D49.2
lower	C47.2-☑	C79.89	—	D36.13	D48.2	D49.2
upper	C47.1-☑	C79.89	—	D36.12	D48.2	D49.2
nates	C47.5	C79.89	—	D36.16	D48.2	D49.2
neck	C47.0	C79.89	—	D36.11	D48.2	D49.2
orbit	C69.6-☑	C79.49	—	D31.6-☑	D48.7	D49.2
pararectal	C47.5	C79.89	—	D36.16	D48.2	D49.2
paraurethral	C47.5	C79.89	—	D36.16	D48.2	D49.2
paravaginal	C47.5	C79.89	—	D36.16	D48.2	D49.2
pelvis (floor)	C47.5	C79.89	—	D36.16	D48.2	D49.2
pelvoabdominal	C47.8	C79.89	—	D36.17	D48.2	D49.2
perineum	C47.5	C79.89	—	D36.16	D48.2	D49.2
perirectal (tissue)	C47.5	C79.89	—	D36.16	D48.2	D49.2
periurethral (tissue)	C47.5	C79.89	—	D36.16	D48.2	D49.2
popliteal fossa or space	C47.2-☑	C79.89	—	D36.13	D48.2	D49.2
presacral	C47.5	C79.89	—	D36.16	D48.2	D49.2
pterygoid fossa	C47.0	C79.89	—	D36.11	D48.2	D49.2
rectovaginal septum or wall	C47.5	C79.89	—	D36.16	D48.2	D49.2
rectovesical	C47.5	C79.89	—	D36.16	D48.2	D49.2
sacrococcygeal region	C47.5	C79.89	—	D36.16	D48.2	D49.2
scalp	C47.0	C79.89	—	D36.11	D48.2	D49.2

Neoplasm, neoplastic	Malignant Primary	Malignant Secondary	Ca in situ	Benign	Uncertain Behavior	Unspecified Behavior
— continued						
nerve — continued						
peripheral — continued						
scapular region	C47.3	C79.89	—	D36.14	D48.2	D49.2
shoulder	C47.1-☑	C79.89	—	D36.12	D48.2	D49.2
submental	C47.0	C79.89	—	D36.11	D48.2	D49.2
supraclavicular region	C47.0	C79.89	—	D36.11	D48.2	D49.2
temple	C47.0	C79.89	—	D36.11	D48.2	D49.2
temporal region	C47.0	C79.89	—	D36.11	D48.2	D49.2
thigh	C47.2-☑	C79.89	—	D36.13	D48.2	D49.2
thoracic (duct) (wall)	C47.3	C79.89	—	D36.14	D48.2	D49.2
thorax	C47.3	C79.89	—	D36.14	D48.2	D49.2
thumb	C47.1-☑	C79.89	—	D36.12	D48.2	D49.2
toe	C47.2-☑	C79.89	—	D36.13	D48.2	D49.2
trunk	C47.6	C79.89	—	D36.17	D48.2	D49.2
umbilicus	C47.4	C79.89	—	D36.15	D48.2	D49.2
vesicorectal	C47.5	C79.89	—	D36.16	D48.2	D49.2
wrist	C47.1-☑	C79.89	—	D36.12	D48.2	D49.2
radial	C47.1-☑	C79.89	—	D36.12	D48.2	D49.2
sacral	C47.5	C79.89	—	D36.16	D48.2	D49.2
sciatic	C47.2-☑	C79.89	—	D36.13	D48.2	D49.2
spinal NEC	C47.9	C79.89	—	D36.10	D48.2	D49.2
accessory	C72.59	C79.49	—	D33.3	D43.3	D49.7
sympathetic NEC — see also Neoplasm, nerve, peripheral	C47.9	C79.89	—	D36.10	D48.2	D49.2
trigeminal	C72.59	C79.49	—	D33.3	D43.3	D49.7
trochlear	C72.59	C79.49	—	D33.3	D43.3	D49.7
ulnar	C47.1-☑	C79.89	—	D36.12	D48.2	D49.2
vagus	C72.59	C79.49	—	D33.3	D43.3	D49.7
nervous system (central)	C72.9	C79.40	—	D33.9	D43.9	D49.7
autonomic — see Neoplasm, nerve, peripheral						
parasympathetic — see Neoplasm, nerve, peripheral						
specified site NEC	—	C79.49	—	D33.7	D43.8	
sympathetic — see Neoplasm, nerve, peripheral						
nevus — see Nevus						
nipple	C50.0-☑	C79.81	D05.-☑	D24.-☑	—	
nose, nasal	C76.0	C79.89	D09.8	D36.7	D48.7	D49.89
ala (external) (nasi) — see also Neoplasm, nose, skin						
skin	C44.301	C79.2	D04.39	D23.39	D48.5	D49.2
bone	C41.0	C79.51	—	D16.4	D48.0	D49.2
cartilage	C30.0	C78.39	D02.3	D14.0	D38.5	D49.1
cavity	C30.0	C78.39	D02.3	D14.0	D38.5	D49.1
choana	C11.3	C79.89	D00.08	D10.6	D37.05	D49.0
external (skin) — see also Neoplasm, nose, skin	C44.301	C79.2	D04.39	D23.39	D48.5	D49.2
fossa	C30.0	C78.39	D02.3	D14.0	D38.5	D49.1
internal	C30.0	C78.39	D02.3	D14.0	D38.5	D49.1
mucosa	C30.0	C78.39	D02.3	D14.0	D38.5	D49.1
septum	C30.0	C78.39	D02.3	D14.0	D38.5	D49.1
posterior margin	C11.3	C79.89	D00.08	D10.6	D37.05	D49.0
sinus — see Neoplasm, sinus						
skin	C44.301	C79.2	D04.39	D23.39	D48.5	D49.2
basal cell carcinoma	C44.311	—	—	—	—	—
specified type NEC	C44.391	—	—	—	—	—
squamous cell carcinoma	C44.321	—	—	—	—	—
turbinate (mucosa)	C30.0	C78.39	D02.3	D14.0	D38.5	D49.1
bone	C41.0	C79.51	—	D16.4	D48.0	D49.2
vestibule	C30.0	C78.39	D02.3	D14.0	D38.5	D49.1

Neoplasm, neoplastic	Malignant Primary	Malignant Secondary	Ca in situ	Benign	Uncertain Behavior	Unspecified Behavior
— continued						
nostril	C30.0	C78.39	D02.3	D14.0	D38.5	D49.1
nucleus pulposus	C41.2	C79.51	—	D16.6	D48.0	D49.2
occipital						
bone	C41.0	C79.51	—	D16.4	D48.0	D49.2
lobe or pole, brain	C71.4	C79.31	—	D33.0	D43.0	D49.6
odontogenic — see Neoplasm, jaw bone						
olfactory nerve or bulb	C72.2-☑	C79.49	—	D33.3	D43.3	D49.7
olive (brain)	C71.7	C79.31	—	D33.1	D43.1	D49.6
omentum	C48.1	C78.6	—	D20.1	D48.4	D49.0
operculum (brain)	C71.0	C79.31	—	D33.0	D43.0	D49.6
optic nerve, chiasm, or tract	C72.3-☑	C79.49	—	D33.3	D43.3	D49.7
oral (cavity)	C06.9	C79.89	D00.00	D10.30	D37.09	D49.0
ill-defined	C14.8	C79.89	D00.00	D10.30	D37.09	D49.0
mucosa	C06.0	C79.89	D00.02	D10.39	D37.09	D49.0
orbit	C69.6-☑	C79.49	D09.2-☑	D31.6-☑	D48.7	D49.89
autonomic nerve	C69.6-☑	C79.49	—	D31.6-☑	D48.7	D49.2
bone	C41.0	C79.51	—	D16.4	D48.0	D49.2
eye	C69.6-☑	C79.49	D09.2-☑	D31.6-☑	D48.7	D49.89
peripheral nerves	C69.6-☑	C79.49	—	D31.6-☑	D48.7	D49.2
soft parts	C69.6-☑	C79.49	D09.2-☑	D31.6-☑	D48.7	D49.89
organ of Zuckerkandl	C75.5	C79.89	—	D35.6	D44.7	D49.7
oropharynx	C10.9	C79.89	D00.08	D10.5	D37.05	D49.0
branchial cleft (vestige)	C10.4	C79.89	D00.08	D10.5	D37.05	D49.0
junctional region	C10.8	C79.89	D00.08	D10.5	D37.05	D49.0
lateral wall	C10.2	C79.89	D00.08	D10.5	D37.05	D49.0
overlapping lesion	C10.8	—	—	—	—	D49.0
pillars or fauces	C09.1	C79.89	D00.08	D10.5	D37.05	D49.0
posterior wall	C10.3	C79.89	D00.08	D10.5	D37.05	D49.0
vallecula	C10.0	C79.89	D00.08	D10.5	D37.05	D49.0
os						
external	C53.1	C79.82	D06.1	D26.0	D39.0	D49.59
internal	C53.0	C79.82	D06.0	D26.0	D39.0	D49.59
ovary	C56.-☑	C79.6-☑	D07.39	D27.-☑	D39.1-☑	D49.59
oviduct	C57.0-☑	C79.82	D07.39	D28.2	D39.8	D49.59
palate	C05.9	C79.89	D00.00	D10.39	D37.09	D49.0
hard	C05.0	C79.89	D00.05	D10.39	D37.09	D49.0
junction of hard and soft palate	C05.9	C79.89	D00.00	D10.39	D37.09	D49.0
overlapping lesions	C05.8	—	—	—	—	—
soft	C05.1	C79.89	D00.04	D10.39	D37.09	D49.0
nasopharyngeal surface	C11.3	C79.89	D00.08	D10.6	D37.05	D49.0
posterior surface	C11.3	C79.89	D00.08	D10.6	D37.05	D49.0
superior surface	C11.3	C79.89	D00.08	D10.6	D37.05	D49.0
palatoglossal arch	C09.1	C79.89	D00.00	D10.5	D37.09	D49.0
palatopharyngeal arch	C09.1	C79.89	D00.00	D10.5	D37.09	D49.0
pallium	C71.0-☑	C79.31	—	D33.0	D43.0	D49.6
palpebra	C44.10-☑	C79.2	D04.1-☑	D23.1-☑	D48.5	D49.2
basal cell carcinoma	C44.11-☑	—	—	—	—	—
sebaceous cell	C44.13-☑	—	—	—	—	—
specified type NEC	C44.19-☑	—	—	—	—	—
squamous cell carcinoma	C44.12-☑	—	—	—	—	—
pancreas	C25.9	C78.89	D01.7	D13.6	D37.8	D49.0
body	C25.1	C78.89	D01.7	D13.6	D37.8	D49.0
duct (of Santorini) (of Wirsung)	C25.3	C78.89	D01.7	D13.6	D37.8	D49.0
ectopic tissue	C25.7	C78.89	—	D13.6	D37.8	D49.0
head	C25.0	C78.89	D01.7	D13.6	D37.8	D49.0
islet cells	C25.4	C78.89	D01.7	D13.7	D37.8	D49.0
neck	C25.7	C78.89	D01.7	D13.6	D37.8	D49.0
overlapping lesion	C25.8	—	—	—	—	—
tail	C25.2	C78.89	D01.7	D13.6	D37.8	D49.0

☑ Additional Character Required — Refer to the Tabular List for Character Selection

Neoplasm Table

Neoplasm, para-aortic body — Neoplasm, rectum

Neoplasm, neoplastic	Malignant Primary	Malignant Secondary	Ca in situ	Benign	Uncertain Behavior	Unspecified Behavior
— continued						
para-aortic body	C75.5	C79.89	—	D35.6	D44.7	D49.7
paraganglion NEC	C75.5	C79.89	—	D35.6	D44.7	D49.7
parametrium	C57.3	C79.82	—	D28.2	D39.8	D49.59
paranephric	C48.0	C78.6	—	D20.0	D48.3	D49.0
pararectal	C76.3	C79.89	—	D36.7	D48.7	D49.89
parasagittal (region)	C76.0	C79.89	D09.8	D36.7	D48.7	D49.89
parasellar	C72.9	C79.49	—	D33.9	D43.8	D49.7
parathyroid (gland)	C75.0	C79.89	D09.3	D35.1	D44.2	D49.7
paraurethral	C76.3	C79.89	—	D36.7	D48.7	D49.89
gland	C68.1	C79.19	D09.19	D30.8	D41.8	D49.59
paravaginal	C76.3	C79.89	—	D36.7	D48.7	D49.89
parenchyma, kidney	C64.-☑	C79.0-☑	D09.19	D30.0-☑	D41.0-☑	D49.51-☑
parietal						
bone	C41.0	C79.51	—	D16.4	D48.0	D49.2
lobe, brain	C71.3	C79.31	—	D33.0	D43.0	D49.6
paroophoron	C57.1-☑	C79.82	D07.39	D28.2	D39.8	D49.59
parotid (duct) (gland)	C07	C79.89	D00.00	D11.0	D37.030	D49.0
parovarium	C57.1-☑	C79.82	D07.39	D28.2	D39.8	D49.59
patella	C40.20	C79.51	—	—	—	—
peduncle, cerebral	C71.7	C79.31	—	D33.1	D43.1	D49.6
pelvirectal junction	C19	C78.5	D01.1	D12.7	D37.5	D49.0
pelvis, pelvic	C76.3	C79.89	D09.8	D36.7	D48.7	D49.89
bone	C41.4	C79.51	—	D16.8	D48.0	D49.2
floor	C76.3	C79.89	D09.8	D36.7	D48.7	D49.89
renal	C65.-☑	C79.0-☑	D09.19	D30.1-☑	D41.1-☑	D49.51-☑
viscera	C76.3	C79.89	D09.8	D36.7	D48.7	D49.89
wall	C76.3	C79.89	D09.8	D36.7	D48.7	D49.89
pelvo-abdominal	C76.8	C79.89	D09.8	D36.7	D48.7	D49.89
penis	C60.9	C79.82	D07.4	D29.0	D40.8	D49.59
body	C60.2	C79.82	D07.4	D29.0	D40.8	D49.59
corpus (cavernosum)	C60.2	C79.82	D07.4	D29.0	D40.8	D49.59
glans	C60.1	C79.82	D07.4	D29.0	D40.8	D49.59
overlapping sites	C60.8	—	—	—	—	—
skin NEC	C60.9	C79.82	D07.4	D29.0	D40.8	D49.59
periadrenal (tissue)	C48.0	C78.6	—	D20.0	D48.3	D49.0
perianal (skin) — see also Neoplasm, anus, skin	C44.500	C79.2	D04.5	D23.5	D48.5	D49.2
pericardium	C38.0	C79.89	—	D15.1	D48.7	D49.89
perinephric	C48.0	C78.6	—	D20.0	D48.3	D49.0
perineum	C76.3	C79.89	D09.8	D36.7	D48.7	D49.89
periodontal tissue NEC	C03.9	C79.89	D00.03	D10.39	D37.09	D49.0
periosteum — see Neoplasm, bone						
peripancreatic	C48.0	C78.6	—	D20.0	D48.3	D49.0
peripheral nerve NEC	C47.9	C79.89	—	D36.10	D48.2	D49.2
perirectal (tissue)	C76.3	C79.89	—	D36.7	D48.7	D49.89
perirenal (tissue)	C48.0	C78.6	—	D20.0	D48.3	D49.0
peritoneum, peritoneal (cavity)	C48.2	C78.6	—	D20.1	D48.4	D49.0
benign mesothelial tissue — see Mesothelioma, benign						
overlapping lesion	C48.8	—	—	—	—	—
with digestive organs	C26.9	—	—	—	—	—
parietal	C48.1	C78.6	—	D20.1	D48.4	D49.0
pelvic	C48.1	C78.6	—	D20.1	D48.4	D49.0
specified part NEC	C48.1	C78.6	—	D20.1	D48.4	D49.0
peritonsillar (tissue)	C76.0	C79.89	D09.8	D36.7	D48.7	D49.89
periurethral tissue	C76.3	C79.89	—	D36.7	D48.7	D49.89
phalanges						
foot	C40.3-☑	C79.51	—	D16.3-☑	—	—
hand	C40.1-☑	C79.51	—	D16.1-☑	—	—
pharynx, pharyngeal	C14.0	C79.89	D00.08	D10.9	D37.05	D49.0
bursa	C11.1	C79.89	D00.08	D10.6	D37.05	D49.0

Neoplasm, neoplastic	Malignant Primary	Malignant Secondary	Ca in situ	Benign	Uncertain Behavior	Unspecified Behavior
— continued						
pharynx, pharyngeal — continued						
fornix	C11.3	C79.89	D00.08	D10.6	D37.05	D49.0
recess	C11.2	C79.89	D00.08	D10.6	D37.05	D49.0
region	C14.0	C79.89	D00.08	D10.9	D37.05	D49.0
tonsil	C11.1	C79.89	D00.08	D10.6	D37.05	D49.0
wall (lateral) (posterior)	C14.0	C79.89	D00.08	D10.9	D37.05	D49.0
pia mater	C70.9	C79.40	—	D32.9	D42.9	D49.7
cerebral	C70.0	C79.32	—	D32.0	D42.0	D49.7
cranial	C70.0	C79.32	—	D32.0	D42.0	D49.7
spinal	C70.1	C79.49	—	D32.1	D42.1	D49.7
pillars of fauces	C09.1	C79.89	D00.08	D10.5	D37.05	D49.0
pineal (body) (gland)	C75.3	C79.89	D09.3	D35.4	D44.5	D49.7
pinna (ear) NEC — see also Neoplasm, skin, ear	C44.20-☑	C79.2	D04.2-☑	D23.2-☑	D48.5	D49.2
piriform fossa or sinus	C12	C79.89	D00.08	D10.7	D37.05	D49.0
pituitary (body) (fossa) (gland) (lobe)	C75.1	C79.89	D09.3	D35.2	D44.3	D49.7
placenta	C58	C79.82	D07.0	D26.7	D39.2	D49.59
pleura, pleural (cavity)	C38.4	C78.2	—	D19.0	D38.2	D49.1
overlapping lesion with heart or mediastinum	C38.8	—	—	—	—	—
parietal	C38.4	C78.2	—	D19.0	D38.2	D49.1
visceral	C38.4	C78.2	—	D19.0	D38.2	D49.1
plexus						
brachial	C47.1-☑	C79.89	—	D36.12	D48.2	D49.2
cervical	C47.0	C79.89	—	D36.11	D48.2	D49.2
choroid	C71.5	C79.31	—	D33.0	D43.0	D49.6
lumbosacral	C47.5	C79.89	—	D36.16	D48.2	D49.2
sacral	C47.5	C79.89	—	D36.16	D48.2	D49.2
pluriendocrine	C75.8	C79.89	D09.3	D35.7	D44.9	D49.7
pole						
frontal	C71.1	C79.31	—	D33.0	D43.0	D49.6
occipital	C71.4	C79.31	—	D33.0	D43.0	D49.6
pons (varolii)	C71.7	C79.31	—	D33.1	D43.1	D49.6
popliteal fossa or space	C76.5-☑	C79.89	D04.7-☑	D36.7	D48.7	D49.89
postcricoid (region)	C13.0	C79.89	D00.08	D10.7	D37.05	D49.0
posterior fossa (cranial)	C71.9	C79.31	—	D33.2	D43.2	D49.6
postnasal space	C11.9	C79.89	D00.08	D10.6	D37.05	D49.0
prepuce	C60.0	C79.82	D07.4	D29.0	D40.8	D49.59
prepylorus	C16.4	C78.89	D00.2	D13.1	D37.1	D49.0
presacral (region)	C76.3	C79.89	—	D36.7	D48.7	D49.89
prostate (gland)	C61	C79.82	D07.5	D29.1	D40.0	D49.59
utricle	C68.0	C79.19	D09.19	D30.4	D41.3	D49.59
pterygoid fossa	C49.0	C79.89	—	D21.0	D48.1	D49.2
pubic bone	C41.4	C79.51	—	D16.8	D48.0	D49.2
pudenda, pudendum (femaie)	C51.9	C79.82	D07.1	D28.0	D39.8	D49.59
pulmonary — see also Neoplasm, lung	C34.9-☑	C78.0-☑	D02.2-☑	D14.3-☑	D38.1	D49.1
putamen	C71.0	C79.31	—	D33.0	D43.0	D49.6
pyloric						
antrum	C16.3	C78.89	D00.2	D13.1	D37.1	D49.0
canal	C16.4	C78.89	D00.2	D13.1	D37.1	D49.0
pylorus	C16.4	C78.89	D00.2	D13.1	D37.1	D49.0
pyramid (brain)	C71.7	C79.31	—	D33.1	D43.1	D49.6
pyriform fossa or sinus	C12	C79.89	D00.08	D10.7	D37.05	D49.0
radius (any part)	C40.0-☑	C79.51	—	D16.0-☑	—	—
Rathke's pouch	C75.1	C79.89	D09.3	D35.2	D44.3	D49.7
rectosigmoid (junction)	C19	C78.5	D01.1	D12.7	D37.5	D49.0
overlapping lesion with anus or rectum	C21.8	—	—	—	—	—
rectouterine pouch	C48.1	C78.6	—	D20.1	D48.4	D49.0
rectovaginal septum or wall	C76.3	C79.89	D09.8	D36.7	D48.7	D49.89
rectovesical septum	C76.3	C79.89	D09.8	D36.7	D48.7	D49.89
rectum (ampulla)	C20	C78.5	D01.2	D12.8	D37.5	D49.0

☑ Additional Character Required — Refer to the Tabular List for Character Selection

Neoplasm, neoplastic — continued	Malignant Primary	Malignant Secondary	Ca in situ	Benign	Uncertain Behavior	Unspecified Behavior
rectum — continued						
and colon	C19	C78.5	D01.1	D12.7	D37.5	D49.0
overlapping lesion with anus or rectosigmoid junction	C21.8	—	—	—	—	—
renal	C64.-☑	C79.0-☑	D09.19	D30.0-☑	D41.0-☑	D49.51-☑
calyx	C65.-☑	C79.0-☑	D09.19	D30.1-☑	D41.1-☑	D49.51-☑
hilus	C65.-☑	C79.0-☑	D09.19	D30.1-☑	D41.1-☑	D49.51-☑
parenchyma	C64.-☑	C79.0-☑	D09.19	D30.0-☑	D41.0-☑	D49.51-☑
pelvis	C65.-☑	C79.0-☑	D09.19	D30.1-☑	D41.1-☑	D49.51-☑
respiratory						
organs or system NEC	C39.9	C78.30	D02.4	D14.4	D38.6	D49.1
tract NEC	C39.9	C78.30	D02.4	D14.4	D38.5	D49.1
upper	C39.0	C78.30	D02.4	D14.4	D38.5	D49.1
retina	C69.2-☑	C79.49	D09.2-☑	D31.2-☑	D48.7	D49.81
retrobulbar	C69.6-☑	C79.49	—	D31.6-☑	D48.7	D49.89
retrocecal	C48.0	C78.6	—	D20.0	D48.3	D49.0
retromolar (area) (triangle) (trigone)	C06.2	C79.89	D00.00	D10.39	D37.09	D49.0
retro-orbital	C76.0	C79.89	D09.8	D36.7	D48.7	D49.89
retroperitoneal (space) (tissue)	C48.0	C78.6	—	D20.0	D48.3	D49.0
retroperitoneum	C48.0	C78.6	—	D20.0	D48.3	D49.0
retropharyngeal	C14.0	C79.89	D00.08	D10.9	D37.05	D49.0
retrovesical (septum)	C76.3	C79.89	D09.8	D36.7	D48.7	D49.89
rhinencephalon	C71.0	C79.31	—	D33.0	D43.0	D49.6
rib	C41.3	C79.51	—	D16.7	D48.0	D49.2
Rosenmuller's fossa	C11.2	C79.89	D00.08	D10.6	D37.05	D49.0
round ligament	C57.2-☑	C79.82	—	D28.2	D39.8	D49.59
sacrococcyx, sacrococcygeal region	C41.4	C79.51	—	D16.8	D48.0	D49.2
	C76.3	C79.89	D09.8	D36.7	D48.7	D49.89
sacrouterine ligament	C57.3	C79.82	—	D28.2	D39.8	D49.59
sacrum, sacral (vertebra)	C41.4	C79.51	—	D16.8	D48.0	D49.2
salivary gland or duct (major)	C08.9	C79.89	D00.00	D11.9	D37.039	D49.0
minor NEC	C06.9	C79.89	D00.00	D10.39	D37.04	D49.0
overlapping lesion	C08.9	—	—	—	—	—
parotid	C07	C79.89	D00.00	D11.0	D37.030	D49.0
pluriglandular	C08.9	C79.89	D00.00	D11.9	D37.039	D49.0
sublingual	C08.1	C79.89	D00.00	D11.7	D37.031	D49.0
submandibular	C08.0	C79.89	D00.00	D11.7	D37.032	D49.0
submaxillary	C08.0	C79.89	D00.00	D11.7	D37.032	D49.0
salpinx (uterine)	C57.0-☑	C79.82	D07.39	D28.2	D39.8	D49.59
Santorini's duct	C25.3	C78.89	D01.7	D13.6	D37.8	D49.0
scalp	C44.40	C79.2	D04.4	D23.4	D48.5	D49.2
basal cell carcinoma	C44.41	—	—	—	—	—
specified type NEC	C44.49	—	—	—	—	—
squamous cell carcinoma	C44.42	—	—	—	—	—
scapula (any part)	C40.0-☑	C79.51	—	D16.0-☑	—	—
scapular region	C76.1	C79.89	D09.8	D36.7	D48.7	D49.89
scar NEC — see also Neoplasm, skin, by site	C44.90	C79.2	D04.9	D23.9	D48.5	D49.2
sciatic nerve	C47.2-☑	C79.89	—	D36.13	D48.2	D49.2
sclera	C69.4-☑	C79.49	D09.2-☑	D31.4-☑	D48.7	D49.89
scrotum (skin)	C63.2	C79.82	D07.61	D29.4	D40.8	D49.59
sebaceous gland — see Neoplasm, skin						
sella turcica	C75.1	C79.89	D09.3	D35.2	D44.3	D49.7
bone	C41.0	C79.51	—	D16.4	D48.0	D49.2
semilunar cartilage (knee)	C40.2-☑	C79.51	—	D16.2-☑	D48.0	D49.2
seminal vesicle	C63.7	C79.82	D07.69	D29.8	D40.8	D49.59
septum						
nasal	C30.0	C78.39	D02.3	D14.0	D38.5	D49.1
posterior margin	C11.3	C79.89	D00.08	D10.6	D37.05	D49.0
rectovaginal	C76.3	C79.89	D09.8	D36.7	D48.7	D49.89
rectovesical	C76.3	C79.89	D09.8	D36.7	D48.7	D49.89

Neoplasm, neoplastic — continued	Malignant Primary	Malignant Secondary	Ca in situ	Benign	Uncertain Behavior	Unspecified Behavior
septum — continued						
urethrovaginal	C57.9	C79.82	D07.30	D28.9	D39.9	D49.59
vesicovaginal	C57.9	C79.82	D07.30	D28.9	D39.9	D49.59
shoulder NEC	C76.4-☑	C79.89	D04.6-☑	D36.7	D48.7	D49.89
sigmoid flexure (lower) (upper)	C18.7	C78.5	D01.0	D12.5	D37.4	D49.0
sinus (accessory)	C31.9	C78.39	D02.3	D14.0	D38.5	D49.1
bone (any)	C41.0	C79.51	—	D16.4	D48.0	D49.2
ethmoidal	C31.1	C78.39	D02.3	D14.0	D38.5	D49.1
frontal	C31.2	C78.39	D02.3	D14.0	D38.5	D49.1
maxillary	C31.0	C78.39	D02.3	D14.0	D38.5	D49.1
nasal, paranasal NEC	C31.9	C78.39	D02.3	D14.0	D38.5	D49.1
overlapping lesion	C31.8	—	—	—	—	—
pyriform	C12	C79.89	D00.08	D10.7	D37.05	D49.0
sphenoid	C31.3	C78.39	D02.3	D14.0	D38.5	D49.1
skeleton, skeletal NEC	C41.9	C79.51	—	D16.9	D48.0	D49.2
Skene's gland	C68.1	C79.19	D09.19	D30.8	D41.8	D49.59
skin NOS	C44.90	C79.2	D04.9	D23.9	D48.5	D49.2
abdominal wall	C44.509	C79.2	D04.5	D23.5	D48.5	D49.2
basal cell carcinoma	C44.519	—	—	—	—	—
specified type NEC	C44.599	—	—	—	—	—
squamous cell carcinoma	C44.529	—	—	—	—	—
ala nasi — see also Neoplasm, nose, skin	C44.301	C79.2	D04.39	D23.39	D48.5	D49.2
ankle — see also Neoplasm, skin, limb, lower	C44.70-☑	C79.2	D04.7-☑	D23.7-☑	D48.5	D49.2
antecubital space — see also Neoplasm, skin, limb, upper	C44.60-☑	C79.2	D04.6-☑	D23.6-☑	D48.5	D49.2
anus	C44.500	C79.2	D04.5	D23.5	D48.5	D49.2
basal cell carcinoma	C44.510	—	—	—	—	—
specified type NEC	C44.590	—	—	—	—	—
squamous cell carcinoma	C44.520	—	—	—	—	—
arm — see also Neoplasm, skin, limb, upper	C44.60-☑	C79.2	D04.6-☑	D23.6-☑	D48.5	D49.2
auditory canal (external) — see also Neoplasm, skin, ear	C44.20-☑	C79.2	D04.2-☑	D23.2-☑	D48.5	D49.2
auricle (ear) — see also Neoplasm, skin, ear	C44.20-☑	C79.2	D04.2-☑	D23.2-☑	D48.5	D49.2
auricular canal (external) — see also Neoplasm, skin, ear	C44.20-☑	C79.2	D04.2-☑	D23.2-☑	D48.5	D49.2
axilla, axillary fold — see also Neoplasm, skin, trunk	C44.509	C79.2	D04.5	D23.5	D48.5	D49.2
back — see also Neoplasm, skin, trunk	C44.509	C79.2	D04.5	D23.5	D48.5	D49.2
basal cell carcinoma	C44.91	—	—	—	—	—
breast	C44.501	C79.2	D04.5	D23.5	D48.5	D49.2
basal cell carcinoma	C44.511	—	—	—	—	—
specified type NEC	C44.591	—	—	—	—	—
squamous cell carcinoma	C44.521	—	—	—	—	—
brow — see also Neoplasm, skin, face	C44.309	C79.2	D04.39	D23.39	D48.5	D49.2
buttock — see also Neoplasm, skin, trunk	C44.509	C79.2	D04.5	D23.5	D48.5	D49.2

☑ Additional Character Required — Refer to the Tabular List for Character Selection

Neoplasm, neoplastic — continued / skin — continued	Malignant Primary	Malignant Secondary	Ca in situ	Benign	Uncertain Behavior	Unspecified Behavior
calf — see also Neoplasm, skin, limb, lower	C44.70-✓	C79.2	D04.7-✓	D23.7-✓	D48.5	D49.2
canthus (eye) (inner) (outer)	C44.10-✓	C79.2	D04.1-✓	D23.1-✓	D48.5	D49.2
basal cell carcinoma	C44.11-✓	—	—	—	—	—
sebaceous cell	C44.13-✓	—	—	—	—	—
specified type NEC	C44.19-✓	—	—	—	—	—
squamous cell carcinoma	C44.12-✓	—	—	—	—	—
cervical region — see also Neoplasm, skin, neck	C44.40	C79.2	D04.4	D23.4	D48.5	D49.2
cheek (external) — see also Neoplasm, skin, face	C44.309	C79.2	D04.39	D23.39	D48.5	D49.2
chest (wall) — see also Neoplasm, skin, trunk	C44.509	C79.2	D04.5	D23.5	D48.5	D49.2
chin — see also Neoplasm, skin, face	C44.309	C79.2	D04.39	D23.39	D48.5	D49.2
clavicular area — see also Neoplasm, skin, trunk	C44.509	C79.2	D04.5	D23.5	D48.5	D49.2
clitoris	C51.2	C79.82	D07.1	D28.0	D39.8	D49.59
columnella — see also Neoplasm, skin, face	C44.309	C79.2	D04.39	D23.39	D48.5	D49.2
concha — see also Neoplasm, skin, ear	C44.20-✓	C79.2	D04.2-✓	D23.2-✓	D48.5	D49.2
ear (external)	C44.20-✓	C79.2	D04.2-✓	D23.2-✓	D48.5	D49.2
basal cell carcinoma	C44.21-✓	—	—	—	—	—
specified type NEC	C44.29-✓	—	—	—	—	—
squamous cell carcinoma	C44.22-✓	—	—	—	—	—
elbow — see also Neoplasm, skin, limb, upper	C44.60-✓	C79.2	D04.6-✓	D23.6-✓	D48.5	D49.2
eyebrow — see also Neoplasm, skin, face	C44.309	C79.2	D04.39	D23.39	D48.5	D49.2
eyelid	C44.10-✓	C79.2	D04.1-✓	D23.1-✓	D48.5	D49.2
basal cell carcinoma	C44.11-✓	—	—	—	—	—
sebaceous cell	C44.13-✓	—	—	—	—	—
specified type NEC	C44.19-✓	—	—	—	—	—
squamous cell carcinoma	C44.12-✓	—	—	—	—	—
face NOS	C44.300	C79.2	D04.30	D23.30	D48.5	D49.2
basal cell carcinoma	C44.310	—	—	—	—	—
specified type NEC	C44.390	—	—	—	—	—
squamous cell carcinoma	C44.320	—	—	—	—	—
female genital organs (external)	C51.9	C79.82	D07.1	D28.0	D39.8	D49.59
clitoris	C51.2	C79.82	D07.1	D28.0	D39.8	D49.59
labium NEC	C51.9	C79.82	D07.1	D28.0	D39.8	D49.59
majus	C51.0	C79.82	D07.1	D28.0	D39.8	D49.59
minus	C51.1	C79.82	D07.1	D28.0	D39.8	D49.59
pudendum	C51.9	C79.82	D07.1	D28.0	D39.8	D49.59
vulva	C51.9	C79.82	D07.1	D28.0	D39.8	D49.59
finger — see also Neoplasm, skin, limb, upper	C44.60-✓	C79.2	D04.6-✓	D23.6-✓	D48.5	D49.2
flank — see also Neoplasm, skin, trunk	C44.509	C79.2	D04.5	D23.5	D48.5	D49.2
foot — see also Neoplasm, skin, limb, lower	C44.70-✓	C79.2	D04.7-✓	D23.7-✓	D48.5	D49.2

Neoplasm, neoplastic — continued / skin — continued	Malignant Primary	Malignant Secondary	Ca in situ	Benign	Uncertain Behavior	Unspecified Behavior
forearm — see also Neoplasm, skin, limb, upper	C44.60-✓	C79.2	D04.6-✓	D23.6-✓	D48.5	D49.2
forehead — see also Neoplasm, skin, face	C44.309	C79.2	D04.39	D23.39	D48.5	D49.2
glabella — see also Neoplasm, skin, face	C44.309	C79.2	D04.39	D23.39	D48.5	D49.2
gluteal region — see also Neoplasm, skin, trunk	C44.509	C79.2	D04.5	D23.5	D48.5	D49.2
groin — see also Neoplasm, skin, trunk	C44.509	C79.2	D04.5	D23.5	D48.5	D49.2
hand — see also Neoplasm, skin, limb, upper	C44.60-✓	C79.2	D04.6-✓	D23.6-✓	D48.5	D49.2
head NEC — see also Neoplasm, skin, scalp	C44.40	C79.2	D04.4	D23.4	D48.5	D49.2
heel — see also Neoplasm, skin, limb, lower	C44.70-✓	C79.2	D04.7-✓	D23.7-✓	D48.5	D49.2
helix — see also Neoplasm, skin, ear	C44.20-✓	C79.2	D04.2-✓	D23.2-✓	D48.5	D49.2
hip — see also Neoplasm, skin, limb, lower	C44.70-✓	C79.2	D04.7-✓	D23.7-✓	D48.5	D49.2
infraclavicular region — see also Neoplasm, skin, trunk	C44.509	C79.2	D04.5	D23.5	D48.5	D49.2
inguinal region — see also Neoplasm, skin, trunk	C44.509	C79.2	D04.5	D23.5	D48.5	D49.2
jaw — see also Neoplasm, skin, face	C44.309	C79.2	D04.39	D23.39	D48.5	D49.2
Kaposi's sarcoma — see Kaposi's, sarcoma, skin						
knee — see also Neoplasm, skin, limb, lower	C44.70-✓	C79.2	D04.7-✓	D23.7-✓	D48.5	D49.2
labia						
majora	C51.0	C79.82	D07.1	D28.0	D39.8	D49.59
minora	C51.1	C79.82	D07.1	D28.0	D39.8	D49.59
leg — see also Neoplasm, skin, limb, lower	C44.70-✓	C79.2	D04.7-✓	D23.7-✓	D48.5	D49.2
lid (lower) (upper)	C44.10-✓	C79.2	D04.1-✓	D23.1-✓	D48.5	D49.2
basal cell carcinoma	C44.11-✓	—	—	—	—	—
sebaceous cell	C44.13-✓	—	—	—	—	—
specified type NEC	C44.19-✓	—	—	—	—	—
squamous cell carcinoma	C44.12-✓	—	—	—	—	—
limb NEC	C44.90	C79.2	D04.9	D23.9	D48.5	D49.2
basal cell carcinoma	C44.91	—	—	—	—	—
lower	C44.70-✓	C79.2	D04.7-✓	D23.7-✓	D48.5	D49.2
basal cell carcinoma	C44.71-✓	—	—	—	—	—
specified type NEC	C44.79-✓	—	—	—	—	—
squamous cell carcinoma	C44.72-✓	—	—	—	—	—
upper	C44.60-✓	C79.2	D04.6-✓	D23.6-✓	D48.5	D49.2
basal cell carcinoma	C44.61-✓	—	—	—	—	—
specified type NEC	C44.69-✓	—	—	—	—	—
squamous cell carcinoma	C44.62-✓	—	—	—	—	—
lip (lower) (upper)	C44.00	C79.2	D04.0	D23.0	D48.5	D49.2

✓ **Additional Character Required — Refer to the Tabular List for Character Selection**

Neoplasm, neoplastic — continued	Malignant Primary	Malignant Secondary	Ca in situ	Benign	Uncertain Behavior	Unspecified Behavior
skin — *continued*						
lip — *continued*						
basal cell carcinoma	C44.01	—	—	—	—	—
specified type NEC	C44.09	—	—	—	—	—
squamous cell carcinoma	C44.02	—	—	—	—	—
male genital organs	C63.9	C79.82	D07.60	D29.9	D40.8	D49.59
penis	C60.9	C79.82	D07.4	D29.0	D40.8	D49.59
prepuce	C60.0	C79.82	D07.4	D29.0	D40.8	D49.59
scrotum	C63.2	C79.82	D07.61	D29.4	D40.8	D49.59
mastectomy site (skin) — *see also* Neoplasm, skin, breast	C44.501	C79.2	—	—	—	—
specified as breast tissue	C50.8-✓	C79.81	—	—	—	—
meatus, acoustic (external) — *see also* Neoplasm, skin, ear	C44.20-✓	C79.2	D04.2-✓	D23.2-✓	D48.5	D49.2
melanotic — *see* Melanoma						
Merkel cell — *see* Carcinoma, Merkel cell						
nates — *see also* Neoplasm, skin, trunk	C44.509	C79.2	D04.5	D23.5	D48.5	D49.2
neck	C44.40	C79.2	D04.4	D23.4	D48.5	D49.2
basal cell carcinoma	C44.41	—	—	—	—	—
specified type NEC	C44.49	—	—	—	—	—
squamous cell carcinoma	C44.42	—	—	—	—	—
nevus — *see* Nevus, skin						
nose (external) — *see also* Neoplasm, nose, skin	C44.301	C79.2	D04.39	D23.39	D48.5	D49.2
overlapping lesion	C44.80	—	—	—	—	—
basal cell carcinoma	C44.81	—	—	—	—	—
specified type NEC	C44.89	—	—	—	—	—
squamous cell carcinoma	C44.82	—	—	—	—	—
palm — *see also* Neoplasm, skin, limb, upper	C44.60-✓	C79.2	D04.6-✓	D23.6-✓	D48.5	D49.2
palpebra	C44.10-✓	C79.2	D04.1-✓	D23.1-✓	D48.5	D49.2
basal cell carcinoma	C44.11-✓	—	—	—	—	—
sebaceous cell	C44.13-✓	—	—	—	—	—
specified type NEC	C44.19-✓	—	—	—	—	—
squamous cell carcinoma	C44.12-✓	—	—	—	—	—
penis NEC	C60.9	C79.82	D07.4	D29.0	D40.8	D49.59
perianal — *see also* Neoplasm, skin, anus	C44.500	C79.2	D04.5	D23.5	D48.5	D49.2
perineum — *see also* Neoplasm, skin, anus	C44.500	C79.2	D04.5	D23.5	D48.5	D49.2
pinna — *see also* Neoplasm, skin, ear	C44.20-✓	C79.2	D04.2-✓	D23.2-✓	D48.5	D49.2
plantar — *see also* Neoplasm, skin, limb, lower	C44.70-✓	C79.2	D04.7-✓	D23.7-✓	D48.5	D49.2
popliteal fossa or space — *see also* Neoplasm, skin, limb, lower	C44.70-✓	C79.2	D04.7-✓	D23.7-✓	D48.5	D49.2
prepuce	C60.0	C79.82	D07.4	D29.0	D40.8	D49.59

Neoplasm, neoplastic — continued	Malignant Primary	Malignant Secondary	Ca in situ	Benign	Uncertain Behavior	Unspecified Behavior
skin — *continued*						
pubes — *see also* Neoplasm, skin, trunk	C44.509	C79.2	D04.5	D23.5	D48.5	D49.2
sacrococcygeal region — *see also* Neoplasm, skin, trunk	C44.509	C79.2	D04.5	D23.5	D48.5	D49.2
scalp	C44.40	C79.2	D04.4	D23.4	D48.5	D49.2
basal cell carcinoma	C44.41	—	—	—	—	—
specified type NEC	C44.49	—	—	—	—	—
squamous cell carcinoma	C44.42	—	—	—	—	—
scapular region — *see also* Neoplasm, skin, trunk	C44.509	C79.2	D04.5	D23.5	D48.5	D49.2
scrotum	C63.2	C79.82	D07.61	D29.4	D40.8	D49.59
shoulder — *see also* Neoplasm, skin, limb, upper	C44.60-✓	C79.2	D04.6-✓	D23.6-✓	D48.5	D49.2
sole (foot) — *see also* Neoplasm, skin, limb, lower	C44.70-✓	C79.2	D04.7-✓	D23.7-✓	D48.5	D49.2
specified sites NEC	C44.80	C79.2	D04.8	D23.9	D48.5	D49.2
basal cell carcinoma	C44.81	—	—	—	—	—
specified type NEC	C44.89	—	—	—	—	—
squamous cell carcinoma	C44.82	—	—	—	—	—
specified type NEC	C44.99	—	—	—	—	—
squamous cell carcinoma	C44.92	—	—	—	—	—
submammary fold — *see also* Neoplasm, skin, trunk	C44.509	C79.2	D04.5	D23.5	D48.5	D49.2
supraclavicular region — *see also* Neoplasm, skin, neck	C44.40	C79.2	D04.4	D23.4	D48.5	D49.2
temple — *see also* Neoplasm, skin, face	C44.309	C79.2	D04.39	D23.39	D48.5	D49.2
thigh — *see also* Neoplasm, skin, limb, lower	C44.70-✓	C79.2	D04.7-✓	D23.7-✓	D48.5	D49.2
thoracic wall — *see also* Neoplasm, skin, trunk	C44.509	C79.2	D04.5	D23.5	D48.5	D49.2
thumb — *see also* Neoplasm, skin, limb, upper	C44.60-✓	C79.2	D04.6-✓	D23.6-✓	D48.5	D49.2
toe — *see also* Neoplasm, skin, limb, lower	C44.70-✓	C79.2	D04.7-✓	D23.7-✓	D48.5	D49.2
tragus — *see also* Neoplasm, skin, ear	C44.20-✓	C79.2	D04.2-✓	D23.2-✓	D48.5	D49.2
trunk	C44.509	C79.2	D04.5	D23.5	D48.5	D49.2
basal cell carcinoma	C44.519	—	—	—	—	—
specified type NEC	C44.599	—	—	—	—	—
squamous cell carcinoma	C44.529	—	—	—	—	—
umbilicus — *see also* Neoplasm, skin, trunk	C44.509	C79.2	D04.5	D23.5	D48.5	D49.2
vulva	C51.9	C79.82	D07.1	D28.0	D39.8	D49.59
overlapping lesion	C51.8	—	—	—	—	—
wrist — *see also* Neoplasm, skin, limb, upper	C44.60-✓	C79.2	D04.6-✓	D23.6-✓	D48.5	D49.2
skull	C41.0	C79.51	—	D16.4	D48.0	D49.2

✓ **Additional Character Required — Refer to the Tabular List for Character Selection**

Neoplasm Table

Neoplasm, neoplastic	Malignant Primary	Malignant Secondary	Ca in situ	Benign	Uncertain Behavior	Unspecified Behavior
— continued						
soft parts or tissues — see Neoplasm, connective tissue						
specified site NEC	C76.8	C79.89	D09.8	D36.7	D48.7	D49.89
spermatic cord	C63.1-☑	C79.89	D07.69	D29.8	D40.8	D49.59
sphenoid	C31.3	C78.39	D02.3	D14.0	D38.5	D49.1
bone	C41.0	C79.51	—	D16.4	D48.0	D49.2
sinus	C31.3	C78.39	D02.3	D14.0	D38.5	D49.1
sphincter						
anal	C21.1	C78.5	D01.3	D12.9	D37.8	D49.0
of Oddi	C24.0	C78.89	D01.5	D13.5	D37.6	D49.0
spine, spinal (column)	C41.2	C79.51	—	D16.6	D48.0	D49.2
bulb	C71.7	C79.31	—	D33.1	D43.1	D49.6
coccyx	C41.4	C79.51	—	D16.8	D48.0	D49.2
cord (cervical) (lumbar) (sacral) (thoracic)	C72.0	C79.49	—	D33.4	D43.4	D49.7
dura mater	C70.1	C79.49	—	D32.1	D42.1	D49.7
lumbosacral	C41.2	C79.51	—	D16.6	D48.0	D49.2
marrow NEC	C96.9	C79.52	—	—	D47.9	D49.89
membrane	C70.1	C79.49	—	D32.1	D42.1	D49.7
meninges	C70.1	C79.49	—	D32.1	D42.1	D49.7
nerve (root)	C47.9	C79.89	—	D36.10	D48.2	D49.2
pia mater	C70.1	C79.49	—	D32.1	D42.1	D49.7
root	C47.9	C79.89	—	D36.10	D48.2	D49.2
sacrum	C41.4	C79.51	—	D16.8	D48.0	D49.2
spleen, splenic NEC	C26.1	C78.89	D01.7	D13.9	D37.8	D49.0
flexure (colon)	C18.5	C78.5	D01.0	D12.3	D37.4	D49.0
stem, brain	C71.7	C79.31	—	D33.1	D43.1	D49.6
Stensen's duct	C07	C79.89	D00.00	D11.0	D37.030	D49.0
sternum	C41.3	C79.51	—	D16.7	D48.0	D49.2
stomach	C16.9	C78.89	D00.2	D13.1	D37.1	D49.0
antrum (pyloric)	C16.3	C78.89	D00.2	D13.1	D37.1	D49.0
body	C16.2	C78.89	D00.2	D13.1	D37.1	D49.0
cardia	C16.0	C78.89	D00.2	D13.1	D37.1	D49.0
cardiac orifice	C16.0	C78.89	D00.2	D13.1	D37.1	D49.0
corpus	C16.2	C78.89	D00.2	D13.1	D37.1	D49.0
fundus	C16.1	C78.89	D00.2	D13.1	D37.1	D49.0
greater curvature NEC	C16.6	C78.89	D00.2	D13.1	D37.1	D49.0
lesser curvature NEC	C16.5	C78.89	D00.2	D13.1	D37.1	D49.0
overlapping lesion	C16.8	—	—	—	—	—
prepylorus	C16.4	C78.89	D00.2	D13.1	D37.1	D49.0
pylorus	C16.4	C78.89	D00.2	D13.1	D37.1	D49.0
wall NEC	C16.9	C78.89	D00.2	D13.1	D37.1	D49.0
anterior NEC	C16.8	C78.89	D00.2	D13.1	D37.1	D49.0
posterior NEC	C16.8	C78.89	D00.2	D13.1	D37.1	D49.0
stroma, endometrial	C54.1	C79.82	D07.0	D26.1	D39.0	D49.59
stump, cervical	C53.8	C79.82	D06.7	D26.0	D39.0	D49.59
subcutaneous (nodule) (tissue) NEC — see Neoplasm, connective tissue						
subdural	C70.9	C79.32	—	D32.9	D42.9	D49.7
subglottis, subglottic	C32.2	C78.39	D02.0	D14.1	D38.0	D49.1
sublingual	C04.9	C79.89	D00.06	D10.2	D37.09	D49.0
gland or duct	C08.1	C79.89	D00.00	D11.7	D37.031	D49.0
submandibular gland	C08.0	C79.89	D00.00	D11.7	D37.032	D49.0
submaxillary gland or duct	C08.0	C79.89	D00.00	D11.7	D37.032	D49.0
submental	C76.0	C79.89	D09.8	D36.7	D48.7	D49.89
subpleural	C34.9-☑	C78.0-☑	D02.2-☑	D14.3-☑	D38.1	D49.1
substernal	C38.1	C78.1	—	D15.2	D38.3	D49.89
sudoriferous, sudoriparous gland, site unspecified	C44.90	C79.2	D04.9	D23.9	D48.5	D49.2
specified site — see Neoplasm, skin						
supraclavicular region	C76.0	C79.89	D09.8	D36.7	D48.7	D49.89
supraglottis	C32.1	C78.39	D02.0	D14.1	D38.0	D49.1
suprarenal	C74.9-☑	C79.7-☑	D09.3	D35.0-☑	D44.1-☑	D49.7
capsule	C74.9-☑	C79.7-☑	D09.3	D35.0-☑	D44.1-☑	D49.7

Neoplasm, neoplastic	Malignant Primary	Malignant Secondary	Ca in situ	Benign	Uncertain Behavior	Unspecified Behavior
— continued						
suprarenal — continued						
cortex	C74.0-☑	C79.7-☑	D09.3	D35.0-☑	D44.1-☑	D49.7
gland	C74.9-☑	C79.7-☑	D09.3	D35.0-☑	D44.1-☑	D49.7
medulla	C74.1-☑	C79.7-☑	D09.3	D35.0-☑	D44.1-☑	D49.7
suprasellar (region)	C71.9	C79.31	—	D33.2	D43.2	D49.6
supratentorial (brain) NEC	C71.0	C79.31	—	D33.0	D43.0	D49.6
sweat gland (apocrine) (eccrine), site unspecified	C44.90	C79.2	D04.9	D23.9	D48.5	D49.2
specified site — see Neoplasm, skin						
sympathetic nerve or nervous system NEC	C47.9	C79.89	—	D36.10	D48.2	D49.2
symphysis pubis	C41.4	C79.51	—	D16.8	D48.0	D49.2
synovial membrane — see Neoplasm, connective tissue						
tapetum, brain	C71.8	C79.31	—	D33.2	D43.2	D49.6
tarsus (any bone)	C40.3-☑	C79.51	—	D16.3-☑	—	—
temple (skin) — see also Neoplasm, skin, face						
face	C44.309	C79.2	D04.39	D23.39	D48.5	D49.2
temporal						
bone	C41.0	C79.51	—	D16.4	D48.0	D49.2
lobe or pole	C71.2	C79.31	—	D33.0	D43.0	D49.6
region	C76.0	C79.89	D09.8	D36.7	D48.7	D49.89
skin — see also Neoplasm, skin, face						
face	C44.309	C79.2	D04.39	D23.39	D48.5	D49.2
tendon (sheath) — see Neoplasm, connective tissue						
tentorium (cerebelli)	C70.0	C79.32	—	D32.0	D42.0	D49.7
testis, testes	C62.9-☑	C79.82	D07.69	D29.2-☑	D40.1-☑	D49.59
descended	C62.1-☑	C79.82	D07.69	D29.2-☑	D40.1-☑	D49.59
ectopic	C62.0-☑	C79.82	D07.69	D29.2-☑	D40.1-☑	D49.59
retained	C62.0-☑	C79.82	D07.69	D29.2-☑	D40.1-☑	D49.59
scrotal	C62.1-☑	C79.82	D07.69	D29.2-☑	D40.1-☑	D49.59
undescended	C62.0-☑	C79.82	D07.69	D29.2-☑	D40.1-☑	D49.59
unspecified whether descended or undescended	C62.9-☑	C79.82	D07.69	D29.2-☑	D40.1-☑	D49.59
thalamus	C71.0	C79.31	—	D33.0	D43.0	D49.6
thigh NEC	C76.5-☑	C79.89	D04.7-☑	D36.7	D48.7	D49.89
thorax, thoracic (cavity) (organs NEC)	C76.1	C79.89	D09.8	D36.7	D48.7	D49.89
duct	C49.3	C79.89	—	D21.3	D48.1	D49.2
wall NEC	C76.1	C79.89	D09.8	D36.7	D48.7	D49.89
throat	C14.0	C79.89	D00.08	D10.9	D37.05	D49.0
thumb NEC	C76.4-☑	C79.89	D04.6-☑	D36.7	D48.7	D49.89
thymus (gland)	C37	C79.89	D09.3	D15.0	D38.4	D49.89
thyroglossal duct	C73	C79.89	D09.3	D34	D44.0	D49.7
thyroid (gland)	C73	C79.89	D09.3	D34	D44.0	D49.7
cartilage	C32.3	C78.39	D02.0	D14.1	D38.0	D49.1
tibia (any part)	C40.2-☑	C79.51	—	D16.2-☑	—	—
toe NEC	C76.5-☑	C79.89	D04.7-☑	D36.7	D48.7	D49.89
tongue	C02.9	C79.89	D00.07	D10.1	D37.02	D49.0
anterior (two-thirds) NEC	C02.3	C79.89	D00.07	D10.1	D37.02	D49.0
dorsal surface	C02.0	C79.89	D00.07	D10.1	D37.02	D49.0
ventral surface	C02.2	C79.89	D00.07	D10.1	D37.02	D49.0
base (dorsal surface)	C01	C79.89	D00.07	D10.1	D37.02	D49.0
border (lateral)	C02.1	C79.89	D00.07	D10.1	D37.02	D49.0
dorsal surface NEC	C02.0	C79.89	D00.07	D10.1	D37.02	D49.0
fixed part NEC	C01	C79.89	D00.07	D10.1	D37.02	D49.0
foramen cecum	C02.0	C79.89	D00.07	D10.1	D37.02	D49.0
frenulum linguae	C02.2	C79.89	D00.07	D10.1	D37.02	D49.0
junctional zone	C02.8	C79.89	D00.07	D10.1	D37.02	D49.0
margin (lateral)	C02.1	C79.89	D00.07	D10.1	D37.02	D49.0
midline NEC	C02.0	C79.89	D00.07	D10.1	D37.02	D49.0
mobile part NEC	C02.3	C79.89	D00.07	D10.1	D37.02	D49.0

☑ Additional Character Required — Refer to the Tabular List for Character Selection

Neoplasm, neoplastic — continued	Malignant Primary	Malignant Secondary	Ca in situ	Benign	Uncertain Behavior	Unspecified Behavior
tongue — continued						
overlapping lesion	C02.8	—	—	—	—	—
posterior (third)	C01	C79.89	D00.07	D10.1	D37.02	D49.0
root	C01	C79.89	D00.07	D10.1	D37.02	D49.0
surface (dorsal)	C02.0	C79.89	D00.07	D10.1	D37.02	D49.0
base	C01	C79.89	D00.07	D10.1	D37.02	D49.0
ventral	C02.2	C79.89	D00.07	D10.1	D37.02	D49.0
tip	C02.1	C79.89	D00.07	D10.1	D37.02	D49.0
tonsil	C02.4	C79.89	D00.07	D10.1	D37.02	D49.0
tonsil	C09.9	C79.89	D00.08	D10.4	D37.05	D49.0
fauces, faucial	C09.9	C79.89	D00.08	D10.4	D37.05	D49.0
lingual	C02.4	C79.89	D00.07	D10.1	D37.02	D49.0
overlapping sites	C09.8	—	—	—	—	—
palatine	C09.9	C79.89	D00.08	D10.4	D37.05	D49.0
pharyngeal	C11.1	C79.89	D00.08	D10.6	D37.05	D49.0
pillar (anterior) (posterior)	C09.1	C79.89	D00.08	D10.5	D37.05	D49.0
tonsillar fossa	C09.0	C79.89	D00.08	D10.5	D37.05	D49.0
tooth socket NEC	C03.9	C79.89	D00.03	D10.39	D37.09	D49.0
trachea (cartilage) (mucosa)	C33	C78.39	D02.1	D14.2	D38.1	D49.1
overlapping lesion with bronchus or lung	C34.8-☑	—	—	—	—	—
tracheobronchial	C34.8-☑	C78.39	D02.1	D14.2	D38.1	D49.1
overlapping lesion with lung	C34.8-☑	—	—	—	—	—
tragus — see also Neoplasm, skin, ear	C44.20-☑	C79.2	D04.2-☑	D23.2-☑	D48.5	D49.2
trunk NEC	C76.8	C79.89	D04.5	D36.7	D48.7	D49.89
tubo-ovarian	C57.8	C79.82	D07.39	D28.7	D39.8	D49.59
tunica vaginalis	C63.7	C79.82	D07.69	D29.8	D40.8	D49.59
turbinate (bone)	C41.0	C79.51	—	D16.4	D48.0	D49.2
nasal	C30.0	C78.39	D02.3	D14.0	D38.5	D49.1
tympanic cavity	C30.1	C78.39	D02.3	D14.0	D38.5	D49.1
ulna (any part)	C40.0-☑	C79.51	—	D16.0-☑	—	—
umbilicus, umbilical — see also Neoplasm, skin, trunk	C44.509	C79.2	D04.5	D23.5	D48.5	D49.2
uncus, brain	C71.2	C79.31	—	D33.0	D43.0	D49.6
unknown site or unspecified	C80.1	C79.9	D09.9	D36.9	D48.9	D49.9
urachus	C67.7	C79.11	D09.0	D30.3	D41.4	D49.4
ureter-bladder (junction)	C67.6	C79.11	D09.0	D30.3	D41.4	D49.4
ureter, ureteral	C66.-☑	C79.19	D09.19	D30.2-☑	D41.2-☑	D49.59
orifice (bladder)	C67.6	C79.11	D09.0	D30.3	D41.4	D49.4
urethra, urethral (gland)	C68.0	C79.19	D09.19	D30.4	D41.3	D49.59
orifice, internal	C67.5	C79.11	D09.0	D30.3	D41.4	D49.4
urethrovaginal (septum)	C57.9	C79.82	D07.30	D28.9	D39.8	D49.59
urinary organ or system	C68.9	C79.10	D09.10	D30.9	D41.9	D49.59
bladder — see Neoplasm, bladder						
overlapping lesion	C68.8	—	—	—	—	—
specified sites NEC	C68.8	C79.19	D09.19	D30.8	D41.8	D49.59
utero-ovarian	C57.8	C79.82	D07.39	D28.7	D39.8	D49.59
ligament	C57.1-☑	C79.82	D07.39	D28.2	D39.8	D49.59
uterosacral ligament	C57.3	C79.82	—	D28.2	D39.8	D49.59
uterus, uteri, uterine	C55	C79.82	D07.0	D26.9	D39.0	D49.59
adnexa NEC	C57.4	C79.82	D07.39	D28.7	D39.8	D49.59
body	C54.9	C79.82	D07.0	D26.1	D39.0	D49.59
cervix	C53.9	C79.82	D06.9	D26.0	D39.0	D49.59
cornu	C54.9	C79.82	D07.0	D26.1	D39.0	D49.59
corpus	C54.9	C79.82	D07.0	D26.1	D39.0	D49.59
endocervix (canal) (gland)	C53.0	C79.82	D06.0	D26.0	D39.0	D49.59
endometrium	C54.1	C79.82	D07.0	D26.1	D39.0	D49.59
exocervix	C53.1	C79.82	D06.1	D26.0	D39.0	D49.59
external os	C53.1	C79.82	D06.1	D26.0	D39.0	D49.59
fundus	C54.3	C79.82	D07.0	D26.1	D39.0	D49.59

Neoplasm, neoplastic — continued	Malignant Primary	Malignant Secondary	Ca in situ	Benign	Uncertain Behavior	Unspecified Behavior
uterus, uteri, uterine — continued						
internal os	C53.0	C79.82	D06.0	D26.0	D39.0	D49.59
isthmus	C54.0	C79.82	D07.0	D26.1	D39.0	D49.59
ligament	C57.3	C79.82	—	D28.2	D39.8	D49.59
broad	C57.1-☑	C79.82	D07.39	D28.2	D39.8	D49.59
round	C57.2-☑	C79.82	—	D28.2	D39.8	D49.59
lower segment	C54.0	C79.82	D07.0	D26.1	D39.0	D49.59
myometrium	C54.2	C79.82	D07.0	D26.1	D39.0	D49.59
overlapping sites	C54.8	—	—	—	—	—
squamocolumnar junction	C53.8	C79.82	D06.7	D26.0	D39.0	D49.59
tube	C57.0-☑	C79.82	D07.39	D28.2	D39.8	D49.59
utricle, prostatic	C68.0	C79.19	D09.19	D30.4	D41.3	D49.59
uveal tract	C69.4-☑	C79.49	D09.2-☑	D31.4-☑	D48.7	D49.89
uvula	C05.2	C79.89	D00.04	D10.39	D37.09	D49.0
vagina, vaginal (fornix) (vault) (wall)	C52	C79.82	D07.2	D28.1	D39.8	D49.59
vaginovesical	C57.9	C79.82	D07.30	D28.9	D39.9	D49.59
septum	C57.9	C79.82	D07.30	D28.9	D39.9	D49.59
vallecula (epigiottis)	C10.0	C79.89	D00.08	D10.5	D37.05	D49.0
vascular — see Neoplasm, connective tissue						
vas deferens	C63.1-☑	C79.82	D07.69	D29.8	D40.8	D49.59
Vater's ampulla	C24.1	C78.89	D01.5	D13.5	D37.6	D49.0
vein, venous — see Neoplasm, connective tissue						
vena cava (abdominal) (inferior)	C49.4	C79.89	—	D21.4	D48.1	D49.2
superior	C49.3	C79.89	—	D21.3	D48.1	D49.2
ventricle (cerebral) (floor) (lateral) (third)	C71.5	C79.31	—	D33.0	D43.0	D49.6
cardiac (left) (right)	C38.0	C79.89	—	D15.1	D48.7	D49.89
fourth	C71.7	C79.31	—	D33.1	D43.1	D49.6
ventricular band of larynx	C32.1	C78.39	D02.0	D14.1	D38.0	D49.1
ventriculus — see Neoplasm, stomach						
vermillion border — see Neoplasm, lip						
vermis, cerebellum	C71.6	C79.31	—	D33.1	D43.1	D49.6
vertebra (column)	C41.2	C79.51	—	D16.6	D48.0	D49.2
coccyx	C41.4	C79.51	—	D16.8	D48.0	D49.2
marrow NEC	C96.9	C79.52	—	—	D47.9	D49.89
sacrum	C41.4	C79.51	—	D16.8	D48.0	D49.2
vesical — see Neoplasm, bladder						
vesicle, seminal	C63.7	C79.82	D07.69	D29.8	D40.8	D49.59
vesicocervical tissue	C57.9	C79.82	D07.30	D28.9	D39.9	D49.59
vesicorectal	C76.3	C79.82	D09.8	D36.7	D48.7	D49.89
vesicovaginal	C57.9	C79.82	D07.30	D28.9	D39.9	D49.59
septum	C57.9	C79.82	D07.30	D28.9	D39.8	D49.59
vessel (blood) — see Neoplasm, connective tissue						
vestibular gland, greater	C51.0	C79.82	D07.1	D28.0	D39.8	D49.59
vestibule						
mouth	C06.1	C79.89	D00.00	D10.39	D37.09	D49.0
nose	C30.0	C78.39	D02.3	D14.0	D38.5	D49.1
Virchow's gland	C77.0	C77.0	—	D36.0	D48.7	D49.89
viscera NEC	C76.8	C79.89	D09.8	D36.7	D48.7	D49.89
vocal cords (true)	C32.0	C78.39	D02.0	D14.1	D38.0	D49.1
false	C32.1	C78.39	D02.0	D14.1	D38.0	D49.1
vomer	C41.0	C79.51	—	D16.4	D48.0	D49.2
vulva	C51.9	C79.82	D07.1	D28.0	D39.8	D49.59
vulvovaginal gland	C51.0	C79.82	D07.1	D28.0	D39.8	D49.59
Waldeyer's ring	C14.2	C79.89	D00.08	D10.9	D37.05	D49.0
Wharton's duct	C08.0	C79.89	D00.00	D11.7	D37.032	D49.0
white matter (central) (cerebral)	C71.0	C79.31	—	D33.0	D43.0	D49.6

☑ Additional Character Required — Refer to the Tabular List for Character Selection

Neoplasm, neoplastic	Malignant Primary	Malignant Secondary	Ca in situ	Benign	Uncertain Behavior	Unspecified Behavior
— continued						
windpipe	C33	C78.39	D02.1	D14.2	D38.1	D49.1
Wirsung's duct	C25.3	C78.89	D01.7	D13.6	D37.8	D49.0
wolffian (body) (duct)						
female	C57.7	C79.82	D07.39	D28.7	D39.8	D49.59
male	C63.7	C79.82	D07.69	D29.8	D40.8	D49.59
womb — *see* Neoplasm, uterus						
wrist NEC	C76.4-☑	C79.89	D04.6-☑	D36.7	D48.7	D49.89
xiphoid process	C41.3	C79.51	—	D16.7	D48.0	D49.2
Zuckerkandl organ	C75.5	C79.89	—	D35.6	D44.7	D49.7

Substance	Poisoning, Accidental (unintentional)	Poisoning, Intentional Self-harm	Poisoning, Assault	Poisoning, Undetermined	Adverse Effect	Under-dosing
14-hydroxydihydro-morphinone	T40.2X1	T40.2X2	T40.2X3	T40.2X4	T40.2X5	T40.2X6
1-Propanol	T51.3X1	T51.3X2	T51.3X3	T51.3X4	—	—
2,3,7,8-Tetrachlorodibenzo-p-dioxin	T53.7X1	T53.7X2	T53.7X3	T53.7X4	—	—
2,4,5-T (trichloro-phenoxyacetic acid)	T60.1X1	T60.1X2	T60.1X3	T60.1X4	—	—
2,4,5-Trichlorophen-oxyacetic acid	T60.3X1	T60.3X2	T60.3X3	T60.3X4	—	—
2,4-D (dichlorophen-oxyacetic acid)	T60.3X1	T60.3X2	T60.3X3	T60.3X4	—	—
2,4-Toluene diisocyanate	T65.0X1	T65.0X2	T65.0X3	T65.0X4	—	—
2-Deoxy-5-fluorouridine	T45.1X1	T45.1X2	T45.1X3	T45.1X4	T45.1X5	T45.1X6
2-Ethoxyethanol	T52.3X1	T52.3X2	T52.3X3	T52.3X4	—	—
2-Methoxyethanol	T52.3X1	T52.3X2	T52.3X3	T52.3X4	—	—
2-Propanol	T51.2X1	T51.2X2	T51.2X3	T51.2X4	—	—
3,4-methylenedioxymeth-amphetamine	T43.641	T43.642	T43.643	T43.644	—	—
4-Aminobutyric acid	T43.8X1	T43.8X2	T43.8X3	T43.8X4	T43.8X5	T43.8X6
4-Aminophenol derivatives	T39.1X1	T39.1X2	T39.1X3	T39.1X4	T39.1X5	T39.1X6
5-Deoxy-5-fluorouridine	T45.1X1	T45.1X2	T45.1X3	T45.1X4	T45.1X5	T45.1X6
5-Methoxypsoralen (5-MOP)	T50.991	T50.992	T50.993	T50.994	T50.995	T50.996
8-Aminoquinoline drugs	T37.2X1	T37.2X2	T37.2X3	T37.2X4	T37.2X5	T37.2X6
8-Methoxypsoralen (8-MOP)	T50.991	T50.992	T50.993	T50.994	T50.995	T50.996
9-hydroxyrisperidone*	T43.591	T43.592	T43.593	T43.594	T43.595	T43.596
ABOB	T37.5X1	T37.5X2	T37.5X3	T37.5X4	T37.5X5	T37.5X6
Abrine	T62.2X1	T62.2X2	T62.2X3	T62.2X4	—	—
Abrus (seed)	T62.2X1	T62.2X2	T62.2X3	T62.2X4	—	—
Absinthe	T51.0X1	T51.0X2	T51.0X3	T51.0X4	—	—
beverage	T51.0X1	T51.0X2	T51.0X3	T51.0X4	—	—
Acaricide	T60.8X1	T60.8X2	T60.8X3	T60.8X4	—	—
Acebutolol	T44.7X1	T44.7X2	T44.7X3	T44.7X4	T44.7X5	T44.7X6
Acecarbromal	T42.6X1	T42.6X2	T42.6X3	T42.6X4	T42.6X5	T42.6X6
Aceclidine	T44.1X1	T44.1X2	T44.1X3	T44.1X4	T44.1X5	T44.1X6
Acedapsone	T37.0X1	T37.0X2	T37.0X3	T37.0X4	T37.0X5	T37.0X6
Acefylline piperazine	T48.6X1	T48.6X2	T48.6X3	T48.6X4	T48.6X5	T48.6X6
Acemorphan	T40.2X1	T40.2X2	T40.2X3	T40.2X4	T40.2X5	T40.2X6
Acenocoumarin	T45.511	T45.512	T45.513	T45.514	T45.515	T45.516
Acenocoumarol	T45.511	T45.512	T45.513	T45.514	T45.515	T45.516
Aceon*	T46.4X1	T46.4X2	T46.4X3	T46.4X4	T46.4X5	T46.4X6
Acepifylline	T48.6X1	T48.6X2	T48.6X3	T48.6X4	T48.6X5	T48.6X6
Acepromazine	T43.3X1	T43.3X2	T43.3X3	T43.3X4	T43.3X5	T43.3X6
Acesulfamethoxypyridazine	T37.0X1	T37.0X2	T37.0X3	T37.0X4	T37.0X5	T37.0X6
Acetal	T52.8X1	T52.8X2	T52.8X3	T52.8X4	—	—
Acetaldehyde (vapor)	T52.8X1	T52.8X2	T52.8X3	T52.8X4	—	—
liquid	T65.891	T65.892	T65.893	T65.894	—	—
Acetaminophen	T39.1X1	T39.1X2	T39.1X3	T39.1X4	T39.1X5	T39.1X6
Acetaminosalol	T39.1X1	T39.1X2	T39.1X3	T39.1X4	T39.1X5	T39.1X6
Acetanilide	T39.1X1	T39.1X2	T39.1X3	T39.1X4	T39.1X5	T39.1X6
Acetarsol	T37.3X1	T37.3X2	T37.3X3	T37.3X4	T37.3X5	T37.3X6
Acetazolamide	T50.2X1	T50.2X2	T50.2X3	T50.2X4	T50.2X5	T50.2X6
Acetiamine	T45.2X1	T45.2X2	T45.2X3	T45.2X4	T45.2X5	T45.2X6
Acetic						
acid	T54.2X1	T54.2X2	T54.2X3	T54.2X4	—	—
with sodium acetate (ointment)	T49.3X1	T49.3X2	T49.3X3	T49.3X4	T49.3X5	T49.3X6
ester (solvent)(vapor)	T52.8X1	T52.8X2	T52.8X3	T52.8X4	—	—
irrigating solution	T50.3X1	T50.3X2	T50.3X3	T50.3X4	T50.3X5	T50.3X6
medicinal (lotion)	T49.2X1	T49.2X2	T49.2X3	T49.2X4	T49.2X5	T49.2X6
anhydride	T65.891	T65.892	T65.893	T65.894	—	—
ether (vapor)	T52.8X1	T52.8X2	T52.8X3	T52.8X4	—	—
Acetohexamide	T38.3X1	T38.3X2	T38.3X3	T38.3X4	T38.3X5	T38.3X6
Acetohydroxamic acid	T50.991	T50.992	T50.993	T50.994	T50.995	T50.996
Acetomenaphthone	T45.7X1	T45.7X2	T45.7X3	T45.7X4	T45.7X5	T45.7X6
Acetomorphine	T40.1X1	T40.1X2	T40.1X3	T40.1X4	—	—
Acetone (oils)	T52.4X1	T52.4X2	T52.4X3	T52.4X4	—	—
chlorinated	T52.4X1	T52.4X2	T52.4X3	T52.4X4	—	—
vapor	T52.4X1	T52.4X2	T52.4X3	T52.4X4	—	—
Acetonitrile	T52.8X1	T52.8X2	T52.8X3	T52.8X4	—	—
Acetophenazine	T43.3X1	T43.3X2	T43.3X3	T43.3X4	T43.3X5	T43.3X6
Acetophenetedin	T39.1X1	T39.1X2	T39.1X3	T39.1X4	T39.1X5	T39.1X6
Acetophenone	T52.4X1	T52.4X2	T52.4X3	T52.4X4	—	—
Acetorphine	T40.2X1	T40.2X2	T40.2X3	T40.2X4	—	—
Acetosulfone (sodium)	T37.1X1	T37.1X2	T37.1X3	T37.1X4	T37.1X5	T37.1X6
Acetrizoate (sodium)	T50.8X1	T50.8X2	T50.8X3	T50.8X4	T50.8X5	T50.8X6
Acetrizoic acid	T50.8X1	T50.8X2	T50.8X3	T50.8X4	T50.8X5	T50.8X6
Acetyl						
bromide	T53.6X1	T53.6X2	T53.6X3	T53.6X4	—	—
chloride	T53.6X1	T53.6X2	T53.6X3	T53.6X4	—	—
Acetylcarbromal	T42.6X1	T42.6X2	T42.6X3	T42.6X4	T42.6X5	T42.6X6
Acetylcholine						

Substance	Poisoning, Accidental (unintentional)	Poisoning, Intentional Self-harm	Poisoning, Assault	Poisoning, Undetermined	Adverse Effect	Under-dosing
Acetylcholine — continued						
chloride	T44.1X1	T44.1X2	T44.1X3	T44.1X4	T44.1X5	T44.1X6
derivative	T44.1X1	T44.1X2	T44.1X3	T44.1X4	T44.1X5	T44.1X6
Acetylcysteine	T48.4X1	T48.4X2	T48.4X3	T48.4X4	T48.4X5	T48.4X6
Acetyldigitoxin	T46.0X1	T46.0X2	T46.0X3	T46.0X4	T46.0X5	T46.0X6
Acetyldigoxin	T46.0X1	T46.0X2	T46.0X3	T46.0X4	T46.0X5	T46.0X6
Acetyldihydrocodeine	T40.2X1	T40.2X2	T40.2X3	T40.2X4	—	—
Acetyldihydrocodeinone	T40.2X1	T40.2X2	T40.2X3	T40.2X4	—	—
Acetylene (gas)	T59.891	T59.892	T59.893	T59.894	—	—
dichloride	T53.6X1	T53.6X2	T53.6X3	T53.6X4	—	—
incomplete combustion of	T58.11	T58.12	T58.13	T58.14	—	—
industrial	T59.891	T59.892	T59.893	T59.894	—	—
tetrachloride	T53.6X1	T53.6X2	T53.6X3	T53.6X4	—	—
vapor	T53.6X1	T53.6X2	T53.6X3	T53.6X4	—	—
Acetylpheneturide	T42.6X1	T42.6X2	T42.6X3	T42.6X4	T42.6X5	T42.6X6
Acetylphenylhydrazine	T39.8X1	T39.8X2	T39.8X3	T39.8X4	T39.8X5	T39.8X6
Acetylsalicylic acid (salts)	T39.011	T39.012	T39.013	T39.014	T39.015	T39.016
enteric coated	T39.011	T39.012	T39.013	T39.014	T39.015	T39.016
Acetylsulfamethoxypyridazine	T37.0X1	T37.0X2	T37.0X3	T37.0X4	T37.0X5	T37.0X6
Achromycin	T36.4X1	T36.4X2	T36.4X3	T36.4X4	T36.4X5	T36.4X6
ophthalmic preparation	T49.5X1	T49.5X2	T49.5X3	T49.5X4	T49.5X5	T49.5X6
topical NEC	T49.0X1	T49.0X2	T49.0X3	T49.0X4	T49.0X5	T49.0X6
Aciclovir	T37.5X1	T37.5X2	T37.5X3	T37.5X4	T37.5X5	T37.5X6
Acidifying agent NEC	T50.901	T50.902	T50.903	T50.904	T50.905	T50.906
Acid (corrosive) NEC	T54.2X1	T54.2X2	T54.2X3	T54.2X4	—	—
AcipHex*	T47.1X1	T47.1X2	T47.1X3	T47.1X4	T47.1X5	T47.1X6
Acipimox	T46.6X1	T46.6X2	T46.6X3	T46.6X4	T46.6X5	T46.6X6
Acitretin	T50.991	T50.992	T50.993	T50.994	T50.995	T50.996
Aclarubicin	T45.1X1	T45.1X2	T45.1X3	T45.1X4	T45.1X5	T45.1X6
Aclatonium napadisilate	T48.1X1	T48.1X2	T48.1X3	T48.1X4	T48.1X5	T48.1X6
Aconite (wild)	T46.991	T46.992	T46.993	T46.994	T46.995	T46.996
Aconitine	T46.991	T46.992	T46.993	T46.994	T46.995	T46.996
Aconitum ferox	T46.991	T46.992	T46.993	T46.994	T46.995	T46.996
Acridine	T65.6X1	T65.6X2	T65.6X3	T65.6X4	—	—
vapor	T59.891	T59.892	T59.893	T59.894	—	—
Acriflavine	T37.91	T37.92	T37.93	T37.94	T37.95	T37.96
Acriflavinium chloride	T49.0X1	T49.0X2	T49.0X3	T49.0X4	T49.0X5	T49.0X6
Acrinol	T49.0X1	T49.0X2	T49.0X3	T49.0X4	T49.0X5	T49.0X6
Acrisorcin	T49.0X1	T49.0X2	T49.0X3	T49.0X4	T49.0X5	T49.0X6
Acrivastine	T45.0X1	T45.0X2	T45.0X3	T45.0X4	T45.0X5	T45.0X6
Acrolein (gas)	T59.891	T59.892	T59.893	T59.894	—	—
liquid	T54.1X1	T54.1X2	T54.1X3	T54.1X4	—	—
Acrylamide	T65.891	T65.892	T65.893	T65.894	—	—
Acrylic resin	T49.3X1	T49.3X2	T49.3X3	T49.3X4	T49.3X5	T49.3X6
Acrylonitrile	T65.891	T65.892	T65.893	T65.894	—	—
Actaea spicata	T62.2X1	T62.2X2	T62.2X3	T62.2X4	—	—
berry	T62.1X1	T62.1X2	T62.1X3	T62.1X4	—	—
Acterol	T37.3X1	T37.3X2	T37.3X3	T37.3X4	T37.3X5	T37.3X6
ACTH	T38.811	T38.812	T38.813	T38.814	T38.815	T38.816
Actinomycin C	T45.1X1	T45.1X2	T45.1X3	T45.1X4	T45.1X5	T45.1X6
Actinomycin D	T45.1X1	T45.1X2	T45.1X3	T45.1X4	T45.1X5	T45.1X6
Activated charcoal — see also Charcoal, medicinal	T47.6X1	T47.6X2	T47.6X3	T47.6X4	T47.6X5	T47.6X6
Activella*	T38.5X1	T38.5X2	T38.5X3	T38.5X4	T38.5X5	T38.5X6
Acyclovir	T37.5X1	T37.5X2	T37.5X3	T37.5X4	T37.5X5	T37.5X6
Adenine	T45.2X1	T45.2X2	T45.2X3	T45.2X4	T45.2X5	T45.2X6
arabinoside	T37.5X1	T37.5X2	T37.5X3	T37.5X4	T37.5X5	T37.5X6
Adenosine (phosphate)	T46.2X1	T46.2X2	T46.2X3	T46.2X4	T46.2X5	T46.2X6
ADH	T38.891	T38.892	T38.893	T38.894	T38.895	T38.896
Adhesive NEC	T65.891	T65.892	T65.893	T65.894	—	—
Adicillin	T36.0X1	T36.0X2	T36.0X3	T36.0X4	T36.0X5	T36.0X6
Adiphenine	T44.3X1	T44.3X2	T44.3X3	T44.3X4	T44.3X5	T44.3X6
Adipiodone	T50.8X1	T50.8X2	T50.8X3	T50.8X4	T50.8X5	T50.8X6
Adjunct, pharmaceutical	T50.901	T50.902	T50.903	T50.904	T50.905	T50.906
Adrenal (extract, cortex or medulla) (glucocorticoids) (hormones) (mineralocorticoids)	T38.0X1	T38.0X2	T38.0X3	T38.0X4	T38.0X5	T38.0X6
ENT agent	T49.6X1	T49.6X2	T49.6X3	T49.6X4	T49.6X5	T49.6X6
ophthalmic preparation	T49.5X1	T49.5X2	T49.5X3	T49.5X4	T49.5X5	T49.5X6
topical NEC	T49.0X1	T49.0X2	T49.0X3	T49.0X4	T49.0X5	T49.0X6
Adrenalin — see Adrenaline						
Adrenaline	T44.5X1	T44.5X2	T44.5X3	T44.5X4	T44.5X5	T44.5X6
Adrenergic NEC	T44.901	T44.902	T44.903	T44.904	T44.905	T44.906
blocking agent NEC	T44.8X1	T44.8X2	T44.8X3	T44.8X4	T44.8X5	T44.8X6
beta, heart	T44.7X1	T44.7X2	T44.7X3	T44.7X4	T44.7X5	T44.7X6
specified NEC	T44.991	T44.992	T44.993	T44.994	T44.995	T44.996
Adrenochrome						
derivative	T46.991	T46.992	T46.993	T46.994	T46.995	T46.996
(mono) semicarbazone	T46.991	T46.992	T46.993	T46.994	T46.995	T46.996
Adrenocorticotrophic hormone	T38.811	T38.812	T38.813	T38.814	T38.815	T38.816
Adrenocorticotrophin	T38.811	T38.812	T38.813	T38.814	T38.815	T38.816

Substance	Poisoning, Accidental (unintentional)	Poisoning, Intentional Self-harm	Poisoning, Assault	Poisoning, Undetermined	Adverse Effect	Under- dosing
Adriamycin	T45.1X1	T45.1X2	T45.1X3	T45.1X4	T45.1X5	T45.1X6
Adrucil*	T45.1X1	T45.1X2	T45.1X3	T45.1X4	T45.1X5	T45.1X6
Aerosol spray NEC	T65.91	T65.92	T65.93	T65.94	—	—
Aerosporin	T36.8X1	T36.8X2	T36.8X3	T36.8X4	T36.8X5	T36.8X6
ENT agent	T49.6X1	T49.6X2	T49.6X3	T49.6X4	T49.6X5	T49.6X6
ophthalmic preparation	T49.5X1	T49.5X2	T49.5X3	T49.5X4	T49.5X5	T49.5X6
topical NEC	T49.0X1	T49.0X2	T49.0X3	T49.0X4	T49.0X5	T49.0X6
Aethusa cynapium	T62.2X1	T62.2X2	T62.2X3	T62.2X4	—	—
Afghanistan black	T40.711	T40.712	T40.713	T40.714	T40.715	T40.716
Aflatoxin	T64.01	T64.02	T64.03	T64.04	—	—
Afloqualone	T42.8X1	T42.8X2	T42.8X3	T42.8X4	T42.8X5	T42.8X6
African boxwood	T62.2X1	T62.2X2	T62.2X3	T62.2X4	—	—
Agar	T47.4X1	T47.4X2	T47.4X3	T47.4X4	T47.4X5	T47.4X6
Agonist						
predominantly						
alpha-adrenoreceptor	T44.4X1	T44.4X2	T44.4X3	T44.4X4	T44.4X5	T44.4X6
beta-adrenoreceptor	T44.5X1	T44.5X2	T44.5X3	T44.5X4	T44.5X5	T44.5X6
Agricultural agent NEC	T65.91	T65.92	T65.93	T65.94	—	—
Agrypnal	T42.3X1	T42.3X2	T42.3X3	T42.3X4	T42.3X5	T42.3X6
AHLG	T50.Z11	T50.Z12	T50.Z13	T50.Z14	T50.Z15	T50.Z16
Air contaminant(s), source/type NOS	T65.91	T65.92	T65.93	T65.94	—	—
Ajmaline	T46.2X1	T46.2X2	T46.2X3	T46.2X4	T46.2X5	T46.2X6
Akee	T62.1X1	T62.1X2	T62.1X3	T62.1X4	—	—
Akne-Mycin*	T49.0X1	T49.0X2	T49.0X3	T49.0X4	T49.0X5	T49.0X6
Akrinol	T49.0X1	T49.0X2	T49.0X3	T49.0X4	T49.0X5	T49.0X6
Akritoin	T37.8X1	T37.8X2	T37.8X3	T37.8X4	T37.8X5	T37.8X6
Alacepril	T46.4X1	T46.4X2	T46.4X3	T46.4X4	T46.4X5	T46.4X6
Alantolactone	T37.4X1	T37.4X2	T37.4X3	T37.4X4	T37.4X5	T37.4X6
Albamycin	T36.8X1	T36.8X2	T36.8X3	T36.8X4	T36.8X5	T36.8X6
Albendazole	T37.4X1	T37.4X2	T37.4X3	T37.4X4	T37.4X5	T37.4X6
Albiglutide*	T38.3X1	T38.3X2	T38.3X3	T38.3X4	T38.3X5	T38.3X6
Albumin						
bovine	T45.8X1	T45.8X2	T45.8X3	T45.8X4	T45.8X5	T45.8X6
human serum	T45.8X1	T45.8X2	T45.8X3	T45.8X4	T45.8X5	T45.8X6
salt-poor	T45.8X1	T45.8X2	T45.8X3	T45.8X4	T45.8X5	T45.8X6
normal human serum	T45.8X1	T45.8X2	T45.8X3	T45.8X4	T45.8X5	T45.8X6
Albuterol	T48.6X1	T48.6X2	T48.6X3	T48.6X4	T48.6X5	T48.6X6
Albutoin	T42.0X1	T42.0X2	T42.0X3	T42.0X4	T42.0X5	T42.0X6
Alclometasone	T49.0X1	T49.0X2	T49.0X3	T49.0X4	T49.0X5	T49.0X6
Alcohol	T51.91	T51.92	T51.93	T51.94	—	—
absolute	T51.0X1	T51.0X2	T51.0X3	T51.0X4	—	—
beverage	T51.0X1	T51.0X2	T51.0X3	T51.0X4	—	—
allyl	T51.8X1	T51.8X2	T51.8X3	T51.8X4	—	—
amyl	T51.3X1	T51.3X2	T51.3X3	T51.3X4	—	—
antifreeze	T51.1X1	T51.1X2	T51.1X3	T51.1X4	—	—
beverage	T51.0X1	T51.0X2	T51.0X3	T51.0X4	—	—
butyl	T51.3X1	T51.3X2	T51.3X3	T51.3X4	—	—
dehydrated	T51.0X1	T51.0X2	T51.0X3	T51.0X4	—	—
beverage	T51.0X1	T51.0X2	T51.0X3	T51.0X4	—	—
denatured	T51.0X1	T51.0X2	T51.0X3	T51.0X4	—	—
deterrent NEC	T50.6X1	T50.6X2	T50.6X3	T50.6X4	T50.6X5	T50.6X6
diagnostic (gastric function)	T50.8X1	T50.8X2	T50.8X3	T50.8X4	T50.8X5	T50.8X6
ethyl	T51.0X1	T51.0X2	T51.0X3	T51.0X4	—	—
beverage	T51.0X1	T51.0X2	T51.0X3	T51.0X4	—	—
grain	T51.0X1	T51.0X2	T51.0X3	T51.0X4	—	—
beverage	T51.0X1	T51.0X2	T51.0X3	T51.0X4	—	—
industrial	T51.0X1	T51.0X2	T51.0X3	T51.0X4	—	—
isopropyl	T51.2X1	T51.2X2	T51.2X3	T51.2X4	—	—
methyl	T51.1X1	T51.1X2	T51.1X3	T51.1X4	—	—
preparation for consumption	T51.0X1	T51.0X2	T51.0X3	T51.0X4	—	—
propyl	T51.3X1	T51.3X2	T51.3X3	T51.3X4	—	—
secondary	T51.2X1	T51.2X2	T51.2X3	T51.2X4	—	—
radiator	T51.1X1	T51.1X2	T51.1X3	T51.1X4	—	—
rubbing	T51.2X1	T51.2X2	T51.2X3	T51.2X4	—	—
specified type NEC	T51.8X1	T51.8X2	T51.8X3	T51.8X4	—	—
surgical	T51.0X1	T51.0X2	T51.0X3	T51.0X4	—	—
vapor (from any type of Alcohol)	T59.891	T59.892	T59.893	T59.894	—	—
wood	T51.1X1	T51.1X2	T51.1X3	T51.1X4	—	—
Alcuronium (chloride)	T48.1X1	T48.1X2	T48.1X3	T48.1X4	T48.1X5	T48.1X6
Aldactone	T50.0X1	T50.0X2	T50.0X3	T50.0X4	T50.0X5	T50.0X6
Aldesulfone sodium	T37.1X1	T37.1X2	T37.1X3	T37.1X4	T37.1X5	T37.1X6
Aldicarb	T60.0X1	T60.0X2	T60.0X3	T60.0X4	—	—
Aldomet	T46.5X1	T46.5X2	T46.5X3	T46.5X4	T46.5X5	T46.5X6
Aldosterone	T50.0X1	T50.0X2	T50.0X3	T50.0X4	T50.0X5	T50.0X6
Aldrin (dust)	T60.1X1	T60.1X2	T60.1X3	T60.1X4	—	—
Aleve — *see* Naproxen						
Alexitol sodium	T47.1X1	T47.1X2	T47.1X3	T47.1X4	T47.1X5	T47.1X6
Alfacalcidol	T45.2X1	T45.2X2	T45.2X3	T45.2X4	T45.2X5	T45.2X6
Alfadolone	T41.1X1	T41.1X2	T41.1X3	T41.1X4	T41.1X5	T41.1X6

Substance	Poisoning, Accidental (unintentional)	Poisoning, Intentional Self-harm	Poisoning, Assault	Poisoning, Undetermined	Adverse Effect	Under- dosing
Alfaxalone	T41.1X1	T41.1X2	T41.1X3	T41.1X4	T41.1X5	T41.1X6
Alfentanil	T40.411	T40.412	T40.413	T40.414	T40.415	T40.416
Alfuzosin (hydrochloride)	T44.8X1	T44.8X2	T44.8X3	T44.8X4	T44.8X5	T44.8X6
Algae (harmful) (toxin)	T65.821	T65.822	T65.823	T65.824	—	—
Algeldrate	T47.1X1	T47.1X2	T47.1X3	T47.1X4	T47.1X5	T47.1X6
Algin	T47.8X1	T47.8X2	T47.8X3	T47.8X4	T47.8X5	T47.8X6
Alglucerase	T45.3X1	T45.3X2	T45.3X3	T45.3X4	T45.3X5	T45.3X6
Alidase	T45.3X1	T45.3X2	T45.3X3	T45.3X4	T45.3X5	T45.3X6
Alimemazine	T43.3X1	T43.3X2	T43.3X3	T43.3X4	T43.3X5	T43.3X6
Aliphatic thiocyanates	T65.0X1	T65.0X2	T65.0X3	T65.0X4	—	—
Alitretinoin*	T49.0X1	T49.0X2	T49.0X3	T49.0X4	T49.0X5	T49.0X6
Alizapride	T45.0X1	T45.0X2	T45.0X3	T45.0X4	T45.0X5	T45.0X6
Alkali (caustic)	T54.3X1	T54.3X2	T54.3X3	T54.3X4	—	—
Alkaline antiseptic solution (aromatic)	T49.6X1	T49.6X2	T49.6X3	T49.6X4	T49.6X5	T49.6X6
Alkalinizing agents (medicinal)	T50.901	T50.902	T50.903	T50.904	T50.905	T50.906
Alkalizing agent NEC	T50.901	T50.902	T50.903	T50.904	T50.905	T50.906
Alka-seltzer	T39.011	T39.012	T39.013	T39.014	T39.015	T39.016
Alkavervir	T46.5X1	T46.5X2	T46.5X3	T46.5X4	T46.5X5	T46.5X6
Alkeran*	T45.1X1	T45.1X2	T45.1X3	T45.1X4	T45.1X5	T45.1X6
Alkonium (bromide)	T49.0X1	T49.0X2	T49.0X3	T49.0X4	T49.0X5	T49.0X6
Alkylating drug NEC	T45.1X1	T45.1X2	T45.1X3	T45.1X4	T45.1X5	T45.1X6
antimyeloproliferative	T45.1X1	T45.1X2	T45.1X3	T45.1X4	T45.1X5	T45.1X6
lymphatic	T45.1X1	T45.1X2	T45.1X3	T45.1X4	T45.1X5	T45.1X6
Alkylisocyanate	T65.0X1	T65.0X2	T65.0X3	T65.0X4	—	—
Allantoin	T49.4X1	T49.4X2	T49.4X3	T49.4X4	T49.4X5	T49.4X6
Allegron	T43.011	T43.012	T43.013	T43.014	T43.015	T43.016
Allethrin	T49.0X1	T49.0X2	T49.0X3	T49.0X4	T49.0X5	T49.0X6
Allobarbital	T42.3X1	T42.3X2	T42.3X3	T42.3X4	T42.3X5	T42.3X6
Allopurinol	T50.4X1	T50.4X2	T50.4X3	T50.4X4	T50.4X5	T50.4X6
Allyl						
alcohol	T51.8X1	T51.8X2	T51.8X3	T51.8X4	—	—
disulfide	T46.6X1	T46.6X2	T46.6X3	T46.6X4	T46.6X5	T46.6X6
Allylestrenol	T38.5X1	T38.5X2	T38.5X3	T38.5X4	T38.5X5	T38.5X6
Allylisopropylacetylurea	T42.6X1	T42.6X2	T42.6X3	T42.6X4	T42.6X5	T42.6X6
Allylisopropylmalonylurea	T42.3X1	T42.3X2	T42.3X3	T42.3X4	T42.3X5	T42.3X6
Allylthiourea	T49.3X1	T49.3X2	T49.3X3	T49.3X4	T49.3X5	T49.3X6
Allyltribromide	T42.6X1	T42.6X2	T42.6X3	T42.6X4	T42.6X5	T42.6X6
Allypropymal	T42.3X1	T42.3X2	T42.3X3	T42.3X4	T42.3X5	T42.3X6
Almagate	T47.1X1	T47.1X2	T47.1X3	T47.1X4	T47.1X5	T47.1X6
Almasilate	T47.1X1	T47.1X2	T47.1X3	T47.1X4	T47.1X5	T47.1X6
Almitrine	T50.7X1	T50.7X2	T50.7X3	T50.7X4	T50.7X5	T50.7X6
Aloes	T47.2X1	T47.2X2	T47.2X3	T47.2X4	T47.2X5	T47.2X6
Aloglutamol	T47.1X1	T47.1X2	T47.1X3	T47.1X4	T47.1X5	T47.1X6
Aloin	T47.2X1	T47.2X2	T47.2X3	T47.2X4	T47.2X5	T47.2X6
Aloxidone	T42.2X1	T42.2X2	T42.2X3	T42.2X4	T42.2X5	T42.2X6
Alpha						
acetyldigoxin	T46.0X1	T46.0X2	T46.0X3	T46.0X4	T46.0X5	T46.0X6
adrenergic blocking drug	T44.6X1	T44.6X2	T44.6X3	T44.6X4	T44.6X5	T44.6X6
amylase	T45.3X1	T45.3X2	T45.3X3	T45.3X4	T45.3X5	T45.3X6
tocoferol (acetate)	T45.2X1	T45.2X2	T45.2X3	T45.2X4	T45.2X5	T45.2X6
tocopherol	T45.2X1	T45.2X2	T45.2X3	T45.2X4	T45.2X5	T45.2X6
Alphadolone	T41.1X1	T41.1X2	T41.1X3	T41.1X4	T41.1X5	T41.1X6
Alphaprodine	T40.491	T40.492	T40.493	T40.494	T40.495	T40.496
Alphaxalone	T41.1X1	T41.1X2	T41.1X3	T41.1X4	T41.1X5	T41.1X6
Alprazolam	T42.4X1	T42.4X2	T42.4X3	T42.4X4	T42.4X5	T42.4X6
Alprenolol	T44.7X1	T44.7X2	T44.7X3	T44.7X4	T44.7X5	T44.7X6
Alprostadil	T46.7X1	T46.7X2	T46.7X3	T46.7X4	T46.7X5	T46.7X6
Alsactide	T38.811	T38.812	T38.813	T38.814	T38.815	T38.816
Alseroxylon	T46.5X1	T46.5X2	T46.5X3	T46.5X4	T46.5X5	T46.5X6
Alteplase	T45.611	T45.612	T45.613	T45.614	T45.615	T45.616
Altizide	T50.2X1	T50.2X2	T50.2X3	T50.2X4	T50.2X5	T50.2X6
Altoprev*	T46.6X1	T46.6X2	T46.6X3	T46.6X4	T46.6X5	T46.6X6
Altretamine	T45.1X1	T45.1X2	T45.1X3	T45.1X4	T45.1X5	T45.1X6
Alum (medicinal)	T49.4X1	T49.4X2	T49.4X3	T49.4X4	T49.4X5	T49.4X6
nonmedicinal (ammonium) (potassium)	T56.891	T56.892	T56.893	T56.894	—	—
Aluminium, aluminum						
acetate	T49.2X1	T49.2X2	T49.2X3	T49.2X4	T49.2X5	T49.2X6
solution	T49.0X1	T49.0X2	T49.0X3	T49.0X4	T49.0X5	T49.0X6
aspirin	T39.011	T39.012	T39.013	T39.014	T39.015	T39.016
bis (acetylsalicylate)	T39.011	T39.012	T39.013	T39.014	T39.015	T39.016
carbonate (gel, basic)	T47.1X1	T47.1X2	T47.1X3	T47.1X4	T47.1X5	T47.1X6
chlorhydroxide-complex	T47.1X1	T47.1X2	T47.1X3	T47.1X4	T47.1X5	T47.1X6
chloride	T49.2X1	T49.2X2	T49.2X3	T49.2X4	T49.2X5	T49.2X6
clofibrate	T46.6X1	T46.6X2	T46.6X3	T46.6X4	T46.6X5	T46.6X6
diacetate	T49.2X1	T49.2X2	T49.2X3	T49.2X4	T49.2X5	T49.2X6
glycinate	T47.1X1	T47.1X2	T47.1X3	T47.1X4	T47.1X5	T47.1X6
hydroxide (gel)	T47.1X1	T47.1X2	T47.1X3	T47.1X4	T47.1X5	T47.1X6
hydroxide-magnesium carb. gel	T47.1X1	T47.1X2	T47.1X3	T47.1X4	T47.1X5	T47.1X6
magnesium silicate	T47.1X1	T47.1X2	T47.1X3	T47.1X4	T47.1X5	T47.1X6

Substance	Poisoning, Accidental (unintentional)	Poisoning, Intentional Self-harm	Poisoning, Assault	Poisoning, Undetermined	Adverse Effect	Under-dosing
Aluminium, aluminum — *continued*						
nicotinate	T46.7X1	T46.7X2	T46.7X3	T46.7X4	T46.7X5	T46.7X6
ointment (surgical) (topical)	T49.3X1	T49.3X2	T49.3X3	T49.3X4	T49.3X5	T49.3X6
phosphate	T47.1X1	T47.1X2	T47.1X3	T47.1X4	T47.1X5	T47.1X6
salicylate	T39.091	T39.092	T39.093	T39.094	T39.095	T39.096
silicate	T47.1X1	T47.1X2	T47.1X3	T47.1X4	T47.1X5	T47.1X6
sodium silicate	T47.1X1	T47.1X2	T47.1X3	T47.1X4	T47.1X5	T47.1X6
subacetate	T49.2X1	T49.2X2	T49.2X3	T49.2X4	T49.2X5	T49.2X6
sulfate	T49.0X1	T49.0X2	T49.0X3	T49.0X4	T49.0X5	T49.0X6
tannate	T47.6X1	T47.6X2	T47.6X3	T47.6X4	T47.6X5	T47.6X6
topical NEC	T49.3X1	T49.3X2	T49.3X3	T49.3X4	T49.3X5	T49.3X6
Alurate	T42.3X1	T42.3X2	T42.3X3	T42.3X4	T42.3X5	T42.3X6
Alverine	T44.3X1	T44.3X2	T44.3X3	T44.3X4	T44.3X5	T44.3X6
Alvodine	T40.2X1	T40.2X2	T40.2X3	T40.2X4	T40.2X5	T40.2X6
Amanita phalloides	T62.0X1	T62.0X2	T62.0X3	T62.0X4	—	—
Amanitine	T62.0X1	T62.0X2	T62.0X3	T62.0X4	—	—
Amantadine	T42.8X1	T42.8X2	T42.8X3	T42.8X4	T42.8X5	T42.8X6
Ambazone	T49.6X1	T49.6X2	T49.6X3	T49.6X4	T49.6X5	T49.6X6
Ambenonium (chloride)	T44.0X1	T44.0X2	T44.0X3	T44.0X4	T44.0X5	T44.0X6
Ambroxol	T48.4X1	T48.4X2	T48.4X3	T48.4X4	T48.4X5	T48.4X6
Ambuphylline	T48.6X1	T48.6X2	T48.6X3	T48.6X4	T48.6X5	T48.6X6
Ambutonium bromide	T44.3X1	T44.3X2	T44.3X3	T44.3X4	T44.3X5	T44.3X6
Amcinonide	T49.0X1	T49.0X2	T49.0X3	T49.0X4	T49.0X5	T49.0X6
Amdinocilline	T36.0X1	T36.0X2	T36.0X3	T36.0X4	T36.0X5	T36.0X6
Americaine*	T41.3X1	T41.3X2	T41.3X3	T41.3X4	T41.3X5	T41.3X6
Ametazole	T50.8X1	T50.8X2	T50.8X3	T50.8X4	T50.8X5	T50.8X6
Amethocaine	T41.3X1	T41.3X2	T41.3X3	T41.3X4	T41.3X5	T41.3X6
regional	T41.3X1	T41.3X2	T41.3X3	T41.3X4	T41.3X5	T41.3X6
spinal	T41.3X1	T41.3X2	T41.3X3	T41.3X4	T41.3X5	T41.3X6
Amethopterin	T45.1X1	T45.1X2	T45.1X3	T45.1X4	T45.1X5	T45.1X6
Amezinium metilsulfate	T44.991	T44.992	T44.993	T44.994	T44.995	T44.996
Amfebutamone	T43.291	T43.292	T43.293	T43.294	T43.295	T43.296
Amfepramone	T50.5X1	T50.5X2	T50.5X3	T50.5X4	T50.5X5	T50.5X6
Amfetamine	T43.621	T43.622	T43.623	T43.624	T43.625	T43.626
Amfetaminil	T43.621	T43.622	T43.623	T43.624	T43.625	T43.626
Amfomycin	T36.8X1	T36.8X2	T36.8X3	T36.8X4	T36.8X5	T36.8X6
Amidefrine mesilate	T48.5X1	T48.5X2	T48.5X3	T48.5X4	T48.5X5	T48.5X6
Amidone	T40.3X1	T40.3X2	T40.3X3	T40.3X4	T40.3X5	T40.3X6
Amidopyrine	T39.2X1	T39.2X2	T39.2X3	T39.2X4	T39.2X5	T39.2X6
Amidotrizoate	T50.8X1	T50.8X2	T50.8X3	T50.8X4	T50.8X5	T50.8X6
Amiflamine	T43.1X1	T43.1X2	T43.1X3	T43.1X4	T43.1X5	T43.1X6
Amikacin	T36.5X1	T36.5X2	T36.5X3	T36.5X4	T36.5X5	T36.5X6
Amikhelline	T46.3X1	T46.3X2	T46.3X3	T46.3X4	T46.3X5	T46.3X6
Amiloride	T50.2X1	T50.2X2	T50.2X3	T50.2X4	T50.2X5	T50.2X6
Aminacrine	T49.0X1	T49.0X2	T49.0X3	T49.0X4	T49.0X5	T49.0X6
Amineptine	T43.011	T43.012	T43.013	T43.014	T43.015	T43.016
Aminitrozole	T37.3X1	T37.3X2	T37.3X3	T37.3X4	T37.3X5	T37.3X6
Aminoacetic acid	T50.3X1	T50.3X2	T50.3X3	T50.3X4	T50.3X5	T50.3X6
(derivatives)						
Amino acids	T50.3X1	T50.3X2	T50.3X3	T50.3X4	T50.3X5	T50.3X6
Aminoacridine	T49.0X1	T49.0X2	T49.0X3	T49.0X4	T49.0X5	T49.0X6
Aminobenzoic acid (-p)	T49.3X1	T49.3X2	T49.3X3	T49.3X4	T49.3X5	T49.3X6
Aminocaproic acid	T45.621	T45.622	T45.623	T45.624	T45.625	T45.626
Aminoethylisothiourium	T45.8X1	T45.8X2	T45.8X3	T45.8X4	T45.8X5	T45.8X6
Aminofenazone	T39.2X1	T39.2X2	T39.2X3	T39.2X4	T39.2X5	T39.2X6
Aminoglutethimide	T45.1X1	T45.1X2	T45.1X3	T45.1X4	T45.1X5	T45.1X6
Aminoglycosides*	T36.5X1	T36.5X2	T36.5X3	T36.5X4	T36.5X5	T36.5X6
Aminohippuric acid	T50.8X1	T50.8X2	T50.8X3	T50.8X4	T50.8X5	T50.8X6
Aminomethylbenzoic acid	T45.691	T45.692	T45.693	T45.694	T45.695	T45.696
Aminometradine	T50.2X1	T50.2X2	T50.2X3	T50.2X4	T50.2X5	T50.2X6
Aminopentamide	T44.3X1	T44.3X2	T44.3X3	T44.3X4	T44.3X5	T44.3X6
Aminophenazone	T39.2X1	T39.2X2	T39.2X3	T39.2X4	T39.2X5	T39.2X6
Aminophenol	T54.0X1	T54.0X2	T54.0X3	T54.0X4	—	—
Aminophenylpyridone	T43.591	T43.592	T43.593	T43.594	T43.595	T43.596
Aminophylline	T48.6X1	T48.6X2	T48.6X3	T48.6X4	T48.6X5	T48.6X6
Aminopterin sodium	T45.1X1	T45.1X2	T45.1X3	T45.1X4	T45.1X5	T45.1X6
Aminopyrine	T39.2X1	T39.2X2	T39.2X3	T39.2X4	T39.2X5	T39.2X6
Aminorex	T50.5X1	T50.5X2	T50.5X3	T50.5X4	T50.5X5	T50.5X6
Aminosalicylic acid	T37.1X1	T37.1X2	T37.1X3	T37.1X4	T37.1X5	T37.1X6
Aminosalylum	T37.1X1	T37.1X2	T37.1X3	T37.1X4	T37.1X5	T37.1X6
Amiodarone	T46.2X1	T46.2X2	T46.2X3	T46.2X4	T46.2X5	T46.2X6
Amiphenazole	T50.7X1	T50.7X2	T50.7X3	T50.7X4	T50.7X5	T50.7X6
Amiquinsin	T46.5X1	T46.5X2	T46.5X3	T46.5X4	T46.5X5	T46.5X6
Amisometradine	T50.2X1	T50.2X2	T50.2X3	T50.2X4	T50.2X5	T50.2X6
Amisulpride	T43.591	T43.592	T43.593	T43.594	T43.595	T43.596
Amitriptyline	T43.011	T43.012	T43.013	T43.014	T43.015	T43.016
Amitriptylinoxide	T43.011	T43.012	T43.013	T43.014	T43.015	T43.016
Amlexanox	T48.6X1	T48.6X2	T48.6X3	T48.6X4	T48.6X5	T48.6X6
Ammonia (fumes) (gas) (vapor)	T59.891	T59.892	T59.893	T59.894	—	—
aromatic spirit	T48.991	T48.992	T48.993	T48.994	T48.995	T48.996

Substance	Poisoning, Accidental (unintentional)	Poisoning, Intentional Self-harm	Poisoning, Assault	Poisoning, Undetermined	Adverse Effect	Under-dosing
Ammonia — *continued*						
liquid (household)	T54.3X1	T54.3X2	T54.3X3	T54.3X4	—	—
Ammoniated mercury	T49.0X1	T49.0X2	T49.0X3	T49.0X4	T49.0X5	T49.0X6
Ammonium						
acid tartrate	T49.5X1	T49.5X2	T49.5X3	T49.5X4	T49.5X5	T49.5X6
bromide	T42.6X1	T42.6X2	T42.6X3	T42.6X4	T42.6X5	T42.6X6
carbonate	T54.3X1	T54.3X2	T54.3X3	T54.3X4	—	—
chloride	T50.991	T50.992	T50.993	T50.994	T50.995	T50.996
expectorant	T48.4X1	T48.4X2	T48.4X3	T48.4X4	T48.4X5	T48.4X6
compounds (household) NEC	T54.3X1	T54.3X2	T54.3X3	T54.3X4	—	—
fumes (any usage)	T59.891	T59.892	T59.893	T59.894	—	—
industrial	T54.3X1	T54.3X2	T54.3X3	T54.3X4	—	—
ichthyosulronate	T49.4X1	T49.4X2	T49.4X3	T49.4X4	T49.4X5	T49.4X6
mandelate	T37.91	T37.92	T37.93	T37.94	T37.95	T37.96
sulfamate	T60.3X1	T60.3X2	T60.3X3	T60.3X4	—	—
sulfonate resin	T47.8X1	T47.8X2	T47.8X3	T47.8X4	T47.8X5	T47.8X6
Amobarbital (sodium)	T42.3X1	T42.3X2	T42.3X3	T42.3X4	T42.3X5	T42.3X6
Amodiaquine	T37.2X1	T37.2X2	T37.2X3	T37.2X4	T37.2X5	T37.2X6
Amopyroquin (e)	T37.2X1	T37.2X2	T37.2X3	T37.2X4	T37.2X5	T37.2X6
Amoxapine	T43.011	T43.012	T43.013	T43.014	T43.015	T43.016
Amoxicillin	T36.0X1	T36.0X2	T36.0X3	T36.0X4	T36.0X5	T36.0X6
Amperozide	T43.591	T43.592	T43.593	T43.594	T43.595	T43.596
Amphenidone	T43.591	T43.592	T43.593	T43.594	T43.595	T43.596
Amphetamine NEC	T43.621	T43.622	T43.623	T43.624	T43.625	T43.626
Amphogel*	T47.1X1	T47.1X2	T47.1X3	T47.1X4	T47.1X5	T47.1X6
Amphomycin	T36.8X1	T36.8X2	T36.8X3	T36.8X4	T36.8X5	T36.8X6
Amphotalide	T37.4X1	T37.4X2	T37.4X3	T37.4X4	T37.4X5	T37.4X6
Amphotericin B	T36.7X1	T36.7X2	T36.7X3	T36.7X4	T36.7X5	T36.7X6
topical	T49.0X1	T49.0X2	T49.0X3	T49.0X4	T49.0X5	T49.0X6
Ampicillin	T36.0X1	T36.0X2	T36.0X3	T36.0X4	T36.0X5	T36.0X6
Amprotropine	T44.3X1	T44.3X2	T44.3X3	T44.3X4	T44.3X5	T44.3X6
Amsacrine	T45.1X1	T45.1X2	T45.1X3	T45.1X4	T45.1X5	T45.1X6
Amygdaline	T62.2X1	T62.2X2	T62.2X3	T62.2X4	—	—
Amyl						
acetate	T52.8X1	T52.8X2	T52.8X3	T52.8X4	—	—
vapor	T59.891	T59.892	T59.893	T59.894	—	—
alcohol	T51.3X1	T51.3X2	T51.3X3	T51.3X4	—	—
chloride	T53.6X1	T53.6X2	T53.6X3	T53.6X4	—	—
formate	T52.8X1	T52.8X2	T52.8X3	T52.8X4	—	—
nitrite	T46.3X1	T46.3X2	T46.3X3	T46.3X4	T46.3X5	T46.3X6
propionate	T65.891	T65.892	T65.893	T65.894	—	—
Amylase	T47.5X1	T47.5X2	T47.5X3	T47.5X4	T47.5X5	T47.5X6
Amyleine, regional	T41.3X1	T41.3X2	T41.3X3	T41.3X4	T41.3X5	T41.3X6
Amylene						
dichloride	T53.6X1	T53.6X2	T53.6X3	T53.6X4	—	—
hydrate	T51.3X1	T51.3X2	T51.3X3	T51.3X4	—	—
Amylmetacresol	T49.6X1	T49.6X2	T49.6X3	T49.6X4	T49.6X5	T49.6X6
Amylobarbitone	T42.3X1	T42.3X2	T42.3X3	T42.3X4	T42.3X5	T42.3X6
Amylocaine, regional	T41.3X1	T41.3X2	T41.3X3	T41.3X4	T41.3X5	T41.3X6
infiltration (subcutaneous)	T41.3X1	T41.3X2	T41.3X3	T41.3X4	T41.3X5	T41.3X6
nerve block (peripheral) (plexus)	T41.3X1	T41.3X2	T41.3X3	T41.3X4	T41.3X5	T41.3X6
spinal	T41.3X1	T41.3X2	T41.3X3	T41.3X4	T41.3X5	T41.3X6
topical (surface)	T41.3X1	T41.3X2	T41.3X3	T41.3X4	T41.3X5	T41.3X6
Amylopectin	T47.6X1	T47.6X2	T47.6X3	T47.6X4	T47.6X5	T47.6X6
Amytal (sodium)	T42.3X1	T42.3X2	T42.3X3	T42.3X4	T42.3X5	T42.3X6
Anabolic steroid	T38.7X1	T38.7X2	T38.7X3	T38.7X4	T38.7X5	T38.7X6
Anacaine*	T41.3X1	T41.3X2	T41.3X3	T41.3X4	T41.3X5	T41.3X6
Analeptic NEC	T50.7X1	T50.7X2	T50.7X3	T50.7X4	T50.7X5	T50.7X6
Analgesic	T39.91	T39.92	T39.93	T39.94	T39.95	T39.96
anti-inflammatory NEC	T39.91	T39.92	T39.93	T39.94	T39.95	T39.96
propionic acid derivative	T39.311	T39.312	T39.313	T39.314	T39.315	T39.316
antirheumatic NEC	T39.4X1	T39.4X2	T39.4X3	T39.4X4	T39.4X5	T39.4X6
aromatic NEC	T39.1X1	T39.1X2	T39.1X3	T39.1X4	T39.1X5	T39.1X6
narcotic NEC	T40.601	T40.602	T40.603	T40.604	T40.605	T40.606
combination	T40.601	T40.602	T40.603	T40.604	T40.605	T40.606
obstetric	T40.601	T40.602	T40.603	T40.604	T40.605	T40.606
non-narcotic NEC	T39.91	T39.92	T39.93	T39.94	T39.95	T39.96
combination	T39.91	T39.92	T39.93	T39.94	T39.95	T39.96
pyrazole	T39.2X1	T39.2X2	T39.2X3	T39.2X4	T39.2X5	T39.2X6
specified NEC	T39.8X1	T39.8X2	T39.8X3	T39.8X4	T39.8X5	T39.8X6
Analgin	T39.2X1	T39.2X2	T39.2X3	T39.2X4	T39.2X5	T39.2X6
Anamirta cocculus	T62.1X1	T62.1X2	T62.1X3	T62.1X4	—	—
Ancillin	T36.0X1	T36.0X2	T36.0X3	T36.0X4	T36.0X5	T36.0X6
Ancrod	T45.691	T45.692	T45.693	T45.694	T45.695	T45.696
Androgen	T38.7X1	T38.7X2	T38.7X3	T38.7X4	T38.7X5	T38.7X6
Androgen-estrogen mixture	T38.7X1	T38.7X2	T38.7X3	T38.7X4	T38.7X5	T38.7X6
Androstalone	T38.7X1	T38.7X2	T38.7X3	T38.7X4	T38.7X5	T38.7X6
Androstanolone	T38.7X1	T38.7X2	T38.7X3	T38.7X4	T38.7X5	T38.7X6
Androsterone	T38.7X1	T38.7X2	T38.7X3	T38.7X4	T38.7X5	T38.7X6
Anemone pulsatilla	T62.2X1	T62.2X2	T62.2X3	T62.2X4	—	—

Substance	Poisoning, Accidental (unintentional)	Poisoning, Intentional Self-harm	Poisoning, Assault	Poisoning, Undetermined	Adverse Effect	Under-dosing
Anesthesia						
caudal	T41.3X1	T41.3X2	T41.3X3	T41.3X4	T41.3X5	T41.3X6
endotracheal	T41.0X1	T41.0X2	T41.0X3	T41.0X4	T41.0X5	T41.0X6
epidural	T41.3X1	T41.3X2	T41.3X3	T41.3X4	T41.3X5	T41.3X6
inhalation	T41.0X1	T41.0X2	T41.0X3	T41.0X4	T41.0X5	T41.0X6
local	T41.3X1	T41.3X2	T41.3X3	T41.3X4	T41.3X5	T41.3X6
mucosal	T41.3X1	T41.3X2	T41.3X3	T41.3X4	T41.3X5	T41.3X6
muscle relaxation	T48.1X1	T48.1X2	T48.1X3	T48.1X4	T48.1X5	T48.1X6
nerve blocking	T41.3X1	T41.3X2	T41.3X3	T41.3X4	T41.3X5	T41.3X6
plexus blocking	T41.3X1	T41.3X2	T41.3X3	T41.3X4	T41.3X5	T41.3X6
potentiated	T41.201	T41.202	T41.203	T41.204	T41.205	T41.206
rectal	T41.201	T41.202	T41.203	T41.204	T41.205	T41.206
general	T41.201	T41.202	T41.203	T41.204	T41.205	T41.206
local	T41.3X1	T41.3X2	T41.3X3	T41.3X4	T41.3X5	T41.3X6
regional	T41.3X1	T41.3X2	T41.3X3	T41.3X4	T41.3X5	T41.3X6
surface	T41.3X1	T41.3X2	T41.3X3	T41.3X4	T41.3X5	T41.3X6
Anesthetic NEC — *see also* Anesthesia	T41.41	T41.42	T41.43	T41.44	T41.45	T41.46
with muscle relaxant	T41.201	T41.202	T41.203	T41.204	T41.205	T41.206
general	T41.201	T41.202	T41.203	T41.204	T41.205	T41.206
local	T41.3X1	T41.3X2	T41.3X3	T41.3X4	T41.3X5	T41.3X6
gaseous NEC	T41.0X1	T41.0X2	T41.0X3	T41.0X4	T41.0X5	T41.0X6
general NEC	T41.201	T41.202	T41.203	T41.204	T41.205	T41.206
halogenated hydrocarbon derivatives NEC	T41.0X1	T41.0X2	T41.0X3	T41.0X4	T41.0X5	T41.0X6
infiltration NEC	T41.3X1	T41.3X2	T41.3X3	T41.3X4	T41.3X5	T41.3X6
intravenous NEC	T41.1X1	T41.1X2	T41.1X3	T41.1X4	T41.1X5	T41.1X6
local NEC	T41.3X1	T41.3X2	T41.3X3	T41.3X4	T41.3X5	T41.3X6
rectal	T41.201	T41.202	T41.203	T41.204	T41.205	T41.206
general	T41.201	T41.202	T41.203	T41.204	T41.205	T41.206
local	T41.3X1	T41.3X2	T41.3X3	T41.3X4	T41.3X5	T41.3X6
regional NEC	T41.3X1	T41.3X2	T41.3X3	T41.3X4	T41.3X5	T41.3X6
spinal NEC	T41.3X1	T41.3X2	T41.3X3	T41.3X4	T41.3X5	T41.3X6
thiobarbiturate	T41.1X1	T41.1X2	T41.1X3	T41.1X4	T41.1X5	T41.1X6
topical	T41.3X1	T41.3X2	T41.3X3	T41.3X4	T41.3X5	T41.3X6
Aneurine	T45.2X1	T45.2X2	T45.2X3	T45.2X4	T45.2X5	T45.2X6
Angeliq*	T38.5X1	T38.5X2	T38.5X3	T38.5X4	T38.5X5	T38.5X6
Angio-Conray	T50.8X1	T50.8X2	T50.8X3	T50.8X4	T50.8X5	T50.8X6
Angiotensin	T44.5X1	T44.5X2	T44.5X3	T44.5X4	T44.5X5	T44.5X6
Angiotensinamide	T44.991	T44.992	T44.993	T44.994	T44.995	T44.996
Anhydrohydroxy-progesterone	T38.5X1	T38.5X2	T38.5X3	T38.5X4	T38.5X5	T38.5X6
Anhydron	T50.2X1	T50.2X2	T50.2X3	T50.2X4	T50.2X5	T50.2X6
Anileridine	T40.491	T40.492	T40.493	T40.494	T40.495	T40.496
Aniline (dye) (liquid)	T65.3X1	T65.3X2	T65.3X3	T65.3X4	—	—
analgesic	T39.1X1	T39.1X2	T39.1X3	T39.1X4	T39.1X5	T39.1X6
derivatives, therapeutic NEC	T39.1X1	T39.1X2	T39.1X3	T39.1X4	T39.1X5	T39.1X6
vapor	T65.3X1	T65.3X2	T65.3X3	T65.3X4	—	—
Aniscoropine	T44.3X1	T44.3X2	T44.3X3	T44.3X4	T44.3X5	T44.3X6
Anise oil	T47.5X1	T47.5X2	T47.5X3	T47.5X4	T47.5X5	T47.5X6
Anisidine	T65.3X1	T65.3X2	T65.3X3	T65.3X4	—	—
Anisindione	T45.511	T45.512	T45.513	T45.514	T45.515	T45.516
Anisotropine	T44.3X1	T44.3X2	T44.3X3	T44.3X4	T44.3X5	T44.3X6
methyl-bromide	T45.611	T45.612	T45.613	T45.614	T45.615	T45.616
Anistreplase	T45.611	T45.612	T45.613	T45.614	T45.615	T45.616
Anorexiant (central)	T50.5X1	T50.5X2	T50.5X3	T50.5X4	T50.5X5	T50.5X6
Anorexic agents	T50.5X1	T50.5X2	T50.5X3	T50.5X4	T50.5X5	T50.5X6
Ansaid*	T39.311	T39.312	T39.313	T39.314	T39.315	T39.316
Ansamycin	T36.6X1	T36.6X2	T36.6X3	T36.6X4	T36.6X5	T36.6X6
Ant (bite) (sting)	T63.421	T63.422	T63.423	T63.424		
Antabuse	T50.6X1	T50.6X2	T50.6X3	T50.6X4	T50.6X5	T50.6X6
Antacid NEC	T47.1X1	T47.1X2	T47.1X3	T47.1X4	T47.1X5	T47.1X6
Antagonist						
Aldosterone	T50.0X1	T50.0X2	T50.0X3	T50.0X4	T50.0X5	T50.0X6
alpha-adrenoreceptor	T44.6X1	T44.6X2	T44.6X3	T44.6X4	T44.6X5	T44.6X6
anticoagulant	T45.7X1	T45.7X2	T45.7X3	T45.7X4	T45.7X5	T45.7X6
beta-adrenoreceptor	T44.7X1	T44.7X2	T44.7X3	T44.7X4	T44.7X5	T44.7X6
extrapyramidal NEC	T44.3X1	T44.3X2	T44.3X3	T44.3X4	T44.3X5	T44.3X6
folic acid	T45.1X1	T45.1X2	T45.1X3	T45.1X4	T45.1X5	T45.1X6
H2 receptor	T47.0X1	T47.0X2	T47.0X3	T47.0X4	T47.0X5	T47.0X6
heavy metal	T45.8X1	T45.8X2	T45.8X3	T45.8X4	T45.8X5	T45.8X6
narcotic analgesic	T50.7X1	T50.7X2	T50.7X3	T50.7X4	T50.7X5	T50.7X6
opiate	T50.7X1	T50.7X2	T50.7X3	T50.7X4	T50.7X5	T50.7X6
pyrimidine	T45.1X1	T45.1X2	T45.1X3	T45.1X4	T45.1X5	T45.1X6
serotonin	T46.5X1	T46.5X2	T46.5X3	T46.5X4	T46.5X5	T46.5X6
Antazolin (e)	T45.0X1	T45.0X2	T45.0X3	T45.0X4	T45.0X5	T45.0X6
Anterior pituitary hormone NEC	T38.811	T38.812	T38.813	T38.814	T38.815	T38.816
Anthelmintic NEC	T37.4X1	T37.4X2	T37.4X3	T37.4X4	T37.4X5	T37.4X6
Anthiolimine	T37.4X1	T37.4X2	T37.4X3	T37.4X4	T37.4X5	T37.4X6
Anthralin	T49.4X1	T49.4X2	T49.4X3	T49.4X4	T49.4X5	T49.4X6
Anthramycin	T45.1X1	T45.1X2	T45.1X3	T45.1X4	T45.1X5	T45.1X6
Antiadrenergic NEC	T44.8X1	T44.8X2	T44.8X3	T44.8X4	T44.8X5	T44.8X6
Antiallergic NEC	T45.0X1	T45.0X2	T45.0X3	T45.0X4	T45.0X5	T45.0X6
Antiandrogen NEC	T38.6X1	T38.6X2	T38.6X3	T38.6X4	T38.6X5	T38.6X6
Anti-anemic (drug) (preparation)	T45.8X1	T45.8X2	T45.8X3	T45.8X4	T45.8X5	T45.8X6
Antianxiety drug NEC	T43.501	T43.502	T43.503	T43.504	T43.505	T43.506
Antiaris toxicaria	T65.891	T65.892	T65.893	T65.894	—	—
Antiarteriosclerotic drug	T46.6X1	T46.6X2	T46.6X3	T46.6X4	T46.6X5	T46.6X6
Antiasthmatic drug NEC	T48.6X1	T48.6X2	T48.6X3	T48.6X4	T48.6X5	T48.6X6
Antibiotic Otic Suspension (Solution)*	T49.6X1	T49.6X2	T49.6X3	T49.6X4	T49.6X5	T49.6X6
Antibiotic NEC	T36.91	T36.92	T36.93	T36.94	T36.95	T36.96
aminoglycoside	T36.5X1	T36.5X2	T36.5X3	T36.5X4	T36.5X5	T36.5X6
anticancer	T45.1X1	T45.1X2	T45.1X3	T45.1X4	T45.1X5	T45.1X6
antifungal	T36.7X1	T36.7X2	T36.7X3	T36.7X4	T36.7X5	T36.7X6
antimycobacterial	T36.5X1	T36.5X2	T36.5X3	T36.5X4	T36.5X5	T36.5X6
antineoplastic	T45.1X1	T45.1X2	T45.1X3	T45.1X4	T45.1X5	T45.1X6
b-lactam NEC	T36.1X1	T36.1X2	T36.1X3	T36.1X4	T36.1X5	T36.1X6
cephalosporin (group)	T36.1X1	T36.1X2	T36.1X3	T36.1X4	T36.1X5	T36.1X6
chloramphenicol (group)	T36.2X1	T36.2X2	T36.2X3	T36.2X4	T36.2X5	T36.2X6
ENT	T49.6X1	T49.6X2	T49.6X3	T49.6X4	T49.6X5	T49.6X6
eye	T49.5X1	T49.5X2	T49.5X3	T49.5X4	T49.5X5	T49.5X6
fungicidal (local)	T49.0X1	T49.0X2	T49.0X3	T49.0X4	T49.0X5	T49.0X6
intestinal	T36.8X1	T36.8X2	T36.8X3	T36.8X4	T36.8X5	T36.8X6
local	T49.0X1	T49.0X2	T49.0X3	T49.0X4	T49.0X5	T49.0X6
macrolides	T36.3X1	T36.3X2	T36.3X3	T36.3X4	T36.3X5	T36.3X6
polypeptide	T36.8X1	T36.8X2	T36.8X3	T36.8X4	T36.8X5	T36.8X6
specified NEC	T36.8X1	T36.8X2	T36.8X3	T36.8X4	T36.8X5	T36.8X6
tetracycline (group)	T36.4X1	T36.4X2	T36.4X3	T36.4X4	T36.4X5	T36.4X6
throat	T49.6X1	T49.6X2	T49.6X3	T49.6X4	T49.6X5	T49.6X6
Anticancer agents NEC	T45.1X1	T45.1X2	T45.1X3	T45.1X4	T45.1X5	T45.1X6
Anticholesterolemic drug NEC	T46.6X1	T46.6X2	T46.6X3	T46.6X4	T46.6X5	T46.6X6
Anticholinergic NEC	T44.3X1	T44.3X2	T44.3X3	T44.3X4	T44.3X5	T44.3X6
Anticholinesterase	T44.0X1	T44.0X2	T44.0X3	T44.0X4	T44.0X5	T44.0X6
organophosphorus insecticide	T60.0X1	T60.0X2	T60.0X3	T60.0X4	—	—
nerve gas	T59.891	T59.892	T59.893	T59.894	—	—
reversible	T44.0X1	T44.0X2	T44.0X3	T44.0X4	T44.0X5	T44.0X6
ophthalmological	T49.5X1	T49.5X2	T49.5X3	T49.5X4	T49.5X5	T49.5X6
Anticoagulant NEC	T45.511	T45.512	T45.513	T45.514	T45.515	T45.516
Antagonist	T45.7X1	T45.7X2	T45.7X3	T45.7X4	T45.7X5	T45.7X6
Anti-common-cold drug NEC	T48.5X1	T48.5X2	T48.5X3	T48.5X4	T48.5X5	T48.5X6
Anticonvulsant	T42.71	T42.72	T42.73	T42.74	T42.75	T42.76
barbiturate	T42.3X1	T42.3X2	T42.3X3	T42.3X4	T42.3X5	T42.3X6
combination (with barbiturate)	T42.3X1	T42.3X2	T42.3X3	T42.3X4	T42.3X5	T42.3X6
hydantoin	T42.0X1	T42.0X2	T42.0X3	T42.0X4	T42.0X5	T42.0X6
hypnotic NEC	T42.6X1	T42.6X2	T42.6X3	T42.6X4	T42.6X5	T42.6X6
oxazolidinedione	T42.2X1	T42.2X2	T42.2X3	T42.2X4	T42.2X5	T42.2X6
pyrimidinedione	T42.6X1	T42.6X2	T42.6X3	T42.6X4	T42.6X5	T42.6X6
specified NEC	T42.6X1	T42.6X2	T42.6X3	T42.6X4	T42.6X5	T42.6X6
succinimide	T42.2X1	T42.2X2	T42.2X3	T42.2X4	T42.2X5	T42.2X6
Antidepressant	T43.201	T43.202	T43.203	T43.204	T43.205	T43.206
monoamine oxidase inhibitor	T43.1X1	T43.1X2	T43.1X3	T43.1X4	T43.1X5	T43.1X6
selective serotonin norepinephrine reuptake inhibitor	T43.211	T43.212	T43.213	T43.214	T43.215	T43.216
selective serotonin reuptake inhibitor	T43.221	T43.222	T43.223	T43.224	T43.225	T43.226
specified NEC	T43.291	T43.292	T43.293	T43.294	T43.295	T43.296
tetracyclic	T43.021	T43.022	T43.023	T43.024	T43.025	T43.026
triazolopyridine	T43.211	T43.212	T43.213	T43.214	T43.215	T43.216
tricyclic	T43.011	T43.012	T43.013	T43.014	T43.015	T43.016
Antidiabetic NEC	T38.3X1	T38.3X2	T38.3X3	T38.3X4	T38.3X5	T38.3X6
biguanide	T38.3X1	T38.3X2	T38.3X3	T38.3X4	T38.3X5	T38.3X6
and sulfonyl combined	T38.3X1	T38.3X2	T38.3X3	T38.3X4	T38.3X5	T38.3X6
combined	T38.3X1	T38.3X2	T38.3X3	T38.3X4	T38.3X5	T38.3X6
sulfonylurea	T38.3X1	T38.3X2	T38.3X3	T38.3X4	T38.3X5	T38.3X6
Antidiarrheal drug NEC	T47.6X1	T47.6X2	T47.6X3	T47.6X4	T47.6X5	T47.6X6
absorbent	T47.6X1	T47.6X2	T47.6X3	T47.6X4	T47.6X5	T47.6X6
Anti-D immunoglobulin (human)	T50.Z11	T50.Z12	T50.Z13	T50.Z14	T50.Z15	T50.Z16
Antidiphtheria serum	T50.Z11	T50.Z12	T50.Z13	T50.Z14	T50.Z15	T50.Z16
Antidiuretic hormone	T38.891	T38.892	T38.893	T38.894	T38.895	T38.896
Antidote NEC	T50.6X1	T50.6X2	T50.6X3	T50.6X4	T50.6X5	T50.6X6
heavy metal	T45.8X1	T45.8X2	T45.8X3	T45.8X4	T45.8X5	T45.8X6
Antidysrhythmic NEC	T46.2X1	T46.2X2	T46.2X3	T46.2X4	T46.2X5	T46.2X6
Antiemetic drug	T45.0X1	T45.0X2	T45.0X3	T45.0X4	T45.0X5	T45.0X6
Antiepilepsy agent	T42.71	T42.72	T42.73	T42.74	T42.75	T42.76
combination	T42.5X1	T42.5X2	T42.5X3	T42.5X4	T42.5X5	T42.5X6
mixed	T42.5X1	T42.5X2	T42.5X3	T42.5X4	T42.5X5	T42.5X6

Substance	Poisoning, Accidental (unintentional)	Poisoning, Intentional Self-harm	Poisoning, Assault	Poisoning, Undetermined	Adverse Effect	Under- dosing
Antiepilepsy agent — continued						
specified, NEC	T42.6X1	T42.6X2	T42.6X3	T42.6X4	T42.6X5	T42.6X6
Antiestrogen NEC	T38.6X1	T38.6X2	T38.6X3	T38.6X4	T38.6X5	T38.6X6
Antifertility pill	T38.4X1	T38.4X2	T38.4X3	T38.4X4	T38.4X5	T38.4X6
Antifibrinolytic drug	T45.621	T45.622	T45.623	T45.624	T45.625	T45.626
Antifilarial drug	T37.4X1	T37.4X2	T37.4X3	T37.4X4	T37.4X5	T37.4X6
Antiflatulent	T47.5X1	T47.5X2	T47.5X3	T47.5X4	T47.5X5	T47.5X6
Antifreeze	T65.91	T65.92	T65.93	T65.94	—	—
alcohol	T51.1X1	T51.1X2	T51.1X3	T51.1X4	—	—
ethylene glycol	T51.8X1	T51.8X2	T51.8X3	T51.8X4	—	—
Antifungal						
antibiotic (systemic)	T36.7X1	T36.7X2	T36.7X3	T36.7X4	T36.7X5	T36.7X6
anti-infective NEC	T37.91	T37.92	T37.93	T37.94	T37.95	T37.96
disinfectant, local	T49.0X1	T49.0X2	T49.0X3	T49.0X4	T49.0X5	T49.0X6
nonmedicinal (spray)	T60.3X1	T60.3X2	T60.3X3	T60.3X4	—	—
topical	T49.0X1	T49.0X2	T49.0X3	T49.0X4	T49.0X5	T49.0X6
Anti-gastric-secretion drug NEC	T47.1X1	T47.1X2	T47.1X3	T47.1X4	T47.1X5	T47.1X6
Antigonadotrophin NEC	T38.6X1	T38.6X2	T38.6X3	T38.6X4	T38.6X5	T38.6X6
Antihallucinogen	T43.501	T43.502	T43.503	T43.504	T43.505	T43.506
Antihelmintics	T37.4X1	T37.4X2	T37.4X3	T37.4X4	T37.4X5	T37.4X6
Antihemophilic						
factor	T45.8X1	T45.8X2	T45.8X3	T45.8X4	T45.8X5	T45.8X6
fraction	T45.8X1	T45.8X2	T45.8X3	T45.8X4	T45.8X5	T45.8X6
globulin concentrate	T45.7X1	T45.7X2	T45.7X3	T45.7X4	T45.7X5	T45.7X6
human plasma	T45.8X1	T45.8X2	T45.8X3	T45.8X4	T45.8X5	T45.8X6
plasma, dried	T45.7X1	T45.7X2	T45.7X3	T45.7X4	T45.7X5	T45.7X6
Antihemorrhoidal preparation	T49.2X1	T49.2X2	T49.2X3	T49.2X4	T49.2X5	T49.2X6
Antiheparin drug	T45.7X1	T45.7X2	T45.7X3	T45.7X4	T45.7X5	T45.7X6
Antihistamine	T45.0X1	T45.0X2	T45.0X3	T45.0X4	T45.0X5	T45.0X6
Antihookworm drug	T37.4X1	T37.4X2	T37.4X3	T37.4X4	T37.4X5	T37.4X6
Anti-human lymphocytic globulin	T50.Z11	T50.Z12	T50.Z13	T50.Z14	T50.Z15	T50.Z16
Antihyperlipidemic drug	T46.6X1	T46.6X2	T46.6X3	T46.6X4	T46.6X5	T46.6X6
Antihypertensive drug NEC	T46.5X1	T46.5X2	T46.5X3	T46.5X4	T46.5X5	T46.5X6
Anti-infective NEC	T37.91	T37.92	T37.93	T37.94	T37.95	T37.96
anthelmintic	T37.4X1	T37.4X2	T37.4X3	T37.4X4	T37.4X5	T37.4X6
antibiotics	T36.91	T36.92	T36.93	T36.94	T36.95	T36.96
specified NEC	T36.8X1	T36.8X2	T36.8X3	T36.8X4	T36.8X5	T36.8X6
antimalarial	T37.2X1	T37.2X2	T37.2X3	T37.2X4	T37.2X5	T37.2X6
antimycobacterial NEC	T37.1X1	T37.1X2	T37.1X3	T37.1X4	T37.1X5	T37.1X6
antibiotics	T36.5X1	T36.5X2	T36.5X3	T36.5X4	T36.5X5	T36.5X6
antiprotozoal NEC	T37.3X1	T37.3X2	T37.3X3	T37.3X4	T37.3X5	T37.3X6
blood	T37.2X1	T37.2X2	T37.2X3	T37.2X4	T37.2X5	T37.2X6
antiviral	T37.5X1	T37.5X2	T37.5X3	T37.5X4	T37.5X5	T37.5X6
arsenical	T37.8X1	T37.8X2	T37.8X3	T37.8X4	T37.8X5	T37.8X6
bismuth, local	T49.0X1	T49.0X2	T49.0X3	T49.0X4	T49.0X5	T49.0X6
ENT	T49.6X1	T49.6X2	T49.6X3	T49.6X4	T49.6X5	T49.6X6
eye NEC	T49.5X1	T49.5X2	T49.5X3	T49.5X4	T49.5X5	T49.5X6
heavy metals NEC	T37.8X1	T37.8X2	T37.8X3	T37.8X4	T37.8X5	T37.8X6
local NEC	T49.0X1	T49.0X2	T49.0X3	T49.0X4	T49.0X5	T49.0X6
specified NEC	T49.0X1	T49.0X2	T49.0X3	T49.0X4	T49.0X5	T49.0X6
mixed	T37.91	T37.92	T37.93	T37.94	T37.95	T37.96
ophthalmic preparation	T49.5X1	T49.5X2	T49.5X3	T49.5X4	T49.5X5	T49.5X6
topical NEC	T49.0X1	T49.0X2	T49.0X3	T49.0X4	T49.0X5	T49.0X6
Anti-inflammatory drug NEC	T39.391	T39.392	T39.393	T39.394	T39.395	T39.396
local	T49.0X1	T49.0X2	T49.0X3	T49.0X4	T49.0X5	T49.0X6
nonsteroidal NEC	T39.391	T39.392	T39.393	T39.394	T39.395	T39.396
propionic acid derivative	T39.311	T39.312	T39.313	T39.314	T39.315	T39.316
specified NEC	T39.391	T39.392	T39.393	T39.394	T39.395	T39.396
Antikaluretic	T50.3X1	T50.3X2	T50.3X3	T50.3X4	T50.3X5	T50.3X6
Antiknock (tetraethyl lead)	T56.0X1	T56.0X2	T56.0X3	T56.0X4	—	—
Antilipemic drug NEC	T46.6X1	T46.6X2	T46.6X3	T46.6X4	T46.6X5	T46.6X6
Antilysin*	T45.621	T45.622	T45.623	T45.624	T45.625	T45.626
Antimalarial	T37.2X1	T37.2X2	T37.2X3	T37.2X4	T37.2X5	T37.2X6
prophylactic NEC	T37.2X1	T37.2X2	T37.2X3	T37.2X4	T37.2X5	T37.2X6
pyrimidine derivative	T37.2X1	T37.2X2	T37.2X3	T37.2X4	T37.2X5	T37.2X6
Antimetabolite	T45.1X1	T45.1X2	T45.1X3	T45.1X4	T45.1X5	T45.1X6
Antimitotic agent	T45.1X1	T45.1X2	T45.1X3	T45.1X4	T45.1X5	T45.1X6
Antimony (compounds) (vapor) NEC	T56.891	T56.892	T56.893	T56.894	—	—
anti-infectives	T37.8X1	T37.8X2	T37.8X3	T37.8X4	T37.8X5	T37.8X6
dimercaptosuccinate	T37.3X1	T37.3X2	T37.3X3	T37.3X4	T37.3X5	T37.3X6
hydride	T56.891	T56.892	T56.893	T56.894	—	—
pesticide (vapor)	T60.8X1	T60.8X2	T60.8X3	T60.8X4	—	—
potassium (sodium) tartrate	T37.8X1	T37.8X2	T37.8X3	T37.8X4	T37.8X5	T37.8X6
sodium dimercaptosuccinate	T37.3X1	T37.3X2	T37.3X3	T37.3X4	T37.3X5	T37.3X6
tartrated	T37.8X1	T37.8X2	T37.8X3	T37.8X4	T37.8X5	T37.8X6

Substance	Poisoning, Accidental (unintentional)	Poisoning, Intentional Self-harm	Poisoning, Assault	Poisoning, Undetermined	Adverse Effect	Under- dosing
Antimuscarinic NEC	T44.3X1	T44.3X2	T44.3X3	T44.3X4	T44.3X5	T44.3X6
Antimycobacterial drug NEC	T37.1X1	T37.1X2	T37.1X3	T37.1X4	T37.1X5	T37.1X6
antibiotics	T36.5X1	T36.5X2	T36.5X3	T36.5X4	T36.5X5	T36.5X6
combination	T37.1X1	T37.1X2	T37.1X3	T37.1X4	T37.1X5	T37.1X6
Antinausea drug	T45.0X1	T45.0X2	T45.0X3	T45.0X4	T45.0X5	T45.0X6
Antinematode drug	T37.4X1	T37.4X2	T37.4X3	T37.4X4	T37.4X5	T37.4X6
Antineoplastic NEC	T45.1X1	T45.1X2	T45.1X3	T45.1X4	T45.1X5	T45.1X6
alkaloidal	T45.1X1	T45.1X2	T45.1X3	T45.1X4	T45.1X5	T45.1X6
antibiotics	T45.1X1	T45.1X2	T45.1X3	T45.1X4	T45.1X5	T45.1X6
combination	T45.1X1	T45.1X2	T45.1X3	T45.1X4	T45.1X5	T45.1X6
estrogen	T38.5X1	T38.5X2	T38.5X3	T38.5X4	T38.5X5	T38.5X6
steroid	T38.7X1	T38.7X2	T38.7X3	T38.7X4	T38.7X5	T38.7X6
Antiparasitic drug (systemic)	T37.91	T37.92	T37.93	T37.94	T37.95	T37.96
local	T49.0X1	T49.0X2	T49.0X3	T49.0X4	T49.0X5	T49.0X6
specified NEC	T37.8X1	T37.8X2	T37.8X3	T37.8X4	T37.8X5	T37.8X6
Antiparkinsonism drug NEC	T42.8X1	T42.8X2	T42.8X3	T42.8X4	T42.8X5	T42.8X6
Antiperspirant NEC	T49.2X1	T49.2X2	T49.2X3	T49.2X4	T49.2X5	T49.2X6
Antiphlogistic NEC	T39.4X1	T39.4X2	T39.4X3	T39.4X4	T39.4X5	T39.4X6
Antiplatyhelmintic drug	T37.4X1	T37.4X2	T37.4X3	T37.4X4	T37.4X5	T37.4X6
Antiprotozoal drug NEC	T37.3X1	T37.3X2	T37.3X3	T37.3X4	T37.3X5	T37.3X6
blood	T37.2X1	T37.2X2	T37.2X3	T37.2X4	T37.2X5	T37.2X6
local	T49.0X1	T49.0X2	T49.0X3	T49.0X4	T49.0X5	T49.0X6
Antipruritic drug NEC	T49.1X1	T49.1X2	T49.1X3	T49.1X4	T49.1X5	T49.1X6
Antipsychotic drug	T43.501	T43.502	T43.503	T43.504	T43.505	T43.506
specified NEC	T43.591	T43.592	T43.593	T43.594	T43.595	T43.596
Antipyretic	T39.91	T39.92	T39.93	T39.94	T39.95	T39.96
specified NEC	T39.8X1	T39.8X2	T39.8X3	T39.8X4	T39.8X5	T39.8X6
Antipyrine	T39.2X1	T39.2X2	T39.2X3	T39.2X4	T39.2X5	T39.2X6
Antirabies hyperimmune serum	T50.Z11	T50.Z12	T50.Z13	T50.Z14	T50.Z15	T50.Z16
Antirheumatic NEC	T39.4X1	T39.4X2	T39.4X3	T39.4X4	T39.4X5	T39.4X6
Antirigidity drug NEC	T42.8X1	T42.8X2	T42.8X3	T42.8X4	T42.8X5	T42.8X6
Antischistosomal drug	T37.4X1	T37.4X2	T37.4X3	T37.4X4	T37.4X5	T37.4X6
Antiscorpion sera	T50.Z11	T50.Z12	T50.Z13	T50.Z14	T50.Z15	T50.Z16
Antiseborrheics	T49.4X1	T49.4X2	T49.4X3	T49.4X4	T49.4X5	T49.4X6
Antiseptics (external) (medicinal)	T49.0X1	T49.0X2	T49.0X3	T49.0X4	T49.0X5	T49.0X6
Antistine				T45.0X3	T45.0X4	T45.0X5	T45.0X6
Antitapeworm drug	T37.4X1	T37.4X2	T37.4X3	T37.4X4	T37.4X5	T37.4X6
Antitetanus immunoglobulin	T50.Z11	T50.Z12	T50.Z13	T50.Z14	T50.Z15	T50.Z16
Antithrombin III*	T45.511	T45.512	T45.513	T45.514	T45.515	T45.516
Antithrombotic	T45.521	T45.522	T45.523	T45.524	T45.525	T45.526
Antithyroid drug NEC	T38.2X1	T38.2X2	T38.2X3	T38.2X4	T38.2X5	T38.2X6
Antitoxin	T50.Z11	T50.Z12	T50.Z13	T50.Z14	T50.Z15	T50.Z16
diphtheria	T50.Z11	T50.Z12	T50.Z13	T50.Z14	T50.Z15	T50.Z16
gas gangrene	T50.Z11	T50.Z12	T50.Z13	T50.Z14	T50.Z15	T50.Z16
tetanus	T50.Z11	T50.Z12	T50.Z13	T50.Z14	T50.Z15	T50.Z16
Antitrichomonal drug	T37.3X1	T37.3X2	T37.3X3	T37.3X4	T37.3X5	T37.3X6
Antituberculars	T37.1X1	T37.1X2	T37.1X3	T37.1X4	T37.1X5	T37.1X6
antibiotics	T36.5X1	T36.5X2	T36.5X3	T36.5X4	T36.5X5	T36.5X6
Antitussive NEC	T48.3X1	T48.3X2	T48.3X3	T48.3X4	T48.3X5	T48.3X6
codeine mixture	T40.2X1	T40.2X2	T40.2X3	T40.2X4	T40.2X5	T40.2X6
opiate	T40.2X1	T40.2X2	T40.2X3	T40.2X4	T40.2X5	T40.2X6
Antivaricose drug	T46.8X1	T46.8X2	T46.8X3	T46.8X4	T46.8X5	T46.8X6
Antivenin, antivenom (sera)	T50.Z11	T50.Z12	T50.Z13	T50.Z14	T50.Z15	T50.Z16
crotaline	T50.Z11	T50.Z12	T50.Z13	T50.Z14	T50.Z15	T50.Z16
spider bite	T50.Z11	T50.Z12	T50.Z13	T50.Z14	T50.Z15	T50.Z16
Antivert*	T45.0X1	T45.0X2	T45.0X3	T45.0X4	T45.0X5	T45.0X6
Antivertigo drug	T45.0X1	T45.0X2	T45.0X3	T45.0X4	T45.0X5	T45.0X6
Antiviral drug NEC	T37.5X1	T37.5X2	T37.5X3	T37.5X4	T37.5X5	T37.5X6
eye	T49.5X1	T49.5X2	T49.5X3	T49.5X4	T49.5X5	T49.5X6
Antiwhipworm drug	T37.4X1	T37.4X2	T37.4X3	T37.4X4	T37.4X5	T37.4X6
Ant poison — see Insecticide						
Antrol — see also by specific chemical substance	T60.91	T60.92	T60.93	T60.94	—	—
fungicide	T60.91	T60.92	T60.93	T60.94	—	—
ANTU (alpha naphthylthiourea)	T60.4X1	T60.4X2	T60.4X3	T60.4X4	—	—
Apalcillin	T36.0X1	T36.0X2	T36.0X3	T36.0X4	T36.0X5	T36.0X6
APC	T48.5X1	T48.5X2	T48.5X3	T48.5X4	T48.5X5	T48.5X6
Aplonidine	T44.4X1	T44.4X2	T44.4X3	T44.4X4	T44.4X5	T44.4X6
Apomorphine	T47.7X1	T47.7X2	T47.7X3	T47.7X4	T47.7X5	T47.7X6
Appetite depressants, central	T50.5X1	T50.5X2	T50.5X3	T50.5X4	T50.5X5	T50.5X6
Apraclonidine (hydrochloride)	T44.4X1	T44.4X2	T44.4X3	T44.4X4	T44.4X5	T44.4X6
Apresoline	T46.5X1	T46.5X2	T46.5X3	T46.5X4	T46.5X5	T46.5X6
Apri*	T38.4X1	T38.4X2	T38.4X3	T38.4X4	T38.4X5	T38.4X6

Substance	Poisoning, Accidental (unintentional)	Poisoning, Intentional Self-harm	Poisoning, Assault	Poisoning, Undetermined	Adverse Effect	Under-dosing
Aprindine	T46.2X1	T46.2X2	T46.2X3	T46.2X4	T46.2X5	T46.2X6
Aprobarbital	T42.3X1	T42.3X2	T42.3X3	T42.3X4	T42.3X5	T42.3X6
Apronalide	T42.6X1	T42.6X2	T42.6X3	T42.6X4	T42.6X5	T42.6X6
Aprotinin	T45.621	T45.622	T45.623	T45.624	T45.625	T45.626
Aptocaine	T41.3X1	T41.3X2	T41.3X3	T41.3X4	T41.3X5	T41.3X6
Aqua fortis	T54.2X1	T54.2X2	T54.2X3	T54.2X4	—	—
Ara-A	T37.5X1	T37.5X2	T37.5X3	T37.5X4	T37.5X5	T37.5X6
Ara-C	T45.1X1	T45.1X2	T45.1X3	T45.1X4	T45.1X5	T45.1X6
Arachis oil	T49.3X1	T49.3X2	T49.3X3	T49.3X4	T49.3X5	T49.3X6
cathartic	T47.4X1	T47.4X2	T47.4X3	T47.4X4	T47.4X5	T47.4X6
Aralen	T37.2X1	T37.2X2	T37.2X3	T37.2X4	T37.2X5	T37.2X6
Arecoline	T44.1X1	T44.1X2	T44.1X3	T44.1X4	T44.1X5	T44.1X6
Arginine	T50.991	T50.992	T50.993	T50.994	T50.995	T50.996
glutamate	T50.991	T50.992	T50.993	T50.994	T50.995	T50.996
Argyrol	T49.0X1	T49.0X2	T49.0X3	T49.0X4	T49.0X5	T49.0X6
ENT agent	T49.6X1	T49.6X2	T49.6X3	T49.6X4	T49.6X5	T49.6X6
ophthalmic preparation	T49.5X1	T49.5X2	T49.5X3	T49.5X4	T49.5X5	T49.5X6
Aristocort	T38.0X1	T38.0X2	T38.0X3	T38.0X4	T38.0X5	T38.0X6
ENT agent	T49.6X1	T49.6X2	T49.6X3	T49.6X4	T49.6X5	T49.6X6
ophthalmic preparation	T49.5X1	T49.5X2	T49.5X3	T49.5X4	T49.5X5	T49.5X6
topical NEC	T49.0X1	T49.0X2	T49.0X3	T49.0X4	T49.0X5	T49.0X6
Aromatics, corrosive	T54.1X1	T54.1X2	T54.1X3	T54.1X4	—	—
disinfectants	T54.1X1	T54.1X2	T54.1X3	T54.1X4	—	—
Arsenate of lead	T57.0X1	T57.0X2	T57.0X3	T57.0X4	—	—
herbicide	T57.0X1	T57.0X2	T57.0X3	T57.0X4	—	—
Arsenic, arsenicals (compounds) (dust) (vapor) **NEC**	T57.0X1	T57.0X2	T57.0X3	T57.0X4	—	—
anti-infectives	T37.8X1	T37.8X2	T37.8X3	T37.8X4	T37.8X5	T37.8X6
pesticide (dust) (fumes)	T57.0X1	T57.0X2	T57.0X3	T57.0X4	—	—
Arsine (gas)	T57.0X1	T57.0X2	T57.0X3	T57.0X4	—	—
Arsobal*	T37.3X1	T37.3X2	T37.3X3	T37.3X4	T37.3X5	T37.3X6
Arsphenamine (silver)	T37.8X1	T37.8X2	T37.8X3	T37.8X4	T37.8X5	T37.8X6
Arsthinol	T37.3X1	T37.3X2	T37.3X3	T37.3X4	T37.3X5	T37.3X6
Artane	T44.3X1	T44.3X2	T44.3X3	T44.3X4	T44.3X5	T44.3X6
Arthropod (venomous) **NEC**	T63.481	T63.482	T63.483	T63.484	—	—
Articaine	T41.3X1	T41.3X2	T41.3X3	T41.3X4	T41.3X5	T41.3X6
Asbestos	T57.8X1	T57.8X2	T57.8X3	T57.8X4	—	—
Ascaridole	T37.4X1	T37.4X2	T37.4X3	T37.4X4	T37.4X5	T37.4X6
Ascorbic acid	T45.2X1	T45.2X2	T45.2X3	T45.2X4	T45.2X5	T45.2X6
Asiaticoside	T49.0X1	T49.0X2	T49.0X3	T49.0X4	T49.0X5	T49.0X6
Asparaginase	T45.1X1	T45.1X2	T45.1X3	T45.1X4	T45.1X5	T45.1X6
Aspidium (oleoresin)	T37.4X1	T37.4X2	T37.4X3	T37.4X4	T37.4X5	T37.4X6
Aspirin (aluminum) (soluble)	T39.011	T39.012	T39.013	T39.014	T39.015	T39.016
Aspoxicillin	T36.0X1	T36.0X2	T36.0X3	T36.0X4	T36.0X5	T36.0X6
Astemizole	T45.0X1	T45.0X2	T45.0X3	T45.0X4	T45.0X5	T45.0X6
Astringent (local)	T49.2X1	T49.2X2	T49.2X3	T49.2X4	T49.2X5	T49.2X6
specified NEC	T49.2X1	T49.2X2	T49.2X3	T49.2X4	T49.2X5	T49.2X6
Astromicin	T36.5X1	T36.5X2	T36.5X3	T36.5X4	T36.5X5	T36.5X6
Ataractic drug NEC	T43.501	T43.502	T43.503	T43.504	T43.505	T43.506
Atenolol	T44.7X1	T44.7X2	T44.7X3	T44.7X4	T44.7X5	T44.7X6
Atonia drug, intestinal	T47.4X1	T47.4X2	T47.4X3	T47.4X4	T47.4X5	T47.4X6
Atophan	T50.4X1	T50.4X2	T50.4X3	T50.4X4	T50.4X5	T50.4X6
Atracurium besilate	T48.1X1	T48.1X2	T48.1X3	T48.1X4	T48.1X5	T48.1X6
Atropine	T44.3X1	T44.3X2	T44.3X3	T44.3X4	T44.3X5	T44.3X6
derivative	T44.3X1	T44.3X2	T44.3X3	T44.3X4	T44.3X5	T44.3X6
methonitrate	T44.3X1	T44.3X2	T44.3X3	T44.3X4	T44.3X5	T44.3X6
Atrovent*	T48.6X1	T48.6X2	T48.6X3	T48.6X4	T48.6X5	T48.6X6
Attapulgite	T47.6X1	T47.6X2	T47.6X3	T47.6X4	T47.6X5	T47.6X6
Auramine	T65.891	T65.892	T65.893	T65.894	—	—
dye	T65.6X1	T65.6X2	T65.6X3	T65.6X4	—	—
fungicide	T60.3X1	T60.3X2	T60.3X3	T60.3X4	—	—
Auranofin	T39.4X1	T39.4X2	T39.4X3	T39.4X4	T39.4X5	T39.4X6
Aurantiin	T46.991	T46.992	T46.993	T46.994	T46.995	T46.996
Aureomycin	T36.4X1	T36.4X2	T36.4X3	T36.4X4	T36.4X5	T36.4X6
ophthalmic preparation	T49.5X1	T49.5X2	T49.5X3	T49.5X4	T49.5X5	T49.5X6
topical NEC	T49.0X1	T49.0X2	T49.0X3	T49.0X4	T49.0X5	T49.0X6
Aurothioglucose	T39.4X1	T39.4X2	T39.4X3	T39.4X4	T39.4X5	T39.4X6
Aurothioglycanide	T39.4X1	T39.4X2	T39.4X3	T39.4X4	T39.4X5	T39.4X6
Aurothiomalate sodium	T39.4X1	T39.4X2	T39.4X3	T39.4X4	T39.4X5	T39.4X6
Aurotioprol	T39.4X1	T39.4X2	T39.4X3	T39.4X4	T39.4X5	T39.4X6
Automobile fuel	T52.0X1	T52.0X2	T52.0X3	T52.0X4	—	—
Autonomic nervous system agent NEC	T44.901	T44.902	T44.903	T44.904	T44.905	T44.906
Avelox*	T36.8X1	T36.8X2	T36.8X3	T36.8X4	T36.8X5	T36.8X6
Avlosulfon	T37.1X1	T37.1X2	T37.1X3	T37.1X4	T37.1X5	T37.1X6
Avomine	T42.6X1	T42.6X2	T42.6X3	T42.6X4	T42.6X5	T42.6X6
Axerophthol	T45.2X1	T45.2X2	T45.2X3	T45.2X4	T45.2X5	T45.2X6
Azacitidine	T45.1X1	T45.1X2	T45.1X3	T45.1X4	T45.1X5	T45.1X6
Azacyclonol	T43.591	T43.592	T43.593	T43.594	T43.595	T43.596
Azadirachta	T60.2X1	T60.2X2	T60.2X3	T60.2X4	—	—
Azanidazole	T37.3X1	T37.3X2	T37.3X3	T37.3X4	T37.3X5	T37.3X6
Azapetine	T46.7X1	T46.7X2	T46.7X3	T46.7X4	T46.7X5	T46.7X6
Azapropazone	T39.2X1	T39.2X2	T39.2X3	T39.2X4	T39.2X5	T39.2X6
Azaribine	T45.1X1	T45.1X2	T45.1X3	T45.1X4	T45.1X5	T45.1X6
Azaserine	T45.1X1	T45.1X2	T45.1X3	T45.1X4	T45.1X5	T45.1X6
Azatadine	T45.0X1	T45.0X2	T45.0X3	T45.0X4	T45.0X5	T45.0X6
Azatepa	T45.1X1	T45.1X2	T45.1X3	T45.1X4	T45.1X5	T45.1X6
Azathioprine	T45.1X1	T45.1X2	T45.1X3	T45.1X4	T45.1X5	T45.1X6
Azelaic acid	T49.0X1	T49.0X2	T49.0X3	T49.0X4	T49.0X5	T49.0X6
Azelastine	T45.0X1	T45.0X2	T45.0X3	T45.0X4	T45.0X5	T45.0X6
Azidocillin	T36.0X1	T36.0X2	T36.0X3	T36.0X4	T36.0X5	T36.0X6
Azidothymidine	T37.5X1	T37.5X2	T37.5X3	T37.5X4	T37.5X5	T37.5X6
Azinphos (ethyl) (methyl)	T60.0X1	T60.0X2	T60.0X3	T60.0X4	—	—
Aziridine (chelating)	T54.1X1	T54.1X2	T54.1X3	T54.1X4	—	—
Azithromycin	T36.3X1	T36.3X2	T36.3X3	T36.3X4	T36.3X5	T36.3X6
Azlocillin	T36.0X1	T36.0X2	T36.0X3	T36.0X4	T36.0X5	T36.0X6
Azobenzene smoke	T65.3X1	T65.3X2	T65.3X3	T65.3X4	—	—
acaricide	T60.8X1	T60.8X2	T60.8X3	T60.8X4	—	—
Azo-Standard*	T49.0X1	T49.0X2	T49.0X3	T49.0X4	T49.0X5	T49.0X6
Azosulfamide	T37.0X1	T37.0X2	T37.0X3	T37.0X4	T37.0X5	T37.0X6
AZT	T37.5X1	T37.5X2	T37.5X3	T37.5X4	T37.5X5	T37.5X6
Aztreonam	T36.1X1	T36.1X2	T36.1X3	T36.1X4	T36.1X5	T36.1X6
Azulfidine	T37.0X1	T37.0X2	T37.0X3	T37.0X4	T37.0X5	T37.0X6
Azuresin	T50.8X1	T50.8X2	T50.8X3	T50.8X4	T50.8X5	T50.8X6
b-acetyldigoxin	T46.0X1	T46.0X2	T46.0X3	T46.0X4	T46.0X5	T46.0X6
P-Acetamidophenol	T39.1X1	T39.1X2	T39.1X3	T39.1X4	T39.1X5	T39.1X6
Bacampicillin	T36.0X1	T36.0X2	T36.0X3	T36.0X4	T36.0X5	T36.0X6
Bacillus						
lactobacillus	T47.8X1	T47.8X2	T47.8X3	T47.8X4	T47.8X5	T47.8X6
subtilis	T47.6X1	T47.6X2	T47.6X3	T47.6X4	T47.6X5	T47.6X6
Bacimycin	T49.0X1	T49.0X2	T49.0X3	T49.0X4	T49.0X5	T49.0X6
ophthalmic preparation	T49.5X1	T49.5X2	T49.5X3	T49.5X4	T49.5X5	T49.5X6
Bacitracin zinc	T49.0X1	T49.0X2	T49.0X3	T49.0X4	T49.0X5	T49.0X6
with neomycin	T49.0X1	T49.0X2	T49.0X3	T49.0X4	T49.0X5	T49.0X6
ENT agent	T49.6X1	T49.6X2	T49.6X3	T49.6X4	T49.6X5	T49.6X6
ophthalmic preparation	T49.5X1	T49.5X2	T49.5X3	T49.5X4	T49.5X5	T49.5X6
topical NEC	T49.0X1	T49.0X2	T49.0X3	T49.0X4	T49.0X5	T49.0X6
Baclofen	T42.8X1	T42.8X2	T42.8X3	T42.8X4	T42.8X5	T42.8X6
Baking soda	T50.991	T50.992	T50.993	T50.994	T50.995	T50.996
BAL	T45.8X1	T45.8X2	T45.8X3	T45.8X4	T45.8X5	T45.8X6
Bambuterol	T48.6X1	T48.6X2	T48.6X3	T48.6X4	T48.6X5	T48.6X6
Bamethan (sulfate)	T46.7X1	T46.7X2	T46.7X3	T46.7X4	T46.7X5	T46.7X6
Bamifylline	T48.6X1	T48.6X2	T48.6X3	T48.6X4	T48.6X5	T48.6X6
Bamipine	T45.0X1	T45.0X2	T45.0X3	T45.0X4	T45.0X5	T45.0X6
Baneberry — see Actaea spicata						
Banewort — see Belladonna						
Barbenyl	T42.3X1	T42.3X2	T42.3X3	T42.3X4	T42.3X5	T42.3X6
Barbexaclone	T42.6X1	T42.6X2	T42.6X3	T42.6X4	T42.6X5	T42.6X6
Barbital	T42.3X1	T42.3X2	T42.3X3	T42.3X4	T42.3X5	T42.3X6
sodium	T42.3X1	T42.3X2	T42.3X3	T42.3X4	T42.3X5	T42.3X6
Barbitone	T42.3X1	T42.3X2	T42.3X3	T42.3X4	T42.3X5	T42.3X6
Barbiturate NEC	T42.3X1	T42.3X2	T42.3X3	T42.3X4	T42.3X5	T42.3X6
with tranquilizer	T42.3X1	T42.3X2	T42.3X3	T42.3X4	T42.3X5	T42.3X6
anesthetic (intravenous)	T41.1X1	T41.1X2	T41.1X3	T41.1X4	T41.1X5	T41.1X6
Barium (carbonate) (chloride) (sulfate)	T57.8X1	T57.8X2	T57.8X3	T57.8X4	—	—
diagnostic agent	T50.8X1	T50.8X2	T50.8X3	T50.8X4	T50.8X5	T50.8X6
pesticide	T60.4X1	T60.4X2	T60.4X3	T60.4X4	—	—
rodenticide	T60.4X1	T60.4X2	T60.4X3	T60.4X4	—	—
sulfate (medicinal)	T50.8X1	T50.8X2	T50.8X3	T50.8X4	T50.8X5	T50.8X6
Barrier cream	T49.3X1	T49.3X2	T49.3X3	T49.3X4	T49.3X5	T49.3X6
Basic fuchsin	T49.0X1	T49.0X2	T49.0X3	T49.0X4	T49.0X5	T49.0X6
Basiliximab*	T45.1X1	T45.1X2	T45.1X3	T45.1X4	T45.1X5	T45.1X6
Battery acid or fluid	T54.2X1	T54.2X2	T54.2X3	T54.2X4	—	—
Bay rum	T51.8X1	T51.8X2	T51.8X3	T51.8X4	—	—
b-benzalbutyramide	T46.6X1	T46.6X2	T46.6X3	T46.6X4	T46.6X5	T46.6X6
BCG (vaccine)	T50.A91	T50.A92	T50.A93	T50.A94	T50.A95	T50.A96
BCNU	T45.1X1	T45.1X2	T45.1X3	T45.1X4	T45.1X5	T45.1X6
Bearsfoot	T62.2X1	T62.2X2	T62.2X3	T62.2X4	—	—
Beclamide	T42.6X1	T42.6X2	T42.6X3	T42.6X4	T42.6X5	T42.6X6
Beclomethasone	T44.5X1	T44.5X2	T44.5X3	T44.5X4	T44.5X5	T44.5X6
Bee (sting) (venom)	T63.441	T63.442	T63.443	T63.444	—	—
Befunolol	T49.5X1	T49.5X2	T49.5X3	T49.5X4	T49.5X5	T49.5X6
Bekanamycin	T36.5X1	T36.5X2	T36.5X3	T36.5X4	T36.5X5	T36.5X6
Belladonna — see also Nightshade						
alkaloids	T44.3X1	T44.3X2	T44.3X3	T44.3X4	T44.3X5	T44.3X6
extract	T44.3X1	T44.3X2	T44.3X3	T44.3X4	T44.3X5	T44.3X6
herb	T44.3X1	T44.3X2	T44.3X3	T44.3X4	T44.3X5	T44.3X6
Belviq*	T50.5X1	T50.5X2	T50.5X3	T50.5X4	T50.5X5	T50.5X6
Bemegride	T50.7X1	T50.7X2	T50.7X3	T50.7X4	T50.7X5	T50.7X6
Benactyzine	T44.3X1	T44.3X2	T44.3X3	T44.3X4	T44.3X5	T44.3X6
Benadryl	T45.0X1	T45.0X2	T45.0X3	T45.0X4	T45.0X5	T45.0X6
Benaprizine	T44.3X1	T44.3X2	T44.3X3	T44.3X4	T44.3X5	T44.3X6
Benazepril	T46.4X1	T46.4X2	T46.4X3	T46.4X4	T46.4X5	T46.4X6

☑ Additional Character May Be Required — Refer to the Tabular List for Character Selection

*Optum Value-Add

Substance	Poisoning, Accidental (unintentional)	Poisoning, Intentional Self-harm	Poisoning, Assault	Poisoning, Undetermined	Adverse Effect	Under-dosing
Bencyclane	T46.7X1	T46.7X2	T46.7X3	T46.7X4	T46.7X5	T46.7X6
Bendazol	T46.3X1	T46.3X2	T46.3X3	T46.3X4	T46.3X5	T46.3X6
Bendrofluazide	T50.2X1	T50.2X2	T50.2X3	T50.2X4	T50.2X5	T50.2X6
Bendroflumethiazide	T50.2X1	T50.2X2	T50.2X3	T50.2X4	T50.2X5	T50.2X6
Benemid	T50.4X1	T50.4X2	T50.4X3	T50.4X4	T50.4X5	T50.4X6
Benethamine penicillin	T36.0X1	T36.0X2	T36.0X3	T36.0X4	T36.0X5	T36.0X6
Benexate	T47.1X1	T47.1X2	T47.1X3	T47.1X4	T47.1X5	T47.1X6
Benfluorex	T46.6X1	T46.6X2	T46.6X3	T46.6X4	T46.6X5	T46.6X6
Benfotiamine	T45.2X1	T45.2X2	T45.2X3	T45.2X4	T45.2X5	T45.2X6
Benisone	T49.0X1	T49.0X2	T49.0X3	T49.0X4	T49.0X5	T49.0X6
Benomyl	T60.0X1	T60.0X2	T60.0X3	T60.0X4	—	—
Benoquin	T49.8X1	T49.8X2	T49.8X3	T49.8X4	T49.8X5	T49.8X6
Benoxinate	T41.3X1	T41.3X2	T41.3X3	T41.3X4	T41.3X5	T41.3X6
Benperidol	T43.4X1	T43.4X2	T43.4X3	T43.4X4	T43.4X5	T43.4X6
Benproperine	T48.3X1	T48.3X2	T48.3X3	T48.3X4	T48.3X5	T48.3X6
Benserazide	T42.8X1	T42.8X2	T42.8X3	T42.8X4	T42.8X5	T42.8X6
Bentazepam	T42.4X1	T42.4X2	T42.4X3	T42.4X4	T42.4X5	T42.4X6
Bentiromide	T50.8X1	T50.8X2	T50.8X3	T50.8X4	T50.8X5	T50.8X6
Bentonite	T49.3X1	T49.3X2	T49.3X3	T49.3X4	T49.3X5	T49.3X6
Benzalbutyramide	T46.6X1	T46.6X2	T46.6X3	T46.6X4	T46.6X5	T46.6X6
Benzalkonium (chloride)	T49.0X1	T49.0X2	T49.0X3	T49.0X4	T49.0X5	T49.0X6
ophthalmic preparation	T49.5X1	T49.5X2	T49.5X3	T49.5X4	T49.5X5	T49.5X6
Benzamidosalicylate	T37.1X1	T37.1X2	T37.1X3	T37.1X4	T37.1X5	T37.1X6
(calcium)						
Benzamine	T41.3X1	T41.3X2	T41.3X3	T41.3X4	T41.3X5	T41.3X6
lactate	T49.1X1	T49.1X2	T49.1X3	T49.1X4	T49.1X5	T49.1X6
Benzamphetamine	T50.5X1	T50.5X2	T50.5X3	T50.5X4	T50.5X5	T50.5X6
Benzapril hydrochloride	T46.5X1	T46.5X2	T46.5X3	T46.5X4	T46.5X5	T46.5X6
Benzathine	T36.0X1	T36.0X2	T36.0X3	T36.0X4	T36.0X5	T36.0X6
benzylpenicillin						
Benzathine penicillin	T36.0X1	T36.0X2	T36.0X3	T36.0X4	T36.0X5	T36.0X6
Benzatropine	T42.8X1	T42.8X2	T42.8X3	T42.8X4	T42.8X5	T42.8X6
Benzbromarone	T50.4X1	T50.4X2	T50.4X3	T50.4X4	T50.4X5	T50.4X6
Benzcarbimine	T45.1X1	T45.1X2	T45.1X3	T45.1X4	T45.1X5	T45.1X6
Benzedrex	T44.991	T44.992	T44.993	T44.994	T44.995	T44.996
Benzedrine (amphetamine)	T43.621	T43.622	T43.623	T43.624	T43.625	T43.626
Benzenamine	T65.3X1	T65.3X2	T65.3X3	T65.3X4	—	—
Benzene	T52.1X1	T52.1X2	T52.1X3	T52.1X4	—	—
homologues (acetyl) (dimethyl)	T52.2X1	T52.2X2	T52.2X3	T52.2X4	—	—
(methyl) (solvent)						
Benzethonium (chloride)	T49.0X1	T49.0X2	T49.0X3	T49.0X4	T49.0X5	T49.0X6
Benzfetamine	T50.5X1	T50.5X2	T50.5X3	T50.5X4	T50.5X5	T50.5X6
Benzhexol	T44.3X1	T44.3X2	T44.3X3	T44.3X4	T44.3X5	T44.3X6
Benzhydramine (chloride)	T45.0X1	T45.0X2	T45.0X3	T45.0X4	T45.0X5	T45.0X6
Benzidine	T65.891	T65.892	T65.893	T65.894	—	—
Benzilonium bromide	T44.3X1	T44.3X2	T44.3X3	T44.3X4	T44.3X5	T44.3X6
Benzimidazole	T60.3X1	T60.3X2	T60.3X3	T60.3X4	—	—
Benzin (e) — see Ligroin						
Benziodarone	T46.3X1	T46.3X2	T46.3X3	T46.3X4	T46.3X5	T46.3X6
Benznidazole	T37.3X1	T37.3X2	T37.3X3	T37.3X4	T37.3X5	T37.3X6
Benzocaine	T41.3X1	T41.3X2	T41.3X3	T41.3X4	T41.3X5	T41.3X6
Benzocol*	T41.3X1	T41.3X2	T41.3X3	T41.3X4	T41.3X5	T41.3X6
Benzodiapin	T42.4X1	T42.4X2	T42.4X3	T42.4X4	T42.4X5	T42.4X6
Benzodiazepine NEC	T42.4X1	T42.4X2	T42.4X3	T42.4X4	T42.4X5	T42.4X6
Benzoic acid	T49.0X1	T49.0X2	T49.0X3	T49.0X4	T49.0X5	T49.0X6
with salicylic acid	T49.0X1	T49.0X2	T49.0X3	T49.0X4	T49.0X5	T49.0X6
Benzoin (tincture)	T48.5X1	T48.5X2	T48.5X3	T48.5X4	T48.5X5	T48.5X6
Benzol (benzene)	T52.1X1	T52.1X2	T52.1X3	T52.1X4	—	—
vapor	T52.0X1	T52.0X2	T52.0X3	T52.0X4	—	—
Benzomorphan	T40.2X1	T40.2X2	T40.2X3	T40.2X4	T40.2X5	T40.2X6
Benzonatate	T48.3X1	T48.3X2	T48.3X3	T48.3X4	T48.3X5	T48.3X6
Benzophenones	T49.3X1	T49.3X2	T49.3X3	T49.3X4	T49.3X5	T49.3X6
Benzopyrone	T46.991	T46.992	T46.993	T46.994	T46.995	T46.996
Benzothiadiazides	T50.2X1	T50.2X2	T50.2X3	T50.2X4	T50.2X5	T50.2X6
Benzoxonium chloride	T49.0X1	T49.0X2	T49.0X3	T49.0X4	T49.0X5	T49.0X6
Benzoylpas calcium	T37.1X1	T37.1X2	T37.1X3	T37.1X4	T37.1X5	T37.1X6
Benzoyl peroxide	T49.0X1	T49.0X2	T49.0X3	T49.0X4	T49.0X5	T49.0X6
Benzperidin	T43.591	T43.592	T43.593	T43.594	T43.595	T43.596
Benzperidol	T43.591	T43.592	T43.593	T43.594	T43.595	T43.596
Benzphetamine	T50.5X1	T50.5X2	T50.5X3	T50.5X4	T50.5X5	T50.5X6
Benzpyrinium bromide	T44.1X1	T44.1X2	T44.1X3	T44.1X4	T44.1X5	T44.1X6
Benzquinamide	T45.0X1	T45.0X2	T45.0X3	T45.0X4	T45.0X5	T45.0X6
Benzthiazide	T50.2X1	T50.2X2	T50.2X3	T50.2X4	T50.2X5	T50.2X6
Benztropine						
anticholinergic	T44.3X1	T44.3X2	T44.3X3	T44.3X4	T44.3X5	T44.3X6
antiparkinson	T42.8X1	T42.8X2	T42.8X3	T42.8X4	T42.8X5	T42.8X6
Benzydamine	T49.0X1	T49.0X2	T49.0X3	T49.0X4	T49.0X5	T49.0X6
Benzyl						
acetate	T52.8X1	T52.8X2	T52.8X3	T52.8X4	—	—
alcohol	T49.0X1	T49.0X2	T49.0X3	T49.0X4	T49.0X5	T49.0X6
benzoate	T49.0X1	T49.0X2	T49.0X3	T49.0X4	T49.0X5	T49.0X6
Benzoic acid	T49.0X1	T49.0X2	T49.0X3	T49.0X4	T49.0X5	T49.0X6
hydroquinone*	T49.4X1	T49.4X2	T49.4X3	T49.4X4	T49.4X5	T49.4X6

Substance	Poisoning, Accidental (unintentional)	Poisoning, Intentional Self-harm	Poisoning, Assault	Poisoning, Undetermined	Adverse Effect	Under-dosing
Benzyl — continued						
morphine	T40.2X1	T40.2X2	T40.2X3	T40.2X4	—	—
nicotinate	T46.6X1	T46.6X2	T46.6X3	T46.6X4	T46.6X5	T46.6X6
penicillin	T36.0X1	T36.0X2	T36.0X3	T36.0X4	T36.0X5	T36.0X6
Benzylhydrochlorthiazide	T50.2X1	T50.2X2	T50.2X3	T50.2X4	T50.2X5	T50.2X6
Benzylpenicillin	T36.0X1	T36.0X2	T36.0X3	T36.0X4	T36.0X5	T36.0X6
Benzylthiouracil	T38.2X1	T38.2X2	T38.2X3	T38.2X4	T38.2X5	T38.2X6
Bephenium	T37.4X1	T37.4X2	T37.4X3	T37.4X4	T37.4X5	T37.4X6
hydroxynaphthoate						
Bepridil	T46.1X1	T46.1X2	T46.1X3	T46.1X4	T46.1X5	T46.1X6
Bergamot oil	T65.891	T65.892	T65.893	T65.894	—	—
Bergapten	T50.991	T50.992	T50.993	T50.994	T50.995	T50.996
Berries, poisonous	T62.1X1	T62.1X2	T62.1X3	T62.1X4	—	—
Beryllium (compounds)	T56.7X1	T56.7X2	T56.7X3	T56.7X4	—	—
beta adrenergic blocking	T44.7X1	T44.7X2	T44.7X3	T44.7X4	T44.7X5	T44.7X6
agent, heart						
Betacarotene	T45.2X1	T45.2X2	T45.2X3	T45.2X4	T45.2X5	T45.2X6
Beta-Chlor	T42.6X1	T42.6X2	T42.6X3	T42.6X4	T42.6X5	T42.6X6
Betahistine	T46.7X1	T46.7X2	T46.7X3	T46.7X4	T46.7X5	T46.7X6
Betaine	T47.5X1	T47.5X2	T47.5X3	T47.5X4	T47.5X5	T47.5X6
Betamethasone	T49.0X1	T49.0X2	T49.0X3	T49.0X4	T49.0X5	T49.0X6
topical	T49.0X1	T49.0X2	T49.0X3	T49.0X4	T49.0X5	T49.0X6
Betamicin	T36.8X1	T36.8X2	T36.8X3	T36.8X4	T36.8X5	T36.8X6
Betanidine	T46.5X1	T46.5X2	T46.5X3	T46.5X4	T46.5X5	T46.5X6
Betaxolol	T44.7X1	T44.7X2	T44.7X3	T44.7X4	T44.7X5	T44.7X6
Betazole	T50.8X1	T50.8X2	T50.8X3	T50.8X4	T50.8X5	T50.8X6
Bethanechol	T44.1X1	T44.1X2	T44.1X3	T44.1X4	T44.1X5	T44.1X6
chloride	T44.1X1	T44.1X2	T44.1X3	T44.1X4	T44.1X5	T44.1X6
Bethanidine	T46.5X1	T46.5X2	T46.5X3	T46.5X4	T46.5X5	T46.5X6
Betoxycaine	T41.3X1	T41.3X2	T41.3X3	T41.3X4	T41.3X5	T41.3X6
Betula oil	T49.3X1	T49.3X2	T49.3X3	T49.3X4	T49.3X5	T49.3X6
Bevantolol	T44.7X1	T44.7X2	T44.7X3	T44.7X4	T44.7X5	T44.7X6
Bevonium metilsulfate	T44.3X1	T44.3X2	T44.3X3	T44.3X4	T44.3X5	T44.3X6
Bezafibrate	T46.6X1	T46.6X2	T46.6X3	T46.6X4	T46.6X5	T46.6X6
Bezitramide	T40.491	T40.492	T40.493	T40.494	T40.495	T40.496
BHA	T50.991	T50.992	T50.993	T50.994	T50.995	T50.996
Bhang	T40.711	T40.712	T40.713	T40.714	T40.715	T40.716
BHC (medicinal)	T49.0X1	T49.0X2	T49.0X3	T49.0X4	T49.0X5	T49.0X6
nonmedicinal (vapor)	T53.6X1	T53.6X2	T53.6X3	T53.6X4	—	—
Bialamicol	T37.3X1	T37.3X2	T37.3X3	T37.3X4	T37.3X5	T37.3X6
Bibenzonium bromide	T48.3X1	T48.3X2	T48.3X3	T48.3X4	T48.3X5	T48.3X6
Bibrocathol	T49.5X1	T49.5X2	T49.5X3	T49.5X4	T49.5X5	T49.5X6
Bichloride of mercury — see						
Mercury, chloride						
Bichromates (calcium)	T57.8X1	T57.8X2	T57.8X3	T57.8X4	—	—
(potassium)(sodium)						
(crystals)						
fumes	T56.2X1	T56.2X2	T56.2X3	T56.2X4	—	—
Biclotymol	T49.6X1	T49.6X2	T49.6X3	T49.6X4	T49.6X5	T49.6X6
BiCNU*	T45.1X1	T45.1X2	T45.1X3	T45.1X4	T45.1X5	T45.1X6
Bicucculine	T50.7X1	T50.7X2	T50.7X3	T50.7X4	T50.7X5	T50.7X6
Bifemelane	T43.291	T43.292	T43.293	T43.294	T43.295	T43.296
Biguanide derivatives,	T38.3X1	T38.3X2	T38.3X3	T38.3X4	T38.3X5	T38.3X6
oral						
Bile salts	T47.5X1	T47.5X2	T47.5X3	T47.5X4	T47.5X5	T47.5X6
Biligrafin	T50.8X1	T50.8X2	T50.8X3	T50.8X4	T50.8X5	T50.8X6
Bilopaque	T50.8X1	T50.8X2	T50.8X3	T50.8X4	T50.8X5	T50.8X6
Binifibrate	T46.6X1	T46.6X2	T46.6X3	T46.6X4	T46.6X5	T46.6X6
Binitrobenzol	T65.3X1	T65.3X2	T65.3X3	T65.3X4	—	—
Bioflavonoid(s)	T46.991	T46.992	T46.993	T46.994	T46.995	T46.996
Biological substance NEC	T50.901	T50.902	T50.903	T50.904	T50.905	T50.906
Biotin	T45.2X1	T45.2X2	T45.2X3	T45.2X4	T45.2X5	T45.2X6
Biperiden	T44.3X1	T44.3X2	T44.3X3	T44.3X4	T44.3X5	T44.3X6
Bisacodyl	T47.2X1	T47.2X2	T47.2X3	T47.2X4	T47.2X5	T47.2X6
Bisbentiamine	T45.2X1	T45.2X2	T45.2X3	T45.2X4	T45.2X5	T45.2X6
Bisbutiamine	T45.2X1	T45.2X2	T45.2X3	T45.2X4	T45.2X5	T45.2X6
Bisdequalinium (salts)	T49.6X1	T49.6X2	T49.6X3	T49.6X4	T49.6X5	T49.6X6
(diacetate)						
Bishydroxycoumarin	T45.511	T45.512	T45.513	T45.514	T45.515	T45.516
Bismarsen	T37.8X1	T37.8X2	T37.8X3	T37.8X4	T37.8X5	T37.8X6
Bismuth salts	T47.6X1	T47.6X2	T47.6X3	T47.6X4	T47.6X5	T47.6X6
aluminate	T47.1X1	T47.1X2	T47.1X3	T47.1X4	T47.1X5	T47.1X6
anti-infectives	T37.8X1	T37.8X2	T37.8X3	T37.8X4	T37.8X5	T37.8X6
formic iodide	T49.0X1	T49.0X2	T49.0X3	T49.0X4	T49.0X5	T49.0X6
glycolylarsenate	T49.0X1	T49.0X2	T49.0X3	T49.0X4	T49.0X5	T49.0X6
nonmedicinal (compounds)	T65.91	T65.92	T65.93	T65.94		
NEC						
subcarbonate	T47.6X1	T47.6X2	T47.6X3	T47.6X4	T47.6X5	T47.6X6
subsalicylate	T37.8X1	T37.8X2	T37.8X3	T37.8X4	T37.8X5	T37.8X6
sulfarsphenamine	T37.8X1	T37.8X2	T37.8X3	T37.8X4	T37.8X5	T37.8X6
Bisoprolol	T44.7X1	T44.7X2	T44.7X3	T44.7X4	T44.7X5	T44.7X6
Bisoxatin	T47.2X1	T47.2X2	T47.2X3	T47.2X4	T47.2X5	T47.2X6
Bisulepin (hydrochloride)	T45.0X1	T45.0X2	T45.0X3	T45.0X4	T45.0X5	T45.0X6

Substance	Poisoning, Accidental (unintentional)	Poisoning, Intentional Self-harm	Poisoning, Assault	Poisoning, Undetermined	Adverse Effect	Under-dosing
Bithionol	T37.8X1	T37.8X2	T37.8X3	T37.8X4	T37.8X5	T37.8X6
anthelminthic	T37.4X1	T37.4X2	T37.4X3	T37.4X4	T37.4X5	T37.4X6
Bitolterol	T48.6X1	T48.6X2	T48.6X3	T48.6X4	T48.6X5	T48.6X6
Bitoscanate	T37.4X1	T37.4X2	T37.4X3	T37.4X4	T37.4X5	T37.4X6
Bitter almond oil	T62.8X1	T62.8X2	T62.8X3	T62.8X4	—	—
Bittersweet	T62.2X1	T62.2X2	T62.2X3	T62.2X4	—	—
Bivalirudin*	T45.511	T45.512	T45.513	T45.514	T45.515	T45.516
Black						
flag	T60.91	T60.92	T60.93	T60.94	—	—
henbane	T62.2X1	T62.2X2	T62.2X3	T62.2X4	—	—
leaf (40)	T60.91	T60.92	T60.93	T60.94	—	—
widow spider (bite)	T63.311	T63.312	T63.313	T63.314	—	—
antivenin	T50.Z11	T50.Z12	T50.Z13	T50.Z14	T50.Z15	T50.Z16
Blast furnace gas (carbon monoxide from)	T58.8X1	T58.8X2	T58.8X3	T58.8X4	—	—
Bleach	T54.91	T54.92	T54.93	T54.94	—	—
Bleaching agent (medicinal)	T49.4X1	T49.4X2	T49.4X3	T49.4X4	T49.4X5	T49.4X6
Bleomycin	T45.1X1	T45.1X2	T45.1X3	T45.1X4	T45.1X5	T45.1X6
Blockain	T41.3X1	T41.3X2	T41.3X3	T41.3X4	T41.3X5	T41.3X6
infiltration (subcutaneous)	T41.3X1	T41.3X2	T41.3X3	T41.3X4	T41.3X5	T41.3X6
nerve block (peripheral) (plexus)	T41.3X1	T41.3X2	T41.3X3	T41.3X4	T41.3X5	T41.3X6
topical (surface)	T41.3X1	T41.3X2	T41.3X3	T41.3X4	T41.3X5	T41.3X6
Blockers, calcium channel	T46.1X1	T46.1X2	T46.1X3	T46.1X4	T46.1X5	T46.1X6
Blood (derivatives) (natural) (plasma) (whole)	T45.8X1	T45.8X2	T45.8X3	T45.8X4	T45.8X5	T45.8X6
dried	T45.8X1	T45.8X2	T45.8X3	T45.8X4	T45.8X5	T45.8X6
drug affecting NEC	T45.91	T45.92	T45.93	T45.94	T45.95	T45.96
expander NEC	T45.8X1	T45.8X2	T45.8X3	T45.8X4	T45.8X5	T45.8X6
fraction NEC	T45.8X1	T45.8X2	T45.8X3	T45.8X4	T45.8X5	T45.8X6
substitute (macromolecular)	T45.8X1	T45.8X2	T45.8X3	T45.8X4	T45.8X5	T45.8X6
Blue velvet	T40.2X1	T40.2X2	T40.2X3	T40.2X4	—	—
Bone meal	T62.8X1	T62.8X2	T62.8X3	T62.8X4	—	—
Bonine	T45.0X1	T45.0X2	T45.0X3	T45.0X4	T45.0X5	T45.0X6
Bontril*	T50.5X1	T50.5X2	T50.5X3	T50.5X4	T50.5X5	T50.5X6
Bopindolol	T44.7X1	T44.7X2	T44.7X3	T44.7X4	T44.7X5	T44.7X6
Boracic acid	T49.0X1	T49.0X2	T49.0X3	T49.0X4	T49.0X5	T49.0X6
ENT agent	T49.6X1	T49.6X2	T49.6X3	T49.6X4	T49.6X5	T49.6X6
ophthalmic preparation	T49.5X1	T49.5X2	T49.5X3	T49.5X4	T49.5X5	T49.5X6
Borane complex	T57.8X1	T57.8X2	T57.8X3	T57.8X4	—	—
Borate(s)	T57.8X1	T57.8X2	T57.8X3	T57.8X4	—	—
buffer	T50.991	T50.992	T50.993	T50.994	T50.995	T50.996
cleanser	T54.91	T54.92	T54.93	T54.94	—	—
sodium	T57.8X1	T57.8X2	T57.8X3	T57.8X4	—	—
Borax (cleanser)	T54.91	T54.92	T54.93	T54.94	—	—
Bordeaux mixture	T60.3X1	T60.3X2	T60.3X3	T60.3X4	—	—
Boric acid	T49.0X1	T49.0X2	T49.0X3	T49.0X4	T49.0X5	T49.0X6
ENT agent	T49.6X1	T49.6X2	T49.6X3	T49.6X4	T49.6X5	T49.6X6
ophthalmic preparation	T49.5X1	T49.5X2	T49.5X3	T49.5X4	T49.5X5	T49.5X6
Bornaprine	T44.3X1	T44.3X2	T44.3X3	T44.3X4	T44.3X5	T44.3X6
Boron	T57.8X1	T57.8X2	T57.8X3	T57.8X4	—	—
hydride NEC	T57.8X1	T57.8X2	T57.8X3	T57.8X4	—	—
fumes or gas	T57.8X1	T57.8X2	T57.8X3	T57.8X4	—	—
trifluoride	T59.891	T59.892	T59.893	T59.894	—	—
Botox	T48.291	T48.292	T48.293	T48.294	T48.295	T48.296
Botulinus anti-toxin (type A, B)	T50.Z11	T50.Z12	T50.Z13	T50.Z14	T50.Z15	T50.Z16
Brake fluid vapor	T59.891	T59.892	T59.893	T59.894	—	—
Brallobarbital	T42.3X1	T42.3X2	T42.3X3	T42.3X4	T42.3X5	T42.3X6
Bran (wheat)	T47.4X1	T47.4X2	T47.4X3	T47.4X4	T47.4X5	T47.4X6
Brass (fumes)	T56.891	T56.892	T56.893	T56.894	—	—
Brasso	T52.0X1	T52.0X2	T52.0X3	T52.0X4	—	—
Bretylium tosilate	T46.2X1	T46.2X2	T46.2X3	T46.2X4	T46.2X5	T46.2X6
Brevital (sodium)	T41.1X1	T41.1X2	T41.1X3	T41.1X4	T41.1X5	T41.1X6
Brinase	T45.3X1	T45.3X2	T45.3X3	T45.3X4	T45.3X5	T45.3X6
British antilewisite	T45.8X1	T45.8X2	T45.8X3	T45.8X4	T45.8X5	T45.8X6
Brodalumab*	T50.991	T50.992	T50.993	T50.994	T50.995	T50.996
Brodifacoum	T60.4X1	T60.4X2	T60.4X3	T60.4X4	—	—
Bromal (hydrate)	T42.6X1	T42.6X2	T42.6X3	T42.6X4	T42.6X5	T42.6X6
Bromazepam	T42.4X1	T42.4X2	T42.4X3	T42.4X4	T42.4X5	T42.4X6
Bromazine	T45.0X1	T45.0X2	T45.0X3	T45.0X4	T45.0X5	T45.0X6
Brombenzylcyanide	T59.3X1	T59.3X2	T59.3X3	T59.3X4	—	—
Bromelains	T45.3X1	T45.3X2	T45.3X3	T45.3X4	T45.3X5	T45.3X6
Bromethalin	T60.4X1	T60.4X2	T60.4X3	T60.4X4	—	—
Bromhexine	T48.4X1	T48.4X2	T48.4X3	T48.4X4	T48.4X5	T48.4X6
Bromide salts	T42.6X1	T42.6X2	T42.6X3	T42.6X4	T42.6X5	T42.6X6
Bromindione	T45.511	T45.512	T45.513	T45.514	T45.515	T45.516
Bromine						
compounds (medicinal)	T42.6X1	T42.6X2	T42.6X3	T42.6X4	T42.6X5	T42.6X6
sedative	T42.6X1	T42.6X2	T42.6X3	T42.6X4	T42.6X5	T42.6X6
vapor	T59.891	T59.892	T59.893	T59.894	—	—
Bromisoval	T42.6X1	T42.6X2	T42.6X3	T42.6X4	T42.6X5	T42.6X6
Bromisovalum	T42.6X1	T42.6X2	T42.6X3	T42.6X4	T42.6X5	T42.6X6
Bromobenzylcyanide	T59.3X1	T59.3X2	T59.3X3	T59.3X4	—	—
Bromochlorosalicylani-lide	T49.0X1	T49.0X2	T49.0X3	T49.0X4	T49.0X5	T49.0X6
Bromocriptine	T42.8X1	T42.8X2	T42.8X3	T42.8X4	T42.8X5	T42.8X6
Bromodiphenhydramine	T45.0X1	T45.0X2	T45.0X3	T45.0X4	T45.0X5	T45.0X6
Bromoform	T42.6X1	T42.6X2	T42.6X3	T42.6X4	T42.6X5	T42.6X6
Bromophenol blue reagent	T50.991	T50.992	T50.993	T50.994	T50.995	T50.996
Bromopride	T47.8X1	T47.8X2	T47.8X3	T47.8X4	T47.8X5	T47.8X6
Bromosalicylchloranitide	T49.0X1	T49.0X2	T49.0X3	T49.0X4	T49.0X5	T49.0X6
Bromosalicylhydroxamic acid	T37.1X1	T37.1X2	T37.1X3	T37.1X4	T37.1X5	T37.1X6
Bromo-seltzer	T39.1X1	T39.1X2	T39.1X3	T39.1X4	T39.1X5	T39.1X6
Bromoxynil	T60.3X1	T60.3X2	T60.3X3	T60.3X4	—	—
Bromperidol	T43.4X1	T43.4X2	T43.4X3	T43.4X4	T43.4X5	T43.4X6
Brompheniramine	T45.0X1	T45.0X2	T45.0X3	T45.0X4	T45.0X5	T45.0X6
Bromsulfophthalein	T50.8X1	T50.8X2	T50.8X3	T50.8X4	T50.8X5	T50.8X6
Bromural	T42.6X1	T42.6X2	T42.6X3	T42.6X4	T42.6X5	T42.6X6
Bromvaletone	T42.6X1	T42.6X2	T42.6X3	T42.6X4	T42.6X5	T42.6X6
Bronchodilator NEC	T48.6X1	T48.6X2	T48.6X3	T48.6X4	T48.6X5	T48.6X6
Brotizolam	T42.4X1	T42.4X2	T42.4X3	T42.4X4	T42.4X5	T42.4X6
Brovincamine	T46.7X1	T46.7X2	T46.7X3	T46.7X4	T46.7X5	T46.7X6
Brown recluse spider (bite) (venom)	T63.331	T63.332	T63.333	T63.334	—	—
Brown spider (bite) (venom)	T63.391	T63.392	T63.393	T63.394	—	—
Broxaterol	T48.6X1	T48.6X2	T48.6X3	T48.6X4	T48.6X5	T48.6X6
Broxuridine	T45.1X1	T45.1X2	T45.1X3	T45.1X4	T45.1X5	T45.1X6
Broxyquinoline	T37.8X1	T37.8X2	T37.8X3	T37.8X4	T37.8X5	T37.8X6
Bruceine	T48.291	T48.292	T48.293	T48.294	T48.295	T48.296
Brucia	T62.2X1	T62.2X2	T62.2X3	T62.2X4	—	—
Brucine	T65.1X1	T65.1X2	T65.1X3	T65.1X4	—	—
Brunswick green — *see* Copper						
Bruten — *see* Ibuprofen						
Bryonia	T47.2X1	T47.2X2	T47.2X3	T47.2X4	T47.2X5	T47.2X6
Buclizine	T45.0X1	T45.0X2	T45.0X3	T45.0X4	T45.0X5	T45.0X6
Buclosamide	T49.0X1	T49.0X2	T49.0X3	T49.0X4	T49.0X5	T49.0X6
Budesonide	T44.5X1	T44.5X2	T44.5X3	T44.5X4	T44.5X5	T44.5X6
Budralazine	T46.5X1	T46.5X2	T46.5X3	T46.5X4	T46.5X5	T46.5X6
Bufferin	T39.011	T39.012	T39.013	T39.014	T39.015	T39.016
Buflomedil	T46.7X1	T46.7X2	T46.7X3	T46.7X4	T46.7X5	T46.7X6
Buformin	T38.3X1	T38.3X2	T38.3X3	T38.3X4	T38.3X5	T38.3X6
Bufotenine	T40.991	T40.992	T40.993	T40.994		
Bufrolin	T48.6X1	T48.6X2	T48.6X3	T48.6X4	T48.6X5	T48.6X6
Bufylline	T48.6X1	T48.6X2	T48.6X3	T48.6X4	T48.6X5	T48.6X6
Bulgaricum IB*	T47.6X1	T47.6X2	T47.6X3	T47.6X4	T47.6X5	T47.6X6
Bulk filler	T50.5X1	T50.5X2	T50.5X3	T50.5X4	T50.5X5	T50.5X6
cathartic	T47.4X1	T47.4X2	T47.4X3	T47.4X4	T47.4X5	T47.4X6
Bumetanide	T50.1X1	T50.1X2	T50.1X3	T50.1X4	T50.1X5	T50.1X6
Bunaftine	T46.2X1	T46.2X2	T46.2X3	T46.2X4	T46.2X5	T46.2X6
Bunamiodyl	T50.8X1	T50.8X2	T50.8X3	T50.8X4	T50.8X5	T50.8X6
Bunazosin	T44.6X1	T44.6X2	T44.6X3	T44.6X4	T44.6X5	T44.6X6
Bunitrolol	T44.7X1	T44.7X2	T44.7X3	T44.7X4	T44.7X5	T44.7X6
Buphenine	T46.7X1	T46.7X2	T46.7X3	T46.7X4	T46.7X5	T46.7X6
Bupivacaine	T41.3X1	T41.3X2	T41.3X3	T41.3X4	T41.3X5	T41.3X6
infiltration (subcutaneous)	T41.3X1	T41.3X2	T41.3X3	T41.3X4	T41.3X5	T41.3X6
nerve block (peripheral) (plexus)	T41.3X1	T41.3X2	T41.3X3	T41.3X4	T41.3X5	T41.3X6
spinal	T41.3X1	T41.3X2	T41.3X3	T41.3X4	T41.3X5	T41.3X6
Bupranolol	T44.7X1	T44.7X2	T44.7X3	T44.7X4	T44.7X5	T44.7X6
Buprenorphine	T40.491	T40.492	T40.493	T40.494	T40.495	T40.496
Bupropion	T43.291	T43.292	T43.293	T43.294	T43.295	T43.296
Burimamide	T47.1X1	T47.1X2	T47.1X3	T47.1X4	T47.1X5	T47.1X6
Buserelin	T38.891	T38.892	T38.893	T38.894	T38.895	T38.896
Buspirone	T43.591	T43.592	T43.593	T43.594	T43.595	T43.596
Busulfan, busulphan	T45.1X1	T45.1X2	T45.1X3	T45.1X4	T45.1X5	T45.1X6
Busulfex*	T45.1X1	T45.1X2	T45.1X3	T45.1X4	T45.1X5	T45.1X6
Butabarbital (sodium)	T42.3X1	T42.3X2	T42.3X3	T42.3X4	T42.3X5	T42.3X6
Butabarbitone	T42.3X1	T42.3X2	T42.3X3	T42.3X4	T42.3X5	T42.3X6
Butabarpal	T42.3X1	T42.3X2	T42.3X3	T42.3X4	T42.3X5	T42.3X6
Butacaine	T41.3X1	T41.3X2	T41.3X3	T41.3X4	T41.3X5	T41.3X6
Butalamine	T46.7X1	T46.7X2	T46.7X3	T46.7X4	T46.7X5	T46.7X6
Butalbital	T42.3X1	T42.3X2	T42.3X3	T42.3X4	T42.3X5	T42.3X6
Butallylonal	T42.3X1	T42.3X2	T42.3X3	T42.3X4	T42.3X5	T42.3X6
Butamben	T41.3X1	T41.3X2	T41.3X3	T41.3X4	T41.3X5	T41.3X6
Butamirate	T48.3X1	T48.3X2	T48.3X3	T48.3X4	T48.3X5	T48.3X6
Butane (distributed in mobile container)	T59.891	T59.892	T59.893	T59.894	—	—
distributed through pipes	T59.891	T59.892	T59.893	T59.894	—	—
incomplete combustion	T58.11	T58.12	T58.13	T58.14		
Butanilicaine	T41.3X1	T41.3X2	T41.3X3	T41.3X4	T41.3X5	T41.3X6
Butanol	T51.3X1	T51.3X2	T51.3X3	T51.3X4		

☑ Additional Character May Be Required — Refer to the Tabular List for Character Selection

*Optum Value-Add

Substance	Poisoning, Accidental (unintentional)	Poisoning, Intentional Self-harm	Poisoning, Assault	Poisoning, Undetermined	Adverse Effect	Under-dosing
Butanone, 2-butanone	T52.4X1	T52.4X2	T52.4X3	T52.4X4	—	—
Butantrone	T49.4X1	T49.4X2	T49.4X3	T49.4X4	T49.4X5	T49.4X6
Butaperazine	T43.3X1	T43.3X2	T43.3X3	T43.3X4	T43.3X5	T43.3X6
Butazolidin	T39.2X1	T39.2X2	T39.2X3	T39.2X4	T39.2X5	T39.2X6
Butetamate	T48.6X1	T48.6X2	T48.6X3	T48.6X4	T48.6X5	T48.6X6
Butethal	T42.3X1	T42.3X2	T42.3X3	T42.3X4	T42.3X5	T42.3X6
Butethamate	T44.3X1	T44.3X2	T44.3X3	T44.3X4	T44.3X5	T44.3X6
Buthalitone (sodium)	T41.1X1	T41.1X2	T41.1X3	T41.1X4	T41.1X5	T41.1X6
Butisol (sodium)	T42.3X1	T42.3X2	T42.3X3	T42.3X4	T42.3X5	T42.3X6
Butizide	T50.2X1	T50.2X2	T50.2X3	T50.2X4	T50.2X5	T50.2X6
Butobarbital	T42.3X1	T42.3X2	T42.3X3	T42.3X4	T42.3X5	T42.3X6
sodium	T42.3X1	T42.3X2	T42.3X3	T42.3X4	T42.3X5	T42.3X6
Butobarbitone	T42.3X1	T42.3X2	T42.3X3	T42.3X4	T42.3X5	T42.3X6
Butoconazole (nitrate)	T49.0X1	T49.0X2	T49.0X3	T49.0X4	T49.0X5	T49.0X6
Butorphanol	T40.491	T40.492	T40.493	T40.494	T40.495	T40.496
Butriptyline	T43.011	T43.012	T43.013	T43.014	T43.015	T43.016
Butropium bromide	T44.3X1	T44.3X2	T44.3X3	T44.3X4	T44.3X5	T44.3X6
Buttercups	T62.2X1	T62.2X2	T62.2X3	T62.2X4	—	—
Butter of antimony — see Antimony						
Butyl						
acetate (secondary)	T52.8X1	T52.8X2	T52.8X3	T52.8X4	—	—
alcohol	T51.3X1	T51.3X2	T51.3X3	T51.3X4	—	—
aminobenzoate	T41.3X1	T41.3X2	T41.3X3	T41.3X4	T41.3X5	T41.3X6
butyrate	T52.8X1	T52.8X2	T52.8X3	T52.8X4	—	—
carbinol	T51.3X1	T51.3X2	T51.3X3	T51.3X4	—	—
carbitol	T52.3X1	T52.3X2	T52.3X3	T52.3X4	—	—
cellosolve	T52.3X1	T52.3X2	T52.3X3	T52.3X4	—	—
chloral (hydrate)	T42.6X1	T42.6X2	T42.6X3	T42.6X4	T42.6X5	T42.6X6
formate	T52.8X1	T52.8X2	T52.8X3	T52.8X4	—	—
lactate	T52.8X1	T52.8X2	T52.8X3	T52.8X4	—	—
propionate	T52.8X1	T52.8X2	T52.8X3	T52.8X4	—	—
scopolamine bromide	T44.3X1	T44.3X2	T44.3X3	T44.3X4	T44.3X5	T44.3X6
thiobarbital sodium	T41.1X1	T41.1X2	T41.1X3	T41.1X4	T41.1X5	T41.1X6
Butylated hydroxyanisole	T50.991	T50.992	T50.993	T50.994	T50.995	T50.996
Butylchloral hydrate	T42.6X1	T42.6X2	T42.6X3	T42.6X4	T42.6X5	T42.6X6
Butyltoluene	T52.2X1	T52.2X2	T52.2X3	T52.2X4	—	—
Butyn	T41.3X1	T41.3X2	T41.3X3	T41.3X4	T41.3X5	T41.3X6
Butyrophenone (-based tranquilizers)	T43.4X1	T43.4X2	T43.4X3	T43.4X4	T43.4X5	T43.4X6
Cabazitaxel*	T45.1X1	T45.1X2	T45.1X3	T45.1X4	T45.1X5	T45.1X6
Cabergoline	T42.8X1	T42.8X2	T42.8X3	T42.8X4	T42.8X5	T42.8X6
Cacodyl, cacodylic acid	T57.0X1	T57.0X2	T57.0X3	T57.0X4	—	—
Cactinomycin	T45.1X1	T45.1X2	T45.1X3	T45.1X4	T45.1X5	T45.1X6
Cade oil	T49.4X1	T49.4X2	T49.4X3	T49.4X4	T49.4X5	T49.4X6
Cadexomer iodine	T49.0X1	T49.0X2	T49.0X3	T49.0X4	T49.0X5	T49.0X6
Cadmium (chloride) (fumes) (oxide)	T56.3X1	T56.3X2	T56.3X3	T56.3X4	—	—
sulfide (medicinal) NEC	T49.4X1	T49.4X2	T49.4X3	T49.4X4	T49.4X5	T49.4X6
Cadralazine	T46.5X1	T46.5X2	T46.5X3	T46.5X4	T46.5X5	T46.5X6
Caffeine	T43.611	T43.612	T43.613	T43.614	T43.615	T43.616
Calabar bean	T62.2X1	T62.2X2	T62.2X3	T62.2X4	—	—
Caladium seguinum	T62.2X1	T62.2X2	T62.2X3	T62.2X4	—	—
Calamine (lotion)	T49.3X1	T49.3X2	T49.3X3	T49.3X4	T49.3X5	T49.3X6
Calcifediol	T45.2X1	T45.2X2	T45.2X3	T45.2X4	T45.2X5	T45.2X6
Calciferol	T45.2X1	T45.2X2	T45.2X3	T45.2X4	T45.2X5	T45.2X6
Calcijex*	T45.2X1	T45.2X2	T45.2X3	T45.2X4	T45.2X5	T45.2X6
Calcitonin	T50.991	T50.992	T50.993	T50.994	T50.995	T50.996
Calcitriol	T45.2X1	T45.2X2	T45.2X3	T45.2X4	T45.2X5	T45.2X6
Calcium	T50.3X1	T50.3X2	T50.3X3	T50.3X4	T50.3X5	T50.3X6
actylsalicylate	T39.011	T39.012	T39.013	T39.014	T39.015	T39.016
benzamidosalicylate	T37.1X1	T37.1X2	T37.1X3	T37.1X4	T37.1X5	T37.1X6
bromide	T42.6X1	T42.6X2	T42.6X3	T42.6X4	T42.6X5	T42.6X6
bromolactobionate	T42.6X1	T42.6X2	T42.6X3	T42.6X4	T42.6X5	T42.6X6
carbaspirin	T39.011	T39.012	T39.013	T39.014	T39.015	T39.016
carbimide	T50.6X1	T50.6X2	T50.6X3	T50.6X4	T50.6X5	T50.6X6
carbonate	T47.1X1	T47.1X2	T47.1X3	T47.1X4	T47.1X5	T47.1X6
chloride	T50.991	T50.992	T50.993	T50.994	T50.995	T50.996
anhydrous	T50.991	T50.992	T50.993	T50.994	T50.995	T50.996
cyanide	T57.8X1	T57.8X2	T57.8X3	T57.8X4	—	—
dioctyl sulfosuccinate	T47.4X1	T47.4X2	T47.4X3	T47.4X4	T47.4X5	T47.4X6
disodium edathamil	T45.8X1	T45.8X2	T45.8X3	T45.8X4	T45.8X5	T45.8X6
disodium edetate	T45.8X1	T45.8X2	T45.8X3	T45.8X4	T45.8X5	T45.8X6
dobesilate	T46.991	T46.992	T46.993	T46.994	T46.995	T46.996
EDTA	T45.8X1	T45.8X2	T45.8X3	T45.8X4	T45.8X5	T45.8X6
ferrous citrate	T45.4X1	T45.4X2	T45.4X3	T45.4X4	T45.4X5	T45.4X6
folinate	T45.8X1	T45.8X2	T45.8X3	T45.8X4	T45.8X5	T45.8X6
glubionate	T50.3X1	T50.3X2	T50.3X3	T50.3X4	T50.3X5	T50.3X6
gluconate	T50.3X1	T50.3X2	T50.3X3	T50.3X4	T50.3X5	T50.3X6
gluconogalactogluconate	T50.3X1	T50.3X2	T50.3X3	T50.3X4	T50.3X5	T50.3X6
hydrate, hydroxide	T54.3X1	T54.3X2	T54.3X3	T54.3X4	—	—
hypochlorite	T54.3X1	T54.3X2	T54.3X3	T54.3X4	—	—
iodide	T48.4X1	T48.4X2	T48.4X3	T48.4X4	T48.4X5	T48.4X6
Calcium — continued						
ipodate	T50.8X1	T50.8X2	T50.8X3	T50.8X4	T50.8X5	T50.8X6
lactate	T50.3X1	T50.3X2	T50.3X3	T50.3X4	T50.3X5	T50.3X6
leucovorin	T45.8X1	T45.8X2	T45.8X3	T45.8X4	T45.8X5	T45.8X6
mandelate	T37.91	T37.92	T37.93	T37.94	T37.95	T37.96
oxide	T54.3X1	T54.3X2	T54.3X3	T54.3X4	—	—
pantothenate	T45.2X1	T45.2X2	T45.2X3	T45.2X4	T45.2X5	T45.2X6
phosphate	T50.3X1	T50.3X2	T50.3X3	T50.3X4	T50.3X5	T50.3X6
salicylate	T39.091	T39.092	T39.093	T39.094	T39.095	T39.096
salts	T50.3X1	T50.3X2	T50.3X3	T50.3X4	T50.3X5	T50.3X6
Calculus-dissolving drug	T50.991	T50.992	T50.993	T50.994	T50.995	T50.996
Calomel	T49.0X1	T49.0X2	T49.0X3	T49.0X4	T49.0X5	T49.0X6
Caloric agent	T50.3X1	T50.3X2	T50.3X3	T50.3X4	T50.3X5	T50.3X6
Calusterone	T38.7X1	T38.7X2	T38.7X3	T38.7X4	T38.7X5	T38.7X6
Camazepam	T42.4X1	T42.4X2	T42.4X3	T42.4X4	T42.4X5	T42.4X6
Camomile	T49.0X1	T49.0X2	T49.0X3	T49.0X4	T49.0X5	T49.0X6
Camoquin	T37.2X1	T37.2X2	T37.2X3	T37.2X4	T37.2X5	T37.2X6
Camphor						
insecticide	T60.2X1	T60.2X2	T60.2X3	T60.2X4	—	—
medicinal	T49.8X1	T49.8X2	T49.8X3	T49.8X4	T49.8X5	T49.8X6
Camylofin	T44.3X1	T44.3X2	T44.3X3	T44.3X4	T44.3X5	T44.3X6
Cancer chemotherapy drug regimen	T45.1X1	T45.1X2	T45.1X3	T45.1X4	T45.1X5	T45.1X6
Candeptin	T49.0X1	T49.0X2	T49.0X3	T49.0X4	T49.0X5	T49.0X6
Candicidin	T49.0X1	T49.0X2	T49.0X3	T49.0X4	T49.0X5	T49.0X6
Cankaid*	T49.6X1	T49.6X2	T49.6X3	T49.6X4	T49.6X5	T49.6X6
Cannabinoids, synthetic	T40.721	T40.722	T40.723	T40.724	T40.725	T40.726
Cannabinol	T40.711	T40.712	T40.713	T40.714	T40.715	T40.716
Cannabis (derivatives)	T40.711	T40.712	T40.713	T40.714	T40.715	T40.716
Canned heat	T51.1X1	T51.1X2	T51.1X3	T51.1X4	—	—
Canrenoic acid	T50.0X1	T50.0X2	T50.0X3	T50.0X4	T50.0X5	T50.0X6
Canrenone	T50.0X1	T50.0X2	T50.0X3	T50.0X4	T50.0X5	T50.0X6
Cantharides, cantharidin, cantharis	T49.8X1	T49.8X2	T49.8X3	T49.8X4	T49.8X5	T49.8X6
Canthaxanthin	T50.991	T50.992	T50.993	T50.994	T50.995	T50.996
Capillary-active drug NEC	T46.901	T46.902	T46.903	T46.904	T46.905	T46.906
Capreomycin	T36.8X1	T36.8X2	T36.8X3	T36.8X4	T36.8X5	T36.8X6
Capresla*	T45.1X1	T45.1X2	T45.1X3	T45.1X4	T45.1X5	T45.1X6
Capsicum	T49.4X1	T49.4X2	T49.4X3	T49.4X4	T49.4X5	T49.4X6
Captafol	T60.3X1	T60.3X2	T60.3X3	T60.3X4	—	—
Captan	T60.3X1	T60.3X2	T60.3X3	T60.3X4	—	—
Captodiame, captodiamine	T43.591	T43.592	T43.593	T43.594	T43.595	T43.596
Captopril	T46.4X1	T46.4X2	T46.4X3	T46.4X4	T46.4X5	T46.4X6
Caramiphen	T44.3X1	T44.3X2	T44.3X3	T44.3X4	T44.3X5	T44.3X6
Carazolol	T44.7X1	T44.7X2	T44.7X3	T44.7X4	T44.7X5	T44.7X6
Carbachol	T44.1X1	T44.1X2	T44.1X3	T44.1X4	T44.1X5	T44.1X6
Carbacrylamine (resin)	T50.3X1	T50.3X2	T50.3X3	T50.3X4	T50.3X5	T50.3X6
Carbamate (insecticide)	T60.0X1	T60.0X2	T60.0X3	T60.0X4	—	—
Carbamate (sedative)	T42.6X1	T42.6X2	T42.6X3	T42.6X4	T42.6X5	T42.6X6
herbicide	T60.0X1	T60.0X2	T60.0X3	T60.0X4	—	—
insecticide	T60.0X1	T60.0X2	T60.0X3	T60.0X4	—	—
Carbamazepine	T42.1X1	T42.1X2	T42.1X3	T42.1X4	T42.1X5	T42.1X6
Carbamide	T47.3X1	T47.3X2	T47.3X3	T47.3X4	T47.3X5	T47.3X6
peroxide	T49.0X1	T49.0X2	T49.0X3	T49.0X4	T49.0X5	T49.0X6
topical	T49.8X1	T49.8X2	T49.8X3	T49.8X4	T49.8X5	T49.8X6
Carbamylcholine chloride	T44.1X1	T44.1X2	T44.1X3	T44.1X4	T44.1X5	T44.1X6
Carbaril	T60.0X1	T60.0X2	T60.0X3	T60.0X4	—	—
Carbarsone	T37.3X1	T37.3X2	T37.3X3	T37.3X4	T37.3X5	T37.3X6
Carbaryl	T60.0X1	T60.0X2	T60.0X3	T60.0X4	—	—
Carbaspirin	T39.011	T39.012	T39.013	T39.014	T39.015	T39.016
Carbastat*	T49.5X1	T49.5X2	T49.5X3	T49.5X4	T49.5X5	T49.5X6
Carbazochrome (salicylate) (sodium sulfonate)	T49.4X1	T49.4X2	T49.4X3	T49.4X4	T49.4X5	T49.4X6
Carbenicillin	T36.0X1	T36.0X2	T36.0X3	T36.0X4	T36.0X5	T36.0X6
Carbenoxolone	T47.1X1	T47.1X2	T47.1X3	T47.1X4	T47.1X5	T47.1X6
Carbetapentane	T48.3X1	T48.3X2	T48.3X3	T48.3X4	T48.3X5	T48.3X6
Carbethyl salicylate	T39.091	T39.092	T39.093	T39.094	T39.095	T39.096
Carbidopa (with levodopa)	T42.8X1	T42.8X2	T42.8X3	T42.8X4	T42.8X5	T42.8X6
Carbimazole	T38.2X1	T38.2X2	T38.2X3	T38.2X4	T38.2X5	T38.2X6
Carbinol	T51.1X1	T51.1X2	T51.1X3	T51.1X4	—	—
Carbinoxamine	T45.0X1	T45.0X2	T45.0X3	T45.0X4	T45.0X5	T45.0X6
Carbiphene	T39.8X1	T39.8X2	T39.8X3	T39.8X4	T39.8X5	T39.8X6
Carbitol	T52.3X1	T52.3X2	T52.3X3	T52.3X4	—	—
Carbocaine	T41.3X1	T41.3X2	T41.3X3	T41.3X4	T41.3X5	T41.3X6
infiltration (subcutaneous)	T41.3X1	T41.3X2	T41.3X3	T41.3X4	T41.3X5	T41.3X6
nerve block (peripheral) (plexus)	T41.3X1	T41.3X2	T41.3X3	T41.3X4	T41.3X5	T41.3X6
topical (surface)	T41.3X1	T41.3X2	T41.3X3	T41.3X4	T41.3X5	T41.3X6
Carbocisteine	T48.4X1	T48.4X2	T48.4X3	T48.4X4	T48.4X5	T48.4X6
Carbocromen	T46.3X1	T46.3X2	T46.3X3	T46.3X4	T46.3X5	T46.3X6
Carbol fuchsin	T49.0X1	T49.0X2	T49.0X3	T49.0X4	T49.0X5	T49.0X6

Table of Drugs and Chemicals

Carbolic acid — Cefotetan

Substance	Poisoning, Accidental (unintentional)	Poisoning, Intentional Self-harm	Poisoning, Assault	Poisoning, Undetermined	Adverse Effect	Under-dosing
Carbolic acid — see also	T54.0X1	T54.0X2	T54.0X3	T54.0X4	—	—
Phenol						
Carbolonium (bromide)	T48.1X1	T48.1X2	T48.1X3	T48.1X4	T48.1X5	T48.1X6
Carbo medicinalis	T47.6X1	T47.6X2	T47.6X3	T47.6X4	T47.6X5	T47.6X6
Carbomycin	T36.8X1	T36.8X2	T36.8X3	T36.8X4	T36.8X5	T36.8X6
Carbon						
bisulfide (liquid)	T65.4X1	T65.4X2	T65.4X3	T65.4X4	—	—
vapor	T65.4X1	T65.4X2	T65.4X3	T65.4X4	—	—
dioxide (gas)	T59.7X1	T59.7X2	T59.7X3	T59.7X4	—	—
medicinal	T41.5X1	T41.5X2	T41.5X3	T41.5X4	T41.5X5	T41.5X6
nonmedicinal	T59.7X1	T59.7X2	T59.7X3	T59.7X4	—	—
snow	T49.4X1	T49.4X2	T49.4X3	T49.4X4	T49.4X5	T49.4X6
disulfide (liquid)	T65.4X1	T65.4X2	T65.4X3	T65.4X4	—	—
vapor	T65.4X1	T65.4X2	T65.4X3	T65.4X4	—	—
monoxide (from incomplete combustion)	T58.91	T58.92	T58.93	T58.94	—	—
blast furnace gas	T58.8X1	T58.8X2	T58.8X3	T58.8X4	—	—
butane (distributed in mobile container)	T58.11	T58.12	T58.13	T58.14	—	—
distributed through pipes	T58.11	T58.12	T58.13	T58.14	—	—
charcoal fumes	T58.2X1	T58.2X2	T58.2X3	T58.2X4	—	—
coal	T58.2X1	T58.2X2	T58.2X3	T58.2X4	—	—
coke (in domestic stoves, fireplaces)	T58.2X1	T58.2X2	T58.2X3	T58.2X4	—	—
exhaust gas (motor) not in transit	T58.01	T58.02	T58.03	T58.04	—	—
combustion engine, any not in watercraft	T58.01	T58.02	T58.03	T58.04	—	—
farm tractor, not in transit	T58.01	T58.02	T58.03	T58.04	—	—
gas engine	T58.01	T58.02	T58.03	T58.04	—	—
motor pump	T58.01	T58.02	T58.03	T58.04	—	—
motor vehicle, not in transit	T58.01	T58.02	T58.03	T58.04	—	—
fuel (in domestic use)	T58.2X1	T58.2X2	T58.2X3	T58.2X4	—	—
gas (piped)	T58.11	T58.12	T58.13	T58.14	—	—
in mobile container	T58.11	T58.12	T58.13	T58.14	—	—
piped (natural)	T58.11	T58.12	T58.13	T58.14	—	—
utility	T58.11	T58.12	T58.13	T58.14	—	—
in mobile container	T58.11	T58.12	T58.13	T58.14	—	—
gas (piped)	T58.11	T58.12	T58.13	T58.14	—	—
illuminating gas	T58.11	T58.12	T58.13	T58.14	—	—
industrial fuels or gases, any	T58.8X1	T58.8X2	T58.8X3	T58.8X4	—	—
kerosene (in domestic stoves, fireplaces)	T58.2X1	T58.2X2	T58.2X3	T58.2X4	—	—
kiln gas or vapor	T58.8X1	T58.8X2	T58.8X3	T58.8X4	—	—
motor exhaust gas, not in transit	T58.01	T58.02	T58.03	T58.04	—	—
piped gas (manufactured) (natural)	T58.11	T58.12	T58.13	T58.14	—	—
producer gas	T58.8X1	T58.8X2	T58.8X3	T58.8X4	—	—
propane (distributed in mobile container)	T58.11	T58.12	T58.13	T58.14	—	—
distributed through pipes	T58.11	T58.12	T58.13	T58.14	—	—
solid (in domestic stoves, fireplaces)	T58.2X1	T58.2X2	T58.2X3	T58.2X4	—	—
specified source NEC	T58.8X1	T58.8X2	T58.8X3	T58.8X4	—	—
stove gas	T58.11	T58.12	T58.13	T58.14	—	—
piped	T58.11	T58.12	T58.13	T58.14	—	—
utility gas	T58.11	T58.12	T58.13	T58.14	—	—
piped	T58.11	T58.12	T58.13	T58.14	—	—
water gas	T58.11	T58.12	T58.13	T58.14	—	—
wood (in domestic stoves, fireplaces)	T58.2X1	T58.2X2	T58.2X3	T58.2X4	—	—
tetrachloride (vapor) NEC	T53.0X1	T53.0X2	T53.0X3	T53.0X4	—	—
liquid (cleansing agent) NEC	T53.0X1	T53.0X2	T53.0X3	T53.0X4	—	—
solvent	T53.0X1	T53.0X2	T53.0X3	T53.0X4	—	—
Carbonic acid gas	T59.7X1	T59.7X2	T59.7X3	T59.7X4	—	—
anhydrase inhibitor NEC	T50.2X1	T50.2X2	T50.2X3	T50.2X4	T50.2X5	T50.2X6
Carbophenothion	T60.0X1	T60.0X2	T60.0X3	T60.0X4	—	—
Carboplatin	T45.1X1	T45.1X2	T45.1X3	T45.1X4	T45.1X5	T45.1X6
Carboprost	T48.0X1	T48.0X2	T48.0X3	T48.0X4	T48.0X5	T48.0X6
Carboquone	T45.1X1	T45.1X2	T45.1X3	T45.1X4	T45.1X5	T45.1X6
Carbowax	T49.3X1	T49.3X2	T49.3X3	T49.3X4	T49.3X5	T49.3X6
Carboxymethylcellulose	T47.4X1	T47.4X2	T47.4X3	T47.4X4	T47.4X5	T47.4X6
Carbrital	T42.3X1	T42.3X2	T42.3X3	T42.3X4	T42.3X5	T42.3X6
Carbromal	T42.6X1	T42.6X2	T42.6X3	T42.6X4	T42.6X5	T42.6X6
Carbutamide	T38.3X1	T38.3X2	T38.3X3	T38.3X4	T38.3X5	T38.3X6
Carbuterol	T48.6X1	T48.6X2	T48.6X3	T48.6X4	T48.6X5	T48.6X6

Substance	Poisoning, Accidental (unintentional)	Poisoning, Intentional Self-harm	Poisoning, Assault	Poisoning, Undetermined	Adverse Effect	Under-dosing
Cardiac						
depressants	T46.2X1	T46.2X2	T46.2X3	T46.2X4	T46.2X5	T46.2X6
rhythm regulator	T46.2X1	T46.2X2	T46.2X3	T46.2X4	T46.2X5	T46.2X6
specified NEC	T46.2X1	T46.2X2	T46.2X3	T46.2X4	T46.2X5	T46.2X6
Cardiografin	T50.8X1	T50.8X2	T50.8X3	T50.8X4	T50.8X5	T50.8X6
Cardiogreen	T50.8X1	T50.8X2	T50.8X3	T50.8X4	T50.8X5	T50.8X6
Cardiotonic (glycoside) NEC	T46.0X1	T46.0X2	T46.0X3	T46.0X4	T46.0X5	T46.0X6
Cardiovascular drug NEC	T46.901	T46.902	T46.903	T46.904	T46.905	T46.906
Cardizem*	T46.1X1	T46.1X2	T46.1X3	T46.1X4	T46.1X5	T46.1X6
Cardrase	T50.2X1	T50.2X2	T50.2X3	T50.2X4	T50.2X5	T50.2X6
Carfecillin	T36.0X1	T36.0X2	T36.0X3	T36.0X4	T36.0X5	T36.0X6
Carfenazine	T43.3X1	T43.3X2	T43.3X3	T43.3X4	T43.3X5	T43.3X6
Carfusin	T49.0X1	T49.0X2	T49.0X3	T49.0X4	T49.0X5	T49.0X6
Carindacillin	T36.0X1	T36.0X2	T36.0X3	T36.0X4	T36.0X5	T36.0X6
Carisoprodol	T42.8X1	T42.8X2	T42.8X3	T42.8X4	T42.8X5	T42.8X6
Carmellose	T47.4X1	T47.4X2	T47.4X3	T47.4X4	T47.4X5	T47.4X6
Carminative	T47.5X1	T47.5X2	T47.5X3	T47.5X4	T47.5X5	T47.5X6
Carmofur	T45.1X1	T45.1X2	T45.1X3	T45.1X4	T45.1X5	T45.1X6
Carmustine	T45.1X1	T45.1X2	T45.1X3	T45.1X4	T45.1X5	T45.1X6
Carotene	T45.2X1	T45.2X2	T45.2X3	T45.2X4	T45.2X5	T45.2X6
Carphenazine	T43.3X1	T43.3X2	T43.3X3	T43.3X4	T43.3X5	T43.3X6
Carpipramine	T42.4X1	T42.4X2	T42.4X3	T42.4X4	T42.4X5	T42.4X6
Carprofen	T39.311	T39.312	T39.313	T39.314	T39.315	T39.316
Carpronium chloride	T44.3X1	T44.3X2	T44.3X3	T44.3X4	T44.3X5	T44.3X6
Carrageenan	T47.8X1	T47.8X2	T47.8X3	T47.8X4	T47.8X5	T47.8X6
Carteolol	T44.7X1	T44.7X2	T44.7X3	T44.7X4	T44.7X5	T44.7X6
Carter's Little Pills	T47.2X1	T47.2X2	T47.2X3	T47.2X4	T47.2X5	T47.2X6
Cartia*	T46.1X1	T46.1X2	T46.1X3	T46.1X4	T46.1X5	T46.1X6
Cascara (sagrada)	T47.2X1	T47.2X2	T47.2X3	T47.2X4	T47.2X5	T47.2X6
Cassava	T62.2X1	T62.2X2	T62.2X3	T62.2X4	—	—
Castellani's paint	T49.0X1	T49.0X2	T49.0X3	T49.0X4	T49.0X5	T49.0X6
Castor						
bean	T62.2X1	T62.2X2	T62.2X3	T62.2X4	—	—
oil	T47.2X1	T47.2X2	T47.2X3	T47.2X4	T47.2X5	T47.2X6
Catalase	T45.3X1	T45.3X2	T45.3X3	T45.3X4	T45.3X5	T45.3X6
Caterpillar (sting)	T63.431	T63.432	T63.433	T63.434	—	—
Catha (edulis) (tea)	T43.691	T43.692	T43.693	T43.694	—	—
Cathartic NEC	T47.4X1	T47.4X2	T47.4X3	T47.4X4	T47.4X5	T47.4X6
anthacene derivative	T47.2X1	T47.2X2	T47.2X3	T47.2X4	T47.2X5	T47.2X6
bulk	T47.4X1	T47.4X2	T47.4X3	T47.4X4	T47.4X5	T47.4X6
contact	T47.2X1	T47.2X2	T47.2X3	T47.2X4	T47.2X5	T47.2X6
emollient NEC	T47.4X1	T47.4X2	T47.4X3	T47.4X4	T47.4X5	T47.4X6
irritant NEC	T47.2X1	T47.2X2	T47.2X3	T47.2X4	T47.2X5	T47.2X6
mucilage	T47.4X1	T47.4X2	T47.4X3	T47.4X4	T47.4X5	T47.4X6
saline	T47.3X1	T47.3X2	T47.3X3	T47.3X4	T47.3X5	T47.3X6
vegetable	T47.2X1	T47.2X2	T47.2X3	T47.2X4	T47.2X5	T47.2X6
Cathine	T50.5X1	T50.5X2	T50.5X3	T50.5X4	T50.5X5	T50.5X6
Cathomycin	T36.8X1	T36.8X2	T36.8X3	T36.8X4	T36.8X5	T36.8X6
Cation exchange resin	T50.3X1	T50.3X2	T50.3X3	T50.3X4	T50.3X5	T50.3X6
Caustic(s) NEC	T54.91	T54.92	T54.93	T54.94	—	—
alkali	T54.3X1	T54.3X2	T54.3X3	T54.3X4	—	—
hydroxide	T54.3X1	T54.3X2	T54.3X3	T54.3X4	—	—
potash	T54.3X1	T54.3X2	T54.3X3	T54.3X4	—	—
soda	T54.3X1	T54.3X2	T54.3X3	T54.3X4	—	—
specified NEC	T54.91	T54.92	T54.93	T54.94	—	—
Ceepryn	T49.0X1	T49.0X2	T49.0X3	T49.0X4	T49.0X5	T49.0X6
ENT agent	T49.6X1	T49.6X2	T49.6X3	T49.6X4	T49.6X5	T49.6X6
lozenges	T49.6X1	T49.6X2	T49.6X3	T49.6X4	T49.6X5	T49.6X6
Cefacetrile	T36.1X1	T36.1X2	T36.1X3	T36.1X4	T36.1X5	T36.1X6
Cefaclor	T36.1X1	T36.1X2	T36.1X3	T36.1X4	T36.1X5	T36.1X6
Cefadroxil	T36.1X1	T36.1X2	T36.1X3	T36.1X4	T36.1X5	T36.1X6
Cefalexin	T36.1X1	T36.1X2	T36.1X3	T36.1X4	T36.1X5	T36.1X6
Cefaloglycin	T36.1X1	T36.1X2	T36.1X3	T36.1X4	T36.1X5	T36.1X6
Cefaloridine	T36.1X1	T36.1X2	T36.1X3	T36.1X4	T36.1X5	T36.1X6
Cefalosporins	T36.1X1	T36.1X2	T36.1X3	T36.1X4	T36.1X5	T36.1X6
Cefalotin	T36.1X1	T36.1X2	T36.1X3	T36.1X4	T36.1X5	T36.1X6
Cefamandole	T36.1X1	T36.1X2	T36.1X3	T36.1X4	T36.1X5	T36.1X6
Cefamycin antibiotic	T36.1X1	T36.1X2	T36.1X3	T36.1X4	T36.1X5	T36.1X6
Cefapirin	T36.1X1	T36.1X2	T36.1X3	T36.1X4	T36.1X5	T36.1X6
Cefatrizine	T36.1X1	T36.1X2	T36.1X3	T36.1X4	T36.1X5	T36.1X6
Cefazedone	T36.1X1	T36.1X2	T36.1X3	T36.1X4	T36.1X5	T36.1X6
Cefazolin	T36.1X1	T36.1X2	T36.1X3	T36.1X4	T36.1X5	T36.1X6
Cefbuperazone	T36.1X1	T36.1X2	T36.1X3	T36.1X4	T36.1X5	T36.1X6
Cefetamet	T36.1X1	T36.1X2	T36.1X3	T36.1X4	T36.1X5	T36.1X6
Cefixime	T36.1X1	T36.1X2	T36.1X3	T36.1X4	T36.1X5	T36.1X6
Cefmenoxime	T36.1X1	T36.1X2	T36.1X3	T36.1X4	T36.1X5	T36.1X6
Cefmetazole	T36.1X1	T36.1X2	T36.1X3	T36.1X4	T36.1X5	T36.1X6
Cefminox	T36.1X1	T36.1X2	T36.1X3	T36.1X4	T36.1X5	T36.1X6
Cefonicid	T36.1X1	T36.1X2	T36.1X3	T36.1X4	T36.1X5	T36.1X6
Cefoperazone	T36.1X1	T36.1X2	T36.1X3	T36.1X4	T36.1X5	T36.1X6
Ceforanide	T36.1X1	T36.1X2	T36.1X3	T36.1X4	T36.1X5	T36.1X6
Cefotaxime	T36.1X1	T36.1X2	T36.1X3	T36.1X4	T36.1X5	T36.1X6
Cefotetan	T36.1X1	T36.1X2	T36.1X3	T36.1X4	T36.1X5	T36.1X6

☑ Additional Character May Be Required — Refer to the Tabular List for Character Selection

*Optum Value-Add

Substance	Poisoning, Accidental (unintentional)	Poisoning, Intentional Self-harm	Poisoning, Assault	Poisoning, Undetermined	Adverse Effect	Under-dosing
Cefotiam	T36.1X1	T36.1X2	T36.1X3	T36.1X4	T36.1X5	T36.1X6
Cefoxitin	T36.1X1	T36.1X2	T36.1X3	T36.1X4	T36.1X5	T36.1X6
Cefpimizole	T36.1X1	T36.1X2	T36.1X3	T36.1X4	T36.1X5	T36.1X6
Cefpiramide	T36.1X1	T36.1X2	T36.1X3	T36.1X4	T36.1X5	T36.1X6
Cefradine	T36.1X1	T36.1X2	T36.1X3	T36.1X4	T36.1X5	T36.1X6
Cefroxadine	T36.1X1	T36.1X2	T36.1X3	T36.1X4	T36.1X5	T36.1X6
Cefsulodin	T36.1X1	T36.1X2	T36.1X3	T36.1X4	T36.1X5	T36.1X6
Ceftazidime	T36.1X1	T36.1X2	T36.1X3	T36.1X4	T36.1X5	T36.1X6
Cefteram	T36.1X1	T36.1X2	T36.1X3	T36.1X4	T36.1X5	T36.1X6
Ceftezole	T36.1X1	T36.1X2	T36.1X3	T36.1X4	T36.1X5	T36.1X6
Ceftin*	T36.1X1	T36.1X2	T36.1X3	T36.1X4	T36.1X5	T36.1X6
Ceftizoxime	T36.1X1	T36.1X2	T36.1X3	T36.1X4	T36.1X5	T36.1X6
Ceftriaxone	T36.1X1	T36.1X2	T36.1X3	T36.1X4	T36.1X5	T36.1X6
Cefuroxime	T36.1X1	T36.1X2	T36.1X3	T36.1X4	T36.1X5	T36.1X6
Cefuzonam	T36.1X1	T36.1X2	T36.1X3	T36.1X4	T36.1X5	T36.1X6
Celestone	T38.0X1	T38.0X2	T38.0X3	T38.0X4	T38.0X5	T38.0X6
topical	T49.0X1	T49.0X2	T49.0X3	T49.0X4	T49.0X5	T49.0X6
Celiprolol	T44.7X1	T44.7X2	T44.7X3	T44.7X4	T44.7X5	T44.7X6
Cellosolve	T52.91	T52.92	T52.93	T52.94		
Cell stimulants and proliferants	T49.8X1	T49.8X2	T49.8X3	T49.8X4	T49.8X5	T49.8X6
Cellulose						
cathartic	T47.4X1	T47.4X2	T47.4X3	T47.4X4	T47.4X5	T47.4X6
hydroxyethyl	T47.4X1	T47.4X2	T47.4X3	T47.4X4	T47.4X5	T47.4X6
nitrates (topical)	T49.3X1	T49.3X2	T49.3X3	T49.3X4	T49.3X5	T49.3X6
oxidized	T49.4X1	T49.4X2	T49.4X3	T49.4X4	T49.4X5	T49.4X6
Centipede (bite)	T63.411	T63.412	T63.413	T63.414	—	—
Central nervous system						
depressants	T42.71	T42.72	T42.73	T42.74	T42.75	T42.76
anesthetic (general) NEC	T41.201	T41.202	T41.203	T41.204	T41.205	T41.206
gases NEC	T41.0X1	T41.0X2	T41.0X3	T41.0X4	T41.0X5	T41.0X6
intravenous	T41.1X1	T41.1X2	T41.1X3	T41.1X4	T41.1X5	T41.1X6
barbiturates	T42.3X1	T42.3X2	T42.3X3	T42.3X4	T42.3X5	T42.3X6
benzodiazepines	T42.4X1	T42.4X2	T42.4X3	T42.4X4	T42.4X5	T42.4X6
bromides	T42.6X1	T42.6X2	T42.6X3	T42.6X4	T42.6X5	T42.6X6
cannabis sativa	T40.711	T40.712	T40.713	T40.714	T40.715	T40.716
chloral hydrate	T42.6X1	T42.6X2	T42.6X3	T42.6X4	T42.6X5	T42.6X6
ethanol	T51.0X1	T51.0X2	T51.0X3	T51.0X4	—	—
hallucinogenics	T40.901	T40.902	T40.903	T40.904	T40.905	T40.906
hypnotics	T42.71	T42.72	T42.73	T42.74	T42.75	T42.76
specified NEC	T42.6X1	T42.6X2	T42.6X3	T42.6X4	T42.6X5	T42.6X6
muscle relaxants	T42.8X1	T42.8X2	T42.8X3	T42.8X4	T42.8X5	T42.8X6
paraldehyde	T42.6X1	T42.6X2	T42.6X3	T42.6X4	T42.6X5	T42.6X6
sedatives; sedative-hypnotics	T42.71	T42.72	T42.73	T42.74	T42.75	T42.76
mixed NEC	T42.6X1	T42.6X2	T42.6X3	T42.6X4	T42.6X5	T42.6X6
specified NEC	T42.6X1	T42.6X2	T42.6X3	T42.6X4	T42.6X5	T42.6X6
muscle-tone depressants	T42.8X1	T42.8X2	T42.8X3	T42.8X4	T42.8X5	T42.8X6
stimulants	T43.601	T43.602	T43.603	T43.604	T43.605	T43.606
amphetamines	T43.621	T43.622	T43.623	T43.624	T43.625	T43.626
analeptics	T50.7X1	T50.7X2	T50.7X3	T50.7X4	T50.7X5	T50.7X6
antidepressants	T43.201	T43.202	T43.203	T43.204	T43.205	T43.206
opiate antagonists	T50.7X1	T50.7X2	T50.7X3	T50.7X4	T50.7X5	T50.7X6
specified NEC	T43.691	T43.692	T43.693	T43.694	T43.695	T43.696
Cepacol*	T41.3X1	T41.3X2	T41.3X3	T41.3X4	T41.3X5	T41.3X6
Cephalexin	T36.1X1	T36.1X2	T36.1X3	T36.1X4	T36.1X5	T36.1X6
Cephaloglycin	T36.1X1	T36.1X2	T36.1X3	T36.1X4	T36.1X5	T36.1X6
Cephaloridine	T36.1X1	T36.1X2	T36.1X3	T36.1X4	T36.1X5	T36.1X6
Cephalosporins	T36.1X1	T36.1X2	T36.1X3	T36.1X4	T36.1X5	T36.1X6
N (adicillin)	T36.0X1	T36.0X2	T36.0X3	T36.0X4	T36.0X5	T36.0X6
Cephalothin	T36.1X1	T36.1X2	T36.1X3	T36.1X4	T36.1X5	T36.1X6
Cephalotin	T36.1X1	T36.1X2	T36.1X3	T36.1X4	T36.1X5	T36.1X6
Cephradine	T36.1X1	T36.1X2	T36.1X3	T36.1X4	T36.1X5	T36.1X6
Cerbera (odallam)	T62.2X1	T62.2X2	T62.2X3	T62.2X4	—	—
Cerberin	T46.0X1	T46.0X2	T46.0X3	T46.0X4	T46.0X5	T46.0X6
Cerebral stimulants	T43.601	T43.602	T43.603	T43.604	T43.605	T43.606
psychotherapeutic	T43.601	T43.602	T43.603	T43.604	T43.605	T43.606
specified NEC	T43.691	T43.692	T43.693	T43.694	T43.695	T43.696
Cerium oxalate	T45.0X1	T45.0X2	T45.0X3	T45.0X4	T45.0X5	T45.0X6
Cerous oxalate	T45.0X1	T45.0X2	T45.0X3	T45.0X4	T45.0X5	T45.0X6
Ceruletide	T50.8X1	T50.8X2	T50.8X3	T50.8X4	T50.8X5	T50.8X6
Cetacort*	T49.0X1	T49.0X2	T49.0X3	T49.0X4	T49.0X5	T49.0X6
Cetalkonium (chloride)	T49.0X1	T49.0X2	T49.0X3	T49.0X4	T49.0X5	T49.0X6
Cethexonium chloride	T49.0X1	T49.0X2	T49.0X3	T49.0X4	T49.0X5	T49.0X6
Cetiedil	T46.7X1	T46.7X2	T46.7X3	T46.7X4	T46.7X5	T46.7X6
Cetirizine	T45.0X1	T45.0X2	T45.0X3	T45.0X4	T45.0X5	T45.0X6
Cetomacrogol	T50.991	T50.992	T50.993	T50.994	T50.995	T50.996
Cetotiamine	T45.2X1	T45.2X2	T45.2X3	T45.2X4	T45.2X5	T45.2X6
Cetoxime	T45.0X1	T45.0X2	T45.0X3	T45.0X4	T45.0X5	T45.0X6
Cetraxate	T47.1X1	T47.1X2	T47.1X3	T47.1X4	T47.1X5	T47.1X6
Cetrimide	T49.0X1	T49.0X2	T49.0X3	T49.0X4	T49.0X5	T49.0X6
Cetrimonium (bromide)	T49.0X1	T49.0X2	T49.0X3	T49.0X4	T49.0X5	T49.0X6
Cetylpyridinium chloride	T49.0X1	T49.0X2	T49.0X3	T49.0X4	T49.0X5	T49.0X6

Substance	Poisoning, Accidental (unintentional)	Poisoning, Intentional Self-harm	Poisoning, Assault	Poisoning, Undetermined	Adverse Effect	Under-dosing
Cetylpyridinium chloride — continued						
ENT agent	T49.6X1	T49.6X2	T49.6X3	T49.6X4	T49.6X5	T49.6X6
lozenges	T49.6X1	T49.6X2	T49.6X3	T49.6X4	T49.6X5	T49.6X6
Cevadilla — see Sabadilla						
Cevitamic acid	T45.2X1	T45.2X2	T45.2X3	T45.2X4	T45.2X5	T45.2X6
Chalk, precipitated	T47.1X1	T47.1X2	T47.1X3	T47.1X4	T47.1X5	T47.1X6
Chamomile	T49.0X1	T49.0X2	T49.0X3	T49.0X4	T49.0X5	T49.0X6
Ch'an su	T46.0X1	T46.0X2	T46.0X3	T46.0X4	T46.0X5	T46.0X6
Charcoal	T47.6X1	T47.6X2	T47.6X3	T47.6X4	T47.6X5	T47.6X6
activated — see also Charcoal, medicinal	T47.6X1	T47.6X2	T47.6X3	T47.6X4	T47.6X5	T47.6X6
fumes (Carbon monoxide)	T58.2X1	T58.2X2	T58.2X3	T58.2X4	—	—
industrial	T58.8X1	T58.8X2	T58.8X3	T58.8X4	—	—
medicinal (activated)	T47.6X1	T47.6X2	T47.6X3	T47.6X4	T47.6X5	T47.6X6
antidiarrheal	T47.6X1	T47.6X2	T47.6X3	T47.6X4	T47.6X5	T47.6X6
poison control	T47.8X1	T47.8X2	T47.8X3	T47.8X4	T47.8X5	T47.8X6
specified use other than for diarrhea	T47.8X1	T47.8X2	T47.8X3	T47.8X4	T47.8X5	T47.8X6
topical	T49.8X1	T49.8X2	T49.8X3	T49.8X4	T49.8X5	T49.8X6
Chaulmosulfone	T37.1X1	T37.1X2	T37.1X3	T37.1X4	T37.1X5	T37.1X6
Chelating agent NEC	T50.6X1	T50.6X2	T50.6X3	T50.6X4	T50.6X5	T50.6X6
Chelidonium majus	T62.2X1	T62.2X2	T62.2X3	T62.2X4	—	—
Chemical substance NEC	T65.91	T65.92	T65.93	T65.94		
Chenodeoxycholic acid	T47.5X1	T47.5X2	T47.5X3	T47.5X4	T47.5X5	T47.5X6
Chenodiol	T47.5X1	T47.5X2	T47.5X3	T47.5X4	T47.5X5	T47.5X6
Chenopodium	T37.4X1	T37.4X2	T37.4X3	T37.4X4	T37.4X5	T37.4X6
Cherry laurel	T62.2X1	T62.2X2	T62.2X3	T62.2X4	—	—
Chiggertox*	T41.3X1	T41.3X2	T41.3X3	T41.3X4	T41.3X5	T41.3X6
Chinidin (e)	T46.2X1	T46.2X2	T46.2X3	T46.2X4	T46.2X5	T46.2X6
Chiniofon	T37.8X1	T37.8X2	T37.8X3	T37.8X4	T37.8X5	T37.8X6
Chlophedianol	T48.3X1	T48.3X2	T48.3X3	T48.3X4	T48.3X5	T48.3X6
Chloral	T42.6X1	T42.6X2	T42.6X3	T42.6X4	T42.6X5	T42.6X6
derivative	T42.6X1	T42.6X2	T42.6X3	T42.6X4	T42.6X5	T42.6X6
hydrate	T42.6X1	T42.6X2	T42.6X3	T42.6X4	T42.6X5	T42.6X6
Chloralamide	T42.6X1	T42.6X2	T42.6X3	T42.6X4	T42.6X5	T42.6X6
Chloralodol	T42.6X1	T42.6X2	T42.6X3	T42.6X4	T42.6X5	T42.6X6
Chloralose	T60.4X1	T60.4X2	T60.4X3	T60.4X4	—	—
Chlorambucil	T45.1X1	T45.1X2	T45.1X3	T45.1X4	T45.1X5	T45.1X6
Chloramine	T57.8X1	T57.8X2	T57.8X3	T57.8X4	—	—
T	T49.0X1	T49.0X2	T49.0X3	T49.0X4	T49.0X5	T49.0X6
topical	T49.0X1	T49.0X2	T49.0X3	T49.0X4	T49.0X5	T49.0X6
Chloramphenicol	T36.2X1	T36.2X2	T36.2X3	T36.2X4	T36.2X5	T36.2X6
ENT agent	T49.6X1	T49.6X2	T49.6X3	T49.6X4	T49.6X5	T49.6X6
ophthalmic preparation	T49.5X1	T49.5X2	T49.5X3	T49.5X4	T49.5X5	T49.5X6
topical NEC	T49.0X1	T49.0X2	T49.0X3	T49.0X4	T49.0X5	T49.0X6
Chlorate (potassium) (sodium) NEC	T60.3X1	T60.3X2	T60.3X3	T60.3X4	—	—
herbicide	T60.3X1	T60.3X2	T60.3X3	T60.3X4	—	—
Chlorazanil	T50.2X1	T50.2X2	T50.2X3	T50.2X4	T50.2X5	T50.2X6
Chlorbenzene, chlorbenzol	T53.7X1	T53.7X2	T53.7X3	T53.7X4	—	—
Chlorbenzoxamine	T44.3X1	T44.3X2	T44.3X3	T44.3X4	T44.3X5	T44.3X6
Chlorbutol	T42.6X1	T42.6X2	T42.6X3	T42.6X4	T42.6X5	T42.6X6
Chlorcyclizine	T45.0X1	T45.0X2	T45.0X3	T45.0X4	T45.0X5	T45.0X6
Chlordan (e) (dust)	T60.1X1	T60.1X2	T60.1X3	T60.1X4	—	—
Chlordantoin	T49.0X1	T49.0X2	T49.0X3	T49.0X4	T49.0X5	T49.0X6
Chlordiazepoxide	T42.4X1	T42.4X2	T42.4X3	T42.4X4	T42.4X5	T42.4X6
Chlordiethyl benzamide	T49.3X1	T49.3X2	T49.3X3	T49.3X4	T49.3X5	T49.3X6
Chloresium	T49.8X1	T49.8X2	T49.8X3	T49.8X4	T49.8X5	T49.8X6
Chlorethiazol	T42.6X1	T42.6X2	T42.6X3	T42.6X4	T42.6X5	T42.6X6
Chlorethyl — see Ethyl, chloride						
Chloretone	T42.6X1	T42.6X2	T42.6X3	T42.6X4	T42.6X5	T42.6X6
Chlorex	T53.6X1	T53.6X2	T53.6X3	T53.6X4	—	—
insecticide	T60.1X1	T60.1X2	T60.1X3	T60.1X4	—	—
Chlorfenvinphos	T60.0X1	T60.0X2	T60.0X3	T60.0X4	—	—
Chlorhexadol	T42.6X1	T42.6X2	T42.6X3	T42.6X4	T42.6X5	T42.6X6
Chlorhexamide	T45.1X1	T45.1X2	T45.1X3	T45.1X4	T45.1X5	T45.1X6
Chlorhexidine	T49.0X1	T49.0X2	T49.0X3	T49.0X4	T49.0X5	T49.0X6
Chlorhexidine Gluconate Oral Rinse*	T49.6X1	T49.6X2	T49.6X3	T49.6X4	T49.6X5	T49.6X6
Chlorhydroxyquinolin	T49.0X1	T49.0X2	T49.0X3	T49.0X4	T49.0X5	T49.0X6
Chloride of lime (bleach)	T54.3X1	T54.3X2	T54.3X3	T54.3X4	—	—
Chlorimipramine	T43.011	T43.012	T43.013	T43.014	T43.015	T43.016
Chlorinated						
camphene	T53.6X1	T53.6X2	T53.6X3	T53.6X4	—	—
diphenyl	T53.7X1	T53.7X2	T53.7X3	T53.7X4	—	—
hydrocarbons NEC	T53.91	T53.92	T53.93	T53.94	—	—
solvents	T53.91	T53.92	T53.93	T53.94	—	—
lime (bleach)	T54.3X1	T54.3X2	T54.3X3	T54.3X4	—	—
and boric acid solution	T49.0X1	T49.0X2	T49.0X3	T49.0X4	T49.0X5	T49.0X6
naphthalene (insecticide)	T60.1X1	T60.1X2	T60.1X3	T60.1X4	—	—

Substance	Poisoning, Accidental (unintentional)	Poisoning, Intentional Self-harm	Poisoning, Assault	Poisoning, Undetermined	Adverse Effect	Under-dosing
Chlorinated — continued						
naphthalene — continued						
industrial (non-pesticide)	T53.7X1	T53.7X2	T53.7X3	T53.7X4	—	—
pesticide NEC	T60.8X1	T60.8X2	T60.8X3	T60.8X4	—	—
soda — see also sodium hypochlorite						
solution	T49.0X1	T49.0X2	T49.0X3	T49.0X4	T49.0X5	T49.0X6
Chlorine (fumes) (gas)	T59.4X1	T59.4X2	T59.4X3	T59.4X4	—	—
bleach	T54.3X1	T54.3X2	T54.3X3	T54.3X4	—	—
compound gas NEC	T59.4X1	T59.4X2	T59.4X3	T59.4X4	—	—
disinfectant	T59.4X1	T59.4X2	T59.4X3	T59.4X4	—	—
releasing agents NEC	T59.4X1	T59.4X2	T59.4X3	T59.4X4	—	—
Chlorisondamine chloride	T46.991	T46.992	T46.993	T46.994	T46.995	T46.996
Chlormadinone	T38.5X1	T38.5X2	T38.5X3	T38.5X4	T38.5X5	T38.5X6
Chlormephos	T60.0X1	T60.0X2	T60.0X3	T60.0X4	—	—
Chlormerodrin	T50.2X1	T50.2X2	T50.2X3	T50.2X4	T50.2X5	T50.2X6
Chlormethiazole	T42.6X1	T42.6X2	T42.6X3	T42.6X4	T42.6X5	T42.6X6
Chlormethine	T45.1X1	T45.1X2	T45.1X3	T45.1X4	T45.1X5	T45.1X6
Chlormethylenecycline	T36.4X1	T36.4X2	T36.4X3	T36.4X4	T36.4X5	T36.4X6
Chlormezanone	T42.6X1	T42.6X2	T42.6X3	T42.6X4	T42.6X5	T42.6X6
Chloroacetic acid	T60.3X1	T60.3X2	T60.3X3	T60.3X4	—	—
Chloroacetone	T59.3X1	T59.3X2	T59.3X3	T59.3X4	—	—
Chloroacetophenone	T59.3X1	T59.3X2	T59.3X3	T59.3X4	—	—
Chloroaniline	T53.7X1	T53.7X2	T53.7X3	T53.7X4	—	—
Chlorobenzene, chlorobenzol	T53.7X1	T53.7X2	T53.7X3	T53.7X4	—	—
Chlorobromomethane (fire extinguisher)	T53.6X1	T53.6X2	T53.6X3	T53.6X4	—	—
Chlorobutanol	T49.0X1	T49.0X2	T49.0X3	T49.0X4	T49.0X5	T49.0X6
Chlorocresol	T49.0X1	T49.0X2	T49.0X3	T49.0X4	T49.0X5	T49.0X6
Chlorodehydromethyltestosterone	T38.7X1	T38.7X2	T38.7X3	T38.7X4	T38.7X5	T38.7X6
Chlorodeoxyadenosine*	T45.1X1	T45.1X2	T45.1X3	T45.1X4	T45.1X5	T45.1X6
Chlorodinitrobenzene	T53.7X1	T53.7X2	T53.7X3	T53.7X4	—	—
dust or vapor	T53.7X1	T53.7X2	T53.7X3	T53.7X4	—	—
Chlorodiphenyl	T53.7X1	T53.7X2	T53.7X3	T53.7X4	—	—
Chloroethane — see Ethyl, chloride						
Chloroethylene	T53.6X1	T53.6X2	T53.6X3	T53.6X4	—	—
Chlorofluorocarbons	T53.5X1	T53.5X2	T53.5X3	T53.5X4	—	—
Chloroform (fumes) (vapor)	T53.1X1	T53.1X2	T53.1X3	T53.1X4	—	—
anesthetic	T41.0X1	T41.0X2	T41.0X3	T41.0X4	T41.0X5	T41.0X6
solvent	T53.1X1	T53.1X2	T53.1X3	T53.1X4	—	—
water, concentrated	T41.0X1	T41.0X2	T41.0X3	T41.0X4	T41.0X5	T41.0X6
Chloroguanide	T37.2X1	T37.2X2	T37.2X3	T37.2X4	T37.2X5	T37.2X6
Chloromycetin	T36.2X1	T36.2X2	T36.2X3	T36.2X4	T36.2X5	T36.2X6
ENT agent	T49.6X1	T49.6X2	T49.6X3	T49.6X4	T49.6X5	T49.6X6
ophthalmic preparation	T49.5X1	T49.5X2	T49.5X3	T49.5X4	T49.5X5	T49.5X6
otic solution	T49.6X1	T49.6X2	T49.6X3	T49.6X4	T49.6X5	T49.6X6
topical NEC	T49.0X1	T49.0X2	T49.0X3	T49.0X4	T49.0X5	T49.0X6
Chloronitrobenzene	T53.7X1	T53.7X2	T53.7X3	T53.7X4	—	—
dust or vapor	T53.7X1	T53.7X2	T53.7X3	T53.7X4	—	—
Chlorophacinone	T60.4X1	T60.4X2	T60.4X3	T60.4X4	—	—
Chlorophenol	T53.7X1	T53.7X2	T53.7X3	T53.7X4	—	—
Chlorophenothane	T60.1X1	T60.1X2	T60.1X3	T60.1X4	—	—
Chlorophyll	T50.991	T50.992	T50.993	T50.994	T50.995	T50.996
Chloropicrin (fumes)	T53.6X1	T53.6X2	T53.6X3	T53.6X4	—	—
fumigant	T60.8X1	T60.8X2	T60.8X3	T60.8X4	—	—
fungicide	T60.3X1	T60.3X2	T60.3X3	T60.3X4	—	—
pesticide	T60.8X1	T60.8X2	T60.8X3	T60.8X4	—	—
Chloroprocaine	T41.3X1	T41.3X2	T41.3X3	T41.3X4	T41.3X5	T41.3X6
infiltration (subcutaneous)	T41.3X1	T41.3X2	T41.3X3	T41.3X4	T41.3X5	T41.3X6
nerve block (peripheral) (plexus)	T41.3X1	T41.3X2	T41.3X3	T41.3X4	T41.3X5	T41.3X6
spinal	T41.3X1	T41.3X2	T41.3X3	T41.3X4	T41.3X5	T41.3X6
Chloroptic	T49.5X1	T49.5X2	T49.5X3	T49.5X4	T49.5X5	T49.5X6
Chloropurine	T45.1X1	T45.1X2	T45.1X3	T45.1X4	T45.1X5	T45.1X6
Chloropyramine	T45.0X1	T45.0X2	T45.0X3	T45.0X4	T45.0X5	T45.0X6
Chloropyrifos	T60.0X1	T60.0X2	T60.0X3	T60.0X4	—	—
Chloropyrilene	T45.0X1	T45.0X2	T45.0X3	T45.0X4	T45.0X5	T45.0X6
Chloroquine	T37.2X1	T37.2X2	T37.2X3	T37.2X4	T37.2X5	T37.2X6
Chlorostat*	T49.0X1	T49.0X2	T49.0X3	T49.0X4	T49.0X5	T49.0X6
Chlorothalonil	T60.3X1	T60.3X2	T60.3X3	T60.3X4	—	—
Chlorothen	T45.0X1	T45.0X2	T45.0X3	T45.0X4	T45.0X5	T45.0X6
Chlorothiazide	T50.2X1	T50.2X2	T50.2X3	T50.2X4	T50.2X5	T50.2X6
Chlorothymol	T49.4X1	T49.4X2	T49.4X3	T49.4X4	T49.4X5	T49.4X6
Chlorotrianisene	T38.5X1	T38.5X2	T38.5X3	T38.5X4	T38.5X5	T38.5X6
Chlorovinyldichloroarsine, not in war	T57.0X1	T57.0X2	T57.0X3	T57.0X4	—	—
Chloroxine	T49.4X1	T49.4X2	T49.4X3	T49.4X4	T49.4X5	T49.4X6
Chloroxylenol	T49.0X1	T49.0X2	T49.0X3	T49.0X4	T49.0X5	T49.0X6
Chlorphenamine	T45.0X1	T45.0X2	T45.0X3	T45.0X4	T45.0X5	T45.0X6
Chlorphenesin	T42.8X1	T42.8X2	T42.8X3	T42.8X4	T42.8X5	T42.8X6
topical (antifungal)	T49.0X1	T49.0X2	T49.0X3	T49.0X4	T49.0X5	T49.0X6
Chlorpheniramine	T45.0X1	T45.0X2	T45.0X3	T45.0X4	T45.0X5	T45.0X6
Chlorphenoxamine	T45.0X1	T45.0X2	T45.0X3	T45.0X4	T45.0X5	T45.0X6
Chlorphentermine	T50.5X1	T50.5X2	T50.5X3	T50.5X4	T50.5X5	T50.5X6
Chlorprocaine — see Chloroprocaine						
Chlorproguanil	T37.2X1	T37.2X2	T37.2X3	T37.2X4	T37.2X5	T37.2X6
Chlorpromazine	T43.3X1	T43.3X2	T43.3X3	T43.3X4	T43.3X5	T43.3X6
Chlorpropamide	T38.3X1	T38.3X2	T38.3X3	T38.3X4	T38.3X5	T38.3X6
Chlorprothixene	T43.4X1	T43.4X2	T43.4X3	T43.4X4	T43.4X5	T43.4X6
Chlorquinaldol	T49.0X1	T49.0X2	T49.0X3	T49.0X4	T49.0X5	T49.0X6
Chlorquinol	T49.0X1	T49.0X2	T49.0X3	T49.0X4	T49.0X5	T49.0X6
Chlortalidone	T50.2X1	T50.2X2	T50.2X3	T50.2X4	T50.2X5	T50.2X6
Chlortetracycline	T36.4X1	T36.4X2	T36.4X3	T36.4X4	T36.4X5	T36.4X6
Chlorthalidone	T50.2X1	T50.2X2	T50.2X3	T50.2X4	T50.2X5	T50.2X6
Chlorthion	T60.0X1	T60.0X2	T60.0X3	T60.0X4	—	—
Chlorthiophos	T60.0X1	T60.0X2	T60.0X3	T60.0X4	—	—
Chlortrianisene	T38.5X1	T38.5X2	T38.5X3	T38.5X4	T38.5X5	T38.5X6
Chlor-Trimeton	T45.0X1	T45.0X2	T45.0X3	T45.0X4	T45.0X5	T45.0X6
Chlorzoxazone	T42.8X1	T42.8X2	T42.8X3	T42.8X4	T42.8X5	T42.8X6
Choke damp	T59.7X1	T59.7X2	T59.7X3	T59.7X4	—	—
Cholagogues	T47.5X1	T47.5X2	T47.5X3	T47.5X4	T47.5X5	T47.5X6
Cholebrine	T50.8X1	T50.8X2	T50.8X3	T50.8X4	T50.8X5	T50.8X6
Cholecalciferol	T45.2X1	T45.2X2	T45.2X3	T45.2X4	T45.2X5	T45.2X6
Cholecystokinin	T50.8X1	T50.8X2	T50.8X3	T50.8X4	T50.8X5	T50.8X6
Cholera vaccine	T50.A91	T50.A92	T50.A93	T50.A94	T50.A95	T50.A96
Choleretic	T47.5X1	T47.5X2	T47.5X3	T47.5X4	T47.5X5	T47.5X6
Cholesterol-lowering agents	T46.6X1	T46.6X2	T46.6X3	T46.6X4	T46.6X5	T46.6X6
Cholestyramine (resin)	T46.6X1	T46.6X2	T46.6X3	T46.6X4	T46.6X5	T46.6X6
Cholic acid	T47.5X1	T47.5X2	T47.5X3	T47.5X4	T47.5X5	T47.5X6
Choline	T48.6X1	T48.6X2	T48.6X3	T48.6X4	T48.6X5	T48.6X6
chloride	T50.991	T50.992	T50.993	T50.994	T50.995	T50.996
dihydrogen citrate	T50.991	T50.992	T50.993	T50.994	T50.995	T50.996
salicylate	T39.091	T39.092	T39.093	T39.094	T39.095	T39.096
theophyllinate	T48.6X1	T48.6X2	T48.6X3	T48.6X4	T48.6X5	T48.6X6
Cholinergic (drug) **NEC**	T44.1X1	T44.1X2	T44.1X3	T44.1X4	T44.1X5	T44.1X6
muscle tone enhancer	T44.1X1	T44.1X2	T44.1X3	T44.1X4	T44.1X5	T44.1X6
organophosphorus	T44.0X1	T44.0X2	T44.0X3	T44.0X4	T44.0X5	T44.0X6
insecticide	T60.0X1	T60.0X2	T60.0X3	T60.0X4	—	—
nerve gas	T59.891	T59.892	T59.893	T59.894	—	—
trimethyl ammonium propanediol	T44.1X1	T44.1X2	T44.1X3	T44.1X4	T44.1X5	T44.1X6
Cholinesterase reactivator	T50.6X1	T50.6X2	T50.6X3	T50.6X4	T50.6X5	T50.6X6
Cholografin	T50.8X1	T50.8X2	T50.8X3	T50.8X4	T50.8X5	T50.8X6
Chorionic gonadotropin	T38.891	T38.892	T38.893	T38.894	T38.895	T38.896
Chromate	T56.2X1	T56.2X2	T56.2X3	T56.2X4	—	—
dust or mist	T56.2X1	T56.2X2	T56.2X3	T56.2X4	—	—
lead — see also lead	T56.0X1	T56.0X2	T56.0X3	T56.0X4	—	—
paint	T56.0X1	T56.0X2	T56.0X3	T56.0X4	—	—
Chromelin*	T49.3X1	T49.3X2	T49.3X3	T49.3X4	T49.3X5	T49.3X6
Chromic						
acid	T56.2X1	T56.2X2	T56.2X3	T56.2X4	—	—
dust or mist	T56.2X1	T56.2X2	T56.2X3	T56.2X4	—	—
phosphate 32P	T45.1X1	T45.1X2	T45.1X3	T45.1X4	T45.1X5	T45.1X6
Chromium	T56.2X1	T56.2X2	T56.2X3	T56.2X4	—	—
compounds — see Chromate						
sesquioxide	T50.8X1	T50.8X2	T50.8X3	T50.8X4	T50.8X5	T50.8X6
Chromomycin A3	T45.1X1	T45.1X2	T45.1X3	T45.1X4	T45.1X5	T45.1X6
Chromonar	T46.3X1	T46.3X2	T46.3X3	T46.3X4	T46.3X5	T46.3X6
Chromyl chloride	T56.2X1	T56.2X2	T56.2X3	T56.2X4	—	—
Chrysarobin	T49.4X1	T49.4X2	T49.4X3	T49.4X4	T49.4X5	T49.4X6
Chrysazin	T47.2X1	T47.2X2	T47.2X3	T47.2X4	T47.2X5	T47.2X6
Chymar	T45.3X1	T45.3X2	T45.3X3	T45.3X4	T45.3X5	T45.3X6
ophthalmic preparation	T49.5X1	T49.5X2	T49.5X3	T49.5X4	T49.5X5	T49.5X6
Chymopapain	T45.3X1	T45.3X2	T45.3X3	T45.3X4	T45.3X5	T45.3X6
Chymotrypsin	T45.3X1	T45.3X2	T45.3X3	T45.3X4	T45.3X5	T45.3X6
ophthalmic preparation	T49.5X1	T49.5X2	T49.5X3	T49.5X4	T49.5X5	T49.5X6
Cianidanol	T50.991	T50.992	T50.993	T50.994	T50.995	T50.996
Cianopramine	T43.011	T43.012	T43.013	T43.014	T43.015	T43.016
Cibenzoline	T46.2X1	T46.2X2	T46.2X3	T46.2X4	T46.2X5	T46.2X6
Ciclacillin	T36.0X1	T36.0X2	T36.0X3	T36.0X4	T36.0X5	T36.0X6
Ciclobarbital — see Hexobarbital						
Ciclonicate	T46.7X1	T46.7X2	T46.7X3	T46.7X4	T46.7X5	T46.7X6
Ciclopirox (olamine)	T49.0X1	T49.0X2	T49.0X3	T49.0X4	T49.0X5	T49.0X6
Ciclosporin	T45.1X1	T45.1X2	T45.1X3	T45.1X4	T45.1X5	T45.1X6
Cicuta maculata or virosa	T62.2X1	T62.2X2	T62.2X3	T62.2X4	—	—
Cicutoxin	T62.2X1	T62.2X2	T62.2X3	T62.2X4	—	—
Cigarette lighter fluid	T52.0X1	T52.0X2	T52.0X3	T52.0X4	—	—
Cigarettes (tobacco)	T65.221	T65.222	T65.223	T65.224	—	—
Ciguatoxin	T61.01	T61.02	T61.03	T61.04	—	—

☑ Additional Character May Be Required — Refer to the Tabular List for Character Selection

*Optum Value-Add

Substance	Poisoning, Accidental (unintentional)	Poisoning, Intentional Self-harm	Poisoning, Assault	Poisoning, Undetermined	Adverse Effect	Under-dosing
Cilazapril	T46.4X1	T46.4X2	T46.4X3	T46.4X4	T46.4X5	T46.4X6
Cimetidine	T47.0X1	T47.0X2	T47.0X3	T47.0X4	T47.0X5	T47.0X6
Cimetropium bromide	T44.3X1	T44.3X2	T44.3X3	T44.3X4	T44.3X5	T44.3X6
Cinchocaine	T41.3X1	T41.3X2	T41.3X3	T41.3X4	T41.3X5	T41.3X6
topical (surface)	T41.3X1	T41.3X2	T41.3X3	T41.3X4	T41.3X5	T41.3X6
Cinchona	T37.2X1	T37.2X2	T37.2X3	T37.2X4	T37.2X5	T37.2X6
Cinchonine alkaloids	T37.2X1	T37.2X2	T37.2X3	T37.2X4	T37.2X5	T37.2X6
Cinchophen	T50.4X1	T50.4X2	T50.4X3	T50.4X4	T50.4X5	T50.4X6
Cinepazide	T46.7X1	T46.7X2	T46.7X3	T46.7X4	T46.7X5	T46.7X6
Cinnamedrine	T48.5X1	T48.5X2	T48.5X3	T48.5X4	T48.5X5	T48.5X6
Cinnarizine	T45.0X1	T45.0X2	T45.0X3	T45.0X4	T45.0X5	T45.0X6
Cinoxacin	T37.8X1	T37.8X2	T37.8X3	T37.8X4	T37.8X5	T37.8X6
Ciprofibrate	T46.6X1	T46.6X2	T46.6X3	T46.6X4	T46.6X5	T46.6X6
Ciprofloxacin	T36.8X1	T36.8X2	T36.8X3	T36.8X4	T36.8X5	T36.8X6
Cisapride	T47.8X1	T47.8X2	T47.8X3	T47.8X4	T47.8X5	T47.8X6
Cisplatin	T45.1X1	T45.1X2	T45.1X3	T45.1X4	T45.1X5	T45.1X6
Citalopram	T43.221	T43.222	T43.223	T43.224	T43.225	T43.226
Citanest	T41.3X1	T41.3X2	T41.3X3	T41.3X4	T41.3X5	T41.3X6
infiltration (subcutaneous)	T41.3X1	T41.3X2	T41.3X3	T41.3X4	T41.3X5	T41.3X6
nerve block (peripheral) (plexus)	T41.3X1	T41.3X2	T41.3X3	T41.3X4	T41.3X5	T41.3X6
Citracel*	T50.3X1	T50.3X2	T50.3X3	T50.3X4	T50.3X5	T50.3X6
Citric acid	T47.5X1	T47.5X2	T47.5X3	T47.5X4	T47.5X5	T47.5X6
Citrovorum (factor)	T45.8X1	T45.8X2	T45.8X3	T45.8X4	T45.8X5	T45.8X6
Claviceps purpurea	T62.2X1	T62.2X2	T62.2X3	T62.2X4	—	—
Clavulanic acid	T36.1X1	T36.1X2	T36.1X3	T36.1X4	T36.1X5	T36.1X6
Cleaner, cleansing agent, type not specified	T65.891	T65.892	T65.893	T65.894	—	—
of paint or varnish	T52.91	T52.92	T52.93	T52.94	—	—
specified type NEC	T65.891	T65.892	T65.893	T65.894	—	—
Clebopride	T47.8X1	T47.8X2	T47.8X3	T47.8X4	T47.8X5	T47.8X6
Clefamide	T37.3X1	T37.3X2	T37.3X3	T37.3X4	T37.3X5	T37.3X6
Clemastine	T45.0X1	T45.0X2	T45.0X3	T45.0X4	T45.0X5	T45.0X6
Clematis vitalba	T62.2X1	T62.2X2	T62.2X3	T62.2X4	—	—
Clemizole	T45.0X1	T45.0X2	T45.0X3	T45.0X4	T45.0X5	T45.0X6
penicillin	T36.0X1	T36.0X2	T36.0X3	T36.0X4	T36.0X5	T36.0X6
Clenbuterol	T48.6X1	T48.6X2	T48.6X3	T48.6X4	T48.6X5	T48.6X6
Clidinium bromide	T44.3X1	T44.3X2	T44.3X3	T44.3X4	T44.3X5	T44.3X6
Clinda-Derm*	T49.0X1	T49.0X2	T49.0X3	T49.0X4	T49.0X5	T49.0X6
Clindamycin	T36.8X1	T36.8X2	T36.8X3	T36.8X4	T36.8X5	T36.8X6
Clinofibrate	T46.6X1	T46.6X2	T46.6X3	T46.6X4	T46.6X5	T46.6X6
Clioquinol	T37.8X1	T37.8X2	T37.8X3	T37.8X4	T37.8X5	T37.8X6
Cliradon	T40.2X1	T40.2X2	T40.2X3	T40.2X4	—	—
Clobazam	T42.4X1	T42.4X2	T42.4X3	T42.4X4	T42.4X5	T42.4X6
Clobenzorex	T50.5X1	T50.5X2	T50.5X3	T50.5X4	T50.5X5	T50.5X6
Clobetasol	T49.0X1	T49.0X2	T49.0X3	T49.0X4	T49.0X5	T49.0X6
Clobetasone	T49.0X1	T49.0X2	T49.0X3	T49.0X4	T49.0X5	T49.0X6
Clobutinol	T48.3X1	T48.3X2	T48.3X3	T48.3X4	T48.3X5	T48.3X6
Clocortolone	T38.0X1	T38.0X2	T38.0X3	T38.0X4	T38.0X5	T38.0X6
Clodantoin	T49.0X1	T49.0X2	T49.0X3	T49.0X4	T49.0X5	T49.0X6
Clodronic acid	T50.991	T50.992	T50.993	T50.994	T50.995	T50.996
Clofazimine	T37.1X1	T37.1X2	T37.1X3	T37.1X4	T37.1X5	T37.1X6
Clofedanol	T48.3X1	T48.3X2	T48.3X3	T48.3X4	T48.3X5	T48.3X6
Clofenamide	T50.2X1	T50.2X2	T50.2X3	T50.2X4	T50.2X5	T50.2X6
Clofenotane	T49.0X1	T49.0X2	T49.0X3	T49.0X4	T49.0X5	T49.0X6
Clofezone	T39.2X1	T39.2X2	T39.2X3	T39.2X4	T39.2X5	T39.2X6
Clofibrate	T46.6X1	T46.6X2	T46.6X3	T46.6X4	T46.6X5	T46.6X6
Clofibride	T46.6X1	T46.6X2	T46.6X3	T46.6X4	T46.6X5	T46.6X6
Cloforex	T50.5X1	T50.5X2	T50.5X3	T50.5X4	T50.5X5	T50.5X6
Clomethiazole	T42.6X1	T42.6X2	T42.6X3	T42.6X4	T42.6X5	T42.6X6
Clometocillin	T36.0X1	T36.0X2	T36.0X3	T36.0X4	T36.0X5	T36.0X6
Clomifene	T38.5X1	T38.5X2	T38.5X3	T38.5X4	T38.5X5	T38.5X6
Clomiphene	T38.5X1	T38.5X2	T38.5X3	T38.5X4	T38.5X5	T38.5X6
Clomipramine	T43.011	T43.012	T43.013	T43.014	T43.015	T43.016
Clomocycline	T36.4X1	T36.4X2	T36.4X3	T36.4X4	T36.4X5	T36.4X6
Clonazepam	T42.4X1	T42.4X2	T42.4X3	T42.4X4	T42.4X5	T42.4X6
Clonidine	T46.5X1	T46.5X2	T46.5X3	T46.5X4	T46.5X5	T46.5X6
Clonixin	T39.8X1	T39.8X2	T39.8X3	T39.8X4	T39.8X5	T39.8X6
Clopamide	T50.2X1	T50.2X2	T50.2X3	T50.2X4	T50.2X5	T50.2X6
Clopenthixol	T43.4X1	T43.4X2	T43.4X3	T43.4X4	T43.4X5	T43.4X6
Cloperastine	T48.3X1	T48.3X2	T48.3X3	T48.3X4	T48.3X5	T48.3X6
Clophedianol	T48.3X1	T48.3X2	T48.3X3	T48.3X4	T48.3X5	T48.3X6
Cloponone	T36.2X1	T36.2X2	T36.2X3	T36.2X4	T36.2X5	T36.2X6
Cloprednol	T38.0X1	T38.0X2	T38.0X3	T38.0X4	T38.0X5	T38.0X6
Cloral betaine	T42.6X1	T42.6X2	T42.6X3	T42.6X4	T42.6X5	T42.6X6
Cloramfenicol	T36.2X1	T36.2X2	T36.2X3	T36.2X4	T36.2X5	T36.2X6
Clorazepate (dipotassium)	T42.4X1	T42.4X2	T42.4X3	T42.4X4	T42.4X5	T42.4X6
Clorexolone	T50.2X1	T50.2X2	T50.2X3	T50.2X4	T50.2X5	T50.2X6
Clorfenamine	T45.0X1	T45.0X2	T45.0X3	T45.0X4	T45.0X5	T45.0X6
Clorgiline	T43.1X1	T43.1X2	T43.1X3	T43.1X4	T43.1X5	T43.1X6
Clorotepine	T44.3X1	T44.3X2	T44.3X3	T44.3X4	T44.3X5	T44.3X6
Clorox (bleach)	T54.91	T54.92	T54.93	T54.94	—	—
Clorprenaline	T48.6X1	T48.6X2	T48.6X3	T48.6X4	T48.6X5	T48.6X6
Clortermine	T50.5X1	T50.5X2	T50.5X3	T50.5X4	T50.5X5	T50.5X6
Clotiapine	T43.591	T43.592	T43.593	T43.594	T43.595	T43.596
Clotiazepam	T42.4X1	T42.4X2	T42.4X3	T42.4X4	T42.4X5	T42.4X6
Clotibric acid	T46.6X1	T46.6X2	T46.6X3	T46.6X4	T46.6X5	T46.6X6
Clotrimazole	T49.0X1	T49.0X2	T49.0X3	T49.0X4	T49.0X5	T49.0X6
Cloxacillin	T36.0X1	T36.0X2	T36.0X3	T36.0X4	T36.0X5	T36.0X6
Cloxazolam	T42.4X1	T42.4X2	T42.4X3	T42.4X4	T42.4X5	T42.4X6
Cloxiquine	T49.0X1	T49.0X2	T49.0X3	T49.0X4	T49.0X5	T49.0X6
Clozapine	T42.4X1	T42.4X2	T42.4X3	T42.4X4	T42.4X5	T42.4X6
Coagulant NEC	T45.7X1	T45.7X2	T45.7X3	T45.7X4	T45.7X5	T45.7X6
Coal (carbon monoxide from) — see also Carbon, monoxide, coal	T58.2X1	T58.2X2	T58.2X3	T58.2X4		
oil — see Kerosene						
tar	T49.1X1	T49.1X2	T49.1X3	T49.1X4	T49.1X5	T49.1X6
fumes	T59.891	T59.892	T59.893	T59.894	—	—
medicinal (ointment)	T49.4X1	T49.4X2	T49.4X3	T49.4X4	T49.4X5	T49.4X6
analgesics NEC	T39.2X1	T39.2X2	T39.2X3	T39.2X4	T39.2X5	T39.2X6
naphtha (solvent)	T52.0X1	T52.0X2	T52.0X3	T52.0X4	—	—
Coartem*	T37.2X1	T37.2X2	T37.2X3	T37.2X4	T37.2X5	T37.2X6
Cobalamine	T45.2X1	T45.2X2	T45.2X3	T45.2X4	T45.2X5	T45.2X6
Cobalt (nonmedicinal) (fumes) (industrial)	T56.891	T56.892	T56.893	T56.894	—	—
medicinal (trace) (chloride)	T45.8X1	T45.8X2	T45.8X3	T45.8X4	T45.8X5	T45.8X6
Cobra (venom)	T63.041	T63.042	T63.043	T63.044	—	—
Coca (leaf)	T40.5X1	T40.5X2	T40.5X3	T40.5X4	T40.5X5	T40.5X6
Cocaine	T40.5X1	T40.5X2	T40.5X3	T40.5X4	T40.5X5	T40.5X6
topical anesthetic	T41.3X1	T41.3X2	T41.3X3	T41.3X4	T41.3X5	T41.3X6
Cocarboxylase	T45.3X1	T45.3X2	T45.3X3	T45.3X4	T45.3X5	T45.3X6
Coccidioidin	T50.8X1	T50.8X2	T50.8X3	T50.8X4	T50.8X5	T50.8X6
Cocculus indicus	T62.1X1	T62.1X2	T62.1X3	T62.1X4	—	—
Cochineal	T65.6X1	T65.6X2	T65.6X3	T65.6X4	—	—
medicinal products	T50.991	T50.992	T50.993	T50.994	T50.995	T50.996
Codeine	T40.2X1	T40.2X2	T40.2X3	T40.2X4	T40.2X5	T40.2X6
Cod-liver oil	T45.2X1	T45.2X2	T45.2X3	T45.2X4	T45.2X5	T45.2X6
Coenzyme A	T50.991	T50.992	T50.993	T50.994	T50.995	T50.996
Coffee	T62.8X1	T62.8X2	T62.8X3	T62.8X4	—	—
Cogalactoisomerase	T50.991	T50.992	T50.993	T50.994	T50.995	T50.996
Cogentin	T44.3X1	T44.3X2	T44.3X3	T44.3X4	T44.3X5	T44.3X6
Coke fumes or gas (carbon monoxide)	T58.2X1	T58.2X2	T58.2X3	T58.2X4		
industrial use	T58.8X1	T58.8X2	T58.8X3	T58.8X4		
Colace	T47.4X1	T47.4X2	T47.4X3	T47.4X4	T47.4X5	T47.4X6
Colaspase	T45.1X1	T45.1X2	T45.1X3	T45.1X4	T45.1X5	T45.1X6
Colazal*	T47.8X1	T47.8X2	T47.8X3	T47.8X4	T47.8X5	T47.8X6
Colchicine	T50.4X1	T50.4X2	T50.4X3	T50.4X4	T50.4X5	T50.4X6
Colchicum	T62.2X1	T62.2X2	T62.2X3	T62.2X4	—	—
Cold cream	T49.3X1	T49.3X2	T49.3X3	T49.3X4	T49.3X5	T49.3X6
Colecalciferol	T45.2X1	T45.2X2	T45.2X3	T45.2X4	T45.2X5	T45.2X6
Colestipol	T46.6X1	T46.6X2	T46.6X3	T46.6X4	T46.6X5	T46.6X6
Colestyramine	T46.6X1	T46.6X2	T46.6X3	T46.6X4	T46.6X5	T46.6X6
Colimycin	T36.8X1	T36.8X2	T36.8X3	T36.8X4	T36.8X5	T36.8X6
Colistimethate	T36.8X1	T36.8X2	T36.8X3	T36.8X4	T36.8X5	T36.8X6
Colistin	T36.8X1	T36.8X2	T36.8X3	T36.8X4	T36.8X5	T36.8X6
sulfate (eye preparation)	T49.5X1	T49.5X2	T49.5X3	T49.5X4	T49.5X5	T49.5X6
Collagen	T50.991	T50.992	T50.993	T50.994	T50.995	T50.996
Collagenase	T49.4X1	T49.4X2	T49.4X3	T49.4X4	T49.4X5	T49.4X6
Collodion	T49.3X1	T49.3X2	T49.3X3	T49.3X4	T49.3X5	T49.3X6
Colocynth	T47.2X1	T47.2X2	T47.2X3	T47.2X4	T47.2X5	T47.2X6
Colophony adhesive	T49.3X1	T49.3X2	T49.3X3	T49.3X4	T49.3X5	T49.3X6
Colorant — see also Dye	T50.991	T50.992	T50.993	T50.994	T50.995	T50.996
Coloring matter — see Dye(s)						
Combustion gas (after combustion) — see Carbon, monoxide						
prior to combustion	T59.891	T59.892	T59.893	T59.894		
Cometriq*	T45.1X1	T45.1X2	T45.1X3	T45.1X4	T45.1X5	T45.1X6
Compazine	T43.3X1	T43.3X2	T43.3X3	T43.3X4	T43.3X5	T43.3X6
Compound						
1080 (sodium fluoroacetate)	T60.4X1	T60.4X2	T60.4X3	T60.4X4	—	—
269 (endrin)	T60.1X1	T60.1X2	T60.1X3	T60.1X4	—	—
3422 (parathion)	T60.0X1	T60.0X2	T60.0X3	T60.0X4	—	—
3911 (phorate)	T60.0X1	T60.0X2	T60.0X3	T60.0X4	—	—
3956 (toxaphene)	T60.1X1	T60.1X2	T60.1X3	T60.1X4	—	—
4049 (malathion)	T60.0X1	T60.0X2	T60.0X3	T60.0X4	—	—
4069 (malathion)	T60.0X1	T60.0X2	T60.0X3	T60.0X4	—	—
4124 (dicapthon)	T60.0X1	T60.0X2	T60.0X3	T60.0X4	—	—
42 (warfarin)	T60.4X1	T60.4X2	T60.4X3	T60.4X4	—	—
497 (dieldrin)	T60.1X1	T60.1X2	T60.1X3	T60.1X4	—	—
E (cortisone)	T38.0X1	T38.0X2	T38.0X3	T38.0X4	T38.0X5	T38.0X6
F (hydrocortisone)	T38.0X1	T38.0X2	T38.0X3	T38.0X4	T38.0X5	T38.0X6
Comvax*	T50.A21	T50.A22	T50.A23	T50.A24	T50.A25	T50.A26

Substance	Poisoning, Accidental (unintentional)	Poisoning, Intentional Self-harm	Poisoning, Assault	Poisoning, Undetermined	Adverse Effect	Under-dosing
Congener, anabolic	T38.7X1	T38.7X2	T38.7X3	T38.7X4	T38.7X5	T38.7X6
Congo red	T50.8X1	T50.8X2	T50.8X3	T50.8X4	T50.8X5	T50.8X6
Coniine, conine	T62.2X1	T62.2X2	T62.2X3	T62.2X4	—	—
Conium (maculatum)	T62.2X1	T62.2X2	T62.2X3	T62.2X4	—	—
Conjugated estrogenic substances	T38.5X1	T38.5X2	T38.5X3	T38.5X4	T38.5X5	T38.5X6
Contac	T48.5X1	T48.5X2	T48.5X3	T48.5X4	T48.5X5	T48.5X6
Contact lens solution	T49.5X1	T49.5X2	T49.5X3	T49.5X4	T49.5X5	T49.5X6
Contraceptive (oral)	T38.4X1	T38.4X2	T38.4X3	T38.4X4	T38.4X5	T38.4X6
vaginal	T49.8X1	T49.8X2	T49.8X3	T49.8X4	T49.8X5	T49.8X6
Contrast medium, radiography	T50.8X1	T50.8X2	T50.8X3	T50.8X4	T50.8X5	T50.8X6
Convallaria glycosides	T46.0X1	T46.0X2	T46.0X3	T46.0X4	T46.0X5	T46.0X6
Convallaria majalis	T62.2X1	T62.2X2	T62.2X3	T62.2X4	—	—
berry	T62.1X1	T62.1X2	T62.1X3	T62.1X4	—	—
Copperhead snake (bite) (venom)	T63.061	T63.062	T63.063	T63.064	—	—
Copper (dust) (fumes) (nonmedicinal) NEC	T56.4X1	T56.4X2	T56.4X3	T56.4X4	—	—
arsenate, arsenite	T57.0X1	T57.0X2	T57.0X3	T57.0X4	—	—
insecticide	T60.2X1	T60.2X2	T60.2X3	T60.2X4	—	—
emetic	T47.7X1	T47.7X2	T47.7X3	T47.7X4	T47.7X5	T47.7X6
fungicide	T60.3X1	T60.3X2	T60.3X3	T60.3X4	—	—
gluconate	T49.0X1	T49.0X2	T49.0X3	T49.0X4	T49.0X5	T49.0X6
insecticide	T60.2X1	T60.2X2	T60.2X3	T60.2X4	—	—
medicinal (trace)	T45.8X1	T45.8X2	T45.8X3	T45.8X4	T45.8X5	T45.8X6
oleate	T49.0X1	T49.0X2	T49.0X3	T49.0X4	T49.0X5	T49.0X6
sulfate	T56.4X1	T56.4X2	T56.4X3	T56.4X4	—	—
cupric	T56.4X1	T56.4X2	T56.4X3	T56.4X4	—	—
fungicide	T60.3X1	T60.3X2	T60.3X3	T60.3X4	—	—
medicinal						
ear	T49.6X1	T49.6X2	T49.6X3	T49.6X4	T49.6X5	T49.6X6
emetic	T47.7X1	T47.7X2	T47.7X3	T47.7X4	T47.7X5	T47.7X6
eye	T49.5X1	T49.5X2	T49.5X3	T49.5X4	T49.5X5	T49.5X6
cuprous	T56.4X1	T56.4X2	T56.4X3	T56.4X4	—	—
fungicide	T60.3X1	T60.3X2	T60.3X3	T60.3X4	—	—
medicinal						
ear	T49.6X1	T49.6X2	T49.6X3	T49.6X4	T49.6X5	T49.6X6
emetic	T47.7X1	T47.7X2	T47.7X3	T47.7X4	T47.7X5	T47.7X6
eye	T49.5X1	T49.5X2	T49.5X3	T49.5X4	T49.5X5	T49.5X6
Coral (sting)	T63.691	T63.692	T63.693	T63.694	—	—
snake (bite) (venom)	T63.021	T63.022	T63.023	T63.024	—	—
Corbadrine	T49.6X1	T49.6X2	T49.6X3	T49.6X4	T49.6X5	T49.6X6
Cordite	T65.891	T65.892	T65.893	T65.894	—	—
vapor	T59.891	T59.892	T59.893	T59.894	—	—
Cordran	T49.0X1	T49.0X2	T49.0X3	T49.0X4	T49.0X5	T49.0X6
Cormax*	T49.0X1	T49.0X2	T49.0X3	T49.0X4	T49.0X5	T49.0X6
Corn cures	T49.4X1	T49.4X2	T49.4X3	T49.4X4	T49.4X5	T49.4X6
Cornhusker's lotion	T49.3X1	T49.3X2	T49.3X3	T49.3X4	T49.3X5	T49.3X6
Corn starch	T49.3X1	T49.3X2	T49.3X3	T49.3X4	T49.3X5	T49.3X6
Coronary vasodilator NEC	T46.3X1	T46.3X2	T46.3X3	T46.3X4	T46.3X5	T46.3X6
Corrosive NEC	T54.91	T54.92	T54.93	T54.94	—	—
acid NEC	T54.2X1	T54.2X2	T54.2X3	T54.2X4	—	—
aromatics	T54.1X1	T54.1X2	T54.1X3	T54.1X4	—	—
disinfectant	T54.1X1	T54.1X2	T54.1X3	T54.1X4	—	—
fumes NEC	T54.91	T54.92	T54.93	T54.94	—	—
specified NEC	T54.91	T54.92	T54.93	T54.94	—	—
sublimate	T56.1X1	T56.1X2	T56.1X3	T56.1X4	—	—
Cortate	T38.0X1	T38.0X2	T38.0X3	T38.0X4	T38.0X5	T38.0X6
Cort-Dome	T38.0X1	T38.0X2	T38.0X3	T38.0X4	T38.0X5	T38.0X6
ENT agent	T49.6X1	T49.6X2	T49.6X3	T49.6X4	T49.6X5	T49.6X6
ophthalmic preparation	T49.5X1	T49.5X2	T49.5X3	T49.5X4	T49.5X5	T49.5X6
topical NEC	T49.0X1	T49.0X2	T49.0X3	T49.0X4	T49.0X5	T49.0X6
Cortef	T38.0X1	T38.0X2	T38.0X3	T38.0X4	T38.0X5	T38.0X6
ENT agent	T49.6X1	T49.6X2	T49.6X3	T49.6X4	T49.6X5	T49.6X6
ophthalmic preparation	T49.5X1	T49.5X2	T49.5X3	T49.5X4	T49.5X5	T49.5X6
topical NEC	T49.0X1	T49.0X2	T49.0X3	T49.0X4	T49.0X5	T49.0X6
Corticosteroid	T38.0X1	T38.0X2	T38.0X3	T38.0X4	T38.0X5	T38.0X6
ENT agent	T49.6X1	T49.6X2	T49.6X3	T49.6X4	T49.6X5	T49.6X6
mineral	T50.0X1	T50.0X2	T50.0X3	T50.0X4	T50.0X5	T50.0X6
ophthalmic	T49.5X1	T49.5X2	T49.5X3	T49.5X4	T49.5X5	T49.5X6
topical NEC	T49.0X1	T49.0X2	T49.0X3	T49.0X4	T49.0X5	T49.0X6
Corticotropin	T38.811	T38.812	T38.813	T38.814	T38.815	T38.816
Cortisol	T49.0X1	T49.0X2	T49.0X3	T49.0X4	T49.0X5	T49.0X6
ENT agent	T49.6X1	T49.6X2	T49.6X3	T49.6X4	T49.6X5	T49.6X6
ophthalmic preparation	T49.5X1	T49.5X2	T49.5X3	T49.5X4	T49.5X5	T49.5X6
topical NEC	T49.0X1	T49.0X2	T49.0X3	T49.0X4	T49.0X5	T49.0X6
Cortisone (acetate)	T38.0X1	T38.0X2	T38.0X3	T38.0X4	T38.0X5	T38.0X6
ENT agent	T49.6X1	T49.6X2	T49.6X3	T49.6X4	T49.6X5	T49.6X6
ophthalmic preparation	T49.5X1	T49.5X2	T49.5X3	T49.5X4	T49.5X5	T49.5X6
topical NEC	T49.0X1	T49.0X2	T49.0X3	T49.0X4	T49.0X5	T49.0X6
Cortisporin*	T49.0X1	T49.0X2	T49.0X3	T49.0X4	T49.0X5	T49.0X6
Cortivazol	T38.0X1	T38.0X2	T38.0X3	T38.0X4	T38.0X5	T38.0X6
Cortogen	T38.0X1	T38.0X2	T38.0X3	T38.0X4	T38.0X5	T38.0X6
ENT agent	T49.6X1	T49.6X2	T49.6X3	T49.6X4	T49.6X5	T49.6X6
ophthalmic preparation	T49.5X1	T49.5X2	T49.5X3	T49.5X4	T49.5X5	T49.5X6
Cortone	T38.0X1	T38.0X2	T38.0X3	T38.0X4	T38.0X5	T38.0X6
ENT agent	T49.6X1	T49.6X2	T49.6X3	T49.6X4	T49.6X5	T49.6X6
ophthalmic preparation	T49.5X1	T49.5X2	T49.5X3	T49.5X4	T49.5X5	T49.5X6
Cortril	T38.0X1	T38.0X2	T38.0X3	T38.0X4	T38.0X5	T38.0X6
ENT agent	T49.6X1	T49.6X2	T49.6X3	T49.6X4	T49.6X5	T49.6X6
ophthalmic preparation	T49.5X1	T49.5X2	T49.5X3	T49.5X4	T49.5X5	T49.5X6
topical NEC	T49.0X1	T49.0X2	T49.0X3	T49.0X4	T49.0X5	T49.0X6
Corynebacterium parvum	T45.1X1	T45.1X2	T45.1X3	T45.1X4	T45.1X5	T45.1X6
Cosmetic preparation	T49.8X1	T49.8X2	T49.8X3	T49.8X4	T49.8X5	T49.8X6
Cosmetics	T49.8X1	T49.8X2	T49.8X3	T49.8X4	T49.8X5	T49.8X6
Cosyntropin	T38.811	T38.812	T38.813	T38.814	T38.815	T38.816
Cotarnine	T45.7X1	T45.7X2	T45.7X3	T45.7X4	T45.7X5	T45.7X6
Co-trimoxazole	T36.8X1	T36.8X2	T36.8X3	T36.8X4	T36.8X5	T36.8X6
Cottonseed oil	T49.3X1	T49.3X2	T49.3X3	T49.3X4	T49.3X5	T49.3X6
Cough mixture (syrup)	T48.4X1	T48.4X2	T48.4X3	T48.4X4	T48.4X5	T48.4X6
containing opiates	T40.2X1	T40.2X2	T40.2X3	T40.2X4	T40.2X5	T40.2X6
expectorants	T48.4X1	T48.4X2	T48.4X3	T48.4X4	T48.4X5	T48.4X6
Coumadin	T45.511	T45.512	T45.513	T45.514	T45.515	T45.516
rodenticide	T60.4X1	T60.4X2	T60.4X3	T60.4X4	—	—
Coumaphos	T60.0X1	T60.0X2	T60.0X3	T60.0X4	—	—
Coumarin	T45.511	T45.512	T45.513	T45.514	T45.515	T45.516
Coumetarol	T45.511	T45.512	T45.513	T45.514	T45.515	T45.516
Cowbane	T62.2X1	T62.2X2	T62.2X3	T62.2X4	—	—
Cozyme	T45.2X1	T45.2X2	T45.2X3	T45.2X4	T45.2X5	T45.2X6
Crack	T40.5X1	T40.5X2	T40.5X3	T40.5X4	—	—
Crataegus extract	T46.0X1	T46.0X2	T46.0X3	T46.0X4	T46.0X5	T46.0X6
Creolin	T54.1X1	T54.1X2	T54.1X3	T54.1X4	—	—
disinfectant	T54.1X1	T54.1X2	T54.1X3	T54.1X4	—	—
Creosol (compound)	T49.0X1	T49.0X2	T49.0X3	T49.0X4	T49.0X5	T49.0X6
Creosote (coal tar) (beechwood)	T49.0X1	T49.0X2	T49.0X3	T49.0X4	T49.0X5	T49.0X6
medicinal (expectorant)	T48.4X1	T48.4X2	T48.4X3	T48.4X4	T48.4X5	T48.4X6
syrup	T48.4X1	T48.4X2	T48.4X3	T48.4X4	T48.4X5	T48.4X6
Cresol(s)	T49.0X1	T49.0X2	T49.0X3	T49.0X4	T49.0X5	T49.0X6
and soap solution	T49.0X1	T49.0X2	T49.0X3	T49.0X4	T49.0X5	T49.0X6
Crestor*	T46.6X1	T46.6X2	T46.6X3	T46.6X4	T46.6X5	T46.6X6
Cresyl acetate	T49.0X1	T49.0X2	T49.0X3	T49.0X4	T49.0X5	T49.0X6
Cresylic acid	T49.0X1	T49.0X2	T49.0X3	T49.0X4	T49.0X5	T49.0X6
Crimidine	T60.4X1	T60.4X2	T60.4X3	T60.4X4	—	—
Croconazole	T37.8X1	T37.8X2	T37.8X3	T37.8X4	T37.8X5	T37.8X6
Cromoglicic acid	T48.6X1	T48.6X2	T48.6X3	T48.6X4	T48.6X5	T48.6X6
Cromolyn	T48.6X1	T48.6X2	T48.6X3	T48.6X4	T48.6X5	T48.6X6
Cromonar	T46.3X1	T46.3X2	T46.3X3	T46.3X4	T46.3X5	T46.3X6
Cropropamide	T39.8X1	T39.8X2	T39.8X3	T39.8X4	T39.8X5	T39.8X6
with crotethamide	T50.7X1	T50.7X2	T50.7X3	T50.7X4	T50.7X5	T50.7X6
Crotamiton	T49.0X1	T49.0X2	T49.0X3	T49.0X4	T49.0X5	T49.0X6
Crotethamide	T39.8X1	T39.8X2	T39.8X3	T39.8X4	T39.8X5	T39.8X6
with cropropamide	T50.7X1	T50.7X2	T50.7X3	T50.7X4	T50.7X5	T50.7X6
Croton (oil)	T47.2X1	T47.2X2	T47.2X3	T47.2X4	T47.2X5	T47.2X6
chloral	T42.6X1	T42.6X2	T42.6X3	T42.6X4	T42.6X5	T42.6X6
Crude oil	T52.0X1	T52.0X2	T52.0X3	T52.0X4	—	—
Cryogenine	T39.8X1	T39.8X2	T39.8X3	T39.8X4	T39.8X5	T39.8X6
Cryolite (vapor)	T60.1X1	T60.1X2	T60.1X3	T60.1X4	—	—
insecticide	T60.1X1	T60.1X2	T60.1X3	T60.1X4	—	—
Cryptenamine (tannates)	T46.5X1	T46.5X2	T46.5X3	T46.5X4	T46.5X5	T46.5X6
Crystal violet	T49.0X1	T49.0X2	T49.0X3	T49.0X4	T49.0X5	T49.0X6
Cuckoopint	T62.2X1	T62.2X2	T62.2X3	T62.2X4	—	—
Cumetharol	T45.511	T45.512	T45.513	T45.514	T45.515	T45.516
Cupric						
acetate	T60.3X1	T60.3X2	T60.3X3	T60.3X4	—	—
acetoarsenite	T57.0X1	T57.0X2	T57.0X3	T57.0X4	—	—
arsenate	T57.0X1	T57.0X2	T57.0X3	T57.0X4	—	—
gluconate	T49.0X1	T49.0X2	T49.0X3	T49.0X4	T49.0X5	T49.0X6
oleate	T49.0X1	T49.0X2	T49.0X3	T49.0X4	T49.0X5	T49.0X6
sulfate	T56.4X1	T56.4X2	T56.4X3	T56.4X4	—	—
Cuprimine*	T50.6X1	T50.6X2	T50.6X3	T50.6X4	T50.6X5	T50.6X6
Cuprous sulfate — see also Copper, sulfate	T56.4X1	T56.4X2	T56.4X3	T56.4X4	—	—
Curare, curarine	T48.1X1	T48.1X2	T48.1X3	T48.1X4	T48.1X5	T48.1X6
Cyamemazine	T43.3X1	T43.3X2	T43.3X3	T43.3X4	T43.3X5	T43.3X6
Cyamopsis tetragonoloba	T46.6X1	T46.6X2	T46.6X3	T46.6X4	T46.6X5	T46.6X6
Cyanacetyl hydrazide	T37.1X1	T37.1X2	T37.1X3	T37.1X4	T37.1X5	T37.1X6
Cyanic acid (gas)	T59.891	T59.892	T59.893	T59.894	—	—
Cyanide(s) (compounds) (potassium) (sodium) NEC	T65.0X1	T65.0X2	T65.0X3	T65.0X4	—	—
dust or gas (inhalation) NEC	T57.3X1	T57.3X2	T57.3X3	T57.3X4	—	—
fumigant	T65.0X1	T65.0X2	T65.0X3	T65.0X4	—	—
hydrogen	T57.3X1	T57.3X2	T57.3X3	T57.3X4	—	—

Substance	Poisoning, Accidental (unintentional)	Poisoning, Intentional Self-harm	Poisoning, Assault	Poisoning, Undetermined	Adverse Effect	Under-dosing
Cyanide(s) (compounds) (potassium) (sodium) NEC — continued						
mercuric — see Mercury						
pesticide (dust) (fumes)	T65.0X1	T65.0X2	T65.0X3	T65.0X4	—	—
Cyanoacrylate adhesive	T49.3X1	T49.3X2	T49.3X3	T49.3X4	T49.3X5	T49.3X6
Cyanocobalamin	T45.8X1	T45.8X2	T45.8X3	T45.8X4	T45.8X5	T45.8X6
Cyanogen (chloride) (gas) NEC	T59.891	T59.892	T59.893	T59.894	—	—
Cyclacillin	T36.0X1	T36.0X2	T36.0X3	T36.0X4	T36.0X5	T36.0X6
Cyclaine	T41.3X1	T41.3X2	T41.3X3	T41.3X4	T41.3X5	T41.3X6
Cyclamate	T50.991	T50.992	T50.993	T50.994	T50.995	T50.996
Cyclamen europaeum	T62.2X1	T62.2X2	T62.2X3	T62.2X4	—	—
Cyclandelate	T46.7X1	T46.7X2	T46.7X3	T46.7X4	T46.7X5	T46.7X6
Cyclazocine	T50.7X1	T50.7X2	T50.7X3	T50.7X4	T50.7X5	T50.7X6
Cyclizine	T45.0X1	T45.0X2	T45.0X3	T45.0X4	T45.0X5	T45.0X6
Cyclobarbital	T42.3X1	T42.3X2	T42.3X3	T42.3X4	T42.3X5	T42.3X6
Cyclobarbitone	T42.3X1	T42.3X2	T42.3X3	T42.3X4	T42.3X5	T42.3X6
Cyclobenzaprine	T48.1X1	T48.1X2	T48.1X3	T48.1X4	T48.1X5	T48.1X6
Cyclodrine	T44.3X1	T44.3X2	T44.3X3	T44.3X4	T44.3X5	T44.3X6
Cycloguanil embonate	T37.2X1	T37.2X2	T37.2X3	T37.2X4	T37.2X5	T37.2X6
Cyclohexane	T52.8X1	T52.8X2	T52.8X3	T52.8X4	—	—
Cyclohexanol	T51.8X1	T51.8X2	T51.8X3	T51.8X4	—	—
Cyclohexanone	T52.4X1	T52.4X2	T52.4X3	T52.4X4	—	—
Cycloheximide	T60.3X1	T60.3X2	T60.3X3	T60.3X4	—	—
Cyclohexyl acetate	T52.8X1	T52.8X2	T52.8X3	T52.8X4	—	—
Cycloleucin	T45.1X1	T45.1X2	T45.1X3	T45.1X4	T45.1X5	T45.1X6
Cyclomethycaine	T41.3X1	T41.3X2	T41.3X3	T41.3X4	T41.3X5	T41.3X6
Cyclopentamine	T44.4X1	T44.4X2	T44.4X3	T44.4X4	T44.4X5	T44.4X6
Cyclopenthiazide	T50.2X1	T50.2X2	T50.2X3	T50.2X4	T50.2X5	T50.2X6
Cyclopentolate	T44.3X1	T44.3X2	T44.3X3	T44.3X4	T44.3X5	T44.3X6
Cyclophosphamide	T45.1X1	T45.1X2	T45.1X3	T45.1X4	T45.1X5	T45.1X6
Cycloplegic drug	T49.5X1	T49.5X2	T49.5X3	T49.5X4	T49.5X5	T49.5X6
Cyclopropane	T41.291	T41.292	T41.293	T41.294	T41.295	T41.296
Cyclopyrabital	T39.8X1	T39.8X2	T39.8X3	T39.8X4	T39.8X5	T39.8X6
Cycloserine	T37.1X1	T37.1X2	T37.1X3	T37.1X4	T37.1X5	T37.1X6
Cyclosporin	T45.1X1	T45.1X2	T45.1X3	T45.1X4	T45.1X5	T45.1X6
Cyclothiazide	T50.2X1	T50.2X2	T50.2X3	T50.2X4	T50.2X5	T50.2X6
Cycrimine	T44.3X1	T44.3X2	T44.3X3	T44.3X4	T44.3X5	T44.3X6
Cyhalothrin	T60.1X1	T60.1X2	T60.1X3	T60.1X4	—	—
Cymarin	T46.0X1	T46.0X2	T46.0X3	T46.0X4	T46.0X5	T46.0X6
Cypermethrin	T60.1X1	T60.1X2	T60.1X3	T60.1X4	—	—
Cyphenothrin	T60.2X1	T60.2X2	T60.2X3	T60.2X4	—	—
Cyproheptadine	T45.0X1	T45.0X2	T45.0X3	T45.0X4	T45.0X5	T45.0X6
Cyproterone	T38.6X1	T38.6X2	T38.6X3	T38.6X4	T38.6X5	T38.6X6
Cystaran*	T49.5X1	T49.5X2	T49.5X3	T49.5X4	T49.5X5	T49.5X6
Cysteamine	T50.6X1	T50.6X2	T50.6X3	T50.6X4	T50.6X5	T50.6X6
Cytarabine	T45.1X1	T45.1X2	T45.1X3	T45.1X4	T45.1X5	T45.1X6
Cytisus						
laburnum	T62.2X1	T62.2X2	T62.2X3	T62.2X4	—	—
scoparius	T62.2X1	T62.2X2	T62.2X3	T62.2X4	—	—
Cytochrome C	T47.5X1	T47.5X2	T47.5X3	T47.5X4	T47.5X5	T47.5X6
Cytomel	T38.1X1	T38.1X2	T38.1X3	T38.1X4	T38.1X5	T38.1X6
Cytosine arabinoside	T45.1X1	T45.1X2	T45.1X3	T45.1X4	T45.1X5	T45.1X6
Cytoxan	T45.1X1	T45.1X2	T45.1X3	T45.1X4	T45.1X5	T45.1X6
Cytozyme	T45.7X1	T45.7X2	T45.7X3	T45.7X4	T45.7X5	T45.7X6
S-Carboxymethylcysteine	T48.4X1	T48.4X2	T48.4X3	T48.4X4	T48.4X5	T48.4X6
Dabigatran*	T45.511	T45.512	T45.513	T45.514	T45.515	T45.516
Dacarbazine	T45.1X1	T45.1X2	T45.1X3	T45.1X4	T45.1X5	T45.1X6
Dactinomycin	T45.1X1	T45.1X2	T45.1X3	T45.1X4	T45.1X5	T45.1X6
DADPS	T37.1X1	T37.1X2	T37.1X3	T37.1X4	T37.1X5	T37.1X6
Dakin's solution	T49.0X1	T49.0X2	T49.0X3	T49.0X4	T49.0X5	T49.0X6
Dalapon (sodium)	T60.3X1	T60.3X2	T60.3X3	T60.3X4	—	—
Dalmane	T42.4X1	T42.4X2	T42.4X3	T42.4X4	T42.4X5	T42.4X6
Danazol	T38.6X1	T38.6X2	T38.6X3	T38.6X4	T38.6X5	T38.6X6
Danilone	T45.511	T45.512	T45.513	T45.514	T45.515	T45.516
Danthron	T47.2X1	T47.2X2	T47.2X3	T47.2X4	T47.2X5	T47.2X6
Dantrolene	T42.8X1	T42.8X2	T42.8X3	T42.8X4	T42.8X5	T42.8X6
Dantron	T47.2X1	T47.2X2	T47.2X3	T47.2X4	T47.2X5	T47.2X6
Daphne (gnidium) (mezereum)	T62.2X1	T62.2X2	T62.2X3	T62.2X4	—	—
berry	T62.1X1	T62.1X2	T62.1X3	T62.1X4	—	—
Dapsone	T37.1X1	T37.1X2	T37.1X3	T37.1X4	T37.1X5	T37.1X6
Daraprim	T37.2X1	T37.2X2	T37.2X3	T37.2X4	T37.2X5	T37.2X6
Darnel	T62.2X1	T62.2X2	T62.2X3	T62.2X4	—	—
Darvon	T39.8X1	T39.8X2	T39.8X3	T39.8X4	T39.8X5	T39.8X6
Daunomycin	T45.1X1	T45.1X2	T45.1X3	T45.1X4	T45.1X5	T45.1X6
Daunorubicin	T45.1X1	T45.1X2	T45.1X3	T45.1X4	T45.1X5	T45.1X6
DBI	T38.3X1	T38.3X2	T38.3X3	T38.3X4	T38.3X5	T38.3X6
D-Con	T60.91	T60.92	T60.93	T60.94	—	—
insecticide	T60.2X1	T60.2X2	T60.2X3	T60.2X4	—	—
rodenticide	T60.4X1	T60.4X2	T60.4X3	T60.4X4	—	—
DDAVP	T38.891	T38.892	T38.893	T38.894	T38.895	T38.896
DDE (bis(chlorophenyl)- dichloroethylene)	T60.2X1	T60.2X2	T60.2X3	T60.2X4	—	—
DDS	T37.1X1	T37.1X2	T37.1X3	T37.1X4	T37.1X5	T37.1X6
DDT (dust)	T60.1X1	T60.1X2	T60.1X3	T60.1X4	—	—
Deadly nightshade — see also Belladonna						
berry	T62.1X1	T62.1X2	T62.1X3	T62.1X4	—	—
Deamino-D-arginine vasopressin	T38.891	T38.892	T38.893	T38.894	T38.895	T38.896
Deanol (aceglumate)	T50.991	T50.992	T50.993	T50.994	T50.995	T50.996
Debrisoquine	T46.5X1	T46.5X2	T46.5X3	T46.5X4	T46.5X5	T46.5X6
Decaborane	T57.8X1	T57.8X2	T57.8X3	T57.8X4	—	—
fumes	T59.891	T59.892	T59.893	T59.894	—	—
Decadron	T38.0X1	T38.0X2	T38.0X3	T38.0X4	T38.0X5	T38.0X6
ENT agent	T49.6X1	T49.6X2	T49.6X3	T49.6X4	T49.6X5	T49.6X6
ophthalmic preparation	T49.5X1	T49.5X2	T49.5X3	T49.5X4	T49.5X5	T49.5X6
topical NEC	T49.0X1	T49.0X2	T49.0X3	T49.0X4	T49.0X5	T49.0X6
Decahydronaphthalene	T52.8X1	T52.8X2	T52.8X3	T52.8X4	—	—
Decalin	T52.8X1	T52.8X2	T52.8X3	T52.8X4	—	—
Decamethonium (bromide)	T48.1X1	T48.1X2	T48.1X3	T48.1X4	T48.1X5	T48.1X6
Decholin	T47.5X1	T47.5X2	T47.5X3	T47.5X4	T47.5X5	T47.5X6
Declomycin	T36.4X1	T36.4X2	T36.4X3	T36.4X4	T36.4X5	T36.4X6
Decongestant, nasal (mucosa)	T48.5X1	T48.5X2	T48.5X3	T48.5X4	T48.5X5	T48.5X6
combination	T48.5X1	T48.5X2	T48.5X3	T48.5X4	T48.5X5	T48.5X6
Deet	T60.8X1	T60.8X2	T60.8X3	T60.8X4	—	—
Deferoxamine	T45.8X1	T45.8X2	T45.8X3	T45.8X4	T45.8X5	T45.8X6
Deflazacort	T38.0X1	T38.0X2	T38.0X3	T38.0X4	T38.0X5	T38.0X6
Deglycyrrhizinized extract of licorice	T48.4X1	T48.4X2	T48.4X3	T48.4X4	T48.4X5	T48.4X6
Dehydrocholic acid	T47.5X1	T47.5X2	T47.5X3	T47.5X4	T47.5X5	T47.5X6
Dehydroemetine	T37.3X1	T37.3X2	T37.3X3	T37.3X4	T37.3X5	T37.3X6
Dekalin	T52.8X1	T52.8X2	T52.8X3	T52.8X4	—	—
Delafloxacin*	T36.8X1	T36.8X2	T36.8X3	T36.8X4	T36.8X5	T36.8X6
Delalutin	T38.5X1	T38.5X2	T38.5X3	T38.5X4	T38.5X5	T38.5X6
Delorazepam	T42.4X1	T42.4X2	T42.4X3	T42.4X4	T42.4X5	T42.4X6
Delphinium	T62.2X1	T62.2X2	T62.2X3	T62.2X4	—	—
Deltacortisone*	T38.0X1	T38.0X2	T38.0X3	T38.0X4	T38.0X5	T38.0X6
Deltamethrin	T60.1X1	T60.1X2	T60.1X3	T60.1X4	—	—
Deltasone	T38.0X1	T38.0X2	T38.0X3	T38.0X4	T38.0X5	T38.0X6
Delta	T38.0X1	T38.0X2	T38.0X3	T38.0X4	T38.0X5	T38.0X6
Delvinal	T42.3X1	T42.3X2	T42.3X3	T42.3X4	T42.3X5	T42.3X6
Demecarium (bromide)	T49.5X1	T49.5X2	T49.5X3	T49.5X4	T49.5X5	T49.5X6
Demeclocycline	T36.4X1	T36.4X2	T36.4X3	T36.4X4	T36.4X5	T36.4X6
Demecolcine	T45.1X1	T45.1X2	T45.1X3	T45.1X4	T45.1X5	T45.1X6
Demegestone	T38.5X1	T38.5X2	T38.5X3	T38.5X4	T38.5X5	T38.5X6
Demelanizing agents	T49.8X1	T49.8X2	T49.8X3	T49.8X4	T49.8X5	T49.8X6
Demephion -O and -S	T60.0X1	T60.0X2	T60.0X3	T60.0X4	—	—
Demerol	T40.2X1	T40.2X2	T40.2X3	T40.2X4	T40.2X5	T40.2X6
Demethylchlortetracycline	T36.4X1	T36.4X2	T36.4X3	T36.4X4	T36.4X5	T36.4X6
Demethyltetracycline	T36.4X1	T36.4X2	T36.4X3	T36.4X4	T36.4X5	T36.4X6
Demeton -O and -S	T60.0X1	T60.0X2	T60.0X3	T60.0X4	—	—
Demulcent (external)	T49.3X1	T49.3X2	T49.3X3	T49.3X4	T49.3X5	T49.3X6
specified NEC	T49.3X1	T49.3X2	T49.3X3	T49.3X4	T49.3X5	T49.3X6
Demulen	T38.4X1	T38.4X2	T38.4X3	T38.4X4	T38.4X5	T38.4X6
Denatured alcohol	T51.0X1	T51.0X2	T51.0X3	T51.0X4	—	—
Dendrid	T49.5X1	T49.5X2	T49.5X3	T49.5X4	T49.5X5	T49.5X6
Dental drug, topical application NEC	T49.7X1	T49.7X2	T49.7X3	T49.7X4	T49.7X5	T49.7X6
Dentifrice	T49.7X1	T49.7X2	T49.7X3	T49.7X4	T49.7X5	T49.7X6
Deodorant spray (feminine hygiene)	T49.8X1	T49.8X2	T49.8X3	T49.8X4	T49.8X5	T49.8X6
Deoxycortone	T50.0X1	T50.0X2	T50.0X3	T50.0X4	T50.0X5	T50.0X6
Deoxyribonuclease (pancreatic)	T45.3X1	T45.3X2	T45.3X3	T45.3X4	T45.3X5	T45.3X6
Depilatory	T49.4X1	T49.4X2	T49.4X3	T49.4X4	T49.4X5	T49.4X6
Deprenalin	T42.8X1	T42.8X2	T42.8X3	T42.8X4	T42.8X5	T42.8X6
Deprenyl	T42.8X1	T42.8X2	T42.8X3	T42.8X4	T42.8X5	T42.8X6
Depressant						
appetite (central)	T50.5X1	T50.5X2	T50.5X3	T50.5X4	T50.5X5	T50.5X6
cardiac	T46.2X1	T46.2X2	T46.2X3	T46.2X4	T46.2X5	T46.2X6
central nervous system (anesthetic) — see also Central nervous system, depressants	T42.71	T42.72	T42.73	T42.74	T42.75	T42.76
general anesthetic	T41.201	T41.202	T41.203	T41.204	T41.205	T41.206
muscle tone	T42.8X1	T42.8X2	T42.8X3	T42.8X4	T42.8X5	T42.8X6
muscle tone, central	T42.8X1	T42.8X2	T42.8X3	T42.8X4	T42.8X5	T42.8X6
psychotherapeutic	T43.501	T43.502	T43.503	T43.504	T43.505	T43.506
Depressant, appetite	T50.5X1	T50.5X2	T50.5X3	T50.5X4	T50.5X5	T50.5X6
Deptropine	T45.0X1	T45.0X2	T45.0X3	T45.0X4	T45.0X5	T45.0X6
Dequalinium (chloride)	T49.0X1	T49.0X2	T49.0X3	T49.0X4	T49.0X5	T49.0X6
Derris root	T60.2X1	T60.2X2	T60.2X3	T60.2X4	—	—

*Optum Value-Add

☑ Additional Character May Be Required — Refer to the Tabular List for Character Selection

Substance	Poisoning, Accidental (unintentional)	Poisoning, Intentional Self-harm	Poisoning, Assault	Poisoning, Undetermined	Adverse Effect	Under-dosing
Deserpidine	T46.5X1	T46.5X2	T46.5X3	T46.5X4	T46.5X5	T46.5X6
Desferrioxamine	T45.8X1	T45.8X2	T45.8X3	T45.8X4	T45.8X5	T45.8X6
Desipramine	T43.011	T43.012	T43.013	T43.014	T43.015	T43.016
Deslanoside	T46.0X1	T46.0X2	T46.0X3	T46.0X4	T46.0X5	T46.0X6
Desloughing agent	T49.4X1	T49.4X2	T49.4X3	T49.4X4	T49.4X5	T49.4X6
Desmethylimipramine	T43.011	T43.012	T43.013	T43.014	T43.015	T43.016
Desmopressin	T38.891	T38.892	T38.893	T38.894	T38.895	T38.896
Desocodeine	T40.2X1	T40.2X2	T40.2X3	T40.2X4	T40.2X5	T40.2X6
Desogestrel	T38.5X1	T38.5X2	T38.5X3	T38.5X4	T38.5X5	T38.5X6
Desomorphine	T40.2X1	T40.2X2	T40.2X3	T40.2X4	—	—
Desonide	T49.0X1	T49.0X2	T49.0X3	T49.0X4	T49.0X5	T49.0X6
Desoximetasone	T49.0X1	T49.0X2	T49.0X3	T49.0X4	T49.0X5	T49.0X6
Desoxycorticosteroid	T50.0X1	T50.0X2	T50.0X3	T50.0X4	T50.0X5	T50.0X6
Desoxycortone	T50.0X1	T50.0X2	T50.0X3	T50.0X4	T50.0X5	T50.0X6
Desoxyephedrine	T43.651	T43.652	T43.652	T43.654	T43.655	T43.656
Detaxtran	T46.6X1	T46.6X2	T46.6X3	T46.6X4	T46.6X5	T46.6X6
Detergent	T49.2X1	T49.2X2	T49.2X3	T49.2X4	T49.2X5	T49.2X6
external medication	T49.2X1	T49.2X2	T49.2X3	T49.2X4	T49.2X5	T49.2X6
local	T49.2X1	T49.2X2	T49.2X3	T49.2X4	T49.2X5	T49.2X6
medicinal	T49.2X1	T49.2X2	T49.2X3	T49.2X4	T49.2X5	T49.2X6
nonmedicinal	T55.1X1	T55.1X2	T55.1X3	T55.1X4	—	—
specified NEC	T55.1X1	T55.1X2	T55.1X3	T55.1X4	—	—
Deterrent, alcohol	T50.6X1	T50.6X2	T50.6X3	T50.6X4	T50.6X5	T50.6X6
Detoxifying agent	T50.6X1	T50.6X2	T50.6X3	T50.6X4	T50.6X5	T50.6X6
Detrothyronine	T38.1X1	T38.1X2	T38.1X3	T38.1X4	T38.1X5	T38.1X6
Dettol (external medication)	T49.0X1	T49.0X2	T49.0X3	T49.0X4	T49.0X5	T49.0X6
Dexamethasone	T38.0X1	T38.0X2	T38.0X3	T38.0X4	T38.0X5	T38.0X6
ENT agent	T49.6X1	T49.6X2	T49.6X3	T49.6X4	T49.6X5	T49.6X6
ophthalmic preparation	T49.5X1	T49.5X2	T49.5X3	T49.5X4	T49.5X5	T49.5X6
topical NEC	T49.0X1	T49.0X2	T49.0X3	T49.0X4	T49.0X5	T49.0X6
Dexamfetamine	T43.621	T43.622	T43.623	T43.624	T43.625	T43.626
Dexamphetamine	T43.621	T43.622	T43.623	T43.624	T43.625	T43.626
Dexbrompheniramine	T45.0X1	T45.0X2	T45.0X3	T45.0X4	T45.0X5	T45.0X6
Dexchlorpheniramine	T45.0X1	T45.0X2	T45.0X3	T45.0X4	T45.0X5	T45.0X6
Dexedrine	T43.621	T43.622	T43.623	T43.624	T43.625	T43.626
Dexetimide	T44.3X1	T44.3X2	T44.3X3	T44.3X4	T44.3X5	T44.3X6
Dexfenfluramine	T50.5X1	T50.5X2	T50.5X3	T50.5X4	T50.5X5	T50.5X6
Dexpanthenol	T45.2X1	T45.2X2	T45.2X3	T45.2X4	T45.2X5	T45.2X6
Dextran (40) (70) (150)	T45.8X1	T45.8X2	T45.8X3	T45.8X4	T45.8X5	T45.8X6
Dextriferron	T45.4X1	T45.4X2	T45.4X3	T45.4X4	T45.4X5	T45.4X6
Dextroamphetamine	T43.621	T43.622	T43.623	T43.624	T43.625	T43.626
Dextro calcium pantothenate	T45.2X1	T45.2X2	T45.2X3	T45.2X4	T45.2X5	T45.2X6
Dextromethorphan	T48.3X1	T48.3X2	T48.3X3	T48.3X4	T48.3X5	T48.3X6
Dextromoramide	T40.491	T40.492	T40.493	T40.494	—	—
topical	T49.8X1	T49.8X2	T49.8X3	T49.8X4	T49.8X5	T49.8X6
Dextro pantothenyl alcohol	T45.2X1	T45.2X2	T45.2X3	T45.2X4	T45.2X5	T45.2X6
Dextropropoxyphene	T40.491	T40.492	T40.493	T40.494	T40.495	T40.496
Dextrorphan	T40.2X1	T40.2X2	T40.2X3	T40.2X4	T40.2X5	T40.2X6
Dextrose	T50.3X1	T50.3X2	T50.3X3	T50.3X4	T50.3X5	T50.3X6
concentrated solution, intravenous	T46.8X1	T46.8X2	T46.8X3	T46.8X4	T46.8X5	T46.8X6
Dextrothyroxin	T38.1X1	T38.1X2	T38.1X3	T38.1X4	T38.1X5	T38.1X6
Dextrothyroxine sodium	T38.1X1	T38.1X2	T38.1X3	T38.1X4	T38.1X5	T38.1X6
DFP	T44.0X1	T44.0X2	T44.0X3	T44.0X4	T44.0X5	T44.0X6
DHE	T37.3X1	T37.3X2	T37.3X3	T37.3X4	T37.3X5	T37.3X6
45	T46.5X1	T46.5X2	T46.5X3	T46.5X4	T46.5X5	T46.5X6
DiaBeta*	T38.3X1	T38.3X2	T38.3X3	T38.3X4	T38.3X5	T38.3X6
Diabinese	T38.3X1	T38.3X2	T38.3X3	T38.3X4	T38.3X5	T38.3X6
Diacetone alcohol	T52.4X1	T52.4X2	T52.4X3	T52.4X4	—	—
Diacetyl monoxime	T50.991	T50.992	T50.993	T50.994	—	—
Diacetylmorphine	T40.1X1	T40.1X2	T40.1X3	T40.1X4	—	—
Diachylon plaster	T49.4X1	T49.4X2	T49.4X3	T49.4X4	T49.4X5	T49.4X6
Diaethylstilboestrolum	T38.5X1	T38.5X2	T38.5X3	T38.5X4	T38.5X5	T38.5X6
Diagnostic agent NEC	T50.8X1	T50.8X2	T50.8X3	T50.8X4	T50.8X5	T50.8X6
Dial (soap)	T49.2X1	T49.2X2	T49.2X3	T49.2X4	T49.2X5	T49.2X6
sedative	T42.3X1	T42.3X2	T42.3X3	T42.3X4	T42.3X5	T42.3X6
Dialkyl carbonate	T52.91	T52.92	T52.93	T52.94	—	—
Diallylbarbituric acid	T42.3X1	T42.3X2	T42.3X3	T42.3X4	T42.3X5	T42.3X6
Diallymal	T42.3X1	T42.3X2	T42.3X3	T42.3X4	T42.3X5	T42.3X6
Dialysis solution (intraperitoneal)	T50.3X1	T50.3X2	T50.3X3	T50.3X4	T50.3X5	T50.3X6
Diaminodiphenylsulfone	T37.1X1	T37.1X2	T37.1X3	T37.1X4	T37.1X5	T37.1X6
Diamorphine	T40.1X1	T40.1X2	T40.1X3	T40.1X4	—	—
Diamox	T50.2X1	T50.2X2	T50.2X3	T50.2X4	T50.2X5	T50.2X6
Diamthazole	T49.0X1	T49.0X2	T49.0X3	T49.0X4	T49.0X5	T49.0X6
Dianthone	T47.2X1	T47.2X2	T47.2X3	T47.2X4	T47.2X5	T47.2X6
Diaphenylsulfone	T37.0X1	T37.0X2	T37.0X3	T37.0X4	T37.0X5	T37.0X6
Diasone (sodium)	T37.1X1	T37.1X2	T37.1X3	T37.1X4	T37.1X5	T37.1X6
Diastase	T47.5X1	T47.5X2	T47.5X3	T47.5X4	T47.5X5	T47.5X6
Diastat*	T42.4X1	T42.4X2	T42.4X3	T42.4X4	T42.4X5	T42.4X6
Diatrizoate	T50.8X1	T50.8X2	T50.8X3	T50.8X4	T50.8X5	T50.8X6

Substance	Poisoning, Accidental (unintentional)	Poisoning, Intentional Self-harm	Poisoning, Assault	Poisoning, Undetermined	Adverse Effect	Under-dosing
Diazepam	T42.4X1	T42.4X2	T42.4X3	T42.4X4	T42.4X5	T42.4X6
Diazinon	T60.0X1	T60.0X2	T60.0X3	T60.0X4	—	—
Diazomethane (gas)	T59.891	T59.892	T59.893	T59.894	—	—
Diazoxide	T46.5X1	T46.5X2	T46.5X3	T46.5X4	T46.5X5	T46.5X6
Dibekacin	T36.5X1	T36.5X2	T36.5X3	T36.5X4	T36.5X5	T36.5X6
Dibenamine	T44.6X1	T44.6X2	T44.6X3	T44.6X4	T44.6X5	T44.6X6
Dibenzepin	T43.011	T43.012	T43.013	T43.014	T43.015	T43.016
Dibenzheptropine	T45.0X1	T45.0X2	T45.0X3	T45.0X4	T45.0X5	T45.0X6
Dibenzyline	T44.6X1	T44.6X2	T44.6X3	T44.6X4	T44.6X5	T44.6X6
Diborane (gas)	T59.891	T59.892	T59.893	T59.894	—	—
Dibromochloropropane	T60.8X1	T60.8X2	T60.8X3	T60.8X4	—	—
Dibromodulcitol	T45.1X1	T45.1X2	T45.1X3	T45.1X4	T45.1X5	T45.1X6
Dibromoethane	T53.6X1	T53.6X2	T53.6X3	T53.6X4	—	—
Dibromomannitol	T45.1X1	T45.1X2	T45.1X3	T45.1X4	T45.1X5	T45.1X6
Dibromopropamidine isethionate	T49.0X1	T49.0X2	T49.0X3	T49.0X4	T49.0X5	T49.0X6
Dibrompropamidine	T49.0X1	T49.0X2	T49.0X3	T49.0X4	T49.0X5	T49.0X6
Dibucaine	T41.3X1	T41.3X2	T41.3X3	T41.3X4	T41.3X5	T41.3X6
topical (surface)	T41.3X1	T41.3X2	T41.3X3	T41.3X4	T41.3X5	T41.3X6
Dibunate sodium	T48.3X1	T48.3X2	T48.3X3	T48.3X4	T48.3X5	T48.3X6
Dibutoline sulfate	T44.3X1	T44.3X2	T44.3X3	T44.3X4	T44.3X5	T44.3X6
Dicamba	T60.3X1	T60.3X2	T60.3X3	T60.3X4	—	—
Dicapthon	T60.0X1	T60.0X2	T60.0X3	T60.0X4	—	—
Dichlobenil	T60.3X1	T60.3X2	T60.3X3	T60.3X4	—	—
Dichlone	T60.3X1	T60.3X2	T60.3X3	T60.3X4	—	—
Dichloralphenozone	T42.6X1	T42.6X2	T42.6X3	T42.6X4	T42.6X5	T42.6X6
Dichlorbenzidine	T65.3X1	T65.3X2	T65.3X3	T65.3X4	—	—
Dichlorhydrin	T52.8X1	T52.8X2	T52.8X3	T52.8X4	—	—
Dichlorhydroxyquinoline	T37.8X1	T37.8X2	T37.8X3	T37.8X4	T37.8X5	T37.8X6
Dichlorobenzene	T53.7X1	T53.7X2	T53.7X3	T53.7X4	—	—
Dichlorobenzyl alcohol	T49.6X1	T49.6X2	T49.6X3	T49.6X4	T49.6X5	T49.6X6
Dichlorodifluoromethane	T53.5X1	T53.5X2	T53.5X3	T53.5X4	—	—
Dichloroethane	T52.8X1	T52.8X2	T52.8X3	T52.8X4	—	—
Dichloroethylene	T53.6X1	T53.6X2	T53.6X3	T53.6X4	—	—
Dichloroethyl sulfide, not in war	T59.891	T59.892	T59.893	T59.894	—	—
Dichloroformoxine, not in war	T59.891	T59.892	T59.893	T59.894	—	—
Dichlorohydrin, alpha-dichlorohydrin	T52.8X1	T52.8X2	T52.8X3	T52.8X4	—	—
Dichloromethane (solvent)	T53.4X1	T53.4X2	T53.4X3	T53.4X4	—	—
vapor	T53.4X1	T53.4X2	T53.4X3	T53.4X4	—	—
Dichloronaphthoquinone	T60.3X1	T60.3X2	T60.3X3	T60.3X4	—	—
Dichlorophen	T37.4X1	T37.4X2	T37.4X3	T37.4X4	T37.4X5	T37.4X6
Dichloropropene	T60.3X1	T60.3X2	T60.3X3	T60.3X4	—	—
Dichloropropionic acid	T60.3X1	T60.3X2	T60.3X3	T60.3X4	—	—
Dichlorphenamide	T50.2X1	T50.2X2	T50.2X3	T50.2X4	T50.2X5	T50.2X6
Dichlorvos	T60.0X1	T60.0X2	T60.0X3	T60.0X4	—	—
Dichysterol*	T45.2X1	T45.2X2	T45.2X3	T45.2X4	T45.2X5	T45.2X6
Diclofenac	T39.391	T39.392	T39.393	T39.394	T39.395	T39.396
Diclofenamide	T50.2X1	T50.2X2	T50.2X3	T50.2X4	T50.2X5	T50.2X6
Diclofensine	T43.291	T43.292	T43.293	T43.294	T43.295	T43.296
Diclonixine	T39.8X1	T39.8X2	T39.8X3	T39.8X4	T39.8X5	T39.8X6
Dicloxacillin	T36.0X1	T36.0X2	T36.0X3	T36.0X4	T36.0X5	T36.0X6
Dicophane	T49.0X1	T49.0X2	T49.0X3	T49.0X4	T49.0X5	T49.0X6
Dicoumarol, dicoumarin, dicumarol	T45.511	T45.512	T45.513	T45.514	T45.515	T45.516
Dicrotophos	T60.0X1	T60.0X2	T60.0X3	T60.0X4	—	—
Dicyanogen (gas)	T65.0X1	T65.0X2	T65.0X3	T65.0X4	—	—
Dicyclomine	T44.3X1	T44.3X2	T44.3X3	T44.3X4	T44.3X5	T44.3X6
Dicycloverine	T44.3X1	T44.3X2	T44.3X3	T44.3X4	T44.3X5	T44.3X6
Didanosine*	T37.5X1	T37.5X2	T37.5X3	T37.5X4	T37.5X5	T37.5X6
Dideoxycytidine	T37.5X1	T37.5X2	T37.5X3	T37.5X4	T37.5X5	T37.5X6
Dideoxyinosine	T37.5X1	T37.5X2	T37.5X3	T37.5X4	T37.5X5	T37.5X6
Dieldrin (vapor)	T60.1X1	T60.1X2	T60.1X3	T60.1X4	—	—
Diemal	T42.3X1	T42.3X2	T42.3X3	T42.3X4	T42.3X5	T42.3X6
Dienestrol	T38.5X1	T38.5X2	T38.5X3	T38.5X4	T38.5X5	T38.5X6
Dienoestrol	T38.5X1	T38.5X2	T38.5X3	T38.5X4	T38.5X5	T38.5X6
Dietetic drug NEC	T50.901	T50.902	T50.903	T50.904	T50.905	T50.906
Diethazine	T42.8X1	T42.8X2	T42.8X3	T42.8X4	T42.8X5	T42.8X6
Diethyl						
barbituric acid	T42.3X1	T42.3X2	T42.3X3	T42.3X4	T42.3X5	T42.3X6
carbamazine	T37.4X1	T37.4X2	T37.4X3	T37.4X4	T37.4X5	T37.4X6
carbinol	T51.3X1	T51.3X2	T51.3X3	T51.3X4	—	—
carbonate	T52.8X1	T52.8X2	T52.8X3	T52.8X4	—	—
ether (vapor) — see also ether	T41.0X1	T41.0X2	T41.0X3	T41.0X4	T41.0X5	T41.0X6
oxide	T52.8X1	T52.8X2	T52.8X3	T52.8X4	—	—
propion	T50.5X1	T50.5X2	T50.5X3	T50.5X4	T50.5X5	T50.5X6
stilbestrol	T38.5X1	T38.5X2	T38.5X3	T38.5X4	T38.5X5	T38.5X6
toluamide (nonmedicinal)	T60.8X1	T60.8X2	T60.8X3	T60.8X4	—	—
medicinal	T49.3X1	T49.3X2	T49.3X3	T49.3X4	T49.3X5	T49.3X6
Diethylcarbamazine	T37.4X1	T37.4X2	T37.4X3	T37.4X4	T37.4X5	T37.4X6

☑ Additional Character May Be Required — Refer to the Tabular List for Character Selection *Optum Value-Add

Substance	Poisoning, Accidental (unintentional)	Poisoning, Intentional Self-harm	Poisoning, Assault	Poisoning, Undetermined	Adverse Effect	Under-dosing
Diethylene						
dioxide	T52.8X1	T52.8X2	T52.8X3	T52.8X4	—	—
glycol (monoacetate) (monobutyl ether) (monoethyl ether)	T52.3X1	T52.3X2	T52.3X3	T52.3X4	—	—
Diethylhexylphthalate	T65.891	T65.892	T65.893	T65.894	—	—
Diethylpropion	T50.5X1	T50.5X2	T50.5X3	T50.5X4	T50.5X5	T50.5X6
Diethylstilbestrol	T38.5X1	T38.5X2	T38.5X3	T38.5X4	T38.5X5	T38.5X6
Diethylstilboestrol	T38.5X1	T38.5X2	T38.5X3	T38.5X4	T38.5X5	T38.5X6
Diethylsulfone-diethyl-methane	T42.6X1	T42.6X2	T42.6X3	T42.6X4	T42.6X5	T42.6X6
Diethyltoluamide	T49.0X1	T49.0X2	T49.0X3	T49.0X4	T49.0X5	T49.0X6
Diethyltryptamine (DET)	T40.991	T40.992	T40.993	T40.994		
Difebarbamate	T42.3X1	T42.3X2	T42.3X3	T42.3X4	T42.3X5	T42.3X6
Difencloxazine	T40.2X1	T40.2X2	T40.2X3	T40.2X4	T40.2X5	T40.2X6
Difenidol	T45.0X1	T45.0X2	T45.0X3	T45.0X4	T45.0X5	T45.0X6
Difenoxin	T47.6X1	T47.6X2	T47.6X3	T47.6X4	T47.6X5	T47.6X6
Difetarsone	T37.3X1	T37.3X2	T37.3X3	T37.3X4	T37.3X5	T37.3X6
Diffusin	T45.3X1	T45.3X2	T45.3X3	T45.3X4	T45.3X5	T45.3X6
Diflorasone	T49.0X1	T49.0X2	T49.0X3	T49.0X4	T49.0X5	T49.0X6
Diflos	T44.0X1	T44.0X2	T44.0X3	T44.0X4	T44.0X5	T44.0X6
Diflubenzuron	T60.1X1	T60.1X2	T60.1X3	T60.1X4	—	—
Diflucortolone	T49.0X1	T49.0X2	T49.0X3	T49.0X4	T49.0X5	T49.0X6
Diflunisal	T39.091	T39.092	T39.093	T39.094	T39.095	T39.096
Difluoromethyldopa	T42.8X1	T42.8X2	T42.8X3	T42.8X4	T42.8X5	T42.8X6
Difluorophate	T44.0X1	T44.0X2	T44.0X3	T44.0X4	T44.0X5	T44.0X6
Digestant NEC	T47.5X1	T47.5X2	T47.5X3	T47.5X4	T47.5X5	T47.5X6
Digitalin (e)	T46.0X1	T46.0X2	T46.0X3	T46.0X4	T46.0X5	T46.0X6
Digitalis (leaf)(glycoside)	T46.0X1	T46.0X2	T46.0X3	T46.0X4	T46.0X5	T46.0X6
lanata	T46.0X1	T46.0X2	T46.0X3	T46.0X4	T46.0X5	T46.0X6
purpurea	T46.0X1	T46.0X2	T46.0X3	T46.0X4	T46.0X5	T46.0X6
Digitoxin	T46.0X1	T46.0X2	T46.0X3	T46.0X4	T46.0X5	T46.0X6
Digitoxose	T46.0X1	T46.0X2	T46.0X3	T46.0X4	T46.0X5	T46.0X6
Digoxin	T46.0X1	T46.0X2	T46.0X3	T46.0X4	T46.0X5	T46.0X6
Digoxine	T46.0X1	T46.0X2	T46.0X3	T46.0X4	T46.0X5	T46.0X6
Dihydralazine	T46.5X1	T46.5X2	T46.5X3	T46.5X4	T46.5X5	T46.5X6
Dihydrazine	T46.5X1	T46.5X2	T46.5X3	T46.5X4	T46.5X5	T46.5X6
Dihydrocodeine	T40.2X1	T40.2X2	T40.2X3	T40.2X4	T40.2X5	T40.2X6
Dihydrocodeinone	T40.2X1	T40.2X2	T40.2X3	T40.2X4	T40.2X5	T40.2X6
Dihydroergocornine	T46.7X1	T46.7X2	T46.7X3	T46.7X4	T46.7X5	T46.7X6
Dihydroergocristine (mesilate)	T46.7X1	T46.7X2	T46.7X3	T46.7X4	T46.7X5	T46.7X6
Dihydroergokryptine	T46.7X1	T46.7X2	T46.7X3	T46.7X4	T46.7X5	T46.7X6
Dihydroergotamine	T46.5X1	T46.5X2	T46.5X3	T46.5X4	T46.5X5	T46.5X6
Dihydroergotoxine	T46.7X1	T46.7X2	T46.7X3	T46.7X4	T46.7X5	T46.7X6
mesilate	T46.7X1	T46.7X2	T46.7X3	T46.7X4	T46.7X5	T46.7X6
Dihydrohydroxycodeinone	T40.2X1	T40.2X2	T40.2X3	T40.2X4	T40.2X5	T40.2X6
Dihydrohydroxymorphinone	T40.2X1	T40.2X2	T40.2X3	T40.2X4	T40.2X5	T40.2X6
Dihydroisocodeine	T40.2X1	T40.2X2	T40.2X3	T40.2X4	T40.2X5	T40.2X6
Dihydromorphine	T40.2X1	T40.2X2	T40.2X3	T40.2X4	—	—
Dihydromorphinone	T40.2X1	T40.2X2	T40.2X3	T40.2X4	T40.2X5	T40.2X6
Dihydrostreptomycin	T36.5X1	T36.5X2	T36.5X3	T36.5X4	T36.5X5	T36.5X6
Dihydrotachysterol	T45.2X1	T45.2X2	T45.2X3	T45.2X4	T45.2X5	T45.2X6
Dihydroxyacetone*	T49.3X1	T49.3X2	T49.3X3	T49.3X4	T49.3X5	T49.3X6
Dihydroxyaluminum aminoacetate	T47.1X1	T47.1X2	T47.1X3	T47.1X4	T47.1X5	T47.1X6
Dihydroxyaluminum sodium carbonate	T47.1X1	T47.1X2	T47.1X3	T47.1X4	T47.1X5	T47.1X6
Dihydroxyanthraquinone	T47.2X1	T47.2X2	T47.2X3	T47.2X4	T47.2X5	T47.2X6
Dihydroxycodeinone	T40.2X1	T40.2X2	T40.2X3	T40.2X4	T40.2X5	T40.2X6
Dihydroxypropyl theophylline	T50.2X1	T50.2X2	T50.2X3	T50.2X4	T50.2X5	T50.2X6
Diiodohydroxyquin	T37.8X1	T37.8X2	T37.8X3	T37.8X4	T37.8X5	T37.8X6
topical	T49.0X1	T49.0X2	T49.0X3	T49.0X4	T49.0X5	T49.0X6
Diiodohydroxyquinoline	T37.8X1	T37.8X2	T37.8X3	T37.8X4	T37.8X5	T37.8X6
Diiodotyrosine	T38.2X1	T38.2X2	T38.2X3	T38.2X4	T38.2X5	T38.2X6
Diisopromine	T44.3X1	T44.3X2	T44.3X3	T44.3X4	T44.3X5	T44.3X6
Diisopropylamine	T46.3X1	T46.3X2	T46.3X3	T46.3X4	T46.3X5	T46.3X6
Diisopropylfluorophos-phonate	T44.0X1	T44.0X2	T44.0X3	T44.0X4	T44.0X5	T44.0X6
Dilantin	T42.0X1	T42.0X2	T42.0X3	T42.0X4	T42.0X5	T42.0X6
Dilatrate*	T46.3X1	T46.3X2	T46.3X3	T46.3X4	T46.3X5	T46.3X6
Dilaudid	T40.2X1	T40.2X2	T40.2X3	T40.2X4	T40.2X5	T40.2X6
Dilazep	T46.3X1	T46.3X2	T46.3X3	T46.3X4	T46.3X5	T46.3X6
Dill	T47.5X1	T47.5X2	T47.5X3	T47.5X4	T47.5X5	T47.5X6
Diloxanide	T37.3X1	T37.3X2	T37.3X3	T37.3X4	T37.3X5	T37.3X6
Diltiazem	T46.1X1	T46.1X2	T46.1X3	T46.1X4	T46.1X5	T46.1X6
Dimazole	T49.0X1	T49.0X2	T49.0X3	T49.0X4	T49.0X5	T49.0X6
Dimefline	T50.7X1	T50.7X2	T50.7X3	T50.7X4	T50.7X5	T50.7X6
Dimefox	T60.0X1	T60.0X2	T60.0X3	T60.0X4		
Dimemorfan	T48.3X1	T48.3X2	T48.3X3	T48.3X4	T48.3X5	T48.3X6
Dimenhydrinate	T45.0X1	T45.0X2	T45.0X3	T45.0X4	T45.0X5	T45.0X6
Dimercaprol (British anti-lewisite)	T45.8X1	T45.8X2	T45.8X3	T45.8X4	T45.8X5	T45.8X6
Dimercaptopropanol	T45.8X1	T45.8X2	T45.8X3	T45.8X4	T45.8X5	T45.8X6
Dimestrol	T38.5X1	T38.5X2	T38.5X3	T38.5X4	T38.5X5	T38.5X6
Dimetane	T45.0X1	T45.0X2	T45.0X3	T45.0X4	T45.0X5	T45.0X6
Dimethicone	T47.1X1	T47.1X2	T47.1X3	T47.1X4	T47.1X5	T47.1X6
Dimethindene	T45.0X1	T45.0X2	T45.0X3	T45.0X4	T45.0X5	T45.0X6
Dimethisoquin	T49.1X1	T49.1X2	T49.1X3	T49.1X4	T49.1X5	T49.1X6
Dimethisterone	T38.5X1	T38.5X2	T38.5X3	T38.5X4	T38.5X5	T38.5X6
Dimethoate	T60.0X1	T60.0X2	T60.0X3	T60.0X4	—	—
Dimethocaine	T41.3X1	T41.3X2	T41.3X3	T41.3X4	T41.3X5	T41.3X6
Dimethoxanate	T48.3X1	T48.3X2	T48.3X3	T48.3X4	T48.3X5	T48.3X6
Dimethyl						
arsine, arsinic acid	T57.0X1	T57.0X2	T57.0X3	T57.0X4	—	—
carbinol	T51.2X1	T51.2X2	T51.2X3	T51.2X4	—	—
carbonate	T52.8X1	T52.8X2	T52.8X3	T52.8X4	—	—
diguanide	T38.3X1	T38.3X2	T38.3X3	T38.3X4	T38.3X5	T38.3X6
ketone	T52.4X1	T52.4X2	T52.4X3	T52.4X4	—	—
vapor	T52.4X1	T52.4X2	T52.4X3	T52.4X4	—	—
meperidine	T40.2X1	T40.2X2	T40.2X3	T40.2X4	T40.2X5	T40.2X6
parathion	T60.0X1	T60.0X2	T60.0X3	T60.0X4	—	—
phthlate	T49.3X1	T49.3X2	T49.3X3	T49.3X4	T49.3X5	T49.3X6
polysiloxane	T47.8X1	T47.8X2	T47.8X3	T47.8X4	T47.8X5	T47.8X6
sulfate (fumes)	T59.891	T59.892	T59.893	T59.894	—	—
liquid	T65.891	T65.892	T65.893	T65.894	—	—
sulfoxide (nonmedicinal)	T52.8X1	T52.8X2	T52.8X3	T52.8X4	—	—
medicinal	T49.4X1	T49.4X2	T49.4X3	T49.4X4	T49.4X5	T49.4X6
tryptamine	T40.991	T40.992	T40.993	T40.994		
tubocurarine	T48.1X1	T48.1X2	T48.1X3	T48.1X4	T48.1X5	T48.1X6
Dimethylamine sulfate	T49.4X1	T49.4X2	T49.4X3	T49.4X4	T49.4X5	T49.4X6
Dimethylcysteine*	T50.6X1	T50.6X2	T50.6X3	T50.6X4	T50.6X5	T50.6X6
Dimethylformamide	T52.8X1	T52.8X2	T52.8X3	T52.8X4	—	—
Dimethyltubocurarinium chloride	T48.1X1	T48.1X2	T48.1X3	T48.1X4	T48.1X5	T48.1X6
Dimeticone	T47.1X1	T47.1X2	T47.1X3	T47.1X4	T47.1X5	T47.1X6
Dimetilan	T60.0X1	T60.0X2	T60.0X3	T60.0X4	—	—
Dimetindene	T45.0X1	T45.0X2	T45.0X3	T45.0X4	T45.0X5	T45.0X6
Dimetotiazine	T43.3X1	T43.3X2	T43.3X3	T43.3X4	T43.3X5	T43.3X6
Dimorpholamine	T50.7X1	T50.7X2	T50.7X3	T50.7X4	T50.7X5	T50.7X6
Dimoxyline	T46.3X1	T46.3X2	T46.3X3	T46.3X4	T46.3X5	T46.3X6
Dinitrobenzene	T65.3X1	T65.3X2	T65.3X3	T65.3X4	—	—
vapor	T59.891	T59.892	T59.893	T59.894	—	—
Dinitrobenzol	T65.3X1	T65.3X2	T65.3X3	T65.3X4	—	—
vapor	T59.891	T59.892	T59.893	T59.894	—	—
Dinitrobutylphenol	T65.3X1	T65.3X2	T65.3X3	T65.3X4	—	—
Dinitro (-ortho-)cresol (pesticide)(spray)	T65.3X1	T65.3X2	T65.3X3	T65.3X4	—	—
Dinitrocyclohexylphenol	T65.3X1	T65.3X2	T65.3X3	T65.3X4	—	—
Dinitrophenol	T65.3X1	T65.3X2	T65.3X3	T65.3X4	—	—
Dinoprost	T48.0X1	T48.0X2	T48.0X3	T48.0X4	T48.0X5	T48.0X6
Dinoprostone	T48.0X1	T48.0X2	T48.0X3	T48.0X4	T48.0X5	T48.0X6
Dinoseb	T60.3X1	T60.3X2	T60.3X3	T60.3X4	—	—
Dioctyl sulfosuccinate (calcium)(sodium)	T47.4X1	T47.4X2	T47.4X3	T47.4X4	T47.4X5	T47.4X6
Diodone	T50.8X1	T50.8X2	T50.8X3	T50.8X4	T50.8X5	T50.8X6
Diodoquin	T37.8X1	T37.8X2	T37.8X3	T37.8X4	T37.8X5	T37.8X6
Dionin	T40.2X1	T40.2X2	T40.2X3	T40.2X4	T40.2X5	T40.2X6
Diosmin	T46.991	T46.992	T46.993	T46.994	T46.995	T46.996
Diovan*	T46.5X1	T46.5X2	T46.5X3	T46.5X4	T46.5X5	T46.5X6
Dioxane	T52.8X1	T52.8X2	T52.8X3	T52.8X4	—	—
Dioxathion	T60.0X1	T60.0X2	T60.0X3	T60.0X4	—	—
Dioxin	T53.7X1	T53.7X2	T53.7X3	T53.7X4	—	—
Dioxopromethazine	T43.3X1	T43.3X2	T43.3X3	T43.3X4	T43.3X5	T43.3X6
Dioxyline	T46.3X1	T46.3X2	T46.3X3	T46.3X4	T46.3X5	T46.3X6
Dipentene	T52.8X1	T52.8X2	T52.8X3	T52.8X4	—	—
Diperodon	T41.3X1	T41.3X2	T41.3X3	T41.3X4	T41.3X5	T41.3X6
Diphacinone	T60.4X1	T60.4X2	T60.4X3	T60.4X4	—	—
Diphemanil	T44.3X1	T44.3X2	T44.3X3	T44.3X4	T44.3X5	T44.3X6
metilsulfate	T44.3X1	T44.3X2	T44.3X3	T44.3X4	T44.3X5	T44.3X6
Diphenadione	T45.511	T45.512	T45.513	T45.514	T45.515	T45.516
rodenticide	T60.4X1	T60.4X2	T60.4X3	T60.4X4	—	—
Diphenhydramine	T45.0X1	T45.0X2	T45.0X3	T45.0X4	T45.0X5	T45.0X6
Diphenidol	T45.0X1	T45.0X2	T45.0X3	T45.0X4	T45.0X5	T45.0X6
Diphenoxylate	T47.6X1	T47.6X2	T47.6X3	T47.6X4	T47.6X5	T47.6X6
Diphenylamine	T65.3X1	T65.3X2	T65.3X3	T65.3X4	—	—
Diphenylbutazone	T39.2X1	T39.2X2	T39.2X3	T39.2X4	T39.2X5	T39.2X6
Diphenylchloroarsine, not in war	T57.0X1	T57.0X2	T57.0X3	T57.0X4	—	—
Diphenylhydantoin	T42.0X1	T42.0X2	T42.0X3	T42.0X4	T42.0X5	T42.0X6
Diphenylmethane dye	T52.1X1	T52.1X2	T52.1X3	T52.1X4	—	—
Diphenylpyraline	T45.0X1	T45.0X2	T45.0X3	T45.0X4	T45.0X5	T45.0X6
Diphtheria						
antitoxin	T50.Z11	T50.Z12	T50.Z13	T50.Z14	T50.Z15	T50.Z16

Substance	Poisoning, Accidental (unintentional)	Poisoning, Intentional Self-harm	Poisoning, Assault	Poisoning, Undetermined	Adverse Effect	Under- dosing
Diphtheria — *continued*						
toxoid	T50.A91	T50.A92	T50.A93	T50.A94	T50.A95	T50.A96
with tetanus toxoid	T50.A21	T50.A22	T50.A23	T50.A24	T50.A25	T50.A26
with pertussis component	T50.A11	T50.A12	T50.A13	T50.A14	T50.A15	T50.A16
vaccine	T50.A91	T50.A92	T50.A93	T50.A94	T50.A95	T50.A96
combination						
without pertussis	T50.A21	T50.A22	T50.A23	T50.A24	T50.A25	T50.A26
including pertussis	T50.A11	T50.A12	T50.A13	T50.A14	T50.A15	T50.A16
Diphylline	T50.2X1	T50.2X2	T50.2X3	T50.2X4	T50.2X5	T50.2X6
Dipipanone	T40.491	T40.492	T40.493	T40.494	—	—
Dipivefrine	T49.5X1	T49.5X2	T49.5X3	T49.5X4	T49.5X5	T49.5X6
Diplovax	T50.B91	T50.B92	T50.B93	T50.B94	T50.B95	T50.B96
Diprophylline	T50.2X1	T50.2X2	T50.2X3	T50.2X4	T50.2X5	T50.2X6
Dipropyline	T48.291	T48.292	T48.293	T48.294	T48.295	T48.296
Dipyridamole	T46.3X1	T46.3X2	T46.3X3	T46.3X4	T46.3X5	T46.3X6
Dipyrone	T39.2X1	T39.2X2	T39.2X3	T39.2X4	T39.2X5	T39.2X6
Diquat (dibromide)	T60.3X1	T60.3X2	T60.3X3	T60.3X4	—	—
Disinfectant	T65.891	T65.892	T65.893	T65.894	—	—
alkaline	T54.3X1	T54.3X2	T54.3X3	T54.3X4	—	—
aromatic	T54.1X1	T54.1X2	T54.1X3	T54.1X4	—	—
intestinal	T37.8X1	T37.8X2	T37.8X3	T37.8X4	T37.8X5	T37.8X6
Disipal	T42.8X1	T42.8X2	T42.8X3	T42.8X4	T42.8X5	T42.8X6
Disodium edetate	T50.6X1	T50.6X2	T50.6X3	T50.6X4	T50.6X5	T50.6X6
Disoprofol	T41.291	T41.292	T41.293	T41.294	T41.295	T41.296
Disopyramide*	T46.2X1	T46.2X2	T46.2X3	T46.2X4	T46.2X5	T46.2X6
Distigmine (bromide)	T44.0X1	T44.0X2	T44.0X3	T44.0X4	T44.0X5	T44.0X6
Disulfamide	T50.2X1	T50.2X2	T50.2X3	T50.2X4	T50.2X5	T50.2X6
Disulfanilamide	T37.0X1	T37.0X2	T37.0X3	T37.0X4	T37.0X5	T37.0X6
Disulfiram	T50.6X1	T50.6X2	T50.6X3	T50.6X4	T50.6X5	T50.6X6
Disulfoton	T60.0X1	T60.0X2	T60.0X3	T60.0X4	—	—
Dithiazanine iodide	T37.4X1	T37.4X2	T37.4X3	T37.4X4	T37.4X5	T37.4X6
Dithiocarbamate	T60.0X1	T60.0X2	T60.0X3	T60.0X4	—	—
Dithranol	T49.4X1	T49.4X2	T49.4X3	T49.4X4	T49.4X5	T49.4X6
Diucardin	T50.2X1	T50.2X2	T50.2X3	T50.2X4	T50.2X5	T50.2X6
Diupres	T50.2X1	T50.2X2	T50.2X3	T50.2X4	T50.2X5	T50.2X6
Diuretic NEC	T50.2X1	T50.2X2	T50.2X3	T50.2X4	T50.2X5	T50.2X6
benzothiadiazine	T50.2X1	T50.2X2	T50.2X3	T50.2X4	T50.2X5	T50.2X6
carbonic acid anhydrase inhibitors	T50.2X1	T50.2X2	T50.2X3	T50.2X4	T50.2X5	T50.2X6
furfuryl NEC	T50.2X1	T50.2X2	T50.2X3	T50.2X4	T50.2X5	T50.2X6
loop (high-ceiling)	T50.1X1	T50.1X2	T50.1X3	T50.1X4	T50.1X5	T50.1X6
mercurial NEC	T50.2X1	T50.2X2	T50.2X3	T50.2X4	T50.2X5	T50.2X6
osmotic	T50.2X1	T50.2X2	T50.2X3	T50.2X4	T50.2X5	T50.2X6
purine NEC	T50.2X1	T50.2X2	T50.2X3	T50.2X4	T50.2X5	T50.2X6
saluretic NEC	T50.2X1	T50.2X2	T50.2X3	T50.2X4	T50.2X5	T50.2X6
sulfonamide	T50.2X1	T50.2X2	T50.2X3	T50.2X4	T50.2X5	T50.2X6
thiazide NEC	T50.2X1	T50.2X2	T50.2X3	T50.2X4	T50.2X5	T50.2X6
xanthine	T50.2X1	T50.2X2	T50.2X3	T50.2X4	T50.2X5	T50.2X6
Diurgin	T50.2X1	T50.2X2	T50.2X3	T50.2X4	T50.2X5	T50.2X6
Diuril	T50.2X1	T50.2X2	T50.2X3	T50.2X4	T50.2X5	T50.2X6
Diuron	T60.3X1	T60.3X2	T60.3X3	T60.3X4	—	—
Divalproex	T42.6X1	T42.6X2	T42.6X3	T42.6X4	T42.6X5	T42.6X6
Divinyl ether	T41.0X1	T41.0X2	T41.0X3	T41.0X4	T41.0X5	T41.0X6
Dixanthogen	T49.0X1	T49.0X2	T49.0X3	T49.0X4	T49.0X5	T49.0X6
Dixyrazine	T43.3X1	T43.3X2	T43.3X3	T43.3X4	T43.3X5	T43.3X6
D-lysergic acid diethylamide	T40.8X1	T40.8X2	T40.8X3	T40.8X4	—	—
DMCT	T36.4X1	T36.4X2	T36.4X3	T36.4X4	T36.4X5	T36.4X6
DMSO — *see* Dimethyl, sulfoxide						
DNBP	T60.3X1	T60.3X2	T60.3X3	T60.3X4	—	—
DNOC	T65.3X1	T65.3X2	T65.3X3	T65.3X4	—	—
Dobutamine	T44.5X1	T44.5X2	T44.5X3	T44.5X4	T44.5X5	T44.5X6
DOCA	T38.0X1	T38.0X2	T38.0X3	T38.0X4	T38.0X5	T38.0X6
Docusate sodium	T47.4X1	T47.4X2	T47.4X3	T47.4X4	T47.4X5	T47.4X6
Dodicin	T49.0X1	T49.0X2	T49.0X3	T49.0X4	T49.0X5	T49.0X6
Dofamium chloride	T49.0X1	T49.0X2	T49.0X3	T49.0X4	T49.0X5	T49.0X6
Dolophine	T40.3X1	T40.3X2	T40.3X3	T40.3X4	T40.3X5	T40.3X6
Doloxene	T39.8X1	T39.8X2	T39.8X3	T39.8X4	T39.8X5	T39.8X6
Domestic gas (after combustion) — *see* Gas, utility						
prior to combustion	T59.891	T59.892	T59.893	T59.894	—	—
Domiodol	T48.4X1	T48.4X2	T48.4X3	T48.4X4	T48.4X5	T48.4X6
Domiphen (bromide)	T49.0X1	T49.0X2	T49.0X3	T49.0X4	T49.0X5	T49.0X6
Domperidone	T45.0X1	T45.0X2	T45.0X3	T45.0X4	T45.0X5	T45.0X6
Donepezil*	T44.0X1	T44.0X2	T44.0X3	T44.0X4	T44.0X5	T44.0X6
Dopa	T42.8X1	T42.8X2	T42.8X3	T42.8X4	T42.8X5	T42.8X6
Dopamine	T44.991	T44.992	T44.993	T44.994	T44.995	T44.996
Doriden	T42.6X1	T42.6X2	T42.6X3	T42.6X4	T42.6X5	T42.6X6
Dormiral	T42.3X1	T42.3X2	T42.3X3	T42.3X4	T42.3X5	T42.3X6
Dormison	T42.6X1	T42.6X2	T42.6X3	T42.6X4	T42.6X5	T42.6X6
Dornase	T48.4X1	T48.4X2	T48.4X3	T48.4X4	T48.4X5	T48.4X6
Dorsacaine	T41.3X1	T41.3X2	T41.3X3	T41.3X4	T41.3X5	T41.3X6

Substance	Poisoning, Accidental (unintentional)	Poisoning, Intentional Self-harm	Poisoning, Assault	Poisoning, Undetermined	Adverse Effect	Under- dosing
Dosulepin	T43.011	T43.012	T43.013	T43.014	T43.015	T43.016
Dothiepin	T43.011	T43.012	T43.013	T43.014	T43.015	T43.016
Doxantrazole	T48.6X1	T48.6X2	T48.6X3	T48.6X4	T48.6X5	T48.6X6
Doxapram	T50.7X1	T50.7X2	T50.7X3	T50.7X4	T50.7X5	T50.7X6
Doxazosin	T44.6X1	T44.6X2	T44.6X3	T44.6X4	T44.6X5	T44.6X6
Doxepin	T43.011	T43.012	T43.013	T43.014	T43.015	T43.016
Doxifluridine	T45.1X1	T45.1X2	T45.1X3	T45.1X4	T45.1X5	T45.1X6
Doxil*	T45.1X1	T45.1X2	T45.1X3	T45.1X4	T45.1X5	T45.1X6
Doxorubicin	T45.1X1	T45.1X2	T45.1X3	T45.1X4	T45.1X5	T45.1X6
Doxycycline	T36.4X1	T36.4X2	T36.4X3	T36.4X4	T36.4X5	T36.4X6
Doxylamine	T45.0X1	T45.0X2	T45.0X3	T45.0X4	T45.0X5	T45.0X6
Dramamine	T45.0X1	T45.0X2	T45.0X3	T45.0X4	T45.0X5	T45.0X6
Drano (drain cleaner)	T54.3X1	T54.3X2	T54.3X3	T54.3X4	—	—
Dressing, live pulp	T49.7X1	T49.7X2	T49.7X3	T49.7X4	T49.7X5	T49.7X6
Drocode	T40.2X1	T40.2X2	T40.2X3	T40.2X4	T40.2X5	T40.2X6
Dromoran	T40.2X1	T40.2X2	T40.2X3	T40.2X4	T40.2X5	T40.2X6
Dromostanolone	T38.7X1	T38.7X2	T38.7X3	T38.7X4	T38.7X5	T38.7X6
Dronabinol	T40.711	T40.712	T40.713	T40.714	T40.715	T40.716
Droperidol	T43.591	T43.592	T43.593	T43.594	T43.595	T43.596
Dropropizine	T48.3X1	T48.3X2	T48.3X3	T48.3X4	T48.3X5	T48.3X6
Drostanolone	T38.7X1	T38.7X2	T38.7X3	T38.7X4	T38.7X5	T38.7X6
Drotaverine	T44.3X1	T44.3X2	T44.3X3	T44.3X4	T44.3X5	T44.3X6
Drotrecogin alfa	T45.511	T45.512	T45.513	T45.514	T45.515	T45.516
Drug NEC	T50.901	T50.902	T50.903	T50.904	T50.905	T50.906
specified NEC	T50.991	T50.992	T50.993	T50.994	T50.995	T50.996
DTIC	T45.1X1	T45.1X2	T45.1X3	T45.1X4	T45.1X5	T45.1X6
Duboisine	T44.3X1	T44.3X2	T44.3X3	T44.3X4	T44.3X5	T44.3X6
Dulcolax	T47.2X1	T47.2X2	T47.2X3	T47.2X4	T47.2X5	T47.2X6
Duponol (C) (EP)	T49.2X1	T49.2X2	T49.2X3	T49.2X4	T49.2X5	T49.2X6
Durabolin	T38.7X1	T38.7X2	T38.7X3	T38.7X4	T38.7X5	T38.7X6
Durezol*	T49.5X1	T49.5X2	T49.5X3	T49.5X4	T49.5X5	T49.5X6
Dyclone	T41.3X1	T41.3X2	T41.3X3	T41.3X4	T41.3X5	T41.3X6
Dyclonine	T41.3X1	T41.3X2	T41.3X3	T41.3X4	T41.3X5	T41.3X6
Dydrogesterone	T38.5X1	T38.5X2	T38.5X3	T38.5X4	T38.5X5	T38.5X6
Dye NEC	T65.6X1	T65.6X2	T65.6X3	T65.6X4	—	—
antiseptic	T49.0X1	T49.0X2	T49.0X3	T49.0X4	T49.0X5	T49.0X6
diagnostic agents	T50.8X1	T50.8X2	T50.8X3	T50.8X4	T50.8X5	T50.8X6
pharmaceutical NEC	T50.901	T50.902	T50.903	T50.904	T50.905	T50.906
Dyflos	T44.0X1	T44.0X2	T44.0X3	T44.0X4	T44.0X5	T44.0X6
Dymelor	T38.3X1	T38.3X2	T38.3X3	T38.3X4	T38.3X5	T38.3X6
Dynamite	T65.3X1	T65.3X2	T65.3X3	T65.3X4	—	—
fumes	T59.891	T59.892	T59.893	T59.894	—	—
Dyphylline	T44.3X1	T44.3X2	T44.3X3	T44.3X4	T44.3X5	T44.3X6
b-eucaine	T49.1X1	T49.1X2	T49.1X3	T49.1X4	T49.1X5	T49.1X6
Ear drug NEC	T49.6X1	T49.6X2	T49.6X3	T49.6X4	T49.6X5	T49.6X6
Ear preparations	T49.6X1	T49.6X2	T49.6X3	T49.6X4	T49.6X5	T49.6X6
Echothiophate, echothiopate, ecothiopate	T49.5X1	T49.5X2	T49.5X3	T49.5X4	T49.5X5	T49.5X6
Econazole	T49.0X1	T49.0X2	T49.0X3	T49.0X4	T49.0X5	T49.0X6
Ecothiopate iodide	T49.5X1	T49.5X2	T49.5X3	T49.5X4	T49.5X5	T49.5X6
Ecstasy	T43.641	T43.642	T43.643	T43.644	—	—
Ectylurea	T42.6X1	T42.6X2	T42.6X3	T42.6X4	T42.6X5	T42.6X6
Edathamil disodium	T45.8X1	T45.8X2	T45.8X3	T45.8X4	T45.8X5	T45.8X6
Edecrin	T50.1X1	T50.1X2	T50.1X3	T50.1X4	T50.1X5	T50.1X6
Edetate, disodium (calcium)	T45.8X1	T45.8X2	T45.8X3	T45.8X4	T45.8X5	T45.8X6
Edoxudine	T49.5X1	T49.5X2	T49.5X3	T49.5X4	T49.5X5	T49.5X6
Edrophonium	T44.0X1	T44.0X2	T44.0X3	T44.0X4	T44.0X5	T44.0X6
chloride	T44.0X1	T44.0X2	T44.0X3	T44.0X4	T44.0X5	T44.0X6
EDTA	T50.6X1	T50.6X2	T50.6X3	T50.6X4	T50.6X5	T50.6X6
Eflornithine	T37.2X1	T37.2X2	T37.2X3	T37.2X4	T37.2X5	T37.2X6
Efloxate	T46.3X1	T46.3X2	T46.3X3	T46.3X4	T46.3X5	T46.3X6
Elase	T49.8X1	T49.8X2	T49.8X3	T49.8X4	T49.8X5	T49.8X6
Elastase	T47.5X1	T47.5X2	T47.5X3	T47.5X4	T47.5X5	T47.5X6
Elaterium	T47.2X1	T47.2X2	T47.2X3	T47.2X4	T47.2X5	T47.2X6
Elcatonin	T50.991	T50.992	T50.993	T50.994	T50.995	T50.996
Elder	T62.2X1	T62.2X2	T62.2X3	T62.2X4	—	—
berry, (unripe)	T62.1X1	T62.1X2	T62.1X3	T62.1X4	—	—
Electrolyte balance drug	T50.3X1	T50.3X2	T50.3X3	T50.3X4	T50.3X5	T50.3X6
Electrolytes NEC	T50.3X1	T50.3X2	T50.3X3	T50.3X4	T50.3X5	T50.3X6
Electrolytic agent NEC	T50.3X1	T50.3X2	T50.3X3	T50.3X4	T50.3X5	T50.3X6
Elemental diet	T50.901	T50.902	T50.903	T50.904	T50.905	T50.906
Elliptinium acetate	T45.1X1	T45.1X2	T45.1X3	T45.1X4	T45.1X5	T45.1X6
Elocon*	T49.0X1	T49.0X2	T49.0X3	T49.0X4	T49.0X5	T49.0X6
Embramine	T45.0X1	T45.0X2	T45.0X3	T45.0X4	T45.0X5	T45.0X6
Emepronium (salts)	T44.3X1	T44.3X2	T44.3X3	T44.3X4	T44.3X5	T44.3X6
bromide	T44.3X1	T44.3X2	T44.3X3	T44.3X4	T44.3X5	T44.3X6
Emetic NEC	T47.7X1	T47.7X2	T47.7X3	T47.7X4	T47.7X5	T47.7X6
Emetine	T37.3X1	T37.3X2	T37.3X3	T37.3X4	T37.3X5	T37.3X6
Emollient NEC	T49.3X1	T49.3X2	T49.3X3	T49.3X4	T49.3X5	T49.3X6
Emorfazone	T39.8X1	T39.8X2	T39.8X3	T39.8X4	T39.8X5	T39.8X6
Emylcamate	T43.591	T43.592	T43.593	T43.594	T43.595	T43.596
Enalapril	T46.4X1	T46.4X2	T46.4X3	T46.4X4	T46.4X5	T46.4X6

Substance	Poisoning, Accidental (unintentional)	Poisoning, Intentional Self-harm	Poisoning, Assault	Poisoning, Undetermined	Adverse Effect	Under-dosing
Enalaprilat	T46.4X1	T46.4X2	T46.4X3	T46.4X4	T46.4X5	T46.4X6
Enbrel*	T39.4X1	T39.4X2	T39.4X3	T39.4X4	T39.4X5	T39.4X6
Encainide	T46.2X1	T46.2X2	T46.2X3	T46.2X4	T46.2X5	T46.2X6
Endocaine	T41.3X1	T41.3X2	T41.3X3	T41.3X4	T41.3X5	T41.3X6
Endosulfan	T60.2X1	T60.2X2	T60.2X3	T60.2X4	—	—
Endothall	T60.3X1	T60.3X2	T60.3X3	T60.3X4	—	—
Endralazine	T46.5X1	T46.5X2	T46.5X3	T46.5X4	T46.5X5	T46.5X6
Endrin	T60.1X1	T60.1X2	T60.1X3	T60.1X4	—	—
Enflurane	T41.0X1	T41.0X2	T41.0X3	T41.0X4	T41.0X5	T41.0X6
Enfuvirtide*	T37.5X1	T37.5X2	T37.5X3	T37.5X4	T37.5X5	T37.5X6
Enhexymal	T42.3X1	T42.3X2	T42.3X3	T42.3X4	T42.3X5	T42.3X6
Enocitabine	T45.1X1	T45.1X2	T45.1X3	T45.1X4	T45.1X5	T45.1X6
Enovid	T38.4X1	T38.4X2	T38.4X3	T38.4X4	T38.4X5	T38.4X6
Enoxacin	T36.8X1	T36.8X2	T36.8X3	T36.8X4	T36.8X5	T36.8X6
Enoxaparin (sodium)	T45.511	T45.512	T45.513	T45.514	T45.515	T45.516
Enpiprazole	T43.591	T43.592	T43.593	T43.594	T43.595	T43.596
Enprofylline	T48.6X1	T48.6X2	T48.6X3	T48.6X4	T48.6X5	T48.6X6
Enprostil	T47.1X1	T47.1X2	T47.1X3	T47.1X4	T47.1X5	T47.1X6
Enterogastrone	T38.891	T38.892	T38.893	T38.894	T38.895	T38.896
ENT preparations (anti-infectives)	T49.6X1	T49.6X2	T49.6X3	T49.6X4	T49.6X5	T49.6X6
Enviomycin	T36.8X1	T36.8X2	T36.8X3	T36.8X4	T36.8X5	T36.8X6
Enzodase	T45.3X1	T45.3X2	T45.3X3	T45.3X4	T45.3X5	T45.3X6
Enzyme NEC	T45.3X1	T45.3X2	T45.3X3	T45.3X4	T45.3X5	T45.3X6
depolymerizing	T49.8X1	T49.8X2	T49.8X3	T49.8X4	T49.8X5	T49.8X6
fibrolytic	T45.3X1	T45.3X2	T45.3X3	T45.3X4	T45.3X5	T45.3X6
gastric	T47.5X1	T47.5X2	T47.5X3	T47.5X4	T47.5X5	T47.5X6
intestinal	T47.5X1	T47.5X2	T47.5X3	T47.5X4	T47.5X5	T47.5X6
local action	T49.4X1	T49.4X2	T49.4X3	T49.4X4	T49.4X5	T49.4X6
proteolytic	T49.4X1	T49.4X2	T49.4X3	T49.4X4	T49.4X5	T49.4X6
thrombolytic	T45.3X1	T45.3X2	T45.3X3	T45.3X4	T45.3X5	T45.3X6
EPAB	T41.3X1	T41.3X2	T41.3X3	T41.3X4	T41.3X5	T41.3X6
Epanutin	T42.0X1	T42.0X2	T42.0X3	T42.0X4	T42.0X5	T42.0X6
Ephedra	T44.991	T44.992	T44.993	T44.994	T44.995	T44.996
Ephedrine	T44.991	T44.992	T44.993	T44.994	T44.995	T44.996
Epichlorhydrin, epichlorohydrin	T52.8X1	T52.8X2	T52.8X3	T52.8X4	—	—
Epicillin	T36.0X1	T36.0X2	T36.0X3	T36.0X4	T36.0X5	T36.0X6
Epiestriol	T38.5X1	T38.5X2	T38.5X3	T38.5X4	T38.5X5	T38.5X6
Epilim — see Sodium, valproate						
Epimestrol	T38.5X1	T38.5X2	T38.5X3	T38.5X4	T38.5X5	T38.5X6
Epinephrine	T44.5X1	T44.5X2	T44.5X3	T44.5X4	T44.5X5	T44.5X6
EpiPen*	T44.5X1	T44.5X2	T44.5X3	T44.5X4	T44.5X5	T44.5X6
Epirubicin	T45.1X1	T45.1X2	T45.1X3	T45.1X4	T45.1X5	T45.1X6
Epitiostanol	T38.7X1	T38.7X2	T38.7X3	T38.7X4	T38.7X5	T38.7X6
Epitizide	T50.2X1	T50.2X2	T50.2X3	T50.2X4	T50.2X5	T50.2X6
EPN	T60.0X1	T60.0X2	T60.0X3	T60.0X4	—	—
EPO	T45.8X1	T45.8X2	T45.8X3	T45.8X4	T45.8X5	T45.8X6
Epoetin alpha	T45.8X1	T45.8X2	T45.8X3	T45.8X4	T45.8X5	T45.8X6
Epomediol	T50.991	T50.992	T50.993	T50.994	T50.995	T50.996
Epoprostenol	T45.521	T45.522	T45.523	T45.524	T45.525	T45.526
Epoxy resin	T65.891	T65.892	T65.893	T65.894	—	—
Eprazinone	T48.4X1	T48.4X2	T48.4X3	T48.4X4	T48.4X5	T48.4X6
Epsilon aminocaproic acid	T45.621	T45.622	T45.623	T45.624	T45.625	T45.626
Epsom salt	T47.3X1	T47.3X2	T47.3X3	T47.3X4	T47.3X5	T47.3X6
Eptazocine	T40.491	T40.492	T40.493	T40.494	T40.495	T40.496
Equanil	T43.591	T43.592	T43.593	T43.594	T43.595	T43.596
Equisetum	T62.2X1	T62.2X2	T62.2X3	T62.2X4	—	—
diuretic	T50.2X1	T50.2X2	T50.2X3	T50.2X4	T50.2X5	T50.2X6
Ergobasine	T48.0X1	T48.0X2	T48.0X3	T48.0X4	T48.0X5	T48.0X6
Ergocalciferol	T45.2X1	T45.2X2	T45.2X3	T45.2X4	T45.2X5	T45.2X6
Ergoloid mesylates	T46.7X1	T46.7X2	T46.7X3	T46.7X4	T46.7X5	T46.7X6
Ergometrine	T48.0X1	T48.0X2	T48.0X3	T48.0X4	T48.0X5	T48.0X6
Ergonovine	T48.0X1	T48.0X2	T48.0X3	T48.0X4	T48.0X5	T48.0X6
Ergotamine	T46.5X1	T46.5X2	T46.5X3	T46.5X4	T46.5X5	T46.5X6
Ergotocine	T48.0X1	T48.0X2	T48.0X3	T48.0X4	T48.0X5	T48.0X6
Ergotrate	T48.0X1	T48.0X2	T48.0X3	T48.0X4	T48.0X5	T48.0X6
Ergot NEC	T64.81	T64.82	T64.83	T64.84	—	—
derivative	T48.0X1	T48.0X2	T48.0X3	T48.0X4	T48.0X5	T48.0X6
medicinal (alkaloids)	T48.0X1	T48.0X2	T48.0X3	T48.0X4	T48.0X5	T48.0X6
prepared	T48.0X1	T48.0X2	T48.0X3	T48.0X4	T48.0X5	T48.0X6
Eritrityl tetranitrate	T46.3X1	T46.3X2	T46.3X3	T46.3X4	T46.3X5	T46.3X6
Erythrityl tetranitrate	T46.3X1	T46.3X2	T46.3X3	T46.3X4	T46.3X5	T46.3X6
Erythrol tetranitrate	T46.3X1	T46.3X2	T46.3X3	T46.3X4	T46.3X5	T46.3X6
Erythromycin (salts)	T36.3X1	T36.3X2	T36.3X3	T36.3X4	T36.3X5	T36.3X6
ophthalmic preparation	T49.5X1	T49.5X2	T49.5X3	T49.5X4	T49.5X5	T49.5X6
topical NEC	T49.0X1	T49.0X2	T49.0X3	T49.0X4	T49.0X5	T49.0X6
Erythropoietin	T45.8X1	T45.8X2	T45.8X3	T45.8X4	T45.8X5	T45.8X6
human	T45.8X1	T45.8X2	T45.8X3	T45.8X4	T45.8X5	T45.8X6
Esbriet*	T48.991	T48.992	T48.993	T48.994	T48.995	T48.996
Escin	T46.991	T46.992	T46.993	T46.994	T46.995	T46.996
Esculin	T45.2X1	T45.2X2	T45.2X3	T45.2X4	T45.2X5	T45.2X6
Esculoside	T45.2X1	T45.2X2	T45.2X3	T45.2X4	T45.2X5	T45.2X6
ESDT (ether-soluble tar distillate)	T49.1X1	T49.1X2	T49.1X3	T49.1X4	T49.1X5	T49.1X6
Eserine	T49.5X1	T49.5X2	T49.5X3	T49.5X4	T49.5X5	T49.5X6
Esflurbiprofen	T39.311	T39.312	T39.313	T39.314	T39.315	T39.316
Eskabarb	T42.3X1	T42.3X2	T42.3X3	T42.3X4	T42.3X5	T42.3X6
Eskalith	T43.8X1	T43.8X2	T43.8X3	T43.8X4	T43.8X5	T43.8X6
Esmolol	T44.7X1	T44.7X2	T44.7X3	T44.7X4	T44.7X5	T44.7X6
Estanozolol	T38.7X1	T38.7X2	T38.7X3	T38.7X4	T38.7X5	T38.7X6
Estazolam	T42.4X1	T42.4X2	T42.4X3	T42.4X4	T42.4X5	T42.4X6
Estradiol	T38.5X1	T38.5X2	T38.5X3	T38.5X4	T38.5X5	T38.5X6
with testosterone	T38.7X1	T38.7X2	T38.7X3	T38.7X4	T38.7X5	T38.7X6
benzoate	T38.5X1	T38.5X2	T38.5X3	T38.5X4	T38.5X5	T38.5X6
Estramustine	T45.1X1	T45.1X2	T45.1X3	T45.1X4	T45.1X5	T45.1X6
Estriol	T38.5X1	T38.5X2	T38.5X3	T38.5X4	T38.5X5	T38.5X6
Estrogen	T38.5X1	T38.5X2	T38.5X3	T38.5X4	T38.5X5	T38.5X6
with progesterone	T38.5X1	T38.5X2	T38.5X3	T38.5X4	T38.5X5	T38.5X6
conjugated	T38.5X1	T38.5X2	T38.5X3	T38.5X4	T38.5X5	T38.5X6
Estrone	T38.5X1	T38.5X2	T38.5X3	T38.5X4	T38.5X5	T38.5X6
Estropipate	T38.5X1	T38.5X2	T38.5X3	T38.5X4	T38.5X5	T38.5X6
Etacrynate sodium	T50.1X1	T50.1X2	T50.1X3	T50.1X4	T50.1X5	T50.1X6
Etacrynic acid	T50.1X1	T50.1X2	T50.1X3	T50.1X4	T50.1X5	T50.1X6
Etafedrine	T48.6X1	T48.6X2	T48.6X3	T48.6X4	T48.6X5	T48.6X6
Etafenone	T46.3X1	T46.3X2	T46.3X3	T46.3X4	T46.3X5	T46.3X6
Etambutol	T37.1X1	T37.1X2	T37.1X3	T37.1X4	T37.1X5	T37.1X6
Etamiphyllin	T48.6X1	T48.6X2	T48.6X3	T48.6X4	T48.6X5	T48.6X6
Etamivan	T50.7X1	T50.7X2	T50.7X3	T50.7X4	T50.7X5	T50.7X6
Etamsylate	T45.7X1	T45.7X2	T45.7X3	T45.7X4	T45.7X5	T45.7X6
Etebenecid	T50.4X1	T50.4X2	T50.4X3	T50.4X4	T50.4X5	T50.4X6
Ethacridine	T49.0X1	T49.0X2	T49.0X3	T49.0X4	T49.0X5	T49.0X6
Ethacrynate*	T50.1X1	T50.1X2	T50.1X3	T50.1X4	T50.1X5	T50.1X6
Ethacrynic acid	T50.1X1	T50.1X2	T50.1X3	T50.1X4	T50.1X5	T50.1X6
Ethadione	T42.2X1	T42.2X2	T42.2X3	T42.2X4	T42.2X5	T42.2X6
Ethambutol	T37.1X1	T37.1X2	T37.1X3	T37.1X4	T37.1X5	T37.1X6
Ethamide	T50.2X1	T50.2X2	T50.2X3	T50.2X4	T50.2X5	T50.2X6
Ethamivan	T50.7X1	T50.7X2	T50.7X3	T50.7X4	T50.7X5	T50.7X6
Ethamsylate	T45.7X1	T45.7X2	T45.7X3	T45.7X4	T45.7X5	T45.7X6
Ethanol	T51.0X1	T51.0X2	T51.0X3	T51.0X4	—	—
beverage	T51.0X1	T51.0X2	T51.0X3	T51.0X4	—	—
Ethanolamine oleate	T46.8X1	T46.8X2	T46.8X3	T46.8X4	T46.8X5	T46.8X6
Ethaverine	T44.3X1	T44.3X2	T44.3X3	T44.3X4	T44.3X5	T44.3X6
Ethchlorvynol	T42.6X1	T42.6X2	T42.6X3	T42.6X4	T42.6X5	T42.6X6
Ethebenecid	T50.4X1	T50.4X2	T50.4X3	T50.4X4	T50.4X5	T50.4X6
Ether (vapor)	T41.0X1	T41.0X2	T41.0X3	T41.0X4	T41.0X5	T41.0X6
anesthetic	T41.0X1	T41.0X2	T41.0X3	T41.0X4	T41.0X5	T41.0X6
divinyl	T41.0X1	T41.0X2	T41.0X3	T41.0X4	T41.0X5	T41.0X6
ethyl (medicinal)	T41.0X1	T41.0X2	T41.0X3	T41.0X4	T41.0X5	T41.0X6
nonmedicinal	T52.8X1	T52.8X2	T52.8X3	T52.8X4	—	—
petroleum — see Ligroin						
solvent	T52.8X1	T52.8X2	T52.8X3	T52.8X4	—	—
Ethiazide	T50.2X1	T50.2X2	T50.2X3	T50.2X4	T50.2X5	T50.2X6
Ethidium chloride (vapor)	T59.891	T59.892	T59.893	T59.894	—	—
Ethinamate	T42.6X1	T42.6X2	T42.6X3	T42.6X4	T42.6X5	T42.6X6
Ethinylestradiol, ethinyloestradiol with	T38.5X1	T38.5X2	T38.5X3	T38.5X4	T38.5X5	T38.5X6
levonorgestrel	T38.4X1	T38.4X2	T38.4X3	T38.4X4	T38.4X5	T38.4X6
norethisterone	T38.4X1	T38.4X2	T38.4X3	T38.4X4	T38.4X5	T38.4X6
Ethiodized oil (131 I)	T50.8X1	T50.8X2	T50.8X3	T50.8X4	T50.8X5	T50.8X6
Ethiofos*	T50.991	T50.992	T50.993	T50.994	T50.995	T50.996
Ethion	T60.0X1	T60.0X2	T60.0X3	T60.0X4	—	—
Ethionamide	T37.1X1	T37.1X2	T37.1X3	T37.1X4	T37.1X5	T37.1X6
Ethioniamide	T37.1X1	T37.1X2	T37.1X3	T37.1X4	T37.1X5	T37.1X6
Ethisterone	T38.5X1	T38.5X2	T38.5X3	T38.5X4	T38.5X5	T38.5X6
Ethobral	T42.3X1	T42.3X2	T42.3X3	T42.3X4	T42.3X5	T42.3X6
Ethocaine (infiltration) (topical)	T41.3X1	T41.3X2	T41.3X3	T41.3X4	T41.3X5	T41.3X6
nerve block (peripheral) (plexus)	T41.3X1	T41.3X2	T41.3X3	T41.3X4	T41.3X5	T41.3X6
spinal	T41.3X1	T41.3X2	T41.3X3	T41.3X4	T41.3X5	T41.3X6
Ethoheptazine	T40.491	T40.492	T40.493	T40.494	T40.495	T40.496
Ethopropazine	T44.3X1	T44.3X2	T44.3X3	T44.3X4	T44.3X5	T44.3X6
Ethosuximide	T42.2X1	T42.2X2	T42.2X3	T42.2X4	T42.2X5	T42.2X6
Ethotoin	T42.0X1	T42.0X2	T42.0X3	T42.0X4	T42.0X5	T42.0X6
Ethoxazene	T37.91	T37.92	T37.93	T37.94	T37.95	T37.96
Ethoxazorutoside	T46.991	T46.992	T46.993	T46.994	T46.995	T46.996
Ethoxzolamide	T50.2X1	T50.2X2	T50.2X3	T50.2X4	T50.2X5	T50.2X6
Ethyl						
acetate	T52.8X1	T52.8X2	T52.8X3	T52.8X4	—	—
alcohol	T51.0X1	T51.0X2	T51.0X3	T51.0X4	—	—
beverage	T51.0X1	T51.0X2	T51.0X3	T51.0X4	—	—
aldehyde (vapor)	T59.891	T59.892	T59.893	T59.894	—	—
liquid	T52.8X1	T52.8X2	T52.8X3	T52.8X4	—	—
aminobenzoate	T41.3X1	T41.3X2	T41.3X3	T41.3X4	T41.3X5	T41.3X6

Substance	Poisoning, Accidental (unintentional)	Poisoning, Intentional Self-harm	Poisoning, Assault	Poisoning, Undetermined	Adverse Effect	Under-dosing
Ethyl — *continued*						
aminophenothiazine	T43.3X1	T43.3X2	T43.3X3	T43.3X4	T43.3X5	T43.3X6
benzoate	T52.8X1	T52.8X2	T52.8X3	T52.8X4	—	—
biscoumacetate	T45.511	T45.512	T45.513	T45.514	T45.515	T45.516
bromide (anesthetic)	T41.0X1	T41.0X2	T41.0X3	T41.0X4	T41.0X5	T41.0X6
carbamate	T45.1X1	T45.1X2	T45.1X3	T45.1X4	T45.1X5	T45.1X6
carbinol	T51.3X1	T51.3X2	T51.3X3	T51.3X4	—	—
carbonate	T52.8X1	T52.8X2	T52.8X3	T52.8X4	—	—
chaulmoograte	T37.1X1	T37.1X2	T37.1X3	T37.1X4	T37.1X5	T37.1X6
chloride (anesthetic)	T41.0X1	T41.0X2	T41.0X3	T41.0X4	T41.0X5	T41.0X6
anesthetic (local)	T41.3X1	T41.3X2	T41.3X3	T41.3X4	T41.3X5	T41.3X6
inhaled	T41.0X1	T41.0X2	T41.0X3	T41.0X4	T41.0X5	T41.0X6
local	T49.4X1	T49.4X2	T49.4X3	T49.4X4	T49.4X5	T49.4X6
solvent	T53.6X1	T53.6X2	T53.6X3	T53.6X4	—	—
dibunate	T48.3X1	T48.3X2	T48.3X3	T48.3X4	T48.3X5	T48.3X6
dichloroarsine (vapor)	T57.0X1	T57.0X2	T57.0X3	T57.0X4	—	—
estranol	T38.7X1	T38.7X2	T38.7X3	T38.7X4	T38.7X5	T38.7X6
ether — *see also* ether						
formate NEC (solvent)	T52.0X1	T52.0X2	T52.0X3	T52.0X4	—	—
fumarate	T49.4X1	T49.4X2	T49.4X3	T49.4X4	T49.4X5	T49.4X6
hydroxyisobutyrate NEC (solvent)	T52.8X1	T52.8X2	T52.8X3	T52.8X4	—	—
iodoacetate	T59.3X1	T59.3X2	T59.3X3	T59.3X4	—	—
lactate NEC (solvent)	T52.8X1	T52.8X2	T52.8X3	T52.8X4	—	—
loflazepate	T42.4X1	T42.4X2	T42.4X3	T42.4X4	T42.4X5	T42.4X6
mercuric chloride	T56.1X1	T56.1X2	T56.1X3	T56.1X4	—	—
methylcarbinol	T51.8X1	T51.8X2	T51.8X3	T51.8X4	—	—
morphine	T40.2X1	T40.2X2	T40.2X3	T40.2X4	T40.2X5	T40.2X6
noradrenaline	T48.6X1	T48.6X2	T48.6X3	T48.6X4	T48.6X5	T48.6X6
oxybutyrate NEC (solvent)	T52.8X1	T52.8X2	T52.8X3	T52.8X4	—	—
Ethylene (gas)	T59.891	T59.892	T59.893	T59.894	—	—
anesthetic (general)	T41.0X1	T41.0X2	T41.0X3	T41.0X4	T41.0X5	T41.0X6
chlorohydrin	T52.8X1	T52.8X2	T52.8X3	T52.8X4	—	—
vapor	T53.6X1	T53.6X2	T53.6X3	T53.6X4	—	—
dichloride	T52.8X1	T52.8X2	T52.8X3	T52.8X4	—	—
vapor	T53.6X1	T53.6X2	T53.6X3	T53.6X4	—	—
dinitrate	T52.3X1	T52.3X2	T52.3X3	T52.3X4	—	—
glycol(s)	T52.8X1	T52.8X2	T52.8X3	T52.8X4	—	—
dinitrate	T52.3X1	T52.3X2	T52.3X3	T52.3X4	—	—
monobutyl ether	T52.3X1	T52.3X2	T52.3X3	T52.3X4	—	—
imine	T54.1X1	T54.1X2	T54.1X3	T54.1X4	—	—
oxide (fumigant) (nonmedicinal)	T59.891	T59.892	T59.893	T59.894	—	—
medicinal	T49.0X1	T49.0X2	T49.0X3	T49.0X4	T49.0X5	T49.0X6
Ethylenediaminetetra-acetic acid	T50.6X1	T50.6X2	T50.6X3	T50.6X4	T50.6X5	T50.6X6
Ethylenediamine theophylline	T48.6X1	T48.6X2	T48.6X3	T48.6X4	T48.6X5	T48.6X6
Ethylenedinitrilotetra-acetate	T50.6X1	T50.6X2	T50.6X3	T50.6X4	T50.6X5	T50.6X6
Ethylestrenol	T38.7X1	T38.7X2	T38.7X3	T38.7X4	T38.7X5	T38.7X6
Ethylhydroxycellulose	T47.4X1	T47.4X2	T47.4X3	T47.4X4	T47.4X5	T47.4X6
Ethylidene						
chloride NEC	T53.6X1	T53.6X2	T53.6X3	T53.6X4	—	—
diacetate	T60.3X1	T60.3X2	T60.3X3	T60.3X4	—	—
dicoumarin	T45.511	T45.512	T45.513	T45.514	T45.515	T45.516
dicoumarol	T45.511	T45.512	T45.513	T45.514	T45.515	T45.516
diethyl ether	T52.0X1	T52.0X2	T52.0X3	T52.0X4	—	—
Ethylmorphine	T40.2X1	T40.2X2	T40.2X3	T40.2X4	T40.2X5	T40.2X6
Ethylnorepinephrine	T48.6X1	T48.6X2	T48.6X3	T48.6X4	T48.6X5	T48.6X6
Ethylparachlorophen-oxyisobutyrate	T46.6X1	T46.6X2	T46.6X3	T46.6X4	T46.6X5	T46.6X6
Ethynodiol	T38.4X1	T38.4X2	T38.4X3	T38.4X4	T38.4X5	T38.4X6
with mestranol diacetate	T38.4X1	T38.4X2	T38.4X3	T38.4X4	T38.4X5	T38.4X6
Ethyol*	T50.991	T50.992	T50.993	T50.994	T50.995	T50.996
Etidocaine	T41.3X1	T41.3X2	T41.3X3	T41.3X4	T41.3X5	T41.3X6
infiltration (subcutaneous)	T41.3X1	T41.3X2	T41.3X3	T41.3X4	T41.3X5	T41.3X6
nerve (peripheral) (plexus)	T41.3X1	T41.3X2	T41.3X3	T41.3X4	T41.3X5	T41.3X6
Etidronate	T50.991	T50.992	T50.993	T50.994	T50.995	T50.996
Etidronic acid (disodium salt)	T50.991	T50.992	T50.993	T50.994	T50.995	T50.996
Etifoxine	T42.6X1	T42.6X2	T42.6X3	T42.6X4	T42.6X5	T42.6X6
Etilefrine	T44.4X1	T44.4X2	T44.4X3	T44.4X4	T44.4X5	T44.4X6
Etilfen	T42.3X1	T42.3X2	T42.3X3	T42.3X4	T42.3X5	T42.3X6
Etinodiol	T38.4X1	T38.4X2	T38.4X3	T38.4X4	T38.4X5	T38.4X6
Etiroxate	T46.6X1	T46.6X2	T46.6X3	T46.6X4	T46.6X5	T46.6X6
Etizolam	T42.4X1	T42.4X2	T42.4X3	T42.4X4	T42.4X5	T42.4X6
Etodolac	T39.391	T39.392	T39.393	T39.394	T39.395	T39.396
Etofamide	T37.3X1	T37.3X2	T37.3X3	T37.3X4	T37.3X5	T37.3X6
Etofibrate	T46.6X1	T46.6X2	T46.6X3	T46.6X4	T46.6X5	T46.6X6
Etofylline	T46.7X1	T46.7X2	T46.7X3	T46.7X4	T46.7X5	T46.7X6
clofibrate	T46.6X1	T46.6X2	T46.6X3	T46.6X4	T46.6X5	T46.6X6
Etoglucid	T45.1X1	T45.1X2	T45.1X3	T45.1X4	T45.1X5	T45.1X6
Etomidate	T41.1X1	T41.1X2	T41.1X3	T41.1X4	T41.1X5	T41.1X6
Etomide	T39.8X1	T39.8X2	T39.8X3	T39.8X4	T39.8X5	T39.8X6
Etomidoline	T44.3X1	T44.3X2	T44.3X3	T44.3X4	T44.3X5	T44.3X6
Etoposide	T45.1X1	T45.1X2	T45.1X3	T45.1X4	T45.1X5	T45.1X6
Etorphine	T40.2X1	T40.2X2	T40.2X3	T40.2X4	T40.2X5	T40.2X6
Etoval	T42.3X1	T42.3X2	T42.3X3	T42.3X4	T42.3X5	T42.3X6
Etozolin	T50.1X1	T50.1X2	T50.1X3	T50.1X4	T50.1X5	T50.1X6
Etravirine*	T37.5X1	T37.5X2	T37.5X3	T37.5X4	T37.5X5	T37.5X6
Etretinate	T50.991	T50.992	T50.993	T50.994	T50.995	T50.996
Etryptamine	T43.691	T43.692	T43.693	T43.694	T43.695	T43.696
Etybenzatropine	T44.3X1	T44.3X2	T44.3X3	T44.3X4	T44.3X5	T44.3X6
Etynodiol	T38.4X1	T38.4X2	T38.4X3	T38.4X4	T38.4X5	T38.4X6
Eucaine	T41.3X1	T41.3X2	T41.3X3	T41.3X4	T41.3X5	T41.3X6
Eucalyptus oil	T49.7X1	T49.7X2	T49.7X3	T49.7X4	T49.7X5	T49.7X6
Eucatropine	T49.5X1	T49.5X2	T49.5X3	T49.5X4	T49.5X5	T49.5X6
Eucodal	T40.2X1	T40.2X2	T40.2X3	T40.2X4	T40.2X5	T40.2X6
Euneryl	T42.3X1	T42.3X2	T42.3X3	T42.3X4	T42.3X5	T42.3X6
Euphthalmine	T44.3X1	T44.3X2	T44.3X3	T44.3X4	T44.3X5	T44.3X6
Eurax	T49.0X1	T49.0X2	T49.0X3	T49.0X4	T49.0X5	T49.0X6
Euresol	T49.4X1	T49.4X2	T49.4X3	T49.4X4	T49.4X5	T49.4X6
Euthroid	T38.1X1	T38.1X2	T38.1X3	T38.1X4	T38.1X5	T38.1X6
Evans blue	T50.8X1	T50.8X2	T50.8X3	T50.8X4	T50.8X5	T50.8X6
Evipal	T42.3X1	T42.3X2	T42.3X3	T42.3X4	T42.3X5	T42.3X6
sodium	T41.1X1	T41.1X2	T41.1X3	T41.1X4	T41.1X5	T41.1X6
Evipan	T42.3X1	T42.3X2	T42.3X3	T42.3X4	T42.3X5	T42.3X6
sodium	T41.1X1	T41.1X2	T41.1X3	T41.1X4	T41.1X5	T41.1X6
Exalamide	T49.0X1	T49.0X2	T49.0X3	T49.0X4	T49.0X5	T49.0X6
Exalgin	T39.1X1	T39.1X2	T39.1X3	T39.1X4	T39.1X5	T39.1X6
Excipients, pharmaceutical	T50.901	T50.902	T50.903	T50.904	T50.905	T50.906
Exhaust gas (engine) (motor vehicle)	T58.01	T58.02	T58.03	T58.04	—	—
Ex-Lax (phenolphthalein)	T47.2X1	T47.2X2	T47.2X3	T47.2X4	T47.2X5	T47.2X6
Expectorant NEC	T48.4X1	T48.4X2	T48.4X3	T48.4X4	T48.4X5	T48.4X6
Extended insulin zinc suspension	T38.3X1	T38.3X2	T38.3X3	T38.3X4	T38.3X5	T38.3X6
External medications (skin) (mucous membrane)	T49.91	T49.92	T49.93	T49.94	T49.95	T49.96
dental agent	T49.7X1	T49.7X2	T49.7X3	T49.7X4	T49.7X5	T49.7X6
ENT agent	T49.6X1	T49.6X2	T49.6X3	T49.6X4	T49.6X5	T49.6X6
ophthalmic preparation	T49.5X1	T49.5X2	T49.5X3	T49.5X4	T49.5X5	T49.5X6
specified NEC	T49.8X1	T49.8X2	T49.8X3	T49.8X4	T49.8X5	T49.8X6
Extina*	T49.0X1	T49.0X2	T49.0X3	T49.0X4	T49.0X5	T49.0X6
Extrapyramidal antagonist NEC	T44.3X1	T44.3X2	T44.3X3	T44.3X4	T44.3X5	T44.3X6
Eye agents (anti-infective)	T49.5X1	T49.5X2	T49.5X3	T49.5X4	T49.5X5	T49.5X6
Eye drug NEC	T49.5X1	T49.5X2	T49.5X3	T49.5X4	T49.5X5	T49.5X6
FAC (fluorouracil + doxorubicin + cyclophosphamide)	T45.1X1	T45.1X2	T45.1X3	T45.1X4	T45.1X5	T45.1X6
Factor						
I (fibrinogen)	T45.8X1	T45.8X2	T45.8X3	T45.8X4	T45.8X5	T45.8X6
III (thromboplastin)	T45.8X1	T45.8X2	T45.8X3	T45.8X4	T45.8X5	T45.8X6
IX complex	T45.7X1	T45.7X2	T45.7X3	T45.7X4	T45.7X5	T45.7X6
human	T45.8X1	T45.8X2	T45.8X3	T45.8X4	T45.8X5	T45.8X6
VIII (antihemophilic Factor) (concentrate)	T45.8X1	T45.8X2	T45.8X3	T45.8X4	T45.8X5	T45.8X6
Famotidine	T47.0X1	T47.0X2	T47.0X3	T47.0X4	T47.0X5	T47.0X6
Fat suspension, intravenous	T50.991	T50.992	T50.993	T50.994	T50.995	T50.996
Fazadinium bromide	T48.1X1	T48.1X2	T48.1X3	T48.1X4	T48.1X5	T48.1X6
Febarbamate	T42.3X1	T42.3X2	T42.3X3	T42.3X4	T42.3X5	T42.3X6
Fecal softener	T47.4X1	T47.4X2	T47.4X3	T47.4X4	T47.4X5	T47.4X6
Fedrilate	T48.3X1	T48.3X2	T48.3X3	T48.3X4	T48.3X5	T48.3X6
Felodipine	T46.1X1	T46.1X2	T46.1X3	T46.1X4	T46.1X5	T46.1X6
Felypressin	T38.891	T38.892	T38.893	T38.894	T38.895	T38.896
Femizol*	T49.0X1	T49.0X2	T49.0X3	T49.0X4	T49.0X5	T49.0X6
Femoxetine	T43.221	T43.222	T43.223	T43.224	T43.225	T43.226
Fenalcomine	T46.3X1	T46.3X2	T46.3X3	T46.3X4	T46.3X5	T46.3X6
Fenamisal	T37.1X1	T37.1X2	T37.1X3	T37.1X4	T37.1X5	T37.1X6
Fenazone	T39.2X1	T39.2X2	T39.2X3	T39.2X4	T39.2X5	T39.2X6
Fenbendazole	T37.4X1	T37.4X2	T37.4X3	T37.4X4	T37.4X5	T37.4X6
Fenbutrazate	T50.5X1	T50.5X2	T50.5X3	T50.5X4	T50.5X5	T50.5X6
Fencamfamine	T43.691	T43.692	T43.693	T43.694	T43.695	T43.696
Fendiline	T46.1X1	T46.1X2	T46.1X3	T46.1X4	T46.1X5	T46.1X6
Fenetylline	T43.691	T43.692	T43.693	T43.694	T43.695	T43.696
Fenflumizole	T39.391	T39.392	T39.393	T39.394	T39.395	T39.396
Fenfluramine	T50.5X1	T50.5X2	T50.5X3	T50.5X4	T50.5X5	T50.5X6
Fenobarbital	T42.3X1	T42.3X2	T42.3X3	T42.3X4	T42.3X5	T42.3X6
Fenofibrate	T46.6X1	T46.6X2	T46.6X3	T46.6X4	T46.6X5	T46.6X6
Fenoprofen	T39.311	T39.312	T39.313	T39.314	T39.315	T39.316
Fenoterol	T48.6X1	T48.6X2	T48.6X3	T48.6X4	T48.6X5	T48.6X6
Fenoverine	T44.3X1	T44.3X2	T44.3X3	T44.3X4	T44.3X5	T44.3X6
Fenoxazoline	T48.5X1	T48.5X2	T48.5X3	T48.5X4	T48.5X5	T48.5X6
Fenproporex	T50.5X1	T50.5X2	T50.5X3	T50.5X4	T50.5X5	T50.5X6

Substance	Poisoning, Accidental (unintentional)	Poisoning, Intentional Self-harm	Poisoning, Assault	Poisoning, Undetermined	Adverse Effect	Under-dosing
Fenquizone	T50.2X1	T50.2X2	T50.2X3	T50.2X4	T50.2X5	T50.2X6
Fentanyl (analogs)	T40.411	T40.412	T40.413	T40.414	T40.415	T40.416
Fentazin	T43.3X1	T43.3X2	T43.3X3	T43.3X4	T43.3X5	T43.3X6
Fenthion	T60.0X1	T60.0X2	T60.0X3	T60.0X4	—	—
Fenticlor	T49.0X1	T49.0X2	T49.0X3	T49.0X4	T49.0X5	T49.0X6
Fenylbutazone	T39.2X1	T39.2X2	T39.2X3	T39.2X4	T39.2X5	T39.2X6
Feprazone	T39.2X1	T39.2X2	T39.2X3	T39.2X4	T39.2X5	T39.2X6
Fer de lance (bite) (venom)	T63.061	T63.062	T63.063	T63.064	—	—
Ferrex*	T45.4X1	T45.4X2	T45.4X3	T45.4X4	T45.4X5	T45.4X6
Ferric — see also Iron						
chloride	T45.4X1	T45.4X2	T45.4X3	T45.4X4	T45.4X5	T45.4X6
citrate	T45.4X1	T45.4X2	T45.4X3	T45.4X4	T45.4X5	T45.4X6
hydroxide						
colloidal	T45.4X1	T45.4X2	T45.4X3	T45.4X4	T45.4X5	T45.4X6
polymaltose	T45.4X1	T45.4X2	T45.4X3	T45.4X4	T45.4X5	T45.4X6
pyrophosphate	T45.4X1	T45.4X2	T45.4X3	T45.4X4	T45.4X5	T45.4X6
Ferritin	T45.4X1	T45.4X2	T45.4X3	T45.4X4	T45.4X5	T45.4X6
Ferrocholinate	T45.4X1	T45.4X2	T45.4X3	T45.4X4	T45.4X5	T45.4X6
Ferrodextrane	T45.4X1	T45.4X2	T45.4X3	T45.4X4	T45.4X5	T45.4X6
Ferropolimaler	T45.4X1	T45.4X2	T45.4X3	T45.4X4	T45.4X5	T45.4X6
Ferrous — see also Iron						
phosphate	T45.4X1	T45.4X2	T45.4X3	T45.4X4	T45.4X5	T45.4X6
salt	T45.4X1	T45.4X2	T45.4X3	T45.4X4	T45.4X5	T45.4X6
with folic acid	T45.4X1	T45.4X2	T45.4X3	T45.4X4	T45.4X5	T45.4X6
Ferrous fumerate, gluconate, lactate, salt NEC, sulfate (medicinal)	T45.4X1	T45.4X2	T45.4X3	T45.4X4	T45.4X5	T45.4X6
Ferrovanadium (fumes)	T59.891	T59.892	T59.893	T59.894	—	—
Ferrum — see Iron						
Fertilizers NEC	T65.891	T65.892	T65.893	T65.894	—	—
with herbicide mixture	T60.3X1	T60.3X2	T60.3X3	T60.3X4	—	—
Fetoxilate	T47.6X1	T47.6X2	T47.6X3	T47.6X4	T47.6X5	T47.6X6
Fiber, dietary	T47.4X1	T47.4X2	T47.4X3	T47.4X4	T47.4X5	T47.4X6
Fiberglass	T65.831	T65.832	T65.833	T65.834	—	—
Fibrinogen (human)	T45.8X1	T45.8X2	T45.8X3	T45.8X4	T45.8X5	T45.8X6
Fibrinolysin (human)	T45.691	T45.692	T45.693	T45.694	T45.695	T45.696
Fibrinolysis						
affecting drug	T45.601	T45.602	T45.603	T45.604	T45.605	T45.606
inhibitor NEC	T45.621	T45.622	T45.623	T45.624	T45.625	T45.626
Fibrinolytic drug	T45.611	T45.612	T45.613	T45.614	T45.615	T45.616
Filix mas	T37.4X1	T37.4X2	T37.4X3	T37.4X4	T37.4X5	T37.4X6
Filtering cream	T49.3X1	T49.3X2	T49.3X3	T49.3X4	T49.3X5	T49.3X6
Finacea*	T49.0X1	T49.0X2	T49.0X3	T49.0X4	T49.0X5	T49.0X6
Fiorinal	T39.011	T39.012	T39.013	T39.014	T39.015	T39.016
Firedamp	T59.891	T59.892	T59.893	T59.894	—	—
Fish, noxious, nonbacterial	T61.91	T61.92	T61.93	T61.94	—	—
ciguatera	T61.01	T61.02	T61.03	T61.04	—	—
scombroid	T61.11	T61.12	T61.13	T61.14	—	—
shell	T61.781	T61.782	T61.783	T61.784	—	—
specified NEC	T61.771	T61.772	T61.773	T61.774	—	—
Flagyl	T37.3X1	T37.3X2	T37.3X3	T37.3X4	T37.3X5	T37.3X6
Flavine adenine dinucleotide	T45.2X1	T45.2X2	T45.2X3	T45.2X4	T45.2X5	T45.2X6
Flavodic acid	T46.991	T46.992	T46.993	T46.994	T46.995	T46.996
Flavoxate	T44.3X1	T44.3X2	T44.3X3	T44.3X4	T44.3X5	T44.3X6
Flaxedil	T48.1X1	T48.1X2	T48.1X3	T48.1X4	T48.1X5	T48.1X6
Flaxseed (medicinal)	T49.3X1	T49.3X2	T49.3X3	T49.3X4	T49.3X5	T49.3X6
Flecainide	T46.2X1	T46.2X2	T46.2X3	T46.2X4	T46.2X5	T46.2X6
Fleroxacin	T36.8X1	T36.8X2	T36.8X3	T36.8X4	T36.8X5	T36.8X6
Floctafenine	T39.8X1	T39.8X2	T39.8X3	T39.8X4	T39.8X5	T39.8X6
Flomax	T44.6X1	T44.6X2	T44.6X3	T44.6X4	T44.6X5	T44.6X6
Flomoxef	T36.1X1	T36.1X2	T36.1X3	T36.1X4	T36.1X5	T36.1X6
Flopropione	T44.3X1	T44.3X2	T44.3X3	T44.3X4	T44.3X5	T44.3X6
FLORAjen*	T47.6X1	T47.6X2	T47.6X3	T47.6X4	T47.6X5	T47.6X6
Florantyrone	T47.5X1	T47.5X2	T47.5X3	T47.5X4	T47.5X5	T47.5X6
Floraquin	T37.8X1	T37.8X2	T37.8X3	T37.8X4	T37.8X5	T37.8X6
Florinef	T38.0X1	T38.0X2	T38.0X3	T38.0X4	T38.0X5	T38.0X6
ENT agent	T49.6X1	T49.6X2	T49.6X3	T49.6X4	T49.6X5	T49.6X6
ophthalmic preparation	T49.5X1	T49.5X2	T49.5X3	T49.5X4	T49.5X5	T49.5X6
topical NEC	T49.0X1	T49.0X2	T49.0X3	T49.0X4	T49.0X5	T49.0X6
Flowers of sulfur	T49.4X1	T49.4X2	T49.4X3	T49.4X4	T49.4X5	T49.4X6
Floxuridine	T45.1X1	T45.1X2	T45.1X3	T45.1X4	T45.1X5	T45.1X6
Fluanisone	T43.4X1	T43.4X2	T43.4X3	T43.4X4	T43.4X5	T43.4X6
Flubendazole	T37.4X1	T37.4X2	T37.4X3	T37.4X4	T37.4X5	T37.4X6
Fluclorolone acetonide	T49.0X1	T49.0X2	T49.0X3	T49.0X4	T49.0X5	T49.0X6
Flucloxacillin	T36.0X1	T36.0X2	T36.0X3	T36.0X4	T36.0X5	T36.0X6
Fluconazole	T37.8X1	T37.8X2	T37.8X3	T37.8X4	T37.8X5	T37.8X6
Flucytosine	T37.8X1	T37.8X2	T37.8X3	T37.8X4	T37.8X5	T37.8X6
Fludeoxyglucose (18F)	T50.8X1	T50.8X2	T50.8X3	T50.8X4	T50.8X5	T50.8X6
Fludiazepam	T42.4X1	T42.4X2	T42.4X3	T42.4X4	T42.4X5	T42.4X6
Fludrocortisone	T50.0X1	T50.0X2	T50.0X3	T50.0X4	T50.0X5	T50.0X6
ENT agent	T49.6X1	T49.6X2	T49.6X3	T49.6X4	T49.6X5	T49.6X6
Fludrocortisone — continued						
ophthalmic preparation	T49.5X1	T49.5X2	T49.5X3	T49.5X4	T49.5X5	T49.5X6
topical NEC	T49.0X1	T49.0X2	T49.0X3	T49.0X4	T49.0X5	T49.0X6
Fludroxycortide	T49.0X1	T49.0X2	T49.0X3	T49.0X4	T49.0X5	T49.0X6
Flufenamic acid	T39.391	T39.392	T39.393	T39.394	T39.395	T39.396
Fluindione	T45.511	T45.512	T45.513	T45.514	T45.515	T45.516
Flumequine	T37.8X1	T37.8X2	T37.8X3	T37.8X4	T37.8X5	T37.8X6
Flumethasone	T49.0X1	T49.0X2	T49.0X3	T49.0X4	T49.0X5	T49.0X6
Flumethiazide	T50.2X1	T50.2X2	T50.2X3	T50.2X4	T50.2X5	T50.2X6
Flumidin	T37.5X1	T37.5X2	T37.5X3	T37.5X4	T37.5X5	T37.5X6
Flunarizine	T46.7X1	T46.7X2	T46.7X3	T46.7X4	T46.7X5	T46.7X6
Flunidazole	T37.8X1	T37.8X2	T37.8X3	T37.8X4	T37.8X5	T37.8X6
Flunisolide	T48.6X1	T48.6X2	T48.6X3	T48.6X4	T48.6X5	T48.6X6
Flunitrazepam	T42.4X1	T42.4X2	T42.4X3	T42.4X4	T42.4X5	T42.4X6
Fluocinolone (acetonide)	T49.0X1	T49.0X2	T49.0X3	T49.0X4	T49.0X5	T49.0X6
Fluocinonide	T49.0X1	T49.0X2	T49.0X3	T49.0X4	T49.0X5	T49.0X6
Fluocortin (butyl)	T49.0X1	T49.0X2	T49.0X3	T49.0X4	T49.0X5	T49.0X6
Fluocortolone	T49.0X1	T49.0X2	T49.0X3	T49.0X4	T49.0X5	T49.0X6
Fluohydrocortisone	T38.0X1	T38.0X2	T38.0X3	T38.0X4	T38.0X5	T38.0X6
ENT agent	T49.6X1	T49.6X2	T49.6X3	T49.6X4	T49.6X5	T49.6X6
ophthalmic preparation	T49.5X1	T49.5X2	T49.5X3	T49.5X4	T49.5X5	T49.5X6
topical NEC	T49.0X1	T49.0X2	T49.0X3	T49.0X4	T49.0X5	T49.0X6
Fluonid	T49.0X1	T49.0X2	T49.0X3	T49.0X4	T49.0X5	T49.0X6
Fluopromazine	T43.3X1	T43.3X2	T43.3X3	T43.3X4	T43.3X5	T43.3X6
Fluoracetate	T60.8X1	T60.8X2	T60.8X3	T60.8X4	—	—
Fluorescein	T50.8X1	T50.8X2	T50.8X3	T50.8X4	T50.8X5	T50.8X6
Fluorhydrocortisone	T50.0X1	T50.0X2	T50.0X3	T50.0X4	T50.0X5	T50.0X6
Fluoride (nonmedicinal) (pesticide) (sodium) NEC	T60.8X1	T60.8X2	T60.8X3	T60.8X4	—	—
hydrogen — see Hydrofluoric acid						
medicinal NEC	T50.991	T50.992	T50.993	T50.994	T50.995	T50.996
dental use	T49.7X1	T49.7X2	T49.7X3	T49.7X4	T49.7X5	T49.7X6
not pesticide NEC	T54.91	T54.92	T54.93	T54.94		
stannous	T49.7X1	T49.7X2	T49.7X3	T49.7X4	T49.7X5	T49.7X6
Fluorigard*	T47.7X1	T47.7X2	T47.7X3	T47.7X4	T47.7X5	T47.7X6
Fluorinated corticosteroids	T38.0X1	T38.0X2	T38.0X3	T38.0X4	T38.0X5	T38.0X6
Fluorine (gas)	T59.5X1	T59.5X2	T59.5X3	T59.5X4	—	—
salt — see Fluoride(s)						
Fluoristan	T49.7X1	T49.7X2	T49.7X3	T49.7X4	T49.7X5	T49.7X6
Fluormetholone	T49.0X1	T49.0X2	T49.0X3	T49.0X4	T49.0X5	T49.0X6
Fluoroacetate	T60.8X1	T60.8X2	T60.8X3	T60.8X4	—	—
Fluorocarbon monomer	T53.6X1	T53.6X2	T53.6X3	T53.6X4	—	—
Fluorocytosine	T37.8X1	T37.8X2	T37.8X3	T37.8X4	T37.8X5	T37.8X6
Fluorodeoxyuridine	T45.1X1	T45.1X2	T45.1X3	T45.1X4	T45.1X5	T45.1X6
Fluorometholone	T49.0X1	T49.0X2	T49.0X3	T49.0X4	T49.0X5	T49.0X6
ophthalmic preparation	T49.5X1	T49.5X2	T49.5X3	T49.5X4	T49.5X5	T49.5X6
Fluorophosphate insecticide	T60.0X1	T60.0X2	T60.0X3	T60.0X4	—	—
Fluorosol	T46.3X1	T46.3X2	T46.3X3	T46.3X4	T46.3X5	T46.3X6
Fluorouracil	T45.1X1	T45.1X2	T45.1X3	T45.1X4	T45.1X5	T45.1X6
Fluorphenylalanine	T49.5X1	T49.5X2	T49.5X3	T49.5X4	T49.5X5	T49.5X6
Fluothane	T41.0X1	T41.0X2	T41.0X3	T41.0X4	T41.0X5	T41.0X6
Fluoxetine	T43.221	T43.222	T43.223	T43.224	T43.225	T43.226
Fluoxymesterone	T38.7X1	T38.7X2	T38.7X3	T38.7X4	T38.7X5	T38.7X6
Flupenthixol	T43.4X1	T43.4X2	T43.4X3	T43.4X4	T43.4X5	T43.4X6
Flupentixol	T43.4X1	T43.4X2	T43.4X3	T43.4X4	T43.4X5	T43.4X6
Fluphenazine	T43.3X1	T43.3X2	T43.3X3	T43.3X4	T43.3X5	T43.3X6
Fluprednidene	T49.0X1	T49.0X2	T49.0X3	T49.0X4	T49.0X5	T49.0X6
Fluprednisolone	T38.0X1	T38.0X2	T38.0X3	T38.0X4	T38.0X5	T38.0X6
Fluradoline	T39.8X1	T39.8X2	T39.8X3	T39.8X4	T39.8X5	T39.8X6
Flurandrenolide	T49.0X1	T49.0X2	T49.0X3	T49.0X4	T49.0X5	T49.0X6
Flurandrenolone	T49.0X1	T49.0X2	T49.0X3	T49.0X4	T49.0X5	T49.0X6
Flurazepam	T42.4X1	T42.4X2	T42.4X3	T42.4X4	T42.4X5	T42.4X6
Flurbiprofen	T39.311	T39.312	T39.313	T39.314	T39.315	T39.316
Flurobate	T49.0X1	T49.0X2	T49.0X3	T49.0X4	T49.0X5	T49.0X6
Fluroxene	T41.0X1	T41.0X2	T41.0X3	T41.0X4	T41.0X5	T41.0X6
Fluspirilene	T43.591	T43.592	T43.593	T43.594	T43.595	T43.596
Flutamide	T38.6X1	T38.6X2	T38.6X3	T38.6X4	T38.6X5	T38.6X6
Flutazolam	T38.0X1	T38.0X2	T38.0X3	T38.0X4	T38.0X5	T38.0X6
Fluticasone propionate	T38.0X1	T38.0X2	T38.0X3	T38.0X4	T38.0X5	T38.0X6
Flutoprazepam	T42.4X1	T42.4X2	T42.4X3	T42.4X4	T42.4X5	T42.4X6
Flutropium bromide	T48.6X1	T48.6X2	T48.6X3	T48.6X4	T48.6X5	T48.6X6
Fluvoxamine	T43.221	T43.222	T43.223	T43.224	T43.225	T43.226
Folacin	T45.8X1	T45.8X2	T45.8X3	T45.8X4	T45.8X5	T45.8X6
Folic acid	T45.8X1	T45.8X2	T45.8X3	T45.8X4	T45.8X5	T45.8X6
with ferrous salt	T45.2X1	T45.2X2	T45.2X3	T45.2X4	T45.2X5	T45.2X6
antagonist	T45.1X1	T45.1X2	T45.1X3	T45.1X4	T45.1X5	T45.1X6
Folinic acid	T45.8X1	T45.8X2	T45.8X3	T45.8X4	T45.8X5	T45.8X6
Folium stramoniae	T48.6X1	T48.6X2	T48.6X3	T48.6X4	T48.6X5	T48.6X6
Follicle-stimulating hormone, human	T38.811	T38.812	T38.813	T38.814	T38.815	T38.816

Substance	Poisoning, Accidental (unintentional)	Poisoning, Intentional Self-harm	Poisoning, Assault	Poisoning, Undetermined	Adverse Effect	Underdosing
Folpet	T60.3X1	T60.3X2	T60.3X3	T60.3X4	—	—
Fomepizole*	T50.6X1	T50.6X2	T50.6X3	T50.6X4	T50.6X5	T50.6X6
Fominoben	T48.3X1	T48.3X2	T48.3X3	T48.3X4	T48.3X5	T48.3X6
Food, foodstuffs, noxious, nonbacterial, NEC	T62.91	T62.92	T62.93	T62.94	—	—
berries	T62.1X1	T62.1X2	T62.1X3	T62.1X4	—	—
fish — see also Fish	T61.91	T61.92	T61.93	T61.94	—	—
mushrooms	T62.0X1	T62.0X2	T62.0X3	T62.0X4	—	—
plants	T62.2X1	T62.2X2	T62.2X3	T62.2X4	—	—
seafood	T61.91	T61.92	T61.93	T61.94	—	—
specified NEC	T61.8X1	T61.8X2	T61.8X3	T61.8X4	—	—
seeds	T62.2X1	T62.2X2	T62.2X3	T62.2X4	—	—
shellfish	T61.781	T61.782	T61.783	T61.784	—	—
specified NEC	T62.8X1	T62.8X2	T62.8X3	T62.8X4	—	—
Fool's parsley	T62.2X1	T62.2X2	T62.2X3	T62.2X4	—	—
Formaldehyde (solution), gas or vapor	T59.2X1	T59.2X2	T59.2X3	T59.2X4	—	—
fungicide	T60.3X1	T60.3X2	T60.3X3	T60.3X4	—	—
Formalin	T59.2X1	T59.2X2	T59.2X3	T59.2X4	—	—
fungicide	T60.3X1	T60.3X2	T60.3X3	T60.3X4	—	—
vapor	T59.2X1	T59.2X2	T59.2X3	T59.2X4	—	—
Formic acid	T54.2X1	T54.2X2	T54.2X3	T54.2X4	—	—
vapor	T59.891	T59.892	T59.893	T59.894	—	—
Formoterol*	T48.6X1	T48.6X2	T48.6X3	T48.6X4	T48.6X5	T48.6X6
Fortaz*	T36.1X1	T36.1X2	T36.1X3	T36.1X4	T36.1X5	T36.1X6
Foscarnet sodium	T37.5X1	T37.5X2	T37.5X3	T37.5X4	T37.5X5	T37.5X6
Fosfestrol	T38.5X1	T38.5X2	T38.5X3	T38.5X4	T38.5X5	T38.5X6
Fosfomycin	T36.8X1	T36.8X2	T36.8X3	T36.8X4	T36.8X5	T36.8X6
Fosfonet sodium	T37.5X1	T37.5X2	T37.5X3	T37.5X4	T37.5X5	T37.5X6
Fosinopril	T46.4X1	T46.4X2	T46.4X3	T46.4X4	T46.4X5	T46.4X6
sodium	T46.4X1	T46.4X2	T46.4X3	T46.4X4	T46.4X5	T46.4X6
Fowler's solution	T57.0X1	T57.0X2	T57.0X3	T57.0X4	—	—
Foxglove	T62.2X1	T62.2X2	T62.2X3	T62.2X4	—	—
Framycetin	T36.5X1	T36.5X2	T36.5X3	T36.5X4	T36.5X5	T36.5X6
Frangula	T47.2X1	T47.2X2	T47.2X3	T47.2X4	T47.2X5	T47.2X6
extract	T47.2X1	T47.2X2	T47.2X3	T47.2X4	T47.2X5	T47.2X6
Frei antigen	T50.8X1	T50.8X2	T50.8X3	T50.8X4	T50.8X5	T50.8X6
Freon	T53.5X1	T53.5X2	T53.5X3	T53.5X4	—	—
Fructose	T50.3X1	T50.3X2	T50.3X3	T50.3X4	T50.3X5	T50.3X6
Frusemide	T50.1X1	T50.1X2	T50.1X3	T50.1X4	T50.1X5	T50.1X6
FSH	T38.811	T38.812	T38.813	T38.814	T38.815	T38.816
Ftorafur	T45.1X1	T45.1X2	T45.1X3	T45.1X4	T45.1X5	T45.1X6
Fuel						
automobile	T52.0X1	T52.0X2	T52.0X3	T52.0X4	—	—
exhaust gas, not in transit	T58.01	T58.02	T58.03	T58.04	—	—
vapor NEC	T52.0X1	T52.0X2	T52.0X3	T52.0X4	—	—
gas (domestic use) — see also Carbon, monoxide, fuel, utility	T59.891	T59.892	T59.893	T59.894	—	—
utility	T59.891	T59.892	T59.893	T59.894	—	—
incomplete combustion of — see Carbon, monoxide, fuel, utility						
in mobile container	T59.891	T59.892	T59.893	T59.894	—	—
piped (natural)	T59.891	T59.892	T59.893	T59.894	—	—
industrial, incomplete combustion	T58.8X1	T58.8X2	T58.8X3	T58.8X4	—	—
Fugillin	T36.8X1	T36.8X2	T36.8X3	T36.8X4	T36.8X5	T36.8X6
Fulminate of mercury	T56.1X1	T56.1X2	T56.1X3	T56.1X4	—	—
Fulvicin	T36.7X1	T36.7X2	T36.7X3	T36.7X4	T36.7X5	T36.7X6
Fumadil	T36.8X1	T36.8X2	T36.8X3	T36.8X4	T36.8X5	T36.8X6
Fumagillin	T36.8X1	T36.8X2	T36.8X3	T36.8X4	T36.8X5	T36.8X6
Fumaric acid	T49.4X1	T49.4X2	T49.4X3	T49.4X4	T49.4X5	T49.4X6
Fumes (from)	T59.91	T59.92	T59.93	T59.94	—	—
carbon monoxide — see Carbon, monoxide						
charcoal (domestic use) — see Charcoal, fumes						
chloroform — see Chloroform						
coke (in domestic stoves, fireplaces) — see Coke fumes						
corrosive NEC	T54.91	T54.92	T54.93	T54.94	—	—
ether — see ether						
freons	T53.5X1	T53.5X2	T53.5X3	T53.5X4	—	—
hydrocarbons	T59.891	T59.892	T59.893	T59.894	—	—
petroleum (liquefied)	T59.891	T59.892	T59.893	T59.894	—	—
distributed through pipes (pure or mixed with air)	T59.891	T59.892	T59.893	T59.894	—	—
lead — see lead						
Fumes — continued						
metal — see Metals, or the specified metal						
nitrogen dioxide	T59.0X1	T59.0X2	T59.0X3	T59.0X4	—	—
pesticides — see Pesticide						
petroleum (liquefied)	T59.891	T59.892	T59.893	T59.894	—	—
distributed through pipes (pure or mixed with air)	T59.891	T59.892	T59.893	T59.894	—	—
polyester	T59.891	T59.892	T59.893	T59.894	—	—
specified source NEC — see also substance specified	T59.891	T59.892	T59.893	T59.894	—	—
sulfur dioxide	T59.1X1	T59.1X2	T59.1X3	T59.1X4	—	—
Fumigant NEC	T60.91	T60.92	T60.93	T60.94	—	—
Fungicide NEC (nonmedicinal)	T60.3X1	T60.3X2	T60.3X3	T60.3X4	—	—
Fungi, noxious, used as food	T62.0X1	T62.0X2	T62.0X3	T62.0X4	—	—
Fungizone	T36.7X1	T36.7X2	T36.7X3	T36.7X4	T36.7X5	T36.7X6
topical	T49.0X1	T49.0X2	T49.0X3	T49.0X4	T49.0X5	T49.0X6
Fungoid*	T49.0X1	T49.0X2	T49.0X3	T49.0X4	T49.0X5	T49.0X6
Furacin	T49.0X1	T49.0X2	T49.0X3	T49.0X4	T49.0X5	T49.0X6
Furadantin	T37.91	T37.92	T37.93	T37.94	T37.95	T37.96
Furazolidone	T37.8X1	T37.8X2	T37.8X3	T37.8X4	T37.8X5	T37.8X6
Furazolium chloride	T49.0X1	T49.0X2	T49.0X3	T49.0X4	T49.0X5	T49.0X6
Furfural	T52.8X1	T52.8X2	T52.8X3	T52.8X4	—	—
Furfural	T52.8X1	T52.8X2	T52.8X3	T52.8X4	—	—
Furnace (coal burning) (domestic), gas from	T58.2X1	T58.2X2	T58.2X3	T58.2X4	—	—
industrial	T58.8X1	T58.8X2	T58.8X3	T58.8X4	—	—
Furniture polish	T65.891	T65.892	T65.893	T65.894	—	—
Furosemide	T50.1X1	T50.1X2	T50.1X3	T50.1X4	T50.1X5	T50.1X6
Furoxone	T37.91	T37.92	T37.93	T37.94	T37.95	T37.96
Fursultiamine	T45.2X1	T45.2X2	T45.2X3	T45.2X4	T45.2X5	T45.2X6
Fusafungine	T36.8X1	T36.8X2	T36.8X3	T36.8X4	T36.8X5	T36.8X6
Fusel oil (any) (amyl) (butyl) (propyl), vapor	T51.3X1	T51.3X2	T51.3X3	T51.3X4	—	—
Fusidate (ethanolamine) (sodium)	T36.8X1	T36.8X2	T36.8X3	T36.8X4	T36.8X5	T36.8X6
Fusidic acid	T36.8X1	T36.8X2	T36.8X3	T36.8X4	T36.8X5	T36.8X6
Fytic acid, nonasodium	T50.6X1	T50.6X2	T50.6X3	T50.6X4	T50.6X5	T50.6X6
b-Galactosidase	T47.5X1	T47.5X2	T47.5X3	T47.5X4	T47.5X5	T47.5X6
GABA	T43.8X1	T43.8X2	T43.8X3	T43.8X4	T43.8X5	T43.8X6
Gabitril*	T42.6X1	T42.6X2	T42.6X3	T42.6X4	T42.6X5	T42.6X6
Gadopentetic acid	T50.8X1	T50.8X2	T50.8X3	T50.8X4	T50.8X5	T50.8X6
Galactose	T50.3X1	T50.3X2	T50.3X3	T50.3X4	T50.3X5	T50.3X6
Galantamine	T44.0X1	T44.0X2	T44.0X3	T44.0X4	T44.0X5	T44.0X6
Gallamine (triethiodide)	T48.1X1	T48.1X2	T48.1X3	T48.1X4	T48.1X5	T48.1X6
Gallium citrate	T50.991	T50.992	T50.993	T50.994	T50.995	T50.996
Gallopamil	T46.1X1	T46.1X2	T46.1X3	T46.1X4	T46.1X5	T46.1X6
Gamboge	T47.2X1	T47.2X2	T47.2X3	T47.2X4	T47.2X5	T47.2X6
Gamimune	T50.Z11	T50.Z12	T50.Z13	T50.Z14	T50.Z15	T50.Z16
Gamma-aminobutyric acid	T43.8X1	T43.8X2	T43.8X3	T43.8X4	T43.8X5	T43.8X6
Gamma-benzene hexachloride (medicinal)	T49.0X1	T49.0X2	T49.0X3	T49.0X4	T49.0X5	T49.0X6
nonmedicinal, vapor	T53.6X1	T53.6X2	T53.6X3	T53.6X4	—	—
Gamma-BHC (medicinal) — see also Gamma-benzene hexachloride	T49.0X1	T49.0X2	T49.0X3	T49.0X4	T49.0X5	T49.0X6
Gamma globulin	T50.Z11	T50.Z12	T50.Z13	T50.Z14	T50.Z15	T50.Z16
Gamulin	T50.Z11	T50.Z12	T50.Z13	T50.Z14	T50.Z15	T50.Z16
Ganciclovir (sodium)	T37.5X1	T37.5X2	T37.5X3	T37.5X4	T37.5X5	T37.5X6
Ganglionic blocking drug NEC	T44.2X1	T44.2X2	T44.2X3	T44.2X4	T44.2X5	T44.2X6
specified NEC	T44.2X1	T44.2X2	T44.2X3	T44.2X4	T44.2X5	T44.2X6
Ganja	T40.711	T40.712	T40.713	T40.714	T40.715	T40.716
Garamycin	T36.5X1	T36.5X2	T36.5X3	T36.5X4	T36.5X5	T36.5X6
ophthalmic preparation	T49.5X1	T49.5X2	T49.5X3	T49.5X4	T49.5X5	T49.5X6
topical NEC	T49.0X1	T49.0X2	T49.0X3	T49.0X4	T49.0X5	T49.0X6
Gardenal	T42.3X1	T42.3X2	T42.3X3	T42.3X4	T42.3X5	T42.3X6
Gardepanyl	T42.3X1	T42.3X2	T42.3X3	T42.3X4	T42.3X5	T42.3X6
Gaseous substance — see Gas						
Gasoline	T52.0X1	T52.0X2	T52.0X3	T52.0X4	—	—
vapor	T52.0X1	T52.0X2	T52.0X3	T52.0X4	—	—
Gastric enzymes	T47.5X1	T47.5X2	T47.5X3	T47.5X4	T47.5X5	T47.5X6
Gastrografin	T50.8X1	T50.8X2	T50.8X3	T50.8X4	T50.8X5	T50.8X6
Gastrointestinal drug	T47.91	T47.92	T47.93	T47.94	T47.95	T47.96
biological	T47.8X1	T47.8X2	T47.8X3	T47.8X4	T47.8X5	T47.8X6
specified NEC	T47.8X1	T47.8X2	T47.8X3	T47.8X4	T47.8X5	T47.8X6
Gas NEC	T59.91	T59.92	T59.93	T59.94	—	—
acetylene	T59.891	T59.892	T59.893	T59.894	—	—
incomplete combustion of	T58.11	T58.12	T58.13	T58.14	—	—

☑ Additional Character May Be Required — Refer to the Tabular List for Character Selection

*Optum Value-Add

Substance	Poisoning, Accidental (unintentional)	Poisoning, Intentional Self-harm	Poisoning, Assault	Poisoning, Undetermined	Adverse Effect	Under-dosing
Gas — *continued*						
air contaminants, source or type not specified	T59.91	T59.92	T59.93	T59.94	—	—
anesthetic	T41.0X1	T41.0X2	T41.0X3	T41.0X4	T41.0X5	T41.0X6
blast furnace	T58.8X1	T58.8X2	T58.8X3	T58.8X4	—	—
butane — *see* butane						
carbon monoxide — *see* Carbon, monoxide						
chlorine	T59.4X1	T59.4X2	T59.4X3	T59.4X4	—	—
coal	T58.2X1	T58.2X2	T58.2X3	T58.2X4	—	—
cyanide	T57.3X1	T57.3X2	T57.3X3	T57.3X4	—	—
dicyanogen	T65.0X1	T65.0X2	T65.0X3	T65.0X4	—	—
domestic — *see* Domestic gas						
exhaust	T58.01	T58.02	T58.03	T58.04		
from utility (for cooking, heating, or lighting) (after combustion) — *see* Carbon, monoxide, fuel, utility						
prior to combustion	T59.891	T59.892	T59.893	T59.894	—	—
from wood- or coal-burning stove or fireplace	T58.2X1	T58.2X2	T58.2X3	T58.2X4	—	—
fuel (domestic use) (after combustion) — *see also* Carbon, monoxide, fuel						
industrial use	T58.8X1	T58.8X2	T58.8X3	T58.8X4	—	—
prior to combustion	T59.891	T59.892	T59.893	T59.894	—	—
utility	T59.891	T59.892	T59.893	T59.894	—	—
incomplete combustion of — *see* Carbon, monoxide, fuel, utility						
in mobile container	T59.891	T59.892	T59.893	T59.894	—	—
piped (natural)	T59.891	T59.892	T59.893	T59.894	—	—
garage	T58.01	T58.02	T58.03	T58.04	—	—
hydrocarbon NEC	T59.891	T59.892	T59.893	T59.894	—	—
incomplete combustion of — *see* Carbon, monoxide, fuel, utility						
liquefied — *see* butane						
piped	T59.891	T59.892	T59.893	T59.894	—	—
hydrocyanic acid	T65.0X1	T65.0X2	T65.0X3	T65.0X4	—	—
illuminating (after combustion)	T58.11	T58.12	T58.13	T58.14	—	—
prior to combustion	T59.891	T59.892	T59.893	T59.894	—	—
incomplete combustion, any — *see* Carbon, monoxide						
kiln	T58.8X1	T58.8X2	T58.8X3	T58.8X4	—	—
lacrimogenic	T59.3X1	T59.3X2	T59.3X3	T59.3X4	—	—
liquefied petroleum — *see* butane						
marsh	T59.891	T59.892	T59.893	T59.894	—	—
motor exhaust, not in transit	T58.01	T58.02	T58.03	T58.04	—	—
mustard, not in war	T59.891	T59.892	T59.893	T59.894	—	—
natural	T59.891	T59.892	T59.893	T59.894	—	—
nerve, not in war	T59.91	T59.92	T59.93	T59.94	—	—
oil	T52.0X1	T52.0X2	T52.0X3	T52.0X4	—	—
petroleum (liquefied) (distributed in mobile containers)	T59.891	T59.892	T59.893	T59.894	—	—
piped (pure or mixed with air)	T59.891	T59.892	T59.893	T59.894	—	—
piped (manufactured) (natural) NEC	T59.891	T59.892	T59.893	T59.894	—	—
producer	T58.8X1	T58.8X2	T58.8X3	T58.8X4	—	—
propane — *see* propane						
refrigerant (chlorofluoro-carbon)	T53.5X1	T53.5X2	T53.5X3	T53.5X4	—	—
not chlorofluoro-carbon	T59.891	T59.892	T59.893	T59.894	—	—
sewer	T59.91	T59.92	T59.93	T59.94	—	—
specified source NEC	T59.91	T59.92	T59.93	T59.94	—	—
stove (after combustion)	T58.11	T58.12	T58.13	T58.14	—	—
prior to combustion	T59.891	T59.892	T59.893	T59.894	—	—
tear	T59.3X1	T59.3X2	T59.3X3	T59.3X4	—	—
therapeutic	T41.5X1	T41.5X2	T41.5X3	T41.5X4	T41.5X5	T41.5X6
utility (for cooking, heating, or lighting) (piped) NEC	T59.891	T59.892	T59.893	T59.894	—	—
incomplete combustion of — *see* Carbon, monoxide, fuel, utility						
in mobile container	T59.891	T59.892	T59.893	T59.894	—	—
piped (natural)	T59.891	T59.892	T59.893	T59.894	—	—
water	T58.11	T58.12	T58.13	T58.14		
Gas — *continued*						
water — *continued*						
incomplete combustion of — *see* Carbon, monoxide, fuel, utility						
Gaultheria procumbens	T62.2X1	T62.2X2	T62.2X3	T62.2X4	—	—
Gaviscon*	T47.1X1	T47.1X2	T47.1X3	T47.1X4	T47.1X5	T47.1X6
Gefarnate	T44.3X1	T44.3X2	T44.3X3	T44.3X4	T44.3X5	T44.3X6
Gelatin (intravenous)	T45.8X1	T45.8X2	T45.8X3	T45.8X4	T45.8X5	T45.8X6
absorbable (sponge)	T45.7X1	T45.7X2	T45.7X3	T45.7X4	T45.7X5	T45.7X6
Gelfilm	T49.8X1	T49.8X2	T49.8X3	T49.8X4	T49.8X5	T49.8X6
Gelfoam	T45.7X1	T45.7X2	T45.7X3	T45.7X4	T45.7X5	T45.7X6
Gelsemine	T50.991	T50.992	T50.993	T50.994	T50.995	T50.996
Gelsemium (sempervirens)	T62.2X1	T62.2X2	T62.2X3	T62.2X4	—	—
Gemeprost	T48.0X1	T48.0X2	T48.0X3	T48.0X4	T48.0X5	T48.0X6
Gemfibrozil	T46.6X1	T46.6X2	T46.6X3	T46.6X4	T46.6X5	T46.6X6
Gemonil	T42.3X1	T42.3X2	T42.3X3	T42.3X4	T42.3X5	T42.3X6
Gentamicin	T36.5X1	T36.5X2	T36.5X3	T36.5X4	T36.5X5	T36.5X6
ophthalmic preparation	T49.5X1	T49.5X2	T49.5X3	T49.5X4	T49.5X5	T49.5X6
topical NEC	T49.0X1	T49.0X2	T49.0X3	T49.0X4	T49.0X5	T49.0X6
Gentasol*	T49.5X1	T49.5X2	T49.5X3	T49.5X4	T49.5X5	T49.5X6
Gentian	T47.5X1	T47.5X2	T47.5X3	T47.5X4	T47.5X5	T47.5X6
violet	T49.0X1	T49.0X2	T49.0X3	T49.0X4	T49.0X5	T49.0X6
Gepefrine	T44.4X1	T44.4X2	T44.4X3	T44.4X4	T44.4X5	T44.4X6
Gestonorone caproate	T38.5X1	T38.5X2	T38.5X3	T38.5X4	T38.5X5	T38.5X6
Gexane	T49.0X1	T49.0X2	T49.0X3	T49.0X4	T49.0X5	T49.0X6
Gila monster (venom)	T63.111	T63.112	T63.113	T63.114	—	—
Ginger	T47.5X1	T47.5X2	T47.5X3	T47.5X4	T47.5X5	T47.5X6
Jamaica — *see* Jamaica, ginger						
Gitalin	T46.0X1	T46.0X2	T46.0X3	T46.0X4	T46.0X5	T46.0X6
amorphous	T46.0X1	T46.0X2	T46.0X3	T46.0X4	T46.0X5	T46.0X6
Gitaloxin	T46.0X1	T46.0X2	T46.0X3	T46.0X4	T46.0X5	T46.0X6
Gitoxin	T46.0X1	T46.0X2	T46.0X3	T46.0X4	T46.0X5	T46.0X6
Glafenine	T39.8X1	T39.8X2	T39.8X3	T39.8X4	T39.8X5	T39.8X6
Glandular extract (medicinal) NEC	T50.Z91	T50.Z92	T50.Z93	T50.Z94	T50.Z95	T50.Z96
Glaucarubin	T37.3X1	T37.3X2	T37.3X3	T37.3X4	T37.3X5	T37.3X6
Glibenclamide	T38.3X1	T38.3X2	T38.3X3	T38.3X4	T38.3X5	T38.3X6
Glibornuride	T38.3X1	T38.3X2	T38.3X3	T38.3X4	T38.3X5	T38.3X6
Gliclazide	T38.3X1	T38.3X2	T38.3X3	T38.3X4	T38.3X5	T38.3X6
Glimidine	T38.3X1	T38.3X2	T38.3X3	T38.3X4	T38.3X5	T38.3X6
Glipizide	T38.3X1	T38.3X2	T38.3X3	T38.3X4	T38.3X5	T38.3X6
Gliquidone	T38.3X1	T38.3X2	T38.3X3	T38.3X4	T38.3X5	T38.3X6
Glisolamide	T38.3X1	T38.3X2	T38.3X3	T38.3X4	T38.3X5	T38.3X6
Glisoxepide	T38.3X1	T38.3X2	T38.3X3	T38.3X4	T38.3X5	T38.3X6
Globin zinc insulin	T38.3X1	T38.3X2	T38.3X3	T38.3X4	T38.3X5	T38.3X6
Globulin						
antilymphocytic	T50.Z11	T50.Z12	T50.Z13	T50.Z14	T50.Z15	T50.Z16
antirhesus	T50.Z11	T50.Z12	T50.Z13	T50.Z14	T50.Z15	T50.Z16
antivenin	T50.Z11	T50.Z12	T50.Z13	T50.Z14	T50.Z15	T50.Z16
antiviral	T50.Z11	T50.Z12	T50.Z13	T50.Z14	T50.Z15	T50.Z16
Glucagon	T38.3X1	T38.3X2	T38.3X3	T38.3X4	T38.3X5	T38.3X6
Glucocorticoids	T38.0X1	T38.0X2	T38.0X3	T38.0X4	T38.0X5	T38.0X6
Glucocorticosteroid	T38.0X1	T38.0X2	T38.0X3	T38.0X4	T38.0X5	T38.0X6
Gluconic acid	T50.991	T50.992	T50.993	T50.994	T50.995	T50.996
Glucosamine sulfate	T39.4X1	T39.4X2	T39.4X3	T39.4X4	T39.4X5	T39.4X6
Glucose	T50.3X1	T50.3X2	T50.3X3	T50.3X4	T50.3X5	T50.3X6
with sodium chloride	T50.3X1	T50.3X2	T50.3X3	T50.3X4	T50.3X5	T50.3X6
Glucosulfone sodium	T37.1X1	T37.1X2	T37.1X3	T37.1X4	T37.1X5	T37.1X6
Glucotrol*	T38.3X1	T38.3X2	T38.3X3	T38.3X4	T38.3X5	T38.3X6
Glucurolactone	T47.8X1	T47.8X2	T47.8X3	T47.8X4	T47.8X5	T47.8X6
Glue NEC	T52.8X1	T52.8X2	T52.8X3	T52.8X4	—	—
Glutamic acid	T47.5X1	T47.5X2	T47.5X3	T47.5X4	T47.5X5	T47.5X6
Glutaral (medicinal)	T49.0X1	T49.0X2	T49.0X3	T49.0X4	T49.0X5	T49.0X6
nonmedicinal	T65.891	T65.892	T65.893	T65.894	—	—
Glutaraldehyde (nonmedicinal)	T65.891	T65.892	T65.893	T65.894	—	—
medicinal	T49.0X1	T49.0X2	T49.0X3	T49.0X4	T49.0X5	T49.0X6
Glutathione	T50.6X1	T50.6X2	T50.6X3	T50.6X4	T50.6X5	T50.6X6
Glutethimide	T42.6X1	T42.6X2	T42.6X3	T42.6X4	T42.6X5	T42.6X6
Glyburide	T38.3X1	T38.3X2	T38.3X3	T38.3X4	T38.3X5	T38.3X6
Glycerin	T47.4X1	T47.4X2	T47.4X3	T47.4X4	T47.4X5	T47.4X6
Glycerol	T47.4X1	T47.4X2	T47.4X3	T47.4X4	T47.4X5	T47.4X6
borax	T49.6X1	T49.6X2	T49.6X3	T49.6X4	T49.6X5	T49.6X6
intravenous	T50.3X1	T50.3X2	T50.3X3	T50.3X4	T50.3X5	T50.3X6
iodinated	T48.4X1	T48.4X2	T48.4X3	T48.4X4	T48.4X5	T48.4X6
Glycerophosphate	T50.991	T50.992	T50.993	T50.994	T50.995	T50.996
Glyceryl						
gualacolate	T48.4X1	T48.4X2	T48.4X3	T48.4X4	T48.4X5	T48.4X6
nitrate	T46.3X1	T46.3X2	T46.3X3	T46.3X4	T46.3X5	T46.3X6
triacetate (topical)	T49.0X1	T49.0X2	T49.0X3	T49.0X4	T49.0X5	T49.0X6
trinitrate	T46.3X1	T46.3X2	T46.3X3	T46.3X4	T46.3X5	T46.3X6
Glycine	T50.3X1	T50.3X2	T50.3X3	T50.3X4	T50.3X5	T50.3X6

*Optum Value-Add   ☑ Additional Character May Be Required — Refer to the Tabular List for Character Selection

Substance	Poisoning, Accidental (unintentional)	Poisoning, Intentional Self-harm	Poisoning, Assault	Poisoning, Undetermined	Adverse Effect	Under-dosing
Glyclopyramide	T38.3X1	T38.3X2	T38.3X3	T38.3X4	T38.3X5	T38.3X6
Glycobiarsol	T37.3X1	T37.3X2	T37.3X3	T37.3X4	T37.3X5	T37.3X6
Glycols (ether)	T52.3X1	T52.3X2	T52.3X3	T52.3X4	—	—
Glyconiazide	T37.1X1	T37.1X2	T37.1X3	T37.1X4	T37.1X5	T37.1X6
Glycopyrrolate	T44.3X1	T44.3X2	T44.3X3	T44.3X4	T44.3X5	T44.3X6
Glycopyrronium	T44.3X1	T44.3X2	T44.3X3	T44.3X4	T44.3X5	T44.3X6
bromide	T44.3X1	T44.3X2	T44.3X3	T44.3X4	T44.3X5	T44.3X6
Glycoside, cardiac (stimulant)	T46.0X1	T46.0X2	T46.0X3	T46.0X4	T46.0X5	T46.0X6
Glycyclamide	T38.3X1	T38.3X2	T38.3X3	T38.3X4	T38.3X5	T38.3X6
Glycyrrhiza extract	T48.4X1	T48.4X2	T48.4X3	T48.4X4	T48.4X5	T48.4X6
Glycyrrhizic acid	T48.4X1	T48.4X2	T48.4X3	T48.4X4	T48.4X5	T48.4X6
Glycyrrhizinate potassium	T48.4X1	T48.4X2	T48.4X3	T48.4X4	T48.4X5	T48.4X6
Glymidine sodium	T38.3X1	T38.3X2	T38.3X3	T38.3X4	T38.3X5	T38.3X6
Glyphosate	T60.3X1	T60.3X2	T60.3X3	T60.3X4	—	—
Glyphylline	T48.6X1	T48.6X2	T48.6X3	T48.6X4	T48.6X5	T48.6X6
Gold						
colloidal (l98Au)	T45.1X1	T45.1X2	T45.1X3	T45.1X4	T45.1X5	T45.1X6
salts	T39.4X1	T39.4X2	T39.4X3	T39.4X4	T39.4X5	T39.4X6
Golden sulfide of antimony	T56.891	T56.892	T56.893	T56.894	—	—
Goldylocks	T62.2X1	T62.2X2	T62.2X3	T62.2X4	—	—
Gonadal tissue extract	T38.901	T38.902	T38.903	T38.904	T38.905	T38.906
female	T38.5X1	T38.5X2	T38.5X3	T38.5X4	T38.5X5	T38.5X6
male	T38.7X1	T38.7X2	T38.7X3	T38.7X4	T38.7X5	T38.7X6
Gonadorelin	T38.891	T38.892	T38.893	T38.894	T38.895	T38.896
Gonadotropin	T38.891	T38.892	T38.893	T38.894	T38.895	T38.896
chorionic	T38.891	T38.892	T38.893	T38.894	T38.895	T38.896
pituitary	T38.811	T38.812	T38.813	T38.814	T38.815	T38.816
Goserelin	T45.1X1	T45.1X2	T45.1X3	T45.1X4	T45.1X5	T45.1X6
Grain alcohol	T51.0X1	T51.0X2	T51.0X3	T51.0X4	—	—
Gralise*	T42.6X1	T42.6X2	T42.6X3	T42.6X4	T42.6X5	T42.6X6
Gramicidin	T49.0X1	T49.0X2	T49.0X3	T49.0X4	T49.0X5	T49.0X6
Granisetron	T45.0X1	T45.0X2	T45.0X3	T45.0X4	T45.0X5	T45.0X6
Gratiola officinalis	T62.2X1	T62.2X2	T62.2X3	T62.2X4	—	—
Grease	T65.891	T65.892	T65.893	T65.894	—	—
Green hellebore	T62.2X1	T62.2X2	T62.2X3	T62.2X4	—	—
Green soap	T49.2X1	T49.2X2	T49.2X3	T49.2X4	T49.2X5	T49.2X6
Grifulvin	T36.7X1	T36.7X2	T36.7X3	T36.7X4	T36.7X5	T36.7X6
Griseofulvin	T36.7X1	T36.7X2	T36.7X3	T36.7X4	T36.7X5	T36.7X6
Growth hormone	T38.811	T38.812	T38.813	T38.814	T38.815	T38.816
Guaiacol derivatives	T48.4X1	T48.4X2	T48.4X3	T48.4X4	T48.4X5	T48.4X6
Guaiac reagent	T50.991	T50.992	T50.993	T50.994	T50.995	T50.996
Guaifenesin	T48.4X1	T48.4X2	T48.4X3	T48.4X4	T48.4X5	T48.4X6
Guaimesal	T48.4X1	T48.4X2	T48.4X3	T48.4X4	T48.4X5	T48.4X6
Guaiphenesin	T48.4X1	T48.4X2	T48.4X3	T48.4X4	T48.4X5	T48.4X6
Guaituss*	T48.4X1	T48.4X2	T48.4X3	T48.4X4	T48.4X5	T48.4X6
Guamecycline	T36.4X1	T36.4X2	T36.4X3	T36.4X4	T36.4X5	T36.4X6
Guanabenz	T46.5X1	T46.5X2	T46.5X3	T46.5X4	T46.5X5	T46.5X6
Guanacline	T46.5X1	T46.5X2	T46.5X3	T46.5X4	T46.5X5	T46.5X6
Guanadrel	T46.5X1	T46.5X2	T46.5X3	T46.5X4	T46.5X5	T46.5X6
Guanatol	T37.2X1	T37.2X2	T37.2X3	T37.2X4	T37.2X5	T37.2X6
Guanethidine	T46.5X1	T46.5X2	T46.5X3	T46.5X4	T46.5X5	T46.5X6
Guanfacine	T46.5X1	T46.5X2	T46.5X3	T46.5X4	T46.5X5	T46.5X6
Guano	T65.891	T65.892	T65.893	T65.894	—	—
Guanochlor	T46.5X1	T46.5X2	T46.5X3	T46.5X4	T46.5X5	T46.5X6
Guanoclor	T46.5X1	T46.5X2	T46.5X3	T46.5X4	T46.5X5	T46.5X6
Guanoctine	T46.5X1	T46.5X2	T46.5X3	T46.5X4	T46.5X5	T46.5X6
Guanoxabenz	T46.5X1	T46.5X2	T46.5X3	T46.5X4	T46.5X5	T46.5X6
Guanoxan	T46.5X1	T46.5X2	T46.5X3	T46.5X4	T46.5X5	T46.5X6
Guar gum (medicinal)	T46.6X1	T46.6X2	T46.6X3	T46.6X4	T46.6X5	T46.6X6
Hachimycin	T36.7X1	T36.7X2	T36.7X3	T36.7X4	T36.7X5	T36.7X6
Hair						
dye	T49.4X1	T49.4X2	T49.4X3	T49.4X4	T49.4X5	T49.4X6
preparation NEC	T49.4X1	T49.4X2	T49.4X3	T49.4X4	T49.4X5	T49.4X6
Halazepam	T42.4X1	T42.4X2	T42.4X3	T42.4X4	T42.4X5	T42.4X6
Halcinolone	T49.0X1	T49.0X2	T49.0X3	T49.0X4	T49.0X5	T49.0X6
Halcinonide	T49.0X1	T49.0X2	T49.0X3	T49.0X4	T49.0X5	T49.0X6
Halethazole	T49.0X1	T49.0X2	T49.0X3	T49.0X4	T49.0X5	T49.0X6
Hallucinogen NOS	T40.901	T40.902	T40.903	T40.904	T40.905	T40.906
specified NEC	T40.991	T40.992	T40.993	T40.994	T40.995	T40.996
Halofantrine	T37.2X1	T37.2X2	T37.2X3	T37.2X4	T37.2X5	T37.2X6
Halofenate	T46.6X1	T46.6X2	T46.6X3	T46.6X4	T46.6X5	T46.6X6
Halometasone	T49.0X1	T49.0X2	T49.0X3	T49.0X4	T49.0X5	T49.0X6
Haloperidol	T43.4X1	T43.4X2	T43.4X3	T43.4X4	T43.4X5	T43.4X6
Haloprogin	T49.0X1	T49.0X2	T49.0X3	T49.0X4	T49.0X5	T49.0X6
Halotex	T49.0X1	T49.0X2	T49.0X3	T49.0X4	T49.0X5	T49.0X6
Halothane	T41.0X1	T41.0X2	T41.0X3	T41.0X4	T41.0X5	T41.0X6
Haloxazolam	T42.4X1	T42.4X2	T42.4X3	T42.4X4	T42.4X5	T42.4X6
Halquinols	T49.0X1	T49.0X2	T49.0X3	T49.0X4	T49.0X5	T49.0X6
Hamamelis	T49.2X1	T49.2X2	T49.2X3	T49.2X4	T49.2X5	T49.2X6
Haptendextran	T45.8X1	T45.8X2	T45.8X3	T45.8X4	T45.8X5	T45.8X6
Harmonyl	T46.5X1	T46.5X2	T46.5X3	T46.5X4	T46.5X5	T46.5X6

Substance	Poisoning, Accidental (unintentional)	Poisoning, Intentional Self-harm	Poisoning, Assault	Poisoning, Undetermined	Adverse Effect	Under-dosing
Hartmann's solution	T50.3X1	T50.3X2	T50.3X3	T50.3X4	T50.3X5	T50.3X6
Hashish	T40.711	T40.712	T40.713	T40.714	T40.715	T40.716
Havrix*	T50.B91	T50.B92	T50.B93	T50.B94	T50.B95	T50.B96
Hawaiian Woodrose seeds	T40.991	T40.992	T40.993	T40.994	—	—
HCB	T60.3X1	T60.3X2	T60.3X3	T60.3X4	—	—
HCH	T53.6X1	T53.6X2	T53.6X3	T53.6X4	—	—
medicinal	T49.0X1	T49.0X2	T49.0X3	T49.0X4	T49.0X5	T49.0X6
HCN	T57.3X1	T57.3X2	T57.3X3	T57.3X4	—	—
Headache cures, drugs, powders NEC	T50.901	T50.902	T50.903	T50.904	T50.905	T50.906
Heavenly Blue (morning glory)	T40.991	T40.992	T40.993	T40.994	—	—
Heavy metal antidote	T45.8X1	T45.8X2	T45.8X3	T45.8X4	T45.8X5	T45.8X6
Hedaquinium	T49.0X1	T49.0X2	T49.0X3	T49.0X4	T49.0X5	T49.0X6
Hedge hyssop	T62.2X1	T62.2X2	T62.2X3	T62.2X4	—	—
Heet	T49.8X1	T49.8X2	T49.8X3	T49.8X4	T49.8X5	T49.8X6
Helenin	T37.4X1	T37.4X2	T37.4X3	T37.4X4	T37.4X5	T37.4X6
Helium (nonmedicinal) **NEC**	T59.891	T59.892	T59.893	T59.894	—	—
medicinal	T48.991	T48.992	T48.993	T48.994	T48.995	T48.996
Hellebore (black) (green) (white)	T62.2X1	T62.2X2	T62.2X3	T62.2X4	—	—
Hematin	T45.8X1	T45.8X2	T45.8X3	T45.8X4	T45.8X5	T45.8X6
Hematinic preparation	T45.8X1	T45.8X2	T45.8X3	T45.8X4	T45.8X5	T45.8X6
Hematological agent	T45.91	T45.92	T45.93	T45.94	T45.95	T45.96
specified NEC	T45.8X1	T45.8X2	T45.8X3	T45.8X4	T45.8X5	T45.8X6
Hemlock	T62.2X1	T62.2X2	T62.2X3	T62.2X4	—	—
Hemostatic	T45.621	T45.622	T45.623	T45.624	T45.625	T45.626
drug, systemic	T45.621	T45.622	T45.623	T45.624	T45.625	T45.626
Hemostyptic	T49.4X1	T49.4X2	T49.4X3	T49.4X4	T49.4X5	T49.4X6
Henbane	T62.2X1	T62.2X2	T62.2X3	T62.2X4	—	—
Heparin (sodium)	T45.511	T45.512	T45.513	T45.514	T45.515	T45.516
action reverser	T45.7X1	T45.7X2	T45.7X3	T45.7X4	T45.7X5	T45.7X6
Heparin-fraction	T45.511	T45.512	T45.513	T45.514	T45.515	T45.516
Heparinoid (systemic)	T45.511	T45.512	T45.513	T45.514	T45.515	T45.516
Hepatic secretion stimulant	T47.8X1	T47.8X2	T47.8X3	T47.8X4	T47.8X5	T47.8X6
Hepatitis A vaccine*	T50.B91	T50.B92	T50.B93	T50.B94	T50.B95	T50.B96
Hepatitis B						
immune globulin	T50.Z11	T50.Z12	T50.Z13	T50.Z14	T50.Z15	T50.Z16
vaccine	T50.B91	T50.B92	T50.B93	T50.B94	T50.B95	T50.B96
Hepronicate	T46.7X1	T46.7X2	T46.7X3	T46.7X4	T46.7X5	T46.7X6
Heptabarb	T42.3X1	T42.3X2	T42.3X3	T42.3X4	T42.3X5	T42.3X6
Heptabarbital	T42.3X1	T42.3X2	T42.3X3	T42.3X4	T42.3X5	T42.3X6
Heptabarbitone	T42.3X1	T42.3X2	T42.3X3	T42.3X4	T42.3X5	T42.3X6
Heptachlor	T60.1X1	T60.1X2	T60.1X3	T60.1X4	—	—
Heptalgin	T40.2X1	T40.2X2	T40.2X3	T40.2X4	T40.2X5	T40.2X6
Heptaminol	T46.3X1	T46.3X2	T46.3X3	T46.3X4	T46.3X5	T46.3X6
Herbicide NEC	T60.3X1	T60.3X2	T60.3X3	T60.3X4	—	—
Heroin	T40.1X1	T40.1X2	T40.1X3	T40.1X4	—	—
Herplex	T49.5X1	T49.5X2	T49.5X3	T49.5X4	T49.5X5	T49.5X6
HES	T45.8X1	T45.8X2	T45.8X3	T45.8X4	T45.8X5	T45.8X6
Hesperidin	T46.991	T46.992	T46.993	T46.994	T46.995	T46.996
Hetacillin	T36.0X1	T36.0X2	T36.0X3	T36.0X4	T36.0X5	T36.0X6
Hetastarch	T45.8X1	T45.8X2	T45.8X3	T45.8X4	T45.8X5	T45.8X6
HETP	T60.0X1	T60.0X2	T60.0X3	T60.0X4	—	—
Hexachlorobenzene (vapor)	T60.3X1	T60.3X2	T60.3X3	T60.3X4	—	—
Hexachlorocyclohexane	T53.6X1	T53.6X2	T53.6X3	T53.6X4	—	—
Hexachlorophene	T49.0X1	T49.0X2	T49.0X3	T49.0X4	T49.0X5	T49.0X6
Hexadiline	T46.3X1	T46.3X2	T46.3X3	T46.3X4	T46.3X5	T46.3X6
Hexadimethrine (bromide)	T45.7X1	T45.7X2	T45.7X3	T45.7X4	T45.7X5	T45.7X6
Hexadylamine	T46.3X1	T46.3X2	T46.3X3	T46.3X4	T46.3X5	T46.3X6
Hexaethyl tetraphosphate	T60.0X1	T60.0X2	T60.0X3	T60.0X4	—	—
Hexafluorenium bromide	T48.1X1	T48.1X2	T48.1X3	T48.1X4	T48.1X5	T48.1X6
Hexafluronium (bromide)	T48.1X1	T48.1X2	T48.1X3	T48.1X4	T48.1X5	T48.1X6
Hexa-germ	T49.2X1	T49.2X2	T49.2X3	T49.2X4	T49.2X5	T49.2X6
Hexahydrobenzol	T52.8X1	T52.8X2	T52.8X3	T52.8X4	—	—
Hexahydrocresol(s)	T51.8X1	T51.8X2	T51.8X3	T51.8X4	—	—
arsenide	T57.0X1	T57.0X2	T57.0X3	T57.0X4	—	—
arseniurated	T57.0X1	T57.0X2	T57.0X3	T57.0X4	—	—
cyanide	T57.3X1	T57.3X2	T57.3X3	T57.3X4	—	—
gas	T59.891	T59.892	T59.893	T59.894	—	—
Fluoride (liquid)	T57.8X1	T57.8X2	T57.8X3	T57.8X4	—	—
vapor	T59.891	T59.892	T59.893	T59.894	—	—
phophorated	T60.0X1	T60.0X2	T60.0X3	T60.0X4	—	—
sulfate	T57.8X1	T57.8X2	T57.8X3	T57.8X4	—	—
sulfide (gas)	T59.6X1	T59.6X2	T59.6X3	T59.6X4	—	—
arseniurated	T57.0X1	T57.0X2	T57.0X3	T57.0X4	—	—
sulfurated	T57.8X1	T57.8X2	T57.8X3	T57.8X4	—	—
Hexahydrophenol	T51.8X1	T51.8X2	T51.8X3	T51.8X4	—	—
Hexalen	T51.8X1	T51.8X2	T51.8X3	T51.8X4	—	—
Hexamethonium bromide	T44.2X1	T44.2X2	T44.2X3	T44.2X4	T44.2X5	T44.2X6
Hexamethylene	T52.8X1	T52.8X2	T52.8X3	T52.8X4	—	—

☑ Additional Character May Be Required — Refer to the Tabular List for Character Selection

*Optum Value-Add

Substance	Poisoning, Accidental (unintentional)	Poisoning, Intentional Self-harm	Poisoning, Assault	Poisoning, Undetermined	Adverse Effect	Under-dosing
Hexamethylmelamine	T45.1X1	T45.1X2	T45.1X3	T45.1X4	T45.1X5	T45.1X6
Hexamidine	T49.0X1	T49.0X2	T49.0X3	T49.0X4	T49.0X5	T49.0X6
Hexamine (mandelate)	T37.8X1	T37.8X2	T37.8X3	T37.8X4	T37.8X5	T37.8X6
Hexanone, 2-hexanone	T52.4X1	T52.4X2	T52.4X3	T52.4X4	—	—
Hexanuorenium	T48.1X1	T48.1X2	T48.1X3	T48.1X4	T48.1X5	T48.1X6
Hexapropymate	T42.6X1	T42.6X2	T42.6X3	T42.6X4	T42.6X5	T42.6X6
Hexasonium iodide	T44.3X1	T44.3X2	T44.3X3	T44.3X4	T44.3X5	T44.3X6
Hexcarbacholine bromide	T48.1X1	T48.1X2	T48.1X3	T48.1X4	T48.1X5	T48.1X6
Hexemal	T42.3X1	T42.3X2	T42.3X3	T42.3X4	T42.3X5	T42.3X6
Hexestrol	T38.5X1	T38.5X2	T38.5X3	T38.5X4	T38.5X5	T38.5X6
Hexethal (sodium)	T42.3X1	T42.3X2	T42.3X3	T42.3X4	T42.3X5	T42.3X6
Hexetidine	T37.8X1	T37.8X2	T37.8X3	T37.8X4	T37.8X5	T37.8X6
Hexobarbital	T42.3X1	T42.3X2	T42.3X3	T42.3X4	T42.3X5	T42.3X6
rectal	T41.291	T41.292	T41.293	T41.294	T41.295	T41.296
sodium	T41.1X1	T41.1X2	T41.1X3	T41.1X4	T41.1X5	T41.1X6
Hexobendine	T46.3X1	T46.3X2	T46.3X3	T46.3X4	T46.3X5	T46.3X6
Hexocyclium	T44.3X1	T44.3X2	T44.3X3	T44.3X4	T44.3X5	T44.3X6
metilsulfate	T44.3X1	T44.3X2	T44.3X3	T44.3X4	T44.3X5	T44.3X6
Hexoestrol	T38.5X1	T38.5X2	T38.5X3	T38.5X4	T38.5X5	T38.5X6
Hexone	T52.4X1	T52.4X2	T52.4X3	T52.4X4	—	—
Hexoprenaline	T48.6X1	T48.6X2	T48.6X3	T48.6X4	T48.6X5	T48.6X6
Hexylcaine	T41.3X1	T41.3X2	T41.3X3	T41.3X4	T41.3X5	T41.3X6
Hexylresorcinol	T52.2X1	T52.2X2	T52.2X3	T52.2X4	—	—
HGH (human growth hormone)	T38.811	T38.812	T38.813	T38.814	T38.815	T38.816
Hibistat*	T49.0X1	T49.0X2	T49.0X3	T49.0X4	T49.0X5	T49.0X6
Hinkle's pills	T47.2X1	T47.2X2	T47.2X3	T47.2X4	T47.2X5	T47.2X6
Histalog	T50.8X1	T50.8X2	T50.8X3	T50.8X4	T50.8X5	T50.8X6
Histamine (phosphate)	T50.8X1	T50.8X2	T50.8X3	T50.8X4	T50.8X5	T50.8X6
Histolyn*	T50.8X1	T50.8X2	T50.8X3	T50.8X4	T50.8X5	T50.8X6
Histoplasmin	T50.8X1	T50.8X2	T50.8X3	T50.8X4	T50.8X5	T50.8X6
Holly berries	T62.2X1	T62.2X2	T62.2X3	T62.2X4	—	—
Homatropine	T44.3X1	T44.3X2	T44.3X3	T44.3X4	T44.3X5	T44.3X6
methylbromide	T44.3X1	T44.3X2	T44.3X3	T44.3X4	T44.3X5	T44.3X6
Homochlorcyclizine	T45.0X1	T45.0X2	T45.0X3	T45.0X4	T45.0X5	T45.0X6
Homosalate	T49.3X1	T49.3X2	T49.3X3	T49.3X4	T49.3X5	T49.3X6
Homo-tet	T50.Z11	T50.Z12	T50.Z13	T50.Z14	T50.Z15	T50.Z16
Hormone	T38.801	T38.802	T38.803	T38.804	T38.805	T38.806
adrenal cortical steroids	T38.0X1	T38.0X2	T38.0X3	T38.0X4	T38.0X5	T38.0X6
androgenic	T38.7X1	T38.7X2	T38.7X3	T38.7X4	T38.7X5	T38.7X6
anterior pituitary NEC	T38.811	T38.812	T38.813	T38.814	T38.815	T38.816
antidiabetic agents	T38.3X1	T38.3X2	T38.3X3	T38.3X4	T38.3X5	T38.3X6
antidiuretic	T38.891	T38.892	T38.893	T38.894	T38.895	T38.896
cancer therapy	T45.1X1	T45.1X2	T45.1X3	T45.1X4	T45.1X5	T45.1X6
follicle stimulating	T38.811	T38.812	T38.813	T38.814	T38.815	T38.816
gonadotropic	T38.891	T38.892	T38.893	T38.894	T38.895	T38.896
pituitary	T38.811	T38.812	T38.813	T38.814	T38.815	T38.816
growth	T38.811	T38.812	T38.813	T38.814	T38.815	T38.816
luteinizing	T38.811	T38.812	T38.813	T38.814	T38.815	T38.816
ovarian	T38.5X1	T38.5X2	T38.5X3	T38.5X4	T38.5X5	T38.5X6
oxytocic	T48.0X1	T48.0X2	T48.0X3	T48.0X4	T48.0X5	T48.0X6
parathyroid (derivatives)	T50.991	T50.992	T50.993	T50.994	T50.995	T50.996
pituitary (posterior) NEC	T38.891	T38.892	T38.893	T38.894	T38.895	T38.896
anterior	T38.811	T38.812	T38.813	T38.814	T38.815	T38.816
specified, NEC	T38.891	T38.892	T38.893	T38.894	T38.895	T38.896
thyroid	T38.1X1	T38.1X2	T38.1X3	T38.1X4	T38.1X5	T38.1X6
Hornet (sting)	T63.451	T63.452	T63.453	T63.454	—	—
Horse anti-human lymphocytic serum	T50.Z11	T50.Z12	T50.Z13	T50.Z14	T50.Z15	T50.Z16
Horticulture agent NEC	T65.91	T65.92	T65.93	T65.94	—	—
with pesticide	T60.91	T60.92	T60.93	T60.94	—	—
Human						
albumin	T45.8X1	T45.8X2	T45.8X3	T45.8X4	T45.8X5	T45.8X6
growth hormone (HGH)	T38.811	T38.812	T38.813	T38.814	T38.815	T38.816
immune serum	T50.Z11	T50.Z12	T50.Z13	T50.Z14	T50.Z15	T50.Z16
Hyaluronidase	T45.3X1	T45.3X2	T45.3X3	T45.3X4	T45.3X5	T45.3X6
Hyazyme	T45.3X1	T45.3X2	T45.3X3	T45.3X4	T45.3X5	T45.3X6
Hycodan	T40.2X1	T40.2X2	T40.2X3	T40.2X4	T40.2X5	T40.2X6
Hydantoin derivative NEC	T42.0X1	T42.0X2	T42.0X3	T42.0X4	T42.0X5	T42.0X6
Hydeltra	T38.0X1	T38.0X2	T38.0X3	T38.0X4	T38.0X5	T38.0X6
Hydergine	T44.6X1	T44.6X2	T44.6X3	T44.6X4	T44.6X5	T44.6X6
Hydrabamine penicillin	T36.0X1	T36.0X2	T36.0X3	T36.0X4	T36.0X5	T36.0X6
Hydralazine	T46.5X1	T46.5X2	T46.5X3	T46.5X4	T46.5X5	T46.5X6
Hydrargaphen	T49.0X1	T49.0X2	T49.0X3	T49.0X4	T49.0X5	T49.0X6
Hydrargyri aminochloridum	T49.0X1	T49.0X2	T49.0X3	T49.0X4	T49.0X5	T49.0X6
Hydrastine	T48.291	T48.292	T48.293	T48.294	T48.295	T48.296
Hydrazine	T54.1X1	T54.1X2	T54.1X3	T54.1X4	—	—
monoamine oxidase inhibitors	T43.1X1	T43.1X2	T43.1X3	T43.1X4	T43.1X5	T43.1X6
Hydrazoic acid, azides	T54.2X1	T54.2X2	T54.2X3	T54.2X4	—	—
Hydriodic acid	T48.4X1	T48.4X2	T48.4X3	T48.4X4	T48.4X5	T48.4X6
Hydrisalic*	T49.4X1	T49.4X2	T49.4X3	T49.4X4	T49.4X5	T49.4X6

Substance	Poisoning, Accidental (unintentional)	Poisoning, Intentional Self-harm	Poisoning, Assault	Poisoning, Undetermined	Adverse Effect	Under-dosing
Hydrocarbon gas	T59.891	T59.892	T59.893	T59.894	—	—
incomplete combustion of — see Carbon, monoxide, fuel, utility						
liquefied (mobile container)	T59.891	T59.892	T59.893	T59.894	—	—
piped (natural)	T59.891	T59.892	T59.893	T59.894	—	—
Hydrochloric acid (liquid)	T54.2X1	T54.2X2	T54.2X3	T54.2X4	—	—
medicinal (digestant)	T47.5X1	T47.5X2	T47.5X3	T47.5X4	T47.5X5	T47.5X6
vapor	T59.891	T59.892	T59.893	T59.894	—	—
Hydrochlorothiazide	T50.2X1	T50.2X2	T50.2X3	T50.2X4	T50.2X5	T50.2X6
Hydrocodone	T40.2X1	T40.2X2	T40.2X3	T40.2X4	T40.2X5	T40.2X6
Hydrocortisone	T38.0X1	T38.0X2	T38.0X3	T38.0X4	T38.0X5	T38.0X6
(derivatives)						
aceponate	T49.0X1	T49.0X2	T49.0X3	T49.0X4	T49.0X5	T49.0X6
ENT agent	T49.6X1	T49.6X2	T49.6X3	T49.6X4	T49.6X5	T49.6X6
ophthalmic preparation	T49.5X1	T49.5X2	T49.5X3	T49.5X4	T49.5X5	T49.5X6
topical NEC	T49.0X1	T49.0X2	T49.0X3	T49.0X4	T49.0X5	T49.0X6
Hydrocortone	T38.0X1	T38.0X2	T38.0X3	T38.0X4	T38.0X5	T38.0X6
ENT agent	T49.6X1	T49.6X2	T49.6X3	T49.6X4	T49.6X5	T49.6X6
ophthalmic preparation	T49.5X1	T49.5X2	T49.5X3	T49.5X4	T49.5X5	T49.5X6
topical NEC	T49.0X1	T49.0X2	T49.0X3	T49.0X4	T49.0X5	T49.0X6
Hydrocyanic acid (liquid)	T57.3X1	T57.3X2	T57.3X3	T57.3X4	—	—
gas	T65.0X1	T65.0X2	T65.0X3	T65.0X4	—	—
Hydroflumethiazide	T50.2X1	T50.2X2	T50.2X3	T50.2X4	T50.2X5	T50.2X6
Hydrofluoric acid (liquid)	T54.2X1	T54.2X2	T54.2X3	T54.2X4	—	—
vapor	T59.891	T59.892	T59.893	T59.894	—	—
Hydrogen	T59.891	T59.892	T59.893	T59.894	—	—
arsenide	T57.0X1	T57.0X2	T57.0X3	T57.0X4	—	—
arseniureted	T57.0X1	T57.0X2	T57.0X3	T57.0X4	—	—
chloride	T57.8X1	T57.8X2	T57.8X3	T57.8X4	—	—
cyanide (salts)	T57.3X1	T57.3X2	T57.3X3	T57.3X4	—	—
gas	T57.3X1	T57.3X2	T57.3X3	T57.3X4	—	—
Fluoride	T59.5X1	T59.5X2	T59.5X3	T59.5X4	—	—
vapor	T59.5X1	T59.5X2	T59.5X3	T59.5X4	—	—
peroxide	T49.0X1	T49.0X2	T49.0X3	T49.0X4	T49.0X5	T49.0X6
phosphureted	T57.1X1	T57.1X2	T57.1X3	T57.1X4	—	—
sulfide	T59.6X1	T59.6X2	T59.6X3	T59.6X4	—	—
arseniureted	T57.0X1	T57.0X2	T57.0X3	T57.0X4	—	—
sulfureted	T59.6X1	T59.6X2	T59.6X3	T59.6X4	—	—
Hydromethylpyridine	T46.7X1	T46.7X2	T46.7X3	T46.7X4	T46.7X5	T46.7X6
Hydromorphinol	T40.2X1	T40.2X2	T40.2X3	T40.2X4	—	—
Hydromorphinone	T40.2X1	T40.2X2	T40.2X3	T40.2X4	T40.2X5	T40.2X6
Hydromorphone	T40.2X1	T40.2X2	T40.2X3	T40.2X4	T40.2X5	T40.2X6
Hydromox	T50.2X1	T50.2X2	T50.2X3	T50.2X4	T50.2X5	T50.2X6
Hydrophilic lotion	T49.3X1	T49.3X2	T49.3X3	T49.3X4	T49.3X5	T49.3X6
Hydroquinidine	T46.2X1	T46.2X2	T46.2X3	T46.2X4	T46.2X5	T46.2X6
Hydroquinone	T52.2X1	T52.2X2	T52.2X3	T52.2X4	—	—
vapor	T59.891	T59.892	T59.893	T59.894	—	—
Hydro-ride*	T50.2X1	T50.2X2	T50.2X3	T50.2X4	T50.2X5	T50.2X6
Hydrosulfuric acid (gas)	T59.6X1	T59.6X2	T59.6X3	T59.6X4	—	—
Hydrotalcite	T47.1X1	T47.1X2	T47.1X3	T47.1X4	T47.1X5	T47.1X6
Hydrous wool fat	T49.3X1	T49.3X2	T49.3X3	T49.3X4	T49.3X5	T49.3X6
Hydroxide, caustic	T54.3X1	T54.3X2	T54.3X3	T54.3X4	—	—
Hydroxocobalamin	T45.8X1	T45.8X2	T45.8X3	T45.8X4	T45.8X5	T45.8X6
Hydroxyamphetamine	T49.5X1	T49.5X2	T49.5X3	T49.5X4	T49.5X5	T49.5X6
Hydroxycarbamide	T45.1X1	T45.1X2	T45.1X3	T45.1X4	T45.1X5	T45.1X6
Hydroxychloroquine	T37.8X1	T37.8X2	T37.8X3	T37.8X4	T37.8X5	T37.8X6
Hydroxydaunorubicin*	T45.1X1	T45.1X2	T45.1X3	T45.1X4	T45.1X5	T45.1X6
Hydroxydihydrocodeinone	T40.2X1	T40.2X2	T40.2X3	T40.2X4	T40.2X5	T40.2X6
Hydroxyestrone	T38.5X1	T38.5X2	T38.5X3	T38.5X4	T38.5X5	T38.5X6
Hydroxyethyl starch	T45.8X1	T45.8X2	T45.8X3	T45.8X4	T45.8X5	T45.8X6
Hydroxymethylpentanone	T52.4X1	T52.4X2	T52.4X3	T52.4X4	—	—
Hydroxyphenamate	T43.591	T43.592	T43.593	T43.594	T43.595	T43.596
Hydroxyphenylbutazone	T39.2X1	T39.2X2	T39.2X3	T39.2X4	T39.2X5	T39.2X6
Hydroxyprogesterone	T38.5X1	T38.5X2	T38.5X3	T38.5X4	T38.5X5	T38.5X6
caproate	T38.5X1	T38.5X2	T38.5X3	T38.5X4	T38.5X5	T38.5X6
Hydroxyquinoline (derivatives) NEC	T37.8X1	T37.8X2	T37.8X3	T37.8X4	T37.8X5	T37.8X6
Hydroxystilbamidine	T37.3X1	T37.3X2	T37.3X3	T37.3X4	T37.3X5	T37.3X6
Hydroxytoluene (nonmedicinal)	T54.0X1	T54.0X2	T54.0X3	T54.0X4	—	—
medicinal	T49.0X1	T49.0X2	T49.0X3	T49.0X4	T49.0X5	T49.0X6
Hydroxyurea	T45.1X1	T45.1X2	T45.1X3	T45.1X4	T45.1X5	T45.1X6
Hydroxyzine	T43.591	T43.592	T43.593	T43.594	T43.595	T43.596
Hyoscine	T44.3X1	T44.3X2	T44.3X3	T44.3X4	T44.3X5	T44.3X6
Hyoscyamine	T44.3X1	T44.3X2	T44.3X3	T44.3X4	T44.3X5	T44.3X6
Hyoscyamus	T44.3X1	T44.3X2	T44.3X3	T44.3X4	T44.3X5	T44.3X6
dry extract	T44.3X1	T44.3X2	T44.3X3	T44.3X4	T44.3X5	T44.3X6
Hypaque	T50.8X1	T50.8X2	T50.8X3	T50.8X4	T50.8X5	T50.8X6
HyperRAB*	T50.Z11	T50.Z12	T50.Z13	T50.Z14	T50.Z15	T50.Z16
Hypertussis	T50.Z11	T50.Z12	T50.Z13	T50.Z14	T50.Z15	T50.Z16
Hypnotic	T42.71	T42.72	T42.73	T42.74	T42.75	T42.76

Hexamethylmelamine — Hypnotic

Substance	Poisoning, Accidental (unintentional)	Poisoning, Intentional Self-harm	Poisoning, Assault	Poisoning, Undetermined	Adverse Effect	Under-dosing
Hypnotic — continued						
anticonvulsant	T42.71	T42.72	T42.73	T42.74	T42.75	T42.76
specified NEC	T42.6X1	T42.6X2	T42.6X3	T42.6X4	T42.6X5	T42.6X6
Hypochlorite	T49.0X1	T49.0X2	T49.0X3	T49.0X4	T49.0X5	T49.0X6
Hypophysis, posterior	T38.891	T38.892	T38.893	T38.894	T38.895	T38.896
Hypotensive NEC	T46.5X1	T46.5X2	T46.5X3	T46.5X4	T46.5X5	T46.5X6
Hypromellose	T49.5X1	T49.5X2	T49.5X3	T49.5X4	T49.5X5	T49.5X6
Ibacitabine	T37.5X1	T37.5X2	T37.5X3	T37.5X4	T37.5X5	T37.5X6
Ibopamine	T44.991	T44.992	T44.993	T44.994	T44.995	T44.996
Ibufenac	T39.311	T39.312	T39.313	T39.314	T39.315	T39.316
Ibuprofen	T39.311	T39.312	T39.313	T39.314	T39.315	T39.316
Ibuproxam	T39.311	T39.312	T39.313	T39.314	T39.315	T39.316
Ibuterol	T48.6X1	T48.6X2	T48.6X3	T48.6X4	T48.6X5	T48.6X6
Ichthammol	T49.0X1	T49.0X2	T49.0X3	T49.0X4	T49.0X5	T49.0X6
Ichthyol	T49.4X1	T49.4X2	T49.4X3	T49.4X4	T49.4X5	T49.4X6
Idarubicin	T45.1X1	T45.1X2	T45.1X3	T45.1X4	T45.1X5	T45.1X6
Idrocilamide	T42.8X1	T42.8X2	T42.8X3	T42.8X4	T42.8X5	T42.8X6
Ifenprodil	T46.7X1	T46.7X2	T46.7X3	T46.7X4	T46.7X5	T46.7X6
Ifosfamide	T45.1X1	T45.1X2	T45.1X3	T45.1X4	T45.1X5	T45.1X6
Iletin	T38.3X1	T38.3X2	T38.3X3	T38.3X4	T38.3X5	T38.3X6
Ilex	T62.2X1	T62.2X2	T62.2X3	T62.2X4	—	—
Illuminating gas (after combustion)	T58.11	T58.12	T58.13	T58.14	—	—
prior to combustion	T59.891	T59.892	T59.893	T59.894	—	—
Ilopan	T45.2X1	T45.2X2	T45.2X3	T45.2X4	T45.2X5	T45.2X6
Iloprost	T46.7X1	T46.7X2	T46.7X3	T46.7X4	T46.7X5	T46.7X6
Ilotycin	T36.3X1	T36.3X2	T36.3X3	T36.3X4	T36.3X5	T36.3X6
ophthalmic preparation	T49.5X1	T49.5X2	T49.5X3	T49.5X4	T49.5X5	T49.5X6
topical NEC	T49.0X1	T49.0X2	T49.0X3	T49.0X4	T49.0X5	T49.0X6
Imdur*	T46.3X1	T46.3X2	T46.3X3	T46.3X4	T46.3X5	T46.3X6
Imidazole-4-carboxamide	T45.1X1	T45.1X2	T45.1X3	T45.1X4	T45.1X5	T45.1X6
Iminostilbene	T42.1X1	T42.1X2	T42.1X3	T42.1X4	T42.1X5	T42.1X6
Imipenem	T36.0X1	T36.0X2	T36.0X3	T36.0X4	T36.0X5	T36.0X6
Imipramine	T43.011	T43.012	T43.013	T43.014	T43.015	T43.016
Immu-G	T50.Z11	T50.Z12	T50.Z13	T50.Z14	T50.Z15	T50.Z16
Immuglobin	T50.Z11	T50.Z12	T50.Z13	T50.Z14	T50.Z15	T50.Z16
Immune						
globulin	T50.Z11	T50.Z12	T50.Z13	T50.Z14	T50.Z15	T50.Z16
serum globulin	T50.Z11	T50.Z12	T50.Z13	T50.Z14	T50.Z15	T50.Z16
Immunoglobin human (intravenous) (normal)	T50.Z11	T50.Z12	T50.Z13	T50.Z14	T50.Z15	T50.Z16
unmodified	T50.Z11	T50.Z12	T50.Z13	T50.Z14	T50.Z15	T50.Z16
Immunosuppressive drug	T45.1X1	T45.1X2	T45.1X3	T45.1X4	T45.1X5	T45.1X6
Immu-tetanus	T50.Z11	T50.Z12	T50.Z13	T50.Z14	T50.Z15	T50.Z16
Indalpine	T43.221	T43.222	T43.223	T43.224	T43.225	T43.226
Indanazoline	T48.5X1	T48.5X2	T48.5X3	T48.5X4	T48.5X5	T48.5X6
Indandione (derivatives)	T45.511	T45.512	T45.513	T45.514	T45.515	T45.516
Indapamide	T46.5X1	T46.5X2	T46.5X3	T46.5X4	T46.5X5	T46.5X6
Indendione (derivatives)	T45.511	T45.512	T45.513	T45.514	T45.515	T45.516
Indenolol	T44.7X1	T44.7X2	T44.7X3	T44.7X4	T44.7X5	T44.7X6
Inderal	T44.7X1	T44.7X2	T44.7X3	T44.7X4	T44.7X5	T44.7X6
Indian						
hemp	T40.711	T40.712	T40.713	T40.714	T40.715	T40.716
tobacco	T62.2X1	T62.2X2	T62.2X3	T62.2X4	—	—
Indigo carmine	T50.8X1	T50.8X2	T50.8X3	T50.8X4	T50.8X5	T50.8X6
Indobufen	T45.521	T45.522	T45.523	T45.524	T45.525	T45.526
Indocin	T39.2X1	T39.2X2	T39.2X3	T39.2X4	T39.2X5	T39.2X6
Indocyanine green	T50.8X1	T50.8X2	T50.8X3	T50.8X4	T50.8X5	T50.8X6
Indometacin	T39.391	T39.392	T39.393	T39.394	T39.395	T39.396
Indomethacin	T39.391	T39.392	T39.393	T39.394	T39.395	T39.396
farnesil	T39.4X1	T39.4X2	T39.4X3	T39.4X4	T39.4X5	T39.4X6
Indoramin	T44.6X1	T44.6X2	T44.6X3	T44.6X4	T44.6X5	T44.6X6
Industrial						
alcohol	T51.0X1	T51.0X2	T51.0X3	T51.0X4	—	—
fumes	T59.891	T59.892	T59.893	T59.894	—	—
solvents (fumes) (vapors)	T52.91	T52.92	T52.93	T52.94	—	—
Inflectra*	T39.4X1	T39.4X2	T39.4X3	T39.4X4	T39.4X5	T39.4X6
Influenza vaccine	T50.B91	T50.B92	T50.B93	T50.B94	T50.B95	T50.B96
Ingested substance NEC	T65.91	T65.92	T65.93	T65.94	—	—
INH	T37.1X1	T37.1X2	T37.1X3	T37.1X4	T37.1X5	T37.1X6
Inhalation, gas (noxious) — see Gas						
Inhibitor						
angiotensin-converting enzyme	T46.4X1	T46.4X2	T46.4X3	T46.4X4	T46.4X5	T46.4X6
carbonic anhydrase	T50.2X1	T50.2X2	T50.2X3	T50.2X4	T50.2X5	T50.2X6
fibrinolysis	T45.621	T45.622	T45.623	T45.624	T45.625	T45.626
monoamine oxidase NEC	T43.1X1	T43.1X2	T43.1X3	T43.1X4	T43.1X5	T43.1X6
hydrazine	T43.1X1	T43.1X2	T43.1X3	T43.1X4	T43.1X5	T43.1X6
postsynaptic	T43.8X1	T43.8X2	T43.8X3	T43.8X4	T43.8X5	T43.8X6
prothrombin synthesis	T45.511	T45.512	T45.513	T45.514	T45.515	T45.516
Ink	T65.891	T65.892	T65.893	T65.894	—	—
Innopran*	T44.7X1	T44.7X2	T44.7X3	T44.7X4	T44.7X5	T44.7X6

Substance	Poisoning, Accidental (unintentional)	Poisoning, Intentional Self-harm	Poisoning, Assault	Poisoning, Undetermined	Adverse Effect	Under-dosing
Inorganic substance NEC	T57.91	T57.92	T57.93	T57.94	—	—
Inosine pranobex	T37.5X1	T37.5X2	T37.5X3	T37.5X4	T37.5X5	T37.5X6
Inositol	T50.991	T50.992	T50.993	T50.994	T50.995	T50.996
nicotinate	T46.7X1	T46.7X2	T46.7X3	T46.7X4	T46.7X5	T46.7X6
Inproquone	T45.1X1	T45.1X2	T45.1X3	T45.1X4	T45.1X5	T45.1X6
Insecticide NEC	T60.91	T60.92	T60.93	T60.94	—	—
carbamate	T60.0X1	T60.0X2	T60.0X3	T60.0X4	—	—
chlorinated	T60.1X1	T60.1X2	T60.1X3	T60.1X4	—	—
mixed	T60.91	T60.92	T60.93	T60.94	—	—
organochlorine	T60.1X1	T60.1X2	T60.1X3	T60.1X4	—	—
organophosphorus	T60.0X1	T60.0X2	T60.0X3	T60.0X4	—	—
Insect (sting), venomous	T63.481	T63.482	T63.483	T63.484	—	—
ant	T63.421	T63.422	T63.423	T63.424	—	—
bee	T63.441	T63.442	T63.443	T63.444	—	—
caterpillar	T63.431	T63.432	T63.433	T63.434	—	—
hornet	T63.451	T63.452	T63.453	T63.454	—	—
wasp	T63.461	T63.462	T63.463	T63.464	—	—
Insular tissue extract	T38.3X1	T38.3X2	T38.3X3	T38.3X4	T38.3X5	T38.3X6
Insulin (amorphous) (globin) (isophane) (Lente) (NPH) (Semilente) (Ultralente)	T38.3X1	T38.3X2	T38.3X3	T38.3X4	T38.3X5	T38.3X6
defalan	T38.3X1	T38.3X2	T38.3X3	T38.3X4	T38.3X5	T38.3X6
human	T38.3X1	T38.3X2	T38.3X3	T38.3X4	T38.3X5	T38.3X6
injection, soluble	T38.3X1	T38.3X2	T38.3X3	T38.3X4	T38.3X5	T38.3X6
biphasic	T38.3X1	T38.3X2	T38.3X3	T38.3X4	T38.3X5	T38.3X6
intermediate acting	T38.3X1	T38.3X2	T38.3X3	T38.3X4	T38.3X5	T38.3X6
protamine zinc	T38.3X1	T38.3X2	T38.3X3	T38.3X4	T38.3X5	T38.3X6
slow acting	T38.3X1	T38.3X2	T38.3X3	T38.3X4	T38.3X5	T38.3X6
zinc						
protamine injection	T38.3X1	T38.3X2	T38.3X3	T38.3X4	T38.3X5	T38.3X6
suspension (amorphous) (crystalline)	T38.3X1	T38.3X2	T38.3X3	T38.3X4	T38.3X5	T38.3X6
Interferon (alpha) (beta) (gamma)	T37.5X1	T37.5X2	T37.5X3	T37.5X4	T37.5X5	T37.5X6
Intestinal motility control drug	T47.6X1	T47.6X2	T47.6X3	T47.6X4	T47.6X5	T47.6X6
biological	T47.8X1	T47.8X2	T47.8X3	T47.8X4	T47.8X5	T47.8X6
Intranarcon	T41.1X1	T41.1X2	T41.1X3	T41.1X4	T41.1X5	T41.1X6
Intravenous						
amino acids	T50.991	T50.992	T50.993	T50.994	T50.995	T50.996
fat suspension	T50.991	T50.992	T50.993	T50.994	T50.995	T50.996
Inulin	T50.8X1	T50.8X2	T50.8X3	T50.8X4	T50.8X5	T50.8X6
Invanz*	T36.1X1	T36.1X2	T36.1X3	T36.1X4	T36.1X5	T36.1X6
Invert sugar	T50.3X1	T50.3X2	T50.3X3	T50.3X4	T50.3X5	T50.3X6
Inza — see Naproxen						
Iobenzamic acid	T50.8X1	T50.8X2	T50.8X3	T50.8X4	T50.8X5	T50.8X6
Iocarmic acid	T50.8X1	T50.8X2	T50.8X3	T50.8X4	T50.8X5	T50.8X6
Iocetamic acid	T50.8X1	T50.8X2	T50.8X3	T50.8X4	T50.8X5	T50.8X6
Iodamide	T50.8X1	T50.8X2	T50.8X3	T50.8X4	T50.8X5	T50.8X6
Iodide NEC — see also Iodine	T49.0X1	T49.0X2	T49.0X3	T49.0X4	T49.0X5	T49.0X6
mercury (ointment)	T49.0X1	T49.0X2	T49.0X3	T49.0X4	T49.0X5	T49.0X6
methylate	T49.0X1	T49.0X2	T49.0X3	T49.0X4	T49.0X5	T49.0X6
potassium (expectorant) NEC	T48.4X1	T48.4X2	T48.4X3	T48.4X4	T48.4X5	T48.4X6
Iodinated						
contrast medium	T50.8X1	T50.8X2	T50.8X3	T50.8X4	T50.8X5	T50.8X6
glycerol	T48.4X1	T48.4X2	T48.4X3	T48.4X4	T48.4X5	T48.4X6
human serum albumin (131I)	T50.8X1	T50.8X2	T50.8X3	T50.8X4	T50.8X5	T50.8X6
Iodine (antiseptic, external) (tincture) **NEC**	T49.0X1	T49.0X2	T49.0X3	T49.0X4	T49.0X5	T49.0X6
125 — see also Radiation sickness, and Exposure to radioactive isotopes						
therapeutic	T50.991	T50.992	T50.993	T50.994	T50.995	T50.996
131 — see also Radiation sickness, and Exposure to radioactive isotopes						
therapeutic	T38.2X1	T38.2X2	T38.2X3	T38.2X4	T38.2X5	T38.2X6
diagnostic	T50.8X1	T50.8X2	T50.8X3	T50.8X4	T50.8X5	T50.8X6
for thyroid conditions (antithyroid)	T38.2X1	T38.2X2	T38.2X3	T38.2X4	T38.2X5	T38.2X6
solution	T49.0X1	T49.0X2	T49.0X3	T49.0X4	T49.0X5	T49.0X6
vapor	T59.891	T59.892	T59.893	T59.894	—	—
Iodipamide	T50.8X1	T50.8X2	T50.8X3	T50.8X4	T50.8X5	T50.8X6
Iodized (poppy seed) oil	T50.8X1	T50.8X2	T50.8X3	T50.8X4	T50.8X5	T50.8X6
Iodobismitol	T37.8X1	T37.8X2	T37.8X3	T37.8X4	T37.8X5	T37.8X6
Iodochlorhydroxyquin	T37.8X1	T37.8X2	T37.8X3	T37.8X4	T37.8X5	T37.8X6
topical	T49.0X1	T49.0X2	T49.0X3	T49.0X4	T49.0X5	T49.0X6
Iodochlorhydroxyquinoline	T37.8X1	T37.8X2	T37.8X3	T37.8X4	T37.8X5	T37.8X6
Iodocholesterol (131I)	T50.8X1	T50.8X2	T50.8X3	T50.8X4	T50.8X5	T50.8X6
Iodoform	T49.0X1	T49.0X2	T49.0X3	T49.0X4	T49.0X5	T49.0X6

☑ **Additional Character May Be Required** — Refer to the Tabular List for Character Selection

*Optum Value-Add

Substance	Poisoning, Accidental (unintentional)	Poisoning, Intentional Self-harm	Poisoning, Assault	Poisoning, Undetermined	Adverse Effect	Under-dosing
Iodohippuric acid	T50.8X1	T50.8X2	T50.8X3	T50.8X4	T50.8X5	T50.8X6
Iodopanoic acid	T50.8X1	T50.8X2	T50.8X3	T50.8X4	T50.8X5	T50.8X6
Iodophthalein (sodium)	T50.8X1	T50.8X2	T50.8X3	T50.8X4	T50.8X5	T50.8X6
Iodopyracet	T50.8X1	T50.8X2	T50.8X3	T50.8X4	T50.8X5	T50.8X6
Iodoquinol	T37.8X1	T37.8X2	T37.8X3	T37.8X4	T37.8X5	T37.8X6
Iodoxamic acid	T50.8X1	T50.8X2	T50.8X3	T50.8X4	T50.8X5	T50.8X6
Iofendylate	T50.8X1	T50.8X2	T50.8X3	T50.8X4	T50.8X5	T50.8X6
Ioglycamic acid	T50.8X1	T50.8X2	T50.8X3	T50.8X4	T50.8X5	T50.8X6
Iohexol	T50.8X1	T50.8X2	T50.8X3	T50.8X4	T50.8X5	T50.8X6
Ion exchange resin						
anion	T47.8X1	T47.8X2	T47.8X3	T47.8X4	T47.8X5	T47.8X6
cation	T50.3X1	T50.3X2	T50.3X3	T50.3X4	T50.3X5	T50.3X6
cholestyramine	T46.6X1	T46.6X2	T46.6X3	T46.6X4	T46.6X5	T46.6X6
intestinal	T47.8X1	T47.8X2	T47.8X3	T47.8X4	T47.8X5	T47.8X6
Iopamidol	T50.8X1	T50.8X2	T50.8X3	T50.8X4	T50.8X5	T50.8X6
Iopanoic acid	T50.8X1	T50.8X2	T50.8X3	T50.8X4	T50.8X5	T50.8X6
Iophenoic acid	T50.8X1	T50.8X2	T50.8X3	T50.8X4	T50.8X5	T50.8X6
Iopodate, sodium	T50.8X1	T50.8X2	T50.8X3	T50.8X4	T50.8X5	T50.8X6
Iopodic acid	T50.8X1	T50.8X2	T50.8X3	T50.8X4	T50.8X5	T50.8X6
Iopromide	T50.8X1	T50.8X2	T50.8X3	T50.8X4	T50.8X5	T50.8X6
Iopydol	T50.8X1	T50.8X2	T50.8X3	T50.8X4	T50.8X5	T50.8X6
Iotalamic acid	T50.8X1	T50.8X2	T50.8X3	T50.8X4	T50.8X5	T50.8X6
Iothalamate	T50.8X1	T50.8X2	T50.8X3	T50.8X4	T50.8X5	T50.8X6
Iothiouracil	T38.2X1	T38.2X2	T38.2X3	T38.2X4	T38.2X5	T38.2X6
Iotrol	T50.8X1	T50.8X2	T50.8X3	T50.8X4	T50.8X5	T50.8X6
Iotrolan	T50.8X1	T50.8X2	T50.8X3	T50.8X4	T50.8X5	T50.8X6
Iotroxate	T50.8X1	T50.8X2	T50.8X3	T50.8X4	T50.8X5	T50.8X6
Iotroxic acid	T50.8X1	T50.8X2	T50.8X3	T50.8X4	T50.8X5	T50.8X6
Ioversol	T50.8X1	T50.8X2	T50.8X3	T50.8X4	T50.8X5	T50.8X6
Ioxaglate	T50.8X1	T50.8X2	T50.8X3	T50.8X4	T50.8X5	T50.8X6
Ioxaglic acid	T50.8X1	T50.8X2	T50.8X3	T50.8X4	T50.8X5	T50.8X6
Ioxitalamic acid	T50.8X1	T50.8X2	T50.8X3	T50.8X4	T50.8X5	T50.8X6
Ipecac	T47.7X1	T47.7X2	T47.7X3	T47.7X4	T47.7X5	T47.7X6
Ipecacuanha	T48.4X1	T48.4X2	T48.4X3	T48.4X4	T48.4X5	T48.4X6
Ipodate, calcium	T50.8X1	T50.8X2	T50.8X3	T50.8X4	T50.8X5	T50.8X6
IPOL*	T50.B91	T50.B92	T50.B93	T50.B94	T50.B95	T50.B96
Ipral	T42.3X1	T42.3X2	T42.3X3	T42.3X4	T42.3X5	T42.3X6
Ipratropium (bromide)	T48.6X1	T48.6X2	T48.6X3	T48.6X4	T48.6X5	T48.6X6
Iproflavone	T46.3X1	T46.3X2	T46.3X3	T46.3X4	T46.3X5	T46.3X6
Iprindole	T43.011	T43.012	T43.013	T43.014	T43.015	T43.016
Iproclozide	T43.1X1	T43.1X2	T43.1X3	T43.1X4	T43.1X5	T43.1X6
Iprofenin	T50.8X1	T50.8X2	T50.8X3	T50.8X4	T50.8X5	T50.8X6
Iproheptine	T49.2X1	T49.2X2	T49.2X3	T49.2X4	T49.2X5	T49.2X6
Iproniazid	T43.1X1	T43.1X2	T43.1X3	T43.1X4	T43.1X5	T43.1X6
Iproplatin	T45.1X1	T45.1X2	T45.1X3	T45.1X4	T45.1X5	T45.1X6
Iproveratril	T46.1X1	T46.1X2	T46.1X3	T46.1X4	T46.1X5	T46.1X6
Irinotecan*	T45.1X1	T45.1X2	T45.1X3	T45.1X4	T45.1X5	T45.1X6
Iron (compounds) (medicinal) NEC	T45.4X1	T45.4X2	T45.4X3	T45.4X4	T45.4X5	T45.4X6
ammonium	T45.4X1	T45.4X2	T45.4X3	T45.4X4	T45.4X5	T45.4X6
dextran injection	T45.4X1	T45.4X2	T45.4X3	T45.4X4	T45.4X5	T45.4X6
nonmedicinal	T56.891	T56.892	T56.893	T56.894	—	—
salts	T45.4X1	T45.4X2	T45.4X3	T45.4X4	T45.4X5	T45.4X6
sorbitex	T45.4X1	T45.4X2	T45.4X3	T45.4X4	T45.4X5	T45.4X6
sorbitol citric acid complex	T45.4X1	T45.4X2	T45.4X3	T45.4X4	T45.4X5	T45.4X6
Irrigating fluid (vaginal)	T49.8X1	T49.8X2	T49.8X3	T49.8X4	T49.8X5	T49.8X6
eye	T49.5X1	T49.5X2	T49.5X3	T49.5X4	T49.5X5	T49.5X6
Isepamicin	T36.5X1	T36.5X2	T36.5X3	T36.5X4	T36.5X5	T36.5X6
Isoaminile (citrate)	T48.3X1	T48.3X2	T48.3X3	T48.3X4	T48.3X5	T48.3X6
Isoamyl nitrite	T46.3X1	T46.3X2	T46.3X3	T46.3X4	T46.3X5	T46.3X6
Isobenzan	T60.1X1	T60.1X2	T60.1X3	T60.1X4	—	—
Isobutyl acetate	T52.8X1	T52.8X2	T52.8X3	T52.8X4	—	—
Isocarboxazid	T43.1X1	T43.1X2	T43.1X3	T43.1X4	T43.1X5	T43.1X6
Isoconazole	T49.0X1	T49.0X2	T49.0X3	T49.0X4	T49.0X5	T49.0X6
Isocyanate	T65.0X1	T65.0X2	T65.0X3	T65.0X4	—	—
Isoephedrine	T44.991	T44.992	T44.993	T44.994	T44.995	T44.996
Isoetarine	T48.6X1	T48.6X2	T48.6X3	T48.6X4	T48.6X5	T48.6X6
Isoethadione	T42.2X1	T42.2X2	T42.2X3	T42.2X4	T42.2X5	T42.2X6
Isoetharine	T44.5X1	T44.5X2	T44.5X3	T44.5X4	T44.5X5	T44.5X6
Isoflurane	T41.0X1	T41.0X2	T41.0X3	T41.0X4	T41.0X5	T41.0X6
Isoflurophate	T44.0X1	T44.0X2	T44.0X3	T44.0X4	T44.0X5	T44.0X6
Isomaltose, ferric complex	T45.4X1	T45.4X2	T45.4X3	T45.4X4	T45.4X5	T45.4X6
Isometheptene	T44.3X1	T44.3X2	T44.3X3	T44.3X4	T44.3X5	T44.3X6
Isoniazid	T37.1X1	T37.1X2	T37.1X3	T37.1X4	T37.1X5	T37.1X6
with						
rifampicin	T36.6X1	T36.6X2	T36.6X3	T36.6X4	T36.6X5	T36.6X6
thioacetazone	T37.1X1	T37.1X2	T37.1X3	T37.1X4	T37.1X5	T37.1X6
Isonicotinic acid hydrazide	T37.1X1	T37.1X2	T37.1X3	T37.1X4	T37.1X5	T37.1X6
Isonipecaine	T40.491	T40.492	T40.493	T40.494	T40.495	T40.496
Isopentaquine	T37.2X1	T37.2X2	T37.2X3	T37.2X4	T37.2X5	T37.2X6
Isophane insulin	T38.3X1	T38.3X2	T38.3X3	T38.3X4	T38.3X5	T38.3X6
Isophorone	T65.891	T65.892	T65.893	T65.894	—	—
Isophosphamide	T45.1X1	T45.1X2	T45.1X3	T45.1X4	T45.1X5	T45.1X6
Isopregnenone	T38.5X1	T38.5X2	T38.5X3	T38.5X4	T38.5X5	T38.5X6
Isoprenaline	T48.6X1	T48.6X2	T48.6X3	T48.6X4	T48.6X5	T48.6X6
Isopromethazine	T43.3X1	T43.3X2	T43.3X3	T43.3X4	T43.3X5	T43.3X6
Isopropamide	T44.3X1	T44.3X2	T44.3X3	T44.3X4	T44.3X5	T44.3X6
iodide	T44.3X1	T44.3X2	T44.3X3	T44.3X4	T44.3X5	T44.3X6
Isopropanol	T51.2X1	T51.2X2	T51.2X3	T51.2X4	—	—
Isopropyl						
acetate	T52.8X1	T52.8X2	T52.8X3	T52.8X4	—	—
alcohol	T51.2X1	T51.2X2	T51.2X3	T51.2X4	—	—
medicinal	T49.4X1	T49.4X2	T49.4X3	T49.4X4	T49.4X5	T49.4X6
ether	T52.8X1	T52.8X2	T52.8X3	T52.8X4	—	—
Isopropylaminophenazone	T39.2X1	T39.2X2	T39.2X3	T39.2X4	T39.2X5	T39.2X6
Isoproterenol	T48.6X1	T48.6X2	T48.6X3	T48.6X4	T48.6X5	T48.6X6
Isosorbide dinitrate	T46.3X1	T46.3X2	T46.3X3	T46.3X4	T46.3X5	T46.3X6
Isothipendyl	T45.0X1	T45.0X2	T45.0X3	T45.0X4	T45.0X5	T45.0X6
Isotretinoin	T50.991	T50.992	T50.993	T50.994	T50.995	T50.996
Isoxazolyl penicillin	T36.0X1	T36.0X2	T36.0X3	T36.0X4	T36.0X5	T36.0X6
Isoxicam	T39.391	T39.392	T39.393	T39.394	T39.395	T39.396
Isoxsuprine	T46.7X1	T46.7X2	T46.7X3	T46.7X4	T46.7X5	T46.7X6
Ispagula	T47.4X1	T47.4X2	T47.4X3	T47.4X4	T47.4X5	T47.4X6
husk	T47.4X1	T47.4X2	T47.4X3	T47.4X4	T47.4X5	T47.4X6
Isradipine	T46.1X1	T46.1X2	T46.1X3	T46.1X4	T46.1X5	T46.1X6
I-thyroxine sodium	T38.1X1	T38.1X2	T38.1X3	T38.1X4	T38.1X5	T38.1X6
Itraconazole	T37.8X1	T37.8X2	T37.8X3	T37.8X4	T37.8X5	T37.8X6
Itramin tosilate	T46.3X1	T46.3X2	T46.3X3	T46.3X4	T46.3X5	T46.3X6
Ivarest*	T41.3X1	T41.3X2	T41.3X3	T41.3X4	T41.3X5	T41.3X6
Ivermectin	T37.4X1	T37.4X2	T37.4X3	T37.4X4	T37.4X5	T37.4X6
Izoniazid	T37.1X1	T37.1X2	T37.1X3	T37.1X4	T37.1X5	T37.1X6
with thioacetazone	T37.1X1	T37.1X2	T37.1X3	T37.1X4	T37.1X5	T37.1X6
Jalap	T47.2X1	T47.2X2	T47.2X3	T47.2X4	T47.2X5	T47.2X6
Jamaica						
dogwood (bark)	T39.8X1	T39.8X2	T39.8X3	T39.8X4	T39.8X5	T39.8X6
ginger	T65.891	T65.892	T65.893	T65.894	—	—
root	T62.2X1	T62.2X2	T62.2X3	T62.2X4	—	—
Jantoven*	T45.511	T45.512	T45.513	T45.514	T45.515	T45.516
Jatropha	T62.2X1	T62.2X2	T62.2X3	T62.2X4	—	—
curcas	T62.2X1	T62.2X2	T62.2X3	T62.2X4	—	—
Jectofer	T45.4X1	T45.4X2	T45.4X3	T45.4X4	T45.4X5	T45.4X6
Jellyfish (sting)	T63.621	T63.622	T63.623	T63.624	—	—
Jequirity (bean)	T62.2X1	T62.2X2	T62.2X3	T62.2X4	—	—
Jimson weed (stramonium)	T62.2X1	T62.2X2	T62.2X3	T62.2X4	—	—
seeds	T62.2X1	T62.2X2	T62.2X3	T62.2X4	—	—
Josamycin	T36.3X1	T36.3X2	T36.3X3	T36.3X4	T36.3X5	T36.3X6
Juniper tar	T49.1X1	T49.1X2	T49.1X3	T49.1X4	T49.1X5	T49.1X6
Kaletra*	T37.5X1	T37.5X2	T37.5X3	T37.5X4	T37.5X5	T37.5X6
Kallidinogenase	T46.7X1	T46.7X2	T46.7X3	T46.7X4	T46.7X5	T46.7X6
Kallikrein	T46.7X1	T46.7X2	T46.7X3	T46.7X4	T46.7X5	T46.7X6
Kanamycin	T36.5X1	T36.5X2	T36.5X3	T36.5X4	T36.5X5	T36.5X6
Kantrex	T36.5X1	T36.5X2	T36.5X3	T36.5X4	T36.5X5	T36.5X6
Kaolin	T47.6X1	T47.6X2	T47.6X3	T47.6X4	T47.6X5	T47.6X6
light	T47.6X1	T47.6X2	T47.6X3	T47.6X4	T47.6X5	T47.6X6
Karaya (gum)	T47.4X1	T47.4X2	T47.4X3	T47.4X4	T47.4X5	T47.4X6
Kebuzone	T39.2X1	T39.2X2	T39.2X3	T39.2X4	T39.2X5	T39.2X6
Kelevan	T60.1X1	T60.1X2	T60.1X3	T60.1X4	—	—
Kemithal	T41.1X1	T41.1X2	T41.1X3	T41.1X4	T41.1X5	T41.1X6
Kenacort	T38.0X1	T38.0X2	T38.0X3	T38.0X4	T38.0X5	T38.0X6
Keratolytic drug NEC	T49.4X1	T49.4X2	T49.4X3	T49.4X4	T49.4X5	T49.4X6
anthracene	T49.4X1	T49.4X2	T49.4X3	T49.4X4	T49.4X5	T49.4X6
Keratoplastic NEC	T49.4X1	T49.4X2	T49.4X3	T49.4X4	T49.4X5	T49.4X6
Kerosene, kerosine (fuel) (solvent) NEC	T52.0X1	T52.0X2	T52.0X3	T52.0X4	—	—
insecticide	T52.0X1	T52.0X2	T52.0X3	T52.0X4	—	—
vapor	T52.0X1	T52.0X2	T52.0X3	T52.0X4	—	—
Ketamine	T41.291	T41.292	T41.293	T41.294	T41.295	T41.296
Ketazolam	T42.4X1	T42.4X2	T42.4X3	T42.4X4	T42.4X5	T42.4X6
Ketazon	T39.2X1	T39.2X2	T39.2X3	T39.2X4	T39.2X5	T39.2X6
Ketobemidone	T40.491	T40.492	T40.493	T40.494	—	—
Ketoconazole	T49.0X1	T49.0X2	T49.0X3	T49.0X4	T49.0X5	T49.0X6
Ketols	T52.4X1	T52.4X2	T52.4X3	T52.4X4	—	—
Ketone oils	T52.4X1	T52.4X2	T52.4X3	T52.4X4	—	—
Ketoprofen	T39.311	T39.312	T39.313	T39.314	T39.315	T39.316
Ketorolac	T39.8X1	T39.8X2	T39.8X3	T39.8X4	T39.8X5	T39.8X6
Ketotifen	T45.0X1	T45.0X2	T45.0X3	T45.0X4	T45.0X5	T45.0X6
Keytruda*	T45.1X1	T45.1X2	T45.1X3	T45.1X4	T45.1X5	T45.1X6
Khat	T43.691	T43.692	T43.693	T43.694	—	—
Khellin	T46.3X1	T46.3X2	T46.3X3	T46.3X4	T46.3X5	T46.3X6
Khelloside	T46.3X1	T46.3X2	T46.3X3	T46.3X4	T46.3X5	T46.3X6
Kiln gas or vapor (carbon monoxide)	T58.8X1	T58.8X2	T58.8X3	T58.8X4	—	—
Kineret*	T39.4X1	T39.4X2	T39.4X3	T39.4X4	T39.4X5	T39.4X6
Kitasamycin	T36.3X1	T36.3X2	T36.3X3	T36.3X4	T36.3X5	T36.3X6
Komgiblyze*	T38.3X1	T38.3X2	T38.3X3	T38.3X4	T38.3X5	T38.3X6
Konsyl	T47.4X1	T47.4X2	T47.4X3	T47.4X4	T47.4X5	T47.4X6

*Optum Value-Add

☑ Additional Character May Be Required — Refer to the Tabular List for Character Selection

Substance	Poisoning, Accidental (unintentional)	Poisoning, Intentional Self-harm	Poisoning, Assault	Poisoning, Undetermined	Adverse Effect	Under-dosing
Kosam seed	T62.2X1	T62.2X2	T62.2X3	T62.2X4	—	—
Krait (venom)	T63.091	T63.092	T63.093	T63.094	—	—
Kwell (insecticide)	T60.1X1	T60.1X2	T60.1X3	T60.1X4	—	—
anti-infective (topical)	T49.0X1	T49.0X2	T49.0X3	T49.0X4	T49.0X5	T49.0X6
Labetalol	T44.8X1	T44.8X2	T44.8X3	T44.8X4	T44.8X5	T44.8X6
Laburnum (seeds)	T62.2X1	T62.2X2	T62.2X3	T62.2X4	—	—
leaves	T62.2X1	T62.2X2	T62.2X3	T62.2X4	—	—
Lachesine	T49.5X1	T49.5X2	T49.5X3	T49.5X4	T49.5X5	T49.5X6
Lacidipine	T46.5X1	T46.5X2	T46.5X3	T46.5X4	T46.5X5	T46.5X6
Lacquer	T65.6X1	T65.6X2	T65.6X3	T65.6X4	—	—
Lacrimogenic gas	T59.3X1	T59.3X2	T59.3X3	T59.3X4	—	—
Lactated potassic saline	T50.3X1	T50.3X2	T50.3X3	T50.3X4	T50.3X5	T50.3X6
Lactic acid	T49.8X1	T49.8X2	T49.8X3	T49.8X4	T49.8X5	T49.8X6
Lactobacillus						
acidophilus	T47.6X1	T47.6X2	T47.6X3	T47.6X4	T47.6X5	T47.6X6
compound	T47.6X1	T47.6X2	T47.6X3	T47.6X4	T47.6X5	T47.6X6
bifidus, lyophilized	T47.6X1	T47.6X2	T47.6X3	T47.6X4	T47.6X5	T47.6X6
bulgaricus	T47.6X1	T47.6X2	T47.6X3	T47.6X4	T47.6X5	T47.6X6
sporogenes	T47.6X1	T47.6X2	T47.6X3	T47.6X4	T47.6X5	T47.6X6
Lactoflavin	T45.2X1	T45.2X2	T45.2X3	T45.2X4	T45.2X5	T45.2X6
Lactose (as excipient)	T50.901	T50.902	T50.903	T50.904	T50.905	T50.906
Lactuca (virosa) (extract)	T42.6X1	T42.6X2	T42.6X3	T42.6X4	T42.6X5	T42.6X6
Lactucarium	T42.6X1	T42.6X2	T42.6X3	T42.6X4	T42.6X5	T42.6X6
Lactulose	T47.3X1	T47.3X2	T47.3X3	T47.3X4	T47.3X5	T47.3X6
Laevo — see Levo-						
Lanatosides	T46.0X1	T46.0X2	T46.0X3	T46.0X4	T46.0X5	T46.0X6
Lanolin	T49.3X1	T49.3X2	T49.3X3	T49.3X4	T49.3X5	T49.3X6
Lanoxin*	T46.0X1	T46.0X2	T46.0X3	T46.0X4	T46.0X5	T46.0X6
Largactil	T43.3X1	T43.3X2	T43.3X3	T43.3X4	T43.3X5	T43.3X6
Larkspur	T62.2X1	T62.2X2	T62.2X3	T62.2X4	—	—
Laroxyl	T43.011	T43.012	T43.013	T43.014	T43.015	T43.016
Lasix	T50.1X1	T50.1X2	T50.1X3	T50.1X4	T50.1X5	T50.1X6
Lassar's paste	T49.4X1	T49.4X2	T49.4X3	T49.4X4	T49.4X5	T49.4X6
Latamoxef	T36.1X1	T36.1X2	T36.1X3	T36.1X4	T36.1X5	T36.1X6
Latex	T65.811	T65.812	T65.813	T65.814	—	—
Lathyrus (seed)	T62.2X1	T62.2X2	T62.2X3	T62.2X4	—	—
Laudanum	T40.0X1	T40.0X2	T40.0X3	T40.0X4	T40.0X5	T40.0X6
Laudexium	T48.1X1	T48.1X2	T48.1X3	T48.1X4	T48.1X5	T48.1X6
Laughing gas	T41.0X1	T41.0X2	T41.0X3	T41.0X4	T41.0X5	T41.0X6
Laurel, black or cherry	T62.2X1	T62.2X2	T62.2X3	T62.2X4	—	—
Laurolinium	T49.0X1	T49.0X2	T49.0X3	T49.0X4	T49.0X5	T49.0X6
Lauryl sulfoacetate	T49.2X1	T49.2X2	T49.2X3	T49.2X4	T49.2X5	T49.2X6
Laxative NEC	T47.4X1	T47.4X2	T47.4X3	T47.4X4	T47.4X5	T47.4X6
osmotic	T47.3X1	T47.3X2	T47.3X3	T47.3X4	T47.3X5	T47.3X6
saline	T47.3X1	T47.3X2	T47.3X3	T47.3X4	T47.3X5	T47.3X6
stimulant	T47.2X1	T47.2X2	T47.2X3	T47.2X4	T47.2X5	T47.2X6
L-dopa	T42.8X1	T42.8X2	T42.8X3	T42.8X4	T42.8X5	T42.8X6
Lead (dust) (fumes) (vapor)	T56.0X1	T56.0X2	T56.0X3	T56.0X4	—	—
NEC	T56.0X1	T56.0X2	T56.0X3	T56.0X4	—	—
acetate	T49.2X1	T49.2X2	T49.2X3	T49.2X4	T49.2X5	T49.2X6
alkyl (fuel additive)	T56.0X1	T56.0X2	T56.0X3	T56.0X4	—	—
anti-infectives	T37.8X1	T37.8X2	T37.8X3	T37.8X4	T37.8X5	T37.8X6
antiknock compound (tetraethyl)	T56.0X1	T56.0X2	T56.0X3	T56.0X4	—	—
arsenate, arsenite (dust)(herbicide) (insecticide) (vapor)	T57.0X1	T57.0X2	T57.0X3	T57.0X4	—	—
carbonate	T56.0X1	T56.0X2	T56.0X3	T56.0X4	—	—
paint	T56.0X1	T56.0X2	T56.0X3	T56.0X4	—	—
chromate	T56.0X1	T56.0X2	T56.0X3	T56.0X4	—	—
paint	T56.0X1	T56.0X2	T56.0X3	T56.0X4	—	—
dioxide	T56.0X1	T56.0X2	T56.0X3	T56.0X4	—	—
inorganic	T56.0X1	T56.0X2	T56.0X3	T56.0X4	—	—
iodide	T56.0X1	T56.0X2	T56.0X3	T56.0X4	—	—
pigment (paint)	T56.0X1	T56.0X2	T56.0X3	T56.0X4	—	—
monoxide (dust)	T56.0X1	T56.0X2	T56.0X3	T56.0X4	—	—
paint	T56.0X1	T56.0X2	T56.0X3	T56.0X4	—	—
organic	T56.0X1	T56.0X2	T56.0X3	T56.0X4	—	—
oxide	T56.0X1	T56.0X2	T56.0X3	T56.0X4	—	—
paint	T56.0X1	T56.0X2	T56.0X3	T56.0X4	—	—
paint	T56.0X1	T56.0X2	T56.0X3	T56.0X4	—	—
salts	T56.0X1	T56.0X2	T56.0X3	T56.0X4	—	—
specified compound NEC	T56.0X1	T56.0X2	T56.0X3	T56.0X4	—	—
tetra-ethyl	T56.0X1	T56.0X2	T56.0X3	T56.0X4	—	—
Lebanese red	T40.711	T40.712	T40.713	T40.714	T40.715	T40.716
Lefetamine	T39.8X1	T39.8X2	T39.8X3	T39.8X4	T39.8X5	T39.8X6
Lenperone	T43.4X1	T43.4X2	T43.4X3	T43.4X4	T43.4X5	T43.4X6
Lente lietin (insulin)	T38.3X1	T38.3X2	T38.3X3	T38.3X4	T38.3X5	T38.3X6
Leptazol	T50.7X1	T50.7X2	T50.7X3	T50.7X4	T50.7X5	T50.7X6
Leptophos	T60.0X1	T60.0X2	T60.0X3	T60.0X4	—	—
Leritine	T40.2X1	T40.2X2	T40.2X3	T40.2X4	T40.2X5	T40.2X6
Lescol*	T46.6X1	T46.6X2	T46.6X3	T46.6X4	T46.6X5	T46.6X6
Letosteine	T48.4X1	T48.4X2	T48.4X3	T48.4X4	T48.4X5	T48.4X6

Substance	Poisoning, Accidental (unintentional)	Poisoning, Intentional Self-harm	Poisoning, Assault	Poisoning, Undetermined	Adverse Effect	Under-dosing
Letter	T38.1X1	T38.1X2	T38.1X3	T38.1X4	T38.1X5	T38.1X6
Lettuce opium	T42.6X1	T42.6X2	T42.6X3	T42.6X4	T42.6X5	T42.6X6
Leucinocaine	T41.3X1	T41.3X2	T41.3X3	T41.3X4	T41.3X5	T41.3X6
Leucocianidol	T46.991	T46.992	T46.993	T46.994	T46.995	T46.996
Leucovorin (factor)	T45.8X1	T45.8X2	T45.8X3	T45.8X4	T45.8X5	T45.8X6
Leukeran	T45.1X1	T45.1X2	T45.1X3	T45.1X4	T45.1X5	T45.1X6
Leuprolide	T38.891	T38.892	T38.893	T38.894	T38.895	T38.896
Levalbuterol	T48.6X1	T48.6X2	T48.6X3	T48.6X4	T48.6X5	T48.6X6
Levallorphan	T50.7X1	T50.7X2	T50.7X3	T50.7X4	T50.7X5	T50.7X6
Levamisole	T37.4X1	T37.4X2	T37.4X3	T37.4X4	T37.4X5	T37.4X6
Levanil	T42.6X1	T42.6X2	T42.6X3	T42.6X4	T42.6X5	T42.6X6
Levarterenol	T44.4X1	T44.4X2	T44.4X3	T44.4X4	T44.4X5	T44.4X6
Levdropropizine	T48.3X1	T48.3X2	T48.3X3	T48.3X4	T48.3X5	T48.3X6
Levobunolol	T49.5X1	T49.5X2	T49.5X3	T49.5X4	T49.5X5	T49.5X6
Levocabastine (hydrochloride)	T45.0X1	T45.0X2	T45.0X3	T45.0X4	T45.0X5	T45.0X6
Levocarnitine	T50.991	T50.992	T50.993	T50.994	T50.995	T50.996
Levodopa	T42.8X1	T42.8X2	T42.8X3	T42.8X4	T42.8X5	T42.8X6
with carbidopa	T42.8X1	T42.8X2	T42.8X3	T42.8X4	T42.8X5	T42.8X6
Levo-dromoran	T40.2X1	T40.2X2	T40.2X3	T40.2X4	T40.2X5	T40.2X6
Levoglutamide	T50.991	T50.992	T50.993	T50.994	T50.995	T50.996
Levoid	T38.1X1	T38.1X2	T38.1X3	T38.1X4	T38.1X5	T38.1X6
Levo-isomethadone	T40.3X1	T40.3X2	T40.3X3	T40.3X4	T40.3X5	T40.3X6
Levomepromazine	T43.3X1	T43.3X2	T43.3X3	T43.3X4	T43.3X5	T43.3X6
Levonordefrin	T49.6X1	T49.6X2	T49.6X3	T49.6X4	T49.6X5	T49.6X6
Levonorgestrel	T38.4X1	T38.4X2	T38.4X3	T38.4X4	T38.4X5	T38.4X6
with ethinylestradiol	T38.5X1	T38.5X2	T38.5X3	T38.5X4	T38.5X5	T38.5X6
Levopromazine	T43.3X1	T43.3X2	T43.3X3	T43.3X4	T43.3X5	T43.3X6
Levoprome	T42.6X1	T42.6X2	T42.6X3	T42.6X4	T42.6X5	T42.6X6
Levopropoxyphene	T40.491	T40.492	T40.493	T40.494	T40.495	T40.496
Levopropylhexedrine	T50.5X1	T50.5X2	T50.5X3	T50.5X4	T50.5X5	T50.5X6
Levoproxyphylline	T48.6X1	T48.6X2	T48.6X3	T48.6X4	T48.6X5	T48.6X6
Levorphanol	T40.491	T40.492	T40.493	T40.494	T40.495	T40.496
Levothroid*	T38.1X1	T38.1X2	T38.1X3	T38.1X4	T38.1X5	T38.1X6
Levothyroxine	T38.1X1	T38.1X2	T38.1X3	T38.1X4	T38.1X5	T38.1X6
sodium	T38.1X1	T38.1X2	T38.1X3	T38.1X4	T38.1X5	T38.1X6
Levsin	T44.3X1	T44.3X2	T44.3X3	T44.3X4	T44.3X5	T44.3X6
Levulose	T50.3X1	T50.3X2	T50.3X3	T50.3X4	T50.3X5	T50.3X6
Lewisite (gas), not in war	T57.0X1	T57.0X2	T57.0X3	T57.0X4	—	—
Librium	T42.4X1	T42.4X2	T42.4X3	T42.4X4	T42.4X5	T42.4X6
Lidex	T49.0X1	T49.0X2	T49.0X3	T49.0X4	T49.0X5	T49.0X6
Lidocaine	T41.3X1	T41.3X2	T41.3X3	T41.3X4	T41.3X5	T41.3X6
regional	T41.3X1	T41.3X2	T41.3X3	T41.3X4	T41.3X5	T41.3X6
spinal	T41.3X1	T41.3X2	T41.3X3	T41.3X4	T41.3X5	T41.3X6
Lidofenin	T50.8X1	T50.8X2	T50.8X3	T50.8X4	T50.8X5	T50.8X6
Lidoflazine	T46.1X1	T46.1X2	T46.1X3	T46.1X4	T46.1X5	T46.1X6
Lighter fluid	T52.0X1	T52.0X2	T52.0X3	T52.0X4	—	—
Lignin hemicellulose	T47.6X1	T47.6X2	T47.6X3	T47.6X4	T47.6X5	T47.6X6
Lignocaine	T41.3X1	T41.3X2	T41.3X3	T41.3X4	T41.3X5	T41.3X6
regional	T41.3X1	T41.3X2	T41.3X3	T41.3X4	T41.3X5	T41.3X6
spinal	T41.3X1	T41.3X2	T41.3X3	T41.3X4	T41.3X5	T41.3X6
Ligroin (e) (solvent)	T52.0X1	T52.0X2	T52.0X3	T52.0X4	—	—
vapor	T59.891	T59.892	T59.893	T59.894	—	—
Ligustrum vulgare	T62.2X1	T62.2X2	T62.2X3	T62.2X4	—	—
Lily of the valley	T62.2X1	T62.2X2	T62.2X3	T62.2X4	—	—
Lime (chloride)	T54.3X1	T54.3X2	T54.3X3	T54.3X4	—	—
Limonene	T52.8X1	T52.8X2	T52.8X3	T52.8X4	—	—
Lincomycin	T36.8X1	T36.8X2	T36.8X3	T36.8X4	T36.8X5	T36.8X6
Lindane (insecticide) (nonmedicinal) (vapor)	T53.6X1	T53.6X2	T53.6X3	T53.6X4	—	—
medicinal	T49.0X1	T49.0X2	T49.0X3	T49.0X4	T49.0X5	T49.0X6
Liniments NEC	T49.91	T49.92	T49.93	T49.94	T49.95	T49.96
Linoleic acid	T46.6X1	T46.6X2	T46.6X3	T46.6X4	T46.6X5	T46.6X6
Linolenic acid	T46.6X1	T46.6X2	T46.6X3	T46.6X4	T46.6X5	T46.6X6
Linseed	T47.4X1	T47.4X2	T47.4X3	T47.4X4	T47.4X5	T47.4X6
Liothyronine	T38.1X1	T38.1X2	T38.1X3	T38.1X4	T38.1X5	T38.1X6
Liotrix	T38.1X1	T38.1X2	T38.1X3	T38.1X4	T38.1X5	T38.1X6
Lipancreatin	T47.5X1	T47.5X2	T47.5X3	T47.5X4	T47.5X5	T47.5X6
Lipo-alprostadil	T46.7X1	T46.7X2	T46.7X3	T46.7X4	T46.7X5	T46.7X6
Lipo-Lutin	T38.5X1	T38.5X2	T38.5X3	T38.5X4	T38.5X5	T38.5X6
Lipotropic drug NEC	T50.901	T50.902	T50.903	T50.904	T50.905	T50.906
Liquefied petroleum gases	T59.891	T59.892	T59.893	T59.894	—	—
piped (pure or mixed with air)	T59.891	T59.892	T59.893	T59.894	—	—
Liquid						
paraffin	T47.4X1	T47.4X2	T47.4X3	T47.4X4	T47.4X5	T47.4X6
petrolatum	T47.4X1	T47.4X2	T47.4X3	T47.4X4	T47.4X5	T47.4X6
topical	T49.3X1	T49.3X2	T49.3X3	T49.3X4	T49.3X5	T49.3X6
specified NEC	T65.891	T65.892	T65.893	T65.894	—	—
substance	T65.91	T65.92	T65.93	T65.94	—	—
Liquor creosolis compositus	T65.891	T65.892	T65.893	T65.894	—	—
Liquorice	T48.4X1	T48.4X2	T48.4X3	T48.4X4	T48.4X5	T48.4X6

☑ Additional Character May Be Required — Refer to the Tabular List for Character Selection

*Optum Value-Add

Substance	Poisoning, Accidental (unintentional)	Poisoning, Intentional Self-harm	Poisoning, Assault	Poisoning, Undetermined	Adverse Effect	Under-dosing
Liquorice — *continued*						
extract	T47.8X1	T47.8X2	T47.8X3	T47.8X4	T47.8X5	T47.8X6
Liraglutide*	T38.3X1	T38.3X2	T38.3X3	T38.3X4	T38.3X5	T38.3X6
Lisinopril	T46.4X1	T46.4X2	T46.4X3	T46.4X4	T46.4X5	T46.4X6
Lisuride	T42.8X1	T42.8X2	T42.8X3	T42.8X4	T42.8X5	T42.8X6
Lithane	T43.8X1	T43.8X2	T43.8X3	T43.8X4	T43.8X5	T43.8X6
Lithium	T56.891	T56.892	T56.893	T56.894	—	—
gluconate	T43.591	T43.592	T43.593	T43.594	T43.595	T43.596
salts (carbonate)	T43.591	T43.592	T43.593	T43.594	T43.595	T43.596
Lithonate	T43.8X1	T43.8X2	T43.8X3	T43.8X4	T43.8X5	T43.8X6
Liver						
extract	T45.8X1	T45.8X2	T45.8X3	T45.8X4	T45.8X5	T45.8X6
for parenteral use	T45.8X1	T45.8X2	T45.8X3	T45.8X4	T45.8X5	T45.8X6
fraction 1	T45.8X1	T45.8X2	T45.8X3	T45.8X4	T45.8X5	T45.8X6
hydrolysate	T45.8X1	T45.8X2	T45.8X3	T45.8X4	T45.8X5	T45.8X6
Lizard (bite) (venom)	T63.121	T63.122	T63.123	T63.124	—	—
LMD	T45.8X1	T45.8X2	T45.8X3	T45.8X4	T45.8X5	T45.8X6
Lobelia	T62.2X1	T62.2X2	T62.2X3	T62.2X4	—	—
Lobeline	T50.7X1	T50.7X2	T50.7X3	T50.7X4	T50.7X5	T50.7X6
Local action drug NEC	T49.8X1	T49.8X2	T49.8X3	T49.8X4	T49.8X5	T49.8X6
Locorten	T49.0X1	T49.0X2	T49.0X3	T49.0X4	T49.0X5	T49.0X6
Lofepramine	T43.011	T43.012	T43.013	T43.014	T43.015	T43.016
Lolium temulentum	T62.2X1	T62.2X2	T62.2X3	T62.2X4	—	—
Lomotil	T47.6X1	T47.6X2	T47.6X3	T47.6X4	T47.6X5	T47.6X6
Lomustine	T45.1X1	T45.1X2	T45.1X3	T45.1X4	T45.1X5	T45.1X6
Lonidamine	T45.1X1	T45.1X2	T45.1X3	T45.1X4	T45.1X5	T45.1X6
LoOvral*	T38.4X1	T38.4X2	T38.4X3	T38.4X4	T38.4X5	T38.4X6
Loperamide	T47.6X1	T47.6X2	T47.6X3	T47.6X4	T47.6X5	T47.6X6
Loprazolam	T42.4X1	T42.4X2	T42.4X3	T42.4X4	T42.4X5	T42.4X6
Lorajmine	T46.2X1	T46.2X2	T46.2X3	T46.2X4	T46.2X5	T46.2X6
Loratidine	T45.0X1	T45.0X2	T45.0X3	T45.0X4	T45.0X5	T45.0X6
Lorazepam	T42.4X1	T42.4X2	T42.4X3	T42.4X4	T42.4X5	T42.4X6
Lorcainide	T46.2X1	T46.2X2	T46.2X3	T46.2X4	T46.2X5	T46.2X6
Lormetazepam	T42.4X1	T42.4X2	T42.4X3	T42.4X4	T42.4X5	T42.4X6
Lotions NEC	T49.91	T49.92	T49.93	T49.94	T49.95	T49.96
Lotrimin*	T49.0X1	T49.0X2	T49.0X3	T49.0X4	T49.0X5	T49.0X6
Lotusate	T42.3X1	T42.3X2	T42.3X3	T42.3X4	T42.3X5	T42.3X6
Lovastatin	T46.6X1	T46.6X2	T46.6X3	T46.6X4	T46.6X5	T46.6X6
Lowila	T49.2X1	T49.2X2	T49.2X3	T49.2X4	T49.2X5	T49.2X6
Loxapine	T43.591	T43.592	T43.593	T43.594	T43.595	T43.596
Lozenges (throat)	T49.6X1	T49.6X2	T49.6X3	T49.6X4	T49.6X5	T49.6X6
LSD	T40.8X1	T40.8X2	T40.8X3	T40.8X4	—	—
L-Tryptophan — *see* amino acid						
Lubricant, eye	T49.5X1	T49.5X2	T49.5X3	T49.5X4	T49.5X5	T49.5X6
Lubricating oil NEC	T52.0X1	T52.0X2	T52.0X3	T52.0X4	—	—
Lucanthone	T37.4X1	T37.4X2	T37.4X3	T37.4X4	T37.4X5	T37.4X6
Luminal	T42.3X1	T42.3X2	T42.3X3	T42.3X4	T42.3X5	T42.3X6
Lung irritant (gas) NEC	T59.91	T59.92	T59.93	T59.94	—	—
Luteinizing hormone	T38.811	T38.812	T38.813	T38.814	T38.815	T38.816
Lutocylol	T38.5X1	T38.5X2	T38.5X3	T38.5X4	T38.5X5	T38.5X6
Lutromone	T38.5X1	T38.5X2	T38.5X3	T38.5X4	T38.5X5	T38.5X6
Lututrin	T48.291	T48.292	T48.293	T48.294	T48.295	T48.296
Luveris*	T38.891	T38.892	T38.893	T38.894	T38.895	T38.896
Lye (concentrated)	T54.3X1	T54.3X2	T54.3X3	T54.3X4	—	—
Lygranum (skin test)	T50.8X1	T50.8X2	T50.8X3	T50.8X4	T50.8X5	T50.8X6
Lymecycline	T36.4X1	T36.4X2	T36.4X3	T36.4X4	T36.4X5	T36.4X6
Lymphogranuloma venereum antigen	T50.8X1	T50.8X2	T50.8X3	T50.8X4	T50.8X5	T50.8X6
Lynestrenol	T38.4X1	T38.4X2	T38.4X3	T38.4X4	T38.4X5	T38.4X6
Lyovac Sodium Edecrin	T50.1X1	T50.1X2	T50.1X3	T50.1X4	T50.1X5	T50.1X6
Lypressin	T38.891	T38.892	T38.893	T38.894	T38.895	T38.896
Lysergic acid diethylamide	T40.8X1	T40.8X2	T40.8X3	T40.8X4	—	—
Lysergide	T40.8X1	T40.8X2	T40.8X3	T40.8X4	—	—
Lysine vasopressin	T38.891	T38.892	T38.893	T38.894	T38.895	T38.896
Lysol	T54.1X1	T54.1X2	T54.1X3	T54.1X4	—	—
Lysozyme	T49.0X1	T49.0X2	T49.0X3	T49.0X4	T49.0X5	T49.0X6
Lytta (vitatta)	T49.8X1	T49.8X2	T49.8X3	T49.8X4	T49.8X5	T49.8X6
Mace	T59.3X1	T59.3X2	T59.3X3	T59.3X4	—	—
Macrogol	T50.991	T50.992	T50.993	T50.994	T50.995	T50.996
Macrolide						
anabolic drug	T38.7X1	T38.7X2	T38.7X3	T38.7X4	T38.7X5	T38.7X6
antibiotic	T36.3X1	T36.3X2	T36.3X3	T36.3X4	T36.3X5	T36.3X6
Mafenide	T49.0X1	T49.0X2	T49.0X3	T49.0X4	T49.0X5	T49.0X6
Magaldrate	T47.1X1	T47.1X2	T47.1X3	T47.1X4	T47.1X5	T47.1X6
Magic mushroom	T40.991	T40.992	T40.993	T40.994	—	—
Magnamycin	T36.8X1	T36.8X2	T36.8X3	T36.8X4	T36.8X5	T36.8X6
Magnesia magma	T47.1X1	T47.1X2	T47.1X3	T47.1X4	T47.1X5	T47.1X6
Magnesium NEC	T56.891	T56.892	T56.893	T56.894	—	—
carbonate	T47.1X1	T47.1X2	T47.1X3	T47.1X4	T47.1X5	T47.1X6
citrate	T47.4X1	T47.4X2	T47.4X3	T47.4X4	T47.4X5	T47.4X6
hydroxide	T47.1X1	T47.1X2	T47.1X3	T47.1X4	T47.1X5	T47.1X6
oxide	T47.1X1	T47.1X2	T47.1X3	T47.1X4	T47.1X5	T47.1X6
peroxide	T49.0X1	T49.0X2	T49.0X3	T49.0X4	T49.0X5	T49.0X6

Substance	Poisoning, Accidental (unintentional)	Poisoning, Intentional Self-harm	Poisoning, Assault	Poisoning, Undetermined	Adverse Effect	Under-dosing
Magnesium — *continued*						
salicylate	T39.091	T39.092	T39.093	T39.094	T39.095	T39.096
silicofluoride	T50.3X1	T50.3X2	T50.3X3	T50.3X4	T50.3X5	T50.3X6
sulfate	T47.4X1	T47.4X2	T47.4X3	T47.4X4	T47.4X5	T47.4X6
thiosulfate	T45.0X1	T45.0X2	T45.0X3	T45.0X4	T45.0X5	T45.0X6
trisilicate	T47.1X1	T47.1X2	T47.1X3	T47.1X4	T47.1X5	T47.1X6
Malathion (medicinal)	T49.0X1	T49.0X2	T49.0X3	T49.0X4	T49.0X5	T49.0X6
insecticide	T60.0X1	T60.0X2	T60.0X3	T60.0X4	—	—
Male fern extract	T37.4X1	T37.4X2	T37.4X3	T37.4X4	T37.4X5	T37.4X6
M-AMSA	T45.1X1	T45.1X2	T45.1X3	T45.1X4	T45.1X5	T45.1X6
Mandelic acid	T37.8X1	T37.8X2	T37.8X3	T37.8X4	T37.8X5	T37.8X6
Manganese (dioxide) (salts)	T57.2X1	T57.2X2	T57.2X3	T57.2X4	—	—
medicinal	T50.991	T50.992	T50.993	T50.994	T50.995	T50.996
Mannitol	T47.3X1	T47.3X2	T47.3X3	T47.3X4	T47.3X5	T47.3X6
hexanitrate	T46.3X1	T46.3X2	T46.3X3	T46.3X4	T46.3X5	T46.3X6
Mannomustine	T45.1X1	T45.1X2	T45.1X3	T45.1X4	T45.1X5	T45.1X6
MAO inhibitors	T43.1X1	T43.1X2	T43.1X3	T43.1X4	T43.1X5	T43.1X6
Mapharsen	T37.8X1	T37.8X2	T37.8X3	T37.8X4	T37.8X5	T37.8X6
Maphenide	T49.0X1	T49.0X2	T49.0X3	T49.0X4	T49.0X5	T49.0X6
Maprotiline	T43.021	T43.022	T43.023	T43.024	T43.025	T43.026
Marcaine	T41.3X1	T41.3X2	T41.3X3	T41.3X4	T41.3X5	T41.3X6
infiltration (subcutaneous)	T41.3X1	T41.3X2	T41.3X3	T41.3X4	T41.3X5	T41.3X6
nerve block (peripheral) (plexus)	T41.3X1	T41.3X2	T41.3X3	T41.3X4	T41.3X5	T41.3X6
Marezine	T45.0X1	T45.0X2	T45.0X3	T45.0X4	T45.0X5	T45.0X6
Marihuana	T40.711	T40.712	T40.713	T40.714	T40.715	T40.716
Marijuana	T40.711	T40.712	T40.713	T40.714	T40.715	T40.716
Marine (sting)	T63.691	T63.692	T63.693	T63.694	—	—
animals (sting)	T63.691	T63.692	T63.693	T63.694	—	—
plants (sting)	T63.711	T63.712	T63.713	T63.714	—	—
Marplan	T43.1X1	T43.1X2	T43.1X3	T43.1X4	T43.1X5	T43.1X6
Marsh gas	T59.891	T59.892	T59.893	T59.894	—	—
Marsilid	T43.1X1	T43.1X2	T43.1X3	T43.1X4	T43.1X5	T43.1X6
Massengill*	T49.0X1	T49.0X2	T49.0X3	T49.0X4	T49.0X5	T49.0X6
Matulane	T45.1X1	T45.1X2	T45.1X3	T45.1X4	T45.1X5	T45.1X6
Mazindol	T50.5X1	T50.5X2	T50.5X3	T50.5X4	T50.5X5	T50.5X6
MCPA	T60.3X1	T60.3X2	T60.3X3	T60.3X4	—	—
MDMA	T43.641	T43.642	T43.643	T43.644	—	—
Meadow saffron	T62.2X1	T62.2X2	T62.2X3	T62.2X4	—	—
Measles virus vaccine (attenuated)	T50.B91	T50.B92	T50.B93	T50.B94	T50.B95	T50.B96
Meat, noxious	T62.8X1	T62.8X2	T62.8X3	T62.8X4	—	—
Meballymal	T42.3X1	T42.3X2	T42.3X3	T42.3X4	T42.3X5	T42.3X6
Mebanazine	T43.1X1	T43.1X2	T43.1X3	T43.1X4	T43.1X5	T43.1X6
Mebaral	T42.3X1	T42.3X2	T42.3X3	T42.3X4	T42.3X5	T42.3X6
Mebendazole	T37.4X1	T37.4X2	T37.4X3	T37.4X4	T37.4X5	T37.4X6
Mebeverine	T44.3X1	T44.3X2	T44.3X3	T44.3X4	T44.3X5	T44.3X6
Mebhydrolin	T45.0X1	T45.0X2	T45.0X3	T45.0X4	T45.0X5	T45.0X6
Mebumal	T42.3X1	T42.3X2	T42.3X3	T42.3X4	T42.3X5	T42.3X6
Mebutamate	T43.591	T43.592	T43.593	T43.594	T43.595	T43.596
Mecamylamine	T44.2X1	T44.2X2	T44.2X3	T44.2X4	T44.2X5	T44.2X6
Mechlorethamine	T45.1X1	T45.1X2	T45.1X3	T45.1X4	T45.1X5	T45.1X6
Mecillinam	T36.0X1	T36.0X2	T36.0X3	T36.0X4	T36.0X5	T36.0X6
Meclizine (hydrochloride)	T45.0X1	T45.0X2	T45.0X3	T45.0X4	T45.0X5	T45.0X6
Meclocycline	T36.4X1	T36.4X2	T36.4X3	T36.4X4	T36.4X5	T36.4X6
Meclofenamate	T39.391	T39.392	T39.393	T39.394	T39.395	T39.396
Meclofenamic acid	T39.391	T39.392	T39.393	T39.394	T39.395	T39.396
Meclofenoxate	T43.691	T43.692	T43.693	T43.694	T43.695	T43.696
Meclozine	T45.0X1	T45.0X2	T45.0X3	T45.0X4	T45.0X5	T45.0X6
Mecobalamin	T45.8X1	T45.8X2	T45.8X3	T45.8X4	T45.8X5	T45.8X6
Mecoprop	T60.3X1	T60.3X2	T60.3X3	T60.3X4	—	—
Mecrilate	T49.3X1	T49.3X2	T49.3X3	T49.3X4	T49.3X5	T49.3X6
Mecystein	T48.4X1	T48.4X2	T48.4X3	T48.4X4	T48.4X5	T48.4X6
Medazepam	T42.4X1	T42.4X2	T42.4X3	T42.4X4	T42.4X5	T42.4X6
Medicament NEC	T50.901	T50.902	T50.903	T50.904	T50.905	T50.906
Medinal	T42.3X1	T42.3X2	T42.3X3	T42.3X4	T42.3X5	T42.3X6
Medomin	T42.3X1	T42.3X2	T42.3X3	T42.3X4	T42.3X5	T42.3X6
Medrogestone	T38.5X1	T38.5X2	T38.5X3	T38.5X4	T38.5X5	T38.5X6
Medroxalol	T44.8X1	T44.8X2	T44.8X3	T44.8X4	T44.8X5	T44.8X6
Medroxyprogesterone acetate (depot)	T38.5X1	T38.5X2	T38.5X3	T38.5X4	T38.5X5	T38.5X6
Medrysone	T49.0X1	T49.0X2	T49.0X3	T49.0X4	T49.0X5	T49.0X6
Mefenamic acid	T39.391	T39.392	T39.393	T39.394	T39.395	T39.396
Mefenorex	T50.5X1	T50.5X2	T50.5X3	T50.5X4	T50.5X5	T50.5X6
Mefloquine	T37.2X1	T37.2X2	T37.2X3	T37.2X4	T37.2X5	T37.2X6
Mefoxin*	T36.1X1	T36.1X2	T36.1X3	T36.1X4	T36.1X5	T36.1X6
Mefruside	T50.2X1	T50.2X2	T50.2X3	T50.2X4	T50.2X5	T50.2X6
Megahallucinogen	T40.901	T40.902	T40.903	T40.904	T40.905	T40.906
Megestrol	T38.5X1	T38.5X2	T38.5X3	T38.5X4	T38.5X5	T38.5X6
Meglumine						
antimoniate	T37.8X1	T37.8X2	T37.8X3	T37.8X4	T37.8X5	T37.8X6
diatrizoate	T50.8X1	T50.8X2	T50.8X3	T50.8X4	T50.8X5	T50.8X6
iodipamide	T50.8X1	T50.8X2	T50.8X3	T50.8X4	T50.8X5	T50.8X6

Substance	Poisoning, Accidental (unintentional)	Poisoning, Intentional Self-harm	Poisoning, Assault	Poisoning, Undetermined	Adverse Effect	Under-dosing
Meglumine — *continued*						
iotroxate	T50.8X1	T50.8X2	T50.8X3	T50.8X4	T50.8X5	T50.8X6
MEK (methyl ethyl ketone)	T52.4X1	T52.4X2	T52.4X3	T52.4X4	—	—
Meladinin	T49.3X1	T49.3X2	T49.3X3	T49.3X4	T49.3X5	T49.3X6
Meladrazine	T44.3X1	T44.3X2	T44.3X3	T44.3X4	T44.3X5	T44.3X6
Melaleuca alternifolia oil	T49.0X1	T49.0X2	T49.0X3	T49.0X4	T49.0X5	T49.0X6
Melanizing agents	T49.3X1	T49.3X2	T49.3X3	T49.3X4	T49.3X5	T49.3X6
Melanocyte-stimulating hormone	T38.891	T38.892	T38.893	T38.894	T38.895	T38.896
Melarsonyl potassium	T37.3X1	T37.3X2	T37.3X3	T37.3X4	T37.3X5	T37.3X6
Melarsoprol	T37.3X1	T37.3X2	T37.3X3	T37.3X4	T37.3X5	T37.3X6
Melia azedarach	T62.2X1	T62.2X2	T62.2X3	T62.2X4	—	—
Melitracen	T43.011	T43.012	T43.013	T43.014	T43.015	T43.016
Mellaril	T43.3X1	T43.3X2	T43.3X3	T43.3X4	T43.3X5	T43.3X6
Meloxicam*	T39.391	T39.392	T39.393	T39.394	T39.395	T39.396
Meloxine	T49.3X1	T49.3X2	T49.3X3	T49.3X4	T49.3X5	T49.3X6
Melperone	T43.4X1	T43.4X2	T43.4X3	T43.4X4	T43.4X5	T43.4X6
Melphalan	T45.1X1	T45.1X2	T45.1X3	T45.1X4	T45.1X5	T45.1X6
Memantine	T43.8X1	T43.8X2	T43.8X3	T43.8X4	T43.8X5	T43.8X6
Menadiol	T45.7X1	T45.7X2	T45.7X3	T45.7X4	T45.7X5	T45.7X6
sodium sulfate	T45.7X1	T45.7X2	T45.7X3	T45.7X4	T45.7X5	T45.7X6
Menadione	T45.7X1	T45.7X2	T45.7X3	T45.7X4	T45.7X5	T45.7X6
sodium bisulfite	T45.7X1	T45.7X2	T45.7X3	T45.7X4	T45.7X5	T45.7X6
Menaphthone	T45.7X1	T45.7X2	T45.7X3	T45.7X4	T45.7X5	T45.7X6
Menaquinone	T45.7X1	T45.7X2	T45.7X3	T45.7X4	T45.7X5	T45.7X6
Menatetrenone	T45.7X1	T45.7X2	T45.7X3	T45.7X4	T45.7X5	T45.7X6
Meningococcal vaccine	T50.A91	T50.A92	T50.A93	T50.A94	T50.A95	T50.A96
Menningovax (-AC) (-C)	T50.A91	T50.A92	T50.A93	T50.A94	T50.A95	T50.A96
Menotropins	T38.811	T38.812	T38.813	T38.814	T38.815	T38.816
Menthol	T48.5X1	T48.5X2	T48.5X3	T48.5X4	T48.5X5	T48.5X6
Mepacrine	T37.2X1	T37.2X2	T37.2X3	T37.2X4	T37.2X5	T37.2X6
Meparfynol	T42.6X1	T42.6X2	T42.6X3	T42.6X4	T42.6X5	T42.6X6
Mepartricin	T36.7X1	T36.7X2	T36.7X3	T36.7X4	T36.7X5	T36.7X6
Mepazine	T43.3X1	T43.3X2	T43.3X3	T43.3X4	T43.3X5	T43.3X6
Mepenzolate	T44.3X1	T44.3X2	T44.3X3	T44.3X4	T44.3X5	T44.3X6
bromide	T44.3X1	T44.3X2	T44.3X3	T44.3X4	T44.3X5	T44.3X6
Meperidine	T40.491	T40.492	T40.493	T40.494	T40.495	T40.496
Mephebarbital	T42.3X1	T42.3X2	T42.3X3	T42.3X4	T42.3X5	T42.3X6
Mephenamin (e)	T42.8X1	T42.8X2	T42.8X3	T42.8X4	T42.8X5	T42.8X6
Mephenesin	T42.8X1	T42.8X2	T42.8X3	T42.8X4	T42.8X5	T42.8X6
Mephenhydramine	T45.0X1	T45.0X2	T45.0X3	T45.0X4	T45.0X5	T45.0X6
Mephenoxalone	T42.8X1	T42.8X2	T42.8X3	T42.8X4	T42.8X5	T42.8X6
Mephentermine	T44.991	T44.992	T44.993	T44.994	T44.995	T44.996
Mephenytoin	T42.0X1	T42.0X2	T42.0X3	T42.0X4	T42.0X5	T42.0X6
with phenobarbital	T42.3X1	T42.3X2	T42.3X3	T42.3X4	T42.3X5	T42.3X6
Mephobarbital	T42.3X1	T42.3X2	T42.3X3	T42.3X4	T42.3X5	T42.3X6
Mephosfolan	T60.0X1	T60.0X2	T60.0X3	T60.0X4	—	—
Mepindolol	T44.7X1	T44.7X2	T44.7X3	T44.7X4	T44.7X5	T44.7X6
Mepiperphenidol	T44.3X1	T44.3X2	T44.3X3	T44.3X4	T44.3X5	T44.3X6
Mepitiostane	T38.7X1	T38.7X2	T38.7X3	T38.7X4	T38.7X5	T38.7X6
Mepivacaine	T41.3X1	T41.3X2	T41.3X3	T41.3X4	T41.3X5	T41.3X6
epidural	T41.3X1	T41.3X2	T41.3X3	T41.3X4	T41.3X5	T41.3X6
Meprednisone	T38.0X1	T38.0X2	T38.0X3	T38.0X4	T38.0X5	T38.0X6
Meprobam	T43.591	T43.592	T43.593	T43.594	T43.595	T43.596
Meprobamate	T43.591	T43.592	T43.593	T43.594	T43.595	T43.596
Meproscillarin	T46.0X1	T46.0X2	T46.0X3	T46.0X4	T46.0X5	T46.0X6
Meprylcaine	T41.3X1	T41.3X2	T41.3X3	T41.3X4	T41.3X5	T41.3X6
Meptazinol	T39.8X1	T39.8X2	T39.8X3	T39.8X4	T39.8X5	T39.8X6
Mepyramine	T45.0X1	T45.0X2	T45.0X3	T45.0X4	T45.0X5	T45.0X6
Mequinol*	T49.8X1	T49.8X2	T49.8X3	T49.8X4	T49.8X5	T49.8X6
Mequitazine	T43.3X1	T43.3X2	T43.3X3	T43.3X4	T43.3X5	T43.3X6
Meralluride	T50.2X1	T50.2X2	T50.2X3	T50.2X4	T50.2X5	T50.2X6
Merbaphen	T50.2X1	T50.2X2	T50.2X3	T50.2X4	T50.2X5	T50.2X6
Merbromin	T49.0X1	T49.0X2	T49.0X3	T49.0X4	T49.0X5	T49.0X6
Mercaptobenzothiazole salts	T49.0X1	T49.0X2	T49.0X3	T49.0X4	T49.0X5	T49.0X6
Mercaptomerin	T50.2X1	T50.2X2	T50.2X3	T50.2X4	T50.2X5	T50.2X6
Mercaptopurine	T45.1X1	T45.1X2	T45.1X3	T45.1X4	T45.1X5	T45.1X6
Mercumatilin	T50.2X1	T50.2X2	T50.2X3	T50.2X4	T50.2X5	T50.2X6
Mercuramide	T50.2X1	T50.2X2	T50.2X3	T50.2X4	T50.2X5	T50.2X6
Mercurochrome	T49.0X1	T49.0X2	T49.0X3	T49.0X4	T49.0X5	T49.0X6
Mercurophylline	T50.2X1	T50.2X2	T50.2X3	T50.2X4	T50.2X5	T50.2X6
Mercury, mercurial, mercuric, mercurous (compounds) (cyanide) (fumes) (nonmedicinal) (vapor) **NEC**	T56.1X1	T56.1X2	T56.1X3	T56.1X4	—	—
ammoniated	T49.0X1	T49.0X2	T49.0X3	T49.0X4	T49.0X5	T49.0X6
anti-infective						
local	T49.0X1	T49.0X2	T49.0X3	T49.0X4	T49.0X5	T49.0X6
systemic	T37.8X1	T37.8X2	T37.8X3	T37.8X4	T37.8X5	T37.8X6
topical	T49.0X1	T49.0X2	T49.0X3	T49.0X4	T49.0X5	T49.0X6
chloride (ammoniated)	T49.0X1	T49.0X2	T49.0X3	T49.0X4	T49.0X5	T49.0X6

Substance	Poisoning, Accidental (unintentional)	Poisoning, Intentional Self-harm	Poisoning, Assault	Poisoning, Undetermined	Adverse Effect	Under-dosing
Mercury, mercurial, mercuric, mercurous (compounds) (cyanide) (fumes) (nonmedicinal) (vapor) **NEC** — *continued*						
chloride — *continued*						
fungicide	T56.1X1	T56.1X2	T56.1X3	T56.1X4	—	—
diuretic NEC	T50.2X1	T50.2X2	T50.2X3	T50.2X4	T50.2X5	T50.2X6
fungicide	T56.1X1	T56.1X2	T56.1X3	T56.1X4	—	—
organic (fungicide)	T56.1X1	T56.1X2	T56.1X3	T56.1X4	—	—
oxide, yellow	T49.0X1	T49.0X2	T49.0X3	T49.0X4	T49.0X5	T49.0X6
Mersalyl	T50.2X1	T50.2X2	T50.2X3	T50.2X4	T50.2X5	T50.2X6
Merthiolate	T49.0X1	T49.0X2	T49.0X3	T49.0X4	T49.0X5	T49.0X6
ophthalmic preparation	T49.5X1	T49.5X2	T49.5X3	T49.5X4	T49.5X5	T49.5X6
Meruvax	T50.B91	T50.B92	T50.B93	T50.B94	T50.B95	T50.B96
Mesalazine	T47.8X1	T47.8X2	T47.8X3	T47.8X4	T47.8X5	T47.8X6
Mescal buttons	T40.991	T40.992	T40.993	T40.994	—	—
Mescaline	T40.991	T40.992	T40.993	T40.994	—	—
Mesna	T48.4X1	T48.4X2	T48.4X3	T48.4X4	T48.4X5	T48.4X6
Mesoglycan	T46.6X1	T46.6X2	T46.6X3	T46.6X4	T46.6X5	T46.6X6
Mesoridazine	T43.3X1	T43.3X2	T43.3X3	T43.3X4	T43.3X5	T43.3X6
Mestanolone	T38.7X1	T38.7X2	T38.7X3	T38.7X4	T38.7X5	T38.7X6
Mesterolone	T38.7X1	T38.7X2	T38.7X3	T38.7X4	T38.7X5	T38.7X6
Mestranol	T38.5X1	T38.5X2	T38.5X3	T38.5X4	T38.5X5	T38.5X6
Mesulergine	T42.8X1	T42.8X2	T42.8X3	T42.8X4	T42.8X5	T42.8X6
Mesulfen	T49.0X1	T49.0X2	T49.0X3	T49.0X4	T49.0X5	T49.0X6
Mesuximide	T42.2X1	T42.2X2	T42.2X3	T42.2X4	T42.2X5	T42.2X6
Metabutethamine	T41.3X1	T41.3X2	T41.3X3	T41.3X4	T41.3X5	T41.3X6
Metactesylacetate	T49.0X1	T49.0X2	T49.0X3	T49.0X4	T49.0X5	T49.0X6
Metacycline	T36.4X1	T36.4X2	T36.4X3	T36.4X4	T36.4X5	T36.4X6
Metaldehyde (snail killer) **NEC**	T60.8X1	T60.8X2	T60.8X3	T60.8X4	—	—
Metals (heavy) (nonmedicinal)	T56.91	T56.92	T56.93	T56.94	—	—
dust, fumes, or vapor NEC	T56.91	T56.92	T56.93	T56.94	—	—
light NEC	T56.91	T56.92	T56.93	T56.94	—	—
dust, fumes, or vapor NEC	T56.91	T56.92	T56.93	T56.94	—	—
specified NEC	T56.891	T56.892	T56.893	T56.894	—	—
thallium	T56.811	T56.812	T56.813	T56.814	—	—
Metamfetamine	T43.651	T43.652	T43.652	T43.654	T43.655	T43.656
Metamizole sodium	T39.2X1	T39.2X2	T39.2X3	T39.2X4	T39.2X5	T39.2X6
Metampicillin	T36.0X1	T36.0X2	T36.0X3	T36.0X4	T36.0X5	T36.0X6
Metamucil	T47.4X1	T47.4X2	T47.4X3	T47.4X4	T47.4X5	T47.4X6
Metandienone	T38.7X1	T38.7X2	T38.7X3	T38.7X4	T38.7X5	T38.7X6
Metandrostenolone	T38.7X1	T38.7X2	T38.7X3	T38.7X4	T38.7X5	T38.7X6
Metaphen	T49.0X1	T49.0X2	T49.0X3	T49.0X4	T49.0X5	T49.0X6
Metaphos	T60.0X1	T60.0X2	T60.0X3	T60.0X4	—	—
Metapramine	T43.011	T43.012	T43.013	T43.014	T43.015	T43.016
Metaproterenol	T48.291	T48.292	T48.293	T48.294	T48.295	T48.296
Metaraminol	T44.4X1	T44.4X2	T44.4X3	T44.4X4	T44.4X5	T44.4X6
Metaxalone	T42.8X1	T42.8X2	T42.8X3	T42.8X4	T42.8X5	T42.8X6
Meted*	T49.4X1	T49.4X2	T49.4X3	T49.4X4	T49.4X5	T49.4X6
Metenolone	T38.7X1	T38.7X2	T38.7X3	T38.7X4	T38.7X5	T38.7X6
Metergoline	T42.8X1	T42.8X2	T42.8X3	T42.8X4	T42.8X5	T42.8X6
Metescufylline	T46.991	T46.992	T46.993	T46.994	T46.995	T46.996
Metetoin	T42.0X1	T42.0X2	T42.0X3	T42.0X4	T42.0X5	T42.0X6
Metformin	T38.3X1	T38.3X2	T38.3X3	T38.3X4	T38.3X5	T38.3X6
Methacholine	T44.1X1	T44.1X2	T44.1X3	T44.1X4	T44.1X5	T44.1X6
Methacycline	T36.4X1	T36.4X2	T36.4X3	T36.4X4	T36.4X5	T36.4X6
Methadone	T40.3X1	T40.3X2	T40.3X3	T40.3X4	T40.3X5	T40.3X6
Methadose*	T40.3X1	T40.3X2	T40.3X3	T40.3X4	T40.3X5	T40.3X6
Methallenestril	T38.5X1	T38.5X2	T38.5X3	T38.5X4	T38.5X5	T38.5X6
Methallenoestril	T38.5X1	T38.5X2	T38.5X3	T38.5X4	T38.5X5	T38.5X6
Methamphetamine	T43.651	T43.652	T43.652	T43.654	T43.655	T43.656
Methampyrone	T39.2X1	T39.2X2	T39.2X3	T39.2X4	T39.2X5	T39.2X6
Methandienone	T38.7X1	T38.7X2	T38.7X3	T38.7X4	T38.7X5	T38.7X6
Methandriol	T38.7X1	T38.7X2	T38.7X3	T38.7X4	T38.7X5	T38.7X6
Methandrostenolone	T38.7X1	T38.7X2	T38.7X3	T38.7X4	T38.7X5	T38.7X6
Methane	T59.891	T59.892	T59.893	T59.894	—	—
Methanethiol	T59.891	T59.892	T59.893	T59.894	—	—
Methaniazide	T37.1X1	T37.1X2	T37.1X3	T37.1X4	T37.1X5	T37.1X6
Methanol (vapor)	T51.1X1	T51.1X2	T51.1X3	T51.1X4	—	—
Methantheline	T44.3X1	T44.3X2	T44.3X3	T44.3X4	T44.3X5	T44.3X6
Methanthelinium bromide	T44.3X1	T44.3X2	T44.3X3	T44.3X4	T44.3X5	T44.3X6
Methaphenilene	T45.0X1	T45.0X2	T45.0X3	T45.0X4	T45.0X5	T45.0X6
Methapyrilene	T45.0X1	T45.0X2	T45.0X3	T45.0X4	T45.0X5	T45.0X6
Methaqualone (compound)	T42.6X1	T42.6X2	T42.6X3	T42.6X4	T42.6X5	T42.6X6
Metharbital	T42.3X1	T42.3X2	T42.3X3	T42.3X4	T42.3X5	T42.3X6
Methazolamide	T50.2X1	T50.2X2	T50.2X3	T50.2X4	T50.2X5	T50.2X6
Methdilazine	T43.3X1	T43.3X2	T43.3X3	T43.3X4	T43.3X5	T43.3X6
Methedrine	T43.651	T43.652	T43.652	T43.654	T43.655	T43.656
Methenamine (mandelate)	T37.8X1	T37.8X2	T37.8X3	T37.8X4	T37.8X5	T37.8X6
Methenolone	T38.7X1	T38.7X2	T38.7X3	T38.7X4	T38.7X5	T38.7X6

☑ **Additional Character May Be Required — Refer to the Tabular List for Character Selection** *Optum Value-Add

Substance	Poisoning, Accidental (unintentional)	Poisoning, Intentional Self-harm	Poisoning, Assault	Poisoning, Undetermined	Adverse Effect	Under-dosing
Methergine	T48.0X1	T48.0X2	T48.0X3	T48.0X4	T48.0X5	T48.0X6
Methetoin	T42.0X1	T42.0X2	T42.0X3	T42.0X4	T42.0X5	T42.0X6
Methiacil	T38.2X1	T38.2X2	T38.2X3	T38.2X4	T38.2X5	T38.2X6
Methicillin	T36.0X1	T36.0X2	T36.0X3	T36.0X4	T36.0X5	T36.0X6
Methimazole	T38.2X1	T38.2X2	T38.2X3	T38.2X4	T38.2X5	T38.2X6
Methiodal sodium	T50.8X1	T50.8X2	T50.8X3	T50.8X4	T50.8X5	T50.8X6
Methionine	T50.991	T50.992	T50.993	T50.994	T50.995	T50.996
Methisazone	T37.5X1	T37.5X2	T37.5X3	T37.5X4	T37.5X5	T37.5X6
Methisoprinol	T37.5X1	T37.5X2	T37.5X3	T37.5X4	T37.5X5	T37.5X6
Methitural	T42.3X1	T42.3X2	T42.3X3	T42.3X4	T42.3X5	T42.3X6
Methixene	T44.3X1	T44.3X2	T44.3X3	T44.3X4	T44.3X5	T44.3X6
Methobarbital, methobarbitone	T42.3X1	T42.3X2	T42.3X3	T42.3X4	T42.3X5	T42.3X6
Methocarbamol	T42.8X1	T42.8X2	T42.8X3	T42.8X4	T42.8X5	T42.8X6
skeletal muscle relaxant	T48.1X1	T48.1X2	T48.1X3	T48.1X4	T48.1X5	T48.1X6
Methohexital	T41.1X1	T41.1X2	T41.1X3	T41.1X4	T41.1X5	T41.1X6
Methohexitone	T41.1X1	T41.1X2	T41.1X3	T41.1X4	T41.1X5	T41.1X6
Methoin	T42.0X1	T42.0X2	T42.0X3	T42.0X4	T42.0X5	T42.0X6
Methopholine	T39.8X1	T39.8X2	T39.8X3	T39.8X4	T39.8X5	T39.8X6
Methopromazine	T43.3X1	T43.3X2	T43.3X3	T43.3X4	T43.3X5	T43.3X6
Methorate	T48.3X1	T48.3X2	T48.3X3	T48.3X4	T48.3X5	T48.3X6
Methoserpidine	T46.5X1	T46.5X2	T46.5X3	T46.5X4	T46.5X5	T46.5X6
Methotrexate	T45.1X1	T45.1X2	T45.1X3	T45.1X4	T45.1X5	T45.1X6
Methotrimeprazine	T43.3X1	T43.3X2	T43.3X3	T43.3X4	T43.3X5	T43.3X6
Methoxa-Dome	T49.3X1	T49.3X2	T49.3X3	T49.3X4	T49.3X5	T49.3X6
Methoxamine	T44.4X1	T44.4X2	T44.4X3	T44.4X4	T44.4X5	T44.4X6
Methoxsalen	T50.991	T50.992	T50.993	T50.994	T50.995	T50.996
Methoxyaniline	T65.3X1	T65.3X2	T65.3X3	T65.3X4	—	—
Methoxybenzyl penicillin	T36.0X1	T36.0X2	T36.0X3	T36.0X4	T36.0X5	T36.0X6
Methoxychlor	T53.7X1	T53.7X2	T53.7X3	T53.7X4	—	—
Methoxy-DDT	T53.7X1	T53.7X2	T53.7X3	T53.7X4	—	—
Methoxyflurane	T41.0X1	T41.0X2	T41.0X3	T41.0X4	T41.0X5	T41.0X6
Methoxyphenamine	T48.6X1	T48.6X2	T48.6X3	T48.6X4	T48.6X5	T48.6X6
Methoxypromazine	T43.3X1	T43.3X2	T43.3X3	T43.3X4	T43.3X5	T43.3X6
Methscopolamine bromide	T44.3X1	T44.3X2	T44.3X3	T44.3X4	T44.3X5	T44.3X6
Methsuximide	T42.2X1	T42.2X2	T42.2X3	T42.2X4	T42.2X5	T42.2X6
Methyclothiazide	T50.2X1	T50.2X2	T50.2X3	T50.2X4	T50.2X5	T50.2X6
Methyl						
acetate	T52.4X1	T52.4X2	T52.4X3	T52.4X4	—	—
acetone	T52.4X1	T52.4X2	T52.4X3	T52.4X4	—	—
acrylate	T65.891	T65.892	T65.893	T65.894	—	—
alcohol	T51.1X1	T51.1X2	T51.1X3	T51.1X4	—	—
aminophenol	T65.3X1	T65.3X2	T65.3X3	T65.3X4	—	—
amphetamine	T43.651	T43.652	T43.652	T43.654	T43.655	T43.656
androstanolone	T38.7X1	T38.7X2	T38.7X3	T38.7X4	T38.7X5	T38.7X6
atropine	T44.3X1	T44.3X2	T44.3X3	T44.3X4	T44.3X5	T44.3X6
benzene	T52.2X1	T52.2X2	T52.2X3	T52.2X4	—	—
benzoate	T52.8X1	T52.8X2	T52.8X3	T52.8X4	—	—
benzol	T52.2X1	T52.2X2	T52.2X3	T52.2X4	—	—
bromide (gas)	T59.891	T59.892	T59.893	T59.894	—	—
fumigant	T60.8X1	T60.8X2	T60.8X3	T60.8X4	—	—
butanol	T51.3X1	T51.3X2	T51.3X3	T51.3X4	—	—
carbinol	T51.1X1	T51.1X2	T51.1X3	T51.1X4	—	—
carbonate	T52.8X1	T52.8X2	T52.8X3	T52.8X4	—	—
CCNU	T45.1X1	T45.1X2	T45.1X3	T45.1X4	T45.1X5	T45.1X6
cellosolve	T52.91	T52.92	T52.93	T52.94	—	—
cellulose	T47.4X1	T47.4X2	T47.4X3	T47.4X4	T47.4X5	T47.4X6
chloride (gas)	T59.891	T59.892	T59.893	T59.894	—	—
chloroformate	T59.3X1	T59.3X2	T59.3X3	T59.3X4	—	—
cyclohexane	T52.8X1	T52.8X2	T52.8X3	T52.8X4	—	—
cyclohexanol	T51.8X1	T51.8X2	T51.8X3	T51.8X4	—	—
cyclohexanone	T52.8X1	T52.8X2	T52.8X3	T52.8X4	—	—
cyclohexyl acetate	T52.8X1	T52.8X2	T52.8X3	T52.8X4	—	—
demeton	T60.0X1	T60.0X2	T60.0X3	T60.0X4	—	—
dihydromorphinone	T40.2X1	T40.2X2	T40.2X3	T40.2X4	T40.2X5	T40.2X6
ergometrine	T48.0X1	T48.0X2	T48.0X3	T48.0X4	T48.0X5	T48.0X6
ergonovine	T48.0X1	T48.0X2	T48.0X3	T48.0X4	T48.0X5	T48.0X6
ethyl ketone	T52.4X1	T52.4X2	T52.4X3	T52.4X4	—	—
glucamine antimonate	T37.8X1	T37.8X2	T37.8X3	T37.8X4	T37.8X5	T37.8X6
hydrazine	T65.891	T65.892	T65.893	T65.894	—	—
iodide	T65.891	T65.892	T65.893	T65.894	—	—
isobutyl ketone	T52.4X1	T52.4X2	T52.4X3	T52.4X4	—	—
isothiocyanate	T60.3X1	T60.3X2	T60.3X3	T60.3X4	—	—
mercaptan	T59.891	T59.892	T59.893	T59.894	—	—
morphine NEC	T40.2X1	T40.2X2	T40.2X3	T40.2X4	T40.2X5	T40.2X6
nicotinate	T49.4X1	T49.4X2	T49.4X3	T49.4X4	T49.4X5	T49.4X6
paraben	T49.0X1	T49.0X2	T49.0X3	T49.0X4	T49.0X5	T49.0X6
parafynol	T42.6X1	T42.6X2	T42.6X3	T42.6X4	T42.6X5	T42.6X6
parathion	T60.0X1	T60.0X2	T60.0X3	T60.0X4	—	—
peridol	T43.4X1	T43.4X2	T43.4X3	T43.4X4	T43.4X5	T43.4X6
phenidate	T43.631	T43.632	T43.633	T43.634	T43.635	T43.636
prednisolone	T38.0X1	T38.0X2	T38.0X3	T38.0X4	T38.0X5	T38.0X6

Substance	Poisoning, Accidental (unintentional)	Poisoning, Intentional Self-harm	Poisoning, Assault	Poisoning, Undetermined	Adverse Effect	Under-dosing
Methyl — continued						
prednisolone — continued						
ENT agent	T49.6X1	T49.6X2	T49.6X3	T49.6X4	T49.6X5	T49.6X6
ophthalmic preparation	T49.5X1	T49.5X2	T49.5X3	T49.5X4	T49.5X5	T49.5X6
topical NEC	T49.0X1	T49.0X2	T49.0X3	T49.0X4	T49.0X5	T49.0X6
propylcarbinol	T51.3X1	T51.3X2	T51.3X3	T51.3X4	—	—
rosaniline NEC	T49.0X1	T49.0X2	T49.0X3	T49.0X4	T49.0X5	T49.0X6
salicylate	T49.2X1	T49.2X2	T49.2X3	T49.2X4	T49.2X5	T49.2X6
sulfate (fumes)	T59.891	T59.892	T59.893	T59.894	—	—
liquid	T52.8X1	T52.8X2	T52.8X3	T52.8X4	—	—
sulfonal	T42.6X1	T42.6X2	T42.6X3	T42.6X4	T42.6X5	T42.6X6
testosterone	T38.7X1	T38.7X2	T38.7X3	T38.7X4	T38.7X5	T38.7X6
thiouracil	T38.2X1	T38.2X2	T38.2X3	T38.2X4	T38.2X5	T38.2X6
Methylacetoxyprogesterone*	T38.5X1	T38.5X2	T38.5X3	T38.5X4	T38.5X5	T38.5X6
Methylamphetamine	T43.651	T43.652	T43.652	T43.654	T43.655	T43.656
Methylated spirit	T51.1X1	T51.1X2	T51.1X3	T51.1X4	—	—
Methylatropine nitrate	T44.3X1	T44.3X2	T44.3X3	T44.3X4	T44.3X5	T44.3X6
Methylbenactyzium bromide	T44.3X1	T44.3X2	T44.3X3	T44.3X4	T44.3X5	T44.3X6
Methylbenzethonium chloride	T49.0X1	T49.0X2	T49.0X3	T49.0X4	T49.0X5	T49.0X6
Methylcellulose	T47.4X1	T47.4X2	T47.4X3	T47.4X4	T47.4X5	T47.4X6
laxative	T47.4X1	T47.4X2	T47.4X3	T47.4X4	T47.4X5	T47.4X6
Methylchlorophenoxyacetic acid	T60.3X1	T60.3X2	T60.3X3	T60.3X4	—	—
Methyldopa	T46.5X1	T46.5X2	T46.5X3	T46.5X4	T46.5X5	T46.5X6
Methyldopate	T46.5X1	T46.5X2	T46.5X3	T46.5X4	T46.5X5	T46.5X6
Methylene						
blue	T50.6X1	T50.6X2	T50.6X3	T50.6X4	T50.6X5	T50.6X6
chloride or dichloride (solvent)	T53.4X1	T53.4X2	T53.4X3	T53.4X4	—	—
NEC						
Methylenedioxyamphetamine	T43.621	T43.622	T43.623	T43.624	T43.625	T43.626
Methylenedioxymeth- amphetamine	T43.641	T43.642	T43.643	T43.644	—	—
Methylergometrine	T48.0X1	T48.0X2	T48.0X3	T48.0X4	T48.0X5	T48.0X6
Methylergonovine	T48.0X1	T48.0X2	T48.0X3	T48.0X4	T48.0X5	T48.0X6
Methylestrenolone	T38.5X1	T38.5X2	T38.5X3	T38.5X4	T38.5X5	T38.5X6
Methylethyl cellulose	T50.991	T50.992	T50.993	T50.994	T50.995	T50.996
Methylhexabital	T42.3X1	T42.3X2	T42.3X3	T42.3X4	T42.3X5	T42.3X6
Methylmorphine	T40.2X1	T40.2X2	T40.2X3	T40.2X4	T40.2X5	T40.2X6
Methylparaben (ophthalmic)	T49.5X1	T49.5X2	T49.5X3	T49.5X4	T49.5X5	T49.5X6
Methylparafynol	T42.6X1	T42.6X2	T42.6X3	T42.6X4	T42.6X5	T42.6X6
Methylpentynol, methylpenthynol	T42.6X1	T42.6X2	T42.6X3	T42.6X4	T42.6X5	T42.6X6
Methylphenidate	T43.631	T43.632	T43.633	T43.634	T43.635	T43.636
Methylphenobarbital	T42.3X1	T42.3X2	T42.3X3	T42.3X4	T42.3X5	T42.3X6
Methylpolysiloxane	T47.1X1	T47.1X2	T47.1X3	T47.1X4	T47.1X5	T47.1X6
Methylprednisolone — see Methyl, prednisolone						
Methylrosaniline	T49.0X1	T49.0X2	T49.0X3	T49.0X4	T49.0X5	T49.0X6
Methylrosanilinium chloride	T49.0X1	T49.0X2	T49.0X3	T49.0X4	T49.0X5	T49.0X6
Methyltestosterone	T38.7X1	T38.7X2	T38.7X3	T38.7X4	T38.7X5	T38.7X6
Methylthionine chloride	T50.6X1	T50.6X2	T50.6X3	T50.6X4	T50.6X5	T50.6X6
Methylthioninine chloride	T50.6X1	T50.6X2	T50.6X3	T50.6X4	T50.6X5	T50.6X6
Methylthiouracil	T38.2X1	T38.2X2	T38.2X3	T38.2X4	T38.2X5	T38.2X6
Methyprylon	T42.6X1	T42.6X2	T42.6X3	T42.6X4	T42.6X5	T42.6X6
Methysergide	T46.5X1	T46.5X2	T46.5X3	T46.5X4	T46.5X5	T46.5X6
Metiamide	T47.1X1	T47.1X2	T47.1X3	T47.1X4	T47.1X5	T47.1X6
Meticillin	T36.0X1	T36.0X2	T36.0X3	T36.0X4	T36.0X5	T36.0X6
Meticrane	T50.2X1	T50.2X2	T50.2X3	T50.2X4	T50.2X5	T50.2X6
Metildigoxin	T46.0X1	T46.0X2	T46.0X3	T46.0X4	T46.0X5	T46.0X6
Metipranolol	T49.5X1	T49.5X2	T49.5X3	T49.5X4	T49.5X5	T49.5X6
Metirosine	T46.5X1	T46.5X2	T46.5X3	T46.5X4	T46.5X5	T46.5X6
Metisazone	T37.5X1	T37.5X2	T37.5X3	T37.5X4	T37.5X5	T37.5X6
Metixene	T44.3X1	T44.3X2	T44.3X3	T44.3X4	T44.3X5	T44.3X6
Metizoline	T48.5X1	T48.5X2	T48.5X3	T48.5X4	T48.5X5	T48.5X6
Metoclopramide	T45.0X1	T45.0X2	T45.0X3	T45.0X4	T45.0X5	T45.0X6
Metofenazate	T43.3X1	T43.3X2	T43.3X3	T43.3X4	T43.3X5	T43.3X6
Metofoline	T39.8X1	T39.8X2	T39.8X3	T39.8X4	T39.8X5	T39.8X6
Metolazone	T50.2X1	T50.2X2	T50.2X3	T50.2X4	T50.2X5	T50.2X6
Metopon	T40.2X1	T40.2X2	T40.2X3	T40.2X4	T40.2X5	T40.2X6
Metoprine	T45.1X1	T45.1X2	T45.1X3	T45.1X4	T45.1X5	T45.1X6
Metoprolol	T44.7X1	T44.7X2	T44.7X3	T44.7X4	T44.7X5	T44.7X6
Metrifonate	T60.0X1	T60.0X2	T60.0X3	T60.0X4	—	—
Metrizamide	T50.8X1	T50.8X2	T50.8X3	T50.8X4	T50.8X5	T50.8X6
Metrizoic acid	T50.8X1	T50.8X2	T50.8X3	T50.8X4	T50.8X5	T50.8X6
Metronidazole	T37.8X1	T37.8X2	T37.8X3	T37.8X4	T37.8X5	T37.8X6
Metycaine	T41.3X1	T41.3X2	T41.3X3	T41.3X4	T41.3X5	T41.3X6
infiltration (subcutaneous)	T41.3X1	T41.3X2	T41.3X3	T41.3X4	T41.3X5	T41.3X6

Substance	Poisoning, Accidental (unintentional)	Poisoning, Intentional Self-harm	Poisoning, Assault	Poisoning, Undetermined	Adverse Effect	Under-dosing
Metycaine — *continued*						
nerve block (peripheral) (plexus)	T41.3X1	T41.3X2	T41.3X3	T41.3X4	T41.3X5	T41.3X6
topical (surface)	T41.3X1	T41.3X2	T41.3X3	T41.3X4	T41.3X5	T41.3X6
Metyrapone	T50.8X1	T50.8X2	T50.8X3	T50.8X4	T50.8X5	T50.8X6
Mevacor*	T46.6X1	T46.6X2	T46.6X3	T46.6X4	T46.6X5	T46.6X6
Mevinphos	T60.0X1	T60.0X2	T60.0X3	T60.0X4	—	—
Mexazolam	T42.4X1	T42.4X2	T42.4X3	T42.4X4	T42.4X5	T42.4X6
Mexenone	T49.3X1	T49.3X2	T49.3X3	T49.3X4	T49.3X5	T49.3X6
Mexiletine	T46.2X1	T46.2X2	T46.2X3	T46.2X4	T46.2X5	T46.2X6
Mezereon	T62.2X1	T62.2X2	T62.2X3	T62.2X4	—	—
berries	T62.1X1	T62.1X2	T62.1X3	T62.1X4	—	—
Mezlocillin	T36.0X1	T36.0X2	T36.0X3	T36.0X4	T36.0X5	T36.0X6
Mianserin	T43.021	T43.022	T43.023	T43.024	T43.025	T43.026
Micatin	T49.0X1	T49.0X2	T49.0X3	T49.0X4	T49.0X5	T49.0X6
Miconazole	T49.0X1	T49.0X2	T49.0X3	T49.0X4	T49.0X5	T49.0X6
Micronomicin	T36.5X1	T36.5X2	T36.5X3	T36.5X4	T36.5X5	T36.5X6
Microzide*	T50.2X1	T50.2X2	T50.2X3	T50.2X4	T50.2X5	T50.2X6
Midazolam	T42.4X1	T42.4X2	T42.4X3	T42.4X4	T42.4X5	T42.4X6
Midecamycin	T36.3X1	T36.3X2	T36.3X3	T36.3X4	T36.3X5	T36.3X6
Mifepristone	T38.6X1	T38.6X2	T38.6X3	T38.6X4	T38.6X5	T38.6X6
Milk of magnesia	T47.1X1	T47.1X2	T47.1X3	T47.1X4	T47.1X5	T47.1X6
Millipede (tropical) (venomous)	T63.411	T63.412	T63.413	T63.414	—	—
Miltown	T43.591	T43.592	T43.593	T43.594	T43.595	T43.596
Milverine	T44.3X1	T44.3X2	T44.3X3	T44.3X4	T44.3X5	T44.3X6
Minaprine	T43.291	T43.292	T43.293	T43.294	T43.295	T43.296
Minaxolone	T41.291	T41.292	T41.293	T41.294	T41.295	T41.296
Mineral						
acids	T54.2X1	T54.2X2	T54.2X3	T54.2X4	—	—
oil (laxative)(medicinal)	T47.4X1	T47.4X2	T47.4X3	T47.4X4	T47.4X5	T47.4X6
emulsion	T47.2X1	T47.2X2	T47.2X3	T47.2X4	T47.2X5	T47.2X6
nonmedicinal	T52.0X1	T52.0X2	T52.0X3	T52.0X4	—	—
topical	T49.3X1	T49.3X2	T49.3X3	T49.3X4	T49.3X5	T49.3X6
salt NEC	T50.3X1	T50.3X2	T50.3X3	T50.3X4	T50.3X5	T50.3X6
spirits	T52.0X1	T52.0X2	T52.0X3	T52.0X4	—	—
Mineralocorticosteroid	T50.0X1	T50.0X2	T50.0X3	T50.0X4	T50.0X5	T50.0X6
Minocycline	T36.4X1	T36.4X2	T36.4X3	T36.4X4	T36.4X5	T36.4X6
Minoxidil	T46.7X1	T46.7X2	T46.7X3	T46.7X4	T46.7X5	T46.7X6
Miokamycin	T36.3X1	T36.3X2	T36.3X3	T36.3X4	T36.3X5	T36.3X6
Miotic drug	T49.5X1	T49.5X2	T49.5X3	T49.5X4	T49.5X5	T49.5X6
Mipafox	T60.0X1	T60.0X2	T60.0X3	T60.0X4	—	—
Mipomerson*	T46.6X1	T46.6X2	T46.6X3	T46.6X4	T46.6X5	T46.6X6
Mirex	T60.1X1	T60.1X2	T60.1X3	T60.1X4	—	—
Mirtazapine	T43.021	T43.022	T43.023	T43.024	T43.025	T43.026
Misonidazole	T37.3X1	T37.3X2	T37.3X3	T37.3X4	T37.3X5	T37.3X6
Misoprostol	T47.1X1	T47.1X2	T47.1X3	T47.1X4	T47.1X5	T47.1X6
Mithramycin	T45.1X1	T45.1X2	T45.1X3	T45.1X4	T45.1X5	T45.1X6
Mitobronitol	T45.1X1	T45.1X2	T45.1X3	T45.1X4	T45.1X5	T45.1X6
Mitoguazone	T45.1X1	T45.1X2	T45.1X3	T45.1X4	T45.1X5	T45.1X6
Mitolactol	T45.1X1	T45.1X2	T45.1X3	T45.1X4	T45.1X5	T45.1X6
Mitomycin	T45.1X1	T45.1X2	T45.1X3	T45.1X4	T45.1X5	T45.1X6
Mitopodozide	T45.1X1	T45.1X2	T45.1X3	T45.1X4	T45.1X5	T45.1X6
Mitotane	T45.1X1	T45.1X2	T45.1X3	T45.1X4	T45.1X5	T45.1X6
Mitoxantrone	T45.1X1	T45.1X2	T45.1X3	T45.1X4	T45.1X5	T45.1X6
Mivacurium chloride	T48.1X1	T48.1X2	T48.1X3	T48.1X4	T48.1X5	T48.1X6
Miyari bacteria	T47.6X1	T47.6X2	T47.6X3	T47.6X4	T47.6X5	T47.6X6
Moclobemide	T43.1X1	T43.1X2	T43.1X3	T43.1X4	T43.1X5	T43.1X6
Moderil	T46.5X1	T46.5X2	T46.5X3	T46.5X4	T46.5X5	T46.5X6
Mofebutazone	T39.2X1	T39.2X2	T39.2X3	T39.2X4	T39.2X5	T39.2X6
Mogadon — *see* Nitrazepam						
Molindone	T43.591	T43.592	T43.593	T43.594	T43.595	T43.596
Molsidomine	T46.3X1	T46.3X2	T46.3X3	T46.3X4	T46.3X5	T46.3X6
Mometasone	T49.0X1	T49.0X2	T49.0X3	T49.0X4	T49.0X5	T49.0X6
Monistat	T49.0X1	T49.0X2	T49.0X3	T49.0X4	T49.0X5	T49.0X6
Monkshood	T62.2X1	T62.2X2	T62.2X3	T62.2X4	—	—
Monoamine oxidase inhibitor NEC	T43.1X1	T43.1X2	T43.1X3	T43.1X4	T43.1X5	T43.1X6
hydrazine	T43.1X1	T43.1X2	T43.1X3	T43.1X4	T43.1X5	T43.1X6
Monobenzone	T49.4X1	T49.4X2	T49.4X3	T49.4X4	T49.4X5	T49.4X6
Monochloroacetic acid	T60.3X1	T60.3X2	T60.3X3	T60.3X4	—	—
Monochlorobenzene	T53.7X1	T53.7X2	T53.7X3	T53.7X4	—	—
Monoethanolamine	T46.8X1	T46.8X2	T46.8X3	T46.8X4	T46.8X5	T46.8X6
oleate	T46.8X1	T46.8X2	T46.8X3	T46.8X4	T46.8X5	T46.8X6
Monooctanoin	T50.991	T50.992	T50.993	T50.994	T50.995	T50.996
Monophenylbutazone	T39.2X1	T39.2X2	T39.2X3	T39.2X4	T39.2X5	T39.2X6
Monopril*	T46.4X1	T46.4X2	T46.4X3	T46.4X4	T46.4X5	T46.4X6
Monosodium glutamate	T65.891	T65.892	T65.893	T65.894	—	—
Monosulfiram	T49.0X1	T49.0X2	T49.0X3	T49.0X4	T49.0X5	T49.0X6
Monoxide, carbon — *see* Carbon, monoxide						
Monoxidine hydrochloride	T46.1X1	T46.1X2	T46.1X3	T46.1X4	T46.1X5	T46.1X6
Monuron	T60.3X1	T60.3X2	T60.3X3	T60.3X4	—	—

Substance	Poisoning, Accidental (unintentional)	Poisoning, Intentional Self-harm	Poisoning, Assault	Poisoning, Undetermined	Adverse Effect	Under-dosing
Moperone	T43.4X1	T43.4X2	T43.4X3	T43.4X4	T43.4X5	T43.4X6
Mopidamol	T45.1X1	T45.1X2	T45.1X3	T45.1X4	T45.1X5	T45.1X6
MOPP (mechloreth-amine + vincristine + prednisone + procarba-zine)	T45.1X1	T45.1X2	T45.1X3	T45.1X4	T45.1X5	T45.1X6
Morfin	T40.2X1	T40.2X2	T40.2X3	T40.2X4	T40.2X5	T40.2X6
Morinamide	T37.1X1	T37.1X2	T37.1X3	T37.1X4	T37.1X5	T37.1X6
Morning glory seeds	T40.991	T40.992	T40.993	T40.994	—	—
Moroxydine	T37.5X1	T37.5X2	T37.5X3	T37.5X4	T37.5X5	T37.5X6
Morphazinamide	T37.1X1	T37.1X2	T37.1X3	T37.1X4	T37.1X5	T37.1X6
Morphine	T40.2X1	T40.2X2	T40.2X3	T40.2X4	T40.2X5	T40.2X6
antagonist	T50.7X1	T50.7X2	T50.7X3	T50.7X4	T50.7X5	T50.7X6
Morpholinylethylmorphine	T40.2X1	T40.2X2	T40.2X3	T40.2X4	—	—
Morsuximide	T42.2X1	T42.2X2	T42.2X3	T42.2X4	T42.2X5	T42.2X6
Mosapramine	T43.591	T43.592	T43.593	T43.594	T43.595	T43.596
Moth balls — *see also* Pesticide	T60.2X1	T60.2X2	T60.2X3	T60.2X4	—	—
naphthalene	T60.2X1	T60.2X2	T60.2X3	T60.2X4	—	—
paradichlorobenzene	T60.1X1	T60.1X2	T60.1X3	T60.1X4	—	—
Motor exhaust gas	T58.01	T58.02	T58.03	T58.04	—	—
Motrin	T39.311	T39.312	T39.313	T39.314	T39.315	T39.316
Mouthwash (antiseptic) (zinc chloride)	T49.6X1	T49.6X2	T49.6X3	T49.6X4	T49.6X5	T49.6X6
Moxastine	T45.0X1	T45.0X2	T45.0X3	T45.0X4	T45.0X5	T45.0X6
Moxaverine	T44.3X1	T44.3X2	T44.3X3	T44.3X4	T44.3X5	T44.3X6
Moxisylyte	T46.7X1	T46.7X2	T46.7X3	T46.7X4	T46.7X5	T46.7X6
Mucilage, plant	T47.4X1	T47.4X2	T47.4X3	T47.4X4	T47.4X5	T47.4X6
Mucolytic drug	T48.4X1	T48.4X2	T48.4X3	T48.4X4	T48.4X5	T48.4X6
Mucomyst	T48.4X1	T48.4X2	T48.4X3	T48.4X4	T48.4X5	T48.4X6
Mucous membrane agents (external)	T49.91	T49.92	T49.93	T49.94	T49.95	T49.96
specified NEC	T49.8X1	T49.8X2	T49.8X3	T49.8X4	T49.8X5	T49.8X6
Multaq*	T46.2X1	T46.2X2	T46.2X3	T46.2X4	T46.2X5	T46.2X6
Multiple unspecified drugs, medicaments and biological substances	T50.911	T50.912	T50.913	T50.914	T50.915	T50.916
Mumps						
immune globulin (human)	T50.Z11	T50.Z12	T50.Z13	T50.Z14	T50.Z15	T50.Z16
skin test antigen	T50.8X1	T50.8X2	T50.8X3	T50.8X4	T50.8X5	T50.8X6
vaccine	T50.B91	T50.B92	T50.B93	T50.B94	T50.B95	T50.B96
Mumpsvax	T50.B91	T50.B92	T50.B93	T50.B94	T50.B95	T50.B96
Mupirocin	T49.0X1	T49.0X2	T49.0X3	T49.0X4	T49.0X5	T49.0X6
Muriatic acid — *see* Hydrochloric acid						
Muromonab-CD3	T45.1X1	T45.1X2	T45.1X3	T45.1X4	T45.1X5	T45.1X6
Muscle-action drug NEC	T48.201	T48.202	T48.203	T48.204	T48.205	T48.206
Muscle affecting agents NEC	T48.201	T48.202	T48.203	T48.204	T48.205	T48.206
oxytocic	T48.0X1	T48.0X2	T48.0X3	T48.0X4	T48.0X5	T48.0X6
relaxants	T48.201	T48.202	T48.203	T48.204	T48.205	T48.206
central nervous system	T42.8X1	T42.8X2	T42.8X3	T42.8X4	T42.8X5	T42.8X6
skeletal	T48.1X1	T48.1X2	T48.1X3	T48.1X4	T48.1X5	T48.1X6
smooth	T44.3X1	T44.3X2	T44.3X3	T44.3X4	T44.3X5	T44.3X6
Muscle relaxant — *see* Relaxant, muscle						
Muscle-tone depressant, central NEC	T42.8X1	T42.8X2	T42.8X3	T42.8X4	T42.8X5	T42.8X6
specified NEC	T42.8X1	T42.8X2	T42.8X3	T42.8X4	T42.8X5	T42.8X6
Mushroom, noxious	T62.0X1	T62.0X2	T62.0X3	T62.0X4	—	—
Mussel, noxious	T61.781	T61.782	T61.783	T61.784	—	—
Mustard (emetic)	T47.7X1	T47.7X2	T47.7X3	T47.7X4	T47.7X5	T47.7X6
black	T47.7X1	T47.7X2	T47.7X3	T47.7X4	T47.7X5	T47.7X6
gas, not in war	T59.91	T59.92	T59.93	T59.94	—	—
nitrogen	T45.1X1	T45.1X2	T45.1X3	T45.1X4	T45.1X5	T45.1X6
Mustine	T45.1X1	T45.1X2	T45.1X3	T45.1X4	T45.1X5	T45.1X6
M-vac	T45.1X1	T45.1X2	T45.1X3	T45.1X4	T45.1X5	T45.1X6
Mycifradin	T36.5X1	T36.5X2	T36.5X3	T36.5X4	T36.5X5	T36.5X6
topical	T49.0X1	T49.0X2	T49.0X3	T49.0X4	T49.0X5	T49.0X6
Mycitracin	T36.8X1	T36.8X2	T36.8X3	T36.8X4	T36.8X5	T36.8X6
ophthalmic preparation	T49.5X1	T49.5X2	T49.5X3	T49.5X4	T49.5X5	T49.5X6
Mycostatin	T36.7X1	T36.7X2	T36.7X3	T36.7X4	T36.7X5	T36.7X6
topical	T49.0X1	T49.0X2	T49.0X3	T49.0X4	T49.0X5	T49.0X6
Mycotoxins	T64.81	T64.82	T64.83	T64.84	—	—
aflatoxin	T64.01	T64.02	T64.03	T64.04	—	—
specified NEC	T64.81	T64.82	T64.83	T64.84	—	—
Mydriacyl	T44.3X1	T44.3X2	T44.3X3	T44.3X4	T44.3X5	T44.3X6
Mydriatic drug	T49.5X1	T49.5X2	T49.5X3	T49.5X4	T49.5X5	T49.5X6
Myelobromal	T45.1X1	T45.1X2	T45.1X3	T45.1X4	T45.1X5	T45.1X6
Myleran	T45.1X1	T45.1X2	T45.1X3	T45.1X4	T45.1X5	T45.1X6
Myochrysin (e)	T39.2X1	T39.2X2	T39.2X3	T39.2X4	T39.2X5	T39.2X6
Myoneural blocking agents	T48.1X1	T48.1X2	T48.1X3	T48.1X4	T48.1X5	T48.1X6
Myrac*	T36.4X1	T36.4X2	T36.4X3	T36.4X4	T36.4X5	T36.4X6

☑ **Additional Character May Be Required** — Refer to the Tabular List for Character Selection

*Optum Value-Add

Substance	Poisoning, Accidental (unintentional)	Poisoning, Intentional Self-harm	Poisoning, Assault	Poisoning, Undetermined	Adverse Effect	Under-dosing
Myralact	T49.0X1	T49.0X2	T49.0X3	T49.0X4	T49.0X5	T49.0X6
Myristica fragrans	T62.2X1	T62.2X2	T62.2X3	T62.2X4	—	—
Myristicin	T65.891	T65.892	T65.893	T65.894	—	—
Mysoline	T42.3X1	T42.3X2	T42.3X3	T42.3X4	T42.3X5	T42.3X6
Nabilone	T40.711	T40.712	T40.713	T40.714	T40.715	T40.716
Nabumetone	T39.391	T39.392	T39.393	T39.394	T39.395	T39.396
Nadolol	T44.7X1	T44.7X2	T44.7X3	T44.7X4	T44.7X5	T44.7X6
Nafcillin	T36.0X1	T36.0X2	T36.0X3	T36.0X4	T36.0X5	T36.0X6
Nafoxidine	T38.6X1	T38.6X2	T38.6X3	T38.6X4	T38.6X5	T38.6X6
Naftazone	T46.991	T46.992	T46.993	T46.994	T46.995	T46.996
Naftidrofuryl (oxalate)	T46.7X1	T46.7X2	T46.7X3	T46.7X4	T46.7X5	T46.7X6
Naftifine	T49.0X1	T49.0X2	T49.0X3	T49.0X4	T49.0X5	T49.0X6
Nail polish remover	T52.91	T52.92	T52.93	T52.94	—	—
Nalbuphine	T40.491	T40.492	T40.493	T40.494	T40.495	T40.496
Naled	T60.0X1	T60.0X2	T60.0X3	T60.0X4	—	—
Nalidixic acid	T37.8X1	T37.8X2	T37.8X3	T37.8X4	T37.8X5	T37.8X6
Nalorphine	T50.7X1	T50.7X2	T50.7X3	T50.7X4	T50.7X5	T50.7X6
Naloxone	T50.7X1	T50.7X2	T50.7X3	T50.7X4	T50.7X5	T50.7X6
Naltrexone	T50.7X1	T50.7X2	T50.7X3	T50.7X4	T50.7X5	T50.7X6
Namenda	T43.8X1	T43.8X2	T43.8X3	T43.8X4	T43.8X5	T43.8X6
Nandrolone	T38.7X1	T38.7X2	T38.7X3	T38.7X4	T38.7X5	T38.7X6
Naphazoline	T48.5X1	T48.5X2	T48.5X3	T48.5X4	T48.5X5	T48.5X6
Naphtha (painters') (petroleum)	T52.0X1	T52.0X2	T52.0X3	T52.0X4	—	—
solvent	T52.0X1	T52.0X2	T52.0X3	T52.0X4	—	—
vapor	T52.0X1	T52.0X2	T52.0X3	T52.0X4	—	—
Naphthalene (non-chlorinated)	T60.2X1	T60.2X2	T60.2X3	T60.2X4	—	—
chlorinated	T60.1X1	T60.1X2	T60.1X3	T60.1X4	—	—
vapor	T60.1X1	T60.1X2	T60.1X3	T60.1X4	—	—
insecticide or moth repellent	T60.2X1	T60.2X2	T60.2X3	T60.2X4	—	—
chlorinated	T60.1X1	T60.1X2	T60.1X3	T60.1X4	—	—
vapor	T60.2X1	T60.2X2	T60.2X3	T60.2X4	—	—
chlorinated	T60.1X1	T60.1X2	T60.1X3	T60.1X4	—	—
Naphthol	T65.891	T65.892	T65.893	T65.894	—	—
Naphthylamine	T65.891	T65.892	T65.893	T65.894	—	—
Naphthylthiourea (ANTU)	T60.4X1	T60.4X2	T60.4X3	T60.4X4	—	—
Naprosyn — see Naproxen						
Naproxen	T39.311	T39.312	T39.313	T39.314	T39.315	T39.316
Narcotic (drug)	T40.601	T40.602	T40.603	T40.604	T40.605	T40.606
analgesic NEC	T40.601	T40.602	T40.603	T40.604	T40.605	T40.606
antagonist	T50.7X1	T50.7X2	T50.7X3	T50.7X4	T50.7X5	T50.7X6
specified NEC	T40.691	T40.692	T40.693	T40.694	T40.695	T40.696
synthetic	T40.491	T40.492	T40.493	T40.494	T40.495	T40.496
Narcotine	T48.3X1	T48.3X2	T48.3X3	T48.3X4	T48.3X5	T48.3X6
Nardil	T43.1X1	T43.1X2	T43.1X3	T43.1X4	T43.1X5	T43.1X6
Nasacort*	T49.5X1	T49.5X2	T49.5X3	T49.5X4	T49.5X5	T49.5X6
Nasal drug NEC	T49.6X1	T49.6X2	T49.6X3	T49.6X4	T49.6X5	T49.6X6
Natamycin	T49.0X1	T49.0X2	T49.0X3	T49.0X4	T49.0X5	T49.0X6
Natrium cyanide — see Cyanide(s)						
Natural						
blood (product)	T45.8X1	T45.8X2	T45.8X3	T45.8X4	T45.8X5	T45.8X6
gas (piped)	T59.891	T59.892	T59.893	T59.894	—	—
incomplete combustion	T58.11	T58.12	T58.13	T58.14	—	—
Nealbarbital	T42.3X1	T42.3X2	T42.3X3	T42.3X4	T42.3X5	T42.3X6
Nectadon	T48.3X1	T48.3X2	T48.3X3	T48.3X4	T48.3X5	T48.3X6
Nedocromil	T48.6X1	T48.6X2	T48.6X3	T48.6X4	T48.6X5	T48.6X6
Nefopam	T39.8X1	T39.8X2	T39.8X3	T39.8X4	T39.8X5	T39.8X6
Nematocyst (sting)	T63.691	T63.692	T63.693	T63.694	—	—
Nembutal	T42.3X1	T42.3X2	T42.3X3	T42.3X4	T42.3X5	T42.3X6
Nemonapride	T43.591	T43.592	T43.593	T43.594	T43.595	T43.596
Neoarsphenamine	T37.8X1	T37.8X2	T37.8X3	T37.8X4	T37.8X5	T37.8X6
Neocinchophen	T50.4X1	T50.4X2	T50.4X3	T50.4X4	T50.4X5	T50.4X6
Neomycin (derivatives)	T36.5X1	T36.5X2	T36.5X3	T36.5X4	T36.5X5	T36.5X6
with bacitracin	T49.0X1	T49.0X2	T49.0X3	T49.0X4	T49.0X5	T49.0X6
neostigmine	T44.0X1	T44.0X2	T44.0X3	T44.0X4	T44.0X5	T44.0X6
ENT agent	T49.6X1	T49.6X2	T49.6X3	T49.6X4	T49.6X5	T49.6X6
ophthalmic preparation	T49.5X1	T49.5X2	T49.5X3	T49.5X4	T49.5X5	T49.5X6
topical NEC	T49.0X1	T49.0X2	T49.0X3	T49.0X4	T49.0X5	T49.0X6
Neonal	T42.3X1	T42.3X2	T42.3X3	T42.3X4	T42.3X5	T42.3X6
Neopham*	T50.3X1	T50.3X2	T50.3X3	T50.3X4	T50.3X5	T50.3X6
Neoprontosil	T37.0X1	T37.0X2	T37.0X3	T37.0X4	T37.0X5	T37.0X6
Neosalvarsan	T37.8X1	T37.8X2	T37.8X3	T37.8X4	T37.8X5	T37.8X6
Neosilversalvarsan	T37.8X1	T37.8X2	T37.8X3	T37.8X4	T37.8X5	T37.8X6
Neosporin	T36.8X1	T36.8X2	T36.8X3	T36.8X4	T36.8X5	T36.8X6
ENT agent	T49.6X1	T49.6X2	T49.6X3	T49.6X4	T49.6X5	T49.6X6
opthalmic preparation	T49.5X1	T49.5X2	T49.5X3	T49.5X4	T49.5X5	T49.5X6
topical NEC	T49.0X1	T49.0X2	T49.0X3	T49.0X4	T49.0X5	T49.0X6
Neostigmine bromide	T44.0X1	T44.0X2	T44.0X3	T44.0X4	T44.0X5	T44.0X6
Neraval	T42.3X1	T42.3X2	T42.3X3	T42.3X4	T42.3X5	T42.3X6

Substance	Poisoning, Accidental (unintentional)	Poisoning, Intentional Self-harm	Poisoning, Assault	Poisoning, Undetermined	Adverse Effect	Under-dosing
Neravan	T42.3X1	T42.3X2	T42.3X3	T42.3X4	T42.3X5	T42.3X6
Nerium oleander	T62.2X1	T62.2X2	T62.2X3	T62.2X4	—	—
Nerlynx*	T45.1X1	T45.1X2	T45.1X3	T45.1X4	T45.1X5	T45.1X6
Nerve gas, not in war	T59.91	T59.92	T59.93	T59.94	—	—
Nesacaine	T41.3X1	T41.3X2	T41.3X3	T41.3X4	T41.3X5	T41.3X6
infiltration (subcutaneous)	T41.3X1	T41.3X2	T41.3X3	T41.3X4	T41.3X5	T41.3X6
nerve block (peripheral) (plexus)	T41.3X1	T41.3X2	T41.3X3	T41.3X4	T41.3X5	T41.3X6
Netilmicin	T36.5X1	T36.5X2	T36.5X3	T36.5X4	T36.5X5	T36.5X6
Neurobarb	T42.3X1	T42.3X2	T42.3X3	T42.3X4	T42.3X5	T42.3X6
Neuroleptic drug NEC	T43.501	T43.502	T43.503	T43.504	T43.505	T43.506
Neuromuscular blocking drug	T48.1X1	T48.1X2	T48.1X3	T48.1X4	T48.1X5	T48.1X6
Neutral insulin injection	T38.3X1	T38.3X2	T38.3X3	T38.3X4	T38.3X5	T38.3X6
Neutral spirits	T51.0X1	T51.0X2	T51.0X3	T51.0X4	—	—
beverage	T51.0X1	T51.0X2	T51.0X3	T51.0X4	—	—
Niacin	T46.7X1	T46.7X2	T46.7X3	T46.7X4	T46.7X5	T46.7X6
Niacinamide	T45.2X1	T45.2X2	T45.2X3	T45.2X4	T45.2X5	T45.2X6
Nialamide	T43.1X1	T43.1X2	T43.1X3	T43.1X4	T43.1X5	T43.1X6
Niaprazine	T42.6X1	T42.6X2	T42.6X3	T42.6X4	T42.6X5	T42.6X6
Nicametate	T46.7X1	T46.7X2	T46.7X3	T46.7X4	T46.7X5	T46.7X6
Nicardipine	T46.1X1	T46.1X2	T46.1X3	T46.1X4	T46.1X5	T46.1X6
Nicergoline	T46.7X1	T46.7X2	T46.7X3	T46.7X4	T46.7X5	T46.7X6
Nickel (carbonyl) (tetra-carbonyl) (fumes) (vapor)	T56.891	T56.892	T56.893	T56.894	—	—
Nickelocene	T56.891	T56.892	T56.893	T56.894	—	—
Niclosamide	T37.4X1	T37.4X2	T37.4X3	T37.4X4	T37.4X5	T37.4X6
Nicofuranose	T46.7X1	T46.7X2	T46.7X3	T46.7X4	T46.7X5	T46.7X6
Nicomorphine	T40.2X1	T40.2X2	T40.2X3	T40.2X4	—	—
Nicorandil	T46.3X1	T46.3X2	T46.3X3	T46.3X4	T46.3X5	T46.3X6
Nicotiana (plant)	T62.2X1	T62.2X2	T62.2X3	T62.2X4	—	—
Nicotinamide	T45.2X1	T45.2X2	T45.2X3	T45.2X4	T45.2X5	T45.2X6
Nicotine (insecticide) (spray) (sulfate) **NEC**	T60.2X1	T60.2X2	T60.2X3	T60.2X4	—	—
from tobacco	T65.291	T65.292	T65.293	T65.294	—	—
cigarettes	T65.221	T65.222	T65.223	T65.224	—	—
not insecticide	T65.291	T65.292	T65.293	T65.294	—	—
Nicotinic acid	T46.7X1	T46.7X2	T46.7X3	T46.7X4	T46.7X5	T46.7X6
Nicotinyl alcohol	T46.7X1	T46.7X2	T46.7X3	T46.7X4	T46.7X5	T46.7X6
Nicoumalone	T45.511	T45.512	T45.513	T45.514	T45.515	T45.516
Nifedipine	T46.1X1	T46.1X2	T46.1X3	T46.1X4	T46.1X5	T46.1X6
Nifenazone	T39.2X1	T39.2X2	T39.2X3	T39.2X4	T39.2X5	T39.2X6
Nifuraldezone	T37.91	T37.92	T37.93	T37.94	T37.95	T37.96
Nifuratel	T37.8X1	T37.8X2	T37.8X3	T37.8X4	T37.8X5	T37.8X6
Nifurtimox	T37.3X1	T37.3X2	T37.3X3	T37.3X4	T37.3X5	T37.3X6
Nifurtoinol	T37.8X1	T37.8X2	T37.8X3	T37.8X4	T37.8X5	T37.8X6
Nightshade, deadly (solanum) — see also Belladonna	T62.2X1	T62.2X2	T62.2X3	T62.2X4	—	—
berry	T62.1X1	T62.1X2	T62.1X3	T62.1X4	—	—
Nikethamide	T50.7X1	T50.7X2	T50.7X3	T50.7X4	T50.7X5	T50.7X6
Nilstat	T36.7X1	T36.7X2	T36.7X3	T36.7X4	T36.7X5	T36.7X6
topical	T49.0X1	T49.0X2	T49.0X3	T49.0X4	T49.0X5	T49.0X6
Nilutamide	T38.6X1	T38.6X2	T38.6X3	T38.6X4	T38.6X5	T38.6X6
Nimesulide	T39.391	T39.392	T39.393	T39.394	T39.395	T39.396
Nimetazepam	T42.4X1	T42.4X2	T42.4X3	T42.4X4	T42.4X5	T42.4X6
Nimodipine	T46.1X1	T46.1X2	T46.1X3	T46.1X4	T46.1X5	T46.1X6
Nimorazole	T37.3X1	T37.3X2	T37.3X3	T37.3X4	T37.3X5	T37.3X6
Nimustine	T45.1X1	T45.1X2	T45.1X3	T45.1X4	T45.1X5	T45.1X6
Nipent*	T45.1X1	T45.1X2	T45.1X3	T45.1X4	T45.1X5	T45.1X6
Niridazole	T37.4X1	T37.4X2	T37.4X3	T37.4X4	T37.4X5	T37.4X6
Nisentil	T40.2X1	T40.2X2	T40.2X3	T40.2X4	T40.2X5	T40.2X6
Nisoldipine	T46.1X1	T46.1X2	T46.1X3	T46.1X4	T46.1X5	T46.1X6
Nitramine	T65.3X1	T65.3X2	T65.3X3	T65.3X4	—	—
Nitrate, organic	T46.3X1	T46.3X2	T46.3X3	T46.3X4	T46.3X5	T46.3X6
Nitrazepam	T42.4X1	T42.4X2	T42.4X3	T42.4X4	T42.4X5	T42.4X6
Nitrefazole	T50.6X1	T50.6X2	T50.6X3	T50.6X4	T50.6X5	T50.6X6
Nitrendipine	T46.1X1	T46.1X2	T46.1X3	T46.1X4	T46.1X5	T46.1X6
Nitric						
acid (liquid)	T54.2X1	T54.2X2	T54.2X3	T54.2X4	—	—
vapor	T59.891	T59.892	T59.893	T59.894	—	—
oxide (gas)	T59.0X1	T59.0X2	T59.0X3	T59.0X4	—	—
Nitrimidazine	T37.3X1	T37.3X2	T37.3X3	T37.3X4	T37.3X5	T37.3X6
Nitrite, amyl (medicinal) (vapor)	T46.3X1	T46.3X2	T46.3X3	T46.3X4	T46.3X5	T46.3X6
Nitroaniline	T65.3X1	T65.3X2	T65.3X3	T65.3X4	—	—
vapor	T59.891	T59.892	T59.893	T59.894	—	—
Nitrobenzene, nitrobenzol	T65.3X1	T65.3X2	T65.3X3	T65.3X4	—	—
vapor	T65.3X1	T65.3X2	T65.3X3	T65.3X4	—	—
Nitrocellulose	T65.891	T65.892	T65.893	T65.894	—	—
lacquer	T65.891	T65.892	T65.893	T65.894	—	—
Nitrodiphenyl	T65.3X1	T65.3X2	T65.3X3	T65.3X4	—	—
Nitrofural	T49.0X1	T49.0X2	T49.0X3	T49.0X4	T49.0X5	T49.0X6
Nitrofurantoin	T37.8X1	T37.8X2	T37.8X3	T37.8X4	T37.8X5	T37.8X6

Table of Drugs and Chemicals

Substance	Poisoning, Accidental (unintentional)	Poisoning, Intentional Self-harm	Poisoning, Assault	Poisoning, Undetermined	Adverse Effect	Under-dosing
Nitrofurazone	T49.0X1	T49.0X2	T49.0X3	T49.0X4	T49.0X5	T49.0X6
Nitrogen	T59.0X1	T59.0X2	T59.0X3	T59.0X4	—	—
mustard	T45.1X1	T45.1X2	T45.1X3	T45.1X4	T45.1X5	T45.1X6
Nitroglycerin, nitroglycerol	T46.3X1	T46.3X2	T46.3X3	T46.3X4	T46.3X5	T46.3X6
(medicinal)						
nonmedicinal	T65.5X1	T65.5X2	T65.5X3	T65.5X4	—	—
fumes	T65.5X1	T65.5X2	T65.5X3	T65.5X4	—	—
Nitroglycol	T52.3X1	T52.3X2	T52.3X3	T52.3X4	—	—
Nitrohydrochloric acid	T54.2X1	T54.2X2	T54.2X3	T54.2X4	—	—
Nitromersol	T49.0X1	T49.0X2	T49.0X3	T49.0X4	T49.0X5	T49.0X6
Nitronaphthalene	T65.891	T65.892	T65.893	T65.894	—	—
Nitrophenol	T54.0X1	T54.0X2	T54.0X3	T54.0X4	—	—
Nitropropane	T52.8X1	T52.8X2	T52.8X3	T52.8X4	—	—
Nitroprusside	T46.5X1	T46.5X2	T46.5X3	T46.5X4	T46.5X5	T46.5X6
Nitrosodimethylamine	T65.3X1	T65.3X2	T65.3X3	T65.3X4	—	—
Nitrothiazol	T37.4X1	T37.4X2	T37.4X3	T37.4X4	T37.4X5	T37.4X6
Nitrotoluene, nitrotoluol	T65.3X1	T65.3X2	T65.3X3	T65.3X4	—	—
vapor	T65.3X1	T65.3X2	T65.3X3	T65.3X4	—	—
Nitrous						
acid (liquid)	T54.2X1	T54.2X2	T54.2X3	T54.2X4	—	—
fumes	T59.891	T59.892	T59.893	T59.894	—	—
ether spirit	T46.3X1	T46.3X2	T46.3X3	T46.3X4	T46.3X5	T46.3X6
oxide	T41.0X1	T41.0X2	T41.0X3	T41.0X4	T41.0X5	T41.0X6
Nitroxoline	T37.8X1	T37.8X2	T37.8X3	T37.8X4	T37.8X5	T37.8X6
Nitrozone	T49.0X1	T49.0X2	T49.0X3	T49.0X4	T49.0X5	T49.0X6
Nizatidine	T47.0X1	T47.0X2	T47.0X3	T47.0X4	T47.0X5	T47.0X6
Nizofenone	T43.8X1	T43.8X2	T43.8X3	T43.8X4	T43.8X5	T43.8X6
Noctec	T42.6X1	T42.6X2	T42.6X3	T42.6X4	T42.6X5	T42.6X6
No Doz*	T43.611	T43.612	T43.613	T43.614	T43.615	T43.616
Noludar	T42.6X1	T42.6X2	T42.6X3	T42.6X4	T42.6X5	T42.6X6
Nomegestrol	T38.5X1	T38.5X2	T38.5X3	T38.5X4	T38.5X5	T38.5X6
Nomifensine	T43.291	T43.292	T43.293	T43.294	T43.295	T43.296
Nonoxinol	T49.8X1	T49.8X2	T49.8X3	T49.8X4	T49.8X5	T49.8X6
Nonylphenoxy	T49.8X1	T49.8X2	T49.8X3	T49.8X4	T49.8X5	T49.8X6
(polyethoxyethanol)						
Noptil	T42.3X1	T42.3X2	T42.3X3	T42.3X4	T42.3X5	T42.3X6
Noradrenaline	T44.4X1	T44.4X2	T44.4X3	T44.4X4	T44.4X5	T44.4X6
Noramidopyrine	T39.2X1	T39.2X2	T39.2X3	T39.2X4	T39.2X5	T39.2X6
methanesulfonate sodium	T39.2X1	T39.2X2	T39.2X3	T39.2X4	T39.2X5	T39.2X6
Norbormide	T60.4X1	T60.4X2	T60.4X3	T60.4X4	—	—
Nordazepam	T42.4X1	T42.4X2	T42.4X3	T42.4X4	T42.4X5	T42.4X6
Norepinephrine	T44.4X1	T44.4X2	T44.4X3	T44.4X4	T44.4X5	T44.4X6
Norethandrolone	T38.7X1	T38.7X2	T38.7X3	T38.7X4	T38.7X5	T38.7X6
Norethindrone	T38.4X1	T38.4X2	T38.4X3	T38.4X4	T38.4X5	T38.4X6
Norethisterone (acetate)	T38.4X1	T38.4X2	T38.4X3	T38.4X4	T38.4X5	T38.4X6
(enantate)						
with ethinylestradiol	T38.5X1	T38.5X2	T38.5X3	T38.5X4	T38.5X5	T38.5X6
Noretynodrel	T38.5X1	T38.5X2	T38.5X3	T38.5X4	T38.5X5	T38.5X6
Norfenefrine	T44.4X1	T44.4X2	T44.4X3	T44.4X4	T44.4X5	T44.4X6
Norfloxacin	T36.8X1	T36.8X2	T36.8X3	T36.8X4	T36.8X5	T36.8X6
Norgestrel	T38.4X1	T38.4X2	T38.4X3	T38.4X4	T38.4X5	T38.4X6
Norgestrienone	T38.4X1	T38.4X2	T38.4X3	T38.4X4	T38.4X5	T38.4X6
Norlestrin	T38.4X1	T38.4X2	T38.4X3	T38.4X4	T38.4X5	T38.4X6
Norlutin	T38.4X1	T38.4X2	T38.4X3	T38.4X4	T38.4X5	T38.4X6
Normal serum albumin	T45.8X1	T45.8X2	T45.8X3	T45.8X4	T45.8X5	T45.8X6
(human), salt-poor						
Normethandrone	T38.5X1	T38.5X2	T38.5X3	T38.5X4	T38.5X5	T38.5X6
Normison — see						
Benzodiazepines						
Normorphine	T40.2X1	T40.2X2	T40.2X3	T40.2X4	—	—
Norpseudoephedrine	T50.5X1	T50.5X2	T50.5X3	T50.5X4	T50.5X5	T50.5X6
Nortestosterone	T38.7X1	T38.7X2	T38.7X3	T38.7X4	T38.7X5	T38.7X6
(furanpropionate)						
Nortriptyline	T43.011	T43.012	T43.013	T43.014	T43.015	T43.016
Norvasc*	T46.1X1	T46.1X2	T46.1X3	T46.1X4	T46.1X5	T46.1X6
Noscapine	T48.3X1	T48.3X2	T48.3X3	T48.3X4	T48.3X5	T48.3X6
Nose preparations	T49.6X1	T49.6X2	T49.6X3	T49.6X4	T49.6X5	T49.6X6
Novobiocin	T36.5X1	T36.5X2	T36.5X3	T36.5X4	T36.5X5	T36.5X6
Novocain (infiltration)	T41.3X1	T41.3X2	T41.3X3	T41.3X4	T41.3X5	T41.3X6
(topical)						
nerve block (peripheral)	T41.3X1	T41.3X2	T41.3X3	T41.3X4	T41.3X5	T41.3X6
(plexus)						
spinal	T41.3X1	T41.3X2	T41.3X3	T41.3X4	T41.3X5	T41.3X6
Noxious foodstuff	T62.91	T62.92	T62.93	T62.94	—	—
specified NEC	T62.8X1	T62.8X2	T62.8X3	T62.8X4	—	—
Noxiptiline	T43.011	T43.012	T43.013	T43.014	T43.015	T43.016
Noxytiolin	T49.0X1	T49.0X2	T49.0X3	T49.0X4	T49.0X5	T49.0X6
NPH Iletin (insulin)	T38.3X1	T38.3X2	T38.3X3	T38.3X4	T38.3X5	T38.3X6
Numorphan	T40.2X1	T40.2X2	T40.2X3	T40.2X4	T40.2X5	T40.2X6
Nunol	T42.3X1	T42.3X2	T42.3X3	T42.3X4	T42.3X5	T42.3X6
Nupercaine (spinal	T41.3X1	T41.3X2	T41.3X3	T41.3X4	T41.3X5	T41.3X6
anesthetic)						
topical (surface)	T41.3X1	T41.3X2	T41.3X3	T41.3X4	T41.3X5	T41.3X6

Substance	Poisoning, Accidental (unintentional)	Poisoning, Intentional Self-harm	Poisoning, Assault	Poisoning, Undetermined	Adverse Effect	Under-dosing
Nutmeg oil (liniment)	T49.3X1	T49.3X2	T49.3X3	T49.3X4	T49.3X5	T49.3X6
Nutrilipid*	T50.991	T50.992	T50.993	T50.994	T50.995	T50.996
Nutritional supplement	T50.901	T50.902	T50.903	T50.904	T50.905	T50.906
Nux vomica	T65.1X1	T65.1X2	T65.1X3	T65.1X4	—	—
Nydrazid	T37.1X1	T37.1X2	T37.1X3	T37.1X4	T37.1X5	T37.1X6
Nylidrin	T46.7X1	T46.7X2	T46.7X3	T46.7X4	T46.7X5	T46.7X6
Nystatin	T36.7X1	T36.7X2	T36.7X3	T36.7X4	T36.7X5	T36.7X6
topical	T49.0X1	T49.0X2	T49.0X3	T49.0X4	T49.0X5	T49.0X6
Nytol	T45.0X1	T45.0X2	T45.0X3	T45.0X4	T45.0X5	T45.0X6
Obidoxime chloride	T50.6X1	T50.6X2	T50.6X3	T50.6X4	T50.6X5	T50.6X6
Octafonium (chloride)	T49.3X1	T49.3X2	T49.3X3	T49.3X4	T49.3X5	T49.3X6
Octamethyl	T60.0X1	T60.0X2	T60.0X3	T60.0X4	—	—
pyrophosphoramide						
Octanoin	T50.991	T50.992	T50.993	T50.994	T50.995	T50.996
Octatropine	T44.3X1	T44.3X2	T44.3X3	T44.3X4	T44.3X5	T44.3X6
methylbromide						
Octotiamine	T45.2X1	T45.2X2	T45.2X3	T45.2X4	T45.2X5	T45.2X6
Octoxinol (9)	T49.8X1	T49.8X2	T49.8X3	T49.8X4	T49.8X5	T49.8X6
Octreotide	T38.991	T38.992	T38.993	T38.994	T38.995	T38.996
Octyl nitrite	T46.3X1	T46.3X2	T46.3X3	T46.3X4	T46.3X5	T46.3X6
Oestradiol	T38.5X1	T38.5X2	T38.5X3	T38.5X4	T38.5X5	T38.5X6
Oestriol	T38.5X1	T38.5X2	T38.5X3	T38.5X4	T38.5X5	T38.5X6
Oestrogen	T38.5X1	T38.5X2	T38.5X3	T38.5X4	T38.5X5	T38.5X6
Oestrone	T38.5X1	T38.5X2	T38.5X3	T38.5X4	T38.5X5	T38.5X6
Ofloxacin	T36.8X1	T36.8X2	T36.8X3	T36.8X4	T36.8X5	T36.8X6
Oil (of)	T65.891	T65.892	T65.893	T65.894		
bitter almond	T62.8X1	T62.8X2	T62.8X3	T62.8X4	—	—
cloves	T49.7X1	T49.7X2	T49.7X3	T49.7X4	T49.7X5	T49.7X6
colors	T65.6X1	T65.6X2	T65.6X3	T65.6X4	—	—
fumes	T59.891	T59.892	T59.893	T59.894	—	—
lubricating	T52.0X1	T52.0X2	T52.0X3	T52.0X4	—	—
Niobe	T52.8X1	T52.8X2	T52.8X3	T52.8X4	—	—
vitriol (liquid)	T54.2X1	T54.2X2	T54.2X3	T54.2X4	—	—
fumes	T54.2X1	T54.2X2	T54.2X3	T54.2X4	—	—
wintergreen (bitter) NEC	T49.3X1	T49.3X2	T49.3X3	T49.3X4	T49.3X5	T49.3X6
Oily preparation (for skin)	T49.3X1	T49.3X2	T49.3X3	T49.3X4	T49.3X5	T49.3X6
Ointment NEC	T49.3X1	T49.3X2	T49.3X3	T49.3X4	T49.3X5	T49.3X6
Olanzapine	T43.591	T43.592	T43.593	T43.594	T43.595	T43.596
Oleander	T62.2X1	T62.2X2	T62.2X3	T62.2X4	—	—
Oleandomycin	T36.3X1	T36.3X2	T36.3X3	T36.3X4	T36.3X5	T36.3X6
Oleandrin	T46.0X1	T46.0X2	T46.0X3	T46.0X4	T46.0X5	T46.0X6
Oleic acid	T46.6X1	T46.6X2	T46.6X3	T46.6X4	T46.6X5	T46.6X6
Oleovitamin A	T45.2X1	T45.2X2	T45.2X3	T45.2X4	T45.2X5	T45.2X6
Oleum ricini	T47.2X1	T47.2X2	T47.2X3	T47.2X4	T47.2X5	T47.2X6
Olive oil (medicinal) NEC	T47.4X1	T47.4X2	T47.4X3	T47.4X4	T47.4X5	T47.4X6
Olivomycin	T45.1X1	T45.1X2	T45.1X3	T45.1X4	T45.1X5	T45.1X6
Olodaterol*	T48.6X1	T48.6X2	T48.6X3	T48.6X4	T48.6X5	T48.6X6
Olsalazine	T47.8X1	T47.8X2	T47.8X3	T47.8X4	T47.8X5	T47.8X6
Omeprazole	T47.1X1	T47.1X2	T47.1X3	T47.1X4	T47.1X5	T47.1X6
OMPA	T60.0X1	T60.0X2	T60.0X3	T60.0X4	—	—
Oncovin	T45.1X1	T45.1X2	T45.1X3	T45.1X4	T45.1X5	T45.1X6
Ondansetron	T45.0X1	T45.0X2	T45.0X3	T45.0X4	T45.0X5	T45.0X6
Ophthaine	T41.3X1	T41.3X2	T41.3X3	T41.3X4	T41.3X5	T41.3X6
Ophthetic	T41.3X1	T41.3X2	T41.3X3	T41.3X4	T41.3X5	T41.3X6
Opiate NEC	T40.601	T40.602	T40.603	T40.604	T40.605	T40.606
antagonists	T50.7X1	T50.7X2	T50.7X3	T50.7X4	T50.7X5	T50.7X6
Opioid NEC	T40.2X1	T40.2X2	T40.2X3	T40.2X4	T40.2X5	T40.2X6
Opipramol	T43.011	T43.012	T43.013	T43.014	T43.015	T43.016
Opium alkaloids (total)	T40.0X1	T40.0X2	T40.0X3	T40.0X4	T40.0X5	T40.0X6
standardized powdered	T40.0X1	T40.0X2	T40.0X3	T40.0X4	T40.0X5	T40.0X6
tincture (camphorated)	T40.0X1	T40.0X2	T40.0X3	T40.0X4	T40.0X5	T40.0X6
Optivar*	T49.5X1	T49.5X2	T49.5X3	T49.5X4	T49.5X5	T49.5X6
Oracon	T38.4X1	T38.4X2	T38.4X3	T38.4X4	T38.4X5	T38.4X6
Oragrafin	T50.8X1	T50.8X2	T50.8X3	T50.8X4	T50.8X5	T50.8X6
Oral contraceptives	T38.4X1	T38.4X2	T38.4X3	T38.4X4	T38.4X5	T38.4X6
Oral rehydration salts	T50.3X1	T50.3X2	T50.3X3	T50.3X4	T50.3X5	T50.3X6
Orazamide	T50.991	T50.992	T50.993	T50.994	T50.995	T50.996
Orciprenaline	T48.291	T48.292	T48.293	T48.294	T48.295	T48.296
Organidin	T48.4X1	T48.4X2	T48.4X3	T48.4X4	T48.4X5	T48.4X6
Organonitrate NEC	T46.3X1	T46.3X2	T46.3X3	T46.3X4	T46.3X5	T46.3X6
Organophosphates	T60.0X1	T60.0X2	T60.0X3	T60.0X4	—	—
Orimune	T50.B91	T50.B92	T50.B93	T50.B94	T50.B95	T50.B96
Orinase	T38.3X1	T38.3X2	T38.3X3	T38.3X4	T38.3X5	T38.3X6
Ormeloxifene	T38.6X1	T38.6X2	T38.6X3	T38.6X4	T38.6X5	T38.6X6
Ornidazole	T37.3X1	T37.3X2	T37.3X3	T37.3X4	T37.3X5	T37.3X6
Ornithine aspartate	T50.991	T50.992	T50.993	T50.994	T50.995	T50.996
Ornoprostil	T47.1X1	T47.1X2	T47.1X3	T47.1X4	T47.1X5	T47.1X6
Orphenadrine	T42.8X1	T42.8X2	T42.8X3	T42.8X4	T42.8X5	T42.8X6
(hydrochloride)						
Ortal (sodium)	T42.3X1	T42.3X2	T42.3X3	T42.3X4	T42.3X5	T42.3X6
Orthoboric acid	T49.0X1	T49.0X2	T49.0X3	T49.0X4	T49.0X5	T49.0X6
ENT agent	T49.6X1	T49.6X2	T49.6X3	T49.6X4	T49.6X5	T49.6X6
ophthalmic preparation	T49.5X1	T49.5X2	T49.5X3	T49.5X4	T49.5X5	T49.5X6

Table of Drugs and Chemicals

Nitrofurazone — Orthoboric acid

Substance	Poisoning, Accidental (unintentional)	Poisoning, Intentional Self-harm	Poisoning, Assault	Poisoning, Undetermined	Adverse Effect	Under-dosing
Orthocaine	T41.3X1	T41.3X2	T41.3X3	T41.3X4	T41.3X5	T41.3X6
Orthodichlorobenzene	T53.7X1	T53.7X2	T53.7X3	T53.7X4	—	—
Ortho-Novum	T38.4X1	T38.4X2	T38.4X3	T38.4X4	T38.4X5	T38.4X6
Orthotolidine (reagent)	T54.2X1	T54.2X2	T54.2X3	T54.2X4	—	—
Osmic acid (liquid)	T54.2X1	T54.2X2	T54.2X3	T54.2X4	—	—
fumes	T54.2X1	T54.2X2	T54.2X3	T54.2X4	—	—
Osmotic diuretics	T50.2X1	T50.2X2	T50.2X3	T50.2X4	T50.2X5	T50.2X6
Otilonium bromide	T44.3X1	T44.3X2	T44.3X3	T44.3X4	T44.3X5	T44.3X6
Otorhinolaryngological drug NEC	T49.6X1	T49.6X2	T49.6X3	T49.6X4	T49.6X5	T49.6X6
Ouabain (e)	T46.0X1	T46.0X2	T46.0X3	T46.0X4	T46.0X5	T46.0X6
Ovarian						
hormone	T38.5X1	T38.5X2	T38.5X3	T38.5X4	T38.5X5	T38.5X6
stimulant	T38.5X1	T38.5X2	T38.5X3	T38.5X4	T38.5X5	T38.5X6
Ovide*	T49.0X1	T49.0X2	T49.0X3	T49.0X4	T49.0X5	T49.0X6
Ovral	T38.4X1	T38.4X2	T38.4X3	T38.4X4	T38.4X5	T38.4X6
Ovulen	T38.4X1	T38.4X2	T38.4X3	T38.4X4	T38.4X5	T38.4X6
Oxacillin	T36.0X1	T36.0X2	T36.0X3	T36.0X4	T36.0X5	T36.0X6
Oxalic acid	T54.2X1	T54.2X2	T54.2X3	T54.2X4	—	—
ammonium salt	T50.991	T50.992	T50.993	T50.994	T50.995	T50.996
Oxamniquine	T37.4X1	T37.4X2	T37.4X3	T37.4X4	T37.4X5	T37.4X6
Oxanamide	T43.591	T43.592	T43.593	T43.594	T43.595	T43.596
Oxandrolone	T38.7X1	T38.7X2	T38.7X3	T38.7X4	T38.7X5	T38.7X6
Oxantel	T37.4X1	T37.4X2	T37.4X3	T37.4X4	T37.4X5	T37.4X6
Oxapium iodide	T44.3X1	T44.3X2	T44.3X3	T44.3X4	T44.3X5	T44.3X6
Oxaprotiline	T43.021	T43.022	T43.023	T43.024	T43.025	T43.026
Oxaprozin	T39.311	T39.312	T39.313	T39.314	T39.315	T39.316
Oxatomide	T45.0X1	T45.0X2	T45.0X3	T45.0X4	T45.0X5	T45.0X6
Oxazepam	T42.4X1	T42.4X2	T42.4X3	T42.4X4	T42.4X5	T42.4X6
Oxazimedrine	T50.5X1	T50.5X2	T50.5X3	T50.5X4	T50.5X5	T50.5X6
Oxazolam	T42.4X1	T42.4X2	T42.4X3	T42.4X4	T42.4X5	T42.4X6
Oxazolidine derivatives	T42.2X1	T42.2X2	T42.2X3	T42.2X4	T42.2X5	T42.2X6
Oxazolidinedione (derivative)	T42.2X1	T42.2X2	T42.2X3	T42.2X4	T42.2X5	T42.2X6
Ox bile extract	T47.5X1	T47.5X2	T47.5X3	T47.5X4	T47.5X5	T47.5X6
Oxcarbazepine	T42.1X1	T42.1X2	T42.1X3	T42.1X4	T42.1X5	T42.1X6
Oxedrine	T44.4X1	T44.4X2	T44.4X3	T44.4X4	T44.4X5	T44.4X6
Oxeladin (citrate)	T48.3X1	T48.3X2	T48.3X3	T48.3X4	T48.3X5	T48.3X6
Oxendolone	T38.5X1	T38.5X2	T38.5X3	T38.5X4	T38.5X5	T38.5X6
Oxetacaine	T41.3X1	T41.3X2	T41.3X3	T41.3X4	T41.3X5	T41.3X6
Oxethazine	T41.3X1	T41.3X2	T41.3X3	T41.3X4	T41.3X5	T41.3X6
Oxetorone	T39.8X1	T39.8X2	T39.8X3	T39.8X4	T39.8X5	T39.8X6
Oxiconazole	T49.0X1	T49.0X2	T49.0X3	T49.0X4	T49.0X5	T49.0X6
Oxidizing agent NEC	T54.91	T54.92	T54.93	T54.94	—	—
Oxipurinol	T50.4X1	T50.4X2	T50.4X3	T50.4X4	T50.4X5	T50.4X6
Oxitriptan	T43.291	T43.292	T43.293	T43.294	T43.295	T43.296
Oxitropium bromide	T48.6X1	T48.6X2	T48.6X3	T48.6X4	T48.6X5	T48.6X6
Oxodipine	T46.1X1	T46.1X2	T46.1X3	T46.1X4	T46.1X5	T46.1X6
Oxolamine	T48.3X1	T48.3X2	T48.3X3	T48.3X4	T48.3X5	T48.3X6
Oxolinic acid	T37.8X1	T37.8X2	T37.8X3	T37.8X4	T37.8X5	T37.8X6
Oxomemazine	T43.3X1	T43.3X2	T43.3X3	T43.3X4	T43.3X5	T43.3X6
Oxophenarsine	T37.3X1	T37.3X2	T37.3X3	T37.3X4	T37.3X5	T37.3X6
Oxprenolol	T44.7X1	T44.7X2	T44.7X3	T44.7X4	T44.7X5	T44.7X6
Oxsoralen	T49.3X1	T49.3X2	T49.3X3	T49.3X4	T49.3X5	T49.3X6
Oxtriphylline	T48.6X1	T48.6X2	T48.6X3	T48.6X4	T48.6X5	T48.6X6
Oxybate sodium	T41.291	T41.292	T41.293	T41.294	T41.295	T41.296
Oxybuprocaine	T41.3X1	T41.3X2	T41.3X3	T41.3X4	T41.3X5	T41.3X6
Oxybutynin	T44.3X1	T44.3X2	T44.3X3	T44.3X4	T44.3X5	T44.3X6
Oxychlorosene	T49.0X1	T49.0X2	T49.0X3	T49.0X4	T49.0X5	T49.0X6
Oxycodone	T40.2X1	T40.2X2	T40.2X3	T40.2X4	T40.2X5	T40.2X6
OxyContin*	T40.2X1	T40.2X2	T40.2X3	T40.2X4	T40.2X5	T40.2X6
Oxyfedrine	T46.3X1	T46.3X2	T46.3X3	T46.3X4	T46.3X5	T46.3X6
Oxygen	T41.5X1	T41.5X2	T41.5X3	T41.5X4	T41.5X5	T41.5X6
Oxylone	T49.0X1	T49.0X2	T49.0X3	T49.0X4	T49.0X5	T49.0X6
ophthalmic preparation	T49.5X1	T49.5X2	T49.5X3	T49.5X4	T49.5X5	T49.5X6
Oxymesterone	T38.7X1	T38.7X2	T38.7X3	T38.7X4	T38.7X5	T38.7X6
Oxymetazoline	T48.5X1	T48.5X2	T48.5X3	T48.5X4	T48.5X5	T48.5X6
Oxymetholone	T38.7X1	T38.7X2	T38.7X3	T38.7X4	T38.7X5	T38.7X6
Oxymorphone	T40.2X1	T40.2X2	T40.2X3	T40.2X4	T40.2X5	T40.2X6
Oxypertine	T43.591	T43.592	T43.593	T43.594	T43.595	T43.596
Oxyphenbutazone	T39.2X1	T39.2X2	T39.2X3	T39.2X4	T39.2X5	T39.2X6
Oxyphencyclimine	T44.3X1	T44.3X2	T44.3X3	T44.3X4	T44.3X5	T44.3X6
Oxyphenisatine	T47.2X1	T47.2X2	T47.2X3	T47.2X4	T47.2X5	T47.2X6
Oxyphenonium bromide	T44.3X1	T44.3X2	T44.3X3	T44.3X4	T44.3X5	T44.3X6
Oxypolygelatin	T45.8X1	T45.8X2	T45.8X3	T45.8X4	T45.8X5	T45.8X6
Oxyquinoline (derivatives)	T37.8X1	T37.8X2	T37.8X3	T37.8X4	T37.8X5	T37.8X6
Oxytetracycline	T36.4X1	T36.4X2	T36.4X3	T36.4X4	T36.4X5	T36.4X6
Oxytocic drug NEC	T48.0X1	T48.0X2	T48.0X3	T48.0X4	T48.0X5	T48.0X6
Oxytocin (synthetic)	T48.0X1	T48.0X2	T48.0X3	T48.0X4	T48.0X5	T48.0X6
Oxytrol*	T44.3X1	T44.3X2	T44.3X3	T44.3X4	T44.3X5	T44.3X6
Ozone	T59.891	T59.892	T59.893	T59.894	—	—
PABA	T49.3X1	T49.3X2	T49.3X3	T49.3X4	T49.3X5	T49.3X6
Packed red cells	T45.8X1	T45.8X2	T45.8X3	T45.8X4	T45.8X5	T45.8X6
Padimate	T49.3X1	T49.3X2	T49.3X3	T49.3X4	T49.3X5	T49.3X6
Paint NEC	T65.6X1	T65.6X2	T65.6X3	T65.6X4	—	—
cleaner	T52.91	T52.92	T52.93	T52.94	—	—
fumes NEC	T59.891	T59.892	T59.893	T59.894	—	—
lead (fumes)	T56.0X1	T56.0X2	T56.0X3	T56.0X4	—	—
solvent NEC	T52.8X1	T52.8X2	T52.8X3	T52.8X4	—	—
stripper	T52.8X1	T52.8X2	T52.8X3	T52.8X4	—	—
Palfium	T40.2X1	T40.2X2	T40.2X3	T40.2X4	—	—
Palm kernel oil	T50.991	T50.992	T50.993	T50.994	T50.995	T50.996
Paludrine	T37.2X1	T37.2X2	T37.2X3	T37.2X4	T37.2X5	T37.2X6
PAM (pralidoxime)	T50.6X1	T50.6X2	T50.6X3	T50.6X4	T50.6X5	T50.6X6
Pamaquine (naphthoute)	T37.2X1	T37.2X2	T37.2X3	T37.2X4	T37.2X5	T37.2X6
Panadol	T39.1X1	T39.1X2	T39.1X3	T39.1X4	T39.1X5	T39.1X6
Pancreatic						
digestive secretion stimulant	T47.8X1	T47.8X2	T47.8X3	T47.8X4	T47.8X5	T47.8X6
dornase	T45.3X1	T45.3X2	T45.3X3	T45.3X4	T45.3X5	T45.3X6
Pancreatin	T47.5X1	T47.5X2	T47.5X3	T47.5X4	T47.5X5	T47.5X6
Pancrelipase	T47.5X1	T47.5X2	T47.5X3	T47.5X4	T47.5X5	T47.5X6
Pancuronium (bromide)	T48.1X1	T48.1X2	T48.1X3	T48.1X4	T48.1X5	T48.1X6
Pangamic acid	T45.2X1	T45.2X2	T45.2X3	T45.2X4	T45.2X5	T45.2X6
Panthenol	T45.2X1	T45.2X2	T45.2X3	T45.2X4	T45.2X5	T45.2X6
topical	T49.8X1	T49.8X2	T49.8X3	T49.8X4	T49.8X5	T49.8X6
Pantopon	T40.0X1	T40.0X2	T40.0X3	T40.0X4	T40.0X5	T40.0X6
Pantoprazole*	T47.1X1	T47.1X2	T47.1X3	T47.1X4	T47.1X5	T47.1X6
Pantothenic acid	T45.2X1	T45.2X2	T45.2X3	T45.2X4	T45.2X5	T45.2X6
Panwarfin	T45.511	T45.512	T45.513	T45.514	T45.515	T45.516
Papain	T47.5X1	T47.5X2	T47.5X3	T47.5X4	T47.5X5	T47.5X6
digestant	T47.5X1	T47.5X2	T47.5X3	T47.5X4	T47.5X5	T47.5X6
Papaveretum	T40.0X1	T40.0X2	T40.0X3	T40.0X4	T40.0X5	T40.0X6
Papaverine	T44.3X1	T44.3X2	T44.3X3	T44.3X4	T44.3X5	T44.3X6
Para-acetamidophenol	T39.1X1	T39.1X2	T39.1X3	T39.1X4	T39.1X5	T39.1X6
Para-aminobenzoic acid	T49.3X1	T49.3X2	T49.3X3	T49.3X4	T49.3X5	T49.3X6
Para-aminophenol derivatives	T39.1X1	T39.1X2	T39.1X3	T39.1X4	T39.1X5	T39.1X6
Para-aminosalicylic acid	T37.1X1	T37.1X2	T37.1X3	T37.1X4	T37.1X5	T37.1X6
Paracetaldehyde	T42.6X1	T42.6X2	T42.6X3	T42.6X4	T42.6X5	T42.6X6
Paracetamol	T39.1X1	T39.1X2	T39.1X3	T39.1X4	T39.1X5	T39.1X6
Parachlorophenol (camphorated)	T49.0X1	T49.0X2	T49.0X3	T49.0X4	T49.0X5	T49.0X6
Paracodin	T40.2X1	T40.2X2	T40.2X3	T40.2X4	T40.2X5	T40.2X6
Paradione	T42.2X1	T42.2X2	T42.2X3	T42.2X4	T42.2X5	T42.2X6
Paraffin(s) (wax)	T52.0X1	T52.0X2	T52.0X3	T52.0X4	—	—
liquid (medicinal)	T47.4X1	T47.4X2	T47.4X3	T47.4X4	T47.4X5	T47.4X6
nonmedicinal	T52.0X1	T52.0X2	T52.0X3	T52.0X4	—	—
Paraformaldehyde	T60.3X1	T60.3X2	T60.3X3	T60.3X4	—	—
Paraldehyde	T42.6X1	T42.6X2	T42.6X3	T42.6X4	T42.6X5	T42.6X6
Paramethadione	T42.2X1	T42.2X2	T42.2X3	T42.2X4	T42.2X5	T42.2X6
Paramethasone	T38.0X1	T38.0X2	T38.0X3	T38.0X4	T38.0X5	T38.0X6
acetate	T49.0X1	T49.0X2	T49.0X3	T49.0X4	T49.0X5	T49.0X6
Paraoxon	T60.0X1	T60.0X2	T60.0X3	T60.0X4	—	—
Paraquat	T60.3X1	T60.3X2	T60.3X3	T60.3X4	—	—
Parasympatholytic NEC	T44.3X1	T44.3X2	T44.3X3	T44.3X4	T44.3X5	T44.3X6
Parasympathomimetic drug NEC	T44.1X1	T44.1X2	T44.1X3	T44.1X4	T44.1X5	T44.1X6
Parathion	T60.0X1	T60.0X2	T60.0X3	T60.0X4	—	—
Parathormone	T50.991	T50.992	T50.993	T50.994	T50.995	T50.996
Parathyroid extract	T50.991	T50.992	T50.993	T50.994	T50.995	T50.996
Parathyphoid vaccine	T50.A91	T50.A92	T50.A93	T50.A94	T50.A95	T50.A96
Paredrine	T44.4X1	T44.4X2	T44.4X3	T44.4X4	T44.4X5	T44.4X6
Paregoric	T40.0X1	T40.0X2	T40.0X3	T40.0X4	T40.0X5	T40.0X6
Pargyline	T46.5X1	T46.5X2	T46.5X3	T46.5X4	T46.5X5	T46.5X6
Paris green	T57.0X1	T57.0X2	T57.0X3	T57.0X4	—	—
insecticide	T57.0X1	T57.0X2	T57.0X3	T57.0X4	—	—
Parnate	T43.1X1	T43.1X2	T43.1X3	T43.1X4	T43.1X5	T43.1X6
Paromomycin	T36.5X1	T36.5X2	T36.5X3	T36.5X4	T36.5X5	T36.5X6
Paroxypropione	T45.1X1	T45.1X2	T45.1X3	T45.1X4	T45.1X5	T45.1X6
Parsabiv*	T50.991	T50.992	T50.993	T50.994	T50.995	T50.996
Parzone	T40.2X1	T40.2X2	T40.2X3	T40.2X4	T40.2X5	T40.2X6
PAS	T37.1X1	T37.1X2	T37.1X3	T37.1X4	T37.1X5	T37.1X6
Pasiniazid	T37.1X1	T37.1X2	T37.1X3	T37.1X4	T37.1X5	T37.1X6
PBB (polybrominated biphenyls)	T65.891	T65.892	T65.893	T65.894	—	—
PCB	T65.891	T65.892	T65.893	T65.894	—	—
PCP						
meaning pentachlorophenol	T60.1X1	T60.1X2	T60.1X3	T60.1X4	—	—
fungicide	T60.3X1	T60.3X2	T60.3X3	T60.3X4	—	—
herbicide	T60.3X1	T60.3X2	T60.3X3	T60.3X4	—	—
insecticide	T60.1X1	T60.1X2	T60.1X3	T60.1X4	—	—
meaning phencyclidine	T40.991	T40.992	T40.993	T40.994	—	—
Peach kernel oil (emulsion)	T47.4X1	T47.4X2	T47.4X3	T47.4X4	T47.4X5	T47.4X6
Peanut oil (emulsion) NEC	T47.4X1	T47.4X2	T47.4X3	T47.4X4	T47.4X5	T47.4X6

Table of Drugs and Chemicals

Peanut oil — Phenbutrazate

Substance	Poisoning, Accidental (unintentional)	Poisoning, Intentional Self-harm	Poisoning, Assault	Poisoning, Undetermined	Adverse Effect	Under-dosing
Peanut oil (emulsion) **NEC** — continued						
topical	T49.3X1	T49.3X2	T49.3X3	T49.3X4	T49.3X5	T49.3X6
Pearly Gates (morning glory seeds)	T40.991	T40.992	T40.993	T40.994	—	—
Pecazine	T43.3X1	T43.3X2	T43.3X3	T43.3X4	T43.3X5	T43.3X6
Pectin	T47.6X1	T47.6X2	T47.6X3	T47.6X4	T47.6X5	T47.6X6
Pediaflor*	T49.7X1	T49.7X2	T49.7X3	T49.7X4	T49.7X5	T49.7X6
Pefloxacin	T37.8X1	T37.8X2	T37.8X3	T37.8X4	T37.8X5	T37.8X6
Pegademase, bovine	T50.Z91	T50.Z92	T50.Z93	T50.Z94	T50.Z95	T50.Z96
Pelletierine tannate	T37.4X1	T37.4X2	T37.4X3	T37.4X4	T37.4X5	T37.4X6
Pemirolast (potassium)	T48.6X1	T48.6X2	T48.6X3	T48.6X4	T48.6X5	T48.6X6
Pemoline	T50.7X1	T50.7X2	T50.7X3	T50.7X4	T50.7X5	T50.7X6
Pempidine	T44.2X1	T44.2X2	T44.2X3	T44.2X4	T44.2X5	T44.2X6
Penamecillin	T36.0X1	T36.0X2	T36.0X3	T36.0X4	T36.0X5	T36.0X6
Penbutolol	T44.7X1	T44.7X2	T44.7X3	T44.7X4	T44.7X5	T44.7X6
Penethamate	T36.0X1	T36.0X2	T36.0X3	T36.0X4	T36.0X5	T36.0X6
Penfluridol	T43.591	T43.592	T43.593	T43.594	T43.595	T43.596
Penflutizide	T50.2X1	T50.2X2	T50.2X3	T50.2X4	T50.2X5	T50.2X6
Pengitoxin	T46.0X1	T46.0X2	T46.0X3	T46.0X4	T46.0X5	T46.0X6
Penicillamine	T50.6X1	T50.6X2	T50.6X3	T50.6X4	T50.6X5	T50.6X6
Penicillin (any)	T36.0X1	T36.0X2	T36.0X3	T36.0X4	T36.0X5	T36.0X6
Penicillinase	T45.3X1	T45.3X2	T45.3X3	T45.3X4	T45.3X5	T45.3X6
Penicilloyl polylysine	T50.8X1	T50.8X2	T50.8X3	T50.8X4	T50.8X5	T50.8X6
Penimepicycline	T36.4X1	T36.4X2	T36.4X3	T36.4X4	T36.4X5	T36.4X6
Pentacel*	T50.A11	T50.A12	T50.A13	T50.A14	T50.A15	T50.A16
Pentachloroethane	T53.6X1	T53.6X2	T53.6X3	T53.6X4	—	—
Pentachloronaphthalene	T53.7X1	T53.7X2	T53.7X3	T53.7X4	—	—
Pentachlorophenol (pesticide)	T60.1X1	T60.1X2	T60.1X3	T60.1X4	—	—
fungicide	T60.3X1	T60.3X2	T60.3X3	T60.3X4	—	—
herbicide	T60.3X1	T60.3X2	T60.3X3	T60.3X4	—	—
insecticide	T60.1X1	T60.1X2	T60.1X3	T60.1X4	—	—
Pentaerythritol	T46.3X1	T46.3X2	T46.3X3	T46.3X4	T46.3X5	T46.3X6
chloral	T42.6X1	T42.6X2	T42.6X3	T42.6X4	T42.6X5	T42.6X6
tetranitrate NEC	T46.3X1	T46.3X2	T46.3X3	T46.3X4	T46.3X5	T46.3X6
Pentaerythrityl tetranitrate	T46.3X1	T46.3X2	T46.3X3	T46.3X4	T46.3X5	T46.3X6
Pentagastrin	T50.8X1	T50.8X2	T50.8X3	T50.8X4	T50.8X5	T50.8X6
Pentalin	T53.6X1	T53.6X2	T53.6X3	T53.6X4	—	—
Pentamethonium bromide	T44.2X1	T44.2X2	T44.2X3	T44.2X4	T44.2X5	T44.2X6
Pentamidine	T37.3X1	T37.3X2	T37.3X3	T37.3X4	T37.3X5	T37.3X6
Pentanol	T51.3X1	T51.3X2	T51.3X3	T51.3X4	—	—
Pentapyrrolinium (bitartrate)	T44.2X1	T44.2X2	T44.2X3	T44.2X4	T44.2X5	T44.2X6
Pentaquine	T37.2X1	T37.2X2	T37.2X3	T37.2X4	T37.2X5	T37.2X6
Pentazocine	T40.491	T40.492	T40.493	T40.494	T40.495	T40.496
Pentetrazole	T50.7X1	T50.7X2	T50.7X3	T50.7X4	T50.7X5	T50.7X6
Penthienate bromide	T44.3X1	T44.3X2	T44.3X3	T44.3X4	T44.3X5	T44.3X6
Pentifylline	T46.7X1	T46.7X2	T46.7X3	T46.7X4	T46.7X5	T46.7X6
Pentobarbital	T42.3X1	T42.3X2	T42.3X3	T42.3X4	T42.3X5	T42.3X6
sodium	T42.3X1	T42.3X2	T42.3X3	T42.3X4	T42.3X5	T42.3X6
Pentobarbitone	T42.3X1	T42.3X2	T42.3X3	T42.3X4	T42.3X5	T42.3X6
Pentolonium tartrate	T44.2X1	T44.2X2	T44.2X3	T44.2X4	T44.2X5	T44.2X6
Pentosan polysulfate (sodium)	T39.8X1	T39.8X2	T39.8X3	T39.8X4	T39.8X5	T39.8X6
Pentostatin	T45.1X1	T45.1X2	T45.1X3	T45.1X4	T45.1X5	T45.1X6
Pentothal	T41.1X1	T41.1X2	T41.1X3	T41.1X4	T41.1X5	T41.1X6
Pentoxifylline	T46.7X1	T46.7X2	T46.7X3	T46.7X4	T46.7X5	T46.7X6
Pentoxyverine	T48.3X1	T48.3X2	T48.3X3	T48.3X4	T48.3X5	T48.3X6
Pentrinat	T46.3X1	T46.3X2	T46.3X3	T46.3X4	T46.3X5	T46.3X6
Pentylenetetrazole	T50.7X1	T50.7X2	T50.7X3	T50.7X4	T50.7X5	T50.7X6
Pentylsalicylamide	T37.1X1	T37.1X2	T37.1X3	T37.1X4	T37.1X5	T37.1X6
Pentymal	T42.3X1	T42.3X2	T42.3X3	T42.3X4	T42.3X5	T42.3X6
Pepcid*	T47.0X1	T47.0X2	T47.0X3	T47.0X4	T47.0X5	T47.0X6
Peplomycin	T45.1X1	T45.1X2	T45.1X3	T45.1X4	T45.1X5	T45.1X6
Peppermint (oil)	T47.5X1	T47.5X2	T47.5X3	T47.5X4	T47.5X5	T47.5X6
Pepsin	T47.5X1	T47.5X2	T47.5X3	T47.5X4	T47.5X5	T47.5X6
digestant	T47.5X1	T47.5X2	T47.5X3	T47.5X4	T47.5X5	T47.5X6
Pepstatin	T47.1X1	T47.1X2	T47.1X3	T47.1X4	T47.1X5	T47.1X6
Peptavlon	T50.8X1	T50.8X2	T50.8X3	T50.8X4	T50.8X5	T50.8X6
Perazine	T43.3X1	T43.3X2	T43.3X3	T43.3X4	T43.3X5	T43.3X6
Percaine (spinal)	T41.3X1	T41.3X2	T41.3X3	T41.3X4	T41.3X5	T41.3X6
topical (surface)	T41.3X1	T41.3X2	T41.3X3	T41.3X4	T41.3X5	T41.3X6
Perchloroethylene	T53.3X1	T53.3X2	T53.3X3	T53.3X4	—	—
medicinal	T37.4X1	T37.4X2	T37.4X3	T37.4X4	T37.4X5	T37.4X6
vapor	T53.3X1	T53.3X2	T53.3X3	T53.3X4	—	—
Percodan	T40.2X1	T40.2X2	T40.2X3	T40.2X4	T40.2X5	T40.2X6
Percogesic — see also acetaminophen	T45.0X1	T45.0X2	T45.0X3	T45.0X4	T45.0X5	T45.0X6
Percorten	T38.0X1	T38.0X2	T38.0X3	T38.0X4	T38.0X5	T38.0X6
Pergolide	T42.8X1	T42.8X2	T42.8X3	T42.8X4	T42.8X5	T42.8X6
Pergonal	T38.811	T38.812	T38.813	T38.814	T38.815	T38.816

Substance	Poisoning, Accidental (unintentional)	Poisoning, Intentional Self-harm	Poisoning, Assault	Poisoning, Undetermined	Adverse Effect	Under-dosing
Perhexilene	T46.3X1	T46.3X2	T46.3X3	T46.3X4	T46.3X5	T46.3X6
Perhexiline (maleate)	T46.3X1	T46.3X2	T46.3X3	T46.3X4	T46.3X5	T46.3X6
Periactin	T45.0X1	T45.0X2	T45.0X3	T45.0X4	T45.0X5	T45.0X6
Periciazine	T43.3X1	T43.3X2	T43.3X3	T43.3X4	T43.3X5	T43.3X6
Periclor	T42.6X1	T42.6X2	T42.6X3	T42.6X4	T42.6X5	T42.6X6
Perindopril	T46.4X1	T46.4X2	T46.4X3	T46.4X4	T46.4X5	T46.4X6
Perisoxal	T39.8X1	T39.8X2	T39.8X3	T39.8X4	T39.8X5	T39.8X6
Peritoneal dialysis solution	T50.3X1	T50.3X2	T50.3X3	T50.3X4	T50.3X5	T50.3X6
Peritrate	T46.3X1	T46.3X2	T46.3X3	T46.3X4	T46.3X5	T46.3X6
Perlapine	T42.4X1	T42.4X2	T42.4X3	T42.4X4	T42.4X5	T42.4X6
Permanganate	T65.891	T65.892	T65.893	T65.894	—	—
Permapen*	T36.0X1	T36.0X2	T36.0X3	T36.0X4	T36.0X5	T36.0X6
Permethrin	T60.1X1	T60.1X2	T60.1X3	T60.1X4	—	—
Pernocton	T42.3X1	T42.3X2	T42.3X3	T42.3X4	T42.3X5	T42.3X6
Pernoston	T42.3X1	T42.3X2	T42.3X3	T42.3X4	T42.3X5	T42.3X6
Peronine	T40.2X1	T40.2X2	T40.2X3	T40.2X4	—	—
Perphenazine	T43.3X1	T43.3X2	T43.3X3	T43.3X4	T43.3X5	T43.3X6
Pertofrane	T43.011	T43.012	T43.013	T43.014	T43.015	T43.016
Pertussis						
immune serum (human)	T50.Z11	T50.Z12	T50.Z13	T50.Z14	T50.Z15	T50.Z16
vaccine (with diphtheria toxoid) (with tetanus toxoid)	T50.A11	T50.A12	T50.A13	T50.A14	T50.A15	T50.A16
Peruvian balsam	T49.0X1	T49.0X2	T49.0X3	T49.0X4	T49.0X5	T49.0X6
Peruvoside	T46.0X1	T46.0X2	T46.0X3	T46.0X4	T46.0X5	T46.0X6
Pesticide (dust) (fumes) (vapor) **NEC**	T60.91	T60.92	T60.93	T60.94	—	—
arsenic	T57.0X1	T57.0X2	T57.0X3	T57.0X4	—	—
chlorinated	T60.1X1	T60.1X2	T60.1X3	T60.1X4	—	—
cyanide	T65.0X1	T65.0X2	T65.0X3	T65.0X4	—	—
kerosene	T52.0X1	T52.0X2	T52.0X3	T52.0X4	—	—
mixture (of compounds)	T60.91	T60.92	T60.93	T60.94	—	—
naphthalene	T60.2X1	T60.2X2	T60.2X3	T60.2X4	—	—
organochlorine (compounds)	T60.1X1	T60.1X2	T60.1X3	T60.1X4	—	—
petroleum (distillate) (products) NEC	T60.8X1	T60.8X2	T60.8X3	T60.8X4	—	—
specified ingredient NEC	T60.8X1	T60.8X2	T60.8X3	T60.8X4	—	—
strychnine	T65.1X1	T65.1X2	T65.1X3	T65.1X4	—	—
thallium	T60.4X1	T60.4X2	T60.4X3	T60.4X4	—	—
Pethidine	T40.491	T40.492	T40.493	T40.494	T40.495	T40.496
Petrichloral	T42.6X1	T42.6X2	T42.6X3	T42.6X4	T42.6X5	T42.6X6
Petrol	T52.0X1	T52.0X2	T52.0X3	T52.0X4	—	—
vapor	T52.0X1	T52.0X2	T52.0X3	T52.0X4	—	—
Petrolatum	T49.3X1	T49.3X2	T49.3X3	T49.3X4	T49.3X5	T49.3X6
hydrophilic	T49.3X1	T49.3X2	T49.3X3	T49.3X4	T49.3X5	T49.3X6
liquid	T47.4X1	T47.4X2	T47.4X3	T47.4X4	T47.4X5	T47.4X6
topical	T49.3X1	T49.3X2	T49.3X3	T49.3X4	T49.3X5	T49.3X6
nonmedicinal	T52.0X1	T52.0X2	T52.0X3	T52.0X4	—	—
red veterinary	T49.3X1	T49.3X2	T49.3X3	T49.3X4	T49.3X5	T49.3X6
white	T49.3X1	T49.3X2	T49.3X3	T49.3X4	T49.3X5	T49.3X6
Petroleum (products) **NEC**	T52.0X1	T52.0X2	T52.0X3	T52.0X4	—	—
benzine(s) — see Ligroin						
ether — see Ligroin						
jelly — see Petrolatum						
naphtha — see Ligroin						
pesticide	T60.8X1	T60.8X2	T60.8X3	T60.8X4	—	—
solids	T52.0X1	T52.0X2	T52.0X3	T52.0X4	—	—
solvents	T52.0X1	T52.0X2	T52.0X3	T52.0X4	—	—
vapor	T52.0X1	T52.0X2	T52.0X3	T52.0X4	—	—
Peyote	T40.991	T40.992	T40.993	T40.994	—	—
Phanodorm, phanodorn	T42.3X1	T42.3X2	T42.3X3	T42.3X4	T42.3X5	T42.3X6
Phanquinone	T37.3X1	T37.3X2	T37.3X3	T37.3X4	T37.3X5	T37.3X6
Phanquone	T37.3X1	T37.3X2	T37.3X3	T37.3X4	T37.3X5	T37.3X6
Pharmaceutical						
adjunct NEC	T50.901	T50.902	T50.903	T50.904	T50.905	T50.906
excipient NEC	T50.901	T50.902	T50.903	T50.904	T50.905	T50.906
sweetener	T50.901	T50.902	T50.903	T50.904	T50.905	T50.906
viscous agent	T50.901	T50.902	T50.903	T50.904	T50.905	T50.906
Phazyme*	T47.1X1	T47.1X2	T47.1X3	T47.1X4	T47.1X5	T47.1X6
Phemitone	T42.3X1	T42.3X2	T42.3X3	T42.3X4	T42.3X5	T42.3X6
Phenacaine	T41.3X1	T41.3X2	T41.3X3	T41.3X4	T41.3X5	T41.3X6
Phenacemide	T42.6X1	T42.6X2	T42.6X3	T42.6X4	T42.6X5	T42.6X6
Phenacetin	T39.1X1	T39.1X2	T39.1X3	T39.1X4	T39.1X5	T39.1X6
Phenadoxone	T40.2X1	T40.2X2	T40.2X3	T40.2X4	—	—
Phenaglycodol	T43.591	T43.592	T43.593	T43.594	T43.595	T43.596
Phenantoin	T42.0X1	T42.0X2	T42.0X3	T42.0X4	T42.0X5	T42.0X6
Phenaphthazine reagent	T50.991	T50.992	T50.993	T50.994	T50.995	T50.996
Phenazocine	T40.491	T40.492	T40.493	T40.494	T40.495	T40.496
Phenazone	T39.2X1	T39.2X2	T39.2X3	T39.2X4	T39.2X5	T39.2X6
Phenazopyridine	T39.8X1	T39.8X2	T39.8X3	T39.8X4	T39.8X5	T39.8X6
Phenbenicillin	T36.0X1	T36.0X2	T36.0X3	T36.0X4	T36.0X5	T36.0X6
Phenbutrazate	T50.5X1	T50.5X2	T50.5X3	T50.5X4	T50.5X5	T50.5X6

☑ Additional Character May Be Required — Refer to the Tabular List for Character Selection   *Optum Value-Add

Substance	Poisoning, Accidental (unintentional)	Poisoning, Intentional Self-harm	Poisoning, Assault	Poisoning, Undetermined	Adverse Effect	Under-dosing
Phencyclidine	T40.991	T40.992	T40.993	T40.994	T40.995	T40.996
Phendimetrazine	T50.5X1	T50.5X2	T50.5X3	T50.5X4	T50.5X5	T50.5X6
Phenelzine	T43.1X1	T43.1X2	T43.1X3	T43.1X4	T43.1X5	T43.1X6
Phenemal	T42.3X1	T42.3X2	T42.3X3	T42.3X4	T42.3X5	T42.3X6
Phenergan	T42.6X1	T42.6X2	T42.6X3	T42.6X4	T42.6X5	T42.6X6
Pheneticillin	T36.0X1	T36.0X2	T36.0X3	T36.0X4	T36.0X5	T36.0X6
Pheneturide	T42.6X1	T42.6X2	T42.6X3	T42.6X4	T42.6X5	T42.6X6
Phenformin	T38.3X1	T38.3X2	T38.3X3	T38.3X4	T38.3X5	T38.3X6
Phenglutarimide	T44.3X1	T44.3X2	T44.3X3	T44.3X4	T44.3X5	T44.3X6
Phenicarbazide	T39.8X1	T39.8X2	T39.8X3	T39.8X4	T39.8X5	T39.8X6
Phenindamine	T45.0X1	T45.0X2	T45.0X3	T45.0X4	T45.0X5	T45.0X6
Phenindione	T45.511	T45.512	T45.513	T45.514	T45.515	T45.516
Pheniprazine	T43.1X1	T43.1X2	T43.1X3	T43.1X4	T43.1X5	T43.1X6
Pheniramine	T45.0X1	T45.0X2	T45.0X3	T45.0X4	T45.0X5	T45.0X6
Phenisatin	T47.2X1	T47.2X2	T47.2X3	T47.2X4	T47.2X5	T47.2X6
Phenmetrazine	T50.5X1	T50.5X2	T50.5X3	T50.5X4	T50.5X5	T50.5X6
Phenobal	T42.3X1	T42.3X2	T42.3X3	T42.3X4	T42.3X5	T42.3X6
Phenobarbital	T42.3X1	T42.3X2	T42.3X3	T42.3X4	T42.3X5	T42.3X6
with						
mephenytoin	T42.3X1	T42.3X2	T42.3X3	T42.3X4	T42.3X5	T42.3X6
phenytoin	T42.3X1	T42.3X2	T42.3X3	T42.3X4	T42.3X5	T42.3X6
sodium	T42.3X1	T42.3X2	T42.3X3	T42.3X4	T42.3X5	T42.3X6
Phenobarbitone	T42.3X1	T42.3X2	T42.3X3	T42.3X4	T42.3X5	T42.3X6
Phenobutiodil	T50.8X1	T50.8X2	T50.8X3	T50.8X4	T50.8X5	T50.8X6
Phenoctide	T49.0X1	T49.0X2	T49.0X3	T49.0X4	T49.0X5	T49.0X6
Phenol	T49.0X1	T49.0X2	T49.0X3	T49.0X4	T49.0X5	T49.0X6
disinfectant	T54.0X1	T54.0X2	T54.0X3	T54.0X4	—	—
in oil injection	T46.8X1	T46.8X2	T46.8X3	T46.8X4	T46.8X5	T46.8X6
medicinal	T49.1X1	T49.1X2	T49.1X3	T49.1X4	T49.1X5	T49.1X6
nonmedicinal NEC	T54.0X1	T54.0X2	T54.0X3	T54.0X4	—	—
pesticide	T60.8X1	T60.8X2	T60.8X3	T60.8X4	—	—
red	T50.8X1	T50.8X2	T50.8X3	T50.8X4	T50.8X5	T50.8X6
Phenolic preparation	T49.1X1	T49.1X2	T49.1X3	T49.1X4	T49.1X5	T49.1X6
Phenolphthalein	T47.2X1	T47.2X2	T47.2X3	T47.2X4	T47.2X5	T47.2X6
Phenolsulfonphthalein	T50.8X1	T50.8X2	T50.8X3	T50.8X4	T50.8X5	T50.8X6
Phenomorphan	T40.2X1	T40.2X2	T40.2X3	T40.2X4	—	—
Phenonyl	T42.3X1	T42.3X2	T42.3X3	T42.3X4	T42.3X5	T42.3X6
Phenoperidine	T40.491	T40.492	T40.493	T40.494	—	—
Phenopyrazone	T46.991	T46.992	T46.993	T46.994	T46.995	T46.996
Phenoquin	T50.4X1	T50.4X2	T50.4X3	T50.4X4	T50.4X5	T50.4X6
Phenothiazine (psychotropic)	T43.3X1	T43.3X2	T43.3X3	T43.3X4	T43.3X5	T43.3X6
NEC						
insecticide	T60.2X1	T60.2X2	T60.2X3	T60.2X4	—	—
Phenothrin	T49.0X1	T49.0X2	T49.0X3	T49.0X4	T49.0X5	T49.0X6
Phenoxybenzamine	T46.7X1	T46.7X2	T46.7X3	T46.7X4	T46.7X5	T46.7X6
Phenoxyethanol	T49.0X1	T49.0X2	T49.0X3	T49.0X4	T49.0X5	T49.0X6
Phenoxymethyl penicillin	T36.0X1	T36.0X2	T36.0X3	T36.0X4	T36.0X5	T36.0X6
Phenprobamate	T42.8X1	T42.8X2	T42.8X3	T42.8X4	T42.8X5	T42.8X6
Phenprocoumon	T45.511	T45.512	T45.513	T45.514	T45.515	T45.516
Phensuximide	T42.2X1	T42.2X2	T42.2X3	T42.2X4	T42.2X5	T42.2X6
Phentermine	T50.5X1	T50.5X2	T50.5X3	T50.5X4	T50.5X5	T50.5X6
Phenthicillin	T36.0X1	T36.0X2	T36.0X3	T36.0X4	T36.0X5	T36.0X6
Phentolamine	T46.7X1	T46.7X2	T46.7X3	T46.7X4	T46.7X5	T46.7X6
Phenyl						
butazone	T39.2X1	T39.2X2	T39.2X3	T39.2X4	T39.2X5	T39.2X6
enediamine	T65.3X1	T65.3X2	T65.3X3	T65.3X4	—	—
hydrazine	T65.3X1	T65.3X2	T65.3X3	T65.3X4	—	—
antineoplastic	T45.1X1	T45.1X2	T45.1X3	T45.1X4	T45.1X5	T45.1X6
mercuric compounds — see Mercury						
salicylate	T49.3X1	T49.3X2	T49.3X3	T49.3X4	T49.3X5	T49.3X6
Phenylalanine mustard	T45.1X1	T45.1X2	T45.1X3	T45.1X4	T45.1X5	T45.1X6
Phenylbutazone	T39.2X1	T39.2X2	T39.2X3	T39.2X4	T39.2X5	T39.2X6
Phenylenediamine	T65.3X1	T65.3X2	T65.3X3	T65.3X4	—	—
Phenylephrine	T44.4X1	T44.4X2	T44.4X3	T44.4X4	T44.4X5	T44.4X6
Phenylethylbiguanide	T38.3X1	T38.3X2	T38.3X3	T38.3X4	T38.3X5	T38.3X6
Phenylmercuric						
acetate	T49.0X1	T49.0X2	T49.0X3	T49.0X4	T49.0X5	T49.0X6
borate	T49.0X1	T49.0X2	T49.0X3	T49.0X4	T49.0X5	T49.0X6
nitrate	T49.0X1	T49.0X2	T49.0X3	T49.0X4	T49.0X5	T49.0X6
Phenylmethylbarbitone	T42.3X1	T42.3X2	T42.3X3	T42.3X4	T42.3X5	T42.3X6
Phenylpropanol	T47.5X1	T47.5X2	T47.5X3	T47.5X4	T47.5X5	T47.5X6
Phenylpropanolamine	T44.991	T44.992	T44.993	T44.994	T44.995	T44.996
Phenylsulfthion	T60.0X1	T60.0X2	T60.0X3	T60.0X4	—	—
Phenyltoloxamine	T45.0X1	T45.0X2	T45.0X3	T45.0X4	T45.0X5	T45.0X6
Phenyramidol, phenyramidon	T39.8X1	T39.8X2	T39.8X3	T39.8X4	T39.8X5	T39.8X6
Phenytek*	T42.0X1	T42.0X2	T42.0X3	T42.0X4	T42.0X5	T42.0X6
Phenytoin	T42.0X1	T42.0X2	T42.0X3	T42.0X4	T42.0X5	T42.0X6
with Phenobarbital	T42.3X1	T42.3X2	T42.3X3	T42.3X4	T42.3X5	T42.3X6
pHisoHex	T49.2X1	T49.2X2	T49.2X3	T49.2X4	T49.2X5	T49.2X6
Pholcodine	T48.3X1	T48.3X2	T48.3X3	T48.3X4	T48.3X5	T48.3X6
Pholedrine	T46.991	T46.992	T46.993	T46.994	T46.995	T46.996

Substance	Poisoning, Accidental (unintentional)	Poisoning, Intentional Self-harm	Poisoning, Assault	Poisoning, Undetermined	Adverse Effect	Under-dosing
Phorate	T60.0X1	T60.0X2	T60.0X3	T60.0X4	—	—
Phosdrin	T60.0X1	T60.0X2	T60.0X3	T60.0X4	—	—
Phosfolan	T60.0X1	T60.0X2	T60.0X3	T60.0X4	—	—
Phosgene (gas)	T59.891	T59.892	T59.893	T59.894	—	—
Phosphamidon	T60.0X1	T60.0X2	T60.0X3	T60.0X4	—	—
Phosphate	T65.891	T65.892	T65.893	T65.894	—	—
laxative	T47.4X1	T47.4X2	T47.4X3	T47.4X4	T47.4X5	T47.4X6
organic	T60.0X1	T60.0X2	T60.0X3	T60.0X4	—	—
solvent	T52.91	T52.92	T52.93	T52.94	—	—
tricresyl	T65.891	T65.892	T65.893	T65.894	—	—
Phosphine	T57.1X1	T57.1X2	T57.1X3	T57.1X4	—	—
fumigant	T57.1X1	T57.1X2	T57.1X3	T57.1X4	—	—
Phospholine	T49.5X1	T49.5X2	T49.5X3	T49.5X4	T49.5X5	T49.5X6
Phosphoric acid	T54.2X1	T54.2X2	T54.2X3	T54.2X4	—	—
Phosphorus (compound) NEC	T57.1X1	T57.1X2	T57.1X3	T57.1X4	—	—
pesticide	T60.0X1	T60.0X2	T60.0X3	T60.0X4	—	—
Photrexa*	T49.5X1	T49.5X2	T49.5X3	T49.5X4	T49.5X5	T49.5X6
Phthalates	T65.891	T65.892	T65.893	T65.894	—	—
Phthalic anhydride	T65.891	T65.892	T65.893	T65.894	—	—
Phthalimidoglutarimide	T42.6X1	T42.6X2	T42.6X3	T42.6X4	T42.6X5	T42.6X6
Phthalylsulfathiazole	T37.0X1	T37.0X2	T37.0X3	T37.0X4	T37.0X5	T37.0X6
Phylloquinone	T45.7X1	T45.7X2	T45.7X3	T45.7X4	T45.7X5	T45.7X6
Physeptone	T40.3X1	T40.3X2	T40.3X3	T40.3X4	T40.3X5	T40.3X6
Physostigma venenosum	T62.2X1	T62.2X2	T62.2X3	T62.2X4	—	—
Physostigmine	T49.5X1	T49.5X2	T49.5X3	T49.5X4	T49.5X5	T49.5X6
Phytolacca decandra	T62.2X1	T62.2X2	T62.2X3	T62.2X4	—	—
berries	T62.1X1	T62.1X2	T62.1X3	T62.1X4	—	—
Phytomenadione	T45.7X1	T45.7X2	T45.7X3	T45.7X4	T45.7X5	T45.7X6
Phytonadione	T45.7X1	T45.7X2	T45.7X3	T45.7X4	T45.7X5	T45.7X6
Picoperine	T48.3X1	T48.3X2	T48.3X3	T48.3X4	T48.3X5	T48.3X6
Picosulfate (sodium)	T47.2X1	T47.2X2	T47.2X3	T47.2X4	T47.2X5	T47.2X6
Picric (acid)	T54.2X1	T54.2X2	T54.2X3	T54.2X4	—	—
Picrotoxin	T50.7X1	T50.7X2	T50.7X3	T50.7X4	T50.7X5	T50.7X6
Piketoprofen	T49.0X1	T49.0X2	T49.0X3	T49.0X4	T49.0X5	T49.0X6
Pilocarpine	T44.1X1	T44.1X2	T44.1X3	T44.1X4	T44.1X5	T44.1X6
Pilocarpus (jaborandi)	T44.1X1	T44.1X2	T44.1X3	T44.1X4	T44.1X5	T44.1X6
extract						
Pilsicainide (hydrochloride)	T46.2X1	T46.2X2	T46.2X3	T46.2X4	T46.2X5	T46.2X6
Pimaricin	T36.7X1	T36.7X2	T36.7X3	T36.7X4	T36.7X5	T36.7X6
Pimeclone	T50.7X1	T50.7X2	T50.7X3	T50.7X4	T50.7X5	T50.7X6
Pimelic ketone	T52.8X1	T52.8X2	T52.8X3	T52.8X4	—	—
Pimethixene	T45.0X1	T45.0X2	T45.0X3	T45.0X4	T45.0X5	T45.0X6
Piminodine	T40.2X1	T40.2X2	T40.2X3	T40.2X4	T40.2X5	T40.2X6
Pimozide	T43.591	T43.592	T43.593	T43.594	T43.595	T43.596
Pinacidil	T46.5X1	T46.5X2	T46.5X3	T46.5X4	T46.5X5	T46.5X6
Pinaverium bromide	T44.3X1	T44.3X2	T44.3X3	T44.3X4	T44.3X5	T44.3X6
Pinazepam	T42.4X1	T42.4X2	T42.4X3	T42.4X4	T42.4X5	T42.4X6
Pindolol	T44.7X1	T44.7X2	T44.7X3	T44.7X4	T44.7X5	T44.7X6
Pindone	T60.4X1	T60.4X2	T60.4X3	T60.4X4	—	—
Pine oil (disinfectant)	T65.891	T65.892	T65.893	T65.894	—	—
Pinkroot	T37.4X1	T37.4X2	T37.4X3	T37.4X4	T37.4X5	T37.4X6
Pipadone	T40.2X1	T40.2X2	T40.2X3	T40.2X4	—	—
Pipamazine	T45.0X1	T45.0X2	T45.0X3	T45.0X4	T45.0X5	T45.0X6
Pipamperone	T43.4X1	T43.4X2	T43.4X3	T43.4X4	T43.4X5	T43.4X6
Pipazetate	T48.3X1	T48.3X2	T48.3X3	T48.3X4	T48.3X5	T48.3X6
Pipemidic acid	T37.8X1	T37.8X2	T37.8X3	T37.8X4	T37.8X5	T37.8X6
Pipenzolate bromide	T44.3X1	T44.3X2	T44.3X3	T44.3X4	T44.3X5	T44.3X6
Piperacetazine	T43.3X1	T43.3X2	T43.3X3	T43.3X4	T43.3X5	T43.3X6
Piperacillin	T36.0X1	T36.0X2	T36.0X3	T36.0X4	T36.0X5	T36.0X6
Piperazine	T37.4X1	T37.4X2	T37.4X3	T37.4X4	T37.4X5	T37.4X6
estrone sulfate	T38.5X1	T38.5X2	T38.5X3	T38.5X4	T38.5X5	T38.5X6
Piper cubeba	T62.2X1	T62.2X2	T62.2X3	T62.2X4	—	—
Piperidione	T48.3X1	T48.3X2	T48.3X3	T48.3X4	T48.3X5	T48.3X6
Piperidolate	T44.3X1	T44.3X2	T44.3X3	T44.3X4	T44.3X5	T44.3X6
Piperocaine	T41.3X1	T41.3X2	T41.3X3	T41.3X4	T41.3X5	T41.3X6
infiltration (subcutaneous)	T41.3X1	T41.3X2	T41.3X3	T41.3X4	T41.3X5	T41.3X6
nerve block (peripheral) (plexus)	T41.3X1	T41.3X2	T41.3X3	T41.3X4	T41.3X5	T41.3X6
topical (surface)	T41.3X1	T41.3X2	T41.3X3	T41.3X4	T41.3X5	T41.3X6
Piperonyl butoxide	T60.8X1	T60.8X2	T60.8X3	T60.8X4	—	—
Pipethanate	T44.3X1	T44.3X2	T44.3X3	T44.3X4	T44.3X5	T44.3X6
Pipobroman	T45.1X1	T45.1X2	T45.1X3	T45.1X4	T45.1X5	T45.1X6
Pipotiazine	T43.3X1	T43.3X2	T43.3X3	T43.3X4	T43.3X5	T43.3X6
Pipoxizine	T45.0X1	T45.0X2	T45.0X3	T45.0X4	T45.0X5	T45.0X6
Pipradrol	T43.691	T43.692	T43.693	T43.694	T43.695	T43.696
Piprinhydrinate	T45.0X1	T45.0X2	T45.0X3	T45.0X4	T45.0X5	T45.0X6
Pirarubicin	T45.1X1	T45.1X2	T45.1X3	T45.1X4	T45.1X5	T45.1X6
Pirazinamide	T37.1X1	T37.1X2	T37.1X3	T37.1X4	T37.1X5	T37.1X6
Pirbuterol	T48.6X1	T48.6X2	T48.6X3	T48.6X4	T48.6X5	T48.6X6
Pirenzepine	T47.1X1	T47.1X2	T47.1X3	T47.1X4	T47.1X5	T47.1X6
Piretanide	T50.1X1	T50.1X2	T50.1X3	T50.1X4	T50.1X5	T50.1X6
Pirfenidone*	T48.991	T48.992	T48.993	T48.994	T48.995	T48.996

Substance	Poisoning, Accidental (unintentional)	Poisoning, Intentional Self-harm	Poisoning, Assault	Poisoning, Undetermined	Adverse Effect	Under-dosing
Piribedil	T42.8X1	T42.8X2	T42.8X3	T42.8X4	T42.8X5	T42.8X6
Piridoxilate	T46.3X1	T46.3X2	T46.3X3	T46.3X4	T46.3X5	T46.3X6
Piritramide	T40.491	T40.492	T40.493	T40.494	—	—
Piromidic acid	T37.8X1	T37.8X2	T37.8X3	T37.8X4	T37.8X5	T37.8X6
Piroxicam	T39.391	T39.392	T39.393	T39.394	T39.395	T39.396
beta-cyclodextrin complex	T39.8X1	T39.8X2	T39.8X3	T39.8X4	T39.8X5	T39.8X6
Pirozadil	T46.6X1	T46.6X2	T46.6X3	T46.6X4	T46.6X5	T46.6X6
Piscidia (bark) (erythrina)	T39.8X1	T39.8X2	T39.8X3	T39.8X4	T39.8X5	T39.8X6
Pitch	T65.891	T65.892	T65.893	T65.894	—	—
Pitkin's solution	T41.3X1	T41.3X2	T41.3X3	T41.3X4	T41.3X5	T41.3X6
Pitocin	T48.0X1	T48.0X2	T48.0X3	T48.0X4	T48.0X5	T48.0X6
Pitressin (tannate)	T38.891	T38.892	T38.893	T38.894	T38.895	T38.896
Pituitary extracts (posterior)	T38.891	T38.892	T38.893	T38.894	T38.895	T38.896
anterior	T38.811	T38.812	T38.813	T38.814	T38.815	T38.816
Pituitrin	T38.891	T38.892	T38.893	T38.894	T38.895	T38.896
Pivampicillin	T36.0X1	T36.0X2	T36.0X3	T36.0X4	T36.0X5	T36.0X6
Pivmecillinam	T36.0X1	T36.0X2	T36.0X3	T36.0X4	T36.0X5	T36.0X6
Placental hormone	T38.891	T38.892	T38.893	T38.894	T38.895	T38.896
Placidyl	T42.6X1	T42.6X2	T42.6X3	T42.6X4	T42.6X5	T42.6X6
Plague vaccine	T50.A91	T50.A92	T50.A93	T50.A94	T50.A95	T50.A96
Plant						
food or fertilizer NEC	T65.891	T65.892	T65.893	T65.894	—	—
containing herbicide	T60.3X1	T60.3X2	T60.3X3	T60.3X4	—	—
noxious, used as food	T62.2X1	T62.2X2	T62.2X3	T62.2X4	—	—
berries	T62.1X1	T62.1X2	T62.1X3	T62.1X4	—	—
seeds	T62.2X1	T62.2X2	T62.2X3	T62.2X4	—	—
specified type NEC	T62.2X1	T62.2X2	T62.2X3	T62.2X4	—	—
Plasma	T45.8X1	T45.8X2	T45.8X3	T45.8X4	T45.8X5	T45.8X6
expander NEC	T45.8X1	T45.8X2	T45.8X3	T45.8X4	T45.8X5	T45.8X6
protein fraction (human)	T45.8X1	T45.8X2	T45.8X3	T45.8X4	T45.8X5	T45.8X6
Plasmanate	T45.8X1	T45.8X2	T45.8X3	T45.8X4	T45.8X5	T45.8X6
Plasminogen (tissue)	T45.611	T45.612	T45.613	T45.614	T45.615	T45.616
activator						
Plaster dressing	T49.3X1	T49.3X2	T49.3X3	T49.3X4	T49.3X5	T49.3X6
Plastic dressing	T49.3X1	T49.3X2	T49.3X3	T49.3X4	T49.3X5	T49.3X6
Plavix*	T45.521	T45.522	T45.523	T45.524	T45.525	T45.526
Plegicil	T43.3X1	T43.3X2	T43.3X3	T43.3X4	T43.3X5	T43.3X6
Plicamycin	T45.1X1	T45.1X2	T45.1X3	T45.1X4	T45.1X5	T45.1X6
Podophyllotoxin	T49.8X1	T49.8X2	T49.8X3	T49.8X4	T49.8X5	T49.8X6
Podophyllum (resin)	T49.4X1	T49.4X2	T49.4X3	T49.4X4	T49.4X5	T49.4X6
Poisonous berries	T62.1X1	T62.1X2	T62.1X3	T62.1X4	—	—
Poison NEC	T65.91	T65.92	T65.93	T65.94	—	—
Pokeweed (any part)	T62.2X1	T62.2X2	T62.2X3	T62.2X4	—	—
Poldine metilsulfate	T44.3X1	T44.3X2	T44.3X3	T44.3X4	T44.3X5	T44.3X6
Polidexide (sulfate)	T46.6X1	T46.6X2	T46.6X3	T46.6X4	T46.6X5	T46.6X6
Polidocanol	T46.8X1	T46.8X2	T46.8X3	T46.8X4	T46.8X5	T46.8X6
Poliomyelitis vaccine	T50.B91	T50.B92	T50.B93	T50.B94	T50.B95	T50.B96
Polish (car) (floor) (furniture) (metal) (porcelain)	T65.891	T65.892	T65.893	T65.894	—	—
(silver)						
abrasive	T65.891	T65.892	T65.893	T65.894	—	—
porcelain	T65.891	T65.892	T65.893	T65.894	—	—
Poloxalkol	T47.4X1	T47.4X2	T47.4X3	T47.4X4	T47.4X5	T47.4X6
Poloxamer	T47.4X1	T47.4X2	T47.4X3	T47.4X4	T47.4X5	T47.4X6
Polyaminostyrene resins	T50.3X1	T50.3X2	T50.3X3	T50.3X4	T50.3X5	T50.3X6
Polycarbophil	T47.4X1	T47.4X2	T47.4X3	T47.4X4	T47.4X5	T47.4X6
Polychlorinated biphenyl	T65.891	T65.892	T65.893	T65.894	—	—
Polycycline	T36.4X1	T36.4X2	T36.4X3	T36.4X4	T36.4X5	T36.4X6
Polyester fumes	T59.891	T59.892	T59.893	T59.894	—	—
Polyester resin hardener	T52.91	T52.92	T52.93	T52.94	—	—
fumes	T59.891	T59.892	T59.893	T59.894	—	—
Polyestradiol phosphate	T38.5X1	T38.5X2	T38.5X3	T38.5X4	T38.5X5	T38.5X6
Polyethanolamine alkyl sulfate	T49.2X1	T49.2X2	T49.2X3	T49.2X4	T49.2X5	T49.2X6
Polyethylene adhesive	T49.3X1	T49.3X2	T49.3X3	T49.3X4	T49.3X5	T49.3X6
Polyferose	T45.4X1	T45.4X2	T45.4X3	T45.4X4	T45.4X5	T45.4X6
Polygeline	T45.8X1	T45.8X2	T45.8X3	T45.8X4	T45.8X5	T45.8X6
Polymyxin	T36.8X1	T36.8X2	T36.8X3	T36.8X4	T36.8X5	T36.8X6
B	T36.8X1	T36.8X2	T36.8X3	T36.8X4	T36.8X5	T36.8X6
ENT agent	T49.6X1	T49.6X2	T49.6X3	T49.6X4	T49.6X5	T49.6X6
ophthalmic preparation	T49.5X1	T49.5X2	T49.5X3	T49.5X4	T49.5X5	T49.5X6
topical NEC	T49.0X1	T49.0X2	T49.0X3	T49.0X4	T49.0X5	T49.0X6
E sulfate (eye preparation)	T49.5X1	T49.5X2	T49.5X3	T49.5X4	T49.5X5	T49.5X6
Polynoxylin	T49.0X1	T49.0X2	T49.0X3	T49.0X4	T49.0X5	T49.0X6
Polyoestradiol phosphate	T38.5X1	T38.5X2	T38.5X3	T38.5X4	T38.5X5	T38.5X6
Polyoxymethyleneurea	T49.0X1	T49.0X2	T49.0X3	T49.0X4	T49.0X5	T49.0X6
Poly-Pred*	T49.5X1	T49.5X2	T49.5X3	T49.5X4	T49.5X5	T49.5X6
Polysilane	T47.8X1	T47.8X2	T47.8X3	T47.8X4	T47.8X5	T47.8X6
Polytetrafluoroethylene (inhaled)	T59.891	T59.892	T59.893	T59.894	—	—
Polythiazide	T50.2X1	T50.2X2	T50.2X3	T50.2X4	T50.2X5	T50.2X6
Polyvidone	T45.8X1	T45.8X2	T45.8X3	T45.8X4	T45.8X5	T45.8X6

Substance	Poisoning, Accidental (unintentional)	Poisoning, Intentional Self-harm	Poisoning, Assault	Poisoning, Undetermined	Adverse Effect	Under-dosing
Polyvinylpyrrolidone	T45.8X1	T45.8X2	T45.8X3	T45.8X4	T45.8X5	T45.8X6
Pontocaine (hydrochloride) (infiltration) (topical)	T41.3X1	T41.3X2	T41.3X3	T41.3X4	T41.3X5	T41.3X6
nerve block (peripheral) (plexus)	T41.3X1	T41.3X2	T41.3X3	T41.3X4	T41.3X5	T41.3X6
spinal	T41.3X1	T41.3X2	T41.3X3	T41.3X4	T41.3X5	T41.3X6
Porfiromycin	T45.1X1	T45.1X2	T45.1X3	T45.1X4	T45.1X5	T45.1X6
Portactant alfa*	T48.991	T48.992	T48.993	T48.994	T48.995	T48.996
Posterior pituitary hormone NEC	T38.891	T38.892	T38.893	T38.894	T38.895	T38.896
Pot	T40.711	T40.712	T40.713	T40.714	T40.715	T40.716
Potash (caustic)	T54.3X1	T54.3X2	T54.3X3	T54.3X4	—	—
Potassic saline injection (lactated)	T50.3X1	T50.3X2	T50.3X3	T50.3X4	T50.3X5	T50.3X6
Potassium (salts) NEC	T50.3X1	T50.3X2	T50.3X3	T50.3X4	T50.3X5	T50.3X6
aminobenzoate	T45.8X1	T45.8X2	T45.8X3	T45.8X4	T45.8X5	T45.8X6
aminosalicylate	T37.1X1	T37.1X2	T37.1X3	T37.1X4	T37.1X5	T37.1X6
antimony ' tartrate'	T37.8X1	T37.8X2	T37.8X3	T37.8X4	T37.8X5	T37.8X6
arsenite (solution)	T57.0X1	T57.0X2	T57.0X3	T57.0X4	—	—
bichromate	T56.2X1	T56.2X2	T56.2X3	T56.2X4	—	—
bisulfate	T47.3X1	T47.3X2	T47.3X3	T47.3X4	T47.3X5	T47.3X6
bromide	T42.6X1	T42.6X2	T42.6X3	T42.6X4	T42.6X5	T42.6X6
canrenoate	T50.0X1	T50.0X2	T50.0X3	T50.0X4	T50.0X5	T50.0X6
carbonate	T54.3X1	T54.3X2	T54.3X3	T54.3X4	—	—
chlorate NEC	T65.891	T65.892	T65.893	T65.894	—	—
chloride	T50.3X1	T50.3X2	T50.3X3	T50.3X4	T50.3X5	T50.3X6
citrate	T50.991	T50.992	T50.993	T50.994	T50.995	T50.996
cyanide	T65.0X1	T65.0X2	T65.0X3	T65.0X4	—	—
ferric hexacyanoferrate (medicinal)	T50.6X1	T50.6X2	T50.6X3	T50.6X4	T50.6X5	T50.6X6
nonmedicinal	T65.891	T65.892	T65.893	T65.894	—	—
Fluoride	T57.8X1	T57.8X2	T57.8X3	T57.8X4	—	—
glucaldrate	T47.1X1	T47.1X2	T47.1X3	T47.1X4	T47.1X5	T47.1X6
hydroxide	T54.3X1	T54.3X2	T54.3X3	T54.3X4	—	—
iodate	T49.0X1	T49.0X2	T49.0X3	T49.0X4	T49.0X5	T49.0X6
iodide	T48.4X1	T48.4X2	T48.4X3	T48.4X4	T48.4X5	T48.4X6
nitrate	T57.8X1	T57.8X2	T57.8X3	T57.8X4	—	—
oxalate	T65.891	T65.892	T65.893	T65.894	—	—
perchlorate (nonmedicinal) NEC	T65.891	T65.892	T65.893	T65.894	—	—
antithyroid	T38.2X1	T38.2X2	T38.2X3	T38.2X4	T38.2X5	T38.2X6
medicinal	T38.2X1	T38.2X2	T38.2X3	T38.2X4	T38.2X5	T38.2X6
Permanganate (nonmedicinal)	T65.891	T65.892	T65.893	T65.894	—	—
medicinal	T49.0X1	T49.0X2	T49.0X3	T49.0X4	T49.0X5	T49.0X6
sulfate	T47.2X1	T47.2X2	T47.2X3	T47.2X4	T47.2X5	T47.2X6
Potassium-removing resin	T50.3X1	T50.3X2	T50.3X3	T50.3X4	T50.3X5	T50.3X6
Potassium-retaining drug	T50.3X1	T50.3X2	T50.3X3	T50.3X4	T50.3X5	T50.3X6
Povidone	T45.8X1	T45.8X2	T45.8X3	T45.8X4	T45.8X5	T45.8X6
iodine	T49.0X1	T49.0X2	T49.0X3	T49.0X4	T49.0X5	T49.0X6
Practolol	T44.7X1	T44.7X2	T44.7X3	T44.7X4	T44.7X5	T44.7X6
Prajmalium bitartrate	T46.2X1	T46.2X2	T46.2X3	T46.2X4	T46.2X5	T46.2X6
Pralidoxime (iodide)	T50.6X1	T50.6X2	T50.6X3	T50.6X4	T50.6X5	T50.6X6
chloride	T50.6X1	T50.6X2	T50.6X3	T50.6X4	T50.6X5	T50.6X6
Pramiverine	T44.3X1	T44.3X2	T44.3X3	T44.3X4	T44.3X5	T44.3X6
Pramlintide*	T38.3X1	T38.3X2	T38.3X3	T38.3X4	T38.3X5	T38.3X6
Pramocaine	T49.1X1	T49.1X2	T49.1X3	T49.1X4	T49.1X5	T49.1X6
Pramoxine	T49.1X1	T49.1X2	T49.1X3	T49.1X4	T49.1X5	T49.1X6
Prasterone	T38.7X1	T38.7X2	T38.7X3	T38.7X4	T38.7X5	T38.7X6
Pravastatin	T46.6X1	T46.6X2	T46.6X3	T46.6X4	T46.6X5	T46.6X6
Prazepam	T42.4X1	T42.4X2	T42.4X3	T42.4X4	T42.4X5	T42.4X6
Praziquantel	T37.4X1	T37.4X2	T37.4X3	T37.4X4	T37.4X5	T37.4X6
Prazitone	T43.291	T43.292	T43.293	T43.294	T43.295	T43.296
Prazosin	T44.6X1	T44.6X2	T44.6X3	T44.6X4	T44.6X5	T44.6X6
Prednicarbate	T49.0X1	T49.0X2	T49.0X3	T49.0X4	T49.0X5	T49.0X6
Prednimustine	T45.1X1	T45.1X2	T45.1X3	T45.1X4	T45.1X5	T45.1X6
Prednisolone	T38.0X1	T38.0X2	T38.0X3	T38.0X4	T38.0X5	T38.0X6
ENT agent	T49.6X1	T49.6X2	T49.6X3	T49.6X4	T49.6X5	T49.6X6
ophthalmic preparation	T49.5X1	T49.5X2	T49.5X3	T49.5X4	T49.5X5	T49.5X6
steaglate	T49.0X1	T49.0X2	T49.0X3	T49.0X4	T49.0X5	T49.0X6
topical NEC	T49.0X1	T49.0X2	T49.0X3	T49.0X4	T49.0X5	T49.0X6
Prednisone	T38.0X1	T38.0X2	T38.0X3	T38.0X4	T38.0X5	T38.0X6
Prednylidene	T38.0X1	T38.0X2	T38.0X3	T38.0X4	T38.0X5	T38.0X6
Pregnandiol	T38.5X1	T38.5X2	T38.5X3	T38.5X4	T38.5X5	T38.5X6
Pregneninolone	T38.5X1	T38.5X2	T38.5X3	T38.5X4	T38.5X5	T38.5X6
Preludin	T43.691	T43.692	T43.693	T43.694	T43.695	T43.696
Premarin	T38.5X1	T38.5X2	T38.5X3	T38.5X4	T38.5X5	T38.5X6
Premedication anesthetic	T41.201	T41.202	T41.203	T41.204	T41.205	T41.206
Prenalterol	T44.5X1	T44.5X2	T44.5X3	T44.5X4	T44.5X5	T44.5X6
Prenoxdiazine	T48.3X1	T48.3X2	T48.3X3	T48.3X4	T48.3X5	T48.3X6
Prenylamine	T46.3X1	T46.3X2	T46.3X3	T46.3X4	T46.3X5	T46.3X6
Preparation H	T49.8X1	T49.8X2	T49.8X3	T49.8X4	T49.8X5	T49.8X6
Preparation, local	T49.4X1	T49.4X2	T49.4X3	T49.4X4	T49.4X5	T49.4X6

☑ Additional Character May Be Required — Refer to the Tabular List for Character Selection

*Optum Value-Add

Table of Drugs and Chemicals

Substance	Poisoning, Accidental (unintentional)	Poisoning, Intentional Self-harm	Poisoning, Assault	Poisoning, Undetermined	Adverse Effect	Under-dosing
Preservative	T65.891	T65.892	T65.893	T65.894	—	—
(nonmedicinal)						
medicinal	T50.901	T50.902	T50.903	T50.904	T50.905	T50.906
wood	T60.91	T60.92	T60.93	T60.94	—	—
Prethcamide	T50.7X1	T50.7X2	T50.7X3	T50.7X4	T50.7X5	T50.7X6
Prevacid*	T47.1X1	T47.1X2	T47.1X3	T47.1X4	T47.1X5	T47.1X6
Pride of China	T62.2X1	T62.2X2	T62.2X3	T62.2X4	—	—
Pridinol	T44.3X1	T44.3X2	T44.3X3	T44.3X4	T44.3X5	T44.3X6
Prifinium bromide	T44.3X1	T44.3X2	T44.3X3	T44.3X4	T44.3X5	T44.3X6
Prilocaine	T41.3X1	T41.3X2	T41.3X3	T41.3X4	T41.3X5	T41.3X6
infiltration (subcutaneous)	T41.3X1	T41.3X2	T41.3X3	T41.3X4	T41.3X5	T41.3X6
nerve block (peripheral) (plexus)	T41.3X1	T41.3X2	T41.3X3	T41.3X4	T41.3X5	T41.3X6
regional	T41.3X1	T41.3X2	T41.3X3	T41.3X4	T41.3X5	T41.3X6
Primaquine	T37.2X1	T37.2X2	T37.2X3	T37.2X4	T37.2X5	T37.2X6
Primidone	T42.6X1	T42.6X2	T42.6X3	T42.6X4	T42.6X5	T42.6X6
Primula (veris)	T62.2X1	T62.2X2	T62.2X3	T62.2X4	—	—
Prinadol	T40.2X1	T40.2X2	T40.2X3	T40.2X4	T40.2X5	T40.2X6
Priscol, Priscoline	T44.6X1	T44.6X2	T44.6X3	T44.6X4	T44.6X5	T44.6X6
Pristinamycin	T36.3X1	T36.3X2	T36.3X3	T36.3X4	T36.3X5	T36.3X6
Pristiq*	T43.211	T43.212	T43.213	T43.214	T43.215	T43.216
Privet	T62.2X1	T62.2X2	T62.2X3	T62.2X4	—	—
berries	T62.1X1	T62.1X2	T62.1X3	T62.1X4	—	—
Privine	T44.4X1	T44.4X2	T44.4X3	T44.4X4	T44.4X5	T44.4X6
Pro-Banthine	T44.3X1	T44.3X2	T44.3X3	T44.3X4	T44.3X5	T44.3X6
Probarbital	T42.3X1	T42.3X2	T42.3X3	T42.3X4	T42.3X5	T42.3X6
Probenecid	T50.4X1	T50.4X2	T50.4X3	T50.4X4	T50.4X5	T50.4X6
Probucol	T46.6X1	T46.6X2	T46.6X3	T46.6X4	T46.6X5	T46.6X6
Procainamide	T46.2X1	T46.2X2	T46.2X3	T46.2X4	T46.2X5	T46.2X6
Procaine	T41.3X1	T41.3X2	T41.3X3	T41.3X4	T41.3X5	T41.3X6
benzylpenicillin	T36.0X1	T36.0X2	T36.0X3	T36.0X4	T36.0X5	T36.0X6
nerve block (periphreal) (plexus)	T41.3X1	T41.3X2	T41.3X3	T41.3X4	T41.3X5	T41.3X6
penicillin G	T36.0X1	T36.0X2	T36.0X3	T36.0X4	T36.0X5	T36.0X6
regional	T41.3X1	T41.3X2	T41.3X3	T41.3X4	T41.3X5	T41.3X6
spinal	T41.3X1	T41.3X2	T41.3X3	T41.3X4	T41.3X5	T41.3X6
Procalmidol	T43.591	T43.592	T43.593	T43.594	T43.595	T43.596
Procarbazine	T45.1X1	T45.1X2	T45.1X3	T45.1X4	T45.1X5	T45.1X6
Procaterol	T44.5X1	T44.5X2	T44.5X3	T44.5X4	T44.5X5	T44.5X6
Prochlorperazine	T43.3X1	T43.3X2	T43.3X3	T43.3X4	T43.3X5	T43.3X6
Procyclidine	T44.3X1	T44.3X2	T44.3X3	T44.3X4	T44.3X5	T44.3X6
Producer gas	T58.8X1	T58.8X2	T58.8X3	T58.8X4	—	—
Profadol	T40.491	T40.492	T40.493	T40.494	T40.495	T40.496
Profenamine	T44.3X1	T44.3X2	T44.3X3	T44.3X4	T44.3X5	T44.3X6
Profenil	T44.3X1	T44.3X2	T44.3X3	T44.3X4	T44.3X5	T44.3X6
Proflavine	T49.0X1	T49.0X2	T49.0X3	T49.0X4	T49.0X5	T49.0X6
Progabide	T42.6X1	T42.6X2	T42.6X3	T42.6X4	T42.6X5	T42.6X6
Progesterone	T38.5X1	T38.5X2	T38.5X3	T38.5X4	T38.5X5	T38.5X6
Progestin	T38.5X1	T38.5X2	T38.5X3	T38.5X4	T38.5X5	T38.5X6
oral contraceptive	T38.4X1	T38.4X2	T38.4X3	T38.4X4	T38.4X5	T38.4X6
Progestogen NEC	T38.5X1	T38.5X2	T38.5X3	T38.5X4	T38.5X5	T38.5X6
Progestone	T38.5X1	T38.5X2	T38.5X3	T38.5X4	T38.5X5	T38.5X6
Proglumide	T47.1X1	T47.1X2	T47.1X3	T47.1X4	T47.1X5	T47.1X6
Prograf*	T45.1X1	T45.1X2	T45.1X3	T45.1X4	T45.1X5	T45.1X6
Proguanil	T37.2X1	T37.2X2	T37.2X3	T37.2X4	T37.2X5	T37.2X6
Prolactin	T38.811	T38.812	T38.813	T38.814	T38.815	T38.816
Prolintane	T43.691	T43.692	T43.693	T43.694	T43.695	T43.696
Proloid	T38.1X1	T38.1X2	T38.1X3	T38.1X4	T38.1X5	T38.1X6
Proluton	T38.5X1	T38.5X2	T38.5X3	T38.5X4	T38.5X5	T38.5X6
Promacetin	T37.1X1	T37.1X2	T37.1X3	T37.1X4	T37.1X5	T37.1X6
Promazine	T43.3X1	T43.3X2	T43.3X3	T43.3X4	T43.3X5	T43.3X6
Promedol	T40.2X1	T40.2X2	T40.2X3	T40.2X4	—	—
Promegestone	T38.5X1	T38.5X2	T38.5X3	T38.5X4	T38.5X5	T38.5X6
Promethazine (teoclate)	T43.3X1	T43.3X2	T43.3X3	T43.3X4	T43.3X5	T43.3X6
Promin	T37.1X1	T37.1X2	T37.1X3	T37.1X4	T37.1X5	T37.1X6
Pronase	T45.3X1	T45.3X2	T45.3X3	T45.3X4	T45.3X5	T45.3X6
Pronestyl (hydrochloride)	T46.2X1	T46.2X2	T46.2X3	T46.2X4	T46.2X5	T46.2X6
Pronetalol	T44.7X1	T44.7X2	T44.7X3	T44.7X4	T44.7X5	T44.7X6
Prontosil	T37.0X1	T37.0X2	T37.0X3	T37.0X4	T37.0X5	T37.0X6
Propachlor	T60.3X1	T60.3X2	T60.3X3	T60.3X4	—	—
Propafenone	T46.2X1	T46.2X2	T46.2X3	T46.2X4	T46.2X5	T46.2X6
Propallylonal	T42.3X1	T42.3X2	T42.3X3	T42.3X4	T42.3X5	T42.3X6
Propamidine	T49.0X1	T49.0X2	T49.0X3	T49.0X4	T49.0X5	T49.0X6
Propane (distributed in mobile container)	T59.891	T59.892	T59.893	T59.894	—	—
distributed through pipes	T59.891	T59.892	T59.893	T59.894	—	—
incomplete combustion	T58.11	T58.12	T58.13	T58.14	—	—
Propanidid	T41.291	T41.292	T41.293	T41.294	T41.295	T41.296
Propanil	T60.3X1	T60.3X2	T60.3X3	T60.3X4	—	—
Propantheline	T44.3X1	T44.3X2	T44.3X3	T44.3X4	T44.3X5	T44.3X6
bromide	T44.3X1	T44.3X2	T44.3X3	T44.3X4	T44.3X5	T44.3X6
Proparacaine	T41.3X1	T41.3X2	T41.3X3	T41.3X4	T41.3X5	T41.3X6
Propatylnitrate	T46.3X1	T46.3X2	T46.3X3	T46.3X4	T46.3X5	T46.3X6

Substance	Poisoning, Accidental (unintentional)	Poisoning, Intentional Self-harm	Poisoning, Assault	Poisoning, Undetermined	Adverse Effect	Under-dosing
Propicillin	T36.0X1	T36.0X2	T36.0X3	T36.0X4	T36.0X5	T36.0X6
Propine*	T49.5X1	T49.5X2	T49.5X3	T49.5X4	T49.5X5	T49.5X6
Propiolactone	T49.0X1	T49.0X2	T49.0X3	T49.0X4	T49.0X5	T49.0X6
Propiomazine	T45.0X1	T45.0X2	T45.0X3	T45.0X4	T45.0X5	T45.0X6
Propionaldehyde (medicinal)	T42.6X1	T42.6X2	T42.6X3	T42.6X4	T42.6X5	T42.6X6
Propionate (calcium) (sodium)	T49.0X1	T49.0X2	T49.0X3	T49.0X4	T49.0X5	T49.0X6
Propion gel	T49.0X1	T49.0X2	T49.0X3	T49.0X4	T49.0X5	T49.0X6
Propitocaine	T41.3X1	T41.3X2	T41.3X3	T41.3X4	T41.3X5	T41.3X6
infiltration (subcutaneous)	T41.3X1	T41.3X2	T41.3X3	T41.3X4	T41.3X5	T41.3X6
nerve block (peripheral) (plexus)	T41.3X1	T41.3X2	T41.3X3	T41.3X4	T41.3X5	T41.3X6
Propofol	T41.291	T41.292	T41.293	T41.294	T41.295	T41.296
Propoxur	T60.0X1	T60.0X2	T60.0X3	T60.0X4	—	—
Propoxycaine	T41.3X1	T41.3X2	T41.3X3	T41.3X4	T41.3X5	T41.3X6
infiltration (subcutaneous)	T41.3X1	T41.3X2	T41.3X3	T41.3X4	T41.3X5	T41.3X6
nerve block (peripheral) (plexus)	T41.3X1	T41.3X2	T41.3X3	T41.3X4	T41.3X5	T41.3X6
topical (surface)	T41.3X1	T41.3X2	T41.3X3	T41.3X4	T41.3X5	T41.3X6
Propoxyphene	T40.491	T40.492	T40.493	T40.494	T40.495	T40.496
Propranolol	T44.7X1	T44.7X2	T44.7X3	T44.7X4	T44.7X5	T44.7X6
Propyl						
alcohol	T51.3X1	T51.3X2	T51.3X3	T51.3X4	—	—
carbinol	T51.3X1	T51.3X2	T51.3X3	T51.3X4	—	—
hexadrine	T44.4X1	T44.4X2	T44.4X3	T44.4X4	T44.4X5	T44.4X6
iodone	T50.8X1	T50.8X2	T50.8X3	T50.8X4	T50.8X5	T50.8X6
thiouracil	T38.2X1	T38.2X2	T38.2X3	T38.2X4	T38.2X5	T38.2X6
Propylaminophenothiazine	T43.3X1	T43.3X2	T43.3X3	T43.3X4	T43.3X5	T43.3X6
Propylene	T59.891	T59.892	T59.893	T59.894	—	—
Propylhexedrine	T48.5X1	T48.5X2	T48.5X3	T48.5X4	T48.5X5	T48.5X6
Propyliodone	T50.8X1	T50.8X2	T50.8X3	T50.8X4	T50.8X5	T50.8X6
Propylparaben (ophthalmic)	T49.5X1	T49.5X2	T49.5X3	T49.5X4	T49.5X5	T49.5X6
Propylthiouracil	T38.2X1	T38.2X2	T38.2X3	T38.2X4	T38.2X5	T38.2X6
Propyphenazone	T39.2X1	T39.2X2	T39.2X3	T39.2X4	T39.2X5	T39.2X6
Proquazone	T39.391	T39.392	T39.393	T39.394	T39.395	T39.396
Proscar*	T38.6X1	T38.6X2	T38.6X3	T38.6X4	T38.6X5	T38.6X6
Proscillaridin	T46.0X1	T46.0X2	T46.0X3	T46.0X4	T46.0X5	T46.0X6
Prostacyclin	T45.521	T45.522	T45.523	T45.524	T45.525	T45.526
Prostaglandin (I2)	T45.521	T45.522	T45.523	T45.524	T45.525	T45.526
E1	T46.7X1	T46.7X2	T46.7X3	T46.7X4	T46.7X5	T46.7X6
E2	T48.0X1	T48.0X2	T48.0X3	T48.0X4	T48.0X5	T48.0X6
F2 alpha	T48.0X1	T48.0X2	T48.0X3	T48.0X4	T48.0X5	T48.0X6
Prostigmin	T44.0X1	T44.0X2	T44.0X3	T44.0X4	T44.0X5	T44.0X6
Prosultiamine	T45.2X1	T45.2X2	T45.2X3	T45.2X4	T45.2X5	T45.2X6
Protamine sulfate	T45.7X1	T45.7X2	T45.7X3	T45.7X4	T45.7X5	T45.7X6
zinc insulin	T38.3X1	T38.3X2	T38.3X3	T38.3X4	T38.3X5	T38.3X6
Protease	T47.5X1	T47.5X2	T47.5X3	T47.5X4	T47.5X5	T47.5X6
Protectant, skin NEC	T49.3X1	T49.3X2	T49.3X3	T49.3X4	T49.3X5	T49.3X6
Protein hydrolysate	T50.991	T50.992	T50.993	T50.994	T50.995	T50.996
Prothiaden — see Dothiepin hydrochloride						
Prothionamide	T37.1X1	T37.1X2	T37.1X3	T37.1X4	T37.1X5	T37.1X6
Prothipendyl	T43.591	T43.592	T43.593	T43.594	T43.595	T43.596
Prothoate	T60.0X1	T60.0X2	T60.0X3	T60.0X4	—	—
Prothrombin						
activator	T45.7X1	T45.7X2	T45.7X3	T45.7X4	T45.7X5	T45.7X6
synthesis inhibitor	T45.511	T45.512	T45.513	T45.514	T45.515	T45.516
Protionamide	T37.1X1	T37.1X2	T37.1X3	T37.1X4	T37.1X5	T37.1X6
Protirelin	T38.891	T38.892	T38.893	T38.894	T38.895	T38.896
Protokylol	T48.6X1	T48.6X2	T48.6X3	T48.6X4	T48.6X5	T48.6X6
Protopam	T50.6X1	T50.6X2	T50.6X3	T50.6X4	T50.6X5	T50.6X6
Protoveratrine(s) (A) (B)	T46.5X1	T46.5X2	T46.5X3	T46.5X4	T46.5X5	T46.5X6
Protriptyline	T43.011	T43.012	T43.013	T43.014	T43.015	T43.016
Proventil*	T48.6X1	T48.6X2	T48.6X3	T48.6X4	T48.6X5	T48.6X6
Provera	T38.5X1	T38.5X2	T38.5X3	T38.5X4	T38.5X5	T38.5X6
Provitamin A	T45.2X1	T45.2X2	T45.2X3	T45.2X4	T45.2X5	T45.2X6
Proxibarbal	T42.3X1	T42.3X2	T42.3X3	T42.3X4	T42.3X5	T42.3X6
Proxymetacaine	T41.3X1	T41.3X2	T41.3X3	T41.3X4	T41.3X5	T41.3X6
Proxyphylline	T48.6X1	T48.6X2	T48.6X3	T48.6X4	T48.6X5	T48.6X6
Prozac — see Fluoxetine hydrochloride						
Prunus						
laurocerasus	T62.2X1	T62.2X2	T62.2X3	T62.2X4	—	—
virginiana	T62.2X1	T62.2X2	T62.2X3	T62.2X4	—	—
Prussian blue						
commercial	T65.891	T65.892	T65.893	T65.894	—	—
therapeutic	T50.6X1	T50.6X2	T50.6X3	T50.6X4	T50.6X5	T50.6X6
Prussic acid	T65.0X1	T65.0X2	T65.0X3	T65.0X4	—	—
vapor	T57.3X1	T57.3X2	T57.3X3	T57.3X4	—	—
Pseudoephedrine	T44.991	T44.992	T44.993	T44.994	T44.995	T44.996
Psilocin	T40.991	T40.992	T40.993	T40.994	—	—

Preservative — Psilocin

Table of Drugs and Chemicals

Psilocybin — Respiratory drug NEC

Substance	Poisoning, Accidental (unintentional)	Poisoning, Intentional Self-harm	Poisoning, Assault	Poisoning, Undetermined	Adverse Effect	Under-dosing
Psilocybin	T40.991	T40.992	T40.993	T40.994	—	—
Psilocybine	T40.991	T40.992	T40.993	T40.994	—	—
Psoralene (nonmedicinal)	T65.891	T65.892	T65.893	T65.894	—	—
Psoralens (medicinal)	T50.991	T50.992	T50.993	T50.994	T50.995	T50.996
PSP	T50.8X1	T50.8X2	T50.8X3	T50.8X4	T50.8X5	T50.8X6
(phenolsulfonphthalein)						
Psychodysleptic drug NOS	T40.901	T40.902	T40.903	T40.904	T40.905	T40.906
specified NEC	T40.991	T40.992	T40.993	T40.994	T40.995	T40.996
Psychostimulant	T43.601	T43.602	T43.603	T43.604	T43.605	T43.606
amphetamine	T43.621	T43.622	T43.623	T43.624	T43.625	T43.626
caffeine	T43.611	T43.612	T43.613	T43.614	T43.615	T43.616
methylphenidate	T43.631	T43.632	T43.633	T43.634	T43.635	T43.636
specified NEC	T43.691	T43.692	T43.693	T43.694	T43.695	T43.696
Psychotherapeutic drug NEC	T43.91	T43.92	T43.93	T43.94	T43.95	T43.96
antidepressants — see also Antidepressant	T43.201	T43.202	T43.203	T43.204	T43.205	T43.206
specified NEC	T43.8X1	T43.8X2	T43.8X3	T43.8X4	T43.8X5	T43.8X6
tranquilizers NEC	T43.501	T43.502	T43.503	T43.504	T43.505	T43.506
Psychotomimetic agents	T40.901	T40.902	T40.903	T40.904	T40.905	T40.906
Psychotropic drug NEC	T43.91	T43.92	T43.93	T43.94	T43.95	T43.96
specified NEC	T43.8X1	T43.8X2	T43.8X3	T43.8X4	T43.8X5	T43.8X6
Psyllium hydrophilic mucilloid	T47.4X1	T47.4X2	T47.4X3	T47.4X4	T47.4X5	T47.4X6
Pteroylglutamic acid	T45.8X1	T45.8X2	T45.8X3	T45.8X4	T45.8X5	T45.8X6
Pteroyltriglutamate	T45.1X1	T45.1X2	T45.1X3	T45.1X4	T45.1X5	T45.1X6
PTFE — see Polytetrafluoroethylene						
Pulmicort*	T44.5X1	T44.5X2	T44.5X3	T44.5X4	T44.5X5	T44.5X6
Pulp						
devitalizing paste	T49.7X1	T49.7X2	T49.7X3	T49.7X4	T49.7X5	T49.7X6
dressing	T49.7X1	T49.7X2	T49.7X3	T49.7X4	T49.7X5	T49.7X6
Pulsatilla	T62.2X1	T62.2X2	T62.2X3	T62.2X4	—	—
Pumpkin seed extract	T37.4X1	T37.4X2	T37.4X3	T37.4X4	T37.4X5	T37.4X6
Purex (bleach)	T54.91	T54.92	T54.93	T54.94	—	—
Purgative NEC — see also Cathartic	T47.4X1	T47.4X2	T47.4X3	T47.4X4	T47.4X5	T47.4X6
Purine analogue (antineoplastic)	T45.1X1	T45.1X2	T45.1X3	T45.1X4	T45.1X5	T45.1X6
Purine diuretics	T50.2X1	T50.2X2	T50.2X3	T50.2X4	T50.2X5	T50.2X6
Purinethol	T45.1X1	T45.1X2	T45.1X3	T45.1X4	T45.1X5	T45.1X6
PVP	T45.8X1	T45.8X2	T45.8X3	T45.8X4	T45.8X5	T45.8X6
Pyrabital	T39.8X1	T39.8X2	T39.8X3	T39.8X4	T39.8X5	T39.8X6
Pyramidon	T39.2X1	T39.2X2	T39.2X3	T39.2X4	T39.2X5	T39.2X6
Pyrantel	T37.4X1	T37.4X2	T37.4X3	T37.4X4	T37.4X5	T37.4X6
Pyrathiazine	T45.0X1	T45.0X2	T45.0X3	T45.0X4	T45.0X5	T45.0X6
Pyrazinamide	T37.1X1	T37.1X2	T37.1X3	T37.1X4	T37.1X5	T37.1X6
Pyrazinoic acid (amide)	T37.1X1	T37.1X2	T37.1X3	T37.1X4	T37.1X5	T37.1X6
Pyrazole (derivatives)	T39.2X1	T39.2X2	T39.2X3	T39.2X4	T39.2X5	T39.2X6
Pyrazolone analgesic NEC	T39.2X1	T39.2X2	T39.2X3	T39.2X4	T39.2X5	T39.2X6
Pyrethrin, pyrethrum (nonmedicinal)	T60.2X1	T60.2X2	T60.2X3	T60.2X4	—	—
Pyrethrum extract	T49.0X1	T49.0X2	T49.0X3	T49.0X4	T49.0X5	T49.0X6
Pyribenzamine	T45.0X1	T45.0X2	T45.0X3	T45.0X4	T45.0X5	T45.0X6
Pyridine	T52.8X1	T52.8X2	T52.8X3	T52.8X4	—	—
aldoxime methiodide	T50.6X1	T50.6X2	T50.6X3	T50.6X4	T50.6X5	T50.6X6
aldoxime methyl chloride	T50.6X1	T50.6X2	T50.6X3	T50.6X4	T50.6X5	T50.6X6
vapor	T59.891	T59.892	T59.893	T59.894	—	—
Pyridium	T39.8X1	T39.8X2	T39.8X3	T39.8X4	T39.8X5	T39.8X6
Pyridostigmine bromide	T44.0X1	T44.0X2	T44.0X3	T44.0X4	T44.0X5	T44.0X6
Pyridoxal phosphate	T45.2X1	T45.2X2	T45.2X3	T45.2X4	T45.2X5	T45.2X6
Pyridoxine	T45.2X1	T45.2X2	T45.2X3	T45.2X4	T45.2X5	T45.2X6
Pyrilamine	T45.0X1	T45.0X2	T45.0X3	T45.0X4	T45.0X5	T45.0X6
Pyrimethamine	T37.2X1	T37.2X2	T37.2X3	T37.2X4	T37.2X5	T37.2X6
with sulfadoxine	T37.2X1	T37.2X2	T37.2X3	T37.2X4	T37.2X5	T37.2X6
Pyrimidine antagonist	T45.1X1	T45.1X2	T45.1X3	T45.1X4	T45.1X5	T45.1X6
Pyriminil	T60.4X1	T60.4X2	T60.4X3	T60.4X4	—	—
Pyrithione zinc	T49.4X1	T49.4X2	T49.4X3	T49.4X4	T49.4X5	T49.4X6
Pyrithyldione	T42.6X1	T42.6X2	T42.6X3	T42.6X4	T42.6X5	T42.6X6
Pyrogallic acid	T49.0X1	T49.0X2	T49.0X3	T49.0X4	T49.0X5	T49.0X6
Pyrogallol	T49.0X1	T49.0X2	T49.0X3	T49.0X4	T49.0X5	T49.0X6
Pyroxylin	T49.3X1	T49.3X2	T49.3X3	T49.3X4	T49.3X5	T49.3X6
Pyrrobutamine	T45.0X1	T45.0X2	T45.0X3	T45.0X4	T45.0X5	T45.0X6
Pyrrolizidine alkaloids	T62.8X1	T62.8X2	T62.8X3	T62.8X4	—	—
Pyrvinium chloride	T37.4X1	T37.4X2	T37.4X3	T37.4X4	T37.4X5	T37.4X6
PZI	T38.3X1	T38.3X2	T38.3X3	T38.3X4	T38.3X5	T38.3X6
Qbrelis*	T46.4X1	T46.4X2	T46.4X3	T46.4X4	T46.4X5	T46.4X6
Quaalude	T42.6X1	T42.6X2	T42.6X3	T42.6X4	T42.6X5	T42.6X6
Quarternary ammonium						
anti-infective	T49.0X1	T49.0X2	T49.0X3	T49.0X4	T49.0X5	T49.0X6
ganglion blocking	T44.2X1	T44.2X2	T44.2X3	T44.2X4	T44.2X5	T44.2X6
parasympatholytic	T44.3X1	T44.3X2	T44.3X3	T44.3X4	T44.3X5	T44.3X6
Quazepam	T42.4X1	T42.4X2	T42.4X3	T42.4X4	T42.4X5	T42.4X6
Quicklime	T54.3X1	T54.3X2	T54.3X3	T54.3X4	—	—
Quilbron-T*	T48.6X1	T48.6X2	T48.6X3	T48.6X4	T48.6X5	T48.6X6
Quillaja extract	T48.4X1	T48.4X2	T48.4X3	T48.4X4	T48.4X5	T48.4X6
Quinacrine	T37.2X1	T37.2X2	T37.2X3	T37.2X4	T37.2X5	T37.2X6
Quinaglute	T46.2X1	T46.2X2	T46.2X3	T46.2X4	T46.2X5	T46.2X6
Quinalbarbital	T42.3X1	T42.3X2	T42.3X3	T42.3X4	T42.3X5	T42.3X6
Quinalbarbitone sodium	T42.3X1	T42.3X2	T42.3X3	T42.3X4	T42.3X5	T42.3X6
Quinalphos	T60.0X1	T60.0X2	T60.0X3	T60.0X4	—	—
Quinapril	T46.4X1	T46.4X2	T46.4X3	T46.4X4	T46.4X5	T46.4X6
Quinestradiol	T38.5X1	T38.5X2	T38.5X3	T38.5X4	T38.5X5	T38.5X6
Quinestradol	T38.5X1	T38.5X2	T38.5X3	T38.5X4	T38.5X5	T38.5X6
Quinestrol	T38.5X1	T38.5X2	T38.5X3	T38.5X4	T38.5X5	T38.5X6
Quinethazone	T50.2X1	T50.2X2	T50.2X3	T50.2X4	T50.2X5	T50.2X6
Quingestanol	T38.4X1	T38.4X2	T38.4X3	T38.4X4	T38.4X5	T38.4X6
Quinidine	T46.2X1	T46.2X2	T46.2X3	T46.2X4	T46.2X5	T46.2X6
Quinine	T37.2X1	T37.2X2	T37.2X3	T37.2X4	T37.2X5	T37.2X6
Quiniobine	T37.8X1	T37.8X2	T37.8X3	T37.8X4	T37.8X5	T37.8X6
Quinisocaine	T49.1X1	T49.1X2	T49.1X3	T49.1X4	T49.1X5	T49.1X6
Quinocide	T37.2X1	T37.2X2	T37.2X3	T37.2X4	T37.2X5	T37.2X6
Quinoline (derivatives) **NEC**	T37.8X1	T37.8X2	T37.8X3	T37.8X4	T37.8X5	T37.8X6
Quinupramine	T43.011	T43.012	T43.013	T43.014	T43.015	T43.016
Quixin*	T49.5X1	T49.5X2	T49.5X3	T49.5X4	T49.5X5	T49.5X6
Quotane	T41.3X1	T41.3X2	T41.3X3	T41.3X4	T41.3X5	T41.3X6
Rabies						
immune globulin (human)	T50.Z11	T50.Z12	T50.Z13	T50.Z14	T50.Z15	T50.Z16
vaccine	T50.B91	T50.B92	T50.B93	T50.B94	T50.B95	T50.B96
Racemoramide	T40.2X1	T40.2X2	T40.2X3	T40.2X4	—	—
Racemorphan	T40.2X1	T40.2X2	T40.2X3	T40.2X4	T40.2X5	T40.2X6
Racepinefrin	T44.5X1	T44.5X2	T44.5X3	T44.5X4	T44.5X5	T44.5X6
Raclopride	T43.591	T43.592	T43.593	T43.594	T43.595	T43.596
Radiator alcohol	T51.1X1	T51.1X2	T51.1X3	T51.1X4	—	—
Radioactive drug NEC	T50.8X1	T50.8X2	T50.8X3	T50.8X4	T50.8X5	T50.8X6
Radio-opaque (drugs) (materials)	T50.8X1	T50.8X2	T50.8X3	T50.8X4	T50.8X5	T50.8X6
Ramifenazone	T39.2X1	T39.2X2	T39.2X3	T39.2X4	T39.2X5	T39.2X6
Ramipril	T46.4X1	T46.4X2	T46.4X3	T46.4X4	T46.4X5	T46.4X6
Ranitidine	T47.0X1	T47.0X2	T47.0X3	T47.0X4	T47.0X5	T47.0X6
Ranunculus	T62.2X1	T62.2X2	T62.2X3	T62.2X4	—	—
Rat poison NEC	T60.4X1	T60.4X2	T60.4X3	T60.4X4	—	—
Rattlesnake (venom)	T63.011	T63.012	T63.013	T63.014	—	—
Raubasine	T46.7X1	T46.7X2	T46.7X3	T46.7X4	T46.7X5	T46.7X6
Raudixin	T46.5X1	T46.5X2	T46.5X3	T46.5X4	T46.5X5	T46.5X6
Rautensin	T46.5X1	T46.5X2	T46.5X3	T46.5X4	T46.5X5	T46.5X6
Rautina	T46.5X1	T46.5X2	T46.5X3	T46.5X4	T46.5X5	T46.5X6
Rautotal	T46.5X1	T46.5X2	T46.5X3	T46.5X4	T46.5X5	T46.5X6
Rauwiloid	T46.5X1	T46.5X2	T46.5X3	T46.5X4	T46.5X5	T46.5X6
Rauwoldin	T46.5X1	T46.5X2	T46.5X3	T46.5X4	T46.5X5	T46.5X6
Rauwolfia (alkaloids)	T46.5X1	T46.5X2	T46.5X3	T46.5X4	T46.5X5	T46.5X6
Razadyne*	T44.0X1	T44.0X2	T44.0X3	T44.0X4	T44.0X5	T44.0X6
Razoxane	T45.1X1	T45.1X2	T45.1X3	T45.1X4	T45.1X5	T45.1X6
Realgar	T57.0X1	T57.0X2	T57.0X3	T57.0X4	—	—
Recombinant (R) — see specific protein						
Red blood cells, packed	T45.8X1	T45.8X2	T45.8X3	T45.8X4	T45.8X5	T45.8X6
Red squill (scilliroside)	T60.4X1	T60.4X2	T60.4X3	T60.4X4	—	—
Reducing agent, industrial NEC	T65.891	T65.892	T65.893	T65.894	—	—
Refrigerant gas (chlorofluorocarbon)	T53.5X1	T53.5X2	T53.5X3	T53.5X4	—	—
not chlorofluorocarbon	T59.891	T59.892	T59.893	T59.894	—	—
Regroton	T50.2X1	T50.2X2	T50.2X3	T50.2X4	T50.2X5	T50.2X6
Rehydration salts (oral)	T50.3X1	T50.3X2	T50.3X3	T50.3X4	T50.3X5	T50.3X6
Rela	T42.8X1	T42.8X2	T42.8X3	T42.8X4	T42.8X5	T42.8X6
Relaxant, muscle						
anesthetic	T48.1X1	T48.1X2	T48.1X3	T48.1X4	T48.1X5	T48.1X6
central nervous system	T42.8X1	T42.8X2	T42.8X3	T42.8X4	T42.8X5	T42.8X6
skeletal NEC	T48.1X1	T48.1X2	T48.1X3	T48.1X4	T48.1X5	T48.1X6
smooth NEC	T44.3X1	T44.3X2	T44.3X3	T44.3X4	T44.3X5	T44.3X6
Remoxipride	T43.591	T43.592	T43.593	T43.594	T43.595	T43.596
Renese	T50.2X1	T50.2X2	T50.2X3	T50.2X4	T50.2X5	T50.2X6
Renografin	T50.8X1	T50.8X2	T50.8X3	T50.8X4	T50.8X5	T50.8X6
Replacement solution	T50.3X1	T50.3X2	T50.3X3	T50.3X4	T50.3X5	T50.3X6
Reproterol	T48.6X1	T48.6X2	T48.6X3	T48.6X4	T48.6X5	T48.6X6
Rescinnamine	T46.5X1	T46.5X2	T46.5X3	T46.5X4	T46.5X5	T46.5X6
Reserpin (e)	T46.5X1	T46.5X2	T46.5X3	T46.5X4	T46.5X5	T46.5X6
Resorcin, resorcinol (nonmedicinal)	T65.891	T65.892	T65.893	T65.894	—	—
medicinal	T49.4X1	T49.4X2	T49.4X3	T49.4X4	T49.4X5	T49.4X6
Respaire	T48.4X1	T48.4X2	T48.4X3	T48.4X4	T48.4X5	T48.4X6
Respiratory drug NEC	T48.901	T48.902	T48.903	T48.904	T48.905	T48.906
antiasthmatic NEC	T48.6X1	T48.6X2	T48.6X3	T48.6X4	T48.6X5	T48.6X6
anti-common-cold NEC	T48.5X1	T48.5X2	T48.5X3	T48.5X4	T48.5X5	T48.5X6
expectorant NEC	T48.4X1	T48.4X2	T48.4X3	T48.4X4	T48.4X5	T48.4X6

☑ **Additional Character May Be Required — Refer to the Tabular List for Character Selection**

*Optum Value-Add

Substance	Poisoning, Accidental (unintentional)	Poisoning, Intentional Self-harm	Poisoning, Assault	Poisoning, Undetermined	Adverse Effect	Under-dosing
Respiratory drug — continued						
stimulant	T48.901	T48.902	T48.903	T48.904	T48.905	T48.906
Restoril*	T42.4X1	T42.4X2	T42.4X3	T42.4X4	T42.4X5	T42.4X6
Retinoic acid	T49.0X1	T49.0X2	T49.0X3	T49.0X4	T49.0X5	T49.0X6
Retinol	T45.2X1	T45.2X2	T45.2X3	T45.2X4	T45.2X5	T45.2X6
Rh (D) immune globulin	T50.Z11	T50.Z12	T50.Z13	T50.Z14	T50.Z15	T50.Z16
(human)						
Rhodine	T39.011	T39.012	T39.013	T39.014	T39.015	T39.016
RhoGAM	T50.Z11	T50.Z12	T50.Z13	T50.Z14	T50.Z15	T50.Z16
Rhubarb						
dry extract	T47.2X1	T47.2X2	T47.2X3	T47.2X4	T47.2X5	T47.2X6
tincture, compound	T47.2X1	T47.2X2	T47.2X3	T47.2X4	T47.2X5	T47.2X6
Ribavirin	T37.5X1	T37.5X2	T37.5X3	T37.5X4	T37.5X5	T37.5X6
Riboflavin	T45.2X1	T45.2X2	T45.2X3	T45.2X4	T45.2X5	T45.2X6
Ribostamycin	T36.5X1	T36.5X2	T36.5X3	T36.5X4	T36.5X5	T36.5X6
Ricin	T62.2X1	T62.2X2	T62.2X3	T62.2X4	—	—
Ricinus communis	T62.2X1	T62.2X2	T62.2X3	T62.2X4	—	—
Rickettsial vaccine NEC	T50.A91	T50.A92	T50.A93	T50.A94	T50.A95	T50.A96
Rifabutin	T36.6X1	T36.6X2	T36.6X3	T36.6X4	T36.6X5	T36.6X6
Rifamide	T36.6X1	T36.6X2	T36.6X3	T36.6X4	T36.6X5	T36.6X6
Rifampicin	T36.6X1	T36.6X2	T36.6X3	T36.6X4	T36.6X5	T36.6X6
with isoniazid	T37.1X1	T37.1X2	T37.1X3	T37.1X4	T37.1X5	T37.1X6
Rifampin	T36.6X1	T36.6X2	T36.6X3	T36.6X4	T36.6X5	T36.6X6
Rifamycin	T36.6X1	T36.6X2	T36.6X3	T36.6X4	T36.6X5	T36.6X6
Rifaximin	T36.6X1	T36.6X2	T36.6X3	T36.6X4	T36.6X5	T36.6X6
Rimantadine	T37.5X1	T37.5X2	T37.5X3	T37.5X4	T37.5X5	T37.5X6
Rimazolium metilsulfate	T39.8X1	T39.8X2	T39.8X3	T39.8X4	T39.8X5	T39.8X6
Rimifon	T37.1X1	T37.1X2	T37.1X3	T37.1X4	T37.1X5	T37.1X6
Rimiterol	T48.6X1	T48.6X2	T48.6X3	T48.6X4	T48.6X5	T48.6X6
Ringer (lactate) **solution**	T50.3X1	T50.3X2	T50.3X3	T50.3X4	T50.3X5	T50.3X6
Risperdal*	T43.591	T43.592	T43.593	T43.594	T43.595	T43.596
Ristocetin	T36.8X1	T36.8X2	T36.8X3	T36.8X4	T36.8X5	T36.8X6
Ritalin	T43.631	T43.632	T43.633	T43.634	T43.635	T43.636
Ritodrine	T44.5X1	T44.5X2	T44.5X3	T44.5X4	T44.5X5	T44.5X6
Roach killer — see Insecticide						
Robitussin*	T48.3X1	T48.3X2	T48.3X3	T48.3X4	T48.3X5	T48.3X6
Rociverine	T44.3X1	T44.3X2	T44.3X3	T44.3X4	T44.3X5	T44.3X6
Rocky Mountain spotted fever vaccine	T50.A91	T50.A92	T50.A93	T50.A94	T50.A95	T50.A96
Rodenticide NEC	T60.4X1	T60.4X2	T60.4X3	T60.4X4	—	—
Rohypnol	T42.4X1	T42.4X2	T42.4X3	T42.4X4	T42.4X5	T42.4X6
Rokitamycin	T36.3X1	T36.3X2	T36.3X3	T36.3X4	T36.3X5	T36.3X6
Rolaids	T47.1X1	T47.1X2	T47.1X3	T47.1X4	T47.1X5	T47.1X6
Rolitetracycline	T36.4X1	T36.4X2	T36.4X3	T36.4X4	T36.4X5	T36.4X6
Romilar	T48.3X1	T48.3X2	T48.3X3	T48.3X4	T48.3X5	T48.3X6
Ronifibrate	T46.6X1	T46.6X2	T46.6X3	T46.6X4	T46.6X5	T46.6X6
Rosaprostol	T47.1X1	T47.1X2	T47.1X3	T47.1X4	T47.1X5	T47.1X6
Rose bengal sodium (131I)	T50.8X1	T50.8X2	T50.8X3	T50.8X4	T50.8X5	T50.8X6
Rose water ointment	T49.3X1	T49.3X2	T49.3X3	T49.3X4	T49.3X5	T49.3X6
Rosoxacin	T37.8X1	T37.8X2	T37.8X3	T37.8X4	T37.8X5	T37.8X6
Rotenone	T60.2X1	T60.2X2	T60.2X3	T60.2X4	—	—
Rotoxamine	T45.0X1	T45.0X2	T45.0X3	T45.0X4	T45.0X5	T45.0X6
Rough-on-rats	T60.4X1	T60.4X2	T60.4X3	T60.4X4	—	—
Roxatidine	T47.0X1	T47.0X2	T47.0X3	T47.0X4	T47.0X5	T47.0X6
Roxithromycin	T36.3X1	T36.3X2	T36.3X3	T36.3X4	T36.3X5	T36.3X6
Rt-PA	T45.611	T45.612	T45.613	T45.614	T45.615	T45.616
Rubbing alcohol	T51.2X1	T51.2X2	T51.2X3	T51.2X4	—	—
Rubefacient	T49.4X1	T49.4X2	T49.4X3	T49.4X4	T49.4X5	T49.4X6
Rubella vaccine	T50.B91	T50.B92	T50.B93	T50.B94	T50.B95	T50.B96
Rubeola vaccine	T50.B91	T50.B92	T50.B93	T50.B94	T50.B95	T50.B96
Rubidium chloride Rb82	T50.8X1	T50.8X2	T50.8X3	T50.8X4	T50.8X5	T50.8X6
Rubidomycin	T45.1X1	T45.1X2	T45.1X3	T45.1X4	T45.1X5	T45.1X6
Rue	T62.2X1	T62.2X2	T62.2X3	T62.2X4	—	—
Rufocromomycin	T45.1X1	T45.1X2	T45.1X3	T45.1X4	T45.1X5	T45.1X6
Russel's viper venin	T45.7X1	T45.7X2	T45.7X3	T45.7X4	T45.7X5	T45.7X6
Ruta (graveolens)	T62.2X1	T62.2X2	T62.2X3	T62.2X4	—	—
Rutinum	T46.991	T46.992	T46.993	T46.994	T46.995	T46.996
Rutoside	T46.991	T46.992	T46.993	T46.994	T46.995	T46.996
b-sitosterol(s)	T46.6X1	T46.6X2	T46.6X3	T46.6X4	T46.6X5	T46.6X6
Sabadilla (plant)	T62.2X1	T62.2X2	T62.2X3	T62.2X4	—	—
pesticide	T60.2X1	T60.2X2	T60.2X3	T60.2X4	—	—
Sabril*	T42.6X1	T42.6X2	T42.6X3	T42.6X4	T42.6X5	T42.6X6
Saccharated iron oxide	T45.8X1	T45.8X2	T45.8X3	T45.8X4	T45.8X5	T45.8X6
Saccharin	T50.901	T50.902	T50.903	T50.904	T50.905	T50.906
Saccharomyces boulardii	T47.6X1	T47.6X2	T47.6X3	T47.6X4	T47.6X5	T47.6X6
Safflower oil	T46.6X1	T46.6X2	T46.6X3	T46.6X4	T46.6X5	T46.6X6
Safrazine	T43.1X1	T43.1X2	T43.1X3	T43.1X4	T43.1X5	T43.1X6
Salazosulfapyridine	T37.0X1	T37.0X2	T37.0X3	T37.0X4	T37.0X5	T37.0X6
Salbutamol	T48.6X1	T48.6X2	T48.6X3	T48.6X4	T48.6X5	T48.6X6
Salicylamide	T39.091	T39.092	T39.093	T39.094	T39.095	T39.096
Salicylate NEC	T39.091	T39.092	T39.093	T39.094	T39.095	T39.096
methyl	T49.3X1	T49.3X2	T49.3X3	T49.3X4	T49.3X5	T49.3X6
theobromine calcium	T50.2X1	T50.2X2	T50.2X3	T50.2X4	T50.2X5	T50.2X6
Salicylazosulfapyridine	T37.0X1	T37.0X2	T37.0X3	T37.0X4	T37.0X5	T37.0X6
Salicylhydroxamic acid	T49.0X1	T49.0X2	T49.0X3	T49.0X4	T49.0X5	T49.0X6
Salicylic acid	T49.4X1	T49.4X2	T49.4X3	T49.4X4	T49.4X5	T49.4X6
with benzoic acid	T49.4X1	T49.4X2	T49.4X3	T49.4X4	T49.4X5	T49.4X6
congeners	T39.091	T39.092	T39.093	T39.094	T39.095	T39.096
derivative	T39.091	T39.092	T39.093	T39.094	T39.095	T39.096
salts	T39.091	T39.092	T39.093	T39.094	T39.095	T39.096
Salinazid	T37.1X1	T37.1X2	T37.1X3	T37.1X4	T37.1X5	T37.1X6
Salmeterol	T48.6X1	T48.6X2	T48.6X3	T48.6X4	T48.6X5	T48.6X6
Salol	T49.3X1	T49.3X2	T49.3X3	T49.3X4	T49.3X5	T49.3X6
Salsalate	T39.091	T39.092	T39.093	T39.094	T39.095	T39.096
Salt-replacing drug	T50.901	T50.902	T50.903	T50.904	T50.905	T50.906
Salt-retaining mineralocorticoid	T50.0X1	T50.0X2	T50.0X3	T50.0X4	T50.0X5	T50.0X6
Salt substitute	T50.901	T50.902	T50.903	T50.904	T50.905	T50.906
Saluretic NEC	T50.2X1	T50.2X2	T50.2X3	T50.2X4	T50.2X5	T50.2X6
Saluron	T50.2X1	T50.2X2	T50.2X3	T50.2X4	T50.2X5	T50.2X6
Salvarsan 606 (neosilver) (silver)	T37.8X1	T37.8X2	T37.8X3	T37.8X4	T37.8X5	T37.8X6
Sambucus canadensis	T62.2X1	T62.2X2	T62.2X3	T62.2X4	—	—
berry	T62.1X1	T62.1X2	T62.1X3	T62.1X4	—	—
Sandril	T46.5X1	T46.5X2	T46.5X3	T46.5X4	T46.5X5	T46.5X6
Sanguinaria canadensis	T62.2X1	T62.2X2	T62.2X3	T62.2X4	—	—
Saniflush (cleaner)	T54.2X1	T54.2X2	T54.2X3	T54.2X4	—	—
Santonin	T37.4X1	T37.4X2	T37.4X3	T37.4X4	T37.4X5	T37.4X6
Santyl	T49.8X1	T49.8X2	T49.8X3	T49.8X4	T49.8X5	T49.8X6
Saralasin	T46.5X1	T46.5X2	T46.5X3	T46.5X4	T46.5X5	T46.5X6
Sarcolysin	T45.1X1	T45.1X2	T45.1X3	T45.1X4	T45.1X5	T45.1X6
Sarilumab*	T39.4X1	T39.4X2	T39.4X3	T39.4X4	T39.4X5	T39.4X6
Sarkomycin	T45.1X1	T45.1X2	T45.1X3	T45.1X4	T45.1X5	T45.1X6
Saroten	T43.011	T43.012	T43.013	T43.014	T43.015	T43.016
Saturnine — see Lead						
Savin (oil)	T49.4X1	T49.4X2	T49.4X3	T49.4X4	T49.4X5	T49.4X6
Scammony	T47.2X1	T47.2X2	T47.2X3	T47.2X4	T47.2X5	T47.2X6
Scarlet red	T49.8X1	T49.8X2	T49.8X3	T49.8X4	T49.8X5	T49.8X6
Scheele's green	T57.0X1	T57.0X2	T57.0X3	T57.0X4	—	—
insecticide	T57.0X1	T57.0X2	T57.0X3	T57.0X4	—	—
Schizontozide (blood) (tissue)	T37.2X1	T37.2X2	T37.2X3	T37.2X4	T37.2X5	T37.2X6
Schradan	T60.0X1	T60.0X2	T60.0X3	T60.0X4	—	—
Schweinfurth green	T57.0X1	T57.0X2	T57.0X3	T57.0X4	—	—
insecticide	T57.0X1	T57.0X2	T57.0X3	T57.0X4	—	—
Scilla, rat poison	T60.4X1	T60.4X2	T60.4X3	T60.4X4	—	—
Scillaren	T60.4X1	T60.4X2	T60.4X3	T60.4X4	—	—
Sclerosing agent	T46.8X1	T46.8X2	T46.8X3	T46.8X4	T46.8X5	T46.8X6
Scombrotoxin	T61.11	T61.12	T61.13	T61.14	—	—
Scopolamine	T44.3X1	T44.3X2	T44.3X3	T44.3X4	T44.3X5	T44.3X6
Scopolia extract	T44.3X1	T44.3X2	T44.3X3	T44.3X4	T44.3X5	T44.3X6
Scouring powder	T65.891	T65.892	T65.893	T65.894	—	—
Sea						
anemone (sting)	T63.631	T63.632	T63.633	T63.634	—	—
cucumber (sting)	T63.691	T63.692	T63.693	T63.694	—	—
snake (bite) (venom)	T63.091	T63.092	T63.093	T63.094	—	—
urchin spine (puncture)	T63.691	T63.692	T63.693	T63.694	—	—
Seafood	T61.91	T61.92	T61.93	T61.94	—	—
specified NEC	T61.8X1	T61.8X2	T61.8X3	T61.8X4	—	—
Secbutabarbital	T42.3X1	T42.3X2	T42.3X3	T42.3X4	T42.3X5	T42.3X6
Secbutabarbitone	T42.3X1	T42.3X2	T42.3X3	T42.3X4	T42.3X5	T42.3X6
Secnidazole	T37.3X1	T37.3X2	T37.3X3	T37.3X4	T37.3X5	T37.3X6
Secobarbital	T42.3X1	T42.3X2	T42.3X3	T42.3X4	T42.3X5	T42.3X6
Seconal	T42.3X1	T42.3X2	T42.3X3	T42.3X4	T42.3X5	T42.3X6
Secretin	T50.8X1	T50.8X2	T50.8X3	T50.8X4	T50.8X5	T50.8X6
Sectral*	T44.7X1	T44.7X2	T44.7X3	T44.7X4	T44.7X5	T44.7X6
Sedative NEC	T42.71	T42.72	T42.73	T42.74	T42.75	T42.76
mixed NEC	T42.6X1	T42.6X2	T42.6X3	T42.6X4	T42.6X5	T42.6X6
Sedormid	T42.6X1	T42.6X2	T42.6X3	T42.6X4	T42.6X5	T42.6X6
Seed disinfectant or dressing	T60.8X1	T60.8X2	T60.8X3	T60.8X4	—	—
Seeds (poisonous)	T62.2X1	T62.2X2	T62.2X3	T62.2X4	—	—
Selegiline	T42.8X1	T42.8X2	T42.8X3	T42.8X4	T42.8X5	T42.8X6
Selenium NEC	T56.891	T56.892	T56.893	T56.894	—	—
disulfide or sulfide	T49.4X1	T49.4X2	T49.4X3	T49.4X4	T49.4X5	T49.4X6
fumes	T59.891	T59.892	T59.893	T59.894	—	—
sulfide	T49.4X1	T49.4X2	T49.4X3	T49.4X4	T49.4X5	T49.4X6
Selenomethionine (75Se)	T50.8X1	T50.8X2	T50.8X3	T50.8X4	T50.8X5	T50.8X6
Selsun	T49.4X1	T49.4X2	T49.4X3	T49.4X4	T49.4X5	T49.4X6
Semustine	T45.1X1	T45.1X2	T45.1X3	T45.1X4	T45.1X5	T45.1X6
Senega syrup	T48.4X1	T48.4X2	T48.4X3	T48.4X4	T48.4X5	T48.4X6
Senna	T47.2X1	T47.2X2	T47.2X3	T47.2X4	T47.2X5	T47.2X6
Sennoside A+B	T47.2X1	T47.2X2	T47.2X3	T47.2X4	T47.2X5	T47.2X6
Septisol	T49.2X1	T49.2X2	T49.2X3	T49.2X4	T49.2X5	T49.2X6
Seractide	T38.811	T38.812	T38.813	T38.814	T38.815	T38.816
Serax	T42.4X1	T42.4X2	T42.4X3	T42.4X4	T42.4X5	T42.4X6

Substance	Poisoning, Accidental (unintentional)	Poisoning, Intentional Self-harm	Poisoning, Assault	Poisoning, Undetermined	Adverse Effect	Under-dosing
Serenesil	T42.6X1	T42.6X2	T42.6X3	T42.6X4	T42.6X5	T42.6X6
Serenium (hydrochloride)	T37.91	T37.92	T37.93	T37.94	T37.95	T37.96
Serepax — see Oxazepam						
Serevent*	T48.6X1	T48.6X2	T48.6X3	T48.6X4	T48.6X5	T48.6X6
Sermorelin	T38.891	T38.892	T38.893	T38.894	T38.895	T38.896
Sernyl	T41.1X1	T41.1X2	T41.1X3	T41.1X4	T41.1X5	T41.1X6
Serotonin	T50.991	T50.992	T50.993	T50.994	T50.995	T50.996
Serpasil	T46.5X1	T46.5X2	T46.5X3	T46.5X4	T46.5X5	T46.5X6
Serrapeptase	T45.3X1	T45.3X2	T45.3X3	T45.3X4	T45.3X5	T45.3X6
Serum						
antibotulinus	T50.Z11	T50.Z12	T50.Z13	T50.Z14	T50.Z15	T50.Z16
anticytotoxic	T50.Z11	T50.Z12	T50.Z13	T50.Z14	T50.Z15	T50.Z16
antidiphtheria	T50.Z11	T50.Z12	T50.Z13	T50.Z14	T50.Z15	T50.Z16
antimeningococcus	T50.Z11	T50.Z12	T50.Z13	T50.Z14	T50.Z15	T50.Z16
anti-Rh	T50.Z11	T50.Z12	T50.Z13	T50.Z14	T50.Z15	T50.Z16
anti-snake-bite	T50.Z11	T50.Z12	T50.Z13	T50.Z14	T50.Z15	T50.Z16
antitetanic	T50.Z11	T50.Z12	T50.Z13	T50.Z14	T50.Z15	T50.Z16
antitoxic	T50.Z11	T50.Z12	T50.Z13	T50.Z14	T50.Z15	T50.Z16
complement (inhibitor)	T45.8X1	T45.8X2	T45.8X3	T45.8X4	T45.8X5	T45.8X6
convalescent	T50.Z11	T50.Z12	T50.Z13	T50.Z14	T50.Z15	T50.Z16
hemolytic complement	T45.8X1	T45.8X2	T45.8X3	T45.8X4	T45.8X5	T45.8X6
immune (human)	T50.Z11	T50.Z12	T50.Z13	T50.Z14	T50.Z15	T50.Z16
protective NEC	T50.Z11	T50.Z12	T50.Z13	T50.Z14	T50.Z15	T50.Z16
Setastine	T45.0X1	T45.0X2	T45.0X3	T45.0X4	T45.0X5	T45.0X6
Setoperone	T43.591	T43.592	T43.593	T43.594	T43.595	T43.596
Sewer gas	T59.91	T59.92	T59.93	T59.94	—	—
Shampoo	T55.0X1	T55.0X2	T55.0X3	T55.0X4	—	—
Shellfish, noxious, nonbacterial	T61.781	T61.782	T61.783	T61.784	—	—
Sildenafil	T46.7X1	T46.7X2	T46.7X3	T46.7X4	T46.7X5	T46.7X6
Silibinin	T50.991	T50.992	T50.993	T50.994	T50.995	T50.996
Silicone NEC	T65.891	T65.892	T65.893	T65.894	—	—
medicinal	T49.3X1	T49.3X2	T49.3X3	T49.3X4	T49.3X5	T49.3X6
Silvadene	T49.0X1	T49.0X2	T49.0X3	T49.0X4	T49.0X5	T49.0X6
Silver	T49.0X1	T49.0X2	T49.0X3	T49.0X4	T49.0X5	T49.0X6
anti-infectives	T49.0X1	T49.0X2	T49.0X3	T49.0X4	T49.0X5	T49.0X6
arsphenamine	T37.8X1	T37.8X2	T37.8X3	T37.8X4	T37.8X5	T37.8X6
colloidal	T49.0X1	T49.0X2	T49.0X3	T49.0X4	T49.0X5	T49.0X6
nitrate	T49.0X1	T49.0X2	T49.0X3	T49.0X4	T49.0X5	T49.0X6
ophthalmic preparation	T49.5X1	T49.5X2	T49.5X3	T49.5X4	T49.5X5	T49.5X6
toughened (keratolytic)	T49.4X1	T49.4X2	T49.4X3	T49.4X4	T49.4X5	T49.4X6
nonmedicinal (dust)	T56.891	T56.892	T56.893	T56.894	—	—
protein	T49.5X1	T49.5X2	T49.5X3	T49.5X4	T49.5X5	T49.5X6
salvarsan	T37.8X1	T37.8X2	T37.8X3	T37.8X4	T37.8X5	T37.8X6
sulfadiazine	T49.4X1	T49.4X2	T49.4X3	T49.4X4	T49.4X5	T49.4X6
Silymarin	T50.991	T50.992	T50.993	T50.994	T50.995	T50.996
Simaldrate	T47.1X1	T47.1X2	T47.1X3	T47.1X4	T47.1X5	T47.1X6
Simazine	T60.3X1	T60.3X2	T60.3X3	T60.3X4	—	—
Simethicone	T47.1X1	T47.1X2	T47.1X3	T47.1X4	T47.1X5	T47.1X6
Simfibrate	T46.6X1	T46.6X2	T46.6X3	T46.6X4	T46.6X5	T46.6X6
Simvastatin	T46.6X1	T46.6X2	T46.6X3	T46.6X4	T46.6X5	T46.6X6
Sincalide	T50.8X1	T50.8X2	T50.8X3	T50.8X4	T50.8X5	T50.8X6
Sinequan	T43.011	T43.012	T43.013	T43.014	T43.015	T43.016
Singoserp	T46.5X1	T46.5X2	T46.5X3	T46.5X4	T46.5X5	T46.5X6
Singulair*	T48.6X1	T48.6X2	T48.6X3	T48.6X4	T48.6X5	T48.6X6
Sintrom	T45.511	T45.512	T45.513	T45.514	T45.515	T45.516
Sisomicin	T36.5X1	T36.5X2	T36.5X3	T36.5X4	T36.5X5	T36.5X6
Sitosterols	T46.6X1	T46.6X2	T46.6X3	T46.6X4	T46.6X5	T46.6X6
Skeletal muscle relaxants	T48.1X1	T48.1X2	T48.1X3	T48.1X4	T48.1X5	T48.1X6
Skin						
agents (external)	T49.91	T49.92	T49.93	T49.94	T49.95	T49.96
specified NEC	T49.8X1	T49.8X2	T49.8X3	T49.8X4	T49.8X5	T49.8X6
test antigen	T50.8X1	T50.8X2	T50.8X3	T50.8X4	T50.8X5	T50.8X6
Sleep-eze	T45.0X1	T45.0X2	T45.0X3	T45.0X4	T45.0X5	T45.0X6
Sleeping draught, pill	T42.71	T42.72	T42.73	T42.74	T42.75	T42.76
Smallpox vaccine	T50.B11	T50.B12	T50.B13	T50.B14	T50.B15	T50.B16
Smelter fumes NEC	T56.91	T56.92	T56.93	T56.94	—	—
Smog	T59.1X1	T59.1X2	T59.1X3	T59.1X4	—	—
Smoke NEC	T59.811	T59.812	T59.813	T59.814	—	—
Smooth muscle relaxant	T44.3X1	T44.3X2	T44.3X3	T44.3X4	T44.3X5	T44.3X6
Snail killer NEC	T60.8X1	T60.8X2	T60.8X3	T60.8X4	—	—
Snake venom or bite	T63.001	T63.002	T63.003	T63.004	—	—
hemocoagulase	T45.7X1	T45.7X2	T45.7X3	T45.7X4	T45.7X5	T45.7X6
Snuff	T65.211	T65.212	T65.213	T65.214	—	—
Soap (powder) (product)	T55.0X1	T55.0X2	T55.0X3	T55.0X4	—	—
enema	T47.4X1	T47.4X2	T47.4X3	T47.4X4	T47.4X5	T47.4X6
medicinal, soft	T49.2X1	T49.2X2	T49.2X3	T49.2X4	T49.2X5	T49.2X6
superfatted	T49.2X1	T49.2X2	T49.2X3	T49.2X4	T49.2X5	T49.2X6
Sobrerol	T48.4X1	T48.4X2	T48.4X3	T48.4X4	T48.4X5	T48.4X6
Soda (caustic)	T54.3X1	T54.3X2	T54.3X3	T54.3X4	—	—
bicarb	T47.1X1	T47.1X2	T47.1X3	T47.1X4	T47.1X5	T47.1X6
chlorinated — see Sodium, hypochlorite						

Substance	Poisoning, Accidental (unintentional)	Poisoning, Intentional Self-harm	Poisoning, Assault	Poisoning, Undetermined	Adverse Effect	Under-dosing
Sodium						
acetosulfone	T37.1X1	T37.1X2	T37.1X3	T37.1X4	T37.1X5	T37.1X6
acetrizoate	T50.8X1	T50.8X2	T50.8X3	T50.8X4	T50.8X5	T50.8X6
acid phosphate	T50.3X1	T50.3X2	T50.3X3	T50.3X4	T50.3X5	T50.3X6
alginate	T47.8X1	T47.8X2	T47.8X3	T47.8X4	T47.8X5	T47.8X6
amidotrizoate	T50.8X1	T50.8X2	T50.8X3	T50.8X4	T50.8X5	T50.8X6
aminohippurate*	T50.8X1	T50.8X2	T50.8X3	T50.8X4	T50.8X5	T50.8X6
aminopterin	T45.1X1	T45.1X2	T45.1X3	T45.1X4	T45.1X5	T45.1X6
amylosulfate	T47.8X1	T47.8X2	T47.8X3	T47.8X4	T47.8X5	T47.8X6
amytal	T42.3X1	T42.3X2	T42.3X3	T42.3X4	T42.3X5	T42.3X6
antimony gluconate	T37.3X1	T37.3X2	T37.3X3	T37.3X4	T37.3X5	T37.3X6
arsenate	T57.0X1	T57.0X2	T57.0X3	T57.0X4	—	—
aurothiomalate	T39.4X1	T39.4X2	T39.4X3	T39.4X4	T39.4X5	T39.4X6
aurothiosulfate	T39.4X1	T39.4X2	T39.4X3	T39.4X4	T39.4X5	T39.4X6
barbiturate	T42.3X1	T42.3X2	T42.3X3	T42.3X4	T42.3X5	T42.3X6
basic phosphate	T47.4X1	T47.4X2	T47.4X3	T47.4X4	T47.4X5	T47.4X6
bicarbonate	T47.1X1	T47.1X2	T47.1X3	T47.1X4	T47.1X5	T47.1X6
bichromate	T57.8X1	T57.8X2	T57.8X3	T57.8X4	—	—
biphosphate	T50.3X1	T50.3X2	T50.3X3	T50.3X4	T50.3X5	T50.3X6
bisulfate	T65.891	T65.892	T65.893	T65.894	—	—
borate						
cleanser	T57.8X1	T57.8X2	T57.8X3	T57.8X4	—	—
eye	T49.5X1	T49.5X2	T49.5X3	T49.5X4	T49.5X5	T49.5X6
therapeutic	T49.8X1	T49.8X2	T49.8X3	T49.8X4	T49.8X5	T49.8X6
bromide	T42.6X1	T42.6X2	T42.6X3	T42.6X4	T42.6X5	T42.6X6
cacodylate (nonmedicinal) NEC	T50.8X1	T50.8X2	T50.8X3	T50.8X4	T50.8X5	T50.8X6
anti-infective	T37.8X1	T37.8X2	T37.8X3	T37.8X4	T37.8X5	T37.8X6
herbicide	T60.3X1	T60.3X2	T60.3X3	T60.3X4	—	—
calcium edetate	T45.8X1	T45.8X2	T45.8X3	T45.8X4	T45.8X5	T45.8X6
carbonate NEC	T54.3X1	T54.3X2	T54.3X3	T54.3X4	—	—
chlorate NEC	T65.891	T65.892	T65.893	T65.894	—	—
herbicide	T54.91	T54.92	T54.93	T54.94	—	—
chloride	T50.3X1	T50.3X2	T50.3X3	T50.3X4	T50.3X5	T50.3X6
with glucose	T50.3X1	T50.3X2	T50.3X3	T50.3X4	T50.3X5	T50.3X6
chromate	T65.891	T65.892	T65.893	T65.894	—	—
citrate	T50.991	T50.992	T50.993	T50.994	T50.995	T50.996
cromoglicate	T48.6X1	T48.6X2	T48.6X3	T48.6X4	T48.6X5	T48.6X6
cyanide	T65.0X1	T65.0X2	T65.0X3	T65.0X4	—	—
cyclamate	T50.3X1	T50.3X2	T50.3X3	T50.3X4	T50.3X5	T50.3X6
dehydrocholate	T45.8X1	T45.8X2	T45.8X3	T45.8X4	T45.8X5	T45.8X6
diatrizoate	T50.8X1	T50.8X2	T50.8X3	T50.8X4	T50.8X5	T50.8X6
dibunate	T48.4X1	T48.4X2	T48.4X3	T48.4X4	T48.4X5	T48.4X6
dioctyl sulfosuccinate	T47.4X1	T47.4X2	T47.4X3	T47.4X4	T47.4X5	T47.4X6
dipantoyl ferrate	T45.8X1	T45.8X2	T45.8X3	T45.8X4	T45.8X5	T45.8X6
edetate	T45.8X1	T45.8X2	T45.8X3	T45.8X4	T45.8X5	T45.8X6
ethacrynate	T50.1X1	T50.1X2	T50.1X3	T50.1X4	T50.1X5	T50.1X6
etidronate*	T50.991	T50.992	T50.993	T50.994	T50.995	T50.996
feredetate	T45.8X1	T45.8X2	T45.8X3	T45.8X4	T45.8X5	T45.8X6
Fluoride — see Fluoride						
fluoroacetate (dust) (pesticide)	T60.4X1	T60.4X2	T60.4X3	T60.4X4	—	—
free salt	T50.3X1	T50.3X2	T50.3X3	T50.3X4	T50.3X5	T50.3X6
fusidate	T36.8X1	T36.8X2	T36.8X3	T36.8X4	T36.8X5	T36.8X6
glucaldrate	T47.1X1	T47.1X2	T47.1X3	T47.1X4	T47.1X5	T47.1X6
glucosulfone	T37.1X1	T37.1X2	T37.1X3	T37.1X4	T37.1X5	T37.1X6
glutamate	T45.8X1	T45.8X2	T45.8X3	T45.8X4	T45.8X5	T45.8X6
hydrogen carbonate	T50.3X1	T50.3X2	T50.3X3	T50.3X4	T50.3X5	T50.3X6
hydroxide	T54.3X1	T54.3X2	T54.3X3	T54.3X4	—	—
hypochlorite (bleach) NEC	T54.3X1	T54.3X2	T54.3X3	T54.3X4	—	—
disinfectant	T54.3X1	T54.3X2	T54.3X3	T54.3X4	—	—
medicinal (anti-infective) (external)	T49.0X1	T49.0X2	T49.0X3	T49.0X4	T49.0X5	T49.0X6
vapor	T54.3X1	T54.3X2	T54.3X3	T54.3X4	—	—
hyposulfite	T49.0X1	T49.0X2	T49.0X3	T49.0X4	T49.0X5	T49.0X6
indigotin disulfonate	T50.8X1	T50.8X2	T50.8X3	T50.8X4	T50.8X5	T50.8X6
iodide	T50.991	T50.992	T50.993	T50.994	T50.995	T50.996
I-131	T50.8X1	T50.8X2	T50.8X3	T50.8X4	T50.8X5	T50.8X6
therapeutic	T38.2X1	T38.2X2	T38.2X3	T38.2X4	T38.2X5	T38.2X6
iodohippurate (131I)	T50.8X1	T50.8X2	T50.8X3	T50.8X4	T50.8X5	T50.8X6
iopodate	T50.8X1	T50.8X2	T50.8X3	T50.8X4	T50.8X5	T50.8X6
iothalamate	T50.8X1	T50.8X2	T50.8X3	T50.8X4	T50.8X5	T50.8X6
iron edetate	T45.4X1	T45.4X2	T45.4X3	T45.4X4	T45.4X5	T45.4X6
lactate (compound solution)	T45.8X1	T45.8X2	T45.8X3	T45.8X4	T45.8X5	T45.8X6
lauryl (sulfate)	T49.2X1	T49.2X2	T49.2X3	T49.2X4	T49.2X5	T49.2X6
L-triiodothyronine	T38.1X1	T38.1X2	T38.1X3	T38.1X4	T38.1X5	T38.1X6
magnesium citrate	T50.991	T50.992	T50.993	T50.994	T50.995	T50.996
mersalate	T50.2X1	T50.2X2	T50.2X3	T50.2X4	T50.2X5	T50.2X6
metasilicate	T65.891	T65.892	T65.893	T65.894	—	—
metrizoate	T50.8X1	T50.8X2	T50.8X3	T50.8X4	T50.8X5	T50.8X6
monofluoroacetate (pesticide)	T60.1X1	T60.1X2	T60.1X3	T60.1X4	—	—

Substance	Poisoning, Accidental (unintentional)	Poisoning, Intentional Self-harm	Poisoning, Assault	Poisoning, Undetermined	Adverse Effect	Under-dosing
Sodium — *continued*						
morrhuate	T46.8X1	T46.8X2	T46.8X3	T46.8X4	T46.8X5	T46.8X6
nafcillin	T36.0X1	T36.0X2	T36.0X3	T36.0X4	T36.0X5	T36.0X6
nitrate (oxidizing agent)	T65.891	T65.892	T65.893	T65.894	—	—
nitrite	T50.6X1	T50.6X2	T50.6X3	T50.6X4	T50.6X5	T50.6X6
nitroferricyanide	T46.5X1	T46.5X2	T46.5X3	T46.5X4	T46.5X5	T46.5X6
nitroprusside	T46.5X1	T46.5X2	T46.5X3	T46.5X4	T46.5X5	T46.5X6
oxalate	T65.891	T65.892	T65.893	T65.894	—	—
oxide/peroxide	T65.891	T65.892	T65.893	T65.894	—	—
oxybate	T41.291	T41.292	T41.293	T41.294	T41.295	T41.296
para-aminohippurate	T50.8X1	T50.8X2	T50.8X3	T50.8X4	T50.8X5	T50.8X6
perborate (nonmedicinal) NEC	T65.891	T65.892	T65.893	T65.894	—	—
medicinal	T49.0X1	T49.0X2	T49.0X3	T49.0X4	T49.0X5	T49.0X6
soap	T55.0X1	T55.0X2	T55.0X3	T55.0X4	—	—
percarbonate — *see* Sodium, perborate						
pertechnetate Tc99m	T50.8X1	T50.8X2	T50.8X3	T50.8X4	T50.8X5	T50.8X6
phosphate						
cellulose	T45.8X1	T45.8X2	T45.8X3	T45.8X4	T45.8X5	T45.8X6
dibasic	T47.2X1	T47.2X2	T47.2X3	T47.2X4	T47.2X5	T47.2X6
monobasic	T47.2X1	T47.2X2	T47.2X3	T47.2X4	T47.2X5	T47.2X6
phytate	T50.6X1	T50.6X2	T50.6X3	T50.6X4	T50.6X5	T50.6X6
picosulfate	T47.2X1	T47.2X2	T47.2X3	T47.2X4	T47.2X5	T47.2X6
polyhydroxyaluminium monocarbonate	T47.1X1	T47.1X2	T47.1X3	T47.1X4	T47.1X5	T47.1X6
polystyrene sulfonate	T50.3X1	T50.3X2	T50.3X3	T50.3X4	T50.3X5	T50.3X6
propionate	T49.0X1	T49.0X2	T49.0X3	T49.0X4	T49.0X5	T49.0X6
propyl hydroxybenzoate	T50.991	T50.992	T50.993	T50.994	T50.995	T50.996
psylliate	T46.8X1	T46.8X2	T46.8X3	T46.8X4	T46.8X5	T46.8X6
removing resins	T50.3X1	T50.3X2	T50.3X3	T50.3X4	T50.3X5	T50.3X6
salicylate	T39.091	T39.092	T39.093	T39.094	T39.095	T39.096
salt NEC	T50.3X1	T50.3X2	T50.3X3	T50.3X4	T50.3X5	T50.3X6
selenate	T60.2X1	T60.2X2	T60.2X3	T60.2X4	—	—
stibogluconate	T37.3X1	T37.3X2	T37.3X3	T37.3X4	T37.3X5	T37.3X6
sulfate	T47.4X1	T47.4X2	T47.4X3	T47.4X4	T47.4X5	T47.4X6
sulfoxone	T37.1X1	T37.1X2	T37.1X3	T37.1X4	T37.1X5	T37.1X6
tetradecyl sulfate	T46.8X1	T46.8X2	T46.8X3	T46.8X4	T46.8X5	T46.8X6
thiopental	T41.1X1	T41.1X2	T41.1X3	T41.1X4	T41.1X5	T41.1X6
thiosalicylate	T39.091	T39.092	T39.093	T39.094	T39.095	T39.096
thiosulfate	T50.6X1	T50.6X2	T50.6X3	T50.6X4	T50.6X5	T50.6X6
tolbutamide	T38.3X1	T38.3X2	T38.3X3	T38.3X4	T38.3X5	T38.3X6
(L)-triiodothyronine	T38.1X1	T38.1X2	T38.1X3	T38.1X4	T38.1X5	T38.1X6
tyropanoate	T50.8X1	T50.8X2	T50.8X3	T50.8X4	T50.8X5	T50.8X6
valproate	T42.6X1	T42.6X2	T42.6X3	T42.6X4	T42.6X5	T42.6X6
versenate	T50.6X1	T50.6X2	T50.6X3	T50.6X4	T50.6X5	T50.6X6
Sodium-free salt	T50.901	T50.902	T50.903	T50.904	T50.905	T50.906
Sodium-removing resin	T50.3X1	T50.3X2	T50.3X3	T50.3X4	T50.3X5	T50.3X6
Soft soap	T55.0X1	T55.0X2	T55.0X3	T55.0X4	—	—
Solanine	T62.2X1	T62.2X2	T62.2X3	T62.2X4	—	—
berries	T62.1X1	T62.1X2	T62.1X3	T62.1X4	—	—
Solanum dulcamara	T62.2X1	T62.2X2	T62.2X3	T62.2X4	—	—
berries	T62.1X1	T62.1X2	T62.1X3	T62.1X4	—	—
Solapsone	T37.1X1	T37.1X2	T37.1X3	T37.1X4	T37.1X5	T37.1X6
Solaquin*	T49.8X1	T49.8X2	T49.8X3	T49.8X4	T49.8X5	T49.8X6
Solar lotion	T49.3X1	T49.3X2	T49.3X3	T49.3X4	T49.3X5	T49.3X6
Solasulfone	T37.1X1	T37.1X2	T37.1X3	T37.1X4	T37.1X5	T37.1X6
Soldering fluid	T65.891	T65.892	T65.893	T65.894	—	—
Solid substance	T65.91	T65.92	T65.93	T65.94	—	—
specified NEC	T65.891	T65.892	T65.893	T65.894	—	—
Solvent, industrial NEC	T52.91	T52.92	T52.93	T52.94	—	—
naphtha	T52.0X1	T52.0X2	T52.0X3	T52.0X4	—	—
petroleum	T52.0X1	T52.0X2	T52.0X3	T52.0X4	—	—
specified NEC	T52.8X1	T52.8X2	T52.8X3	T52.8X4	—	—
Soma	T42.8X1	T42.8X2	T42.8X3	T42.8X4	T42.8X5	T42.8X6
Somatorelin	T38.891	T38.892	T38.893	T38.894	T38.895	T38.896
Somatostatin	T38.991	T38.992	T38.993	T38.994	T38.995	T38.996
Somatotropin	T38.811	T38.812	T38.813	T38.814	T38.815	T38.816
Somatrem	T38.811	T38.812	T38.813	T38.814	T38.815	T38.816
Somatropin	T38.811	T38.812	T38.813	T38.814	T38.815	T38.816
Sominex	T45.0X1	T45.0X2	T45.0X3	T45.0X4	T45.0X5	T45.0X6
Somnos	T42.6X1	T42.6X2	T42.6X3	T42.6X4	T42.6X5	T42.6X6
Somonal	T42.3X1	T42.3X2	T42.3X3	T42.3X4	T42.3X5	T42.3X6
Soneryl	T42.3X1	T42.3X2	T42.3X3	T42.3X4	T42.3X5	T42.3X6
Soothing syrup	T50.901	T50.902	T50.903	T50.904	T50.905	T50.906
Sopor	T42.6X1	T42.6X2	T42.6X3	T42.6X4	T42.6X5	T42.6X6
Soporific	T42.71	T42.72	T42.73	T42.74	T42.75	T42.76
Soporific drug	T42.71	T42.72	T42.73	T42.74	T42.75	T42.76
specified type NEC	T42.6X1	T42.6X2	T42.6X3	T42.6X4	T42.6X5	T42.6X6
Sorbide nitrate	T46.3X1	T46.3X2	T46.3X3	T46.3X4	T46.3X5	T46.3X6
Sorbitol	T47.4X1	T47.4X2	T47.4X3	T47.4X4	T47.4X5	T47.4X6
Sotalol	T44.7X1	T44.7X2	T44.7X3	T44.7X4	T44.7X5	T44.7X6
Sotradecol	T46.8X1	T46.8X2	T46.8X3	T46.8X4	T46.8X5	T46.8X6

Substance	Poisoning, Accidental (unintentional)	Poisoning, Intentional Self-harm	Poisoning, Assault	Poisoning, Undetermined	Adverse Effect	Under-dosing
Soysterol	T46.6X1	T46.6X2	T46.6X3	T46.6X4	T46.6X5	T46.6X6
Spacoline	T44.3X1	T44.3X2	T44.3X3	T44.3X4	T44.3X5	T44.3X6
Spanish fly	T49.8X1	T49.8X2	T49.8X3	T49.8X4	T49.8X5	T49.8X6
Sparine	T43.3X1	T43.3X2	T43.3X3	T43.3X4	T43.3X5	T43.3X6
Sparteine	T48.0X1	T48.0X2	T48.0X3	T48.0X4	T48.0X5	T48.0X6
Spasmolytic						
anticholinergics	T44.3X1	T44.3X2	T44.3X3	T44.3X4	T44.3X5	T44.3X6
autonomic	T44.3X1	T44.3X2	T44.3X3	T44.3X4	T44.3X5	T44.3X6
bronchial NEC	T48.6X1	T48.6X2	T48.6X3	T48.6X4	T48.6X5	T48.6X6
quaternary ammonium	T44.3X1	T44.3X2	T44.3X3	T44.3X4	T44.3X5	T44.3X6
skeletal muscle NEC	T48.1X1	T48.1X2	T48.1X3	T48.1X4	T48.1X5	T48.1X6
Spectinomycin	T36.5X1	T36.5X2	T36.5X3	T36.5X4	T36.5X5	T36.5X6
Spectracef*	T36.1X1	T36.1X2	T36.1X3	T36.1X4	T36.1X5	T36.1X6
Speed	T43.651	T43.652	T43.653	T43.654	T43.655	T43.656
Spermicide	T49.8X1	T49.8X2	T49.8X3	T49.8X4	T49.8X5	T49.8X6
Spider (bite) (venom)	T63.391	T63.392	T63.393	T63.394	—	—
antivenin	T50.Z11	T50.Z12	T50.Z13	T50.Z14	T50.Z15	T50.Z16
Spigelia (root)	T37.4X1	T37.4X2	T37.4X3	T37.4X4	T37.4X5	T37.4X6
Spindle inactivator	T50.4X1	T50.4X2	T50.4X3	T50.4X4	T50.4X5	T50.4X6
Spiperone	T43.4X1	T43.4X2	T43.4X3	T43.4X4	T43.4X5	T43.4X6
Spiramycin	T36.3X1	T36.3X2	T36.3X3	T36.3X4	T36.3X5	T36.3X6
Spirapril	T46.4X1	T46.4X2	T46.4X3	T46.4X4	T46.4X5	T46.4X6
Spirilene	T43.591	T43.592	T43.593	T43.594	T43.595	T43.596
Spirit(s) (neutral) NEC	T51.0X1	T51.0X2	T51.0X3	T51.0X4	—	—
beverage	T51.0X1	T51.0X2	T51.0X3	T51.0X4	—	—
industrial	T51.0X1	T51.0X2	T51.0X3	T51.0X4	—	—
mineral	T52.0X1	T52.0X2	T52.0X3	T52.0X4	—	—
of salt — *see* Hydrochloric acid						
surgical	T51.0X1	T51.0X2	T51.0X3	T51.0X4	—	—
Spiriva*	T44.3X1	T44.3X2	T44.3X3	T44.3X4	T44.3X5	T44.3X6
Spironolactone	T50.0X1	T50.0X2	T50.0X3	T50.0X4	T50.0X5	T50.0X6
Spiroperidol	T43.4X1	T43.4X2	T43.4X3	T43.4X4	T43.4X5	T43.4X6
Sponge, absorbable (gelatin)	T45.7X1	T45.7X2	T45.7X3	T45.7X4	T45.7X5	T45.7X6
Sporostacin	T49.0X1	T49.0X2	T49.0X3	T49.0X4	T49.0X5	T49.0X6
Spray (aerosol)	T65.91	T65.92	T65.93	T65.94	—	—
cosmetic	T65.891	T65.892	T65.893	T65.894	—	—
medicinal NEC	T50.901	T50.902	T50.903	T50.904	T50.905	T50.906
pesticides — *see* Pesticide						
specified content — *see* specific substance						
Spurge flax	T62.2X1	T62.2X2	T62.2X3	T62.2X4	—	—
Spurges	T62.2X1	T62.2X2	T62.2X3	T62.2X4	—	—
Sputum viscosity-lowering drug	T48.4X1	T48.4X2	T48.4X3	T48.4X4	T48.4X5	T48.4X6
Squill	T46.0X1	T46.0X2	T46.0X3	T46.0X4	T46.0X5	T46.0X6
rat poison	T60.4X1	T60.4X2	T60.4X3	T60.4X4	—	—
Squirting cucumber (cathartic)	T47.2X1	T47.2X2	T47.2X3	T47.2X4	T47.2X5	T47.2X6
Stains	T65.6X1	T65.6X2	T65.6X3	T65.6X4	—	—
Stannous fluoride	T49.7X1	T49.7X2	T49.7X3	T49.7X4	T49.7X5	T49.7X6
Stanolone	T38.7X1	T38.7X2	T38.7X3	T38.7X4	T38.7X5	T38.7X6
Stanozolol	T38.7X1	T38.7X2	T38.7X3	T38.7X4	T38.7X5	T38.7X6
Staphisagria or stavesacre (pediculicide)	T49.0X1	T49.0X2	T49.0X3	T49.0X4	T49.0X5	T49.0X6
Starch	T50.901	T50.902	T50.903	T50.904	T50.905	T50.906
Stavzor*	T42.6X1	T42.6X2	T42.6X3	T42.6X4	T42.6X5	T42.6X6
Stelazine	T43.3X1	T43.3X2	T43.3X3	T43.3X4	T43.3X5	T43.3X6
Stemetil	T43.3X1	T43.3X2	T43.3X3	T43.3X4	T43.3X5	T43.3X6
Stepronin	T48.4X1	T48.4X2	T48.4X3	T48.4X4	T48.4X5	T48.4X6
Sterculia	T47.4X1	T47.4X2	T47.4X3	T47.4X4	T47.4X5	T47.4X6
Sternutator gas	T59.891	T59.892	T59.893	T59.894	—	—
Steroid	T38.0X1	T38.0X2	T38.0X3	T38.0X4	T38.0X5	T38.0X6
anabolic	T38.7X1	T38.7X2	T38.7X3	T38.7X4	T38.7X5	T38.7X6
androgenic	T38.7X1	T38.7X2	T38.7X3	T38.7X4	T38.7X5	T38.7X6
antineoplastic, hormone	T38.7X1	T38.7X2	T38.7X3	T38.7X4	T38.7X5	T38.7X6
estrogen	T38.5X1	T38.5X2	T38.5X3	T38.5X4	T38.5X5	T38.5X6
ENT agent	T49.6X1	T49.6X2	T49.6X3	T49.6X4	T49.6X5	T49.6X6
ophthalmic preparation	T49.5X1	T49.5X2	T49.5X3	T49.5X4	T49.5X5	T49.5X6
topical NEC	T49.0X1	T49.0X2	T49.0X3	T49.0X4	T49.0X5	T49.0X6
Stibine	T56.891	T56.892	T56.893	T56.894	—	—
Stibogluconate	T37.3X1	T37.3X2	T37.3X3	T37.3X4	T37.3X5	T37.3X6
Stibophen	T37.4X1	T37.4X2	T37.4X3	T37.4X4	T37.4X5	T37.4X6
Stilbamidine (isetionate)	T37.3X1	T37.3X2	T37.3X3	T37.3X4	T37.3X5	T37.3X6
Stilbestrol	T38.5X1	T38.5X2	T38.5X3	T38.5X4	T38.5X5	T38.5X6
Stilboestrol	T38.5X1	T38.5X2	T38.5X3	T38.5X4	T38.5X5	T38.5X6
Stimulant						
central nervous system — *see also* Psychostimulant	T43.601	T43.602	T43.603	T43.604	T43.605	T43.606
analeptics	T50.7X1	T50.7X2	T50.7X3	T50.7X4	T50.7X5	T50.7X6
opiate antagonist	T50.7X1	T50.7X2	T50.7X3	T50.7X4	T50.7X5	T50.7X6

Table of Drugs and Chemicals

Sodium — Stimulant

Substance	Poisoning, Accidental (unintentional)	Poisoning, Intentional Self-harm	Poisoning, Assault	Poisoning, Undetermined	Adverse Effect	Under-dosing
Stimulant — continued						
central nervous system — see also Psychostimulant — continued						
psychotherapeutic NEC — see also Psychotherapeutic drug	T43.601	T43.602	T43.603	T43.604	T43.605	T43.606
specified NEC	T43.691	T43.692	T43.693	T43.694	T43.695	T43.696
respiratory	T48.901	T48.902	T48.903	T48.904	T48.905	T48.906
Stone-dissolving drug	T50.901	T50.902	T50.903	T50.904	T50.905	T50.906
Storage battery (cells) (acid)	T54.2X1	T54.2X2	T54.2X3	T54.2X4	—	—
Stovaine	T41.3X1	T41.3X2	T41.3X3	T41.3X4	T41.3X5	T41.3X6
infiltration (subcutaneous)	T41.3X1	T41.3X2	T41.3X3	T41.3X4	T41.3X5	T41.3X6
nerve block (peripheral) (plexus)	T41.3X1	T41.3X2	T41.3X3	T41.3X4	T41.3X5	T41.3X6
spinal	T41.3X1	T41.3X2	T41.3X3	T41.3X4	T41.3X5	T41.3X6
topical (surface)	T41.3X1	T41.3X2	T41.3X3	T41.3X4	T41.3X5	T41.3X6
Stovarsal	T37.8X1	T37.8X2	T37.8X3	T37.8X4	T37.8X5	T37.8X6
Stove gas — see Gas, stove						
Stoxil	T49.5X1	T49.5X2	T49.5X3	T49.5X4	T49.5X5	T49.5X6
Stramonium	T48.6X1	T48.6X2	T48.6X3	T48.6X4	T48.6X5	T48.6X6
natural state	T62.2X1	T62.2X2	T62.2X3	T62.2X4	—	—
Streptodornase	T45.3X1	T45.3X2	T45.3X3	T45.3X4	T45.3X5	T45.3X6
Streptoduocin	T36.5X1	T36.5X2	T36.5X3	T36.5X4	T36.5X5	T36.5X6
Streptokinase	T45.611	T45.612	T45.613	T45.614	T45.615	T45.616
Streptomycin (derivative)	T36.5X1	T36.5X2	T36.5X3	T36.5X4	T36.5X5	T36.5X6
Streptonivicin	T36.5X1	T36.5X2	T36.5X3	T36.5X4	T36.5X5	T36.5X6
Streptovarycin	T36.5X1	T36.5X2	T36.5X3	T36.5X4	T36.5X5	T36.5X6
Streptozocin	T45.1X1	T45.1X2	T45.1X3	T45.1X4	T45.1X5	T45.1X6
Streptozotocin	T45.1X1	T45.1X2	T45.1X3	T45.1X4	T45.1X5	T45.1X6
Stripper (paint) (solvent)	T52.8X1	T52.8X2	T52.8X3	T52.8X4	—	—
Strobane	T60.1X1	T60.1X2	T60.1X3	T60.1X4	—	—
Strofantina	T46.0X1	T46.0X2	T46.0X3	T46.0X4	T46.0X5	T46.0X6
Stromectol*	T37.4X1	T37.4X2	T37.4X3	T37.4X4	T37.4X5	T37.4X6
Strophanthin (g) (k)	T46.0X1	T46.0X2	T46.0X3	T46.0X4	T46.0X5	T46.0X6
Strophanthus	T46.0X1	T46.0X2	T46.0X3	T46.0X4	T46.0X5	T46.0X6
Strophantin	T46.0X1	T46.0X2	T46.0X3	T46.0X4	T46.0X5	T46.0X6
Strophantin-g	T46.0X1	T46.0X2	T46.0X3	T46.0X4	T46.0X5	T46.0X6
Strychnine (nonmedicinal) (pesticide) (salts)	T65.1X1	T65.1X2	T65.1X3	T65.1X4	—	—
medicinal	T48.291	T48.292	T48.293	T48.294	T48.295	T48.296
Strychnos (ignatii) — see Strychnine						
Styramate	T42.8X1	T42.8X2	T42.8X3	T42.8X4	T42.8X5	T42.8X6
Styrene	T65.891	T65.892	T65.893	T65.894	—	—
Succinimide, antiepileptic or anticonvulsant	T42.2X1	T42.2X2	T42.2X3	T42.2X4	T42.2X5	T42.2X6
mercuric — see Mercury						
Succinylcholine	T48.1X1	T48.1X2	T48.1X3	T48.1X4	T48.1X5	T48.1X6
Succinylsulfathiazole	T37.0X1	T37.0X2	T37.0X3	T37.0X4	T37.0X5	T37.0X6
Sucralfate	T47.1X1	T47.1X2	T47.1X3	T47.1X4	T47.1X5	T47.1X6
Sucrose	T50.3X1	T50.3X2	T50.3X3	T50.3X4	T50.3X5	T50.3X6
Sufentanil	T40.411	T40.412	T40.413	T40.414	T40.415	T40.416
Sulbactam	T36.0X1	T36.0X2	T36.0X3	T36.0X4	T36.0X5	T36.0X6
Sulbenicillin	T36.0X1	T36.0X2	T36.0X3	T36.0X4	T36.0X5	T36.0X6
Sulbentine	T49.0X1	T49.0X2	T49.0X3	T49.0X4	T49.0X5	T49.0X6
Sulconazole*	T49.0X1	T49.0X2	T49.0X3	T49.0X4	T49.0X5	T49.0X6
Sulfacetamide	T49.0X1	T49.0X2	T49.0X3	T49.0X4	T49.0X5	T49.0X6
ophthalmic preparation	T49.5X1	T49.5X2	T49.5X3	T49.5X4	T49.5X5	T49.5X6
Sulfachlorpyridazine	T37.0X1	T37.0X2	T37.0X3	T37.0X4	T37.0X5	T37.0X6
Sulfacitine	T37.0X1	T37.0X2	T37.0X3	T37.0X4	T37.0X5	T37.0X6
Sulfadiasulfone sodium	T37.0X1	T37.0X2	T37.0X3	T37.0X4	T37.0X5	T37.0X6
Sulfadiazine	T37.0X1	T37.0X2	T37.0X3	T37.0X4	T37.0X5	T37.0X6
silver (topical)	T49.0X1	T49.0X2	T49.0X3	T49.0X4	T49.0X5	T49.0X6
Sulfadimethoxine	T37.0X1	T37.0X2	T37.0X3	T37.0X4	T37.0X5	T37.0X6
Sulfadimidine	T37.0X1	T37.0X2	T37.0X3	T37.0X4	T37.0X5	T37.0X6
Sulfadoxine	T37.0X1	T37.0X2	T37.0X3	T37.0X4	T37.0X5	T37.0X6
with pyrimethamine	T37.2X1	T37.2X2	T37.2X3	T37.2X4	T37.2X5	T37.2X6
Sulfaethidole	T37.0X1	T37.0X2	T37.0X3	T37.0X4	T37.0X5	T37.0X6
Sulfafurazole	T37.0X1	T37.0X2	T37.0X3	T37.0X4	T37.0X5	T37.0X6
Sulfaguanidine	T37.0X1	T37.0X2	T37.0X3	T37.0X4	T37.0X5	T37.0X6
Sulfalene	T37.0X1	T37.0X2	T37.0X3	T37.0X4	T37.0X5	T37.0X6
Sulfaloxate	T37.0X1	T37.0X2	T37.0X3	T37.0X4	T37.0X5	T37.0X6
Sulfaloxic acid	T37.0X1	T37.0X2	T37.0X3	T37.0X4	T37.0X5	T37.0X6
Sulfamazone	T39.2X1	T39.2X2	T39.2X3	T39.2X4	T39.2X5	T39.2X6
Sulfamerazine	T37.0X1	T37.0X2	T37.0X3	T37.0X4	T37.0X5	T37.0X6
Sulfameter	T37.0X1	T37.0X2	T37.0X3	T37.0X4	T37.0X5	T37.0X6
Sulfamethazine	T37.0X1	T37.0X2	T37.0X3	T37.0X4	T37.0X5	T37.0X6
Sulfamethizole	T37.0X1	T37.0X2	T37.0X3	T37.0X4	T37.0X5	T37.0X6
Sulfamethoxazole	T37.0X1	T37.0X2	T37.0X3	T37.0X4	T37.0X5	T37.0X6
with trimethoprim	T36.8X1	T36.8X2	T36.8X3	T36.8X4	T36.8X5	T36.8X6
Sulfamethoxydiazine	T37.0X1	T37.0X2	T37.0X3	T37.0X4	T37.0X5	T37.0X6
Sulfamethoxypyridazine	T37.0X1	T37.0X2	T37.0X3	T37.0X4	T37.0X5	T37.0X6
Sulfamethylthiazole	T37.0X1	T37.0X2	T37.0X3	T37.0X4	T37.0X5	T37.0X6
Sulfametoxydiazine	T37.0X1	T37.0X2	T37.0X3	T37.0X4	T37.0X5	T37.0X6
Sulfamidopyrine	T39.2X1	T39.2X2	T39.2X3	T39.2X4	T39.2X5	T39.2X6
Sulfamonomethoxine	T37.0X1	T37.0X2	T37.0X3	T37.0X4	T37.0X5	T37.0X6
Sulfamoxole	T37.0X1	T37.0X2	T37.0X3	T37.0X4	T37.0X5	T37.0X6
Sulfamylon	T49.0X1	T49.0X2	T49.0X3	T49.0X4	T49.0X5	T49.0X6
Sulfan blue (diagnostic dye)	T50.8X1	T50.8X2	T50.8X3	T50.8X4	T50.8X5	T50.8X6
Sulfanilamide	T37.0X1	T37.0X2	T37.0X3	T37.0X4	T37.0X5	T37.0X6
Sulfanilylguanidine	T37.0X1	T37.0X2	T37.0X3	T37.0X4	T37.0X5	T37.0X6
Sulfaperin	T37.0X1	T37.0X2	T37.0X3	T37.0X4	T37.0X5	T37.0X6
Sulfaphenazole	T37.0X1	T37.0X2	T37.0X3	T37.0X4	T37.0X5	T37.0X6
Sulfaphenylthiazole	T37.0X1	T37.0X2	T37.0X3	T37.0X4	T37.0X5	T37.0X6
Sulfaproxyline	T37.0X1	T37.0X2	T37.0X3	T37.0X4	T37.0X5	T37.0X6
Sulfapyridine	T37.0X1	T37.0X2	T37.0X3	T37.0X4	T37.0X5	T37.0X6
Sulfapyrimidine	T37.0X1	T37.0X2	T37.0X3	T37.0X4	T37.0X5	T37.0X6
Sulfarsphenamine	T37.8X1	T37.8X2	T37.8X3	T37.8X4	T37.8X5	T37.8X6
Sulfasalazine	T37.0X1	T37.0X2	T37.0X3	T37.0X4	T37.0X5	T37.0X6
Sulfasuxidine	T37.0X1	T37.0X2	T37.0X3	T37.0X4	T37.0X5	T37.0X6
Sulfasymazine	T37.0X1	T37.0X2	T37.0X3	T37.0X4	T37.0X5	T37.0X6
Sulfated amylopectin	T47.8X1	T47.8X2	T47.8X3	T47.8X4	T47.8X5	T47.8X6
Sulfathiazole	T37.0X1	T37.0X2	T37.0X3	T37.0X4	T37.0X5	T37.0X6
Sulfatostearate	T49.2X1	T49.2X2	T49.2X3	T49.2X4	T49.2X5	T49.2X6
Sulfatrim*	T36.8X1	T36.8X2	T36.8X3	T36.8X4	T36.8X5	T36.8X6
Sulfinpyrazone	T50.4X1	T50.4X2	T50.4X3	T50.4X4	T50.4X5	T50.4X6
Sulfiram	T49.0X1	T49.0X2	T49.0X3	T49.0X4	T49.0X5	T49.0X6
Sulfisomidine	T37.0X1	T37.0X2	T37.0X3	T37.0X4	T37.0X5	T37.0X6
Sulfisoxazole	T37.0X1	T37.0X2	T37.0X3	T37.0X4	T37.0X5	T37.0X6
ophthalmic preparation	T49.5X1	T49.5X2	T49.5X3	T49.5X4	T49.5X5	T49.5X6
Sulfobromophthalein (sodium)	T50.8X1	T50.8X2	T50.8X3	T50.8X4	T50.8X5	T50.8X6
Sulfobromphthalein	T50.8X1	T50.8X2	T50.8X3	T50.8X4	T50.8X5	T50.8X6
Sulfogaiacol	T48.4X1	T48.4X2	T48.4X3	T48.4X4	T48.4X5	T48.4X6
Sulfomyxin	T36.8X1	T36.8X2	T36.8X3	T36.8X4	T36.8X5	T36.8X6
Sulfonal	T42.6X1	T42.6X2	T42.6X3	T42.6X4	T42.6X5	T42.6X6
Sulfonamide NEC	T37.0X1	T37.0X2	T37.0X3	T37.0X4	T37.0X5	T37.0X6
eye	T49.5X1	T49.5X2	T49.5X3	T49.5X4	T49.5X5	T49.5X6
Sulfonazide	T37.1X1	T37.1X2	T37.1X3	T37.1X4	T37.1X5	T37.1X6
Sulfones	T37.1X1	T37.1X2	T37.1X3	T37.1X4	T37.1X5	T37.1X6
Sulfonethylmethane	T42.6X1	T42.6X2	T42.6X3	T42.6X4	T42.6X5	T42.6X6
Sulfonmethane	T42.6X1	T42.6X2	T42.6X3	T42.6X4	T42.6X5	T42.6X6
Sulfonphthal, sulfonphthol	T50.8X1	T50.8X2	T50.8X3	T50.8X4	T50.8X5	T50.8X6
Sulfonylurea derivatives, oral	T38.3X1	T38.3X2	T38.3X3	T38.3X4	T38.3X5	T38.3X6
Sulforidazine	T43.3X1	T43.3X2	T43.3X3	T43.3X4	T43.3X5	T43.3X6
Sulfoxone	T37.1X1	T37.1X2	T37.1X3	T37.1X4	T37.1X5	T37.1X6
Sulfuric acid	T54.2X1	T54.2X2	T54.2X3	T54.2X4	—	—
Sulfur, sulfurated, sulfuric, sulfurous, sulfuryl (compounds NEC) (medicinal)	T49.4X1	T49.4X2	T49.4X3	T49.4X4	T49.4X5	T49.4X6
acid	T54.2X1	T54.2X2	T54.2X3	T54.2X4	—	—
dioxide (gas)	T59.1X1	T59.1X2	T59.1X3	T59.1X4	—	—
ether — see Ether(s)						
hydrogen	T59.6X1	T59.6X2	T59.6X3	T59.6X4	—	—
medicinal (keratolytic) (ointment) NEC	T49.4X1	T49.4X2	T49.4X3	T49.4X4	T49.4X5	T49.4X6
ointment	T49.0X1	T49.0X2	T49.0X3	T49.0X4	T49.0X5	T49.0X6
pesticide (vapor)	T60.91	T60.92	T60.93	T60.94	—	—
vapor NEC	T59.891	T59.892	T59.893	T59.894	—	—
Sulglicotide	T47.1X1	T47.1X2	T47.1X3	T47.1X4	T47.1X5	T47.1X6
Sulindac	T39.391	T39.392	T39.393	T39.394	T39.395	T39.396
Sulisatin	T47.2X1	T47.2X2	T47.2X3	T47.2X4	T47.2X5	T47.2X6
Sulisobenzone	T49.3X1	T49.3X2	T49.3X3	T49.3X4	T49.3X5	T49.3X6
Sulkowitch's reagent	T50.8X1	T50.8X2	T50.8X3	T50.8X4	T50.8X5	T50.8X6
Sulmetozine	T44.3X1	T44.3X2	T44.3X3	T44.3X4	T44.3X5	T44.3X6
Suloctidil	T46.7X1	T46.7X2	T46.7X3	T46.7X4	T46.7X5	T46.7X6
Sulph- — see also Sulf-						
Sulphadiazine	T37.0X1	T37.0X2	T37.0X3	T37.0X4	T37.0X5	T37.0X6
Sulphadimethoxine	T37.0X1	T37.0X2	T37.0X3	T37.0X4	T37.0X5	T37.0X6
Sulphadimidine	T37.0X1	T37.0X2	T37.0X3	T37.0X4	T37.0X5	T37.0X6
Sulphadione	T37.1X1	T37.1X2	T37.1X3	T37.1X4	T37.1X5	T37.1X6
Sulphafurazole	T37.0X1	T37.0X2	T37.0X3	T37.0X4	T37.0X5	T37.0X6
Sulphamethizole	T37.0X1	T37.0X2	T37.0X3	T37.0X4	T37.0X5	T37.0X6
Sulphamethoxazole	T37.0X1	T37.0X2	T37.0X3	T37.0X4	T37.0X5	T37.0X6
Sulphan blue	T50.8X1	T50.8X2	T50.8X3	T50.8X4	T50.8X5	T50.8X6
Sulphaphenazole	T37.0X1	T37.0X2	T37.0X3	T37.0X4	T37.0X5	T37.0X6
Sulphapyridine	T37.0X1	T37.0X2	T37.0X3	T37.0X4	T37.0X5	T37.0X6
Sulphasalazine	T37.0X1	T37.0X2	T37.0X3	T37.0X4	T37.0X5	T37.0X6
Sulphinpyrazone	T50.4X1	T50.4X2	T50.4X3	T50.4X4	T50.4X5	T50.4X6
Sulpiride	T43.591	T43.592	T43.593	T43.594	T43.595	T43.596
Sulprostone	T48.0X1	T48.0X2	T48.0X3	T48.0X4	T48.0X5	T48.0X6

☑ Additional Character May Be Required — Refer to the Tabular List for Character Selection

*Optum Value-Add

Substance	Poisoning, Accidental (unintentional)	Poisoning, Intentional Self-harm	Poisoning, Assault	Poisoning, Undetermined	Adverse Effect	Under-dosing
Sulpyrine	T39.2X1	T39.2X2	T39.2X3	T39.2X4	T39.2X5	T39.2X6
Sultamicillin	T36.0X1	T36.0X2	T36.0X3	T36.0X4	T36.0X5	T36.0X6
Sulthiame	T42.6X1	T42.6X2	T42.6X3	T42.6X4	T42.6X5	T42.6X6
Sultiame	T42.6X1	T42.6X2	T42.6X3	T42.6X4	T42.6X5	T42.6X6
Sultopride	T43.591	T43.592	T43.593	T43.594	T43.595	T43.596
Sumatriptan	T39.8X1	T39.8X2	T39.8X3	T39.8X4	T39.8X5	T39.8X6
Sumavel*	T39.8X1	T39.8X2	T39.8X3	T39.8X4	T39.8X5	T39.8X6
Sunflower seed oil	T46.6X1	T46.6X2	T46.6X3	T46.6X4	T46.6X5	T46.6X6
Superinone	T48.4X1	T48.4X2	T48.4X3	T48.4X4	T48.4X5	T48.4X6
Suprofen	T39.311	T39.312	T39.313	T39.314	T39.315	T39.316
Suramin (sodium)	T37.4X1	T37.4X2	T37.4X3	T37.4X4	T37.4X5	T37.4X6
Surfacaine	T41.3X1	T41.3X2	T41.3X3	T41.3X4	T41.3X5	T41.3X6
Surital	T41.1X1	T41.1X2	T41.1X3	T41.1X4	T41.1X5	T41.1X6
Sutilains	T45.3X1	T45.3X2	T45.3X3	T45.3X4	T45.3X5	T45.3X6
Suxamethonium (chloride)	T48.1X1	T48.1X2	T48.1X3	T48.1X4	T48.1X5	T48.1X6
Suxethonium (chloride)	T48.1X1	T48.1X2	T48.1X3	T48.1X4	T48.1X5	T48.1X6
Suxibuzone	T39.2X1	T39.2X2	T39.2X3	T39.2X4	T39.2X5	T39.2X6
Sweetener	T50.901	T50.902	T50.903	T50.904	T50.905	T50.906
Sweet niter spirit	T46.3X1	T46.3X2	T46.3X3	T46.3X4	T46.3X5	T46.3X6
Sweet oil (birch)	T49.3X1	T49.3X2	T49.3X3	T49.3X4	T49.3X5	T49.3X6
Sylvant*	T45.1X1	T45.1X2	T45.1X3	T45.1X4	T45.1X5	T45.1X6
Sym-dichloroethyl ether	T53.6X1	T53.6X2	T53.6X3	T53.6X4	—	—
Sympatholytic NEC	T44.8X1	T44.8X2	T44.8X3	T44.8X4	T44.8X5	T44.8X6
haloalkylamine	T44.8X1	T44.8X2	T44.8X3	T44.8X4	T44.8X5	T44.8X6
Sympathomimetic NEC	T44.901	T44.902	T44.903	T44.904	T44.905	T44.906
anti-common-cold	T48.5X1	T48.5X2	T48.5X3	T48.5X4	T48.5X5	T48.5X6
bronchodilator	T48.6X1	T48.6X2	T48.6X3	T48.6X4	T48.6X5	T48.6X6
specified NEC	T44.991	T44.992	T44.993	T44.994	T44.995	T44.996
Synagis	T50.B91	T50.B92	T50.B93	T50.B94	T50.B95	T50.B96
Synalar	T49.0X1	T49.0X2	T49.0X3	T49.0X4	T49.0X5	T49.0X6
Synthetic cannabinoids	T40.721	T40.722	T40.723	T40.724	T40.725	T40.726
Synthroid	T38.1X1	T38.1X2	T38.1X3	T38.1X4	T38.1X5	T38.1X6
Syntocinon	T48.0X1	T48.0X2	T48.0X3	T48.0X4	T48.0X5	T48.0X6
Syrosingopine	T46.5X1	T46.5X2	T46.5X3	T46.5X4	T46.5X5	T46.5X6
Systemic drug	T45.91	T45.92	T45.93	T45.94	T45.95	T45.96
specified NEC	T45.8X1	T45.8X2	T45.8X3	T45.8X4	T45.8X5	T45.8X6
Tablets — see also specified substance	T50.901	T50.902	T50.903	T50.904	T50.905	T50.906
Tace	T38.5X1	T38.5X2	T38.5X3	T38.5X4	T38.5X5	T38.5X6
Tacrine	T44.0X1	T44.0X2	T44.0X3	T44.0X4	T44.0X5	T44.0X6
Tadalafil	T46.7X1	T46.7X2	T46.7X3	T46.7X4	T46.7X5	T46.7X6
Talampicillin	T36.0X1	T36.0X2	T36.0X3	T36.0X4	T36.0X5	T36.0X6
Talbutal	T42.3X1	T42.3X2	T42.3X3	T42.3X4	T42.3X5	T42.3X6
Talc powder	T49.3X1	T49.3X2	T49.3X3	T49.3X4	T49.3X5	T49.3X6
Talcum	T49.3X1	T49.3X2	T49.3X3	T49.3X4	T49.3X5	T49.3X6
Taleranol	T38.6X1	T38.6X2	T38.6X3	T38.6X4	T38.6X5	T38.6X6
Taltz*	T39.391	T39.392	T39.393	T39.394	T39.395	T39.396
Tamoxifen	T38.6X1	T38.6X2	T38.6X3	T38.6X4	T38.6X5	T38.6X6
Tamsulosin	T44.6X1	T44.6X2	T44.6X3	T44.6X4	T44.6X5	T44.6X6
Tandearil, tanderil	T39.2X1	T39.2X2	T39.2X3	T39.2X4	T39.2X5	T39.2X6
Tannic acid	T49.2X1	T49.2X2	T49.2X3	T49.2X4	T49.2X5	T49.2X6
medicinal (astringent)	T49.2X1	T49.2X2	T49.2X3	T49.2X4	T49.2X5	T49.2X6
Tannin — see Tannic acid						
Tansy	T62.2X1	T62.2X2	T62.2X3	T62.2X4	—	—
TAO	T36.3X1	T36.3X2	T36.3X3	T36.3X4	T36.3X5	T36.3X6
Tapazole	T38.2X1	T38.2X2	T38.2X3	T38.2X4	T38.2X5	T38.2X6
Taractan	T43.591	T43.592	T43.593	T43.594	T43.595	T43.596
Tarantula (venomous)	T63.321	T63.322	T63.323	T63.324	—	—
Tartar emetic	T37.8X1	T37.8X2	T37.8X3	T37.8X4	T37.8X5	T37.8X6
Tartaric acid	T65.891	T65.892	T65.893	T65.894	—	—
Tartrated antimony	T37.8X1	T37.8X2	T37.8X3	T37.8X4	T37.8X5	T37.8X6
(anti-infective)						
Tartrate, laxative	T47.4X1	T47.4X2	T47.4X3	T47.4X4	T47.4X5	T47.4X6
Tar NEC	T52.0X1	T52.0X2	T52.0X3	T52.0X4	—	—
camphor	T60.1X1	T60.1X2	T60.1X3	T60.1X4	—	—
distillate	T49.1X1	T49.1X2	T49.1X3	T49.1X4	T49.1X5	T49.1X6
fumes	T59.891	T59.892	T59.893	T59.894	—	—
medicinal	T49.1X1	T49.1X2	T49.1X3	T49.1X4	T49.1X5	T49.1X6
ointment	T49.1X1	T49.1X2	T49.1X3	T49.1X4	T49.1X5	T49.1X6
Tauromustine	T45.1X1	T45.1X2	T45.1X3	T45.1X4	T45.1X5	T45.1X6
TCA — see Trichloroacetic acid						
TCDD	T53.7X1	T53.7X2	T53.7X3	T53.7X4	—	—
TDI (vapor)	T65.0X1	T65.0X2	T65.0X3	T65.0X4	—	—
Tear						
gas	T59.3X1	T59.3X2	T59.3X3	T59.3X4	—	—
solution	T49.5X1	T49.5X2	T49.5X3	T49.5X4	T49.5X5	T49.5X6
Tecentriq*	T45.1X1	T45.1X2	T45.1X3	T45.1X4	T45.1X5	T45.1X6
Teclothiazide	T50.2X1	T50.2X2	T50.2X3	T50.2X4	T50.2X5	T50.2X6
Teclozan	T37.3X1	T37.3X2	T37.3X3	T37.3X4	T37.3X5	T37.3X6
Tegafur	T45.1X1	T45.1X2	T45.1X3	T45.1X4	T45.1X5	T45.1X6
Tegretol	T42.1X1	T42.1X2	T42.1X3	T42.1X4	T42.1X5	T42.1X6
Teicoplanin	T36.8X1	T36.8X2	T36.8X3	T36.8X4	T36.8X5	T36.8X6
Telepaque	T50.8X1	T50.8X2	T50.8X3	T50.8X4	T50.8X5	T50.8X6
Tellurium	T56.891	T56.892	T56.893	T56.894	—	—
fumes	T56.891	T56.892	T56.893	T56.894	—	—
TEM	T45.1X1	T45.1X2	T45.1X3	T45.1X4	T45.1X5	T45.1X6
Temazepam	T42.4X1	T42.4X2	T42.4X3	T42.4X4	T42.4X5	T42.4X6
Temocillin	T36.0X1	T36.0X2	T36.0X3	T36.0X4	T36.0X5	T36.0X6
Tenamfetamine	T43.621	T43.622	T43.623	T43.624	T43.625	T43.626
Tenecteplase*	T45.611	T45.612	T45.613	T45.614	T45.615	T45.616
Teniposide	T45.1X1	T45.1X2	T45.1X3	T45.1X4	T45.1X5	T45.1X6
Tenitramine	T46.3X1	T46.3X2	T46.3X3	T46.3X4	T46.3X5	T46.3X6
Tenoglicin	T48.4X1	T48.4X2	T48.4X3	T48.4X4	T48.4X5	T48.4X6
Tenonitrozole	T37.3X1	T37.3X2	T37.3X3	T37.3X4	T37.3X5	T37.3X6
Tenoxicam	T39.391	T39.392	T39.393	T39.394	T39.395	T39.396
TEPA	T45.1X1	T45.1X2	T45.1X3	T45.1X4	T45.1X5	T45.1X6
TEPP	T60.0X1	T60.0X2	T60.0X3	T60.0X4	—	—
Teprotide	T46.5X1	T46.5X2	T46.5X3	T46.5X4	T46.5X5	T46.5X6
Terazosin	T44.6X1	T44.6X2	T44.6X3	T44.6X4	T44.6X5	T44.6X6
Terbufos	T60.0X1	T60.0X2	T60.0X3	T60.0X4	—	—
Terbutaline	T48.6X1	T48.6X2	T48.6X3	T48.6X4	T48.6X5	T48.6X6
Terconazole	T49.0X1	T49.0X2	T49.0X3	T49.0X4	T49.0X5	T49.0X6
Terfenadine	T45.0X1	T45.0X2	T45.0X3	T45.0X4	T45.0X5	T45.0X6
Teriparatide (acetate)	T50.991	T50.992	T50.993	T50.994	T50.995	T50.996
Terizidone	T37.1X1	T37.1X2	T37.1X3	T37.1X4	T37.1X5	T37.1X6
Terlipressin	T38.891	T38.892	T38.893	T38.894	T38.895	T38.896
Terodiline	T46.3X1	T46.3X2	T46.3X3	T46.3X4	T46.3X5	T46.3X6
Teroxalene	T37.4X1	T37.4X2	T37.4X3	T37.4X4	T37.4X5	T37.4X6
Terpin (cis) **hydrate**	T48.4X1	T48.4X2	T48.4X3	T48.4X4	T48.4X5	T48.4X6
Terramycin	T36.4X1	T36.4X2	T36.4X3	T36.4X4	T36.4X5	T36.4X6
Tertatolol	T44.7X1	T44.7X2	T44.7X3	T44.7X4	T44.7X5	T44.7X6
Tessalon	T48.3X1	T48.3X2	T48.3X3	T48.3X4	T48.3X5	T48.3X6
Testolactone	T38.7X1	T38.7X2	T38.7X3	T38.7X4	T38.7X5	T38.7X6
Testosterone	T38.7X1	T38.7X2	T38.7X3	T38.7X4	T38.7X5	T38.7X6
Tetanus toxoid or vaccine	T50.A91	T50.A92	T50.A93	T50.A94	T50.A95	T50.A96
antitoxin	T50.Z11	T50.Z12	T50.Z13	T50.Z14	T50.Z15	T50.Z16
immune globulin (human)	T50.Z11	T50.Z12	T50.Z13	T50.Z14	T50.Z15	T50.Z16
toxoid	T50.A91	T50.A92	T50.A93	T50.A94	T50.A95	T50.A96
with diphtheria toxoid	T50.A21	T50.A22	T50.A23	T50.A24	T50.A25	T50.A26
with pertussis	T50.A11	T50.A12	T50.A13	T50.A14	T50.A15	T50.A16
Tetrabenazine	T43.591	T43.592	T43.593	T43.594	T43.595	T43.596
Tetracaine	T41.3X1	T41.3X2	T41.3X3	T41.3X4	T41.3X5	T41.3X6
nerve block (peripheral) (plexus)	T41.3X1	T41.3X2	T41.3X3	T41.3X4	T41.3X5	T41.3X6
regional	T41.3X1	T41.3X2	T41.3X3	T41.3X4	T41.3X5	T41.3X6
spinal	T41.3X1	T41.3X2	T41.3X3	T41.3X4	T41.3X5	T41.3X6
Tetrachlorethylene — see Tetrachloroethylene						
Tetrachlormethiazide	T50.2X1	T50.2X2	T50.2X3	T50.2X4	T50.2X5	T50.2X6
Tetrachloroethane	T53.6X1	T53.6X2	T53.6X3	T53.6X4	—	—
vapor	T53.6X1	T53.6X2	T53.6X3	T53.6X4	—	—
paint or varnish	T53.6X1	T53.6X2	T53.6X3	T53.6X4	—	—
Tetrachloroethylene (liquid)	T53.3X1	T53.3X2	T53.3X3	T53.3X4	—	—
medicinal	T37.4X1	T37.4X2	T37.4X3	T37.4X4	T37.4X5	T37.4X6
vapor	T53.3X1	T53.3X2	T53.3X3	T53.3X4	—	—
Tetrachloromethane — see Carbon tetrachloride						
Tetracosactide	T38.811	T38.812	T38.813	T38.814	T38.815	T38.816
Tetracosactrin	T38.811	T38.812	T38.813	T38.814	T38.815	T38.816
Tetracycline	T36.4X1	T36.4X2	T36.4X3	T36.4X4	T36.4X5	T36.4X6
ophthalmic preparation	T49.5X1	T49.5X2	T49.5X3	T49.5X4	T49.5X5	T49.5X6
topical NEC	T49.0X1	T49.0X2	T49.0X3	T49.0X4	T49.0X5	T49.0X6
Tetradifon	T60.8X1	T60.8X2	T60.8X3	T60.8X4	—	—
Tetradotoxin	T61.771	T61.772	T61.773	T61.774	—	—
Tetraethyl						
lead	T56.0X1	T56.0X2	T56.0X3	T56.0X4	—	—
pyrophosphate	T60.0X1	T60.0X2	T60.0X3	T60.0X4	—	—
Tetraethylammonium chloride	T44.2X1	T44.2X2	T44.2X3	T44.2X4	T44.2X5	T44.2X6
Tetraethylthiuram disulfide	T50.6X1	T50.6X2	T50.6X3	T50.6X4	T50.6X5	T50.6X6
Tetrahydroaminoacridine	T44.0X1	T44.0X2	T44.0X3	T44.0X4	T44.0X5	T44.0X6
Tetrahydrocannabinol	T40.711	T40.712	T40.713	T40.714	T40.715	T40.716
Tetrahydrofuran	T52.8X1	T52.8X2	T52.8X3	T52.8X4	—	—
Tetrahydrolipstatin*	T47.8X1	T47.8X2	T47.8X3	T47.8X4	T47.8X5	T47.8X6
Tetrahydronaphthalene	T52.8X1	T52.8X2	T52.8X3	T52.8X4	—	—
Tetrahydrozoline	T49.5X1	T49.5X2	T49.5X3	T49.5X4	T49.5X5	T49.5X6
Tetralin	T52.8X1	T52.8X2	T52.8X3	T52.8X4	—	—
Tetramethrin	T60.2X1	T60.2X2	T60.2X3	T60.2X4	—	—
Tetramethylthiuram (disulfide) **NEC**	T60.3X1	T60.3X2	T60.3X3	T60.3X4	—	—
medicinal	T49.0X1	T49.0X2	T49.0X3	T49.0X4	T49.0X5	T49.0X6
Tetramisole	T37.4X1	T37.4X2	T37.4X3	T37.4X4	T37.4X5	T37.4X6
Tetranicotinoyl fructose	T46.7X1	T46.7X2	T46.7X3	T46.7X4	T46.7X5	T46.7X6
Tetrazepam	T42.4X1	T42.4X2	T42.4X3	T42.4X4	T42.4X5	T42.4X6

Substance	Poisoning, Accidental (unintentional)	Poisoning, Intentional Self-harm	Poisoning, Assault	Poisoning, Undetermined	Adverse Effect	Under-dosing
Tetronal	T42.6X1	T42.6X2	T42.6X3	T42.6X4	T42.6X5	T42.6X6
Tetryl	T65.3X1	T65.3X2	T65.3X3	T65.3X4	—	—
Tetrylammonium chloride	T44.2X1	T44.2X2	T44.2X3	T44.2X4	T44.2X5	T44.2X6
Tetryzoline	T49.5X1	T49.5X2	T49.5X3	T49.5X4	T49.5X5	T49.5X6
Thalidomide	T45.1X1	T45.1X2	T45.1X3	T45.1X4	T45.1X5	T45.1X6
Thallium (compounds) (dust) **NEC**	T56.811	T56.812	T56.813	T56.814	—	—
pesticide	T60.4X1	T60.4X2	T60.4X3	T60.4X4	—	—
THC	T40.711	T40.712	T40.713	T40.714	T40.715	T40.716
Thebacon	T48.3X1	T48.3X2	T48.3X3	T48.3X4	T48.3X5	T48.3X6
Thebaine	T40.2X1	T40.2X2	T40.2X3	T40.2X4	T40.2X5	T40.2X6
Thenoic acid	T49.6X1	T49.6X2	T49.6X3	T49.6X4	T49.6X5	T49.6X6
Thenyldiamine	T45.0X1	T45.0X2	T45.0X3	T45.0X4	T45.0X5	T45.0X6
Theobromine (calcium salicylate)	T48.6X1	T48.6X2	T48.6X3	T48.6X4	T48.6X5	T48.6X6
sodium salicylate	T48.6X1	T48.6X2	T48.6X3	T48.6X4	T48.6X5	T48.6X6
Theolair*	T48.6X1	T48.6X2	T48.6X3	T48.6X4	T48.6X5	T48.6X6
Theophyllamine	T48.6X1	T48.6X2	T48.6X3	T48.6X4	T48.6X5	T48.6X6
Theophylline	T48.6X1	T48.6X2	T48.6X3	T48.6X4	T48.6X5	T48.6X6
aminobenzoic acid	T48.6X1	T48.6X2	T48.6X3	T48.6X4	T48.6X5	T48.6X6
ethylenediamine	T48.6X1	T48.6X2	T48.6X3	T48.6X4	T48.6X5	T48.6X6
piperazine	T48.6X1	T48.6X2	T48.6X3	T48.6X4	T48.6X5	T48.6X6
p-amino-benzoate						
Therevac*	T47.4X1	T47.4X2	T47.4X3	T47.4X4	T47.4X5	T47.4X6
Thiabendazole	T37.4X1	T37.4X2	T37.4X3	T37.4X4	T37.4X5	T37.4X6
Thialbarbital	T41.1X1	T41.1X2	T41.1X3	T41.1X4	T41.1X5	T41.1X6
Thiamazole	T38.2X1	T38.2X2	T38.2X3	T38.2X4	T38.2X5	T38.2X6
Thiambutosine	T37.1X1	T37.1X2	T37.1X3	T37.1X4	T37.1X5	T37.1X6
Thiamine	T45.2X1	T45.2X2	T45.2X3	T45.2X4	T45.2X5	T45.2X6
Thiamphenicol	T36.2X1	T36.2X2	T36.2X3	T36.2X4	T36.2X5	T36.2X6
Thiamylal	T41.1X1	T41.1X2	T41.1X3	T41.1X4	T41.1X5	T41.1X6
sodium	T41.1X1	T41.1X2	T41.1X3	T41.1X4	T41.1X5	T41.1X6
Thiazesim	T43.291	T43.292	T43.293	T43.294	T43.295	T43.296
Thiazides (diuretics)	T50.2X1	T50.2X2	T50.2X3	T50.2X4	T50.2X5	T50.2X6
Thiazinamium metilsulfate	T43.3X1	T43.3X2	T43.3X3	T43.3X4	T43.3X5	T43.3X6
Thiethylperazine	T43.3X1	T43.3X2	T43.3X3	T43.3X4	T43.3X5	T43.3X6
Thimerosal	T49.0X1	T49.0X2	T49.0X3	T49.0X4	T49.0X5	T49.0X6
ophthalmic preparation	T49.5X1	T49.5X2	T49.5X3	T49.5X4	T49.5X5	T49.5X6
Thioacetazone	T37.1X1	T37.1X2	T37.1X3	T37.1X4	T37.1X5	T37.1X6
with isoniazid	T37.1X1	T37.1X2	T37.1X3	T37.1X4	T37.1X5	T37.1X6
Thiobarbital sodium	T41.1X1	T41.1X2	T41.1X3	T41.1X4	T41.1X5	T41.1X6
Thiobarbiturate anesthetic	T41.1X1	T41.1X2	T41.1X3	T41.1X4	T41.1X5	T41.1X6
Thiobismol	T37.8X1	T37.8X2	T37.8X3	T37.8X4	T37.8X5	T37.8X6
Thiobutabarbital sodium	T41.1X1	T41.1X2	T41.1X3	T41.1X4	T41.1X5	T41.1X6
Thiocarbamate (insecticide)	T60.0X1	T60.0X2	T60.0X3	T60.0X4	—	—
Thiocarbamide	T38.2X1	T38.2X2	T38.2X3	T38.2X4	T38.2X5	T38.2X6
Thiocarbarsone	T37.8X1	T37.8X2	T37.8X3	T37.8X4	T37.8X5	T37.8X6
Thiocarlide	T37.1X1	T37.1X2	T37.1X3	T37.1X4	T37.1X5	T37.1X6
Thioctamide	T50.991	T50.992	T50.993	T50.994	T50.995	T50.996
Thioctic acid	T50.991	T50.992	T50.993	T50.994	T50.995	T50.996
Thiofos	T60.0X1	T60.0X2	T60.0X3	T60.0X4	—	—
Thioglycolate	T49.4X1	T49.4X2	T49.4X3	T49.4X4	T49.4X5	T49.4X6
Thioglycolic acid	T65.891	T65.892	T65.893	T65.894	—	—
Thioguanine	T45.1X1	T45.1X2	T45.1X3	T45.1X4	T45.1X5	T45.1X6
Thiomercaptomerin	T50.2X1	T50.2X2	T50.2X3	T50.2X4	T50.2X5	T50.2X6
Thiomerin	T50.2X1	T50.2X2	T50.2X3	T50.2X4	T50.2X5	T50.2X6
Thiomersal	T49.0X1	T49.0X2	T49.0X3	T49.0X4	T49.0X5	T49.0X6
Thionazin	T60.0X1	T60.0X2	T60.0X3	T60.0X4	—	—
Thiopental (sodium)	T41.1X1	T41.1X2	T41.1X3	T41.1X4	T41.1X5	T41.1X6
Thiopentone (sodium)	T41.1X1	T41.1X2	T41.1X3	T41.1X4	T41.1X5	T41.1X6
Thiopropazate	T43.3X1	T43.3X2	T43.3X3	T43.3X4	T43.3X5	T43.3X6
Thioproperazine	T43.3X1	T43.3X2	T43.3X3	T43.3X4	T43.3X5	T43.3X6
Thioridazine	T43.3X1	T43.3X2	T43.3X3	T43.3X4	T43.3X5	T43.3X6
Thiosinamine	T49.3X1	T49.3X2	T49.3X3	T49.3X4	T49.3X5	T49.3X6
Thiotepa	T45.1X1	T45.1X2	T45.1X3	T45.1X4	T45.1X5	T45.1X6
Thiothixene	T43.4X1	T43.4X2	T43.4X3	T43.4X4	T43.4X5	T43.4X6
Thiouracil (benzyl) (methyl) (propyl)	T38.2X1	T38.2X2	T38.2X3	T38.2X4	T38.2X5	T38.2X6
Thiourea	T38.2X1	T38.2X2	T38.2X3	T38.2X4	T38.2X5	T38.2X6
Thiphenamil	T44.3X1	T44.3X2	T44.3X3	T44.3X4	T44.3X5	T44.3X6
Thiram	T60.3X1	T60.3X2	T60.3X3	T60.3X4	—	—
medicinal	T49.2X1	T49.2X2	T49.2X3	T49.2X4	T49.2X5	T49.2X6
Thonzylamine (systemic)	T45.0X1	T45.0X2	T45.0X3	T45.0X4	T45.0X5	T45.0X6
mucosal decongestant	T48.5X1	T48.5X2	T48.5X3	T48.5X4	T48.5X5	T48.5X6
Thorazine	T43.3X1	T43.3X2	T43.3X3	T43.3X4	T43.3X5	T43.3X6
Thorium dioxide suspension	T50.8X1	T50.8X2	T50.8X3	T50.8X4	T50.8X5	T50.8X6
Thornapple	T62.2X1	T62.2X2	T62.2X3	T62.2X4	—	—
Throat drug NEC	T49.6X1	T49.6X2	T49.6X3	T49.6X4	T49.6X5	T49.6X6
Thrombate 111*	T45.511	T45.512	T45.513	T45.514	T45.515	T45.516

Substance	Poisoning, Accidental (unintentional)	Poisoning, Intentional Self-harm	Poisoning, Assault	Poisoning, Undetermined	Adverse Effect	Under-dosing
Thrombin	T45.7X1	T45.7X2	T45.7X3	T45.7X4	T45.7X5	T45.7X6
Thrombolysin	T45.611	T45.612	T45.613	T45.614	T45.615	T45.616
Thromboplastin	T45.7X1	T45.7X2	T45.7X3	T45.7X4	T45.7X5	T45.7X6
Thurfyl nicotinate	T46.7X1	T46.7X2	T46.7X3	T46.7X4	T46.7X5	T46.7X6
Thymol	T49.0X1	T49.0X2	T49.0X3	T49.0X4	T49.0X5	T49.0X6
Thymopentin	T37.5X1	T37.5X2	T37.5X3	T37.5X4	T37.5X5	T37.5X6
Thymoxamine	T46.7X1	T46.7X2	T46.7X3	T46.7X4	T46.7X5	T46.7X6
Thymus extract	T38.891	T38.892	T38.893	T38.894	T38.895	T38.896
Thyreotrophic hormone	T38.811	T38.812	T38.813	T38.814	T38.815	T38.816
Thyroglobulin	T38.1X1	T38.1X2	T38.1X3	T38.1X4	T38.1X5	T38.1X6
Thyroid (hormone)	T38.1X1	T38.1X2	T38.1X3	T38.1X4	T38.1X5	T38.1X6
Thyrolar	T38.1X1	T38.1X2	T38.1X3	T38.1X4	T38.1X5	T38.1X6
Thyrotrophin	T38.811	T38.812	T38.813	T38.814	T38.815	T38.816
Thyrotropic hormone	T38.811	T38.812	T38.813	T38.814	T38.815	T38.816
Thyroxine	T38.1X1	T38.1X2	T38.1X3	T38.1X4	T38.1X5	T38.1X6
Tiabendazole	T37.4X1	T37.4X2	T37.4X3	T37.4X4	T37.4X5	T37.4X6
Tiamizide	T50.2X1	T50.2X2	T50.2X3	T50.2X4	T50.2X5	T50.2X6
Tianeptine	T43.291	T43.292	T43.293	T43.294	T43.295	T43.296
Tiapamil	T46.1X1	T46.1X2	T46.1X3	T46.1X4	T46.1X5	T46.1X6
Tiapride	T43.591	T43.592	T43.593	T43.594	T43.595	T43.596
Tiaprofenic acid	T39.311	T39.312	T39.313	T39.314	T39.315	T39.316
Tiaramide	T39.8X1	T39.8X2	T39.8X3	T39.8X4	T39.8X5	T39.8X6
Ticagrelor*	T45.521	T45.522	T45.523	T45.524	T45.525	T45.526
Ticarcillin	T36.0X1	T36.0X2	T36.0X3	T36.0X4	T36.0X5	T36.0X6
Ticlatone	T49.0X1	T49.0X2	T49.0X3	T49.0X4	T49.0X5	T49.0X6
Ticlopidine	T45.521	T45.522	T45.523	T45.524	T45.525	T45.526
Ticrynafen	T50.1X1	T50.1X2	T50.1X3	T50.1X4	T50.1X5	T50.1X6
Tidiacic	T50.991	T50.992	T50.993	T50.994	T50.995	T50.996
Tiemonium	T44.3X1	T44.3X2	T44.3X3	T44.3X4	T44.3X5	T44.3X6
iodide	T44.3X1	T44.3X2	T44.3X3	T44.3X4	T44.3X5	T44.3X6
Tienilic acid	T50.1X1	T50.1X2	T50.1X3	T50.1X4	T50.1X5	T50.1X6
Tifenamil	T44.3X1	T44.3X2	T44.3X3	T44.3X4	T44.3X5	T44.3X6
Tigan	T45.0X1	T45.0X2	T45.0X3	T45.0X4	T45.0X5	T45.0X6
Tigloidine	T44.3X1	T44.3X2	T44.3X3	T44.3X4	T44.3X5	T44.3X6
Tilactase	T47.5X1	T47.5X2	T47.5X3	T47.5X4	T47.5X5	T47.5X6
Tiletamine	T41.291	T41.292	T41.293	T41.294	T41.295	T41.296
Tilidine	T40.491	T40.492	T40.493	T40.494	—	—
Timepidium bromide	T44.3X1	T44.3X2	T44.3X3	T44.3X4	T44.3X5	T44.3X6
Timiperone	T43.4X1	T43.4X2	T43.4X3	T43.4X4	T43.4X5	T43.4X6
Timolol	T44.7X1	T44.7X2	T44.7X3	T44.7X4	T44.7X5	T44.7X6
Tincture, iodine — see Iodine						
Tindal	T43.3X1	T43.3X2	T43.3X3	T43.3X4	T43.3X5	T43.3X6
Tinidazole	T37.3X1	T37.3X2	T37.3X3	T37.3X4	T37.3X5	T37.3X6
Tin (chloride) (dust) (oxide) **NEC**	T56.6X1	T56.6X2	T56.6X3	T56.6X4	—	—
anti-infectives	T37.8X1	T37.8X2	T37.8X3	T37.8X4	T37.8X5	T37.8X6
Tinoridine	T39.8X1	T39.8X2	T39.8X3	T39.8X4	T39.8X5	T39.8X6
Tiocarlide	T37.1X1	T37.1X2	T37.1X3	T37.1X4	T37.1X5	T37.1X6
Tioclomarol	T45.511	T45.512	T45.513	T45.514	T45.515	T45.516
Tioconazole	T49.0X1	T49.0X2	T49.0X3	T49.0X4	T49.0X5	T49.0X6
Tioguanine	T45.1X1	T45.1X2	T45.1X3	T45.1X4	T45.1X5	T45.1X6
Tiopronin	T50.991	T50.992	T50.993	T50.994	T50.995	T50.996
Tiotixene	T43.4X1	T43.4X2	T43.4X3	T43.4X4	T43.4X5	T43.4X6
Tioxolone	T49.4X1	T49.4X2	T49.4X3	T49.4X4	T49.4X5	T49.4X6
Tipepidine	T48.3X1	T48.3X2	T48.3X3	T48.3X4	T48.3X5	T48.3X6
Tiquizium bromide	T44.3X1	T44.3X2	T44.3X3	T44.3X4	T44.3X5	T44.3X6
Tiratricol	T38.1X1	T38.1X2	T38.1X3	T38.1X4	T38.1X5	T38.1X6
Tisopurine	T50.4X1	T50.4X2	T50.4X3	T50.4X4	T50.4X5	T50.4X6
Titanium (compounds) (vapor)	T56.891	T56.892	T56.893	T56.894	—	—
dioxide	T49.3X1	T49.3X2	T49.3X3	T49.3X4	T49.3X5	T49.3X6
ointment	T49.3X1	T49.3X2	T49.3X3	T49.3X4	T49.3X5	T49.3X6
oxide	T49.3X1	T49.3X2	T49.3X3	T49.3X4	T49.3X5	T49.3X6
tetrachloride	T56.891	T56.892	T56.893	T56.894	—	—
Titanocene	T56.891	T56.892	T56.893	T56.894	—	—
Titroid	T38.1X1	T38.1X2	T38.1X3	T38.1X4	T38.1X5	T38.1X6
Tizanidine	T42.8X1	T42.8X2	T42.8X3	T42.8X4	T42.8X5	T42.8X6
TMTD	T60.3X1	T60.3X2	T60.3X3	T60.3X4	—	—
TNT (fumes)	T65.3X1	T65.3X2	T65.3X3	T65.3X4	—	—
Toadstool	T62.0X1	T62.0X2	T62.0X3	T62.0X4	—	—
Tobacco NEC	T65.291	T65.292	T65.293	T65.294	—	—
cigarettes	T65.221	T65.222	T65.223	T65.224	—	—
Indian	T62.2X1	T62.2X2	T62.2X3	T62.2X4	—	—
smoke, second-hand	T65.221	T65.222	T65.223	T65.224	—	—
Tobraflex*	T49.5X1	T49.5X2	T49.5X3	T49.5X4	T49.5X5	T49.5X6
Tobramycin	T36.5X1	T36.5X2	T36.5X3	T36.5X4	T36.5X5	T36.5X6
Tocainide	T46.2X1	T46.2X2	T46.2X3	T46.2X4	T46.2X5	T46.2X6
Tocoferol	T45.2X1	T45.2X2	T45.2X3	T45.2X4	T45.2X5	T45.2X6
Tocopherol	T45.2X1	T45.2X2	T45.2X3	T45.2X4	T45.2X5	T45.2X6
acetate	T45.2X1	T45.2X2	T45.2X3	T45.2X4	T45.2X5	T45.2X6
Tocosamine	T48.0X1	T48.0X2	T48.0X3	T48.0X4	T48.0X5	T48.0X6
Todralazine	T46.5X1	T46.5X2	T46.5X3	T46.5X4	T46.5X5	T46.5X6
Tofisopam	T42.4X1	T42.4X2	T42.4X3	T42.4X4	T42.4X5	T42.4X6

☑ Additional Character May Be Required — Refer to the Tabular List for Character Selection

*Optum Value-Add

Substance	Poisoning, Accidental (unintentional)	Poisoning, Intentional Self-harm	Poisoning, Assault	Poisoning, Undetermined	Adverse Effect	Under-dosing
Tofranil	T43.011	T43.012	T43.013	T43.014	T43.015	T43.016
Toilet deodorizer	T65.891	T65.892	T65.893	T65.894	—	—
Tolamolol	T44.7X1	T44.7X2	T44.7X3	T44.7X4	T44.7X5	T44.7X6
Tolazamide	T38.3X1	T38.3X2	T38.3X3	T38.3X4	T38.3X5	T38.3X6
Tolazoline	T46.7X1	T46.7X2	T46.7X3	T46.7X4	T46.7X5	T46.7X6
Tolbutamide (sodium)	T38.3X1	T38.3X2	T38.3X3	T38.3X4	T38.3X5	T38.3X6
Tolciclate	T49.0X1	T49.0X2	T49.0X3	T49.0X4	T49.0X5	T49.0X6
Tolmetin	T39.391	T39.392	T39.393	T39.394	T39.395	T39.396
Tolnaftate	T49.0X1	T49.0X2	T49.0X3	T49.0X4	T49.0X5	T49.0X6
Tolonidine	T46.5X1	T46.5X2	T46.5X3	T46.5X4	T46.5X5	T46.5X6
Toloxatone	T42.6X1	T42.6X2	T42.6X3	T42.6X4	T42.6X5	T42.6X6
Tolperisone	T44.3X1	T44.3X2	T44.3X3	T44.3X4	T44.3X5	T44.3X6
Tolserol	T42.8X1	T42.8X2	T42.8X3	T42.8X4	T42.8X5	T42.8X6
Toluene (liquid)	T52.2X1	T52.2X2	T52.2X3	T52.2X4	—	—
diisocyanate	T65.0X1	T65.0X2	T65.0X3	T65.0X4	—	—
Toluidine	T65.891	T65.892	T65.893	T65.894	—	—
vapor	T59.891	T59.892	T59.893	T59.894	—	—
Toluol (liquid)	T52.2X1	T52.2X2	T52.2X3	T52.2X4	—	—
vapor	T52.2X1	T52.2X2	T52.2X3	T52.2X4	—	—
Toluylenediamine	T65.3X1	T65.3X2	T65.3X3	T65.3X4	—	—
Tolylene-2,4-diisocyanate	T65.0X1	T65.0X2	T65.0X3	T65.0X4	—	—
Tonic NEC	T50.901	T50.902	T50.903	T50.904	T50.905	T50.906
Topical action drug NEC	T49.91	T49.92	T49.93	T49.94	T49.95	T49.96
ear, nose or throat	T49.6X1	T49.6X2	T49.6X3	T49.6X4	T49.6X5	T49.6X6
eye	T49.5X1	T49.5X2	T49.5X3	T49.5X4	T49.5X5	T49.5X6
skin	T49.91	T49.92	T49.93	T49.94	T49.95	T49.96
specified NEC	T49.8X1	T49.8X2	T49.8X3	T49.8X4	T49.8X5	T49.8X6
Toprol*	T44.7X1	T44.7X2	T44.7X3	T44.7X4	T44.7X5	T44.7X6
Toquizine	T44.3X1	T44.3X2	T44.3X3	T44.3X4	T44.3X5	T44.3X6
Toremifene	T38.6X1	T38.6X2	T38.6X3	T38.6X4	T38.6X5	T38.6X6
Tosylchloramide sodium	T49.8X1	T49.8X2	T49.8X3	T49.8X4	T49.8X5	T49.8X6
Toxaphene (dust) (spray)	T60.1X1	T60.1X2	T60.1X3	T60.1X4	—	—
Toxin, diphtheria (Schick Test)	T50.8X1	T50.8X2	T50.8X3	T50.8X4	T50.8X5	T50.8X6
Toxoid						
combined	T50.A21	T50.A22	T50.A23	T50.A24	T50.A25	T50.A26
diphtheria	T50.A91	T50.A92	T50.A93	T50.A94	T50.A95	T50.A96
tetanus	T50.A91	T50.A92	T50.A93	T50.A94	T50.A95	T50.A96
Trace element NEC	T45.8X1	T45.8X2	T45.8X3	T45.8X4	T45.8X5	T45.8X6
Tractor fuel NEC	T52.0X1	T52.0X2	T52.0X3	T52.0X4	—	—
Tragacanth	T50.991	T50.992	T50.993	T50.994	T50.995	T50.996
Tramadol	T40.421	T40.422	T40.423	T40.424	T40.425	T40.426
Tramazoline	T48.5X1	T48.5X2	T48.5X3	T48.5X4	T48.5X5	T48.5X6
Tranexamic acid	T45.621	T45.622	T45.623	T45.624	T45.625	T45.626
Tranilast	T45.0X1	T45.0X2	T45.0X3	T45.0X4	T45.0X5	T45.0X6
Tranquilizer NEC	T43.501	T43.502	T43.503	T43.504	T43.505	T43.506
with hypnotic or sedative	T42.6X1	T42.6X2	T42.6X3	T42.6X4	T42.6X5	T42.6X6
benzodiazepine NEC	T42.4X1	T42.4X2	T42.4X3	T42.4X4	T42.4X5	T42.4X6
butyrophenone NEC	T43.4X1	T43.4X2	T43.4X3	T43.4X4	T43.4X5	T43.4X6
carbamate	T43.591	T43.592	T43.593	T43.594	T43.595	T43.596
dimethylamine	T43.3X1	T43.3X2	T43.3X3	T43.3X4	T43.3X5	T43.3X6
ethylamine	T43.3X1	T43.3X2	T43.3X3	T43.3X4	T43.3X5	T43.3X6
hydroxyzine	T43.591	T43.592	T43.593	T43.594	T43.595	T43.596
major NEC	T43.501	T43.502	T43.503	T43.504	T43.505	T43.506
penothiazine NEC	T43.3X1	T43.3X2	T43.3X3	T43.3X4	T43.3X5	T43.3X6
phenothiazine-based	T43.3X1	T43.3X2	T43.3X3	T43.3X4	T43.3X5	T43.3X6
piperazine NEC	T43.3X1	T43.3X2	T43.3X3	T43.3X4	T43.3X5	T43.3X6
piperidine	T43.3X1	T43.3X2	T43.3X3	T43.3X4	T43.3X5	T43.3X6
propylamine	T43.3X1	T43.3X2	T43.3X3	T43.3X4	T43.3X5	T43.3X6
specified NEC	T43.591	T43.592	T43.593	T43.594	T43.595	T43.596
thioxanthene NEC	T43.591	T43.592	T43.593	T43.594	T43.595	T43.596
Tranxene	T42.4X1	T42.4X2	T42.4X3	T42.4X4	T42.4X5	T42.4X6
Tranylcypromine	T43.1X1	T43.1X2	T43.1X3	T43.1X4	T43.1X5	T43.1X6
Trapidil	T46.3X1	T46.3X2	T46.3X3	T46.3X4	T46.3X5	T46.3X6
Trasentine	T44.3X1	T44.3X2	T44.3X3	T44.3X4	T44.3X5	T44.3X6
Travert	T50.3X1	T50.3X2	T50.3X3	T50.3X4	T50.3X5	T50.3X6
Trazodone	T43.211	T43.212	T43.213	T43.214	T43.215	T43.216
Treanda*	T45.1X1	T45.1X2	T45.1X3	T45.1X4	T45.1X5	T45.1X6
Trecator	T37.1X1	T37.1X2	T37.1X3	T37.1X4	T37.1X5	T37.1X6
Treosulfan	T45.1X1	T45.1X2	T45.1X3	T45.1X4	T45.1X5	T45.1X6
Tretamine	T45.1X1	T45.1X2	T45.1X3	T45.1X4	T45.1X5	T45.1X6
Tretinoin	T49.0X1	T49.0X2	T49.0X3	T49.0X4	T49.0X5	T49.0X6
Tretoquinol	T48.6X1	T48.6X2	T48.6X3	T48.6X4	T48.6X5	T48.6X6
Triacetin	T49.0X1	T49.0X2	T49.0X3	T49.0X4	T49.0X5	T49.0X6
Triacetoxyanthracene	T49.4X1	T49.4X2	T49.4X3	T49.4X4	T49.4X5	T49.4X6
Triacetyloleandomycin	T36.3X1	T36.3X2	T36.3X3	T36.3X4	T36.3X5	T36.3X6
Triamcinolone	T38.0X1	T38.0X2	T38.0X3	T38.0X4	T38.0X5	T38.0X6
ENT agent	T49.6X1	T49.6X2	T49.6X3	T49.6X4	T49.6X5	T49.6X6
hexacetonide	T49.0X1	T49.0X2	T49.0X3	T49.0X4	T49.0X5	T49.0X6
ophthalmic preparation	T49.5X1	T49.5X2	T49.5X3	T49.5X4	T49.5X5	T49.5X6
topical NEC	T49.0X1	T49.0X2	T49.0X3	T49.0X4	T49.0X5	T49.0X6
Triampyzine	T44.3X1	T44.3X2	T44.3X3	T44.3X4	T44.3X5	T44.3X6
Triamterene	T50.2X1	T50.2X2	T50.2X3	T50.2X4	T50.2X5	T50.2X6
Triazine (herbicide)	T60.3X1	T60.3X2	T60.3X3	T60.3X4	—	—
Triaziquone	T45.1X1	T45.1X2	T45.1X3	T45.1X4	T45.1X5	T45.1X6
Triazolam	T42.4X1	T42.4X2	T42.4X3	T42.4X4	T42.4X5	T42.4X6
Triazole (herbicide)	T60.3X1	T60.3X2	T60.3X3	T60.3X4	—	—
Tribavirin*	T37.5X1	T37.5X2	T37.5X3	T37.5X4	T37.5X5	T37.5X6
Tribenoside	T46.991	T46.992	T46.993	T46.994	T46.995	T46.996
Tribromacetaldehyde	T42.6X1	T42.6X2	T42.6X3	T42.6X4	T42.6X5	T42.6X6
Tribromoethanol, rectal	T41.291	T41.292	T41.293	T41.294	T41.295	T41.296
Tribromomethane	T42.6X1	T42.6X2	T42.6X3	T42.6X4	T42.6X5	T42.6X6
Trichlorethane	T53.2X1	T53.2X2	T53.2X3	T53.2X4	—	—
Trichlorethylene	T53.2X1	T53.2X2	T53.2X3	T53.2X4	—	—
Trichlorfon	T60.0X1	T60.0X2	T60.0X3	T60.0X4	—	—
Trichlormethiazide	T50.2X1	T50.2X2	T50.2X3	T50.2X4	T50.2X5	T50.2X6
Trichlormethine	T45.1X1	T45.1X2	T45.1X3	T45.1X4	T45.1X5	T45.1X6
Trichloroacetic acid, Trichloracetic acid	T54.2X1	T54.2X2	T54.2X3	T54.2X4		
medicinal	T49.4X1	T49.4X2	T49.4X3	T49.4X4	T49.4X5	T49.4X6
Trichloroethane	T53.2X1	T53.2X2	T53.2X3	T53.2X4	—	—
Trichloroethanol	T42.6X1	T42.6X2	T42.6X3	T42.6X4	T42.6X5	T42.6X6
Trichloroethylene (liquid) (vapor)	T53.2X1	T53.2X2	T53.2X3	T53.2X4	—	—
anesthetic (gas)	T41.0X1	T41.0X2	T41.0X3	T41.0X4	T41.0X5	T41.0X6
vapor NEC	T53.2X1	T53.2X2	T53.2X3	T53.2X4	—	—
Trichloroethyl phosphate	T42.6X1	T42.6X2	T42.6X3	T42.6X4	T42.6X5	T42.6X6
Trichlorofluoromethane NEC	T53.5X1	T53.5X2	T53.5X3	T53.5X4	—	—
Trichloronate	T60.0X1	T60.0X2	T60.0X3	T60.0X4	—	—
Trichloropropane	T53.6X1	T53.6X2	T53.6X3	T53.6X4	—	—
Trichlorotriethylamine	T45.1X1	T45.1X2	T45.1X3	T45.1X4	T45.1X5	T45.1X6
Trichomonacides NEC	T37.3X1	T37.3X2	T37.3X3	T37.3X4	T37.3X5	T37.3X6
Trichomycin	T36.7X1	T36.7X2	T36.7X3	T36.7X4	T36.7X5	T36.7X6
Triclobisonium chloride	T49.0X1	T49.0X2	T49.0X3	T49.0X4	T49.0X5	T49.0X6
Triclocarban	T49.0X1	T49.0X2	T49.0X3	T49.0X4	T49.0X5	T49.0X6
Triclofos	T42.6X1	T42.6X2	T42.6X3	T42.6X4	T42.6X5	T42.6X6
Triclosan	T49.0X1	T49.0X2	T49.0X3	T49.0X4	T49.0X5	T49.0X6
Tricosal*	T39.091	T39.092	T39.093	T39.094	T39.095	T39.096
Tricresyl phosphate	T65.891	T65.892	T65.893	T65.894	—	—
solvent	T52.91	T52.92	T52.93	T52.94	—	—
Tricyclamol chloride	T44.3X1	T44.3X2	T44.3X3	T44.3X4	T44.3X5	T44.3X6
Tridesilon	T49.0X1	T49.0X2	T49.0X3	T49.0X4	T49.0X5	T49.0X6
Tridihexethyl iodide	T44.3X1	T44.3X2	T44.3X3	T44.3X4	T44.3X5	T44.3X6
Tridione	T42.2X1	T42.2X2	T42.2X3	T42.2X4	T42.2X5	T42.2X6
Trientine	T45.8X1	T45.8X2	T45.8X3	T45.8X4	T45.8X5	T45.8X6
Triethanolamine NEC	T54.3X1	T54.3X2	T54.3X3	T54.3X4	—	—
detergent	T54.3X1	T54.3X2	T54.3X3	T54.3X4	—	—
trinitrate (biphosphate)	T46.3X1	T46.3X2	T46.3X3	T46.3X4	T46.3X5	T46.3X6
Triethanomelamine	T45.1X1	T45.1X2	T45.1X3	T45.1X4	T45.1X5	T45.1X6
Triethylenemelamine	T45.1X1	T45.1X2	T45.1X3	T45.1X4	T45.1X5	T45.1X6
Triethylenephosphoramide	T45.1X1	T45.1X2	T45.1X3	T45.1X4	T45.1X5	T45.1X6
Triethylenethiophosphoramide	T45.1X1	T45.1X2	T45.1X3	T45.1X4	T45.1X5	T45.1X6
Trifluoperazine	T43.3X1	T43.3X2	T43.3X3	T43.3X4	T43.3X5	T43.3X6
Trifluoroethyl vinyl ether	T41.0X1	T41.0X2	T41.0X3	T41.0X4	T41.0X5	T41.0X6
Trifluperidol	T43.4X1	T43.4X2	T43.4X3	T43.4X4	T43.4X5	T43.4X6
Triflupromazine	T43.3X1	T43.3X2	T43.3X3	T43.3X4	T43.3X5	T43.3X6
Trifluridine	T37.5X1	T37.5X2	T37.5X3	T37.5X4	T37.5X5	T37.5X6
Triflusal	T45.521	T45.522	T45.523	T45.524	T45.525	T45.526
Trihexyphenidyl	T44.3X1	T44.3X2	T44.3X3	T44.3X4	T44.3X5	T44.3X6
Triiodothyronine	T38.1X1	T38.1X2	T38.1X3	T38.1X4	T38.1X5	T38.1X6
Trilene	T41.0X1	T41.0X2	T41.0X3	T41.0X4	T41.0X5	T41.0X6
Trilostane	T38.991	T38.992	T38.993	T38.994	T38.995	T38.996
Trimebutine	T44.3X1	T44.3X2	T44.3X3	T44.3X4	T44.3X5	T44.3X6
Trimecaine	T41.3X1	T41.3X2	T41.3X3	T41.3X4	T41.3X5	T41.3X6
Trimeprazine (tartrate)	T44.3X1	T44.3X2	T44.3X3	T44.3X4	T44.3X5	T44.3X6
Trimetaphan camsilate	T44.2X1	T44.2X2	T44.2X3	T44.2X4	T44.2X5	T44.2X6
Trimetazidine	T46.7X1	T46.7X2	T46.7X3	T46.7X4	T46.7X5	T46.7X6
Trimethadione	T42.2X1	T42.2X2	T42.2X3	T42.2X4	T42.2X5	T42.2X6
Trimethaphan	T44.2X1	T44.2X2	T44.2X3	T44.2X4	T44.2X5	T44.2X6
Trimethidinium	T44.2X1	T44.2X2	T44.2X3	T44.2X4	T44.2X5	T44.2X6
Trimethobenzamide	T45.0X1	T45.0X2	T45.0X3	T45.0X4	T45.0X5	T45.0X6
Trimethoprim	T37.8X1	T37.8X2	T37.8X3	T37.8X4	T37.8X5	T37.8X6
with sulfamethoxazole	T36.8X1	T36.8X2	T36.8X3	T36.8X4	T36.8X5	T36.8X6
Trimethylcarbinol	T51.3X1	T51.3X2	T51.3X3	T51.3X4	—	—
Trimethylpsoralen	T49.3X1	T49.3X2	T49.3X3	T49.3X4	T49.3X5	T49.3X6
Trimeton	T45.0X1	T45.0X2	T45.0X3	T45.0X4	T45.0X5	T45.0X6
Trimetrexate	T45.1X1	T45.1X2	T45.1X3	T45.1X4	T45.1X5	T45.1X6
Trimipramine	T43.011	T43.012	T43.013	T43.014	T43.015	T43.016
Trimox*	T36.0X1	T36.0X2	T36.0X3	T36.0X4	T36.0X5	T36.0X6
Trimustine	T45.1X1	T45.1X2	T45.1X3	T45.1X4	T45.1X5	T45.1X6
Trinitrin	T46.3X1	T46.3X2	T46.3X3	T46.3X4	T46.3X5	T46.3X6
Trinitrobenzol	T65.3X1	T65.3X2	T65.3X3	T65.3X4	—	—
Trinitrophenol	T65.3X1	T65.3X2	T65.3X3	T65.3X4	—	—
Trinitrotoluene (fumes)	T65.3X1	T65.3X2	T65.3X3	T65.3X4	—	—

Table of Drugs and Chemicals

Substance	Poisoning, Accidental (unintentional)	Poisoning, Intentional Self-harm	Poisoning, Assault	Poisoning, Undetermined	Adverse Effect	Under-dosing
Trional	T42.6X1	T42.6X2	T42.6X3	T42.6X4	T42.6X5	T42.6X6
Triorthocresyl phosphate	T65.891	T65.892	T65.893	T65.894	—	—
Trioxide of arsenic	T57.0X1	T57.0X2	T57.0X3	T57.0X4	—	—
Trioxysalen	T49.4X1	T49.4X2	T49.4X3	T49.4X4	T49.4X5	T49.4X6
Tripamide	T50.2X1	T50.2X2	T50.2X3	T50.2X4	T50.2X5	T50.2X6
Triparanol	T46.6X1	T46.6X2	T46.6X3	T46.6X4	T46.6X5	T46.6X6
Tripelennamine	T45.0X1	T45.0X2	T45.0X3	T45.0X4	T45.0X5	T45.0X6
Triperiden	T44.3X1	T44.3X2	T44.3X3	T44.3X4	T44.3X5	T44.3X6
Triperidol	T43.4X1	T43.4X2	T43.4X3	T43.4X4	T43.4X5	T43.4X6
Triphenylphosphate	T65.891	T65.892	T65.893	T65.894	—	—
Triple						
bromides	T42.6X1	T42.6X2	T42.6X3	T42.6X4	T42.6X5	T42.6X6
carbonate	T47.1X1	T47.1X2	T47.1X3	T47.1X4	T47.1X5	T47.1X6
vaccine						
DPT	T50.A11	T50.A12	T50.A13	T50.A14	T50.A15	T50.A16
including pertussis	T50.A11	T50.A12	T50.A13	T50.A14	T50.A15	T50.A16
MMR	T50.B91	T50.B92	T50.B93	T50.B94	T50.B95	T50.B96
Triprolidine	T45.0X1	T45.0X2	T45.0X3	T45.0X4	T45.0X5	T45.0X6
Trisodium hydrogen edetate	T50.6X1	T50.6X2	T50.6X3	T50.6X4	T50.6X5	T50.6X6
Trisoralen	T49.3X1	T49.3X2	T49.3X3	T49.3X4	T49.3X5	T49.3X6
Trisulfapyrimidines	T37.0X1	T37.0X2	T37.0X3	T37.0X4	T37.0X5	T37.0X6
Trithiozine	T44.3X1	T44.3X2	T44.3X3	T44.3X4	T44.3X5	T44.3X6
Tritiozine	T44.3X1	T44.3X2	T44.3X3	T44.3X4	T44.3X5	T44.3X6
Tritoqualine	T45.0X1	T45.0X2	T45.0X3	T45.0X4	T45.0X5	T45.0X6
Trizivir*	T37.5X1	T37.5X2	T37.5X3	T37.5X4	T37.5X5	T37.5X6
Trofosfamide	T45.1X1	T45.1X2	T45.1X3	T45.1X4	T45.1X5	T45.1X6
Troleandomycin	T36.3X1	T36.3X2	T36.3X3	T36.3X4	T36.3X5	T36.3X6
Trolnitrate (phosphate)	T46.3X1	T46.3X2	T46.3X3	T46.3X4	T46.3X5	T46.3X6
Tromantadine	T37.5X1	T37.5X2	T37.5X3	T37.5X4	T37.5X5	T37.5X6
Trometamol	T50.2X1	T50.2X2	T50.2X3	T50.2X4	T50.2X5	T50.2X6
Tromethamine	T50.2X1	T50.2X2	T50.2X3	T50.2X4	T50.2X5	T50.2X6
Tronothane	T41.3X1	T41.3X2	T41.3X3	T41.3X4	T41.3X5	T41.3X6
Tropacine	T44.3X1	T44.3X2	T44.3X3	T44.3X4	T44.3X5	T44.3X6
Tropatepine	T44.3X1	T44.3X2	T44.3X3	T44.3X4	T44.3X5	T44.3X6
Tropicamide	T44.3X1	T44.3X2	T44.3X3	T44.3X4	T44.3X5	T44.3X6
Trospium chloride	T44.3X1	T44.3X2	T44.3X3	T44.3X4	T44.3X5	T44.3X6
Troxerutin	T46.991	T46.992	T46.993	T46.994	T46.995	T46.996
Troxidone	T42.2X1	T42.2X2	T42.2X3	T42.2X4	T42.2X5	T42.2X6
Tryparsamide	T37.3X1	T37.3X2	T37.3X3	T37.3X4	T37.3X5	T37.3X6
Trypsin	T45.3X1	T45.3X2	T45.3X3	T45.3X4	T45.3X5	T45.3X6
Tryptizol	T43.011	T43.012	T43.013	T43.014	T43.015	T43.016
TSH	T38.811	T38.812	T38.813	T38.814	T38.815	T38.816
Tuaminoheptane	T48.5X1	T48.5X2	T48.5X3	T48.5X4	T48.5X5	T48.5X6
Tuberculin, purified protein derivative (PPD)	T50.8X1	T50.8X2	T50.8X3	T50.8X4	T50.8X5	T50.8X6
Tubocurare	T48.1X1	T48.1X2	T48.1X3	T48.1X4	T48.1X5	T48.1X6
Tubocurarine (chloride)	T48.1X1	T48.1X2	T48.1X3	T48.1X4	T48.1X5	T48.1X6
Tulobuterol	T48.6X1	T48.6X2	T48.6X3	T48.6X4	T48.6X5	T48.6X6
Turpentine (spirits of)	T52.8X1	T52.8X2	T52.8X3	T52.8X4	—	—
vapor	T52.8X1	T52.8X2	T52.8X3	T52.8X4	—	—
Twinrix*	T50.B91	T50.B92	T50.B93	T50.B94	T50.B95	T50.B96
Tybamate	T43.591	T43.592	T43.593	T43.594	T43.595	T43.596
Tygacil*	T36.4X1	T36.4X2	T36.4X3	T36.4X4	T36.4X5	T36.4X6
Tyloxapol	T48.4X1	T48.4X2	T48.4X3	T48.4X4	T48.4X5	T48.4X6
Tymazoline	T48.5X1	T48.5X2	T48.5X3	T48.5X4	T48.5X5	T48.5X6
Tymlos*	T50.991	T50.992	T50.993	T50.994	T50.995	T50.996
Typhoid-paratyphoid vaccine	T50.A91	T50.A92	T50.A93	T50.A94	T50.A95	T50.A96
Typhus vaccine	T50.A91	T50.A92	T50.A93	T50.A94	T50.A95	T50.A96
Tyropanoate	T50.8X1	T50.8X2	T50.8X3	T50.8X4	T50.8X5	T50.8X6
Tyrothricin	T49.6X1	T49.6X2	T49.6X3	T49.6X4	T49.6X5	T49.6X6
ENT agent	T49.6X1	T49.6X2	T49.6X3	T49.6X4	T49.6X5	T49.6X6
ophthalmic preparation	T49.5X1	T49.5X2	T49.5X3	T49.5X4	T49.5X5	T49.5X6
Ufenamate	T39.391	T39.392	T39.393	T39.394	T39.395	T39.396
Ultraviolet light protectant	T49.3X1	T49.3X2	T49.3X3	T49.3X4	T49.3X5	T49.3X6
Unasyn*	T36.0X1	T36.0X2	T36.0X3	T36.0X4	T36.0X5	T36.0X6
Undecenoic acid	T49.0X1	T49.0X2	T49.0X3	T49.0X4	T49.0X5	T49.0X6
Undecoylium	T49.0X1	T49.0X2	T49.0X3	T49.0X4	T49.0X5	T49.0X6
Undecylenic acid (derivatives)	T49.0X1	T49.0X2	T49.0X3	T49.0X4	T49.0X5	T49.0X6
Unna's boot	T49.3X1	T49.3X2	T49.3X3	T49.3X4	T49.3X5	T49.3X6
Unsaturated fatty acid	T46.6X1	T46.6X2	T46.6X3	T46.6X4	T46.6X5	T46.6X6
Uracil mustard	T45.1X1	T45.1X2	T45.1X3	T45.1X4	T45.1X5	T45.1X6
Uramustine	T45.1X1	T45.1X2	T45.1X3	T45.1X4	T45.1X5	T45.1X6
Urapidil	T46.5X1	T46.5X2	T46.5X3	T46.5X4	T46.5X5	T46.5X6
Urari	T48.1X1	T48.1X2	T48.1X3	T48.1X4	T48.1X5	T48.1X6
Urate oxidase	T50.4X1	T50.4X2	T50.4X3	T50.4X4	T50.4X5	T50.4X6
Urea	T47.3X1	T47.3X2	T47.3X3	T47.3X4	T47.3X5	T47.3X6
peroxide	T49.0X1	T49.0X2	T49.0X3	T49.0X4	T49.0X5	T49.0X6
stibamine	T37.4X1	T37.4X2	T37.4X3	T37.4X4	T37.4X5	T37.4X6
topical	T49.8X1	T49.8X2	T49.8X3	T49.8X4	T49.8X5	T49.8X6
Ureaphil*	T48.0X1	T48.0X2	T48.0X3	T48.0X4	T48.0X5	T48.0X6
Urethane	T45.1X1	T45.1X2	T45.1X3	T45.1X4	T45.1X5	T45.1X6
Urginea (maritima) (scilla) — see Squill						
Uric acid metabolism drug NEC	T50.4X1	T50.4X2	T50.4X3	T50.4X4	T50.4X5	T50.4X6
Uricosuric agent	T50.4X1	T50.4X2	T50.4X3	T50.4X4	T50.4X5	T50.4X6
Urinary anti-infective	T37.8X1	T37.8X2	T37.8X3	T37.8X4	T37.8X5	T37.8X6
Urofollitropin	T38.811	T38.812	T38.813	T38.814	T38.815	T38.816
Urokinase	T45.611	T45.612	T45.613	T45.614	T45.615	T45.616
Urokon	T50.8X1	T50.8X2	T50.8X3	T50.8X4	T50.8X5	T50.8X6
Ursodeoxycholic acid	T50.991	T50.992	T50.993	T50.994	T50.995	T50.996
Ursodiol	T50.991	T50.992	T50.993	T50.994	T50.995	T50.996
Urtica	T62.2X1	T62.2X2	T62.2X3	T62.2X4	—	—
Utility gas — see Gas, utility						
Vaccine NEC	T50.Z91	T50.Z92	T50.Z93	T50.Z94	T50.Z95	T50.Z96
antineoplastic	T50.Z91	T50.Z92	T50.Z93	T50.Z94	T50.Z95	T50.Z96
bacterial NEC	T50.A91	T50.A92	T50.A93	T50.A94	T50.A95	T50.A96
with						
other bacterial component	T50.A21	T50.A22	T50.A23	T50.A24	T50.A25	T50.A26
pertussis component	T50.A11	T50.A12	T50.A13	T50.A14	T50.A15	T50.A16
viral-rickettsial component	T50.A21	T50.A22	T50.A23	T50.A24	T50.A25	T50.A26
mixed NEC	T50.A21	T50.A22	T50.A23	T50.A24	T50.A25	T50.A26
BCG	T50.A91	T50.A92	T50.A93	T50.A94	T50.A95	T50.A96
cholera	T50.A91	T50.A92	T50.A93	T50.A94	T50.A95	T50.A96
diphtheria	T50.A91	T50.A92	T50.A93	T50.A94	T50.A95	T50.A96
with tetanus	T50.A21	T50.A22	T50.A23	T50.A24	T50.A25	T50.A26
and pertussis	T50.A11	T50.A12	T50.A13	T50.A14	T50.A15	T50.A16
influenza	T50.B91	T50.B92	T50.B93	T50.B94	T50.B95	T50.B96
measles	T50.B91	T50.B92	T50.B93	T50.B94	T50.B95	T50.B96
with mumps and rubella	T50.B91	T50.B92	T50.B93	T50.B94	T50.B95	T50.B96
meningococcal	T50.A91	T50.A92	T50.A93	T50.A94	T50.A95	T50.A96
mumps	T50.B91	T50.B92	T50.B93	T50.B94	T50.B95	T50.B96
paratyphoid	T50.A91	T50.A92	T50.A93	T50.A94	T50.A95	T50.A96
pertussis	T50.A11	T50.A12	T50.A13	T50.A14	T50.A15	T50.A16
with diphtheria	T50.A11	T50.A12	T50.A13	T50.A14	T50.A15	T50.A16
and tetanus	T50.A11	T50.A12	T50.A13	T50.A14	T50.A15	T50.A16
with other component	T50.A11	T50.A12	T50.A13	T50.A14	T50.A15	T50.A16
plague	T50.A91	T50.A92	T50.A93	T50.A94	T50.A95	T50.A96
poliomyelitis	T50.B91	T50.B92	T50.B93	T50.B94	T50.B95	T50.B96
poliovirus	T50.B91	T50.B92	T50.B93	T50.B94	T50.B95	T50.B96
rabies	T50.B91	T50.B92	T50.B93	T50.B94	T50.B95	T50.B96
respiratory syncytial virus	T50.B91	T50.B92	T50.B93	T50.B94	T50.B95	T50.B96
rickettsial NEC	T50.A91	T50.A92	T50.A93	T50.A94	T50.A95	T50.A96
with bacterial component	T50.A21	T50.A22	T50.A23	T50.A24	T50.A25	T50.A26
Rocky Mountain spotted fever	T50.A91	T50.A92	T50.A93	T50.A94	T50.A95	T50.A96
rubella	T50.B91	T50.B92	T50.B93	T50.B94	T50.B95	T50.B96
sabin oral	T50.B91	T50.B92	T50.B93	T50.B94	T50.B95	T50.B96
smallpox	T50.B11	T50.B12	T50.B13	T50.B14	T50.B15	T50.B16
TAB	T50.A91	T50.A92	T50.A93	T50.A94	T50.A95	T50.A96
tetanus	T50.A91	T50.A92	T50.A93	T50.A94	T50.A95	T50.A96
typhoid	T50.A91	T50.A92	T50.A93	T50.A94	T50.A95	T50.A96
typhus	T50.A91	T50.A92	T50.A93	T50.A94	T50.A95	T50.A96
viral NEC	T50.B91	T50.B92	T50.B93	T50.B94	T50.B95	T50.B96
yellow fever	T50.B91	T50.B92	T50.B93	T50.B94	T50.B95	T50.B96
Vaccinia immune globulin	T50.Z11	T50.Z12	T50.Z13	T50.Z14	T50.Z15	T50.Z16
Vaginal contraceptives	T49.8X1	T49.8X2	T49.8X3	T49.8X4	T49.8X5	T49.8X6
Valacyclovir*	T37.5X1	T37.5X2	T37.5X3	T37.5X4	T37.5X5	T37.5X6
Valerian						
root	T42.6X1	T42.6X2	T42.6X3	T42.6X4	T42.6X5	T42.6X6
tincture	T42.6X1	T42.6X2	T42.6X3	T42.6X4	T42.6X5	T42.6X6
Valethamate bromide	T44.3X1	T44.3X2	T44.3X3	T44.3X4	T44.3X5	T44.3X6
Valisone	T49.0X1	T49.0X2	T49.0X3	T49.0X4	T49.0X5	T49.0X6
Valium	T42.4X1	T42.4X2	T42.4X3	T42.4X4	T42.4X5	T42.4X6
Valmid	T42.6X1	T42.6X2	T42.6X3	T42.6X4	T42.6X5	T42.6X6
Valnoctamide	T42.6X1	T42.6X2	T42.6X3	T42.6X4	T42.6X5	T42.6X6
Valproate (sodium)	T42.6X1	T42.6X2	T42.6X3	T42.6X4	T42.6X5	T42.6X6
Valproic acid	T42.6X1	T42.6X2	T42.6X3	T42.6X4	T42.6X5	T42.6X6
Valpromide	T42.6X1	T42.6X2	T42.6X3	T42.6X4	T42.6X5	T42.6X6
Vanadium	T56.891	T56.892	T56.893	T56.894	—	—
Vancomycin	T36.8X1	T36.8X2	T36.8X3	T36.8X4	T36.8X5	T36.8X6
Vandazole*	T49.0X1	T49.0X2	T49.0X3	T49.0X4	T49.0X5	T49.0X6
Vapor — see also Gas	T59.91	T59.92	T59.93	T59.94	—	—
kiln (carbon monoxide)	T58.8X1	T58.8X2	T58.8X3	T58.8X4	—	—
lead — see lead						
specified source NEC	T59.891	T59.892	T59.893	T59.894	—	—
Vardenafil	T46.7X1	T46.7X2	T46.7X3	T46.7X4	T46.7X5	T46.7X6
Varicose reduction drug	T46.8X1	T46.8X2	T46.8X3	T46.8X4	T46.8X5	T46.8X6
Varnish	T65.4X1	T65.4X2	T65.4X3	T65.4X4	—	—

Substance	Poisoning, Accidental (unintentional)	Poisoning, Intentional Self-harm	Poisoning, Assault	Poisoning, Undetermined	Adverse Effect	Under-dosing
Varnish — *continued*						
cleaner	T52.91	T52.92	T52.93	T52.94	—	—
Vaseline	T49.3X1	T49.3X2	T49.3X3	T49.3X4	T49.3X5	T49.3X6
Vasodilan	T46.7X1	T46.7X2	T46.7X3	T46.7X4	T46.7X5	T46.7X6
Vasodilator						
coronary NEC	T46.3X1	T46.3X2	T46.3X3	T46.3X4	T46.3X5	T46.3X6
peripheral NEC	T46.7X1	T46.7X2	T46.7X3	T46.7X4	T46.7X5	T46.7X6
Vasopressin	T38.891	T38.892	T38.893	T38.894	T38.895	T38.896
Vasopressor drugs	T38.891	T38.892	T38.893	T38.894	T38.895	T38.896
Vecuronium bromide	T48.1X1	T48.1X2	T48.1X3	T48.1X4	T48.1X5	T48.1X6
Vegetable extract, astringent	T49.2X1	T49.2X2	T49.2X3	T49.2X4	T49.2X5	T49.2X6
Venlafaxine	T43.211	T43.212	T43.213	T43.214	T43.215	T43.216
Venom, venomous (bite) (sting)	T63.91	T63.92	T63.93	T63.94	—	—
amphibian NEC	T63.831	T63.832	T63.833	T63.834	—	—
animal NEC	T63.891	T63.892	T63.893	T63.894	—	—
ant	T63.421	T63.422	T63.423	T63.424	—	—
arthropod NEC	T63.481	T63.482	T63.483	T63.484	—	—
bee	T63.441	T63.442	T63.443	T63.444	—	—
centipede	T63.411	T63.412	T63.413	T63.414	—	—
fish	T63.591	T63.592	T63.593	T63.594	—	—
frog	T63.811	T63.812	T63.813	T63.814	—	—
hornet	T63.451	T63.452	T63.453	T63.454	—	—
insect NEC	T63.481	T63.482	T63.483	T63.484	—	—
lizard	T63.121	T63.122	T63.123	T63.124	—	—
marine						
animals	T63.691	T63.692	T63.693	T63.694	—	—
bluebottle	T63.611	T63.612	T63.613	T63.614	—	—
jellyfish NEC	T63.621	T63.622	T63.623	T63.624	—	—
Portuguese Man-o-war	T63.611	T63.612	T63.613	T63.614	—	—
sea anemone	T63.631	T63.632	T63.633	T63.634	—	—
specified NEC	T63.691	T63.692	T63.693	T63.694	—	—
fish	T63.591	T63.592	T63.593	T63.594	—	—
plants	T63.711	T63.712	T63.713	T63.714	—	—
sting ray	T63.511	T63.512	T63.513	T63.514	—	—
millipede (tropical)	T63.411	T63.412	T63.413	T63.414	—	—
plant NEC	T63.791	T63.792	T63.793	T63.794	—	—
marine	T63.711	T63.712	T63.713	T63.714	—	—
reptile	T63.191	T63.192	T63.193	T63.194	—	—
gila monster	T63.111	T63.112	T63.113	T63.114	—	—
lizard NEC	T63.121	T63.122	T63.123	T63.124	—	—
scorpion	T63.2X1	T63.2X2	T63.2X3	T63.2X4	—	—
snake	T63.001	T63.002	T63.003	T63.004	—	—
African NEC	T63.081	T63.082	T63.083	T63.084	—	—
American (North) (South) NEC	T63.061	T63.062	T63.063	T63.064	—	—
Asian	T63.081	T63.082	T63.083	T63.084	—	—
Australian	T63.071	T63.072	T63.073	T63.074	—	—
cobra	T63.041	T63.042	T63.043	T63.044	—	—
coral snake	T63.021	T63.022	T63.023	T63.024	—	—
rattlesnake	T63.011	T63.012	T63.013	T63.014	—	—
specified NEC	T63.091	T63.092	T63.093	T63.094	—	—
taipan	T63.031	T63.032	T63.033	T63.034	—	—
specified NEC	T63.891	T63.892	T63.893	T63.894	—	—
spider	T63.301	T63.302	T63.303	T63.304	—	—
black widow	T63.311	T63.312	T63.313	T63.314	—	—
brown recluse	T63.331	T63.332	T63.333	T63.334	—	—
specified NEC	T63.391	T63.392	T63.393	T63.394	—	—
tarantula	T63.321	T63.322	T63.323	T63.324	—	—
sting ray	T63.511	T63.512	T63.513	T63.514	—	—
toad	T63.821	T63.822	T63.823	T63.824	—	—
wasp	T63.461	T63.462	T63.463	T63.464	—	—
Venous sclerosing drug NEC	T46.8X1	T46.8X2	T46.8X3	T46.8X4	T46.8X5	T46.8X6
Ventavis*	T46.7X1	T46.7X2	T46.7X3	T46.7X4	T46.7X5	T46.7X6
Ventolin — *see* Albuterol						
Veramon	T42.3X1	T42.3X2	T42.3X3	T42.3X4	T42.3X5	T42.3X6
Verapamil	T46.1X1	T46.1X2	T46.1X3	T46.1X4	T46.1X5	T46.1X6
Veratrine	T46.5X1	T46.5X2	T46.5X3	T46.5X4	T46.5X5	T46.5X6
Veratrum						
album	T62.2X1	T62.2X2	T62.2X3	T62.2X4	—	—
alkaloids	T46.5X1	T46.5X2	T46.5X3	T46.5X4	T46.5X5	T46.5X6
viride	T62.2X1	T62.2X2	T62.2X3	T62.2X4	—	—
Verdigris	T60.3X1	T60.3X2	T60.3X3	T60.3X4	—	—
Veronal	T42.3X1	T42.3X2	T42.3X3	T42.3X4	T42.3X5	T42.3X6
Veroxil	T37.4X1	T37.4X2	T37.4X3	T37.4X4	T37.4X5	T37.4X6
Versenate	T50.6X1	T50.6X2	T50.6X3	T50.6X4	T50.6X5	T50.6X6
Versidyne	T39.8X1	T39.8X2	T39.8X3	T39.8X4	T39.8X5	T39.8X6
Vetrabutine	T48.0X1	T48.0X2	T48.0X3	T48.0X4	T48.0X5	T48.0X6
Vexol*	T49.5X1	T49.5X2	T49.5X3	T49.5X4	T49.5X5	T49.5X6
Victrelis*	T37.5X1	T37.5X2	T37.5X3	T37.5X4	T37.5X5	T37.5X6
Vidarabine	T37.5X1	T37.5X2	T37.5X3	T37.5X4	T37.5X5	T37.5X6

Substance	Poisoning, Accidental (unintentional)	Poisoning, Intentional Self-harm	Poisoning, Assault	Poisoning, Undetermined	Adverse Effect	Under-dosing
Vienna						
green	T57.0X1	T57.0X2	T57.0X3	T57.0X4	—	—
insecticide	T60.2X1	T60.2X2	T60.2X3	T60.2X4	—	—
red	T57.0X1	T57.0X2	T57.0X3	T57.0X4	—	—
pharmaceutical dye	T50.991	T50.992	T50.993	T50.994	T50.995	T50.996
Vigabatrin	T42.6X1	T42.6X2	T42.6X3	T42.6X4	T42.6X5	T42.6X6
Viloxazine	T43.291	T43.292	T43.293	T43.294	T43.295	T43.296
Viminol	T39.8X1	T39.8X2	T39.8X3	T39.8X4	T39.8X5	T39.8X6
Vinbarbital, vinbarbitone	T42.3X1	T42.3X2	T42.3X3	T42.3X4	T42.3X5	T42.3X6
Vinblastine	T45.1X1	T45.1X2	T45.1X3	T45.1X4	T45.1X5	T45.1X6
Vinburnine	T46.7X1	T46.7X2	T46.7X3	T46.7X4	T46.7X5	T46.7X6
Vincamine	T45.1X1	T45.1X2	T45.1X3	T45.1X4	T45.1X5	T45.1X6
Vincristine	T45.1X1	T45.1X2	T45.1X3	T45.1X4	T45.1X5	T45.1X6
Vindesine	T45.1X1	T45.1X2	T45.1X3	T45.1X4	T45.1X5	T45.1X6
Vinesthene, vinethene	T41.0X1	T41.0X2	T41.0X3	T41.0X4	T41.0X5	T41.0X6
Vinorelbine tartrate	T45.1X1	T45.1X2	T45.1X3	T45.1X4	T45.1X5	T45.1X6
Vinpocetine	T46.7X1	T46.7X2	T46.7X3	T46.7X4	T46.7X5	T46.7X6
Vinyl						
acetate	T65.891	T65.892	T65.893	T65.894	—	—
bital	T42.3X1	T42.3X2	T42.3X3	T42.3X4	T42.3X5	T42.3X6
bromide	T65.891	T65.892	T65.893	T65.894	—	—
chloride	T59.891	T59.892	T59.893	T59.894	—	—
ether	T41.0X1	T41.0X2	T41.0X3	T41.0X4	T41.0X5	T41.0X6
Vinylbital	T42.3X1	T42.3X2	T42.3X3	T42.3X4	T42.3X5	T42.3X6
Vinylidene chloride	T65.891	T65.892	T65.893	T65.894	—	—
Vioform	T37.8X1	T37.8X2	T37.8X3	T37.8X4	T37.8X5	T37.8X6
topical	T49.0X1	T49.0X2	T49.0X3	T49.0X4	T49.0X5	T49.0X6
Viokase*	T47.5X1	T47.5X2	T47.5X3	T47.5X4	T47.5X5	T47.5X6
Viomycin	T36.8X1	T36.8X2	T36.8X3	T36.8X4	T36.8X5	T36.8X6
Viosterol	T45.2X1	T45.2X2	T45.2X3	T45.2X4	T45.2X5	T45.2X6
Viper (venom)	T63.091	T63.092	T63.093	T63.094	—	—
Viprynium	T37.4X1	T37.4X2	T37.4X3	T37.4X4	T37.4X5	T37.4X6
Viquidil	T46.7X1	T46.7X2	T46.7X3	T46.7X4	T46.7X5	T46.7X6
Viral vaccine NEC	T50.B91	T50.B92	T50.B93	T50.B94	T50.B95	T50.B96
Virginiamycin	T36.8X1	T36.8X2	T36.8X3	T36.8X4	T36.8X5	T36.8X6
Virugon	T37.5X1	T37.5X2	T37.5X3	T37.5X4	T37.5X5	T37.5X6
Viscous agent	T50.901	T50.902	T50.903	T50.904	T50.905	T50.906
Visine	T49.5X1	T49.5X2	T49.5X3	T49.5X4	T49.5X5	T49.5X6
Visnadine	T46.3X1	T46.3X2	T46.3X3	T46.3X4	T46.3X5	T46.3X6
Vitamin NEC	T45.2X1	T45.2X2	T45.2X3	T45.2X4	T45.2X5	T45.2X6
A	T45.2X1	T45.2X2	T45.2X3	T45.2X4	T45.2X5	T45.2X6
B1	T45.2X1	T45.2X2	T45.2X3	T45.2X4	T45.2X5	T45.2X6
B2	T45.2X1	T45.2X2	T45.2X3	T45.2X4	T45.2X5	T45.2X6
B6	T45.2X1	T45.2X2	T45.2X3	T45.2X4	T45.2X5	T45.2X6
B12	T45.2X1	T45.2X2	T45.2X3	T45.2X4	T45.2X5	T45.2X6
B15	T45.2X1	T45.2X2	T45.2X3	T45.2X4	T45.2X5	T45.2X6
B NEC	T45.2X1	T45.2X2	T45.2X3	T45.2X4	T45.2X5	T45.2X6
nicotinic acid	T46.7X1	T46.7X2	T46.7X3	T46.7X4	T46.7X5	T46.7X6
C	T45.2X1	T45.2X2	T45.2X3	T45.2X4	T45.2X5	T45.2X6
D	T45.2X1	T45.2X2	T45.2X3	T45.2X4	T45.2X5	T45.2X6
D2	T45.2X1	T45.2X2	T45.2X3	T45.2X4	T45.2X5	T45.2X6
D3	T45.2X1	T45.2X2	T45.2X3	T45.2X4	T45.2X5	T45.2X6
E	T45.2X1	T45.2X2	T45.2X3	T45.2X4	T45.2X5	T45.2X6
E acetate	T45.2X1	T45.2X2	T45.2X3	T45.2X4	T45.2X5	T45.2X6
hematopoietic	T45.8X1	T45.8X2	T45.8X3	T45.8X4	T45.8X5	T45.8X6
K1	T45.7X1	T45.7X2	T45.7X3	T45.7X4	T45.7X5	T45.7X6
K2	T45.7X1	T45.7X2	T45.7X3	T45.7X4	T45.7X5	T45.7X6
K NEC	T45.7X1	T45.7X2	T45.7X3	T45.7X4	T45.7X5	T45.7X6
PP	T45.2X1	T45.2X2	T45.2X3	T45.2X4	T45.2X5	T45.2X6
ulceroprotectant	T47.1X1	T47.1X2	T47.1X3	T47.1X4	T47.1X5	T47.1X6
Vleminckx's solution	T49.4X1	T49.4X2	T49.4X3	T49.4X4	T49.4X5	T49.4X6
Voltaren — *see* Diclofenac sodium						
Voraxaze*	T50.6X1	T50.6X2	T50.6X3	T50.6X4	T50.6X5	T50.6X6
Warfarin	T45.511	T45.512	T45.513	T45.514	T45.515	T45.516
rodenticide	T60.4X1-	T60.4X2-	T60.4X3-	T60.4X4-	—	—
sodium	T45.511	T45.512	T45.513	T45.514	T45.515	T45.516
Wasp (sting)	T63.461	T63.462	T63.463	T63.464	—	—
Water						
balance drug	T50.3X1	T50.3X2	T50.3X3	T50.3X4	T50.3X5	T50.3X6
distilled	T50.3X1	T50.3X2	T50.3X3	T50.3X4	T50.3X5	T50.3X6
gas — *see* Gas, water						
incomplete combustion of — *see* Carbon, monoxide, fuel, utility						
hemlock	T62.2X1	T62.2X2	T62.2X3	T62.2X4	—	—
moccasin (venom)	T63.061	T63.062	T63.063	T63.064	—	—
purified	T50.3X1	T50.3X2	T50.3X3	T50.3X4	T50.3X5	T50.3X6
Wax (paraffin) (petroleum)	T52.0X1	T52.0X2	T52.0X3	T52.0X4	—	—
automobile	T65.891	T65.892	T65.893	T65.894	—	—
floor	T52.0X1	T52.0X2	T52.0X3	T52.0X4	—	—
Weed killers NEC	T60.3X1	T60.3X2	T60.3X3	T60.3X4	—	—
Wellbutrin*	T43.291	T43.292	T43.293	T43.294	T43.295	T43.296

Table of Drugs and Chemicals

Substance	Poisoning, Accidental (unintentional)	Poisoning, Intentional Self-harm	Poisoning, Assault	Poisoning, Undetermined	Adverse Effect	Under-dosing
Welldorm	T42.6X1	T42.6X2	T42.6X3	T42.6X4	T42.6X5	T42.6X6
Westcort*	T49.0X1	T49.0X2	T49.0X3	T49.0X4	T49.0X5	T49.0X6
White						
arsenic	T57.0X1	T57.0X2	T57.0X3	T57.0X4	—	—
hellebore	T62.2X1	T62.2X2	T62.2X3	T62.2X4	—	—
lotion (keratolytic)	T49.4X1	T49.4X2	T49.4X3	T49.4X4	T49.4X5	T49.4X6
spirit	T52.0X1	T52.0X2	T52.0X3	T52.0X4	—	—
Whitewash	T65.891	T65.892	T65.893	T65.894	—	—
Whole blood (human)	T45.8X1	T45.8X2	T45.8X3	T45.8X4	T45.8X5	T45.8X6
Wild						
black cherry	T62.2X1	T62.2X2	T62.2X3	T62.2X4	—	—
poisonous plants NEC	T62.2X1	T62.2X2	T62.2X3	T62.2X4	—	—
Window cleaning fluid	T65.891	T65.892	T65.893	T65.894	—	—
Wintergreen (oil)	T49.3X1	T49.3X2	T49.3X3	T49.3X4	T49.3X5	T49.3X6
Wisterine	T62.2X1	T62.2X2	T62.2X3	T62.2X4	—	—
Witch hazel	T49.2X1	T49.2X2	T49.2X3	T49.2X4	T49.2X5	T49.2X6
Wood alcohol or spirit	T51.1X1	T51.1X2	T51.1X3	T51.1X4	—	—
Wool fat (hydrous)	T49.3X1	T49.3X2	T49.3X3	T49.3X4	T49.3X5	T49.3X6
Woorali	T48.1X1	T48.1X2	T48.1X3	T48.1X4	T48.1X5	T48.1X6
Wormseed, American	T37.4X1	T37.4X2	T37.4X3	T37.4X4	T37.4X5	T37.4X6
Xamoterol	T44.5X1	T44.5X2	T44.5X3	T44.5X4	T44.5X5	T44.5X6
Xanax*	T42.4X1	T42.4X2	T42.4X3	T42.4X4	T42.4X5	T42.4X6
Xanthine diuretics	T50.2X1	T50.2X2	T50.2X3	T50.2X4	T50.2X5	T50.2X6
Xanthinol nicotinate	T46.7X1	T46.7X2	T46.7X3	T46.7X4	T46.7X5	T46.7X6
Xanthotoxin	T49.3X1	T49.3X2	T49.3X3	T49.3X4	T49.3X5	T49.3X6
Xantinol nicotinate	T46.7X1	T46.7X2	T46.7X3	T46.7X4	T46.7X5	T46.7X6
Xantocillin	T36.0X1	T36.0X2	T36.0X3	T36.0X4	T36.0X5	T36.0X6
Xenon (127Xe) (133Xe)	T50.8X1	T50.8X2	T50.8X3	T50.8X4	T50.8X5	T50.8X6
Xenysalate	T49.4X1	T49.4X2	T49.4X3	T49.4X4	T49.4X5	T49.4X6
Xibornol	T37.8X1	T37.8X2	T37.8X3	T37.8X4	T37.8X5	T37.8X6
Xigris	T45.511	T45.512	T45.513	T45.514	T45.515	T45.516
Xipamide	T50.2X1	T50.2X2	T50.2X3	T50.2X4	T50.2X5	T50.2X6
Xylene (vapor)	T52.2X1	T52.2X2	T52.2X3	T52.2X4	—	—
Xylocaine (infiltration) (topical)	T41.3X1	T41.3X2	T41.3X3	T41.3X4	T41.3X5	T41.3X6
nerve block (peripheral) (plexus)	T41.3X1	T41.3X2	T41.3X3	T41.3X4	T41.3X5	T41.3X6
spinal	T41.3X1	T41.3X2	T41.3X3	T41.3X4	T41.3X5	T41.3X6
Xylol (vapor)	T52.2X1	T52.2X2	T52.2X3	T52.2X4	—	—
Xylometazoline	T48.5X1	T48.5X2	T48.5X3	T48.5X4	T48.5X5	T48.5X6
Xylose*	T50.8X1	T50.8X2	T50.8X3	T50.8X4	T50.8X5	T50.8X6
Yaz*	T38.4X1	T38.4X2	T38.4X3	T38.4X4	T38.4X5	T38.4X6
Yeast	T45.2X1	T45.2X2	T45.2X3	T45.2X4	T45.2X5	T45.2X6
dried	T45.2X1	T45.2X2	T45.2X3	T45.2X4	T45.2X5	T45.2X6
Yellow						
fever vaccine	T50.B91	T50.B92	T50.B93	T50.B94	T50.B95	T50.B96
jasmine	T62.2X1	T62.2X2	T62.2X3	T62.2X4	—	—
phenolphthalein	T47.2X1	T47.2X2	T47.2X3	T47.2X4	T47.2X5	T47.2X6
Yervoy*	T45.1X1	T45.1X2	T45.1X3	T45.1X4	T45.1X5	T45.1X6
Yew	T62.2X1	T62.2X2	T62.2X3	T62.2X4	—	—
Yohimbic acid	T40.991	T40.992	T40.993	T40.994	T40.995	T40.996
Zactane	T39.8X1	T39.8X2	T39.8X3	T39.8X4	T39.8X5	T39.8X6
Zalcitabine	T37.5X1	T37.5X2	T37.5X3	T37.5X4	T37.5X5	T37.5X6
Zanaflex*	T48.1X1	T48.1X2	T48.1X3	T48.1X4	T48.1X5	T48.1X6
Zaroxolyn	T50.2X1	T50.2X2	T50.2X3	T50.2X4	T50.2X5	T50.2X6
Zephiran (topical)	T49.0X1	T49.0X2	T49.0X3	T49.0X4	T49.0X5	T49.0X6
ophthalmic preparation	T49.5X1	T49.5X2	T49.5X3	T49.5X4	T49.5X5	T49.5X6
Zeranol	T38.7X1	T38.7X2	T38.7X3	T38.7X4	T38.7X5	T38.7X6
Zerone	T51.1X1	T51.1X2	T51.1X3	T51.1X4	—	—
Zidovudine	T37.5X1	T37.5X2	T37.5X3	T37.5X4	T37.5X5	T37.5X6
Zilactin*	T41.3X1	T41.3X2	T41.3X3	T41.3X4	T41.3X5	T41.3X6
Zimeldine	T43.221	T43.222	T43.223	T43.224	T43.225	T43.226
Zinc (compounds) (fumes) (vapor)	T56.5X1	T56.5X2	T56.5X3	T56.5X4	—	—
NEC						
anti-infectives	T49.0X1	T49.0X2	T49.0X3	T49.0X4	T49.0X5	T49.0X6
antivaricose	T46.8X1	T46.8X2	T46.8X3	T46.8X4	T46.8X5	T46.8X6
bacitracin	T49.0X1	T49.0X2	T49.0X3	T49.0X4	T49.0X5	T49.0X6
chloride (mouthwash)	T49.6X1	T49.6X2	T49.6X3	T49.6X4	T49.6X5	T49.6X6
chromate	T56.5X1	T56.5X2	T56.5X3	T56.5X4	—	—
gelatin	T49.3X1	T49.3X2	T49.3X3	T49.3X4	T49.3X5	T49.3X6
oxide	T49.3X1	T49.3X2	T49.3X3	T49.3X4	T49.3X5	T49.3X6
plaster	T49.3X1	T49.3X2	T49.3X3	T49.3X4	T49.3X5	T49.3X6
peroxide	T49.0X1	T49.0X2	T49.0X3	T49.0X4	T49.0X5	T49.0X6
pesticides	T56.5X1	T56.5X2	T56.5X3	T56.5X4	—	—
phosphide	T60.4X1	T60.4X2	T60.4X3	T60.4X4	—	—
pyrithionate	T49.4X1	T49.4X2	T49.4X3	T49.4X4	T49.4X5	T49.4X6
stearate	T49.3X1	T49.3X2	T49.3X3	T49.3X4	T49.3X5	T49.3X6
sulfate	T49.5X1	T49.5X2	T49.5X3	T49.5X4	T49.5X5	T49.5X6
ENT agent	T49.6X1	T49.6X2	T49.6X3	T49.6X4	T49.6X5	T49.6X6
ophthalmic solution	T49.5X1	T49.5X2	T49.5X3	T49.5X4	T49.5X5	T49.5X6
topical NEC	T49.0X1	T49.0X2	T49.0X3	T49.0X4	T49.0X5	T49.0X6
undecylenate	T49.0X1	T49.0X2	T49.0X3	T49.0X4	T49.0X5	T49.0X6
Zineb	T60.0X1	T60.0X2	T60.0X3	T60.0X4	—	—

Substance	Poisoning, Accidental (unintentional)	Poisoning, Intentional Self-harm	Poisoning, Assault	Poisoning, Undetermined	Adverse Effect	Under-dosing
Zinostatin	T45.1X1	T45.1X2	T45.1X3	T45.1X4	T45.1X5	T45.1X6
Zipeprol	T48.3X1	T48.3X2	T48.3X3	T48.3X4	T48.3X5	T48.3X6
Zofenopril	T46.4X1	T46.4X2	T46.4X3	T46.4X4	T46.4X5	T46.4X6
Zolpidem	T42.6X1	T42.6X2	T42.6X3	T42.6X4	T42.6X5	T42.6X6
Zomepirac	T39.391	T39.392	T39.393	T39.394	T39.395	T39.396
Zopiclone	T42.6X1	T42.6X2	T42.6X3	T42.6X4	T42.6X5	T42.6X6
Zorubicin	T45.1X1	T45.1X2	T45.1X3	T45.1X4	T45.1X5	T45.1X6
Zotepine	T43.591	T43.592	T43.593	T43.594	T43.595	T43.596
Zovant	T45.511	T45.512	T45.513	T45.514	T45.515	T45.516
Zoxazolamine	T42.8X1	T42.8X2	T42.8X3	T42.8X4	T42.8X5	T42.8X6
Zuclopenthixol	T43.4X1	T43.4X2	T43.4X3	T43.4X4	T43.4X5	T43.4X6
Zyflo*	T48.6X1	T48.6X2	T48.6X3	T48.6X4	T48.6X5	T48.6X6
Zygadenus (venenosus)	T62.2X1	T62.2X2	T62.2X3	T62.2X4	—	—
Zyprexa	T43.591	T43.592	T43.593	T43.594	T43.595	T43.596
Zyzal*	T45.0X1	T45.0X2	T45.0X3	T45.0X4	T45.0X5	T45.0X6

A

Abandonment (causing exposure to weather conditions) (with intent to injure or kill) NEC X58 ☑
Abuse (adult) (child) (mental) (physical) (sexual) X58 ☑
Accident (to) X58 ☑
  aircraft (in transit) (powered) — *see also* Accident, transport, aircraft
    due to, caused by cataclysm — *see* Forces of nature, by type
  animal-drawn vehicle — *see* Accident, transport, animal-drawn vehicle occupant
  animal-rider — *see* Accident, transport, animal-rider
  automobile — *see* Accident, transport, car occupant
  bare foot water skier V94.4 ☑
  boat, boating — *see also* Accident, watercraft
    striking swimmer
      powered V94.11 ☑
      unpowered V94.12 ☑
  bus — *see* Accident, transport, bus occupant
  cable car, not on rails V98.0 ☑
    on rails — *see* Accident, transport, streetcar occupant
  car — *see* Accident, transport, car occupant
  caused by, due to
    animal NEC W64 ☑
    chain hoist W24.0 ☑
    cold (excessive) — *see* Exposure, cold
    corrosive liquid, substance — *see* Table of Drugs and Chemicals
    cutting or piercing instrument — *see* Contact, with, by type of instrument
    drive belt W24.0 ☑
    electric
      current — *see* Exposure, electric current
      motor — *see also* Contact, with, by type of machine W31.3 ☑
      current (of) W86.8 ☑
    environmental factor NEC X58 ☑
    explosive material — *see* Explosion
    fire, flames — *see* Exposure, fire
    firearm missile — *see* Discharge, firearm by type
    heat (excessive) — *see* Heat
    hot — *see* Contact, with, hot
    ignition — *see* Ignition
    lifting device W24.0 ☑
    lightning — *see* subcategory T75.0 ☑
      causing fire — *see* Exposure, fire
    machine, machinery — *see* Contact, with, by type of machine
    natural factor NEC X58 ☑
    pulley (block) W24.0 ☑
    radiation — *see* Radiation
    steam X13.1 ☑
      inhalation X13.0 ☑
      pipe X16 ☑
    thunderbolt — *see* subcategory T75.0 ☑
      causing fire — *see* Exposure, fire
    transmission device W24.1 ☑
  coach — *see* Accident, transport, bus occupant
  coal car — *see* Accident, transport, industrial vehicle occupant
  diving — *see also* Fall, into, water
    with
      drowning or submersion — *see* Drowning
  forklift — *see* Accident, transport, industrial vehicle occupant
  heavy transport vehicle NOS — *see* Accident, transport, truck occupant
  ice yacht V98.2 ☑
  in
    medical, surgical procedure
      as, or due to misadventure — *see* Misadventure
      causing an abnormal reaction or later complication without mention of misadventure — *see also* Complication of or following, by type of procedure Y84.9
  land yacht V98.1 ☑
  late effect of — *see* W00-X58 with 7th character S
  logging car — *see* Accident, transport, industrial vehicle occupant
  machine, machinery — *see also* Contact, with, by type of machine
    on board watercraft V93.69 ☑
      explosion — *see* Explosion, in, watercraft

Accident — *continued*
  machine, machinery — *see also* Contact, with, by type of machine — *continued*
    on board watercraft — *continued*
      fire — *see* Burn, on board watercraft
      powered craft V93.63 ☑
        ferry boat V93.61 ☑
        fishing boat V93.62 ☑
        jetskis V93.63 ☑
        liner V93.61 ☑
        merchant ship V93.60 ☑
        passenger ship V93.61 ☑
        sailboat V93.64 ☑
  mine tram — *see* Accident, transport, industrial vehicle occupant
  mobility scooter (motorized) — *see* Accident, transport, pedestrian, conveyance, specified type NEC
  motor scooter — *see* Accident, transport, motorcyclist
  motor vehicle NOS (traffic) — *see also* Accident, transport V89.2 ☑
    nontraffic V89.0 ☑
    three-wheeled NOS — *see* Accident, transport, three-wheeled motor vehicle occupant
  motorcycle NOS — *see* Accident, transport, motorcyclist
  nonmotor vehicle NOS (nontraffic) — *see also* Accident, transport V89.1 ☑
    traffic NOS V89.3 ☑
  nontraffic (victim's mode of transport NOS) V88.9 ☑
    collision (between) V88.7 ☑
      bus and truck V88.5 ☑
      car and:
        bus V88.3 ☑
        pickup V88.2 ☑
        three-wheeled motor vehicle V88.0 ☑
        train V88.6 ☑
        truck V88.4 ☑
        two-wheeled motor vehicle V88.0 ☑
        van V88.2 ☑
      specified vehicle NEC and:
        three-wheeled motor vehicle V88.1 ☑
        two-wheeled motor vehicle V88.1 ☑
    known mode of transport — *see* Accident, transport, by type of vehicle
    noncollision V88.8 ☑
  on board watercraft V93.89 ☑
    powered craft V93.83 ☑
      ferry boat V93.81 ☑
      fishing boat V93.82 ☑
      jetskis V93.83 ☑
      liner V93.81 ☑
      merchant ship V93.80 ☑
      passenger ship V93.81 ☑
    unpowered craft V93.88 ☑
      canoe V93.85 ☑
      inflatable V93.86 ☑
        in tow
          recreational V94.31 ☑
          specified NEC V94.32 ☑
      kayak V93.85 ☑
      sailboat V93.84 ☑
      surf-board V93.88 ☑
      water skis V93.87 ☑
      windsurfer V93.88 ☑
  parachutist V97.29 ☑
    entangled in object V97.21 ☑
    injured on landing V97.22 ☑
  pedal cycle — *see* Accident, transport, pedal cyclist
  pedestrian (on foot)
    with
      another pedestrian W51 ☑
        on pedestrian conveyance NEC V00.09 ☑
        with fall W03 ☑
          due to ice or snow W00.0 ☑
      rider of
        hoverboard V00.038 ☑
        Segway V00.038 ☑
        standing
          electric scooter V00.031 ☑
          micro-mobility pedestrian conveyance NEC V00.038 ☑
      roller skater (in-line) V00.01 ☑
      skate boarder V00.02 ☑
      transport vehicle — *see* Accident, transport
    on pedestrian conveyance — *see* Accident, transport, pedestrian, conveyance

Accident — *continued*
  pick-up truck or van — *see* Accident, transport, pickup truck occupant
  quarry truck — *see* Accident, transport, industrial vehicle occupant
  railway vehicle (any) (in motion) — *see* Accident, transport, railway vehicle occupant
    due to cataclysm — *see* Forces of nature, by type
  scooter (non-motorized) — *see* Accident, transport, pedestrian, conveyance, scooter
  sequelae of — *see* categories W00-X58 with 7th character S
  skateboard — *see* Accident, transport, pedestrian, conveyance, skateboard
  ski(ing) — *see* Accident, transport, pedestrian, conveyance
    lift V98.3 ☑
  specified cause NEC X58 ☑
  streetcar — *see* Accident, transport, streetcar occupant
  traffic (victim's mode of transport NOS) V87.9 ☑
    collision (between) V87.7 ☑
      bus and truck V87.5 ☑
      car and:
        bus V87.3 ☑
        pickup V87.2 ☑
        three-wheeled motor vehicle V87.0 ☑
        train V87.6 ☑
        truck V87.4 ☑
        two-wheeled motor vehicle V87.0 ☑
        van V87.2 ☑
      specified vehicle NEC V86.39 ☑
        and
          three-wheeled motor vehicle V87.1 ☑
          two-wheeled motor vehicle V87.1 ☑
        driver V86.09 ☑
        passenger V86.19 ☑
        person on outside V86.29 ☑
        while boarding or alighting V86.49 ☑
    known mode of transport — *see* Accident, transport, by type of vehicle
    noncollision V87.8 ☑
  transport (involving injury to) V99 ☑
    18 wheeler — *see* Accident, transport, truck occupant
    agricultural vehicle occupant (nontraffic) V84.9 ☑
      driver V84.5 ☑
      hanger-on V84.7 ☑
      passenger V84.6 ☑
      traffic V84.3 ☑
        driver V84.0 ☑
        hanger-on V84.2 ☑
        passenger V84.1 ☑
      while boarding or alighting V84.4 ☑
    aircraft NEC V97.89 ☑
      military NEC V97.818 ☑
        civilian injured by V97.811 ☑
        with civilian aircraft V97.810 ☑
      occupant injured (in)
        nonpowered craft accident V96.9 ☑
          balloon V96.00 ☑
            collision V96.03 ☑
            crash V96.01 ☑
            explosion V96.05 ☑
            fire V96.04 ☑
            forced landing V96.02 ☑
            specified type NEC V96.09 ☑
          glider V96.20 ☑
            collision V96.23 ☑
            crash V96.21 ☑
            explosion V96.25 ☑
            fire V96.24 ☑
            forced landing V96.22 ☑
            specified type NEC V96.29 ☑
          hang glider V96.10 ☑
            collision V96.13 ☑
            crash V96.11 ☑
            explosion V96.15 ☑
            fire V96.14 ☑
            forced landing V96.12 ☑
            specified type NEC V96.19 ☑
          specified craft NEC V96.8 ☑
        powered craft accident V95.9 ☑
          fixed wing NEC
            commercial V95.30 ☑
              collision V95.33 ☑
              crash V95.31 ☑

External Causes Index

Accident — *continued*
  transport — *continued*
    aircraft — *continued*
      occupant injured — *continued*
        powered craft accident — *continued*
          fixed wing — *continued*
            commercial — *continued*
              explosion V95.35 ☑
              fire V95.34 ☑
              forced landing V95.32 ☑
              specified type NEC V95.39 ☑
            private V95.20 ☑
              collision V95.23 ☑
              crash V95.21 ☑
              explosion V95.25 ☑
              fire V95.24 ☑
              forced landing V95.22 ☑
              specified type NEC V95.29 ☑
          glider V95.10 ☑
            collision V95.13 ☑
            crash V95.11 ☑
            explosion V95.15 ☑
            fire V95.14 ☑
            forced landing V95.12 ☑
            specified type NEC V95.19 ☑
          helicopter V95.00 ☑
            collision V95.03 ☑
            crash V95.01 ☑
            explosion V95.05 ☑
            fire V95.04 ☑
            forced landing V95.02 ☑
            specified type NEC V95.09 ☑
          spacecraft V95.40 ☑
            collision V95.43 ☑
            crash V95.41 ☑
            explosion V95.45 ☑
            fire V95.44 ☑
            forced landing V95.42 ☑
            specified type NEC V95.49 ☑
          specified craft NEC V95.8 ☑
          ultralight V95.10 ☑
            collision V95.13 ☑
            crash V95.11 ☑
            explosion V95.15 ☑
            fire V95.14 ☑
            forced landing V95.12 ☑
            specified type NEC V95.19 ☑
        specified accident NEC V97.0 ☑
        while boarding or alighting V97.1 ☑
      person (injured by)
        falling from, in or on aircraft V97.0 ☑
        machinery on aircraft V97.89 ☑
        on ground with aircraft involvement V97.39 ☑
        rotating propeller V97.32 ☑
        struck by object falling from aircraft V97.31 ☑
        sucked into aircraft jet V97.33 ☑
        while boarding or alighting aircraft V97.1 ☑
    airport (battery-powered) passenger vehicle — *see* Accident, transport, industrial vehicle occupant
    all-terrain vehicle occupant (nontraffic) V86.95 ☑
      driver V86.55 ☑
      dune buggy — *see* Accident, transport, dune buggy occupant
      hanger-on V86.75 ☑
      passenger V86.65 ☑
      snowmobile — *see* Accident, transport, snowmobile occupant
      specified type NEC V86.99 ☑
        driver V86.59 ☑
        passenger V86.69 ☑
        person on outside V86.79 ☑
      traffic V86.35 ☑
        driver V86.05 ☑
        hanger-on V86.25 ☑
        passenger V86.15 ☑
      while boarding or alighting V86.45 ☑
    ambulance occupant (traffic) V86.31 ☑
      driver V86.01 ☑
      hanger-on V86.21 ☑
      nontraffic V86.91 ☑
        driver V86.51 ☑
        hanger-on V86.71 ☑
        passenger V86.61 ☑
      passenger V86.11 ☑

Accident — *continued*
  transport — *continued*
    ambulance occupant — *continued*
      while boarding or alighting V86.41 ☑
    animal-drawn vehicle occupant (in) V80.929 ☑
      collision (with)
        animal V80.12 ☑
          being ridden V80.711 ☑
        animal-drawn vehicle V80.721 ☑
        bus V80.42 ☑
        car V80.42 ☑
        fixed or stationary object V80.82 ☑
        military vehicle V80.920 ☑
        nonmotor vehicle V80.791 ☑
        pedal cycle V80.22 ☑
        pedestrian V80.12 ☑
        pickup V80.42 ☑
        railway train or vehicle V80.62 ☑
        specified motor vehicle NEC V80.52 ☑
        streetcar V80.731 ☑
        truck V80.42 ☑
        two- or three-wheeled motor vehicle V80.32 ☑
        van V80.42 ☑
      noncollision V80.02 ☑
      specified circumstance NEC V80.928 ☑
    animal-rider V80.919 ☑
      collision (with)
        animal V80.11 ☑
          being ridden V80.710 ☑
        animal-drawn vehicle V80.720 ☑
        bus V80.41 ☑
        car V80.41 ☑
        fixed or stationary object V80.81 ☑
        military vehicle V80.910 ☑
        nonmotor vehicle V80.790 ☑
        pedal cycle V80.21 ☑
        pedestrian V80.11 ☑
        pickup V80.41 ☑
        railway train or vehicle V80.61 ☑
        specified motor vehicle NEC V80.51 ☑
        streetcar V80.730 ☑
        truck V80.41 ☑
        two- or three-wheeled motor vehicle V80.31 ☑
        van V80.41 ☑
      noncollision V80.018 ☑
        specified as horse rider V80.010 ☑
      specified circumstance NEC V80.918 ☑
    armored car — *see* Accident, transport, truck occupant
    battery-powered truck (baggage) (mail) — *see* Accident, transport, industrial vehicle occupant
    bus occupant V79.9 ☑
      collision (with)
        animal (traffic) V70.9 ☑
          being ridden (traffic) V76.9 ☑
            nontraffic V76.3 ☑
            while boarding or alighting V76.4 ☑
          nontraffic V70.3 ☑
          while boarding or alighting V70.4 ☑
        animal-drawn vehicle (traffic) V76.9 ☑
          nontraffic V76.3 ☑
          while boarding or alighting V76.4 ☑
        bus (traffic) V74.9 ☑
          nontraffic V74.3 ☑
          while boarding or alighting V74.4 ☑
        car (traffic) V73.9 ☑
          nontraffic V73.3 ☑
          while boarding or alighting V73.4 ☑
        motor vehicle NOS (traffic) V79.60 ☑
          nontraffic V79.20 ☑
          specified type NEC (traffic) V79.69 ☑
            nontraffic V79.29 ☑
        pedal cycle (traffic) V71.9 ☑
          nontraffic V71.3 ☑
          while boarding or alighting V71.4 ☑
        pickup truck (traffic) V73.9 ☑
          nontraffic V73.3 ☑
          while boarding or alighting V73.4 ☑
        railway vehicle (traffic) V75.9 ☑
          nontraffic V75.3 ☑
          while boarding or alighting V75.4 ☑
        specified vehicle NEC (traffic) V76.9 ☑
          nontraffic V76.3 ☑
          while boarding or alighting V76.4 ☑

Accident — *continued*
  transport — *continued*
    bus occupant — *continued*
      collision — *continued*
        stationary object (traffic) V77.9 ☑
          nontraffic V77.3 ☑
          while boarding or alighting V77.4 ☑
        streetcar (traffic) V76.9 ☑
          nontraffic V76.3 ☑
          while boarding or alighting V76.4 ☑
        three wheeled motor vehicle (traffic) V72.9 ☑
          nontraffic V72.3 ☑
          while boarding or alighting V72.4 ☑
        truck (traffic) V74.9 ☑
          nontraffic V74.3 ☑
          while boarding or alighting V74.4 ☑
        two wheeled motor vehicle (traffic) V72.9 ☑
          nontraffic V72.3 ☑
          while boarding or alighting V72.4 ☑
        van (traffic) V73.9 ☑
          nontraffic V73.3 ☑
          while boarding or alighting V73.4 ☑
      driver
        collision (with)
          animal (traffic) V70.5 ☑
            being ridden (traffic) V76.5 ☑
              nontraffic V76.0 ☑
            nontraffic V70.0 ☑
          animal-drawn vehicle (traffic) V76.5 ☑
            nontraffic V76.0 ☑
          bus (traffic) V74.5 ☑
            nontraffic V74.0 ☑
          car (traffic) V73.5 ☑
            nontraffic V73.0 ☑
          motor vehicle NOS (traffic) V79.40 ☑
            nontraffic V79.00 ☑
            specified type NEC (traffic) V79.49 ☑
              nontraffic V79.09 ☑
          pedal cycle (traffic) V71.5 ☑
            nontraffic V71.0 ☑
          pickup truck (traffic) V73.5 ☑
            nontraffic V73.0 ☑
          railway vehicle (traffic) V75.5 ☑
            nontraffic V75.0 ☑
          specified vehicle NEC (traffic) V76.5 ☑
            nontraffic V76.0 ☑
          stationary object (traffic) V77.5 ☑
            nontraffic V77.0 ☑
          streetcar (traffic) V76.5 ☑
            nontraffic V76.0 ☑
          three wheeled motor vehicle (traffic) V72.5 ☑
            nontraffic V72.0 ☑
          truck (traffic) V74.5 ☑
            nontraffic V74.0 ☑
          two wheeled motor vehicle (traffic) V72.5 ☑
            nontraffic V72.0 ☑
          van (traffic) V73.5 ☑
            nontraffic V73.0 ☑
        noncollision accident (traffic) V78.5 ☑
          nontraffic V78.0 ☑
      hanger-on
        collision (with)
          animal (traffic) V70.7 ☑
            being ridden (traffic) V76.7 ☑
              nontraffic V76.2 ☑
            nontraffic V70.2 ☑
          animal-drawn vehicle (traffic) V76.7 ☑
            nontraffic V76.2 ☑
          bus (traffic) V74.7 ☑
            nontraffic V74.2 ☑
          car (traffic) V73.7 ☑
            nontraffic V73.2 ☑
          pedal cycle (traffic) V71.7 ☑
            nontraffic V71.2 ☑
          pickup truck (traffic) V73.7 ☑
            nontraffic V73.2 ☑
          railway vehicle (traffic) V75.7 ☑
            nontraffic V75.2 ☑
          specified vehicle NEC (traffic) V76.7 ☑
            nontraffic V76.2 ☑
          stationary object (traffic) V77.7 ☑
            nontraffic V77.2 ☑
          streetcar (traffic) V76.7 ☑
            nontraffic V76.2 ☑

Accident — Accident

Accident — *continued*
  transport — *continued*
    bus occupant — *continued*
      hanger-on — *continued*
        collision — *continued*
          three wheeled motor vehicle (traffic) V72.7 ☑
            nontraffic V72.2 ☑
          truck (traffic) V74.7 ☑
            nontraffic V74.2 ☑
          two wheeled motor vehicle (traffic) V72.7 ☑
            nontraffic V72.2 ☑
          van (traffic) V73.7 ☑
            nontraffic V73.2 ☑
        noncollision accident (traffic) V78.7 ☑
          nontraffic V78.2 ☑
      noncollision accident (traffic) V78.9 ☑
        nontraffic V78.3 ☑
        while boarding or alighting V78.4 ☑
      nontraffic V79.3 ☑
      passenger
        collision (with)
          animal (traffic) V70.6 ☑
            being ridden (traffic) V76.6 ☑
              nontraffic V76.1 ☑
            nontraffic V70.1 ☑
          animal-drawn vehicle (traffic) V76.6 ☑
            nontraffic V76.1 ☑
          bus (traffic) V74.6 ☑
            nontraffic V74.1 ☑
          car (traffic) V73.6 ☑
            nontraffic V73.1 ☑
          motor vehicle NOS (traffic) V79.50 ☑
            nontraffic V79.10 ☑
            specified type NEC (traffic) V79.59 ☑
              nontraffic V79.19 ☑
          pedal cycle (traffic) V71.6 ☑
            nontraffic V71.1 ☑
          pickup truck (traffic) V73.6 ☑
            nontraffic V73.1 ☑
          railway vehicle (traffic) V75.6 ☑
            nontraffic V75.1 ☑
          specified vehicle NEC (traffic) V76.6 ☑
            nontraffic V76.1 ☑
          stationary object (traffic) V77.6 ☑
            nontraffic V77.1 ☑
          streetcar (traffic) V76.6 ☑
            nontraffic V76.1 ☑
          three wheeled motor vehicle (traffic) V72.6 ☑
            nontraffic V72.1 ☑
          truck (traffic) V74.6 ☑
            nontraffic V74.1 ☑
          two wheeled motor vehicle (traffic) V72.6 ☑
            nontraffic V72.1 ☑
          van (traffic) V73.6 ☑
            nontraffic V73.1 ☑
        noncollision accident (traffic) V78.6 ☑
          nontraffic V78.1 ☑
      specified type NEC V79.88 ☑
      military vehicle V79.81 ☑
    cable car, not on rails V98.0 ☑
      on rails — *see* Accident, transport, streetcar occupant
    car occupant V49.9 ☑
      ambulance occupant — *see* Accident, transport, ambulance occupant
      collision (with)
        animal (traffic) V40.9 ☑
          being ridden (traffic) V46.9 ☑
            nontraffic V46.3 ☑
            while boarding or alighting V46.4 ☑
          nontraffic V40.3 ☑
          while boarding or alighting V40.4 ☑
        animal-drawn vehicle (traffic) V46.9 ☑
          nontraffic V46.3 ☑
          while boarding or alighting V46.4 ☑
        bus (traffic) V44.9 ☑
          nontraffic V44.3 ☑
          while boarding or alighting V44.4 ☑
        car (traffic) V43.92 ☑
          nontraffic V43.32 ☑
          while boarding or alighting V43.42 ☑
        motor vehicle NOS (traffic) V49.60 ☑

Accident — *continued*
  transport — *continued*
    car occupant — *continued*
      collision — *continued*
        motor vehicle — *continued*
          nontraffic V49.20 ☑
          specified type NEC (traffic) V49.69 ☑
            nontraffic V49.29 ☑
        pedal cycle (traffic) V41.9 ☑
          nontraffic V41.3 ☑
          while boarding or alighting V41.4 ☑
        pickup truck (traffic) V43.93 ☑
          nontraffic V43.33 ☑
          while boarding or alighting V43.43 ☑
        railway vehicle (traffic) V45.9 ☑
          nontraffic V45.3 ☑
          while boarding or alighting V45.4 ☑
        specified vehicle NEC (traffic) V46.9 ☑
          nontraffic V46.3 ☑
          while boarding or alighting V46.4 ☑
        sport utility vehicle (traffic) V43.91 ☑
          nontraffic V43.31 ☑
          while boarding or alighting V43.41 ☑
        stationary object (traffic) V47.9 ☑
          nontraffic V47.3 ☑
          while boarding or alighting V47.4 ☑
        streetcar (traffic) V46.9 ☑
          nontraffic V46.3 ☑
          while boarding or alighting V46.4 ☑
        three wheeled motor vehicle (traffic) V42.9 ☑
          nontraffic V42.3 ☑
          while boarding or alighting V42.4 ☑
        truck (traffic) V44.9 ☑
          nontraffic V44.3 ☑
          while boarding or alighting V44.4 ☑
        two wheeled motor vehicle (traffic) V42.9 ☑
          nontraffic V42.3 ☑
          while boarding or alighting V42.4 ☑
        van (traffic) V43.94 ☑
          nontraffic V43.34 ☑
          while boarding or alighting V43.44 ☑
      driver
        collision (with)
          animal (traffic) V40.5 ☑
            being ridden (traffic) V46.5 ☑
              nontraffic V46.0 ☑
            nontraffic V40.0 ☑
          animal-drawn vehicle (traffic) V46.5 ☑
            nontraffic V46.0 ☑
          bus (traffic) V44.5 ☑
            nontraffic V44.0 ☑
          car (traffic) V43.52 ☑
            nontraffic V43.02 ☑
          motor vehicle NOS (traffic) V49.40 ☑
            nontraffic V49.00 ☑
            specified type NEC (traffic) V49.49 ☑
              nontraffic V49.09 ☑
          pedal cycle (traffic) V41.5 ☑
            nontraffic V41.0 ☑
          pickup truck (traffic) V43.53 ☑
            nontraffic V43.03 ☑
          railway vehicle (traffic) V45.5 ☑
            nontraffic V45.0 ☑
          specified vehicle NEC (traffic) V46.5 ☑
            nontraffic V46.0 ☑
          sport utility vehicle (traffic) V43.51 ☑
            nontraffic V43.01 ☑
          stationary object (traffic) V47.5 ☑
            nontraffic V47.0 ☑
          streetcar (traffic) V46.5 ☑
            nontraffic V46.0 ☑
          three wheeled motor vehicle (traffic) V42.5 ☑
            nontraffic V42.0 ☑
          truck (traffic) V44.5 ☑
            nontraffic V44.0 ☑
          two wheeled motor vehicle (traffic) V42.5 ☑
            nontraffic V42.0 ☑
          van (traffic) V43.54 ☑
            nontraffic V43.04 ☑
        noncollision accident (traffic) V48.5 ☑
          nontraffic V48.0 ☑
      hanger-on
        collision (with)
          animal (traffic) V40.7 ☑

Accident — *continued*
  transport — *continued*
    car occupant — *continued*
      hanger-on — *continued*
        collision — *continued*
          animal — *continued*
            being ridden (traffic) V46.7 ☑
              nontraffic V46.2 ☑
            nontraffic V40.2 ☑
          animal-drawn vehicle (traffic) V46.7 ☑
            nontraffic V46.2 ☑
          bus (traffic) V44.7 ☑
            nontraffic V44.2 ☑
          car (traffic) V43.72 ☑
            nontraffic V43.22 ☑
          pedal cycle (traffic) V41.7 ☑
            nontraffic V41.2 ☑
          pickup truck (traffic) V43.73 ☑
            nontraffic V43.23 ☑
          railway vehicle (traffic) V45.7 ☑
            nontraffic V45.2 ☑
          specified vehicle NEC (traffic) V46.7 ☑
            nontraffic V46.2 ☑
          sport utility vehicle (traffic) V43.71 ☑
            nontraffic V43.21 ☑
          stationary object (traffic) V47.7 ☑
            nontraffic V47.2 ☑
          streetcar (traffic) V46.7 ☑
            nontraffic V46.2 ☑
          three wheeled motor vehicle (traffic) V42.7 ☑
            nontraffic V42.2 ☑
          truck (traffic) V44.7 ☑
            nontraffic V44.2 ☑
          two wheeled motor vehicle (traffic) V42.7 ☑
            nontraffic V42.2 ☑
          van (traffic) V43.74 ☑
            nontraffic V43.24 ☑
        noncollision accident (traffic) V48.7 ☑
          nontraffic V48.2 ☑
      noncollision accident (traffic) V48.9 ☑
        nontraffic V48.3 ☑
        while boarding or alighting V48.4 ☑
      nontraffic V49.3 ☑
      passenger
        collision (with)
          animal (traffic) V40.6 ☑
            being ridden (traffic) V46.6 ☑
              nontraffic V46.1 ☑
            nontraffic V40.1 ☑
          animal-drawn vehicle (traffic) V46.6 ☑
            nontraffic V46.1 ☑
          bus (traffic) V44.6 ☑
            nontraffic V44.1 ☑
          car (traffic) V43.62 ☑
            nontraffic V43.12 ☑
          motor vehicle NOS (traffic) V49.50 ☑
            nontraffic V49.10 ☑
            specified type NEC (traffic) V49.59 ☑
              nontraffic V49.19 ☑
          pedal cycle (traffic) V41.6 ☑
            nontraffic V41.1 ☑
          pickup truck (traffic) V43.63 ☑
            nontraffic V43.13 ☑
          railway vehicle (traffic) V45.6 ☑
            nontraffic V45.1 ☑
          specified vehicle NEC (traffic) V46.6 ☑
            nontraffic V46.1 ☑
          sport utility vehicle (traffic) V43.61 ☑
            nontraffic V43.11 ☑
          stationary object (traffic) V47.6 ☑
            nontraffic V47.1 ☑
          streetcar (traffic) V46.6 ☑
            nontraffic V46.1 ☑
          three wheeled motor vehicle (traffic) V42.6 ☑
            nontraffic V42.1 ☑
          truck (traffic) V44.6 ☑
            nontraffic V44.1 ☑
          two wheeled motor vehicle (traffic) V42.6 ☑
            nontraffic V42.1 ☑
          van (traffic) V43.64 ☑
            nontraffic V43.14 ☑
        noncollision accident (traffic) V48.6 ☑

☑ **Additional Character Required — Refer to the Tabular List for Character Selection**

Accident — *continued*
  transport — *continued*
    car occupant — *continued*
      passenger — *continued*
        noncollision accident — *continued*
          nontraffic V48.1
        specified type NEC V49.88 ☑
        military vehicle V49.81 ☑
      coal car — *see* Accident, transport, industrial vehicle
        occupant
      construction vehicle occupant (nontraffic) V85.9 ☑
        driver V85.5 ☑
        hanger-on V85.7 ☑
        passenger V85.6 ☑
        traffic V85.3 ☑
          driver V85.0 ☑
          hanger-on V85.2 ☑
          passenger V85.1 ☑
        while boarding or alighting V85.4 ☑
      dirt bike rider (nontraffic) V86.96 ☑
        driver V86.56 ☑
        hanger-on V86.76 ☑
        passenger V86.66 ☑
        traffic V86.36 ☑
          driver V86.06 ☑
          hanger-on V86.26 ☑
          passenger V86.16 ☑
        while boarding or alighting V86.46 ☑
      due to cataclysm — *see* Forces of nature, by type
      dune buggy occupant (nontraffic) V86.93 ☑
        driver V86.53 ☑
        hanger-on V86.73 ☑
        passenger V86.63 ☑
        traffic V86.33 ☑
          driver V86.03 ☑
          hanger-on V86.23 ☑
          passenger V86.13 ☑
        while boarding or alighting V86.43 ☑
      e-bicycle — *see* Accident, transport, electric (assisted) bicyclist
      e-bike — *see* Accident, transport, electric (assisted) bicyclist
      electric (assisted) bicyclist V29.91 ☑
        collision (with)
          animal (traffic) V20.91 ☑
            being ridden (traffic) V26.91 ☑
              nontraffic V26.21 ☑
                while boarding or alighting V26.31 ☑
            nontraffic V20.21 ☑
              while boarding or alighting V20.31 ☑
          animal-drawn vehicle (traffic) V26.91 ☑
            nontraffic V26.21 ☑
              while boarding or alighting V26.31 ☑
          bus (traffic) V24.91 ☑
            nontraffic V24.21 ☑
              while boarding or alighting V24.31 ☑
          car (traffic) V23.91 ☑
            nontraffic V23.21 ☑
              while boarding or alighting V23.31 ☑
          motor vehicle NOS (traffic) V29.601 ☑
            nontraffic V29.201 ☑
            specified type NEC (traffic) V29.691 ☑
              nontraffic V29.291 ☑
          pedal cycle (traffic) V21.91 ☑
            nontraffic V21.21 ☑
              while boarding or alighting V21.31 ☑
          pedestrian V20.91 ☑
            nontraffic V20.01 ☑
              while boarding or alighting V20.31 ☑
          pickup truck (traffic) V23.91 ☑
            nontraffic V23.21 ☑
              while boarding or alighting V23.31 ☑
          railway vehicle (traffic) V25.91 ☑
            nontraffic V25.21 ☑
              while boarding or alighting V25.31 ☑
          specified vehicle NEC (traffic) V26.91 ☑
            nontraffic V26.21 ☑
              while boarding or alighting V26.31 ☑
          stationary object (traffic) V27.91 ☑
            nontraffic V27.21 ☑
              while boarding or alighting V27.31 ☑
          streetcar (traffic) V26.91 ☑
            nontraffic V26.21 ☑
              while boarding or alighting V26.31 ☑
          three wheeled motor vehicle (traffic)
            V22.91 ☑

Accident — *continued*
  transport — *continued*
    electric bicyclist — *continued*
      collision — *continued*
        three wheeled motor vehicle — *continued*
          nontraffic V22.21 ☑
          while boarding or alighting V22.31 ☑
        truck (traffic) V24.91 ☑
          nontraffic V24.21 ☑
          while boarding or alighting V24.31 ☑
        two wheeled motor vehicle (traffic) V22.91 ☑
          nontraffic V22.21 ☑
          while boarding or alighting V22.31 ☑
        van (traffic) V23.91 ☑
          nontraffic V23.21 ☑
          while boarding or alighting V23.31 ☑
      driver
        collision (with)
          animal (traffic) V20.41 ☑
            being ridden (traffic) V26.41 ☑
              nontraffic V26.01 ☑
            nontraffic V20.01 ☑
          animal-drawn vehicle (traffic) V26.41 ☑
            nontraffic V26.01 ☑
          bus (traffic) V24.41 ☑
            nontraffic V24.01 ☑
          car (traffic) V23.41 ☑
            nontraffic V23.01 ☑
          motor vehicle NOS (traffic) V29.401 ☑
            nontraffic V29.001 ☑
            specified type NEC (traffic) V29.491 ☑
              nontraffic V29.091 ☑
          pedal cycle (traffic) V21.41 ☑
            nontraffic V21.01 ☑
          pedestrian
            nontraffic V20.01 ☑
            traffic V20.41 ☑
          pickup truck (traffic) V23.41 ☑
            nontraffic V23.01 ☑
          railway vehicle (traffic) V25.41 ☑
            nontraffic V25.01 ☑
          specified vehicle NEC (traffic) V26.41 ☑
            nontraffic V26.01 ☑
          stationary object (traffic) V27.41 ☑
            nontraffic V27.01 ☑
          streetcar (traffic) V26.41 ☑
            nontraffic V26.01 ☑
          three wheeled motor vehicle (traffic)
            V22.41 ☑
            nontraffic V22.01 ☑
          truck (traffic) V24.41 ☑
            nontraffic V24.01 ☑
          two wheeled motor vehicle (traffic)
            V22.41 ☑
            nontraffic V22.01 ☑
          van (traffic) V23.41 ☑
            nontraffic V23.01 ☑
        noncollision accident (traffic) V28.41 ☑
          nontraffic V28.01 ☑
      noncollision accident (traffic) V28.91 ☑
        nontraffic V28.21 ☑
        while boarding or alighting V28.31 ☑
      nontraffic V29.31 ☑
      passenger
        collision (with)
          animal (traffic) V20.51 ☑
            being ridden (traffic) V26.51 ☑
              nontraffic V26.11 ☑
            nontraffic V20.11 ☑
          animal-drawn vehicle (traffic) V26.51 ☑
            nontraffic V26.11 ☑
          bus (traffic) V24.51 ☑
            nontraffic V24.11 ☑
          car (traffic) V23.51 ☑
            nontraffic V23.11 ☑
          motor vehicle NOS (traffic) V29.501 ☑
            nontraffic V29.101 ☑
            specified type NEC (traffic) V29.591 ☑
              nontraffic V29.191 ☑
          pedal cycle (traffic) V21.51 ☑
            nontraffic V21.11 ☑
          pedestrian
            nontraffic V20.11 ☑
            traffic V20.51 ☑
          pickup truck (traffic) V23.51 ☑
            nontraffic V23.11 ☑

Accident — *continued*
  transport — *continued*
    electric bicyclist — *continued*
      passenger — *continued*
        collision — *continued*
          railway vehicle (traffic) V25.51 ☑
            nontraffic V25.11 ☑
          specified vehicle NEC (traffic) V26.51 ☑
            nontraffic V26.11 ☑
          stationary object (traffic) V27.51 ☑
            nontraffic V27.11 ☑
          streetcar (traffic) V26.51 ☑
            nontraffic V26.11 ☑
          three wheeled motor vehicle (traffic)
            V22.51 ☑
            nontraffic V22.11 ☑
          truck (traffic) V24.51 ☑
            nontraffic V24.11 ☑
          two wheeled motor vehicle (traffic)
            V22.51 ☑
            nontraffic V22.11 ☑
          van (traffic) V23.51 ☑
            nontraffic V23.11 ☑
        noncollision accident (traffic) V28.51 ☑
          nontraffic V28.11 ☑
      specified type NEC V29.881 ☑
      military vehicle V29.811 ☑
    forklift — *see* Accident, transport, industrial vehicle
      occupant
    go cart — *see* Accident, transport, all-terrain vehicle
      occupant
    golf cart — *see* Accident, transport, all-terrain vehicle occupant
    heavy transport vehicle occupant — *see* Accident,
      transport, truck occupant
    hoverboard V00.848 ☑
    ice yacht V98.2 ☑
    industrial vehicle occupant (nontraffic) V83.9 ☑
      driver V83.5 ☑
      hanger-on V83.7 ☑
      passenger V83.6 ☑
      traffic V83.3 ☑
        driver V83.0 ☑
        hanger-on V83.2 ☑
        passenger V83.1 ☑
      while boarding or alighting V83.4 ☑
    interurban electric car — *see* Accident, transport,
      streetcar
    land yacht V98.1 ☑
    logging car — *see* Accident, transport, industrial
      vehicle occupant
    military vehicle occupant (traffic) V86.34 ☑
      driver V86.04 ☑
      hanger-on V86.24 ☑
      nontraffic V86.94 ☑
        driver V86.54 ☑
        hanger-on V86.74 ☑
        passenger V86.64 ☑
      passenger V86.14 ☑
      while boarding or alighting V86.44 ☑
    mine tram — *see* Accident, transport, industrial vehicle occupant
    motor vehicle NEC occupant (traffic) V89.2 ☑
    motorcoach — *see* Accident, transport, bus occupant
    motor/cross bike rider — *see also* Accident, transport, dirt bike rider V86.96 ☑
    motorcyclist V29.99 ☑
      collision (with)
        animal (traffic) V20.99 ☑
          being ridden (traffic) V26.99 ☑
            nontraffic V26.29 ☑
            while boarding or alighting V26.39 ☑
          nontraffic V20.29 ☑
            while boarding or alighting V20.39 ☑
        animal-drawn vehicle (traffic) V26.99 ☑
          nontraffic V26.29 ☑
            while boarding or alighting V26.39 ☑
        bus (traffic) V24.99 ☑
          nontraffic V24.29 ☑
            while boarding or alighting V24.39 ☑
        car (traffic) V23.99 ☑
          nontraffic V23.29 ☑
            while boarding or alighting V23.39 ☑
        motor vehicle NOS (traffic) V29.608 ☑
          nontraffic V29.208 ☑

☑ Additional Character Required — Refer to the Tabular List for Character Selection

Accident — *continued*
    transport — *continued*
        motorcyclist — *continued*
            collision — *continued*
                motor vehicle — *continued*
                    specified type NEC (traffic) V29.698 ☑
                    nontraffic V29.298 ☑
                    pedal cycle (traffic) V21.99 ☑
                        nontraffic V21.29 ☑
                        while boarding or alighting V21.39 ☑
                    pickup truck (traffic) V23.99 ☑
                        nontraffic V23.29 ☑
                        while boarding or alighting V23.39 ☑
                    railway vehicle (traffic) V25.99 ☑
                        nontraffic V25.29 ☑
                        while boarding or alighting V25.39 ☑
                    specified vehicle NEC (traffic) V26.99 ☑
                        nontraffic V26.29 ☑
                        while boarding or alighting V26.39 ☑
                    stationary object (traffic) V27.99 ☑
                        nontraffic V27.29 ☑
                        while boarding or alighting V27.39 ☑
                    streetcar (traffic) V26.99 ☑
                        nontraffic V26.29 ☑
                        while boarding or alighting V26.39 ☑
                    three wheeled motor vehicle (traffic) V22.99 ☑
                        nontraffic V22.29 ☑
                        while boarding or alighting V22.39 ☑
                    truck (traffic) V24.99 ☑
                        nontraffic V24.29 ☑
                        while boarding or alighting V24.39 ☑
                    two wheeled motor vehicle (traffic) V22.99 ☑
                        nontraffic V22.29 ☑
                        while boarding or alighting V22.39 ☑
                    van (traffic) V23.99 ☑
                        nontraffic V23.29 ☑
                        while boarding or alighting V23.39 ☑
            driver
                collision (with)
                    animal (traffic) V20.49 ☑
                        being ridden (traffic) V26.49 ☑
                            nontraffic V26.09 ☑
                        nontraffic V20.09 ☑
                    animal-drawn vehicle (traffic) V26.49 ☑
                        nontraffic V26.09 ☑
                    bus (traffic) V24.49 ☑
                        nontraffic V24.09 ☑
                    car (traffic) V23.49 ☑
                        nontraffic V23.09 ☑
                    motor vehicle NOS (traffic) V29.408 ☑
                        nontraffic V29.008 ☑
                        specified type NEC (traffic) V29.498 ☑
                            nontraffic V29.098 ☑
                    pedal cycle (traffic) V21.49 ☑
                        nontraffic V21.09 ☑
                    pedestrian
                        nontraffic V20.09 ☑
                        traffic V20.49 ☑
                    pickup truck (traffic) V23.49 ☑
                        nontraffic V23.09 ☑
                    railway vehicle (traffic) V25.49 ☑
                        nontraffic V25.09 ☑
                    specified vehicle NEC (traffic) V26.49 ☑
                        nontraffic V26.09 ☑
                    stationary object (traffic) V27.49 ☑
                        nontraffic V27.09 ☑
                    streetcar (traffic) V26.49 ☑
                        nontraffic V26.09 ☑
                    three wheeled motor vehicle (traffic) V22.49 ☑
                        nontraffic V22.09 ☑
                    truck (traffic) V24.49 ☑
                        nontraffic V24.09 ☑
                    two wheeled motor vehicle (traffic) V22.49 ☑
                        nontraffic V22.09 ☑
                    van (traffic) V23.49 ☑
                        nontraffic V23.09 ☑
                noncollision accident (traffic) V28.49 ☑
                    nontraffic V28.09 ☑
            noncollision accident (traffic) V28.99 ☑
                nontraffic V28.29 ☑
                while boarding or alighting V28.39 ☑
            nontraffic V29.39 ☑

Accident — *continued*
    transport — *continued*
        motorcyclist — *continued*
            passenger
                collision (with)
                    animal (traffic) V20.59 ☑
                        being ridden (traffic) V26.59 ☑
                            nontraffic V26.19 ☑
                        nontraffic V20.19 ☑
                    animal-drawn vehicle (traffic) V26.59 ☑
                        nontraffic V26.19 ☑
                    bus (traffic) V24.59 ☑
                        nontraffic V24.19 ☑
                    car (traffic) V23.59 ☑
                        nontraffic V23.19 ☑
                    motor vehicle NOS (traffic) V29.508 ☑
                        nontraffic V29.108 ☑
                        specified type NEC (traffic) V29.598 ☑
                            nontraffic V29.198 ☑
                    pedal cycle (traffic) V21.59 ☑
                        nontraffic V21.19 ☑
                    pedestrian
                        nontraffic V20.19 ☑
                        traffic V20.59 ☑
                    pickup truck (traffic) V23.59 ☑
                        nontraffic V23.19 ☑
                    railway vehicle (traffic) V25.59 ☑
                        nontraffic V25.19 ☑
                    specified vehicle NEC (traffic) V26.59 ☑
                        nontraffic V26.19 ☑
                    stationary object (traffic) V27.59 ☑
                        nontraffic V27.19 ☑
                    streetcar (traffic) V26.59 ☑
                        nontraffic V26.19 ☑
                    three wheeled motor vehicle (traffic) V22.59 ☑
                        nontraffic V22.19 ☑
                    truck (traffic) V24.59 ☑
                        nontraffic V24.19 ☑
                    two wheeled motor vehicle (traffic) V22.59 ☑
                        nontraffic V22.19 ☑
                    van (traffic) V23.59 ☑
                        nontraffic V23.19 ☑
                noncollision accident (traffic) V28.59 ☑
                    nontraffic V28.19 ☑
            specified type NEC V29.888 ☑
            military vehicle V29.818 ☑
        occupant (of)
            aircraft (powered) V95.9 ☑
                fixed wing
                    commercial — *see* Accident, transport, aircraft, occupant, powered, fixed wing, commercial
                    private — *see* Accident, transport, aircraft, occupant, powered, fixed wing, private
                nonpowered V96.9 ☑
                specified NEC V95.8 ☑
            airport battery-powered vehicle — *see* Accident, transport, industrial vehicle occupant
            all-terrain vehicle (ATV) — *see* Accident, transport, all-terrain vehicle occupant
            animal-drawn vehicle — *see* Accident, transport, animal-drawn vehicle occupant
            automobile — *see* Accident, transport, car occupant
            balloon V96.00 ☑
            battery-powered vehicle — *see* Accident, transport, industrial vehicle occupant
            bicycle — *see* Accident, transport, pedal cyclist
                motorized — *see* Accident, transport, motorcycle rider
            boat NEC — *see* Accident, watercraft
            bulldozer — *see* Accident, transport, construction vehicle occupant
            bus — *see* Accident, transport, bus occupant
            cable car (on rails) — *see also* Accident, transport, streetcar occupant
                not on rails V98.0 ☑
            car — *see also* Accident, transport, car occupant
                cable (on rails) — *see also* Accident, transport, streetcar occupant
                not on rails V98.0 ☑
            coach — *see* Accident, transport, bus occupant

Accident — *continued*
    transport — *continued*
        occupant — *continued*
            coal-car — *see* Accident, transport, industrial vehicle occupant
            digger — *see* Accident, transport, construction vehicle occupant
            dump truck — *see* Accident, transport, construction vehicle occupant
            earth-leveler — *see* Accident, transport, construction vehicle occupant
            farm machinery (self-propelled) — *see* Accident, transport, agricultural vehicle occupant
            forklift — *see* Accident, transport, industrial vehicle occupant
            glider (unpowered) V96.20 ☑
                hang V96.10 ☑
                powered (microlight) (ultralight) — *see* Accident, transport, aircraft, occupant, powered, glider
            glider (unpowered) NEC V96.20 ☑
            hang-glider V96.10 ☑
            harvester — *see* Accident, transport, agricultural vehicle occupant
            heavy (transport) vehicle — *see* Accident, transport, truck occupant
            helicopter — *see* Accident, transport, aircraft, occupant, helicopter
            ice-yacht V98.2 ☑
            kite (carrying person) V96.8 ☑
            land-yacht V98.1 ☑
            logging car — *see* Accident, transport, industrial vehicle occupant
            mechanical shovel — *see* Accident, transport, construction vehicle occupant
            microlight — *see* Accident, transport, aircraft, occupant, powered, glider
            minibus — *see* Accident, transport, pickup truck occupant
            minivan — *see* Accident, transport, pickup truck occupant
            moped — *see* Accident, transport, motorcycle
            motor scooter — *see* Accident, transport, motorcycle
            motorcycle (with sidecar) — *see* Accident, transport, motorcycle
            off-road motor-vehicle — *see also* Accident, transport, all-terrain vehicle occupant V86.99 ☑
            pedal cycle — *see also* Accident, transport, pedal cyclist
            pick-up (truck) — *see* Accident, transport, pickup truck occupant
            railway (train) (vehicle) (subterranean) (elevated) — *see* Accident, transport, railway vehicle occupant
            rickshaw — *see* Accident, transport, pedal cycle
                motorized — *see* Accident, transport, three-wheeled motor vehicle
                pedal driven — *see* Accident, transport, pedal cyclist
            road-roller — *see* Accident, transport, construction vehicle occupant
            ship NOS V94.9 ☑
            ski-lift (chair) (gondola) V98.3 ☑
            snowmobile — *see* Accident, transport, snowmobile occupant
            spacecraft, spaceship — *see* Accident, transport, aircraft, occupant, spacecraft
            sport utility vehicle — *see* Accident, transport, pickup truck occupant
            streetcar (interurban) (operating on public street or highway) — *see* Accident, transport, streetcar occupant
            SUV — *see* Accident, transport, pickup truck occupant
            téléférique V98.0 ☑
            three-wheeled vehicle (motorized) — *see also* Accident, transport, three-wheeled motor vehicle occupant
                nonmotorized — *see* Accident, transport, pedal cycle
            tractor (farm) (and trailer) — *see* Accident, transport, agricultural vehicle occupant
            train — *see* Accident, transport, railway vehicle occupant

☑ **Additional Character Required — Refer to the Tabular List for Character Selection**

Accident — *continued*
  transport — *continued*
    occupant — *continued*
      tram — *see* Accident, transport, streetcar occupant
        in mine or quarry — *see* Accident, transport, industrial vehicle occupant
      tricycle — *see* Accident, transport, pedal cycle
        motorized — *see* Accident, transport, three-wheeled motor vehicle
      trolley — *see* Accident, transport, streetcar occupant
        in mine or quarry — *see* Accident, transport, industrial vehicle occupant
      tub, in mine or quarry — *see* Accident, transport, industrial vehicle occupant
      ultralight — *see* Accident, transport, aircraft, occupant, powered, glider
      van — *see* Accident, transport, van occupant
      vehicle NEC V89.9 ☑
        heavy transport — *see* Accident, transport, truck occupant
        motor (traffic) NEC V89.2 ☑
        nontraffic NEC V89.0 ☑
      watercraft NOS V94.9 ☑
        causing drowning — *see* Drowning, resulting from accident to boat
      off-road motor-vehicle — *see also* Accident, transport, all-terrain vehicle occupant V86.99 ☑
  parachutist V97.29 ☑
    after accident to aircraft — *see* Accident, transport, aircraft
    entangled in object V97.21 ☑
    injured on landing V97.22 ☑
  pedal cyclist V19.9 ☑
    collision (with)
      animal (traffic) V10.9 ☑
        being ridden (traffic) V16.9 ☑
          nontraffic V16.2 ☑
            while boarding or alighting V16.3 ☑
        nontraffic V10.2 ☑
          while boarding or alighting V10.3 ☑
      animal-drawn vehicle (traffic) V16.9 ☑
        nontraffic V16.2 ☑
          while boarding or alighting V16.3 ☑
      bus (traffic) V14.9 ☑
        nontraffic V14.2 ☑
          while boarding or alighting V14.3 ☑
      car (traffic) V13.9 ☑
        nontraffic V13.2 ☑
          while boarding or alighting V13.3 ☑
      motor vehicle NOS (traffic) V19.60 ☑
        nontraffic V19.20 ☑
        specified type NEC (traffic) V19.69 ☑
          nontraffic V19.29 ☑
      pedal cycle (traffic) V11.9 ☑
        nontraffic V11.2 ☑
          while boarding or alighting V11.3 ☑
      pickup truck (traffic) V13.9 ☑
        nontraffic V13.2 ☑
          while boarding or alighting V13.3 ☑
      railway vehicle (traffic) V15.9 ☑
        nontraffic V15.2 ☑
          while boarding or alighting V15.3 ☑
      specified vehicle NEC (traffic) V16.9 ☑
        nontraffic V16.2 ☑
          while boarding or alighting V16.3 ☑
      stationary object (traffic) V17.9 ☑
        nontraffic V17.2 ☑
          while boarding or alighting V17.3 ☑
      streetcar (traffic) V16.9 ☑
        nontraffic V16.2 ☑
          while boarding or alighting V16.3 ☑
      three wheeled motor vehicle (traffic) V12.9 ☑
        nontraffic V12.2 ☑
          while boarding or alighting V12.3 ☑
      truck (traffic) V14.9 ☑
        nontraffic V14.2 ☑
          while boarding or alighting V14.3 ☑
      two wheeled motor vehicle (traffic) V12.9 ☑
        nontraffic V12.2 ☑
          while boarding or alighting V12.3 ☑
      van (traffic) V13.9 ☑
        nontraffic V13.2 ☑
          while boarding or alighting V13.3 ☑

Accident — *continued*
  transport — *continued*
    pedal cyclist — *continued*
      driver
        collision (with)
          animal (traffic) V10.4 ☑
            being ridden (traffic) V16.4 ☑
              nontraffic V16.0 ☑
            nontraffic V10.0 ☑
          animal-drawn vehicle (traffic) V16.4 ☑
            nontraffic V16.0 ☑
          bus (traffic) V14.4 ☑
            nontraffic V14.0 ☑
          car (traffic) V13.4 ☑
            nontraffic V13.0 ☑
          motor vehicle NOS (traffic) V19.40 ☑
            nontraffic V19.00 ☑
            specified type NEC (traffic) V19.49 ☑
              nontraffic V19.09 ☑
          pedal cycle (traffic) V11.4 ☑
            nontraffic V11.0 ☑
          pickup truck (traffic) V13.4 ☑
            nontraffic V13.0 ☑
          railway vehicle (traffic) V15.4 ☑
            nontraffic V15.0 ☑
          specified vehicle NEC (traffic) V16.4 ☑
            nontraffic V16.0 ☑
          stationary object (traffic) V17.4 ☑
            nontraffic V17.0 ☑
          streetcar (traffic) V16.4 ☑
            nontraffic V16.0 ☑
          three wheeled motor vehicle (traffic) V12.4 ☑
            nontraffic V12.0 ☑
          truck (traffic) V14.4 ☑
            nontraffic V14.0 ☑
          two wheeled motor vehicle (traffic) V12.4 ☑
            nontraffic V12.0 ☑
          van (traffic) V13.4 ☑
            nontraffic V13.0 ☑
        noncollision accident (traffic) V18.4 ☑
          nontraffic V18.0 ☑
      noncollision accident (traffic) V18.9 ☑
        nontraffic V18.2 ☑
          while boarding or alighting V18.3 ☑
      nontraffic V19.3 ☑
      passenger
        collision (with)
          animal (traffic) V10.5 ☑
            being ridden (traffic) V16.5 ☑
              nontraffic V16.1 ☑
            nontraffic V10.1 ☑
          animal-drawn vehicle (traffic) V16.5 ☑
            nontraffic V16.1 ☑
          bus (traffic) V14.5 ☑
            nontraffic V14.1 ☑
          car (traffic) V13.5 ☑
            nontraffic V13.1 ☑
          motor vehicle NOS (traffic) V19.50 ☑
            nontraffic V19.10 ☑
            specified type NEC (traffic) V19.59 ☑
              nontraffic V19.19 ☑
          pedal cycle (traffic) V11.5 ☑
            nontraffic V11.1 ☑
          pickup truck (traffic) V13.5 ☑
            nontraffic V13.1 ☑
          railway vehicle (traffic) V15.5 ☑
            nontraffic V15.1 ☑
          specified vehicle NEC (traffic) V16.5 ☑
            nontraffic V16.1 ☑
          stationary object (traffic) V17.5 ☑
            nontraffic V17.1 ☑
          streetcar (traffic) V16.5 ☑
            nontraffic V16.1 ☑
          three wheeled motor vehicle (traffic) V12.5 ☑
            nontraffic V12.1 ☑
          truck (traffic) V14.5 ☑
            nontraffic V14.1 ☑
          two wheeled motor vehicle (traffic) V12.5 ☑
            nontraffic V12.1 ☑
          van (traffic) V13.5 ☑
            nontraffic V13.1 ☑
        noncollision accident (traffic) V18.5 ☑

Accident — *continued*
  transport — *continued*
    pedal cyclist — *continued*
      passenger — *continued*
        noncollision accident — *continued*
          nontraffic V18.1 ☑
        specified type NEC V19.88 ☑
        military vehicle V19.81 ☑
  pedestrian
    conveyance (occupant) V09.9 ☑
      baby stroller V00.828 ☑
        collision (with) V09.9 ☑
          animal being ridden or animal drawn vehicle V06.99 ☑
            nontraffic V06.09 ☑
            traffic V06.19 ☑
          bus or heavy transport V04.99 ☑
            nontraffic V04.09 ☑
            traffic V04.19 ☑
          car V03.99 ☑
            nontraffic V03.09 ☑
            traffic V03.19 ☑
          pedal cycle V01.99 ☑
            nontraffic V01.09 ☑
            traffic V01.19 ☑
          pick-up truck or van V03.99 ☑
            nontraffic V03.09 ☑
            traffic V03.19 ☑
          railway (train) (vehicle) V05.99 ☑
            nontraffic V05.09 ☑
            traffic V05.19 ☑
          stationary object V00.822 ☑
          streetcar V06.99 ☑
            nontraffic V06.09 ☑
            traffic V06.19 ☑
          two- or three-wheeled motor vehicle V02.99 ☑
            nontraffic V02.09 ☑
            traffic V02.19 ☑
          vehicle V09.9 ☑
            animal-drawn V06.99 ☑
              nontraffic V06.09 ☑
              traffic V06.19 ☑
            motor
              nontraffic V09.00 ☑
              traffic V09.20 ☑
        fall V00.821 ☑
        nontraffic V09.1 ☑
          involving motor vehicle NEC V09.00 ☑
        traffic V09.3 ☑
          involving motor vehicle NEC V09.20 ☑
      flat-bottomed NEC V00.388 ☑
        collision (with) V09.9 ☑
          animal being ridden or animal drawn vehicle V06.99 ☑
            nontraffic V06.09 ☑
            traffic V06.19 ☑
          bus or heavy transport V04.99 ☑
            nontraffic V04.09 ☑
            traffic V04.19 ☑
          car V03.99 ☑
            nontraffic V03.09 ☑
            traffic V03.19 ☑
          pedal cycle V01.99 ☑
            nontraffic V01.09 ☑
            traffic V01.19 ☑
          pick-up truck or van V03.99 ☑
            nontraffic V03.09 ☑
            traffic V03.19 ☑
          railway (train) (vehicle) V05.99 ☑
            nontraffic V05.09 ☑
            traffic V05.19 ☑
          stationary object V00.382 ☑
          streetcar V06.99 ☑
            nontraffic V06.09 ☑
            traffic V06.19 ☑
          two- or three-wheeled motor vehicle V02.99 ☑
            nontraffic V02.09 ☑
            traffic V02.19 ☑
          vehicle V09.9 ☑
            animal-drawn V06.99 ☑
              nontraffic V06.09 ☑
              traffic V06.19 ☑
            motor
              nontraffic V09.00 ☑

☑ **Additional Character Required — Refer to the Tabular List for Character Selection**

Accident — *continued*
  transport — *continued*
    pedestrian — *continued*
      conveyance — *continued*
        flat-bottomed — *continued*
          collision — *continued*
            vehicle — *continued*
              motor — *continued*
                traffic V09.20 ☑
          fall V00.381 ☑
          nontraffic V09.1 ☑
            involving motor vehicle NEC V09.00 ☑
          snow
            board — *see* Accident, transport, pedestrian, conveyance, snow board
            ski — *see* Accident, transport, pedestrian, conveyance, skis (snow)
          traffic V09.3 ☑
            involving motor vehicle NEC V09.20 ☑
        gliding type NEC V00.288 ☑
          collision (with) V09.9 ☑
            animal being ridden or animal drawn vehicle V06.99 ☑
              nontraffic V06.09 ☑
              traffic V06.19 ☑
            bus or heavy transport V04.99 ☑
              nontraffic V04.09 ☑
              traffic V04.19 ☑
            car V03.99 ☑
              nontraffic V03.09 ☑
              traffic V03.19 ☑
            pedal cycle V01.99 ☑
              nontraffic V01.09 ☑
              traffic V01.19 ☑
            pick-up truck or van V03.99 ☑
              nontraffic V03.09 ☑
              traffic V03.19 ☑
            railway (train) (vehicle) V05.99 ☑
              nontraffic V05.09 ☑
              traffic V05.19 ☑
            stationary object V00.282 ☑
            streetcar V06.99 ☑
              nontraffic V06.09 ☑
              traffic V02.19 ☑
            two- or three-wheeled motor vehicle V02.99 ☑
              nontraffic V02.09 ☑
              traffic V02.19 ☑
            vehicle V09.9 ☑
              animal-drawn V06.99 ☑
                nontraffic V06.09 ☑
                traffic V06.19 ☑
              motor
                nontraffic V09.00 ☑
                traffic V09.20 ☑
          fall V00.281 ☑
        heelies — *see* Accident, transport, pedestrian, conveyance, heelies
        ice skate — *see* Accident, transport, pedestrian, conveyance, ice skate
        nontraffic V09.1 ☑
          involving motor vehicle NEC V09.00 ☑
        sled — *see* Accident, transport, pedestrian, conveyance, sled
        traffic V09.3 ☑
          involving motor vehicle NEC V09.20 ☑
        wheelies — *see* Accident, transport, pedestrian, conveyance, heelies
      heelies V00.158 ☑
        colliding with stationary object V00.152 ☑
        fall V00.151 ☑
      hoverboard
        collision with
          animal being ridden or animal drawn vehicle V06.938 ☑
            nontraffic V06.038 ☑
            traffic V06.138 ☑
          bus or heavy transport V04.938 ☑
            nontraffic V04.038 ☑
            traffic V04.138 ☑
          car V03.938 ☑
            nontraffic V03.038 ☑
            traffic V03.138 ☑
          pedal cycle V01.938 ☑

Accident — *continued*
  transport — *continued*
    pedestrian — *continued*
      conveyance — *continued*
        hoverboard — *continued*
          collision with — *continued*
            pedal cycle — *continued*
              nontraffic V01.038 ☑
              traffic V01.138 ☑
            pick-up or van V03.938 ☑
              nontraffic V03.038 ☑
              traffic V03.138 ☑
            railway (train) (vehicle) V05.938 ☑
              nontraffic V05.038 ☑
              traffic V05.138 ☑
            streetcar V06.938 ☑
              nontraffic V06.038 ☑
              traffic V06.138 ☑
            three-wheeled motor vehicle V02.938 ☑
              nontraffic V02.038 ☑
              traffic V02.138 ☑
            two-wheeled motor vehicle V02.938 ☑
              nontraffic V02.038 ☑
              traffic V02.138 ☑
            vehicle, nonmotor, specified NEC V06.938 ☑
              nontraffic V06.038 ☑
              traffic V06.138 ☑
          fall V00.848 ☑
        ice skates V00.218 ☑
          collision (with) V09.9 ☑
            animal being ridden or animal drawn vehicle V06.99 ☑
              nontraffic V06.09 ☑
              traffic V06.19 ☑
            bus or heavy transport V04.99 ☑
              nontraffic V04.09 ☑
              traffic V04.19 ☑
            car V03.99 ☑
              nontraffic V03.09 ☑
              traffic V03.19 ☑
            pedal cycle V01.99 ☑
              nontraffic V01.09 ☑
              traffic V01.19 ☑
            pick-up truck or van V03.99 ☑
              nontraffic V03.09 ☑
              traffic V03.19 ☑
            railway (train) (vehicle) V05.99 ☑
              nontraffic V05.09 ☑
              traffic V05.19 ☑
            stationary object V00.212 ☑
            streetcar V06.99 ☑
              nontraffic V06.09 ☑
              traffic V06.19 ☑
            two- or three-wheeled motor vehicle V02.99 ☑
              nontraffic V02.09 ☑
              traffic V02.19 ☑
            vehicle V09.9 ☑
              animal-drawn V06.99 ☑
                nontraffic V06.09 ☑
                traffic V06.19 ☑
              motor
                nontraffic V09.00 ☑
                traffic V09.20 ☑
          fall V00.211 ☑
          nontraffic V09.1 ☑
            involving motor vehicle NEC V09.00 ☑
          traffic V09.3 ☑
            involving motor vehicle NEC V09.20 ☑
        motorized mobility scooter V00.838 ☑
          collision with stationary object V00.832 ☑
          fall from V00.831 ☑
        nontraffic V09.1 ☑
          involving motor vehicle V09.00 ☑
            military V09.01 ☑
            specified type NEC V09.09 ☑
        roller skates (non in-line) V00.128 ☑
          collision (with) V09.9 ☑
            animal being ridden or animal drawn vehicle V06.91 ☑
              nontraffic V06.01 ☑
              traffic V06.11 ☑

Accident — *continued*
  transport — *continued*
    pedestrian — *continued*
      conveyance — *continued*
        roller skates — *continued*
          collision — *continued*
            bus or heavy transport V04.91 ☑
              nontraffic V04.01 ☑
              traffic V04.11 ☑
            car V03.91 ☑
              nontraffic V03.01 ☑
              traffic V03.11 ☑
            pedal cycle V01.91 ☑
              nontraffic V01.01 ☑
              traffic V01.11 ☑
            pick-up truck or van V03.91 ☑
              nontraffic V03.01 ☑
              traffic V03.11 ☑
            railway (train) (vehicle) V05.91 ☑
              nontraffic V05.01 ☑
              traffic V05.11 ☑
            stationary object V00.122 ☑
            streetcar V06.91 ☑
              nontraffic V06.01 ☑
              traffic V06.11 ☑
            two- or three-wheeled motor vehicle V02.91 ☑
              nontraffic V02.01 ☑
              traffic V02.11 ☑
            vehicle V09.9 ☑
              animal-drawn V06.91 ☑
                nontraffic V06.01 ☑
                traffic V06.11 ☑
              motor
                nontraffic V09.00 ☑
                traffic V09.20 ☑
          fall V00.121 ☑
          in-line V00.118 ☑
            collision — *see* also Accident, transport, pedestrian, conveyance occupant, roller skates, collision with stationary object V00.112 ☑
            fall V00.111 ☑
          nontraffic V09.1 ☑
            involving motor vehicle NEC V09.00 ☑
          traffic V09.3 ☑
            involving motor vehicle NEC V09.20 ☑
        rolling shoes V00.158 ☑
          colliding with stationary object V00.152 ☑
          fall V00.151 ☑
        rolling type NEC V00.188 ☑
          collision (with) V09.9 ☑
            animal being ridden or animal drawn vehicle V06.99 ☑
              nontraffic V06.09 ☑
              traffic V06.19 ☑
            bus or heavy transport V04.99 ☑
              nontraffic V04.09 ☑
              traffic V04.19 ☑
            car V03.99 ☑
              nontraffic V03.09 ☑
              traffic V03.19 ☑
            pedal cycle V01.99 ☑
              nontraffic V01.09 ☑
              traffic V01.19 ☑
            pick-up truck or van V03.99 ☑
              nontraffic V03.09 ☑
              traffic V03.19 ☑
            railway (train) (vehicle) V05.99 ☑
              nontraffic V05.09 ☑
              traffic V05.19 ☑
            stationary object V00.182 ☑
            streetcar V06.99 ☑
              nontraffic V06.09 ☑
              traffic V06.19 ☑
            two- or three-wheeled motor vehicle V02.99 ☑
              nontraffic V02.09 ☑
              traffic V02.19 ☑
            vehicle V09.9 ☑
              animal-drawn V06.99 ☑
                nontraffic V06.09 ☑
                traffic V06.19 ☑
              motor
                nontraffic V09.00 ☑

Accident — *continued*
  transport — *continued*
    pedestrian — *continued*
      conveyance — *continued*
        rolling type — *continued*
          collision — *continued*
            vehicle — *continued*
              motor — *continued*
                traffic V09.20 ☑
          fall V00.181 ☑
          in-line roller skate — *see* Accident, transport, pedestrian, conveyance, roller skate, in-line
          nontraffic V09.1 ☑
            involving motor vehicle NEC V09.00 ☑
          roller skate — *see* Accident, transport, pedestrian, conveyance, roller skate
          scooter (non-motorized) — *see* Accident, transport, pedestrian, conveyance, scooter
          skateboard — *see* Accident, transport, pedestrian, conveyance, skateboard
          traffic V09.3 ☑
            involving motor vehicle NEC V09.20 ☑
        scooter (non-motorized) V00.148 ☑
          collision (with) V09.9 ☑
            animal being ridden or animal drawn vehicle V06.99 ☑
              nontraffic V06.09 ☑
              traffic V06.19 ☑
            bus or heavy transport V04.99 ☑
              nontraffic V04.09 ☑
              traffic V04.19 ☑
            car V03.99 ☑
              nontraffic V03.09 ☑
              traffic V03.19 ☑
            pedal cycle V01.99 ☑
              nontraffic V01.09 ☑
              traffic V01.19 ☑
            pick-up truck or van V03.99 ☑
              nontraffic V03.09 ☑
              traffic V03.19 ☑
            railway (train) (vehicle) V05.99 ☑
              nontraffic V05.09 ☑
              traffic V05.19 ☑
            stationary object V00.142 ☑
            streetcar V06.99 ☑
              nontraffic V06.09 ☑
              traffic V06.19 ☑
            two- or three-wheeled motor vehicle V02.99 ☑
              nontraffic V02.09 ☑
              traffic V02.19 ☑
            vehicle V09.9 ☑
              animal-drawn V06.99 ☑
                nontraffic V06.09 ☑
                traffic V06.19 ☑
              motor
                nontraffic V09.00 ☑
                traffic V09.20 ☑
          fall V00.141 ☑
          nontraffic V09.1 ☑
            involving motor vehicle NEC V09.00 ☑
          traffic V09.3 ☑
            involving motor vehicle NEC V09.20 ☑
        Segway
          collision with
            animal being ridden or animal drawn vehicle V06.938 ☑
              nontraffic V06.038 ☑
              traffic V06.138 ☑
            bus or heavy transport V04.938 ☑
              nontraffic V04.038 ☑
              traffic V04.138 ☑
            car V03.938 ☑
              nontraffic V03.038 ☑
              traffic V03.138 ☑
            pedal cycle V01.938 ☑
              nontraffic V01.038 ☑
              traffic V01.138 ☑
            pick-up or van V03.938 ☑
              nontraffic V03.038 ☑
              traffic V03.138 ☑
            railway (train) (vehicle) V05.938 ☑

Accident — *continued*
  transport — *continued*
    pedestrian — *continued*
      conveyance — *continued*
        Segway — *continued*
          collision with — *continued*
            railway — *continued*
              nontraffic V05.038 ☑
              traffic V05.138 ☑
            streetcar V06.938 ☑
              nontraffic V06.038 ☑
              traffic V06.138 ☑
            three-wheeled vehicle V02.938 ☑
              nontraffic V02.038 ☑
              traffic V02.138 ☑
            two-wheeled vehicle V02.938 ☑
              nontraffic V02.038 ☑
              traffic V02.138 ☑
            vehicle, nonmotor, specified NEC V06.938 ☑
              nontraffic V06.038 ☑
              traffic V06.138 ☑
          fall V00.848 ☑
        skateboard V00.138 ☑
          collision (with) V09.9 ☑
            animal being ridden or animal drawn vehicle V06.92 ☑
              nontraffic V06.02 ☑
              traffic V06.12 ☑
            bus or heavy transport V04.92 ☑
              nontraffic V04.02 ☑
              traffic V04.12 ☑
            car V03.92 ☑
              nontraffic V03.02 ☑
              traffic V03.12 ☑
            pedal cycle V01.92 ☑
              nontraffic V01.02 ☑
              traffic V01.12 ☑
            pick-up truck or van V03.92 ☑
              nontraffic V03.02 ☑
              traffic V03.12 ☑
            railway (train) (vehicle) V05.92 ☑
              nontraffic V05.02 ☑
              traffic V05.12 ☑
            stationary object V00.132 ☑
            streetcar V06.92 ☑
              nontraffic V06.02 ☑
              traffic V06.12 ☑
            two- or three-wheeled motor vehicle V02.92 ☑
              nontraffic V02.02 ☑
              traffic V02.12 ☑
            vehicle V09.9 ☑
              animal-drawn V06.92 ☑
                nontraffic V06.02 ☑
                traffic V06.12 ☑
              motor
                nontraffic V09.00 ☑
                traffic V09.20 ☑
          fall V00.131 ☑
          nontraffic V09.1 ☑
            involving motor vehicle NEC V09.00 ☑
          traffic V09.3 ☑
            involving motor vehicle NEC V09.20 ☑
        skis (snow) V00.328 ☑
          collision (with) V09.9 ☑
            animal being ridden or animal drawn vehicle V06.99 ☑
              nontraffic V06.09 ☑
              traffic V06.19 ☑
            bus or heavy transport V04.99 ☑
              nontraffic V04.09 ☑
              traffic V04.19 ☑
            car V03.99 ☑
              nontraffic V03.09 ☑
              traffic V03.19 ☑
            pedal cycle V01.99 ☑
              nontraffic V01.09 ☑
              traffic V01.19 ☑
            pick-up truck or van V03.99 ☑
              nontraffic V03.09 ☑
              traffic V03.19 ☑
            railway (train) (vehicle) V05.99 ☑
              nontraffic V05.09 ☑
              traffic V05.19 ☑
            stationary object V00.322 ☑

Accident — *continued*
  transport — *continued*
    pedestrian — *continued*
      conveyance — *continued*
        skis — *continued*
          collision — *continued*
            streetcar V06.99 ☑
              nontraffic V06.09 ☑
              traffic V06.19 ☑
            two- or three-wheeled motor vehicle V02.99 ☑
              nontraffic V02.09 ☑
              traffic V02.19 ☑
            vehicle V09.9 ☑
              animal-drawn V06.99 ☑
                nontraffic V06.09 ☑
                traffic V06.19 ☑
              motor
                nontraffic V09.00 ☑
                traffic V09.20 ☑
          fall V00.321 ☑
          nontraffic V09.1 ☑
            involving motor vehicle NEC V09.00 ☑
          traffic V09.3 ☑
            involving motor vehicle NEC V09.20 ☑
        sled V00.228 ☑
          collision (with) V09.9 ☑
            animal being ridden or animal drawn vehicle V06.99 ☑
              nontraffic V06.09 ☑
              traffic V06.19 ☑
            bus or heavy transport V04.99 ☑
              nontraffic V04.09 ☑
              traffic V04.19 ☑
            car V03.99 ☑
              nontraffic V03.09 ☑
              traffic V03.19 ☑
            pedal cycle V01.99 ☑
              nontraffic V01.09 ☑
              traffic V01.19 ☑
            pick-up truck or van V03.99 ☑
              nontraffic V03.09 ☑
              traffic V03.19 ☑
            railway (train) (vehicle) V05.99 ☑
              nontraffic V05.09 ☑
              traffic V05.19 ☑
            stationary object V00.222 ☑
            streetcar V06.99 ☑
              nontraffic V06.09 ☑
              traffic V06.19 ☑
            two- or three-wheeled motor vehicle V02.99 ☑
              nontraffic V02.09 ☑
              traffic V02.19 ☑
            vehicle V09.9 ☑
              animal-drawn V06.99 ☑
                nontraffic V06.09 ☑
                traffic V06.19 ☑
              motor
                nontraffic V09.00 ☑
                traffic V09.20 ☑
          fall V00.221 ☑
          nontraffic V09.1 ☑
            involving motor vehicle NEC V09.00 ☑
          traffic V09.3 ☑
            involving motor vehicle NEC V09.20 ☑
        snow board V00.318 ☑
          collision (with) V06.99 ☑
            animal being ridden or animal drawn vehicle V06.99 ☑
              nontraffic V06.09 ☑
              traffic V06.19 ☑
            bus or heavy transport V04.99 ☑
              nontraffic V04.09 ☑
              traffic V04.19 ☑
            car V03.99 ☑
              nontraffic V03.09 ☑
              traffic V03.19 ☑
            pedal cycle V01.99 ☑
              nontraffic V01.09 ☑
              traffic V01.19 ☑
            pick-up truck or van V03.99 ☑
              nontraffic V03.09 ☑
              traffic V03.19 ☑
            railway (train) (vehicle) V05.99 ☑
              nontraffic V05.09 ☑

Accident — *continued*
  transport — *continued*
    pedestrian — *continued*
      conveyance — *continued*
        snow board — *continued*
          collision — *continued*
            railway — *continued*
              traffic V05.19 ☑
            stationary object V05.312 ☑
            streetcar V06.99 ☑
              nontraffic V06.09 ☑
              traffic V06.19 ☑
            two- or three-wheeled motor vehicle
              V02.99 ☑
              nontraffic V02.09 ☑
              traffic V02.19 ☑
            vehicle V09.9 ☑
              animal-drawn V06.99 ☑
                nontraffic V06.09 ☑
                traffic V06.19 ☑
              motor
                nontraffic V09.00 ☑
                traffic V09.20 ☑
           fall V00.311 ☑
          nontraffic V09.1 ☑
            involving motor vehicle NEC V09.00 ☑
          traffic V09.3 ☑
            involving motor vehicle NEC V09.20 ☑
        specified type NEC V00.898 ☑
          collision (with) V09.9 ☑
            animal being ridden or animal drawn
              vehicle V06.99 ☑
              nontraffic V06.09 ☑
              traffic V06.19 ☑
            bus or heavy transport V04.99 ☑
              nontraffic V04.09 ☑
              traffic V04.19 ☑
            car V03.99 ☑
              nontraffic V03.09 ☑
              traffic V03.19 ☑
            pedal cycle V01.99 ☑
              nontraffic V01.09 ☑
              traffic V01.19 ☑
            pick-up truck or van V03.99 ☑
              nontraffic V03.09 ☑
              traffic V03.19 ☑
            railway (train) (vehicle) V05.99 ☑
              nontraffic V05.09 ☑
              traffic V05.19 ☑
            stationary object V00.892 ☑
            streetcar V06.99 ☑
              nontraffic V06.09 ☑
              traffic V06.19 ☑
            two- or three-wheeled motor vehicle
              V02.99 ☑
              nontraffic V02.09 ☑
              traffic V02.19 ☑
            vehicle V09.9 ☑
              animal-drawn V06.99 ☑
                nontraffic V06.09 ☑
                traffic V06.19 ☑
              motor
                nontraffic V09.00 ☑
                traffic V09.20 ☑
         fall V00.891 ☑
        nontraffic V09.1 ☑
          involving motor vehicle NEC V09.00 ☑
        traffic V09.3 ☑
          involving motor vehicle NEC V09.20 ☑
      standing
        electric scooter
          collision with
            animal being ridden or animal
              drawn vehicle V06.931 ☑
              nontraffic V06.031 ☑
              traffic V06.131 ☑
            bus or heavy transport V04.931 ☑
              nontraffic V04.031 ☑
              traffic V04.131 ☑
            car V03.931 ☑
              nontraffic V04.031 ☑
              traffic V04.131 ☑
            pedal cycle V01.931 ☑
              nontraffic V01.031 ☑
              traffic V01.131 ☑
            pick-up or van V03.931 ☑

Accident — *continued*
  transport — *continued*
    pedestrian — *continued*
      conveyance — *continued*
        standing — *continued*
          electric scooter — *continued*
            collision with — *continued*
              pick-up or van — *continued*
                nontraffic V03.031 ☑
                traffic V03.131 ☑
              railway (train) (vehicle) V05.931 ☑
                nontraffic V05.031 ☑
                traffic V05.131 ☑
              streetcar V06.931 ☑
                nontraffic V06.031 ☑
                traffic V06.131 ☑
              three-wheeled motor vehicle
                V02.931 ☑
                nontraffic V02.031 ☑
                traffic V02.131 ☑
              two-wheeled motor vehicle
                V02.931 ☑
                nontraffic V02.031 ☑
                traffic V02.131 ☑
              vehicle, nonmotor, specified NEC
                V06.931 ☑
                nontraffic V06.031 ☑
                traffic V06.131 ☑
           fall V00.841 ☑
        micro-mobility pedestrian conveyance
          collision with
            animal being ridden or animal
              drawn vehicle V06.938 ☑
              nontraffic V06.038 ☑
              traffic V06.138 ☑
            bus or heavy transport V04.938 ☑
              nontraffic V04.038 ☑
              traffic V04.138 ☑
            car V03.938 ☑
              nontraffic V03.038 ☑
              traffic V03.138 ☑
            pedal cycle V01.938 ☑
              nontraffic V01.038 ☑
              traffic V01.138 ☑
            pick-up or van V03.938 ☑
              nontraffic V03.038 ☑
              traffic V03.138 ☑
            railway (train) (vehicle) V05.938 ☑
              nontraffic V05.038 ☑
              traffic V05.138 ☑
            stationary object V00.842 ☑
            streetcar V06.938 ☑
              nontraffic V06.038 ☑
              traffic V06.138 ☑
            three-wheeled motor vehicle
              V02.938 ☑
              nontraffic V02.038 ☑
              traffic V02.138 ☑
            two-wheeled motor vehicle
              V02.938 ☑
              nontraffic V02.038 ☑
              traffic V02.138 ☑
            vehicle, nonmotor, specified NEC
              V06.938 ☑
              nontraffic V06.038 ☑
              traffic V06.138 ☑
          fall V00.848 ☑
    traffic V09.3 ☑
      involving motor vehicle V09.20 ☑
        military V09.21 ☑
        specified type NEC V09.29 ☑
    wheelchair (powered) V00.818 ☑
      collision (with) V09.9 ☑
        animal being ridden or animal drawn
          vehicle V06.99 ☑
          nontraffic V06.09 ☑
          traffic V06.19 ☑
        bus or heavy transport V04.99 ☑
          nontraffic V04.09 ☑
          traffic V04.19 ☑
        car V03.99 ☑
          nontraffic V03.09 ☑
          traffic V03.19 ☑
        pedal cycle V01.99 ☑
          nontraffic V01.09 ☑
          traffic V01.19 ☑

Accident — *continued*
  transport — *continued*
    pedestrian — *continued*
      conveyance — *continued*
        wheelchair — *continued*
          collision — *continued*
            pick-up truck or van V03.99 ☑
              nontraffic V03.09 ☑
              traffic V03.19 ☑
            railway (train) (vehicle) V05.99 ☑
              nontraffic V05.09 ☑
              traffic V05.19 ☑
            stationary object V00.812 ☑
            streetcar V06.99 ☑
              nontraffic V06.09 ☑
              traffic V06.19 ☑
            two- or three-wheeled motor vehicle
              V02.99 ☑
              nontraffic V02.09 ☑
              traffic V02.19 ☑
            vehicle V09.9 ☑
              animal-drawn V06.99 ☑
                nontraffic V06.09 ☑
                traffic V06.19 ☑
              motor
                nontraffic V09.00 ☑
                traffic V09.20 ☑
          fall V00.811 ☑
        nontraffic V09.1 ☑
          involving motor vehicle NEC V09.00 ☑
        traffic V09.3 ☑
          involving motor vehicle NEC V09.20 ☑
      wheeled shoe V00.158 ☑
        colliding with stationary object
          V00.152 ☑
        fall V00.151 ☑
    on foot — *see also* Accident, pedestrian
      collision (with)
        animal being ridden or animal drawn ve-
          hicle V06.90 ☑
          nontraffic V06.00 ☑
          traffic V06.10 ☑
        bus or heavy transport V04.90 ☑
          nontraffic V04.00 ☑
          traffic V04.10 ☑
        car V03.90 ☑
          nontraffic V03.00 ☑
          traffic V03.10 ☑
        pedal cycle V01.90 ☑
          nontraffic V01.00 ☑
          traffic V01.10 ☑
        pick-up truck or van V03.90 ☑
          nontraffic V03.00 ☑
          traffic V03.10 ☑
        railway (train) (vehicle) V05.90 ☑
          nontraffic V05.00 ☑
          traffic V05.10 ☑
        streetcar V06.90 ☑
          nontraffic V06.00 ☑
          traffic V06.10 ☑
        two- or three-wheeled motor vehicle
          V02.90 ☑
          nontraffic V02.00 ☑
          traffic V02.10 ☑
        vehicle V09.9 ☑
          animal-drawn V06.90 ☑
            nontraffic V06.00 ☑
            traffic V06.10 ☑
          motor
        nontraffic V09.1 ☑
          involving motor vehicle V09.00 ☑
            military V09.01 ☑
            specified type NEC V09.09 ☑
        traffic V09.3 ☑
          involving motor vehicle V09.20 ☑
            military V09.21 ☑
            specified type NEC V09.29 ☑
  person NEC (unknown way or transportation) V99 ☑
    collision (between)
      bus (with)
        heavy transport vehicle (traffic) V87.5 ☑
          nontraffic V88.5 ☑
      car (with)
        bus (traffic) V87.3 ☑
          nontraffic V88.3 ☑
        heavy transport vehicle (traffic) V87.4 ☑

☑ Additional Character Required — Refer to the Tabular List for Character Selection

Accident — *continued*
  transport — *continued*
    person — *continued*
      collision — *continued*
        car — *continued*
          heavy transport vehicle — *continued*
            nontraffic V88.4 ☑
            nontraffic V88.5 ☑
          pick-up truck or van (traffic) V87.2 ☑
            nontraffic V88.2 ☑
          train or railway vehicle (traffic) V87.6 ☑
            nontraffic V88.6 ☑
          two-or three-wheeled motor vehicle
            (traffic) V87.0 ☑
            nontraffic V88.0 ☑
        motor vehicle (traffic) NEC V87.7 ☑
          nontraffic V88.7 ☑
        two-or three-wheeled vehicle (with) (traffic)
          motor vehicle NEC V87.1 ☑
          nontraffic V88.1 ☑
        nonmotor vehicle (collision) (noncollision) (traffic) V87.9 ☑
          nontraffic V88.9 ☑
    pickup truck occupant V59.9 ☑
      collision (with)
        animal (traffic) V50.9 ☑
          being ridden (traffic) V56.9 ☑
            nontraffic V56.3 ☑
              while boarding or alighting V56.4 ☑
          nontraffic V50.3 ☑
          while boarding or alighting V50.4 ☑
        animal-drawn vehicle (traffic) V56.9 ☑
          nontraffic V56.3 ☑
          while boarding or alighting V56.4 ☑
        bus (traffic) V54.9 ☑
          nontraffic V54.3 ☑
          while boarding or alighting V54.4 ☑
        car (traffic) V53.9 ☑
          nontraffic V53.3 ☑
          while boarding or alighting V53.4 ☑
        motor vehicle NOS (traffic) V59.60 ☑
          nontraffic V59.20 ☑
          specified type NEC (traffic) V59.69 ☑
            nontraffic V59.29 ☑
        pedal cycle (traffic) V51.9 ☑
          nontraffic V51.3 ☑
          while boarding or alighting V51.4 ☑
        pickup truck (traffic) V53.9 ☑
          nontraffic V53.3 ☑
          while boarding or alighting V53.4 ☑
        railway vehicle (traffic) V55.9 ☑
          nontraffic V55.3 ☑
          while boarding or alighting V55.4 ☑
        specified vehicle NEC (traffic) V56.9 ☑
          nontraffic V56.3 ☑
          while boarding or alighting V56.4 ☑
        stationary object (traffic) V57.9 ☑
          nontraffic V57.3 ☑
          while boarding or alighting V57.4 ☑
        streetcar (traffic) V56.9 ☑
          nontraffic V56.3 ☑
          while boarding or alighting V56.4 ☑
        three wheeled motor vehicle (traffic) V52.9 ☑
          nontraffic V52.3 ☑
          while boarding or alighting V52.4 ☑
        truck (traffic) V54.9 ☑
          nontraffic V54.3 ☑
          while boarding or alighting V54.4 ☑
        two wheeled motor vehicle (traffic) V52.9 ☑
          nontraffic V52.3 ☑
          while boarding or alighting V52.4 ☑
        van (traffic) V53.9 ☑
          nontraffic V53.3 ☑
          while boarding or alighting V53.4 ☑
      driver
        collision (with)
          animal (traffic) V50.5 ☑
            being ridden (traffic) V56.5 ☑
              nontraffic V56.0 ☑
            nontraffic V50.0 ☑
          animal-drawn vehicle (traffic) V56.5 ☑
            nontraffic V56.0 ☑
          bus (traffic) V54.5 ☑
            nontraffic V54.0 ☑
          car (traffic) V53.5 ☑
            nontraffic V53.0 ☑

Accident — *continued*
  transport — *continued*
    pickup truck occupant — *continued*
      driver — *continued*
        collision — *continued*
          motor vehicle NOS (traffic) V59.40 ☑
            nontraffic V59.00 ☑
            specified type NEC (traffic) V59.49 ☑
              nontraffic V59.09 ☑
          pedal cycle (traffic) V51.5 ☑
            nontraffic V51.0 ☑
          pickup truck (traffic) V53.5 ☑
            nontraffic V53.0 ☑
          railway vehicle (traffic) V55.5 ☑
            nontraffic V55.0 ☑
          specified vehicle NEC (traffic) V56.5 ☑
            nontraffic V56.0 ☑
          stationary object (traffic) V57.5 ☑
            nontraffic V57.0 ☑
          streetcar (traffic) V56.5 ☑
            nontraffic V56.0 ☑
          three wheeled motor vehicle (traffic)
            V52.5 ☑
            nontraffic V52.0 ☑
          truck (traffic) V54.5 ☑
            nontraffic V54.0 ☑
          two wheeled motor vehicle (traffic)
            V52.5 ☑
            nontraffic V52.0 ☑
          van (traffic) V53.5 ☑
            nontraffic V53.0 ☑
        noncollision accident (traffic) V58.5 ☑
          nontraffic V58.0 ☑
      hanger-on
        collision (with)
          animal (traffic) V50.7 ☑
            being ridden (traffic) V56.7 ☑
              nontraffic V56.2 ☑
            nontraffic V50.2 ☑
          animal-drawn vehicle (traffic) V56.7 ☑
            nontraffic V56.2 ☑
          bus (traffic) V54.7 ☑
            nontraffic V54.2 ☑
          car (traffic) V53.7 ☑
            nontraffic V53.2 ☑
          pedal cycle (traffic) V51.7 ☑
            nontraffic V51.2 ☑
          pickup truck (traffic) V53.7 ☑
            nontraffic V53.2 ☑
          railway vehicle (traffic) V55.7 ☑
            nontraffic V55.2 ☑
          specified vehicle NEC (traffic) V56.7 ☑
            nontraffic V56.2 ☑
          stationary object (traffic) V57.7 ☑
            nontraffic V57.2 ☑
          streetcar (traffic) V56.7 ☑
            nontraffic V56.2 ☑
          three wheeled motor vehicle (traffic)
            V52.7 ☑
            nontraffic V52.2 ☑
          truck (traffic) V54.7 ☑
            nontraffic V54.2 ☑
          two wheeled motor vehicle (traffic)
            V52.7 ☑
            nontraffic V52.2 ☑
          van (traffic) V53.7 ☑
            nontraffic V53.2 ☑
        noncollision accident (traffic) V58.7 ☑
          nontraffic V58.2 ☑
      noncollision accident (traffic) V58.9 ☑
        nontraffic V58.3 ☑
        while boarding or alighting V58.4 ☑
      nontraffic V59.3 ☑
      passenger
        collision (with)
          animal (traffic) V50.6 ☑
            being ridden (traffic) V56.6 ☑
              nontraffic V56.1 ☑
            nontraffic V50.1 ☑
          animal-drawn vehicle (traffic) V56.6 ☑
            nontraffic V56.1 ☑
          bus (traffic) V54.6 ☑
            nontraffic V54.1 ☑
          car (traffic) V53.6 ☑
            nontraffic V53.1 ☑
          motor vehicle NOS (traffic) V59.50 ☑

Accident — *continued*
  transport — *continued*
    pickup truck occupant — *continued*
      passenger — *continued*
        collision — *continued*
          motor vehicle — *continued*
            nontraffic V59.10 ☑
            specified type NEC (traffic) V59.59 ☑
              nontraffic V59.19 ☑
          pedal cycle (traffic) V51.6 ☑
            nontraffic V51.1 ☑
          pickup truck (traffic) V53.6 ☑
            nontraffic V53.1 ☑
          railway vehicle (traffic) V55.6 ☑
            nontraffic V55.1 ☑
          specified vehicle NEC (traffic) V56.6 ☑
            nontraffic V56.1 ☑
          stationary object (traffic) V57.6 ☑
            nontraffic V57.1 ☑
          streetcar (traffic) V56.6 ☑
            nontraffic V56.1 ☑
          three wheeled motor vehicle (traffic)
            V52.6 ☑
            nontraffic V52.1 ☑
          truck (traffic) V54.6 ☑
            nontraffic V54.1 ☑
          two wheeled motor vehicle (traffic)
            V52.6 ☑
            nontraffic V52.1 ☑
          van (traffic) V53.6 ☑
            nontraffic V53.1 ☑
        noncollision accident (traffic) V58.6 ☑
          nontraffic V58.1 ☑
      specified type NEC V59.88 ☑
      military vehicle V59.81 ☑
    quarry truck — *see* Accident, transport, industrial
      vehicle occupant
    race car — *see* Accident, transport, motor vehicle
      NEC occupant
    railway vehicle occupant V81.9 ☑
      collision (with) V81.3 ☑
        motor vehicle (non-military) (traffic) V81.1 ☑
          military V81.83 ☑
          nontraffic V81.0 ☑
        rolling stock V81.2 ☑
        specified object NEC V81.3 ☑
      during derailment V81.7 ☑
        with antecedent collision — *see* Accident,
          transport, railway vehicle occupant,
          collision
      explosion V81.81 ☑
      fall (in railway vehicle) V81.5 ☑
        during derailment V81.7 ☑
          with antecedent collision — *see* Accident,
            transport, railway vehicle occupant,
            collision
        from railway vehicle V81.6 ☑
          during derailment V81.7 ☑
            with antecedent collision — *see* Accident, transport, railway vehicle
              occupant, collision
        while boarding or alighting V81.4 ☑
      fire V81.81 ☑
      object falling onto train V81.82 ☑
      specified type NEC V81.89 ☑
      while boarding or alighting V81.4 ☑
    Segway V00.848 ☑
    ski lift V98.3 ☑
    snowmobile occupant (nontraffic) V86.92 ☑
      driver V86.52 ☑
      hanger-on V86.72 ☑
      passenger V86.62 ☑
      traffic V86.32 ☑
        driver V86.02 ☑
        hanger-on V86.22 ☑
        passenger V86.12 ☑
      while boarding or alighting V86.42 ☑
    specified NEC V98.8 ☑
    sport utility vehicle occupant — *see also* Accident,
      transport, pickup truck occupant
    streetcar occupant V82.9 ☑
      collision (with) V82.3 ☑
        motor vehicle (traffic) V82.1 ☑
          nontraffic V82.0 ☑
        rolling stock V82.2 ☑
      during derailment V82.7 ☑

Accident — *continued*
transport — *continued*
streetcar occupant — *continued*
during derailment — *continued*
with antecedent collision — *see* Accident,
transport, streetcar occupant, collision
fall (in streetcar) V82.5
during derailment V82.7
with antecedent collision — *see* Accident,
transport, streetcar occupant, collision
from streetcar V82.6
during derailment V82.7
with antecedent collision — *see* Accident, transport, streetcar occupant, collision
while boarding or alighting V82.4
while boarding or alighting V82.4
specified type NEC V82.8
while boarding or alighting V82.4
three-wheeled motor vehicle occupant V39.9
collision (with)
animal (traffic) V30.9
being ridden (traffic) V36.9
nontraffic V36.3
while boarding or alighting V36.4
nontraffic V30.3
while boarding or alighting V30.4
animal-drawn vehicle (traffic) V36.9
nontraffic V36.3
while boarding or alighting V36.4
bus (traffic) V34.9
nontraffic V34.3
while boarding or alighting V34.4
car (traffic) V33.9
nontraffic V33.3
while boarding or alighting V33.4
motor vehicle NOS (traffic) V39.60
nontraffic V39.20
specified type NEC (traffic) V39.69
nontraffic V39.29
pedal cycle (traffic) V31.9
nontraffic V31.3
while boarding or alighting V31.4
pickup truck (traffic) V33.9
nontraffic V33.3
while boarding or alighting V33.4
railway vehicle (traffic) V35.9
nontraffic V35.3
while boarding or alighting V35.4
specified vehicle NEC (traffic) V36.9
nontraffic V36.3
while boarding or alighting V36.4
stationary object (traffic) V37.9
nontraffic V37.3
while boarding or alighting V37.4
streetcar (traffic) V36.9
nontraffic V36.3
while boarding or alighting V36.4
three wheeled motor vehicle (traffic) V32.9
nontraffic V32.3
while boarding or alighting V32.4
truck (traffic) V34.9
nontraffic V34.3
while boarding or alighting V34.4
two wheeled motor vehicle (traffic) V32.9
nontraffic V32.3
while boarding or alighting V32.4
van (traffic) V33.9
nontraffic V33.3
while boarding or alighting V33.4
driver
collision (with)
animal (traffic) V30.5
being ridden (traffic) V36.5
nontraffic V36.0
nontraffic V30.0
animal-drawn vehicle (traffic) V36.5
nontraffic V36.0
bus (traffic) V34.5
nontraffic V34.0
car (traffic) V33.5
nontraffic V33.0
motor vehicle NOS (traffic) V39.40
nontraffic V39.00
specified type NEC (traffic) V39.49

Accident — *continued*
transport — *continued*
three-wheeled motor vehicle occupant — *continued*
driver — *continued*
collision — *continued*
motor vehicle — *continued*
specified type — *continued*
nontraffic V39.09
pedal cycle (traffic) V31.5
nontraffic V31.0
pickup truck (traffic) V33.5
nontraffic V33.0
railway vehicle (traffic) V35.5
nontraffic V35.0
specified vehicle NEC (traffic) V36.5
nontraffic V36.0
stationary object (traffic) V37.5
nontraffic V37.0
streetcar (traffic) V36.5
nontraffic V36.0
three wheeled motor vehicle (traffic) V32.5
nontraffic V32.0
truck (traffic) V34.5
nontraffic V34.0
two wheeled motor vehicle (traffic) V32.5
nontraffic V32.0
van (traffic) V33.5
nontraffic V33.0
noncollision accident (traffic) V38.5
nontraffic V38.0
hanger-on
collision (with)
animal (traffic) V30.7
being ridden (traffic) V36.7
nontraffic V36.2
nontraffic V30.2
animal-drawn vehicle (traffic) V36.7
nontraffic V36.2
bus (traffic) V34.7
nontraffic V34.2
car (traffic) V33.7
nontraffic V33.2
pedal cycle (traffic) V31.7
nontraffic V31.2
pickup truck (traffic) V33.7
nontraffic V33.2
railway vehicle (traffic) V35.7
nontraffic V35.2
specified vehicle NEC (traffic) V36.7
nontraffic V36.2
stationary object (traffic) V37.7
nontraffic V37.2
streetcar (traffic) V36.7
nontraffic V36.2
three wheeled motor vehicle (traffic) V32.7
nontraffic V32.2
truck (traffic) V34.7
nontraffic V34.2
two wheeled motor vehicle (traffic) V32.7
nontraffic V32.2
van (traffic) V33.7
nontraffic V33.2
noncollision accident (traffic) V38.7
nontraffic V38.2
noncollision accident (traffic) V38.9
nontraffic V38.3
while boarding or alighting V38.4
nontraffic V39.3
passenger
collision (with)
animal (traffic) V30.6
being ridden (traffic) V36.6
nontraffic V36.1
nontraffic V30.1
animal-drawn vehicle (traffic) V36.6
nontraffic V36.1
bus (traffic) V34.6
nontraffic V34.1
car (traffic) V33.6
nontraffic V33.1
motor vehicle NOS (traffic) V39.50

Accident — *continued*
transport — *continued*
three-wheeled motor vehicle occupant — *continued*
passenger — *continued*
collision — *continued*
motor vehicle — *continued*
nontraffic V39.10
specified type NEC (traffic) V39.59
nontraffic V39.19
pedal cycle (traffic) V31.6
nontraffic V31.1
pickup truck (traffic) V33.6
nontraffic V33.1
railway vehicle (traffic) V35.6
nontraffic V35.1
specified vehicle NEC (traffic) V36.6
nontraffic V36.1
stationary object (traffic) V37.6
nontraffic V37.1
streetcar (traffic) V36.6
nontraffic V36.1
three wheeled motor vehicle (traffic) V32.6
nontraffic V32.1
truck (traffic) V34.6
nontraffic V34.1
two wheeled motor vehicle (traffic) V32.6
nontraffic V32.1
van (traffic) V33.6
nontraffic V33.1
noncollision accident (traffic) V38.6
nontraffic V38.1
specified type NEC V39.89
military vehicle V39.81
tractor (farm) (and trailer) — *see* Accident, transport, agricultural vehicle occupant
tram — *see* Accident, transport, streetcar
in mine or quarry — *see* Accident, transport, industrial vehicle occupant
trolley — *see* Accident, transport, streetcar
in mine or quarry — *see* Accident, transport, industrial vehicle occupant
truck (heavy) occupant V69.9
collision (with)
animal (traffic) V60.9
being ridden (traffic) V66.9
nontraffic V66.3
while boarding or alighting V66.4
nontraffic V60.3
while boarding or alighting V60.4
animal-drawn vehicle (traffic) V66.9
nontraffic V66.3
while boarding or alighting V66.4
bus (traffic) V64.9
nontraffic V64.3
while boarding or alighting V64.4
car (traffic) V63.9
nontraffic V63.3
while boarding or alighting V63.4
motor vehicle NOS (traffic) V69.60
nontraffic V69.20
specified type NEC (traffic) V69.69
nontraffic V69.29
pedal cycle (traffic) V61.9
nontraffic V61.3
while boarding or alighting V61.4
pickup truck (traffic) V63.9
nontraffic V63.3
while boarding or alighting V63.4
railway vehicle (traffic) V65.9
nontraffic V65.3
while boarding or alighting V65.4
specified vehicle NEC (traffic) V66.9
nontraffic V66.3
while boarding or alighting V66.4
stationary object (traffic) V67.9
nontraffic V67.3
while boarding or alighting V67.4
streetcar (traffic) V66.9
nontraffic V66.3
while boarding or alighting V66.4
three wheeled motor vehicle (traffic) V62.9
nontraffic V62.3
while boarding or alighting V62.4

Accident — *continued*
  transport — *continued*
    truck occupant — *continued*
      collision — *continued*
        truck (traffic) V64.9 ☑
          nontraffic V64.3 ☑
          while boarding or alighting V64.4 ☑
        two wheeled motor vehicle (traffic) V62.9 ☑
          nontraffic V62.3 ☑
          while boarding or alighting V62.4 ☑
        van (traffic) V63.9 ☑
          nontraffic V63.3 ☑
          while boarding or alighting V63.4 ☑
      driver
        collision (with)
          animal (traffic) V60.5 ☑
            being ridden (traffic) V66.5 ☑
              nontraffic V66.0 ☑
            nontraffic V60.0 ☑
          animal-drawn vehicle (traffic) V66.5 ☑
            nontraffic V66.0 ☑
          bus (traffic) V64.5 ☑
            nontraffic V64.0 ☑
          car (traffic) V63.5 ☑
            nontraffic V63.0 ☑
          motor vehicle NOS (traffic) V69.40 ☑
            nontraffic V69.00 ☑
            specified type NEC (traffic) V69.49 ☑
              nontraffic V69.09 ☑
          pedal cycle (traffic) V61.5 ☑
            nontraffic V61.0 ☑
          pickup truck (traffic) V63.5 ☑
            nontraffic V63.0 ☑
          railway vehicle (traffic) V65.5 ☑
            nontraffic V65.0 ☑
          specified vehicle NEC (traffic) V66.5 ☑
            nontraffic V66.0 ☑
          stationary object (traffic) V67.5 ☑
            nontraffic V67.0 ☑
          streetcar (traffic) V66.5 ☑
            nontraffic V66.0 ☑
          three wheeled motor vehicle (traffic)
            V62.5 ☑
            nontraffic V62.0 ☑
          truck (traffic) V64.5 ☑
            nontraffic V64.0 ☑
          two wheeled motor vehicle (traffic)
            V62.5 ☑
            nontraffic V62.0 ☑
          van (traffic) V63.5 ☑
            nontraffic V63.0 ☑
        noncollision accident (traffic) V68.5 ☑
          nontraffic V68.0 ☑
      dump — *see* Accident, transport, construction
        vehicle occupant
      hanger-on
        collision (with)
          animal (traffic) V60.7 ☑
            being ridden (traffic) V66.7 ☑
              nontraffic V66.2 ☑
            nontraffic V60.2 ☑
          animal-drawn vehicle (traffic) V66.7 ☑
            nontraffic V66.2 ☑
          bus (traffic) V64.7 ☑
            nontraffic V64.2 ☑
          car (traffic) V63.7 ☑
            nontraffic V63.2 ☑
          pedal cycle (traffic) V61.7 ☑
            nontraffic V61.2 ☑
          pickup truck (traffic) V63.7 ☑
            nontraffic V63.2 ☑
          railway vehicle (traffic) V65.7 ☑
            nontraffic V65.2 ☑
          specified vehicle NEC (traffic) V66.7 ☑
            nontraffic V66.2 ☑
          stationary object (traffic) V67.7 ☑
            nontraffic V67.2 ☑
          streetcar (traffic) V66.7 ☑
            nontraffic V66.2 ☑
          three wheeled motor vehicle (traffic)
            V62.7 ☑
            nontraffic V62.2 ☑
          truck (traffic) V64.7 ☑
            nontraffic V64.2 ☑
          two wheeled motor vehicle (traffic)
            V62.7 ☑

Accident — *continued*
  transport — *continued*
    truck occupant — *continued*
      hanger-on — *continued*
        collision — *continued*
          two wheeled motor vehicle — *continued*
            nontraffic V62.2 ☑
          van (traffic) V63.7 ☑
            nontraffic V63.2 ☑
        noncollision accident (traffic) V68.7 ☑
          nontraffic V68.2 ☑
      noncollision accident (traffic) V68.9 ☑
        nontraffic V68.3 ☑
        while boarding or alighting V68.4 ☑
      nontraffic V69.3 ☑
      passenger
        collision (with)
          animal (traffic) V60.6 ☑
            being ridden (traffic) V66.6 ☑
              nontraffic V66.1-
            nontraffic V60.1 ☑
          animal-drawn vehicle (traffic) V66.6 ☑
            nontraffic V66.1 ☑
          bus (traffic) V64.6 ☑
            nontraffic V64.1 ☑
          car (traffic) V63.6 ☑
            nontraffic V63.1 ☑
          motor vehicle NOS (traffic) V69.50 ☑
            nontraffic V69.10 ☑
            specified type NEC (traffic) V69.59 ☑
              nontraffic V69.19 ☑
          pedal cycle (traffic) V61.6 ☑
            nontraffic V61.1 ☑
          pickup truck (traffic) V63.6 ☑
            nontraffic V63.1 ☑
          railway vehicle (traffic) V65.6 ☑
            nontraffic V65.1 ☑
          specified vehicle NEC (traffic) V66.6 ☑
            nontraffic V66.1 ☑
          stationary object (traffic) V67.6 ☑
            nontraffic V67.1 ☑
          streetcar (traffic) V66.6 ☑
            nontraffic V66.1 ☑
          three wheeled motor vehicle (traffic)
            V62.6 ☑
            nontraffic V62.1 ☑
          truck (traffic) V64.6 ☑
            nontraffic V64.1 ☑
          two wheeled motor vehicle (traffic)
            V62.6 ☑
            nontraffic V62.1 ☑
          van (traffic) V63.6 ☑
            nontraffic V63.1 ☑
        noncollision accident (traffic) V68.6 ☑
          nontraffic V68.1 ☑
      pickup — *see* Accident, transport, pickup truck
        occupant
      specified type NEC V69.88 ☑
        military vehicle V69.81 ☑
    van occupant V59.9 ☑
      collision (with)
        animal (traffic) V50.9 ☑
          being ridden (traffic) V56.9 ☑
            nontraffic V56.3 ☑
            while boarding or alighting V56.4 ☑
          nontraffic V50.3 ☑
          while boarding or alighting V50.4 ☑
        animal-drawn vehicle (traffic) V56.9 ☑
          nontraffic V56.3 ☑
          while boarding or alighting V56.4 ☑
        bus (traffic) V54.9 ☑
          nontraffic V54.3 ☑
          while boarding or alighting V54.4 ☑
        car (traffic) V53.9 ☑
          nontraffic V53.3 ☑
          while boarding or alighting V53.4 ☑
        motor vehicle NOS (traffic) V59.60 ☑
          nontraffic V59.20 ☑
          specified type NEC (traffic) V59.69 ☑
            nontraffic V59.29 ☑
        pedal cycle (traffic) V51.9 ☑
          nontraffic V51.3 ☑
          while boarding or alighting V51.4 ☑
        pickup truck (traffic) V53.9 ☑
          nontraffic V53.3 ☑

Accident — *continued*
  transport — *continued*
    van occupant — *continued*
      collision — *continued*
        pickup truck — *continued*
          while boarding or alighting V53.4 ☑
        railway vehicle (traffic) V55.9 ☑
          nontraffic V55.3 ☑
          while boarding or alighting V55.4 ☑
        specified vehicle NEC (traffic) V56.9 ☑
          nontraffic V56.3 ☑
          while boarding or alighting V56.4 ☑
        stationary object (traffic) V57.9 ☑
          nontraffic V57.3 ☑
          while boarding or alighting V57.4 ☑
        streetcar (traffic) V56.9 ☑
          nontraffic V56.3 ☑
          while boarding or alighting V56.4 ☑
        three wheeled motor vehicle (traffic) V52.9 ☑
          nontraffic V52.3 ☑
          while boarding or alighting V52.4 ☑
        truck (traffic) V54.9 ☑
          nontraffic V54.3 ☑
          while boarding or alighting V54.4 ☑
        two wheeled motor vehicle (traffic) V52.9 ☑
          nontraffic V52.3 ☑
          while boarding or alighting V52.4 ☑
        van (traffic) V53.9 ☑
          nontraffic V53.3 ☑
          while boarding or alighting V53.4 ☑
      driver
        collision (with)
          animal (traffic) V50.5 ☑
            being ridden (traffic) V56.5 ☑
              nontraffic V56.0 ☑
            nontraffic V50.0 ☑
          animal-drawn vehicle (traffic) V56.5 ☑
            nontraffic V56.0 ☑
          bus (traffic) V54.5 ☑
            nontraffic V54.0 ☑
          car (traffic) V53.5 ☑
            nontraffic V53.0 ☑
          motor vehicle NOS (traffic) V59.40 ☑
            nontraffic V59.00 ☑
            specified type NEC (traffic) V59.49 ☑
              nontraffic V59.09 ☑
          pedal cycle (traffic) V51.5 ☑
            nontraffic V51.0 ☑
          pickup truck (traffic) V53.5 ☑
            nontraffic V53.0 ☑
          railway vehicle (traffic) V55.5 ☑
            nontraffic V55.0 ☑
          specified vehicle NEC (traffic) V56.5 ☑
            nontraffic V56.0 ☑
          stationary object (traffic) V57.5 ☑
            nontraffic V57.0 ☑
          streetcar (traffic) V56.5 ☑
            nontraffic V56.0 ☑
          three wheeled motor vehicle (traffic)
            V52.5 ☑
            nontraffic V52.0 ☑
          truck (traffic) V54.5 ☑
            nontraffic V54.0 ☑
          two wheeled motor vehicle (traffic)
            V52.5 ☑
            nontraffic V52.0 ☑
          van (traffic) V53.5 ☑
            nontraffic V53.0 ☑
        noncollision accident (traffic) V58.5 ☑
          nontraffic V58.0 ☑
      hanger-on
        collision (with)
          animal (traffic) V50.7 ☑
            being ridden (traffic) V56.7 ☑
              nontraffic V56.2 ☑
            nontraffic V50.2 ☑
          animal-drawn vehicle (traffic) V56.7 ☑
            nontraffic V56.2 ☑
          bus (traffic) V54.7 ☑
            nontraffic V54.2 ☑
          car (traffic) V53.7 ☑
            nontraffic V53.2 ☑
          pedal cycle (traffic) V51.7 ☑
            nontraffic V51.2 ☑
          pickup truck (traffic) V53.7 ☑
            nontraffic V53.2 ☑

Accident — *continued*
  transport — *continued*
    van occupant — *continued*
      hanger-on — *continued*
        collision — *continued*
          railway vehicle (traffic) V55.7 ☑
            nontraffic V55.2 ☑
          specified vehicle NEC (traffic) V56.7 ☑
            nontraffic V56.2 ☑
          stationary object (traffic) V57.7 ☑
            nontraffic V57.2 ☑
          streetcar (traffic) V56.7 ☑
            nontraffic V56.2 ☑
          three wheeled motor vehicle (traffic) V52.7 ☑
            nontraffic V52.2 ☑
          truck (traffic) V54.7 ☑
            nontraffic V54.2 ☑
          two wheeled motor vehicle (traffic) V52.7 ☑
            nontraffic V52.2 ☑
          van (traffic) V53.7 ☑
            nontraffic V53.2 ☑
        noncollision accident (traffic) V58.7 ☑
          nontraffic V58.2 ☑
        noncollision accident (traffic) V58.9 ☑
          nontraffic V58.3 ☑
        while boarding or alighting V58.4 ☑
      nontraffic V59.3 ☑
      passenger
        collision (with)
          animal (traffic) V50.6 ☑
            being ridden (traffic) V56.6 ☑
              nontraffic V56.1 ☑
            nontraffic V50.1 ☑
          animal-drawn vehicle (traffic) V56.6 ☑
            nontraffic V56.1 ☑
          bus (traffic) V54.6 ☑
            nontraffic V54.1 ☑
          car (traffic) V53.6 ☑
            nontraffic V53.1 ☑
          motor vehicle NOS (traffic) V59.50 ☑
            nontraffic V59.10 ☑
            specified type NEC (traffic) V59.59 ☑
              nontraffic V59.19 ☑
          pedal cycle (traffic) V51.6 ☑
            nontraffic V51.1 ☑
          pickup truck (traffic) V53.6 ☑
            nontraffic V53.1 ☑
          railway vehicle (traffic) V55.6 ☑
            nontraffic V55.1 ☑
          specified vehicle NEC (traffic) V56.6 ☑
            nontraffic V56.1 ☑
          stationary object (traffic) V57.6 ☑
            nontraffic V57.1 ☑
          streetcar (traffic) V56.6 ☑
            nontraffic V56.1 ☑
          three wheeled motor vehicle (traffic) V52.6 ☑
            nontraffic V52.1 ☑
          truck (traffic) V54.6 ☑
            nontraffic V54.1 ☑
          two wheeled motor vehicle (traffic) V52.6 ☑
            nontraffic V52.1 ☑
          van (traffic) V53.6 ☑
            nontraffic V53.1 ☑
        noncollision accident (traffic) V58.6 ☑
          nontraffic V58.1 ☑
      specified type NEC V59.88 ☑
      military vehicle V59.81 ☑
    watercraft occupant — *see* Accident, watercraft
  vehicle NEC V89.9 ☑
    animal-drawn NEC — *see* Accident, transport, animal-drawn vehicle occupant
    special
      agricultural — *see* Accident, transport, agricultural vehicle occupant
      construction — *see* Accident, transport, construction vehicle occupant
      industrial — *see* Accident, transport, industrial vehicle occupant
    three-wheeled NEC (motorized) — *see* Accident, transport, three-wheeled motor vehicle occupant
  watercraft V94.9 ☑

Accident — *continued*
  watercraft — *continued*
    causing
      drowning — *see* Drowning, due to, accident to, watercraft
      injury NEC V91.89 ☑
        crushed between craft and object V91.19 ☑
          powered craft V91.13 ☑
            ferry boat V91.11 ☑
            fishing boat V91.12 ☑
            jetskis V91.13 ☑
            liner V91.11 ☑
            merchant ship V91.10 ☑
            passenger ship V91.11 ☑
          unpowered craft V91.18 ☑
            canoe V91.15 ☑
            inflatable V91.16 ☑
            kayak V91.15 ☑
            sailboat V91.14 ☑
            surf-board V91.18 ☑
            windsurfer V91.18 ☑
        fall on board V91.29 ☑
          powered craft V91.23 ☑
            ferry boat V91.21 ☑
            fishing boat V91.22 ☑
            jetskis V91.23 ☑
            liner V91.21 ☑
            merchant ship V91.20 ☑
            passenger ship V91.21 ☑
          unpowered craft
            canoe V91.25 ☑
            inflatable V91.26 ☑
            kayak V91.25 ☑
            sailboat V91.24 ☑
        fire on board causing burn V91.09 ☑
          powered craft V91.03 ☑
            ferry boat V91.01 ☑
            fishing boat V91.02 ☑
            jetskis V91.03 ☑
            liner V91.01 ☑
            merchant ship V91.00 ☑
            passenger ship V91.01 ☑
          unpowered craft V91.08 ☑
            canoe V91.05 ☑
            inflatable V91.06 ☑
            kayak V91.05 ☑
            sailboat V91.04 ☑
            surf-board V91.08 ☑
            water skis V91.07 ☑
            windsurfer V91.08 ☑
        hit by falling object V91.39 ☑
          powered craft V91.33 ☑
            ferry boat V91.31 ☑
            fishing boat V91.32 ☑
            jetskis V91.33 ☑
            liner V91.31 ☑
            merchant ship V91.30 ☑
            passenger ship V91.31 ☑
          unpowered craft V91.38 ☑
            canoe V91.35 ☑
            inflatable V91.36 ☑
            kayak V91.35 ☑
            sailboat V91.34 ☑
            surf-board V91.38 ☑
            water skis V91.37 ☑
            windsurfer V91.38 ☑
        specified type NEC V91.89 ☑
          powered craft V91.83 ☑
            ferry boat V91.81 ☑
            fishing boat V91.82 ☑
            jetskis V91.83 ☑
            liner V91.81 ☑
            merchant ship V91.80 ☑
            passenger ship V91.81 ☑
          unpowered craft V91.88 ☑
            canoe V91.85 ☑
            inflatable V91.86 ☑
            kayak V91.85 ☑
            sailboat V91.84 ☑
            surf-board V91.88 ☑
            water skis V91.87 ☑
            windsurfer V91.88 ☑
      due to, caused by cataclysm — *see* Forces of nature, by type
      military NEC V94.818 ☑
        civilian in water injured by V94.811 ☑

Accident — *continued*
  watercraft — *continued*
    military — *continued*
      with civilian watercraft V94.810 ☑
    nonpowered, struck by
      nonpowered vessel V94.22 ☑
      powered vessel V94.21 ☑
      specified type NEC V94.89 ☑
    striking swimmer
      powered V94.11 ☑
      unpowered V94.12 ☑
Acid throwing (assault) Y08.89 ☑
Activity (involving) (of victim at time of event) Y93.9
  aerobic and step exercise (class) Y93.A3 (*following* Y93.7)
  alpine skiing Y93.23
  animal care NEC Y93.K9 (*following* Y93.7)
  arts and handcrafts NEC Y93.D9 (*following* Y93.7)
  athletics played as a team or group NEC Y93.69
  athletics played individually NEC Y93.59
  athletics NEC Y93.79
  baking Y93.G3 (*following* Y93.7)
  ballet Y93.41
  barbells Y93.B3 (*following* Y93.7)
  BASE (Building, Antenna, Span, Earth) jumping Y93.33
  baseball Y93.64
  basketball Y93.67
  bathing (personal) Y93.E1 (*following* Y93.7)
  beach volleyball Y93.68
  bike riding Y93.55
  blackout game Y93.85
  boogie boarding Y93.18
  bowling Y93.54
  boxing Y93.71
  brass instrument playing Y93.J4 (*following* Y93.7)
  building construction Y93.H3 (*following* Y93.7)
  bungee jumping Y93.34
  calisthenics Y93.A2 (*following* Y93.7)
  canoeing (in calm and turbulent water) Y93.16
  capture the flag Y93.6A
  cardiorespiratory exercise NEC Y93.A9 (*following* Y93.7)
  caregiving (providing) NEC Y93.F9 (*following* Y93.7)
    bathing Y93.F1 (*following* Y93.7)
    lifting Y93.F2 (*following* Y93.7)
  cellular
    communication device Y93.C2 (*following* Y93.7)
    telephone Y93.C2 (*following* Y93.7)
  challenge course Y93.A5 (*following* Y93.7)
  cheerleading Y93.45
  choking game Y93.85
  circuit training Y93.A4 (*following* Y93.7)
  cleaning
    floor Y93.E5 (*following* Y93.7)
  climbing NEC Y93.39
    mountain Y93.31
    rock Y93.31
    wall Y93.31
  clothing care and maintenance NEC Y93.E9 (*following* Y93.7)
  combatives Y93.75
  computer
    keyboarding Y93.C1 (*following* Y93.7)
    technology NEC Y93.C9 (*following* Y93.7)
  confidence course Y93.A5 (*following* Y93.7)
  construction (building) Y93.H3 (*following* Y93.7)
  cooking and baking Y93.G3 (*following* Y93.7)
  cool down exercises Y93.A2 (*following* Y93.7)
  cricket Y93.69
  crocheting Y93.D1 (*following* Y93.7)
  cross country skiing Y93.24
  dancing (all types) Y93.41
  digging
    dirt Y93.H1 (*following* Y93.7)
  dirt digging Y93.H1 (*following* Y93.7)
  dishwashing Y93.G1 (*following* Y93.7)
  diving (platform) (springboard) Y93.12
    underwater Y93.15
  dodge ball Y93.6A
  downhill skiing Y93.23
  drum playing Y93.J2 (*following* Y93.7)
  dumbbells Y93.B3 (*following* Y93.7)
  electronic
    devices NEC Y93.C9 (*following* Y93.7)
      hand held interactive Y93.C2 (*following* Y93.7)
    game playing (using) (with)
      interactive device Y93.C2 (*following* Y93.7)
      keyboard or other stationary device Y93.C1 (*following* Y93.7)

Activity — *continued*
elliptical machine Y93.A1 (*following* Y93.7)
exercise(s)
  machines ((primarily) for)
    cardiorespiratory conditioning Y93.A1 (*following* Y93.7)
    muscle strengthening Y93.B1 (*following* Y93.7)
    muscle strengthening (non-machine) NEC Y93.B9 (*following* Y93.7)
external motion NEC Y93.I9 (*following* Y93.7)
  rollercoaster Y93.I1 (*following* Y93.7)
fainting game Y93.85
field hockey Y93.65
figure skating (pairs) (singles) Y93.21
flag football Y93.62
floor mopping and cleaning Y93.E5 (*following* Y93.7)
food preparation and clean up Y93.G1 (*following* Y93.7)
football (American) NOS Y93.61
  flag Y93.62
  tackle Y93.61
  touch Y93.62
four square Y93.6A
free weights Y93.B3 (*following* Y93.7)
frisbee (ultimate) Y93.74
furniture
  building Y93.D3 (*following* Y93.7)
  finishing Y93.D3 (*following* Y93.7)
  repair Y93.D3 (*following* Y93.7)
game playing (electronic)
  using interactive device Y93.C2 (*following* Y93.7)
  using keyboard or other stationary device Y93.C1 (*following* Y93.7)
gardening Y93.H2 (*following* Y93.7)
golf Y93.53
grass drills Y93.A6 (*following* Y93.7)
grilling and smoking food Y93.G2 (*following* Y93.7)
grooming and shearing an animal Y93.K3 (*following* Y93.7)
guerilla drills Y93.A6 (*following* Y93.7)
gymnastics (rhythmic) Y93.43
hand held interactive electronic device Y93.C2 (*following* Y93.7)
handball Y93.73
handcrafts NEC Y93.D9 (*following* Y93.7)
hang gliding Y93.35
hiking (on level or elevated terrain) Y93.01
hockey (ice) Y93.22
  field Y93.65
horseback riding Y93.52
household (interior) maintenance NEC Y93.E9 (*following* Y93.7)
ice NEC Y93.29
  dancing Y93.21
  hockey Y93.22
  skating Y93.21
inline roller skating Y93.51
ironing Y93.E4 (*following* Y93.7)
judo Y93.75
jumping jacks Y93.A2 (*following* Y93.7)
jumping rope Y93.56
jumping (off) NEC Y93.39
  BASE (Building, Antenna, Span, Earth) Y93.33
  bungee Y93.34
  jacks Y93.A2 (*following* Y93.7)
  rope Y93.56
karate Y93.75
kayaking (in calm and turbulent water) Y93.16
keyboarding (computer) Y93.C1 (*following* Y93.7)
kickball Y93.6A
knitting Y93.D1 (*following* Y93.7)
lacrosse Y93.65
land maintenance NEC Y93.H9 (*following* Y93.7)
landscaping Y93.H2 (*following* Y93.7)
laundry Y93.E2 (*following* Y93.7)
machines (exercise)
  primarily for cardiorespiratory conditioning Y93.A1 (*following* Y93.7)
  primarily for muscle strengthening Y93.B1 (*following* Y93.7)
maintenance
  exterior building NEC Y93.H9 (*following* Y93.7)
  household (interior) NEC Y93.E9 (*following* Y93.7)
  land Y93.H9 (*following* Y93.7)
  property Y93.H9 (*following* Y93.7)
marching (on level or elevated terrain) Y93.01
martial arts Y93.75
microwave oven Y93.G3 (*following* Y93.7)
milking an animal Y93.K2 (*following* Y93.7)
mopping (floor) Y93.E5 (*following* Y93.7)

Activity — *continued*
mountain climbing Y93.31
muscle strengthening
  exercises (non-machine) NEC Y93.B9 (*following* Y93.7)
  machines Y93.B1 (*following* Y93.7)
musical keyboard (electronic) playing Y93.J1 (*following* Y93.7)
nordic skiing Y93.24
obstacle course Y93.A5 (*following* Y93.7)
oven (microwave) Y93.G3 (*following* Y93.7)
packing up and unpacking in moving to a new residence Y93.E6 (*following* Y93.7)
parasailing Y93.19
pass out game Y93.85
percussion instrument playing NEC Y93.J2 (*following* Y93.7)
personal
  bathing and showering Y93.E1 (*following* Y93.7)
  hygiene NEC Y93.E8 (*following* Y93.7)
  showering Y93.E1 (*following* Y93.7)
physical games generally associated with school recess, summer camp and children Y93.6A
physical training NEC Y93.A9 (*following* Y93.7)
piano playing Y93.J1 (*following* Y93.7)
pilates Y93.B4 (*following* Y93.7)
platform diving Y93.12
playing musical instrument
  brass instrument Y93.J4 (*following* Y93.7)
  drum Y93.J2 (*following* Y93.7)
  musical keyboard (electronic) Y93.J1 (*following* Y93.7)
  percussion instrument NEC Y93.J2 (*following* Y93.7)
  piano Y93.J1 (*following* Y93.7)
  string instrument Y93.J3 (*following* Y93.7)
  winds instrument Y93.J4 (*following* Y93.7)
property maintenance
  exterior NEC Y93.H9 (*following* Y93.7)
  interior NEC Y93.E9 (*following* Y93.7)
pruning (garden and lawn) Y93.H2 (*following* Y93.7)
pull-ups Y93.B2 (*following* Y93.7)
push-ups Y93.B2 (*following* Y93.7)
racquetball Y93.73
rafting (in calm and turbulent water) Y93.16
raking (leaves) Y93.H1 (*following* Y93.7)
rappelling Y93.32
refereeing a sports activity Y93.81
residential relocation Y93.E6 (*following* Y93.7)
rhythmic gymnastics Y93.43
rhythmic movement NEC Y93.49
riding
  horseback Y93.52
  rollercoaster Y93.I1 (*following* Y93.7)
rock climbing Y93.31
roller skating (inline) Y93.51
rollercoaster riding Y93.I1 (*following* Y93.7)
rough housing and horseplay Y93.83
rowing (in calm and turbulent water) Y93.16
rugby Y93.63
running Y93.02
SCUBA diving Y93.15
sewing Y93.D2 (*following* Y93.7)
shoveling Y93.H1 (*following* Y93.7)
  dirt Y93.H1 (*following* Y93.7)
  snow Y93.H1 (*following* Y93.7)
showering (personal) Y93.E1 (*following* Y93.7)
sit-ups Y93.B2 (*following* Y93.7)
skateboarding Y93.51
skating (ice) Y93.21
  roller Y93.51
skiing (alpine) (downhill) Y93.23
  cross country Y93.24
  nordic Y93.24
  water Y93.17
sledding (snow) Y93.23
sleeping (sleep) Y93.84
smoking and grilling food Y93.G2 (*following* Y93.7)
snorkeling Y93.15
snow NEC Y93.29
  boarding Y93.23
  shoveling Y93.H1 (*following* Y93.7)
  sledding Y93.23
  tubing Y93.23
soccer Y93.66
softball Y93.64
specified NEC Y93.89
spectator at an event Y93.82
sports NEC Y93.79
  sports played as a team or group NEC Y93.69

Activity — *continued*
sports — *continued*
  sports played individually NEC Y93.59
springboard diving Y93.12
squash Y93.73
stationary bike Y93.A1 (*following* Y93.7)
step (stepping) exercise (class) Y93.A3 (*following* Y93.7)
stepper machine Y93.A1 (*following* Y93.7)
stove Y93.G3 (*following* Y93.7)
string instrument playing Y93.J3 (*following* Y93.7)
surfing Y93.18
  wind Y93.18
swimming Y93.11
tackle football Y93.61
tap dancing Y93.41
tennis Y93.73
tobogganing Y93.23
touch football Y93.62
track and field events (non-running) Y93.57
  running Y93.02
trampoline Y93.44
treadmill Y93.A1 (*following* Y93.7)
trimming shrubs Y93.H2 (*following* Y93.7)
tubing (in calm and turbulent water) Y93.16
  snow Y93.23
ultimate frisbee Y93.74
underwater diving Y93.15
unpacking in moving to a new residence Y93.E6 (*following* Y93.7)
use of stove, oven and microwave oven Y93.G3 (*following* Y93.7)
vacuuming Y93.E3 (*following* Y93.7)
volleyball (beach) (court) Y93.68
wake boarding Y93.17
walking (on level or elevated terrain) Y93.01
  an animal Y93.K1 (*following* Y93.7)
walking an animal Y93.K1 (*following* Y93.7)
wall climbing Y93.31
warm up and cool down exercises Y93.A2 (*following* Y93.7)
water NEC Y93.19
  aerobics Y93.14
  craft NEC Y93.19
  exercise Y93.14
  polo Y93.13
  skiing Y93.17
  sliding Y93.18
  survival training and testing Y93.19
weeding (garden and lawn) Y93.H2 (*following* Y93.7)
wind instrument playing Y93.J4 (*following* Y93.7)
windsurfing Y93.18
wrestling Y93.72
yoga Y93.42
Adverse effect of drugs — *see* Table of Drugs and Chemicals
Aerosinusitis — *see* Air, pressure
After-effect, late — *see* Sequelae
Air
blast in war operations — *see* War operations, air blast
pressure
  change, rapid
    during
      ascent W94.29 ☑
        while (in) (surfacing from)
          aircraft W94.23 ☑
          deep water diving W94.21 ☑
          underground W94.22 ☑
      descent W94.39 ☑
        in
          aircraft W94.31 ☑
          water W94.32 ☑
  high, prolonged W94.0 ☑
  low, prolonged W94.12 ☑
    due to residence or long visit at high altitude W94.11 ☑
Alpine sickness W94.11 ☑
Altitude sickness W94.11 ☑
Anaphylactic shock, anaphylaxis — *see* Table of Drugs and Chemicals
Andes disease W94.11 ☑
Arachnidism, arachnoidism X58 ☑
Arson (with intent to injure or kill) X97 ☑
Asphyxia, asphyxiation
by
  food (bone) (seed) — *see* categories T17 and T18 ☑
  gas — *see also* Table of Drugs and Chemicals
    legal
      execution — *see* Legal, intervention, gas

Asphyxia, asphyxiation — *continued*
  by — *continued*
    gas — *see also* Table of Drugs and Chemicals —
      continued
      legal — *continued*
        intervention — *see* Legal, intervention, gas
  from
    fire — *see also* Exposure, fire
      in war operations — *see* War operations, fire
    ignition — *see* Ignition
    vomitus T17.81 ☑
  in war operations — *see* War operations, restriction of
    airway
Aspiration
  food (any type) (into respiratory tract) (with asphyxia,
    obstruction respiratory tract, suffocation) — *see*
    categories T17 and T18
  foreign body — *see* Foreign body, aspiration
  vomitus (with asphyxia, obstruction respiratory tract,
    suffocation) T17.81 ☑
Assassination (attempt) — *see* Assault
Assault (homicidal) (by) (in) Y09
  arson X97 ☑
  bite (of human being) Y04.1 ☑
  bodily force Y04.8 ☑
    bite Y04.1 ☑
    bumping into Y04.2 ☑
    sexual — *see* subcategories T74.0, T76.0 ☑
    unarmed fight Y04.0 ☑
  bomb X96.9 ☑
    antipersonnel X96.0 ☑
    fertilizer X96.3 ☑
    gasoline X96.1 ☑
    letter X96.2 ☑
    petrol X96.1 ☑
    pipe X96.3 ☑
    specified NEC X96.8 ☑
  brawl (hand) (fists) (foot) (unarmed) Y04.0 ☑
  burning, burns (by fire) NEC X97 ☑
    acid Y08.89 ☑
    caustic, corrosive substance Y08.89 ☑
    chemical from swallowing caustic, corrosive sub-
      stance — *see* Table of Drugs and Chemicals
    cigarette(s) X97 ☑
    hot object X98.9 ☑
      fluid NEC X98.2 ☑
      household appliance X98.3 ☑
      specified NEC X98.8 ☑
      steam X98.0 ☑
      tap water X98.1 ☑
      vapors X98.0 ☑
    scalding — *see* Assault, burning
    steam X98.0 ☑
    vitriol Y08.89 ☑
  caustic, corrosive substance (gas) Y08.89 ☑
  crashing of
    aircraft Y08.81 ☑
    motor vehicle Y03.8 ☑
      pushed in front of Y02.0 ☑
      run over Y03.0 ☑
      specified NEC Y03.8 ☑
  cutting or piercing instrument X99.9 ☑
    dagger X99.2 ☑
    glass X99.0 ☑
    knife X99.1 ☑
    specified NEC X99.8 ☑
    sword X99.2 ☑
  dagger X99.2 ☑
  drowning (in) X92.9 ☑
    bathtub X92.0 ☑
    natural water X92.3 ☑
    specified NEC X92.8 ☑
    swimming pool X92.1 ☑
      following fall X92.2 ☑
  dynamite X96.8 ☑
  explosive(s) (material) X96.9 ☑
  fight (hand) (fists) (foot) (unarmed) Y04.0 ☑
    with weapon — *see* Assault, by type of weapon
  fire X97 ☑
  firearm X95.9 ☑
    airgun X95.01 ☑
    handgun X93
    hunting rifle X94.1 ☑
    larger X94.9 ☑
      specified NEC X94.8 ☑
    machine gun X94.2 ☑

Assault — *continued*
  firearm — *continued*
    shotgun X94.0 ☑
    specified NEC X95.8 ☑
  from high place Y01 ☑
  gunshot (wound) NEC — *see* Assault, firearm, by type
  incendiary device X97 ☑
  injury Y09
    to child due to criminal abortion attempt NEC
      Y08.89 ☑
  knife X99.1 ☑
  late effect of — *see* categories X92-Y08 with 7th char-
    acter S
  placing before moving object NEC Y02.8 ☑
    motor vehicle Y02.0 ☑
  poisoning — *see* categories T36-T65 with 7th character
    S
  puncture, any part of body — *see* Assault, cutting or
    piercing instrument
  pushing
    before moving object NEC Y02.8 ☑
      motor vehicle Y02.0 ☑
      subway train Y02.1 ☑
      train Y02.1 ☑
    from high place Y01 ☑
  rape T74.2- ☑
  scalding — *see* Assault, burning
  sequelae of — *see* categories X92-Y08 with 7th charac-
    ter S
  sexual (by bodily force) T74.2- ☑
  shooting — *see* Assault, firearm
  specified means NEC Y08.89 ☑
  stab, any part of body — *see* Assault, cutting or piercing
    instrument
  steam X98.0 ☑
  striking against
    other person Y04.2 ☑
    sports equipment Y08.09 ☑
      baseball bat Y08.02 ☑
      hockey stick Y08.01 ☑
  struck by
    sports equipment Y08.09 ☑
      baseball bat Y08.02 ☑
      hockey stick Y08.01 ☑
  submersion — *see* Assault, drowning
  violence Y09
  weapon Y09
    blunt Y00 ☑
    cutting or piercing — *see* Assault, cutting or piercing
      instrument
    firearm — *see* Assault, firearm
  wound Y09
    cutting — *see* Assault, cutting or piercing instru-
      ment
    gunshot — *see* Assault, firearm
    knife X99.1 ☑
    piercing — *see* Assault, cutting or piercing instru-
      ment
    puncture — *see* Assault, cutting or piercing instru-
      ment
    stab — *see* Assault, cutting or piercing instrument
Attack by mammals NEC W55.89 ☑
Avalanche — *see* Landslide
Aviator's disease — *see* Air, pressure

B

Barotitis, barodontalgia, barosinusitis, barotrauma
  (otitic) (sinus) — *see* Air, pressure
Battered (baby) (child) (person) (syndrome) X58 ☑
Bayonet wound W26.1 ☑
  in
    legal intervention — *see* Legal, intervention, sharp
      object, bayonet
    war operations — *see* War operations, combat
  stated as undetermined whether accidental or inten-
    tional Y28.8 ☑
  suicide (attempt) X78.2 ☑
Bean in nose — *see* categories T17 and T18 ☑
Bed set on fire NEC — *see* Exposure, fire, uncontrolled,
  building, bed
Beheading (by guillotine)
  homicide X99.9 ☑
  legal execution — *see* Legal, intervention
Bending, injury in (prolonged) (static) X50.1 ☑
Bends — *see* Air, pressure, change

Bite, bitten by
  alligator W58.01 ☑
  arthropod (nonvenomous) NEC W57 ☑
  bull W55.21 ☑
  cat W55.01 ☑
  cow W55.21 ☑
  crocodile W58.11 ☑
  dog W54.0 ☑
  goat W55.31 ☑
  hoof stock NEC W55.31 ☑
  horse W55.11 ☑
  human being (accidentally) W50.3 ☑
    with intent to injure or kill Y04.1 ☑
    as, or caused by, a crowd or human stampede (with
      fall) W52 ☑
    assault Y04.1 ☑
    homicide (attempt) Y04.1 ☑
    in
      fight Y04.1 ☑
  insect (nonvenomous) W57 ☑
  lizard (nonvenomous) W59.01 ☑
  mammal NEC W55.81 ☑
    marine W56.31 ☑
  marine animal (nonvenomous) W56.81 ☑
  millipede W57 ☑
  moray eel W56.51 ☑
  mouse W53.01 ☑
  person(s) (accidentally) W50.3 ☑
    with intent to injure or kill Y04.1 ☑
    as, or caused by, a crowd or human stampede (with
      fall) W52 ☑
    assault Y04.1 ☑
    homicide (attempt) Y04.1 ☑
    in
      fight Y04.1 ☑
  pig W55.41 ☑
  raccoon W55.51 ☑
  rat W53.11 ☑
  reptile W59.81 ☑
    lizard W59.01 ☑
    snake W59.11 ☑
    turtle W59.21 ☑
      terrestrial W59.81 ☑
  rodent W53.81 ☑
    mouse W53.01 ☑
    rat W53.11 ☑
    specified NEC W53.81 ☑
    squirrel W53.21 ☑
  shark W56.41 ☑
  sheep W55.31 ☑
  snake (nonvenomous) W59.11 ☑
  spider (nonvenomous) W57 ☑
  squirrel W53.21 ☑
Blast (air) in war operations — *see* War operations, blast
Blizzard X37.2 ☑
Blood alcohol level Y90.9
  less than 20mg/100ml Y90.0
  presence in blood, level not specified Y90.9
  20-39mg/100ml Y90.1
  40-59mg/100ml Y90.2
  60-79mg/100ml Y90.3
  80-99mg/100ml Y90.4
  100-119mg/100ml Y90.5
  120-199mg/100ml Y90.6
  200-239mg/100ml Y90.7
Blow X58 ☑
  by law-enforcing agent, police (on duty) — *see* Legal,
    intervention, manhandling
  blunt object — *see* Legal, intervention, blunt object
Blowing up — *see* Explosion
Brawl (hand) (fists) (foot) Y04.0 ☑
Breakage (accidental) (part of)
  ladder (causing fall) W11
  scaffolding (causing fall) W12 ☑
Broken
  glass, contact with — *see* Contact, with, glass
  power line (causing electric shock) W85 ☑
Bumping against, into (accidentally)
  object NEC W22.8 ☑
    caused by crowd or human stampede (with fall)
      W52 ☑
    sports equipment W21.9 ☑
    with fall — *see* Fall, due to, bumping against, object
  person(s) W51 ☑
    with fall W03 ☑
      due to ice or snow W00.0 ☑

Bumping against, into — *continued*
 person(s) — *continued*
  assault Y04.2 ☑
  caused by, a crowd or human stampede (with fall) W52 ☑
  homicide (attempt) Y04.2 ☑
 sports equipment W21.9 ☑

Burn, burned, burning (accidental) (by) (from) (on)
 acid NEC — *see* Table of Drugs and Chemicals
 bed linen — *see* Exposure, fire, uncontrolled, in building, bed
 blowtorch X08.8 ☑
  with ignition of clothing NEC X06.2 ☑
   nightwear X05 ☑
 bonfire, campfire (controlled) — *see also* Exposure, fire, controlled, not in building
  uncontrolled — *see* Exposure, fire, uncontrolled, not in building
 candle X08.8 ☑
  with ignition of clothing NEC X06.2 ☑
   nightwear X05 ☑
 caustic liquid, substance (external) (internal) NEC — *see* Table of Drugs and Chemicals
 chemical (external) (internal) — *see also* Table of Drugs and Chemicals
  in war operations — *see* War operations. fire
 cigar(s) or cigarette(s) X08.8 ☑
  with ignition of clothing NEC X06.2 ☑
   nightwear X05 ☑
 clothes, clothing NEC (from controlled fire) X06.2 ☑
  with conflagration — *see* Exposure, fire, uncontrolled, building
   not in building or structure — *see* Exposure, fire, uncontrolled, not in building
 cooker (hot) X15.8 ☑
  stated as undetermined whether accidental or intentional Y27.3 ☑
  suicide (attempt) X77.3 ☑
 electric blanket X16 ☑
 engine (hot) X17 ☑
 fire, flames — *see* Exposure, fire
 flare, Very pistol — *see* Discharge, firearm NEC
 heat
  from appliance (electrical) (household) X15.8 ☑
   cooker X15.8 ☑
   hotplate X15.2 ☑
   kettle X15.8 ☑
   light bulb X15.8 ☑
   saucepan X15.3 ☑
   skillet X15.3 ☑
   stated as undetermined whether accidental or intentional Y27.3 ☑
   stove X15.0 ☑
   suicide (attempt) X77.3 ☑
   toaster X15.1 ☑
  in local application or packing during medical or surgical procedure Y63.5
 heating
  appliance, radiator or pipe X16 ☑
 homicide (attempt) — *see* Assault, burning
 hot
  air X14.1 ☑
  cooker X15.8 ☑
  drink X10.0 ☑
  engine X17 ☑
  fat X10.2 ☑
  fluid NEC X12 ☑
  food X10.1 ☑
  gases X14.1 ☑
  heating appliance X16 ☑
  household appliance NEC X15.8 ☑
  kettle X15.8 ☑
  liquid NEC X12 ☑
  machinery X17 ☑
  metal (molten) (liquid) NEC X18 ☑
  object (not producing fire or flames) NEC X19 ☑
  oil (cooking) X10.2 ☑
  pipe(s) X16 ☑
  radiator X16 ☑
  saucepan (glass) (metal) X15.3 ☑
  stove (kitchen) X15.0 ☑
  substance NEC X19 ☑
   caustic or corrosive NEC — *see* Table of Drugs and Chemicals
  toaster X15.1 ☑
  tool X17 ☑

Burn, burned, burning — *continued*
 hot — *continued*
  vapor X13.1 ☑
  water (tap) — *see* Contact, with, hot, tap water
 hotplate X15.2 ☑
  suicide (attempt) X77.3 ☑
 ignition — *see* Ignition
 in war operations — *see* War operations, fire
 inflicted by other person X97 ☑
  by hot objects, hot vapor, and steam — *see* Assault, burning, hot object
 internal, from swallowed caustic, corrosive liquid, substance — *see* Table of Drugs and Chemicals
 iron (hot) X15.8 ☑
  stated as undetermined whether accidental or intentional Y27.3 ☑
  suicide (attempt) X77.3 ☑
 kettle (hot) X15.8 ☑
  stated as undetermined whether accidental or intentional Y27.3 ☑
  suicide (attempt) X77.3 ☑
 lamp (flame) X08.8 ☑
  with ignition of clothing NEC X06.2 ☑
   nightwear X05 ☑
 lighter (cigar) (cigarette) X08.8 ☑
  with ignition of clothing NEC X06.2 ☑
   nightwear X05 ☑
 lightning — *see* subcategory T75.0 ☑
  causing fire — *see* Exposure, fire
 liquid (boiling) (hot) NEC X12 ☑
  stated as undetermined whether accidental or intentional Y27.2 ☑
  suicide (attempt) X77.2 ☑
 local application of externally applied substance in medical or surgical care Y63.5
 machinery (hot) X17 ☑
 matches X08.8 ☑
  with ignition of clothing NEC X06.2 ☑
   nightwear X05 ☑
 mattress — *see* Exposure, fire, uncontrolled, building, bed
 medicament, externally applied Y63.5
 metal (hot) (liquid) (molten) NEC X18 ☑
 nightwear (nightclothes, nightdress, gown, pajamas, robe) X05 ☑
 object (hot) NEC X19 ☑
 on board watercraft
  due to
   accident to watercraft V91.09 ☑
    powered craft V91.03 ☑
     ferry boat V91.01 ☑
     fishing boat V91.02 ☑
     jetskis V91.03 ☑
     liner V91.01 ☑
     merchant ship V91.00 ☑
     passenger ship V91.01 ☑
    unpowered craft V91.08 ☑
     canoe V91.05 ☑
     inflatable V91.06 ☑
     kayak V91.05 ☑
     sailboat V91.04 ☑
     surf-board V91.08 ☑
     water skis V91.07 ☑
     windsurfer V91.08 ☑
   fire on board V93.09 ☑
    ferry boat V93.01 ☑
    fishing boat V93.02 ☑
    jetskis V93.03 ☑
    liner V93.01 ☑
    merchant ship V93.00 ☑
    passenger ship V93.01 ☑
    powered craft NEC V93.03 ☑
    sailboat V93.04 ☑
   specified heat source NEC on board V93.19 ☑
    ferry boat V93.11 ☑
    fishing boat V93.12 ☑
    jetskis V93.13 ☑
    liner V93.11 ☑
    merchant ship V93.10 ☑
    passenger ship V93.11 ☑
    powered craft NEC V93.13 ☑
    sailboat V93.14 ☑
 pipe (hot) X16 ☑
  smoking X08.8 ☑
   with ignition of clothing NEC X06.2 ☑
    nightwear X05 ☑

Burn, burned, burning — *continued*
 powder — *see* Powder burn
 radiator (hot) X16 ☑
 saucepan (hot) (glass) (metal) X15.3 ☑
  stated as undetermined whether accidental or intentional Y27.3 ☑
  suicide (attempt) X77.3 ☑
 self-inflicted X76 ☑
  stated as undetermined whether accidental or intentional Y26 ☑
 stated as undetermined whether accidental or intentional Y27.0 ☑
 steam X13.1 ☑
  pipe X16 ☑
   stated as undetermined whether accidental or intentional Y27.8 ☑
  stated as undetermined whether accidental or intentional Y27.0 ☑
  suicide (attempt) X77.0 ☑
 stove (hot) (kitchen) X15.0 ☑
  stated as undetermined whether accidental or intentional Y27.3 ☑
  suicide (attempt) X77.3 ☑
 substance (hot) NEC X19 ☑
  boiling X12 ☑
   stated as undetermined whether accidental or intentional Y27.2 ☑
   suicide (attempt) X77.2 ☑
  molten (metal) X18 ☑
 suicide (attempt) NEC X76 ☑
  hot
   household appliance X77.3 ☑
   object X77.9 ☑
 therapeutic misadventure
  heat in local application or packing during medical or surgical procedure Y63.5
  overdose of radiation Y63.2
 toaster (hot) X15.1 ☑
  stated as undetermined whether accidental or intentional Y27.3 ☑
  suicide (attempt) X77.3 ☑
 tool (hot) X17 ☑
 torch, welding X08.8 ☑
  with ignition of clothing NEC X06.2 ☑
   nightwear X05 ☑
 trash fire (controlled) — *see* Exposure, fire, controlled, not in building
  uncontrolled — *see* Exposure, fire, uncontrolled, not in building
 vapor (hot) X13.1 ☑
  stated as undetermined whether accidental or intentional Y27.0 ☑
  suicide (attempt) X77.0 ☑
 Very pistol — *see* Discharge, firearm NEC

Butted by animal W55.82 ☑
 bull W55.22 ☑
 cow W55.22 ☑
 goat W55.32 ☑
 horse W55.12 ☑
 pig W55.42 ☑
 sheep W55.32 ☑

C

Caisson disease — *see* Air, pressure, change
Campfire (exposure to) (controlled) — *see also* Exposure, fire, controlled, not in building
 uncontrolled — *see* Exposure, fire, uncontrolled, not in building
Capital punishment (any means) — *see* Legal, intervention
Car sickness T75.3 ☑
Casualty (not due to war) NEC X58 ☑
 war — *see* War operations
Cat
 bite W55.01 ☑
 scratch W55.03 ☑
Cataclysm, cataclysmic (any injury) NEC — *see* Forces of nature
Catching fire — *see* Exposure, fire
Caught
 between
  folding object W23.0 ☑
  objects (moving) W23.0 ☑

External Causes Index

Caught — *continued*
 between — *continued*
  objects — *continued*
   and
    machinery — *see* Contact, with, by type of machine
    stationary
    stationary W23.1 ☑
     and moving
    sliding door and door frame W23.0 ☑
 by, in
  machinery (moving parts of) — *see* Contact, with, by type of machine
  washing-machine wringer W23.0 ☑
 under packing crate (due to losing grip) W23.1 ☑
Cave-in caused by cataclysmic earth surface movement or eruption — *see* Landslide
Change(s) in air pressure — *see* Air, pressure, change
Choked, choking (on) (any object except food or vomitus)
 food (bone) (seed) — *see* categories T17 and T18 ☑
 vomitus T17.81- ☑
Civil insurrection — *see* War operations
Cloudburst (any injury) X37.8 ☑
Cold, exposure to (accidental) (excessive) (extreme) (natural) (place) NEC — *see* Exposure, cold
Collapse
 building W20.1 ☑
  burning (uncontrolled fire) X00.2 ☑
 dam or man-made structure (causing earth movement) X36.0 ☑
 machinery — *see* Contact, with, by type of machine
 structure W20.1 ☑
  burning (uncontrolled fire) X00.2 ☑
Collision (accidental) NEC — *see also* Accident, transport V89.9 ☑
 pedestrian W51 ☑
  with fall W03 ☑
   due to ice or snow W00.0 ☑
   involving pedestrian conveyance — *see* Accident, transport, pedestrian, conveyance
   and
    crowd or human stampede (with fall) W52 ☑
    object W22.8 ☑
     with fall — *see* Fall, due to, bumping against, object
  person(s) — *see* Collision, pedestrian
 transport vehicle NEC V89.9 ☑
  and
   avalanche, fallen or not moving — *see* Accident, transport
    falling or moving — *see* Landslide
   landslide, fallen or not moving — *see* Accident, transport
    falling or moving — *see* Landslide
 due to cataclysm — *see* Forces of nature, by type
 intentional, purposeful suicide (attempt) — *see* Suicide, collision
Combustion, spontaneous — *see* Ignition
Complication (delayed) **of or following** (medical or surgical procedure) Y84.9
 with misadventure — *see* Misadventure
 amputation of limb(s) Y83.5
 anastomosis (arteriovenous) (blood vessel) (gastrojejunal) (tendon) (natural or artificial material) Y83.2
 aspiration (of fluid) Y84.4
  tissue Y84.8
 biopsy Y84.8
 blood
  sampling Y84.7
  transfusion
   procedure Y84.8
 bypass Y83.2
 catheterization (urinary) Y84.6
  cardiac Y84.0
 colostomy Y83.3
 cystostomy Y83.3
 dialysis (kidney) Y84.1
 drug — *see* Table of Drugs and Chemicals
 due to misadventure — *see* Misadventure
 duodenostomy Y83.3
 electroshock therapy Y84.3
 external stoma, creation of Y83.3
 formation of external stoma Y83.3
 gastrostomy Y83.3
 graft Y83.2
 hypothermia (medically-induced) Y84.8

Complication (delayed) **of or following** — *continued*
 implant, implantation (of)
  artificial
   internal device (cardiac pacemaker) (electrodes in brain) (heart valve prosthesis) (orthopedic) Y83.1
   material or tissue (for anastomosis or bypass) Y83.2
    with creation of external stoma Y83.3
   natural tissues (for anastomosis or bypass) Y83.2
    with creation of external stoma Y83.3
 infusion
  procedure Y84.8
 injection — *see* Table of Drugs and Chemicals
  procedure Y84.8
 insertion of gastric or duodenal sound Y84.5
 insulin-shock therapy Y84.3
 paracentesis (abdominal) (thoracic) (aspirative) Y84.4
 procedures other than surgical operation — *see* Complication of or following, by type of procedure
 radiological procedure or therapy Y84.2
 removal of organ (partial) (total) NEC Y83.6
 sampling
  blood Y84.7
  fluid NEC Y84.4
  tissue Y84.8
 shock therapy Y84.3
 surgical operation NEC — *see also* Complication of or following, by type of operation Y83.9
  reconstructive NEC Y83.4
   with
    anastomosis, bypass or graft Y83.2
    formation of external stoma Y83.3
  specified NEC Y83.8
 transfusion — *see also* Table of Drugs and Chemicals
  procedure Y84.8
 transplant, transplantation (heart) (kidney) (liver) (whole organ, any) Y83.0
  partial organ Y83.4
 ureterostomy Y83.3
 vaccination — *see also* Table of Drugs and Chemicals
  procedure Y84.8
Compression
 divers' squeeze — *see* Air, pressure, change
 trachea by
  food (lodged in esophagus) — *see* categories T17 and T18 ☑
  vomitus (lodged in esophagus) T17.81- ☑
Conflagration — *see* Exposure, fire, uncontrolled
Constriction (external)
 hair W49.01 ☑
 jewelry W49.04 ☑
 ring W49.04 ☑
 rubber band W49.03 ☑
 specified item NEC W49.09 ☑
 string W49.02 ☑
 thread W49.02 ☑
Contact (accidental)
 with
  abrasive wheel (metalworking) W31.1 ☑
  alligator W58.09 ☑
   bite W58.01 ☑
   crushing W58.03 ☑
   strike W58.02 ☑
  amphibian W62.9 ☑
   frog W62.0 ☑
   toad W62.1 ☑
  animal (nonvenomous) NEC W64 ☑
   marine W56.89 ☑
    bite W56.81 ☑
    dolphin — *see* Contact, with, dolphin
    fish NEC — *see* Contact, with, fish
    mammal — *see* Contact, with, mammal, marine
    orca — *see* Contact, with, orca
    sea lion — *see* Contact, with, sea lion
    shark — *see* Contact, with, shark
    strike W56.82 ☑
  animate mechanical force NEC W64 ☑
  arrow W21.89 ☑
   not thrown, projected or falling W45.8 ☑
  arthropods (nonvenomous) W57 ☑
  axe W27.0 ☑
  band-saw (industrial) W31.2 ☑
  bayonet — *see* Bayonet wound
  bee(s) X58 ☑

Contact — *continued*
 with — *continued*
  bench-saw (industrial) W31.2 ☑
  bird W61.99 ☑
   bite W61.91 ☑
   chicken — *see* Contact, with, chicken
   duck — *see* Contact, with, duck
   goose — *see* Contact, with, goose
   macaw — *see* Contact, with, macaw
   parrot — *see* Contact, with, parrot
   psittacine — *see* Contact, with, psittacine
   strike W61.92 ☑
   turkey — *see* Contact, with, turkey
  blender W29.0 ☑
  boiling water X12 ☑
   stated as undetermined whether accidental or intentional Y27.2 ☑
   suicide (attempt) X77.2 ☑
  bore, earth-drilling or mining (land) (seabed) W31.0 ☑
  buffalo — *see* Contact, with, hoof stock NEC
  bull W55.29 ☑
   bite W55.21 ☑
   gored W55.22 ☑
   strike W55.22 ☑
  bumper cars W31.81 ☑
  camel — *see* Contact, with, hoof stock NEC
  can
   lid W26.8 ☑
   opener W27.4 ☑
    powered W29.0 ☑
  cat W55.09 ☑
   bite W55.01 ☑
   scratch W55.03 ☑
  caterpillar (venomous) X58 ☑
  centipede (venomous) X58 ☑
  chain
   hoist W24.0 ☑
    agricultural operations W30.89 ☑
   saw W29.3 ☑
  chicken W61.39 ☑
   peck W61.33 ☑
   strike W61.32 ☑
  chisel W27.0 ☑
  circular saw W31.2 ☑
  cobra X58 ☑
  combine (harvester) W30.0 ☑
  conveyer belt W24.1 ☑
  cooker (hot) X15.8 ☑
   stated as undetermined whether accidental or intentional Y27.3 ☑
   suicide (attempt) X77.3 ☑
  coral X58 ☑
  cotton gin W31.82 ☑
  cow W55.29 ☑
   bite W55.21 ☑
   strike W55.22 ☑
  crane W24.0 ☑
   agricultural operations W30.89 ☑
  crocodile W58.19 ☑
   bite W58.11 ☑
   crushing W58.13 ☑
   strike W58.12 ☑
  dagger W26.1 ☑
   stated as undetermined whether accidental or intentional Y28.2 ☑
   suicide (attempt) X78.2 ☑
  dairy equipment W31.82 ☑
  dart W21.89 ☑
   not thrown, projected or falling W45.8 ☑
  deer — *see* Contact, with, hoof stock NEC
  derrick W24.0 ☑
   agricultural operations W30.89 ☑
    hay W30.2 ☑
  dog W54.8 ☑
   bite W54.0 ☑
   strike W54.1 ☑
  dolphin W56.09 ☑
   bite W56.01 ☑
   strike W56.02 ☑
  donkey — *see* Contact, with, hoof stock NEC
  drill (powered) W29.8 ☑
   earth (land) (seabed) W31.0 ☑
   nonpowered W27.8 ☑
  drive belt W24.0 ☑
   agricultural operations W30.89 ☑

Caught — Contact

Contact — *continued*
  with — *continued*
    dry ice — *see* Exposure, cold, man-made
    dryer (clothes) (powered) (spin) W29.2 ☑
    duck W61.69 ☑
      bite W61.61 ☑
      strike W61.62 ☑
    earth (-)
      drilling machine (industrial) W31.0 ☑
      scraping machine in stationary use W31.83 ☑
    edge of stiff paper W26.2 ☑
    electric
      beater W29.0 ☑
      blanket X16 ☑
      fan W29.2 ☑
        commercial W31.82 ☑
      knife W29.1 ☑
      mixer W29.0 ☑
    elevator (building) W24.0 ☑
      agricultural operations W30.89 ☑
        grain W30.3 ☑
    engine(s), hot NEC X17 ☑
    excavating machine W31.0 ☑
    farm machine W30.9 ☑
    feces — *see* Contact, with, by type of animal
    fer de lance X58 ☑
    fish W56.59 ☑
      bite W56.51 ☑
      shark — *see* Contact, with, shark
      strike W56.52 ☑
    flying horses W31.81 ☑
    forging (metalworking) machine W31.1 ☑
    fork W27.4 ☑
    forklift (truck) W24.0 ☑
      agricultural operations W30.89 ☑
    frog W62.0 ☑
    garden
      cultivator (powered) W29.3 ☑
        riding W30.89 ☑
      fork W27.1 ☑
    gas turbine W31.3 ☑
    Gila monster X58 ☑
    giraffe — *see* Contact, with, hoof stock NEC
    glass (sharp) (broken) W25 ☑
      assault X99.0 ☑
      due to fall — *see* Fall, by type
      stated as undetermined whether accidental or
        intentional Y28.0 ☑
      suicide (attempt) X78.0 ☑
      with subsequent fall W18.02 ☑
    goat W55.39 ☑
      bite W55.31 ☑
      strike W55.32 ☑
    goose W61.59 ☑
      bite W61.51 ☑
      strike W61.52 ☑
    hand
      saw W27.0 ☑
      tool (not powered) NEC W27.8 ☑
        powered W29.8 ☑
    harvester W30.0 ☑
    hay-derrick W30.2 ☑
    heating
      appliance (hot) X16 ☑
      pad (electric) X16 ☑
    heat NEC X19 ☑
      from appliance (electrical) (household) — *see*
        Contact, with, hot, household appliance
        heating appliance X16 ☑
    hedge-trimmer (powered) W29.3 ☑
    hoe W27.1 ☑
    hoist (chain) (shaft) NEC W24.0 ☑
      agricultural W30.89 ☑
    hoof stock NEC W55.39 ☑
      bite W55.31 ☑
      strike W55.32 ☑
    hornet(s) X58 ☑
    horse W55.19 ☑
      bite W55.11 ☑
      strike W55.12 ☑
    hot
      air X14.1 ☑
        inhalation X14.0 ☑
      cooker X15.8 ☑
      cooking
        pan X15.3 ☑

Contact — *continued*
  with — *continued*
    hot — *continued*
      cooking — *continued*
        pot X15.3 ☑
      drinks X10.0 ☑
      engine X17 ☑
      fats X10.2 ☑
      fluids NEC X12 ☑
        assault X98.2 ☑
        suicide (attempt) X77.2 ☑
        undetermined whether accidental or inten-
          tional Y27.2 ☑
      food X10.1 ☑
      gases X14.1 ☑
        inhalation X14.0 ☑
      heating appliance X16 ☑
      household appliance X15.8 ☑
        assault X98.3 ☑
        cooker X15.8 ☑
        hotplate X15.2 ☑
        kettle X15.8 ☑
        light bulb X15.8 ☑
        object NEC X19 ☑
          assault X98.8 ☑
          stated as undetermined whether acciden-
            tal or intentional Y27.9 ☑
          suicide (attempt) X77.8 ☑
        saucepan X15.3 ☑
        skillet X15.3 ☑
        stated as undetermined whether accidental
          or intentional Y27.3 ☑
        stove X15.0 ☑
        suicide (attempt) X77.3 ☑
        toaster X15.1 ☑
      kettle X15.8 ☑
      light bulb X15.8 ☑
      liquid NEC — *see also* Burn X12 ☑
        drinks X10.0 ☑
        stated as undetermined whether accidental
          or intentional Y27.2 ☑
        suicide (attempt) X77.2 ☑
        tap water X11.8 ☑
          stated as undetermined whether acciden-
            tal or intentional Y27.1 ☑
          suicide (attempt) X77.1 ☑
      machinery X17 ☑
      metal (molten) (liquid) NEC X18 ☑
      object (not producing fire or flames) NEC X19 ☑
      oil (cooking) X10.2 ☑
      pipe X16 ☑
      plate X15.2 ☑
      radiator X16 ☑
      saucepan (glass) (metal) X15.3 ☑
      skillet X15.3 ☑
      stove (kitchen) X15.0 ☑
      substance NEC X19 ☑
      tap-water X11.8 ☑
        assault X98.1 ☑
        heated on stove X12 ☑
          stated as undetermined whether acciden-
            tal or intentional Y27.2 ☑
          suicide (attempt) X77.2 ☑
        in bathtub X11.0 ☑
        running X11.1 ☑
        stated as undetermined whether accidental
          or intentional Y27.1 ☑
        suicide (attempt) X77.1 ☑
      toaster X15.1 ☑
      tool X17 ☑
      vapors X13.1 ☑
        inhalation X13.0 ☑
      water (tap) X11.8 ☑
        boiling X12 ☑
          stated as undetermined whether acciden-
            tal or intentional Y27.2 ☑
          suicide (attempt) X77.2 ☑
        heated on stove X12 ☑
          stated as undetermined whether acciden-
            tal or intentional Y27.2 ☑
          suicide (attempt) X77.2 ☑
        in bathtub X11.0 ☑
        running X11.1 ☑
        stated as undetermined whether accidental
          or intentional Y27.1 ☑
        suicide (attempt) X77.1 ☑

Contact — *continued*
  with — *continued*
    hotplate X15.2 ☑
    ice-pick W27.4 ☑
    insect (nonvenomous) NEC W57 ☑
    kettle (hot) X15.8 ☑
    knife W26.0 ☑
      assault X99.1 ☑
      electric W29.1 ☑
      stated as undetermined whether accidental or
        intentional Y28.1 ☑
      suicide (attempt) X78.1 ☑
    lathe (metalworking) W31.1 ☑
      turnings W45.8 ☑
      woodworking W31.2 ☑
    lawnmower (powered) (ridden) W28 ☑
      causing electrocution W86.8 ☑
        suicide (attempt) X83.1 ☑
      unpowered W27.1 ☑
    lift, lifting (devices) W24.0 ☑
      agricultural operations W30.89 ☑
      shaft W24.0 ☑
    liquefied gas — *see* Exposure, cold, man-made
    liquid air, hydrogen, nitrogen — *see* Exposure, cold,
      man-made
    lizard (nonvenomous) W59.09 ☑
      bite W59.01 ☑
      strike W59.02 ☑
    llama — *see* Contact, with, hoof stock NEC
    macaw W61.19 ☑
      bite W61.11 ☑
      strike W61.12 ☑
    machine, machinery W31.9 ☑
      abrasive wheel W31.1 ☑
      agricultural including animal-powered W30.9 ☑
        combine harvester W30.0 ☑
        grain storage elevator W30.3 ☑
        hay derrick W30.2 ☑
        power take-off device W30.1 ☑
        reaper W30.0 ☑
        specified NEC W30.89 ☑
        thresher W30.0 ☑
        transport vehicle, stationary W30.81 ☑
      band saw W31.2 ☑
      bench saw W31.2 ☑
      circular saw W31.2 ☑
      commercial NEC W31.82 ☑
      drilling, metal (industrial) W31.1 ☑
      earth-drilling W31.0 ☑
      earthmoving or scraping W31.89 ☑
      excavating W31.89 ☑
      forging machine W31.1 ☑
      gas turbine W31.3 ☑
      hot X17 ☑
      internal combustion engine W31.3 ☑
      land drill W31.0 ☑
      lathe W31.1 ☑
      lifting (devices) W24.0 ☑
      metal drill W31.1 ☑
      metalworking (industrial) W31.1 ☑
      milling, metal W31.1 ☑
      mining W31.0 ☑
      molding W31.2 ☑
      overhead plane W31.2 ☑
      power press, metal W31.1 ☑
      prime mover W31.3 ☑
      printing W31.89 ☑
      radial saw W31.2 ☑
      recreational W31.81 ☑
      roller-coaster W31.81 ☑
      rolling mill, metal W31.1 ☑
      sander W31.2 ☑
      seabed drill W31.0 ☑
      shaft
        hoist W31.0 ☑
        lift W31.0 ☑
      specified NEC W31.89 ☑
      spinning W31.89 ☑
      steam engine W31.3 ☑
      transmission W24.1 ☑
      undercutter W31.0 ☑
      water driven turbine W31.3 ☑
      weaving W31.89 ☑
      woodworking or forming (industrial) W31.2 ☑
    mammal (feces) (urine) W55.89 ☑
      bull — *see* Contact, with, bull

☑ Additional Character Required — Refer to the Tabular List for Character Selection

Contact — Contact / External Causes Index

Contact — *continued*
  with — *continued*
    mammal — *continued*
      cat — *see* Contact, with, cat
      cow — *see* Contact, with, cow
      goat — *see* Contact, with, goat
      hoof stock — *see* Contact, with, hoof stock
      horse — *see* Contact, with, horse
      marine W56.39 ☑
        dolphin — *see* Contact, with, dolphin
        orca — *see* Contact, with, orca
        sea lion — *see* Contact, with, sea lion
        specified NEC W56.39 ☑
          bite W56.31 ☑
          strike W56.32 ☑
      pig — *see* Contact, with, pig
      raccoon — *see* Contact, with, raccoon
      rodent — *see* Contact, with, rodent
      sheep — *see* Contact, with, sheep
      specified NEC W55.89 ☑
        bite W55.81 ☑
        strike W55.82 ☑
    marine
      animal W56.89 ☑
        bite W56.81 ☑
        dolphin — *see* Contact, with, dolphin
        fish NEC — *see* Contact, with, fish
        mammal — *see* Contact, with, mammal, marine
        orca — *see* Contact, with, orca
        sea lion — *see* Contact, with, sea lion
        shark — *see* Contact, with, shark
        strike W56.82 ☑
    meat
      grinder (domestic) W29.0 ☑
        industrial W31.82 ☑
        nonpowered W27.4 ☑
      slicer (domestic) W29.0 ☑
        industrial W31.82 ☑
    merry go round W31.81 ☑
    metal, hot (liquid) (molten) NEC X18 ☑
    millipede W57 ☑
    nail W45.0 ☑
      gun W29.4 ☑
    needle (sewing) W27.3 ☑
      hypodermic W46.0 ☑
        contaminated W46.1 ☑
    object (blunt) NEC
      hot NEC X19 ☑
      legal intervention — *see* Legal, intervention, blunt object
      sharp NEC W45.8 ☑
        inflicted by other person NEC W45.8 ☑
          stated as
            intentional homicide (attempt) — *see* Assault, cutting or piercing instrument
        legal intervention — *see* Legal, intervention, sharp object
        self-inflicted X78.9 ☑
    orca W56.29 ☑
      bite W56.21 ☑
      strike W56.22 ☑
    overhead plane W31.2 ☑
    paper (as sharp object) W26.2 ☑
    paper-cutter W27.5 ☑
    parrot W61.09 ☑
      bite W61.01 ☑
      strike W61.02 ☑
    pig W55.49 ☑
      bite W55.41 ☑
      strike W55.42 ☑
    pipe, hot X16 ☑
    pitchfork W27.1 ☑
    plane (metal) (wood) W27.0 ☑
      overhead W31.2 ☑
    plant thorns, spines, sharp leaves or other mechanisms W60 ☑
    powered
      garden cultivator W29.3 ☑
      household appliance, implement, or machine W29.8 ☑
      saw (industrial) W31.2 ☑
        hand W29.8 ☑
    printing machine W31.89 ☑
    psittacine bird W61.29 ☑

Contact — *continued*
  with — *continued*
    psittacine bird — *continued*
      bite W61.21 ☑
      macaw — *see* Contact, with, macaw
      parrot — *see* Contact, with, parrot
      strike W61.22 ☑
    pulley (block) (transmission) W24.0 ☑
      agricultural operations W30.89 ☑
    raccoon W55.59 ☑
      bite W55.51 ☑
      strike W55.52 ☑
    radial-saw (industrial) W31.2 ☑
    radiator (hot) X16 ☑
    rake W27.1 ☑
    rattlesnake X58 ☑
    reaper W30.0 ☑
    reptile W59.89 ☑
      lizard — *see* Contact, with, lizard
      snake — *see* Contact, with, snake
      specified NEC W59.89 ☑
        bite W59.81 ☑
        crushing W59.83 ☑
        strike W59.82 ☑
      turtle — *see* Contact, with, turtle
    rivet gun (powered) W29.4 ☑
    road scraper — *see* Accident, transport, construction vehicle
    rodent (feces) (urine) W53.89 ☑
      bite W53.81 ☑
      mouse W53.09 ☑
        bite W53.01 ☑
      rat W53.19 ☑
        bite W53.11 ☑
      specified NEC W53.89 ☑
        bite W53.81 ☑
      squirrel W53.29 ☑
        bite W53.21 ☑
    roller coaster W31.81 ☑
    rope NEC W24.0 ☑
      agricultural operations W30.89 ☑
    saliva — *see* Contact, with, by type of animal
    sander W29.8 ☑
      industrial W31.2 ☑
    saucepan (hot) (glass) (metal) X15.3 ☑
    saw W27.0 ☑
      band (industrial) W31.2 ☑
      bench (industrial) W31.2 ☑
      chain W29.3 ☑
      hand W27.0 ☑
    sawing machine, metal W31.1 ☑
    scissors W27.2 ☑
    scorpion X58 ☑
    screwdriver W27.0 ☑
      powered W29.8 ☑
    sea
      anemone, cucumber or urchin (spine) X58 ☑
      lion W56.19 ☑
        bite W56.11 ☑
        strike W56.12 ☑
    serpent — *see* Contact, with, snake, by type
    sewing-machine (electric) (powered) W29.2 ☑
      not powered W27.8 ☑
    shaft (hoist) (lift) (transmission) NEC W24.0 ☑
      agricultural W30.89 ☑
    shark W56.49 ☑
      bite W56.41 ☑
      strike W56.42 ☑
    sharp object(s) W26.9 ☑
      specified NEC W26.8 ☑
    shears (hand) W27.2 ☑
      powered (industrial) W31.1 ☑
        domestic W29.2 ☑
    sheep W55.39 ☑
      bite W55.31 ☑
      strike W55.32 ☑
    shovel W27.8 ☑
      steam — *see* Accident, transport, construction vehicle
    snake (nonvenomous) W59.19 ☑
      bite W59.11 ☑
      crushing W59.13 ☑
      strike W59.12 ☑
    spade W27.1 ☑
    spider (venomous) X58 ☑
    spin-drier W29.2 ☑

Contact — *continued*
  with — *continued*
    spinning machine W31.89 ☑
    splinter W45.8 ☑
    sports equipment W21.9 ☑
    staple gun (powered) W29.8 ☑
    steam X13.1 ☑
      engine W31.3 ☑
      inhalation X13.0 ☑
      pipe X16 ☑
      shovel W31.89 ☑
    stove (hot) (kitchen) X15.0 ☑
    substance, hot NEC X19 ☑
      molten (metal) X18 ☑
    sword W26.1 ☑
      assault X99.2 ☑
      stated as undetermined whether accidental or intentional Y28.2 ☑
      suicide (attempt) X78.2 ☑
    tarantula X58 ☑
    thresher W30.0 ☑
    tin can lid W26.8 ☑
    toad W62.1 ☑
    toaster (hot) X15.1 ☑
    tool W27.8 ☑
      hand (not powered) W27.8 ☑
        auger W27.0 ☑
        axe W27.0 ☑
        can opener W27.4 ☑
        chisel W27.0 ☑
        fork W27.4 ☑
        garden W27.1 ☑
        handsaw W27.0 ☑
        hoe W27.1 ☑
        ice-pick W27.4 ☑
        kitchen utensil W27.4 ☑
        manual
          lawn mower W27.1 ☑
          sewing machine W27.8 ☑
        meat grinder W27.4 ☑
        needle (sewing) W27.3 ☑
          hypodermic W46.0 ☑
            contaminated W46.1 ☑
        paper cutter W27.5 ☑
        pitchfork W27.1 ☑
        rake W27.1 ☑
        scissors W27.2 ☑
        screwdriver W27.0 ☑
        specified NEC W27.8 ☑
        workbench W27.0 ☑
      hot X17 ☑
      powered W29.8 ☑
        blender W29.0 ☑
          commercial W31.82 ☑
        can opener W29.0 ☑
          commercial W31.82 ☑
        chainsaw W29.3 ☑
        clothes dryer W29.2 ☑
          commercial W31.82 ☑
        dishwasher W29.2 ☑
          commercial W31.82 ☑
        edger W29.3 ☑
        electric fan W29.2 ☑
          commercial W31.82 ☑
        electric knife W29.1 ☑
        food processor W29.0 ☑
          commercial W31.82 ☑
        garbage disposal W29.0 ☑
          commercial W31.82 ☑
        garden tool W29.3 ☑
        hedge trimmer W29.3 ☑
        ice maker W29.0 ☑
          commercial W31.82 ☑
        kitchen appliance W29.0 ☑
          commercial W31.82 ☑
        lawn mower W28 ☑
        meat grinder W29.0 ☑
          commercial W31.82 ☑
        mixer W29.0 ☑
          commercial W31.82 ☑
        rototiller W29.3 ☑
        sewing machine W29.2 ☑
          commercial W31.82 ☑
        washing machine W29.2 ☑
          commercial W31.82 ☑

Contact — *continued*
  with — *continued*
    transmission device (belt, cable, chain, gear, pinion, shaft) W24.1 ☑
      agricultural operations W30.89 ☑
    turbine (gas) (water-driven) W31.3 ☑
    turkey W61.49 ☑
      peck W61.43 ☑
      strike W61.42 ☑
    turtle (nonvenomous) W59.29 ☑
      bite W59.21 ☑
      strike W59.22 ☑
      terrestrial W59.89 ☑
        bite W59.81 ☑
        crushing W59.83 ☑
        strike W59.82 ☑
    under-cutter W31.0 ☑
    urine — *see* Contact, with, by type of animal
    vehicle
      agricultural use (transport) — *see* Accident, transport, agricultural vehicle
        not on public highway W30.81 ☑
      industrial use (transport) — *see* Accident, transport, industrial vehicle
        not on public highway W31.83 ☑
      off-road use (transport) — *see* Accident, transport, all-terrain or off-road vehicle
        not on public highway W31.83 ☑
      special construction use (transport) — *see* Accident, transport, construction vehicle
        not on public highway W31.83 ☑
    venomous
      animal X58 ☑
      arthropods X58 ☑
      lizard X58 ☑
      marine animal NEC X58 ☑
      marine plant NEC X58 ☑
      millipedes (tropical) X58 ☑
      plant(s) X58 ☑
      snake X58 ☑
      spider X58 ☑
    viper X58 ☑
    washing-machine (powered) W29.2 ☑
    wasp X58 ☑
    weaving-machine W31.89 ☑
    winch W24.0 ☑
      agricultural operations W30.89 ☑
    wire NEC W24.0 ☑
      agricultural operations W30.89 ☑
    wood slivers W45.8 ☑
    yellow jacket X58 ☑
    zebra — *see* Contact, with, hoof stock NEC
  pressure X50.9 ☑
  stress X50.9 ☑
Coup de soleil X32 ☑
Crash
  aircraft (in transit) (powered) V95.9 ☑
    balloon V96.01 ☑
    fixed wing NEC (private) V95.21 ☑
      commercial V95.31 ☑
    glider V96.21 ☑
      hang V96.11 ☑
      powered V95.11 ☑
    helicopter V95.01 ☑
    in war operations — *see* War operations, destruction of aircraft
    microlight V95.11 ☑
    nonpowered V96.9 ☑
      specified NEC V96.8 ☑
    powered NEC V95.8 ☑
    stated as
      homicide (attempt) Y08.81 ☑
      suicide (attempt) X83.0 ☑
    ultralight V95.11 ☑
  spacecraft V95.41 ☑
  transport vehicle NEC — *see also* Accident, transport V89.9 ☑
    homicide (attempt) Y03.8 ☑
    motor NEC (traffic) V89.2 ☑
      homicide (attempt) Y03.8 ☑
      suicide (attempt) — *see* Suicide, collision
Cruelty (mental) (physical) (sexual) X58 ☑
Crushed (accidentally) X58 ☑
  between objects (moving) (stationary and moving) W23.0 ☑
    stationary W23.1 ☑

Crushed — *continued*
  by
    alligator W58.03 ☑
    avalanche NEC — *see* Landslide
    cave-in W20.0 ☑
      caused by cataclysmic earth surface movement — *see* Landslide
    crocodile W58.13 ☑
    crowd or human stampede W52 ☑
    falling
      aircraft V97.39 ☑
        in war operations — *see* War operations, destruction of aircraft
      earth, material W20.0 ☑
        caused by cataclysmic earth surface movement — *see* Landslide
      object NEC W20.8 ☑
    landslide NEC — *see* Landslide
    lizard (nonvenomous) W59.09 ☑
    machinery — *see* Contact, with, by type of machine
    reptile NEC W59.89 ☑
    snake (nonvenomous) W59.13 ☑
  in
    machinery — *see* Contact, with, by type of machine
Cut, cutting (any part of body) (accidental) — *see also* Contact, with, by object or machine
  during medical or surgical treatment as misadventure — *see* Index to Diseases and Injuries, Complications
  homicide (attempt) — *see* Assault, cutting or piercing instrument
  inflicted by other person — *see* Assault, cutting or piercing instrument
  legal
    execution — *see* Legal, intervention
    intervention — *see* Legal, intervention, sharp object
  machine NEC — *see also* Contact, with, by type of machine W31.9 ☑
  self-inflicted — *see* Suicide, cutting or piercing instrument
  suicide (attempt) — *see* Suicide, cutting or piercing instrument
Cyclone (any injury) X37.1 ☑

D

Decapitation (accidental circumstances) NEC X58 ☑
  homicide X99.9 ☑
  legal execution — *see* Legal, intervention
Dehydration from lack of water X58 ☑
Deprivation X58 ☑
Derailment (accidental)
  railway (rolling stock) (train) (vehicle) (without antecedent collision) V81.7 ☑
    with antecedent collision — *see* Accident, transport, railway vehicle occupant
  streetcar (without antecedent collision) V82.7 ☑
    with antecedent collision — *see* Accident, transport, streetcar occupant
Descent
  parachute (voluntary) (without accident to aircraft) V97.29 ☑
    due to accident to aircraft — *see* Accident, transport, aircraft
Desertion X58 ☑
Destitution X58 ☑
Disability, late effect or sequela of injury — *see* Sequelae
Discharge (accidental)
  airgun W34.010 ☑
    assault X95.01 ☑
    homicide (attempt) X95.01 ☑
    stated as undetermined whether accidental or intentional Y24.0 ☑
    suicide (attempt) X74.01 ☑
  BB gun — *see* Discharge, airgun
  firearm (accidental) W34.00 ☑
    assault X95.9 ☑
    handgun (pistol) (revolver) W32.0 ☑
      assault X93 ☑
      homicide (attempt) X93 ☑
      legal intervention — *see* Legal, intervention, firearm, handgun
      stated as undetermined whether accidental or intentional Y22 ☑
      suicide (attempt) X72 ☑

Discharge — *continued*
  firearm — *continued*
    homicide (attempt) X95.9 ☑
    hunting rifle W33.02 ☑
      assault X94.1 ☑
      homicide (attempt) X94.1 ☑
      legal intervention
        injuring
          bystander Y35.032 ☑
          law enforcement personnel Y35.031 ☑
          suspect Y35.033 ☑
          unspecified person Y35.039 ☑
      stated as undetermined whether accidental or intentional Y23.1 ☑
      suicide (attempt) X73.1 ☑
    larger W33.00 ☑
      assault X94.9 ☑
      homicide (attempt) X94.9 ☑
      hunting rifle — *see* Discharge, firearm, hunting rifle
      legal intervention — *see* Legal, intervention, firearm by type of firearm
      machine gun — *see* Discharge, firearm, machine gun
      shotgun — *see* Discharge, firearm, shotgun
      specified NEC W33.09 ☑
        assault X94.8 ☑
        homicide (attempt) X94.8 ☑
        legal intervention
          injuring
            bystander Y35.092 ☑
            law enforcement personnel Y35.091 ☑
            suspect Y35.093 ☑
            unspecified person Y35.099 ☑
        stated as undetermined whether accidental or intentional Y23.8 ☑
        suicide (attempt) X73.8 ☑
      stated as undetermined whether accidental or intentional Y23.9 ☑
      suicide (attempt) X73.9 ☑
    legal intervention
      injuring
        bystander Y35.002 ☑
        law enforcement personnel Y35.001 ☑
        suspect Y35.03 ☑
        unspecified person Y35.009 ☑
      using rubber bullet
        injuring
          bystander Y35.042 ☑
          law enforcement personnel Y35.041 ☑
          suspect Y35.043 ☑
          unspecified person Y35.049 ☑
    machine gun W33.03 ☑
      assault X94.2 ☑
      homicide (attempt) X94.2 ☑
      legal intervention — *see* Legal, intervention, firearm, machine gun
      stated as undetermined whether accidental or intentional Y23.3 ☑
      suicide (attempt) X73.2 ☑
    pellet gun — *see* Discharge, airgun
    shotgun W33.01 ☑
      assault X94.0 ☑
      homicide (attempt) X94.0 ☑
      legal intervention — *see* Legal, intervention, firearm, specified NEC
      stated as undetermined whether accidental or intentional Y23.0 ☑
      suicide (attempt) X73.0 ☑
    specified NEC W34.09 ☑
      assault X95.8 ☑
      homicide (attempt) X95.8 ☑
      legal intervention — *see* Legal, intervention, firearm, specified NEC
      stated as undetermined whether accidental or intentional Y24.8 ☑
      suicide (attempt) X74.8 ☑
    stated as undetermined whether accidental or intentional Y24.9 ☑
    suicide (attempt) X74.9 ☑
    Very pistol W34.09 ☑
      assault X95.8 ☑
      homicide (attempt) X95.8 ☑
      stated as undetermined whether accidental or intentional Y24.8 ☑

Discharge — *continued*
  firearm — *continued*
    Very pistol — *continued*
      suicide (attempt) X74.8 ☑
  firework(s) W39 ☑
    stated as undetermined whether accidental or intentional Y25 ☑
  gas-operated gun NEC W34.018 ☑
    airgun — *see* Discharge, airgun
    assault X95.09 ☑
    homicide (attempt) X95.09 ☑
    paintball gun — *see* Discharge, paintball gun
    stated as undetermined whether accidental or intentional Y24.8 ☑
    suicide (attempt) X74.09 ☑
  gun NEC — *see also* Discharge, firearm NEC
    air — *see* Discharge, airgun
    BB — *see* Discharge, airgun
    for single hand use — *see* Discharge, firearm, handgun
    hand — *see* Discharge, firearm, handgun
    machine — *see* Discharge, firearm, machine gun
    other specified — *see* Discharge, firearm NEC
    paintball — *see* Discharge, paintball gun
    pellet — *see* Discharge, airgun
  handgun — *see* Discharge, firearm, handgun
  machine gun — *see* Discharge, firearm, machine gun
  paintball gun W34.011 ☑
    assault X95.02 ☑
    homicide (attempt) X95.02 ☑
    stated as undetermined whether accidental or intentional Y24.8 ☑
    suicide (attempt) X74.02 ☑
  pistol — *see* Discharge, firearm, handgun
    flare — *see* Discharge, firearm, Very pistol
    pellet — *see* Discharge, airgun
    Very — *see* Discharge, firearm, Very pistol
  revolver — *see* Discharge, firearm, handgun
  rifle (hunting) — *see* Discharge, firearm, hunting rifle
  shotgun — *see* Discharge, firearm, shotgun
  spring-operated gun NEC W34.018 ☑
    assault X95.09 ☑
    homicide (attempt) X95.09 ☑
    stated as undetermined whether accidental or intentional Y24.8 ☑
    suicide (attempt) X74.09 ☑
Disease
  Andes W94.11 ☑
  aviator's — *see* Air, pressure
  range W94.11 ☑
Diver's disease, palsy, paralysis, squeeze — *see* Air, pressure
Diving (into water) — *see* Accident, diving
Dog bite W54.0 ☑
Dragged by transport vehicle NEC — *see also* Accident, transport V09.9 ☑
Drinking poison (accidental) — *see* Table of Drugs and Chemicals
Dropped (accidentally) **while being carried or supported by other person** W04 ☑
Drowning (accidental) W74 ☑
  assault X92.9 ☑
  due to
    accident (to)
      machinery — *see* Contact, with, by type of machine
      watercraft V90.89 ☑
        burning V90.29 ☑
          powered V90.23 ☑
            fishing boat V90.22 ☑
            jetskis V90.23 ☑
            merchant ship V90.20 ☑
            passenger ship V90.21 ☑
          unpowered V90.28 ☑
            canoe V90.25 ☑
            inflatable V90.26 ☑
            kayak V90.25 ☑
            sailboat V90.24 ☑
            water skis V90.27 ☑
        crushed V90.39 ☑
          powered V90.33 ☑
            fishing boat V90.32 ☑
            jetskis V90.33 ☑
            merchant ship V90.30 ☑
            passenger ship V90.31 ☑
          unpowered V90.38 ☑

Drowning — *continued*
  due to — *continued*
    accident — *continued*
      watercraft — *continued*
        crushed — *continued*
          unpowered — *continued*
            canoe V90.35 ☑
            inflatable V90.36 ☑
            kayak V90.35 ☑
            sailboat V90.34 ☑
            water skis V90.37 ☑
        overturning V90.09 ☑
          powered V90.03 ☑
            fishing boat V90.02 ☑
            jetskis V90.03 ☑
            merchant ship V90.00 ☑
            passenger ship V90.01 ☑
          unpowered V90.08 ☑
            canoe V90.05 ☑
            inflatable V90.06 ☑
            kayak V90.05 ☑
            sailboat V90.04 ☑
        sinking V90.19 ☑
          powered V90.13 ☑
            fishing boat V90.12 ☑
            jetskis V90.13 ☑
            merchant ship V90.10 ☑
            passenger ship V90.11 ☑
          unpowered V90.18 ☑
            canoe V90.15 ☑
            inflatable V90.16 ☑
            kayak V90.15 ☑
            sailboat V90.14 ☑
        specified type NEC V90.89 ☑
          powered V90.83 ☑
            fishing boat V90.82 ☑
            jetskis V90.83 ☑
            merchant ship V90.80 ☑
            passenger ship V90.81 ☑
          unpowered V90.88 ☑
            canoe V90.85 ☑
            inflatable V90.86 ☑
            kayak V90.85 ☑
            sailboat V90.84 ☑
            water skis V90.87 ☑
  avalanche — *see* Landslide
  cataclysmic
    earth surface movement NEC — *see* Forces of nature, earth movement
    storm — *see* Forces of nature, cataclysmic storm
  cloudburst X37.8 ☑
  cyclone X37.1 ☑
  fall overboard (from) V92.09 ☑
    powered craft V92.03 ☑
      ferry boat V92.01 ☑
      fishing boat V92.02 ☑
      jetskis V92.03 ☑
      liner V92.01 ☑
      merchant ship V92.00 ☑
      passenger ship V92.01 ☑
    resulting from
      accident to watercraft — *see* Drowning, due to, accident to, watercraft
      being washed overboard (from) V92.29 ☑
        powered craft V92.23 ☑
          ferry boat V92.21 ☑
          fishing boat V92.22 ☑
          jetskis V92.23 ☑
          liner V92.21 ☑
          merchant ship V92.20 ☑
          passenger ship V92.21 ☑
        unpowered craft V92.28 ☑
          canoe V92.25 ☑
          inflatable V92.26 ☑
          kayak V92.25 ☑
          sailboat V92.24 ☑
          surf-board V92.28 ☑
          water skis V92.27 ☑
          windsurfer V92.28 ☑
      motion of watercraft V92.19 ☑
        powered craft V92.13 ☑
          ferry boat V92.11 ☑
          fishing boat V92.12 ☑
          jetskis V92.13 ☑
          liner V92.11 ☑
          merchant ship V92.10 ☑

Drowning — *continued*
  due to — *continued*
    fall overboard — *continued*
      resulting from — *continued*
        motion of watercraft — *continued*
          powered craft — *continued*
            passenger ship V92.11 ☑
          unpowered craft
            canoe V92.15 ☑
            inflatable V92.16 ☑
            kayak V92.15 ☑
            sailboat V92.14 ☑
      unpowered craft V92.08 ☑
        canoe V92.05 ☑
        inflatable V92.06 ☑
        kayak V92.05 ☑
        sailboat V92.04 ☑
        surf-board V92.08 ☑
        water skis V92.07 ☑
        windsurfer V92.08 ☑
  hurricane X37.0 ☑
  jumping into water from watercraft (involved in accident) — *see also* Drowning, due to, accident to, watercraft
    without accident to or on watercraft W16.711 ☑
  tidal wave NEC — *see* Forces of nature, tidal wave
  torrential rain X37.8 ☑
  following
    fall
      into
        bathtub W16.211 ☑
        bucket W16.221 ☑
        fountain — *see* Drowning, following, fall, into, water, specified NEC
        quarry — *see* Drowning, following, fall, into, water, specified NEC
        reservoir — *see* Drowning, following, fall, into, water, specified NEC
        swimming-pool W16.011 ☑
          stated as undetermined whether accidental or intentional Y21.3 ☑
          striking
            bottom W16.021 ☑
            wall W16.031 ☑
          suicide (attempt) X71.2 ☑
        water NOS W16.41 ☑
          natural (lake) (open sea) (river) (stream) (pond) W16.111 ☑
            striking
              bottom W16.121 ☑
              side W16.131 ☑
          specified NEC W16.311 ☑
            striking
              bottom W16.321 ☑
              wall W16.331 ☑
    overboard NEC — *see* Drowning, due to, fall overboard
  jump or dive
    from boat W16.711 ☑
      striking bottom W16.721 ☑
    into
      fountain — *see* Drowning, following, jump or dive, into, water, specified NEC
      quarry — *see* Drowning, following, jump or dive, into, water, specified NEC
      reservoir — *see* Drowning, following, jump or dive, into, water, specified NEC
      swimming-pool W16.511 ☑
        striking
          bottom W16.521 ☑
          wall W16.531 ☑
        suicide (attempt) X71.2 ☑
      water NOS W16.91 ☑
        natural (lake) (open sea) (river) (stream) (pond) W16.611 ☑
        specified NEC W16.811 ☑
          bottom W16.821 ☑
          striking
            bottom W16.821 ☑
            wall W16.831 ☑
        striking
          bottom W16.821 ☑
          wall W16.831 ☑
        striking bottom W16.621 ☑
  homicide (attempt) X92.9 ☑
  in
    bathtub (accidental) W65 ☑

Drowning — *continued*
  in — *continued*
    bathtub — *continued*
      assault X92.0 ☑
      following fall W16.211 ☑
        stated as undetermined whether accidental
          or intentional Y21.1 ☑
      stated as undetermined whether accidental or
        intentional Y21.0 ☑
      suicide (attempt) X71.0 ☑
    lake — *see* Drowning, in, natural water
    natural water (lake) (open sea) (river) (stream)
      (pond) W69 ☑
      assault X92.3 ☑
      following
        dive or jump W16.611 ☑
          striking bottom W16.621 ☑
        fall W16.111 ☑
          striking
            bottom W16.121 ☑
            side W16.131 ☑
      stated as undetermined whether accidental or
        intentional Y21.4 ☑
      suicide (attempt) X71.3 ☑
    quarry — *see* Drowning, in, specified place NEC
    quenching tank — *see* Drowning, in, specified place
      NEC
    reservoir — *see* Drowning, in, specified place NEC
    river — *see* Drowning, in, natural water
    sea — *see* Drowning, in, natural water
    specified place NEC W73 ☑
      assault X92.8 ☑
      following
        dive or jump W16.811 ☑
          striking
            bottom W16.821 ☑
            wall W16.831 ☑
        fall W16.311 ☑
          striking
            bottom W16.321 ☑
            wall W16.331 ☑
      stated as undetermined whether accidental or
        intentional Y21.8 ☑
      suicide (attempt) X71.8 ☑
    stream — *see* Drowning, in, natural water
    swimming-pool W67 ☑
      assault X92.1 ☑
        following fall X92.2 ☑
      following
        dive or jump W16.511 ☑
          striking
            bottom W16.521 ☑
            wall W16.531 ☑
        fall W16.011 ☑
          striking
            bottom W16.021 ☑
            wall W16.031 ☑
      stated as undetermined whether accidental or
        intentional Y21.2 ☑
      following fall Y21.3 ☑
      suicide (attempt) X71.1 ☑
        following fall X71.2 ☑
  war operations — *see* War operations, restriction
    of airway
  resulting from accident to watercraft — *see* Drowning,
    due to, accident, watercraft
  self-inflicted X71.9 ☑
  stated as undetermined whether accidental or inten-
    tional Y21.9 ☑
  suicide (attempt) X71.9 ☑

E

Earth falling (on) W20.0 ☑
  caused by cataclysmic earth surface movement or
    eruption — *see* Landslide
Earth (surface) **movement NEC** — *see* Forces of nature,
  earth movement
Earthquake (any injury) X34 ☑
Effect(s) (adverse) **of**
  air pressure (any) — *see* Air, pressure
  cold, excessive (exposure to) — *see* Exposure, cold
  heat (excessive) — *see* Heat
  hot place (weather) — *see* Heat
  insolation X30 ☑
  late — *see* Sequelae

Effect(s) (adverse) **of** — *continued*
  motion — *see* Motion
  nuclear explosion or weapon in war operations — *see*
    War operations, nuclear weapon
  radiation — *see* Radiation
  travel — *see* Travel
Electric shock (accidental) (by) (in) — *see* Exposure,
  electric current
Electrocution (accidental) — *see* Exposure, electric current
Endotracheal tube wrongly placed during anesthetic
  procedure
Entanglement
  in
    bed linen, causing suffocation T71 ☑
    wheel of pedal cycle V19.88 ☑
Entry of foreign body or material — *see* Foreign body
Environmental pollution related condition — *see*
  category Z57 ☑
Execution, legal (any method) — *see* Legal, intervention
Exhaustion
  cold — *see* Exposure, cold
  due to excessive exertion — *see also* Overexertion
    X50.9 ☑
  heat — *see* Heat
Explosion (accidental) (of) (with secondary fire) W40.9 ☑
  acetylene W40.1 ☑
  aerosol can W36.1 ☑
  air tank (compressed) (in machinery) W36.2 ☑
  aircraft (in transit) (powered) NEC V95.9 ☑
    balloon V96.05 ☑
    fixed wing NEC (private) V95.25 ☑
      commercial V95.35 ☑
    glider V96.25 ☑
      hang V96.15 ☑
      powered V95.15 ☑
    helicopter V95.05 ☑
    in war operations — *see* War operations, destruction
      of aircraft
    microlight V95.15 ☑
    nonpowered V96.9 ☑
      specified NEC V96.8 ☑
    powered NEC V95.8 ☑
    stated as
      homicide (attempt) Y03.8 ☑
      suicide (attempt) X83.0 ☑
    ultralight V95.15 ☑
  anesthetic gas in operating room W40.1 ☑
  antipersonnel bomb W40.8 ☑
    assault X96.0 ☑
    homicide (attempt) X96.0 ☑
    suicide (attempt) X75 ☑
  assault X96.9 ☑
  bicycle tire W37.0 ☑
  blasting (cap) (materials) W40.0 ☑
  boiler (machinery), not on transport vehicle W35 ☑
    on watercraft — *see* Explosion, in, watercraft
  butane W40.1 ☑
  caused by other person X96.9 ☑
  coal gas W40.1 ☑
  detonator W40.0 ☑
  dump (munitions) W40.8 ☑
  dynamite W40.0 ☑
    in
      assault X96.8 ☑
      homicide (attempt) X96.8 ☑
      legal intervention
        injuring
          bystander Y35.112 ☑
          law enforcement personnel Y35.111 ☑
          suspect Y35.113 ☑
          unspecified person Y35.119 ☑
      suicide (attempt) X75 ☑
  explosive (material) W40.9 ☑
    gas W40.1 ☑
    in blasting operation W40.0 ☑
    specified NEC W40.8 ☑
      in
        assault X96.8 ☑
        homicide (attempt) X96.8 ☑
        legal intervention
          injuring
            bystander Y35.192 ☑
            law enforcement personnel
              Y35.191 ☑
            suspect Y35.193 ☑

Explosion — *continued*
  explosive — *continued*
    specified — *continued*
      in — *continued*
        legal intervention — *continued*
          injuring — *continued*
            unspecified person Y35.199 ☑
        suicide (attempt) X75 ☑
  factory (munitions) W40.8 ☑
  fertilizer bomb W40.8 ☑
    assault X96.3 ☑
    homicide (attempt) X96.3 ☑
    suicide (attempt) X75 ☑
  firearm (parts) NEC W34.19 ☑
    airgun W34.110 ☑
    BB gun W34.110 ☑
    gas, air or spring-operated gun NEC W34.118 ☑
    hangun W32.1 ☑
    hunting rifle W33.12 ☑
    larger firearm W33.10 ☑
      specified NEC W33.19 ☑
    machine gun W33.13 ☑
    paintball gun W34.111 ☑
    pellet gun W34.110 ☑
    shotgun W33.11 ☑
    Very pistol [flare] W34.19 ☑
  fire-damp W40.1 ☑
  fireworks W39 ☑
  gas (coal) (explosive) W40.1 ☑
    cylinder W36.9 ☑
      aerosol can W36.1 ☑
      air tank W36.2 ☑
      pressurized W36.3 ☑
      specified NEC W36.8 ☑
  gasoline (fumes) (tank) not in moving motor vehicle
    W40.1 ☑
    bomb W40.8 ☑
      assault X96.1 ☑
      homicide (attempt) X96.1 ☑
      suicide (attempt) X75 ☑
    in motor vehicle — *see* Accident, transport, by type
      of vehicle
  grain store W40.8 ☑
  grenade W40.8 ☑
    in
      assault X96.8 ☑
      homicide (attempt) X96.8 ☑
      legal intervention
        injuring
          bystander Y35.192 ☑
          law enforcement personnel Y35.191 ☑
          suspect Y35.193 ☑
          unspecified person Y35.199 ☑
      suicide (attempt) X75 ☑
  handgun (parts) — *see* Explosion, firearm, hangun
    (parts)
  homicide (attempt) X96.9 ☑
    antipersonnel bomb — *see* Explosion, antipersonnel
      bomb
    fertilizer bomb — *see* Explosion, fertilizer bomb
    gasoline bomb — *see* Explosion, gasoline bomb
    letter bomb — *see* Explosion, letter bomb
    pipe bomb — *see* Explosion, pipe bomb
    specified NEC X96.8 ☑
  hose, pressurized W37.8 ☑
  hot water heater, tank (in machinery) W35 ☑
    on watercraft — *see* Explosion, in, watercraft
  in, on
    dump W40.8 ☑
    factory W40.8 ☑
    mine (of explosive gases) NEC W40.1 ☑
    watercraft V93.59 ☑
      powered craft V93.53 ☑
        ferry boat V93.51 ☑
        fishing boat V93.52 ☑
        jetskis V93.53 ☑
        liner V93.51 ☑
        merchant ship V93.50 ☑
        passenger ship V93.51 ☑
        sailboat V93.54 ☑
  letter bomb W40.8 ☑
    assault X96.2 ☑
    homicide (attempt) X96.2 ☑
    suicide (attempt) X75 ☑
  machinery — *see also* Contact, with, by type of ma-
    chine

Explosion — *continued*
  machinery — *see also* Contact, with, by type of machine — *continued*
    on board watercraft — *see* Explosion, in, watercraft
    pressure vessel — *see* Explosion, by type of vessel
  methane W40.1 ☑
  mine W40.1 ☑
  missile NEC W40.8 ☑
  mortar bomb W40.8 ☑
    in
      assault X96.8 ☑
      homicide (attempt) X96.8 ☑
      legal intervention
        injuring
          bystander Y35.192 ☑
          law enforcement personnel Y35.191 ☑
          suspect Y35.193 ☑
          unspecified person Y35.199 ☑
      suicide (attempt) X75 ☑
  munitions (dump) (factory) W40.8 ☑
  pipe, pressurized W37.8 ☑
    bomb W40.8 ☑
      assault X96.4 ☑
      homicide (attempt) X96.4 ☑
      suicide (attempt) X75 ☑
  pressure, pressurized
    cooker W38 ☑
    gas tank (in machinery) W36.3 ☑
    hose W37.8 ☑
    pipe W37.8 ☑
    specified device NEC W38 ☑
    tire W37.8 ☑
      bicycle W37.0 ☑
    vessel (in machinery) W38 ☑
  propane W40.1 ☑
  self-inflicted X75 ☑
  shell (artillery) NEC W40.8 ☑
    during war operations — *see* War operations, explosion
    in
      legal intervention
        injuring
          bystander Y35.122 ☑
          law enforcement personnel Y35.121 ☑
          suspect Y35.123 ☑
          unspecified person Y35.129 ☑
      war — *see* War operations, explosion
  spacecraft V95.45 ☑
  stated as undetermined whether accidental or intentional Y25 ☑
  steam or water lines (in machinery) W37.8 ☑
  stove W40.9 ☑
  suicide (attempt) X75 ☑
  tire, pressurized W37.8 ☑
    bicycle W37.0 ☑
  undetermined whether accidental or intentional Y25 ☑
  vehicle tire NEC W37.8 ☑
    bicycle W37.0 ☑
  war operations — *see* War operations, explosion
Exposure (to) X58 ☑
  air pressure change — *see* Air, pressure
  cold (accidental) (excessive) (extreme) (natural) (place) X31 ☑
    assault Y08.89 ☑
    due to
      man-made conditions W93.8 ☑
        dry ice (contact) W93.01 ☑
          inhalation W93.02 ☑
        liquid air (contact) (hydrogen) (nitrogen) W93.11 ☑
          inhalation W93.12 ☑
        refrigeration unit (deep freeze) W93.2 ☑
      suicide (attempt) X83.2 ☑
      weather (conditions) X31 ☑
    homicide (attempt) Y08.89 ☑
    self-inflicted X83.2 ☑
  due to abandonment or neglect X58 ☑
  electric current W86.8 ☑
    appliance (faulty) W86.8 ☑
      domestic W86.0 ☑
    caused by other person Y08.89 ☑
    conductor (faulty) W86.1 ☑
    control apparatus (faulty) W86.1 ☑
    electric power generating plant, distribution station W86.1 ☑

Exposure — *continued*
  electric current — *continued*
    electroshock gun — *see* Exposure, electric current, taser
    high-voltage cable W85 ☑
    homicide (attempt) Y08.89 ☑
    legal execution — *see* Legal, intervention, specified means NEC
    lightning — *see* subcategory T75.0 ☑
    live rail W86.8 ☑
    misadventure in medical or surgical procedure in electroshock therapy Y63.4
    motor (electric) (faulty) W86.8 ☑
      domestic W86.0 ☑
    self-inflicted X83.1 ☑
    specified NEC W86.8 ☑
      domestic W86.0 ☑
    stun gun — *see* Exposure, electric current, taser
    suicide (attempt) X83.1 ☑
    taser W86.8 ☑
      assault Y08.89 ☑
      legal intervention — *see* category Y35
      self-harm (intentional) X83.8 ☑
      undetermined intent Y33 ☑
    third rail W86.8 ☑
    transformer (faulty) W86.1 ☑
    transmission lines W85 ☑
  environmental tobacco smoke X58 ☑
  excessive
    cold — *see* Exposure, cold
    heat (natural) NEC X30 ☑
      man-made W92 ☑
  factor(s) NOS X58 ☑
    environmental NEC X58 ☑
    man-made NEC W99 ☑
    natural NEC — *see* Forces of nature
    specified NEC X58 ☑
  fire, flames (accidental) X08.8 ☑
    assault X97 ☑
    campfire — *see* Exposure, fire, controlled, not in building
    controlled (in)
      with ignition (of) clothing — *see also* Ignition, clothes X06.2 ☑
        nightwear X05 ☑
      bonfire — *see* Exposure, fire, controlled, not in building
      brazier (in building or structure) — *see also* Exposure, fire, controlled, building
        not in building or structure — *see* Exposure, fire, controlled, not in building
      building or structure X02.0 ☑
        with
          fall from building X02.3 ☑
          from building X02.5 ☑
          injury due to building collapse X02.2 ☑
          smoke inhalation X02.1 ☑
        hit by object from building X02.4 ☑
        specified mode of injury NEC X02.8 ☑
      fireplace, furnace or stove — *see* Exposure, fire, controlled, building
      not in building or structure X03.0 ☑
        with
          fall X03.3 ☑
          smoke inhalation X03.1 ☑
        hit by object X03.4 ☑
        specified mode of injury NEC X03.8 ☑
      trash — *see* Exposure, fire, controlled, not in building
    fireplace — *see* Exposure, fire, controlled, building
    fittings or furniture (in building or structure) (uncontrolled) — *see* Exposure, fire, uncontrolled, building
    forest (uncontrolled) — *see* Exposure, fire, uncontrolled, not in building
    grass (uncontrolled) — *see* Exposure, fire, uncontrolled, not in building
    hay (uncontrolled) — *see* Exposure, fire, uncontrolled, not in building
    homicide (attempt) X97 ☑
    ignition of highly flammable material X04 ☑
    in, of, on, starting in
      machinery — *see* Contact, with, by type of machine

Exposure — *continued*
  fire, flames — *continued*
    in, of, on, starting in — *continued*
      motor vehicle (in motion) — *see also* Accident, transport, occupant by type of vehicle V87.8 ☑
        with collision — *see* Collision
      railway rolling stock, train, vehicle V81.81 ☑
        with collision — *see* Accident, transport, railway vehicle occupant
      street car (in motion) V82.8 ☑
        with collision — *see* Accident, transport, streetcar occupant
      transport vehicle NEC — *see also* Accident, transport
        with collision — *see* Collision
      war operations — *see also* War operations, fire from nuclear explosion — *see* War operations, nuclear weapons
      watercraft (in transit) (not in transit) V91.09 ☑
        localized — *see* Burn, on board watercraft, due to, fire on board
        powered craft V91.03 ☑
          ferry boat V91.01 ☑
          fishing boat V91.02 ☑
          jet skis V91.03 ☑
          liner V91.01 ☑
          merchant ship V91.00 ☑
          passenger ship V91.01 ☑
        unpowered craft V91.08 ☑
          canoe V91.05 ☑
          inflatable V91.06 ☑
          kayak V91.05 ☑
          sailboat V91.04 ☑
          surf-board V91.08 ☑
          waterskis V91.07 ☑
          windsurfer V91.08 ☑
    lumber (uncontrolled) — *see* Exposure, fire, uncontrolled, not in building
    mine (uncontrolled) — *see* Exposure, fire, uncontrolled, not in building
    prairie (uncontrolled) — *see* Exposure, fire, uncontrolled, not in building
    resulting from
      explosion — *see* Explosion
      lightning X08.8 ☑
    self-inflicted X76 ☑
    specified NEC X08.8 ☑
    started by other person X97 ☑
    stated as undetermined whether accidental or intentional Y26 ☑
    stove — *see* Exposure, fire, controlled, building
    suicide (attempt) X76 ☑
    tunnel (uncontrolled) — *see* Exposure, fire, uncontrolled, not in building
    uncontrolled
      in building or structure X00.0 ☑
        with
          fall from building X00.3 ☑
          injury due to building collapse X00.2 ☑
          jump from building X00.5 ☑
          smoke inhalation X00.1 ☑
        bed X08.00 ☑
          due to
            cigarette X08.01 ☑
            specified material NEC X08.09 ☑
        furniture NEC X08.20 ☑
          due to
            cigarette X08.21 ☑
            specified material NEC X08.29 ☑
        hit by object from building X00.4 ☑
        sofa X08.10 ☑
          due to
            cigarette X08.11 ☑
            specified material NEC X08.19 ☑
        specified mode of injury NEC X00.8 ☑
      not in building or structure (any) X01.0 ☑
        with
          fall X01.3 ☑
          smoke inhalation X01.1 ☑
        hit by object X01.4 ☑
        specified mode of injury NEC X01.8 ☑
    undetermined whether accidental or intentional Y26 ☑
  forces of nature NEC — *see* Forces of nature
  G-forces (abnormal) W49.9 ☑

Exposure — *continued*
  gravitational forces (abnormal) W49.9 ☑
  heat (natural) NEC — *see* Heat
  high-pressure jet (hydraulic) (pneumatic) W49.9 ☑
  hydraulic jet W49.9 ☑
  inanimate mechanical force W49.9 ☑
  jet, high-pressure (hydraulic) (pneumatic) W49.9 ☑
  lightning — *see* subcategory T75.0 ☑
    causing fire — *see* Exposure, fire
  mechanical forces NEC W49.9 ☑
    animate NEC W64 ☑
    inanimate NEC W49.9 ☑
  noise W42.9 ☑
    supersonic W42.0 ☑
  noxious substance — *see* Table of Drugs and Chemicals
  pneumatic jet W49.9 ☑
  prolonged in deep-freeze unit or refrigerator W93.2 ☑
  radiation — *see* Radiation
  smoke — *see also* Exposure, fire
    tobacco, second hand Z77.22
  specified factors NEC X58 ☑
  sunlight X32 ☑
    man-made (sun lamp) W89.8 ☑
      tanning bed W89.1 ☑
  supersonic waves W42.0 ☑
  transmission line(s), electric W85 ☑
  vibration W49.9 ☑
  waves
    infrasound W49.9 ☑
    sound W42.9 ☑
    supersonic W42.0 ☑
  weather NEC — *see* Forces of nature
External cause status Y99.9
  child assisting in compensated work for family Y99.8
  civilian activity done for financial or other compensation Y99.0
  civilian activity done for income or pay Y99.0
  family member assisting in compensated work for other family member Y99.8
  hobby not done for income Y99.8
  leisure activity Y99.8
  military activity Y99.1
  off-duty activity of military personnel Y99.8
  recreation or sport not for income or while a student Y99.8
  specified NEC Y99.8
  student activity Y99.8
  volunteer activity Y99.2

F

Factors, supplemental
  alcohol
    blood level
      less than 20mg/100ml Y90.0
      presence in blood, level not specified Y90.9
      20-39mg/100ml Y90.1
      40-59mg/100ml Y90.2
      60-79mg/100ml Y90.3
      80-99mg/100ml Y90.4
      100-119mg/100ml Y90.5
      120-199mg/100ml Y90.6
      200-239mg/100ml Y90.7
      240mg/100ml or more Y90.8
    presence in blood, but level not specified Y90.9
  environmental-pollution-related condition- see Z57 ☑
  nosocomial condition Y95
  work-related condition Y99.0
Failure
  in suture or ligature during surgical procedure Y65.2
  mechanical, of instrument or apparatus (any) (during any medical or surgical procedure) Y65.8
  sterile precautions (during medical and surgical care) — *see* Misadventure, failure, sterile precautions, by type of procedure
  to
    introduce tube or instrument Y65.4
      endotracheal tube during anesthesia Y65.3
    make curve (transport vehicle) NEC — *see* Accident, transport
    remove tube or instrument Y65.4
Fall, falling (accidental) W19 ☑
  building W20.1 ☑
    burning (uncontrolled fire) X00.3 ☑
  down
    embankment W17.81 ☑
    escalator W10.0 ☑

Fall, falling — *continued*
  down — *continued*
    hill W17.81 ☑
    ladder W11 ☑
    ramp W10.2 ☑
    stairs, steps W10.9 ☑
  due to
    bumping against
      object W18.00 ☑
        sharp glass W18.02 ☑
        specified NEC W18.09 ☑
        sports equipment W18.01 ☑
      person W03 ☑
        due to ice or snow W00.0 ☑
        on pedestrian conveyance — *see* Accident, transport, pedestrian, conveyance
    collision with another person W03 ☑
      due to ice or snow W00.0 ☑
      involving pedestrian conveyance — *see* Accident, transport, pedestrian, conveyance
    grocery cart tipping over W17.82 ☑
    ice or snow W00.9 ☑
      from one level to another W00.2 ☑
        on stairs or steps W00.1 ☑
      involving pedestrian conveyance — *see* Accident, transport, pedestrian, conveyance
      on same level W00.0 ☑
    slipping (on moving sidewalk) W01.0 ☑
      with subsequent striking against object W01.10 ☑
        furniture W01.190 ☑
        sharp object W01.119 ☑
          glass W01.110 ☑
          power tool or machine W01.111 ☑
          specified NEC W01.118 ☑
        specified NEC W01.198 ☑
    striking against
      object W18.00 ☑
        sharp glass W18.02 ☑
        specified NEC W18.09 ☑
        sports equipment W18.01 ☑
      person W03 ☑
        due to ice or snow W00.0 ☑
        on pedestrian conveyance — *see* Accident, transport, pedestrian, conveyance
  earth (with asphyxia or suffocation (by pressure)) — *see* Earth, falling
  from, off, out of
    aircraft NEC (with accident to aircraft NEC) V97.0 ☑
      while boarding or alighting V97.1 ☑
    balcony W13.0 ☑
    bed W06 ☑
    boat, ship, watercraft NEC (with drowning or submersion) — *see* Drowning, due to, fall overboard
      with hitting bottom or object V94.0 ☑
    bridge W13.1 ☑
    building W13.9 ☑
      burning (uncontrolled fire) X00.3 ☑
    cavity W17.2 ☑
    chair W07 ☑
    cherry picker W17.89 ☑
    cliff W15 ☑
    dock W17.4 ☑
    embankment W17.81 ☑
    escalator W10.0 ☑
    flagpole W13.8 ☑
    furniture NEC W08 ☑
    grocery cart W17.82 ☑
    haystack W17.89 ☑
    high place NEC W17.89 ☑
      stated as undetermined whether accidental or intentional Y30 ☑
    hole W17.2 ☑
    incline W10.2 ☑
    ladder W11 ☑
    lifting device W17.89 ☑
    machine, machinery — *see also* Contact, with, by type of machine
      not in operation W17.89 ☑
    manhole W17.1 ☑
    mobile elevated work platform [MEWP] W17.89 ☑
    motorized mobility scooter W05.2 ☑
    one level to another NEC W17.89 ☑
      intentional, purposeful, suicide (attempt) X80 ☑

Fall, falling — *continued*
  from, off, out of — *continued*
    one level to another — *continued*
      stated as undetermined whether accidental or intentional Y30 ☑
    pit W17.2 ☑
    playground equipment W09.8 ☑
      jungle gym W09.2 ☑
      slide W09.0 ☑
      swing W09.1 ☑
    quarry W17.89 ☑
    railing W13.9 ☑
    ramp W10.2 ☑
    roof W13.2 ☑
    scaffolding W12 ☑
    scooter (nonmotorized) W05.1 ☑
      motorized mobility W05.2 ☑
    sky lift W17.89 ☑
    stairs, steps W10.9 ☑
      curb W10.1 ☑
      due to ice or snow W00.1 ☑
      escalator W10.0 ☑
      incline W10.2 ☑
      ramp W10.2 ☑
      sidewalk curb W10.1 ☑
      specified NEC W10.8 ☑
      standing
        electric scooter V00.841 ☑
        micro-mobility pedestrian conveyance V00.848 ☑
    stepladder W11 ☑
    stool W08 ☑
    storm drain W17.1 ☑
    streetcar NEC V82.6 ☑
      while boarding or alighting V82.4 ☑
      with antecedent collision — *see* Accident, transport, streetcar occupant
    structure NEC W13.8 ☑
      burning (uncontrolled fire) X00.3 ☑
    table W08 ☑
    toilet W18.11 ☑
      with subsequent striking against object W18.12 ☑
    train NEC V81.6 ☑
      during derailment (without antecedent collision) V81.7 ☑
        with antecedent collision — *see* Accident, transport, railway vehicle occupant
      while boarding or alighting V81.4 ☑
    transport vehicle after collision — *see* Accident, transport, by type of vehicle, collision
    tree W14 ☑
    vehicle (in motion) NEC — *see also* Accident, transport V89.9 ☑
      motor NEC — *see also* Accident, transport, occupant, by type of vehicle V87.8 ☑
      stationary W17.89 ☑
        while boarding or alighting — *see* Accident, transport, by type of vehicle, while boarding or alighting
    viaduct W13.8 ☑
    wall W13.8 ☑
    watercraft — *see also* Drowning, due to, fall overboard
      with hitting bottom or object V94.0 ☑
    well W17.0 ☑
    wheelchair, non-moving W05.0 ☑
      powered — *see* Accident, transport, pedestrian, conveyance occupant, specified type NEC
    window W13.4 ☑
  in, on
    aircraft NEC V97.0 ☑
      while boarding or alighting V97.1 ☑
      with accident to aircraft V97.0 ☑
    bathtub (empty) W18.2 ☑
      filled W16.212 ☑
        causing drowning W16.211 ☑
    escalator W10.0 ☑
    incline W10.2 ☑
    ladder W11 ☑
    machine, machinery — *see* Contact, with, by type of machine
    object, edged, pointed or sharp (with cut) — *see* Fall, by type
    playground equipment W09.8 ☑
      jungle gym W09.2 ☑

Fall, falling — continued
- in, on — continued
  - playground equipment — continued
    - slide W09.0 ☑
    - swing W09.1 ☑
  - ramp W10.2 ☑
  - scaffolding W12 ☑
  - shower W18.2 ☑
    - causing drowning W16.211 ☑
  - staircase, stairs, steps W10.9 ☑
    - curb W10.1 ☑
    - due to ice or snow W00.1 ☑
    - escalator W10.0 ☑
    - incline W10.2 ☑
    - specified NEC W10.8 ☑
  - streetcar (without antecedent collision) V82.5 ☑
    - with antecedent collision — see Accident, transport, streetcar occupant
    - while boarding or alighting V82.4 ☑
  - train (without antecedent collision) V81.5 ☑
    - with antecedent collision — see Accident, transport, railway vehicle occupant
    - during derailment (without antecedent collision) V81.7 ☑
      - with antecedent collision — see Accident, transport, railway vehicle occupant
    - while boarding or alighting V81.4 ☑
  - transport vehicle after collision — see Accident, transport, by type of vehicle, collision
  - watercraft V93.39 ☑
    - due to
      - accident to craft V91.29 ☑
        - powered craft V91.23 ☑
          - ferry boat V91.21 ☑
          - fishing boat V91.22 ☑
          - jetskis V91.23 ☑
          - liner V91.21 ☑
          - merchant ship V91.20 ☑
          - passenger ship V91.21 ☑
        - unpowered craft
          - canoe V91.25 ☑
          - inflatable V91.26 ☑
          - kayak V91.25 ☑
          - sailboat V91.24 ☑
    - powered craft V93.33 ☑
      - ferry boat V93.31 ☑
      - fishing boat V93.32 ☑
      - jetskis V93.33 ☑
      - liner V93.31 ☑
      - merchant ship V93.30 ☑
      - passenger ship V93.31 ☑
    - unpowered craft V93.38 ☑
      - canoe V93.35 ☑
      - inflatable V93.36 ☑
      - kayak V93.35 ☑
      - sailboat V93.34 ☑
      - surf-board V93.38 ☑
      - windsurfer V93.38 ☑
- into
  - cavity W17.2 ☑
  - dock W17.4 ☑
  - fire — see Exposure, fire, by type
  - haystack W17.89 ☑
  - hole W17.2 ☑
  - lake — see Fall, into, water
  - manhole W17.1 ☑
  - moving part of machinery — see Contact, with, by type of machine
  - ocean — see Fall, into, water
  - opening in surface NEC W17.89 ☑
  - pit W17.2 ☑
  - pond — see Fall, into, water
  - quarry W17.89 ☑
  - river — see Fall, into, water
  - shaft W17.89 ☑
  - storm drain W17.1 ☑
  - stream — see Fall, into, water
  - swimming pool — see also Fall, into, water, in, swimming pool
    - empty W17.3 ☑
  - tank W17.89 ☑
  - water W16.42 ☑
    - causing drowning W16.41 ☑
    - from watercraft — see Drowning, due to, fall overboard
    - hitting diving board W21.4 ☑

Fall, falling — continued
- into — continued
  - water — continued
    - in
      - bathtub W16.212 ☑
        - causing drowning W16.211 ☑
      - bucket W16.222 ☑
        - causing drowning W16.221 ☑
      - natural body of water W16.112 ☑
        - causing drowning W16.111 ☑
        - striking
          - bottom W16.122 ☑
            - causing drowning W16.121 ☑
          - side W16.132 ☑
            - causing drowning W16.131 ☑
      - specified water NEC W16.312 ☑
        - causing drowning W16.311 ☑
        - striking
          - bottom W16.322 ☑
            - causing drowning W16.321 ☑
          - wall W16.332 ☑
            - causing drowning W16.331 ☑
      - swimming pool W16.012 ☑
        - causing drowning W16.011 ☑
        - striking
          - bottom W16.022 ☑
            - causing drowning W16.031 ☑
          - wall W16.032 ☑
            - causing drowning W16.021 ☑
      - utility bucket W16.222 ☑
        - causing drowning W16.221 ☑
  - well W17.0 ☑
- involving
  - bed W06 ☑
  - chair W07 ☑
  - furniture NEC W08 ☑
  - glass — see Fall, by type
  - playground equipment W09.8 ☑
    - jungle gym W09.2 ☑
    - slide W09.0 ☑
    - swing W09.1 ☑
  - roller blades — see Accident, transport, pedestrian, conveyance
  - skateboard(s) — see Accident, transport, pedestrian, conveyance
  - skates (ice) (in line) (roller) — see Accident, transport, pedestrian, conveyance
  - skis — see Accident, transport, pedestrian, conveyance
  - table W08 ☑
  - wheelchair, non-moving W05.0 ☑
    - powered — see Accident, transport, pedestrian, conveyance, specified type NEC
- object — see Struck by, object, falling
- off
  - toilet W18.11 ☑
    - with subsequent striking against object W18.12 ☑
  - on same level W18.30 ☑
    - due to
      - specified NEC W18.39 ☑
      - stepping on an object W18.31 ☑
- out of
  - bed W06 ☑
  - building NEC W13.8 ☑
  - chair W07 ☑
  - furniture NEC W08 ☑
  - wheelchair, non-moving W05.0 ☑
    - powered — see Accident, transport, pedestrian, conveyance, specified type NEC
  - window W13.4 ☑
- over
  - animal W01.0 ☑
  - cliff W15 ☑
  - embankment W17.81 ☑
  - small object W01.0 ☑
- rock W20.8 ☑
- same level W18.30 ☑
  - from
    - being crushed, pushed, or stepped on by a crowd or human stampede W52 ☑
    - collision, pushing, shoving, by or with other person W03 ☑
    - slipping, stumbling, tripping W01.0 ☑
  - involving ice or snow W00.0 ☑

Fall, falling — continued
- same level — continued
  - involving ice or snow — continued
    - involving skates (ice) (roller), skateboard, skis — see Accident, transport, pedestrian, conveyance
  - snowslide (avalanche) — see Landslide
  - stone W20.8 ☑
  - structure W20.1 ☑
    - burning (uncontrolled fire) X00.3 ☑
- through
  - bridge W13.1 ☑
  - floor W13.3 ☑
  - roof W13.2 ☑
  - wall W13.8 ☑
  - window W13.4 ☑
  - timber W20.8 ☑
  - tree (caused by lightning) W20.8 ☑
- while being carried or supported by other person(s) W04 ☑

Fallen on by
- animal (not being ridden) NEC W55.89 ☑

Felo-de-se — see Suicide

Fight (hand) (fists) (foot) — see Assault, fight

Fire (accidental) — see Exposure, fire

Firearm discharge — see Discharge, firearm

Fireball effects from nuclear explosion in war operations — see War operations, nuclear weapons

Fireworks (explosion) W39 ☑

Flash burns from explosion — see Explosion

Flood (any injury) (caused by) X38 ☑
- collapse of man-made structure causing earth movement X36.0 ☑
- tidal wave — see Forces of nature, tidal wave

Food (any type) **in**
- air passages (with asphyxia, obstruction, or suffocation) — see categories T17 and T18
- alimentary tract causing asphyxia (due to compression of trachea) — see categories T17 and T18 ☑

Forces of nature X39.8 ☑
- avalanche X36.1 ☑
  - causing transport accident — see Accident, transport, by type of vehicle
- blizzard X37.2 ☑
- cataclysmic storm X37.9 ☑
  - with flood X38 ☑
  - blizzard X37.2 ☑
  - cloudburst X37.8 ☑
  - cyclone X37.1 ☑
  - dust storm X37.3 ☑
  - hurricane X37.0 ☑
  - specified storm NEC X37.8 ☑
  - storm surge X37.0 ☑
  - tornado X37.1 ☑
  - twister X37.1 ☑
  - typhoon X37.0 ☑
- cloudburst X37.8 ☑
- cold (natural) X31 ☑
- cyclone X37.1 ☑
- dam collapse causing earth movement X36.0 ☑
- dust storm X37.3 ☑
- earth movement X36.1 ☑
  - caused by dam or structure collapse X36.0 ☑
  - earthquake X34 ☑
- earthquake X34 ☑
- flood (caused by) X38 ☑
  - dam collapse X36.0 ☑
  - tidal wave — see Forces of nature, tidal wave
- heat (natural) X30 ☑
- hurricane X37.0 ☑
- landslide X36.1 ☑
  - causing transport accident — see Accident, transport, by type of vehicle
- lightning — see subcategory T75.0 ☑
  - causing fire — see Exposure, fire
- mudslide X36.1 ☑
  - causing transport accident — see Accident, transport, by type of vehicle
- radiation (natural) X39.08 ☑
  - radon X39.01 ☑
- radon X39.01 ☑
- specified force NEC X39.8 ☑
- storm surge X37.0 ☑
- structure collapse causing earth movement X36.0 ☑
- sunlight X32 ☑
- tidal wave X37.41 ☑

Forces of nature — *continued*
  tidal wave — *continued*
    due to
      earthquake X37.41 ☑
      landslide X37.43 ☑
      storm X37.42 ☑
      volcanic eruption X37.41 ☑
    tornado X37.1 ☑
    tsunami X37.41 ☑
    twister X37.1 ☑
    typhoon X37.0 ☑
    volcanic eruption X35 ☑
Foreign body
  aspiration — *see* Index to Diseases and Injuries, Foreign
    body, respiratory tract
  embedded in skin W45 ☑
  entering through skin W45.8 ☑
    can lid W26.8 ☑
    nail W45.0 ☑
    paper W26.2 ☑
    specified NEC W45.8 ☑
    splinter W45.8 ☑
Forest fire (exposure to) — *see* Exposure, fire, uncontrolled, not in building
Found injured X58 ☑
  from exposure (to) — *see* Exposure
  on
    highway, road(way), street V89.9 ☑
    railway right of way V81.9 ☑
Fracture (circumstances unknown or unspecified) X58 ☑
  due to specified cause NEC X58 ☑
Freezing — *see* Exposure, cold
Frostbite X31 ☑
  due to man-made conditions — *see* Exposure, cold, man-made
Frozen — *see* Exposure, cold

G

Gored by bull W55.22 ☑
Gunshot wound W34.00 ☑

H

Hailstones, injured by X39.8 ☑
Hanged herself or himself — *see* Hanging, self-inflicted
Hanging (accidental) — *see also* category T71 ☑
  legal execution — *see* Legal, intervention, specified means NEC
Heat (effects of) (excessive) X30 ☑
  due to
    man-made conditions W92 ☑
      on board watercraft V93.29 ☑
        fishing boat V93.22 ☑
        merchant ship V93.20 ☑
        passenger ship V93.21 ☑
        sailboat V93.24 ☑
        specified powered craft NEC V93.23 ☑
    weather (conditions) X30 ☑
  from
    electric heating apparatus causing burning X16 ☑
    nuclear explosion in war operations — *see* War operations, nuclear weapons
  inappropriate in local application or packing in medical or surgical procedure Y63.5
Hemorrhage
  delayed following medical or surgical treatment without mention of misadventure — *see* Index to Diseases and Injuries, Complication(s)
  during medical or surgical treatment as misadventure — *see* Index to Diseases and Injuries, Complication(s)
High
  altitude (effects) — *see* Air, pressure, low
  level of radioactivity, effects — *see* Radiation
  pressure (effects) — *see* Air, pressure, high
  temperature, effects — *see* Heat
Hit, hitting (accidental) by — *see* Struck by
Hitting against — *see* Striking against
Homicide (attempt) (justifiable) — *see* Assault
Hot
  place, effects — *see also* Heat
  weather, effects X30 ☑
House fire (uncontrolled) — *see* Exposure, fire, uncontrolled, building
Humidity, causing problem X39.8 ☑

Hunger X58 ☑
Hurricane (any injury) X37.0 ☑
Hypobarism, hypobaropathy — *see* Air, pressure, low

I

Ictus
  caloris — *see also* Heat
  solaris X30 ☑
Ignition (accidental) — *see also* Exposure, fire X08.8 ☑
  anesthetic gas in operating room W40.1 ☑
  apparel X06.2 ☑
    from highly flammable material X04 ☑
    nightwear X05 ☑
  bed linen (sheets) (spreads) (pillows) (mattress) — *see* Exposure, fire, uncontrolled, building, bed
  benzine X04 ☑
  clothes, clothing NEC (from controlled fire) X06.2 ☑
    from
      highly flammable material X04 ☑
  ether X04 ☑
    in operating room W40.1 ☑
  explosive material — *see* Explosion
  gasoline X04 ☑
  jewelry (plastic) (any) X06.0 ☑
  kerosene X04 ☑
  material
    explosive — *see* Explosion
    highly flammable with secondary explosion X04 ☑
  nightwear X05 ☑
  paraffin X04 ☑
  petrol X04 ☑
Immersion (accidental) — *see also* Drowning
  hand or foot due to cold (excessive) X31 ☑
Implantation of quills of porcupine W55.89 ☑
Inanition (from) (hunger) X58 ☑
  thirst X58 ☑
Inappropriate operation performed
  correct operation on wrong side or body part (wrong side) (wrong site) Y65.53
  operation intended for another patient done on wrong patient Y65.52
  wrong operation performed on correct patient Y65.51
Inattention after, at birth (homicidal intent) (infanticidal intent) X58 ☑
Incident, adverse
  device
    anesthesiology Y70.8
      accessory Y70.2
      diagnostic Y70.0
      miscellaneous Y70.8
      monitoring Y70.0
      prosthetic Y70.2
      rehabilitative Y70.1
      surgical Y70.3
      therapeutic Y70.1
    cardiovascular Y71.8
      accessory Y71.2
      diagnostic Y71.0
      miscellaneous Y71.8
      monitoring Y71.0
      prosthetic Y71.2
      rehabilitative Y71.1
      surgical Y71.3
      therapeutic Y71.1
    gastroenterology Y73.8
      accessory Y73.2
      diagnostic Y73.0
      miscellaneous Y73.8
      monitoring Y73.0
      prosthetic Y73.2
      rehabilitative Y73.1
      surgical Y73.3
      therapeutic Y73.1
    general
      hospital Y74.8
        accessory Y74.2
        diagnostic Y74.0
        miscellaneous Y74.8
        monitoring Y74.0
        prosthetic Y74.2
        rehabilitative Y74.1
        surgical Y74.3
        therapeutic Y74.1
      surgical Y81.8
        accessory Y81.2
        diagnostic Y81.0

Incident, adverse — *continued*
  device — *continued*
    general — *continued*
      surgical — *continued*
        miscellaneous Y81.8
        monitoring Y81.0
        prosthetic Y81.2
        rehabilitative Y81.1
        surgical Y81.3
        therapeutic Y81.1
    gynecological Y76.8
      accessory Y76.2
      diagnostic Y76.0
      miscellaneous Y76.8
      monitoring Y76.0
      prosthetic Y76.2
      rehabilitative Y76.1
      surgical Y76.3
      therapeutic Y76.1
    medical Y82.9
      specified type NEC Y82.8
    neurological Y75.8
      accessory Y75.2
      diagnostic Y75.0
      miscellaneous Y75.8
      monitoring Y75.0
      prosthetic Y75.2
      rehabilitative Y75.1
      surgical Y75.3
      therapeutic Y75.1
    obstetrical Y76.8
      accessory Y76.2
      diagnostic Y76.0
      miscellaneous Y76.8
      monitoring Y76.0
      prosthetic Y76.2
      rehabilitative Y76.1
      surgical Y76.3
      therapeutic Y76.1
    ophthalmic Y77.8
      accessory Y77.2
      contact lens (rigid gas permeable) (soft (hydrophilic)) Y77.11
      diagnostic Y77.0
      miscellaneous Y77.8
      monitoring Y77.0
      prosthetic Y77.2
      rehabilitative Y77.19
      surgical Y77.3
      therapeutic Y77.19
    orthopedic Y79.8
      accessory Y79.2
      diagnostic Y79.0
      miscellaneous Y79.8
      monitoring Y79.0
      prosthetic Y79.2
      rehabilitative Y79.1
      surgical Y79.3
      therapeutic Y79.1
    otorhinolaryngological Y72.8
      accessory Y72.2
      diagnostic Y72.0
      miscellaneous Y72.8
      monitoring Y72.0
      prosthetic Y72.2
      rehabilitative Y72.1
      surgical Y72.3
      therapeutic Y72.1
    personal use Y74.8
      accessory Y74.2
      diagnostic Y74.0
      miscellaneous Y74.8
      monitoring Y74.0
      prosthetic Y74.2
      rehabilitative Y74.1
      surgical Y74.3
      therapeutic Y74.1
    physical medicine Y80.8
      accessory Y80.2
      diagnostic Y80.0
      miscellaneous Y80.8
      monitoring Y80.0
      prosthetic Y80.2
      rehabilitative Y80.1
      surgical Y80.3
      therapeutic Y80.1
    plastic surgical Y81.8
      accessory Y81.2
      diagnostic Y81.0

Incident, adverse — *continued*
  device — *continued*
    plastic surgical — *continued*
      miscellaneous Y81.8
      monitoring Y81.0
      prosthetic Y81.2
      rehabilitative Y81.1
      surgical Y81.3
      therapeutic Y81.1
    radiological Y78.8
      accessory Y78.2
      diagnostic Y78.0
      miscellaneous Y78.8
      monitoring Y78.0
      prosthetic Y78.2
      rehabilitative Y78.1
      surgical Y78.3
      therapeutic Y78.1
    urology Y73.8
      accessory Y73.2
      diagnostic Y73.0
      miscellaneous Y73.8
      monitoring Y73.0
      prosthetic Y73.2
      rehabilitative Y73.1
      surgical Y73.3
      therapeutic Y73.1
Incineration (accidental) — *see* Exposure, fire
Infanticide — *see* Assault
Infrasound waves (causing injury) W49.9 ☑
Ingestion
  foreign body (causing injury) (with obstruction) — *see* Foreign body, alimentary canal
  poisonous
    plant(s) X58 ☑
    substance NEC — *see* Table of Drugs and Chemicals
Inhalation
  excessively cold substance, man-made — *see* Exposure, cold, man-made
  food (any type) (into respiratory tract) (with asphyxia, obstruction respiratory tract, suffocation) — *see* categories T17 and T18 ☑
  foreign body — *see* Foreign body, aspiration
  gastric contents (with asphyxia, obstruction respiratory passage, suffocation) T17.81- ☑
  hot air or gases X14.0 ☑
  liquid air, hydrogen, nitrogen W93.12 ☑
    suicide (attempt) X83.2 ☑
  steam X13.0 ☑
    assault X98.0 ☑
    stated as undetermined whether accidental or intentional Y27.0 ☑
    suicide (attempt) X77.0 ☑
  toxic gas — *see* Table of Drugs and Chemicals
  vomitus (with asphyxia, obstruction respiratory passage, suffocation) T17.81- ☑
Injury, injured (accidental(ly)) NOS X58 ☑
  by, caused by, from
    assault — *see* Assault
    law-enforcing agent, police, in course of legal intervention — *see* Legal intervention
    suicide (attempt) X83.8 ☑
  due to, in
    civil insurrection — *see* War operations
    fight — *see also* Assault, fight Y04.0 ☑
    war operations — *see* War operations
  homicide — *see also* Assault Y09
  inflicted (by)
    in course of arrest (attempted), suppression of disturbance, maintenance of order, by law-enforcing agents — *see* Legal intervention
    other person
      stated as
        accidental X58 ☑
        intentional, homicide (attempt) — *see* Assault
        undetermined whether accidental or intentional Y33 ☑
  purposely (inflicted) by other person(s) — *see* Assault
  self-inflicted X83.8 ☑
    stated as accidental X58 ☑
  specified cause NEC X58 ☑
  undetermined whether accidental or intentional Y33 ☑
Insolation, effects X30 ☑
Insufficient nourishment X58 ☑
Interruption of respiration (by)
  food (lodged in esophagus) — *see* categories T17 and T18 ☑

Interruption of respiration — *continued*
  vomitus (lodged in esophagus) T17.81- ☑
Intervention, legal — *see* Legal intervention
Intoxication
  drug — *see* Table of Drugs and Chemicals
  poison — *see* Table of Drugs and Chemicals

J

Jammed (accidentally)
  between objects (moving) (stationary and moving) W23.0 ☑
  stationary W23.1 ☑
Jumped, jumping
  before moving object NEC X81.8 ☑
    motor vehicle X81.0 ☑
    subway train X81.1 ☑
    train X81.1 ☑
    undetermined whether accidental or intentional Y31 ☑
  from
    boat (into water) voluntarily, without accident (to or on boat) W16.712 ☑
      striking bottom W16.722 ☑
        causing drowning W16.721 ☑
      with
        accident to or on boat — *see* Accident, watercraft
        drowning or submersion W16.711 ☑
          suicide (attempt) X71.3 ☑
    building — *see also* Jumped, from, high place W13.9 ☑
      burning (uncontrolled fire) X00.5 ☑
    high place NEC W17.89 ☑
      suicide (attempt) X80 ☑
      undetermined whether accidental or intentional Y30 ☑
    structure — *see also* Jumped, from, high place W13.9 ☑
      burning (uncontrolled fire) X00.5 ☑
  into water W16.92 ☑
    causing drowning W16.91 ☑
    from, off watercraft — *see* Jumped, from, boat
    in
      natural body W16.612 ☑
        causing drowning W16.611 ☑
        striking bottom W16.622 ☑
          causing drowning W16.621 ☑
      specified place NEC W16.812 ☑
        causing drowning W16.811 ☑
        striking
          bottom W16.822 ☑
            causing drowning W16.821 ☑
          wall W16.832 ☑
            causing drowning W16.831 ☑
      swimming pool W16.512 ☑
        causing drowning W16.511 ☑
        striking
          bottom W16.522 ☑
            causing drowning W16.521 ☑
          wall W16.532 ☑
            causing drowning W16.531 ☑
    suicide (attempt) X71.3 ☑

K

Kicked by
  animal NEC W55.82 ☑
  person(s) (accidentally) W50.1 ☑
    with intent to injure or kill Y04.0 ☑
    as, or caused by, a crowd or human stampede (with fall) W52 ☑
    assault Y04.0 ☑
    homicide (attempt) Y04.0 ☑
    in
      fight Y04.0 ☑
      legal intervention
        injuring
          bystander Y35.812 ☑
          law enforcement personnel Y35.811 ☑
          suspect Y35.813 ☑
          unspecified person Y35.819 ☑
Kicking
  against
    object W22.8 ☑
      sports equipment W21.9 ☑

Kicking — *continued*
  against — *continued*
    object — *continued*
      stationary W22.09 ☑
        sports equipment W21.89 ☑
      person — *see* Striking against, person
      sports equipment W21.9 ☑
  carpet stretcher with knee X50.3 ☑
Killed, killing (accidentally) NOS — *see also* Injury X58 ☑
  in
    action — *see* War operations
    brawl, fight (hand) (fists) (foot) Y04.0 ☑
      by weapon — *see also* Assault
        cutting, piercing — *see* Assault, cutting or piercing instrument
        firearm — *see* Discharge, firearm, by type, homicide
  self
    stated as
      accident NOS X58 ☑
      suicide — *see* Suicide
      undetermined whether accidental or intentional Y33 ☑
Kneeling (prolonged (static)) X50.1 ☑
Knocked down (accidentally) (by) NOS X58 ☑
  animal (not being ridden) NEC — *see also* Struck by, by type of animal
  crowd or human stampede W52 ☑
  person W51 ☑
    in brawl, fight Y04.0 ☑
  transport vehicle NEC — *see also* Accident, transport V09.9 ☑

L

Laceration NEC — *see* Injury
Lack of
  care (helpless person) (infant) (newborn) X58 ☑
  food except as result of abandonment or neglect X58 ☑
    due to abandonment or neglect X58 ☑
  water except as result of transport accident X58 ☑
    due to transport accident — *see* Accident, transport, by type
  helpless person, infant, newborn X58 ☑
Landslide (falling on transport vehicle) X36.1 ☑
  caused by collapse of man-made structure X36.0 ☑
Late effect — *see* Sequelae
Legal
  execution (any method) — *see* Legal, intervention
  intervention (by)
    baton — *see* Legal, intervention, blunt object, baton
    bayonet — *see* Legal, intervention, sharp object, bayonet
    blow — *see* Legal, intervention, manhandling
    blunt object
      baton
        injuring
          bystander Y35.312 ☑
          law enforcement personnel Y35.311 ☑
          suspect Y35.313 ☑
          unspecified person Y35.319 ☑
        injuring
          bystander Y35.302 ☑
          law enforcement personnel Y35.301 ☑
          suspect Y35.303 ☑
          unspecified person Y35.309 ☑
      specified NEC
        injuring
          bystander Y35.392 ☑
          law enforcement personnel Y35.391 ☑
          suspect Y35.393 ☑
          unspecified person Y35.399 ☑
      stave
        injuring
          bystander Y35.392 ☑
          law enforcement personnel Y35.391 ☑
          suspect Y35.393 ☑
          unspecified person Y35.399 ☑
    bomb — *see* Legal, intervention, explosive
    conducted energy device
      injuring
        bystander Y35.832 ☑
        law enforcement personnel Y35.831 ☑
        suspect Y35.833 ☑
        unspecified person Y35.839 ☑

Legal — *continued*
    intervention — *continued*
        cutting or piercing instrument — *see* Legal, inter-
            vention, sharp object
        dynamite — *see* Legal, intervention, explosive, dy-
            namite
        electroshock device (taser)
            injuring
                bystander Y35.832 ☑
                law enforcement personnel Y35.831 ☑
                suspect Y35.833 ☑
                unspecified person Y35.839 ☑
        explosive(s)
            dynamite
                injuring
                    bystander Y35.112 ☑
                    law enforcement personnel Y35.111 ☑
                    suspect Y35.113 ☑
                    unspecified person Y35.119 ☑
            grenade
                injuring
                    bystander Y35.192 ☑
                    law enforcement personnel Y35.191 ☑
                    suspect Y35.193 ☑
                    unspecified person Y35.199 ☑
            injuring
                bystander Y35.102 ☑
                law enforcement personnel Y35.101 ☑
                suspect Y35.103 ☑
                unspecified person Y35.109 ☑
            mortar bomb
                injuring
                    bystander Y35.192 ☑
                    law enforcement personnel Y35.191 ☑
                    suspect Y35.193 ☑
                    unspecified person Y35.199 ☑
            shell
                injuring
                    bystander Y35.122 ☑
                    law enforcement personnel Y35.121 ☑
                    suspect Y35.123 ☑
                    unspecified person Y35.129 ☑
            specified NEC
                injuring
                    bystander Y35.192 ☑
                    law enforcement personnel Y35.191 ☑
                    suspect Y35.193 ☑
                    unspecified person Y35.199 ☑
        firearm(s) (discharge)
            handgun
                injuring
                    bystander Y35.022 ☑
                    law enforcement personnel Y35.021 ☑
                    suspect Y35.023 ☑
                    unspecified person Y35.029 ☑
            injuring
                bystander Y35.002 ☑
                law enforcement personnel Y35.001 ☑
                suspect Y35.003 ☑
                unspecified person Y35.009 ☑
            machine gun
                injuring
                    bystander Y35.012 ☑
                    law enforcement personnel Y35.011 ☑
                    suspect Y35.013 ☑
                    unspecified person Y35.019 ☑
            rifle pellet
                injuring
                    bystander Y35.032 ☑
                    law enforcement personnel Y35.031 ☑
                    suspect Y35.033 ☑
                    unspecified person Y35.039 ☑
            rubber bullet
                injuring
                    bystander Y35.042 ☑
                    law enforcement personnel Y35.041 ☑
                    suspect Y35.043 ☑
                    unspecified person Y35.049 ☑
            shotgun — *see* Legal, intervention, firearm,
                specified NEC
            specified NEC
                injuring
                    bystander Y35.092 ☑
                    law enforcement personnel Y35.091 ☑
                    suspect Y35.093 ☑
                    unspecified person Y35.099 ☑

Legal — *continued*
    intervention — *continued*
        gas (asphyxiation) (poisoning)
            injuring
                 bystander Y35.202 ☑
                law enforcement personnel Y35.201 ☑
                suspect Y35.203 ☑
                unspecified person Y35.209 ☑
            specified NEC
                injuring
                    bystander Y35.292 ☑
                    law enforcement personnel Y35.291 ☑
                    suspect Y35.293 ☑
                    unspecified person Y35.299 ☑
            tear gas
                injuring
                    bystander Y35.212 ☑
                    law enforcement personnel Y35.211 ☑
                    suspect Y35.213 ☑
                    unspecified person Y35.219 ☑
        grenade — *see* Legal, intervention, explosive,
            grenade
        injuring
            bystander Y35.92 ☑
            law enforcement personnel Y35.91 ☑
            suspect Y35.93 ☑
            unspecified person Y35.99 ☑
        late effect (of) — *see* with 7th character S Y35 ☑
        manhandling
            injuring
                 bystander Y35.812 ☑
                law enforcement personnel Y35.811 ☑
                suspect Y35.813 ☑
                unspecified person Y35.819 ☑
        sequelae (of) — *see* with 7th character S Y35 ☑
        sharp objects
            bayonet
                injuring
                    bystander Y35.412 ☑
                    law enforcement personnel Y35.411 ☑
                    suspect Y35.413 ☑
                    unspecified person Y35.419 ☑
            injuring
                bystander Y35.402 ☑
                law enforcement personnel Y35.401 ☑
                suspect Y35.403 ☑
                unspecified person Y35.409 ☑
            specified NEC
                injuring
                    bystander Y35.492 ☑
                    law enforcement personnel Y35.491 ☑
                    suspect Y35.493 ☑
                    unspecified person Y35.499 ☑
        specified means NEC
            injuring
                bystander Y35.892 ☑
                law enforcement personnel Y35.891 ☑
                suspect Y35.893 ☑
                unspecified person Y35.899 ☑
        stabbing — *see* Legal, intervention, sharp object
        stave — *see* Legal, intervention, blunt object, stave
        stun gun
            injuring
                bystander Y35.832 ☑
                law enforcement personnel Y35.831 ☑
                suspect Y35.833 ☑
                unspecified person Y35.839 ☑
        taser
            injuring
                bystander Y35.832 ☑
                law enforcement personnel Y35.831 ☑
                suspect Y35.833 ☑
                unspecified person Y35.839 ☑
        tear gas — *see* Legal, intervention, gas, tear gas
        truncheon — *see* Legal, intervention, blunt object,
            stave
Lifting — *see also* Overexertion
    heavy objects X50.0 ☑
    weights X50.0 ☑
Lightning (shock) (stroke) (struck by) — *see* subcategory
    T75.0 ☑
    causing fire — *see* Exposure, fire
Loss of control (transport vehicle) NEC — *see* Accident,
    transport
Lost at sea NOS — *see* Drowning, due to, fall overboard

Low
    pressure (effects) — *see* Air, pressure, low
    temperature (effects) — *see* Exposure, cold
Lying before train, vehicle or other moving object
    X81.8 ☑
    subway train X81.1 ☑
    train X81.1 ☑
    undetermined whether accidental or intentional Y31 ☑
Lynching — *see* Assault

M

Malfunction (mechanism or component) (of)
    firearm W34.10 ☑
        airgun W34.110 ☑
        BB gun W34.110 ☑
        gas, air or spring-operated gun NEC W34.118 ☑
        handgun W32.1 ☑
        hunting rifle W33.12 ☑
        larger firearm W33.10 ☑
            specified NEC W33.19 ☑
        machine gun W33.13 ☑
        paintball gun W34.111 ☑
        pellet gun W34.110 ☑
        shotgun W33.11 ☑
        specified NEC W34.19 ☑
        Very pistol [flare] W34.19 ☑
    handgun — *see* Malfunction, firearm, handgun
Maltreatment — *see* Perpetrator
Mangled (accidentally) NOS X58 ☑
Manhandling (in brawl, fight) Y04.0 ☑
    legal intervention — *see* Legal, intervention, manhan-
        dling
Manslaughter (nonaccidental) — *see* Assault
Mauled by animal NEC W55.89 ☑
Medical procedure, complication of (delayed or as an
    abnormal reaction without mention of misadven-
    ture) — *see* Complication of or following, by speci-
    fied type of procedure
    due to or as a result of misadventure — *see* Misadven-
        ture
Melting (due to fire) — *see also* Exposure, fire
    apparel NEC X06.3 ☑
    clothes, clothing NEC X06.3 ☑
        nightwear X05 ☑
    fittings or furniture (burning building) (uncontrolled
        fire) X00.8 ☑
    nightwear X05 ☑
    plastic jewelry X06.1 ☑
Mental cruelty X58 ☑
Military operations (injuries to military and civilians
    occuring during peacetime on military property and
    during routine military exercises and operations)
    (by) (from) (involving) Y37.90- ☑
    air blast Y37.20- ☑
    aircraft
        destruction — *see* Military operations, destruction
            of aircraft
        airway restriction — *see* Military operations, restriction
            of airways
        asphyxiation — *see* Military operations, restriction of
            airways
    biological weapons Y37.6X- ☑
    blast Y37.20- ☑
    blast fragments Y37.20- ☑
    blast wave Y37.20- ☑
    blast wind Y37.20- ☑
    bomb Y37.20- ☑
        dirty Y37.50- ☑
        gasoline Y37.31- ☑
        incendiary Y37.31- ☑
        petrol Y37.31- ☑
    bullet Y37.43- ☑
        incendiary Y37.32- ☑
        rubber Y37.41- ☑
    chemical weapons Y37.7X- ☑
    combat
        hand to hand (unarmed) combat Y37.44- ☑
        using blunt or piercing object Y37.45- ☑
    conflagration — *see* Military operations, fire
    conventional warfare NEC Y37.49- ☑
    depth-charge Y37.01- ☑
    destruction of aircraft Y37.10- ☑
        due to
            air to air missile Y37.11- ☑
            collision with other aircraft Y37.12- ☑

Military operations — *continued*
  destruction of aircraft — *continued*
    due to — *continued*
      detonation (accidental) of onboard munitions
        and explosives Y37.14- ☑
      enemy fire or explosives Y37.11- ☑
      explosive placed on aircraft Y37.11- ☑
      onboard fire Y37.13- ☑
      rocket propelled grenade [RPG] Y37.11- ☑
      small arms fire Y37.11- ☑
      surface to air missile Y37.11- ☑
    specified NEC Y37.19- ☑
  detonation (accidental) of
    onboard marine weapons Y37.05- ☑
    own munitions or munitions launch device
      Y37.24- ☑
  dirty bomb Y37.50- ☑
  explosion (of) Y37.20- ☑
    aerial bomb Y37.21- ☑
    bomb NOS — *see also* Military operations, bomb(s)
      Y37.20- ☑
    fragments Y37.20- ☑
    grenade Y37.29- ☑
    guided missile Y37.22- ☑
    improvised explosive device [IED] (person-borne)
      (roadside) (vehicle-borne) Y37.23- ☑
    land mine Y37.29- ☑
    marine mine (at sea) (in harbor) Y37.02- ☑
    marine weapon Y37.00- ☑
      specified NEC Y37.09- ☑
    own munitions or munitions launch device (acciden-
      tal) Y37.24- ☑
    sea-based artillery shell Y37.03- ☑
    specified NEC Y37.29- ☑
    torpedo Y37.04- ☑
  fire Y37.30- ☑
    specified NEC Y37.39- ☑
  firearms
    discharge Y37.43- ☑
    pellets Y37.42- ☑
  flamethrower Y37.33- ☑
  fragments (from) (of)
    improvised explosive device [IED] (person-borne)
      (roadside) (vehicle-borne) Y37.26- ☑
    munitions Y37.25- ☑
    specified NEC Y37.29- ☑
    weapons Y37.27- ☑
  friendly fire Y37.92- ☑
  hand to hand (unarmed) combat Y37.44- ☑
  hot substances — *see* Military operations, fire
  incendiary bullet Y37.32- ☑
  nuclear weapon (effects of) Y37.50- ☑
    acute radiation exposure Y37.54- ☑
    blast pressure Y37.51- ☑
    direct blast Y37.51- ☑
    direct heat Y37.53- ☑
    fallout exposure Y37.54- ☑
    fireball Y37.53- ☑
    indirect blast (struck or crushed by blast debris)
      (being thrown by blast) Y37.52- ☑
    ionizing radiation (immediate exposure) Y37.54- ☑
    nuclear radiation Y37.54- ☑
    radiation
      ionizing (immediate exposure) Y37.54- ☑
      nuclear Y37.54- ☑
      thermal Y37.53- ☑
    secondary effects Y37.54- ☑
    specified NEC Y37.59- ☑
    thermal radiation Y37.53- ☑
  restriction of air (airway)
    intentional Y37.46- ☑
    unintentional Y37.47- ☑
  rubber bullets Y37.41- ☑
  shrapnel NOS Y37.29- ☑
  suffocation — *see* Military operations, restriction of
    airways
  unconventional warfare NEC Y37.7X- ☑
  underwater blast NOS Y37.00- ☑
  warfare
    conventional NEC Y37.49- ☑
    unconventional NEC Y37.7X- ☑
  weapon of mass destruction [WMD] Y37.91- ☑
  weapons
    biological weapons Y37.6X- ☑
    chemical Y37.7X- ☑
    nuclear (effects of) Y37.50- ☑

Military operations — *continued*
  weapons — *continued*
    nuclear — *continued*
      acute radiation exposure Y37.54- ☑
      blast pressure Y37.51- ☑
      direct blast Y37.51- ☑
      direct heat Y37.53- ☑
      fallout exposure Y37.54- ☑
      fireball Y37.53- ☑
      radiation
        ionizing (immediate exposure) Y37.54- ☑
        nuclear Y37.54- ☑
        thermal Y37.53- ☑
      secondary effects Y37.54- ☑
      specified NEC Y37.59- ☑
    of mass destruction [WMD] Y37.91- ☑
Misadventure(s) **to patient**(s) **during surgical or
medical care** Y69
  contaminated medical or biological substance (blood,
    drug, fluid) Y64.9
    administered (by) NEC Y64.9
      immunization Y64.1
      infusion Y64.0
      injection Y64.1
      specified means NEC Y64.8
      transfusion Y64.0
      vaccination Y64.1
  excessive amount of blood or other fluid during trans-
    fusion or infusion Y63.0
  failure
    in dosage Y63.9
      electroshock therapy Y63.4
      inappropriate temperature (too hot or too cold)
        in local application and packing Y63.5
      infusion
        excessive amount of fluid Y63.0
        incorrect dilution of fluid Y63.1
      insulin-shock therapy Y63.4
      nonadministration of necessary drug or biologi-
        cal substance Y63.6
      overdose — *see* Table of Drugs and Chemicals
        radiation, in therapy Y63.2
      radiation
        overdose Y63.2
      specified procedure NEC Y63.8
      transfusion
        excessive amount of blood Y63.0
    mechanical, of instrument or apparatus (any) (during
      any procedure) Y65.8
    sterile precautions (during procedure) Y62.9
      aspiration of fluid or tissue (by puncture or
        catheterization, except heart) Y62.6
      biopsy (except needle aspiration) Y62.8
        needle (aspirating) Y62.6
      blood sampling Y62.6
      catheterization Y62.6
        heart Y62.5
      dialysis (kidney) Y62.2
      endoscopic examination Y62.4
      enema Y62.8
      immunization Y62.3
      infusion Y62.1
      injection Y62.3
      needle biopsy Y62.6
      paracentesis (abdominal) (thoracic) Y62.6
      perfusion Y62.2
      puncture (lumbar) Y62.6
      removal of catheter or packing Y62.8
      specified procedure NEC Y62.8
      surgical operation Y62.0
      transfusion Y62.1
      vaccination Y62.3
    suture or ligature during surgical procedure Y65.2
    to introduce or to remove tube or instrument —
      see Failure, to
  hemorrhage — *see* Index to Diseases and Injuries,
    Complication(s)
  inadvertent exposure of patient to radiation Y63.3
  inappropriate
    operation performed — *see* Inappropriate operation
      performed
    temperature (too hot or too cold) in local application
      or packing Y63.5
  infusion — *see also* Misadventure, by type, infusion
    Y69
    excessive amount of fluid Y63.0
    incorrect dilution of fluid Y63.1
    wrong fluid Y65.1

Misadventure(s) **to patient**(s) **during surgical or
medical care** — *continued*
  mismatched blood in transfusion Y65.0
  nonadministration of necessary drug or biological
    substance Y63.6
  overdose — *see* Table of Drugs and Chemicals
    radiation (in therapy) Y63.2
  perforation — *see* Index to Diseases and Injuries,
    Complication(s)
  performance of inappropriate operation — *see* Inap-
    propriate operation performed
  puncture — *see* Index to Diseases and Injuries, Compli-
    cation(s)
  specified type NEC Y65.8
    failure
      suture or ligature during surgical operation Y65.2
      to introduce or to remove tube or instrument —
        see Failure, to
    infusion of wrong fluid Y65.1
    performance of inappropriate operation — *see* In-
      appropriate operation performed
    transfusion of mismatched blood Y65.0
    wrong
      fluid in infusion Y65.1
      placement of endotracheal tube during anesthet-
        ic procedure Y65.3
  transfusion — *see* Misadventure, by type, transfusion
    excessive amount of blood Y63.0
    mismatched blood Y65.0
  wrong
    drug given in error — *see* Table of Drugs and
      Chemicals
    fluid in infusion Y65.1
    placement of endotracheal tube during anesthetic
      procedure Y65.3
Mismatched blood in transfusion Y65.0
Motion sickness T75.3 ☑
Mountain sickness W94.11 ☑
Mudslide (of cataclysmic nature) — *see* Landslide
Murder (attempt) — *see* Assault

N

Nail
  contact with W45.0 ☑
    gun W29.4 ☑
  embedded in skin W45.0 ☑
Neglect (criminal) (homicidal intent) X58 ☑
Noise (causing injury) (pollution) W42.9 ☑
  supersonic W42.0 ☑
Nonadministration (of)
  drug or biological substance (necessary) Y63.6
  surgical and medical care Y66
Nosocomial condition Y95

O

Object
  falling
    from, in, on, hitting
      machinery — *see* Contact, with, by type of ma-
        chine
  set in motion by
    accidental explosion or rupture of pressure vessel
      W38 ☑
    firearm — *see* Discharge, firearm, by type
    machine(ry) — *see* Contact, with, by type of ma-
      chine
Overdose (drug) — *see* Table of Drugs and Chemicals
  radiation Y63.2
Overexertion X50.9 ☑
  from
    prolonged static or awkward postures X50.1 ☑
    repetitive movements X50.3 ☑
    specified strenuous movements or postures NEC
      X50.9 ☑
    strenuous movement or load X50.0 ☑
Overexposure (accidental) (to)
  cold — *see also* Exposure, cold X31 ☑
    due to man-made conditions — *see* Exposure, cold,
      man-made
  heat — *see also* Heat X30 ☑
  radiation — *see* Radiation
  radioactivity W88.0 ☑
  sun (sunburn) X32 ☑
  weather NEC — *see* Forces of nature
  wind NEC — *see* Forces of nature

Overheated — see Heat
Overturning (accidental)
  machinery — see Contact, with, by type of machine
  transport vehicle NEC — see also Accident, transport
    V89.9 ☑
  watercraft (causing drowning, submersion) — see also
    Drowning, due to, accident to, watercraft, over-
    turning
    causing injury except drowning or submersion —
      see Accident, watercraft, causing, injury NEC

P

Parachute descent (voluntary) (without accident to aircraft) V97.29 ☑
  due to accident to aircraft — see Accident, transport,
    aircraft
Pecked by bird W61.99 ☑
**Perforation during medical or surgical treatment as
  misadventure** — see Index to Diseases and Injuries, Complication(s)
**Perpetrator, perpetration, of assault, maltreatment
  and neglect** (by) Y07.9
boyfriend Y07.03
brother Y07.410
  stepbrother Y07.435
coach Y07.53
cousin
  female Y07.491
  male Y07.490
daycare provider Y07.519
  at-home
    adult care Y07.512
    childcare Y07.510
  care center
    adult care Y07.513
    childcare Y07.511
family member NEC Y07.499
father Y07.11
  adoptive Y07.13
  foster Y07.420
  stepfather Y07.430
foster father Y07.420
foster mother Y07.421
girl friend Y07.04
healthcare provider Y07.529
  mental health Y07.521
  specified NEC Y07.528
husband Y07.01
instructor Y07.53
mother Y07.12
  adoptive Y07.14
  foster Y07.421
  stepmother Y07.433
multiple perpetrators Y07.6
nonfamily member Y07.50
  specified NEC Y07.59
nurse Y07.528
occupational therapist Y07.528
partner of parent
  female Y07.434
  male Y07.432
physical therapist Y07.528
sister Y07.411
speech therapist Y07.528
stepbrother Y07.435
stepfather Y07.430
stepmother Y07.433
stepsister Y07.436
teacher Y07.53
wife Y07.02
Piercing — see Contact, with, by type of object or machine
Pinched
  between objects (moving) (stationary and moving)
    W23.0 ☑
    stationary W23.1 ☑
Pinned under machine(ry) — see Contact, with, by type
  of machine
Place of occurrence Y92.9
abandoned house Y92.89
airplane Y92.813
airport Y92.520
ambulatory health services establishment NEC Y92.538
ambulatory surgery center Y92.530
amusement park Y92.831
apartment (co-op) — see Place of occurrence, residence, apartment

Place of occurrence — continued
assembly hall Y92.29
bank Y92.510
barn Y92.71
baseball field Y92.320
basketball court Y92.310
beach Y92.832
boarding house — see Place of occurrence, residence,
  boarding house
boat Y92.814
bowling alley Y92.39
bridge Y92.89
building under construction Y92.61
bus Y92.811
  station Y92.521
cafe Y92.511
campsite Y92.833
campus — see Place of occurrence, school
canal Y92.89
car Y92.810
casino Y92.59
children's home — see Place of occurrence, residence,
  institutional, orphanage
church Y92.22
cinema Y92.26
clubhouse Y92.29
coal pit Y92.64
college (community) Y92.214
condominium — see Place of occurrence, residence,
  apartment
construction area — see Place of occurrence, industrial
  and construction area
convalescent home — see Place of occurrence, residence, institutional, nursing home
court-house Y92.240
cricket ground Y92.328
cultural building Y92.258
  art gallery Y92.250
  museum Y92.251
  music hall Y92.252
  opera house Y92.253
  specified NEC Y92.258
  theater Y92.254
dancehall Y92.252
day nursery Y92.210
dentist office Y92.531
derelict house Y92.89
desert Y92.820
dockyard Y92.62
dock NOS Y92.89
doctor's office Y92.531
dormitory — see Place of occurrence, residence, institutional, school dormitory
dry dock Y92.62
factory (building) (premises) Y92.63
farm (land under cultivation) (outbuildings) Y92.79
  barn Y92.71
  chicken coop Y92.72
  field Y92.73
  hen house Y92.72
  house — see Place of occurrence, residence, house
  orchard Y92.74
  specified NEC Y92.79
football field Y92.321
forest Y92.821
freeway Y92.411
gallery Y92.250
garage (commercial) Y92.59
  boarding house Y92.044
  military base Y92.135
  mobile home Y92.025
  nursing home Y92.124
  orphanage Y92.114
  private house Y92.015
  reform school Y92.155
gas station Y92.524
gasworks Y92.69
golf course Y92.39
gravel pit Y92.64
grocery Y92.512
gymnasium Y92.39
handball court Y92.318
harbor Y92.89
harness racing course Y92.39
healthcare provider office Y92.531
highway Y92.410
  interstate Y92.411
hill Y92.828

Place of occurrence — continued
hockey rink Y92.330
home — see Place of occurrence, residence
hospice — see Place of occurrence, residence, institutional, nursing home
hospital Y92.239
  cafeteria Y92.233
  corridor Y92.232
  operating room Y92.234
  patient
    bathroom Y92.231
    room Y92.230
  specified NEC Y92.238
hotel Y92.59
house — see also Place of occurrence, residence
  abandoned Y92.89
  under construction Y92.61
industrial and construction area (yard) Y92.69
  building under construction Y92.61
  dock Y92.62
  dry dock Y92.62
  factory Y92.63
  gasworks Y92.69
  mine Y92.64
  oil rig Y92.65
  pit Y92.64
  power station Y92.69
  shipyard Y92.62
  specified NEC Y92.69
  tunnel under construction Y92.69
  workshop Y92.69
interstate Y92.411
kindergarten Y92.211
lacrosse field Y92.328
lake Y92.838
  wilderness Y92.828
library Y92.241
mall Y92.59
market Y92.512
marsh Y92.828
military
  base — see Place of occurrence, residence, institu-
    tional, military base
  training ground Y92.84
mine Y92.64
mosque Y92.22
motel Y92.59
motorway (interstate) Y92.411
mountain Y92.828
movie-house Y92.26
museum Y92.251
music-hall Y92.252
not applicable Y92.9
nuclear power station Y92.69
nursing home — see Place of occurrence, residence,
  institutional, nursing home
office building Y92.59
offshore installation Y92.65
oil rig Y92.65
old people's home — see Place of occurrence, residence, institutional, specified NEC
opera-house Y92.253
orphanage — see Place of occurrence, residence, institutional, orphanage
outpatient surgery center Y92.530
park (public) Y92.830
  amusement Y92.831
parking garage Y92.89
  lot Y92.481
pavement Y92.480
physician office Y92.531
polo field Y92.328
pond Y92.828
post office Y92.242
power station Y92.69
prairie Y92.828
prison — see Place of occurrence, residence, institutional, prison
public
  administration building Y92.248
    city hall Y92.243
    courthouse Y92.240
    library Y92.241
    post office Y92.242
    specified NEC Y92.248
  building NEC Y92.29
  hall Y92.29
  place NOS Y92.89

Place of occurrence — *continued*
- race course Y92.39
- radio station Y92.59
- railway line (bridge) Y92.85
- ranch (outbuildings) — *see* Place of occurrence, farm
- recreation area Y92.838
  - amusement park Y92.831
  - beach Y92.832
  - campsite Y92.833
  - park (public) Y92.830
  - seashore Y92.832
  - specified NEC Y92.838
- reform school - — *see* Place of occurrence, residence, institutional, reform school
- religious institution Y92.22
- residence (non-institutional) (private) Y92.009
  - apartment Y92.039
    - bathroom Y92.031
    - bedroom Y92.032
    - kitchen Y92.030
    - specified NEC Y92.038
  - bathroom Y92.002
  - bedroom Y92.003
  - boarding house Y92.049
    - bathroom Y92.041
    - bedroom Y92.042
    - driveway Y92.043
    - garage Y92.044
    - garden Y92.046
    - kitchen Y92.040
    - specified NEC Y92.048
    - swimming pool Y92.045
    - yard Y92.046
  - dining room Y92.001
  - garden Y92.007
  - home Y92.009
  - house, single family Y92.019
    - bathroom Y92.012
    - bedroom Y92.013
    - dining room Y92.011
    - driveway Y92.014
    - garage Y92.015
    - garden Y92.017
    - kitchen Y92.010
    - specified NEC Y92.018
    - swimming pool Y92.016
    - yard Y92.017
  - institutional Y92.10
    - children's home — *see* Place of occurrence, residence, institutional, orphanage
    - hospice — *see* Place of occurrence, residence, institutional, nursing home
    - military base Y92.139
      - barracks Y92.133
      - garage Y92.135
      - garden Y92.137
      - kitchen Y92.130
      - mess hall Y92.131
      - specified NEC Y92.138
      - swimming pool Y92.136
      - yard Y92.137
    - nursing home Y92.129
      - bathroom Y92.121
      - bedroom Y92.122
      - driveway Y92.123
      - garage Y92.124
      - garden Y92.126
      - kitchen Y92.120
      - specified NEC Y92.128
      - swimming pool Y92.125
      - yard Y92.126
    - orphanage Y92.119
      - bathroom Y92.111
      - bedroom Y92.112
      - driveway Y92.113
      - garage Y92.114
      - garden Y92.116
      - kitchen Y92.110
      - specified NEC Y92.118
      - swimming pool Y92.115
      - yard Y92.116
    - prison Y92.149
      - bathroom Y92.142
      - cell Y92.143
      - courtyard Y92.147
      - dining room Y92.141
      - kitchen Y92.140
      - specified NEC Y92.148
      - swimming pool Y92.146

Place of occurrence — *continued*
- residence — *continued*
  - institutional — *continued*
    - reform school Y92.159
      - bathroom Y92.152
      - bedroom Y92.153
      - dining room Y92.151
      - driveway Y92.154
      - garage Y92.155
      - garden Y92.157
      - kitchen Y92.150
      - specified NEC Y92.158
      - swimming pool Y92.156
      - yard Y92.157
    - school dormitory Y92.169
      - bathroom Y92.162
      - bedroom Y92.163
      - dining room Y92.161
      - kitchen Y92.160
      - specified NEC Y92.168
    - specified NEC Y92.199
      - bathroom Y92.192
      - bedroom Y92.193
      - dining room Y92.191
      - driveway Y92.194
      - garage Y92.195
      - garden Y92.197
      - kitchen Y92.190
      - specified NEC Y92.198
      - swimming pool Y92.196
      - yard Y92.197
  - kitchen Y92.000
  - mobile home Y92.029
    - bathroom Y92.022
    - bedroom Y92.023
    - dining room Y92.021
    - driveway Y92.024
    - garage Y92.025
    - garden Y92.027
    - kitchen Y92.020
    - specified NEC Y92.028
    - swimming pool Y92.026
    - yard Y92.027
  - specified place in residence NEC Y92.008
  - specified residence type NEC Y92.099
    - bathroom Y92.091
    - bedroom Y92.092
    - driveway Y92.093
    - garage Y92.094
    - garden Y92.096
    - kitchen Y92.090
    - specified NEC Y92.098
    - swimming pool Y92.095
    - yard Y92.096
- restaurant Y92.511
- riding school Y92.39
- river Y92.828
- road Y92.410
- rodeo ring Y92.39
- rugby field Y92.328
- same day surgery center Y92.530
- sand pit Y92.64
- school (private) (public) (state) Y92.219
  - college Y92.214
  - daycare center Y92.210
  - elementary school Y92.211
  - high school Y92.213
  - kindergarten Y92.211
  - middle school Y92.212
  - specified NEC Y92.218
  - trace school Y92.215
  - university Y92.214
  - vocational school Y92.215
- sea (shore) Y92.832
- senior citizen center Y92.29
- service area
  - airport Y92.520
  - bus station Y92.521
  - gas station Y92.524
  - highway rest stop Y92.523
  - railway station Y92.522
- shipyard Y92.62
- shop (commercial) Y92.513
- sidewalk Y92.480
- silo Y92.79
- skating rink (roller) Y92.331
  - ice Y92.330
- slaughter house Y92.86
- soccer field Y92.322

Place of occurrence — *continued*
- specified place NEC Y92.89
- sports area Y92.39
  - athletic
    - court Y92.318
      - basketball Y92.310
      - specified NEC Y92.318
      - squash Y92.311
      - tennis Y92.312
    - field Y92.328
      - baseball Y92.320
      - cricket ground Y92.328
      - football Y92.321
      - hockey Y92.328
      - soccer Y92.322
      - specified NEC Y92.328
  - golf course Y92.39
  - gymnasium Y92.39
  - riding school Y92.39
  - skating rink (roller) Y92.331
    - ice Y92.330
  - stadium Y92.39
  - swimming pool Y92.34
- squash court Y92.311
- stadium Y92.39
- steeplechasing course Y92.39
- store Y92.512
- stream Y92.828
- street and highway Y92.410
  - bike path Y92.482
  - freeway Y92.411
  - highway ramp Y92.415
  - interstate highway Y92.411
  - local residential or business street Y92.414
  - motorway Y92.411
  - parking lot Y92.481
  - parkway Y92.412
  - sidewalk Y92.480
  - specified NEC Y92.488
  - state road Y92.413
- subway car Y92.816
- supermarket Y92.512
- swamp Y92.828
- swimming pool (public) Y92.34
  - private (at) Y92.095
    - boarding house Y92.045
    - military base Y92.136
    - mobile home Y92.026
    - nursing home Y92.125
    - orphanage Y92.115
    - prison Y92.146
    - reform school Y92.156
    - single family residence Y92.016
- synagogue Y92.22
- television station Y92.59
- tennis court Y92.312
- theater Y92.254
- trade area Y92.59
  - bank Y92.510
  - cafe Y92.511
  - casino Y92.59
  - garage Y92.59
  - hotel Y92.59
  - market Y92.512
  - office building Y92.59
  - radio station Y92.59
  - restaurant Y92.511
  - shop Y92.513
  - shopping mall Y92.59
  - store Y92.512
  - supermarket Y92.512
  - television station Y92.59
  - warehouse Y92.59
- trailer park, residential — *see* Place of occurrence, residence, mobile home
- trailer site NOS Y92.89
- train Y92.815
  - station Y92.522
- truck Y92.812
- tunnel under construction Y92.69
- university Y92.214
- urgent (health) care center Y92.532
- vehicle (transport) Y92.818
  - airplane Y92.813
  - boat Y92.814
  - bus Y92.811
  - car Y92.810
  - specified NEC Y92.818
  - subway car Y92.816

Place of occurrence — continued
vehicle — continued
   train Y92.815
   truck Y92.812
warehouse Y92.59
water reservoir Y92.89
wilderness area Y92.828
   desert Y92.820
   forest Y92.821
   marsh Y92.828
   mountain Y92.828
   prairie Y92.828
   specified NEC Y92.828
   swamp Y92.828
workshop Y92.69
yard, private Y92.096
   boarding house Y92.046
   mobile home Y92.027
   single family house Y92.017
youth center Y92.29
zoo (zoological garden) Y92.834
Plumbism — see Table of Drugs and Chemicals, lead
Poisoning (accidental) (by) — see also Table of Drugs
   and Chemicals
by plant, thorns, spines, sharp leaves or other mechanisms NEC X58 ☑
carbon monoxide
   generated by
      motor vehicle — see Accident, transport
      watercraft (in transit) (not in transit) V93.89 ☑
         ferry boat V93.81 ☑
         fishing boat V93.82 ☑
         jet skis V93.83 ☑
         liner V93.81 ☑
         merchant ship V93.80 ☑
         passenger ship V93.81 ☑
         powered craft NEC V93.83 ☑
caused by injection of poisons into skin by plant thorns,
   spines, sharp leaves X58 ☑
   marine or sea plants (venomous) X58 ☑
execution — see Legal, intervention, gas
   intervention
      by gas — see Legal, intervention, gas
      other specified means — see Legal, intervention,
         specified means NEC
exhaust gas
   generated by
      motor vehicle — see Accident, transport
      watercraft (in transit) (not in transit) V93.89 ☑
         ferry boat V93.81 ☑
         fishing boat V93.82 ☑
         jet skis V93.83 ☑
         liner V93.81 ☑
         merchant ship V93.80 ☑
         passenger ship V93.81 ☑
         powered craft NEC V93.83 ☑
fumes or smoke due to
   explosion — see also Explosion W40.9 ☑
   fire — see Exposure, fire
   ignition — see Ignition
gas
   in legal intervention — see Legal, intervention, gas
   legal execution — see Legal, intervention, gas
in war operations — see War operations
legal
Powder burn (by) (from)
airgun W34.110 ☑
BB gun W34.110 ☑
firearm NEC W34.19 ☑
gas, air or spring-operated gun NEC W34.118 ☑
handgun W32.1 ☑
hunting rifle W33.12 ☑
larger firearm W33.10 ☑
   specified NEC W33.19 ☑
machine gun W33.13 ☑
paintball gun W34.111 ☑
pellet gun W34.110 ☑
shotgun W33.11 ☑
Very pistol [flare] W34.19 ☑
Premature cessation (of) **surgical and medical care**
   Y66
Privation (food) (water) X58 ☑
Procedure (operation)
correct, on wrong side or body part (wrong side)
   (wrong site) Y65.53
intended for another patient done on wrong patient
   Y65.52

Procedure — continued
performed on patient not scheduled for surgery Y65.52
performed on wrong patient Y65.52
wrong, performed on correct patient Y65.51
Prolonged
sitting in transport vehicle — see Travel, by type of
   vehicle
stay in
   high altitude as cause of anoxia, barodontalgia,
      barotitis or hypoxia W94.11 ☑
   weightless environment X52 ☑
Pulling, excessive — see also Overexertion X50.9-
Puncture, puncturing — see also Contact, with, by type
   of object or machine
by
   plant thorns, spines, sharp leaves or other mecha-
      nisms NEC W60 ☑
during medical or surgical treatment as misadventure
   — see Index to Diseases and Injuries, Complica-
   tion(s)
Pushed, pushing (accidental) (injury in)
by other person(s) (accidental) W51 ☑
   as, or caused by, a crowd or human stampede (with
      fall) W52 ☑
   before moving object NEC Y02.8 ☑
      motor vehicle Y02.0 ☑
      subway train Y02.1 ☑
      train Y02.1 ☑
   from
      high place NEC
         in accidental circumstances W17.89 ☑
         stated as
            intentional, homicide (attempt) Y01 ☑
            undetermined whether accidental or in-
               tentional Y30 ☑
         transport vehicle NEC — see also Accident,
            transport V89.9 ☑
         stated as
            intentional, homicide (attempt) Y08.89 ☑
   with fall W03 ☑
   due to ice or snow W00.0 ☑
overexertion X50.9 ☑

R

Radiation (exposure to)
arc lamps W89.0 ☑
atomic power plant (malfunction) NEC W88.1 ☑
complication of or abnormal reaction to medical radiotherapy Y84.2
electromagnetic, ionizing W88.0 ☑
gamma rays W88.1 ☑
in
   war operations (from or following nuclear explosion)
      — see War operations
inadvertent exposure of patient (receiving test or
   therapy) Y63.3
infrared (heaters and lamps) W90.1 ☑
   excessive heat from W92 ☑
ionized, ionizing (particles, artificially accelerated)
   radioisotopes W88.1 ☑
   specified NEC W88.8 ☑
   x-rays W88.0 ☑
isotopes, radioactive — see Radiation, radioactive isotopes
laser(s) W90.2 ☑
   in war operations — see War operations
   misadventure in medical care Y63.2
light sources (man-made visible and ultraviolet)
   W89.9 ☑
   natural X32 ☑
   specified NEC W89.8 ☑
   tanning bed W89.1 ☑
   welding light W89.0 ☑
man-made visible light W89.9 ☑
   specified NEC W89.8 ☑
   tanning bed W89.1 ☑
   welding light W89.0 ☑
microwave W90.8 ☑
misadventure in medical or surgical procedure Y63.2
natural NEC X39.08 ☑
   radon X39.01 ☑
overdose (in medical or surgical procedure) Y63.2
radar W90.0 ☑
radioactive isotopes (any) W88.1 ☑
   atomic power plant malfunction W88.1 ☑
   misadventure in medical or surgical treatment Y63.2

Radiation — continued
radiofrequency W90.0 ☑
radium NEC W88.1 ☑
sun X32 ☑
ultraviolet (light) (man-made) W89.9 ☑
   natural X32 ☑
   specified NEC W89.8 ☑
   tanning bed W89.1 ☑
   welding light W89.0 ☑
welding arc, torch, or light W89.0 ☑
   excessive heat from W92 ☑
x-rays (hard) (soft) W88.0 ☑
Range disease W94.11 ☑
Rape (attempted) T74.2-
Rat bite W53.11 ☑
Reaching (prolonged) (static) X50.1 ☑
Reaction, abnormal to medical procedure — see also
   Complication of or following, by type of procedure
   Y84.9
biologicals — see Table of Drugs and Chemicals
drugs — see Table of Drugs and Chemicals
vaccine — see Table of Drugs and Chemicals
with misadventure — see Misadventure
Recoil
airgun W34.110 ☑
BB gun W34.110 ☑
firearm NEC W34.19 ☑
gas, air or spring-operated gun NEC W34.118 ☑
handgun W32.1 ☑
hunting rifle W33.12 ☑
larger firearm W33.10 ☑
   specified NEC W33.19 ☑
machine gun W33.13 ☑
paintball gun W34.111 ☑
pellet W34.110 ☑
shotgun W33.11 ☑
Very pistol [flare] W34.19 ☑
Reduction in
atmospheric pressure — see Air, pressure, change
Rock falling on or hitting (accidentally) (person)
   W20.8 ☑
in cave-in W20.0 ☑
Run over (accidentally) (by)
animal (not being ridden) NEC W55.89 ☑
machinery — see Contact, with, by specified type of
   machine
transport vehicle NEC — see also Accident, transport
   V09.9 ☑
   intentional homicide (attempt) Y03.0 ☑
   motor NEC V09.20 ☑
      intentional homicide (attempt) Y03.0 ☑
Running
before moving object X81.8 ☑
   motor vehicle X81.0 ☑
Running off, away
animal (being ridden) — see also Accident, transport
   V80.918 ☑
   not being ridden W55.89 ☑
animal-drawn vehicle NEC — see also Accident, transport V80.928 ☑
highway, road(way), street
   transport vehicle NEC — see also Accident, transport
      V89.9 ☑
Rupture pressurized devices — see Explosion, by type
   of device

S

Saturnism — see Table of Drugs and Chemicals, lead
Scald, scalding (accidental) (by) (from) (in) X19 ☑
air (hot) X14.1 ☑
gases (hot) X14.1 ☑
homicide (attempt) — see Assault, burning, hot object
inflicted by other person
   stated as intentional, homicide (attempt) — see
      Assault, burning, hot object
liquid (boiling) (hot) NEC X12 ☑
   stated as undetermined whether accidental or inten-
      tional X27.2 ☑
   suicide (attempt) X77.2 ☑
local application of externally applied substance in
   medical or surgical care Y63.5
metal (molten) (liquid) (hot) NEC X18 ☑
self-inflicted X77.9 ☑
stated as undetermined whether accidental or intentional Y27.8 ☑

Scald, scalding — *continued*
  steam X13.1 ☑
    assault X98.0 ☑
    stated as undetermined whether accidental or intentional Y27.0 ☑
    suicide (attempt) X77.0 ☑
  suicide (attempt) X77.9 ☑
  vapor (hot) X13.1 ☑
    assault X98.0 ☑
    stated as undetermined whether accidental or intentional Y27.0 ☑
    suicide (attempt) X77.0 ☑
Scratched by
  cat W55.03 ☑
  person(s) (accidentally) W50.4 ☑
    with intent to injure or kill Y04.0 ☑
    as, or caused by, a crowd or human stampede (with fall) W52 ☑
    assault Y04.0 ☑
    homicide (attempt) Y04.0 ☑
    in
      fight Y04.0 ☑
      legal intervention
        injuring
          bystander Y35.892 ☑
          law enforcement personnel Y35.891 ☑
          suspect Y35.893 ☑
          unspecified person Y35.899 ☑
Seasickness T75.3 ☑
Self-harm NEC — *see also* External cause by type, undetermined whether accidental or intentional
  intentional — *see* Suicide
  poisoning NEC — *see* Table of Drugs and Chemicals, poisoning, accidental
Self-inflicted (injury) **NEC** — *see also* External cause by type, undetermined whether accidental or intentional
  intentional — *see* Suicide
  poisoning NEC — *see* Table of Drugs and Chemicals, poisoning, accidental
Sequelae (of)
  accident NEC — *see* W00-X58 with 7th character S
  assault (homicidal) (any means) — *see* X92-Y08 with 7th character S
  homicide, attempt (any means) — *see* X92-Y08 with 7th character S
  injury undetermined whether accidentally or purposely inflicted — *see* Y21-Y33 with 7th character S
  intentional self-harm (classifiable to X71-X83) — *see* X71-X83 with 7th character S
  legal intervention — *see* with 7th character S Y35 ☑
  motor vehicle accident — *see* V00-V99 with 7th character S
  suicide, attempt (any means) — *see* X71-X83 with 7th character S
  transport accident — *see* V00-V99 with 7th character S
  war operations — *see* War operations
Shock
  electric — *see* Exposure, electric current
  from electric appliance (any) (faulty) W86.8 ☑
    domestic W86.0 ☑
    suicide (attempt) X83.1 ☑
Shooting, shot (accidental(ly)) — *see also* Discharge, firearm, by type
  herself or himself — *see* Discharge, firearm by type, self-inflicted
  homicide (attempt) — *see* Discharge, firearm by type, homicide
  in war operations — *see* War operations
  inflicted by other person — *see* Discharge, firearm by type, homicide
    accidental — *see* Discharge, firearm, by type of firearm
  legal
    execution — *see* Legal, intervention, firearm
    intervention — *see* Legal, intervention, firearm
  self-inflicted — *see* Discharge, firearm by type, suicide
    accidental — *see* Discharge, firearm, by type of firearm
  suicide (attempt) — *see* Discharge, firearm by type, suicide
Shoving (accidentally) **by other person** — *see* Pushed, by other person
Sickness
  alpine W94.11 ☑
  motion — *see* Motion

Sickness — *continued*
  mountain W94.11 ☑
Sinking (accidental)
  watercraft (causing drowning, submersion) — *see also* Drowning, due to, accident to, watercraft, sinking
    causing injury except drowning or submersion — *see* Accident, watercraft, causing, injury NEC
Siriasis X32 ☑
Sitting (prolonged) (static) X50.1 ☑
Slashed wrists — *see* Cut, self-inflicted
Slipping (accidental) (on same level) (with fall) W01.0 ☑
  on
    ice W00.0 ☑
      with skates — *see* Accident, transport, pedestrian, conveyance
    mud W01.0 ☑
    oil W01.0 ☑
    snow W00.0 ☑
      with skis — *see* Accident, transport, pedestrian, conveyance
    surface (slippery) (wet) NEC W01.0 ☑
  without fall W18.40 ☑
    due to
      specified NEC W18.49 ☑
      stepping from one level to another W18.43 ☑
      stepping into hole or opening W18.42 ☑
      stepping on object W18.41 ☑
Sliver, wood, contact with W45.8 ☑
Smoldering (due to fire) — *see* Exposure, fire
Sodomy (attempted) **by force** T74.2 ☑
Sound waves (causing injury) W42.9 ☑
  supersonic W42.0 ☑
Splinter, contact with W45.8 ☑
Stab, stabbing — *see* Cut
Standing (prolonged) (static) X50.1 ☑
Starvation X58 ☑
Status of external cause Y99.9
  child assisting in compensated work for family Y99.8
  civilian activity done for financial or other compensation Y99.0
  civilian activity done for income or pay Y99.0
  family member assisting in compensated work for other family member Y99.8
  hobby not done for income Y99.8
  leisure activity Y99.8
  military activity Y99.1
  off-duty activity of military personnel Y99.8
  recreation or sport not for income or while a student Y99.8
  specified NEC Y99.8
  student activity Y99.8
  volunteer activity Y99.2
Stepped on
  by
    animal (not being ridden) NEC W55.89 ☑
    crowd or human stampede W52 ☑
    person W50.0 ☑
Stepping on
  object W22.8 ☑
    sports equipment W21.9 ☑
    stationary W22.09 ☑
      sports equipment W21.89 ☑
    with fall W18.31 ☑
  person W51 ☑
    by crowd or human stampede W52 ☑
  sports equipment W21.9 ☑
Sting
  arthropod, nonvenomous W57 ☑
  insect, nonvenomous W57 ☑
Storm (cataclysmic) — *see* Forces of nature, cataclysmic storm
Straining, excessive — *see also* Overexertion X50.9 ☑
Strangling — *see* Strangulation
Strangulation (accidental) T71 ☑
Strenuous movements — *see also* Overexertion X50.9 ☑
Striking against
  airbag (automobile) W22.10 ☑
    driver side W22.11 ☑
    front passenger side W22.12 ☑
    specified NEC W22.19 ☑
  bottom when
    diving or jumping into water (in) W16.822 ☑
      causing drowning W16.821 ☑
      from boat W16.722 ☑
        causing drowning W16.721 ☑

Striking against — *continued*
  bottom when — *continued*
    diving or jumping into water — *continued*
      natural body W16.622 ☑
        causing drowning W16.821 ☑
      swimming pool W16.522 ☑
        causing drowning W16.521 ☑
    falling into water (in) W16.322 ☑
      causing drowning W16.321 ☑
      fountain — *see* Striking against, bottom when, falling into water, specified NEC
      natural body W16.122 ☑
        causing drowning W16.121 ☑
      reservoir — *see* Striking against, bottom when, falling into water, specified NEC
      specified NEC W16.322 ☑
        causing drowning W16.321 ☑
      swimming pool W16.022 ☑
        causing drowning W16.021 ☑
  diving board (swimming-pool) W21.4 ☑
  object W22.8 ☑
    caused by crowd or human stampede (with fall) W52 ☑
    furniture W22.03 ☑
    lamppost W22.02 ☑
    sports equipment W21.9 ☑
    stationary W22.09 ☑
      sports equipment W21.89 ☑
    wall W22.01 ☑
    with
      drowning or submersion — *see* Drowning
      fall — *see* Fall, due to, bumping against, object
  person(s) W51 ☑
    as, or caused by, a crowd or human stampede (with fall) W52 ☑
    assault Y04.0 ☑
    homicide (attempt) Y04.2 ☑
    with fall W03 ☑
      due to ice or snow W00.0 ☑
  sports equipment W21.9 ☑
  wall (when) W22.01 ☑
    diving or jumping into water (in) W16.832 ☑
      causing drowning W16.831 ☑
      swimming pool W16.532 ☑
        causing drowning W16.531 ☑
    falling into water (in) W16.332 ☑
      causing drowning W16.331 ☑
      fountain — *see* Striking against, wall when, falling into water, specified NEC
      natural body W16.132 ☑
        causing drowning W16.131 ☑
      reservoir — *see* Striking against, wall when, falling into water, specified NEC
      specified NEC W16.332 ☑
        causing drowning W16.331 ☑
      swimming pool W16.032 ☑
        causing drowning W16.031 ☑
    swimming pool (when) W22.042 ☑
      causing drowning W22.041 ☑
      diving or jumping into water W16.532 ☑
        causing drowning W16.531 ☑
      falling into water W16.032 ☑
        causing drowning W16.031 ☑
Struck (accidentally) **by**
  airbag (automobile) W22.10 ☑
    driver side W22.11 ☑
    front passenger side W22.12 ☑
    specified NEC W22.19 ☑
  alligator W58.02 ☑
  animal (not being ridden) NEC W55.89 ☑
  avalanche — *see* Landslide
  ball (hit) (thrown) W21.00 ☑
    assault Y08.09 ☑
    baseball W21.03 ☑
    basketball W21.05 ☑
    football W21.01 ☑
    golf ball W21.04 ☑
    soccer W21.02 ☑
    softball W21.07 ☑
    specified NEC W21.09 ☑
    volleyball W21.06 ☑
  bat or racquet
    baseball bat W21.11 ☑
      assault Y08.02 ☑
    golf club W21.13 ☑
      assault Y08.09 ☑

Struck (accidentally) **by** — *continued*
- bat or racquet — *continued*
    - specified NEC W21.19 ☑
        - assault Y08.09 ☑
    - tennis racquet W21.12 ☑
        - assault Y08.09 ☑
- bullet — *see also* Discharge, firearm by type
    - in war operations — *see* War operations
- crocodile W58.12 ☑
- dog W54.1 ☑
- flare, Very pistol — *see* Discharge, firearm NEC
- hailstones X39.8 ☑
- hockey (ice)
    - field
        - puck W21.221 ☑
        - stick W21.211 ☑
    - puck W21.220 ☑
    - stick W21.210 ☑
        - assault Y08.01 ☑
- landslide — *see* Landslide
- law-enforcement agent (on duty) — *see* Legal, intervention, manhandling
    - with blunt object — *see* Legal, intervention, blunt object
- lightning T75.0 ☑
    - causing fire — *see* Exposure, fire
- machine — *see* Contact, with, by type of machine
- mammal NEC W55.89 ☑
    - marine W56.32 ☑
- marine animal W56.82 ☑
- missile
    - firearm — *see* Discharge, firearm by type
    - in war operations — *see* War operations, missile
- object W22.8 ☑
    - blunt W22.8 ☑
        - assault Y00 ☑
        - suicide (attempt) X79 ☑
        - undetermined whether accidental or intentional Y29 ☑
    - falling W20.8 ☑
        - from, in, on
            - building W20.1 ☑
                - burning (uncontrolled fire) X00.4 ☑
            - cataclysmic
                - earth surface movement NEC — *see* Landslide
                - storm — *see* Forces of nature, cataclysmic storm
            - cave-in W20.0 ☑
            - earthquake X34 ☑
            - machine (in operation) — *see* Contact, with, by type of machine
            - structure W20.1 ☑
                - burning X00.4 ☑
            - transport vehicle (in motion) — *see* Accident, transport, by type of vehicle
            - watercraft V93.49 ☑
                - due to
                    - accident to craft V91.39 ☑
                        - powered craft V91.33 ☑
                            - ferry boat V91.31 ☑
                            - fishing boat V91.32 ☑
                            - jetskis V91.33 ☑
                            - liner V91.31 ☑
                            - merchant ship V91.30 ☑
                            - passenger ship V91.31 ☑
                        - unpowered craft V91.38 ☑
                            - canoe V91.35 ☑
                            - inflatable V91.36 ☑
                            - kayak V91.35 ☑
                            - sailboat V91.34 ☑
                            - surf-board V91.38 ☑
                            - windsurfer V91.38 ☑
                    - powered craft V93.43 ☑
                        - ferry boat V93.41 ☑
                        - fishing boat V93.42 ☑
                        - jetskis V93.43 ☑
                        - liner V93.41 ☑
                        - merchant ship V93.40 ☑
                        - passenger ship V93.41 ☑
                    - unpowered craft V93.48 ☑
                        - sailboat V93.44 ☑
                        - surf-board V93.48 ☑
                        - windsurfer V93.48 ☑
    - moving NEC W20.8 ☑
    - projected W20.8 ☑

Struck (accidentally) **by** — *continued*
- object — *continued*
    - projected — *continued*
        - assault Y00 ☑
        - in sports W21.9 ☑
            - assault Y08.09 ☑
            - ball W21.00 ☑
                - baseball W21.03 ☑
                - basketball W21.05 ☑
                - football W21.01 ☑
                - golf ball W21.04 ☑
                - soccer W21.02 ☑
                - softball W21.07 ☑
                - specified NEC W21.09 ☑
                - volleyball W21.06 ☑
            - bat or racquet
                - baseball bat W21.11 ☑
                    - assault Y08.02 ☑
                - golf club W21.13 ☑
                    - assault Y08.09 ☑
                - specified NEC W21.19 ☑
                    - assault Y08.09 ☑
                - tennis racquet W21.12 ☑
                    - assault Y08.09 ☑
            - hockey (ice)
                - field
                    - puck W21.221 ☑
                    - stick W21.211 ☑
                - puck W21.220 ☑
                - stick W21.210 ☑
                    - assault Y08.01 ☑
            - specified NEC W21.89 ☑
        - set in motion by explosion — *see* Explosion
    - thrown W20.8 ☑
        - assault Y00 ☑
        - in sports W21.9 ☑
            - assault Y08.09 ☑
            - ball W21.00 ☑
                - baseball W21.03 ☑
                - basketball W21.05 ☑
                - football W21.01 ☑
                - golf ball W21.04 ☑
                - soccer W21.02 ☑
                - soft ball W21.07 ☑
                - specified NEC W21.09 ☑
                - volleyball W21.06 ☑
            - bat or racquet
                - baseball bat W21.11 ☑
                    - assault Y08.02 ☑
                - golf club W21.13 ☑
                    - assault Y08.09 ☑
                - specified NEC W21.19 ☑
                    - assault Y08.09 ☑
                - tennis racquet W21.12 ☑
                    - assault Y08.09 ☑
            - hockey (ice)
                - field
                    - puck W21.221 ☑
                    - stick W21.211 ☑
                - puck W21.220 ☑
                - stick W21.210 ☑
                    - assault Y08.01 ☑
            - specified NEC W21.89 ☑
- other person(s) W50.0 ☑
    - with
        - blunt object W22.8 ☑
            - intentional, homicide (attempt) Y00 ☑
            - sports equipment W21.9 ☑
            - undetermined whether accidental or intentional Y29 ☑
        - fall W03 ☑
            - due to ice or snow W00.0 ☑
        - as, or caused by, a crowd or human stampede (with fall) W52 ☑
    - assault Y04.2 ☑
    - homicide (attempt) Y04.2 ☑
    - in legal intervention
        - injuring
            - bystander Y35.812 ☑
            - law enforcement personnel Y35.811 ☑
            - suspect Y35.813 ☑
            - unspecified person Y35.819 ☑
    - sports equipment W21.9 ☑
- police (on duty) — *see* Legal, intervention, manhandling

Struck (accidentally) **by** — *continued*
- police — *see* Legal, intervention, manhandling — *continued*
    - with blunt object — *see* Legal, intervention, blunt object
- sports equipment W21.9 ☑
    - assault Y08.09 ☑
    - ball W21.00 ☑
        - baseball W21.03 ☑
        - basketball W21.05 ☑
        - football W21.01 ☑
        - golf ball W21.04 ☑
        - soccer W21.02 ☑
        - soft ball W21.07 ☑
        - specified NEC W21.09 ☑
        - volleyball W21.06 ☑
    - bat or racquet
        - baseball bat W21.11 ☑
            - assault Y08.02 ☑
        - golf club W21.13 ☑
            - assault Y08.09 ☑
        - specified NEC W21.19 ☑
        - tennis racquet W21.12 ☑
            - assault Y08.09 ☑
    - cleats (shoe) W21.31 ☑
    - foot wear NEC W21.39 ☑
    - football helmet W21.81 ☑
    - hockey (ice)
        - field
            - puck W21.221 ☑
            - stick W21.211 ☑
        - puck W21.220 ☑
        - stick W21.210 ☑
            - assault Y08.01 ☑
    - skate blades W21.32 ☑
    - specified NEC W21.89 ☑
        - assault Y08.09 ☑
- thunderbolt — *see* subcategory T75.0 ☑
    - causing fire — *see* Exposure, fire
- transport vehicle NEC — *see also* Accident, transport V09.9 ☑
    - intentional, homicide (attempt) Y03.0 ☑
    - motor NEC — *see also* Accident, transport V09.20 ☑
        - homicide Y03.0 ☑
- vehicle (transport) NEC — *see* Accident, transport, by type of vehicle
    - stationary (falling from jack, hydraulic lift, ramp) W20.8 ☑

Stumbling
- over
    - animal NEC W01.0 ☑
        - with fall W18.09 ☑
    - carpet, rug or (small) object W22.8 ☑
        - with fall W18.09 ☑
    - person W51 ☑
        - with fall W03 ☑
            - due to ice or snow W00.0 ☑
- without fall W18.40 ☑
    - due to
        - specified NEC W18.49 ☑
        - stepping from one level to another W18.43 ☑
        - stepping into hole or opening W18.42 ☑
        - stepping on object W18.41 ☑

Submersion (accidental) — *see* Drowning

Suffocation (accidental) (by external means) (by pressure) (mechanical) — *see also* category T71 ☑
- due to, by
    - avalanche — *see* Landslide
    - explosion — *see* Explosion
    - fire — *see* Exposure, fire
    - food, any type (aspiration) (ingestion) (inhalation) — *see* categories T17 and T18 ☑
    - ignition — *see* Ignition
    - landslide — *see* Landslide
    - machine(ry) — *see* Contact, with, by type of machine
    - vomitus (aspiration) (inhalation) T17.81- ☑
- in
    - burning building X00.8 ☑

Suicide, suicidal (attempted) (by) X83.8 ☑
- blunt object X79 ☑
- burning, burns X76 ☑
    - hot object X77.9 ☑
        - fluid NEC X77.2 ☑
        - household appliance X77.3 ☑
        - specified NEC X77.8 ☑

Suicide, suicidal — *continued*
  burning, burns — *continued*
    hot object — *continued*
      steam X77.0 ☑
      tap water X77.1 ☑
      vapors X77.0 ☑
    caustic substance — *see* Table of Drugs and Chemicals
  cold, extreme X83.2 ☑
  collision of motor vehicle with
    motor vehicle X82.0 ☑
    specified NEC X82.8 ☑
    train X82.1 ☑
    tree X82.2 ☑
  crashing of aircraft X83.0 ☑
  cut (any part of body) X78.9 ☑
  cutting or piercing instrument X78.9 ☑
    dagger X78.2 ☑
    glass X78.0 ☑
    knife X78.1 ☑
    specified NEC X78.8 ☑
    sword X78.2 ☑
  drowning (in) X71.9 ☑
    bathtub X71.0 ☑
    natural water X71.3 ☑
    specified NEC X71.8 ☑
    swimming pool X71.1 ☑
      following fall X71.2 ☑
  electrocution X83.1 ☑
  explosive(s) (material) X75 ☑
  fire, flames X76 ☑
  firearm X74.9 ☑
    airgun X74.01 ☑
    handgun X72 ☑
    hunting rifle X73.1 ☑
    larger X73.9 ☑
      specified NEC X73.8 ☑
    machine gun X73.2 ☑
    shotgun X73.0 ☑
    specified NEC X74.8 ☑
  hanging X83.8 ☑
  hot object — *see* Suicide, burning, hot object
  jumping
    before moving object X81.8 ☑
      motor vehicle X81.0 ☑
      subway train X81.1 ☑
      train X81.1 ☑
    from high place X80 ☑
  late effect of attempt — *see* X71-X83 with 7th character S
  lying before moving object, train, vehicle X81.8 ☑
  poisoning — *see* Table of Drugs and Chemicals
  puncture (any part of body) — *see* Suicide, cutting or piercing instrument
  scald — *see* Suicide, burning, hot object
  sequelae of attempt — *see* X71-X83 with 7th character S
  sharp object (any) — *see* Suicide, cutting or piercing instrument
  shooting — *see* Suicide, firearm
  specified means NEC X83.8 ☑
  stab (any part of body) — *see* Suicide, cutting or piercing instrument
  steam, hot vapors X77.0 ☑
  strangulation X83.8 ☑
  submersion — *see* Suicide, drowning
  suffocation X83.8 ☑
  wound NEC X83.8 ☑
Sunstroke X32 ☑
Supersonic waves (causing injury) W42.0 ☑
Surgical procedure, complication of (delayed or as an abnormal reaction without mention of misadventure) — *see also* Complication of or following, by type of procedure
  due to or as a result of misadventure — *see* Misadventure
Swallowed, swallowing
  foreign body — *see* Foreign body, alimentary canal
  poison — *see* Table of Drugs and Chemicals
  substance
    caustic or corrosive — *see* Table of Drugs and Chemicals
    poisonous — *see* Table of Drugs and Chemicals

T

Tackle in sport W03 ☑

Terrorism (involving) Y38.80 ☑
  biological weapons Y38.6X- ☑
  chemical weapons Y38.7X- ☑
  conflagration Y38.3X- ☑
  drowning and submersion Y38.89- ☑
  explosion Y38.2X- ☑
    destruction of aircraft Y38.1X- ☑
    marine weapons Y38.0X- ☑
  fire Y38.3X- ☑
  firearms Y38.4X- ☑
  hot substances Y38.3X- ☑
  lasers Y38.89- ☑
  nuclear weapons Y38.5X- ☑
  piercing or stabbing instruments Y38.89- ☑
  secondary effects Y38.9X- ☑
  specified method NEC Y38.89- ☑
  suicide bomber Y38.81- ☑
Thirst X58 ☑
Threat to breathing
  aspiration — *see* Aspiration
  due to cave-in, falling earth or substance NEC T71 ☑
Thrown (accidentally)
  against part (any) of or object in transport vehicle (in motion) NEC — *see also* Accident, transport
  from
    high place, homicide (attempt) Y01 ☑
    machinery — *see* Contact, with, by type of machine
    transport vehicle NEC — *see also* Accident, transport V89.9 ☑
  off — *see* Thrown, from
Thunderbolt — *see* subcategory T75.0 ☑
  causing fire — *see* Exposure, fire
Tidal wave (any injury) **NEC** — *see* Forces of nature, tidal wave
Took
  overdose (drug) — *see* Table of Drugs and Chemicals
  poison — *see* Table of Drugs and Chemicals
Tornado (any injury) X37.1 ☑
Torrential rain (any injury) X37.8 ☑
Torture X58 ☑
Trampled by animal NEC W55.89 ☑
Trapped (accidentally)
  between objects (moving) (stationary and moving) — *see* Caught
  by part (any) of
    electric (assisted) bicycle V29.881 ☑
    motorcycle V29.888 ☑
    pedal cycle V19.88 ☑
    transport vehicle NEC — *see also* Accident, transport V89.9 ☑
Travel (effects) (sickness) T75.3 ☑
Tree falling on or hitting (accidentally) (person) W20.8 ☑
Tripping
  over
    animal W01.0 ☑
      with fall W01.0 ☑
    carpet, rug or (small) object W22.8 ☑
      with fall W18.09 ☑
    person W51 ☑
      with fall W03 ☑
        due to ice or snow W00.0 ☑
    without fall W18.40 ☑
      due to
        specified NEC W18.49 ☑
        stepping from one level to another W18.43 ☑
        stepping into hole or opening W18.42 ☑
        stepping on object W18.41 ☑
Twisted by person(s) (accidentally) W50.2 ☑
  with intent to injure or kill Y04.0 ☑
  as, or caused by, a crowd or human stampede (with fall) W52 ☑
  assault Y04.0 ☑
  homicide (attempt) Y04.0 ☑
  in
    fight Y04.0 ☑
    legal intervention — *see* Legal, intervention, manhandling
Twisting (prolonged) (static) X50.1- ☑

U

Underdosing of necessary drugs, medicaments or biological substances Y63.6
Undetermined intent (contact) (exposure)
  automobile collision Y32 ☑

Undetermined intent — *continued*
  blunt object Y29 ☑
  drowning (submersion) (in) Y21.9 ☑
    bathtub Y21.0 ☑
      after fall Y21.1 ☑
    natural water (lake) (ocean) (pond) (river) (stream) Y21.4 ☑
    specified place NEC Y21.8 ☑
    swimming pool Y21.2 ☑
      after fall Y21.3 ☑
  explosive material Y25 ☑
  fall, jump or push from high place Y30 ☑
  falling, lying or running before moving object Y31 ☑
  fire Y26 ☑
  firearm discharge Y24.9 ☑
    airgun (BB) (pellet) Y24.0 ☑
    handgun (pistol) (revolver) Y22 ☑
    hunting rifle Y23.1 ☑
    larger Y23.9 ☑
      hunting rifle Y23.1 ☑
      machine gun Y23.3 ☑
      military Y23.2 ☑
      shotgun Y23.0 ☑
      specified type NEC Y23.8 ☑
    machine gun Y23.3 ☑
    military Y23.2 ☑
    shotgun Y23.0 ☑
    specified type NEC Y24.8 ☑
    Very pistol Y24.8 ☑
  hot object Y27.9 ☑
    fluid NEC Y27.2 ☑
    household appliance Y27.3 ☑
    specified object NEC Y27.8 ☑
    steam Y27.0 ☑
    tap water Y27.1 ☑
    vapor Y27.0 ☑
  jump, fall or push from high place Y30 ☑
  lying, falling or running before moving object Y31 ☑
  motor vehicle crash Y32 ☑
  push, fall or jump from high place Y30 ☑
  running, falling or lying before moving object Y31 ☑
  sharp object Y28.9 ☑
    dagger Y28.2 ☑
    glass Y28.0 ☑
    knife Y28.1 ☑
    specified object NEC Y28.8 ☑
    sword Y28.2 ☑
  smoke Y26 ☑
  specified event NEC Y33 ☑
Use of hand as hammer X50.3 ☑

V

Vibration (causing injury) W49.9 ☑
Victim (of)
  avalanche — *see* Landslide
  earth movements NEC — *see* Forces of nature, earth movement
  earthquake X34 ☑
  flood — *see* Flood
  landslide — *see* Landslide
  lightning — *see* subcategory T75.0 ☑
    causing fire — *see* Exposure, fire
  storm (cataclysmic) NEC — *see* Forces of nature, cataclysmic storm
  volcanic eruption X35 ☑
Volcanic eruption (any injury) X35 ☑
Vomitus, gastric contents in air passages (with asphyxia, obstruction or suffocation) T17.81- ☑

W

Walked into stationary object (any) W22.09 ☑
  furniture W22.03 ☑
  lamppost W22.02 ☑
  wall W22.01 ☑
War operations (injuries to military personnel and civilians during war, civil insurrection and peacekeeping missions) (by) (from) (involving) Y36.90 ☑
  after cessation of hostilities Y36.89- ☑
    explosion (of)
      bomb placed during war operations Y36.82- ☑
      mine placed during war operations Y36.81- ☑
    specified NEC Y36.88- ☑
  air blast Y36.20- ☑

War operations — *continued*
  aircraft
    destruction — *see* War operations, destruction of aircraft
    airway restriction — *see* War operations, restriction of airways
    asphyxiation — *see* War operations, restriction of airways
  biological weapons Y36.6X- ☑
  blast Y36.20- ☑
  blast fragments Y36.20- ☑
  blast wave Y36.20- ☑
  blast wind Y36.20- ☑
  bomb Y36.20- ☑
    dirty Y36.50- ☑
    gasoline Y36.31- ☑
    incendiary Y36.31- ☑
    petrol Y36.31- ☑
  bullet Y36.43- ☑
    incendiary Y36.32- ☑
    rubber Y36.41- ☑
  chemical weapons Y36.7X- ☑
  combat
    hand to hand (unarmed) combat Y36.44- ☑
    using blunt or piercing object Y36.45- ☑
  conflagration — *see* War operations, fire
  conventional warfare NEC Y36.0̸1- ☑
  depth-charge Y36.0̸1- ☑
  destruction of aircraft Y36.10̸- ☑
    due to
      air to air missile Y36.11- ☑
      collision with other aircraft Y36.12- ☑
      detonation (accidental) of onboard munitions and explosives Y36.14- ☑
      enemy fire or explosives Y36.11- ☑
      explosive placed on aircraft Y36.11- ☑
      onboard fire Y36.13- ☑
      rocket propelled grenade [RPG] Y36.11- ☑
      small arms fire Y36.11- ☑
      surface to air missile Y36.11- ☑
    specified NEC Y36.19- ☑
  detonation (accidental) of
    onboard marine weapons Y36.0̸5- ☑
    own munitions or munitions launch device Y36.24- ☑
  dirty bomb Y36.50̸- ☑
  explosion (of) Y36.20̸- ☑
    aerial bomb Y36.21- ☑
    after cessation of hostilities
      bomb placed during war operations Y36.82- ☑
      mine placed during war operations Y36.81- ☑

War operations — *continued*
  explosion — *continued*
    bomb NOS — *see also* War operations, bomb(s) Y36.20̸- ☑
    fragments Y36.20̸- ☑
    grenade Y36.29- ☑
    guided missile Y36.22- ☑
    improvised explosive device [IED] (person-borne) (roadside) (vehicle-borne) Y36.23- ☑
    land mine Y36.29- ☑
    marine mine (at sea) (in harbor) Y36.0̸2- ☑
    marine weapon Y36.0̸0̸- ☑
      specified NEC Y36.0̸9- ☑
    own munitions or munitions launch device (accidental) Y36.24- ☑
    sea-based artillery shell Y36.0̸3- ☑
    specified NEC Y36.29- ☑
    torpedo Y36.0̸4- ☑
  fire Y36.30̸- ☑
    specified NEC Y36.39- ☑
  firearms
    discharge Y36.43- ☑
    pellets Y36.42- ☑
  flamethrower Y36.33- ☑
  fragments (from) (of)
    improvised explosive device [IED] (person-borne) (roadside) (vehicle-borne) Y36.26- ☑
    munitions Y36.25- ☑
    specified NEC Y36.29- ☑
    weapons Y36.27- ☑
  friendly fire Y36.92
  hand to hand (unarmed) combat Y36.44- ☑
  hot substances — *see* War operations, fire
  incendiary bullet Y36.32- ☑
  nuclear weapon (effects of) Y36.50̸- ☑
    acute radiation exposure Y36.54- ☑
    blast pressure Y36.51- ☑
    direct blast Y36.51- ☑
    direct heat Y36.53- ☑
    fallout exposure Y36.54- ☑
    fireball Y36.53- ☑
    indirect blast (struck or crushed by blast debris) (being thrown by blast) Y36.52- ☑
    ionizing radiation (immediate exposure) Y36.54- ☑
    nuclear radiation Y36.54- ☑
    radiation
      ionizing (immediate exposure) Y36.54- ☑
      nuclear Y36.54- ☑
      thermal Y36.53- ☑
    secondary effects Y36.54- ☑

War operations — *continued*
  nuclear weapon — *continued*
    specified NEC Y36.59- ☑
    thermal radiation Y36.53- ☑
  restriction of air (airway)
    intentional Y36.46- ☑
    unintentional Y36.47- ☑
  rubber bullets Y36.41- ☑
  shrapnel NOS Y36.29- ☑
  suffocation — *see* War operations, restriction of airways
  unconventional warfare NEC Y36.7X- ☑
  underwater blast NOS Y36.0̸0̸- ☑
  warfare
    conventional NEC Y36.49- ☑
    unconventional NEC Y36.7X- ☑
  weapon of mass destruction [WMD] Y36.91 ☑
  weapons
    biological weapons Y36.6X- ☑
    chemical Y36.7X- ☑
    nuclear (effects of) Y36.50̸- ☑
      acute radiation exposure Y36.54- ☑
      blast pressure Y36.51- ☑
      direct blast Y36.51- ☑
      direct heat Y36.53- ☑
      fallout exposure Y36.54- ☑
      fireball Y36.53- ☑
      radiation
        ionizing (immediate exposure) Y36.54- ☑
        nuclear Y36.54- ☑
        thermal Y36.53- ☑
      secondary effects Y36.54- ☑
      specified NEC Y36.59- ☑
    of mass destruction [WMD] Y36.91 ☑
Washed
  away by flood — *see* Flood
  off road by storm (transport vehicle) — *see* Forces of nature, cataclysmic storm
Weather exposure NEC — *see* Forces of nature
Weightlessness (causing injury) (effects of) (in spacecraft, real or simulated) X52 ☑
Work related condition Y99.0̸
Wound (accidental) NEC — *see also* Injury X58 ☑
  battle — *see also* War operations Y36.90̸
  gunshot — *see* Discharge, firearm by type
Wreck transport vehicle NEC — *see also* Accident, transport V89.9 ☑
Wrong
  device implanted into correct surgical site Y65.51
  fluid in infusion Y65.1
  patient, procedure performed on Y65.52
  procedure (operation) on correct patient Y65.51

☑ **Additional Character Required — Refer to the Tabular List for Character Selection**

ICD-10-CM Tabular List of Diseases and Injuries

Chapter 1. Certain Infectious and Parasitic Diseases (A00–B99)

Chapter-specific Guidelines with Coding Examples

The chapter-specific guidelines from the ICD-10-CM Official Guidelines for Coding and Reporting have been provided below. Along with these guidelines are coding examples, contained in the shaded boxes, that have been developed to help illustrate the coding and/or sequencing guidance found in these guidelines.

a. Human immunodeficiency virus (HIV) infections

1) Code only confirmed cases

Code only confirmed cases of HIV infection/illness. This is an exception to the hospital inpatient guideline Section II, H.

In this context, "confirmation" does not require documentation of positive serology or culture for HIV; the provider's diagnostic statement that the patient is HIV positive or has an HIV-related illness is sufficient.

> Patient being seen for hypothyroidism with possible HIV infection
>
> **E03.9   Hypothyroidism, unspecified**
>
> *Explanation:* Only the hypothyroidism is coded in this scenario because it has not been confirmed that an HIV infection is present.

2) Selection and sequencing of HIV codes

(a) Patient admitted for HIV-related condition

If a patient is admitted for an HIV-related condition, the principal diagnosis should be B20, Human immunodeficiency virus [HIV] disease followed by additional diagnosis codes for all reported HIV-related conditions.

An exception to this guideline is if the reason for admission is hemolytic-uremic syndrome associated with HIV disease. Assign code D59.31, Infection-associated hemolytic-uremic syndrome, followed by code B20, Human immunodeficiency virus [HIV] disease.

> HIV with CMV
>
> **B20   Human immunodeficiency virus [HIV] disease**
>
> **B25.9   Cytomegaloviral disease, unspecified**
>
> *Explanation:* Cytomegaloviral infection is an HIV related condition, so the HIV diagnosis code is reported first, followed by the code for the CMV.

(b) Patient with HIV disease admitted for unrelated condition

If a patient with HIV disease is admitted for an unrelated condition (such as a traumatic injury), the code for the unrelated condition (e.g., the nature of injury code) should be the principal diagnosis. Other diagnoses would be B20 followed by additional diagnosis codes for all reported HIV-related conditions.

> Sprain of the internal collateral ligament, right ankle; HIV
>
> **S93.491A   Sprain of other ligament of right ankle, initial encounter**
>
> **B20   Human immunodeficiency virus [HIV] disease**
>
> *Explanation:* The ankle sprain is not related to HIV, so it is the first-listed diagnosis code, and HIV is reported secondarily.

(c) Whether the patient is newly diagnosed

Whether the patient is newly diagnosed or has had previous admissions/encounters for HIV conditions is irrelevant to the sequencing decision.

> Newly diagnosed multiple cutaneous Kaposi's sarcoma lesions in previously diagnosed HIV disease
>
> **B20   Human immunodeficiency virus [HIV] disease**
>
> **C46.0   Kaposi's sarcoma of skin**
>
> *Explanation:* Even though the HIV was diagnosed on a previous encounter, it is still sequenced first when coded with an HIV-related condition. Kaposi's sarcoma is an HIV-related condition.

(d) Asymptomatic human immunodeficiency virus

Z21, Asymptomatic human immunodeficiency virus [HIV] infection status, is to be applied when the patient without any documentation of symptoms is listed as being "HIV positive," "known HIV," "HIV test positive," or similar terminology. Do not use this code if the term "AIDS" or "HIV disease" is used or if the patient is treated for any HIV-related illness or is described as having any condition(s) resulting from his/her HIV positive status; use B20 in these cases.

(e) Patients with inconclusive HIV serology

Patients with inconclusive HIV serology, but no definitive diagnosis or manifestations of the illness, may be assigned code R75, Inconclusive laboratory evidence of human immunodeficiency virus [HIV].

(f) Previously diagnosed HIV-related illness

Patients with any known prior diagnosis of an HIV-related illness should be coded to B20. Once a patient has developed an HIV-related illness, the patient should always be assigned code B20 on every subsequent admission/encounter. Patients previously diagnosed with any HIV illness (B20) should never be assigned to R75 or Z21, Asymptomatic human immunodeficiency virus [HIV] infection status.

(g) HIV infection in pregnancy, childbirth and the puerperium

During pregnancy, childbirth or the puerperium, a patient admitted (or presenting for a health care encounter) because of an HIV-related illness should receive a principal diagnosis code of O98.7-, Human immunodeficiency [HIV] disease complicating pregnancy, childbirth and the puerperium, followed by B20 and the code(s) for the HIV-related illness(es). Codes from Chapter 15 always take sequencing priority.

Patients with asymptomatic HIV infection status admitted (or presenting for a health care encounter) during pregnancy, childbirth, or the puerperium should receive codes of O98.7- and Z21.

(h) Encounters for testing for HIV

If a patient is being seen to determine his/her HIV status, use code Z11.4, Encounter for screening for human immunodeficiency virus [HIV]. Use additional codes for any associated high-risk behavior, if applicable.

If a patient with signs or symptoms is being seen for HIV testing, code the signs and symptoms. An additional counseling code Z71.7, Human immunodeficiency virus [HIV] counseling, may be used if counseling is provided during the encounter for the test.

When a patient returns to be informed of his/her HIV test results and the test result is negative, use code Z71.7, Human immunodeficiency virus [HIV] counseling.

If the results are positive, see previous guidelines and assign codes as appropriate.

(i) HIV managed by antiretroviral medication

If a patient with documented HIV disease, **HIV-related illness or AIDS** is currently managed on antiretroviral medications, assign code B20, Human immunodeficiency virus [HIV] disease. Code Z79.899, Other long term (current) drug therapy, may be assigned as an additional code to identify the long-term (current) use of antiretroviral medications.

b. Infectious agents as the cause of diseases classified to other chapters

Certain infections are classified in chapters other than Chapter 1 and no organism is identified as part of the infection code. In these instances, it is necessary to use an additional code from Chapter 1 to identify the organism. A code from category B95, Streptococcus, Staphylococcus, and Enterococcus as the cause of diseases classified to other chapters, B96, Other bacterial agents as the cause of diseases classified to other chapters, or B97, Viral agents as the cause of diseases classified to other chapters, is to be used as an additional code to identify the organism. An instructional note will be found at the infection code advising that an additional organism code is required.

> Acute *E. coli* cystitis
>
> **N30.00   Acute cystitis without hematuria**
>
> **B96.20   Unspecified Escherichia coli [E.coli] as the cause of diseases classified elsewhere**
>
> *Explanation:* An instructional note under the category for the cystitis indicates to code also the specific organism.

c. Infections resistant to antibiotics

Many bacterial infections are resistant to current antibiotics. It is necessary to identify all infections documented as antibiotic resistant. Assign a code from category Z16, Resistance to antimicrobial drugs, following the infection code only if the infection code does not identify drug resistance.

Penicillin-resistant *Streptococcus pneumoniae* pneumonia

J13	Pneumonia due to Streptococcus pneumoniae
Z16.11	Resistance to penicillins

Explanation: Code Z16.11 is assigned as a secondary code to represent the penicillin resistance. This code includes resistance to amoxicillin and ampicillin.

d. Sepsis, severe sepsis, and septic shock

1) Coding of Sepsis and Severe Sepsis

(a) Sepsis

For a diagnosis of sepsis, assign the appropriate code for the underlying systemic infection. If the type of infection or causal organism is not further specified, assign code A41.9, Sepsis, unspecified organism.

A code from subcategory R65.2, Severe sepsis, should not be assigned unless severe sepsis or an associated acute organ dysfunction is documented.

Gram-negative sepsis

A41.50	Gram-negative sepsis, unspecified

Staphylococcal sepsis

A41.2	Sepsis due to unspecified staphylococcus

Explanation: In both examples above the organism causing the sepsis is identified, therefore A41.9 Sepsis, unspecified organism, would not be appropriate as this code would not capture the highest degree of specificity found in the documentation. Do not use an additional code for severe sepsis unless an acute organ dysfunction was also documented as "associated with" or "due to" the sepsis or the sepsis was documented as "severe."

(i) Negative or inconclusive blood cultures and sepsis

Negative or inconclusive blood cultures do not preclude a diagnosis of sepsis in patients with clinical evidence of the condition; however, the provider should be queried.

(ii) Urosepsis

The term urosepsis is a nonspecific term. It is not to be considered synonymous with sepsis. It has no default code in the Alphabetic Index. Should a provider use this term, he/she must be queried for clarification.

(iii) Sepsis with organ dysfunction

If a patient has sepsis and associated acute organ dysfunction or multiple organ dysfunction (MOD), follow the instructions for coding severe sepsis.

(iv) Acute organ dysfunction that is not clearly associated with the sepsis

If a patient has sepsis and an acute organ dysfunction, but the medical record documentation indicates that the acute organ dysfunction is related to a medical condition other than the sepsis, do not assign a code from subcategory R65.2, Severe sepsis. An acute organ dysfunction must be associated with the sepsis in order to assign the severe sepsis code. If the documentation is not clear as to whether an acute organ dysfunction is related to the sepsis or another medical condition, query the provider.

Sepsis and acute respiratory failure due to COPD exacerbation

A41.9	Sepsis, unspecified organism
J44.1	Chronic obstructive pulmonary disease with (acute) exacerbation
J96.00	Acute respiratory failure, unspecified whether with hypoxia or hypercapnia

Explanation: Although acute organ dysfunction is present in the form of acute respiratory failure, severe sepsis (R65.2) is not coded in this example, as the acute respiratory failure is attributed to the COPD exacerbation rather than the sepsis. Sequencing of these codes would be determined by the reason for the encounter.

(b) Severe sepsis

The coding of severe sepsis requires a minimum of 2 codes: first a code for the underlying systemic infection, followed by a code from subcategory R65.2, Severe sepsis. If the causal organism is not documented, assign code A41.9, Sepsis, unspecified organism, for the infection. Additional code(s) for the associated acute organ dysfunction are also required.

Due to the complex nature of severe sepsis, some cases may require querying the provider prior to assignment of the codes.

2) Septic shock

Septic shock generally refers to circulatory failure associated with severe sepsis, and therefore, it represents a type of acute organ dysfunction.

For cases of septic shock, the code for the systemic infection should be sequenced first, followed by code R65.21, Severe sepsis with septic shock or code T81.12, Postprocedural septic shock. Any additional codes for the other acute organ dysfunctions should also be assigned. As noted in the sequencing instructions in the Tabular List, the code for septic shock cannot be assigned as a principal diagnosis.

Sepsis with septic shock

A41.9	Sepsis, unspecified organism
R65.21	Severe sepsis with septic shock

Explanation: Documentation of septic shock automatically implies severe sepsis as it is a form of acute organ dysfunction. Septic shock is not coded as the first-listed diagnosis; it is always preceded by the code for the systemic infection.

3) Sequencing of severe sepsis

If severe sepsis is present on admission, and meets the definition of principal diagnosis, the underlying systemic infection should be assigned as principal diagnosis followed by the appropriate code from subcategory R65.2 as required by the sequencing rules in the Tabular List. A code from subcategory R65.2 can never be assigned as a principal diagnosis.

When severe sepsis develops during an encounter (it was not present on admission), the underlying systemic infection and the appropriate code from subcategory R65.2 should be assigned as secondary diagnoses.

Severe sepsis may be present on admission, but the diagnosis may not be confirmed until sometime after admission. If the documentation is not clear whether severe sepsis was present on admission, the provider should be queried.

For infection-associated hemolytic-uremic syndrome with severe sepsis, see guideline I.C.1.d.9.

4) Sepsis or severe sepsis with a localized infection

If the reason for admission is sepsis or severe sepsis and a localized infection, such as pneumonia or cellulitis, a code(s) for the underlying systemic infection should be assigned first and the code for the localized infection should be assigned as a secondary diagnosis. If the patient has severe sepsis, a code from subcategory R65.2 should also be assigned as a secondary diagnosis. If the patient is admitted with a localized infection, such as pneumonia, and sepsis/severe sepsis doesn't develop until after admission, the localized infection should be assigned first, followed by the appropriate sepsis/severe sepsis codes.

For hemolytic-uremic syndrome associated with sepsis, see guideline I. C.1.d.9.

Patient presents with acute renal failure due to severe sepsis from *Pseudomonas pneumonia*

A41.52	Sepsis due to Pseudomonas
J15.1	Pneumonia due to Pseudomonas
R65.20	Severe sepsis without septic shock
N17.9	Acute kidney failure, unspecified

Explanation: If all conditions are present, the systemic infection (sepsis) is sequenced first followed by the codes for the localized infection (pneumonia), severe sepsis and any organ dysfunction.

5) Sepsis due to a postprocedural infection

(a) Documentation of causal relationship

As with all postprocedural complications, code assignment is based on the provider's documentation of the relationship between the infection and the procedure.

(b) Sepsis due to a postprocedural infection

For infections following a procedure, a code from T81.40, to T81.43 Infection following a procedure, or a code from O86.00 to O86.03, Infection of obstetric surgical wound, that identifies the site of the infection should be coded first, if known. Assign an additional code for sepsis following a procedure (T81.44) or sepsis following an obstetrical procedure (O86.04). Use an additional code to identify the infectious agent. If the patient has severe sepsis, the appropriate code from subcategory R65.2 should also be assigned with the additional code(s) for any acute organ dysfunction.

For infections following infusion, transfusion, therapeutic injection, or immunization, a code from subcategory T80.2, Infections following infusion, transfusion, and therapeutic injection, or code T88.0-,

Infection following immunization, should be coded first, followed by the code for the specific infection. If the patient has severe sepsis, the appropriate code from subcategory R65.2 should also be assigned, with the additional codes(s) for any acute organ dysfunction.

(c) Postprocedural infection and postprocedural septic shock

If a postprocedural infection has resulted in postprocedural septic shock, assign the codes indicated above for sepsis due to a postprocedural infection, followed by code T81.12-, Postprocedural septic shock. Do not assign code R65.21, Severe sepsis with septic shock. Additional code(s) should be assigned for any acute organ dysfunction.

6) Sepsis and severe sepsis associated with a noninfectious process (condition)

In some cases, a noninfectious process (condition) such as trauma, may lead to an infection which can result in sepsis or severe sepsis. If sepsis or severe sepsis is documented as associated with a noninfectious condition, such as a burn or serious injury, and this condition meets the definition for principal diagnosis, the code for the noninfectious condition should be sequenced first, followed by the code for the resulting infection. If severe sepsis is present, a code from subcategory R65.2 should also be assigned with any associated organ dysfunction(s) codes. It is not necessary to assign a code from subcategory R65.1, Systemic inflammatory response syndrome (SIRS) of non-infectious origin, for these cases.

If the infection meets the definition of principal diagnosis, it should be sequenced before the non-infectious condition. When both the associated non-infectious condition and the infection meet the definition of principal diagnosis, either may be assigned as principal diagnosis.

Only one code from category R65, Symptoms and signs specifically associated with systemic inflammation and infection, should be assigned. Therefore, when a non-infectious condition leads to an infection resulting in severe sepsis, assign the appropriate code from subcategory R65.2, Severe sepsis. Do not additionally assign a code from subcategory R65.1, Systemic inflammatory response syndrome (SIRS) of non-infectious origin.

See Section I.C.18. SIRS due to non-infectious process

7) Sepsis and septic shock complicating abortion, pregnancy, childbirth, and the puerperium

See Section I.C.15. Sepsis and septic shock complicating abortion, pregnancy, childbirth and the puerperium

8) Newborn sepsis

See Section I.C.16. f. Bacterial sepsis of Newborn

9) Hemolytic-uremic syndrome associated with sepsis

If the reason for admission is hemolytic-uremic syndrome that is associated with sepsis, assign code D59.31, Infection-associated hemolytic-uremic syndrome, as the principal diagnosis. Codes for the underlying systemic infection and any other conditions (such as severe sepsis) should be assigned as secondary diagnoses.

e. Methicillin resistant Staphylococcus aureus (MRSA) conditions

1) Selection and sequencing of MRSA codes

(a) Combination codes for MRSA infection

When a patient is diagnosed with an infection that is due to methicillin resistant *Staphylococcus aureus* (MRSA), and that infection has a combination code that includes the causal organism (e.g., sepsis, pneumonia) assign the appropriate combination code for the condition (e.g., code A41.02, Sepsis due to Methicillin resistant Staphylococcus aureus or code J15.212, Pneumonia due to Methicillin resistant Staphylococcus aureus). Do not assign code B95.62, Methicillin resistant Staphylococcus aureus infection as the cause of diseases classified elsewhere, as an additional code, because the combination code includes the type of infection and the MRSA organism. Do not assign a code from subcategory Z16.11, Resistance to penicillins, as an additional diagnosis.

See Section C.1. for instructions on coding and sequencing of sepsis and severe sepsis.

(b) Other codes for MRSA infection

When there is documentation of a current infection (e.g., wound infection, stitch abscess, urinary tract infection) due to MRSA, and that infection does not have a combination code that includes the causal organism, assign the appropriate code to identify the condition along with code B95.62, Methicillin resistant Staphylococcus aureus infection as the cause of diseases classified elsewhere for the MRSA infection. Do not assign a code from subcategory Z16.11, Resistance to penicillins.

(c) Methicillin susceptible Staphylococcus aureus (MSSA) and MRSA colonization

The condition or state of being colonized or carrying MSSA or MRSA is called colonization or carriage, while an individual person is described as being colonized or being a carrier.

Colonization means that MSSA or MSRA is present on or in the body without necessarily causing illness. A positive MRSA colonization test might be documented by the provider as "MRSA screen positive" or "MRSA nasal swab positive".

Assign code Z22.322, Carrier or suspected carrier of Methicillin resistant Staphylococcus aureus, for patients documented as having MRSA colonization. Assign code Z22.321, Carrier or suspected carrier of Methicillin susceptible Staphylococcus aureus, for patients documented as having MSSA colonization. Colonization is not necessarily indicative of a disease process or as the cause of a specific condition the patient may have unless documented as such by the provider.

(d) MRSA colonization and infection

If a patient is documented as having both MRSA colonization and infection during a hospital admission, code Z22.322, Carrier or suspected carrier of Methicillin resistant Staphylococcus aureus, and a code for the MRSA infection may both be assigned.

f. Zika virus infections

1) Code only confirmed cases

Code only a confirmed diagnosis of Zika virus (A92.5, Zika virus disease) as documented by the provider. This is an exception to the hospital inpatient guideline Section II, H. In this context, "confirmation" does not require documentation of the type of test performed; the provider's diagnostic statement that the condition is confirmed is sufficient. This code should be assigned regardless of the stated mode of transmission.

If the provider documents "suspected", "possible" or "probable" Zika, do not assign code A92.5. Assign a code(s) explaining the reason for encounter (such as fever, rash, or joint pain) or Z20.821, Contact with and (suspected) exposure to Zika virus.

g. Coronavirus infections

1) COVID-19 infection (infection due to SARS-CoV-2)

(a) Code only confirmed cases

Code only a confirmed diagnosis of the 2019 novel coronavirus disease (COVID-19) as documented by the provider, or documentation of a positive COVID-19 test result. For a confirmed diagnosis, assign code U07.1, COVID-19. This is an exception to the hospital inpatient guideline Section II, H. In this context, "confirmation" does not require documentation of a positive test result for COVID-19; the provider's documentation that the individual has COVID-19 is sufficient.

> Physician documentation states the patient has tested positive for the 2019 novel coronavirus disease.
>
> **U07.1**   **COVID-19**
>
> *Explanation*: The type of test is not required; physician documentation that states the patient has COVID-19 or a documented positive COVID-19 test result is sufficient.

If the provider documents "suspected," "possible," "probable," or "inconclusive" COVID-19, do not assign code U07.1. Instead, code the signs and symptoms reported. See guideline I.C.1.g.1.g.

> Patient presents with cough and a slight fever and fear they were exposed to the coronavirus. The provider documents cough, temperature of 99.4, lungs clear, rule out COVID-19.
>
> **R50.9**   **Fever, unspecified**
>
> **R05.9**   **Cough, unspecified**
>
> **Z20.822**   **Contact with and (suspected) exposure to COVID-19**
>
> *Explanation*: For patients who have been exposed or fear they have been exposed to coronavirus, report codes for signs and symptoms, followed by the Z code. Report U07.1 COVID-19, only when the diagnosis is confirmed through provider documentation or a documented positive test result.

(b) Sequencing of codes

When COVID-19 meets the definition of principal diagnosis, code U07.1, COVID-19, should be sequenced first, followed by the appropriate codes for associated manifestations, except when another guideline requires that certain codes be sequenced first, such as obstetrics, sepsis, or transplant complications.

For a COVID-19 infection that progresses to sepsis, see Section I.C.1.d. Sepsis, Severe Sepsis, and Septic Shock

See Section I.C.15.s. for COVID-19 infection in pregnancy, childbirth, and the puerperium

See Section I.C.16.h. for COVID-19 infection in newborn

For a COVID-19 infection in a lung transplant patient, see Section I.C.1g.3.a. Transplant complications other than kidney.

(c) Acute respiratory manifestations of COVID-19

When the reason for the encounter/admission is a respiratory manifestation of COVID-19, assign code U07.1, COVID-19, as the principal/first-listed diagnosis and assign code(s) for the respiratory manifestation(s) as additional diagnoses.

The following conditions are examples of common respiratory manifestations of COVID-19.

(i) Pneumonia

For a patient with pneumonia confirmed as due to COVID-19, assign codes U07.1, COVID-19, and J12.82, Pneumonia due to coronavirus disease 2019.

(ii) Acute bronchitis

For a patient with acute bronchitis confirmed as due to COVID-19, assign codes U07.1, and J20.8, Acute bronchitis due to other specified organisms.

Bronchitis not otherwise specified (NOS) due to COVID-19 should be coded using code U07.1 and J40, Bronchitis, not specified as acute or chronic.

(iii) Lower respiratory infection

If the COVID-19 is documented as being associated with a lower respiratory infection, not otherwise specified (NOS), or an acute respiratory infection, NOS, codes U07.1 and J22, Unspecified acute lower respiratory infection, should be assigned.

If the COVID-19 is documented as being associated with a respiratory infection, NOS, codes U07.1 and J98.8, Other specified respiratory disorders, should be assigned.

(iv) Acute respiratory distress syndrome

For acute respiratory distress syndrome (ARDS) due to COVID-19, assign codes U07.1, and J80, Acute respiratory distress syndrome.

(v) Acute respiratory failure

For acute respiratory failure due to COVID-19, assign code U07.1, and code J96.0-, Acute respiratory failure.

(d) Non-respiratory manifestations of COVID-19

When the reason for the encounter/admission is a non-respiratory manifestation (e.g., viral enteritis) of COVID-19, assign code U07.1, COVID-19, as the principal/first-listed diagnosis and assign code(s) for the manifestation(s) as additional diagnoses.

(e) Exposure to COVID-19

For asymptomatic individuals with actual or suspected exposure to COVID-19, assign code Z20.822, Contact with and (suspected) exposure to COVID-19.

For symptomatic individuals with actual or suspected exposure to COVID-19 and the infection has been ruled out, or test results are inconclusive or unknown, assign code Z20.822, Contact with and (suspected) exposure to COVID-19. See guideline I.C.21.c.1, Contact/Exposure, for additional guidance regarding the use of category Z20 codes.

If COVID-19 is confirmed, see guideline I.C.1.g.1.a.

Patient was exposed to COVID-19 by a family member. They are asymptomatic and their test result is negative.

Z20.822   Contact with and (suspected) exposure to COVID-19

Explanation: Report Z20.822 for patients who have a negative test result but have known exposure to someone who has tested positive for COVID-19.

(f) Screening for COVID-19

During the COVID-19 pandemic, a screening code is generally not appropriate. Do not assign code Z11.52, Encounter for screening for COVID-19. For encounters for COVID-19 testing, including preoperative testing, code as exposure to COVID-19 (guideline I.C.1.g.1.e).

Coding guidance will be updated as new information concerning any changes in the pandemic status becomes available.

(g) Signs and symptoms without definitive diagnosis of COVID-19

For patients presenting with any signs/symptoms associated with COVID-19 (such as fever, etc.) but a definitive diagnosis has not been established, assign the appropriate code(s) for each of the presenting signs and symptoms such as:

- R05.1, Acute cough, or R05.9, Cough, unspecified
- R06.02 Shortness of breath
- R50.9 Fever, unspecified

If a patient with signs/symptoms associated with COVID-19 also has an actual or suspected contact with or exposure to COVID-19, assign Z20.822, Contact with and (suspected) exposure to COVID19, as an additional code.

(h) Asymptomatic individuals who test positive for COVID-19

For asymptomatic individuals who test positive for COVID-19, see guideline I.C.1.g.1.a. Although the individual is asymptomatic, the individual has tested positive and is considered to have the COVID-19 infection.

(i) Personal history of COVID-19

For patients with a history of COVID-19, assign code Z86.16, Personal history of COVID-19.

(j) Follow-up visits after COVID-19 infection has resolved

For individuals who previously had COVID-19, without residual symptom(s) or condition(s), and are being seen for follow-up evaluation, and COVID-19 test results are negative, assign codes Z09, Encounter for follow-up examination after completed treatment for conditions other than malignant neoplasm, and Z86.16, Personal history of COVID-19.

For follow-up visits for individuals with symptom(s) or condition(s) related to a previous COVID-19 infection, see guideline I.C.1.g.1.m.

See Section I.C.21.c.8, Factors influencing health states and contact with health services, Follow-up

(k) Encounter for antibody testing

For an encounter for antibody testing that is not being performed to confirm a current COVID-19 infection, nor is a follow-up test after resolution of COVID-19, assign Z01.84, Encounter for antibody response examination.

Follow the applicable guidelines above if the individual is being tested to confirm a current COVID-19 infection.

For follow-up testing after a COVID-19 infection, see guideline I.C.1.g.1.j.

(l) Multisystem inflammatory syndrome

For individuals with multisystem inflammatory syndrome (MIS) and COVID-19, assign code U07.1, COVID-19, as the principal/first-listed diagnosis and assign code M35.81, Multisystem inflammatory syndrome, as an additional diagnosis.

If an individual with a history of COVID-19 develops MIS, assign codes M35.81, Multisystem inflammatory syndrome, and U09.9, Post COVID-19 condition, unspecified.

If an individual with a known or suspected exposure to COVID- 19, and no current COVID-19 infection or history of COVID-19, develops MIS, assign codes M35.81, Multisystem inflammatory syndrome, and Z20.822, Contact with and (suspected) exposure to COVID-19.

Additional codes should be assigned for any associated complications of MIS.

(m) Post COVID-19 condition

For sequela of COVID-19, or associated symptoms or conditions that develop following a previous COVID-19 infection, assign a code(s) for the specific symptom(s) or condition(s) related to the previous COVID-19 infection, if known, and code U09.9, Post COVID-19 condition, unspecified.

Code U09.9 should not be assigned for manifestations of an active (current) COVID-19 infection.

If a patient has a condition(s) associated with a previous COVID-19 infection and develops a new active (current) COVID-19 infection, code U09.9 may be assigned in conjunction with code U07.1, COVID-19, to identify that the patient also has a condition(s) associated with a previous COVID-19 infection. Code(s) for the specific condition(s) associated with the previous COVID-19 infection and code(s) for manifestation(s) of the new active (current) COVID-19 infection should also be assigned.

(n) Underimmunization for COVID-19 Status

Code Z28.310, Unvaccinated for COVID-19, may be assigned when the patient has not received a COVID-19 vaccine of any type. Code Z28.311, Partially vaccinated for COVID-19, may be assigned when the patient has been partially vaccinated for COVID-19 as per the recommendations of the Centers for Disease Control and Prevention (CDC) in place at the time of the encounter. For information, visit the CDC's website https://www.cdc.gov/coronavirus/2019-ncov/vaccines/.

See Section I.B.14. for underimmunization documentation by clinicians other than patient's provider.

Chapter 1. Certain Infectious and Parasitic Diseases (A00-B99)

INCLUDES   diseases generally recognized as communicable or transmissible

Use additional code to identify resistance to antimicrobial drugs (Z16.-)

EXCLUDES 1   *certain localized infections - see body system-related chapters*

EXCLUDES 2   *carrier or suspected carrier of infectious disease (Z22.-)*

infectious and parasitic diseases complicating pregnancy, childbirth and the puerperium (O98.-)

infectious and parasitic diseases specific to the perinatal period (P35-P39)

influenza and other acute respiratory infections (J00-J22)

This chapter contains the following blocks:

A00-A09	Intestinal infectious diseases
A15-A19	Tuberculosis
A20-A28	Certain zoonotic bacterial diseases
A30-A49	Other bacterial diseases
A50-A64	Infections with a predominantly sexual mode of transmission
A65-A69	Other spirochetal diseases
A70-A74	Other diseases caused by chlamydiae
A75-A79	Rickettsioses
A80-A89	Viral and prion infections of the central nervous system
A90-A99	Arthropod-borne viral fevers and viral hemorrhagic fevers
B00-B09	Viral infections characterized by skin and mucous membrane lesions
B10	Other human herpesviruses
B15-B19	Viral hepatitis
B20	Human immunodeficiency virus [HIV] disease
B25-B34	Other viral diseases
B35-B49	Mycoses
B50-B64	Protozoal diseases
B65-B83	Helminthiases
B85-B89	Pediculosis, acariasis and other infestations
B90-B94	Sequelae of infectious and parasitic diseases
B95-B97	Bacterial and viral infectious agents
B99	Other infectious diseases

Intestinal infectious diseases (A00-A09)

✓4ᵗʰ **A00 Cholera**

DEF: Acute infection of the bowel due to *Vibrio cholerae* that presents with profuse diarrhea, cramps, and vomiting, resulting in severe dehydration, electrolyte imbalance, and death. It is spread through ingestion of food or water contaminated with feces of infected persons.

  A00.0 Cholera due to Vibrio cholerae 01, biovar cholerae
    Classical cholera

  A00.1 Cholera due to Vibrio cholerae 01, biovar eltor
    Cholera eltor

  A00.9 Cholera, unspecified

✓4ᵗʰ **A01 Typhoid and paratyphoid fevers**

DEF: Typhoid fever: Acute generalized illness caused by *Salmonella typhi*. Clinical features include fever, headache, abdominal pain, cough, toxemia, leukopenia, abnormal pulse, rose spots on the skin, bacteremia, hyperplasia of intestinal lymph nodes, mesenteric lymphadenopathy, and Peyer's patches in the intestines.

DEF: Paratyphoid fever: Prolonged febrile illness, caused by *Salmonella* serotypes other than *S. typhi*, especially *S. enterica* serotypes paratyphi A, B, and C.

  ✓5ᵗʰ **A01.0 Typhoid fever**
    Infection due to Salmonella typhi

    A01.00 Typhoid fever, unspecified

    A01.01 Typhoid meningitis   COM

    A01.02 Typhoid fever with heart involvement   COM
      Typhoid endocarditis
      Typhoid myocarditis

    A01.03 Typhoid pneumonia   HCC ESR

    A01.04 Typhoid arthritis   HCC ESR COM

    A01.05 Typhoid osteomyelitis   HCC ESR COM

    A01.09 Typhoid fever with other complications

  A01.1 Paratyphoid fever A

  A01.2 Paratyphoid fever B

  A01.3 Paratyphoid fever C

  A01.4 Paratyphoid fever, unspecified
    Infection due to Salmonella paratyphi NOS

✓4ᵗʰ **A02 Other salmonella infections**

  INCLUDES   infection or foodborne intoxication due to any Salmonella species other than S. typhi and S. paratyphi

  A02.0 Salmonella enteritis
    Salmonellosis
    TIP: Dehydration (E86.0) is a complication of salmonella enteritis and may be reported separately.

  A02.1 Salmonella sepsis   HCC ESR COM

  ✓5ᵗʰ **A02.2 Localized salmonella infections**

    A02.20 Localized salmonella infection, unspecified

    A02.21 Salmonella meningitis   COM

    A02.22 Salmonella pneumonia   HCC ESR

    A02.23 Salmonella arthritis   HCC ESR COM

    A02.24 Salmonella osteomyelitis   HCC ESR COM

    A02.25 Salmonella pyelonephritis
      Salmonella tubulo-interstitial nephropathy

    A02.29 Salmonella with other localized infection

  A02.8 Other specified salmonella infections

  A02.9 Salmonella infection, unspecified

✓4ᵗʰ **A03 Shigellosis**

DEF: Infection caused by the genus *Shigella*, of the family *Enterobacteriaceae* that is known to cause an acute dysenteric infection of the bowel with fever, drowsiness, anorexia, nausea, vomiting, bloody diarrhea, abdominal cramps, and distention.

  A03.0 Shigellosis due to Shigella dysenteriae
    Group A shigellosis [Shiga-Kruse dysentery]

  A03.1 Shigellosis due to Shigella flexneri
    Group B shigellosis

  A03.2 Shigellosis due to Shigella boydii
    Group C shigellosis

  A03.3 Shigellosis due to Shigella sonnei
    Group D shigellosis

  A03.8 Other shigellosis

  A03.9 Shigellosis, unspecified
    Bacillary dysentery NOS

✓4ᵗʰ **A04 Other bacterial intestinal infections**

  EXCLUDES 1   *bacterial foodborne intoxications, NEC (A05.-)*
         tuberculous enteritis (A18.32)

DEF: *Escherichia coli*: Gram-negative, anaerobic bacteria of the family *Enterobacteriaceae* found in the large intestine of warm-blooded animals, generally as a nonpathologic entity aiding in digestion. They become pathogenic when an opportunity to grow somewhere outside this relationship presents itself, such as ingestion of fecal-contaminated food or water.

  A04.0 Enteropathogenic Escherichia coli infection

  A04.1 Enterotoxigenic Escherichia coli infection

  A04.2 Enteroinvasive Escherichia coli infection

  A04.3 Enterohemorrhagic Escherichia coli infection
    DEF: *E. coli* infection penetrating the intestinal mucosa, producing microscopic ulceration and bleeding.

  A04.4 Other intestinal Escherichia coli infections
    Escherichia coli enteritis NOS

  A04.5 Campylobacter enteritis
    TIP: For Guillain-Barre syndrome occurring as a sequela of *Campylobacter enteritis*, assign code G61.0 as the first-listed diagnosis followed by B94.8 for the sequelae.

  A04.6 Enteritis due to Yersinia enterocolitica
    EXCLUDES 1   *extraintestinal yersiniosis (A28.2)*

  ✓5ᵗʰ **A04.7 Enterocolitis due to Clostridium difficile**
    Foodborne intoxication by Clostridium difficile
    Pseudomembranous colitis
    AHA: 2017,4Q,4

    A04.71 Enterocolitis due to Clostridium difficile, recurrent
      AHA: 2020,1Q,18

    A04.72 Enterocolitis due to Clostridium difficile, not specified as recurrent

  A04.8 Other specified bacterial intestinal infections

  A04.9 Bacterial intestinal infection, unspecified
    Bacterial enteritis NOS

✓ Additional Character Required   ✓x7ᵗʰ Placeholder Alert   Manifestation   Unspecified Dx   Q QPP   UPD Unacceptable PDx

Chapter 1. Certain Infectious and Parasitic Diseases

✓4ᵗʰ **A05** **Other bacterial foodborne intoxications, not elsewhere classified**

EXCLUDES 1   Clostridium difficile foodborne intoxication and infection (A04.7-)

Escherichia coli infection (A04.0-A04.4)

listeriosis (A32.-)

salmonella foodborne intoxication and infection (A02.-)

toxic effect of noxious foodstuffs (T61-T62)

A05.0 **Foodborne staphylococcal intoxication**

TIP: Assign code A04.8 to report a staphylococcal infection when it is caused by the ingestion of contaminated food but not caused by S. aureus toxins.

A05.1 **Botulism food poisoning**

Botulism NOS

Classical foodborne intoxication due to Clostridium botulinum

EXCLUDES 1   infant botulism (A48.51)

wound botulism (A48.52)

DEF: Muscle-paralyzing neurotoxic disease caused by ingesting pre-formed toxin from the bacterium Clostridium botulinum. It causes vomiting and diarrhea, vision problems, slurred speech, difficulty swallowing, paralysis, and death.

A05.2 **Foodborne Clostridium perfringens [Clostridium welchii] intoxication**

Enteritis necroticans

Pig-bel

A05.3 **Foodborne Vibrio parahaemolyticus intoxication**

A05.4 **Foodborne Bacillus cereus intoxication**

A05.5 **Foodborne Vibrio vulnificus intoxication**

A05.8 **Other specified bacterial foodborne intoxications**

A05.9 **Bacterial foodborne intoxication, unspecified**

✓4ᵗʰ **A06** **Amebiasis**

INCLUDES   infection due to Entamoeba histolytica

EXCLUDES 1   other protozoal intestinal diseases (A07.-)

EXCLUDES 2   acanthamebiasis (B60.1-)

Naegleriasis (B60.2)

DEF: Infection with a single cell protozoan known as the amoeba. Transmission occurs through ingestion of feces, contaminated food or water, use of human feces as fertilizer, or person-to-person contact.

A06.0 **Acute amebic dysentery**

Acute amebiasis

Intestinal amebiasis NOS

A06.1 **Chronic intestinal amebiasis**

A06.2 **Amebic nondysenteric colitis**

A06.3 **Ameboma of intestine**

Ameboma NOS

A06.4 **Amebic liver abscess**   COM

Hepatic amebiasis

A06.5 **Amebic lung abscess**   HCC ESR COM

Amebic abscess of lung (and liver)

A06.6 **Amebic brain abscess**   COM

Amebic abscess of brain (and liver) (and lung)

A06.7 **Cutaneous amebiasis**

✓5ᵗʰ **A06.8** **Amebic infection of other sites**

A06.81 **Amebic cystitis**

A06.82 **Other amebic genitourinary infections**

Amebic balanitis

Amebic vesiculitis

Amebic vulvovaginitis

A06.89 **Other amebic infections**

Amebic appendicitis

Amebic splenic abscess

A06.9 **Amebiasis, unspecified**

✓4ᵗʰ **A07** **Other protozoal intestinal diseases**

DEF: Protozoa: Group comprised of the simplest, single celled organisms, ranging in size from micro to macroscopic. They can live alone or in colonies, and do not show any differentiation in tissues. Most are motile and can live free in nature, but some are parasitic, causing disease in the variety of hosts they inhabit.

A07.0 **Balantidiasis**

Balantidial dysentery

A07.1 **Giardiasis [lambliasis]**

DEF: Infection caused by the flagellate protozoan Giardia lamblia causing gastrointestinal problems such as vomiting, chronic diarrhea, and weight loss. The most common parasite in the U.S., this is usually transmitted by ingesting contaminated water while in the cyst state, after which it latches onto the wall of the small intestine.

A07.2 **Cryptosporidiosis**   HCC Rx ESR COM

DEF: Microscopic parasite found in water and one of the most common causes of waterborne gastrointestinal infectious disease in the United States. It is usually transmitted by ingesting contaminated drinking water or recreational water and causes profuse watery diarrhea, flatulence, abdominal pain, and cramping.

A07.3 **Isosporiasis**

Infection due to Isospora belli and Isospora hominis

Intestinal coccidiosis

Isosporosis

A07.4 **Cyclosporiasis**

A07.8 **Other specified protozoal intestinal diseases**

Intestinal microsporidiosis

Intestinal trichomoniasis

Sarcocystosis

Sarcosporidiosis

A07.9 **Protozoal intestinal disease, unspecified**

Flagellate diarrhea

Protozoal colitis

Protozoal diarrhea

Protozoal dysentery

✓4ᵗʰ **A08** **Viral and other specified intestinal infections**

EXCLUDES 1   influenza with involvement of gastrointestinal tract (J09.X3, J10.2, J11.2)

A08.0 **Rotaviral enteritis**

✓5ᵗʰ **A08.1** **Acute gastroenteropathy due to Norwalk agent and other small round viruses**

A08.11 **Acute gastroenteropathy due to Norwalk agent**

Acute gastroenteropathy due to Norovirus

Acute gastroenteropathy due to Norwalk-like agent

A08.19 **Acute gastroenteropathy due to other small round viruses**

Acute gastroenteropathy due to small round virus [SRV] NOS

A08.2 **Adenoviral enteritis**

✓5ᵗʰ **A08.3** **Other viral enteritis**

A08.31 **Calicivirus enteritis**

A08.32 **Astrovirus enteritis**

A08.39 **Other viral enteritis**

Coxsackie virus enteritis

Echovirus enteritis

Enterovirus enteritis NEC

Torovirus enteritis

A08.4 **Viral intestinal infection, unspecified**

Viral enteritis NOS

Viral gastroenteritis NOS

Viral gastroenteropathy NOS

AHA: 2016,3Q,12

A08.8 **Other specified intestinal infections**

A09 **Infectious gastroenteritis and colitis, unspecified**

Infectious colitis NOS

Infectious enteritis NOS

Infectious gastroenteritis NOS

EXCLUDES 1   colitis NOS (K52.9)

diarrhea NOS (R19.7)

enteritis NOS (K52.9)

gastroenteritis NOS (K52.9)

noninfective gastroenteritis and colitis, unspecified (K52.9)

DEF: Colitis: Inflammation of mucous membranes of the colon.

DEF: Enteritis: Inflammation of mucous membranes of the small intestine.

DEF: Gastroenteritis: Inflammation of mucous membranes of the stomach and intestines.

Tuberculosis (A15-A19)

INCLUDES	infections due to Mycobacterium tuberculosis and Mycobacterium bovis
EXCLUDES 1	congenital tuberculosis (P37.0)
	nonspecific reaction to test for tuberculosis without active tuberculosis (R76.1-)
	pneumoconiosis associated with tuberculosis, any type in A15 (J65)
	positive PPD (R76.11)
	positive tuberculin skin test without active tuberculosis (R76.11)
	sequelae of tuberculosis (B90.-)
	silicotuberculosis (J65)

DEF: Bacterial infection that typically spreads by inhalation of an airborne agent that usually attacks the lungs, but may also affect other organs.

✓4ᵗʰ A15 Respiratory tuberculosis

A15.0 Tuberculosis of lung
Tuberculous bronchiectasis
Tuberculous fibrosis of lung
Tuberculous pneumonia
Tuberculous pneumothorax

Tuberculosis of Lung

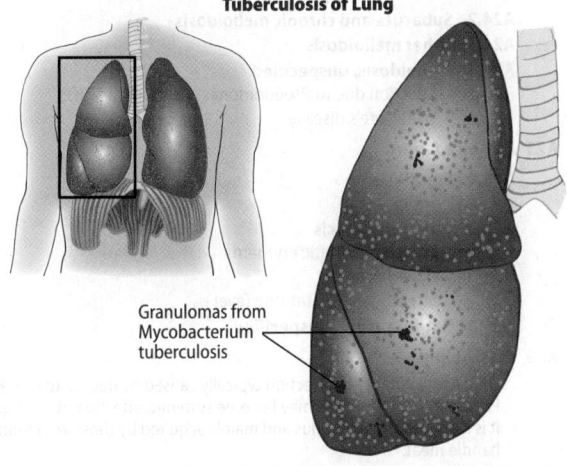

Granulomas from Mycobacterium tuberculosis

A15.4 Tuberculosis of intrathoracic lymph nodes
Tuberculosis of hilar lymph nodes
Tuberculosis of mediastinal lymph nodes
Tuberculosis of tracheobronchial lymph nodes
EXCLUDES 1   tuberculosis specified as primary (A15.7)

A15.5 Tuberculosis of larynx, trachea and bronchus
Tuberculosis of bronchus
Tuberculosis of glottis
Tuberculosis of larynx
Tuberculosis of trachea

A15.6 Tuberculous pleurisy
Tuberculosis of pleura Tuberculous empyema
EXCLUDES 1   primary respiratory tuberculosis (A15.7)

A15.7 Primary respiratory tuberculosis

A15.8 Other respiratory tuberculosis
Mediastinal tuberculosis
Nasopharyngeal tuberculosis
Tuberculosis of nose
Tuberculosis of sinus [any nasal]

A15.9 Respiratory tuberculosis unspecified

✓4ᵗʰ A17 Tuberculosis of nervous system

A17.0 Tuberculous meningitis   COM
Tuberculosis of meninges (cerebral)(spinal)
Tuberculous leptomeningitis
EXCLUDES 1   tuberculous meningoencephalitis (A17.82)

A17.1 Meningeal tuberculoma   COM
Tuberculoma of meninges (cerebral) (spinal)
EXCLUDES 2   tuberculoma of brain and spinal cord (A17.81)

✓5ᵗʰ A17.8 Other tuberculosis of nervous system

    A17.81 Tuberculoma of brain and spinal cord   COM
    Tuberculous abscess of brain and spinal cord

    A17.82 Tuberculous meningoencephalitis   COM
    Tuberculous myelitis

    A17.83 Tuberculous neuritis   COM
    Tuberculous mononeuropathy

    A17.89 Other tuberculosis of nervous system   COM
    Tuberculous polyneuropathy

A17.9 Tuberculosis of nervous system, unspecified   COM

✓4ᵗʰ A18 Tuberculosis of other organs

✓5ᵗʰ A18.0 Tuberculosis of bones and joints

    A18.01 Tuberculosis of spine
    Pott's disease or curvature of spine
    Tuberculous arthritis
    Tuberculous osteomyelitis of spine
    Tuberculous spondylitis

    A18.02 Tuberculous arthritis of other joints
    Tuberculosis of hip (joint)
    Tuberculosis of knee (joint)

    A18.03 Tuberculosis of other bones
    Tuberculous mastoiditis
    Tuberculous osteomyelitis

    A18.09 Other musculoskeletal tuberculosis
    Tuberculous myositis
    Tuberculous synovitis
    Tuberculous tenosynovitis

✓5ᵗʰ A18.1 Tuberculosis of genitourinary system

    A18.10 Tuberculosis of genitourinary system, unspecified
    A18.11 Tuberculosis of kidney and ureter
    A18.12 Tuberculosis of bladder
    A18.13 Tuberculosis of other urinary organs
    Tuberculous urethritis
    A18.14 Tuberculosis of prostate   A ♂
    A18.15 Tuberculosis of other male genital organs   ♂
    A18.16 Tuberculosis of cervix   ♀
    A18.17 Tuberculous female pelvic inflammatory disease   ♀
    Tuberculous endometritis
    Tuberculous oophoritis and salpingitis

    A18.18 Tuberculosis of other female genital organs   ♀
    Tuberculous ulceration of vulva

A18.2 Tuberculous peripheral lymphadenopathy
Tuberculous adenitis
EXCLUDES 2   tuberculosis of bronchial and mediastinal lymph nodes (A15.4)
        tuberculosis of mesenteric and retroperitoneal lymph nodes (A18.39)
        tuberculous tracheobronchial adenopathy (A15.4)

✓5ᵗʰ A18.3 Tuberculosis of intestines, peritoneum and mesenteric glands

    A18.31 Tuberculous peritonitis
    Tuberculous ascites
    DEF: Tuberculous inflammation of the membrane lining the abdomen.

    A18.32 Tuberculous enteritis
    Tuberculosis of anus and rectum
    Tuberculosis of intestine (large) (small)

    A18.39 Retroperitoneal tuberculosis
    Tuberculosis of mesenteric glands
    Tuberculosis of retroperitoneal (lymph glands)

A18.4 Tuberculosis of skin and subcutaneous tissue
Erythema induratum, tuberculous
Lupus excedens
Lupus vulgaris NOS
Lupus vulgaris of eyelid
Scrofuloderma
Tuberculosis of external ear
EXCLUDES 2   lupus erythematosus (L93.-)
        systemic lupus erythematosus (M32.-)

✓5ᵗʰ A18.5 Tuberculosis of eye
EXCLUDES 2   lupus vulgaris of eyelid (A18.4)

    A18.50 Tuberculosis of eye, unspecified
    A18.51 Tuberculous episcleritis
    A18.52 Tuberculous keratitis
    Tuberculous interstitial keratitis
    Tuberculous keratoconjunctivitis (interstitial) (phlyctenular)

    A18.53 Tuberculous chorioretinitis
    A18.54 Tuberculous iridocyclitis
    A18.59 Other tuberculosis of eye
    Tuberculous conjunctivitis

A18.6 Tuberculosis of (inner) (middle) ear
Tuberculous otitis media
EXCLUDES 2   *tuberculosis of external ear (A18.4)*
      tuberculous mastoiditis (A18.03)

A18.7 Tuberculosis of adrenal glands
Tuberculous Addison's disease

✓5ᵗʰ **A18.8 Tuberculosis of other specified organs**

A18.81 Tuberculosis of thyroid gland

A18.82 Tuberculosis of other endocrine glands
Tuberculosis of pituitary gland
Tuberculosis of thymus gland

A18.83 Tuberculosis of digestive tract organs, not elsewhere classified
EXCLUDES 1   *tuberculosis of intestine (A18.32)*

A18.84 Tuberculosis of heart
Tuberculous cardiomyopathy
Tuberculous endocarditis
Tuberculous myocarditis
Tuberculous pericarditis

A18.85 Tuberculosis of spleen

A18.89 Tuberculosis of other sites
Tuberculosis of muscle
Tuberculous cerebral arteritis

✓4ᵗʰ **A19 Miliary tuberculosis**
INCLUDES   disseminated tuberculosis
     generalized tuberculosis
     tuberculous polyserositis

A19.0 Acute miliary tuberculosis of a single specified site

A19.1 Acute miliary tuberculosis of multiple sites

A19.2 Acute miliary tuberculosis, unspecified

A19.8 Other miliary tuberculosis

A19.9 Miliary tuberculosis, unspecified

Certain zoonotic bacterial diseases (A20-A28)

✓4ᵗʰ **A20 Plague**
INCLUDES   infection due to Yersinia pestis

A20.0 Bubonic plague

A20.1 Cellulocutaneous plague

A20.2 Pneumonic plague   HCC ESR

A20.3 Plague meningitis   COM

A20.7 Septicemic plague   HCC ESR COM

A20.8 Other forms of plague
Abortive plague
Asymptomatic plague
Pestis minor

A20.9 Plague, unspecified

✓4ᵗʰ **A21 Tularemia**
INCLUDES   deer-fly fever
     infection due to Francisella tularensis
     rabbit fever
DEF: Febrile disease transmitted to humans by the bites of deer flies, fleas, and ticks, by inhaling aerosolized *F. tularensis*, or by ingesting contaminated food or water. Patients quickly develop fever, chills, weakness, headache, backache, and malaise.

A21.0 Ulceroglandular tularemia

A21.1 Oculoglandular tularemia
Ophthalmic tularemia

A21.2 Pulmonary tularemia   HCC ESR

A21.3 Gastrointestinal tularemia
Abdominal tularemia

A21.7 Generalized tularemia

A21.8 Other forms of tularemia

A21.9 Tularemia, unspecified

✓4ᵗʰ **A22 Anthrax**
INCLUDES   infection due to Bacillus anthracis

A22.0 Cutaneous anthrax
Malignant carbuncle
Malignant pustule

A22.1 Pulmonary anthrax   HCC ESR
Inhalation anthrax
Ragpicker's disease
Woolsorter's disease

A22.2 Gastrointestinal anthrax

A22.7 Anthrax sepsis   HCC ESR COM

A22.8 Other forms of anthrax
Anthrax meningitis

A22.9 Anthrax, unspecified

✓4ᵗʰ **A23 Brucellosis**
INCLUDES   Malta fever
     Mediterranean fever
     undulant fever

A23.0 Brucellosis due to Brucella melitensis

A23.1 Brucellosis due to Brucella abortus

A23.2 Brucellosis due to Brucella suis

A23.3 Brucellosis due to Brucella canis

A23.8 Other brucellosis

A23.9 Brucellosis, unspecified

✓4ᵗʰ **A24 Glanders and melioidosis**

A24.0 Glanders
Infection due to Pseudomonas mallei
Malleus

A24.1 Acute and fulminating melioidosis
Melioidosis pneumonia
Melioidosis sepsis

A24.2 Subacute and chronic melioidosis

A24.3 Other melioidosis

A24.9 Melioidosis, unspecified
Infection due to Pseudomonas pseudomallei NOS
Whitmore's disease

✓4ᵗʰ **A25 Rat-bite fevers**

A25.0 Spirillosis
Sodoku

A25.1 Streptobacillosis
Epidemic arthritic erythema
Haverhill fever
Streptobacillary rat-bite fever

A25.9 Rat-bite fever, unspecified

✓4ᵗʰ **A26 Erysipeloid**
DEF: Acute cutaneous infection typically caused by trauma to the skin. Presenting as cellulitis, it may become systemic, affecting other organs. It is a gram-positive bacillus and mainly acquired by those who routinely handle meat.

A26.0 Cutaneous erysipeloid
Erythema migrans

A26.7 Erysipelothrix sepsis   HCC ESR COM

A26.8 Other forms of erysipeloid

A26.9 Erysipeloid, unspecified

✓4ᵗʰ **A27 Leptospirosis**

A27.0 Leptospirosis icterohemorrhagica
Leptospiral or spirochetal jaundice (hemorrhagic)
Weil's disease

✓5ᵗʰ **A27.8 Other forms of leptospirosis**

A27.81 Aseptic meningitis in leptospirosis   COM

A27.89 Other forms of leptospirosis

A27.9 Leptospirosis, unspecified

✓4ᵗʰ **A28 Other zoonotic bacterial diseases, not elsewhere classified**

A28.0 Pasteurellosis

A28.1 Cat-scratch disease
Cat-scratch fever

A28.2 Extraintestinal yersiniosis
EXCLUDES 1   *enteritis due to Yersinia enterocolitica (A04.6)*
     plague (A20.-)

A28.8 Other specified zoonotic bacterial diseases, not elsewhere classified

A28.9 Zoonotic bacterial disease, unspecified

Other bacterial diseases (A30-A49)

AHA: 2016,3Q,8-14

✓4ᵗʰ **A30 Leprosy [Hansen's disease]**
INCLUDES   infection due to Mycobacterium leprae
EXCLUDES 1   *sequelae of leprosy (B92)*

A30.0 Indeterminate leprosy
I leprosy

A30.1 Tuberculoid leprosy
TT leprosy

A30.2 **Borderline tuberculoid leprosy**
BT leprosy

A30.3 **Borderline leprosy**
BB leprosy

A30.4 **Borderline lepromatous leprosy**
BL leprosy

A30.5 **Lepromatous leprosy**
LL leprosy

A30.8 **Other forms of leprosy**

A30.9 **Leprosy, unspecified**

✓4th **A31** **Infection due to other mycobacteria**
EXCLUDES 2   *leprosy (A30.-)*
tuberculosis (A15-A19)

A31.0 **Pulmonary mycobacterial infection**   HCC Rx ESR COM
Infection due to Mycobacterium avium
Infection due to Mycobacterium intracellulare [Battey bacillus]
Infection due to Mycobacterium kansasii

A31.1 **Cutaneous mycobacterial infection**
Buruli ulcer
Infection due to Mycobacterium marinum
Infection due to Mycobacterium ulcerans

A31.2 **Disseminated mycobacterium avium-intracellulare complex (DMAC)**   HCC Rx ESR COM
MAC sepsis

A31.8 **Other mycobacterial infections**

A31.9 **Mycobacterial infection, unspecified**
Atypical mycobacterial infection NOS
Mycobacteriosis NOS

✓4th **A32** **Listeriosis**
INCLUDES   listerial foodborne infection
EXCLUDES 1   *neonatal (disseminated) listeriosis (P37.2)*

A32.0 **Cutaneous listeriosis**

✓5th **A32.1** **Listerial meningitis and meningoencephalitis**

    A32.11 **Listerial meningitis**   COM

    A32.12 **Listerial meningoencephalitis**   COM

A32.7 **Listerial sepsis**   HCC ESR COM

✓5th **A32.8** **Other forms of listeriosis**

    A32.81 **Oculoglandular listeriosis**

    A32.82 **Listerial endocarditis**   COM

    A32.89 **Other forms of listeriosis**
Listerial cerebral arteritis

A32.9 **Listeriosis, unspecified**

A33 **Tetanus neonatorum**   N

A34 **Obstetrical tetanus**   COM M ♀

A35 **Other tetanus**   COM
Tetanus NOS
EXCLUDES 1   *obstetrical tetanus (A34)*
tetanus neonatorum (A33)
DEF: Tetanus: Acute, often fatal, infectious disease caused by the anaerobic, spore-forming bacillus *Clostridium tetani*. The bacillus enters the body through a contaminated wound, burns, surgical wounds, or cutaneous ulcers. Symptoms include lockjaw, spasms, seizures, and paralysis.

✓4th **A36** **Diphtheria**

A36.0 **Pharyngeal diphtheria**
Diphtheritic membranous angina
Tonsillar diphtheria

A36.1 **Nasopharyngeal diphtheria**

A36.2 **Laryngeal diphtheria**
Diphtheritic laryngotracheitis

A36.3 **Cutaneous diphtheria**
EXCLUDES 2   *erythrasma (L08.1)*

✓5th **A36.8** **Other diphtheria**

    A36.81 **Diphtheritic cardiomyopathy**   HCC Rx ESR COM
Diphtheritic myocarditis

    A36.82 **Diphtheritic radiculomyelitis**

    A36.83 **Diphtheritic polyneuritis**

    A36.84 **Diphtheritic tubulo-interstitial nephropathy**

    A36.85 **Diphtheritic cystitis**

    A36.86 **Diphtheritic conjunctivitis**

    A36.89 **Other diphtheritic complications**
Diphtheritic peritonitis

A36.9 **Diphtheria, unspecified**

✓4th **A37** **Whooping cough**
DEF: Acute, highly contagious respiratory tract infection caused by *Bordetella pertussis* and *B. bronchiseptica*. Whooping cough is known by its characteristic paroxysmal cough.

✓5th **A37.0** **Whooping cough due to Bordetella pertussis**

    A37.00 **Whooping cough due to Bordetella pertussis without pneumonia**
Paroxysmal cough due to Bordetella pertussis without pneumonia

    A37.01 **Whooping cough due to Bordetella pertussis with pneumonia**
Paroxysmal cough due to Bordetella pertussis with pneumonia

✓5th **A37.1** **Whooping cough due to Bordetella parapertussis**

    A37.10 **Whooping cough due to Bordetella parapertussis without pneumonia**

    A37.11 **Whooping cough due to Bordetella parapertussis with pneumonia**

✓5th **A37.8** **Whooping cough due to other Bordetella species**

    A37.80 **Whooping cough due to other Bordetella species without pneumonia**

    A37.81 **Whooping cough due to other Bordetella species with pneumonia**

✓5th **A37.9** **Whooping cough, unspecified species**

    A37.90 **Whooping cough, unspecified species without pneumonia**

    A37.91 **Whooping cough, unspecified species with pneumonia**

✓4th **A38** **Scarlet fever**
INCLUDES   scarlatina
EXCLUDES 2   *streptococcal sore throat (J02.0)*
DEF: Acute contagious disease caused by Group A bacteria, the same bacterium that causes strep throat. Individuals with strep throat can develop scarlet fever particularly if the infection is not treated with antibiotics. It is characterized by a red blush to the skin of the chest and abdomen and swelling of the nose, throat, and mouth.

A38.0 **Scarlet fever with otitis media**

A38.1 **Scarlet fever with myocarditis**   COM

A38.8 **Scarlet fever with other complications**

A38.9 **Scarlet fever, uncomplicated**
Scarlet fever, NOS

✓4th **A39** **Meningococcal infection**
DEF: Condition caused by *Neisseria meningitidis*, a bacteria that may invade the spinal cord, brain, heart, joints, optic nerve, or bloodstream.

A39.0 **Meningococcal meningitis**   COM

A39.1 **Waterhouse-Friderichsen syndrome**   HCC Rx ESR COM
Meningococcal hemorrhagic adrenalitis
Meningococcic adrenal syndrome

A39.2 **Acute meningococcemia**   HCC ESR COM

A39.3 **Chronic meningococcemia**   HCC ESR COM

A39.4 **Meningococcemia, unspecified**   HCC ESR COM

✓5th **A39.5** **Meningococcal heart disease**

    A39.50 **Meningococcal carditis, unspecified**   COM

    A39.51 **Meningococcal endocarditis**   COM

    A39.52 **Meningococcal myocarditis**   COM

    A39.53 **Meningococcal pericarditis**   COM

✓5th **A39.8** **Other meningococcal infections**

    A39.81 **Meningococcal encephalitis**   COM

    A39.82 **Meningococcal retrobulbar neuritis**

    A39.83 **Meningococcal arthritis**   HCC ESR COM

    A39.84 **Postmeningococcal arthritis**   HCC ESR COM

    A39.89 **Other meningococcal infections**
Meningococcal conjunctivitis

A39.9 **Meningococcal infection, unspecified**
Meningococcal disease NOS

Chapter 1. Certain Infectious and Parasitic Diseases

☑4ᵗʰ **A40 Streptococcal sepsis**
Code first:
postprocedural streptococcal sepsis (T81.4-)
streptococcal sepsis during labor (O75.3)
streptococcal sepsis following abortion or ectopic or molar pregnancy (O03-O07, O08.0)
streptococcal sepsis following immunization (T88.0)
streptococcal sepsis following infusion, transfusion or therapeutic injection (T80.2-)
EXCLUDES 1   neonatal (P36.0-P36.1)
     puerperal sepsis (O85)
     sepsis due to Streptococcus, group D (A41.81)
AHA: 2020,2Q,8,28; 2019,4Q,65; 2018,4Q,89; 2018,1Q,16; 2016,1Q,32

A40.0 Sepsis due to streptococcus, group A   HCC ESR COM

A40.1 Sepsis due to streptococcus, group B   HCC ESR COM
AHA: 2019,1Q,14

A40.3 Sepsis due to Streptococcus pneumoniae   HCC ESR COM
Pneumococcal sepsis

A40.8 Other streptococcal sepsis   HCC ESR COM

A40.9 Streptococcal sepsis, unspecified   HCC ESR COM

☑4ᵗʰ **A41 Other sepsis**
Code first:
postprocedural sepsis (T81.4-)
sepsis during labor (O75.3)
sepsis following abortion, ectopic or molar pregnancy (O03-O07, O08.0)
sepsis following immunization (T88.0)
sepsis following infusion, transfusion or therapeutic injection (T80.2-)
EXCLUDES 1   bacteremia NOS (R78.81)
     neonatal (P36.-)
     puerperal sepsis (O85)
     streptococcal sepsis (A40.-)
EXCLUDES 2   sepsis (due to) (in) actinomycotic (A42.7)
     sepsis (due to) (in) anthrax (A22.7)
     sepsis (due to) (in) candidal (B37.7)
     sepsis (due to) (in) Erysipelothrix (A26.7)
     sepsis (due to) (in) extraintestinal yersiniosis (A28.2)
     sepsis (due to) (in) gonococcal (A54.86)
     sepsis (due to) (in) herpesviral (B00.7)
     sepsis (due to) (in) listerial (A32.7)
     sepsis (due to) (in) melioidosis (A24.1)
     sepsis (due to) (in) meningococcal (A39.2-A39.4)
     sepsis (due to) (in) plague (A20.7)
     sepsis (due to) (in) tularemia (A21.7)
     toxic shock syndrome (A48.3)
AHA: 2020,2Q,8,28; 2019,4Q,65; 2019,3Q,17; 2018,4Q,18; 2018,1Q,16; 2016,1Q,32; 2014,2Q,13

☑5ᵗʰ **A41.0 Sepsis due to Staphylococcus aureus**

A41.01 Sepsis due to Methicillin susceptible Staphylococcus aureus   HCC ESR COM
MSSA sepsis
Staphylococcus aureus sepsis NOS
AHA: 2020,2Q,17

A41.02 Sepsis due to Methicillin resistant Staphylococcus aureus   HCC ESR COM

A41.1 Sepsis due to other specified staphylococcus   HCC ESR COM
Coagulase negative staphylococcus sepsis

A41.2 Sepsis due to unspecified staphylococcus   HCC ESR COM

A41.3 Sepsis due to Hemophilus influenzae   HCC ESR COM

A41.4 Sepsis due to anaerobes   HCC ESR COM
EXCLUDES 1   gas gangrene (A48.0)

☑5ᵗʰ **A41.5 Sepsis due to other Gram-negative organisms**

A41.50 Gram-negative sepsis, unspecified   HCC ESR COM
Gram-negative sepsis NOS
AHA: 2020,2Q,28

A41.51 Sepsis due to Escherichia coli [E. coli]   HCC ESR COM
AHA: 2020,2Q,17

A41.52 Sepsis due to Pseudomonas   HCC ESR COM
Pseudomonas aeroginosa

A41.53 Sepsis due to Serratia   HCC ESR COM

A41.59 Other Gram-negative sepsis   HCC ESR COM

☑5ᵗʰ **A41.8 Other specified sepsis**

A41.81 Sepsis due to Enterococcus   HCC ESR COM
TIP: *E. faecium,* is a species of *Enterococcus* that is highly resistant to multiple antibiotics. Assign a code from category Z16 when resistance to antimicrobial drugs is documented.

A41.89 Other specified sepsis   HCC ESR COM
AHA: 2020,2Q,8; 2017,1Q,51; 2016,3Q,8-14

A41.9 Sepsis, unspecified organism   HCC ESR COM
Septicemia NOS
AHA: 2022,2Q,5; 2022,1Q,35; 2020,2Q,28

☑4ᵗʰ **A42 Actinomycosis**
EXCLUDES 1   actinomycetoma (B47.1)

A42.0 Pulmonary actinomycosis   HCC ESR

A42.1 Abdominal actinomycosis

A42.2 Cervicofacial actinomycosis

A42.7 Actinomycotic sepsis   HCC ESR COM

☑5ᵗʰ **A42.8 Other forms of actinomycosis**

A42.81 Actinomycotic meningitis   COM

A42.82 Actinomycotic encephalitis   COM

A42.89 Other forms of actinomycosis

A42.9 Actinomycosis, unspecified

☑4ᵗʰ **A43 Nocardiosis**
DEF: Rare bacterial infection occurring most often in those with weakened immune systems. Can be acquired in soil, decaying plants, or standing water. It typically begins in the lungs and has a tendency to spread to other body systems.

A43.0 Pulmonary nocardiosis   HCC ESR

A43.1 Cutaneous nocardiosis

A43.8 Other forms of nocardiosis

A43.9 Nocardiosis, unspecified

☑4ᵗʰ **A44 Bartonellosis**

A44.0 Systemic bartonellosis
Oroya fever

A44.1 Cutaneous and mucocutaneous bartonellosis
Verruga peruana

A44.8 Other forms of bartonellosis

A44.9 Bartonellosis, unspecified

A46 Erysipelas
EXCLUDES 1   postpartum or puerperal erysipelas (O86.89)
DEF: Skin infection affecting the upper dermis and superficial dermal lymphatics. Lesion edges are well-demarcated with distinct raised borders. It is often caused by group A *Streptococci.*

☑4ᵗʰ **A48 Other bacterial diseases, not elsewhere classified**
EXCLUDES 1   actinomycetoma (B47.1)

A48.0 Gas gangrene   HCC ESR COM
Clostridial cellulitis
Clostridial myonecrosis
AHA: 2017,4Q,102

A48.1 Legionnaires' disease   HCC ESR COM
DEF: Severe and often fatal infection by *Legionella pneumophila.* Symptoms include high fever, gastrointestinal pain, headache, myalgia, dry cough, and pneumonia and it is usually transmitted through airborne water droplets via air conditioning systems or hot tubs.

A48.2 Nonpneumonic Legionnaires' disease [Pontiac fever]

A48.3 Toxic shock syndrome   HCC ESR COM
Use additional code to identify the organism (B95, B96)
EXCLUDES 1   endotoxic shock NOS (R57.8)
     sepsis NOS (A41.9)
AHA: 2022,1Q,35
DEF: Bacteria producing an endotoxin, such as *Staphylococci,* flood the body with the toxins producing a high fever, vomiting and diarrhea, decreasing blood pressure, a skin rash, and shock.
Synonym(s): TSS.

A48.4 Brazilian purpuric fever
Systemic Hemophilus aegyptius infection

☑5ᵗʰ **A48.5 Other specified botulism**
Non-foodborne intoxication due to toxins of Clostridium botulinum [C. botulinum]
EXCLUDES 1   food poisoning due to toxins of Clostridium botulinum (A05.1)

A48.51 Infant botulism   P

A48.52   Wound **botulism**
     Non-foodborne botulism NOS
     Use additional code for associated wound

A48.8   **Other specified bacterial diseases**

✔4ᵗʰ **A49**   **Bacterial infection of unspecified site**
     EXCLUDES 1   *bacterial agents as the cause of diseases classified elsewhere (B95-B96)*
           chlamydial infection NOS (A74.9)
           meningococcal infection NOS (A39.9)
           rickettsial infection NOS (A79.9)
           spirochetal infection NOS (A69.9)

   ✔5ᵗʰ **A49.0**   **Staphylococcal infection, unspecified site**
       A49.01   **Methicillin susceptible Staphylococcus aureus infection, unspecified site**
           Methicillin susceptible Staphylococcus aureus (MSSA) infection
           Staphylococcus aureus infection NOS
       A49.02   **Methicillin resistant Staphylococcus aureus infection, unspecified site**
           Methicillin resistant Staphylococcus aureus (MRSA) infection

   A49.1   **Streptococcal infection, unspecified site**

   A49.2   **Hemophilus influenzae infection, unspecified site**

   A49.3   **Mycoplasma infection, unspecified site**

   A49.8   **Other bacterial infections of unspecified site**

   A49.9   **Bacterial infection, unspecified**
       EXCLUDES 1   *bacteremia NOS (R78.81)*

Infections with a predominantly sexual mode of transmission (A50-A64)

   EXCLUDES 1   *human immunodeficiency virus [HIV] disease (B20)*
           nonspecific and nongonococcal urethritis (N34.1)
           Reiter's disease (M02.3-)

   AHA: 2021,2Q,6

✔4ᵗʰ **A50**   **Congenital syphilis**

   ✔5ᵗʰ **A50.0**   **Early congenital syphilis, symptomatic**
       Any congenital syphilitic condition specified as early or manifest less than two years after birth.
       A50.01   **Early congenital syphilitic oculopathy**
       A50.02   **Early congenital syphilitic osteochondropathy**
       A50.03   **Early congenital syphilitic pharyngitis**
           Early congenital syphilitic laryngitis
       A50.04   **Early congenital syphilitic pneumonia**   COM
       A50.05   **Early congenital syphilitic rhinitis**
       A50.06   **Early cutaneous congenital syphilis**
       A50.07   **Early mucocutaneous congenital syphilis**
       A50.08   **Early visceral congenital syphilis**
       A50.09   **Other early congenital syphilis, symptomatic**

   A50.1   **Early congenital syphilis, latent**
       Congenital syphilis without clinical manifestations, with positive serological reaction and negative spinal fluid test, less than two years after birth.

   A50.2   **Early congenital syphilis, unspecified**
       Congenital syphilis NOS less than two years after birth.

   ✔5ᵗʰ **A50.3**   **Late congenital syphilitic oculopathy**
       EXCLUDES 1   *Hutchinson's triad (A50.53)*
       A50.30   **Late congenital syphilitic oculopathy, unspecified**
       A50.31   **Late congenital syphilitic interstitial keratitis**
       A50.32   **Late congenital syphilitic chorioretinitis**
       A50.39   **Other late congenital syphilitic oculopathy**

   ✔5ᵗʰ **A50.4**   **Late congenital neurosyphilis [juvenile neurosyphilis]**
       Use additional code to identify any associated mental disorder
       EXCLUDES 1   *Hutchinson's triad (A50.53)*
       A50.40   **Late congenital neurosyphilis, unspecified**   COM
           Juvenile neurosyphilis NOS
       A50.41   **Late congenital syphilitic meningitis**   COM
       A50.42   **Late congenital syphilitic encephalitis**   COM
       A50.43   **Late congenital syphilitic polyneuropathy**   COM
       A50.44   **Late congenital syphilitic optic nerve atrophy**   COM
       A50.45   **Juvenile general paresis**   COM
           Dementia paralytica juvenilis
           Juvenile tabetoparetic neurosyphilis

       A50.49   **Other late congenital neurosyphilis**   COM
           Juvenile tabes dorsalis

   ✔5ᵗʰ **A50.5**   **Other late congenital syphilis, symptomatic**
       Any congenital syphilitic condition specified as late or manifest two years or more after birth.
       A50.51   **Clutton's joints**
       A50.52   **Hutchinson's teeth**
       A50.53   **Hutchinson's triad**
       A50.54   **Late congenital cardiovascular syphilis**   COM
       A50.55   **Late congenital syphilitic arthropathy**   HCC ESR COM
       A50.56   **Late congenital syphilitic osteochondropathy**
       A50.57   **Syphilitic saddle nose**
       A50.59   **Other late congenital syphilis, symptomatic**

   A50.6   **Late congenital syphilis, latent**
       Congenital syphilis without clinical manifestations, with positive serological reaction and negative spinal fluid test, two years or more after birth.

   A50.7   **Late congenital syphilis, unspecified**
       Congenital syphilis NOS two years or more after birth.

   A50.9   **Congenital syphilis, unspecified**

✔4ᵗʰ **A51**   **Early syphilis**
     DEF: Syphilis: Sexually transmitted disease caused by the *Treponema pallidum* spirochete. Syphilis usually exhibits cutaneous manifestations and may exist for years without symptoms.

   A51.0   **Primary genital syphilis**
       Syphilitic chancre NOS

   A51.1   **Primary anal syphilis**

   A51.2   **Primary syphilis of other sites**

   ✔5ᵗʰ **A51.3**   **Secondary syphilis of skin and mucous membranes**
       DEF: Transitory or chronic cutaneous eruptions that present within two to 10 weeks following an initial syphilis infection that may include nontender lymphadenopathy along with alopecia and condylomata lata.
       A51.31   **Condyloma latum**
       A51.32   **Syphilitic alopecia**
       A51.39   **Other secondary syphilis of skin**
           Syphilitic leukoderma
           Syphilitic mucous patch
           EXCLUDES 1   *late syphilitic leukoderma (A52.79)*

   ✔5ᵗʰ **A51.4**   **Other secondary syphilis**
       A51.41   **Secondary syphilitic meningitis**   COM
       A51.42   **Secondary syphilitic female pelvic disease**   ♀
       A51.43   **Secondary syphilitic oculopathy**
           Secondary syphilitic chorioretinitis
           Secondary syphilitic iridocyclitis, iritis
           Secondary syphilitic uveitis
       A51.44   **Secondary syphilitic nephritis**
       A51.45   **Secondary syphilitic hepatitis**
       A51.46   **Secondary syphilitic osteopathy**
       A51.49   **Other secondary syphilitic conditions**
           Secondary syphilitic lymphadenopathy
           Secondary syphilitic myositis

   A51.5   **Early syphilis, latent**
       Syphilis (acquired) without clinical manifestations, with positive serological reaction and negative spinal fluid test, less than two years after infection.

   A51.9   **Early syphilis, unspecified**

✔4ᵗʰ **A52**   **Late syphilis**

   ✔5ᵗʰ **A52.0**   **Cardiovascular and cerebrovascular syphilis**
       A52.00   **Cardiovascular syphilis, unspecified**   COM
       A52.01   **Syphilitic aneurysm of aorta**   COM
       A52.02   **Syphilitic aortitis**   COM
       A52.03   **Syphilitic endocarditis**   COM
           Syphilitic aortic valve incompetence or stenosis
           Syphilitic mitral valve stenosis
           Syphilitic pulmonary valve regurgitation
       A52.04   **Syphilitic cerebral arteritis**
       A52.05   **Other cerebrovascular syphilis**   COM
           Syphilitic cerebral aneurysm (ruptured) (non-ruptured)
           Syphilitic cerebral thrombosis

A52.06 **Other syphilitic heart involvement** `COM`
Syphilitic coronary artery disease
Syphilitic myocarditis
Syphilitic pericarditis

A52.09 **Other cardiovascular syphilis** `COM`

✓5ᵗʰ **A52.1** **Symptomatic neurosyphilis**

A52.10 **Symptomatic neurosyphilis, unspecified** `COM`

A52.11 **Tabes dorsalis** `COM`
Locomotor ataxia (progressive)
Tabetic neurosyphilis

A52.12 **Other cerebrospinal syphilis** `COM`

A52.13 **Late syphilitic meningitis** `COM`

A52.14 **Late syphilitic encephalitis** `COM`

A52.15 **Late syphilitic neuropathy** `COM`
Late syphilitic acoustic neuritis
Late syphilitic optic (nerve) atrophy
Late syphilitic polyneuropathy
Late syphilitic retrobulbar neuritis

A52.16 **Charcôt's arthropathy (tabetic)** `COM`
DEF: Progressive neurologic arthropathy in which chronic degeneration of joints in the weight-bearing areas with peripheral hypertrophy occurs as a complication of a neuropathy disorder. Supporting structures relax from a loss of sensation resulting in chronic joint instability.

A52.17 **General paresis** `COM`
Dementia paralytica

A52.19 **Other symptomatic neurosyphilis** `COM`
Syphilitic parkinsonism

A52.2 **Asymptomatic neurosyphilis** `COM`

A52.3 **Neurosyphilis, unspecified** `COM`
Gumma (syphilitic)
Syphilis (late)
Syphiloma
AHA: 2021,2Q,6

✓5ᵗʰ **A52.7** **Other symptomatic late syphilis**

A52.71 **Late syphilitic oculopathy**
Late syphilitic chorioretinitis
Late syphilitic episcleritis

A52.72 **Syphilis of lung and bronchus**

A52.73 **Symptomatic late syphilis of other respiratory organs**

A52.74 **Syphilis of liver and other viscera**
Late syphilitic peritonitis

A52.75 **Syphilis of kidney and ureter**
Syphilitic glomerular disease

A52.76 **Other genitourinary symptomatic late syphilis**
Late syphilitic female pelvic inflammatory disease

A52.77 **Syphilis of bone and joint**

A52.78 **Syphilis of other musculoskeletal tissue**
Late syphilitic bursitis
Syphilis [stage unspecified] of bursa
Syphilis [stage unspecified] of muscle
Syphilis [stage unspecified] of synovium
Syphilis [stage unspecified] of tendon

A52.79 **Other symptomatic late syphilis**
Late syphilitic leukoderma
Syphilis of adrenal gland
Syphilis of pituitary gland
Syphilis of thyroid gland
Syphilitic splenomegaly
EXCLUDES 1 syphilitic leukoderma (secondary) (A51.39)

A52.8 **Late syphilis, latent**
Syphilis (acquired) without clinical manifestations, with positive serological reaction and negative spinal fluid test, two years or more after infection

A52.9 **Late syphilis, unspecified**

✓4ᵗʰ **A53** **Other and unspecified syphilis**

A53.0 **Latent syphilis, unspecified as early or late**
Latent syphilis NOS
Positive serological reaction for syphilis

A53.9 **Syphilis, unspecified**
Infection due to Treponema pallidum NOS
Syphilis (acquired) NOS
EXCLUDES 1 syphilis NOS under two years of age (A50.2)

✓4ᵗʰ **A54** **Gonococcal infection**
DEF: Sexually transmitted bacterial infection caused by *Neisseria gonorrhoeae*. Women are often asymptomatic, while men tend to develop urinary symptoms quickly.

✓5ᵗʰ **A54.0** **Gonococcal infection of lower genitourinary tract without periurethral or accessory gland abscess**
EXCLUDES 1 gonococcal infection with genitourinary gland abscess (A54.1)
gonococcal infection with periurethral abscess (A54.1)

A54.00 **Gonococcal infection of lower genitourinary tract, unspecified**

A54.01 **Gonococcal cystitis and urethritis, unspecified**

A54.02 **Gonococcal vulvovaginitis, unspecified** ♀

A54.03 **Gonococcal cervicitis, unspecified** ♀

A54.09 **Other gonococcal infection of lower genitourinary tract**

A54.1 **Gonococcal infection of lower genitourinary tract with periurethral and accessory gland abscess**
Gonococcal Bartholin's gland abscess

✓5ᵗʰ **A54.2** **Gonococcal pelviperitonitis and other gonococcal genitourinary infection**

A54.21 **Gonococcal infection of kidney and ureter**

A54.22 **Gonococcal prostatitis** ♂

A54.23 **Gonococcal infection of other male genital organs** ♂
Gonococcal epididymitis
Gonococcal orchitis

A54.24 **Gonococcal female pelvic inflammatory disease** ♀
Gonococcal pelviperitonitis
EXCLUDES 1 gonococcal peritonitis (A54.85)

A54.29 **Other gonococcal genitourinary infections**

✓5ᵗʰ **A54.3** **Gonococcal infection of eye**

A54.30 **Gonococcal infection of eye, unspecified**

A54.31 **Gonococcal conjunctivitis**
Ophthalmia neonatorum due to gonococcus

A54.32 **Gonococcal iridocyclitis**

A54.33 **Gonococcal keratitis**

A54.39 **Other gonococcal eye infection**
Gonococcal endophthalmia

✓5ᵗʰ **A54.4** **Gonococcal infection of musculoskeletal system**

A54.40 **Gonococcal infection of musculoskeletal system, unspecified** `HCC` `ESR` `COM`

A54.41 **Gonococcal spondylopathy** `HCC` `ESR` `COM`

A54.42 **Gonococcal arthritis** `HCC` `ESR` `COM`
EXCLUDES 2 gonococcal infection of spine (A54.41)

A54.43 **Gonococcal osteomyelitis** `HCC` `ESR` `COM`
EXCLUDES 2 gonococcal infection of spine (A54.41)

A54.49 **Gonococcal infection of other musculoskeletal tissue** `HCC` `ESR` `COM`
Gonococcal bursitis
Gonococcal myositis
Gonococcal synovitis
Gonococcal tenosynovitis

A54.5 **Gonococcal pharyngitis**

A54.6 **Gonococcal infection of anus and rectum**

✓5ᵗʰ **A54.8** **Other gonococcal infections**

A54.81 **Gonococcal meningitis** `COM`

A54.82 **Gonococcal brain abscess** `COM`

A54.83 **Gonococcal heart infection** `COM`
Gonococcal endocarditis
Gonococcal myocarditis
Gonococcal pericarditis

A54.84 **Gonococcal pneumonia** `HCC` `ESR`

A54.85 **Gonococcal peritonitis** `HCC` `ESR` `COM`
EXCLUDES 1 gonococcal pelviperitonitis (A54.24)

A54.86 **Gonococcal sepsis** `HCC` `ESR` `COM`

A54.89 **Other gonococcal infections**
Gonococcal keratoderma
Gonococcal lymphadenitis

A54.9 **Gonococcal infection, unspecified**

A55 Chlamydial lymphogranuloma (venereum)
Climatic or tropical bubo
Durand-Nicolas-Favre disease
Esthiomene
Lymphogranuloma inguinale

✓4ᵗʰ **A56 Other sexually transmitted chlamydial diseases**

INCLUDES   sexually transmitted diseases due to Chlamydia trachomatis

EXCLUDES 1   neonatal chlamydial conjunctivitis (P39.1)
neonatal chlamydial pneumonia (P23.1)

EXCLUDES 2   chlamydial lymphogranuloma (A55)
conditions classified to A74.-

DEF: *Chlamydia trachomatis:* Bacterium that causes a common venereal disease. Symptoms of chlamydia are usually mild or absent, however, serious complications may cause irreversible damage, including cystitis, pelvic inflammatory disease, and infertility in women and discharge from the penis, prostatitis, and infertility in men. Genital chlamydial infection can cause arthritis, skin lesions, and inflammation of the eye and urethra.
Synonym(s): *Reiter's syndrome.*

✓5ᵗʰ **A56.0 Chlamydial infection of** lower genitourinary tract

    A56.00 Chlamydial infection of lower genitourinary tract, unspecified

    A56.01 Chlamydial cystitis and urethritis

    A56.02 Chlamydial vulvovaginitis   ♀

    A56.09 Other chlamydial infection of lower genitourinary tract
Chlamydial cervicitis

✓5ᵗʰ **A56.1 Chlamydial infection of** pelviperitoneum **and other genitourinary organs**

    A56.11 Chlamydial female pelvic inflammatory disease   ♀

    A56.19 Other chlamydial genitourinary infection
Chlamydial epididymitis
Chlamydial orchitis

  A56.2 Chlamydial infection of genitourinary tract, unspecified

  A56.3 Chlamydial infection of anus and rectum

  A56.4 Chlamydial infection of pharynx

  A56.8 Sexually transmitted chlamydial infection of other sites

A57 Chancroid
Ulcus molle
DEF: Localized infection by *Haemophilus ducreyi,* causing genital ulcers and infecting the inguinal lymph nodes.

A58 Granuloma inguinale
Donovanosis

✓4ᵗʰ **A59 Trichomoniasis**

EXCLUDES 2   intestinal trichomoniasis (A07.8)

DEF: Infection with the parasitic, flagellated protozoa of the genus *Trichomonas.* This protozoon is found in the intestinal and genitourinary tracts of humans and in the mouth around tartar, cavities, and areas of periodontal disease.

✓5ᵗʰ **A59.0 Urogenital trichomoniasis**

    A59.00 Urogenital trichomoniasis, unspecified
Fluor (vaginalis) due to Trichomonas
Leukorrhea (vaginalis) due to Trichomonas

    A59.01 Trichomonal vulvovaginitis   ♀

    A59.02 Trichomonal prostatitis   ♂

    A59.03 Trichomonal cystitis and urethritis

    A59.09 Other urogenital trichomoniasis
Trichomonas cervicitis

  A59.8 Trichomoniasis of other sites

  A59.9 Trichomoniasis, unspecified

✓4ᵗʰ **A60 Anogenital herpesviral [herpes simplex] infections**

✓5ᵗʰ **A60.0 Herpesviral infection of** genitalia and urogenital tract

    A60.00 Herpesviral infection of urogenital system, unspecified

    A60.01 Herpesviral infection of penis   ♂

    A60.02 Herpesviral infection of other male genital organs   ♂

    A60.03 Herpesviral cervicitis   ♀

    A60.04 Herpesviral vulvovaginitis   ♀
Herpesviral [herpes simplex] ulceration
Herpesviral [herpes simplex] vaginitis
Herpesviral [herpes simplex] vulvitis

    A60.09 Herpesviral infection of other urogenital tract
AHA: 2020,1Q,20

  A60.1 Herpesviral infection of perianal skin and rectum

  A60.9 Anogenital herpesviral infection, unspecified

✓4ᵗʰ **A63 Other predominantly sexually transmitted diseases, not elsewhere classified**

EXCLUDES 2   molluscum contagiosum (B08.1)
papilloma of cervix (D26.0)

  A63.0 Anogenital (venereal) warts
Anogenital warts due to (human) papillomavirus [HPV]
Condyloma acuminatum

  A63.8 Other specified predominantly sexually transmitted diseases

A64 Unspecified sexually transmitted disease

Other spirochetal diseases (A65-A69)

EXCLUDES 2   leptospirosis (A27.-)
syphilis (A50-A53)

A65 Nonvenereal syphilis
Bejel
Endemic syphilis
Njovera

✓4ᵗʰ **A66 Yaws**

INCLUDES   bouba
frambesia (tropica)
pian

  A66.0 Initial lesions of yaws
Chancre of yaws
Frambesia, initial or primary
Initial frambesial ulcer
Mother yaw

  A66.1 Multiple papillomata and wet crab yaws
Frambesioma
Pianoma
Plantar or palmar papilloma of yaws

  A66.2 Other early skin lesions of yaws
Cutaneous yaws, less than five years after infection
Early yaws (cutaneous) (macular) (maculopapular) (micropapular) (papular)
Frambeside of early yaws

  A66.3 Hyperkeratosis of yaws
Ghoul hand
Hyperkeratosis, palmar or plantar (early) (late) due to yaws
Worm-eaten soles

  A66.4 Gummata and ulcers of yaws
Gummatous frambeside
Nodular late yaws (ulcerated)

  A66.5 Gangosa
Rhinopharyngitis mutilans

  A66.6 Bone and joint lesions of yaws   HCC ESR COM
Yaws ganglion
Yaws goundou
Yaws gumma, bone
Yaws gummatous osteitis or periostitis
Yaws hydrarthrosis
Yaws osteitis
Yaws periostitis (hypertrophic)

  A66.7 Other manifestations of yaws
Juxta-articular nodules of yaws
Mucosal yaws

  A66.8 Latent yaws
Yaws without clinical manifestations, with positive serology

  A66.9 Yaws, unspecified

✓4ᵗʰ **A67 Pinta [carate]**

  A67.0 Primary lesions of pinta
Chancre (primary) of pinta
Papule (primary) of pinta

  A67.1 Intermediate lesions of pinta
Erythematous plaques of pinta
Hyperchromic lesions of pinta
Hyperkeratosis of pinta
Pintids

  A67.2 Late lesions of pinta
Achromic skin lesions of pinta
Cicatricial skin lesions of pinta
Dyschromic skin lesions of pinta

  A67.3 Mixed lesions of pinta
Achromic with hyperchromic skin lesions of pinta [carate]

  A67.9 Pinta, unspecified

✓4ᵗʰ **A68 Relapsing fevers**

INCLUDES recurrent fever
EXCLUDES 2 Lyme disease (A69.2-)

A68.0 Louse-borne relapsing fever
Relapsing fever due to Borrelia recurrentis

A68.1 Tick-borne relapsing fever
Relapsing fever due to any Borrelia species other than Borrelia recurrentis

A68.9 Relapsing fever, unspecified

✓4ᵗʰ **A69 Other spirochetal infections**

A69.0 Necrotizing ulcerative stomatitis
Cancrum oris
Fusospirochetal gangrene
Noma
Stomatitis gangrenosa

A69.1 Other Vincent's infections
Fusospirochetal pharyngitis
Necrotizing ulcerative (acute) gingivitis
Necrotizing ulcerative (acute) gingivostomatitis
Spirochetal stomatitis
Trench mouth
Vincent's angina
Vincent's gingivitis

✓5ᵗʰ **A69.2 Lyme disease**
Erythema chronicum migrans due to Borrelia burgdorferi
DEF: Recurrent multisystem disorder through tick bites that begins with lesions of erythema chronicum migrans and is followed by arthritis of the large joints, myalgia, malaise, and neurological and cardiac manifestations.

A69.20 Lyme disease, unspecified
AHA: 2021,4Q,5

A69.21 Meningitis due to Lyme disease COM

A69.22 Other neurologic disorders in Lyme disease
Cranial neuritis
Meningoencephalitis
Polyneuropathy

A69.23 Arthritis due to Lyme disease HCC ESR COM

A69.29 Other conditions associated with Lyme disease
Myopericarditis due to Lyme disease
AHA: 2016,3Q,12

A69.8 Other specified spirochetal infections

A69.9 Spirochetal infection, unspecified

Other diseases caused by chlamydiae (A70-A74)

EXCLUDES 1 sexually transmitted chlamydial diseases (A55-A56)

A70 Chlamydia psittaci infections
Ornithosis
Parrot fever
Psittacosis

✓4ᵗʰ **A71 Trachoma**

EXCLUDES 1 sequelae of trachoma (B94.0)

A71.0 Initial stage of trachoma
Trachoma dubium

A71.1 Active stage of trachoma
Granular conjunctivitis (trachomatous)
Trachomatous follicular conjunctivitis
Trachomatous pannus

A71.9 Trachoma, unspecified

✓4ᵗʰ **A74 Other diseases caused by chlamydiae**

EXCLUDES 1 neonatal chlamydial conjunctivitis (P39.1)
neonatal chlamydial pneumonia (P23.1)
Reiter's disease (M02.3-)
sexually transmitted chlamydial diseases (A55-A56)
EXCLUDES 2 chlamydial pneumonia (J16.0)

A74.0 Chlamydial conjunctivitis
Paratrachoma

✓5ᵗʰ **A74.8 Other chlamydial diseases**

A74.81 Chlamydial peritonitis

A74.89 Other chlamydial diseases

A74.9 Chlamydial infection, unspecified
Chlamydiosis NOS

Rickettsioses (A75-A79)

DEF: Rickettsia: Condition caused by bacteria that live in lice/ticks transmitted to humans through bites.

✓4ᵗʰ **A75 Typhus fever**

EXCLUDES 1 rickettsiosis due to Ehrlichia sennetsu (A79.81)

A75.0 Epidemic louse-borne typhus fever due to Rickettsia prowazekii
Classical typhus (fever)
Epidemic (louse-borne) typhus

A75.1 Recrudescent typhus [Brill's disease]
Brill-Zinsser disease

A75.2 Typhus fever due to Rickettsia typhi
Murine (flea-borne) typhus

A75.3 Typhus fever due to Rickettsia tsutsugamushi
Scrub (mite-borne) typhus
Tsutsugamushi fever
Typhus fever due to Orientia Tsutsugamushi (scrub typhus)

A75.9 Typhus fever, unspecified
Typhus (fever) NOS

✓4ᵗʰ **A77 Spotted fever [tick-borne rickettsioses]**

A77.0 Spotted fever due to Rickettsia rickettsii
Rocky Mountain spotted fever
Sao Paulo fever

A77.1 Spotted fever due to Rickettsia conorii
African tick typhus
Boutonneuse fever
India tick typhus
Kenya tick typhus
Marseilles fever
Mediterranean tick fever

A77.2 Spotted fever due to Rickettsia siberica
North Asian tick fever
Siberian tick typhus

A77.3 Spotted fever due to Rickettsia australis
Queensland tick typhus

✓5ᵗʰ **A77.4 Ehrlichiosis**

EXCLUDES 1 anaplasmosis [A. phagocytophilum] (A79.82)
rickettsiosis due to Ehrlichia sennetsu (A79.81)
AHA: 2021,4Q,5

A77.40 Ehrlichiosis, unspecified

A77.41 Ehrlichiosis chafeensis [E. chafeensis]

A77.49 Other ehrlichiosis
Ehrlichiosis due to E. ewingii
Ehrlichiosis due to E. muris euclairensis

A77.8 Other spotted fevers
Rickettsia 364D/R. philipii (Pacific Coast tick fever)
Spotted fever due to Rickettsia africae (African tick bite fever)
Spotted fever due to Rickettsia parkeri

A77.9 Spotted fever, unspecified
Tick-borne typhus NOS

A78 Q fever
Infection due to Coxiella burnetii
Nine Mile fever
Quadrilateral fever

✓4ᵗʰ **A79 Other rickettsioses**

A79.0 Trench fever
Quintan fever
Wolhynian fever

A79.1 Rickettsialpox due to Rickettsia akari
Kew Garden fever
Vesicular rickettsiosis

✓5ᵗʰ **A79.8 Other specified rickettsioses**

A79.81 Rickettsiosis due to Ehrlichia sennetsu
Rickettsiosis due to Neorickettsia sennetsu

A79.82 Anaplasmosis [A. phagocytophilum]
Transfusion transmitted A. phagocytophilum
AHA: 2021,4Q,4-5

A79.89 Other specified rickettsioses

A79.9 Rickettsiosis, unspecified
Rickettsial infection NOS

Viral and prion infections of the central nervous system (A80-A89)

EXCLUDES 1   *postpolio syndrome (G14)*
sequelae of poliomyelitis (B91)
sequelae of viral encephalitis (B94.1)

✓4ᵗʰ **A80 Acute poliomyelitis**

    EXCLUDES 1   *acute flaccid myelitis (G04.82)*

   A80.0   **Acute paralytic poliomyelitis, vaccine-associated**   COM

   A80.1   **Acute paralytic poliomyelitis, wild virus, imported**   COM

   A80.2   **Acute paralytic poliomyelitis, wild virus, indigenous**   COM

   ✓5ᵗʰ **A80.3**   **Acute paralytic poliomyelitis, other and unspecified**

     A80.30   **Acute paralytic poliomyelitis, unspecified**   COM

     A80.39   **Other acute paralytic poliomyelitis**   COM

   A80.4   **Acute nonparalytic poliomyelitis**   COM

   A80.9   **Acute poliomyelitis, unspecified**   COM

✓4ᵗʰ **A81 Atypical virus infections of central nervous system**

    INCLUDES   diseases of the central nervous system caused by prions

   ▶Use additional code, if applicable, to identify:◀

    ▶dementia with anxiety (F02.84, F02.A4, F02.B4, F02.C4)◀
    dementia with behavioral disturbance ▶(F02.81-, F02.A1-, F02.B1-, F02.C1-)◀
    ▶dementia with mood disturbance (F02.83, F02.A3, F02.B3, F02.C3)◀
    ▶dementia with psychotic disturbance (F02.82, F02.A2, F02.B2, F02.C2)◀
    dementia without behavioral disturbance ▶(F02.80, F02.A0, F02.B0, F02.C0)◀
    ▶mild neurocognitive disorder due to known physiological condition (F06.7-)◀

   ✓5ᵗʰ **A81.0**   **Creutzfeldt-Jakob disease**

    DEF: Communicable, rare spongiform encephalopathy occurring later in life with progressive destruction of the pyramidal and extrapyramidal systems eventually leading to death. Progressive dementia, wasting of muscles, tremor, and other symptoms are present.

     A81.00   **Creutzfeldt-Jakob disease, unspecified**   HCC Rx ESR
      Jakob-Creutzfeldt disease, unspecified

     A81.01   **Variant Creutzfeldt-Jakob disease**   HCC Rx ESR
      vCJD

     A81.09   **Other Creutzfeldt-Jakob disease**   HCC Rx ESR
      CJD
      Familial Creutzfeldt-Jakob disease
      Iatrogenic Creutzfeldt-Jakob disease
      Sporadic Creutzfeldt-Jakob disease
      Subacute spongiform encephalopathy (with dementia)

   A81.1   **Subacute sclerosing panencephalitis**   HCC Rx ESR
    Dawson's inclusion body encephalitis
    Van Bogaert's sclerosing leukoencephalopathy

   A81.2   **Progressive multifocal leukoencephalopathy**   HCC Rx ESR
    Multifocal leukoencephalopathy NOS

   ✓5ᵗʰ **A81.8**   **Other atypical virus infections of central nervous system**

     A81.81   **Kuru**   HCC Rx ESR

     A81.82   **Gerstmann-Sträussler-Scheinker syndrome**   HCC Rx ESR
      GSS syndrome

     A81.83   **Fatal familial insomnia**   HCC Rx ESR
      FFI

     A81.89   **Other atypical virus infections of central nervous system**   HCC Rx ESR

   A81.9   **Atypical virus infection of central nervous system, unspecified**   HCC Rx ESR
    Prion diseases of the central nervous system NOS

✓4ᵗʰ **A82 Rabies**

   A82.0   **Sylvatic rabies**   COM

   A82.1   **Urban rabies**   COM

   A82.9   **Rabies, unspecified**   COM

✓4ᵗʰ **A83 Mosquito-borne viral encephalitis**

    INCLUDES   mosquito-borne viral meningoencephalitis

    EXCLUDES 2   *Venezuelan equine encephalitis (A92.2)*
      West Nile fever (A92.3-)
      West Nile virus (A92.3-)

   A83.0   **Japanese encephalitis**   COM

   A83.1   **Western equine encephalitis**   COM

   A83.2   **Eastern equine encephalitis**   COM

   A83.3   **St Louis encephalitis**   COM

   A83.4   **Australian encephalitis**   COM
    Kunjin virus disease

   A83.5   **California encephalitis**   COM
    California meningoencephalitis
    La Crosse encephalitis

   A83.6   **Rocio virus disease**   COM

   A83.8   **Other mosquito-borne viral encephalitis**   COM

   A83.9   **Mosquito-borne viral encephalitis, unspecified**   COM

✓4ᵗʰ **A84 Tick-borne viral encephalitis**

    INCLUDES   tick-borne viral meningoencephalitis

   A84.0   **Far Eastern tick-borne encephalitis [Russian spring-summer encephalitis]**   COM

   A84.1   **Central European tick-borne encephalitis**   COM

   ✓5ᵗʰ **A84.8**   **Other tick-borne viral encephalitis**

     AHA: 2020,4Q,4-5

     A84.81   **Powassan virus disease**   COM

     A84.89   **Other tick-borne viral encephalitis**   COM
      Louping ill
      Code first, if applicable, transfusion related infection (T80.22-)

   A84.9   **Tick-borne viral encephalitis, unspecified**   COM

✓4ᵗʰ **A85 Other viral encephalitis, not elsewhere classified**

    INCLUDES   specified viral encephalomyelitis NEC
      specified viral meningoencephalitis NEC

    EXCLUDES 1   *benign myalgic encephalomyelitis (G93.3)*
     encephalitis due to cytomegalovirus (B25.8)
     encephalitis due to herpesvirus NEC (B10.0-)
     encephalitis due to herpesvirus [herpes simplex] (B00.4)
     encephalitis due to measles virus (B05.0)
     encephalitis due to mumps virus (B26.2)
     encephalitis due to poliomyelitis virus (A80.-)
     encephalitis due to zoster (B02.0)
     lymphocytic choriomeningitis (A87.2)
     ▶*myalgic encephalomyelitis (G93.32)*◀

   A85.0   **Enteroviral encephalitis**   COM
    Enteroviral encephalomyelitis

   A85.1   **Adenoviral encephalitis**   COM
    Adenoviral meningoencephalitis

   A85.2   **Arthropod-borne viral encephalitis, unspecified**   COM
    EXCLUDES 1   *West nile virus with encephalitis (A92.31)*

   A85.8   **Other specified viral encephalitis**   COM
    Encephalitis lethargica
    Von Economo-Cruchet disease

A86 Unspecified viral encephalitis   COM
   Viral encephalomyelitis NOS
   Viral meningoencephalitis NOS

✓4ᵗʰ **A87 Viral meningitis**

    EXCLUDES 1   *meningitis due to herpesvirus [herpes simplex] (B00.3)*
     meningitis due to measles virus (B05.1)
     meningitis due to mumps virus (B26.1)
     meningitis due to poliomyelitis virus (A80.-)
     meningitis due to zoster (B02.1)

   DEF: Meningitis: Inflammation of the meningeal layers of the brain and spine.

   A87.0   **Enteroviral meningitis**   COM
    Coxsackievirus meningitis
    Echovirus meningitis

   A87.1   **Adenoviral meningitis**   COM

   A87.2   **Lymphocytic choriomeningitis**   COM
    Lymphocytic meningoencephalitis

   A87.8   **Other viral meningitis**   COM

   A87.9   **Viral meningitis, unspecified**   COM

✓4ᵗʰ **A88** **Other viral infections of central nervous system, not elsewhere classified**
     EXCLUDES 1   *viral encephalitis NOS (A86)*
                  viral meningitis NOS (A87.9)

     A88.0 **Enteroviral exanthematous fever [Boston exanthem]** `COM`
     A88.1 **Epidemic vertigo**
     A88.8 **Other specified viral infections of central nervous system** `COM`

A89 **Unspecified viral infection of central nervous system** `COM`

Arthropod-borne viral fevers and viral hemorrhagic fevers (A90-A99)

A90 **Dengue fever [classical dengue]**
     EXCLUDES 1   *dengue hemorrhagic fever (A91)*
     AHA: 2016,3Q,13

A91 **Dengue hemorrhagic fever**

✓4ᵗʰ **A92** **Other mosquito-borne viral fevers**
     EXCLUDES 1   *Ross River disease (B33.1)*

     A92.0 **Chikungunya virus disease**
           Chikungunya (hemorrhagic) fever

     A92.1 **O'nyong-nyong fever**

     A92.2 **Venezuelan equine fever** `COM`
           Venezuelan equine encephalitis
           Venezuelan equine encephalomyelitis virus disease

     ✓5ᵗʰ **A92.3** **West Nile virus infection**
           West Nile fever
           AHA: 2016,3Q,12

         A92.30 **West Nile virus infection, unspecified** `COM`
              West Nile fever NOS
              West Nile fever without complications
              West Nile virus NOS

         A92.31 **West Nile virus infection with encephalitis** `COM`
              West Nile encephalitis
              West Nile encephalomyelitis

         A92.32 **West Nile virus infection with other neurologic manifestation** `COM`
              Use additional code to specify the neurologic manifestation

         A92.39 **West Nile virus infection with other complications** `COM`
              Use additional code to specify the other conditions

     A92.4 **Rift Valley fever**

     A92.5 **Zika virus disease**
           Zika virus fever
           Zika virus infection
           Zika NOS
           EXCLUDES 1   *congenital Zika virus disease (P35.4)*
           AHA: 2016,4Q,4-7
           DEF: Virus transmitted via a bite from an infected Aedes species mosquito. Common symptoms of the virus include fever, rash, joint pain, and conjunctivitis; they are usually mild in nature and may last from several days to a week. Most people who have the Zika virus do not require medical attention; however, in pregnant women, the Zika virus can cause a serious birth defect called microcephaly, as well as other severe fetal brain defects.
           TIP: Assign code Z71.1, when a patient requests testing for Zika virus but in the absence of symptoms or recent exposure to the virus.
           TIP: Code only confirmed diagnoses of Zika virus; documentation by the physician that the disease is confirmed is sufficient.

     A92.8 **Other specified mosquito-borne viral fevers**
     A92.9 **Mosquito-borne viral fever, unspecified**

✓4ᵗʰ **A93** **Other arthropod-borne viral fevers, not elsewhere classified**

     A93.0 **Oropouche virus disease**
           Oropouche fever

     A93.1 **Sandfly fever**
           Pappataci fever
           Phlebotomus fever

     A93.2 **Colorado tick fever**

     A93.8 **Other specified arthropod-borne viral fevers**
           Piry virus disease
           Vesicular stomatitis virus disease [Indiana fever]

A94 **Unspecified arthropod-borne viral fever**
     Arboviral fever NOS
     Arbovirus infection NOS

✓4ᵗʰ **A95** **Yellow fever**

     A95.0 **Sylvatic yellow fever**
           Jungle yellow fever

     A95.1 **Urban yellow fever**

     A95.9 **Yellow fever, unspecified**

✓4ᵗʰ **A96** **Arenaviral hemorrhagic fever**

     A96.0 **Junin hemorrhagic fever**
           Argentinian hemorrhagic fever

     A96.1 **Machupo hemorrhagic fever**
           Bolivian hemorrhagic fever

     A96.2 **Lassa fever**

     A96.8 **Other arenaviral hemorrhagic fevers**

     A96.9 **Arenaviral hemorrhagic fever, unspecified**

✓4ᵗʰ **A98** **Other viral hemorrhagic fevers, not elsewhere classified**
     EXCLUDES 1   *chikungunya hemorrhagic fever (A92.0)*
                  dengue hemorrhagic fever (A91)

     A98.0 **Crimean-Congo hemorrhagic fever**
           Central Asian hemorrhagic fever

     A98.1 **Omsk hemorrhagic fever**

     A98.2 **Kyasanur Forest disease**

     A98.3 **Marburg virus disease**

     A98.4 **Ebola virus disease**

     A98.5 **Hemorrhagic fever with renal syndrome**
           Epidemic hemorrhagic fever
           Korean hemorrhagic fever
           Russian hemorrhagic fever
           Hantaan virus disease
           Hantavirus disease with renal manifestations
           Nephropathia epidemica
           Songo fever
           EXCLUDES 1   *hantavirus (cardio)-pulmonary syndrome (B33.4)*

     A98.8 **Other specified viral hemorrhagic fevers**

A99 **Unspecified viral hemorrhagic fever**

Viral infections characterized by skin and mucous membrane lesions (B00-B09)

✓4ᵗʰ **B00** **Herpesviral [herpes simplex] infections**
     EXCLUDES 1   *congenital herpesviral infections (P35.2)*
     EXCLUDES 2   *anogenital herpesviral infection (A60.-)*
                  gammaherpesviral mononucleosis (B27.0-)
                  herpangina (B08.5)

     B00.0 **Eczema herpeticum**
           Kaposi's varicelliform eruption

     B00.1 **Herpesviral vesicular dermatitis**
           Herpes simplex facialis
           Herpes simplex labialis
           Herpes simplex otitis externa
           Vesicular dermatitis of ear
           Vesicular dermatitis of lip

     B00.2 **Herpesviral gingivostomatitis and pharyngotonsillitis**
           Herpesviral pharyngitis

     B00.3 **Herpesviral meningitis** `COM`

     B00.4 **Herpesviral encephalitis** `COM`
           Herpesviral meningoencephalitis
           Simian B disease
           EXCLUDES 1   *herpesviral encephalitis due to herpesvirus 6 and 7 (B10.01, B10.09)*
                  non-simplex herpesviral encephalitis (B10.0-)

     ✓5ᵗʰ **B00.5** **Herpesviral ocular disease**

         B00.50 **Herpesviral ocular disease, unspecified**

         B00.51 **Herpesviral iridocyclitis**
              Herpesviral iritis
              Herpesviral uveitis, anterior

         B00.52 **Herpesviral keratitis**
              Herpesviral keratoconjunctivitis

         B00.53 **Herpesviral conjunctivitis**

         B00.59 **Other herpesviral disease of eye**
              Herpesviral dermatitis of eyelid

     B00.7 **Disseminated herpesviral disease** `HCC` `ESR` `COM`
           Herpesviral sepsis

`HCC` CMS-HCC   `Rx` Rx HCC   `ESH` ESRD HCC   `COM` Commercial HCC   N Newborn: 0   P Pediatric: 0-17   M Maternity: 9-64   A Adult: 15-124

462

ICD-10-CM 2023

√5ᵗʰ B00.8 Other forms of herpesviral infections

    B00.81 Herpesviral hepatitis

    B00.82 Herpes simplex myelitis `HCC` `Rx` `ESR` `COM`

    B00.89 Other herpesviral infection
        Herpesviral whitlow

B00.9 Herpesviral infection, unspecified
    Herpes simplex infection NOS

√4ᵗʰ B01 Varicella [chickenpox]

    B01.0 Varicella meningitis `COM`

    √5ᵗʰ B01.1 Varicella encephalitis, myelitis and encephalomyelitis
        Postchickenpox encephalitis, myelitis and encephalomyelitis

        B01.11 Varicella encephalitis and encephalomyelitis `COM`
            Postchickenpox encephalitis and encephalomyelitis

        B01.12 Varicella myelitis `HCC` `Rx` `ESR` `COM`
            Postchickenpox myelitis

    B01.2 Varicella pneumonia

    √5ᵗʰ B01.8 Varicella with other complications

        B01.81 Varicella keratitis

        B01.89 Other varicella complications

    B01.9 Varicella without complication
        Varicella NOS

√4ᵗʰ B02 Zoster [herpes zoster]

    `INCLUDES`   shingles
              zona

    B02.0 Zoster encephalitis `COM`
        Zoster meningoencephalitis

    B02.1 Zoster meningitis `COM`
        AHA: 2019,1Q,18

    √5ᵗʰ B02.2 Zoster with other nervous system involvement

        B02.21 Postherpetic geniculate ganglionitis `Rx`

        B02.22 Postherpetic trigeminal neuralgia `Rx`

        B02.23 Postherpetic polyneuropathy `Rx`

        B02.24 Postherpetic myelitis `HCC` `Rx` `ESR` `COM`
            Herpes zoster myelitis

        B02.29 Other postherpetic nervous system involvement `Rx`
            Postherpetic radiculopathy

    √5ᵗʰ B02.3 Zoster ocular disease

        B02.30 Zoster ocular disease, unspecified

        B02.31 Zoster conjunctivitis

        B02.32 Zoster iridocyclitis

        B02.33 Zoster keratitis
            Herpes zoster keratoconjunctivitis

        B02.34 Zoster scleritis

        B02.39 Other herpes zoster eye disease
            Zoster blepharitis

    B02.7 Disseminated zoster

    B02.8 Zoster with other complications
        Herpes zoster otitis externa

    B02.9 Zoster without complications
        Zoster NOS

B03 Smallpox

    `NOTE`   In 1980 the 33rd World Health Assembly declared that smallpox had been eradicated.

         The classification is maintained for surveillance purposes.

B04 Monkeypox

√4ᵗʰ B05 Measles

    `INCLUDES`   morbilli
    `EXCLUDES 1`   subacute sclerosing panencephalitis (A81.1)

    B05.0 Measles complicated by encephalitis `COM`
        Postmeasles encephalitis

    B05.1 Measles complicated by meningitis `COM`
        Postmeasles meningitis

    B05.2 Measles complicated by pneumonia
        Postmeasles pneumonia

    B05.3 Measles complicated by otitis media
        Postmeasles otitis media

    B05.4 Measles with intestinal complications

    √5ᵗʰ B05.8 Measles with other complications

        B05.81 Measles keratitis and keratoconjunctivitis

        B05.89 Other measles complications

B05.9 Measles without complication
    Measles NOS

√4ᵗʰ B06 Rubella [German measles]

    `EXCLUDES 1`   congenital rubella (P35.0)
    DEF: Highly contagious virus in which the symptoms are mild and short-lived in most people. Rubella during pregnancy, however, can result in abortion, stillbirth, or congenital defects.

    √5ᵗʰ B06.0 Rubella with neurological complications

        B06.00 Rubella with neurological complication, unspecified

        B06.01 Rubella encephalitis `COM`
            Rubella meningoencephalitis

        B06.02 Rubella meningitis `COM`

        B06.09 Other neurological complications of rubella

    √5ᵗʰ B06.8 Rubella with other complications

        B06.81 Rubella pneumonia

        B06.82 Rubella arthritis `HCC` `ESR` `COM`

        B06.89 Other rubella complications

    B06.9 Rubella without complication
        Rubella NOS

√4ᵗʰ B07 Viral warts

    `INCLUDES`   verruca simplex
              verruca vulgaris
              viral warts due to human papillomavirus
    `EXCLUDES 2`   anogenital (venereal) warts (A63.0)
              papilloma of bladder (D41.4)
              papilloma of cervix (D26.0)
              papilloma larynx (D14.1)

    B07.0 Plantar wart
        Verruca plantaris

    B07.8 Other viral warts
        Common wart
        Flat wart
        Verruca plana

    B07.9 Viral wart, unspecified

√4ᵗʰ B08 Other viral infections characterized by skin and mucous membrane lesions, not elsewhere classified

    `EXCLUDES 1`   vesicular stomatitis virus disease (A93.8)

    √5ᵗʰ B08.0 Other orthopoxvirus infections

        `EXCLUDES 2`   monkeypox (B04)

        √6ᵗʰ B08.01 Cowpox and vaccinia not from vaccine

            B08.010 Cowpox
                DEF: Disease contracted by milking infected cows. The vesicles usually appear on the fingers, hands, and adjacent areas and usually disappear without scarring. Other symptoms include local edema, lymphangitis, and regional lymphadenitis with or without fever.

            B08.011 Vaccinia not from vaccine
                `EXCLUDES 1`   vaccinia (from vaccination) (generalized) (T88.1)

        B08.02 Orf virus disease
            Contagious pustular dermatitis
            Ecthyma contagiosum

        B08.03 Pseudocowpox [milker's node]

        B08.04 Paravaccinia, unspecified

        B08.09 Other orthopoxvirus infections
            Orthopoxvirus infection NOS

    B08.1 Molluscum contagiosum
        DEF: Benign poxvirus infection causing small bumps on the skin or conjunctiva, transmitted by close contact.

    √5ᵗʰ B08.2 Exanthema subitum [sixth disease]
        Roseola infantum

        B08.20 Exanthema subitum [sixth disease], unspecified `P`
            Roseola infantum, unspecified

        B08.21 Exanthema subitum [sixth disease] due to human herpesvirus 6 `P`
            Roseola infantum due to human herpesvirus 6

        B08.22 Exanthema subitum [sixth disease] due to human herpesvirus 7 `P`
            Roseola infantum due to human herpesvirus 7

B08.3 Erythema infectiosum [fifth disease]
DEF: Infection with human parvovirus B19, mainly occurring in children. Symptoms include a low-grade fever, malaise, or a "cold" a few days before the appearance of a mild rash illness that presents as a "slapped-cheek" rash on the face and a lacy red rash on the trunk and limbs.

B08.4 Enteroviral vesicular stomatitis with exanthem
Hand, foot and mouth disease

B08.5 Enteroviral vesicular pharyngitis
Herpangina
DEF: Acute infectious Coxsackie virus infection causing throat lesions, fever, and vomiting that generally affects children in the summer.

✓5ᵗʰ **B08.6 Parapoxvirus infections**
    B08.60 Parapoxvirus infection, unspecified
    B08.61 Bovine stomatitis
    B08.62 Sealpox
    B08.69 Other parapoxvirus infections

✓5ᵗʰ **B08.7 Yatapoxvirus infections**
    B08.70 Yatapoxvirus infection, unspecified
    B08.71 Tanapox virus disease
    B08.72 Yaba pox virus disease
        Yaba monkey tumor disease
    B08.79 Other yatapoxvirus infections

B08.8 Other specified viral infections characterized by skin and mucous membrane lesions
Enteroviral lymphonodular pharyngitis
Foot-and-mouth disease
Poxvirus NEC

B09 Unspecified viral infection characterized by skin and mucous membrane lesions
Viral enanthema NOS
Viral exanthema NOS

Other human herpesviruses (B10)

✓4ᵗʰ **B10 Other human herpesviruses**
    EXCLUDES 2   cytomegalovirus (B25.9)
        Epstein-Barr virus (B27.0-)
        herpes NOS (B00.9)
        herpes simplex (B00.-)
        herpes zoster (B02.-)
        human herpesvirus NOS (B00.-)
        human herpesvirus 1 and 2 (B00.-)
        human herpesvirus 3 (B01.-, B02.-)
        human herpesvirus 4 (B27.0-)
        human herpesvirus 5 (B25.-)
        varicella (B01.-)
        zoster (B02.-)

✓5ᵗʰ **B10.0 Other human herpesvirus encephalitis**
    EXCLUDES 2   herpes encephalitis NOS (B00.4)
        herpes simplex encephalitis (B00.4)
        human herpesvirus encephalitis (B00.4)
        simian B herpes virus encephalitis (B00.4)
    B10.01 Human herpesvirus 6 encephalitis   COM
    B10.09 Other human herpesvirus encephalitis   COM
        Human herpesvirus 7 encephalitis

✓5ᵗʰ **B10.8 Other human herpesvirus infection**
    B10.81 Human herpesvirus 6 infection
    B10.82 Human herpesvirus 7 infection
    B10.89 Other human herpesvirus infection
        Human herpesvirus 8 infection
        Kaposi's sarcoma-associated herpesvirus infection

Viral hepatitis (B15-B19)

EXCLUDES 1   *sequelae of viral hepatitis (B94.2)*
EXCLUDES 2   *cytomegaloviral hepatitis (B25.1)*
        herpesviral [herpes simplex] hepatitis (B00.81)

DEF: Hepatitis A: HAV infection that is self-limiting with flulike symptoms. Transmission is fecal-oral.
DEF: Hepatitis B: HBV infection that can be chronic and systemic. Transmission is bodily fluids.
DEF: Hepatitis C: HCV infection that can be chronic and systemic. Transmission is blood transfusion and unidentified agents.
DEF: Hepatitis D (delta): HDV that occurs only in the presence of hepatitis B virus. Transmission is contaminated blood in contact with mucous membranes.
DEF: Hepatitis E: HEV is an epidemic form. Transmission is fecal-oral, most often from contaminated water.

✓4ᵗʰ **B15 Acute hepatitis A**
    B15.0 Hepatitis A with hepatic coma   COM
    B15.9 Hepatitis A without hepatic coma
        Hepatitis A (acute)(viral) NOS

✓4ᵗʰ **B16 Acute hepatitis B**
    AHA: 2016,3Q,13
    B16.0 Acute hepatitis B with delta-agent with hepatic coma   COM
    B16.1 Acute hepatitis B with delta-agent without hepatic coma
    B16.2 Acute hepatitis B without delta-agent with hepatic coma   COM
    B16.9 Acute hepatitis B without delta-agent and without hepatic coma
        Hepatitis B (acute) (viral) NOS

✓4ᵗʰ **B17 Other acute viral hepatitis**
    B17.0 Acute delta-(super) infection of hepatitis B carrier
    ✓5ᵗʰ **B17.1 Acute hepatitis C**
        B17.10 Acute hepatitis C without hepatic coma   Rx
            Acute hepatitis C NOS
        B17.11 Acute hepatitis C with hepatic coma   Rx COM
    B17.2 Acute hepatitis E
    B17.8 Other specified acute viral hepatitis
        Hepatitis non-A non-B (acute) (viral) NEC
    B17.9 Acute viral hepatitis, unspecified
        Acute hepatitis NOS
        Acute infectious hepatitis NOS

✓4ᵗʰ **B18 Chronic viral hepatitis**
    INCLUDES   carrier of viral hepatitis
    AHA: 2017,1Q,41
    B18.0 Chronic viral hepatitis B with delta-agent   HCC Rx ESR COM
    B18.1 Chronic viral hepatitis B without delta-agent   HCC Rx ESR COM
        Carrier of viral hepatitis B
        Chronic (viral) hepatitis B
    B18.2 Chronic viral hepatitis C   HCC Rx ESR COM
        Carrier of viral hepatitis C
        AHA: 2018,1Q,4
    B18.8 Other chronic viral hepatitis   HCC Rx ESR COM
        Carrier of other viral hepatitis
    B18.9 Chronic viral hepatitis, unspecified   HCC ESR COM
        Carrier of unspecified viral hepatitis

✓4ᵗʰ **B19 Unspecified viral hepatitis**
    B19.0 Unspecified viral hepatitis with hepatic coma   COM
    ✓5ᵗʰ **B19.1 Unspecified viral hepatitis B**
        B19.10 Unspecified viral hepatitis B without hepatic coma
            Unspecified viral hepatitis B NOS
        B19.11 Unspecified viral hepatitis B with hepatic coma   COM
    ✓5ᵗʰ **B19.2 Unspecified viral hepatitis C**
        B19.20 Unspecified viral hepatitis C without hepatic coma   Rx
            Viral hepatitis C NOS
        B19.21 Unspecified viral hepatitis C with hepatic coma   Rx COM
    B19.9 Unspecified viral hepatitis without hepatic coma
        Viral hepatitis NOS

Human immunodeficiency virus [HIV] disease (B20)

B20 Human immunodeficiency virus [HIV] disease `HCC` `Rx` `ESR` `COM`

[INCLUDES] acquired immune deficiency syndrome [AIDS]
AIDS-related complex [ARC]
HIV infection, symptomatic

Code first Human immunodeficiency virus [HIV] disease complicating pregnancy, childbirth and the puerperium, if applicable (O98.7-)

Use additional code(s) to identify all manifestations of HIV infection

[EXCLUDES 1] *asymptomatic human immunodeficiency virus [HIV] infection status (Z21)*
exposure to HIV virus (Z20.6)
inconclusive serologic evidence of HIV (R75)

AHA: 2022,1Q,36; 2021,2Q,6; 2021,1Q,52; 2020,4Q,97; 2020,2Q,12; 2019,1Q,8-11

Other viral diseases (B25-B34)

✓4th **B25 Cytomegaloviral disease**

[EXCLUDES 1] *congenital cytomegalovirus infection (P35.1)*
cytomegaloviral mononucleosis (B27.1-)

B25.0 Cytomegaloviral pneumonitis `HCC` `Rx` `ESR` `COM`
B25.1 Cytomegaloviral hepatitis `HCC` `Rx` `ESR` `COM`
B25.2 Cytomegaloviral pancreatitis `HCC` `Rx` `ESR` `COM`
B25.8 Other cytomegaloviral diseases `HCC` `Rx` `ESR` `COM`
    Cytomegaloviral encephalitis
B25.9 Cytomegaloviral disease, unspecified `HCC` `Rx` `ESR` `COM`

✓4th **B26 Mumps**

[INCLUDES] epidemic parotitis
infectious parotitis

B26.0 Mumps orchitis ♂
B26.1 Mumps meningitis `COM`
B26.2 Mumps encephalitis `COM`
B26.3 Mumps pancreatitis `COM`
✓5th **B26.8 Mumps with other complications**
    B26.81 Mumps hepatitis
    B26.82 Mumps myocarditis `COM`
    B26.83 Mumps nephritis
    B26.84 Mumps polyneuropathy
    B26.85 Mumps arthritis `HCC` `ESR` `COM`
    B26.89 Other mumps complications
B26.9 Mumps without complication
    Mumps NOS
    Mumps parotitis NOS

✓4th **B27 Infectious mononucleosis**

[INCLUDES] glandular fever
monocytic angina
Pfeiffer's disease

✓5th **B27.0 Gammaherpesviral mononucleosis**
    Mononucleosis due to Epstein-Barr virus
    B27.00 Gammaherpesviral mononucleosis without complication
    B27.01 Gammaherpesviral mononucleosis with polyneuropathy
    B27.02 Gammaherpesviral mononucleosis with meningitis `COM`
    B27.09 Gammaherpesviral mononucleosis with other complications
        Hepatomegaly in gammaherpesviral mononucleosis
✓5th **B27.1 Cytomegaloviral mononucleosis**
    B27.10 Cytomegaloviral mononucleosis without complications
    B27.11 Cytomegaloviral mononucleosis with polyneuropathy
    B27.12 Cytomegaloviral mononucleosis with meningitis `COM`
    B27.19 Cytomegaloviral mononucleosis with other complication
        Hepatomegaly in cytomegaloviral mononucleosis
✓5th **B27.8 Other infectious mononucleosis**
    B27.80 Other infectious mononucleosis without complication
    B27.81 Other infectious mononucleosis with polyneuropathy

    B27.82 Other infectious mononucleosis with meningitis `COM`
    B27.89 Other infectious mononucleosis with other complication
        Hepatomegaly in other infectious mononucleosis
✓5th **B27.9 Infectious mononucleosis, unspecified**
    B27.90 Infectious mononucleosis, unspecified without complication
    B27.91 Infectious mononucleosis, unspecified with polyneuropathy
    B27.92 Infectious mononucleosis, unspecified with meningitis `COM`
    B27.99 Infectious mononucleosis, unspecified with other complication
        Hepatomegaly in unspecified infectious mononucleosis

✓4th **B30 Viral conjunctivitis**

[EXCLUDES 1] *herpesviral [herpes simplex] ocular disease (B00.5)*
ocular zoster (B02.3)

Viral Conjunctivitis

Inflamed conjunctiva

Normal conjunctiva

B30.0 Keratoconjunctivitis due to adenovirus
    Epidemic keratoconjunctivitis
    Shipyard eye
B30.1 Conjunctivitis due to adenovirus
    Acute adenoviral follicular conjunctivitis
    Swimming-pool conjunctivitis
B30.2 Viral pharyngoconjunctivitis
B30.3 Acute epidemic hemorrhagic conjunctivitis (enteroviral)
    Conjunctivitis due to coxsackievirus 24
    Conjunctivitis due to enterovirus 70
    Hemorrhagic conjunctivitis (acute)(epidemic)
B30.8 Other viral conjunctivitis
    Newcastle conjunctivitis
B30.9 Viral conjunctivitis, unspecified

✓4th **B33 Other viral diseases, not elsewhere classified**

B33.0 Epidemic myalgia
    Bornholm disease
B33.1 Ross River disease
    Epidemic polyarthritis and exanthema
    Ross River fever
✓5th **B33.2 Viral carditis**
    Coxsackie (virus) carditis
    B33.20 Viral carditis, unspecified `COM`
    B33.21 Viral endocarditis `COM`
    B33.22 Viral myocarditis `COM`
    B33.23 Viral pericarditis `COM`
    B33.24 Viral cardiomyopathy `HCC` `Rx` `ESR` `COM`
B33.3 Retrovirus infections, not elsewhere classified
    Retrovirus infection NOS
B33.4 Hantavirus (cardio)-pulmonary syndrome [HPS] [HCPS]
    Hantavirus disease with pulmonary manifestations
    Sin nombre virus disease
    Use additional code to identify any associated acute kidney failure (N17.9)
    [EXCLUDES 1] *hantavirus disease with renal manifestations (A98.5)*
        hemorrhagic fever with renal manifestations (A98.5)
B33.8 Other specified viral diseases
    [EXCLUDES 1] *anogenital human papillomavirus infection (A63.0)*
        viral warts due to human papillomavirus infection (B07)

✓4ᵗʰ **B34 Viral infection of unspecified site**
   EXCLUDES 1   anogenital human papillomavirus infection (A63.0)
                cytomegaloviral disease NOS (B25.9)
                herpesvirus [herpes simplex] infection NOS (B00.9)
                retrovirus infection NOS (B33.3)
                viral agents as the cause of diseases classified elsewhere
                   (B97.-)
                viral warts due to human papillomavirus infection (B07)

   B34.0 Adenovirus infection, unspecified
   B34.1 Enterovirus infection, unspecified
            Coxsackievirus infection NOS
            Echovirus infection NOS
   B34.2 Coronavirus infection, unspecified
       EXCLUDES 1   COVID-19 (U07.1)
                    pneumonia due to SARS-associated coronavirus
                       (J12.81)
            AHA: 2020,1Q,34-36
   B34.3 Parvovirus infection, unspecified
   B34.4 Papovavirus infection, unspecified
   B34.8 Other viral infections of unspecified site
   B34.9 Viral infection, unspecified
            Viremia NOS
            AHA: 2016,3Q,10

Mycoses (B35-B49)

   EXCLUDES 2   hypersensitivity pneumonitis due to organic dust (J67.-)
                mycosis fungoides (C84.0-)

✓4ᵗʰ **B35 Dermatophytosis**
   INCLUDES   favus
              infections due to species of Epidermophyton, Micro-sporum
                 and Trichophyton
              tinea, any type except those in B36.-
   DEF: Contagious superficial fungal infection of the skin that invades and
   grows in dead keratin.

   B35.0 Tinea barbae and tinea capitis
            Beard ringworm
            Kerion
            Scalp ringworm
            Sycosis, mycotic
   B35.1 Tinea unguium
            Dermatophytic onychia
            Dermatophytosis of nail
            Onychomycosis
            Ringworm of nails
   B35.2 Tinea manuum
            Dermatophytosis of hand
            Hand ringworm
   B35.3 Tinea pedis
            Athlete's foot
            Dermatophytosis of foot
            Foot ringworm
   B35.4 Tinea corporis
            Ringworm of the body
   B35.5 Tinea imbricata
            Tokelau
   B35.6 Tinea cruris
            Dhobi itch
            Groin ringworm
            Jock itch
   B35.8 Other dermatophytoses
            Disseminated dermatophytosis
            Granulomatous dermatophytosis
   B35.9 Dermatophytosis, unspecified
            Ringworm NOS

✓4ᵗʰ **B36 Other superficial mycoses**
   B36.0 Pityriasis versicolor
            Tinea flava
            Tinea versicolor
   B36.1 Tinea nigra
            Keratomycosis nigricans palmaris
            Microsporosis nigra
            Pityriasis nigra
   B36.2 White piedra
            Tinea blanca
   B36.3 Black piedra
   B36.8 Other specified superficial mycoses

   B36.9 Superficial mycosis, unspecified

✓4ᵗʰ **B37 Candidiasis**
   INCLUDES   candidosis
              moniliasis
       EXCLUDES 1   neonatal candidiasis (P37.5)
   DEF: Candida: Genus of yeast-like fungi that are commonly found in the
   mouth, skin, intestinal tract, and vagina. It may cause a white, cheesy
   discharge.

   B37.0 Candidal stomatitis
            Oral thrush
   B37.1 Pulmonary candidiasis   HCC Rx ESR COM
            Candidal bronchitis
            Candidal pneumonia
   B37.2 Candidiasis of skin and nail
            Candidal onychia
            Candidal paronychia
       EXCLUDES 2   diaper dermatitis (L22)
▲ ✓5ᵗʰ **B37.3 Candidiasis of vulva and vagina**
            Candidal vulvovaginitis
            Monilial vulvovaginitis
            Vaginal thrush
●   **B37.31 Acute candidiasis of vulva and vagina**
                     Candidiasis of vulva and vagina NOS
●   **B37.32 Chronic candidiasis of vulva and vagina**
                     Recurrent candidiasis of vulva and vagina
   ✓5ᵗʰ **B37.4 Candidiasis of other urogenital sites**
            B37.41 Candidal cystitis and urethritis
            B37.42 Candidal balanitis   ♂
            B37.49 Other urogenital candidiasis
                     Candidal pyelonephritis
   B37.5 Candidal meningitis   COM
   B37.6 Candidal endocarditis   COM
   B37.7 Candidal sepsis   HCC Rx ESR COM
            Disseminated candidiasis
            Systemic candidiasis
            AHA: 2014,4Q,46
            TIP: This code is assigned when sepsis is documented as due to
            any Candida type. If the nonspecific term "non-Candida albicans"
            is documented, code B48.8 Other specified mycoses, is assigned.
   ✓5ᵗʰ **B37.8 Candidiasis of other sites**
            B37.81 Candidal esophagitis   HCC Rx ESR COM
            B37.82 Candidal enteritis
                     Candidal proctitis
            B37.83 Candidal cheilitis
            B37.84 Candidal otitis externa
            B37.89 Other sites of candidiasis
                     Candidal osteomyelitis
   B37.9 Candidiasis, unspecified
            Thrush NOS

✓4ᵗʰ **B38 Coccidioidomycosis**
   B38.0 Acute pulmonary coccidioidomycosis   HCC ESR COM
   B38.1 Chronic pulmonary coccidioidomycosis   HCC ESR COM
   B38.2 Pulmonary coccidioidomycosis, unspecified HCC ESR COM
   B38.3 Cutaneous coccidioidomycosis
   B38.4 Coccidioidomycosis meningitis   COM
            DEF: Coccidioides immitis infection of the lining of the brain and/or
            spinal cord.
   B38.7 Disseminated coccidioidomycosis
            Generalized coccidioidomycosis
   ✓5ᵗʰ **B38.8 Other forms of coccidioidomycosis**
            B38.81 Prostatic coccidioidomycosis   ♂
            B38.89 Other forms of coccidioidomycosis
   B38.9 Coccidioidomycosis, unspecified

✓4ᵗʰ **B39 Histoplasmosis**

Code first associated AIDS (B20)
Use additional code for any associated manifestations, such as:
    endocarditis (I39)
    meningitis (G02)
    pericarditis (I32)
    retinitis (H32)
DEF: Type of lung infection caused by breathing in fungal spores often found in the droppings of bats and birds or soil contaminated by their droppings.

Histoplasmosis

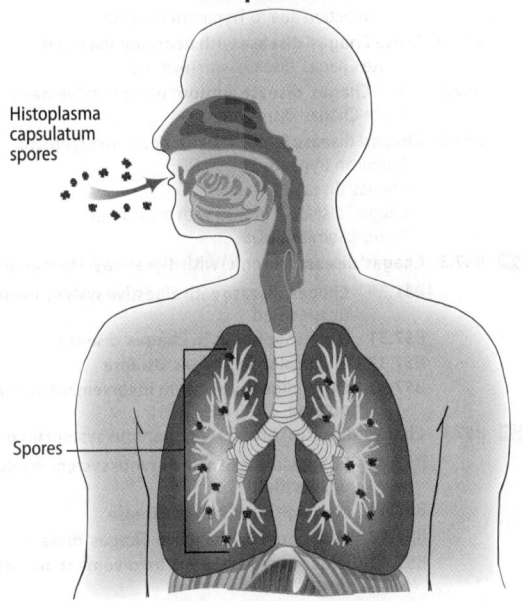

Histoplasma capsulatum spores

Spores

B39.0	Acute pulmonary **histoplasmosis capsulati**	HCC ESR COM
B39.1	Chronic pulmonary **histoplasmosis capsulati**	HCC ESR COM
B39.2	Pulmonary **histoplasmosis capsulati, unspecified**	HCC ESR COM
B39.3	Disseminated **histoplasmosis capsulati**	
	Generalized histoplasmosis capsulati	
B39.4	**Histoplasmosis capsulati, unspecified**	
	American histoplasmosis	
B39.5	**Histoplasmosis duboisii**	
	African histoplasmosis	
B39.9	**Histoplasmosis, unspecified**	

✓4ᵗʰ **B40 Blastomycosis**

EXCLUDES 1   *Brazilian blastomycosis (B41.-)*
                  keloidal blastomycosis (B48.0)

B40.0	Acute pulmonary **blastomycosis**	HCC ESR COM
B40.1	Chronic pulmonary **blastomycosis**	HCC ESR COM
B40.2	Pulmonary **blastomycosis, unspecified**	HCC ESR COM
B40.3	Cutaneous **blastomycosis**	
B40.7	Disseminated **blastomycosis**	
	Generalized blastomycosis	

✓5ᵗʰ **B40.8** Other forms of blastomycosis

B40.81	**Blastomycotic meningoencephalitis**	COM
	Meningomyelitis due to blastomycosis	
B40.89	Other forms of blastomycosis	

B40.9 **Blastomycosis, unspecified**

✓4ᵗʰ **B41 Paracoccidioidomycosis**

INCLUDES   Brazilian blastomycosis
                Lutz' disease

B41.0	Pulmonary **paracoccidioidomycosis**	HCC ESR COM
B41.7	Disseminated **paracoccidioidomycosis**	
	Generalized paracoccidioidomycosis	
B41.8	Other forms of paracoccidioidomycosis	
B41.9	Paracoccidioidomycosis, unspecified	

✓4ᵗʰ **B42 Sporotrichosis**

B42.0	Pulmonary **sporotrichosis**
B42.1	Lymphocutaneous **sporotrichosis**

B42.7	Disseminated **sporotrichosis**	
	Generalized sporotrichosis	

✓5ᵗʰ **B42.8** Other forms of sporotrichosis

B42.81	**Cerebral sporotrichosis**	COM
	Meningitis due to sporotrichosis	
B42.82	**Sporotrichosis arthritis**	HCC ESR COM
B42.89	Other forms of sporotrichosis	

B42.9 **Sporotrichosis, unspecified**

✓4ᵗʰ **B43 Chromomycosis and pheomycotic abscess**

B43.0	Cutaneous **chromomycosis**	
	Dermatitis verrucosa	
B43.1	Pheomycotic **brain abscess**	COM
	Cerebral chromomycosis	
B43.2	Subcutaneous **pheomycotic abscess and cyst**	
B43.8	Other forms of chromomycosis	
B43.9	**Chromomycosis, unspecified**	

✓4ᵗʰ **B44 Aspergillosis**

INCLUDES   aspergilloma

B44.0	Invasive pulmonary **aspergillosis**	HCC Rx ESR COM
B44.1	Other pulmonary **aspergillosis**	HCC Rx ESR COM
B44.2	Tonsillar **aspergillosis**	HCC Rx ESR COM
B44.7	Disseminated **aspergillosis**	HCC Rx ESR COM
	Generalized aspergillosis	

✓5ᵗʰ **B44.8** Other forms of aspergillosis

B44.81	Allergic bronchopulmonary aspergillosis	HCC Rx ESR COM
B44.89	Other forms of aspergillosis	HCC Rx ESR COM

B44.9 **Aspergillosis, unspecified**   HCC Rx ESR COM

✓4ᵗʰ **B45 Cryptococcosis**

B45.0	Pulmonary **cryptococcosis**	HCC Rx ESR COM
B45.1	Cerebral **cryptococcosis**	HCC Rx ESR COM
	Cryptococcal meningitis	
	Cryptococcosis meningocerebralis	
B45.2	Cutaneous **cryptococcosis**	HCC Rx ESR COM
B45.3	Osseous **cryptococcosis**	HCC Rx ESR COM
B45.7	Disseminated **cryptococcosis**	HCC Rx ESR COM
	Generalized cryptococcosis	
B45.8	Other forms of cryptococcosis	HCC Rx ESR COM
B45.9	**Cryptococcosis, unspecified**	HCC Rx ESR COM

✓4ᵗʰ **B46 Zygomycosis**

B46.0	Pulmonary **mucormycosis**	HCC Rx ESR COM
B46.1	Rhinocerebral **mucormycosii**	HCC Rx ESR COM
B46.2	Gastrointestinal **mucormycosis**	HCC Rx ESR COM
B46.3	Cutaneous **mucormycosis**	HCC Rx ESR COM
	Subcutaneous mucormycosis	
B46.4	Disseminated **mucormycosis**	HCC Rx ESR COM
	Generalized mucormycosis	
B46.5	**Mucormycosis, unspecified**	HCC Rx ESR COM
B46.8	Other zygomycoses	HCC Rx ESR COM
	Entomophthoromycosis	
B46.9	**Zygomycosis, unspecified**	HCC Rx ESR COM
	Phycomycosis NOS	

✓4ᵗʰ **B47 Mycetoma**

B47.0	**Eumycetoma**
	Madura foot, mycotic
	Maduromycosis
B47.1	**Actinomycetoma**
B47.9	**Mycetoma, unspecified**
	Madura foot NOS

✓4ᵗʰ **B48 Other mycoses, not elsewhere classified**

B48.0	**Lobomycosis**
	Keloidal blastomycosis
	Lobo's disease
B48.1	**Rhinosporidiosis**
B48.2	**Allescheriasis**
	Infection due to Pseudallescheria boydii
	EXCLUDES 1 *eumycetoma (B47.0)*
B48.3	**Geotrichosis**
	Geotrichum stomatitis

B48.4 Penicillosis `HCC` `Rx` `ESR` `COM`
Talaromycosis

B48.8 Other specified mycoses `HCC` `Rx` `ESR` `COM`
Adiaspiromycosis
Infection of tissue and organs by Alternaria
Infection of tissue and organs by Drechslera
Infection of tissue and organs by Fusarium
Infection of tissue and organs by saprophytic fungi NEC
AHA: 2014,4Q,46; 2014,2Q,13
TIP: This code is assigned when the nonspecific term
"non-*Candida albicans*" sepsis is documented. If sepsis is
documented as due to any *Candida* type, code B37.7 Candidal
sepsis, is assigned.

B49 Unspecified mycosis
Fungemia NOS

Protozoal diseases (B50-B64)

EXCLUDES 1   amebiasis (A06.-)
other protozoal intestinal diseases (A07.-)

☑4ᵗʰ B50 Plasmodium falciparum malaria
INCLUDES   mixed infections of Plasmodium falciparum with any other
Plasmodium species

B50.0 Plasmodium falciparum malaria with cerebral complications
Cerebral malaria NOS

B50.8 Other severe and complicated Plasmodium falciparum malaria
Severe or complicated Plasmodium falciparum malaria NOS

B50.9 Plasmodium falciparum malaria, unspecified

☑4ᵗʰ B51 Plasmodium vivax malaria
INCLUDES   mixed infections of Plasmodium vivax with other
Plasmodium species, except Plasmodium falciparum
EXCLUDES 1   Plasmodium vivax with Plasmodium falciparum (B50.-)

B51.0 Plasmodium vivax malaria with rupture of spleen
B51.8 Plasmodium vivax malaria with other complications
B51.9 Plasmodium vivax malaria without complication
Plasmodium vivax malaria NOS

☑4ᵗʰ B52 Plasmodium malariae malaria
INCLUDES   mixed infections of Plasmodium malariae with other
Plasmodium species, except Plasmodium falciparum
and Plasmodium vivax
EXCLUDES 1   Plasmodium falciparum (B50.-)
Plasmodium vivax (B51.-)

B52.0 Plasmodium malariae malaria with nephropathy
B52.8 Plasmodium malariae malaria with other complications
B52.9 Plasmodium malariae malaria without complication
Plasmodium malariae malaria NOS

☑4ᵗʰ B53 Other specified malaria
B53.0 Plasmodium ovale malaria
EXCLUDES 1   Plasmodium ovale with Plasmodium falciparum (B50.-)
Plasmodium ovale with Plasmodium malariae (B52.-)
Plasmodium ovale with Plasmodium vivax (B51.-)

B53.1 Malaria due to simian plasmodia
EXCLUDES 1   malaria due to simian plasmodia with Plasmodium falciparum (B50.-)
malaria due to simian plasmodia with Plasmodium malariae (B52.-)
malaria due to simian plasmodia with Plasmodium ovale (B53.0)
malaria due to simian plasmodia with Plasmodium vivax (B51.-)

B53.8 Other malaria, not elsewhere classified

B54 Unspecified malaria

☑4ᵗʰ B55 Leishmaniasis
B55.0 Visceral leishmaniasis
Kala-azar
Post-kala-azar dermal leishmaniasis
B55.1 Cutaneous leishmaniasis
B55.2 Mucocutaneous leishmaniasis
B55.9 Leishmaniasis, unspecified

☑4ᵗʰ B56 African trypanosomiasis
B56.0 Gambiense trypanosomiasis
Infection due to Trypanosoma brucei gambiense
West African sleeping sickness
B56.1 Rhodesiense trypanosomiasis
East African sleeping sickness
Infection due to Trypanosoma brucei rhodesiense
B56.9 African trypanosomiasis, unspecified
Sleeping sickness NOS

☑4ᵗʰ B57 Chagas' disease
INCLUDES   American trypanosomiasis
infection due to Trypanosoma cruzi
B57.0 Acute Chagas' disease with heart involvement
Acute Chagas' disease with myocarditis
B57.1 Acute Chagas' disease without heart involvement
Acute Chagas' disease NOS
B57.2 Chagas' disease (chronic) with heart involvement
American trypanosomiasis NOS
Chagas' disease (chronic) NOS
Chagas' disease (chronic) with myocarditis
Trypanosomiasis NOS
☑5ᵗʰ B57.3 Chagas' disease (chronic) with digestive system involvement
B57.30 Chagas' disease with digestive system involvement, unspecified
B57.31 Megaesophagus in Chagas' disease
B57.32 Megacolon in Chagas' disease
B57.39 Other digestive system involvement in Chagas' disease
☑5ᵗʰ B57.4 Chagas' disease (chronic) with nervous system involvement
B57.40 Chagas' disease with nervous system involvement, unspecified
B57.41 Meningitis in Chagas' disease `COM`
B57.42 Meningoencephalitis in Chagas' disease `COM`
B57.49 Other nervous system involvement in Chagas' disease
B57.5 Chagas' disease (chronic) with other organ involvement

☑4ᵗʰ B58 Toxoplasmosis
INCLUDES   infection due to Toxoplasma gondii
EXCLUDES 1   congenital toxoplasmosis (P37.1)
☑5ᵗʰ B58.0 Toxoplasma oculopathy
B58.00 Toxoplasma oculopathy, unspecified
B58.01 Toxoplasma chorioretinitis
B58.09 Other toxoplasma oculopathy
Toxoplasma uveitis
B58.1 Toxoplasma hepatitis
B58.2 Toxoplasma meningoencephalitis `HCC` `Rx` `ESR` `COM`
B58.3 Pulmonary toxoplasmosis `HCC` `Rx` `ESR` `COM`
☑5ᵗʰ B58.8 Toxoplasmosis with other organ involvement
B58.81 Toxoplasma myocarditis `COM`
B58.82 Toxoplasma myositis
B58.83 Toxoplasma tubulo-interstitial nephropathy
Toxoplasma pyelonephritis
B58.89 Toxoplasmosis with other organ involvement
B58.9 Toxoplasmosis, unspecified

B59 Pneumocystosis `HCC` `Rx` `ESR` `COM`
Pneumonia due to Pneumocystis carinii
Pneumonia due to Pneumocystis jiroveci

☑4ᵗʰ B60 Other protozoal diseases, not elsewhere classified
EXCLUDES 1   cryptosporidiosis (A07.2)
intestinal microsporidiosis (A07.8)
isosporiasis (A07.3)
☑5ᵗʰ B60.0 Babesiosis
AHA: 2020,4Q,5-6
B60.00 Babesiosis, unspecified
Babesiosis due to unspecified Babesia species
Piroplasmosis, unspecified
B60.01 Babesiosis due to Babesia microti
Infection due to B. microti
B60.02 Babesiosis due to Babesia duncani
Infection due to B. duncani and B. duncani-type species

B60.03   **Babesiosis due to Babesia divergens**
Babesiosis due to Babesia MO-1
Infection due to B. divergens and B. divergens-like strains

B60.09   **Other babesiosis**
Babesiosis due to Babesia KO-1
Babesiosis due to Babesia venatorum
Infection due to other Babesia species
Infection due to other protozoa of the order Piroplasmida
Other piroplasmosis

√5ᵗʰ **B60.1**   **Acanthamebiasis**

B60.10   **Acanthamebiasis, unspecified**

B60.11   **Meningoencephalitis due to Acanthamoeba (culbertsoni)**   `COM`

B60.12   **Conjunctivitis due to Acanthamoeba**

B60.13   **Keratoconjunctivitis due to Acanthamoeba**

B60.19   **Other acanthamebic disease**

B60.2   **Naegleriasis**
Primary amebic meningoencephalitis

B60.8   **Other specified protozoal diseases**
Microsporidiosis

B64   **Unspecified protozoal disease**

Helminthiases (B65-B83)

√4ᵗʰ **B65**   **Schistosomiasis [bilharziasis]**

    `INCLUDES`   snail fever

B65.0   **Schistosomiasis due to Schistosoma haematobium [urinary schistosomiasis]**

B65.1   **Schistosomiasis due to Schistosoma mansoni [intestinal schistosomiasis]**

B65.2   **Schistosomiasis due to Schistosoma japonicum**
Asiatic schistosomiasis

B65.3   **Cercarial dermatitis**
Swimmer's itch

B65.8   **Other schistosomiasis**
Infection due to Schistosoma intercalatum
Infection due to Schistosoma mattheei
Infection due to Schistosoma mekongi

B65.9   **Schistosomiasis, unspecified**

√4ᵗʰ **B66**   **Other fluke infections**

B66.0   **Opisthorchiasis**
Infection due to cat liver fluke
Infection due to Opisthorchis (felineus)(viverrini)

B66.1   **Clonorchiasis**
Chinese liver fluke disease
Infection due to Clonorchis sinensis
Oriental liver fluke disease

B66.2   **Dicroceliasis**
Infection due to Dicrocoelium dendriticum
Lancet fluke infection

B66.3   **Fascioliasis**
Infection due to Fasciola gigantica
Infection due to Fasciola hepatica
Infection due to Fasciola indica
Sheep liver fluke disease

B66.4   **Paragonimiasis**   `HCC` `ESR` `COM`
Infection due to Paragonimus species
Lung fluke disease
Pulmonary distomiasis

B66.5   **Fasciolopsiasis**
Infection due to Fasciolopsis buski
Intestinal distomiasis

B66.8   **Other specified fluke infections**
Echinostomiasis
Heterophyiasis
Metagonimiasis
Nanophyetiasis
Watsoniasis

B66.9   **Fluke infection, unspecified**

√4ᵗʰ **B67**   **Echinococcosis**

    `INCLUDES`   hydatidosis

B67.0   **Echinococcus granulosus infection of liver**

B67.1   **Echinococcus granulosus infection of lung**   `HCC` `ESR` `COM`

B67.2   **Echinococcus granulosus infection of bone**

√5ᵗʰ **B67.3**   **Echinococcus granulosus infection, other and multiple sites**

B67.31   **Echinococcus granulosus infection, thyroid gland**

B67.32   **Echinococcus granulosus infection, multiple sites**

B67.39   **Echinococcus granulosus infection, other sites**

B67.4   **Echinococcus granulosus infection, unspecified**
Dog tapeworm (infection)

B67.5   **Echinococcus multilocularis infection of liver**

√5ᵗʰ **B67.6**   **Echinococcus multilocularis infection, other and multiple sites**

B67.61   **Echinococcus multilocularis infection, multiple sites**

B67.69   **Echinococcus multilocularis infection, other sites**

B67.7   **Echinococcus multilocularis infection, unspecified**

B67.8   **Echinococcosis, unspecified, of liver**

√5ᵗʰ **B67.9**   **Echinococcosis, other and unspecified**

B67.90   **Echinococcosis, unspecified**
Echinococcosis NOS

B67.99   **Other echinococcosis**

√4ᵗʰ **B68**   **Taeniasis**

    `EXCLUDES 1`   cysticercosis (B69.-)

B68.0   **Taenia solium taeniasis**
Pork tapeworm (infection)

B68.1   **Taenia saginata taeniasis**
Beef tapeworm (infection)
Infection due to adult tapeworm Taenia saginata

B68.9   **Taeniasis, unspecified**

√4ᵗʰ **B69**   **Cysticercosis**

    `INCLUDES`   cysticerciasis infection due to larval form of Taenia solium
    DEF: Condition that is developed when larvae or eggs of the tapeworm Taenia solium are ingested, most commonly in fecally contaminated water or undercooked pork.

B69.0   **Cysticercosis of central nervous system**

B69.1   **Cysticercosis of eye**

√5ᵗʰ **B69.8**   **Cysticercosis of other sites**

B69.81   **Myositis in cysticercosis**

B69.89   **Cysticercosis of other sites**

B69.9   **Cysticercosis, unspecified**

√4ᵗʰ **B70**   **Diphyllobothriasis and sparganosis**

B70.0   **Diphyllobothriasis**
Diphyllobothrium (adult) (latum) (pacificum) infection
Fish tapeworm (infection)
    `EXCLUDES 2`   larval diphyllobothriasis (B70.1)

B70.1   **Sparganosis**
Infection due to Sparganum (mansoni) (proliferum)
Infection due to Spirometra larva
Larval diphyllobothriasis
Spirometrosis

√4ᵗʰ **B71**   **Other cestode infections**

B71.0   **Hymenolepiasis**
Dwarf tapeworm infection
Rat tapeworm (infection)

B71.1   **Dipylidiasis**

B71.8   **Other specified cestode infections**
Coenurosis

B71.9   **Cestode infection, unspecified**
Tapeworm (infection) NOS

B72   **Dracunculiasis**

    `INCLUDES`   guinea worm infection
                infection due to Dracunculus medinensis

√4ᵗʰ **B73**   **Onchocerciasis**

    `INCLUDES`   onchocerca volvulus infection
                onchocercosis
                river blindness

√5ᵗʰ **B73.0**   **Onchocerciasis with eye disease**

B73.00   **Onchocerciasis with eye involvement, unspecified**

B73.01   **Onchocerciasis with endophthalmitis**

B73.02   **Onchocerciasis with glaucoma**

B73.09   **Onchocerciasis with other eye involvement**
Infestation of eyelid due to onchocerciasis

B73.1   **Onchocerciasis without eye disease**

✓4th B74 Filariasis

> EXCLUDES 2   onchocerciasis (B73)
> tropical (pulmonary) eosinophilia NOS (J82.89)

B74.0 Filariasis due to Wuchereria bancrofti
Bancroftian elephantiasis
Bancroftian filariasis

B74.1 Filariasis due to Brugia malayi

B74.2 Filariasis due to Brugia timori

B74.3 Loiasis
Calabar swelling
Eyeworm disease of Africa
Loa loa infection

B74.4 Mansonelliasis
Infection due to Mansonella ozzardi
Infection due to Mansonella perstans
Infection due to Mansonella streptocerca

B74.8 Other filariases
Dirofilariasis

B74.9 Filariasis, unspecified

B75 Trichinellosis

> INCLUDES   infection due to Trichinella species
> trichiniasis

DEF: Infection by *Trichinella spiralis,* the smallest of the parasitic nematodes, that is transmitted by eating undercooked pork or bear meat.
Synonym(s): Trichinosis.

✓4th B76 Hookworm diseases

> INCLUDES   uncinariasis

B76.0 Ancylostomiasis
Infection due to Ancylostoma species

B76.1 Necatoriasis
Infection due to Necator americanus

B76.8 Other hookworm diseases

B76.9 Hookworm disease, unspecified
Cutaneous larva migrans NOS

✓4th B77 Ascariasis

> INCLUDES   ascaridiasis
> roundworm infection

B77.0 Ascariasis with intestinal complications

✓5th B77.8 Ascariasis with other complications

    B77.81 Ascariasis pneumonia

    B77.89 Ascariasis with other complications

B77.9 Ascariasis, unspecified

✓4th B78 Strongyloidiasis

> EXCLUDES 1   trichostrongyliasis (B81.2)

B78.0 Intestinal strongyloidiasis

B78.1 Cutaneous strongyloidiasis

B78.7 Disseminated strongyloidiasis

B78.9 Strongyloidiasis, unspecified

B79 Trichuriasis

> INCLUDES   trichocephaliasis
> whipworm (disease)(infection)

B80 Enterobiasis

> INCLUDES   oxyuriasis
> pinworm infection
> threadworm infection

✓4th B81 Other intestinal helminthiases, not elsewhere classified

> EXCLUDES 1   angiostrongyliasis due to:
>   angiostrongylus cantonensis (B83.2)
>   parastrongylus cantonensis (B83.2)

B81.0 Anisakiasis
Infection due to Anisakis larva

B81.1 Intestinal capillariasis
Capillariasis NOS
Infection due to Capillaria philippinensis

> EXCLUDES 2   hepatic capillariasis (B83.8)

B81.2 Trichostrongyliasis

B81.3 Intestinal angiostrongyliasis
Angiostrongyliasis due to:
Angiostrongylus costaricensis
Parastrongylus costaricensis

B81.4 Mixed intestinal helminthiases
Infection due to intestinal helminths classified to more than one of the categories B65.0-B81.3 and B81.8
Mixed helminthiasis NOS

B81.8 Other specified intestinal helminthiases
Infection due to Oesophagostomum species [esophagostomiasis]
Infection due to Ternidens diminutus [ternidensiasis]

✓4th B82 Unspecified intestinal parasitism

B82.0 Intestinal helminthiasis, unspecified

B82.9 Intestinal parasitism, unspecified

✓4th B83 Other helminthiases

> EXCLUDES 1   capillariasis NOS (B81.1)
> EXCLUDES 2   intestinal capillariasis (B81.1)

B83.0 Visceral larva migrans
Toxocariasis

B83.1 Gnathostomiasis
Wandering swelling

B83.2 Angiostrongyliasis due to Parastrongylus cantonensis
Eosinophilic meningoencephalitis due to Parastrongylus cantonensis

> EXCLUDES 2   intestinal angiostrongyliasis (B81.3)

B83.3 Syngamiasis
Syngamosis

B83.4 Internal hirudiniasis

> EXCLUDES 2   external hirudiniasis (B88.3)

B83.8 Other specified helminthiases
Acanthocephaliasis
Gongylonemiasis
Hepatic capillariasis
Metastrongyliasis
Thelaziasis

B83.9 Helminthiasis, unspecified
Worms NOS

> EXCLUDES 1   intestinal helminthiasis NOS (B82.0)

Pediculosis, acariasis and other infestations (B85-B89)

✓4th B85 Pediculosis and phthiriasis

B85.0 Pediculosis due to Pediculus humanus capitis
Head-louse infestation

B85.1 Pediculosis due to Pediculus humanus corporis
Body-louse infestation

B85.2 Pediculosis, unspecified

B85.3 Phthiriasis
Infestation by crab-louse
Infestation by Phthirus pubis

B85.4 Mixed pediculosis and phthiriasis
Infestation classifiable to more than one of the categories B85.0-B85.3

B86 Scabies
Sarcoptic itch
DEF: Mite infestation that is caused by *Sarcoptes scabiei.* Scabies causes intense itching and sometimes secondary infection.

✓4th B87 Myiasis

> INCLUDES   infestation by larva of flies

B87.0 Cutaneous myiasis
Creeping myiasis

B87.1 Wound myiasis
Traumatic myiasis

B87.2 Ocular myiasis

B87.3 Nasopharyngeal myiasis
Laryngeal myiasis

B87.4 Aural myiasis

✓5th B87.8 Myiasis of other sites

    B87.81 Genitourinary myiasis

    B87.82 Intestinal myiasis

    B87.89 Myiasis of other sites

B87.9 Myiasis, unspecified

✓4th B88 Other infestations

B88.0 Other acariasis
Acarine dermatitis
Dermatitis due to Demodex species
Dermatitis due to Dermanyssus gallinae
Dermatitis due to Liponyssoides sanguineus
Trombiculosis
EXCLUDES 2   scabies (B86)

B88.1 Tungiasis [sandflea infestation]

B88.2 Other arthropod infestations
Scarabiasis

B88.3 External hirudiniasis
Leech infestation NOS
EXCLUDES 2   internal hirudiniasis (B83.4)

B88.8 Other specified infestations
Ichthyoparasitism due to Vandellia cirrhosa
Linguatulosis
Porocephaliasis

B88.9 Infestation, unspecified
Infestation (skin) NOS
Infestation by mites NOS
Skin parasites NOS

B89 Unspecified parasitic disease

Sequelae of infectious and parasitic diseases (B90-B94)

NOTE   Categories B90-B94 are to be used to indicate conditions in categories A00-B89 as the cause of sequelae, which are themselves classified elsewhere. The "sequelae" include conditions specified as such; they also include residuals of diseases classifiable to the above categories if there is evidence that the disease itself is no longer present. Codes from these categories are not to be used for chronic infections. Code chronic current infections to active infectious disease as appropriate.

Code first condition resulting from (sequela) the infectious or parasitic disease

✓4th B90 Sequelae of tuberculosis

B90.0 Sequelae of central nervous system tuberculosis

B90.1 Sequelae of genitourinary tuberculosis

B90.2 Sequelae of tuberculosis of bones and joints

B90.8 Sequelae of tuberculosis of other organs
EXCLUDES 2   sequelae of respiratory tuberculosis (B90.9)

B90.9 Sequelae of respiratory and unspecified tuberculosis
Sequelae of tuberculosis NOS

B91 Sequelae of poliomyelitis
EXCLUDES 1   postpolio syndrome (G14)

B92 Sequelae of leprosy

✓4th B94 Sequelae of other and unspecified infectious and parasitic diseases

B94.0 Sequelae of trachoma

B94.1 Sequelae of viral encephalitis

B94.2 Sequelae of viral hepatitis

B94.8 Sequelae of other specified infectious and parasitic diseases
AHA: 2021,1Q,25-30,31-49; 2020,3Q,10-14; 2017,4Q,109

B94.9 Sequelae of unspecified infectious and parasitic disease
EXCLUDES 2   post COVID-19 condition (U09.9)

Bacterial and viral infectious agents (B95-B97)

NOTE   These categories are provided for use as supplementary or additional codes to identify the infectious agent(s) in diseases classified elsewhere.

AHA: 2020,2Q,18; 2018,4Q,34; 2018,1Q,16

✓4th B95 Streptococcus, Staphylococcus, and Enterococcus as the cause of diseases classified elsewhere

B95.0 Streptococcus, group A, as the cause of diseases classified elsewhere UPD

B95.1 Streptococcus, group B, as the cause of diseases classified elsewhere UPD
AHA: 2020,1Q,10; 2019,2Q,8-10

B95.2 Enterococcus as the cause of diseases classified elsewhere UPD

B95.3 Streptococcus pneumoniae as the cause of diseases classified elsewhere UPD

B95.4 Other streptococcus as the cause of diseases classified elsewhere UPD

B95.5 Unspecified streptococcus as the cause of diseases classified elsewhere UPD

✓5th B95.6 Staphylococcus aureus as the cause of diseases classified elsewhere

B95.61 Methicillin susceptible Staphylococcus aureus infection as the cause of diseases classified elsewhere UPD
Methicillin susceptible Staphylococcus aureus (MSSA) infection as the cause of diseases classified elsewhere
Staphylococcus aureus infection NOS as the cause of diseases classified elsewhere

B95.62 Methicillin resistant Staphylococcus aureus infection as the cause of diseases classified elsewhere UPD
Methicillin resistant staphylococcus aureus (MRSA) infection as the cause of diseases classified elsewhere
AHA: 2016,1Q,12

B95.7 Other staphylococcus as the cause of diseases classified elsewhere UPD

B95.8 Unspecified staphylococcus as the cause of diseases classified elsewhere UPD

✓4th B96 Other bacterial agents as the cause of diseases classified elsewhere

B96.0 Mycoplasma pneumoniae [M. pneumoniae] as the cause of diseases classified elsewhere UPD
Pleuro-pneumonia-like-organism [PPLO]

B96.1 Klebsiella pneumoniae [K. pneumoniae] as the cause of diseases classified elsewhere UPD

✓5th B96.2 Escherichia coli [E. coli] as the cause of diseases classified elsewhere
AHA: 2022,1Q,31

B96.20 Unspecified Escherichia coli [E. coli] as the cause of diseases classified elsewhere UPD
Escherichia coli [E. coli] NOS

B96.21 Shiga toxin-producing Escherichia coli [E. coli] [STEC] O157 as the cause of diseases classified elsewhere UPD
E. coli O157:H- (nonmotile) with confirmation of Shiga toxin
E. coli O157 with confirmation of Shiga toxin when H antigen is unknown, or is not H7
O157:H7 Escherichia coli [E.coli] with or without confirmation of Shiga toxin-production
Shiga toxin-producing Escherichia coli [E.coli] O157:H7 with or without confirmation of Shiga toxin-production
STEC O157:H7 with or without confirmation of Shiga toxin-production

B96.22 Other specified Shiga toxin-producing Escherichia coli [E. coli] [STEC] as the cause of diseases classified elsewhere UPD
Non-O157 Shiga toxin-producing Escherichia coli [E.coli]
Non-O157 Shiga toxin-producing Escherichia coli [E.coli] with known O group

B96.23 Unspecified Shiga toxin-producing Escherichia coli [E. coli] [STEC] as the cause of diseases classified elsewhere UPD
Shiga toxin-producing Escherichia coli [E. coli] with unspecified O group
STEC NOS

B96.29 Other Escherichia coli [E. coli] as the cause of diseases classified elsewhere UPD
Non-Shiga toxin-producing E. coli

B96.3 Hemophilus influenzae [H. influenzae] as the cause of diseases classified elsewhere UPD

B96.4 Proteus (mirabilis) (morganii) as the cause of diseases classified elsewhere UPD

B96.5 Pseudomonas (aeruginosa) (mallei) (pseudomallei) as the cause of diseases classified elsewhere UPD
AHA: 2015,1Q,18

B96.6 Bacteroides fragilis [B. fragilis] as the cause of diseases classified elsewhere UPD

B96.7 Clostridium perfringens [C. perfringens] as the cause of diseases classified elsewhere UPD

✓5th B96.8 Other specified bacterial agents as the cause of diseases classified elsewhere

B96.81 Helicobacter pylori [H. pylori] as the cause of diseases classified elsewhere UPD

    B96.82   **Vibrio vulnificus** as the cause of diseases classified elsewhere `UPD`

    B96.89   **Other specified bacterial agents** as the cause of diseases classified elsewhere `UPD`

✓4ᵗʰ **B97 Viral agents as the cause of diseases classified elsewhere**

    AHA: 2016,3Q,8-10,14

    B97.0   **Adenovirus** as the cause of diseases classified elsewhere `UPD`

    ✓5ᵗʰ **B97.1**   **Enterovirus** as the cause of diseases classified elsewhere

        B97.10   **Unspecified enterovirus** as the cause of diseases classified elsewhere `UPD`

        B97.11   **Coxsackievirus** as the cause of diseases classified elsewhere `UPD`

        B97.12   **Echovirus** as the cause of diseases classified elsewhere `UPD`

        B97.19   **Other enterovirus** as the cause of diseases classified elsewhere `UPD`

    ✓5ᵗʰ **B97.2**   **Coronavirus** as the cause of diseases classified elsewhere

        TIP: Do not report a code from this subcategory for COVID-19; refer to U07.1.

        B97.21   **SARS-associated** coronavirus as the cause of diseases classified elsewhere `UPD`

             EXCLUDES 1   pneumonia due to SARS-associated coronavirus (J12.81)

        B97.29   **Other coronavirus** as the cause of diseases classified elsewhere `UPD`

             AHA: 2020,2Q,5; 2020,1Q,34-36

    ✓5ᵗʰ **B97.3**   **Retrovirus** as the cause of diseases classified elsewhere

        EXCLUDES 1   human immunodeficiency virus [HIV] disease (B20)

        B97.30   **Unspecified retrovirus** as the cause of diseases classified elsewhere `UPD`

        B97.31   **Lentivirus** as the cause of diseases classified elsewhere `UPD`

        B97.32   **Oncovirus** as the cause of diseases classified elsewhere `UPD`

        B97.33   **Human T-cell lymphotrophic virus, type I [HTLV-I]** as the cause of diseases classified elsewhere `UPD`

        B97.34   **Human T-cell lymphotrophic virus, type II [HTLV-II]** as the cause of diseases classified elsewhere `UPD`

        B97.35   **Human immunodeficiency virus, type 2 [HIV 2]** as the cause of diseases classified elsewhere `HCC` `Rx` `ESR` `COM` `UPD`

        B97.39   **Other retrovirus** as the cause of diseases classified elsewhere `UPD`

    B97.4   **Respiratory syncytial** virus as the cause of diseases classified elsewhere `UPD`

        RSV as the cause of diseases classified elsewhere

        Code first related disorders, such as:

            otitis media (H65.-)

            upper respiratory infection (J06.9)

        EXCLUDES 1   acute bronchiolitis due to respiratory syncytial virus (RSV) (J21.0)

                 acute bronchitis due to respiratory syncytial virus (RSV) (J20.5)

                 respiratory syncytial virus (RSV) pneumonia (J12.1)

    B97.5   **Reovirus** as the cause of diseases classified elsewhere `UPD`

    B97.6   **Parvovirus** as the cause of diseases classified elsewhere `UPD`

    B97.7   **Papillomavirus** as the cause of diseases classified elsewhere `UPD`

    ✓5ᵗʰ **B97.8**   **Other viral agents** as the cause of diseases classified elsewhere

        B97.81   **Human metapneumovirus** as the cause of diseases classified elsewhere `UPD`

        B97.89   **Other viral agents** as the cause of diseases classified elsewhere `UPD`

Other infectious diseases (B99)

✓4ᵗʰ **B99 Other and unspecified infectious diseases**

    B99.8   **Other infectious disease**

    B99.9   **Unspecified infectious disease**

`HCC` CMS-HCC   `Rx` Rx HCC   `ESR` ESRD HCC   `COM` Commercial HCC   `N` Newborn: 0   `P` Pediatric: 0-17   `M` Maternity: 9-64   `A` Adult: 15-124

472   ICD-10-CM 2023

Chapter 2. Neoplasms (C00–D49)

Chapter-specific Guidelines with Coding Examples

The chapter-specific guidelines from the ICD-10-CM Official Guidelines for Coding and Reporting have been provided below. Along with these guidelines are coding examples, contained in the shaded boxes, that have been developed to help illustrate the coding and/or sequencing guidance found in these guidelines.

General guidelines

Chapter 2 of the ICD-10-CM contains the codes for most benign and all malignant neoplasms. Certain benign neoplasms, such as prostatic adenomas, may be found in the specific body system chapters. To properly code a neoplasm, it is necessary to determine from the record if the neoplasm is benign, in-situ, malignant, or of uncertain histologic behavior. If malignant, any secondary (metastatic) sites should also be determined.

Primary malignant neoplasms overlapping site boundaries

A primary malignant neoplasm that overlaps two or more contiguous (next to each other) sites should be classified to the subcategory/code .8 ('overlapping lesion'), unless the combination is specifically indexed elsewhere. For multiple neoplasms of the same site that are not contiguous such as tumors in different quadrants of the same breast, codes for each site should be assigned.

> A 62-year-old female with a malignant lesion of the upper lip that extends from the lipstick area to the labial frenulum
>
> **C00.8**   **Malignant neoplasm of overlapping sites of lip**
>
> *Explanation*: Because this is a single lesion that overlaps two contiguous sites, a single code for overlapping sites is assigned.

> A 74-year-old male is treated for two distinct malignant lesions, one in the mucosa of the upper lip and a second in the mucosa of the lower lip.
>
> **C00.3**   **Malignant neoplasm of upper lip, inner aspect**
>
> **C00.4**   **Malignant neoplasm of lower lip, inner aspect**
>
> *Explanation*: This patient has two distinct malignant lesions of the upper and lower lips. Because the lesions are not contiguous, two codes are reported.

Malignant neoplasm of ectopic tissue

Malignant neoplasms of ectopic tissue are to be coded to the site of origin mentioned, e.g., ectopic pancreatic malignant neoplasms involving the stomach are coded to malignant neoplasm of pancreas, unspecified (C25.9).

The neoplasm table in the Alphabetic Index should be referenced first. However, if the histological term is documented, that term should be referenced first, rather than going immediately to the Neoplasm Table, in order to determine which column in the Neoplasm Table is appropriate. For example, if the documentation indicates "adenoma," refer to the term in the Alphabetic Index to review the entries under this term and the instructional note to "see also neoplasm, by site, benign." The table provides the proper code based on the type of neoplasm and the site. It is important to select the proper column in the table that corresponds to the type of neoplasm. The Tabular List should then be referenced to verify that the correct code has been selected from the table and that a more specific site code does not exist.

See Section I.C.21. Factors influencing health status and contact with health services, Status, for information regarding Z15.0, codes for genetic susceptibility to cancer.

a. Admission/Encounter for treatment of primary site

If the malignancy **is chiefly responsible for occasioning the patient admission/encounter and treatment is directed at the primary site**, designate the **primary** malignancy as the principal/**first-listed** diagnosis.

The only exception to this guideline is if the administration of chemotherapy, immunotherapy or external beam radiation therapy **is chiefly responsible for occasioning the admission/encounter. In that case**, assign the appropriate Z51.-- code as the first-listed or principal diagnosis, and the **underlying** diagnosis or problem for which the service is being performed as a secondary diagnosis.

b. Admission/Encounter for treatment of secondary site

When a patient is admitted because of a primary neoplasm with metastasis and treatment is directed toward the secondary site only, the secondary neoplasm is designated as the principal diagnosis even though the primary malignancy is still present.

> Patient with primary prostate cancer with metastasis to lungs presents for wedge resection of mass in right lung
>
> **C78.01**   **Secondary malignant neoplasm of right lung**
>
> **C61**   **Malignant neoplasm of prostate**
>
> *Explanation*: Since the encounter is for treatment of the lung metastasis, the secondary lung metastasis is sequenced before the primary prostate cancer.

c. Coding and sequencing of complications

Coding and sequencing of complications associated with the malignancies or with the therapy thereof are subject to the following guidelines:

1) Anemia associated with malignancy

When admission/encounter is for management of an anemia associated with the malignancy, and the treatment is only for anemia, the appropriate code for the malignancy is sequenced as the principal or first-listed diagnosis followed by the appropriate code for the anemia (such as code D63.0, Anemia in neoplastic disease).

> Patient is seen for treatment of anemia in advanced primary liver cancer
>
> **C22.8**   **Malignant neoplasm of liver, primary, unspecified as to type**
>
> **D63.0**   **Anemia in neoplastic disease**
>
> *Explanation*: Even though the admission was solely to treat the anemia, this guideline indicates that the code for the malignancy is sequenced first.

2) Anemia associated with chemotherapy, immunotherapy and radiation therapy

When the admission/encounter is for management of an anemia associated with an adverse effect of the administration of chemotherapy or immunotherapy and the only treatment is for the anemia, the anemia code is sequenced first followed by the appropriate codes for the neoplasm and the adverse effect (T45.1X5, Adverse effect of antineoplastic and immunosuppressive drugs).

When the admission/encounter is for management of an anemia associated with an adverse effect of radiotherapy, the anemia code should be sequenced first, followed by the appropriate neoplasm code and code Y84.2, Radiological procedure and radiotherapy as the cause of abnormal reaction of the patient, or of later complication, without mention of misadventure at the time of the procedure.

> A 55-year-old male with a large malignant rectal tumor has been receiving external radiation therapy to shrink the tumor prior to planned surgery. He is referred today for a blood transfusion to treat anemia related to radiation therapy.
>
> **D64.89**   **Other specified anemias**
>
> **C20**   **Malignant neoplasm of rectum**
>
> **Y84.2**   **Radiological procedure and radiotherapy as the cause of abnormal reaction of the patient, or of later complication, without mention of misadventure at the time of the procedure**
>
> *Explanation*: The code for the anemia is sequenced first, followed by the code for the malignancy, and lastly the code for the abnormal reaction due to radiotherapy.

3) Management of dehydration due to the malignancy

When the admission/encounter is for management of dehydration due to the malignancy and only the dehydration is being treated (intravenous rehydration), the dehydration is sequenced first, followed by the code(s) for the malignancy.

4) Treatment of a complication resulting from a surgical procedure

When the admission/encounter is for treatment of a complication resulting from a surgical procedure, designate the complication as the principal or first-listed diagnosis if treatment is directed at resolving the complication.

d. Primary malignancy previously excised

When a primary malignancy has been previously excised or eradicated from its site and there is no further treatment directed to that site and there is no evidence of any existing primary malignancy at that site, a code from category Z85, Personal history of malignant neoplasm, should be used to indicate the former site of the malignancy. Any mention of extension, invasion, or metastasis to another site is coded as a secondary malignant neoplasm to that site. The secondary site may be the principal or first-listed diagnosis with the Z85 code used as a secondary code.

See section I.C.2.t. Secondary malignant neoplasm of lymphoid tissue.

History of lung cancer, left upper lobectomy 18 months ago with no current treatment; MRI of the brain shows metastatic disease in the brain

C79.31	Secondary malignant neoplasm of brain
Z85.118	Personal history of other malignant neoplasm of bronchus and lung

Explanation: The patient has undergone a diagnostic procedure that revealed metastatic lung cancer in the brain. The code for the secondary (metastatic) site is sequenced first, followed by a personal history code to identify the former site of the primary malignancy.

e. Admissions/encounters involving chemotherapy, immunotherapy and radiation therapy

1) Episode of care involves surgical removal of neoplasm

When an episode of care involves the surgical removal of a neoplasm, primary or secondary site, followed by adjunct chemotherapy or radiation treatment during the same episode of care, the code for the neoplasm should be assigned as principal or first-listed diagnosis.

2) Patient admission/encounter solely for administration of chemotherapy, immunotherapy and radiation therapy

If a patient admission/encounter is solely for the administration of chemotherapy, immunotherapy or external beam radiation therapy assign code Z51.0, Encounter for antineoplastic radiation therapy, or Z51.11, Encounter for antineoplastic chemotherapy, or Z51.12, Encounter for antineoplastic immunotherapy as the first-listed or principal diagnosis. If a patient receives more than one of these therapies during the same admission more than one of these codes may be assigned, in any sequence.

The malignancy for which the therapy is being administered should be assigned as a secondary diagnosis.

If a patient admission/encounter is for the insertion or implantation of radioactive elements (e.g., brachytherapy) the appropriate code for the malignancy is sequenced as the principal or first-listed diagnosis. Code Z51.0 should not be assigned.

Patient presents for second round of rituximab and fludarabine for his chronic B cell lymphocytic leukemia

Z51.11	Encounter for antineoplastic chemotherapy
Z51.12	Encounter for antineoplastic immunotherapy
C91.10	Chronic lymphocytic leukemia of B-cell type not having achieved remission

Explanation: Rituximab is an antineoplastic immunotherapy while fludarabine is an antineoplastic chemotherapy. The two treatments are often used together. The encounter was solely for the purpose of administering this treatment and either can be sequenced first, before the neoplastic condition.

3) Patient admitted for radiation therapy, chemotherapy or immunotherapy and develops complications

When a patient is admitted for the purpose of external beam radiotherapy, immunotherapy or chemotherapy and develops complications such as uncontrolled nausea and vomiting or dehydration, the principal or first-listed diagnosis is Z51.0, Encounter for antineoplastic radiation therapy, or Z51.11, Encounter for antineoplastic chemotherapy, or Z51.12, Encounter for antineoplastic immunotherapy followed by any codes for the complications.

When a patient is admitted for the purpose of insertion or implantation of radioactive elements (e.g., brachytherapy) and develops complications such as uncontrolled nausea and vomiting or dehydration, the principal or first-listed diagnosis is the appropriate code for the malignancy followed by any codes for the complications.

f. Admission/encounter to determine extent of malignancy

When the reason for admission/encounter is to determine the extent of the malignancy, or for a procedure such as paracentesis or thoracentesis, the primary malignancy or appropriate metastatic site is designated as the principal or first-listed diagnosis, even though chemotherapy or radiotherapy is administered.

Patient with left lung cancer with malignant pleural effusion being seen for paracentesis and initiation/administration of chemotherapy

C34.92	Malignant neoplasm of unspecified part of left bronchus or lung
J91.0	Malignant pleural effusion
Z51.11	Encounter for antineoplastic chemotherapy

Explanation: The lung cancer is sequenced before the chemotherapy in this instance because the paracentesis for the malignant effusion is also being performed. An instructional note under the malignant effusion instructs that the lung cancer be sequenced first.

g. Symptoms, signs, and abnormal findings listed in Chapter 18 associated with neoplasms

Symptoms, signs, and ill-defined conditions listed in Chapter 18 characteristic of, or associated with, an existing primary or secondary site malignancy cannot be used to replace the malignancy as principal or first-listed diagnosis, regardless of the number of admissions or encounters for treatment and care of the neoplasm.

See Section I.C.21. Factors influencing health status and contact with health services, Encounter for prophylactic organ removal.

h. Admission/encounter for pain control/management

See Section I.C.6. for information on coding admission/encounter for pain control/management.

i. Malignancy in two or more noncontiguous sites

A patient may have more than one malignant tumor in the same organ. These tumors may represent different primaries or metastatic disease, depending on the site. Should the documentation be unclear, the provider should be queried as to the status of each tumor so that the correct codes can be assigned.

j. Disseminated malignant neoplasm, unspecified

Code C80.0, Disseminated malignant neoplasm, unspecified, is for use only in those cases where the patient has advanced metastatic disease and no known primary or secondary sites are specified. It should not be used in place of assigning codes for the primary site and all known secondary sites.

k. Malignant neoplasm without specification of site

Code C80.1, Malignant (primary) neoplasm, unspecified, equates to Cancer, unspecified. This code should only be used when no determination can be made as to the primary site of a malignancy. This code should rarely be used in the inpatient setting.

Evaluation of painful hip leads to diagnosis of a metastatic bone lesion from an unknown primary neoplasm source

C79.51	Secondary malignant neoplasm of bone
C80.1	Malignant (primary) neoplasm, unspecified

Explanation: If only the secondary site is known, use code C80.1 for the unknown primary site.

l. Sequencing of neoplasm codes

1) Encounter for treatment of primary malignancy

If the reason for the encounter is for treatment of a primary malignancy, assign the malignancy as the principal/first-listed diagnosis. The primary site is to be sequenced first, followed by any metastatic sites.

2) Encounter for treatment of secondary malignancy

When an encounter is for a primary malignancy with metastasis and treatment is directed toward the metastatic (secondary) site(s) only, the metastatic site(s) is designated as the principal/first-listed diagnosis. The primary malignancy is coded as an additional code.

Patient has primary colon cancer with metastasis to rib and is evaluated for possible excision of portion of rib bone

C79.51   **Secondary malignant neoplasm of bone**

C18.9   **Malignant neoplasm of colon, unspecified**

Explanation: The treatment for this encounter is focused on the metastasis to the rib bone rather than the primary colon cancer, thus indicating that the bone metastasis is sequenced as the first-listed code.

3) Malignant neoplasm in a pregnant patient

When a pregnant patient has a malignant neoplasm, a code from subcategory O9A.1-, Malignant neoplasm complicating pregnancy, childbirth, and the puerperium, should be sequenced first, followed by the appropriate code from Chapter 2 to indicate the type of neoplasm.

A 30-year-old pregnant female in first trimester evaluated for pituitary gland malignancy

O9A.111   **Malignant neoplasm complicating pregnancy, first trimester**

C75.1   **Malignant neoplasm of pituitary gland**

Explanation: Codes from chapter 15 describing complications of pregnancy are sequenced as first-listed codes, further specified by codes from other chapters such as neoplastic, unless the pregnancy is documented as incidental to the condition. See also guideline 1.C.15.a.1.

4) Encounter for complication associated with a neoplasm

When an encounter is for management of a complication associated with a neoplasm, such as dehydration, and the treatment is only for the complication, the complication is coded first, followed by the appropriate code(s) for the neoplasm.

The exception to this guideline is anemia. When the admission/encounter is for management of an anemia associated with the malignancy, and the treatment is only for anemia, the appropriate code for the malignancy is sequenced as the principal or first-listed diagnosis followed by code D63.0, Anemia in neoplastic disease.

Patient with pancreatic cancer is seen for initiation of TPN for cancer-related moderate protein-calorie malnutrition

E44.0   **Moderate protein-calorie malnutrition**

C25.9   **Malignant neoplasm of pancreas, unspecified**

Explanation: The encounter is to initiate treatment for malnutrition, a common complication of many types of neoplasms, and is sequenced first.

5) Complication from surgical procedure for treatment of a neoplasm

When an encounter is for treatment of a complication resulting from a surgical procedure performed for the treatment of the neoplasm, designate the complication as the principal/first-listed diagnosis. See the guideline regarding the coding of a current malignancy versus personal history to determine if the code for the neoplasm should also be assigned.

6) Pathologic fracture due to a neoplasm

When an encounter is for a pathological fracture due to a neoplasm, and the focus of treatment is the fracture, a code from subcategory M84.5, Pathological fracture in neoplastic disease, should be sequenced first, followed by the code for the neoplasm.

If the focus of treatment is the neoplasm with an associated pathological fracture, the neoplasm code should be sequenced first, followed by a code from M84.5 for the pathological fracture.

m. Current malignancy versus personal history of malignancy

When a primary malignancy has been excised but further treatment, such as an additional surgery for the malignancy, radiation therapy or chemotherapy is directed to that site, the primary malignancy code should be used until treatment is completed.

Female patient with ongoing chemotherapy after right mastectomy for breast cancer

C50.911   **Malignant neoplasm of unspecified site of right female breast**

Z90.11   **Acquired absence of right breast and nipple**

Explanation: Even though the breast has been removed, the breast cancer is still being treated with chemotherapy and therefore is still coded as a current condition rather than personal history.

When a primary malignancy has been previously excised or eradicated from its site, there is no further treatment (of the malignancy) directed to that site, and there is no evidence of any existing primary malignancy at that site, a code from category Z85, Personal history of malignant neoplasm, should be used to indicate the former site of the malignancy.

Codes from subcategories Z85.0 – Z85.85 should only be assigned for the former site of a primary malignancy, not the site of a secondary malignancy. Code Z85.89 may be assigned for the former site(s) of either a primary or secondary malignancy.

See Section I.C.21. Factors influencing health status and contact with health services, History (of)

n. Leukemia, multiple myeloma, and malignant plasma cell neoplasms in remission versus personal history

The categories for leukemia, and category C90, Multiple myeloma and malignant plasma cell neoplasms, have codes indicating whether or not the leukemia has achieved remission. There are also codes Z85.6, Personal history of leukemia, and Z85.79, Personal history of other malignant neoplasms of lymphoid, hematopoietic and related tissues. If the documentation is unclear as to whether the leukemia has achieved remission, the provider should be queried.

See Section I.C.21. Factors influencing health status and contact with health services, History (of)

o. Aftercare following surgery for neoplasm

See Section I.C.21. Factors influencing health status and contact with health services, Aftercare

p. Follow-up care for completed treatment of a malignancy

See Section I.C.21. Factors influencing health status and contact with health services, Follow-up

q. Prophylactic organ removal for prevention of malignancy

See Section I.C. 21, Factors influencing health status and contact with health services, Prophylactic organ removal

r. Malignant neoplasm associated with transplanted organ

A malignant neoplasm of a transplanted organ should be coded as a transplant complication. Assign first the appropriate code from category T86.-, Complications of transplanted organs and tissue, followed by code C80.2, Malignant neoplasm associated with transplanted organ. Use an additional code for the specific malignancy.

s. Breast implant associated anaplastic large cell lymphoma

Breast implant associated anaplastic large cell lymphoma (BIA-ALCL) is a type of lymphoma that can develop around breast implants. Assign code C84.7A, Anaplastic large cell lymphoma, ALK-negative, breast, for BIA-ALCL. Do not assign a complication code from chapter 19.

t. Secondary malignant neoplasm of lymphoid tissue

When a malignant neoplasm of lymphoid tissue metastasizes beyond the lymph nodes, a code from categories C81-C85 with a final character "9" should be assigned identifying "extranodal and solid organ sites" rather than a code for the secondary neoplasm of the affected solid organ. For example, for metastasis of B-cell lymphoma to the lung, brain and left adrenal gland, assign code C83.39, Diffuse large B-cell lymphoma, extranodal and solid organ sites.

Chapter 2. Neoplasms (C00-D49)

NOTE

Functional activity
All neoplasms are classified in this chapter, whether they are functionally active or not. An additional code from Chapter 4 may be used, to identify functional activity associated with any neoplasm.

Morphology [Histology]
Chapter 2 classifies neoplasms primarily by site (topography), with broad groupings for behavior, malignant, in situ, benign, etc. The Table of Neoplasms should be used to identify the correct topography code. In a few cases, such as for malignant melanoma and certain neuroendocrine tumors, the morphology (histologic type) is included in the category and codes.

Primary malignant neoplasms overlapping site boundaries
A primary malignant neoplasm that overlaps two or more contiguous (next to each other) sites should be classified to the subcategory/code .8 ("overlapping lesion"), unless the combination is specifically indexed elsewhere. For multiple neoplasms of the same site that are not contiguous, such as tumors in different quadrants of the same breast, codes for each site should be assigned.

Malignant neoplasm of ectopic tissue
Malignant neoplasms of ectopic tissue are to be coded to the site mentioned, e.g., ectopic pancreatic malignant neoplasms are coded to pancreas, unspecified (C25.9).

AHA: 2017,4Q,103; 2017,1Q,4,5-6,8

This chapter contains the following blocks:

C00-C14	Malignant neoplasms of lip, oral cavity and pharynx
C15-C26	Malignant neoplasms of digestive organs
C30-C39	Malignant neoplasms of respiratory and intrathoracic organs
C40-C41	Malignant neoplasms of bone and articular cartilage
C43-C44	Melanoma and other malignant neoplasms of skin
C45-C49	Malignant neoplasms of mesothelial and soft tissue
C50	Malignant neoplasms of breast
C51-C58	Malignant neoplasms of female genital organs
C60-C63	Malignant neoplasms of male genital organs
C64-C68	Malignant neoplasms of urinary tract
C69-C72	Malignant neoplasms of eye, brain and other parts of central nervous system
C73-C75	Malignant neoplasms of thyroid and other endocrine glands
C7A	Malignant neuroendocrine tumors
C7B	Secondary neuroendocrine tumors
C76-C80	Malignant neoplasms of ill-defined, other secondary and unspecified sites
C81-C96	Malignant neoplasms of lymphoid, hematopoietic and related tissue
D00-D09	In situ neoplasms
D10-D36	Benign neoplasms, except benign neuroendocrine tumors
D3A	Benign neuroendocrine tumors
D37-D48	Neoplasms of uncertain behavior, polycythemia vera and myelodysplastic syndromes
D49	Neoplasms of unspecified behavior

MALIGNANT NEOPLASMS (C00-C96)

Malignant neoplasms, stated or presumed to be primary (of specified sites), and certain specified histologies, except neuroendocrine, and of lymphoid, hematopoietic and related tissue (C00-C75)

AHA: 2022,1Q,16

TIP: Codes from this code block can be assigned for outpatient encounters based on the diagnosis listed in a pathology or cytology report when authenticated by a pathologist and available at the time of code assignment.

Malignant neoplasms of lip, oral cavity and pharynx (C00-C14)

☑4ᵗʰ C00 Malignant neoplasm of lip

Use additional code to identify:
 alcohol abuse and dependence (F10.-)
 history of tobacco dependence (Z87.891)
 tobacco dependence (F17.-)
 tobacco use (Z72.0)

 EXCLUDES 1
  malignant melanoma of lip (C43.0)
  Merkel cell carcinoma of lip (C4A.0)
  other and unspecified malignant neoplasm of skin of lip (C44.0-)

C00.0 Malignant neoplasm of external upper lip
 Malignant neoplasm of lipstick area of upper lip
 Malignant neoplasm of upper lip NOS
 Malignant neoplasm of vermilion border of upper lip

C00.1 Malignant neoplasm of external lower lip
 Malignant neoplasm of lower lip NOS
 Malignant neoplasm of lipstick area of lower lip
 Malignant neoplasm of vermilion border of lower lip

C00.2 Malignant neoplasm of external lip, unspecified
 Malignant neoplasm of vermilion border of lip NOS

C00.3 Malignant neoplasm of upper lip, inner aspect
 Malignant neoplasm of buccal aspect of upper lip
 Malignant neoplasm of frenulum of upper lip
 Malignant neoplasm of mucosa of upper lip
 Malignant neoplasm of oral aspect of upper lip

C00.4 Malignant neoplasm of lower lip, inner aspect
 Malignant neoplasm of buccal aspect of lower lip
 Malignant neoplasm of frenulum of lower lip
 Malignant neoplasm of mucosa of lower lip
 Malignant neoplasm of oral aspect of lower lip

C00.5 Malignant neoplasm of lip, unspecified, inner aspect
 Malignant neoplasm of buccal aspect of lip, unspecified
 Malignant neoplasm of frenulum of lip, unspecified
 Malignant neoplasm of mucosa of lip, unspecified
 Malignant neoplasm of oral aspect of lip, unspecified

C00.6 Malignant neoplasm of commissure of lip, unspecified

C00.8 Malignant neoplasm of overlapping sites of lip

C00.9 Malignant neoplasm of lip, unspecified

C01 Malignant neoplasm of base of tongue   HCC Rx ESR COM
 Malignant neoplasm of dorsal surface of base of tongue
 Malignant neoplasm of fixed part of tongue NOS
 Malignant neoplasm of posterior third of tongue
 Use additional code to identify:
  alcohol abuse and dependence (F10.-)
  history of tobacco dependence (Z87.891)
  tobacco dependence (F17.-)
  tobacco use (Z72.0)

Malignant Neoplasm of Tongue

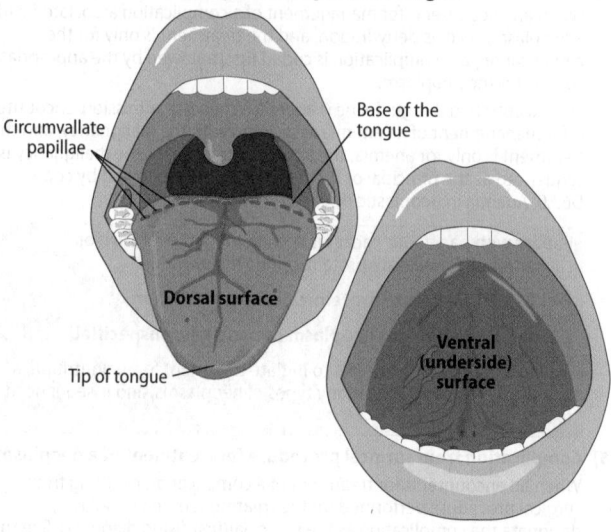

Circumvallate papillae — Base of the tongue — Dorsal surface — Tip of tongue — Ventral (underside) surface

☑4ᵗʰ C02 Malignant neoplasm of other and unspecified parts of tongue

Use additional code to identify:
 alcohol abuse and dependence (F10.-)
 history of tobacco dependence (Z87.891)
 tobacco dependence (F17.-)
 tobacco use (Z72.0)

C02.0 Malignant neoplasm of dorsal surface of tongue   HCC Rx ESR COM
 Malignant neoplasm of anterior two-thirds of tongue, dorsal surface
 EXCLUDES 2   malignant neoplasm of dorsal surface of base of tongue (C01)

C02.1 Malignant neoplasm of border of tongue   HCC Rx ESR COM
 Malignant neoplasm of tip of tongue

C02.2 Malignant neoplasm of ventral surface of tongue   HCC Rx ESR COM
 Malignant neoplasm of anterior two-thirds of tongue, ventral surface
 Malignant neoplasm of frenulum linguae

C02.3 Malignant neoplasm of anterior two-thirds of tongue, part unspecified   HCC Rx ESR COM
 Malignant neoplasm of middle third of tongue NOS
 Malignant neoplasm of mobile part of tongue NOS

C02.4 **Malignant neoplasm of** lingual tonsil   HCC Rx ESR COM
    EXCLUDES 2   *malignant neoplasm of tonsil NOS (C09.9)*

C02.8 **Malignant neoplasm of** overlapping sites of tongue   HCC Rx ESR COM
    Malignant neoplasm of two or more contiguous sites of tongue

C02.9 **Malignant neoplasm of tongue, unspecified**   HCC Rx ESR COM

✓4th **C03** **Malignant neoplasm of** gum
    INCLUDES   malignant neoplasm of alveolar (ridge) mucosa
                      malignant neoplasm of gingiva
    Use additional code to identify:
        alcohol abuse and dependence (F10.-)
        history of tobacco dependence (Z87.891)
        tobacco dependence (F17.-)
        tobacco use (Z72.0)
    EXCLUDES 2   *malignant odontogenic neoplasms (C41.0-C41.1)*

C03.0 **Malignant neoplasm of** upper gum   HCC Rx ESR COM
C03.1 **Malignant neoplasm of** lower gum   HCC Rx ESR COM
C03.9 **Malignant neoplasm of** gum, unspecified   HCC Rx ESR COM

✓4th **C04** **Malignant neoplasm of** floor of mouth
    Use additional code to identify:
        alcohol abuse and dependence (F10.-)
        history of tobacco dependence (Z87.891)
        tobacco dependence (F17.-)
        tobacco use (Z72.0)

C04.0 **Malignant neoplasm of** anterior **floor of mouth**   HCC Rx ESR COM
    Malignant neoplasm of anterior to the premolar-canine junction

C04.1 **Malignant neoplasm of** lateral **floor of mouth**   HCC Rx ESR COM

C04.8 **Malignant neoplasm of** overlapping sites **of floor of mouth**   HCC Rx ESR COM

C04.9 **Malignant neoplasm of floor of mouth, unspecified**   HCC Rx ESR COM

✓4th **C05** **Malignant neoplasm of** palate
    Use additional code to identify:
        alcohol abuse and dependence (F10.-)
        history of tobacco dependence (Z87.891)
        tobacco dependence (F17.-)
        tobacco use (Z72.0)
    EXCLUDES 1   *Kaposi's sarcoma of palate (C46.2)*

C05.0 **Malignant neoplasm of** hard **palate**   HCC Rx ESR COM
C05.1 **Malignant neoplasm of** soft **palate**   HCC Rx ESR COM
    EXCLUDES 2   *malignant neoplasm of nasopharyngeal surface of soft palate (C11.3)*
C05.2 **Malignant neoplasm of** uvula   HCC Rx ESR COM
C05.8 **Malignant neoplasm of** overlapping sites of **palate**   HCC Rx ESR COM
C05.9 **Malignant neoplasm of palate, unspecified**   HCC Rx ESR COM
    Malignant neoplasm of roof of mouth

✓4th **C06** **Malignant neoplasm of** other and unspecified parts of mouth
    Use additional code to identify:
        alcohol abuse and dependence (F10.-)
        history of tobacco dependence (Z87.891)
        tobacco dependence (F17.-)
        tobacco use (Z72.0)

C06.0 **Malignant neoplasm of** cheek mucosa   HCC Rx ESR COM
    Malignant neoplasm of buccal mucosa NOS
    Malignant neoplasm of internal cheek

C06.1 **Malignant neoplasm of** vestibule **of mouth**   HCC Rx ESR COM
    Malignant neoplasm of buccal sulcus (upper) (lower)
    Malignant neoplasm of labial sulcus (upper) (lower)

C06.2 **Malignant neoplasm of** retromolar area   HCC Rx ESR COM

✓5th **C06.8** **Malignant neoplasm of** overlapping sites **of other and unspecified parts of mouth**

    C06.80 **Malignant neoplasm of overlapping sites of unspecified parts of mouth**   HCC Rx ESR COM

    C06.89 **Malignant neoplasm of overlapping sites of other parts of mouth**   HCC Rx ESR COM
        "book leaf" neoplasm [ventral surface of tongue and floor of mouth]

C06.9 **Malignant neoplasm of mouth, unspecified**   HCC Rx ESR COM
    Malignant neoplasm of minor salivary gland, unspecified site
    Malignant neoplasm of oral cavity NOS

C07 **Malignant neoplasm of** parotid gland   HCC Rx ESR COM
    Use additional code to identify:
        alcohol abuse and dependence (F10.-)
        exposure to environmental tobacco smoke (Z77.22)
        exposure to tobacco smoke in the perinatal period (P96.81)
        history of tobacco dependence (Z87.891)
        occupational exposure to environmental tobacco smoke (Z57.31)
        tobacco dependence (F17.-)
        tobacco use (Z72.0)

✓4th **C08** **Malignant neoplasm of** other and unspecified major salivary glands
    INCLUDES   malignant neoplasm of salivary ducts
    Use additional code to identify:
        alcohol abuse and dependence (F10.-)
        exposure to environmental tobacco smoke (Z77.22)
        exposure to tobacco smoke in the perinatal period (P96.81)
        history of tobacco dependence (Z87.891)
        occupational exposure to environmental tobacco smoke (Z57.31)
        tobacco dependence (F17.-)
        tobacco use (Z72.0)
    EXCLUDES 1   *malignant neoplasms of specified minor salivary glands which are classified according to their anatomical location*
    EXCLUDES 2   *malignant neoplasms of minor salivary glands NOS (C06.9)*
                   malignant neoplasm of parotid gland (C07)

C08.0 **Malignant neoplasm of** submandibular **gland**   HCC Rx ESR COM
    Malignant neoplasm of submaxillary gland

C08.1 **Malignant neoplasm of** sublingual **gland**   HCC Rx ESR COM

C08.9 **Malignant neoplasm of** major salivary gland, **unspecified**   HCC Rx ESR COM
    Malignant neoplasm of salivary gland (major) NOS

✓4th **C09** **Malignant neoplasm of** tonsil
    Use additional code to identify:
        alcohol abuse and dependence (F10.-)
        exposure to environmental tobacco smoke (Z77.22)
        exposure to tobacco smoke in the perinatal period (P96.81)
        history of tobacco dependence (Z87.891)
        occupational exposure to environmental tobacco smoke (Z57.31)
        tobacco dependence (F17.-)
        tobacco use (Z72.0)
    EXCLUDES 2   *malignant neoplasm of lingual tonsil (C02.4)*
                   malignant neoplasm of pharyngeal tonsil (C11.1)

C09.0 **Malignant neoplasm of** tonsillar fossa   HCC ESR COM
C09.1 **Malignant neoplasm of** tonsillar pillar (anterior) (posterior)   HCC ESR COM
C09.8 **Malignant neoplasm of** overlapping sites of **tonsil**   HCC ESR COM
C09.9 **Malignant neoplasm of tonsil, unspecified**   HCC ESR COM
    Malignant neoplasm of tonsil NOS
    Malignant neoplasm of faucial tonsils
    Malignant neoplasm of palatine tonsils

✓4th **C10** **Malignant neoplasm of** oropharynx
    Use additional code to identify:
        alcohol abuse and dependence (F10.-)
        exposure to environmental tobacco smoke (Z77.22)
        exposure to tobacco smoke in the perinatal period (P96.81)
        history of tobacco dependence (Z87.891)
        occupational exposure to environmental tobacco smoke (Z57.31)
        tobacco dependence (F17.-)
        tobacco use (Z72.0)
    EXCLUDES 2   *malignant neoplasm of tonsil (C09.-)*
    DEF: Oropharynx: Middle portion of pharynx (throat); communicates with the oral cavity, nasopharynx and laryngopharynx.

C10.0 **Malignant neoplasm of** vallecula   HCC ESR COM
C10.1 **Malignant neoplasm of** anterior surface of **epiglottis**   HCC ESR COM
    Malignant neoplasm of epiglottis, free border [margin]
    Malignant neoplasm of glossoepiglottic fold(s)
    EXCLUDES 2   *malignant neoplasm of epiglottis (suprahyoid portion) NOS (C32.1)*

C10.2 **Malignant neoplasm of** lateral wall **of oropharynx**   HCC ESR COM
C10.3 **Malignant neoplasm of** posterior wall **of oropharynx**   HCC ESR COM

Chapter 2. Neoplasms

C02.4–C10.3

C10.4 **Malignant neoplasm of** branchial cleft   `HCC` `ESR` `COM`
     Malignant neoplasm of branchial cyst [site of neoplasm]

C10.8 **Malignant neoplasm of** overlapping sites of oropharynx   `HCC` `ESR` `COM`
     Malignant neoplasm of junctional region of oropharynx

C10.9 **Malignant neoplasm of oropharynx, unspecified**   `HCC` `ESR` `COM`

✓4ᵗʰ **C11** **Malignant neoplasm of** nasopharynx
     Use additional code to identify:
       exposure to environmental tobacco smoke (Z77.22)
       exposure to tobacco smoke in the perinatal period (P96.81)
       history of tobacco dependence (Z87.891)
       occupational exposure to environmental tobacco smoke (Z57.31)
       tobacco dependence (F17.-)
       tobacco use (Z72.0)
     DEF: Nasopharynx: Upper portion of pharynx (throat); communicates with the nasal cavities, oropharynx and tympanic cavities.

C11.0 **Malignant neoplasm of** superior wall of nasopharynx   `HCC` `ESR` `COM`
     Malignant neoplasm of roof of nasopharynx

C11.1 **Malignant neoplasm of** posterior wall of nasopharynx   `HCC` `ESR` `COM`
     Malignant neoplasm of adenoid
     Malignant neoplasm of pharyngeal tonsil

C11.2 **Malignant neoplasm of** lateral wall of nasopharynx   `HCC` `ESR` `COM`
     Malignant neoplasm of fossa of Rosenmüller
     Malignant neoplasm of opening of auditory tube
     Malignant neoplasm of pharyngeal recess

C11.3 **Malignant neoplasm of** anterior wall of nasopharynx   `HCC` `ESR` `COM`
     Malignant neoplasm of floor of nasopharynx
     Malignant neoplasm of nasopharyngeal (anterior) (posterior) surface of soft palate
     Malignant neoplasm of posterior margin of nasal choana
     Malignant neoplasm of posterior margin of nasal septum

C11.8 **Malignant neoplasm of** overlapping sites of nasopharynx   `HCC` `ESR` `COM`

C11.9 **Malignant neoplasm of nasopharynx, unspecified**   `HCC` `ESR` `COM`
     Malignant neoplasm of nasopharyngeal wall NOS

C12 **Malignant neoplasm of** pyriform sinus   `HCC` `ESR` `COM`
     Malignant neoplasm of pyriform fossa
     Use additional code to identify:
       exposure to environmental tobacco smoke (Z77.22)
       exposure to tobacco smoke in the perinatal period (P96.81)
       history of tobacco dependence (Z87.891)
       occupational exposure to environmental tobacco smoke (Z57.31)
       tobacco dependence (F17.-)
       tobacco use (Z72.0)

✓4ᵗʰ **C13** **Malignant neoplasm of** hypopharynx
     Use additional code to identify:
       exposure to environmental tobacco smoke (Z77.22)
       exposure to tobacco smoke in the perinatal period (P96.81)
       history of tobacco dependence (Z87.891)
       occupational exposure to environmental tobacco smoke (Z57.31)
       tobacco dependence (F17.-)
       tobacco use (Z72.0)
     EXCLUDES 2   malignant neoplasm of pyriform sinus (C12)
     DEF: Hypopharynx: Lower portion of pharynx (throat); communicates with the oropharynx and the esophagus. **Synonym(s):** laryngopharynx.

C13.0 **Malignant neoplasm of** postcricoid region   `HCC` `ESR` `COM`

C13.1 **Malignant neoplasm of** aryepiglottic fold, hypopharyngeal aspect   `HCC` `ESR` `COM`
     Malignant neoplasm of aryepiglottic fold, marginal zone
     Malignant neoplasm of aryepiglottic fold NOS
     Malignant neoplasm of interarytenoid fold, marginal zone
     Malignant neoplasm of interarytenoid fold NOS
     EXCLUDES 2   malignant neoplasm of aryepiglottic fold or interarytenoid fold, laryngeal aspect (C32.1)

C13.2 **Malignant neoplasm of** posterior wall of hypopharynx   `HCC` `ESR` `COM`

C13.8 **Malignant neoplasm of** overlapping sites of hypopharynx   `HCC` `ESR` `COM`

C13.9 **Malignant neoplasm of hypopharynx, unspecified**   `HCC` `ESR` `COM`
     Malignant neoplasm of hypopharyngeal wall NOS

✓4ᵗʰ **C14** **Malignant neoplasm of** other and ill-defined sites in the lip, oral cavity and pharynx
     Use additional code to identify:
       alcohol abuse and dependence (F10.-)
       exposure to environmental tobacco smoke (Z77.22)
       exposure to tobacco smoke in the perinatal period (P96.81)
       history of tobacco dependence (Z87.891)
       occupational exposure to environmental tobacco smoke (Z57.31)
       tobacco dependence (F17.-)
       tobacco use (Z72.0)
     EXCLUDES 1   malignant neoplasm of oral cavity NOS (C06.9)

C14.0 **Malignant neoplasm of pharynx, unspecified**   `HCC` `ESR` `COM`

C14.2 **Malignant neoplasm of** Waldeyer's ring   `HCC` `ESR` `COM`
     DEF: Waldeyer's ring: Ring of lymphoid tissue that is made up of the two palatine tonsils, the pharyngeal tonsil (adenoid), and the lingual tonsil. It functions as the defense against infection and assists with the development of the immune system.

C14.8 **Malignant neoplasm of** overlapping sites of lip, oral cavity and pharynx   `HCC` `ESR` `COM`
     Primary malignant neoplasm of two or more contiguous sites of lip, oral cavity and pharynx
     EXCLUDES 1   "book leaf" neoplasm [ventral surface of tongue and floor of mouth] (C06.89)

Malignant neoplasms of digestive organs (C15-C26)

     EXCLUDES 1   Kaposi's sarcoma of gastrointestinal sites (C46.4)
     EXCLUDES 2   gastrointestinal stromal tumors (C49.A-)

✓4ᵗʰ **C15** **Malignant neoplasm of** esophagus
     Use additional code to identify:
       alcohol abuse and dependence (F10.-)

C15.3 **Malignant neoplasm of** upper third of esophagus   `HCC` `ESR` `COM`

C15.4 **Malignant neoplasm of** middle third of esophagus   `HCC` `ESR` `COM`

C15.5 **Malignant neoplasm of** lower third of esophagus   `HCC` `ESR` `COM`
     EXCLUDES 1   malignant neoplasm of cardio-esophageal junction (C16.0)

C15.8 **Malignant neoplasm of** overlapping sites of esophagus   `HCC` `ESR` `COM`

C15.9 **Malignant neoplasm of esophagus, unspecified**   `HCC` `ESR` `COM`

✓4ᵗʰ **C16** **Malignant neoplasm of** stomach
     Use additional code to identify:
       alcohol abuse and dependence (F10.-)
     EXCLUDES 2   malignant carcinoid tumor of the stomach (C7A.092)

C16.0 **Malignant neoplasm of** cardia   `HCC` `Rx` `ESR` `COM`
     Malignant neoplasm of cardiac orifice
     Malignant neoplasm of cardio-esophageal junction
     Malignant neoplasm of esophagus and stomach
     Malignant neoplasm of gastro-esophageal junction

C16.1 **Malignant neoplasm of** fundus of stomach   `HCC` `Rx` `ESR` `COM`

C16.2 **Malignant neoplasm of** body of stomach   `HCC` `Rx` `ESR` `COM`

C16.3 **Malignant neoplasm of** pyloric antrum   `HCC` `Rx` `ESR` `COM`
     Malignant neoplasm of gastric antrum

C16.4 **Malignant neoplasm of** pylorus   `HCC` `Rx` `ESR` `COM`
     Malignant neoplasm of prepylorus
     Malignant neoplasm of pyloric canal

C16.5 **Malignant neoplasm of** lesser curvature of stomach, unspecified   `HCC` `Rx` `ESR` `COM`
     Malignant neoplasm of lesser curvature of stomach, not classifiable to C16.1-C16.4

C16.6 **Malignant neoplasm of** greater curvature of stomach, unspecified   `HCC` `Rx` `ESR` `COM`
     Malignant neoplasm of greater curvature of stomach, not classifiable to C16.0-C16.4

C16.8 **Malignant neoplasm of** overlapping sites of stomach   `HCC` `Rx` `ESR` `COM`

C16.9 **Malignant neoplasm of stomach, unspecified**   `HCC` `Rx` `ESR` `COM`
     Gastric cancer NOS

`HCC` CMS-HCC   `Rx` Rx HCC   `ESR` ESRD HCC   `COM` Commercial HCC   `N` Newborn: 0   `P` Pediatric: 0-17   `M` Maternity: 9-64   `A` Adult: 15-124

478   ICD-10-CM 2023

☑4ᵗʰ **C17** **Malignant neoplasm of** small intestine
> *EXCLUDES 1*   *malignant carcinoid tumors of the small intestine (C7A.01)*
> **AHA:** 2016,1Q,19

C17.0   **Malignant neoplasm of** duodenum   HCC Rx ESR COM

C17.1   **Malignant neoplasm of** jejunum   HCC Rx ESR COM

C17.2   **Malignant neoplasm of** ileum   HCC Rx ESR COM
> *EXCLUDES 1*   *malignant neoplasm of ileocecal valve (C18.0)*

C17.3   **Meckel's diverticulum, malignant**   HCC Rx ESR COM
> *EXCLUDES 1*   *Meckel's diverticulum, congenital (Q43.0)*
> **DEF:** Congenital, abnormal remnant of embryonic digestive system development that leaves a sacculation or outpouching from the wall of the small intestine near the terminal part of the ileum made of acid-secreting tissue as in the stomach.

C17.8   **Malignant neoplasm of** overlapping sites **of small intestine**   HCC Rx ESR COM

C17.9   **Malignant neoplasm of small intestine, unspecified**   HCC Rx ESR COM

☑4ᵗʰ **C18** **Malignant neoplasm of** colon
> *EXCLUDES 1*   *malignant carcinoid tumors of the colon (C7A.02-)*

Colon

Anatomical distribution of large bowel cancers

C18.0   **Malignant neoplasm of** cecum   HCC ESR COM
> Malignant neoplasm of ileocecal valve

C18.1   **Malignant neoplasm of** appendix   HCC ESR COM

C18.2   **Malignant neoplasm of** ascending colon   HCC ESR COM

C18.3   **Malignant neoplasm of** hepatic flexure   HCC ESR COM

C18.4   **Malignant neoplasm of** transverse colon   HCC ESR COM

C18.5   **Malignant neoplasm of** splenic flexure   HCC ESR COM

C18.6   **Malignant neoplasm of** descending colon   HCC ESR COM

C18.7   **Malignant neoplasm of** sigmoid colon   HCC ESR COM
> Malignant neoplasm of sigmoid (flexure)
> *EXCLUDES 1*   *malignant neoplasm of rectosigmoid junction (C19)*

C18.8   **Malignant neoplasm of** overlapping sites **of colon**   HCC ESR COM

C18.9   **Malignant neoplasm of colon, unspecified**   HCC ESR COM
> Malignant neoplasm of large intestine NOS

C19   **Malignant neoplasm of** rectosigmoid junction   HCC ESR COM
> Malignant neoplasm of colon with rectum
> Malignant neoplasm of rectosigmoid (colon)
> *EXCLUDES 1*   *malignant carcinoid tumors of the colon (C7A.02-)*

C20   **Malignant neoplasm of** rectum   HCC ESR COM
> Malignant neoplasm of rectal ampulla
> *EXCLUDES 1*   *malignant carcinoid tumor of the rectum (C7A.026)*

☑4ᵗʰ **C21** **Malignant neoplasm of** anus and anal canal
> *EXCLUDES 2*   *malignant carcinoid tumors of the colon (C7A.02-)*
> *malignant melanoma of anal margin (C43.51)*
> *malignant melanoma of anal skin (C43.51)*
> *malignant melanoma of perianal skin (C43.51)*
> *other and unspecified malignant neoplasm of anal margin (C44.500, C44.510, C44.520, C44.590)*
> *other and unspecified malignant neoplasm of anal skin (C44.500, C44.510, C44.520, C44.590)*
> *other and unspecified malignant neoplasm of perianal skin (C44.500, C44.510, C44.520, C44.590)*

C21.0   **Malignant neoplasm of** anus, unspecified   HCC ESR COM

C21.1   **Malignant neoplasm of** anal canal   HCC ESR COM
> Malignant neoplasm of anal sphincter

C21.2   **Malignant neoplasm of** cloacogenic zone   HCC ESR COM

C21.8   **Malignant neoplasm of** overlapping sites **of rectum, anus and anal canal**   HCC ESR COM
> Malignant neoplasm of anorectal junction
> Malignant neoplasm of anorectum
> Primary malignant neoplasm of two or more contiguous sites of rectum, anus and anal canal

☑4ᵗʰ **C22** **Malignant neoplasm of** liver and intrahepatic bile ducts
> *EXCLUDES 1*   *malignant neoplasm of biliary tract NOS (C24.9)*
> *secondary malignant neoplasm of liver and intrahepatic bile duct (C78.7)*
> Use additional code to identify:
> alcohol abuse and dependence (F10.-)
> hepatitis B (B16.-, B18.0-B18.1)
> hepatitis C (B17.1-, B18.2)

C22.0   **Liver cell carcinoma**   HCC Rx ESR COM
> Hepatocellular carcinoma
> Hepatoma
> **AHA:** 2016,1Q,18

C22.1   **Intrahepatic bile duct carcinoma**   HCC Rx ESR COM
> Cholangiocarcinoma
> *EXCLUDES 1*   *malignant neoplasm of hepatic duct (C24.0)*

C22.2   **Hepatoblastoma**   HCC Rx ESR COM

C22.3   **Angiosarcoma of liver**   HCC Rx ESR COM
> Kupffer cell sarcoma

C22.4   **Other sarcomas of liver**   HCC Rx ESR COM

C22.7   **Other specified carcinomas of liver**   HCC Rx ESR COM

C22.8   **Malignant neoplasm of liver, primary, unspecified as to type**   HCC Rx ESR COM

C22.9   **Malignant neoplasm of liver, not specified as primary or secondary**   HCC Rx ESR COM

C23   **Malignant neoplasm of** gallbladder   HCC Rx ESR COM

☑4ᵗʰ **C24** **Malignant neoplasm of** other and unspecified parts of biliary tract
> *EXCLUDES 1*   *malignant neoplasm of intrahepatic bile duct (C22.1)*

C24.0   **Malignant neoplasm of** extrahepatic bile duct   HCC Rx ESR COM
> Malignant neoplasm of biliary duct or passage NOS
> Malignant neoplasm of common bile duct
> Malignant neoplasm of cystic duct
> Malignant neoplasm of hepatic duct

C24.1   **Malignant neoplasm of** ampulla of Vater   HCC Rx ESR COM
> **DEF:** Malignant neoplasm in the area of dilation at the juncture of the common bile and pancreatic ducts near the opening into the lumen of the duodenum.

C24.8   **Malignant neoplasm of** overlapping sites **of biliary tract**   HCC Rx ESR COM
> Malignant neoplasm involving both intrahepatic and extrahepatic bile ducts
> Primary malignant neoplasm of two or more contiguous sites of biliary tract

C24.9   **Malignant neoplasm of biliary tract, unspecified**   HCC Rx ESR COM

☑ Additional Character Required   ☑x7ᵗʰ Placeholder Alert   Manifestation   Unspecified Dx   🄌 QPP   UPD Unacceptable PDx

Chapter 2. Neoplasms

C25–C33

✓4ᵗʰ **C25 Malignant neoplasm of pancreas**

    Code also if applicable exocrine pancreatic insufficiency (K86.81)
    Use additional code to identify:
       alcohol abuse and dependence (F10.-)

Pancreas

  C25.0 Malignant neoplasm of head of pancreas `HCC` `Rx` `ESR` `COM`
  C25.1 Malignant neoplasm of body of pancreas `HCC` `Rx` `ESR` `COM`
  C25.2 Malignant neoplasm of tail of pancreas `HCC` `Rx` `ESR` `COM`
  C25.3 Malignant neoplasm of pancreatic duct `HCC` `Rx` `ESR` `COM`
  C25.4 Malignant neoplasm of endocrine pancreas `HCC` `Rx` `ESR`
      Malignant neoplasm of islets of Langerhans
      Use additional code to identify any functional activity
  C25.7 Malignant neoplasm of other parts of pancreas `HCC` `Rx` `ESR` `COM`
      Malignant neoplasm of neck of pancreas
  C25.8 Malignant neoplasm of overlapping sites of pancreas `HCC` `Rx` `ESR` `COM`
  C25.9 Malignant neoplasm of pancreas, unspecified `HCC` `Rx` `ESR` `COM`

✓4ᵗʰ **C26 Malignant neoplasm of other and ill-defined digestive organs**
    EXCLUDES 1   malignant neoplasm of peritoneum and retroperitoneum (C48.-)
  C26.0 Malignant neoplasm of intestinal tract, part unspecified `HCC` `ESR` `COM`
      Malignant neoplasm of intestine NOS
  C26.1 Malignant neoplasm of spleen `HCC` `ESR` `COM`
    EXCLUDES 1   Hodgkin lymphoma (C81.-)
                 non-Hodgkin lymphoma (C82-C85)
  C26.9 Malignant neoplasm of ill-defined sites within the digestive system `HCC` `ESR` `COM`
      Malignant neoplasm of alimentary canal or tract NOS
      Malignant neoplasm of gastrointestinal tract NOS
    EXCLUDES 1   malignant neoplasm of abdominal NOS (C76.2)
                 malignant neoplasm of intra-abdominal NOS (C76.2)

Malignant neoplasms of respiratory and intrathoracic organs (C30-C39)

  INCLUDES   malignant neoplasm of middle ear
  EXCLUDES 1   mesothelioma (C45.-)

✓4ᵗʰ **C30 Malignant neoplasm of nasal cavity and middle ear**

  C30.0 Malignant neoplasm of nasal cavity `HCC` `Rx` `ESR` `COM`
      Malignant neoplasm of cartilage of nose
      Malignant neoplasm of nasal concha
      Malignant neoplasm of internal nose
      Malignant neoplasm of septum of nose
      Malignant neoplasm of vestibule of nose
    EXCLUDES 1   malignant neoplasm of nasal bone (C41.0)
                 malignant neoplasm of nose NOS (C76.0)
                 malignant neoplasm of olfactory bulb (C72.2-)
                 malignant neoplasm of posterior margin of nasal septum and choana (C11.3)
                 malignant melanoma of skin of nose (C43.31)
                 malignant neoplasm of turbinates (C41.0)
                 other and unspecified malignant neoplasm of skin of nose (C44.301, C44.311, C44.321, C44.391)

  C30.1 Malignant neoplasm of middle ear `HCC` `Rx` `ESR` `COM`
      Malignant neoplasm of antrum tympanicum
      Malignant neoplasm of auditory tube
      Malignant neoplasm of eustachian tube
      Malignant neoplasm of inner ear
      Malignant neoplasm of mastoid air cells
      Malignant neoplasm of tympanic cavity
    EXCLUDES 1   malignant neoplasm of auricular canal (external) (C43.2-,C44.2-)
                 malignant neoplasm of bone of ear (meatus) (C41.0)
                 malignant neoplasm of cartilage of ear (C49.0)
                 malignant melanoma of skin of (external) ear (C43.2-)
                 other and unspecified malignant neoplasm of skin of (external) ear (C44.2-)

✓4ᵗʰ **C31 Malignant neoplasm of accessory sinuses**

  C31.0 Malignant neoplasm of maxillary sinus `HCC` `Rx` `ESR` `COM`
      Malignant neoplasm of antrum (Highmore) (maxillary)
  C31.1 Malignant neoplasm of ethmoidal sinus `HCC` `Rx` `ESR` `COM`
  C31.2 Malignant neoplasm of frontal sinus `HCC` `Rx` `ESR` `COM`
  C31.3 Malignant neoplasm of sphenoid sinus `HCC` `Rx` `ESR` `COM`
  C31.8 Malignant neoplasm of overlapping sites of accessory sinuses `HCC` `Rx` `ESR` `COM`
  C31.9 Malignant neoplasm of accessory sinus, unspecified `HCC` `Rx` `ESR` `COM`

✓4ᵗʰ **C32 Malignant neoplasm of larynx**

    Use additional code to identify:
      alcohol abuse and dependence (F10.-)
      exposure to environmental tobacco smoke (Z77.22)
      exposure to tobacco smoke in the perinatal period (P96.81)
      history of tobacco dependence (Z87.891)
      occupational exposure to environmental tobacco smoke (Z57.31)
      tobacco dependence (F17.-)
      tobacco use (Z72.0)

  C32.0 Malignant neoplasm of glottis `HCC` `ESR` `COM`
      Malignant neoplasm of intrinsic larynx
      Malignant neoplasm of laryngeal commissure (anterior)(posterior)
      Malignant neoplasm of vocal cord (true) NOS
  C32.1 Malignant neoplasm of supraglottis `HCC` `ESR` `COM`
      Malignant neoplasm of aryepiglottic fold or interarytenoid fold, laryngeal aspect
      Malignant neoplasm of epiglottis (suprahyoid portion) NOS
      Malignant neoplasm of extrinsic larynx
      Malignant neoplasm of false vocal cord
      Malignant neoplasm of posterior (laryngeal) surface of epiglottis
      Malignant neoplasm of ventricular bands
    EXCLUDES 2   malignant neoplasm of anterior surface of epiglottis (C10.1)
                 malignant neoplasm of aryepiglottic fold or interarytenoid fold, hypopharyngeal aspect (C13.1)
                 malignant neoplasm of aryepiglottic fold or interarytenoid fold, marginal zone (C13.1)
                 malignant neoplasm of aryepiglottic fold or interarytenoid fold NOS (C13.1)

  C32.2 Malignant neoplasm of subglottis `HCC` `ESR` `COM`
  C32.3 Malignant neoplasm of laryngeal cartilage `HCC` `ESR` `COM`
  C32.8 Malignant neoplasm of overlapping sites of larynx `HCC` `ESR` `COM`
  C32.9 Malignant neoplasm of larynx, unspecified `HCC` `ESR` `COM`

C33 Malignant neoplasm of trachea `HCC` `Rx` `ESR` `COM`
    Use additional code to identify:
      exposure to environmental tobacco smoke (Z77.22)
      exposure to tobacco smoke in the perinatal period (P96.81)
      history of tobacco dependence (Z87.891)
      occupational exposure to environmental tobacco smoke (Z57.31)
      tobacco dependence (F17.-)
      tobacco use (Z72.0)

`HCC` CMS-HCC   `Rx` Rx HCC   `ESR` ESRD HCC   `COM` Commercial HCC   `N` Newborn: 0   `P` Pediatric: 0-17   `M` Maternity: 9-64   `A` Adult: 15-124

480   ICD-10-CM 2023

✓4th **C34 Malignant neoplasm of bronchus and lung**

Use additional code to identify:
exposure to environmental tobacco smoke (Z77.22)
exposure to tobacco smoke in the perinatal period (P96.81)
history of tobacco dependence (Z87.891)
occupational exposure to environmental tobacco smoke (Z57.31)
tobacco dependence (F17.-)
tobacco use (Z72.0)

EXCLUDES 1   Kaposi's sarcoma of lung (C46.5-)
malignant carcinoid tumor of the bronchus and lung (C7A.090)

AHA: 2019,1Q,16

TIP: When documented, assign code I31.3 for associated malignant pericardial effusion. If the sole reason for admission is to treat the effusion with no treatment of the lung malignancy rendered, code I31.3 may be sequenced first.

✓5th **C34.0 Malignant neoplasm of main bronchus**
Malignant neoplasm of carina
Malignant neoplasm of hilus (of lung)

    C34.00 Malignant neoplasm of unspecified main bronchus HCC Rx ESR COM Q

    C34.01 Malignant neoplasm of right main bronchus HCC Rx ESR COM Q

    C34.02 Malignant neoplasm of left main bronchus HCC Rx ESR COM Q

✓5th **C34.1 Malignant neoplasm of upper lobe, bronchus or lung**

    C34.10 Malignant neoplasm of upper lobe, unspecified bronchus or lung HCC Rx ESR COM Q

    C34.11 Malignant neoplasm of upper lobe, right bronchus or lung HCC Rx ESR COM Q

    C34.12 Malignant neoplasm of upper lobe, left bronchus or lung HCC Rx ESR COM Q

  C34.2 Malignant neoplasm of middle lobe, bronchus or lung HCC Rx ESR COM Q

✓5th **C34.3 Malignant neoplasm of lower lobe, bronchus or lung**

    C34.30 Malignant neoplasm of lower lobe, unspecified bronchus or lung HCC Rx ESR COM Q

    C34.31 Malignant neoplasm of lower lobe, right bronchus or lung HCC Rx ESR COM Q

    C34.32 Malignant neoplasm of lower lobe, left bronchus or lung HCC Rx ESR COM Q

✓5th **C34.8 Malignant neoplasm of overlapping sites of bronchus and lung**

    C34.80 Malignant neoplasm of overlapping sites of unspecified bronchus and lung HCC Rx ESR COM Q

    C34.81 Malignant neoplasm of overlapping sites of right bronchus and lung HCC Rx ESR COM Q

    C34.82 Malignant neoplasm of overlapping sites of left bronchus and lung HCC Rx ESR COM Q

✓5th **C34.9 Malignant neoplasm of unspecified part of bronchus or lung**

    C34.90 Malignant neoplasm of unspecified part of unspecified bronchus or lung HCC Rx ESR COM Q
Lung cancer NOS

    C34.91 Malignant neoplasm of unspecified part of right bronchus or lung HCC Rx ESR COM Q

    C34.92 Malignant neoplasm of unspecified part of left bronchus or lung HCC Rx ESR COM Q

C37 Malignant neoplasm of thymus HCC Rx ESR COM
EXCLUDES 1   malignant carcinoid tumor of the thymus (C7A.091)

✓4th **C38 Malignant neoplasm of heart, mediastinum and pleura**
EXCLUDES 1   mesothelioma (C45.-)

  C38.0 Malignant neoplasm of heart HCC Rx ESR COM
Malignant neoplasm of pericardium
EXCLUDES 1   malignant neoplasm of great vessels (C49.3)

  C38.1 Malignant neoplasm of anterior mediastinum HCC Rx ESR COM

  C38.2 Malignant neoplasm of posterior mediastinum HCC Rx ESR COM

  C38.3 Malignant neoplasm of mediastinum, part unspecified HCC Rx ESR COM

  C38.4 Malignant neoplasm of pleura HCC Rx ESR COM

  C38.8 Malignant neoplasm of overlapping sites of heart, mediastinum and pleura HCC Rx ESR COM

✓4th **C39 Malignant neoplasm of other and ill-defined sites in the respiratory system and intrathoracic organs**

Use additional code to identify:
exposure to environmental tobacco smoke (Z77.22)
exposure to tobacco smoke in the perinatal period (P96.81)
history of tobacco dependence (Z87.891)
occupational exposure to environmental tobacco smoke (Z57.31)
tobacco dependence (F17.-)
tobacco use (Z72.0)

EXCLUDES 1   intrathoracic malignant neoplasm NOS (C76.1)
thoracic malignant neoplasm NOS (C76.1)

  C39.0 Malignant neoplasm of upper respiratory tract, part unspecified HCC Rx ESR COM

  C39.9 Malignant neoplasm of lower respiratory tract, part unspecified HCC Rx ESR COM
Malignant neoplasm of respiratory tract NOS

Malignant neoplasms of bone and articular cartilage (C40-C41)

INCLUDES   malignant neoplasm of cartilage (articular) (joint)
malignant neoplasm of periosteum

EXCLUDES 1   malignant neoplasm of bone marrow NOS (C96.9)
malignant neoplasm of synovia (C49.-)

✓4th **C40 Malignant neoplasm of bone and articular cartilage of limbs**

Use additional code to identify major osseous defect, if applicable (M89.7-)

✓5th **C40.0 Malignant neoplasm of scapula and long bones of upper limb**

    C40.00 Malignant neoplasm of scapula and long bones of unspecified upper limb HCC Rx ESR COM

    C40.01 Malignant neoplasm of scapula and long bones of right upper limb HCC Rx ESR COM

    C40.02 Malignant neoplasm of scapula and long bones of left upper limb HCC Rx ESR COM

✓5th **C40.1 Malignant neoplasm of short bones of upper limb**

    C40.10 Malignant neoplasm of short bones of unspecified upper limb HCC Rx ESR COM

    C40.11 Malignant neoplasm of short bones of right upper limb HCC Rx ESR COM

    C40.12 Malignant neoplasm of short bones of left upper limb HCC Rx ESR COM

✓5th **C40.2 Malignant neoplasm of long bones of lower limb**

    C40.20 Malignant neoplasm of long bones of unspecified lower limb HCC Rx ESR COM

    C40.21 Malignant neoplasm of long bones of right lower limb HCC Rx ESR COM

    C40.22 Malignant neoplasm of long bones of left lower limb HCC Rx ESR COM

✓5th **C40.3 Malignant neoplasm of short bones of lower limb**

    C40.30 Malignant neoplasm of short bones of unspecified lower limb HCC Rx ESR COM

    C40.31 Malignant neoplasm of short bones of right lower limb HCC Rx ESR COM

    C40.32 Malignant neoplasm of short bones of left lower limb HCC Rx ESR COM

✓5th **C40.8 Malignant neoplasm of overlapping sites of bone and articular cartilage of limb**

    C40.80 Malignant neoplasm of overlapping sites of bone and articular cartilage of unspecified limb HCC Rx ESR COM

    C40.81 Malignant neoplasm of overlapping sites of bone and articular cartilage of right limb HCC Rx ESR COM

    C40.82 Malignant neoplasm of overlapping sites of bone and articular cartilage of left limb HCC Rx ESR COM

✓5th **C40.9 Malignant neoplasm of unspecified bones and articular cartilage of limb**

    C40.90 Malignant neoplasm of unspecified bones and articular cartilage of unspecified limb HCC Rx ESR COM

    C40.91 Malignant neoplasm of unspecified bones and articular cartilage of right limb HCC Rx ESR COM

    C40.92 Malignant neoplasm of unspecified bones and articular cartilage of left limb HCC Rx ESR COM

Chapter 2. Neoplasms

☑4ᵗʰ **C41** **Malignant neoplasm of bone and articular cartilage of other and unspecified sites**
    EXCLUDES 1   *malignant neoplasm of bones of limbs (C40.-)*
          malignant neoplasm of cartilage of ear (C49.0)
          malignant neoplasm of cartilage of eyelid (C49.0)
          malignant neoplasm of cartilage of larynx (C32.3)
          malignant neoplasm of cartilage of limbs (C40.-)
          malignant neoplasm of cartilage of nose (C30.0)

C41.0 **Malignant neoplasm of bones of skull and face**   HCC Rx ESR COM
    Malignant neoplasm of maxilla (superior)
    Malignant neoplasm of orbital bone
    EXCLUDES 2   *carcinoma, any type except intraosseous or odontogenic of:*
          maxillary sinus (C31.0)
          upper jaw (C03.0)
          malignant neoplasm of jaw bone (lower) (C41.1)

C41.1 **Malignant neoplasm of mandible**   HCC Rx ESR COM
    Malignant neoplasm of inferior maxilla
    Malignant neoplasm of lower jaw bone
    EXCLUDES 2   *carcinoma, any type except intraosseous or odontogenic of:*
          jaw NOS (C03.9)
          lower (C03.1)
          malignant neoplasm of upper jaw bone (C41.0)

C41.2 **Malignant neoplasm of vertebral column**   HCC Rx ESR COM
    EXCLUDES 1   *malignant neoplasm of sacrum and coccyx (C41.4)*

C41.3 **Malignant neoplasm of ribs, sternum and clavicle**   HCC Rx ESR COM

C41.4 **Malignant neoplasm of pelvic bones, sacrum and coccyx**   HCC Rx ESR COM

C41.9 **Malignant neoplasm of bone and articular cartilage, unspecified**   HCC Rx ESR COM

Melanoma and other malignant neoplasms of skin (C43-C44)

☑4ᵗʰ **C43** **Malignant melanoma of skin**
    EXCLUDES 1   *melanoma in situ (D03.-)*
    EXCLUDES 2   *malignant melanoma of skin of genital organs (C51-C52, C60.-, C63.-)*
          Merkel cell carcinoma (C4A.-)
          sites other than skin - code to malignant neoplasm of the site

C43.0 **Malignant melanoma of lip**   HCC Rx ESR COM Q
    EXCLUDES 1   *malignant neoplasm of vermilion border of lip (C00.0-C00.2)*

☑5ᵗʰ **C43.1** **Malignant melanoma of eyelid, including canthus**
    AHA: 2018,4Q,4
    C43.10 **Malignant melanoma of unspecified eyelid, including canthus**   HCC Rx ESR COM Q
    ☑6ᵗʰ **C43.11** **Malignant melanoma of right eyelid, including canthus**
        C43.111 **Malignant melanoma of right upper eyelid, including canthus**   HCC Rx ESR COM
        C43.112 **Malignant melanoma of right lower eyelid, including canthus**   HCC Rx ESR COM
    ☑6ᵗʰ **C43.12** **Malignant melanoma of left eyelid, including canthus**
        C43.121 **Malignant melanoma of left upper eyelid, including canthus**   HCC Rx ESR COM
        C43.122 **Malignant melanoma of left lower eyelid, including canthus**   HCC Rx ESR COM

☑5ᵗʰ **C43.2** **Malignant melanoma of ear and external auricular canal**
    C43.20 **Malignant melanoma of unspecified ear and external auricular canal**   HCC Rx ESR COM Q
    C43.21 **Malignant melanoma of right ear and external auricular canal**   HCC Rx ESR COM Q
    C43.22 **Malignant melanoma of left ear and external auricular canal**   HCC Rx ESR COM Q

☑5ᵗʰ **C43.3** **Malignant melanoma of other and unspecified parts of face**
    C43.30 **Malignant melanoma of unspecified part of face**   HCC Rx ESR COM Q
    C43.31 **Malignant melanoma of nose**   HCC Rx ESR COM Q
    C43.39 **Malignant melanoma of other parts of face**   HCC Rx ESR COM Q

C43.4 **Malignant melanoma of scalp and neck**   HCC Rx ESR COM Q

☑5ᵗʰ **C43.5** **Malignant melanoma of trunk**
    EXCLUDES 2   *malignant neoplasm of anus NOS (C21.0)*
          malignant neoplasm of scrotum (C63.2)
    C43.51 **Malignant melanoma of anal skin**   HCC Rx ESR COM Q
        Malignant melanoma of anal margin
        Malignant melanoma of perianal skin
    C43.52 **Malignant melanoma of skin of breast**   HCC Rx ESR COM Q
    C43.59 **Malignant melanoma of other part of trunk**   HCC Rx ESR COM Q

☑5ᵗʰ **C43.6** **Malignant melanoma of upper limb, including shoulder**
    C43.60 **Malignant melanoma of unspecified upper limb, including shoulder**   HCC Rx ESR COM Q
    C43.61 **Malignant melanoma of right upper limb, including shoulder**   HCC Rx ESR COM Q
    C43.62 **Malignant melanoma of left upper limb, including shoulder**   HCC Rx ESR COM Q

☑5ᵗʰ **C43.7** **Malignant melanoma of lower limb, including hip**
    C43.70 **Malignant melanoma of unspecified lower limb, including hip**   HCC Rx ESR COM Q
    C43.71 **Malignant melanoma of right lower limb, including hip**   HCC Rx ESR COM Q
    C43.72 **Malignant melanoma of left lower limb, including hip**   HCC Rx ESR COM Q

C43.8 **Malignant melanoma of overlapping sites of skin**   HCC Rx ESR COM Q

C43.9 **Malignant melanoma of skin, unspecified**   HCC Rx ESR COM Q
    Malignant melanoma of unspecified site of skin
    Melanoma (malignant) NOS

☑4ᵗʰ **C4A** **Merkel cell carcinoma**
    DEF: Malignant cutaneous cancer predominantly found in elderly patients with sun exposure that usually presents as a flesh-colored or bluish-red lump typically seen on the neck, head, and face.

C4A.0 **Merkel cell carcinoma of lip**   HCC Rx ESR COM
    EXCLUDES 1   *malignant neoplasm of vermilion border of lip (C00.0-C00.2)*

☑5ᵗʰ **C4A.1** **Merkel cell carcinoma of eyelid, including canthus**
    AHA: 2018,4Q,4
    C4A.10 **Merkel cell carcinoma of unspecified eyelid, including canthus**   HCC Rx ESR COM
    ☑6ᵗʰ **C4A.11** **Merkel cell carcinoma of right eyelid, including canthus**
        C4A.111 **Merkel cell carcinoma of right upper eyelid, including canthus**   HCC Rx ESR COM
        C4A.112 **Merkel cell carcinoma of right lower eyelid, including canthus**   HCC Rx ESR COM
    ☑6ᵗʰ **C4A.12** **Merkel cell carcinoma of left eyelid, including canthus**
        C4A.121 **Merkel cell carcinoma of left upper eyelid, including canthus**   HCC Rx ESR COM
        C4A.122 **Merkel cell carcinoma of left lower eyelid, including canthus**   HCC Rx ESR COM

☑5ᵗʰ **C4A.2** **Merkel cell carcinoma of ear and external auricular canal**
    C4A.20 **Merkel cell carcinoma of unspecified ear and external auricular canal**   HCC Rx ESR COM
    C4A.21 **Merkel cell carcinoma of right ear and external auricular canal**   HCC Rx ESR COM
    C4A.22 **Merkel cell carcinoma of left ear and external auricular canal**   HCC Rx ESR COM

☑5ᵗʰ **C4A.3** **Merkel cell carcinoma of other and unspecified parts of face**
    C4A.30 **Merkel cell carcinoma of unspecified part of face**   HCC Rx ESR COM
    C4A.31 **Merkel cell carcinoma of nose**   HCC Rx ESR COM
    C4A.39 **Merkel cell carcinoma of other parts of face**   HCC Rx ESR COM

C4A.4 **Merkel cell carcinoma of scalp and neck**   HCC Rx ESR COM

√5ᵗʰ **C4A.5　Merkel cell carcinoma of trunk**

　　　EXCLUDES 2　*malignant neoplasm of anus NOS (C21.0)*
　　　　　　　　malignant neoplasm of scrotum (C63.2)

　　C4A.51　Merkel cell carcinoma of anal skin HCC Rx ESR COM
　　　　Merkel cell carcinoma of anal margin
　　　　Merkel cell carcinoma of perianal skin

　　C4A.52　Merkel cell carcinoma of skin of breast HCC Rx ESR COM

　　C4A.59　Merkel cell carcinoma of other part of trunk HCC Rx ESR COM

√5ᵗʰ **C4A.6　Merkel cell carcinoma of upper limb, including shoulder**

　　C4A.60　Merkel cell carcinoma of unspecified upper limb, including shoulder HCC Rx ESR COM

　　C4A.61　Merkel cell carcinoma of right upper limb, including shoulder HCC Rx ESR COM

　　C4A.62　Merkel cell carcinoma of left upper limb, including shoulder HCC Rx ESR COM

√5ᵗʰ **C4A.7　Merkel cell carcinoma of lower limb, including hip**

　　C4A.70　Merkel cell carcinoma of unspecified lower limb, including hip HCC Rx ESR COM

　　C4A.71　Merkel cell carcinoma of right lower limb, including hip HCC Rx ESR COM

　　C4A.72　Merkel cell carcinoma of left lower limb, including hip HCC Rx ESR COM

C4A.8　Merkel cell carcinoma of overlapping sites HCC Rx ESR COM

C4A.9　Merkel cell carcinoma, unspecified HCC Rx ESR COM
　　Merkel cell carcinoma of unspecified site
　　Merkel cell carcinoma NOS

√4ᵗʰ **C44　Other and unspecified malignant neoplasm of skin**

　　INCLUDES　malignant neoplasm of sebaceous glands
　　　　　　malignant neoplasm of sweat glands

　　EXCLUDES 1　*Kaposi's sarcoma of skin (C46.0)*
　　　　　　malignant melanoma of skin (C43.-)
　　　　　　malignant neoplasm of skin of genital organs (C51-C52, C60.-, C63.2)
　　　　　　Merkel cell carcinoma (C4A.-)

　　DEF: Basal cell carcinoma: Abnormal growth of skin cells that arises from the deepest layer of the epidermis and may present as an open sore, red patches, pink growth, or scar. Typically caused by sun exposure, it is one of the most common forms of skin cancer.

　　DEF: Squamous cell carcinoma: Uncontrolled growth of abnormal skin cells that arises from the outer layers of the skin (epidermis) and may present as an open sore. It is characterized by a firm, red nodule, elevated growth with a central depression, or a flat sore with a scaly crust.

√5ᵗʰ **C44.0　Other and unspecified malignant neoplasm of skin of lip**

　　EXCLUDES 1　*malignant neoplasm of lip (C00.-)*

　　C44.00　Unspecified malignant neoplasm of skin of lip

　　C44.01　Basal cell carcinoma of skin of lip

　　C44.02　Squamous cell carcinoma of skin of lip

　　C44.09　Other specified malignant neoplasm of skin of lip

√5ᵗʰ **C44.1　Other and unspecified malignant neoplasm of skin of eyelid, including canthus**

　　EXCLUDES 1　*connective tissue of eyelid (C49.0)*

　　AHA: 2018,4Q,4

　　√6ᵗʰ **C44.10　Unspecified malignant neoplasm of skin of eyelid, including canthus**

　　　　C44.101　Unspecified malignant neoplasm of skin of unspecified eyelid, including canthus

　　　　√7ᵗʰ **C44.102　Unspecified malignant neoplasm of skin of right eyelid, including canthus**

　　　　　　C44.1021　Unspecified malignant neoplasm of skin of right upper eyelid, including canthus

　　　　　　C44.1022　Unspecified malignant neoplasm of skin of right lower eyelid, including canthus

　　　　√7ᵗʰ **C44.109　Unspecified malignant neoplasm of skin of left eyelid, including canthus**

　　　　　　C44.1091　Unspecified malignant neoplasm of skin of left upper eyelid, including canthus

　　　　　　C44.1092　Unspecified malignant neoplasm of skin of left lower eyelid, including canthus

　　√6ᵗʰ **C44.11　Basal cell carcinoma of skin of eyelid, including canthus**

　　　　C44.111　Basal cell carcinoma of skin of unspecified eyelid, including canthus

　　　　√7ᵗʰ **C44.112　Basal cell carcinoma of skin of right eyelid, including canthus**

　　　　　　C44.1121　Basal cell carcinoma of skin of right upper eyelid, including canthus

　　　　　　C44.1122　Basal cell carcinoma of skin of right lower eyelid, including canthus

　　　　√7ᵗʰ **C44.119　Basal cell carcinoma of skin of left eyelid, including canthus**

　　　　　　C44.1191　Basal cell carcinoma of skin of left upper eyelid, including canthus

　　　　　　C44.1192　Basal cell carcinoma of skin of left lower eyelid, including canthus

　　√6ᵗʰ **C44.12　Squamous cell carcinoma of skin of eyelid, including canthus**

　　　　C44.121　Squamous cell carcinoma of skin of unspecified eyelid, including canthus

　　　　√7ᵗʰ **C44.122　Squamous cell carcinoma of skin of right eyelid, including canthus**

　　　　　　C44.1221　Squamous cell carcinoma of skin of right upper eyelid, including canthus

　　　　　　C44.1222　Squamous cell carcinoma of skin of right lower eyelid, including canthus

　　　　√7ᵗʰ **C44.129　Squamous cell carcinoma of skin of left eyelid, including canthus**

　　　　　　C44.1291　Squamous cell carcinoma of skin of left upper eyelid, including canthus

　　　　　　C44.1292　Squamous cell carcinoma of skin of left lower eyelid, including canthus

　　√6ᵗʰ **C44.13　Sebaceous cell carcinoma of skin of eyelid, including canthus**

　　　　C44.131　Sebaceous cell carcinoma of skin of unspecified eyelid, including canthus

　　　　√7ᵗʰ **C44.132　Sebaceous cell carcinoma of skin of right eyelid, including canthus**

　　　　　　C44.1321　Sebaceous cell carcinoma of skin of right upper eyelid, including canthus

　　　　　　C44.1322　Sebaceous cell carcinoma of skin of right lower eyelid, including canthus

　　　　√7ᵗʰ **C44.139　Sebaceous cell carcinoma of skin of left eyelid, including canthus**

　　　　　　C44.1391　Sebaceous cell carcinoma of skin of left upper eyelid, including canthus

　　　　　　C44.1392　Sebaceous cell carcinoma of skin of left lower eyelid, including canthus

　　√6ᵗʰ **C44.19　Other specified malignant neoplasm of skin of eyelid, including canthus**

　　　　C44.191　Other specified malignant neoplasm of skin of unspecified eyelid, including canthus

　　　　√7ᵗʰ **C44.192　Other specified malignant neoplasm of skin of right eyelid, including canthus**

　　　　　　C44.1921　Other specified malignant neoplasm of skin of right upper eyelid, including canthus

　　　　　　C44.1922　Other specified malignant neoplasm of skin of right lower eyelid, including canthus

　　　　√7ᵗʰ **C44.199　Other specified malignant neoplasm of skin of left eyelid, including canthus**

　　　　　　C44.1991　Other specified malignant neoplasm of skin of left upper eyelid, including canthus

　　　　　　C44.1992　Other specified malignant neoplasm of skin of left lower eyelid, including canthus

☑ Additional Character Required　　　√x7ᵗʰ Placeholder Alert　　　Manifestation　　　Unspecified Dx　　　ℚ QPP　　　UPD Unacceptable PDx

Chapter 2. Neoplasms

☑5ᵗʰ **C44.2 Other and unspecified malignant neoplasm of skin of ear and external auricular canal**

    EXCLUDES 1   connective tissue of ear (C49.0)

☑6ᵗʰ **C44.20 Unspecified malignant neoplasm of skin of ear and external auricular canal**

    C44.201 Unspecified malignant neoplasm of skin of unspecified ear and external auricular canal

    C44.202 Unspecified malignant neoplasm of skin of right ear and external auricular canal

    C44.209 Unspecified malignant neoplasm of skin of left ear and external auricular canal

☑6ᵗʰ **C44.21 Basal cell carcinoma of skin of ear and external auricular canal**

    C44.211 Basal cell carcinoma of skin of unspecified ear and external auricular canal

    C44.212 Basal cell carcinoma of skin of right ear and external auricular canal

    C44.219 Basal cell carcinoma of skin of left ear and external auricular canal

☑6ᵗʰ **C44.22 Squamous cell carcinoma of skin of ear and external auricular canal**

    C44.221 Squamous cell carcinoma of skin of unspecified ear and external auricular canal

    C44.222 Squamous cell carcinoma of skin of right ear and external auricular canal

    C44.229 Squamous cell carcinoma of skin of left ear and external auricular canal

☑6ᵗʰ **C44.29 Other specified malignant neoplasm of skin of ear and external auricular canal**

    C44.291 Other specified malignant neoplasm of skin of unspecified ear and external auricular canal

    C44.292 Other specified malignant neoplasm of skin of right ear and external auricular canal

    C44.299 Other specified malignant neoplasm of skin of left ear and external auricular canal

☑5ᵗʰ **C44.3 Other and unspecified malignant neoplasm of skin of other and unspecified parts of face**

☑6ᵗʰ **C44.30 Unspecified malignant neoplasm of skin of other and unspecified parts of face**

    C44.300 Unspecified malignant neoplasm of skin of unspecified part of face

    C44.301 Unspecified malignant neoplasm of skin of nose

    C44.309 Unspecified malignant neoplasm of skin of other parts of face

☑6ᵗʰ **C44.31 Basal cell carcinoma of skin of other and unspecified parts of face**

    C44.310 Basal cell carcinoma of skin of unspecified parts of face

    C44.311 Basal cell carcinoma of skin of nose

    C44.319 Basal cell carcinoma of skin of other parts of face

☑6ᵗʰ **C44.32 Squamous cell carcinoma of skin of other and unspecified parts of face**

    C44.320 Squamous cell carcinoma of skin of unspecified parts of face

    C44.321 Squamous cell carcinoma of skin of nose

    C44.329 Squamous cell carcinoma of skin of other parts of face

☑6ᵗʰ **C44.39 Other specified malignant neoplasm of skin of other and unspecified parts of face**

    C44.390 Other specified malignant neoplasm of skin of unspecified parts of face

    C44.391 Other specified malignant neoplasm of skin of nose

    C44.399 Other specified malignant neoplasm of skin of other parts of face

☑5ᵗʰ **C44.4 Other and unspecified malignant neoplasm of skin of scalp and neck**

    C44.40 Unspecified malignant neoplasm of skin of scalp and neck

    C44.41 Basal cell carcinoma of skin of scalp and neck

    C44.42 Squamous cell carcinoma of skin of scalp and neck

    C44.49 Other specified malignant neoplasm of skin of scalp and neck

☑5ᵗʰ **C44.5 Other and unspecified malignant neoplasm of skin of trunk**

    EXCLUDES 1   anus NOS (C21.0)

           scrotum (C63.2)

☑6ᵗʰ **C44.50 Unspecified malignant neoplasm of skin of trunk**

    C44.500 Unspecified malignant neoplasm of anal skin

         Unspecified malignant neoplasm of anal margin

         Unspecified malignant neoplasm of perianal skin

    C44.501 Unspecified malignant neoplasm of skin of breast

    C44.509 Unspecified malignant neoplasm of skin of other part of trunk

☑6ᵗʰ **C44.51 Basal cell carcinoma of skin of trunk**

    C44.510 Basal cell carcinoma of anal skin

         Basal cell carcinoma of anal margin

         Basal cell carcinoma of perianal skin

    C44.511 Basal cell carcinoma of skin of breast

    C44.519 Basal cell carcinoma of skin of other part of trunk

☑6ᵗʰ **C44.52 Squamous cell carcinoma of skin of trunk**

    C44.520 Squamous cell carcinoma of anal skin

         Squamous cell carcinoma of anal margin

         Squamous cell carcinoma of perianal skin

    C44.521 Squamous cell carcinoma of skin of breast

    C44.529 Squamous cell carcinoma of skin of other part of trunk

☑6ᵗʰ **C44.59 Other specified malignant neoplasm of skin of trunk**

    C44.590 Other specified malignant neoplasm of anal skin

         Other specified malignant neoplasm of anal margin

         Other specified malignant neoplasm of perianal skin

    C44.591 Other specified malignant neoplasm of skin of breast

    C44.599 Other specified malignant neoplasm of skin of other part of trunk

☑5ᵗʰ **C44.6 Other and unspecified malignant neoplasm of skin of upper limb, including shoulder**

☑6ᵗʰ **C44.60 Unspecified malignant neoplasm of skin of upper limb, including shoulder**

    C44.601 Unspecified malignant neoplasm of skin of unspecified upper limb, including shoulder

    C44.602 Unspecified malignant neoplasm of skin of right upper limb, including shoulder

    C44.609 Unspecified malignant neoplasm of skin of left upper limb, including shoulder

☑6ᵗʰ **C44.61 Basal cell carcinoma of skin of upper limb, including shoulder**

    C44.611 Basal cell carcinoma of skin of unspecified upper limb, including shoulder

    C44.612 Basal cell carcinoma of skin of right upper limb, including shoulder

    C44.619 Basal cell carcinoma of skin of left upper limb, including shoulder

☑6ᵗʰ **C44.62 Squamous cell carcinoma of skin of upper limb, including shoulder**

    C44.621 Squamous cell carcinoma of skin of unspecified upper limb, including shoulder

    C44.622 Squamous cell carcinoma of skin of right upper limb, including shoulder

    C44.629 Squamous cell carcinoma of skin of left upper limb, including shoulder

☑6ᵗʰ **C44.69 Other specified malignant neoplasm of skin of upper limb, including shoulder**

    C44.691 Other specified malignant neoplasm of skin of unspecified upper limb, including shoulder

    C44.692 Other specified malignant neoplasm of skin of right upper limb, including shoulder

    C44.699 Other specified malignant neoplasm of skin of left upper limb, including shoulder

HCC CMS-HCC   **Rx** Rx HCC   **ESR** ESRD HCC   **COM** Commercial HCC   **N** Newborn: 0   **P** Pediatric: 0-17   **M** Maternity: 9-64   **A** Adult: 15-124

484   ICD-10-CM 2023

√5th **C44.7** **Other and unspecified malignant neoplasm of skin of lower limb, including hip**

  √6th **C44.70** **Unspecified malignant neoplasm of skin of lower limb, including hip**

    C44.701 Unspecified malignant neoplasm of skin of unspecified lower limb, including hip

    C44.702 Unspecified malignant neoplasm of skin of right lower limb, including hip

    C44.709 Unspecified malignant neoplasm of skin of left lower limb, including hip

  √6th **C44.71** **Basal cell carcinoma of skin of lower limb, including hip**

    C44.711 Basal cell carcinoma of skin of unspecified lower limb, including hip

    C44.712 Basal cell carcinoma of skin of right lower limb, including hip

    C44.719 Basal cell carcinoma of skin of left lower limb, including hip

  √6th **C44.72** **Squamous cell carcinoma of skin of lower limb, including hip**

    C44.721 Squamous cell carcinoma of skin of unspecified lower limb, including hip

    C44.722 Squamous cell carcinoma of skin of right lower limb, including hip

    C44.729 Squamous cell carcinoma of skin of left lower limb, including hip

  √6th **C44.79** **Other specified malignant neoplasm of skin of lower limb, including hip**

    C44.791 Other specified malignant neoplasm of skin of unspecified lower limb, including hip

    C44.792 Other specified malignant neoplasm of skin of right lower limb, including hip

    C44.799 Other specified malignant neoplasm of skin of left lower limb, including hip

√5th **C44.8** **Other and unspecified malignant neoplasm of overlapping sites of skin**

  C44.80 Unspecified malignant neoplasm of overlapping sites of skin

  C44.81 Basal cell carcinoma of overlapping sites of skin

  C44.82 Squamous cell carcinoma of overlapping sites of skin

  C44.89 Other specified malignant neoplasm of overlapping sites of skin

√5th **C44.9** **Other and unspecified malignant neoplasm of skin, unspecified**

  C44.90 Unspecified malignant neoplasm of skin, unspecified

    Malignant neoplasm of unspecified site of skin

  C44.91 Basal cell carcinoma of skin, unspecified

  C44.92 Squamous cell carcinoma of skin, unspecified

  C44.99 Other specified malignant neoplasm of skin, unspecified

Malignant neoplasms of mesothelial and soft tissue (C45-C49)

√4th **C45** **Mesothelioma**

DEF: Rare type of cancer that forms in the thin layer of protective tissue that covers the majority of internal organs (mesothelium).

  C45.0 **Mesothelioma of pleura**   HCC Rx ESR COM

    EXCLUDES 1   other malignant neoplasm of pleura (C38.4)

    AHA: 2017,2Q,11

    TIP: For pleural mesothelioma that has metastasized to the chest wall, assign this code for the primary site along with C79.89 for metastatic cancer in the chest wall.

  C45.1 **Mesothelioma of peritoneum**   HCC Rx ESR COM

    Mesothelioma of cul-de-sac

    Mesothelioma of mesentery

    Mesothelioma of mesocolon

    Mesothelioma of omentum

    Mesothelioma of peritoneum (parietal) (pelvic)

    EXCLUDES 1   other malignant neoplasm of soft tissue of peritoneum (C48.-)

  C45.2 **Mesothelioma of pericardium**   HCC Rx ESR COM

    EXCLUDES 1   other malignant neoplasm of pericardium (C38.0)

  C45.7 **Mesothelioma of other sites**   HCC Rx ESR COM

  C45.9 **Mesothelioma, unspecified**   HCC Rx ESR COM

√4th **C46** **Kaposi's sarcoma**

Code first any human immunodeficiency virus [HIV] disease (B20)

DEF: Malignant neoplasm that causes patches of abnormal tissue to grow under the skin, in the lining of the mouth, nose, and throat, in lymph nodes, or in other visceral organs. Kaposi's sarcoma is caused by human herpesvirus8 (HHV8).

  C46.0 **Kaposi's sarcoma of skin**   HCC Rx ESR COM

  C46.1 **Kaposi's sarcoma of soft tissue**   HCC Rx ESR COM

    Kaposi's sarcoma of blood vessel

    Kaposi's sarcoma of connective tissue

    Kaposi's sarcoma of fascia

    Kaposi's sarcoma of ligament

    Kaposi's sarcoma of lymphatic(s) NEC

    Kaposi's sarcoma of muscle

    EXCLUDES 2   Kaposi's sarcoma of lymph glands and nodes (C46.3)

  C46.2 **Kaposi's sarcoma of palate**   HCC Rx ESR COM

  C46.3 **Kaposi's sarcoma of lymph nodes**   HCC Rx ESR COM

  C46.4 **Kaposi's sarcoma of gastrointestinal sites**   HCC Rx ESR COM

√5th **C46.5** **Kaposi's sarcoma of lung**

    AHA: 2019,1Q,16

    TIP: When associated malignant pericardial effusion is documented, assign code I31.3. If the sole reason for admission is to treat the effusion with no treatment of the lung malignancy rendered, code I31.3 may be sequenced first.

    C46.50 Kaposi's sarcoma of unspecified lung   HCC Rx ESR COM

    C46.51 Kaposi's sarcoma of right lung   HCC Rx ESR COM

    C46.52 Kaposi's sarcoma of left lung   HCC Rx ESR COM

  C46.7 **Kaposi's sarcoma of other sites**   HCC Rx ESR COM

  C46.9 **Kaposi's sarcoma, unspecified**   HCC Rx ESR COM

    Kaposi's sarcoma of unspecified site

√4th **C47** **Malignant neoplasm of peripheral nerves and autonomic nervous system**

    INCLUDES   malignant neoplasm of sympathetic and parasympathetic nerves and ganglia

    EXCLUDES 1   Kaposi's sarcoma of soft tissue (C46.1)

  C47.0 **Malignant neoplasm of peripheral nerves of head, face and neck**   HCC Rx ESR COM

    EXCLUDES 1   malignant neoplasm of peripheral nerves of orbit (C69.6-)

√5th **C47.1** **Malignant neoplasm of peripheral nerves of upper limb, including shoulder**

    C47.10 Malignant neoplasm of peripheral nerves of unspecified upper limb, including shoulder   HCC Rx ESR COM

    C47.11 Malignant neoplasm of peripheral nerves of right upper limb, including shoulder   HCC Rx ESR COM

    C47.12 Malignant neoplasm of peripheral nerves of left upper limb, including shoulder   HCC Rx ESR COM

√5th **C47.2** **Malignant neoplasm of peripheral nerves of lower limb, including hip**

    C47.20 Malignant neoplasm of peripheral nerves of unspecified lower limb, including hip   HCC Rx ESR COM

    C47.21 Malignant neoplasm of peripheral nerves of right lower limb, including hip   HCC Rx ESR COM

    C47.22 Malignant neoplasm of peripheral nerves of left lower limb, including hip   HCC Rx ESR COM

  C47.3 **Malignant neoplasm of peripheral nerves of thorax**   HCC Rx ESR COM

  C47.4 **Malignant neoplasm of peripheral nerves of abdomen**   HCC Rx ESR COM

  C47.5 **Malignant neoplasm of peripheral nerves of pelvis**   HCC Rx ESR COM

  C47.6 **Malignant neoplasm of peripheral nerves of trunk, unspecified**   HCC Rx ESR COM

    Malignant neoplasm of peripheral nerves of unspecified part of trunk

  C47.8 **Malignant neoplasm of overlapping sites of peripheral nerves and autonomic nervous system**   HCC Rx ESR COM

  C47.9 **Malignant neoplasm of peripheral nerves and autonomic nervous system, unspecified**   HCC Rx ESR COM

    Malignant neoplasm of unspecified site of peripheral nerves and autonomic nervous system

Chapter 2. Neoplasms

☑4ᵗʰ **C48 Malignant neoplasm of retroperitoneum and peritoneum**

> EXCLUDES 1   *Kaposi's sarcoma of connective tissue (C46.1)*
> *mesothelioma (C45.-)*

C48.0 Malignant neoplasm of retroperitoneum HCC Rx ESR COM

C48.1 Malignant neoplasm of specified parts of peritoneum HCC Rx ESR COM
> Malignant neoplasm of cul-de-sac
> Malignant neoplasm of mesentery
> Malignant neoplasm of mesocolon
> Malignant neoplasm of omentum
> Malignant neoplasm of parietal peritoneum
> Malignant neoplasm of pelvic peritoneum

C48.2 Malignant neoplasm of peritoneum, unspecified HCC Rx ESR COM

C48.8 Malignant neoplasm of overlapping sites of retroperitoneum and peritoneum HCC Rx ESR COM

☑4ᵗʰ **C49 Malignant neoplasm of other connective and soft tissue**

> INCLUDES   malignant neoplasm of blood vessel
> malignant neoplasm of bursa
> malignant neoplasm of cartilage
> malignant neoplasm of fascia
> malignant neoplasm of fat
> malignant neoplasm of ligament, except uterine
> malignant neoplasm of lymphatic vessel
> malignant neoplasm of muscle
> malignant neoplasm of synovia
> malignant neoplasm of tendon (sheath)

> EXCLUDES 1   *malignant neoplasm of cartilage (of):*
> *articular (C40-C41)*
> *larynx (C32.3)*
> *nose (C30.0)*
> *malignant neoplasm of connective tissue of breast (C50.-)*

> EXCLUDES 2   *Kaposi's sarcoma of soft tissue (C46.1)*
> *malignant neoplasm of heart (C38.0)*
> *malignant neoplasm of peripheral nerves and autonomic nervous system (C47.-)*
> *malignant neoplasm of peritoneum (C48.2)*
> *malignant neoplasm of retroperitoneum (C48.0)*
> *malignant neoplasm of uterine ligament (C57.3)*
> *mesothelioma (C45.-)*

C49.0 Malignant neoplasm of connective and soft tissue of head, face and neck HCC Rx ESR COM
> Malignant neoplasm of connective tissue of ear
> Malignant neoplasm of connective tissue of eyelid
> > EXCLUDES 1   *connective tissue of orbit (C69.6-)*

☑5ᵗʰ **C49.1 Malignant neoplasm of connective and soft tissue of upper limb, including shoulder**

> **C49.10 Malignant neoplasm of connective and soft tissue of unspecified upper limb, including shoulder** HCC Rx ESR COM
> **C49.11 Malignant neoplasm of connective and soft tissue of right upper limb, including shoulder** HCC Rx ESR COM
> **C49.12 Malignant neoplasm of connective and soft tissue of left upper limb, including shoulder** HCC Rx ESR COM

☑5ᵗʰ **C49.2 Malignant neoplasm of connective and soft tissue of lower limb, including hip**

> **C49.20 Malignant neoplasm of connective and soft tissue of unspecified lower limb, including hip** HCC Rx ESR COM
> **C49.21 Malignant neoplasm of connective and soft tissue of right lower limb, including hip** HCC Rx ESR COM
> **C49.22 Malignant neoplasm of connective and soft tissue of left lower limb, including hip** HCC Rx ESR COM

C49.3 Malignant neoplasm of connective and soft tissue of thorax HCC Rx ESR COM
> Malignant neoplasm of axilla
> Malignant neoplasm of diaphragm
> Malignant neoplasm of great vessels
> > EXCLUDES 1   *malignant neoplasm of breast (C50.-)*
> > *malignant neoplasm of heart (C38.0)*
> > *malignant neoplasm of mediastinum (C38.1-C38.3)*
> > *malignant neoplasm of thymus (C37)*
> **AHA:** 2015,3Q,19

C49.4 Malignant neoplasm of connective and soft tissue of abdomen HCC Rx ESR COM
> Malignant neoplasm of abdominal wall
> Malignant neoplasm of hypochondrium

C49.5 Malignant neoplasm of connective and soft tissue of pelvis HCC Rx ESR COM
> Malignant neoplasm of buttock
> Malignant neoplasm of groin
> Malignant neoplasm of perineum

C49.6 Malignant neoplasm of connective and soft tissue of trunk, unspecified HCC Rx ESR COM
> Malignant neoplasm of back NOS

C49.8 Malignant neoplasm of overlapping sites of connective and soft tissue HCC Rx ESR COM
> Primary malignant neoplasm of two or more contiguous sites of connective and soft tissue

C49.9 Malignant neoplasm of connective and soft tissue, unspecified HCC Rx ESR COM

☑5ᵗʰ **C49.A Gastrointestinal stromal tumor**

> **AHA:** 2016,4Q,8
> **DEF:** Uncommon malignant tumor found in the GI tract that originates from interstitial cells of the autonomic nervous system. Most occur in the stomach or small intestine but can originate anywhere in the GI tract.

> **C49.A0 Gastrointestinal stromal tumor, unspecified site** HCC Rx ESR COM
> **C49.A1 Gastrointestinal stromal tumor of esophagus** HCC Rx ESR COM
> **C49.A2 Gastrointestinal stromal tumor of stomach** HCC Rx ESR COM
> **C49.A3 Gastrointestinal stromal tumor of small intestine** HCC Rx ESR COM
> **C49.A4 Gastrointestinal stromal tumor of large intestine** HCC Rx ESR COM
> **C49.A5 Gastrointestinal stromal tumor of rectum** HCC Rx ESR COM
> **C49.A9 Gastrointestinal stromal tumor of other sites** HCC Rx ESR COM

Malignant neoplasms of breast (C50)

☑4ᵗʰ **C50 Malignant neoplasm of breast**

> INCLUDES   connective tissue of breast
> Paget's disease of breast
> Paget's disease of nipple
> Use additional code to identify estrogen receptor status (Z17.0, Z17.1)
> > EXCLUDES 1   *skin of breast (C44.501, C44.511, C44.521, C44.591)*
> **AHA:** 2017,4Q,19

Female Breast

☑5ᵗʰ **C50.0 Malignant neoplasm of nipple and areola**

> ☑6ᵗʰ **C50.01 Malignant neoplasm of nipple and areola, female**
> > **C50.011 Malignant neoplasm of nipple and areola, right female breast** HCC Rx ESR COM ♀
> > **C50.012 Malignant neoplasm of nipple and areola, left female breast** HCC Rx ESR COM ♀

C50.019   **Malignant neoplasm of nipple and areola, unspecified female breast** `HCC` `Rx` `ESR` `COM` ♀

✓6ᵗʰ   C50.02   **Malignant neoplasm of nipple and areola,** male

     C50.021   **Malignant neoplasm of nipple and areola, right male breast** `HCC` `Rx` `ESR` `COM` ♂

     C50.022   **Malignant neoplasm of nipple and areola, left male breast** `HCC` `Rx` `ESR` `COM` ♂

     C50.029   **Malignant neoplasm of nipple and areola, unspecified male breast** `HCC` `Rx` `ESR` `COM` ♂

✓5ᵗʰ   C50.1   **Malignant neoplasm of** central portion **of breast**

✓6ᵗʰ   C50.11   **Malignant neoplasm of central portion of breast,** female

     C50.111   **Malignant neoplasm of central portion of** right **female breast** `HCC` `Rx` `ESR` `COM` ♀

     C50.112   **Malignant neoplasm of central portion of** left **female breast** `HCC` `Rx` `ESR` `COM` ♀

     C50.119   **Malignant neoplasm of central portion of unspecified female breast** `HCC` `Rx` `ESR` `COM` ♀

✓6ᵗʰ   C50.12   **Malignant neoplasm of central portion of breast,** male

     C50.121   **Malignant neoplasm of central portion of** right **male breast** `HCC` `Rx` `ESR` `COM` ♂

     C50.122   **Malignant neoplasm of central portion of** left **male breast** `HCC` `Rx` `ESR` `COM` ♂

     C50.129   **Malignant neoplasm of central portion of unspecified male breast** `HCC` `Rx` `ESR` `COM` ♂

✓5ᵗʰ   C50.2   **Malignant neoplasm of** upper-inner quadrant **of breast**

✓6ᵗʰ   C50.21   **Malignant neoplasm of upper-inner quadrant of breast,** female

     C50.211   **Malignant neoplasm of upper-inner quadrant of** right **female breast** `HCC` `Rx` `ESR` `COM` ♀

     C50.212   **Malignant neoplasm of upper-inner quadrant of** left **female breast** `HCC` `Rx` `ESR` `COM` ♀

     C50.219   **Malignant neoplasm of upper-inner quadrant of unspecified female breast** `HCC` `Rx` `ESR` `COM` ♀

✓6ᵗʰ   C50.22   **Malignant neoplasm of upper-inner quadrant of breast,** male

     C50.221   **Malignant neoplasm of upper-inner quadrant of** right **male breast** `HCC` `Rx` `ESR` `COM` ♂

     C50.222   **Malignant neoplasm of upper-inner quadrant of** left **male breast** `HCC` `Rx` `ESR` `COM` ♂

     C50.229   **Malignant neoplasm of upper-inner quadrant of unspecified male breast** `HCC` `Rx` `ESR` `COM` ♂

✓5ᵗʰ   C50.3   **Malignant neoplasm of** lower-inner quadrant **of breast**

✓6ᵗʰ   C50.31   **Malignant neoplasm of lower-inner quadrant of breast,** female

     C50.311   **Malignant neoplasm of lower-inner quadrant of** right **female breast** `HCC` `Rx` `ESR` `COM` ♀

     C50.312   **Malignant neoplasm of lower-inner quadrant of** left **female breast** `HCC` `Rx` `ESR` `COM` ♀

     C50.319   **Malignant neoplasm of lower-inner quadrant of unspecified female breast** `HCC` `Rx` `ESR` `COM` ♀

✓6ᵗʰ   C50.32   **Malignant neoplasm of lower-inner quadrant of breast,** male

     C50.321   **Malignant neoplasm of lower-inner quadrant of** right **male breast** `HCC` `Rx` `ESR` `COM` ♂

     C50.322   **Malignant neoplasm of lower-inner quadrant of** left **male breast** `HCC` `Rx` `ESR` `COM` ♂

     C50.329   **Malignant neoplasm of lower-inner quadrant of unspecified male breast** `HCC` `Rx` `ESR` `COM` ♂

✓5ᵗʰ   C50.4   **Malignant neoplasm of** upper-outer quadrant **of breast**

✓6ᵗʰ   C50.41   **Malignant neoplasm of upper-outer quadrant of breast,** female

     C50.411   **Malignant neoplasm of upper-outer quadrant of** right **female breast** `HCC` `Rx` `ESR` `COM` ♀

     C50.412   **Malignant neoplasm of upper-outer quadrant of** left **female breast** `HCC` `Rx` `ESR` `COM` ♀

     C50.419   **Malignant neoplasm of upper-outer quadrant of unspecified female breast** `HCC` `Rx` `ESR` `COM` ♀

✓6ᵗʰ   C50.42   **Malignant neoplasm of upper-outer quadrant of breast,** male

     C50.421   **Malignant neoplasm of upper-outer quadrant of** right **male breast** `HCC` `Rx` `ESR` `COM` ♂

     C50.422   **Malignant neoplasm of upper-outer quadrant of** left **male breast** `HCC` `Rx` `ESR` `COM` ♂

     C50.429   **Malignant neoplasm of upper-outer quadrant of unspecified male breast** `HCC` `Rx` `ESR` `COM` ♂

✓5ᵗʰ   C50.5   **Malignant neoplasm of** lower-outer quadrant **of breast**

✓6ᵗʰ   C50.51   **Malignant neoplasm of lower-outer quadrant of breast,** female

     C50.511   **Malignant neoplasm of lower-outer quadrant of** right **female breast** `HCC` `Rx` `ESR` `COM` ♀

     C50.512   **Malignant neoplasm of lower-outer quadrant of** left **female breast** `HCC` `Rx` `ESR` `COM` ♀

     C50.519   **Malignant neoplasm of lower-outer quadrant of unspecified female breast** `HCC` `Rx` `ESR` `COM` ♀

✓6ᵗʰ   C50.52   **Malignant neoplasm of lower-outer quadrant of breast,** male

     C50.521   **Malignant neoplasm of lower-outer quadrant of** right **male breast** `HCC` `Rx` `ESR` `COM` ♂

     C50.522   **Malignant neoplasm of lower-outer quadrant of** left **male breast** `HCC` `Rx` `ESR` `COM` ♂

     C50.529   **Malignant neoplasm of lower-outer quadrant of unspecified male breast** `HCC` `Rx` `ESR` `COM` ♂

✓5ᵗʰ   C50.6   **Malignant neoplasm of** axillary tail **of breast**

✓6ᵗʰ   C50.61   **Malignant neoplasm of axillary tail of breast,** female

     C50.611   **Malignant neoplasm of axillary tail of** right **female breast** `HCC` `Rx` `ESR` `COM` ♀

     C50.612   **Malignant neoplasm of axillary tail of** left **female breast** `HCC` `Rx` `ESR` `COM` ♀

     C50.619   **Malignant neoplasm of axillary tail of unspecified female breast** `HCC` `Rx` `ESR` `COM` ♀

✓6ᵗʰ   C50.62   **Malignant neoplasm of axillary tail of breast,** male

     C50.621   **Malignant neoplasm of axillary tail of** right **male breast** `HCC` `Rx` `ESR` `COM` ♂

     C50.622   **Malignant neoplasm of axillary tail of** left **male breast** `HCC` `Rx` `ESR` `COM` ♂

     C50.629   **Malignant neoplasm of axillary tail of unspecified male breast** `HCC` `Rx` `ESR` `COM` ♂

✓5ᵗʰ   C50.8   **Malignant neoplasm of** overlapping sites **of breast**

✓6ᵗʰ   C50.81   **Malignant neoplasm of overlapping sites of breast,** female

     C50.811   **Malignant neoplasm of overlapping sites of** right **female breast** `HCC` `Rx` `ESR` `COM` ♀

     C50.812   **Malignant neoplasm of overlapping sites of** left **female breast** `HCC` `Rx` `ESR` `COM` ♀

     C50.819   **Malignant neoplasm of overlapping sites of unspecified female breast** `HCC` `Rx` `ESR` `COM` ♀

✓6ᵗʰ   C50.82   **Malignant neoplasm of overlapping sites of breast,** male

     C50.821   **Malignant neoplasm of overlapping sites of** right **male breast** `HCC` `Rx` `ESR` `COM` ♂

     C50.822   **Malignant neoplasm of overlapping sites of** left **male breast** `HCC` `Rx` `ESR` `COM` ♂

☑ Additional Character Required   ✓x7ᵗʰ Placeholder Alert   Manifestation   Unspecified Dx   Ⓠ QPP   `UPD` Unacceptable PDx

C50.829 Malignant neoplasm of overlapping sites of unspecified male breast   HCC Rx ESR COM ♂

√5ᵗʰ **C50.9** Malignant neoplasm of breast of unspecified site

√6ᵗʰ **C50.91** Malignant neoplasm of breast of unspecified site, female

C50.911 Malignant neoplasm of unspecified site of right female breast   HCC Rx ESR COM ♀

C50.912 Malignant neoplasm of unspecified site of left female breast   HCC Rx ESR COM ♀

C50.919 Malignant neoplasm of unspecified site of unspecified female breast   HCC Rx ESR COM ♀

√6ᵗʰ **C50.92** Malignant neoplasm of breast of unspecified site, male

C50.921 Malignant neoplasm of unspecified site of right male breast   HCC Rx ESR COM ♂

C50.922 Malignant neoplasm of unspecified site of left male breast   HCC Rx ESR COM ♂

C50.929 Malignant neoplasm of unspecified site of unspecified male breast   HCC Rx ESR COM ♂

Malignant neoplasms of female genital organs (C51-C58)

INCLUDES   malignant neoplasm of skin of female genital organs

√4ᵗʰ **C51** Malignant neoplasm of vulva

EXCLUDES 1   carcinoma in situ of vulva (D07.1)

C51.0 Malignant neoplasm of labium majus   HCC ESR COM ♀
Malignant neoplasm of Bartholin's [greater vestibular] gland

C51.1 Malignant neoplasm of labium minus   HCC ESR COM ♀

C51.2 Malignant neoplasm of clitoris   HCC ESR COM ♀

C51.8 Malignant neoplasm of overlapping sites of vulva   HCC ESR COM ♀

C51.9 Malignant neoplasm of vulva, unspecified   HCC ESR COM ♀
Malignant neoplasm of external female genitalia NOS
Malignant neoplasm of pudendum

C52 Malignant neoplasm of vagina   HCC ESR COM ♀
EXCLUDES 1   carcinoma in situ of vagina (D07.2)

√4ᵗʰ **C53** Malignant neoplasm of cervix uteri
EXCLUDES 1   carcinoma in situ of cervix uteri (D06.-)
AHA: 2017,4Q,103

C53.0 Malignant neoplasm of endocervix   HCC ESR COM ♀

C53.1 Malignant neoplasm of exocervix   HCC ESR COM ♀

C53.8 Malignant neoplasm of overlapping sites of cervix uteri   HCC ESR COM ♀

C53.9 Malignant neoplasm of cervix uteri, unspecified   HCC ESR COM ♀

√4ᵗʰ **C54** Malignant neoplasm of corpus uteri

C54.0 Malignant neoplasm of isthmus uteri   HCC ESR COM ♀
Malignant neoplasm of lower uterine segment

C54.1 Malignant neoplasm of endometrium   HCC ESR COM ♀

C54.2 Malignant neoplasm of myometrium   HCC ESR COM ♀

C54.3 Malignant neoplasm of fundus uteri   HCC ESR COM ♀

C54.8 Malignant neoplasm of overlapping sites of corpus uteri   HCC ESR COM ♀

C54.9 Malignant neoplasm of corpus uteri, unspecified   HCC ESR COM ♀

C55 Malignant neoplasm of uterus, part unspecified   HCC ESR COM ♀

√4ᵗʰ **C56** Malignant neoplasm of ovary
Use additional code to identify any functional activity

C56.1 Malignant neoplasm of right ovary   HCC Rx ESR COM ♀

C56.2 Malignant neoplasm of left ovary   HCC Rx ESR COM ♀

C56.3 Malignant neoplasm of bilateral ovaries   HCC Rx ESR COM ♀

C56.9 Malignant neoplasm of unspecified ovary   HCC Rx ESR COM ♀

√4ᵗʰ **C57** Malignant neoplasm of other and unspecified female genital organs

√5ᵗʰ **C57.0** Malignant neoplasm of fallopian tube
Malignant neoplasm of oviduct
Malignant neoplasm of uterine tube

C57.00 Malignant neoplasm of unspecified fallopian tube   HCC Rx ESR COM ♀

C57.01 Malignant neoplasm of right fallopian tube   HCC Rx ESR COM ♀

C57.02 Malignant neoplasm of left fallopian tube   HCC Rx ESR COM ♀

√5ᵗʰ **C57.1** Malignant neoplasm of broad ligament

C57.10 Malignant neoplasm of unspecified broad ligament   HCC Rx ESR COM ♀

C57.11 Malignant neoplasm of right broad ligament   HCC Rx ESR COM ♀

C57.12 Malignant neoplasm of left broad ligament   HCC Rx ESR COM ♀

√5ᵗʰ **C57.2** Malignant neoplasm of round ligament

C57.20 Malignant neoplasm of unspecified round ligament   HCC Rx ESR COM ♀

C57.21 Malignant neoplasm of right round ligament   HCC Rx ESR COM ♀

C57.22 Malignant neoplasm of left round ligament   HCC Rx ESR COM ♀

C57.3 Malignant neoplasm of parametrium   HCC Rx ESR COM ♀
Malignant neoplasm of uterine ligament NOS

C57.4 Malignant neoplasm of uterine adnexa, unspecified   HCC Rx ESR COM ♀

C57.7 Malignant neoplasm of other specified female genital organs   HCC ESR COM ♀
Malignant neoplasm of wolffian body or duct

C57.8 Malignant neoplasm of overlapping sites of female genital organs   HCC ESR COM ♀
Primary malignant neoplasm of two or more contiguous sites of the female genital organs whose point of origin cannot be determined
Primary tubo-ovarian malignant neoplasm whose point of origin cannot be determined
Primary utero-ovarian malignant neoplasm whose point of origin cannot be determined

C57.9 Malignant neoplasm of female genital organ, unspecified   HCC ESR COM ♀
Malignant neoplasm of female genitourinary tract NOS

C58 Malignant neoplasm of placenta   HCC Rx ESR COM M ♀
INCLUDES   choriocarcinoma NOS
chorionepithelioma NOS
EXCLUDES 1   chorioadenoma (destruens) (D39.2)
hydatidiform mole NOS (O01.9)
invasive hydatidiform mole (D39.2)
male choriocarcinoma NOS (C62.9-)
malignant hydatidiform mole (D39.2)

Malignant neoplasms of male genital organs (C60-C63)

INCLUDES   malignant neoplasm of skin of male genital organs

√4ᵗʰ **C60** Malignant neoplasm of penis

C60.0 Malignant neoplasm of prepuce   HCC Rx ESR COM ♂
Malignant neoplasm of foreskin

C60.1 Malignant neoplasm of glans penis   HCC Rx ESR COM ♂

C60.2 Malignant neoplasm of body of penis   HCC Rx ESR COM ♂
Malignant neoplasm of corpus cavernosum

C60.8 Malignant neoplasm of overlapping sites of penis   HCC Rx ESR COM ♂

C60.9 Malignant neoplasm of penis, unspecified   HCC Rx ESR COM ♂
Malignant neoplasm of skin of penis NOS

C61 Malignant neoplasm of prostate   HCC Rx ESR COM 0 ♂
▶Use additional code, if applicable, to identify:◀
hormone sensitivity status (Z19.1-Z19.2)
rising PSA following treatment for malignant neoplasm of prostate (R97.21)
EXCLUDES 1   malignant neoplasm of seminal vesicle (C63.7)
AHA: 2017,1Q,17

√4ᵗʰ **C62** Malignant neoplasm of testis
Use additional code to identify any functional activity

√5ᵗʰ **C62.0** Malignant neoplasm of undescended testis
Malignant neoplasm of ectopic testis
Malignant neoplasm of retained testis

C62.00 Malignant neoplasm of unspecified undescended testis   HCC Rx ESR COM ♂

C62.01 Malignant neoplasm of undescended right testis   HCC Rx ESR COM ♂

HCC CMS-HCC   Rx Rx HCC   ESR ESRD HCC   COM Commercial HCC   N Newborn: 0   P Pediatric: 0-17   M Maternity: 9-64   A Adult: 15-124

✓4th **C92 Myeloid leukemia**

INCLUDES   granulocytic leukemia
       myelogenous leukemia

EXCLUDES 1   *personal history of leukemia (Z85.6)*

AHA: 2020,1Q,13; 2019,1Q,16

DEF: Cancer that develops in immature myelocytes called myeloblasts. These are the cells that become white blood cells (except lymphocytes), red blood cells, or platelet-making cells. Can be acute (AML) or chronic (CML).

TIP: Pancytopenia, although common in some types of myeloid leukemias, is not always inherent. When it is documented, code D61.818 can be assigned in addition to a code from this category.

✓5th **C92.0 Acute myeloblastic leukemia**

Acute myeloblastic leukemia, minimal differentiation
Acute myeloblastic leukemia (with maturation)
Acute myeloblastic leukemia 1/ETO
Acute myeloblastic leukemia MØ
Acute myeloblastic leukemia M1
Acute myeloblastic leukemia M2
Acute myeloblastic leukemia with t(8;21)
Acute myeloblastic leukemia (without a FAB classification) NOS
Refractory anemia with excess blasts in transformation [RAEBT]

EXCLUDES 1   *acute exacerbation of chronic myeloid leukemia (C92.10)*
                  refractory anemia with excess of blasts not in transformation (D46.2-)

AHA: 2018,4Q,87

C92.00 Acute myeloblastic leukemia, not having achieved remission HCC Rx ESR COM

Acute myeloblastic leukemia with failed remission
Acute myeloblastic leukemia NOS

C92.01 Acute myeloblastic leukemia, in remission HCC Rx ESR COM

AHA: 2021,3Q,4

C92.02 Acute myeloblastic leukemia, in relapse HCC Rx ESR COM

✓5th **C92.1 Chronic myeloid leukemia, BCR/ABL-positive**

Chronic myelogenous leukemia, Philadelphia chromosome (Ph1) positive
Chronic myelogenous leukemia, t(9;22) (q34;q11)
Chronic myelogenous leukemia with crisis of blast cells

EXCLUDES 1   *atypical chronic myeloid leukemia BCR/ABL-negative (C92.2-)*
                  chronic myelomonocytic leukemia (C93.1-)
                  chronic myeloproliferative disease (D47.1)

C92.10 Chronic myeloid leukemia, BCR/ABL-positive, not having achieved remission HCC Rx ESR COM

Chronic myeloid leukemia, BCR/ABL-positive with failed remission
Chronic myeloid leukemia, BCR/ABL-positive NOS

C92.11 Chronic myeloid leukemia, BCR/ABL-positive, in remission HCC Rx ESR COM

C92.12 Chronic myeloid leukemia, BCR/ABL-positive, in relapse HCC Rx ESR COM

✓5th **C92.2 Atypical chronic myeloid leukemia, BCR/ABL-negative**

C92.20 Atypical chronic myeloid leukemia, BCR/ABL-negative, not having achieved remission HCC Rx ESR COM

Atypical chronic myeloid leukemia, BCR/ABL-negative with failed remission
Atypical chronic myeloid leukemia, BCR/ABL-negative NOS

C92.21 Atypical chronic myeloid leukemia, BCR/ABL-negative, in remission HCC Rx ESR COM

C92.22 Atypical chronic myeloid leukemia, BCR/ABL-negative, in relapse HCC Rx ESR COM

✓5th **C92.3 Myeloid sarcoma**

A malignant tumor of immature myeloid cells
Chloroma
Granulocytic sarcoma

C92.30 Myeloid sarcoma, not having achieved remission HCC Rx ESR COM

Myeloid sarcoma with failed remission
Myeloid sarcoma NOS

C92.31 Myeloid sarcoma, in remission HCC Rx ESR COM

C92.32 Myeloid sarcoma, in relapse HCC Rx ESR COM

✓5th **C92.4 Acute promyelocytic leukemia**

AML M3
AML Me with t(15;17) and variants

C92.40 Acute promyelocytic leukemia, not having achieved remission HCC Rx ESR COM

Acute promyelocytic leukemia with failed remission
Acute promyelocytic leukemia NOS

C92.41 Acute promyelocytic leukemia, in remission HCC Rx ESR COM

C92.42 Acute promyelocytic leukemia, in relapse HCC Rx ESR COM

✓5th **C92.5 Acute myelomonocytic leukemia**

AML M4
AML M4 Eo with inv(16) or t(16;16)

C92.50 Acute myelomonocytic leukemia, not having achieved remission HCC Rx ESR COM

Acute myelomonocytic leukemia with failed remission
Acute myelomonocytic leukemia NOS

C92.51 Acute myelomonocytic leukemia, in remission HCC Rx ESR COM

C92.52 Acute myelomonocytic leukemia, in relapse HCC Rx ESR COM

✓5th **C92.6 Acute myeloid leukemia with 11q23-abnormality**

Acute myeloid leukemia with variation of MLL-gene

C92.60 Acute myeloid leukemia with 11q23-abnormality not having achieved remission HCC Rx ESR COM

Acute myeloid leukemia with 11q23-abnormality with failed remission
Acute myeloid leukemia with 11q23-abnormality NOS

C92.61 Acute myeloid leukemia with 11q23-abnormality in remission HCC Rx ESR COM

C92.62 Acute myeloid leukemia with 11q23-abnormality in relapse HCC Rx ESR COM

✓5th **C92.A Acute myeloid leukemia with multilineage dysplasia**

Acute myeloid leukemia with dysplasia of remaining hematopoesis and/or myelodysplastic disease in its history

C92.AØ Acute myeloid leukemia with multilineage dysplasia, not having achieved remission HCC Rx ESR COM

Acute myeloid leukemia with multilineage dysplasia with failed remission
Acute myeloid leukemia with multilineage dysplasia NOS

C92.A1 Acute myeloid leukemia with multilineage dysplasia, in remission HCC Rx ESR COM

C92.A2 Acute myeloid leukemia with multilineage dysplasia, in relapse HCC Rx ESR COM

✓5th **C92.Z Other myeloid leukemia**

C92.ZØ Other myeloid leukemia not having achieved remission HCC Rx ESR COM

Myeloid leukemia NEC with failed remission
Myeloid leukemia NEC

C92.Z1 Other myeloid leukemia, in remission HCC Rx ESR COM

C92.Z2 Other myeloid leukemia, in relapse HCC Rx ESR COM

✓5th **C92.9 Myeloid leukemia, unspecified**

C92.90 Myeloid leukemia, unspecified, not having achieved remission HCC Rx ESR COM

Myeloid leukemia, unspecified with failed remission
Myeloid leukemia, unspecified NOS

C92.91 Myeloid leukemia, unspecified in remission HCC Rx ESR COM

C92.92 Myeloid leukemia, unspecified in relapse HCC Rx ESR COM

Chapter 2. Neoplasms

C93–C95.02

✓4ᵗʰ **C93** **Monocytic leukemia**

> INCLUDES   monocytoid leukemia
> EXCLUDES 1   *personal history of leukemia (Z85.6)*
> **AHA:** 2020,1Q,13

✓5ᵗʰ **C93.0** **Acute monoblastic/monocytic leukemia**
> AML M5
> AML M5a
> AML M5b

     C93.00 **Acute monoblastic/monocytic leukemia, not having achieved remission** `HCC` `Rx` `ESR` `COM`
> Acute monoblastic/monocytic leukemia with failed remission
> Acute monoblastic/monocytic leukemia NOS

     C93.01 **Acute monoblastic/monocytic leukemia, in remission** `HCC` `Rx` `ESR` `COM`

     C93.02 **Acute monoblastic/monocytic leukemia, in relapse** `HCC` `Rx` `ESR` `COM`

✓5ᵗʰ **C93.1** **Chronic myelomonocytic leukemia**
> Chronic monocytic leukemia
> CMML-1
> CMML-2
> CMML with eosinophilia
> Code also, if applicable, eosinophilia (D72.18)

     C93.10 **Chronic myelomonocytic leukemia not having achieved remission** `HCC` `Rx` `ESR` `COM`
> Chronic myelomonocytic leukemia with failed remission
> Chronic myelomonocytic leukemia NOS

     C93.11 **Chronic myelomonocytic leukemia, in remission** `HCC` `Rx` `ESR` `COM`

     C93.12 **Chronic myelomonocytic leukemia, in relapse** `HCC` `Rx` `ESR` `COM`

✓5ᵗʰ **C93.3** **Juvenile myelomonocytic leukemia**

     C93.30 **Juvenile myelomonocytic leukemia, not having achieved remission** `HCC` `Rx` `ESR` `COM` `P`
> Juvenile myelomonocytic leukemia with failed remission
> Juvenile myelomonocytic leukemia NOS

     C93.31 **Juvenile myelomonocytic leukemia, in remission** `HCC` `Rx` `ESR` `COM` `P`

     C93.32 **Juvenile myelomonocytic leukemia, in relapse** `HCC` `Rx` `ESR` `COM` `P`

✓5ᵗʰ **C93.Z** **Other monocytic leukemia**

     C93.Z0 **Other monocytic leukemia, not having achieved remission** `HCC` `Rx` `ESR` `COM`
> Other monocytic leukemia NOS

     C93.Z1 **Other monocytic leukemia, in remission** `HCC` `Rx` `ESR` `COM`

     C93.Z2 **Other monocytic leukemia, in relapse** `HCC` `Rx` `ESR` `COM`

✓5ᵗʰ **C93.9** **Monocytic leukemia, unspecified**

     C93.90 **Monocytic leukemia, unspecified, not having achieved remission** `HCC` `Rx` `ESR` `COM`
> Monocytic leukemia, unspecified with failed remission
> Monocytic leukemia, unspecified NOS

     C93.91 **Monocytic leukemia, unspecified in remission** `HCC` `Rx` `ESR` `COM`

     C93.92 **Monocytic leukemia, unspecified in relapse** `HCC` `Rx` `ESR` `COM`

✓4ᵗʰ **C94** **Other leukemias of specified cell type**

> EXCLUDES 1   *leukemic reticuloendotheliosis (C91.4-)*
> *myelodysplastic syndromes (D46.-)*
> *personal history of leukemia (Z85.6)*
> *plasma cell leukemia (C90.1-)*
> **AHA:** 2020,1Q,13

✓5ᵗʰ **C94.0** **Acute erythroid leukemia**
> Acute myeloid leukemia M6(a)(b)
> Erythroleukemia
> **DEF:** Erythroleukemia: Malignant blood dyscrasia (a myeloproliferative disorder).

     C94.00 **Acute erythroid leukemia, not having achieved remission** `HCC` `Rx` `ESR` `COM`
> Acute erythroid leukemia with failed remission
> Acute erythroid leukemia NOS

     C94.01 **Acute erythroid leukemia, in remission** `HCC` `Rx` `ESR` `COM`

     C94.02 **Acute erythroid leukemia, in relapse** `HCC` `Rx` `ESR` `COM`

✓5ᵗʰ **C94.2** **Acute megakaryoblastic leukemia**
> Acute myeloid leukemia M7
> Acute megakaryocytic leukemia

     C94.20 **Acute megakaryoblastic leukemia not having achieved remission** `HCC` `Rx` `ESR` `COM`
> Acute megakaryoblastic leukemia with failed remission
> Acute megakaryoblastic leukemia NOS

     C94.21 **Acute megakaryoblastic leukemia, in remission** `HCC` `Rx` `ESR` `COM`

     C94.22 **Acute megakaryoblastic leukemia, in relapse** `HCC` `Rx` `ESR` `COM`

✓5ᵗʰ **C94.3** **Mast cell leukemia**
> **AHA:** 2017,4Q,5

     C94.30 **Mast cell leukemia not having achieved remission** `HCC` `Rx` `ESR` `COM`
> Mast cell leukemia with failed remission
> Mast cell leukemia NOS

     C94.31 **Mast cell leukemia, in remission** `HCC` `Rx` `ESR` `COM`

     C94.32 **Mast cell leukemia, in relapse** `HCC` `Rx` `ESR` `COM`

✓5ᵗʰ **C94.4** **Acute panmyelosis with myelofibrosis**
> Acute myelofibrosis
> EXCLUDES 1   *myelofibrosis NOS (D75.81)*
> *secondary myelofibrosis NOS (D75.81)*

     C94.40 **Acute panmyelosis with myelofibrosis not having achieved remission** `HCC` `Rx` `ESR` `COM`
> Acute myelofibrosis NOS
> Acute panmyelosis with myelofibrosis with failed remission
> Acute panmyelosis NOS

     C94.41 **Acute panmyelosis with myelofibrosis, in remission** `HCC` `Rx` `ESR` `COM`

     C94.42 **Acute panmyelosis with myelofibrosis, in relapse** `HCC` `Rx` `ESR` `COM`

▲ **C94.6** **Myelodysplastic disease, not elsewhere classified** `HCC` `Rx` `ESR` `COM`
> ▶Myelodysplastic/myeloproliferative neoplasm, unclassifiable◀
> ▶Myeloproliferative disease, not elsewhere classified◀

✓5ᵗʰ **C94.8** **Other specified leukemias**
> Aggressive NK-cell leukemia
> Acute basophilic leukemia

     C94.80 **Other specified leukemias not having achieved remission** `HCC` `Rx` `ESR` `COM`
> Other specified leukemia with failed remission
> Other specified leukemias NOS

     C94.81 **Other specified leukemias, in remission** `HCC` `Rx` `ESR` `COM`

     C94.82 **Other specified leukemias, in relapse** `HCC` `Rx` `ESR` `COM`

✓4ᵗʰ **C95** **Leukemia of unspecified cell type**

> EXCLUDES 1   *personal history of leukemia (Z85.6)*
> **AHA:** 2020,1Q,13

✓5ᵗʰ **C95.0** **Acute leukemia of unspecified cell type**
> Acute bilineal leukemia
> Acute mixed lineage leukemia
> Biphenotypic acute leukemia
> Stem cell leukemia of unclear lineage
> EXCLUDES 1   *acute exacerbation of unspecified chronic leukemia (C95.10)*

     C95.00 **Acute leukemia of unspecified cell type not having achieved remission** `HCC` `Rx` `ESR` `COM`
> Acute leukemia of unspecified cell type with failed remission
> Acute leukemia NOS

     C95.01 **Acute leukemia of unspecified cell type, in remission** `HCC` `Rx` `ESR` `COM`

     C95.02 **Acute leukemia of unspecified cell type, in relapse** `HCC` `Rx` `ESR` `COM`

`HCC` CMS-HCC   `Rx` Rx HCC   `ESR` ESRD HCC   `COM` Commercial HCC   `N` Newborn: 0   `P` Pediatric: 0-17   `M` Maternity: 9-64   `A` Adult: 15-124

502   ICD-10-CM 2023

☑5ʰ C95.1 Chronic **leukemia of unspecified cell type**

     C95.10 Chronic **leukemia of unspecified cell type** not having achieved remission   `HCC` `Rx` `ESR` `COM`
         Chronic leukemia of unspecified cell type with failed remission
         Chronic leukemia NOS

     C95.11 Chronic **leukemia of unspecified cell type,** in remission   `HCC` `Rx` `ESR` `COM`

     C95.12 Chronic **leukemia of unspecified cell type,** in relapse   `HCC` `Rx` `ESR` `COM`

☑5ʰ C95.9 Leukemia, unspecified

     C95.90 **Leukemia, unspecified** not having achieved remission   `HCC` `Rx` `ESR` `COM`
         Leukemia, unspecified with failed remission
         Leukemia NOS

     C95.91 **Leukemia, unspecified,** in remission   `HCC` `Rx` `ESR` `COM`

     C95.92 **Leukemia, unspecified,** in relapse   `HCC` `Rx` `ESR` `COM`

☑4ʰ C96 **Other and unspecified malignant neoplasms of lymphoid, hematopoietic and related tissue**

     EXCLUDES 1   personal history of other malignant neoplasms of lymphoid, hematopoietic and related tissues (Z85.79)

   C96.0 **Multifocal and multisystemic (disseminated) Langerhans-cell histiocytosis**   `HCC` `Rx` `ESR` `COM`
     Histiocytosis X, multisystemic
     Letterer-Siwe disease
     EXCLUDES 1   adult pulmonary Langerhans cell histiocytosis (J84.82)
              multifocal and unisystemic Langerhans-cell histiocytosis (C96.5)
              unifocal Langerhans-cell histiocytosis (C96.6)

   ☑5ʰ C96.2 **Malignant mast cell neoplasm**
     EXCLUDES 1   indolent mastocytosis (D47.02)
              mast cell leukemia (C94.30)
              mastocytosis (congenital) (cutaneous) (Q82.2)
     AHA: 2017,4Q,5
     DEF: Mast cell: Type of white blood cell found in the loose connective tissue of blood vessels and bronchioles responsible for acute hypersensitivity reactions, including anaphylactic shock. The IgE receptors on these cells bind with allergens causing cell degranulation and diffuse, widespread histamine release that results in airway constriction and vasodilation with decreased systemic blood pressure.

     C96.20 **Malignant mast cell neoplasm, unspecified**   `HCC` `Rx` `ESR` `COM`

     C96.21 **Aggressive systemic mastocytosis**   `HCC` `Rx` `ESR` `COM`

     C96.22 **Mast cell sarcoma**   `HCC` `Rx` `ESR` `COM`

     C96.29 **Other malignant mast cell neoplasm**   `HCC` `Rx` `ESR` `COM`

   C96.4 **Sarcoma of dendritic cells (accessory cells)**   `HCC` `Rx` `ESR` `COM`
     Follicular dendritic cell sarcoma
     Interdigitating dendritic cell sarcoma
     Langerhans cell sarcoma

   C96.5 **Multifocal and unisystemic Langerhans-cell histiocytosis**   `HCC` `Rx` `ESR` `COM`
     Hand-Schüller-Christian disease
     Histiocytosis X, multifocal
     EXCLUDES 1   multifocal and multisystemic (disseminated) Langerhans-cell histiocytosis (C96.0)
              unifocal Langerhans-cell histiocytosis (C96.6)

   C96.6 **Unifocal Langerhans-cell histiocytosis**   `HCC` `Rx` `ESR` `COM`
     Eosinophilic granuloma
     Histiocytosis X, unifocal
     Histiocytosis X NOS
     Langerhans-cell histiocytosis NOS
     EXCLUDES 1   multifocal and multisysemic (disseminated) Langerhans-cell histiocytosis (C96.0)
              multifocal and unisystemic Langerhans-cell histiocytosis (C96.5)

   C96.A **Histiocytic sarcoma**   `HCC` `Rx` `ESR` `COM`
     Malignant histiocytosis

   C96.Z **Other specified malignant neoplasms of lymphoid, hematopoietic and related tissue**   `HCC` `Rx` `ESR` `COM`

   C96.9 **Malignant neoplasm of lymphoid, hematopoietic and related tissue, unspecified**   `HCC` `Rx` `ESR` `COM`

In situ neoplasms (D00-D09)

`INCLUDES`   Bowen's disease
           erythroplasia
           grade III intraepithelial neoplasia
           Queyrat's erythroplasia

☑4ʰ D00 **Carcinoma in situ of oral cavity, esophagus and stomach**
     EXCLUDES 1   melanoma in situ (D03.-)

   ☑5ʰ D00.0 **Carcinoma in situ of lip, oral cavity and pharynx**
     Use additional code to identify:
         exposure to environmental tobacco smoke (Z77.22)
         exposure to tobacco smoke in the perinatal period (P96.81)
         history of tobacco dependence (Z87.891)
         occupational exposure to environmental tobacco smoke (Z57.31)
         tobacco dependence (F17.-)
         tobacco use (Z72.0)
     EXCLUDES 1   carcinoma in situ of aryepiglottic fold or interarytenoid fold, laryngeal aspect (D02.0)
              carcinoma in situ of epiglottis NOS (D02.0)
              carcinoma in situ of epiglottis suprahyoid portion (D02.0)
              carcinoma in situ of skin of lip (D03.0, D04.0)

     D00.00 **Carcinoma in situ of oral cavity, unspecified site**
     D00.01 **Carcinoma in situ of labial mucosa and vermilion border**
     D00.02 **Carcinoma in situ of buccal mucosa**
     D00.03 **Carcinoma in situ of gingiva and edentulous alveolar ridge**
     D00.04 **Carcinoma in situ of soft palate**
     D00.05 **Carcinoma in situ of hard palate**
     D00.06 **Carcinoma in situ of floor of mouth**
     D00.07 **Carcinoma in situ of tongue**
     D00.08 **Carcinoma in situ of pharynx**
         Carcinoma in situ of aryepiglottic fold NOS
         Carcinoma in situ of hypopharyngeal aspect of aryepiglottic fold
         Carcinoma in situ of marginal zone of aryepiglottic fold

   D00.1 **Carcinoma in situ of esophagus**

   D00.2 **Carcinoma in situ of stomach**

☑4ʰ D01 **Carcinoma in situ of other and unspecified digestive organs**
     EXCLUDES 1   melanoma in situ (D03.-)

   D01.0 **Carcinoma in situ of colon**
     EXCLUDES 1   carcinoma in situ of rectosigmoid junction (D01.1)

   D01.1 **Carcinoma in situ of rectosigmoid junction**

   D01.2 **Carcinoma in situ of rectum**

   D01.3 **Carcinoma in situ of anus and anal canal**
     Anal intraepithelial neoplasia III [AIN III]
     Severe dysplasia of anus
     EXCLUDES 1   anal intraepithelial neoplasia I and II [AIN I and AIN II] (K62.82)
              carcinoma in situ of anal margin (D04.5)
              carcinoma in situ of anal skin (D04.5)
              carcinoma in situ of perianal skin (D04.5)

   ☑5ʰ D01.4 **Carcinoma in situ of other and unspecified parts of intestine**
     EXCLUDES 1   carcinoma in situ of ampulla of Vater (D01.5)

     D01.40 **Carcinoma in situ of unspecified part of intestine**
     D01.49 **Carcinoma in situ of other parts of intestine**

   D01.5 **Carcinoma in situ of liver, gallbladder and bile ducts**
     Carcinoma in situ of ampulla of Vater

   D01.7 **Carcinoma in situ of other specified digestive organs**
     Carcinoma in situ of pancreas

   D01.9 **Carcinoma in situ of digestive organ, unspecified**

✓4ᵗʰ **D02 Carcinoma in situ of** middle ear and respiratory system
Use additional code to identify:
exposure to environmental tobacco smoke (Z77.22)
exposure to tobacco smoke in the perinatal period (P96.81)
history of tobacco dependence (Z87.891)
occupational exposure to environmental tobacco smoke (Z57.31)
tobacco dependence (F17.-)
tobacco use (Z72.0)
EXCLUDES 1   melanoma in situ (D03.-)

D02.0 Carcinoma in situ of larynx
Carcinoma in situ of aryepiglottic fold or interarytenoid fold, laryngeal aspect
Carcinoma in situ of epiglottis (suprahyoid portion)
EXCLUDES 1   carcinoma in situ of aryepiglottic fold or interarytenoid fold NOS (D00.08)
carcinoma in situ of hypopharyngeal aspect (D00.08)
carcinoma in situ of marginal zone (D00.08)

D02.1 Carcinoma in situ of trachea

✓5ᵗʰ **D02.2 Carcinoma in situ of** bronchus and lung
D02.20 Carcinoma in situ of unspecified bronchus and lung
D02.21 Carcinoma in situ of right **bronchus and lung**
D02.22 Carcinoma in situ of left **bronchus and lung**

D02.3 Carcinoma in situ of other parts of respiratory system
Carcinoma in situ of accessory sinuses
Carcinoma in situ of middle ear
Carcinoma in situ of nasal cavities
EXCLUDES 1   carcinoma in situ of ear (external) (skin) (D04.2-)
carcinoma in situ of nose NOS (D09.8)
carcinoma in situ of skin of nose (D04.3)

D02.4 Carcinoma in situ of respiratory system, unspecified

✓4ᵗʰ **D03** Melanoma in situ

D03.0 Melanoma in situ of lip   HCC Rx ESR COM

✓5ᵗʰ **D03.1 Melanoma in situ of** eyelid, including canthus
AHA: 2018,4Q,4
D03.10 Melanoma in situ of unspecified eyelid, including canthus   HCC Rx ESR COM
✓6ᵗʰ **D03.11 Melanoma in situ of** right **eyelid, including canthus**
D03.111 Melanoma in situ of right upper **eyelid, including canthus**   HCC Rx ESR COM
D03.112 Melanoma in situ of right lower **eyelid, including canthus**   HCC Rx ESR COM
✓6ᵗʰ **D03.12 Melanoma in situ of** left **eyelid, including canthus**
D03.121 Melanoma in situ of left upper **eyelid, including canthus**
D03.122 Melanoma in situ of left lower **eyelid, including canthus**   HCC Rx ESR COM

✓5ᵗʰ **D03.2 Melanoma in situ of** ear and external auricular canal
D03.20 Melanoma in situ of unspecified ear and external auricular canal   HCC Rx ESR COM
D03.21 Melanoma in situ of right **ear and external auricular canal**   HCC Rx ESR COM
D03.22 Melanoma in situ of left **ear and external auricular canal**   HCC Rx ESR COM

✓5ᵗʰ **D03.3 Melanoma in situ of other and unspecified parts of** face
D03.30 Melanoma in situ of unspecified part of face   HCC Rx ESR COM
D03.39 Melanoma in situ of other parts of face   HCC Rx ESR COM

D03.4 Melanoma in situ of scalp and neck   HCC Rx ESR COM

✓5ᵗʰ **D03.5 Melanoma in situ of** trunk
D03.51 Melanoma in situ of anal skin   HCC Rx ESR COM
Melanoma in situ of anal margin
Melanoma in situ of perianal skin
D03.52 Melanoma in situ of breast (skin) (soft tissue)   HCC Rx ESR COM
D03.59 Melanoma in situ of other part of trunk   HCC Rx ESR COM

✓5ᵗʰ **D03.6 Melanoma in situ of** upper limb, including shoulder
D03.60 Melanoma in situ of unspecified upper limb, including shoulder   HCC Rx ESR COM
D03.61 Melanoma in situ of right **upper limb, including shoulder**   HCC Rx ESR COM
D03.62 Melanoma in situ of left **upper limb, including shoulder**   HCC Rx ESR COM

✓5ᵗʰ **D03.7 Melanoma in situ of** lower limb, including hip
D03.70 Melanoma in situ of unspecified lower limb, including hip   HCC Rx ESR COM
D03.71 Melanoma in situ of right **lower limb, including hip**   HCC Rx ESR COM
D03.72 Melanoma in situ of left **lower limb, including hip**   HCC Rx ESR COM

D03.8 Melanoma in situ of other sites   HCC Rx ESR COM
Melanoma in situ of scrotum
EXCLUDES 1   carcinoma in situ of scrotum (D07.61)

D03.9 Melanoma in situ, unspecified   HCC Rx ESR COM

✓4ᵗʰ **D04 Carcinoma in situ of** skin
EXCLUDES 1   erythroplasia of Queyrat (penis) NOS (D07.4)
melanoma in situ (D03.-)

D04.0 Carcinoma in situ of skin of lip
EXCLUDES 2   carcinoma in situ of vermilion border of lip (D00.01)

✓5ᵗʰ **D04.1 Carcinoma in situ of skin of** eyelid, including canthus
AHA: 2018,4Q,4
D04.10 Carcinoma in situ of skin of unspecified eyelid, including canthus
✓6ᵗʰ **D04.11 Carcinoma in situ of skin of** right **eyelid, including canthus**
D04.111 Carcinoma in situ of skin of right upper **eyelid, including canthus**
D04.112 Carcinoma in situ of skin of right lower **eyelid, including canthus**
✓6ᵗʰ **D04.12 Carcinoma in situ of skin of** left **eyelid, including canthus**
D04.121 Carcinoma in situ of skin of left upper **eyelid, including canthus**
D04.122 Carcinoma in situ of skin of left lower **eyelid, including canthus**

✓5ᵗʰ **D04.2 Carcinoma in situ of skin of** ear and external auricular canal
D04.20 Carcinoma in situ of skin of unspecified ear and external auricular canal
D04.21 Carcinoma in situ of skin of right **ear and external auricular canal**
D04.22 Carcinoma in situ of skin of left **ear and external auricular canal**

✓5ᵗʰ **D04.3 Carcinoma in situ of skin of other and unspecified** parts of face
D04.30 Carcinoma in situ of skin of unspecified part of face
D04.39 Carcinoma in situ of skin of other parts of face

D04.4 Carcinoma in situ of skin of scalp and neck

D04.5 Carcinoma in situ of skin of trunk
Carcinoma in situ of anal margin
Carcinoma in situ of anal skin
Carcinoma in situ of perianal skin
Carcinoma in situ of skin of breast
EXCLUDES 1   carcinoma in situ of anus NOS (D01.3)
carcinoma in situ of scrotum (D07.61)
carcinoma in situ of skin of genital organs (D07.-)

✓5ᵗʰ **D04.6 Carcinoma in situ of skin of** upper limb, including shoulder
D04.60 Carcinoma in situ of skin of unspecified upper limb, including shoulder
D04.61 Carcinoma in situ of skin of right **upper limb, including shoulder**
D04.62 Carcinoma in situ of skin of left **upper limb, including shoulder**

✓5ᵗʰ **D04.7 Carcinoma in situ of skin of** lower limb, including hip
D04.70 Carcinoma in situ of skin of unspecified lower limb, including hip
D04.71 Carcinoma in situ of skin of right **lower limb, including hip**
D04.72 Carcinoma in situ of skin of left **lower limb, including hip**

D04.8 Carcinoma in situ of skin of other sites

D04.9 Carcinoma in situ of skin, unspecified

✓4ᵗʰ **D05 Carcinoma in situ of** breast
EXCLUDES 1   carcinoma in situ of skin of breast (D04.5)
melanoma in situ of breast (skin) (D03.5)
Paget's disease of breast or nipple (C50.-)

✓5ᵗʰ **D05.0** Lobular **carcinoma in situ of breast**
D05.00 Lobular carcinoma in situ of unspecified breast
D05.01 Lobular carcinoma in situ of right **breast**
D05.02 Lobular carcinoma in situ of left **breast**

✓5ᵗʰ **D05.1 Intraductal carcinoma in situ of breast**

     D05.10 Intraductal carcinoma in situ of unspecified breast

     D05.11 Intraductal carcinoma in situ of right breast

     D05.12 Intraductal carcinoma in situ of left breast

✓5ᵗʰ **D05.8 Other specified type of carcinoma in situ of breast**

     D05.80 Other specified type of carcinoma in situ of unspecified breast

     D05.81 Other specified type of carcinoma in situ of right breast

     D05.82 Other specified type of carcinoma in situ of left breast

✓5ᵗʰ **D05.9 Unspecified type of carcinoma in situ of breast**

     D05.90 Unspecified type of carcinoma in situ of unspecified breast

     D05.91 Unspecified type of carcinoma in situ of right breast

     D05.92 Unspecified type of carcinoma in situ of left breast

✓4ᵗʰ **D06 Carcinoma in situ of cervix uteri**

     INCLUDES   cervical adenocarcinoma in situ
            cervical intraepithelial glandular neoplasia
            cervical intraepithelial neoplasia III [CIN III]
            severe dysplasia of cervix uteri

     EXCLUDES 1   *cervical intraepithelial neoplasia II [CIN II] (N87.1)*
            cytologic evidence of malignancy of cervix without histologic confirmation (R87.614)
            high grade squamous intraepithelial lesion (HGSIL) of cervix (R87.613)
            melanoma in situ of cervix (D03.5)
            moderate cervical dysplasia (N87.1)

     D06.0 Carcinoma in situ of endocervix   ♀

     D06.1 Carcinoma in situ of exocervix   ♀

     D06.7 Carcinoma in situ of other parts of cervix   ♀

     D06.9 Carcinoma in situ of cervix, unspecified   ♀

✓4ᵗʰ **D07 Carcinoma in situ of other and unspecified genital organs**

     EXCLUDES 1   *melanoma in situ of trunk (D03.5)*

     D07.0 Carcinoma in situ of endometrium   ♀

     D07.1 Carcinoma in situ of vulva   ♀
         Severe dysplasia of vulva
         Vulvar intraepithelial neoplasia III [VIN III]
         EXCLUDES 1   *moderate dysplasia of vulva (N90.1)*
                 vulvar intraepithelial neoplasia II [VIN II] (N90.1)

     D07.2 Carcinoma in situ of vagina   ♀
         Severe dysplasia of vagina
         Vaginal intraepithelial neoplasia III [VAIN III]
         EXCLUDES 1   *moderate dysplasia of vagina (N89.1)*
                 vaginal intraepithelial neoplasia II [VIN II] (N89.1)

✓5ᵗʰ **D07.3 Carcinoma in situ of other and unspecified female genital organs**

     D07.30 Carcinoma in situ of unspecified female genital organs   ♀

     D07.39 Carcinoma in situ of other female genital organs   ♀

     D07.4 Carcinoma in situ of penis   ♂
         Erythroplasia of Queyrat NOS

     D07.5 Carcinoma in situ of prostate   ♂
         Prostatic intraepithelial neoplasia III (PIN III)
         Severe dysplasia of prostate
         EXCLUDES 1   *dysplasia (mild) (moderate) of prostate (N42.3-)*
                 prostatic intraepithelial neoplasia II [PIN II] (N42.3-)

✓5ᵗʰ **D07.6 Carcinoma in situ of other and unspecified male genital organs**

     D07.60 Carcinoma in situ of unspecified male genital organs   ♂

     D07.61 Carcinoma in situ of scrotum   ♂

     D07.69 Carcinoma in situ of other male genital organs   ♂

✓4ᵗʰ **D09 Carcinoma in situ of other and unspecified sites**

     EXCLUDES 1   *melanoma in situ (D03.-)*

     D09.0 Carcinoma in situ of bladder

✓5ᵗʰ **D09.1 Carcinoma in situ of other and unspecified urinary organs**

     D09.10 Carcinoma in situ of unspecified urinary organ

     D09.19 Carcinoma in situ of other urinary organs

✓5ᵗʰ **D09.2 Carcinoma in situ of eye**

     EXCLUDES 1   *carcinoma in situ of skin of eyelid (D04.1-)*

     D09.20 Carcinoma in situ of unspecified eye

     D09.21 Carcinoma in situ of right eye

     D09.22 Carcinoma in situ of left eye

     D09.3 Carcinoma in situ of thyroid and other endocrine glands

     EXCLUDES 1   *carcinoma in situ of endocrine pancreas (D01.7)*
            carcinoma in situ of ovary (D07.39)
            carcinoma in situ of testis (D07.69)

     D09.8 Carcinoma in situ of other specified sites

     D09.9 Carcinoma in situ, unspecified

Benign neoplasms, except benign neuroendocrine tumors (D10-D36)

✓4ᵗʰ **D10 Benign neoplasm of mouth and pharynx**

     D10.0 Benign neoplasm of lip
         Benign neoplasm of lip (frenulum) (inner aspect) (mucosa) (vermilion border)
         EXCLUDES 1   *benign neoplasm of skin of lip (D22.0, D23.0)*

     D10.1 Benign neoplasm of tongue
         Benign neoplasm of lingual tonsil

     D10.2 Benign neoplasm of floor of mouth

✓5ᵗʰ **D10.3 Benign neoplasm of other and unspecified parts of mouth**

     D10.30 Benign neoplasm of unspecified part of mouth

     D10.39 Benign neoplasm of other parts of mouth
         Benign neoplasm of minor salivary gland NOS
         EXCLUDES 1   *benign odontogenic neoplasms (D16.4-D16.5)*
                 benign neoplasm of mucosa of lip (D10.0)
                 benign neoplasm of nasopharyngeal surface of soft palate (D10.6)

     D10.4 Benign neoplasm of tonsil
         Benign neoplasm of tonsil (faucial) (palatine)
         EXCLUDES 1   *benign neoplasm of lingual tonsil (D10.1)*
                 benign neoplasm of pharyngeal tonsil (D10.6)
                 benign neoplasm of tonsillar fossa (D10.5)
                 benign neoplasm of tonsillar pillars (D10.5)

     D10.5 Benign neoplasm of other parts of oropharynx
         Benign neoplasm of epiglottis, anterior aspect
         Benign neoplasm of tonsillar fossa
         Benign neoplasm of tonsillar pillars
         Benign neoplasm of vallecula
         EXCLUDES 1   *benign neoplasm of epiglottis NOS (D14.1)*
                 benign neoplasm of epiglottis, suprahyoid portion (D14.1)
         DEF: Oropharynx: Middle portion of pharynx (throat); communicates with the oral cavity, nasopharynx and laryngopharynx.

     D10.6 Benign neoplasm of nasopharynx
         Benign neoplasm of pharyngeal tonsil
         Benign neoplasm of posterior margin of septum and choanae
         DEF: Nasopharynx: Upper portion of pharynx (throat); communicates with the nasal cavities, oropharynx and tympanic cavities.

     D10.7 Benign neoplasm of hypopharynx
         DEF: Hypopharynx: Lower portion of pharynx (throat); communicates with the oropharynx and the esophagus.
         Synonym(s): laryngopharynx.

     D10.9 Benign neoplasm of pharynx, unspecified

✓4ᵗʰ **D11 Benign neoplasm of major salivary glands**

     EXCLUDES 1   *benign neoplasms of specified minor salivary glands which are classified according to their anatomical location*
            benign neoplasms of minor salivary glands NOS (D10.39)

     D11.0 Benign neoplasm of parotid gland

     D11.7 Benign neoplasm of other major salivary glands
         Benign neoplasm of sublingual salivary gland
         Benign neoplasm of submandibular salivary gland

     D11.9 Benign neoplasm of major salivary gland, unspecified

✓4ᵗʰ **D12 Benign neoplasm of colon, rectum, anus and anal canal**

     EXCLUDES 1   *benign carcinoid tumors of the large intestine, and rectum (D3A.02-)*
            polyp of colon NOS (K63.5)

     AHA: 2018,2Q,14; 2017,1Q,15; 2015,2Q,14

     TIP: Code K63.5 Polyp of colon, is assigned when documentation states hyperplastic colon polyps, regardless of the site in the colon. Slow-growing, hyperplastic polyps are not precancerous and are classified differently from benign or adenomatous polyps.

     D12.0 Benign neoplasm of cecum
         Benign neoplasm of ileocecal valve

Chapter 2. Neoplasms

D12.1–D17.20

D12.1 Benign neoplasm of appendix
> EXCLUDES 1   *benign carcinoid tumor of the appendix (D3A.020)*

D12.2 Benign neoplasm of ascending colon

D12.3 Benign neoplasm of transverse colon
Benign neoplasm of hepatic flexure
Benign neoplasm of splenic flexure
AHA: 2017,1Q,16

D12.4 Benign neoplasm of descending colon

D12.5 Benign neoplasm of sigmoid colon

D12.6 Benign neoplasm of colon, unspecified
Adenomatosis of colon
Benign neoplasm of large intestine NOS
Polyposis (hereditary) of colon
> EXCLUDES 1   *inflammatory polyp of colon (K51.4-)*

D12.7 Benign neoplasm of rectosigmoid junction

D12.8 Benign neoplasm of rectum
> EXCLUDES 1   *benign carcinoid tumor of the rectum (D3A.026)*

AHA: 2018,1Q,6

D12.9 Benign neoplasm of anus and anal canal
Benign neoplasm of anus NOS
> EXCLUDES 1   *benign neoplasm of anal margin (D22.5, D23.5)*
> *benign neoplasm of anal skin (D22.5, D23.5)*
> *benign neoplasm of perianal skin (D22.5, D23.5)*

✓4ᵗʰ **D13 Benign neoplasm of other and ill-defined parts of digestive system**
> EXCLUDES 1   *benign stromal tumors of digestive system (D21.4)*

D13.0 Benign neoplasm of esophagus

D13.1 Benign neoplasm of stomach
> EXCLUDES 1   *benign carcinoid tumor of the stomach (D3A.092)*

D13.2 Benign neoplasm of duodenum
> EXCLUDES 1   *benign carcinoid tumor of the duodenum (D3A.010)*

✓5ᵗʰ **D13.3 Benign neoplasm of other and unspecified parts of small intestine**
> EXCLUDES 1   *benign carcinoid tumors of the small intestine (D3A.01-)*
> *benign neoplasm of ileocecal valve (D12.0)*

     D13.30 Benign neoplasm of unspecified part of small intestine

     D13.39 Benign neoplasm of other parts of small intestine

D13.4 Benign neoplasm of liver
Benign neoplasm of intrahepatic bile ducts

D13.5 Benign neoplasm of extrahepatic bile ducts

D13.6 Benign neoplasm of pancreas
> EXCLUDES 1   *benign neoplasm of endocrine pancreas (D13.7)*

D13.7 Benign neoplasm of endocrine pancreas
Benign neoplasm of islets of Langerhans
Islet cell tumor
Use additional code to identify any functional activity

D13.9 Benign neoplasm of ill-defined sites within the digestive system
Benign neoplasm of digestive system NOS
Benign neoplasm of intestine NOS
Benign neoplasm of spleen

✓4ᵗʰ **D14 Benign neoplasm of middle ear and respiratory system**

D14.0 Benign neoplasm of middle ear, nasal cavity and accessory sinuses
Benign neoplasm of cartilage of nose
> EXCLUDES 1   *benign neoplasm of auricular canal (external) (D22.2-, D23.2-)*
> *benign neoplasm of bone of ear (D16.4)*
> *benign neoplasm of bone of nose (D16.4)*
> *benign neoplasm of cartilage of ear (D21.0)*
> *benign neoplasm of ear (external)(skin) (D22.2-, D23.2-)*
> *benign neoplasm of nose NOS (D36.7)*
> *benign neoplasm of skin of nose (D22.39, D23.39)*
> *benign neoplasm of olfactory bulb (D33.3)*
> *benign neoplasm of posterior margin of septum and choanae (D10.6)*
> *polyp of accessory sinus (J33.8)*
> *polyp of ear (middle) (H74.4)*
> *polyp of nasal (cavity) (J33.-)*

D14.1 Benign neoplasm of larynx
Adenomatous polyp of larynx
Benign neoplasm of epiglottis (suprahyoid portion)
> EXCLUDES 1   *benign neoplasm of epiglottis, anterior aspect (D10.5)*
> *polyp (nonadenomatous) of vocal cord or larynx (J38.1)*

D14.2 Benign neoplasm of trachea

✓5ᵗʰ **D14.3 Benign neoplasm of bronchus and lung**
> EXCLUDES 1   *benign carcinoid tumor of the bronchus and lung (D3A.090)*

     D14.30 Benign neoplasm of unspecified bronchus and lung
     D14.31 Benign neoplasm of right bronchus and lung
     D14.32 Benign neoplasm of left bronchus and lung
D14.4 Benign neoplasm of respiratory system, unspecified

✓4ᵗʰ **D15 Benign neoplasm of other and unspecified intrathoracic organs**
> EXCLUDES 1   *benign neoplasm of mesothelial tissue (D19.-)*

D15.0 Benign neoplasm of thymus
> EXCLUDES 1   *benign carcinoid tumor of the thymus (D3A.091)*

D15.1 Benign neoplasm of heart   COM
> EXCLUDES 1   *benign neoplasm of great vessels (D21.3)*

D15.2 Benign neoplasm of mediastinum

D15.7 Benign neoplasm of other specified intrathoracic organs

D15.9 Benign neoplasm of intrathoracic organ, unspecified

✓4ᵗʰ **D16 Benign neoplasm of bone and articular cartilage**
> EXCLUDES 1   *benign neoplasm of connective tissue of ear (D21.0)*
> *benign neoplasm of connective tissue of eyelid (D21.0)*
> *benign neoplasm of connective tissue of larynx (D14.1)*
> *benign neoplasm of connective tissue of nose (D14.0)*
> *benign neoplasm of synovia (D21.-)*

✓5ᵗʰ **D16.0 Benign neoplasm of scapula and long bones of upper limb**
     D16.00 Benign neoplasm of scapula and long bones of unspecified upper limb
     D16.01 Benign neoplasm of scapula and long bones of right upper limb
     D16.02 Benign neoplasm of scapula and long bones of left upper limb

✓5ᵗʰ **D16.1 Benign neoplasm of short bones of upper limb**
     D16.10 Benign neoplasm of short bones of unspecified upper limb
     D16.11 Benign neoplasm of short bones of right upper limb
     D16.12 Benign neoplasm of short bones of left upper limb

✓5ᵗʰ **D16.2 Benign neoplasm of long bones of lower limb**
     D16.20 Benign neoplasm of long bones of unspecified lower limb
     D16.21 Benign neoplasm of long bones of right lower limb
     D16.22 Benign neoplasm of long bones of left lower limb

✓5ᵗʰ **D16.3 Benign neoplasm of short bones of lower limb**
     D16.30 Benign neoplasm of short bones of unspecified lower limb
     D16.31 Benign neoplasm of short bones of right lower limb
     D16.32 Benign neoplasm of short bones of left lower limb

D16.4 Benign neoplasm of bones of skull and face
Benign neoplasm of maxilla (superior)
Benign neoplasm of orbital bone
Keratocyst of maxilla
Keratocystic odontogenic tumor of maxilla
> EXCLUDES 2   *benign neoplasm of lower jaw bone (D16.5)*

D16.5 Benign neoplasm of lower jaw bone
Keratocyst of mandible
Keratocystic odontogenic tumor of mandible

D16.6 Benign neoplasm of vertebral column
> EXCLUDES 1   *benign neoplasm of sacrum and coccyx (D16.8)*

D16.7 Benign neoplasm of ribs, sternum and clavicle

D16.8 Benign neoplasm of pelvic bones, sacrum and coccyx

D16.9 Benign neoplasm of bone and articular cartilage, unspecified

✓4ᵗʰ **D17 Benign lipomatous neoplasm**

D17.0 Benign lipomatous neoplasm of skin and subcutaneous tissue of head, face and neck

D17.1 Benign lipomatous neoplasm of skin and subcutaneous tissue of trunk

✓5ᵗʰ **D17.2 Benign lipomatous neoplasm of skin and subcutaneous tissue of limb**
     D17.20 Benign lipomatous neoplasm of skin and subcutaneous tissue of unspecified limb

---

HCC CMS-HCC   Rx Rx HCC   ESR ESRD HCC   COM Commercial HCC   N Newborn: 0   P Pediatric: 0-17   M Maternity: 9-64   A Adult: 15-124

D17.21   **Benign lipomatous neoplasm of skin and subcutaneous tissue of** right arm

D17.22   **Benign lipomatous neoplasm of skin and subcutaneous tissue of** left arm

D17.23   **Benign lipomatous neoplasm of skin and subcutaneous tissue of** right leg

D17.24   **Benign lipomatous neoplasm of skin and subcutaneous tissue of** left leg

✓5th **D17.3**   **Benign lipomatous neoplasm of** skin and subcutaneous tissue **of other and unspecified sites**

D17.30   **Benign lipomatous neoplasm of skin and subcutaneous tissue of unspecified sites**

D17.39   **Benign lipomatous neoplasm of skin and subcutaneous tissue of other sites**

D17.4   **Benign lipomatous neoplasm of** intrathoracic organs

D17.5   **Benign lipomatous neoplasm of** intra-abdominal organs

EXCLUDES 1   *benign lipomatous neoplasm of peritoneum and retroperitoneum (D17.79)*

D17.6   **Benign lipomatous neoplasm of** spermatic cord   ♂

✓5th **D17.7**   **Benign lipomatous neoplasm of other sites**

D17.71   **Benign lipomatous neoplasm of** kidney

D17.72   **Benign lipomatous neoplasm of other** genitourinary organ

D17.79   **Benign lipomatous neoplasm of other sites**
Benign lipomatous neoplasm of peritoneum
Benign lipomatous neoplasm of retroperitoneum

D17.9   **Benign lipomatous neoplasm, unspecified**
Lipoma NOS

✓4th **D18**   **Hemangioma and lymphangioma, any site**

EXCLUDES 1   *benign neoplasm of glomus jugulare (D35.6)*
blue or pigmented nevus (D22.-)
nevus NOS (D22.-)
vascular nevus (Q82.5)

✓5th **D18.0**   **Hemangioma**
Angioma NOS
Cavernous nevus
DEF: Common benign tumor usually occurring in infancy that is composed of newly formed blood vessels due to malformation of the angioblastic tissue.

D18.00   **Hemangioma unspecified site**

D18.01   **Hemangioma of** skin and subcutaneous tissue

D18.02   **Hemangioma of** intracranial structures   HCC Rx ESR COM

D18.03   **Hemangioma of** intra-abdominal structures

D18.09   **Hemangioma of other sites**

D18.1   **Lymphangioma, any site**
AHA: 2018,3Q,31; 2018,2Q,13

✓4th **D19**   **Benign neoplasm of** mesothelial tissue

D19.0   **Benign neoplasm of mesothelial tissue of** pleura

D19.1   **Benign neoplasm of mesothelial tissue of** peritoneum

D19.7   **Benign neoplasm of mesothelial tissue of other sites**

D19.9   **Benign neoplasm of mesothelial tissue, unspecified**
Benign mesothelioma NOS

✓4th **D20**   **Benign neoplasm of soft tissue of** retroperitoneum and peritoneum

EXCLUDES 1   *benign lipomatous neoplasm of peritoneum and retroperitoneum (D17.79)*
benign neoplasm of mesothelial tissue (D19.-)

D20.0   **Benign neoplasm of soft tissue of** retroperitoneum

D20.1   **Benign neoplasm of soft tissue of** peritoneum

✓4th **D21**   **Other benign neoplasms of** connective and other soft tissue

INCLUDES   benign neoplasm of blood vessel
benign neoplasm of bursa
benign neoplasm of cartilage
benign neoplasm of fascia
benign neoplasm of fat
benign neoplasm of ligament, except uterine
benign neoplasm of lymphatic channel
benign neoplasm of muscle
benign neoplasm of synovia
benign neoplasm of tendon (sheath)
benign stromal tumors

EXCLUDES 1   *benign neoplasm of articular cartilage (D16.-)*
benign neoplasm of cartilage of larynx (D14.1)
benign neoplasm of cartilage of nose (D14.0)
benign neoplasm of connective tissue of breast (D24.-)
benign neoplasm of peripheral nerves and autonomic nervous system (D36.1-)
benign neoplasm of peritoneum (D20.1)
benign neoplasm of retroperitoneum (D20.0)
benign neoplasm of uterine ligament, any (D28.2)
benign neoplasm of vascular tissue (D18.-)
hemangioma (D18.0-)
lipomatous neoplasm (D17.-)
lymphangioma (D18.1)
uterine leiomyoma (D25.-)

D21.0   **Benign neoplasm of connective and other soft tissue of** head, face and neck
Benign neoplasm of connective tissue of ear
Benign neoplasm of connective tissue of eyelid

EXCLUDES 1   *benign neoplasm of connective tissue of orbit (D31.6-)*

✓5th **D21.1**   **Benign neoplasm of connective and other soft tissue of** upper limb, including shoulder

D21.10   **Benign neoplasm of connective and other soft tissue of unspecified upper limb, including shoulder**

D21.11   **Benign neoplasm of connective and other soft tissue of** right upper limb, including shoulder

D21.12   **Benign neoplasm of connective and other soft tissue of** left upper limb, including shoulder

✓5th **D21.2**   **Benign neoplasm of connective and other soft tissue of** lower limb, including hip

D21.20   **Benign neoplasm of connective and other soft tissue of unspecified lower limb, including hip**

D21.21   **Benign neoplasm of connective and other soft tissue of** right lower limb, including hip

D21.22   **Benign neoplasm of connective and other soft tissue of** left lower limb, including hip

D21.3   **Benign neoplasm of connective and other soft tissue of** thorax
Benign neoplasm of axilla
Benign neoplasm of diaphragm
Benign neoplasm of great vessels

EXCLUDES 1   *benign neoplasm of heart (D15.1)*
benign neoplasm of mediastinum (D15.2)
benign neoplasm of thymus (D15.0)

D21.4   **Benign neoplasm of connective and other soft tissue of** abdomen
Benign stromal tumors of abdomen

D21.5   **Benign neoplasm of connective and other soft tissue of** pelvis

EXCLUDES 1   *benign neoplasm of any uterine ligament (D28.2)*
uterine leiomyoma (D25.-)

D21.6   **Benign neoplasm of connective and other soft tissue of** trunk, unspecified
Benign neoplasm of connective and other soft tissue of back NOS

D21.9   **Benign neoplasm of connective and other soft tissue, unspecified**

✓4th **D22**   **Melanocytic nevi**

INCLUDES   atypical nevus
blue hairy pigmented nevus
nevus NOS

D22.0   **Melanocytic nevi of** lip

✓5th **D22.1**   **Melanocytic nevi of** eyelid, including canthus
AHA: 2018,4Q,4

D22.10   **Melanocytic nevi of unspecified eyelid, including canthus**

✓6ᵗʰ **D22.11 Melanocytic nevi of** right **eyelid, including canthus**
     D22.111 Melanocytic nevi of right upper **eyelid, including canthus**
     D22.112 Melanocytic nevi of right lower **eyelid, including canthus**

✓6ᵗʰ **D22.12 Melanocytic nevi of** left **eyelid, including canthus**
     D22.121 Melanocytic nevi of left upper **eyelid, including canthus**
     D22.122 Melanocytic nevi of left lower **eyelid, including canthus**

✓5ᵗʰ **D22.2 Melanocytic nevi of** ear and external auricular canal
     D22.20 Melanocytic nevi of unspecified ear and external auricular canal
     D22.21 Melanocytic nevi of right **ear and external auricular canal**
     D22.22 Melanocytic nevi of left **ear and external auricular canal**

✓5ᵗʰ **D22.3 Melanocytic nevi of other and unspecified** parts of face
     D22.30 Melanocytic nevi of unspecified part of face
     D22.39 Melanocytic nevi of other parts of face

D22.4 Melanocytic nevi of scalp and neck

D22.5 Melanocytic nevi of trunk
     Melanocytic nevi of anal margin
     Melanocytic nevi of anal skin
     Melanocytic nevi of perianal skin
     Melanocytic nevi of skin of breast

✓5ᵗʰ **D22.6 Melanocytic nevi of** upper limb, including shoulder
     D22.60 Melanocytic nevi of unspecified upper limb, including shoulder
     D22.61 Melanocytic nevi of right **upper limb, including shoulder**
     D22.62 Melanocytic nevi of left **upper limb, including shoulder**

✓5ᵗʰ **D22.7 Melanocytic nevi of** lower limb, including hip
     D22.70 Melanocytic nevi of unspecified lower limb, including hip
     D22.71 Melanocytic nevi of right **lower limb, including hip**
     D22.72 Melanocytic nevi of left **lower limb, including hip**

D22.9 Melanocytic nevi, unspecified

✓4ᵗʰ **D23 Other benign neoplasms of** skin
     INCLUDES   benign neoplasm of hair follicles
         benign neoplasm of sebaceous glands
         benign neoplasm of sweat glands
     EXCLUDES 1   *benign lipomatous neoplasms of skin (D17.0-D17.3)*
     EXCLUDES 2   *melanocytic nevi (D22.-)*

D23.0 Other benign neoplasm of skin of lip
     EXCLUDES 1   *benign neoplasm of vermilion border of lip (D10.0)*

✓5ᵗʰ **D23.1 Other benign neoplasm of skin of** eyelid, including canthus
     AHA: 2018,4Q,4
     D23.10 Other benign neoplasm of skin of unspecified eyelid, including canthus
     ✓6ᵗʰ **D23.11 Other benign neoplasm of skin of** right **eyelid, including canthus**
         D23.111 Other benign neoplasm of skin of right upper **eyelid, including canthus**
         D23.112 Other benign neoplasm of skin of right lower **eyelid, including canthus**
     ✓6ᵗʰ **D23.12 Other benign neoplasm of skin of** left **eyelid, including canthus**
         D23.121 Other benign neoplasm of skin of left upper **eyelid, including canthus**
         D23.122 Other benign neoplasm of skin of left lower **eyelid, including canthus**

✓5ᵗʰ **D23.2 Other benign neoplasm of skin of** ear and external auricular canal
     D23.20 Other benign neoplasm of skin of unspecified ear and external auricular canal
     D23.21 Other benign neoplasm of skin of right **ear and external auricular canal**
     D23.22 Other benign neoplasm of skin of left **ear and external auricular canal**

✓5ᵗʰ **D23.3 Other benign neoplasm of skin of other and unspecified parts of** face
     D23.30 Other benign neoplasm of skin of unspecified part of face
     D23.39 Other benign neoplasm of skin of other parts of face

D23.4 Other benign neoplasm of skin of scalp and neck

D23.5 Other benign neoplasm of skin of trunk
     Other benign neoplasm of anal margin
     Other benign neoplasm of anal skin
     Other benign neoplasm of perianal skin
     Other benign neoplasm of skin of breast
     EXCLUDES 1   *benign neoplasm of anus NOS (D12.9)*

✓5ᵗʰ **D23.6 Other benign neoplasm of skin of** upper limb, including shoulder
     D23.60 Other benign neoplasm of skin of unspecified upper limb, including shoulder
     D23.61 Other benign neoplasm of skin of right **upper limb, including shoulder**
     D23.62 Other benign neoplasm of skin of left **upper limb, including shoulder**

✓6ᵗʰ **D23.7 Other benign neoplasm of skin of** lower limb, including hip
     D23.70 Other benign neoplasm of skin of unspecified lower limb, including hip
     D23.71 Other benign neoplasm of skin of right **lower limb, including hip**
     D23.72 Other benign neoplasm of skin of left **lower limb, including hip**

D23.9 Other benign neoplasm of skin, unspecified

✓4ᵗʰ **D24 Benign neoplasm of** breast
     INCLUDES   benign neoplasm of connective tissue of breast
         benign neoplasm of soft parts of breast
         fibroadenoma of breast
     EXCLUDES 2   *adenofibrosis of breast (N60.2)*
         benign cyst of breast (N60.-)
         benign mammary dysplasia (N60.-)
         benign neoplasm of skin of breast (D22.5, D23.5)
         fibrocystic disease of breast (N60.-)

D24.1 Benign neoplasm of right **breast**

D24.2 Benign neoplasm of left **breast**

D24.9 Benign neoplasm of unspecified breast

✓4ᵗʰ **D25 Leiomyoma of uterus**
     INCLUDES   uterine fibroid
         uterine fibromyoma
         uterine myoma

Uterine Leiomyomas (Fibroids)

D25.0 Submucous leiomyoma of uterus ♀

D25.1 Intramural leiomyoma of uterus ♀
     Interstitial leiomyoma of uterus

D25.2 Subserosal leiomyoma of uterus ♀
     Subperitoneal leiomyoma of uterus

D25.9 Leiomyoma of uterus, unspecified ♀

✓4ᵗʰ **D26 Other benign neoplasms of** uterus

D26.0 Other benign neoplasm of cervix uteri ♀

D26.1 Other benign neoplasm of corpus uteri ♀

D26.7 Other benign neoplasm of other parts of uterus ♀

D26.9 Other benign neoplasm of uterus, unspecified ♀

Chapter 2. Neoplasms

☑4ᵗʰ D27 Benign neoplasm of ovary
Use additional code to identify any functional activity
EXCLUDES 2   corpus albicans cyst (N83.2-)
     corpus luteum cyst (N83.1-)
     endometrial cyst ▶(N80.1-)◀
     follicular (atretic) cyst (N83.0-)
     graafian follicle cyst (N83.0-)
     ovarian cyst NEC (N83.2-)
     ovarian retention cyst (N83.2-)

   D27.0 Benign neoplasm of right ovary   ♀
   D27.1 Benign neoplasm of left ovary   ♀
   D27.9 Benign neoplasm of unspecified ovary   ♀

☑4ᵗʰ D28 Benign neoplasm of other and unspecified female genital organs
INCLUDES   adenomatous polyp
     benign neoplasm of skin of female genital organs
     benign teratoma
EXCLUDES 1   epoophoron cyst (Q50.5)
     fimbrial cyst (Q50.4)
     Gartner's duct cyst (Q52.4)
     parovarian cyst (Q50.5)

   D28.0 Benign neoplasm of vulva   ♀
   D28.1 Benign neoplasm of vagina   ♀
   D28.2 Benign neoplasm of uterine tubes and ligaments   ♀
     Benign neoplasm of fallopian tube
     Benign neoplasm of uterine ligament (broad) (round)
   D28.7 Benign neoplasm of other specified female genital organs   ♀
   D28.9 Benign neoplasm of female genital organ, unspecified   ♀

☑4ᵗʰ D29 Benign neoplasm of male genital organs
INCLUDES   benign neoplasm of skin of male genital organs

   D29.0 Benign neoplasm of penis   ♂
   D29.1 Benign neoplasm of prostate   ♂
     EXCLUDES 1   enlarged prostate (N40.-)
   ☑5ᵗʰ D29.2 Benign neoplasm of testis
     Use additional code to identify any functional activity
     D29.20 Benign neoplasm of unspecified testis   ♂
     D29.21 Benign neoplasm of right testis   ♂
     D29.22 Benign neoplasm of left testis   ♂
   ☑5ᵗʰ D29.3 Benign neoplasm of epididymis
     D29.30 Benign neoplasm of unspecified epididymis   ♂
     D29.31 Benign neoplasm of right epididymis   ♂
     D29.32 Benign neoplasm of left epididymis   ♂
   D29.4 Benign neoplasm of scrotum   ♂
     Benign neoplasm of skin of scrotum
   D29.8 Benign neoplasm of other specified male genital organs   ♂
     Benign neoplasm of seminal vesicle
     Benign neoplasm of spermatic cord
     Benign neoplasm of tunica vaginalis
   D29.9 Benign neoplasm of male genital organ, unspecified   ♂

☑4ᵗʰ D30 Benign neoplasm of urinary organs
   ☑5ᵗʰ D30.0 Benign neoplasm of kidney
     EXCLUDES 1   benign carcinoid tumor of the kidney (D3A.093)
       benign neoplasm of renal calyces (D30.1-)
       benign neoplasm of renal pelvis (D30.1-)
     D30.00 Benign neoplasm of unspecified kidney
     D30.01 Benign neoplasm of right kidney
     D30.02 Benign neoplasm of left kidney
   ☑5ᵗʰ D30.1 Benign neoplasm of renal pelvis
     D30.10 Benign neoplasm of unspecified renal pelvis
     D30.11 Benign neoplasm of right renal pelvis
     D30.12 Benign neoplasm of left renal pelvis
   ☑5ᵗʰ D30.2 Benign neoplasm of ureter
     EXCLUDES 1   benign neoplasm of ureteric orifice of bladder (D30.3)
     D30.20 Benign neoplasm of unspecified ureter
     D30.21 Benign neoplasm of right ureter
     D30.22 Benign neoplasm of left ureter
   D30.3 Benign neoplasm of bladder
     Benign neoplasm of ureteric orifice of bladder
     Benign neoplasm of urethral orifice of bladder

   D30.4 Benign neoplasm of urethra
     EXCLUDES 1   benign neoplasm of urethral orifice of bladder (D30.3)
   D30.8 Benign neoplasm of other specified urinary organs
     Benign neoplasm of paraurethral glands
   D30.9 Benign neoplasm of urinary organ, unspecified
     Benign neoplasm of urinary system NOS

☑4ᵗʰ D31 Benign neoplasm of eye and adnexa
   EXCLUDES 1   benign neoplasm of connective tissue of eyelid (D21.0)
     benign neoplasm of optic nerve (D33.3)
     benign neoplasm of skin of eyelid (D22.1-, D23.1-)
   ☑5ᵗʰ D31.0 Benign neoplasm of conjunctiva
     D31.00 Benign neoplasm of unspecified conjunctiva
     D31.01 Benign neoplasm of right conjunctiva
     D31.02 Benign neoplasm of left conjunctiva
   ☑5ᵗʰ D31.1 Benign neoplasm of cornea
     D31.10 Benign neoplasm of unspecified cornea
     D31.11 Benign neoplasm of right cornea
     D31.12 Benign neoplasm of left cornea
   ☑5ᵗʰ D31.2 Benign neoplasm of retina
     EXCLUDES 1   dark area on retina (D49.81)
       hemangioma of retina (D49.81)
       neoplasm of unspecified behavior of retina and choroid (D49.81)
       retinal freckle (D49.81)
     D31.20 Benign neoplasm of unspecified retina
     D31.21 Benign neoplasm of right retina
     D31.22 Benign neoplasm of left retina
   ☑5ᵗʰ D31.3 Benign neoplasm of choroid
     D31.30 Benign neoplasm of unspecified choroid
     D31.31 Benign neoplasm of right choroid
     D31.32 Benign neoplasm of left choroid
   ☑5ᵗʰ D31.4 Benign neoplasm of ciliary body
     D31.40 Benign neoplasm of unspecified ciliary body
     D31.41 Benign neoplasm of right ciliary body
     D31.42 Benign neoplasm of left ciliary body
   ☑5ᵗʰ D31.5 Benign neoplasm of lacrimal gland and duct
     Benign neoplasm of lacrimal sac
     Benign neoplasm of nasolacrimal duct
     D31.50 Benign neoplasm of unspecified lacrimal gland and duct
     D31.51 Benign neoplasm of right lacrimal gland and duct
     D31.52 Benign neoplasm of left lacrimal gland and duct
   ☑5ᵗʰ D31.6 Benign neoplasm of unspecified site of orbit
     Benign neoplasm of connective tissue of orbit
     Benign neoplasm of extraocular muscle
     Benign neoplasm of peripheral nerves of orbit
     Benign neoplasm of retrobulbar tissue
     Benign neoplasm of retro-ocular tissue
     EXCLUDES 1   benign neoplasm of orbital bone (D16.4)
     D31.60 Benign neoplasm of unspecified site of unspecified orbit
     D31.61 Benign neoplasm of unspecified site of right orbit
     D31.62 Benign neoplasm of unspecified site of left orbit
   ☑5ᵗʰ D31.9 Benign neoplasm of unspecified part of eye
     Benign neoplasm of eyeball
     D31.90 Benign neoplasm of unspecified part of unspecified eye
     D31.91 Benign neoplasm of unspecified part of right eye
     D31.92 Benign neoplasm of unspecified part of left eye

☑4ᵗʰ D32 Benign neoplasm of meninges
   D32.0 Benign neoplasm of cerebral meninges   HCC   Rx   ESR   COM
   D32.1 Benign neoplasm of spinal meninges   HCC   Rx   ESR   COM
   D32.9 Benign neoplasm of meninges, unspecified   HCC   Rx   ESR   COM
     Meningioma NOS

☑ Additional Character Required   ☑x7ᵗʰ Placeholder Alert   Manifestation   Unspecified Dx   Q QPP   UPD Unacceptable PDx
ICD-10-CM 2023
509

Chapter 2. Neoplasms

D27–D32.9

Chapter 2. Neoplasms

D33–D3A.8

✓4ᵗʰ **D33** **Benign neoplasm of** brain and other parts of central nervous system
   EXCLUDES 1   angioma (D18.0-)
          benign neoplasm of meninges (D32.-)
          benign neoplasm of peripheral nerves and autonomic nervous system (D36.1-)
          hemangioma (D18.0-)
          neurofibromatosis (Q85.0-)
          retro-ocular benign neoplasm (D31.6-)

D33.0 **Benign neoplasm of** brain, supratentorial   HCC Rx ESR COM
   Benign neoplasm of cerebral ventricle
   Benign neoplasm of cerebrum
   Benign neoplasm of frontal lobe
   Benign neoplasm of occipital lobe
   Benign neoplasm of parietal lobe
   Benign neoplasm of temporal lobe
   EXCLUDES 1   benign neoplasm of fourth ventricle (D33.1)

D33.1 **Benign neoplasm of** brain, infratentorial   HCC Rx ESR COM
   Benign neoplasm of brain stem
   Benign neoplasm of cerebellum
   Benign neoplasm of fourth ventricle

D33.2 **Benign neoplasm of** brain, unspecified   HCC Rx ESR COM

D33.3 **Benign neoplasm of** cranial nerves   HCC Rx ESR COM
   Benign neoplasm of olfactory bulb

D33.4 **Benign neoplasm of** spinal cord   HCC Rx ESR COM

D33.7 **Benign neoplasm of** other specified parts of central nervous system   HCC Rx ESR COM

D33.9 **Benign neoplasm of** central nervous system, unspecified   HCC Rx ESR COM
   Benign neoplasm of nervous system (central) NOS

D34 **Benign neoplasm of** thyroid gland
   Use additional code to identify any functional activity

✓4ᵗʰ **D35** **Benign neoplasm of** other and unspecified endocrine glands
   Use additional code to identify any functional activity
   EXCLUDES 1   benign neoplasm of endocrine pancreas (D13.7)
          benign neoplasm of ovary (D27.-)
          benign neoplasm of testis (D29.2.-)
          benign neoplasm of thymus (D15.0)

   ✓5ᵗʰ **D35.0** **Benign neoplasm of** adrenal gland
      D35.00 **Benign neoplasm of** unspecified adrenal gland
      D35.01 **Benign neoplasm of** right adrenal gland
      D35.02 **Benign neoplasm of** left adrenal gland

   D35.1 **Benign neoplasm of** parathyroid gland

   D35.2 **Benign neoplasm of** pituitary gland   HCC Rx ESR COM
      AHA: 2014,3Q,22

   D35.3 **Benign neoplasm of** craniopharyngeal duct   HCC Rx ESR COM

   D35.4 **Benign neoplasm of** pineal gland   HCC Rx ESR COM

   D35.5 **Benign neoplasm of** carotid body

   D35.6 **Benign neoplasm of** aortic body and other paraganglia
      Benign tumor of glomus jugulare

   D35.7 **Benign neoplasm of** other specified endocrine glands

   D35.9 **Benign neoplasm of** endocrine gland, unspecified
      Benign neoplasm of unspecified endocrine gland

✓4ᵗʰ **D36** **Benign neoplasm of** other and unspecified sites

   D36.0 **Benign neoplasm of** lymph nodes
      EXCLUDES 1   lymphangioma (D18.1)

   ✓5ᵗʰ **D36.1** **Benign neoplasm of** peripheral nerves and autonomic nervous system
      EXCLUDES 1   benign neoplasm of peripheral nerves of orbit (D31.6-)
            neurofibromatosis (Q85.0-)

      D36.10 **Benign neoplasm of** peripheral nerves and autonomic nervous system, unspecified

      D36.11 **Benign neoplasm of** peripheral nerves and autonomic nervous system of face, head, and neck

      D36.12 **Benign neoplasm of** peripheral nerves and autonomic nervous system, upper limb, including shoulder

      D36.13 **Benign neoplasm of** peripheral nerves and autonomic nervous system of lower limb, including hip

      D36.14 **Benign neoplasm of** peripheral nerves and autonomic nervous system of thorax

      D36.15 **Benign neoplasm of** peripheral nerves and autonomic nervous system of abdomen

      D36.16 **Benign neoplasm of** peripheral nerves and autonomic nervous system of pelvis

      D36.17 **Benign neoplasm of** peripheral nerves and autonomic nervous system of trunk, unspecified

   D36.7 **Benign neoplasm of** other specified sites
      Benign neoplasm of back NOS
      Benign neoplasm of nose NOS

   D36.9 **Benign neoplasm,** unspecified site

Benign neuroendocrine tumors (D3A)

✓4ᵗʰ **D3A** **Benign** neuroendocrine tumors
   Code also any associated multiple endocrine neoplasia [MEN] syndromes (E31.2-)
   Use additional code to identify any associated endocrine syndrome, such as:
   carcinoid syndrome (E34.0)
   EXCLUDES 2   benign pancreatic islet cell tumors (D13.7)

   ✓5ᵗʰ **D3A.0** **Benign** carcinoid tumors
      DEF: Specific type of slow-growing neuroendocrine tumors. Carcinoid tumors occur most commonly in the hormone producing cells of the gastrointestinal tracts and can also occur in the pancreas, testes, ovaries, or lungs.

      D3A.00 **Benign carcinoid tumor of** unspecified site   Rx
        Carcinoid tumor NOS

      ✓6ᵗʰ **D3A.01** **Benign carcinoid tumors of the** small intestine

        D3A.010 **Benign carcinoid tumor of the** duodenum   Rx

        D3A.011 **Benign carcinoid tumor of the** jejunum   Rx

        D3A.012 **Benign carcinoid tumor of the** ileum   Rx

        D3A.019 **Benign carcinoid tumor of the** small intestine, unspecified portion   Rx

      ✓6ᵗʰ **D3A.02** **Benign carcinoid tumors of the** appendix, large intestine, and rectum

        D3A.020 **Benign carcinoid tumor of the** appendix   Rx

        D3A.021 **Benign carcinoid tumor of the** cecum   Rx

        D3A.022 **Benign carcinoid tumor of the** ascending colon   Rx

        D3A.023 **Benign carcinoid tumor of the** transverse colon   Rx

        D3A.024 **Benign carcinoid tumor of the** descending colon   Rx

        D3A.025 **Benign carcinoid tumor of the** sigmoid colon   Rx

        D3A.026 **Benign carcinoid tumor of the** rectum   Rx

        D3A.029 **Benign carcinoid tumor of the** large intestine, unspecified portion   Rx
          Benign carcinoid tumor of the colon NOS

      ✓6ᵗʰ **D3A.09** **Benign carcinoid tumors of** other sites

        D3A.090 **Benign carcinoid tumor of the** bronchus and lung   Rx

        D3A.091 **Benign carcinoid tumor of the** thymus   Rx

        D3A.092 **Benign carcinoid tumor of the** stomach   Rx

        D3A.093 **Benign carcinoid tumor of the** kidney   Rx

        D3A.094 **Benign carcinoid tumor of the** foregut, unspecified   Rx

        D3A.095 **Benign carcinoid tumor of the** midgut, unspecified   Rx

        D3A.096 **Benign carcinoid tumor of the** hindgut, unspecified   Rx

        D3A.098 **Benign carcinoid tumors of** other sites   Rx

   D3A.8 **Other benign neuroendocrine tumors**   Rx
      Neuroendocrine tumor NOS

Neoplasms of uncertain behavior, polycythemia vera and myelodysplastic syndromes (D37-D48)

NOTE Categories D37-D44, and D48 classify by site neoplasms of uncertain behavior, i.e., histologic confirmation whether the neoplasm is malignant or benign cannot be made.

EXCLUDES 1 *neoplasms of unspecified behavior (D49.-)*

✓4ᵗʰ **D37 Neoplasm of uncertain behavior of** oral cavity and digestive organs

> **EXCLUDES 1** *stromal tumors of uncertain behavior of digestive system (D48.1)*

✓5ᵗʰ **D37.0 Neoplasm of uncertain behavior of** lip, oral cavity and pharynx

> **EXCLUDES 1** *neoplasm of uncertain behavior of aryepiglottic fold or interarytenoid fold, laryngeal aspect (D38.0)*
> *neoplasm of uncertain behavior of epiglottis NOS (D38.0)*
> *neoplasm of uncertain behavior of skin of lip (D48.5)*
> *neoplasm of uncertain behavior of suprahyoid portion of epiglottis (D38.0)*

D37.01 Neoplasm of uncertain behavior of lip
Neoplasm of uncertain behavior of vermilion border of lip

D37.02 Neoplasm of uncertain behavior of tongue

✓6ᵗʰ **D37.03 Neoplasm of uncertain behavior of the** major salivary glands

D37.030 Neoplasm of uncertain behavior of the parotid **salivary glands**

D37.031 Neoplasm of uncertain behavior of the sublingual **salivary glands**

D37.032 Neoplasm of uncertain behavior of the submandibular **salivary glands**

D37.039 Neoplasm of uncertain behavior of the major salivary glands, unspecified

D37.04 Neoplasm of uncertain behavior of the minor salivary glands
Neoplasm of uncertain behavior of submucosal salivary glands of lip
Neoplasm of uncertain behavior of submucosal salivary glands of cheek
Neoplasm of uncertain behavior of submucosal salivary glands of hard palate
Neoplasm of uncertain behavior of submucosal salivary glands of soft palate

D37.05 Neoplasm of uncertain behavior of pharynx
Neoplasm of uncertain behavior of aryepiglottic fold of pharynx NOS
Neoplasm of uncertain behavior of hypopharyngeal aspect of aryepiglottic fold of pharynx
Neoplasm of uncertain behavior of marginal zone of aryepiglottic fold of pharynx

D37.09 Neoplasm of uncertain behavior of other specified sites of the oral cavity

D37.1 Neoplasm of uncertain behavior of stomach

D37.2 Neoplasm of uncertain behavior of small intestine

D37.3 Neoplasm of uncertain behavior of appendix

D37.4 Neoplasm of uncertain behavior of colon

D37.5 Neoplasm of uncertain behavior of rectum
Neoplasm of uncertain behavior of rectosigmoid junction

D37.6 Neoplasm of uncertain behavior of liver, gallbladder and bile ducts
Neoplasm of uncertain behavior of ampulla of Vater

D37.8 Neoplasm of uncertain behavior of other specified digestive organs
Neoplasm of uncertain behavior of anal canal
Neoplasm of uncertain behavior of anal sphincter
Neoplasm of uncertain behavior of anus NOS
Neoplasm of uncertain behavior of esophagus
Neoplasm of uncertain behavior of intestine NOS
Neoplasm of uncertain behavior of pancreas

> **EXCLUDES 1** *neoplasm of uncertain behavior of anal margin (D48.5)*
> *neoplasm of uncertain behavior of anal skin (D48.5)*
> *neoplasm of uncertain behavior of perianal skin (D48.5)*

D37.9 Neoplasm of uncertain behavior of digestive organ, unspecified

✓4ᵗʰ **D38 Neoplasm of uncertain behavior of** middle ear and respiratory and intrathoracic organs

> **EXCLUDES 1** *neoplasm of uncertain behavior of heart (D48.7)*

D38.0 Neoplasm of uncertain behavior of larynx
Neoplasm of uncertain behavior of aryepiglottic fold or interarytenoid fold, laryngeal aspect
Neoplasm of uncertain behavior of epiglottis (suprahyoid portion)

> **EXCLUDES 1** *neoplasm of uncertain behavior of aryepiglottic fold or interarytenoid fold NOS (D37.05)*
> *neoplasm of uncertain behavior of hypopharyngeal aspect of aryepiglottic fold (D37.05)*
> *neoplasm of uncertain behavior of marginal zone of aryepiglottic fold (D37.05)*

D38.1 Neoplasm of uncertain behavior of trachea, bronchus and lung

D38.2 Neoplasm of uncertain behavior of pleura

D38.3 Neoplasm of uncertain behavior of mediastinum

D38.4 Neoplasm of uncertain behavior of thymus

D38.5 Neoplasm of uncertain behavior of other respiratory organs
Neoplasm of uncertain behavior of accessory sinuses
Neoplasm of uncertain behavior of cartilage of nose
Neoplasm of uncertain behavior of middle ear
Neoplasm of uncertain behavior of nasal cavities

> **EXCLUDES 1** *neoplasm of uncertain behavior of ear (external) (skin) (D48.5)*
> *neoplasm of uncertain behavior of nose NOS (D48.7)*
> *neoplasm of uncertain behavior of skin of nose (D48.5)*

D38.6 Neoplasm of uncertain behavior of respiratory organ, unspecified

✓4ᵗʰ **D39 Neoplasm of uncertain behavior of** female genital organs

D39.0 Neoplasm of uncertain behavior of uterus ♀

✓5ᵗʰ **D39.1 Neoplasm of uncertain behavior of** ovary
Use additional code to identify any functional activity

D39.10 Neoplasm of uncertain behavior of unspecified ovary ♀

D39.11 Neoplasm of uncertain behavior of right **ovary** ♀

D39.12 Neoplasm of uncertain behavior of left **ovary** ♀

D39.2 Neoplasm of uncertain behavior of placenta Ⓜ ♀
Chorioadenoma destruens
Invasive hydatidiform mole
Malignant hydatidiform mole

> **EXCLUDES 1** *hydatidiform mole NOS (O01.9)*

D39.8 Neoplasm of uncertain behavior of other specified female genital organs ♀
Neoplasm of uncertain behavior of skin of female genital organs

D39.9 Neoplasm of uncertain behavior of female genital organ, unspecified ♀

✓4ᵗʰ **D40 Neoplasm of uncertain behavior of** male genital organs

D40.0 Neoplasm of uncertain behavior of prostate ♂

✓5ᵗʰ **D40.1 Neoplasm of uncertain behavior of** testis

D40.10 Neoplasm of uncertain behavior of unspecified testis ♂

D40.11 Neoplasm of uncertain behavior of right **testis** ♂

D40.12 Neoplasm of uncertain behavior of left **testis** ♂

D40.8 Neoplasm of uncertain behavior of other specified male genital organs ♂
Neoplasm of uncertain behavior of skin of male genital organs

D40.9 Neoplasm of uncertain behavior of male genital organ, unspecified ♂

✓4ᵗʰ **D41 Neoplasm of uncertain behavior of** urinary organs

✓5ᵗʰ **D41.0 Neoplasm of uncertain behavior of** kidney

> **EXCLUDES 1** *neoplasm of uncertain behavior of renal pelvis (D41.1-)*

D41.00 Neoplasm of uncertain behavior of unspecified kidney

D41.01 Neoplasm of uncertain behavior of right **kidney**

D41.02 Neoplasm of uncertain behavior of left **kidney**

✓5ᵗʰ **D41.1 Neoplasm of uncertain behavior of** renal pelvis

D41.10 Neoplasm of uncertain behavior of unspecified renal pelvis

D41.11 Neoplasm of uncertain behavior of right renal pelvis

D41.12 Neoplasm of uncertain behavior of left renal pelvis

Chapter 2. Neoplasms

D41.2–D47.Ø1

☑5ᵗʰ **D41.2 Neoplasm of uncertain behavior of** ureter

     D41.2Ø Neoplasm of uncertain behavior of unspecified ureter

     D41.21 Neoplasm of uncertain behavior of right **ureter**

     D41.22 Neoplasm of uncertain behavior of left **ureter**

D41.3 Neoplasm of uncertain behavior of urethra

D41.4 Neoplasm of uncertain behavior of bladder

D41.8 Neoplasm of uncertain behavior of other specified urinary organs

D41.9 Neoplasm of uncertain behavior of unspecified urinary organ

☑4ᵗʰ **D42 Neoplasm of uncertain behavior of** meninges

D42.Ø Neoplasm of uncertain behavior of cerebral **meninges** HCC Rx ESR COM

D42.1 Neoplasm of uncertain behavior of spinal **meninges** HCC Rx ESR COM

D42.9 Neoplasm of uncertain behavior of meninges, unspecified HCC Rx ESR COM

☑4ᵗʰ **D43 Neoplasm of uncertain behavior of** brain and central nervous system

     EXCLUDES 1   *neoplasm of uncertain behavior of peripheral nerves and autonomic nervous system (D48.2)*

D43.Ø Neoplasm of uncertain behavior of brain, supratentorial HCC Rx ESR COM

     Neoplasm of uncertain behavior of cerebral ventricle

     Neoplasm of uncertain behavior of cerebrum

     Neoplasm of uncertain behavior of frontal lobe

     Neoplasm of uncertain behavior of occipital lobe

     Neoplasm of uncertain behavior of parietal lobe

     Neoplasm of uncertain behavior of temporal lobe

     EXCLUDES 1   *neoplasm of uncertain behavior of fourth ventricle (D43.1)*

D43.1 Neoplasm of uncertain behavior of brain, infratentorial HCC Rx ESR COM

     Neoplasm of uncertain behavior of brain stem

     Neoplasm of uncertain behavior of cerebellum

     Neoplasm of uncertain behavior of fourth ventricle

D43.2 Neoplasm of uncertain behavior of brain, unspecified HCC Rx ESR COM

D43.3 Neoplasm of uncertain behavior of cranial nerves HCC Rx ESR COM

D43.4 Neoplasm of uncertain behavior of spinal cord HCC Rx ESR COM

D43.8 Neoplasm of uncertain behavior of other specified parts of central nervous system HCC Rx ESR COM

D43.9 Neoplasm of uncertain behavior of central nervous system, unspecified HCC Rx ESR COM

     Neoplasm of uncertain behavior of nervous system (central) NOS

☑4ᵗʰ **D44 Neoplasm of uncertain behavior of** endocrine glands

     EXCLUDES 1   *multiple endocrine adenomatosis (E31.2-)*

          multiple endocrine neoplasia (E31.2-)

          neoplasm of uncertain behavior of endocrine pancreas (D37.8)

          neoplasm of uncertain behavior of ovary (D39.1-)

          neoplasm of uncertain behavior of testis (D40.1-)

          neoplasm of uncertain behavior of thymus (D38.4)

D44.Ø Neoplasm of uncertain behavior of thyroid gland

☑6ᵗʰ **D44.1 Neoplasm of uncertain behavior of** adrenal gland

     Use additional code to identify any functional activity

     D44.1Ø Neoplasm of uncertain behavior of unspecified adrenal gland

     D44.11 Neoplasm of uncertain behavior of right **adrenal gland**

     D44.12 Neoplasm of uncertain behavior of left **adrenal gland**

D44.2 Neoplasm of uncertain behavior of parathyroid gland

D44.3 Neoplasm of uncertain behavior of pituitary gland HCC Rx ESR COM

     Use additional code to identify any functional activity

D44.4 Neoplasm of uncertain behavior of craniopharyngeal duct HCC Rx ESR COM

D44.5 Neoplasm of uncertain behavior of pineal gland HCC Rx ESR COM

D44.6 Neoplasm of uncertain behavior of carotid body HCC Rx ESR COM

D44.7 Neoplasm of uncertain behavior of aortic body and other paraganglia HCC Rx ESR COM

     AHA: 2021,2Q,7; 2016,4Q,26

D44.9 Neoplasm of uncertain behavior of unspecified endocrine gland

D45 Polycythemia vera HCC Rx ESR COM

     EXCLUDES 1   *familial polycythemia (D75.Ø)*

          secondary polycythemia (D75.1)

     DEF: Abnormal proliferation of all bone marrow elements, increased red cell mass, and total blood volume. The etiology is unknown, but it is frequently associated with splenomegaly, leukocytosis, and thrombocythemia.

☑4ᵗʰ **D46 Myelodysplastic syndromes**

     Use additional code for adverse effect, if applicable, to identify drug (T36-T5Ø with fifth or sixth character 5)

     EXCLUDES 2   *drug-induced aplastic anemia (D61.1)*

D46.Ø Refractory anemia without ring sideroblasts, **so stated** HCC Rx ESR COM

     Refractory anemia without sideroblasts, without excess of blasts

D46.1 Refractory anemia with ring sideroblasts HCC Rx ESR COM

     RARS

☑5ᵗʰ **D46.2 Refractory anemia** with excess of blasts [RAEB]

     D46.2Ø Refractory anemia with excess of blasts, unspecified HCC Rx ESR COM

         RAEB NOS

     D46.21 Refractory anemia with excess of blasts 1 HCC Rx ESR COM

         RAEB 1

     D46.22 Refractory anemia with excess of blasts 2 HCC Rx ESR COM

         RAEB 2

D46.A Refractory cytopenia with multilineage dysplasia HCC Rx ESR COM

D46.B Refractory cytopenia with multilineage dysplasia and ring sideroblasts HCC Rx ESR COM

     RCMD RS

D46.C Myelodysplastic syndrome with isolated del(5q) chromosomal abnormality HCC Rx ESR COM

     Myelodysplastic syndrome with 5q deletion

     5q minus syndrome NOS

D46.4 Refractory anemia, unspecified HCC Rx ESR COM

D46.Z Other myelodysplastic syndromes HCC Rx ESR COM

     EXCLUDES 1   *chronic myelomonocytic leukemia (C93.1-)*

D46.9 Myelodysplastic syndrome, unspecified HCC Rx ESR COM

     Myelodysplasia NOS

☑4ᵗʰ **D47 Other neoplasms of uncertain behavior of** lymphoid, hematopoietic and related tissue

☑5ᵗʰ **D47.Ø Mast cell neoplasms of uncertain behavior**

     EXCLUDES 1   *congenital cutaneous mastocytosis (Q82.2)*

          histiocytic neoplasms of uncertain behavior (D47.Z9)

          malignant mast cell neoplasm (C96.2-)

     AHA: 2017,4Q,5

     D47.Ø1 Cutaneous mastocytosis Rx

         Diffuse cutaneous mastocytosis

         Maculopapular cutaneous mastocytosis

         Solitary mastocytoma

         Telangiectasia macularis eruptiva perstans

         Urticaria pigmentosa

         EXCLUDES 1   *congenital (diffuse) (maculopapular) cutaneous mastocytosis (Q82.2)*

                congenital urticaria pigmentosa (Q82.2)

                extracutaneous mastocytoma (D47.Ø9)

D47.02 **Systemic mastocytosis** `Rx`
Indolent systemic mastocytosis
Isolated bone marrow mastocytosis
Smoldering systemic mastocytosis
Systemic mastocytosis, with an associated hematological non-mast cell lineage disease (SM-AHNMD)
Code also, if applicable, any associated hematological non-mast cell lineage disease, such as:
acute myeloid leukemia (C92.6-, C92.A-)
chronic myelomonocytic leukemia (C93.1-)
essential thrombocytosis (D47.3)
hypereosinophilic syndrome (D72.1)
myelodysplastic syndrome (D46.9)
myeloproliferative syndrome (D47.1)
non-Hodgkin lymphoma (C82-C85)
plasma cell myeloma (C90.0-)
polycythemia vera (D45)
EXCLUDES 1   *aggressive systemic mastocytosis (C96.21)*
mast cell leukemia (C94.3-)

D47.09 **Other mast cell neoplasms of uncertain behavior** `Rx`
Extracutaneous mastocytoma
Mast cell tumor NOS
Mastocytoma NOS
Mastocytosis NOS

D47.1 **Chronic myeloproliferative disease** `HCC` `Rx` `ESR` `COM`
Chronic neutrophilic leukemia
Myeloproliferative disease, unspecified
EXCLUDES 1   *atypical chronic myeloid leukemia BCR/ABL-negative (C92.2-)*
chronic myeloid leukemia BCR/ABL-positive (C92.1-)
myelofibrosis NOS (D75.81)
myelophthisic anemia (D61.82)
myelophthisis (D61.82)
secondary myelofibrosis NOS (D75.81)

D47.2 **Monoclonal gammopathy**
Monoclonal gammopathy of undetermined significance [MGUS]
AHA: 2021,3Q,5
TIP: Smoldering multiple myeloma (SMM) is coded here.

D47.3 **Essential (hemorrhagic) thrombocythemia** `HCC` `Rx` `ESR` `COM`
Essential thrombocytosis
Idiopathic hemorrhagic thrombocythemia
Primary thrombocytosis
EXCLUDES 2   *reactive thrombocytosis (D75.838)*
secondary thrombocytosis (D75.838)
thrombocythemia NOS (D75.839)
thrombocytosis NOS (D75.839)
DEF: Chronic myeloproliferative neoplasm involving production of excess blood platelets that may result in abnormal clotting or hemorrhaging.

D47.4 **Osteomyelofibrosis** `HCC` `Rx` `ESR` `COM`
Chronic idiopathic myelofibrosis
Myelofibrosis (idiopathic) (with myeloid metaplasia)
Myelosclerosis (megakaryocytic) with myeloid metaplasia
Secondary myelofibrosis in myeloproliferative disease
EXCLUDES 1   *acute myelofibrosis (C94.4-)*

✓5ᵗʰ **D47.Z** **Other specified neoplasms of uncertain behavior of lymphoid, hematopoietic and related tissue**
AHA: 2016,4Q,8

D47.Z1 **Post-transplant lymphoproliferative disorder (PTLD)** `HCC` `ESR` `COM` `UPD`
Code first complications of transplanted organs and tissue (T86.-)
DEF: Excessive proliferation of B-cell lymphocytes following Epstein-Barr virus infection in organ transplant patients. It may progress to non-Hodgkin lymphoma.

D47.Z2 **Castleman disease** `HCC` `Rx` `ESR` `COM`
Code also, if applicable, human herpesvirus 8 infection (B10.89)
EXCLUDES 2   *Kaposi's sarcoma (C46.-)*
DEF: Rare disease of the lymph nodes and lymphoid tissues that closely mimics lymphoma.

D47.Z9 **Other specified neoplasms of uncertain behavior of lymphoid, hematopoietic and related tissue** `HCC` `Rx` `ESR` `COM`
Histiocytic tumors of uncertain behavior

D47.9 **Neoplasm of uncertain behavior of lymphoid, hematopoietic and related tissue, unspecified** `HCC` `Rx` `ESR` `COM`
Lymphoproliferative disease NOS

✓4ᵗʰ **D48** **Neoplasm of uncertain behavior of other and unspecified sites**
EXCLUDES 1   *neurofibromatosis (nonmalignant) (Q85.0-)*

D48.0 **Neoplasm of uncertain behavior of bone and articular cartilage**
EXCLUDES 1   *neoplasm of uncertain behavior of cartilage of ear (D48.1)*
neoplasm of uncertain behavior of cartilage of larynx (D38.0)
neoplasm of uncertain behavior of cartilage of nose (D38.5)
neoplasm of uncertain behavior of connective tissue of eyelid (D48.1)
neoplasm of uncertain behavior of synovia (D48.1)

D48.1 **Neoplasm of uncertain behavior of connective and other soft tissue**
Neoplasm of uncertain behavior of connective tissue of ear
Neoplasm of uncertain behavior of connective tissue of eyelid
Stromal tumors of uncertain behavior of digestive system
EXCLUDES 1   *neoplasm of uncertain behavior of articular cartilage (D48.0)*
neoplasm of uncertain behavior of cartilage of larynx (D38.0)
neoplasm of uncertain behavior of cartilage of nose (D38.5)
neoplasm of uncertain behavior of connective tissue of breast (D48.6-)

D48.2 **Neoplasm of uncertain behavior of peripheral nerves and autonomic nervous system**
EXCLUDES 1   *neoplasm of uncertain behavior of peripheral nerves of orbit (D48.7)*

D48.3 **Neoplasm of uncertain behavior of retroperitoneum**

D48.4 **Neoplasm of uncertain behavior of peritoneum**

D48.5 **Neoplasm of uncertain behavior of skin**
Neoplasm of uncertain behavior of anal margin
Neoplasm of uncertain behavior of anal skin
Neoplasm of uncertain behavior of perianal skin
Neoplasm of uncertain behavior of skin of breast
EXCLUDES 1   *neoplasm of uncertain behavior of anus NOS (D37.8)*
neoplasm of uncertain behavior of skin of genital organs (D39.8, D40.8)
neoplasm of uncertain behavior of vermilion border of lip (D37.0)

✓5ᵗʰ **D48.6** **Neoplasm of uncertain behavior of breast**
Neoplasm of uncertain behavior of connective tissue of breast
Cystosarcoma phyllodes
EXCLUDES 1   *neoplasm of uncertain behavior of skin of breast (D48.5)*

D48.60 **Neoplasm of uncertain behavior of unspecified breast**
D48.61 **Neoplasm of uncertain behavior of right breast**
D48.62 **Neoplasm of uncertain behavior of left breast**

D48.7 **Neoplasm of uncertain behavior of other specified sites**
Neoplasm of uncertain behavior of eye
Neoplasm of uncertain behavior of heart
Neoplasm of uncertain behavior of peripheral nerves of orbit
EXCLUDES 1   *neoplasm of uncertain behavior of connective tissue (D48.1)*
neoplasm of uncertain behavior of skin of eyelid (D48.5)

D48.9 **Neoplasm of uncertain behavior, unspecified**

☑ Additional Character Required   ✓x7ᵗʰ Placeholder Alert   Manifestation   Unspecified Dx   Q QPP   UPD Unacceptable PDx
ICD-10-CM 2023   513

D47.02–D48.9

Neoplasms of unspecified behavior (D49)

√4ᵗʰ **D49   Neoplasms of unspecified behavior**

> **NOTE**   Category D49 classifies by site neoplasms of unspecified morphology and behavior. The term "mass", unless otherwise stated, is not to be regarded as a neoplastic growth.
>
> **INCLUDES**   "growth" NOS
> neoplasm NOS
> new growth NOS
> tumor NOS
>
> **EXCLUDES 1**   *neoplasms of uncertain behavior (D37-D44, D48)*

D49.0   Neoplasm of unspecified behavior of digestive system

> **EXCLUDES 1**   *neoplasm of unspecified behavior of margin of anus (D49.2)*
> *neoplasm of unspecified behavior of perianal skin (D49.2)*
> *neoplasm of unspecified behavior of skin of anus (D49.2)*

D49.1   Neoplasm of unspecified behavior of respiratory system

D49.2   Neoplasm of unspecified behavior of bone, soft tissue, and skin

> **EXCLUDES 1**   *neoplasm of unspecified behavior of anal canal (D49.0)*
> *neoplasm of unspecified behavior of anus NOS (D49.0)*
> *neoplasm of unspecified behavior of bone marrow (D49.89)*
> *neoplasm of unspecified behavior of cartilage of larynx (D49.1)*
> *neoplasm of unspecified behavior of cartilage of nose (D49.1)*
> *neoplasm of unspecified behavior of connective tissue of breast (D49.3)*
> *neoplasm of unspecified behavior of skin of genital organs (D49.59)*
> *neoplasm of unspecified behavior of vermilion border of lip (D49.0)*

D49.3   Neoplasm of unspecified behavior of breast

> **EXCLUDES 1**   *neoplasm of unspecified behavior of skin of breast (D49.2)*

D49.4   Neoplasm of unspecified behavior of bladder

√5ᵗʰ **D49.5   Neoplasm of unspecified behavior of** other genitourinary organs

> **AHA:** 2016,4Q,9

√6ᵗʰ **D49.51   Neoplasm of unspecified behavior of** kidney

> **D49.511   Neoplasm of unspecified behavior of** right **kidney**
>
> **D49.512   Neoplasm of unspecified behavior of** left **kidney**
>
> **D49.519   Neoplasm of unspecified behavior of unspecified kidney**

D49.59   Neoplasm of unspecified behavior of other genitourinary organ

D49.6   Neoplasm of unspecified behavior of brain   HCC Rx ESR COM

> **EXCLUDES 1**   *neoplasm of unspecified behavior of cerebral meninges (D49.7)*
> *neoplasm of unspecified behavior of cranial nerves (D49.7)*

D49.7   Neoplasm of unspecified behavior of endocrine glands and other parts of nervous system

> **EXCLUDES 1**   *neoplasm of unspecified behavior of peripheral, sympathetic, and parasympathetic nerves and ganglia (D49.2)*

√5ᵗʰ **D49.8   Neoplasm of unspecified behavior of other specified sites**

> **EXCLUDES 1**   *neoplasm of unspecified behavior of eyelid (skin) (D49.2)*
> *neoplasm of unspecified behavior of eyelid cartilage (D49.2)*
> *neoplasm of unspecified behavior of great vessels (D49.2)*
> *neoplasm of unspecified behavior of optic nerve (D49.7)*

D49.81   Neoplasm of unspecified behavior of retina and choroid

> Dark area on retina
> Retinal freckle

D49.89   Neoplasm of unspecified behavior of other specified sites

D49.9   Neoplasm of unspecified behavior of unspecified site

Chapter 3. Disease of the Blood and Blood-Forming Organs and Certain Disorders Involving the Immune Mechanism (D50–D89)

Chapter-specific Guidelines with Coding Examples
Reserved for future guideline expansion.

Chapter 3. Diseases of the Blood and Blood-forming Organs and Certain Disorders Involving the Immune Mechanism (D50-D89)

EXCLUDES 2   *autoimmune disease (systemic) NOS (M35.9)*
certain conditions originating in the perinatal period (P00-P96)
complications of pregnancy, childbirth and the puerperium (O00-O9A)
congenital malformations, deformations and chromosomal abnormalities (Q00-Q99)
endocrine, nutritional and metabolic diseases (E00-E88)
human immunodeficiency virus [HIV] disease (B20)
injury, poisoning and certain other consequences of external causes (S00-T88)
neoplasms (C00-D49)
symptoms, signs and abnormal clinical and laboratory findings, not elsewhere classified (R00-R94)

This chapter contains the following blocks:

D50-D53   Nutritional anemias
D55-D59   Hemolytic anemias
D60-D64   Aplastic and other anemias and other bone marrow failure syndromes
D65-D69   Coagulation defects, purpura and other hemorrhagic conditions
D70-D77   Other disorders of blood and blood-forming organs
D78   Intraoperative and postprocedural complications of the spleen
D80-D89   Certain disorders involving the immune mechanism

Nutritional anemias (D50-D53)

DEF: Nutritional anemia: The result of inadequate intake or absorption of a vitamin or mineral that impacts the production of red blood cells or causes them to develop abnormally affecting the size and shape.

TIP: Documentation must identify a link between anemia and the nutritional deficiency; low levels of a particular nutrient may occur concurrently with anemia but not cause the anemia.

✓4th D50   Iron deficiency anemia

INCLUDES   asiderotic anemia
hypochromic anemia

D50.0   Iron deficiency anemia secondary to blood loss (chronic)
Posthemorrhagic anemia (chronic)
     EXCLUDES 1   *acute posthemorrhagic anemia (D62)*
                   congenital anemia from fetal blood loss (P61.3)
     AHA: 2019,3Q,17

D50.1   Sideropenic dysphagia
Kelly-Paterson syndrome
Plummer-Vinson syndrome

D50.8   Other iron deficiency anemias
Iron deficiency anemia due to inadequate dietary iron intake

D50.9   Iron deficiency anemia, unspecified

✓4th D51   Vitamin B12 deficiency anemia

EXCLUDES 1   *vitamin B12 deficiency (E53.8)*

D51.0   Vitamin B12 deficiency anemia due to intrinsic factor deficiency
Addison anemia
Biermer anemia
Pernicious (congenital) anemia
Congenital intrinsic factor deficiency
DEF: Chronic progressive anemia due to vitamin B12 malabsorption, caused by lack of secretion of intrinsic factor, which is produced by the gastric mucosa of the stomach.

D51.1   Vitamin B12 deficiency anemia due to selective vitamin B12 malabsorption with proteinuria
Imerslund (Gräsbeck) syndrome
Megaloblastic hereditary anemia

D51.2   Transcobalamin II deficiency

D51.3   Other dietary vitamin B12 deficiency anemia
Vegan anemia

D51.8   Other vitamin B12 deficiency anemias

D51.9   Vitamin B12 deficiency anemia, unspecified

✓4th D52   Folate deficiency anemia

EXCLUDES 1   *folate deficiency without anemia (E53.8)*
DEF: Deficiency in a B complex vitamin needed for the production of healthy red blood cells. Lack of folate, or folic acid, and other absorption conditions can cause anemia resulting in large, misshapen red blood cells called megaloblasts.

D52.0   Dietary folate deficiency anemia
Nutritional megaloblastic anemia
DEF: Result of a poor diet with inadequate intake of folate, which is needed to produce healthy red blood cells.

D52.1   Drug-induced folate deficiency anemia
Use additional code for adverse effect, if applicable, to identify drug (T36-T50 with fifth or sixth character 5)

D52.8   Other folate deficiency anemias

D52.9   Folate deficiency anemia, unspecified
Folic acid deficiency anemia NOS

✓4th D53   Other nutritional anemias

INCLUDES   megaloblastic anemia unresponsive to vitamin B12 or folate therapy

D53.0   Protein deficiency anemia
Amino-acid deficiency anemia
Orotaciduric anemia
     EXCLUDES 1   *Lesch-Nyhan syndrome (E79.1)*

D53.1   Other megaloblastic anemias, not elsewhere classified
Megaloblastic anemia NOS
     EXCLUDES 1   *Di Guglielmo's disease (C94.0)*

D53.2   Scorbutic anemia
     EXCLUDES 1   *scurvy (E54)*

D53.8   Other specified nutritional anemias
Anemia associated with deficiency of copper
Anemia associated with deficiency of molybdenum
Anemia associated with deficiency of zinc
     EXCLUDES 1   *nutritional deficiencies without anemia, such as:*
                   copper deficiency NOS (E61.0)
                   molybdenum deficiency NOS (E61.5)
                   zinc deficiency NOS (E60)

D53.9   Nutritional anemia, unspecified
Simple chronic anemia
     EXCLUDES 1   *anemia NOS (D64.9)*
     AHA: 2018,4Q,88

Hemolytic anemias (D55-D59)

✓4th D55   Anemia due to enzyme disorders

EXCLUDES 1   *drug-induced enzyme deficiency anemia (D59.2)*

D55.0   Anemia due to glucose-6-phosphate dehydrogenase [G6PD] deficiency   HCC ESR
Favism
G6PD deficiency anemia
     EXCLUDES 1   *glucose-6-phosphate dehydrogenase (G6PD) deficiency without anemia (D75.A)*

D55.1   Anemia due to other disorders of glutathione metabolism   HCC ESR
Anemia (due to) enzyme deficiencies, except G6PD, related to the hexose monophosphate [HMP] shunt pathway
Anemia (due to) hemolytic nonspherocytic (hereditary), type I

✓5th D55.2   Anemia due to disorders of glycolytic enzymes
     EXCLUDES 1   *disorders of glycolysis not associated with anemia (E74.81-)*
     AHA: 2021,4Q,6-7

     D55.21   Anemia due to pyruvate kinase deficiency   HCC ESR
         PK deficiency anemia
         Pyruvate kinase deficiency anemia

     D55.29   Anemia due to other disorders of glycolytic enzymes   HCC ESR
         Hexokinase deficiency anemia
         Triose-phosphate isomerase deficiency anemia

D55.3   Anemia due to disorders of nucleotide metabolism   HCC ESR

D55.8   Other anemias due to enzyme disorders   HCC ESR

D55.9   Anemia due to enzyme disorder, unspecified   HCC ESR

✓4ᵗʰ D56 Thalassemia

EXCLUDES 1 *sickle-cell thalassemia (D57.4-)*

DEF: Group of inherited disorders of hemoglobin metabolism causing mild to severe anemia. It is usually found in people of Mediterranean, African, Chinese, or Asian descent.

Thalassemia

Misshapen RBC

Misshapen RBC   Healthy RBC

D56.0 Alpha thalassemia   HCC ESR

Alpha thalassemia major
Hemoglobin H Constant Spring
Hemoglobin H disease
Hydrops fetalis due to alpha thalassemia
Severe alpha thalassemia
Triple gene defect alpha thalassemia
Use additional code, if applicable, for hydrops fetalis due to alpha thalassemia (P56.99)

EXCLUDES 1 *alpha thalassemia trait or minor (D56.3)*
asymptomatic alpha thalassemia (D56.3)
hydrops fetalis due to isoimmunization (P56.0)
hydrops fetalis not due to immune hemolysis (P83.2)

DEF: HBA1 and HBA2 genetic variant of chromosome 16 prevalent among those of African and Southeast Asian descent. Alpha thalassemia is associated with a wide spectrum of anemic presentation and includes hemoglobin H disease subtypes.

D56.1 Beta thalassemia   HCC ESR COM

Beta thalassemia major
Cooley's anemia
Homozygous beta thalassemia
Severe beta thalassemia
Thalassemia intermedia
Thalassemia major

EXCLUDES 1 *beta thalassemia minor (D56.3)*
beta thalassemia trait (D56.3)
delta-beta thalassemia (D56.2)
hemoglobin E-beta thalassemia (D56.5)
sickle-cell beta thalassemia (D57.4-)

D56.2 Delta-beta thalassemia   HCC ESR COM

Homozygous delta-beta thalassemia

EXCLUDES 1 *delta-beta thalassemia minor (D56.3)*
delta-beta thalassemia trait (D56.3)

D56.3 Thalassemia minor

Alpha thalassemia minor
Alpha thalassemia silent carrier
Alpha thalassemia trait
Beta thalassemia minor
Beta thalassemia trait
Delta-beta thalassemia minor
Delta-beta thalassemia trait
Thalassemia trait NOS

EXCLUDES 1 *alpha thalassemia (D56.0)*
beta thalassemia (D56.1)
delta-beta thalassemia (D56.2)
hemoglobin E-beta thalassemia (D56.5)
sickle-cell trait (D57.3)

DEF: Solitary abnormal gene that identifies a carrier of the disease, yet with an absence of symptoms or a clinically mild anemic presentation.

D56.4 Hereditary persistence of fetal hemoglobin [HPFH]   HCC ESR

D56.5 Hemoglobin E-beta thalassemia   HCC ESR COM

EXCLUDES 1 *beta thalassemia (D56.1)*
beta thalassemia minor (D56.3)
beta thalassemia trait (D56.3)
delta-beta thalassemia (D56.2)
delta-beta thalassemia trait (D56.3)
hemoglobin E disease (D58.2)
other hemoglobinopathies (D58.2)
sickle-cell beta thalassemia (D57.4-)

D56.8 Other thalassemias   HCC ESR

Dominant thalassemia
Hemoglobin C thalassemia
Mixed thalassemia
Thalassemia with other hemoglobinopathy

EXCLUDES 1 *hemoglobin C disease (D58.2)*
hemoglobin E disease (D58.2)
other hemoglobinopathies (D58.2)
sickle-cell anemia (D57.-)
sickle-cell thalassemia (D57.4)

D56.9 Thalassemia, unspecified

Mediterranean anemia (with other hemoglobinopathy)

✓4ᵗʰ D57 Sickle-cell disorders

Use additional code for any associated fever (R50.81)

EXCLUDES 1 *other hemoglobinopathies (D58.-)*

AHA: 2022,2Q,28

DEF: Severe, chronic inherited diseases caused by a genetic variation in hemoglobin protein of the red blood cell. The gene mutation causes the red blood cell to become hard, sticky, and crescent or sickle shaped, making it harder for red blood cells to travel through the bloodstream, disrupting blood flow and decreasing oxygen transport to tissues.

Sickle cell

Sickle cells

Normal RBCs

✓5ᵗʰ D57.0 Hb-SS disease with crisis

Sickle-cell disease with crisis
Hb-SS disease with vasoocclusive pain

AHA: 2020,4Q,6-7

D57.00 Hb-SS disease with crisis, unspecified   HCC Rx ESR COM

Hb-SS disease with (painful) crisis NOS
Hb-SS disease with vasoocclusive pain NOS

D57.01 Hb-SS disease with acute chest syndrome   HCC Rx ESR COM

D57.02 Hb-SS disease with splenic sequestration   HCC Rx ESR COM

D57.03 Hb-SS disease with cerebral vascular involvement   HCC Rx ESR COM

Code also, if applicable, cerebral infarction (I63.-)

D57.09 Hb-SS disease with crisis with other specified complication   HCC Rx ESR COM

Use additional code to identify complications, such as:
cholelithiasis (K80.-)
priapism (N48.32)

D57.1 Sickle-cell disease without crisis   HCC Rx ESR COM

Hb-SS disease without crisis
Sickle-cell anemia NOS
Sickle-cell disease NOS
Sickle-cell disorder NOS

✓5ᵗʰ D57.2 Sickle-cell/Hb-C disease

Hb-SC disease
Hb-S/Hb-C disease

AHA: 2020,4Q,6-7

D57.20 Sickle-cell/Hb-C disease without crisis   HCC ESR

Chapter 3. Diseases of the Blood and Blood-forming Organs

☑6ᵗʰ **D57.21** **Sickle-cell/Hb-C disease** with crisis

    D57.211 **Sickle-cell/Hb-C disease** with acute chest syndrome `HCC` `ESR`

    D57.212 **Sickle-cell/Hb-C disease** with splenic sequestration `HCC` `ESR`

    D57.213 **Sickle-cell/Hb-C disease** with cerebral vascular involvement `HCC` `ESR`

        Code also, if applicable, cerebral infarction (I63.-)

    D57.218 **Sickle-cell/Hb-C disease with crisis with other specified complication** `HCC` `ESR`

        Use additional code to identify complications, such as:
        cholelithiasis (K8Ø.-)
        priapism (N48.32)

    D57.219 **Sickle-cell/Hb-C disease with crisis, unspecified** `HCC` `ESR`

        Sickle-cell/Hb-C disease with crisis NOS
        Sickle-cell/Hb-C disease with vasoocclusive pain NOS

D57.3 **Sickle-cell** trait `HCC` `ESR`

    Hb-S trait
    Heterozygous hemoglobin S
    DEF: Heterozygous genetic makeup characterized by one gene for normal hemoglobin and one for sickle-cell hemoglobin. The clinical disease is rarely present.

☑5ᵗʰ **D57.4** **Sickle-cell** thalassemia

    Sickle-cell beta thalassemia
    Thalassemia Hb-S disease
    AHA: 2020,4Q,6-7

    D57.4Ø **Sickle-cell thalassemia** without crisis `HCC` `ESR`
        Microdrepanocytosis
        Sickle-cell thalassemia NOS

☑6ᵗʰ **D57.41** **Sickle-cell thalassemia, unspecified, with crisis**

    Sickle-cell thalassemia with (painful) crisis NOS
    Sickle-cell thalassemia with vasoocclusive pain NOS

    D57.411 **Sickle-cell thalassemia, unspecified,** with acute chest syndrome `HCC` `ESR`

    D57.412 **Sickle-cell thalassemia, unspecified,** with splenic sequestration `HCC` `ESR`

    D57.413 **Sickle-cell thalassemia, unspecified,** with cerebral vascular involvement `HCC` `ESR`
        Code also, if applicable cerebral infarction (I63.-)

    D57.418 **Sickle-cell thalassemia, unspecified, with crisis with other specified complication** `HCC` `ESR`
        Use additional code to identify complications, such as:
        cholelithiasis (K8Ø.-)
        priapism (N48.32)

    D57.419 **Sickle-cell thalassemia, unspecified, with crisis** `HCC` `ESR`
        Sickle-cell thalassemia with (painful) crisis NOS
        Sickle-cell thalassemia with vasoocclusive pain NOS

D57.42 **Sickle-cell thalassemia** beta zero without crisis `HCC` `Rx` `ESR` `COM`
    HbS-beta zero without crisis
    Sickle-cell beta zero without crisis

☑6ᵗʰ **D57.43** **Sickle-cell thalassemia** beta zero with crisis
    HbS-beta zero with crisis
    Sickle-cell beta zero with crisis

    D57.431 **Sickle-cell thalassemia beta zero** with acute chest syndrome `HCC` `Rx` `ESR` `COM`
        HbS-beta zero with acute chest syndrome
        Sickle-cell beta zero with acute chest syndrome

    D57.432 **Sickle-cell thalassemia beta zero** with splenic sequestration `HCC` `Rx` `ESR` `COM`
        HbS-beta zero with splenic sequestration
        Sickle-cell beta zero with splenic sequestration

D57.433 **Sickle-cell thalassemia beta zero** with cerebral vascular involvement `HCC` `Rx` `ESR` `COM`
    HbS-beta zero with cerebral vascular involvement
    Sickle-cell beta zero with cerebral vascular involvement
    Code also, if applicable cerebral infarction (I63.-)

D57.438 **Sickle-cell thalassemia beta zero with crisis with other specified complication** `HCC` `Rx` `ESR` `COM`
    HbS-beta zero with other specified complication
    Sickle-cell beta zero with other specified complication
    Use additional code to identify complications, such as:
    cholelithiasis (K8Ø.-)
    priapism (N48.32)

D57.439 **Sickle-cell thalassemia beta zero with crisis, unspecified** `HCC` `Rx` `ESR` `COM`
    HbS-beta zero with other specified complication
    Sickle-cell beta zero with crisis unspecified
    Sickle-cell thalassemia beta zero with (painful) crisis NOS
    Sickle-cell thalassemia beta zero with vasoocclusive pain NOS

D57.44 **Sickle-cell thalassemia** beta plus without crisis `HCC` `ESR`
    HbS-beta plus without crisis
    Sickle-cell beta plus without crisis

☑6ᵗʰ **D57.45** **Sickle-cell thalassemia** beta plus with crisis
    HbS-beta plus with crisis
    Sickle-cell beta plus with crisis

    D57.451 **Sickle-cell thalassemia beta plus** with acute chest syndrome `HCC` `ESR`
        HbS-beta plus with acute chest syndrome
        Sickle-cell beta plus with acute chest syndrome

    D57.452 **Sickle-cell thalassemia beta plus** with splenic sequestration `HCC` `ESR`
        HbS-beta plus with splenic sequestration
        Sickle-cell beta plus with splenic sequestration

    D57.453 **Sickle-cell thalassemia beta plus** with cerebral vascular involvement `HCC` `ESR`
        HbS-beta plus with cerebral vascular involvement
        Sickle-cell beta plus with cerebral vascular involvement
        Code also, if applicable cerebral infarction (I63.-)

    D57.458 **Sickle-cell thalassemia beta plus with crisis with other specified complication** `HCC` `ESR`
        HbS-beta plus with crisis with other specified complication
        Sickle-cell beta plus with crisis with other specified complication
        Use additional code to identify complications, such as:
        cholelithiasis (K8Ø.-)
        priapism (N48.32)

    D57.459 **Sickle-cell thalassemia beta plus with crisis, unspecified** `HCC` `ESR`
        HbS-beta plus with crisis with unspecified complication
        Sickle-cell beta plus with crisis with unspecified complication
        Sickle-cell thalassemia beta plus with (painful) crisis NOS
        Sickle-cell thalassemia beta plus with vasoocclusive pain NOS

`HCC` CMS-HCC   `Rx` Rx HCC   `ESR` ESRD HCC   `COM` Commercial HCC   `N` Newborn: 0   `P` Pediatric: 0-17   `M` Maternity: 9-64   `A` Adult: 15-124

518   ICD-10-CM 2023

☑5ᵗʰ **D57.8** **Other sickle-cell disorders**
Hb-SD disease
Hb-SE disease
AHA: 2020,4Q,6-7

D57.80 **Other sickle-cell disorders** without crisis   HCC ESR

☑6ᵗʰ **D57.81** **Other sickle-cell disorders** with crisis

D57.811 **Other sickle-cell disorders** with acute
chest syndrome   HCC ESR

D57.812 **Other sickle-cell disorders** with splenic
sequestration   HCC ESR

D57.813 **Other sickle-cell disorders** with cerebral
vascular involvement   HCC ESR
Code also, if applicable: cerebral infarction
(I63.-)

D57.818 **Other sickle-cell disorders with crisis with
other specified complication**   HCC ESR
Use additional code to identify
complications, such as:
cholelithiasis (K80.-)
priapism (N48.32)

D57.819 **Other sickle-cell disorders with crisis,
unspecified**   HCC ESR
Other sickle-cell disorders with crisis NOS
Other sickle-cell disorders with
vasoocclusive pain NOS

☑4ᵗʰ **D58** **Other hereditary hemolytic anemias**
EXCLUDES 1   hemolytic anemia of the newborn (P55.-)

D58.0 **Hereditary spherocytosis**   HCC ESR
Acholuric (familial) jaundice
Congenital (spherocytic) hemolytic icterus
Minkowski-Chauffard syndrome
DEF: Inherited condition caused by mutations to genes
responsible for the production of proteins that form the
membranes of red blood cells. The shape and flexibility of the red
blood cell membrane is altered, diminishing the cell's ability to
traverse the spleen, therefore becoming trapped and destroyed
before the red blood cell has reached maturity.

D58.1 **Hereditary elliptocytosis**   HCC ESR
Elliptocytosis (congenital)
Ovalocytosis (congenital) (hereditary)

D58.2 **Other hemoglobinopathies**   HCC ESR
Abnormal hemoglobin NOS
Congenital Heinz body anemia
Hb-C disease
Hb-D disease
Hb-E disease
Hemoglobinopathy NOS
Unstable hemoglobin hemolytic disease
EXCLUDES 1   familial polycythemia (D75.0)
Hb-M disease (D74.0)
hemoglobin E-beta thalassemia (D56.5)
hereditary persistence of fetal hemoglobin [HPFH]
(D56.4)
high-altitude polycythemia (D75.1)
methemoglobinemia (D74.-)
other hemoglobinopathies with thalassemia (D56.8)

D58.8 **Other specified hereditary hemolytic anemias**   HCC ESR
Stomatocytosis

D58.9 **Hereditary hemolytic anemia, unspecified**   HCC ESR

☑4ᵗʰ **D59** **Acquired hemolytic anemia**
DEF: Non-hereditary anemia characterized by premature destruction of
red blood cells caused by infectious organisms, poisons, and physical
agents.

D59.0 **Drug-induced autoimmune hemolytic
anemia**   HCC Rx ESR COM
Use additional code for adverse effect, if applicable, to identify
drug (T36-T50 with fifth or sixth character 5)

☑5ᵗʰ **D59.1** **Other autoimmune hemolytic anemias**
EXCLUDES 2   Evans syndrome (D69.41)
hemolytic disease of newborn (P55.-)
paroxysmal cold hemoglobinuria (D59.6)
AHA: 2020,4Q,7-8

D59.10 **Autoimmune hemolytic anemia,
unspecified**   HCC Rx ESR COM

D59.11 **Warm autoimmune hemolytic
anemia**   HCC Rx ESR COM
Warm type (primary) (secondary) (symptomatic)
autoimmune hemolytic anemia
Warm type autoimmune hemolytic disease

D59.12 **Cold autoimmune hemolytic
anemia**   HCC Rx ESR COM
Chronic cold hemagglutinin disease
Cold agglutinin disease
Cold agglutinin hemoglobinuria
Cold type (primary) (secondary) (symptomatic)
autoimmune hemolytic anemia
Cold type autoimmune hemolytic disease

D59.13 **Mixed type autoimmune hemolytic
anemia**   HCC Rx ESR COM
Mixed type autoimmune hemolytic disease
Mixed type, cold and warm, (primary) (secondary)
(symptomatic) autoimmune hemolytic anemia

D59.19 **Other autoimmune hemolytic
anemia**   HCC Rx ESR COM

D59.2 **Drug-induced nonautoimmune hemolytic
anemia**   HCC Rx ESR COM
Drug-induced enzyme deficiency anemia
Use additional code for adverse effect, if applicable, to identify
drug (T36-T50 with fifth or sixth character 5)

▲ ☑5ᵗʰ **D59.3** **Hemolytic-uremic syndrome**
Use additional code to identify associated:
E. coli infection (B96.2-)
Pneumococcal pneumonia (J13)
Shigella dysenteriae (A03.9)
▶Code also, if applicable, any associated:◀
▶acute kidney failure (N17.-)◀
▶chronic kidney disease (N18.-)◀
DEF: Condition typically precipitated by infection causing low
platelets and destruction of red blood cells resulting in hemolytic
anemia. This cell damage and blockage of renal capillaries lead
to kidney failure. Mainly affects children.

● **D59.30** **Hemolytic-uremic syndrome, unspecified**
Hemolytic-uremic syndrome NOS

● **D59.31** **Infection-associated hemolytic-uremic syndrome**
Shiga toxin-producing E. coli [STEC] related hemolytic
uremic syndrome
Typical hemolytic uremic syndrome
Use additional code to identify associated infection,
such as:
E. coli infection (B96.2-)
human immunodeficiency virus [HIV] disease (B20)
pneumococcal meningitis (G00.1)
pneumococcal pneumonia (J13)
sepsis due to Streptococcus pneumoniae (A40.3)
Shigella dysenteriae (A03.9)
streptococcus pneumoniae as the cause of diseases
classified elsewhere (B95.3)

● **D59.32** **Hereditary hemolytic-uremic syndrome**
Atypical hemolytic uremic syndrome with an
identified genetic cause
Code also, if applicable:
defects in the complement system (D84.1)
methylmalonic acidemia (E71.120)

● **D59.39** **Other hemolytic-uremic syndrome**
Atypical (nongenetic) hemolytic uremic syndrome
Secondary hemolytic-uremic syndrome
Code first, if applicable, any associated:
COVID-19 (U07.1)
complications of kidney transplant (T86.1-)
complications of heart transplant (T86.2-)
complications of liver transplant (T86.4-)
Code also, if applicable, any associated condition,
such as:
hypertensive emergency (I16.1)
malignant neoplasm (C00-C96)
systemic lupus erythematosus (M32.-)
Use additional code, if applicable, for adverse effect
to identify drug (T36-T50 with fifth or sixth
character 5)

D59.4 **Other** **nonautoimmune** **hemolytic anemias** `HCC` `Rx` `ESR` `COM`
Mechanical hemolytic anemia
Microangiopathic hemolytic anemia
Toxic hemolytic anemia

D59.5 **Paroxysmal nocturnal hemoglobinuria [Marchiafava-Micheli]** `HCC` `Rx` `ESR` `COM`
EXCLUDES 1   *hemoglobinuria NOS (R82.3)*

D59.6 **Hemoglobinuria** **due to hemolysis from other external causes** `HCC` `Rx` `ESR` `COM`
Hemoglobinuria from exertion
March hemoglobinuria
Paroxysmal cold hemoglobinuria
Use additional code (Chapter 20) to identify external cause
EXCLUDES 1   *hemoglobinuria NOS (R82.3)*

D59.8 **Other acquired hemolytic anemias** `HCC` `Rx` `ESR` `COM`

D59.9 **Acquired hemolytic anemia, unspecified** `HCC` `Rx` `ESR` `COM`
Idiopathic hemolytic anemia, chronic

Aplastic and other anemias and other bone marrow failure syndromes (D60-D64)

✓4ᵗʰ **D60** **Acquired pure red cell aplasia [erythroblastopenia]**
INCLUDES   red cell aplasia (acquired) (adult) (with thymoma)
EXCLUDES 1   *congenital red cell aplasia (D61.01)*
DEF: Bone marrow failure characterized by underproduction of red blood cells while white blood cell and platelet production remains normal.

D60.0 **Chronic** **acquired pure red cell aplasia** `HCC` `Rx` `ESR` `COM`

D60.1 **Transient** **acquired pure red cell aplasia** `HCC` `Rx` `ESR` `COM`

D60.8 **Other acquired pure red cell aplasias** `HCC` `Rx` `ESR` `COM`

D60.9 **Acquired pure red cell aplasia, unspecified** `HCC` `Rx` `ESR` `COM`

✓4ᵗʰ **D61** **Other aplastic anemias and other bone marrow failure syndromes**
EXCLUDES 2   *neutropenia (D70.-)*
AHA: 2020,3Q,22; 2014,4Q,22
DEF: Aplastic anemia: Bone marrow failure characterized by underproduction of red bloods cells, white blood cells and platelets.

✓5ᵗʰ **D61.0** **Constitutional** **aplastic anemia**

D61.01 **Constitutional (pure)** **red blood cell aplasia** `HCC` `Rx` `ESR` `COM`
Blackfan-Diamond syndrome
Congenital (pure) red cell aplasia
Familial hypoplastic anemia
Primary (pure) red cell aplasia
Red cell (pure) aplasia of infants
EXCLUDES 1   *acquired red cell aplasia (D60.9)*

D61.09 **Other constitutional aplastic anemia** `HCC` `Rx` `ESR` `COM`
Fanconi's anemia
Pancytopenia with malformations

D61.1 **Drug-induced** **aplastic anemia** `HCC` `Rx` `ESR` `COM`
Use additional code for adverse effect, if applicable, to identify drug (T36-T50 with fifth or sixth character 5)

D61.2 **Aplastic anemia due to other** **external agents** `HCC` `Rx` `ESR` `COM`
Code first, if applicable, toxic effects of substances chiefly nonmedicinal as to source (T51-T65)

D61.3 **Idiopathic** **aplastic anemia** `HCC` `Rx` `ESR` `COM`

✓5ᵗʰ **D61.8** **Other specified aplastic anemias and other bone marrow failure syndromes**

✓6ᵗʰ **D61.81** **Pancytopenia**
EXCLUDES 1   *pancytopenia (due to) (with) aplastic anemia (D61.9)*
pancytopenia (due to) (with) bone marrow infiltration (D61.82)
pancytopenia (due to) (with) congenital (pure) red cell aplasia (D61.01)
pancytopenia (due to) (with) hairy cell leukemia (C91.4-)
pancytopenia (due to) (with) human immunodeficiency virus disease (B20)
pancytopenia (due to) (with) leukoerythroblastic anemia (D61.82)
pancytopenia (due to) (with) myeloproliferative disease (D47.1)
EXCLUDES 2   *pancytopenia (due to) (with) myelodysplastic syndromes (D46.-)*
DEF: Shortage of all three blood cells: white, red, and platelets.

D61.810 **Antineoplastic chemotherapy** **induced pancytopenia** `HCC` `ESR`
EXCLUDES 2   *aplastic anemia due to antineoplastic chemotherapy (D61.1)*
AHA: 2020,3Q,22

D61.811 **Other drug-induced pancytopenia** `HCC` `ESR`
EXCLUDES 2   *aplastic anemia due to drugs (D61.1)*

D61.818 **Other pancytopenia** `HCC` `ESR`
AHA: 2020,3Q,24; 2019,1Q,16
TIP: Assign this code in addition to myeloid leukemia codes (C92.-) when pancytopenia is documented. Although common in some types of myeloid leukemia, pancytopenia is not always inherent.

D61.82 **Myelophthisis** `HCC` `Rx` `ESR` `COM`
Leukoerythroblastic anemia
Myelophthisic anemia
Panmyelophthisis
Code also the underlying disorder, such as:
  malignant neoplasm of breast (C50.-)
  tuberculosis (A15.-)
EXCLUDES 1   *idiopathic myelofibrosis (D47.1)*
myelofibrosis NOS (D75.81)
myelofibrosis with myeloid metaplasia (D47.4)
primary myelofibrosis (D47.1)
secondary myelofibrosis (D75.81)
DEF: Condition that occurs when normal hematopoietic tissue in the bone marrow is replaced with abnormal tissue, such as fibrous tissue or tumors. Most commonly seen during the advanced stages of cancer.

D61.89 **Other specified aplastic anemias and other bone marrow failure syndromes** `HCC` `Rx` `ESR` `COM`

D61.9 **Aplastic anemia, unspecified** `HCC` `Rx` `ESR` `COM`
Hypoplastic anemia NOS
Medullary hypoplasia

D62 **Acute posthemorrhagic anemia**
EXCLUDES 1   *anemia due to chronic blood loss (D50.0)*
blood loss anemia NOS (D50.0)
congenital anemia from fetal blood loss (P61.3)
AHA: 2019,3Q,11,17

✓4ᵗʰ **D63** **Anemia in chronic diseases classified elsewhere**

D63.0 **Anemia in** **neoplastic disease**
Code first neoplasm (C00-D49)
EXCLUDES 1   *aplastic anemia due to antineoplastic chemotherapy (D61.1)*
EXCLUDES 2   *anemia due to antineoplastic chemotherapy (D64.81)*

D63.1 **Anemia in** **chronic kidney disease**
Erythropoietin resistant anemia (EPO resistant anemia)
Code first underlying chronic kidney disease (CKD) (N18.-)

D63.8 *Anemia in other chronic diseases classified elsewhere*
Code first underlying disease, such as:
diphyllobothriasis (B70.0)
hookworm disease (B76.0-B76.9)
hypothyroidism (E00.0-E03.9)
malaria (B50.0-B54)
symptomatic late syphilis (A52.79)
tuberculosis (A18.89)

✓4ᵗʰ **D64 Other anemias**

EXCLUDES 1 *refractory anemia (D46.-)*
refractory anemia with excess blasts in transformation [RAEB T] (C92.0-)

DEF: Sideroblastic anemia: Hereditary or secondary disorder in which the red blood cells cannot effectively use iron, a nutrient needed to make hemoglobin. Although the iron can enter the red blood cell it is not assimilated into the hemoglobin molecule and builds up ringed sideroblasts around the cell nucleus.

D64.0 Hereditary sideroblastic anemia `HCC` `Rx` `ESR` `COM`
Sex-linked hypochromic sideroblastic anemia

D64.1 *Secondary sideroblastic anemia due to disease* `HCC` `Rx` `ESR` `COM`
Code first underlying disease

D64.2 Secondary sideroblastic anemia due to drugs and toxins `HCC` `Rx` `ESR` `COM`
Code first poisoning due to drug or toxin, if applicable (T36-T65 with fifth or sixth character 1-4 or 6)
Use additional code for adverse effect, if applicable, to identify drug (T36-T50 with fifth or sixth character 5)

D64.3 Other sideroblastic anemias `HCC` `Rx` `ESR` `COM`
Sideroblastic anemia NOS
Pyridoxine-responsive sideroblastic anemia NEC

D64.4 Congenital dyserythropoietic anemia
Dyshematopoietic anemia (congenital)
EXCLUDES 1 *Blackfan-Diamond syndrome (D61.01)*
Di Guglielmo's disease (C94.0)

✓5ᵗʰ **D64.8 Other specified anemias**

D64.81 Anemia due to antineoplastic chemotherapy
Antineoplastic chemotherapy induced anemia
EXCLUDES 2 *anemia in neoplastic disease (D63.0)*
aplastic anemia due to antineoplastic chemotherapy (D61.1)
AHA: 2021,3Q,4; 2014,4Q,22

D64.89 Other specified anemias
Infantile pseudoleukemia

D64.9 Anemia, unspecified
AHA: 2020,3Q,24; 2018,4Q,88; 2017,1Q,7

Coagulation defects, purpura and other hemorrhagic conditions (D65-D69)

D65 Disseminated intravascular coagulation [defibrination syndrome] `HCC` `ESR` `COM`
Afibrinogenemia, acquired
Consumption coagulopathy
Diffuse or disseminated intravascular coagulation [DIC]
Fibrinolytic hemorrhage, acquired
Fibrinolytic purpura
Purpura fulminans
EXCLUDES 1 *disseminated intravascular coagulation (complicating):*
abortion or ectopic or molar pregnancy (O00-O07, O08.1)
in newborn (P60)
pregnancy, childbirth and the puerperium (O45.0, O46.0, O67.0, O72.3)
AHA: 2021,1Q,39

Coagulation

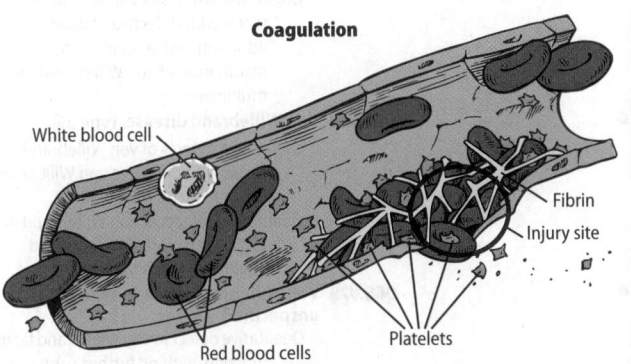

White blood cell
Fibrin
Injury site
Platelets
Red blood cells

D66 Hereditary factor VIII deficiency `HCC` `ESR` `COM`
Classical hemophilia
Deficiency factor VIII (with functional defect)
Hemophilia NOS
Hemophilia A
EXCLUDES 1 *factor VIII deficiency with vascular defect ▶(D68.0-)◀*
DEF: Hereditary, sex-linked lack of antihemophilic globulin (AHG) (factor VIII) that causes abnormal coagulation characterized by increased bleeding; large bruises of skin; bleeding in the mouth, nose, and gastrointestinal tract; and hemorrhages into joints, resulting in swelling and impaired function.

D67 Hereditary factor IX deficiency `HCC` `ESR` `COM`
Christmas disease
Factor IX deficiency (with functional defect)
Hemophilia B
Plasma thromboplastin component [PTC] deficiency

✓4ᵗʰ **D68 Other coagulation defects**
EXCLUDES 1 ▶*abnormal coagulation profile NOS◀ (R79.1)*
coagulation defects complicating abortion or ectopic or molar pregnancy (O00-O07, O08.1)
coagulation defects complicating pregnancy, childbirth and the puerperium (O45.0, O46.0, O67.0, O72.3)
EXCLUDES 2 ▶*coagulation defects complicating abortion or ectopic or molar pregnancy (O00-O07, O08.1)◀*
▶*coagulation defects complicating pregnancy, childbirth and the puerperium (O45.0, O46.0, O67.0, O72.3)◀*
AHA: 2016,1Q,14

▲ ✓5ᵗʰ **D68.0 Von Willebrand disease**
Angiohemophilia
Factor VIII deficiency with vascular defect
Vascular hemophilia
EXCLUDES 1 *capillary fragility (hereditary) (D69.8)*
factor VIII deficiency NOS (D66)
factor VIII deficiency with functional defect (D66)
DEF: Congenital, abnormal blood coagulation caused by deficient blood factor VII. Symptoms include excess or prolonged bleeding.

● **D68.00 Von Willebrand disease, unspecified**

● **D68.01 Von Willebrand disease, type 1**
Partial quantitative deficiency of von Willebrand factor
Type 1C von Willebrand disease

Chapter 3. Diseases of the Blood and Blood-forming Organs

D68.02–D68.52

- ✓6ᵗʰ **D68.02 Von Willebrand disease, type 2**
  Qualitative defects of von Willebrand factor
  - **D68.020 Von Willebrand disease, type 2A**
    Qualitative defects of von Willebrand factor with decreased platelet adhesion and selective deficiency of high-molecular-weight multimers
  - **D68.021 Von Willebrand disease, type 2B**
    Qualitative defects of von Willebrand factor with high-molecular-weight von Willebrand factor loss
    Qualitative defects of von Willebrand factor with hyper-adhesive forms
    Qualitative defects of von Willebrand factor with increased affinity for platelet glycoprotein Ib
  - **D68.022 Von Willebrand disease, type 2M**
    Qualitative defects of von Willebrand factor with defective platelet adhesion with a normal size distribution of von Willebrand factor multimers
  - **D68.023 Von Willebrand disease, type 2N**
    Qualitative defects of von Willebrand factor with defective von Willebrand factor to factor VIII binding
    Qualitative defects of von Willebrand factor with markedly decreased affinity for factor VIII
  - **D68.029 Von Willebrand disease, type 2, unspecified**
    Qualitative defect in von Willebrand factor function, with no further subtyping
- **D68.03 Von Willebrand disease, type 3**
  (Near) complete absence of von Willebrand factor
  Total quantitative deficiency of von Willebrand factor
- **D68.04 Acquired von Willebrand disease**
  Acquired von Willebrand syndrome
- **D68.09 Other von Willebrand disease**
  Platelet-type von Willebrand disease
  Pseudo-von Willebrand disease
  Code also, if applicable, qualitative platelet defects (D69.1)
- **D68.1 Hereditary factor XI deficiency**   HCC ESR COM
  Hemophilia C
  Plasma thromboplastin antecedent [PTA] deficiency
  Rosenthal's disease
- **D68.2 Hereditary deficiency of other clotting factors**   HCC ESR COM
  AC globulin deficiency
  Congenital afibrinogenemia
  Deficiency of factor I [fibrinogen]
  Deficiency of factor II [prothrombin]
  Deficiency of factor V [labile]
  Deficiency of factor VII [stable]
  Deficiency of factor X [Stuart-Prower]
  Deficiency of factor XII [Hageman]
  Deficiency of factor XIII [fibrin stabilizing]
  Dysfibrinogenemia (congenital)
  Hypoproconvertinemia
  Owren's disease
  Proaccelerin deficiency
- ✓5ᵗʰ **D68.3 Hemorrhagic disorder due to circulating anticoagulants**
  - ✓6ᵗʰ **D68.31 Hemorrhagic disorder due to intrinsic circulating anticoagulants, antibodies, or inhibitors**
    - **D68.311 Acquired hemophilia**   HCC ESR COM
      Autoimmune hemophilia
      Autoimmune inhibitors to clotting factors
      Secondary hemophilia

- **D68.312 Antiphospholipid antibody with hemorrhagic disorder**   HCC ESR COM
  Lupus anticoagulant (LAC) with hemorrhagic disorder
  Systemic lupus erythematosus [SLE] inhibitor with hemorrhagic disorder
  EXCLUDES 1   *antiphospholipid antibody, finding without diagnosis (R76.0)*
  antiphospholipid antibody syndrome (D68.61)
  antiphospholipid antibody with hypercoagulable state (D68.61)
  lupus anticoagulant (LAC) finding without diagnosis (R76.0)
  lupus anticoagulant (LAC) with hypercoagulable state (D68.62)
  systemic lupus erythematosus [SLE] inhibitor finding without diagnosis (R76.0)
  systemic lupus erythematosus [SLE] inhibitor with hypercoagulable state (D68.62)
- **D68.318 Other hemorrhagic disorder due to intrinsic circulating anticoagulants, antibodies, or inhibitors**   HCC ESR COM
  Antithromboplastinemia
  Antithromboplastinogenemia
  Hemorrhagic disorder due to intrinsic increase in antithrombin
  Hemorrhagic disorder due to intrinsic increase in anti-VIIIa
  Hemorrhagic disorder due to intrinsic increase in anti-IXa
  Hemorrhagic disorder due to intrinsic increase in anti-XIa
- **D68.32 Hemorrhagic disorder due to extrinsic circulating anticoagulants**   HCC ESR COM
  Drug-induced hemorrhagic disorder
  Hemorrhagic disorder due to increase in anti-IIa
  Hemorrhagic disorder due to increase in anti-Xa
  Hyperheparinemia
  Use additional code for adverse effect, if applicable, to identify drug (T45.515, T45.525)
  AHA: 2021,1Q,4; 2016,1Q,14-15
  TIP: Do not assign to identify routine therapeutic anticoagulation effects; assign only for documented adverse effects.
- **D68.4 Acquired coagulation factor deficiency**   HCC ESR COM
  Deficiency of coagulation factor due to liver disease
  Deficiency of coagulation factor due to vitamin K deficiency
  EXCLUDES 1   *vitamin K deficiency of newborn (P53)*
- ✓5ᵗʰ **D68.5 Primary thrombophilia**
  Primary hypercoagulable states
  EXCLUDES 1   *antiphospholipid syndrome (D68.61)*
  lupus anticoagulant (D68.62)
  secondary activated protein C resistance (D68.69)
  secondary antiphospholipid antibody syndrome (D68.69)
  secondary lupus anticoagulant with hypercoagulable state (D68.69)
  secondary systemic lupus erythematosus [SLE] inhibitor with hypercoagulable state (D68.69)
  systemic lupus erythematosus [SLE] inhibitor finding without diagnosis (R76.0)
  systemic lupus erythematosus [SLE] inhibitor with hemorrhagic disorder (D68.312)
  thrombotic thrombocytopenic purpura (M31.19)
  DEF: Thrombophilia: Increased tendency of the blood to clot, which can lead to thrombus or embolus formation.
  - **D68.51 Activated protein C resistance**   HCC ESR COM
    Factor V Leiden mutation
  - **D68.52 Prothrombin gene mutation**   HCC ESR COM

D68.59 **Other primary thrombophilia** `HCC` `ESR` `COM`
Antithrombin III deficiency
Hypercoagulable state NOS
Primary hypercoagulable state NEC
Primary thrombophilia NEC
Protein C deficiency
Protein S deficiency
Thrombophilia NOS
AHA: 2021,2Q,8

D68.6 **Other thrombophilia** ✓5th
Other hypercoagulable states
EXCLUDES 1   *diffuse or disseminated intravascular coagulation [DIC] (D65)*
heparin induced thrombocytopenia (HIT) ▶*(D75.82-)*◀
hyperhomocysteinemia (E72.11)

D68.61 **Antiphospholipid syndrome** `HCC` `ESR` `COM`
Anticardiolipin syndrome
Antiphospholipid antibody syndrome
EXCLUDES 1   *anti-phospholipid antibody, finding without diagnosis (R76.0)*
anti-phospholipid antibody with hemorrhagic disorder (D68.312)
lupus anticoagulant syndrome (D68.62)

D68.62 **Lupus anticoagulant syndrome** `HCC` `ESR` `COM`
Lupus anticoagulant
Presence of systemic lupus erythematosus [SLE] inhibitor
EXCLUDES 1   *anticardiolipin syndrome (D68.61)*
antiphospholipid syndrome (D68.61)
lupus anticoagulant (LAC) finding without diagnosis (R76.0)
lupus anticoagulant (LAC) with hemorrhagic disorder (D68.312)

D68.69 **Other thrombophilia** `HCC` `ESR` `COM`
Hypercoagulable states NEC
Secondary hypercoagulable state NOS
AHA: 2021,2Q,8

D68.8 **Other specified coagulation defects** `HCC` `ESR` `COM`
EXCLUDES 1   *hemorrhagic disease of newborn (P53)*
AHA: 2021,1Q,39

D68.9 **Coagulation defect, unspecified** `HCC` `ESR` `COM`

D69 **Purpura and other hemorrhagic conditions** ✓4th
EXCLUDES 1   *benign hypergammaglobulinemic purpura (D89.0)*
cryoglobulinemic purpura (D89.1)
essential (hemorrhagic) thrombocythemia (D47.3)
hemorrhagic thrombocythemia (D47.3)
purpura fulminans (D65)
thrombotic thrombocytopenic purpura (M31.19)
Waldenström hypergammaglobulinemic purpura (D89.0)

D69.0 **Allergic purpura** `HCC` `ESR`
Allergic vasculitis
Nonthrombocytopenic hemorrhagic purpura
Nonthrombocytopenic idiopathic purpura
Purpura anaphylactoid
Purpura Henoch(-Schönlein)
Purpura rheumatica
Vascular purpura
EXCLUDES 1   *thrombocytopenic hemorrhagic purpura (D69.3)*
AHA: 2020,3Q,26
DEF: Any hemorrhagic condition, thrombocytic or nonthrombocytopenic in origin, caused by a presumed allergic reaction.

D69.1 **Qualitative platelet defects** `HCC` `ESR` `COM`
Bernard-Soulier [giant platelet] syndrome
Glanzmann's disease
Grey platelet syndrome
Thromboasthenia (hemorrhagic) (hereditary)
Thrombocytopathy
EXCLUDES 1   ▶*hemolytic-uremic syndrome (D59.3-)*◀
von Willebrand's disease (D68.0)
EXCLUDES 2   ▶*von Willebrand disease (D68.0-)*◀

D69.2 **Other nonthrombocytopenic purpura** `HCC` `ESR`
Purpura NOS
Purpura simplex
Senile purpura

D69.3 **Immune thrombocytopenic purpura** `HCC` `Rx` `ESR` `COM`
Hemorrhagic (thrombocytopenic) purpura
Idiopathic thrombocytopenic purpura
Tidal platelet dysgenesis
DEF: Tidal platelet dysgenesis: Fluctuation of platelet counts from normal to very low within periods of 20 to 40 days and may involve autoimmune platelet destruction.

D69.4 **Other primary thrombocytopenia** ✓5th
EXCLUDES 1   *transient neonatal thrombocytopenia (P61.0)*
Wiskott-Aldrich syndrome (D82.0)

D69.41 **Evans syndrome** `HCC` `ESR` `COM`
D69.42 **Congenital and hereditary thrombocytopenia purpura** `HCC` `ESR` `COM`
Congenital thrombocytopenia
Hereditary thrombocytopenia
Code first congenital or hereditary disorder, such as:
thrombocytopenia with absent radius (TAR syndrome) (Q87.2)

D69.49 **Other primary thrombocytopenia** `HCC` `ESR` `COM`
Megakaryocytic hypoplasia
Primary thrombocytopenia NOS

D69.5 **Secondary thrombocytopenia** ✓5th
EXCLUDES 1   *heparin induced thrombocytopenia (HIT)* ▶*(D75.82-)*◀
transient thrombocytopenia of newborn (P61.0)

D69.51 **Posttransfusion purpura**
Posttransfusion purpura from whole blood (fresh) or blood products
PTP

D69.59 **Other secondary thrombocytopenia**
AHA: 2014,4Q,22

D69.6 **Thrombocytopenia, unspecified** `HCC` `ESR`
AHA: 2020,3Q,24

D69.8 **Other specified hemorrhagic conditions** `HCC` `ESR`
Capillary fragility (hereditary)
Vascular pseudohemophilia

D69.9 **Hemorrhagic condition, unspecified** `HCC` `ESR`

Other disorders of blood and blood-forming organs (D70-D77)

D70 **Neutropenia** ✓4th
INCLUDES   agranulocytosis
decreased absolute neurophile count (ANC)
Use additional code for any associated:
fever (R50.81)
mucositis (J34.81, K12.3-, K92.81, N76.81)
EXCLUDES 1   *neutropenic splenomegaly (D73.81)*
transient neonatal neutropenia (P61.5)
DEF: Abnormally low number of neutrophils. Neutrophils are phagocytic, meaning they surround and consume harmful pathogens, primarily bacteria. When neutrophil counts decrease the risk of infection increases.

D70.0 **Congenital agranulocytosis** `HCC` `ESR` `COM`
Congenital neutropenia
Infantile genetic agranulocytosis
Kostmann's disease

D70.1 **Agranulocytosis secondary to cancer chemotherapy** `HCC` `ESR`
Code also underlying neoplasm
Use additional code for adverse effect, if applicable, to identify drug (T45.1X5)
AHA: 2020,3Q,22; 2014,4Q,22

D70.2 **Other drug-induced agranulocytosis** `HCC` `ESR`
Use additional code for adverse effect, if applicable, to identify drug (T36-T50 with fifth or sixth character 5)

D70.3 **Neutropenia due to infection** `HCC` `ESR`

D70.4 **Cyclic neutropenia** `HCC` `ESR` `COM`
Cyclic hematopoiesis
Periodic neutropenia

D70.8 **Other neutropenia** `HCC` `ESR`

D70.9 **Neutropenia, unspecified** `HCC` `ESR`
AHA: 2020,3Q,24

Chapter 3. Diseases of the Blood and Blood-forming Organs

D71 Functional disorders of polymorphonuclear neutrophils   `HCC` `ESR` `COM`
Cell membrane receptor complex [CR3] defect
Chronic (childhood) granulomatous disease
Congenital dysphagocytosis
Progressive septic granulomatosis

✓4ᵗʰ D72 Other disorders of white blood cells
   EXCLUDES 1   basophilia (D72.824)
       immunity disorders (D80-D89)
       neutropenia (D70)
       preleukemia (syndrome) (D46.9)

D72.0 Genetic anomalies of leukocytes   `HCC` `ESR` `COM`
Alder (granulation) (granulocyte) anomaly
Alder syndrome
Hereditary leukocytic hypersegmentation
Hereditary leukocytic hyposegmentation
Hereditary leukomelanopathy
May-Hegglin (granulation) (granulocyte) anomaly
May-Hegglin syndrome
Pelger-Huët (granulation) (granulocyte) anomaly
Pelger-Huët syndrome
   EXCLUDES 1   Chédiak (-Steinbrinck)-Higashi syndrome (E70.330)

✓5ᵗʰ D72.1 Eosinophilia
   EXCLUDES 2   Löffler's syndrome (J82.89)
       pulmonary eosinophilia (J82.-)
   AHA: 2020,4Q,8-10
   DEF: Abnormally large accumulation or formation of eosinophils (nucleated, granular leukocytes) in the blood, characteristic of allergic states and infection.

   D72.10 Eosinophilia, unspecified
✓6ᵗʰ D72.11 Hypereosinophilic syndrome [HES]
     D72.110 Idiopathic hypereosinophilic syndrome [IHES]
     D72.111 Lymphocytic Variant Hypereosinophilic Syndrome [LHES]
        Lymphocyte variant hypereosinophilia
        Code also, if applicable, any associated lymphocytic neoplastic disorder
     D72.118 Other hypereosinophilic syndrome
        Episodic angioedema with eosinophilia
        Gleich's syndrome
     D72.119 Hypereosinophilic syndrome [HES], unspecified
   D72.12 Drug rash with eosinophilia and systemic symptoms syndrome
      DRESS syndrome
      Use additional code for adverse effect, if applicable, to identify drug (T36-T50 with fifth or sixth character 5)
   D72.18 Eosinophilia in diseases classified elsewhere
      Code first underlying disease, such as:
      chronic myelomonocytic leukemia (C93.1-)
   D72.19 Other eosinophilia
      Familial eosinophilia
      Hereditary eosinophilia

✓5ᵗʰ D72.8 Other specified disorders of white blood cells
   EXCLUDES 1   leukemia (C91-C95)
✓6ᵗʰ D72.81 Decreased white blood cell count
     EXCLUDES 1   neutropenia (D70.-)
     D72.810 Lymphocytopenia
        Decreased lymphocytes
     D72.818 Other decreased white blood cell count
        Basophilic leukopenia
        Eosinophilic leukopenia
        Monocytopenia
        Other decreased leukocytes
        Plasmacytopenia
     D72.819 Decreased white blood cell count, unspecified
        Decreased leukocytes, unspecified
        Leukocytopenia, unspecified
        Leukopenia
       EXCLUDES 1   malignant leukopenia (D70.9)

✓6ᵗʰ D72.82 Elevated white blood cell count
   EXCLUDES 1   eosinophilia (D72.1)
   D72.820 Lymphocytosis (symptomatic)
      Elevated lymphocytes
   D72.821 Monocytosis (symptomatic)
     EXCLUDES 1   infectious mononucleosis (B27.-)
   D72.822 Plasmacytosis
   D72.823 Leukemoid reaction
      Basophilic leukemoid reaction
      Leukemoid reaction NOS
      Lymphocytic leukemoid reaction
      Monocytic leukemoid reaction
      Myelocytic leukemoid reaction
      Neutrophilic leukemoid reaction
   D72.824 Basophilia
      DEF: Increase in the basophils of the blood, a type of white blood cell, often seen in conjunction with neoplastic disorders.
   D72.825 Bandemia
      Bandemia without diagnosis of specific infection
     EXCLUDES 1   confirmed infection - code to infection
        leukemia (C91.-, C92.-, C93.-, C94.-, C95.-)
      DEF: Increase in early neutrophil cells, called band cells, that may indicate infection.
   D72.828 Other elevated white blood cell count
   D72.829 Elevated white blood cell count, unspecified
      Elevated leukocytes, unspecified
      Leukocytosis, unspecified
   D72.89 Other specified disorders of white blood cells
      Abnormality of white blood cells NEC
  D72.9 Disorder of white blood cells, unspecified
     Abnormal leukocyte differential NOS

✓4ᵗʰ D73 Diseases of spleen
  D73.0 Hyposplenism
     Atrophy of spleen
   EXCLUDES 1   asplenia (congenital) (Q89.01)
       postsurgical absence of spleen (Z90.81)
  D73.1 Hypersplenism
   EXCLUDES 1   neutropenic splenomegaly (D73.81)
       primary splenic neutropenia (D73.81)
       splenitis, splenomegaly in late syphilis (A52.79)
       splenitis, splenomegaly in tuberculosis (A18.85)
       splenomegaly NOS (R16.1)
       splenomegaly congenital (Q89.0)
  D73.2 Chronic congestive splenomegaly
  D73.3 Abscess of spleen
  D73.4 Cyst of spleen
  D73.5 Infarction of spleen
     Splenic rupture, nontraumatic
     Torsion of spleen
   EXCLUDES 1   rupture of spleen due to Plasmodium vivax malaria (B51.0)
       traumatic rupture of spleen (S36.03-)
✓5ᵗʰ D73.8 Other diseases of spleen
   D73.81 Neutropenic splenomegaly
      Werner-Schultz disease
   D73.89 Other diseases of spleen
      Fibrosis of spleen NOS
      Perisplenitis
      Splenitis NOS
  D73.9 Disease of spleen, unspecified

✓4ᵗʰ D74 Methemoglobinemia
  D74.0 Congenital methemoglobinemia
     Congenital NADH-methemoglobin reductase deficiency
     Hemoglobin-M [Hb-M] disease
     Methemoglobinemia, hereditary
  D74.8 Other methemoglobinemias
     Acquired methemoglobinemia (with sulfhemoglobinemia)
     Toxic methemoglobinemia
  D74.9 Methemoglobinemia, unspecified

✓4ᵗʰ **D75　Other and unspecified diseases of blood and blood-forming organs**

　　EXCLUDES 2　*acute lymphadenitis (L04.-)*
　　　　　　　chronic lymphadenitis (I88.1)
　　　　　　　enlarged lymph nodes (R59.-)
　　　　　　　hypergammaglobulinemia NOS (D89.2)
　　　　　　　lymphadenitis NOS (I88.9)
　　　　　　　mesenteric lymphadenitis (acute) (chronic) (I88.0)

　D75.0　Familial erythrocytosis
　　　Benign polycythemia
　　　Familial polycythemia
　　　EXCLUDES 1　*hereditary ovalocytosis (D58.1)*

　D75.1　Secondary polycythemia
　　　Acquired polycythemia
　　　Emotional polycythemia
　　　Erythrocytosis NOS
　　　Hypoxemic polycythemia
　　　Nephrogenous polycythemia
　　　Polycythemia due to erythropoietin
　　　Polycythemia due to fall in plasma volume
　　　Polycythemia due to high altitude
　　　Polycythemia due to stress
　　　Polycythemia NOS
　　　Relative polycythemia
　　　EXCLUDES 1　*polycythemia neonatorum (P61.1)*
　　　　　　　polycythemia vera (D45)
　　　DEF: Elevated number of red blood cells in circulating blood as a result of reduced oxygen supply to the tissues.

✓5ᵗʰ **D75.8　Other specified diseases of blood and blood-forming organs**

　　D75.81　*Myelofibrosis* 　HCC Rx ESR COM
　　　Myelofibrosis NOS
　　　Secondary myelofibrosis NOS
　　　Code first the underlying disorder, such as:
　　　　malignant neoplasm of breast (C50.-)
　　　Use additional code, if applicable, for associated therapy-related myelodysplastic syndrome (D46.-)
　　　Use additional code for adverse effect, if applicable, to identify drug (T45.1X5)
　　　EXCLUDES 1　*acute myelofibrosis (C94.4-)*
　　　　　　　idiopathic myelofibrosis (D47.1)
　　　　　　　leukoerythroblastic anemia (D61.82)
　　　　　　　myelofibrosis with myeloid metaplasia (D47.4)
　　　　　　　myelophthisic anemia (D61.82)
　　　　　　　myelophthisis (D61.82)
　　　　　　　primary myelofibrosis (D47.1)

▲　✓6ᵗʰ **D75.82　Heparin induced thrombocytopenia (HIT)**
　　　▶Use additional code, if applicable, for adverse effect of heparin (T45.515-)◀
　　　DEF: Immune-mediated reaction to heparin therapy causing an abrupt fall in platelet count and serious complications such as pulmonary embolism, stroke, AMI, or DVT.

　　●**D75.821　Non-immune heparin-induced thrombocytopenia**
　　　Non-immune HIT
　　　Type 1 heparin-induced thrombocytopenia

　　●**D75.822　Immune-mediated heparin-induced thrombocytopenia**
　　　Immune-mediated HIT
　　　Type 2 heparin-induced thrombocytopenia

　　●**D75.828　Other heparin-induced thrombocytopenia syndrome**
　　　Autoimmune heparin-induced thrombocytopenia syndrome
　　　Delayed-onset heparin-induced thrombocytopenia
　　　Persisting heparin-induced thrombocytopenia

　　●**D75.829　Heparin-induced thrombocytopenia, unspecified**

　　✓6ᵗʰ **D75.83　Thrombocytosis**
　　　EXCLUDES 2　*essential thrombocythemia (D47.3)*
　　　AHA: 2021,4Q,7-8
　　　D75.838　Other thrombocytosis
　　　　Reactive thrombocytosis
　　　　Secondary thrombocytosis
　　　　Code also underlying condition, if known and applicable
　　　D75.839　Thrombocytosis, unspecified
　　　　Thrombocythemia NOS
　　　　Thrombocytosis NOS

　●**D75.84　Other platelet-activating anti-PF4 disorders**
　　　Spontaneous heparin-induced thrombocytopenia syndrome (without heparin exposure)
　　　Thrombosis with thrombocytopenia syndrome
　　　Vaccine-induced thrombotic thrombocytopenia
　　　Use additional code, if applicable, for adverse effect of other viral vaccine (T50.B95-)

　　D75.89　Other specified diseases of blood and blood-forming organs

　D75.9　Disease of blood and blood-forming organs, unspecified

　D75.A　Glucose-6-phosphate dehydrogenase (G6PD) deficiency without anemia
　　　EXCLUDES 1　*glucose-6-phosphate dehydrogenase (G6PD) deficiency with anemia (D55.0)*
　　　AHA: 2019,4Q,4-5

✓4ᵗʰ **D76　Other specified diseases with participation of lymphoreticular and reticulohistiocytic tissue**

　　EXCLUDES 1　*(Abt-) Letterer-Siwe disease (C96.0)*
　　　　　　　eosinophilic granuloma (C96.6)
　　　　　　　Hand-Schüller-Christian disease (C96.5)
　　　　　　　histiocytic medullary reticulosis (C96.9)
　　　　　　　histiocytic sarcoma (C96.A)
　　　　　　　histiocytosis X, multifocal (C96.5)
　　　　　　　histiocytosis X, unifocal (C96.6)
　　　　　　　Langerhans-cell histiocytosis, multifocal (C96.5)
　　　　　　　Langerhans-cell histiocytosis NOS (C96.6)
　　　　　　　Langerhans-cell histiocytosis, unifocal (C96.6)
　　　　　　　leukemic reticuloendotheliosis (C91.4-)
　　　　　　　lipomelanotic reticulosis (I89.8)
　　　　　　　malignant histiocytosis (C96.A)
　　　　　　　malignant reticulosis (C86.0)
　　　　　　　nonlipid reticuloendotheliosis (C96.0)

　D76.1　Hemophagocytic lymphohistiocytosis　HCC ESR COM
　　　Familial hemophagocytic reticulosis
　　　Histiocytoses of mononuclear phagocytes

　D76.2　Hemophagocytic syndrome, infection-associated　HCC ESR COM
　　　Use additional code to identify infectious agent or disease

　D76.3　Other histiocytosis syndromes　HCC ESR COM
　　　Reticulohistiocytoma (giant-cell)
　　　Sinus histiocytosis with massive lymphadenopathy
　　　Xanthogranuloma

D77　*Other disorders of blood and blood-forming organs in diseases classified elsewhere*
　　Code first underlying disease, such as:
　　　amyloidosis (E85.-)
　　　congenital early syphilis (A50.0)
　　　echinococcosis (B67.0-B67.9)
　　　malaria (B50.0-B54)
　　　schistosomiasis [bilharziasis] (B65.0-B65.9)
　　　vitamin C deficiency (E54)
　　　EXCLUDES 1　*rupture of spleen due to Plasmodium vivax malaria (B51.0)*
　　　　　　　splenitis, splenomegaly in late syphilis (A52.79)
　　　　　　　splenitis, splenomegaly in tuberculosis (A18.85)

Intraoperative and postprocedural complications of the spleen (D78)

☑4th D78 Intraoperative and postprocedural complications of the spleen
AHA: 2016,4Q,9-10

☑5th D78.0 Intraoperative hemorrhage and hematoma of the spleen complicating a procedure
EXCLUDES 1   intraoperative hemorrhage and hematoma of the spleen due to accidental puncture or laceration during a procedure (D78.1-)

D78.01 Intraoperative hemorrhage and hematoma of the spleen complicating a procedure on the spleen

D78.02 Intraoperative hemorrhage and hematoma of the spleen complicating other procedure

☑5th D78.1 Accidental puncture and laceration of the spleen during a procedure

D78.11 Accidental puncture and laceration of the spleen during a procedure on the spleen

D78.12 Accidental puncture and laceration of the spleen during other procedure
AHA: 2022,1Q,22

☑5th D78.2 Postprocedural hemorrhage of the spleen following a procedure

D78.21 Postprocedural hemorrhage of the spleen following a procedure on the spleen

D78.22 Postprocedural hemorrhage of the spleen following other procedure

☑5th D78.3 Postprocedural hematoma and seroma of the spleen following a procedure

D78.31 Postprocedural hematoma of the spleen following a procedure on the spleen

D78.32 Postprocedural hematoma of the spleen following other procedure

D78.33 Postprocedural seroma of the spleen following a procedure on the spleen

D78.34 Postprocedural seroma of the spleen following other procedure

☑5th D78.8 Other intraoperative and postprocedural complications of the spleen
Use additional code, if applicable, to further specify disorder

D78.81 Other intraoperative complications of the spleen

D78.89 Other postprocedural complications of the spleen

Certain disorders involving the immune mechanism (D80-D89)

INCLUDES   defects in the complement system
immunodeficiency disorders, except human immunodeficiency virus [HIV] disease
sarcoidosis

EXCLUDES 1   autoimmune disease (systemic) NOS (M35.9)
functional disorders of polymorphonuclear neutrophils (D71)
human immunodeficiency virus [HIV] disease (B20)

☑4th D80 Immunodeficiency with predominantly antibody defects

D80.0 Hereditary hypogammaglobulinemia   HCC Rx ESR COM
Autosomal recessive agammaglobulinemia (Swiss type)
X-linked agammaglobulinemia [Bruton] (with growth hormone deficiency)

D80.1 Nonfamilial hypogammaglobulinemia   HCC Rx ESR COM
Agammaglobulinemia with immunoglobulin-bearing B-lymphocytes
Common variable agammaglobulinemia [CVAgamma]
Hypogammaglobulinemia NOS

D80.2 Selective deficiency of immunoglobulin A [IgA]   HCC Rx ESR COM

D80.3 Selective deficiency of immunoglobulin G [IgG] subclasses   HCC Rx ESR COM

D80.4 Selective deficiency of immunoglobulin M [IgM]   HCC Rx ESR COM

D80.5 Immunodeficiency with increased immunoglobulin M [IgM]   HCC Rx ESR COM

D80.6 Antibody deficiency with near-normal immunoglobulins or with hyperimmunoglobulinemia   HCC Rx ESR COM

D80.7 Transient hypogammaglobulinemia of infancy   HCC Rx ESR COM

D80.8 Other immunodeficiencies with predominantly antibody defects   HCC Rx ESR COM
Kappa light chain deficiency

D80.9 Immunodeficiency with predominantly antibody defects, unspecified   HCC Rx ESR COM

☑4th D81 Combined immunodeficiencies
EXCLUDES 1   autosomal recessive agammaglobulinemia (Swiss type) (D80.0)

D81.0 Severe combined immunodeficiency [SCID] with reticular dysgenesis   HCC Rx ESR COM

D81.1 Severe combined immunodeficiency [SCID] with low T- and B-cell numbers   HCC Rx ESR COM

D81.2 Severe combined immunodeficiency [SCID] with low or normal B-cell numbers   HCC Rx ESR COM

☑5th D81.3 Adenosine deaminase [ADA] deficiency
AHA: 2019,4Q,5-6

D81.30 Adenosine deaminase deficiency, unspecified   HCC Rx ESR COM
ADA deficiency NOS

D81.31 Severe combined immunodeficiency due to adenosine deaminase deficiency   HCC Rx ESR COM
ADA deficiency with SCID
Adenosine deaminase [ADA] deficiency with severe combined immunodeficiency

D81.32 Adenosine deaminase 2 deficiency   HCC Rx ESR COM
ADA2 deficiency
Adenosine deaminase deficiency type 2
Code also, if applicable, any associated manifestations, such as:
polyarteritis nodosa (M30.0)
stroke (I63.-)

D81.39 Other adenosine deaminase deficiency   HCC Rx ESR COM
Adenosine deaminase [ADA] deficiency type 1, NOS
Adenosine deaminase [ADA] deficiency type 1, without SCID
Adenosine deaminase [ADA] deficiency type 1, without severe combined immunodeficiency
Partial ADA deficiency (type 1)
Partial adenosine deaminase deficiency (type 1)

D81.4 Nezelof's syndrome   HCC Rx ESR COM

D81.5 Purine nucleoside phosphorylase [PNP] deficiency   HCC Rx ESR COM

D81.6 Major histocompatibility complex class I deficiency   HCC Rx ESR COM
Bare lymphocyte syndrome

D81.7 Major histocompatibility complex class II deficiency   HCC Rx ESR COM

☑5th D81.8 Other combined immunodeficiencies

☑6th D81.81 Biotin-dependent carboxylase deficiency
Multiple carboxylase deficiency
EXCLUDES 1   biotin-dependent carboxylase deficiency due to dietary deficiency of biotin (E53.8)

D81.810 Biotinidase deficiency

D81.818 Other biotin-dependent carboxylase deficiency
Holocarboxylase synthetase deficiency
Other multiple carboxylase deficiency

D81.819 Biotin-dependent carboxylase deficiency, unspecified
Multiple carboxylase deficiency, unspecified

D81.82 Activated Phosphoinositide 3-kinase Delta Syndrome [APDS]
p110d-activating mutation causing senescent T cells, lymphadenopathy, and immunodeficiency [PASLI] disease
Code also, if applicable, any associated manifestations, such as:
bronchiectasis (J47.-)
herpes virus infections (B00.-)
other acute respiratory tract infections (J00-J06; J20-J22)
other infections (A00-B99)
pneumonia (J12-J18)

D81.89 Other combined immunodeficiencies   HCC Rx ESR COM

D81.9 Combined immunodeficiency, unspecified   HCC Rx ESR COM
Severe combined immunodeficiency disorder [SCID] NOS

✓4ᵗʰ D82 Immunodeficiency associated with other major defects

> EXCLUDES 1   ataxia telangiectasia [Louis-Bar] (G11.3)

D82.0 Wiskott-Aldrich syndrome   HCC Rx ESR COM
> Immunodeficiency with thrombocytopenia and eczema

D82.1 Di George's syndrome   HCC Rx ESR COM
> Pharyngeal pouch syndrome
> Thymic alymphoplasia
> Thymic aplasia or hypoplasia with immunodeficiency
> AHA: 2019,3Q,14

D82.2 Immunodeficiency with short-limbed stature   HCC Rx ESR COM

D82.3 Immunodeficiency following hereditary defective response to Epstein-Barr virus   HCC Rx ESR COM
> X-linked lymphoproliferative disease

D82.4 Hyperimmunoglobulin E [IgE] syndrome   HCC Rx ESR COM

D82.8 Immunodeficiency associated with other specified major defects   HCC Rx ESR COM

D82.9 Immunodeficiency associated with major defect, unspecified   HCC Rx ESR COM

✓4ᵗʰ D83 Common variable immunodeficiency

D83.0 Common variable immunodeficiency with predominant abnormalities of B-cell numbers and function   HCC Rx ESR COM

D83.1 Common variable immunodeficiency with predominant immunoregulatory T-cell disorders   HCC Rx ESR COM

D83.2 Common variable immunodeficiency with autoantibodies to B- or T-cells   HCC Rx ESR COM

D83.8 Other common variable immunodeficiencies   HCC Rx ESR COM

D83.9 Common variable immunodeficiency, unspecified   HCC Rx ESR COM

✓4ᵗʰ D84 Other immunodeficiencies

D84.0 Lymphocyte function antigen-1 [LFA-1] defect   HCC Rx ESR COM

D84.1 Defects in the complement system   HCC Rx ESR COM
> C1 esterase inhibitor [C1-INH] deficiency

✓5ᵗʰ D84.8 Other specified immunodeficiencies
> AHA: 2020,4Q,10-12

D84.81 Immunodeficiency due to conditions classified elsewhere   HCC Rx ESR COM
> Code first underlying condition, such as:
> chromosomal abnormalities (Q90-Q99)
> diabetes mellitus (E08-E13)
> malignant neoplasms (C00-C96)
>> EXCLUDES 1   certain disorders involving the immune mechanism (D80-D83, D84.0, D84.1, D84.9)
>> human immunodeficiency virus [HIV] disease (B20)
>
> AHA: 2021,1Q,52

✓6ᵗʰ D84.82 Immunodeficiency due to drugs and external causes

D84.821 Immunodeficiency due to drugs   HCC Rx ESR COM
> Immunodeficiency due to (current or past) medication
> Use additional code for adverse effect if applicable, to identify adverse effect of drug (T36-T50 with fifth or six character 5)
> Use additional code, if applicable, for associated long term (current) drug therapy drug or medication such as:
> long term (current) drug therapy systemic steroids (Z79.52)
> other long term (current) drug therapy (Z79.899)

D84.822 Immunodeficiency due to external causes   HCC Rx ESR COM
> Code also, if applicable, radiological procedure and radiotherapy (Y84.2)
> Use additional code for external cause such as:
> exposure to ionizing radiation (W88)

D84.89 Other immunodeficiencies   HCC Rx ESR COM

D84.9 Immunodeficiency, unspecified   HCC Rx ESR COM
> Immunocompromised NOS
> Immunodeficient NOS
> Immunosuppressed NOS
> AHA: 2020,4Q,10

✓4ᵗʰ D86 Sarcoidosis

> DEF: Clustering of immune cells resulting in granuloma formation. Often affects the lungs and lymphatic system but can occur in other body sites.

D86.0 Sarcoidosis of lung   HCC Rx ESR COM

D86.1 Sarcoidosis of lymph nodes

D86.2 Sarcoidosis of lung with sarcoidosis of lymph nodes   HCC Rx ESR COM

D86.3 Sarcoidosis of skin

✓5ᵗʰ D86.8 Sarcoidosis of other sites

D86.81 Sarcoid meningitis   COM

D86.82 Multiple cranial nerve palsies in sarcoidosis   HCC Rx ESR COM

D86.83 Sarcoid iridocyclitis

D86.84 Sarcoid pyelonephritis
> Tubulo-interstitial nephropathy in sarcoidosis

D86.85 Sarcoid myocarditis   COM

D86.86 Sarcoid arthropathy
> Polyarthritis in sarcoidosis

D86.87 Sarcoid myositis

D86.89 Sarcoidosis of other sites
> Hepatic granuloma
> Uveoparotid fever [Heerfordt]

D86.9 Sarcoidosis, unspecified

✓4ᵗʰ D89 Other disorders involving the immune mechanism, not elsewhere classified

> EXCLUDES 1   hyperglobulinemia NOS (R77.1)
> monoclonal gammopathy (of undetermined significance) (D47.2)
> EXCLUDES 2   transplant failure and rejection (T86.-)

D89.0 Polyclonal hypergammaglobulinemia   Rx
> Benign hypergammaglobulinemic purpura
> Polyclonal gammopathy NOS

D89.1 Cryoglobulinemia   HCC Rx ESR
> Cryoglobulinemic purpura
> Cryoglobulinemic vasculitis
> Essential cryoglobulinemia
> Idiopathic cryoglobulinemia
> Mixed cryoglobulinemia
> Primary cryoglobulinemia
> Secondary cryoglobulinemia

D89.2 Hypergammaglobulinemia, unspecified

D89.3 Immune reconstitution syndrome   HCC Rx ESR COM
> Immune reconstitution inflammatory syndrome [IRIS]
> Use additional code for adverse effect, if applicable, to identify drug (T36-T50 with fifth or sixth character 5)

✓5ᵗʰ D89.4 Mast cell activation syndrome and related disorders

> EXCLUDES 1   aggressive systemic mastocytosis (C96.21)
> congenital cutaneous mastocytosis (Q82.2)
> (non-congenital) cutaneous mastocytosis (D47.01)
> (indolent) systemic mastocytosis (D47.02)
> malignant mast cell neoplasm (C96.2-)
> malignant mastocytoma (C96.29)
> mast cell leukemia (C94.3-)
> mast cell sarcoma (C96.22)
> mastocytoma NOS (D47.09)
> other mast cell neoplasms of uncertain behavior (D47.09)
> systemic mastocytosis associated with a clonal hematologic non-mast cell lineage disease (SM-AHNMD) (D47.02)
>
> AHA: 2016,4Q,11

D89.40 Mast cell activation, unspecified   HCC Rx ESR COM
> Mast cell activation disorder, unspecified
> Mast cell activation syndrome, NOS

D89.41 Monoclonal mast cell activation syndrome   HCC Rx ESR COM

D89.42 Idiopathic mast cell activation syndrome   HCC Rx ESR COM

D89.43 **Secondary mast cell activation** `HCC` `Rx` `ESR` `COM`
Secondary mast cell activation syndrome
Code also underlying etiology, if known

D89.44 **Hereditary alpha tryptasemia** `HCC` `Rx` `ESR` `COM`
Use additional code, if applicable, for:
allergy status, other than to drugs and biological
substances (Z91.0-)
personal history of anaphylaxis (Z87.892)
AHA: 2021,4Q,8

D89.49 **Other mast cell activation disorder** `HCC` `Rx` `ESR` `COM`
Other mast cell activation syndrome

✓5ᵗʰ **D89.8** **Other specified disorders involving the immune mechanism, not elsewhere classified**

✓6ᵗʰ **D89.81** **Graft-versus-host disease**
Code first underlying cause, such as:
complications of transplanted organs and tissue
(T86.-)
complications of blood transfusion (T80.89)
Use additional code to identify associated
manifestations, such as:
desquamative dermatitis (L30.8)
diarrhea (R19.7)
elevated bilirubin (R17)
hair loss (L65.9)

D89.810 **Acute graft-versus-host disease** `HCC` `Rx` `ESR` `COM` `UPD`

D89.811 **Chronic graft-versus-host disease** `HCC` `Rx` `ESR` `COM` `UPD`

D89.812 **Acute on chronic graft-versus-host disease** `HCC` `Rx` `ESR` `COM` `UPD`

D89.813 **Graft-versus-host disease, unspecified** `HCC` `Rx` `ESR` `COM` `UPD`

D89.82 **Autoimmune lymphoproliferative syndrome [ALPS]** `HCC` `ESR` `COM`
DEF: Rare genetic alteration of the Fas protein that
impairs normal cellular apoptosis (normal cell death),
causing abnormal accumulation of lymphocytes in the
lymph glands, liver, and spleen. Symptoms include
neutropenia, anemia, and thrombocytopenia.

✓6ᵗʰ **D89.83** **Cytokine release syndrome**
Code first underlying cause, such as:
complications following infusion, transfusion and
therapeutic injection (T80.89-)
complications of transplanted organs and tissue
(T86.-)
Use additional code to identify associated
manifestations
AHA: 2020,4Q,12-15
DEF: Form of systemic inflammatory response
syndrome (SIRS) in which immune substances
(cytokines) are released rapidly and in large amounts
from the affected immune cells into the blood. The
severity of associated symptoms or manifestations
varies based on the underlying cause. This syndrome
occurs as a complication of a disease, infection, or drug
(often an adverse effect of immunotherapy in the form
of treatment receiving monoclonal antibodies or
Chimeric Antigen Receptor T [CAR-T] cells).

D89.831 **Cytokine release syndrome, grade 1** `UPD`

D89.832 **Cytokine release syndrome, grade 2** `UPD`

D89.833 **Cytokine release syndrome, grade 3** `UPD`

D89.834 **Cytokine release syndrome, grade 4** `UPD`

D89.835 **Cytokine release syndrome, grade 5** `UPD`

D89.839 **Cytokine release syndrome, grade unspecified** `UPD`

D89.89 **Other specified disorders involving the immune mechanism, not elsewhere classified** `HCC` `Rx` `ESR` `COM`
`EXCLUDES 1`   *human immunodeficiency virus disease (B20)*
AHA: 2017,4Q,109

D89.9 **Disorder involving the immune mechanism, unspecified** `HCC` `Rx` `ESR` `COM`
Immune disease NOS
AHA: 2015,3Q,22

`HCC` CMS-HCC   `Rx` Rx HCC   `ESR` ESRD HCC   `COM` Commercial HCC   `N` Newborn: 0   `P` Pediatric: 0-17   `M` Maternity: 9-64   `A` Adult: 15-124

528   ICD-10-CM 2023

Chapter 4. Endocrine, Nutritional, and Metabolic Diseases (E00–E89)

Chapter-specific Guidelines with Coding Examples

The chapter-specific guidelines from the ICD-10-CM Official Guidelines for Coding and Reporting have been provided below. Along with these guidelines are coding examples, contained in the shaded boxes, that have been developed to help illustrate the coding and/or sequencing guidance found in these guidelines.

a. Diabetes mellitus

The diabetes mellitus codes are combination codes that include the type of diabetes mellitus, the body system affected, and the complications affecting that body system. As many codes within a particular category as are necessary to describe all of the complications of the disease may be used. They should be sequenced based on the reason for a particular encounter. Assign as many codes from categories E08–E13 as needed to identify all of the associated conditions that the patient has.

> Patient is seen for uncontrolled diabetes, type 2, with hyperglycemia diabetic nephropathy, and diabetic gastroparesis
>
> **E11.65**   **Type 2 diabetes mellitus with hyperglycemia**
>
> **E11.21**   **Type 2 diabetes mellitus with diabetic nephropathy**
>
> **E11.43**   **Type 2 diabetes mellitus with diabetic autonomic (poly)neuropathy**
>
> **K31.84**   **Gastroparesis**
>
> *Explanation*: Use as many codes to describe the diabetic complications as needed. Many are combination codes that describe more than one condition. Code first the reason for the encounter. The term "uncontrolled" can refer to either hyperglycemia or hypoglycemia. In this case, "uncontrolled" is described as "with hyperglycemia."

1) Type of diabetes

The age of a patient is not the sole determining factor, though most type 1 diabetics develop the condition before reaching puberty. For this reason, type 1 diabetes mellitus is also referred to as juvenile diabetes.

> A 45-year-old patient is diagnosed with type 1 diabetes
>
> **E10.9**   **Type 1 diabetes mellitus without complications**
>
> *Explanation*: Although most type 1 diabetics are diagnosed in childhood or adolescence, it can also begin in adults.

2) Type of diabetes mellitus not documented

If the type of diabetes mellitus is not documented in the medical record the default is E11.-, Type 2 diabetes mellitus.

> Office visit lists diabetic retinopathy with macular edema and hypertension on patient problem list
>
> **E11.311**   **Type 2 diabetes mellitus with unspecified diabetic retinopathy with macular edema**
>
> **I10**   **Essential (primary) hypertension**
>
> *Explanation*: Since the type of diabetes was not documented, default to category E11.

3) Diabetes mellitus and the use of insulin, oral hypoglycemics, and injectable non-insulin drugs

If the documentation in a medical record does not indicate the type of diabetes but does indicate that the patient uses insulin, code E11-, Type 2 diabetes mellitus, should be assigned. Additional code(s) should be assigned from category Z79 to identify the long-term (current) use of insulin, oral hypoglycemic drugs, or injectable non-insulin antidiabetic, as follows:

> If the patient is treated with both oral **hypoglycemic drugs** and insulin, both code Z79.4, Long term (current) use of insulin, and code Z79.84, Long term (current) use of oral hypoglycemic drugs, should be assigned.
>
> If the patient is treated with both insulin and an injectable non-insulin antidiabetic drug, assign codes Z79.4, Long term (current) use of insulin, and **Z79.85, Long-term (current) use of injectable non-insulin antidiabetic drugs.**

If the patient is treated with both oral hypoglycemic drugs and an injectable non-insulin antidiabetic drug, assign codes Z79.84, Long term (current) use of oral hypoglycemic drugs, and **Z79.85, Long-term (current) use of injectable non-insulin antidiabetic drugs.**

Code Z79.4 should not be assigned if insulin is given temporarily to bring a type 2 patient's blood sugar under control during an encounter.

> Office visit lists chronic diabetes with daily insulin use on patient problem list
>
> **E11.9**   **Type 2 diabetes mellitus without complications**
>
> **Z79.4**   **Long term (current) use of insulin**
>
> *Explanation*: Do not assume that a patient on insulin must have type 1 diabetes. The default for diabetes without further specification defaults to type 2. Add the code for long term use of insulin.

4) Diabetes mellitus in pregnancy and gestational diabetes

See Section I.C.15. Diabetes mellitus in pregnancy.

See Section I.C.15. Gestational (pregnancy induced) diabetes

5) Complications due to insulin pump malfunction

(a) Underdose of insulin due to insulin pump failure

An underdose of insulin due to an insulin pump failure should be assigned to a code from subcategory T85.6, Mechanical complication of other specified internal and external prosthetic devices, implants and grafts, that specifies the type of pump malfunction, as the principal or first-listed code, followed by code T38.3X6-, Underdosing of insulin and oral hypoglycemic [antidiabetic] drugs. Additional codes for the type of diabetes mellitus and any associated complications due to the underdosing should also be assigned.

> A 24-year-old type 1 diabetic male treated in for hyperglycemia; insulin pump found to be malfunctioning and underdosing
>
> **T85.614A**   **Breakdown (mechanical) of insulin pump, initial encounter**
>
> **T38.3X6A**   **Underdosing of insulin and oral hypoglycemic [antidiabetic] drugs, initial encounter**
>
> **E10.65**   **Type 1 diabetes mellitus with hyperglycemia**
>
> *Explanation*: The complication code for the mechanical breakdown of the pump is sequenced first, followed by the underdosing code and type of diabetes with complication. Code all other diabetic complication codes necessary to describe the patient's condition.

(b) Overdose of insulin due to insulin pump failure

The principal or first-listed code for an encounter due to an insulin pump malfunction resulting in an overdose of insulin, should also be T85.6-, Mechanical complication of other specified internal and external prosthetic devices, implants and grafts, followed by code T38.3X1-, Poisoning by insulin and oral hypoglycemic [antidiabetic] drugs, accidental (unintentional).

> A 24-year-old type 1 diabetic male found down with diabetic coma, brought into ED and treated for hypoglycemia; insulin pump found to be malfunctioning and overdosing
>
> **T85.614A**   **Breakdown (mechanical) of insulin pump, initial encounter**
>
> **T38.3X1A**   **Poisoning by insulin and oral hypoglycemic [antidiabetic] drugs, accidental (unintentional), initial encounter**
>
> **E10.641**   **Type 1 diabetes mellitus with hypoglycemia with coma**
>
> *Explanation*: The complication code for the mechanical breakdown of the pump is sequenced first, followed by the poisoning code and type of diabetes with complication. All the characters in the combination code must be used to form a valid code and to fully describe the type of diabetes, the hypoglycemia, and the coma.

6) Secondary diabetes mellitus

Codes under categories E08, Diabetes mellitus due to underlying condition, E09, Drug or chemical induced diabetes mellitus, and E13, Other specified diabetes mellitus, identify complications/manifestations associated with secondary diabetes mellitus. Secondary diabetes is always caused by another condition or event (e.g., cystic fibrosis, malignant neoplasm of pancreas, pancreatectomy, adverse effect of drug, or poisoning).

(a) Secondary diabetes mellitus and the use of insulin or oral hypoglycemic drugs

For patients with secondary diabetes mellitus who routinely use insulin, oral hypoglycemic drugs, or injectable non-insulin drugs, additional code(s) from category Z79 should be assigned to identify the long-term (current) use of insulin, oral hypoglycemic drugs, or non-injectable non-insulin drugs as follows:

If the patient is treated with both oral **hypoglycemic drugs** and insulin, both code Z79.4, Long term (current) use of insulin, and code Z79.84, Long term (current) use of oral hypoglycemic drugs, should be assigned.

If the patient is treated with both insulin and an injectable non-insulin antidiabetic drug, assign codes Z79.4, Long-term (current) use of insulin, and **Z79.85, Long-term (current) use of injectable non-insulin antidiabetic drugs**.

If the patient is treated with both oral hypoglycemic drugs and an injectable non-insulin antidiabetic drug, assign codes Z79.84, Long-term (current) use of oral hypoglycemic drugs, and **Z79.85, Long-term (current) use of injectable non-insulin antidiabetic drugs.**

Code Z79.4 should not be assigned if insulin is given temporarily to bring a secondary diabetic patient's blood sugar under control during an encounter.

Type 2 diabetic with no complications, normally only on oral metformin, is given insulin for three days to maintain glucose control while in the hospital recovering from surgery

E11.9	**Type 2 diabetes mellitus without complications**
Z79.84	**Long term (current) use of oral hypoglycemic drugs**

Explanation: Although the patient was given insulin for a short time during his hospital stay, the intent was only to maintain the patient's glucose levels while off his regular oral hypoglycemic medication, not for long term use. No code is needed for long term use of insulin, but a Z code for long term use of an oral hypoglycemic should be added to identify the chronic use of this drug.

Type 2 diabetic with diabetic polyneuropathy on insulin

E11.42	**Type 2 diabetes mellitus with diabetic polyneuropathy**
Z79.4	**Long term (current) use of insulin**

Explanation: Add a Z code for the long term use of insulin and the long term use of metformin because both are taken chronically.

(b) Assigning and sequencing secondary diabetes codes and its causes

The sequencing of the secondary diabetes codes in relationship to codes for the cause of the diabetes is based on the Tabular List instructions for categories E08, E09 and E13.

(i) Secondary diabetes mellitus due to pancreatectomy

For postpancreatectomy diabetes mellitus (lack of insulin due to the surgical removal of all or part of the pancreas), assign code E89.1, Postprocedural hypoinsulinemia. Assign a code from category E13 and a code from subcategory Z90.41-, Acquired absence of pancreas, as additional codes.

Patient with newly diagnosed diabetes after surgical removal of part of pancreas

E89.1	**Postprocedural hypoinsulinemia**
E13.9	**Other specified diabetes mellitus without complications**
Z90.411	**Acquired partial absence of pancreas**

Explanation: Sequence the postprocedural complication of the hypoinsulinemia due to the partial removal of the pancreas as the first-listed code, followed by codes for other specified diabetes (NEC) without complications and partial acquired absence of the pancreas.

(ii) Secondary diabetes due to drugs

Secondary diabetes may be caused by an adverse effect of correctly administered medications, poisoning or sequela of poisoning.

See section I.C.19.e. for coding of adverse effects and poisoning, and section I.C.20 for external cause code reporting.

Initial encounter for corticosteroid-induced diabetes mellitus

E09.9	**Drug or chemical induced diabetes mellitus without complications**
T38.0X5A	**Adverse effect of glucocorticoids and synthetic analogues, initial encounter**

Explanation: If the diabetes is caused by an adverse effect of a drug, the diabetic condition is coded first. If it occurs from a poisoning or overdose, the poisoning code causing the diabetes is sequenced first.

Chapter 4. Endocrine, Nutritional and Metabolic Diseases (E00-E89)

NOTE All neoplasms, whether functionally active or not, are classified in Chapter 2. Appropriate codes in this chapter (i.e. E05.8, E07.0, E16-E31, E34.-) may be used as additional codes to indicate either functional activity by neoplasms and ectopic endocrine tissue or hyperfunction and hypofunction of endocrine glands associated with neoplasms and other conditions classified elsewhere.

EXCLUDES 1   *transitory endocrine and metabolic disorders specific to newborn (P70-P74)*

AHA: 2018,2Q,6

This chapter contains the following blocks:

E00-E07	Disorders of thyroid gland
E08-E13	Diabetes mellitus
E15-E16	Other disorders of glucose regulation and pancreatic internal secretion
E20-E35	Disorders of other endocrine glands
E36	Intraoperative complications of endocrine system
E40-E46	Malnutrition
E50-E64	Other nutritional deficiencies
E65-E68	Overweight, obesity and other hyperalimentation
E70-E88	Metabolic disorders
E89	Postprocedural endocrine and metabolic complications and disorders, not elsewhere classified

Disorders of thyroid gland (E00-E07)

✓4ᵗʰ E00 Congenital iodine-deficiency syndrome

Use additional code (F70-F79) to identify associated intellectual disabilities

EXCLUDES 1   *subclinical iodine-deficiency hypothyroidism (E02)*

E00.0 Congenital iodine-deficiency syndrome, neurological type `Rx`

Endemic cretinism, neurological type

E00.1 Congenital iodine-deficiency syndrome, myxedematous type `Rx`

Endemic hypothyroid cretinism

Endemic cretinism, myxedematous type

E00.2 Congenital iodine-deficiency syndrome, mixed type `Rx`

Endemic cretinism, mixed type

E00.9 Congenital iodine-deficiency syndrome, unspecified `Rx`

Congenital iodine-deficiency hypothyroidism NOS

Endemic cretinism NOS

✓4ᵗʰ E01 Iodine-deficiency related thyroid disorders and allied conditions

EXCLUDES 1   *congenital iodine-deficiency syndrome (E00.-)*
subclinical iodine-deficiency hypothyroidism (E02)

E01.0 Iodine-deficiency related diffuse (endemic) goiter `Rx`

E01.1 Iodine-deficiency related multinodular (endemic) goiter `Rx`

Iodine-deficiency related nodular goiter

E01.2 Iodine-deficiency related (endemic) goiter, unspecified `Rx`

Endemic goiter NOS

E01.8 Other iodine-deficiency related thyroid disorders and allied conditions `Rx`

Acquired iodine-deficiency hypothyroidism NOS

E02 Subclinical iodine-deficiency hypothyroidism `Rx`

AHA: 2021,1Q,8

✓4ᵗʰ E03 Other hypothyroidism

EXCLUDES 1   *iodine-deficiency related hypothyroidism (E00-E02)*
postprocedural hypothyroidism (E89.0)

DEF: Hypothyroidism: Underproduction of thyroid hormone.

E03.0 Congenital hypothyroidism with diffuse goiter `Rx`

Congenital parenchymatous goiter (nontoxic)

Congenital goiter (nontoxic) NOS

EXCLUDES 1   *transitory congenital goiter with normal function (P72.0)*

E03.1 Congenital hypothyroidism without goiter `Rx`

Aplasia of thyroid (with myxedema)

Congenital atrophy of thyroid

Congenital hypothyroidism NOS

E03.2 Hypothyroidism due to medicaments and other exogenous substances `Rx`

Code first poisoning due to drug or toxin, if applicable (T36-T65 with fifth or sixth character 1-4 or 6)

Use additional code for adverse effect, if applicable, to identify drug (T36-T50 with fifth or sixth character 5)

E03.3 Postinfectious hypothyroidism `Rx`

E03.4 Atrophy of thyroid (acquired) `Rx`

EXCLUDES 1   *congenital atrophy of thyroid (E03.1)*

E03.5 Myxedema coma `HCC` `Rx` `ESR` `COM`

E03.8 Other specified hypothyroidism `Rx`

AHA: 2021,1Q,8

E03.9 Hypothyroidism, unspecified `Rx`

Myxedema NOS

✓4ᵗʰ E04 Other nontoxic goiter

EXCLUDES 1   *congenital goiter (NOS) (diffuse) (parenchymatous) (E03.0)*
iodine-deficiency related goiter (E00-E02)

E04.0 Nontoxic diffuse goiter `Rx`

Diffuse (colloid) nontoxic goiter

Simple nontoxic goiter

E04.1 Nontoxic single thyroid nodule `Rx`

Colloid nodule (cystic) (thyroid)

Nontoxic uninodular goiter

Thyroid (cystic) nodule NOS

DEF: Enlarged thyroid, commonly due to decreased thyroid production, with a single nodule. No clinical hypothyroidism.

E04.2 Nontoxic multinodular goiter `Rx`

Cystic goiter NOS

Multinodular (cystic) goiter NOS

DEF: Enlarged thyroid, commonly due to decreased thyroid production with multiple nodules. No clinical hypothyroidism.

E04.8 Other specified nontoxic goiter `Rx`

E04.9 Nontoxic goiter, unspecified `Rx`

Goiter NOS

Nodular goiter (nontoxic) NOS

✓4ᵗʰ E05 Thyrotoxicosis [hyperthyroidism]

EXCLUDES 1   *chronic thyroiditis with transient thyrotoxicosis (E06.2)*
neonatal thyrotoxicosis (P72.1)

DEF: Excessive quantities of hormones from the thyroid gland caused by overproduction or loss of storage ability.

✓5ᵗʰ E05.0 Thyrotoxicosis with diffuse goiter

Exophthalmic or toxic goiter NOS

Graves' disease

Toxic diffuse goiter

DEF: Diffuse thyroid enlargement accompanied by hyperthyroidism, bulging eyes, and dermopathy.

E05.00 Thyrotoxicosis with diffuse goiter without thyrotoxic crisis or storm `Rx`

E05.01 Thyrotoxicosis with diffuse goiter with thyrotoxic crisis or storm `Rx`

Goiter

Pyramidal lobe

Thyroid cartilage

(- - - -) Healthy thyroid

Goiter (hyperfunctioning thyroid)

✓5ᵗʰ E05.1 Thyrotoxicosis with toxic single thyroid nodule

Thyrotoxicosis with toxic uninodular goiter

DEF: Symptomatic hyperthyroidism with a single nodule on the enlarged thyroid gland. Onset of symptoms can be abrupt and include extreme nervousness, insomnia, weight loss, tremors, and psychosis or coma.

E05.10 Thyrotoxicosis with toxic single thyroid nodule without thyrotoxic crisis or storm `Rx`

E05.11 Thyrotoxicosis with toxic single thyroid nodule with thyrotoxic crisis or storm `Rx`

✓5ᵗʰ E05.2 Thyrotoxicosis with toxic multinodular goiter

Toxic nodular goiter NOS

E05.20 Thyrotoxicosis with toxic multinodular goiter without thyrotoxic crisis or storm `Rx`

E05.21 Thyrotoxicosis with toxic multinodular goiter with thyrotoxic crisis or storm `Rx` `ESR`

☑5ᵗʰ **E05.3 Thyrotoxicosis** from ectopic thyroid tissue

    E05.30 Thyrotoxicosis from ectopic thyroid tissue without thyrotoxic crisis or storm   **Rx**

    E05.31 Thyrotoxicosis from ectopic thyroid tissue with thyrotoxic crisis or storm   **Rx**

☑5ᵗʰ **E05.4 Thyrotoxicosis factitia**

    E05.40 Thyrotoxicosis factitia without thyrotoxic crisis or storm   **Rx**

    E05.41 Thyrotoxicosis factitia with thyrotoxic crisis or storm   **Rx**

☑5ᵗʰ **E05.8 Other thyrotoxicosis**

    Overproduction of thyroid-stimulating hormone

    E05.80 Other thyrotoxicosis without thyrotoxic crisis or storm   **Rx**

    E05.81 Other thyrotoxicosis with thyrotoxic crisis or storm   **Rx**

☑5ᵗʰ **E05.9 Thyrotoxicosis, unspecified**

    Hyperthyroidism NOS

    E05.90 Thyrotoxicosis, unspecified without thyrotoxic crisis or storm   **Rx**

    E05.91 Thyrotoxicosis, unspecified with thyrotoxic crisis or storm   **Rx**

☑4ᵗʰ **E06 Thyroiditis**

    EXCLUDES 1 postpartum thyroiditis (O90.5)

    DEF: Inflammation of the thyroid gland.

    E06.0 Acute thyroiditis   **Rx**

      Abscess of thyroid

      Pyogenic thyroiditis

      Suppurative thyroiditis

      Use additional code (B95-B97) to identify infectious agent

    E06.1 Subacute thyroiditis   **Rx**

      de Quervain thyroiditis

      Giant-cell thyroiditis

      Granulomatous thyroiditis

      Nonsuppurative thyroiditis

      Viral thyroiditis

      EXCLUDES 1 autoimmune thyroiditis (E06.3)

    E06.2 Chronic thyroiditis with transient thyrotoxicosis   **Rx**

      EXCLUDES 1 autoimmune thyroiditis (E06.3)

    E06.3 Autoimmune thyroiditis   **Rx**

      Hashimoto's thyroiditis

      Hashitoxicosis (transient)

      Lymphadenoid goiter

      Lymphocytic thyroiditis

      Struma lymphomatosa

    E06.4 Drug-induced thyroiditis   **Rx**

      Use additional code for adverse effect, if applicable, to identify drug (T36-T50 with fifth or sixth character 5)

    E06.5 Other chronic thyroiditis   **Rx**

      Chronic fibrous thyroiditis

      Chronic thyroiditis NOS

      Ligneous thyroiditis

      Riedel thyroiditis

    E06.9 Thyroiditis, unspecified   **Rx**

☑4ᵗʰ **E07 Other disorders of thyroid**

    E07.0 Hypersecretion of calcitonin   **Rx**

      C-cell hyperplasia of thyroid

      Hypersecretion of thyrocalcitonin

    E07.1 Dyshormogenetic goiter   **Rx**

      Familial dyshormogenetic goiter

      Pendred's syndrome

      EXCLUDES 1 transitory congenital goiter with normal function (P72.0)

☑5ᵗʰ **E07.8 Other specified disorders of thyroid**

    E07.81 Sick-euthyroid syndrome

      Euthyroid sick-syndrome

      DEF: Thyroid dysfunction caused by abnormal levels of thyroid hormones T3 and/or T4. This syndrome is often associated with starvation or critical illness.

    E07.89 Other specified disorders of thyroid   **Rx**

      Abnormality of thyroid-binding globulin

      Hemorrhage of thyroid

      Infarction of thyroid

    E07.9 Disorder of thyroid, unspecified   **Rx**

Diabetes mellitus (E08-E13)

AHA: 2020,1Q,12; 2018,2Q,6; 2017,4Q,100-101; 2016,2Q,36; 2016,1Q,11-13; 2013,4Q,114; 2013,3Q,20

TIP: There is no default code for diabetes mellitus documented only as uncontrolled. The provider must indicate whether the diabetic patient is hypoglycemic or hyperglycemic to determine the appropriate code.

☑4ᵗʰ **E08 Diabetes mellitus** due to underlying condition

    Code first the underlying condition, such as:

      congenital rubella (P35.0)

      Cushing's syndrome (E24.-)

      cystic fibrosis (E84.-)

      malignant neoplasm (C00-C96)

      malnutrition (E40-E46)

      pancreatitis and other diseases of the pancreas (K85-K86.-)

    Use additional code to identify control using:

      insulin (Z79.4)

      oral antidiabetic drugs (Z79.84)

      oral hypoglycemic drugs (Z79.84)

    EXCLUDES 1 drug or chemical induced diabetes mellitus (E09.-)

        gestational diabetes (O24.4-)

        neonatal diabetes mellitus (P70.2)

        postpancreatectomy diabetes mellitus (E13.-)

        postprocedural diabetes mellitus (E13.-)

        secondary diabetes mellitus NEC (E13.-)

        type 1 diabetes mellitus (E10.-)

        type 2 diabetes mellitus (E11.-)

☑5ᵗʰ **E08.0 Diabetes mellitus due to underlying condition with hyperosmolarity**

    DEF: Diabetic hyperosmolarity: Extremely high levels of glucose in the blood without ketones.

    E08.00 Diabetes mellitus due to underlying condition with hyperosmolarity without nonketotic hyperglycemic-hyperosmolar coma (NKHHC)   **HCC Rx ESR COM**

    E08.01 Diabetes mellitus due to underlying condition with hyperosmolarity with coma   **HCC Rx ESR COM**

☑5ᵗʰ **E08.1 Diabetes mellitus due to underlying condition with ketoacidosis**

    DEF: Diabetic ketoacidosis: Potentially life-threatening complication due to a shortage of insulin in which the body switches to burning fatty acids and producing acidic ketone bodies.

    E08.10 Diabetes mellitus due to underlying condition with ketoacidosis without coma   **HCC Rx ESR COM**

    E08.11 Diabetes mellitus due to underlying condition with ketoacidosis with coma   **HCC Rx ESR COM**

☑5ᵗʰ **E08.2 Diabetes mellitus due to underlying condition with kidney complications**

    AHA: 2019,3Q,3; 2018,4Q,88

    E08.21 Diabetes mellitus due to underlying condition with diabetic nephropathy   **HCC Rx ESR COM**

      Diabetes mellitus due to underlying condition with intercapillary glomerulosclerosis

      Diabetes mellitus due to underlying condition with intracapillary glomerulonephrosis

      Diabetes mellitus due to underlying condition with Kimmelstiel-Wilson disease

    E08.22 Diabetes mellitus due to underlying condition with diabetic chronic kidney disease   **HCC Rx ESR COM**

      Use additional code to identify stage of chronic kidney disease (N18.1-N18.6)

    E08.29 Diabetes mellitus due to underlying condition with other diabetic kidney complication   **HCC Rx ESR COM**

      Renal tubular degeneration in diabetes mellitus due to underlying condition

HCC CMS-HCC   **Rx** Rx HCC   **ESR** ESRD HCC   **COM** Commercial HCC   **N** Newborn: 0   **P** Pediatric: 0-17   **M** Maternity: 9-64   **A** Adult: 15-124

532   ICD-10-CM 2023

√6ᵗʰ **E08.3 Diabetes mellitus due to underlying condition with ophthalmic complications**
AHA: 2016,4Q,11-13

One of the following 7th characters is to be assigned to codes in subcategories E08.32, E08.33, E08.34, E08.35, and E08.37 to designate laterality of the disease:
1   right eye
2   left eye
3   bilateral
9   unspecified eye

√6ᵗʰ **E08.31 Diabetes mellitus due to underlying condition with unspecified diabetic retinopathy**
DEF: Diabetic retinopathy: Diabetic complication from damage to the retinal vessels resulting in vision problems that can progress to blindness.

E08.311 Diabetes mellitus due to underlying condition with unspecified diabetic retinopathy with macular edema HCC Rx ESR COM

E08.319 Diabetes mellitus due to underlying condition with unspecified diabetic retinopathy without macular edema HCC Rx ESR COM

√6ᵗʰ **E08.32 Diabetes mellitus due to underlying condition with mild nonproliferative diabetic retinopathy**
Diabetes mellitus due to underlying condition with nonproliferative diabetic retinopathy NOS

√7ᵗʰ *E08.321 Diabetes mellitus due to underlying condition with mild nonproliferative diabetic retinopathy with macular edema* HCC Rx ESR COM

√7ᵗʰ *E08.329 Diabetes mellitus due to underlying condition with mild nonproliferative diabetic retinopathy without macular edema* HCC Rx ESR COM

√6ᵗʰ **E08.33 Diabetes mellitus due to underlying condition with moderate nonproliferative diabetic retinopathy**

√7ᵗʰ *E08.331 Diabetes mellitus due to underlying condition with moderate nonproliferative diabetic retinopathy with macular edema* HCC Rx ESR COM

√7ᵗʰ *E08.339 Diabetes mellitus due to underlying condition with moderate nonproliferative diabetic retinopathy without macular edema* HCC Rx ESR COM

√6ᵗʰ **E08.34 Diabetes mellitus due to underlying condition with severe nonproliferative diabetic retinopathy**

√7ᵗʰ *E08.341 Diabetes mellitus due to underlying condition with severe nonproliferative diabetic retinopathy with macular edema* HCC Rx ESR COM

√7ᵗʰ *E08.349 Diabetes mellitus due to underlying condition with severe nonproliferative diabetic retinopathy without macular edema* HCC Rx ESR COM

√6ᵗʰ **E08.35 Diabetes mellitus due to underlying condition with proliferative diabetic retinopathy**

√7ᵗʰ *E08.351 Diabetes mellitus due to underlying condition with proliferative diabetic retinopathy with macular edema* HCC Rx ESR COM

√7ᵗʰ *E08.352 Diabetes mellitus due to underlying condition with proliferative diabetic retinopathy with traction retinal detachment involving the macula* HCC Rx ESR COM

√7ᵗʰ *E08.353 Diabetes mellitus due to underlying condition with proliferative diabetic retinopathy with traction retinal detachment not involving the macula* HCC Rx ESR COM

√7ᵗʰ *E08.354 Diabetes mellitus due to underlying condition with proliferative diabetic retinopathy with combined traction retinal detachment and rhegmatogenous retinal detachment* HCC Rx ESR COM

√7ᵗʰ *E08.355 Diabetes mellitus due to underlying condition with stable proliferative diabetic retinopathy* HCC Rx ESR COM

√7ᵗʰ *E08.359 Diabetes mellitus due to underlying condition with proliferative diabetic retinopathy without macular edema* HCC Rx ESR COM

E08.36 *Diabetes mellitus due to underlying condition with diabetic cataract* HCC Rx ESR COM
AHA: 2019,2Q,30-31; 2016,4Q,142

√x7ᵗʰ **E08.37 *Diabetes mellitus due to underlying condition with diabetic macular edema, resolved following treatment*** HCC Rx ESR COM

E08.39 *Diabetes mellitus due to underlying condition with other diabetic ophthalmic complication* HCC Rx ESR COM
Use additional code to identify manifestation, such as:
diabetic glaucoma (H40-H42)

√5ᵗʰ **E08.4 Diabetes mellitus due to underlying condition with neurological complications**

E08.40 Diabetes mellitus due to underlying condition with diabetic neuropathy, unspecified HCC Rx ESR COM

E08.41 Diabetes mellitus due to underlying condition with diabetic mononeuropathy HCC Rx ESR COM

E08.42 Diabetes mellitus due to underlying condition with diabetic polyneuropathy HCC Rx ESR COM
Diabetes mellitus due to underlying condition with diabetic neuralgia

E08.43 Diabetes mellitus due to underlying condition with diabetic autonomic (poly)neuropathy HCC Rx ESR COM
Diabetes mellitus due to underlying condition with diabetic gastroparesis
AHA: 2013,4Q,114

E08.44 Diabetes mellitus due to underlying condition with diabetic amyotrophy HCC Rx ESR COM

E08.49 Diabetes mellitus due to underlying condition with other diabetic neurological complication HCC Rx ESR COM

√5ᵗʰ **E08.5 Diabetes mellitus due to underlying condition with circulatory complications**

E08.51 Diabetes mellitus due to underlying condition with diabetic peripheral angiopathy without gangrene HCC Rx ESR COM
AHA: 2018,3Q,3-4; 2018,2Q,7

E08.52 Diabetes mellitus due to underlying condition with diabetic peripheral angiopathy with gangrene HCC Rx ESR COM
Diabetes mellitus due to underlying condition with diabetic gangrene
AHA: 2020,2Q,18; 2018,3Q,3; 2018,2Q,7; 2017,4Q,102

E08.59 Diabetes mellitus due to underlying condition with other circulatory complications HCC Rx ESR COM

√5ᵗʰ **E08.6 Diabetes mellitus due to underlying condition with other specified complications**

√6ᵗʰ **E08.61 Diabetes mellitus due to underlying condition with diabetic arthropathy**

E08.610 Diabetes mellitus due to underlying condition with diabetic neuropathic arthropathy HCC Rx ESR COM
Diabetes mellitus due to underlying condition with Charcôt's joints
DEF: Charcot's joint: Progressive neurologic arthropathy in which chronic degeneration of joints in the weight-bearing areas with peripheral hypertrophy occurs as a complication of a neuropathy disorder. Supporting structures relax from a loss of sensation resulting in chronic joint instability.

E08.618 Diabetes mellitus due to underlying condition with other diabetic arthropathy HCC Rx ESR COM
AHA: 2018,2Q,6

√6ᵗʰ **E08.62 Diabetes mellitus due to underlying condition with skin complications**

E08.620 Diabetes mellitus due to underlying condition with diabetic dermatitis HCC Rx ESR COM
Diabetes mellitus due to underlying condition with diabetic necrobiosis lipoidica

---

☑ Additional Character Required   √x7ᵗʰ Placeholder Alert   Manifestation   Unspecified Dx   Q QPP   UPD Unacceptable PDx

E08.621 *Diabetes mellitus due to underlying condition with* foot ulcer   `HCC` `Rx` `ESR` `COM`

Use additional code to identify site of ulcer (L97.4-, L97.5-)

AHA: 2020,2Q,19

TIP: Do not assign a code for diabetic ulcer when the ulcer is closed/resolved or to report history of diabetic ulcers; Z86.31 Personal history of diabetic foot ulcer, may be assigned.

E08.622 *Diabetes mellitus due to underlying condition with other skin ulcer*   `HCC` `Rx` `ESR` `COM`

Use additional code to identify site of ulcer (L97.1-L97.9, L98.41-L98.49)

AHA: 2021,1Q,7; 2017,4Q,17

E08.628 *Diabetes mellitus due to underlying condition with other skin complications*   `HCC` `Rx` `ESR` `COM`

√6ᵗʰ **E08.63** **Diabetes mellitus due to underlying condition with oral complications**

E08.630 *Diabetes mellitus due to underlying condition with* periodontal disease   `HCC` `Rx` `ESR` `COM`

E08.638 *Diabetes mellitus due to underlying condition with other oral complications*   `HCC` `Rx` `ESR` `COM`

√6ᵗʰ **E08.64** **Diabetes mellitus due to underlying condition with** hypoglycemia

AHA: 2017,1Q,42

E08.641 *Diabetes mellitus due to underlying condition with hypoglycemia with* coma   `HCC` `Rx` `ESR` `COM`

E08.649 *Diabetes mellitus due to underlying condition with hypoglycemia without* coma   `HCC` `Rx` `ESR` `COM`

AHA: 2016,3Q,42; 2015,3Q,21

E08.65 *Diabetes mellitus due to underlying condition with* hyperglycemia   `HCC` `Rx` `ESR` `COM`

AHA: 2017,1Q,42; 2013,3Q,20

E08.69 *Diabetes mellitus due to underlying condition with other specified complication*   `HCC` `Rx` `ESR` `COM`

Use additional code to identify complication

AHA: 2016,4Q,141; 2016,1Q,13

E08.8 *Diabetes mellitus due to underlying condition with unspecified complications*   `HCC` `Rx` `ESR` `COM`

E08.9 *Diabetes mellitus due to underlying condition* without complications   `HCC` `Rx` `ESR` `COM`

AHA: 2020,2Q,18

√4ᵗʰ **E09** **Drug or chemical induced** **diabetes mellitus**

Code first poisoning due to drug or toxin, if applicable (T36-T65 with fifth or sixth character 1-4 or 6)

Use additional code for adverse effect, if applicable, to identify drug (T36-T50 with fifth or sixth character 5)

Use additional code to identify control using:
insulin (Z79.4)
oral antidiabetic drugs (Z79.84)
oral hypoglycemic drugs (Z79.84)

EXCLUDES 1   *diabetes mellitus due to underlying condition (E08.-)*
gestational diabetes (O24.4-)
neonatal diabetes mellitus (P70.2)
postpancreatectomy diabetes mellitus (E13.-)
postprocedural diabetes mellitus (E13.-)
secondary diabetes mellitus NEC (E13.-)
type 1 diabetes mellitus (E10.-)
type 2 diabetes mellitus (E11.-)

√5ᵗʰ **E09.0** **Drug or chemical induced diabetes mellitus with** hyperosmolarity

DEF: Diabetic hyperosmolarity: Extremely high levels of glucose in the blood without ketones.

E09.00 **Drug or chemical induced diabetes mellitus with hyperosmolarity** without nonketotic hyperglycemic-hyperosmolar coma (NKHHC)   `HCC` `Rx` `ESR` `COM`

E09.01 **Drug or chemical induced diabetes mellitus with hyperosmolarity** with coma   `HCC` `Rx` `ESR` `COM`

√5ᵗʰ **E09.1** **Drug or chemical induced diabetes mellitus with** ketoacidosis

DEF: Diabetic ketoacidosis: Potentially life-threatening complication due to a shortage of insulin in which the body switches to burning fatty acids and producing acidic ketone bodies.

E09.10 **Drug or chemical induced diabetes mellitus with ketoacidosis** without coma   `HCC` `Rx` `ESR` `COM`

E09.11 **Drug or chemical induced diabetes mellitus with ketoacidosis** with coma   `HCC` `Rx` `ESR` `COM`

√5ᵗʰ **E09.2** **Drug or chemical induced diabetes mellitus with** kidney complications

AHA: 2019,3Q,3; 2018,4Q,88

E09.21 **Drug or chemical induced diabetes mellitus with diabetic** nephropathy   `HCC` `Rx` `ESR` `COM`

Drug or chemical induced diabetes mellitus with intercapillary glomerulosclerosis

Drug or chemical induced diabetes mellitus with intracapillary glomerulonephrosis

Drug or chemical induced diabetes mellitus with Kimmelstiel-Wilson disease

E09.22 **Drug or chemical induced diabetes mellitus with diabetic** chronic kidney disease   `HCC` `Rx` `ESR` `COM`

Use additional code to identify stage of chronic kidney disease (N18.1-N18.6)

E09.29 **Drug or chemical induced diabetes mellitus with other diabetic kidney complication**   `HCC` `Rx` `ESR` `COM`

Drug or chemical induced diabetes mellitus with renal tubular degeneration

√5ᵗʰ **E09.3** **Drug or chemical induced diabetes mellitus with** ophthalmic complications

AHA: 2016,4Q,11-13

One of the following 7th characters is to be assigned to codes in subcategories E09.32, E09.33, E09.34, E09.35, and E09.37 to designate laterality of the disease:

1   right eye
2   left eye
3   bilateral
9   unspecified eye

√6ᵗʰ **E09.31** **Drug or chemical induced diabetes mellitus with unspecified diabetic** retinopathy

DEF: Diabetic retinopathy: Diabetic complication from damage to the retinal vessels resulting in vision problems that can progress to blindness.

E09.311 **Drug or chemical induced diabetes mellitus with unspecified diabetic retinopathy** with macular edema   `HCC` `Rx` `ESR` `COM`

E09.319 **Drug or chemical induced diabetes mellitus with unspecified diabetic retinopathy** without macular edema   `HCC` `Rx` `ESR` `COM`

√6ᵗʰ **E09.32** **Drug or chemical induced diabetes mellitus with** mild nonproliferative **diabetic** retinopathy

Drug or chemical induced diabetes mellitus with nonproliferative diabetic retinopathy NOS

√7ᵗʰ **E09.321** **Drug or chemical induced diabetes mellitus with mild nonproliferative diabetic retinopathy** with macular edema   `HCC` `Rx` `ESR` `COM`

√7ᵗʰ **E09.329** **Drug or chemical induced diabetes mellitus with mild nonproliferative diabetic retinopathy** without macular edema   `HCC` `Rx` `ESR` `COM`

√6ᵗʰ **E09.33** **Drug or chemical induced diabetes mellitus with** moderate nonproliferative **diabetic** retinopathy

√7ᵗʰ **E09.331** **Drug or chemical induced diabetes mellitus with moderate nonproliferative diabetic retinopathy** with macular edema   `HCC` `Rx` `ESR` `COM`

√7ᵗʰ **E09.339** **Drug or chemical induced diabetes mellitus with moderate nonproliferative diabetic retinopathy** without macular edema   `HCC` `Rx` `ESR` `COM`

√6ᵗʰ **E09.34** **Drug or chemical induced diabetes mellitus with** severe nonproliferative **diabetic** retinopathy

√7ᵗʰ **E09.341** **Drug or chemical induced diabetes mellitus with severe nonproliferative diabetic retinopathy** with macular edema   `HCC` `Rx` `ESR` `COM`

`HCC` CMS-HCC   `Rx` Rx HCC   `ESR` ESRD HCC   `COM` Commercial HCC   N Newborn: 0   P Pediatric: 0-17   M Maternity: 9-64   A Adult: 15-124

534   ICD-10-CM 2023

☑7ᵗʰ **E09.349** **Drug or chemical induced diabetes mellitus with severe nonproliferative diabetic retinopathy** without macular edema `HCC` `Rx` `ESR` `COM`

☑6ᵗʰ **E09.35** **Drug or chemical induced diabetes mellitus with** proliferative diabetic retinopathy

☑7ᵗʰ **E09.351** **Drug or chemical induced diabetes mellitus with proliferative diabetic retinopathy** with macular edema `HCC` `Rx` `ESR` `COM`

☑7ᵗʰ **E09.352** **Drug or chemical induced diabetes mellitus with proliferative diabetic retinopathy** with traction retinal detachment involving the macula `HCC` `Rx` `ESR` `COM`

☑7ᵗʰ **E09.353** **Drug or chemical induced diabetes mellitus with proliferative diabetic retinopathy** with traction retinal detachment not involving the macula `HCC` `Rx` `ESR` `COM`

☑7ᵗʰ **E09.354** **Drug or chemical induced diabetes mellitus with proliferative diabetic retinopathy** with combined traction retinal detachment and rhegmatogenous retinal detachment `HCC` `Rx` `ESR` `COM`

☑7ᵗʰ **E09.355** **Drug or chemical induced diabetes mellitus** with stable **proliferative diabetic retinopathy** `HCC` `Rx` `ESR` `COM`

☑7ᵗʰ **E09.359** **Drug or chemical induced diabetes mellitus with proliferative diabetic retinopathy** without macular edema `HCC` `Rx` `ESR` `COM`

E09.36 **Drug or chemical induced diabetes mellitus with diabetic** cataract `HCC` `Rx` `ESR` `COM`
    AHA: 2019,2Q,30-31; 2016,4Q,142

☑x7ᵗʰ **E09.37** **Drug or chemical induced diabetes mellitus with diabetic** macular edema, resolved following treatment `HCC` `Rx` `ESR` `COM`

E09.39 **Drug or chemical induced diabetes mellitus with other diabetic ophthalmic complication** `HCC` `Rx` `ESR` `COM`
    Use additional code to identify manifestation, such as:
      diabetic glaucoma (H40-H42)

☑5ᵗʰ **E09.4** **Drug or chemical induced diabetes mellitus with** neurological complications

E09.40 **Drug or chemical induced diabetes mellitus with neurological complications with diabetic** neuropathy, unspecified `HCC` `Rx` `ESR` `COM`

E09.41 **Drug or chemical induced diabetes mellitus with neurological complications with diabetic** mononeuropathy `HCC` `Rx` `ESR` `COM`

E09.42 **Drug or chemical induced diabetes mellitus with neurological complications with diabetic** polyneuropathy `HCC` `Rx` `ESR` `COM`
    Drug or chemical induced diabetes mellitus with diabetic neuralgia

E09.43 **Drug or chemical induced diabetes mellitus with neurological complications with diabetic** autonomic (poly)neuropathy `HCC` `Rx` `ESR` `COM`
    Drug or chemical induced diabetes mellitus with diabetic gastroparesis
    AHA: 2013,4Q,114

E09.44 **Drug or chemical induced diabetes mellitus with neurological complications with diabetic** amyotrophy `HCC` `Rx` `ESR` `COM`

E09.49 **Drug or chemical induced diabetes mellitus with neurological complications with other diabetic neurological complication** `HCC` `Rx` `ESR` `COM`

☑5ᵗʰ **E09.5** **Drug or chemical induced diabetes mellitus with** circulatory complications

E09.51 **Drug or chemical induced diabetes mellitus with diabetic** peripheral angiopathy without gangrene `HCC` `Rx` `ESR` `COM`
    AHA: 2018,3Q,3-4; 2018,2Q,7

E09.52 **Drug or chemical induced diabetes mellitus with diabetic** peripheral angiopathy with gangrene `HCC` `Rx` `ESR` `COM`
    Drug or chemical induced diabetes mellitus with diabetic gangrene
    AHA: 2020,2Q,18; 2018,3Q,3; 2018,2Q,7; 2017,4Q,102

E09.59 **Drug or chemical induced diabetes mellitus with other circulatory complications** `HCC` `Rx` `ESR` `COM`

☑5ᵗʰ **E09.6** **Drug or chemical induced diabetes mellitus with other specified complications**

☑6ᵗʰ **E09.61** **Drug or chemical induced diabetes mellitus with** diabetic arthropathy

E09.610 **Drug or chemical induced diabetes mellitus with diabetic** neuropathic arthropathy `HCC` `Rx` `ESR` `COM`
    Drug or chemical induced diabetes mellitus with Charcôt's joints
    DEF: Charcot's joint: Progressive neurologic arthropathy in which chronic degeneration of joints in the weight-bearing areas with peripheral hypertrophy occurs as a complication of a neuropathy disorder. Supporting structures relax from a loss of sensation resulting in chronic joint instability.

E09.618 **Drug or chemical induced diabetes mellitus with other diabetic arthropathy** `HCC` `Rx` `ESR` `COM`
    AHA: 2018,2Q,6

☑6ᵗʰ **E09.62** **Drug or chemical induced diabetes mellitus with** skin complications

E09.620 **Drug or chemical induced diabetes mellitus with** diabetic dermatitis `HCC` `Rx` `ESR` `COM`
    Drug or chemical induced diabetes mellitus with diabetic necrobiosis lipoidica

E09.621 **Drug or chemical induced diabetes mellitus with** foot ulcer `HCC` `Rx` `ESR` `COM`
    Use additional code to identify site of ulcer (L97.4-, L97.5-)
    AHA: 2020,2Q,19
    TIP: Do not assign a code for diabetic ulcer when the ulcer is closed/resolved or to report history of diabetic ulcers; Z86.31 Personal history of diabetic foot ulcer, may be assigned.

E09.622 **Drug or chemical induced diabetes mellitus with other skin ulcer** `HCC` `Rx` `ESR` `COM`
    Use additional code to identify site of ulcer (L97.1-L97.9, L98.41-L98.49)
    AHA: 2021,1Q,7; 2017,4Q,17

E09.628 **Drug or chemical induced diabetes mellitus with other skin complications** `HCC` `Rx` `ESR` `COM`

☑6ᵗʰ **E09.63** **Drug or chemical induced diabetes mellitus with** oral complications

E09.630 **Drug or chemical induced diabetes mellitus with** periodontal disease `HCC` `Rx` `ESR` `COM`

E09.638 **Drug or chemical induced diabetes mellitus with other oral complications** `HCC` `Rx` `ESR` `COM`

☑6ᵗʰ **E09.64** **Drug or chemical induced diabetes mellitus with** hypoglycemia
    AHA: 2017,1Q,42

E09.641 **Drug or chemical induced diabetes mellitus with hypoglycemia** with coma `HCC` `Rx` `ESR` `COM`

E09.649 **Drug or chemical induced diabetes mellitus with hypoglycemia** without coma `HCC` `Rx` `ESR` `COM`
    AHA: 2016,3Q,42; 2015,3Q,21

E09.65 **Drug or chemical induced diabetes mellitus with** hyperglycemia `HCC` `Rx` `ESR` `COM`
    AHA: 2017,1Q,42; 2013,3Q,20

E09.69 **Drug or chemical induced diabetes mellitus with other specified complication** `HCC` `Rx` `ESR` `COM`
    Use additional code to identify complication
    AHA: 2016,4Q,141; 2016,1Q,13

E09.8 **Drug or chemical induced diabetes mellitus with unspecified complications** `HCC` `Rx` `ESR` `COM`

E09.9 **Drug or chemical induced diabetes mellitus** without complications `HCC` `Rx` `ESR` `COM`
    AHA: 2020,2Q,18

☑ Additional Character Required   ☑x7ᵗʰ Placeholder Alert   Manifestation   Unspecified Dx   **Q** QPP   **UPD** Unacceptable PDx

Chapter 4. Endocrine, Nutritional and Metabolic Diseases

E10–E10.59

✓4ᵗʰ **E10**   Type 1 diabetes mellitus

INCLUDES   brittle diabetes (mellitus)
diabetes (mellitus) due to autoimmune process
diabetes (mellitus) due to immune mediated pancreatic islet beta-cell destruction
idiopathic diabetes (mellitus)
juvenile onset diabetes (mellitus)
ketosis-prone diabetes (mellitus)

EXCLUDES 1   *diabetes mellitus due to underlying condition (E08.-)*
drug or chemical induced diabetes mellitus (E09.-)
gestational diabetes (O24.4-)
hyperglycemia NOS (R73.9)
neonatal diabetes mellitus (P70.2)
postpancreatectomy diabetes mellitus (E13.-)
postprocedural diabetes mellitus (E13.-)
secondary diabetes mellitus NEC (E13.-)
type 2 diabetes mellitus (E11.-)

AHA: 2020,3Q,30

✓5ᵗʰ **E10.1**   Type 1 diabetes mellitus with ketoacidosis

AHA: 2013,3Q,20

DEF: Diabetic ketoacidosis: Potentially life-threatening complication due to a shortage of insulin in which the body switches to burning fatty acids and producing acidic ketone bodies.

E10.10   Type 1 diabetes mellitus with ketoacidosis without coma   HCC Rx ESR COM Q

E10.11   Type 1 diabetes mellitus with ketoacidosis with coma   HCC Rx ESR COM Q

✓5ᵗʰ **E10.2**   Type 1 diabetes mellitus with kidney complications

AHA: 2019,3Q,3; 2018,4Q,88

E10.21   Type 1 diabetes mellitus with diabetic nephropathy   HCC Rx ESR COM Q

Type 1 diabetes mellitus with intercapillary glomerulosclerosis
Type 1 diabetes mellitus with intracapillary glomerulonephrosis
Type 1 diabetes mellitus with Kimmelstiel-Wilson disease

E10.22   Type 1 diabetes mellitus with diabetic chronic kidney disease   HCC Rx ESR COM Q

Use additional code to identify stage of chronic kidney disease (N18.1-N18.6)

E10.29   Type 1 diabetes mellitus with other diabetic kidney complication   HCC Rx ESR COM Q

Type 1 diabetes mellitus with renal tubular degeneration

AHA: 2016,1Q,13

✓5ᵗʰ **E10.3**   Type 1 diabetes mellitus with ophthalmic complications

AHA: 2016,4Q,11-13

One of the following 7th characters is to be assigned to codes in subcategories E10.32, E10.33, E10.34, E10.35, and E10.37 to designate laterality of the disease:
1   right eye
2   left eye
3   bilateral
9   unspecified eye

✓6ᵗʰ **E10.31**   Type 1 diabetes mellitus with unspecified diabetic retinopathy

DEF: Diabetic retinopathy: Diabetic complication from damage to the retinal vessels resulting in vision problems that can progress to blindness.

E10.311   Type 1 diabetes mellitus with unspecified diabetic retinopathy with macular edema   HCC Rx ESR COM Q

E10.319   Type 1 diabetes mellitus with unspecified diabetic retinopathy without macular edema   HCC Rx ESR COM Q

✓6ᵗʰ **E10.32**   Type 1 diabetes mellitus with mild nonproliferative diabetic retinopathy

Type 1 diabetes mellitus with nonproliferative diabetic retinopathy NOS

E10.321   Type 1 diabetes mellitus with mild nonproliferative diabetic retinopathy with macular edema   HCC Rx ESR COM Q

E10.329   Type 1 diabetes mellitus with mild nonproliferative diabetic retinopathy without macular edema   HCC Rx ESR COM Q

✓6ᵗʰ **E10.33**   Type 1 diabetes mellitus with moderate nonproliferative diabetic retinopathy

E10.331   Type 1 diabetes mellitus with moderate nonproliferative diabetic retinopathy with macular edema   HCC Rx ESR COM Q

E10.339   Type 1 diabetes mellitus with moderate nonproliferative diabetic retinopathy without macular edema   HCC Rx ESR COM Q

✓6ᵗʰ **E10.34**   Type 1 diabetes mellitus with severe nonproliferative diabetic retinopathy

E10.341   Type 1 diabetes mellitus with severe nonproliferative diabetic retinopathy with macular edema   HCC Rx ESR COM Q

E10.349   Type 1 diabetes mellitus with severe nonproliferative diabetic retinopathy without macular edema   HCC Rx ESR COM Q

✓6ᵗʰ **E10.35**   Type 1 diabetes mellitus with proliferative diabetic retinopathy

E10.351   Type 1 diabetes mellitus with proliferative diabetic retinopathy with macular edema   HCC Rx ESR COM Q

E10.352   Type 1 diabetes mellitus with proliferative diabetic retinopathy with traction retinal detachment involving the macula   HCC Rx ESR COM Q

E10.353   Type 1 diabetes mellitus with proliferative diabetic retinopathy with traction retinal detachment not involving the macula   HCC Rx ESR COM Q

E10.354   Type 1 diabetes mellitus with proliferative diabetic retinopathy with combined traction retinal detachment and rhegmatogenous retinal detachment   HCC Rx ESR COM Q

E10.355   Type 1 diabetes mellitus with stable proliferative diabetic retinopathy   HCC Rx ESR COM Q

E10.359   Type 1 diabetes mellitus with proliferative diabetic retinopathy without macular edema   HCC Rx ESR COM Q

E10.36   Type 1 diabetes mellitus with diabetic cataract   HCC Rx ESR COM Q

AHA: 2019,2Q,30-31; 2016,4Q,142

✓x7ᵗʰ **E10.37**   Type 1 diabetes mellitus with diabetic macular edema, resolved following treatment   HCC Rx ESR COM Q

E10.39   Type 1 diabetes mellitus with other diabetic ophthalmic complication   HCC Rx ESR COM Q

Use additional code to identify manifestation, such as:
diabetic glaucoma (H40-H42)

✓5ᵗʰ **E10.4**   Type 1 diabetes mellitus with neurological complications

E10.40   Type 1 diabetes mellitus with diabetic neuropathy, unspecified   HCC Rx ESR COM Q

E10.41   Type 1 diabetes mellitus with diabetic mononeuropathy   HCC Rx ESR COM Q

E10.42   Type 1 diabetes mellitus with diabetic polyneuropathy   HCC Rx ESR COM Q

Type 1 diabetes mellitus with diabetic neuralgia

E10.43   Type 1 diabetes mellitus with diabetic autonomic (poly)neuropathy   HCC Rx ESR COM Q

Type 1 diabetes mellitus with diabetic gastroparesis

AHA: 2013,4Q,114

E10.44   Type 1 diabetes mellitus with diabetic amyotrophy   HCC Rx ESR COM Q

E10.49   Type 1 diabetes mellitus with other diabetic neurological complication   HCC Rx ESR COM Q

✓5ᵗʰ **E10.5**   Type 1 diabetes mellitus with circulatory complications

E10.51   Type 1 diabetes mellitus with diabetic peripheral angiopathy without gangrene   HCC Rx ESR COM Q

AHA: 2018,3Q,3-4; 2018,2Q,7

E10.52   Type 1 diabetes mellitus with diabetic peripheral angiopathy with gangrene   HCC Rx ESR COM Q

Type 1 diabetes mellitus with diabetic gangrene

AHA: 2020,2Q,18; 2018,3Q,3; 2018,2Q,7; 2017,4Q,102

E10.59   Type 1 diabetes mellitus with other circulatory complications   HCC Rx ESR COM Q

✓5ᵗʰ **E10.6 Type 1 diabetes mellitus with other specified complications**

✓6ᵗʰ   **E10.61 Type 1 diabetes mellitus with diabetic** arthropathy

E10.610 Type 1 diabetes mellitus with diabetic neuropathic arthropathy `HCC` `Rx` `ESR` `COM` `Q`
Type 1 diabetes mellitus with Charcôt's joints
DEF: Charcot's joint: Progressive neurologic arthropathy in which chronic degeneration of joints in the weight-bearing areas with peripheral hypertrophy occurs as a complication of a neuropathy disorder. Supporting structures relax from a loss of sensation resulting in chronic joint instability.

E10.618 Type 1 diabetes mellitus with other diabetic arthropathy `HCC` `Rx` `ESR` `COM` `Q`
AHA: 2018,2Q,6

✓6ᵗʰ   **E10.62 Type 1 diabetes mellitus with** skin complications

E10.620 Type 1 diabetes mellitus with diabetic dermatitis `HCC` `Rx` `ESR` `COM` `Q`
Type 1 diabetes mellitus with diabetic necrobiosis lipoidica

E10.621 Type 1 diabetes mellitus with foot ulcer `HCC` `Rx` `ESR` `COM` `Q`
Use additional code to identify site of ulcer (L97.4-, L97.5-)
AHA: 2020,2Q,19
TIP: Do not assign a code for diabetic ulcer when the ulcer is closed/resolved or to report history of diabetic ulcers; Z86.31 Personal history of diabetic foot ulcer, may be assigned.

E10.622 Type 1 diabetes mellitus with other skin ulcer `HCC` `Rx` `ESR` `COM` `Q`
Use additional code to identify site of ulcer (L97.1-L97.9, L98.41-L98.49)
AHA: 2021,1Q,7; 2017,4Q,17

E10.628 Type 1 diabetes mellitus with other skin complications `HCC` `Rx` `ESR` `COM` `Q`

✓6ᵗʰ   **E10.63 Type 1 diabetes mellitus with** oral complications

E10.630 Type 1 diabetes mellitus with periodontal disease `HCC` `Rx` `ESR` `COM` `Q`

E10.638 Type 1 diabetes mellitus with other oral complications `HCC` `Rx` `ESR` `COM` `Q`

✓6ᵗʰ   **E10.64 Type 1 diabetes mellitus with** hypoglycemia
AHA: 2017,1Q,42

E10.641 Type 1 diabetes mellitus with hypoglycemia with **coma** `HCC` `Rx` `ESR` `COM` `Q`

E10.649 Type 1 diabetes mellitus with hypoglycemia without **coma** `HCC` `Rx` `ESR` `COM` `Q`
AHA: 2016,3Q,42; 2016,1Q,13; 2015,3Q,21

E10.65 Type 1 diabetes mellitus with hyperglycemia `HCC` `Rx` `ESR` `COM` `Q`
AHA: 2022,1Q,28; 2017,1Q,42; 2013,3Q,20

E10.69 Type 1 diabetes mellitus with other specified complication `HCC` `Rx` `ESR` `COM` `Q`
Use additional code to identify complication
AHA: 2022,1Q,28; 2016,4Q,141; 2016,1Q,13

E10.8 Type 1 diabetes mellitus with unspecified complications `HCC` `Rx` `ESR` `COM` `Q`

E10.9 Type 1 diabetes mellitus without **complications** `HCC` `Rx` `ESR` `COM` `Q`
AHA: 2020,2Q,18

✓4ᵗʰ **E11 Type 2 diabetes mellitus**

`INCLUDES` diabetes (mellitus) due to insulin secretory defect
diabetes NOS
insulin resistant diabetes (mellitus)
Use additional code to identify control using:
insulin (Z79.4)
oral antidiabetic drugs (Z79.84)
oral hypoglycemic drugs (Z79.84)

`EXCLUDES 1` diabetes mellitus due to underlying condition (E08.-)
drug or chemical induced diabetes mellitus (E09.-)
gestational diabetes (O24.4-)
neonatal diabetes mellitus (P70.2)
postpancreatectomy diabetes mellitus (E13.-)
postprocedural diabetes mellitus (E13.-)
secondary diabetes mellitus NEC (E13.-)
type 1 diabetes mellitus (E10.-)
AHA: 2020,3Q,30; 2020,1Q,12; 2016,2Q,10; 2013,1Q,26

✓5ᵗʰ **E11.0 Type 2 diabetes mellitus with** hyperosmolarity
DEF: Diabetic hyperosmolarity: Extremely high levels of glucose in the blood without ketones.

E11.00 Type 2 diabetes mellitus with hyperosmolarity without nonketotic hyperglycemic-hyperosmolar coma (NKHHC) `HCC` `Rx` `ESR` `COM` `Q`
AHA: 2022,1Q,28

E11.01 Type 2 diabetes mellitus with hyperosmolarity with coma `HCC` `Rx` `ESR` `COM` `Q`

✓5ᵗʰ **E11.1 Type 2 diabetes mellitus with** ketoacidosis
AHA: 2017,4Q,6
DEF: Diabetic ketoacidosis: Potentially life-threatening complication due to a shortage of insulin in which the body switches to burning fatty acids and producing acidic ketone bodies.

E11.10 Type 2 diabetes mellitus with ketoacidosis without coma `HCC` `Rx` `ESR` `COM`

E11.11 Type 2 diabetes mellitus with ketoacidosis with coma `HCC` `Rx` `ESR` `COM`

✓5ᵗʰ **E11.2 Type 2 diabetes mellitus with** kidney complications
AHA: 2019,3Q,3; 2018,4Q,88

E11.21 Type 2 diabetes mellitus with diabetic nephropathy `HCC` `Rx` `ESR` `COM` `Q`
Type 2 diabetes mellitus with intercapillary glomerulosclerosis
Type 2 diabetes mellitus with intracapillary glomerulonephrosis
Type 2 diabetes mellitus with Kimmelstiel-Wilson disease

E11.22 Type 2 diabetes mellitus with diabetic chronic kidney disease `HCC` `Rx` `ESR` `COM` `Q`
Use additional code to identify stage of chronic kidney disease (N18.1-N18.6)

E11.29 Type 2 diabetes mellitus with other diabetic kidney complication `HCC` `Rx` `ESR` `COM` `Q`
Type 2 diabetes mellitus with renal tubular degeneration

✓5ᵗʰ **E11.3 Type 2 diabetes mellitus with** ophthalmic complications
AHA: 2016,4Q,11-13

One of the following 7th characters is to be assigned to codes in subcategories E11.32, E11.33, E11.34, E11.35, and E11.37 to designate laterality of the disease:
1   right eye
2   left eye
3   bilateral
9   unspecified eye

✓6ᵗʰ **E11.31 Type 2 diabetes mellitus with unspecified diabetic retinopathy**
DEF: Diabetic retinopathy: Diabetic complication from damage to the retinal vessels resulting in vision problems that can progress to blindness.

E11.311 Type 2 diabetes mellitus with unspecified diabetic retinopathy with macular **edema** `HCC` `Rx` `ESR` `COM` `Q`

E11.319 Type 2 diabetes mellitus with unspecified diabetic retinopathy without macular **edema** `HCC` `Rx` `ESR` `COM` `Q`

Chapter 4. Endocrine, Nutritional and Metabolic Diseases

E11.32–E11.9

✓6ᵗʰ **E11.32 Type 2 diabetes mellitus with mild nonproliferative diabetic retinopathy**
Type 2 diabetes mellitus with nonproliferative diabetic retinopathy NOS

   ✓7ᵗʰ **E11.321 Type 2 diabetes mellitus with mild nonproliferative diabetic retinopathy with macular edema** HCC Rx ESR COM Q

   ✓7ᵗʰ **E11.329 Type 2 diabetes mellitus with mild nonproliferative diabetic retinopathy without macular edema** HCC Rx ESR COM Q

✓6ᵗʰ **E11.33 Type 2 diabetes mellitus with moderate nonproliferative diabetic retinopathy**

   ✓7ᵗʰ **E11.331 Type 2 diabetes mellitus with moderate nonproliferative diabetic retinopathy with macular edema** HCC Rx ESR COM Q

   ✓7ᵗʰ **E11.339 Type 2 diabetes mellitus with moderate nonproliferative diabetic retinopathy without macular edema** HCC Rx ESR COM Q

✓6ᵗʰ **E11.34 Type 2 diabetes mellitus with severe nonproliferative diabetic retinopathy**

   ✓7ᵗʰ **E11.341 Type 2 diabetes mellitus with severe nonproliferative diabetic retinopathy with macular edema** HCC Rx ESR COM Q

   ✓7ᵗʰ **E11.349 Type 2 diabetes mellitus with severe nonproliferative diabetic retinopathy without macular edema** HCC Rx ESR COM Q

✓6ᵗʰ **E11.35 Type 2 diabetes mellitus with proliferative diabetic retinopathy**

   ✓7ᵗʰ **E11.351 Type 2 diabetes mellitus with proliferative diabetic retinopathy with macular edema** HCC Rx ESR COM Q

   ✓7ᵗʰ **E11.352 Type 2 diabetes mellitus with proliferative diabetic retinopathy with traction retinal detachment involving the macula** HCC Rx ESR COM Q

   ✓7ᵗʰ **E11.353 Type 2 diabetes mellitus with proliferative diabetic retinopathy with traction retinal detachment not involving the macula** HCC Rx ESR COM Q

   ✓7ᵗʰ **E11.354 Type 2 diabetes mellitus with proliferative diabetic retinopathy with combined traction retinal detachment and rhegmatogenous retinal detachment** HCC Rx ESR COM Q

   ✓7ᵗʰ **E11.355 Type 2 diabetes mellitus with stable proliferative diabetic retinopathy** HCC Rx ESR COM Q

   ✓7ᵗʰ **E11.359 Type 2 diabetes mellitus with proliferative diabetic retinopathy without macular edema** HCC Rx ESR COM Q

E11.36 Type 2 diabetes mellitus with diabetic cataract HCC Rx ESR COM Q
AHA: 2019,2Q,30-31; 2016,4Q,142

✓x7ᵗʰ **E11.37 Type 2 diabetes mellitus with diabetic macular edema, resolved following treatment** HCC Rx ESR COM Q

E11.39 Type 2 diabetes mellitus with other diabetic ophthalmic complication HCC Rx ESR COM Q
Use additional code to identify manifestation, such as:
   diabetic glaucoma (H40-H42)

✓5ᵗʰ **E11.4 Type 2 diabetes mellitus with neurological complications**

E11.40 Type 2 diabetes mellitus with diabetic neuropathy, unspecified HCC Rx ESR COM Q
AHA: 2013,4Q,129

E11.41 Type 2 diabetes mellitus with diabetic mononeuropathy HCC Rx ESR COM Q

E11.42 Type 2 diabetes mellitus with diabetic polyneuropathy HCC Rx ESR COM Q
Type 2 diabetes mellitus with diabetic neuralgia
AHA: 2020,1Q,12

E11.43 Type 2 diabetes mellitus with diabetic autonomic (poly)neuropathy HCC Rx ESR COM Q
Type 2 diabetes mellitus with diabetic gastroparesis
AHA: 2013,4Q,114

E11.44 Type 2 diabetes mellitus with diabetic amyotrophy HCC Rx ESR COM Q

E11.49 Type 2 diabetes mellitus with other diabetic neurological complication HCC Rx ESR COM Q

✓5ᵗʰ **E11.5 Type 2 diabetes mellitus with circulatory complications**

E11.51 Type 2 diabetes mellitus with diabetic peripheral angiopathy without gangrene HCC Rx ESR COM Q
AHA: 2018,3Q,3-4; 2018,2Q,7

E11.52 Type 2 diabetes mellitus with diabetic peripheral angiopathy with gangrene HCC Rx ESR COM Q
Type 2 diabetes mellitus with diabetic gangrene
AHA: 2020,2Q,18; 2018,3Q,3; 2018,2Q,7; 2017,4Q,102

E11.59 Type 2 diabetes mellitus with other circulatory complications HCC Rx ESR COM Q

✓5ᵗʰ **E11.6 Type 2 diabetes mellitus with other specified complications**

✓6ᵗʰ **E11.61 Type 2 diabetes mellitus with diabetic arthropathy**

E11.610 Type 2 diabetes mellitus with diabetic neuropathic arthropathy HCC Rx ESR COM Q
Type 2 diabetes mellitus with Charcôt's joints
DEF: Charcot's joint: Progressive neurologic arthropathy in which chronic degeneration of joints in the weight-bearing areas with peripheral hypertrophy occurs as a complication of a neuropathy disorder. Supporting structures relax from a loss of sensation resulting in chronic joint instability.

E11.618 Type 2 diabetes mellitus with other diabetic arthropathy HCC Rx ESR COM Q
AHA: 2018,2Q,6

✓6ᵗʰ **E11.62 Type 2 diabetes mellitus with skin complications**

E11.620 Type 2 diabetes mellitus with diabetic dermatitis HCC Rx ESR COM Q
Type 2 diabetes mellitus with diabetic necrobiosis lipoidica

E11.621 Type 2 diabetes mellitus with foot ulcer HCC Rx ESR COM Q
Use additional code to identify site of ulcer (L97.4-, L97.5-)
AHA: 2020,2Q,19; 2020,1Q,12
TIP: Do not assign a code for diabetic ulcer when the ulcer is closed/resolved or to report history of diabetic ulcers; Z86.31 Personal history of diabetic foot ulcer, may be assigned.

E11.622 Type 2 diabetes mellitus with other skin ulcer HCC Rx ESR COM Q
Use additional code to identify site of ulcer (L97.1-L97.9, L98.41-L98.49)
AHA: 2021,1Q,7; 2017,4Q,17

E11.628 Type 2 diabetes mellitus with other skin complications HCC Rx ESR COM Q

✓6ᵗʰ **E11.63 Type 2 diabetes mellitus with oral complications**

E11.630 Type 2 diabetes mellitus with periodontal disease HCC Rx ESR COM Q

E11.638 Type 2 diabetes mellitus with other oral complications HCC Rx ESR COM Q

✓6ᵗʰ **E11.64 Type 2 diabetes mellitus with hypoglycemia**
AHA: 2017,1Q,42

E11.641 Type 2 diabetes mellitus with hypoglycemia with coma HCC Rx ESR COM Q

E11.649 Type 2 diabetes mellitus with hypoglycemia without coma HCC Rx ESR COM Q
AHA: 2016,3Q,42; 2015,3Q,21

E11.65 Type 2 diabetes mellitus with hyperglycemia HCC Rx ESR COM Q
AHA: 2022,1Q,28; 2017,1Q,42; 2013,3Q,20

E11.69 Type 2 diabetes mellitus with other specified complication HCC Rx ESR COM Q
Use additional code to identify complication
AHA: 2020,1Q,12; 2016,4Q,141; 2016,1Q,13

E11.8 Type 2 diabetes mellitus with unspecified complications HCC Rx ESR COM Q

E11.9 Type 2 diabetes mellitus without complications HCC Rx ESR COM Q
AHA: 2020,2Q,18

HCC CMS-HCC   Rx Rx HCC   ESR ESRD HCC   COM Commercial HCC   N Newborn: 0   P Pediatric: 0-17   M Maternity: 9-64   A Adult: 15-124

☑4ᵗʰ **E13 Other specified diabetes mellitus**

INCLUDES   diabetes mellitus due to genetic defects of beta-cell function
diabetes mellitus due to genetic defects in insulin action
postpancreatectomy diabetes mellitus
postprocedural diabetes mellitus
secondary diabetes mellitus NEC

Use additional code to identify control using:
insulin (Z79.4)
oral antidiabetic drugs (Z79.84)
oral hypoglycemic drugs (Z79.84)

EXCLUDES 1   diabetes (mellitus) due to autoimmune process (E10.-)
diabetes (mellitus) due to immune mediated pancreatic islet beta-cell destruction (E10.-)
diabetes mellitus due to underlying condition (E08.-)
drug or chemical induced diabetes mellitus (E09.-)
gestational diabetes (O24.4-)
neonatal diabetes mellitus (P70.2)
type 1 diabetes mellitus (E10.-)

AHA: 2018,3Q,4; 2016,1Q,11-13

TIP: Use this category when the diabetes is documented as diabetes type 1.5. Synonymous terms used in the documentation may also include combined diabetes type 1 and type 2, latent autoimmune diabetes of adults (LADA), slow-progressing type 1 diabetes, or double diabetes.

TIP: When postprocedural or postpancreatectomy hypoinsulinemia (E89.1) is documented with postprocedural or postpancreatectomy diabetes mellitus (E13.-), code E89.1 should be sequenced first.

☑5ᵗʰ **E13.0 Other specified diabetes mellitus with** hyperosmolarity
    DEF: Diabetic hyperosmolarity: Extremely high levels of glucose in the blood without ketones.

    E13.00 Other specified diabetes mellitus with hyperosmolarity without nonketotic hyperglycemic-hyperosmolar coma (NKHHC)   HCC Rx ESR COM Q
        EXCLUDES 2   type 2 diabetes mellitus (E11.-)

    E13.01 Other specified diabetes mellitus with hyperosmolarity with coma   HCC Rx ESR COM Q

☑5ᵗʰ **E13.1 Other specified diabetes mellitus with** ketoacidosis
    AHA: 2016,2Q,10; 2013,1Q,26
    DEF: Diabetic ketoacidosis: Potentially life-threatening complication due to a shortage of insulin in which the body switches to burning fatty acids and producing acidic ketone bodies.

    E13.10 Other specified diabetes mellitus with ketoacidosis without coma   HCC Rx ESR COM Q

    E13.11 Other specified diabetes mellitus with ketoacidosis with coma   HCC Rx ESR COM Q

☑5ᵗʰ **E13.2 Other specified diabetes mellitus with** kidney complications
    AHA: 2019,3Q,3; 2018,4Q,88

    E13.21 Other specified diabetes mellitus with diabetic nephropathy   HCC Rx ESR COM Q
        Other specified diabetes mellitus with intercapillary glomerulosclerosis
        Other specified diabetes mellitus with intracapillary glomerulonephrosis
        Other specified diabetes mellitus with Kimmelstiel-Wilson disease

    E13.22 Other specified diabetes mellitus with diabetic chronic kidney disease   HCC Rx ESR COM Q
        Use additional code to identify stage of chronic kidney disease (N18.1-N18.6)

    E13.29 Other specified diabetes mellitus with other diabetic kidney complication   HCC Rx ESR COM Q
        Other specified diabetes mellitus with renal tubular degeneration

☑5ᵗʰ **E13.3 Other specified diabetes mellitus with** ophthalmic complications
    AHA: 2016,4Q,11-13

One of the following 7th characters is to be assigned to codes in subcategories E13.32, E13.33, E13.34, E13.35, and E13.37 to designate laterality of the disease:
1   right eye
2   left eye
3   bilateral
9   unspecified eye

☑6ᵗʰ **E13.31 Other specified diabetes mellitus with unspecified diabetic** retinopathy
    DEF: Diabetic retinopathy: Diabetic complication from damage to the retinal vessels resulting in vision problems that can progress to blindness.

    E13.311 Other specified diabetes mellitus with unspecified diabetic retinopathy with macular edema   HCC Rx ESR COM Q

    E13.319 Other specified diabetes mellitus with unspecified diabetic retinopathy without macular edema   HCC Rx ESR COM Q

☑6ᵗʰ **E13.32 Other specified diabetes mellitus with** mild nonproliferative diabetic retinopathy
    Other specified diabetes mellitus with nonproliferative diabetic retinopathy NOS

    ☑7ᵗʰ **E13.321 Other specified diabetes mellitus with mild nonproliferative diabetic retinopathy** with macular edema   HCC Rx ESR COM Q

    ☑7ᵗʰ **E13.329 Other specified diabetes mellitus with mild nonproliferative diabetic retinopathy** without macular edema   HCC Rx ESR COM Q

☑6ᵗʰ **E13.33 Other specified diabetes mellitus with** moderate nonproliferative diabetic retinopathy

    ☑7ᵗʰ **E13.331 Other specified diabetes mellitus with moderate nonproliferative diabetic retinopathy** with macular edema   HCC Rx ESR COM Q

    ☑7ᵗʰ **E13.339 Other specified diabetes mellitus with moderate nonproliferative diabetic retinopathy** without macular edema   HCC Rx ESR COM Q

☑6ᵗʰ **E13.34 Other specified diabetes mellitus with** severe nonproliferative diabetic retinopathy

    ☑7ᵗʰ **E13.341 Other specified diabetes mellitus with severe nonproliferative diabetic retinopathy** with macular edema   HCC Rx ESR COM Q

    ☑7ᵗʰ **E13.349 Other specified diabetes mellitus with severe nonproliferative diabetic retinopathy** without macular edema   HCC Rx ESR COM Q

☑6ᵗʰ **E13.35 Other specified diabetes mellitus with** proliferative diabetic retinopathy

    ☑7ᵗʰ **E13.351 Other specified diabetes mellitus with proliferative diabetic retinopathy** with macular edema   HCC Rx ESR COM Q

    ☑7ᵗʰ **E13.352 Other specified diabetes mellitus with proliferative diabetic retinopathy** with traction retinal detachment involving the macula   HCC Rx ESR COM Q

    ☑7ᵗʰ **E13.353 Other specified diabetes mellitus with proliferative diabetic retinopathy** with traction retinal detachment not involving the macula   HCC Rx ESR COM Q

    ☑7ᵗʰ **E13.354 Other specified diabetes mellitus with proliferative diabetic retinopathy** with combined traction retinal detachment and rhegmatogenous retinal detachment   HCC Rx ESR COM Q

    ☑7ᵗʰ **E13.355 Other specified diabetes mellitus with** stable proliferative diabetic retinopathy   HCC Rx ESR COM Q

    ☑7ᵗʰ **E13.359 Other specified diabetes mellitus with proliferative diabetic retinopathy** without macular edema   HCC Rx ESR COM Q

    E13.36 Other specified diabetes mellitus with diabetic cataract   HCC Rx ESR COM Q
        AHA: 2019,2Q,30-31; 2016,4Q,142

√x7ᵗʰ **E13.37 Other specified diabetes mellitus with diabetic macular edema, resolved following treatment** `HCC` `Rx` `ESR` `COM` `Q`

E13.39 Other specified diabetes mellitus with other diabetic ophthalmic complication `HCC` `Rx` `ESR` `COM` `Q`
Use additional code to identify manifestation, such as:
diabetic glaucoma (H40-H42)

√5ᵗʰ **E13.4 Other specified diabetes mellitus with neurological complications**

E13.40 Other specified diabetes mellitus with diabetic neuropathy, unspecified `HCC` `Rx` `ESR` `COM` `Q`

E13.41 Other specified diabetes mellitus with diabetic mononeuropathy `HCC` `Rx` `ESR` `COM` `Q`

E13.42 Other specified diabetes mellitus with diabetic polyneuropathy `HCC` `Rx` `ESR` `COM` `Q`
Other specified diabetes mellitus with diabetic neuralgia

E13.43 Other specified diabetes mellitus with diabetic autonomic (poly)neuropathy `HCC` `Rx` `ESR` `COM` `Q`
Other specified diabetes mellitus with diabetic gastroparesis
AHA: 2013,4Q,114

E13.44 Other specified diabetes mellitus with diabetic amyotrophy `HCC` `Rx` `ESR` `COM` `Q`

E13.49 Other specified diabetes mellitus with other diabetic neurological complication `HCC` `Rx` `ESR` `COM` `Q`

√5ᵗʰ **E13.5 Other specified diabetes mellitus with circulatory complications**

E13.51 Other specified diabetes mellitus with diabetic peripheral angiopathy without gangrene `HCC` `Rx` `ESR` `COM` `Q`
AHA: 2018,3Q,3-4; 2018,2Q,7

E13.52 Other specified diabetes mellitus with diabetic peripheral angiopathy with gangrene `HCC` `Rx` `ESR` `COM` `Q`
Other specified diabetes mellitus with diabetic gangrene
AHA: 2020,2Q,18; 2018,3Q,3; 2018,2Q,7; 2017,4Q,102

E13.59 Other specified diabetes mellitus with other circulatory complications `HCC` `Rx` `ESR` `COM` `Q`

√5ᵗʰ **E13.6 Other specified diabetes mellitus with other specified complications**

√6ᵗʰ **E13.61 Other specified diabetes mellitus with diabetic arthropathy**

E13.610 Other specified diabetes mellitus with diabetic neuropathic arthropathy `HCC` `Rx` `ESR` `COM` `Q`
Other specified diabetes mellitus with Charcôt's joints
DEF: Charcot's joint: Progressive neurologic arthropathy in which chronic degeneration of joints in the weight-bearing areas with peripheral hypertrophy occurs as a complication of a neuropathy disorder. Supporting structures relax from a loss of sensation resulting in chronic joint instability.

E13.618 Other specified diabetes mellitus with other diabetic arthropathy `HCC` `Rx` `ESR` `COM` `Q`
AHA: 2018,2Q,6

√6ᵗʰ **E13.62 Other specified diabetes mellitus with skin complications**

E13.620 Other specified diabetes mellitus with diabetic dermatitis `HCC` `Rx` `ESR` `COM` `Q`
Other specified diabetes mellitus with diabetic necrobiosis lipoidica

E13.621 Other specified diabetes mellitus with foot ulcer `HCC` `Rx` `ESR` `COM` `Q`
Use additional code to identify site of ulcer (L97.4-, L97.5-)
AHA: 2020,2Q,19
TIP: Do not assign a code for diabetic ulcer when the ulcer is closed/resolved or to report history of diabetic ulcers; Z86.31 Personal history of diabetic foot ulcer, may be assigned.

E13.622 Other specified diabetes mellitus with other skin ulcer `HCC` `Rx` `ESR` `COM` `Q`
Use additional code to identify site of ulcer (L97.1-L97.9, L98.41-L98.49)
AHA: 2021,1Q,7; 2017,4Q,17

E13.628 Other specified diabetes mellitus with other skin complications `HCC` `Rx` `ESR` `COM` `Q`

√6ᵗʰ **E13.63 Other specified diabetes mellitus with oral complications**

E13.630 Other specified diabetes mellitus with periodontal disease `HCC` `Rx` `ESR` `COM` `Q`

E13.638 Other specified diabetes mellitus with other oral complications `HCC` `Rx` `ESR` `COM` `Q`

√6ᵗʰ **E13.64 Other specified diabetes mellitus with hypoglycemia**
AHA: 2017,1Q,42

E13.641 Other specified diabetes mellitus with hypoglycemia with coma `HCC` `Rx` `ESR` `COM` `Q`

E13.649 Other specified diabetes mellitus with hypoglycemia without coma `HCC` `Rx` `ESR` `COM` `Q`
AHA: 2016,3Q,42; 2015,3Q,21

E13.65 Other specified diabetes mellitus with hyperglycemia `HCC` `Rx` `ESR` `COM` `Q`
AHA: 2017,1Q,42; 2013,3Q,20

E13.69 Other specified diabetes mellitus with other specified complication `HCC` `Rx` `ESR` `COM` `Q`
Use additional code to identify complication
AHA: 2016,4Q,141; 2016,1Q,13

E13.8 Other specified diabetes mellitus with unspecified complications `HCC` `Rx` `ESR` `COM` `Q`

E13.9 Other specified diabetes mellitus without complications `HCC` `Rx` `ESR` `COM` `Q`
AHA: 2020,2Q,18

Other disorders of glucose regulation and pancreatic internal secretion (E15-E16)

E15 Nondiabetic hypoglycemic coma `HCC` `ESR` `COM`
`INCLUDES` drug-induced insulin coma in nondiabetic
hyperinsulinism with hypoglycemic coma
hypoglycemic coma NOS

√4ᵗʰ **E16 Other disorders of pancreatic internal secretion**

E16.0 Drug-induced hypoglycemia without coma
`EXCLUDES 1` *diabetes with hypoglycemia without coma (E09.649)*
Use additional code for adverse effect, if applicable, to identify drug (T36-T50 with fifth or sixth character 5)

E16.1 Other hypoglycemia
Functional hyperinsulinism
Functional nonhyperinsulinemic hypoglycemia
Hyperinsulinism NOS
Hyperplasia of pancreatic islet beta cells NOS
`EXCLUDES 1` *diabetes with hypoglycemia (E08.649, E10.649, E11.649, E13.649)*
hypoglycemia in infant of diabetic mother (P70.1)
neonatal hypoglycemia (P70.4)

E16.2 Hypoglycemia, unspecified
`EXCLUDES 1` *diabetes with hypoglycemia (E08.649, E10.649, E11.649, E13.649)*
AHA: 2016,3Q,42
TIP: Assign for nondiabetic hypoglycemic encephalopathy not further clarified in the documentation.

E16.3 Increased secretion of glucagon `Rx`
Hyperplasia of pancreatic endocrine cells with glucagon excess

E16.4 Increased secretion of gastrin `Rx`
Hypergastrinemia
Hyperplasia of pancreatic endocrine cells with gastrin excess
Zollinger-Ellison syndrome

`HCC` CMS-HCC   `Rx` Rx HCC   `ESR` ESRD HCC   `COM` Commercial HCC   `N` Newborn: 0   `P` Pediatric: 0-17   `M` Maternity: 9-64   `A` Adult: 15-124

540   ICD-10-CM 2023

E16.8 Other specified disorders of pancreatic internal secretion `Rx`
Increased secretion from endocrine pancreas of growth hormone-releasing hormone
Increased secretion from endocrine pancreas of pancreatic polypeptide
Increased secretion from endocrine pancreas of somatostatin
Increased secretion from endocrine pancreas of vasoactive-intestinal polypeptide

E16.9 Disorder of pancreatic internal secretion, unspecified `Rx`
Islet-cell hyperplasia NOS
Pancreatic endocrine cell hyperplasia NOS

Disorders of other endocrine glands (E20-E35)

EXCLUDES 1   *galactorrhea (N64.3)*
gynecomastia (N62)

✓4th **E20 Hypoparathyroidism**
EXCLUDES 1   *Di George's syndrome (D82.1)*
postprocedural hypoparathyroidism (E89.2)
tetany NOS (R29.0)
transitory neonatal hypoparathyroidism (P71.4)

E20.0 Idiopathic hypoparathyroidism `HCC` `Rx` `ESR` `COM`
DEF: Abnormally low secretion of parathyroid hormones, with unknown cause, which triggers decreased calcium and increased phosphorus in the blood that can result in cataracts, muscle cramps, tetany, tingling, or burning in the lips, fingers, and toes.

E20.1 Pseudohypoparathyroidism

E20.8 Other hypoparathyroidism `HCC` `Rx` `ESR` `COM`

E20.9 Hypoparathyroidism, unspecified `HCC` `Rx` `ESR` `COM`
Parathyroid tetany

✓4th **E21 Hyperparathyroidism and other disorders of parathyroid gland**
EXCLUDES 1   *adult osteomalacia (M83.-)*
ectopic hyperparathyroidism (E34.2)
hungry bone syndrome (E83.81)
infantile and juvenile osteomalacia (E55.0)
EXCLUDES 2   *familial hypocalciuric hypercalcemia (E83.52)*

E21.0 Primary hyperparathyroidism `HCC` `Rx` `ESR` `COM`
Hyperplasia of parathyroid
Osteitis fibrosa cystica generalisata [von Recklinghausen's disease of bone]
DEF: Parathyroid dysfunction commonly caused by hyperplasia of two or more glands. Symptoms include hypercalcemia and increased parathyroid hormone levels.

E21.1 Secondary hyperparathyroidism, not elsewhere classified `HCC` `Rx` `ESR` `COM`
EXCLUDES 1   *secondary hyperparathyroidism of renal origin (N25.81)*

E21.2 Other hyperparathyroidism `HCC` `Rx` `ESR` `COM`
Tertiary hyperparathyroidism
EXCLUDES 1   *familial hypocalciuric hypercalcemia (E83.52)*

E21.3 Hyperparathyroidism, unspecified `HCC` `Rx` `ESR` `COM`

E21.4 Other specified disorders of parathyroid gland `HCC` `Rx` `ESR` `COM`

E21.5 Disorder of parathyroid gland, unspecified `HCC` `Rx` `ESR` `COM`

✓4th **E22 Hyperfunction of pituitary gland**
EXCLUDES 1   *Cushing's syndrome (E24.-)*
Nelson's syndrome (E24.1)
overproduction of ACTH not associated with Cushing's disease (E27.0)
overproduction of pituitary ACTH (E24.0)
overproduction of thyroid-stimulating hormone (E05.8-)

E22.0 Acromegaly and pituitary gigantism `HCC` `Rx` `ESR` `COM`
Overproduction of growth hormone
EXCLUDES 1   *constitutional gigantism (E34.4)*
constitutional tall stature (E34.4)
increased secretion from endocrine pancreas of growth hormone-releasing hormone (E16.8)
DEF: Acromegaly: Chronic condition caused by overproduction of the pituitary growth hormone resulting in enlarged skeletal parts and facial features.

E22.1 Hyperprolactinemia `HCC` `Rx` `ESR` `COM`
Use additional code for adverse effect, if applicable, to identify drug (T36-T50 with fifth or sixth character 5)

E22.2 Syndrome of inappropriate secretion of antidiuretic hormone `HCC` `Rx` `ESR` `COM`

E22.8 Other hyperfunction of pituitary gland `HCC` `Rx` `ESR` `COM`
Central precocious puberty

E22.9 Hyperfunction of pituitary gland, unspecified `HCC` `Rx` `ESR` `COM`

✓4th **E23 Hypofunction and other disorders of the pituitary gland**
INCLUDES   the listed conditions whether the disorder is in the pituitary or the hypothalamus
EXCLUDES 1   *postprocedural hypopituitarism (E89.3)*
▶*short stature due to endocrine disorder (E34.3-)*◄

E23.0 Hypopituitarism `HCC` `Rx` `ESR` `COM`
Fertile eunuch syndrome
Hypogonadotropic hypogonadism
Idiopathic growth hormone deficiency
Isolated deficiency of gonadotropin
Isolated deficiency of growth hormone
Isolated deficiency of pituitary hormone
Kallmann's syndrome
Lorain-Levi short stature
Necrosis of pituitary gland (postpartum)
Panhypopituitarism
Pituitary cachexia
Pituitary insufficiency NOS
Pituitary short stature
Sheehan's syndrome
Simmonds' disease

E23.1 Drug-induced hypopituitarism `HCC` `Rx` `ESR` `COM`
Use additional code for adverse effect, if applicable, to identify drug (T36-T50 with fifth or sixth character 5)

E23.2 Diabetes insipidus `HCC` `Rx` `ESR` `COM`
EXCLUDES 1   *nephrogenic diabetes insipidus (N25.1)*

E23.3 Hypothalamic dysfunction, not elsewhere classified `HCC` `Rx` `ESR` `COM`
EXCLUDES 1   *Prader-Willi syndrome (Q87.11)*
Russell-Silver syndrome (Q87.19)

E23.6 Other disorders of pituitary gland `HCC` `Rx` `ESR` `COM`
Abscess of pituitary
Adiposogenital dystrophy

E23.7 Disorder of pituitary gland, unspecified `HCC` `Rx` `ESR` `COM`

✓4th **E24 Cushing's syndrome**
EXCLUDES 1   *congenital adrenal hyperplasia (E25.0)*
DEF: Abdominal striae, acne, hypertension, decreased carbohydrate tolerance, moon face, obesity, protein catabolism, and psychiatric disturbances resulting from increased adrenocortical secretion of cortisol caused by ACTH-dependent adrenocortical hyperplasia or tumor, or by steroid effects.

E24.0 Pituitary-dependent Cushing's disease `HCC` `Rx` `ESR` `COM`
Overproduction of pituitary ACTH
Pituitary-dependent hypercorticalism

E24.1 Nelson's syndrome `HCC` `Rx` `ESR` `COM`

E24.2 Drug-induced Cushing's syndrome `HCC` `Rx` `ESR` `COM`
Use additional code for adverse effect, if applicable, to identify drug (T36-T50 with fifth or sixth character 5)

E24.3 Ectopic ACTH syndrome `HCC` `Rx` `ESR` `COM`

E24.4 Alcohol-induced pseudo-Cushing's syndrome `HCC` `Rx` `ESR` `COM`

E24.8 Other Cushing's syndrome `HCC` `Rx` `ESR` `COM`

E24.9 Cushing's syndrome, unspecified `HCC` `Rx` `ESR` `COM`

Chapter 4. Endocrine, Nutritional and Metabolic Diseases

✓4ᵗʰ **E25** **Adrenogenital disorders**

INCLUDES   adrenogenital syndromes, virilizing or feminizing, whether acquired or due to adrenal hyperplasia
consequent on inborn enzyme defects in hormone synthesis
female adrenal pseudohermaphroditism
female heterosexual precocious pseudopuberty
male isosexual precocious pseudopuberty
male macrogenitosomia praecox
male sexual precocity with adrenal hyperplasia
male virilization (female)

EXCLUDES 1   *indeterminate sex and pseudohermaphroditism (Q56)*
chromosomal abnormalities (Q90-Q99)

E25.0   **Congenital adrenogenital disorders associated with enzyme deficiency**   HCC Rx ESR COM
Congenital adrenal hyperplasia
21-Hydroxylase deficiency
Salt-losing congenital adrenal hyperplasia

E25.8   **Other adrenogenital disorders**   HCC Rx ESR COM
Idiopathic adrenogenital disorder
Use additional code for adverse effect, if applicable, to identify drug (T36-T50 with fifth or sixth character 5)

E25.9   **Adrenogenital disorder, unspecified**   HCC Rx ESR COM
Adrenogenital syndrome NOS

✓4ᵗʰ **E26** **Hyperaldosteronism**

✓5ᵗʰ **E26.0**   **Primary hyperaldosteronism**

    E26.01   **Conn's syndrome**   HCC Rx ESR COM
Code also adrenal adenoma (D35.0-)

    E26.02   **Glucocorticoid-remediable aldosteronism**   HCC Rx ESR COM
Familial aldosteronism type I
DEF: Rare autosomal dominant familial form of primary aldosteronism in which the secretion of aldosterone is under the influence of adrenocorticotrophic hormone (ACTH) rather than the renin-angiotensin mechanism. Moderate hypersecretion of aldosterone and suppressed plasma renin activity that are rapidly reversed by administration of glucosteroids. Symptoms include hypertension and mild hypokalemia.

    E26.09   **Other primary hyperaldosteronism**   HCC Rx ESR COM
Primary aldosteronism due to adrenal hyperplasia (bilateral)

E26.1   **Secondary hyperaldosteronism**   HCC Rx ESR COM

✓5ᵗʰ **E26.8**   **Other hyperaldosteronism**

    E26.81   **Bartter's syndrome**   HCC Rx ESR COM

    E26.89   **Other hyperaldosteronism**   HCC Rx ESR COM

E26.9   **Hyperaldosteronism, unspecified**   HCC Rx ESR COM
Aldosteronism NOS
Hyperaldosteronism NOS

✓4ᵗʰ **E27** **Other disorders of adrenal gland**

E27.0   **Other adrenocortical overactivity**   HCC Rx ESR COM
Overproduction of ACTH, not associated with Cushing's disease
Premature adrenarche
EXCLUDES 1   *Cushing's syndrome (E24.-)*

E27.1   **Primary adrenocortical insufficiency**   HCC Rx ESR COM
Addison's disease
Autoimmune adrenalitis
EXCLUDES 1   *Addison only phenotype adrenoleukodystrophy (E71.528)*
amyloidosis (E85.-)
tuberculous Addison's disease (A18.7)
Waterhouse-Friderichsen syndrome (A39.1)

E27.2   **Addisonian crisis**   HCC Rx ESR COM
Adrenal crisis
Adrenocortical crisis
DEF: Life-threatening condition that occurs when there is not enough cortisol excreted from the adrenal glands. This condition may be due to injury to the adrenal glands or to the pituitary gland, which controls adrenal hormone secretion, or when a patient stops hydrocortisone treatment too quickly or too early.

E27.3   **Drug-induced adrenocortical insufficiency**   HCC Rx ESR COM
Use additional code for adverse effect, if applicable, to identify drug (T36-T50 with fifth or sixth character 5)

✓5ᵗʰ **E27.4**   **Other and unspecified adrenocortical insufficiency**
EXCLUDES 1   *adrenoleukodystrophy [Addison-Schilder] (E71.528)*
Waterhouse-Friderichsen syndrome (A39.1)

    E27.40   **Unspecified adrenocortical insufficiency**   HCC Rx ESR COM
Adrenocortical insufficiency NOS
Hypoaldosteronism

    E27.49   **Other adrenocortical insufficiency**   HCC Rx ESR COM
Adrenal hemorrhage
Adrenal infarction

E27.5   **Adrenomedullary hyperfunction**   HCC Rx ESR COM
Adrenomedullary hyperplasia
Catecholamine hypersecretion

E27.8   **Other specified disorders of adrenal gland**   HCC Rx ESR COM
Abnormality of cortisol-binding globulin

E27.9   **Disorder of adrenal gland, unspecified**   HCC Rx ESR COM

✓4ᵗʰ **E28** **Ovarian dysfunction**
EXCLUDES 1   *isolated gonadotropin deficiency (E23.0)*
postprocedural ovarian failure (E89.4-)

E28.0   **Estrogen excess**   ♀
Use additional code for adverse effect, if applicable, to identify drug (T36-T50 with fifth or sixth character 5)

E28.1   **Androgen excess**   ♀
Hypersecretion of ovarian androgens
Use additional code for adverse effect, if applicable, to identify drug (T36-T50 with fifth or sixth character 5)

E28.2   **Polycystic ovarian syndrome**   ♀
Sclerocystic ovary syndrome
Stein-Leventhal syndrome
AHA: 2022,2Q,16
DEF: Common hormonal disorder among women of reproductive age that involves enlarged ovaries with numerous small cysts located along the outer ovarian edge.

✓5ᵗʰ **E28.3**   **Primary ovarian failure**
EXCLUDES 1   *pure gonadal dysgenesis (Q99.1)*
Turner's syndrome (Q96.-)

    ✓6ᵗʰ **E28.31**   **Premature menopause**

       E28.310   **Symptomatic premature menopause**   A ♀
Symptoms such as flushing, sleeplessness, headache, lack of concentration, associated with premature menopause

       E28.319   **Asymptomatic premature menopause**   A ♀
Premature menopause NOS

    E28.39   **Other primary ovarian failure**   ♀
Decreased estrogen
Resistant ovary syndrome

E28.8   **Other ovarian dysfunction**   ♀
Ovarian hyperfunction NOS
EXCLUDES 1   *postprocedural ovarian failure (E89.4-)*

E28.9   **Ovarian dysfunction, unspecified**   ♀

✓4ᵗʰ **E29** **Testicular dysfunction**
EXCLUDES 1   *androgen insensitivity syndrome (E34.5-)*
azoospermia or oligospermia NOS (N46.0-N46.1)
isolated gonadotropin deficiency (E23.0)
Klinefelter's syndrome (Q98.0-Q98.1, Q98.4)

E29.0   **Testicular hyperfunction**   ♂
Hypersecretion of testicular hormones

E29.1   **Testicular hypofunction**   ♂
Defective biosynthesis of testicular androgen NOS
5-delta-Reductase deficiency (with male pseudohermaphroditism)
Testicular hypogonadism NOS
Use additional code for adverse effect, if applicable, to identify drug (T36-T50 with fifth or sixth character 5)
EXCLUDES 1   *postprocedural testicular hypofunction (E89.5)*

E29.8   **Other testicular dysfunction**   ♂

E29.9   **Testicular dysfunction, unspecified**   ♂

Chapter 4. Endocrine, Nutritional and Metabolic Diseases

E30–E34.9

✓4ᵗʰ E30 Disorders of puberty, not elsewhere classified

E30.0 Delayed puberty
Constitutional delay of puberty
Delayed sexual development

E30.1 Precocious puberty   P
Precocious menstruation
> EXCLUDES 1   Albright (-McCune) (-Sternberg) syndrome (Q78.1)
> central precocious puberty (E22.8)
> congenital adrenal hyperplasia (E25.0)
> female heterosexual precocious pseudopuberty (E25.-)
> male isosexual precocious pseudopuberty (E25.-)

E30.8 Other disorders of puberty   P
Premature thelarche

E30.9 Disorder of puberty, unspecified

✓4ᵗʰ E31 Polyglandular dysfunction
> EXCLUDES 1   ataxia telangiectasia [Louis-Bar] (G11.3)
> dystrophia myotonica [Steinert] (G71.11)
> pseudohypoparathyroidism (E20.1)

E31.0 Autoimmune polyglandular failure   HCC Rx ESR COM
Schmidt's syndrome

E31.1 Polyglandular hyperfunction   HCC Rx ESR COM
> EXCLUDES 1   multiple endocrine adenomatosis (E31.2-)
> multiple endocrine neoplasia (E31.2-)

✓5ᵗʰ E31.2 Multiple endocrine neoplasia [MEN] syndromes
Multiple endocrine adenomatosis
Code also any associated malignancies and other conditions associated with the syndromes
DEF: Group of conditions in which several endocrine glands grow excessively (such as in adenomatous hyperplasia) and/or develop benign or malignant tumors. Tumors and hyperplasia associated with MEN often produce excess hormones, which impede normal physiology. There is no comprehensive cure known for MEN syndrome. Treatment is directed at the hyperplasia or tumors in each individual gland. Tumors are usually surgically removed and oral medications or hormonal injections are used to correct hormone imbalances.

E31.20 Multiple endocrine neoplasia [MEN] syndrome, unspecified   HCC Rx ESR COM
Multiple endocrine adenomatosis NOS
Multiple endocrine neoplasia [MEN] syndrome NOS

E31.21 Multiple endocrine neoplasia [MEN] type I   HCC Rx ESR COM
Wermer's syndrome

E31.22 Multiple endocrine neoplasia [MEN] type IIA   HCC Rx ESR COM
Sipple's syndrome

E31.23 Multiple endocrine neoplasia [MEN] type IIB   HCC Rx ESR COM

E31.8 Other polyglandular dysfunction   HCC Rx ESR COM

E31.9 Polyglandular dysfunction, unspecified   HCC Rx ESR COM

✓4ᵗʰ E32 Diseases of thymus
> EXCLUDES 1   aplasia or hypoplasia of thymus with immunodeficiency (D82.1)
> myasthenia gravis (G70.0)

E32.0 Persistent hyperplasia of thymus   HCC Rx ESR COM
Hypertrophy of thymus

E32.1 Abscess of thymus   HCC Rx ESR COM

E32.8 Other diseases of thymus   HCC Rx ESR COM
> EXCLUDES 1   aplasia or hypoplasia with immunodeficiency (D82.1)
> thymoma (D15.0)

E32.9 Disease of thymus, unspecified   HCC Rx ESR COM

✓4ᵗʰ E34 Other endocrine disorders
> EXCLUDES 1   pseudohypoparathyroidism (E20.1)

E34.0 Carcinoid syndrome   HCC Rx ESR COM
> NOTE   May be used as an additional code to identify functional activity associated with a carcinoid tumor.

E34.1 Other hypersecretion of intestinal hormones

E34.2 Ectopic hormone secretion, not elsewhere classified
> EXCLUDES 1   ectopic ACTH syndrome (E24.3)

▲ ✓5ᵗʰ E34.3 Short stature due to endocrine disorder
~~Constitutional short stature~~
~~Laron-type short stature~~
> EXCLUDES 1   achondroplastic short stature (Q77.4)
> hypochondroplastic short stature (Q77.4)
> nutritional short stature (E45)
> pituitary short stature (E23.0)
> progeria (E34.8)
> renal short stature (N25.0)
> Russell-Silver syndrome (Q87.19)
> short-limbed stature with immunodeficiency (D82.2)
> ►short stature (child) (R62.52)◄
> short stature in specific dysmorphic syndromes - code to syndrome - see Alphabetical Index
> short stature NOS (R62.52)

● #### E34.30 Short stature due to endocrine disorder, unspecified

● #### E34.31 Constitutional short stature
Constitutional delay of growth, puberty, or maturation

● ### ✓6ᵗʰ E34.32 Genetic causes of short stature

● ##### E34.321 Primary insulin-like growth factor-1 (IGF-1) deficiency
Acid-labile subunit gene (IGFALS) defect
Growth hormone gene 1 (GH1) defect with growth hormone neutralizing antibodies
Growth hormone insensitivity syndrome (GHIS)
Insulin-like growth factor 1 gene (IGF1) defect
Laron type short stature
Severe primary insulin-like growth factor-1 deficiency (SPIGFD)
Signal transducer and activator of transcription 5B gene (STAT5b) defect

● ##### E34.322 Insulin-like growth factor-1 (IGF-1) resistance
Genetic syndrome with resistance to insulin-like growth factor-1
Insulin-like growth factor-1 receptor (IGF-1R) defect
Post-insulin-like growth factor-1 receptor signaling defect

● ##### E34.328 Other genetic causes of short stature
Short stature due to ACAN gene variant
Short stature due to aggrecan deficiency
Short stature due to NPR-2 gene variant

● ##### E34.329 Unspecified genetic causes of short stature

● #### E34.39 Other short stature due to endocrine disorder

E34.4 Constitutional tall stature   HCC Rx ESR COM
Constitutional gigantism

✓5ᵗʰ E34.5 Androgen insensitivity syndrome
DEF: X-linked recessive condition in which individuals that are chromosomally male fail to develop normal male external genitalia due to an abnormality on the X chromosome that prohibits the body, completely or in part, from recognizing the androgens produced. **Synonym(s):** AIS

E34.50 Androgen insensitivity syndrome, unspecified
Androgen insensitivity NOS

E34.51 Complete androgen insensitivity syndrome
Complete androgen insensitivity
de Quervain syndrome
Goldberg-Maxwell syndrome

E34.52 Partial androgen insensitivity syndrome
Partial androgen insensitivity
Reifenstein syndrome

E34.8 Other specified endocrine disorders
Pineal gland dysfunction
Progeria
> EXCLUDES 2   pseudohypoparathyroidism (E20.1)

E34.9 Endocrine disorder, unspecified
Endocrine disturbance NOS
Hormone disturbance NOS

E35 Disorders of endocrine glands in diseases classified elsewhere

Code first underlying disease, such as:
late congenital syphilis of thymus gland [Dubois disease] (A50.5)

Use additional code, if applicable, to identify:
sequelae of tuberculosis of other organs (B90.8)

EXCLUDES 1   Echinococcus granulosus infection of thyroid gland (B67.3)
meningococcal hemorrhagic adrenalitis (A39.1)
syphilis of endocrine gland (A52.79)
tuberculosis of adrenal gland, except calcification (A18.7)
tuberculosis of endocrine gland NEC (A18.82)
tuberculosis of thyroid gland (A18.81)
Waterhouse-Friderichsen syndrome (A39.1)

Intraoperative complications of endocrine system (E36)

E36 Intraoperative complications of endocrine system

EXCLUDES 2   postprocedural endocrine and metabolic complications and disorders, not elsewhere classified (E89.-)

E36.0 Intraoperative hemorrhage and hematoma of an endocrine system organ or structure complicating a procedure

EXCLUDES 1   intraoperative hemorrhage and hematoma of an endocrine system organ or structure due to accidental puncture or laceration during a procedure (E36.1-)

E36.01 Intraoperative hemorrhage and hematoma of an endocrine system organ or structure complicating an endocrine system procedure
AHA: 2020,1Q,19

E36.02 Intraoperative hemorrhage and hematoma of an endocrine system organ or structure complicating other procedure

E36.1 Accidental puncture and laceration of an endocrine system organ or structure during a procedure

E36.11 Accidental puncture and laceration of an endocrine system organ or structure during an endocrine system procedure

E36.12 Accidental puncture and laceration of an endocrine system organ or structure during other procedure

E36.8 Other intraoperative complications of endocrine system
Use additional code, if applicable, to further specify disorder

Malnutrition (E40-E46)

EXCLUDES 1   intestinal malabsorption (K90.-)
sequelae of protein-calorie malnutrition (E64.0)

EXCLUDES 2   nutritional anemias (D50-D53)
starvation (T73.0)

AHA: 2020,1Q,4-7; 2017,4Q,108; 2017,3Q,25
TIP: Assign additional code for BMI from category Z68, when documented. BMI can be based on documentation from clinicians who are not the patient's provider.
TIP: Malnutrition is not considered integral to cancer; assign the appropriate code in addition to the code for the specific type of cancer.

E40 Kwashiorkor   HCC ESR COM
Severe malnutrition with nutritional edema with dyspigmentation of skin and hair
EXCLUDES 1   marasmic kwashiorkor (E42)

E41 Nutritional marasmus   HCC ESR COM
Severe malnutrition with marasmus
EXCLUDES 1   marasmic kwashiorkor (E42)
AHA: 2017,3Q,24
DEF: Protein-calorie malabsorption or malnutrition in children characterized by tissue wasting, dehydration, and subcutaneous fat depletion. It may occur with infectious disease.

E42 Marasmic kwashiorkor   HCC ESR COM
Intermediate form severe protein-calorie malnutrition
Severe protein-calorie malnutrition with signs of both kwashiorkor and marasmus

E43 Unspecified severe protein-calorie malnutrition   HCC ESR COM
Starvation edema
AHA: 2022,1Q,13; 2020,1Q,5,6; 2017,4Q,108
TIP: Assign code R64 when emaciation is documented without documentation of malnutrition.

E44 Protein-calorie malnutrition of moderate and mild degree
AHA: 2020,1Q,5
E44.0 Moderate protein-calorie malnutrition   HCC ESR COM
E44.1 Mild protein-calorie malnutrition   HCC ESR COM

E45 Retarded development following protein-calorie malnutrition   HCC ESR COM
Nutritional short stature
Nutritional stunting
Physical retardation due to malnutrition

E46 Unspecified protein-calorie malnutrition   HCC ESR COM
Malnutrition NOS
Protein-calorie imbalance NOS
EXCLUDES 1   nutritional deficiency NOS (E63.9)
AHA: 2018,4Q,82

Other nutritional deficiencies (E50-E64)

EXCLUDES 2   nutritional anemias (D50-D53)

E50 Vitamin A deficiency
EXCLUDES 1   sequelae of vitamin A deficiency (E64.1)
E50.0 Vitamin A deficiency with conjunctival xerosis
E50.1 Vitamin A deficiency with Bitot's spot and conjunctival xerosis
Bitot's spot in the young child
DEF: Vitamin A deficiency with conjunctival dryness and superficial spots of keratinized epithelium.
E50.2 Vitamin A deficiency with corneal xerosis
E50.3 Vitamin A deficiency with corneal ulceration and xerosis
E50.4 Vitamin A deficiency with keratomalacia
DEF: Vitamin A deficiency creating corneal dryness that progresses to corneal insensitivity, softness, and necrosis. It is usually bilateral.
E50.5 Vitamin A deficiency with night blindness
E50.6 Vitamin A deficiency with xerophthalmic scars of cornea
E50.7 Other ocular manifestations of vitamin A deficiency
Xerophthalmia NOS
E50.8 Other manifestations of vitamin A deficiency
Follicular keratosis
Xeroderma
E50.9 Vitamin A deficiency, unspecified
Hypovitaminosis A NOS

E51 Thiamine deficiency
EXCLUDES 1   sequelae of thiamine deficiency (E64.8)
E51.1 Beriberi
E51.11 Dry beriberi
Beriberi NOS
Beriberi with polyneuropathy
E51.12 Wet beriberi
Beriberi with cardiovascular manifestations
Cardiovascular beriberi
Shoshin disease
E51.2 Wernicke's encephalopathy
DEF: Deficiency of vitamin B1 resulting in a triad of acute mental confusion, ataxia, and ophthalmoplegia. The vast majority of affected patients are alcoholics.
E51.8 Other manifestations of thiamine deficiency
E51.9 Thiamine deficiency, unspecified

E52 Niacin deficiency [pellagra]
Niacin (-tryptophan) deficiency
Nicotinamide deficiency
Pellagra (alcoholic)
EXCLUDES 1   sequelae of niacin deficiency (E64.8)

E53 Deficiency of other B group vitamins
EXCLUDES 1   sequelae of vitamin B deficiency (E64.8)
E53.0 Riboflavin deficiency
Ariboflavinosis
Vitamin B2 deficiency
E53.1 Pyridoxine deficiency
Vitamin B6 deficiency
EXCLUDES 1   pyridoxine-responsive sideroblastic anemia (D64.3)
E53.8 Deficiency of other specified B group vitamins
Biotin deficiency
Cyanocobalamin deficiency
Folate deficiency
Folic acid deficiency
Pantothenic acid deficiency
Vitamin B12 deficiency
EXCLUDES 1   folate deficiency anemia (D52.-)
vitamin B12 deficiency anemia (D51.-)
E53.9 Vitamin B deficiency, unspecified

E54 **Ascorbic acid deficiency**
Deficiency of vitamin C
Scurvy
EXCLUDES 1   *scorbutic anemia (D53.2)*
sequelae of vitamin C deficiency (E64.2)
DEF: Vitamin C deficiency causing swollen gums, myalgia, weight loss, and weakness.

✓4ᵗʰ **E55** **Vitamin D deficiency**
EXCLUDES 1   *adult osteomalacia (M83.-)*
osteoporosis (M80.-)
sequelae of rickets (E64.3)

     E55.0 **Rickets, active**   Rx
Infantile osteomalacia
Juvenile osteomalacia
EXCLUDES 1   *celiac rickets (K90.0)*
Crohn's rickets (K50.-)
hereditary vitamin D-dependent rickets (E83.32)
inactive rickets (E64.3)
renal rickets (N25.0)
sequelae of rickets (E64.3)
vitamin D-resistant rickets (E83.31)
DEF: Rickets: Softening or weakening of the bones due to a lack of vitamin D, calcium, and phosphate.
     E55.9 **Vitamin D deficiency, unspecified**
Avitaminosis D

✓4ᵗʰ **E56** **Other vitamin deficiencies**
EXCLUDES 1   *sequelae of other vitamin deficiencies (E64.8)*

     E56.0 **Deficiency of vitamin E**
     E56.1 **Deficiency of vitamin K**
EXCLUDES 1   *deficiency of coagulation factor due to vitamin K deficiency (D68.4)*
vitamin K deficiency of newborn (P53)

     E56.8 **Deficiency of other vitamins**
     E56.9 **Vitamin deficiency, unspecified**

E58 **Dietary calcium deficiency**
EXCLUDES 1   *disorders of calcium metabolism (E83.5-)*
sequelae of calcium deficiency (E64.8)

E59 **Dietary selenium deficiency**
Keshan disease
EXCLUDES 1   *sequelae of selenium deficiency (E64.8)*

E60 **Dietary zinc deficiency**

✓4ᵗʰ **E61** **Deficiency of other nutrient elements**
Use additional code for adverse effect, if applicable, to identify drug (T36-T50 with fifth or sixth character 5)
EXCLUDES 1   *disorders of mineral metabolism (E83.-)*
iodine deficiency related thyroid disorders (E00-E02)
sequelae of malnutrition and other nutritional deficiencies (E64.-)

     E61.0 **Copper deficiency**
     E61.1 **Iron deficiency**
EXCLUDES 1   *iron deficiency anemia (D50.-)*

     E61.2 **Magnesium deficiency**
     E61.3 **Manganese deficiency**
     E61.4 **Chromium deficiency**
     E61.5 **Molybdenum deficiency**
     E61.6 **Vanadium deficiency**
     E61.7 **Deficiency of multiple nutrient elements**
     E61.8 **Deficiency of other specified nutrient elements**
     E61.9 **Deficiency of nutrient element, unspecified**

✓4ᵗʰ **E63** **Other nutritional deficiencies**
EXCLUDES 2   *dehydration (E86.0)*
failure to thrive, adult (R62.7)
failure to thrive, child (R62.51)
feeding problems in newborn (P92.-)
sequelae of malnutrition and other nutritional deficiencies (E64.-)

     E63.0 **Essential fatty acid [EFA] deficiency**
     E63.1 **Imbalance of constituents of food intake**
     E63.8 **Other specified nutritional deficiencies**
     E63.9 **Nutritional deficiency, unspecified**

✓4ᵗʰ **E64** **Sequelae of malnutrition and other nutritional deficiencies**
NOTE   This category is to be used to indicate conditions in categories E43, E44, E46, E50-E63 as the cause of sequelae, which are themselves classified elsewhere. The 'sequelae' include conditions specified as such; they also include the late effects of diseases classifiable to the above categories if the disease itself is no longer present
Code first condition resulting from (sequela) of malnutrition and other nutritional deficiencies

     E64.0 **Sequelae of protein-calorie malnutrition**   HCC ESR
EXCLUDES 2   *retarded development following protein-calorie malnutrition (E45)*

     E64.1 **Sequelae of vitamin A deficiency**
     E64.2 **Sequelae of vitamin C deficiency**
     E64.3 **Sequelae of rickets**
     E64.8 **Sequelae of other nutritional deficiencies**
     E64.9 **Sequelae of unspecified nutritional deficiency**

Overweight, obesity and other hyperalimentation (E65-E68)

E65 **Localized adiposity**
Fat pad

✓4ᵗʰ **E66** **Overweight and obesity**
Code first obesity complicating pregnancy, childbirth and the puerperium, if applicable (O99.21-)
Use additional code to identify body mass index (BMI), if known (Z68.-)
EXCLUDES 1   *adiposogenital dystrophy (E23.6)*
lipomatosis NOS (E88.2)
lipomatosis dolorosa [Dercum] (E88.2)
Prader-Willi syndrome (Q87.11)
AHA: 2018,4Q,77,79-80
TIP: Do not assign a BMI code (Z68.-) when a pregnant patient is documented as being overweight or obese. Only a code from subcategory O99.21- and a code from this category should be assigned.

✓5ᵗʰ **E66.0** **Obesity due to excess calories**
     E66.01 **Morbid (severe) obesity due to excess calories**   HCC ESR
EXCLUDES 1   *morbid (severe) obesity with alveolar hypoventilation (E66.2)*
AHA: 2022,2Q,9
     E66.09 **Other obesity due to excess calories**
     E66.1 **Drug-induced obesity**
Use additional code for adverse effect, if applicable, to identify drug (T36-T50 with fifth or sixth character 5)
     E66.2 **Morbid (severe) obesity with alveolar hypoventilation**   HCC ESR
Obesity hypoventilation syndrome (OHS)
Pickwickian syndrome
     E66.3 **Overweight**
AHA: 2018,4Q,78
     E66.8 **Other obesity**
     E66.9 **Obesity, unspecified**
Obesity NOS
AHA: 2021,2Q,10

✓4ᵗʰ **E67** **Other hyperalimentation**
EXCLUDES 1   *hyperalimentation NOS (R63.2)*
sequelae of hyperalimentation (E68)

     E67.0 **Hypervitaminosis A**
     E67.1 **Hypercarotenemia**
DEF: Elevated blood carotene level as a result of excessive carotenoid ingestion or an inability to convert carotenoids to vitamin A. Characteristics often include yellow discoloration of the skin, which may follow overeating of carotenoid-rich foods such as carrots, sweet potatoes, or squash.
     E67.2 **Megavitamin-B6 syndrome**
     E67.3 **Hypervitaminosis D**
     E67.8 **Other specified hyperalimentation**

E68 **Sequelae of hyperalimentation**
Code first condition resulting from (sequela) of hyperalimentation

Chapter 4. Endocrine, Nutritional and Metabolic Diseases

E70–E71.448

Metabolic disorders (E70-E88)

EXCLUDES 1   *androgen insensitivity syndrome (E34.5-)*
congenital adrenal hyperplasia (E25.0)
hemolytic anemias attributable to enzyme disorders (D55.-)
Marfan's syndrome (Q87.4)
5-alpha-reductase deficiency (E29.1)
EXCLUDES 2   *Ehlers-Danlos syndromes (Q79.6-)*
AHA: 2018,2Q,6

✓4ᵗʰ **E70 Disorders of aromatic amino-acid metabolism**

E70.0   **Classical** phenylketonuria   HCC Rx ESR COM

E70.1   **Other** hyperphenylalaninemias   HCC Rx ESR COM

✓5ᵗʰ **E70.2**   **Disorders of** tyrosine metabolism

      EXCLUDES 1   *transitory tyrosinemia of newborn (P74.5)*

      E70.20   **Disorder of tyrosine metabolism, unspecified**   HCC Rx ESR COM

      E70.21   **Tyrosinemia**   HCC Rx ESR COM
          Hypertyrosinemia

      E70.29   **Other disorders of tyrosine metabolism**   HCC Rx ESR COM
          Alkaptonuria
          Ochronosis

✓5ᵗʰ **E70.3**   Albinism

      DEF: Absence of pigment in skin, hair, and eyes. This genetic condition is often accompanied by astigmatism, photophobia, and nystagmus.

      E70.30   **Albinism, unspecified**   HCC Rx ESR COM

   ✓6ᵗʰ **E70.31**   Ocular albinism

      E70.310   **X-linked** ocular albinism   HCC Rx ESR COM

      E70.311   **Autosomal recessive** ocular albinism   HCC Rx ESR COM

      E70.318   **Other ocular albinism**   HCC Rx ESR COM

      E70.319   **Ocular albinism, unspecified**   HCC Rx ESR COM

   ✓6ᵗʰ **E70.32**   Oculocutaneous albinism

      EXCLUDES 1   *Chediak-Higashi syndrome (E70.330)*
            Hermansky-Pudlak syndrome (E70.331)

      E70.320   **Tyrosinase negative** oculocutaneous albinism   HCC Rx ESR COM
          Albinism I
          Oculocutaneous albinism ty-neg

      E70.321   **Tyrosinase positive** oculocutaneous albinism   HCC Rx ESR COM
          Albinism II
          Oculocutaneous albinism ty-pos

      E70.328   **Other oculocutaneous albinism**   HCC Rx ESR COM
          Cross syndrome

      E70.329   **Oculocutaneous albinism, unspecified**   HCC Rx ESR COM

   ✓6ᵗʰ **E70.33**   Albinism with hematologic abnormality

      E70.330   **Chediak-Higashi syndrome**   HCC Rx ESR COM

      E70.331   **Hermansky-Pudlak syndrome**   HCC Rx ESR COM

      E70.338   **Other albinism with hematologic abnormality**   HCC Rx ESR COM

      E70.339   **Albinism with hematologic abnormality, unspecified**   HCC Rx ESR COM

      E70.39   **Other specified albinism**   HCC Rx ESR COM
          Piebaldism

✓5ᵗʰ **E70.4**   **Disorders of** histidine metabolism

      E70.40   **Disorders of histidine metabolism, unspecified**   HCC Rx ESR COM

      E70.41   **Histidinemia**   HCC Rx ESR COM

      E70.49   **Other disorders of histidine metabolism**   HCC Rx ESR COM

E70.5   **Disorders of** tryptophan metabolism   HCC Rx ESR COM

✓5ᵗʰ **E70.8**   **Other disorders of aromatic amino-acid metabolism**

      AHA: 2020,4Q,15-16

      E70.81   **Aromatic L-amino acid decarboxylase deficiency**   HCC Rx ESR COM
          AADC deficiency

      E70.89   **Other disorders of aromatic amino-acid metabolism**   HCC Rx ESR COM

E70.9   **Disorder of aromatic amino-acid metabolism, unspecified**   HCC Rx ESR COM

✓4ᵗʰ **E71 Disorders of branched-chain amino-acid metabolism and fatty-acid metabolism**

E71.0   **Maple-syrup-urine** disease   HCC Rx ESR COM

✓5ᵗʰ **E71.1**   **Other disorders of** branched-chain amino-acid **metabolism**

   ✓6ᵗʰ **E71.11**   Branched-chain organic acidurias

      E71.110   **Isovaleric** acidemia   HCC Rx ESR COM

      E71.111   **3-methylglutaconic aciduria**   HCC Rx ESR COM

      E71.118   **Other branched-chain organic acidurias**   HCC Rx ESR COM

   ✓6ᵗʰ **E71.12**   Disorders of propionate metabolism

      E71.120   **Methylmalonic acidemia**   HCC Rx ESR COM

      E71.121   **Propionic acidemia**   HCC Rx ESR COM

      E71.128   **Other disorders of propionate metabolism**   HCC Rx ESR COM

      E71.19   **Other disorders of branched-chain amino-acid metabolism**   HCC Rx ESR COM
          Hyperleucine-isoleucinemia
          Hypervalinemia

E71.2   **Disorder of branched-chain amino-acid metabolism, unspecified**   HCC Rx ESR COM

✓5ᵗʰ **E71.3**   **Disorders of fatty-acid metabolism**

      EXCLUDES 1   *peroxisomal disorders (E71.5)*
            Refsum's disease (G60.1)
            Schilder's disease (G37.0)
      EXCLUDES 2   *carnitine deficiency due to inborn error of metabolism (E71.42)*

      E71.30   **Disorder of fatty-acid metabolism, unspecified**   Rx COM

   ✓6ᵗʰ **E71.31**   Disorders of fatty-acid oxidation

      E71.310   **Long chain/very long chain** acyl CoA dehydrogenase deficiency   HCC Rx ESR COM
          LCAD
          VLCAD

      E71.311   **Medium chain** acyl CoA dehydrogenase deficiency   HCC Rx ESR COM
          MCAD

      E71.312   **Short chain** acyl CoA dehydrogenase deficiency   HCC Rx ESR COM
          SCAD

      E71.313   **Glutaric aciduria type II**   HCC Rx ESR COM
          Glutaric aciduria type II A
          Glutaric aciduria type II B
          Glutaric aciduria type II C
          EXCLUDES 1   *glutaric aciduria (type 1) NOS (E72.3)*

      E71.314   **Muscle carnitine palmitoyltransferase deficiency**   HCC Rx ESR COM

      E71.318   **Other disorders of fatty-acid oxidation**   HCC Rx ESR COM

      E71.32   **Disorders of** ketone metabolism   HCC Rx ESR COM

      E71.39   **Other disorders of fatty-acid metabolism**   HCC Rx ESR COM

✓5ᵗʰ **E71.4**   **Disorders of** carnitine metabolism

      EXCLUDES 1   *muscle carnitine palmitoyltransferase deficiency (E71.314)*

      E71.40   **Disorder of carnitine metabolism, unspecified**   HCC Rx ESR COM

      E71.41   **Primary carnitine deficiency**   HCC Rx ESR COM

      E71.42   **Carnitine deficiency due to** inborn errors of metabolism   HCC Rx ESR COM
          Code also associated inborn error or metabolism

      E71.43   **Iatrogenic carnitine deficiency**   HCC Rx ESR COM
          Carnitine deficiency due to hemodialysis
          Carnitine deficiency due to Valproic acid therapy

   ✓6ᵗʰ **E71.44**   Other secondary carnitine deficiency

      E71.440   **Ruvalcaba-Myhre-Smith syndrome**   HCC Rx ESR COM

      E71.448   **Other secondary carnitine deficiency**   HCC Rx ESR COM

HCC CMS-HCC   Rx Rx HCC   ESR ESRD HCC   COM Commercial HCC   N Newborn: 0   P Pediatric: 0-17   M Maternity: 9-64   A Adult: 15-124

✓5ᵗʰ **E71.5 Peroxisomal disorders**
> EXCLUDES 1   Schilder's disease (G37.0)

E71.50 Peroxisomal disorder, unspecified `HCC` `Rx` `ESR` `COM`

✓6ᵗʰ **E71.51 Disorders of peroxisome biogenesis**
Group 1 peroxisomal disorders
> EXCLUDES 1   Refsum's disease (G60.1)

E71.510 Zellweger syndrome `HCC` `Rx` `ESR` `COM`

E71.511 Neonatal adrenoleukodystrophy `HCC` `Rx` `ESR` `COM`
> EXCLUDES 1   X-linked adrenoleukodystrophy (E71.42-)

E71.518 Other disorders of peroxisome biogenesis `HCC` `Rx` `ESR` `COM`

✓6ᵗʰ **E71.52 X-linked adrenoleukodystrophy**

E71.520 Childhood cerebral X-linked adrenoleukodystrophy `HCC` `Rx` `ESR` `COM`

E71.521 Adolescent X-linked adrenoleukodystrophy `HCC` `Rx` `ESR` `COM`

E71.522 Adrenomyeloneuropathy `HCC` `Rx` `ESR` `COM`

E71.528 Other X-linked adrenoleukodystrophy
Addison only phenotype adrenoleukodystrophy
Addison-Schilder adrenoleukodystrophy

E71.529 X-linked adrenoleukodystrophy, unspecified type `HCC` `Rx` `ESR` `COM`

E71.53 Other group 2 peroxisomal disorders `HCC` `Rx` `ESR` `COM`

✓6ᵗʰ **E71.54 Other peroxisomal disorders**

E71.540 Rhizomelic chondrodysplasia punctata `HCC` `Rx` `ESR` `COM`
> EXCLUDES 1   chondrodysplasia punctata NOS (Q77.3)

E71.541 Zellweger-like syndrome `HCC` `Rx` `ESR` `COM`

E71.542 Other group 3 peroxisomal disorders `HCC` `Rx` `ESR` `COM`

E71.548 Other peroxisomal disorders `HCC` `Rx` `ESR` `COM`

✓4ᵗʰ **E72 Other disorders of amino-acid metabolism**
> EXCLUDES 1   disorders of:
> aromatic amino-acid metabolism (E70.-)
> branched-chain amino-acid metabolism (E71.0-E71.2)
> fatty-acid metabolism (E71.3)
> purine and pyrimidine metabolism (E79.-)
> gout (M1A.-, M10.-)

✓5ᵗʰ **E72.0 Disorders of amino-acid transport**
> EXCLUDES 1   disorders of tryptophan metabolism (E70.5)

E72.00 Disorders of amino-acid transport, unspecified `HCC` `Rx` `ESR` `COM`

E72.01 Cystinuria `HCC` `Rx` `ESR` `COM`

E72.02 Hartnup's disease `HCC` `Rx` `ESR` `COM`

E72.03 Lowe's syndrome `HCC` `Rx` `ESR` `COM`
Use additional code for associated glaucoma (H42)

E72.04 Cystinosis `HCC` `Rx` `ESR` `COM`
Fanconi (-de Toni) (-Debré) syndrome with cystinosis
> EXCLUDES 1   Fanconi (-de Toni) (-Debré) syndrome without cystinosis (E72.09)

E72.09 Other disorders of amino-acid transport `HCC` `Rx` `ESR` `COM`
Fanconi (-de Toni) (-Debré) syndrome, unspecified

✓5ᵗʰ **E72.1 Disorders of sulfur-bearing amino-acid metabolism**
> EXCLUDES 1   cystinosis (E72.04)
> cystinuria (E72.01)
> transcobalamin II deficiency (D51.2)

E72.10 Disorders of sulfur-bearing amino-acid metabolism, unspecified `HCC` `Rx` `ESR` `COM`

E72.11 Homocystinuria `HCC` `Rx` `ESR` `COM`
Cystathionine synthase deficiency
AHA: 2021,4Q,28

E72.12 Methylenetetrahydrofolate reductase deficiency `HCC` `Rx` `ESR` `COM`

E72.19 Other disorders of sulfur-bearing amino-acid metabolism `HCC` `Rx` `ESR` `COM`
Cystathioninuria
Methioninemia
Sulfite oxidase deficiency

✓5ᵗʰ **E72.2 Disorders of urea cycle metabolism**
> EXCLUDES 1   disorders of ornithine metabolism (E72.4)

E72.20 Disorder of urea cycle metabolism, unspecified `HCC` `Rx` `ESR` `COM`
Hyperammonemia
> EXCLUDES 1   hyperammonemia- hyperornithinemia-homocitrullinemia syndrome E72.4
> transient hyperammonemia of newborn (P74.6)

E72.21 Argininemia `HCC` `Rx` `ESR` `COM`

E72.22 Arginosuccinic aciduria `HCC` `Rx` `ESR` `COM`

E72.23 Citrullinemia `HCC` `Rx` `ESR` `COM`

E72.29 Other disorders of urea cycle metabolism `HCC` `Rx` `ESR` `COM`

E72.3 Disorders of lysine and hydroxylysine metabolism `HCC` `Rx` `ESR` `COM`
Glutaric aciduria NOS
Glutaric aciduria (type I)
Hydroxylysinemia
Hyperlysinemia
> EXCLUDES 1   glutaric aciduria type II (E71.313)
> Refsum's disease (G60.1)
> Zellweger syndrome (E71.510)

E72.4 Disorders of ornithine metabolism `HCC` `Rx` `ESR` `COM`
Hyperammonemia-Hyperornithinemia-Homocitrullinemia syndrome
Ornithinemia (types I, II)
Ornithine transcarbamylase deficiency
> EXCLUDES 1   hereditary choroidal dystrophy (H31.2-)

✓5ᵗʰ **E72.5 Disorders of glycine metabolism**

E72.50 Disorder of glycine metabolism, unspecified `HCC` `Rx` `ESR` `COM`

E72.51 Non-ketotic hyperglycinemia `HCC` `Rx` `ESR` `COM`

E72.52 Trimethylaminuria `HCC` `Rx` `ESR` `COM`

E72.53 Primary hyperoxaluria `HCC` `Rx` `ESR` `COM`
Oxalosis
Oxaluria
AHA: 2018,4Q,29

E72.59 Other disorders of glycine metabolism `HCC` `Rx` `ESR` `COM`
D-glycericacidemia
Hyperhydroxyprolinemia
Hyperprolinemia (types I, II)
Sarcosinemia

✓5ᵗʰ **E72.8 Other specified disorders of amino-acid metabolism**
AHA: 2018,4Q,5

E72.81 Disorders of gamma aminobutyric acid metabolism `HCC` `Rx` `ESR` `COM`
4-hydroxybutyric aciduria
Disorders of GABA metabolism
GABA metabolic defect
GABA transaminase deficiency
GABA-T deficiency
Gamma-hydroxybutyric aciduria
SSADHD
Succinic semialdehyde dehydrogenase deficiency

E72.89 Other specified disorders of amino-acid metabolism `HCC` `Rx` `ESR` `COM`
Disorders of beta-amino-acid metabolism
Disorders of gamma-glutamyl cycle

E72.9 Disorder of amino-acid metabolism, unspecified `HCC` `Rx` `ESR` `COM`

✓4ᵗʰ **E73 Lactose intolerance**
DEF: Inability to break down sugar in dairy products due to a deficiency in the enzyme lactase.

E73.0 Congenital lactase deficiency

E73.1 Secondary lactase deficiency

E73.8 Other lactose intolerance

E73.9 Lactose intolerance, unspecified

| ☑ Additional Character Required | ✓x7ᵗʰ Placeholder Alert | Manifestation | Unspecified Dx | ◪ QPP | UPD Unacceptable PDx |

ICD-10-CM 2023   547

√4ᵗʰ **E74 Other disorders of carbohydrate metabolism**
  EXCLUDES 1 diabetes mellitus (E08-E13)
    hypoglycemia NOS (E16.2)
    increased secretion of glucagon (E16.3)
    mucopolysaccharidosis (E76.0-E76.3)

√5ᵗʰ **E74.0 Glycogen storage disease**

  E74.00 Glycogen storage disease, unspecified HCC Rx ESR COM

  E74.01 von Gierke disease HCC Rx ESR COM
    Type I glycogen storage disease

  E74.02 Pompe disease HCC Rx ESR COM
    Cardiac glycogenosis
    Type II glycogen storage disease

  E74.03 Cori disease HCC Rx ESR COM
    Forbes disease
    Type III glycogen storage disease

  E74.04 McArdle disease HCC Rx ESR COM
    Type V glycogen storage disease

  E74.09 Other glycogen storage disease HCC Rx ESR COM
    Andersen disease
    Hers disease
    Tauri disease
    Glycogen storage disease, types 0, IV, VI-XI
    Liver phosphorylase deficiency
    Muscle phosphofructokinase deficiency

√5ᵗʰ **E74.1 Disorders of fructose metabolism**
  EXCLUDES 1 muscle phosphofructokinase deficiency (E74.09)

  E74.10 Disorder of fructose metabolism, unspecified

  E74.11 Essential fructosuria
    Fructokinase deficiency

  E74.12 Hereditary fructose intolerance
    Fructosemia

  E74.19 Other disorders of fructose metabolism
    Fructose-1, 6-diphosphatase deficiency

√5ᵗʰ **E74.2 Disorders of galactose metabolism**

  E74.20 Disorders of galactose metabolism, unspecified HCC Rx ESR COM

  E74.21 Galactosemia HCC Rx ESR COM
    DEF: Any of three genetic disorders caused by a defective galactose metabolism. Symptoms include failure to thrive in infancy, jaundice, liver and spleen damage, cataracts, and mental retardation.

  E74.29 Other disorders of galactose metabolism HCC Rx ESR COM
    Galactokinase deficiency

√5ᵗʰ **E74.3 Other disorders of intestinal carbohydrate absorption**
  EXCLUDES 2 lactose intolerance (E73.-)

  E74.31 Sucrase-isomaltase deficiency Rx

  E74.39 Other disorders of intestinal carbohydrate absorption
    Disorder of intestinal carbohydrate absorption NOS
    Glucose-galactose malabsorption
    Sucrase deficiency

E74.4 Disorders of pyruvate metabolism and gluconeogenesis HCC Rx ESR COM
    Deficiency of phosphoenolpyruvate carboxykinase
    Deficiency of pyruvate carboxylase
    Deficiency of pyruvate dehydrogenase
  EXCLUDES 1 disorders of pyruvate metabolism and gluconeogenesis with anemia (D55.-)
    Leigh's syndrome (G31.82)

√5ᵗʰ **E74.8 Other specified disorders of carbohydrate metabolism**
    AHA: 2020,4Q,16

√6ᵗʰ **E74.81 Disorders of glucose transport, not elsewhere classified**

  E74.810 Glucose transporter protein type 1 deficiency HCC Rx ESR COM
    De Vivo syndrome
    Glucose transport defect, blood-brain barrier
    Glut1 deficiency
    GLUT1 deficiency syndrome 1, infantile onset
    GLUT1 deficiency syndrome 2, childhood onset

  E74.818 Other disorders of glucose transport HCC Rx ESR COM
    (Familial) renal glycosuria

  E74.819 Disorders of glucose transport, unspecified HCC Rx ESR COM

  E74.89 Other specified disorders of carbohydrate metabolism HCC Rx ESR COM
    Essential pentosuria

E74.9 Disorder of carbohydrate metabolism, unspecified HCC Rx ESR COM

√4ᵗʰ **E75 Disorders of sphingolipid metabolism and other lipid storage disorders**
  EXCLUDES 1 mucolipidosis, types I-III (E77.0-E77.1)
    Refsum's disease (G60.1)

√5ᵗʰ **E75.0 GM2 gangliosidosis**

  E75.00 GM2 gangliosidosis, unspecified HCC Rx ESR COM

  E75.01 Sandhoff disease HCC Rx ESR COM

  E75.02 Tay-Sachs disease HCC Rx ESR COM
    DEF: Genetic mutation of the HEXA gene that inhibits the breakdown of a toxic substance called ganglioside. The accumulation of ganglioside results in destruction of the neurons in the brain and spinal cord.

Tay-Sachs Disease

Healthy neuron
Lysosome
Neuron affected by Tay-Sachs
Bulging lysosome

  E75.09 Other GM2 gangliosidosis HCC Rx ESR COM
    Adult GM2 gangliosidosis
    Juvenile GM2 gangliosidosis

√5ᵗʰ **E75.1 Other and unspecified gangliosidosis**

  E75.10 Unspecified gangliosidosis HCC Rx ESR COM
    Gangliosidosis NOS

  E75.11 Mucolipidosis IV HCC Rx ESR COM

  E75.19 Other gangliosidosis HCC Rx ESR COM
    GM1 gangliosidosis
    GM3 gangliosidosis

√5ᵗʰ **E75.2 Other sphingolipidosis**
  EXCLUDES 1 adrenoleukodystrophy [Addison-Schilder] (E71.528)

  E75.21 Fabry (-Anderson) disease HCC Rx ESR COM

  E75.22 Gaucher disease HCC Rx ESR COM

  E75.23 Krabbe disease HCC Rx ESR COM

√6ᵗʰ **E75.24 Niemann-Pick disease**
    Acid sphingomyelinase deficiency (ASMD)

  E75.240 Niemann-Pick disease type A HCC Rx ESR COM
    Acid sphingomyelinase deficiency type A (ASMD type A)
    Infantile neurovisceral acid sphingomyelinase deficiency

  E75.241 Niemann-Pick disease type B HCC Rx ESR COM
    Acid sphingomyelinase deficiency type B (ASMD type B)
    Chronic visceral acid sphingomyelinase deficiency

E75.242 **Niemann-Pick disease** type **C** `HCC` `Rx` `ESR` `COM`

E75.243 **Niemann-Pick disease** type **D** `HCC` `Rx` `ESR` `COM`

E75.244 **Niemann-Pick disease** type **A/B** `HCC` `Rx` `ESR` `COM`
Acid sphingomyelinase deficiency type A/B (ASMD type A/B)
Chronic neurovisceral acid sphingomyelinase deficiency
AHA: 2021,4Q,8-9

E75.248 **Other Niemann-Pick disease** `HCC` `Rx` `ESR` `COM`

E75.249 **Niemann-Pick disease, unspecified** `HCC` `Rx` `ESR` `COM`
Acid sphingomyelinase deficiency (ASMD) NOS

E75.25 **Metachromatic leukodystrophy** `HCC` `Rx` `ESR` `COM`

E75.26 **Sulfatase deficiency** `HCC` `Rx` `ESR` `COM`
Multiple sulfatase deficiency (MSD)
AHA: 2018,4Q,5-6

E75.29 **Other sphingolipidosis** `HCC` `Rx` `ESR` `COM`
Farber's syndrome
Sulfatide lipidosis

E75.3 **Sphingolipidosis, unspecified** `HCC` `Rx` `ESR` `COM`

E75.4 **Neuronal ceroid lipofuscinosis** `HCC` `Rx` `ESR` `COM`
Batten disease
Bielschowsky-Jansky disease
Kufs disease
Spielmeyer-Vogt disease

E75.5 **Other lipid storage disorders** `Rx`
Cerebrotendinous cholesterosis [van Bogaert-Scherer-Epstein]
Wolman's disease

E75.6 **Lipid storage disorder, unspecified** `Rx`

☑4ᵗʰ **E76 Disorders of glycosaminoglycan metabolism**

☑5ᵗʰ **E76.0 Mucopolysaccharidosis, type I**

E76.01 **Hurler's syndrome** `HCC` `Rx` `ESR` `COM`

E76.02 **Hurler-Scheie syndrome** `HCC` `Rx` `ESR` `COM`

E76.03 **Scheie's syndrome** `HCC` `Rx` `ESR` `COM`

E76.1 **Mucopolysaccharidosis, type II** `HCC` `Rx` `ESR` `COM`
Hunter's syndrome

☑5ᵗʰ **E76.2 Other mucopolysaccharidoses**

☑6ᵗʰ E76.21 **Morquio mucopolysaccharidoses**

E76.210 **Morquio A mucopolysaccharidoses** `HCC` `Rx` `ESR` `COM`
Classic Morquio syndrome
Morquio syndrome A
Mucopolysaccharidosis, type IVA

E76.211 **Morquio B mucopolysaccharidoses** `HCC` `Rx` `ESR` `COM`
Morquio-like mucopolysaccharidoses
Morquio-like syndrome
Morquio syndrome B
Mucopolysaccharidosis, type IVB

E76.219 **Morquio mucopolysaccharidoses, unspecified** `HCC` `Rx` `ESR` `COM`
Morquio syndrome
Mucopolysaccharidosis, type IV

E76.22 **Sanfilippo mucopolysaccharidoses** `HCC` `Rx` `ESR` `COM`
Mucopolysaccharidosis, type III (A) (B) (C) (D)
Sanfilippo A syndrome
Sanfilippo B syndrome
Sanfilippo C syndrome
Sanfilippo D syndrome

E76.29 **Other mucopolysaccharidoses** `HCC` `Rx` `ESR` `COM`
beta-Glucuronidase deficiency
Maroteaux-Lamy (mild) (severe) syndrome
Mucopolysaccharidosis, types VI, VII

E76.3 **Mucopolysaccharidosis, unspecified** `HCC` `Rx` `ESR` `COM`

E76.8 **Other disorders of glucosaminoglycan metabolism** `HCC` `Rx` `ESR` `COM`

E76.9 **Glucosaminoglycan metabolism disorder, unspecified** `HCC` `Rx` `ESR` `COM`

☑4ᵗʰ **E77 Disorders of glycoprotein metabolism**

E77.0 **Defects in post-translational modification of lysosomal enzymes** `HCC` `Rx` `ESR` `COM`
Mucolipidosis II [I-cell disease]
Mucolipidosis III [pseudo-Hurler polydystrophy]

E77.1 **Defects in glycoprotein degradation** `HCC` `Rx` `ESR` `COM`
Aspartylglucosaminuria
Fucosidosis
Mannosidosis
Sialidosis [mucolipidosis I]

E77.8 **Other disorders of glycoprotein metabolism** `HCC` `Rx` `ESR` `COM`

E77.9 **Disorder of glycoprotein metabolism, unspecified** `HCC` `Rx` `ESR` `COM`

☑4ᵗʰ **E78 Disorders of lipoprotein metabolism and other lipidemias**
EXCLUDES 1 sphingolipidosis (E75.0-E75.3)

☑5ᵗʰ **E78.0 Pure hypercholesterolemia**
AHA: 2016,4Q,13-14

E78.00 **Pure hypercholesterolemia, unspecified** `Rx`
Fredrickson's hyperlipoproteinemia, type IIa
Hyperbetalipoproteinemia
Low-density-lipoprotein-type [LDL] hyperlipoproteinemia
(Pure) hypercholesterolemia NOS
AHA: 2022,2Q,5-6

E78.01 **Familial hypercholesterolemia** `Rx`

E78.1 **Pure hyperglyceridemia** `Rx`
Elevated fasting triglycerides
Endogenous hyperglyceridemia
Fredrickson's hyperlipoproteinemia, type IV
Hyperlipidemia, group B
Hyperprebetalipoproteinemia
Very-low-density-lipoprotein-type [VLDL] hyperlipoproteinemia

E78.2 **Mixed hyperlipidemia** `Rx`
Broad- or floating-betalipoproteinemia
Combined hyperlipidemia NOS
Elevated cholesterol with elevated triglycerides NEC
Fredrickson's hyperlipoproteinemia, type IIb or III
Hyperbetalipoproteinemia with prebetalipoproteinemia
Hypercholesteremia with endogenous hyperglyceridemia
Hyperlipidemia, group C
Tubo-eruptive xanthoma
Xanthoma tuberosum
EXCLUDES 1 cerebrotendinous cholesterosis [van Bogaert-Scherer-Epstein] (E75.5)
familial combined hyperlipidemia (E78.49)
AHA: 2022,2Q,6

E78.3 **Hyperchylomicronemia** `Rx`
Chylomicron retention disease
Fredrickson's hyperlipoproteinemia, type I or V
Hyperlipidemia, group D
Mixed hyperglyceridemia

☑5ᵗʰ **E78.4 Other hyperlipidemia**
AHA: 2018,4Q,6

E78.41 **Elevated Lipoprotein(a)** `Rx`
Elevated Lp(a)

E78.49 **Other hyperlipidemia** `Rx`
Familial combined hyperlipidemia

E78.5 **Hyperlipidemia, unspecified** `Rx`
AHA: 2022,2Q,5

E78.6 **Lipoprotein deficiency** `Rx`
Abetalipoproteinemia
Depressed HDL cholesterol
High-density lipoprotein deficiency
Hypoalphalipoproteinemia
Hypobetalipoproteinemia (familial)
Lecithin cholesterol acyltransferase deficiency
Tangier disease

☑5ᵗʰ **E78.7 Disorders of bile acid and cholesterol metabolism**
EXCLUDES 1 Niemann-Pick disease type C (E75.242)

E78.70 **Disorder of bile acid and cholesterol metabolism, unspecified** `Rx`

E78.71 **Barth syndrome** `COM`

E78.72 **Smith-Lemli-Opitz syndrome** `COM`

☑ Additional Character Required   √x7ᵗʰ Placeholder Alert   Manifestation   Unspecified Dx   Ⓠ QPP   UPD Unacceptable PDx

E78.79   **Other disorders of bile acid and cholesterol metabolism** `Rx`

✓5ᵗʰ **E78.8   Other disorders of lipoprotein metabolism**

     E78.81   **Lipoid dermatoarthritis** `Rx`

     E78.89   **Other lipoprotein metabolism disorders** `Rx`

E78.9   Disorder of lipoprotein metabolism, unspecified `Rx`

✓4ᵗʰ **E79   Disorders of purine and pyrimidine metabolism**

     EXCLUDES 1   *Ataxia-telangiectasia (Q87.19)*
          Bloom's syndrome (Q82.8)
          Cockayne's syndrome (Q87.19)
          calculus of kidney (N20.0)
          combined immunodeficiency disorders (D81.-)
          Fanconi's anemia (D61.09)
          gout (M1A.-, M10.-)
          orotaciduric anemia (D53.0)
          progeria (E34.8)
          Werner's syndrome (E34.8)
          xeroderma pigmentosum (Q82.1)

E79.0   Hyperuricemia without signs of inflammatory arthritis and tophaceous disease
     Asymptomatic hyperuricemia

E79.1   Lesch-Nyhan syndrome `HCC` `Rx` `ESR` `COM`
     HGPRT deficiency

E79.2   Myoadenylate deaminase deficiency `HCC` `Rx` `ESR` `COM`

E79.8   Other disorders of purine and pyrimidine metabolism `HCC` `Rx` `ESR` `COM`
     Hereditary xanthinuria

E79.9   Disorder of purine and pyrimidine metabolism, unspecified `HCC` `Rx` `ESR` `COM`

✓4ᵗʰ **E80   Disorders of porphyrin and bilirubin metabolism**

     INCLUDES   defects of catalase and peroxidase

E80.0   Hereditary erythropoietic porphyria `HCC` `Rx` `ESR` `COM`
     Congenital erythropoietic porphyria
     Erythropoietic protoporphyria

E80.1   Porphyria cutanea tarda `HCC` `Rx` `ESR` `COM`

✓5ᵗʰ **E80.2   Other and unspecified porphyria**

     E80.20   **Unspecified porphyria** `HCC` `Rx` `ESR` `COM`
          Porphyria NOS

     E80.21   **Acute intermittent (hepatic) porphyria** `HCC` `Rx` `ESR` `COM`

     E80.29   **Other porphyria** `HCC` `Rx` `ESR` `COM`
          Hereditary coproporphyria

E80.3   Defects of catalase and peroxidase `HCC` `Rx` `ESR` `COM`
     Acatalasia [Takahara]

E80.4   Gilbert syndrome

E80.5   Crigler-Najjar syndrome

E80.6   Other disorders of bilirubin metabolism
     Dubin-Johnson syndrome
     Rotor's syndrome

E80.7   Disorder of bilirubin metabolism, unspecified

✓4ᵗʰ **E83   Disorders of mineral metabolism**

     EXCLUDES 1   *dietary mineral deficiency (E58-E61)*
          parathyroid disorders (E20-E21)
          vitamin D deficiency (E55.-)

✓5ᵗʰ **E83.0   Disorders of copper metabolism**

     E83.00   **Disorder of copper metabolism, unspecified** `Rx` `COM`

     E83.01   **Wilson's disease** `Rx` `COM`
          Code also associated Kayser Fleischer ring (H18.04-)

     E83.09   **Other disorders of copper metabolism** `Rx` `COM`
          Menkes' (kinky hair) (steely hair) disease

✓5ᵗʰ **E83.1   Disorders of iron metabolism**

     EXCLUDES 1   *iron deficiency anemia (D50.-)*
          sideroblastic anemia (D64.0-D64.3)

     E83.10   **Disorder of iron metabolism, unspecified** `Rx`

✓6ᵗʰ   E83.11   **Hemochromatosis**

     EXCLUDES 1   *GALD (P78.84)*
          gestational alloimmune liver disease (P78.84)
          neonatal hemochromatosis (P78.84)

     E83.110   **Hereditary hemochromatosis** `HCC` `Rx` `ESR`
          Bronzed diabetes
          Pigmentary cirrhosis (of liver)
          Primary (hereditary) hemochromatosis

     E83.111   **Hemochromatosis due to repeated red blood cell transfusions**
          Iron overload due to repeated red blood cell transfusions
          Transfusion (red blood cell) associated hemochromatosis

     E83.118   **Other hemochromatosis** `Rx`

     E83.119   **Hemochromatosis, unspecified** `Rx`

     E83.19   **Other disorders of iron metabolism** `Rx`
          Use additional code, if applicable, for idiopathic pulmonary hemosiderosis (J84.03)

E83.2   Disorders of zinc metabolism
     Acrodermatitis enteropathica

✓5ᵗʰ **E83.3   Disorders of phosphorus metabolism and phosphatases**

     EXCLUDES 1   *adult osteomalacia (M83.-)*
          osteoporosis (M80.-)

     E83.30   **Disorder of phosphorus metabolism, unspecified** `Rx`

     E83.31   **Familial hypophosphatemia** `Rx`
          Vitamin D-resistant osteomalacia
          Vitamin D-resistant rickets
          EXCLUDES 1   *vitamin D-deficiency rickets (E55.0)*

     E83.32   **Hereditary vitamin D-dependent rickets (type 1) (type 2)** `Rx`
          25-hydroxyvitamin D 1-alpha-hydroxylase deficiency
          Pseudovitamin D deficiency
          Vitamin D receptor defect

     E83.39   **Other disorders of phosphorus metabolism** `Rx`
          Acid phosphatase deficiency
          Hypophosphatasia

✓5ᵗʰ **E83.4   Disorders of magnesium metabolism**

     E83.40   **Disorders of magnesium metabolism, unspecified**

     E83.41   **Hypermagnesemia**
          AHA: 2016,4Q,54

     E83.42   **Hypomagnesemia**

     E83.49   **Other disorders of magnesium metabolism**

✓5ᵗʰ **E83.5   Disorders of calcium metabolism**

     EXCLUDES 1   *chondrocalcinosis (M11.1-M11.2)*
          hungry bone syndrome (E83.81)
          hyperparathyroidism (E21.0-E21.3)

     E83.50   **Unspecified disorder of calcium metabolism**

     E83.51   **Hypocalcemia**

     E83.52   **Hypercalcemia**
          Familial hypocalciuric hypercalcemia

     E83.59   **Other disorders of calcium metabolism**

✓5ᵗʰ **E83.8   Other disorders of mineral metabolism**

     E83.81   **Hungry bone syndrome**

     E83.89   **Other disorders of mineral metabolism**

E83.9   Disorder of mineral metabolism, unspecified

✓4ᵗʰ **E84   Cystic fibrosis**

     INCLUDES   mucoviscidosis

     Code also exocrine pancreatic insufficiency (K86.81)

     DEF: Genetic disorder affecting the respiratory, digestive, and reproductive systems in infants to young adults by disturbing exocrine gland function and causing chronic pulmonary disease with excess mucus production and pancreatic deficiency.

E84.0   Cystic fibrosis with pulmonary manifestations `HCC` `Rx` `ESR` `COM`
     Use additional code to identify any infectious organism present, such as:
     Pseudomonas (B96.5)
     AHA: 2021,1Q,23

`HCC` CMS-HCC   `Rx` Rx HCC   `ESR` ESRD HCC   `COM` Commercial HCC   N Newborn: 0   P Pediatric: 0-17   M Maternity: 9-64   A Adult: 15-124

550   ICD-10-CM 2023

√5ᵗʰ **E84.1 Cystic fibrosis with intestinal manifestations**

  E84.11 Meconium ileus in cystic fibrosis   HCC Rx ESR COM N

    EXCLUDES 1   *meconium ileus not due to cystic fibrosis (P76.0)*

  E84.19 Cystic fibrosis with other intestinal manifestations   HCC Rx ESR COM

    Distal intestinal obstruction syndrome

  E84.8 Cystic fibrosis with other manifestations   HCC Rx ESR COM

  E84.9 Cystic fibrosis, unspecified   HCC Rx ESR COM

√4ᵗʰ **E85 Amyloidosis**

  EXCLUDES 2   *Alzheimer's disease (G30.0-)*

  DEF: Conditions of diverse etiologies characterized by the accumulation of insoluble fibrillar proteins (amyloid) in various organs and tissues of the body, compromising vital functions.

  E85.0 Non-neuropathic heredofamilial amyloidosis   HCC ESR COM

    Hereditary amyloid nephropathy

    Code also associated disorders, such as:

      autoinflammatory syndromes (M04.-)

    EXCLUDES 2   *transthyretin-related (ATTR) familial amyloid cardiomyopathy (E85.4)*

  E85.1 Neuropathic heredofamilial amyloidosis   HCC ESR COM

    Amyloid polyneuropathy (Portuguese)

    Transthyretin-related (ATTR) familial amyloid polyneuropathy

    AHA: 2012,4Q,99

  E85.2 Heredofamilial amyloidosis, unspecified   HCC ESR COM

  E85.3 Secondary systemic amyloidosis   HCC ESR COM

    Hemodialysis-associated amyloidosis

  E85.4 Organ-limited amyloidosis   HCC ESR COM

    Localized amyloidosis

    Transthyretin-related (ATTR) familial amyloid cardiomyopathy

√5ᵗʰ **E85.8 Other amyloidosis**

    AHA: 2017,4Q,7

  E85.81 Light chain (AL) amyloidosis   HCC ESR COM

  E85.82 Wild-type transthyretin-related (ATTR) amyloidosis   HCC ESR COM

    Senile systemic amyloidosis (SSA)

  E85.89 Other amyloidosis   HCC ESR COM

  E85.9 Amyloidosis, unspecified   HCC ESR COM

√4ᵗʰ **E86 Volume depletion**

  Use additional code(s) for any associated disorders of electrolyte and acid-base balance (E87.-)

  EXCLUDES 1   *dehydration of newborn (P74.1)*

      postprocedural hypovolemic shock (T81.19)

      traumatic hypovolemic shock (T79.4)

  EXCLUDES 2   *hypovolemic shock NOS (R57.1)*

  AHA: 2019,2Q,7; 2018,2Q,6

  E86.0 Dehydration

    AHA: 2019,2Q,7; 2019,1Q,12; 2014,1Q,7

    TIP: Can be assigned in addition to hypernatremia (E87.0) or hyponatremia (E87.1), when documented.

  E86.1 Hypovolemia

    Depletion of volume of plasma

  E86.9 Volume depletion, unspecified

    DEF: Depletion of total body water (dehydration) and/or contraction of total intravascular plasma (hypovolemia).

√4ᵗʰ **E87 Other disorders of fluid, electrolyte and acid-base balance**

  EXCLUDES 1   *diabetes insipidus (E23.2)*

      electrolyte imbalance associated with hyperemesis gravidarum (O21.1)

      electrolyte imbalance following ectopic or molar pregnancy (O08.5)

      familial periodic paralysis (G72.3)

  AHA: 2018,2Q,6

  E87.0 Hyperosmolality and hypernatremia

    Sodium [Na] excess

    Sodium [Na] overload

    AHA: 2022,1Q,28; 2014,1Q,7

    TIP: Assign an additional code for dehydration (E86.0), when documented.

  E87.1 Hypo-osmolality and hyponatremia

    Sodium [Na] deficiency

    EXCLUDES 1   *syndrome of inappropriate secretion of antidiuretic hormone (E22.2)*

    AHA: 2014,1Q,7

    TIP: Assign an additional code for dehydration (E86.0), when documented.

▲ √5ᵗʰ **E87.2 Acidosis**

    ~~Acidosis NOS~~

    ~~Lactic acidosis~~

    ~~Metabolic acidosis~~

    ~~Respiratory acidosis~~

    EXCLUDES 1   *diabetic acidosis - see categories E08-E10, E11, E13 with ketoacidosis*

    AHA: 2020,3Q,30

    DEF: Reduction of alkaline in the blood and tissues caused by an increase in acid and decrease in bicarbonate.

●   **E87.20 Acidosis, unspecified**

    Lactic acidosis NOS

    Metabolic acidosis NOS

    Code also, if applicable, respiratory failure with hypercapnia (J96. with 5th character 2)

●   **E87.21 Acute metabolic acidosis**

    Acute lactic acidosis

●   **E87.22 Chronic metabolic acidosis**

    Chronic lactic acidosis

    Code first underlying etiology, if applicable

●   **E87.29 Other acidosis**

    Respiratory acidosis NOS

    EXCLUDES 2   *acute respiratory acidosis (J96.02)*

      chronic respiratory acidosis (J96.12)

  E87.3 Alkalosis

    Alkalosis NOS

    Metabolic alkalosis

    Respiratory alkalosis

  E87.4 Mixed disorder of acid-base balance

  E87.5 Hyperkalemia

    Potassium [K] excess

    Potassium [K] overload

  E87.6 Hypokalemia

    Potassium [K] deficiency

√5ᵗʰ **E87.7 Fluid overload**

    EXCLUDES 1   *edema NOS (R60.9)*

      fluid retention (R60.9)

  E87.70 Fluid overload, unspecified

  E87.71 Transfusion associated circulatory overload

    Fluid overload due to transfusion (blood) (blood components)

    TACO

  E87.79 Other fluid overload

  E87.8 Other disorders of electrolyte and fluid balance, not elsewhere classified

    Electrolyte imbalance NOS

    Hyperchloremia

    Hypochloremia

√4ᵗʰ **E88 Other and unspecified metabolic disorders**

  Use additional codes for associated conditions

  EXCLUDES 1   *histiocytosis X (chronic) (C96.6)*

√5ᵗʰ **E88.0 Disorders of plasma-protein metabolism, not elsewhere classified**

    EXCLUDES 1   *monoclonal gammopathy (of undetermined significance) (D47.2)*

      polyclonal hypergammaglobulinemia (D89.0)

      Waldenström macroglobulinemia (C88.0)

    EXCLUDES 2   *disorder of lipoprotein metabolism (E78.-)*

  E88.01 Alpha-1-antitrypsin deficiency   HCC Rx ESR COM

    AAT deficiency

Chapter 4. Endocrine, Nutritional and Metabolic Diseases

E88.02   Plasminogen deficiency
Dysplasminogenemia
Hypoplasminogenemia
Type 1 plasminogen deficiency
Type 2 plasminogen deficiency
Code also, if applicable, ligneous conjunctivitis
(H10.51)
Use additional code for associated findings, such as:
hydrocephalus (G91.4)
otitis media (H67.-)
respiratory disorder related to plasminogen
deficiency (J99)
AHA: 2018,4Q,6-7

E88.09   Other disorders of plasma-protein metabolism, not elsewhere classified
Bisalbuminemia

E88.1   Lipodystrophy, not elsewhere classified
Lipodystrophy NOS
   EXCLUDES 1   Whipple's disease (K90.81)

E88.2   Lipomatosis, not elsewhere classified   `Rx`
Lipomatosis NOS
Lipomatosis (Check) dolorosa [Dercum]

E88.3   Tumor lysis syndrome   `COM`
Tumor lysis syndrome (spontaneous)
Tumor lysis syndrome following antineoplastic drug
chemotherapy
Use additional code for adverse effect, if applicable, to identify
drug (T45.1X5)
AHA: 2020,1Q,37; 2019,2Q,24
DEF: Potentially fatal metabolic complication of tumor necrosis
caused by spontaneous or treatment-related accumulation of
byproducts from dying cancer cells. Symptoms include
hyperkalemia, hyperphosphatemia, hypocalcemia, hyperuricemia,
and hyperuricosuria.

√5ᵗʰ E88.4   Mitochondrial metabolism disorders
   EXCLUDES 1   disorders of pyruvate metabolism (E74.4)
Kearns-Sayre syndrome (H49.81)
Leber's disease (H47.22)
Leigh's encephalopathy (G31.82)
mitochondrial myopathy, NEC (G71.3)
Reye's syndrome (G93.7)

E88.40   Mitochondrial metabolism disorder, unspecified   `HCC` `Rx` `ESR` `COM`

E88.41   MELAS syndrome   `HCC` `Rx` `ESR` `COM`
Mitochondrial myopathy, encephalopathy, lactic
acidosis and stroke-like episodes

E88.42   MERRF syndrome   `HCC` `Rx` `ESR` `COM`
Myoclonic epilepsy associated with ragged-red fibers
Code also progressive myoclonic epilepsy (G40.3-)

E88.49   Other mitochondrial metabolism disorders   `HCC` `Rx` `ESR` `COM`

√5ᵗʰ E88.8   Other specified metabolic disorders

E88.81   Metabolic syndrome
Dysmetabolic syndrome X
Use additional codes for associated manifestations,
such as:
obesity (E66.-)
DEF: Group of health risks that increase the likelihood
of developing heart disease, stroke, and diabetes. These
risks include certain parameters for blood pressure,
cholesterol, and glucose levels.

E88.89   Other specified metabolic disorders   `HCC` `Rx` `ESR` `COM`
Launois-Bensaude adenolipomatosis
   EXCLUDES 1   adult pulmonary Langerhans cell
histiocytosis (J84.82)

E88.9   Metabolic disorder, unspecified

Postprocedural endocrine and metabolic complications and disorders, not elsewhere classified (E89)

√4ᵗʰ E89   Postprocedural endocrine and metabolic complications and disorders, not elsewhere classified
   EXCLUDES 2   intraoperative complications of endocrine system organ or
structure (E36.0-, E36.1-, E36.8)

E89.0   Postprocedural hypothyroidism   `Rx`
Postirradiation hypothyroidism
Postsurgical hypothyroidism

E89.1   Postprocedural hypoinsulinemia
Postpancreatectomy hyperglycemia
Postsurgical hypoinsulinemia
Use additional code, if applicable, to identify:
acquired absence of pancreas (Z90.41-)
diabetes mellitus (postpancreatectomy) (postprocedural)
(E13.-)
insulin use (Z79.4)
   EXCLUDES 1   transient postprocedural hyperglycemia (R73.9)
transient postprocedural hypoglycemia (E16.2)

E89.2   Postprocedural hypoparathyroidism   `HCC` `Rx` `ESR` `COM`
Parathyroprival tetany

E89.3   Postprocedural hypopituitarism   `HCC` `Rx` `ESR` `COM`
Postirradiation hypopituitarism

√5ᵗʰ E89.4   Postprocedural ovarian failure

E89.40   Asymptomatic postprocedural ovarian failure   ♀
Postprocedural ovarian failure NOS

E89.41   Symptomatic postprocedural ovarian failure   ♀
Symptoms such as flushing, sleeplessness, headache,
lack of concentration, associated with
postprocedural menopause

E89.5   Postprocedural testicular hypofunction   ♂

E89.6   Postprocedural adrenocortical (-medullary) hypofunction   `HCC` `Rx` `ESR` `COM`

√5ᵗʰ E89.8   Other postprocedural endocrine and metabolic complications and disorders
AHA: 2016,4Q,9-10

√6ᵗʰ E89.81   Postprocedural hemorrhage of an endocrine system organ or structure following a procedure

E89.810   Postprocedural hemorrhage of an endocrine system organ or structure following an endocrine system procedure

E89.811   Postprocedural hemorrhage of an endocrine system organ or structure following other procedure

√6ᵗʰ E89.82   Postprocedural hematoma and seroma of an endocrine system organ or structure

E89.820   Postprocedural hematoma of an endocrine system organ or structure following an endocrine system procedure

E89.821   Postprocedural hematoma of an endocrine system organ or structure following other procedure

E89.822   Postprocedural seroma of an endocrine system organ or structure following an endocrine system procedure

E89.823   Postprocedural seroma of an endocrine system organ or structure following other procedure

E89.89   Other postprocedural endocrine and metabolic complications and disorders
Use additional code, if applicable, to further specify
disorder

`HCC` CMS-HCC   `Rx` Rx HCC   `ESR` ESRD HCC   `COM` Commercial HCC   `N` Newborn: 0   `P` Pediatric: 0-17   `M` Maternity: 9-64   `A` Adult: 15-124

552   ICD-10-CM 2023

Chapter 5. Mental, Behavioral and Neurodevelopmental Disorders (F01–F99)

Chapter-specific Guidelines with Coding Examples

The chapter-specific guidelines from the ICD-10-CM Official Guidelines for Coding and Reporting have been provided below. Along with these guidelines are coding examples, contained in the shaded boxes, that have been developed to help illustrate the coding and/or sequencing guidance found in these guidelines.

a. Pain disorders related to psychological factors

Assign code F45.41, for pain that is exclusively related to psychological disorders. As indicated by the Excludes 1 note under category G89, a code from category G89 should not be assigned with code F45.41.

> Chest pain determined to be persistent somatoform pain disorder
>
> **F45.41   Pain disorder exclusively related to psychological factors**
>
> *Explanation*: This pain was diagnosed as being exclusively psychological; therefore, no code from category G89 is added.

Code F45.42, Pain disorders with related psychological factors, should be used with a code from category G89, Pain, not elsewhere classified, if there is documentation of a psychological component for a patient with acute or chronic pain.
See Section I.C.6. Pain

b. Mental and behavioral disorders due to psychoactive substance use

1) In remission

Selection of codes **describing** "in remission" for categories F10-F19, Mental and behavioral disorders due to psychoactive substance use (categories F10-F19 with -.11, -.21, **-.91**) requires the provider's clinical judgment **and** are assigned only on the basis of provider documentation (as defined in the Official Guidelines for Coding and Reporting), unless otherwise instructed by the classification.

Mild substance use disorders in early or sustained remission are classified to the appropriate codes for substance abuse in remission, and moderate or severe substance use disorders in early or sustained remission are classified to the appropriate codes for substance dependence in remission.

> Physician documentation indicates the patient is seen to monitor progress on quitting cigarette smoking. The problem list indicates mild tobacco use disorder that is currently in remission.
>
> **F17.211   Nicotine dependence, cigarettes, in remission**
>
> *Explanation*: According to the index, Disorder, tobacco use, cigarettes (mild) (moderate) (severe), in remission (early) (sustained) is categorized to dependence (F17.211). Since the physician clearly documents mild cigarette use "disorder" and that the disorder is in remission, a code for nicotine dependence "in remission" is appropriate.

2) Psychoactive substance use, abuse and dependence

When the provider documentation refers to use, abuse and dependence of the same substance (e.g. alcohol, opioid, cannabis, etc.), only one code should be assigned to identify the pattern of use based on the following hierarchy:

- If both use and abuse are documented, assign only the code for abuse
- If both abuse and dependence are documented, assign only the code for dependence
- If use, abuse and dependence are all documented, assign only the code for dependence
- If both use and dependence are documented, assign only the code for dependence.

> History and physical notes cannabis dependence and ongoing cannabis abuse
>
> **F12.20   Cannabis dependence, uncomplicated**
>
> *Explanation*: In the hierarchy, the dependence code is used if both abuse and dependence are documented.

> Current problem list indicates daily opioid use with opioid abuse.
>
> **F11.10   Opioid abuse, uncomplicated**
>
> *Explanation*: In the hierarchy, the abuse code is used if both abuse and use are documented.

3) Psychoactive substance use, unspecified

As with all other unspecified diagnoses, the codes for unspecified psychoactive substance use (F10.9-, F11.9-, F12.9-, F13.9-, F14.9-, F15.9-, F16.9-, F18.9-, F19.9-) should only be assigned based on provider documentation and when they meet the definition of a reportable diagnosis (see Section III, Reporting Additional Diagnoses). These codes are to be used only when the psychoactive substance use is associated with a substance related disorder (chapter 5 disorders such as sexual dysfunction, sleep disorder, or a mental or behavioral disorder) or medical condition, and such a relationship is documented by the provider.

4) Medical conditions due to psychoactive substance use, abuse and dependence

Medical conditions due to substance use, abuse, and dependence are not classified as substance-induced disorders. Assign the diagnosis code for the medical condition as directed by the Alphabetical Index along with the appropriate psychoactive substance use, abuse or dependence code. For example, for alcoholic pancreatitis due to alcohol dependence, assign the appropriate code from subcategory K85.2, Alcohol induced acute pancreatitis, and the appropriate code from subcategory F10.2, such as code F10.20, Alcohol dependence, uncomplicated. It would not be appropriate to assign code F10.288, Alcohol dependence with other alcohol-induced disorder.

5) Blood alcohol level

A code from category Y90, Evidence of alcohol involvement determined by blood alcohol level, may be assigned when this information is documented and the patient's provider has documented a condition classifiable to category F10, Alcohol related disorders. The blood alcohol level does not need to be documented by the patient's provider in order for it to be coded.

See Section I.B.14. for blood alcohol level documentation by clinicians other than patient's provider.

c. Factitious disorder

Factitious disorder imposed on self or Munchausen's syndrome is a disorder in which a person falsely reports or causes his or her own physical or psychological signs or symptoms. For patients with documented factitious disorder on self or Munchausen's syndrome, assign the appropriate code from subcategory F68.1-, Factitious disorder imposed on self.

Munchausen's syndrome by proxy (MSBP) is a disorder in which a caregiver (perpetrator) falsely reports or causes an illness or injury in another person (victim) under his or her care, such as a child, an elderly adult, or a person who has a disability. The condition is also referred to as "factitious disorder imposed on another" or "factitious disorder by proxy." The perpetrator, not the victim, receives this diagnosis. Assign code F68.A, Factitious disorder imposed on another, to the perpetrator's record. For the victim of a patient suffering from MSBP, assign the appropriate code from categories T74, Adult and child abuse, neglect and other maltreatment, confirmed, or T76, Adult and child abuse, neglect and other maltreatment, suspected.

See Section I.C.19.f. Adult and child abuse, neglect and other maltreatment

d. Dementia

The ICD-10-CM classifies dementia (categories F01, F02, and F03) on the basis of the etiology and severity (unspecified, mild, moderate or severe). Selection of the appropriate severity level requires the provider's clinical judgment and codes should be assigned only on the basis of provider documentation (as defined in the *Official Guidelines for Coding and Reporting*), unless otherwise instructed by the classification. If the documentation does not provide information about the severity of the dementia, assign the appropriate code for unspecified severity.

If a patient is admitted to an inpatient acute care hospital or other inpatient facility setting with dementia at one severity level and it progresses to a higher severity level, assign one code for the highest severity level reported during the stay.

Chapter 5. Mental, Behavioral and Neurodevelopmental Disorders (F01-F99)

INCLUDES   disorders of psychological development

EXCLUDES 2   *symptoms, signs and abnormal clinical laboratory findings, not elsewhere classified (R00-R99)*

This chapter contains the following blocks:

F01-F09	Mental disorders due to known physiological conditions
F10-F19	Mental and behavioral disorders due to psychoactive substance use
F20-F29	Schizophrenia, schizotypal, delusional, and other non-mood psychotic disorders
F30-F39	Mood [affective] disorders
F40-F48	Anxiety, dissociative, stress-related, somatoform and other nonpsychotic mental disorders
F50-F59	Behavioral syndromes associated with physiological disturbances and physical factors
F60-F69	Disorders of adult personality and behavior
F70-F79	Intellectual disabilities
F80-F89	Pervasive and specific developmental disorders
F90-F98	Behavioral and emotional disorders with onset usually occurring in childhood and adolescence
F99	Unspecified mental disorder

Mental disorders due to known physiological conditions (F01-F09)

NOTE   This block comprises a range of mental disorders grouped together on the basis of their having in common a demonstrable etiology in cerebral disease, brain injury, or other insult leading to cerebral dysfunction. The dysfunction may be primary, as in diseases, injuries, and insults that affect the brain directly and selectively; or secondary, as in systemic diseases and disorders that attack the brain only as one of the multiple organs or systems of the body that are involved.

✓4ᵗʰ F01 Vascular dementia

Vascular dementia as a result of infarction of the brain due to vascular disease, including hypertensive cerebrovascular disease.

INCLUDES   arteriosclerotic dementia
- ►major neurocognitive disorder due to vascular disease◄
- ►multi-infarct dementia◄

Code first the underlying physiological condition or sequelae of cerebrovascular disease.

▲   **✓5ᵗʰ F01.5 Vascular dementia, unspecified severity**

▲   **F01.50 Vascular dementia, unspecified severity, without behavioral disturbance, psychotic disturbance, mood disturbance, and anxiety**   **HCC Rx ESR A**
- ►Major neurocognitive disorder due to vascular disease NOS◄
- ►Vascular dementia NOS◄
  AHA: 2021,2Q,4

▲   **✓6ᵗʰ F01.51 Vascular dementia, unspecified severity, with behavioral disturbance**

~~Major neurocognitive disorder due to vascular disease, with behavioral disturbance~~
~~Major neurocognitive disorder with aggressive behavior~~
~~Major neurocognitive disorder with combative behavior~~
~~Major neurocognitive disorder with violent behavior~~
~~Vascular dementia with aggressive behavior~~
~~Vascular dementia with combative behavior~~
~~Vascular dementia with violent behavior~~
~~Use additional code, if applicable, to identify wandering in vascular dementia (Z91.83)~~

●   **F01.511 Vascular dementia, unspecified severity, with agitation**

Major neurocognitive disorder due to vascular disease, unspecified severity, with aberrant motor behavior such as restlessness, rocking, pacing, or exit-seeking

Major neurocognitive disorder due to vascular disease, unspecified severity, with verbal or physical behaviors such as profanity, shouting, threatening, anger, aggression, combativeness, or violence

Vascular dementia, unspecified severity, with aberrant motor behavior such as restlessness, rocking, pacing, or exit-seeking

Vascular dementia, unspecified severity, with verbal or physical behaviors such as profanity, shouting, threatening, anger, aggression, combativeness, or violence

●   **F01.518 Vascular dementia, unspecified severity, with other behavioral disturbance**

Major neurocognitive disorder due to vascular disease, unspecified severity, with behavioral disturbances such as sleep disturbance, social disinhibition, or sexual disinhibition

Vascular dementia, unspecified severity, with behavioral disturbances such as sleep disturbance, social disinhibition, or sexual disinhibition

Use additional code, if applicable, to identify wandering in vascular dementia (Z91.83)

●   **F01.52 Vascular dementia, unspecified severity, with psychotic disturbance**

Major neurocognitive disorder due to vascular disease, unspecified severity, with psychotic disturbance such as hallucinations, paranoia, suspiciousness, or delusional state

Vascular dementia, unspecified severity, with psychotic disturbance such as hallucinations, paranoia, suspiciousness, or delusional state

●   **F01.53 Vascular dementia, unspecified severity, with mood disturbance**

Major neurocognitive disorder due to vascular disease, unspecified severity, with mood disturbance such as depression, apathy, or anhedonia

Vascular dementia, unspecified severity, with mood disturbance such as depression, apathy, or anhedonia

●   **F01.54 Vascular dementia, unspecified severity, with anxiety**

Major neurocognitive disorder due to vascular disease, unspecified severity, with anxiety

- ✓5ᵗʰ **F01.A**   **Vascular dementia, mild**
  - EXCLUDES 1   *mild neurocognitive disorder due to known physiological condition with or without behavioral disturbance (F06.7-)*
-     **F01.A0**   **Vascular dementia, mild, without behavioral disturbance, psychotic disturbance, mood disturbance, and anxiety**
  - Major neurocognitive disorder due to vascular disease, mild, NOS
  - Vascular dementia, mild, NOS
- ✓6ᵗʰ **F01.A1**   **Vascular dementia, mild, with behavioral disturbance**
-     **F01.A11**   **Vascular dementia, mild, with agitation**
  - Major neurocognitive disorder due to vascular disease, mild, with aberrant motor behavior such as restlessness, rocking, pacing, or exit-seeking
  - Major neurocognitive disorder due to vascular disease, mild, with verbal or physical behaviors such as profanity, shouting, threatening, anger, aggression, combativeness, or violence
  - Vascular dementia, mild, with aberrant motor behavior such as restlessness, rocking, pacing, or exit-seeking
  - Vascular dementia, mild, with verbal or physical behaviors such as profanity, shouting, threatening, anger, aggression, combativeness, or violence
-     **F01.A18**   **Vascular dementia, mild, with other behavioral disturbance**
  - Major neurocognitive disorder due to vascular disease, mild, with behavioral disturbances such as sleep disturbance, social disinhibition, or sexual disinhibition
  - Vascular dementia, mild, with behavioral disturbances such as sleep disturbance, social disinhibition, or sexual disinhibition
  - Use additional code, if applicable, to identify wandering in vascular dementia (Z91.83)
-     **F01.A2**   **Vascular dementia, mild, with psychotic disturbance**
  - Major neurocognitive disorder due to vascular disease, mild, with psychotic disturbance such as hallucinations, paranoia, suspiciousness, or delusional state
  - Vascular dementia, mild, with psychotic disturbance such as hallucinations, paranoia, suspiciousness, or delusional state
-     **F01.A3**   **Vascular dementia, mild, with mood disturbance**
  - Major neurocognitive disorder due to vascular disease, mild, with mood disturbance such as depression, apathy, or anhedonia
  - Vascular dementia, mild, with mood disturbance such as depression, apathy, or anhedonia
-     **F01.A4**   **Vascular dementia, mild, with anxiety**
  - Major neurocognitive disorder due to vascular disease, mild, with anxiety
- ✓5ᵗʰ **F01.B**   **Vascular dementia, moderate**
-     **F01.B0**   **Vascular dementia, moderate, without behavioral disturbance, psychotic disturbance, mood disturbance, and anxiety**
  - Major neurocognitive disorder due to vascular disease, moderate, NOS
  - Vascular dementia, moderate, NOS

- ✓6ᵗʰ **F01.B1**   **Vascular dementia, moderate, with behavioral disturbance**
-     **F01.B11**   **Vascular dementia, moderate, with agitation**
  - Major neurocognitive disorder due to vascular disease, moderate, with aberrant motor behavior such as restlessness, rocking, pacing, or exit-seeking
  - Major neurocognitive disorder due to vascular disease, moderate, with verbal or physical behaviors such as profanity, shouting, threatening, anger, aggression, combativeness, or violence
  - Vascular dementia, moderate, with aberrant motor behavior such as restlessness, rocking, pacing, or exit-seeking
  - Vascular dementia, moderate, with verbal or physical behaviors such as profanity, shouting, threatening, anger, aggression, combativeness, or violence
-     **F01.B18**   **Vascular dementia, moderate, with other behavioral disturbance**
  - Major neurocognitive disorder due to vascular disease, moderate, with behavioral disturbances such as sleep disturbance, social disinhibition, or sexual disinhibition
  - Vascular dementia, moderate, with behavioral disturbances such as sleep disturbance, social disinhibition, or sexual disinhibition
  - Use additional code, if applicable, to identify wandering in vascular dementia (Z91.83)
-     **F01.B2**   **Vascular dementia, moderate, with psychotic disturbance**
  - Major neurocognitive disorder due to vascular disease, moderate, with psychotic disturbance such as hallucinations, paranoia, suspiciousness, or delusional state
  - Vascular dementia, moderate, with psychotic disturbance such as hallucinations, paranoia, suspiciousness, or delusional state
-     **F01.B3**   **Vascular dementia, moderate, with mood disturbance**
  - Major neurocognitive disorder due to vascular disease, moderate, with mood disturbance such as depression, apathy, or anhedonia
  - Vascular dementia, moderate, with mood disturbance such as depression, apathy, or anhedonia
-     **F01.B4**   **Vascular dementia, moderate, with anxiety**
  - Major neurocognitive disorder due to vascular disease, moderate, with anxiety
- ✓5ᵗʰ **F01.C**   **Vascular dementia, severe**
-     **F01.C0**   **Vascular dementia, severe, without behavioral disturbance, psychotic disturbance, mood disturbance, and anxiety**
  - Major neurocognitive disorder due to vascular disease, severe, NOS
  - Vascular dementia, severe, NOS

☑ Additional Character Required   ✓x7ᵗʰ Placeholder Alert   Manifestation   Unspecified Dx   Q QPP   UPD Unacceptable PDx

Chapter 5. Mental, Behavioral and Neurodevelopmental Disorders

- ✓6ᵗʰ **F01.C1 Vascular dementia, severe, with behavioral disturbance**
  - **F01.C11 Vascular dementia, severe, with agitation**

    Major neurocognitive disorder due to vascular disease, severe, with aberrant motor behavior such as restlessness, rocking, pacing, or exit-seeking

    Major neurocognitive disorder due to vascular disease, severe, with verbal or physical behaviors such as profanity, shouting, threatening, anger, aggression, combativeness, or violence

    Vascular dementia, severe, with aberrant motor behavior such as restlessness, rocking, pacing, or exit-seeking

    Vascular dementia, severe, with verbal or physical behaviors such as profanity, shouting, threatening, anger, aggression, combativeness, or violence

- **F01.C18 Vascular dementia, severe, with other behavioral disturbance**

    Major neurocognitive disorder due to vascular disease, severe, with behavioral disturbances such as sleep disturbance, social disinhibition, or sexual disinhibition

    Vascular dementia, severe, with behavioral disturbances such as sleep disturbance, social disinhibition, or sexual disinhibition

    Use additional code, if applicable, to identify wandering in vascular dementia (Z91.83)

- **F01.C2 Vascular dementia, severe, with psychotic disturbance**

    Major neurocognitive disorder due to vascular disease, severe, with psychotic disturbance such as hallucinations, paranoia, suspiciousness, or delusional state

    Vascular dementia, severe, with psychotic disturbance such as hallucinations, paranoia, suspiciousness, or delusional state

- **F01.C3 Vascular dementia, severe, with mood disturbance**

    Major neurocognitive disorder due to vascular disease, severe, with mood disturbance such as depression, apathy, or anhedonia

    Vascular dementia, severe, with mood disturbance such as depression, apathy, or anhedonia

- **F01.C4 Vascular dementia, severe, with anxiety**

    Major neurocognitive disorder due to vascular disease, severe, with anxiety

- ✓4ᵗʰ **F02 Dementia in other diseases classified elsewhere**

  INCLUDES   major neurocognitive disorder in other diseases classified elsewhere

  Code first the underlying physiological condition, such as:
  - Alzheimer's (G30.-)
  - cerebral lipidosis (E75.4)
  - Creutzfeldt-Jakob disease (A81.0-)
  - dementia with Lewy bodies (G31.83)
  - dementia with Parkinsonism (G31.83)
  - epilepsy and recurrent seizures (G40.-)
  - frontotemporal dementia (G31.09)
  - hepatolenticular degeneration (E83.0)
  - human immunodeficiency virus [HIV] disease (B20)
  - Huntington's disease (G10)
  - hypercalcemia (E83.52)
  - hypothyroidism, acquired (E00-E03.-)
  - intoxications (T36-T65)
  - Jakob-Creutzfeldt disease (A81.0-)
  - multiple sclerosis (G35)
  - neurosyphilis (A52.17)
  - niacin deficiency [pellagra] (E52)
  - Parkinson's disease (G20)
  - Pick's disease (G31.01)
  - polyarteritis nodosa (M30.0)
  - prion disease (A81.9)
  - systemic lupus erythematosus (M32.-)
  - traumatic brain injury (S06.-)
  - trypanosomiasis (B56.-, B57.-)
  - vitamin B deficiency (E53.8)

  EXCLUDES 1   ▶mild neurocognitive disorder due to known physiological condition with or without behavioral disturbance (F06.7-)◀

  EXCLUDES 2   dementia in alcohol and psychoactive substance disorders (F10-F19, with .17, .27, .97)

           vascular dementia ▶(F01.5-, F01.A-, F01.B-, F01.C-)◀

- ▲ ✓5ᵗʰ **F02.8 Dementia in other diseases classified elsewhere, unspecified severity**

    AHA: 2022,1Q,25; 2017,2Q,7; 2016,4Q,141; 2016,2Q,6

    TIP: A code from this subcategory should always be assigned with a code from category G30 when Alzheimer's disease is documented, even in the absence of documented dementia.

- ▲ **F02.80 _Dementia in other diseases classified elsewhere, unspecified severity, without behavioral disturbance, psychotic disturbance, mood disturbance, and anxiety_** HCC Rx ESR

    Dementia in other diseases classified elsewhere NOS

    ▶Major neurocognitive disorder in other diseases classified elsewhere NOS◀

▲ ✓6ᵗʰ **F02.81 Dementia in other diseases classified elsewhere, unspecified severity, with behavioral disturbance**
~~Dementia in other diseases classified elsewhere with aggressive behavior~~
~~Dementia in other diseases classified elsewhere with combative behavior~~
~~Dementia in other diseases classified elsewhere with violent behavior~~
~~Major neurocognitive disorder in other diseases classified elsewhere with aggressive behavior~~
~~Major neurocognitive disorder in other diseases classified elsewhere with combative behavior~~
~~Major neurocognitive disorder in other diseases classified elsewhere with violent behavior~~
~~Use additional code, if applicable, to identify wandering in dementia in conditions classified elsewhere (Z91.83)~~

● **F02.811 Dementia in other diseases classified elsewhere, unspecified severity, with agitation**
Dementia in other diseases classified elsewhere, unspecified severity, with aberrant motor behavior such as restlessness, rocking, pacing, or exit-seeking
Dementia in other diseases classified elsewhere, unspecified severity, with verbal or physical behaviors such as profanity, shouting, threatening, anger, aggression, combativeness, or violence
Major neurocognitive disorder in other diseases classified elsewhere, unspecified severity, with aberrant motor behavior such as restlessness, rocking, pacing, or exit-seeking
Major neurocognitive disorder in other diseases classified elsewhere, unspecified severity, with verbal or physical behaviors such as profanity, shouting, threatening, anger, aggression, combativeness, or violence

● **F02.818 Dementia in other diseases classified elsewhere, unspecified severity, with other behavioral disturbance**
Dementia in other diseases classified elsewhere with sleep disturbance, social disinhibition, or sexual disinhibition
Major neurocognitive disorder in other diseases classified elsewhere with sleep disturbance, social disinhibition, or sexual disinhibition
Use additional code, if applicable, to identify wandering in dementia in conditions classified elsewhere (Z91.83)

● **F02.82 Dementia in other diseases classified elsewhere, unspecified severity, with psychotic disturbance**
Dementia in other diseases classified elsewhere, unspecified severity, with psychotic disturbance such as hallucinations, paranoia, suspiciousness, or delusional state
Major neurocognitive disorder in other diseases classified elsewhere, unspecified, with psychotic disturbance such as hallucinations, paranoia, suspiciousness, or delusional state

● **F02.83 Dementia in other diseases classified elsewhere, unspecified severity, with mood disturbance**
Dementia in other diseases classified elsewhere, unspecified severity, with mood disturbance such as depression, apathy, or anhedonia
Major neurocognitive disorder in other diseases classified elsewhere unspecified severity, with mood disturbance such as with depression, apathy, or anhedonia

● **F02.84 Dementia in other diseases classified elsewhere, unspecified severity, with anxiety**
Major neurocognitive disorder in other diseases classified elsewhere unspecified severity, with anxiety

● ✓5ᵗʰ **F02.A Dementia in other diseases classified elsewhere, mild**
EXCLUDES 1 *mild neurocognitive disorder due to known physiological condition with or without behavioral disturbance (F06.7-)*

● **F02.A0 Dementia in other diseases classified elsewhere, mild, without behavioral disturbance, psychotic disturbance, mood disturbance, and anxiety**
Dementia in other diseases classified elsewhere, mild, NOS
Major neurocognitive disorder in other diseases classified elsewhere, mild, NOS

✓6ᵗʰ **F02.A1 Dementia in other diseases classified elsewhere, mild, with behavioral disturbance**
F02.A11 Dementia in other diseases classified elsewhere, mild, with agitation
Dementia in other diseases classified elsewhere, mild, with aberrant motor behavior such as restlessness, rocking, pacing, or exit-seeking
Dementia in other diseases classified elsewhere, mild, with verbal or physical behaviors such as profanity, shouting, threatening, anger, aggression, combativeness, or violence
Major neurocognitive disorder in other diseases classified elsewhere, mild, with aberrant motor behavior such as restlessness, rocking, pacing, or exit-seeking
Major neurocognitive disorder in other diseases classified elsewhere, mild, with verbal or physical behaviors such as profanity, shouting, threatening, anger, aggression, combativeness, or violence

● **F02.A18 Dementia in other diseases classified elsewhere, mild, with other behavioral disturbance**
Dementia in other diseases classified elsewhere, mild, with behavioral disturbances such as sleep disturbance, social disinhibition, or sexual disinhibition
Major neurocognitive disorder in other diseases classified elsewhere, mild, with behavioral disturbances such as sleep disturbance, social disinhibition, or sexual disinhibition
Use additional code, if applicable, to identify wandering in dementia in conditions classified elsewhere (Z91.83)

● **F02.A2 Dementia in other diseases classified elsewhere, mild, with psychotic disturbance**
Dementia in other diseases classified elsewhere, mild, with psychotic disturbance such as hallucinations, paranoia, suspiciousness, or delusional state
Major neurocognitive disorder in other diseases classified elsewhere, mild, with psychotic disturbance such as hallucinations, paranoia, suspiciousness, or delusional state

● **F02.A3 Dementia in other diseases classified elsewhere, mild, with mood disturbance**
Dementia in other diseases classified elsewhere, mild, with mood disturbance such as depression, apathy, or anhedonia
Major neurocognitive disorder in other diseases classified elsewhere, mild, with mood disturbance such as depression, apathy, or anhedonia

●   **F02.A4**   **Dementia in other diseases classified elsewhere, mild, with anxiety**
Major neurocognitive disorder in other diseases classified elsewhere, mild, with anxiety

●   ✓5ᵗʰ **F02.B**   **Dementia in other diseases classified elsewhere, moderate**

●   **F02.B0**   **Dementia in other diseases classified elsewhere, moderate, without behavioral disturbance, psychotic disturbance, mood disturbance, and anxiety**
Dementia in other diseases classified elsewhere, moderate, NOS
Major neurocognitive disorder in other diseases classified elsewhere, moderate, NOS

●   ✓6ᵗʰ **F02.B1**   **Dementia in other diseases classified elsewhere, moderate, with behavioral disturbance**

●   **F02.B11**   **Dementia in other diseases classified elsewhere, moderate, with agitation**
Dementia in other diseases classified elsewhere, moderate, with aberrant motor behavior such as restlessness, rocking, pacing, or exit-seeking
Dementia in other diseases classified elsewhere, moderate, with verbal or physical behaviors such as profanity, shouting, threatening, anger, aggression, combativeness, or violence
Major neurocognitive disorder in other diseases classified elsewhere, moderate, with aberrant motor behavior such as restlessness, rocking, pacing, or exit-seeking
Major neurocognitive disorder in other diseases classified elsewhere, moderate, with verbal or physical behaviors such as profanity, shouting, threatening, anger, aggression, combativeness, or violence

     F02.B18   **Dementia in other diseases classified elsewhere, moderate, with other behavioral disturbance**
Dementia in other diseases classified elsewhere, moderate, with behavioral disturbances such as sleep disturbance, social disinhibition, or sexual disinhibition
Major neurocognitive disorder in other diseases classified elsewhere, moderate, with behavioral disturbance such as sleep disturbance, social disinhibition, or sexual disinhibition
Use additional code, if applicable, to identify wandering in dementia in conditions classified elsewhere (Z91.83)

●   **F02.B2**   **Dementia in other diseases classified elsewhere, moderate, with psychotic disturbance**
Dementia in other diseases classified elsewhere, moderate, with psychotic disturbance such as hallucinations, paranoia, suspiciousness, or delusional state
Major neurocognitive disorder in other diseases classified elsewhere, moderate, with psychotic disturbance such as hallucinations, paranoia, suspiciousness, or delusional state

●   **F02.B3**   **Dementia in other diseases classified elsewhere, moderate, with mood disturbance**
Dementia in other diseases classified elsewhere, moderate, with mood disturbance such as depression, apathy, or anhedonia
Major neurocognitive disorder in other diseases classified elsewhere, moderate, with mood disturbance such as depression, apathy, or anhedonia

●   **F02.B4**   **Dementia in other diseases classified elsewhere, moderate, with anxiety**
Major neurocognitive disorder in other diseases classified elsewhere, moderate, with anxiety

●   ✓5ᵗʰ **F02.C**   **Dementia in other diseases classified elsewhere, severe**

●   **F02.C0**   **Dementia in other diseases classified elsewhere, severe, without behavioral disturbance, psychotic disturbance, mood disturbance, and anxiety**
Dementia in other diseases classified elsewhere, severe, NOS
Major neurocognitive disorder in other diseases classified elsewhere, severe, NOS

●   ✓6ᵗʰ **F02.C1**   **Dementia in other diseases classified elsewhere, severe, with behavioral disturbance**

     F02.C11   **Dementia in other diseases classified elsewhere, severe, with agitation**
Dementia in other diseases classified elsewhere, severe, with aberrant motor behavior such as restlessness, rocking, pacing, or exit-seeking
Dementia in other diseases classified elsewhere, severe, with verbal or physical behaviors such as profanity, shouting, threatening, anger, aggression, combativeness, or violence
Major neurocognitive disorder in other diseases classified elsewhere, severe, with aberrant motor behavior such as restlessness, rocking, pacing, or exit-seeking
Major neurocognitive disorder in other diseases classified elsewhere, severe, with verbal or physical behaviors such as profanity, shouting, threatening, anger, aggression, combativeness, or violence

     F02.C18   **Dementia in other diseases classified elsewhere, severe, with other behavioral disturbance**
Dementia in other diseases classified elsewhere, severe, with behavioral disturbances such as sleep disturbance, social disinhibition, or sexual disinhibition
Major neurocognitive disorder in other diseases classified elsewhere, severe, with behavioral disturbances such as sleep disturbance, social disinhibition, or sexual disinhibition
Use additional code, if applicable, to identify wandering in dementia in conditions classified elsewhere (Z91.83)

●   **F02.C2**   **Dementia in other diseases classified elsewhere, severe, with psychotic disturbance**
Dementia in other diseases classified elsewhere, severe, with psychotic disturbance such as hallucinations, paranoia, suspiciousness, or delusional state
Major neurocognitive disorder in other diseases classified elsewhere, severe, with psychotic disturbance such as hallucinations, paranoia, suspiciousness, or delusional state

●   **F02.C3**   **Dementia in other diseases classified elsewhere, severe, with mood disturbance**
Dementia in other diseases classified elsewhere, severe, with mood disturbance such as depression, apathy, or anhedonia
Major neurocognitive disorder in other diseases classified elsewhere, severe, with mood disturbance such as depression, apathy, or anhedonia

●   **F02.C4**   **Dementia in other diseases classified elsewhere, severe, with anxiety**
Major neurocognitive disorder in other diseases classified elsewhere, severe, with anxiety

✓4ᵗʰ F03   **Unspecified dementia**
> ▶Major neurocognitive disorder NOS◀
> Presenile dementia NOS
> Presenile psychosis NOS
> Primary degenerative dementia NOS
> Senile dementia NOS
> Senile dementia depressed or paranoid type
> Senile psychosis NOS
> > EXCLUDES 1   senility NOS (R41.81)
> > EXCLUDES 2   mild memory disturbance due to known physiological condition (F06.8)
> >   senile dementia with delirium or acute confusional state (F05)

▲   ✓5ᵗʰ   **F03.9**   **Unspecified dementia, unspecified severity**

▲   **F03.90**   **Unspecified dementia, unspecified severity, without behavioral disturbance, psychotic disturbance, mood disturbance, and anxiety**   HCC Rx ESR A
> Dementia NOS
> AHA: 2021,2Q,4; 2012,4Q,92

▲   ✓6ᵗʰ   **F03.91**   **Unspecified dementia, unspecified severity, with behavioral disturbance**
> Unspecified dementia with aggressive behavior
> Unspecified dementia with combative behavior
> Unspecified dementia with violent behavior
> Use additional code, if applicable, to identify wandering in unspecified dementia (Z91.83)

>   **F03.911**   **Unspecified dementia, unspecified severity, with agitation**
> > Unspecified dementia, unspecified severity, with aberrant motor behavior such as restlessness, rocking, pacing, or exit-seeking
> > Unspecified dementia, unspecified severity, with verbal or physical behaviors such as profanity, shouting, threatening, anger, aggression, combativeness, or violence

>   **F03.918**   **Unspecified dementia, unspecified severity, with other behavioral disturbance**
> > Unspecified dementia, unspecified severity, with behavioral disturbances such as sleep disturbance, social disinhibition, or sexual disinhibition
> > Use additional code, if applicable, to identify wandering in unspecified dementia (Z91.83)

>   **F03.92**   **Unspecified dementia, unspecified severity, with psychotic disturbance**
> > Unspecified dementia, unspecified severity, with psychotic disturbance such as hallucinations, paranoia, suspiciousness, or delusional state

>   **F03.93**   **Unspecified dementia, unspecified severity, with mood disturbance**
> > Unspecified dementia, unspecified severity, with mood disturbance such as depression, apathy, or anhedonia

>   **F03.94**   **Unspecified dementia, unspecified severity, with anxiety**

✓5ᵗʰ   **F03.A**   **Unspecified dementia, mild**
> > EXCLUDES 1   mild neurocognitive disorder due to known physiological condition with or without behavioral disturbance (F06.7-)

>   **F03.A0**   **Unspecified dementia, mild, without behavioral disturbance, psychotic disturbance, mood disturbance, and anxiety**
> > Dementia, mild, NOS

>   ✓6ᵗʰ   **F03.A1**   **Unspecified dementia, mild, with behavioral disturbance**

>   **F03.A11**   **Unspecified dementia, mild, with agitation**
> > > Unspecified dementia, mild, with aberrant motor behavior such as restlessness, rocking, pacing, or exit-seeking
> > > Unspecified dementia, mild, with verbal or physical behaviors such as profanity, shouting, threatening, anger, aggression, combativeness, or violence

>   **F03.A18**   **Unspecified dementia, mild, with other behavioral disturbance**
> > > Unspecified dementia, mild, with behavioral disturbances such as sleep disturbance, social disinhibition, or sexual disinhibition
> > > Use additional code, if applicable, to identify wandering in unspecified dementia (Z91.83)

>   **F03.A2**   **Unspecified dementia, mild, with psychotic disturbance**
> > Unspecified dementia, mild, with psychotic disturbance such as hallucinations, paranoia, suspiciousness, or delusional state

>   **F03.A3**   **Unspecified dementia, mild, with mood disturbance**
> > Unspecified dementia, mild, with mood disturbance such as depression, apathy, or anhedonia

>   **F03.A4**   **Unspecified dementia, mild, with anxiety**

✓5ᵗʰ   **F03.B**   **Unspecified dementia, moderate**

>   **F03.B0**   **Unspecified dementia, moderate, without behavioral disturbance, psychotic disturbance, mood disturbance, and anxiety**
> > Dementia, moderate, NOS

>   ✓6ᵗʰ   **F03.B1**   **Unspecified dementia, moderate, with behavioral disturbance**

>   **F03.B11**   **Unspecified dementia, moderate, with agitation**
> > > Unspecified dementia, moderate, with aberrant motor behavior such as restlessness, rocking, pacing, or exit-seeking
> > > Unspecified dementia, moderate, with verbal or physical behaviors such as profanity, shouting, threatening, anger, aggression, combativeness, or violence

>   **F03.B18**   **Unspecified dementia, moderate, with other behavioral disturbance**
> > > Unspecified dementia, moderate, with behavioral disturbances such as sleep disturbance, social disinhibition, or sexual disinhibition
> > > Use additional code, if applicable, to identify wandering in unspecified dementia (Z91.83)

>   **F03.B2**   **Unspecified dementia, moderate, with psychotic disturbance**
> > Unspecified dementia, moderate, with psychotic disturbance such as hallucinations, paranoia, suspiciousness, or delusional state

>   **F03.B3**   **Unspecified dementia, moderate, with mood disturbance**
> > Unspecified dementia, moderate, with mood disturbance such as depression, apathy, or anhedonia

>   **F03.B4**   **Unspecified dementia, moderate, with anxiety**

✓5ᵗʰ   **F03.C**   **Unspecified dementia, severe**

>   **F03.C0**   **Unspecified dementia, severe, without behavioral disturbance, psychotic disturbance, mood disturbance, and anxiety**
> > Dementia, severe, NOS

>   ✓6ᵗʰ   **F03.C1**   **Unspecified dementia, severe, with behavioral disturbance**

>   **F03.C11**   **Unspecified dementia, severe, with agitation**
> > > Unspecified dementia, severe, with aberrant motor behavior such as restlessness, rocking, pacing, or exit-seeking
> > > Unspecified dementia, severe, with verbal or physical behaviors such as profanity, shouting, threatening, anger, aggression, combativeness, or violence

F03.C18 Unspecified dementia, severe, with other behavioral disturbance
Unspecified dementia, severe, with behavioral disturbances such as sleep disturbance, social disinhibition, or sexual disinhibition
Use additional code, if applicable, to identify wandering in unspecified dementia (Z91.83)

F03.C2 Unspecified dementia, severe, with psychotic disturbance
Unspecified dementia, severe, with psychotic disturbance such as hallucinations, paranoia, suspiciousness, or delusional state

F03.C3 Unspecified dementia, severe, with mood disturbance
Unspecified dementia, severe, with mood disturbance such as depression, apathy, or anhedonia

F03.C4 Unspecified dementia, severe, with anxiety

F04 Amnestic disorder due to known physiological condition   HCC Rx ESR
Korsakov's psychosis or syndrome, nonalcoholic
Code first the underlying physiological condition
EXCLUDES 1   *amnesia NOS (R41.3)*
   anterograde amnesia (R41.1)
   dissociative amnesia (F44.0)
   retrograde amnesia (R41.2)
EXCLUDES 2   *alcohol-induced or unspecified Korsakov's syndrome (F10.26, F10.96)*
   Korsakov's syndrome induced by other psychoactive substances (F13.26, F13.96, F19.16, F19.26, F19.96)

F05 Delirium due to known physiological condition
Acute or subacute brain syndrome
Acute or subacute confusional state (nonalcoholic)
Acute or subacute infective psychosis
Acute or subacute organic reaction
Acute or subacute psycho-organic syndrome
Delirium of mixed etiology
Delirium superimposed on dementia
Sundowning
Code first the underlying physiological condition
EXCLUDES 1   *delirium NOS (R41.0)*
EXCLUDES 2   *delirium tremens alcohol-induced or unspecified (F10.231, F10.921)*
AHA: 2019,2Q,34

✓4th **F06 Other mental disorders due to known physiological condition**
INCLUDES   mental disorders due to endocrine disorder
   mental disorders due to exogenous hormone
   mental disorders due to exogenous toxic substance
   mental disorders due to primary cerebral disease
   mental disorders due to somatic illness
   mental disorders due to systemic disease affecting the brain
Code first the underlying physiological condition
EXCLUDES 1   *unspecified dementia (F03)*
EXCLUDES 2   *delirium due to known physiological condition (F05)*
   dementia as classified in F01-F02
   other mental disorders associated with alcohol and other psychoactive substances (F10-F19)

F06.0 Psychotic disorder with hallucinations due to known physiological condition
Organic hallucinatory state (nonalcoholic)
EXCLUDES 2   *hallucinations and perceptual disturbance induced by alcohol and other psychoactive substances (F10-F19 with .151, .251, .951)*
   schizophrenia (F20.-)

F06.1 Catatonic disorder due to known physiological condition
Catatonia associated with another mental disorder
Catatonia NOS
EXCLUDES 1   *catatonic stupor (R40.1)*
   stupor NOS (R40.1)
EXCLUDES 2   *catatonic schizophrenia (F20.2)*
   dissociative stupor (F44.2)
DEF: Catatonic: Abnormal neuropsychiatric state characterized by stupor, immobility or purposeless movements, or unresponsiveness in a person who otherwise appears awake.

F06.2 Psychotic disorder with delusions due to known physiological condition
Paranoid and paranoid-hallucinatory organic states
Schizophrenia-like psychosis in epilepsy
EXCLUDES 2   *alcohol and drug-induced psychotic disorder (F10-F19 with .150, .250, .950)*
   brief psychotic disorder (F23)
   delusional disorder (F22)
   schizophrenia (F20.-)

✓5th **F06.3 Mood disorder due to known physiological condition**
EXCLUDES 2   *mood disorders due to alcohol and other psychoactive substances (F10-F19 with .14, .24, .94)*
   mood disorders, not due to known physiological condition or unspecified (F30-F39)

F06.30 Mood disorder due to known physiological condition, unspecified

F06.31 Mood disorder due to known physiological condition with depressive features
Depressive disorder due to known physiological condition, with depressive features

F06.32 Mood disorder due to known physiological condition with major depressive-like episode
Depressive disorder due to known physiological condition, with major depressive-like episode

F06.33 Mood disorder due to known physiological condition with manic features
Bipolar and related disorder due to a known physiological condition, with manic features
Bipolar and related disorder due to known physiological condition, with manic- or hypomanic-like episodes

F06.34 Mood disorder due to known physiological condition with mixed features
Bipolar and related disorder due to known physiological condition, with mixed features
Depressive disorder due to known physiological condition, with mixed features

F06.4 Anxiety disorder due to known physiological condition
EXCLUDES 2   *anxiety disorders due to alcohol and other psychoactive substances (F10-F19 with .180, .280, .980)*
   anxiety disorders, not due to known physiological condition or unspecified (F40.-, F41.-)

✓5th **F06.7 Mild neurocognitive disorder due to known physiological condition**
Mild neurocognitive impairment due to a known physiological condition
Code first the underlying physiological condition, such as:
   Alzheimer's disease (G30.-)
   frontotemporal neurocognitive disorder (G31.09)
   human immunodeficiency virus [HIV] disease (B20)
   Huntington's disease (G10)
   neurocognitive disorder with Lewy bodies (G31.83)
   Parkinson's disease (G20)
   systemic lupus erythematosus (M32.-)
   traumatic brain injury (S06.-)
   vitamin B deficiency (E53-)
EXCLUDES 1   *age related cognitive decline (R41.81)*
   altered mental status (R41.82)
   cerebral degeneration (G31.9)
   change in mental status (R41.82)
   cognitive deficits following (sequelae of) cerebral hemorrhage or infarction (I69.01-I69.11-, I69.21-I69.31-, I69.81- I69.91-)
   dementia (F01.-, F02.-, F03)
   mild cognitive impairment due to unknown or unspecified etiology (G31.84)
   neurologic neglect syndrome (R41.4)
   personality change, nonpsychotic (F68.8)

F06.70 Mild neurocognitive disorder due to known physiological condition without behavioral disturbance
Mild neurocognitive disorder due to known physiological condition, NOS

F06.71 Mild neurocognitive disorder due to known physiological condition with behavioral disturbance

F06.8 Other specified mental disorders due to known physiological condition
     Epileptic psychosis NOS
     Obsessive-compulsive and related disorder due to a known physiological condition
     Organic dissociative disorder
     Organic emotionally labile [asthenic] disorder

✓4ᵗʰ **F07 Personality and behavioral disorders due to known physiological condition**
     Code first the underlying physiological condition

     F07.0 Personality change due to known physiological condition
         Frontal lobe syndrome
         Limbic epilepsy personality syndrome
         Lobotomy syndrome
         Organic personality disorder
         Organic pseudopsychopathic personality
         Organic pseudoretarded personality
         Postleucotomy syndrome
         Code first underlying physiological condition
         EXCLUDES 1   mild cognitive impairment (G31.84)
                 postconcussional syndrome (F07.81)
                 postencephalitic syndrome (F07.89)
                 signs and symptoms involving emotional state (R45.-)
         EXCLUDES 2   specific personality disorder (F60.-)

     ✓5ᵗʰ **F07.8 Other personality and behavioral disorders due to known physiological condition**
         F07.81 Postconcussional syndrome
             Postcontusional syndrome (encephalopathy)
             Post-traumatic brain syndrome, nonpsychotic
             Use additional code to identify associated post-traumatic headache, if applicable (G44.3-)
             EXCLUDES 1   current concussion (brain) (S06.0-)
                    postencephalitic syndrome (F07.89)
             DEF: Concussion symptoms that persist for weeks or months after a head injury. These symptoms may include headache, giddiness, fatigue, insomnia, mood fluctuation, and a subjective feeling of impaired intellectual function with extreme reaction to normal stressors.
         F07.89 Other personality and behavioral disorders due to known physiological condition
             Postencephalitic syndrome
             Right hemispheric organic affective disorder

     F07.9 Unspecified personality and behavioral disorder due to known physiological condition
         Organic psychosyndrome

F09 Unspecified mental disorder due to known physiological condition
     Mental disorder NOS due to known physiological condition
     Organic brain syndrome NOS
     Organic mental disorder NOS
     Organic psychosis NOS
     Symptomatic psychosis NOS
     Code first the underlying physiological condition
     EXCLUDES 1   ▶mild neurocognitive disorder due to known physiological condition (F06.7-)◀
                 psychosis NOS (F29)

Mental and behavioral disorders due to psychoactive substance use (F10-F19)

AHA: 2022,1Q,34; 2020,1Q,9; 2018,4Q,69-70; 2017,4Q,8; 2017,2Q,27
TIP: Psychoactive substance withdrawal can occur in individuals who do not have a diagnosis of dependence but who use the substance regularly (i.e., use or abuse) and then reduce or cease the use.

✓4ᵗʰ **F10 Alcohol related disorders**
     Use additional code for blood alcohol level, if applicable (Y90.-)
     AHA: 2019,3Q,8

     ✓5ᵗʰ **F10.1 Alcohol abuse**
         EXCLUDES 1   alcohol dependence (F10.2-)
                 alcohol use, unspecified (F10.9-)
         AHA: 2018,1Q,16; 2015,2Q,15
         F10.10 Alcohol abuse, uncomplicated
             Alcohol use disorder, mild
         F10.11 Alcohol abuse, in remission
             Alcohol use disorder, mild, in early remission
             Alcohol use disorder, mild, in sustained remission
             AHA: 2022,1Q,25

✓6ᵗʰ **F10.12 Alcohol abuse with intoxication**
     F10.120 Alcohol abuse with intoxication, uncomplicated HCC ESR
     F10.121 Alcohol abuse with intoxication delirium HCC ESR
     F10.129 Alcohol abuse with intoxication, unspecified HCC ESR

✓6ᵗʰ **F10.13 Alcohol abuse, with withdrawal**
     AHA: 2020,4Q,16-17
     F10.130 Alcohol abuse with withdrawal, uncomplicated HCC ESR COM
     F10.131 Alcohol abuse with withdrawal delirium HCC ESR COM
     F10.132 Alcohol abuse with withdrawal with perceptual disturbance HCC ESR COM
     F10.139 Alcohol abuse with withdrawal, unspecified HCC ESR COM

     F10.14 Alcohol abuse with alcohol-induced mood disorder HCC ESR COM
         Alcohol use disorder, mild, with alcohol-induced bipolar or related disorder
         Alcohol use disorder, mild, with alcohol-induced depressive disorder

✓6ᵗʰ **F10.15 Alcohol abuse with alcohol-induced psychotic disorder**
     F10.150 Alcohol abuse with alcohol-induced psychotic disorder with delusions HCC ESR COM
     F10.151 Alcohol abuse with alcohol-induced psychotic disorder with hallucinations HCC ESR COM
         DEF: Psychosis lasting less than six months with slight or no clouding of consciousness in which auditory hallucinations predominate.
     F10.159 Alcohol abuse with alcohol-induced psychotic disorder, unspecified HCC ESR COM

✓6ᵗʰ **F10.18 Alcohol abuse with other alcohol-induced disorders**
     AHA: 2022,1Q,33
     F10.180 Alcohol abuse with alcohol-induced anxiety disorder HCC ESR COM
         AHA: 2022,1Q,25,33
     F10.181 Alcohol abuse with alcohol-induced sexual dysfunction HCC ESR COM
     F10.182 Alcohol abuse with alcohol-induced sleep disorder HCC ESR COM
     F10.188 Alcohol abuse with other alcohol-induced disorder HCC ESR COM
         AHA: 2022,1Q,25

     F10.19 Alcohol abuse with unspecified alcohol-induced disorder HCC ESR

✓5ᵗʰ **F10.2 Alcohol dependence**
     EXCLUDES 1   alcohol abuse (F10.1-)
                 alcohol use, unspecified (F10.9-)
     EXCLUDES 2   toxic effect of alcohol (T51.0-)
     F10.20 Alcohol dependence, uncomplicated HCC ESR COM
         Alcohol use disorder, moderate
         Alcohol use disorder, severe
         AHA: 2020,1Q,9
     F10.21 Alcohol dependence, in remission HCC ESR COM
         Alcohol use disorder, moderate, in early remission
         Alcohol use disorder, moderate, in sustained remission
         Alcohol use disorder, severe, in early remission
         Alcohol use disorder, severe, in sustained remission

✓6ᵗʰ **F10.22 Alcohol dependence with intoxication**
     Acute drunkenness (in alcoholism)
     EXCLUDES 2   alcohol dependence with withdrawal (F10.23-)
     F10.220 Alcohol dependence with intoxication, uncomplicated HCC ESR COM
     F10.221 Alcohol dependence with intoxication delirium HCC ESR COM
     F10.229 Alcohol dependence with intoxication, unspecified HCC ESR COM

Chapter 5. Mental, Behavioral and Neurodevelopmental Disorders

F10.23–F10.982

✓6ᵗʰ **F10.23** **Alcohol dependence with** withdrawal

EXCLUDES 2   *alcohol dependence with intoxication (F10.22-)*

AHA: 2018,1Q,16; 2015,2Q,15

F10.230 **Alcohol dependence with withdrawal,** uncomplicated   HCC ESR COM

F10.231 **Alcohol dependence with withdrawal** delirium   HCC ESR COM

F10.232 **Alcohol dependence with withdrawal with** perceptual disturbance   HCC ESR COM

F10.239 **Alcohol dependence with withdrawal,** unspecified   HCC ESR COM

F10.24 **Alcohol dependence with alcohol-induced** mood disorder   HCC ESR COM

Alcohol use disorder, moderate, with alcohol-induced bipolar or related disorder

Alcohol use disorder, moderate, with alcohol-induced depressive disorder

Alcohol use disorder, severe, with alcohol-induced bipolar or related disorder

Alcohol use disorder, severe, with alcohol-induced depressive disorder

✓6ᵗʰ **F10.25** **Alcohol dependence with alcohol-induced** psychotic disorder

F10.250 **Alcohol dependence with alcohol-induced psychotic disorder with** delusions   HCC ESR COM

F10.251 **Alcohol dependence with alcohol-induced psychotic disorder with** hallucinations   HCC ESR COM

F10.259 **Alcohol dependence with alcohol-induced psychotic disorder,** unspecified   HCC ESR COM

F10.26 **Alcohol dependence with alcohol-induced** persisting amnestic disorder   HCC ESR COM

Alcohol use disorder, moderate, with alcohol-induced major neurocognitive disorder, amnestic-confabulatory type

Alcohol use disorder, severe, with alcohol-induced major neurocognitive disorder, amnestic-confabulatory type

DEF: Prominent and lasting reduced memory span and disordered time appreciation and confabulation that occurs in alcoholics as sequel to acute alcoholic psychosis.

F10.27 **Alcohol dependence with alcohol-induced** persisting dementia   HCC ESR COM

Alcohol use disorder, moderate, with alcohol-induced major neurocognitive disorder, nonamnestic-confabulatory type

Alcohol use disorder, severe, with alcohol-induced major neurocognitive disorder, nonamnestic-confabulatory type

✓6ᵗʰ **F10.28** **Alcohol dependence with other alcohol-induced disorders**

F10.280 **Alcohol dependence with alcohol-induced** anxiety disorder   HCC ESR COM

F10.281 **Alcohol dependence with alcohol-induced** sexual dysfunction   HCC ESR COM

F10.282 **Alcohol dependence with alcohol-induced** sleep disorder   HCC ESR COM

F10.288 **Alcohol dependence with other alcohol-induced disorder**   HCC ESR COM

Alcohol use disorder, moderate, with alcohol-induced mild neurocognitive disorder

Alcohol use disorder, severe, with alcohol-induced mild neurocognitive disorder

AHA: 2020,1Q,9

F10.29 **Alcohol dependence with unspecified alcohol-induced disorder**   HCC ESR COM

✓5ᵗʰ **F10.9** **Alcohol** use, **unspecified**

EXCLUDES 1   *alcohol abuse (F10.1-)*

alcohol dependence (F10.2-)

AHA: 2018,2Q,10-11

TIP: Assign a substance use code only when the provider documents a relationship between the use and an associated physical, mental, or behavioral disorder. As with all diagnoses, substance use codes must meet the definition of a reportable diagnosis.

● **F10.90** **Alcohol use, unspecified,** uncomplicated

● **F10.91** **Alcohol use, unspecified,** in remission

✓6ᵗʰ **F10.92** **Alcohol use, unspecified with** intoxication

F10.920 **Alcohol use, unspecified with intoxication,** uncomplicated   HCC ESR

AHA: 2018,2Q,10-11

F10.921 **Alcohol use, unspecified with intoxication** delirium   HCC ESR

F10.929 **Alcohol use, unspecified with intoxication, unspecified**   HCC ESR

✓6ᵗʰ **F10.93** **Alcohol use, unspecified with** withdrawal

AHA: 2020,4Q,16-17

F10.930 **Alcohol use, unspecified with withdrawal,** uncomplicated   HCC ESR COM

F10.931 **Alcohol use, unspecified with withdrawal** delirium   HCC ESR COM

F10.932 **Alcohol use, unspecified with withdrawal with** perceptual disturbance   HCC ESR COM

F10.939 **Alcohol use, unspecified with withdrawal, unspecified**   HCC ESR COM

F10.94 **Alcohol use, unspecified with alcohol-induced** mood disorder   HCC ESR COM

Alcohol induced bipolar or related disorder, without use disorder

Alcohol induced depressive disorder, without use disorder

✓6ᵗʰ **F10.95** **Alcohol use, unspecified with alcohol-induced** psychotic disorder

F10.950 **Alcohol use, unspecified with alcohol-induced psychotic disorder with** delusions   HCC ESR COM

F10.951 **Alcohol use, unspecified with alcohol-induced psychotic disorder with** hallucinations   HCC ESR COM

F10.959 **Alcohol use, unspecified with alcohol-induced psychotic disorder,** unspecified   HCC ESR COM

Alcohol-induced psychotic disorder without use disorder

F10.96 **Alcohol use, unspecified with alcohol-induced** persisting amnestic disorder   HCC ESR COM

Alcohol-induced major neurocognitive disorder, amnestic-confabulatory type, without use disorder

F10.97 **Alcohol use, unspecified with alcohol-induced** persisting dementia   HCC ESR COM

Alcohol-induced major neurocognitive disorder, nonamnestic-confabulatory type, without use disorder

✓6ᵗʰ **F10.98** **Alcohol use, unspecified with other alcohol-induced disorders**

F10.980 **Alcohol use, unspecified with alcohol-induced** anxiety disorder   HCC ESR COM

Alcohol induced anxiety disorder, without use disorder

F10.981 **Alcohol use, unspecified with alcohol-induced** sexual dysfunction   HCC ESR COM

Alcohol induced sexual dysfunction, without use disorder

F10.982 **Alcohol use, unspecified with alcohol-induced** sleep disorder   HCC ESR COM

Alcohol induced sleep disorder, without use disorder

F10.988 Alcohol use, unspecified with other alcohol-induced disorder `HCC` `ESR` `COM`
Alcohol induced mild neurocognitive disorder, without use disorder

F10.99 Alcohol use, unspecified with unspecified alcohol-induced disorder `HCC` `ESR`

☑️4ᵗʰ **F11** **Opioid** related disorders

☑️5ᵗʰ **F11.1** **Opioid** abuse

EXCLUDES 1 opioid dependence (F11.2-)
opioid use, unspecified (F11.9-)

F11.10 Opioid abuse, uncomplicated `HCC` `ESR`
Opioid use disorder, mild

F11.11 Opioid abuse, in remission `HCC` `ESR`
Opioid use disorder, mild, in early remission
Opioid use disorder, mild, in sustained remission

☑️6ᵗʰ **F11.12** Opioid abuse with intoxication

F11.120 Opioid abuse with intoxication, uncomplicated `HCC` `ESR` `COM`

F11.121 Opioid abuse with intoxication delirium `HCC` `ESR` `COM`

F11.122 Opioid abuse with intoxication with perceptual disturbance `HCC` `ESR` `COM`

F11.129 Opioid abuse with intoxication, unspecified `HCC` `ESR` `COM`

F11.13 Opioid abuse with withdrawal `HCC` `ESR` `COM`
AHA: 2020,4Q,16-17

F11.14 Opioid abuse with opioid-induced mood disorder `HCC` `ESR` `COM`
Opioid use disorder, mild, with opioid-induced depressive disorder

☑️6ᵗʰ **F11.15** Opioid abuse with opioid-induced psychotic disorder

F11.150 Opioid abuse with opioid-induced psychotic disorder with delusions `HCC` `ESR` `COM`

F11.151 Opioid abuse with opioid-induced psychotic disorder with hallucinations `HCC` `ESR` `COM`

F11.159 Opioid abuse with opioid-induced psychotic disorder, unspecified `HCC` `ESR` `COM`

☑️6ᵗʰ **F11.18** Opioid abuse with other opioid-induced disorder

F11.181 Opioid abuse with opioid-induced sexual dysfunction `HCC` `ESR` `COM`

F11.182 Opioid abuse with opioid-induced sleep disorder `HCC` `ESR` `COM`

F11.188 Opioid abuse with other opioid-induced disorder `HCC` `ESR` `COM`

F11.19 Opioid abuse with unspecified opioid-induced disorder `HCC` `ESR` `COM`

☑️5ᵗʰ **F11.2** **Opioid** dependence

EXCLUDES 1 opioid abuse (F11.1-)
opioid use, unspecified (F11.9-)
EXCLUDES 2 opioid poisoning (T40.0-T40.2-)

F11.20 Opioid dependence, uncomplicated `HCC` `ESR` `COM`
Opioid use disorder, moderate
Opioid use disorder, severe

F11.21 Opioid dependence, in remission `HCC` `ESR` `COM`
Opioid use disorder, moderate, in early remission
Opioid use disorder, moderate, in sustained remission
Opioid use disorder, severe, in early remission
Opioid use disorder, severe, in sustained remission

☑️6ᵗʰ **F11.22** Opioid dependence with intoxication

EXCLUDES 1 opioid dependence with withdrawal (F11.23)

F11.220 Opioid dependence with intoxication, uncomplicated `HCC` `ESR` `COM`

F11.221 Opioid dependence with intoxication delirium `HCC` `ESR` `COM`

F11.222 Opioid dependence with intoxication with perceptual disturbance `HCC` `ESR` `COM`

F11.229 Opioid dependence with intoxication, unspecified `HCC` `ESR` `COM`

F11.23 Opioid dependence with withdrawal `HCC` `ESR` `COM`

EXCLUDES 1 opioid dependence with intoxication (F11.22-)

F11.24 Opioid dependence with opioid-induced mood disorder `HCC` `ESR` `COM`
Opioid use disorder, moderate, with opioid induced depressive disorder

☑️6ᵗʰ **F11.25** Opioid dependence with opioid-induced psychotic disorder

F11.250 Opioid dependence with opioid-induced psychotic disorder with delusions `HCC` `ESR` `COM`

F11.251 Opioid dependence with opioid-induced psychotic disorder with hallucinations `HCC` `ESR` `COM`

F11.259 Opioid dependence with opioid-induced psychotic disorder, unspecified `HCC` `ESR` `COM`

☑️6ᵗʰ **F11.28** Opioid dependence with other opioid-induced disorder

F11.281 Opioid dependence with opioid-induced sexual dysfunction `HCC` `ESR` `COM`

F11.282 Opioid dependence with opioid-induced sleep disorder `HCC` `ESR` `COM`

F11.288 Opioid dependence with other opioid-induced disorder `HCC` `ESR` `COM`

F11.29 Opioid dependence with unspecified opioid-induced disorder `HCC` `ESR` `COM`

☑️5ᵗʰ **F11.9** **Opioid** use, unspecified

EXCLUDES 1 opioid abuse (F11.1-)
opioid dependence (F11.2-)

TIP: Assign a substance use code only when the provider documents a relationship between the use and an associated physical, mental, or behavioral disorder. As with all diagnoses, substance use codes must meet the definition of a reportable diagnosis.

F11.90 Opioid use, unspecified, uncomplicated
AHA: 2018,2Q,10-11

● **F11.91** Opioid use, unspecified, in remission

☑️6ᵗʰ **F11.92** Opioid use, unspecified with intoxication

EXCLUDES 1 opioid use, unspecified with withdrawal (F11.93)

F11.920 Opioid use, unspecified with intoxication, uncomplicated `HCC` `ESR` `COM`

F11.921 Opioid use, unspecified with intoxication delirium `HCC` `ESR` `COM`
Opioid-induced delirium

F11.922 Opioid use, unspecified with intoxication with perceptual disturbance `HCC` `ESR` `COM`

F11.929 Opioid use, unspecified with intoxication, unspecified `HCC` `ESR` `COM`

F11.93 Opioid use, unspecified with withdrawal `HCC` `ESR` `COM`

EXCLUDES 1 opioid use, unspecified with intoxication (F11.92-)

F11.94 Opioid use, unspecified with opioid-induced mood disorder `HCC` `ESR` `COM`
Opioid induced depressive disorder, without use disorder

☑️6ᵗʰ **F11.95** Opioid use, unspecified with opioid-induced psychotic disorder

F11.950 Opioid use, unspecified with opioid-induced psychotic disorder with delusions `HCC` `ESR` `COM`

F11.951 Opioid use, unspecified with opioid-induced psychotic disorder with hallucinations `HCC` `ESR` `COM`

F11.959 Opioid use, unspecified with opioid-induced psychotic disorder, unspecified `HCC` `ESR` `COM`

☑️6ᵗʰ **F11.98** Opioid use, unspecified with other specified opioid-induced disorder

F11.981 Opioid use, unspecified with opioid-induced sexual dysfunction `HCC` `ESR` `COM`
Opioid induced sexual dysfunction, without use disorder

F11.982   **Opioid use, unspecified with opioid-induced** sleep **disorder** `HCC` `ESR` `COM`
   Opioid induced sleep disorder, without use disorder

F11.988   **Opioid use, unspecified with other opioid-induced disorder** `HCC` `ESR` `COM`
   Opioid induced anxiety disorder, without use disorder

F11.99   **Opioid use, unspecified with unspecified opioid-induced disorder** `HCC` `ESR` `COM`

✓4ᵗʰ **F12**   Cannabis **related disorders**
    INCLUDES   marijuana
    AHA: 2020,1Q,8

✓5ᵗʰ **F12.1**   **Cannabis** abuse
    EXCLUDES 1   cannabis dependence (F12.2-)
             cannabis use, unspecified (F12.9-)

   F12.10   **Cannabis abuse,** uncomplicated
      Cannabis use disorder, mild

   F12.11   **Cannabis abuse,** in remission
      Cannabis use disorder, mild, in early remission
      Cannabis use disorder, mild, in sustained remission

✓6ᵗʰ **F12.12**   **Cannabis abuse with** intoxication
    F12.120   **Cannabis abuse with intoxication,** uncomplicated `HCC` `ESR` `COM`
    F12.121   **Cannabis abuse with intoxication** delirium `HCC` `ESR` `COM`
    F12.122   **Cannabis abuse with intoxication with** perceptual disturbance `HCC` `ESR` `COM`
    F12.129   **Cannabis abuse with intoxication, unspecified** `HCC` `ESR` `COM`

   F12.13   **Cannabis abuse with** withdrawal `HCC` `ESR` `COM`
      AHA: 2020,4Q,16-17

✓6ᵗʰ **F12.15**   **Cannabis abuse with** psychotic disorder
    F12.150   **Cannabis abuse with psychotic disorder with** delusions `HCC` `ESR` `COM`
    F12.151   **Cannabis abuse with psychotic disorder with** hallucinations `HCC` `ESR` `COM`
    F12.159   **Cannabis abuse with psychotic disorder, unspecified** `HCC` `ESR` `COM`

✓6ᵗʰ **F12.18**   **Cannabis abuse with other cannabis-induced disorder**
    F12.180   **Cannabis abuse with cannabis-induced** anxiety disorder `HCC` `ESR` `COM`
    F12.188   **Cannabis abuse with other cannabis-induced disorder** `HCC` `ESR` `COM`
      Cannabis use disorder, mild, with cannabis-induced sleep disorder

   F12.19   **Cannabis abuse with unspecified cannabis-induced disorder** `HCC` `ESR` `COM`

✓5ᵗʰ **F12.2**   **Cannabis** dependence
    EXCLUDES 1   cannabis abuse (F12.1-)
             cannabis use, unspecified (F12.9-)
    EXCLUDES 2   cannabis poisoning (T40.7-)

   F12.20   **Cannabis dependence,** uncomplicated `HCC` `ESR` `COM`
      Cannabis use disorder, moderate
      Cannabis use disorder, severe

   F12.21   **Cannabis dependence,** in remission `HCC` `ESR` `COM`
      Cannabis use disorder, moderate, in early remission
      Cannabis use disorder, moderate, in sustained remission
      Cannabis use disorder, severe, in early remission
      Cannabis use disorder, severe, in sustained remission

✓6ᵗʰ **F12.22**   **Cannabis dependence with** intoxication
    F12.220   **Cannabis dependence with intoxication,** uncomplicated `HCC` `ESR` `COM`
    F12.221   **Cannabis dependence with intoxication** delirium `HCC` `ESR` `COM`
    F12.222   **Cannabis dependence with intoxication with** perceptual disturbance `HCC` `ESR` `COM`
    F12.229   **Cannabis dependence with intoxication, unspecified** `HCC` `ESR` `COM`

F12.23   **Cannabis dependence with** withdrawal `HCC` `ESR` `COM`
    AHA: 2018,4Q,7

✓6ᵗʰ **F12.25**   **Cannabis dependence with** psychotic disorder
    F12.250   **Cannabis dependence with psychotic disorder with** delusions `HCC` `ESR` `COM`
    F12.251   **Cannabis dependence with psychotic disorder with** hallucinations `HCC` `ESR` `COM`
    F12.259   **Cannabis dependence with psychotic disorder, unspecified** `HCC` `ESR` `COM`

✓6ᵗʰ **F12.28**   **Cannabis dependence with other cannabis-induced disorder**
    F12.280   **Cannabis dependence with cannabis-induced** anxiety disorder `HCC` `ESR` `COM`
    F12.288   **Cannabis dependence with other cannabis-induced disorder** `HCC` `ESR` `COM`
      Cannabis use disorder, moderate, with cannabis-induced sleep disorder
      Cannabis use disorder, severe, with cannabis-induced sleep disorder

F12.29   **Cannabis dependence with unspecified cannabis-induced disorder** `HCC` `ESR` `COM`

✓5ᵗʰ **F12.9**   **Cannabis use, unspecified**
    EXCLUDES 1   cannabis abuse (F12.1-)
             cannabis dependence (F12.2-)
    TIP: Assign a substance use code only when the provider documents a relationship between the use and an associated physical, mental, or behavioral disorder. As with all diagnoses, substance use codes must meet the definition of a reportable diagnosis.

F12.90   **Cannabis use, unspecified,** uncomplicated
    AHA: 2018,2Q,10-11

F12.91   **Cannabis use, unspecified,** in remission

✓6ᵗʰ **F12.92**   **Cannabis use, unspecified with** intoxication
    F12.920   **Cannabis use, unspecified with intoxication,** uncomplicated `HCC` `ESR` `COM`
    F12.921   **Cannabis use, unspecified with intoxication** delirium `HCC` `ESR` `COM`
    F12.922   **Cannabis use, unspecified with intoxication with** perceptual disturbance `HCC` `ESR` `COM`
    F12.929   **Cannabis use, unspecified with intoxication, unspecified** `HCC` `ESR` `COM`

F12.93   **Cannabis use, unspecified with** withdrawal `HCC` `ESR` `COM`
    AHA: 2018,4Q,7

✓6ᵗʰ **F12.95**   **Cannabis use, unspecified with** psychotic disorder
    F12.950   **Cannabis use, unspecified with psychotic disorder with** delusions `HCC` `ESR` `COM`
    F12.951   **Cannabis use, unspecified with psychotic disorder with** hallucinations `HCC` `ESR` `COM`
    F12.959   **Cannabis use, unspecified with psychotic disorder, unspecified** `HCC` `ESR` `COM`
      Cannabis induced psychotic disorder, without use disorder

✓6ᵗʰ **F12.98**   **Cannabis use, unspecified with other cannabis-induced disorder**
    F12.980   **Cannabis use, unspecified with** anxiety disorder `HCC` `ESR` `COM`
      Cannabis induced anxiety disorder, without use disorder
    F12.988   **Cannabis use, unspecified with other cannabis-induced disorder** `HCC` `ESR` `COM`
      Cannabis induced sleep disorder, without use disorder

F12.99   **Cannabis use, unspecified with unspecified cannabis-induced disorder** `HCC` `ESR` `COM`

`HCC` CMS-HCC   `Rx` Rx HCC   `ESR` ESRD HCC   `COM` Commercial HCC   `N` Newborn: 0   `P` Pediatric: 0-17   `M` Maternity: 9-64   `A` Adult: 15-124

564   ICD-10-CM 2023

✓4th **F13** Sedative, hypnotic, or anxiolytic **related disorders**

✓5th **F13.1** Sedative, hypnotic or anxiolytic-related **abuse**

EXCLUDES 1   *sedative, hypnotic or anxiolytic-related dependence (F13.2-)*
sedative, hypnotic, or anxiolytic use, unspecified (F13.9-)

F13.10 Sedative, hypnotic or anxiolytic abuse, uncomplicated   HCC ESR
Sedative, hypnotic, or anxiolytic use disorder, mild

F13.11 Sedative, hypnotic or anxiolytic abuse, in remission   HCC ESR
Sedative, hypnotic or anxiolytic use disorder, mild, in early remission
Sedative, hypnotic or anxiolytic use disorder, mild, in sustained remission

✓6th **F13.12** Sedative, hypnotic or anxiolytic abuse with intoxication

F13.120 Sedative, hypnotic or anxiolytic abuse with intoxication, uncomplicated   HCC ESR COM

F13.121 Sedative, hypnotic or anxiolytic abuse with intoxication delirium   HCC ESR COM

F13.129 Sedative, hypnotic or anxiolytic abuse with intoxication, unspecified   HCC ESR COM

✓6th **F13.13** Sedative, hypnotic or anxiolytic abuse with withdrawal
AHA: 2020,4Q,16-17

F13.130 Sedative, hypnotic or anxiolytic abuse with withdrawal, uncomplicated   HCC ESR COM

F13.131 Sedative, hypnotic or anxiolytic abuse with withdrawal delirium   HCC ESR COM

F13.132 Sedative, hypnotic or anxiolytic abuse with withdrawal with perceptual disturbance   HCC ESR COM

F13.139 Sedative, hypnotic or anxiolytic abuse with withdrawal, unspecified   HCC ESR COM

F13.14 Sedative, hypnotic or anxiolytic abuse with sedative, hypnotic or anxiolytic-induced **mood** disorder   HCC ESR COM
Sedative, hypnotic, or anxiolytic use disorder, mild, with sedative, hypnotic, or anxiolytic-induced bipolar or related disorder
Sedative, hypnotic, or anxiolytic use disorder, mild, with sedative, hypnotic, or anxiolytic-induced depressive disorder

✓6th **F13.15** Sedative, hypnotic or anxiolytic abuse with sedative, hypnotic or anxiolytic-induced **psychotic** disorder

F13.150 Sedative, hypnotic or anxiolytic abuse with sedative, hypnotic or anxiolytic-induced psychotic disorder with **delusions**   HCC ESR COM

F13.151 Sedative, hypnotic or anxiolytic abuse with sedative, hypnotic or anxiolytic-induced psychotic disorder with **hallucinations**   HCC ESR COM

F13.159 Sedative, hypnotic or anxiolytic abuse with sedative, hypnotic or anxiolytic-induced psychotic disorder, unspecified   HCC ESR COM

✓6th **F13.18** Sedative, hypnotic or anxiolytic abuse with other sedative, hypnotic or anxiolytic-induced disorders

F13.180 Sedative, hypnotic or anxiolytic abuse with sedative, hypnotic or anxiolytic-induced **anxiety** disorder   HCC ESR COM

F13.181 Sedative, hypnotic or anxiolytic abuse with sedative, hypnotic or anxiolytic-induced **sexual** dysfunction   HCC ESR COM

F13.182 Sedative, hypnotic or anxiolytic abuse with sedative, hypnotic or anxiolytic-induced **sleep** disorder   HCC ESR COM

F13.188 Sedative, hypnotic or anxiolytic abuse with other sedative, hypnotic or anxiolytic-induced disorder   HCC ESR COM

F13.19 Sedative, hypnotic or anxiolytic abuse with unspecified sedative, hypnotic or anxiolytic-induced disorder   HCC ESR COM

✓5th **F13.2** Sedative, hypnotic or anxiolytic-related **dependence**

EXCLUDES 1   *sedative, hypnotic or anxiolytic-related abuse (F13.1-)*
sedative, hypnotic, or anxiolytic use, unspecified (F13.9-)

EXCLUDES 2   *sedative, hypnotic, or anxiolytic poisoning (T42.-)*

F13.20 Sedative, hypnotic or anxiolytic dependence, uncomplicated   HCC ESR COM

F13.21 Sedative, hypnotic or anxiolytic dependence, in remission   HCC ESR COM
Sedative, hypnotic or anxiolytic use disorder, moderate, in early remission
Sedative, hypnotic or anxiolytic use disorder, moderate, in sustained remission
Sedative, hypnotic or anxiolytic use disorder, severe, in early remission
Sedative, hypnotic or anxiolytic use disorder, severe, in sustained remission

✓6th **F13.22** Sedative, hypnotic or anxiolytic dependence with intoxication

EXCLUDES 1   *sedative, hypnotic or anxiolytic dependence with withdrawal (F13.23-)*

F13.220 Sedative, hypnotic or anxiolytic dependence with intoxication, uncomplicated   HCC ESR COM

F13.221 Sedative, hypnotic or anxiolytic dependence with intoxication delirium   HCC ESR COM

F13.229 Sedative, hypnotic or anxiolytic dependence with intoxication, unspecified   HCC ESR COM

✓6th **F13.23** Sedative, hypnotic or anxiolytic dependence with withdrawal
Sedative, hypnotic, or anxiolytic use disorder, moderate
Sedative, hypnotic, or anxiolytic use disorder, severe

EXCLUDES 1   *sedative, hypnotic or anxiolytic dependence with intoxication (F13.22-)*

F13.230 Sedative, hypnotic or anxiolytic dependence with withdrawal, uncomplicated   HCC ESR COM

F13.231 Sedative, hypnotic or anxiolytic dependence with withdrawal delirium   HCC ESR COM

F13.232 Sedative, hypnotic or anxiolytic dependence with withdrawal with perceptual disturbance   HCC ESR COM
Sedative, hypnotic, or anxiolytic withdrawal with perceptual disturbances

F13.239 Sedative, hypnotic or anxiolytic dependence with withdrawal, unspecified   HCC ESR COM
Sedative, hypnotic, or anxiolytic withdrawal without perceptual disturbances

F13.24 Sedative, hypnotic or anxiolytic dependence with sedative, hypnotic or anxiolytic-induced **mood** disorder   HCC ESR COM
Sedative, hypnotic, or anxiolytic use disorder, moderate, with sedative, hypnotic, or anxiolytic-induced bipolar or related disorder
Sedative, hypnotic, or anxiolytic use disorder, moderate, with sedative, hypnotic, or anxiolytic-induced depressive disorder
Sedative, hypnotic, or anxiolytic use disorder, severe, with sedative, hypnotic, or anxiolytic-induced bipolar or related disorder
Sedative, hypnotic, or anxiolytic use disorder, severe, with sedative, hypnotic, or anxiolytic-induced depressive disorder

√6th **F13.25** **Sedative, hypnotic or anxiolytic dependence with sedative, hypnotic or anxiolytic-induced** psychotic disorder

F13.250 **Sedative, hypnotic or anxiolytic dependence with sedative, hypnotic or anxiolytic-induced psychotic disorder with** delusions `HCC` `ESR` `COM`

F13.251 **Sedative, hypnotic or anxiolytic dependence with sedative, hypnotic or anxiolytic-induced psychotic disorder with** hallucinations `HCC` `ESR` `COM`

F13.259 **Sedative, hypnotic or anxiolytic dependence with sedative, hypnotic or anxiolytic-induced psychotic disorder, unspecified** `HCC` `ESR` `COM`

F13.26 **Sedative, hypnotic or anxiolytic dependence with sedative, hypnotic or anxiolytic-induced** persisting amnestic disorder `HCC` `ESR` `COM`

F13.27 **Sedative, hypnotic or anxiolytic dependence with sedative, hypnotic or anxiolytic-induced** persisting dementia `HCC` `ESR` `COM`

Sedative, hypnotic, or anxiolytic use disorder, moderate, with sedative, hypnotic, or anxiolytic induced major neurocognitive disorder

Sedative, hypnotic, or anxiolytic use disorder, severe, with sedative, hypnotic, or anxiolytic-induced major neurocognitive disorder

√6th **F13.28** **Sedative, hypnotic or anxiolytic dependence with other sedative, hypnotic or anxiolytic-induced disorders**

F13.280 **Sedative, hypnotic or anxiolytic dependence with sedative, hypnotic or anxiolytic-induced** anxiety disorder `HCC` `ESR` `COM`

F13.281 **Sedative, hypnotic or anxiolytic dependence with sedative, hypnotic or anxiolytic-induced** sexual dysfunction `HCC` `ESR` `COM`

F13.282 **Sedative, hypnotic or anxiolytic dependence with sedative, hypnotic or anxiolytic-induced** sleep disorder `HCC` `ESR` `COM`

F13.288 **Sedative, hypnotic or anxiolytic dependence with other sedative, hypnotic or anxiolytic-induced disorder** `HCC` `ESR` `COM`

Sedative, hypnotic, or anxiolytic use disorder, moderate, with sedative, hypnotic, or anxiolytic-induced mild neurocognitive disorder

Sedative, hypnotic, or anxiolytic use disorder, severe, with sedative, hypnotic, or anxiolytic-induced mild neurocognitive disorder

F13.29 **Sedative, hypnotic or anxiolytic dependence with unspecified sedative, hypnotic or anxiolytic-induced disorder** `HCC` `ESR` `COM`

√5th **F13.9** **Sedative, hypnotic or anxiolytic-related use, unspecified**

EXCLUDES 1 *sedative, hypnotic or anxiolytic-related abuse (F13.1-)*
sedative, hypnotic or anxiolytic-related dependence (F13.2-)

TIP: Assign a substance use code only when the provider documents a relationship between the use and an associated physical, mental, or behavioral disorder. As with all diagnoses, substance use codes must meet the definition of a reportable diagnosis.

F13.90 **Sedative, hypnotic, or anxiolytic use, unspecified, uncomplicated**
AHA: 2018,2Q,10-11

F13.91 **Sedative, hypnotic or anxiolytic use, unspecified, in remission**

√6th **F13.92** **Sedative, hypnotic or anxiolytic use, unspecified with** intoxication

EXCLUDES 1 *sedative, hypnotic or anxiolytic use, unspecified with withdrawal (F13.93-)*

F13.920 **Sedative, hypnotic or anxiolytic use, unspecified with intoxication, uncomplicated** `HCC` `ESR` `COM`

F13.921 **Sedative, hypnotic or anxiolytic use, unspecified with intoxication** delirium `HCC` `ESR` `COM`

Sedative, hypnotic, or anxiolytic-induced delirium

F13.929 **Sedative, hypnotic or anxiolytic use, unspecified with intoxication, unspecified** `HCC` `ESR` `COM`

√6th **F13.93** **Sedative, hypnotic or anxiolytic use, unspecified with** withdrawal

EXCLUDES 1 *sedative, hypnotic or anxiolytic use, unspecified with intoxication (F13.92-)*

F13.930 **Sedative, hypnotic or anxiolytic use, unspecified with withdrawal, uncomplicated** `HCC` `ESR` `COM`

F13.931 **Sedative, hypnotic or anxiolytic use, unspecified with withdrawal** delirium `HCC` `ESR` `COM`

F13.932 **Sedative, hypnotic or anxiolytic use, unspecified with withdrawal with** perceptual disturbances `HCC` `ESR` `COM`

F13.939 **Sedative, hypnotic or anxiolytic use, unspecified with withdrawal, unspecified** `HCC` `ESR` `COM`

F13.94 **Sedative, hypnotic or anxiolytic use, unspecified with sedative, hypnotic or anxiolytic-induced** mood disorder `HCC` `ESR` `COM`

Sedative, hypnotic, or anxiolytic-induced bipolar or related disorder, without use disorder

Sedative, hypnotic, or anxiolytic-induced depressive disorder, without use disorder

√6th **F13.95** **Sedative, hypnotic or anxiolytic use, unspecified with sedative, hypnotic or anxiolytic-induced psychotic disorder**

F13.950 **Sedative, hypnotic or anxiolytic use, unspecified with sedative, hypnotic or anxiolytic-induced psychotic disorder with** delusions `HCC` `ESR` `COM`

F13.951 **Sedative, hypnotic or anxiolytic use, unspecified with sedative, hypnotic or anxiolytic-induced psychotic disorder with** hallucinations `HCC` `ESR` `COM`

F13.959 **Sedative, hypnotic or anxiolytic use, unspecified with sedative, hypnotic or anxiolytic-induced psychotic disorder, unspecified** `HCC` `ESR` `COM`

Sedative, hypnotic, or anxiolytic-induced psychotic disorder, without use disorder

F13.96 **Sedative, hypnotic or anxiolytic use, unspecified with sedative, hypnotic or anxiolytic-induced** persisting amnestic disorder `HCC` `ESR` `COM`

F13.97 **Sedative, hypnotic or anxiolytic use, unspecified with sedative, hypnotic or anxiolytic-induced** persisting dementia `HCC` `ESR` `COM`

Sedative, hypnotic, or anxiolytic-induced major neurocognitive disorder, without use disorder

√6th **F13.98** **Sedative, hypnotic or anxiolytic use, unspecified with other sedative, hypnotic or anxiolytic-induced disorders**

F13.980 **Sedative, hypnotic or anxiolytic use, unspecified with sedative, hypnotic or anxiolytic-induced** anxiety disorder `HCC` `ESR` `COM`

Sedative, hypnotic, or anxiolytic-induced anxiety disorder, without use disorder

F13.981 **Sedative, hypnotic or anxiolytic use, unspecified with sedative, hypnotic or anxiolytic-induced** sexual dysfunction `HCC` `ESR` `COM`

Sedative, hypnotic, or anxiolytic-induced sexual dysfunction disorder, without use disorder

F13.982 **Sedative, hypnotic or anxiolytic use, unspecified with sedative, hypnotic or anxiolytic-induced** sleep disorder `HCC` `ESR` `COM`

Sedative, hypnotic, or anxiolytic-induced sleep disorder, without use disorder

F13.988 Sedative, hypnotic or anxiolytic use, unspecified with other sedative, hypnotic or anxiolytic-induced disorder `HCC` `ESR` `COM`
    Sedative, hypnotic, or anxiolytic-induced mild neurocognitive disorder

F13.99 Sedative, hypnotic or anxiolytic use, unspecified with unspecified sedative, hypnotic or anxiolytic-induced disorder `HCC` `ESR` `COM`

√4th **F14** **Cocaine related disorders**
    EXCLUDES 2   *other stimulant-related disorders (F15.-)*

√5th **F14.1** **Cocaine abuse**
    EXCLUDES 1   *cocaine dependence (F14.2-)*
                cocaine use, unspecified (F14.9-)

F14.10 **Cocaine abuse, uncomplicated** `HCC` `ESR`
    Cocaine use disorder, mild

F14.11 **Cocaine abuse, in remission** `HCC` `ESR`
    Cocaine use disorder, mild, in early remission
    Cocaine use disorder, mild, in sustained remission

√6th **F14.12** **Cocaine abuse with intoxication**

F14.120 **Cocaine abuse with intoxication, uncomplicated** `HCC` `ESR` `COM`

F14.121 **Cocaine abuse with intoxication with delirium** `HCC` `ESR` `COM`

F14.122 **Cocaine abuse with intoxication with perceptual disturbance** `HCC` `ESR` `COM`

F14.129 **Cocaine abuse with intoxication, unspecified** `HCC` `ESR` `COM`

F14.13 **Cocaine abuse, unspecified with withdrawal** `HCC` `ESR` `COM`
    AHA: 2020,4Q,16-17

F14.14 **Cocaine abuse with cocaine-induced mood disorder** `HCC` `ESR` `COM`
    Cocaine use disorder, mild, with cocaine-induced bipolar or related disorder
    Cocaine use disorder, mild, with cocaine-induced depressive disorder

√6th **F14.15** **Cocaine abuse with cocaine-induced psychotic disorder**

F14.150 **Cocaine abuse with cocaine-induced psychotic disorder with delusions** `HCC` `ESR` `COM`

F14.151 **Cocaine abuse with cocaine-induced psychotic disorder with hallucinations** `HCC` `ESR` `COM`

F14.159 **Cocaine abuse with cocaine-induced psychotic disorder, unspecified** `HCC` `ESR` `COM`

√6th **F14.18** **Cocaine abuse with other cocaine-induced disorder**

F14.180 **Cocaine abuse with cocaine-induced anxiety disorder** `HCC` `ESR` `COM`

F14.181 **Cocaine abuse with cocaine-induced sexual dysfunction** `HCC` `ESR` `COM`

F14.182 **Cocaine abuse with cocaine-induced sleep disorder** `HCC` `ESR` `COM`

F14.188 **Cocaine abuse with other cocaine-induced disorder** `HCC` `ESR` `COM`
    Cocaine use disorder, mild, with cocaine-induced obsessive compulsive or related disorder

F14.19 **Cocaine abuse with unspecified cocaine-induced disorder** `HCC` `ESR` `COM`

√5th **F14.2** **Cocaine dependence**
    EXCLUDES 1   *cocaine abuse (F14.1-)*
                cocaine use, unspecified (F14.9-)
    EXCLUDES 2   *cocaine poisoning (T40.5-)*

F14.20 **Cocaine dependence, uncomplicated** `HCC` `ESR` `COM`
    Cocaine use disorder, moderate
    Cocaine use disorder, severe

F14.21 **Cocaine dependence, in remission** `HCC` `ESR` `COM`
    Cocaine use disorder, moderate, in early remission
    Cocaine use disorder, moderate, in sustained remission
    Cocaine use disorder, severe, in early remission
    Cocaine use disorder, severe, in sustained remission

√6th **F14.22** **Cocaine dependence with intoxication**
    EXCLUDES 1   *cocaine dependence with withdrawal (F14.23)*

F14.220 **Cocaine dependence with intoxication, uncomplicated** `HCC` `ESR` `COM`

F14.221 **Cocaine dependence with intoxication delirium** `HCC` `ESR` `COM`

F14.222 **Cocaine dependence with intoxication with perceptual disturbance** `HCC` `ESR` `COM`

F14.229 **Cocaine dependence with intoxication, unspecified** `HCC` `ESR` `COM`

F14.23 **Cocaine dependence with withdrawal** `HCC` `ESR` `COM`
    EXCLUDES 1   *cocaine dependence with intoxication (F14.22-)*

F14.24 **Cocaine dependence with cocaine-induced mood disorder** `HCC` `ESR` `COM`
    Cocaine use disorder, moderate, with cocaine-induced bipolar or related disorder
    Cocaine use disorder, moderate, with cocaine-induced depressive disorder
    Cocaine use disorder, severe, with cocaine-induced bipolar or related disorder
    Cocaine use disorder, severe, with cocaine-induced depressive disorder

√6th **F14.25** **Cocaine dependence with cocaine-induced psychotic disorder**

F14.250 **Cocaine dependence with cocaine-induced psychotic disorder with delusions** `HCC` `ESR` `COM`

F14.251 **Cocaine dependence with cocaine-induced psychotic disorder with hallucinations** `HCC` `ESR` `COM`

F14.259 **Cocaine dependence with cocaine-induced psychotic disorder, unspecified** `HCC` `ESR` `COM`

√6th **F14.28** **Cocaine dependence with other cocaine-induced disorder**

F14.280 **Cocaine dependence with cocaine-induced anxiety disorder** `HCC` `ESR` `COM`

F14.281 **Cocaine dependence with cocaine-induced sexual dysfunction** `HCC` `ESR` `COM`

F14.282 **Cocaine dependence with cocaine-induced sleep disorder** `HCC` `ESR` `COM`

F14.288 **Cocaine dependence with other cocaine-induced disorder** `HCC` `ESR` `COM`
    Cocaine use disorder, moderate, with cocaine-induced obsessive compulsive or related disorder
    Cocaine use disorder, severe, with cocaine-induced obsessive compulsive or related disorder

F14.29 **Cocaine dependence with unspecified cocaine-induced disorder** `HCC` `ESR` `COM`

√5th **F14.9** **Cocaine use, unspecified**
    EXCLUDES 1   *cocaine abuse (F14.1-)*
                cocaine dependence (F14.2-)
    TIP: Assign a substance use code only when the provider documents a relationship between the use and an associated physical, mental, or behavioral disorder. As with all diagnoses, substance use codes must meet the definition of a reportable diagnosis.

F14.90 **Cocaine use, unspecified, uncomplicated**
    AHA: 2018,2Q,10-11

● **F14.91** **Cocaine use, unspecified, in remission**

√6th **F14.92** **Cocaine use, unspecified with intoxication**

F14.920 **Cocaine use, unspecified with intoxication, uncomplicated** `HCC` `ESR` `COM`

F14.921 **Cocaine use, unspecified with intoxication delirium** `HCC` `ESR` `COM`

F14.922 **Cocaine use, unspecified with intoxication with perceptual disturbance** `HCC` `ESR` `COM`

F14.929 **Cocaine use, unspecified with intoxication, unspecified** `HCC` `ESR` `COM`

F14.93 Cocaine use, unspecified with withdrawal HCC ESR COM
AHA: 2020,4Q,16-17

F14.94 Cocaine use, unspecified with cocaine-induced mood disorder HCC ESR COM
Cocaine induced bipolar or related disorder, without use disorder
Cocaine induced depressive disorder, without use disorder

✓6th **F14.95 Cocaine use, unspecified with cocaine-induced psychotic disorder**
F14.950 Cocaine use, unspecified with cocaine-induced psychotic disorder with delusions HCC ESR COM
F14.951 Cocaine use, unspecified with cocaine-induced psychotic disorder with hallucinations HCC ESR COM
F14.959 Cocaine use, unspecified with cocaine-induced psychotic disorder, unspecified HCC ESR COM
Cocaine induced psychotic disorder, without use disorder

✓6th **F14.98 Cocaine use, unspecified with other specified cocaine-induced disorder**
F14.980 Cocaine use, unspecified with cocaine-induced anxiety disorder HCC ESR COM
Cocaine induced anxiety disorder, without use disorder
F14.981 Cocaine use, unspecified with cocaine-induced sexual dysfunction HCC ESR COM
Cocaine induced sexual dysfunction, without use disorder
F14.982 Cocaine use, unspecified with cocaine-induced sleep disorder HCC ESR COM
Cocaine induced sleep disorder, without use disorder
F14.988 Cocaine use, unspecified with other cocaine-induced disorder HCC ESR COM
Cocaine induced obsessive compulsive or related disorder

F14.99 Cocaine use, unspecified with unspecified cocaine-induced disorder HCC ESR COM

✓4th **F15 Other stimulant related disorders**
INCLUDES   amphetamine-related disorders
caffeine
EXCLUDES 2   cocaine-related disorders (F14.-)

✓5th **F15.1 Other stimulant abuse**
EXCLUDES 1   other stimulant dependence (F15.2-)
other stimulant use, unspecified (F15.9-)

F15.10 Other stimulant abuse, uncomplicated HCC ESR
Amphetamine type substance use disorder, mild
Other or unspecified stimulant use disorder, mild

F15.11 Other stimulant abuse, in remission HCC ESR
Amphetamine type substance use disorder, mild, in early remission
Amphetamine type substance use disorder, mild, in sustained remission
Other or unspecified stimulant use disorder, mild, in early remission
Other or unspecified stimulant use disorder, mild, in sustained remission
AHA: 2021,3Q,8

✓6th **F15.12 Other stimulant abuse with intoxication**
F15.120 Other stimulant abuse with intoxication, uncomplicated HCC ESR COM
F15.121 Other stimulant abuse with intoxication delirium HCC ESR COM
F15.122 Other stimulant abuse with intoxication with perceptual disturbance HCC ESR COM
Amphetamine or other stimulant use disorder, mild, with amphetamine or other stimulant intoxication, with perceptual disturbances

F15.129 Other stimulant abuse with intoxication, unspecified HCC ESR COM
Amphetamine or other stimulant use disorder, mild, with amphetamine or other stimulant intoxication, without perceptual disturbances

F15.13 Other stimulant abuse with withdrawal HCC ESR COM
AHA: 2020,4Q,16-17

F15.14 Other stimulant abuse with stimulant-induced mood disorder HCC ESR COM
Amphetamine or other stimulant use disorder, mild, with amphetamine or other stimulant induced bipolar or related disorder
Amphetamine or other stimulant use disorder, mild, with amphetamine or other stimulant induced depressive disorder

✓6th **F15.15 Other stimulant abuse with stimulant-induced psychotic disorder**
F15.150 Other stimulant abuse with stimulant-induced psychotic disorder with delusions HCC ESR COM
F15.151 Other stimulant abuse with stimulant-induced psychotic disorder with hallucinations HCC ESR COM
F15.159 Other stimulant abuse with stimulant-induced psychotic disorder, unspecified HCC ESR COM

✓6th **F15.18 Other stimulant abuse with other stimulant-induced disorder**
F15.180 Other stimulant abuse with stimulant-induced anxiety disorder HCC ESR COM
F15.181 Other stimulant abuse with stimulant-induced sexual dysfunction HCC ESR COM
F15.182 Other stimulant abuse with stimulant-induced sleep disorder HCC ESR COM
F15.188 Other stimulant abuse with other stimulant-induced disorder HCC ESR COM
Amphetamine or other stimulant use disorder, mild, with amphetamine or other stimulant induced obsessive-compulsive or related disorder

F15.19 Other stimulant abuse with unspecified stimulant-induced disorder HCC ESR COM

✓5th **F15.2 Other stimulant dependence**
EXCLUDES 1   other stimulant abuse (F15.1-)
other stimulant use, unspecified (F15.9-)

F15.20 Other stimulant dependence, uncomplicated HCC ESR COM
Amphetamine type substance use disorder, moderate
Amphetamine type substance use disorder, severe
Other or unspecified stimulant use disorder, moderate
Other or unspecified stimulant use disorder, severe

F15.21 Other stimulant dependence, in remission HCC ESR COM
Amphetamine type substance use disorder, moderate, in early remission
Amphetamine type substance use disorder, moderate, in sustained remission
Amphetamine type substance use disorder, severe, in early remission
Amphetamine type substance use disorder, severe, in sustained remission
Other or unspecified stimulant use disorder, moderate, in early remission
Other or unspecified stimulant use disorder, moderate, in sustained remission
Other or unspecified stimulant use disorder, severe, in early remission
Other or unspecified stimulant use disorder, severe, in sustained remission

✓6ᵗʰ **F15.22** **Other stimulant dependence with intoxication**

> EXCLUDES 1   *other stimulant dependence with withdrawal (F15.23)*

F15.220 **Other stimulant dependence with intoxication, uncomplicated** `HCC` `ESR` `COM`

F15.221 **Other stimulant dependence with intoxication delirium** `HCC` `ESR` `COM`

F15.222 **Other stimulant dependence with intoxication with perceptual disturbance** `HCC` `ESR` `COM`
> Amphetamine or other stimulant use disorder, moderate, with amphetamine or other stimulant intoxication, with perceptual disturbances
> Amphetamine or other stimulant use disorder, severe, with amphetamine or other stimulant intoxication, with perceptual disturbances

F15.229 **Other stimulant dependence with intoxication, unspecified** `HCC` `ESR` `COM`
> Amphetamine or other stimulant use disorder, moderate, with amphetamine or other stimulant intoxication, without perceptual disturbances
> Amphetamine or other stimulant use disorder, severe, with amphetamine or other stimulant intoxication, without perceptual disturbances

F15.23 **Other stimulant dependence with withdrawal** `HCC` `ESR` `COM`
> Amphetamine or other stimulant withdrawal
> EXCLUDES 1   *other stimulant dependence with intoxication (F15.22-)*

F15.24 **Other stimulant dependence with stimulant-induced mood disorder** `HCC` `ESR` `COM`
> Amphetamine or other stimulant use disorder, moderate, with amphetamine or other stimulant-induced bipolar or related disorder
> Amphetamine or other stimulant use disorder, moderate, with amphetamine or other stimulant induced depressive disorder
> Amphetamine or other stimulant use disorder, severe, with amphetamine or other stimulant-induced bipolar or related disorder
> Amphetamine or other stimulant use disorder, severe, with amphetamine or other stimulant-induced depressive disorder

✓6ᵗʰ **F15.25** **Other stimulant dependence with stimulant-induced psychotic disorder**

F15.250 **Other stimulant dependence with stimulant-induced psychotic disorder with delusions** `HCC` `ESR` `COM`

F15.251 **Other stimulant dependence with stimulant-induced psychotic disorder with hallucinations** `HCC` `ESR` `COM`

F15.259 **Other stimulant dependence with stimulant-induced psychotic disorder, unspecified** `HCC` `ESR` `COM`

✓6ᵗʰ **F15.28** **Other stimulant dependence with other stimulant-induced disorder**

F15.280 **Other stimulant dependence with stimulant-induced anxiety disorder** `HCC` `ESR` `COM`

F15.281 **Other stimulant dependence with stimulant-induced sexual dysfunction** `HCC` `ESR` `COM`

F15.282 **Other stimulant dependence with stimulant-induced sleep disorder** `HCC` `ESR` `COM`

F15.288 **Other stimulant dependence with other stimulant-induced disorder** `HCC` `ESR` `COM`
> Amphetamine or other stimulant use disorder, moderate, with amphetamine orother stimulant induced obsessive compulsive or related disorder
> Amphetamine or other stimulant use disorder, severe, with amphetamine or otherstimulant induced obsessive compulsive or related disorder

F15.29 **Other stimulant dependence with unspecified stimulant-induced disorder** `HCC` `ESR` `COM`

✓5ᵗʰ **F15.9** **Other stimulant use, unspecified**
> EXCLUDES 1   *other stimulant abuse (F15.1-)*
> *other stimulant dependence (F15.2-)*

TIP: Assign a substance use code only when the provider documents a relationship between the use and an associated physical, mental, or behavioral disorder. As with all diagnoses, substance use codes must meet the definition of a reportable diagnosis.

F15.90 **Other stimulant use, unspecified, uncomplicated**
> AHA: 2018,2Q,10-11

F15.91 **Other stimulant use, unspecified, in remission**

✓6ᵗʰ **F15.92** **Other stimulant use, unspecified with intoxication**
> EXCLUDES 1   *other stimulant use, unspecified with withdrawal (F15.93)*

F15.920 **Other stimulant use, unspecified with intoxication, uncomplicated** `HCC` `ESR` `COM`

F15.921 **Other stimulant use, unspecified with intoxication delirium** `HCC` `ESR` `COM`
> Amphetamine or other stimulant-induced delirium

F15.922 **Other stimulant use, unspecified with intoxication with perceptual disturbance** `HCC` `ESR` `COM`

F15.929 **Other stimulant use, unspecified with intoxication, unspecified** `HCC` `ESR` `COM`
> Caffeine intoxication

F15.93 **Other stimulant use, unspecified with withdrawal** `HCC` `ESR` `COM`
> Caffeine withdrawal
> EXCLUDES 1   *other stimulant use, unspecified with intoxication (F15.92-)*

F15.94 **Other stimulant use, unspecified with stimulant-induced mood disorder** `HCC` `ESR` `COM`
> Amphetamine or other stimulant-induced bipolar or related disorder, without use disorder
> Amphetamine or other stimulant-induced depressive disorder, without use disorder

✓6ᵗʰ **F15.95** **Other stimulant use, unspecified with stimulant-induced psychotic disorder**

F15.950 **Other stimulant use, unspecified with stimulant-induced psychotic disorder with delusions** `HCC` `ESR` `COM`

F15.951 **Other stimulant use, unspecified with stimulant-induced psychotic disorder with hallucinations** `HCC` `ESR` `COM`

F15.959 **Other stimulant use, unspecified with stimulant-induced psychotic disorder, unspecified** `HCC` `ESR` `COM`
> Amphetamine or other stimulant-induced psychotic disorder, without use disorder

✓6ᵗʰ **F15.98** **Other stimulant use, unspecified with other stimulant-induced disorder**

F15.980 **Other stimulant use, unspecified with stimulant-induced anxiety disorder** `HCC` `ESR` `COM`
> Amphetamine or other stimulant-induced anxiety disorder, without use disorder
> Caffeine induced anxiety disorder, without use disorder

F15.981 Other stimulant use, unspecified with stimulant-induced **sexual dysfunction** `HCC` `ESR` `COM`
  Amphetamine or other stimulant-induced sexual dysfunction, without use disorder

F15.982 Other stimulant use, unspecified with stimulant-induced **sleep disorder** `HCC` `ESR` `COM`
  Amphetamine or other stimulant-induced sleep disorder, without use disorder
  Caffeine induced sleep disorder, without use disorder

F15.988 Other stimulant use, unspecified with other stimulant-induced disorder `HCC` `ESR` `COM`
  Amphetamine or other stimulant-induced obsessive compulsive or related disorder, without use disorder

F15.99 Other stimulant use, unspecified with unspecified stimulant-induced disorder `HCC` `ESR` `COM`

✓4ᵗʰ **F16** **Hallucinogen** related disorders
  `INCLUDES` ecstasy
    PCP
    phencyclidine
  AHA: 2018,4Q,31

✓5ᵗʰ **F16.1** **Hallucinogen** abuse
  `EXCLUDES 1` *hallucinogen dependence (F16.2-)*
    hallucinogen use, unspecified (F16.9-)

  F16.10 **Hallucinogen abuse, uncomplicated** `HCC` `ESR`
    Other hallucinogen use disorder, mild
    Phencyclidine use disorder, mild

  F16.11 **Hallucinogen abuse, in remission** `HCC` `ESR`
    Other hallucinogen use disorder, mild, in early remission
    Other hallucinogen use disorder, mild, in sustained remission
    Phencyclidine use disorder, mild, in early remission
    Phencyclidine use disorder, mild, in sustained remission

  ✓6ᵗʰ **F16.12** **Hallucinogen abuse with intoxication**
    F16.120 **Hallucinogen abuse with intoxication, uncomplicated** `HCC` `ESR` `COM`
    F16.121 **Hallucinogen abuse with intoxication with delirium** `HCC` `ESR` `COM`
    F16.122 **Hallucinogen abuse with intoxication with perceptual disturbance** `HCC` `ESR` `COM`
    F16.129 **Hallucinogen abuse with intoxication, unspecified** `HCC` `ESR` `COM`

  F16.14 **Hallucinogen abuse with hallucinogen-induced mood disorder** `HCC` `ESR` `COM`
    Other hallucinogen use disorder, mild, with other hallucinogen induced bipolar or related disorder
    Other hallucinogen use disorder, mild, with other hallucinogen induced depressive disorder
    Phencyclidine use disorder, mild, with phencyclidine induced bipolar or related disorder
    Phencyclidine use disorder, mild, with phencyclidine induced depressive disorder

  ✓6ᵗʰ **F16.15** **Hallucinogen abuse with hallucinogen-induced psychotic disorder**
    F16.150 **Hallucinogen abuse with hallucinogen-induced psychotic disorder with delusions** `HCC` `ESR` `COM`
    F16.151 **Hallucinogen abuse with hallucinogen-induced psychotic disorder with hallucinations** `HCC` `ESR` `COM`
    F16.159 **Hallucinogen abuse with hallucinogen-induced psychotic disorder, unspecified** `HCC` `ESR` `COM`

  ✓6ᵗʰ **F16.18** **Hallucinogen abuse with other hallucinogen-induced disorder**
    F16.180 **Hallucinogen abuse with hallucinogen-induced anxiety disorder** `HCC` `ESR` `COM`
    F16.183 **Hallucinogen abuse with hallucinogen persisting perception disorder (flashbacks)** `HCC` `ESR` `COM`

F16.188 **Hallucinogen abuse with other hallucinogen-induced disorder** `HCC` `ESR` `COM`

F16.19 **Hallucinogen abuse with unspecified hallucinogen-induced disorder** `HCC` `ESR` `COM`

✓5ᵗʰ **F16.2** **Hallucinogen** dependence
  `EXCLUDES 1` *hallucinogen abuse (F16.1-)*
    hallucinogen use, unspecified (F16.9-)

  F16.20 **Hallucinogen dependence, uncomplicated** `HCC` `ESR` `COM`
    Other hallucinogen use disorder, moderate
    Other hallucinogen use disorder, severe
    Phencyclidine use disorder, moderate
    Phencyclidine use disorder, severe

  F16.21 **Hallucinogen dependence, in remission** `HCC` `ESR` `COM`
    Other hallucinogen use disorder, moderate, in early remission
    Other hallucinogen use disorder, moderate, in sustained remission
    Other hallucinogen use disorder, severe, in early remission
    Other hallucinogen use disorder, severe, in sustained remission
    Phencyclidine use disorder, moderate, in early remission
    Phencyclidine use disorder, moderate, in sustained remission
    Phencyclidine use disorder, severe, in early remission
    Phencyclidine use disorder, severe, in sustained remission

  ✓6ᵗʰ **F16.22** **Hallucinogen dependence with intoxication**
    F16.220 **Hallucinogen dependence with intoxication, uncomplicated** `HCC` `ESR` `COM`
    F16.221 **Hallucinogen dependence with intoxication with delirium** `HCC` `ESR` `COM`
    F16.229 **Hallucinogen dependence with intoxication, unspecified** `HCC` `ESR` `COM`

  F16.24 **Hallucinogen dependence with hallucinogen-induced mood disorder** `HCC` `ESR` `COM`
    Other hallucinogen use disorder, moderate, with other hallucinogen induced bipolar or related disorder
    Other hallucinogen use disorder, moderate, with other hallucinogen induced depressive disorder
    Other hallucinogen use disorder, severe, with other hallucinogen-induced bipolar or related disorder
    Other hallucinogen use disorder, severe, with other hallucinogen-induced depressive disorder
    Phencyclidine use disorder, moderate, with phencyclidine induced bipolar or related disorder
    Phencyclidine use disorder, moderate, with phencyclidine induced depressive disorder
    Phencyclidine use disorder, severe, with phencyclidine induced bipolar or related disorder
    Phencyclidine use disorder, severe, with phencyclidine-induced depressive disorder

  ✓6ᵗʰ **F16.25** **Hallucinogen dependence with hallucinogen-induced psychotic disorder**
    F16.250 **Hallucinogen dependence with hallucinogen-induced psychotic disorder with delusions** `HCC` `ESR` `COM`
    F16.251 **Hallucinogen dependence with hallucinogen-induced psychotic disorder with hallucinations** `HCC` `ESR` `COM`
    F16.259 **Hallucinogen dependence with hallucinogen-induced psychotic disorder, unspecified** `HCC` `ESR` `COM`

  ✓6ᵗʰ **F16.28** **Hallucinogen dependence with other hallucinogen-induced disorder**
    F16.280 **Hallucinogen dependence with hallucinogen-induced anxiety disorder** `HCC` `ESR` `COM`
    F16.283 **Hallucinogen dependence with hallucinogen persisting perception disorder (flashbacks)** `HCC` `ESR` `COM`

F16.288 Hallucinogen dependence with other hallucinogen-induced disorder `HCC` `ESR` `COM`

F16.29 Hallucinogen dependence with unspecified hallucinogen-induced disorder `HCC` `ESR` `COM`

✓6ᵗʰ **F16.9 Hallucinogen use, unspecified**

     EXCLUDES 1   hallucinogen abuse (F16.1-)
                 hallucinogen dependence (F16.2-)

     TIP: Assign a substance use code only when the provider documents a relationship between the use and an associated physical, mental, or behavioral disorder. As with all diagnoses, substance use codes must meet the definition of a reportable diagnosis.

     F16.90 Hallucinogen use, unspecified, uncomplicated
         AHA: 2018,2Q,10-11

     F16.91 Hallucinogen use, unspecified, in remission

✓6ᵗʰ **F16.92 Hallucinogen use, unspecified with intoxication**

     F16.920 Hallucinogen use, unspecified with intoxication, uncomplicated `HCC` `ESR` `COM`

     F16.921 Hallucinogen use, unspecified with intoxication with delirium `HCC` `ESR` `COM`
         Other hallucinogen intoxication delirium

     F16.929 Hallucinogen use, unspecified with intoxication, unspecified `HCC` `ESR` `COM`

     F16.94 Hallucinogen use, unspecified with hallucinogen-induced mood disorder `HCC` `ESR` `COM`
         Other hallucinogen induced bipolar or related disorder, without use disorder
         Other hallucinogen induced depressive disorder, without use disorder
         Phencyclidine induced bipolar or related disorder, without use disorder
         Phencyclidine induced depressive disorder, without use disorder

✓6ᵗʰ **F16.95 Hallucinogen use, unspecified with hallucinogen-induced psychotic disorder**

     F16.950 Hallucinogen use, unspecified with hallucinogen-induced psychotic disorder with delusions `HCC` `ESR` `COM`

     F16.951 Hallucinogen use, unspecified with hallucinogen-induced psychotic disorder with hallucinations `HCC` `ESR` `COM`

     F16.959 Hallucinogen use, unspecified with hallucinogen-induced psychotic disorder, unspecified `HCC` `ESR` `COM`
         Other hallucinogen induced psychotic disorder, without use disorder
         Phencyclidine induced psychotic disorder, without use disorder

✓6ᵗʰ **F16.98 Hallucinogen use, unspecified with other specified hallucinogen-induced disorder**

     F16.980 Hallucinogen use, unspecified with hallucinogen-induced anxiety disorder `HCC` `ESR` `COM`
         Other hallucinogen-induced anxiety disorder, without use disorder
         Phencyclidine induced anxiety disorder, without use disorder

     F16.983 Hallucinogen use, unspecified with hallucinogen persisting perception disorder (flashbacks) `HCC` `ESR` `COM`

     F16.988 Hallucinogen use, unspecified with other hallucinogen-induced disorder `HCC` `ESR` `COM`

     F16.99 Hallucinogen use, unspecified with unspecified hallucinogen-induced disorder `HCC` `ESR` `COM`

✓4ᵗʰ **F17 Nicotine dependence**

     EXCLUDES 1   history of tobacco dependence (Z87.891)
                 tobacco use NOS (Z72.0)

     EXCLUDES 2   tobacco use (smoking) during pregnancy, childbirth and the puerperium (O99.33-)
                 toxic effect of nicotine (T65.2-)

     AHA: 2013,4Q,108-109

✓5ᵗʰ **F17.2 Nicotine dependence**

✓6ᵗʰ **F17.20 Nicotine dependence, unspecified**

     F17.200 Nicotine dependence, unspecified, uncomplicated
         Tobacco use disorder, mild
         Tobacco use disorder, moderate
         Tobacco use disorder, severe
         AHA: 2016,1Q,36
         TIP: Assign when provider documentation indicates "smoker" without further specification.

     F17.201 Nicotine dependence, unspecified, in remission
         Tobacco use disorder, mild, in early remission
         Tobacco use disorder, mild, in sustained remission
         Tobacco use disorder, moderate, in early remission
         Tobacco use disorder, moderate, in sustained remission
         Tobacco use disorder, severe, in early remission
         Tobacco use disorder, severe, in sustained remission

     F17.203 Nicotine dependence unspecified, with withdrawal
         Tobacco withdrawal

     F17.208 Nicotine dependence, unspecified, with other nicotine-induced disorders

     F17.209 Nicotine dependence, unspecified, with unspecified nicotine-induced disorders

✓6ᵗʰ **F17.21 Nicotine dependence, cigarettes**

     F17.210 Nicotine dependence, cigarettes, uncomplicated
         AHA: 2017,2Q,28-29

     F17.211 Nicotine dependence, cigarettes, in remission
         Tobacco use disorder, cigarettes, mild, in early remission
         Tobacco use disorder, cigarettes, mild, in sustained remission
         Tobacco use disorder, cigarettes, moderate, in early remission
         Tobacco use disorder, cigarettes, moderate, in sustained remission
         Tobacco use disorder, cigarettes, severe, in early remission
         Tobacco use disorder, cigarettes, severe, in sustained remission

     F17.213 Nicotine dependence, cigarettes, with withdrawal

     F17.218 Nicotine dependence, cigarettes, with other nicotine-induced disorders

     F17.219 Nicotine dependence, cigarettes, with unspecified nicotine-induced disorders

✓6ᵗʰ **F17.22 Nicotine dependence, chewing tobacco**

     F17.220 Nicotine dependence, chewing tobacco, uncomplicated

---

Chapter 5. Mental, Behavioral and Neurodevelopmental Disorders

F17.221   **Nicotine dependence, chewing tobacco, in remission**
Tobacco use disorder, chewing tobacco, mild, in early remission
Tobacco use disorder, chewing tobacco, mild, in sustained remission
Tobacco use disorder, chewing tobacco, moderate, in early remission
Tobacco use disorder, chewing tobacco, moderate, in sustained remission
Tobacco use disorder, chewing tobacco, severe, in early remission
Tobacco use disorder, chewing tobacco, severe, in sustained remission

F17.223   **Nicotine dependence, chewing tobacco, with withdrawal**

F17.228   **Nicotine dependence, chewing tobacco, with other nicotine-induced disorders**

F17.229   **Nicotine dependence, chewing tobacco, with unspecified nicotine-induced disorders**

✓6ᵗʰ   **F17.29**   **Nicotine dependence, other tobacco product**

F17.290   **Nicotine dependence, other tobacco product, uncomplicated**
AHA: 2017,2Q,28-29

F17.291   **Nicotine dependence, other tobacco product, in remission**
Tobacco use disorder, other tobacco product, mild, in early remission
Tobacco use disorder, other tobacco product, mild, in sustained remission
Tobacco use disorder, other tobacco product, moderate, in early remission
Tobacco use disorder, other tobacco product, moderate, in sustained remission
Tobacco use disorder, other tobacco product, severe, in early remission
Tobacco use disorder, other tobacco product, severe, in sustained remission

F17.293   **Nicotine dependence, other tobacco product, with withdrawal**

F17.298   **Nicotine dependence, other tobacco product, with other nicotine-induced disorders**

F17.299   **Nicotine dependence, other tobacco product, with unspecified nicotine-induced disorders**

✓4ᵗʰ   **F18**   **Inhalant related disorders**
INCLUDES   volatile solvents

✓5ᵗʰ   **F18.1**   **Inhalant abuse**
EXCLUDES 1   inhalant dependence (F18.2-)
inhalant use, unspecified (F18.9-)

F18.10   **Inhalant abuse, uncomplicated**   HCC ESR
Inhalant use disorder, mild

F18.11   **Inhalant abuse, in remission**   HCC ESR
Inhalant use disorder, mild, in early remission
Inhalant use disorder, mild, in sustained remission

✓6ᵗʰ   **F18.12**   **Inhalant abuse with intoxication**

F18.120   **Inhalant abuse with intoxication, uncomplicated**   HCC ESR COM

F18.121   **Inhalant abuse with intoxication delirium**   HCC ESR COM

F18.129   **Inhalant abuse with intoxication, unspecified**   HCC ESR COM

F18.14   **Inhalant abuse with inhalant-induced mood disorder**   HCC ESR COM
Inhalant use disorder, mild, with inhalant induced depressive disorder

✓6ᵗʰ   **F18.15**   **Inhalant abuse with inhalant-induced psychotic disorder**

F18.150   **Inhalant abuse with inhalant-induced psychotic disorder with delusions**   HCC ESR COM

F18.151   **Inhalant abuse with inhalant-induced psychotic disorder with hallucinations**   HCC ESR COM

F18.159   **Inhalant abuse with inhalant-induced psychotic disorder, unspecified**   HCC ESR COM

F18.17   **Inhalant abuse with inhalant-induced dementia**   HCC ESR COM
Inhalant use disorder, mild, with inhalant induced major neurocognitive disorder

✓6ᵗʰ   **F18.18**   **Inhalant abuse with other inhalant-induced disorders**

F18.180   **Inhalant abuse with inhalant-induced anxiety disorder**   HCC ESR COM

F18.188   **Inhalant abuse with other inhalant-induced disorder**   HCC ESR COM
Inhalant use disorder, mild, with inhalant induced mild neurocognitive disorder

F18.19   **Inhalant abuse with unspecified inhalant-induced disorder**   HCC ESR COM

✓5ᵗʰ   **F18.2**   **Inhalant dependence**
EXCLUDES 1   inhalant abuse (F18.1-)
inhalant use, unspecified (F18.9-)

F18.20   **Inhalant dependence, uncomplicated**   HCC ESR COM
Inhalant use disorder, moderate
Inhalant use disorder, severe

F18.21   **Inhalant dependence, in remission**   HCC ESR COM
Inhalant use disorder, moderate, in early remission
Inhalant use disorder, moderate, in sustained remission
Inhalant use disorder, severe, in early remission
Inhalant use disorder, severe, in sustained remission

✓6ᵗʰ   **F18.22**   **Inhalant dependence with intoxication**

F18.220   **Inhalant dependence with intoxication, uncomplicated**   HCC ESR COM

F18.221   **Inhalant dependence with intoxication delirium**   HCC ESR COM

F18.229   **Inhalant dependence with intoxication, unspecified**   HCC ESR COM

F18.24   **Inhalant dependence with inhalant-induced mood disorder**   HCC ESR COM
Inhalant use disorder, moderate, with inhalant induced depressive disorder
Inhalant use disorder, severe, with inhalant induced depressive disorder

✓6ᵗʰ   **F18.25**   **Inhalant dependence with inhalant-induced psychotic disorder**

F18.250   **Inhalant dependence with inhalant-induced psychotic disorder with delusions**   HCC ESR COM

F18.251   **Inhalant dependence with inhalant-induced psychotic disorder with hallucinations**   HCC ESR COM

F18.259   **Inhalant dependence with inhalant-induced psychotic disorder, unspecified**   HCC ESR COM

F18.27   **Inhalant dependence with inhalant-induced dementia**   HCC ESR COM
Inhalant use disorder, moderate, with inhalant induced major neurocognitive disorder
Inhalant use disorder, severe, with inhalant induced major neurocognitive disorder

✓6ᵗʰ   **F18.28**   **Inhalant dependence with other inhalant-induced disorders**

F18.280   **Inhalant dependence with inhalant-induced anxiety disorder**   HCC ESR COM

F18.288   **Inhalant dependence with other inhalant-induced disorder**   HCC ESR COM
Inhalant use disorder, moderate, with inhalant-induced mild neurocognitive disorder
Inhalant use disorder, severe, with inhalant-induced mild neurocognitive disorder

F18.29   **Inhalant dependence with unspecified inhalant-induced disorder**   HCC ESR COM

✓5ᵗʰ F18.9 Inhalant use, unspecified

> EXCLUDES 1   *inhalant abuse (F18.1-)*
> *inhalant dependence (F18.2-)*

> **TIP:** Assign a substance use code only when the provider documents a relationship between the use and an associated physical, mental, or behavioral disorder. As with all diagnoses, substance use codes must meet the definition of a reportable diagnosis.

> **F18.90 Inhalant use, unspecified, uncomplicated**
> AHA: 2018,2Q,10-11

● **F18.91 Inhalant use, unspecified, in remission**

✓6ᵗʰ F18.92 Inhalant use, unspecified with intoxication
> **F18.920 Inhalant use, unspecified with intoxication, uncomplicated** HCC ESR COM
> **F18.921 Inhalant use, unspecified with intoxication with delirium** HCC ESR COM
> **F18.929 Inhalant use, unspecified with intoxication, unspecified** HCC ESR COM

F18.94 Inhalant use, unspecified with inhalant-induced mood disorder HCC ESR COM
> Inhalant induced depressive disorder

✓6ᵗʰ F18.95 Inhalant use, unspecified with inhalant-induced psychotic disorder
> **F18.950 Inhalant use, unspecified with inhalant-induced psychotic disorder with delusions** HCC ESR COM
> **F18.951 Inhalant use, unspecified with inhalant-induced psychotic disorder with hallucinations** HCC ESR COM
> **F18.959 Inhalant use, unspecified with inhalant-induced psychotic disorder, unspecified** HCC ESR COM

F18.97 Inhalant use, unspecified with inhalant-induced persisting dementia HCC ESR COM
> Inhalant-induced major neurocognitive disorder

✓6ᵗʰ F18.98 Inhalant use, unspecified with other inhalant-induced disorders
> **F18.980 Inhalant use, unspecified with inhalant-induced anxiety disorder** HCC ESR COM
> **F18.988 Inhalant use, unspecified with other inhalant-induced disorder** HCC ESR COM
> > Inhalant-induced mild neurocognitive disorder

F18.99 Inhalant use, unspecified with unspecified inhalant-induced disorder HCC ESR COM

✓4ᵗʰ F19 Other psychoactive substance related disorders
> INCLUDES   polysubstance drug use (indiscriminate drug use)

✓5ᵗʰ F19.1 Other psychoactive substance abuse
> EXCLUDES 1   *other psychoactive substance dependence (F19.2-)*
> *other psychoactive substance use, unspecified (F19.9-)*

> **F19.10 Other psychoactive substance abuse, uncomplicated** HCC ESR
> > Other (or unknown) substance use disorder, mild

> **F19.11 Other psychoactive substance abuse, in remission** HCC ESR
> > Other (or unknown) substance use disorder, mild, in early remission
> > Other (or unknown) substance use disorder, mild, in sustained remission

✓6ᵗʰ F19.12 Other psychoactive substance abuse with intoxication
> **F19.120 Other psychoactive substance abuse with intoxication, uncomplicated** HCC ESR COM
> **F19.121 Other psychoactive substance abuse with intoxication delirium** HCC ESR COM
> **F19.122 Other psychoactive substance abuse with intoxication with perceptual disturbances** HCC ESR COM
> **F19.129 Other psychoactive substance abuse with intoxication, unspecified** HCC ESR COM

✓6ᵗʰ F19.13 Other psychoactive substance abuse with withdrawal
> AHA: 2020,4Q,16-17
> **F19.130 Other psychoactive substance abuse with withdrawal, uncomplicated** HCC ESR COM
> **F19.131 Other psychoactive substance abuse with withdrawal delirium** HCC ESR COM
> **F19.132 Other psychoactive substance abuse with withdrawal with perceptual disturbance** HCC ESR COM
> **F19.139 Other psychoactive substance abuse with withdrawal, unspecified** HCC ESR COM

F19.14 Other psychoactive substance abuse with psychoactive substance-induced mood disorder HCC ESR COM
> Other (or unknown) substance use disorder, mild, with other (or unknown) substance-induced bipolar or related disorder
> Other (or unknown) substance use disorder, mild, with other (or unknown) substance-induced depressive disorder

✓6ᵗʰ F19.15 Other psychoactive substance abuse with psychoactive substance-induced psychotic disorder
> **F19.150 Other psychoactive substance abuse with psychoactive substance-induced psychotic disorder with delusions** HCC ESR COM
> **F19.151 Other psychoactive substance abuse with psychoactive substance-induced psychotic disorder with hallucinations** HCC ESR COM
> **F19.159 Other psychoactive substance abuse with psychoactive substance-induced psychotic disorder, unspecified** HCC ESR COM

F19.16 Other psychoactive substance abuse with psychoactive substance-induced persisting amnestic disorder HCC ESR COM

F19.17 Other psychoactive substance abuse with psychoactive substance-induced persisting dementia HCC ESR COM
> Other (or unknown) substance use disorder, mild, with other (or unknown) substance-induced major neurocognitive disorder

✓6ᵗʰ F19.18 Other psychoactive substance abuse with other psychoactive substance-induced disorders
> **F19.180 Other psychoactive substance abuse with psychoactive substance-induced anxiety disorder** HCC ESR COM
> **F19.181 Other psychoactive substance abuse with psychoactive substance-induced sexual dysfunction** HCC ESR COM
> **F19.182 Other psychoactive substance abuse with psychoactive substance-induced sleep disorder** HCC ESR COM
> **F19.188 Other psychoactive substance abuse with other psychoactive substance-induced disorder** HCC ESR COM
> > Other (or unknown) substance use disorder, mild, with other (or unknown) substance induced mild neurocognitive disorder
> > Other (or unknown) substance use disorder, mild, with other (or unknown) substance induced obsessive-compulsive or related disorder

F19.19 Other psychoactive substance abuse with unspecified psychoactive substance-induced disorder HCC ESR COM

✓5ᵗʰ F19.2 Other psychoactive substance dependence
> EXCLUDES 1   *other psychoactive substance abuse (F19.1-)*
> *other psychoactive substance use, unspecified (F19.9-)*

> **F19.20 Other psychoactive substance dependence, uncomplicated** HCC ESR COM
> > Other (or unknown) substance use disorder, moderate
> > Other (or unknown) substance use disorder, severe

Chapter 5. Mental, Behavioral and Neurodevelopmental Disorders

F19.21 Other psychoactive substance dependence, in remission HCC ESR COM
Other (or unknown) substance use disorder, moderate, in early remission
Other (or unknown) substance use disorder, moderate, in sustained remission
Other (or unknown) substance use disorder, severe, in early remission
Other (or unknown) substance use disorder, severe, in sustained remission

√6ᵗʰ **F19.22 Other psychoactive substance dependence with intoxication**
EXCLUDES 1 other psychoactive substance dependence with withdrawal (F19.23-)
F19.220 Other psychoactive substance dependence with intoxication, uncomplicated HCC ESR COM
F19.221 Other psychoactive substance dependence with intoxication delirium HCC ESR COM
F19.222 Other psychoactive substance dependence with intoxication with perceptual disturbance HCC ESR COM
F19.229 Other psychoactive substance dependence with intoxication, unspecified HCC ESR COM

√6ᵗʰ **F19.23 Other psychoactive substance dependence with withdrawal**
EXCLUDES 1 other psychoactive substance dependence with intoxication (F19.22-)
F19.230 Other psychoactive substance dependence with withdrawal, uncomplicated HCC ESR COM
F19.231 Other psychoactive substance dependence with withdrawal delirium HCC ESR COM
F19.232 Other psychoactive substance dependence with withdrawal with perceptual disturbance HCC ESR COM
F19.239 Other psychoactive substance dependence with withdrawal, unspecified HCC ESR COM

F19.24 Other psychoactive substance dependence with psychoactive substance-induced mood disorder HCC ESR COM
Other (or unknown) substance use disorder, moderate, with other (or unknown) substance induced bipolar or related disorder
Other (or unknown) substance use disorder, moderate, with other (or unknown) substance induced depressive disorder
Other (or unknown) substance use disorder, severe, with other (or unknown) substance induced bipolar or related disorder
Other (or unknown) substance use disorder, severe, with other (or unknown) substance induced depressive disorder

√6ᵗʰ **F19.25 Other psychoactive substance dependence with psychoactive substance-induced psychotic disorder**
F19.250 Other psychoactive substance dependence with psychoactive substance-induced psychotic disorder with delusions HCC ESR COM
F19.251 Other psychoactive substance dependence with psychoactive substance-induced psychotic disorder with hallucinations HCC ESR COM
F19.259 Other psychoactive substance dependence with psychoactive substance-induced psychotic disorder, unspecified HCC ESR COM

F19.26 Other psychoactive substance dependence with psychoactive substance-induced persisting amnestic disorder HCC ESR COM

F19.27 Other psychoactive substance dependence with psychoactive substance-induced persisting dementia HCC ESR COM
Other (or unknown) substance use disorder, moderate, with other (or unknown) substance induced major neurocognitive disorder
Other (or unknown) substance use disorder, severe, with other (or unknown) substance induced major neurocognitive disorder

√6ᵗʰ **F19.28 Other psychoactive substance dependence with other psychoactive substance-induced disorders**
F19.280 Other psychoactive substance dependence with psychoactive substance-induced anxiety disorder HCC ESR COM
F19.281 Other psychoactive substance dependence with psychoactive substance-induced sexual dysfunction HCC ESR COM
F19.282 Other psychoactive substance dependence with psychoactive substance-induced sleep disorder HCC ESR COM
F19.288 Other psychoactive substance dependence with other psychoactive substance-induced disorder HCC ESR COM
Other (or unknown) substance use disorder, moderate, with other (or unknown) substance induced mild neurocognitive disorder
Other (or unknown) substance use disorder, severe, with other (or unknown) substance induced mild neurocognitive disorder
Other (or unknown) substance use disorder, moderate, with other (or unknown) substance induced obsessive compulsive or related disorder
Other (or unknown) substance use disorder, severe, with other (or unknown) substance induced obsessive-compulsive or related disorder

F19.29 Other psychoactive substance dependence with unspecified psychoactive substance-induced disorder HCC ESR COM

√5ᵗʰ **F19.9 Other psychoactive substance use, unspecified**
EXCLUDES 1 other psychoactive substance abuse (F19.1-)
other psychoactive substance dependence (F19.2-)
TIP: Assign a substance use code only when the provider documents a relationship between the use and an associated physical, mental, or behavioral disorder. As with all diagnoses, substance use codes must meet the definition of a reportable diagnosis.
F19.90 Other psychoactive substance use, unspecified, uncomplicated
AHA: 2018,2Q,10-11
F19.91 Other psychoactive substance use, unspecified, in remission
√6ᵗʰ **F19.92 Other psychoactive substance use, unspecified with intoxication**
EXCLUDES 1 other psychoactive substance use, unspecified with withdrawal (F19.93)
F19.920 Other psychoactive substance use, unspecified with intoxication, uncomplicated HCC ESR COM
F19.921 Other psychoactive substance use, unspecified with intoxication with delirium HCC ESR COM
Other (or unknown) substance-induced delirium
F19.922 Other psychoactive substance use, unspecified with intoxication with perceptual disturbance HCC ESR COM
F19.929 Other psychoactive substance use, unspecified with intoxication, unspecified HCC ESR COM

√6ᵗʰ **F19.93** **Other psychoactive substance use, unspecified with withdrawal**

> *EXCLUDES 1*   *other psychoactive substance use, unspecified with intoxication (F19.92-)*

    F19.930 **Other psychoactive substance use, unspecified with withdrawal, uncomplicated** `HCC` `ESR` `COM`

    F19.931 **Other psychoactive substance use, unspecified with withdrawal delirium** `HCC` `ESR` `COM`

    F19.932 **Other psychoactive substance use, unspecified with withdrawal with perceptual disturbance** `HCC` `ESR` `COM`

    F19.939 **Other psychoactive substance use, unspecified with withdrawal, unspecified** `HCC` `ESR` `COM`

F19.94 **Other psychoactive substance use, unspecified with psychoactive substance-induced mood disorder**
> Other (or unknown) substance-induced bipolar or related disorder, without use disorder
> Other (or unknown) substance-induced depressive disorder, without use disorder

√6ᵗʰ **F19.95** **Other psychoactive substance use, unspecified with psychoactive substance-induced psychotic disorder**

    F19.950 **Other psychoactive substance use, unspecified with psychoactive substance-induced psychotic disorder with delusions** `HCC` `ESR` `COM`

    F19.951 **Other psychoactive substance use, unspecified with psychoactive substance-induced psychotic disorder with hallucinations** `HCC` `ESR` `COM`

    F19.959 **Other psychoactive substance use, unspecified with psychoactive substance-induced psychotic disorder, unspecified** `HCC` `ESR` `COM`
> Other or unknown substance-induced psychotic disorder, without use disorder

F19.96 **Other psychoactive substance use, unspecified with psychoactive substance-induced persisting amnestic disorder** `HCC` `ESR` `COM`

F19.97 **Other psychoactive substance use, unspecified with psychoactive substance-induced persisting dementia** `HCC` `ESR` `COM`
> Other (or unknown) substance-induced major neurocognitive disorder, without use disorder

√6ᵗʰ **F19.98** **Other psychoactive substance use, unspecified with other psychoactive substance-induced disorders**

    F19.980 **Other psychoactive substance use, unspecified with psychoactive substance-induced anxiety disorder** `HCC` `ESR` `COM`
> Other (or unknown) substance-induced anxiety disorder, without use disorder

    F19.981 **Other psychoactive substance use, unspecified with psychoactive substance-induced sexual dysfunction** `HCC` `ESR` `COM`
> Other (or unknown) substance-induced sexual dysfunction, without use disorder

    F19.982 **Other psychoactive substance use, unspecified with psychoactive substance-induced sleep disorder** `HCC` `ESR` `COM`
> Other (or unknown) substance-induced sleep disorder, without use disorder

    F19.988 **Other psychoactive substance use, unspecified with other psychoactive substance-induced disorder** `HCC` `ESR` `COM`
> Other (or unknown) substance-induced mild neurocognitive disorder, without use disorder
> Other (or unknown) substance-induced obsessive-compulsive or related disorder, without use disorder

F19.99 **Other psychoactive substance use, unspecified with unspecified psychoactive substance-induced disorder** `HCC` `ESR` `COM`

Schizophrenia, schizotypal, delusional, and other non-mood psychotic disorders (F20-F29)

√4ᵗʰ **F20** **Schizophrenia**

> *EXCLUDES 1*   *brief psychotic disorder (F23)*
> *cyclic schizophrenia (F25.0)*
> *mood [affective] disorders with psychotic symptoms (F30.2, F31.2, F31.5, F31.64, F32.3, F33.3)*
> *schizoaffective disorder (F25.-)*
> *schizophrenic reaction NOS (F23)*

> *EXCLUDES 2*   *schizophrenic reaction in:*
>   *alcoholism (F10.15-, F10.25-, F10.95-)*
>   *brain disease (F06.2)*
>   *epilepsy (F06.2)*
>   *psychoactive drug use (F11-F19 with .15, .25, .95)*
>   *schizotypal disorder (F21)*

DEF: Group of disorders with disturbances in thought (delusions, hallucinations), mood (blunted, flattened, inappropriate affect), and sense of self. Schizophrenia also includes bizarre, purposeless behavior, repetitive activity, or inactivity.

F20.0 **Paranoid schizophrenia** `HCC` `Rx` `ESR` `COM`
> Paraphrenic schizophrenia
> *EXCLUDES 1*   *involutional paranoid state (F22)*
>   *paranoia (F22)*

DEF: Preoccupied with delusional suspicions and auditory hallucinations related to a single theme. This type of schizophrenia is usually hostile, grandiose, threatening, persecutory, and occasionally hypochondriacal.

F20.1 **Disorganized schizophrenia** `HCC` `Rx` `ESR` `COM`
> Hebephrenic schizophrenia
> Hebephrenia

F20.2 **Catatonic schizophrenia** `HCC` `Rx` `ESR` `COM`
> Schizophrenic catalepsy
> Schizophrenic catatonia
> Schizophrenic flexibilitas cerea
> *EXCLUDES 1*   *catatonic stupor (R40.1)*

DEF: Extreme changes in motor activity. One extreme is a decreased response or reaction to the environment and the other is spontaneous activity.

F20.3 **Undifferentiated schizophrenia** `HCC` `Rx` `ESR` `COM`
> Atypical schizophrenia
> *EXCLUDES 1*   *acute schizophrenia-like psychotic disorder (F23)*
> *EXCLUDES 2*   *post-schizophrenic depression (F32.89)*

F20.5 **Residual schizophrenia** `HCC` `Rx` `ESR` `COM`
> Restzustand (schizophrenic)
> Schizophrenic residual state

√5ᵗʰ **F20.8** **Other schizophrenia**

    F20.81 **Schizophreniform disorder** `HCC` `Rx` `ESR` `COM`
> Schizophreniform psychosis NOS

    F20.89 **Other schizophrenia** `HCC` `Rx` `ESR` `COM`
> Cenesthopathic schizophrenia
> Simple schizophrenia

F20.9 **Schizophrenia, unspecified** `HCC` `Rx` `ESR` `COM`
> **AHA:** 2019,2Q,32

F21 **Schizotypal disorder** `HCC` `Rx` `ESR` `COM`
> Borderline schizophrenia
> Latent schizophrenia
> Latent schizophrenic reaction
> Prepsychotic schizophrenia
> Prodromal schizophrenia
> Pseudoneurotic schizophrenia
> Pseudopsychopathic schizophrenia
> Schizotypal personality disorder
> *EXCLUDES 2*   *Asperger's syndrome (F84.5)*
>   *schizoid personality disorder (F60.1)*

DEF: Disorder characterized by various oddities of thinking, perception, communication, and behavior that may be manifested as magical thinking, ideas of reference, paranoid ideation, recurrent illusions and derealization (depersonalization), or social isolation.

F22 Delusional disorders `HCC` `Rx` `ESR` `COM`
Delusional dysmorphophobia
Involutional paranoid state
Paranoia
Paranoia querulans
Paranoid psychosis
Paranoid state
Paraphrenia (late)
Sensitiver Beziehungswahn
- **EXCLUDES 1** *mood [affective] disorders with psychotic symptoms (F30.2, F31.2, F31.5, F31.64, F32.3, F33.3)*
  paranoid schizophrenia (F20.0)
- **EXCLUDES 2** *paranoid personality disorder (F60.0)*
  paranoid psychosis, psychogenic (F23)
  paranoid reaction (F23)

F23 Brief psychotic disorder `HCC` `Rx` `ESR` `COM`
Paranoid reaction
Psychogenic paranoid psychosis
- **EXCLUDES 2** *mood [affective] disorders with psychotic symptoms (F30.2, F31.2, F31.5, F31.64, F32.3, F33.3)*
- **AHA:** 2019,2Q,32

F24 Shared psychotic disorder `HCC` `Rx` `ESR` `COM`
Folie à deux
Induced paranoid disorder
Induced psychotic disorder

✓4ᵗʰ F25 Schizoaffective disorders
- **EXCLUDES 1** *mood [affective] disorders with psychotic symptoms (F30.2, F31.2, F31.5, F31.64, F32.3, F33.3)*
  schizophrenia (F20.-)

F25.0 Schizoaffective disorder, bipolar type `HCC` `Rx` `ESR` `COM`
Cyclic schizophrenia
Schizoaffective disorder, manic type
Schizoaffective disorder, mixed type
Schizoaffective psychosis, bipolar type

F25.1 Schizoaffective disorder, depressive type `HCC` `Rx` `ESR` `COM`
Schizoaffective psychosis, depressive type

F25.8 Other schizoaffective disorders `HCC` `Rx` `ESR` `COM`

F25.9 Schizoaffective disorder, unspecified `HCC` `Rx` `ESR` `COM`
Schizoaffective psychosis NOS

F28 Other psychotic disorder not due to a substance or known physiological condition `HCC` `Rx` `ESR` `COM`
Chronic hallucinatory psychosis
Other specified schizophrenia spectrum and other psychotic disorder

F29 Unspecified psychosis not due to a substance or known physiological condition `HCC` `Rx` `ESR` `COM`
Psychosis NOS
Unspecified schizophrenia spectrum and other psychotic disorder
- **EXCLUDES 1** *mental disorder NOS (F99)*
  unspecified mental disorder due to known physiological condition (F09)

Mood [affective] disorders (F30-F39)

✓4ᵗʰ F30 Manic episode
- **INCLUDES** bipolar disorder, single manic episode
  mixed affective episode
- **EXCLUDES 1** *bipolar disorder (F31.-)*
  major depressive disorder, recurrent (F33.-)
  major depressive disorder, single episode (F32.-)
- **DEF:** Mania: Characterized by abnormal states of elation or excitement out of keeping with the individual's circumstances and varying from enhanced liveliness (hypomania) to violent, almost uncontrollable, excitement. Aggression and anger, flight of ideas, distractibility, impaired judgment, and grandiose ideas are common.

✓5ᵗʰ F30.1 Manic episode without psychotic symptoms
F30.10 Manic episode without psychotic symptoms, unspecified `HCC` `Rx` `ESR` `COM`
F30.11 Manic episode without psychotic symptoms, mild `HCC` `Rx` `ESR` `COM`
F30.12 Manic episode without psychotic symptoms, moderate `HCC` `Rx` `ESR` `COM`
F30.13 Manic episode, severe, without psychotic symptoms `HCC` `Rx` `ESR` `COM`

F30.2 Manic episode, severe with psychotic symptoms `HCC` `Rx` `ESR` `COM`
Manic stupor
Mania with mood-congruent psychotic symptoms
Mania with mood-incongruent psychotic symptoms

F30.3 Manic episode in partial remission `HCC` `Rx` `ESR` `COM`
F30.4 Manic episode in full remission `HCC` `Rx` `ESR` `COM`
F30.8 Other manic episodes `HCC` `Rx` `ESR` `COM`
Hypomania
F30.9 Manic episode, unspecified `HCC` `Rx` `ESR` `COM`
Mania NOS

✓4ᵗʰ F31 Bipolar disorder
- **INCLUDES** bipolar I disorder
  bipolar type I disorder
  manic-depressive illness
  manic-depressive psychosis
  manic-depressive reaction
  ►seasonal bipolar disorder◄
- **EXCLUDES 1** *bipolar disorder, single manic episode (F30.-)*
  major depressive disorder, recurrent (F33.-)
  major depressive disorder, single episode (F32.-)
- **EXCLUDES 2** *cyclothymia (F34.0)*
- **AHA:** 2020,1Q,23

F31.0 Bipolar disorder, current episode hypomanic `HCC` `Rx` `ESR` `COM`

✓5ᵗʰ F31.1 Bipolar disorder, current episode manic without psychotic features
F31.10 Bipolar disorder, current episode manic without psychotic features, unspecified `HCC` `Rx` `ESR` `COM` `Q`
F31.11 Bipolar disorder, current episode manic without psychotic features, mild `HCC` `Rx` `ESR` `COM` `Q`
F31.12 Bipolar disorder, current episode manic without psychotic features, moderate `HCC` `Rx` `ESR` `COM` `Q`
F31.13 Bipolar disorder, current episode manic without psychotic features, severe `HCC` `Rx` `ESR` `COM` `Q`

F31.2 Bipolar disorder, current episode manic severe with psychotic features `HCC` `Rx` `ESR` `COM` `Q`
Bipolar disorder, current episode manic with mood-congruent psychotic symptoms
Bipolar disorder, current episode manic with mood-incongruent psychotic symptoms
Bipolar I disorder, current or most recent episode manic with psychotic features

✓5ᵗʰ F31.3 Bipolar disorder, current episode depressed, mild or moderate severity
F31.30 Bipolar disorder, current episode depressed, mild or moderate severity, unspecified `HCC` `Rx` `ESR` `COM` `Q`
F31.31 Bipolar disorder, current episode depressed, mild `HCC` `Rx` `ESR` `COM` `Q`
F31.32 Bipolar disorder, current episode depressed, moderate `HCC` `Rx` `ESR` `COM` `Q`

F31.4 Bipolar disorder, current episode depressed, severe, without psychotic features `HCC` `Rx` `ESR` `COM` `Q`

F31.5 Bipolar disorder, current episode depressed, severe, with psychotic features `HCC` `Rx` `ESR` `COM` `Q`
Bipolar disorder, current episode depressed with mood-congruent psychotic symptoms
Bipolar disorder, current episode depressed with mood-incongruent psychotic symptoms
Bipolar I disorder, current or most recent episode depressed, with psychotic features

✓5ᵗʰ F31.6 Bipolar disorder, current episode mixed
F31.60 Bipolar disorder, current episode mixed, unspecified `HCC` `Rx` `ESR` `COM` `Q`
F31.61 Bipolar disorder, current episode mixed, mild `HCC` `Rx` `ESR` `COM` `Q`
F31.62 Bipolar disorder, current episode mixed, moderate `HCC` `Rx` `ESR` `COM` `Q`
F31.63 Bipolar disorder, current episode mixed, severe, without psychotic features `HCC` `Rx` `ESR` `COM` `Q`

F31.64   **Bipolar disorder, current episode mixed,** severe, with psychotic features   `HCC` `Rx` `ESR` `COM` `Q`
>> Bipolar disorder, current episode mixed with mood-congruent psychotic symptoms
>> Bipolar disorder, current episode mixed with mood-incongruent psychotic symptoms

✓5ᵗʰ **F31.7**   **Bipolar disorder, currently** in remission

> **F31.70**   **Bipolar disorder, currently in remission, most recent episode unspecified**   `HCC` `Rx` `ESR` `COM` `Q`

> **F31.71**   **Bipolar disorder,** in partial remission, **most recent episode** hypomanic   `HCC` `Rx` `ESR` `COM` `Q`

> **F31.72**   **Bipolar disorder,** in full remission, **most recent episode** hypomanic   `HCC` `Rx` `ESR` `COM` `Q`

> **F31.73**   **Bipolar disorder,** in partial remission, **most recent episode** manic   `HCC` `Rx` `ESR` `COM` `Q`

> **F31.74**   **Bipolar disorder,** in full remission, **most recent episode** manic   `HCC` `Rx` `ESR` `COM` `Q`

> **F31.75**   **Bipolar disorder,** in partial remission, **most recent episode** depressed   `HCC` `Rx` `ESR` `COM` `Q`

> **F31.76**   **Bipolar disorder,** in full remission, **most recent episode** depressed   `HCC` `Rx` `ESR` `COM` `Q`

> **F31.77**   **Bipolar disorder,** in partial remission, **most recent episode** mixed   `HCC` `Rx` `ESR` `COM` `Q`

> **F31.78**   **Bipolar disorder,** in full remission, **most recent episode** mixed   `HCC` `Rx` `ESR` `COM` `Q`

✓5ᵗʰ **F31.8**   **Other bipolar disorders**

> **F31.81**   **Bipolar II disorder**   `HCC` `Rx` `ESR` `COM` `Q`
>> Bipolar disorder, type 2

> **F31.89**   **Other bipolar disorder**   `HCC` `Rx` `ESR` `COM` `Q`
>> Recurrent manic episodes NOS

F31.9   **Bipolar disorder, unspecified**   `HCC` `Rx` `ESR` `COM` `Q`
> Manic depression
> **AHA:** 2020,1Q,23

✓4ᵗʰ **F32**   **Depressive episode**

> `INCLUDES`   single episode of agitated depression
>> single episode of depressive reaction
>> single episode of major depression
>> single episode of psychogenic depression
>> single episode of reactive depression
>> single episode of vital depression

> `EXCLUDES 1`   bipolar disorder (F31.-)
>> manic episode (F30.-)
>> recurrent depressive disorder (F33.-)

> `EXCLUDES 2`   adjustment disorder (F43.2)

> **AHA:** 2020,1Q,23
> **DEF:** Mood disorder that produces depression that may exhibit as sadness, low self-esteem, or guilt feelings. Other manifestations may be withdrawal from friends and family and interrupted sleep.

F32.0   **Major depressive disorder, single episode, mild**   `HCC` `Rx` `ESR` `Q`

F32.1   **Major depressive disorder, single episode, moderate**   `HCC` `Rx` `ESR` `Q`

F32.2   **Major depressive disorder, single episode, severe without psychotic features**   `HCC` `Rx` `ESR` `COM` `Q`

F32.3   **Major depressive disorder, single episode, severe with psychotic features**   `HCC` `Rx` `ESR` `COM` `Q`
> Single episode of major depression with mood-congruent psychotic symptoms
> Single episode of major depression with mood-incongruent psychotic symptoms
> Single episode of major depression with psychotic symptoms
> Single episode of psychogenic depressive psychosis
> Single episode of psychotic depression
> Single episode of reactive depressive psychosis

F32.4   **Major depressive disorder, single episode, in partial remission**   `HCC` `Rx` `ESR` `Q`

F32.5   **Major depressive disorder, single episode, in full remission**   `HCC` `Rx` `ESR` `Q`

✓5ᵗʰ **F32.8**   **Other depressive episodes**
> **AHA:** 2016,4Q,14

> **F32.81**   **Premenstrual dysphoric disorder**   `Rx` ♀
>> `EXCLUDES 1`   premenstrual tension syndrome (N94.3)
>> **DEF:** Severe manifestation of premenstrual syndrome (PMS) that can be disabling and destructive to day-to-day activities. It can exacerbate pre-existing emotional disorders, like depression and anxiety, and cause feelings of loss of control, fatigue, and irritability.

> **F32.89**   **Other specified depressive episodes**   `Rx` `Q`
>> Atypical depression
>> Post-schizophrenic depression
>> Single episode of 'masked' depression NOS

F32.9   **Major depressive disorder, single episode, unspecified**   `Rx` `Q`
> Major depression NOS
> **AHA:** 2021,4Q,10; 2021,1Q,10; 2013,4Q,107

F32.A   **Depression, unspecified**   `Rx` `Q`
> Depression NOS
> Depressive disorder NOS
> **AHA:** 2021,4Q,9-10

✓4ᵗʰ **F33**   **Major depressive disorder,** recurrent

> `INCLUDES`   recurrent episodes of depressive reaction
>> recurrent episodes of endogenous depression
>> recurrent episodes of major depression
>> recurrent episodes of psychogenic depression
>> recurrent episodes of reactive depression
>> ▶recurrent episodes of seasonal affective disorder◀
>> recurrent episodes of seasonal depressive disorder
>> recurrent episodes of vital depression

> `EXCLUDES 1`   bipolar disorder (F31.-)
>> manic episode (F30.-)

> **AHA:** 2020,1Q,23
> **DEF:** Mood disorder that produces depression that may exhibit as sadness, low self-esteem, or guilt feelings. Other manifestations may be withdrawal from friends and family and interrupted sleep.

F33.0   **Major depressive disorder, recurrent,** mild   `HCC` `Rx` `ESR` `Q`

F33.1   **Major depressive disorder, recurrent, moderate**   `HCC` `Rx` `ESR` `Q`

F33.2   **Major depressive disorder, recurrent, severe without psychotic features**   `HCC` `Rx` `ESR` `COM` `Q`

F33.3   **Major depressive disorder, recurrent, severe with psychotic symptoms**   `HCC` `Rx` `ESR` `COM` `Q`
> Endogenous depression with psychotic symptoms
> Major depressive disorder, recurrent, with psychotic features
> Recurrent severe episodes of major depression with mood-congruent psychotic symptoms
> Recurrent severe episodes of major depression with mood-incongruent psychotic symptoms
> Recurrent severe episodes of major depression with psychotic symptoms
> Recurrent severe episodes of psychogenic depressive psychosis
> Recurrent severe episodes of psychotic depression
> Recurrent severe episodes of reactive depressive psychosis

✓5ᵗʰ **F33.4**   **Major depressive disorder, recurrent,** in remission

> **F33.40**   **Major depressive disorder, recurrent, in remission, unspecified**   `HCC` `Rx` `ESR` `Q`

> **F33.41**   **Major depressive disorder, recurrent, in** partial **remission**   `HCC` `Rx` `ESR` `Q`

> **F33.42**   **Major depressive disorder, recurrent, in** full **remission**   `HCC` `Rx` `ESR` `Q`

F33.8   **Other recurrent depressive disorders**   `HCC` `Rx` `ESR` `Q`
> Recurrent brief depressive episodes

F33.9   **Major depressive disorder, recurrent, unspecified**   `HCC` `Rx` `ESR` `Q`
> Monopolar depression NOS

✓4ᵗʰ **F34**   **Persistent mood [affective] disorders**

> **F34.0**   **Cyclothymic disorder**   `Rx`
>> Affective personality disorder
>> Cycloid personality
>> Cyclothymia
>> Cyclothymic personality
>> **DEF:** Mood disorder characterized by fast and repeated alterations between hypomanic and depressed moods.

Chapter 5. Mental, Behavioral and Neurodevelopmental Disorders *(left margin)*

F34.1–F43.12 *(left margin)*

F34.1 Dysthymic disorder   Rx Q
- Depressive neurosis
- Depressive personality disorder
- Dysthymia
- Neurotic depression
- Persistent anxiety depression
- Persistent depressive disorder
  - EXCLUDES 2   *anxiety depression (mild or not persistent) (F41.8)*
  - **DEF:** Depression without psychosis. It is a less severe but persistent depression and is considered a mild to moderate chronic form of depression.

√5ᵗʰ **F34.8 Other persistent mood [affective] disorders**
- **AHA:** 2016,4Q,14
  - **F34.81 Disruptive mood dysregulation disorder**   HCC Rx ESR COM Q
  - **F34.89 Other specified persistent mood disorders**   HCC Rx ESR Q

F34.9 Persistent mood [affective] disorder, unspecified   HCC Rx ESR

F39 Unspecified mood [affective] disorder   HCC Rx ESR
- Affective psychosis NOS

Anxiety, dissociative, stress-related, somatoform and other nonpsychotic mental disorders (F40-F48)

√4ᵗʰ **F40 Phobic anxiety disorders**
- **DEF:** Phobia: Broad-range anxiety with abnormally intense dread of certain objects or specific situations that would not normally have that effect.

√5ᵗʰ **F40.0 Agoraphobia**
- **DEF:** Profound anxiety or fear of leaving familiar settings like home, or being in unfamiliar locations or with strangers or crowds. Agoraphobia may or may not be preceded by recurrent panic attacks.
  - **F40.00 Agoraphobia, unspecified**   Rx
  - **F40.01 Agoraphobia with panic disorder**   Rx
    - Panic disorder with agoraphobia
    - EXCLUDES 1   *panic disorder without agoraphobia (F41.0)*
  - **F40.02 Agoraphobia without panic disorder**   Rx

√5ᵗʰ **F40.1 Social phobias**
- Anthropophobia
- Social anxiety disorder
- Social anxiety disorder of childhood
- Social neurosis
  - **F40.10 Social phobia, unspecified**   Rx
  - **F40.11 Social phobia, generalized**   Rx

√5ᵗʰ **F40.2 Specific (isolated) phobias**
- EXCLUDES 2   *dysmorphophobia (nondelusional) (F45.22)*
  - *nosophobia (F45.22)*
  - √6ᵗʰ **F40.21 Animal type phobia**
    - **F40.210 Arachnophobia**   Rx
      - Fear of spiders
    - **F40.218 Other animal type phobia**   Rx
  - √6ᵗʰ **F40.22 Natural environment type phobia**
    - **F40.220 Fear of thunderstorms**   Rx
    - **F40.228 Other natural environment type phobia**   Rx
  - √6ᵗʰ **F40.23 Blood, injection, injury type phobia**
    - **F40.230 Fear of blood**   Rx
    - **F40.231 Fear of injections and transfusions**   Rx
    - **F40.232 Fear of other medical care**   Rx
    - **F40.233 Fear of injury**   Rx
  - √6ᵗʰ **F40.24 Situational type phobia**
    - **F40.240 Claustrophobia**   Rx
    - **F40.241 Acrophobia**   Rx
    - **F40.242 Fear of bridges**   Rx
    - **F40.243 Fear of flying**   Rx
    - **F40.248 Other situational type phobia**   Rx
  - √6ᵗʰ **F40.29 Other specified phobia**
    - **F40.290 Androphobia**   Rx
      - Fear of men
    - **F40.291 Gynephobia**   Rx
      - Fear of women
    - **F40.298 Other specified phobia**   Rx

F40.8 Other phobic anxiety disorders   Rx
- Phobic anxiety disorder of childhood

F40.9 Phobic anxiety disorder, unspecified   Rx
- Phobia NOS
- Phobic state NOS

√4ᵗʰ **F41 Other anxiety disorders**
- EXCLUDES 2   *anxiety in:*
  - *acute stress reaction (F43.0)*
  - *neurasthenia (F48.8)*
  - *psychophysiologic disorders (F45.-)*
  - *transient adjustment reaction (F43.2)*
  - *separation anxiety (F93.0)*

F41.0 Panic disorder [episodic paroxysmal anxiety]   Rx
- Panic attack
- Panic state
  - EXCLUDES 1   *panic disorder with agoraphobia (F40.01)*
  - **DEF:** Neurotic disorder characterized by recurrent panic or anxiety, apprehension, fear, or terror. Symptoms include shortness of breath, palpitations, dizziness, and shakiness; fear of dying may persist.

F41.1 Generalized anxiety disorder   Rx
- Anxiety neurosis
- Anxiety reaction
- Anxiety state
- Overanxious disorder
  - EXCLUDES 2   *neurasthenia (F48.8)*

F41.3 Other mixed anxiety disorders

F41.8 Other specified anxiety disorders
- Anxiety depression (mild or not persistent)
- Anxiety hysteria
- Mixed anxiety and depressive disorder
- **AHA:** 2021,1Q,10

F41.9 Anxiety disorder, unspecified
- Anxiety NOS
- **AHA:** 2021,1Q,10

√4ᵗʰ **F42 Obsessive-compulsive disorder**
- EXCLUDES 2   *obsessive-compulsive personality (disorder) (F60.5)*
  - *obsessive-compulsive symptoms occurring in depression (F32-F33)*
  - *obsessive-compulsive symptoms occurring in schizophrenia (F20.-)*
- **AHA:** 2016,4Q,14-15

F42.2 Mixed obsessional thoughts and acts   Rx

F42.3 Hoarding disorder   Rx

F42.4 Excoriation (skin-picking) disorder   Rx
- EXCLUDES 1   *factitial dermatitis (L98.1)*
  - *other specified behavioral and emotional disorders with onset usually occurring in early childhood and adolescence (F98.8)*

F42.8 Other obsessive-compulsive disorder   Rx
- Anancastic neurosis
- Obsessive-compulsive neurosis

F42.9 Obsessive-compulsive disorder, unspecified   Rx

√4ᵗʰ **F43 Reaction to severe stress, and adjustment disorders**

F43.0 Acute stress reaction
- Acute crisis reaction
- Acute reaction to stress
- Combat and operational stress reaction
- Combat fatigue
- Crisis state
- Psychic shock

√5ᵗʰ **F43.1 Post-traumatic stress disorder (PTSD)**
- Traumatic neurosis
- **DEF:** Preoccupation with traumatic events beyond normal experience (i.e., rape, personal assault, etc.) that may also include recurring flashbacks of the trauma. Symptoms include difficulty remembering, sleeping, or concentrating, and guilt feelings for surviving.
  - **F43.10 Post-traumatic stress disorder, unspecified**   Rx
  - **F43.11 Post-traumatic stress disorder, acute**   Rx
  - **F43.12 Post-traumatic stress disorder, chronic**   Rx

✓5th **F43.2 Adjustment disorders**
Culture shock
Grief reaction
Hospitalism in children
EXCLUDES 2   *separation anxiety disorder of childhood (F93.0)*

     F43.20 Adjustment disorder, unspecified   Rx

     F43.21 Adjustment disorder with depressed mood   Rx 🔘
         AHA: 2014,1Q,25

     F43.22 Adjustment disorder with anxiety   Rx

     F43.23 Adjustment disorder with mixed anxiety and depressed mood   Rx 🔘

     F43.24 Adjustment disorder with disturbance of conduct   Rx

     F43.25 Adjustment disorder with mixed disturbance of emotions and conduct   Rx

     F43.29 Adjustment disorder with other symptoms   Rx

▲ ✓5th **F43.8 Other reactions to severe stress**
Other specified trauma and stressor-related disorder

●   **F43.81 Prolonged grief disorder**
Complicated grief
Complicated grief disorder
Persistent complex bereavement disorder

●   **F43.89 Other reactions to severe stress**

F43.9 Reaction to severe stress, unspecified
Trauma and stressor-related disorder, NOS
▶Unspecified trauma and stressor-related disorder◀

✓4th **F44 Dissociative and conversion disorders**
INCLUDES   conversion hysteria
conversion reaction
hysteria
hysterical psychosis
EXCLUDES 2   *malingering [conscious simulation] (Z76.5)*

F44.0 Dissociative amnesia   HCC Rx ESR COM
EXCLUDES 1   *amnesia NOS (R41.3)*
anterograde amnesia (R41.1)
dissociative amnesia with dissociative fugue (F44.1)
retrograde amnesia (R41.2)
EXCLUDES 2   *alcohol-or other psychoactive substance-induced amnestic disorder (F10, F13, F19 with .26, .96)*
amnestic disorder due to known physiological condition (F04)
postictal amnesia in epilepsy (G40.-)

F44.1 Dissociative fugue   HCC Rx ESR COM
Dissociative amnesia with dissociative fugue
EXCLUDES 2   *postictal fugue in epilepsy (G40.-)*
DEF: Dissociative hysteria identified by memory loss and flight from familiar surroundings to a completely separate environment. Episodes may last hours or days. Conscious activity is not associated with perception of surroundings and there is no later memory of the episode.

F44.2 Dissociative stupor   Rx
EXCLUDES 1   *catatonic stupor (R40.1)*
stupor NOS (R40.1)
EXCLUDES 2   *catatonic disorder due to known physiological condition (F06.1)*
depressive stupor (F32, F33)
manic stupor (F30, F31)

F44.4 Conversion disorder with motor symptom or deficit   Rx
Conversion disorder with abnormal movement
Conversion disorder with speech symptoms
Conversion disorder with swallowing symptoms
Conversion disorder with weakness/paralysis
Dissociative motor disorders
Psychogenic aphonia
Psychogenic dysphonia

F44.5 Conversion disorder with seizures or convulsions   Rx
Conversion disorder with attacks or seizures
Dissociative convulsions
AHA: 2021,1Q,3; 2019,1Q,19

F44.6 Conversion disorder with sensory symptom or deficit   Rx
Conversion disorder with anesthesia or sensory loss
Conversion disorder with special sensory symptoms
Dissociative anesthesia and sensory loss
Psychogenic deafness

F44.7 Conversion disorder with mixed symptom presentation   Rx

✓5th **F44.8 Other dissociative and conversion disorders**

     F44.81 Dissociative identity disorder   HCC Rx ESR COM
Multiple personality disorder

     F44.89 Other dissociative and conversion disorders   Rx
Ganser's syndrome
Psychogenic confusion
Psychogenic twilight state
Trance and possession disorders

F44.9 Dissociative and conversion disorder, unspecified   Rx
Dissociative disorder NOS

✓4th **F45 Somatoform disorders**
EXCLUDES 2   *dissociative and conversion disorders (F44.-)*
factitious disorders (F68.1-, F68.A)
hair-plucking (F63.3)
lalling (F80.0)
lisping (F80.0)
malingering [conscious simulation] (Z76.5)
nail-biting (F98.8)
psychological or behavioral factors associated with disorders or diseases classified elsewhere (F54)
sexual dysfunction, not due to a substance or known physiological condition (F52.-)
thumb-sucking (F98.8)
tic disorders (in childhood and adolescence) (F95.-)
Tourette's syndrome (F95.2)
trichotillomania (F63.3)
DEF: Types of disorders causing inconsistent physical symptoms that cannot be explained.

F45.0 Somatization disorder   Rx
Briquet's disorder
Multiple psychosomatic disorder

F45.1 Undifferentiated somatoform disorder   Rx
Somatic symptom disorder
Undifferentiated psychosomatic disorder

✓5th **F45.2 Hypochondriacal disorders**
EXCLUDES 2   *delusional dysmorphophobia (F22)*
fixed delusions about bodily functions or shape (F22)

     F45.20 Hypochondriacal disorder, unspecified   Rx

     F45.21 Hypochondriasis   Rx
Hypochondriacal neurosis
Illness anxiety disorder

     F45.22 Body dysmorphic disorder   Rx
Dysmorphophobia (nondelusional)
Nosophobia

     F45.29 Other hypochondriacal disorders   Rx

✓5th **F45.4 Pain disorders related to psychological factors**
EXCLUDES 1   *pain NOS (R52)*

     F45.41 Pain disorder exclusively related to psychological factors
Somatoform pain disorder (persistent)

     F45.42 Pain disorder with related psychological factors
Code also associated acute or chronic pain (G89.-)

F45.8 Other somatoform disorders   Rx
Psychogenic dysmenorrhea
Psychogenic dysphagia, including 'globus hystericus'
Psychogenic pruritus
Psychogenic torticollis
Somatoform autonomic dysfunction
Teeth grinding
EXCLUDES 1   *sleep related teeth grinding (G47.63)*

F45.9 Somatoform disorder, unspecified   Rx
Psychosomatic disorder NOS

✓4th **F48 Other nonpsychotic mental disorders**

     F48.1 Depersonalization-derealization syndrome   HCC Rx ESR COM

     F48.2 Pseudobulbar affect
Involuntary emotional expression disorder
Code first underlying cause, if known, such as:
amyotrophic lateral sclerosis (G12.21)
multiple sclerosis (G35)
sequelae of cerebrovascular disease (I69.-)
sequelae of traumatic intracranial injury (S06.-)

F48.8 **Other specified nonpsychotic mental disorders**
Dhat syndrome
Neurasthenia
Occupational neurosis, including writer's cramp
Psychasthenia
Psychasthenic neurosis
Psychogenic syncope

F48.9 **Nonpsychotic mental disorder, unspecified**
Neurosis NOS

Behavioral syndromes associated with physiological disturbances and physical factors (F50-F59)

✓4ᵗʰ **F50** **Eating disorders**
   EXCLUDES 1   anorexia NOS (R63.0)
                feeding problems of newborn (P92.-)
                polyphagia (R63.2)
   EXCLUDES 2   feeding difficulties (R63.3)
                feeding disorder in infancy or childhood (F98.2-)
   AHA: 2022,1Q,13; 2018,4Q,82
   TIP: Assign additional code for BMI from category Z68, when documented. BMI can be based on documentation from clinicians who are not the patient's provider.

✓5ᵗʰ **F50.0** **Anorexia nervosa**
      EXCLUDES 1   loss of appetite (R63.0)
                   psychogenic loss of appetite (F50.89)
      DEF: Psychological eating disorder characterized by an intense fear of gaining weight and an unrealistic perception of body image that perpetuates the feeling of being fat or having too much fat. Avoidance of food and restrictive or unhealthy eating are common.

      F50.00 **Anorexia nervosa, unspecified**   Rx COM
      F50.01 **Anorexia nervosa, restricting type**   Rx COM
      F50.02 **Anorexia nervosa, binge eating/purging type**   Rx COM
                 EXCLUDES 1   bulimia nervosa (F50.2)

   F50.2 **Bulimia nervosa**   Rx COM
      Bulimia NOS
      Hyperorexia nervosa
      EXCLUDES 1   anorexia nervosa, binge eating/purging type (F50.02)
      DEF: Episodic pattern of overeating (binge eating) followed by purging or extreme exercise accompanied by an awareness of the abnormal eating pattern with a fear of not being able to stop eating.

✓5ᵗʰ **F50.8** **Other eating disorders**
      EXCLUDES 2   pica of infancy and childhood (F98.3)
      AHA: 2017,4Q,9; 2016,4Q,15-16

      F50.81 **Binge eating disorder**   Rx
      F50.82 **Avoidant/restrictive food intake disorder**   Rx
      F50.89 **Other specified eating disorder**   Rx
                 Pica in adults
                 Psychogenic loss of appetite

   F50.9 **Eating disorder, unspecified**   Rx
      Atypical anorexia nervosa
      Atypical bulimia nervosa
      Feeding or eating disorder, unspecified
      Other specified feeding disorder

✓4ᵗʰ **F51** **Sleep disorders not due to a substance or known physiological condition**
      EXCLUDES 2   organic sleep disorders (G47.-)

✓5ᵗʰ **F51.0** **Insomnia not due to a substance or known physiological condition**
      EXCLUDES 2   alcohol related insomnia (F10.182, F10.282, F10.982)
                   drug-related insomnia (F11.182, F11.282, F11.982, F13.182, F13.282, F13.982, F14.182, F14.282, F14.982, F15.182, F15.282, F15.982, F19.182, F19.282, F19.982)
                   insomnia NOS (G47.0-)
                   insomnia due to known physiological condition (G47.0-)
                   organic insomnia (G47.0-)
                   sleep deprivation (Z72.820)

      F51.01 **Primary insomnia**
                 Idiopathic insomnia
      F51.02 **Adjustment insomnia**
      F51.03 **Paradoxical insomnia**
      F51.04 **Psychophysiologic insomnia**

      F51.05 **Insomnia due to other mental disorder**
                 Code also associated mental disorder
      F51.09 **Other insomnia not due to a substance or known physiological condition**

✓5ᵗʰ **F51.1** **Hypersomnia not due to a substance or known physiological condition**
      EXCLUDES 2   alcohol related hypersomnia (F10.182, F10.282, F10.982)
                   drug-related hypersomnia (F11.182, F11.282, F11.982, F13.182, F13.282, F13.982, F14.182, F14.282, F14.982, F15.182, F15.282, F15.982, F19.182, F19.282, F19.982)
                   hypersomnia NOS (G47.10)
                   hypersomnia due to known physiological condition (G47.10)
                   idiopathic hypersomnia (G47.11, G47.12)
                   narcolepsy (G47.4-)

      F51.11 **Primary hypersomnia**
      F51.12 **Insufficient sleep syndrome**
                 EXCLUDES 1   sleep deprivation (Z72.820)
      F51.13 **Hypersomnia due to other mental disorder**
                 Code also associated mental disorder
      F51.19 **Other hypersomnia not due to a substance or known physiological condition**

   F51.3 **Sleepwalking [somnambulism]**
      Non-rapid eye movement sleep arousal disorders, sleepwalking type

   F51.4 **Sleep terrors [night terrors]**
      Non-rapid eye movement sleep arousal disorders, sleep terror type

   F51.5 **Nightmare disorder**
      Dream anxiety disorder

   F51.8 **Other sleep disorders not due to a substance or known physiological condition**

   F51.9 **Sleep disorder not due to a substance or known physiological condition, unspecified**
      Emotional sleep disorder NOS

✓4ᵗʰ **F52** **Sexual dysfunction not due to a substance or known physiological condition**
      EXCLUDES 2   Dhat syndrome (F48.8)

   F52.0 **Hypoactive sexual desire disorder**
      Lack or loss of sexual desire
      Male hypoactive sexual desire disorder
      Sexual anhedonia
      EXCLUDES 1   decreased libido (R68.82)

   F52.1 **Sexual aversion disorder**
      Sexual aversion and lack of sexual enjoyment

✓5ᵗʰ **F52.2** **Sexual arousal disorders**
      Failure of genital response

      F52.21 **Male erectile disorder**   ♂
                 Erectile disorder
                 Psychogenic impotence
                 EXCLUDES 1   impotence of organic origin (N52.-)
                              impotence NOS (N52.-)
      F52.22 **Female sexual arousal disorder**   ♀
                 Female sexual interest/arousal disorder

✓5ᵗʰ **F52.3** **Orgasmic disorder**
      Inhibited orgasm
      Psychogenic anorgasmy
      F52.31 **Female orgasmic disorder**   ♀
      F52.32 **Male orgasmic disorder**   ♂
                 Delayed ejaculation

   F52.4 **Premature ejaculation**   ♂

   F52.5 **Vaginismus not due to a substance or known physiological condition**   ♀
      Psychogenic vaginismus
      EXCLUDES 2   vaginismus (due to a known physiological condition) (N94.2)
      DEF: Psychogenic response resulting in painful contractions of the vaginal canal muscles. This condition can be severe enough to prevent sexual intercourse.

F52.6 Dyspareunia not due to a substance or known physiological condition
Genito-pelvic pain penetration disorder
Psychogenic dyspareunia
> EXCLUDES 2   *dyspareunia (due to a known physiological condition) (N94.1-)*

F52.8 Other sexual dysfunction not due to a substance or known physiological condition
Excessive sexual drive
Nymphomania
Satyriasis

F52.9 Unspecified sexual dysfunction not due to a substance or known physiological condition
Sexual dysfunction NOS

✓4ᵗʰ **F53 Mental and behavioral disorders associated with the puerperium, not elsewhere classified**
> EXCLUDES 1   *mood disorders with psychotic features (F30.2, F31.2, F31.5, F31.64, F32.3, F33.3)*
> *postpartum dysphoria (O90.6)*
> *psychosis in schizophrenia, schizotypal, delusional, and other psychotic disorders (F20-F29)*

AHA: 2018,4Q,8

F53.0 Postpartum depression   `Rx` `Q` `M` ♀
Postnatal depression, NOS
Postpartum depression, NOS

F53.1 Puerperal psychosis   `HCC` `Rx` `ESR` `COM` `Q` `M` ♀
Postpartum psychosis
Puerperal psychosis, NOS

F54 *Psychological and behavioral factors associated with disorders or diseases classified elsewhere*
Psychological factors affecting physical conditions
Code first the associated physical disorder, such as:
asthma (J45.-)
dermatitis (L23-L25)
gastric ulcer (K25.-)
mucous colitis (K58.-)
ulcerative colitis (K51.-)
urticaria (L50.-)
> EXCLUDES 2   *tension-type headache (G44.2)*

✓4ᵗʰ **F55 Abuse of non-psychoactive substances**
> EXCLUDES 2   *abuse of psychoactive substances (F10-F19)*

F55.0 Abuse of antacids
F55.1 Abuse of herbal or folk remedies
F55.2 Abuse of laxatives
F55.3 Abuse of steroids or hormones
F55.4 Abuse of vitamins
F55.8 Abuse of other non-psychoactive substances

F59 Unspecified behavioral syndromes associated with physiological disturbances and physical factors
Psychogenic physiological dysfunction NOS

Disorders of adult personality and behavior (F60-F69)

✓4ᵗʰ **F60 Specific personality disorders**

F60.0 Paranoid personality disorder   `HCC` `Rx` `ESR` `COM`
Expansive paranoid personality (disorder)
Fanatic personality (disorder)
Paranoid personality (disorder)
Querulant personality (disorder)
Sensitive paranoid personality (disorder)
> EXCLUDES 2   *paranoia (F22)*
> *paranoia querulans (F22)*
> *paranoid psychosis (F22)*
> *paranoid schizophrenia (F20.0)*
> *paranoid state (F22)*

F60.1 Schizoid personality disorder   `HCC` `Rx` `ESR` `COM`
> EXCLUDES 2   *Asperger's syndrome (F84.5)*
> *delusional disorder (F22)*
> *schizoid disorder of childhood (F84.5)*
> *schizophrenia (F20.-)*
> *schizotypal disorder (F21)*

F60.2 Antisocial personality disorder   `HCC` `Rx` `ESR` `COM`
Amoral personality (disorder)
Asocial personality (disorder)
Dissocial personality disorder
Psychopathic personality (disorder)
Sociopathic personality (disorder)
> EXCLUDES 1   *conduct disorders (F91.-)*
> EXCLUDES 2   *borderline personality disorder (F60.3)*

F60.3 Borderline personality disorder   `HCC` `Rx` `ESR` `COM`
Aggressive personality (disorder)
Emotionally unstable personality disorder
Explosive personality (disorder)
> EXCLUDES 2   *antisocial personality disorder (F60.2)*

F60.4 Histrionic personality disorder   `HCC` `Rx` `ESR` `COM`
Hysterical personality (disorder)
Psychoinfantile personality (disorder)

F60.5 Obsessive-compulsive personality disorder   `HCC` `Rx` `ESR` `COM`
Anankastic personality (disorder)
Compulsive personality (disorder)
Obsessional personality (disorder)
> EXCLUDES 2   *obsessive-compulsive disorder (F42.-)*

F60.6 Avoidant personality disorder   `HCC` `Rx` `ESR` `COM`
Anxious personality disorder

F60.7 Dependent personality disorder   `HCC` `Rx` `ESR` `COM`
Asthenic personality (disorder)
Inadequate personality (disorder)
Passive personality (disorder)
DEF: Lack of self-confidence, fear of abandonment, and an obsessive need to be taken care of.

✓5ᵗʰ **F60.8 Other specific personality disorders**

F60.81 Narcissistic personality disorder   `HCC` `Rx` `ESR` `COM`
F60.89 Other specific personality disorders   `HCC` `Rx` `ESR` `COM`
Eccentric personality disorder
"Haltlose" type personality disorder
Immature personality disorder
Passive-aggressive personality disorder
Psychoneurotic personality disorder
Self-defeating personality disorder

F60.9 Personality disorder, unspecified   `HCC` `Rx` `ESR` `COM`
Character disorder NOS
Character neurosis NOS
Pathological personality NOS

✓4ᵗʰ **F63 Impulse disorders**
> EXCLUDES 2   *habitual excessive use of alcohol or psychoactive substances (F10-F19)*
> *impulse disorders involving sexual behavior (F65.-)*

F63.0 Pathological gambling   `Rx`
Compulsive gambling
Gambling disorder
> EXCLUDES 1   *gambling and betting NOS (Z72.6)*
> EXCLUDES 2   *excessive gambling by manic patients (F30, F31)*
> *gambling in antisocial personality disorder (F60.2)*

F63.1 Pyromania   `Rx`
Pathological fire-setting
> EXCLUDES 2   *fire-setting (by) (in):*
> *adult with antisocial personality disorder (F60.2)*
> *alcohol or psychoactive substance intoxication (F10-F19)*
> *conduct disorders (F91.-)*
> *mental disorders due to known physiological condition (F01-F09)*
> *schizophrenia (F20.-)*

F63.2 Kleptomania   `Rx`
Pathological stealing
> EXCLUDES 1   *shoplifting as the reason for observation for suspected mental disorder (Z03.8)*
> EXCLUDES 2   *depressive disorder with stealing (F31-F33)*
> *stealing due to underlying mental condition - code to mental condition*
> *stealing in mental disorders due to known physiological condition (F01-F09)*

Chapter 5. Mental, Behavioral and Neurodevelopmental Disorders

F63.3   **Trichotillomania**   `Rx`
    Hair plucking
    EXCLUDES 2   *other stereotyped movement disorder (F98.4)*

✓5ᵗʰ **F63.8**   **Other impulse disorders**
    F63.81   **Intermittent explosive disorder**   `Rx`
    F63.89   **Other impulse disorders**   `Rx`

F63.9   **Impulse disorder, unspecified**   `Rx`
    Impulse control disorder NOS

✓4ᵗʰ **F64**   **Gender identity disorders**
    AHA: 2016,4Q,16

F64.0   **Transsexualism**
    Gender identity disorder in adolescence and adulthood
    Gender dysphoria in adolescents and adults

F64.1   **Dual role transvestism**
    Use additional code to identify sex reassignment status (Z87.890)
    EXCLUDES 1   *gender identity disorder in childhood (F64.2)*
    EXCLUDES 2   *fetishistic transvestism (F65.1)*

F64.2   **Gender identity disorder of childhood**   `P`
    Gender dysphoria in children
    EXCLUDES 1   *gender identity disorder in adolescence and adulthood (F64.0)*
    EXCLUDES 2   *sexual maturation disorder (F66)*

F64.8   **Other gender identity disorders**
    Other specified gender dysphoria

F64.9   **Gender identity disorder, unspecified**
    Gender dysphoria, unspecified
    Gender-role disorder NOS

✓4ᵗʰ **F65**   **Paraphilias**

F65.0   **Fetishism**
    Fetishistic disorder

F65.1   **Transvestic fetishism**
    Fetishistic transvestism
    Transvestic disorder

F65.2   **Exhibitionism**
    Exhibitionistic disorder

F65.3   **Voyeurism**
    Voyeuristic disorder

F65.4   **Pedophilia**
    Pedophilic disorder

✓5ᵗʰ **F65.5**   **Sadomasochism**
    F65.50   **Sadomasochism, unspecified**
    F65.51   **Sexual masochism**
        Sexual masochism disorder
    F65.52   **Sexual sadism**
        Sexual sadism disorder

✓5ᵗʰ **F65.8**   **Other paraphilias**
    F65.81   **Frotteurism**
        Frotteuristic disorder
    F65.89   **Other paraphilias**
        Necrophilia
        Other specified paraphilic disorder

F65.9   **Paraphilia, unspecified**
    Paraphilic disorder, unspecified
    Sexual deviation NOS

F66   **Other sexual disorders**
    Sexual maturation disorder
    Sexual relationship disorder

✓4ᵗʰ **F68**   **Other disorders of adult personality and behavior**
    AHA: 2018,4Q,9,65

✓5ᵗʰ **F68.1**   **Factitious disorder** imposed on self
    Compensation neurosis
    Elaboration of physical symptoms for psychological reasons
    Hospital hopper syndrome
    Münchausen's syndrome
    Peregrinating patient
    EXCLUDES 2   *factitial dermatitis (L98.1)*
            person feigning illness (with obvious motivation) (Z76.5)
    F68.10   **Factitious disorder imposed on self, unspecified**   `Rx`
    F68.11   **Factitious disorder imposed on self, with predominantly psychological signs and symptoms**   `Rx`

F68.12   **Factitious disorder imposed on self, with predominantly physical signs and symptoms**   `Rx`
F68.13   **Factitious disorder imposed on self, with combined psychological and physical signs and symptoms**   `Rx`

F68.A   **Factitious disorder** imposed on another   `Rx`
    Factitious disorder by proxy
    Münchausen's by proxy

F68.8   **Other specified disorders of adult personality and behavior**

F69   **Unspecified disorder of adult personality and behavior**   `A`

Intellectual disabilities (F70-F79)

Code first any associated physical or developmental disorders
    EXCLUDES 1   *borderline intellectual functioning, IQ above 70 to 84 (R41.83)*

F70   **Mild** intellectual disabilities   `Rx`
    IQ level 50-55 to approximately 70
    Mild mental subnormality

F71   **Moderate** intellectual disabilities   `Rx`
    IQ level 35-40 to 50-55
    Moderate mental subnormality

F72   **Severe** intellectual disabilities   `Rx`
    IQ 20-25 to 35-40
    Severe mental subnormality

F73   **Profound** intellectual disabilities   `Rx`
    IQ level below 20-25
    Profound mental subnormality

✓4ᵗʰ **F78**   **Other intellectual disabilities**   `Rx`

✓5ᵗʰ **F78.A**   **Other genetic related intellectual disabilities**
    AHA: 2021,4Q,10-11
    F78.A1   **SYNGAP1-related** intellectual disability   `Rx`
        Code also, if applicable, any associated:
            autism spectrum disorder (F84.0)
            autistic disorder (F84.0)
            encephalopathy (G93.4-)
            epilepsy and recurrent seizures (G40.-)
            other pervasive developmental disorders (F84.8)
            pervasive developmental disorder, NOS (F84.9)

    F78.A9   **Other genetic related intellectual disability**   `Rx`
        Code also, if applicable, any associated disorders

F79   **Unspecified intellectual disabilities**   `Rx`
    Mental deficiency NOS
    Mental subnormality NOS

Pervasive and specific developmental disorders (F80-F89)

✓4ᵗʰ **F80**   **Specific developmental disorders of speech and language**

F80.0   **Phonological** disorder
    Dyslalia
    Functional speech articulation disorder
    Lalling
    Lisping
    Phonological developmental disorder
    Speech articulation developmental disorder
    Speech-sound disorder
    EXCLUDES 1   *speech articulation impairment due to aphasia NOS (R47.01)*
            speech articulation impairment due to apraxia (R48.2)
    EXCLUDES 2   *speech articulation impairment due to hearing loss (F80.4)*
            speech articulation impairment due to intellectual disabilities (F70-F79)
            speech articulation impairment with expressive language developmental disorder (F80.1)
            speech articulation impairment with mixed receptive expressive language developmental disorder (F80.2)

`HCC` CMS-HCC   `Rx` Rx HCC   `ESR` ESRD HCC   `COM` Commercial HCC   `N` Newborn: 0   `P` Pediatric: 0-17   `M` Maternity: 9-64   `A` Adult: 15-124

582   ICD-10-CM 2023

F80.1 **Expressive language** disorder

Developmental dysphasia or aphasia, expressive type

EXCLUDES 1   *mixed receptive-expressive language disorder (F80.2)*
           dysphasia and aphasia NOS (R47.-)

EXCLUDES 2   *acquired aphasia with epilepsy [Landau-Kleffner]*
           (G40.80-)
           selective mutism (F94.0)
           intellectual disabilities (F70-F79)
           pervasive developmental disorders (F84.-)

F80.2 **Mixed receptive-expressive language** disorder

Developmental dysphasia or aphasia, receptive type

Developmental Wernicke's aphasia

EXCLUDES 1   *central auditory processing disorder (H93.25)*
           dysphasia or aphasia NOS (R47.-)
           expressive language disorder (F80.1)
           expressive type dysphasia or aphasia (F80.1)
           word deafness (H93.25)

EXCLUDES 2   *acquired aphasia with epilepsy [Landau-Kleffner]*
           (G40.80-)
           pervasive developmental disorders (F84.-)
           selective mutism (F94.0)
           intellectual disabilities (F70-F79)

F80.4 **Speech and language development delay** due to hearing loss

Code also type of hearing loss (H90.-, H91.-)

✓5th **F80.8** **Other developmental disorders of speech and language**

AHA: 2017, 1Q, 27

F80.81 **Childhood onset fluency disorder**

Cluttering NOS

Stuttering NOS

EXCLUDES 1   *adult onset fluency disorder (F98.5)*
           fluency disorder in conditions classified
           elsewhere (R47.82)
           fluency disorder (stuttering) following
           cerebrovascular disease (I69. with
           final characters -23)

F80.82 **Social pragmatic communication disorder**

EXCLUDES 1   *Asperger's syndrome (F84.5)*
           autistic disorder (F84.0)

AHA: 2016, 4Q, 16

F80.89 **Other developmental disorders of speech and language**

F80.9 **Developmental disorder of speech and language, unspecified**

Communication disorder NOS

Language disorder NOS

✓4th **F81** **Specific developmental disorders of** scholastic skills

F81.0 **Specific reading disorder**

"Backward reading"

Developmental dyslexia

Specific learning disorder, with impairment in reading

Specific reading retardation

EXCLUDES 1   *alexia NOS (R48.0)*
           dyslexia NOS (R48.0)

DEF: Serious impairment of reading skills unexplained in relation to general intelligence and teaching processes.

F81.2 **Mathematics disorder**

Developmental acalculia

Developmental arithmetical disorder

Developmental Gerstmann's syndrome

Specific learning disorder, with impairment in mathematics

EXCLUDES 1   *acalculia NOS (R48.8)*

EXCLUDES 2   *arithmetical difficulties associated with a reading*
           disorder (F81.0)
           arithmetical difficulties associated with a spelling
           disorder (F81.81)
           arithmetical difficulties due to inadequate teaching
           (Z55.8)

✓5th **F81.8** **Other developmental disorders of scholastic skills**

F81.81 **Disorder of written expression**

Specific learning disorder, with impairment in written expression

Specific spelling disorder

F81.89 **Other developmental disorders of** scholastic skills

F81.9 **Developmental disorder of scholastic skills, unspecified**

Knowledge acquisition disability NOS

Learning disability NOS

Learning disorder NOS

F82 **Specific developmental disorder of motor function**

Clumsy child syndrome

Developmental coordination disorder

Developmental dyspraxia

EXCLUDES 1   *abnormalities of gait and mobility (R26.-)*
           lack of coordination (R27.-)

EXCLUDES 2   *lack of coordination secondary to intellectual disabilities*
           (F70-F79)

✓4th **F84** **Pervasive developmental disorders**

Code also any associated medical condition and intellectual disabilities

F84.0 **Autistic disorder**   Rx COM

Autism spectrum disorder

Infantile autism

Infantile psychosis

Kanner's syndrome

EXCLUDES 1   *Asperger's syndrome (F84.5)*

AHA: 2017, 1Q, 27

TIP: When the encounter is focused on treatment of conditions related to autism spectrum disorder, first assign codes to identify the problem or manifestation receiving therapeutic services.

F84.2 **Rett's syndrome**   Rx COM

EXCLUDES 1   *Asperger's syndrome (F84.5)*
           autistic disorder (F84.0)
           other childhood disintegrative disorder (F84.3)

F84.3 **Other childhood disintegrative disorder**   Rx COM P

Dementia infantilis

Disintegrative psychosis

Heller's syndrome

Symbiotic psychosis

Use additional code to identify any associated neurological condition

EXCLUDES 1   *Asperger's syndrome (F84.5)*
           autistic disorder (F84.0)
           Rett's syndrome (F84.2)

F84.5 **Asperger's syndrome**   Rx COM

Asperger's disorder

Autistic psychopathy

Schizoid disorder of childhood

DEF: High-functioning form of autism. Children with this syndrome usually develop speech on schedule, are generally very intelligent, and communicate well, but have considerable social shortcomings. *Synonym(s): AS.*

F84.8 **Other pervasive developmental disorders**   Rx COM

Overactive disorder associated with intellectual disabilities and stereotyped movements

F84.9 **Pervasive developmental disorder, unspecified**   Rx COM

Atypical autism

F88 **Other disorders of psychological development**

Developmental agnosia

Global developmental delay

Other specified neurodevelopmental disorder

F89 **Unspecified disorder of psychological development**

Developmental disorder NOS

Neurodevelopmental disorder NOS

Behavioral and emotional disorders with onset usually occurring in childhood and adolescence (F90-F98)

NOTE Codes within categories F90-F98 may be used regardless of the age of a patient. These disorders generally have onset within the childhood or adolescent years, but may continue throughout life or not be diagnosed until adulthood

✓4ᵗʰ **F90 Attention-deficit hyperactivity disorders**

INCLUDES attention deficit disorder with hyperactivity
attention deficit syndrome with hyperactivity

EXCLUDES 2 anxiety disorders (F40.-, F41.-)
mood [affective] disorders (F30-F39)
pervasive developmental disorders (F84.-)
schizophrenia (F20.-)

F90.0 Attention-deficit hyperactivity disorder, predominantly inattentive type `Rx`
Attention-deficit/hyperactivity disorder, predominantly inattentive presentation

F90.1 Attention-deficit hyperactivity disorder, predominantly hyperactive type `Rx`
Attention-deficit/hyperactivity disorder, predominantly hyperactive impulsive presentation

F90.2 Attention-deficit hyperactivity disorder, combined type `Rx`
Attention-deficit/hyperactivity disorder, combined presentation

F90.8 Attention-deficit hyperactivity disorder, other type `Rx`

F90.9 Attention-deficit hyperactivity disorder, unspecified type `Rx`
Attention-deficit hyperactivity disorder of childhood or adolescence NOS
Attention-deficit hyperactivity disorder NOS

✓4ᵗʰ **F91 Conduct disorders**

EXCLUDES 1 antisocial behavior (Z72.81-)
antisocial personality disorder (F60.2)

EXCLUDES 2 conduct problems associated with attention-deficit hyperactivity disorder (F90.-)
mood [affective] disorders (F30-F39)
pervasive developmental disorders (F84.-)
schizophrenia (F20.-)

F91.0 Conduct disorder confined to family context `Rx`

F91.1 Conduct disorder, childhood-onset type `Rx`
Unsocialized conduct disorder
Conduct disorder, solitary aggressive type
Unsocialized aggressive disorder

F91.2 Conduct disorder, adolescent-onset type `Rx`
Socialized conduct disorder
Conduct disorder, group type

F91.3 Oppositional defiant disorder `Rx`

F91.8 Other conduct disorders `Rx`
Other specified conduct disorder
Other specified disruptive disorder

F91.9 Conduct disorder, unspecified `Rx`
Behavioral disorder NOS
Conduct disorder NOS
Disruptive behavior disorder NOS
Disruptive disorder NOS

✓4ᵗʰ **F93 Emotional disorders with onset specific to childhood**

F93.0 Separation anxiety disorder of childhood `Rx`
EXCLUDES 2 mood [affective] disorders (F30-F39)
nonpsychotic mental disorders (F40-F48)
phobic anxiety disorder of childhood (F40.8)
social phobia (F40.1)

F93.8 Other childhood emotional disorders
Identity disorder
EXCLUDES 2 gender identity disorder of childhood (F64.2)

F93.9 Childhood emotional disorder, unspecified

✓4ᵗʰ **F94 Disorders of social functioning with onset specific to childhood and adolescence**

F94.0 Selective mutism
Elective mutism
EXCLUDES 2 pervasive developmental disorders (F84.-)
schizophrenia (F20.-)
specific developmental disorders of speech and language (F80.-)
transient mutism as part of separation anxiety in young children (F93.0)

F94.1 Reactive attachment disorder of childhood
Use additional code to identify any associated failure to thrive or growth retardation
EXCLUDES 1 disinhibited attachment disorder of childhood (F94.2)
normal variation in pattern of selective attachment
EXCLUDES 2 Asperger's syndrome (F84.5)
maltreatment syndromes (T74.-)
sexual or physical abuse in childhood, resulting in psychosocial problems (Z62.81-)

F94.2 Disinhibited attachment disorder of childhood
Affectionless psychopathy
Institutional syndrome
EXCLUDES 1 reactive attachment disorder of childhood (F94.1)
EXCLUDES 2 Asperger's syndrome (F84.5)
attention-deficit hyperactivity disorders (F90.-)
hospitalism in children (F43.2-)

F94.8 Other childhood disorders of social functioning

F94.9 Childhood disorder of social functioning, unspecified

✓4ᵗʰ **F95 Tic disorder**

F95.0 Transient tic disorder `Rx`
Provisional tic disorder

F95.1 Chronic motor or vocal tic disorder `Rx`

F95.2 Tourette's disorder `Rx`
Combined vocal and multiple motor tic disorder [de la Tourette]
Tourette's syndrome

F95.8 Other tic disorders `Rx`

F95.9 Tic disorder, unspecified `Rx`
Tic NOS

✓4ᵗʰ **F98 Other behavioral and emotional disorders with onset usually occurring in childhood and adolescence**
EXCLUDES 2 breath-holding spells (R06.89)
gender identity disorder of childhood (F64.2)
Kleine-Levin syndrome (G47.13)
obsessive-compulsive disorder (F42.-)
sleep disorders not due to a substance or known physiological condition (F51.-)

F98.0 Enuresis not due to a substance or known physiological condition
Enuresis (primary) (secondary) of nonorganic origin
Functional enuresis
Psychogenic enuresis
Urinary incontinence of nonorganic origin
EXCLUDES 1 enuresis NOS (R32)

F98.1 Encopresis not due to a substance or known physiological condition
Functional encopresis
Incontinence of feces of nonorganic origin
Psychogenic encopresis
Use additional code to identify the cause of any coexisting constipation
EXCLUDES 1 encopresis NOS (R15.-)

✓5ᵗʰ **F98.2 Other feeding disorders of infancy and childhood**
EXCLUDES 2 anorexia nervosa and other eating disorders (F50.-)
feeding difficulties (R63.3)
feeding problems of newborn (P92.-)
pica of infancy or childhood (F98.3)

F98.21 Rumination disorder of infancy `Rx`
F98.29 Other feeding disorders of infancy and early childhood `Rx`

F98.3 Pica of infancy and childhood `Rx`

F98.4 Stereotyped movement disorders [Rx]
Stereotype/habit disorder
> EXCLUDES 1   *abnormal involuntary movements (R25.-)*
> EXCLUDES 2   *compulsions in obsessive-compulsive disorder (F42.-)*
> *hair plucking (F63.3)*
> *movement disorders of organic origin (G20-G25)*
> *nail-biting (F98.8)*
> *nose-picking (F98.8)*
> *stereotypies that are part of a broader psychiatric condition (F01-F95)*
> *thumb-sucking (F98.8)*
> *tic disorders (F95.-)*
> *trichotillomania (F63.3)*

F98.5 Adult onset fluency disorder
> EXCLUDES 1   *childhood onset fluency disorder (F80.81)*
> *dysphasia (R47.02)*
> *fluency disorder in conditions classified elsewhere (R47.82)*
> *fluency disorder (stuttering) following cerebrovascular disease (I69. with final characters -23)*
> *tic disorders (F95.-)*

F98.8 Other specified behavioral and emotional disorders with onset usually occurring in childhood and adolescence
Excessive masturbation
Nail-biting
Nose-picking
Thumb-sucking

F98.9 Unspecified behavioral and emotional disorders with onset usually occurring in childhood and adolescence

Unspecified mental disorder (F99)

F99 Mental disorder, not otherwise specified
Mental illness NOS
> EXCLUDES 1   *unspecified mental disorder due to known physiological condition (F09)*

Chapter 6. Diseases of the Nervous System (G00-G99)

Chapter-specific Guidelines with Coding Examples

The chapter-specific guidelines from the ICD-10-CM Official Guidelines for Coding and Reporting have been provided below. Along with these guidelines are coding examples, contained in the shaded boxes, that have been developed to help illustrate the coding and/or sequencing guidance found in these guidelines.

a. Dominant/nondominant side

Codes from category G81, Hemiplegia and hemiparesis, and subcategories G83.1, Monoplegia of lower limb, G83.2, Monoplegia of upper limb, and G83.3, Monoplegia, unspecified, identify whether the dominant or nondominant side is affected. Should the affected side be documented, but not specified as dominant or nondominant, and the classification system does not indicate a default, code selection is as follows:

- For ambidextrous patients, the default should be dominant.
- If the left side is affected, the default is non-dominant.
- If the right side is affected, the default is dominant.

> Hemiplegia affecting left side of ambidextrous patient
>
> **G81.92 Hemiplegia, unspecified affecting left dominant side**
>
> *Explanation*: Documentation states that the left side is affected and dominant is used for ambidextrous persons.

> Right spastic hemiplegia, unknown whether patient is right- or left-handed
>
> **G81.11 Spastic hemiplegia affecting right dominant side**
>
> *Explanation*: Since it is unknown whether the patient is right- or left-handed, if the right side is affected, the default is dominant.

b. Pain—Category G89

1) General coding information

Codes in category G89, Pain, not elsewhere classified, may be used in conjunction with codes from other categories and chapters to provide more detail about acute or chronic pain and neoplasm-related pain, unless otherwise indicated below.

If the pain is not specified as acute or chronic, post-thoracotomy, postprocedural, or neoplasm-related, do not assign codes from category G89.

A code from category G89 should not be assigned if the underlying (definitive) diagnosis is known, unless the reason for the encounter is pain control/ management and not management of the underlying condition.

When an admission or encounter is for a procedure aimed at treating the underlying condition (e.g., spinal fusion, kyphoplasty), a code for the underlying condition (e.g., vertebral fracture, spinal stenosis) should be assigned as the principal diagnosis. No code from category G89 should be assigned.

> Elderly patient with back pain is admitted for outpatient kyphoplasty for age-related osteopathic compression fracture at vertebra T3
>
> **M80.08XA Age-related osteoporosis with current pathological fracture, vertebra(e), initial encounter for fracture**
>
> *Explanation*: No code is assigned for the pain as it is inherent in the underlying condition being treated.

(a) Category G89 codes as principal or first-listed diagnosis

Category G89 codes are acceptable as principal diagnosis or the first-listed code:

- When pain control or pain management is the reason for the admission/encounter (e.g., a patient with displaced intervertebral disc, nerve impingement and severe back pain presents for injection of steroid into the spinal canal). The underlying cause of the pain should be reported as an additional diagnosis, if known.

> Patient presents for steroid injection in the right elbow due to chronic pain associated with primary degenerative joint disease.
>
> **G89.29 Other chronic pain**
>
> **M19.021 Primary osteoarthritis, right elbow**
>
> *Explanation*: Since the encounter is for control of pain, not treating the underlying condition, the pain code is sequenced first followed by the underlying condition. The M25 pain code is not necessary as the underlying condition code represents the specific site.

- When a patient is admitted for the insertion of a neurostimulator for pain control, assign the appropriate pain code as the principal or first-listed diagnosis. When an admission or encounter is for a procedure aimed at treating the underlying condition and a neurostimulator is inserted for pain control during the same admission/encounter, a code for the underlying condition should be assigned as the principal diagnosis and the appropriate pain code should be assigned as a secondary diagnosis.

(b) Use of category G89 codes in conjunction with site specific pain codes

(i) Assigning category G89 and site-specific pain codes

Codes from category G89 may be used in conjunction with codes that identify the site of pain (including codes from chapter 18) if the category G89 code provides additional information. For example, if the code describes the site of the pain, but does not fully describe whether the pain is acute or chronic, then both codes should be assigned.

> Patient is seen to evaluate chronic right knee pain
>
> **M25.561 Pain in right knee**
>
> **G89.29 Other chronic pain**
>
> *Explanation*: No underlying condition has been determined yet so the pain would be the reason for the visit. The M25 pain code in this instance does not fully describe the condition as it does not represent that the pain is chronic. The G89 chronic pain code is assigned to provide specificity.

(ii) Sequencing of category G89 codes with site-specific pain codes

The sequencing of category G89 codes with site-specific pain codes (including chapter 18 codes), is dependent on the circumstances of the encounter/admission as follows:

- If the encounter is for pain control or pain management, assign the code from category G89 followed by the code identifying the specific site of pain (e.g., encounter for pain management for acute neck pain from trauma is assigned code G89.11, Acute pain due to trauma, followed by code M54.2, Cervicalgia, to identify the site of pain).

> Management of acute, traumatic left shoulder pain
>
> **G89.11 Acute pain due to trauma**
>
> **M25.512 Pain in left shoulder**
>
> *Explanation*: The reason for the encounter is to manage or control the pain, not to treat or evaluate an underlying condition. The G89 pain code is assigned as the first-listed diagnosis but in this instance does not fully describe the condition as it does not include the site and laterality. The M25 pain code is added to provide this information.

- If the encounter is for any other reason except pain control or pain management, and a related definitive diagnosis has not been established (confirmed) by the provider, assign the code for the specific site of pain first, followed by the appropriate code from category G89.

> Tests are performed to investigate the source of the patient's chronic epigastric abdominal pain
>
> **R10.13**   **Epigastric pain**
>
> **G89.29**   **Other chronic pain**
>
> *Explanation*: In this instance the patient's epigastric pain is not being treated; rather the source of the pain is being investigated. A code from chapter 18 for epigastric pain is sequenced before the additional specificity of the G89 code for the chronic pain.

2) Pain due to devices, implants and grafts

See Section I.C.19. Pain due to medical devices

3) Postoperative Pain

The provider's documentation should be used to guide the coding of postoperative pain, as well as *Section III. Reporting Additional Diagnoses* and *Section IV. Diagnostic Coding and Reporting in the Outpatient Setting.*

The default for post-thoracotomy and other postoperative pain not specified as acute or chronic is the code for the acute form.

Routine or expected postoperative pain immediately after surgery should not be coded.

> Pain pump dose is increased for the patient's unexpected, extreme pain post-thoracotomy
>
> **G89.12**   **Acute post-thoracotomy pain**
>
> *Explanation*: When acute or chronic is not documented, default to acute. The use of "unexpected, extreme" and the increase of medication dosage indicate that the pain was more than routine or expected.

(a) Postoperative pain not associated with specific postoperative complication

Postoperative pain not associated with a specific postoperative complication is assigned to the appropriate postoperative pain code in category G89.

(b) Postoperative pain associated with specific postoperative complication

Postoperative pain associated with a specific postoperative complication (such as painful wire sutures) is assigned to the appropriate code(s) found in Chapter 19, Injury, poisoning, and certain other consequences of external causes. If appropriate, use additional code(s) from category G89 to identify acute or chronic pain (G89.18 or G89.28).

4) Chronic pain

Chronic pain is classified to subcategory G89.2. There is no time frame defining when pain becomes chronic pain. The provider's documentation should be used to guide use of these codes.

5) Neoplasm related pain

Code G89.3 is assigned to pain documented as being related, associated or due to cancer, primary or secondary malignancy, or tumor. This code is assigned regardless of whether the pain is acute or chronic.

This code may be assigned as the principal or first-listed code when the stated reason for the admission/encounter is documented as pain control/pain management. The underlying neoplasm should be reported as an additional diagnosis.

> Patient referred today for pain management due to acute pain related to malignancy of the right breast.
>
> **G89.3**   **Neoplasm related pain (acute)(chronic)**
>
> **C50.911**   **Malignant neoplasm of unspecified site of right female breast**
>
> *Explanation*: Since the encounter was for pain medication management, the pain, rather than the neoplasm, was the reason for the encounter and is sequenced first. This "neoplasm-related pain" code includes both acute and chronic pain.

When the reason for the admission/encounter is management of the neoplasm and the pain associated with the neoplasm is also documented, code G89.3 may be assigned as an additional diagnosis. It is not necessary to assign an additional code for the site of the pain.

See Section I.C.2. for instructions on the sequencing of neoplasms for all other stated reasons or the admission/encounter (except for pain control/pain management).

> Patient with lung cancer presents with acute hip pain and is evaluated and found to have iliac bone metastasis
>
> **C79.51**   **Secondary malignant neoplasm of bone**
>
> **C34.90**   **Malignant neoplasm of unspecified part of unspecified bronchus or lung**
>
> **G89.3**   **Neoplasm related pain (acute)(chronic)**
>
> *Explanation*: The reason for the encounter was the evaluation and diagnosis of the bone metastasis, whose code would be assigned as first-listed, followed by codes for the primary neoplasm and the pain due to the iliac bone metastasis.

6) Chronic pain syndrome

Central pain syndrome (G89.0) and chronic pain syndrome (G89.4) are different than the term "chronic pain," and therefore codes should only be used when the provider has specifically documented this condition.

See Section I.C.5. Pain disorders related to psychological factors

Chapter 6. Diseases of the Nervous System (G00–G99)

EXCLUDES 2   certain conditions originating in the perinatal period (P04-P96)
certain infectious and parasitic diseases (A00-B99)
complications of pregnancy, childbirth and the puerperium (O00-O9A)
congenital malformations, deformations, and chromosomal abnormalities (Q00-Q99)
endocrine, nutritional and metabolic diseases (E00-E88)
injury, poisoning and certain other consequences of external causes (S00-T88)
neoplasms (C00-D49)
symptoms, signs and abnormal clinical and laboratory findings, not elsewhere classified (R00-R94)

This chapter contains the following blocks:

G00-G09   Inflammatory diseases of the central nervous system
G10-G14   Systemic atrophies primarily affecting the central nervous system
G20-G26   Extrapyramidal and movement disorders
G30-G32   Other degenerative diseases of the nervous system
G35-G37   Demyelinating diseases of the central nervous system
G40-G47   Episodic and paroxysmal disorders
G50-G59   Nerve, nerve root and plexus disorders
G60-G65   Polyneuropathies and other disorders of the peripheral nervous system
G70-G73   Diseases of myoneural junction and muscle
G80-G83   Cerebral palsy and other paralytic syndromes
G89-G99   Other disorders of the nervous system

Inflammatory diseases of the central nervous system (G00-G09)

✓4ᵗʰ G00 Bacterial meningitis, not elsewhere classified

INCLUDES   bacterial arachnoiditis
bacterial leptomeningitis
bacterial meningitis
bacterial pachymeningitis

EXCLUDES 1   bacterial meningoencephalitis (G04.2)
bacterial meningomyelitis (G04.2)

DEF: Inflammation of meningeal layers of the brain and spinal cord due to a bacterial infection.

G00.0 Hemophilus meningitis   COM
Meningitis due to Hemophilus influenzae

G00.1 Pneumococcal meningitis   COM
Meningtitis due to Streptococcal pneumoniae

G00.2 Streptococcal meningitis   COM
Use additional code to further identify organism (B95.0-B95.5)

G00.3 Staphylococcal meningitis   COM
Use additional code to further identify organism (B95.61-B95.8)

G00.8 Other bacterial meningitis   COM
Meningitis due to Escherichia coli
Meningitis due to Friedländer's bacillus
Meningitis due to Klebsiella
Use additional code to further identify organism (B96.-)

G00.9 Bacterial meningitis, unspecified   COM
Meningitis due to gram-negative bacteria, unspecified
Purulent meningitis NOS
Pyogenic meningitis NOS
Suppurative meningitis NOS

G01 Meningitis in bacterial diseases classified elsewhere   COM
Code first underlying disease

EXCLUDES 1   meningitis (in):
gonococcal (A54.81)
leptospirosis (A27.81)
listeriosis (A32.11)
Lyme disease (A69.21)
meningococcal (A39.0)
neurosyphilis (A52.13)
tuberculosis (A17.0)
meningoencephalitis and meningomyelitis in bacterial diseases classified elsewhere (G05)

G02 Meningitis in other infectious and parasitic diseases classified elsewhere   COM
Code first underlying disease, such as:
African trypanosomiasis (B56.-)
poliovirus infection (A80.-)

EXCLUDES 1   candidal meningitis (B37.5)
coccidioidomycosis meningitis (B38.4)
cryptococcal meningitis (B45.1)
herpesviral [herpes simplex] meningitis (B00.3)
infectious mononucleosis complicated by meningitis (B27.- with fifth character 2)
measles complicated by meningitis (B05.1)
meningoencephalitis and meningomyelitis in other infectious and parasitic diseases classified elsewhere (G05)
mumps meningitis (B26.1)
rubella meningitis (B06.02)
varicella [chickenpox] meningitis (B01.0)
zoster meningitis (B02.1)

✓4ᵗʰ G03 Meningitis due to other and unspecified causes

INCLUDES   arachnoiditis NOS
leptomeningitis NOS
meningitis NOS
pachymeningitis NOS

EXCLUDES 1   meningoencephalitis (G04.-)
meningomyelitis (G04.-)

G03.0 Nonpyogenic meningitis   COM
Aseptic meningitis
Nonbacterial meningitis
DEF: Type of meningitis where no bacterial, viral, or other infectious source exists that explains the meningitis symptomology.

G03.1 Chronic meningitis   COM

G03.2 Benign recurrent meningitis [Mollaret]   COM
DEF: Aseptic or noninfectious inflammation of the meninges with the presence of Mollaret cells in the spinal fluid. The patient experiences recurrent bouts of inflammation, lasting anywhere from two to five days.

G03.8 Meningitis due to other specified causes   COM

G03.9 Meningitis, unspecified   COM
Arachnoiditis (spinal) NOS

✓4ᵗʰ G04 Encephalitis, myelitis and encephalomyelitis

INCLUDES   acute ascending myelitis
meningoencephalitis
meningomyelitis

EXCLUDES 1   encephalopathy NOS (G93.40)

EXCLUDES 2   acute transverse myelitis (G37.3-)
alcoholic encephalopathy (G31.2)
~~benign myalgic encephalomyelitis (G93.3)~~
multiple sclerosis (G35)
▶myalgic encephalomyelitis (G93.32)◀
subacute necrotizing myelitis (G37.4)
toxic encephalitis (G92.8)
toxic encephalopathy (G92.8)

DEF: Encephalitis: Inflammation of the brain, often caused by viral or bacterial infection.
DEF: Encephalomyelitis: Inflammatory disease, often viral in nature, that affects the brain and spinal cord.
DEF: Myelitis: Inflammation of the spinal cord.

✓5ᵗʰ G04.0 Acute disseminated encephalitis and encephalomyelitis (ADEM)

EXCLUDES 1   acute necrotizing hemorrhagic encephalopathy (G04.3-)
other noninfectious acute disseminated encephalomyelitis (noninfectious ADEM) (G04.81)

G04.00 Acute disseminated encephalitis and encephalomyelitis, unspecified   COM

G04.01 Postinfectious acute disseminated encephalitis and encephalomyelitis (postinfectious ADEM)   COM

EXCLUDES 1   post chickenpox encephalitis (B01.1)
post measles encephalitis (B05.0)
post measles myelitis (B05.1)

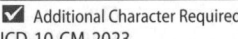

G04.02 **Postimmunization** **acute disseminated encephalitis, myelitis and encephalomyelitis** `COM`
Encephalitis, post immunization
Encephalomyelitis, post immunization
Use additional code to identify the vaccine (T50.A-, T50.B-, T50.Z-)

G04.1 **Tropical spastic paraplegia** `HCC` `Rx` `ESR` `COM`

G04.2 **Bacterial meningoencephalitis and meningomyelitis, not elsewhere classified** `COM`

✓5ᵗʰ **G04.3** **Acute necrotizing hemorrhagic encephalopathy**

EXCLUDES 1 *acute disseminated encephalitis and encephalomyelitis (G04.0-)*

G04.30 **Acute necrotizing hemorrhagic encephalopathy, unspecified** `COM`

G04.31 **Postinfectious** **acute necrotizing hemorrhagic encephalopathy** `COM`

G04.32 **Postimmunization** **acute necrotizing hemorrhagic encephalopathy** `COM`
Use additional code to identify the vaccine (T50.A-, T50.B-, T50.Z-)

G04.39 **Other acute necrotizing hemorrhagic encephalopathy** `COM`
Code also underlying etiology, if applicable

✓5ᵗʰ **G04.8** **Other encephalitis, myelitis and encephalomyelitis**
Code also any associated seizure (G40.-, R56.9)

G04.81 **Other encephalitis and encephalomyelitis** `COM`
Noninfectious acute disseminated encephalomyelitis (noninfectious ADEM)

G04.82 **Acute flaccid myelitis** `HCC` `Rx` `ESR` `COM`
EXCLUDES 1 *transverse myelitis (G37.3)*
AHA: 2021,4Q,11

G04.89 **Other myelitis** `HCC` `Rx` `ESR` `COM`
AHA: 2020,1Q,14

✓5ᵗʰ **G04.9** **Encephalitis, myelitis and encephalomyelitis, unspecified**

G04.90 **Encephalitis and encephalomyelitis, unspecified** `COM`
Ventriculitis (cerebral) NOS

G04.91 **Myelitis, unspecified** `HCC` `Rx` `ESR` `COM`

✓4ᵗʰ **G05** **Encephalitis, myelitis and encephalomyelitis in diseases classified elsewhere**
Code first underlying disease, such as:
congenital toxoplasmosis encephalitis, myelitis and encephalomyelitis (P37.1)
cytomegaloviral encephalitis, myelitis and encephalomyelitis (B25.8)
encephalitis, myelitis and encephalomyelitis (in) systemic lupus erythematosus (M32.19)
eosinophilic meningoencephalitis (B83.2)
human immunodeficiency virus [HIV] disease (B20)
poliovirus (A80.-)
suppurative otitis media (H66.01-H66.4)
trichinellosis (B75)

EXCLUDES 1 *adenoviral encephalitis, myelitis and encephalomyelitis (A85.1)*
encephalitis, myelitis and encephalomyelitis (in) measles (B05.0)
enteroviral encephalitis, myelitis and encephalomyelitis (A85.0)
herpesviral [herpes simplex] encephalitis, myelitis and encephalomyelitis (B00.4)
listerial encephalitis, myelitis and encephalomyelitis (A32.12)
meningococcal encephalitis, myelitis and encephalomyelitis (A39.81)
mumps encephalitis, myelitis and encephalomyelitis (B26.2)
postchickenpox encephalitis, myelitis and encephalomyelitis (B01.1-)
rubella encephalitis, myelitis and encephalomyelitis (B06.01)
toxoplasmosis encephalitis, myelitis and encephalomyelitis (B58.2)
zoster encephalitis, myelitis and encephalomyelitis (B02.0)

G05.3 *Encephalitis and encephalomyelitis in diseases classified elsewhere* `COM`
Meningoencephalitis in diseases classified elsewhere

G05.4 *Myelitis in diseases classified elsewhere* `HCC` `Rx` `ESR` `COM`
Meningomyelitis in diseases classified elsewhere

✓4ᵗʰ **G06** **Intracranial and intraspinal abscess and granuloma**
Use additional code (B95-B97) to identify infectious agent
DEF: Abscess: Circumscribed collection of pus resulting from bacteria, frequently associated with swelling and other signs of inflammation.
DEF: Granuloma: Abnormal, dense collections of cells forming a mass or nodule of chronically inflamed tissue with granulations that is usually associated with an infective process.

G06.0 **Intracranial** **abscess and granuloma** `COM`
Brain [any part] abscess (embolic)
Cerebellar abscess (embolic)
Cerebral abscess (embolic)
Intracranial epidural abscess or granuloma
Intracranial extradural abscess or granuloma
Intracranial subdural abscess or granuloma
Otogenic abscess (embolic)
EXCLUDES 1 *tuberculous intracranial abscess and granuloma (A17.81)*

G06.1 **Intraspinal** **abscess and granuloma** `COM`
Abscess (embolic) of spinal cord [any part]
Intraspinal epidural abscess or granuloma
Intraspinal extradural abscess or granuloma
Intraspinal subdural abscess or granuloma
EXCLUDES 1 *tuberculous intraspinal abscess and granuloma (A17.81)*

G06.2 **Extradural and subdural abscess, unspecified** `COM`

G07 *Intracranial and intraspinal abscess and granuloma in diseases classified elsewhere* `COM`
Code first underlying disease, such as:
schistosomiasis granuloma of brain (B65.-)
EXCLUDES 1 *abscess of brain:*
amebic (A06.6)
chromomycotic (B43.1)
gonococcal (A54.82)
tuberculous (A17.81)
tuberculoma of meninges (A17.1)

G08 **Intracranial and intraspinal phlebitis and thrombophlebitis** `COM`
Septic embolism of intracranial or intraspinal venous sinuses and veins
Septic endophlebitis of intracranial or intraspinal venous sinuses and veins
Septic phlebitis of intracranial or intraspinal venous sinuses and veins
Septic thrombophlebitis of intracranial or intraspinal venous sinuses and veins
Septic thrombosis of intracranial or intraspinal venous sinuses and veins
EXCLUDES 1 *intracranial phlebitis and thrombophlebitis complicating:*
abortion, ectopic or molar pregnancy (O00-O07, O08.7)
pregnancy, childbirth and the puerperium (O22.5, O87.3)
nonpyogenic intracranial phlebitis and thrombophlebitis (I67.6)
EXCLUDES 2 *intracranial phlebitis and thrombophlebitis complicating nonpyogenic intraspinal phlebitis and thrombophlebitis (G95.1)*
DEF: Inflammation and formation of a blood clot in a vein within the brain or spine, or their linings.

G09 **Sequelae of inflammatory diseases of central nervous system**
NOTE Category G09 is to be used to indicate conditions whose primary classification is to G00-G08 as the cause of sequelae, themselves classifiable elsewhere. The "sequelae" include conditions specified as residuals.
Code first condition resulting from (sequela) of inflammatory diseases of central nervous system

Systemic atrophies primarily affecting the central nervous system (G10-G14)

G10 Huntington's disease HCC Rx ESR COM
Huntington's chorea
Huntington's dementia
▶Use additional code, if applicable, to identify:◀
▶dementia with anxiety (F02.84, F02.A4, F02.B4, F02.C4)◀
▶dementia with behavioral disturbance (F02.81-, F02.A1-, F02.B1-, F02.C1-)◀
▶dementia with mood disturbance (F02.83, F02.A3, F02.B3, F02.C3)◀
▶dementia with psychotic disturbance (F02.82, F02.A2, F02.B2, F02.C2)◀
▶dementia without behavioral disturbance (F02.80, F02.A0, F02.B0, F02.C0)◀
▶mild neurocognitive disorder due to known physiological condition (F06.7-)◀
Code also dementia in other diseases classified elsewhere without behavioral disturbance (F02.80)
DEF: Genetic disease caused by degeneration of nerve cells in the brain, characterized by chronic progressive mental deterioration. Dementia and death occur within 15 to 20 years of onset.

✓4ᵗʰ G11 Hereditary ataxia
EXCLUDES 2   cerebral palsy (G80.-)
hereditary and idiopathic neuropathy (G60.-)
metabolic disorders (E70-E88)
DEF: Ataxia: Defect in muscular control or coordination due to a central nervous system disorder, particularly when voluntary muscular movements are attempted.
G11.0 Congenital nonprogressive ataxia HCC ESR COM
✓5ᵗʰ G11.1 Early-onset cerebellar ataxia
AHA: 2020,4Q,17-18
G11.10 Early-onset cerebellar ataxia, unspecified HCC ESR COM
G11.11 Friedreich ataxia HCC ESR COM
Autosomal recessive Friedreich ataxia
Friedreich ataxia with retained reflexes
G11.19 Other early-onset cerebellar ataxia HCC ESR COM
Early-onset cerebellar ataxia with essential tremor
Early-onset cerebellar ataxia with myoclonus [Hunt's ataxia]
Early-onset cerebellar ataxia with retained tendon reflexes
X-linked recessive spinocerebellar ataxia
G11.2 Late-onset cerebellar ataxia HCC ESR COM A
G11.3 Cerebellar ataxia with defective DNA repair HCC ESR COM
Ataxia telangiectasia [Louis-Bar]
EXCLUDES 2   Cockayne's syndrome (Q87.19)
other disorders of purine and pyrimidine metabolism (E79.-)
xeroderma pigmentosum (Q82.1)
G11.4 Hereditary spastic paraplegia HCC ESR COM
G11.8 Other hereditary ataxias HCC ESR COM
G11.9 Hereditary ataxia, unspecified HCC ESR COM
Hereditary cerebellar ataxia NOS
Hereditary cerebellar degeneration
Hereditary cerebellar disease
Hereditary cerebellar syndrome

✓4ᵗʰ G12 Spinal muscular atrophy and related syndromes
G12.0 Infantile spinal muscular atrophy, type I [Werdnig-Hoffman] HCC Rx ESR COM
G12.1 Other inherited spinal muscular atrophy HCC Rx ESR COM
Adult form spinal muscular atrophy
Childhood form, type II spinal muscular atrophy
Distal spinal muscular atrophy
Juvenile form, type III spinal muscular atrophy [Kugelberg-Welander]
Progressive bulbar palsy of childhood [Fazio-Londe]
Scapuloperoneal form spinal muscular atrophy
✓5ᵗʰ G12.2 Motor neuron disease
AHA: 2017,4Q,9-10
G12.20 Motor neuron disease, unspecified HCC Rx ESR COM
G12.21 Amyotrophic lateral sclerosis HCC Rx ESR COM A
G12.22 Progressive bulbar palsy HCC Rx ESR COM
G12.23 Primary lateral sclerosis HCC Rx ESR COM
G12.24 Familial motor neuron disease HCC Rx ESR COM
G12.25 Progressive spinal muscle atrophy HCC Rx ESR COM
G12.29 Other motor neuron disease HCC Rx ESR COM
G12.8 Other spinal muscular atrophies and related syndromes HCC Rx ESR COM
G12.9 Spinal muscular atrophy, unspecified HCC Rx ESR COM

✓4ᵗʰ G13 Systemic atrophies primarily affecting central nervous system in diseases classified elsewhere
G13.0 Paraneoplastic neuromyopathy and neuropathy HCC Rx ESR COM
Carcinomatous neuromyopathy
Sensorial paraneoplastic neuropathy [Denny Brown]
Code first underlying neoplasm (C00-D49)
G13.1 Other systemic atrophy primarily affecting central nervous system in neoplastic disease HCC Rx ESR COM
Paraneoplastic limbic encephalopathy
Code first underlying neoplasm (C00-D49)
G13.2 Systemic atrophy primarily affecting the central nervous system in myxedema HCC Rx ESR
Code first underlying disease, such as:
hypothyroidism (E03.-)
myxedematous congenital iodine deficiency (E00.1)
G13.8 Systemic atrophy primarily affecting central nervous system in other diseases classified elsewhere HCC Rx ESR
Code first underlying disease

G14 Postpolio syndrome
INCLUDES   postpolio myelitic syndrome
EXCLUDES 1   sequelae of poliomyelitis (B91)

Extrapyramidal and movement disorders (G20-G26)

G20 Parkinson's disease HCC Rx ESR COM
Hemiparkinsonism
Idiopathic Parkinsonism or Parkinson's disease
Paralysis agitans
Parkinsonism or Parkinson's disease NOS
Primary Parkinsonism or Parkinson's disease
▶Use additional code, if applicable, to identify:◀
▶dementia with anxiety (F02.84, F02.A4, F02.B4, F02.C4)◀
dementia with behavioral disturbance ▶(F02.81-, F02.A1-, F02.B1-, F02.C1-)◀
▶dementia with mood disturbance (F02.83, F02.A3, F02.B3, F02.C3)◀
▶dementia with psychotic disturbance (F02.82, F02.A2, F02.B2, F02.C2)◀
dementia without behavioral disturbance ▶(F02.80, F02.A0, F02.B0, F02.C0)◀
▶mild neurocognitive disorder due to known physiological condition (F06.7-)◀
EXCLUDES 1   dementia with Parkinsonism (G31.83)
AHA: 2017,2Q,7; 2016,2Q,6
TIP: Repeated falls (R29.6) are not integral to Parkinson's disease and can be separately coded.

✓4ᵗʰ G21 Secondary parkinsonism
EXCLUDES 1   dementia with Parkinsonism (G31.83)
Huntington's disease (G10)
Shy-Drager syndrome (G90.3)
syphilitic Parkinsonism (A52.19)
G21.0 Malignant neuroleptic syndrome
Use additional code for adverse effect, if applicable, to identify drug (T43.3X5, T43.4X5, T43.505, T43.595)
EXCLUDES 1   neuroleptic induced parkinsonism (G21.11)
✓5ᵗʰ G21.1 Other drug-induced secondary parkinsonism
G21.11 Neuroleptic induced parkinsonism HCC Rx ESR COM
Use additional code for adverse effect, if applicable, to identify drug (T43.3X5, T43.4X5, T43.505, T43.595)
EXCLUDES 1   malignant neuroleptic syndrome (G21.0)
G21.19 Other drug induced secondary parkinsonism HCC Rx ESR COM
Other medication-induced parkinsonism
Use additional code for adverse effect, if applicable, to identify drug (T36-T50 with fifth or sixth character 5)

G21.2 Secondary parkinsonism due to other external agents `HCC` `Rx` `ESR` `COM`
Code first (T51-T65) to identify external agent

G21.3 Postencephalitic **parkinsonism** `HCC` `Rx` `ESR` `COM`

G21.4 Vascular **parkinsonism** `HCC` `Rx` `ESR` `COM`

G21.8 Other secondary parkinsonism `HCC` `Rx` `ESR` `COM`

G21.9 Secondary parkinsonism, unspecified `HCC` `Rx` `ESR` `COM`

✓4ᵗʰ **G23** Other degenerative diseases of basal ganglia
> `EXCLUDES 2` *multi-system degeneration of the autonomic nervous system (G90.3)*

G23.0 Hallervorden-Spatz disease `HCC` `Rx` `ESR` `COM`
Pigmentary pallidal degeneration

G23.1 Progressive supranuclear ophthalmoplegia [Steele-Richardson-Olszewski] `HCC` `Rx` `ESR` `COM`
Progressive supranuclear palsy

G23.2 Striatonigral degeneration `HCC` `Rx` `ESR` `COM`

G23.8 Other specified degenerative diseases of basal ganglia `HCC` `Rx` `ESR` `COM`
Calcification of basal ganglia

G23.9 Degenerative disease of basal ganglia, unspecified `HCC` `Rx` `ESR` `COM`

✓4ᵗʰ **G24** Dystonia
> `INCLUDES` dyskinesia
> `EXCLUDES 2` *athetoid cerebral palsy (G80.3)*

DEF: Disorder of abnormal muscle tone, excessive or inadequate. Involuntary movements and prolonged muscle contractions result in tremors, abnormalities in posture, and twisting body motions that affect an isolated area or the whole body.

✓5ᵗʰ **G24.0** Drug induced **dystonia**
Use additional code for adverse effect, if applicable, to identify drug (T36-T50 with fifth or sixth character 5)

G24.01 Drug induced subacute dyskinesia
Drug induced blepharospasm
Drug induced orofacial dyskinesia
Neuroleptic induced tardive dyskinesia
Tardive dyskinesia

G24.02 Drug induced acute dystonia
Acute dystonic reaction to drugs
Neuroleptic induced acute dystonia

G24.09 Other drug induced dystonia

G24.1 Genetic torsion **dystonia**
Dystonia deformans progressiva
Dystonia musculorum deformans
Familial torsion dystonia
Idiopathic familial dystonia
Idiopathic (torsion) dystonia NOS
(Schwalbe-) Ziehen-Oppenheim disease

G24.2 Idiopathic nonfamilial **dystonia**

G24.3 Spasmodic torticollis
> `EXCLUDES 1` *congenital torticollis (Q68.0)*
> *hysterical torticollis (F44.4)*
> *ocular torticollis (R29.891)*
> *psychogenic torticollis (F45.8)*
> *torticollis NOS (M43.6)*
> *traumatic recurrent torticollis (S13.4)*

DEF: Twisted, unnatural position of the neck due to contracted cervical muscles that pull the head to one side or cause involuntary shaking of the head.

G24.4 Idiopathic orofacial **dystonia**
Orofacial dyskinesia
> `EXCLUDES 1` *drug induced orofacial dyskinesia (G24.01)*

G24.5 Blepharospasm
> `EXCLUDES 1` *drug induced blepharospasm (G24.01)*

DEF: Involuntary contraction of the orbicularis oculi muscle, resulting in the eyelids being completely closed.

G24.8 Other dystonia
Acquired torsion dystonia NOS

G24.9 Dystonia, unspecified
Dyskinesia NOS

✓4ᵗʰ **G25** Other extrapyramidal and movement disorders
> `EXCLUDES 2` *sleep related movement disorders (G47.6-)*

G25.0 Essential tremor
Familial tremor
> `EXCLUDES 1` *tremor NOS (R25.1)*

G25.1 Drug-induced **tremor**
Use additional code for adverse effect, if applicable, to identify drug (T36-T50 with fifth or sixth character 5)

G25.2 Other specified forms of tremor
Intention tremor

G25.3 Myoclonus
Drug-induced myoclonus
Palatal myoclonus
Use additional code for adverse effect, if applicable, to identify drug (T36-T50 with fifth or sixth character 5)
> `EXCLUDES 1` *facial myokymia (G51.4)*
> *myoclonic epilepsy (G40.-)*

DEF: Spasmodic, brief, involuntary muscle contractions that can be due to an undetermined etiology, drug-induced, or caused by a disease process.

G25.4 Drug-induced chorea
Use additional code for adverse effect, if applicable, to identify drug (T36-T50 with fifth or sixth character 5)

G25.5 Other chorea
Chorea NOS
> `EXCLUDES 1` *chorea NOS with heart involvement (I02.0)*
> *Huntington's chorea (G10)*
> *rheumatic chorea (I02.-)*
> *Sydenham's chorea (I02.-)*

✓5ᵗʰ **G25.6** Drug induced tics and other tics of organic origin

G25.61 Drug induced tics
Use additional code for adverse effect, if applicable, to identify drug (T36-T50 with fifth or sixth character 5)

G25.69 Other tics of organic origin
> `EXCLUDES 1` *habit spasm (F95.9)*
> *tic NOS (F95.9)*
> *Tourette's syndrome (F95.2)*

✓5ᵗʰ **G25.7** Other and unspecified drug induced movement disorders
Use additional code for adverse effect, if applicable, to identify drug (T36-T50 with fifth or sixth character 5)

G25.70 Drug induced movement disorder, unspecified

G25.71 Drug induced akathisia
Drug induced acathisia
Neuroleptic induced acute akathisia
Tardive akathisia

G25.79 Other drug induced movement disorders

✓5ᵗʰ **G25.8** Other specified extrapyramidal and movement disorders

G25.81 Restless legs syndrome
DEF: Neurological disorder of unknown etiology creating an irresistible urge to move the legs, which may temporarily relieve the symptoms. This syndrome is accompanied by motor restlessness and sensations of pain, burning, prickling, or tingling.

G25.82 Stiff-man syndrome

G25.83 Benign shuddering attacks

G25.89 Other specified extrapyramidal and movement disorders

G25.9 Extrapyramidal and movement disorder, unspecified

G26 *Extrapyramidal and movement disorders in diseases classified elsewhere*
Code first underlying disease

`HCC` CMS-HCC   `Rx` Rx HCC   `ESR` ESRD HCC   `COM` Commercial HCC   `N` Newborn: 0   `P` Pediatric: 0-17   `M` Maternity: 9-64   `A` Adult: 15-124

592   ICD-10-CM 2023

Other degenerative diseases of the nervous system (G30-G32)

✅4ᵗʰ G30 Alzheimer's disease

INCLUDES   Alzheimer's dementia senile and presenile forms

▶Use additional code, if applicable, to identify:◀

delirium, if applicable (F05)

▶dementia with anxiety (F02.84, F02.A4, F02.B4, F02.C4)◀

dementia with behavioral disturbance ▶(F02.81-, F02.A1-, F02.B1-, F02.C1-)◀

▶dementia with mood disturbance (F02.83, F02.A3, F02.B3, F02.C3)◀

▶dementia with psychotic disturbance (F02.82, F02.A2, F02.B2, F02.C2)◀

dementia without behavioral disturbance ▶(F02.80, F02.A0, F02.B0, F02.C0)◀

▶mild neurocognitive disorder due to known physiological condition (F06.7-)◀

EXCLUDES 1   *senile degeneration of brain NEC (G31.1)*

senile dementia NOS (F03)

senility NOS (R41.81)

AHA: 2017,1Q,43

TIP: A code from subcategory F02.8 should always be assigned with a code from this category, even in the absence of documented dementia.

TIP: Functional quadriplegia (R53.2) is not integral to Alzheimer's disease and can be coded in addition to codes from category G30.

G30.0 Alzheimer's disease with early onset   HCC Rx ESR

G30.1 Alzheimer's disease with late onset   HCC Rx ESR A

G30.8 Other Alzheimer's disease   HCC Rx ESR

G30.9 Alzheimer's disease, unspecified   HCC Rx ESR

       AHA: 2016,2Q,6; 2012,4Q,95

✅4ᵗʰ G31 Other degenerative diseases of nervous system, not elsewhere classified

For codes G31.0 - G31.83, G31.85 - G31.9, use additional code, if applicable, to identify:

▶dementia with anxiety (F02.84, F02.A4, F02.B4, F02.C4)◀

dementia with behavioral disturbance ▶(F02.81-, F02.A1-, F02.B1-, F02.C1-)◀

▶dementia with mood disturbance (F02.83, F02.A3, F02.B3, F02.C3)◀

▶dementia with psychotic disturbance (F02.82, F02.A2, F02.B2, F02.C2)◀

dementia without behavioral disturbance ▶(F02.80, F02.A0, F02.B0, F02.C0)◀

▶mild neurocognitive disorder due to known physiological condition (F06.7-)◀

EXCLUDES 2   *Reye's syndrome (G93.7)*

✅5ᵗʰ G31.0 Frontotemporal dementia

G31.01 Pick's disease   HCC Rx ESR

Primary progressive aphasia

Progressive isolated aphasia

DEF: Progressive frontotemporal dementia with asymmetrical atrophy of the frontal and temporal regions of the cerebral cortex and abnormal rounded brain cells called Pick cells with the presence of abnormal staining of protein (called tau). Symptoms include prominent apathy, behavioral changes such as disinhibition and restlessness, echolalia, impairment of language, memory, and intellect, increased carelessness, poor personal hygiene, and decreased attention span.

▲ G31.09 Other frontotemporal neurocognitive disorder   HCC Rx ESR

Frontal dementia

▶Use additional code, if applicable, to identify mild neurocognitive disorders due to known physiological condition (F06.7-)◀

G31.1 Senile degeneration of brain, not elsewhere classified   HCC Rx ESR

EXCLUDES 1   *Alzheimer's disease (G30.-)*

senility NOS (R41.81)

G31.2 Degeneration of nervous system due to alcohol   HCC Rx ESR

Alcoholic cerebellar ataxia

Alcoholic cerebellar degeneration

Alcoholic cerebral degeneration

Alcoholic encephalopathy

Dysfunction of the autonomic nervous system due to alcohol

Code also associated alcoholism (F10.-)

✅5ᵗʰ G31.8 Other specified degenerative diseases of nervous system

G31.81 Alpers disease   HCC Rx ESR COM

Grey-matter degeneration

G31.82 Leigh's disease   HCC Rx ESR COM

Subacute necrotizing encephalopathy

▲ G31.83 Neurocognitive disorder with Lewy bodies   HCC Rx ESR

~~Dementia with Parkinsonism~~

Lewy body dementia

Lewy body disease

▶Use additional code, if applicable, to identify mild neurocognitive disorders due to known physiological condition (F06.7-)◀

AHA: 2017,2Q,7; 2016,4Q,141

DEF: Cerebral dementia with neurophysiologic changes, increased hippocampal volume, hypoperfusion in the occipital lobes, beta amyloid deposits with neurofibrillary tangles, and atrophy of the cortex and brainstem. Hallmark neuropsychological characteristics include fluctuating cognition with pronounced variation in attention and alertness, recurrent hallucinations, and Parkinsonism.

▲ G31.84 Mild cognitive impairment of uncertain or unknown etiology

▶Mild cognitive disorder NOS◀

~~Mild neurocognitive disorder~~

▶Mild neurocognitive disorder of uncertain or unknown etiology◀

▶Use additional code to identify presence of:◀

▶alcohol abuse and dependence (F10.-)◀

▶exposure to environmental tobacco smoke (Z77.22)◀

▶history of tobacco dependence (Z87.891)◀

▶hypertension (I10-I16)◀

▶occupational exposure to environmental tobacco smoke (Z57.31)◀

▶tobacco dependence (F17.-)◀

▶tobacco use (Z72.0)◀

EXCLUDES 1   *age related cognitive decline (R41.81)*

altered mental status (R41.82)

cerebral degeneration (G31.9)

▶*cerebrovascular diseases (I60-I69)*◀

change in mental status (R41.82)

cognitive deficits following (sequelae of) cerebral hemorrhage or infarction (I69.0-, I69.11-, I69.21-, I69.31-, I69.81-, I69.91-)

cognitive impairment due to intracranial or head injury (S06.-)

dementia (F01.-, F02.-, F03)

~~*mild memory disturbance (F06.8)*~~

▶*mild neurocognitive disorder due to a known physiological condition (F06.7-)*◀

neurologic neglect syndrome (R41.4)

personality change, nonpsychotic (F68.8)

AHA: 2021,3Q,3

G31.85 Corticobasal degeneration   HCC Rx ESR

G31.89 Other specified degenerative diseases of nervous system   HCC Rx ESR

G31.9 Degenerative disease of nervous system, unspecified   HCC Rx ESR

AHA: 2021,3Q,3

✅4ᵗʰ G32 Other degenerative disorders of nervous system in diseases classified elsewhere

G32.0 *Subacute combined degeneration of spinal cord in diseases classified elsewhere*   HCC Rx ESR COM

Dana-Putnam syndrome

Sclerosis of spinal cord (combined) (dorsolateral) (posterolateral)

Code first underlying disease, such as:

anemia (D51.9)

dietary (D51.3)

pernicious (D51.0)

vitamin B12 deficiency (E53.8)

EXCLUDES 1   *syphilitic combined degeneration of spinal cord (A52.11)*

☑5ᵗʰ **G32.8 Other specified degenerative disorders of nervous system in diseases classified elsewhere**
Code first underlying disease, such as:
amyloidosis cerebral degeneration (E85.-)
cerebral degeneration (due to) hypothyroidism (E00.0-E03.9)
cerebral degeneration (due to) neoplasm (C00-D49)
cerebral degeneration (due to) vitamin B deficiency, except thiamine (E52-E53.-)

EXCLUDES 1   *superior hemorrhagic polioencephalitis [Wernicke's encephalopathy] (E51.2)*

G32.81 *Cerebellar ataxia in diseases classified elsewhere*   HCC ESR COM
Code first underlying disease, such as:
celiac disease (with gluten ataxia) (K90.0)
cerebellar ataxia (in) neoplastic disease (paraneoplastic cerebellar degeneration) (C00-D49)
non-celiac gluten ataxia (M35.9)

EXCLUDES 1   *systemic atrophy primarily affecting the central nervous system in alcoholic cerebellar ataxia (G31.2)*
systemic atrophy primarily affecting the central nervous system in myxedema (G13.2)

G32.89 *Other specified degenerative disorders of nervous system in diseases classified elsewhere*
Degenerative encephalopathy in diseases classified elsewhere

Demyelinating diseases of the central nervous system (G35-G37)

G35 Multiple sclerosis   HCC Rx ESR COM
Disseminated multiple sclerosis
Generalized multiple sclerosis
Multiple sclerosis NOS
Multiple sclerosis of brain stem
Multiple sclerosis of cord
AHA: 2021,1Q,7

☑4ᵗʰ **G36 Other acute disseminated demyelination**

EXCLUDES 1   *postinfectious encephalitis and encephalomyelitis NOS (G04.01)*

DEF: Demyelination: Abnormal loss of myelin, the protective white matter that insulates nerve endings and facilitates neuroreception and neurotransmission. When this substance is damaged, the nerve is short-circuited, resulting in impaired or loss of function.

G36.0 Neuromyelitis optica [Devic]   HCC Rx ESR COM
Demyelination in optic neuritis

EXCLUDES 1   *optic neuritis NOS (H46)*

G36.1 Acute and subacute hemorrhagic leukoencephalitis [Hurst]   HCC ESR

G36.8 Other specified acute disseminated demyelination   HCC ESR

G36.9 Acute disseminated demyelination, unspecified   HCC ESR

☑4ᵗʰ **G37 Other demyelinating diseases of central nervous system**

G37.0 Diffuse sclerosis of central nervous system   HCC Rx ESR COM
Periaxial encephalitis
Schilder's disease

EXCLUDES 1   *X linked adrenoleukodystrophy (E71.52-)*

G37.1 Central demyelination of corpus callosum   HCC ESR

G37.2 Central pontine myelinolysis   HCC ESR
AHA: 2022,2Q,10

G37.3 Acute transverse myelitis in demyelinating disease of central nervous system   HCC Rx ESR COM
Acute transverse myelitis NOS
Acute transverse myelopathy

EXCLUDES 1   *acute flaccid myelitis (G04.82)*
multiple sclerosis (G35)
neuromyelitis optica [Devic] (G36.0)

G37.4 Subacute necrotizing myelitis of central nervous system   HCC Rx ESR COM

G37.5 Concentric sclerosis [Balo] of central nervous system   HCC Rx ESR COM

G37.8 Other specified demyelinating diseases of central nervous system   HCC ESR

G37.9 Demyelinating disease of central nervous system, unspecified   HCC ESR

Episodic and paroxysmal disorders (G40-G47)

☑4ᵗʰ **G40 Epilepsy and recurrent seizures**

NOTE   The following terms are to be considered equivalent to intractable: pharmacoresistant (pharmacologically resistant), treatment resistant, refractory (medically) and poorly controlled

EXCLUDES 1   *conversion disorder with seizures (F44.5)*
convulsions NOS (R56.9)
post traumatic seizures (R56.1)
seizure (convulsive) NOS (R56.9)
seizure of newborn (P90)

EXCLUDES 2   *hippocampal sclerosis (G93.81)*
mesial temporal sclerosis (G93.81)
temporal sclerosis (G93.81)
Todd's paralysis (G83.84)

☑5ᵗʰ **G40.0 Localization-related (focal) (partial) idiopathic epilepsy and epileptic syndromes with seizures of localized onset**
Benign childhood epilepsy with centrotemporal EEG spikes
Childhood epilepsy with occipital EEG paroxysms

EXCLUDES 1   *adult onset localization-related epilepsy (G40.1-, G40.2-)*

☑6ᵗʰ **G40.00 Localization-related (focal) (partial) idiopathic epilepsy and epileptic syndromes with seizures of localized onset, not intractable**
Localization-related (focal) (partial) idiopathic epilepsy and epileptic syndromes with seizures of localized onset without intractability

G40.001 Localization-related (focal) (partial) idiopathic epilepsy and epileptic syndromes with seizures of localized onset, not intractable, with status epilepticus   HCC Rx ESR COM

G40.009 Localization-related (focal) (partial) idiopathic epilepsy and epileptic syndromes with seizures of localized onset, not intractable, without status epilepticus   HCC Rx ESR COM
Localization-related (focal) (partial) idiopathic epilepsy and epileptic syndromes with seizures of localized onset NOS

☑6ᵗʰ **G40.01 Localization-related (focal) (partial) idiopathic epilepsy and epileptic syndromes with seizures of localized onset, intractable**

G40.011 Localization-related (focal) (partial) idiopathic epilepsy and epileptic syndromes with seizures of localized onset, intractable, with status epilepticus   HCC Rx ESR COM

G40.019 Localization-related (focal) (partial) idiopathic epilepsy and epileptic syndromes with seizures of localized onset, intractable, without status epilepticus   HCC Rx ESR COM

☑5ᵗʰ **G40.1 Localization-related (focal) (partial) symptomatic epilepsy and epileptic syndromes with simple partial seizures**
Attacks without alteration of consciousness
Epilepsia partialis continua [Kozhevnikof]
Simple partial seizures developing into secondarily generalized seizures

☑6ᵗʰ **G40.10 Localization-related (focal) (partial) symptomatic epilepsy and epileptic syndromes with simple partial seizures, not intractable**
Localization-related (focal) (partial) symptomatic epilepsy and epileptic syndromes with simple partial seizures without intractability

G40.101 Localization-related (focal) (partial) symptomatic epilepsy and epileptic syndromes with simple partial seizures, not intractable, with status epilepticus   HCC Rx ESR COM

G40.109 **Localization-related (focal) (partial) symptomatic epilepsy and epileptic syndromes with simple partial seizures, not intractable, without status epilepticus** `HCC` `Rx` `ESR` `COM`

Localization-related (focal) (partial) symptomatic epilepsy and epileptic syndromes with simple partial seizures NOS

✓6ᵗʰ **G40.11** **Localization-related (focal) (partial) symptomatic epilepsy and epileptic syndromes with simple partial seizures, intractable**

G40.111 **Localization-related (focal) (partial) symptomatic epilepsy and epileptic syndromes with simple partial seizures, intractable, with status epilepticus** `HCC` `Rx` `ESR` `COM`

G40.119 **Localization-related (focal) (partial) symptomatic epilepsy and epileptic syndromes with simple partial seizures, intractable, without status epilepticus** `HCC` `Rx` `ESR` `COM`

✓5ᵗʰ **G40.2** **Localization-related (focal) (partial) symptomatic epilepsy and epileptic syndromes with complex partial seizures**

Attacks with alteration of consciousness, often with automatisms

Complex partial seizures developing into secondarily generalized seizures

✓6ᵗʰ **G40.20** **Localization-related (focal) (partial) symptomatic epilepsy and epileptic syndromes with complex partial seizures, not intractable**

Localization-related (focal) (partial) symptomatic epilepsy and epileptic syndromes with complex partial seizures without intractability

G40.201 **Localization-related (focal) (partial) symptomatic epilepsy and epileptic syndromes with complex partial seizures, not intractable, with status epilepticus** `HCC` `Rx` `ESR` `COM`

G40.209 **Localization-related (focal) (partial) symptomatic epilepsy and epileptic syndromes with complex partial seizures, not intractable, without status epilepticus** `HCC` `Rx` `ESR` `COM`

Localization-related (focal) (partial) symptomatic epilepsy and epileptic syndromes with complex partial seizures NOS

✓6ᵗʰ **G40.21** **Localization-related (focal) (partial) symptomatic epilepsy and epileptic syndromes with complex partial seizures, intractable**

G40.211 **Localization-related (focal) (partial) symptomatic epilepsy and epileptic syndromes with complex partial seizures, intractable, with status epilepticus** `HCC` `Rx` `ESR` `COM`

G40.219 **Localization-related (focal) (partial) symptomatic epilepsy and epileptic syndromes with complex partial seizures, intractable, without status epilepticus** `HCC` `Rx` `ESR` `COM`

✓5ᵗʰ **G40.3** **Generalized idiopathic epilepsy and epileptic syndromes**

Code also MERRF syndrome, if applicable (E88.42)

✓6ᵗʰ **G40.30** **Generalized idiopathic epilepsy and epileptic syndromes, not intractable**

Generalized idiopathic epilepsy and epileptic syndromes without intractability

G40.301 **Generalized idiopathic epilepsy and epileptic syndromes, not intractable, with status epilepticus** `HCC` `Rx` `ESR` `COM`

G40.309 **Generalized idiopathic epilepsy and epileptic syndromes, not intractable, without status epilepticus** `HCC` `Rx` `ESR` `COM`

Generalized idiopathic epilepsy and epileptic syndromes NOS

✓6ᵗʰ **G40.31** **Generalized idiopathic epilepsy and epileptic syndromes, intractable**

G40.311 **Generalized idiopathic epilepsy and epileptic syndromes, intractable, with status epilepticus** `HCC` `Rx` `ESR` `COM`

G40.319 **Generalized idiopathic epilepsy and epileptic syndromes, intractable, without status epilepticus** `HCC` `Rx` `ESR` `COM`

✓5ᵗʰ **G40.A** **Absence epileptic syndrome**

Childhood absence epilepsy [pyknolepsy]
Juvenile absence epilepsy
Absence epileptic syndrome, NOS

✓6ᵗʰ **G40.A0** **Absence epileptic syndrome, not intractable**

G40.A01 **Absence epileptic syndrome, not intractable, with status epilepticus** `HCC` `Rx` `ESR` `COM`

G40.A09 **Absence epileptic syndrome, not intractable, without status epilepticus** `HCC` `Rx` `ESR` `COM`

✓6ᵗʰ **G40.A1** **Absence epileptic syndrome, intractable**

G40.A11 **Absence epileptic syndrome, intractable, with status epilepticus** `HCC` `Rx` `ESR` `COM`

G40.A19 **Absence epileptic syndrome, intractable, without status epilepticus** `HCC` `Rx` `ESR` `COM`

✓5ᵗʰ **G40.B** **Juvenile myoclonic epilepsy [impulsive petit mal]**

✓6ᵗʰ **G40.B0** **Juvenile myoclonic epilepsy, not intractable**

G40.B01 **Juvenile myoclonic epilepsy, not intractable, with status epilepticus** `HCC` `Rx` `ESR` `COM`

G40.B09 **Juvenile myoclonic epilepsy, not intractable, without status epilepticus** `HCC` `Rx` `ESR` `COM`

✓6ᵗʰ **G40.B1** **Juvenile myoclonic epilepsy, intractable**

G40.B11 **Juvenile myoclonic epilepsy, intractable, with status epilepticus** `HCC` `Rx` `ESR` `COM`

G40.B19 **Juvenile myoclonic epilepsy, intractable, without status epilepticus** `HCC` `Rx` `ESR` `COM`

✓5ᵗʰ **G40.4** **Other generalized epilepsy and epileptic syndromes**

Epilepsy with grand mal seizures on awakening
Epilepsy with myoclonic absences
Epilepsy with myoclonic-astatic seizures
Grand mal seizure NOS
Nonspecific atonic epileptic seizures
Nonspecific clonic epileptic seizures
Nonspecific myoclonic epileptic seizures
Nonspecific tonic epileptic seizures
Nonspecific tonic-clonic epileptic seizures
Symptomatic early myoclonic encephalopathy

✓6ᵗʰ **G40.40** **Other generalized epilepsy and epileptic syndromes, not intractable**

Other generalized epilepsy and epileptic syndromes without intractability

Other generalized epilepsy and epileptic syndromes NOS

G40.401 **Other generalized epilepsy and epileptic syndromes, not intractable, with status epilepticus** `HCC` `Rx` `ESR` `COM`

G40.409 **Other generalized epilepsy and epileptic syndromes, not intractable, without status epilepticus** `HCC` `Rx` `ESR` `COM`

✓6ᵗʰ **G40.41** **Other generalized epilepsy and epileptic syndromes, intractable**

G40.411 **Other generalized epilepsy and epileptic syndromes, intractable, with status epilepticus** `HCC` `Rx` `ESR` `COM`

G40.419 **Other generalized epilepsy and epileptic syndromes, intractable, without status epilepticus** `HCC` `Rx` `ESR` `COM`

G40.42 **Cyclin-Dependent Kinase-Like 5 Deficiency Disorder** `HCC` `Rx` `ESR` `COM`

CDKL5

Use additional code, if known, to identify associated manifestations, such as:
cortical blindness (H47.61-)
global development delay (F88)

AHA: 2020,4Q,18-19

√5ᵗʰ **G40.5 Epileptic seizures related to** external causes
Epileptic seizures related to alcohol
Epileptic seizures related to drugs
Epileptic seizures related to hormonal changes
Epileptic seizures related to sleep deprivation
Epileptic seizures related to stress
Code also, if applicable, associated epilepsy and recurrent seizures (G40.-)
Use additional code for adverse effect, if applicable, to identify drug (T36-T50 with fifth or sixth character 5)

√6ᵗʰ **G40.50 Epileptic seizures related to external causes,** not intractable
G40.501 Epileptic seizures related to external causes, not intractable, with status epilepticus HCC Rx ESR COM
G40.509 Epileptic seizures related to external causes, not intractable, without status epilepticus HCC Rx ESR COM
Epileptic seizures related to external causes, NOS

√5ᵗʰ **G40.8 Other epilepsy and recurrent seizures**
Epilepsies and epileptic syndromes undetermined as to whether they are focal or generalized
Landau-Kleffner syndrome

√6ᵗʰ **G40.80 Other epilepsy**
G40.801 Other epilepsy, not intractable, with status epilepticus HCC Rx ESR COM
Other epilepsy without intractability with status epilepticus
G40.802 Other epilepsy, not intractable, without status epilepticus HCC Rx ESR COM
Other epilepsy NOS
Other epilepsy without intractability without status epilepticus
G40.803 Other epilepsy, intractable, with status epilepticus HCC Rx ESR COM
G40.804 Other epilepsy, intractable, without status epilepticus HCC Rx ESR COM

√6ᵗʰ **G40.81 Lennox-Gastaut syndrome**
DEF: Severe form of epilepsy with usual onset in early childhood. Seizures are frequent and difficult to treat, causing falls and intellectual impairment.
G40.811 Lennox-Gastaut syndrome, not intractable, with status epilepticus HCC Rx ESR COM
G40.812 Lennox-Gastaut syndrome, not intractable, without status epilepticus HCC Rx ESR COM
G40.813 Lennox-Gastaut syndrome, intractable, with status epilepticus HCC Rx ESR COM
G40.814 Lennox-Gastaut syndrome, intractable, without status epilepticus HCC Rx ESR COM

√6ᵗʰ **G40.82 Epileptic spasms**
Infantile spasms
Salaam attacks
West's syndrome
G40.821 Epileptic spasms, not intractable, with status epilepticus HCC Rx ESR COM
G40.822 Epileptic spasms, not intractable, without status epilepticus HCC Rx ESR COM
G40.823 Epileptic spasms, intractable, with status epilepticus HCC Rx ESR COM
G40.824 Epileptic spasms, intractable, without status epilepticus HCC Rx ESR COM

√6ᵗʰ **G40.83 Dravet syndrome**
Polymorphic epilepsy in infancy (PMEI)
Severe myoclonic epilepsy in infancy (SMEI)
AHA: 2020,4Q,19
G40.833 Dravet syndrome, intractable, with status epilepticus HCC Rx ESR COM
G40.834 Dravet syndrome, intractable, without status epilepticus HCC Rx ESR COM
Dravet syndrome NOS

G40.89 Other seizures HCC Rx ESR COM
EXCLUDES 1 post traumatic seizures (R56.1)
recurrent seizures NOS (G40.909)
seizure NOS (R56.9)

√5ᵗʰ **G40.9 Epilepsy, unspecified**
AHA: 2019,1Q,19
√6ᵗʰ **G40.90 Epilepsy, unspecified,** not intractable
Epilepsy, unspecified, without intractability
G40.901 Epilepsy, unspecified, not intractable, with status epilepticus HCC Rx ESR COM
G40.909 Epilepsy, unspecified, not intractable, without status epilepticus HCC Rx ESR COM
Epilepsy NOS
Epileptic convulsions NOS
Epileptic fits NOS
Epileptic seizures NOS
Recurrent seizures NOS
Seizure disorder NOS
AHA: 2021,2Q,3; 2021,1Q,3

√6ᵗʰ **G40.91 Epilepsy, unspecified,** intractable
Intractable seizure disorder NOS
G40.911 Epilepsy, unspecified, intractable, with status epilepticus HCC Rx ESR COM
G40.919 Epilepsy, unspecified, intractable, without status epilepticus HCC Rx ESR COM

√4ᵗʰ **G43 Migraine**
NOTE The following terms are to be considered equivalent to intractable: pharmacoresistant (pharmacologically resistant), treatment resistant, refractory (medically) and poorly controlled
Use additional code for adverse effect, if applicable, to identify drug (T36-T50 with fifth or sixth character 5)
EXCLUDES 1 headache NOS (R51.9)
lower half migraine (G44.00)
EXCLUDES 2 headache syndromes (G44.-)
DEF: Headaches that occur periodically on one or both sides of the head that may be associated with nausea and vomiting, sensitivity to light and sound, dizziness, distorted vision, and cognitive disturbances.

√5ᵗʰ **G43.0 Migraine** without aura
Common migraine
EXCLUDES 1 chronic migraine without aura (G43.7-)
√6ᵗʰ **G43.00 Migraine without aura,** not intractable
Migraine without aura without mention of refractory migraine
G43.001 Migraine without aura, not intractable, with status migrainosus Rx
G43.009 Migraine without aura, not intractable, without status migrainosus Rx
Migraine without aura NOS
√6ᵗʰ **G43.01 Migraine without aura,** intractable
Migraine without aura with refractory migraine
G43.011 Migraine without aura, intractable, with status migrainosus Rx
G43.019 Migraine without aura, intractable, without status migrainosus Rx

√5ᵗʰ **G43.1 Migraine** with aura
Basilar migraine
Classical migraine
Migraine equivalents
Migraine preceded or accompanied by transient focal neurological phenomena
Migraine triggered seizures
Migraine with acute-onset aura
Migraine with aura without headache (migraine equivalents)
Migraine with prolonged aura
Migraine with typical aura
Retinal migraine
Code also any associated seizure (G40.-, R56.9)
EXCLUDES 1 persistent migraine aura (G43.5-, G43.6-)
√6ᵗʰ **G43.10 Migraine with aura,** not intractable
Migraine with aura without mention of refractory migraine
G43.101 Migraine with aura, not intractable, with status migrainosus Rx

G43.109 Migraine with aura, not intractable, without status migrainosus `Rx`
Migraine with aura NOS

✓6ᵗʰ **G43.11** Migraine with aura, intractable
Migraine with aura with refractory migraine

G43.111 Migraine with aura, intractable, with status migrainosus `Rx`

G43.119 Migraine with aura, intractable, without status migrainosus `Rx`

✓5ᵗʰ **G43.4** Hemiplegic migraine
Familial migraine
Sporadic migraine

✓6ᵗʰ **G43.40** Hemiplegic migraine, not intractable
Hemiplegic migraine without refractory migraine

G43.401 Hemiplegic migraine, not intractable, with status migrainosus `Rx`

G43.409 Hemiplegic migraine, not intractable, without status migrainosus `Rx`
Hemiplegic migraine NOS

✓6ᵗʰ **G43.41** Hemiplegic migraine, intractable
Hemiplegic migraine with refractory migraine

G43.411 Hemiplegic migraine, intractable, with status migrainosus `Rx`

G43.419 Hemiplegic migraine, intractable, without status migrainosus `Rx`

✓5ᵗʰ **G43.5** Persistent migraine aura without cerebral infarction

✓6ᵗʰ **G43.50** Persistent migraine aura without cerebral infarction, not intractable
Persistent migraine aura without cerebral infarction, without refractory migraine

G43.501 Persistent migraine aura without cerebral infarction, not intractable, with status migrainosus `Rx`

G43.509 Persistent migraine aura without cerebral infarction, not intractable, without status migrainosus `Rx`
Persistent migraine aura NOS

✓6ᵗʰ **G43.51** Persistent migraine aura without cerebral infarction, intractable
Persistent migraine aura without cerebral infarction, with refractory migraine

G43.511 Persistent migraine aura without cerebral infarction, intractable, with status migrainosus `Rx`

G43.519 Persistent migraine aura without cerebral infarction, intractable, without status migrainosus `Rx`

✓5ᵗʰ **G43.6** Persistent migraine aura with cerebral infarction
Code also the type of cerebral infarction (I63.-)

✓6ᵗʰ **G43.60** Persistent migraine aura with cerebral infarction, not intractable
Persistent migraine aura with cerebral infarction, without refractory migraine

G43.601 Persistent migraine aura with cerebral infarction, not intractable, with status migrainosus `Rx`

G43.609 Persistent migraine aura with cerebral infarction, not intractable, without status migrainosus `Rx`

✓6ᵗʰ **G43.61** Persistent migraine aura with cerebral infarction, intractable
Persistent migraine aura with cerebral infarction, with refractory migraine

G43.611 Persistent migraine aura with cerebral infarction, intractable, with status migrainosus `Rx`

G43.619 Persistent migraine aura with cerebral infarction, intractable, without status migrainosus `Rx`

✓5ᵗʰ **G43.7** Chronic migraine without aura
Transformed migraine
EXCLUDES 1 migraine without aura (G43.0-)

✓6ᵗʰ **G43.70** Chronic migraine without aura, not intractable
Chronic migraine without aura, without refractory migraine

G43.701 Chronic migraine without aura, not intractable, with status migrainosus `Rx`

G43.709 Chronic migraine without aura, not intractable, without status migrainosus `Rx`
Chronic migraine without aura NOS

✓6ᵗʰ **G43.71** Chronic migraine without aura, intractable
Chronic migraine without aura, with refractory migraine

G43.711 Chronic migraine without aura, intractable, with status migrainosus `Rx`

G43.719 Chronic migraine without aura, intractable, without status migrainosus `Rx`

✓5ᵗʰ **G43.A** Cyclical vomiting
EXCLUDES 1 cyclical vomiting syndrome unrelated to migraine (R11.15)
AHA: 2019,4Q,15

G43.A0 Cyclical vomiting, in migraine, not intractable `Rx`
Cyclical vomiting, without refractory migraine

G43.A1 Cyclical vomiting, in migraine, intractable `Rx`
Cyclical vomiting, with refractory migraine

✓5ᵗʰ **G43.B** Ophthalmoplegic migraine

G43.B0 Ophthalmoplegic migraine, not intractable `Rx`
Ophthalmoplegic migraine, without refractory migraine

G43.B1 Ophthalmoplegic migraine, intractable `Rx`
Ophthalmoplegic migraine, with refractory migraine

✓5ᵗʰ **G43.C** Periodic headache syndromes in child or adult

G43.C0 Periodic headache syndromes in child or adult, not intractable `Rx`
Periodic headache syndromes in child or adult, without refractory migraine

G43.C1 Periodic headache syndromes in child or adult, intractable `Rx`
Periodic headache syndromes in child or adult, with refractory migraine

✓5ᵗʰ **G43.D** Abdominal migraine

G43.D0 Abdominal migraine, not intractable `Rx`
Abdominal migraine, without refractory migraine

G43.D1 Abdominal migraine, intractable `Rx`
Abdominal migraine, with refractory migraine

✓5ᵗʰ **G43.8** Other migraine

✓6ᵗʰ **G43.80** Other migraine, not intractable
Other migraine, without refractory migraine

G43.801 Other migraine, not intractable, with status migrainosus `Rx`

G43.809 Other migraine, not intractable, without status migrainosus `Rx`

✓6ᵗʰ **G43.81** Other migraine, intractable
Other migraine, with refractory migraine

G43.811 Other migraine, intractable, with status migrainosus `Rx`

G43.819 Other migraine, intractable, without status migrainosus `Rx`

✓6ᵗʰ **G43.82** Menstrual migraine, not intractable
Menstrual headache, not intractable
Menstrual migraine, without refractory migraine
Menstrually related migraine, not intractable
Pre-menstrual headache, not intractable
Pre-menstrual migraine, not intractable
Pure menstrual migraine, not intractable
Code also associated premenstrual tension syndrome (N94.3)

G43.821 Menstrual migraine, not intractable, with status migrainosus `Rx` ♀

G43.829 Menstrual migraine, not intractable, without status migrainosus `Rx` ♀
Menstrual migraine NOS

Chapter 6. Diseases of the Nervous System

✓6ᵗʰ **G43.83** **Menstrual migraine, intractable**

Menstrual headache, intractable
Menstrual migraine, with refractory migraine
Menstrually related migraine, intractable
Pre-menstrual headache, intractable
Pre-menstrual migraine, intractable
Pure menstrual migraine, intractable
Code also associated premenstrual tension syndrome (N94.3)

G43.831 **Menstrual migraine, intractable, with status migrainosus** Rx ♀

G43.839 **Menstrual migraine, intractable, without status migrainosus** Rx ♀

✓5ᵗʰ **G43.9** **Migraine, unspecified**

✓6ᵗʰ **G43.90** **Migraine, unspecified, not intractable**

Migraine, unspecified, without refractory migraine

G43.901 **Migraine, unspecified, not intractable, with status migrainosus** Rx
Status migrainosus NOS

G43.909 **Migraine, unspecified, not intractable, without status migrainosus** Rx
Migraine NOS

✓6ᵗʰ **G43.91** **Migraine, unspecified, intractable**

Migraine, unspecified, with refractory migraine

G43.911 **Migraine, unspecified, intractable, with status migrainosus** Rx

G43.919 **Migraine, unspecified, intractable, without status migrainosus** Rx

✓4ᵗʰ **G44** **Other headache syndromes**

EXCLUDES 1　headache NOS (R51.9)

EXCLUDES 2　atypical facial pain (G50.1)
headache due to lumbar puncture (G97.1)
migraines (G43.-)
trigeminal neuralgia (G50.0)

✓5ᵗʰ **G44.0** **Cluster headaches and other trigeminal autonomic cephalgias (TAC)**

DEF: Cluster headache: Characteristic grouping or clustering of headaches that can last for a number of weeks or months and then completely disappear for months or years. They are typically not associated with gastrointestinal upset or light sensitivity as experienced in migraines.

✓6ᵗʰ **G44.00** **Cluster headache syndrome, unspecified**

Ciliary neuralgia
Cluster headache NOS
Histamine cephalgia
Lower half migraine
Migrainous neuralgia

G44.001 **Cluster headache syndrome, unspecified, intractable**

G44.009 **Cluster headache syndrome, unspecified, not intractable**
Cluster headache syndrome NOS

✓6ᵗʰ **G44.01** **Episodic cluster headache**

G44.011 **Episodic cluster headache, intractable**

G44.019 **Episodic cluster headache, not intractable**
Episodic cluster headache NOS

✓6ᵗʰ **G44.02** **Chronic cluster headache**

G44.021 **Chronic cluster headache, intractable**

G44.029 **Chronic cluster headache, not intractable**
Chronic cluster headache NOS

✓6ᵗʰ **G44.03** **Episodic paroxysmal hemicrania**

Paroxysmal hemicrania NOS

G44.031 **Episodic paroxysmal hemicrania, intractable**

G44.039 **Episodic paroxysmal hemicrania, not intractable**
Episodic paroxysmal hemicrania NOS

✓6ᵗʰ **G44.04** **Chronic paroxysmal hemicrania**

G44.041 **Chronic paroxysmal hemicrania, intractable**

G44.049 **Chronic paroxysmal hemicrania, not intractable**
Chronic paroxysmal hemicrania NOS

✓6ᵗʰ **G44.05** **Short lasting unilateral neuralgiform headache with conjunctival injection and tearing (SUNCT)**

G44.051 **Short lasting unilateral neuralgiform headache with conjunctival injection and tearing (SUNCT), intractable**

G44.059 **Short lasting unilateral neuralgiform headache with conjunctival injection and tearing (SUNCT), not intractable**
Short lasting unilateral neuralgiform headache with conjunctival injection and tearing (SUNCT) NOS

✓6ᵗʰ **G44.09** **Other trigeminal autonomic cephalgias (TAC)**

G44.091 **Other trigeminal autonomic cephalgias (TAC), intractable**

G44.099 **Other trigeminal autonomic cephalgias (TAC), not intractable**

G44.1 **Vascular headache, not elsewhere classified**

EXCLUDES 2　cluster headache (G44.0)
complicated headache syndromes (G44.5-)
drug-induced headache (G44.4-)
migraine (G43.-)
other specified headache syndromes (G44.8-)
post-traumatic headache (G44.3-)
tension-type headache (G44.2-)

✓5ᵗʰ **G44.2** **Tension-type headache**

✓6ᵗʰ **G44.20** **Tension-type headache, unspecified**

G44.201 **Tension-type headache, unspecified, intractable**

G44.209 **Tension-type headache, unspecified, not intractable**
Tension headache NOS

✓6ᵗʰ **G44.21** **Episodic tension-type headache**

G44.211 **Episodic tension-type headache, intractable**

G44.219 **Episodic tension-type headache, not intractable**
Episodic tension-type headache NOS

✓6ᵗʰ **G44.22** **Chronic tension-type headache**

G44.221 **Chronic tension-type headache, intractable**

G44.229 **Chronic tension-type headache, not intractable**
Chronic tension-type headache NOS

✓5ᵗʰ **G44.3** **Post-traumatic headache**

✓6ᵗʰ **G44.30** **Post-traumatic headache, unspecified**

G44.301 **Post-traumatic headache, unspecified, intractable**

G44.309 **Post-traumatic headache, unspecified, not intractable**
Post-traumatic headache NOS

✓6ᵗʰ **G44.31** **Acute post-traumatic headache**

G44.311 **Acute post-traumatic headache, intractable**

G44.319 **Acute post-traumatic headache, not intractable**
Acute post-traumatic headache NOS

✓6ᵗʰ **G44.32** **Chronic post-traumatic headache**

G44.321 **Chronic post-traumatic headache, intractable**

G44.329 **Chronic post-traumatic headache, not intractable**
Chronic post-traumatic headache NOS

✓5ᵗʰ **G44.4** **Drug-induced headache, not elsewhere classified**

Medication overuse headache
Use additional code for adverse effect, if applicable, to identify drug (T36-T50 with fifth or sixth character 5)

G44.40 **Drug-induced headache, not elsewhere classified, not intractable**

G44.41 **Drug-induced headache, not elsewhere classified, intractable**

✓5ᵗʰ **G44.5** **Complicated headache syndromes**

G44.51 **Hemicrania continua**
DEF: Persistent primary headache of unknown causation occurring on one side of the face and head. May last for more than three months, with daily and continuous pain of moderate intensity with severe exacerbations.

G44.52 **New daily persistent headache (NDPH)**

G44.53   **Primary thunderclap headache**

G44.59   **Other complicated headache syndrome**

✓5ᵗʰ   G44.8   **Other specified headache syndromes**

> EXCLUDES 2   *headache with orthostatic or positional component, not elsewhere classifed (R51.0)*

G44.81   **Hypnic headache**

G44.82   **Headache associated with sexual activity**
Orgasmic headache
Preorgasmic headache

G44.83   **Primary cough headache**

G44.84   **Primary exertional headache**

G44.85   **Primary stabbing headache**

G44.86   **Cervicogenic headache**
Code also associated cervical spinal condition, if known
AHA: 2021,4Q,11-12

G44.89   **Other headache syndrome**

✓4ᵗʰ   **G45   Transient cerebral ischemic attacks and related syndromes**

> EXCLUDES 1   *neonatal cerebral ischemia (P91.0)*
> *transient retinal artery occlusion (H34.0-)*

AHA: 2018,2Q,9
DEF: Transient cerebral ischemic attack: Intermittent or brief cerebral dysfunction from lack of oxygenation with no persistent neurological deficits associated with occlusive vascular disease. TIA may denote an impending cerebrovascular accident.

G45.0   **Vertebro-basilar artery syndrome**

G45.1   **Carotid artery syndrome (hemispheric)**

G45.2   **Multiple and bilateral precerebral artery syndromes**

G45.3   **Amaurosis fugax**

G45.4   **Transient global amnesia**

> EXCLUDES 1   *amnesia NOS (R41.3)*

G45.8   **Other transient cerebral ischemic attacks and related syndromes**

G45.9   **Transient cerebral ischemic attack, unspecified**
Spasm of cerebral artery
TIA
Transient cerebral ischemia NOS

✓4ᵗʰ   **G46   Vascular syndromes of brain in cerebrovascular diseases**
Code first underlying cerebrovascular disease (I60-I69)

G46.0   **Middle cerebral artery syndrome**

G46.1   **Anterior cerebral artery syndrome**

G46.2   **Posterior cerebral artery syndrome**

G46.3   **Brain stem stroke syndrome**
Benedikt syndrome
Claude syndrome
Foville syndrome
Millard-Gubler syndrome
Wallenberg syndrome
Weber syndrome

G46.4   **Cerebellar stroke syndrome**

G46.5   **Pure motor lacunar syndrome**

G46.6   **Pure sensory lacunar syndrome**

G46.7   **Other lacunar syndromes**

G46.8   **Other vascular syndromes of brain in cerebrovascular diseases**

✓4ᵗʰ   **G47   Sleep disorders**

> EXCLUDES 2   *nightmares (F51.5)*
> *nonorganic sleep disorders (F51.-)*
> *sleep terrors (F51.4)*
> *sleepwalking (F51.3)*

✓5ᵗʰ   G47.0   **Insomnia**

> EXCLUDES 2   *alcohol related insomnia (F10.182, F10.282, F10.982)*
> *drug-related insomnia (F11.182, F11.282, F11.982, F13.182, F13.282, F13.982, F14.182, F14.282, F14.982, F15.182, F15.282, F15.982, F19.182, F19.282, F19.982)*
> *idiopathic insomnia (F51.01)*
> *insomnia due to a mental disorder (F51.05)*
> *insomnia not due to a substance or known physiological condition (F51.0-)*
> *nonorganic insomnia (F51.0-)*
> *primary insomnia (F51.01)*
> *sleep apnea (G47.3-)*

G47.00   **Insomnia, unspecified**
Insomnia NOS

G47.01   **Insomnia due to medical condition**
Code also associated medical condition

G47.09   **Other insomnia**

✓5ᵗʰ   G47.1   **Hypersomnia**

> EXCLUDES 2   *alcohol-related hypersomnia (F10.182, F10.282, F10.982)*
> *drug-related hypersomnia (F11.182, F11.282, F11.982, F13.182, F13.282, F13.982, F14.182, F14.282, F14.982, F15.182, F15.282, F15.982, F19.182, F19.282, F19.982)*
> *hypersomnia due to a mental disorder (F51.13)*
> *hypersomnia not due to a substance or known physiological condition (F51.1-)*
> *primary hypersomnia (F51.11)*
> *sleep apnea (G47.3-)*

G47.10   **Hypersomnia, unspecified**
Hypersomnia NOS

G47.11   **Idiopathic hypersomnia with long sleep time**
Idiopathic hypersomnia NOS

G47.12   **Idiopathic hypersomnia without long sleep time**

G47.13   **Recurrent hypersomnia**
Kleine-Levin syndrome
Menstrual related hypersomnia

G47.14   **Hypersomnia due to medical condition**
Code also associated medical condition

G47.19   **Other hypersomnia**

✓5ᵗʰ   G47.2   **Circadian rhythm sleep disorders**

Disorders of the sleep wake schedule
Inversion of nyctohemeral rhythm
Inversion of sleep rhythm
DEF: Circadian rhythm: Daily cycle (24-hour period) of physical, mental, and behavioral changes. It is largely influenced by environmental cues, such as changes in light or temperature. *Synonym(s):* sleep/wake cycle.

G47.20   **Circadian rhythm sleep disorder, unspecified type**
Sleep wake schedule disorder NOS

G47.21   **Circadian rhythm sleep disorder, delayed sleep phase type**
Delayed sleep phase syndrome

G47.22   **Circadian rhythm sleep disorder, advanced sleep phase type**

G47.23   **Circadian rhythm sleep disorder, irregular sleep wake type**
Irregular sleep-wake pattern

G47.24   **Circadian rhythm sleep disorder, free running type**
Circadian rhythm sleep disorder, non-24-hour sleep-wake type

G47.25   **Circadian rhythm sleep disorder, jet lag type**

G47.26   **Circadian rhythm sleep disorder, shift work type**

G47.27   ***Circadian rhythm sleep disorder in conditions classified elsewhere***
Code first underlying condition

G47.29   **Other circadian rhythm sleep disorder**

Chapter 6. Diseases of the Nervous System

G47.3–G53

✓5ᵗʰ **G47.3 Sleep apnea**
    Code also any associated underlying condition
    EXCLUDES 1   *apnea NOS (R06.81)*
        Cheyne-Stokes breathing (R06.3)
        pickwickian syndrome (E66.2)
        sleep apnea of newborn ▶*(P28.3-)*◀

    G47.30 Sleep apnea, unspecified
        Sleep apnea NOS

    G47.31 Primary central sleep apnea
        Idiopathic central sleep apnea

    G47.32 High altitude periodic breathing

    G47.33 Obstructive sleep apnea (adult) (pediatric)
        Obstructive sleep apnea hypopnea
        EXCLUDES 1   *obstructive sleep apnea of newborn*
            ▶*(P28.3-)*◀

    G47.34 Idiopathic sleep related nonobstructive alveolar hypoventilation
        Sleep related hypoxia

    G47.35 Congenital central alveolar hypoventilation syndrome

    G47.36 *Sleep related hypoventilation in conditions classified elsewhere*
        Sleep related hypoxemia in conditions classified elsewhere
        Code first underlying condition

    G47.37 *Central sleep apnea in conditions classified elsewhere*
        Code first underlying condition

    G47.39 Other sleep apnea

✓5ᵗʰ **G47.4 Narcolepsy and cataplexy**

  ✓6ᵗʰ **G47.41 Narcolepsy**
      G47.411 Narcolepsy with cataplexy Rx COM
      G47.419 Narcolepsy without cataplexy Rx COM
          Narcolepsy NOS

  ✓6ᵗʰ **G47.42 Narcolepsy in conditions classified elsewhere**
      Code first underlying condition
      G47.421 *Narcolepsy in conditions classified elsewhere with cataplexy* Rx COM
      G47.429 *Narcolepsy in conditions classified elsewhere without cataplexy* Rx COM

✓5ᵗʰ **G47.5 Parasomnia**
    EXCLUDES 1   *alcohol induced parasomnia (F10.182, F10.282, F10.982)*
        drug induced parasomnia (F11.182, F11.282, F11.982, F13.182, F13.282, F13.982, F14.182, F14.282, F14.982, F15.182, F15.282, F15.982, F19.182, F19.282, F19.982)
        parasomnia not due to a substance or known physiological condition (F51.8)

    G47.50 Parasomnia, unspecified
        Parasomnia NOS

    G47.51 Confusional arousals
    G47.52 REM sleep behavior disorder
    G47.53 Recurrent isolated sleep paralysis
    G47.54 *Parasomnia in conditions classified elsewhere*
        Code first underlying condition
    G47.59 Other parasomnia

✓5ᵗʰ **G47.6 Sleep related movement disorders**
    EXCLUDES 2   *restless legs syndrome (G25.81)*
    G47.61 Periodic limb movement disorder
    G47.62 Sleep related leg cramps
    G47.63 Sleep related bruxism
        EXCLUDES 1   *psychogenic bruxism (F45.8)*
    G47.69 Other sleep related movement disorders

G47.8 Other sleep disorders
    Other specified sleep-wake disorder

G47.9 Sleep disorder, unspecified
    Sleep disorder NOS
    Unspecified sleep-wake disorder

Nerve, nerve root and plexus disorders (G50-G59)

EXCLUDES 1   *current traumatic nerve, nerve root and plexus disorders - see Injury, nerve by body region*
    neuralgia NOS (M79.2)
    neuritis NOS (M79.2)
    peripheral neuritis in pregnancy (O26.82-)
    radiculitis NOS (M54.1-)

✓4ᵗʰ **G50 Disorders of trigeminal nerve**
    INCLUDES   disorders of 5th cranial nerve

    G50.0 Trigeminal neuralgia   Rx
        Syndrome of paroxysmal facial pain
        Tic douloureux

    G50.1 Atypical facial pain   Rx
    G50.8 Other disorders of trigeminal nerve   Rx
    G50.9 Disorder of trigeminal nerve, unspecified   Rx

✓4ᵗʰ **G51 Facial nerve disorders**
    INCLUDES   disorders of 7th cranial nerve

    G51.0 Bell's palsy
        Facial palsy

    G51.1 Geniculate ganglionitis
        EXCLUDES 1   *postherpetic geniculate ganglionitis (B02.21)*

    G51.2 Melkersson's syndrome
        Melkersson-Rosenthal syndrome

  ✓5ᵗʰ **G51.3 Clonic hemifacial spasm**
      AHA: 2018,4Q,10
      G51.31 Clonic hemifacial spasm, right
      G51.32 Clonic hemifacial spasm, left
      G51.33 Clonic hemifacial spasm, bilateral
      G51.39 Clonic hemifacial spasm, unspecified

    G51.4 Facial myokymia
    G51.8 Other disorders of facial nerve
    G51.9 Disorder of facial nerve, unspecified

✓4ᵗʰ **G52 Disorders of other cranial nerves**
    EXCLUDES 2   *disorders of acoustic [8th] nerve (H93.3)*
        disorders of optic [2nd] nerve (H46, H47.0)
        paralytic strabismus due to nerve palsy (H49.0-H49.2)

    G52.0 Disorders of olfactory nerve
        Disorders of 1st cranial nerve

    G52.1 Disorders of glossopharyngeal nerve
        Disorder of 9th cranial nerve
        Glossopharyngeal neuralgia

    G52.2 Disorders of vagus nerve
        Disorders of pneumogastric [10th] nerve

    G52.3 Disorders of hypoglossal nerve
        Disorders of 12th cranial nerve

    G52.7 Disorders of multiple cranial nerves
        Polyneuritis cranialis

    G52.8 Disorders of other specified cranial nerves
    G52.9 Cranial nerve disorder, unspecified

G53 *Cranial nerve disorders in diseases classified elsewhere*
    Code first underlying disease, such as:
    neoplasm (C00-D49)
    EXCLUDES 1   *multiple cranial nerve palsy in sarcoidosis (D86.82)*
        multiple cranial nerve palsy in syphilis (A52.15)
        postherpetic geniculate ganglionitis (B02.21)
        postherpetic trigeminal neuralgia (B02.22)

✓4th G54 Nerve root and plexus disorders

EXCLUDES 1   current traumatic nerve root and plexus disorders - see nerve injury by body region
intervertebral disc disorders (M50-M51)
neuralgia or neuritis NOS (M79.2)
neuritis or radiculitis brachial NOS (M54.13)
neuritis or radiculitis lumbar NOS (M54.16)
neuritis or radiculitis lumbosacral NOS (M54.17)
neuritis or radiculitis thoracic NOS (M54.14)
radiculitis NOS (M54.10)
radiculopathy NOS (M54.10)
spondylosis (M47.-)

G54.0   Brachial plexus disorders
Thoracic outlet syndrome
DEF: Acquired disorder affecting the spinal nerves that send signals to the shoulder, arm, and hand, causing corresponding motor and sensory dysfunction. This disorder is characterized by regional paresthesia, pain, muscle weakness, and in severe cases paralysis.

G54.1   Lumbosacral plexus disorders

G54.2   Cervical root disorders, not elsewhere classified

G54.3   Thoracic root disorders, not elsewhere classified

G54.4   Lumbosacral root disorders, not elsewhere classified

G54.5   Neuralgic amyotrophy
Parsonage-Aldren-Turner syndrome
Shoulder-girdle neuritis
EXCLUDES 1   neuralgic amyotrophy in diabetes mellitus (E08-E13 with .44)

G54.6   Phantom limb syndrome with pain   HCC ESR COM

G54.7   Phantom limb syndrome without pain   HCC ESR COM
Phantom limb syndrome NOS

G54.8   Other nerve root and plexus disorders

G54.9   Nerve root and plexus disorder, unspecified

G55 Nerve root and plexus compressions in diseases classified elsewhere

Code first underlying disease, such as:
neoplasm (C00-D49)
EXCLUDES 1   nerve root compression (due to) (in) ankylosing spondylitis (M45.-)
nerve root compression (due to) (in) dorsopathies (M53.-, M54.-)
nerve root compression (due to) (in) intervertebral disc disorders (M50.1.-, M51.1.-)
nerve root compression (due to) (in) spondylopathies (M46.-, M48.-)
nerve root compression (due to) (in) spondylosis (M47.0-, M47.2-)

✓4th G56 Mononeuropathies of upper limb

EXCLUDES 1   current traumatic nerve disorder - see nerve injury by body region
AHA: 2016,4Q,17-18

✓5th G56.0 Carpal tunnel syndrome

DEF: Swelling and inflammation in the tendons or bursa surrounding the median nerve caused by repetitive activity. The resulting compression on the nerve causes pain, numbness, and tingling especially to the palm, index, middle finger, and thumb.

G56.00   Carpal tunnel syndrome, unspecified upper limb
G56.01   Carpal tunnel syndrome, right upper limb
G56.02   Carpal tunnel syndrome, left upper limb
G56.03   Carpal tunnel syndrome, bilateral upper limbs

✓5th G56.1 Other lesions of median nerve

G56.10   Other lesions of median nerve, unspecified upper limb
G56.11   Other lesions of median nerve, right upper limb
G56.12   Other lesions of median nerve, left upper limb
G56.13   Other lesions of median nerve, bilateral upper limbs

✓5th G56.2 Lesion of ulnar nerve

Tardy ulnar nerve palsy

G56.20   Lesion of ulnar nerve, unspecified upper limb
G56.21   Lesion of ulnar nerve, right upper limb
G56.22   Lesion of ulnar nerve, left upper limb
G56.23   Lesion of ulnar nerve, bilateral upper limbs

✓5th G56.3 Lesion of radial nerve

G56.30   Lesion of radial nerve, unspecified upper limb
G56.31   Lesion of radial nerve, right upper limb
G56.32   Lesion of radial nerve, left upper limb
G56.33   Lesion of radial nerve, bilateral upper limbs

✓5th G56.4 Causalgia of upper limb

Complex regional pain syndrome II of upper limb
EXCLUDES 1   complex regional pain syndrome I of lower limb (G90.52-)
complex regional pain syndrome I of upper limb (G90.51-)
complex regional pain syndrome II of lower limb (G57.7-)
reflex sympathetic dystrophy of lower limb (G90.52-)
reflex sympathetic dystrophy of upper limb (G90.51-)

G56.40   Causalgia of unspecified upper limb
G56.41   Causalgia of right upper limb
G56.42   Causalgia of left upper limb
G56.43   Causalgia of bilateral upper limbs

✓5th G56.8 Other specified mononeuropathies of upper limb

Interdigital neuroma of upper limb

G56.80   Other specified mononeuropathies of unspecified upper limb
G56.81   Other specified mononeuropathies of right upper limb
G56.82   Other specified mononeuropathies of left upper limb
G56.83   Other specified mononeuropathies of bilateral upper limbs

✓5th G56.9 Unspecified mononeuropathy of upper limb

G56.90   Unspecified mononeuropathy of unspecified upper limb
G56.91   Unspecified mononeuropathy of right upper limb
G56.92   Unspecified mononeuropathy of left upper limb
G56.93   Unspecified mononeuropathy of bilateral upper limbs

✓4th G57 Mononeuropathies of lower limb

EXCLUDES 1   current traumatic nerve disorder - see nerve injury by body region
AHA: 2016,4Q,17-18

✓5th G57.0 Lesion of sciatic nerve

EXCLUDES 1   sciatica NOS (M54.3-)
EXCLUDES 2   sciatica attributed to intervertebral disc disorder (M51.1.-)

G57.00   Lesion of sciatic nerve, unspecified lower limb
G57.01   Lesion of sciatic nerve, right lower limb
G57.02   Lesion of sciatic nerve, left lower limb
G57.03   Lesion of sciatic nerve, bilateral lower limbs

✓5th G57.1 Meralgia paresthetica

Lateral cutaneous nerve of thigh syndrome

G57.10   Meralgia paresthetica, unspecified lower limb
G57.11   Meralgia paresthetica, right lower limb
G57.12   Meralgia paresthetica, left lower limb
G57.13   Meralgia paresthetica, bilateral lower limbs

✓5th G57.2 Lesion of femoral nerve

G57.20   Lesion of femoral nerve, unspecified lower limb
G57.21   Lesion of femoral nerve, right lower limb
G57.22   Lesion of femoral nerve, left lower limb
G57.23   Lesion of femoral nerve, bilateral lower limbs

✓5th G57.3 Lesion of lateral popliteal nerve

Peroneal nerve palsy
AHA: 2020,3Q,12

G57.30   Lesion of lateral popliteal nerve, unspecified lower limb
G57.31   Lesion of lateral popliteal nerve, right lower limb
G57.32   Lesion of lateral popliteal nerve, left lower limb
G57.33   Lesion of lateral popliteal nerve, bilateral lower limbs

✓5th G57.4 Lesion of medial popliteal nerve

G57.40   Lesion of medial popliteal nerve, unspecified lower limb
G57.41   Lesion of medial popliteal nerve, right lower limb
G57.42   Lesion of medial popliteal nerve, left lower limb
G57.43   Lesion of medial popliteal nerve, bilateral lower limbs

✓5th G57.5 Tarsal tunnel syndrome

G57.50   Tarsal tunnel syndrome, unspecified lower limb
G57.51   Tarsal tunnel syndrome, right lower limb
G57.52   Tarsal tunnel syndrome, left lower limb
G57.53   Tarsal tunnel syndrome, bilateral lower limbs

Chapter 6. Diseases of the Nervous System

G57.6–G65.2

√5ᵗʰ **G57.6 Lesion of plantar nerve**
Morton's metatarsalgia

G57.60 Lesion of plantar nerve, unspecified lower limb
G57.61 Lesion of plantar nerve, right lower limb
G57.62 Lesion of plantar nerve, left lower limb
G57.63 Lesion of plantar nerve, bilateral lower limbs

√5ᵗʰ **G57.7 Causalgia of lower limb**
Complex regional pain syndrome II of lower limb

EXCLUDES 1   *complex regional pain syndrome I of lower limb (G90.52-)*
complex regional pain syndrome I of upper limb (G90.51-)
complex regional pain syndrome II of upper limb (G56.4-)
reflex sympathetic dystrophy of lower limb (G90.52-)
reflex sympathetic dystrophy of upper limb (G90.51-)

G57.70 Causalgia of unspecified lower limb
G57.71 Causalgia of right lower limb
G57.72 Causalgia of left lower limb
G57.73 Causalgia of bilateral lower limbs

√5ᵗʰ **G57.8 Other specified mononeuropathies of lower limb**
Interdigital neuroma of lower limb

G57.80 Other specified mononeuropathies of unspecified lower limb
G57.81 Other specified mononeuropathies of right lower limb
G57.82 Other specified mononeuropathies of left lower limb
G57.83 Other specified mononeuropathies of bilateral lower limbs

√5ᵗʰ **G57.9 Unspecified mononeuropathy of lower limb**

G57.90 Unspecified mononeuropathy of unspecified lower limb
G57.91 Unspecified mononeuropathy of right lower limb
G57.92 Unspecified mononeuropathy of left lower limb
G57.93 Unspecified mononeuropathy of bilateral lower limbs

√4ᵗʰ **G58 Other mononeuropathies**

G58.0 Intercostal neuropathy
G58.7 Mononeuritis multiplex
G58.8 Other specified mononeuropathies
G58.9 Mononeuropathy, unspecified

G59 *Mononeuropathy in diseases classified elsewhere*
Code first underlying disease

EXCLUDES 1   *diabetic mononeuropathy (E08-E13 with .41)*
syphilitic nerve paralysis (A52.19)
syphilitic neuritis (A52.15)
tuberculous mononeuropathy (A17.83)

Polyneuropathies and other disorders of the peripheral nervous system (G60-G65)

EXCLUDES 1   *neuralgia NOS (M79.2)*
neuritis NOS (M79.2)
peripheral neuritis in pregnancy (O26.82-)
radiculitis NOS (M54.10)

√4ᵗʰ **G60 Hereditary and idiopathic neuropathy**

G60.0 Hereditary motor and sensory neuropathy
Charcôt-Marie-Tooth disease
Déjérine-Sottas disease
Hereditary motor and sensory neuropathy, types I-IV
Hypertrophic neuropathy of infancy
Peroneal muscular atrophy (axonal type) (hypertrophic type)
Roussy-Levy syndrome

G60.1 Refsum's disease
Infantile Refsum disease
DEF: Genetic disorder of the lipid metabolism characterized by retinitis pigmentosa, degenerative nerve disease, ataxia, and dry, rough, scaly skin.

G60.2 Neuropathy in association with hereditary ataxia
G60.3 Idiopathic progressive neuropathy
G60.8 Other hereditary and idiopathic neuropathies
Dominantly inherited sensory neuropathy
Morvan's disease
Nelaton's syndrome
Recessively inherited sensory neuropathy

G60.9 Hereditary and idiopathic neuropathy, unspecified

√4ᵗʰ **G61 Inflammatory polyneuropathy**

G61.0 Guillain-Barre syndrome   HCC Rx ESR COM
Acute (post-)infective polyneuritis
Miller Fisher syndrome
AHA: 2020,3Q,12; 2014,2Q,4
DEF: Autoimmune disorder due to an immune response to foreign antigens with paraplegia of limbs, flaccid paralysis, ophthalmoplegia, ataxia, and areflexia. In most cases, this disorder is triggered by a mild viral infection, surgery, or following an immunization.
TIP: Guillain-Barre syndrome can occur as a sequela of *Campylobacter* enteritis. Assign code B94.8 for the sequelae as an additional diagnosis.

G61.1 Serum neuropathy   HCC Rx ESR COM
Use additional code for adverse effect, if applicable, to identify serum (T50.-)

√5ᵗʰ **G61.8 Other inflammatory polyneuropathies**

G61.81 Chronic inflammatory demyelinating polyneuritis   HCC Rx ESR COM
G61.82 Multifocal motor neuropathy   HCC Rx ESR COM
MMN
AHA: 2016,4Q,18
G61.89 Other inflammatory polyneuropathies   HCC Rx ESR COM

G61.9 Inflammatory polyneuropathy, unspecified   HCC Rx ESR COM

√4ᵗʰ **G62 Other and unspecified polyneuropathies**

G62.0 Drug-induced polyneuropathy   HCC Rx ESR COM
Use additional code for adverse effect, if applicable, to identify drug (T36-T50 with fifth or sixth character 5)

G62.1 Alcoholic polyneuropathy   HCC Rx ESR COM
AHA: 2019,3Q,8

G62.2 Polyneuropathy due to other toxic agents   HCC Rx ESR COM
Code first (T51-T65) to identify toxic agent

√5ᵗʰ **G62.8 Other specified polyneuropathies**

G62.81 Critical illness polyneuropathy   HCC Rx ESR COM
Acute motor neuropathy
G62.82 Radiation-induced polyneuropathy   HCC Rx ESR COM
Use additional external cause code (W88-W90, X39.0-) to identify cause
G62.89 Other specified polyneuropathies
AHA: 2016,2Q,11

G62.9 Polyneuropathy, unspecified
Neuropathy NOS

G63 *Polyneuropathy in diseases classified elsewhere*   HCC Rx ESR COM
Code first underlying disease, such as:
amyloidosis (E85.-)
endocrine disease, except diabetes (E00-E07, E15-E16, E20-E34)
metabolic diseases (E70-E88)
neoplasm (C00-D49)
nutritional deficiency (E40-E64)

EXCLUDES 1   *polyneuropathy (in):*
diabetes mellitus (E08-E13 with .42)
diphtheria (A36.83)
infectious mononucleosis complicated by polyneuropathy (B27.0-B27.9 with fifth character 1)
Lyme disease (A69.22)
mumps (B26.84)
postherpetic (B02.23)
rheumatoid arthritis (M05.5-)
scleroderma (M34.83)
systemic lupus erythematosus (M32.19)

AHA: 2021,1Q,7; 2012,4Q,99

G64 Other disorders of peripheral nervous system
Disorder of peripheral nervous system NOS

√4ᵗʰ **G65 Sequelae of inflammatory and toxic polyneuropathies**
Code first condition resulting from (sequela) of inflammatory and toxic polyneuropathies

G65.0 Sequelae of Guillain-Barré syndrome   HCC Rx ESR COM
G65.1 Sequelae of other inflammatory polyneuropathy   HCC Rx ESR COM
G65.2 Sequelae of toxic polyneuropathy   HCC Rx ESR COM

Diseases of myoneural junction and muscle (G70-G73)

✓4ᵗʰ **G70 Myasthenia gravis and other myoneural disorders**

    EXCLUDES 1   botulism (A05.1, A48.51-A48.52)
           transient neonatal myasthenia gravis (P94.0)

✓5ᵗʰ **G70.0 Myasthenia gravis**

    DEF: Autoimmune neuromuscular disorder caused by antibodies to the acetylcholine receptors at the neuromuscular junction, interfering with proper binding of the neurotransmitter from the neuron to the target muscle, causing muscle weakness, fatigue, and exhaustion, without pain or atrophy.

    G70.00 Myasthenia gravis without (acute) exacerbation   HCC Rx ESR COM
         Myasthenia gravis NOS

    G70.01 Myasthenia gravis with (acute) exacerbation   HCC Rx ESR COM
         Myasthenia gravis in crisis

  G70.1 Toxic myoneural disorders   HCC Rx ESR COM
     Code first (T51-T65) to identify toxic agent

  G70.2 Congenital and developmental myasthenia   HCC Rx ESR COM

✓5ᵗʰ **G70.8 Other specified myoneural disorders**

    G70.80 Lambert-Eaton syndrome, unspecified   HCC Rx ESR COM
         Lambert-Eaton syndrome NOS

    G70.81 *Lambert-Eaton syndrome in disease classified elsewhere*   HCC Rx ESR COM
         Code first underlying disease
           EXCLUDES 1   Lambert-Eaton syndrome in neoplastic disease (G73.1)

    G70.89 Other specified myoneural disorders   HCC Rx ESR COM

  G70.9 Myoneural disorder, unspecified   HCC Rx ESR COM

✓4ᵗʰ **G71 Primary disorders of muscles**

    EXCLUDES 2   arthrogryposis multiplex congenita (Q74.3)
           metabolic disorders (E70-E88)
           myositis (M60.-)

✓5ᵗʰ **G71.0 Muscular dystrophy**

    AHA: 2018,4Q,11-12

    G71.00 Muscular dystrophy, unspecified   HCC ESR COM

    G71.01 Duchenne or Becker muscular dystrophy   HCC ESR COM
         Autosomal recessive, childhood type, muscular dystrophy resembling Duchenne or Becker muscular dystrophy
         Benign [Becker] muscular dystrophy
         Severe [Duchenne] muscular dystrophy

    G71.02 Facioscapulohumeral muscular dystrophy   HCC ESR COM
         Scapulohumeral muscular dystrophy

    ✓6ᵗʰ **G71.03 Limb girdle muscular dystrophies**

        G71.031 Autosomal dominant limb girdle muscular dystrophy
           LGMD D4 calpain-3-related
           LGMD D5 collagen 6-related
           Limb girdle muscular dystrophy type 1

        G71.032 Autosomal recessive limb girdle muscular dystrophy due to calpain-3 dysfunction
           Limb girdle muscular dystrophy type 2A
           LGMD R1 calpain-3-related
           Primary calpainopathy

        G71.033 Limb girdle muscular dystrophy due to dysferlin dysfunction
           Dysferlinopathy
           LGMD R2 dysferlin-related
           Limb girdle muscular dystrophy type 2B
           Miyoshi Myopathy type 1

        ✓7ᵗʰ **G71.034 Limb girdle muscular dystrophy due to sarcoglycan dysfunction**
            G71.0340 Limb girdle muscular dystrophy due to sarcoglycan dysfunction, unspecified
               Sarcoglycanopathy, NOS

            G71.0341 Limb girdle muscular dystrophy due to alpha sarcoglycan dysfunction
               Alpha sarcoglycanopathy
               Limb-girdle muscular dystrophy due to alpha-sarcoglycan deficiency
               Limb girdle muscular dystrophy type 2D

            G71.0342 Limb girdle muscular dystrophy due to beta sarcoglycan dysfunction
               Beta sarcoglycanopathy
               Limb girdle muscular dystrophy due to beta-sarcoglycan deficiency
               Limb girdle muscular dystrophy type 2E

            G71.0349 Limb girdle muscular dystrophy due to other sarcoglycan dysfunction
               Delta sarcoglycanopathy
               Delta-sarcoglycan-related LGMD R6
               Gamma sarcoglycanopathy
               Gamma-sarcoglycan-related LGMD R5
               Limb girdle muscular dystrophy type 2C
               Limb girdle muscular dystrophy type 2F

        G71.035 Limb girdle muscular dystrophy due to anoctamin-5 dysfunction
           Anoctamin-5-related LGMD R12
           Anoctaminopathy
           Autosomal recessive limb girdle muscular dystrophy type 2L
           Miyoshi myopathy type 3

        G71.038 Other limb girdle muscular dystrophy
           LGMD R9 FKRP-related
           LGMD R22 collagen 6-related
           Limb girdle muscular dystrophy due to fukutin related protein dysfunction
           Limb girdle muscular dystrophy type 2I
           Other autosomal recessive limb girdle muscular dystrophy

        G71.039 Limb girdle muscular dystrophy, unspecified

    G71.09 Other specified muscular dystrophies   HCC ESR COM
         Benign scapuloperoneal muscular dystrophy with early contractures [Emery-Dreifuss]
         Congenital muscular dystrophy NOS
         Congenital muscular dystrophy with specific morphological abnormalities of the muscle fiber
         Distal muscular dystrophy
         ~~Limb-girdle muscular dystrophy~~
         Ocular muscular dystrophy
         Oculopharyngeal muscular dystrophy
         Scapuloperoneal muscular dystrophy

✓5ᵗʰ **G71.1 Myotonic disorders**

    G71.11 Myotonic muscular dystrophy   HCC ESR COM
         Dystrophia myotonica [Steinert]
         Myotonia atrophica
         Myotonic dystrophy
         Proximal myotonic myopathy (PROMM)
         Steinert disease

    G71.12 Myotonia congenita
         Acetazolamide responsive myotonia congenita
         Dominant myotonia congenita [Thomsen disease]
         Myotonia levior
         Recessive myotonia congenita [Becker disease]

    G71.13 Myotonic chondrodystrophy
         Chondrodystrophic myotonia
         Congenital myotonic chondrodystrophy
         Schwartz-Jampel disease

G71.14 Drug induced myotonia
Use additional code for adverse effect, if applicable, to identify drug (T36-T50 with fifth or sixth character 5)

G71.19 Other specified myotonic disorders
Myotonia fluctuans
Myotonia permanens
Neuromyotonia [Isaacs]
Paramyotonia congenita (of von Eulenburg)
Pseudomyotonia
Symptomatic myotonia

√5ᵗʰ **G71.2 Congenital myopathies**
> EXCLUDES 2   *arthrogryposis multiplex congenita (Q74.3)*
> AHA: 2020,4Q,19-21

G71.20 Congenital myopathy, unspecified HCC ESR COM

G71.21 Nemaline myopathy HCC ESR COM

√6ᵗʰ **G71.22 Centronuclear myopathy**

G71.220 X-linked myotubular myopathy HCC ESR COM
Myotubular (centronuclear) myopathy

G71.228 Other centronuclear myopathy HCC ESR COM
Autosomal centronuclear myopathy
Autosomal dominant centronuclear myopathy
Autosomal recessive centronuclear myopathy
Centronuclear myopathy, NOS

G71.29 Other congenital myopathy HCC ESR COM
Central core disease
Minicore disease
Multicore disease
Multiminicore disease

G71.3 Mitochondrial myopathy, not elsewhere classified
> EXCLUDES 1   *Kearns-Sayre syndrome (H49.81)*
> *Leber's disease (H47.21)*
> *Leigh's encephalopathy (G31.82)*
> *mitochondrial metabolism disorders (E88.4.-)*
> *Reye's syndrome (G93.7)*

G71.8 Other primary disorders of muscles

G71.9 Primary disorder of muscle, unspecified
Hereditary myopathy NOS

√4ᵗʰ **G72 Other and unspecified myopathies**
> EXCLUDES 1   *arthrogryposis multiplex congenita (Q74.3)*
> *dermatopolymyositis (M33.-)*
> *ischemic infarction of muscle (M62.2-)*
> *myositis (M60.-)*
> *polymyositis (M33.2.-)*

G72.0 Drug-induced myopathy
Use additional code for adverse effect, if applicable, to identify drug (T36-T50 with fifth or sixth character 5)

G72.1 Alcoholic myopathy
Use additional code to identify alcoholism (F10.-)

G72.2 Myopathy due to other toxic agents
Code first (T51-T65) to identify toxic agent

G72.3 Periodic paralysis
Familial periodic paralysis
Hyperkalemic periodic paralysis (familial)
Hypokalemic periodic paralysis (familial)
Myotonic periodic paralysis (familial)
Normokalemic paralysis (familial)
Potassium sensitive periodic paralysis
> EXCLUDES 1   *paramyotonia congenita (of von Eulenburg) (G71.19)*

√5ᵗʰ **G72.4 Inflammatory and immune myopathies, not elsewhere classified**

G72.41 Inclusion body myositis [IBM]

G72.49 Other inflammatory and immune myopathies, not elsewhere classified
Inflammatory myopathy NOS

√5ᵗʰ **G72.8 Other specified myopathies**

G72.81 Critical illness myopathy
Acute necrotizing myopathy
Acute quadriplegic myopathy
Intensive care (ICU) myopathy
Myopathy of critical illness
AHA: 2020,3Q,12

G72.89 Other specified myopathies

G72.9 Myopathy, unspecified

√4ᵗʰ **G73 Disorders of myoneural junction and muscle in diseases classified elsewhere**

G73.1 Lambert-Eaton syndrome in neoplastic disease HCC Rx ESR COM UPD
Code first underlying neoplasm (C00-D49)
> EXCLUDES 1   *Lambert-Eaton syndrome not associated with neoplasm (G70.80-G70.81)*

G73.3 Myasthenic syndromes in other diseases classified elsewhere HCC Rx ESR COM
Code first underlying disease, such as:
neoplasm (C00-D49)
thyrotoxicosis (E05.-)

G73.7 Myopathy in diseases classified elsewhere
Code first underlying disease, such as:
hyperparathyroidism (E21.0, E21.3)
hypoparathyroidism (E20.-)
glycogen storage disease (E74.0)
lipid storage disorders (E75.-)
> EXCLUDES 1   *myopathy in:*
> *rheumatoid arthritis (M05.32)*
> *sarcoidosis (D86.87)*
> *scleroderma (M34.82)*
> *Sjögren syndrome (M35.03)*
> *systemic lupus erythematosus (M32.19)*

Cerebral palsy and other paralytic syndromes (G80-G83)

√4ᵗʰ **G80 Cerebral palsy**
> EXCLUDES 1   *hereditary spastic paraplegia (G11.4)*

G80.0 Spastic quadriplegic cerebral palsy HCC ESR COM
Congenital spastic paralysis (cerebral)

G80.1 Spastic diplegic cerebral palsy HCC ESR COM
Spastic cerebral palsy NOS

G80.2 Spastic hemiplegic cerebral palsy HCC ESR COM

G80.3 Athetoid cerebral palsy HCC ESR COM
Double athetosis (syndrome)
Dyskinetic cerebral palsy
Dystonic cerebral palsy
Vogt disease

G80.4 Ataxic cerebral palsy HCC ESR COM

G80.8 Other cerebral palsy HCC ESR COM
Mixed cerebral palsy syndromes

G80.9 Cerebral palsy, unspecified HCC ESR COM
Cerebral palsy NOS

√4ᵗʰ **G81 Hemiplegia and hemiparesis**
> NOTE   This category is to be used only when hemiplegia (complete)(incomplete) is reported without further specification, or is stated to be old or longstanding but of unspecified cause. The category is also for use in multiple coding to identify these types of hemiplegia resulting from any cause.
> EXCLUDES 1   *congenital cerebral palsy (G80.-)*
> *hemiplegia and hemiparesis due to sequela of cerebrovascular disease (I69.05-, I69.15-, I69.25-, I69.35-, I69.85-, I69.95-)*

AHA: 2015,1Q,25
TIP: If the documentation specifies the affected side but not whether it is the dominant or nondominant side, the default is as follows: for ambidextrous patients, the default is dominant; when the left side is affected, the default is nondominant; and when the right side is affected, the default is dominant.

√5ᵗʰ **G81.0 Flaccid hemiplegia**

G81.00 Flaccid hemiplegia affecting unspecified side HCC ESR COM

G81.01 Flaccid hemiplegia affecting right dominant side HCC ESR COM

G81.02 Flaccid hemiplegia affecting left dominant side HCC ESR COM

G81.Ø3 Flaccid hemiplegia affecting right nondominant side HCC ESR COM

G81.Ø4 Flaccid hemiplegia affecting left nondominant side HCC ESR COM

√5ᵗʰ **G81.1 Spastic hemiplegia**

G81.1Ø Spastic hemiplegia affecting unspecified side HCC Rx ESR COM

G81.11 Spastic hemiplegia affecting right dominant side HCC Rx ESR COM

G81.12 Spastic hemiplegia affecting left dominant side HCC Rx ESR COM

G81.13 Spastic hemiplegia affecting right nondominant side HCC Rx ESR COM

G81.14 Spastic hemiplegia affecting left nondominant side HCC Rx ESR COM

√5ᵗʰ **G81.9 Hemiplegia, unspecified**

AHA: 2014,1Q,23

G81.9Ø Hemiplegia, unspecified affecting unspecified side HCC ESR COM

G81.91 Hemiplegia, unspecified affecting right dominant side HCC ESR COM

G81.92 Hemiplegia, unspecified affecting left dominant side HCC ESR COM

G81.93 Hemiplegia, unspecified affecting right nondominant side HCC ESR COM

G81.94 Hemiplegia, unspecified affecting left nondominant side HCC ESR COM

√4ᵗʰ **G82 Paraplegia (paraparesis) and quadriplegia (quadriparesis)**

NOTE This category is to be used only when the listed conditions are reported without further specification, or are stated to be old or longstanding but of unspecified cause. The category is also for use in multiple coding to identify these conditions resulting from any cause

EXCLUDES 1 congenital cerebral palsy (G8Ø.-)
functional quadriplegia (R53.2)
hysterical paralysis (F44.4)

√6ᵗʰ **G82.2 Paraplegia**

Paralysis of both lower limbs NOS
Paraparesis (lower) NOS
Paraplegia (lower) NOS
AHA: 2017,3Q,3

G82.2Ø Paraplegia, unspecified HCC ESR COM
G82.21 Paraplegia, complete HCC ESR COM
G82.22 Paraplegia, incomplete HCC ESR COM

√6ᵗʰ **G82.5 Quadriplegia**

G82.5Ø Quadriplegia, unspecified HCC ESR COM
G82.51 Quadriplegia, C1-C4 complete HCC ESR COM
G82.52 Quadriplegia, C1-C4 incomplete HCC ESR COM
G82.53 Quadriplegia, C5-C7 complete HCC ESR COM
G82.54 Quadriplegia, C5-C7 incomplete HCC ESR COM

√4ᵗʰ **G83 Other paralytic syndromes**

NOTE This category is to be used only when the listed conditions are reported without further specification, or are stated to be old or longstanding but of unspecified cause. The category is also for use in multiple coding to identify these conditions resulting from any cause.

INCLUDES paralysis (complete) (incomplete), except as in G8Ø-G82

G83.Ø Diplegia of upper limbs HCC ESR COM
Diplegia (upper)
Paralysis of both upper limbs

√5ᵗʰ **G83.1 Monoplegia of lower limb**

Paralysis of lower limb
EXCLUDES 1 monoplegia of lower limbs due to sequela of cerebrovascular disease (I69.Ø4-, I69.14-, I69.24-, I69.34-, I69.84-, I69.94-)

TIP: If the documentation specifies the affected side but not whether it is the dominant or nondominant side, the default is as follows: for ambidextrous patients, the default is dominant; when the left side is affected, the default is nondominant; and when the right side is affected, the default is dominant.

G83.1Ø Monoplegia of lower limb affecting unspecified side HCC ESR COM

G83.11 Monoplegia of lower limb affecting right dominant side HCC ESR COM

G83.12 Monoplegia of lower limb affecting left dominant side HCC ESR COM

G83.13 Monoplegia of lower limb affecting right nondominant side HCC ESR COM

G83.14 Monoplegia of lower limb affecting left nondominant side HCC ESR COM

√5ᵗʰ **G83.2 Monoplegia of upper limb**

Paralysis of upper limb
EXCLUDES 1 monoplegia of upper limbs due to sequela of cerebrovascular disease (I69.Ø3-, I69.13-, I69.23-, I69.33-, I69.83-, I69.93-)

TIP: If the documentation specifies the affected side but not whether it is the dominant or nondominant side, the default is as follows: for ambidextrous patients, the default is dominant; when the left side is affected, the default is nondominant; and when the right side is affected, the default is dominant.

G83.2Ø Monoplegia of upper limb affecting unspecified side HCC ESR COM

G83.21 Monoplegia of upper limb affecting right dominant side HCC ESR COM

G83.22 Monoplegia of upper limb affecting left dominant side HCC ESR COM

G83.23 Monoplegia of upper limb affecting right nondominant side HCC ESR COM

G83.24 Monoplegia of upper limb affecting left nondominant side HCC ESR COM

√5ᵗʰ **G83.3 Monoplegia, unspecified**

TIP: If the documentation specifies the affected side but not whether it is the dominant or nondominant side, the default is as follows: for ambidextrous patients, the default is dominant; when the left side is affected, the default is nondominant; and when the right side is affected, the default is dominant.

G83.3Ø Monoplegia, unspecified affecting unspecified side HCC ESR COM

G83.31 Monoplegia, unspecified affecting right dominant side HCC ESR COM

G83.32 Monoplegia, unspecified affecting left dominant side HCC ESR COM

G83.33 Monoplegia, unspecified affecting right nondominant side HCC ESR COM

G83.34 Monoplegia, unspecified affecting left nondominant side HCC ESR COM

G83.4 Cauda equina syndrome HCC Rx ESR COM
Neurogenic bladder due to cauda equina syndrome
EXCLUDES 1 cord bladder NOS (G95.89)
neurogenic bladder NOS (N31.9)

AHA: 2020,3Q,24
DEF: Compression of the spinal nerve roots presenting with pain and tingling radiating down the buttocks, back of the thigh and calf, and into the foot in a sciatic manner with aching in the bladder, perineum, and sacrum. Loss of bowel and bladder control may also occur.

G83.5 Locked-in state HCC ESR COM
AHA: 2022,2Q,10

√5ᵗʰ **G83.8 Other specified paralytic syndromes**

EXCLUDES 1 paralytic syndromes due to current spinal cord injury - code to spinal cord injury (S14, S24, S34)

G83.81 Brown-Séquard syndrome HCC ESR COM
G83.82 Anterior cord syndrome HCC ESR COM
G83.83 Posterior cord syndrome HCC ESR COM
G83.84 Todd's paralysis (postepileptic) HCC ESR COM
G83.89 Other specified paralytic syndromes HCC ESR COM

G83.9 Paralytic syndrome, unspecified HCC ESR COM

Other disorders of the nervous system (G89-G99)

✓4th G89   Pain, not elsewhere classified

Code also related psychological factors associated with pain (F45.42)

EXCLUDES 1   *generalized pain NOS (R52)*
pain disorders exclusively related to psychological factors (F45.41)
pain NOS (R52)

EXCLUDES 2   *atypical face pain (G50.1)*
headache syndromes (G44.-)
localized pain, unspecified type - code to pain by site, such as:
abdomen pain (R10.-)
back pain (M54.9)
breast pain (N64.4)
chest pain (R07.1-R07.9)
ear pain (H92.0-)
eye pain (H57.1)
headache (R51.9)
joint pain (M25.5-)
limb pain (M79.6-)
lumbar region pain (M54.5-)
painful urination (R30.9)
pelvic and perineal pain (R10.2)
renal colic (N23)
shoulder pain (M25.51-)
spine pain (M54.-)
throat pain (R07.0)
tongue pain (K14.6)
tooth pain (K08.8)
migraines (G43.-)
myalgia (M79.1-)
pain from prosthetic devices, implants, and grafts (T82.84, T83.84, T84.84, T85.84-)
phantom limb syndrome with pain (G54.6)
vulvar vestibulitis (N94.810)
vulvodynia (N94.81-)

G89.0   Central pain syndrome
Déjérine-Roussy syndrome
Myelopathic pain syndrome
Thalamic pain syndrome (hyperesthetic)

✓5th G89.1   Acute pain, not elsewhere classified

G89.11   Acute pain due to trauma

G89.12   Acute post-thoracotomy pain
Post-thoracotomy pain NOS

G89.18   Other acute postprocedural pain
Postoperative pain NOS
Postprocedural pain NOS

✓5th G89.2   Chronic pain, not elsewhere classified

EXCLUDES 1   *causalgia, lower limb (G57.7-)*
causalgia, upper limb (G56.4-)
central pain syndrome (G89.0)
chronic pain syndrome (G89.4)
complex regional pain syndrome II, lower limb (G57.7-)
complex regional pain syndrome II, upper limb (G56.4-)
neoplasm related chronic pain (G89.3)
reflex sympathetic dystrophy (G90.5-)

G89.21   Chronic pain due to trauma

G89.22   Chronic post-thoracotomy pain

G89.28   Other chronic postprocedural pain
Other chronic postoperative pain

G89.29   Other chronic pain

G89.3   Neoplasm related pain (acute) (chronic)
Cancer associated pain
Pain due to malignancy (primary) (secondary)
Tumor associated pain

G89.4   Chronic pain syndrome
Chronic pain associated with significant psychosocial dysfunction

✓4th G90   Disorders of autonomic nervous system

EXCLUDES 1   *dysfunction of the autonomic nervous system due to alcohol (G31.2)*

✓5th G90.0   Idiopathic peripheral autonomic neuropathy

G90.01   Carotid sinus syncope
Carotid sinus syndrome
DEF: Vagal activation caused by pressure on the carotid sinus baroreceptors. Sympathetic nerve impulses may cause sinus arrest or AV block.

G90.09   Other idiopathic peripheral autonomic neuropathy
Idiopathic peripheral autonomic neuropathy NOS

G90.1   Familial dysautonomia [Riley-Day]   HCC Rx ESR COM

G90.2   Horner's syndrome
Bernard(-Horner) syndrome
Cervical sympathetic dystrophy or paralysis

G90.3   Multi-system degeneration of the autonomic nervous system   HCC Rx ESR COM
Neurogenic orthostatic hypotension [Shy-Drager]
EXCLUDES 1   *orthostatic hypotension NOS (I95.1)*

G90.4   Autonomic dysreflexia
Use additional code to identify the cause, such as:
fecal impaction (K56.41)
pressure ulcer (pressure area) (L89.-)
urinary tract infection (N39.0)

✓5th G90.5   Complex regional pain syndrome I (CRPS I)

Reflex sympathetic dystrophy
EXCLUDES 1   *causalgia of lower limb (G57.7-)*
causalgia of upper limb (G56.4-)
complex regional pain syndrome II of lower limb (G57.7-)
complex regional pain syndrome II of upper limb (G56.4-)

G90.50   Complex regional pain syndrome I, unspecified

✓6th G90.51   Complex regional pain syndrome I of upper limb

G90.511   Complex regional pain syndrome I of right upper limb

G90.512   Complex regional pain syndrome I of left upper limb

G90.513   Complex regional pain syndrome I of upper limb, bilateral

G90.519   Complex regional pain syndrome I of unspecified upper limb

✓6th G90.52   Complex regional pain syndrome I of lower limb

G90.521   Complex regional pain syndrome I of right lower limb

G90.522   Complex regional pain syndrome I of left lower limb

G90.523   Complex regional pain syndrome I of lower limb, bilateral

G90.529   Complex regional pain syndrome I of unspecified lower limb

G90.59   Complex regional pain syndrome I of other specified site

G90.8   Other disorders of autonomic nervous system

G90.9   Disorder of the autonomic nervous system, unspecified

G90.A   Postural orthostatic tachycardia syndrome [POTS]
Chronic orthostatic intolerance
Postural tachycardia syndrome

✓4th **G91 Hydrocephalus**

> INCLUDES   acquired hydrocephalus
> EXCLUDES 1   *Arnold-Chiari syndrome with hydrocephalus (Q07.-)*
> *congenital hydrocephalus (Q03.-)*
> *spina bifida with hydrocephalus (Q05.-)*
> **DEF:** Abnormal buildup of cerebrospinal fluid in the brain causing dilation of the ventricles.

Hydrocephalus (Acquired)

Normal ventricles   Hydrocephalic ventricles

G91.0 Communicating hydrocephalus   HCC ESR COM
     Secondary normal pressure hydrocephalus

G91.1 Obstructive hydrocephalus   HCC ESR COM
     DEF: Obstruction of the cerebrospinal fluid passage from the brain into the spinal canal characterized by headaches, drowsiness, poor coordination, urinary incontinence, nausea, vomiting, and papilledema.

G91.2 (Idiopathic) normal pressure hydrocephalus   HCC ESR COM
     Normal pressure hydrocephalus NOS

G91.3 Post-traumatic hydrocephalus, unspecified   HCC ESR COM

G91.4 Hydrocephalus in diseases classified elsewhere   HCC ESR COM
     Code first underlying condition, such as:
       congenital syphilis (A50.4-)
       neoplasm (C00-D49)
       plasminogen deficiency (E88.02)
     EXCLUDES 1   *hydrocephalus due to congenital toxoplasmosis (P37.1)*
     AHA: 2014,3Q,3

G91.8 Other hydrocephalus   HCC ESR COM

G91.9 Hydrocephalus, unspecified   HCC ESR COM

✓4th **G92 Toxic encephalopathy**
     AHA: 2022,1Q,52; 2021,4Q,12-14; 2021,1Q,13; 2017,1Q,39-40
     DEF: Brain tissue degeneration due to a toxic substance.

   ✓5th **G92.0 Immune effector cell-associated neurotoxicity syndrome**
     Code first underlying cause such as:
       complications of immune effector cellular therapy (T80.82)
     Code also associated signs and symptoms, such as seizures and cerebral edema
     Code also, if applicable:
       cerebral edema (G93.6)
       unspecified convulsions (R56.9)

     G92.00 Immune effector cell-associated neurotoxicity syndrome, grade unspecified   UPD
       ICANS, grade unspecified

     G92.01 Immune effector cell-associated neurotoxicity syndrome, grade 1   UPD
       ICANS, grade 1

     G92.02 Immune effector cell-associated neurotoxicity syndrome, grade 2   UPD
       ICANS, grade 2

     G92.03 Immune effector cell-associated neurotoxicity syndrome, grade 3   UPD
       ICANS, grade 3

     G92.04 Immune effector cell-associated neurotoxicity syndrome, grade 4   UPD
       ICANS, grade 4

     G92.05 Immune effector cell-associated neurotoxicity syndrome, grade 5   UPD
       ICANS, grade 5

   G92.8 Other toxic encephalopathy
     Toxic encephalitis
     Toxic metabolic encephalopathy
     Code first poisoning due to drug or toxin, if applicable, (T36-T65 with fifth or sixth character 1-4 or 6)
     Use additional code for adverse effect, if applicable, to identify drug (T36-T50 with fifth or sixth character 5)
     AHA: 2022,1Q,52

   G92.9 Unspecified toxic encephalopathy
     Code first poisoning due to drug or toxin, if applicable, (T36-T65 with fifth or sixth character 1-4 or 6)
     Use additional code for adverse effect, if applicable, to identify drug (T36-T50 with fifth or sixth character 5)

✓4th **G93 Other disorders of brain**

   G93.0 Cerebral cysts
     Arachnoid cyst
     Porencephalic cyst, acquired
     EXCLUDES 1   *acquired periventricular cysts of newborn (P91.1)*
                congenital cerebral cysts (Q04.6)

   G93.1 Anoxic brain damage, not elsewhere classified   HCC ESR COM
     EXCLUDES 1   *cerebral anoxia due to anesthesia during labor and delivery (O74.3)*
                cerebral anoxia due to anesthesia during the puerperium (O89.2)
                neonatal anoxia (P84)
     DEF: Brain injury not resulting from birth trauma that is due to lack of oxygen. Brain cells, when deprived of oxygen, begin to expire after four minutes.

   G93.2 Benign intracranial hypertension
     Pseudotumor
     EXCLUDES 1   *hypertensive encephalopathy (I67.4)*
                obstructive hydrocephalus (G91.1)

▲   ✓5th **G93.3 Postviral and related fatigue syndromes**
     ~~Benign myalgic encephalomyelitis~~
     ►Use additional code, if applicable, for post COVID-19 condition, unspecified (U09.9)◄
     EXCLUDES 1   *chronic fatigue syndrome NOS (R53.82)*
                ►*neurasthenia (F48.8)*◄

   ●   **G93.31 Postviral fatigue syndrome**

   ●   **G93.32 Myalgic encephalomyelitis/chronic fatigue syndrome**
     Chronic fatigue syndrome
     ME/CFS
     Myalgic encephalomyelitis

   ●   **G93.39 Other post infection and related fatigue syndromes**

   ✓5th **G93.4 Other and unspecified encephalopathy**
     EXCLUDES 1   *alcoholic encephalopathy (G31.2)*
                encephalopathy in diseases classified elsewhere (G94)
                hypertensive encephalopathy (I67.4)
     EXCLUDES 2   *toxic (metabolic) encephalopathy (G92.8)*

     G93.40 Encephalopathy, unspecified
       AHA: 2017,2Q,8

     G93.41 Metabolic encephalopathy
       Septic encephalopathy
       AHA: 2017,2Q,8; 2016,3Q,42; 2015,3Q,21
       TIP: Assign separately when documented with diabetic hypoglycemia (E08.649, E09.649, E10.649, E11.649, E13.649).

     G93.49 Other encephalopathy
       Encephalopathy NEC
       AHA: 2021,2Q,3; 2018,4Q,16; 2018,2Q,22,24; 2017,2Q,9

   G93.5 Compression of brain   HCC ESR COM
     Arnold-Chiari type 1 compression of brain
     Compression of brain (stem)
     Herniation of brain (stem)
     EXCLUDES 1   *traumatic compression of brain (S06.A-)*
     AHA: 2020,2Q,31

   G93.6 Cerebral edema   HCC ESR COM
     EXCLUDES 1   *cerebral edema due to birth injury (P11.0)*
                traumatic cerebral edema (S06.1-)

✓ Additional Character Required   ✓x7th Placeholder Alert   Manifestation   Unspecified Dx   ⓠ QPP   UPD Unacceptable PDx

Chapter 6. Diseases of the Nervous System *(left margin)*

G93.7 Reye's syndrome `HCC` `Rx` `ESR` `COM` `P`
　Code first poisoning due to salicylates, if applicable (T39.0-, with sixth character 1-4)
　Use additional code for adverse effect due to salicylates, if applicable (T39.0-, with sixth character 5)
　DEF: Rare childhood illness often developed after a viral upper respiratory infection. Symptoms include vomiting, elevated serum transaminase, brain swelling, disturbances of consciousness, seizures, and changes in liver and other viscera; it can be fatal.

✓5ᵗʰ **G93.8 Other specified disorders of brain**

　G93.81 Temporal sclerosis
　　Hippocampal sclerosis
　　Mesial temporal sclerosis

　G93.82 Brain death

　G93.89 Other specified disorders of brain
　　Postradiation encephalopathy
　　AHA: 2020,2Q,24; 2019,3Q,8

G93.9 Disorder of brain, unspecified

G94 *Other disorders of brain in diseases classified elsewhere*
　Code first underlying disease
　EXCLUDES 1 *encephalopathy in congenital syphilis (A50.49)*
　　　encephalopathy in influenza (J09.X9, J10.81, J11.81)
　　　encephalopathy in syphilis (A52.19)
　　　hydrocephalus in diseases classified elsewhere (G91.4)
　AHA: 2018,2Q,22; 2017,2Q,8-9

✓4ᵗʰ **G95 Other and unspecified diseases of spinal cord**
　EXCLUDES 2 *myelitis (G04.-)*

　G95.0 Syringomyelia and syringobulbia `HCC` `Rx` `ESR` `COM`

✓5ᵗʰ **G95.1 Vascular myelopathies**
　EXCLUDES 2 *intraspinal phlebitis and thrombophlebitis, except non-pyogenic (G08)*

　G95.11 Acute infarction of spinal cord (embolic) (nonembolic) `HCC` `Rx` `ESR` `COM`
　　Anoxia of spinal cord
　　Arterial thrombosis of spinal cord

　G95.19 Other vascular myelopathies `HCC` `Rx` `ESR` `COM`
　　Edema of spinal cord
　　Hematomyelia
　　Nonpyogenic intraspinal phlebitis and thrombophlebitis
　　Subacute necrotic myelopathy

✓5ᵗʰ **G95.2 Other and unspecified cord compression**
　G95.20 Unspecified cord compression `HCC` `Rx` `ESR` `COM`
　G95.29 Other cord compression `HCC` `Rx` `ESR` `COM`

✓5ᵗʰ **G95.8 Other specified diseases of spinal cord**
　EXCLUDES 1 *neurogenic bladder NOS (N31.9)*
　　　neurogenic bladder due to cauda equina syndrome (G83.4)
　　　neuromuscular dysfunction of bladder without spinal cord lesion (N31.-)

　G95.81 Conus medullaris syndrome `HCC` `Rx` `ESR` `COM`

　G95.89 Other specified diseases of spinal cord `HCC` `Rx` `ESR` `COM`
　　Cord bladder NOS
　　Drug-induced myelopathy
　　Radiation-induced myelopathy
　　EXCLUDES 1 *myelopathy NOS (G95.9)*

G95.9 Disease of spinal cord, unspecified `HCC` `Rx` `ESR` `COM`
　Myelopathy NOS

✓4ᵗʰ **G96 Other disorders of central nervous system**

✓5ᵗʰ **G96.0 Cerebrospinal fluid leak**
　Code also if applicable:
　　intracranial hypotension (G96.81-)
　EXCLUDES 1 *cerebrospinal fluid leak from spinal puncture (G97.0)*
　AHA: 2020,4Q,21-22; 2018,2Q,13

　G96.00 Cerebrospinal fluid leak, unspecified
　　Code also if applicable:
　　　head injury ▶(S00–S09)◀

　G96.01 Cranial cerebrospinal fluid leak, spontaneous
　　Otorrhea due to spontaneous cerebrospinal fluid CSF leak
　　Rhinorrhea due to spontaneous cerebrospinal fluid CSF leak
　　Spontaneous cerebrospinal fluid leak from skull base

　G96.02 Spinal cerebrospinal fluid leak, spontaneous
　　Spontaneous cerebrospinal fluid leak from spine

　G96.08 Other cranial cerebrospinal fluid leak
　　Postoperative cranial cerebrospinal fluid leak
　　Traumatic cranial cerebrospinal fluid leak
　　Code also if applicable:
　　　head injury (S00.- to S09.-)

　G96.09 Other spinal cerebrospinal fluid leak
　　Other spinal CSF leak
　　Postoperative spinal cerebrospinal fluid leak
　　Traumatic spinal cerebrospinal fluid leak
　　Code also if applicable:
　　　head injury (S00.- to S09.-)

✓6ᵗʰ **G96.1 Disorders of meninges, not elsewhere classified**

　G96.11 Dural tear
　　Code also intracranial hypotension, if applicable (G96.81-)
　　EXCLUDES 1 *accidental puncture or laceration of dura during a procedure (G97.41)*
　　AHA: 2014,4Q,24

　G96.12 Meningeal adhesions (cerebral) (spinal)

✓6ᵗʰ **G96.19 Other disorders of meninges, not elsewhere classified**
　　AHA: 2020,4Q,22
　　G96.191 Perineural cyst
　　　Cervical nerve root cyst
　　　Lumbar nerve root cyst
　　　Sacral nerve root cyst
　　　Tarlov cyst
　　　Thoracic nerve root cyst
　　G96.198 Other disorders of meninges, not elsewhere classified

✓6ᵗʰ **G96.8 Other specified disorders of central nervous system**
　AHA: 2020,4Q,21,23-24

✓6ᵗʰ **G96.81 Intracranial hypotension**
　　Code also any associated diagnoses, such as:
　　　brachial amyotrophy (G54.5)
　　　cerebrospinal fluid leak from spine (G96.02)
　　　cranial nerve disorders in diseases classified elsewhere (G53)
　　　nerve root and compressions in diseases classified elsewhere (G55)
　　　nonpyogenic thrombosis of intracranial venous system (I67.6)
　　　nontraumatic intracerebral hemorrhage (I61.-)
　　　nontraumatic subdural hemorrhage (I62.0-)
　　　other and unspecified cord compression (G95.2-)
　　　other secondary parkinsonism (G21.8)
　　　reversible cerebrovascular vasoconstriction syndrome (I67.841)
　　　spinal cord herniation (G95.89)
　　　stroke (I63.-)
　　　syringomyelia (G95.0)
　　DEF: Central nervous system disorder resulting from a loss of cerebrospinal fluid (CSF) volume. More often associated with CSF leak at the level of the spine rather than the skull base, causes can be spontaneous, iatrogenic or traumatic spinal dura defects or holes, or overdrainage of CSF shunt devices. The most common symptom is headache.
　　G96.810 Intracranial hypotension, unspecified
　　G96.811 Intracranial hypotension, spontaneous
　　G96.819 Other intracranial hypotension

　G96.89 Other specified disorders of central nervous system

G96.9 Disorder of central nervous system, unspecified

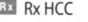
`HCC` CMS-HCC   `Rx` Rx HCC   `ESR` ESRD HCC   `COM` Commercial HCC   `N` Newborn: 0   `P` Pediatric: 0-17   `M` Maternity: 9-64   `A` Adult: 15-124

608   ICD-10-CM 2023

✓4ᵗʰ **G97 Intraoperative and postprocedural complications and disorders of nervous system, not elsewhere classified**

> EXCLUDES 2   *intraoperative and postprocedural cerebrovascular infarction (I97.81-, I97.82-)*
>
> **AHA:** 2016,4Q,9-10

G97.0 Cerebrospinal fluid leak from spinal puncture
> Code also any associated diagnoses or complications, such as: intracranial hypotension following a procedure (G97.83-G97.84)

Spinal Puncture

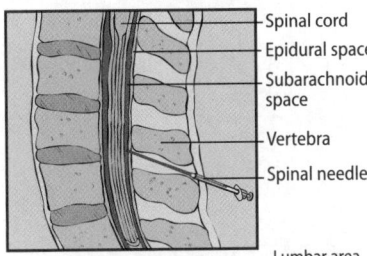

- Spinal cord
- Epidural space
- Subarachnoid space
- Vertebra
- Spinal needle

Lumbar area

G97.1 Other reaction to spinal and lumbar puncture
> Headache due to lumbar puncture
> Other reaction to spinal dural puncture
> Code also, if applicable, any associated headache with orthostatic component (R51.0)

G97.2 Intracranial hypotension following ventricular shunting
> Code also any associated diagnoses or complications

✓5ᵗʰ **G97.3 Intraoperative hemorrhage and hematoma of a nervous system organ or structure complicating a procedure**
> EXCLUDES 1   *intraoperative hemorrhage and hematoma of a nervous system organ or structure due to accidental puncture and laceration during a procedure (G97.4-)*

   G97.31 Intraoperative hemorrhage and hematoma of a nervous system organ or structure complicating a nervous system procedure

   G97.32 Intraoperative hemorrhage and hematoma of a nervous system organ or structure complicating other procedure

✓5ᵗʰ **G97.4 Accidental puncture and laceration of a nervous system organ or structure during a procedure**

   G97.41 Accidental puncture or laceration of dura during a procedure
> Incidental (inadvertent) durotomy
> Code also any associated diagnoses or complications
> **AHA:** 2014,4Q,24

   G97.48 Accidental puncture and laceration of other nervous system organ or structure during a nervous system procedure

   G97.49 Accidental puncture and laceration of other nervous system organ or structure during other procedure

✓5ᵗʰ **G97.5 Postprocedural hemorrhage of a nervous system organ or structure following a procedure**

   G97.51 Postprocedural hemorrhage of a nervous system organ or structure following a nervous system procedure

   G97.52 Postprocedural hemorrhage of a nervous system organ or structure following other procedure

✓5ᵗʰ **G97.6 Postprocedural hematoma and seroma of a nervous system organ or structure following a procedure**

   G97.61 Postprocedural hematoma of a nervous system organ or structure following a nervous system procedure
> **AHA:** 2020,3Q,24

   G97.62 Postprocedural hematoma of a nervous system organ or structure following other procedure

   G97.63 Postprocedural seroma of a nervous system organ or structure following a nervous system procedure

   G97.64 Postprocedural seroma of a nervous system organ or structure following other procedure

✓5ᵗʰ **G97.8 Other intraoperative and postprocedural complications and disorders of nervous system**
> Use additional code to further specify disorder
> **AHA:** 2020,4Q,23

   G97.81 Other intraoperative complications of nervous system

   G97.82 Other postprocedural complications and disorders of nervous system
> **AHA:** 2022,1Q,34

   G97.83 Intracranial hypotension following lumbar cerebrospinal fluid shunting
> Code also any associated diagnoses or complications

   G97.84 Intracranial hypotension following other procedure
> Code also, if applicable:
> accidental puncture or laceration of dura during a procedure (G97.41)
> cerebrospinal fluid leak from spinal puncture (G97.0)

✓4ᵗʰ **G98 Other disorders of nervous system not elsewhere classified**
> INCLUDES   nervous system disorder NOS

G98.0 Neurogenic arthritis, not elsewhere classified
> Nonsyphilitic neurogenic arthropathy NEC
> Nonsyphilitic neurogenic spondylopathy NEC
> EXCLUDES 1   *spondylopathy (in):*
> *syringomyelia and syringobulbia (G95.0)*
> *tabes dorsalis (A52.11)*

G98.8 Other disorders of nervous system
> Nervous system disorder NOS

✓4ᵗʰ **G99 Other disorders of nervous system in diseases classified elsewhere**

G99.0 *Autonomic neuropathy in diseases classified elsewhere*
> Code first underlying disease, such as:
> amyloidosis (E85.-)
> gout (M1A.-, M10.-)
> hyperthyroidism (E05.-)
> EXCLUDES 1   *diabetic autonomic neuropathy (E08-E13 with .43)*

G99.2 *Myelopathy in diseases classified elsewhere* HCC Rx ESR COM
> Code first underlying disease, such as:
> neoplasm (C00-D49)
> EXCLUDES 1   *myelopathy in:*
> *intervertebral disease (M50.0-, M51.0-)*
> *spondylosis (M47.0-, M47.1-)*
>
> **AHA:** 2018,3Q,18-19
> **TIP:** Use this code in addition to a spondylolisthesis code (M43.1-) or a spinal stenosis code (M48.0-) when either of these disorders is documented as the cause of the myelopathy.

G99.8 *Other specified disorders of nervous system in diseases classified elsewhere*
> Code first underlying disorder, such as:
> amyloidosis (E85.-)
> avitaminosis (E56.9)
> EXCLUDES 1   *nervous system involvement in:*
> *cysticercosis (B69.0)*
> *rubella (B06.0-)*
> *syphilis (A52.1-)*

☑ Additional Character Required   ✓x7ᵗʰ Placeholder Alert   Manifestation   Unspecified Dx   Q QPP   UPD Unacceptable PDx

Chapter 7. Diseases of the Eye and Adnexa (H00–H59)

Chapter-specific Guidelines with Coding Examples

The chapter-specific guidelines from the ICD-10-CM Official Guidelines for Coding and Reporting have been provided below. Along with these guidelines are coding examples, contained in the shaded boxes, that have been developed to help illustrate the coding and/or sequencing guidance found in these guidelines.

a. Glaucoma

1) **Assigning glaucoma codes**

   Assign as many codes from category H40, Glaucoma, as needed to identify the type of glaucoma, the affected eye, and the glaucoma stage.

2) **Bilateral glaucoma with same type and stage**

   When a patient has bilateral glaucoma and both eyes are documented as being the same type and stage, and there is a code for bilateral glaucoma, report only the code for the type of glaucoma, bilateral, with the seventh character for the stage.

   > Bilateral mild stage primary open-angle glaucoma
   >
   > **H40.1131   Primary open-angle glaucoma, bilateral, mild stage**
   >
   > *Explanation*: In this scenario, the patient has the same type and stage of glaucoma in both eyes. As this type of glaucoma has a code for bilateral, assign only the code for the bilateral glaucoma with the seventh character for the stage.

   When a patient has bilateral glaucoma and both eyes are documented as being the same type and stage, and the classification does not provide a code for bilateral glaucoma (i.e. subcategories H40.10 and H40.20) report only one code for the type of glaucoma with the appropriate seventh character for the stage.

   > Bilateral open-angle glaucoma, severe stage; not specified as to type
   >
   > **H40.10X3   Unspecified open-angle glaucoma, severe stage**
   >
   > *Explanation*: In this scenario, the patient has glaucoma of the same type and stage of both eyes, but there is no code specifically for bilateral glaucoma. Only one code is assigned with the appropriate seventh character for the stage.

3) **Bilateral glaucoma stage with different types or stages**

   When a patient has bilateral glaucoma and each eye is documented as having a different type or stage, and the classification distinguishes laterality, assign the appropriate code for each eye rather than the code for bilateral glaucoma.

   > Bilateral chronic angle-closure glaucoma; right eye is documented as mild stage and left eye as moderate stage
   >
   > **H40.2211   Chronic angle-closure glaucoma, right eye, mild stage**
   >
   > **H40.2222   Chronic angle-closure glaucoma, left eye, moderate stage**
   >
   > *Explanation*: In this scenario the patient has the same type of glaucoma in both eyes, but each eye is at a different stage. Because the subcategory for this condition identifies laterality, one code is assigned for the right eye and one code is assigned for the left eye, each with the appropriate seventh character for the stage appended.

When a patient has bilateral glaucoma and each eye is documented as having a different type, and the classification does not distinguish laterality (i.e. subcategories H40.10 and H40.20), assign one code for each type of glaucoma with the appropriate seventh character for the stage.

> Documentation relates mild, unspecified primary angle-closure glaucoma of the left eye with mild unspecified open-angle glaucoma of the right eye
>
> **H40.20X1   Unspecified primary angle-closure glaucoma, mild stage**
>
> **H40.10X1   Unspecified open-angle glaucoma, mild stage**
>
> *Explanation*: In this scenario the patient has a different type of glaucoma in each eye and the classification does not distinguish laterality. A code for each type of glaucoma is assigned, each with the appropriate seventh character for the stage.

When a patient has bilateral glaucoma and each eye is documented as having the same type, but different stage, and the classification does not distinguish laterality (i.e. subcategories H40.10 and H40.20), assign a code for the type of glaucoma for each eye with the seventh character for the specific glaucoma stage documented for each eye.

> Bilateral open-angle glaucoma, not specified as to type; the right eye is documented to be in mild stage and the left eye as being in moderate stage
>
> **H40.10X1   Unspecified open-angle glaucoma, mild stage**
>
> **H40.10X2   Unspecified open-angle glaucoma, moderate stage**
>
> *Explanation*: In this scenario the patient has the same type of glaucoma in each eye but each eye is at a different stage, and the classification does not distinguish laterality at this subcategory level. Two codes are assigned; both codes represent the same type of glaucoma but each has a different seventh character identifying the appropriate stage for each eye.

4) **Patient admitted with glaucoma and stage evolves during the admission**

   If a patient is admitted with glaucoma and the stage progresses during the admission, assign the code for highest stage documented.

5) **Indeterminate stage glaucoma**

   Assignment of the seventh character "4" for "indeterminate stage" should be based on the clinical documentation. The seventh character "4" is used for glaucomas whose stage cannot be clinically determined. This seventh character should not be confused with the seventh character "0", unspecified, which should be assigned when there is no documentation regarding the stage of the glaucoma.

b. Blindness

If "blindness" or "low vision" of both eyes is documented but the visual impairment category is not documented, assign code H54.3, Unqualified visual loss, both eyes. If "blindness" or "low vision" in one eye is documented but the visual impairment category is not documented, assign a code from H54.6-, Unqualified visual loss, one eye. If "blindness" or "visual loss" is documented without any information about whether one or both eyes are affected, assign code H54.7, Unspecified visual loss.

> Patient assessment indicates moderately impaired/low vision in the left eye with no visual impairments in the right eye
>
> **H54.62   Unqualified visual loss, left eye, normal vision right eye**
>
> Report unqualified visual loss when the visual impairment category is not specified. In this case, only the left eye is impacted by visual loss with normal vision of the right eye documented.

Chapter 7. Diseases of the Eye and Adnexa (H00-H59)

NOTE Use an external cause code following the code for the eye condition, if applicable, to identify the cause of the eye condition

EXCLUDES 2　certain conditions originating in the perinatal period (P04-P96)
certain infectious and parasitic diseases (A00-B99)
complications of pregnancy, childbirth and the puerperium (O00-O9A)
congenital malformations, deformations, and chromosomal abnormalities (Q00-Q99)
diabetes mellitus related eye conditions (E09.3-, E10.3-, E11.3-, E13.3-)
endocrine, nutritional and metabolic diseases (E00-E88)
injury (trauma) of eye and orbit (S05.-)
injury, poisoning and certain other consequences of external causes (S00-T88)
neoplasms (C00-D49)
symptoms, signs and abnormal clinical and laboratory findings, not elsewhere classified (R00-R94)
syphilis related eye disorders (A50.01, A50.3-, A51.43, A52.71)

This chapter contains the following blocks:
H00-H05　Disorders of eyelid, lacrimal system and orbit
H10-H11　Disorders of conjunctiva
H15-H22　Disorders of sclera, cornea, iris and ciliary body
H25-H28　Disorders of lens
H30-H36　Disorders of choroid and retina
H40-H42　Glaucoma
H43-H44　Disorders of vitreous body and globe
H46-H47　Disorders of optic nerve and visual pathways
H49-H52　Disorders of ocular muscles, binocular movement, accommodation and refraction
H53-H54　Visual disturbances and blindness
H55-H57　Other disorders of eye and adnexa
H59　Intraoperative and postprocedural complications and disorders of eye and adnexa, not elsewhere classified

Disorders of eyelid, lacrimal system and orbit (H00-H05)

EXCLUDES 2　open wound of eyelid (S01.1-)
superficial injury of eyelid (S00.1-, S00.2-)

✓4ᵗʰ **H00　Hordeolum and chalazion**

　✓5ᵗʰ **H00.0　Hordeolum (externum) (internum) of eyelid**
　　　　DEF: Acute localized infection of the gland of Zeis (external hordeolum) or Molt or of the meibomian glands (internal hordeolum) of the orbit.

　　✓6ᵗʰ **H00.01　Hordeolum externum**
　　　　Hordeolum NOS
　　　　Stye
　　　　H00.011　Hordeolum externum right upper eyelid
　　　　H00.012　Hordeolum externum right lower eyelid
　　　　H00.013　Hordeolum externum right eye, unspecified eyelid
　　　　H00.014　Hordeolum externum left upper eyelid
　　　　H00.015　Hordeolum externum left lower eyelid
　　　　H00.016　Hordeolum externum left eye, unspecified eyelid
　　　　H00.019　Hordeolum externum unspecified eye, unspecified eyelid

　　✓6ᵗʰ **H00.02　Hordeolum internum**
　　　　Infection of meibomian gland
　　　　H00.021　Hordeolum internum right upper eyelid
　　　　H00.022　Hordeolum internum right lower eyelid
　　　　H00.023　Hordeolum internum right eye, unspecified eyelid
　　　　H00.024　Hordeolum internum left upper eyelid
　　　　H00.025　Hordeolum internum left lower eyelid
　　　　H00.026　Hordeolum internum left eye, unspecified eyelid
　　　　H00.029　Hordeolum internum unspecified eye, unspecified eyelid

　　✓6ᵗʰ **H00.03　Abscess of eyelid**
　　　　Furuncle of eyelid
　　　　H00.031　Abscess of right upper eyelid
　　　　H00.032　Abscess of right lower eyelid
　　　　H00.033　Abscess of eyelid right eye, unspecified eyelid
　　　　H00.034　Abscess of left upper eyelid
　　　　H00.035　Abscess of left lower eyelid
　　　　H00.036　Abscess of eyelid left eye, unspecified eyelid
　　　　H00.039　Abscess of eyelid unspecified eye, unspecified eyelid

　✓5ᵗʰ **H00.1　Chalazion**
　　　Meibomian (gland) cyst
　　　EXCLUDES 2　infected meibomian gland (H00.02-)
　　　DEF: Noninfectious, obstructive mass in the oil gland of the eyelid that results in a small chronic lump or inflammation.
　　　H00.11　Chalazion right upper eyelid
　　　H00.12　Chalazion right lower eyelid
　　　H00.13　Chalazion right eye, unspecified eyelid
　　　H00.14　Chalazion left upper eyelid
　　　H00.15　Chalazion left lower eyelid
　　　H00.16　Chalazion left eye, unspecified eyelid
　　　H00.19　Chalazion unspecified eye, unspecified eyelid

✓4ᵗʰ **H01　Other inflammation of eyelid**

　✓5ᵗʰ **H01.0　Blepharitis**
　　　EXCLUDES 1　blepharoconjunctivitis (H10.5-)

　　✓6ᵗʰ **H01.00　Unspecified blepharitis**
　　　　AHA: 2018,4Q,13
　　　　H01.001　Unspecified blepharitis right upper eyelid
　　　　H01.002　Unspecified blepharitis right lower eyelid
　　　　H01.003　Unspecified blepharitis right eye, unspecified eyelid
　　　　H01.004　Unspecified blepharitis left upper eyelid
　　　　H01.005　Unspecified blepharitis left lower eyelid
　　　　H01.006　Unspecified blepharitis left eye, unspecified eyelid
　　　　H01.009　Unspecified blepharitis unspecified eye, unspecified eyelid
　　　　H01.00A　Unspecified blepharitis right eye, upper and lower eyelids
　　　　H01.00B　Unspecified blepharitis left eye, upper and lower eyelids

　　✓6ᵗʰ **H01.01　Ulcerative blepharitis**
　　　　AHA: 2018,4Q,13
　　　　H01.011　Ulcerative blepharitis right upper eyelid
　　　　H01.012　Ulcerative blepharitis right lower eyelid
　　　　H01.013　Ulcerative blepharitis right eye, unspecified eyelid
　　　　H01.014　Ulcerative blepharitis left upper eyelid
　　　　H01.015　Ulcerative blepharitis left lower eyelid
　　　　H01.016　Ulcerative blepharitis left eye, unspecified eyelid
　　　　H01.019　Ulcerative blepharitis unspecified eye, unspecified eyelid
　　　　H01.01A　Ulcerative blepharitis right eye, upper and lower eyelids
　　　　H01.01B　Ulcerative blepharitis left eye, upper and lower eyelids

　　✓6ᵗʰ **H01.02　Squamous blepharitis**
　　　　AHA: 2018,4Q,13
　　　　H01.021　Squamous blepharitis right upper eyelid
　　　　H01.022　Squamous blepharitis right lower eyelid
　　　　H01.023　Squamous blepharitis right eye, unspecified eyelid
　　　　H01.024　Squamous blepharitis left upper eyelid
　　　　H01.025　Squamous blepharitis left lower eyelid
　　　　H01.026　Squamous blepharitis left eye, unspecified eyelid
　　　　H01.029　Squamous blepharitis unspecified eye, unspecified eyelid
　　　　H01.02A　Squamous blepharitis right eye, upper and lower eyelids
　　　　H01.02B　Squamous blepharitis left eye, upper and lower eyelids

　✓5ᵗʰ **H01.1　Noninfectious dermatoses of eyelid**

　　✓6ᵗʰ **H01.11　Allergic dermatitis of eyelid**
　　　　Contact dermatitis of eyelid
　　　　H01.111　Allergic dermatitis of right upper eyelid
　　　　H01.112　Allergic dermatitis of right lower eyelid
　　　　H01.113　Allergic dermatitis of right eye, unspecified eyelid
　　　　H01.114　Allergic dermatitis of left upper eyelid
　　　　H01.115　Allergic dermatitis of left lower eyelid
　　　　H01.116　Allergic dermatitis of left eye, unspecified eyelid
　　　　H01.119　Allergic dermatitis of unspecified eye, unspecified eyelid

✓6ᵗʰ **H01.12 Discoid lupus erythematosus of eyelid**

    H01.121 Discoid lupus erythematosus of right upper eyelid Rx

    H01.122 Discoid lupus erythematosus of right lower eyelid Rx

    H01.123 Discoid lupus erythematosus of right eye, unspecified eyelid Rx

    H01.124 Discoid lupus erythematosus of left upper eyelid Rx

    H01.125 Discoid lupus erythematosus of left lower eyelid

    H01.126 Discoid lupus erythematosus of left eye, unspecified eyelid Rx

    H01.129 Discoid lupus erythematosus of unspecified eye, unspecified eyelid Rx

✓6ᵗʰ **H01.13 Eczematous dermatitis of eyelid**

    H01.131 Eczematous dermatitis of right upper eyelid

    H01.132 Eczematous dermatitis of right lower eyelid

    H01.133 Eczematous dermatitis of right eye, unspecified eyelid

    H01.134 Eczematous dermatitis of left upper eyelid

    H01.135 Eczematous dermatitis of left lower eyelid

    H01.136 Eczematous dermatitis of left eye, unspecified eyelid

    H01.139 Eczematous dermatitis of unspecified eye, unspecified eyelid

✓6ᵗʰ **H01.14 Xeroderma of eyelid**

    H01.141 Xeroderma of right upper eyelid

    H01.142 Xeroderma of right lower eyelid

    H01.143 Xeroderma of right eye, unspecified eyelid

    H01.144 Xeroderma of left upper eyelid

    H01.145 Xeroderma of left lower eyelid

    H01.146 Xeroderma of left eye, unspecified eyelid

    H01.149 Xeroderma of unspecified eye, unspecified eyelid

H01.8 Other specified inflammations of eyelid

H01.9 Unspecified inflammation of eyelid

    Inflammation of eyelid NOS

✓4ᵗʰ **H02 Other disorders of eyelid**

    EXCLUDES 1   *congenital malformations of eyelid (Q10.0-Q10.3)*

Entropion and Ectropion

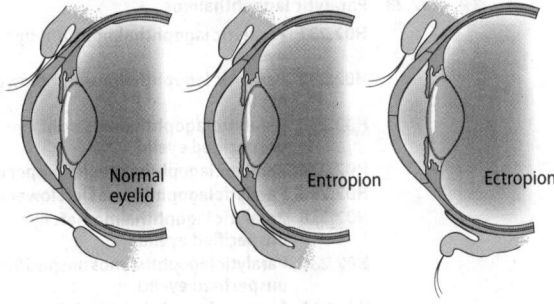

Normal eyelid   Entropion   Ectropion

✓5ᵗʰ **H02.0 Entropion and trichiasis of eyelid**

    DEF: Entropion: Inversion of the eyelid, turning the edge in toward the eyeball and causing irritation from contact of the lashes with the surface of the eye.

    DEF: Trichiasis: Condition wherein the eyelid is in a normal position but lashes are ingrown or misdirected in their growth so that they irritate the tissues of the eye.

✓6ᵗʰ **H02.00 Unspecified entropion of eyelid**

    H02.001 Unspecified entropion of right upper eyelid

    H02.002 Unspecified entropion of right lower eyelid

    H02.003 Unspecified entropion of right eye, unspecified eyelid

    H02.004 Unspecified entropion of left upper eyelid

    H02.005 Unspecified entropion of left lower eyelid

    H02.006 Unspecified entropion of left eye, unspecified eyelid

    H02.009 Unspecified entropion of unspecified eye, unspecified eyelid

✓6ᵗʰ **H02.01 Cicatricial entropion of eyelid**

    H02.011 Cicatricial entropion of right upper eyelid

    H02.012 Cicatricial entropion of right lower eyelid

    H02.013 Cicatricial entropion of right eye, unspecified eyelid

    H02.014 Cicatricial entropion of left upper eyelid

    H02.015 Cicatricial entropion of left lower eyelid

    H02.016 Cicatricial entropion of left eye, unspecified eyelid

    H02.019 Cicatricial entropion of unspecified eye, unspecified eyelid

✓6ᵗʰ **H02.02 Mechanical entropion of eyelid**

    H02.021 Mechanical entropion of right upper eyelid

    H02.022 Mechanical entropion of right lower eyelid

    H02.023 Mechanical entropion of right eye, unspecified eyelid

    H02.024 Mechanical entropion of left upper eyelid

    H02.025 Mechanical entropion of left lower eyelid

    H02.026 Mechanical entropion of left eye, unspecified eyelid

    H02.029 Mechanical entropion of unspecified eye, unspecified eyelid

✓6ᵗʰ **H02.03 Senile entropion of eyelid**

    H02.031 Senile entropion of right upper eyelid A

    H02.032 Senile entropion of right lower eyelid A

    H02.033 Senile entropion of right eye, unspecified eyelid A

    H02.034 Senile entropion of left upper eyelid A

    H02.035 Senile entropion of left lower eyelid A

    H02.036 Senile entropion of left eye, unspecified eyelid A

    H02.039 Senile entropion of unspecified eye, unspecified eyelid A

✓6ᵗʰ **H02.04 Spastic entropion of eyelid**

    H02.041 Spastic entropion of right upper eyelid

    H02.042 Spastic entropion of right lower eyelid

    H02.043 Spastic entropion of right eye, unspecified eyelid

    H02.044 Spastic entropion of left upper eyelid

    H02.045 Spastic entropion of left lower eyelid

    H02.046 Spastic entropion of left eye, unspecified eyelid

    H02.049 Spastic entropion of unspecified eye, unspecified eyelid

✓6ᵗʰ **H02.05 Trichiasis without entropion**

    H02.051 Trichiasis without entropion right upper eyelid

    H02.052 Trichiasis without entropion right lower eyelid

    H02.053 Trichiasis without entropion right eye, unspecified eyelid

    H02.054 Trichiasis without entropion left upper eyelid

    H02.055 Trichiasis without entropion left lower eyelid

    H02.056 Trichiasis without entropion left eye, unspecified eyelid

    H02.059 Trichiasis without entropion unspecified eye, unspecified eyelid

✓5ᵗʰ **H02.1 Ectropion of eyelid**

    DEF: Drooping of the lower eyelid away from the eye or outward turning or eversion of the edge of the eye, exposing the palpebral conjunctiva and causing irritation.

✓6ᵗʰ **H02.10 Unspecified ectropion of eyelid**

    H02.101 Unspecified ectropion of right upper eyelid

    H02.102 Unspecified ectropion of right lower eyelid

    H02.103 Unspecified ectropion of right eye, unspecified eyelid

    H02.104 Unspecified ectropion of left upper eyelid

    H02.105 Unspecified ectropion of left lower eyelid

    H02.106 Unspecified ectropion of left eye, unspecified eyelid

H02.109 Unspecified ectropion of unspecified eye, unspecified eyelid

✓6ᵗʰ **H02.11** Cicatricial ectropion of eyelid

    H02.111 Cicatricial ectropion of right upper eyelid

    H02.112 Cicatricial ectropion of right lower eyelid

    H02.113 Cicatricial ectropion of right eye, unspecified eyelid

    H02.114 Cicatricial ectropion of left upper eyelid

    H02.115 Cicatricial ectropion of left lower eyelid

    H02.116 Cicatricial ectropion of left eye, unspecified eyelid

    H02.119 Cicatricial ectropion of unspecified eye, unspecified eyelid

✓6ᵗʰ **H02.12** Mechanical ectropion of eyelid

    H02.121 Mechanical ectropion of right upper eyelid

    H02.122 Mechanical ectropion of right lower eyelid

    H02.123 Mechanical ectropion of right eye, unspecified eyelid

    H02.124 Mechanical ectropion of left upper eyelid

    H02.125 Mechanical ectropion of left lower eyelid

    H02.126 Mechanical ectropion of left eye, unspecified eyelid

    H02.129 Mechanical ectropion of unspecified eye, unspecified eyelid

✓6ᵗʰ **H02.13** Senile ectropion of eyelid

    H02.131 Senile ectropion of right upper eyelid   **A**

    H02.132 Senile ectropion of right lower eyelid   **A**

    H02.133 Senile ectropion of right eye, unspecified eyelid   **A**

    H02.134 Senile ectropion of left upper eyelid   **A**

    H02.135 Senile ectropion of left lower eyelid   **A**

    H02.136 Senile ectropion of left eye, unspecified eyelid   **A**

    H02.139 Senile ectropion of unspecified eye, unspecified eyelid   **A**

✓6ᵗʰ **H02.14** Spastic ectropion of eyelid

    H02.141 Spastic ectropion of right upper eyelid

    H02.142 Spastic ectropion of right lower eyelid

    H02.143 Spastic ectropion of right eye, unspecified eyelid

    H02.144 Spastic ectropion of left upper eyelid

    H02.145 Spastic ectropion of left lower eyelid

    H02.146 Spastic ectropion of left eye, unspecified eyelid

    H02.149 Spastic ectropion of unspecified eye, unspecified eyelid

✓6ᵗʰ **H02.15** Paralytic ectropion of eyelid

    AHA: 2018,4Q,13

    H02.151 Paralytic ectropion of right upper eyelid

    H02.152 Paralytic ectropion of right lower eyelid

    H02.153 Paralytic ectropion of right eye, unspecified eyelid

    H02.154 Paralytic ectropion of left upper eyelid

    H02.155 Paralytic ectropion of left lower eyelid

    H02.156 Paralytic ectropion of left eye, unspecified eyelid

    H02.159 Paralytic ectropion of unspecified eye, unspecified eyelid

✓5ᵗʰ **H02.2** Lagophthalmos

    AHA: 2018,4Q,14

    DEF: Condition of the eye that prevents it from closing completely.

✓6ᵗʰ **H02.20** Unspecified lagophthalmos

    H02.201 Unspecified lagophthalmos right upper eyelid

    H02.202 Unspecified lagophthalmos right lower eyelid

    H02.203 Unspecified lagophthalmos right eye, unspecified eyelid

    H02.204 Unspecified lagophthalmos left upper eyelid

    H02.205 Unspecified lagophthalmos left lower eyelid

    H02.206 Unspecified lagophthalmos left eye, unspecified eyelid

    H02.209 Unspecified lagophthalmos unspecified eye, unspecified eyelid

    H02.20A Unspecified lagophthalmos right eye, upper and lower eyelids

    H02.20B Unspecified lagophthalmos left eye, upper and lower eyelids

    H02.20C Unspecified lagophthalmos, bilateral, upper and lower eyelids

✓6ᵗʰ **H02.21** Cicatricial lagophthalmos

    H02.211 Cicatricial lagophthalmos right upper eyelid

    H02.212 Cicatricial lagophthalmos right lower eyelid

    H02.213 Cicatricial lagophthalmos right eye, unspecified eyelid

    H02.214 Cicatricial lagophthalmos left upper eyelid

    H02.215 Cicatricial lagophthalmos left lower eyelid

    H02.216 Cicatricial lagophthalmos left eye, unspecified eyelid

    H02.219 Cicatricial lagophthalmos unspecified eye, unspecified eyelid

    H02.21A Cicatricial lagophthalmos right eye, upper and lower eyelids

    H02.21B Cicatricial lagophthalmos left eye, upper and lower eyelids

    H02.21C Cicatricial lagophthalmos, bilateral, upper and lower eyelids

✓6ᵗʰ **H02.22** Mechanical lagophthalmos

    H02.221 Mechanical lagophthalmos right upper eyelid

    H02.222 Mechanical lagophthalmos right lower eyelid

    H02.223 Mechanical lagophthalmos right eye, unspecified eyelid

    H02.224 Mechanical lagophthalmos left upper eyelid

    H02.225 Mechanical lagophthalmos left lower eyelid

    H02.226 Mechanical lagophthalmos left eye, unspecified eyelid

    H02.229 Mechanical lagophthalmos unspecified eye, unspecified eyelid

    H02.22A Mechanical lagophthalmos right eye, upper and lower eyelids

    H02.22B Mechanical lagophthalmos left eye, upper and lower eyelids

    H02.22C Mechanical lagophthalmos, bilateral, upper and lower eyelids

✓6ᵗʰ **H02.23** Paralytic lagophthalmos

    H02.231 Paralytic lagophthalmos right upper eyelid

    H02.232 Paralytic lagophthalmos right lower eyelid

    H02.233 Paralytic lagophthalmos right eye, unspecified eyelid

    H02.234 Paralytic lagophthalmos left upper eyelid

    H02.235 Paralytic lagophthalmos left lower eyelid

    H02.236 Paralytic lagophthalmos left eye, unspecified eyelid

    H02.239 Paralytic lagophthalmos unspecified eye, unspecified eyelid

    H02.23A Paralytic lagophthalmos right eye, upper and lower eyelids

    H02.23B Paralytic lagophthalmos left eye, upper and lower eyelids

    H02.23C Paralytic lagophthalmos, bilateral, upper and lower eyelids

✓5ᵗʰ **H02.3** Blepharochalasis

    Pseudoptosis

    DEF: Loss of elasticity and relaxation of skin of the eyelid, thickened or indurated skin on the eyelid associated with recurrent episodes of edema, and intracellular atrophy.

    H02.30 Blepharochalasis unspecified eye, unspecified eyelid

    H02.31 Blepharochalasis right upper eyelid

    H02.32 Blepharochalasis right lower eyelid

    H02.33 Blepharochalasis right eye, unspecified eyelid

    H02.34 Blepharochalasis left upper eyelid

    H02.35 Blepharochalasis left lower eyelid

    H02.36 Blepharochalasis left eye, unspecified eyelid

 HCC CMS-HCC   **Rx** Rx HCC   **ESR** ESRD HCC   **COM** Commercial HCC   **N** Newborn: 0   **P** Pediatric: 0-17   **M** Maternity: 9-64   **A** Adult: 15-124

614   ICD-10-CM 2023

✓5ᵗʰ **H02.4 Ptosis of eyelid**
  ✓6ᵗʰ **H02.40 Unspecified ptosis of eyelid**
      H02.401 Unspecified ptosis of right eyelid
      H02.402 Unspecified ptosis of left eyelid
      H02.403 Unspecified ptosis of bilateral eyelids
      H02.409 Unspecified ptosis of unspecified eyelid
  ✓6ᵗʰ **H02.41 Mechanical ptosis of eyelid**
      H02.411 Mechanical ptosis of right eyelid
      H02.412 Mechanical ptosis of left eyelid
      H02.413 Mechanical ptosis of bilateral eyelids
      H02.419 Mechanical ptosis of unspecified eyelid
  ✓6ᵗʰ **H02.42 Myogenic ptosis of eyelid**
      H02.421 Myogenic ptosis of right eyelid
      H02.422 Myogenic ptosis of left eyelid
      H02.423 Myogenic ptosis of bilateral eyelids
      H02.429 Myogenic ptosis of unspecified eyelid
  ✓6ᵗʰ **H02.43 Paralytic ptosis of eyelid**
      Neurogenic ptosis of eyelid
      H02.431 Paralytic ptosis of right eyelid
      H02.432 Paralytic ptosis of left eyelid
      H02.433 Paralytic ptosis of bilateral eyelids
      H02.439 Paralytic ptosis unspecified eyelid
✓5ᵗʰ **H02.5 Other disorders affecting eyelid function**
      EXCLUDES 2 blepharospasm (G24.5)
              organic tic (G25.69)
              psychogenic tic (F95.-)
  ✓6ᵗʰ **H02.51 Abnormal innervation syndrome**
      H02.511 Abnormal innervation syndrome right upper eyelid
      H02.512 Abnormal innervation syndrome right lower eyelid
      H02.513 Abnormal innervation syndrome right eye, unspecified eyelid
      H02.514 Abnormal innervation syndrome left upper eyelid
      H02.515 Abnormal innervation syndrome left lower eyelid
      H02.516 Abnormal innervation syndrome left eye, unspecified eyelid
      H02.519 Abnormal innervation syndrome unspecified eye, unspecified eyelid
  ✓6ᵗʰ **H02.52 Blepharophimosis**
      Ankyloblepharon
      H02.521 Blepharophimosis right upper eyelid
      H02.522 Blepharophimosis right lower eyelid
      H02.523 Blepharophimosis right eye, unspecified eyelid
      H02.524 Blepharophimosis left upper eyelid
      H02.525 Blepharophimosis left lower eyelid
      H02.526 Blepharophimosis left eye, unspecified eyelid
      H02.529 Blepharophimosis unspecified eye, unspecified lid
  ✓6ᵗʰ **H02.53 Eyelid retraction**
      Eyelid lag
      H02.531 Eyelid retraction right upper eyelid
      H02.532 Eyelid retraction right lower eyelid
      H02.533 Eyelid retraction right eye, unspecified eyelid
      H02.534 Eyelid retraction left upper eyelid
      H02.535 Eyelid retraction left lower eyelid
      H02.536 Eyelid retraction left eye, unspecified eyelid
      H02.539 Eyelid retraction unspecified eye, unspecified lid
  H02.59 Other disorders affecting eyelid function
      Deficient blink reflex
      Sensory disorders
✓5ᵗʰ **H02.6 Xanthelasma of eyelid**
      DEF: Condition in which there are small yellow tumors that occur on the eyelid, usually appearing near the nose.
      H02.60 Xanthelasma of unspecified eye, unspecified eyelid
      H02.61 Xanthelasma of right upper eyelid
      H02.62 Xanthelasma of right lower eyelid
      H02.63 Xanthelasma of right eye, unspecified eyelid
      H02.64 Xanthelasma of left upper eyelid
      H02.65 Xanthelasma of left lower eyelid
      H02.66 Xanthelasma of left eye, unspecified eyelid

✓5ᵗʰ **H02.7 Other and unspecified degenerative disorders of eyelid and periocular area**
      H02.70 Unspecified degenerative disorders of eyelid and periocular area
  ✓6ᵗʰ **H02.71 Chloasma of eyelid and periocular area**
      Dyspigmentation of eyelid
      Hyperpigmentation of eyelid
      H02.711 Chloasma of right upper eyelid and periocular area
      H02.712 Chloasma of right lower eyelid and periocular area
      H02.713 Chloasma of right eye, unspecified eyelid and periocular area
      H02.714 Chloasma of left upper eyelid and periocular area
      H02.715 Chloasma of left lower eyelid and periocular area
      H02.716 Chloasma of left eye, unspecified eyelid and periocular area
      H02.719 Chloasma of unspecified eye, unspecified eyelid and periocular area
  ✓6ᵗʰ **H02.72 Madarosis of eyelid and periocular area**
      Hypotrichosis of eyelid
      H02.721 Madarosis of right upper eyelid and periocular area
      H02.722 Madarosis of right lower eyelid and periocular area
      H02.723 Madarosis of right eye, unspecified eyelid and periocular area
      H02.724 Madarosis of left upper eyelid and periocular area
      H02.725 Madarosis of left lower eyelid and periocular area
      H02.726 Madarosis of left eye, unspecified eyelid and periocular area
      H02.729 Madarosis of unspecified eye, unspecified eyelid and periocular area
  ✓6ᵗʰ **H02.73 Vitiligo of eyelid and periocular area**
      Hypopigmentation of eyelid
      H02.731 Vitiligo of right upper eyelid and periocular area
      H02.732 Vitiligo of right lower eyelid and periocular area
      H02.733 Vitiligo of right eye, unspecified eyelid and periocular area
      H02.734 Vitiligo of left upper eyelid and periocular area
      H02.735 Vitiligo of left lower eyelid and periocular area
      H02.736 Vitiligo of left eye, unspecified eyelid and periocular area
      H02.739 Vitiligo of unspecified eye, unspecified eyelid and periocular area
      H02.79 Other degenerative disorders of eyelid and periocular area
✓5ᵗʰ **H02.8 Other specified disorders of eyelid**
  ✓6ᵗʰ **H02.81 Retained foreign body in eyelid**
      Use additional code to identify the type of retained foreign body (Z18.-)
      EXCLUDES 1 laceration of eyelid with foreign body (S01.12-)
              retained intraocular foreign body (H44.6-, H44.7-)
              superficial foreign body of eyelid and periocular area (S00.25-)
      H02.811 Retained foreign body in right upper eyelid
      H02.812 Retained foreign body in right lower eyelid
      H02.813 Retained foreign body in right eye, unspecified eyelid
      H02.814 Retained foreign body in left upper eyelid
      H02.815 Retained foreign body in left lower eyelid
      H02.816 Retained foreign body in left eye, unspecified eyelid
      H02.819 Retained foreign body in unspecified eye, unspecified eyelid
  ✓6ᵗʰ **H02.82 Cysts of eyelid**
      Sebaceous cyst of eyelid
      H02.821 Cysts of right upper eyelid
      H02.822 Cysts of right lower eyelid

☑ Additional Character Required   ✓x7ᵗʰ Placeholder Alert   Manifestation   Unspecified Dx   ⚕ QPP   UPD Unacceptable PDx

H02.823 Cysts of right eye, unspecified eyelid
H02.824 Cysts of left upper eyelid
H02.825 Cysts of left lower eyelid
H02.826 Cysts of left eye, unspecified eyelid
H02.829 Cysts of unspecified eye, unspecified eyelid

☑6th **H02.83** Dermatochalasis of eyelid

DEF: Acquired form of connective tissue disorder associated with decreased elastic tissue and abnormal elastin formation, resulting in loss of elasticity of the skin of the eyelid. It is generally associated with aging.

H02.831 Dermatochalasis of right upper eyelid
H02.832 Dermatochalasis of right lower eyelid
H02.833 Dermatochalasis of right eye, unspecified eyelid
H02.834 Dermatochalasis of left upper eyelid
H02.835 Dermatochalasis of left lower eyelid
H02.836 Dermatochalasis of left eye, unspecified eyelid
H02.839 Dermatochalasis of unspecified eye, unspecified eyelid

☑6th **H02.84** Edema of eyelid

Hyperemia of eyelid

H02.841 Edema of right upper eyelid
H02.842 Edema of right lower eyelid
H02.843 Edema of right eye, unspecified eyelid
H02.844 Edema of left upper eyelid
H02.845 Edema of left lower eyelid
H02.846 Edema of left eye, unspecified eyelid
H02.849 Edema of unspecified eye, unspecified eyelid

☑6th **H02.85** Elephantiasis of eyelid

H02.851 Elephantiasis of right upper eyelid
H02.852 Elephantiasis of right lower eyelid
H02.853 Elephantiasis of right eye, unspecified eyelid
H02.854 Elephantiasis of left upper eyelid
H02.855 Elephantiasis of left lower eyelid
H02.856 Elephantiasis of left eye, unspecified eyelid
H02.859 Elephantiasis of unspecified eye, unspecified eyelid

☑6th **H02.86** Hypertrichosis of eyelid

H02.861 Hypertrichosis of right upper eyelid
H02.862 Hypertrichosis of right lower eyelid
H02.863 Hypertrichosis of right eye, unspecified eyelid
H02.864 Hypertrichosis of left upper eyelid
H02.865 Hypertrichosis of left lower eyelid
H02.866 Hypertrichosis of left eye, unspecified eyelid
H02.869 Hypertrichosis of unspecified eye, unspecified eyelid

☑6th **H02.87** Vascular anomalies of eyelid

H02.871 Vascular anomalies of right upper eyelid
H02.872 Vascular anomalies of right lower eyelid
H02.873 Vascular anomalies of right eye, unspecified eyelid
H02.874 Vascular anomalies of left upper eyelid
H02.875 Vascular anomalies of left lower eyelid
H02.876 Vascular anomalies of left eye, unspecified eyelid
H02.879 Vascular anomalies of unspecified eye, unspecified eyelid

☑6th **H02.88** Meibomian gland dysfunction of eyelid

AHA: 2018,4Q,14-15

H02.881 Meibomian gland dysfunction right upper eyelid
H02.882 Meibomian gland dysfunction right lower eyelid
H02.883 Meibomian gland dysfunction of right eye, unspecified eyelid
H02.884 Meibomian gland dysfunction left upper eyelid
H02.885 Meibomian gland dysfunction left lower eyelid
H02.886 Meibomian gland dysfunction of left eye, unspecified eyelid
H02.889 Meibomian gland dysfunction of unspecified eye, unspecified eyelid

H02.88A Meibomian gland dysfunction right eye, upper and lower eyelids
H02.88B Meibomian gland dysfunction left eye, upper and lower eyelids

H02.89 Other specified disorders of eyelid

Hemorrhage of eyelid

H02.9 Unspecified disorder of eyelid

Disorder of eyelid NOS

☑4th **H04** **Disorders of lacrimal system**

EXCLUDES 1   *congenital malformations of lacrimal system (Q10.4-Q10.6)*

☑5th **H04.0** Dacryoadenitis

DEF: Inflammation of the lacrimal gland.

☑6th **H04.00** Unspecified dacryoadenitis

H04.001 Unspecified dacryoadenitis, right lacrimal gland
H04.002 Unspecified dacryoadenitis, left lacrimal gland
H04.003 Unspecified dacryoadenitis, bilateral lacrimal glands
H04.009 Unspecified dacryoadenitis, unspecified lacrimal gland

☑6th **H04.01** Acute dacryoadenitis

H04.011 Acute dacryoadenitis, right lacrimal gland
H04.012 Acute dacryoadenitis, left lacrimal gland
H04.013 Acute dacryoadenitis, bilateral lacrimal glands
H04.019 Acute dacryoadenitis, unspecified lacrimal gland

☑6th **H04.02** Chronic dacryoadenitis

H04.021 Chronic dacryoadenitis, right lacrimal gland
H04.022 Chronic dacryoadenitis, left lacrimal gland
H04.023 Chronic dacryoadenitis, bilateral lacrimal gland
H04.029 Chronic dacryoadenitis, unspecified lacrimal gland

☑6th **H04.03** Chronic enlargement of lacrimal gland

H04.031 Chronic enlargement of right lacrimal gland
H04.032 Chronic enlargement of left lacrimal gland
H04.033 Chronic enlargement of bilateral lacrimal glands
H04.039 Chronic enlargement of unspecified lacrimal gland

☑5th **H04.1** Other disorders of lacrimal gland

☑6th **H04.11** Dacryops

H04.111 Dacryops of right lacrimal gland
H04.112 Dacryops of left lacrimal gland
H04.113 Dacryops of bilateral lacrimal glands
H04.119 Dacryops of unspecified lacrimal gland

☑6th **H04.12** Dry eye syndrome

Tear film insufficiency, NOS

H04.121 Dry eye syndrome of right lacrimal gland
H04.122 Dry eye syndrome of left lacrimal gland
H04.123 Dry eye syndrome of bilateral lacrimal glands
H04.129 Dry eye syndrome of unspecified lacrimal gland

☑6th **H04.13** Lacrimal cyst

Lacrimal cystic degeneration

H04.131 Lacrimal cyst, right lacrimal gland
H04.132 Lacrimal cyst, left lacrimal gland
H04.133 Lacrimal cyst, bilateral lacrimal glands
H04.139 Lacrimal cyst, unspecified lacrimal gland

☑6th **H04.14** Primary lacrimal gland atrophy

H04.141 Primary lacrimal gland atrophy, right lacrimal gland
H04.142 Primary lacrimal gland atrophy, left lacrimal gland
H04.143 Primary lacrimal gland atrophy, bilateral lacrimal glands
H04.149 Primary lacrimal gland atrophy, unspecified lacrimal gland

☑6th **H04.15** Secondary lacrimal gland atrophy

H04.151 Secondary lacrimal gland atrophy, right lacrimal gland

H04.152   Secondary lacrimal gland atrophy, left lacrimal gland

H04.153   Secondary lacrimal gland atrophy, bilateral lacrimal glands

H04.159   Secondary lacrimal gland atrophy, unspecified lacrimal gland

√6ᵗʰ **H04.16**   **Lacrimal gland dislocation**

H04.161   Lacrimal gland dislocation, right lacrimal gland

H04.162   Lacrimal gland dislocation, left lacrimal gland

H04.163   Lacrimal gland dislocation, bilateral lacrimal glands

H04.169   Lacrimal gland dislocation, unspecified lacrimal gland

H04.19   **Other specified disorders of lacrimal gland**

√5ᵗʰ **H04.2**   **Epiphora**

DEF: Excessive tearing or overflow of tears down the cheeks often due to a stricture in the lacrimal passages but can be caused by other conditions.

√6ᵗʰ **H04.20**   **Unspecified epiphora**

H04.201   Unspecified epiphora, right side

H04.202   Unspecified epiphora, left side

H04.203   Unspecified epiphora, bilateral

H04.209   Unspecified epiphora, unspecified side

√6ᵗʰ **H04.21**   **Epiphora due to excess lacrimation**

H04.211   Epiphora due to excess lacrimation, right lacrimal gland

H04.212   Epiphora due to excess lacrimation, left lacrimal gland

H04.213   Epiphora due to excess lacrimation, bilateral lacrimal glands

H04.219   Epiphora due to excess lacrimation, unspecified lacrimal gland

√6ᵗʰ **H04.22**   **Epiphora due to insufficient drainage**

H04.221   Epiphora due to insufficient drainage, right side

H04.222   Epiphora due to insufficient drainage, left side

H04.223   Epiphora due to insufficient drainage, bilateral

H04.229   Epiphora due to insufficient drainage, unspecified side

√5ᵗʰ **H04.3**   **Acute and unspecified inflammation of lacrimal passages**

EXCLUDES 1   neonatal dacryocystitis (P39.1)

√6ᵗʰ **H04.30**   **Unspecified dacryocystitis**

H04.301   Unspecified dacryocystitis of right lacrimal passage

H04.302   Unspecified dacryocystitis of left lacrimal passage

H04.303   Unspecified dacryocystitis of bilateral lacrimal passages

H04.309   Unspecified dacryocystitis of unspecified lacrimal passage

√6ᵗʰ **H04.31**   **Phlegmonous dacryocystitis**

H04.311   Phlegmonous dacryocystitis of right lacrimal passage

H04.312   Phlegmonous dacryocystitis of left lacrimal passage

H04.313   Phlegmonous dacryocystitis of bilateral lacrimal passages

H04.319   Phlegmonous dacryocystitis of unspecified lacrimal passage

√6ᵗʰ **H04.32**   **Acute dacryocystitis**

Acute dacryopericystitis

H04.321   Acute dacryocystitis of right lacrimal passage

H04.322   Acute dacryocystitis of left lacrimal passage

H04.323   Acute dacryocystitis of bilateral lacrimal passages

H04.329   Acute dacryocystitis of unspecified lacrimal passage

√6ᵗʰ **H04.33**   **Acute lacrimal canaliculitis**

H04.331   Acute lacrimal canaliculitis of right lacrimal passage

H04.332   Acute lacrimal canaliculitis of left lacrimal passage

H04.333   Acute lacrimal canaliculitis of bilateral lacrimal passages

H04.339   Acute lacrimal canaliculitis of unspecified lacrimal passage

√5ᵗʰ **H04.4**   **Chronic inflammation of lacrimal passages**

√6ᵗʰ **H04.41**   **Chronic dacryocystitis**

H04.411   Chronic dacryocystitis of right lacrimal passage

H04.412   Chronic dacryocystitis of left lacrimal passage

H04.413   Chronic dacryocystitis of bilateral lacrimal passages

H04.419   Chronic dacryocystitis of unspecified lacrimal passage

√6ᵗʰ **H04.42**   **Chronic lacrimal canaliculitis**

H04.421   Chronic lacrimal canaliculitis of right lacrimal passage

H04.422   Chronic lacrimal canaliculitis of left lacrimal passage

H04.423   Chronic lacrimal canaliculitis of bilateral lacrimal passages

H04.429   Chronic lacrimal canaliculitis of unspecified lacrimal passage

√6ᵗʰ **H04.43**   **Chronic lacrimal mucocele**

H04.431   Chronic lacrimal mucocele of right lacrimal passage

H04.432   Chronic lacrimal mucocele of left lacrimal passage

H04.433   Chronic lacrimal mucocele of bilateral lacrimal passages

H04.439   Chronic lacrimal mucocele of unspecified lacrimal passage

√5ᵗʰ **H04.5**   **Stenosis and insufficiency of lacrimal passages**

√6ᵗʰ **H04.51**   **Dacryolith**

H04.511   Dacryolith of right lacrimal passage

H04.512   Dacryolith of left lacrimal passage

H04.513   Dacryolith of bilateral lacrimal passages

H04.519   Dacryolith of unspecified lacrimal passage

√6ᵗʰ **H04.52**   **Eversion of lacrimal punctum**

H04.521   Eversion of right lacrimal punctum

H04.522   Eversion of left lacrimal punctum

H04.523   Eversion of bilateral lacrimal punctum

H04.529   Eversion of unspecified lacrimal punctum

√6ᵗʰ **H04.53**   **Neonatal obstruction of nasolacrimal duct**

EXCLUDES 1   congenital stenosis and stricture of lacrimal duct (Q10.5)

H04.531   Neonatal obstruction of right nasolacrimal duct   N

H04.532   Neonatal obstruction of left nasolacrimal duct   N

H04.533   Neonatal obstruction of bilateral nasolacrimal duct   N

H04.539   Neonatal obstruction of unspecified nasolacrimal duct   N

√6ᵗʰ **H04.54**   **Stenosis of lacrimal canaliculi**

H04.541   Stenosis of right lacrimal canaliculi

H04.542   Stenosis of left lacrimal canaliculi

H04.543   Stenosis of bilateral lacrimal canaliculi

H04.549   Stenosis of unspecified lacrimal canaliculi

√6ᵗʰ **H04.55**   **Acquired stenosis of nasolacrimal duct**

H04.551   Acquired stenosis of right nasolacrimal duct

H04.552   Acquired stenosis of left nasolacrimal duct

H04.553   Acquired stenosis of bilateral nasolacrimal duct

H04.559   Acquired stenosis of unspecified nasolacrimal duct

√6ᵗʰ **H04.56**   **Stenosis of lacrimal punctum**

H04.561   Stenosis of right lacrimal punctum

H04.562   Stenosis of left lacrimal punctum

H04.563   Stenosis of bilateral lacrimal punctum

H04.569   Stenosis of unspecified lacrimal punctum

√6ᵗʰ **H04.57**   **Stenosis of lacrimal sac**

H04.571   Stenosis of right lacrimal sac

H04.572   Stenosis of left lacrimal sac

H04.573   Stenosis of bilateral lacrimal sac

H04.579   Stenosis of unspecified lacrimal sac

✓5ᵗʰ **H04.6**   **Other changes of lacrimal passages**

     ✓6ᵗʰ **H04.61**   **Lacrimal** *fistula*

         H04.611   **Lacrimal fistula** right **lacrimal passage**

         H04.612   **Lacrimal fistula** left **lacrimal passage**

         H04.613   **Lacrimal fistula** bilateral **lacrimal passages**

         H04.619   **Lacrimal fistula unspecified lacrimal passage**

         H04.69   **Other changes of lacrimal passages**

✓5ᵗʰ **H04.8**   **Other disorders of lacrimal system**

     ✓6ᵗʰ **H04.81**   **Granuloma of lacrimal passages**

         H04.811   **Granuloma of** right **lacrimal passage**

         H04.812   **Granuloma of** left **lacrimal passage**

         H04.813   **Granuloma of** bilateral **lacrimal passages**

         H04.819   **Granuloma of unspecified lacrimal passage**

         H04.89   **Other disorders of lacrimal system**

     H04.9   **Disorder of lacrimal system, unspecified**

✓4ᵗʰ **H05**   **Disorders of orbit**

     EXCLUDES 1   *congenital malformation of orbit (Q10.7)*

✓5ᵗʰ **H05.0**   **Acute inflammation of orbit**

     H05.00   **Unspecified acute inflammation of orbit**

     ✓6ᵗʰ **H05.01**   **Cellulitis of orbit**

         Abscess of orbit

         H05.011   **Cellulitis of** right **orbit**

         H05.012   **Cellulitis of** left **orbit**

         H05.013   **Cellulitis of** bilateral **orbits**

         H05.019   **Cellulitis of unspecified orbit**

     ✓6ᵗʰ **H05.02**   **Osteomyelitis of orbit**

         H05.021   **Osteomyelitis of** right **orbit**

         H05.022   **Osteomyelitis of** left **orbit**

         H05.023   **Osteomyelitis of** bilateral **orbits**

         H05.029   **Osteomyelitis of unspecified orbit**

     ✓6ᵗʰ **H05.03**   **Periostitis of orbit**

         H05.031   **Periostitis of** right **orbit**

         H05.032   **Periostitis of** left **orbit**

         H05.033   **Periostitis of** bilateral **orbits**

         H05.039   **Periostitis of unspecified orbit**

     ✓6ᵗʰ **H05.04**   **Tenonitis of orbit**

         H05.041   **Tenonitis of** right **orbit**

         H05.042   **Tenonitis of** left **orbit**

         H05.043   **Tenonitis of** bilateral **orbits**

         H05.049   **Tenonitis of unspecified orbit**

✓5ᵗʰ **H05.1**   **Chronic inflammatory disorders of orbit**

     H05.10   **Unspecified chronic inflammatory disorders of orbit**

     ✓6ᵗʰ **H05.11**   **Granuloma of orbit**

         Pseudotumor (inflammatory) of orbit

         H05.111   **Granuloma of** right **orbit**

         H05.112   **Granuloma of** left **orbit**

         H05.113   **Granuloma of** bilateral **orbits**

         H05.119   **Granuloma of unspecified orbit**

     ✓6ᵗʰ **H05.12**   **Orbital** *myositis*

         H05.121   **Orbital myositis,** right **orbit**

         H05.122   **Orbital myositis,** left **orbit**

         H05.123   **Orbital myositis,** bilateral

         H05.129   **Orbital myositis, unspecified orbit**

✓5ᵗʰ **H05.2**   **Exophthalmic conditions**

     H05.20   **Unspecified exophthalmos**

     ✓6ᵗʰ **H05.21**   **Displacement (lateral) of globe**

         H05.211   **Displacement (lateral) of globe,** right **eye**

         H05.212   **Displacement (lateral) of globe,** left **eye**

         H05.213   **Displacement (lateral) of globe,** bilateral

         H05.219   **Displacement (lateral) of globe, unspecified eye**

     ✓6ᵗʰ **H05.22**   **Edema of orbit**

         Orbital congestion

         H05.221   **Edema of** right **orbit**

         H05.222   **Edema of** left **orbit**

         H05.223   **Edema of** bilateral **orbit**

         H05.229   **Edema of unspecified orbit**

     ✓6ᵗʰ **H05.23**   **Hemorrhage of orbit**

         H05.231   **Hemorrhage of** right **orbit**

         H05.232   **Hemorrhage of** left **orbit**

         H05.233   **Hemorrhage of** bilateral **orbit**

         H05.239   **Hemorrhage of unspecified orbit**

     ✓6ᵗʰ **H05.24**   **Constant exophthalmos**

         H05.241   **Constant exophthalmos,** right **eye**

         H05.242   **Constant exophthalmos,** left **eye**

         H05.243   **Constant exophthalmos,** bilateral

         H05.249   **Constant exophthalmos, unspecified eye**

     ✓6ᵗʰ **H05.25**   **Intermittent exophthalmos**

         H05.251   **Intermittent exophthalmos,** right **eye**

         H05.252   **Intermittent exophthalmos,** left **eye**

         H05.253   **Intermittent exophthalmos,** bilateral

         H05.259   **Intermittent exophthalmos, unspecified eye**

     ✓6ᵗʰ **H05.26**   **Pulsating exophthalmos**

         H05.261   **Pulsating exophthalmos,** right **eye**

         H05.262   **Pulsating exophthalmos,** left **eye**

         H05.263   **Pulsating exophthalmos,** bilateral

         H05.269   **Pulsating exophthalmos, unspecified eye**

✓5ᵗʰ **H05.3**   **Deformity of orbit**

     EXCLUDES 1   *congenital deformity of orbit (Q10.7)*

               hypertelorism (Q75.2)

     H05.30   **Unspecified deformity of orbit**

     ✓6ᵗʰ **H05.31**   **Atrophy of orbit**

         H05.311   **Atrophy of** right **orbit**

         H05.312   **Atrophy of** left **orbit**

         H05.313   **Atrophy of** bilateral **orbit**

         H05.319   **Atrophy of unspecified orbit**

     ✓6ᵗʰ **H05.32**   **Deformity of orbit** due to bone disease

         Code also associated bone disease

         H05.321   **Deformity of** right **orbit due to bone disease**

         H05.322   **Deformity of** left **orbit due to bone disease**

         H05.323   **Deformity of** bilateral **orbits due to bone disease**

         H05.329   **Deformity of unspecified orbit due to bone disease**

     ✓6ᵗʰ **H05.33**   **Deformity of orbit** due to trauma or surgery

         H05.331   **Deformity of** right **orbit due to trauma or surgery**

         H05.332   **Deformity of** left **orbit due to trauma or surgery**

         H05.333   **Deformity of** bilateral **orbits due to trauma or surgery**

         H05.339   **Deformity of unspecified orbit due to trauma or surgery**

     ✓6ᵗʰ **H05.34**   **Enlargement of orbit**

         H05.341   **Enlargement of** right **orbit**

         H05.342   **Enlargement of** left **orbit**

         H05.343   **Enlargement of** bilateral **orbits**

         H05.349   **Enlargement of unspecified orbit**

     ✓6ᵗʰ **H05.35**   **Exostosis of orbit**

         H05.351   **Exostosis of** right **orbit**

         H05.352   **Exostosis of** left **orbit**

         H05.353   **Exostosis of** bilateral **orbits**

         H05.359   **Exostosis of unspecified orbit**

✓5ᵗʰ **H05.4**   **Enophthalmos**

     ✓6ᵗʰ **H05.40**   **Unspecified enophthalmos**

         H05.401   **Unspecified enophthalmos,** right **eye**

         H05.402   **Unspecified enophthalmos,** left **eye**

         H05.403   **Unspecified enophthalmos,** bilateral

         H05.409   **Unspecified enophthalmos, unspecified eye**

     ✓6ᵗʰ **H05.41**   **Enophthalmos** due to atrophy of orbital tissue

         H05.411   **Enophthalmos due to atrophy of orbital tissue,** right **eye**

         H05.412   **Enophthalmos due to atrophy of orbital tissue,** left **eye**

         H05.413   **Enophthalmos due to atrophy of orbital tissue,** bilateral

         H05.419   **Enophthalmos due to atrophy of orbital tissue, unspecified eye**

     ✓6ᵗʰ **H05.42**   **Enophthalmos** due to trauma or surgery

         H05.421   **Enophthalmos due to trauma or surgery,** right **eye**

         H05.422   **Enophthalmos due to trauma or surgery,** left **eye**

         H05.423   **Enophthalmos due to trauma or surgery,** bilateral

---

HCC CMS-HCC   **Rx** Rx HCC   **ESR** ESRD HCC   **COM** Commercial HCC   **N** Newborn: 0   **P** Pediatric: 0-17   **M** Maternity: 9-64   **A** Adult: 15-124

618   ICD-10-CM 2023

H05.429   **Enophthalmos due to trauma or surgery,** unspecified eye

✓5ᵗʰ **H05.5**   **Retained (old) foreign body following penetrating wound of orbit**
    Retrobulbar foreign body
    Use additional code to identify the type of retained foreign body (Z18.-)
    EXCLUDES 1   current penetrating wound of orbit (S05.4-)
    EXCLUDES 2   retained foreign body of eyelid (H02.81-)
                  retained intraocular foreign body (H44.6-, H44.7-)

     H05.50   **Retained (old) foreign body following penetrating wound of unspecified orbit**
     H05.51   **Retained (old) foreign body following penetrating wound of right orbit**
     H05.52   **Retained (old) foreign body following penetrating wound of left orbit**
     H05.53   **Retained (old) foreign body following penetrating wound of bilateral orbits**

✓5ᵗʰ **H05.8**   **Other disorders of orbit**
     ✓6ᵗʰ **H05.81**   **Cyst of orbit**
         Encephalocele of orbit
         H05.811   **Cyst of right orbit**
         H05.812   **Cyst of left orbit**
         H05.813   **Cyst of bilateral orbits**
         H05.819   **Cyst of unspecified orbit**
     ✓6ᵗʰ **H05.82**   **Myopathy of extraocular muscles**
         H05.821   **Myopathy of extraocular muscles, right orbit**
         H05.822   **Myopathy of extraocular muscles, left orbit**
         H05.823   **Myopathy of extraocular muscles, bilateral**
         H05.829   **Myopathy of extraocular muscles, unspecified orbit**
     H05.89   **Other disorders of orbit**
   H05.9   **Unspecified disorder of orbit**

Disorders of conjunctiva (H10-H11)

✓4ᵗʰ **H10**   **Conjunctivitis**
    EXCLUDES 1   keratoconjunctivitis (H16.2-)

   ✓5ᵗʰ **H10.0**   **Mucopurulent conjunctivitis**
     ✓6ᵗʰ **H10.01**   **Acute follicular conjunctivitis**
         H10.011   **Acute follicular conjunctivitis, right eye**
         H10.012   **Acute follicular conjunctivitis, left eye**
         H10.013   **Acute follicular conjunctivitis, bilateral**
         H10.019   **Acute follicular conjunctivitis, unspecified eye**
     ✓6ᵗʰ **H10.02**   **Other mucopurulent conjunctivitis**
         H10.021   **Other mucopurulent conjunctivitis, right eye**
         H10.022   **Other mucopurulent conjunctivitis, left eye**
         H10.023   **Other mucopurulent conjunctivitis, bilateral**
         H10.029   **Other mucopurulent conjunctivitis, unspecified eye**

   ✓5ᵗʰ **H10.1**   **Acute atopic conjunctivitis**
    Acute papillary conjunctivitis
     H10.10   **Acute atopic conjunctivitis, unspecified eye**
     H10.11   **Acute atopic conjunctivitis, right eye**
     H10.12   **Acute atopic conjunctivitis, left eye**
     H10.13   **Acute atopic conjunctivitis, bilateral**

   ✓5ᵗʰ **H10.2**   **Other acute conjunctivitis**
     ✓6ᵗʰ **H10.21**   **Acute toxic conjunctivitis**
        Acute chemical conjunctivitis
        Code first (T51-T65) to identify chemical and intent
        EXCLUDES 1   burn and corrosion of eye and adnexa (T26.-)
         H10.211   **Acute toxic conjunctivitis, right eye**
         H10.212   **Acute toxic conjunctivitis, left eye**
         H10.213   **Acute toxic conjunctivitis, bilateral**
         H10.219   **Acute toxic conjunctivitis, unspecified eye**
     ✓6ᵗʰ **H10.22**   **Pseudomembranous conjunctivitis**
         H10.221   **Pseudomembranous conjunctivitis, right eye**

H10.222   **Pseudomembranous conjunctivitis, left eye**
H10.223   **Pseudomembranous conjunctivitis, bilateral**
H10.229   **Pseudomembranous conjunctivitis, unspecified eye**

   ✓6ᵗʰ **H10.23**   **Serous conjunctivitis, except viral**
    EXCLUDES 1   viral conjunctivitis (B30.-)
     H10.231   **Serous conjunctivitis, except viral, right eye**
     H10.232   **Serous conjunctivitis, except viral, left eye**
     H10.233   **Serous conjunctivitis, except viral, bilateral**
     H10.239   **Serous conjunctivitis, except viral, unspecified eye**

   ✓5ᵗʰ **H10.3**   **Unspecified acute conjunctivitis**
    EXCLUDES 1   ophthalmia neonatorum NOS (P39.1)
     H10.30   **Unspecified acute conjunctivitis, unspecified eye**
     H10.31   **Unspecified acute conjunctivitis, right eye**
     H10.32   **Unspecified acute conjunctivitis, left eye**
     H10.33   **Unspecified acute conjunctivitis, bilateral**

   ✓5ᵗʰ **H10.4**   **Chronic conjunctivitis**
     ✓6ᵗʰ **H10.40**   **Unspecified chronic conjunctivitis**
         H10.401   **Unspecified chronic conjunctivitis, right eye**
         H10.402   **Unspecified chronic conjunctivitis, left eye**
         H10.403   **Unspecified chronic conjunctivitis, bilateral**
         H10.409   **Unspecified chronic conjunctivitis, unspecified eye**
     ✓6ᵗʰ **H10.41**   **Chronic giant papillary conjunctivitis**
         H10.411   **Chronic giant papillary conjunctivitis, right eye**
         H10.412   **Chronic giant papillary conjunctivitis, left eye**
         H10.413   **Chronic giant papillary conjunctivitis, bilateral**
         H10.419   **Chronic giant papillary conjunctivitis, unspecified eye**
     ✓6ᵗʰ **H10.42**   **Simple chronic conjunctivitis**
         H10.421   **Simple chronic conjunctivitis, right eye**
         H10.422   **Simple chronic conjunctivitis, left eye**
         H10.423   **Simple chronic conjunctivitis, bilateral**
         H10.429   **Simple chronic conjunctivitis, unspecified eye**
     ✓6ᵗʰ **H10.43**   **Chronic follicular conjunctivitis**
         H10.431   **Chronic follicular conjunctivitis, right eye**
         H10.432   **Chronic follicular conjunctivitis, left eye**
         H10.433   **Chronic follicular conjunctivitis, bilateral**
         H10.439   **Chronic follicular conjunctivitis, unspecified eye**
     H10.44   **Vernal conjunctivitis**
        EXCLUDES 1   vernal keratoconjunctivitis with limbar and corneal involvement (H16.26-)
     H10.45   **Other chronic allergic conjunctivitis**

   ✓6ᵗʰ **H10.5**   **Blepharoconjunctivitis**
     ✓6ᵗʰ **H10.50**   **Unspecified blepharoconjunctivitis**
         H10.501   **Unspecified blepharoconjunctivitis, right eye**
         H10.502   **Unspecified blepharoconjunctivitis, left eye**
         H10.503   **Unspecified blepharoconjunctivitis, bilateral**
         H10.509   **Unspecified blepharoconjunctivitis, unspecified eye**
     ✓6ᵗʰ **H10.51**   **Ligneous conjunctivitis**
        Code also underlying condition if known, such as: plasminogen deficiency (E88.02)
         H10.511   **Ligneous conjunctivitis, right eye**
         H10.512   **Ligneous conjunctivitis, left eye**
         H10.513   **Ligneous conjunctivitis, bilateral**
         H10.519   **Ligneous conjunctivitis, unspecified eye**
     ✓6ᵗʰ **H10.52**   **Angular blepharoconjunctivitis**
         H10.521   **Angular blepharoconjunctivitis, right eye**
         H10.522   **Angular blepharoconjunctivitis, left eye**
         H10.523   **Angular blepharoconjunctivitis, bilateral**

H10.529   Angular blepharoconjunctivitis, unspecified eye

✓6ᵗʰ **H10.53**   Contact blepharoconjunctivitis

     H10.531   Contact blepharoconjunctivitis, right eye

     H10.532   Contact blepharoconjunctivitis, left eye

     H10.533   Contact blepharoconjunctivitis, bilateral

     H10.539   Contact blepharoconjunctivitis, unspecified eye

✓5ᵗʰ **H10.8**   Other conjunctivitis

   ✓5ᵗʰ **H10.81**   Pingueculitis

     EXCLUDES 1   pinguecula (H11.15-)

     H10.811   Pingueculitis, right eye

     H10.812   Pingueculitis, left eye

     H10.813   Pingueculitis, bilateral

     H10.819   Pingueculitis, unspecified eye

   ✓6ᵗʰ **H10.82**   Rosacea conjunctivitis

     Code first underlying rosacea dermatitis (L71.-)

     AHA: 2018,4Q,15

     H10.821   Rosacea conjunctivitis, right eye

     H10.822   Rosacea conjunctivitis, left eye

     H10.823   Rosacea conjunctivitis, bilateral

     H10.829   Rosacea conjunctivitis, unspecified eye

     H10.89   Other conjunctivitis

   H10.9   Unspecified conjunctivitis

✓4ᵗʰ **H11**   Other disorders of conjunctiva

     EXCLUDES 1   keratoconjunctivitis (H16.2-)

   ✓5ᵗʰ **H11.0**   Pterygium of eye

     EXCLUDES 1   pseudopterygium (H11.81-)

     DEF: Benign, wedge-shaped, conjunctival thickening that advances from the inner corner of the eye toward the cornea.

Pterygium

Pterygium

   ✓6ᵗʰ **H11.00**   Unspecified pterygium of eye

     H11.001   Unspecified pterygium of right eye

     H11.002   Unspecified pterygium of left eye

     H11.003   Unspecified pterygium of eye, bilateral

     H11.009   Unspecified pterygium of unspecified eye

   ✓6ᵗʰ **H11.01**   Amyloid pterygium

     H11.011   Amyloid pterygium of right eye

     H11.012   Amyloid pterygium of left eye

     H11.013   Amyloid pterygium of eye, bilateral

     H11.019   Amyloid pterygium of unspecified eye

   ✓6ᵗʰ **H11.02**   Central pterygium of eye

     H11.021   Central pterygium of right eye

     H11.022   Central pterygium of left eye

     H11.023   Central pterygium of eye, bilateral

     H11.029   Central pterygium of unspecified eye

   ✓6ᵗʰ **H11.03**   Double pterygium of eye

     H11.031   Double pterygium of right eye

     H11.032   Double pterygium of left eye

     H11.033   Double pterygium of eye, bilateral

     H11.039   Double pterygium of unspecified eye

   ✓6ᵗʰ **H11.04**   Peripheral pterygium of eye, stationary

     H11.041   Peripheral pterygium, stationary, right eye

     H11.042   Peripheral pterygium, stationary, left eye

     H11.043   Peripheral pterygium, stationary, bilateral

     H11.049   Peripheral pterygium, stationary, unspecified eye

   ✓6ᵗʰ **H11.05**   Peripheral pterygium of eye, progressive

     H11.051   Peripheral pterygium, progressive, right eye

     H11.052   Peripheral pterygium, progressive, left eye

     H11.053   Peripheral pterygium, progressive, bilateral

     H11.059   Peripheral pterygium, progressive, unspecified eye

   ✓6ᵗʰ **H11.06**   Recurrent pterygium of eye

     H11.061   Recurrent pterygium of right eye

     H11.062   Recurrent pterygium of left eye

     H11.063   Recurrent pterygium of eye, bilateral

     H11.069   Recurrent pterygium of unspecified eye

   ✓5ᵗʰ **H11.1**   Conjunctival degenerations and deposits

     EXCLUDES 2   pseudopterygium (H11.81)

     H11.10   Unspecified conjunctival degenerations

   ✓6ᵗʰ **H11.11**   Conjunctival deposits

     H11.111   Conjunctival deposits, right eye

     H11.112   Conjunctival deposits, left eye

     H11.113   Conjunctival deposits, bilateral

     H11.119   Conjunctival deposits, unspecified eye

   ✓6ᵗʰ **H11.12**   Conjunctival concretions

     H11.121   Conjunctival concretions, right eye

     H11.122   Conjunctival concretions, left eye

     H11.123   Conjunctival concretions, bilateral

     H11.129   Conjunctival concretions, unspecified eye

   ✓6ᵗʰ **H11.13**   Conjunctival pigmentations

     Conjunctival argyrosis [argyria]

     H11.131   Conjunctival pigmentations, right eye

     H11.132   Conjunctival pigmentations, left eye

     H11.133   Conjunctival pigmentations, bilateral

     H11.139   Conjunctival pigmentations, unspecified eye

   ✓6ᵗʰ **H11.14**   Conjunctival xerosis, unspecified

     EXCLUDES 1   xerosis of conjunctiva due to vitamin A deficiency (E50.0, E50.1)

     DEF: Abnormal dryness of the conjunctiva due to lack of sufficient tears or conjunctival secretions.

     H11.141   Conjunctival xerosis, unspecified, right eye

     H11.142   Conjunctival xerosis, unspecified, left eye

     H11.143   Conjunctival xerosis, unspecified, bilateral

     H11.149   Conjunctival xerosis, unspecified, unspecified eye

   ✓6ᵗʰ **H11.15**   Pinguecula

     EXCLUDES 1   pingueculitis (H10.81-)

     DEF: Proliferation on the conjunctiva near the sclerocorneal junction, usually of the side of the nose and usually in older patients.

Pinguecula

Pinguecula

     H11.151   Pinguecula, right eye

     H11.152   Pinguecula, left eye

     H11.153   Pinguecula, bilateral

     H11.159   Pinguecula, unspecified eye

   ✓5ᵗʰ **H11.2**   Conjunctival scars

   ✓6ᵗʰ **H11.21**   Conjunctival adhesions and strands (localized)

     H11.211   Conjunctival adhesions and strands (localized), right eye

     H11.212   Conjunctival adhesions and strands (localized), left eye

     H11.213   Conjunctival adhesions and strands (localized), bilateral

     H11.219   Conjunctival adhesions and strands (localized), unspecified eye

   ✓6ᵗʰ **H11.22**   Conjunctival granuloma

     H11.221   Conjunctival granuloma, right eye

     H11.222   Conjunctival granuloma, left eye

HCC CMS-HCC   **Rx** Rx HCC   **ESR** ESRD HCC   **COM** Commercial HCC   **N** Newborn: 0   **P** Pediatric: 0-17   **M** Maternity: 9-64   **A** Adult: 15-124

620   ICD-10-CM 2023

H11.223 Conjunctival granuloma, bilateral
H11.229 Conjunctival granuloma, unspecified
√6ᵗʰ H11.23 Symblepharon
H11.231 Symblepharon, right eye
H11.232 Symblepharon, left eye
H11.233 Symblepharon, bilateral
H11.239 Symblepharon, unspecified eye
√6ᵗʰ H11.24 Scarring of conjunctiva
H11.241 Scarring of conjunctiva, right eye
H11.242 Scarring of conjunctiva, left eye
H11.243 Scarring of conjunctiva, bilateral
H11.249 Scarring of conjunctiva, unspecified eye
√5ᵗʰ H11.3 Conjunctival hemorrhage
Subconjunctival hemorrhage
H11.30 Conjunctival hemorrhage, unspecified eye
H11.31 Conjunctival hemorrhage, right eye
H11.32 Conjunctival hemorrhage, left eye
H11.33 Conjunctival hemorrhage, bilateral
√5ᵗʰ H11.4 Other conjunctival vascular disorders and cysts
√6ᵗʰ H11.41 Vascular abnormalities of conjunctiva
Conjunctival aneurysm
H11.411 Vascular abnormalities of conjunctiva, right eye
H11.412 Vascular abnormalities of conjunctiva, left eye
H11.413 Vascular abnormalities of conjunctiva, bilateral
H11.419 Vascular abnormalities of conjunctiva, unspecified eye
√6ᵗʰ H11.42 Conjunctival edema
H11.421 Conjunctival edema, right eye
H11.422 Conjunctival edema, left eye
H11.423 Conjunctival edema, bilateral
H11.429 Conjunctival edema, unspecified eye
√6ᵗʰ H11.43 Conjunctival hyperemia
H11.431 Conjunctival hyperemia, right eye
H11.432 Conjunctival hyperemia, left eye
H11.433 Conjunctival hyperemia, bilateral
H11.439 Conjunctival hyperemia, unspecified eye
√6ᵗʰ H11.44 Conjunctival cysts
H11.441 Conjunctival cysts, right eye
H11.442 Conjunctival cysts, left eye
H11.443 Conjunctival cysts, bilateral
H11.449 Conjunctival cysts, unspecified eye
√5ᵗʰ H11.8 Other specified disorders of conjunctiva
√6ᵗʰ H11.81 Pseudopterygium of conjunctiva
H11.811 Pseudopterygium of conjunctiva, right eye
H11.812 Pseudopterygium of conjunctiva, left eye
H11.813 Pseudopterygium of conjunctiva, bilateral
H11.819 Pseudopterygium of conjunctiva, unspecified eye
√6ᵗʰ H11.82 Conjunctivochalasis
H11.821 Conjunctivochalasis, right eye
H11.822 Conjunctivochalasis, left eye
H11.823 Conjunctivochalasis, bilateral
H11.829 Conjunctivochalasis, unspecified eye
H11.89 Other specified disorders of conjunctiva
H11.9 Unspecified disorder of conjunctiva

Disorders of sclera, cornea, iris and ciliary body (H15-H22)

√4ᵗʰ H15 Disorders of sclera
√5ᵗʰ H15.0 Scleritis
√6ᵗʰ H15.00 Unspecified scleritis
H15.001 Unspecified scleritis, right eye
H15.002 Unspecified scleritis, left eye
H15.003 Unspecified scleritis, bilateral
H15.009 Unspecified scleritis, unspecified eye
√6ᵗʰ H15.01 Anterior scleritis
H15.011 Anterior scleritis, right eye
H15.012 Anterior scleritis, left eye
H15.013 Anterior scleritis, bilateral
H15.019 Anterior scleritis, unspecified eye

√6ᵗʰ H15.02 Brawny scleritis
H15.021 Brawny scleritis, right eye
H15.022 Brawny scleritis, left eye
H15.023 Brawny scleritis, bilateral
H15.029 Brawny scleritis, unspecified eye
√6ᵗʰ H15.03 Posterior scleritis
Sclerotenonitis
H15.031 Posterior scleritis, right eye
H15.032 Posterior scleritis, left eye
H15.033 Posterior scleritis, bilateral
H15.039 Posterior scleritis, unspecified eye
√6ᵗʰ H15.04 Scleritis with corneal involvement
H15.041 Scleritis with corneal involvement, right eye
H15.042 Scleritis with corneal involvement, left eye
H15.043 Scleritis with corneal involvement, bilateral
H15.049 Scleritis with corneal involvement, unspecified eye
√6ᵗʰ H15.05 Scleromalacia perforans
H15.051 Scleromalacia perforans, right eye
H15.052 Scleromalacia perforans, left eye
H15.053 Scleromalacia perforans, bilateral
H15.059 Scleromalacia perforans, unspecified eye
√6ᵗʰ H15.09 Other scleritis
Scleral abscess
H15.091 Other scleritis, right eye
H15.092 Other scleritis, left eye
H15.093 Other scleritis, bilateral
H15.099 Other scleritis, unspecified eye
√5ᵗʰ H15.1 Episcleritis
√6ᵗʰ H15.10 Unspecified episcleritis
H15.101 Unspecified episcleritis, right eye
H15.102 Unspecified episcleritis, left eye
H15.103 Unspecified episcleritis, bilateral
H15.109 Unspecified episcleritis, unspecified eye
√6ᵗʰ H15.11 Episcleritis periodica fugax
H15.111 Episcleritis periodica fugax, right eye
H15.112 Episcleritis periodica fugax, left eye
H15.113 Episcleritis periodica fugax, bilateral
H15.119 Episcleritis periodica fugax, unspecified eye
√6ᵗʰ H15.12 Nodular episcleritis
H15.121 Nodular episcleritis, right eye
H15.122 Nodular episcleritis, left eye
H15.123 Nodular episcleritis, bilateral
H15.129 Nodular episcleritis, unspecified eye
√5ᵗʰ H15.8 Other disorders of sclera
EXCLUDES 2   blue sclera (Q13.5)
degenerative myopia (H44.2-)
√6ᵗʰ H15.81 Equatorial staphyloma
H15.811 Equatorial staphyloma, right eye
H15.812 Equatorial staphyloma, left eye
H15.813 Equatorial staphyloma, bilateral
H15.819 Equatorial staphyloma, unspecified eye
√6ᵗʰ H15.82 Localized anterior staphyloma
H15.821 Localized anterior staphyloma, right eye
H15.822 Localized anterior staphyloma, left eye
H15.823 Localized anterior staphyloma, bilateral
H15.829 Localized anterior staphyloma, unspecified eye
√6ᵗʰ H15.83 Staphyloma posticum
H15.831 Staphyloma posticum, right eye
H15.832 Staphyloma posticum, left eye
H15.833 Staphyloma posticum, bilateral
H15.839 Staphyloma posticum, unspecified eye
√6ᵗʰ H15.84 Scleral ectasia
H15.841 Scleral ectasia, right eye
H15.842 Scleral ectasia, left eye
H15.843 Scleral ectasia, bilateral
H15.849 Scleral ectasia, unspecified eye
√6ᵗʰ H15.85 Ring staphyloma
H15.851 Ring staphyloma, right eye
H15.852 Ring staphyloma, left eye
H15.853 Ring staphyloma, bilateral

H15.859   Ring staphyloma, unspecified eye
H15.89   Other disorders of sclera
H15.9   Unspecified disorder of sclera

✓4ᵗʰ **H16   Keratitis**
    DEF: Condition in which the cornea becomes inflamed and irritated.

✓5ᵗʰ   **H16.0   Corneal ulcer**

✓6ᵗʰ   **H16.00   Unspecified corneal ulcer**
     H16.001   Unspecified corneal ulcer, right eye
     H16.002   Unspecified corneal ulcer, left eye
     H16.003   Unspecified corneal ulcer, bilateral
     H16.009   Unspecified corneal ulcer, unspecified eye

✓6ᵗʰ   **H16.01   Central corneal ulcer**
     H16.011   Central corneal ulcer, right eye
     H16.012   Central corneal ulcer, left eye
     H16.013   Central corneal ulcer, bilateral
     H16.019   Central corneal ulcer, unspecified eye

✓6ᵗʰ   **H16.02   Ring corneal ulcer**
     H16.021   Ring corneal ulcer, right eye
     H16.022   Ring corneal ulcer, left eye
     H16.023   Ring corneal ulcer, bilateral
     H16.029   Ring corneal ulcer, unspecified eye

✓6ᵗʰ   **H16.03   Corneal ulcer with hypopyon**
     H16.031   Corneal ulcer with hypopyon, right eye
     H16.032   Corneal ulcer with hypopyon, left eye
     H16.033   Corneal ulcer with hypopyon, bilateral
     H16.039   Corneal ulcer with hypopyon, unspecified eye

✓6ᵗʰ   **H16.04   Marginal corneal ulcer**
     H16.041   Marginal corneal ulcer, right eye
     H16.042   Marginal corneal ulcer, left eye
     H16.043   Marginal corneal ulcer, bilateral
     H16.049   Marginal corneal ulcer, unspecified eye

✓6ᵗʰ   **H16.05   Mooren's corneal ulcer**
     H16.051   Mooren's corneal ulcer, right eye
     H16.052   Mooren's corneal ulcer, left eye
     H16.053   Mooren's corneal ulcer, bilateral
     H16.059   Mooren's corneal ulcer, unspecified eye

✓6ᵗʰ   **H16.06   Mycotic corneal ulcer**
     H16.061   Mycotic corneal ulcer, right eye
     H16.062   Mycotic corneal ulcer, left eye
     H16.063   Mycotic corneal ulcer, bilateral
     H16.069   Mycotic corneal ulcer, unspecified eye

✓6ᵗʰ   **H16.07   Perforated corneal ulcer**
     H16.071   Perforated corneal ulcer, right eye
     H16.072   Perforated corneal ulcer, left eye
     H16.073   Perforated corneal ulcer, bilateral
     H16.079   Perforated corneal ulcer, unspecified eye

✓5ᵗʰ   **H16.1   Other and unspecified superficial keratitis without conjunctivitis**

✓6ᵗʰ   **H16.10   Unspecified superficial keratitis**
     H16.101   Unspecified superficial keratitis, right eye
     H16.102   Unspecified superficial keratitis, left eye
     H16.103   Unspecified superficial keratitis, bilateral
     H16.109   Unspecified superficial keratitis, unspecified eye

✓6ᵗʰ   **H16.11   Macular keratitis**
     Areolar keratitis
     Nummular keratitis
     Stellate keratitis
     Striate keratitis
     H16.111   Macular keratitis, right eye
     H16.112   Macular keratitis, left eye
     H16.113   Macular keratitis, bilateral
     H16.119   Macular keratitis, unspecified eye

✓6ᵗʰ   **H16.12   Filamentary keratitis**
     H16.121   Filamentary keratitis, right eye
     H16.122   Filamentary keratitis, left eye
     H16.123   Filamentary keratitis, bilateral
     H16.129   Filamentary keratitis, unspecified eye

✓6ᵗʰ   **H16.13   Photokeratitis**
     Snow blindness
     Welders keratitis
     H16.131   Photokeratitis, right eye
     H16.132   Photokeratitis, left eye
     H16.133   Photokeratitis, bilateral

H16.139   Photokeratitis, unspecified eye

✓6ᵗʰ   **H16.14   Punctate keratitis**
     H16.141   Punctate keratitis, right eye
     H16.142   Punctate keratitis, left eye
     H16.143   Punctate keratitis, bilateral
     H16.149   Punctate keratitis, unspecified eye

✓5ᵗʰ   **H16.2   Keratoconjunctivitis**

✓6ᵗʰ   **H16.20   Unspecified keratoconjunctivitis**
     Superficial keratitis with conjunctivitis NOS
     H16.201   Unspecified keratoconjunctivitis, right eye
     H16.202   Unspecified keratoconjunctivitis, left eye
     H16.203   Unspecified keratoconjunctivitis, bilateral
     H16.209   Unspecified keratoconjunctivitis, unspecified eye

✓6ᵗʰ   **H16.21   Exposure keratoconjunctivitis**
     H16.211   Exposure keratoconjunctivitis, right eye
     H16.212   Exposure keratoconjunctivitis, left eye
     H16.213   Exposure keratoconjunctivitis, bilateral
     H16.219   Exposure keratoconjunctivitis, unspecified eye

✓6ᵗʰ   **H16.22   Keratoconjunctivitis sicca, not specified as Sjögren's**
     EXCLUDES 1   *Sjögren's syndrome (M35.01)*
     H16.221   Keratoconjunctivitis sicca, not specified as Sjögren's, right eye
     H16.222   Keratoconjunctivitis sicca, not specified as Sjögren's, left eye
     H16.223   Keratoconjunctivitis sicca, not specified as Sjögren's, bilateral
     H16.229   Keratoconjunctivitis sicca, not specified as Sjögren's, unspecified eye

✓6ᵗʰ   **H16.23   Neurotrophic keratoconjunctivitis**
     H16.231   Neurotrophic keratoconjunctivitis, right eye
     H16.232   Neurotrophic keratoconjunctivitis, left eye
     H16.233   Neurotrophic keratoconjunctivitis, bilateral
     H16.239   Neurotrophic keratoconjunctivitis, unspecified eye

✓6ᵗʰ   **H16.24   Ophthalmia nodosa**
     H16.241   Ophthalmia nodosa, right eye
     H16.242   Ophthalmia nodosa, left eye
     H16.243   Ophthalmia nodosa, bilateral
     H16.249   Ophthalmia nodosa, unspecified eye

✓6ᵗʰ   **H16.25   Phlyctenular keratoconjunctivitis**
     H16.251   Phlyctenular keratoconjunctivitis, right eye
     H16.252   Phlyctenular keratoconjunctivitis, left eye
     H16.253   Phlyctenular keratoconjunctivitis, bilateral
     H16.259   Phlyctenular keratoconjunctivitis, unspecified eye

✓6ᵗʰ   **H16.26   Vernal keratoconjunctivitis, with limbar and corneal involvement**
     EXCLUDES 1   *vernal conjunctivitis without limbar and corneal involvement (H10.44)*
     H16.261   Vernal keratoconjunctivitis, with limbar and corneal involvement, right eye
     H16.262   Vernal keratoconjunctivitis, with limbar and corneal involvement, left eye
     H16.263   Vernal keratoconjunctivitis, with limbar and corneal involvement, bilateral
     H16.269   Vernal keratoconjunctivitis, with limbar and corneal involvement, unspecified eye

✓6ᵗʰ   **H16.29   Other keratoconjunctivitis**
     H16.291   Other keratoconjunctivitis, right eye
     H16.292   Other keratoconjunctivitis, left eye
     H16.293   Other keratoconjunctivitis, bilateral
     H16.299   Other keratoconjunctivitis, unspecified eye

✓5ᵗʰ   **H16.3   Interstitial and deep keratitis**

✓6ᵗʰ   **H16.30   Unspecified interstitial keratitis**
     H16.301   Unspecified interstitial keratitis, right eye
     H16.302   Unspecified interstitial keratitis, left eye
     H16.303   Unspecified interstitial keratitis, bilateral

HCC CMS-HCC   **Rx** Rx HCC   **ESR** ESRD HCC   **COM** Commercial HCC   **N** Newborn: 0   **P** Pediatric: 0-17   **M** Maternity: 9-64   **A** Adult: 15-124

622   ICD-10-CM 2023

H16.309   Unspecified interstitial keratitis, unspecified eye

√6ᵗʰ **H16.31**   Corneal **abscess**

H16.311   **Corneal abscess,** right eye
H16.312   **Corneal abscess,** left eye
H16.313   **Corneal abscess,** bilateral
H16.319   **Corneal abscess,** unspecified eye

√6ᵗʰ **H16.32**   Diffuse **interstitial keratitis**

Cogan's syndrome
H16.321   **Diffuse interstitial keratitis,** right eye
H16.322   **Diffuse interstitial keratitis,** left eye
H16.323   **Diffuse interstitial keratitis,** bilateral
H16.329   **Diffuse interstitial keratitis,** unspecified eye

√6ᵗʰ **H16.33**   Sclerosing **keratitis**

H16.331   **Sclerosing keratitis,** right eye
H16.332   **Sclerosing keratitis,** left eye
H16.333   **Sclerosing keratitis,** bilateral
H16.339   **Sclerosing keratitis,** unspecified eye

√6ᵗʰ **H16.39**   **Other interstitial and deep keratitis**

H16.391   **Other interstitial and deep keratitis,** right eye
H16.392   **Other interstitial and deep keratitis,** left eye
H16.393   **Other interstitial and deep keratitis,** bilateral
H16.399   **Other interstitial and deep keratitis,** unspecified eye

√5ᵗʰ **H16.4**   Corneal **neovascularization**

√6ᵗʰ **H16.40**   **Unspecified corneal neovascularization**

H16.401   **Unspecified corneal neovascularization,** right eye
H16.402   **Unspecified corneal neovascularization,** left eye
H16.403   **Unspecified corneal neovascularization,** bilateral
H16.409   **Unspecified corneal neovascularization,** unspecified eye

√6ᵗʰ **H16.41**   Ghost vessels **(corneal)**

H16.411   **Ghost vessels (corneal),** right eye
H16.412   **Ghost vessels (corneal),** left eye
H16.413   **Ghost vessels (corneal),** bilateral
H16.419   **Ghost vessels (corneal),** unspecified eye

√6ᵗʰ **H16.42**   Pannus **(corneal)**

H16.421   **Pannus (corneal),** right eye
H16.422   **Pannus (corneal),** left eye
H16.423   **Pannus (corneal),** bilateral
H16.429   **Pannus (corneal),** unspecified eye

√6ᵗʰ **H16.43**   Localized vascularization **of cornea**

H16.431   **Localized vascularization of cornea,** right eye
H16.432   **Localized vascularization of cornea,** left eye
H16.433   **Localized vascularization of cornea,** bilateral
H16.439   **Localized vascularization of cornea,** unspecified eye

√6ᵗʰ **H16.44**   Deep vascularization **of cornea**

H16.441   **Deep vascularization of cornea,** right eye
H16.442   **Deep vascularization of cornea,** left eye
H16.443   **Deep vascularization of cornea,** bilateral
H16.449   **Deep vascularization of cornea,** unspecified eye

H16.8   **Other keratitis**

H16.9   **Unspecified keratitis**

√4ᵗʰ **H17**   **Corneal scars and opacities**

√6ᵗʰ **H17.0**   **Adherent leukoma**

H17.00   **Adherent leukoma,** unspecified eye
H17.01   **Adherent leukoma,** right eye
H17.02   **Adherent leukoma,** left eye
H17.03   **Adherent leukoma,** bilateral

√5ᵗʰ **H17.1**   **Central corneal opacity**

H17.10   **Central corneal opacity,** unspecified eye
H17.11   **Central corneal opacity,** right eye
H17.12   **Central corneal opacity,** left eye
H17.13   **Central corneal opacity,** bilateral

√5ᵗʰ **H17.8**   **Other corneal scars and opacities**

√6ᵗʰ **H17.81**   Minor **opacity of cornea**

Corneal nebula
H17.811   **Minor opacity of cornea,** right eye
H17.812   **Minor opacity of cornea,** left eye
H17.813   **Minor opacity of cornea,** bilateral
H17.819   **Minor opacity of cornea,** unspecified eye

√6ᵗʰ **H17.82**   Peripheral **opacity of cornea**

H17.821   **Peripheral opacity of cornea,** right eye
H17.822   **Peripheral opacity of cornea,** left eye
H17.823   **Peripheral opacity of cornea,** bilateral
H17.829   **Peripheral opacity of cornea,** unspecified eye

H17.89   **Other corneal scars and opacities**

H17.9   **Unspecified corneal scar and opacity**

√4ᵗʰ **H18**   **Other disorders of cornea**

√5ᵗʰ **H18.0**   **Corneal pigmentations and deposits**

√6ᵗʰ **H18.00**   **Unspecified corneal deposit**

H18.001   **Unspecified corneal deposit,** right eye
H18.002   **Unspecified corneal deposit,** left eye
H18.003   **Unspecified corneal deposit,** bilateral
H18.009   **Unspecified corneal deposit,** unspecified eye

√6ᵗʰ **H18.01**   Anterior **corneal pigmentations**

Staehli's line
H18.011   **Anterior corneal pigmentations,** right eye
H18.012   **Anterior corneal pigmentations,** left eye
H18.013   **Anterior corneal pigmentations,** bilateral
H18.019   **Anterior corneal pigmentations,** unspecified eye

√6ᵗʰ **H18.02**   Argentous **corneal deposits**

H18.021   **Argentous corneal deposits,** right eye
H18.022   **Argentous corneal deposits,** left eye
H18.023   **Argentous corneal deposits,** bilateral
H18.029   **Argentous corneal deposits,** unspecified eye

√6ᵗʰ **H18.03**   **Corneal deposits in metabolic disorders**

Code also associated metabolic disorder
H18.031   **Corneal deposits in metabolic disorders,** right eye
H18.032   **Corneal deposits in metabolic disorders,** left eye
H18.033   **Corneal deposits in metabolic disorders,** bilateral
H18.039   **Corneal deposits in metabolic disorders,** unspecified eye

√6ᵗʰ **H18.04**   Kayser-Fleischer **ring**

Code also associated Wilson's disease (E83.01)
H18.041   **Kayser-Fleischer ring,** right eye
H18.042   **Kayser-Fleischer ring,** left eye
H18.043   **Kayser-Fleischer ring,** bilateral
H18.049   **Kayser-Fleischer ring,** unspecified eye

√6ᵗʰ **H18.05**   Posterior **corneal pigmentations**

Krukenberg's spindle
H18.051   **Posterior corneal pigmentations,** right eye
H18.052   **Posterior corneal pigmentations,** left eye
H18.053   **Posterior corneal pigmentations,** bilateral
H18.059   **Posterior corneal pigmentations,** unspecified eye

√6ᵗʰ **H18.06**   Stromal **corneal pigmentations**

Hematocornea
H18.061   **Stromal corneal pigmentations,** right eye
H18.062   **Stromal corneal pigmentations,** left eye
H18.063   **Stromal corneal pigmentations,** bilateral
H18.069   **Stromal corneal pigmentations,** unspecified eye

√5ᵗʰ **H18.1**   **Bullous keratopathy**

DEF: Corneal swelling due to a damaged corneal endothelium. Bullous keratopathy is characterized by recurring, rupturing epithelial blisters causing glaucoma, iridocyclitis, and Fuchs' dystrophy.
H18.10   **Bullous keratopathy,** unspecified eye
H18.11   **Bullous keratopathy,** right eye
H18.12   **Bullous keratopathy,** left eye
H18.13   **Bullous keratopathy,** bilateral

✓5ᵗʰ **H18.2** **Other and unspecified corneal edema**

    H18.20 **Unspecified corneal edema**

    ✓6ᵗʰ **H18.21** **Corneal edema** secondary to contact lens

        EXCLUDES 2 *other corneal disorders due to contact lens (H18.82-)*

        H18.211 **Corneal edema secondary to contact lens, right eye**

        H18.212 **Corneal edema secondary to contact lens, left eye**

        H18.213 **Corneal edema secondary to contact lens, bilateral**

        H18.219 **Corneal edema secondary to contact lens, unspecified eye**

    ✓6ᵗʰ **H18.22** **Idiopathic corneal edema**

        H18.221 **Idiopathic corneal edema, right eye**

        H18.222 **Idiopathic corneal edema, left eye**

        H18.223 **Idiopathic corneal edema, bilateral**

        H18.229 **Idiopathic corneal edema, unspecified eye**

    ✓6ᵗʰ **H18.23** **Secondary corneal edema**

        H18.231 **Secondary corneal edema, right eye**

        H18.232 **Secondary corneal edema, left eye**

        H18.233 **Secondary corneal edema, bilateral**

        H18.239 **Secondary corneal edema, unspecified eye**

✓5ᵗʰ **H18.3** **Changes of corneal membranes**

    H18.30 **Unspecified corneal membrane change**

    ✓6ᵗʰ **H18.31** **Folds and rupture in** Bowman's membrane

        H18.311 **Folds and rupture in Bowman's membrane, right eye**

        H18.312 **Folds and rupture in Bowman's membrane, left eye**

        H18.313 **Folds and rupture in Bowman's membrane, bilateral**

        H18.319 **Folds and rupture in Bowman's membrane, unspecified eye**

    ✓6ᵗʰ **H18.32** **Folds in** Descemet's membrane

        H18.321 **Folds in Descemet's membrane, right eye**

        H18.322 **Folds in Descemet's membrane, left eye**

        H18.323 **Folds in Descemet's membrane, bilateral**

        H18.329 **Folds in Descemet's membrane, unspecified eye**

    ✓6ᵗʰ **H18.33** **Rupture in** Descemet's membrane

        H18.331 **Rupture in Descemet's membrane, right eye**

        H18.332 **Rupture in Descemet's membrane, left eye**

        H18.333 **Rupture in Descemet's membrane, bilateral**

        H18.339 **Rupture in Descemet's membrane, unspecified eye**

✓5ᵗʰ **H18.4** **Corneal degeneration**

        EXCLUDES 1 *Mooren's ulcer (H16.0-)*

                      recurrent erosion of cornea (H18.83-)

    H18.40 **Unspecified corneal degeneration**

    ✓6ᵗʰ **H18.41** **Arcus senilis**

        Senile corneal changes

        H18.411 **Arcus senilis, right eye**

        H18.412 **Arcus senilis, left eye**

        H18.413 **Arcus senilis, bilateral**

        H18.419 **Arcus senilis, unspecified eye**

    ✓6ᵗʰ **H18.42** **Band keratopathy**

        H18.421 **Band keratopathy, right eye**

        H18.422 **Band keratopathy, left eye**

        H18.423 **Band keratopathy, bilateral**

        H18.429 **Band keratopathy, unspecified eye**

    H18.43 **Other calcerous corneal degeneration**

    ✓6ᵗʰ **H18.44** **Keratomalacia**

        EXCLUDES 1 *keratomalacia due to vitamin A deficiency (E50.4)*

        H18.441 **Keratomalacia, right eye**

        H18.442 **Keratomalacia, left eye**

        H18.443 **Keratomalacia, bilateral**

        H18.449 **Keratomalacia, unspecified eye**

    ✓6ᵗʰ **H18.45** **Nodular corneal degeneration**

        H18.451 **Nodular corneal degeneration, right eye**

        H18.452 **Nodular corneal degeneration, left eye**

        H18.453 **Nodular corneal degeneration,** bilateral

        H18.459 **Nodular corneal degeneration, unspecified eye**

    ✓6ᵗʰ **H18.46** **Peripheral corneal degeneration**

        H18.461 **Peripheral corneal degeneration,** right eye

        H18.462 **Peripheral corneal degeneration,** left eye

        H18.463 **Peripheral corneal degeneration, bilateral**

        H18.469 **Peripheral corneal degeneration, unspecified eye**

    H18.49 **Other corneal degeneration**

✓5ᵗʰ **H18.5** **Hereditary corneal dystrophies**

    AHA: 2020,4Q,24

    ✓6ᵗʰ **H18.50** **Unspecified hereditary corneal dystrophies**

        H18.501 **Unspecified hereditary corneal dystrophies, right eye**

        H18.502 **Unspecified hereditary corneal dystrophies, left eye**

        H18.503 **Unspecified hereditary corneal dystrophies, bilateral**

        H18.509 **Unspecified hereditary corneal dystrophies, unspecified eye**

    ✓6ᵗʰ **H18.51** **Endothelial corneal dystrophy**

        Fuchs' dystrophy

        H18.511 **Endothelial corneal dystrophy,** right eye

        H18.512 **Endothelial corneal dystrophy,** left eye

        H18.513 **Endothelial corneal dystrophy,** bilateral

        H18.519 **Endothelial corneal dystrophy, unspecified eye**

    ✓6ᵗʰ **H18.52** **Epithelial (juvenile) corneal dystrophy**

        H18.521 **Epithelial (juvenile) corneal dystrophy, right eye**

        H18.522 **Epithelial (juvenile) corneal dystrophy,** left eye

        H18.523 **Epithelial (juvenile) corneal dystrophy,** bilateral

        H18.529 **Epithelial (juvenile) corneal dystrophy, unspecified eye**

    ✓6ᵗʰ **H18.53** **Granular corneal dystrophy**

        H18.531 **Granular corneal dystrophy,** right eye

        H18.532 **Granular corneal dystrophy,** left eye

        H18.533 **Granular corneal dystrophy,** bilateral

        H18.539 **Granular corneal dystrophy, unspecified eye**

    ✓6ᵗʰ **H18.54** **Lattice corneal dystrophy**

        H18.541 **Lattice corneal dystrophy,** right eye

        H18.542 **Lattice corneal dystrophy,** left eye

        H18.543 **Lattice corneal dystrophy,** bilateral

        H18.549 **Lattice corneal dystrophy, unspecified eye**

    ✓6ᵗʰ **H18.55** **Macular corneal dystrophy**

        H18.551 **Macular corneal dystrophy,** right eye

        H18.552 **Macular corneal dystrophy,** left eye

        H18.553 **Macular corneal dystrophy,** bilateral

        H18.559 **Macular corneal dystrophy, unspecified eye**

    ✓6ᵗʰ **H18.59** **Other hereditary corneal dystrophies**

        H18.591 **Other hereditary corneal dystrophies, right eye**

        H18.592 **Other hereditary corneal dystrophies,** left eye

        H18.593 **Other hereditary corneal dystrophies, bilateral**

        H18.599 **Other hereditary corneal dystrophies, unspecified eye**

✓5ᵗʰ **H18.6** **Keratoconus**

    ✓6ᵗʰ **H18.60** **Keratoconus, unspecified**

        H18.601 **Keratoconus, unspecified, right eye**

        H18.602 **Keratoconus, unspecified, left eye**

        H18.603 **Keratoconus, unspecified, bilateral**

        H18.609 **Keratoconus, unspecified, unspecified eye**

    ✓6ᵗʰ **H18.61** **Keratoconus,** stable

        H18.611 **Keratoconus, stable, right eye**

        H18.612 **Keratoconus, stable, left eye**

        H18.613 **Keratoconus, stable, bilateral**

        H18.619 **Keratoconus, stable, unspecified eye**

HCC CMS-HCC   **Rx** Rx HCC   **ESR** ESRD HCC   **COM** Commercial HCC   **N** Newborn: 0   **P** Pediatric: 0-17   **M** Maternity: 9-64   **A** Adult: 15-124

624   ICD-10-CM 2023

√6ᵗʰ **H18.62 Keratoconus, unstable**
     Acute hydrops
     H18.621 Keratoconus, unstable, right eye
     H18.622 Keratoconus, unstable, left eye
     H18.623 Keratoconus, unstable, bilateral
     H18.629 Keratoconus, unstable, unspecified eye

√5ᵗʰ **H18.7 Other and unspecified corneal deformities**
     EXCLUDES 1   *congenital malformations of cornea (Q13.3-Q13.4)*
     H18.70 Unspecified corneal deformity

√6ᵗʰ **H18.71 Corneal ectasia**
     H18.711 Corneal ectasia, right eye
     H18.712 Corneal ectasia, left eye
     H18.713 Corneal ectasia, bilateral
     H18.719 Corneal ectasia, unspecified eye

√6ᵗʰ **H18.72 Corneal staphyloma**
     H18.721 Corneal staphyloma, right eye
     H18.722 Corneal staphyloma, left eye
     H18.723 Corneal staphyloma, bilateral
     H18.729 Corneal staphyloma, unspecified eye

√6ᵗʰ **H18.73 Descemetocele**
     H18.731 Descemetocele, right eye
     H18.732 Descemetocele, left eye
     H18.733 Descemetocele, bilateral
     H18.739 Descemetocele, unspecified eye

√6ᵗʰ **H18.79 Other corneal deformities**
     H18.791 Other corneal deformities, right eye
     H18.792 Other corneal deformities, left eye
     H18.793 Other corneal deformities, bilateral
     H18.799 Other corneal deformities, unspecified eye

√5ᵗʰ **H18.8 Other specified disorders of cornea**

√6ᵗʰ **H18.81 Anesthesia and hypoesthesia of cornea**
     H18.811 Anesthesia and hypoesthesia of cornea, right eye
     H18.812 Anesthesia and hypoesthesia of cornea, left eye
     H18.813 Anesthesia and hypoesthesia of cornea, bilateral
     H18.819 Anesthesia and hypoesthesia of cornea, unspecified eye

√6ᵗʰ **H18.82 Corneal disorder due to contact lens**
     EXCLUDES 2   *corneal edema due to contact lens (H18.21-)*
     H18.821 Corneal disorder due to contact lens, right eye
     H18.822 Corneal disorder due to contact lens, left eye
     H18.823 Corneal disorder due to contact lens, bilateral
     H18.829 Corneal disorder due to contact lens, unspecified eye

√6ᵗʰ **H18.83 Recurrent erosion of cornea**
     H18.831 Recurrent erosion of cornea, right eye
     H18.832 Recurrent erosion of cornea, left eye
     H18.833 Recurrent erosion of cornea, bilateral
     H18.839 Recurrent erosion of cornea, unspecified eye

√6ᵗʰ **H18.89 Other specified disorders of cornea**
     H18.891 Other specified disorders of cornea, right eye
     H18.892 Other specified disorders of cornea, left eye
     H18.893 Other specified disorders of cornea, bilateral
     H18.899 Other specified disorders of cornea, unspecified eye

H18.9 Unspecified disorder of cornea

√4ᵗʰ **H20 Iridocyclitis**

√5ᵗʰ **H20.0 Acute and subacute iridocyclitis**
     Acute anterior uveitis
     Acute cyclitis
     Acute iritis
     Subacute anterior uveitis
     Subacute cyclitis
     Subacute iritis
     EXCLUDES 1   *iridocyclitis, iritis, uveitis (due to) (in) diabetes mellitus (E08-E13 with .39)*
                 iridocyclitis, iritis, uveitis (due to) (in) diphtheria (A36.89)
                 iridocyclitis, iritis, uveitis (due to) (in) gonococcal (A54.32)
                 iridocyclitis, iritis, uveitis (due to) (in) herpes (simplex) (B00.51)
                 iridocyclitis, iritis, uveitis (due to) (in) herpes zoster (B02.32)
                 iridocyclitis, iritis, uveitis (due to) (in) late congenital syphilis (A50.39)
                 iridocyclitis, iritis, uveitis (due to) (in) late syphilis (A52.71)
                 iridocyclitis, iritis, uveitis (due to) (in) sarcoidosis (D86.83)
                 iridocyclitis, iritis, uveitis (due to) (in) syphilis (A51.43)
                 iridocyclitis, iritis, uveitis (due to) (in) toxoplasmosis (B58.09)
                 iridocyclitis, iritis, uveitis (due to) (in) tuberculosis (A18.54)
     H20.00 Unspecified acute and subacute iridocyclitis

√6ᵗʰ **H20.01 Primary iridocyclitis**
     H20.011 Primary iridocyclitis, right eye
     H20.012 Primary iridocyclitis, left eye
     H20.013 Primary iridocyclitis, bilateral
     H20.019 Primary iridocyclitis, unspecified eye

√6ᵗʰ **H20.02 Recurrent acute iridocyclitis**
     H20.021 Recurrent acute iridocyclitis, right eye
     H20.022 Recurrent acute iridocyclitis, left eye
     H20.023 Recurrent acute iridocyclitis, bilateral
     H20.029 Recurrent acute iridocyclitis, unspecified eye

√6ᵗʰ **H20.03 Secondary infectious iridocyclitis**
     H20.031 Secondary infectious iridocyclitis, right eye
     H20.032 Secondary infectious iridocyclitis, left eye
     H20.033 Secondary infectious iridocyclitis, bilateral
     H20.039 Secondary infectious iridocyclitis, unspecified eye

√6ᵗʰ **H20.04 Secondary noninfectious iridocyclitis**
     H20.041 Secondary noninfectious iridocyclitis, right eye
     H20.042 Secondary noninfectious iridocyclitis, left eye
     H20.043 Secondary noninfectious iridocyclitis, bilateral
     H20.049 Secondary noninfectious iridocyclitis, unspecified eye

√6ᵗʰ **H20.05 Hypopyon**
     H20.051 Hypopyon, right eye
     H20.052 Hypopyon, left eye
     H20.053 Hypopyon, bilateral
     H20.059 Hypopyon, unspecified eye

√5ᵗʰ **H20.1 Chronic iridocyclitis**
     Use additional code for any associated cataract (H26.21-)
     EXCLUDES 2   *posterior cyclitis (H30.2-)*
     H20.10 Chronic iridocyclitis, unspecified eye
     H20.11 Chronic iridocyclitis, right eye
     H20.12 Chronic iridocyclitis, left eye
     H20.13 Chronic iridocyclitis, bilateral

√5ᵗʰ **H20.2 Lens-induced iridocyclitis**
     H20.20 Lens-induced iridocyclitis, unspecified eye
     H20.21 Lens-induced iridocyclitis, right eye
     H20.22 Lens-induced iridocyclitis, left eye
     H20.23 Lens-induced iridocyclitis, bilateral

✓6ᵗʰ **H20.8 Other iridocyclitis**
> EXCLUDES 2   *glaucomatocyclitis crises (H40.4-)*
> *posterior cyclitis (H30.2-)*
> *sympathetic uveitis (H44.13-)*

  ✓6ᵗʰ **H20.81 Fuchs' heterochromic cyclitis**
    H20.811 Fuchs' heterochromic cyclitis, right eye
    H20.812 Fuchs' heterochromic cyclitis, left eye
    H20.813 Fuchs' heterochromic cyclitis, bilateral
    H20.819 Fuchs' heterochromic cyclitis, unspecified eye

  ✓6ᵗʰ **H20.82 Vogt-Koyanagi syndrome**
    H20.821 Vogt-Koyanagi syndrome, right eye
    H20.822 Vogt-Koyanagi syndrome, left eye
    H20.823 Vogt-Koyanagi syndrome, bilateral
    H20.829 Vogt-Koyanagi syndrome, unspecified eye

H20.9 Unspecified iridocyclitis
  Uveitis NOS

✓4ᵗʰ **H21 Other disorders of iris and ciliary body**
> EXCLUDES 2   *sympathetic uveitis (H44.1-)*

✓5ᵗʰ **H21.0 Hyphema**
> EXCLUDES 1   *traumatic hyphema (S05.1-)*

Hyphema

- Iris
- Cornea
- Hyphema

H21.00 Hyphema, unspecified eye
H21.01 Hyphema, right eye
H21.02 Hyphema, left eye
H21.03 Hyphema, bilateral

✓5ᵗʰ **H21.1 Other vascular disorders of iris and ciliary body**
  Neovascularization of iris or ciliary body
  Rubeosis iridis
  Rubeosis of iris

  ✓6ᵗʰ **H21.1X Other vascular disorders of iris and ciliary body**
    H21.1X1 Other vascular disorders of iris and ciliary body, right eye
    H21.1X2 Other vascular disorders of iris and ciliary body, left eye
    H21.1X3 Other vascular disorders of iris and ciliary body, bilateral
    H21.1X9 Other vascular disorders of iris and ciliary body, unspecified eye

✓5ᵗʰ **H21.2 Degeneration of iris and ciliary body**

  ✓6ᵗʰ **H21.21 Degeneration of chamber angle**
    H21.211 Degeneration of chamber angle, right eye
    H21.212 Degeneration of chamber angle, left eye
    H21.213 Degeneration of chamber angle, bilateral
    H21.219 Degeneration of chamber angle, unspecified eye

  ✓6ᵗʰ **H21.22 Degeneration of ciliary body**
    H21.221 Degeneration of ciliary body, right eye
    H21.222 Degeneration of ciliary body, left eye
    H21.223 Degeneration of ciliary body, bilateral
    H21.229 Degeneration of ciliary body, unspecified eye

  ✓6ᵗʰ **H21.23 Degeneration of iris (pigmentary)**
    Translucency of iris
    H21.231 Degeneration of iris (pigmentary), right eye
    H21.232 Degeneration of iris (pigmentary), left eye
    H21.233 Degeneration of iris (pigmentary), bilateral

H21.239 Degeneration of iris (pigmentary), unspecified eye

✓6ᵗʰ **H21.24 Degeneration of pupillary margin**
  H21.241 Degeneration of pupillary margin, right eye
  H21.242 Degeneration of pupillary margin, left eye
  H21.243 Degeneration of pupillary margin, bilateral
  H21.249 Degeneration of pupillary margin, unspecified eye

✓6ᵗʰ **H21.25 Iridoschisis**
  H21.251 Iridoschisis, right eye
  H21.252 Iridoschisis, left eye
  H21.253 Iridoschisis, bilateral
  H21.259 Iridoschisis, unspecified eye

✓6ᵗʰ **H21.26 Iris atrophy (essential) (progressive)**
  H21.261 Iris atrophy (essential) (progressive), right eye
  H21.262 Iris atrophy (essential) (progressive), left eye
  H21.263 Iris atrophy (essential) (progressive), bilateral
  H21.269 Iris atrophy (essential) (progressive), unspecified eye

✓6ᵗʰ **H21.27 Miotic pupillary cyst**
  H21.271 Miotic pupillary cyst, right eye
  H21.272 Miotic pupillary cyst, left eye
  H21.273 Miotic pupillary cyst, bilateral
  H21.279 Miotic pupillary cyst, unspecified eye

H21.29 Other iris atrophy

✓5ᵗʰ **H21.3 Cyst of iris, ciliary body and anterior chamber**
> EXCLUDES 2   *miotic pupillary cyst (H21.27-)*

  ✓6ᵗʰ **H21.30 Idiopathic cysts of iris, ciliary body or anterior chamber**
    Cyst of iris, ciliary body or anterior chamber NOS
    H21.301 Idiopathic cysts of iris, ciliary body or anterior chamber, right eye
    H21.302 Idiopathic cysts of iris, ciliary body or anterior chamber, left eye
    H21.303 Idiopathic cysts of iris, ciliary body or anterior chamber, bilateral
    H21.309 Idiopathic cysts of iris, ciliary body or anterior chamber, unspecified eye

  ✓6ᵗʰ **H21.31 Exudative cysts of iris or anterior chamber**
    H21.311 Exudative cysts of iris or anterior chamber, right eye
    H21.312 Exudative cysts of iris or anterior chamber, left eye
    H21.313 Exudative cysts of iris or anterior chamber, bilateral
    H21.319 Exudative cysts of iris or anterior chamber, unspecified eye

  ✓6ᵗʰ **H21.32 Implantation cysts of iris, ciliary body or anterior chamber**
    H21.321 Implantation cysts of iris, ciliary body or anterior chamber, right eye
    H21.322 Implantation cysts of iris, ciliary body or anterior chamber, left eye
    H21.323 Implantation cysts of iris, ciliary body or anterior chamber, bilateral
    H21.329 Implantation cysts of iris, ciliary body or anterior chamber, unspecified eye

  ✓6ᵗʰ **H21.33 Parasitic cyst of iris, ciliary body or anterior chamber**
    H21.331 Parasitic cyst of iris, ciliary body or anterior chamber, right eye
    H21.332 Parasitic cyst of iris, ciliary body or anterior chamber, left eye
    H21.333 Parasitic cyst of iris, ciliary body or anterior chamber, bilateral
    H21.339 Parasitic cyst of iris, ciliary body or anterior chamber, unspecified eye

  ✓6ᵗʰ **H21.34 Primary cyst of pars plana**
    H21.341 Primary cyst of pars plana, right eye
    H21.342 Primary cyst of pars plana, left eye
    H21.343 Primary cyst of pars plana, bilateral
    H21.349 Primary cyst of pars plana, unspecified eye

✓6th **H21.35 Exudative cyst of pars plana**

DEF: Protein, fatty-filled bullous elevation of the nonpigmented outermost ciliary epithelium of pars plana, due to fluid leak from blood vessels.

H21.351 Exudative cyst of pars plana, **right eye**
H21.352 Exudative cyst of pars plana, **left eye**
H21.353 Exudative cyst of pars plana, **bilateral**
H21.359 Exudative cyst of pars plana, **unspecified eye**

✓5th **H21.4 Pupillary membranes**

Iris bombé
Pupillary occlusion
Pupillary seclusion

EXCLUDES 1   congenital pupillary membranes (Q13.8)

H21.40 Pupillary membranes, **unspecified eye**
H21.41 Pupillary membranes, **right eye**
H21.42 Pupillary membranes, **left eye**
H21.43 Pupillary membranes, **bilateral**

✓5th **H21.5 Other and unspecified adhesions and disruptions of iris and ciliary body**

EXCLUDES 1   corectopia (Q13.2)

✓6th **H21.50 Unspecified adhesions of iris**

Synechia (iris) NOS

H21.501 Unspecified adhesions of iris, **right eye**
H21.502 Unspecified adhesions of iris, **left eye**
H21.503 Unspecified adhesions of iris, **bilateral**
H21.509 Unspecified adhesions of iris and ciliary body, **unspecified eye**

✓6th **H21.51 Anterior synechiae (iris)**

H21.511 Anterior synechiae (iris), **right eye**
H21.512 Anterior synechiae (iris), **left eye**
H21.513 Anterior synechiae (iris), **bilateral**
H21.519 Anterior synechiae (iris), **unspecified eye**

✓6th **H21.52 Goniosynechiae**

H21.521 Goniosynechiae, **right eye**
H21.522 Goniosynechiae, **left eye**
H21.523 Goniosynechiae, **bilateral**
H21.529 Goniosynechiae, **unspecified eye**

✓6th **H21.53 Iridodialysis**

H21.531 Iridodialysis, **right eye**
H21.532 Iridodialysis, **left eye**
H21.533 Iridodialysis, **bilateral**
H21.539 Iridodialysis, **unspecified eye**

✓6th **H21.54 Posterior synechiae (iris)**

H21.541 Posterior synechiae (iris), **right eye**
H21.542 Posterior synechiae (iris), **left eye**
H21.543 Posterior synechiae (iris), **bilateral**
H21.549 Posterior synechiae (iris), **unspecified eye**

✓6th **H21.55 Recession of chamber angle**

H21.551 Recession of chamber angle, **right eye**
H21.552 Recession of chamber angle, **left eye**
H21.553 Recession of chamber angle, **bilateral**
H21.559 Recession of chamber angle, **unspecified eye**

✓6th **H21.56 Pupillary abnormalities**

Deformed pupil
Ectopic pupil
Rupture of sphincter, pupil

EXCLUDES 1   congenital deformity of pupil (Q13.2-)

H21.561 Pupillary abnormality, **right eye**
H21.562 Pupillary abnormality, **left eye**
H21.563 Pupillary abnormality, **bilateral**
H21.569 Pupillary abnormality, **unspecified eye**

✓5th **H21.8 Other specified disorders of iris and ciliary body**

H21.81 Floppy iris syndrome

Intraoperative floppy iris syndrome (IFIS)
Use additional code for adverse effect, if applicable, to identify drug (T36-T50 with fifth or sixth character 5)

H21.82 Plateau iris syndrome (post-iridectomy) (postprocedural)

H21.89 Other specified disorders of iris and ciliary body

H21.9 Unspecified disorder of iris and ciliary body

H22 *Disorders of iris and ciliary body in diseases classified elsewhere*

Code first underlying disease, such as:
gout (M1A.-, M10.-)
leprosy (A30.-)
parasitic disease (B89)

Disorders of lens (H25-H28)

✓4th **H25 Age-related cataract**

Senile cataract

EXCLUDES 2   capsular glaucoma with pseudoexfoliation of lens (H40.1-)

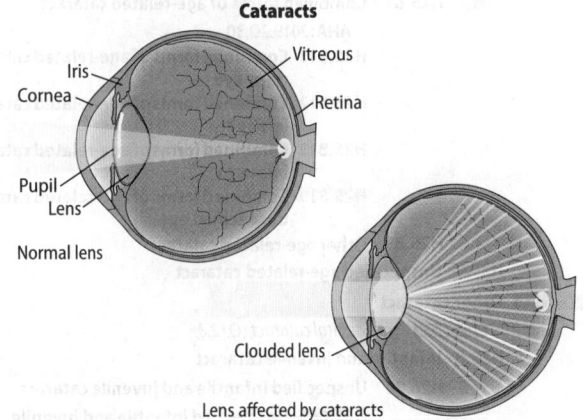

Cataracts

Iris — Vitreous
Cornea —
— Retina
Pupil —
Lens —
Normal lens

Clouded lens

Lens affected by cataracts

✓5th **H25.0 Age-related incipient cataract**

✓6th **H25.01 Cortical age-related cataract**

H25.011 Cortical age-related cataract, **right eye**   A
H25.012 Cortical age-related cataract, **left eye**   A
H25.013 Cortical age-related cataract, **bilateral**   A
H25.019 Cortical age-related cataract, **unspecified eye**   A

✓6th **H25.03 Anterior subcapsular polar age-related cataract**

H25.031 Anterior subcapsular polar age-related cataract, **right eye**   A
H25.032 Anterior subcapsular polar age-related cataract, **left eye**   A
H25.033 Anterior subcapsular polar age-related cataract, **bilateral**   A
H25.039 Anterior subcapsular polar age-related cataract, **unspecified eye**   A

✓6th **H25.04 Posterior subcapsular polar age-related cataract**

H25.041 Posterior subcapsular polar age-related cataract, **right eye**   A
H25.042 Posterior subcapsular polar age-related cataract, **left eye**   A
H25.043 Posterior subcapsular polar age-related cataract, **bilateral**   A
H25.049 Posterior subcapsular polar age-related cataract, **unspecified eye**   A

✓6th **H25.09 Other age-related incipient cataract**

Coronary age-related cataract
Punctate age-related cataract
Water clefts

H25.091 Other age-related incipient cataract, **right eye**   A
H25.092 Other age-related incipient cataract, **left eye**   A
H25.093 Other age-related incipient cataract, **bilateral**   A
H25.099 Other age-related incipient cataract, **unspecified eye**   A

✓5th **H25.1 Age-related nuclear cataract**

Cataracta brunescens
Nuclear sclerosis cataract
AHA: 2019,2Q,31; 2016,1Q,32

H25.10 Age-related nuclear cataract, **unspecified eye**   A
H25.11 Age-related nuclear cataract, **right eye**   A
H25.12 Age-related nuclear cataract, **left eye**   A
H25.13 Age-related nuclear cataract, **bilateral**   A

Chapter 7. Diseases of the Eye and Adnexa

H25.2–H26.33

✓5ᵗʰ **H25.2 Age-related cataract,** morgagnian type
    Age-related hypermature cataract

  H25.20 Age-related cataract, morgagnian type, unspecified eye Ⓐ

  H25.21 Age-related cataract, morgagnian type, right **eye** Ⓐ

  H25.22 Age-related cataract, morgagnian type, left **eye** Ⓐ

  H25.23 Age-related cataract, morgagnian type, bilateral Ⓐ

✓5ᵗʰ **H25.8 Other age-related cataract**

  ✓6ᵗʰ **H25.81 Combined forms of age-related cataract**
      AHA: 2019,2Q,30

    H25.811 Combined forms of age-related cataract, right **eye** Ⓐ

    H25.812 Combined forms of age-related cataract, left **eye** Ⓐ

    H25.813 Combined forms of age-related cataract, bilateral Ⓐ

    H25.819 Combined forms of age-related cataract, unspecified eye Ⓐ

  H25.89 Other age-related cataract Ⓐ

✓6ᵗʰ **H25.9 Unspecified age-related cataract** Ⓐ

✓4ᵗʰ **H26 Other cataract**

  EXCLUDES 1   congenital cataract (Q12.0)

  ✓5ᵗʰ **H26.0 Infantile and juvenile cataract**

    ✓6ᵗʰ **H26.00 Unspecified infantile and juvenile cataract**

      H26.001 Unspecified infantile and juvenile cataract, right **eye** Ⓟ

      H26.002 Unspecified infantile and juvenile cataract, left **eye** Ⓟ

      H26.003 Unspecified infantile and juvenile cataract, bilateral Ⓟ

      H26.009 Unspecified infantile and juvenile cataract, unspecified eye Ⓟ

    ✓6ᵗʰ **H26.01 Infantile and juvenile** cortical, lamellar, or zonular **cataract**

      H26.011 Infantile and juvenile cortical, lamellar, or zonular cataract, right **eye** Ⓟ

      H26.012 Infantile and juvenile cortical, lamellar, or zonular cataract, left **eye** Ⓟ

      H26.013 Infantile and juvenile cortical, lamellar, or zonular cataract, bilateral Ⓟ

      H26.019 Infantile and juvenile cortical, lamellar, or zonular cataract, unspecified eye Ⓟ

    ✓6ᵗʰ **H26.03 Infantile and juvenile** nuclear **cataract**

      H26.031 Infantile and juvenile nuclear cataract, right **eye** Ⓟ

      H26.032 Infantile and juvenile nuclear cataract, left **eye** Ⓟ

      H26.033 Infantile and juvenile nuclear cataract, bilateral Ⓟ

      H26.039 Infantile and juvenile nuclear cataract, unspecified eye Ⓟ

    ✓6ᵗʰ **H26.04 Anterior subcapsular polar infantile and juvenile cataract**

      H26.041 Anterior subcapsular polar infantile and juvenile cataract, right **eye** Ⓟ

      H26.042 Anterior subcapsular polar infantile and juvenile cataract, left **eye** Ⓟ

      H26.043 Anterior subcapsular polar infantile and juvenile cataract, bilateral Ⓟ

      H26.049 Anterior subcapsular polar infantile and juvenile cataract, unspecified eye Ⓟ

    ✓6ᵗʰ **H26.05 Posterior subcapsular polar infantile and juvenile cataract**

      H26.051 Posterior subcapsular polar infantile and juvenile cataract, right **eye** Ⓟ

      H26.052 Posterior subcapsular polar infantile and juvenile cataract, left **eye** Ⓟ

      H26.053 Posterior subcapsular polar infantile and juvenile cataract, bilateral Ⓟ

      H26.059 Posterior subcapsular polar infantile and juvenile cataract, unspecified eye Ⓟ

    ✓6ᵗʰ **H26.06 Combined forms of infantile and juvenile cataract**

      H26.061 Combined forms of infantile and juvenile cataract, right **eye** Ⓟ

      H26.062 Combined forms of infantile and juvenile cataract, left **eye** Ⓟ

      H26.063 Combined forms of infantile and juvenile cataract, bilateral Ⓟ

      H26.069 Combined forms of infantile and juvenile cataract, unspecified eye Ⓟ

    H26.09 Other infantile and juvenile cataract Ⓟ

  ✓5ᵗʰ **H26.1 Traumatic cataract**
    Use additional code (Chapter 20) to identify external cause

    ✓6ᵗʰ **H26.10 Unspecified traumatic cataract**

      H26.101 Unspecified traumatic cataract, right **eye**

      H26.102 Unspecified traumatic cataract, left **eye**

      H26.103 Unspecified traumatic cataract, bilateral

      H26.109 Unspecified traumatic cataract, unspecified eye

    ✓6ᵗʰ **H26.11 Localized traumatic opacities**

      H26.111 Localized traumatic opacities, right **eye**

      H26.112 Localized traumatic opacities, left **eye**

      H26.113 Localized traumatic opacities, bilateral

      H26.119 Localized traumatic opacities, unspecified eye

    ✓6ᵗʰ **H26.12 Partially resolved traumatic cataract**

      H26.121 Partially resolved traumatic cataract, right **eye**

      H26.122 Partially resolved traumatic cataract, left **eye**

      H26.123 Partially resolved traumatic cataract, bilateral

      H26.129 Partially resolved traumatic cataract, unspecified eye

    ✓6ᵗʰ **H26.13 Total traumatic cataract**

      H26.131 Total traumatic cataract, right **eye**

      H26.132 Total traumatic cataract, left **eye**

      H26.133 Total traumatic cataract, bilateral

      H26.139 Total traumatic cataract, unspecified eye

  ✓5ᵗʰ **H26.2 Complicated cataract**

    H26.20 Unspecified complicated cataract
      Cataracta complicata NOS

    ✓6ᵗʰ **H26.21 Cataract with neovascularization**
      Code also associated condition, such as:
        chronic iridocyclitis (H20.1-)

      H26.211 Cataract with neovascularization, right **eye**

      H26.212 Cataract with neovascularization, left **eye**

      H26.213 Cataract with neovascularization, bilateral

      H26.219 Cataract with neovascularization, unspecified eye

    ✓6ᵗʰ **H26.22 Cataract secondary to ocular disorders (degenerative) (inflammatory)**
      Code also associated ocular disorder

      H26.221 Cataract secondary to ocular disorders (degenerative) (inflammatory), right **eye**

      H26.222 Cataract secondary to ocular disorders (degenerative) (inflammatory), left **eye**

      H26.223 Cataract secondary to ocular disorders (degenerative) (inflammatory), bilateral

      H26.229 Cataract secondary to ocular disorders (degenerative) (inflammatory), unspecified eye

    ✓6ᵗʰ **H26.23 Glaucomatous flecks (subcapsular)**
      Code first underlying glaucoma (H40-H42)

      H26.231 Glaucomatous flecks (subcapsular), right **eye**

      H26.232 Glaucomatous flecks (subcapsular), left **eye**

      H26.233 Glaucomatous flecks (subcapsular), bilateral

      H26.239 Glaucomatous flecks (subcapsular), unspecified eye

  ✓5ᵗʰ **H26.3 Drug-induced cataract**
    Toxic cataract
    Use additional code for adverse effect, if applicable, to identify drug (T36-T50 with fifth or sixth character 5)

    H26.30 Drug-induced cataract, unspecified eye

    H26.31 Drug-induced cataract, right **eye**

    H26.32 Drug-induced cataract, left **eye**

    H26.33 Drug-induced cataract, bilateral

☑5ᵗʰ **H26.4 Secondary cataract**

    H26.40 Unspecified secondary cataract

    ☑6ᵗʰ **H26.41 Soemmering's ring**

        H26.411 Soemmering's ring, right eye

        H26.412 Soemmering's ring, left eye

        H26.413 Soemmering's ring, bilateral

        H26.419 Soemmering's ring, unspecified eye

    ☑6ᵗʰ **H26.49 Other secondary cataract**

        AHA: 2018,2Q,14

        H26.491 Other secondary cataract, right eye

        H26.492 Other secondary cataract, left eye

        H26.493 Other secondary cataract, bilateral

        H26.499 Other secondary cataract, unspecified eye

H26.8 Other specified cataract

H26.9 Unspecified cataract

☑4ᵗʰ **H27 Other disorders of lens**

    EXCLUDES 1   *congenital lens malformations (Q12.-)*

           mechanical complications of intraocular lens implant (T85.2)

           pseudophakia (Z96.1)

    ☑5ᵗʰ **H27.0 Aphakia**

        Acquired absence of lens

        Acquired aphakia

        Aphakia due to trauma

        EXCLUDES 1   *cataract extraction status (Z98.4-)*

              congenital absence of lens (Q12.3)

              congenital aphakia (Q12.3)

        H27.00 Aphakia, unspecified eye

        H27.01 Aphakia, right eye

        H27.02 Aphakia, left eye

        H27.03 Aphakia, bilateral

    ☑5ᵗʰ **H27.1 Dislocation of lens**

        H27.10 Unspecified dislocation of lens

        ☑6ᵗʰ **H27.11 Subluxation of lens**

            H27.111 Subluxation of lens, right eye

            H27.112 Subluxation of lens, left eye

            H27.113 Subluxation of lens, bilateral

            H27.119 Subluxation of lens, unspecified eye

        ☑6ᵗʰ **H27.12 Anterior dislocation of lens**

            H27.121 Anterior dislocation of lens, right eye

            H27.122 Anterior dislocation of lens, left eye

            H27.123 Anterior dislocation of lens, bilateral

            H27.129 Anterior dislocation of lens, unspecified eye

        ☑6ᵗʰ **H27.13 Posterior dislocation of lens**

            H27.131 Posterior dislocation of lens, right eye

            H27.132 Posterior dislocation of lens, left eye

            H27.133 Posterior dislocation of lens, bilateral

            H27.139 Posterior dislocation of lens, unspecified eye

    H27.8 Other specified disorders of lens

    H27.9 Unspecified disorder of lens

H28 Cataract in diseases classified elsewhere

    Code first underlying disease, such as:

      hypoparathyroidism (E20.-)

      myotonia (G71.1-)

      myxedema (E03.-)

      protein-calorie malnutrition (E40-E46)

    EXCLUDES 1   *cataract in diabetes mellitus (E08.36, E09.36, E10.36, E11.36, E13.36)*

Disorders of choroid and retina (H30-H36)

☑4ᵗʰ **H30 Chorioretinal inflammation**

    ☑5ᵗʰ **H30.0 Focal chorioretinal inflammation**

        Focal chorioretinitis

        Focal choroiditis

        Focal retinitis

        Focal retinochoroiditis

        ☑6ᵗʰ **H30.00 Unspecified focal chorioretinal inflammation**

            Focal chorioretinitis NOS

            Focal choroiditis NOS

            Focal retinitis NOS

            Focal retinochoroiditis NOS

            H30.001 Unspecified focal chorioretinal inflammation, right eye

            H30.002 Unspecified focal chorioretinal inflammation, left eye

            H30.003 Unspecified focal chorioretinal inflammation, bilateral

            H30.009 Unspecified focal chorioretinal inflammation, unspecified eye

        ☑6ᵗʰ **H30.01 Focal chorioretinal inflammation, juxtapapillary**

            H30.011 Focal chorioretinal inflammation, juxtapapillary, right eye

            H30.012 Focal chorioretinal inflammation, juxtapapillary, left eye

            H30.013 Focal chorioretinal inflammation, juxtapapillary, bilateral

            H30.019 Focal chorioretinal inflammation, juxtapapillary, unspecified eye

        ☑6ᵗʰ **H30.02 Focal chorioretinal inflammation of posterior pole**

            H30.021 Focal chorioretinal inflammation of posterior pole, right eye

            H30.022 Focal chorioretinal inflammation of posterior pole, left eye

            H30.023 Focal chorioretinal inflammation of posterior pole, bilateral

            H30.029 Focal chorioretinal inflammation of posterior pole, unspecified eye

        ☑6ᵗʰ **H30.03 Focal chorioretinal inflammation, peripheral**

            H30.031 Focal chorioretinal inflammation, peripheral, right eye

            H30.032 Focal chorioretinal inflammation, peripheral, left eye

            H30.033 Focal chorioretinal inflammation, peripheral, bilateral

            H30.039 Focal chorioretinal inflammation, peripheral, unspecified eye

        ☑6ᵗʰ **H30.04 Focal chorioretinal inflammation, macular or paramacular**

            H30.041 Focal chorioretinal inflammation, macular or paramacular, right eye

            H30.042 Focal chorioretinal inflammation, macular or paramacular, left eye

            H30.043 Focal chorioretinal inflammation, macular or paramacular, bilateral

            H30.049 Focal chorioretinal inflammation, macular or paramacular, unspecified eye

    ☑5ᵗʰ **H30.1 Disseminated chorioretinal inflammation**

        Disseminated chorioretinitis

        Disseminated choroiditis

        Disseminated retinitis

        Disseminated retinochoroiditis

        EXCLUDES 2   *exudative retinopathy (H35.02-)*

        ☑6ᵗʰ **H30.10 Unspecified disseminated chorioretinal inflammation**

            Disseminated chorioretinitis NOS

            Disseminated choroiditis NOS

            Disseminated retinitis NOS

            Disseminated retinochoroiditis NOS

            H30.101 Unspecified disseminated chorioretinal inflammation, right eye

            H30.102 Unspecified disseminated chorioretinal inflammation, left eye

            H30.103 Unspecified disseminated chorioretinal inflammation, bilateral

            H30.109 Unspecified disseminated chorioretinal inflammation, unspecified eye

        ☑6ᵗʰ **H30.11 Disseminated chorioretinal inflammation of posterior pole**

            H30.111 Disseminated chorioretinal inflammation of posterior pole, right eye

            H30.112 Disseminated chorioretinal inflammation of posterior pole, left eye

            H30.113 Disseminated chorioretinal inflammation of posterior pole, bilateral

            H30.119 Disseminated chorioretinal inflammation of posterior pole, unspecified eye

        ☑6ᵗʰ **H30.12 Disseminated chorioretinal inflammation, peripheral**

            H30.121 Disseminated chorioretinal inflammation, peripheral right eye

            H30.122 Disseminated chorioretinal inflammation, peripheral, left eye

            H30.123 Disseminated chorioretinal inflammation, peripheral, bilateral

H30.129   Disseminated chorioretinal inflammation, peripheral, unspecified eye

☑6ᵗʰ H30.13   Disseminated chorioretinal inflammation, generalized

H30.131   Disseminated chorioretinal inflammation, generalized, right eye

H30.132   Disseminated chorioretinal inflammation, generalized, left eye

H30.133   Disseminated chorioretinal inflammation, generalized, bilateral

H30.139   Disseminated chorioretinal inflammation, generalized, unspecified eye

☑6ᵗʰ H30.14   Acute posterior multifocal placoid pigment epitheliopathy

H30.141   Acute posterior multifocal placoid pigment epitheliopathy, right eye

H30.142   Acute posterior multifocal placoid pigment epitheliopathy, left eye

H30.143   Acute posterior multifocal placoid pigment epitheliopathy, bilateral

H30.149   Acute posterior multifocal placoid pigment epitheliopathy, unspecified eye

☑5ᵗʰ H30.2   Posterior cyclitis

Pars planitis

H30.20   Posterior cyclitis, unspecified eye

H30.21   Posterior cyclitis, right eye

H30.22   Posterior cyclitis, left eye

H30.23   Posterior cyclitis, bilateral

☑5ᵗʰ H30.8   Other chorioretinal inflammations

☑6ᵗʰ H30.81   Harada's disease

H30.811   Harada's disease, right eye

H30.812   Harada's disease, left eye

H30.813   Harada's disease, bilateral

H30.819   Harada's disease, unspecified eye

☑6ᵗʰ H30.89   Other chorioretinal inflammations

H30.891   Other chorioretinal inflammations, right eye

H30.892   Other chorioretinal inflammations, left eye

H30.893   Other chorioretinal inflammations, bilateral

H30.899   Other chorioretinal inflammations, unspecified eye

☑5ᵗʰ H30.9   Unspecified chorioretinal inflammation

Chorioretinitis NOS

Choroiditis NOS

Neuroretinitis NOS

Retinitis NOS

Retinochoroiditis NOS

H30.90   Unspecified chorioretinal inflammation, unspecified eye

H30.91   Unspecified chorioretinal inflammation, right eye

H30.92   Unspecified chorioretinal inflammation, left eye

H30.93   Unspecified chorioretinal inflammation, bilateral

☑4ᵗʰ **H31   Other disorders of choroid**

☑5ᵗʰ H31.0   Chorioretinal scars

    EXCLUDES 2   postsurgical chorioretinal scars (H59.81-)

☑6ᵗʰ H31.00   Unspecified chorioretinal scars

H31.001   Unspecified chorioretinal scars, right eye

H31.002   Unspecified chorioretinal scars, left eye

H31.003   Unspecified chorioretinal scars, bilateral

H31.009   Unspecified chorioretinal scars, unspecified eye

☑6ᵗʰ H31.01   Macula scars of posterior pole (postinflammatory) (post-traumatic)

    EXCLUDES 1   postprocedural chorioretinal scar (H59.81-)

H31.011   Macula scars of posterior pole (postinflammatory) (post-traumatic), right eye

H31.012   Macula scars of posterior pole (postinflammatory) (post-traumatic), left eye

H31.013   Macula scars of posterior pole (postinflammatory) (post-traumatic), bilateral

H31.019   Macula scars of posterior pole (postinflammatory) (post-traumatic), unspecified eye

☑6ᵗʰ H31.02   Solar retinopathy

H31.021   Solar retinopathy, right eye

H31.022   Solar retinopathy, left eye

H31.023   Solar retinopathy, bilateral

H31.029   Solar retinopathy, unspecified eye

☑6ᵗʰ H31.09   Other chorioretinal scars

H31.091   Other chorioretinal scars, right eye

H31.092   Other chorioretinal scars, left eye

H31.093   Other chorioretinal scars, bilateral

H31.099   Other chorioretinal scars, unspecified eye

☑5ᵗʰ H31.1   Choroidal degeneration

    EXCLUDES 2   angioid streaks of macula (H35.33)

☑6ᵗʰ H31.10   Unspecified choroidal degeneration

Choroidal sclerosis NOS

H31.101   Choroidal degeneration, unspecified, right eye

H31.102   Choroidal degeneration, unspecified, left eye

H31.103   Choroidal degeneration, unspecified, bilateral

H31.109   Choroidal degeneration, unspecified, unspecified eye

☑6ᵗʰ H31.11   Age-related choroidal atrophy

H31.111   Age-related choroidal atrophy, right eye   Ⓐ

H31.112   Age-related choroidal atrophy, left eye   Ⓐ

H31.113   Age-related choroidal atrophy, bilateral   Ⓐ

H31.119   Age-related choroidal atrophy, unspecified eye   Ⓐ

☑6ᵗʰ H31.12   Diffuse secondary atrophy of choroid

H31.121   Diffuse secondary atrophy of choroid, right eye

H31.122   Diffuse secondary atrophy of choroid, left eye

H31.123   Diffuse secondary atrophy of choroid, bilateral

H31.129   Diffuse secondary atrophy of choroid, unspecified eye

☑5ᵗʰ H31.2   Hereditary choroidal dystrophy

    EXCLUDES 2   hyperornithinemia (E72.4)

           ornithinemia (E72.4)

H31.20   Hereditary choroidal dystrophy, unspecified

H31.21   Choroideremia

H31.22   Choroidal dystrophy (central areolar) (generalized) (peripapillary)

H31.23   Gyrate atrophy, choroid

H31.29   Other hereditary choroidal dystrophy

☑5ᵗʰ H31.3   Choroidal hemorrhage and rupture

☑6ᵗʰ H31.30   Unspecified choroidal hemorrhage

H31.301   Unspecified choroidal hemorrhage, right eye

H31.302   Unspecified choroidal hemorrhage, left eye

H31.303   Unspecified choroidal hemorrhage, bilateral

H31.309   Unspecified choroidal hemorrhage, unspecified eye

☑6ᵗʰ H31.31   Expulsive choroidal hemorrhage

H31.311   Expulsive choroidal hemorrhage, right eye

H31.312   Expulsive choroidal hemorrhage, left eye

H31.313   Expulsive choroidal hemorrhage, bilateral

H31.319   Expulsive choroidal hemorrhage, unspecified eye

☑6ᵗʰ H31.32   Choroidal rupture

H31.321   Choroidal rupture, right eye

H31.322   Choroidal rupture, left eye

H31.323   Choroidal rupture, bilateral

H31.329   Choroidal rupture, unspecified eye

☑5ᵗʰ H31.4   Choroidal detachment

☑6ᵗʰ H31.40   Unspecified choroidal detachment

H31.401   Unspecified choroidal detachment, right eye

H31.402   Unspecified choroidal detachment, left eye

       H31.403 **Unspecified choroidal detachment,** **bilateral**

       H31.409 **Unspecified choroidal detachment, unspecified eye**

✓6ᵗʰ **H31.41 Hemorrhagic choroidal detachment**

       H31.411 **Hemorrhagic choroidal detachment, right eye**

       H31.412 **Hemorrhagic choroidal detachment, left eye**

       H31.413 **Hemorrhagic choroidal detachment, bilateral**

       H31.419 **Hemorrhagic choroidal detachment, unspecified eye**

✓6ᵗʰ **H31.42 Serous choroidal detachment**

       H31.421 **Serous choroidal detachment, right eye**
       H31.422 **Serous choroidal detachment, left eye**
       H31.423 **Serous choroidal detachment, bilateral**
       H31.429 **Serous choroidal detachment, unspecified eye**

H31.8 Other specified disorders of choroid

H31.9 Unspecified disorder of choroid

H32 *Chorioretinal disorders in diseases classified elsewhere*

Code first underlying disease, such as:
congenital toxoplasmosis (P37.1)
histoplasmosis (B39.-)
leprosy (A30.-)

EXCLUDES 1   *chorioretinitis (in):*
       toxoplasmosis (acquired) (B58.01)
       tuberculosis (A18.53)

✓4ᵗʰ **H33 Retinal detachments and breaks**

EXCLUDES 1   *detachment of retinal pigment epithelium (H35.72-, H35.73-)*

Retinal Detachment

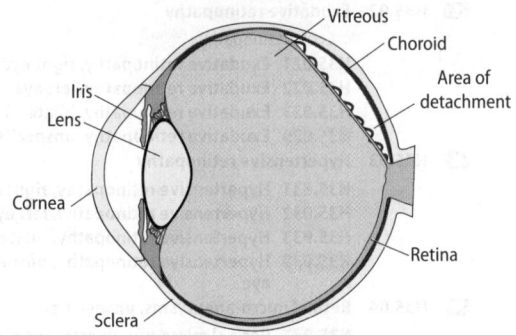

✓5ᵗʰ **H33.0 Retinal detachment with retinal break**

Rhegmatogenous retinal detachment

EXCLUDES 1   *serous retinal detachment (without retinal break) (H33.2-)*

✓6ᵗʰ **H33.00 Unspecified retinal detachment with retinal break**

       H33.001 **Unspecified retinal detachment with retinal break, right eye**

       H33.002 **Unspecified retinal detachment with retinal break, left eye**

       H33.003 **Unspecified retinal detachment with retinal break, bilateral**

       H33.009 **Unspecified retinal detachment with retinal break, unspecified eye**

✓6ᵗʰ **H33.01 Retinal detachment with single break**

       H33.011 **Retinal detachment with single break, right eye**

       H33.012 **Retinal detachment with single break, left eye**

       H33.013 **Retinal detachment with single break, bilateral**

       H33.019 **Retinal detachment with single break, unspecified eye**

✓6ᵗʰ **H33.02 Retinal detachment with multiple breaks**

       H33.021 **Retinal detachment with multiple breaks, right eye**

       H33.022 **Retinal detachment with multiple breaks, left eye**

       H33.023 **Retinal detachment with multiple breaks, bilateral**

       H33.029 **Retinal detachment with multiple breaks, unspecified eye**

✓6ᵗʰ **H33.03 Retinal detachment with giant retinal tear**

       H33.031 **Retinal detachment with giant retinal tear, right eye**

       H33.032 **Retinal detachment with giant retinal tear, left eye**

       H33.033 **Retinal detachment with giant retinal tear, bilateral**

       H33.039 **Retinal detachment with giant retinal tear, unspecified eye**

✓6ᵗʰ **H33.04 Retinal detachment with retinal dialysis**

       H33.041 **Retinal detachment with retinal dialysis, right eye**

       H33.042 **Retinal detachment with retinal dialysis, left eye**

       H33.043 **Retinal detachment with retinal dialysis, bilateral**

       H33.049 **Retinal detachment with retinal dialysis, unspecified eye**

✓6ᵗʰ **H33.05 Total retinal detachment**

       H33.051 **Total retinal detachment, right eye**
       H33.052 **Total retinal detachment, left eye**
       H33.053 **Total retinal detachment, bilateral**
       H33.059 **Total retinal detachment, unspecified eye**

✓5ᵗʰ **H33.1 Retinoschisis and retinal cysts**

EXCLUDES 1   *congenital retinoschisis (Q14.1)*
       microcystoid degeneration of retina (H35.42-)

✓6ᵗʰ **H33.10 Unspecified retinoschisis**

       H33.101 **Unspecified retinoschisis, right eye**
       H33.102 **Unspecified retinoschisis, left eye**
       H33.103 **Unspecified retinoschisis, bilateral**
       H33.109 **Unspecified retinoschisis, unspecified eye**

✓6ᵗʰ **H33.11 Cyst of ora serrata**

       H33.111 **Cyst of ora serrata, right eye**
       H33.112 **Cyst of ora serrata, left eye**
       H33.113 **Cyst of ora serrata, bilateral**
       H33.119 **Cyst of ora serrata, unspecified eye**

✓6ᵗʰ **H33.12 Parasitic cyst of retina**

       H33.121 **Parasitic cyst of retina, right eye**
       H33.122 **Parasitic cyst of retina, left eye**
       H33.123 **Parasitic cyst of retina, bilateral**
       H33.129 **Parasitic cyst of retina, unspecified eye**

✓6ᵗʰ **H33.19 Other retinoschisis and retinal cysts**

Pseudocyst of retina

       H33.191 **Other retinoschisis and retinal cysts, right eye**

       H33.192 **Other retinoschisis and retinal cysts, left eye**

       H33.193 **Other retinoschisis and retinal cysts, bilateral**

       H33.199 **Other retinoschisis and retinal cysts, unspecified eye**

✓5ᵗʰ **H33.2 Serous retinal detachment**

Retinal detachment NOS
Retinal detachment without retinal break

EXCLUDES 1   *central serous chorioretinopathy (H35.71-)*

       H33.20 **Serous retinal detachment, unspecified eye**
       H33.21 **Serous retinal detachment, right eye**
       H33.22 **Serous retinal detachment, left eye**
       H33.23 **Serous retinal detachment, bilateral**

✓5ᵗʰ **H33.3 Retinal breaks without detachment**

EXCLUDES 1   *chorioretinal scars after surgery for detachment (H59.81-)*
       peripheral retinal degeneration without break (H35.4-)

✓6ᵗʰ **H33.30 Unspecified retinal break**

       H33.301 **Unspecified retinal break, right eye**
       H33.302 **Unspecified retinal break, left eye**
       H33.303 **Unspecified retinal break, bilateral**
       H33.309 **Unspecified retinal break, unspecified eye**

✓6ᵗʰ **H33.31 Horseshoe tear of retina without detachment**

Operculum of retina without detachment

       H33.311 **Horseshoe tear of retina without detachment, right eye**

       H33.312 **Horseshoe tear of retina without detachment, left eye**

H33.313 Horseshoe tear of retina without detachment, bilateral
H33.319 Horseshoe tear of retina without detachment, unspecified eye
√6ᵗʰ **H33.32 Round hole** of retina without detachment
H33.321 Round hole, right eye
H33.322 Round hole, left eye
H33.323 Round hole, bilateral
H33.329 Round hole, unspecified eye
√6ᵗʰ **H33.33 Multiple defects** of retina without detachment
H33.331 Multiple defects of retina without detachment, right eye
H33.332 Multiple defects of retina without detachment, left eye
H33.333 Multiple defects of retina without detachment, bilateral
H33.339 Multiple defects of retina without detachment, unspecified eye
√5ᵗʰ **H33.4 Traction detachment of retina**
Proliferative vitreo-retinopathy with retinal detachment
H33.40 Traction detachment of retina, unspecified eye
H33.41 Traction detachment of retina, right eye
H33.42 Traction detachment of retina, left eye
H33.43 Traction detachment of retina, bilateral
H33.8 Other retinal detachments
√4ᵗʰ **H34 Retinal vascular occlusions**
EXCLUDES 1 amaurosis fugax (G45.3)
√5ᵗʰ **H34.0 Transient retinal artery occlusion**
H34.00 Transient retinal artery occlusion, unspecified eye
H34.01 Transient retinal artery occlusion, right eye
H34.02 Transient retinal artery occlusion, left eye
H34.03 Transient retinal artery occlusion, bilateral
√5ᵗʰ **H34.1 Central retinal artery occlusion**
H34.10 Central retinal artery occlusion, unspecified eye
H34.11 Central retinal artery occlusion, right eye
H34.12 Central retinal artery occlusion, left eye
H34.13 Central retinal artery occlusion, bilateral
√5ᵗʰ **H34.2 Other retinal artery occlusions**
√6ᵗʰ **H34.21 Partial retinal artery occlusion**
Hollenhorst's plaque
Retinal microembolism
H34.211 Partial retinal artery occlusion, right eye
H34.212 Partial retinal artery occlusion, left eye
H34.213 Partial retinal artery occlusion, bilateral
H34.219 Partial retinal artery occlusion, unspecified eye
√6ᵗʰ **H34.23 Retinal artery branch occlusion**
H34.231 Retinal artery branch occlusion, right eye
H34.232 Retinal artery branch occlusion, left eye
H34.233 Retinal artery branch occlusion, bilateral
H34.239 Retinal artery branch occlusion, unspecified eye
√5ᵗʰ **H34.8 Other retinal vascular occlusions**
AHA: 2016,4Q,19
√6ᵗʰ **H34.81 Central retinal vein occlusion**
One of the following 7th characters is to be assigned to codes in subcategory H34.81 to designate the severity of the occlusion:
Ø   with macular edema
1   with retinal neovascularization
2   stable
old central retinal vein occlusion
√7ᵗʰ **H34.811 Central retinal vein occlusion, right eye**
√7ᵗʰ **H34.812 Central retinal vein occlusion, left eye**
√7ᵗʰ **H34.813 Central retinal vein occlusion, bilateral**
√7ᵗʰ **H34.819 Central retinal vein occlusion, unspecified eye**
√6ᵗʰ **H34.82 Venous engorgement**
Incipient retinal vein occlusion
Partial retinal vein occlusion
H34.821 Venous engorgement, right eye
H34.822 Venous engorgement, left eye
H34.823 Venous engorgement, bilateral
H34.829 Venous engorgement, unspecified eye

√6ᵗʰ **H34.83 Tributary (branch) retinal vein occlusion**
One of the following 7th characters is to be assigned to codes in subcategory H34.83 to designate the severity of the occlusion:
Ø   with macular edema
1   with retinal neovascularization
2   stable
old tributary (branch) retinal vein occlusion
√7ᵗʰ **H34.831 Tributary (branch) retinal vein occlusion, right eye**
√7ᵗʰ **H34.832 Tributary (branch) retinal vein occlusion, left eye**
√7ᵗʰ **H34.833 Tributary (branch) retinal vein occlusion, bilateral**
√7ᵗʰ **H34.839 Tributary (branch) retinal vein occlusion, unspecified eye**
H34.9 Unspecified retinal vascular occlusion
√4ᵗʰ **H35 Other retinal disorders**
EXCLUDES 2 diabetic retinal disorders (E08.311-E08.359, E09.311-E09.359, E10.311-E10.359, E11.311-E11.359, E13.311-E13.359)
√5ᵗʰ **H35.0 Background retinopathy and retinal vascular changes**
Code also any associated hypertension (I10)
H35.00 Unspecified background retinopathy
√6ᵗʰ **H35.01 Changes in retinal vascular appearance**
Retinal vascular sheathing
H35.011 Changes in retinal vascular appearance, right eye
H35.012 Changes in retinal vascular appearance, left eye
H35.013 Changes in retinal vascular appearance, bilateral
H35.019 Changes in retinal vascular appearance, unspecified eye
√6ᵗʰ **H35.02 Exudative retinopathy**
Coats retinopathy
H35.021 Exudative retinopathy, right eye
H35.022 Exudative retinopathy, left eye
H35.023 Exudative retinopathy, bilateral
H35.029 Exudative retinopathy, unspecified eye
√6ᵗʰ **H35.03 Hypertensive retinopathy**
H35.031 Hypertensive retinopathy, right eye
H35.032 Hypertensive retinopathy, left eye
H35.033 Hypertensive retinopathy, bilateral
H35.039 Hypertensive retinopathy, unspecified eye
√6ᵗʰ **H35.04 Retinal micro-aneurysms, unspecified**
H35.041 Retinal micro-aneurysms, unspecified, right eye
H35.042 Retinal micro-aneurysms, unspecified, left eye
H35.043 Retinal micro-aneurysms, unspecified, bilateral
H35.049 Retinal micro-aneurysms, unspecified, unspecified eye
√6ᵗʰ **H35.05 Retinal neovascularization, unspecified**
H35.051 Retinal neovascularization, unspecified, right eye
H35.052 Retinal neovascularization, unspecified, left eye
H35.053 Retinal neovascularization, unspecified, bilateral
H35.059 Retinal neovascularization, unspecified, unspecified eye
√6ᵗʰ **H35.06 Retinal vasculitis**
Eales disease
Retinal perivasculitis
DEF: Sight-threatening intraocular inflammation of the retinal blood vessels that causes minimal, partial, or even complete blindness.
H35.061 Retinal vasculitis, right eye
H35.062 Retinal vasculitis, left eye
H35.063 Retinal vasculitis, bilateral
H35.069 Retinal vasculitis, unspecified eye
√6ᵗʰ **H35.07 Retinal telangiectasis**
H35.071 Retinal telangiectasis, right eye
H35.072 Retinal telangiectasis, left eye
H35.073 Retinal telangiectasis, bilateral
H35.079 Retinal telangiectasis, unspecified eye

H35.09   **Other intraretinal microvascular abnormalities**
Retinal varices

✓5ᵗʰ **H35.1**   **Retinopathy of prematurity**

✓6ᵗʰ **H35.10**   **Retinopathy of prematurity, unspecified**
Retinopathy of prematurity NOS

    H35.101   **Retinopathy of prematurity, unspecified, right eye**

    H35.102   **Retinopathy of prematurity, unspecified, left eye**

    H35.103   **Retinopathy of prematurity, unspecified, bilateral**

    H35.109   **Retinopathy of prematurity, unspecified, unspecified eye**

✓6ᵗʰ **H35.11**   **Retinopathy of prematurity, stage 0**

    H35.111   **Retinopathy of prematurity, stage 0, right eye**

    H35.112   **Retinopathy of prematurity, stage 0, left eye**

    H35.113   **Retinopathy of prematurity, stage 0, bilateral**

    H35.119   **Retinopathy of prematurity, stage 0, unspecified eye**

✓6ᵗʰ **H35.12**   **Retinopathy of prematurity, stage 1**

    H35.121   **Retinopathy of prematurity, stage 1, right eye**

    H35.122   **Retinopathy of prematurity, stage 1, left eye**

    H35.123   **Retinopathy of prematurity, stage 1, bilateral**

    H35.129   **Retinopathy of prematurity, stage 1, unspecified eye**

✓6ᵗʰ **H35.13**   **Retinopathy of prematurity, stage 2**

    H35.131   **Retinopathy of prematurity, stage 2, right eye**

    H35.132   **Retinopathy of prematurity, stage 2, left eye**

    H35.133   **Retinopathy of prematurity, stage 2, bilateral**

    H35.139   **Retinopathy of prematurity, stage 2, unspecified eye**

✓6ᵗʰ **H35.14**   **Retinopathy of prematurity, stage 3**

    H35.141   **Retinopathy of prematurity, stage 3, right eye**

    H35.142   **Retinopathy of prematurity, stage 3, left eye**

    H35.143   **Retinopathy of prematurity, stage 3, bilateral**

    H35.149   **Retinopathy of prematurity, stage 3, unspecified eye**

✓6ᵗʰ **H35.15**   **Retinopathy of prematurity, stage 4**

    H35.151   **Retinopathy of prematurity, stage 4, right eye**

    H35.152   **Retinopathy of prematurity, stage 4, left eye**

    H35.153   **Retinopathy of prematurity, stage 4, bilateral**

    H35.159   **Retinopathy of prematurity, stage 4, unspecified eye**

✓6ᵗʰ **H35.16**   **Retinopathy of prematurity, stage 5**

    H35.161   **Retinopathy of prematurity, stage 5, right eye**

    H35.162   **Retinopathy of prematurity, stage 5, left eye**

    H35.163   **Retinopathy of prematurity, stage 5, bilateral**

    H35.169   **Retinopathy of prematurity, stage 5, unspecified eye**

✓6ᵗʰ **H35.17**   **Retrolental fibroplasia**

    H35.171   **Retrolental fibroplasia, right eye**

    H35.172   **Retrolental fibroplasia, left eye**

    H35.173   **Retrolental fibroplasia, bilateral**

    H35.179   **Retrolental fibroplasia, unspecified eye**

✓6ᵗʰ **H35.2**   **Other non-diabetic proliferative retinopathy**
Proliferative vitreo-retinopathy
  EXCLUDES 1   *proliferative vitreo-retinopathy with retinal detachment (H33.4-)*

    H35.20   **Other non-diabetic proliferative retinopathy, unspecified eye**

    H35.21   **Other non-diabetic proliferative retinopathy, right eye**

H35.22   **Other non-diabetic proliferative retinopathy, left eye**

H35.23   **Other non-diabetic proliferative retinopathy, bilateral**

✓5ᵗʰ **H35.3**   **Degeneration of macula and posterior pole**

    H35.30   **Unspecified macular degeneration**   A
Age-related macular degeneration

✓6ᵗʰ **H35.31**   **Nonexudative age-related macular degeneration**
Atrophic age-related macular degeneration
Dry age-related macular degeneration
AHA: 2016,4Q,20-21

> One of the following 7th characters is to be assigned to each code in subcategory H35.31 to designate the stage of the disease:
> 0   stage unspecified
> 1   early dry stage
> 2   intermediate dry stage
> 3   advanced atrophic without subfoveal involvement
>   advanced dry stage
> 4   advanced atrophic with subfoveal involvement

   ✓7ᵗʰ **H35.311**   **Nonexudative age-related macular degeneration, right eye**   A

   ✓7ᵗʰ **H35.312**   **Nonexudative age-related macular degeneration, left eye**   A

   ✓7ᵗʰ **H35.313**   **Nonexudative age-related macular degeneration, bilateral**   A

   ✓7ᵗʰ **H35.319**   **Nonexudative age-related macular degeneration, unspecified eye**   A

✓6ᵗʰ **H35.32**   **Exudative age-related macular degeneration**
Wet age-related macular degeneration
AHA: 2016,4Q,20-21

> One of the following 7th characters is to be assigned to each code in subcategory H35.32 to designate the stage of the disease:
> 0   stage unspecified
> 1   with active choroidal neovascularization
> 2   with inactive choroidal neovascularization
>   with involuted or regressed neovascularization
> 3   with inactive scar

   ✓7ᵗʰ **H35.321**   **Exudative age-related macular degeneration, right eye**   HCC ESR COM A

   ✓7ᵗʰ **H35.322**   **Exudative age-related macular degeneration, left eye**   HCC ESR COM A

   ✓7ᵗʰ **H35.323**   **Exudative age-related macular degeneration, bilateral**   HCC ESR COM A

   ✓7ᵗʰ **H35.329**   **Exudative age-related macular degeneration, unspecified eye**   HCC ESR COM A

    H35.33   **Angioid streaks of macula**
DEF: Degeneration of the choroid, characterized by broad, irregular, dark brown streaks radiating from the optic disc; occurs with pseudoxanthoma elasticum or Paget's disease.

✓6ᵗʰ **H35.34**   **Macular cyst, hole, or pseudohole**

    H35.341   **Macular cyst, hole, or pseudohole, right eye**

    H35.342   **Macular cyst, hole, or pseudohole, left eye**

    H35.343   **Macular cyst, hole, or pseudohole, bilateral**

    H35.349   **Macular cyst, hole, or pseudohole, unspecified eye**

✓6ᵗʰ **H35.35**   **Cystoid macular degeneration**
  EXCLUDES 1   *cystoid macular edema following cataract surgery (H59.03-)*

    H35.351   **Cystoid macular degeneration, right eye**

    H35.352   **Cystoid macular degeneration, left eye**

    H35.353   **Cystoid macular degeneration, bilateral**

    H35.359   **Cystoid macular degeneration, unspecified eye**

✓6ᵗʰ **H35.36**   **Drusen (degenerative) of macula**
AHA: 2017,1Q,51; 2016,4Q,21

    H35.361   **Drusen (degenerative) of macula, right eye**

    H35.362   **Drusen (degenerative) of macula, left eye**

    H35.363   **Drusen (degenerative) of macula, bilateral**

H35.369 **Drusen (degenerative) of macula, unspecified eye**

√6ᵗʰ H35.37 **Puckering of macula**

H35.371 **Puckering of macula, right eye**
H35.372 **Puckering of macula, left eye**
H35.373 **Puckering of macula, bilateral**
H35.379 **Puckering of macula, unspecified eye**

√6ᵗʰ H35.38 **Toxic maculopathy**

Code first poisoning due to drug or toxin, if applicable (T36-T65 with fifth or sixth character 1-4 or 6)
Use additional code for adverse effect, if applicable, to identify drug (T36-T50 with fifth or sixth character 5)

H35.381 **Toxic maculopathy, right eye**
H35.382 **Toxic maculopathy, left eye**
H35.383 **Toxic maculopathy, bilateral**
H35.389 **Toxic maculopathy, unspecified eye**

√5ᵗʰ H35.4 **Peripheral retinal degeneration**

EXCLUDES 1   *hereditary retinal degeneration (dystrophy) (H35.5-)*
peripheral retinal degeneration with retinal break (H33.3-)

H35.40 **Unspecified peripheral retinal degeneration**

√6ᵗʰ H35.41 **Lattice degeneration of retina**

Palisade degeneration of retina
DEF: Degeneration of the retina, often bilateral, that is usually benign. It is characterized by lines intersecting at irregular intervals in the peripheral retina. Retinal thinning and retinal holes may occur.

H35.411 **Lattice degeneration of retina, right eye**
H35.412 **Lattice degeneration of retina, left eye**
H35.413 **Lattice degeneration of retina, bilateral**
H35.419 **Lattice degeneration of retina, unspecified eye**

√6ᵗʰ H35.42 **Microcystoid degeneration of retina**

H35.421 **Microcystoid degeneration of retina, right eye**
H35.422 **Microcystoid degeneration of retina, left eye**
H35.423 **Microcystoid degeneration of retina, bilateral**
H35.429 **Microcystoid degeneration of retina, unspecified eye**

√6ᵗʰ H35.43 **Paving stone degeneration of retina**

H35.431 **Paving stone degeneration of retina, right eye**
H35.432 **Paving stone degeneration of retina, left eye**
H35.433 **Paving stone degeneration of retina, bilateral**
H35.439 **Paving stone degeneration of retina, unspecified eye**

√6ᵗʰ H35.44 **Age-related reticular degeneration of retina**

H35.441 **Age-related reticular degeneration of retina, right eye**   A
H35.442 **Age-related reticular degeneration of retina, left eye**   A
H35.443 **Age-related reticular degeneration of retina, bilateral**   A
H35.449 **Age-related reticular degeneration of retina, unspecified eye**   A

√6ᵗʰ H35.45 **Secondary pigmentary degeneration**

H35.451 **Secondary pigmentary degeneration, right eye**
H35.452 **Secondary pigmentary degeneration, left eye**
H35.453 **Secondary pigmentary degeneration, bilateral**
H35.459 **Secondary pigmentary degeneration, unspecified eye**

√6ᵗʰ H35.46 **Secondary vitreoretinal degeneration**

H35.461 **Secondary vitreoretinal degeneration, right eye**
H35.462 **Secondary vitreoretinal degeneration, left eye**
H35.463 **Secondary vitreoretinal degeneration, bilateral**
H35.469 **Secondary vitreoretinal degeneration, unspecified eye**

√5ᵗʰ H35.5 **Hereditary retinal dystrophy**

EXCLUDES 1   *dystrophies primarily involving Bruch's membrane (H31.1-)*

H35.50 **Unspecified hereditary retinal dystrophy**
H35.51 **Vitreoretinal dystrophy**
H35.52 **Pigmentary retinal dystrophy**

Albipunctate retinal dystrophy
Retinitis pigmentosa
Tapetoretinal dystrophy

H35.53 **Other dystrophies primarily involving the sensory retina**

Stargardt's disease

H35.54 **Dystrophies primarily involving the retinal pigment epithelium**

Vitelliform retinal dystrophy

√5ᵗʰ H35.6 **Retinal hemorrhage**

H35.60 **Retinal hemorrhage, unspecified eye**
H35.61 **Retinal hemorrhage, right eye**
H35.62 **Retinal hemorrhage, left eye**
H35.63 **Retinal hemorrhage, bilateral**

√5ᵗʰ H35.7 **Separation of retinal layers**

EXCLUDES 1   *retinal detachment (serous) (H33.2-)*
rhegmatogenous retinal detachment (H33.0-)

H35.70 **Unspecified separation of retinal layers**

√6ᵗʰ H35.71 **Central serous chorioretinopathy**

H35.711 **Central serous chorioretinopathy, right eye**
H35.712 **Central serous chorioretinopathy, left eye**
H35.713 **Central serous chorioretinopathy, bilateral**
H35.719 **Central serous chorioretinopathy, unspecified eye**

√6ᵗʰ H35.72 **Serous detachment of retinal pigment epithelium**

H35.721 **Serous detachment of retinal pigment epithelium, right eye**
H35.722 **Serous detachment of retinal pigment epithelium, left eye**
H35.723 **Serous detachment of retinal pigment epithelium, bilateral**
H35.729 **Serous detachment of retinal pigment epithelium, unspecified eye**

√6ᵗʰ H35.73 **Hemorrhagic detachment of retinal pigment epithelium**

H35.731 **Hemorrhagic detachment of retinal pigment epithelium, right eye**
H35.732 **Hemorrhagic detachment of retinal pigment epithelium, left eye**
H35.733 **Hemorrhagic detachment of retinal pigment epithelium, bilateral**
H35.739 **Hemorrhagic detachment of retinal pigment epithelium, unspecified eye**

√5ᵗʰ H35.8 **Other specified retinal disorders**

EXCLUDES 2   *retinal hemorrhage (H35.6-)*

H35.81 **Retinal edema**

Retinal cotton wool spots

H35.82 **Retinal ischemia**
H35.89 **Other specified retinal disorders**

H35.9 **Unspecified retinal disorder**

H36   *Retinal disorders in diseases classified elsewhere*

Code first underlying disease, such as:
lipid storage disorders (E75.-)
sickle-cell disorders (D57.-)

EXCLUDES 1   *arteriosclerotic retinopathy (H35.0-)*
diabetic retinopathy (E08.3-, E09.3-, E10.3-, E11.3-, E13.3-)

Glaucoma (H40-H42)

✓4th **H40 Glaucoma**

EXCLUDES 1   *absolute glaucoma (H44.51-)*
congenital glaucoma (Q15.0)
traumatic glaucoma due to birth injury (P15.3)

Open Angle/Angle Closure Glaucoma

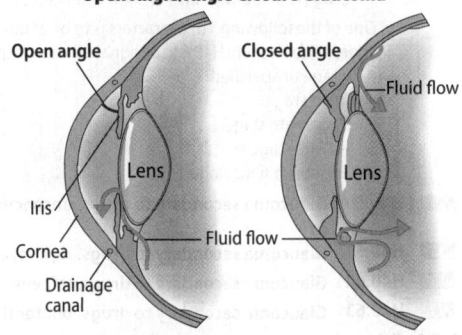

✓5th **H40.0 Glaucoma** suspect

✓6th **H40.00 Preglaucoma, unspecified**

- **H40.001 Preglaucoma, unspecified, right eye**
- **H40.002 Preglaucoma, unspecified, left eye**
- **H40.003 Preglaucoma, unspecified, bilateral**
- **H40.009 Preglaucoma, unspecified, unspecified eye**

✓6th **H40.01 Open angle** with borderline findings, low risk

Open angle, low risk

- **H40.011 Open angle with borderline findings, low risk, right eye**
- **H40.012 Open angle with borderline findings, low risk, left eye**
- **H40.013 Open angle with borderline findings, low risk, bilateral**
- **H40.019 Open angle with borderline findings, low risk, unspecified eye**

✓6th **H40.02 Open angle** with borderline findings, high risk

Open angle, high risk

- **H40.021 Open angle with borderline findings, high risk, right eye**
- **H40.022 Open angle with borderline findings, high risk, left eye**
- **H40.023 Open angle with borderline findings, high risk, bilateral**
- **H40.029 Open angle with borderline findings, high risk, unspecified eye**

✓6th **H40.03 Anatomical narrow** angle

Primary angle closure suspect

- **H40.031 Anatomical narrow angle, right eye**
- **H40.032 Anatomical narrow angle, left eye**
- **H40.033 Anatomical narrow angle, bilateral**
- **H40.039 Anatomical narrow angle, unspecified eye**

✓6th **H40.04 Steroid responder**

- **H40.041 Steroid responder, right eye**
- **H40.042 Steroid responder, left eye**
- **H40.043 Steroid responder, bilateral**
- **H40.049 Steroid responder, unspecified eye**

✓6th **H40.05 Ocular hypertension**

- **H40.051 Ocular hypertension, right eye**
- **H40.052 Ocular hypertension, left eye**
- **H40.053 Ocular hypertension, bilateral**
- **H40.059 Ocular hypertension, unspecified eye**

✓6th **H40.06 Primary angle closure** without glaucoma damage

- **H40.061 Primary angle closure without glaucoma damage, right eye**
- **H40.062 Primary angle closure without glaucoma damage, left eye**
- **H40.063 Primary angle closure without glaucoma damage, bilateral**
- **H40.069 Primary angle closure without glaucoma damage, unspecified eye**

✓5th **H40.1 Open-angle glaucoma**

One of the following 7th characters is to be assigned to each code in subcategories H40.10, H40.11, H40.12, H40.13, and H40.14 to designate the stage of glaucoma.
- 0   stage unspecified
- 1   mild stage
- 2   moderate stage
- 3   severe stage
- 4   indeterminate stage

✓x7th **H40.10 Unspecified open-angle glaucoma**   Rx

TIP: Only one code from this subcategory should be assigned when both left and right eyes are the same stage.

✓6th **H40.11 Primary open-angle glaucoma**

Chronic simple glaucoma
AHA: 2016,4Q,22

- ✓7th **H40.111 Primary open-angle glaucoma, right eye**   Rx Q
- ✓7th **H40.112 Primary open-angle glaucoma, left eye**   Rx Q
- ✓7th **H40.113 Primary open-angle glaucoma, bilateral**   Rx Q
- ✓7th **H40.119 Primary open-angle glaucoma, unspecified eye**   Rx

✓6th **H40.12 Low-tension glaucoma**

- ✓7th **H40.121 Low-tension glaucoma, right eye**   Rx Q
- ✓7th **H40.122 Low-tension glaucoma, left eye**   Rx Q
- ✓7th **H40.123 Low-tension glaucoma, bilateral**   Rx Q
- ✓7th **H40.129 Low-tension glaucoma, unspecified eye**   Rx

✓6th **H40.13 Pigmentary glaucoma**

- ✓7th **H40.131 Pigmentary glaucoma, right eye**   Rx
- ✓7th **H40.132 Pigmentary glaucoma, left eye**   Rx
- ✓7th **H40.133 Pigmentary glaucoma, bilateral**   Rx
- ✓7th **H40.139 Pigmentary glaucoma, unspecified eye**   Rx

✓6th **H40.14 Capsular glaucoma with pseudoexfoliation** of lens

- ✓7th **H40.141 Capsular glaucoma with pseudoexfoliation of lens, right eye**   Rx
- ✓7th **H40.142 Capsular glaucoma with pseudoexfoliation of lens, left eye**   Rx
- ✓7th **H40.143 Capsular glaucoma with pseudoexfoliation of lens, bilateral**   Rx
- ✓7th **H40.149 Capsular glaucoma with pseudoexfoliation of lens, unspecified eye**   Rx

✓6th **H40.15 Residual stage** of open-angle glaucoma

- **H40.151 Residual stage of open-angle glaucoma, right eye**   Rx Q
- **H40.152 Residual stage of open-angle glaucoma, left eye**   Rx Q
- **H40.153 Residual stage of open-angle glaucoma, bilateral**   Rx Q
- **H40.159 Residual stage of open-angle glaucoma, unspecified eye**   Rx

✓5th **H40.2 Primary angle-closure glaucoma**

EXCLUDES 1   *aqueous misdirection (H40.83-)*
malignant glaucoma (H40.83-)

One of the following 7th characters is to be assigned to code H40.20 and H40.22 to designate the stage of glaucoma.
- 0   stage unspecified
- 1   mild stage
- 2   moderate stage
- 3   severe stage
- 4   indeterminate stage

✓x7th **H40.20 Unspecified primary angle-closure glaucoma**   Rx

TIP: Only one code from this subcategory should be assigned when both left and right eyes are the same stage.

✓6th **H40.21 Acute angle-closure glaucoma**

Acute angle-closure glaucoma attack
Acute angle-closure glaucoma crisis

- **H40.211 Acute angle-closure glaucoma, right eye**
- **H40.212 Acute angle-closure glaucoma, left eye**

Chapter 7. Diseases of the Eye and Adnexa

H40.213 Acute angle-closure glaucoma, bilateral
H40.219 Acute angle-closure glaucoma, unspecified eye

✓6ᵗʰ **H40.22** Chronic angle-closure glaucoma
    Chronic primary angle closure glaucoma

✓7ᵗʰ **H40.221** Chronic angle-closure glaucoma, right eye   Rx
✓7ᵗʰ **H40.222** Chronic angle-closure glaucoma, left eye   Rx
✓7ᵗʰ **H40.223** Chronic angle-closure glaucoma, bilateral   Rx
✓7ᵗʰ **H40.229** Chronic angle-closure glaucoma, unspecified eye   Rx

✓6ᵗʰ **H40.23** Intermittent angle-closure glaucoma

H40.231 Intermittent angle-closure glaucoma, right eye   Rx
H40.232 Intermittent angle-closure glaucoma, left eye   Rx
H40.233 Intermittent angle-closure glaucoma, bilateral   Rx
H40.239 Intermittent angle-closure glaucoma, unspecified eye   Rx

✓6ᵗʰ **H40.24** Residual stage of angle-closure glaucoma

H40.241 Residual stage of angle-closure glaucoma, right eye   Rx
H40.242 Residual stage of angle-closure glaucoma, left eye   Rx
H40.243 Residual stage of angle-closure glaucoma, bilateral   Rx
H40.249 Residual stage of angle-closure glaucoma, unspecified eye   Rx

✓5ᵗʰ **H40.3** Glaucoma secondary to eye trauma
    Code also underlying condition

> One of the following 7th characters is to be assigned to each code in subcategory H40.3 to designate the stage of glaucoma.
> 0   stage unspecified
> 1   mild stage
> 2   moderate stage
> 3   severe stage
> 4   indeterminate stage

✓x7ᵗʰ **H40.30** Glaucoma secondary to eye trauma, unspecified eye   Rx
✓x7ᵗʰ **H40.31** Glaucoma secondary to eye trauma, right eye   Rx
✓x7ᵗʰ **H40.32** Glaucoma secondary to eye trauma, left eye   Rx
✓x7ᵗʰ **H40.33** Glaucoma secondary to eye trauma, bilateral   Rx

✓5ᵗʰ **H40.4** Glaucoma secondary to eye inflammation
    Code also underlying condition

> One of the following 7th characters is to be assigned to each code in subcategory H40.4 to designate the stage of glaucoma.
> 0   stage unspecified
> 1   mild stage
> 2   moderate stage
> 3   severe stage
> 4   indeterminate stage

✓x7ᵗʰ **H40.40** Glaucoma secondary to eye inflammation, unspecified eye   Rx
✓x7ᵗʰ **H40.41** Glaucoma secondary to eye inflammation, right eye   Rx
✓x7ᵗʰ **H40.42** Glaucoma secondary to eye inflammation, left eye   Rx
✓x7ᵗʰ **H40.43** Glaucoma secondary to eye inflammation, bilateral   Rx

✓5ᵗʰ **H40.5** Glaucoma secondary to other eye disorders
    Code also underlying eye disorder

> One of the following 7th characters is to be assigned to each code in subcategory H40.5 to designate the stage of glaucoma.
> 0   stage unspecified
> 1   mild stage
> 2   moderate stage
> 3   severe stage
> 4   indeterminate stage

✓x7ᵗʰ **H40.50** Glaucoma secondary to other eye disorders, unspecified eye   Rx

✓x7ᵗʰ **H40.51** Glaucoma secondary to other eye disorders, right eye   Rx
✓x7ᵗʰ **H40.52** Glaucoma secondary to other eye disorders, left eye   Rx
✓x7ᵗʰ **H40.53** Glaucoma secondary to other eye disorders, bilateral   Rx

✓5ᵗʰ **H40.6** Glaucoma secondary to drugs
    Use additional code for adverse effect, if applicable, to identify drug (T36-T50 with fifth or sixth character 5)

> One of the following 7th characters is to be assigned to each code in subcategory H40.6 to designate the stage of glaucoma
> 0   stage unspecified
> 1   mild stage
> 2   moderate stage
> 3   severe stage
> 4   indeterminate stage

✓x7ᵗʰ **H40.60** Glaucoma secondary to drugs, unspecified eye   Rx
✓x7ᵗʰ **H40.61** Glaucoma secondary to drugs, right eye   Rx
✓x7ᵗʰ **H40.62** Glaucoma secondary to drugs, left eye   Rx
✓x7ᵗʰ **H40.63** Glaucoma secondary to drugs, bilateral   Rx

✓5ᵗʰ **H40.8** Other glaucoma

✓6ᵗʰ **H40.81** Glaucoma with increased episcleral venous pressure

H40.811 Glaucoma with increased episcleral venous pressure, right eye   Rx
H40.812 Glaucoma with increased episcleral venous pressure, left eye   Rx
H40.813 Glaucoma with increased episcleral venous pressure, bilateral   Rx
H40.819 Glaucoma with increased episcleral venous pressure, unspecified eye   Rx

✓6ᵗʰ **H40.82** Hypersecretion glaucoma

H40.821 Hypersecretion glaucoma, right eye   Rx
H40.822 Hypersecretion glaucoma, left eye   Rx
H40.823 Hypersecretion glaucoma, bilateral   Rx
H40.829 Hypersecretion glaucoma, unspecified eye   Rx

✓6ᵗʰ **H40.83** Aqueous misdirection
    Malignant glaucoma

H40.831 Aqueous misdirection, right eye   Rx
H40.832 Aqueous misdirection, left eye   Rx
H40.833 Aqueous misdirection, bilateral   Rx
H40.839 Aqueous misdirection, unspecified eye   Rx

H40.89 Other specified glaucoma   Rx

H40.9 Unspecified glaucoma   Rx

H42 *Glaucoma in diseases classified elsewhere*   Rx
    Code first underlying condition, such as:
      amyloidosis (E85.-)
      aniridia (Q13.1)
      glaucoma (in) diabetes mellitus (E08.39, E09.39, E10.39, E11.39, E13.39)
      Lowe's syndrome (E72.03)
      Reiger's anomaly (Q13.81)
      specified metabolic disorder (E70-E88)
    EXCLUDES 1   *glaucoma (in) onchocerciasis (B73.02)*
               glaucoma (in) syphilis (A52.71)
               glaucoma (in) tuberculous (A18.59)

Disorders of vitreous body and globe (H43-H44)

✓4ᵗʰ **H43** Disorders of vitreous body

✓5ᵗʰ **H43.0** Vitreous prolapse
    EXCLUDES 1   *traumatic vitreous prolapse (S05.2-)*
               vitreous syndrome following cataract surgery (H59.0-)

H43.00 Vitreous prolapse, unspecified eye
H43.01 Vitreous prolapse, right eye
H43.02 Vitreous prolapse, left eye
H43.03 Vitreous prolapse, bilateral

✓5ᵗʰ **H43.1** Vitreous hemorrhage

H43.10 Vitreous hemorrhage, unspecified eye   HCC ESR
H43.11 Vitreous hemorrhage, right eye   HCC ESR
H43.12 Vitreous hemorrhage, left eye   HCC ESR

H43.13   **Vitreous hemorrhage,** bilateral   `HCC` `ESR`

✓5ᵗʰ **H43.2   Crystalline deposits** in vitreous body

     H43.20   **Crystalline deposits in vitreous body, unspecified eye**

     H43.21   **Crystalline deposits in vitreous body, right eye**

     H43.22   **Crystalline deposits in vitreous body, left eye**

     H43.23   **Crystalline deposits in vitreous body, bilateral**

✓5ᵗʰ **H43.3   Other vitreous opacities**

   ✓6ᵗʰ **H43.31   Vitreous** membranes and strands

     H43.311   **Vitreous membranes and strands,** right eye

     H43.312   **Vitreous membranes and strands,** left eye

     H43.313   **Vitreous membranes and strands, bilateral**

     H43.319   **Vitreous membranes and strands, unspecified eye**

   ✓6ᵗʰ **H43.39   Other vitreous opacities**

     Vitreous floaters

     H43.391   **Other vitreous opacities, right eye**

     H43.392   **Other vitreous opacities, left eye**

     H43.393   **Other vitreous opacities, bilateral**

     H43.399   **Other vitreous opacities, unspecified eye**

✓5ᵗʰ **H43.8   Other disorders of vitreous body**

   `EXCLUDES 1`   *proliferative vitreo-retinopathy with retinal detachment (H33.4-)*

   `EXCLUDES 2`   *vitreous abscess (H44.02-)*

   ✓6ᵗʰ **H43.81   Vitreous** degeneration

     Vitreous detachment

     H43.811   **Vitreous degeneration,** right eye

     H43.812   **Vitreous degeneration,** left eye

     H43.813   **Vitreous degeneration, bilateral**

     H43.819   **Vitreous degeneration, unspecified eye**

   ✓6ᵗʰ **H43.82   Vitreomacular** adhesion

     Vitreomacular traction

     H43.821   **Vitreomacular adhesion,** right eye   `A`

     H43.822   **Vitreomacular adhesion,** left eye   `A`

     H43.823   **Vitreomacular adhesion, bilateral**   `A`

     H43.829   **Vitreomacular adhesion, unspecified eye**   `A`

     H43.89   **Other disorders of vitreous body**

  H43.9   **Unspecified disorder of vitreous body**

✓4ᵗʰ **H44   Disorders of globe**

   `INCLUDES`   disorders affecting multiple structures of eye

✓5ᵗʰ **H44.0   Purulent endophthalmitis**

     Use additional code to identify organism

   `EXCLUDES 1`   *bleb associated endophthalmitis (H59.4-)*

   ✓6ᵗʰ **H44.00   Unspecified purulent endophthalmitis**

     H44.001   **Unspecified purulent endophthalmitis, right eye**

     H44.002   **Unspecified purulent endophthalmitis, left eye**

     H44.003   **Unspecified purulent endophthalmitis, bilateral**

     H44.009   **Unspecified purulent endophthalmitis, unspecified eye**

   ✓6ᵗʰ **H44.01   Panophthalmitis (acute)**

     H44.011   **Panophthalmitis (acute),** right eye

     H44.012   **Panophthalmitis (acute),** left eye

     H44.013   **Panophthalmitis (acute), bilateral**

     H44.019   **Panophthalmitis (acute), unspecified eye**

   ✓6ᵗʰ **H44.02   Vitreous abscess (chronic)**

     H44.021   **Vitreous abscess (chronic),** right eye

     H44.022   **Vitreous abscess (chronic),** left eye

     H44.023   **Vitreous abscess (chronic), bilateral**

     H44.029   **Vitreous abscess (chronic), unspecified eye**

✓5ᵗʰ **H44.1   Other endophthalmitis**

   `EXCLUDES 1`   *bleb associated endophthalmitis (H59.4-)*

   `EXCLUDES 2`   *ophthalmia nodosa (H16.2-)*

   ✓6ᵗʰ **H44.11   Panuveitis**

     DEF: Inflammation of all layers of the uvea of the eye, including the choroid, iris, and ciliary body. It also typically involves the lens, retina, optic nerve, and vitreous and causes reduced vision or blindness.

     H44.111   **Panuveitis,** right eye

     H44.112   **Panuveitis,** left eye

     H44.113   **Panuveitis,** bilateral

     H44.119   **Panuveitis, unspecified eye**

   ✓6ᵗʰ **H44.12   Parasitic endophthalmitis, unspecified**

     H44.121   **Parasitic endophthalmitis, unspecified, right eye**

     H44.122   **Parasitic endophthalmitis, unspecified, left eye**

     H44.123   **Parasitic endophthalmitis, unspecified, bilateral**

     H44.129   **Parasitic endophthalmitis, unspecified, unspecified eye**

   ✓6ᵗʰ **H44.13   Sympathetic uveitis**

     H44.131   **Sympathetic uveitis,** right eye

     H44.132   **Sympathetic uveitis,** left eye

     H44.133   **Sympathetic uveitis,** bilateral

     H44.139   **Sympathetic uveitis, unspecified eye**

     H44.19   **Other endophthalmitis**

✓5ᵗʰ **H44.2   Degenerative myopia**

     Malignant myopia

     AHA: 2017,4Q,10-11

     H44.20   **Degenerative myopia, unspecified eye**

     H44.21   **Degenerative myopia, right eye**

     H44.22   **Degenerative myopia, left eye**

     H44.23   **Degenerative myopia, bilateral**

   ✓6ᵗʰ **H44.2A   Degenerative myopia with** choroidal neovascularization

     Use additional code for any associated choroid disorders (H31.-)

     H44.2A1   **Degenerative myopia with choroidal neovascularization,** right eye

     H44.2A2   **Degenerative myopia with choroidal neovascularization,** left eye

     H44.2A3   **Degenerative myopia with choroidal neovascularization, bilateral eye**

     H44.2A9   **Degenerative myopia with choroidal neovascularization, unspecified eye**

   ✓6ᵗʰ **H44.2B   Degenerative myopia** with macular hole

     H44.2B1   **Degenerative myopia with macular hole, right eye**

     H44.2B2   **Degenerative myopia with macular hole, left eye**

     H44.2B3   **Degenerative myopia with macular hole, bilateral eye**

     H44.2B9   **Degenerative myopia with macular hole, unspecified eye**

   ✓6ᵗʰ **H44.2C   Degenerative myopia** with retinal detachment

     Use additional code to identify the retinal detachment (H33.-)

     H44.2C1   **Degenerative myopia with retinal detachment,** right eye

     H44.2C2   **Degenerative myopia with retinal detachment,** left eye

     H44.2C3   **Degenerative myopia with retinal detachment, bilateral eye**

     H44.2C9   **Degenerative myopia with retinal detachment, unspecified eye**

   ✓6ᵗʰ **H44.2D   Degenerative myopia** with foveoschisis

     H44.2D1   **Degenerative myopia with foveoschisis, right eye**

     H44.2D2   **Degenerative myopia with foveoschisis, left eye**

     H44.2D3   **Degenerative myopia with foveoschisis, bilateral eye**

     H44.2D9   **Degenerative myopia with foveoschisis, unspecified eye**

   ✓6ᵗʰ **H44.2E   Degenerative myopia with other maculopathy**

     H44.2E1   **Degenerative myopia with other maculopathy,** right eye

     H44.2E2   **Degenerative myopia with other maculopathy,** left eye

     H44.2E3   **Degenerative myopia with other maculopathy,** bilateral eye

     H44.2E9   **Degenerative myopia with other maculopathy, unspecified eye**

✓5ᵗʰ **H44.3   Other and unspecified degenerative disorders of globe**

     H44.30   **Unspecified degenerative disorder of globe**

   ✓6ᵗʰ **H44.31   Chalcosis**

     H44.311   **Chalcosis,** right eye

     H44.312   **Chalcosis,** left eye

Chapter 7. Diseases of the Eye and Adnexa

H44.313 Chalcosis, bilateral
H44.319 Chalcosis, unspecified eye

✓6ᵗʰ **H44.32** Siderosis of eye
> **DEF:** Iron pigment deposits within tissue of the eyeball caused by high iron content of the blood. Symptoms include cataracts, rust-colored anterior subcapsular deposits, iris heterochromia, pupillary mydriasis, and depressed electroretinogram amplitudes.

H44.321 Siderosis of eye, right eye
H44.322 Siderosis of eye, left eye
H44.323 Siderosis of eye, bilateral
H44.329 Siderosis of eye, unspecified eye

✓6ᵗʰ **H44.39** Other degenerative disorders of globe
H44.391 Other degenerative disorders of globe, right eye
H44.392 Other degenerative disorders of globe, left eye
H44.393 Other degenerative disorders of globe, bilateral
H44.399 Other degenerative disorders of globe, unspecified eye

✓5ᵗʰ **H44.4** Hypotony of eye
H44.40 Unspecified hypotony of eye

✓6ᵗʰ **H44.41** Flat anterior chamber hypotony of eye
H44.411 Flat anterior chamber hypotony of right eye
H44.412 Flat anterior chamber hypotony of left eye
H44.413 Flat anterior chamber hypotony of eye, bilateral
H44.419 Flat anterior chamber hypotony of unspecified eye

✓6ᵗʰ **H44.42** Hypotony of eye due to ocular fistula
H44.421 Hypotony of right eye due to ocular fistula
H44.422 Hypotony of left eye due to ocular fistula
H44.423 Hypotony of eye due to ocular fistula, bilateral
H44.429 Hypotony of unspecified eye due to ocular fistula

✓6ᵗʰ **H44.43** Hypotony of eye due to other ocular disorders
H44.431 Hypotony of eye due to other ocular disorders, right eye
H44.432 Hypotony of eye due to other ocular disorders, left eye
H44.433 Hypotony of eye due to other ocular disorders, bilateral
H44.439 Hypotony of eye due to other ocular disorders, unspecified eye

✓6ᵗʰ **H44.44** Primary hypotony of eye
H44.441 Primary hypotony of right eye
H44.442 Primary hypotony of left eye
H44.443 Primary hypotony of eye, bilateral
H44.449 Primary hypotony of unspecified eye

✓5ᵗʰ **H44.5** Degenerated conditions of globe
H44.50 Unspecified degenerated conditions of globe

✓6ᵗʰ **H44.51** Absolute glaucoma
H44.511 Absolute glaucoma, right eye
H44.512 Absolute glaucoma, left eye
H44.513 Absolute glaucoma, bilateral
H44.519 Absolute glaucoma, unspecified eye

✓6ᵗʰ **H44.52** Atrophy of globe
> Phthisis bulbi

H44.521 Atrophy of globe, right eye
H44.522 Atrophy of globe, left eye
H44.523 Atrophy of globe, bilateral
H44.529 Atrophy of globe, unspecified eye

✓6ᵗʰ **H44.53** Leucocoria
H44.531 Leucocoria, right eye
H44.532 Leucocoria, left eye
H44.533 Leucocoria, bilateral
H44.539 Leucocoria, unspecified eye

✓5ᵗʰ **H44.6** Retained (old) intraocular foreign body, magnetic
> Use additional code to identify magnetic foreign body (Z18.11)
> *EXCLUDES 1* current intraocular foreign body (S05.-)
> *EXCLUDES 2* retained foreign body in eyelid (H02.81-)
> retained (old) foreign body following penetrating wound of orbit (H05.5-)
> retained (old) intraocular foreign body, nonmagnetic (H44.7-)

✓6ᵗʰ **H44.60** Unspecified retained (old) intraocular foreign body, magnetic
H44.601 Unspecified retained (old) intraocular foreign body, magnetic, right eye
H44.602 Unspecified retained (old) intraocular foreign body, magnetic, left eye
H44.603 Unspecified retained (old) intraocular foreign body, magnetic, bilateral
H44.609 Unspecified retained (old) intraocular foreign body, magnetic, unspecified eye

✓6ᵗʰ **H44.61** Retained (old) magnetic foreign body in anterior chamber
H44.611 Retained (old) magnetic foreign body in anterior chamber, right eye
H44.612 Retained (old) magnetic foreign body in anterior chamber, left eye
H44.613 Retained (old) magnetic foreign body in anterior chamber, bilateral
H44.619 Retained (old) magnetic foreign body in anterior chamber, unspecified eye

✓6ᵗʰ **H44.62** Retained (old) magnetic foreign body in iris or ciliary body
H44.621 Retained (old) magnetic foreign body in iris or ciliary body, right eye
H44.622 Retained (old) magnetic foreign body in iris or ciliary body, left eye
H44.623 Retained (old) magnetic foreign body in iris or ciliary body, bilateral
H44.629 Retained (old) magnetic foreign body in iris or ciliary body, unspecified eye

✓6ᵗʰ **H44.63** Retained (old) magnetic foreign body in lens
H44.631 Retained (old) magnetic foreign body in lens, right eye
H44.632 Retained (old) magnetic foreign body in lens, left eye
H44.633 Retained (old) magnetic foreign body in lens, bilateral
H44.639 Retained (old) magnetic foreign body in lens, unspecified eye

✓6ᵗʰ **H44.64** Retained (old) magnetic foreign body in posterior wall of globe
H44.641 Retained (old) magnetic foreign body in posterior wall of globe, right eye
H44.642 Retained (old) magnetic foreign body in posterior wall of globe, left eye
H44.643 Retained (old) magnetic foreign body in posterior wall of globe, bilateral
H44.649 Retained (old) magnetic foreign body in posterior wall of globe, unspecified eye

✓6ᵗʰ **H44.65** Retained (old) magnetic foreign body in vitreous body
H44.651 Retained (old) magnetic foreign body in vitreous body, right eye
H44.652 Retained (old) magnetic foreign body in vitreous body, left eye
H44.653 Retained (old) magnetic foreign body in vitreous body, bilateral
H44.659 Retained (old) magnetic foreign body in vitreous body, unspecified eye

✓6ᵗʰ **H44.69** Retained (old) intraocular foreign body, magnetic, in other or multiple sites
H44.691 Retained (old) intraocular foreign body, magnetic, in other or multiple sites, right eye
H44.692 Retained (old) intraocular foreign body, magnetic, in other or multiple sites, left eye
H44.693 Retained (old) intraocular foreign body, magnetic, in other or multiple sites, bilateral
H44.699 Retained (old) intraocular foreign body, magnetic, in other or multiple sites, unspecified eye

✓5ᵗʰ **H44.7 Retained (old) intraocular foreign body, nonmagnetic**
Use additional code to identify nonmagnetic foreign body (Z18.01-Z18.10, Z18.12, Z18.2-Z18.9)

EXCLUDES 1   *current intraocular foreign body (S05.-)*
EXCLUDES 2   *retained foreign body in eyelid (H02.81-)*
retained foreign body following penetrating wound of orbit (H05.5-)
retained (old) intraocular foreign body, magnetic (H44.6-)

✓6ᵗʰ **H44.70 Unspecified retained (old) intraocular foreign body, nonmagnetic**

- **H44.701** Unspecified retained (old) intraocular foreign body, nonmagnetic, right eye
- **H44.702** Unspecified retained (old) intraocular foreign body, nonmagnetic, left eye
- **H44.703** Unspecified retained (old) intraocular foreign body, nonmagnetic, bilateral
- **H44.709** Unspecified retained (old) intraocular foreign body, nonmagnetic, unspecified eye
  - Retained (old) intraocular foreign body NOS

✓6ᵗʰ **H44.71 Retained (nonmagnetic) (old) foreign body in anterior chamber**

- **H44.711** Retained (nonmagnetic) (old) foreign body in anterior chamber, right eye
- **H44.712** Retained (nonmagnetic) (old) foreign body in anterior chamber, left eye
- **H44.713** Retained (nonmagnetic) (old) foreign body in anterior chamber, bilateral
- **H44.719** Retained (nonmagnetic) (old) foreign body in anterior chamber, unspecified eye

✓6ᵗʰ **H44.72 Retained (nonmagnetic) (old) foreign body in iris or ciliary body**

- **H44.721** Retained (nonmagnetic) (old) foreign body in iris or ciliary body, right eye
- **H44.722** Retained (nonmagnetic) (old) foreign body in iris or ciliary body, left eye
- **H44.723** Retained (nonmagnetic) (old) foreign body in iris or ciliary body, bilateral
- **H44.729** Retained (nonmagnetic) (old) foreign body in iris or ciliary body, unspecified eye

✓6ᵗʰ **H44.73 Retained (nonmagnetic) (old) foreign body in lens**

- **H44.731** Retained (nonmagnetic) (old) foreign body in lens, right eye
- **H44.732** Retained (nonmagnetic) (old) foreign body in lens, left eye
- **H44.733** Retained (nonmagnetic) (old) foreign body in lens, bilateral
- **H44.739** Retained (nonmagnetic) (old) foreign body in lens, unspecified eye

✓6ᵗʰ **H44.74 Retained (nonmagnetic) (old) foreign body in posterior wall of globe**

- **H44.741** Retained (nonmagnetic) (old) foreign body in posterior wall of globe, right eye
- **H44.742** Retained (nonmagnetic) (old) foreign body in posterior wall of globe, left eye
- **H44.743** Retained (nonmagnetic) (old) foreign body in posterior wall of globe, bilateral
- **H44.749** Retained (nonmagnetic) (old) foreign body in posterior wall of globe, unspecified eye

✓6ᵗʰ **H44.75 Retained (nonmagnetic) (old) foreign body in vitreous body**

- **H44.751** Retained (nonmagnetic) (old) foreign body in vitreous body, right eye
- **H44.752** Retained (nonmagnetic) (old) foreign body in vitreous body, left eye
- **H44.753** Retained (nonmagnetic) (old) foreign body in vitreous body, bilateral
- **H44.759** Retained (nonmagnetic) (old) foreign body in vitreous body, unspecified eye

✓6ᵗʰ **H44.79 Retained (old) intraocular foreign body, nonmagnetic, in other or multiple sites**

- **H44.791** Retained (old) intraocular foreign body, nonmagnetic, in other or multiple sites, right eye
- **H44.792** Retained (old) intraocular foreign body, nonmagnetic, in other or multiple sites, left eye
- **H44.793** Retained (old) intraocular foreign body, nonmagnetic, in other or multiple sites, bilateral
- **H44.799** Retained (old) intraocular foreign body, nonmagnetic, in other or multiple sites, unspecified eye

✓5ᵗʰ **H44.8 Other disorders of globe**

✓6ᵗʰ **H44.81 Hemophthalmos**
DEF: Pool of blood within the eyeball, not from a current injury.
- **H44.811** Hemophthalmos, right eye
- **H44.812** Hemophthalmos, left eye
- **H44.813** Hemophthalmos, bilateral
- **H44.819** Hemophthalmos, unspecified eye

✓6ᵗʰ **H44.82 Luxation of globe**
- **H44.821** Luxation of globe, right eye
- **H44.822** Luxation of globe, left eye
- **H44.823** Luxation of globe, bilateral
- **H44.829** Luxation of globe, unspecified eye

H44.89 Other disorders of globe
AHA: 2022,1Q,33

H44.9 Unspecified disorder of globe

Disorders of optic nerve and visual pathways (H46-H47)

✓4ᵗʰ **H46 Optic neuritis**
EXCLUDES 2   *ischemic optic neuropathy (H47.01-)*
neuromyelitis optica [Devic] (G36.0)

✓5ᵗʰ **H46.0 Optic papillitis**
- **H46.00** Optic papillitis, unspecified eye
- **H46.01** Optic papillitis, right eye
- **H46.02** Optic papillitis, left eye
- **H46.03** Optic papillitis, bilateral

✓5ᵗʰ **H46.1 Retrobulbar neuritis**
Retrobulbar neuritis NOS
EXCLUDES 1   *syphilitic retrobulbar neuritis (A52.15)*
- **H46.10** Retrobulbar neuritis, unspecified eye
- **H46.11** Retrobulbar neuritis, right eye
- **H46.12** Retrobulbar neuritis, left eye
- **H46.13** Retrobulbar neuritis, bilateral

H46.2 Nutritional optic neuropathy

H46.3 Toxic optic neuropathy
Code first (T51-T65) to identify cause

H46.8 Other optic neuritis

H46.9 Unspecified optic neuritis

✓4ᵗʰ **H47 Other disorders of optic [2nd] nerve and visual pathways**

✓5ᵗʰ **H47.0 Disorders of optic nerve, not elsewhere classified**

✓6ᵗʰ **H47.01 Ischemic optic neuropathy**
- **H47.011** Ischemic optic neuropathy, right eye
- **H47.012** Ischemic optic neuropathy, left eye
- **H47.013** Ischemic optic neuropathy, bilateral
- **H47.019** Ischemic optic neuropathy, unspecified eye

✓6ᵗʰ **H47.02 Hemorrhage in optic nerve sheath**
- **H47.021** Hemorrhage in optic nerve sheath, right eye
- **H47.022** Hemorrhage in optic nerve sheath, left eye
- **H47.023** Hemorrhage in optic nerve sheath, bilateral
- **H47.029** Hemorrhage in optic nerve sheath, unspecified eye

✓6ᵗʰ **H47.03 Optic nerve hypoplasia**
- **H47.031** Optic nerve hypoplasia, right eye
- **H47.032** Optic nerve hypoplasia, left eye
- **H47.033** Optic nerve hypoplasia, bilateral
- **H47.039** Optic nerve hypoplasia, unspecified eye

✓6ᵗʰ **H47.09 Other disorders of optic nerve, not elsewhere classified**
Compression of optic nerve
- **H47.091** Other disorders of optic nerve, not elsewhere classified, right eye
- **H47.092** Other disorders of optic nerve, not elsewhere classified, left eye
- **H47.093** Other disorders of optic nerve, not elsewhere classified, bilateral

H47.Ø99 **Other disorders of optic nerve, not elsewhere classified, unspecified eye**

✓5ᵗʰ **H47.1 Papilledema**

> **DEF:** Swelling of the optic papilla, the raised area connected to the optic disk made up of nerves that enter the eyeball. It may be caused by increased intracranial pressure, decreased ocular pressure, or a retinal disorder.

H47.1Ø **Unspecified papilledema**

H47.11 **Papilledema associated with** increased intracranial pressure

H47.12 **Papilledema associated with** decreased ocular pressure

H47.13 **Papilledema associated with** retinal disorder

✓6ᵗʰ H47.14 **Foster-Kennedy syndrome**

H47.141 **Foster-Kennedy syndrome,** right eye

H47.142 **Foster-Kennedy syndrome,** left eye

H47.143 **Foster-Kennedy syndrome,** bilateral

H47.149 **Foster-Kennedy syndrome, unspecified eye**

✓5ᵗʰ **H47.2 Optic atrophy**

H47.2Ø **Unspecified optic atrophy**

✓6ᵗʰ H47.21 **Primary** optic atrophy

H47.211 **Primary optic atrophy,** right eye

H47.212 **Primary optic atrophy,** left eye

H47.213 **Primary optic atrophy,** bilateral

H47.219 **Primary optic atrophy, unspecified eye**

H47.22 **Hereditary** optic atrophy

> Leber's optic atrophy

✓6ᵗʰ H47.23 **Glaucomatous** optic atrophy

H47.231 **Glaucomatous optic atrophy,** right eye

H47.232 **Glaucomatous optic atrophy,** left eye

H47.233 **Glaucomatous optic atrophy,** bilateral

H47.239 **Glaucomatous optic atrophy, unspecified eye**

✓6ᵗʰ H47.29 **Other optic atrophy**

> Temporal pallor of optic disc

H47.291 **Other optic atrophy,** right eye

H47.292 **Other optic atrophy,** left eye

H47.293 **Other optic atrophy,** bilateral

H47.299 **Other optic atrophy, unspecified eye**

✓5ᵗʰ **H47.3 Other disorders of optic disc**

✓6ᵗʰ H47.31 **Coloboma** of optic disc

H47.311 **Coloboma of optic disc,** right eye

H47.312 **Coloboma of optic disc,** left eye

H47.313 **Coloboma of optic disc,** bilateral

H47.319 **Coloboma of optic disc, unspecified eye**

✓6ᵗʰ H47.32 **Drusen** of optic disc

H47.321 **Drusen of optic disc,** right eye

H47.322 **Drusen of optic disc,** left eye

H47.323 **Drusen of optic disc,** bilateral

H47.329 **Drusen of optic disc, unspecified eye**

✓6ᵗʰ H47.33 **Pseudopapilledema** of optic disc

H47.331 **Pseudopapilledema of optic disc,** right eye

H47.332 **Pseudopapilledema of optic disc,** left eye

H47.333 **Pseudopapilledema of optic disc,** bilateral

H47.339 **Pseudopapilledema of optic disc, unspecified eye**

✓6ᵗʰ H47.39 **Other disorders of optic disc**

H47.391 **Other disorders of optic disc,** right eye

H47.392 **Other disorders of optic disc,** left eye

H47.393 **Other disorders of optic disc,** bilateral

H47.399 **Other disorders of optic disc, unspecified eye**

✓5ᵗʰ **H47.4 Disorders of optic chiasm**

> Code also underlying condition

H47.41 **Disorders of optic chiasm in (due to)** inflammatory disorders

H47.42 **Disorders of optic chiasm in (due to)** neoplasm

H47.43 **Disorders of optic chiasm in (due to)** vascular disorders

H47.49 **Disorders of optic chiasm in (due to) other disorders**

✓5ᵗʰ **H47.5 Disorders of other visual pathways**

> Disorders of optic tracts, geniculate nuclei and optic radiations
> Code also underlying condition

✓6ᵗʰ H47.51 **Disorders of visual pathways in (due to)** inflammatory disorders

H47.511 **Disorders of visual pathways in (due to) inflammatory disorders,** right side

H47.512 **Disorders of visual pathways in (due to) inflammatory disorders,** left side

H47.519 **Disorders of visual pathways in (due to) inflammatory disorders, unspecified side**

✓6ᵗʰ H47.52 **Disorders of visual pathways in (due to)** neoplasm

H47.521 **Disorders of visual pathways in (due to) neoplasm,** right side

H47.522 **Disorders of visual pathways in (due to) neoplasm,** left side

H47.529 **Disorders of visual pathways in (due to) neoplasm, unspecified side**

✓6ᵗʰ H47.53 **Disorders of visual pathways in (due to)** vascular disorders

H47.531 **Disorders of visual pathways in (due to) vascular disorders,** right side

H47.532 **Disorders of visual pathways in (due to) vascular disorders,** left side

H47.539 **Disorders of visual pathways in (due to) vascular disorders, unspecified side**

✓5ᵗʰ **H47.6 Disorders of visual cortex**

> Code also underlying condition
>
> EXCLUDES 1   injury to visual cortex SØ4.Ø4-

✓6ᵗʰ H47.61 **Cortical blindness**

H47.611 **Cortical blindness,** right side of brain

H47.612 **Cortical blindness,** left side of brain

H47.619 **Cortical blindness, unspecified side of brain**

✓6ᵗʰ H47.62 **Disorders of visual cortex in (due to)** inflammatory disorders

H47.621 **Disorders of visual cortex in (due to) inflammatory disorders,** right side of brain

H47.622 **Disorders of visual cortex in (due to) inflammatory disorders,** left side of brain

H47.629 **Disorders of visual cortex in (due to) inflammatory disorders, unspecified side of brain**

✓6ᵗʰ H47.63 **Disorders of visual cortex in (due to)** neoplasm

H47.631 **Disorders of visual cortex in (due to) neoplasm,** right side of brain

H47.632 **Disorders of visual cortex in (due to) neoplasm,** left side of brain

H47.639 **Disorders of visual cortex in (due to) neoplasm, unspecified side of brain**

✓6ᵗʰ H47.64 **Disorders of visual cortex in (due to)** vascular disorders

H47.641 **Disorders of visual cortex in (due to) vascular disorders,** right side of brain

H47.642 **Disorders of visual cortex in (due to) vascular disorders,** left side of brain

H47.649 **Disorders of visual cortex in (due to) vascular disorders, unspecified side of brain**

H47.9 **Unspecified disorder of visual pathways**

Disorders of ocular muscles, binocular movement, accommodation and refraction (H49-H52)

> EXCLUDES 2   nystagmus and other irregular eye movements (H55)

✓4ᵗʰ **H49 Paralytic strabismus**

> EXCLUDES 2   internal ophthalmoplegia (H52.51-)
> internuclear ophthalmoplegia (H51.2-)
> progressive supranuclear ophthalmoplegia (G23.1)
>
> **DEF:** Strabismus: Misalignment of the eyes with the inability to move and focus in the same direction due to conditions affecting the muscles controlling them.

✓5ᵗʰ **H49.Ø Third [oculomotor] nerve palsy**

H49.ØØ **Third [oculomotor] nerve palsy, unspecified eye**

H49.Ø1 **Third [oculomotor] nerve palsy,** right eye

H49.Ø2 **Third [oculomotor] nerve palsy,** left eye

H49.Ø3 **Third [oculomotor] nerve palsy,** bilateral

✓5ᵗʰ **H49.1 Fourth [trochlear] nerve palsy**

H49.1Ø **Fourth [trochlear] nerve palsy, unspecified eye**

H49.11   Fourth [trochlear] nerve palsy, right eye
H49.12   Fourth [trochlear] nerve palsy, left eye
H49.13   Fourth [trochlear] nerve palsy, bilateral

√5ᵗʰ H49.2   Sixth [abducent] nerve palsy
H49.20   Sixth [abducent] nerve palsy, unspecified eye
H49.21   Sixth [abducent] nerve palsy, right eye
H49.22   Sixth [abducent] nerve palsy, left eye
H49.23   Sixth [abducent] nerve palsy, bilateral

√5ᵗʰ H49.3   Total (external) ophthalmoplegia
H49.30   Total (external) ophthalmoplegia, unspecified eye
H49.31   Total (external) ophthalmoplegia, right eye
H49.32   Total (external) ophthalmoplegia, left eye
H49.33   Total (external) ophthalmoplegia, bilateral

√5ᵗʰ H49.4   Progressive external ophthalmoplegia
     EXCLUDES 1   Kearns-Sayre syndrome (H49.81-)
H49.40   Progressive external ophthalmoplegia, unspecified eye
H49.41   Progressive external ophthalmoplegia, right eye
H49.42   Progressive external ophthalmoplegia, left eye
H49.43   Progressive external ophthalmoplegia, bilateral

√5ᵗʰ H49.8   Other paralytic strabismus
  √6ᵗʰ H49.81   Kearns-Sayre syndrome
     Progressive external ophthalmoplegia with pigmentary retinopathy
     Use additional code for other manifestation, such as: heart block (I45.9)
     H49.811   Kearns-Sayre syndrome, right eye   HCC Rx ESR COM
     H49.812   Kearns-Sayre syndrome, left eye   HCC Rx ESR COM
     H49.813   Kearns-Sayre syndrome, bilateral   HCC Rx ESR COM
     H49.819   Kearns-Sayre syndrome, unspecified eye   HCC Rx ESR COM
  √6ᵗʰ H49.88   Other paralytic strabismus
     External ophthalmoplegia NOS
     H49.881   Other paralytic strabismus, right eye
     H49.882   Other paralytic strabismus, left eye
     H49.883   Other paralytic strabismus, bilateral
     H49.889   Other paralytic strabismus, unspecified eye

H49.9   Unspecified paralytic strabismus

√4ᵗʰ H50   Other strabismus
     DEF: Strabismus: Misalignment of the eyes with the inability to move and focus in the same direction due to conditions affecting the muscles controlling them.

√5ᵗʰ H50.0   Esotropia
     Convergent concomitant strabismus
     EXCLUDES 1   intermittent esotropia (H50.31-, H50.32)
     H50.00   Unspecified esotropia
  √6ᵗʰ H50.01   Monocular esotropia
     H50.011   Monocular esotropia, right eye
     H50.012   Monocular esotropia, left eye
  √6ᵗʰ H50.02   Monocular esotropia with A pattern
     H50.021   Monocular esotropia with A pattern, right eye
     H50.022   Monocular esotropia with A pattern, left eye
  √6ᵗʰ H50.03   Monocular esotropia with V pattern
     H50.031   Monocular esotropia with V pattern, right eye
     H50.032   Monocular esotropia with V pattern, left eye
  √6ᵗʰ H50.04   Monocular esotropia with other noncomitancies
     H50.041   Monocular esotropia with other noncomitancies, right eye
     H50.042   Monocular esotropia with other noncomitancies, left eye
     H50.05   Alternating esotropia
     H50.06   Alternating esotropia with A pattern
     H50.07   Alternating esotropia with V pattern

H50.08   Alternating esotropia with other noncomitancies

Eye Muscle Diseases

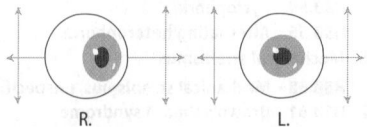
R.   L.
Monocular (one eye only) esotropia (inward)

Monocular exotropia (outward)

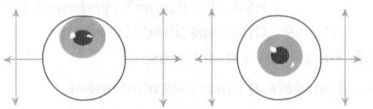
Monocular hypertropia (upward)

√5ᵗʰ H50.1   Exotropia
     Divergent concomitant strabismus
     EXCLUDES 1   intermittent exotropia (H50.33-, H50.34)
     H50.10   Unspecified exotropia
  √6ᵗʰ H50.11   Monocular exotropia
     H50.111   Monocular exotropia, right eye
     H50.112   Monocular exotropia, left eye
  √6ᵗʰ H50.12   Monocular exotropia with A pattern
     H50.121   Monocular exotropia with A pattern, right eye
     H50.122   Monocular exotropia with A pattern, left eye
  √6ᵗʰ H50.13   Monocular exotropia with V pattern
     H50.131   Monocular exotropia with V pattern, right eye
     H50.132   Monocular exotropia with V pattern, left eye
  √6ᵗʰ H50.14   Monocular exotropia with other noncomitancies
     H50.141   Monocular exotropia with other noncomitancies, right eye
     H50.142   Monocular exotropia with other noncomitancies, left eye
     H50.15   Alternating exotropia
     H50.16   Alternating exotropia with A pattern
     H50.17   Alternating exotropia with V pattern
     H50.18   Alternating exotropia with other noncomitancies

√5ᵗʰ H50.2   Vertical strabismus
     Hypertropia
     H50.21   Vertical strabismus, right eye
     H50.22   Vertical strabismus, left eye

√5ᵗʰ H50.3   Intermittent heterotropia
     H50.30   Unspecified intermittent heterotropia
  √6ᵗʰ H50.31   Intermittent monocular esotropia
     H50.311   Intermittent monocular esotropia, right eye
     H50.312   Intermittent monocular esotropia, left eye
     H50.32   Intermittent alternating esotropia
  √6ᵗʰ H50.33   Intermittent monocular exotropia
     H50.331   Intermittent monocular exotropia, right eye
     H50.332   Intermittent monocular exotropia, left eye
     H50.34   Intermittent alternating exotropia

√5ᵗʰ H50.4   Other and unspecified heterotropia
     H50.40   Unspecified heterotropia
  √6ᵗʰ H50.41   Cyclotropia
     H50.411   Cyclotropia, right eye
     H50.412   Cyclotropia, left eye
     H50.42   Monofixation syndrome
     H50.43   Accommodative component in esotropia

√5ᵗʰ H50.5   Heterophoria
     H50.50   Unspecified heterophoria

H50.51 **Esophoria**

H50.52 **Exophoria**

H50.53 **Vertical** heterophoria

H50.54 **Cyclophoria**

H50.55 **Alternating** heterophoria

✓5ᵗʰ **H50.6 Mechanical strabismus**

     H50.60 **Mechanical strabismus, unspecified**

     ✓6ᵗʰ H50.61 **Brown's sheath syndrome**

         H50.611 **Brown's sheath syndrome, right eye**

         H50.612 **Brown's sheath syndrome, left eye**

     H50.69 **Other mechanical strabismus**
         Strabismus due to adhesions
         Traumatic limitation of duction of eye muscle

✓5ᵗʰ **H50.8 Other specified strabismus**

     ✓6ᵗʰ H50.81 **Duane's syndrome**

         H50.811 **Duane's syndrome, right eye**

         H50.812 **Duane's syndrome, left eye**

     H50.89 **Other specified strabismus**

H50.9 **Unspecified strabismus**

✓4ᵗʰ **H51 Other disorders of binocular movement**

H51.0 **Palsy (spasm) of conjugate gaze**

✓5ᵗʰ **H51.1 Convergence insufficiency and excess**

     H51.11 **Convergence insufficiency**

     H51.12 **Convergence excess**

✓5ᵗʰ **H51.2 Internuclear ophthalmoplegia**

     H51.20 **Internuclear ophthalmoplegia, unspecified eye**

     H51.21 **Internuclear ophthalmoplegia, right eye**

     H51.22 **Internuclear ophthalmoplegia, left eye**

     H51.23 **Internuclear ophthalmoplegia, bilateral**

H51.8 **Other specified disorders of binocular movement**

H51.9 **Unspecified disorder of binocular movement**

✓4ᵗʰ **H52 Disorders of refraction and accommodation**

✓5ᵗʰ **H52.0 Hypermetropia**

     H52.00 **Hypermetropia, unspecified eye**

     H52.01 **Hypermetropia, right eye**

     H52.02 **Hypermetropia, left eye**

     H52.03 **Hypermetropia, bilateral**

✓5ᵗʰ **H52.1 Myopia**

     EXCLUDES 1   *degenerative myopia (H44.2-)*

     H52.10 **Myopia, unspecified eye**

     H52.11 **Myopia, right eye**

     H52.12 **Myopia, left eye**

     H52.13 **Myopia, bilateral**

✓5ᵗʰ **H52.2 Astigmatism**

     ✓6ᵗʰ H52.20 **Unspecified astigmatism**

         H52.201 **Unspecified astigmatism, right eye**

         H52.202 **Unspecified astigmatism, left eye**

         H52.203 **Unspecified astigmatism, bilateral**

         H52.209 **Unspecified astigmatism, unspecified eye**

     ✓6ᵗʰ H52.21 **Irregular astigmatism**

         H52.211 **Irregular astigmatism, right eye**

         H52.212 **Irregular astigmatism, left eye**

         H52.213 **Irregular astigmatism, bilateral**

         H52.219 **Irregular astigmatism, unspecified eye**

     ✓6ᵗʰ H52.22 **Regular astigmatism**

         H52.221 **Regular astigmatism, right eye**

         H52.222 **Regular astigmatism, left eye**

         H52.223 **Regular astigmatism, bilateral**

         H52.229 **Regular astigmatism, unspecified eye**

✓5ᵗʰ **H52.3 Anisometropia and aniseikonia**

     H52.31 **Anisometropia**

     H52.32 **Aniseikonia**

H52.4 **Presbyopia**

✓5ᵗʰ **H52.5 Disorders of accommodation**

     ✓6ᵗʰ H52.51 **Internal ophthalmoplegia (complete) (total)**

         H52.511 **Internal ophthalmoplegia (complete) (total), right eye**

         H52.512 **Internal ophthalmoplegia (complete) (total), left eye**

         H52.513 **Internal ophthalmoplegia (complete) (total), bilateral**

         H52.519 **Internal ophthalmoplegia (complete) (total), unspecified eye**

     ✓6ᵗʰ H52.52 **Paresis of accommodation**

         H52.521 **Paresis of accommodation, right eye**

         H52.522 **Paresis of accommodation, left eye**

         H52.523 **Paresis of accommodation, bilateral**

         H52.529 **Paresis of accommodation, unspecified eye**

     ✓6ᵗʰ H52.53 **Spasm of accommodation**

         H52.531 **Spasm of accommodation, right eye**

         H52.532 **Spasm of accommodation, left eye**

         H52.533 **Spasm of accommodation, bilateral**

         H52.539 **Spasm of accommodation, unspecified eye**

H52.6 **Other disorders of refraction**

H52.7 **Unspecified disorder of refraction**

Visual disturbances and blindness (H53-H54)

✓4ᵗʰ **H53 Visual disturbances**

✓5ᵗʰ **H53.0 Amblyopia ex anopsia**

     EXCLUDES 1   *amblyopia due to vitamin A deficiency (E50.5)*

     ✓6ᵗʰ H53.00 **Unspecified amblyopia**

         H53.001 **Unspecified amblyopia, right eye**

         H53.002 **Unspecified amblyopia, left eye**

         H53.003 **Unspecified amblyopia, bilateral**

         H53.009 **Unspecified amblyopia, unspecified eye**

     ✓6ᵗʰ H53.01 **Deprivation amblyopia**

         H53.011 **Deprivation amblyopia, right eye**

         H53.012 **Deprivation amblyopia, left eye**

         H53.013 **Deprivation amblyopia, bilateral**

         H53.019 **Deprivation amblyopia, unspecified eye**

     ✓6ᵗʰ H53.02 **Refractive amblyopia**

         H53.021 **Refractive amblyopia, right eye**

         H53.022 **Refractive amblyopia, left eye**

         H53.023 **Refractive amblyopia, bilateral**

         H53.029 **Refractive amblyopia, unspecified eye**

     ✓6ᵗʰ H53.03 **Strabismic amblyopia**

         EXCLUDES 1   *strabismus (H50.-)*

         H53.031 **Strabismic amblyopia, right eye**

         H53.032 **Strabismic amblyopia, left eye**

         H53.033 **Strabismic amblyopia, bilateral**

         H53.039 **Strabismic amblyopia, unspecified eye**

     ✓6ᵗʰ H53.04 **Amblyopia suspect**

         AHA: 2016,4Q,22-23

         H53.041 **Amblyopia suspect, right eye**

         H53.042 **Amblyopia suspect, left eye**

         H53.043 **Amblyopia suspect, bilateral**

         H53.049 **Amblyopia suspect, unspecified eye**

✓5ᵗʰ **H53.1 Subjective visual disturbances**

     EXCLUDES 1   *subjective visual disturbances due to vitamin A deficiency (E50.5)*
                    visual hallucinations (R44.1)

     H53.10 **Unspecified subjective visual disturbances**

     H53.11 **Day blindness**
         Hemeralopia

     ✓6ᵗʰ H53.12 **Transient visual loss**
         Scintillating scotoma
         EXCLUDES 1   *amaurosis fugax (G45.3-)*
                    transient retinal artery occlusion (H34.0-)
         AHA: 2022,1Q,30

         H53.121 **Transient visual loss, right eye**

         H53.122 **Transient visual loss, left eye**

         H53.123 **Transient visual loss, bilateral**

         H53.129 **Transient visual loss, unspecified eye**

     ✓6ᵗʰ H53.13 **Sudden visual loss**

         H53.131 **Sudden visual loss, right eye**

         H53.132 **Sudden visual loss, left eye**

         H53.133 **Sudden visual loss, bilateral**

         H53.139 **Sudden visual loss, unspecified eye**

     ✓6ᵗʰ H53.14 **Visual discomfort**
         Asthenopia
         Photophobia

         H53.141 **Visual discomfort, right eye**

         H53.142 **Visual discomfort, left eye**

         H53.143 **Visual discomfort, bilateral**

         H53.149 **Visual discomfort, unspecified**

H53.15 Visual distortions of shape and size
Metamorphopsia

H53.16 Psychophysical visual disturbances

H53.19 Other subjective visual disturbances
Visual halos
AHA: 2022,1Q,30

H53.2 Diplopia
Double vision

H53.3 Other and unspecified disorders of binocular vision

H53.30 Unspecified disorder of binocular vision

H53.31 Abnormal retinal correspondence

H53.32 Fusion with defective stereopsis

H53.33 Simultaneous visual perception without fusion

H53.34 Suppression of binocular vision

H53.4 Visual field defects

H53.40 Unspecified visual field defects

H53.41 Scotoma involving central area
Central scotoma
AHA: 2022,1Q,30

    H53.411 Scotoma involving central area, right eye
    H53.412 Scotoma involving central area, left eye
    H53.413 Scotoma involving central area, bilateral
    H53.419 Scotoma involving central area, unspecified eye

H53.42 Scotoma of blind spot area
Enlarged blind spot

    H53.421 Scotoma of blind spot area, right eye
    H53.422 Scotoma of blind spot area, left eye
    H53.423 Scotoma of blind spot area, bilateral
    H53.429 Scotoma of blind spot area, unspecified eye

H53.43 Sector or arcuate defects
Arcuate scotoma
Bjerrum scotoma

    H53.431 Sector or arcuate defects, right eye
    H53.432 Sector or arcuate defects, left eye
    H53.433 Sector or arcuate defects, bilateral
    H53.439 Sector or arcuate defects, unspecified eye

H53.45 Other localized visual field defect
Peripheral visual field defect
Ring scotoma NOS
Scotoma NOS

    H53.451 Other localized visual field defect, right eye
    H53.452 Other localized visual field defect, left eye
    H53.453 Other localized visual field defect, bilateral
    H53.459 Other localized visual field defect, unspecified eye

H53.46 Homonymous bilateral field defects
Homonymous hemianopia
Homonymous hemianopsia
Quadrant anopia
Quadrant anopsia

    H53.461 Homonymous bilateral field defects, right side
    H53.462 Homonymous bilateral field defects, left side
    H53.469 Homonymous bilateral field defects, unspecified side
       Homonymous bilateral field defects NOS

H53.47 Heteronymous bilateral field defects
Heteronymous hemianop(s)ia

H53.48 Generalized contraction of visual field

    H53.481 Generalized contraction of visual field, right eye
    H53.482 Generalized contraction of visual field, left eye
    H53.483 Generalized contraction of visual field, bilateral
    H53.489 Generalized contraction of visual field, unspecified eye

H53.5 Color vision deficiencies
Color blindness
EXCLUDES 2   *day blindness (H53.11)*

H53.50 Unspecified color vision deficiencies
Color blindness NOS

H53.51 Achromatopsia
DEF: Nonprogressive genetic visual disorder characterized by complete color blindness, decreased vision, and light sensitivity.

H53.52 Acquired color vision deficiency

H53.53 Deuteranomaly
Deuteranopia
DEF: Male-only genetic disorder causing difficulty in distinguishing green and red; no shortened spectrum.

H53.54 Protanomaly
Protanopia

H53.55 Tritanomaly
Tritanopia

H53.59 Other color vision deficiencies

H53.6 Night blindness
EXCLUDES 1   *night blindness due to vitamin A deficiency (E50.5)*

H53.60 Unspecified night blindness

H53.61 Abnormal dark adaptation curve

H53.62 Acquired night blindness

H53.63 Congenital night blindness

H53.69 Other night blindness

H53.7 Vision sensitivity deficiencies

H53.71 Glare sensitivity

H53.72 Impaired contrast sensitivity

H53.8 Other visual disturbances

H53.9 Unspecified visual disturbance

H54 Blindness and low vision

NOTE   For definition of visual impairment categories see table below

Code first any associated underlying cause of the blindness
EXCLUDES 1   *amaurosis fugax (G45.3)*
AHA: 2017,4Q,11-12

H54.0 Blindness, both eyes
Visual impairment categories 3, 4, 5 in both eyes.

H54.0X Blindness, both eyes, different category levels

    H54.0X3 Blindness right eye, category 3

       H54.0X33 Blindness right eye category 3, blindness left eye category 3
       H54.0X34 Blindness right eye category 3, blindness left eye category 4
       H54.0X35 Blindness right eye category 3, blindness left eye category 5

    H54.0X4 Blindness right eye, category 4

       H54.0X43 Blindness right eye category 4, blindness left eye category 3
       H54.0X44 Blindness right eye category 4, blindness left eye category 4
       H54.0X45 Blindness right eye category 4, blindness left eye category 5

    H54.0X5 Blindness right eye, category 5

       H54.0X53 Blindness right eye category 5, blindness left eye category 3
       H54.0X54 Blindness right eye category 5, blindness left eye category 4
       H54.0X55 Blindness right eye category 5, blindness left eye category 5

H54.1 Blindness, one eye, low vision other eye
Visual impairment categories 3, 4, 5 in one eye, with categories 1 or 2 in the other eye.

H54.10 Blindness, one eye, low vision other eye, unspecified eyes

H54.11 Blindness, right eye, low vision left eye

    H54.113 Blindness right eye category 3, low vision left eye

       H54.1131 Blindness right eye category 3, low vision left eye category 1
       H54.1132 Blindness right eye category 3, low vision left eye category 2

    H54.114 Blindness right eye category 4, low vision left eye

       H54.1141 Blindness right eye category 4, low vision left eye category 1

✔ Additional Character Required   ✔x7ᵗʰ Placeholder Alert   Manifestation   Unspecified Dx   Q QPP   UPD Unacceptable PDx

Chapter 7. Diseases of the Eye and Adnexa

H53.15–H54.1141

Chapter 7. Diseases of the Eye and Adnexa

H54.1142–H54.8

H54.1142 **Blindness right eye category 4, low vision left eye category 2**

✓7ᵗʰ H54.115 **Blindness right eye category 5, low vision left eye**

    H54.1151 **Blindness right eye category 5, low vision left eye category 1**

    H54.1152 **Blindness right eye category 5, low vision left eye category 2**

✓6ᵗʰ H54.12 Blindness, left eye, low vision right eye

✓7ᵗʰ H54.121 **Low vision right eye category 1, blindness left eye**

    H54.1213 **Low vision right eye category 1, blindness left eye category 3**

    H54.1214 **Low vision right eye category 1, blindness left eye category 4**

    H54.1215 **Low vision right eye category 1, blindness left eye category 5**

✓7ᵗʰ H54.122 **Low vision right eye category 2, blindness left eye**

    H54.1223 **Low vision right eye category 2, blindness left eye category 3**

    H54.1224 **Low vision right eye category 2, blindness left eye category 4**

    H54.1225 **Low vision right eye category 2, blindness left eye category 5**

✓5ᵗʰ H54.2 Low vision, **both eyes**

Visual impairment categories 1 or 2 in both eyes.

✓6ᵗʰ H54.2X Low vision, both eyes, different category levels

✓7ᵗʰ H54.2X1 **Low vision, right eye, category 1**

    H54.2X11 **Low vision right eye category 1, low vision left eye category 1**

    H54.2X12 **Low vision right eye category 1, low vision left eye category 2**

✓7ᵗʰ H54.2X2 **Low vision, right eye, category 2**

    H54.2X21 **Low vision right eye category 2, low vision left eye category 1**

    H54.2X22 **Low vision right eye category 2, low vision left eye category 2**

H54.3 Unqualified **visual loss, both eyes**

Visual impairment category 9 in both eyes.

TIP: Assign only when both eyes are documented as affected by blindness or low vision but the visual impairment category is not documented.

✓5ᵗʰ H54.4 Blindness, **one eye**

Visual impairment categories 3, 4, 5 in one eye [normal vision in other eye]

H54.40 **Blindness, one eye, unspecified eye**

✓6ᵗʰ H54.41 Blindness, right eye, normal vision left eye

✓7ᵗʰ H54.413 **Blindness, right eye, category 3**

    H54.413A **Blindness right eye category 3, normal vision left eye**

✓7ᵗʰ H54.414 **Blindness, right eye, category 4**

    H54.414A **Blindness right eye category 4, normal vision left eye**

✓7ᵗʰ H54.415 **Blindness, right eye, category 5**

    H54.415A **Blindness right eye category 5, normal vision left eye**

✓6ᵗʰ H54.42 Blindness, left eye, normal vision right eye

✓7ᵗʰ H54.42A **Blindness, left eye, category 3-5**

    H54.42A3 **Blindness left eye category 3, normal vision right eye**

    H54.42A4 **Blindness left eye category 4, normal vision right eye**

    H54.42A5 **Blindness left eye category 5, normal vision right eye**

✓5ᵗʰ H54.5 Low vision, **one eye**

Visual impairment categories 1 or 2 in one eye [normal vision in other eye].

H54.50 **Low vision, one eye, unspecified eye**

✓6ᵗʰ H54.51 Low vision, right eye, normal vision left eye

✓7ᵗʰ H54.511 **Low vision, right eye, category 1-2**

    H54.511A **Low vision right eye category 1, normal vision left eye**

    H54.512A **Low vision right eye category 2, normal vision left eye**

✓7ᵗʰ H54.52 Low vision, left eye, normal vision right eye

✓7ᵗʰ H54.52A **Low vision, left eye, category 1-2**

    H54.52A1 **Low vision left eye category 1, normal vision right eye**

    H54.52A2 **Low vision left eye category 2, normal vision right eye**

✓5ᵗʰ H54.6 Unqualified **visual loss, one eye**

Visual impairment category 9 in one eye [normal vision in other eye].

TIP: Assign a code from this category only when one eye is documented as affected by blindness or low vision but the visual impairment category is not documented.

H54.60 **Unqualified visual loss, one eye, unspecified**

H54.61 **Unqualified visual loss, right eye, normal vision left eye**

H54.62 **Unqualified visual loss, left eye, normal vision right eye**

H54.7 Unspecified visual loss

Visual impairment category 9 NOS

TIP: Assign only when documentation specifies blindness, visual loss, or low vision but not whether one or both eyes are affected or the visual impairment category.

H54.8 Legal blindness, as defined in USA

Blindness NOS according to USA definition

EXCLUDES 1   legal blindness with specification of impairment level (H54.0-H54.7)

NOTE   The table below gives a classification of severity of visual impairment recommended by a WHO Study Group on the Prevention of Blindness, Geneva, 6-10 November 1972.

The term "low vision" in category H54 comprises categories 1 and 2 of the table, the term "blindness" categories 3, 4 and 5, and the term "unqualified visual loss" category 9.

If the extent of the visual field is taken into account, patients with a field no greater than 10 but greater than 5 around central fixation should be placed in category 3 and patients with a field no greater than 5 around central fixation should be placed in category 4, even if the central acuity is not impaired.

Category of visual impairment	Visual acuity with best possible correction	
	Maximum less than:	**Minimum equal to or better than:**
1	6/18 3/10 (0.3) 20/70	6/60 1/10 (0.1) 20/200
2	6/60 1/10 (0.1) 20/200	3/60 1/20 (0.05) 20/400
3	3/60 1/200 (0.05) 20/400	1/60 (finger counting at one meter) 1/50 (0.02) 5/300 (20/1200)
4	1/60 (finger counting at one meter) 1/50 (0.02) 5/300	Light perception
5	No light perception	
9	Undetermined or unspecified	

Other disorders of eye and adnexa (H55-H57)

✓4ᵗʰ **H55 Nystagmus and other** irregular eye movements

  ✓5ᵗʰ **H55.0 Nystagmus**

    DEF: Rapid, rhythmic, involuntary movements of the eyeball in vertical, horizontal, rotational, or mixed directions.

    H55.00 Unspecified nystagmus

    H55.01 Congenital nystagmus

    H55.02 Latent nystagmus

    H55.03 Visual deprivation nystagmus

    H55.04 Dissociated nystagmus

    H55.09 Other forms of nystagmus

  ✓5ᵗʰ **H55.8 Other irregular eye movements**

    AHA: 2020,4Q,25

    H55.81 Deficient saccadic eye movements

    H55.82 Deficient smooth pursuit eye movements

    H55.89 Other irregular eye movements

✓4ᵗʰ **H57 Other disorders of eye and adnexa**

  ✓5ᵗʰ **H57.0 Anomalies of pupillary function**

    H57.00 Unspecified anomaly of pupillary function

    H57.01 Argyll Robertson pupil, atypical

      EXCLUDES 1   *syphilitic Argyll Robertson pupil (A52.19)*

    H57.02 Anisocoria

    H57.03 Miosis

    H57.04 Mydriasis

    ✓6ᵗʰ **H57.05 Tonic pupil**

      H57.051 Tonic pupil, right eye

      H57.052 Tonic pupil, left eye

      H57.053 Tonic pupil, bilateral

      H57.059 Tonic pupil, unspecified eye

    H57.09 Other anomalies of pupillary function

  ✓5ᵗʰ **H57.1 Ocular pain**

    H57.10 Ocular pain, unspecified eye

    H57.11 Ocular pain, right eye

    H57.12 Ocular pain, left eye

    H57.13 Ocular pain, bilateral

  ✓5ᵗʰ **H57.8 Other specified disorders of eye and adnexa**

    AHA: 2018,4Q,15-16

    ✓6ᵗʰ **H57.81 Brow ptosis**

      H57.811 Brow ptosis, right

      H57.812 Brow ptosis, left

      H57.813 Brow ptosis, bilateral

      H57.819 Brow ptosis, unspecified

    H57.89 Other specified disorders of eye and adnexa

  H57.9 Unspecified disorder of eye and adnexa

Intraoperative and postprocedural complications and disorders of eye and adnexa, not elsewhere classified (H59)

✓4ᵗʰ **H59 Intraoperative and postprocedural complications and disorders of eye and adnexa, not elsewhere classified**

    EXCLUDES 1   *mechanical complication of intraocular lens (T85.2)*

           mechanical complication of other ocular prosthetic devices, implants and grafts (T85.3)

           pseudophakia (Z96.1)

           secondary cataracts (H26.4-)

  ✓5ᵗʰ **H59.0 Disorders of the eye** following cataract surgery

    ✓6ᵗʰ **H59.01 Keratopathy (bullous aphakic) following cataract surgery**

      Vitreal corneal syndrome

      Vitreous (touch) syndrome

      H59.011 Keratopathy (bullous aphakic) following cataract surgery, right eye

      H59.012 Keratopathy (bullous aphakic) following cataract surgery, left eye

      H59.013 Keratopathy (bullous aphakic) following cataract surgery, bilateral

      H59.019 Keratopathy (bullous aphakic) following cataract surgery, unspecified eye

    ✓6ᵗʰ **H59.02 Cataract (lens) fragments in eye following cataract surgery**

      H59.021 Cataract (lens) fragments in eye following cataract surgery, right eye

      H59.022 Cataract (lens) fragments in eye following cataract surgery, left eye

      H59.023 Cataract (lens) fragments in eye following cataract surgery, bilateral

      H59.029 Cataract (lens) fragments in eye following cataract surgery, unspecified eye

    ✓6ᵗʰ **H59.03 Cystoid macular edema following cataract surgery**

      H59.031 Cystoid macular edema following cataract surgery, right eye

      H59.032 Cystoid macular edema following cataract surgery, left eye

      H59.033 Cystoid macular edema following cataract surgery, bilateral

      H59.039 Cystoid macular edema following cataract surgery, unspecified eye

    ✓6ᵗʰ **H59.09 Other disorders of the eye following cataract surgery**

      H59.091 Other disorders of the right eye following cataract surgery

      H59.092 Other disorders of the left eye following cataract surgery

      H59.093 Other disorders of the eye following cataract surgery, bilateral

      H59.099 Other disorders of unspecified eye following cataract surgery

  ✓5ᵗʰ **H59.1 Intraoperative hemorrhage and hematoma of eye and adnexa complicating a procedure**

    EXCLUDES 1   *intraoperative hemorrhage and hematoma of eye and adnexa due to accidental puncture or laceration during a procedure (H59.2-)*

    ✓6ᵗʰ **H59.11 Intraoperative hemorrhage and hematoma of eye and adnexa complicating an ophthalmic procedure**

      H59.111 Intraoperative hemorrhage and hematoma of right eye and adnexa complicating an ophthalmic procedure

      H59.112 Intraoperative hemorrhage and hematoma of left eye and adnexa complicating an ophthalmic procedure

      H59.113 Intraoperative hemorrhage and hematoma of eye and adnexa complicating an ophthalmic procedure, bilateral

      H59.119 Intraoperative hemorrhage and hematoma of unspecified eye and adnexa complicating an ophthalmic procedure

    ✓6ᵗʰ **H59.12 Intraoperative hemorrhage and hematoma of eye and adnexa complicating other procedure**

      H59.121 Intraoperative hemorrhage and hematoma of right eye and adnexa complicating other procedure

      H59.122 Intraoperative hemorrhage and hematoma of left eye and adnexa complicating other procedure

      H59.123 Intraoperative hemorrhage and hematoma of eye and adnexa complicating other procedure, bilateral

      H59.129 Intraoperative hemorrhage and hematoma of unspecified eye and adnexa complicating other procedure

  ✓5ᵗʰ **H59.2 Accidental puncture and laceration of eye and adnexa during a procedure**

    ✓6ᵗʰ **H59.21 Accidental puncture and laceration of eye and adnexa during an ophthalmic procedure**

      H59.211 Accidental puncture and laceration of right eye and adnexa during an ophthalmic procedure

      H59.212 Accidental puncture and laceration of left eye and adnexa during an ophthalmic procedure

      H59.213 Accidental puncture and laceration of eye and adnexa during an ophthalmic procedure, bilateral

      H59.219 Accidental puncture and laceration of unspecified eye and adnexa during an ophthalmic procedure

    ✓6ᵗʰ **H59.22 Accidental puncture and laceration of eye and adnexa during other procedure**

      H59.221 Accidental puncture and laceration of right eye and adnexa during other procedure

      H59.222 Accidental puncture and laceration of left eye and adnexa during other procedure

      H59.223 Accidental puncture and laceration of eye and adnexa during other procedure, bilateral

Chapter 7. Diseases of the Eye and Adnexa

H59.229 Accidental puncture and laceration of unspecified eye and adnexa during other procedure

✓5ᵗʰ **H59.3** Postprocedural hemorrhage, hematoma, and seroma of eye and adnexa following a procedure
AHA: 2016,4Q,9-10

✓6ᵗʰ **H59.31** Postprocedural hemorrhage of eye and adnexa following an ophthalmic procedure

H59.311 Postprocedural hemorrhage of right eye and adnexa following an ophthalmic procedure

H59.312 Postprocedural hemorrhage of left eye and adnexa following an ophthalmic procedure

H59.313 Postprocedural hemorrhage of eye and adnexa following an ophthalmic procedure, bilateral

H59.319 Postprocedural hemorrhage of unspecified eye and adnexa following an ophthalmic procedure

✓6ᵗʰ **H59.32** Postprocedural hemorrhage of eye and adnexa following other procedure

H59.321 Postprocedural hemorrhage of right eye and adnexa following other procedure

H59.322 Postprocedural hemorrhage of left eye and adnexa following other procedure

H59.323 Postprocedural hemorrhage of eye and adnexa following other procedure, bilateral

H59.329 Postprocedural hemorrhage of unspecified eye and adnexa following other procedure

✓6ᵗʰ **H59.33** Postprocedural hematoma of eye and adnexa following an ophthalmic procedure

H59.331 Postprocedural hematoma of right eye and adnexa following an ophthalmic procedure

H59.332 Postprocedural hematoma of left eye and adnexa following an ophthalmic procedure

H59.333 Postprocedural hematoma of eye and adnexa following an ophthalmic procedure, bilateral

H59.339 Postprocedural hematoma of unspecified eye and adnexa following an ophthalmic procedure

✓6ᵗʰ **H59.34** Postprocedural hematoma of eye and adnexa following other procedure

H59.341 Postprocedural hematoma of right eye and adnexa following other procedure

H59.342 Postprocedural hematoma of left eye and adnexa following other procedure

H59.343 Postprocedural hematoma of eye and adnexa following other procedure, bilateral

H59.349 Postprocedural hematoma of unspecified eye and adnexa following other procedure

✓6ᵗʰ **H59.35** Postprocedural seroma of eye and adnexa following an ophthalmic procedure

H59.351 Postprocedural seroma of right eye and adnexa following an ophthalmic procedure

H59.352 Postprocedural seroma of left eye and adnexa following an ophthalmic procedure

H59.353 Postprocedural seroma of eye and adnexa following an ophthalmic procedure, bilateral

H59.359 Postprocedural seroma of unspecified eye and adnexa following an ophthalmic procedure

✓6ᵗʰ **H59.36** Postprocedural seroma of eye and adnexa following other procedure

H59.361 Postprocedural seroma of right eye and adnexa following other procedure

H59.362 Postprocedural seroma of left eye and adnexa following other procedure

H59.363 Postprocedural seroma of eye and adnexa following other procedure, bilateral

H59.369 Postprocedural seroma of unspecified eye and adnexa following other procedure

✓5ᵗʰ **H59.4** Inflammation (infection) of postprocedural bleb
Postprocedural blebitis
EXCLUDES 1   filtering (vitreous) bleb after glaucoma surgery status (Z98.83)

H59.40 Inflammation (infection) of postprocedural bleb, unspecified

H59.41 Inflammation (infection) of postprocedural bleb, stage 1

H59.42 Inflammation (infection) of postprocedural bleb, stage 2

H59.43 Inflammation (infection) of postprocedural bleb, stage 3
Bleb endophthalmitis

✓5ᵗʰ **H59.8** Other intraoperative and postprocedural complications and disorders of eye and adnexa, not elsewhere classified

✓6ᵗʰ **H59.81** Chorioretinal scars after surgery for detachment

H59.811 Chorioretinal scars after surgery for detachment, right eye

H59.812 Chorioretinal scars after surgery for detachment, left eye

H59.813 Chorioretinal scars after surgery for detachment, bilateral

H59.819 Chorioretinal scars after surgery for detachment, unspecified eye

H59.88 Other intraoperative complications of eye and adnexa, not elsewhere classified

H59.89 Other postprocedural complications and disorders of eye and adnexa, not elsewhere classified
AHA: 2020,3Q,29

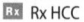 HCC CMS-HCC | Rx Rx HCC | ESR ESRD HCC | COM Commercial HCC | N Newborn: 0 | P Pediatric: 0-17 | M Maternity: 9-64 | A Adult: 15-124

646

ICD-10-CM 2023

Chapter 8. Diseases of the Ear and Mastoid Process (H60–H95)

Chapter-specific Guidelines with Coding Examples
Reserved for future guideline expansion.

Chapter 8. Diseases of the Ear and Mastoid Process

Chapter 8. Diseases of the Ear and Mastoid Process

H60–H60.91

Chapter 8. Diseases of the Ear and Mastoid Process (H60-H95)

NOTE   Use an external cause code following the code for the ear condition, if applicable, to identify the cause of the ear condition

EXCLUDES 2   *certain conditions originating in the perinatal period (P04-P96)*
certain infectious and parasitic diseases (A00-B99)
complications of pregnancy, childbirth and the puerperium (O00-O9A)
congenital malformations, deformations and chromosomal abnormalities (Q00-Q99)
endocrine, nutritional and metabolic diseases (E00-E88)
injury, poisoning and certain other consequences of external causes (S00-T88)
neoplasms (C00-D49)
symptoms, signs and abnormal clinical and laboratory findings, not elsewhere classified (R00-R94)

This chapter contains the following blocks:
H60-H62   Diseases of external ear
H65-H75   Diseases of middle ear and mastoid
H80-H83   Diseases of inner ear
H90-H94   Other disorders of ear
H95   Intraoperative and postprocedural complications and disorders of ear and mastoid process, not elsewhere classified

Diseases of external ear (H60-H62)

√4ᵗʰ **H60   Otitis externa**

     TIP: When the specific infectious agent is identified, a code from Chapter 1 is assigned instead of a code from this category.

√5ᵗʰ **H60.0   Abscess of external ear**
     Boil of external ear
     Carbuncle of auricle or external auditory canal
     Furuncle of external ear
     H60.00   Abscess of external ear, unspecified ear
     H60.01   Abscess of right external ear
     H60.02   Abscess of left external ear
     H60.03   Abscess of external ear, bilateral

√5ᵗʰ **H60.1   Cellulitis of external ear**
     Cellulitis of auricle
     Cellulitis of external auditory canal
     H60.10   Cellulitis of external ear, unspecified ear
     H60.11   Cellulitis of right external ear
     H60.12   Cellulitis of left external ear
     H60.13   Cellulitis of external ear, bilateral

√5ᵗʰ **H60.2   Malignant otitis externa**
     H60.20   Malignant otitis externa, unspecified ear
     H60.21   Malignant otitis externa, right ear
     H60.22   Malignant otitis externa, left ear
     H60.23   Malignant otitis externa, bilateral

√5ᵗʰ **H60.3   Other infective otitis externa**

     √6ᵗʰ **H60.31   Diffuse otitis externa**
         H60.311   Diffuse otitis externa, right ear
         H60.312   Diffuse otitis externa, left ear
         H60.313   Diffuse otitis externa, bilateral
         H60.319   Diffuse otitis externa, unspecified ear

     √6ᵗʰ **H60.32   Hemorrhagic otitis externa**
         H60.321   Hemorrhagic otitis externa, right ear
         H60.322   Hemorrhagic otitis externa, left ear
         H60.323   Hemorrhagic otitis externa, bilateral
         H60.329   Hemorrhagic otitis externa, unspecified ear

     √6ᵗʰ **H60.33   Swimmer's ear**
         DEF: Commonly occurs when water gets trapped in the ear after swimming.
         H60.331   Swimmer's ear, right ear
         H60.332   Swimmer's ear, left ear
         H60.333   Swimmer's ear, bilateral
         H60.339   Swimmer's ear, unspecified ear

     √6ᵗʰ **H60.39   Other infective otitis externa**
         H60.391   Other infective otitis externa, right ear
         H60.392   Other infective otitis externa, left ear
         H60.393   Other infective otitis externa, bilateral
         H60.399   Other infective otitis externa, unspecified ear

√5ᵗʰ **H60.4   Cholesteatoma of external ear**
     Keratosis obturans of external ear (canal)
     EXCLUDES 2   *cholesteatoma of middle ear (H71.-)*
         recurrent cholesteatoma of postmastoidectomy cavity (H95.0-)
     DEF: Cholesteatoma: Noncancerous cyst-like mass of cell debris, including cholesterol and epithelial cells resulting from trauma, repeated or improperly healed infections, and congenital enclosure of epidermal cells.
     H60.40   Cholesteatoma of external ear, unspecified ear
     H60.41   Cholesteatoma of right external ear
     H60.42   Cholesteatoma of left external ear
     H60.43   Cholesteatoma of external ear, bilateral

√5ᵗʰ **H60.5   Acute noninfective otitis externa**

     √6ᵗʰ **H60.50   Unspecified acute noninfective otitis externa**
         Acute otitis externa NOS
         H60.501   Unspecified acute noninfective otitis externa, right ear
         H60.502   Unspecified acute noninfective otitis externa, left ear
         H60.503   Unspecified acute noninfective otitis externa, bilateral
         H60.509   Unspecified acute noninfective otitis externa, unspecified ear

     √6ᵗʰ **H60.51   Acute actinic otitis externa**
         H60.511   Acute actinic otitis externa, right ear
         H60.512   Acute actinic otitis externa, left ear
         H60.513   Acute actinic otitis externa, bilateral
         H60.519   Acute actinic otitis externa, unspecified ear

     √6ᵗʰ **H60.52   Acute chemical otitis externa**
         H60.521   Acute chemical otitis externa, right ear
         H60.522   Acute chemical otitis externa, left ear
         H60.523   Acute chemical otitis externa, bilateral
         H60.529   Acute chemical otitis externa, unspecified ear

     √6ᵗʰ **H60.53   Acute contact otitis externa**
         H60.531   Acute contact otitis externa, right ear
         H60.532   Acute contact otitis externa, left ear
         H60.533   Acute contact otitis externa, bilateral
         H60.539   Acute contact otitis externa, unspecified ear

     √6ᵗʰ **H60.54   Acute eczematoid otitis externa**
         H60.541   Acute eczematoid otitis externa, right ear
         H60.542   Acute eczematoid otitis externa, left ear
         H60.543   Acute eczematoid otitis externa, bilateral
         H60.549   Acute eczematoid otitis externa, unspecified ear

     √6ᵗʰ **H60.55   Acute reactive otitis externa**
         H60.551   Acute reactive otitis externa, right ear
         H60.552   Acute reactive otitis externa, left ear
         H60.553   Acute reactive otitis externa, bilateral
         H60.559   Acute reactive otitis externa, unspecified ear

     √6ᵗʰ **H60.59   Other noninfective acute otitis externa**
         H60.591   Other noninfective acute otitis externa, right ear
         H60.592   Other noninfective acute otitis externa, left ear
         H60.593   Other noninfective acute otitis externa, bilateral
         H60.599   Other noninfective acute otitis externa, unspecified ear

√5ᵗʰ **H60.6   Unspecified chronic otitis externa**
     H60.60   Unspecified chronic otitis externa, unspecified ear
     H60.61   Unspecified chronic otitis externa, right ear
     H60.62   Unspecified chronic otitis externa, left ear
     H60.63   Unspecified chronic otitis externa, bilateral

√5ᵗʰ **H60.8   Other otitis externa**
     √6ᵗʰ **H60.8X   Other otitis externa**
         H60.8X1   Other otitis externa, right ear
         H60.8X2   Other otitis externa, left ear
         H60.8X3   Other otitis externa, bilateral
         H60.8X9   Other otitis externa, unspecified ear

√5ᵗʰ **H60.9   Unspecified otitis externa**
     H60.90   Unspecified otitis externa, unspecified ear
     H60.91   Unspecified otitis externa, right ear

HCC CMS-HCC   **Rx** Rx HCC   **ESR** ESRD HCC   **COM** Commercial HCC   **N** Newborn: 0   **P** Pediatric: 0-17   **M** Maternity: 9-64   **A** Adult: 15-124

648   ICD-10-CM 2023

H60.92   **Unspecified otitis externa, left ear**
H60.93   **Unspecified otitis externa, bilateral**

☑️4ᵗʰ **H61 Other disorders of external ear**

✓5ᵗʰ **H61.0 Chondritis and perichondritis of external ear**

Chondrodermatitis nodularis chronica helicis
Perichondritis of auricle
Perichondritis of pinna

✓6ᵗʰ **H61.00 Unspecified perichondritis of external ear**

H61.001 Unspecified perichondritis of right external ear
H61.002 Unspecified perichondritis of left ear
H61.003 Unspecified perichondritis of external ear, bilateral
H61.009 Unspecified perichondritis of external ear, unspecified ear

✓6ᵗʰ **H61.01 Acute perichondritis of external ear**

H61.011 Acute perichondritis of right external ear
H61.012 Acute perichondritis of left external ear
H61.013 Acute perichondritis of external ear, bilateral
H61.019 Acute perichondritis of external ear, unspecified ear

✓6ᵗʰ **H61.02 Chronic perichondritis of external ear**

H61.021 Chronic perichondritis of right external ear
H61.022 Chronic perichondritis of left external ear
H61.023 Chronic perichondritis of external ear, bilateral
H61.029 Chronic perichondritis of external ear, unspecified ear

✓6ᵗʰ **H61.03 Chondritis of external ear**

Chondritis of auricle
Chondritis of pinna
AHA: 2015,1Q,18
DEF: Infection that has progressed into the cartilage and presents as indurated and edematous skin over the pinna. Vascular compromise occurs with tissue necrosis and deformity.

H61.031 Chondritis of right external ear
H61.032 Chondritis of left external ear
H61.033 Chondritis of external ear, bilateral
H61.039 Chondritis of external ear, unspecified ear

✓5ᵗʰ **H61.1 Noninfective disorders of pinna**

EXCLUDES 2   *cauliflower ear (M95.1-)*
gouty tophi of ear (M1A.-)

✓6ᵗʰ **H61.10 Unspecified noninfective disorders of pinna**

Disorder of pinna NOS

H61.101 Unspecified noninfective disorders of pinna, right ear
H61.102 Unspecified noninfective disorders of pinna, left ear
H61.103 Unspecified noninfective disorders of pinna, bilateral
H61.109 Unspecified noninfective disorders of pinna, unspecified ear

✓6ᵗʰ **H61.11 Acquired deformity of pinna**

Acquired deformity of auricle
EXCLUDES 2   *cauliflower ear (M95.1-)*

H61.111 Acquired deformity of pinna, right ear
H61.112 Acquired deformity of pinna, left ear
H61.113 Acquired deformity of pinna, bilateral
H61.119 Acquired deformity of pinna, unspecified ear

✓6ᵗʰ **H61.12 Hematoma of pinna**

Hematoma of auricle

H61.121 Hematoma of pinna, right ear
H61.122 Hematoma of pinna, left ear
H61.123 Hematoma of pinna, bilateral
H61.129 Hematoma of pinna, unspecified ear

✓6ᵗʰ **H61.19 Other noninfective disorders of pinna**

H61.191 Noninfective disorders of pinna, right ear
H61.192 Noninfective disorders of pinna, left ear
H61.193 Noninfective disorders of pinna, bilateral
H61.199 Noninfective disorders of pinna, unspecified ear

✓5ᵗʰ **H61.2 Impacted cerumen**

Wax in ear

H61.20 Impacted cerumen, unspecified ear
H61.21 Impacted cerumen, right ear
H61.22 Impacted cerumen, left ear
H61.23 Impacted cerumen, bilateral

✓5ᵗʰ **H61.3 Acquired stenosis of external ear canal**

Collapse of external ear canal
EXCLUDES 1   *postprocedural stenosis of external ear canal (H95.81-)*

✓6ᵗʰ **H61.30 Acquired stenosis of external ear canal, unspecified**

H61.301 Acquired stenosis of right external ear canal, unspecified
H61.302 Acquired stenosis of left external ear canal, unspecified
H61.303 Acquired stenosis of external ear canal, unspecified, bilateral
H61.309 Acquired stenosis of external ear canal, unspecified, unspecified ear

✓6ᵗʰ **H61.31 Acquired stenosis of external ear canal secondary to trauma**

H61.311 Acquired stenosis of right external ear canal secondary to trauma
H61.312 Acquired stenosis of left external ear canal secondary to trauma
H61.313 Acquired stenosis of external ear canal secondary to trauma, bilateral
H61.319 Acquired stenosis of external ear canal secondary to trauma, unspecified ear

✓6ᵗʰ **H61.32 Acquired stenosis of external ear canal secondary to inflammation and infection**

DEF: Narrowing of the external ear canal due to chronic inflammation or infection.

H61.321 Acquired stenosis of right external ear canal secondary to inflammation and infection
H61.322 Acquired stenosis of left external ear canal secondary to inflammation and infection
H61.323 Acquired stenosis of external ear canal secondary to inflammation and infection, bilateral
H61.329 Acquired stenosis of external ear canal secondary to inflammation and infection, unspecified ear

✓6ᵗʰ **H61.39 Other acquired stenosis of external ear canal**

H61.391 Other acquired stenosis of right external ear canal
H61.392 Other acquired stenosis of left external ear canal
H61.393 Other acquired stenosis of external ear canal, bilateral
H61.399 Other acquired stenosis of external ear canal, unspecified ear

✓5ᵗʰ **H61.8 Other specified disorders of external ear**

✓6ᵗʰ **H61.81 Exostosis of external canal**

H61.811 Exostosis of right external canal
H61.812 Exostosis of left external canal
H61.813 Exostosis of external canal, bilateral
H61.819 Exostosis of external canal, unspecified ear

✓6ᵗʰ **H61.89 Other specified disorders of external ear**

H61.891 Other specified disorders of right external ear
H61.892 Other specified disorders of left external ear
H61.893 Other specified disorders of external ear, bilateral
H61.899 Other specified disorders of external ear, unspecified ear

✓5ᵗʰ **H61.9 Disorder of external ear, unspecified**

H61.90 Disorder of external ear, unspecified, unspecified ear
H61.91 Disorder of right external ear, unspecified
H61.92 Disorder of left external ear, unspecified
H61.93 Disorder of external ear, unspecified, bilateral

✓4ᵗʰ **H62 Disorders of external ear in diseases classified elsewhere**

  ✓5ᵗʰ **H62.4 Otitis externa in other diseases classified elsewhere**

    Code first underlying disease, such as:
      erysipelas (A46)
      impetigo (L01.0)

      EXCLUDES 1   otitis externa (in):
        candidiasis (B37.84)
        herpes viral [herpes simplex] (B00.1)
        herpes zoster (B02.8)

    H62.40 Otitis externa in other diseases classified elsewhere, unspecified ear

    H62.41 Otitis externa in other diseases classified elsewhere, right ear

    H62.42 Otitis externa in other diseases classified elsewhere, left ear

    H62.43 Otitis externa in other diseases classified elsewhere, bilateral

  ✓5ᵗʰ **H62.8 Other disorders of external ear in diseases classified elsewhere**

    Code first underlying disease, such as:
      gout (M1A.-, M10.-)

    ✓6ᵗʰ **H62.8X Other disorders of external ear in diseases classified elsewhere**

      H62.8X1 Other disorders of right external ear in diseases classified elsewhere

      H62.8X2 Other disorders of left external ear in diseases classified elsewhere

      H62.8X3 Other disorders of external ear in diseases classified elsewhere, bilateral

      H62.8X9 Other disorders of external ear in diseases classified elsewhere, unspecified ear

Diseases of middle ear and mastoid (H65-H75)

✓4ᵗʰ **H65 Nonsuppurative otitis media**

  INCLUDES   nonsuppurative otitis media with myringitis

  Use additional code for any associated perforated tympanic membrane (H72.-)

  Use additional code, if applicable, to identify:
    exposure to environmental tobacco smoke (Z77.22)
    exposure to tobacco smoke in the perinatal period (P96.81)
    history of tobacco dependence (Z87.891)
    infectious agent (B95-B97)
    occupational exposure to environmental tobacco smoke (Z57.31)
    tobacco dependence (F17.-)
    tobacco use (Z72.0)

  ✓5ᵗʰ **H65.0 Acute serous otitis media**

    Acute and subacute secretory otitis

    H65.00 Acute serous otitis media, unspecified ear
    H65.01 Acute serous otitis media, right ear
    H65.02 Acute serous otitis media, left ear
    H65.03 Acute serous otitis media, bilateral
    H65.04 Acute serous otitis media, recurrent, right ear
    H65.05 Acute serous otitis media, recurrent, left ear
    H65.06 Acute serous otitis media, recurrent, bilateral
    H65.07 Acute serous otitis media, recurrent, unspecified ear

  ✓5ᵗʰ **H65.1 Other acute nonsuppurative otitis media**

    EXCLUDES 1   otitic barotrauma (T70.0)
        otitis media (acute) NOS (H66.9)

    ✓6ᵗʰ **H65.11 Acute and subacute allergic otitis media (mucoid) (sanguinous) (serous)**

      H65.111 Acute and subacute allergic otitis media (mucoid) (sanguinous) (serous), right ear
      H65.112 Acute and subacute allergic otitis media (mucoid) (sanguinous) (serous), left ear
      H65.113 Acute and subacute allergic otitis media (mucoid) (sanguinous) (serous), bilateral
      H65.114 Acute and subacute allergic otitis media (mucoid) (sanguinous) (serous), recurrent, right ear
      H65.115 Acute and subacute allergic otitis media (mucoid) (sanguinous) (serous), recurrent, left ear
      H65.116 Acute and subacute allergic otitis media (mucoid) (sanguinous) (serous), recurrent, bilateral
      H65.117 Acute and subacute allergic otitis media (mucoid) (sanguinous) (serous), recurrent, unspecified ear

      H65.119 Acute and subacute allergic otitis media (mucoid) (sanguinous) (serous), unspecified ear

    ✓6ᵗʰ **H65.19 Other acute nonsuppurative otitis media**

      Acute and subacute mucoid otitis media
      Acute and subacute nonsuppurative otitis media NOS
      Acute and subacute sanguinous otitis media
      Acute and subacute seromucinous otitis media

      H65.191 Other acute nonsuppurative otitis media, right ear
      H65.192 Other acute nonsuppurative otitis media, left ear
      H65.193 Other acute nonsuppurative otitis media, bilateral
      H65.194 Other acute nonsuppurative otitis media, recurrent, right ear
      H65.195 Other acute nonsuppurative otitis media, recurrent, left ear
      H65.196 Other acute nonsuppurative otitis media, recurrent, bilateral
      H65.197 Other acute nonsuppurative otitis media recurrent, unspecified ear
      H65.199 Other acute nonsuppurative otitis media, unspecified ear

  ✓5ᵗʰ **H65.2 Chronic serous otitis media**

    Chronic tubotympanic catarrh

    H65.20 Chronic serous otitis media, unspecified ear
    H65.21 Chronic serous otitis media, right ear
    H65.22 Chronic serous otitis media, left ear
    H65.23 Chronic serous otitis media, bilateral

  ✓5ᵗʰ **H65.3 Chronic mucoid otitis media**

    Chronic mucinous otitis media
    Chronic secretory otitis media
    Chronic transudative otitis media
    Glue ear

    EXCLUDES 1   adhesive middle ear disease (H74.1)

    H65.30 Chronic mucoid otitis media, unspecified ear
    H65.31 Chronic mucoid otitis media, right ear
    H65.32 Chronic mucoid otitis media, left ear
    H65.33 Chronic mucoid otitis media, bilateral

  ✓5ᵗʰ **H65.4 Other chronic nonsuppurative otitis media**

    ✓6ᵗʰ **H65.41 Chronic allergic otitis media**

      H65.411 Chronic allergic otitis media, right ear
      H65.412 Chronic allergic otitis media, left ear
      H65.413 Chronic allergic otitis media, bilateral
      H65.419 Chronic allergic otitis media, unspecified ear

    ✓6ᵗʰ **H65.49 Other chronic nonsuppurative otitis media**

      Chronic exudative otitis media
      Chronic nonsuppurative otitis media NOS
      Chronic otitis media with effusion (nonpurulent)
      Chronic seromucinous otitis media

      H65.491 Other chronic nonsuppurative otitis media, right ear
      H65.492 Other chronic nonsuppurative otitis media, left ear
      H65.493 Other chronic nonsuppurative otitis media, bilateral
      H65.499 Other chronic nonsuppurative otitis media, unspecified ear

  ✓5ᵗʰ **H65.9 Unspecified nonsuppurative otitis media**

    Allergic otitis media NOS
    Catarrhal otitis media NOS
    Exudative otitis media NOS
    Mucoid otitis media NOS
    Otitis media with effusion (nonpurulent) NOS
    Secretory otitis media NOS
    Seromucinous otitis media NOS
    Serous otitis media NOS
    Transudative otitis media NOS

    H65.90 Unspecified nonsuppurative otitis media, unspecified ear
    H65.91 Unspecified nonsuppurative otitis media, right ear
    H65.92 Unspecified nonsuppurative otitis media, left ear
    H65.93 Unspecified nonsuppurative otitis media, bilateral

☑4ᵗʰ **H66 Suppurative and unspecified otitis media**

    INCLUDES   suppurative and unspecified otitis media with myringitis

    Use additional code to identify:

      exposure to environmental tobacco smoke (Z77.22)

      exposure to tobacco smoke in the perinatal period (P96.81)

      history of tobacco dependence (Z87.891)

      occupational exposure to environmental tobacco smoke (Z57.31)

      tobacco dependence (F17.-)

      tobacco use (Z72.0)

    AHA: 2016,1Q,34

☑5ᵗʰ   **H66.0**   Acute suppurative **otitis media**

    ☑6ᵗʰ   **H66.00**   **Acute suppurative otitis media** without spontaneous rupture of ear drum

      H66.001   Acute suppurative otitis media without spontaneous rupture of ear drum, right ear

      H66.002   Acute suppurative otitis media without spontaneous rupture of ear drum, left ear

      H66.003   Acute suppurative otitis media without spontaneous rupture of ear drum, bilateral

      H66.004   Acute suppurative otitis media without spontaneous rupture of ear drum, recurrent, right ear

      H66.005   Acute suppurative otitis media without spontaneous rupture of ear drum, recurrent, left ear

      H66.006   Acute suppurative otitis media without spontaneous rupture of ear drum, recurrent, bilateral

      H66.007   Acute suppurative otitis media without spontaneous rupture of ear drum, recurrent, unspecified ear

      H66.009   Acute suppurative otitis media without spontaneous rupture of ear drum, unspecified ear

    ☑6ᵗʰ   **H66.01**   **Acute suppurative otitis media** with spontaneous rupture of ear drum

      DEF: Sudden, severe inflammation of the middle ear, causing pressure that perforates the ear drum tissue.

      H66.011   Acute suppurative otitis media with spontaneous rupture of ear drum, right ear

      H66.012   Acute suppurative otitis media with spontaneous rupture of ear drum, left ear

      H66.013   Acute suppurative otitis media with spontaneous rupture of ear drum, bilateral

      H66.014   Acute suppurative otitis media with spontaneous rupture of ear drum, recurrent, right ear

      H66.015   Acute suppurative otitis media with spontaneous rupture of ear drum, recurrent, left ear

      H66.016   Acute suppurative otitis media with spontaneous rupture of ear drum, recurrent, bilateral

      H66.017   Acute suppurative otitis media with spontaneous rupture of ear drum, recurrent, unspecified ear

      H66.019   Acute suppurative otitis media with spontaneous rupture of ear drum, unspecified ear

☑5ᵗʰ   **H66.1**   Chronic tubotympanic suppurative **otitis media**

    Benign chronic suppurative otitis media

    Chronic tubotympanic disease

    Use additional code for any associated perforated tympanic membrane (H72.-)

    H66.10   Chronic tubotympanic suppurative otitis media, unspecified

    H66.11   Chronic tubotympanic suppurative otitis media, right ear

    H66.12   Chronic tubotympanic suppurative otitis media, left ear

    H66.13   Chronic tubotympanic suppurative otitis media, bilateral

☑5ᵗʰ   **H66.2**   Chronic atticoantral suppurative **otitis media**

    Chronic atticoantral disease

    Use additional code for any associated perforated tympanic membrane (H72.-)

    H66.20   Chronic atticoantral suppurative otitis media, unspecified ear

    H66.21   Chronic atticoantral suppurative otitis media, right ear

    H66.22   Chronic atticoantral suppurative otitis media, left ear

    H66.23   Chronic atticoantral suppurative otitis media, bilateral

☑5ᵗʰ   **H66.3**   Other chronic suppurative otitis media

    Chronic suppurative otitis media NOS

    Use additional code for any associated perforated tympanic membrane (H72.-)

    EXCLUDES 1   tuberculous otitis media (A18.6)

    ☑6ᵗʰ   **H66.3X**   Other chronic suppurative otitis media

      H66.3X1   Other chronic suppurative otitis media, right ear

      H66.3X2   Other chronic suppurative otitis media, left ear

      H66.3X3   Other chronic suppurative otitis media, bilateral

      H66.3X9   Other chronic suppurative otitis media, unspecified ear

☑5ᵗʰ   **H66.4**   Suppurative otitis media, unspecified

    Purulent otitis media NOS

    Use additional code for any associated perforated tympanic membrane (H72.-)

    H66.40   Suppurative otitis media, unspecified, unspecified ear

    H66.41   Suppurative otitis media, unspecified, right ear

    H66.42   Suppurative otitis media, unspecified, left ear

    H66.43   Suppurative otitis media, unspecified, bilateral

☑5ᵗʰ   **H66.9**   Otitis media, unspecified

    Otitis media NOS

    Acute otitis media NOS

    Chronic otitis media NOS

    Use additional code for any associated perforated tympanic membrane (H72.-)

    H66.90   Otitis media, unspecified, unspecified ear

    H66.91   Otitis media, unspecified, right ear

    H66.92   Otitis media, unspecified, left ear

    H66.93   Otitis media, unspecified, bilateral

☑4ᵗʰ **H67 Otitis media in diseases classified elsewhere**

    Code first underlying disease, such as:

      plasminogen deficiency (E88.02)

      viral disease NEC (B00-B34)

    Use additional code for any associated perforated tympanic membrane (H72.-)

    EXCLUDES 1   otitis media in:

      influenza (J09.X9, J10.83, J11.83)

      measles (B05.3)

      scarlet fever (A38.0)

      tuberculosis (A18.6)

    H67.1   *Otitis media in diseases classified elsewhere, right ear*

    H67.2   *Otitis media in diseases classified elsewhere, left ear*

    H67.3   *Otitis media in diseases classified elsewhere, bilateral*

    H67.9   *Otitis media in diseases classified elsewhere, unspecified ear*

☑4ᵗʰ **H68 Eustachian salpingitis and obstruction**

    DEF: Eustachian tube: Internal channel between the tympanic cavity and the nasopharynx that equalizes internal pressure to the outside pressure and drains mucous production from the middle ear.

☑5ᵗʰ   **H68.0**   Eustachian salpingitis

    ☑6ᵗʰ   **H68.00**   Unspecified Eustachian salpingitis

      H68.001   Unspecified Eustachian salpingitis, right ear

      H68.002   Unspecified Eustachian salpingitis, left ear

      H68.003   Unspecified Eustachian salpingitis, bilateral

      H68.009   Unspecified Eustachian salpingitis, unspecified ear

    ☑6ᵗʰ   **H68.01**   Acute Eustachian salpingitis

      H68.011   Acute Eustachian salpingitis, right ear

      H68.012   Acute Eustachian salpingitis, left ear

      H68.013   Acute Eustachian salpingitis, bilateral

      H68.019   Acute Eustachian salpingitis, unspecified ear

    ☑6ᵗʰ   **H68.02**   Chronic Eustachian salpingitis

      H68.021   Chronic Eustachian salpingitis, right ear

      H68.022   Chronic Eustachian salpingitis, left ear

☑ Additional Character Required   ☑x7ᵗʰ Placeholder Alert   Manifestation   Unspecified Dx   ❶ QPP   UPD Unacceptable PDx

H68.023　Chronic Eustachian salpingitis, bilateral

H68.029　Chronic Eustachian salpingitis, unspecified ear

√5ᵗʰ **H68.1**　Obstruction of Eustachian tube
Stenosis of Eustachian tube
Stricture of Eustachian tube

√6ᵗʰ **H68.10**　Unspecified obstruction of Eustachian tube

H68.101　Unspecified obstruction of Eustachian tube, right ear

H68.102　Unspecified obstruction of Eustachian tube, left ear

H68.103　Unspecified obstruction of Eustachian tube, bilateral

H68.109　Unspecified obstruction of Eustachian tube, unspecified ear

√6ᵗʰ **H68.11**　Osseous obstruction of Eustachian tube

H68.111　Osseous obstruction of Eustachian tube, right ear

H68.112　Osseous obstruction of Eustachian tube, left ear

H68.113　Osseous obstruction of Eustachian tube, bilateral

H68.119　Osseous obstruction of Eustachian tube, unspecified ear

√6ᵗʰ **H68.12**　Intrinsic cartilagenous obstruction of Eustachian tube

H68.121　Intrinsic cartilagenous obstruction of Eustachian tube, right ear

H68.122　Intrinsic cartilagenous obstruction of Eustachian tube, left ear

H68.123　Intrinsic cartilagenous obstruction of Eustachian tube, bilateral

H68.129　Intrinsic cartilagenous obstruction of Eustachian tube, unspecified ear

√6ᵗʰ **H68.13**　Extrinsic cartilagenous obstruction of Eustachian tube
Compression of Eustachian tube

H68.131　Extrinsic cartilagenous obstruction of Eustachian tube, right ear

H68.132　Extrinsic cartilagenous obstruction of Eustachian tube, left ear

H68.133　Extrinsic cartilagenous obstruction of Eustachian tube, bilateral

H68.139　Extrinsic cartilagenous obstruction of Eustachian tube, unspecified ear

√4ᵗʰ **H69**　Other and unspecified disorders of Eustachian tube

DEF: Eustachian tube: Internal channel between the tympanic cavity and the nasopharynx that equalizes internal pressure to the outside pressure and drains mucous production from the middle ear.

√5ᵗʰ **H69.0**　Patulous Eustachian tube

H69.00　Patulous Eustachian tube, unspecified ear

H69.01　Patulous Eustachian tube, right ear

H69.02　Patulous Eustachian tube, left ear

H69.03　Patulous Eustachian tube, bilateral

√5ᵗʰ **H69.8**　Other specified disorders of Eustachian tube

H69.80　Other specified disorders of Eustachian tube, unspecified ear

H69.81　Other specified disorders of Eustachian tube, right ear

H69.82　Other specified disorders of Eustachian tube, left ear

H69.83　Other specified disorders of Eustachian tube, bilateral

√5ᵗʰ **H69.9**　Unspecified Eustachian tube disorder

H69.90　Unspecified Eustachian tube disorder, unspecified ear

H69.91　Unspecified Eustachian tube disorder, right ear

H69.92　Unspecified Eustachian tube disorder, left ear

H69.93　Unspecified Eustachian tube disorder, bilateral

√4ᵗʰ **H70**　Mastoiditis and related conditions

√5ᵗʰ **H70.0**　Acute mastoiditis
Abscess of mastoid
Empyema of mastoid

√6ᵗʰ **H70.00**　Acute mastoiditis without complications

H70.001　Acute mastoiditis without complications, right ear

H70.002　Acute mastoiditis without complications, left ear

H70.003　Acute mastoiditis without complications, bilateral

H70.009　Acute mastoiditis without complications, unspecified ear

√6ᵗʰ **H70.01**　Subperiosteal abscess of mastoid

H70.011　Subperiosteal abscess of mastoid, right ear

H70.012　Subperiosteal abscess of mastoid, left ear

H70.013　Subperiosteal abscess of mastoid, bilateral

H70.019　Subperiosteal abscess of mastoid, unspecified ear

√6ᵗʰ **H70.09**　Acute mastoiditis with other complications

H70.091　Acute mastoiditis with other complications, right ear

H70.092　Acute mastoiditis with other complications, left ear

H70.093　Acute mastoiditis with other complications, bilateral

H70.099　Acute mastoiditis with other complications, unspecified ear

√5ᵗʰ **H70.1**　Chronic mastoiditis
Caries of mastoid
Fistula of mastoid
EXCLUDES 1　tuberculous mastoiditis (A18.03)

H70.10　Chronic mastoiditis, unspecified ear

H70.11　Chronic mastoiditis, right ear

H70.12　Chronic mastoiditis, left ear

H70.13　Chronic mastoiditis, bilateral

√5ᵗʰ **H70.2**　Petrositis
Inflammation of petrous bone

√6ᵗʰ **H70.20**　Unspecified petrositis

H70.201　Unspecified petrositis, right ear

H70.202　Unspecified petrositis, left ear

H70.203　Unspecified petrositis, bilateral

H70.209　Unspecified petrositis, unspecified ear

√6ᵗʰ **H70.21**　Acute petrositis

DEF: Sudden, severe inflammation of the petrous temporal bone behind the ear, associated with a middle ear infection.

H70.211　Acute petrositis, right ear

H70.212　Acute petrositis, left ear

H70.213　Acute petrositis, bilateral

H70.219　Acute petrositis, unspecified ear

√6ᵗʰ **H70.22**　Chronic petrositis

H70.221　Chronic petrositis, right ear

H70.222　Chronic petrositis, left ear

H70.223　Chronic petrositis, bilateral

H70.229　Chronic petrositis, unspecified ear

√5ᵗʰ **H70.8**　Other mastoiditis and related conditions

EXCLUDES 1　preauricular sinus and cyst (Q18.1)
sinus, fistula, and cyst of branchial cleft (Q18.0)

√6ᵗʰ **H70.81**　Postauricular fistula

H70.811　Postauricular fistula, right ear

H70.812　Postauricular fistula, left ear

H70.813　Postauricular fistula, bilateral

H70.819　Postauricular fistula, unspecified ear

√6ᵗʰ **H70.89**　Other mastoiditis and related conditions

H70.891　Other mastoiditis and related conditions, right ear

H70.892　Other mastoiditis and related conditions, left ear

H70.893　Other mastoiditis and related conditions, bilateral

H70.899　Other mastoiditis and related conditions, unspecified ear

√5ᵗʰ **H70.9**　Unspecified mastoiditis

H70.90　Unspecified mastoiditis, unspecified ear

H70.91　Unspecified mastoiditis, right ear

H70.92　Unspecified mastoiditis, left ear

H70.93　Unspecified mastoiditis, bilateral

| HCC CMS-HCC | Rx Rx HCC | ESR ESRD HCC | COM Commercial HCC | N Newborn: 0 | P Pediatric: 0-17 | M Maternity: 9-64 | A Adult: 15-124 |

652
ICD-10-CM 2023

✓4ᵗʰ H71 Cholesteatoma of middle ear

EXCLUDES 2 cholesteatoma of external ear (H60.4-)
recurrent cholesteatoma of postmastoidectomy cavity
(H95.0-)

AHA: 2021,3Q,8
DEF: Cholesteatoma: Noncancerous cyst-like mass of cell debris, including cholesterol and epithelial cells resulting from trauma, repeated or improperly healed infections, and congenital enclosure of epidermal cells.

Cholesteatoma of Middle Ear

Middle ear chamber
Ear drum
Cholesteatoma sac

✓5ᵗʰ H71.0 Cholesteatoma of attic

H71.00 Cholesteatoma of attic, unspecified ear
H71.01 Cholesteatoma of attic, right ear
H71.02 Cholesteatoma of attic, left ear
H71.03 Cholesteatoma of attic, bilateral

✓5ᵗʰ H71.1 Cholesteatoma of tympanum

H71.10 Cholesteatoma of tympanum, unspecified ear
H71.11 Cholesteatoma of tympanum, right ear
H71.12 Cholesteatoma of tympanum, left ear
H71.13 Cholesteatoma of tympanum, bilateral

✓5ᵗʰ H71.2 Cholesteatoma of mastoid

H71.20 Cholesteatoma of mastoid, unspecified ear
H71.21 Cholesteatoma of mastoid, right ear
H71.22 Cholesteatoma of mastoid, left ear
H71.23 Cholesteatoma of mastoid, bilateral

✓5ᵗʰ H71.3 Diffuse cholesteatosis

AHA: 2021,3Q,8

H71.30 Diffuse cholesteatosis, unspecified ear
H71.31 Diffuse cholesteatosis, right ear
H71.32 Diffuse cholesteatosis, left ear
H71.33 Diffuse cholesteatosis, bilateral

✓5ᵗʰ H71.9 Unspecified cholesteatoma

H71.90 Unspecified cholesteatoma, unspecified ear
H71.91 Unspecified cholesteatoma, right ear
H71.92 Unspecified cholesteatoma, left ear
H71.93 Unspecified cholesteatoma, bilateral

✓4ᵗʰ H72 Perforation of tympanic membrane

INCLUDES persistent post-traumatic perforation of ear drum
postinflammatory perforation of ear drum
Code first any associated otitis media (H65.-, H66.1-, H66.2-, H66.3-, H66.4-, H66.9-, H67.-)

EXCLUDES 1 acute suppurative otitis media with rupture of the tympanic
membrane (H66.01-)
traumatic rupture of ear drum (S09.2-)

✓5ᵗʰ H72.0 Central perforation of tympanic membrane

H72.00 Central perforation of tympanic membrane, unspecified ear
H72.01 Central perforation of tympanic membrane, right ear
H72.02 Central perforation of tympanic membrane, left ear
H72.03 Central perforation of tympanic membrane, bilateral

✓5ᵗʰ H72.1 Attic perforation of tympanic membrane

Perforation of pars flaccida
H72.10 Attic perforation of tympanic membrane, unspecified ear
H72.11 Attic perforation of tympanic membrane, right ear
H72.12 Attic perforation of tympanic membrane, left ear

H72.13 Attic perforation of tympanic membrane, bilateral

✓5ᵗʰ H72.2 Other marginal perforations of tympanic membrane

✓6ᵗʰ H72.2X Other marginal perforations of tympanic membrane

H72.2X1 Other marginal perforations of tympanic membrane, right ear
H72.2X2 Other marginal perforations of tympanic membrane, left ear
H72.2X3 Other marginal perforations of tympanic membrane, bilateral
H72.2X9 Other marginal perforations of tympanic membrane, unspecified ear

✓5ᵗʰ H72.8 Other perforations of tympanic membrane

✓6ᵗʰ H72.81 Multiple perforations of tympanic membrane

H72.811 Multiple perforations of tympanic membrane, right ear
H72.812 Multiple perforations of tympanic membrane, left ear
H72.813 Multiple perforations of tympanic membrane, bilateral
H72.819 Multiple perforations of tympanic membrane, unspecified ear

✓6ᵗʰ H72.82 Total perforations of tympanic membrane

H72.821 Total perforations of tympanic membrane, right ear
H72.822 Total perforations of tympanic membrane, left ear
H72.823 Total perforations of tympanic membrane, bilateral
H72.829 Total perforations of tympanic membrane, unspecified ear

✓5ᵗʰ H72.9 Unspecified perforation of tympanic membrane

H72.90 Unspecified perforation of tympanic membrane, unspecified ear
H72.91 Unspecified perforation of tympanic membrane, right ear
H72.92 Unspecified perforation of tympanic membrane, left ear
H72.93 Unspecified perforation of tympanic membrane, bilateral

✓4ᵗʰ H73 Other disorders of tympanic membrane

✓5ᵗʰ H73.0 Acute myringitis

EXCLUDES 1 acute myringitis with otitis media (H65, H66)

✓6ᵗʰ H73.00 Unspecified acute myringitis

Acute tympanitis NOS
H73.001 Acute myringitis, right ear
H73.002 Acute myringitis, left ear
H73.003 Acute myringitis, bilateral
H73.009 Acute myringitis, unspecified ear

✓6ᵗʰ H73.01 Bullous myringitis

DEF: Bacterial or viral otitis media that is characterized by the appearance of serous or hemorrhagic blebs on the ear drum and sudden onset of severe pain in ear.

H73.011 Bullous myringitis, right ear
H73.012 Bullous myringitis, left ear
H73.013 Bullous myringitis, bilateral
H73.019 Bullous myringitis, unspecified ear

✓6ᵗʰ H73.09 Other acute myringitis

H73.091 Other acute myringitis, right ear
H73.092 Other acute myringitis, left ear
H73.093 Other acute myringitis, bilateral
H73.099 Other acute myringitis, unspecified ear

✓5ᵗʰ H73.1 Chronic myringitis

Chronic tympanitis
EXCLUDES 1 chronic myringitis with otitis media (H65, H66)

H73.10 Chronic myringitis, unspecified ear
H73.11 Chronic myringitis, right ear
H73.12 Chronic myringitis, left ear
H73.13 Chronic myringitis, bilateral

✓5ᵗʰ H73.2 Unspecified myringitis

H73.20 Unspecified myringitis, unspecified ear
H73.21 Unspecified myringitis, right ear
H73.22 Unspecified myringitis, left ear
H73.23 Unspecified myringitis, bilateral

✓5ᵗʰ H73.8 Other specified disorders of tympanic membrane

✓6ᵗʰ H73.81 Atrophic flaccid tympanic membrane

H73.811 Atrophic flaccid tympanic membrane, right ear

☑ Additional Character Required   ✓x7ᵗʰ Placeholder Alert   Manifestation   Unspecified Dx   Q QPP   UPD Unacceptable PDx

Chapter 8. Diseases of the Ear and Mastoid Process

H73.812   Atrophic flaccid tympanic membrane, left ear

H73.813   Atrophic flaccid tympanic membrane, bilateral

H73.819   Atrophic flaccid tympanic membrane, unspecified ear

√6ᵗʰ **H73.82**   Atrophic nonflaccid tympanic membrane

H73.821   Atrophic nonflaccid tympanic membrane, right ear

H73.822   Atrophic nonflaccid tympanic membrane, left ear

H73.823   Atrophic nonflaccid tympanic membrane, bilateral

H73.829   Atrophic nonflaccid tympanic membrane, unspecified ear

√6ᵗʰ **H73.89**   Other specified disorders of tympanic membrane

H73.891   Other specified disorders of tympanic membrane, right ear

H73.892   Other specified disorders of tympanic membrane, left ear

H73.893   Other specified disorders of tympanic membrane, bilateral

H73.899   Other specified disorders of tympanic membrane, unspecified ear

√5ᵗʰ **H73.9**   Unspecified disorder of tympanic membrane

H73.90   Unspecified disorder of tympanic membrane, unspecified ear

H73.91   Unspecified disorder of tympanic membrane, right ear

H73.92   Unspecified disorder of tympanic membrane, left ear

H73.93   Unspecified disorder of tympanic membrane, bilateral

√4ᵗʰ **H74**   **Other disorders of middle ear mastoid**

EXCLUDES 2   mastoiditis (H70.-)

√5ᵗʰ **H74.0**   Tympanosclerosis

DEF: Calcification of tissue in the ear drum, middle ear bones, and middle ear canal.

H74.01   Tympanosclerosis, right ear

H74.02   Tympanosclerosis, left ear

H74.03   Tympanosclerosis, bilateral

H74.09   Tympanosclerosis, unspecified ear

√5ᵗʰ **H74.1**   Adhesive middle ear disease

Adhesive otitis

EXCLUDES 1   glue ear (H65.3-)

H74.11   Adhesive right middle ear disease

H74.12   Adhesive left middle ear disease

H74.13   Adhesive middle ear disease, bilateral

H74.19   Adhesive middle ear disease, unspecified ear

√5ᵗʰ **H74.2**   Discontinuity and dislocation of ear ossicles

H74.20   Discontinuity and dislocation of ear ossicles, unspecified ear

H74.21   Discontinuity and dislocation of right ear ossicles

H74.22   Discontinuity and dislocation of left ear ossicles

H74.23   Discontinuity and dislocation of ear ossicles, bilateral

√5ᵗʰ **H74.3**   Other acquired abnormalities of ear ossicles

√6ᵗʰ **H74.31**   Ankylosis of ear ossicles

H74.311   Ankylosis of ear ossicles, right ear

H74.312   Ankylosis of ear ossicles, left ear

H74.313   Ankylosis of ear ossicles, bilateral

H74.319   Ankylosis of ear ossicles, unspecified ear

√6ᵗʰ **H74.32**   Partial loss of ear ossicles

H74.321   Partial loss of ear ossicles, right ear

H74.322   Partial loss of ear ossicles, left ear

H74.323   Partial loss of ear ossicles, bilateral

H74.329   Partial loss of ear ossicles, unspecified ear

√6ᵗʰ **H74.39**   Other acquired abnormalities of ear ossicles

H74.391   Other acquired abnormalities of right ear ossicles

H74.392   Other acquired abnormalities of left ear ossicles

H74.393   Other acquired abnormalities of ear ossicles, bilateral

H74.399   Other acquired abnormalities of ear ossicles, unspecified ear

√5ᵗʰ **H74.4**   Polyp of middle ear

H74.40   Polyp of middle ear, unspecified ear

H74.41   Polyp of right middle ear

H74.42   Polyp of left middle ear

H74.43   Polyp of middle ear, bilateral

√5ᵗʰ **H74.8**   Other specified disorders of middle ear and mastoid

√6ᵗʰ **H74.8X**   Other specified disorders of middle ear and mastoid

H74.8X1   Other specified disorders of right middle ear and mastoid

H74.8X2   Other specified disorders of left middle ear and mastoid

H74.8X3   Other specified disorders of middle ear and mastoid, bilateral

H74.8X9   Other specified disorders of middle ear and mastoid, unspecified ear

√5ᵗʰ **H74.9**   Unspecified disorder of middle ear and mastoid

H74.90   Unspecified disorder of middle ear and mastoid, unspecified ear

H74.91   Unspecified disorder of right middle ear and mastoid

H74.92   Unspecified disorder of left middle ear and mastoid

H74.93   Unspecified disorder of middle ear and mastoid, bilateral

√4ᵗʰ **H75**   **Other disorders of middle ear and mastoid in diseases classified elsewhere**

Code first underlying disease

√5ᵗʰ **H75.0**   Mastoiditis in infectious and parasitic diseases classified elsewhere

EXCLUDES 1   mastoiditis (in):

syphilis (A52.77)

tuberculosis (A18.03)

H75.00   Mastoiditis in infectious and parasitic diseases classified elsewhere, unspecified ear

H75.01   Mastoiditis in infectious and parasitic diseases classified elsewhere, right ear

H75.02   Mastoiditis in infectious and parasitic diseases classified elsewhere, left ear

H75.03   Mastoiditis in infectious and parasitic diseases classified elsewhere, bilateral

√5ᵗʰ **H75.8**   Other specified disorders of middle ear and mastoid in diseases classified elsewhere

H75.80   Other specified disorders of middle ear and mastoid in diseases classified elsewhere, unspecified ear

H75.81   Other specified disorders of right middle ear and mastoid in diseases classified elsewhere

H75.82   Other specified disorders of left middle ear and mastoid in diseases classified elsewhere

H75.83   Other specified disorders of middle ear and mastoid in diseases classified elsewhere, bilateral

Diseases of inner ear (H80-H83)

√4ᵗʰ **H80**   **Otosclerosis**

INCLUDES   otospongiosis

√5ᵗʰ **H80.0**   Otosclerosis involving oval window, nonobliterative

H80.00   Otosclerosis involving oval window, nonobliterative, unspecified ear

H80.01   Otosclerosis involving oval window, nonobliterative, right ear

H80.02   Otosclerosis involving oval window, nonobliterative, left ear

H80.03   Otosclerosis involving oval window, nonobliterative, bilateral

√5ᵗʰ **H80.1**   Otosclerosis involving oval window, obliterative

H80.10   Otosclerosis involving oval window, obliterative, unspecified ear

H80.11   Otosclerosis involving oval window, obliterative, right ear

H80.12   Otosclerosis involving oval window, obliterative, left ear

H80.13   Otosclerosis involving oval window, obliterative, bilateral

√5ᵗʰ **H80.2**   Cochlear otosclerosis

Otosclerosis involving otic capsule

Otosclerosis involving round window

H80.20   Cochlear otosclerosis, unspecified ear

H80.21   Cochlear otosclerosis, right ear

H80.22   Cochlear otosclerosis, left ear

H80.23   Cochlear otosclerosis, bilateral

✓5ᵗʰ **H80.8 Other otosclerosis**
     H80.80 **Other otosclerosis, unspecified ear**
     H80.81 **Other otosclerosis, right ear**
     H80.82 **Other otosclerosis, left ear**
     H80.83 **Other otosclerosis, bilateral**

✓5ᵗʰ **H80.9 Unspecified otosclerosis**
     H80.90 **Unspecified otosclerosis, unspecified ear**
     H80.91 **Unspecified otosclerosis, right ear**
     H80.92 **Unspecified otosclerosis, left ear**
     H80.93 **Unspecified otosclerosis, bilateral**

✓4ᵗʰ **H81 Disorders of vestibular function**
     EXCLUDES 1   epidemic vertigo (A88.1)
                  vertigo NOS (R42)

✓5ᵗʰ **H81.0 Ménière's disease**
     Labyrinthine hydrops
     Ménière's syndrome or vertigo
     DEF: Distended membranous labyrinth of the middle ear from fluctuating pressure of fluid (hydrops) that causes vertigo, tinnitus, pressure, and hearing loss that may last on and off for several hours. Episodes may occur in clusters or may subside for weeks, months, or even years.
     H81.01 **Ménière's disease, right ear**
     H81.02 **Ménière's disease, left ear**
     H81.03 **Ménière's disease, bilateral**
     H81.09 **Ménière's disease, unspecified ear**

✓5ᵗʰ **H81.1 Benign paroxysmal vertigo**
     H81.10 **Benign paroxysmal vertigo, unspecified ear** ◘
     H81.11 **Benign paroxysmal vertigo, right ear** ◘
     H81.12 **Benign paroxysmal vertigo, left ear** ◘
     H81.13 **Benign paroxysmal vertigo, bilateral** ◘

✓5ᵗʰ **H81.2 Vestibular neuronitis**
     DEF: Transient benign vertigo caused by inflammation of the vestibular nerve. It is characterized by response to caloric stimulation on one side and nystagmus with rhythmic movement of the eyes. Normal auditory function is present.
     H81.20 **Vestibular neuronitis, unspecified ear**
     H81.21 **Vestibular neuronitis, right ear**
     H81.22 **Vestibular neuronitis, left ear**
     H81.23 **Vestibular neuronitis, bilateral**

✓5ᵗʰ **H81.3 Other peripheral vertigo**
     ✓6ᵗʰ **H81.31 Aural vertigo**
         H81.311 **Aural vertigo, right ear**
         H81.312 **Aural vertigo, left ear**
         H81.313 **Aural vertigo, bilateral**
         H81.319 **Aural vertigo, unspecified ear**
     ✓6ᵗʰ **H81.39 Other peripheral vertigo**
         Lermoyez' syndrome
         Otogenic vertigo
         Peripheral vertigo NOS
         H81.391 **Other peripheral vertigo, right ear**
         H81.392 **Other peripheral vertigo, left ear**
         H81.393 **Other peripheral vertigo, bilateral**
         H81.399 **Other peripheral vertigo, unspecified ear**

H81.4 Vertigo of central origin
     Central positional nystagmus

✓5ᵗʰ **H81.8 Other disorders of vestibular function**
     ✓6ᵗʰ **H81.8X Other disorders of vestibular function**
         H81.8X1 **Other disorders of vestibular function, right ear**
         H81.8X2 **Other disorders of vestibular function, left ear**
         H81.8X3 **Other disorders of vestibular function, bilateral**
         H81.8X9 **Other disorders of vestibular function, unspecified ear**
         AHA: 2022,2Q,12

✓5ᵗʰ **H81.9 Unspecified disorder of vestibular function**
     Vertiginous syndrome NOS
     H81.90 **Unspecified disorder of vestibular function, unspecified ear**
     H81.91 **Unspecified disorder of vestibular function, right ear**
     H81.92 **Unspecified disorder of vestibular function, left ear**
     H81.93 **Unspecified disorder of vestibular function, bilateral**

✓4ᵗʰ **H82 Vertiginous syndromes in diseases classified elsewhere**
     Code first underlying disease
     EXCLUDES 1   epidemic vertigo (A88.1)
     H82.1 *Vertiginous syndromes in diseases classified elsewhere, right ear*
     H82.2 *Vertiginous syndromes in diseases classified elsewhere, left ear*
     H82.3 *Vertiginous syndromes in diseases classified elsewhere, bilateral*
     H82.9 *Vertiginous syndromes in diseases classified elsewhere, unspecified ear*

✓4ᵗʰ **H83 Other diseases of inner ear**
     ✓5ᵗʰ **H83.0 Labyrinthitis**
         DEF: Inflammation of the inner ear, or labyrinth, characterized by pus, vertigo, dizziness, nausea, and hearing loss.
         H83.01 **Labyrinthitis, right ear**
         H83.02 **Labyrinthitis, left ear**
         H83.03 **Labyrinthitis, bilateral**
         H83.09 **Labyrinthitis, unspecified ear**
     ✓5ᵗʰ **H83.1 Labyrinthine fistula**
         H83.11 **Labyrinthine fistula, right ear**
         H83.12 **Labyrinthine fistula, left ear**
         H83.13 **Labyrinthine fistula, bilateral**
         H83.19 **Labyrinthine fistula, unspecified ear**
     ✓5ᵗʰ **H83.2 Labyrinthine dysfunction**
         Labyrinthine hypersensitivity
         Labyrinthine hypofunction
         Labyrinthine loss of function
         DEF: Decreased function of the labyrinth sensors.
         ✓6ᵗʰ **H83.2X Labyrinthine dysfunction**
             H83.2X1 **Labyrinthine dysfunction, right ear**
             H83.2X2 **Labyrinthine dysfunction, left ear**
             H83.2X3 **Labyrinthine dysfunction, bilateral**
             H83.2X9 **Labyrinthine dysfunction, unspecified ear**
     ✓5ᵗʰ **H83.3 Noise effects on inner ear**
         Acoustic trauma of inner ear
         Noise-induced hearing loss of inner ear
         ✓6ᵗʰ **H83.3X Noise effects on inner ear**
             H83.3X1 **Noise effects on right inner ear**
             H83.3X2 **Noise effects on left inner ear**
             H83.3X3 **Noise effects on inner ear, bilateral**
             H83.3X9 **Noise effects on inner ear, unspecified ear**
     ✓5ᵗʰ **H83.8 Other specified diseases of inner ear**
         ✓6ᵗʰ **H83.8X Other specified diseases of inner ear**
             H83.8X1 **Other specified diseases of right inner ear**
             H83.8X2 **Other specified diseases of left inner ear**
             H83.8X3 **Other specified diseases of inner ear, bilateral**
             H83.8X9 **Other specified diseases of inner ear, unspecified ear**
     ✓5ᵗʰ **H83.9 Unspecified disease of inner ear**
         H83.90 **Unspecified disease of inner ear, unspecified ear**
         H83.91 **Unspecified disease of right inner ear**
         H83.92 **Unspecified disease of left inner ear**
         H83.93 **Unspecified disease of inner ear, bilateral**

Other disorders of ear (H90-H94)

✓4ᵗʰ **H90 Conductive and sensorineural hearing loss**
     EXCLUDES 1   deaf nonspeaking NEC (H91.3)
                deafness NOS (H91.9-)
                hearing loss NOS (H91.9-)
                noise-induced hearing loss (H83.3-)
                ototoxic hearing loss (H91.0-)
                sudden (idiopathic) hearing loss (H91.2-)
     AHA: 2015,2Q,7
     DEF: Conductive hearing loss: Hearing loss due to the inability of soundwaves to move from the outer (external) ear to the inner ear.
     DEF: Sensorineural hearing loss: Hearing loss that occurs from damage to the hair cells of the inner ear or problems with the nerve pathways from the inner ear to the brain.
     H90.0 Conductive hearing loss, bilateral

Chapter 8. Diseases of the Ear and Mastoid Process

H90.1–H93.A3

✓5ᵗʰ **H90.1** Conductive hearing loss, unilateral with unrestricted hearing on the contralateral side

    H90.11 Conductive hearing loss, unilateral, right ear, with unrestricted hearing on the contralateral side

    H90.12 Conductive hearing loss, unilateral, left ear, with unrestricted hearing on the contralateral side

H90.2 Conductive hearing loss, unspecified

    Conductive deafness NOS

H90.3 Sensorineural hearing loss, bilateral

✓5ᵗʰ **H90.4** Sensorineural hearing loss, unilateral with unrestricted hearing on the contralateral side

    H90.41 Sensorineural hearing loss, unilateral, right ear, with unrestricted hearing on the contralateral side

    H90.42 Sensorineural hearing loss, unilateral, left ear, with unrestricted hearing on the contralateral side

H90.5 Unspecified sensorineural hearing loss

    Central hearing loss NOS

    Congenital deafness NOS

    Neural hearing loss NOS

    Perceptive hearing loss NOS

    Sensorineural deafness NOS

    Sensory hearing loss NOS

    EXCLUDES 1   abnormal auditory perception (H93.2-)

                 psychogenic deafness (F44.6)

H90.6 Mixed conductive and sensorineural hearing loss, bilateral

    AHA: 2015,2Q,7

✓5ᵗʰ **H90.7** Mixed conductive and sensorineural hearing loss, unilateral with unrestricted hearing on the contralateral side

    H90.71 Mixed conductive and sensorineural hearing loss, unilateral, right ear, with unrestricted hearing on the contralateral side

    H90.72 Mixed conductive and sensorineural hearing loss, unilateral, left ear, with unrestricted hearing on the contralateral side

H90.8 Mixed conductive and sensorineural hearing loss, unspecified

✓5ᵗʰ **H90.A** Conductive and sensorineural hearing loss with restricted hearing on the contralateral side

    AHA: 2016,4Q,23-25

  ✓6ᵗʰ **H90.A1** Conductive hearing loss, unilateral, with restricted hearing on the contralateral side

      H90.A11 Conductive hearing loss, unilateral, right ear with restricted hearing on the contralateral side

      H90.A12 Conductive hearing loss, unilateral, left ear with restricted hearing on the contralateral side

  ✓6ᵗʰ **H90.A2** Sensorineural hearing loss, unilateral, with restricted hearing on the contralateral side

      H90.A21 Sensorineural hearing loss, unilateral, right ear, with restricted hearing on the contralateral side

      H90.A22 Sensorineural hearing loss, unilateral, left ear, with restricted hearing on the contralateral side

  ✓6ᵗʰ **H90.A3** Mixed conductive and sensorineural hearing loss, unilateral with restricted hearing on the contralateral side

      H90.A31 Mixed conductive and sensorineural hearing loss, unilateral, right ear with restricted hearing on the contralateral side

      H90.A32 Mixed conductive and sensorineural hearing, unilateral, left ear with restricted hearing on the contralateral side

✓4ᵗʰ **H91** Other and unspecified hearing loss

    EXCLUDES 1   abnormal auditory perception (H93.2-)

                 hearing loss as classified in H90.-

                 impacted cerumen (H61.2-)

                 noise-induced hearing loss (H83.3-)

                 psychogenic deafness (F44.6)

                 transient ischemic deafness (H93.01-)

  ✓5ᵗʰ **H91.0** Ototoxic hearing loss

    Code first poisoning due to drug or toxin, if applicable (T36-T65 with fifth or sixth character 1-4 or 6)

    Use additional code for adverse effect, if applicable, to identify drug (T36-T50 with fifth or sixth character 5)

    H91.01 Ototoxic hearing loss, right ear

    H91.02 Ototoxic hearing loss, left ear

    H91.03 Ototoxic hearing loss, bilateral

    H91.09 Ototoxic hearing loss, unspecified ear

✓5ᵗʰ **H91.1** Presbycusis

    Presbyacusia

    H91.10 Presbycusis, unspecified ear

    H91.11 Presbycusis, right ear

    H91.12 Presbycusis, left ear

    H91.13 Presbycusis, bilateral

✓5ᵗʰ **H91.2** Sudden idiopathic hearing loss

    Sudden hearing loss NOS

    H91.20 Sudden idiopathic hearing loss, unspecified ear

    H91.21 Sudden idiopathic hearing loss, right ear

    H91.22 Sudden idiopathic hearing loss, left ear

    H91.23 Sudden idiopathic hearing loss, bilateral

H91.3 Deaf nonspeaking, not elsewhere classified

✓5ᵗʰ **H91.8** Other specified hearing loss

  ✓6ᵗʰ **H91.8X** Other specified hearing loss

    H91.8X1 Other specified hearing loss, right ear

    H91.8X2 Other specified hearing loss, left ear

    H91.8X3 Other specified hearing loss, bilateral

    H91.8X9 Other specified hearing loss, unspecified ear

✓5ᵗʰ **H91.9** Unspecified hearing loss

    Deafness NOS

    High frequency deafness

    Low frequency deafness

    H91.90 Unspecified hearing loss, unspecified ear

    H91.91 Unspecified hearing loss, right ear

    H91.92 Unspecified hearing loss, left ear

    H91.93 Unspecified hearing loss, bilateral

✓4ᵗʰ **H92** Otalgia and effusion of ear

  ✓5ᵗʰ **H92.0** Otalgia

    H92.01 Otalgia, right ear

    H92.02 Otalgia, left ear

    H92.03 Otalgia, bilateral

    H92.09 Otalgia, unspecified ear

  ✓5ᵗʰ **H92.1** Otorrhea

    EXCLUDES 1   leakage of cerebrospinal fluid through ear (G96.0)

    H92.10 Otorrhea, unspecified ear

    H92.11 Otorrhea, right ear

    H92.12 Otorrhea, left ear

    H92.13 Otorrhea, bilateral

  ✓5ᵗʰ **H92.2** Otorrhagia

    EXCLUDES 1   traumatic otorrhagia - code to injury

    H92.20 Otorrhagia, unspecified ear

    H92.21 Otorrhagia, right ear

    H92.22 Otorrhagia, left ear

    H92.23 Otorrhagia, bilateral

✓4ᵗʰ **H93** Other disorders of ear, not elsewhere classified

  ✓5ᵗʰ **H93.0** Degenerative and vascular disorders of ear

    EXCLUDES 1   presbycusis (H91.1)

    ✓6ᵗʰ **H93.01** Transient ischemic deafness

      H93.011 Transient ischemic deafness, right ear

      H93.012 Transient ischemic deafness, left ear

      H93.013 Transient ischemic deafness, bilateral

      H93.019 Transient ischemic deafness, unspecified ear

    ✓6ᵗʰ **H93.09** Unspecified degenerative and vascular disorders of ear

      H93.091 Unspecified degenerative and vascular disorders of right ear

      H93.092 Unspecified degenerative and vascular disorders of left ear

      H93.093 Unspecified degenerative and vascular disorders of ear, bilateral

      H93.099 Unspecified degenerative and vascular disorders of unspecified ear

  ✓5ᵗʰ **H93.1** Tinnitus

    H93.11 Tinnitus, right ear

    H93.12 Tinnitus, left ear

    H93.13 Tinnitus, bilateral

    H93.19 Tinnitus, unspecified ear

  ✓5ᵗʰ **H93.A** Pulsatile tinnitus

    AHA: 2016,4Q,25-26

    H93.A1 Pulsatile tinnitus, right ear

    H93.A2 Pulsatile tinnitus, left ear

    H93.A3 Pulsatile tinnitus, bilateral

HCC CMS-HCC   **Rx** Rx HCC   **ESR** ESRD HCC   **COM** Commercial HCC   **N** Newborn: 0   **P** Pediatric: 0-17   **M** Maternity: 9-64   **A** Adult: 15-124

656   ICD-10-CM 2023

H93.A9   **Pulsatile tinnitus, unspecified ear**

✓5ᵗʰ **H93.2**   **Other abnormal auditory perceptions**
- EXCLUDES 2   auditory hallucinations (R44.Ø)

✓6ᵗʰ **H93.21**   **Auditory recruitment**
- H93.211   **Auditory recruitment, right ear**
- H93.212   **Auditory recruitment, left ear**
- H93.213   **Auditory recruitment, bilateral**
- H93.219   **Auditory recruitment, unspecified ear**

✓6ᵗʰ **H93.22**   **Diplacusis**
- H93.221   **Diplacusis, right ear**
- H93.222   **Diplacusis, left ear**
- H93.223   **Diplacusis, bilateral**
- H93.229   **Diplacusis, unspecified ear**

✓6ᵗʰ **H93.23**   **Hyperacusis**
- **DEF:** Exceptionally acute sense of hearing caused by such conditions as Bell's palsy. This term may also refer to painful sensitivity to sounds.
- H93.231   **Hyperacusis, right ear**
- H93.232   **Hyperacusis, left ear**
- H93.233   **Hyperacusis, bilateral**
- H93.239   **Hyperacusis, unspecified ear**

✓6ᵗʰ **H93.24**   **Temporary auditory threshold shift**
- H93.241   **Temporary auditory threshold shift, right ear**
- H93.242   **Temporary auditory threshold shift, left ear**
- H93.243   **Temporary auditory threshold shift, bilateral**
- H93.249   **Temporary auditory threshold shift, unspecified ear**

H93.25   **Central auditory processing disorder**
- Congenital auditory imperception
- Word deafness
- EXCLUDES 1   mixed receptive-expressive language disorder (F8Ø.2)

✓6ᵗʰ **H93.29**   **Other abnormal auditory perceptions**
- H93.291   **Other abnormal auditory perceptions, right ear**
- H93.292   **Other abnormal auditory perceptions, left ear**
- H93.293   **Other abnormal auditory perceptions, bilateral**
- H93.299   **Other abnormal auditory perceptions, unspecified ear**

✓5ᵗʰ **H93.3**   **Disorders of acoustic nerve**
- Disorder of 8th cranial nerve
- EXCLUDES 1   acoustic neuroma (D33.3)
-      syphilitic acoustic neuritis (A52.15)

✓6ᵗʰ **H93.3X**   **Disorders of acoustic nerve**
- H93.3X1   **Disorders of right acoustic nerve**
- H93.3X2   **Disorders of left acoustic nerve**
- H93.3X3   **Disorders of bilateral acoustic nerves**
- H93.3X9   **Disorders of unspecified acoustic nerve**

✓5ᵗʰ **H93.8**   **Other specified disorders of ear**

✓6ᵗʰ **H93.8X**   **Other specified disorders of ear**
- H93.8X1   **Other specified disorders of right ear**
- H93.8X2   **Other specified disorders of left ear**
- H93.8X3   **Other specified disorders of ear, bilateral**
- H93.8X9   **Other specified disorders of ear, unspecified ear**

✓5ᵗʰ **H93.9**   **Unspecified disorder of ear**
- H93.9Ø   **Unspecified disorder of ear, unspecified ear**
- H93.91   **Unspecified disorder of right ear**
- H93.92   **Unspecified disorder of left ear**
- H93.93   **Unspecified disorder of ear, bilateral**

✓4ᵗʰ **H94**   **Other disorders of ear in diseases classified elsewhere**

✓5ᵗʰ **H94.Ø**   **Acoustic neuritis in infectious and parasitic diseases classified elsewhere**
- Code first underlying disease, such as:
- parasitic disease (B65-B89)
- EXCLUDES 1   acoustic neuritis (in):
-      herpes zoster (BØ2.29)
-      syphilis (A52.15)
- H94.ØØ   *Acoustic neuritis in infectious and parasitic diseases classified elsewhere, unspecified ear*
- H94.Ø1   *Acoustic neuritis in infectious and parasitic diseases classified elsewhere, right ear*

- H94.Ø2   *Acoustic neuritis in infectious and parasitic diseases classified elsewhere, left ear*
- H94.Ø3   *Acoustic neuritis in infectious and parasitic diseases classified elsewhere, bilateral*

✓5ᵗʰ **H94.8**   **Other specified disorders of ear in diseases classified elsewhere**
- Code first underlying disease, such as:
- congenital syphilis (A5Ø.Ø)
- EXCLUDES 1   aural myiasis (B87.4)
-      syphilitic labyrinthitis (A52.79)
- H94.8Ø   *Other specified disorders of ear in diseases classified elsewhere, unspecified ear*
- H94.81   *Other specified disorders of right ear in diseases classified elsewhere*
- H94.82   *Other specified disorders of left ear in diseases classified elsewhere*
- H94.83   *Other specified disorders of ear in diseases classified elsewhere, bilateral*

Intraoperative and postprocedural complications and disorders of ear and mastoid process, not elsewhere classified (H95)

✓4ᵗʰ **H95**   **Intraoperative and postprocedural complications and disorders of ear and mastoid process, not elsewhere classified**
- AHA: 2016,4Q,9-10

✓5ᵗʰ **H95.Ø**   **Recurrent cholesteatoma of postmastoidectomy cavity**
- H95.ØØ   **Recurrent cholesteatoma of postmastoidectomy cavity, unspecified ear**
- H95.Ø1   **Recurrent cholesteatoma of postmastoidectomy cavity, right ear**
- H95.Ø2   **Recurrent cholesteatoma of postmastoidectomy cavity, left ear**
- H95.Ø3   **Recurrent cholesteatoma of postmastoidectomy cavity, bilateral ears**

✓5ᵗʰ **H95.1**   **Other disorders of ear and mastoid process following mastoidectomy**

✓6ᵗʰ **H95.11**   **Chronic inflammation of postmastoidectomy cavity**
- H95.111   **Chronic inflammation of postmastoidectomy cavity, right ear**
- H95.112   **Chronic inflammation of postmastoidectomy cavity, left ear**
- H95.113   **Chronic inflammation of postmastoidectomy cavity, bilateral ears**
- H95.119   **Chronic inflammation of postmastoidectomy cavity, unspecified ear**

✓6ᵗʰ **H95.12**   **Granulation of postmastoidectomy cavity**
- H95.121   **Granulation of postmastoidectomy cavity, right ear**
- H95.122   **Granulation of postmastoidectomy cavity, left ear**
- H95.123   **Granulation of postmastoidectomy cavity, bilateral ears**
- H95.129   **Granulation of postmastoidectomy cavity, unspecified ear**

✓6ᵗʰ **H95.13**   **Mucosal cyst of postmastoidectomy cavity**
- H95.131   **Mucosal cyst of postmastoidectomy cavity, right ear**
- H95.132   **Mucosal cyst of postmastoidectomy cavity, left ear**
- H95.133   **Mucosal cyst of postmastoidectomy cavity, bilateral ears**
- H95.139   **Mucosal cyst of postmastoidectomy cavity, unspecified ear**

✓6ᵗʰ **H95.19**   **Other disorders following mastoidectomy**
- H95.191   **Other disorders following mastoidectomy, right ear**
- H95.192   **Other disorders following mastoidectomy, left ear**
- H95.193   **Other disorders following mastoidectomy, bilateral ears**
- H95.199   **Other disorders following mastoidectomy, unspecified ear**

Chapter 8. Diseases of the Ear and Mastoid Process

✓5ᵗʰ **H95.2** Intraoperative hemorrhage and hematoma of ear and mastoid process complicating a procedure

> EXCLUDES 1   intraoperative hemorrhage and hematoma of ear and mastoid process due to accidental puncture or laceration during a procedure (H95.3-)

     H95.21 Intraoperative hemorrhage and hematoma of ear and mastoid process complicating a procedure on the ear and mastoid process

     H95.22 Intraoperative hemorrhage and hematoma of ear and mastoid process complicating other procedure

✓5ᵗʰ **H95.3** Accidental puncture and laceration of ear and mastoid process during a procedure

     H95.31 Accidental puncture and laceration of the ear and mastoid process during a procedure on the ear and mastoid process

     H95.32 Accidental puncture and laceration of the ear and mastoid process during other procedure

✓6ᵗʰ **H95.4** Postprocedural hemorrhage of ear and mastoid process following a procedure

     H95.41 Postprocedural hemorrhage of ear and mastoid process following a procedure on the ear and mastoid process

     H95.42 Postprocedural hemorrhage of ear and mastoid process following other procedure

✓5ᵗʰ **H95.5** Postprocedural hematoma and seroma of ear and mastoid process following a procedure

     H95.51 Postprocedural hematoma of ear and mastoid process following a procedure on the ear and mastoid process

     H95.52 Postprocedural hematoma of ear and mastoid process following other procedure

     H95.53 Postprocedural seroma of ear and mastoid process following a procedure on the ear and mastoid process

     H95.54 Postprocedural seroma of ear and mastoid process following other procedure

✓5ᵗʰ **H95.8** Other intraoperative and postprocedural complications and disorders of the ear and mastoid process, not elsewhere classified

> EXCLUDES 2   postprocedural complications and disorders following mastoidectomy (H95.0-, H95.1-)

     ✓6ᵗʰ **H95.81** Postprocedural stenosis of external ear canal

         H95.811 Postprocedural stenosis of right external ear canal

         H95.812 Postprocedural stenosis of left external ear canal

         H95.813 Postprocedural stenosis of external ear canal, bilateral

         H95.819 Postprocedural stenosis of unspecified external ear canal

     H95.88 Other intraoperative complications and disorders of the ear and mastoid process, not elsewhere classified

         Use additional code, if applicable, to further specify disorder

     H95.89 Other postprocedural complications and disorders of the ear and mastoid process, not elsewhere classified

         Use additional code, if applicable, to further specify disorder

Chapter 9. Diseases of the Circulatory System (I00–I99)

Chapter-specific Guidelines with Coding Examples

The chapter-specific guidelines from the ICD-10-CM Official Guidelines for Coding and Reporting have been provided below. Along with these guidelines are coding examples, contained in the shaded boxes, that have been developed to help illustrate the coding and/or sequencing guidance found in these guidelines.

a. Hypertension

The classification presumes a causal relationship between hypertension and heart involvement and between hypertension and kidney involvement, as the two conditions are linked by the term "with" in the Alphabetic Index. These conditions should be coded as related even in the absence of provider documentation explicitly linking them, unless the documentation clearly states the conditions are unrelated.

For hypertension and conditions not specifically linked by relational terms such as "with," "associated with" or "due to" in the classification, provider documentation must link the conditions in order to code them as related.

1) Hypertension with heart disease

Hypertension with heart conditions classified to I50.- or I51.4-I51.7, I51.89, I51.9, are assigned to a code from category I11, Hypertensive heart disease. Use additional code(s) from category I50, Heart failure, to identify the type(s) of heart failure in those patients with heart failure.

The same heart conditions (I50.-, I51.4-I51.7, I51.89, I51.9) with hypertension are coded separately if the provider has documented they are unrelated to the hypertension. Sequence according to the circumstances of the admission/encounter.

2) Hypertensive chronic kidney disease

Assign codes from category I12, Hypertensive chronic kidney disease, when both hypertension and a condition classifiable to category N18, Chronic kidney disease (CKD), are present. CKD should not be coded as hypertensive if the provider indicates the CKD is not related to the hypertension.

The appropriate code from category N18 should be used as a secondary code with a code from category I12 to identify the stage of chronic kidney disease.

See Section I.C.14. Chronic kidney disease.

If a patient has hypertensive chronic kidney disease and acute renal failure, the acute renal failure should also be coded. Sequence according to the circumstances of the admission/encounter.

> Patient is admitted with stage IV chronic kidney disease (CKD) due to polycystic kidney disease. Patient also is on lisinopril for hypertension.
>
> | N18.4 | Chronic kidney disease, stage 4 (severe) |
> |---|---|
> | Q61.3 | Polycystic kidney, unspecified |
> | I10 | Essential (primary) hypertension |
>
> *Explanation*: A combination code describing a relationship between hypertension and CKD is not used because the physician documentation identifies the polycystic kidney disease as the cause for the CKD.

3) Hypertensive heart and chronic kidney disease

Assign codes from combination category I13, Hypertensive heart and chronic kidney disease, when there is hypertension with both heart and kidney involvement. If heart failure is present, assign an additional code from category I50 to identify the type of heart failure.

The appropriate code from category N18, Chronic kidney disease, should be used as a secondary code with a code from category I13 to identify the stage of chronic kidney disease.

See Section I.C.14. Chronic kidney disease.

The codes in category I13, Hypertensive heart and chronic kidney disease, are combination codes that include hypertension, heart disease and chronic kidney disease. The Includes note at I13 specifies that the conditions included at I11 and I12 are included together in I13. If a patient has hypertension, heart disease and chronic kidney disease, then a code from I13 should be used, not individual codes for hypertension, heart disease and chronic kidney disease, or codes from I11 or I12.

For patients with both acute renal failure and chronic kidney disease, the acute renal failure should also be coded. Sequence according to the circumstances of the admission/encounter.

> Hypertensive heart and kidney disease with congestive heart failure and stage 2 chronic kidney disease
>
> | I13.0 | Hypertensive heart and chronic kidney disease with heart failure and stage 1 through stage 4 chronic kidney disease, or unspecified chronic kidney disease |
> |---|---|
> | I50.9 | Heart failure, unspecified |
> | N18.2 | Chronic kidney disease, stage 2 (mild) |
>
> *Explanation*: Combination codes in category I13 are used to report conditions classifiable to *both* categories I11 and I12. Do not report conditions classifiable to I11 and I12 separately. Use additional codes to report type of heart failure and stage of CKD.

4) Hypertensive cerebrovascular disease

For hypertensive cerebrovascular disease, first assign the appropriate code from categories I60-I69, followed by the appropriate hypertension code.

> Rupture of cerebral aneurysm caused by malignant hypertension
>
> | I60.7 | Nontraumatic subarachnoid hemorrhage from unspecified intracranial artery |
> |---|---|
> | I10 | Essential (primary) hypertension |
>
> *Explanation*: Hypertensive cerebrovascular disease requires two codes: the appropriate I60–I69 code followed by the appropriate hypertension code.

5) Hypertensive retinopathy

Subcategory H35.0, Background retinopathy and retinal vascular changes, should be used along with a code from categories I10-I15, in the Hypertensive diseases section, to include the systemic hypertension. The sequencing is based on the reason for the encounter.

6) Hypertension, secondary

Secondary hypertension is due to an underlying condition. Two codes are required: one to identify the underlying etiology and one from category I15 to identify the hypertension. Sequencing of codes is determined by the reason for admission/encounter.

> Renovascular hypertension due to renal artery atherosclerosis
>
> | I15.0 | Renovascular hypertension |
> |---|---|
> | I70.1 | Atherosclerosis of renal artery |
>
> *Explanation*: Secondary hypertension requires two codes: a code to identify the etiology and the appropriate I15 code.

7) Hypertension, transient

Assign code R03.0, Elevated blood pressure reading without diagnosis of hypertension, unless patient has an established diagnosis of hypertension. Assign code O13.-, Gestational [pregnancy-induced] hypertension without significant proteinuria, or O14.-, Pre-eclampsia, for transient hypertension of pregnancy.

8) Hypertension, controlled

This diagnostic statement usually refers to an existing state of hypertension under control by therapy. Assign the appropriate code from categories I10-I15, Hypertensive diseases.

9) Hypertension, uncontrolled

Uncontrolled hypertension may refer to untreated hypertension or hypertension not responding to current therapeutic regimen. In either case, assign the appropriate code from categories I10-I15, Hypertensive diseases.

10) Hypertensive crisis

Assign a code from category I16, Hypertensive crisis, for documented hypertensive urgency, hypertensive emergency or unspecified hypertensive crisis. Code also any identified hypertensive disease (I10-I15). The sequencing is based on the reason for the encounter.

11) Pulmonary hypertension

Pulmonary hypertension is classified to category I27, Other pulmonary heart diseases. For secondary pulmonary hypertension (I27.1, I27.2-), code also any associated conditions or adverse effects of drugs or toxins. The sequencing is based on the reason for the encounter, except for adverse effects of drugs (See Section I.C.19.e.).

b. Atherosclerotic coronary artery disease and angina

ICD-10-CM has combination codes for atherosclerotic heart disease with angina pectoris. The subcategories for these codes are I25.11, Atherosclerotic heart disease of native coronary artery with angina pectoris and I25.7, Atherosclerosis of coronary artery bypass graft(s) and coronary artery of transplanted heart with angina pectoris.

When using one of these combination codes it is not necessary to use an additional code for angina pectoris. A causal relationship can be assumed in a patient with both atherosclerosis and angina pectoris, unless the documentation indicates the angina is due to something other than the atherosclerosis.

If a patient with coronary artery disease is admitted due to an acute myocardial infarction (AMI), the AMI should be sequenced before the coronary artery disease.

See Section I.C.9. Acute myocardial infarction (AMI)

Patient is being seen for spastic angina pectoris. She also has a documented history of progressive coronary artery disease of the native vessels.

I25.111   Atherosclerotic heart disease of native coronary artery with angina pectoris with documented spasm

Explanation: Report the combination code for atherosclerotic heart disease (coronary artery disease) with angina pectoris. A causal relationship is assumed in a patient with both atherosclerosis and angina pectoris, unless the documentation indicates the angina is due to something other than the atherosclerosis. When using one of these combination codes, it is not necessary to use an additional code for angina pectoris.

c. Intraoperative and postprocedural cerebrovascular accident

Medical record documentation should clearly specify the cause- and- effect relationship between the medical intervention and the cerebrovascular accident in order to assign a code for intraoperative or postprocedural cerebrovascular accident.

Proper code assignment depends on whether it was an infarction or hemorrhage and whether it occurred intraoperatively or postoperatively. If it was a cerebral hemorrhage, code assignment depends on the type of procedure performed.

Embolic cerebral infarction of the right middle cerebral artery that occurred during hip replacement surgery. The surgeon documented as due to the surgery.

I97.811   Intraoperative cerebrovascular infarction during other surgery

I63.411   Cerebral infarction due to embolism of right middle cerebral artery

Explanation: Code assignment for intraoperative or postprocedural cerebrovascular accident is based on the provider's documentation of a cause-and-effect relationship between the condition and the procedure. Proper code assignment also depends on whether the cerebrovascular accident was an infarction or hemorrhage, occurred intraoperatively or postoperatively, and the type of procedure performed.

d. Sequelae of cerebrovascular disease

1) Category I69, Sequelae of cerebrovascular disease

Category I69 is used to indicate conditions classifiable to categories I60-I67 as the causes of sequela (neurologic deficits), themselves classified elsewhere. These "late effects" include neurologic deficits that persist after initial onset of conditions classifiable to categories I60-I67. The neurologic deficits caused by cerebrovascular disease may be present from the onset or may arise at any time after the onset of the condition classifiable to categories I60-I67.

Codes from category I69, Sequelae of cerebrovascular disease, that specify hemiplegia, hemiparesis and monoplegia identify whether the dominant or nondominant side is affected. Should the affected side be documented, but not specified as dominant or nondominant, and the classification system does not indicate a default, code selection is as follows:

- For ambidextrous patients, the default should be dominant.
- If the left side is affected, the default is non-dominant.
- If the right side is affected, the default is dominant.

2) Codes from category I69 with codes from I60–I67

Codes from category I69 may be assigned on a health care record with codes from I60-I67, if the patient has a current cerebrovascular disease and deficits from an old cerebrovascular disease.

3) Codes from category I69 and personal history of transient ischemic attack (TIA) and cerebral infarction (Z86.73)

Codes from category I69 should not be assigned if the patient does not have neurologic deficits.

See Section I.C.21. 4. History (of) for use of personal history codes

e. Acute myocardial infarction (AMI)

1) Type 1 ST elevation myocardial infarction (STEMI) and non-ST elevation myocardial infarction (NSTEMI)

The ICD-10-CM codes for type 1 acute myocardial infarction (AMI) identify the site, such as anterolateral wall or true posterior wall. Subcategories I21.Ø-I21.2 and code I21.3 are used for type 1 ST elevation myocardial infarction (STEMI). Code I21.4, Non-ST elevation (NSTEMI) myocardial infarction, is used for type 1 non-ST elevation myocardial infarction (NSTEMI) and nontransmural MIs.

If a type 1 NSTEMI evolves to STEMI, assign the STEMI code. If a type 1 STEMI converts to NSTEMI due to thrombolytic therapy, it is still coded as STEMI.

For encounters occurring while the myocardial infarction is equal to, or less than, four weeks old, including transfers to another acute setting or a postacute setting, and the myocardial infarction meets the definition for "other diagnoses" (see Section III, Reporting Additional Diagnoses), codes from category I21 may continue to be reported. For encounters after the 4-week time frame and the patient is still receiving care related to the myocardial infarction, the appropriate aftercare code should be assigned, rather than a code from category I21. For old or healed myocardial infarctions not requiring further care, code I25.2, Old myocardial infarction, may be assigned.

2) Acute myocardial infarction, unspecified

Code I21.9, Acute myocardial infarction, unspecified, is the default for unspecified acute myocardial infarction or unspecified type. If only type 1 STEMI or transmural MI without the site is documented, assign code I21.3, ST elevation (STEMI) myocardial infarction of unspecified site.

3) AMI documented as nontransmural or subendocardial but site provided

If an AMI is documented as nontransmural or subendocardial, but the site is provided, it is still coded as subendocardial AMI.

See Section I.C.21.3.for information on coding status post administration of tPA in a different facility within the last 24 hours.

Acute inferior subendocardial myocardial infarction (NSTEMI)

I21.4   Non-ST elevation (NSTEMI) myocardial infarction

Explanation: An AMI documented as subendocardial or nontransmural is coded as such (I21.4, I22.2), even if the site of infarction is specified.

4) Subsequent acute myocardial infarction

A code from category I22, Subsequent ST elevation (STEMI) and non-ST elevation (NSTEMI) myocardial infarction, is to be used when a patient who has suffered a type 1 or unspecified AMI has a new AMI within the 4-week time frame of the initial AMI. A code from category I22 must be used in conjunction with a code from category I21. The sequencing of the I22 and I21 codes depends on the circumstances of the encounter.

Do not assign code I22 for subsequent myocardial infarctions other than type 1 or unspecified. For subsequent type 2 AMI assign only code I21.A1. For subsequent type 4 or type 5 AMI, assign only code I21.A9.

If a subsequent myocardial infarction of one type occurs within 4 weeks of a myocardial infarction of a different type, assign the appropriate codes from category I21 to identify each type. Do not assign a code from I22. Codes from category I22 should only be assigned if both the initial and subsequent myocardial infarctions are type 1 or unspecified.

Patient suffered an acute NSTEMI 14 days ago and is now seen for an inferior STEMI.

I22.1   Subsequent ST elevation (STEMI) myocardial infarction of inferior wall

I21.4   Non-ST elevation (NSTEMI) myocardial infarction

Explanation: Both MIs were type 1, and the current MI occurred within the four-week time frame; therefore a code for the current/subsequent STEMI (I22.1) is reported as well as a code for the previous NSTEMI (I21.4).

5) Other Types of Myocardial Infarction

The ICD-10-CM provides codes for different types of myocardial infarction. Type 1 myocardial infarctions are assigned to codes I21.Ø-I21.4.

Type 2 myocardial infarction (myocardial infarction due to demand ischemia or secondary to ischemic imbalance) is assigned to code I21.A1, Myocardial infarction type 2 with the underlying cause coded first. Do not assign code I24.8, Other forms of acute ischemic heart disease, for the demand ischemia. If a type 2 AMI is described as NSTEMI or STEMI, only assign code I21.A1. Codes I21.Ø1-I21.4 should only be assigned for type 1 AMIs.

Acute myocardial infarctions type 3, 4a, 4b, 4c and 5 are assigned to code I21.A9, Other myocardial infarction type.

The "Code also" and "Code first" notes should be followed related to complications, and for coding of postprocedural myocardial infarctions during or following cardiac surgery.

Chapter 9. Diseases of the Circulatory System (I00-I99)

EXCLUDES 2   certain conditions originating in the perinatal period (P04-P96)
certain infectious and parasitic diseases (A00-B99)
complications of pregnancy, childbirth and the puerperium (O00-O9A)
congenital malformations, deformations, and chromosomal abnormalities (Q00-Q99)
endocrine, nutritional and metabolic diseases (E00-E88)
injury, poisoning and certain other consequences of external causes (S00-T88)
neoplasms (C00-D49)
symptoms, signs and abnormal clinical and laboratory findings, not elsewhere classified (R00-R94)
systemic connective tissue disorders (M30-M36)
transient cerebral ischemic attacks and related syndromes (G45.-)

This chapter contains the following blocks:

I00-I02   Acute rheumatic fever
I05-I09   Chronic rheumatic heart diseases
I10-I16   Hypertensive diseases
I20-I25   Ischemic heart diseases
I26-I28   Pulmonary heart disease and diseases of pulmonary circulation
I30-I5A   Other forms of heart disease
I60-I69   Cerebrovascular diseases
I70-I79   Diseases of arteries, arterioles and capillaries
I80-I89   Diseases of veins, lymphatic vessels and lymph nodes, not elsewhere classified
I95-I99   Other and unspecified disorders of the circulatory system

Acute rheumatic fever (I00-I02)

DEF: Rheumatic fever: Inflammatory disease that can follow a throat infection by group A *streptococci*. Complications can involve the joints (arthritis), subcutaneous tissue (nodules), skin (erythema marginatum), heart (carditis), or brain (chorea).

I00   **Rheumatic fever without heart involvement**
     INCLUDES   arthritis, rheumatic, acute or subacute
     EXCLUDES 1   rheumatic fever with heart involvement (I01.0-I01.9)

√4ᵗʰ **I01**   **Rheumatic fever with heart involvement**
     EXCLUDES 1   chronic diseases of rheumatic origin (I05-I09) unless rheumatic fever is also present or there is evidence of reactivation or activity of the rheumatic process

   I01.0   **Acute rheumatic pericarditis**
     Any condition in I00 with pericarditis
     Rheumatic pericarditis (acute)
     EXCLUDES 1   acute pericarditis not specified as rheumatic (I30.-)

   I01.1   **Acute rheumatic endocarditis**
     Any condition in I00 with endocarditis or valvulitis
     Acute rheumatic valvulitis

   I01.2   **Acute rheumatic myocarditis**
     Any condition in I00 with myocarditis

   I01.8   **Other acute rheumatic heart disease**
     Any condition in I00 with other or multiple types of heart involvement
     Acute rheumatic pancarditis

   I01.9   **Acute rheumatic heart disease, unspecified**
     Any condition in I00 with unspecified type of heart involvement
     Rheumatic carditis, acute
     Rheumatic heart disease, active or acute

√4ᵗʰ **I02**   **Rheumatic chorea**
     INCLUDES   Sydenham's chorea
     EXCLUDES 1   chorea NOS (G25.5)
                Huntington's chorea (G10)

   I02.0   **Rheumatic chorea with heart involvement**
     Chorea NOS with heart involvement
     Rheumatic chorea with heart involvement of any type classifiable under I01.-

   I02.9   **Rheumatic chorea without heart involvement**
     Rheumatic chorea NOS

Chronic rheumatic heart diseases (I05-I09)

√4ᵗʰ **I05**   **Rheumatic mitral valve diseases**
     INCLUDES   conditions classifiable to both I05.0 and I05.2-I05.9, whether specified as rheumatic or not
     EXCLUDES 1   mitral valve disease specified as nonrheumatic (I34.-)
                mitral valve disease with aortic and/or tricuspid valve involvement (I08.-)

   I05.0   **Rheumatic mitral stenosis**
     Mitral (valve) obstruction (rheumatic)

   I05.1   **Rheumatic mitral insufficiency**
     Rheumatic mitral incompetence
     Rheumatic mitral regurgitation
     EXCLUDES 1   mitral insufficiency not specified as rheumatic (I34.0)

   I05.2   **Rheumatic mitral stenosis with insufficiency**
     Rheumatic mitral stenosis with incompetence or regurgitation

   I05.8   **Other rheumatic mitral valve diseases**
     Rheumatic mitral (valve) failure

   I05.9   **Rheumatic mitral valve disease, unspecified**
     Rheumatic mitral (valve) disorder (chronic) NOS

√4ᵗʰ **I06**   **Rheumatic aortic valve diseases**
     EXCLUDES 1   aortic valve disease not specified as rheumatic (I35.-)
                aortic valve disease with mitral and/or tricuspid valve involvement (I08.-)

   I06.0   **Rheumatic aortic stenosis**
     Rheumatic aortic (valve) obstruction

   I06.1   **Rheumatic aortic insufficiency**
     Rheumatic aortic incompetence
     Rheumatic aortic regurgitation

   I06.2   **Rheumatic aortic stenosis with insufficiency**
     Rheumatic aortic stenosis with incompetence or regurgitation

   I06.8   **Other rheumatic aortic valve diseases**

   I06.9   **Rheumatic aortic valve disease, unspecified**
     Rheumatic aortic (valve) disease NOS

√4ᵗʰ **I07**   **Rheumatic tricuspid valve diseases**
     INCLUDES   rheumatic tricuspid valve diseases specified as rheumatic or unspecified
     EXCLUDES 1   tricuspid valve disease specified as nonrheumatic (I36.-)
                tricuspid valve disease with aortic and/or mitral valve involvement (I08.-)

   I07.0   **Rheumatic tricuspid stenosis**
     Tricuspid (valve) stenosis (rheumatic)

   I07.1   **Rheumatic tricuspid insufficiency**
     Tricuspid (valve) insufficiency (rheumatic)

   I07.2   **Rheumatic tricuspid stenosis and insufficiency**

   I07.8   **Other rheumatic tricuspid valve diseases**

   I07.9   **Rheumatic tricuspid valve disease, unspecified**
     Rheumatic tricuspid valve disorder NOS

√4ᵗʰ **I08**   **Multiple valve diseases**
     INCLUDES   multiple valve diseases specified as rheumatic or unspecified
     EXCLUDES 1   endocarditis, valve unspecified (I38)
                multiple valve disease specified a nonrheumatic (I34.-, I35.-, I36.-, I37.-, I38.-, Q22.-, Q23.-, Q24.8-)
                rheumatic valve disease NOS (I09.1)

   I08.0   **Rheumatic disorders of both mitral and aortic valves**
     Involvement of both mitral and aortic valves specified as rheumatic or unspecified
     AHA: 2019,2Q,5

   I08.1   **Rheumatic disorders of both mitral and tricuspid valves**

   I08.2   **Rheumatic disorders of both aortic and tricuspid valves**

   I08.3   **Combined rheumatic disorders of mitral, aortic and tricuspid valves**

   I08.8   **Other rheumatic multiple valve diseases**

   I08.9   **Rheumatic multiple valve disease, unspecified**

√4ᵗʰ **I09**   **Other rheumatic heart diseases**

   I09.0   **Rheumatic myocarditis**
     EXCLUDES 1   myocarditis not specified as rheumatic (I51.4)

   I09.1   **Rheumatic diseases of endocardium, valve unspecified**
     Rheumatic endocarditis (chronic)
     Rheumatic valvulitis (chronic)
     EXCLUDES 1   endocarditis, valve unspecified (I38)

   I09.2   **Chronic rheumatic pericarditis**
     Adherent pericardium, rheumatic
     Chronic rheumatic mediastinopericarditis
     Chronic rheumatic myopericarditis
     EXCLUDES 1   chronic pericarditis not specified as rheumatic (I31.-)

√5ᵗʰ **I09.8**   **Other specified rheumatic heart diseases**

     I09.81   **Rheumatic heart failure**   HCC Rx ESR COM
         Use additional code to identify type of heart failure (I50.-)

     I09.89   **Other specified rheumatic heart diseases**
         Rheumatic disease of pulmonary valve

I09.9 Rheumatic heart disease, unspecified
Rheumatic carditis
EXCLUDES 1   rheumatoid carditis (M05.31)

Hypertensive diseases (I10-I16)

Use additional code to identify:
exposure to environmental tobacco smoke (Z77.22)
history of tobacco dependence (Z87.891)
occupational exposure to environmental tobacco smoke (Z57.31)
tobacco dependence (F17.-)
tobacco use (Z72.0)
EXCLUDES 1   neonatal hypertension (P29.2)
       primary pulmonary hypertension (I27.0)
EXCLUDES 2   hypertensive disease complicating pregnancy, childbirth and the puerperium (O10-O11, O13-O16)

I10 Essential (primary) hypertension   `Rx` `Q`
INCLUDES   high blood pressure
       hypertension (arterial) (benign) (essential) (malignant) (primary) (systemic)
EXCLUDES 1   hypertensive disease complicating pregnancy, childbirth and the puerperium (O10-O11, O13-O16)
EXCLUDES 2   essential (primary) hypertension involving vessels of brain (I60-I69)
       essential (primary) hypertension involving vessels of eye (H35.0-)
AHA: 2022,1Q,36; 2020,1Q,12; 2018,2Q,9; 2016,4Q,27

✓4ᵗʰ I11 Hypertensive heart disease
INCLUDES   any condition in I50.- or I51.4-I51.7, I51.89, I51.9 due to hypertension
AHA: 2018,2Q,9
TIP: Do not assign a code from this category when provider documentation indicates the heart disease is attributable to another cause.

I11.0 Hypertensive heart disease with heart failure   `HCC` `Rx` `ESR` `COM`
Hypertensive heart failure
Use additional code to identify type of heart failure (I50.-)
AHA: 2017,1Q,47

I11.9 Hypertensive heart disease without heart failure   `Rx`
Hypertensive heart disease NOS

✓4ᵗʰ I12 Hypertensive chronic kidney disease
INCLUDES   any condition in N18 and N26 — due to hypertension
       arteriosclerosis of kidney
       arteriosclerotic nephritis (chronic) (interstitial)
       hypertensive nephropathy
       nephrosclerosis
EXCLUDES 1   hypertension due to kidney disease (I15.0, I15.1)
       renovascular hypertension (I15.0)
       secondary hypertension (I15.-)
EXCLUDES 2   acute kidney failure (N17.-)
AHA: 2019,3Q,3; 2018,4Q,88; 2016,3Q,22
TIP: Do not assign a code from this category when provider documentation indicates the chronic kidney disease (CKD) is attributable to another cause.

I12.0 Hypertensive chronic kidney disease with stage 5 chronic kidney disease or end stage renal disease   `HCC` `Rx` `ESR` `COM`
Use additional code to identify the stage of chronic kidney disease (N18.5, N18.6)

I12.9 Hypertensive chronic kidney disease with stage 1 through stage 4 chronic kidney disease, or unspecified chronic kidney disease   `Rx`
Hypertensive chronic kidney disease NOS
Hypertensive renal disease NOS
Use additional code to identify the stage of chronic kidney disease (N18.1-N18.4, N18.9)

✓4ᵗʰ I13 Hypertensive heart and chronic kidney disease
INCLUDES   any condition in I11.- with any condition in I12.-
       cardiorenal disease
       cardiovascular renal disease
TIP: Do not assign a code from this category when provider documentation indicates the heart and/or chronic kidney disease is attributable to another cause.

I13.0 Hypertensive heart and chronic kidney disease with heart failure and stage 1 through stage 4 chronic kidney disease, or unspecified chronic kidney disease   `HCC` `Rx` `ESR` `COM`
Use additional code to identify type of heart failure (I50.-)
Use additional code to identify stage of chronic kidney disease (N18.1-N18.4, N18.9)

✓5ᵗʰ I13.1 Hypertensive heart and chronic kidney disease without heart failure

I13.10 Hypertensive heart and chronic kidney disease without heart failure, with stage 1 through stage 4 chronic kidney disease, or unspecified chronic kidney disease   `Rx`
Hypertensive heart disease and hypertensive chronic kidney disease NOS
Use additional code to identify the stage of chronic kidney disease (N18.1-N18.4, N18.9)

I13.11 Hypertensive heart and chronic kidney disease without heart failure, with stage 5 chronic kidney disease, or end stage renal disease   `HCC` `Rx` `ESR` `COM`
Use additional code to identify the stage of chronic kidney disease (N18.5, N18.6)

I13.2 Hypertensive heart and chronic kidney disease with heart failure and with stage 5 chronic kidney disease, or end stage renal disease   `HCC` `Rx` `ESR` `COM`
Use additional code to identify type of heart failure (I50.-)
Use additional code to identify the stage of chronic kidney disease (N18.5, N18.6)

✓4ᵗʰ I15 Secondary hypertension
Code also underlying condition
EXCLUDES 1   postprocedural hypertension (I97.3)
EXCLUDES 2   secondary hypertension involving vessels of brain (I60-I69)
       secondary hypertension involving vessels of eye (H35.0-)

I15.0 Renovascular hypertension   `Rx`
I15.1 Hypertension secondary to other renal disorders   `Rx`
AHA: 2016,3Q,22
I15.2 Hypertension secondary to endocrine disorders   `Rx`
I15.8 Other secondary hypertension   `Rx`
I15.9 Secondary hypertension, unspecified   `Rx`

✓4ᵗʰ I16 Hypertensive crisis
Code also any identified hypertensive disease (I10-I15)
AHA: 2016,4Q,26-28
I16.0 Hypertensive urgency   `Rx`
I16.1 Hypertensive emergency   `Rx`
I16.9 Hypertensive crisis, unspecified   `Rx`

Ischemic heart diseases (I20-I25)

Code also the presence of hypertension (I10-I16)

✓4ᵗʰ I20 Angina pectoris
Use additional code to identify:
exposure to environmental tobacco smoke (Z77.22)
history of tobacco dependence (Z87.891)
occupational exposure to environmental tobacco smoke (Z57.31)
tobacco dependence (F17.-)
tobacco use (Z72.0)
EXCLUDES 1   angina pectoris with atherosclerotic heart disease of native coronary arteries (I25.1-)
       atherosclerosis of coronary artery bypass graft(s) and coronary artery of transplanted heart with angina pectoris (I25.7-)
       postinfarction angina (I23.7)
DEF: Chest pain due to reduced blood flow resulting in a lack of oxygen to the heart muscles.

I20.0 Unstable angina   `HCC` `Rx` `ESR` `COM`
Accelerated angina
Crescendo angina
De novo effort angina
Intermediate coronary syndrome
Preinfarction syndrome
Worsening effort angina

I20.1 Angina pectoris with documented spasm   `HCC` `Rx` `ESR`
Angiospastic angina
Prinzmetal angina
Spasm-induced angina
Variant angina

● **I20.2 Refractory angina pectoris**

`HCC` CMS-HCC   `Rx` Rx HCC   `ESR` ESRD HCC   `COM` Commercial HCC   `N` Newborn: 0   `P` Pediatric: 0-17   `M` Maternity: 9-64   `A` Adult: 15-124

662   ICD-10-CM 2023

I20.8 **Other forms of angina pectoris**   `HCC` `Rx` `ESR`
     Angina equivalent
     Angina of effort
     Coronary slow flow syndrome
     Stable angina
     Stenocardia
     Use additional code(s) for symptoms associated with angina
         equivalent

I20.9 **Angina pectoris, unspecified**   `HCC` `Rx` `ESR`
     Angina NOS
     Anginal syndrome
     Cardiac angina
     Ischemic chest pain

☑4ᵗʰ **I21 Acute myocardial infarction**
     `INCLUDES`   cardiac infarction
         coronary (artery) embolism
         coronary (artery) occlusion
         coronary (artery) rupture
         coronary (artery) thrombosis
         infarction of heart, myocardium, or ventricle
         myocardial infarction specified as acute or with a stated
             duration of 4 weeks (28 days) or less from onset
     Use additional code, if applicable, to identify:
     exposure to environmental tobacco smoke (Z77.22)
     history of tobacco dependence (Z87.891)
     occupational exposure to environmental tobacco smoke (Z57.31)
     status post administration of tPA (rtPA) in a different facility within
         the last 24 hours prior to admission to current facility (Z92.82)
     tobacco dependence (F17.-)
     tobacco use (Z72.0)
     `EXCLUDES 2`   old myocardial infarction (I25.2)
         postmyocardial infarction syndrome (I24.1)
         subsequent type 1 myocardial infarction (I22.-)
     AHA: 2019,2Q,5; 2018,4Q,68; 2018,3Q,5; 2017,4Q,12-14; 2017,1Q,44-45;
     2016,4Q,140; 2015,2Q,16; 2013,1Q,25; 2012,4Q,96,102-103
     TIP: When chronic total occlusion and myocardial infarction are
     documented as being in different vessels, assign code I25.82 Chronic total
     occlusion of coronary artery, in addition to the myocardial infarction code.

☑5ᵗʰ **I21.0 ST elevation (STEMI) myocardial infarction of** anterior wall
     Type 1 ST elevation myocardial infarction of anterior wall
     DEF: ST elevation myocardial infarction: Complete obstruction
     of one or more coronary arteries causing decreased blood flow
     (ischemia) and necrosis of myocardial muscle cells.

     **I21.01 ST elevation (STEMI) myocardial infarction
         involving** left main **coronary
         artery**   `HCC` `Rx` `ESR` `COM`

     **I21.02 ST elevation (STEMI) myocardial infarction
         involving** left anterior descending **coronary
         artery**   `HCC` `Rx` `ESR` `COM`
         ST elevation (STEMI) myocardial infarction involving
            diagonal coronary artery
         AHA: 2013,1Q,25

     **I21.09 ST elevation (STEMI) myocardial infarction
         involving** other **coronary artery of anterior
         wall**   `HCC` `Rx` `ESR` `COM`
         Acute transmural myocardial infarction of anterior
            wall
         Anteroapical transmural (Q wave) infarction (acute)
         Anterolateral transmural (Q wave) infarction (acute)
         Anteroseptal transmural (Q wave) infarction (acute)
         Transmural (Q wave) infarction (acute) (of) anterior
            (wall) NOS
         AHA: 2012,4Q,102-103

☑5ᵗʰ **I21.1 ST elevation (STEMI) myocardial infarction of** inferior wall
     Type 1 ST elevation myocardial infarction of inferior wall
     DEF: ST elevation myocardial infarction: Complete obstruction
     of one or more coronary arteries causing decreased blood flow
     (ischemia) and necrosis of myocardial muscle cells.

     **I21.11 ST elevation (STEMI) myocardial infarction
         involving** right **coronary artery**   `HCC` `Rx` `ESR` `COM`
         Inferoposterior transmural (Q wave) infarction (acute)

     **I21.19 ST elevation (STEMI) myocardial infarction
         involving** other **coronary artery of inferior
         wall**   `HCC` `Rx` `ESR` `COM`
         Acute transmural myocardial infarction of inferior
            wall
         Inferolateral transmural (Q wave) infarction (acute)
         Transmural (Q wave) infarction (acute) (of)
            diaphragmatic wall
         Transmural (Q wave) infarction (acute) (of) inferior
            (wall) NOS
         `EXCLUDES 2`   ST elevation (STEMI) myocardial infarction
               involving left circumflex coronary
               artery (I21.21)
         AHA: 2012,4Q,96

☑5ᵗʰ **I21.2 ST elevation (STEMI) myocardial infarction of other sites**
     Type 1 ST elevation myocardial infarction of other sites
     DEF: ST elevation myocardial infarction: Complete obstruction
     of one or more coronary arteries causing decreased blood flow
     (ischemia) and necrosis of myocardial muscle cells.

     **I21.21 ST elevation (STEMI) myocardial infarction
         involving** left circumflex **coronary
         artery**   `HCC` `Rx` `ESR` `COM`
         ST elevation (STEMI) myocardial infarction involving
            oblique marginal coronary artery

     **I21.29 ST elevation (STEMI) myocardial infarction
         involving other sites**   `HCC` `Rx` `ESR` `COM`
         Acute transmural myocardial infarction of other sites
         Apical-lateral transmural (Q wave) infarction (acute)
         Basal-lateral transmural (Q wave) infarction (acute)
         High lateral transmural (Q wave) infarction (acute)
         Lateral (wall) NOS transmural (Q wave) infarction
            (acute)
         Posterior (true) transmural (Q wave) infarction (acute)
         Posterobasal transmural (Q wave) infarction (acute)
         Posterolateral transmural (Q wave) infarction (acute)
         Posteroseptal transmural (Q wave) infarction (acute)
         Septal transmural (Q wave) infarction (acute) NOS

**I21.3 ST elevation (STEMI) myocardial infarction of unspecified
site**   `HCC` `Rx` `ESR` `COM`
     Acute transmural myocardial infarction of unspecified site
     Transmural (Q wave) myocardial infarction NOS
     Type 1 ST elevation myocardial infarction of unspecified site
     DEF: ST elevation myocardial infarction: Complete obstruction
     of one or more coronary arteries causing decreased blood flow
     (ischemia) and necrosis of myocardial muscle cells.

**I21.4 Non-ST elevation (NSTEMI) myocardial
infarction**   `HCC` `Rx` `ESR` `COM`
     Acute subendocardial myocardial infarction
     Non-Q wave myocardial infarction NOS
     Nontransmural myocardial infarction NOS
     Type 1 non-ST elevation myocardial infarction
     AHA: 2021,3Q,6; 2019,2Q,33; 2017,1Q,44-45
     DEF: Partial obstruction of one or more coronary arteries that
     causes decreased blood flow (ischemia) and may cause partial
     thickness necrosis of myocardial muscle cells.

I21.9 Acute myocardial infarction, unspecified   `HCC` `Rx` `ESR` `COM`
     Myocardial infarction (acute) NOS

☑5ᵗʰ **I21.A Other type of myocardial infarction**
     AHA: 2019,2Q,5

     I21.A1 Myocardial infarction type 2   `HCC` `Rx` `ESR` `COM`
         Myocardial infarction due to demand ischemia
         Myocardial infarction secondary to ischemic
            imbalance
         Code first the underlying cause, such as:
            anemia (D50.0-D64.9)
            chronic obstructive pulmonary disease (J44.-)
            paroxysmal tachycardia (I47.0-I47.9)
            shock (R57.0-R57.9)
         AHA: 2019,4Q,53; 2017,4Q,13-14
         DEF: Often referred to as due to demand ischemia,
         myocardial infarction (MI) type 2 refers to an MI due to
         ischemia and necrosis resulting from an oxygen
         imbalance to the heart. This mismatch between oxygen
         decreased supply and increased demand is caused by
         conditions other than coronary artery disease such as
         vasospasm, embolism, anemia, hypertension,
         hypotension, or arrhythmias.

I21.A9 Other myocardial infarction type HCC Rx ESR COM

Myocardial infarction associated with revascularization procedure
Myocardial infarction type 3
Myocardial infarction type 4a
Myocardial infarction type 4b
Myocardial infarction type 4c
Myocardial infarction type 5

Code first, if applicable, postprocedural myocardial infarction following cardiac surgery (I97.190), or postprocedural myocardial infarction during cardiac surgery (I97.790)

Code also complication, if known and applicable, such as:
(acute) stent occlusion (T82.897-)
(acute) stent stenosis (T82.855-)
(acute) stent thrombosis (T82.867-)
cardiac arrest due to underlying cardiac condition (I46.2)
complication of percutaneous coronary intervention (PCI) (I97.89)
occlusion of coronary artery bypass graft (T82.218-)
AHA: 2021,3Q,6; 2019,2Q,33

✓4ᵗʰ I22 Subsequent ST elevation (STEMI) and non-ST elevation (NSTEMI) myocardial infarction

INCLUDES acute myocardial infarction occurring within four weeks (28 days) of a previous acute myocardial infarction, regardless of site
cardiac infarction
coronary (artery) embolism
coronary (artery) occlusion
coronary (artery) rupture
coronary (artery) thrombosis
infarction of heart, myocardium, or ventricle
recurrent myocardial infarction
reinfarction of myocardium
rupture of heart, myocardium, or ventricle
subsequent type 1 myocardial infarction

Use additional code, if applicable, to identify:
exposure to environmental tobacco smoke (Z77.22)
history of tobacco dependence (Z87.891)
occupational exposure to environmental tobacco smoke (Z57.31)
status post administration of tPA (rtPA) in a different facility within the last 24 hours prior to admission to current facility (Z92.82)
tobacco dependence (F17.-)
tobacco use (Z72.0)

EXCLUDES 1 subsequent myocardial infarction, type 2 (I21.A1)
subsequent myocardial infarction of other type (type 3) (type 4) (type 5) (I21.A9)

AHA: 2018,4Q,68; 2018,3Q,5; 2017,4Q,12-13; 2017,2Q,11; 2013,1Q,25; 2012,4Q,97,102-103
DEF: Non-ST elevation myocardial infarction: Partial obstruction of one or more coronary arteries that causes decreased blood flow (ischemia) and may cause partial thickness necrosis of myocardial muscle cells.
DEF: ST elevation myocardial infarction: Complete obstruction of one or more coronary arteries causing decreased blood flow (ischemia) and necrosis of myocardial muscle cells.
TIP: When chronic total occlusion and myocardial infarction are documented as being in different vessels, assign code I25.82 Chronic total occlusion of coronary artery, in addition to the myocardial infarction code.

I22.0 Subsequent ST elevation (STEMI) myocardial infarction of anterior wall HCC Rx ESR COM
Subsequent acute transmural myocardial infarction of anterior wall
Subsequent transmural (Q wave) infarction (acute)(of) anterior (wall) NOS
Subsequent anteroapical transmural (Q wave) infarction (acute)
Subsequent anterolateral transmural (Q wave) infarction (acute)
Subsequent anteroseptal transmural (Q wave) infarction (acute)

I22.1 Subsequent ST elevation (STEMI) myocardial infarction of inferior wall HCC Rx ESR COM
Subsequent acute transmural myocardial infarction of inferior wall
Subsequent transmural (Q wave) infarction (acute)(of) diaphragmatic wall
Subsequent transmural (Q wave) infarction (acute)(of) inferior (wall) NOS
Subsequent inferolateral transmural (Q wave) infarction (acute)
Subsequent inferoposterior transmural (Q wave) infarction (acute)
AHA: 2012,4Q,102

I22.2 Subsequent non-ST elevation (NSTEMI) myocardial infarction HCC Rx ESR COM
Subsequent acute subendocardial myocardial infarction
Subsequent non-Q wave myocardial infarction NOS
Subsequent nontransmural myocardial infarction NOS

I22.8 Subsequent ST elevation (STEMI) myocardial infarction of other sites HCC Rx ESR COM
Subsequent acute transmural myocardial infarction of other sites
Subsequent apical-lateral transmural (Q wave) myocardial infarction (acute)
Subsequent basal-lateral transmural (Q wave) myocardial infarction (acute)
Subsequent high lateral transmural (Q wave) myocardial infarction (acute)
Subsequent transmural (Q wave) myocardial infarction (acute)(of) lateral (wall) NOS
Subsequent posterior (true) transmural (Q wave) myocardial infarction (acute)
Subsequent posterobasal transmural (Q wave) myocardial infarction (acute)
Subsequent posterolateral transmural (Q wave) myocardial infarction (acute)
Subsequent posteroseptal transmural (Q wave) myocardial infarction (acute)
Subsequent septal NOS transmural (Q wave) myocardial infarction (acute)

I22.9 Subsequent ST elevation (STEMI) myocardial infarction of unspecified site HCC Rx ESR COM
Subsequent acute myocardial infarction of unspecified site
Subsequent myocardial infarction (acute) NOS

✓4ᵗʰ I23 Certain current complications following ST elevation (STEMI) and non-ST elevation (NSTEMI) myocardial infarction (within the 28 day period)
AHA: 2017,2Q,11
DEF: ST elevation myocardial infarction: Complete obstruction of one or more coronary arteries causing decreased blood flow (ischemia) and necrosis of myocardial muscle cells.
DEF: Non-ST elevation myocardial infarction: Partial obstruction of one or more coronary arteries that causes decreased blood flow (ischemia) and may cause partial thickness necrosis of myocardial muscle cells.

I23.0 Hemopericardium as current complication following acute myocardial infarction HCC Rx ESR COM A
EXCLUDES 1 hemopericardium not specified as current complication following acute myocardial infarction (I31.2)

I23.1 Atrial septal defect as current complication following acute myocardial infarction HCC Rx ESR COM A
EXCLUDES 1 acquired atrial septal defect not specified as current complication following acute myocardial infarction (I51.0)

I23.2 Ventricular septal defect as current complication following acute myocardial infarction HCC Rx ESR COM A
EXCLUDES 1 acquired ventricular septal defect not specified as current complication following acute myocardial infarction (I51.0)

I23.3 Rupture of cardiac wall without hemopericardium as current complication following acute myocardial infarction HCC Rx ESR COM A

I23.4 Rupture of chordae tendineae as current complication following acute myocardial infarction HCC Rx ESR COM
EXCLUDES 1 rupture of chordae tendineae not specified as current complication following acute myocardial infarction (I51.1)

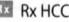

I23.5 Rupture of papillary muscle as current complication following acute myocardial infarction `HCC` `Rx` `ESR` `COM`
> *EXCLUDES 1*   rupture of papillary muscle not specified as current complication following acute myocardial infarction (I51.2)

I23.6 Thrombosis of atrium, auricular appendage, and ventricle as current complications following acute myocardial infarction `HCC` `Rx` `ESR` `COM` `A`
> *EXCLUDES 1*   thrombosis of atrium, auricular appendage, and ventricle not specified as current complication following acute myocardial infarction (I51.3)

I23.7 Postinfarction angina `HCC` `Rx` `ESR` `COM` `A`
> **AHA:** 2015,2Q,16
>
> **TIP:** When postinfarction angina occurs with atherosclerotic coronary artery disease, code both I23.7 and I25.118 for atherosclerotic disease with other forms of angina pectoris.

I23.8 Other current complications following acute myocardial infarction `HCC` `Rx` `ESR` `COM` `A`

✓4ᵗʰ I24 Other acute ischemic heart diseases
> *EXCLUDES 1*   angina pectoris (I20.-)
> transient myocardial ischemia in newborn (P29.4)
> *EXCLUDES 2*   non-ischemic myocardial injury (I5A)

I24.0 Acute coronary thrombosis not resulting in myocardial infarction `HCC` `Rx` `ESR` `COM`
> Acute coronary (artery) (vein) embolism not resulting in myocardial infarction
> Acute coronary (artery) (vein) occlusion not resulting in myocardial infarction
> Acute coronary (artery) (vein) thromboembolism not resulting in myocardial infarction
> *EXCLUDES 1*   atherosclerotic heart disease (I25.1-)
>
> **AHA:** 2013,1Q,24

I24.1 Dressler's syndrome `HCC` `Rx` `ESR` `COM`
> Postmyocardial infarction syndrome
> *EXCLUDES 1*   postinfarction angina (I23.7)
>
> **DEF:** Fever, leukocytosis, chest pain, evidence of pericarditis, pleurisy, and pneumonia occurring days or weeks after a myocardial infarction.

I24.8 Other forms of acute ischemic heart disease `HCC` `Rx` `ESR` `COM`
> *EXCLUDES 1*   myocardial infarction due to demand ischemia (I21.A1)
>
> **AHA:** 2019,4Q,53; 2017,4Q,13

I24.9 Acute ischemic heart disease, unspecified `HCC` `Rx` `ESR` `COM`
> *EXCLUDES 1*   ischemic heart disease (chronic) NOS (I25.9)

✓4ᵗʰ I25 Chronic ischemic heart disease
> Use additional code to identify:
> chronic total occlusion of coronary artery (I25.82)
> exposure to environmental tobacco smoke (Z77.22)
> history of tobacco dependence (Z87.891)
> occupational exposure to environmental tobacco smoke (Z57.31)
> tobacco dependence (F17.-)
> tobacco use (Z72.0)
> *EXCLUDES 2*   non-ischemic myocardial injury (I5A)

✓5ᵗʰ I25.1 Atherosclerotic heart disease of native coronary artery
> Atherosclerotic cardiovascular disease
> Coronary (artery) atheroma
> Coronary (artery) atherosclerosis
> Coronary (artery) disease
> Coronary (artery) sclerosis
> Use additional code, if applicable, to identify:
> coronary atherosclerosis due to calcified coronary lesion (I25.84)
> coronary atherosclerosis due to lipid rich plaque (I25.83)
> *EXCLUDES 2*   atheroembolism (I75.-)
> atherosclerosis of coronary artery bypass graft(s) and transplanted heart (I25.7-)

Atheromas

Atheromas (fatty tissue and/or plaque)   Lumen

I25.10 Atherosclerotic heart disease of native coronary artery without angina pectoris `Rx` `A`
> Atherosclerotic heart disease NOS
> **AHA:** 2021,3Q,6-7; 2015,2Q,16; 2012,4Q,92

✓6ᵗʰ I25.11 Atherosclerotic heart disease of native coronary artery with angina pectoris

   I25.110 Atherosclerotic heart disease of native coronary artery with unstable angina pectoris `HCC` `Rx` `ESR` `COM` `A`
> *EXCLUDES 1*   unstable angina without atherosclerotic heart disease (I20.0)

   I25.111 Atherosclerotic heart disease of native coronary artery with angina pectoris with documented spasm `HCC` `Rx` `ESR` `A`
> *EXCLUDES 1*   angina pectoris with documented spasm without atherosclerotic heart disease (I20.1)

   I25.112 Atherosclerosic heart disease of native coronary artery with refractory angina pectoris

   I25.118 Atherosclerotic heart disease of native coronary artery with other forms of angina pectoris `HCC` `Rx` `ESR` `A`
> *EXCLUDES 1*   other forms of angina pectoris without atherosclerotic heart disease (I20.8)
>
> **AHA:** 2015,2Q,16
> **TIP:** When postinfarction angina occurs with atherosclerotic coronary artery disease, code both I23.7 and I25.118 for atherosclerotic disease with other forms of angina pectoris.

   I25.119 Atherosclerotic heart disease of native coronary artery with unspecified angina pectoris `HCC` `Rx` `ESR` `A`
> Atherosclerotic heart disease with angina NOS
> Atherosclerotic heart disease with ischemic chest pain
> *EXCLUDES 1*   unspecified angina pectoris without atherosclerotic heart disease (I20.9)

I25.2 Old myocardial infarction `Rx`
Healed myocardial infarction
Past myocardial infarction diagnosed by ECG or other
investigation, but currently presenting no symptoms

I25.3 Aneurysm of heart `Rx`
Mural aneurysm
Ventricular aneurysm

√5ᵗʰ **I25.4 Coronary artery aneurysm and dissection**

I25.41 Coronary artery aneurysm `Rx`
Coronary arteriovenous fistula, acquired
> *EXCLUDES 1*   congenital coronary (artery) aneurysm
> (Q24.5)

I25.42 Coronary artery dissection `Rx`
DEF: Tear in the intimal arterial wall of a coronary artery
resulting in the sudden intrusion of blood within the
layers of the wall.

I25.5 Ischemic cardiomyopathy `Rx`
> *EXCLUDES 2*   coronary atherosclerosis (I25.1-, I25.7-)

I25.6 Silent myocardial ischemia `Rx`

√5ᵗʰ **I25.7 Atherosclerosis of coronary artery bypass graft(s) and
coronary artery of transplanted heart with angina pectoris**
Use additional code, if applicable, to identify:
coronary atherosclerosis due to calcified coronary lesion
(I25.84)
coronary atherosclerosis due to lipid rich plaque (I25.83)
> *EXCLUDES 1*   atherosclerosis of bypass graft(s) of transplanted
> heart without angina pectoris (I25.812)
> atherosclerosis of coronary artery bypass graft(s)
> without angina pectoris (I25.810)
> atherosclerosis of native coronary artery of
> transplanted heart without angina pectoris
> (I25.811)

√6ᵗʰ **I25.70 Atherosclerosis of coronary artery bypass graft(s),
unspecified, with angina pectoris**

**I25.700 Atherosclerosis of coronary artery bypass
graft(s), unspecified, with unstable
angina pectoris** `HCC` `Rx` `ESR` `COM` `A`
> *EXCLUDES 1*   unstable angina pectoris
> without atherosclerosis of
> coronary artery bypass
> graft (I20.0)

**I25.701 Atherosclerosis of coronary artery bypass
graft(s), unspecified, with angina pectoris
with documented spasm** `HCC` `Rx` `ESR` `A`
> *EXCLUDES 1*   angina pectoris with
> documented spasm
> without atherosclerosis of
> coronary artery bypass
> graft (I20.1)

**I25.702 Atherosclerosis of coronary artery bypass
graft(s), unspecified, with refractory
angina pectoris**

**I25.708 Atherosclerosis of coronary artery bypass
graft(s), unspecified, with other forms of
angina pectoris** `HCC` `Rx` `ESR` `A`
> *EXCLUDES 1*   other forms of angina pectoris
> without atherosclerosis of
> coronary artery bypass
> graft (I20.8)

**I25.709 Atherosclerosis of coronary artery bypass
graft(s), unspecified, with unspecified
angina pectoris** `HCC` `Rx` `ESR` `A`
> *EXCLUDES 1*   unspecified angina pectoris
> without atherosclerosis of
> coronary artery bypass
> graft (I20.9)

√6ᵗʰ **I25.71 Atherosclerosis of autologous vein coronary artery
bypass graft(s) with angina pectoris**

**I25.710 Atherosclerosis of autologous vein
coronary artery bypass graft(s) with
unstable angina
pectoris** `HCC` `Rx` `ESR` `COM` `A`
> *EXCLUDES 1*   unstable angina without
> atherosclerosis of
> autologous vein coronary
> artery bypass graft(s)
> (I20.0)
> *EXCLUDES 2*   embolism or thrombus of
> coronary artery bypass
> graft(s) (T82.8-)

**I25.711 Atherosclerosis of autologous vein
coronary artery bypass graft(s) with
angina pectoris with documented
spasm** `HCC` `Rx` `ESR` `A`
> *EXCLUDES 1*   angina pectoris with
> documented spasm
> without atherosclerosis of
> autologous vein coronary
> artery bypass graft(s)
> (I20.1)

**I25.712 Atherosclerosis of autologous vein
coronary artery bypass graft(s) with
refractory angina pectoris**

**I25.718 Atherosclerosis of autologous vein
coronary artery bypass graft(s) with other
forms of angina pectoris** `HCC` `Rx` `ESR` `A`
> *EXCLUDES 1*   other forms of angina pectoris
> without atherosclerosis of
> autologous vein coronary
> artery bypass graft(s)
> (I20.8)

**I25.719 Atherosclerosis of autologous vein
coronary artery bypass graft(s) with
unspecified angina
pectoris** `HCC` `Rx` `ESR` `A`
> *EXCLUDES 1*   unspecified angina pectoris
> without atherosclerosis of
> autologous vein coronary
> artery bypass graft(s)
> (I20.9)

√6ᵗʰ **I25.72 Atherosclerosis of autologous artery coronary
artery bypass graft(s) with angina pectoris**
Atherosclerosis of internal mammary artery graft with
angina pectoris

**I25.720 Atherosclerosis of autologous artery
coronary artery bypass graft(s) with
unstable angina
pectoris** `HCC` `Rx` `ESR` `COM` `A`
> *EXCLUDES 1*   unstable angina without
> atherosclerosis of
> autologous artery
> coronary artery bypass
> graft(s) (I20.0)

**I25.721 Atherosclerosis of autologous artery
coronary artery bypass graft(s) with
angina pectoris with documented
spasm** `HCC` `Rx` `ESR` `A`
> *EXCLUDES 1*   angina pectoris with
> documented spasm
> without atherosclerosis of
> autologous artery
> coronary artery bypass
> graft(s) (I20.1)

**I25.722 Atherosclerosis of autologous artery
coronary artery bypass graft(s) with
refractory angina pectoris**

**I25.728 Atherosclerosis of autologous artery
coronary artery bypass graft(s) with other
forms of angina pectoris** `HCC` `Rx` `ESR` `A`
> *EXCLUDES 1*   other forms of angina pectoris
> without atherosclerosis of
> autologous artery
> coronary artery bypass
> graft(s) (I20.8)

`HCC` CMS-HCC   `Rx` Rx HCC   `ESR` ESRD HCC   `COM` Commercial HCC   `N` Newborn: 0   `P` Pediatric: 0-17   `M` Maternity: 9-64   `A` Adult: 15-124

666   ICD-10-CM 2023

I25.729 Atherosclerosis of autologous artery coronary artery bypass graft(s) with unspecified angina pectoris `HCC` `Rx` `ESR` `A`

    EXCLUDES 1   *unspecified angina pectoris without atherosclerosis of autologous artery coronary artery bypass graft(s) (I20.9)*

✓6th **I25.73** Atherosclerosis of nonautologous biological coronary artery bypass graft(s) with angina pectoris

I25.730 Atherosclerosis of nonautologous biological coronary artery bypass graft(s) with unstable angina pectoris `HCC` `Rx` `ESR` `COM` `A`

    EXCLUDES 1   *unstable angina without atherosclerosis of nonautologous biological coronary artery bypass graft(s) (I20.0)*

I25.731 Atherosclerosis of nonautologous biological coronary artery bypass graft(s) with angina pectoris with documented spasm `HCC` `Rx` `ESR` `A`

    EXCLUDES 1   *angina pectoris with documented spasm without atherosclerosis of nonautologous biological coronary artery bypass graft(s) (I20.1)*

I25.732 Atherosclerosis of nonautologous biological coronary artery bypass graft(s) with refractory angina pectoris

I25.738 Atherosclerosis of nonautologous biological coronary artery bypass graft(s) with other forms of angina pectoris `HCC` `Rx` `ESR` `A`

    EXCLUDES 1   *other forms of angina pectoris without atherosclerosis of nonautologous biological coronary artery bypass graft(s) (I20.8)*

I25.739 Atherosclerosis of nonautologous biological coronary artery bypass graft(s) with unspecified angina pectoris `HCC` `Rx` `ESR` `A`

    EXCLUDES 1   *unspecified angina pectoris without atherosclerosis of nonautologous biological coronary artery bypass graft(s) (I20.9)*

✓6th **I25.75** Atherosclerosis of native coronary artery of transplanted heart with angina pectoris

    EXCLUDES 1   *atherosclerosis of native coronary artery of transplanted heart without angina pectoris (I25.811)*

I25.750 Atherosclerosis of native coronary artery of transplanted heart with unstable angina `HCC` `Rx` `ESR` `COM`

I25.751 Atherosclerosis of native coronary artery of transplanted heart with angina pectoris with documented spasm `HCC` `Rx` `ESR`

I25.752 Atherosclerosis of native coronary artery of transplanted heart with refractory angina pectoris

I25.758 Atherosclerosis of native coronary artery of transplanted heart with other forms of angina pectoris `HCC` `Rx` `ESR`

I25.759 Atherosclerosis of native coronary artery of transplanted heart with unspecified angina pectoris `HCC` `Rx` `ESR`

✓6th **I25.76** Atherosclerosis of bypass graft of coronary artery of transplanted heart with angina pectoris

    EXCLUDES 1   *atherosclerosis of bypass graft of coronary artery of transplanted heart without angina pectoris (I25.812)*

I25.760 Atherosclerosis of bypass graft of coronary artery of transplanted heart with unstable angina `HCC` `Rx` `ESR` `COM` `A`

I25.761 Atherosclerosis of bypass graft of coronary artery of transplanted heart with angina pectoris with documented spasm `HCC` `Rx` `ESR` `A`

I25.762 Atherosclerosis of bypass graft of coronary artery of transplanted heart with refractory angina pectoris

I25.768 Atherosclerosis of bypass graft of coronary artery of transplanted heart with other forms of angina pectoris `HCC` `Rx` `ESR` `A`

I25.769 Atherosclerosis of bypass graft of coronary artery of transplanted heart with unspecified angina pectoris `HCC` `Rx` `ESR` `A`

✓6th **I25.79** Atherosclerosis of other coronary artery bypass graft(s) with angina pectoris

I25.790 Atherosclerosis of other coronary artery bypass graft(s) with unstable angina pectoris `HCC` `Rx` `ESR` `COM` `A`

    EXCLUDES 1   *unstable angina without atherosclerosis of other coronary artery bypass graft(s) (I20.0)*

I25.791 Atherosclerosis of other coronary artery bypass graft(s) with angina pectoris with documented spasm `HCC` `Rx` `ESR` `A`

    EXCLUDES 1   *angina pectoris with documented spasm without atherosclerosis of other coronary artery bypass graft(s) (I20.1)*

I25.792 Atherosclerosis of other coronary artery bypass graft(s) with refractory angina pectoris

I25.798 Atherosclerosis of other coronary artery bypass graft(s) with other forms of angina pectoris `HCC` `Rx` `ESR` `A`

    EXCLUDES 1   *other forms of angina pectoris without atherosclerosis of other coronary artery bypass graft(s) (I20.8)*

I25.799 Atherosclerosis of other coronary artery bypass graft(s) with unspecified angina pectoris `HCC` `Rx` `ESR` `A`

    EXCLUDES 1   *unspecified angina pectoris without atherosclerosis of other coronary artery bypass graft(s) (I20.9)*

✓5th **I25.8** Other forms of chronic ischemic heart disease

✓6th **I25.81** Atherosclerosis of other coronary vessels without angina pectoris

    Use additional code, if applicable, to identify:

    coronary atherosclerosis due to calcified coronary lesion (I25.84)

    coronary atherosclerosis due to lipid rich plaque (I25.83)

    EXCLUDES 2   *atherosclerotic heart disease of native coronary artery without angina pectoris (I25.10)*

I25.810 Atherosclerosis of coronary artery bypass graft(s) without angina pectoris `Rx` `A`

    Atherosclerosis of coronary artery bypass graft NOS

    EXCLUDES 1   *atherosclerosis of coronary bypass graft(s) with angina pectoris (I25.70-I25.73-, I25.79-)*

I25.811 Atherosclerosis of native coronary artery of transplanted heart without angina pectoris `Rx`

    Atherosclerosis of native coronary artery of transplanted heart NOS

    EXCLUDES 1   *atherosclerosis of native coronary artery of transplanted heart with angina pectoris (I25.75-)*

Chapter 9. Diseases of the Circulatory System

I25.812   **Atherosclerosis of bypass graft of coronary artery of transplanted heart without angina pectoris** `Rx` `A`

Atherosclerosis of bypass graft of transplanted heart NOS

EXCLUDES 1   *atherosclerosis of bypass graft of transplanted heart with angina pectoris (I25.76)*

I25.82   **Chronic total occlusion of coronary artery** `Rx` `UPD`

Complete occlusion of coronary artery

Total occlusion of coronary artery

Code first coronary atherosclerosis (I25.1-, I25.7-, I25.81-)

EXCLUDES 1   *acute coronary occlusion with myocardial infarction (I21.0-I21.9, I22.-)*

acute coronary occlusion without myocardial infarction (I24.0)

AHA: 2018,3Q,5

DEF: Complete blockage of the coronary artery due to plaque accumulation over an extended period of time, resulting in substantial reduction of blood flow. Symptoms include angina or chest pain.

TIP: Report this code in addition to a code from category I21 or I22 when the chronic total occlusion and the myocardial infarction are documented as being in different vessels.

I25.83   **Coronary atherosclerosis due to lipid rich plaque** `Rx` `UPD` `A`

Code first coronary atherosclerosis (I25.1-, I25.7-, I25.81-)

I25.84   **Coronary atherosclerosis due to calcified coronary lesion** `Rx` `UPD`

Coronary atherosclerosis due to severely calcified coronary lesion

Code first coronary atherosclerosis (I25.1-, I25.7-, I25.81-)

I25.89   **Other forms of chronic ischemic heart disease** `Rx`

I25.9   **Chronic ischemic heart disease, unspecified** `Rx`

Ischemic heart disease (chronic) NOS

Pulmonary heart disease and diseases of pulmonary circulation (I26-I28)

`✓4ᵗʰ` **I26**   **Pulmonary embolism**

INCLUDES   pulmonary (acute)(artery)(vein) infarction

pulmonary (acute) (artery)(vein) thromboembolism

pulmonary (acute)(artery)(vein) thrombosis

EXCLUDES 2   *chronic pulmonary embolism (I27.82)*

personal history of pulmonary embolism (Z86.711)

pulmonary embolism complicating abortion, ectopic or molar pregnancy (O00-O07, O08.2)

pulmonary embolism complicating pregnancy, childbirth and the puerperium (O88.-)

pulmonary embolism due to trauma (T79.0, T79.1)

pulmonary embolism due to complications of surgical and medical care (T80.0, T81.7-, T82.8-)

septic (non-pulmonary) arterial embolism (I76)

`✓5ᵗʰ` **I26.0**   **Pulmonary embolism with acute cor pulmonale**

DEF: Cor pulmonale: Heart-lung disease appearing in identifiable forms as chronic or acute. The chronic form of this heart-lung disease is marked by dilation, hypertrophy and failure of the right ventricle due to a disease that has affected the function of the lungs, excluding congenital or left heart diseases and is also called chronic cardiopulmonary disease. The acute form is an overload of the right ventricle from a rapid onset of pulmonary hypertension, usually arising from a pulmonary embolism.

I26.01   **Septic pulmonary embolism with acute cor pulmonale** `HCC` `Rx` `ESR` `COM` `UPD`

Code first underlying infection

I26.02   **Saddle embolus of pulmonary artery with acute cor pulmonale** `HCC` `Rx` `ESR` `COM`

I26.09   **Other pulmonary embolism with acute cor pulmonale** `HCC` `Rx` `ESR` `COM`

Acute cor pulmonale NOS

AHA: 2014,4Q,21

`✓5ᵗʰ` **I26.9**   **Pulmonary embolism without acute cor pulmonale**

I26.90   **Septic pulmonary embolism without acute cor pulmonale** `HCC` `Rx` `ESR` `COM` `UPD`

Code first underlying infection

I26.92   **Saddle embolus of pulmonary artery without acute cor pulmonale** `HCC` `Rx` `ESR` `COM`

I26.93   **Single subsegmental pulmonary embolism without acute cor pulmonale** `HCC` `Rx` `ESR` `COM`

Subsegmental pulmonary embolism NOS

AHA: 2021,2Q,9; 2019,4Q,6-7

I26.94   **Multiple subsegmental pulmonary emboli without acute cor pulmonale** `HCC` `Rx` `ESR` `COM`

AHA: 2022,2Q,13; 2021,2Q,9; 2019,4Q,6-7

I26.99   **Other pulmonary embolism without acute cor pulmonale** `HCC` `Rx` `ESR` `COM`

Acute pulmonary embolism NOS

Pulmonary embolism NOS

AHA: 2022,2Q,13; 2020,3Q,10-11; 2019,2Q,22

`✓4ᵗʰ` **I27**   **Other pulmonary heart diseases**

I27.0   **Primary pulmonary hypertension** `HCC` `Rx` `ESR` `COM`

Heritable pulmonary arterial hypertension

Idiopathic pulmonary arterial hypertension

Primary group 1 pulmonary hypertension

Primary pulmonary arterial hypertension

EXCLUDES 1   *persistent pulmonary hypertension of newborn (P29.30)*

pulmonary hypertension NOS (I27.20)

secondary pulmonary arterial hypertension (I27.21)

secondary pulmonary hypertension (I27.29)

DEF: Condition that occurs when pressure within the pulmonary artery is elevated and vascular resistance is observed in the lungs.

I27.1   **Kyphoscoliotic heart disease** `HCC` `Rx` `ESR` `COM`

`✓5ᵗʰ` **I27.2**   **Other secondary pulmonary hypertension**

Code also associated underlying condition

EXCLUDES 1   *Eisenmenger's syndrome (I27.83)*

AHA: 2017,4Q,14-15; 2014,4Q,21

DEF: Condition that occurs when pressure within the pulmonary artery is elevated and vascular resistance is observed in the lungs.

I27.20   **Pulmonary hypertension, unspecified** `HCC` `Rx` `ESR` `COM`

Pulmonary hypertension NOS

I27.21   **Secondary pulmonary arterial hypertension** `HCC` `Rx` `ESR` `COM`

(Associated) (drug-induced) (toxin-induced) pulmonary arterial hypertension NOS

(Associated) (drug-induced) (toxin-induced) (secondary) group 1 pulmonary hypertension

Code also associated conditions if applicable, or adverse effects of drugs or toxins, such as:

adverse effect of appetite depressants (T50.5X5)

congenital heart disease (Q20-Q28)

human immunodeficiency virus [HIV] disease (B20)

polymyositis (M33.2-)

portal hypertension (K76.6)

rheumatoid arthritis (M05.-)

schistosomiasis (B65.-)

Sjögren syndrome (M35.0-)

systemic sclerosis (M34.-)

I27.22   **Pulmonary hypertension due to left heart disease** `HCC` `Rx` `ESR` `COM`

Group 2 pulmonary hypertension

Code also associated left heart disease, if known, such as:

multiple valve disease (I08.-)

rheumatic aortic valve diseases (I06.-)

rheumatic mitral valve diseases (I05.-)

I27.23   **Pulmonary hypertension due to lung diseases and hypoxia** `HCC` `Rx` `ESR` `COM`

Group 3 pulmonary hypertension

Code also associated lung disease, if known, such as:

bronchiectasis (J47.-)

cystic fibrosis with pulmonary manifestations (E84.0)

interstitial lung disease (J84.-)

pleural effusion (J90)

sleep apnea (G47.3-)

`HCC` CMS-HCC   `Rx` Rx HCC   `ESR` ESRD HCC   `COM` Commercial HCC   `N` Newborn: 0   `P` Pediatric: 0-17   `M` Maternity: 9-64   `A` Adult: 15-124

668   ICD-10-CM 2023

I27.24 **Chronic thromboembolic pulmonary hypertension** `HCC` `Rx` `ESR` `COM`
Group 4 pulmonary hypertension
Code also associated pulmonary embolism, if applicable (I26.-, I27.82)

I27.29 **Other secondary pulmonary hypertension** `HCC` `Rx` `ESR` `COM`
Group 5 pulmonary hypertension
Pulmonary hypertension with unclear multifactorial mechanisms
Pulmonary hypertension due to hematologic disorders
Pulmonary hypertension due to metabolic disorders
Pulmonary hypertension due to other systemic disorders
Code also other associated disorders, if known, such as:
chronic myeloid leukemia (C92.10-C92.22)
essential thrombocythemia (D47.3)
Gaucher disease (E75.22)
hypertensive chronic kidney disease with end stage renal disease (I12.0, I13.11, I13.2)
hyperthyroidism (E05.-)
hypothyroidism (E00-E03)
polycythemia vera (D45)
sarcoidosis (D86.-)
AHA: 2016,2Q,8

✓6ᵗʰ **I27.8** **Other specified pulmonary heart diseases**

I27.81 **Cor pulmonale (chronic)** `HCC` `Rx` `ESR` `COM`
Cor pulmonale NOS
EXCLUDES 1   *acute cor pulmonale (I26.0-)*
AHA: 2014,4Q,21
DEF: Heart-lung disease appearing in identifiable forms as chronic or acute. The chronic form of this heart-lung disease is marked by dilation, hypertrophy and failure of the right ventricle due to a disease that has affected the function of the lungs, excluding congenital or left heart diseases and is also called chronic cardiopulmonary disease. The acute form is an overload of the right ventricle from a rapid onset of pulmonary hypertension, usually arising from a pulmonary embolism.

I27.82 **Chronic pulmonary embolism** `HCC` `Rx` `ESR` `COM`
Use additional code, if applicable, for associated long-term (current) use of anticoagulants (Z79.01)
EXCLUDES 1   *personal history of pulmonary embolism (Z86.711)*
AHA: 2021,2Q,9
DEF: Long-standing condition commonly associated with pulmonary hypertension in which small blood clots travel to the lungs repeatedly over many weeks, months, or years, requiring continuation of established anticoagulant or thrombolytic therapy.

I27.83 **Eisenmenger's syndrome** `HCC` `Rx` `ESR` `COM`
Eisenmenger's complex
(Irreversible) Eisenmenger's disease
Pulmonary hypertension with right to left shunt related to congenital heart disease
Code also underlying heart defect, if known, such as:
atrial septal defect ▶(Q21.1-)◀
Eisenmenger's defect (Q21.8)
patent ductus arteriosus (Q25.0)
ventricular septal defect (Q21.0)
DEF: Pulmonary hypertension with congenital communication between two circulations resulting in a right to left shunt. This causes reduced oxygen saturation in the arterial blood, leading to cyanosis and organ damage. Once it develops, this life-threating condition is irreversible.

I27.89 **Other specified pulmonary heart diseases** `HCC` `Rx` `ESR` `COM`

I27.9 **Pulmonary heart disease, unspecified** `HCC` `Rx` `ESR` `COM`
Chronic cardiopulmonary disease

✓4ᵗʰ **I28** **Other diseases of pulmonary vessels**

I28.0 **Arteriovenous fistula of pulmonary vessels** `HCC` `Rx` `ESR` `COM`
EXCLUDES 1   *congenital arteriovenous fistula (Q25.72)*

I28.1 **Aneurysm of pulmonary artery** `HCC` `Rx` `ESR` `COM`
EXCLUDES 1   *congenital aneurysm (Q25.79)*
congenital arteriovenous aneurysm (Q25.72)

I28.8 **Other diseases of pulmonary vessels** `HCC` `Rx` `ESR` `COM`
Pulmonary arteritis
Pulmonary endarteritis
Rupture of pulmonary vessels
Stenosis of pulmonary vessels
Stricture of pulmonary vessels

I28.9 **Disease of pulmonary vessels, unspecified** `HCC` `Rx` `ESR` `COM`

Other forms of heart disease (I30-I5A)

✓4ᵗʰ **I30** **Acute pericarditis**
INCLUDES   acute mediastinopericarditis
acute myopericarditis
acute pericardial effusion
acute pleuropericarditis
acute pneumopericarditis
EXCLUDES 1   *Dressler's syndrome (I24.1)*
rheumatic pericarditis (acute) (I01.0)
viral pericarditis due to Coxsakie virus (B33.23)
DEF: Pericarditis: Inflammation affecting the pericardium, the fibroserous membrane that surrounds the heart.

I30.0 **Acute nonspecific idiopathic pericarditis** `COM`

I30.1 **Infective pericarditis** `COM`
Pneumococcal pericarditis
Pneumopyopericardium
Purulent pericarditis
Pyopericarditis
Pyopericardium
Pyopneumopericardium
Staphylococcal pericarditis
Streptococcal pericarditis
Suppurative pericarditis
Viral pericarditis
Use additional code (B95-B97) to identify infectious agent

I30.8 **Other forms of acute pericarditis** `COM`

I30.9 **Acute pericarditis, unspecified** `COM`

✓4ᵗʰ **I31** **Other diseases of pericardium**
EXCLUDES 1   *diseases of pericardium specified as rheumatic (I09.2)*
postcardiotomy syndrome (I97.0)
traumatic injury to pericardium (S26.-)

I31.0 **Chronic adhesive pericarditis** `COM`
Accretio cordis
Adherent pericardium
Adhesive mediastinopericarditis

I31.1 **Chronic constrictive pericarditis** `COM`
Concretio cordis
Pericardial calcification

I31.2 **Hemopericardium, not elsewhere classified** `COM`
EXCLUDES 1   *hemopericardium as current complication following acute myocardial infarction (I23.0)*
▶*malignant pericardial effusion (I31.31)*◀
DEF: Presence of blood in the pericardial sac (pericardium). It can lead to potentially fatal cardiac tamponade if enough blood enters the pericardial cavity.

▲ ✓5ᵗʰ **I31.3** **Pericardial effusion (noninflammatory)**
~~Chylopericardium~~
EXCLUDES 1   *acute pericardial effusion (I30.9)*
AHA: 2019,1Q,16

● **I31.31** **Malignant pericardial effusion in diseases classified elsewhere**
Code first underlying neoplasm (C00-D49)

● **I31.39** **Other pericardial effusion (noninflammatory)**
Chylopericardium

I31.4 **Cardiac tamponade** `COM` `UPD`
Code first underlying cause
DEF: Life-threatening condition in which fluid or blood accumulates in the space between the muscle of the heart (myocardium) and the outer sac that covers the heart (pericardium), resulting in compression of the heart.

Cardiac Tamponade

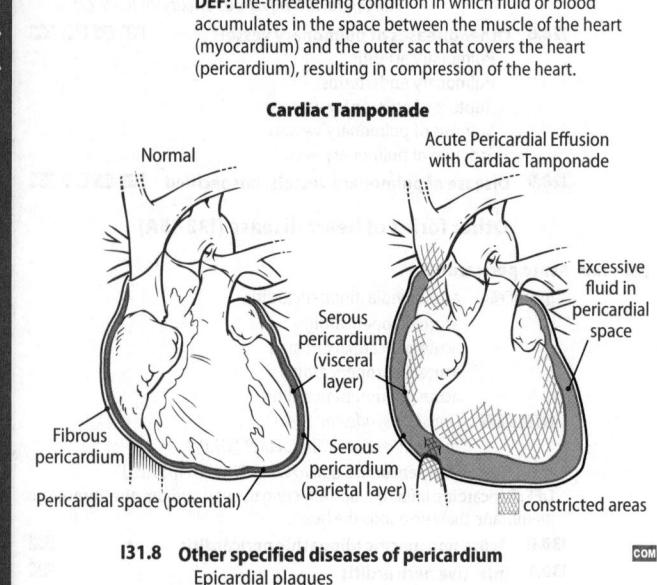

Normal

Acute Pericardial Effusion with Cardiac Tamponade

Excessive fluid in pericardial space

Serous pericardium (visceral layer)

Fibrous pericardium

Serous pericardium (parietal layer)

Pericardial space (potential)

constricted areas

I31.8 **Other specified diseases of pericardium** `COM`
Epicardial plaques
Focal pericardial adhesions

I31.9 **Disease of pericardium, unspecified** `COM`
Pericarditis (chronic) NOS

I32 *Pericarditis in diseases classified elsewhere* `COM`
Code first underlying disease
EXCLUDES 1 *pericarditis (in):*
coxsackie (virus) (B33.23)
gonococcal (A54.83)
meningococcal (A39.53)
rheumatoid (arthritis) (M05.31)
syphilitic (A52.06)
systemic lupus erythematosus (M32.12)
tuberculosis (A18.84)
DEF: Pericarditis: Inflammation affecting the pericardium, the fibroserous membrane that surrounds the heart.

√4ᵗʰ **I33** **Acute and subacute endocarditis**
EXCLUDES 1 *acute rheumatic endocarditis (I01.1)*
endocarditis NOS (I38)
DEF: Endocarditis: Inflammatory disease of the interior lining of the heart chamber and heart valves.

I33.0 **Acute and subacute infective endocarditis** `COM`
Bacterial endocarditis (acute) (subacute)
Infective endocarditis (acute) (subacute) NOS
Endocarditis lenta (acute) (subacute)
Malignant endocarditis (acute) (subacute)
Purulent endocarditis (acute) (subacute)
Septic endocarditis (acute) (subacute)
Ulcerative endocarditis (acute) (subacute)
Vegetative endocarditis (acute) (subacute)
Use additional code (B95-B97) to identify infectious agent

I33.9 **Acute and subacute endocarditis, unspecified** `COM`
Acute endocarditis NOS
Acute myoendocarditis NOS
Acute periendocarditis NOS
Subacute endocarditis NOS
Subacute myoendocarditis NOS
Subacute periendocarditis NOS

√4ᵗʰ **I34** **Nonrheumatic mitral valve disorders**
EXCLUDES 1 *mitral valve disease (I05.9)*
mitral valve failure (I05.8)
mitral valve stenosis (I05.0)
mitral valve disorder of unspecified cause with diseases of aortic and/or tricuspid valve(s) (I08.-)
mitral valve disorder of unspecified cause with mitral stenosis or obstruction (I05.0)
mitral valve disorder specified as congenital (Q23.2, Q23.9)
mitral valve disorder specified as rheumatic (I05.-)

I34.0 **Nonrheumatic mitral (valve) insufficiency**
Nonrheumatic mitral (valve) incompetence NOS
Nonrheumatic mitral (valve) regurgitation NOS
►Code also, if applicable:◄
►nonrheumatic mitral (valve) annulus calcification (I34.81)◄

I34.1 **Nonrheumatic mitral (valve) prolapse**
Floppy nonrheumatic mitral valve syndrome
EXCLUDES 1 *Marfan's syndrome (Q87.4-)*

I34.2 **Nonrheumatic mitral (valve) stenosis**
►Code also, if applicable:◄
►nonrheumatic mitral (valve) annulus calcification (I34.81)◄

▲ **√5ᵗʰ** **I34.8** **Other nonrheumatic mitral valve disorders**
● **I34.81** **Nonrheumatic mitral (valve) annulus calcification**
Nonrheumatic mitral (valve) annular calcification
Mitral (valve) annulus calcification NOS
Code also, if applicable:
nonrheumatic mitral (valve) insufficiency (I34.0)
nonrheumatic mitral (valve) stenosis (I34.2)
● **I34.89** **Other nonrheumatic mitral valve disorders**
I34.9 **Nonrheumatic mitral valve disorder, unspecified**

√4ᵗʰ **I35** **Nonrheumatic aortic valve disorders**
EXCLUDES 1 *aortic valve disorder of unspecified cause but with diseases of mitral and/or tricuspid valve(s) (I08.-)*
aortic valve disorder specified as congenital (Q23.0, Q23.1)
aortic valve disorder specified as rheumatic (I06.-)
hypertrophic subaortic stenosis (I42.1)

I35.0 **Nonrheumatic aortic (valve) stenosis**
I35.1 **Nonrheumatic aortic (valve) insufficiency**
Nonrheumatic aortic (valve) incompetence NOS
Nonrheumatic aortic (valve) regurgitation NOS
I35.2 **Nonrheumatic aortic (valve) stenosis with insufficiency**
I35.8 **Other nonrheumatic aortic valve disorders**
I35.9 **Nonrheumatic aortic valve disorder, unspecified**

√4ᵗʰ **I36** **Nonrheumatic tricuspid valve disorders**
EXCLUDES 1 *tricuspid valve disorders of unspecified cause (I07.-)*
tricuspid valve disorders specified as congenital (Q22.4, Q22.8, Q22.9)
tricuspid valve disorders specified as rheumatic (I07.-)
tricuspid valve disorders with aortic and/or mitral valve involvement (I08.-)

I36.0 **Nonrheumatic tricuspid (valve) stenosis**
I36.1 **Nonrheumatic tricuspid (valve) insufficiency**
Nonrheumatic tricuspid (valve) incompetence
Nonrheumatic tricuspid (valve) regurgitation
I36.2 **Nonrheumatic tricuspid (valve) stenosis with insufficiency**
I36.8 **Other nonrheumatic tricuspid valve disorders**
I36.9 **Nonrheumatic tricuspid valve disorder, unspecified**

√4ᵗʰ **I37** **Nonrheumatic pulmonary valve disorders**
EXCLUDES 1 *pulmonary valve disorder specified as congenital (Q22.1, Q22.2, Q22.3)*
pulmonary valve disorder specified as rheumatic (I09.89)

I37.0 **Nonrheumatic pulmonary valve stenosis**
I37.1 **Nonrheumatic pulmonary valve insufficiency**
Nonrheumatic pulmonary valve incompetence
Nonrheumatic pulmonary valve regurgitation
I37.2 **Nonrheumatic pulmonary valve stenosis with insufficiency**
I37.8 **Other nonrheumatic pulmonary valve disorders**
I37.9 **Nonrheumatic pulmonary valve disorder, unspecified**

I38 Endocarditis, valve unspecified

INCLUDES   endocarditis (chronic) NOS
valvular incompetence NOS
valvular insufficiency NOS
valvular regurgitation NOS
valvular stenosis NOS
valvulitis (chronic) NOS

EXCLUDES 1   congenital insufficiency of cardiac valve NOS (Q24.8)
congenital stenosis of cardiac valve NOS (Q24.8)
endocardial fibroelastosis (I42.4)
endocarditis specified as rheumatic (I09.1)

DEF: Endocarditis: Inflammatory disease of the interior lining of the heart chamber and heart valves.

I39 Endocarditis and heart valve disorders in diseases classified elsewhere

Code first underlying disease, such as:
Q fever (A78)

EXCLUDES 1   endocardial involvement in:
candidiasis (B37.6)
gonococcal infection (A54.83)
Libman-Sacks disease (M32.11)
listerosis (A32.82)
meningococcal infection (A39.51)
rheumatoid arthritis (M05.31)
syphilis (A52.03)
tuberculosis (A18.84)
typhoid fever (A01.02)

DEF: Endocarditis: Inflammatory disease of the interior lining of the heart chamber and heart valves.

✓4ᵗʰ I40 Acute myocarditis

INCLUDES   subacute myocarditis
EXCLUDES 1   acute rheumatic myocarditis (I01.2)
DEF: Myocarditis: Inflammation of the middle layer of the heart, which is composed of muscle tissue.

I40.0 Infective myocarditis   COM
Septic myocarditis
Use additional code (B95-B97) to identify infectious agent

I40.1 Isolated myocarditis   COM
Fiedler's myocarditis
Giant cell myocarditis
Idiopathic myocarditis

I40.8 Other acute myocarditis   COM

I40.9 Acute myocarditis, unspecified   COM

I41 Myocarditis in diseases classified elsewhere   COM

Code first underlying disease, such as:
typhus (A75.0-A75.9)

EXCLUDES 1   myocarditis (in):
Chagas' disease (chronic) (B57.2)
acute (B57.0)
coxsackie (virus) infection (B33.22)
diphtheritic (A36.81)
gonococcal (A54.83)
influenzal (J09.X9, J10.82, J11.82)
meningococcal (A39.52)
mumps (B26.82)
rheumatoid arthritis (M05.31)
sarcoid (D86.85)
syphilis (A52.06)
toxoplasmosis (B58.81)
tuberculous (A18.84)

DEF: Myocarditis: Inflammation of the middle layer of the heart, which is composed of muscle tissue.

✓4ᵗʰ I42 Cardiomyopathy

INCLUDES   myocardiopathy
Code first pre-existing cardiomyopathy complicating pregnancy and puerperium (O99.4)
EXCLUDES 2   ischemic cardiomyopathy (I25.5)
peripartum cardiomyopathy (O90.3)
ventricular hypertrophy (I51.7)

I42.0 Dilated cardiomyopathy   HCC Rx ESR COM
Congestive cardiomyopathy

I42.1 Obstructive hypertrophic cardiomyopathy   HCC Rx ESR COM
Hypertrophic subaortic stenosis (idiopathic)
DEF: Cardiomyopathy marked by left ventricle hypertrophy and an enlarged septum that result in obstructed blood flow, arrhythmias, mitral regurgitation, and sudden cardiac death.
TIP: When this condition is described as inherited, assign code Q24.8.

I42.2 Other hypertrophic cardiomyopathy   HCC Rx ESR COM
Nonobstructive hypertrophic cardiomyopathy

I42.3 Endomyocardial (eosinophilic) disease   HCC Rx ESR COM
Endomyocardial (tropical) fibrosis
Löffler's endocarditis

I42.4 Endocardial fibroelastosis   HCC Rx ESR COM
Congenital cardiomyopathy
Elastomyofibrosis

I42.5 Other restrictive cardiomyopathy   HCC Rx ESR COM
Constrictive cardiomyopathy NOS

I42.6 Alcoholic cardiomyopathy   HCC Rx ESR COM
Code also presence of alcoholism (F10.-)

I42.7 Cardiomyopathy due to drug and external agent   HCC Rx ESR COM
Code first poisoning due to drug or toxin, if applicable (T36-T65 with fifth or sixth character 1-4 or 6)
Use additional code for adverse effect, if applicable, to identify drug (T36-T50 with fifth or sixth character 5)
AHA: 2021,3Q,8

I42.8 Other cardiomyopathies   HCC Rx ESR COM

I42.9 Cardiomyopathy, unspecified   HCC Rx ESR COM
Cardiomyopathy (primary) (secondary) NOS

I43 Cardiomyopathy in diseases classified elsewhere   HCC Rx ESR COM
Code first underlying disease, such as:
amyloidosis (E85.-)
glycogen storage disease (E74.0)
gout (M10.0-)
thyrotoxicosis (E05.0-E05.9-)

EXCLUDES 1   cardiomyopathy (in):
coxsackie (virus) (B33.24)
diphtheria (A36.81)
sarcoidosis (D86.85)
tuberculosis (A18.84)

✓4ᵗʰ I44 Atrioventricular and left bundle-branch block

I44.0 Atrioventricular block, first degree

I44.1 Atrioventricular block, second degree
Atrioventricular block, type I and II
Möbitz block, type I and II
Second degree block, type I and II
Wenckebach's block

I44.2 Atrioventricular block, complete   HCC ESR COM
Complete heart block NOS
Third degree block
AHA: 2019,2Q,4

✓5ᵗʰ I44.3 Other and unspecified atrioventricular block
Atrioventricular block NOS

I44.30 Unspecified atrioventricular block

I44.39 Other atrioventricular block

I44.4 Left anterior fascicular block

I44.5 Left posterior fascicular block

✓5ᵗʰ I44.6 Other and unspecified fascicular block

I44.60 Unspecified fascicular block
Left bundle-branch hemiblock NOS

I44.69 Other fascicular block

I44.7　Left bundle-branch block, unspecified

Conduction Disorders

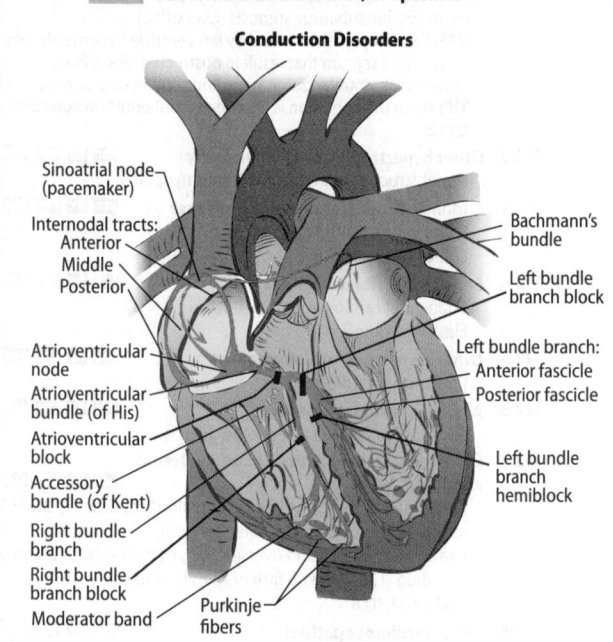

Sinoatrial node (pacemaker)
Internodal tracts:
　Anterior
　Middle
　Posterior
Atrioventricular node
Atrioventricular bundle (of His)
Atrioventricular block
Accessory bundle (of Kent)
Right bundle branch
Right bundle branch block
Moderator band
Purkinje fibers

Bachmann's bundle
Left bundle branch block
Left bundle branch:
　Anterior fascicle
　Posterior fascicle
Left bundle branch hemiblock

✓4th **I45**　Other conduction disorders

　I45.0　Right fascicular block

✓5th **I45.1**　Other and unspecified right bundle-branch block

　　I45.10　Unspecified right bundle-branch block
　　　　Right bundle-branch block NOS

　　I45.19　Other right bundle-branch block

　I45.2　Bifascicular block

　I45.3　Trifascicular block

　I45.4　Nonspecific intraventricular block
　　　Bundle-branch block NOS

　I45.5　Other specified heart block
　　　Sinoatrial block
　　　Sinoauricular block
　　　EXCLUDES 1　heart block NOS (I45.9)

　I45.6　Pre-excitation syndrome
　　　Accelerated atrioventricular conduction
　　　Accessory atrioventricular conduction
　　　Anomalous atrioventricular excitation
　　　Lown-Ganong-Levine syndrome
　　　Pre-excitation atrioventricular conduction
　　　Wolff-Parkinson-White syndrome

✓5th **I45.8**　Other specified conduction disorders

　　I45.81　Long QT syndrome
　　　DEF: Condition characterized by recurrent syncope, malignant arrhythmias, and sudden death. This syndrome has a characteristic prolonged Q-T interval on an electrocardiogram.

　　I45.89　Other specified conduction disorders
　　　Atrioventricular [AV] dissociation
　　　Interference dissociation
　　　Isorhythmic dissociation
　　　Nonparoxysmal AV nodal tachycardia
　　　AHA: 2013,2Q,31

　I45.9　Conduction disorder, unspecified
　　　Heart block NOS
　　　Stokes-Adams syndrome

✓4th **I46**　Cardiac arrest
　　　EXCLUDES 2　cardiogenic shock (R57.0)
　　　AHA: 2019,2Q,4-5

　I46.2　Cardiac arrest due to underlying cardiac condition　HCC ESR COM UPD
　　　Code first underlying cardiac condition

　I46.8　Cardiac arrest due to other underlying condition　HCC ESR COM UPD
　　　Code first underlying condition

　I46.9　Cardiac arrest, cause unspecified　HCC ESR COM
　　　AHA: 2020,3Q,26

✓4th **I47**　Paroxysmal tachycardia
　　Code first tachycardia complicating:
　　　abortion or ectopic or molar pregnancy (O00-O07, O08.8)
　　　obstetric surgery and procedures (O75.4)
　　　EXCLUDES 1　tachycardia NOS (R00.0)
　　　　　sinoauricular tachycardia NOS (R00.0)
　　　　　sinus [sinusal] tachycardia NOS (R00.0)

　I47.0　Re-entry ventricular arrhythmia　HCC ESR COM

　I47.1　Supraventricular tachycardia　HCC Rx ESR COM
　　　Atrial (paroxysmal) tachycardia
　　　Atrioventricular [AV] (paroxysmal) tachycardia
　　　Atrioventricular re-entrant (nodal) tachycardia [AVNRT] [AVRT]
　　　Junctional (paroxysmal) tachycardia
　　　Nodal (paroxysmal) tachycardia

▲ ✓5th **I47.2**　Ventricular tachycardia
　　　AHA: 2021,3Q,11; 2013,3Q,23

● 　　**I47.20**　Ventricular tachycardia, unspecified

● 　　**I47.21**　Torsades de pointes
　　　Code also, if applicable, long QT syndrome (I45.81)
　　　Use additional code for adverse effect, if applicable, to identify drug (T36-T50 with fifth or sixth character 5)
　　　DEF: Torsades de pointes (TdP): Accelerated heart rhythm, anywhere between 150 and 300 beats per minute, that initiates in the lower chambers of the heart (ventricles). Most commonly occurs in the setting of inherited or medication-induced long QT syndrome.

● 　　**I47.29**　Other ventricular tachycardia

　I47.9　Paroxysmal tachycardia, unspecified　HCC Rx ESR COM
　　　Bouveret (-Hoffman) syndrome

✓4th **I48**　Atrial fibrillation and flutter

　I48.0　Paroxysmal atrial fibrillation　HCC Rx ESR COM
　　　AHA: 2021,2Q,8; 2018,3Q,6

✓5th **I48.1**　Persistent atrial fibrillation
　　　EXCLUDES 1　permanent atrial fibrillation (I48.21)
　　　AHA: 2021,2Q,8; 2019,4Q,7; 2019,2Q,3; 2018,3Q,6

　　I48.11　Longstanding persistent atrial fibrillation　HCC Rx ESR COM

　　I48.19　Other persistent atrial fibrillation　HCC Rx ESR COM
　　　Chronic persistent atrial fibrillation
　　　Persistent atrial fibrillation, NOS
　　　AHA: 2019,4Q,7

✓5th **I48.2**　Chronic atrial fibrillation
　　　AHA: 2021,2Q,8; 2019,4Q,7; 2019,2Q,3; 2018,3Q,6

　　I48.20　Chronic atrial fibrillation, unspecified　HCC Rx ESR COM
　　　EXCLUDES 1　chronic persistent atrial fibrillation (I48.19)

　　I48.21　Permanent atrial fibrillation　HCC Rx ESR COM

　I48.3　Typical atrial flutter　HCC Rx ESR COM
　　　Type I atrial flutter

　I48.4　Atypical atrial flutter　HCC Rx ESR COM
　　　Type II atrial flutter

✓5th **I48.9**　Unspecified atrial fibrillation and atrial flutter

　　I48.91　Unspecified atrial fibrillation　HCC Rx ESR COM

　　I48.92　Unspecified atrial flutter　HCC Rx ESR COM

✓4th **I49**　Other cardiac arrhythmias
　　Code first cardiac arrhythmia complicating:
　　　abortion or ectopic or molar pregnancy (O00-O07, O08.8)
　　　obstetric surgery and procedures (O75.4)
　　　EXCLUDES 1　neonatal dysrhythmia (P29.1-)
　　　　　sinoatrial bradycardia (R00.1)
　　　　　sinus bradycardia (R00.1)
　　　　　vagal bradycardia (R00.1)
　　　EXCLUDES 2　bradycardia NOS (R00.1)

✓5th **I49.0**　Ventricular fibrillation and flutter

　　I49.01　Ventricular fibrillation　HCC ESR COM
　　　AHA: 2022,2Q,14

　　I49.02　Ventricular flutter　HCC ESR COM

　I49.1　Atrial premature depolarization　HCC Rx ESR COM
　　　Atrial premature beats

　I49.2　Junctional premature depolarization　HCC Rx ESR COM

I49.3   **Ventricular** premature **depolarization**
    AHA: 2020,2Q,23

☑5ᵗʰ   **I49.4**   **Other and unspecified premature depolarization**

    I49.40   **Unspecified premature depolarization**
      Premature beats NOS

    I49.49   **Other premature depolarization**
      Ectopic beats
      Extrasystoles
      Extrasystolic arrhythmias
      Premature contractions

I49.5   **Sick sinus syndrome**   `HCC` `ESR` `COM`
    Tachycardia-bradycardia syndrome
    AHA: 2019,1Q,33
    TIP: The presence of a pacemaker controls but does not cure sick sinus syndrome and therefore is considered a reportable chronic condition. When a pacemaker is evaluated by a provider, this code and code Z95.0 Presence of cardiac pacemaker, should be reported, even in the absence of any notable changes or management.

I49.8   **Other specified cardiac arrhythmias**
    Brugada syndrome
    Coronary sinus rhythm disorder
    Ectopic rhythm disorder
    Nodal rhythm disorder

I49.9   **Cardiac arrhythmia, unspecified**
    Arrhythmia (cardiac) NOS

☑4ᵗʰ   **I50**   **Heart failure**
    Code first:
     heart failure complicating abortion or ectopic or molar pregnancy (O00-O07, O08.8)
     heart failure due to hypertension (I11.0)
     heart failure due to hypertension with chronic kidney disease (I13.-)
     heart failure following surgery (I97.13-)
     obstetric surgery and procedures (O75.4)
     rheumatic heart failure (I09.81)
    EXCLUDES 2   *cardiac arrest (I46.-)*
              neonatal cardiac failure (P29.0)
    AHA: 2018,4Q,67; 2018,2Q,9; 2017,1Q,47; 2014,1Q,25; 2013,2Q,33

    I50.1   **Left ventricular** failure, unspecified   `HCC` `Rx` `ESR` `COM`
     Cardiac asthma
     Edema of lung with heart disease NOS
     Edema of lung with heart failure
     Left heart failure
     Pulmonary edema with heart disease NOS
     Pulmonary edema with heart failure
     EXCLUDES 1   *edema of lung without heart disease or heart failure (J81.-)*
               pulmonary edema without heart disease or failure (J81.-)

☑5ᵗʰ   **I50.2**   **Systolic (congestive) heart failure**
     Heart failure with reduced ejection fraction [HFrEF]
     Systolic left ventricular heart failure
     Code also end stage heart failure, if applicable (I50.84)
     EXCLUDES 1   *combined systolic (congestive) and diastolic (congestive) heart failure (I50.4-)*
     AHA: 2020,3Q,32; 2017,1Q,46; 2016,1Q,10

    I50.20   **Unspecified systolic (congestive) heart failure**   `HCC` `Rx` `ESR` `COM`

    I50.21   **Acute systolic (congestive) heart failure**   `HCC` `Rx` `ESR` `COM`

    I50.22   **Chronic systolic (congestive) heart failure**   `HCC` `Rx` `ESR` `COM`

    I50.23   **Acute on chronic** systolic **(congestive) heart failure**   `HCC` `Rx` `ESR` `COM`

☑5ᵗʰ   **I50.3**   **Diastolic (congestive) heart failure**
     Diastolic left ventricular heart failure
     Heart failure with normal ejection fraction
     Heart failure with preserved ejection fraction [HFpEF]
     Code also end stage heart failure, if applicable (I50.84)
     EXCLUDES 1   *combined systolic (congestive) and diastolic (congestive) heart failure (I50.4-)*
     AHA: 2020,3Q,32; 2017,1Q,46; 2016,1Q,10

    I50.30   **Unspecified diastolic (congestive) heart failure**   `HCC` `Rx` `ESR` `COM`

    I50.31   **Acute diastolic (congestive) heart failure**   `HCC` `Rx` `ESR` `COM`

    I50.32   **Chronic diastolic (congestive) heart failure**   `HCC` `Rx` `ESR` `COM`

    I50.33   **Acute on chronic diastolic (congestive) heart failure**   `HCC` `Rx` `ESR` `COM`

☑5ᵗʰ   **I50.4**   **Combined systolic (congestive) and diastolic (congestive) heart failure**
     Combined systolic and diastolic left ventricular heart failure
     Heart failure with reduced ejection fraction and diastolic dysfunction
     Code also end stage heart failure, if applicable (I50.84)
     AHA: 2017,1Q,46; 2016,1Q,10

    I50.40   **Unspecified combined systolic (congestive) and diastolic (congestive) heart failure**   `HCC` `Rx` `ESR` `COM`

    I50.41   **Acute combined systolic (congestive) and diastolic (congestive) heart failure**   `HCC` `Rx` `ESR` `COM`

    I50.42   **Chronic combined systolic (congestive) and diastolic (congestive) heart failure**   `HCC` `Rx` `ESR` `COM`

    I50.43   **Acute on chronic combined** systolic **(congestive) and diastolic (congestive) heart failure**   `HCC` `Rx` `ESR` `COM`

☑5ᵗʰ   **I50.8**   **Other heart failure**
    AHA: 2017,4Q,15-16

☑6ᵗʰ   **I50.81**   **Right** heart failure
     Right ventricular failure

    I50.810   **Right heart failure, unspecified**   `HCC` `Rx` `ESR` `COM`
      Right heart failure without mention of left heart failure
      Right ventricular failure NOS

    I50.811   **Acute right heart failure**   `HCC` `Rx` `ESR` `COM`
      Acute isolated right heart failure
      Acute (isolated) right ventricular failure

    I50.812   **Chronic right heart failure**   `HCC` `Rx` `ESR` `COM`
      Chronic isolated right heart failure
      Chronic (isolated) right ventricular failure

    I50.813   **Acute on chronic right heart failure**   `HCC` `Rx` `ESR` `COM`
      Acute on chronic isolated right heart failure
      Acute on chronic (isolated) right ventricular failure
      Acute decompensation of chronic (isolated) right ventricular failure
      Acute exacerbation of chronic (isolated) right ventricular failure

    I50.814   **Right heart failure due to left heart failure**   `HCC` `Rx` `ESR` `COM`
      Right ventricular failure secondary to left ventricular failure
      Code also the type of left ventricular failure, if known (I50.2-I50.43)
      EXCLUDES 1   *right heart failure with but not due to left heart failure (I50.82)*

    I50.82   **Biventricular** heart failure   `HCC` `Rx` `ESR` `COM`
     Code also the type of left ventricular failure as systolic, diastolic, or combined, if known (I50.2-I50.43)

    I50.83   **High output** heart failure   `HCC` `Rx` `ESR` `COM`
     DEF: Occurs when the high demand for blood exceeds the capacity of a normally functioning heart to meet the demand.

    I50.84   **End stage** heart failure   `HCC` `Rx` `ESR` `COM`
     Stage D heart failure
     Code also the type of heart failure as systolic, diastolic, or combined, if known (I50.2-I50.43)

    I50.89   **Other heart failure**   `HCC` `Rx` `ESR` `COM`

    I50.9   **Heart failure, unspecified**   `HCC` `Rx` `ESR` `COM`
     Cardiac, heart or myocardial failure NOS
     Congestive heart disease
     Congestive heart failure NOS
     EXCLUDES 2   *fluid overload unrelated to congestive heart failure (E87.70)*
     AHA: 2017,4Q,15-16; 2017,1Q,45-46; 2014,4Q,21; 2012,4Q,92

☑ Additional Character Required   ✓x 7ᵗʰ Placeholder Alert   Manifestation   Unspecified Dx   Q QPP   UPD Unacceptable PDx

Chapter 9. Diseases of the Circulatory System

I51–I60.4

✓4ᵗʰ **I51 Complications and ill-defined descriptions of heart disease**

> EXCLUDES 1   *any condition in I51.4-I51.9 due to hypertension (I11.-)*
>
> *any condition in I51.4-I51.9 due to hypertension and chronic kidney disease (I13.-)*
>
> *heart disease specified as rheumatic (I00-I09)*

I51.0 Cardiac septal defect, acquired   A

Acquired septal atrial defect (old)

Acquired septal auricular defect (old)

Acquired septal ventricular defect (old)

> EXCLUDES 1   *cardiac septal defect as current complication following acute myocardial infarction (I23.1, I23.2)*

DEF: Abnormal communication between opposite heart chambers due to a defect of the septum. It is not present at birth.

I51.1 Rupture of chordae tendineae, not elsewhere classified   HCC Rx ESR COM

> EXCLUDES 1   *rupture of chordae tendineae as current complication following acute myocardial infarction (I23.4)*

I51.2 Rupture of papillary muscle, not elsewhere classified   HCC Rx ESR COM

> EXCLUDES 1   *rupture of papillary muscle as current complication following acute myocardial infarction (I23.5)*

I51.3 Intracardiac thrombosis, not elsewhere classified

Apical thrombosis (old)

Atrial thrombosis (old)

Auricular thrombosis (old)

Mural thrombosis (old)

Ventricular thrombosis (old)

> EXCLUDES 1   *intracardiac thrombosis as current complication following acute myocardial infarction (I23.6)*

AHA: 2013,1Q,24

I51.4 Myocarditis, unspecified   HCC Rx ESR COM

Chronic (interstitial) myocarditis

Myocardial fibrosis

Myocarditis NOS

> EXCLUDES 1   *acute or subacute myocarditis (I40.-)*

AHA: 2018,4Q,67; 2018,2Q,9

I51.5 Myocardial degeneration   HCC Rx ESR COM

Fatty degeneration of heart or myocardium

Myocardial disease

Senile degeneration of heart or myocardium

AHA: 2018,4Q,67; 2018,2Q,9

I51.7 Cardiomegaly

Cardiac dilatation

Cardiac hypertrophy

Ventricular dilatation

AHA: 2018,4Q,67; 2018,2Q,9

✓5ᵗʰ **I51.8 Other ill-defined heart diseases**

AHA: 2018,2Q,9

I51.81 Takotsubo syndrome

Reversible left ventricular dysfunction following sudden emotional stress

Stress induced cardiomyopathy

Takotsubo cardiomyopathy

Transient left ventricular apical ballooning syndrome

DEF: Complex of symptoms mimicking myocardial infarct in absence of heart disease, with the majority of cases occurring in postmenopausal women. Heart muscles are temporarily weakened, and a sudden, massive surge of adrenalin stuns the heart, greatly reducing the ability to pump blood.

I51.89 Other ill-defined heart diseases

Carditis (acute)(chronic)

Pancarditis (acute)(chronic)

AHA: 2019,2Q,5; 2018,4Q,67

I51.9 Heart disease, unspecified

AHA: 2018,4Q,67; 2018,2Q,9

I52 Other heart disorders in diseases classified elsewhere

Code first underlying disease, such as:

congenital syphilis (A50.5)

mucopolysaccharidosis (E76.3)

schistosomiasis (B65.0-B65.9)

> EXCLUDES 1   *heart disease (in):*
>
> *gonococcal infection (A54.83)*
>
> *meningococcal infection (A39.50)*
>
> *rheumatoid arthritis (M05.31)*
>
> *syphilis (A52.06)*

I5A Non-ischemic myocardial injury (non-traumatic)

Acute (non-ischemic) myocardial injury

Chronic (non-ischemic) myocardial injury

Unspecified (non-ischemic) myocardial injury

Code first the underlying cause, if known and applicable, such as:

acute kidney failure (N17.-)

acute myocarditis (I40.-)

cardiomyopathy (I42.-)

chronic kidney disease (CKD) (N18.-)

heart failure (I50.-)

hypertensive urgency (I16.0)

nonrheumatic aortic valve disorders (I35.-)

paroxysmal tachycardia (I47.-)

pulmonary embolism (I26.-)

pulmonary hypertension (I27.0, I27.2-)

sepsis (A41.-)

takotsubo syndrome (I51.81)

> EXCLUDES 1   *acute myocardial infarction (I21.-)*
>
> *injury of heart (S26.-)*

> EXCLUDES 2   *other acute ischemic heart diseases (I24.-)*

AHA: 2021,4Q,14-15

Cerebrovascular diseases (I60-I69)

Use additional code to identify presence of:

alcohol abuse and dependence (F10.-)

exposure to environmental tobacco smoke (Z77.22)

history of tobacco dependence (Z87.891)

hypertension (I10-I16)

occupational exposure to environmental tobacco smoke (Z57.31)

tobacco dependence (F17.-)

tobacco use (Z72.0)

> EXCLUDES 1   *traumatic intracranial hemorrhage (S06.-)*

AHA: 2014,3Q,5; 2012,4Q,91-92

✓4ᵗʰ **I60 Nontraumatic subarachnoid hemorrhage**

> EXCLUDES 1   *syphilitic ruptured cerebral aneurysm (A52.05)*

> EXCLUDES 2   *sequelae of subarachnoid hemorrhage (I69.0-)*

✓5ᵗʰ **I60.0 Nontraumatic subarachnoid hemorrhage from carotid siphon and bifurcation**

I60.00 Nontraumatic subarachnoid hemorrhage from unspecified carotid siphon and bifurcation   HCC ESR COM

I60.01 Nontraumatic subarachnoid hemorrhage from right carotid siphon and bifurcation   HCC ESR COM

I60.02 Nontraumatic subarachnoid hemorrhage from left carotid siphon and bifurcation   HCC ESR COM

✓5ᵗʰ **I60.1 Nontraumatic subarachnoid hemorrhage from middle cerebral artery**

I60.10 Nontraumatic subarachnoid hemorrhage from unspecified middle cerebral artery   HCC ESR COM

I60.11 Nontraumatic subarachnoid hemorrhage from right middle cerebral artery   HCC ESR COM

I60.12 Nontraumatic subarachnoid hemorrhage from left middle cerebral artery   HCC ESR COM

I60.2 Nontraumatic subarachnoid hemorrhage from anterior communicating artery   HCC ESR COM

✓5ᵗʰ **I60.3 Nontraumatic subarachnoid hemorrhage from posterior communicating artery**

I60.30 Nontraumatic subarachnoid hemorrhage from unspecified posterior communicating artery   HCC ESR COM

I60.31 Nontraumatic subarachnoid hemorrhage from right posterior communicating artery   HCC ESR COM

I60.32 Nontraumatic subarachnoid hemorrhage from left posterior communicating artery   HCC ESR COM

I60.4 Nontraumatic subarachnoid hemorrhage from basilar artery   HCC ESR COM

✓5ᵗʰ I60.5 **Nontraumatic subarachnoid hemorrhage from** vertebral artery

     I60.50 **Nontraumatic subarachnoid hemorrhage from** unspecified vertebral artery   HCC ESR COM

     I60.51 **Nontraumatic subarachnoid hemorrhage from** right vertebral artery   HCC ESR COM

     I60.52 **Nontraumatic subarachnoid hemorrhage from** left vertebral artery   HCC ESR COM

I60.6 **Nontraumatic subarachnoid hemorrhage from other intracranial arteries**   HCC ESR COM

I60.7 **Nontraumatic subarachnoid hemorrhage from unspecified intracranial artery**   HCC ESR COM

     Ruptured (congenital) berry aneurysm

     Ruptured (congenital) cerebral aneurysm

     Subarachnoid hemorrhage (nontraumatic) from cerebral artery NOS

     Subarachnoid hemorrhage (nontraumatic) from communicating artery NOS

     EXCLUDES 1   berry aneurysm, nonruptured (I67.1)

I60.8 **Other nontraumatic subarachnoid hemorrhage**   HCC ESR COM

     Meningeal hemorrhage

     Rupture of cerebral arteriovenous malformation

I60.9 **Nontraumatic subarachnoid hemorrhage, unspecified**   HCC ESR COM

✓4ᵗʰ I61 **Nontraumatic intracerebral hemorrhage**

     EXCLUDES 2   sequelae of intracerebral hemorrhage (I69.1-)

     AHA: 2017,2Q,9-10

I61.0 **Nontraumatic intracerebral hemorrhage in** hemisphere, subcortical   HCC ESR COM

     Deep intracerebral hemorrhage (nontraumatic)

     AHA: 2016,4Q,27

I61.1 **Nontraumatic intracerebral hemorrhage in** hemisphere, cortical   HCC ESR COM

     Cerebral lobe hemorrhage (nontraumatic)

     Superficial intracerebral hemorrhage (nontraumatic)

I61.2 **Nontraumatic intracerebral hemorrhage in** hemisphere, unspecified   HCC ESR COM

I61.3 **Nontraumatic intracerebral hemorrhage in** brain stem   HCC ESR COM

I61.4 **Nontraumatic intracerebral hemorrhage in** cerebellum   HCC ESR COM

I61.5 **Nontraumatic intracerebral hemorrhage,** intraventricular   HCC ESR COM

I61.6 **Nontraumatic intracerebral hemorrhage,** multiple localized   HCC ESR COM

I61.8 **Other nontraumatic intracerebral hemorrhage**   HCC ESR COM

I61.9 **Nontraumatic intracerebral hemorrhage, unspecified**   HCC ESR COM

✓4ᵗʰ I62 **Other and unspecified** nontraumatic intracranial **hemorrhage**

     EXCLUDES 2   sequelae of intracranial hemorrhage (I69.2)

✓5ᵗʰ I62.0 **Nontraumatic** subdural **hemorrhage**

     I62.00 **Nontraumatic subdural hemorrhage, unspecified**   HCC ESR COM

     I62.01 **Nontraumatic** acute subdural **hemorrhage**   HCC ESR COM

     I62.02 **Nontraumatic** subacute subdural **hemorrhage**   HCC ESR COM

     I62.03 **Nontraumatic** chronic subdural **hemorrhage**   HCC ESR COM

I62.1 **Nontraumatic** extradural **hemorrhage**   HCC ESR COM

     Nontraumatic epidural hemorrhage

I62.9 **Nontraumatic intracranial hemorrhage, unspecified**   HCC ESR COM

✓4ᵗʰ I63 **Cerebral infarction**

     INCLUDES   occlusion and stenosis of cerebral and precerebral arteries, resulting in cerebral infarction

     Use additional code, if applicable, to identify status post administration of tPA (rtPA) in a different facility within the last 24 hours prior to admission to current facility (Z92.82)

     Use additional code, if known, to indicate National Institutes of Health Stroke Scale (NIHSS) score (R29.7-)

     EXCLUDES 1   neonatal cerebral infarction (P91.82-)

     EXCLUDES 2   sequelae of cerebral infarction (I69.3-)

     AHA: 2017,2Q,9-10; 2016,4Q,28,61-62; 2015,1Q,25; 2014,1Q,23

     TIP: Weakness on one side of the body documented as secondary to stroke is synonymous with hemiparesis/hemiplegia (G81.-). Weakness of one limb documented as secondary to stroke is synonymous with monoplegia (G83.1-, G83.2-, G83.3-).

✓5ᵗʰ I63.0 **Cerebral infarction due to** thrombosis of precerebral **arteries**

     I63.00 **Cerebral infarction due to thrombosis of unspecified precerebral artery**   HCC ESR COM

     ✓6ᵗʰ I63.01 **Cerebral infarction due to thrombosis of** vertebral artery

       I63.011 **Cerebral infarction due to thrombosis of** right vertebral artery   HCC ESR COM

       I63.012 **Cerebral infarction due to thrombosis of** left vertebral artery   HCC ESR COM

       I63.013 **Cerebral infarction due to thrombosis of** bilateral vertebral arteries   HCC ESR COM

       I63.019 **Cerebral infarction due to thrombosis of** unspecified vertebral artery   HCC ESR COM

     I63.02 **Cerebral infarction due to thrombosis of** basilar artery   HCC ESR COM

     ✓6ᵗʰ I63.03 **Cerebral infarction due to thrombosis of** carotid artery

       I63.031 **Cerebral infarction due to thrombosis of** right carotid artery   HCC ESR COM

       I63.032 **Cerebral infarction due to thrombosis of** left carotid artery   HCC ESR COM

       I63.033 **Cerebral infarction due to thrombosis of** bilateral carotid arteries   HCC ESR COM

       I63.039 **Cerebral infarction due to thrombosis of** unspecified carotid artery   HCC ESR COM

     I63.09 **Cerebral infarction due to thrombosis of other precerebral artery**   HCC ESR COM

✓5ᵗʰ I63.1 **Cerebral infarction due to** embolism of precerebral **arteries**

     I63.10 **Cerebral infarction due to embolism of unspecified precerebral artery**   HCC ESR COM

     ✓6ᵗʰ I63.11 **Cerebral infarction due to embolism of** vertebral artery

       I63.111 **Cerebral infarction due to embolism of** right vertebral artery   HCC ESR COM

       I63.112 **Cerebral infarction due to embolism of** left vertebral artery   HCC ESR COM

       I63.113 **Cerebral infarction due to embolism of** bilateral vertebral arteries   HCC ESR COM

       I63.119 **Cerebral infarction due to embolism of** unspecified vertebral artery   HCC ESR COM

     I63.12 **Cerebral infarction due to embolism of** basilar artery   HCC ESR COM

     ✓6ᵗʰ I63.13 **Cerebral infarction due to embolism of** carotid artery

       I63.131 **Cerebral infarction due to embolism of** right carotid artery   HCC ESR COM

       I63.132 **Cerebral infarction due to embolism of** left carotid artery   HCC ESR COM

       I63.133 **Cerebral infarction due to embolism of** bilateral carotid arteries   HCC ESR COM

       I63.139 **Cerebral infarction due to embolism of** unspecified carotid artery   HCC ESR COM

     I63.19 **Cerebral infarction due to embolism of other precerebral artery**   HCC ESR COM

✓5ᵗʰ I63.2 **Cerebral infarction due to unspecified** occlusion or stenosis of precerebral **arteries**

     AHA: 2020,3Q,27-28

     I63.20 **Cerebral infarction due to unspecified occlusion or stenosis of unspecified precerebral arteries**   HCC ESR COM

I63.21 Cerebral infarction due to unspecified occlusion or stenosis of vertebral arteries ✓6th

I63.211 Cerebral infarction due to unspecified occlusion or stenosis of right vertebral artery HCC ESR COM

I63.212 Cerebral infarction due to unspecified occlusion or stenosis of left vertebral artery HCC ESR COM

I63.213 Cerebral infarction due to unspecified occlusion or stenosis of bilateral vertebral arteries HCC ESR COM

I63.219 Cerebral infarction due to unspecified occlusion or stenosis of unspecified vertebral artery HCC ESR COM

I63.22 Cerebral infarction due to unspecified occlusion or stenosis of basilar artery HCC ESR COM

I63.23 Cerebral infarction due to unspecified occlusion or stenosis of carotid arteries ✓6th

I63.231 Cerebral infarction due to unspecified occlusion or stenosis of right carotid arteries HCC ESR COM

I63.232 Cerebral infarction due to unspecified occlusion or stenosis of left carotid arteries HCC ESR COM

I63.233 Cerebral infarction due to unspecified occlusion or stenosis of bilateral carotid arteries HCC ESR COM

I63.239 Cerebral infarction due to unspecified occlusion or stenosis of unspecified carotid artery HCC ESR COM

I63.29 Cerebral infarction due to unspecified occlusion or stenosis of other precerebral arteries HCC ESR COM

I63.3 Cerebral infarction due to thrombosis of cerebral arteries ✓5th

I63.30 Cerebral infarction due to thrombosis of unspecified cerebral artery HCC ESR COM

I63.31 Cerebral infarction due to thrombosis of middle cerebral artery ✓6th

I63.311 Cerebral infarction due to thrombosis of right middle cerebral artery HCC ESR COM

I63.312 Cerebral infarction due to thrombosis of left middle cerebral artery HCC ESR COM

I63.313 Cerebral infarction due to thrombosis of bilateral middle cerebral arteries HCC ESR COM

I63.319 Cerebral infarction due to thrombosis of unspecified middle cerebral artery HCC ESR COM

I63.32 Cerebral infarction due to thrombosis of anterior cerebral artery ✓6th

I63.321 Cerebral infarction due to thrombosis of right anterior cerebral artery HCC ESR COM

I63.322 Cerebral infarction due to thrombosis of left anterior cerebral artery HCC ESR COM

I63.323 Cerebral infarction due to thrombosis of bilateral anterior cerebral arteries HCC ESR COM

I63.329 Cerebral infarction due to thrombosis of unspecified anterior cerebral artery HCC ESR COM

I63.33 Cerebral infarction due to thrombosis of posterior cerebral artery ✓6th

I63.331 Cerebral infarction due to thrombosis of right posterior cerebral artery HCC ESR COM

I63.332 Cerebral infarction due to thrombosis of left posterior cerebral artery HCC ESR COM

I63.333 Cerebral infarction due to thrombosis of bilateral posterior cerebral arteries HCC ESR COM

I63.339 Cerebral infarction due to thrombosis of unspecified posterior cerebral artery HCC ESR COM

I63.34 Cerebral infarction due to thrombosis of cerebellar artery ✓6th

I63.341 Cerebral infarction due to thrombosis of right cerebellar artery HCC ESR COM

I63.342 Cerebral infarction due to thrombosis of left cerebellar artery HCC ESR COM

I63.343 Cerebral infarction due to thrombosis of bilateral cerebellar arteries HCC ESR COM

I63.349 Cerebral infarction due to thrombosis of unspecified cerebellar artery HCC ESR COM

I63.39 Cerebral infarction due to thrombosis of other cerebral artery HCC ESR COM

I63.4 Cerebral infarction due to embolism of cerebral arteries ✓5th

I63.40 Cerebral infarction due to embolism of unspecified cerebral artery HCC ESR COM

I63.41 Cerebral infarction due to embolism of middle cerebral artery ✓6th

I63.411 Cerebral infarction due to embolism of right middle cerebral artery HCC ESR COM

I63.412 Cerebral infarction due to embolism of left middle cerebral artery HCC ESR COM

I63.413 Cerebral infarction due to embolism of bilateral middle cerebral arteries HCC ESR COM

I63.419 Cerebral infarction due to embolism of unspecified middle cerebral artery HCC ESR COM

I63.42 Cerebral infarction due to embolism of anterior cerebral artery ✓6th

I63.421 Cerebral infarction due to embolism of right anterior cerebral artery HCC ESR COM

I63.422 Cerebral infarction due to embolism of left anterior cerebral artery HCC ESR COM

I63.423 Cerebral infarction due to embolism of bilateral anterior cerebral arteries HCC ESR COM

I63.429 Cerebral infarction due to embolism of unspecified anterior cerebral artery HCC ESR COM

I63.43 Cerebral infarction due to embolism of posterior cerebral artery ✓6th

I63.431 Cerebral infarction due to embolism of right posterior cerebral artery HCC ESR COM

I63.432 Cerebral infarction due to embolism of left posterior cerebral artery HCC ESR COM

I63.433 Cerebral infarction due to embolism of bilateral posterior cerebral arteries HCC ESR COM

I63.439 Cerebral infarction due to embolism of unspecified posterior cerebral artery HCC ESR COM

I63.44 Cerebral infarction due to embolism of cerebellar artery ✓6th

I63.441 Cerebral infarction due to embolism of right cerebellar artery HCC ESR COM

I63.442 Cerebral infarction due to embolism of left cerebellar artery HCC ESR COM

I63.443 Cerebral infarction due to embolism of bilateral cerebellar arteries HCC ESR COM

I63.449 Cerebral infarction due to embolism of unspecified cerebellar artery HCC ESR COM

I63.49 Cerebral infarction due to embolism of other cerebral artery HCC ESR COM

I63.5 Cerebral infarction due to unspecified occlusion or stenosis of cerebral arteries ✓5th

I63.50 Cerebral infarction due to unspecified occlusion or stenosis of unspecified cerebral artery HCC ESR COM

I63.51 Cerebral infarction due to unspecified occlusion or stenosis of middle cerebral artery ✓6th

I63.511 Cerebral infarction due to unspecified occlusion or stenosis of right middle cerebral artery HCC ESR COM

I63.512 Cerebral infarction due to unspecified occlusion or stenosis of left middle cerebral artery HCC ESR COM

I63.513 Cerebral infarction due to unspecified occlusion or stenosis of bilateral middle cerebral arteries `HCC` `ESR` `COM`

I63.519 Cerebral infarction due to unspecified occlusion or stenosis of unspecified middle cerebral artery `HCC` `ESR` `COM`

√6ᵗʰ **I63.52** Cerebral infarction due to unspecified occlusion or stenosis of anterior cerebral artery

I63.521 Cerebral infarction due to unspecified occlusion or stenosis of right anterior cerebral artery `HCC` `ESR` `COM`

I63.522 Cerebral infarction due to unspecified occlusion or stenosis of left anterior cerebral artery `HCC` `ESR` `COM`

I63.523 Cerebral infarction due to unspecified occlusion or stenosis of bilateral anterior cerebral arteries `HCC` `ESR` `COM`

I63.529 Cerebral infarction due to unspecified occlusion or stenosis of unspecified anterior cerebral artery `HCC` `ESR` `COM`

√6ᵗʰ **I63.53** Cerebral infarction due to unspecified occlusion or stenosis of posterior cerebral artery

I63.531 Cerebral infarction due to unspecified occlusion or stenosis of right posterior cerebral artery `HCC` `ESR` `COM`

I63.532 Cerebral infarction due to unspecified occlusion or stenosis of left posterior cerebral artery `HCC` `ESR` `COM`

I63.533 Cerebral infarction due to unspecified occlusion or stenosis of bilateral posterior cerebral arteries `HCC` `ESR` `COM`

I63.539 Cerebral infarction due to unspecified occlusion or stenosis of unspecified posterior cerebral artery `HCC` `ESR` `COM`

√6ᵗʰ **I63.54** Cerebral infarction due to unspecified occlusion or stenosis of cerebellar artery

I63.541 Cerebral infarction due to unspecified occlusion or stenosis of right cerebellar artery `HCC` `ESR` `COM`

I63.542 Cerebral infarction due to unspecified occlusion or stenosis of left cerebellar artery `HCC` `ESR` `COM`

I63.543 Cerebral infarction due to unspecified occlusion or stenosis of bilateral cerebellar arteries `HCC` `ESR` `COM`

I63.549 Cerebral infarction due to unspecified occlusion or stenosis of unspecified cerebellar artery `HCC` `ESR` `COM`

I63.59 Cerebral infarction due to unspecified occlusion or stenosis of other cerebral artery `HCC` `ESR` `COM`

I63.6 Cerebral infarction due to cerebral venous thrombosis, nonpyogenic `HCC` `ESR` `COM`

√5ᵗʰ **I63.8** Other cerebral infarction
AHA: 2018,4Q,16

I63.81 Other cerebral infarction due to occlusion or stenosis of small artery `HCC` `ESR` `COM`
Lacunar infarction
AHA: 2020,3Q,27

I63.89 Other cerebral infarction `HCC` `ESR` `COM`
AHA: 2022,1Q,25

I63.9 Cerebral infarction, unspecified `HCC` `ESR` `COM`
Stroke NOS
EXCLUDES 2 transient cerebral ischemic attacks and related syndromes (G45.-)
AHA: 2020,2Q,29
TIP: When provider documentation does not identify the location of an infarction, imaging reports can be used to pinpoint the location and lead to a more specific infarction code.

√4ᵗʰ **I65** Occlusion and stenosis of precerebral arteries, not resulting in cerebral infarction
INCLUDES embolism of precerebral artery
narrowing of precerebral artery
obstruction (complete) (partial) of precerebral artery
thrombosis of precerebral artery
EXCLUDES 1 insufficiency, NOS, of precerebral artery (G45.-)
insufficiency of precerebral arteries causing cerebral infarction (I63.0-I63.2)
AHA: 2018,2Q,9

√5ᵗʰ **I65.0** Occlusion and stenosis of vertebral artery

I65.01 Occlusion and stenosis of right vertebral artery

I65.02 Occlusion and stenosis of left vertebral artery

I65.03 Occlusion and stenosis of bilateral vertebral arteries

I65.09 Occlusion and stenosis of unspecified vertebral artery

I65.1 Occlusion and stenosis of basilar artery

√5ᵗʰ **I65.2** Occlusion and stenosis of carotid artery
AHA: 2021,1Q,4; 2020,3Q,28

I65.21 Occlusion and stenosis of right carotid artery

I65.22 Occlusion and stenosis of left carotid artery

I65.23 Occlusion and stenosis of bilateral carotid arteries

I65.29 Occlusion and stenosis of unspecified carotid artery

I65.8 Occlusion and stenosis of other precerebral arteries

I65.9 Occlusion and stenosis of unspecified precerebral artery
Occlusion and stenosis of precerebral artery NOS

√4ᵗʰ **I66** Occlusion and stenosis of cerebral arteries, not resulting in cerebral infarction
INCLUDES embolism of cerebral artery
narrowing of cerebral artery
obstruction (complete) (partial) of cerebral artery
thrombosis of cerebral artery
EXCLUDES 1 occlusion and stenosis of cerebral artery causing cerebral infarction (I63.3-I63.5)

√5ᵗʰ **I66.0** Occlusion and stenosis of middle cerebral artery

I66.01 Occlusion and stenosis of right middle cerebral artery

I66.02 Occlusion and stenosis of left middle cerebral artery

I66.03 Occlusion and stenosis of bilateral middle cerebral arteries

I66.09 Occlusion and stenosis of unspecified middle cerebral artery

√5ᵗʰ **I66.1** Occlusion and stenosis of anterior cerebral artery

I66.11 Occlusion and stenosis of right anterior cerebral artery

I66.12 Occlusion and stenosis of left anterior cerebral artery

I66.13 Occlusion and stenosis of bilateral anterior cerebral arteries

I66.19 Occlusion and stenosis of unspecified anterior cerebral artery

√5ᵗʰ **I66.2** Occlusion and stenosis of posterior cerebral artery

I66.21 Occlusion and stenosis of right posterior cerebral artery

I66.22 Occlusion and stenosis of left posterior cerebral artery

I66.23 Occlusion and stenosis of bilateral posterior cerebral arteries

I66.29 Occlusion and stenosis of unspecified posterior cerebral artery

I66.3 Occlusion and stenosis of cerebellar arteries

I66.8 Occlusion and stenosis of other cerebral arteries
Occlusion and stenosis of perforating arteries

I66.9 Occlusion and stenosis of unspecified cerebral artery

√4ᵗʰ **I67** Other cerebrovascular diseases
EXCLUDES 2 sequelae of the listed conditions (I69.8)

I67.0 Dissection of cerebral arteries, nonruptured `HCC` `ESR` `COM`
EXCLUDES 1 ruptured cerebral arteries (I60.7)
AHA: 2021,3Q,5
DEF: Dissecting aneurysm: Tear within an arterial wall that allows blood to accumulate between the outer and middle layers, creating a false lumen.

Chapter 9. Diseases of the Circulatory System

I67.1   **Cerebral aneurysm, nonruptured**   `COM`
Cerebral aneurysm NOS
Cerebral arteriovenous fistula, acquired
Internal carotid artery aneurysm, intracranial portion
Internal carotid artery aneurysm, NOS

> **EXCLUDES 1**   *congenital cerebral aneurysm, nonruptured (Q28.-)*
> *ruptured cerebral aneurysm (I60.7)*

AHA: 2021,3Q,5
TIP: A diagnosis of dissecting aneurysm should be coded to the dissection code, I67.0. The bulging/aneurysm, although present, occurred secondary to the dissection. The dissection represents the most significant problem.

Berry Aneurysm

Berry aneurysms form at the site of a weakness in an arterial wall, often at a junction

Berry aneurysm

Anterior communicating artery
Anterior cerebral artery
40%
34%
Internal carotid
20%
Middle cerebral artery
4%
Posterior cerebral artery
Posterior communicating artery
Basilar artery

Common sites of berry aneurysms in the circle of Willis arteries

I67.2   **Cerebral atherosclerosis**   `A`
Atheroma of cerebral and precerebral arteries

I67.3   **Progressive vascular leukoencephalopathy**   `HCC` `Rx` `ESR`
Binswanger's disease

I67.4   **Hypertensive encephalopathy**   `Rx`

> **EXCLUDES 2**   *insufficiency, NOS, of precerebral arteries (G45.2)*

I67.5   **Moyamoya disease**
DEF: Cerebrovascular ischemia. Vessels occlude and rupture, causing tiny hemorrhages at the base of brain. It affects predominantly Japanese people.

I67.6   **Nonpyogenic thrombosis of intracranial venous system**
Nonpyogenic thrombosis of cerebral vein
Nonpyogenic thrombosis of intracranial venous sinus

> **EXCLUDES 1**   *nonpyogenic thrombosis of intracranial venous system causing infarction (I63.6)*

I67.7   **Cerebral arteritis, not elsewhere classified**
Granulomatous angiitis of the nervous system

> **EXCLUDES 1**   *allergic granulomatous angiitis (M30.1)*

✓5ᵗʰ **I67.8**   **Other specified cerebrovascular diseases**

   I67.81   **Acute cerebrovascular insufficiency**
Acute cerebrovascular insufficiency unspecified as to location or reversibility

   I67.82   **Cerebral ischemia**
Chronic cerebral ischemia

   I67.83   **Posterior reversible encephalopathy syndrome**
PRES

✓6ᵗʰ **I67.84**   **Cerebral vasospasm and vasoconstriction**

    I67.841   **Reversible cerebrovascular vasoconstriction syndrome**
Call-Fleming syndrome
Code first underlying condition, if applicable, such as eclampsia (O15.00-O15.9)

    I67.848   **Other cerebrovascular vasospasm and vasoconstriction**

✓6ᵗʰ **I67.85**   **Hereditary cerebrovascular diseases**
AHA: 2018,4Q,17

   I67.850   **Cerebral autosomal dominant arteriopathy with subcortical infarcts and leukoencephalopathy**
CADASIL
Code also any associated diagnoses, such as:
epilepsy (G40.-)
stroke (I63.-)
vascular dementia (F01.-)

   I67.858   **Other hereditary cerebrovascular disease**

I67.89   **Other cerebrovascular disease**

I67.9   **Cerebrovascular disease, unspecified**

✓4ᵗʰ **I68**   **Cerebrovascular disorders in diseases classified elsewhere**

I68.0   *Cerebral amyloid angiopathy*
Code first underlying amyloidosis (E85.-)

I68.2   *Cerebral arteritis in other diseases classified elsewhere*
Code first underlying disease

> **EXCLUDES 1**   *cerebral arteritis (in):*
> *listerosis (A32.89)*
> *syphilis (A52.04)*
> *systemic lupus erythematosus (M32.19)*
> *tuberculosis (A18.89)*

I68.8   *Other cerebrovascular disorders in diseases classified elsewhere*
Code first underlying disease

> **EXCLUDES 1**   *syphilitic cerebral aneurysm (A52.05)*

✓4ᵗʰ **I69**   **Sequelae of cerebrovascular disease**

> **NOTE**   Category I69 is to be used to indicate conditions in I60-I67 as the cause of sequelae. The "sequelae" include conditions specified as such or as residuals which may occur at any time after the onset of the causal condition

> **EXCLUDES 1**   *personal history of cerebral infarction without residual deficit (Z86.73)*
> *personal history of prolonged reversible ischemic neurologic deficit (PRIND) (Z86.73)*
> *personal history of reversible ischemic neurologcial deficit (RIND) (Z86.73)*
> *sequelae of traumatic intracranial injury (S06.-)*

AHA: 2020,2Q,29; 2017,1Q,47; 2016,4Q,28; 2015,1Q,25; 2012,4Q,106
TIP: Weakness on one side of the body (unilateral weakness) documented as secondary to old cerebrovascular disease is synonymous with hemiparesis/hemiplegia. Weakness of one limb documented as secondary to old cerebrovascular disease is synonymous with monoplegia.
TIP: For codes describing hemiplegia, hemiparesis, and monoplegia; if the documentation identifies the affected side but not whether it is the dominant or nondominant side, the default is as follows: for ambidextrous patients, the default is dominant; when the left side is affected, the default is nondominant; and when the right side is affected, the default is dominant.

✓5ᵗʰ **I69.0**   **Sequelae of nontraumatic subarachnoid hemorrhage**

   I69.00   **Unspecified sequelae of nontraumatic subarachnoid hemorrhage**

✓6ᵗʰ   **I69.01**   **Cognitive deficits following nontraumatic subarachnoid hemorrhage**

    I69.010   **Attention and concentration deficit following nontraumatic subarachnoid hemorrhage**

    I69.011   **Memory deficit following nontraumatic subarachnoid hemorrhage**

    I69.012   **Visuospatial deficit and spatial neglect following nontraumatic subarachnoid hemorrhage**

    I69.013   **Psychomotor deficit following nontraumatic subarachnoid hemorrhage**

    I69.014   **Frontal lobe and executive function deficit following nontraumatic subarachnoid hemorrhage**

    I69.015   **Cognitive social or emotional deficit following nontraumatic subarachnoid hemorrhage**

    I69.018   **Other symptoms and signs involving cognitive functions following nontraumatic subarachnoid hemorrhage**

    I69.019   **Unspecified symptoms and signs involving cognitive functions following nontraumatic subarachnoid hemorrhage**

√6ᵗʰ **I69.02** **Speech and language deficits** following nontraumatic subarachnoid hemorrhage

    I69.020 **Aphasia** following nontraumatic subarachnoid hemorrhage

    I69.021 **Dysphasia** following nontraumatic subarachnoid hemorrhage

    I69.022 **Dysarthria** following nontraumatic subarachnoid hemorrhage

    I69.023 **Fluency disorder** following nontraumatic subarachnoid hemorrhage

        Stuttering following nontraumatic subarachnoid hemorrhage

    I69.028 **Other speech and language deficits** following nontraumatic subarachnoid hemorrhage

√6ᵗʰ **I69.03** Monoplegia of upper limb following nontraumatic subarachnoid hemorrhage

    AHA: 2017,1Q,47

    I69.031 **Monoplegia of upper limb** following nontraumatic subarachnoid hemorrhage affecting right dominant side   HCC ESR COM

    I69.032 **Monoplegia of upper limb** following nontraumatic subarachnoid hemorrhage affecting left dominant side   HCC ESR COM

    I69.033 **Monoplegia of upper limb** following nontraumatic subarachnoid hemorrhage affecting right non-dominant side   HCC ESR COM

    I69.034 **Monoplegia of upper limb** following nontraumatic subarachnoid hemorrhage affecting left non-dominant side   HCC ESR COM

    I69.039 **Monoplegia of upper limb** following nontraumatic subarachnoid hemorrhage affecting unspecified side   HCC ESR COM

√6ᵗʰ **I69.04** Monoplegia of lower limb following nontraumatic subarachnoid hemorrhage

    AHA: 2017,1Q,47

    I69.041 **Monoplegia of lower limb** following nontraumatic subarachnoid hemorrhage affecting right dominant side   HCC ESR COM

    I69.042 **Monoplegia of lower limb** following nontraumatic subarachnoid hemorrhage affecting left dominant side   HCC ESR COM

    I69.043 **Monoplegia of lower limb** following nontraumatic subarachnoid hemorrhage affecting right non-dominant side   HCC ESR COM

    I69.044 **Monoplegia of lower limb** following nontraumatic subarachnoid hemorrhage affecting left non-dominant side   HCC ESR COM

    I69.049 **Monoplegia of lower limb** following nontraumatic subarachnoid hemorrhage affecting unspecified side   HCC ESR COM

√6ᵗʰ **I69.05** Hemiplegia and hemiparesis following nontraumatic subarachnoid hemorrhage

    AHA: 2015,1Q,25

    I69.051 **Hemiplegia and hemiparesis** following nontraumatic subarachnoid hemorrhage affecting right dominant side   HCC ESR COM

    I69.052 **Hemiplegia and hemiparesis** following nontraumatic subarachnoid hemorrhage affecting left dominant side   HCC ESR COM

    I69.053 **Hemiplegia and hemiparesis** following nontraumatic subarachnoid hemorrhage affecting right non-dominant side   HCC ESR COM

    I69.054 **Hemiplegia and hemiparesis** following nontraumatic subarachnoid hemorrhage affecting left non-dominant side   HCC ESR COM

    I69.059 **Hemiplegia and hemiparesis** following nontraumatic subarachnoid hemorrhage affecting unspecified side   HCC ESR COM

√6ᵗʰ **I69.06** Other paralytic syndrome following nontraumatic subarachnoid hemorrhage

    Use additional code to identify type of paralytic syndrome, such as:

    locked-in state (G83.5)

    quadriplegia (G82.5-)

    EXCLUDES 1   *hemiplegia/hemiparesis following nontraumatic subarachnoid hemorrhage (I69.05-)*

        monoplegia of lower limb following nontraumatic subarachnoid hemorrhage (I69.04-)

        monoplegia of upper limb following nontraumatic subarachnoid hemorrhage (I69.03-)

    I69.061 **Other paralytic syndrome** following nontraumatic subarachnoid hemorrhage affecting right dominant side   HCC ESR COM

    I69.062 **Other paralytic syndrome** following nontraumatic subarachnoid hemorrhage affecting left dominant side   HCC ESR COM

    I69.063 **Other paralytic syndrome** following nontraumatic subarachnoid hemorrhage affecting right non-dominant side   HCC ESR COM

    I69.064 **Other paralytic syndrome** following nontraumatic subarachnoid hemorrhage affecting left non-dominant side   HCC ESR COM

    I69.065 **Other paralytic syndrome** following nontraumatic subarachnoid hemorrhage, bilateral   HCC ESR COM

    I69.069 **Other paralytic syndrome** following nontraumatic subarachnoid hemorrhage affecting unspecified side   HCC ESR COM

√6ᵗʰ **I69.09** Other sequelae of nontraumatic subarachnoid hemorrhage

    I69.090 **Apraxia** following nontraumatic subarachnoid hemorrhage

    I69.091 **Dysphagia** following nontraumatic subarachnoid hemorrhage

        Use additional code to identify the type of dysphagia, if known ▶(R13.11-R13.19)◀

    I69.092 **Facial weakness** following nontraumatic subarachnoid hemorrhage

        Facial droop following nontraumatic subarachnoid hemorrhage

    I69.093 **Ataxia** following nontraumatic subarachnoid hemorrhage

    I69.098 **Other sequelae** following nontraumatic subarachnoid hemorrhage

        Alterations of sensation following nontraumatic subarachnoid hemorrhage

        Disturbance of vision following nontraumatic subarachnoid hemorrhage

        Use additional code to identify the sequelae

√5ᵗʰ **I69.1** Sequelae of nontraumatic intracerebral hemorrhage

    I69.10 Unspecified sequelae of nontraumatic intracerebral hemorrhage

√6ᵗʰ **I69.11** Cognitive deficits following nontraumatic intracerebral hemorrhage

    I69.110 **Attention and concentration deficit** following nontraumatic intracerebral hemorrhage

    I69.111 **Memory deficit** following nontraumatic intracerebral hemorrhage

    I69.112 **Visuospatial deficit and spatial neglect** following nontraumatic intracerebral hemorrhage

    I69.113 **Psychomotor deficit** following nontraumatic intracerebral hemorrhage

    I69.114 **Frontal lobe and executive function deficit** following nontraumatic intracerebral hemorrhage

---

✔ Additional Character Required   ✔x7ᵗʰ Placeholder Alert   Manifestation   Unspecified Dx   Q QPP   UPD Unacceptable PDx

Chapter 9. Diseases of the Circulatory System

I69.115–I69.212

I69.115 Cognitive social or emotional **deficit following nontraumatic intracerebral hemorrhage**

I69.118 **Other symptoms and signs involving cognitive functions following nontraumatic intracerebral hemorrhage**

I69.119 **Unspecified symptoms and signs involving cognitive functions following nontraumatic intracerebral hemorrhage**

✓6ᵗʰ **I69.12** Speech and language deficits **following nontraumatic intracerebral hemorrhage**

I69.120 Aphasia **following nontraumatic intracerebral hemorrhage**

I69.121 Dysphasia **following nontraumatic intracerebral hemorrhage**

I69.122 Dysarthria **following nontraumatic intracerebral hemorrhage**

I69.123 Fluency disorder **following nontraumatic intracerebral hemorrhage**

Stuttering following nontraumatic intracerebral hemorrhage

I69.128 **Other speech and language deficits following nontraumatic intracerebral hemorrhage**

✓6ᵗʰ **I69.13** Monoplegia of upper limb **following nontraumatic intracerebral hemorrhage**
AHA: 2017,1Q,47

I69.131 **Monoplegia of upper limb following nontraumatic intracerebral hemorrhage affecting** right dominant **side** HCC ESR COM

I69.132 **Monoplegia of upper limb following nontraumatic intracerebral hemorrhage affecting** left dominant **side** HCC ESR COM

I69.133 **Monoplegia of upper limb following nontraumatic intracerebral hemorrhage affecting** right non-dominant **side** HCC ESR COM

I69.134 **Monoplegia of upper limb following nontraumatic intracerebral hemorrhage affecting** left non-dominant **side** HCC ESR COM

I69.139 **Monoplegia of upper limb following nontraumatic intracerebral hemorrhage affecting unspecified side** HCC ESR COM

✓6ᵗʰ **I69.14** Monoplegia of lower limb **following nontraumatic intracerebral hemorrhage**
AHA: 2017,1Q,47

I69.141 **Monoplegia of lower limb following nontraumatic intracerebral hemorrhage affecting** right dominant **side** HCC ESR COM

I69.142 **Monoplegia of lower limb following nontraumatic intracerebral hemorrhage affecting** left dominant **side** HCC ESR COM

I69.143 **Monoplegia of lower limb following nontraumatic intracerebral hemorrhage affecting** right non-dominant **side** HCC ESR COM

I69.144 **Monoplegia of lower limb following nontraumatic intracerebral hemorrhage affecting** left non-dominant **side** HCC ESR COM

I69.149 **Monoplegia of lower limb following nontraumatic intracerebral hemorrhage affecting unspecified side** HCC ESR COM

✓6ᵗʰ **I69.15** Hemiplegia and hemiparesis **following nontraumatic intracerebral hemorrhage**
AHA: 2015,1Q,25

I69.151 **Hemiplegia and hemiparesis following nontraumatic intracerebral hemorrhage affecting** right dominant **side** HCC ESR COM

I69.152 **Hemiplegia and hemiparesis following nontraumatic intracerebral hemorrhage affecting** left dominant **side** HCC ESR COM

I69.153 **Hemiplegia and hemiparesis following nontraumatic intracerebral hemorrhage affecting** right non-dominant **side** HCC ESR COM

I69.154 **Hemiplegia and hemiparesis following nontraumatic intracerebral hemorrhage affecting** left non-dominant **side** HCC ESR COM

I69.159 **Hemiplegia and hemiparesis following nontraumatic intracerebral hemorrhage affecting unspecified side** HCC ESR COM

✓6ᵗʰ **I69.16** **Other** paralytic syndrome **following nontraumatic intracerebral hemorrhage**

Use additional code to identify type of paralytic syndrome, such as:

locked-in state (G83.5)

quadriplegia (G82.5-)

EXCLUDES 1 *hemiplegia/hemiparesis following nontraumatic intracerebral hemorrhage (I69.15-)*

monoplegia of lower limb following nontraumatic intracerebral hemorrhage (I69.14-)

monoplegia of upper limb following nontraumatic intracerebral hemorrhage (I69.13-)

I69.161 **Other paralytic syndrome following nontraumatic intracerebral hemorrhage affecting** right dominant **side** HCC ESR COM

I69.162 **Other paralytic syndrome following nontraumatic intracerebral hemorrhage affecting** left dominant **side** HCC ESR COM

I69.163 **Other paralytic syndrome following nontraumatic intracerebral hemorrhage affecting** right non-dominant **side** HCC ESR COM

I69.164 **Other paralytic syndrome following nontraumatic intracerebral hemorrhage affecting** left non-dominant **side** HCC ESR COM

I69.165 **Other paralytic syndrome following nontraumatic intracerebral hemorrhage, bilateral** HCC ESR COM

I69.169 **Other paralytic syndrome following nontraumatic intracerebral hemorrhage affecting unspecified side** HCC ESR COM

✓6ᵗʰ **I69.19** **Other sequelae of nontraumatic intracerebral hemorrhage**

I69.190 Apraxia **following nontraumatic intracerebral hemorrhage**

I69.191 Dysphagia **following nontraumatic intracerebral hemorrhage**

Use additional code to identify the type of dysphagia, if known

▶(R13.11-R13.19)◀

I69.192 Facial weakness **following nontraumatic intracerebral hemorrhage**

Facial droop following nontraumatic intracerebral hemorrhage

I69.193 Ataxia **following nontraumatic intracerebral hemorrhage**

I69.198 **Other sequelae of nontraumatic intracerebral hemorrhage**

Alteration of sensations following nontraumatic intracerebral hemorrhage

Disturbance of vision following nontraumatic intracerebral hemorrhage

Use additional code to identify the sequelae

✓5ᵗʰ **I69.2** Sequelae of other nontraumatic intracranial **hemorrhage**

I69.20 **Unspecified sequelae of other nontraumatic intracranial hemorrhage**

✓6ᵗʰ **I69.21** Cognitive deficits **following other nontraumatic intracranial hemorrhage**

I69.210 Attention and concentration **deficit following other nontraumatic intracranial hemorrhage**

I69.211 Memory **deficit following other nontraumatic intracranial hemorrhage**

I69.212 Visuospatial **deficit and** spatial neglect **following other nontraumatic intracranial hemorrhage**

I69.213 **Psychomotor deficit following other nontraumatic intracranial hemorrhage**

I69.214 **Frontal lobe and executive function deficit following other nontraumatic intracranial hemorrhage**

I69.215 **Cognitive social or emotional deficit following other nontraumatic intracranial hemorrhage**

I69.218 **Other symptoms and signs involving cognitive functions following other nontraumatic intracranial hemorrhage**

I69.219 **Unspecified symptoms and signs involving cognitive functions following other nontraumatic intracranial hemorrhage**

✓6ᵗʰ I69.22 **Speech and language deficits following other nontraumatic intracranial hemorrhage**

I69.220 **Aphasia following other nontraumatic intracranial hemorrhage**

I69.221 **Dysphasia following other nontraumatic intracranial hemorrhage**

I69.222 **Dysarthria following other nontraumatic intracranial hemorrhage**

I69.223 **Fluency disorder following other nontraumatic intracranial hemorrhage**
Stuttering following other nontraumatic intracranial hemorrhage

I69.228 **Other speech and language deficits following other nontraumatic intracranial hemorrhage**

✓6ᵗʰ I69.23 **Monoplegia of upper limb following other nontraumatic intracranial hemorrhage**
AHA: 2017,1Q,47

I69.231 **Monoplegia of upper limb following other nontraumatic intracranial hemorrhage affecting right dominant side** HCC ESR COM

I69.232 **Monoplegia of upper limb following other nontraumatic intracranial hemorrhage affecting left dominant side** HCC ESR COM

I69.233 **Monoplegia of upper limb following other nontraumatic intracranial hemorrhage affecting right non-dominant side** HCC ESR COM

I69.234 **Monoplegia of upper limb following other nontraumatic intracranial hemorrhage affecting left non-dominant side** HCC ESR COM

I69.239 **Monoplegia of upper limb following other nontraumatic intracranial hemorrhage affecting unspecified side** HCC ESR COM

✓6ᵗʰ I69.24 **Monoplegia of lower limb following other nontraumatic intracranial hemorrhage**
AHA: 2017,1Q,47

I69.241 **Monoplegia of lower limb following other nontraumatic intracranial hemorrhage affecting right dominant side** HCC ESR COM

I69.242 **Monoplegia of lower limb following other nontraumatic intracranial hemorrhage affecting left dominant side** HCC ESR COM

I69.243 **Monoplegia of lower limb following other nontraumatic intracranial hemorrhage affecting right non-dominant side** HCC ESR COM

I69.244 **Monoplegia of lower limb following other nontraumatic intracranial hemorrhage affecting left non-dominant side** HCC ESR COM

I69.249 **Monoplegia of lower limb following other nontraumatic intracranial hemorrhage affecting unspecified side** HCC ESR COM

✓6ᵗʰ I69.25 **Hemiplegia and hemiparesis following other nontraumatic intracranial hemorrhage**
AHA: 2015,1Q,25

I69.251 **Hemiplegia and hemiparesis following other nontraumatic intracranial hemorrhage affecting right dominant side** HCC ESR COM

I69.252 **Hemiplegia and hemiparesis following other nontraumatic intracranial hemorrhage affecting left dominant side** HCC ESR COM

I69.253 **Hemiplegia and hemiparesis following other nontraumatic intracranial hemorrhage affecting right non-dominant side** HCC ESR COM

I69.254 **Hemiplegia and hemiparesis following other nontraumatic intracranial hemorrhage affecting left non-dominant side** HCC ESR COM

I69.259 **Hemiplegia and hemiparesis following other nontraumatic intracranial hemorrhage affecting unspecified side** HCC ESR COM

✓6ᵗʰ I69.26 **Other paralytic syndrome following other nontraumatic intracranial hemorrhage**
Use additional code to identify type of paralytic syndrome, such as:
locked-in state (G83.5)
quadriplegia (G82.5-)
EXCLUDES 1   *hemiplegia/hemiparesis following other nontraumatic intracranial hemorrhage (I69.25-)*
monoplegia of lower limb following other nontraumatic intracranial hemorrhage (I69.24-)
monoplegia of upper limb following other nontraumatic intracranial hemorrhage (I69.23-)

I69.261 **Other paralytic syndrome following other nontraumatic intracranial hemorrhage affecting right dominant side** HCC ESR COM

I69.262 **Other paralytic syndrome following other nontraumatic intracranial hemorrhage affecting left dominant side** HCC ESR COM

I69.263 **Other paralytic syndrome following other nontraumatic intracranial hemorrhage affecting right non-dominant side** HCC ESR COM

I69.264 **Other paralytic syndrome following other nontraumatic intracranial hemorrhage affecting left non-dominant side** HCC ESR COM

I69.265 **Other paralytic syndrome following other nontraumatic intracranial hemorrhage, bilateral** HCC ESR COM

I69.269 **Other paralytic syndrome following other nontraumatic intracranial hemorrhage affecting unspecified side** HCC ESR COM

✓6ᵗʰ I69.29 **Other sequelae of other nontraumatic intracranial hemorrhage**

I69.290 **Apraxia following other nontraumatic intracranial hemorrhage**

I69.291 **Dysphagia following other nontraumatic intracranial hemorrhage**
Use additional code to identify the type of dysphagia, if known
▶(R13.11-R13.19)◄

I69.292 **Facial weakness following other nontraumatic intracranial hemorrhage**
Facial droop following other nontraumatic intracranial hemorrhage

I69.293 **Ataxia following other nontraumatic intracranial hemorrhage**

I69.298 **Other sequelae of other nontraumatic intracranial hemorrhage**
Alteration of sensation following other nontraumatic intracranial hemorrhage
Disturbance of vision following other nontraumatic intracranial hemorrhage
Use additional code to identify the sequelae

Chapter 9. Diseases of the Circulatory System

I69.3–I69.815

✓5ᵗʰ **I69.3 Sequelae of** cerebral infarction
     Sequelae of stroke NOS
     AHA: 2013,4Q,127-128; 2012,4Q,92,94

     I69.30 Unspecified sequelae of cerebral infarction

✓6ᵗʰ **I69.31 Cognitive** deficits following cerebral infarction

     I69.310 Attention and concentration deficit following cerebral infarction

     I69.311 Memory deficit following cerebral infarction

     I69.312 Visuospatial deficit and spatial neglect **following cerebral infarction**

     I69.313 Psychomotor deficit following cerebral infarction

     I69.314 Frontal lobe and executive function deficit following cerebral infarction

     I69.315 Cognitive social or emotional deficit following cerebral infarction

     I69.318 Other symptoms and signs involving cognitive functions following cerebral infarction

     I69.319 Unspecified symptoms and signs involving cognitive functions following cerebral infarction

✓6ᵗʰ **I69.32 Speech and language deficits** following cerebral infarction

     I69.320 Aphasia following cerebral infarction

     I69.321 Dysphasia following cerebral infarction
         AHA: 2012,4Q,91

     I69.322 Dysarthria following cerebral infarction
         EXCLUDES 2   transient ischemic attack (TIA) (G45.9)

     I69.323 Fluency disorder following cerebral infarction
         Stuttering following cerebral infarction

     I69.328 Other speech and language deficits following cerebral infarction

✓6ᵗʰ **I69.33 Monoplegia of upper limb** following cerebral infarction
     AHA: 2017,1Q,47

     I69.331 Monoplegia of upper limb following cerebral infarction affecting right **dominant side** HCC ESR COM

     I69.332 Monoplegia of upper limb following cerebral infarction affecting left **dominant side** HCC ESR COM

     I69.333 Monoplegia of upper limb following cerebral infarction affecting right **non-dominant side** HCC ESR COM

     I69.334 Monoplegia of upper limb following cerebral infarction affecting left **non-dominant side** HCC ESR COM

     I69.339 Monoplegia of upper limb following cerebral infarction affecting unspecified side HCC ESR COM

✓6ᵗʰ **I69.34 Monoplegia of lower limb** following cerebral infarction
     AHA: 2017,1Q,47

     I69.341 Monoplegia of lower limb following cerebral infarction affecting right **dominant side** HCC ESR COM

     I69.342 Monoplegia of lower limb following cerebral infarction affecting left **dominant side** HCC ESR COM

     I69.343 Monoplegia of lower limb following cerebral infarction affecting right **non-dominant side** HCC ESR COM

     I69.344 Monoplegia of lower limb following cerebral infarction affecting left **non-dominant side** HCC ESR COM

     I69.349 Monoplegia of lower limb following cerebral infarction affecting unspecified side HCC ESR COM

✓6ᵗʰ **I69.35 Hemiplegia and hemiparesis** following cerebral infarction
     AHA: 2015,1Q,25

     I69.351 Hemiplegia and hemiparesis following cerebral infarction affecting right **dominant side** HCC ESR COM
         EXCLUDES 2   transient ischemic attack (TIA) (G45.9)

     I69.352 Hemiplegia and hemiparesis following cerebral infarction affecting left **dominant side** HCC ESR COM

     I69.353 Hemiplegia and hemiparesis following cerebral infarction affecting right **non-dominant side** HCC ESR COM

     I69.354 Hemiplegia and hemiparesis following cerebral infarction affecting left **non-dominant side** HCC ESR COM
         AHA: 2012,4Q,91

     I69.359 Hemiplegia and hemiparesis following cerebral infarction affecting unspecified side HCC ESR COM

✓6ᵗʰ **I69.36 Other** paralytic syndrome **following cerebral infarction**
     Use additional code to identify type of paralytic syndrome, such as:
     locked-in state (G83.5)
     quadriplegia (G82.5-)
     EXCLUDES 1   hemiplegia/hemiparesis following cerebral infarction (I69.35-)
         monoplegia of lower limb following cerebral infarction (I69.34-)
         monoplegia of upper limb following cerebral infarction (I69.33-)

     I69.361 Other paralytic syndrome following cerebral infarction affecting right **dominant side** HCC ESR COM

     I69.362 Other paralytic syndrome following cerebral infarction affecting left **dominant side** HCC ESR COM

     I69.363 Other paralytic syndrome following cerebral infarction affecting right **non-dominant side** HCC ESR COM

     I69.364 Other paralytic syndrome following cerebral infarction affecting left **non-dominant side** HCC ESR COM

     I69.365 Other paralytic syndrome following cerebral infarction, bilateral HCC ESR COM

     I69.369 Other paralytic syndrome following cerebral infarction affecting unspecified side HCC ESR COM

✓6ᵗʰ **I69.39 Other sequelae of cerebral infarction**

     I69.390 Apraxia following cerebral infarction

     I69.391 Dysphagia following cerebral infarction
         Use additional code to identify the type of dysphagia, if known
         ▶(R13.11-R13.19)◀

     I69.392 Facial weakness following cerebral infarction
         Facial droop following cerebral infarction

     I69.393 Ataxia following cerebral infarction

     I69.398 Other sequelae of cerebral infarction
         Alteration of sensation following cerebral infarction
         Disturbance of vision following cerebral infarction
         Use additional code to identify the sequelae
         AHA: 2020,2Q,29

✓5ᵗʰ **I69.8 Sequelae of other** cerebrovascular diseases
     EXCLUDES 1   sequelae of traumatic intracranial injury (S06.-)

     I69.80 Unspecified sequelae of other cerebrovascular disease

✓6ᵗʰ **I69.81 Cognitive deficits following other cerebrovascular disease**

     I69.810 Attention and concentration deficit following other cerebrovascular disease

     I69.811 Memory deficit following other cerebrovascular disease

     I69.812 Visuospatial deficit and spatial neglect **following other cerebrovascular disease**

     I69.813 Psychomotor deficit following other cerebrovascular disease

     I69.814 Frontal lobe and executive function deficit following other cerebrovascular disease

     I69.815 Cognitive social or emotional deficit following other cerebrovascular disease

I69.818 Other symptoms and signs involving cognitive functions following other cerebrovascular disease

I69.819 Unspecified symptoms and signs involving cognitive functions following other cerebrovascular disease

√6ᵗʰ **I69.82** Speech and language deficits following other cerebrovascular disease

    I69.820 Aphasia following other cerebrovascular disease

    I69.821 Dysphasia following other cerebrovascular disease

    I69.822 Dysarthria following other cerebrovascular disease

    I69.823 Fluency disorder following other cerebrovascular disease

        Stuttering following other cerebrovascular disease

    I69.828 Other speech and language deficits following other cerebrovascular disease

        AHA: 2019,3Q,8

√6ᵗʰ **I69.83** Monoplegia of upper limb following other cerebrovascular disease

    AHA: 2017,1Q,47

    I69.831 Monoplegia of upper limb following other cerebrovascular disease affecting right dominant side   HCC ESR COM

    I69.832 Monoplegia of upper limb following other cerebrovascular disease affecting left dominant side   HCC ESR COM

    I69.833 Monoplegia of upper limb following other cerebrovascular disease affecting right non-dominant side   HCC ESR COM

    I69.834 Monoplegia of upper limb following other cerebrovascular disease affecting left non-dominant side   HCC ESR COM

    I69.839 Monoplegia of upper limb following other cerebrovascular disease affecting unspecified side   HCC ESR COM

√6ᵗʰ **I69.84** Monoplegia of lower limb following other cerebrovascular disease

    AHA: 2017,1Q,47

    I69.841 Monoplegia of lower limb following other cerebrovascular disease affecting right dominant side   HCC ESR COM

    I69.842 Monoplegia of lower limb following other cerebrovascular disease affecting left dominant side   HCC ESR COM

    I69.843 Monoplegia of lower limb following other cerebrovascular disease affecting right non-dominant side   HCC ESR COM

    I69.844 Monoplegia of lower limb following other cerebrovascular disease affecting left non-dominant side   HCC ESR COM

    I69.849 Monoplegia of lower limb following other cerebrovascular disease affecting unspecified side   HCC ESR COM

√6ᵗʰ **I69.85** Hemiplegia and hemiparesis following other cerebrovascular disease

    AHA: 2015,1Q,25

    I69.851 Hemiplegia and hemiparesis following other cerebrovascular disease affecting right dominant side   HCC ESR COM

    I69.852 Hemiplegia and hemiparesis following other cerebrovascular disease affecting left dominant side   HCC ESR COM

    I69.853 Hemiplegia and hemiparesis following other cerebrovascular disease affecting right non-dominant side   HCC ESR COM

    I69.854 Hemiplegia and hemiparesis following other cerebrovascular disease affecting left non-dominant side   HCC ESR COM

    I69.859 Hemiplegia and hemiparesis following other cerebrovascular disease affecting unspecified side   HCC ESR COM

√6ᵗʰ **I69.86** Other paralytic syndrome following other cerebrovascular disease

    Use additional code to identify type of paralytic syndrome, such as:

    locked-in state (G83.5)

    quadriplegia (G82.5-)

    EXCLUDES 1 hemiplegia/hemiparesis following other cerebrovascular disease (I69.85-)

        monoplegia of lower limb following other cerebrovascular disease (I69.84-)

        monoplegia of upper limb following other cerebrovascular disease (I69.83-)

    I69.861 Other paralytic syndrome following other cerebrovascular disease affecting right dominant side   HCC ESR COM

    I69.862 Other paralytic syndrome following other cerebrovascular disease affecting left dominant side   HCC ESR COM

    I69.863 Other paralytic syndrome following other cerebrovascular disease affecting right non-dominant side   HCC ESR COM

    I69.864 Other paralytic syndrome following other cerebrovascular disease affecting left non-dominant side   HCC ESR COM

    I69.865 Other paralytic syndrome following other cerebrovascular disease, bilateral   HCC ESR COM

    I69.869 Other paralytic syndrome following other cerebrovascular disease affecting unspecified side   HCC ESR COM

√6ᵗʰ **I69.89** Other sequelae of other cerebrovascular disease

    I69.890 Apraxia following other cerebrovascular disease

    I69.891 Dysphagia following other cerebrovascular disease

        Use additional code to identify the type of dysphagia, if known

        ▶(R13.11-R13.19)◀

    I69.892 Facial weakness following other cerebrovascular disease

        Facial droop following other cerebrovascular disease

    I69.893 Ataxia following other cerebrovascular disease

    I69.898 Other sequelae of other cerebrovascular disease

        Alteration of sensation following other cerebrovascular disease

        Disturbance of vision following other cerebrovascular disease

        Use additional code to identify the sequelae

√5ᵗʰ **I69.9** Sequelae of unspecified cerebrovascular diseases

    EXCLUDES 1 sequelae of stroke (I69.3)

        sequelae of traumatic intracranial injury (S06.-)

    I69.90 Unspecified sequelae of unspecified cerebrovascular disease

√6ᵗʰ **I69.91** Cognitive deficits following unspecified cerebrovascular disease

    I69.910 Attention and concentration deficit following unspecified cerebrovascular disease

    I69.911 Memory deficit following unspecified cerebrovascular disease

    I69.912 Visuospatial deficit and spatial neglect following unspecified cerebrovascular disease

    I69.913 Psychomotor deficit following unspecified cerebrovascular disease

    I69.914 Frontal lobe and executive function deficit following unspecified cerebrovascular disease

    I69.915 Cognitive social or emotional deficit following unspecified cerebrovascular disease

    I69.918 Other symptoms and signs involving cognitive functions following unspecified cerebrovascular disease

    I69.919 Unspecified symptoms and signs involving cognitive functions following unspecified cerebrovascular disease

✓6ᵗʰ **I69.92** Speech and language deficits following unspecified cerebrovascular disease

I69.920 Aphasia following unspecified cerebrovascular disease

I69.921 Dysphasia following unspecified cerebrovascular disease

I69.922 Dysarthria following unspecified cerebrovascular disease

I69.923 Fluency disorder following unspecified cerebrovascular disease
Stuttering following unspecified cerebrovascular disease

I69.928 Other speech and language deficits following unspecified cerebrovascular disease

✓6ᵗʰ **I69.93** Monoplegia of upper limb following unspecified cerebrovascular disease
AHA: 2017,1Q,47

I69.931 Monoplegia of upper limb following unspecified cerebrovascular disease affecting right dominant side HCC ESR COM

I69.932 Monoplegia of upper limb following unspecified cerebrovascular disease affecting left dominant side HCC ESR COM

I69.933 Monoplegia of upper limb following unspecified cerebrovascular disease affecting right non-dominant side HCC ESR COM

I69.934 Monoplegia of upper limb following unspecified cerebrovascular disease affecting left non-dominant side HCC ESR COM

I69.939 Monoplegia of upper limb following unspecified cerebrovascular disease affecting unspecified side HCC ESR COM

✓6ᵗʰ **I69.94** Monoplegia of lower limb following unspecified cerebrovascular disease
AHA: 2017,1Q,47

I69.941 Monoplegia of lower limb following unspecified cerebrovascular disease affecting right dominant side HCC ESR COM

I69.942 Monoplegia of lower limb following unspecified cerebrovascular disease affecting left dominant side HCC ESR COM

I69.943 Monoplegia of lower limb following unspecified cerebrovascular disease affecting right non-dominant side HCC ESR COM

I69.944 Monoplegia of lower limb following unspecified cerebrovascular disease affecting left non-dominant side HCC ESR COM

I69.949 Monoplegia of lower limb following unspecified cerebrovascular disease affecting unspecified side HCC ESR COM

✓6ᵗʰ **I69.95** Hemiplegia and hemiparesis following unspecified cerebrovascular disease
AHA: 2015,1Q,25

I69.951 Hemiplegia and hemiparesis following unspecified cerebrovascular disease affecting right dominant side HCC ESR COM

I69.952 Hemiplegia and hemiparesis following unspecified cerebrovascular disease affecting left dominant side HCC ESR COM

I69.953 Hemiplegia and hemiparesis following unspecified cerebrovascular disease affecting right non-dominant side HCC ESR COM

I69.954 Hemiplegia and hemiparesis following unspecified cerebrovascular disease affecting left non-dominant side HCC ESR COM

I69.959 Hemiplegia and hemiparesis following unspecified cerebrovascular disease affecting unspecified side HCC ESR COM

✓6ᵗʰ **I69.96** Other paralytic syndrome following unspecified cerebrovascular disease
Use additional code to identify type of paralytic syndrome, such as:
locked-in state (G83.5)
quadriplegia (G82.5-)
EXCLUDES 1 hemiplegia/hemiparesis following unspecified cerebrovascular disease (I69.95-)
monoplegia of lower limb following unspecified cerebrovascular disease (I69.94-)
monoplegia of upper limb following unspecified cerebrovascular disease (I69.93-)

I69.961 Other paralytic syndrome following unspecified cerebrovascular disease affecting right dominant side HCC ESR COM

I69.962 Other paralytic syndrome following unspecified cerebrovascular disease affecting left dominant side HCC ESR COM

I69.963 Other paralytic syndrome following unspecified cerebrovascular disease affecting right non-dominant side HCC ESR COM

I69.964 Other paralytic syndrome following unspecified cerebrovascular disease affecting left non-dominant side HCC ESR COM

I69.965 Other paralytic syndrome following unspecified cerebrovascular disease, bilateral HCC ESR COM

I69.969 Other paralytic syndrome following unspecified cerebrovascular disease affecting unspecified side HCC ESR COM

✓6ᵗʰ **I69.99** Other sequelae of unspecified cerebrovascular disease

I69.990 Apraxia following unspecified cerebrovascular disease

I69.991 Dysphagia following unspecified cerebrovascular disease
Use additional code to identify the type of dysphagia, if known
▶(R13.11-R13.19)◀

I69.992 Facial weakness following unspecified cerebrovascular disease
Facial droop following unspecified cerebrovascular disease

I69.993 Ataxia following unspecified cerebrovascular disease

I69.998 Other sequelae following unspecified cerebrovascular disease
Alteration in sensation following unspecified cerebrovascular disease
Disturbance of vision following unspecified cerebrovascular disease
Use additional code to identify the sequelae

Diseases of arteries, arterioles and capillaries (I70-I79)

☑4ᵗʰ **I70 Atherosclerosis**

    INCLUDES   arterial degeneration
              arteriolosclerosis
              arteriosclerosis
              arteriosclerotic vascular disease
              arteriovascular degeneration
              atheroma
              endarteritis deformans or obliterans
              senile arteritis
              senile endarteritis
              vascular degeneration
    Use additional code to identify:
      exposure to environmental tobacco smoke (Z77.22)
      history of tobacco dependence (Z87.891)
      occupational exposure to environmental tobacco smoke (Z57.31)
      tobacco dependence (F17.-)
      tobacco use (Z72.0)
     EXCLUDES 2   *arteriosclerotic cardiovascular disease (I25.1-)*
              arteriosclerotic heart disease (I25.1-)
              atheroembolism (I75.-)
              cerebral atherosclerosis (I67.2)
              coronary atherosclerosis (I25.1-)
              mesenteric atherosclerosis (K55.1)
              precerebral atherosclerosis (I67.2)
              primary pulmonary atherosclerosis (I27.0)

    I70.0 Atherosclerosis of aorta   HCC ESR A

    I70.1 Atherosclerosis of renal artery   HCC ESR A
       Goldblatt's kidney
         EXCLUDES 2   *atherosclerosis of renal arterioles (I12.-)*

☑5ᵗʰ **I70.2 Atherosclerosis of native arteries of the extremities**
       Mönckeberg's (medial) sclerosis
       Use additional code, if applicable, to identify chronic total
         occlusion of artery of extremity (I70.92)
         EXCLUDES 2   *atherosclerosis of bypass graft of extremities*
                (I70.30-I70.79)
       AHA: 2020,4Q,98; 2018,3Q,4; 2018,2Q,7

     ☑6ᵗʰ **I70.20 Unspecified atherosclerosis of native arteries of extremities**

       I70.201 Unspecified atherosclerosis of native arteries of extremities, right leg   HCC ESR A

       I70.202 Unspecified atherosclerosis of native arteries of extremities, left leg   HCC ESR A

       I70.203 Unspecified atherosclerosis of native arteries of extremities, bilateral legs   HCC ESR A

       I70.208 Unspecified atherosclerosis of native arteries of extremities, other extremity   HCC ESR A

       I70.209 Unspecified atherosclerosis of native arteries of extremities, unspecified extremity   HCC ESR A

     ☑6ᵗʰ **I70.21 Atherosclerosis of native arteries of extremities with intermittent claudication**

       I70.211 Atherosclerosis of native arteries of extremities with intermittent claudication, right leg   HCC ESR A

       I70.212 Atherosclerosis of native arteries of extremities with intermittent claudication, left leg   HCC ESR A

       I70.213 Atherosclerosis of native arteries of extremities with intermittent claudication, bilateral legs   HCC ESR A

       I70.218 Atherosclerosis of native arteries of extremities with intermittent claudication, other extremity   HCC ESR A

       I70.219 Atherosclerosis of native arteries of extremities with intermittent claudication, unspecified extremity   HCC ESR A

     ☑6ᵗʰ **I70.22 Atherosclerosis of native arteries of extremities with rest pain**
       INCLUDES   any condition classifiable to I70.21-
            chronic limb-threatening ischemia NOS of native arteries of extremities
            chronic limb-threatening ischemia of native arteries of extremities with rest pain
            critical limb ischemia NOS of native arteries of extremities
            critical limb ischemia of native arteries of extremities with rest pain

       I70.221 Atherosclerosis of native arteries of extremities with rest pain, right leg   HCC ESR A

       I70.222 Atherosclerosis of native arteries of extremities with rest pain, left leg   HCC ESR A

       I70.223 Atherosclerosis of native arteries of extremities with rest pain, bilateral legs   HCC ESR A

       I70.228 Atherosclerosis of native arteries of extremities with rest pain, other extremity   HCC ESR A

       I70.229 Atherosclerosis of native arteries of extremities with rest pain, unspecified extremity   HCC ESR A

     ☑6ᵗʰ **I70.23 Atherosclerosis of native arteries of right leg with ulceration**
       INCLUDES   any condition classifiable to I70.211 and I70.221
            chronic limb-threatening ischemia of native arteries of right leg with ulceration
            critical limb ischemia of native arteries of right leg with ulceration
       Use additional code to identify severity of ulcer (L97.-)

       I70.231 Atherosclerosis of native arteries of right leg with ulceration of thigh   HCC Rx ESR COM A

       I70.232 Atherosclerosis of native arteries of right leg with ulceration of calf   HCC Rx ESR COM A

       I70.233 Atherosclerosis of native arteries of right leg with ulceration of ankle   HCC Rx ESR COM A

       I70.234 Atherosclerosis of native arteries of right leg with ulceration of heel and midfoot   HCC Rx ESR COM A
          Atherosclerosis of native arteries of right leg with ulceration of plantar surface of midfoot

       I70.235 Atherosclerosis of native arteries of right leg with ulceration of other part of foot   HCC Rx ESR COM A
          Atherosclerosis of native arteries of right leg extremities with ulceration of toe

       I70.238 Atherosclerosis of native arteries of right leg with ulceration of other part of lower leg   HCC Rx ESR COM A

       I70.239 Atherosclerosis of native arteries of right leg with ulceration of unspecified site   HCC Rx ESR COM A

     ☑6ᵗʰ **I70.24 Atherosclerosis of native arteries of left leg with ulceration**
       INCLUDES   any condition classifiable to I70.212 and I70.222
            chronic limb-threatening ischemia of native arteries of left leg with ulceration
            critical limb ischemia of native arteries of left leg with ulceration
       Use additional code to identify severity of ulcer (L97.-)

       I70.241 Atherosclerosis of native arteries of left leg with ulceration of thigh   HCC Rx ESR COM A

       I70.242 Atherosclerosis of native arteries of left leg with ulceration of calf   HCC Rx ESR COM A

I70.243 Atherosclerosis of native arteries of left leg with ulceration of ankle HCC Rx ESR COM A

I70.244 Atherosclerosis of native arteries of left leg with ulceration of heel and midfoot HCC Rx ESR COM A

Atherosclerosis of native arteries of left leg with ulceration of plantar surface of midfoot

I70.245 Atherosclerosis of native arteries of left leg with ulceration of other part of foot HCC Rx ESR COM A

Atherosclerosis of native arteries of left leg extremities with ulceration of toe

I70.248 Atherosclerosis of native arteries of left leg with ulceration of other part of lower leg HCC Rx ESR COM A

I70.249 Atherosclerosis of native arteries of left leg with ulceration of unspecified site HCC Rx ESR COM A

I70.25 Atherosclerosis of native arteries of other extremities with ulceration HCC Rx ESR COM A

INCLUDES any condition classifiable to I70.218 and I70.228

Use additional code to identify the severity of the ulcer (L98.49-)

✓6th **I70.26 Atherosclerosis of native arteries of extremities with gangrene**

INCLUDES any condition classifiable to I70.21-, I70.22-, I70.23-, I70.24-, and I70.25-

chronic limb-threatening ischemia of native arteries of extremities with gangrene

critical limb ischemia of native arteries of extremities with gangrene

Use additional code to identify the severity of any ulcer (L97.-, L98.49-), if applicable

I70.261 Atherosclerosis of native arteries of extremities with gangrene, right leg HCC ESR COM A

I70.262 Atherosclerosis of native arteries of extremities with gangrene, left leg HCC ESR COM A

I70.263 Atherosclerosis of native arteries of extremities with gangrene, bilateral legs HCC ESR COM A

I70.268 Atherosclerosis of native arteries of extremities with gangrene, other extremity HCC ESR COM A

I70.269 Atherosclerosis of native arteries of extremities with gangrene, unspecified extremity HCC ESR COM A

✓6th **I70.29 Other atherosclerosis of native arteries of extremities**

I70.291 Other atherosclerosis of native arteries of extremities, right leg HCC ESR A

I70.292 Other atherosclerosis of native arteries of extremities, left leg HCC ESR A

I70.293 Other atherosclerosis of native arteries of extremities, bilateral legs HCC ESR A

I70.298 Other atherosclerosis of native arteries of extremities, other extremity HCC ESR A

I70.299 Other atherosclerosis of native arteries of extremities, unspecified extremity HCC ESR A

✓5th **I70.3 Atherosclerosis of unspecified type of bypass graft(s) of the extremities**

Use additional code, if applicable, to identify chronic total occlusion of artery of extremity (I70.92)

EXCLUDES 1 embolism or thrombus of bypass graft(s) of extremities (T82.8-)

AHA: 2020,4Q,98

✓6th **I70.30 Unspecified atherosclerosis of unspecified type of bypass graft(s) of the extremities**

I70.301 Unspecified atherosclerosis of unspecified type of bypass graft(s) of the extremities, right leg HCC ESR A

I70.302 Unspecified atherosclerosis of unspecified type of bypass graft(s) of the extremities, left leg HCC ESR A

I70.303 Unspecified atherosclerosis of unspecified type of bypass graft(s) of the extremities, bilateral legs HCC ESR A

I70.308 Unspecified atherosclerosis of unspecified type of bypass graft(s) of the extremities, other extremity HCC ESR A

I70.309 Unspecified atherosclerosis of unspecified type of bypass graft(s) of the extremities, unspecified extremity HCC ESR A

✓6th **I70.31 Atherosclerosis of unspecified type of bypass graft(s) of the extremities with intermittent claudication**

I70.311 Atherosclerosis of unspecified type of bypass graft(s) of the extremities with intermittent claudication, right leg HCC ESR A

I70.312 Atherosclerosis of unspecified type of bypass graft(s) of the extremities with intermittent claudication, left leg HCC ESR A

I70.313 Atherosclerosis of unspecified type of bypass graft(s) of the extremities with intermittent claudication, bilateral legs HCC ESR A

I70.318 Atherosclerosis of unspecified type of bypass graft(s) of the extremities with intermittent claudication, other extremity HCC ESR A

I70.319 Atherosclerosis of unspecified type of bypass graft(s) of the extremities with intermittent claudication, unspecified extremity HCC ESR A

✓6th **I70.32 Atherosclerosis of unspecified type of bypass graft(s) of the extremities with rest pain**

INCLUDES any condition classifiable to I70.31-

chronic limb-threatening ischemia NOS of unspecified type of bypass graft(s) of the extremities

▶chronic limb-threatening ischemia of unspecified type of bypass graft(s) of the extremities with rest pain◀

critical limb ischemia NOS of unspecified type of bypass graft(s) of the extremities

critical limb ischemia of unspecified type of bypass graft(s) of the extremities with rest pain

I70.321 Atherosclerosis of unspecified type of bypass graft(s) of the extremities with rest pain, right leg HCC ESR A

I70.322 Atherosclerosis of unspecified type of bypass graft(s) of the extremities with rest pain, left leg HCC ESR A

I70.323 Atherosclerosis of unspecified type of bypass graft(s) of the extremities with rest pain, bilateral legs HCC ESR A

I70.328 Atherosclerosis of unspecified type of bypass graft(s) of the extremities with rest pain, other extremity HCC ESR A

I70.329 Atherosclerosis of unspecified type of bypass graft(s) of the extremities with rest pain, unspecified extremity HCC ESR A

✓6th **I70.33 Atherosclerosis of unspecified type of bypass graft(s) of the right leg with ulceration**

INCLUDES any condition classifiable to I70.311 and I70.321

chronic limb-threatening ischemia of unspecified type of bypass graft(s) of the right leg with ulceration

critical limb ischemia of unspecified type of bypass graft(s) of the right leg with ulceration

Use additional code to identify severity of ulcer (L97.-)

I70.331 Atherosclerosis of unspecified type of bypass graft(s) of the right leg with ulceration of thigh HCC Rx ESR COM A

I70.332 Atherosclerosis of unspecified type of bypass graft(s) of the right leg with ulceration of calf `HCC` `Rx` `ESR` `COM` `A`

I70.333 Atherosclerosis of unspecified type of bypass graft(s) of the right leg with ulceration of ankle `HCC` `Rx` `ESR` `COM` `A`

I70.334 Atherosclerosis of unspecified type of bypass graft(s) of the right leg with ulceration of heel and midfoot `HCC` `Rx` `ESR` `COM` `A`

Atherosclerosis of unspecified type of bypass graft(s) of right leg with ulceration of plantar surface of midfoot

I70.335 Atherosclerosis of unspecified type of bypass graft(s) of the right leg with ulceration of other part of foot `HCC` `Rx` `ESR` `COM` `A`

Atherosclerosis of unspecified type of bypass graft(s) of the right leg with ulceration of toe

I70.338 Atherosclerosis of unspecified type of bypass graft(s) of the right leg with ulceration of other part of lower leg `HCC` `Rx` `ESR` `COM` `A`

I70.339 Atherosclerosis of unspecified type of bypass graft(s) of the right leg with ulceration of unspecified site `HCC` `Rx` `ESR` `COM` `A`

✓6ᵗʰ **I70.34** Atherosclerosis of unspecified type of bypass graft(s) of the left leg with ulceration

INCLUDES   any condition classifiable to I70.312 and I70.322

chronic limb-threatening ischemia of unspecified type of bypass graft(s) of the left leg with ulceration

critical limb ischemia of unspecified type of bypass graft(s) of the left leg with ulceration

Use additional code to identify severity of ulcer (L97.-)

I70.341 Atherosclerosis of unspecified type of bypass graft(s) of the left leg with ulceration of thigh `HCC` `Rx` `ESR` `COM` `A`

I70.342 Atherosclerosis of unspecified type of bypass graft(s) of the left leg with ulceration of calf `HCC` `Rx` `ESR` `COM` `A`

I70.343 Atherosclerosis of unspecified type of bypass graft(s) of the left leg with ulceration of ankle `HCC` `Rx` `ESR` `COM` `A`

I70.344 Atherosclerosis of unspecified type of bypass graft(s) of the left leg with ulceration of heel and midfoot `HCC` `Rx` `ESR` `COM` `A`

Atherosclerosis of unspecified type of bypass graft(s) of left leg with ulceration of plantar surface of midfoot

I70.345 Atherosclerosis of unspecified type of bypass graft(s) of the left leg with ulceration of other part of foot `HCC` `Rx` `ESR` `COM` `A`

Atherosclerosis of unspecified type of bypass graft(s) of the left leg with ulceration of toe

I70.348 Atherosclerosis of unspecified type of bypass graft(s) of the left leg with ulceration of other part of lower leg `HCC` `Rx` `ESR` `COM` `A`

I70.349 Atherosclerosis of unspecified type of bypass graft(s) of the left leg with ulceration of unspecified site `HCC` `Rx` `ESR` `COM` `A`

I70.35 Atherosclerosis of unspecified type of bypass graft(s) of other extremity with ulceration `HCC` `Rx` `ESR` `COM` `A`

INCLUDES   any condition classifiable to I70.318 and I70.328

Use additional code to identify severity of ulcer (L98.49-)

✓6ᵗʰ **I70.36** Atherosclerosis of unspecified type of bypass graft(s) of the extremities with gangrene

INCLUDES   any condition classifiable to I70.31-, I70.32-, I70.33-, I70.34-, I70.35

chronic limb-threatening ischemia of unspecified type of bypass graft(s) of the extremities with gangrene

critical limb ischemia of unspecified type of bypass graft(s) of the extremities with gangrene

Use additional code to identify the severity of any ulcer (L97.-, L98.49-), if applicable

I70.361 Atherosclerosis of unspecified type of bypass graft(s) of the extremities with gangrene, right leg `HCC` `ESR` `COM` `A`

I70.362 Atherosclerosis of unspecified type of bypass graft(s) of the extremities with gangrene, left leg `HCC` `ESR` `COM` `A`

I70.363 Atherosclerosis of unspecified type of bypass graft(s) of the extremities with gangrene, bilateral legs `HCC` `ESR` `COM` `A`

I70.368 Atherosclerosis of unspecified type of bypass graft(s) of the extremities with gangrene, other extremity `HCC` `ESR` `COM` `A`

I70.369 Atherosclerosis of unspecified type of bypass graft(s) of the extremities with gangrene, unspecified extremity `HCC` `ESR` `COM` `A`

✓6ᵗʰ **I70.39** Other atherosclerosis of unspecified type of bypass graft(s) of the extremities

I70.391 Other atherosclerosis of unspecified type of bypass graft(s) of the extremities, right leg `HCC` `ESR` `A`

I70.392 Other atherosclerosis of unspecified type of bypass graft(s) of the extremities, left leg `HCC` `ESR` `A`

I70.393 Other atherosclerosis of unspecified type of bypass graft(s) of the extremities, bilateral legs `HCC` `ESR` `A`

I70.398 Other atherosclerosis of unspecified type of bypass graft(s) of the extremities, other extremity `HCC` `ESR` `A`

I70.399 Other atherosclerosis of unspecified type of bypass graft(s) of the extremities, unspecified extremity `HCC` `ESR` `A`

✓5ᵗʰ **I70.4** Atherosclerosis of autologous vein bypass graft(s) of the extremities

Use additional code, if applicable, to identify chronic total occlusion of artery of extremity (I70.92)

AHA: 2020,4Q,98

✓6ᵗʰ **I70.40** Unspecified atherosclerosis of autologous vein bypass graft(s) of the extremities

I70.401 Unspecified atherosclerosis of autologous vein bypass graft(s) of the extremities, right leg `HCC` `ESR` `A`

I70.402 Unspecified atherosclerosis of autologous vein bypass graft(s) of the extremities, left leg `HCC` `ESR` `A`

I70.403 Unspecified atherosclerosis of autologous vein bypass graft(s) of the extremities, bilateral legs `HCC` `ESR` `A`

I70.408 Unspecified atherosclerosis of autologous vein bypass graft(s) of the extremities, other extremity `HCC` `ESR` `A`

I70.409 Unspecified atherosclerosis of autologous vein bypass graft(s) of the extremities, unspecified extremity `HCC` `ESR` `A`

✓6ᵗʰ **I70.41** Atherosclerosis of autologous vein bypass graft(s) of the extremities with intermittent claudication

I70.411 Atherosclerosis of autologous vein bypass graft(s) of the extremities with intermittent claudication, right leg `HCC` `ESR` `A`

I70.412 Atherosclerosis of autologous vein bypass graft(s) of the extremities with intermittent claudication, left leg `HCC` `ESR` `A`

I70.413 Atherosclerosis of autologous vein bypass graft(s) of the extremities with intermittent claudication, bilateral legs `HCC` `ESR` `A`

I70.418 Atherosclerosis of autologous vein bypass graft(s) of the extremities with intermittent claudication, other extremity `HCC` `ESR` `A`

I70.419 Atherosclerosis of autologous vein bypass graft(s) of the extremities with intermittent claudication, unspecified extremity `HCC` `ESR` `A`

✓6ᵗʰ **I70.42** Atherosclerosis of autologous vein bypass graft(s) of the extremities with rest pain

INCLUDES   any condition classifiable to I70.41-
chronic limb-threatening ischemia NOS of autologous vein bypass graft(s) of the extremities
chronic limb-threatening ischemia of autologous vein bypass graft(s) of the extremities with rest pain
critical limb ischemia NOS of autologous vein bypass graft(s) of the extremities
critical limb ischemia of autologous vein bypass graft(s) of the extremities with rest pain

I70.421 Atherosclerosis of autologous vein bypass graft(s) of the extremities with rest pain, right leg `HCC` `ESR` `A`

I70.422 Atherosclerosis of autologous vein bypass graft(s) of the extremities with rest pain, left leg `HCC` `ESR` `A`

I70.423 Atherosclerosis of autologous vein bypass graft(s) of the extremities with rest pain, bilateral legs `HCC` `ESR` `A`

I70.428 Atherosclerosis of autologous vein bypass graft(s) of the extremities with rest pain, other extremity `HCC` `ESR` `A`

I70.429 Atherosclerosis of autologous vein bypass graft(s) of the extremities with rest pain, unspecified extremity `HCC` `ESR` `A`

✓6ᵗʰ **I70.43** Atherosclerosis of autologous vein bypass graft(s) of the right leg with ulceration

INCLUDES   any condition classifiable to I70.411 and I70.421
chronic limb-threatening ischemia of autologous vein bypass graft(s) of the right leg with ulceration
critical limb ischemia of autologous vein bypass graft(s) of the right leg with ulceration
Use additional code to identify severity of ulcer (L97.-)

I70.431 Atherosclerosis of autologous vein bypass graft(s) of the right leg with ulceration of thigh `HCC` `Rx` `ESR` `COM` `A`

I70.432 Atherosclerosis of autologous vein bypass graft(s) of the right leg with ulceration of calf `HCC` `Rx` `ESR` `COM` `A`

I70.433 Atherosclerosis of autologous vein bypass graft(s) of the right leg with ulceration of ankle `HCC` `Rx` `ESR` `COM` `A`

I70.434 Atherosclerosis of autologous vein bypass graft(s) of the right leg with ulceration of heel and midfoot `HCC` `Rx` `ESR` `COM` `A`
Atherosclerosis of autologous vein bypass graft(s) of right leg with ulceration of plantar surface of midfoot

I70.435 Atherosclerosis of autologous vein bypass graft(s) of the right leg with ulceration of other part of foot `HCC` `Rx` `ESR` `COM` `A`
Atherosclerosis of autologous vein bypass graft(s) of right leg with ulceration of toe

I70.438 Atherosclerosis of autologous vein bypass graft(s) of the right leg with ulceration of other part of lower leg `HCC` `Rx` `ESR` `COM` `A`

I70.439 Atherosclerosis of autologous vein bypass graft(s) of the right leg with ulceration of unspecified site `HCC` `Rx` `ESR` `COM` `A`

✓6ᵗʰ **I70.44** Atherosclerosis of autologous vein bypass graft(s) of the left leg with ulceration

INCLUDES   any condition classifiable to I70.412 and I70.422
chronic limb-threatening ischemia of autologous vein bypass graft(s) of the left leg with ulceration
critical limb ischemia of autologous vein bypass graft(s) of the left leg with ulceration
Use additional code to identify severity of ulcer (L97.-)

I70.441 Atherosclerosis of autologous vein bypass graft(s) of the left leg with ulceration of thigh `HCC` `Rx` `ESR` `COM` `A`

I70.442 Atherosclerosis of autologous vein bypass graft(s) of the left leg with ulceration of calf `HCC` `Rx` `ESR` `COM` `A`

I70.443 Atherosclerosis of autologous vein bypass graft(s) of the left leg with ulceration of ankle `HCC` `Rx` `ESR` `COM` `A`

I70.444 Atherosclerosis of autologous vein bypass graft(s) of the left leg with ulceration of heel and midfoot `HCC` `Rx` `ESR` `COM` `A`
Atherosclerosis of autologous vein bypass graft(s) of left leg with ulceration of plantar surface of midfoot

I70.445 Atherosclerosis of autologous vein bypass graft(s) of the left leg with ulceration of other part of foot `HCC` `Rx` `ESR` `COM` `A`
Atherosclerosis of autologous vein bypass graft(s) of left leg with ulceration of toe

I70.448 Atherosclerosis of autologous vein bypass graft(s) of the left leg with ulceration of other part of lower leg `HCC` `Rx` `ESR` `COM` `A`

I70.449 Atherosclerosis of autologous vein bypass graft(s) of the left leg with ulceration of unspecified site `HCC` `Rx` `ESR` `COM` `A`

I70.45 Atherosclerosis of autologous vein bypass graft(s) of other extremity with ulceration `HCC` `Rx` `ESR` `COM` `A`

INCLUDES   any condition classifiable to I70.418, I70.428, and I70.438
Use additional code to identify severity of ulcer (L98.49)

✓6ᵗʰ **I70.46** Atherosclerosis of autologous vein bypass graft(s) of the extremities with gangrene

INCLUDES   any condition classifiable to I70.41-, I70.42-, and I70.43-, I70.44-, I70.45
chronic limb-threatening ischemia of autologous vein bypass graft(s) of the extremities with gangrene
critical limb ischemia of autologous vein bypass graft(s) of the extremities with gangrene
Use additional code to identify the severity of any ulcer (L97.-, L98.49-), if applicable

I70.461 Atherosclerosis of autologous vein bypass graft(s) of the extremities with gangrene, right leg `HCC` `ESR` `COM` `A`

I70.462 Atherosclerosis of autologous vein bypass graft(s) of the extremities with gangrene, left leg `HCC` `ESR` `COM` `A`

I70.463 Atherosclerosis of autologous vein bypass graft(s) of the extremities with gangrene, bilateral legs `HCC` `ESR` `COM` `A`

I70.468 Atherosclerosis of autologous vein bypass graft(s) of the extremities with gangrene, other extremity `HCC` `ESR` `COM` `A`

I70.469 Atherosclerosis of autologous vein bypass graft(s) of the extremities with gangrene, unspecified extremity `HCC` `ESR` `COM` `A`

✓6ᵗʰ **I70.49** Other atherosclerosis of autologous vein bypass graft(s) of the extremities

I70.491 Other atherosclerosis of autologous vein bypass graft(s) of the extremities, right leg `HCC` `ESR` `A`

I70.492 Other atherosclerosis of autologous vein bypass graft(s) of the extremities, left leg `HCC` `ESR` `A`

`HCC` CMS-HCC   `Rx` Rx HCC   `ESR` ESRD HCC   `COM` Commercial HCC   `N` Newborn: 0   `P` Pediatric: 0-17   `M` Maternity: 9-64   `A` Adult: 15-124

688   ICD-10-CM 2023

I70.493   **Other atherosclerosis of autologous vein bypass graft(s) of the extremities, bilateral legs** `HCC` `ESR` `A`

I70.498   **Other atherosclerosis of autologous vein bypass graft(s) of the extremities, other extremity** `HCC` `ESR` `A`

I70.499   **Other atherosclerosis of autologous vein bypass graft(s) of the extremities, unspecified extremity** `HCC` `ESR` `A`

✓5ᵗʰ **I70.5**   **Atherosclerosis of nonautologous biological bypass graft(s) of the extremities**

    Use additional code, if applicable, to identify chronic total occlusion of artery of extremity (I70.92)

    AHA: 2020,4Q,98

✓6ᵗʰ **I70.50**   **Unspecified atherosclerosis of nonautologous biological bypass graft(s) of the extremities**

I70.501   **Unspecified atherosclerosis of nonautologous biological bypass graft(s) of the extremities, right leg** `HCC` `ESR` `A`

I70.502   **Unspecified atherosclerosis of nonautologous biological bypass graft(s) of the extremities, left leg** `HCC` `ESR` `A`

I70.503   **Unspecified atherosclerosis of nonautologous biological bypass graft(s) of the extremities, bilateral legs** `HCC` `ESR` `A`

I70.508   **Unspecified atherosclerosis of nonautologous biological bypass graft(s) of the extremities, other extremity** `HCC` `ESR` `A`

I70.509   **Unspecified atherosclerosis of nonautologous biological bypass graft(s) of the extremities, unspecified extremity** `HCC` `ESR` `A`

✓6ᵗʰ **I70.51**   **Atherosclerosis of nonautologous biological bypass graft(s) of the extremities intermittent claudication**

I70.511   **Atherosclerosis of nonautologous biological bypass graft(s) of the extremities with intermittent claudication, right leg** `HCC` `ESR` `A`

I70.512   **Atherosclerosis of nonautologous biological bypass graft(s) of the extremities with intermittent claudication, left leg** `HCC` `ESR` `A`

I70.513   **Atherosclerosis of nonautologous biological bypass graft(s) of the extremities with intermittent claudication, bilateral legs** `HCC` `ESR` `A`

I70.518   **Atherosclerosis of nonautologous biological bypass graft(s) of the extremities with intermittent claudication, other extremity** `HCC` `ESR` `A`

I70.519   **Atherosclerosis of nonautologous biological bypass graft(s) of the extremities with intermittent claudication, unspecified extremity** `HCC` `ESR` `A`

✓6ᵗʰ **I70.52**   **Atherosclerosis of nonautologous biological bypass graft(s) of the extremities with rest pain**

    `INCLUDES`   any condition classifiable to I70.51-
       chronic limb-threatening ischemia NOS of nonautologous biological bypass graft(s) of the extremities
       chronic limb-threatening ischemia of nonautologous biological bypass graft(s) of the extremities with rest pain
       critical limb ischemia NOS of nonautologous biological bypass graft(s) of the extremities
       critical limb ischemia of nonautologous biological bypass graft(s) of the extremities with rest pain

I70.521   **Atherosclerosis of nonautologous biological bypass graft(s) of the extremities with rest pain, right leg** `HCC` `ESR` `A`

I70.522   **Atherosclerosis of nonautologous biological bypass graft(s) of the extremities with rest pain, left leg** `HCC` `ESR` `A`

I70.523   **Atherosclerosis of nonautologous biological bypass graft(s) of the extremities with rest pain, bilateral legs** `HCC` `ESR` `A`

I70.528   **Atherosclerosis of nonautologous biological bypass graft(s) of the extremities with rest pain, other extremity** `HCC` `ESR` `A`

I70.529   **Atherosclerosis of nonautologous biological bypass graft(s) of the extremities with rest pain, unspecified extremity** `HCC` `ESR` `A`

✓6ᵗʰ **I70.53**   **Atherosclerosis of nonautologous biological bypass graft(s) of the right leg with ulceration**

    `INCLUDES`   any condition classifiable to I70.511 and I70.521
       chronic limb-threatening ischemia of nonautologous biological bypass graft(s) of the right leg with ulceration
       critical limb ischemia of nonautologous biological bypass graft(s) of the right leg with ulceration

    Use additional code to identify severity of ulcer (L97.-)

I70.531   **Atherosclerosis of nonautologous biological bypass graft(s) of the right leg with ulceration of thigh** `HCC` `Rx` `ESR` `COM` `A`

I70.532   **Atherosclerosis of nonautologous biological bypass graft(s) of the right leg with ulceration of calf** `HCC` `Rx` `ESR` `COM` `A`

I70.533   **Atherosclerosis of nonautologous biological bypass graft(s) of the right leg with ulceration of ankle** `HCC` `Rx` `ESR` `COM` `A`

I70.534   **Atherosclerosis of nonautologous biological bypass graft(s) of the right leg with ulceration of heel and midfoot** `HCC` `Rx` `ESR` `COM` `A`

    Atherosclerosis of nonautologous biological bypass graft(s) of right leg with ulceration of plantar surface of midfoot

I70.535   **Atherosclerosis of nonautologous biological bypass graft(s) of the right leg with ulceration of other part of foot** `HCC` `Rx` `ESR` `COM` `A`

    Atherosclerosis of nonautologous biological bypass graft(s) of the right leg with ulceration of toe

I70.538   **Atherosclerosis of nonautologous biological bypass graft(s) of the right leg with ulceration of other part of lower leg** `HCC` `Rx` `ESR` `COM` `A`

I70.539   **Atherosclerosis of nonautologous biological bypass graft(s) of the right leg with ulceration of unspecified site** `HCC` `Rx` `ESR` `COM` `A`

✓6ᵗʰ **I70.54**   **Atherosclerosis of nonautologous biological bypass graft(s) of the left leg with ulceration**

    `INCLUDES`   any condition classifiable to I70.512 and I70.522
       chronic limb-threatening ischemia of nonautologous biological bypass graft(s) of the left leg with ulceration
       critical limb ischemia of nonautologous biological bypass graft(s) of the left leg with ulceration

    Use additional code to identify severity of ulcer (L97.-)

I70.541   **Atherosclerosis of nonautologous biological bypass graft(s) of the left leg with ulceration of thigh** `HCC` `Rx` `ESR` `COM` `A`

I70.542   **Atherosclerosis of nonautologous biological bypass graft(s) of the left leg with ulceration of calf** `HCC` `Rx` `ESR` `COM` `A`

✅ Additional Character Required   ✓x7ᵗʰ Placeholder Alert   Manifestation   Unspecified Dx   🆀 QPP   🆄🅿🅳 Unacceptable PDx

I70.543 Atherosclerosis of nonautologous biological bypass graft(s) of the left leg with ulceration of ankle `HCC` `Rx` `ESR` `COM` `A`

I70.544 Atherosclerosis of nonautologous biological bypass graft(s) of the left leg with ulceration of heel and midfoot `HCC` `Rx` `ESR` `COM` `A`

Atherosclerosis of nonautologous biological bypass graft(s) of left leg with ulceration of plantar surface of midfoot

I70.545 Atherosclerosis of nonautologous biological bypass graft(s) of the left leg with ulceration of other part of foot `HCC` `Rx` `ESR` `COM` `A`

Atherosclerosis of nonautologous biological bypass graft(s) of the left leg with ulceration of toe

I70.548 Atherosclerosis of nonautologous biological bypass graft(s) of the left leg with ulceration of other part of lower leg `HCC` `Rx` `ESR` `COM` `A`

I70.549 Atherosclerosis of nonautologous biological bypass graft(s) of the left leg with ulceration of unspecified site `HCC` `Rx` `ESR` `COM` `A`

I70.55 Atherosclerosis of nonautologous biological bypass graft(s) of other extremity with ulceration `HCC` `Rx` `ESR` `COM` `A`

> INCLUDES   any condition classifiable to I70.518, I70.528, and I70.538

Use additional code to identify severity of ulcer (L98.49)

✓6ᵗʰ **I70.56** Atherosclerosis of nonautologous biological bypass graft(s) of the extremities with gangrene

> INCLUDES   any condition classifiable to I70.51-, I70.52-, and I70.53-, I70.54-, I70.55
> chronic limb-threatening ischemia of nonautologous biological bypass graft(s) of the extremities with gangrene
> critical limb ischemia of nonautologous biological bypass graft(s) of the extremities with gangrene

Use additional code to identify the severity of any ulcer (L97.-, L98.49-), if applicable

I70.561 Atherosclerosis of nonautologous biological bypass graft(s) of the extremities with gangrene, right leg `HCC` `ESR` `COM` `A`

I70.562 Atherosclerosis of nonautologous biological bypass graft(s) of the extremities with gangrene, left leg `HCC` `ESR` `COM` `A`

I70.563 Atherosclerosis of nonautologous biological bypass graft(s) of the extremities with gangrene, bilateral legs `HCC` `ESR` `COM` `A`

I70.568 Atherosclerosis of nonautologous biological bypass graft(s) of the extremities with gangrene, other extremity `HCC` `ESR` `COM` `A`

I70.569 Atherosclerosis of nonautologous biological bypass graft(s) of the extremities with gangrene, unspecified extremity `HCC` `ESR` `COM` `A`

✓6ᵗʰ **I70.59** Other atherosclerosis of nonautologous biological bypass graft(s) of the extremities

I70.591 Other atherosclerosis of nonautologous biological bypass graft(s) of the extremities, right leg `HCC` `ESR` `A`

I70.592 Other atherosclerosis of nonautologous biological bypass graft(s) of the extremities, left leg `HCC` `ESR` `A`

I70.593 Other atherosclerosis of nonautologous biological bypass graft(s) of the extremities, bilateral legs `HCC` `ESR` `A`

I70.598 Other atherosclerosis of nonautologous biological bypass graft(s) of the extremities, other extremity `HCC` `ESR` `A`

I70.599 Other atherosclerosis of nonautologous biological bypass graft(s) of the extremities, unspecified extremity `HCC` `ESR` `A`

✓5ᵗʰ **I70.6** Atherosclerosis of nonbiological bypass graft(s) of the extremities

Use additional code, if applicable, to identify chronic total occlusion of artery of extremity (I70.92)

AHA: 2020,4Q,98

✓6ᵗʰ **I70.60** Unspecified atherosclerosis of nonbiological bypass graft(s) of the extremities

I70.601 Unspecified atherosclerosis of nonbiological bypass graft(s) of the extremities, right leg `HCC` `ESR` `A`

I70.602 Unspecified atherosclerosis of nonbiological bypass graft(s) of the extremities, left leg `HCC` `ESR` `A`

I70.603 Unspecified atherosclerosis of nonbiological bypass graft(s) of the extremities, bilateral legs `HCC` `ESR` `A`

I70.608 Unspecified atherosclerosis of nonbiological bypass graft(s) of the extremities, other extremity `HCC` `ESR` `A`

I70.609 Unspecified atherosclerosis of nonbiological bypass graft(s) of the extremities, unspecified extremity `HCC` `ESR` `A`

✓6ᵗʰ **I70.61** Atherosclerosis of nonbiological bypass graft(s) of the extremities with intermittent claudication

I70.611 Atherosclerosis of nonbiological bypass graft(s) of the extremities with intermittent claudication, right leg `HCC` `ESR` `A`

I70.612 Atherosclerosis of nonbiological bypass graft(s) of the extremities with intermittent claudication, left leg `HCC` `ESR` `A`

I70.613 Atherosclerosis of nonbiological bypass graft(s) of the extremities with intermittent claudication, bilateral legs `HCC` `ESR` `A`

I70.618 Atherosclerosis of nonbiological bypass graft(s) of the extremities with intermittent claudication, other extremity `HCC` `ESR` `A`

I70.619 Atherosclerosis of nonbiological bypass graft(s) of the extremities with intermittent claudication, unspecified extremity `HCC` `ESR` `A`

✓6ᵗʰ **I70.62** Atherosclerosis of nonbiological bypass graft(s) of the extremities with rest pain

> INCLUDES   any condition classifiable to I70.61-
> chronic limb-threatening ischemia NOS of nonbiological bypass graft(s) of the extremities
> chronic limb-threatening ischemia of nonbiological bypass graft(s) of the extremities with rest pain
> critical limb ischemia NOS of nonbiological bypass graft(s) of the extremities
> critical limb ischemia of nonbiological bypass graft(s) of the extremities with rest pain

I70.621 Atherosclerosis of nonbiological bypass graft(s) of the extremities with rest pain, right leg `HCC` `ESR` `A`

I70.622 Atherosclerosis of nonbiological bypass graft(s) of the extremities with rest pain, left leg `HCC` `ESR` `A`

I70.623 Atherosclerosis of nonbiological bypass graft(s) of the extremities with rest pain, bilateral legs `HCC` `ESR` `A`

I70.628 Atherosclerosis of nonbiological bypass graft(s) of the extremities with rest pain, other extremity `HCC` `ESR` `A`

I70.629 Atherosclerosis of nonbiological bypass graft(s) of the extremities with rest pain, unspecified extremity `HCC` `ESR` `A`

`HCC` CMS-HCC   `Rx` Rx HCC   `ESR` ESRD HCC   `COM` Commercial HCC   `N` Newborn: 0   `P` Pediatric: 0-17   `M` Maternity: 9-64   `A` Adult: 15-124

690   ICD-10-CM 2023

√6ᵗʰ **I70.63** **Atherosclerosis of nonbiological bypass graft(s) of the right leg with ulceration**

> INCLUDES   any condition classifiable to I70.611 and I70.621
> chronic limb-threatening ischemia of nonbiological bypass graft(s) of the right leg with ulceration
> critical limb ischemia of nonbiological bypass graft(s) of the right leg with ulceration
> Use additional code to identify severity of ulcer (L97.-)

I70.631 Atherosclerosis of nonbiological bypass graft(s) of the right leg with ulceration of thigh   HCC Rx ESR COM A

I70.632 Atherosclerosis of nonbiological bypass graft(s) of the right leg with ulceration of calf   HCC Rx ESR COM A

I70.633 Atherosclerosis of nonbiological bypass graft(s) of the right leg with ulceration of ankle   HCC Rx ESR COM A

I70.634 Atherosclerosis of nonbiological bypass graft(s) of the right leg with ulceration of heel and midfoot   HCC Rx ESR COM A
> Atherosclerosis of nonbiological bypass graft(s) of right leg with ulceration of plantar surface of midfoot

I70.635 Atherosclerosis of nonbiological bypass graft(s) of the right leg with ulceration of other part of foot   HCC Rx ESR COM A
> Atherosclerosis of nonbiological bypass graft(s) of the right leg with ulceration of toe

I70.638 Atherosclerosis of nonbiological bypass graft(s) of the right leg with ulceration of other part of lower leg   HCC Rx ESR COM A

I70.639 Atherosclerosis of nonbiological bypass graft(s) of the right leg with ulceration of unspecified site   HCC Rx ESR COM A

√6ᵗʰ **I70.64** **Atherosclerosis of nonbiological bypass graft(s) of the left leg with ulceration**

> INCLUDES   any condition classifiable to I70.612 and I70.622
> chronic limb-threatening ischemia of nonbiological bypass graft(s) of the left leg with ulceration
> critical limb ischemia of nonbiological bypass graft(s) of the left leg with ulceration
> Use additional code to identify severity of ulcer (L97.-)

I70.641 Atherosclerosis of nonbiological bypass graft(s) of the left leg with ulceration of thigh   HCC Rx ESR COM A

I70.642 Atherosclerosis of nonbiological bypass graft(s) of the left leg with ulceration of calf   HCC Rx ESR COM A

I70.643 Atherosclerosis of nonbiological bypass graft(s) of the left leg with ulceration of ankle   HCC Rx ESR COM A

I70.644 Atherosclerosis of nonbiological bypass graft(s) of the left leg with ulceration of heel and midfoot   HCC Rx ESR COM A
> Atherosclerosis of nonbiological bypass graft(s) of left leg with ulceration of plantar surface of midfoot

I70.645 Atherosclerosis of nonbiological bypass graft(s) of the left leg with ulceration of other part of foot   HCC Rx ESR COM A
> Atherosclerosis of nonbiological bypass graft(s) of the left leg with ulceration of toe

I70.648 Atherosclerosis of nonbiological bypass graft(s) of the left leg with ulceration of other part of lower leg   HCC Rx ESR COM A

I70.649 Atherosclerosis of nonbiological bypass graft(s) of the left leg with ulceration of unspecified site   HCC Rx ESR COM A

I70.65 **Atherosclerosis of nonbiological bypass graft(s) of other extremity with ulceration**   HCC Rx ESR COM A

> INCLUDES   any condition classifiable to I70.618 and I70.628
> Use additional code to identify severity of ulcer (L98.49)

√6ᵗʰ **I70.66** **Atherosclerosis of nonbiological bypass graft(s) of the extremities with gangrene**

> INCLUDES   any condition classifiable to I70.61-, I70.62-, I70.63-, I70.64-, I70.65
> chronic limb-threatening ischemia of nonbiological bypass graft(s) of the extremities with gangrene
> critical limb ischemia of nonbiological bypass graft(s) of the extremities with gangrene
> Use additional code to identify the severity of any ulcer (L97.-, L98.49-), if applicable

I70.661 Atherosclerosis of nonbiological bypass graft(s) of the extremities with gangrene, right leg   HCC ESR COM A

I70.662 Atherosclerosis of nonbiological bypass graft(s) of the extremities with gangrene, left leg   HCC ESR COM A

I70.663 Atherosclerosis of nonbiological bypass graft(s) of the extremities with gangrene, bilateral legs   HCC ESR COM A

I70.668 Atherosclerosis of nonbiological bypass graft(s) of the extremities with gangrene, other extremity   HCC ESR COM A

I70.669 Atherosclerosis of nonbiological bypass graft(s) of the extremities with gangrene, unspecified extremity   HCC ESR COM A

√6ᵗʰ **I70.69** **Other atherosclerosis of nonbiological bypass graft(s) of the extremities**

I70.691 Other atherosclerosis of nonbiological bypass graft(s) of the extremities, right leg   HCC ESR

I70.692 Other atherosclerosis of nonbiological bypass graft(s) of the extremities, left leg   HCC ESR

I70.693 Other atherosclerosis of nonbiological bypass graft(s) of the extremities, bilateral legs   HCC ESR

I70.698 Other atherosclerosis of nonbiological bypass graft(s) of the extremities, other extremity   HCC ESR

I70.699 Other atherosclerosis of nonbiological bypass graft(s) of the extremities, unspecified extremity   HCC ESR

√5ᵗʰ **I70.7** **Atherosclerosis of other type of bypass graft(s) of the extremities**
> Use additional code, if applicable, to identify chronic total occlusion of artery of extremity (I70.92)
> **AHA:** 2020,4Q,98

√6ᵗʰ **I70.70** **Unspecified atherosclerosis of other type of bypass graft(s) of the extremities**

I70.701 Unspecified atherosclerosis of other type of bypass graft(s) of the extremities, right leg   HCC ESR A

I70.702 Unspecified atherosclerosis of other type of bypass graft(s) of the extremities, left leg   HCC ESR A

I70.703 Unspecified atherosclerosis of other type of bypass graft(s) of the extremities, bilateral legs   HCC ESR A

I70.708 Unspecified atherosclerosis of other type of bypass graft(s) of the extremities, other extremity   HCC ESR A

I70.709 Unspecified atherosclerosis of other type of bypass graft(s) of the extremities, unspecified extremity   HCC ESR A

√6ᵗʰ **I70.71** **Atherosclerosis of other type of bypass graft(s) of the extremities with intermittent claudication**

I70.711 Atherosclerosis of other type of bypass graft(s) of the extremities with intermittent claudication, right leg   HCC ESR A

Chapter 9. Diseases of the Circulatory System

I70.712–I70.791

I70.712 Atherosclerosis of other type of bypass graft(s) of the extremities with intermittent claudication, left leg   HCC ESR A

I70.713 Atherosclerosis of other type of bypass graft(s) of the extremities with intermittent claudication, bilateral legs   HCC ESR A

I70.718 Atherosclerosis of other type of bypass graft(s) of the extremities with intermittent claudication, other extremity   HCC ESR A

I70.719 Atherosclerosis of other type of bypass graft(s) of the extremities with intermittent claudication, unspecified extremity   HCC ESR A

✓6ᵗʰ I70.72 Atherosclerosis of other type of bypass graft(s) of the extremities with rest pain
   INCLUDES   any condition classifiable to I70.71-
     chronic limb-threatening ischemia NOS of other type of bypass graft(s) of the extremities
     chronic limb-threatening ischemia of other type of bypass graft(s) of the extremities with rest pain
     critical limb ischemia NOS of other type of bypass graft(s) of the extremities
     critical limb ischemia of other type of bypass graft(s) of the extremities with rest pain

I70.721 Atherosclerosis of other type of bypass graft(s) of the extremities with rest pain, right leg   HCC ESR A

I70.722 Atherosclerosis of other type of bypass graft(s) of the extremities with rest pain, left leg   HCC ESR A

I70.723 Atherosclerosis of other type of bypass graft(s) of the extremities with rest pain, bilateral legs   HCC ESR A

I70.728 Atherosclerosis of other type of bypass graft(s) of the extremities with rest pain, other extremity   HCC ESR A

I70.729 Atherosclerosis of other type of bypass graft(s) of the extremities with rest pain, unspecified extremity   HCC ESR A

✓6ᵗʰ I70.73 Atherosclerosis of other type of bypass graft(s) of the right leg with ulceration
   INCLUDES   any condition classifiable to I70.711 and I70.721
     chronic limb-threatening ischemia of other type of bypass graft(s) of the right leg with ulceration
     critical limb ischemia of other type of bypass graft(s) of the right leg with ulceration
   Use additional code to identify severity of ulcer (L97.-)

I70.731 Atherosclerosis of other type of bypass graft(s) of the right leg with ulceration of thigh   HCC Rx ESR COM A

I70.732 Atherosclerosis of other type of bypass graft(s) of the right leg with ulceration of calf   HCC Rx ESR COM A

I70.733 Atherosclerosis of other type of bypass graft(s) of the right leg with ulceration of ankle   HCC Rx ESR COM A

I70.734 Atherosclerosis of other type of bypass graft(s) of the right leg with ulceration of heel and midfoot   HCC Rx ESR COM A
     Atherosclerosis of other type of bypass graft(s) of right leg with ulceration of plantar surface of midfoot

I70.735 Atherosclerosis of other type of bypass graft(s) of the right leg with ulceration of other part of foot   HCC Rx ESR COM A
     Atherosclerosis of other type of bypass graft(s) of right leg with ulceration of toe

I70.738 Atherosclerosis of other type of bypass graft(s) of the right leg with ulceration of other part of lower leg   HCC Rx ESR COM A

I70.739 Atherosclerosis of other type of bypass graft(s) of the right leg with ulceration of unspecified site   HCC Rx ESR COM A

✓6ᵗʰ I70.74 Atherosclerosis of other type of bypass graft(s) of the left leg with ulceration
   INCLUDES   any condition classifiable to I70.712 and I70.722
     chronic limb-threatening ischemia of other type of bypass graft(s) of the left leg with ulceration
     critical limb ischemia of other type of bypass graft(s) of the left leg with ulceration
   Use additional code to identify severity of ulcer (L97.-)

I70.741 Atherosclerosis of other type of bypass graft(s) of the left leg with ulceration of thigh   HCC Rx ESR COM A

I70.742 Atherosclerosis of other type of bypass graft(s) of the left leg with ulceration of calf   HCC Rx ESR COM A

I70.743 Atherosclerosis of other type of bypass graft(s) of the left leg with ulceration of ankle   HCC Rx ESR COM A

I70.744 Atherosclerosis of other type of bypass graft(s) of the left leg with ulceration of heel and midfoot   HCC Rx ESR COM A
     Atherosclerosis of other type of bypass graft(s) of left leg with ulceration of plantar surface of midfoot

I70.745 Atherosclerosis of other type of bypass graft(s) of the left leg with ulceration of other part of foot   HCC Rx ESR COM A
     Atherosclerosis of other type of bypass graft(s) of left leg with ulceration of toe

I70.748 Atherosclerosis of other type of bypass graft(s) of the left leg with ulceration of other part of lower leg   HCC Rx ESR COM A

I70.749 Atherosclerosis of other type of bypass graft(s) of the left leg with ulceration of unspecified site   HCC Rx ESR COM A

I70.75 Atherosclerosis of other type of bypass graft(s) of other extremity with ulceration   HCC Rx ESR COM A
   INCLUDES   any condition classifiable to I70.718 and I70.728
   Use additional code to identify severity of ulcer (L98.49)

✓6ᵗʰ I70.76 Atherosclerosis of other type of bypass graft(s) of the extremities with gangrene
   INCLUDES   any condition classifiable to I70.71-, I70.72-, I70.73-, I70.74-, I70.75
     chronic limb-threatening ischemia of other type of bypass graft(s) of the extremities with gangrene
     critical limb ischemia of other type of bypass graft(s) of the extremities with gangrene
   Use additional code to identify the severity of any ulcer (L97.-, L98.49-), if applicable

I70.761 Atherosclerosis of other type of bypass graft(s) of the extremities with gangrene, right leg   HCC ESR COM A

I70.762 Atherosclerosis of other type of bypass graft(s) of the extremities with gangrene, left leg   HCC ESR COM A

I70.763 Atherosclerosis of other type of bypass graft(s) of the extremities with gangrene, bilateral legs   HCC ESR COM A

I70.768 Atherosclerosis of other type of bypass graft(s) of the extremities with gangrene, other extremity   HCC ESR COM A

I70.769 Atherosclerosis of other type of bypass graft(s) of the extremities with gangrene, unspecified extremity   HCC ESR COM A

✓6ᵗʰ I70.79 Other atherosclerosis of other type of bypass graft(s) of the extremities

I70.791 Other atherosclerosis of other type of bypass graft(s) of the extremities, right leg   HCC ESR A

I70.792 Other atherosclerosis of other type of bypass graft(s) of the extremities, left leg `HCC` `ESR` `A`

I70.793 Other atherosclerosis of other type of bypass graft(s) of the extremities, bilateral legs `HCC` `ESR` `A`

I70.798 Other atherosclerosis of other type of bypass graft(s) of the extremities, other extremity `HCC` `ESR` `A`

I70.799 Other atherosclerosis of other type of bypass graft(s) of the extremities, unspecified extremity `HCC` `ESR` `A`

I70.8 Atherosclerosis of other arteries `A`
    TIP: Arteriosclerosis of the iliac arteries is coded here.

√6ᵗʰ **I70.9** Other and unspecified atherosclerosis

    I70.90 Unspecified atherosclerosis `A`

    I70.91 Generalized atherosclerosis `A`

    I70.92 Chronic total occlusion of artery of the extremities `HCC` `ESR` `UPD` `A`
        Complete occlusion of artery of the extremities
        Total occlusion of artery of the extremities
        Code first atherosclerosis of arteries of the extremities (I70.2-, I70.3-, I70.4-, I70.5-, I70.6-, I70.7-)

√4ᵗʰ **I71 Aortic aneurysm and dissection**

    `EXCLUDES 1` aortic ectasia (I77.81-)
        syphilitic aortic aneurysm (A52.01)
        traumatic aortic aneurysm (S25.09, S35.09)

    ▶Code first, if applicable:◀
    ▶syphilitic aortic aneurysm (A52.01)◀
    ▶traumatic aortic aneurysm (S25.09, S35.09)◀

√5ᵗʰ **I71.0** Dissection of aorta

    I71.00 Dissection of unspecified site of aorta `HCC` `ESR` `COM`

▲ √6ᵗʰ   **I71.01** Dissection of thoracic aorta
●   **I71.010** Dissection of ascending aorta
●   **I71.011** Dissection of aortic arch
●   **I71.012** Dissection of descending thoracic aorta
●   **I71.019** Dissection of thoracic aorta, unspecified

    I71.02 Dissection of abdominal aorta `HCC` `ESR` `COM`

    I71.03 Dissection of thoracoabdominal aorta `HCC` `ESR` `COM`

▲ √5ᵗʰ **I71.1** Thoracic aortic aneurysm, ruptured
●   **I71.10** Thoracic aortic aneurysm, ruptured, unspecified
●   **I71.11** Aneurysm of the ascending aorta, ruptured
●   **I71.12** Aneurysm of the aortic arch, ruptured
●   **I71.13** Aneurysm of the descending thoracic aorta, ruptured

▲ √5ᵗʰ **I71.2** Thoracic aortic aneurysm, without rupture
●   **I71.20** Thoracic aortic aneurysm, without rupture, unspecified
●   **I71.21** Aneurysm of the ascending aorta, without rupture
●   **I71.22** Aneurysm of the aortic arch, without rupture
●   **I71.23** Aneurysm of the descending thoracic aorta, without rupture

▲ √5ᵗʰ **I71.3** Abdominal aortic aneurysm, ruptured
●   **I71.30** Abdominal aortic aneurysm, ruptured, unspecified
●   **I71.31** Pararenal abdominal aortic aneurysm, ruptured
●   **I71.32** Juxtarenal abdominal aortic aneurysm, ruptured
●   **I71.33** Infrarenal abdominal aortic aneurysm, ruptured

▲ √5ᵗʰ **I71.4** Abdominal aortic aneurysm, without rupture
●   **I71.40** Abdominal aortic aneurysm, without rupture, unspecified
●   **I71.41** Pararenal abdominal aortic aneurysm, without rupture
●   **I71.42** Juxtarenal abdominal aortic aneurysm, without rupture
●   **I71.43** Infrarenal abdominal aortic aneurysm, without rupture

▲ √6ᵗʰ **I71.5** Thoracoabdominal aortic aneurysm, ruptured
●   **I71.50** Thoracoabdominal aortic aneurysm, ruptured, unspecified
●   **I71.51** Supraceliac aneurysm of the abdominal aorta, ruptured

    I71.52 Paravisceral aneurysm of the abdominal aorta, ruptured

▲ √5ᵗʰ **I71.6** Thoracoabdominal aortic aneurysm, without rupture
●   **I71.60** Thoracoabdominal aortic aneurysm, without rupture, unspecified
●   **I71.61** Supraceliac aneurysm of the abdominal aorta, without rupture
●   **I71.62** Paravisceral aneurysm of the abdominal aorta, without rupture

    I71.8 Aortic aneurysm of unspecified site, ruptured `HCC` `ESR` `COM`
        Rupture of aorta NOS

    I71.9 Aortic aneurysm of unspecified site, without rupture `HCC` `ESR`
        Aneurysm of aorta
        Dilatation of aorta
        Hyaline necrosis of aorta

√4ᵗʰ **I72 Other aneurysm**

    `INCLUDES`   aneurysm (cirsoid) (false) (ruptured)
    `EXCLUDES 2`   acquired aneurysm (I77.0)
        aneurysm (of) aorta (I71.-)
        aneurysm (of) arteriovenous NOS (Q27.3-)
        carotid artery dissection (I77.71)
        cerebral (nonruptured) aneurysm (I67.1)
        coronary aneurysm (I25.4)
        coronary artery dissection (I25.42)
        dissection of artery NEC (I77.79)
        dissection of precerebral artery, congenital (nonruptured) (Q28.1)
        heart aneurysm (I25.3)
        iliac artery dissection (I77.72)
        precerebral artery, congenital (nonruptured) (Q28.1)
        pulmonary artery aneurysm (I28.1)
        renal artery dissection (I77.73)
        retinal aneurysm (H35.0)
        ruptured cerebral aneurysm (I60.7)
        varicose aneurysm (I77.0)
        vertebral artery dissection (I77.74)

    AHA: 2016,4Q,28-29

    I72.0 Aneurysm of carotid artery `HCC` `ESR`
        Aneurysm of common carotid artery
        Aneurysm of external carotid artery
        Aneurysm of internal carotid artery, extracranial portion
        `EXCLUDES 1`   aneurysm of internal carotid artery, intracranial portion (I67.1)
            aneurysm of internal carotid artery NOS (I67.1)

    I72.1 Aneurysm of artery of upper extremity `HCC` `ESR`

    I72.2 Aneurysm of renal artery `HCC` `ESR`

    I72.3 Aneurysm of iliac artery `HCC` `ESR`

    I72.4 Aneurysm of artery of lower extremity `HCC` `ESR`
        AHA: 2019,2Q,21

    I72.5 Aneurysm of other precerebral arteries `HCC` `ESR`
        Aneurysm of basilar artery (trunk)
        `EXCLUDES 2`   aneurysm of carotid artery (I72.0)
            aneurysm of vertebral artery (I72.6)
            dissection of carotid artery (I77.71)
            dissection of other precerebral arteries (I77.75)
            dissection of vertebral artery (I77.74)

    I72.6 Aneurysm of vertebral artery `HCC` `ESR`
        `EXCLUDES 2`   dissection of vertebral artery (I77.74)

    I72.8 Aneurysm of other specified arteries `HCC` `ESR`

I72.9 **Aneurysm of unspecified site**   HCC ESR

Aneurysm

Outer layer

Layers of muscular and elastic tissue

Inner layer

Aneurysm

✓4ᵗʰ **I73** **Other peripheral vascular diseases**
 EXCLUDES 2   chilblains (T69.1)
      frostbite (T33-T34)
      immersion hand or foot (T69.0-)
      spasm of cerebral artery (G45.9)
 AHA: 2018,4Q,87

✓5ᵗʰ **I73.0** **Raynaud's syndrome**
      Raynaud's disease
      Raynaud's phenomenon (secondary)
      DEF: Constriction of the arteries of the digits caused by cold or by nerve or arterial damage and can be prompted by stress or emotion. Blood cannot reach the skin and soft tissues and the skin turns white with blue mottling.
   I73.00 **Raynaud's syndrome** without gangrene
   I73.01 **Raynaud's syndrome** with gangrene   HCC ESR COM

I73.1 **Thromboangiitis obliterans [Buerger's disease]**   HCC ESR
      DEF: Inflammatory disease of the extremity blood vessels, mainly the lower blood vessels. This disease is associated with heavy tobacco use. The arteries are more affected than veins. It occurs primarily in young men and leads to tissue ischemia and gangrene.

✓5ᵗʰ **I73.8** **Other specified peripheral vascular diseases**
 EXCLUDES 1   diabetic (peripheral) angiopathy (E08-E13 with .51-.52)
   I73.81 **Erythromelalgia**   HCC ESR
   I73.89 **Other specified peripheral vascular diseases**   HCC ESR
      Acrocyanosis
      Erythrocyanosis
      Simple acroparesthesia [Schultze's type]
      Vasomotor acroparesthesia [Nothnagel's type]

I73.9 **Peripheral vascular disease, unspecified**   HCC ESR
      Intermittent claudication
      Peripheral angiopathy NOS
      Spasm of artery
 EXCLUDES 1   atherosclerosis of the extremities (I70.2-I70.7-)
 AHA: 2018,2Q,7

✓4ᵗʰ **I74** **Arterial embolism and thrombosis**
 INCLUDES   embolic infarction
      embolic occlusion
      thrombotic infarction
      thrombotic occlusion
 Code first:
      embolism and thrombosis complicating abortion or ectopic or molar pregnancy (O00-O07, O08.2)
      embolism and thrombosis complicating pregnancy, childbirth and the puerperium (O88.-)
 EXCLUDES 2   atheroembolism (I75.-)
      basilar embolism and thrombosis (I63.0-I63.2, I65.1)
      carotid embolism and thrombosis (I63.0-I63.2, I65.2)
      cerebral embolism and thrombosis (I63.3-I63.5, I66.-)
      coronary embolism and thrombosis (I21-I25)
      mesenteric embolism and thrombosis (K55.0-)
      ophthalmic embolism and thrombosis (H34.-)
      precerebral embolism and thrombosis NOS (I63.0-I63.2, I65.9)
      pulmonary embolism and thrombosis (I26.-)
      renal embolism and thrombosis (N28.0)
      retinal embolism and thrombosis (H34.-)
      septic embolism and thrombosis (I76)
      vertebral embolism and thrombosis (I63.0-I63.2, I65.0)

✓5ᵗʰ **I74.0** **Embolism and thrombosis of** abdominal aorta
   I74.01 **Saddle embolus of abdominal aorta**   HCC ESR COM
   I74.09 **Other arterial embolism and thrombosis of abdominal aorta**   HCC ESR COM
      Aortic bifurcation syndrome
      Aortoiliac obstruction
      Leriche's syndrome

✓5ᵗʰ **I74.1** **Embolism and thrombosis of other and unspecified parts of aorta**
   I74.10 **Embolism and thrombosis of unspecified parts of aorta**   HCC ESR COM
   I74.11 **Embolism and thrombosis of** thoracic aorta   HCC ESR COM
   I74.19 **Embolism and thrombosis of other parts of aorta**   HCC ESR COM

I74.2 **Embolism and thrombosis of arteries of the** upper extremities   HCC ESR COM

I74.3 **Embolism and thrombosis of arteries of the** lower extremities   HCC ESR COM

I74.4 **Embolism and thrombosis of arteries of extremities, unspecified**   HCC ESR COM
      Peripheral arterial embolism NOS

I74.5 **Embolism and thrombosis of** iliac artery   HCC ESR COM

I74.8 **Embolism and thrombosis of other arteries**   HCC ESR COM

I74.9 **Embolism and thrombosis of unspecified artery**   HCC ESR COM

✓4ᵗʰ **I75** **Atheroembolism**
 INCLUDES   atherothrombotic microembolism
      cholesterol embolism

✓5ᵗʰ **I75.0** **Atheroembolism of** extremities
 ✓6ᵗʰ **I75.01** **Atheroembolism of** upper extremity
   I75.011 **Atheroembolism of** right upper extremity   HCC ESR COM
   I75.012 **Atheroembolism of** left upper extremity   HCC ESR COM
   I75.013 **Atheroembolism of** bilateral upper extremities   HCC ESR COM
   I75.019 **Atheroembolism of unspecified upper extremity**   HCC ESR COM
 ✓6ᵗʰ **I75.02** **Atheroembolism of** lower extremity
   I75.021 **Atheroembolism of** right lower extremity   HCC ESR COM
   I75.022 **Atheroembolism of** left lower extremity   HCC ESR COM
   I75.023 **Atheroembolism of** bilateral lower extremities   HCC ESR COM
   I75.029 **Atheroembolism of unspecified lower extremity**   HCC ESR COM

✓5ᵗʰ **I75.8** **Atheroembolism of other sites**
   I75.81 **Atheroembolism of** kidney   HCC ESR COM
      Use additional code for any associated acute kidney failure and chronic kidney disease (N17.-, N18.-)
   I75.89 **Atheroembolism of other site**   HCC ESR COM

I76 Septic arterial embolism `HCC` `ESR` `COM` `UPD`

Code first underlying infection, such as:
infective endocarditis (I33.0)
lung abscess (J85.-)
Use additional code to identify the site of the embolism (I74.-)

EXCLUDES 2   *septic pulmonary embolism (I26.01, I26.90)*

✓4ᵗʰ I77 Other disorders of arteries and arterioles

EXCLUDES 2   *collagen (vascular) diseases (M30-M36)*
hypersensitivity angiitis (M31.0)
pulmonary artery (I28.-)

I77.0 Arteriovenous fistula, acquired `HCC` `ESR`
Aneurysmal varix
Arteriovenous aneurysm, acquired

EXCLUDES 1   *arteriovenous aneurysm NOS (Q27.3-)*
presence of arteriovenous shunt (fistula) for dialysis (Z99.2)
traumatic - see injury of blood vessel by body region

EXCLUDES 2   *cerebral (I67.1)*
coronary (I25.4)

DEF: Communication between an artery and vein caused by trauma or invasive procedures.

I77.1 Stricture of artery `HCC` `ESR`
Narrowing of artery
AHA: 2021,3Q,12

I77.2 Rupture of artery `HCC` `ESR`
Erosion of artery
Fistula of artery
Ulcer of artery

EXCLUDES 1   *traumatic rupture of artery - see injury of blood vessel by body region*

I77.3 Arterial fibromuscular dysplasia `HCC` `ESR`
Fibromuscular hyperplasia (of) carotid artery
Fibromuscular hyperplasia (of) renal artery

I77.4 Celiac artery compression syndrome `HCC` `ESR`
AHA: 2021,3Q,12

I77.5 Necrosis of artery `HCC` `ESR`

I77.6 Arteritis, unspecified `HCC` `ESR`
Aortitis NOS
Endarteritis NOS

EXCLUDES 1   *arteritis or endarteritis:*
aortic arch (M31.4)
cerebral NEC (I67.7)
coronary (I25.89)
deformans (I70.-)
giant cell (M31.5, M31.6)
obliterans (I70.-)
senile (I70.-)

✓5ᵗʰ I77.7 Other arterial dissection

EXCLUDES 2   *dissection of aorta (I71.0-)*
dissection of coronary artery (I25.42)

AHA: 2016,4Q,28-29

I77.70 Dissection of unspecified artery `HCC` `ESR` `COM`
I77.71 Dissection of carotid artery `HCC` `ESR` `COM`
I77.72 Dissection of iliac artery `HCC` `ESR` `COM`
I77.73 Dissection of renal artery `HCC` `ESR` `COM`
I77.74 Dissection of vertebral artery `HCC` `ESR` `COM`

EXCLUDES 2   *aneurysm of vertebral artery (I72.6)*

I77.75 Dissection of other precerebral arteries `HCC` `ESR` `COM`
Dissection of basilar artery (trunk)

EXCLUDES 2   *aneurysm of carotid artery (I72.0)*
aneurysm of other precerebral arteries (I72.5)
aneurysm of vertebral artery (I72.6)
dissection of carotid artery (I77.71)
dissection of vertebral artery (I77.74)

I77.76 Dissection of artery of upper extremity `HCC` `ESR` `COM`
I77.77 Dissection of artery of lower extremity `HCC` `ESR` `COM`
I77.79 Dissection of other specified artery `HCC` `ESR` `COM`

✓5ᵗʰ I77.8 Other specified disorders of arteries and arterioles

✓6ᵗʰ I77.81 Aortic ectasia
Ectasis aorta

EXCLUDES 1   *aortic aneurysm and dissection ▶(I71.-)◄*

I77.810 Thoracic aortic ectasia `HCC` `ESR`
I77.811 Abdominal aortic ectasia `HCC` `ESR`
I77.812 Thoracoabdominal aortic ectasia `HCC` `ESR`
I77.819 Aortic ectasia, unspecified site `HCC` `ESR`

I77.82 Antineutrophilic cytoplasmic antibody [ANCA] vasculitis
ANCA associated vasculitis
ANCA positive vasculitis

EXCLUDES 2   *eosinophilic granulomatosis with polyangiitis (M30.1)*
granulomatosis with polyangiitis (M31.3-)
microscopic polyangiitis (M31.7)

I77.89 Other specified disorders of arteries and arterioles `HCC` `ESR`
AHA: 2021,1Q,23

I77.9 Disorder of arteries and arterioles, unspecified `HCC` `ESR`
AHA: 2021,1Q,4; 2018,2Q,7

✓4ᵗʰ I78 Diseases of capillaries

I78.0 Hereditary hemorrhagic telangiectasia `HCC` `ESR`
Rendu-Osler-Weber disease

I78.1 Nevus, non-neoplastic
Araneus nevus
Senile nevus
Spider nevus
Stellar nevus

EXCLUDES 1   *nevus NOS (D22.-)*
vascular NOS (Q82.5)

EXCLUDES 2   *blue nevus (D22.-)*
flammeus nevus (Q82.5)
hairy nevus (D22.-)
melanocytic nevus (D22.-)
pigmented nevus (D22.-)
portwine nevus (Q82.5)
sanguineous nevus (Q82.5)
strawberry nevus (Q82.5)
verrucous nevus (Q82.5)

AHA: 2019,1Q,21

I78.8 Other diseases of capillaries
I78.9 Disease of capillaries, unspecified

✓4ᵗʰ I79 Disorders of arteries, arterioles and capillaries in diseases classified elsewhere

I79.0 Aneurysm of aorta in diseases classified elsewhere `HCC` `ESR`
Code first underlying disease

EXCLUDES 1   *syphilitic aneurysm (A52.01)*

I79.1 Aortitis in diseases classified elsewhere `HCC` `ESR`
Code first underlying disease

EXCLUDES 1   *syphilitic aortitis (A52.02)*

I79.8 Other disorders of arteries, arterioles and capillaries in diseases classified elsewhere `HCC` `ESR`
Code first underlying disease, such as:
amyloidosis (E85.-)

EXCLUDES 1   *diabetic (peripheral) angiopathy (E08-E13 with .51-.52)*
syphilitic endarteritis (A52.09)
tuberculous endarteritis (A18.89)

☑ Additional Character Required   ✓x7ᵗʰ Placeholder Alert   Manifestation   Unspecified Dx   Ⓠ QPP   `UPD` Unacceptable PDx

Chapter 9. Diseases of the Circulatory System

Diseases of veins, lymphatic vessels and lymph nodes, not elsewhere classified (I80-I89)

✓4ᵗʰ **I80 Phlebitis and thrombophlebitis**

INCLUDES endophlebitis
inflammation, vein
periphlebitis
suppurative phlebitis

Code first:
phlebitis and thrombophlebitis complicating abortion, ectopic or molar pregnancy (O00-O07, O08.7)
phlebitis and thrombophlebitis complicating pregnancy, childbirth and the puerperium (O22.-, O87.-)

EXCLUDES 1 venous embolism and thrombosis of lower extremities (I82.4-, I82.5-, I82.81-)

✓5ᵗʰ **I80.0 Phlebitis and thrombophlebitis of superficial vessels of lower extremities**
Phlebitis and thrombophlebitis of femoropopliteal vein

    I80.00 Phlebitis and thrombophlebitis of superficial vessels of unspecified lower extremity

    I80.01 Phlebitis and thrombophlebitis of superficial vessels of right lower extremity

    I80.02 Phlebitis and thrombophlebitis of superficial vessels of left lower extremity

    I80.03 Phlebitis and thrombophlebitis of superficial vessels of lower extremities, bilateral

✓5ᵗʰ **I80.1 Phlebitis and thrombophlebitis of femoral vein**
Phlebitis and thrombophlebitis of common femoral vein
Phlebitis and thrombophlebitis of deep femoral vein

    I80.10 Phlebitis and thrombophlebitis of unspecified femoral vein HCC Rx ESR COM

    I80.11 Phlebitis and thrombophlebitis of right femoral vein HCC Rx ESR COM

    I80.12 Phlebitis and thrombophlebitis of left femoral vein HCC Rx ESR COM

    I80.13 Phlebitis and thrombophlebitis of femoral vein, bilateral HCC Rx ESR COM

✓5ᵗʰ **I80.2 Phlebitis and thrombophlebitis of other and unspecified deep vessels of lower extremities**

✓6ᵗʰ   **I80.20 Phlebitis and thrombophlebitis of unspecified deep vessels of lower extremities**

    I80.201 Phlebitis and thrombophlebitis of unspecified deep vessels of right lower extremity HCC Rx ESR COM

    I80.202 Phlebitis and thrombophlebitis of unspecified deep vessels of left lower extremity HCC Rx ESR COM

    I80.203 Phlebitis and thrombophlebitis of unspecified deep vessels of lower extremities, bilateral HCC Rx ESR COM

    I80.209 Phlebitis and thrombophlebitis of unspecified deep vessels of unspecified lower extremity HCC Rx ESR COM

✓6ᵗʰ   **I80.21 Phlebitis and thrombophlebitis of iliac vein**
Phlebitis and thrombophlebitis of common iliac vein
Phlebitis and thrombophlebitis of external iliac vein
Phlebitis and thrombophlebitis of internal iliac vein

    I80.211 Phlebitis and thrombophlebitis of right iliac vein HCC Rx ESR COM

    I80.212 Phlebitis and thrombophlebitis of left iliac vein HCC Rx ESR COM

    I80.213 Phlebitis and thrombophlebitis of iliac vein, bilateral HCC Rx ESR COM

    I80.219 Phlebitis and thrombophlebitis of unspecified iliac vein HCC Rx ESR COM

✓6ᵗʰ   **I80.22 Phlebitis and thrombophlebitis of popliteal vein**

    I80.221 Phlebitis and thrombophlebitis of right popliteal vein HCC Rx ESR COM

    I80.222 Phlebitis and thrombophlebitis of left popliteal vein HCC Rx ESR COM

    I80.223 Phlebitis and thrombophlebitis of popliteal vein, bilateral HCC Rx ESR COM

    I80.229 Phlebitis and thrombophlebitis of unspecified popliteal vein HCC Rx ESR COM

✓6ᵗʰ **I80.23 Phlebitis and thrombophlebitis of tibial vein**
Phlebitis and thrombophlebitis of anterior tibial vein
Phlebitis and thrombophlebitis of posterior tibial vein

    I80.231 Phlebitis and thrombophlebitis of right tibial vein HCC Rx ESR COM

    I80.232 Phlebitis and thrombophlebitis of left tibial vein HCC Rx ESR COM

    I80.233 Phlebitis and thrombophlebitis of tibial vein, bilateral HCC Rx ESR COM

    I80.239 Phlebitis and thrombophlebitis of unspecified tibial vein HCC Rx ESR COM

✓6ᵗʰ **I80.24 Phlebitis and thrombophlebitis of peroneal vein**
AHA: 2019,4Q,8

    I80.241 Phlebitis and thrombophlebitis of right peroneal vein HCC Rx ESR COM

    I80.242 Phlebitis and thrombophlebitis of left peroneal vein HCC Rx ESR COM

    I80.243 Phlebitis and thrombophlebitis of peroneal vein, bilateral HCC Rx ESR COM

    I80.249 Phlebitis and thrombophlebitis of unspecified peroneal vein HCC Rx ESR COM

✓6ᵗʰ **I80.25 Phlebitis and thrombophlebitis of calf muscular vein**
Phlebitis and thrombophlebitis of calf muscular vein, NOS
Phlebitis and thrombophlebitis of gastrocnemial vein
Phlebitis and thrombophlebitis of soleal vein
AHA: 2019,4Q,8

    I80.251 Phlebitis and thrombophlebitis of right calf muscular vein HCC Rx ESR COM

    I80.252 Phlebitis and thrombophlebitis of left calf muscular vein HCC Rx ESR COM

    I80.253 Phlebitis and thrombophlebitis of calf muscular vein, bilateral HCC Rx ESR COM

    I80.259 Phlebitis and thrombophlebitis of unspecified calf muscular vein HCC Rx ESR COM

✓6ᵗʰ **I80.29 Phlebitis and thrombophlebitis of other deep vessels of lower extremities**

    I80.291 Phlebitis and thrombophlebitis of other deep vessels of right lower extremity HCC Rx ESR COM

    I80.292 Phlebitis and thrombophlebitis of other deep vessels of left lower extremity HCC Rx ESR COM

    I80.293 Phlebitis and thrombophlebitis of other deep vessels of lower extremity, bilateral HCC Rx ESR COM

    I80.299 Phlebitis and thrombophlebitis of other deep vessels of unspecified lower extremity HCC Rx ESR COM

I80.3 Phlebitis and thrombophlebitis of lower extremities, unspecified

I80.8 Phlebitis and thrombophlebitis of other sites

I80.9 Phlebitis and thrombophlebitis of unspecified site

I81 Portal vein thrombosis
Portal (vein) obstruction

EXCLUDES 2 hepatic vein thrombosis (I82.0)
phlebitis of portal vein (K75.1)

AHA: 2019,4Q,68

☑4ᵗʰ **I82 Other venous embolism and thrombosis**

Code first venous embolism and thrombosis complicating:
abortion, ectopic or molar pregnancy (O00-O07, O08.7)
pregnancy, childbirth and the puerperium (O22.-, O87.-)

EXCLUDES 2   *venous embolism and thrombosis (of):*
       cerebral (I63.6, I67.6)
       coronary (I21-I25)
       intracranial and intraspinal, septic or NOS (G08)
       intracranial, nonpyogenic (I67.6)
       intraspinal, nonpyogenic (G95.1)
       mesenteric (K55.0-)
       portal (I81)
       pulmonary (I26.-)

I82.0 Budd-Chiari syndrome   HCC Rx ESR COM
Hepatic vein thrombosis
DEF: Thrombosis or other obstruction of the hepatic veins. Symptoms include an enlarged liver, extensive collateral vessels, intractable ascites, and severe portal hypertension.

I82.1 Thrombophlebitis migrans

☑5ᵗʰ **I82.2 Embolism and thrombosis of** vena cava **and other** thoracic **veins**

☑6ᵗʰ **I82.21 Embolism and thrombosis of** superior vena cava

     I82.210 Acute embolism and thrombosis of superior vena cava   HCC Rx ESR COM
       Embolism and thrombosis of superior vena cava NOS

     I82.211 Chronic embolism and thrombosis of superior vena cava   HCC Rx ESR COM

☑6ᵗʰ **I82.22 Embolism and thrombosis of** inferior vena cava

     I82.220 Acute embolism and thrombosis of inferior vena cava   HCC Rx ESR COM
       Embolism and thrombosis of inferior vena cava NOS

     I82.221 Chronic embolism and thrombosis of inferior vena cava   HCC Rx ESR COM

☑6ᵗʰ **I82.29 Embolism and thrombosis of other thoracic veins**
     Embolism and thrombosis of brachiocephalic (innominate) vein

     I82.290 Acute embolism and thrombosis of other thoracic veins   HCC Rx ESR COM

     I82.291 Chronic embolism and thrombosis of other thoracic veins   HCC Rx ESR COM

I82.3 Embolism and thrombosis of renal vein   HCC Rx ESR COM

☑5ᵗʰ **I82.4** Acute **embolism and thrombosis of** deep veins of lower extremity

☑6ᵗʰ **I82.40 Acute embolism and thrombosis of unspecified deep veins of** lower extremity
     Deep vein thrombosis NOS
     DVT NOS

     EXCLUDES 1   *acute embolism and thrombosis of unspecified deep veins of distal lower extremity (I82.4Z-)*
         acute embolism and thrombosis of unspecified deep veins of proximal lower extremity (I82.4Y-)

     I82.401 Acute embolism and thrombosis of unspecified deep veins of right **lower extremity**   HCC Rx ESR COM

     I82.402 Acute embolism and thrombosis of unspecified deep veins of left **lower extremity**   HCC Rx ESR COM

     I82.403 Acute embolism and thrombosis of unspecified deep veins of lower extremity, bilateral   HCC Rx ESR COM

     I82.409 Acute embolism and thrombosis of unspecified deep veins of unspecified lower extremity   HCC Rx ESR COM

☑6ᵗʰ **I82.41 Acute embolism and thrombosis of** femoral vein
     Acute embolism and thrombosis of common femoral vein
     Acute embolism and thrombosis of deep femoral vein

     I82.411 Acute embolism and thrombosis of right **femoral vein**   HCC Rx ESR COM

     I82.412 Acute embolism and thrombosis of left **femoral vein**   HCC Rx ESR COM

     I82.413 Acute embolism and thrombosis of femoral vein, bilateral   HCC Rx ESR COM

     I82.419 Acute embolism and thrombosis of unspecified femoral vein   HCC Rx ESR COM

☑6ᵗʰ **I82.42 Acute embolism and thrombosis of** iliac vein
     Acute embolism and thrombosis of common iliac vein
     Acute embolism and thrombosis of external iliac vein
     Acute embolism and thrombosis of internal iliac vein

     I82.421 Acute embolism and thrombosis of right **iliac vein**   HCC Rx ESR COM

     I82.422 Acute embolism and thrombosis of left **iliac vein**   HCC Rx ESR COM

     I82.423 Acute embolism and thrombosis of iliac vein, bilateral   HCC Rx ESR COM

     I82.429 Acute embolism and thrombosis of unspecified iliac vein   HCC Rx ESR COM

☑6ᵗʰ **I82.43 Acute embolism and thrombosis of** popliteal vein

     I82.431 Acute embolism and thrombosis of right **popliteal vein**   HCC Rx ESR COM

     I82.432 Acute embolism and thrombosis of left **popliteal vein**   HCC Rx ESR COM

     I82.433 Acute embolism and thrombosis of popliteal vein, bilateral   HCC Rx ESR COM

     I82.439 Acute embolism and thrombosis of unspecified popliteal vein   HCC Rx ESR COM

☑6ᵗʰ **I82.44 Acute embolism and thrombosis of** tibial vein
     Acute embolism and thrombosis of anterior tibial vein
     Acute embolism and thrombosis of posterior tibial vein

     I82.441 Acute embolism and thrombosis of right **tibial vein**   HCC Rx ESR COM

     I82.442 Acute embolism and thrombosis of left **tibial vein**   HCC Rx ESR COM

     I82.443 Acute embolism and thrombosis of tibial vein, bilateral   HCC Rx ESR COM

     I82.449 Acute embolism and thrombosis of unspecified tibial vein   HCC Rx ESR COM

☑6ᵗʰ **I82.45 Acute embolism and thrombosis of** peroneal vein
     AHA: 2019,4Q,8-10

     I82.451 Acute embolism and thrombosis of right **peroneal vein**   HCC Rx ESR COM

     I82.452 Acute embolism and thrombosis of left **peroneal vein**   HCC Rx ESR COM

     I82.453 Acute embolism and thrombosis of peroneal vein, bilateral   HCC Rx ESR COM

     I82.459 Acute embolism and thrombosis of unspecified peroneal vein   HCC Rx ESR COM

☑6ᵗʰ **I82.46 Acute embolism and thrombosis of** calf muscular vein
     Acute embolism and thrombosis of calf muscular vein, NOS
     Acute embolism and thrombosis of gastrocnemial vein
     Acute embolism and thrombosis of soleal vein
     AHA: 2019,4Q,8-10

     I82.461 Acute embolism and thrombosis of right **calf muscular vein**   HCC Rx ESR COM

     I82.462 Acute embolism and thrombosis of left **calf muscular vein**   HCC Rx ESR COM

     I82.463 Acute embolism and thrombosis of calf muscular vein, bilateral   HCC Rx ESR COM

     I82.469 Acute embolism and thrombosis of unspecified calf muscular vein   HCC Rx ESR COM

☑6ᵗʰ **I82.49 Acute embolism and thrombosis of other specified deep vein of lower extremity**

     I82.491 Acute embolism and thrombosis of other specified deep vein of right **lower extremity**   HCC Rx ESR COM

     I82.492 Acute embolism and thrombosis of other specified deep vein of left **lower extremity**   HCC Rx ESR COM

     I82.493 Acute embolism and thrombosis of other specified deep vein of lower extremity, bilateral   HCC Rx ESR COM

     I82.499 Acute embolism and thrombosis of other specified deep vein of unspecified lower extremity   HCC Rx ESR COM

✓6ᵗʰ I82.4Y Acute embolism and thrombosis of unspecified deep veins of proximal lower extremity
Acute embolism and thrombosis of deep vein of thigh NOS
Acute embolism and thrombosis of deep vein of upper leg NOS

I82.4Y1 Acute embolism and thrombosis of unspecified deep veins of right proximal lower extremity HCC Rx ESR COM
I82.4Y2 Acute embolism and thrombosis of unspecified deep veins of left proximal lower extremity HCC Rx ESR COM
I82.4Y3 Acute embolism and thrombosis of unspecified deep veins of proximal lower extremity, bilateral HCC Rx ESR COM
I82.4Y9 Acute embolism and thrombosis of unspecified deep veins of unspecified proximal lower extremity HCC Rx ESR COM

✓6ᵗʰ I82.4Z Acute embolism and thrombosis of unspecified deep veins of distal lower extremity
Acute embolism and thrombosis of deep vein of calf NOS
Acute embolism and thrombosis of deep vein of lower leg NOS

I82.4Z1 Acute embolism and thrombosis of unspecified deep veins of right distal lower extremity HCC Rx ESR COM
I82.4Z2 Acute embolism and thrombosis of unspecified deep veins of left distal lower extremity HCC Rx ESR COM
I82.4Z3 Acute embolism and thrombosis of unspecified deep veins of distal lower extremity, bilateral HCC Rx ESR COM
I82.4Z9 Acute embolism and thrombosis of unspecified deep veins of unspecified distal lower extremity HCC Rx ESR COM

✓5ᵗʰ I82.5 Chronic embolism and thrombosis of deep veins of lower extremity
Use additional code, if applicable, for associated long-term (current) use of anticoagulants (Z79.01)
EXCLUDES 1   personal history of venous embolism and thrombosis (Z86.718)
AHA: 2020,2Q,20

✓6ᵗʰ I82.50 Chronic embolism and thrombosis of unspecified deep veins of lower extremity
EXCLUDES 1   chronic embolism and thrombosis of unspecified deep veins of distal lower extremity (I82.5Z-)
chronic embolism and thrombosis of unspecified deep veins of proximal lower extremity (I82.5Y-)

I82.501 Chronic embolism and thrombosis of unspecified deep veins of right lower extremity HCC Rx ESR COM
I82.502 Chronic embolism and thrombosis of unspecified deep veins of left lower extremity HCC Rx ESR COM
I82.503 Chronic embolism and thrombosis of unspecified deep veins of lower extremity, bilateral HCC Rx ESR COM
I82.509 Chronic embolism and thrombosis of unspecified deep veins of unspecified lower extremity HCC Rx ESR COM

✓6ᵗʰ I82.51 Chronic embolism and thrombosis of femoral vein
Chronic embolism and thrombosis of common femoral vein
Chronic embolism and thrombosis of deep femoral vein

I82.511 Chronic embolism and thrombosis of right femoral vein HCC Rx ESR COM
I82.512 Chronic embolism and thrombosis of left femoral vein HCC Rx ESR COM
I82.513 Chronic embolism and thrombosis of femoral vein, bilateral HCC Rx ESR COM
I82.519 Chronic embolism and thrombosis of unspecified femoral vein HCC Rx ESR COM

✓6ᵗʰ I82.52 Chronic embolism and thrombosis of iliac vein
Chronic embolism and thrombosis of common iliac vein
Chronic embolism and thrombosis of external iliac vein
Chronic embolism and thrombosis of internal iliac vein

I82.521 Chronic embolism and thrombosis of right iliac vein HCC Rx ESR COM
I82.522 Chronic embolism and thrombosis of left iliac vein HCC Rx ESR COM
I82.523 Chronic embolism and thrombosis of iliac vein, bilateral HCC Rx ESR COM
I82.529 Chronic embolism and thrombosis of unspecified iliac vein HCC Rx ESR COM

✓6ᵗʰ I82.53 Chronic embolism and thrombosis of popliteal vein
I82.531 Chronic embolism and thrombosis of right popliteal vein HCC Rx ESR COM
I82.532 Chronic embolism and thrombosis of left popliteal vein HCC Rx ESR COM
I82.533 Chronic embolism and thrombosis of popliteal vein, bilateral HCC Rx ESR COM
I82.539 Chronic embolism and thrombosis of unspecified popliteal vein HCC Rx ESR COM

✓6ᵗʰ I82.54 Chronic embolism and thrombosis of tibial vein
Chronic embolism and thrombosis of anterior tibial vein
Chronic embolism and thrombosis of posterior tibial vein

I82.541 Chronic embolism and thrombosis of right tibial vein HCC Rx ESR COM
I82.542 Chronic embolism and thrombosis of left tibial vein HCC Rx ESR COM
I82.543 Chronic embolism and thrombosis of tibial vein, bilateral HCC Rx ESR COM
I82.549 Chronic embolism and thrombosis of unspecified tibial vein HCC Rx ESR COM

✓6ᵗʰ I82.55 Chronic embolism and thrombosis of peroneal vein
AHA: 2019,4Q,8-10
I82.551 Chronic embolism and thrombosis of right peroneal vein HCC Rx ESR COM
I82.552 Chronic embolism and thrombosis of left peroneal vein HCC Rx ESR COM
I82.553 Chronic embolism and thrombosis of peroneal vein, bilateral HCC Rx ESR COM
I82.559 Chronic embolism and thrombosis of unspecified peroneal vein HCC Rx ESR COM

✓6ᵗʰ I82.56 Chronic embolism and thrombosis of calf muscular vein
Chronic embolism and thrombosis of calf muscular vein NOS
Chronic embolism and thrombosis of gastrocnemial vein
Chronic embolism and thrombosis of soleal vein
AHA: 2019,4Q,8-10
I82.561 Chronic embolism and thrombosis of right calf muscular vein HCC Rx ESR COM
I82.562 Chronic embolism and thrombosis of left calf muscular vein HCC Rx ESR COM
I82.563 Chronic embolism and thrombosis of calf muscular vein, bilateral HCC Rx ESR COM
I82.569 Chronic embolism and thrombosis of unspecified calf muscular vein HCC Rx ESR COM

✓6ᵗʰ I82.59 Chronic embolism and thrombosis of other specified deep vein of lower extremity
I82.591 Chronic embolism and thrombosis of other specified deep vein of right lower extremity HCC Rx ESR COM
I82.592 Chronic embolism and thrombosis of other specified deep vein of left lower extremity HCC Rx ESR COM
I82.593 Chronic embolism and thrombosis of other specified deep vein of lower extremity, bilateral HCC Rx ESR COM
I82.599 Chronic embolism and thrombosis of other specified deep vein of unspecified lower extremity HCC Rx ESR COM

✓6ᵗʰ   **I82.5Y**   **Chronic embolism and thrombosis of unspecified deep veins of proximal lower extremity**
Chronic embolism and thrombosis of deep veins of thigh NOS
Chronic embolism and thrombosis of deep veins of upper leg NOS

     I82.5Y1   **Chronic embolism and thrombosis of unspecified deep veins of right proximal lower extremity**   HCC Rx ESR COM

     I82.5Y2   **Chronic embolism and thrombosis of unspecified deep veins of left proximal lower extremity**   HCC Rx ESR COM

     I82.5Y3   **Chronic embolism and thrombosis of unspecified deep veins of proximal lower extremity, bilateral**   HCC Rx ESR COM

     I82.5Y9   **Chronic embolism and thrombosis of unspecified deep veins of unspecified proximal lower extremity**   HCC Rx ESR COM

✓6ᵗʰ   **I82.5Z**   **Chronic embolism and thrombosis of unspecified deep veins of distal lower extremity**
Chronic embolism and thrombosis of deep veins of calf NOS
Chronic embolism and thrombosis of deep veins of lower leg NOS

     I82.5Z1   **Chronic embolism and thrombosis of unspecified deep veins of right distal lower extremity**   HCC Rx ESR COM

     I82.5Z2   **Chronic embolism and thrombosis of unspecified deep veins of left distal lower extremity**   HCC Rx ESR COM

     I82.5Z3   **Chronic embolism and thrombosis of unspecified deep veins of distal lower extremity, bilateral**   HCC Rx ESR COM

     I82.5Z9   **Chronic embolism and thrombosis of unspecified deep veins of unspecified distal lower extremity**   HCC Rx ESR COM

✓5ᵗʰ   **I82.6**   **Acute embolism and thrombosis of veins of upper extremity**

✓6ᵗʰ   **I82.60**   **Acute embolism and thrombosis of unspecified veins of upper extremity**

     I82.601   **Acute embolism and thrombosis of unspecified veins of right upper extremity**

     I82.602   **Acute embolism and thrombosis of unspecified veins of left upper extremity**

     I82.603   **Acute embolism and thrombosis of unspecified veins of upper extremity, bilateral**

     I82.609   **Acute embolism and thrombosis of unspecified veins of unspecified upper extremity**

✓6ᵗʰ   **I82.61**   **Acute embolism and thrombosis of superficial veins of upper extremity**
Acute embolism and thrombosis of antecubital vein
Acute embolism and thrombosis of basilic vein
Acute embolism and thrombosis of cephalic vein

     I82.611   **Acute embolism and thrombosis of superficial veins of right upper extremity**

     I82.612   **Acute embolism and thrombosis of superficial veins of left upper extremity**

     I82.613   **Acute embolism and thrombosis of superficial veins of upper extremity, bilateral**

     I82.619   **Acute embolism and thrombosis of superficial veins of unspecified upper extremity**

✓6ᵗʰ   **I82.62**   **Acute embolism and thrombosis of deep veins of upper extremity**
Acute embolism and thrombosis of brachial vein
Acute embolism and thrombosis of radial vein
Acute embolism and thrombosis of ulnar vein

     I82.621   **Acute embolism and thrombosis of deep veins of right upper extremity**   HCC Rx ESR COM

     I82.622   **Acute embolism and thrombosis of deep veins of left upper extremity**   HCC Rx ESR COM

     I82.623   **Acute embolism and thrombosis of deep veins of upper extremity, bilateral**   HCC Rx ESR COM

     I82.629   **Acute embolism and thrombosis of deep veins of unspecified upper extremity**   HCC Rx ESR COM

✓5ᵗʰ   **I82.7**   **Chronic embolism and thrombosis of veins of upper extremity**
Use additional code, if applicable, for associated long-term (current) use of anticoagulants (Z79.01)
   EXCLUDES 1   *personal history of venous embolism and thrombosis (Z86.718)*

✓6ᵗʰ   **I82.70**   **Chronic embolism and thrombosis of unspecified veins of upper extremity**

     I82.701   **Chronic embolism and thrombosis of unspecified veins of right upper extremity**

     I82.702   **Chronic embolism and thrombosis of unspecified veins of left upper extremity**

     I82.703   **Chronic embolism and thrombosis of unspecified veins of upper extremity, bilateral**

     I82.709   **Chronic embolism and thrombosis of unspecified veins of unspecified upper extremity**

✓6ᵗʰ   **I82.71**   **Chronic embolism and thrombosis of superficial veins of upper extremity**
Chronic embolism and thrombosis of antecubital vein
Chronic embolism and thrombosis of basilic vein
Chronic embolism and thrombosis of cephalic vein

     I82.711   **Chronic embolism and thrombosis of superficial veins of right upper extremity**

     I82.712   **Chronic embolism and thrombosis of superficial veins of left upper extremity**

     I82.713   **Chronic embolism and thrombosis of superficial veins of upper extremity, bilateral**

     I82.719   **Chronic embolism and thrombosis of superficial veins of unspecified upper extremity**

✓6ᵗʰ   **I82.72**   **Chronic embolism and thrombosis of deep veins of upper extremity**
Chronic embolism and thrombosis of brachial vein
Chronic embolism and thrombosis of radial vein
Chronic embolism and thrombosis of ulnar vein

     I82.721   **Chronic embolism and thrombosis of deep veins of right upper extremity**   HCC Rx ESR COM

     I82.722   **Chronic embolism and thrombosis of deep veins of left upper extremity**   HCC Rx ESR COM

     I82.723   **Chronic embolism and thrombosis of deep veins of upper extremity, bilateral**   HCC Rx ESR COM

     I82.729   **Chronic embolism and thrombosis of deep veins of unspecified upper extremity**   HCC Rx ESR COM

✓5ᵗʰ   **I82.A**   **Embolism and thrombosis of axillary vein**

✓6ᵗʰ   **I82.A1**   **Acute embolism and thrombosis of axillary vein**

     I82.A11   **Acute embolism and thrombosis of right axillary vein**   HCC Rx ESR COM

     I82.A12   **Acute embolism and thrombosis of left axillary vein**   HCC Rx ESR COM

     I82.A13   **Acute embolism and thrombosis of axillary vein, bilateral**   HCC Rx ESR COM

     I82.A19   **Acute embolism and thrombosis of unspecified axillary vein**   HCC Rx ESR COM

✓6ᵗʰ   **I82.A2**   **Chronic embolism and thrombosis of axillary vein**

     I82.A21   **Chronic embolism and thrombosis of right axillary vein**   HCC Rx ESR COM

     I82.A22   **Chronic embolism and thrombosis of left axillary vein**   HCC Rx ESR COM

     I82.A23   **Chronic embolism and thrombosis of axillary vein, bilateral**   HCC Rx ESR COM

     I82.A29   **Chronic embolism and thrombosis of unspecified axillary vein**   HCC Rx ESR COM

✓5ᵗʰ   **I82.B**   **Embolism and thrombosis of subclavian vein**

✓6ᵗʰ   **I82.B1**   **Acute embolism and thrombosis of subclavian vein**

     I82.B11   **Acute embolism and thrombosis of right subclavian vein**   HCC Rx ESR COM

     I82.B12   **Acute embolism and thrombosis of left subclavian vein**   HCC Rx ESR COM

✓ Additional Character Required   ✓x /ⁿ Placeholder Alert   Manifestation   Unspecified Dx   Q QPP   UPD Unacceptable PDx

I82.B13 Acute embolism and thrombosis of subclavian vein, bilateral `HCC` `Rx` `ESR` `COM`

I82.B19 Acute embolism and thrombosis of unspecified subclavian vein `HCC` `Rx` `ESR` `COM`

√6ᵗʰ **I82.B2** Chronic embolism and thrombosis of subclavian vein

I82.B21 Chronic embolism and thrombosis of right subclavian vein `HCC` `Rx` `ESR` `COM`

I82.B22 Chronic embolism and thrombosis of left subclavian vein `HCC` `Rx` `ESR` `COM`

I82.B23 Chronic embolism and thrombosis of subclavian vein, bilateral `HCC` `Rx` `ESR` `COM`

I82.B29 Chronic embolism and thrombosis of unspecified subclavian vein `HCC` `Rx` `ESR` `COM`

√5ᵗʰ **I82.C** Embolism and thrombosis of internal jugular vein

√6ᵗʰ **I82.C1** Acute embolism and thrombosis of internal jugular vein

I82.C11 Acute embolism and thrombosis of right internal jugular vein `HCC` `Rx` `ESR` `COM`

I82.C12 Acute embolism and thrombosis of left internal jugular vein `HCC` `Rx` `ESR` `COM`

I82.C13 Acute embolism and thrombosis of internal jugular vein, bilateral `HCC` `Rx` `ESR` `COM`

I82.C19 Acute embolism and thrombosis of unspecified internal jugular vein `HCC` `Rx` `ESR` `COM`

√6ᵗʰ **I82.C2** Chronic embolism and thrombosis of internal jugular vein

I82.C21 Chronic embolism and thrombosis of right internal jugular vein `HCC` `Rx` `ESR` `COM`

I82.C22 Chronic embolism and thrombosis of left internal jugular vein `HCC` `Rx` `ESR` `COM`

I82.C23 Chronic embolism and thrombosis of internal jugular vein, bilateral `HCC` `Rx` `ESR` `COM`

I82.C29 Chronic embolism and thrombosis of unspecified internal jugular vein `HCC` `Rx` `ESR` `COM`

√5ᵗʰ **I82.8** Embolism and thrombosis of other specified veins

Use additional code, if applicable, for associated long-term (current) use of anticoagulants (Z79.01)

√6ᵗʰ **I82.81** Embolism and thrombosis of superficial veins of lower extremities

Embolism and thrombosis of saphenous vein (greater) (lesser)

I82.811 Embolism and thrombosis of superficial veins of right lower extremity

I82.812 Embolism and thrombosis of superficial veins of left lower extremity

I82.813 Embolism and thrombosis of superficial veins of lower extremities, bilateral

I82.819 Embolism and thrombosis of superficial veins of unspecified lower extremity

√6ᵗʰ **I82.89** Embolism and thrombosis of other specified veins

I82.890 Acute embolism and thrombosis of other specified veins

I82.891 Chronic embolism and thrombosis of other specified veins

√5ᵗʰ **I82.9** Embolism and thrombosis of unspecified vein

I82.90 Acute embolism and thrombosis of unspecified vein
Embolism of vein NOS
Thrombosis (vein) NOS

I82.91 Chronic embolism and thrombosis of unspecified vein

√4ᵗʰ **I83** Varicose veins of lower extremities

EXCLUDES 2   varicose veins complicating pregnancy (O22.0-)
varicose veins complicating the puerperium (O87.4)

√5ᵗʰ **I83.0** Varicose veins of lower extremities with ulcer

Use additional code to identify severity of ulcer (L97.-)

√6ᵗʰ **I83.00** Varicose veins of unspecified lower extremity with ulcer

I83.001 Varicose veins of unspecified lower extremity with ulcer of thigh `HCC` `ESR` `COM` `A`

I83.002 Varicose veins of unspecified lower extremity with ulcer of calf `HCC` `ESR` `COM` `A`

I83.003 Varicose veins of unspecified lower extremity with ulcer of ankle `HCC` `ESR` `COM` `A`

I83.004 Varicose veins of unspecified lower extremity with ulcer of heel and midfoot `HCC` `ESR` `COM` `A`
Varicose veins of unspecified lower extremity with ulcer of plantar surface of midfoot

I83.005 Varicose veins of unspecified lower extremity with ulcer other part of foot `HCC` `ESR` `COM` `A`
Varicose veins of unspecified lower extremity with ulcer of toe

I83.008 Varicose veins of unspecified lower extremity with ulcer other part of lower leg `HCC` `ESR` `COM` `A`

I83.009 Varicose veins of unspecified lower extremity with ulcer of unspecified site `HCC` `ESR` `COM` `A`

√6ᵗʰ **I83.01** Varicose veins of right lower extremity with ulcer

I83.011 Varicose veins of right lower extremity with ulcer of thigh `HCC` `ESR` `COM` `A`

I83.012 Varicose veins of right lower extremity with ulcer of calf `HCC` `ESR` `COM` `A`

I83.013 Varicose veins of right lower extremity with ulcer of ankle `HCC` `ESR` `COM` `A`

I83.014 Varicose veins of right lower extremity with ulcer of heel and midfoot `HCC` `ESR` `COM` `A`
Varicose veins of right lower extremity with ulcer of plantar surface of midfoot

I83.015 Varicose veins of right lower extremity with ulcer other part of foot `HCC` `ESR` `COM` `A`
Varicose veins of right lower extremity with ulcer of toe

I83.018 Varicose veins of right lower extremity with ulcer other part of lower leg `HCC` `ESR` `COM` `A`

I83.019 Varicose veins of right lower extremity with ulcer of unspecified site `HCC` `ESR` `COM` `A`

√6ᵗʰ **I83.02** Varicose veins of left lower extremity with ulcer

I83.021 Varicose veins of left lower extremity with ulcer of thigh `HCC` `ESR` `COM` `A`

I83.022 Varicose veins of left lower extremity with ulcer of calf `HCC` `ESR` `COM` `A`

I83.023 Varicose veins of left lower extremity with ulcer of ankle `HCC` `ESR` `COM` `A`

I83.024 Varicose veins of left lower extremity with ulcer of heel and midfoot `HCC` `ESR` `COM` `A`
Varicose veins of left lower extremity with ulcer of plantar surface of midfoot

I83.025 Varicose veins of left lower extremity with ulcer other part of foot `HCC` `ESR` `COM` `A`
Varicose veins of left lower extremity with ulcer of toe

I83.028 Varicose veins of left lower extremity with ulcer other part of lower leg `HCC` `ESR` `COM` `A`

I83.029 Varicose veins of left lower extremity with ulcer of unspecified site `HCC` `ESR` `COM` `A`

√5ᵗʰ **I83.1** Varicose veins of lower extremities with inflammation

I83.10 Varicose veins of unspecified lower extremity with inflammation `A`

I83.11 Varicose veins of right lower extremity with inflammation `A`

I83.12 Varicose veins of left lower extremity with inflammation `A`

`HCC` CMS-HCC   `Rx` Rx HCC   `ESR` ESRD HCC   `COM` Commercial HCC   `N` Newborn: 0   `P` Pediatric: 0-17   `M` Maternity: 9-64   `A` Adult: 15-124

700
ICD-10-CM 2023

✓5ᵗʰ **I83.2 Varicose veins of lower extremities with both** ulcer and inflammation
    Use additional code to identify severity of ulcer (L97.-)

✓6ᵗʰ **I83.20 Varicose veins of** unspecified **lower extremity with both ulcer and inflammation**

    I83.201 Varicose veins of unspecified lower extremity with both ulcer of thigh **and inflammation** `HCC` `ESR` `COM` `A`

    I83.202 Varicose veins of unspecified lower extremity with both ulcer of calf **and inflammation** `HCC` `ESR` `COM` `A`

    I83.203 Varicose veins of unspecified lower extremity with both ulcer of ankle **and inflammation** `HCC` `ESR` `COM` `A`

    I83.204 Varicose veins of unspecified lower extremity with both ulcer of heel and midfoot **and inflammation** `HCC` `ESR` `COM` `A`
        Varicose veins of unspecified lower extremity with both ulcer of plantar surface of midfoot and inflammation

    I83.205 Varicose veins of unspecified lower extremity with both ulcer of other part of foot and inflammation `HCC` `ESR` `COM` `A`
        Varicose veins of unspecified lower extremity with both ulcer of toe and inflammation

    I83.208 Varicose veins of unspecified lower extremity with both ulcer of other part of lower extremity and inflammation `HCC` `ESR` `COM` `A`

    I83.209 Varicose veins of unspecified lower extremity with both ulcer of unspecified site and inflammation `HCC` `ESR` `COM` `A`

✓6ᵗʰ **I83.21 Varicose veins of** right **lower extremity with both ulcer and inflammation**

    I83.211 Varicose veins of right lower extremity with both ulcer of thigh **and inflammation** `HCC` `ESR` `COM` `A`

    I83.212 Varicose veins of right lower extremity with both ulcer of calf **and inflammation** `HCC` `ESR` `COM` `A`

    I83.213 Varicose veins of right lower extremity with both ulcer of ankle **and inflammation** `HCC` `ESR` `COM` `A`

    I83.214 Varicose veins of right lower extremity with both ulcer of heel and midfoot **and inflammation** `HCC` `ESR` `COM` `A`
        Varicose veins of right lower extremity with both ulcer of plantar surface of midfoot and inflammation

    I83.215 Varicose veins of right lower extremity with both ulcer other part of foot and inflammation `HCC` `ESR` `COM` `A`
        Varicose veins of right lower extremity with both ulcer of toe and inflammation

    I83.218 Varicose veins of right lower extremity with both ulcer of other part of lower extremity and inflammation `HCC` `ESR` `COM` `A`

    I83.219 Varicose veins of right lower extremity with both ulcer of unspecified site and inflammation `HCC` `ESR` `COM` `A`

✓6ᵗʰ **I83.22 Varicose veins of** left **lower extremity with both ulcer and inflammation**

    I83.221 Varicose veins of left lower extremity with both ulcer of thigh **and inflammation** `HCC` `ESR` `COM` `A`

    I83.222 Varicose veins of left lower extremity with both ulcer of calf **and inflammation** `HCC` `ESR` `COM` `A`

    I83.223 Varicose veins of left lower extremity with both ulcer of ankle **and inflammation** `HCC` `ESR` `COM` `A`

    I83.224 Varicose veins of left lower extremity with both ulcer of heel and midfoot **and inflammation** `HCC` `ESR` `COM` `A`
        Varicose veins of left lower extremity with both ulcer of plantar surface of midfoot and inflammation

    I83.225 Varicose veins of left lower extremity with both ulcer other part of foot and inflammation `HCC` `ESR` `COM` `A`
        Varicose veins of left lower extremity with both ulcer of toe and inflammation

    I83.228 Varicose veins of left lower extremity with both ulcer of other part of lower extremity and inflammation `HCC` `ESR` `COM` `A`

    I83.229 Varicose veins of left lower extremity with both ulcer of unspecified site and inflammation `HCC` `ESR` `COM` `A`

✓5ᵗʰ **I83.8 Varicose veins of lower extremities with other complications**

✓6ᵗʰ **I83.81 Varicose veins of lower extremities with** pain

    I83.811 Varicose veins of right **lower extremity with pain** `A`

    I83.812 Varicose veins of left **lower extremity with pain** `A`

    I83.813 Varicose veins of bilateral **lower extremities with pain** `A`

    I83.819 Varicose veins of unspecified lower extremity with pain `A`

✓6ᵗʰ **I83.89 Varicose veins of lower extremities with other complications**
    Varicose veins of lower extremities with edema
    Varicose veins of lower extremities with swelling

    I83.891 Varicose veins of right **lower extremity with other complications** `A`

    I83.892 Varicose veins of left **lower extremity with other complications** `A`

    I83.893 Varicose veins of bilateral **lower extremities with other complications** `A`

    I83.899 Varicose veins of unspecified lower extremity with other complications `A`

✓5ᵗʰ **I83.9 Asymptomatic varicose veins of lower extremities**
    Phlebectasia of lower extremities
    Varicose veins of lower extremities
    Varix of lower extremities

    I83.90 Asymptomatic varicose veins of unspecified lower extremity `A`
        Varicose veins NOS

    I83.91 Asymptomatic varicose veins of right **lower extremity** `A`

    I83.92 Asymptomatic varicose veins of left **lower extremity** `A`

    I83.93 Asymptomatic varicose veins of bilateral **lower extremities** `A`

✓4ᵗʰ **I85 Esophageal varices**
    Use additional code to identify:
    alcohol abuse and dependence (F10.-)

✓5ᵗʰ **I85.0 Esophageal varices**
    Idiopathic esophageal varices
    Primary esophageal varices

    I85.00 Esophageal varices without **bleeding** `HCC` `ESR` `COM`
        Esophageal varices NOS

    I85.01 Esophageal varices with bleeding `HCC` `ESR` `COM`

✓5ᵗʰ **I85.1 Secondary esophageal varices**
    Esophageal varices secondary to alcoholic liver disease
    Esophageal varices secondary to cirrhosis of liver
    Esophageal varices secondary to schistosomiasis
    Esophageal varices secondary to toxic liver disease
    Code first underlying disease

    I85.10 Secondary esophageal varices without **bleeding** `HCC` `ESR` `COM`

    I85.11 Secondary esophageal varices with **bleeding** `HCC` `ESR` `COM`

✓4ᵗʰ **I86 Varicose veins of other sites**
    EXCLUDES 1   varicose veins of unspecified site (I83.9-)
    EXCLUDES 2   retinal varices (H35.0-)

    I86.0 Sublingual varices
        DEF: Distended, tortuous veins beneath the tongue.

    I86.1 Scrotal varices ♂
        Varicocele

    I86.2 Pelvic varices

Chapter 9. Diseases of the Circulatory System *(side tab)*

I86.3 Vulval varices ♀
　EXCLUDES 1　vulval varices complicating childbirth and the puerperium (O87.8)
　　vulval varices complicating pregnancy (O22.1-)

I86.4 Gastric varices

I86.8 Varicose veins of other specified sites ▲
　Varicose ulcer of nasal septum

I87 Other disorders of veins

I87.0 Postthrombotic syndrome
　Chronic venous hypertension due to deep vein thrombosis
　Postphlebitic syndrome
　EXCLUDES 1　chronic venous hypertension without deep vein thrombosis (I87.3-)

　I87.00 Postthrombotic syndrome without complications
　　Asymptomatic postthrombotic syndrome
　　I87.001 Postthrombotic syndrome without complications of right lower extremity
　　I87.002 Postthrombotic syndrome without complications of left lower extremity
　　I87.003 Postthrombotic syndrome without complications of bilateral lower extremity
　　I87.009 Postthrombotic syndrome without complications of unspecified extremity
　　　Postthrombotic syndrome NOS

　I87.01 Postthrombotic syndrome with ulcer
　　Use additional code to specify site and severity of ulcer (L97.-)
　　I87.011 Postthrombotic syndrome with ulcer of right lower extremity HCC ESR COM
　　I87.012 Postthrombotic syndrome with ulcer of left lower extremity HCC ESR COM
　　I87.013 Postthrombotic syndrome with ulcer of bilateral lower extremity HCC ESR COM
　　I87.019 Postthrombotic syndrome with ulcer of unspecified lower extremity HCC ESR COM

　I87.02 Postthrombotic syndrome with inflammation
　　I87.021 Postthrombotic syndrome with inflammation of right lower extremity
　　I87.022 Postthrombotic syndrome with inflammation of left lower extremity
　　I87.023 Postthrombotic syndrome with inflammation of bilateral lower extremity
　　I87.029 Postthrombotic syndrome with inflammation of unspecified lower extremity

　I87.03 Postthrombotic syndrome with ulcer and inflammation
　　Use additional code to specify site and severity of ulcer (L97.-)
　　I87.031 Postthrombotic syndrome with ulcer and inflammation of right lower extremity HCC ESR COM
　　I87.032 Postthrombotic syndrome with ulcer and inflammation of left lower extremity HCC ESR COM
　　I87.033 Postthrombotic syndrome with ulcer and inflammation of bilateral lower extremity HCC ESR COM
　　I87.039 Postthrombotic syndrome with ulcer and inflammation of unspecified lower extremity HCC ESR COM

　I87.09 Postthrombotic syndrome with other complications
　　I87.091 Postthrombotic syndrome with other complications of right lower extremity
　　I87.092 Postthrombotic syndrome with other complications of left lower extremity
　　I87.093 Postthrombotic syndrome with other complications of bilateral lower extremity
　　I87.099 Postthrombotic syndrome with other complications of unspecified lower extremity

I87.1 Compression of vein
　Stricture of vein
　Vena cava syndrome (inferior) (superior)
　EXCLUDES 2　compression of pulmonary vein (I28.8)

I87.2 Venous insufficiency (chronic) (peripheral)
　Stasis dermatitis
　EXCLUDES 1　stasis dermatitis with varicose veins of lower extremities (I83.1-, I83.2-)
　DEF: Insufficient drainage of venous blood in any part of the body that results in edema or dermatosis.

I87.3 Chronic venous hypertension (idiopathic)
　Stasis edema
　EXCLUDES 1　chronic venous hypertension due to deep vein thrombosis (I87.0-)
　　varicose veins of lower extremities (I83.-)

　I87.30 Chronic venous hypertension (idiopathic) without complications
　　Asymptomatic chronic venous hypertension (idiopathic)
　　I87.301 Chronic venous hypertension (idiopathic) without complications of right lower extremity
　　I87.302 Chronic venous hypertension (idiopathic) without complications of left lower extremity
　　I87.303 Chronic venous hypertension (idiopathic) without complications of bilateral lower extremity
　　I87.309 Chronic venous hypertension (idiopathic) without complications of unspecified lower extremity
　　　Chronic venous hypertension NOS

　I87.31 Chronic venous hypertension (idiopathic) with ulcer
　　Use additional code to specify site and severity of ulcer (L97.-)
　　I87.311 Chronic venous hypertension (idiopathic) with ulcer of right lower extremity HCC ESR COM
　　I87.312 Chronic venous hypertension (idiopathic) with ulcer of left lower extremity HCC ESR COM
　　I87.313 Chronic venous hypertension (idiopathic) with ulcer of bilateral lower extremity HCC ESR COM
　　I87.319 Chronic venous hypertension (idiopathic) with ulcer of unspecified lower extremity HCC ESR COM

　I87.32 Chronic venous hypertension (idiopathic) with inflammation
　　I87.321 Chronic venous hypertension (idiopathic) with inflammation of right lower extremity
　　I87.322 Chronic venous hypertension (idiopathic) with inflammation of left lower extremity
　　I87.323 Chronic venous hypertension (idiopathic) with inflammation of bilateral lower extremity
　　I87.329 Chronic venous hypertension (idiopathic) with inflammation of unspecified lower extremity

　I87.33 Chronic venous hypertension (idiopathic) with ulcer and inflammation
　　Use additional code to specify site and severity of ulcer (L97.-)
　　I87.331 Chronic venous hypertension (idiopathic) with ulcer and inflammation of right lower extremity HCC ESR COM
　　I87.332 Chronic venous hypertension (idiopathic) with ulcer and inflammation of left lower extremity HCC ESR COM
　　I87.333 Chronic venous hypertension (idiopathic) with ulcer and inflammation of bilateral lower extremity HCC ESR COM
　　I87.339 Chronic venous hypertension (idiopathic) with ulcer and inflammation of unspecified lower extremity HCC ESR COM

　I87.39 Chronic venous hypertension (idiopathic) with other complications
　　I87.391 Chronic venous hypertension (idiopathic) with other complications of right lower extremity
　　I87.392 Chronic venous hypertension (idiopathic) with other complications of left lower extremity

I87.393 Chronic venous hypertension (idiopathic) with other complications of bilateral lower extremity

I87.399 Chronic venous hypertension (idiopathic) with other complications of unspecified lower extremity

I87.8 Other specified disorders of veins
Phlebosclerosis
Venofibrosis

I87.9 Disorder of vein, unspecified

✔4ᵗʰ **I88** Nonspecific lymphadenitis
EXCLUDES 1   *acute lymphadenitis, except mesenteric (L04.-)*
enlarged lymph nodes NOS (R59.-)
human immunodeficiency virus [HIV] disease resulting in generalized lymphadenopathy (B20)

I88.0 Nonspecific mesenteric lymphadenitis
Mesenteric lymphadenitis (acute)(chronic)

I88.1 Chronic lymphadenitis, except mesenteric
Adenitis
Lymphadenitis

I88.8 Other nonspecific lymphadenitis

I88.9 Nonspecific lymphadenitis, unspecified
Lymphadenitis NOS

✔4ᵗʰ **I89** Other noninfective disorders of lymphatic vessels and lymph nodes
EXCLUDES 1   *chylocele, tunica vaginalis (nonfilarial) NOS (N50.89)*
enlarged lymph nodes NOS (R59.-)
filarial chylocele (B74.-)
hereditary lymphedema (Q82.0)

I89.0 Lymphedema, not elsewhere classified
Elephantiasis (nonfilarial) NOS
Lymphangiectasis
Obliteration, lymphatic vessel
Praecox lymphedema
Secondary lymphedema
EXCLUDES 1   *postmastectomy lymphedema (I97.2)*

I89.1 Lymphangitis
Chronic lymphangitis
Lymphangitis NOS
Subacute lymphangitis
EXCLUDES 1   *acute lymphangitis (L03.-)*

I89.8 Other specified noninfective disorders of lymphatic vessels and lymph nodes
Chylocele (nonfilarial)
Chylous ascites
Chylous cyst
Lipomelanotic reticulosis
Lymph node or vessel fistula
Lymph node or vessel infarction
Lymph node or vessel rupture

I89.9 Noninfective disorder of lymphatic vessels and lymph nodes, unspecified
Disease of lymphatic vessels NOS

Other and unspecified disorders of the circulatory system (I95-I99)

✔4ᵗʰ **I95** Hypotension
EXCLUDES 1   *cardiovascular collapse (R57.9) (~R57.9)*
maternal hypotension syndrome (O26.5-)
nonspecific low blood pressure reading NOS (R03.1)

I95.0 Idiopathic hypotension

I95.1 Orthostatic hypotension
Hypotension, postural
EXCLUDES 1   *neurogenic orthostatic hypotension [Shy-Drager] (G90.3)*
orthostatic hypotension due to drugs (I95.2)

I95.2 Hypotension due to drugs
Orthostatic hypotension due to drugs
Use additional code for adverse effect, if applicable, to identify drug (T36-T50 with fifth or sixth character 5)

I95.3 Hypotension of hemodialysis
Intra-dialytic hypotension

✔5ᵗʰ **I95.8** Other hypotension

I95.81 Postprocedural hypotension

I95.89 Other hypotension
Chronic hypotension

I95.9 Hypotension, unspecified

I96 Gangrene, not elsewhere classified   HCC ESR COM
Gangrenous cellulitis
EXCLUDES 1   *gangrene in atherosclerosis of native arteries of the extremities (I70.26)*
gangrene in hernia (K40.1, K40.4, K41.1, K41.4, K42.1, K43.1-, K44.1, K45.1, K46.1)
gangrene in other peripheral vascular diseases (I73.-)
gangrene of certain specified sites - see Alphabetical Index
gas gangrene (A48.0)
pyoderma gangrenosum (L88)
EXCLUDES 2   *gangrene in diabetes mellitus (E08-E13 with .52)*
AHA: 2018,4Q,87; 2018,3Q,3; 2017,3Q,6; 2013,2Q,34

✔4ᵗʰ **I97** Intraoperative and postprocedural complications and disorders of circulatory system, not elsewhere classified
EXCLUDES 2   *postprocedural shock (T81.1-)*
AHA: 2021,1Q,13; 2019,2Q,21

I97.0 Postcardiotomy syndrome

✔5ᵗʰ **I97.1** Other postprocedural cardiac functional disturbances
EXCLUDES 2   *acute pulmonary insufficiency following thoracic surgery (J95.1)*
intraoperative cardiac functional disturbances (I97.7-)

✔6ᵗʰ **I97.11** Postprocedural cardiac insufficiency

I97.110 Postprocedural cardiac insufficiency following cardiac surgery

I97.111 Postprocedural cardiac insufficiency following other surgery

✔6ᵗʰ **I97.12** Postprocedural cardiac arrest

I97.120 Postprocedural cardiac arrest following cardiac surgery

I97.121 Postprocedural cardiac arrest following other surgery

✔6ᵗʰ **I97.13** Postprocedural heart failure
Use additional code to identify the heart failure (I50.-)

I97.130 Postprocedural heart failure following cardiac surgery

I97.131 Postprocedural heart failure following other surgery

✔6ᵗʰ **I97.19** Other postprocedural cardiac functional disturbances
Use additional code, if applicable, to further specify disorder

I97.190 Other postprocedural cardiac functional disturbances following cardiac surgery
Use additional code, if applicable, for type 4 or type 5 myocardial infarction, to further specify disorder
AHA: 2019,2Q,33

I97.191 Other postprocedural cardiac functional disturbances following other surgery

I97.2 Postmastectomy lymphedema syndrome   A
Elephantiasis due to mastectomy
Obliteration of lymphatic vessels

I97.3 Postprocedural hypertension

✔5ᵗʰ **I97.4** Intraoperative hemorrhage and hematoma of a circulatory system organ or structure complicating a procedure
EXCLUDES 1   *intraoperative hemorrhage and hematoma of a circulatory system organ or structure due to accidental puncture and laceration during a procedure (I97.5-)*
EXCLUDES 2   *intraoperative cerebrovascular hemorrhage complicating a procedure (G97.3-)*

✔6ᵗʰ **I97.41** Intraoperative hemorrhage and hematoma of a circulatory system organ or structure complicating a circulatory system procedure

I97.410 Intraoperative hemorrhage and hematoma of a circulatory system organ or structure complicating a cardiac catheterization

I97.411 Intraoperative hemorrhage and hematoma of a circulatory system organ or structure complicating a cardiac bypass

Chapter 9. Diseases of the Circulatory System

I97.418   **Intraoperative hemorrhage and hematoma of a circulatory system organ or structure complicating** other **circulatory system procedure**

I97.42   **Intraoperative hemorrhage and hematoma of a circulatory system organ or structure complicating** other **procedure**
AHA: 2020,1Q,19

✓5th I97.5   Accidental puncture and laceration **of a circulatory system organ or structure during a procedure**
EXCLUDES 2   *accidental puncture and laceration of brain during a procedure (G97.4-)*

I97.51   **Accidental puncture and laceration of a circulatory system organ or structure during a** circulatory system procedure
AHA: 2019,2Q,24

I97.52   **Accidental puncture and laceration of a circulatory system organ or structure during** other procedure

✓5th I97.6   Postprocedural hemorrhage, hematoma and seroma **of a circulatory system organ or structure following a procedure**
EXCLUDES 2   *postprocedural cerebrovascular hemorrhage complicating a procedure (G97.5-)*
AHA: 2016,4Q,9-10

✓6th I97.61   Postprocedural hemorrhage **of a circulatory system organ or structure following a** circulatory system procedure

I97.610   **Postprocedural hemorrhage of a circulatory system organ or structure following a** cardiac catheterization

I97.611   **Postprocedural hemorrhage of a circulatory system organ or structure following** cardiac bypass

I97.618   **Postprocedural hemorrhage of a circulatory system organ or structure following** other circulatory system procedure

✓6th I97.62   Postprocedural hemorrhage, hematoma and seroma **of a circulatory system organ or structure following** other procedure

I97.620   **Postprocedural** hemorrhage **of a circulatory system organ or structure following other procedure**

I97.621   **Postprocedural** hematoma **of a circulatory system organ or structure following other procedure**

I97.622   **Postprocedural** seroma **of a circulatory system organ or structure following other procedure**

✓6th I97.63   Postprocedural hematoma **of a circulatory system organ or structure following a** circulatory system procedure

I97.630   **Postprocedural hematoma of a circulatory system organ or structure following a** cardiac catheterization

I97.631   **Postprocedural hematoma of a circulatory system organ or structure following** cardiac bypass

I97.638   **Postprocedural hematoma of a circulatory system organ or structure following** other circulatory system procedure

✓6th I97.64   Postprocedural seroma **of a circulatory system organ or structure following a circulatory system procedure**

I97.640   **Postprocedural seroma of a circulatory system organ or structure following a** cardiac catheterization

I97.641   **Postprocedural seroma of a circulatory system organ or structure following** cardiac bypass

I97.648   **Postprocedural seroma of a circulatory system organ or structure following other circulatory system procedure**

✓5th I97.7   Intraoperative cardiac functional disturbances
EXCLUDES 2   *acute pulmonary insufficiency following thoracic surgery (J95.1)*
postprocedural cardiac functional disturbances (I97.1-)

✓6th I97.71   Intraoperative cardiac arrest

I97.710   **Intraoperative cardiac arrest during** cardiac surgery

I97.711   **Intraoperative cardiac arrest during** other surgery

✓6th I97.79   **Other intraoperative cardiac functional disturbances**
Use additional code, if applicable, to further specify disorder

I97.790   **Other intraoperative cardiac functional disturbances during** cardiac surgery

I97.791   **Other intraoperative cardiac functional disturbances during** other surgery

✓5th I97.8   Other intraoperative and postprocedural complications and disorders of the circulatory system, not elsewhere classified
Use additional code, if applicable, to further specify disorder

✓6th I97.81   Intraoperative cerebrovascular infarction

I97.810   **Intraoperative cerebrovascular infarction during** cardiac surgery   HCC ESR

I97.811   **Intraoperative cerebrovascular infarction during** other surgery   HCC ESR

✓6th I97.82   Postprocedural cerebrovascular infarction

I97.820   **Postprocedural cerebrovascular infarction following** cardiac surgery   HCC ESR

I97.821   **Postprocedural cerebrovascular infarction following** other surgery   HCC ESR

I97.88   **Other intraoperative complications of the circulatory system, not elsewhere classified**

I97.89   **Other postprocedural complications and disorders of the circulatory system, not elsewhere classified**
AHA: 2021,3Q,33; 2020,3Q,3-8; 2019,2Q,33

✓4th I99   Other and unspecified disorders of circulatory system

I99.8   **Other disorder of circulatory system**
AHA: 2020,4Q,98

I99.9   **Unspecified disorder of circulatory system**

Chapter 10. Diseases of the Respiratory System (J00–J99)

Chapter-specific Guidelines with Coding Examples

The chapter-specific guidelines from the ICD-10-CM Official Guidelines for Coding and Reporting have been provided below. Along with these guidelines are coding examples, contained in the shaded boxes, that have been developed to help illustrate the coding and/or sequencing guidance found in these guidelines.

a. Chronic obstructive pulmonary disease [COPD] and asthma

1) Acute exacerbation of chronic obstructive bronchitis and asthma

The codes in categories J44 and J45 distinguish between uncomplicated cases and those in acute exacerbation. An acute exacerbation is a worsening or a decompensation of a chronic condition. An acute exacerbation is not equivalent to an infection superimposed on a chronic condition, though an exacerbation may be triggered by an infection.

Acute streptococcal bronchitis with acute exacerbation of COPD

J20.2   **Acute bronchitis due to streptococcus**

J44.0   **Chronic obstructive pulmonary disease with (acute) lower respiratory infection**

J44.1   **Chronic obstructive pulmonary disease with (acute) exacerbation**

Explanation: ICD-10-CM uses combination codes to create organism-specific classifications for acute bronchitis. Category J44 codes include combination codes with severity components, which differentiate between COPD with acute lower respiratory infection (acute bronchitis), COPD with acute exacerbation, and COPD without mention of a complication (unspecified).

An acute exacerbation is a worsening or a decompensation of a chronic condition. An acute exacerbation is not equivalent to an infection superimposed on a chronic condition, though an exacerbation may be triggered by an infection, as in this example.

Exacerbation of moderate persistent asthma with status asthmaticus

J45.42   **Moderate persistent asthma with status asthmaticus**

Explanation: Category J45 Asthma includes severity-specific subcategories and fifth-character codes to distinguish between uncomplicated cases, those in acute exacerbation, and those with status asthmaticus.

---

b. Acute respiratory failure

1) Acute respiratory failure as principal diagnosis

A code from subcategory J96.0, Acute respiratory failure, or subcategory J96.2, Acute and chronic respiratory failure, may be assigned as a principal diagnosis when it is the condition established after study to be chiefly responsible for occasioning the admission to the hospital, and the selection is supported by the Alphabetic Index and Tabular List. However, chapter-specific coding guidelines (such as obstetrics, poisoning, HIV, newborn) that provide sequencing direction take precedence.

Acute hypoxic respiratory failure due to exacerbation of chronic obstructive bronchitis

J96.01   **Acute respiratory failure with hypoxia**

J44.1   **Chronic obstructive pulmonary disease with (acute) exacerbation**

Explanation: Category J96 classifies respiratory failure with combination codes that designate the severity and the presence of hypoxia and hypercapnia. Code J96.01 is sequenced as the first-listed diagnosis, as the reason for the encounter. Respiratory failure may be assigned as a principal diagnosis when it is the condition established after study to be chiefly responsible for occasioning the encounter and the selection is supported by the Alphabetic Index and Tabular List.

---

2) Acute respiratory failure as secondary diagnosis

Respiratory failure may be listed as a secondary diagnosis if it occurs after admission, or if it is present on admission, but does not meet the definition of principal diagnosis.

Acute respiratory failure due to accidental oxycodone overdose

T40.2X1A   **Poisoning by other opioids, accidental (unintentional), initial encounter**

J96.00   **Acute respiratory failure, unspecified whether with hypoxia or hypercapnia**

Explanation: Respiratory failure may be assigned as a principal diagnosis when it is the condition established after study to be chiefly responsible for occasioning the encounter, and the selection is supported by the Alphabetic Index and Tabular List. However, chapter-specific coding guidelines, such as poisoning, that provide sequencing direction take precedence. When coding a poisoning or reaction to the improper use of a medication (e.g., overdose, wrong substance given or taken in error, wrong route of administration), first assign the appropriate code from categories T36–T50. Use additional code(s) for all manifestations of the poisoning. In this instance, the respiratory failure is a manifestation of the poisoning and is sequenced as a secondary diagnosis.

---

3) Sequencing of acute respiratory failure and another acute condition

When a patient is admitted with respiratory failure and another acute condition, (e.g., myocardial infarction, cerebrovascular accident, aspiration pneumonia), the principal diagnosis will not be the same in every situation. This applies whether the other acute condition is a respiratory or nonrespiratory condition. Selection of the principal diagnosis will be dependent on the circumstances of admission. If both the respiratory failure and the other acute condition are equally responsible for occasioning the admission to the hospital, and there are no chapter-specific sequencing rules, the guideline regarding two or more diagnoses that equally meet the definition for principal diagnosis (*Section II, C.*) may be applied in these situations.

If the documentation is not clear as to whether acute respiratory failure and another condition are equally responsible for occasioning the admission, query the provider for clarification.

Patient presents with acute pneumococcal pneumonia and acute respiratory failure

J96.00   **Acute respiratory failure, unspecified whether with hypoxia or hypercapnia**

J13   **Pneumonia due to Streptococcus pneumoniae**

Explanation: When a patient is seen for respiratory failure and another acute condition, such as a bacterial pneumonia, the principal or first-listed diagnosis is not the same in every situation. This applies whether the other acute condition is a respiratory or nonrespiratory condition. The principal diagnosis depends on the problem chiefly responsible for the encounter.

---

c. Influenza due to certain identified influenza viruses

Code only confirmed cases of influenza due to certain identified influenza viruses (category J09), and due to other identified influenza virus (category J10). This is an exception to the hospital inpatient guideline Section II, H. (Uncertain Diagnosis).

In this context, "confirmation" does not require documentation of positive laboratory testing specific for avian or other novel influenza A or other identified influenza virus. However, coding should be based on the provider's diagnostic statement that the patient has avian influenza, or other novel influenza A, for category J09, or has another particular identified strain of influenza, such as H1N1 or H3N2, but not identified as novel or variant, for category J10.

If the provider records "suspected" or "possible" or "probable" avian influenza, or novel influenza, or other identified influenza, then the appropriate influenza code from category J11, Influenza due to unidentified influenza virus, should be assigned. A code from category J09, Influenza due to certain identified influenza viruses, should not be assigned nor should a code from category J10, Influenza due to other identified influenza virus.

Influenza due to avian influenza virus with pneumonia

J09.X1 Influenza due to identified novel influenza A virus with pneumonia

Explanation: Codes in category J09 Influenza due to certain identified influenza viruses should be assigned only for confirmed cases. "Confirmation" does not require positive laboratory testing of a specific influenza virus but does need to be based on the provider's diagnostic statement, which should not include terms such as "possible," "probable," or "suspected."

d. Ventilator associated pneumonia

1) Documentation of ventilator associated pneumonia

As with all procedural or postprocedural complications, code assignment is based on the provider's documentation of the relationship between the condition and the procedure.

Code J95.851, Ventilator associated pneumonia, should be assigned only when the provider has documented ventilator associated pneumonia (VAP). An additional code to identify the organism (e.g., Pseudomonas aeruginosa, code B96.5) should also be assigned. Do not assign an additional code from categories J12-J18 to identify the type of pneumonia.

Code J95.851 should not be assigned for cases where the patient has pneumonia and is on a mechanical ventilator and the provider has not specifically stated that the pneumonia is ventilator-associated pneumonia. If the documentation is unclear as to whether the patient has a pneumonia that is a complication attributable to the mechanical ventilator, query the provider.

2) Ventilator associated pneumonia develops after admission

A patient may be admitted with one type of pneumonia (e.g., code J13, Pneumonia due to Streptococcus pneumonia) and subsequently develop VAP. In this instance, the principal diagnosis would be the appropriate code from categories J12-J18 for the pneumonia diagnosed at the time of admission. Code J95.851, Ventilator associated pneumonia, would be assigned as an additional diagnosis when the provider has also documented the presence of ventilator associated pneumonia.

e. Vaping-related disorders

For patients presenting with condition(s) related to vaping, assign code U07.0, Vaping-related disorder, as the principal diagnosis. For lung injury due to vaping, assign only code U07.0. Assign additional codes for other manifestations, such as acute respiratory failure (subcategory J96.0-) or pneumonitis (code J68.0).

Associated respiratory signs and symptoms due to vaping, such as cough, shortness of breath, etc., are not coded separately, when a definitive diagnosis has been established. However, it would be appropriate to code separately any gastrointestinal symptoms, such as diarrhea and abdominal pain.

See Section I.C.1.g.1.c.i. for Pneumonia confirmed as due to COVID-19

Chapter 10. Diseases of the Respiratory System
(J00–J99)

NOTE When a respiratory condition is described as occurring in more than one site and is not specifically indexed, it should be classified to the lower anatomic site (e.g., tracheobronchitis to bronchitis in J40).

Use additional code, where applicable, to identify:
- exposure to environmental tobacco smoke (Z77.22)
- exposure to tobacco smoke in the perinatal period (P96.81)
- history of tobacco dependence (Z87.891)
- occupational exposure to environmental tobacco smoke (Z57.31)
- tobacco dependence (F17.-)
- tobacco use (Z72.0)

EXCLUDES 2
- certain conditions originating in the perinatal period (P04-P96)
- certain infectious and parasitic diseases (A00-B99)
- complications of pregnancy, childbirth and the puerperium (O00-O9A)
- congenital malformations, deformations and chromosomal abnormalities (Q00-Q99)
- endocrine, nutritional and metabolic diseases (E00-E88)
- injury, poisoning and certain other consequences of external causes (S00-T88)
- neoplasms (C00-D49)
- smoke inhalation (T59.81-)
- symptoms, signs and abnormal clinical and laboratory findings, not elsewhere classified (R00-R94)

This chapter contains the following blocks:
- J00-J06 Acute upper respiratory infections
- J09-J18 Influenza and pneumonia
- J20-J22 Other acute lower respiratory infections
- J30-J39 Other diseases of upper respiratory tract
- J40-J47 Chronic lower respiratory diseases
- J60-J70 Lung diseases due to external agents
- J80-J84 Other respiratory diseases principally affecting the interstitium
- J85-J86 Suppurative and necrotic conditions of the lower respiratory tract
- J90-J94 Other diseases of the pleura
- J95 Intraoperative and postprocedural complications and disorders of respiratory system, not elsewhere classified
- J96-J99 Other diseases of the respiratory system

Acute upper respiratory infections (J00-J06)

EXCLUDES 1 chronic obstructive pulmonary disease with acute lower respiratory infection (J44.0)

J00 Acute nasopharyngitis [common cold]
Acute rhinitis
Coryza (acute)
Infective nasopharyngitis NOS
Infective rhinitis
Nasal catarrh, acute
Nasopharyngitis NOS
EXCLUDES 1 acute pharyngitis (J02.-)
acute sore throat NOS (J02.9)
influenza virus with other respiratory manifestations (J09.X2, J10.1, J11.1)
pharyngitis NOS (J02.9)
rhinitis NOS (J31.0)
sore throat NOS (J02.9)
EXCLUDES 2 allergic rhinitis (J30.1-J30.9)
chronic pharyngitis (J31.2)
chronic rhinitis (J31.0)
chronic sore throat (J31.2)
nasopharyngitis, chronic (J31.1)
vasomotor rhinitis (J30.0)

✓4ᵗʰ J01 Acute sinusitis
INCLUDES acute abscess of sinus
acute empyema of sinus
acute infection of sinus
acute inflammation of sinus
acute suppuration of sinus
Use additional code (B95-B97) to identify infectious agent
EXCLUDES 1 sinusitis NOS (J32.9)
EXCLUDES 2 chronic sinusitis (J32.0-J32.8)

✓5ᵗʰ J01.0 Acute maxillary sinusitis
Acute antritis
  J01.00 Acute maxillary sinusitis, unspecified
  J01.01 Acute recurrent maxillary sinusitis
✓5ᵗʰ J01.1 Acute frontal sinusitis
  J01.10 Acute frontal sinusitis, unspecified
  J01.11 Acute recurrent frontal sinusitis

✓5ᵗʰ J01.2 Acute ethmoidal sinusitis
  J01.20 Acute ethmoidal sinusitis, unspecified
  J01.21 Acute recurrent ethmoidal sinusitis
✓5ᵗʰ J01.3 Acute sphenoidal sinusitis
  J01.30 Acute sphenoidal sinusitis, unspecified
  J01.31 Acute recurrent sphenoidal sinusitis
✓5ᵗʰ J01.4 Acute pansinusitis
  J01.40 Acute pansinusitis, unspecified
  J01.41 Acute recurrent pansinusitis
✓5ᵗʰ J01.8 Other acute sinusitis
  J01.80 Other acute sinusitis
Acute sinusitis involving more than one sinus but not pansinusitis
  J01.81 Other acute recurrent sinusitis
Acute recurrent sinusitis involving more than one sinus but not pansinusitis
✓5ᵗʰ J01.9 Acute sinusitis, unspecified
  J01.90 Acute sinusitis, unspecified
  J01.91 Acute recurrent sinusitis, unspecified

✓4ᵗʰ J02 Acute pharyngitis
INCLUDES acute sore throat
EXCLUDES 1 acute laryngopharyngitis (J06.0)
peritonsillar abscess (J36)
pharyngeal abscess (J39.1)
retropharyngeal abscess (J39.0)
EXCLUDES 2 chronic pharyngitis (J31.2)

J02.0 Streptococcal pharyngitis
Septic pharyngitis
Streptococcal sore throat
EXCLUDES 2 scarlet fever (A38.-)
J02.8 Acute pharyngitis due to other specified organisms
Use additional code (B95-B97) to identify infectious agent
EXCLUDES 1 acute pharyngitis due to coxsackie virus (B08.5)
acute pharyngitis due to gonococcus (A54.5)
acute pharyngitis due to herpes [simplex] virus (B00.2)
acute pharyngitis due to infectious mononucleosis (B27.-)
enteroviral vesicular pharyngitis (B08.5)
J02.9 Acute pharyngitis, unspecified
Gangrenous pharyngitis (acute)
Infective pharyngitis (acute) NOS
Pharyngitis (acute) NOS
Sore throat (acute) NOS
Suppurative pharyngitis (acute)
Ulcerative pharyngitis (acute)
EXCLUDES 1 influenza virus with other respiratory manifestations (J09.X2, J10.1, J11.1)

✓4ᵗʰ J03 Acute tonsillitis
EXCLUDES 1 acute sore throat (J02.-)
hypertrophy of tonsils (J35.1)
peritonsillar abscess (J36)
sore throat NOS (J02.9)
streptococcal sore throat (J02.0)
EXCLUDES 2 chronic tonsillitis (J35.0)
✓5ᵗʰ J03.0 Streptococcal tonsillitis
  J03.00 Acute streptococcal tonsillitis, unspecified
  J03.01 Acute recurrent streptococcal tonsillitis
✓5ᵗʰ J03.8 Acute tonsillitis due to other specified organisms
Use additional code (B95-B97) to identify infectious agent
EXCLUDES 1 diphtheritic tonsillitis (A36.0)
herpesviral pharyngotonsillitis (B00.2)
streptococcal tonsillitis (J03.0)
tuberculous tonsillitis (A15.8)
Vincent's tonsillitis (A69.1)
  J03.80 Acute tonsillitis due to other specified organisms
  J03.81 Acute recurrent tonsillitis due to other specified organisms

√5ᵗʰ J03.9 Acute tonsillitis, unspecified

Follicular tonsillitis (acute)

Gangrenous tonsillitis (acute)

Infective tonsillitis (acute)

Tonsillitis (acute) NOS

Ulcerative tonsillitis (acute)

> *EXCLUDES 1*   *influenza virus with other respiratory manifestations (J09.X2, J10.1, J11.1)*

J03.90   Acute tonsillitis, unspecified

J03.91   Acute recurrent tonsillitis, unspecified

√4ᵗʰ J04   Acute laryngitis and tracheitis

Code also influenza, if present, such as:

influenza due to identified novel influenza A virus with other respiratory manifestations (J09.X2)

influenza due to other identified influenza virus with other respiratory manifestations (J10.1)

influenza due to unidentified influenza virus with other respiratory manifestations (J11.1)

Use additional code (B95-B97) to identify infectious agent

> *EXCLUDES 1*   *acute obstructive laryngitis [croup] and epiglottitis (J05.-)*
>
> *EXCLUDES 2*   *laryngismus (stridulus) (J38.5)*

J04.0   Acute laryngitis

Edematous laryngitis (acute)

Laryngitis (acute) NOS

Subglottic laryngitis (acute)

Suppurative laryngitis (acute)

Ulcerative laryngitis (acute)

> *EXCLUDES 1*   *acute obstructive laryngitis (J05.0)*
>
> *EXCLUDES 2*   *chronic laryngitis (J37.0)*

√6ᵗʰ J04.1   Acute tracheitis

Acute viral tracheitis

Catarrhal tracheitis (acute)

Tracheitis (acute) NOS

> *EXCLUDES 2*   *chronic tracheitis (J42)*

J04.10   Acute tracheitis without obstruction

J04.11   Acute tracheitis with obstruction

J04.2   Acute laryngotracheitis

Laryngotracheitis NOS

Tracheitis (acute) with laryngitis (acute)

> *EXCLUDES 1*   *acute obstructive laryngotracheitis (J05.0)*
>
> *EXCLUDES 2*   *chronic laryngotracheitis (J37.1)*

√5ᵗʰ J04.3   Supraglottitis, unspecified

J04.30   Supraglottitis, unspecified, without obstruction

J04.31   Supraglottitis, unspecified, with obstruction

√4ᵗʰ J05   Acute obstructive laryngitis [croup] and epiglottitis

Code also, influenza, if present, such as:

influenza due to identified novel influenza A virus with other respiratory manifestations (J09.X2)

influenza due to other identified influenza virus with other respiratory manifestations (J10.1)

influenza due to unidentified influenza virus with other respiratory manifestations (J11.1)

Use additional code (B95-B97) to identify infectious agent

J05.0   Acute obstructive laryngitis [croup]

Obstructive laryngitis (acute) NOS

Obstructive laryngotracheitis NOS

DEF: Acute laryngeal obstruction due to allergies, foreign bodies, or in the majority of cases a viral infection. Symptoms include a harsh, barking cough, hoarseness, and a persistent, high-pitched respiratory sound (stridor).

√6ᵗʰ J05.1   Acute epiglottitis

> *EXCLUDES 2*   *epiglottitis, chronic (J37.0)*

J05.10   Acute epiglottitis without obstruction

Epiglottitis NOS

J05.11   Acute epiglottitis with obstruction

√4ᵗʰ J06   Acute upper respiratory infections of multiple and unspecified sites

> *EXCLUDES 1*   *acute respiratory infection NOS (J22)*
>
> *influenza virus with other respiratory manifestations (J09.X2, J10.1, J11.1)*
>
> *streptococcal pharyngitis (J02.0)*

J06.0   Acute laryngopharyngitis

J06.9   Acute upper respiratory infection, unspecified

Upper respiratory disease, acute

Upper respiratory infection NOS

Use additional code (B95-B97) to identify infectious agent, if known, such as:

respiratory syncytial virus (RSV) (B97.4)

AHA: 2020,1Q,22

Influenza and pneumonia (J09-J18)

> *EXCLUDES 2*   *allergic or eosinophilic pneumonia (J82)*
>
> *aspiration pneumonia NOS (J69.0)*
>
> *meconium pneumonia (P24.01)*
>
> *neonatal aspiration pneumonia (P24.-)*
>
> *pneumonia due to solids and liquids (J69.-)*
>
> *congenital pneumonia (P23.9)*
>
> *lipid pneumonia (J69.1)*
>
> *rheumatic pneumonia (I00)*
>
> *ventilator associated pneumonia (J95.851)*

AHA: 2017,4Q,96

TIP: Hemoptysis (R04.2) is not customarily associated with pneumonia and may be reported separately.

√4ᵗʰ J09   Influenza due to certain identified influenza viruses

> *EXCLUDES 1*   *influenza A/H1N1 (J10.-)*
>
> *influenza due to other identified influenza virus (J10.-)*
>
> *influenza due to unidentified influenza virus (J11.-)*
>
> *seasonal influenza due to other identified influenza virus (J10.-)*
>
> *seasonal influenza due to unidentified influenza virus (J11.-)*

√5ᵗʰ J09.X   Influenza due to identified novel influenza A virus

Avian influenza

Bird influenza

Influenza A/H5N1

Influenza of other animal origin, not bird or swine

Swine influenza virus (viruses that normally cause infections in pigs)

AHA: 2016,3Q,10

J09.X1   Influenza due to identified novel influenza A virus with pneumonia

Code also, if applicable, associated:

lung abscess (J85.1)

other specified type of pneumonia

J09.X2   Influenza due to identified novel influenza A virus with other respiratory manifestations

Influenza due to identified novel influenza A virus NOS

Influenza due to identified novel influenza A virus with laryngitis

Influenza due to identified novel influenza A virus with pharyngitis

Influenza due to identified novel influenza A virus with upper respiratory symptoms

Use additional code, if applicable, for associated:

pleural effusion (J91.8)

sinusitis (J01.-)

J09.X3   Influenza due to identified novel influenza A virus with gastrointestinal manifestations

Influenza due to identified novel influenza A virus gastroenteritis

> *EXCLUDES 1*   *'intestinal flu' [viral gastroenteritis] (A08.-)*

J09.X9   Influenza due to identified novel influenza A virus with other manifestations

Influenza due to identified novel influenza A virus with encephalopathy

Influenza due to identified novel influenza A virus with myocarditis

Influenza due to identified novel influenza A virus with otitis media

Use additional code to identify manifestation

√4ᵗʰ J10 Influenza due to other identified influenza virus

INCLUDES   influenza A (non-novel)
       influenza B
       influenza C

EXCLUDES 1   *influenza due to avian influenza virus (J09.X-)*
       influenza due to swine flu (J09.X-)
       influenza due to unidentifed influenza virus (J11.-)

√5ᵗʰ J10.0 Influenza due to other identified influenza virus with pneumonia

Code also associated lung abscess, if applicable (J85.1)

J10.00 Influenza due to other identified influenza virus with unspecified type of pneumonia

J10.01 Influenza due to other identified influenza virus with the same other identified influenza virus pneumonia

J10.08 Influenza due to other identified influenza virus with other specified pneumonia

Code also other specified type of pneumonia

J10.1 Influenza due to other identified influenza virus with other respiratory manifestations

Influenza due to other identified influenza virus NOS
Influenza due to other identified influenza virus with laryngitis
Influenza due to other identified influenza virus with pharyngitis
Influenza due to other identified influenza virus with upper respiratory symptoms

Use additional code for associated pleural effusion, if applicable (J91.8)
Use additional code for associated sinusitis, if applicable (J01.-)

AHA: 2016,3Q,10-11

J10.2 Influenza due to other identified influenza virus with gastrointestinal manifestations

Influenza due to other identified influenza virus gastroenteritis

EXCLUDES 1   *"intestinal flu" [viral gastroenteritis] (A08.-)*

√5ᵗʰ J10.8 Influenza due to other identified influenza virus with other manifestations

J10.81 Influenza due to other identified influenza virus with encephalopathy

J10.82 Influenza due to other identified influenza virus with myocarditis

J10.83 Influenza due to other identified influenza virus with otitis media

Use additional code for any associated perforated tympanic membrane (H72.-)

J10.89 Influenza due to other identified influenza virus with other manifestations

Use additional codes to identify the manifestations

√4ᵗʰ J11 Influenza due to unidentified influenza virus

√5ᵗʰ J11.0 Influenza due to unidentified influenza virus with pneumonia

Code also associated lung abscess, if applicable (J85.1)

AHA: 2016,3Q,11

J11.00 Influenza due to unidentified influenza virus with unspecified type of pneumonia

Influenza with pneumonia NOS

J11.08 Influenza due to unidentified influenza virus with specified pneumonia

Code also other specified type of pneumonia

J11.1 Influenza due to unidentified influenza virus with other respiratory manifestations

Influenza NOS
Influenzal laryngitis NOS
Influenzal pharyngitis NOS
Influenza with upper respiratory symptoms NOS

Use additional code for associated pleural effusion, if applicable (J91.8)
Use additional code for associated sinusitis, if applicable (J01.-)

J11.2 Influenza due to unidentified influenza virus with gastrointestinal manifestations

Influenza gastroenteritis NOS

EXCLUDES 1   *"intestinal flu" [viral gastroenteritis] (A08.-)*

√5ᵗʰ J11.8 Influenza due to unidentified influenza virus with other manifestations

J11.81 Influenza due to unidentified influenza virus with encephalopathy

Influenzal encephalopathy NOS

J11.82 Influenza due to unidentified influenza virus with myocarditis

Influenzal myocarditis NOS

J11.83 Influenza due to unidentified influenza virus with otitis media

Influenzal otitis media NOS

Use additional code for any associated perforated tympanic membrane (H72.-)

J11.89 Influenza due to unidentified influenza virus with other manifestations

Use additional codes to identify the manifestations

√4ᵗʰ J12 Viral pneumonia, not elsewhere classified

INCLUDES   bronchopneumonia due to viruses other than influenza viruses

Code first associated influenza, if applicable (J09.X1, J10.0-, J11.0-)
Code also associated abscess, if applicable (J85.1)

EXCLUDES 1   *aspiration pneumonia due to anesthesia during labor and delivery (O74.0)*
       aspiration pneumonia due to anesthesia during pregnancy (O29)
       aspiration pneumonia due to anesthesia during puerperium (O89.0)
       aspiration pneumonia due to solids and liquids (J69.-)
       aspiration pneumonia NOS (J69.0)
       congenital pneumonia (P23.0)
       congenital rubella pneumonitis (P35.0)
       interstitial pneumonia NOS (J84.9)
       lipid pneumonia (J69.1)
       neonatal aspiration pneumonia (P24.-)

AHA: 2020,2Q,28; 2019,1Q,35; 2018,3Q,24; 2016,3Q,15; 2013,4Q,118

J12.0 Adenoviral pneumonia

J12.1 Respiratory syncytial virus pneumonia

RSV pneumonia

J12.2 Parainfluenza virus pneumonia

J12.3 Human metapneumovirus pneumonia

√5ᵗʰ J12.8 Other viral pneumonia

J12.81 Pneumonia due to SARS-associated coronavirus

Severe acute respiratory syndrome NOS

DEF: Inflammation of the lungs with consolidation, caused by the severe adult respiratory syndrome (SARS)-associated coronavirus or SARS-CoV. This pneumonia should not be confused with that caused by SARS-CoV-2 (COVID-19).

J12.82 Pneumonia due to coronavirus disease 2019 UPD

Pneumonia due to 2019 novel coronavirus (SARS-CoV-2)
Pneumonia due to COVID-19
Code first COVID-19 (U07.1)

AHA: 2021,1Q,25-30,31-49

J12.89 Other viral pneumonia

AHA: 2021,1Q,33-34; 2020,2Q,8,11; 2020,1Q,34-36

J12.9 Viral pneumonia, unspecified

J13 Pneumonia due to Streptococcus pneumoniae   HCC ESR

Bronchopneumonia due to S. pneumoniae
Code first associated influenza, if applicable (J09.X1, J10.0-, J11.0-)
Code also associated abscess, if applicable (J85.1)

EXCLUDES 1   *congenital pneumonia due to S. pneumoniae (P23.6)*
       lobar pneumonia, unspecified organism (J18.1)
       pneumonia due to other streptococci (J15.3-J15.4)

AHA: 2020,2Q,28; 2019,1Q,35; 2018,3Q,24; 2016,3Q,15; 2013,4Q,118

J14 Pneumonia due to Hemophilus influenzae   HCC ESR

Bronchopneumonia due to H. influenzae
Code first associated influenza, if applicable (J09.X1, J10.0-, J11.0-)
Code also associated abscess, if applicable (J85.1)

EXCLUDES 1   *congenital pneumonia due to H. influenzae (P23.6)*

AHA: 2020,2Q,28; 2019,1Q,35; 2018,3Q,24; 2016,3Q,15; 2013,4Q,118

√4ᵗʰ J15 Bacterial pneumonia, not elsewhere classified

INCLUDES   Bronchopneumonia due to bacteria other than S. pneumoniae and H. influenzae

Code first associated influenza, if applicable (J09.X1, J10.0-, -J11.0-)
Code also associated abscess, if applicable (J85.1)

EXCLUDES 1   *chlamydial pneumonia (J16.0)*
       congenital pneumonia (P23.-)
       Legionnaires' disease (A48.1)
       spirochetal pneumonia (A69.8)

AHA: 2020,2Q,28; 2019,1Q,35; 2018,3Q,24; 2016,3Q,15; 2013,4Q,118

J15.0 Pneumonia due to Klebsiella pneumoniae   HCC ESR COM

J15.1 Pneumonia due to Pseudomonas   HCC ESR COM

Chapter 10. Diseases of the Respiratory System

J15.2–J18.9

✓6ᵗʰ **J15.2** **Pneumonia due to** staphylococcus

    J15.20 **Pneumonia due to staphylococcus, unspecified** `HCC` `ESR` `COM`

    ✓6ᵗʰ **J15.21** **Pneumonia due to Staphylococcus** aureus

        J15.211 **Pneumonia due to** methicillin susceptible **Staphylococcus aureus** `HCC` `ESR` `COM`
            MSSA pneumonia
            Pneumonia due to Staphylococcus aureus NOS

        J15.212 **Pneumonia due to** methicillin resistant **Staphylococcus aureus** `HCC` `ESR` `COM`

    J15.29 **Pneumonia due to other staphylococcus** `HCC` `ESR` `COM`

J15.3 **Pneumonia due to streptococcus,** group B `HCC` `ESR`

J15.4 **Pneumonia due to other streptococci** `HCC` `ESR`

    EXCLUDES 1   pneumonia due to streptococcus, group B (J15.3)
                pneumonia due to Streptococcus pneumoniae (J13)

J15.5 **Pneumonia due to** Escherichia coli `HCC` `ESR` `COM`

J15.6 **Pneumonia due to** other Gram-negative bacteria `HCC` `ESR` `COM`
    Pneumonia due to other aerobic Gram-negative bacteria
    Pneumonia due to Serratia marcescens
    AHA: 2020,2Q,28

J15.7 **Pneumonia due to** Mycoplasma pneumoniae

J15.8 **Pneumonia due to other specified bacteria** `HCC` `ESR` `COM`

J15.9 **Unspecified bacterial pneumonia**
    Pneumonia due to gram-positive bacteria

✓4ᵗʰ **J16** **Pneumonia due to other infectious organisms, not elsewhere classified**
    Code first associated influenza, if applicable (J09.X1, J10.0-, J11.0-)
    Code also associated abscess, if applicable (J85.1)
    EXCLUDES 1   congenital pneumonia (P23.-)
                ornithosis (A70)
                pneumocystosis (B59)
                pneumonia NOS (J18.9)
    AHA: 2020,2Q,28; 2019,1Q,35; 2018,3Q,24; 2016,3Q,15; 2013,4Q,118

    J16.0 **Chlamydial** **pneumonia**

    J16.8 **Pneumonia due to other specified infectious organisms**

J17 *Pneumonia in diseases classified elsewhere*
    Code first underlying disease, such as:
    Q fever (A78)
    rheumatic fever (I00)
    schistosomiasis (B65.0-B65.9)
    EXCLUDES 1   candidial pneumonia (B37.1)
                chlamydial pneumonia (J16.0)
                gonorrheal pneumonia (A54.84)
                histoplasmosis pneumonia (B39.0-B39.2)
                measles pneumonia (B05.2)
                nocardiosis pneumonia (A43.0)
                pneumocystosis (B59)
                pneumonia due to Pneumocystis carinii (B59)
                pneumonia due to Pneumocystis jiroveci (B59)
                pneumonia in actinomycosis (A42.0)
                pneumonia in anthrax (A22.1)
                pneumonia in ascariasis (B77.81)
                pneumonia in aspergillosis (B44.0-B44.1)
                pneumonia in coccidioidomycosis (B38.0-B38.2)
                pneumonia in cytomegalovirus disease (B25.0)
                pneumonia in toxoplasmosis (B58.3)
                rubella pneumonia (B06.81)
                salmonella pneumonia (A02.22)
                spirochetal infection NEC with pneumonia (A69.8)
                tularemia pneumonia (A21.2)
                typhoid fever with pneumonia (A01.03)
                varicella pneumonia (B01.2)
                whooping cough with pneumonia (A37 with fifth character 1)
    AHA: 2020,2Q,28; 2019,1Q,35; 2016,3Q,15; 2013,4Q,118

✓4ᵗʰ **J18** **Pneumonia, unspecified organism**
    Code first associated influenza, if applicable (J09.X1, J10.0-, J11.0-)
    EXCLUDES 1   abscess of lung with pneumonia (J85.1)
                aspiration pneumonia due to anesthesia during labor and delivery (O74.0)
                aspiration pneumonia due to anesthesia during pregnancy (O29)
                aspiration pneumonia due to anesthesia during puerperium (O89.0)
                aspiration pneumonia due to solids and liquids (J69.-)
                aspiration pneumonia NOS (J69.0)
                congenital pneumonia (P23.0)
                drug-induced interstitial lung disorder (J70.2-J70.4)
                interstitial pneumonia NOS (J84.9)
                lipid pneumonia (J69.1)
                neonatal aspiration pneumonia (P24.-)
                pneumonitis due to external agents (J67-J70)
                pneumonitis due to fumes and vapors (J68.0)
                usual interstitial pneumonia (J84.178)
    AHA: 2020,2Q,28; 2019,1Q,35; 2016,3Q,15; 2013,4Q,118

    J18.0 **Bronchopneumonia,** **unspecified organism**
        EXCLUDES 1   hypostatic bronchopneumonia (J18.2)
                lipid pneumonia (J69.1)
        EXCLUDES 2   acute bronchiolitis (J21.-)
                chronic bronchiolitis (J44.9)

    J18.1 **Lobar** **pneumonia, unspecified organism** `HCC` `ESR`
        AHA: 2019,3Q,37; 2018,3Q,24
        DEF: Lobar pneumonia is characterized by consolidated inflammation confined or localized to only one or a few lobes of the lung. The consolidation affects primarily the alveolar air spaces, unlike bronchopneumonia, which arises from the bronchi or bronchioles and affects a wide area without any localization.
        TIP: Documentation of right upper lobe, left upper lobe, right lower lobe, left lower lobe, or right middle lobe pneumonia alone is not synonymous with "lobar pneumonia," nor should a diagnosis of lobar pneumonia be assumed based on an imaging report that identifies pneumonia in a specific lobe. Assign J18.1 only when the provider specifically documents "lobar pneumonia" without specifying a causal organism.

    J18.2 **Hypostatic** **pneumonia, unspecified organism** `COM`
        Hypostatic bronchopneumonia
        Passive pneumonia

    J18.8 **Other pneumonia, unspecified organism**

    J18.9 **Pneumonia, unspecified organism**
        AHA: 2020,2Q,28; 2019,3Q,15; 2019,2Q,28; 2014,3Q,4; 2013,4Q,119; 2012,4Q,94

`HCC` CMS-HCC   `Rx` Rx HCC   `ESR` ESRD HCC   `COM` Commercial HCC   Newborn: 0   Pediatric: 0-17   M Maternity: 9-64   A Adult: 15-124

710   ICD-10-CM 2023

Other acute lower respiratory infections (J20-J22)

EXCLUDES 2   *chronic obstructive pulmonary disease with acute lower respiratory infection (J44.0)*

✓4th J20 Acute bronchitis

INCLUDES   acute and subacute bronchitis (with) bronchospasm
acute and subacute bronchitis (with) tracheitis
acute and subacute bronchitis (with) tracheobronchitis, acute
acute and subacute fibrinous bronchitis
acute and subacute membranous bronchitis
acute and subacute purulent bronchitis
acute and subacute septic bronchitis

EXCLUDES 1   *bronchitis NOS (J40)*
tracheobronchitis NOS (J40)

EXCLUDES 2   *acute bronchitis with bronchiectasis (J47.0)*
acute bronchitis with chronic obstructive asthma (J44.0)
acute bronchitis with chronic obstructive pulmonary disease (J44.0)
allergic bronchitis NOS (J45.909-)
bronchitis due to chemicals, fumes and vapors (J68.0)
chronic bronchitis NOS (J42)
chronic mucopurulent bronchitis (J41.1)
chronic obstructive bronchitis (J44.-)
chronic obstructive tracheobronchitis (J44.-)
chronic simple bronchitis (J41.0)
chronic tracheobronchitis (J42)

AHA: 2019,1Q,35; 2016,3Q,10,16

DEF: Acute inflammation of the main branches of the bronchial tree due to infectious or irritant agents. Symptoms include cough with a varied production of sputum, fever, substernal soreness, and lung rales. Bronchitis usually lasts three to 10 days.

J20.0   Acute bronchitis due to Mycoplasma pneumoniae

J20.1   Acute bronchitis due to Hemophilus influenzae

J20.2   Acute bronchitis due to streptococcus

J20.3   Acute bronchitis due to coxsackievirus

J20.4   Acute bronchitis due to parainfluenza virus

J20.5   Acute bronchitis due to respiratory syncytial virus
Acute bronchitis due to RSV

J20.6   Acute bronchitis due to rhinovirus

J20.7   Acute bronchitis due to echovirus

J20.8   Acute bronchitis due to other specified organisms
AHA: 2020,1Q,34-36
TIP: Assign as a secondary code for a patient with acute bronchitis confirmed as due to COVID-19; assign U07.1 as the principal or first-listed code.

J20.9   Acute bronchitis, unspecified

✓4th J21 Acute bronchiolitis

INCLUDES   acute bronchiolitis with bronchospasm
EXCLUDES 2   *respiratory bronchiolitis interstitial lung disease (J84.115)*

J21.0   Acute bronchiolitis due to respiratory syncytial virus
Acute bronchiolitis due to RSV

J21.1   Acute bronchiolitis due to human metapneumovirus

J21.8   Acute bronchiolitis due to other specified organisms

J21.9   Acute bronchiolitis, unspecified
Bronchiolitis (acute)
EXCLUDES 1   *chronic bronchiolitis (J44.-)*

J22 Unspecified acute lower respiratory infection
Acute (lower) respiratory (tract) infection NOS
EXCLUDES 1   *upper respiratory infection (acute) (J06.9)*

AHA: 2020,1Q,22,34-36
TIP: Assign as a secondary code for a patient with a respiratory infection specified as acute or lower that is documented as being associated with COVID-19; assign U07.1 as the principal or first-listed code. If the respiratory infection documentation does not specify acute or lower, assign J98.8.

Other diseases of upper respiratory tract (J30-J39)

✓4th J30 Vasomotor and allergic rhinitis

INCLUDES   spasmodic rhinorrhea
EXCLUDES 1   *allergic rhinitis with asthma (bronchial) (J45.909)*
rhinitis NOS (J31.0)

J30.0   Vasomotor rhinitis
DEF: Noninfectious and nonallergic type of rhinitis for which the cause is often unknown. Symptoms often mimic those of allergic rhinitis with a diagnosis of vasomotor rhinitis typically made after ruling out allergens as the cause.

J30.1   Allergic rhinitis due to pollen
Allergy NOS due to pollen
Hay fever
Pollinosis

J30.2   Other seasonal allergic rhinitis

J30.5   Allergic rhinitis due to food

✓5th J30.8 Other allergic rhinitis

J30.81   Allergic rhinitis due to animal (cat) (dog) hair and dander

J30.89   Other allergic rhinitis
Perennial allergic rhinitis

J30.9   Allergic rhinitis, unspecified

✓4th J31 Chronic rhinitis, nasopharyngitis and pharyngitis

Use additional code to identify:
exposure to environmental tobacco smoke (Z77.22)
exposure to tobacco smoke in the perinatal period (P96.81)
history of tobacco dependence (Z87.891)
occupational exposure to environmental tobacco smoke (Z57.31)
tobacco dependence (F17.-)
tobacco use (Z72.0)

J31.0   Chronic rhinitis
Atrophic rhinitis (chronic)
Granulomatous rhinitis (chronic)
Hypertrophic rhinitis (chronic)
Obstructive rhinitis (chronic)
Ozena
Purulent rhinitis (chronic)
Rhinitis (chronic) NOS
Ulcerative rhinitis (chronic)
EXCLUDES 1   *allergic rhinitis (J30.1-J30.9)*
vasomotor rhinitis (J30.0)
DEF: Persistent inflammation of the mucous membranes of the nose, characterized by a postnasal drip.

J31.1   Chronic nasopharyngitis
EXCLUDES 2   *acute nasopharyngitis (J00)*
DEF: Persistent inflammation of the mucous membranes extending from the nares to the pharynx. It is characterized by constant irritation in the nasopharynx and postnasal drip.

J31.2   Chronic pharyngitis
Atrophic pharyngitis (chronic)
Chronic sore throat
Granular pharyngitis (chronic)
Hypertrophic pharyngitis (chronic)
EXCLUDES 2   *acute pharyngitis (J02.9)*

✓4th J32 Chronic sinusitis

INCLUDES   sinus abscess
sinus empyema
sinus infection
sinus suppuration
Use additional code to identify:
exposure to environmental tobacco smoke (Z77.22)
exposure to tobacco smoke in the perinatal period (P96.81)
history of tobacco dependence (Z87.891)
infectious agent (B95-B97)
occupational exposure to environmental tobacco smoke (Z57.31)
tobacco dependence (F17.-)
tobacco use (Z72.0)
EXCLUDES 2   *acute sinusitis (J01.-)*

J32.0   Chronic maxillary sinusitis
Antritis (chronic)
Maxillary sinusitis NOS

J32.1   Chronic frontal sinusitis
Frontal sinusitis NOS

J32.2   **Chronic** ethmoidal **sinusitis**
Ethmoidal sinusitis NOS
> EXCLUDES 1   *Woakes' ethmoiditis (J33.1)*

J32.3   **Chronic** sphenoidal **sinusitis**
Sphenoidal sinusitis NOS

J32.4   **Chronic** pansinusitis
Pansinusitis NOS

J32.8   **Other chronic sinusitis**
Sinusitis (chronic) involving more than one sinus but not pansinusitis

J32.9   **Chronic sinusitis, unspecified**
Sinusitis (chronic) NOS

✓4ᵗʰ **J33**   **Nasal polyp**
Use additional code to identify:
exposure to environmental tobacco smoke (Z77.22)
exposure to tobacco smoke in the perinatal period (P96.81)
history of tobacco dependence (Z87.891)
occupational exposure to environmental tobacco smoke (Z57.31)
tobacco dependence (F17.-)
tobacco use (Z72.0)
> EXCLUDES 1   *adenomatous polyps (D14.0)*

J33.0   **Polyp of nasal cavity**
Choanal polyp
Nasopharyngeal polyp

J33.1   **Polypoid sinus degeneration**
Woakes' syndrome or ethmoiditis

J33.8   **Other polyp of sinus**
Accessory polyp of sinus
Ethmoidal polyp of sinus
Maxillary polyp of sinus
Sphenoidal polyp of sinus

J33.9   **Nasal polyp, unspecified**

✓4ᵗʰ **J34**   **Other and unspecified disorders of nose and nasal sinuses**
> EXCLUDES 2   *varicose ulcer of nasal septum (I86.8)*

J34.0   **Abscess, furuncle and carbuncle of nose**
Cellulitis of nose
Necrosis of nose
Ulceration of nose

J34.1   **Cyst and mucocele of nose and nasal sinus**

J34.2   **Deviated nasal septum**
Deflection or deviation of septum (nasal) (acquired)
> EXCLUDES 1   *congenital deviated nasal septum (Q67.4)*

DEF: Condition in which the nasal septum, a thin wall composed of cartilage and bone that separates the two nostrils, is crooked or displaced from the midline.

J34.3   **Hypertrophy of nasal turbinates**
DEF: Overgrowth of bones within the nasal turbinate, which are ridges of bone and soft tissue that project from the sidewalls of the nasal passages. Hypertrophy can cause obstruction of the nasal passages.

✓5ᵗʰ **J34.8**   **Other specified disorders of nose and nasal sinuses**

     J34.81   **Nasal mucositis (ulcerative)**
Code also type of associated therapy, such as:
antineoplastic and immunosuppressive drugs (T45.1X-)
radiological procedure and radiotherapy (Y84.2)
> EXCLUDES 2   *gastrointestinal mucositis (ulcerative) (K92.81)*
> *mucositis (ulcerative) of vagina and vulva (N76.81)*
> *oral mucositis (ulcerative) (K12.3-)*

     J34.89   **Other specified disorders of nose and nasal sinuses**
Perforation of nasal septum NOS
Rhinolith

J34.9   **Unspecified disorder of nose and nasal sinuses**

✓4ᵗʰ **J35**   **Chronic diseases of tonsils and adenoids**
Use additional code to identify:
exposure to environmental tobacco smoke (Z77.22)
exposure to tobacco smoke in the perinatal period (P96.81)
history of tobacco dependence (Z87.891)
occupational exposure to environmental tobacco smoke (Z57.31)
tobacco dependence (F17.-)
tobacco use (Z72.0)

✓5ᵗʰ **J35.0**   **Chronic tonsillitis and adenoiditis**
> EXCLUDES 2   *acute tonsillitis (J03.-)*

     J35.01   **Chronic** tonsillitis

     J35.02   **Chronic** adenoiditis

     J35.03   **Chronic** tonsillitis and adenoiditis

J35.1   **Hypertrophy of** tonsils
Enlargement of tonsils
> EXCLUDES 1   *hypertrophy of tonsils with tonsillitis (J35.0-)*

J35.2   **Hypertrophy of** adenoids
Enlargement of adenoids
> EXCLUDES 1   *hypertrophy of adenoids with adenoiditis (J35.0-)*

J35.3   **Hypertrophy of** tonsils with hypertrophy of adenoids
> EXCLUDES 1   *hypertrophy of tonsils and adenoids with tonsillitis and adenoiditis (J35.03)*

J35.8   **Other chronic diseases of tonsils and adenoids**
Adenoid vegetations
Amygdalolith
Calculus, tonsil
Cicatrix of tonsil (and adenoid)
Tonsillar tag
Ulcer of tonsil

J35.9   **Chronic disease of tonsils and adenoids, unspecified**
Disease (chronic) of tonsils and adenoids NOS

J36   **Peritonsillar abscess**
> INCLUDES   abscess of tonsil
> peritonsillar cellulitis
> quinsy

Use additional code (B95-B97) to identify infectious agent
> EXCLUDES 1   *acute tonsillitis (J03.-)*
> *chronic tonsillitis (J35.0)*
> *retropharyngeal abscess (J39.0)*
> *tonsillitis NOS (J03.9-)*

✓4ᵗʰ **J37**   **Chronic laryngitis and laryngotracheitis**
Use additional code to identify:
exposure to environmental tobacco smoke (Z77.22)
exposure to tobacco smoke in the perinatal period (P96.81)
history of tobacco dependence (Z87.891)
infectious agent (B95-B97)
occupational exposure to environmental tobacco smoke (Z57.31)
tobacco dependence (F17.-)
tobacco use (Z72.0)

J37.0   **Chronic** laryngitis
Catarrhal laryngitis
Hypertrophic laryngitis
Sicca laryngitis
> EXCLUDES 2   *acute laryngitis (J04.0)*
> *obstructive (acute) laryngitis (J05.0)*

J37.1   **Chronic** laryngotracheitis
Laryngitis, chronic, with tracheitis (chronic)
Tracheitis, chronic, with laryngitis
> EXCLUDES 1   *chronic tracheitis (J42)*
> EXCLUDES 2   *acute laryngotracheitis (J04.2)*
> *acute tracheitis (J04.1)*

✓4ᵗʰ **J38**   **Diseases of vocal cords and larynx, not elsewhere classified**
Use additional code to identify:
exposure to environmental tobacco smoke (Z77.22)
exposure to tobacco smoke in the perinatal period (P96.81)
history of tobacco dependence (Z87.891)
occupational exposure to environmental tobacco smoke (Z57.31)
tobacco dependence (F17.-)
tobacco use (Z72.0)
> EXCLUDES 1   *congenital laryngeal stridor (P28.89)*
> *obstructive laryngitis (acute) (J05.0)*
> *postprocedural subglottic stenosis (J95.5)*
> *stridor (R06.1)*
> *ulcerative laryngitis (J04.0)*

✓5ᵗʰ **J38.0**   **Paralysis of vocal cords and larynx**
Laryngoplegia
Paralysis of glottis

     J38.00   **Paralysis of vocal cords and larynx, unspecified**

     J38.01   **Paralysis of vocal cords and larynx,** unilateral

     J38.02   **Paralysis of vocal cords and larynx,** bilateral

J38.1   **Polyp** of vocal cord and larynx
> EXCLUDES 1   *adenomatous polyps (D14.1)*

J38.2   **Nodules of vocal cords**
Chorditis (fibrinous)(nodosa)(tuberosa)
Singer's nodes
Teacher's nodes

J38.3   **Other diseases of vocal cords**
Abscess of vocal cords
Cellulitis of vocal cords
Granuloma of vocal cords
Leukokeratosis of vocal cords
Leukoplakia of vocal cords

J38.4   **Edema of larynx**
Edema (of) glottis
Subglottic edema
Supraglottic edema
> EXCLUDES 1   *acute obstructive laryngitis [croup] (J05.0)*
> *edematous laryngitis (J04.0)*

J38.5   **Laryngeal spasm**
Laryngismus (stridulus)

J38.6   **Stenosis of larynx**

J38.7   **Other diseases of larynx**
Abscess of larynx
Cellulitis of larynx
Disease of larynx NOS
Necrosis of larynx
Pachyderma of larynx
Perichondritis of larynx
Ulcer of larynx

✓4ᵗʰ J39   Other diseases of upper respiratory tract
> EXCLUDES 1   *acute respiratory infection NOS (J22)*
> *acute upper respiratory infection (J06.9)*
> *upper respiratory inflammation due to chemicals, gases, fumes or vapors (J68.2)*

J39.0   **Retropharyngeal and parapharyngeal abscess**
Peripharyngeal abscess
> EXCLUDES 1   *peritonsillar abscess (J36)*

DEF: Purulent infection behind the pharynx and the front of the precerebral fascia, characterized by neck stiffness, cervical lymphadenopathy, sore throat, fever, and stridor.

J39.1   **Other abscess of pharynx**
Cellulitis of pharynx
Nasopharyngeal abscess

J39.2   **Other diseases of pharynx**
Cyst of pharynx
Edema of pharynx
> EXCLUDES 2   *chronic pharyngitis (J31.2)*
> *ulcerative pharyngitis (J02.9)*

J39.3   **Upper respiratory tract hypersensitivity reaction, site unspecified**
> EXCLUDES 1   *hypersensitivity reaction of upper respiratory tract, such as:*
> *extrinsic allergic alveolitis (J67.9)*
> *pneumoconiosis (J60-J67.9)*

J39.8   **Other specified diseases of upper respiratory tract**

J39.9   **Disease of upper respiratory tract, unspecified**

Chronic lower respiratory diseases (J40-J47)

> EXCLUDES 1   *bronchitis due to chemicals, gases, fumes and vapors (J68.0)*
> EXCLUDES 2   *cystic fibrosis (E84.-)*

J40   Bronchitis, not specified as acute or chronic
Bronchitis NOS
Bronchitis with tracheitis NOS
Catarrhal bronchitis
Tracheobronchitis NOS
Use additional code to identify:
exposure to environmental tobacco smoke (Z77.22)
exposure to tobacco smoke in the perinatal period (P96.81)
history of tobacco dependence (Z87.891)
occupational exposure to environmental tobacco smoke (Z57.31)
tobacco dependence (F17.-)
tobacco use (Z72.0)
> EXCLUDES 1   *acute bronchitis (J20.-)*
> *allergic bronchitis NOS (J45.909-)*
> *asthmatic bronchitis NOS (J45.9-)*
> *bronchitis due to chemicals, gases, fumes and vapors (J68.0)*

AHA: 2020,1Q,34-36
TIP: Assign as a secondary code for a patient with bronchitis of unspecified acuity due to COVID-19; assign U07.1 as the principal or first-listed code.

✓4ᵗʰ J41   Simple and mucopurulent chronic bronchitis
Use additional code to identify:
exposure to environmental tobacco smoke (Z77.22)
exposure to tobacco smoke in the perinatal period (P96.81)
history of tobacco dependence (Z87.891)
occupational exposure to environmental tobacco smoke (Z57.31)
tobacco dependence (F17.-)
tobacco use (Z72.0)
> EXCLUDES 1   *chronic bronchitis NOS (J42)*
> *chronic obstructive bronchitis (J44.-)*

J41.0   **Simple chronic bronchitis**   HCC Rx ESR COM

J41.1   **Mucopurulent chronic bronchitis**   HCC Rx ESR COM

J41.8   **Mixed simple and mucopurulent chronic bronchitis**   HCC Rx ESR COM

J42   Unspecified chronic bronchitis   HCC Rx ESR COM
Chronic bronchitis NOS
Chronic tracheitis
Chronic tracheobronchitis
Use additional code to identify:
exposure to environmental tobacco smoke (Z77.22)
exposure to tobacco smoke in the perinatal period (P96.81)
history of tobacco dependence (Z87.891)
occupational exposure to environmental tobacco smoke (Z57.31)
tobacco dependence (F17.-)
tobacco use (Z72.0)
> EXCLUDES 1   *chronic asthmatic bronchitis (J44.-)*
> *chronic bronchitis with airways obstruction (J44.-)*
> *chronic emphysematous bronchitis (J44.-)*
> *chronic obstructive pulmonary disease NOS (J44.9)*
> *simple and mucopurulent chronic bronchitis (J41.-)*

✓4ᵗʰ J43 Emphysema

Use additional code to identify:
exposure to environmental tobacco smoke (Z77.22)
history of tobacco dependence (Z87.891)
occupational exposure to environmental tobacco smoke (Z57.31)
tobacco dependence (F17.-)
tobacco use (Z72.0)

EXCLUDES 1   compensatory emphysema (J98.3)
emphysema due to inhalation of chemicals, gases, fumes or vapors (J68.4)
emphysema with chronic (obstructive) bronchitis (J44.-)
emphysematous (obstructive) bronchitis (J44.-)
interstitial emphysema (J98.2)
mediastinal emphysema (J98.2)
neonatal interstitial emphysema (P25.0)
surgical (subcutaneous) emphysema (T81.82)

EXCLUDES 2   traumatic subcutaneous emphysema (T79.7)

DEF: Pathological condition in which there is destructive enlargement of the air sacs in the lungs resulting in damage and lack of elasticity to the alveolar walls, commonly seen in long-term smokers.

Emphysema

Healthy alveoli
Patent bronchiole
Well-vascularized
Dilated alveoli
Excess mucus

Alveoli w/ Emphysema
Collapsed bronchiole
Broken/fewer capillaries
Enlarged alveoli
Alveolar membranes break down

J43.0   **Unilateral pulmonary emphysema [MacLeod's syndrome]**   HCC Rx ESR COM
Swyer-James syndrome
Unilateral emphysema
Unilateral hyperlucent lung
Unilateral pulmonary artery functional hypoplasia
Unilateral transparency of lung

J43.1   **Panlobular emphysema**   HCC Rx ESR COM
Panacinar emphysema

J43.2   **Centrilobular emphysema**   HCC Rx ESR COM

J43.8   **Other emphysema**   HCC Rx ESR COM

J43.9   **Emphysema, unspecified**   HCC Rx ESR COM
Bullous emphysema (lung)(pulmonary)
Emphysema (lung)(pulmonary) NOS
Emphysematous bleb
Vesicular emphysema (lung)(pulmonary)
AHA: 2019,1Q,34-36; 2017,4Q,97-98

✓4ᵗʰ J44 Other chronic obstructive pulmonary disease

INCLUDES   asthma with chronic obstructive pulmonary disease
chronic asthmatic (obstructive) bronchitis
chronic bronchitis with airway obstruction
chronic bronchitis with emphysema
chronic emphysematous bronchitis
chronic obstructive asthma
chronic obstructive bronchitis
chronic obstructive tracheobronchitis

Code also type of asthma, if applicable (J45.-)
Use additional code to identify:
exposure to environmental tobacco smoke (Z77.22)
history of tobacco dependence (Z87.891)
occupational exposure to environmental tobacco smoke (Z57.31)
tobacco dependence (F17.-)
tobacco use (Z72.0)

EXCLUDES 1   bronchiectasis (J47.-)
chronic bronchitis NOS (J42)
chronic simple and mucopurulent bronchitis (J41.-)
chronic tracheitis (J42)
chronic tracheobronchitis (J42)
emphysema without chronic bronchitis (J43.-)

AHA: 2019,1Q,34-36; 2017,4Q,97-98; 2017,1Q,25-26; 2016,3Q,15-16; 2013,4Q,109

J44.0   **Chronic obstructive pulmonary disease with (acute) lower respiratory infection**   HCC Rx ESR COM
Code also to identify the infection
AHA: 2019,1Q,35; 2017,4Q,96; 2017,1Q,24-25
TIP: Do not assign when only aspiration pneumonia is present. Aspiration pneumonia is not classified as a respiratory infection.

J44.1   **Chronic obstructive pulmonary disease with (acute) exacerbation**   HCC Rx ESR COM
Decompensated COPD
Decompensated COPD with (acute) exacerbation
EXCLUDES 2   chronic obstructive pulmonary disease [COPD] with acute bronchitis (J44.0)
lung diseases due to external agents (J60-J70)
AHA: 2019,1Q,34; 2017,4Q,96; 2017,1Q,26; 2016,1Q,36
TIP: Exacerbation of COPD should not be assumed based upon worsening of a concomitant respiratory disease or when COPD is described as end-stage.
TIP: Assign J43.9 when COPD exacerbation with emphysema is documented.

J44.9   **Chronic obstructive pulmonary disease, unspecified**   HCC Rx ESR COM
Chronic obstructive airway disease NOS
Chronic obstructive lung disease NOS
EXCLUDES 2   lung diseases due to external agents (J60-J70)
AHA: 2019,1Q,36; 2017,4Q,96-97; 2016,1Q,36; 2014,4Q,21; 2013,4Q,109

✓4th **J45 Asthma**

INCLUDES   allergic (predominantly) asthma
allergic bronchitis NOS
allergic rhinitis with asthma
atopic asthma
extrinsic allergic asthma
hay fever with asthma
idiosyncratic asthma
intrinsic nonallergic asthma
nonallergic asthma

Use additional code to identify:
eosinophilic asthma (J82.83)
exposure to environmental tobacco smoke (Z77.22)
exposure to tobacco smoke in the perinatal period (P96.81)
history of tobacco dependence (Z87.891)
occupational exposure to environmental tobacco smoke (Z57.31)
tobacco dependence (F17.-)
tobacco use (Z72.0)

EXCLUDES 1   detergent asthma (J69.8)
~~eosinophilic asthma (J82)~~
miner's asthma (J60)
wheezing NOS (R06.2)
wood asthma (J67.8)

EXCLUDES 2   asthma with chronic obstructive pulmonary disease (J44.9)
chronic asthmatic (obstructive) bronchitis (J44.9)
chronic obstructive asthma (J44.9)

AHA: 2019,1Q,36; 2017,1Q,25-26; 2012,4Q,99
DEF: Status asthmaticus: Severe, intractable episode of asthma that is unresponsive to normal therapeutic measures.

✓5th **J45.2 Mild intermittent asthma**

J45.20 Mild intermittent asthma, uncomplicated Rx COM
Mild intermittent asthma NOS

J45.21 Mild intermittent asthma with (acute) exacerbation Rx COM

J45.22 Mild intermittent asthma with status asthmaticus Rx COM

✓5th **J45.3 Mild persistent asthma**

J45.30 Mild persistent asthma, uncomplicated Rx COM
Mild persistent asthma NOS

J45.31 Mild persistent asthma with (acute) exacerbation Rx COM
AHA: 2016,1Q,35

J45.32 Mild persistent asthma with status asthmaticus Rx COM

✓5th **J45.4 Moderate persistent asthma**

J45.40 Moderate persistent asthma, uncomplicated Rx COM
Moderate persistent asthma NOS

J45.41 Moderate persistent asthma with (acute) exacerbation Rx COM
AHA: 2017,1Q,26

J45.42 Moderate persistent asthma with status asthmaticus Rx COM

✓5th **J45.5 Severe persistent asthma**

J45.50 Severe persistent asthma, uncomplicated Rx COM
Severe persistent asthma NOS

J45.51 Severe persistent asthma with (acute) exacerbation Rx COM

J45.52 Severe persistent asthma with status asthmaticus Rx COM

✓5th **J45.9 Other and unspecified asthma**

✓6th **J45.90 Unspecified asthma**
Asthmatic bronchitis NOS
Childhood asthma NOS
Late onset asthma
AHA: 2017,4Q,96; 2017,1Q,25

J45.901 Unspecified asthma with (acute) exacerbation Rx COM

J45.902 Unspecified asthma with status asthmaticus Rx COM

J45.909 Unspecified asthma, uncomplicated Rx COM
Asthma NOS
EXCLUDES 2   lung diseases due to external agents (J60-J70)
AHA: 2017,1Q,25

✓6th **J45.99 Other asthma**

J45.990 Exercise induced bronchospasm Rx COM

J45.991 Cough variant asthma Rx COM

J45.998 Other asthma Rx COM

✓4th **J47 Bronchiectasis**

INCLUDES   bronchiolectasis
Use additional code to identify:
exposure to environmental tobacco smoke (Z77.22)
exposure to tobacco smoke in the perinatal period (P96.81)
history of tobacco dependence (Z87.891)
occupational exposure to environmental tobacco smoke (Z57.31)
tobacco dependence (F17.-)
tobacco use (Z72.0)

EXCLUDES 1   congenital bronchiectasis (Q33.4)
tuberculous bronchiectasis (current disease) (A15.0)

DEF: Dilation of the bronchi with mucus production and persistent cough due to infection or chronic conditions that causes diminished lung capacity and frequent infections of the lung.

J47.0 Bronchiectasis with acute lower respiratory infection HCC Rx ESR COM
Bronchiectasis with acute bronchitis
Code also to identify infection, if applicable

J47.1 Bronchiectasis with (acute) exacerbation HCC Rx ESR COM
AHA: 2021,1Q,23

J47.9 Bronchiectasis, uncomplicated HCC Rx ESR COM
Bronchiectasis NOS

Lung diseases due to external agents (J60-J70)

EXCLUDES 2   asthma (J45.-)
malignant neoplasm of bronchus and lung (C34.-)

DEF: Pneumoconiosis: Condition caused by inhaling inorganic dust particles, typically associated with occupations that require regular exposure to mineral dusts. A form of interstitial lung disease that contributes to the inflammation of the air sacs, causing the lung tissue to harden.

J60 Coalworker's pneumoconiosis HCC ESR COM A
Anthracosilicosis
Anthracosis
Black lung disease
Coalworker's lung
EXCLUDES 1   coalworker pneumoconiosis with tuberculosis, any type in A15 (J65)

J61 Pneumoconiosis due to asbestos and other mineral fibers HCC ESR COM A
Asbestosis
EXCLUDES 1   pleural plaque with asbestosis (J92.0)
pneumoconiosis with tuberculosis, any type in A15 (J65)

✓4th **J62 Pneumoconiosis due to dust containing silica**
INCLUDES   silicotic fibrosis (massive) of lung
EXCLUDES 1   pneumoconiosis with tuberculosis, any type in A15 (J65)

J62.0 Pneumoconiosis due to talc dust HCC ESR COM

J62.8 Pneumoconiosis due to other dust containing silica HCC ESR COM
Silicosis NOS

✓4th **J63 Pneumoconiosis due to other inorganic dusts**
EXCLUDES 1   pneumoconiosis with tuberculosis, any type in A15 (J65)

J63.0 Aluminosis (of lung) HCC ESR COM

J63.1 Bauxite fibrosis (of lung) HCC ESR COM

J63.2 Berylliosis HCC ESR COM

J63.3 Graphite fibrosis (of lung) HCC ESR COM

J63.4 Siderosis HCC ESR COM
AHA: 2019,3Q,8

J63.5 Stannosis HCC ESR COM

J63.6 Pneumoconiosis due to other specified inorganic dusts HCC ESR COM

J64 Unspecified pneumoconiosis HCC ESR COM
EXCLUDES 1   pneumoconiosis with tuberculosis, any type in A15 (J65)

J65 **Pneumoconiosis** associated with tuberculosis   `HCC` `ESR` `COM`
Any condition in J60-J64 with tuberculosis, any type in A15
Silicotuberculosis

✓4th **J66** **Airway disease due to specific** organic dust
    `EXCLUDES 2`   allergic alveolitis (J67.-)
            asbestosis (J61)
            bagassosis (J67.1)
            farmer's lung (J67.0)
            hypersensitivity pneumonitis due to organic dust (J67.-)
            reactive airways dysfunction syndrome (J68.3)

   J66.0 **Byssinosis**   `HCC` `ESR` `COM`
       Airway disease due to cotton dust

   J66.1 **Flax-dressers' disease**   `HCC` `ESR` `COM`

   J66.2 **Cannabinosis**   `HCC` `ESR` `COM`

   J66.8 **Airway disease due to other specific organic dusts**   `HCC` `ESR` `COM`

✓4th **J67** **Hypersensitivity pneumonitis due to organic dust**
    `INCLUDES`   allergic alveolitis and pneumonitis due to inhaled organic dust and particles of fungal, actinomycetic or other origin
    `EXCLUDES 1`   pneumonitis due to inhalation of chemicals, gases, fumes or vapors (J68.0)

   J67.0 **Farmer's lung**   `HCC` `ESR` `COM`
       Harvester's lung
       Haymaker's lung
       Moldy hay disease

   J67.1 **Bagassosis**   `HCC` `ESR` `COM`
       Bagasse disease
       Bagasse pneumonitis

   J67.2 **Bird fancier's lung**   `HCC` `ESR` `COM`
       Budgerigar fancier's disease or lung
       Pigeon fancier's disease or lung

   J67.3 **Suberosis**   `HCC` `ESR` `COM`
       Corkhandler's disease or lung
       Corkworker's disease or lung

   J67.4 **Maltworker's lung**   `HCC` `ESR` `COM`
       Alveolitis due to Aspergillus clavatus

   J67.5 **Mushroom-worker's lung**   `HCC` `ESR` `COM`

   J67.6 **Maple-bark-stripper's lung**   `HCC` `ESR` `COM`
       Alveolitis due to Cryptostroma corticale
       Cryptostromosis

   J67.7 **Air conditioner and humidifier lung**   `HCC` `ESR` `COM`
       Allergic alveolitis due to fungal, thermophilic actinomycetes and other organisms growing in ventilation [air conditioning] systems

   J67.8 **Hypersensitivity pneumonitis due to other organic dusts**   `HCC` `ESR` `COM`
       Cheese-washer's lung
       Coffee-worker's lung
       Fish-meal worker's lung
       Furrier's lung
       Sequoiosis

   J67.9 **Hypersensitivity pneumonitis due to unspecified organic dust**   `HCC` `ESR` `COM`
       Allergic alveolitis (extrinsic) NOS
       Hypersensitivity pneumonitis NOS

✓4th **J68** **Respiratory conditions due to inhalation of chemicals, gases, fumes and vapors**
    Code first (T51-T65) to identify cause
    Use additional code to identify associated respiratory conditions, such as:
    acute respiratory failure (J96.0-)

   J68.0 **Bronchitis and pneumonitis due to chemicals, gases, fumes and vapors**   `HCC` `ESR` `COM`
       Chemical bronchitis (acute)
       AHA: 2019,2Q,31

   J68.1 **Pulmonary edema due to chemicals, gases, fumes and vapors**   `HCC` `ESR` `COM`
       Chemical pulmonary edema (acute) (chronic)
      `EXCLUDES 1`   pulmonary edema (acute) (chronic) NOS (J81.-)

   J68.2 **Upper respiratory inflammation due to chemicals, gases, fumes and vapors, not elsewhere classified**   `HCC` `ESR` `COM`

   J68.3 **Other** acute and subacute respiratory conditions **due to chemicals, gases, fumes and vapors**   `HCC` `ESR` `COM`
       Reactive airways dysfunction syndrome

   J68.4 **Chronic respiratory conditions due to chemicals, gases, fumes and vapors**   `HCC` `ESR` `COM`
       Emphysema (diffuse) (chronic) due to inhalation of chemicals, gases, fumes and vapors
       Obliterative bronchiolitis (chronic) (subacute) due to inhalation of chemicals, gases, fumes and vapors
       Pulmonary fibrosis (chronic) due to inhalation of chemicals, gases, fumes and vapors
      `EXCLUDES 1`   chronic pulmonary edema due to chemicals, gases, fumes and vapors (J68.1)

   J68.8 **Other respiratory conditions due to chemicals, gases, fumes and vapors**   `HCC` `ESR` `COM`

   J68.9 **Unspecified respiratory condition due to chemicals, gases, fumes and vapors**   `HCC` `ESR` `COM`

✓4th **J69** **Pneumonitis due to solids and liquids**
    `EXCLUDES 1`   neonatal aspiration syndromes (P24.-)
            postprocedural pneumonitis (J95.4)
    AHA: 2017,1Q,24
    DEF: Pneumonitis: Noninfectious inflammation of the walls of the alveoli in the lung tissue due to inhalation of food, vomit, oils, essences, or other solids or liquids.

   J69.0 **Pneumonitis due to** inhalation of food and vomit   `HCC` `ESR` `COM`
       Aspiration pneumonia NOS
       Aspiration pneumonia (due to) food (regurgitated)
       Aspiration pneumonia (due to) gastric secretions
       Aspiration pneumonia (due to) milk
       Aspiration pneumonia (due to) vomit
       Code also any associated foreign body in respiratory tract (T17.-)
      `EXCLUDES 1`   chemical pneumonitis due to anesthesia (J95.4)
                obstetric aspiration pneumonia (O74.0)
       AHA: 2020,2Q,11,28; 2019,3Q,17; 2019,2Q,6,31

   J69.1 **Pneumonitis due to** inhalation of oils and essences
       Exogenous lipoid pneumonia   `HCC` `ESR` `COM`
       Lipid pneumonia NOS
       Code first (T51-T65) to identify substance
      `EXCLUDES 1`   endogenous lipoid pneumonia (J84.89)

   J69.8 **Pneumonitis due to inhalation of other solids and liquids**   `HCC` `ESR` `COM`
       Pneumonitis due to aspiration of blood
       Pneumonitis due to aspiration of detergent
       Code first (T51-T65) to identify substance

✓4th **J70** **Respiratory conditions due to other external agents**

   J70.0 **Acute pulmonary manifestations due to radiation**   `HCC` `ESR` `COM`
       Radiation pneumonitis
       Use additional code (W88-W90, X39.0-) to identify the external cause

   J70.1 **Chronic and other pulmonary manifestations due to radiation**   `HCC` `ESR` `COM`
       Fibrosis of lung following radiation
       Use additional code (W88-W90, X39.0-) to identify the external cause

   J70.2 **Acute drug-induced interstitial lung disorders**   `HCC` `ESR`
       Use additional code for adverse effect, if applicable, to identify drug (T36-T50 with fifth or sixth character 5)
      `EXCLUDES 1`   interstitial pneumonia NOS (J84.9)
                lymphoid interstitial pneumonia (J84.2)
       AHA: 2019,2Q,28

   J70.3 **Chronic drug-induced interstitial lung disorders**   `HCC` `ESR`
       Use additional code for adverse effect, if applicable, to identify drug (T36-T50 with fifth or sixth character 5)
      `EXCLUDES 1`   interstitial pneumonia NOS (J84.9)
                lymphoid interstitial pneumonia (J84.2)

   J70.4 **Drug-induced interstitial lung disorders, unspecified**   `HCC` `ESR`
       Use additional code for adverse effect, if applicable, to identify drug (T36-T50 with fifth or sixth character 5)
      `EXCLUDES 1`   interstitial pneumonia NOS (J84.9)
                lymphoid interstitial pneumonia (J84.2)
       AHA: 2019,2Q,28

`HCC` CMS-HCC   `Rx` Rx HCC   `ESR` ESRD HCC   `COM` Commercial HCC   `N` Newborn: 0   `P` Pediatric: 0-17   `M` Maternity: 9-64   `A` Adult: 15-124

716   ICD 10 CM 2023

J70.5 **Respiratory conditions due to** smoke inhalation   `HCC` `ESR`
Code first smoke inhalation (T59.81-)
> EXCLUDES 2   *smoke inhalation due to chemicals, gases, fumes and vapors (J68.9)*

AHA: 2013,4Q,121

J70.8 **Respiratory conditions due to other specified external agents**   `HCC` `ESR`
Code first (T51-T65) to identify the external agent

J70.9 **Respiratory conditions due to unspecified external agent**   `HCC` `ESR`
Code first (T51-T65) to identify the external agent

Other respiratory diseases principally affecting the interstitium (J80-J84)

J80 **Acute respiratory distress syndrome**   `HCC` `ESR` `COM`
Acute respiratory distress syndrome in adult or child
Adult hyaline membrane disease
> EXCLUDES 1   *respiratory distress syndrome in newborn (perinatal) (P22.0)*

AHA: 2021,1Q,23; 2020,4Q,96; 2020,1Q,34-36; 2017,1Q,26
DEF: Lung inflammation or injury resulting in a build-up of fluid in the air sacs, preventing the passage of oxygen from the air into the bloodstream.
TIP: Assign as a secondary code for a patient with acute respiratory distress syndrome (ARDS) due to COVID-19; assign code U07.1 as the principal or first-listed code.

✓4ᵗʰ J81 **Pulmonary edema**
Use additional code to identify:
exposure to environmental tobacco smoke (Z77.22)
history of tobacco dependence (Z87.891)
occupational exposure to environmental tobacco smoke (Z57.31)
tobacco dependence (F17.-)
tobacco use (Z72.0)
> EXCLUDES 1   *chemical (acute) pulmonary edema (J68.1)*
> *hypostatic pneumonia (J18.2)*
> *passive pneumonia (J18.2)*
> *pulmonary edema due to external agents (J60-J70)*
> *pulmonary edema with heart disease NOS (I50.1)*
> *pulmonary edema with heart failure (I50.1)*

DEF: Accumulation of fluid in the air sacs of the lungs, making it difficult to breathe.

J81.0 **Acute pulmonary edema**   `HCC` `ESR` `COM`
Acute edema of lung
AHA: 2020,3Q,27

J81.1 **Chronic pulmonary edema**   `COM`
Pulmonary congestion (chronic) (passive)
Pulmonary edema NOS

✓4ᵗʰ J82 **Pulmonary eosinophilia, not elsewhere classified**
> EXCLUDES 2   *pulmonary eosinophilia due to aspergillosis (B44.-)*
> *pulmonary eosinophilia due to drugs (J70.2-J70.4)*
> *pulmonary eosinophilia due to specified parasitic infection (B50-B83)*
> *pulmonary eosinophilia due to systemic connective tissue disorders (M30-M36)*
> *pulmonary infiltrate NOS (R91.8)*

DEF: Infiltration of eosinophils (white blood cells of the immune system) into the parenchyma of the lungs, resulting in cough, fever, and dyspnea.

✓5ᵗʰ J82.8 **Pulmonary eosinophilia, not elsewhere classified**
AHA: 2020,4Q,25-27

J82.81 **Chronic eosinophilic pneumonia**   `HCC` `Rx` `ESR` `COM`
Eosinophilic pneumonia, NOS

J82.82 **Acute eosinophilic pneumonia**

J82.83 **Eosinophilic asthma**   `Rx` `COM`
Code first asthma, by type, such as:
mild intermittent asthma (J45.2-)
mild persistent asthma (J45.3-)
moderate persistent asthma (J45.4-)
severe persistent asthma (J45.5-)

J82.89 **Other pulmonary eosinophilia, not elsewhere classified**   `HCC` `ESR` `COM`
Allergic pneumonia
Löffler's pneumonia
Tropical (pulmonary) eosinophilia NOS

✓4ᵗʰ J84 **Other** interstitial **pulmonary diseases**
> EXCLUDES 1   *drug-induced interstitial lung disorders (J70.2-J70.4)*
> *interstitial emphysema (J98.2)*
> EXCLUDES 2   *lung diseases due to external agents (J60-J70)*

DEF: Interstitial: Within the small spaces or gaps occurring in tissue or organs.

✓5ᵗʰ J84.0 **Alveolar and parieto-alveolar conditions**

J84.01 **Alveolar proteinosis**   `HCC` `Rx` `ESR` `COM`
DEF: Reduced ventilation due to proteinaceous deposits on alveoli. Symptoms include dyspnea, cough, chest pain, weakness, weight loss, and hemoptysis.

J84.02 **Pulmonary alveolar microlithiasis**   `HCC` `Rx` `ESR` `COM`

J84.03 *Idiopathic pulmonary hemosiderosis*   `HCC` `Rx` `ESR` `COM`
Essential brown induration of lung
Code first underlying disease, such as:
disorders of iron metabolism (E83.1-)
> EXCLUDES 1   *acute idiopathic pulmonary hemorrhage in infants [AIPHI] (R04.81)*

DEF: Fibrosis of the alveolar walls marked by abnormal accumulation of iron as hemosiderin in the lungs. It primarily affects children and symptoms include anemia, fluid in the lungs, and blood in the sputum. Etiology is unknown.

J84.09 **Other alveolar and parieto-alveolar conditions**   `HCC` `Rx` `ESR` `COM`

✓5ᵗʰ J84.1 **Other interstitial pulmonary diseases with fibrosis**
> EXCLUDES 1   *pulmonary fibrosis (chronic) due to inhalation of chemicals, gases, fumes or vapors (J68.4)*
> *pulmonary fibrosis (chronic) following radiation (J70.1)*

J84.10 **Pulmonary fibrosis, unspecified**   `HCC` `Rx` `ESR` `COM`
Capillary fibrosis of lung
Cirrhosis of lung (chronic) NOS
Fibrosis of lung (atrophic) (chronic) (confluent) (massive) (perialveolar) (peribronchial) NOS
Induration of lung (chronic) NOS
Postinflammatory pulmonary fibrosis

✓6ᵗʰ J84.11 **Idiopathic interstitial pneumonia**
> EXCLUDES 1   *lymphoid interstitial pneumonia (J84.2)*
> *pneumocystis pneumonia (B59)*

J84.111 **Idiopathic interstitial pneumonia, not otherwise specified**   `HCC` `Rx` `ESR` `COM`

J84.112 **Idiopathic pulmonary fibrosis**   `HCC` `Rx` `ESR` `COM`
Cryptogenic fibrosing alveolitis
Idiopathic fibrosing alveolitis

J84.113 **Idiopathic non-specific interstitial pneumonitis**   `HCC` `Rx` `ESR` `COM`
> EXCLUDES 1   *non-specific interstitial pneumonia NOS, or due to known underlying cause (J84.89)*

J84.114 **Acute interstitial pneumonitis**   `HCC` `Rx` `ESR` `COM`
Hamman-Rich syndrome
> EXCLUDES 1   *pneumocystis pneumonia (B59)*

J84.115 **Respiratory bronchiolitis interstitial lung disease**   `HCC` `Rx` `ESR` `COM`

J84.116 **Cryptogenic organizing pneumonia**   `HCC` `Rx` `ESR` `COM`
> EXCLUDES 1   *organizing pneumonia NOS, or due to known underlying cause (J84.89)*

J84.117 **Desquamative interstitial pneumonia**   `HCC` `Rx` `ESR` `COM`

√6ᵗʰ **J84.17 Other interstitial pulmonary diseases with fibrosis in diseases classified elsewhere**
AHA: 2020,4Q,27-28

J84.170 Interstitial lung disease with progressive fibrotic phenotype in diseases classified elsewhere HCC Rx ESR COM
Progressive fibrotic interstitial lung disease
Code first underlying disease, such as:
lung diseases due to external agents (J60-J70)
rheumatoid arthritis (M05.00-M06.9)
sarcoidosis (D86)
systemic connective tissue disorders (M30-M36)

J84.178 Other interstitial pulmonary diseases with fibrosis in diseases classified elsewhere HCC Rx ESR COM
Interstitial pneumonia (nonspecific) (usual) due to collagen vascular disease
Interstitial pneumonia (nonspecific) (usual) in diseases classified elsewhere
Organizing pneumonia due to collagen vascular disease
Organizing pneumonia in diseases classified elsewhere
Code first underlying disease, such as:
progressive systemic sclerosis (M34.0)
rheumatoid arthritis (M05.00-M06.9)
systemic lupus erythematosis (M32.0-M32.9)

J84.2 Lymphoid interstitial pneumonia HCC Rx ESR COM
Lymphoid interstitial pneumonitis

√5ᵗʰ **J84.8 Other specified interstitial pulmonary diseases**
EXCLUDES 1   *exogenous lipoid pneumonia (J69.1)*
unspecified lipoid pneumonia (J69.1)

J84.81 Lymphangioleiomyomatosis HCC Rx ESR COM
Lymphangiomyomatosis

J84.82 Adult pulmonary Langerhans cell histiocytosis HCC Rx ESR COM A
Adult PLCH

J84.83 Surfactant mutations of the lung HCC Rx ESR COM
DEF: Genetic disorder resulting in insufficient secretion of a complex mixture of phospholipids and proteins that reduce surface tension in the alveoli following the onset of breathing to facilitate lung expansion in the newborn. It is the leading indication for pediatric lung transplantation.

√6ᵗʰ **J84.84 Other interstitial lung diseases of childhood**

J84.841 Neuroendocrine cell hyperplasia of infancy HCC Rx ESR COM

J84.842 Pulmonary interstitial glycogenosis HCC Rx ESR COM

J84.843 Alveolar capillary dysplasia with vein misalignment HCC Rx ESR COM

J84.848 Other interstitial lung diseases of childhood HCC Rx ESR COM

J84.89 Other specified interstitial pulmonary diseases HCC Rx ESR COM
Endogenous lipoid pneumonia
Interstitial pneumonitis
Non-specific interstitial pneumonitis NOS
Organizing pneumonia NOS
Code first, if applicable:
poisoning due to drug or toxin (T51-T65 with fifth or sixth character to indicate intent), for toxic pneumonopathy
underlying cause of pneumonopathy, if known
Use additional code, for adverse effect, to identify drug (T36-T50 with fifth or sixth character 5), if drug-induced
EXCLUDES 1   *cryptogenic organizing pneumonia (J84.116)*
idiopathic non-specific interstitial pneumonitis (J84.113)
lymphoid interstitial pneumonia (J84.2)
lipoid pneumonia, exogenous or unspecified (J69.1)
AHA: 2021,4Q,106; 2021,1Q,48; 2019,2Q,28

J84.9 Interstitial pulmonary disease, unspecified HCC Rx ESR COM
Interstitial pneumonia NOS

Suppurative and necrotic conditions of the lower respiratory tract (J85-J86)

√4ᵗʰ **J85 Abscess of lung and mediastinum**
Use additional code (B95-B97) to identify infectious agent

J85.0 Gangrene and necrosis of lung HCC ESR COM

J85.1 Abscess of lung with pneumonia HCC ESR COM
Code also the type of pneumonia

J85.2 Abscess of lung without pneumonia HCC ESR COM
Abscess of lung NOS

J85.3 Abscess of mediastinum HCC ESR COM

√4ᵗʰ **J86 Pyothorax**
Use additional code (B95-B97) to identify infectious agent
EXCLUDES 1   *abscess of lung (J85.-)*
pyothorax due to tuberculosis (A15.6)
DEF: Collection of pus in the pleural space that is commonly caused by an infection that spreads from the lung, such as bacterial pneumonia or a lung abscess.

J86.0 Pyothorax with fistula HCC ESR COM
Bronchocutaneous fistula
Bronchopleural fistula
Hepatopleural fistula
Mediastinal fistula
Pleural fistula
Thoracic fistula
Any condition classifiable to J86.9 with fistula
DEF: Purulent infection of the respiratory cavity, with communication from a cavity to another structure.

J86.9 Pyothorax without fistula HCC ESR COM
Abscess of pleura
Abscess of thorax
Empyema (chest) (lung) (pleura)
Fibrinopurulent pleurisy
Purulent pleurisy
Pyopneumothorax
Septic pleurisy
Seropurulent pleurisy
Suppurative pleurisy

Other diseases of the pleura (J90-J94)

J90 Pleural effusion, not elsewhere classified
Encysted pleurisy
Pleural effusion NOS
Pleurisy with effusion (exudative) (serous)
EXCLUDES 1   *chylous (pleural) effusion (J94.0)*
malignant pleural effusion (J91.0)
pleurisy NOS (R09.1)
tuberculous pleural effusion (A15.6)
DEF: Collection of lymph and other fluid within the pleural space.

☑️4ᵗʰ **J91 Pleural effusion in conditions classified elsewhere**

> EXCLUDES 2   *pleural effusion in heart failure (I50.-)*
> *pleural effusion in systemic lupus erythematosus (M32.13)*

DEF: Collection of lymph and other fluid within the pleural space.

J91.0 *Malignant pleural effusion*
> Code first underlying neoplasm ▶(C00-D49)◀

J91.8 *Pleural effusion in other conditions classified elsewhere*
> Code first underlying disease, such as:
> filariasis (B74.0-B74.9)
> influenza (J09.X2, J10.1, J11.1)
> **AHA:** 2015,2Q,15
> **TIP:** Assign this code as a secondary diagnosis to congestive heart failure (I50.-) only if pleural effusion is specifically evaluated or treated.

Pleural Effusion

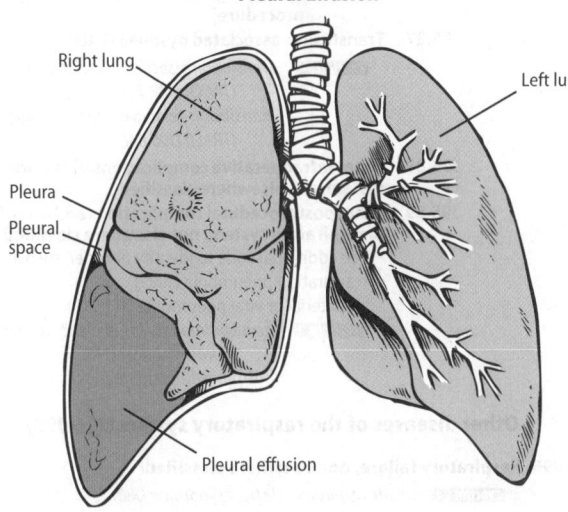

Right lung

Left lung

Pleura

Pleural space

Pleural effusion

☑️4ᵗʰ **J92 Pleural plaque**

> INCLUDES   pleural thickening

DEF: Areas of fibrous thickening that form on the parietal or visceral pleura, the membranes that line the ribs and lungs.

J92.0 Pleural plaque with presence of asbestos

J92.9 Pleural plaque without asbestos
> Pleural plaque NOS

☑️4ᵗʰ **J93 Pneumothorax and air leak**

> EXCLUDES 1   *congenital or perinatal pneumothorax (P25.1)*
> *postprocedural air leak (J95.812)*
> *postprocedural pneumothorax (J95.811)*
> *pyopneumothorax (J86.-)*
> *traumatic pneumothorax (S27.0)*
> *tuberculous (current disease) pneumothorax (A15.-)*

DEF: Pneumothorax: Lung displacement due to abnormal leakage of air or gas that is trapped in the pleural space formed by the membrane that encloses the lungs and lines the thoracic cavity.

J93.0 Spontaneous tension pneumothorax
> **DEF:** Leaking air from the lung into the lining, causing collapse.

☑️5ᵗʰ **J93.1 Other** spontaneous **pneumothorax**

     J93.11 Primary spontaneous pneumothorax

     J93.12 Secondary spontaneous pneumothorax   UPD
> Code first underlying condition, such as:
> catamenial pneumothorax due to endometriosis ▶(N80.B-)◀
> cystic fibrosis (E84.-)
> eosinophilic pneumonia (J82)
> lymphangioleiomyomatosis (J84.81)
> malignant neoplasm of bronchus and lung (C34.-)
> Marfan's syndrome (Q87.4)
> pneumonia due to Pneumocystis carinii (B59)
> secondary malignant neoplasm of lung (C78.0-)
> spontaneous rupture of the esophagus (K22.3)

☑️5ᵗʰ **J93.8 Other** pneumothorax and air leak

     J93.81 Chronic pneumothorax

     J93.82 Other air leak
> Persistent air leak

     J93.83 Other pneumothorax
> Acute pneumothorax
> Spontaneous pneumothorax NOS
> **AHA:** 2020,3Q,9-10

J93.9 Pneumothorax, unspecified
> Pneumothorax NOS

☑️4ᵗʰ **J94 Other pleural conditions**

> EXCLUDES 1   *pleurisy NOS (R09.1)*
> *traumatic hemopneumothorax (S27.2)*
> *traumatic hemothorax (S27.1)*
> *tuberculous pleural conditions (current disease) (A15.-)*

J94.0 Chylous effusion
> Chyliform effusion
> **DEF:** Fluid within the pleural space due to the leaking of lymph contents into the space, usually as a result of thoracic duct damage or injury or mediastinal lymphoma.

J94.1 Fibrothorax
> **DEF:** Fibrosis within the pleural lining of the lungs commonly seen as a stiff layer surrounding the lung typically attributed to traumatic hemothorax or pleural effusion.

J94.2 Hemothorax
> Hemopneumothorax

J94.8 Other specified pleural conditions
> Hydropneumothorax
> Hydrothorax
> **AHA:** 2021,1Q,48

J94.9 Pleural condition, unspecified

Intraoperative and postprocedural complications and disorders of respiratory system, not elsewhere classified (J95)

☑️4ᵗʰ **J95 Intraoperative and postprocedural complications and disorders of respiratory system, not elsewhere classified**

> EXCLUDES 2   *aspiration pneumonia (J69.-)*
> *emphysema (subcutaneous) resulting from a procedure (T81.82)*
> *hypostatic pneumonia (J18.2)*
> *pulmonary manifestations due to radiation (J70.0-J70.1)*

☑️5ᵗʰ **J95.0 Tracheostomy complications**
> **DEF:** Tracheostomy: Formation of a tracheal opening on the neck surface with tube insertion to allow for respiration in cases of obstruction or decreased patency. A tracheostomy may be planned or performed on an emergency basis for temporary or long-term use.

     J95.00 Unspecified tracheostomy complication   HCC ESR COM

     J95.01 Hemorrhage from tracheostomy stoma   HCC ESR COM

     J95.02 Infection of tracheostomy stoma   HCC ESR COM
> Use additional code to identify type of infection, such as:
> cellulitis of neck (L03.221)
> sepsis (A40, A41.-)

     J95.03 Malfunction of tracheostomy stoma   HCC ESR COM
> Mechanical complication of tracheostomy stoma
> Obstruction of tracheostomy airway
> Tracheal stenosis due to tracheostomy

     J95.04 Tracheo-esophageal fistula following tracheostomy   HCC ESR COM

     J95.09 Other tracheostomy complication   HCC ESR COM

J95.1 Acute pulmonary insufficiency following thoracic surgery   HCC ESR
> EXCLUDES 2   *functional disturbances following cardiac surgery (I97.0, I97.1-)*

J95.2 Acute pulmonary insufficiency following nonthoracic surgery   HCC ESR
> EXCLUDES 2   *functional disturbances following cardiac surgery (I97.0, I97.1-)*

J95.3 Chronic pulmonary insufficiency following surgery   HCC ESR
> EXCLUDES 2   *functional disturbances following cardiac surgery (I97.0, I97.1-)*

Chapter 10. Diseases of the Respiratory System

J95.4 **Chemical pneumonitis due to anesthesia**
Mendelson's syndrome
Postprocedural aspiration pneumonia
Use additional code for adverse effect, if applicable, to identify drug (T41.- with fifth or sixth character 5)
> EXCLUDES 1   *aspiration pneumonitis due to anesthesia complicating labor and delivery (O74.0)*
> *aspiration pneumonitis due to anesthesia complicating pregnancy (O29)*
> *aspiration pneumonitis due to anesthesia complicating the puerperium (O89.01)*

J95.5 **Postprocedural subglottic stenosis**

✓5ᵗʰ J95.6 **Intraoperative hemorrhage and hematoma of a respiratory system organ or structure complicating a procedure**
> EXCLUDES 1   *intraoperative hemorrhage and hematoma of a respiratory system organ or structure due to accidental puncture and laceration during procedure (J95.7-)*

   J95.61 **Intraoperative hemorrhage and hematoma of a respiratory system organ or structure complicating a respiratory system procedure**

   J95.62 **Intraoperative hemorrhage and hematoma of a respiratory system organ or structure complicating other procedure**

✓5ᵗʰ J95.7 **Accidental puncture and laceration of a respiratory system organ or structure during a procedure**
> EXCLUDES 2   *postprocedural pneumothorax (J95.811)*

   J95.71 **Accidental puncture and laceration of a respiratory system organ or structure during a respiratory system procedure**

   J95.72 **Accidental puncture and laceration of a respiratory system organ or structure during other procedure**

✓5ᵗʰ J95.8 **Other intraoperative and postprocedural complications and disorders of respiratory system, not elsewhere classified**
AHA: 2016,4Q,9-10

   ✓6ᵗʰ J95.81 **Postprocedural pneumothorax and air leak**

     J95.811 **Postprocedural pneumothorax**
AHA: 2021,1Q,48

     J95.812 **Postprocedural air leak**

   ✓6ᵗʰ J95.82 **Postprocedural respiratory failure**
> EXCLUDES 1   *respiratory failure in other conditions (J96.-)*

     J95.821 **Acute postprocedural respiratory failure** `HCC` `ESR`
Postprocedural respiratory failure NOS

     J95.822 **Acute and chronic postprocedural respiratory failure** `HCC` `ESR`

   ✓6ᵗʰ J95.83 **Postprocedural hemorrhage of a respiratory system organ or structure following a procedure**

     J95.830 **Postprocedural hemorrhage of a respiratory system organ or structure following a respiratory system procedure**

     J95.831 **Postprocedural hemorrhage of a respiratory system organ or structure following other procedure**

   J95.84 **Transfusion-related acute lung injury (TRALI)**
DEF: Relatively rare, but serious, pulmonary complication of blood transfusion, with acute respiratory distress, noncardiogenic pulmonary edema, cyanosis, hypoxemia, hypotension, fever, and chills.

   ✓6ᵗʰ J95.85 **Complication of respirator [ventilator]**

     J95.850 **Mechanical complication of respirator** `HCC` `ESR` `COM`
> EXCLUDES 1   *encounter for respirator [ventilator] dependence during power failure (Z99.12)*

     J95.851 **Ventilator associated pneumonia** `HCC` `ESR`
Ventilator associated pneumonitis
Use additional code to identify the organism, if known (B95.-, B96.-, B97.-)
> EXCLUDES 1   *ventilator lung in newborn (P27.8)*
AHA: 2020,2Q,17; 2017,1Q,25

     J95.859 **Other complication of respirator [ventilator]** `HCC` `ESR` `COM`
AHA: 2021,1Q,48

   ✓6ᵗʰ J95.86 **Postprocedural hematoma and seroma of a respiratory system organ or structure following a procedure**

     J95.860 **Postprocedural hematoma of a respiratory system organ or structure following a respiratory system procedure**

     J95.861 **Postprocedural hematoma of a respiratory system organ or structure following other procedure**

     J95.862 **Postprocedural seroma of a respiratory system organ or structure following a respiratory system procedure**

     J95.863 **Postprocedural seroma of a respiratory system organ or structure following other procedure**

   ● J95.87 **Transfusion-associated dyspnea (TAD)**
> EXCLUDES 1   *transfusion associated circulatory overload (TACO) (E87.71)*
> *transfusion-related acute lung injury (TRALI) (J95.84)*

   J95.88 **Other intraoperative complications of respiratory system, not elsewhere classified**

   J95.89 **Other postprocedural complications and disorders of respiratory system, not elsewhere classified**
Use additional code to identify disorder, such as:
   aspiration pneumonia (J69.-)
   bacterial or viral pneumonia (J12-J18)
> EXCLUDES 2   *acute pulmonary insufficiency following thoracic surgery (J95.1)*
> *postprocedural subglottic stenosis (J95.5)*

Other diseases of the respiratory system (J96-J99)

✓4ᵗʰ J96 **Respiratory failure, not elsewhere classified**
> EXCLUDES 1   *acute respiratory distress syndrome (J80)*
> *cardiorespiratory failure (R09.2)*
> *newborn respiratory distress syndrome (P22.0)*
> *postprocedural respiratory failure (J95.82-)*
> *respiratory arrest (R09.2)*
> *respiratory arrest of newborn (P28.81)*
> *respiratory failure of newborn (P28.5)*
AHA: 2021,1Q,27,44-45; 2020,4Q,96

   ✓5ᵗʰ J96.0 **Acute respiratory failure**

     J96.00 **Acute respiratory failure, unspecified whether with hypoxia or hypercapnia** `HCC` `ESR` `COM`
AHA: 2016,3Q,14; 2013,4Q,121

     J96.01 **Acute respiratory failure with hypoxia** `HCC` `ESR` `COM`
AHA: 2020,3Q,12

     J96.02 **Acute respiratory failure with hypercapnia** `HCC` `ESR` `COM`
▶Acute respiratory acidosis◀

   ✓5ᵗʰ J96.1 **Chronic respiratory failure**

     J96.10 **Chronic respiratory failure, unspecified whether with hypoxia or hypercapnia** `HCC` `ESR` `COM`
AHA: 2016,1Q,38; 2015,1Q,21

     J96.11 **Chronic respiratory failure with hypoxia** `HCC` `ESR` `COM`
AHA: 2013,4Q,129

     J96.12 **Chronic respiratory failure with hypercapnia** `HCC` `ESR` `COM`
▶Chronic respiratory acidosis◀

   ✓5ᵗʰ J96.2 **Acute and chronic respiratory failure**
Acute on chronic respiratory failure

     J96.20 **Acute and chronic respiratory failure, unspecified whether with hypoxia or hypercapnia** `HCC` `ESR` `COM`

     J96.21 **Acute and chronic respiratory failure with hypoxia** `HCC` `ESR` `COM`

     J96.22 **Acute and chronic respiratory failure with hypercapnia** `HCC` `ESR` `COM`

   ✓5ᵗʰ J96.9 **Respiratory failure, unspecified**

     J96.90 **Respiratory failure, unspecified, unspecified whether with hypoxia or hypercapnia** `HCC` `ESR` `COM`

`HCC` CMS-HCC   `Rx` Rx HCC   `ESR` ESRD HCC   `COM` Commercial HCC   `N` Newborn: 0   `P` Pediatric: 0-17   `M` Maternity: 9-64   `A` Adult: 15-124

720   ICD-10-CM 2023

J96.91   **Respiratory failure, unspecified with hypoxia**   `HCC` `ESR` `COM`

J96.92   **Respiratory failure, unspecified with hypercapnia**   `HCC` `ESR` `COM`

√4ᵗʰ **J98**   **Other respiratory disorders**

Use additional code to identify:

exposure to environmental tobacco smoke (Z77.22)

exposure to tobacco smoke in the perinatal period (P96.81)

history of tobacco dependence (Z87.891)

occupational exposure to environmental tobacco smoke (Z57.31)

tobacco dependence (F17.-)

tobacco use (Z72.0)

EXCLUDES 1   *newborn apnea ▶(P28.4-)◀*

       newborn sleep apnea ▶(P28.3-)◀

EXCLUDES 2   *apnea NOS (R06.81)*

       sleep apnea (G47.3-)

√5ᵗʰ **J98.0**   **Diseases of bronchus, not elsewhere classified**

J98.01   **Acute bronchospasm**

EXCLUDES 1   *acute bronchiolitis with bronchospasm (J21.-)*

       acute bronchitis with bronchospasm (J20.-)

       asthma (J45.-)

       exercise induced bronchospasm (J45.990)

J98.09   **Other diseases of bronchus, not elsewhere classified**

Broncholithiasis

Calcification of bronchus

Stenosis of bronchus

Tracheobronchial collapse

Tracheobronchial dyskinesia

Ulcer of bronchus

√5ᵗʰ **J98.1**   **Pulmonary collapse**

EXCLUDES 1   *therapeutic collapse of lung status (Z98.3)*

J98.11   **Atelectasis**

EXCLUDES 1   *newborn atelectasis*

       tuberculous atelectasis (current disease) (A15)

DEF: Collapse of lung tissue affecting part or all of one lung, preventing normal oxygen absorption to healthy tissues.

J98.19   **Other pulmonary collapse**

J98.2   **Interstitial emphysema**   `HCC` `Rx` `ESR` `COM`

Mediastinal emphysema

EXCLUDES 1   *emphysema NOS (J43.9)*

       emphysema in newborn (P25.0)

       surgical emphysema (subcutaneous) (T81.82)

       traumatic subcutaneous emphysema (T79.7)

J98.3   **Compensatory emphysema**   `HCC` `Rx` `ESR` `COM`

DEF: Distention of all or part of the lung caused by disease processes or surgical intervention that decreased volume in another part of the lung, causing an overcompensation reaction. Compensatory emphysema occurs in association with pneumonias, pleural effusions, atelectasis, empyema, and pneumothorax.

J98.4   **Other disorders of lung**

Calcification of lung

Cystic lung disease (acquired)

Lung disease NOS

Pulmolithiasis

EXCLUDES 1   *acute interstitial pneumonitis (J84.114)*

       pulmonary insufficiency following surgery (J95.1-J95.2)

√5ᵗʰ **J98.5**   **Diseases of mediastinum, not elsewhere classified**

EXCLUDES 2   *abscess of mediastinum (J85.3)*

AHA: 2016,4Q,29

J98.51   **Mediastinitis**

Code first underlying condition, if applicable, such as postoperative mediastinitis (T81.-)

J98.59   **Other diseases of mediastinum, not elsewhere classified**

Fibrosis of mediastinum

Hernia of mediastinum

Retraction of mediastinum

J98.6   **Disorders of diaphragm**

Diaphragmatitis

Paralysis of diaphragm

Relaxation of diaphragm

EXCLUDES 1   *congenital malformation of diaphragm NEC (Q79.1)*

       congenital diaphragmatic hernia (Q79.0)

EXCLUDES 2   *diaphragmatic hernia (K44.-)*

J98.8   **Other specified respiratory disorders**

AHA: 2020,1Q,34-36

TIP: Assign as a secondary code for a patient with a respiratory infection that is not further specified but is documented as being associated with COVID-19; assign U07.1 as the principal or first-listed code. If the respiratory infection documentation specifies acute or lower respiratory infection (NOS), assign J22 instead.

J98.9   **Respiratory disorder, unspecified**

Respiratory disease (chronic) NOS

J99   ***Respiratory disorders in diseases classified elsewhere***   `HCC` `Rx` `ESR` `COM`

Code first underlying disease, such as:

amyloidosis (E85.-)

ankylosing spondylitis (M45)

congenital syphilis (A50.5)

cryoglobulinemia (D89.1)

early congenital syphilis (A50.0)

plasminogen deficiency (E88.02)

schistosomiasis (B65.0-B65.9)

EXCLUDES 1   *respiratory disorders in:*

       amebiasis (A06.5)

       blastomycosis (B40.0-B40.2)

       candidiasis (B37.1)

       coccidioidomycosis (B38.0-B38.2)

       cystic fibrosis with pulmonary manifestations (E84.0)

       dermatomyositis (M33.01, M33.11)

       histoplasmosis (B39.0-B39.2)

       late syphilis (A52.72, A52.73)

       polymyositis (M33.21)

       Sjögren syndrome (M35.02)

       systemic lupus erythematosus (M32.13)

       systemic sclerosis (M34.81)

       Wegener's granulomatosis (M31.30-M31.31)

☑ Additional Character Required   √x7ᵗʰ Placeholder Alert   Manifestation   Unspecified Dx   ◑ QPP   UPD Unacceptable PDx

Chapter 11. Diseases of the Digestive System (K00–K95)

Chapter-specific Guidelines with Coding Examples
Reserved for future guideline expansion.

Chapter 11. Diseases of the Digestive System (K00-K95)

> EXCLUDES 2   certain conditions originating in the perinatal period (P04-P96)
> certain infectious and parasitic diseases (A00-B99)
> complications of pregnancy, childbirth and the puerperium (O00-O9A)
> congenital malformations, deformations and chromosomal abnormalities (Q00-Q99)
> endocrine, nutritional and metabolic diseases (E00-E88)
> injury, poisoning and certain other consequences of external causes (S00-T88)
> neoplasms (C00-D49)
> symptoms, signs and abnormal clinical and laboratory findings, not elsewhere classified (R00-R94)

This chapter contains the following blocks:

K00-K14   Diseases of oral cavity and salivary glands
K20-K31   Diseases of esophagus, stomach and duodenum
K35-K38   Diseases of appendix
K40-K46   Hernia
K50-K52   Noninfective enteritis and colitis
K55-K64   Other diseases of intestines
K65-K68   Diseases of peritoneum and retroperitoneum
K70-K77   Diseases of liver
K80-K87   Disorders of gallbladder, biliary tract and pancreas
K90-K95   Other diseases of the digestive system

Diseases of oral cavity and salivary glands (K00-K14)

K00   Disorders of tooth development and eruption
> EXCLUDES 2   embedded and impacted teeth (K01.-)

K00.0   Anodontia
Hypodontia
Oligodontia
> EXCLUDES 1   acquired absence of teeth (K08.1-)

DEF: Partial or complete absence of teeth due to a congenital defect involving the tooth bud.

K00.1   Supernumerary teeth
Distomolar
Fourth molar
Mesiodens
Paramolar
Supplementary teeth
> EXCLUDES 2   supernumerary roots (K00.2)

K00.2   Abnormalities of size and form of teeth
Concrescence of teeth
Fusion of teeth
Gemination of teeth
Dens evaginatus
Dens in dente
Dens invaginatus
Enamel pearls
Macrodontia
Microdontia
Peg-shaped [conical] teeth
Supernumerary roots
Taurodontism
Tuberculum paramolare
> EXCLUDES 1   abnormalities of teeth due to congenital syphilis (A50.5)
> tuberculum Carabelli, which is regarded as a normal variation and should not be coded

K00.3   Mottled teeth
Dental fluorosis
Mottling of enamel
Nonfluoride enamel opacities
> EXCLUDES 2   deposits [accretions] on teeth (K03.6)

K00.4   Disturbances in tooth formation
Aplasia and hypoplasia of cementum
Dilaceration of tooth
Enamel hypoplasia (neonatal) (postnatal) (prenatal)
Regional odontodysplasia
Turner's tooth
> EXCLUDES 1   Hutchinson's teeth and mulberry molars in congenital syphilis (A50.5)
> EXCLUDES 2   mottled teeth (K00.3)

K00.5   Hereditary disturbances in tooth structure, not elsewhere classified
Amelogenesis imperfecta
Dentinogenesis imperfecta
Odontogenesis imperfecta
Dentinal dysplasia
Shell teeth

K00.6   Disturbances in tooth eruption
Dentia praecox
Natal tooth
Neonatal tooth
Premature eruption of tooth
Premature shedding of primary [deciduous] tooth
Prenatal teeth
Retained [persistent] primary tooth
> EXCLUDES 2   embedded and impacted teeth (K01.-)

K00.7   Teething syndrome

K00.8   Other disorders of tooth development
Color changes during tooth formation
Intrinsic staining of teeth NOS
> EXCLUDES 2   posteruptive color changes (K03.7)

K00.9   Disorder of tooth development, unspecified
Disorder of odontogenesis NOS

K01   Embedded and impacted teeth
> EXCLUDES 1   abnormal position of fully erupted teeth (M26.3-)

K01.0   Embedded teeth
K01.1   Impacted teeth

K02   Dental caries
> INCLUDES   caries of dentine
> dental cavities
> early childhood caries
> pre-eruptive caries
> recurrent caries (dentino enamel junction) (enamel) (to the pulp)
> tooth decay

Tooth Anatomy

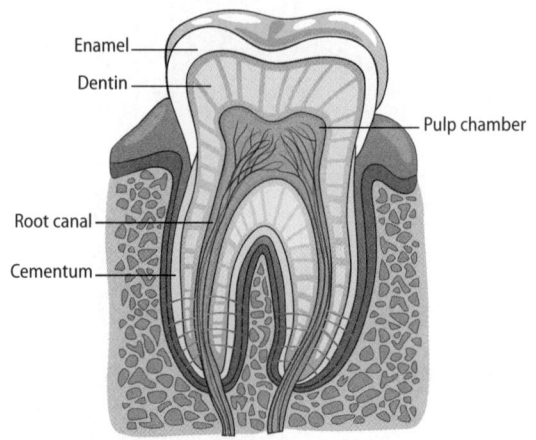

K02.3   Arrested dental caries
Arrested coronal and root caries

K02.5   Dental caries on pit and fissure surface
Dental caries on chewing surface of tooth

K02.51   Dental caries on pit and fissure surface limited to enamel
White spot lesions [initial caries] on pit and fissure surface of tooth

K02.52   Dental caries on pit and fissure surface penetrating into dentin
Primary dental caries, cervical origin

K02.53   Dental caries on pit and fissure surface penetrating into pulp

K02.6   Dental caries on smooth surface

K02.61   Dental caries on smooth surface limited to enamel
White spot lesions [initial caries] on smooth surface of tooth

K02.62   Dental caries on smooth surface penetrating into dentin

K02.63   Dental caries on smooth surface penetrating into pulp

K02.7 **Dental** root **caries**

K02.9 **Dental caries, unspecified**

✓4ᵗʰ **K03 Other diseases of hard tissues of teeth**

> EXCLUDES 2   *bruxism (F45.8)*
> *dental caries (K02.-)*
> *teeth-grinding NOS (F45.8)*

K03.0 **Excessive attrition of teeth**
> Approximal wear of teeth
> Occlusal wear of teeth
> **DEF:** Attrition: In dentistry, wearing away or erosion of tooth surface from abrasive food or grinding teeth.

K03.1 **Abrasion of teeth**
> Dentifrice abrasion of teeth
> Habitual abrasion of teeth
> Occupational abrasion of teeth
> Ritual abrasion of teeth
> Traditional abrasion of teeth
> Wedge defect NOS

K03.2 **Erosion of teeth**
> Erosion of teeth due to diet
> Erosion of teeth due to drugs and medicaments
> Erosion of teeth due to persistent vomiting
> Erosion of teeth NOS
> Idiopathic erosion of teeth
> Occupational erosion of teeth

K03.3 **Pathological resorption of teeth**
> Internal granuloma of pulp
> Resorption of teeth (external)

K03.4 **Hypercementosis**
> Cementation hyperplasia

K03.5 **Ankylosis of teeth**

K03.6 **Deposits [accretions] on teeth**
> Betel deposits [accretions] on teeth
> Black deposits [accretions] on teeth
> Extrinsic staining of teeth NOS
> Green deposits [accretions] on teeth
> Materia alba deposits [accretions] on teeth
> Orange deposits [accretions] on teeth
> Staining of teeth NOS
> Subgingival dental calculus
> Supragingival dental calculus
> Tobacco deposits [accretions] on teeth

K03.7 **Posteruptive color changes of dental hard tissues**
> EXCLUDES 2   *deposits [accretions] on teeth (K03.6)*

✓5ᵗʰ **K03.8 Other specified diseases of hard tissues of teeth**

> K03.81 **Cracked tooth**
> > EXCLUDES 1   *asymptomatic craze lines in enamel - omit code*
> > *broken or fractured tooth due to trauma (S02.5)*
>
> K03.89 **Other specified diseases of hard tissues of teeth**

K03.9 **Disease of hard tissues of teeth, unspecified**

✓4ᵗʰ **K04 Diseases of pulp and periapical tissues**
> **AHA:** 2016,4Q,29-30

✓5ᵗʰ **K04.0** Pulpitis
> Acute pulpitis
> Chronic (hyperplastic) (ulcerative) pulpitis
> K04.01 Reversible **pulpitis**
> K04.02 Irreversible **pulpitis**

K04.1 **Necrosis of pulp**
> Pulpal gangrene

K04.2 **Pulp degeneration**
> Denticles
> Pulpal calcifications
> Pulpal stones

K04.3 **Abnormal hard tissue formation in pulp**
> Secondary or irregular dentine

K04.4 **Acute apical periodontitis of pulpal origin**
> Acute apical periodontitis NOS
> EXCLUDES 1   *acute periodontitis (K05.2-)*
> **DEF:** Severe inflammation of the area surrounding the tip of a tooth's root that is often secondary to infection or trauma.

K04.5 **Chronic apical periodontitis**
> Apical or periapical granuloma
> Apical periodontitis NOS
> EXCLUDES 1   *chronic periodontitis (K05.3-)*

K04.6 **Periapical abscess with sinus**
> Dental abscess with sinus
> Dentoalveolar abscess with sinus

K04.7 **Periapical abscess without sinus**
> Dental abscess without sinus
> Dentoalveolar abscess without sinus

K04.8 **Radicular cyst**
> Apical (periodontal) cyst
> Periapical cyst
> Residual radicular cyst
> EXCLUDES 2   *lateral periodontal cyst (K09.0)*
> **DEF:** Most common odontogenic cyst in tissue around the tooth apex due to chronic inflammation of dental pulp.

✓5ᵗʰ **K04.9 Other and unspecified diseases of pulp and periapical tissues**

> K04.90 **Unspecified diseases of pulp and periapical tissues**
> K04.99 **Other diseases of pulp and periapical tissues**

✓4ᵗʰ **K05 Gingivitis and periodontal diseases**
> Use additional code to identify:
> alcohol abuse and dependence (F10.-)
> exposure to environmental tobacco smoke (Z77.22)
> exposure to tobacco smoke in the perinatal period (P96.81)
> history of tobacco dependence (Z87.891)
> occupational exposure to environmental tobacco smoke (Z57.31)
> tobacco dependence (F17.-)
> tobacco use (Z72.0)
> **AHA:** 2016,4Q,29-30

✓5ᵗʰ **K05.0 Acute gingivitis**
> > EXCLUDES 1   *acute necrotizing ulcerative gingivitis (A69.1)*
> > *herpesviral [herpes simplex] gingivostomatitis (B00.2)*
>
> K05.00 **Acute gingivitis,** plaque induced
> > Acute gingivitis NOS
> > Plaque induced gingival disease
> K05.01 **Acute gingivitis,** non-plaque induced

✓5ᵗʰ **K05.1 Chronic gingivitis**
> Desquamative gingivitis (chronic)
> Gingivitis (chronic) NOS
> Hyperplastic gingivitis (chronic)
> Pregnancy associated gingivitis
> Simple marginal gingivitis (chronic)
> Ulcerative gingivitis (chronic)
> Code first, if applicable, diseases of the digestive system complicating pregnacy (O99.61-)
>
> K05.10 **Chronic gingivitis,** plaque induced
> > Chronic gingivitis NOS
> > Gingivitis NOS
> K05.11 **Chronic gingivitis,** non-plaque induced

✓5ᵗʰ **K05.2 Aggressive periodontitis**
> Acute pericoronitis
> EXCLUDES 1   *acute apical periodontitis (K04.4)*
> *periapical abscess (K04.7)*
> *periapical abscess with sinus (K04.6)*
>
> K05.20 **Aggressive periodontitis, unspecified**
>
> ✓6ᵗʰ K05.21 **Aggressive periodontitis,** localized
> > Periodontal abscess
> > K05.211 **Aggressive periodontitis, localized,** slight
> > K05.212 **Aggressive periodontitis, localized, moderate**
> > K05.213 **Aggressive periodontitis, localized, severe**
> > K05.219 **Aggressive periodontitis, localized, unspecified severity**
>
> ✓6ᵗʰ K05.22 **Aggressive periodontitis,** generalized
> > K05.221 **Aggressive periodontitis, generalized, slight**
> > K05.222 **Aggressive periodontitis, generalized, moderate**
> > K05.223 **Aggressive periodontitis, generalized, severe**
> > K05.229 **Aggressive periodontitis, generalized, unspecified severity**

☑ Additional Character Required   ✓x7ᵗʰ Placeholder Alert   Manifestation   Unspecified Dx   🔲 QPP   UPD Unacceptable PDx

✓5ᵗʰ K05.3 Chronic periodontitis
Chronic pericoronitis
Complex periodontitis
Periodontitis NOS
Simplex periodontitis
EXCLUDES 1   *chronic apical periodontitis (K04.5)*

K05.30 Chronic periodontitis, unspecified

✓6ᵗʰ K05.31 Chronic periodontitis, localized
K05.311 Chronic periodontitis, localized, slight
K05.312 Chronic periodontitis, localized, moderate
K05.313 Chronic periodontitis, localized, severe
K05.319 Chronic periodontitis, localized, unspecified severity

✓6ᵗʰ K05.32 Chronic periodontitis, generalized
K05.321 Chronic periodontitis, generalized, slight
K05.322 Chronic periodontitis, generalized, moderate
K05.323 Chronic periodontitis, generalized, severe
K05.329 Chronic periodontitis, generalized, unspecified

K05.4 Periodontosis
Juvenile periodontosis

K05.5 Other periodontal diseases
Combined periodontic-endodontic lesion
Narrow gingival width (of periodontal soft tissue)
EXCLUDES 2   *leukoplakia of gingiva (K13.21)*

K05.6 Periodontal disease, unspecified

✓4ᵗʰ K06 Other disorders of gingiva and edentulous alveolar ridge
EXCLUDES 2   *acute gingivitis (K05.0)*
atrophy of edentulous alveolar ridge (K08.2)
chronic gingivitis (K05.1)
gingivitis NOS (K05.1)
AHA: 2016,4Q,29-30

✓5ᵗʰ K06.0 Gingival recession
Gingival recession (postinfective) (postprocedural)
AHA: 2017,4Q,16

✓6ᵗʰ K06.01 Gingival recession, localized
K06.010 Localized gingival recession, unspecified
Localized gingival recession, NOS
K06.011 Localized gingival recession, minimal
K06.012 Localized gingival recession, moderate
K06.013 Localized gingival recession, severe

✓6ᵗʰ K06.02 Gingival recession, generalized
K06.020 Generalized gingival recession, unspecified
Generalized gingival recession, NOS
K06.021 Generalized gingival recession, minimal
K06.022 Generalized gingival recession, moderate
K06.023 Generalized gingival recession, severe

K06.1 Gingival enlargement
Gingival fibromatosis

K06.2 Gingival and edentulous alveolar ridge lesions associated with trauma
Irritative hyperplasia of edentulous ridge [denture hyperplasia]
Use additional code (Chapter 20) to identify external cause or denture status (Z97.2)

K06.3 Horizontal alveolar bone loss

K06.8 Other specified disorders of gingiva and edentulous alveolar ridge
Fibrous epulis
Flabby alveolar ridge
Giant cell epulis
Peripheral giant cell granuloma of gingiva
Pyogenic granuloma of gingiva
Vertical ridge deficiency
EXCLUDES 2   *gingival cyst (K09.0)*

K06.9 Disorder of gingiva and edentulous alveolar ridge, unspecified

✓4ᵗʰ K08 Other disorders of teeth and supporting structures
EXCLUDES 2   *dentofacial anomalies [including malocclusion] (M26.-)*
disorders of jaw (M27.-)
AHA: 2016,4Q,29-30

K08.0 Exfoliation of teeth due to systemic causes
Code also underlying systemic condition

✓5ᵗʰ K08.1 Complete loss of teeth
Acquired loss of teeth, complete
EXCLUDES 1   *congenital absence of teeth (K00.0)*
exfoliation of teeth due to systemic causes (K08.0)
partial loss of teeth (K08.4-)

✓6ᵗʰ K08.10 Complete loss of teeth, unspecified cause
K08.101 Complete loss of teeth, unspecified cause, class I
K08.102 Complete loss of teeth, unspecified cause, class II
K08.103 Complete loss of teeth, unspecified cause, class III
K08.104 Complete loss of teeth, unspecified cause, class IV
K08.109 Complete loss of teeth, unspecified cause, unspecified class
Edentulism NOS

✓6ᵗʰ K08.11 Complete loss of teeth due to trauma
K08.111 Complete loss of teeth due to trauma, class I
K08.112 Complete loss of teeth due to trauma, class II
K08.113 Complete loss of teeth due to trauma, class III
K08.114 Complete loss of teeth due to trauma, class IV
K08.119 Complete loss of teeth due to trauma, unspecified class

✓6ᵗʰ K08.12 Complete loss of teeth due to periodontal diseases
K08.121 Complete loss of teeth due to periodontal diseases, class I
K08.122 Complete loss of teeth due to periodontal diseases, class II
K08.123 Complete loss of teeth due to periodontal diseases, class III
K08.124 Complete loss of teeth due to periodontal diseases, class IV
K08.129 Complete loss of teeth due to periodontal diseases, unspecified class

✓6ᵗʰ K08.13 Complete loss of teeth due to caries
K08.131 Complete loss of teeth due to caries, class I
K08.132 Complete loss of teeth due to caries, class II
K08.133 Complete loss of teeth due to caries, class III
K08.134 Complete loss of teeth due to caries, class IV
K08.139 Complete loss of teeth due to caries, unspecified class

✓6ᵗʰ K08.19 Complete loss of teeth due to other specified cause
K08.191 Complete loss of teeth due to other specified cause, class I
K08.192 Complete loss of teeth due to other specified cause, class II
K08.193 Complete loss of teeth due to other specified cause, class III
K08.194 Complete loss of teeth due to other specified cause, class IV
K08.199 Complete loss of teeth due to other specified cause, unspecified class

✓5ᵗʰ K08.2 Atrophy of edentulous alveolar ridge
K08.20 Unspecified atrophy of edentulous alveolar ridge
Atrophy of the mandible NOS
Atrophy of the maxilla NOS
K08.21 Minimal atrophy of the mandible
Minimal atrophy of the edentulous mandible
K08.22 Moderate atrophy of the mandible
Moderate atrophy of the edentulous mandible
K08.23 Severe atrophy of the mandible
Severe atrophy of the edentulous mandible
K08.24 Minimal atrophy of maxilla
Minimal atrophy of the edentulous maxilla
K08.25 Moderate atrophy of the maxilla
Moderate atrophy of the edentulous maxilla
K08.26 Severe atrophy of the maxilla
Severe atrophy of the edentulous maxilla

K08.3 Retained dental root

✓5ᵗʰ **K08.4 Partial loss of teeth**
Acquired loss of teeth, partial
EXCLUDES 1   *complete loss of teeth (K08.1-)*
           congenital absence of teeth (K00.0)
EXCLUDES 2   *exfoliation of teeth due to systemic causes (K08.0)*

✓6ᵗʰ **K08.40 Partial loss of teeth, unspecified cause**
K08.401 Partial loss of teeth, unspecified cause, class I
K08.402 Partial loss of teeth, unspecified cause, class II
K08.403 Partial loss of teeth, unspecified cause, class III
K08.404 Partial loss of teeth, unspecified cause, class IV
K08.409 Partial loss of teeth, unspecified cause, unspecified class
       Tooth extraction status NOS

✓6ᵗʰ **K08.41 Partial loss of teeth due to trauma**
K08.411 Partial loss of teeth due to trauma, class I
K08.412 Partial loss of teeth due to trauma, class II
K08.413 Partial loss of teeth due to trauma, class III
K08.414 Partial loss of teeth due to trauma, class IV
K08.419 Partial loss of teeth due to trauma, unspecified class

✓6ᵗʰ **K08.42 Partial loss of teeth due to periodontal diseases**
K08.421 Partial loss of teeth due to periodontal diseases, class I
K08.422 Partial loss of teeth due to periodontal diseases, class II
K08.423 Partial loss of teeth due to periodontal diseases, class III
K08.424 Partial loss of teeth due to periodontal diseases, class IV
K08.429 Partial loss of teeth due to periodontal diseases, unspecified class

✓6ᵗʰ **K08.43 Partial loss of teeth due to caries**
K08.431 Partial loss of teeth due to caries, class I
K08.432 Partial loss of teeth due to caries, class II
K08.433 Partial loss of teeth due to caries, class III
K08.434 Partial loss of teeth due to caries, class IV
K08.439 Partial loss of teeth due to caries, unspecified class

✓6ᵗʰ **K08.49 Partial loss of teeth due to other specified cause**
K08.491 Partial loss of teeth due to other specified cause, class I
K08.492 Partial loss of teeth due to other specified cause, class II
K08.493 Partial loss of teeth due to other specified cause, class III
K08.494 Partial loss of teeth due to other specified cause, class IV
K08.499 Partial loss of teeth due to other specified cause, unspecified class

✓5ᵗʰ **K08.5 Unsatisfactory restoration of tooth**
Defective bridge, crown, filling
Defective dental restoration
EXCLUDES 1   *dental restoration status (Z98.811)*
EXCLUDES 2   *endosseous dental implant failure (M27.6-)*
           unsatisfactory endodontic treatment (M27.5-)

K08.50 Unsatisfactory restoration of tooth, unspecified
Defective dental restoration NOS

K08.51 Open restoration margins of tooth
Dental restoration failure of marginal integrity
Open margin on tooth restoration
Poor gingival margin to tooth restoration

K08.52 Unrepairable overhanging of dental restorative materials
Overhanging of tooth restoration

✓6ᵗʰ **K08.53 Fractured dental restorative material**
EXCLUDES 1   *cracked tooth (K03.81)*
           traumatic fracture of tooth (S02.5)

K08.530 Fractured dental restorative material without loss of material
K08.531 Fractured dental restorative material with loss of material

K08.539 Fractured dental restorative material, unspecified

K08.54 Contour of existing restoration of tooth biologically incompatible with oral health
Dental restoration failure of periodontal anatomical integrity
Unacceptable contours of existing restoration of tooth
Unacceptable morphology of existing restoration of tooth

K08.55 Allergy to existing dental restorative material
Use additional code to identify the specific type of allergy

K08.56 Poor aesthetic of existing restoration of tooth
Dental restoration aesthetically inadequate or displeasing

K08.59 Other unsatisfactory restoration of tooth
Other defective dental restoration

✓5ᵗʰ **K08.8 Other specified disorders of teeth and supporting structures**
K08.81 Primary occlusal trauma
K08.82 Secondary occlusal trauma
K08.89 Other specified disorders of teeth and supporting structures
Enlargement of alveolar ridge NOS
Insufficient anatomic crown height
Insufficient clinical crown length
Irregular alveolar process
Toothache NOS

K08.9 Disorder of teeth and supporting structures, unspecified

✓4ᵗʰ **K09 Cysts of oral region, not elsewhere classified**
INCLUDES   lesions showing histological features both of aneurysmal cyst and of another fibro-osseous lesion
EXCLUDES 2   *cysts of jaw (M27.0-, M27.4-)*
           radicular cyst (K04.8)

K09.0 Developmental odontogenic cysts
Dentigerous cyst
Eruption cyst
Follicular cyst
Gingival cyst
Lateral periodontal cyst
Primordial cyst
EXCLUDES 2   *keratocysts (D16.4, D16.5)*
           odontogenic keratocystic tumors (D16.4, D16.5)

K09.1 Developmental (nonodontogenic) cysts of oral region
Cyst (of) incisive canal
Cyst (of) palatine of papilla
Globulomaxillary cyst
Median palatal cyst
Nasoalveolar cyst
Nasolabial cyst
Nasopalatine duct cyst

K09.8 Other cysts of oral region, not elsewhere classified
Dermoid cyst
Epidermoid cyst
Lymphoepithelial cyst
Epstein's pearl

K09.9 Cyst of oral region, unspecified

✓4ᵗʰ **K11 Diseases of salivary glands**
Use additional code to identify:
alcohol abuse and dependence (F10.-)
exposure to environmental tobacco smoke (Z77.22)
exposure to tobacco smoke in the perinatal period (P96.81)
history of tobacco dependence (Z87.891)
occupational exposure to environmental tobacco smoke (Z57.31)
tobacco dependence (F17.-)
tobacco use (Z72.0)

K11.0 Atrophy of salivary gland
K11.1 Hypertrophy of salivary gland
DEF: Overgrowth of or enlarged salivary gland tissue caused by infection, salivary duct blockage, autoimmune diseases, and benign and malignant tumors.

✓5ᵗʰ **K11.2 Sialoadenitis**
Parotitis
EXCLUDES 1   *epidemic parotitis (B26.-)*
           mumps (B26.-)
           uveoparotid fever [Heerfordt] (D86.89)
DEF: Inflammation of the salivary gland.

K11.20 Sialoadenitis, unspecified

K11.21   Acute **sialoadenitis**
> EXCLUDES 1   *acute recurrent sialoadenitis (K11.22)*

K11.22   Acute recurrent **sialoadenitis**

K11.23   Chronic **sialoadenitis**

K11.3   **Abscess** of salivary gland

K11.4   **Fistula** of salivary gland
> EXCLUDES 1   *congenital fistula of salivary gland (Q38.4)*

K11.5   **Sialolithiasis**
Calculus of salivary gland or duct
Stone of salivary gland or duct

K11.6   **Mucocele** of salivary gland
Mucous extravasation cyst of salivary gland
Mucous retention cyst of salivary gland
Ranula

K11.7   **Disturbances of salivary** secretion
Hypoptyalism
Ptyalism
Xerostomia
> EXCLUDES 2   *dry mouth NOS (R68.2)*

K11.8   **Other diseases of salivary glands**
Benign lymphoepithelial lesion of salivary gland
Mikulicz' disease
Necrotizing sialometaplasia
Sialectasia
Stenosis of salivary duct
Stricture of salivary duct
> EXCLUDES 1   *Sjögren syndrome (M35.0-)*

K11.9   **Disease of salivary gland, unspecified**
Sialoadenopathy NOS

✓4ᵗʰ **K12**   **Stomatitis and related lesions**
Use additional code to identify:
   alcohol abuse and dependence (F10.-)
   exposure to environmental tobacco smoke (Z77.22)
   exposure to tobacco smoke in the perinatal period (P96.81)
   history of tobacco dependence (Z87.891)
   occupational exposure to environmental tobacco smoke (Z57.31)
   tobacco dependence (F17.-)
   tobacco use (Z72.0)
> EXCLUDES 1   *cancrum oris (A69.0)*
> *cheilitis (K13.0)*
> *gangrenous stomatitis (A69.0)*
> *herpesviral [herpes simplex] gingivostomatitis (B00.2)*
> *noma (A69.0)*

K12.0   **Recurrent oral aphthae**
Aphthous stomatitis (major) (minor)
Bednar's aphthae
Periadenitis mucosa necrotica recurrens
Recurrent aphthous ulcer
Stomatitis herpetiformis
DEF: Disorder of unknown etiology with small oval or round painful ulcers of the mouth marked by a grayish exudate and a red halo effect.

K12.1   **Other forms of stomatitis**
Stomatitis NOS
Denture stomatitis
Ulcerative stomatitis
Vesicular stomatitis
> EXCLUDES 1   *acute necrotizing ulcerative stomatitis (A69.1)*
> *Vincent's stomatitis (A69.1)*

K12.2   **Cellulitis and abscess of mouth**
Cellulitis of mouth (floor)
Submandibular abscess
> EXCLUDES 2   *abscess of salivary gland (K11.3)*
> *abscess of tongue (K14.0)*
> *periapical abscess (K04.6-K04.7)*
> *periodontal abscess (K05.21)*
> *peritonsillar abscess (J36)*

✓5ᵗʰ **K12.3**   **Oral mucositis (ulcerative)**
Mucositis (oral) (oropharyneal)
> EXCLUDES 2   *gastrointestinal mucositis (ulcerative) (K92.81)*
> *mucositis (ulcerative) of vagina and vulva (N76.81)*
> *nasal mucositis (ulcerative) (J34.81)*

K12.30   **Oral mucositis (ulcerative), unspecified**

K12.31   **Oral mucositis (ulcerative) due to** antineoplastic therapy
Use additional code for adverse effect, if applicable, to identify antineoplastic and immunosuppressive drugs (T45.1X5)
Use additional code for other antineoplastic therapy, such as:
   radiological procedure and radiotherapy (Y84.2)

K12.32   **Oral mucositis (ulcerative) due to other drugs**
Use additional code for adverse effect, if applicable, to identify drug (T36-T50 with fifth or sixth character 5)

K12.33   **Oral mucositis (ulcerative) due to** radiation
Use additional external cause code (W88-W90, X39.0-) to identify cause

K12.39   **Other oral mucositis (ulcerative)**
Viral oral mucositis (ulcerative)

✓4ᵗʰ **K13**   **Other diseases of lip and oral mucosa**
> INCLUDES   epithelial disturbances of tongue

Use additional code to identify:
   alcohol abuse and dependence (F10.-)
   exposure to environmental tobacco smoke (Z77.22)
   exposure to tobacco smoke in the perinatal period (P96.81)
   history of tobacco dependence (Z87.891)
   occupational exposure to environmental tobacco smoke (Z57.31)
   tobacco dependence (F17.-)
   tobacco use (Z72.0)
> EXCLUDES 2   *certain disorders of gingiva and edentulous alveolar ridge (K05-K06)*
> *cysts of oral region (K09.-)*
> *diseases of tongue (K14.-)*
> *stomatitis and related lesions (K12.-)*

K13.0   **Diseases of lips**
Abscess of lips
Angular cheilitis
Cellulitis of lips
Cheilitis NOS
Cheilodynia
Cheilosis
Exfoliative cheilitis
Fistula of lips
Glandular cheilitis
Hypertrophy of lips
Perlèche NEC
> EXCLUDES 1   *ariboflavinosis (E53.0)*
> *cheilitis due to radiation-related disorders (L55-L59)*
> *congenital fistula of lips (Q38.0)*
> *congenital hypertrophy of lips (Q18.6)*
> *perlèche due to candidiasis (B37.83)*
> *perlèche due to riboflavin deficiency (E53.0)*

K13.1   **Cheek and lip biting**

✓5ᵗʰ **K13.2**   **Leukoplakia and other disturbances of oral epithelium, including tongue**
> EXCLUDES 1   *carcinoma in situ of oral epithelium (D00.0-)*
> *hairy leukoplakia (K13.3)*

DEF: Leukoplakia: Thickened white patches or lesions appearing on a mucous membrane, such as oral mucosa or tongue.

K13.21   **Leukoplakia of** oral mucosa, **including tongue**
Leukokeratosis of oral mucosa
Leukoplakia of gingiva, lips, tongue
> EXCLUDES 1   *hairy leukoplakia (K13.3)*
> *leukokeratosis nicotina palati (K13.24)*

K13.22   **Minimal keratinized residual ridge mucosa**
Minimal keratinization of alveolar ridge mucosa

K13.23   **Excessive keratinized residual ridge mucosa**
Excessive keratinization of alveolar ridge mucosa

K13.24   **Leukokeratosis nicotina palati**
Smoker's palate

K13.29   **Other disturbances of oral epithelium, including tongue**
Erythroplakia of mouth or tongue
Focal epithelial hyperplasia of mouth or tongue
Leukoedema of mouth or tongue
Other oral epithelium disturbances

K13.3   **Hairy leukoplakia**

K13.4 Granuloma and granuloma-like lesions of oral mucosa
    Eosinophilic granuloma
    Granuloma pyogenicum
    Verrucous xanthoma

K13.5 Oral submucous fibrosis
    Submucous fibrosis of tongue

K13.6 Irritative hyperplasia of oral mucosa
    EXCLUDES 2   *irritative hyperplasia of edentulous ridge [denture hyperplasia] (K06.2)*

√5ᵗʰ K13.7 Other and unspecified lesions of oral mucosa
    K13.70 Unspecified lesions of oral mucosa
    K13.79 Other lesions of oral mucosa
        Focal oral mucinosis
        AHA: 2022,2Q,7

√4ᵗʰ K14 Diseases of tongue
    Use additional code to identify:
      alcohol abuse and dependence (F10.-)
      exposure to environmental tobacco smoke (Z77.22)
      history of tobacco dependence (Z87.891)
      occupational exposure to environmental tobacco smoke (Z57.31)
      tobacco dependence (F17.-)
      tobacco use (Z72.0)
    EXCLUDES 2   *erythroplakia (K13.29)*
        focal epithelial hyperplasia (K13.29)
        leukedema of tongue (K13.29)
        leukoplakia of tongue (K13.21)
        hairy leukoplakia (K13.3)
        macroglossia (congenital) (Q38.2)
        submucous fibrosis of tongue (K13.5)

K14.0 Glossitis
    Abscess of tongue
    Ulceration (traumatic) of tongue
    EXCLUDES 1   *atrophic glossitis (K14.4)*
    DEF: Inflammation and swelling of the tongue that may be associated with infection, adverse drug reactions, smoking, or injury.

K14.1 Geographic tongue
    Benign migratory glossitis
    Glossitis areata exfoliativa

K14.2 Median rhomboid glossitis

K14.3 Hypertrophy of tongue papillae
    Black hairy tongue
    Coated tongue
    Hypertrophy of foliate papillae
    Lingua villosa nigra

K14.4 Atrophy of tongue papillae
    Atrophic glossitis

K14.5 Plicated tongue
    Fissured tongue
    Furrowed tongue
    Scrotal tongue
    EXCLUDES 1   *fissured tongue, congenital (Q38.3)*

K14.6 Glossodynia
    Glossopyrosis
    Painful tongue

K14.8 Other diseases of tongue
    Atrophy of tongue
    Crenated tongue
    Enlargement of tongue
    Glossocele
    Glossoptosis
    Hypertrophy of tongue

K14.9 Disease of tongue, unspecified
    Glossopathy NOS

Diseases of esophagus, stomach and duodenum (K20-K31)

EXCLUDES 2   *hiatus hernia (K44.-)*

√4ᵗʰ K20 Esophagitis
    Use additional code to identify:
      alcohol abuse and dependence (F10.-)
    EXCLUDES 1   *erosion of esophagus (K22.1-)*
        esophagitis with gastro-esophageal reflux disease (K21.0-)
        reflux esophagitis (K21.0-)
        ulcerative esophagitis (K22.1-)
    EXCLUDES 2   *eosinophilic gastritis or gastroenteritis (K52.81)*

    K20.0 Eosinophilic esophagitis
        AHA: 2020,4Q,9
    √5ᵗʰ K20.8 Other esophagitis
        AHA: 2020,4Q,28-29
        K20.80 Other esophagitis without bleeding
            Abscess of esophagus
            Other esophagitis NOS
        K20.81 Other esophagitis with bleeding
    √5ᵗʰ K20.9 Esophagitis, unspecified
        AHA: 2020,4Q,28-29
        K20.90 Esophagitis, unspecified without bleeding
            Esophagitis NOS
        K20.91 Esophagitis, unspecified with bleeding

√4ᵗʰ K21 Gastro-esophageal reflux disease
    EXCLUDES 1   *newborn esophageal reflux (P78.83)*
    √5ᵗʰ K21.0 Gastro-esophageal reflux disease with esophagitis
        AHA: 2020,4Q,28-29
        K21.00 Gastro-esophageal reflux disease with esophagitis, without bleeding
            Reflux esophagitis
        K21.01 Gastro-esophageal reflux disease with esophagitis, with bleeding
    K21.9 Gastro-esophageal reflux disease without esophagitis
        Esophageal reflux NOS
        AHA: 2016,1Q,18

√4ᵗʰ K22 Other diseases of esophagus
    EXCLUDES 2   *esophageal varices (I85.-)*
    K22.0 Achalasia of cardia
        Achalasia NOS
        Cardiospasm
        EXCLUDES 1   *congenital cardiospasm (Q39.5)*
        DEF: Esophageal motility disorder that is caused by absence of the esophageal peristalsis and impaired relaxation of the lower esophageal sphincter. It is characterized by dysphagia, regurgitation, and heartburn.
    √5ᵗʰ K22.1 Ulcer of esophagus
        Barrett's ulcer
        Erosion of esophagus
        Fungal ulcer of esophagus
        Peptic ulcer of esophagus
        Ulcer of esophagus due to ingestion of chemicals
        Ulcer of esophagus due to ingestion of drugs and medicaments
        Ulcerative esophagitis
        Code first poisoning due to drug or toxin, if applicable (T36-T65 with fifth or sixth character 1-4 or 6)
        Use additional code for adverse effect, if applicable, to identify drug (T36-T50 with fifth or sixth character 5)
        EXCLUDES 1   *Barrett's esophagus (K22.7-)*
        AHA: 2018,3Q,22; 2017,3Q,27
        TIP: Assign a code for "with bleeding" when an esophageal ulcer and bleeding (hematemesis) are documented. The ICD-10-CM classification assumes the two are related without the provider linking the two conditions. Evidence of bleeding during a procedure is not required.
        K22.10 Ulcer of esophagus without bleeding
            Ulcer of esophagus NOS
        K22.11 Ulcer of esophagus with bleeding
            EXCLUDES 2   *bleeding esophageal varices (I85.01, I85.11)*
            TIP: For bleeding esophageal ulcers resulting from anticoagulant therapy, assign this code, code D68.32 Hemorrhagic disorder due to extrinsic circulating anticoagulant, and adverse effect code T45.515- with the appropriate seventh character.

Chapter 11. Diseases of the Digestive System

K22.2 Esophageal obstruction
    Compression of esophagus
    Constriction of esophagus
    Stenosis of esophagus
    Stricture of esophagus
    EXCLUDES 1   *congenital stenosis or stricture of esophagus (Q39.3)*

K22.3 Perforation of esophagus
    Rupture of esophagus
    EXCLUDES 1   *traumatic perforation of (thoracic) esophagus (S27.8-)*

K22.4 Dyskinesia of esophagus
    Corkscrew esophagus
    Diffuse esophageal spasm
    Spasm of esophagus
    EXCLUDES 1   *cardiospasm (K22.0)*

K22.5 Diverticulum of esophagus, acquired
    Esophageal pouch, acquired
    EXCLUDES 1   *diverticulum of esophagus (congenital) (Q39.6)*

K22.6 Gastro-esophageal laceration-hemorrhage syndrome
    Mallory-Weiss syndrome

√5ᵗʰ **K22.7 Barrett's esophagus**
    Barrett's disease
    Barrett's syndrome
    EXCLUDES 1   *Barrett's ulcer (K22.1)*
                 malignant neoplasm of esophagus (C15.-)
    DEF: Metaplastic disorder in which specialized columnar epithelial cells replace the normal squamous epithelial cells. Secondary to chronic gastroesophageal reflux damage to the mucosa, this disorder increases the risk of developing adenocarcinoma.
    K22.70 Barrett's esophagus without dysplasia   **Q**
        Barrett's esophagus NOS
    √6ᵗʰ **K22.71 Barrett's esophagus with dysplasia**
        K22.710 Barrett's esophagus with low grade dysplasia   **Q**
        K22.711 Barrett's esophagus with high grade dysplasia   **Q**
        K22.719 Barrett's esophagus with dysplasia, unspecified   **Q**

√5ᵗʰ **K22.8 Other specified diseases of esophagus**
    EXCLUDES 2   *esophageal varices (I85.-)*
                  Paterson-Kelly syndrome (D50.1)
    AHA: 2021,4Q,15; 2020,1Q,16
    K22.81 Esophageal polyp
        EXCLUDES 1   *benign neoplasm of esophagus (D13.0)*
    K22.82 Esophagogastric junction polyp
        EXCLUDES 1   *benign neoplasm of stomach (D13.1)*
    K22.89 Other specified disease of esophagus
        Hemorrhage of esophagus NOS

K22.9 Disease of esophagus, unspecified

K23 *Disorders of esophagus in diseases classified elsewhere*
    Code first underlying disease, such as:
      congenital syphilis (A50.5)
    EXCLUDES 1   *late syphilis (A52.79)*
                  megaesophagus due to Chagas' disease (B57.31)
                  tuberculosis (A18.83)

√4ᵗʰ **K25 Gastric ulcer**
    INCLUDES   erosion (acute) of stomach
               pylorus ulcer (peptic)
               stomach ulcer (peptic)
    Use additional code to identify:
      alcohol abuse and dependence (F10.-)
    EXCLUDES 1   *acute gastritis (K29.0-)*
                  peptic ulcer NOS (K27.-)
    AHA: 2021,1Q,9,11; 2017,3Q,27
    TIP: Assign a code for "with hemorrhage" when a gastric ulcer and GI bleeding are documented. The ICD-10-CM classification assumes the two are related without the provider linking the two conditions. Evidence of bleeding during a procedure is not required.
    TIP: For bleeding ulcers resulting from anticoagulant therapy, assign the appropriate "with hemorrhage" ulcer code from this category, code D68.32 Hemorrhagic disorder due to extrinsic circulating anticoagulant, and adverse effect code T45.515- with the appropriate seventh character.
    K25.0 Acute gastric ulcer with hemorrhage
    K25.1 Acute gastric ulcer with perforation   HCC ESR COM
    K25.2 Acute gastric ulcer with both hemorrhage and perforation   HCC ESR COM

K25.3 Acute gastric ulcer without hemorrhage or perforation
K25.4 Chronic or unspecified gastric ulcer with hemorrhage
K25.5 Chronic or unspecified gastric ulcer with perforation   HCC ESR COM
K25.6 Chronic or unspecified gastric ulcer with both hemorrhage and perforation   HCC ESR COM
K25.7 Chronic gastric ulcer without hemorrhage or perforation
K25.9 Gastric ulcer, unspecified as acute or chronic, without hemorrhage or perforation

Gastrointestinal Ulcers

√4ᵗʰ **K26 Duodenal ulcer**
    INCLUDES   erosion (acute) of duodenum
               duodenum ulcer (peptic)
               postpyloric ulcer (peptic)
    Use additional code to identify:
      alcohol abuse and dependence (F10.-)
    EXCLUDES 1   *peptic ulcer NOS (K27.-)*
    AHA: 2017,3Q,27
    TIP: Assign a code for "with hemorrhage" when a duodenal ulcer and GI bleeding are documented. The ICD-10-CM classification assumes the two are related without the provider linking the two conditions. Evidence of bleeding during a procedure is not required.
    TIP: For bleeding ulcers resulting from anticoagulant therapy, assign the appropriate "with hemorrhage" ulcer code from this category, code D68.32 Hemorrhagic disorder due to extrinsic circulating anticoagulant, and adverse effect code T45.515- with the appropriate seventh character.
    K26.0 Acute duodenal ulcer with hemorrhage
    K26.1 Acute duodenal ulcer with perforation   HCC ESR COM
    K26.2 Acute duodenal ulcer with both hemorrhage and perforation   HCC ESR COM
    K26.3 Acute duodenal ulcer without hemorrhage or perforation
    K26.4 Chronic or unspecified duodenal ulcer with hemorrhage
        AHA: 2016,1Q,14
    K26.5 Chronic or unspecified duodenal ulcer with perforation   HCC ESR COM
    K26.6 Chronic or unspecified duodenal ulcer with both hemorrhage and perforation   HCC ESR COM
    K26.7 Chronic duodenal ulcer without hemorrhage or perforation
    K26.9 Duodenal ulcer, unspecified as acute or chronic, without hemorrhage or perforation

√4ᵗʰ **K27 Peptic ulcer, site unspecified**
    INCLUDES   gastroduodenal ulcer NOS
               peptic ulcer NOS
    Use additional code to identify:
      alcohol abuse and dependence (F10.-)
    EXCLUDES 1   *peptic ulcer of newborn (P78.82)*
    AHA: 2017,3Q,27
    TIP: Assign a code for "with hemorrhage" when a peptic ulcer and GI bleeding are documented. The ICD-10-CM classification assumes the two are related without the provider linking the two conditions. Evidence of bleeding during a procedure is not required.
    TIP: For bleeding ulcers resulting from anticoagulant therapy, assign the appropriate "with hemorrhage" ulcer code from this category, code D68.32 Hemorrhagic disorder due to extrinsic circulating anticoagulant, and adverse effect code T45.515- with the appropriate seventh character.
    K27.0 Acute peptic ulcer, site unspecified, with hemorrhage
    K27.1 Acute peptic ulcer, site unspecified, with perforation   HCC ESR COM
    K27.2 Acute peptic ulcer, site unspecified, with both hemorrhage and perforation   HCC ESR COM

K27.3 Acute peptic ulcer, site unspecified, without hemorrhage or perforation

K27.4 Chronic or unspecified peptic ulcer, site unspecified, with hemorrhage

K27.5 Chronic or unspecified peptic ulcer, site unspecified, with perforation   HCC ESR COM

K27.6 Chronic or unspecified peptic ulcer, site unspecified, with both hemorrhage and perforation   HCC ESR COM

K27.7 Chronic peptic ulcer, site unspecified, without hemorrhage or perforation

K27.9 Peptic ulcer, site unspecified, unspecified as acute or chronic, without hemorrhage or perforation

☑4ᵗʰ K28 Gastrojejunal ulcer

INCLUDES   anastomotic ulcer (peptic) or erosion
gastrocolic ulcer (peptic) or erosion
gastrointestinal ulcer (peptic) or erosion
gastrojejunal ulcer (peptic) or erosion
jejunal ulcer (peptic) or erosion
marginal ulcer (peptic) or erosion
stomal ulcer (peptic) or erosion

Use additional code to identify:
alcohol abuse and dependence (F10.-)

EXCLUDES 1   primary ulcer of small intestine (K63.3)

AHA: 2017,3Q,27

TIP: Assign a code for "with hemorrhage" when a gastrojejunal ulcer and GI bleeding are documented. The ICD-10-CM classification assumes the two are related without the provider linking the two conditions. Evidence of bleeding during a procedure is not required.

TIP: For bleeding ulcers resulting from anticoagulant therapy, assign the appropriate "with hemorrhage" ulcer code from this category, code D68.32 Hemorrhagic disorder due to extrinsic circulating anticoagulant, and adverse effect code T45.515- with the appropriate seventh character.

K28.0 Acute gastrojejunal ulcer with hemorrhage

K28.1 Acute gastrojejunal ulcer with perforation   HCC ESR COM

K28.2 Acute gastrojejunal ulcer with both hemorrhage and perforation   HCC ESR COM

K28.3 Acute gastrojejunal ulcer without hemorrhage or perforation

K28.4 Chronic or unspecified gastrojejunal ulcer with hemorrhage

K28.5 Chronic or unspecified gastrojejunal ulcer with perforation   HCC ESR COM

K28.6 Chronic or unspecified gastrojejunal ulcer with both hemorrhage and perforation   HCC ESR COM

K28.7 Chronic gastrojejunal ulcer without hemorrhage or perforation

K28.9 Gastrojejunal ulcer, unspecified as acute or chronic, without hemorrhage or perforation

☑4ᵗʰ K29 Gastritis and duodenitis

EXCLUDES 1   eosinophilic gastritis or gastroenteritis (K52.81)
Zollinger-Ellison syndrome (E16.4)

AHA: 2018,3Q,22

TIP: Assign a code for "with bleeding" when gastritis or duodenitis and GI bleeding are documented. The ICD-10-CM classification assumes the two are related without the provider linking the two conditions. Evidence of bleeding during a procedure is not required.

TIP: For bleeding ulcers resulting from anticoagulant therapy, assign the appropriate "with hemorrhage" ulcer code from this category, code D68.32 Hemorrhagic disorder due to extrinsic circulating anticoagulant, and adverse effect code T45.515- with the appropriate seventh character.

☑5ᵗʰ K29.0 Acute gastritis

Use additional code to identify:
alcohol abuse and dependence (F10.-)
EXCLUDES 1   erosion (acute) of stomach (K25.-)

K29.00 Acute gastritis without bleeding
K29.01 Acute gastritis with bleeding

☑5ᵗʰ K29.2 Alcoholic gastritis

Use additional code to identify:
alcohol abuse and dependence (F10.-)

K29.20 Alcoholic gastritis without bleeding
K29.21 Alcoholic gastritis with bleeding

☑5ᵗʰ K29.3 Chronic superficial gastritis

K29.30 Chronic superficial gastritis without bleeding
K29.31 Chronic superficial gastritis with bleeding

☑5ᵗʰ K29.4 Chronic atrophic gastritis

Gastric atrophy

K29.40 Chronic atrophic gastritis without bleeding
K29.41 Chronic atrophic gastritis with bleeding

☑5ᵗʰ K29.5 Unspecified chronic gastritis

Chronic antral gastritis
Chronic fundal gastritis

K29.50 Unspecified chronic gastritis without bleeding
K29.51 Unspecified chronic gastritis with bleeding

☑5ᵗʰ K29.6 Other gastritis

Giant hypertrophic gastritis
Granulomatous gastritis
Ménétrier's disease

K29.60 Other gastritis without bleeding
K29.61 Other gastritis with bleeding

☑5ᵗʰ K29.7 Gastritis, unspecified

K29.70 Gastritis, unspecified, without bleeding
K29.71 Gastritis, unspecified, with bleeding

☑5ᵗʰ K29.8 Duodenitis

K29.80 Duodenitis without bleeding
K29.81 Duodenitis with bleeding

☑5ᵗʰ K29.9 Gastroduodenitis, unspecified

K29.90 Gastroduodenitis, unspecified, without bleeding
K29.91 Gastroduodenitis, unspecified, with bleeding

K30 Functional dyspepsia

Indigestion

EXCLUDES 1   dyspepsia NOS (R10.13)
heartburn (R12)
nervous dyspepsia (F45.8)
neurotic dyspepsia (F45.8)
psychogenic dyspepsia (F45.8)

☑4ᵗʰ K31 Other diseases of stomach and duodenum

INCLUDES   functional disorders of stomach
EXCLUDES 2   diabetic gastroparesis (E08.43, E09.43, E10.43, E11.43, E13.43)
diverticulum of duodenum (K57.00-K57.13)

K31.0 Acute dilatation of stomach
Acute distention of stomach

K31.1 Adult hypertrophic pyloric stenosis   COM A
Pyloric stenosis NOS
EXCLUDES 1   congenital or infantile pyloric stenosis (Q40.0)

K31.2 Hourglass stricture and stenosis of stomach
EXCLUDES 1   congenital hourglass stomach (Q40.2)
hourglass contraction of stomach (K31.89)

K31.3 Pylorospasm, not elsewhere classified   COM
EXCLUDES 1   congenital or infantile pylorospasm (Q40.0)
neurotic pylorospasm (F45.8)
psychogenic pylorospasm (F45.8)

K31.4 Gastric diverticulum
EXCLUDES 1   congenital diverticulum of stomach (Q40.2)

K31.5 Obstruction of duodenum   COM
Constriction of duodenum
Duodenal ileus (chronic)
Stenosis of duodenum
Stricture of duodenum
Volvulus of duodenum
EXCLUDES 1   congenital stenosis of duodenum (Q41.0)

K31.6 Fistula of stomach and duodenum
Gastrocolic fistula
Gastrojejunocolic fistula

K31.7 Polyp of stomach and duodenum
EXCLUDES 1   adenomatous polyp of stomach (D13.1)
AHA: 2020,1Q,16

☑5ᵗʰ K31.8 Other specified diseases of stomach and duodenum

☑6ᵗʰ K31.81 Angiodysplasia of stomach and duodenum

TIP: Assign a code for "with bleeding" when angiodysplasia of the stomach or the duodenum and GI bleeding are documented. The ICD-10-CM classification assumes the two are related without the provider linking the two conditions. Evidence of bleeding during a procedure is not required.

K31.811 Angiodysplasia of stomach and duodenum with bleeding

K31.819 Angiodysplasia of stomach and duodenum without bleeding
Angiodysplasia of stomach and duodenum NOS

Chapter 11. Diseases of the Digestive System

K31.82 **Dieulafoy lesion (hemorrhagic) of stomach and duodenum**
     EXCLUDES 2   *Dieulafoy lesion of intestine (K63.81)*
     DEF: Abnormally large submucosal artery protruding through a defect in the stomach mucosa or intestines that can cause massive and life-threatening hemorrhaging.

K31.83 **Achlorhydria**
     DEF: Absence of hydrochloric acid in gastric secretions due to gastric mucosa atrophy. Achlorhydria is unresponsive to histamines.

K31.84 **Gastroparesis**
     Gastroparalysis
     Code first underlying disease, if known, such as:
         anorexia nervosa (F50.0-)
         diabetes mellitus (E08.43, E09.43, E10.43, E11.43, E13.43)
         scleroderma (M34.-)
     AHA: 2013,4Q,114

K31.89 **Other diseases of stomach and duodenum**
     AHA: 2020,1Q,15; 2017,1Q,28

K31.9 **Disease of stomach and duodenum, unspecified**

✓5ᵗʰ **K31.A** **Gastric intestinal** metaplasia
     AHA: 2021,4Q,15-16

     K31.A0 **Gastric intestinal metaplasia, unspecified**
         Gastric intestinal metaplasia indefinite for dysplasia
         Gastric intestinal metaplasia NOS

     ✓6ᵗʰ **K31.A1** **Gastric intestinal metaplasia** without dysplasia

         K31.A11 **Gastric intestinal metaplasia without dysplasia,** involving the antrum
         K31.A12 **Gastric intestinal metaplasia without dysplasia,** involving the body **(corpus)**
         K31.A13 **Gastric intestinal metaplasia without dysplasia,** involving the fundus
         K31.A14 **Gastric intestinal metaplasia without dysplasia,** involving the cardia
         K31.A15 **Gastric intestinal metaplasia without dysplasia,** involving multiple sites
         K31.A19 **Gastric intestinal metaplasia without dysplasia,** unspecified site

     ✓6ᵗʰ **K31.A2** **Gastric intestinal metaplasia** with dysplasia

         K31.A21 **Gastric intestinal metaplasia with** low grade **dysplasia**
         K31.A22 **Gastric intestinal metaplasia with** high grade **dysplasia**
         K31.A29 **Gastric intestinal metaplasia with dysplasia,** unspecified

Diseases of appendix (K35-K38)

✓4ᵗʰ **K35** **Acute** appendicitis
     AHA: 2018,4Q,17-18

     ✓5ᵗʰ **K35.2** **Acute appendicitis** with generalized peritonitis
         Appendicitis (acute) with generalized (diffuse) peritonitis following rupture or perforation of appendix

         K35.20 **Acute appendicitis with generalized peritonitis,** without abscess
            (Acute) appendicitis with generalized peritonitis NOS
         K35.21 **Acute appendicitis with generalized peritonitis,** with abscess

     ✓5ᵗʰ **K35.3** **Acute appendicitis** with localized peritonitis

         K35.30 **Acute appendicitis with localized peritonitis,** without perforation or gangrene
            Acute appendicitis with localized peritonitis NOS
         K35.31 **Acute appendicitis with localized peritonitis and gangrene,** without perforation
▲   **K35.32** **Acute appendicitis with perforation, localized peritonitis, and gangrene,** without abscess
            (Acute) appendicitis with perforation NOS
            Perforated appendix NOS
            Ruptured appendix (with localized peritonitis) NOS
            AHA: 2020,1Q,16
▲   **K35.33** **Acute appendicitis with perforation, localized peritonitis, and gangrene,** with abscess
            (Acute) appendicitis with (peritoneal) abscess NOS
            Ruptured appendix with localized peritonitis and abscess

     ✓5ᵗʰ **K35.8** **Other and unspecified acute appendicitis**

         K35.80 **Unspecified acute appendicitis**
            Acute appendicitis NOS
            Acute appendicitis without (localized) (generalized) peritonitis

         ✓6ᵗʰ **K35.89** **Other acute appendicitis**
            AHA: 2020,1Q,16

            K35.890 **Other acute appendicitis** without perforation or gangrene
            K35.891 **Other acute appendicitis** without perforation, with gangrene
              (Acute) appendicitis with gangrene NOS

K36 **Other appendicitis**
     Chronic appendicitis
     Recurrent appendicitis

K37 **Unspecified appendicitis**
     EXCLUDES 1   unspecified appendicitis with peritonitis (K35.2-, K35.3-)

✓4ᵗʰ **K38** **Other diseases of appendix**

     K38.0 **Hyperplasia of appendix**

     K38.1 **Appendicular concretions**
         Fecalith of appendix
         Stercolith of appendix

     K38.2 **Diverticulum of appendix**

     K38.3 **Fistula of appendix**

     K38.8 **Other specified diseases of appendix**
         Intussusception of appendix

     K38.9 **Disease of appendix, unspecified**

Hernia (K40-K46)

NOTE   Hernia with both gangrene and obstruction is classified to hernia with gangrene.

INCLUDES   acquired hernia
         congenital [except diaphragmatic or hiatus] hernia
         recurrent hernia
AHA: 2021,3Q,30-31
TIP: Do not assign a code for bilateral hernia when the right and left sides have differing pathology. For example, two codes would be assigned for bilateral femoral hernia in which the left side is incarcerated (with obstruction) but the right side is not incarcerated; the code for bilateral would not apply in this case.

✓4ᵗʰ **K40** **Inguinal** hernia

     INCLUDES   bubonocele
         direct inguinal hernia
         double inguinal hernia
         indirect inguinal hernia
         inguinal hernia NOS
         oblique inguinal hernia
         scrotal hernia
     DEF: Within the groin region.

     ✓5ᵗʰ **K40.0** **Bilateral** inguinal hernia, with obstruction, without gangrene
         Inguinal hernia (bilateral) causing obstruction without gangrene
         Incarcerated inguinal hernia (bilateral) without gangrene
         Irreducible inguinal hernia (bilateral) without gangrene
         Strangulated inguinal hernia (bilateral) without gangrene

         K40.00 **Bilateral inguinal hernia, with obstruction, without gangrene,** not specified as recurrent
            Bilateral inguinal hernia, with obstruction, without gangrene NOS
         K40.01 **Bilateral inguinal hernia, with obstruction, without gangrene,** recurrent

     ✓5ᵗʰ **K40.1** **Bilateral** inguinal hernia, with gangrene

         K40.10 **Bilateral inguinal hernia, with gangrene,** not specified as recurrent
            Bilateral inguinal hernia, with gangrene NOS
         K40.11 **Bilateral inguinal hernia, with gangrene,** recurrent

     ✓5ᵗʰ **K40.2** **Bilateral** inguinal hernia, without obstruction or gangrene

         K40.20 **Bilateral inguinal hernia, without obstruction or gangrene,** not specified as recurrent
            Bilateral inguinal hernia NOS
         K40.21 **Bilateral inguinal hernia, without obstruction or gangrene,** recurrent

✅5ᵗʰ **K40.3** Unilateral **inguinal hernia, with obstruction, without gangrene**
Inguinal hernia (unilateral) causing obstruction without gangrene
Incarcerated inguinal hernia (unilateral) without gangrene
Irreducible inguinal hernia (unilateral) without gangrene
Strangulated inguinal hernia (unilateral) without gangrene

     K40.30 **Unilateral inguinal hernia, with obstruction, without gangrene, not specified as recurrent**
Inguinal hernia, with obstruction NOS
Unilateral inguinal hernia, with obstruction, without gangrene NOS

     K40.31 **Unilateral inguinal hernia, with obstruction, without gangrene, recurrent**

✅5ᵗʰ **K40.4** Unilateral **inguinal hernia, with gangrene**

     K40.40 **Unilateral inguinal hernia, with gangrene, not specified as recurrent**
Inguinal hernia with gangrene NOS
Unilateral inguinal hernia with gangrene NOS

     K40.41 **Unilateral inguinal hernia, with gangrene, recurrent**

✅5ᵗʰ **K40.9** Unilateral **inguinal hernia, without obstruction or gangrene**

     K40.90 **Unilateral inguinal hernia, without obstruction or gangrene, not specified as recurrent**
Inguinal hernia NOS
Unilateral inguinal hernia NOS

     K40.91 **Unilateral inguinal hernia, without obstruction or gangrene, recurrent**

Hernia Sites

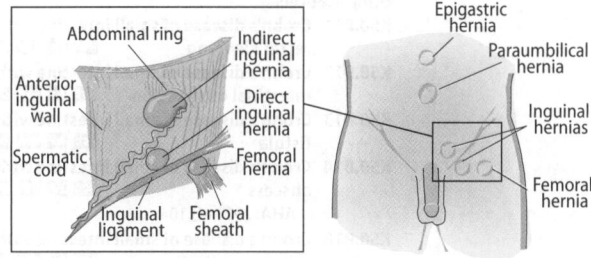

✅4ᵗʰ **K41** Femoral **hernia**

✅5ᵗʰ **K41.0** Bilateral **femoral hernia, with obstruction, without gangrene**
Femoral hernia (bilateral) causing obstruction, without gangrene
Incarcerated femoral hernia (bilateral), without gangrene
Irreducible femoral hernia (bilateral), without gangrene
Strangulated femoral hernia (bilateral), without gangrene

     K41.00 **Bilateral femoral hernia, with obstruction, without gangrene, not specified as recurrent**
Bilateral femoral hernia, with obstruction, without gangrene NOS

     K41.01 **Bilateral femoral hernia, with obstruction, without gangrene, recurrent**

✅5ᵗʰ **K41.1** Bilateral **femoral hernia, with gangrene**

     K41.10 **Bilateral femoral hernia, with gangrene, not specified as recurrent**
Bilateral femoral hernia, with gangrene NOS

     K41.11 **Bilateral femoral hernia, with gangrene, recurrent**

✅5ᵗʰ **K41.2** Bilateral **femoral hernia, without obstruction or gangrene**

     K41.20 **Bilateral femoral hernia, without obstruction or gangrene, not specified as recurrent**
Bilateral femoral hernia NOS

     K41.21 **Bilateral femoral hernia, without obstruction or gangrene, recurrent**

✅5ᵗʰ **K41.3** Unilateral **femoral hernia, with obstruction, without gangrene**
Femoral hernia (unilateral) causing obstruction, without gangrene
Incarcerated femoral hernia (unilateral), without gangrene
Irreducible femoral hernia (unilateral), without gangrene
Strangulated femoral hernia (unilateral), without gangrene

     K41.30 **Unilateral femoral hernia, with obstruction, without gangrene, not specified as recurrent**
Femoral hernia, with obstruction NOS
Unilateral femoral hernia, with obstruction NOS

     K41.31 **Unilateral femoral hernia, with obstruction, without gangrene, recurrent**

✅5ᵗʰ **K41.4** Unilateral **femoral hernia, with gangrene**

     K41.40 **Unilateral femoral hernia, with gangrene, not specified as recurrent**
Femoral hernia, with gangrene NOS
Unilateral femoral hernia, with gangrene NOS

     K41.41 **Unilateral femoral hernia, with gangrene, recurrent**

✅5ᵗʰ **K41.9** Unilateral **femoral hernia, without obstruction or gangrene**

     K41.90 **Unilateral femoral hernia, without obstruction or gangrene, not specified as recurrent**
Femoral hernia NOS
Unilateral femoral hernia NOS

     K41.91 **Unilateral femoral hernia, without obstruction or gangrene, recurrent**

✅4ᵗʰ **K42** Umbilical **hernia**

     INCLUDES   paraumbilical hernia
     EXCLUDES 1   *omphalocele (Q79.2)*

     K42.0 **Umbilical hernia** with obstruction, without gangrene
Umbilical hernia causing obstruction, without gangrene
Incarcerated umbilical hernia, without gangrene
Irreducible umbilical hernia, without gangrene
Strangulated umbilical hernia, without gangrene

     K42.1 **Umbilical hernia** with gangrene
Gangrenous umbilical hernia

     K42.9 **Umbilical hernia** without obstruction or gangrene
Umbilical hernia NOS

✅4ᵗʰ **K43** Ventral **hernia**
DEF: Condition in which a loop of bowel protrudes through a weakness in the abdominal wall muscles that may occur as a birth defect, past surgical site (incisional), or form at a stomal site (parastomal).

     K43.0 **Incisional hernia** with obstruction, without gangrene
Incisional hernia causing obstruction, without gangrene
Incarcerated incisional hernia, without gangrene
Irreducible incisional hernia, without gangrene
Strangulated incisional hernia, without gangrene

     K43.1 **Incisional hernia** with gangrene
Gangrenous incisional hernia
AHA: 2020,2Q,22

     K43.2 **Incisional hernia** without obstruction or gangrene
Incisional hernia NOS

     K43.3 **Parastomal hernia** with obstruction, without gangrene
Incarcerated parastomal hernia, without gangrene
Irreducible parastomal hernia, without gangrene
Parastomal hernia causing obstruction, without gangrene
Strangulated parastomal hernia, without gangrene

     K43.4 **Parastomal hernia** with gangrene
Gangrenous parastomal hernia

     K43.5 **Parastomal hernia** without obstruction or gangrene
Parastomal hernia NOS

     K43.6 **Other and unspecified ventral hernia with obstruction, without gangrene**
Epigastric hernia causing obstruction, without gangrene
Hypogastric hernia causing obstruction, without gangrene
Incarcerated epigastric hernia without gangrene
Incarcerated hypogastric hernia without gangrene
Incarcerated midline hernia without gangrene
Incarcerated spigelian hernia without gangrene
Incarcerated subxiphoid hernia without gangrene
Irreducible epigastric hernia without gangrene
Irreducible hypogastric hernia without gangrene
Irreducible midline hernia without gangrene
Irreducible spigelian hernia without gangrene
Irreducible subxiphoid hernia without gangrene
Midline hernia causing obstruction, without gangrene
Spigelian hernia causing obstruction, without gangrene
Strangulated epigastric hernia without gangrene
Strangulated hypogastric hernia without gangrene
Strangulated midline hernia without gangrene
Strangulated spigelian hernia without gangrene
Strangulated subxiphoid hernia without gangrene
Subxiphoid hernia causing obstruction, without gangrene

     K43.7 **Other and unspecified ventral hernia** with gangrene
Any condition listed under K43.6 specified as gangrenous

     K43.9 **Ventral hernia** without obstruction or gangrene
Epigastric hernia
Ventral hernia NOS

✓4ᵗʰ **K44 Diaphragmatic hernia**

> INCLUDES   hiatus hernia (esophageal) (sliding)
> paraesophageal hernia
> EXCLUDES 1   *congenital diaphragmatic hernia (Q79.0)*
> *congenital hiatus hernia (Q40.1)*

DEF: Protrusion of an abdominal organ, usually the stomach, through the esophageal opening within the diaphragm and occurring in two types: the sliding hiatal hernia and the paraesophageal hernia.

Hiatal Hernia

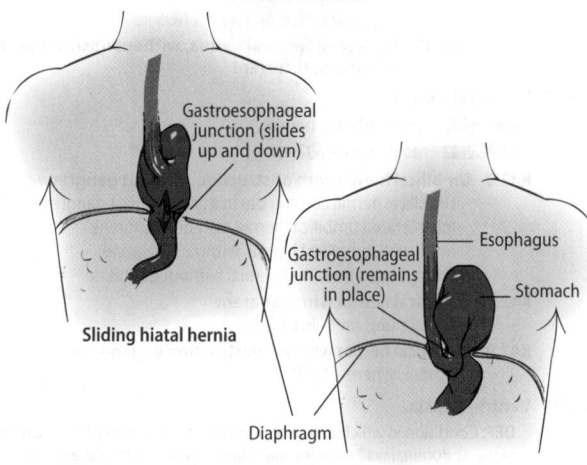

Gastroesophageal junction (slides up and down)

Sliding hiatal hernia

Gastroesophageal junction (remains in place)

Esophagus

Stomach

Diaphragm

Paraesophageal hiatal hernia

K44.0 Diaphragmatic hernia with obstruction, without gangrene
Diaphragmatic hernia causing obstruction
Incarcerated diaphragmatic hernia
Irreducible diaphragmatic hernia
Strangulated diaphragmatic hernia
AHA: 2022,2Q,13

K44.1 Diaphragmatic hernia with gangrene
Gangrenous diaphragmatic hernia

K44.9 Diaphragmatic hernia without obstruction or gangrene
Diaphragmatic hernia NOS

✓4ᵗʰ **K45 Other abdominal hernia**

> INCLUDES   abdominal hernia, specified site NEC
> lumbar hernia
> obturator hernia
> pudendal hernia
> retroperitoneal hernia
> sciatic hernia

K45.0 Other specified abdominal hernia with obstruction, without gangrene
Other specified abdominal hernia causing obstruction
Other specified incarcerated abdominal hernia
Other specified irreducible abdominal hernia
Other specified strangulated abdominal hernia

K45.1 Other specified abdominal hernia with gangrene
Any condition listed under K45 specified as gangrenous

K45.8 Other specified abdominal hernia without obstruction or gangrene

✓4ᵗʰ **K46 Unspecified abdominal hernia**

> INCLUDES   enterocele
> epiplocele
> hernia NOS
> interstitial hernia
> intestinal hernia
> intra-abdominal hernia
> EXCLUDES 1   *vaginal enterocele (N81.5)*

K46.0 Unspecified abdominal hernia with obstruction, without gangrene
Unspecified abdominal hernia causing obstruction
Unspecified incarcerated abdominal hernia
Unspecified irreducible abdominal hernia
Unspecified strangulated abdominal hernia

K46.1 Unspecified abdominal hernia with gangrene
Any condition listed under K46 specified as gangrenous

K46.9 Unspecified abdominal hernia without obstruction or gangrene
Abdominal hernia NOS

Noninfective enteritis and colitis (K50-K52)

> INCLUDES   noninfective inflammatory bowel disease
> EXCLUDES 1   *irritable bowel syndrome (K58.-)*
> *megacolon (K59.3-)*

✓4ᵗʰ **K50 Crohn's disease [regional enteritis]**

> INCLUDES   granulomatous enteritis
> Use additional code to identify manifestations, such as:
> pyoderma gangrenosum (L88)
> EXCLUDES 1   *ulcerative colitis (K51.-)*

AHA: 2019,3Q,5; 2012,4Q,104
DEF: Chronic inflammation of the gastrointestinal tract characterized by chronic granulomatous disease, most commonly affecting the intestines and the terminal ileum.

✓5ᵗʰ **K50.0 Crohn's disease of small intestine**
Crohn's disease [regional enteritis] of duodenum
Crohn's disease [regional enteritis] of ileum
Crohn's disease [regional enteritis] of jejunum
Regional ileitis
Terminal ileitis

> EXCLUDES 1   *Crohn's disease of both small and large intestine (K50.8-)*

K50.00 Crohn's disease of small intestine without complications HCC Rx ESR COM

✓6ᵗʰ **K50.01 Crohn's disease of small intestine with complications**

K50.011 Crohn's disease of small intestine with rectal bleeding HCC Rx ESR COM

K50.012 Crohn's disease of small intestine with intestinal obstruction HCC Rx ESR COM

K50.013 Crohn's disease of small intestine with fistula HCC Rx ESR COM

K50.014 Crohn's disease of small intestine with abscess HCC Rx ESR COM
AHA: 2012,4Q,104

K50.018 Crohn's disease of small intestine with other complication HCC Rx ESR COM

K50.019 Crohn's disease of small intestine with unspecified complications HCC Rx ESR COM

✓5ᵗʰ **K50.1 Crohn's disease of large intestine**
Crohn's disease [regional enteritis] of colon
Crohn's disease [regional enteritis] of large bowel
Crohn's disease [regional enteritis] of rectum
Granulomatous colitis
Regional colitis

> EXCLUDES 1   *Crohn's disease of both small and large intestine (K50.8)*

K50.10 Crohn's disease of large intestine without complications HCC Rx ESR COM

✓6ᵗʰ **K50.11 Crohn's disease of large intestine with complications**

K50.111 Crohn's disease of large intestine with rectal bleeding HCC Rx ESR COM

K50.112 Crohn's disease of large intestine with intestinal obstruction HCC Rx ESR COM

K50.113 Crohn's disease of large intestine with fistula HCC Rx ESR COM

K50.114 Crohn's disease of large intestine with abscess HCC Rx ESR COM

K50.118 Crohn's disease of large intestine with other complication HCC Rx ESR COM

K50.119 Crohn's disease of large intestine with unspecified complications HCC Rx ESR COM

✓5ᵗʰ **K50.8 Crohn's disease of both small and large intestine**

K50.80 Crohn's disease of both small and large intestine without complications HCC Rx ESR COM

✓6ᵗʰ **K50.81 Crohn's disease of both small and large intestine with complications**

K50.811 Crohn's disease of both small and large intestine with rectal bleeding HCC Rx ESR COM

K50.812 Crohn's disease of both small and large intestine with intestinal obstruction `HCC` `Rx` `ESR` `COM`

K50.813 Crohn's disease of both small and large intestine with fistula `HCC` `Rx` `ESR` `COM`

K50.814 Crohn's disease of both small and large intestine with abscess `HCC` `Rx` `ESR` `COM`

K50.818 Crohn's disease of both small and large intestine with other complication `HCC` `Rx` `ESR` `COM`

K50.819 Crohn's disease of both small and large intestine with unspecified complications `HCC` `Rx` `ESR` `COM`

✓5th **K50.9** Crohn's disease, unspecified

K50.90 Crohn's disease, unspecified, without complications `HCC` `Rx` `ESR` `COM`
Crohn's disease NOS
Regional enteritis NOS

✓6th **K50.91** Crohn's disease, unspecified, with complications

K50.911 Crohn's disease, unspecified, with rectal bleeding `HCC` `Rx` `ESR` `COM`

K50.912 Crohn's disease, unspecified, with intestinal obstruction `HCC` `Rx` `ESR` `COM`

K50.913 Crohn's disease, unspecified, with fistula `HCC` `Rx` `ESR` `COM`

K50.914 Crohn's disease, unspecified, with abscess `HCC` `Rx` `ESR` `COM`

K50.918 Crohn's disease, unspecified, with other complication `HCC` `Rx` `ESR` `COM`

K50.919 Crohn's disease, unspecified, with unspecified complications `HCC` `Rx` `ESR` `COM`

✓4th **K51** Ulcerative colitis

Use additional code to identify manifestations, such as:
pyoderma gangrenosum (L88)
EXCLUDES 1   Crohn's disease [regional enteritis] (K50.-)

✓5th **K51.0** Ulcerative (chronic) pancolitis
Backwash ileitis

K51.00 Ulcerative (chronic) pancolitis without complications `HCC` `Rx` `ESR` `COM`
Ulcerative (chronic) pancolitis NOS

✓6th **K51.01** Ulcerative (chronic) pancolitis with complications

K51.011 Ulcerative (chronic) pancolitis with rectal bleeding `HCC` `Rx` `ESR` `COM`

K51.012 Ulcerative (chronic) pancolitis with intestinal obstruction `HCC` `Rx` `ESR` `COM`

K51.013 Ulcerative (chronic) pancolitis with fistula `HCC` `Rx` `ESR` `COM`

K51.014 Ulcerative (chronic) pancolitis with abscess `HCC` `Rx` `ESR` `COM`

K51.018 Ulcerative (chronic) pancolitis with other complication `HCC` `Rx` `ESR` `COM`

K51.019 Ulcerative (chronic) pancolitis with unspecified complications `HCC` `Rx` `ESR` `COM`

✓5th **K51.2** Ulcerative (chronic) proctitis

K51.20 Ulcerative (chronic) proctitis without complications `HCC` `Rx` `ESR` `COM`
Ulcerative (chronic) proctitis NOS

✓6th **K51.21** Ulcerative (chronic) proctitis with complications

K51.211 Ulcerative (chronic) proctitis with rectal bleeding `HCC` `Rx` `ESR` `COM`

K51.212 Ulcerative (chronic) proctitis with intestinal obstruction `HCC` `Rx` `ESR` `COM`

K51.213 Ulcerative (chronic) proctitis with fistula `HCC` `Rx` `ESR` `COM`

K51.214 Ulcerative (chronic) proctitis with abscess `HCC` `Rx` `ESR` `COM`

K51.218 Ulcerative (chronic) proctitis with other complication `HCC` `Rx` `ESR` `COM`

K51.219 Ulcerative (chronic) proctitis with unspecified complications `HCC` `Rx` `ESR` `COM`

✓5th **K51.3** Ulcerative (chronic) rectosigmoiditis

K51.30 Ulcerative (chronic) rectosigmoiditis without complications `HCC` `Rx` `ESR` `COM`
Ulcerative (chronic) rectosigmoiditis NOS

✓6th **K51.31** Ulcerative (chronic) rectosigmoiditis with complications

K51.311 Ulcerative (chronic) rectosigmoiditis with rectal bleeding `HCC` `Rx` `ESR` `COM`

K51.312 Ulcerative (chronic) rectosigmoiditis with intestinal obstruction `HCC` `Rx` `ESR` `COM`

K51.313 Ulcerative (chronic) rectosigmoiditis with fistula `HCC` `Rx` `ESR` `COM`

K51.314 Ulcerative (chronic) rectosigmoiditis with abscess `HCC` `Rx` `ESR` `COM`

K51.318 Ulcerative (chronic) rectosigmoiditis with other complication `HCC` `Rx` `ESR` `COM`

K51.319 Ulcerative (chronic) rectosigmoiditis with unspecified complications `HCC` `Rx` `ESR` `COM`

✓5th **K51.4** Inflammatory polyps of colon
EXCLUDES 1   adenomatous polyp of colon (D12.6)
polyposis of colon (D12.6)
polyps of colon NOS (K63.5)

K51.40 Inflammatory polyps of colon without complications `HCC` `Rx` `ESR` `COM`
Inflammatory polyps of colon NOS

✓6th **K51.41** Inflammatory polyps of colon with complications

K51.411 Inflammatory polyps of colon with rectal bleeding `HCC` `Rx` `ESR` `COM`

K51.412 Inflammatory polyps of colon with intestinal obstruction `HCC` `Rx` `ESR` `COM`

K51.413 Inflammatory polyps of colon with fistula `HCC` `Rx` `ESR` `COM`

K51.414 Inflammatory polyps of colon with abscess `HCC` `Rx` `ESR` `COM`

K51.418 Inflammatory polyps of colon with other complication `HCC` `Rx` `ESR` `COM`

K51.419 Inflammatory polyps of colon with unspecified complications `HCC` `Rx` `ESR` `COM`

✓5th **K51.5** Left sided colitis
Left hemicolitis

K51.50 Left sided colitis without complications `HCC` `Rx` `ESR` `COM`
Left sided colitis NOS

✓6th **K51.51** Left sided colitis with complications

K51.511 Left sided colitis with rectal bleeding `HCC` `Rx` `ESR` `COM`

K51.512 Left sided colitis with intestinal obstruction `HCC` `Rx` `ESR` `COM`

K51.513 Left sided colitis with fistula `HCC` `Rx` `ESR` `COM`

K51.514 Left sided colitis with abscess `HCC` `Rx` `ESR` `COM`

K51.518 Left sided colitis with other complication `HCC` `Rx` `ESR` `COM`

K51.519 Left sided colitis with unspecified complications `HCC` `Rx` `ESR` `COM`

✓5th **K51.8** Other ulcerative colitis

K51.80 Other ulcerative colitis without complications `HCC` `Rx` `ESR` `COM`

✓6th **K51.81** Other ulcerative colitis with complications

K51.811 Other ulcerative colitis with rectal bleeding `HCC` `Rx` `ESR` `COM`

K51.812 Other ulcerative colitis with intestinal obstruction `HCC` `Rx` `ESR` `COM`

K51.813 Other ulcerative colitis with fistula `HCC` `Rx` `ESR` `COM`

K51.814 Other ulcerative colitis with abscess `HCC` `Rx` `ESR` `COM`

K51.818 Other ulcerative colitis with other complication `HCC` `Rx` `ESR` `COM`

K51.819 Other ulcerative colitis with unspecified complications `HCC` `Rx` `ESR` `COM`

✓5th **K51.9** Ulcerative colitis, unspecified

K51.90 Ulcerative colitis, unspecified, without complications `HCC` `Rx` `ESR` `COM`

✓6th **K51.91** Ulcerative colitis, unspecified, with complications

K51.911 Ulcerative colitis, unspecified with rectal bleeding `HCC` `Rx` `ESR` `COM`

K51.912 Ulcerative colitis, unspecified with intestinal obstruction `HCC` `Rx` `ESR` `COM`

K51.913   Ulcerative colitis, unspecified with fistula   `HCC` `Rx` `ESR` `COM`

K51.914   Ulcerative colitis, unspecified with abscess   `HCC` `Rx` `ESR` `COM`

K51.918   Ulcerative colitis, unspecified with other complication   `HCC` `Rx` `ESR` `COM`

K51.919   Ulcerative colitis, unspecified with unspecified complications   `HCC` `Rx` `ESR` `COM`

✓4ᵗʰ **K52**   **Other and unspecified noninfective gastroenteritis and colitis**

     AHA: 2016,4Q,30-31

K52.Ø   **Gastroenteritis and colitis due to** radiation

K52.1   Toxic **gastroenteritis and colitis**

     Drug-induced gastroenteritis and colitis

     Code first (T51-T65) to identify toxic agent

     Use additional code for adverse effect, if applicable, to identify drug (T36-T5Ø with fifth or sixth character 5)

     AHA: 2019,1Q,17

✓5ᵗʰ **K52.2**   Allergic and dietetic **gastroenteritis and colitis**

     Food hypersensitivity gastroenteritis or colitis

     Use additional code to identify type of food allergy (Z91.Ø1-, Z91.Ø2-)

     EXCLUDES 2   *allergic eosinophilic colitis (K52.82)*

               allergic eosinophilic esophagitis (K2Ø.Ø)

               allergic eosinophilic gastritis (K52.81)

               allergic eosinophilic gastroenteritis (K52.81)

     DEF: True immunoglobulin E (IgE)-mediated allergic reaction of the lining of the stomach, intestines, or colon to food proteins. It causes nausea, vomiting, diarrhea, and abdominal cramping.

K52.21   **Food protein-induced** enterocolitis syndrome

     FPIES

     Use additional code for hypovolemic shock, if present (R57.1)

K52.22   **Food protein-induced** enteropathy

K52.29   **Other allergic and dietetic gastroenteritis and colitis**

     Allergic proctocolitis

     Food hypersensitivity gastroenteritis or colitis

     Food-induced eosinophilic proctocolitis

     Food protein-induced proctocolitis

     Immediate gastrointestinal hypersensitivity

     Milk protein-induced proctocolitis

K52.3   Indeterminate **colitis**

     Colonic inflammatory bowel disease unclassified (IBDU)

     EXCLUDES 1   *unspecified colitis (K52.9)*

✓5ᵗʰ **K52.8**   **Other specified noninfective gastroenteritis and colitis**

K52.81   **Eosinophilic gastritis or gastroenteritis**

     Eosinophilic enteritis

     EXCLUDES 2   *eosinophilic esophagitis (K2Ø.Ø)*

     DEF: Disorder involving the accumulation of eosinophil in the lining of the stomach or multiple levels of the gastrointestinal tract, but without a known cause such as connective tissue disease, drug reaction, malignancy, or parasitic infection.

K52.82   **Eosinophilic colitis**

     EXCLUDES 2   *allergic proctocolitis (K52.29)*

               food-induced eosinophilic proctocolitis (K52.29)

               food protein-induced enterocolitis syndrome (FPIES) (K52.21)

               food protein-induced proctocolitis (K52.29)

               milk protein-induced proctocolitis (K52.29)

     DEF: Disorder involving the accumulation of eosinophil in the tissues lining the colon, but without a known cause such as connective tissue disease, drug reaction, malignancy, or parasitic infection. The resultant inflammation may cause extreme abdominal pain, diarrhea, or bloody stool.

✓6ᵗʰ **K52.83**   **Microscopic colitis**

K52.831   Collagenous **colitis**   `Rx`

K52.832   Lymphocytic **colitis**   `Rx`

K52.838   **Other microscopic colitis**   `Rx`

K52.839   **Microscopic colitis, unspecified**   `Rx`

K52.89   **Other specified noninfective gastroenteritis and colitis**

     AHA: 2019,1Q,20

K52.9   **Noninfective gastroenteritis and colitis, unspecified**

     Colitis NOS

     Enteritis NOS

     Gastroenteritis NOS

     Ileitis NOS

     Jejunitis NOS

     Sigmoiditis NOS

     EXCLUDES 1   *diarrhea NOS (R19.7)*

               functional diarrhea (K59.1)

               infectious gastroenteritis and colitis NOS (AØ9)

               neonatal diarrhea (noninfective) (P78.3)

               psychogenic diarrhea (F45.8)

     AHA: 2021,3Q,3

Other diseases of intestines (K55-K64)

✓4ᵗʰ **K55**   **Vascular disorders of intestine**

     EXCLUDES 1   *necrotizing enterocolitis of newborn (P77.-)*

     AHA: 2016,4Q,32

✓5ᵗʰ **K55.Ø**   Acute **vascular disorders of intestine**

     Infarction of appendices epiploicae

     Mesenteric (artery) (vein) embolism

     Mesenteric (artery) (vein) infarction

     Mesenteric (artery) (vein) thrombosis

     AHA: 2019,4Q,68

✓6ᵗʰ **K55.Ø1**   **Acute (reversible)** ischemia of small intestine

K55.Ø11   **Focal (segmental) acute (reversible) ischemia of small intestine**   `HCC` `ESR` `COM`

K55.Ø12   **Diffuse acute (reversible) ischemia of small intestine**   `HCC` `ESR` `COM`

K55.Ø19   **Acute (reversible) ischemia of small intestine, extent unspecified**   `HCC` `ESR` `COM`

✓6ᵗʰ **K55.Ø2**   **Acute** infarction of small intestine

     Gangrene of small intestine

     Necrosis of small intestine

K55.Ø21   **Focal (segmental) acute infarction of small intestine**   `HCC` `ESR` `COM`

K55.Ø22   **Diffuse acute infarction of small intestine**   `HCC` `ESR` `COM`

K55.Ø29   **Acute infarction of small intestine, extent unspecified**   `HCC` `ESR` `COM`

✓6ᵗʰ **K55.Ø3**   **Acute (reversible)** ischemia of large intestine

     Acute fulminant ischemic colitis

     Subacute ischemic colitis

K55.Ø31   **Focal (segmental) acute (reversible) ischemia of large intestine**   `HCC` `ESR` `COM`

K55.Ø32   **Diffuse acute (reversible) ischemia of large intestine**   `HCC` `ESR` `COM`

K55.Ø39   **Acute (reversible) ischemia of large intestine, extent unspecified**   `HCC` `ESR` `COM`

     AHA: 2019,4Q,68

✓6ᵗʰ **K55.Ø4**   **Acute** infarction of large intestine

     Gangrene of large intestine

     Necrosis of large intestine

K55.Ø41   **Focal (segmental) acute infarction of large intestine**   `HCC` `ESR` `COM`

K55.Ø42   **Diffuse acute infarction of large intestine**   `HCC` `ESR` `COM`

K55.Ø49   **Acute infarction of large intestine, extent unspecified**   `HCC` `ESR` `COM`

✓6ᵗʰ **K55.Ø5**   **Acute (reversible)** ischemia of intestine, part unspecified

K55.Ø51   **Focal (segmental) acute (reversible) ischemia of intestine, part unspecified**   `HCC` `ESR` `COM`

K55.Ø52   **Diffuse acute (reversible) ischemia of intestine, part unspecified**   `HCC` `ESR` `COM`

K55.Ø59   **Acute (reversible) ischemia of intestine, part and extent unspecified**   `HCC` `ESR` `COM`

`HCC` CMS-HCC   `Rx` Rx HCC   `ESR` ESRD HCC   `COM` Commercial HCC   `N` Newborn: 0   `P` Pediatric: 0-17   `M` Maternity: 9-64   `A` Adult: 15-124

736   ICD-10-CM 2023

√6ᵗʰ **K55.06** **Acute infarction of intestine, part unspecified**
Acute intestinal infarction
Gangrene of intestine
Necrosis of intestine

    K55.061 **Focal (segmental) acute infarction of intestine, part unspecified** `HCC` `ESR` `COM`

    K55.062 **Diffuse acute infarction of intestine, part unspecified** `HCC` `ESR` `COM`

    K55.069 **Acute infarction of intestine, part and extent unspecified** `HCC` `ESR` `COM`

K55.1 **Chronic vascular disorders of intestine** `HCC` `ESR` `COM`
Chronic ischemic colitis
Chronic ischemic enteritis
Chronic ischemic enterocolitis
Ischemic stricture of intestine
Mesenteric atherosclerosis
Mesenteric vascular insufficiency

√5ᵗʰ **K55.2** **Angiodysplasia of colon**

AHA: 2018,3Q,21

TIP: Assign a code for "with hemorrhage" when angiodysplasia and GI bleeding are documented. The ICD-10-CM classification assumes the two are related without the provider linking the two conditions. Evidence of bleeding during a procedure is not required.

    K55.20 **Angiodysplasia of colon without hemorrhage**

    K55.21 **Angiodysplasia of colon with hemorrhage**
      DEF: Small vascular abnormalities due to fragile blood vessels in the colon, resulting in blood loss from the gastrointestinal (GI) tract.

√5ᵗʰ **K55.3** **Necrotizing enterocolitis**
    EXCLUDES 1   *necrotizing enterocolitis of newborn (P77.-)*
    EXCLUDES 2   *necrotizing enterocolitis due to Clostridium difficile (A04.7-)*

    K55.30 **Necrotizing enterocolitis, unspecified** `HCC` `ESR` `COM`
      Necrotizing enterocolitis, NOS

    K55.31 **Stage 1 necrotizing enterocolitis** `HCC` `ESR` `COM`
      Necrotizing enterocolitis without pneumatosis, without perforation

    K55.32 **Stage 2 necrotizing enterocolitis** `HCC` `ESR` `COM`
      Necrotizing enterocolitis with pneumatosis, without perforation

    K55.33 **Stage 3 necrotizing enterocolitis** `HCC` `ESR` `COM`
      Necrotizing enterocolitis with perforation
      Necrotizing enterocolitis with pneumatosis and perforation

K55.8 **Other vascular disorders of intestine** `HCC` `ESR` `COM`

K55.9 **Vascular disorder of intestine, unspecified** `HCC` `ESR` `COM`
Ischemic colitis
Ischemic enteritis
Ischemic enterocolitis

√4ᵗʰ **K56** **Paralytic ileus and intestinal obstruction without hernia**
    EXCLUDES 1   *congenital stricture or stenosis of intestine (Q41-Q42)*
      cystic fibrosis with meconium ileus (E84.11)
      ischemic stricture of intestine (K55.1)
      meconium ileus NOS (P76.0)
      neonatal intestinal obstructions classifiable to P76.-
      obstruction of duodenum (K31.5)
      postprocedural intestinal obstruction (K91.3-)
    EXCLUDES 2   *stenosis of anus or rectum (K62.4)*

K56.0 **Paralytic ileus** `HCC` `ESR` `COM`
Paralysis of bowel
Paralysis of colon
Paralysis of intestine
    EXCLUDES 1   *gallstone ileus (K56.3)*
      ileus NOS (K56.7)
      obstructive ileus NOS (K56.69-)
    DEF: Intestinal obstruction due to paralysis of bowel motility or peristalsis.

K56.1 **Intussusception** `HCC` `ESR` `COM`
Intussusception or invagination of bowel
Intussusception or invagination of colon
Intussusception or invagination of intestine
Intussusception or invagination of rectum
    EXCLUDES 2   *intussusception of appendix (K38.8)*
    DEF: Intestinal obstruction due to prolapse of a bowel section into an adjacent section. It occurs primarily in children and symptoms include acute abdominal pain, vomiting, and passage of blood and mucus from the rectum.

K56.2 **Volvulus** `HCC` `ESR` `COM`
Strangulation of colon or intestine
Torsion of colon or intestine
Twist of colon or intestine
    EXCLUDES 2   *volvulus of duodenum (K31.5)*
    DEF: Twisting, knotting, or entanglement of the bowel on itself that may quickly compromise oxygen supply to the intestinal tissues. A volvulus usually occurs at the sigmoid and ileocecal areas of the intestines.

Volvulus

Knotted intestine (volvulus)

K56.3 **Gallstone ileus** `HCC` `ESR` `COM`
Obstruction of intestine by gallstone

√5ᵗʰ **K56.4** **Other impaction of intestine**

    K56.41 **Fecal impaction** `HCC` `ESR` `COM`
      EXCLUDES 1   *constipation (K59.0-)*
           incomplete defecation (R15.0)

    K56.49 **Other impaction of intestine** `HCC` `ESR` `COM`

√5ᵗʰ **K56.5** **Intestinal adhesions [bands] with obstruction (postinfection)**
Abdominal hernia due to adhesions with obstruction
Peritoneal adhesions [bands] with intestinal obstruction (postinfection)
AHA: 2017,4Q,16-17

    K56.50 **Intestinal adhesions [bands], unspecified as to partial versus complete obstruction** `HCC` `ESR` `COM`
      Intestinal adhesions with obstruction NOS

    K56.51 **Intestinal adhesions [bands], with partial obstruction** `HCC` `ESR` `COM`
      Intestinal adhesions with incomplete obstruction

    K56.52 **Intestinal adhesions [bands] with complete obstruction** `HCC` `ESR` `COM`

√5ᵗʰ **K56.6** **Other and unspecified intestinal obstruction**
AHA: 2017,4Q,16-17; 2017,2Q,12

  √6ᵗʰ **K56.60** **Unspecified intestinal obstruction**

    K56.600 **Partial intestinal obstruction, unspecified as to cause** `HCC` `ESR` `COM`
      Incomplete intestinal obstruction, NOS

    K56.601 **Complete intestinal obstruction, unspecified as to cause** `HCC` `ESR` `COM`

    K56.609 **Unspecified intestinal obstruction, unspecified as to partial versus complete obstruction** `HCC` `ESR` `COM`
      Intestinal obstruction NOS

√6ᵗʰ **K56.69 Other intestinal obstruction**
     Enterostenosis NOS
     Obstructive ileus NOS
     Occlusion of colon or intestine NOS
     Stenosis of colon or intestine NOS
     Stricture of colon or intestine NOS
     EXCLUDES 1   *intestinal obstruction due to specified condition - code to condition*

K56.690 Other partial intestinal obstruction HCC ESR COM
     Other incomplete intestinal obstruction

K56.691 Other complete intestinal obstruction HCC ESR COM

K56.699 Other intestinal obstruction unspecified as to partial versus complete obstruction HCC ESR COM
     Other intestinal obstruction, NEC

K56.7 Ileus, unspecified HCC ESR COM
     EXCLUDES 1   *obstructive ileus (K56.69-)*
     EXCLUDES 2   *intestinal obstruction with hernia (K40-K46)*
     AHA: 2017,1Q,40

√4ᵗʰ **K57 Diverticular disease of intestine**
     Code also if applicable peritonitis K65.-
     EXCLUDES 1   *congenital diverticulum of intestine (Q43.8)*
               Meckel's diverticulum (Q43.0)
     EXCLUDES 2   *diverticulum of appendix (K38.2)*
     AHA: 2022,1Q,26-27; 2021,1Q,9,11; 2018,3Q,21
     TIP: Assign a code for "with bleeding" when diverticular disease of the intestine and GI bleeding are documented. The ICD-10-CM classification assumes the two are related without the provider linking the two conditions. Evidence of bleeding during a procedure is not required.

√5ᵗʰ **K57.0 Diverticulitis of small intestine with perforation and abscess**
     EXCLUDES 1   *diverticulitis of both small and large intestine with perforation and abscess (K57.4-)*

K57.00 Diverticulitis of small intestine with perforation and abscess without bleeding

K57.01 Diverticulitis of small intestine with perforation and abscess with bleeding

√5ᵗʰ **K57.1 Diverticular disease of small intestine without perforation or abscess**
     EXCLUDES 1   *diverticular disease of both small and large intestine without perforation or abscess (K57.5-)*

K57.10 Diverticulosis of small intestine without perforation or abscess without bleeding
     Diverticular disease of small intestine NOS

K57.11 Diverticulosis of small intestine without perforation or abscess with bleeding

K57.12 Diverticulitis of small intestine without perforation or abscess without bleeding

K57.13 Diverticulitis of small intestine without perforation or abscess with bleeding

√5ᵗʰ **K57.2 Diverticulitis of large intestine with perforation and abscess**
     EXCLUDES 1   *diverticulitis of both small and large intestine with perforation and abscess (K57.4-)*

K57.20 Diverticulitis of large intestine with perforation and abscess without bleeding

K57.21 Diverticulitis of large intestine with perforation and abscess with bleeding

√5ᵗʰ **K57.3 Diverticular disease of large intestine without perforation or abscess**
     EXCLUDES 1   *diverticular disease of both small and large intestine without perforation or abscess (K57.5-)*

K57.30 Diverticulosis of large intestine without perforation or abscess without bleeding
     Diverticular disease of colon NOS

K57.31 Diverticulosis of large intestine without perforation or abscess with bleeding

K57.32 Diverticulitis of large intestine without perforation or abscess without bleeding

K57.33 Diverticulitis of large intestine without perforation or abscess with bleeding

√5ᵗʰ **K57.4 Diverticulitis of both small and large intestine with perforation and abscess**

K57.40 Diverticulitis of both small and large intestine with perforation and abscess without bleeding

K57.41 Diverticulitis of both small and large intestine with perforation and abscess with bleeding

√5ᵗʰ **K57.5 Diverticular disease of both small and large intestine without perforation or abscess**

K57.50 Diverticulosis of both small and large intestine without perforation or abscess without bleeding
     Diverticular disease of both small and large intestine NOS

K57.51 Diverticulosis of both small and large intestine without perforation or abscess with bleeding

K57.52 Diverticulitis of both small and large intestine without perforation or abscess without bleeding

K57.53 Diverticulitis of both small and large intestine without perforation or abscess with bleeding

√5ᵗʰ **K57.8 Diverticulitis of intestine, part unspecified, with perforation and abscess**

K57.80 Diverticulitis of intestine, part unspecified, with perforation and abscess without bleeding

K57.81 Diverticulitis of intestine, part unspecified, with perforation and abscess with bleeding

√5ᵗʰ **K57.9 Diverticular disease of intestine, part unspecified, without perforation or abscess**

K57.90 Diverticulosis of intestine, part unspecified, without perforation or abscess without bleeding
     Diverticular disease of intestine NOS

K57.91 Diverticulosis of intestine, part unspecified, without perforation or abscess with bleeding

K57.92 Diverticulitis of intestine, part unspecified, without perforation or abscess without bleeding

K57.93 Diverticulitis of intestine, part unspecified, without perforation or abscess with bleeding

√4ᵗʰ **K58 Irritable bowel syndrome**
     INCLUDES   irritable colon
               spastic colon
     AHA: 2016,4Q,32-33

K58.0 Irritable bowel syndrome with diarrhea

K58.1 Irritable bowel syndrome with constipation

K58.2 Mixed irritable bowel syndrome

K58.8 Other irritable bowel syndrome

K58.9 Irritable bowel syndrome without diarrhea
     Irritable bowel syndrome NOS

√4ᵗʰ **K59 Other functional intestinal disorders**
     EXCLUDES 1   *change in bowel habit NOS (R19.4)*
               intestinal malabsorption (K90.-)
               psychogenic intestinal disorders (F45.8)
     EXCLUDES 2   *functional disorders of stomach (K31.-)*

√5ᵗʰ **K59.0 Constipation**
     EXCLUDES 1   *fecal impaction (K56.41)*
               incomplete defecation (R15.0)
     AHA: 2016,4Q,33

K59.00 Constipation, unspecified

K59.01 Slow transit constipation
     DEF: Delay in the transit of fecal material through the colon secondary to smooth muscle dysfunction or decreased peristaltic contractions along the colon.

K59.02 Outlet dysfunction constipation

K59.03 Drug induced constipation
     Use additional code for adverse effect, if applicable, to identify drug (T36-T50 with fifth or sixth character 5)

K59.04 Chronic idiopathic constipation
     Functional constipation

K59.09 Other constipation
     Chronic constipation

K59.1 Functional diarrhea
     EXCLUDES 1   *diarrhea NOS (R19.7)*
               irritable bowel syndrome with diarrhea (K58.0)

K59.2 Neurogenic bowel, not elsewhere classified
     DEF: Disorder of bowel due to a spinal cord lesion because of injury or as a complication of conditions such as multiple sclerosis (MS) or spina bifida. Loss of bowel control is the primary symptom, manifested as constipation or bowel incontinence.

✓5ᵗʰ **K59.3　Megacolon, not elsewhere classified**
　　　　Dilatation of colon
　　　　Code first, if applicable (T51-T65) to identify toxic agent
　　　　EXCLUDES 1　*congenital megacolon (aganglionic) (Q43.1)*
　　　　　　　　　　megacolon (due to) (in) Chagas' disease (B57.32)
　　　　　　　　　　megacolon (due to) (in) Clostridium difficile (A04.7-)
　　　　　　　　　　megacolon (due to) (in) Hirschsprung's disease
　　　　　　　　　　　(Q43.1)
　　　　AHA: 2016,4Q,33-34
　　K59.31　Toxic megacolon　　　　　HCC ESR COM
　　K59.39　Other megacolon
　　　　　　　Megacolon NOS
K59.4　Anal spasm
　　　　Proctalgia fugax
✓5ᵗʰ **K59.8　Other specified functional intestinal disorders**
　　　　AHA: 2020,4Q,29-30
　　K59.81　Ogilvie syndrome
　　　　　　　Acute colonic pseudo-obstruction (ACPO)
　　K59.89　Other specified functional intestinal disorders
　　　　　　　Atony of colon
　　　　　　　Pseudo-obstruction (acute) (chronic) of intestine
K59.9　Functional intestinal disorder, unspecified

✓4ᵗʰ **K60　Fissure and fistula of anal and rectal regions**
　　　　EXCLUDES 1　*fissure and fistula of anal and rectal regions with abscess or*
　　　　　　　　　　cellulitis (K61.-)
　　　　EXCLUDES 2　*anal sphincter tear (healed) (nontraumatic) (old) (K62.81)*
　　K60.0　Acute anal fissure
　　K60.1　Chronic anal fissure
　　K60.2　Anal fissure, unspecified
　　K60.3　Anal fistula
　　K60.4　Rectal fistula
　　　　　　　Fistula of rectum to skin
　　　　　　EXCLUDES 1　*rectovaginal fistula (N82.3)*
　　　　　　　　　　　vesicorectal fistual (N32.1)
　　K60.5　Anorectal fistula

✓4ᵗʰ **K61　Abscess of anal and rectal regions**
　　　　INCLUDES　abscess of anal and rectal regions
　　　　　　　　　cellulitis of anal and rectal regions
　　K61.0　Anal abscess
　　　　　　　Perianal abscess
　　　　　　EXCLUDES 2　*intrasphincteric abscess (K61.4)*
　　K61.1　Rectal abscess
　　　　　　　Perirectal abscess
　　　　　　EXCLUDES 1　*ischiorectal abscess (K61.39)*
　　　　　　AHA: 2012,4Q,104
　　K61.2　Anorectal abscess
✓5ᵗʰ **K61.3　Ischiorectal abscess**
　　　　　　AHA: 2018,4Q,19
　　K61.31　Horseshoe abscess
　　K61.39　Other ischiorectal abscess
　　　　　　　Abscess of ischiorectal fossa
　　　　　　　Ischiorectal abscess, NOS
　　K61.4　Intrasphincteric abscess
　　　　　　　Intersphincteric abscess
　　K61.5　Supralevator abscess
　　　　　　AHA: 2018,4Q,19

✓4ᵗʰ **K62　Other diseases of anus and rectum**
　　　　INCLUDES　anal canal
　　　　EXCLUDES 2　*colostomy and enterostomy malfunction (K94.0-, K94.1-)*
　　　　　　　　　　fecal incontinence (R15.-)
　　　　　　　　　　hemorrhoids (K64.-)
　　K62.0　Anal polyp
　　K62.1　Rectal polyp
　　　　　　EXCLUDES 1　*adenomatous polyp (D12.8)*
　　　　　　AHA: 2018,1Q,6
　　K62.2　Anal prolapse
　　　　　　　Prolapse of anal canal
　　K62.3　Rectal prolapse
　　　　　　　Prolapse of rectal mucosa
　　K62.4　Stenosis of anus and rectum
　　　　　　　Stricture of anus (sphincter)
　　　　　　AHA: 2019,2Q,13

K62.5　Hemorrhage of anus and rectum
　　　　EXCLUDES 1　*gastrointestinal bleeding NOS (K92.2)*
　　　　　　　　　　melena (K92.1)
　　　　　　　　　　neonatal rectal hemorrhage (P54.2)
　　　　AHA: 2019,1Q,21
K62.6　Ulcer of anus and rectum
　　　　Solitary ulcer of anus and rectum
　　　　Stercoral ulcer of anus and rectum
　　　　EXCLUDES 1　*fissure and fistula of anus and rectum (K60.-)*
　　　　　　　　　　ulcerative colitis (K51.-)
K62.7　Radiation proctitis
　　　　Use additional code to identify the type of radiation (W88.-) or
　　　　　radiation therapy (Y84.2)
　　　　AHA: 2019,1Q,21
✓5ᵗʰ **K62.8　Other specified diseases of anus and rectum**
　　　　EXCLUDES 2　*ulcerative proctitis (K51.2)*
　　K62.81　Anal sphincter tear (healed) (nontraumatic) (old)
　　　　　　　Tear of anus, nontraumatic
　　　　　　　Use additional code for any associated fecal
　　　　　　　　incontinence (R15.-)
　　　　　　EXCLUDES 2　*anal fissure (K60.-)*
　　　　　　　　　　　anal sphincter tear (healed) (old)
　　　　　　　　　　　　complicating delivery (O34.7-)
　　　　　　　　　　　traumatic tear of anal sphincter (S31.831)
　　K62.82　Dysplasia of anus
　　　　　　　Anal intraepithelial neoplasia I and II (AIN I and II)
　　　　　　　　(histologically confirmed)
　　　　　　　Dysplasia of anus NOS
　　　　　　　Mild and moderate dysplasia of anus (histologically
　　　　　　　　confirmed)
　　　　　　EXCLUDES 1　*abnormal results from anal cytologic*
　　　　　　　　　　　examination without histologic
　　　　　　　　　　　confirmation (R85.61-)
　　　　　　　　　　　anal intraepithelial neoplasia III (D01.3)
　　　　　　　　　　　carcinoma in situ of anus (D01.3)
　　　　　　　　　　　HGSIL of anus (R85.613)
　　　　　　　　　　　severe dysplasia of anus (D01.3)
　　K62.89　Other specified diseases of anus and rectum
　　　　　　　Proctitis NOS
　　　　　　　Use additional code for any associated fecal
　　　　　　　　incontinence (R15.-)
K62.9　Disease of anus and rectum, unspecified

✓4ᵗʰ **K63　Other diseases of intestine**
　　K63.0　Abscess of intestine
　　　　　　EXCLUDES 1　*abscess of intestine with Crohn's disease (K50.014,*
　　　　　　　　　　　K50.114, K50.814, K50.914)
　　　　　　　　　　　abscess of intestine with diverticular disease (K57.0,
　　　　　　　　　　　K57.2, K57.4, K57.8)
　　　　　　　　　　　abscess of intestine with ulcerative colitis (K51.014,
　　　　　　　　　　　K51.214, K51.314, K51.414, K51.514, K51.814,
　　　　　　　　　　　K51.914)
　　　　　　EXCLUDES 2　*abscess of anal and rectal regions (K61.-)*
　　　　　　　　　　　abscess of appendix (K35.3-)
　　K63.1　Perforation of intestine (nontraumatic)　　　HCC ESR COM
　　　　　　　Perforation (nontraumatic) of rectum
　　　　　　EXCLUDES 1　*perforation (nontraumatic) of duodenum (K26.-)*
　　　　　　　　　　　perforation (nontraumatic) of intestine with
　　　　　　　　　　　diverticular disease (K57.0, K57.2, K57.4, K57.8)
　　　　　　EXCLUDES 2　*perforation (nontraumatic) of appendix (K35.2-,*
　　　　　　　　　　　K35.3-)
　　　　　　AHA: 2020,2Q,22
　　K63.2　Fistula of intestine
　　　　　　EXCLUDES 1　*fistula of duodenum (K31.6)*
　　　　　　　　　　　fistula of intestine with Crohn's disease (K50.013,
　　　　　　　　　　　K50.113, K50.813, K50.913)
　　　　　　　　　　　fistula of intestine with ulcerative colitis (K51.013,
　　　　　　　　　　　K51.213, K51.313, K51.413, K51.513, K51.813,
　　　　　　　　　　　K51.913)
　　　　　　EXCLUDES 2　*fistula of anal and rectal regions (K60.-)*
　　　　　　　　　　　fistula of appendix (K38.3)
　　　　　　　　　　　intestinal-genital fistula, female (N82.2-N82.4)
　　　　　　　　　　　vesicointestinal fistula (N32.1)
　　　　　　AHA: 2017,3Q,4

K63.3 **Ulcer of intestine**
Primary ulcer of small intestine
> EXCLUDES 1 *duodenal ulcer (K26.-)*
> *gastrointestinal ulcer (K28.-)*
> *gastrojejunal ulcer (K28.-)*
> *jejunal ulcer (K28.-)*
> *peptic ulcer, site unspecified (K27.-)*
> *ulcer of intestine with perforation (K63.1)*
> *ulcer of anus or rectum (K62.6)*
> *ulcerative colitis (K51.-)*

K63.4 **Enteroptosis**

K63.5 **Polyp of colon**
> EXCLUDES 1 *adenomatous polyp of colon (D12.-)*
> *inflammatory polyp of colon (K51.4-)*
> *polyposis of colon (D12.6)*

AHA: 2019,1Q,33; 2018,2Q,14; 2017,1Q,15; 2015,2Q,14
TIP: Assign this code when documentation states hyperplastic colon polyp regardless of the site in the colon. Slow-growing, hyperplastic polyps are not precancerous and are classified differently from benign or adenomatous polyps.

✓5ᵗʰ **K63.8** **Other specified diseases of intestine**

K63.81 **Dieulafoy lesion of intestine**
> EXCLUDES 2 *Dieulafoy lesion of stomach and duodenum (K31.82)*

DEF: Abnormally large submucosal artery protruding through a defect in the stomach mucosa or intestines that can cause massive and life-threatening hemorrhaging.

K63.89 **Other specified diseases of intestine**
AHA: 2013,2Q,31

K63.9 **Disease of intestine, unspecified**

✓4ᵗʰ **K64** **Hemorrhoids and perianal venous thrombosis**
> INCLUDES piles
> EXCLUDES 1 *hemorrhoids complicating childbirth and the puerperium (O87.2)*
> *hemorrhoids complicating pregnancy (O22.4)*

Hemorrhoids

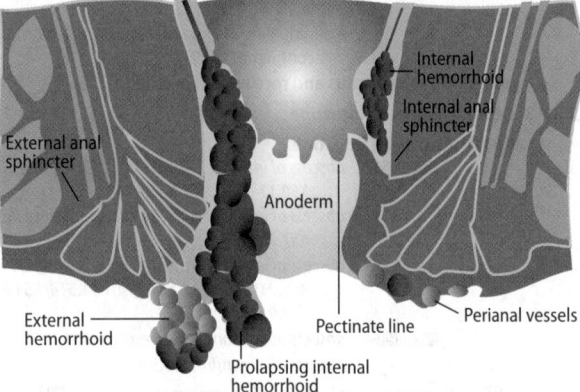

K64.0 **First degree hemorrhoids**
Grade/stage I hemorrhoids
Hemorrhoids (bleeding) without prolapse outside of anal canal

K64.1 **Second degree hemorrhoids**
Grade/stage II hemorrhoids
Hemorrhoids (bleeding) that prolapse with straining, but retract spontaneously

K64.2 **Third degree hemorrhoids**
Grade/stage III hemorrhoids
Hemorrhoids (bleeding) that prolapse with straining and require manual replacement back inside anal canal

K64.3 **Fourth degree hemorrhoids**
Grade/stage IV hemorrhoids
Hemorrhoids (bleeding) with prolapsed tissue that cannot be manually replaced

K64.4 **Residual hemorrhoidal skin tags**
External hemorrhoids, NOS
Skin tags of anus

K64.5 **Perianal venous thrombosis**
External hemorrhoids with thrombosis
Perianal hematoma
Thrombosed hemorrhoids NOS

K64.8 **Other hemorrhoids**
Internal hemorrhoids, without mention of degree
Prolapsed hemorrhoids, degree not specified

K64.9 **Unspecified hemorrhoids**
Hemorrhoids (bleeding) NOS
Hemorrhoids (bleeding) without mention of degree

Diseases of peritoneum and retroperitoneum (K65-K68)

✓4ᵗʰ **K65** **Peritonitis**
Use additional code (B95-B97), to identify infectious agent, if known
Code also if applicable diverticular disease of intestine (K57.-)
> EXCLUDES 1 *acute appendicitis with generalized peritonitis (K35.2-)*
> *aseptic peritonitis (T81.6)*
> *benign paroxysmal peritonitis (E85.0)*
> *chemical peritonitis (T81.6)*
> *gonococcal peritonitis (A54.85)*
> *neonatal peritonitis (P78.0-P78.1)*
> *pelvic peritonitis, female (N73.3-N73.5)*
> *periodic familial peritonitis (E85.0)*
> *peritonitis due to talc or other foreign substance (T81.6)*
> *peritonitis in chlamydia (A74.81)*
> *peritonitis in diphtheria (A36.89)*
> *peritonitis in syphilis (late) (A52.74)*
> *peritonitis in tuberculosis (A18.31)*
> *peritonitis with or following abortion or ectopic or molar pregnancy (O00-O07, O08.0)*
> *peritonitis with or following appendicitis (K35.-)*
> *puerperal peritonitis (O85)*
> *retroperitoneal infections (K68.-)*

K65.0 **Generalized (acute) peritonitis** HCC ESR COM
Pelvic peritonitis (acute), male
Subphrenic peritonitis (acute)
Suppurative peritonitis (acute)

K65.1 **Peritoneal abscess** HCC ESR COM
Abdominopelvic abscess
Abscess (of) omentum
Abscess (of) peritoneum
Mesenteric abscess
Retrocecal abscess
Subdiaphragmatic abscess
Subhepatic abscess
Subphrenic abscess
AHA: 2022,1Q,26; 2019,1Q,15

K65.2 **Spontaneous bacterial peritonitis** HCC ESR COM
> EXCLUDES 1 *bacterial peritonitis NOS (K65.9)*

K65.3 **Choleperitonitis** HCC ESR COM
Peritonitis due to bile
DEF: Inflammation of the peritoneum due to leakage of bile into the peritoneal cavity resulting from rupture of the bile passages or gallbladder.

K65.4 **Sclerosing mesenteritis** HCC ESR COM
Fat necrosis of peritoneum
(Idiopathic) sclerosing mesenteric fibrosis
Mesenteric lipodystrophy
Mesenteric panniculitis
Retractile mesenteritis

K65.8 **Other peritonitis** HCC ESR COM
Chronic proliferative peritonitis
Peritonitis due to urine

K65.9 **Peritonitis, unspecified** HCC ESR COM
Bacterial peritonitis NOS
AHA: 2022,1Q,27; 2013,2Q,31

✓4ᵗʰ K66 Other disorders of peritoneum

EXCLUDES 2　ascites (R18.-)

peritoneal effusion (chronic) (R18.8)

K66.0 Peritoneal adhesions (postprocedural) (postinfection)

Adhesions (of) abdominal (wall)

Adhesions (of) diaphragm

Adhesions (of) intestine

Adhesions (of) male pelvis

Adhesions (of) omentum

Adhesions (of) stomach

Adhesive bands

Mesenteric adhesions

EXCLUDES 1　female pelvic adhesions [bands] (N73.6)

peritoneal adhesions with intestinal obstruction (K56.5-)

K66.1 Hemoperitoneum

EXCLUDES 1　traumatic hemoperitoneum (S36.8-)

AHA: 2022,1Q,22-23

K66.8 Other specified disorders of peritoneum

K66.9 Disorder of peritoneum, unspecified

K67 *Disorders of peritoneum in infectious diseases classified elsewhere*　HCC ESR COM

Code first underlying disease, such as:

congenital syphilis (A50.0)

helminthiasis (B65.0-B83.9)

EXCLUDES 1　peritonitis in chlamydia (A74.81)

peritonitis in diphtheria (A36.89)

peritonitis in gonococcal (A54.85)

peritonitis in syphilis (late) (A52.74)

peritonitis in tuberculosis (A18.31)

✓4ᵗʰ K68 Disorders of retroperitoneum

✓5ᵗʰ K68.1 Retroperitoneal abscess

K68.11 Postprocedural retroperitoneal abscess

EXCLUDES 2　infection following procedure (T81.4-)

K68.12 Psoas muscle abscess　HCC ESR COM

K68.19 Other retroperitoneal abscess　HCC ESR COM

AHA: 2019,1Q,15

TIP: This code should be used for a diagnosis of internal presacral abscess. If an intra-abdominal abscess is also present, code K65.1 can also be assigned; sequencing depends on the circumstances of admission.

K68.9 Other disorders of retroperitoneum

Diseases of liver (K70-K77)

EXCLUDES 1　jaundice NOS (R17)

EXCLUDES 2　hemochromatosis (E83.11-)

Reye's syndrome (G93.7)

viral hepatitis (B15-B19)

Wilson's disease (E83.0)

✓4ᵗʰ K70 Alcoholic liver disease

Use additional code to identify:

alcohol abuse and dependence (F10.-)

K70.0 Alcoholic fatty liver　A

✓5ᵗʰ K70.1 Alcoholic hepatitis

K70.10 Alcoholic hepatitis without ascites　COM A

K70.11 Alcoholic hepatitis with ascites　COM A

K70.2 Alcoholic fibrosis and sclerosis of liver　A

✓5ᵗʰ K70.3 Alcoholic cirrhosis of liver

Alcoholic cirrhosis NOS

K70.30 Alcoholic cirrhosis of liver without ascites　HCC ESR COM A

K70.31 Alcoholic cirrhosis of liver with ascites　HCC ESR COM A

AHA: 2018,1Q,4

✓5ᵗʰ K70.4 Alcoholic hepatic failure

Acute alcoholic hepatic failure

Alcoholic hepatic failure NOS

Chronic alcoholic hepatic failure

Subacute alcoholic hepatic failure

K70.40 Alcoholic hepatic failure without coma　HCC ESR COM A

K70.41 Alcoholic hepatic failure with coma　HCC ESR COM A

K70.9 Alcoholic liver disease, unspecified　HCC ESR

✓4ᵗʰ K71 Toxic liver disease

INCLUDES　drug-induced idiosyncratic (unpredictable) liver disease

drug-induced toxic (predictable) liver disease

Code first poisoning due to drug or toxin, if applicable (T36-T65 with fifth or sixth character 1-4 or 6)

Use additional code for adverse effect, if applicable, to identify drug (T36-T50 with fifth or sixth character 5)

EXCLUDES 2　alcoholic liver disease (K70.-)

Budd-Chiari syndrome (I82.0)

K71.0 Toxic liver disease with cholestasis

Cholestasis with hepatocyte injury

"Pure" cholestasis

✓5ᵗʰ K71.1 Toxic liver disease with hepatic necrosis

Hepatic failure (acute) (chronic) due to drugs

K71.10 Toxic liver disease with hepatic necrosis, without coma　COM

K71.11 Toxic liver disease with hepatic necrosis, with coma　HCC ESR COM

K71.2 Toxic liver disease with acute hepatitis

K71.3 Toxic liver disease with chronic persistent hepatitis　COM

K71.4 Toxic liver disease with chronic lobular hepatitis　COM

✓5ᵗʰ K71.5 Toxic liver disease with chronic active hepatitis

Toxic liver disease with lupoid hepatitis

K71.50 Toxic liver disease with chronic active hepatitis without ascites　COM

K71.51 Toxic liver disease with chronic active hepatitis with ascites　COM

AHA: 2018,1Q,4

K71.6 Toxic liver disease with hepatitis, not elsewhere classified

K71.7 Toxic liver disease with fibrosis and cirrhosis of liver　COM

K71.8 Toxic liver disease with other disorders of liver

Toxic liver disease with focal nodular hyperplasia

Toxic liver disease with hepatic granulomas

Toxic liver disease with peliosis hepatis

Toxic liver disease with veno-occlusive disease of liver

K71.9 Toxic liver disease, unspecified

✓4ᵗʰ K72 Hepatic failure, not elsewhere classified

INCLUDES　fulminant hepatitis NEC, with hepatic failure

~~hepatic encephalopathy NOS~~

liver (cell) necrosis with hepatic failure

malignant hepatitis NEC, with hepatic failure

yellow liver atrophy or dystrophy

EXCLUDES 1　alcoholic hepatic failure (K70.4)

hepatic failure with toxic liver disease (K71.1-)

icterus of newborn (P55-P59)

postprocedural hepatic failure (K91.82)

EXCLUDES 2　hepatic failure complicating abortion or ectopic or molar pregnancy (O00-O07, O08.8)

hepatic failure complicating pregnancy, childbirth and the puerperium (O26.6-)

viral hepatitis with hepatic coma (B15-B19)

AHA: 2017,1Q,41

✓5ᵗʰ K72.0 Acute and subacute hepatic failure

Acute non-viral hepatitis NOS

AHA: 2015,2Q,17; 2014,2Q,13

K72.00 Acute and subacute hepatic failure without coma　COM

AHA: 2021,1Q,13

K72.01 Acute and subacute hepatic failure with coma　HCC ESR COM

✓5ᵗʰ K72.1 Chronic hepatic failure

End stage liver disease

K72.10 Chronic hepatic failure without coma　HCC ESR COM

AHA: 2021,1Q,13

K72.11 Chronic hepatic failure with coma　HCC ESR COM

✓5ᵗʰ K72.9 Hepatic failure, unspecified

K72.90 Hepatic failure, unspecified without coma　HCC ESR COM

AHA: 2022,1Q,52; 2018,4Q,20; 2016,2Q,35

K72.91 Hepatic failure, unspecified with coma　HCC ESR COM

Hepatic coma NOS

Chapter 11. Diseases of the Digestive System

☑4ᵗʰ **K73 Chronic hepatitis, not elsewhere classified**
> **EXCLUDES 1**   *alcoholic hepatitis (chronic) (K70.1-)*
> *drug-induced hepatitis (chronic) (K71.-)*
> *granulomatous hepatitis (chronic) NEC (K75.3)*
> *reactive, nonspecific hepatitis (chronic) (K75.2)*
> *viral hepatitis (chronic) (B15-B19)*

  K73.0 Chronic persistent hepatitis, not elsewhere classified   HCC ESR COM

  K73.1 Chronic lobular hepatitis, not elsewhere classified   HCC ESR COM

  K73.2 Chronic active hepatitis, not elsewhere classified   HCC ESR COM

  K73.8 Other chronic hepatitis, not elsewhere classified   HCC ESR COM

  K73.9 Chronic hepatitis, unspecified   HCC ESR COM

☑4ᵗʰ **K74 Fibrosis and cirrhosis of liver**
> Code also, if applicable, viral hepatitis (acute) (chronic) (B15-B19)
> **EXCLUDES 1**   *alcoholic cirrhosis (of liver) (K70.3)*
> *alcoholic fibrosis of liver (K70.2)*
> *cardiac sclerosis of liver (K76.1)*
> *cirrhosis (of liver) with toxic liver disease (K71.7)*
> *congenital cirrhosis (of liver) (P78.81)*
> *pigmentary cirrhosis (of liver) (E83.110)*

☑5ᵗʰ **K74.0 Hepatic fibrosis**
> Code first underlying liver disease, such as:
> nonalcoholic steatohepatitis (NASH) (K75.81)
> **AHA:** 2020,4Q,30-31

    K74.00 Hepatic fibrosis, unspecified

    K74.01 Hepatic fibrosis, early fibrosis
> Hepatic fibrosis, stage F1 or stage F2

    K74.02 Hepatic fibrosis, advanced fibrosis
> Hepatic fibrosis, stage F3
> **EXCLUDES 1**   *cirrhosis of liver (K74.6-)*
> *hepatic fibrosis, stage F4 (K74.6-)*

  K74.1 Hepatic sclerosis

  K74.2 Hepatic fibrosis with hepatic sclerosis

  K74.3 Primary biliary cirrhosis   HCC Rx ESR COM
> Chronic nonsuppurative destructive cholangitis
> Primary biliary cholangitis
> **EXCLUDES 2**   *primary sclerosing cholangitis (K83.01)*

  K74.4 Secondary biliary cirrhosis   HCC ESR COM

  K74.5 Biliary cirrhosis, unspecified   HCC ESR COM

☑5ᵗʰ **K74.6 Other and unspecified cirrhosis of liver**
> **AHA:** 2020,4Q,30-31

    K74.60 Unspecified cirrhosis of liver   HCC ESR COM
> Cirrhosis (of liver) NOS
> **AHA:** 2018,1Q,4

    K74.69 Other cirrhosis of liver   HCC ESR COM
> Cryptogenic cirrhosis (of liver)
> Macronodular cirrhosis (of liver)
> Micronodular cirrhosis (of liver)
> Mixed type cirrhosis (of liver)
> Portal cirrhosis (of liver)
> Postnecrotic cirrhosis (of liver)

☑4ᵗʰ **K75 Other inflammatory liver diseases**
> **EXCLUDES 2**   *toxic liver disease (K71.-)*

  K75.0 Abscess of liver   COM
> Cholangitic hepatic abscess
> Hematogenic hepatic abscess
> Hepatic abscess NOS
> Lymphogenic hepatic abscess
> Pylephlebitic hepatic abscess
> **EXCLUDES 1**   *amebic liver abscess (A06.4)*
> *cholangitis without liver abscess (K83.09)*
> *pylephlebitis without liver abscess (K75.1)*
> **EXCLUDES 2**   *acute or subacute hepatitis NOS (B17.9)*
> *acute or subacute non-viral hepatitis (K72.0)*
> *chronic hepatitis NEC (K73.8)*

  K75.1 Phlebitis of portal vein   COM
> Pylephlebitis
> **EXCLUDES 1**   *pylephlebitic liver abscess (K75.0)*
> **DEF:** Inflammation of the portal vein or branches due to diverticulitis, perforated appendicitis, or peritonitis. Symptoms include fever, chills, jaundice, sweating, and abscess in various body parts.

  K75.2 Nonspecific reactive hepatitis
> **EXCLUDES 1**   *acute or subacute hepatitis (K72.0-)*
> *chronic hepatitis NEC (K73.-)*
> *viral hepatitis (B15-B19)*

  K75.3 Granulomatous hepatitis, not elsewhere classified
> **EXCLUDES 1**   *acute or subacute hepatitis (K72.0-)*
> *chronic hepatitis NEC (K73.-)*
> *viral hepatitis (B15-B19)*

  K75.4 Autoimmune hepatitis   HCC ESR COM
> Lupoid hepatitis NEC

☑5ᵗʰ **K75.8 Other specified inflammatory liver diseases**

    K75.81 Nonalcoholic steatohepatitis (NASH)
> Use additional code, if applicable, hepatic fibrosis (K74.0-)

    K75.89 Other specified inflammatory liver diseases

  K75.9 Inflammatory liver disease, unspecified
> Hepatitis NOS
> **EXCLUDES 1**   *acute or subacute hepatitis (K72.0-)*
> *chronic hepatitis NEC (K73.-)*
> *viral hepatitis (B15-B19)*
> **AHA:** 2015,2Q,17

☑4ᵗʰ **K76 Other diseases of liver**
> **EXCLUDES 2**   *alcoholic liver disease (K70.-)*
> *amyloid degeneration of liver (E85.-)*
> *cystic disease of liver (congenital) (Q44.6)*
> *hepatic vein thrombosis (I82.0)*
> *hepatomegaly NOS (R16.0)*
> *pigmentary cirrhosis (of liver) (E83.110)*
> *portal vein thrombosis (I81)*
> *toxic liver disease (K71.-)*

  K76.0 Fatty (change of) liver, not elsewhere classified
> Nonalcoholic fatty liver disease (NAFLD)
> **EXCLUDES 2**   *nonalcoholic steatohepatitis (NASH) (K75.81)*

  K76.1 Chronic passive congestion of liver
> Cardiac cirrhosis
> Cardiac sclerosis

  K76.2 Central hemorrhagic necrosis of liver   COM
> **EXCLUDES 1**   *liver necrosis with hepatic failure (K72.-)*

  K76.3 Infarction of liver   COM

  K76.4 Peliosis hepatis
> Hepatic angiomatosis

  K76.5 Hepatic veno-occlusive disease
> **EXCLUDES 1**   *Budd-Chiari syndrome (I82.0)*

  K76.6 Portal hypertension   HCC ESR COM
> Use additional code for any associated complications, such as:
> portal hypertensive gastropathy (K31.89)
> **AHA:** 2020,1Q,15

  K76.7 Hepatorenal syndrome   HCC ESR COM
> **EXCLUDES 1**   *hepatorenal syndrome following labor and delivery (O90.4)*
> *postprocedural hepatorenal syndrome (K91.83)*

☑5ᵗʰ **K76.8 Other specified diseases of liver**

    K76.81 Hepatopulmonary syndrome   HCC ESR COM
> Code first underlying liver disease, such as:
> alcoholic cirrhosis of liver (K70.3-)
> cirrhosis of liver without mention of alcohol (K74.6-)

●   **K76.82**   **Hepatic encephalopathy**

       Hepatic encephalopathy, NOS

       Hepatic encephalopathy without coma

       Hepatocerebral intoxication

       Portal-systemic encephalopathy

       Code also underlying liver disease, such as:

         acute and subacute hepatic failure without coma (K72.00)

         alcoholic hepatic failure without coma (K70.40)

         chronic hepatic failure without coma (K72.10)

         hepatic failure with toxic liver disease without coma (K71.10)

         hepatic failure without coma (K72.90)

         icterus of newborn (P55-P59)

         postprocedural hepatic failure (K91.82)

         viral hepatitis without hepatic coma (B15.9, B16.1, B16.9, B17.10, B19.10, B19.20, B19.9)

         EXCLUDES 1   *acute and subacute hepatic failure with coma (K72.01)*

               alcoholic hepatic failure with coma (K70.41)

               chronic hepatic failure with coma (K72.11)

               hepatic failure with coma (K72.91)

     K76.89   **Other specified diseases of liver**

       Cyst (simple) of liver

       Focal nodular hyperplasia of liver

       Hepatoptosis

K76.9   **Liver disease, unspecified**

K77   *Liver disorders in diseases classified elsewhere*

     Code first underlying disease, such as:

       amyloidosis (E85.-)

       congenital syphilis (A50.0, A50.5)

       congenital toxoplasmosis (P37.1)

       infectious mononucleosis with liver disease ▶(B27.0-B27.9 with fifth character 9)◀

       schistosomiasis (B65.0-B65.9)

       EXCLUDES 1   *alcoholic hepatitis (K70.1-)*

               alcoholic liver disease (K70.-)

               cytomegaloviral hepatitis (B25.1)

               herpesviral [herpes simplex] hepatitis (B00.81)

               mumps hepatitis (B26.81)

               sarcoidosis with liver disease (D86.89)

               secondary syphilis with liver disease (A51.45)

               syphilis (late) with liver disease (A52.74)

               toxoplasmosis (acquired) hepatitis (B58.1)

               tuberculosis with liver disease (A18.83)

Disorders of gallbladder, biliary tract and pancreas (K80-K87)

✓4ᵗʰ **K80**   **Cholelithiasis**

     EXCLUDES 1   *retained cholelithiasis following cholecystectomy (K91.86)*

     AHA: 2018,4Q,20

     DEF: Presence or formation of concretions (calculi or "gallstones") in the gallbladder. The stones contain cholesterol, calcium carbonate, or calcium bilirubinate in pure forms or in various combinations.

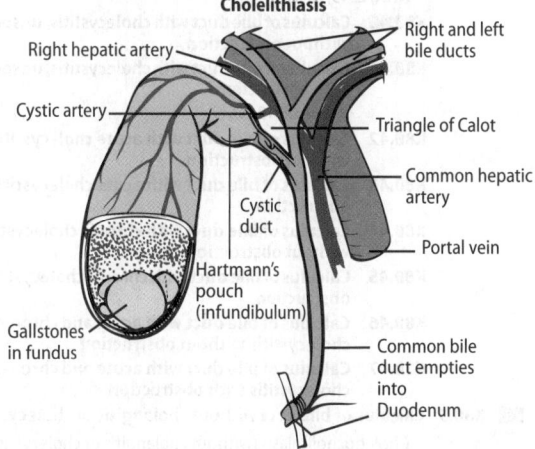

Cholelithiasis

Right hepatic artery — ; Right and left bile ducts; Cystic artery —; Triangle of Calot; Common hepatic artery; Cystic duct; Portal vein; Hartmann's pouch (infundibulum); Gallstones in fundus; Common bile duct empties into Duodenum

✓5ᵗʰ **K80.0**   **Calculus of** gallbladder **with acute cholecystitis**

     Any condition listed in K80.2 with acute cholecystitis

     Use additional code if applicable for associated gangrene of gallbladder (K82.A1), or perforation of gallbladder (K82.A2)

     K80.00   **Calculus of gallbladder with acute cholecystitis without obstruction**

     K80.01   **Calculus of gallbladder with acute cholecystitis with obstruction**

✓5ᵗʰ **K80.1**   **Calculus of** gallbladder **with other cholecystitis**

     Use additional code if applicable for associated gangrene of gallbladder (K82.A1), or perforation of gallbladder (K82.A2)

     K80.10   **Calculus of gallbladder with** chronic **cholecystitis without obstruction**

       Cholelithiasis with cholecystitis NOS

     K80.11   **Calculus of gallbladder with** chronic **cholecystitis with obstruction**

     K80.12   **Calculus of gallbladder with** acute and chronic **cholecystitis without obstruction**

     K80.13   **Calculus of gallbladder with** acute and chronic **cholecystitis with obstruction**

     K80.18   **Calculus of gallbladder with other cholecystitis without obstruction**

     K80.19   **Calculus of gallbladder with other cholecystitis** with **obstruction**

✓5ᵗʰ **K80.2**   **Calculus of** gallbladder **without cholecystitis**

     Cholecystolithiasis without cholecystitis

     Cholelithiasis (without cholecystitis)

     Colic (recurrent) of gallbladder (without cholecystitis)

     Gallstone (impacted) of cystic duct (without cholecystitis)

     Gallstone (impacted) of gallbladder (without cholecystitis)

     K80.20   **Calculus of gallbladder without cholecystitis without obstruction**

     K80.21   **Calculus of gallbladder without cholecystitis with obstruction**

✓5ᵗʰ **K80.3**   **Calculus of** bile duct **with cholangitis**

     Any condition listed in K80.5 with cholangitis

     DEF: Cholangitis: Inflammation of the bile ducts.

     K80.30   **Calculus of bile duct with cholangitis, unspecified, without obstruction**

     K80.31   **Calculus of bile duct with cholangitis, unspecified, with obstruction**

     K80.32   **Calculus of bile duct with** acute **cholangitis** without **obstruction**

     K80.33   **Calculus of bile duct with** acute **cholangitis with obstruction**

     K80.34   **Calculus of bile duct with** chronic **cholangitis without obstruction**

     K80.35   **Calculus of bile duct with** chronic **cholangitis with obstruction**

K80.36 Calculus of bile duct with acute and chronic cholangitis without obstruction

K80.37 Calculus of bile duct with acute and chronic cholangitis with obstruction

✓5ᵗʰ **K80.4** Calculus of bile duct with cholecystitis
Any condition listed in K80.5 with cholecystitis (with cholangitis)
▶Code also fistula of bile duct◀ (K83.3)
Use additional code if applicable for associated gangrene of gallbladder (K82.A1), or perforation of gallbladder (K82.A2)
AHA: 2019,1Q,17

K80.40 Calculus of bile duct with cholecystitis, unspecified, without obstruction

K80.41 Calculus of bile duct with cholecystitis, unspecified, with obstruction
AHA: 2019,1Q,17

K80.42 Calculus of bile duct with acute cholecystitis without obstruction

K80.43 Calculus of bile duct with acute cholecystitis with obstruction

K80.44 Calculus of bile duct with chronic cholecystitis without obstruction

K80.45 Calculus of bile duct with chronic cholecystitis with obstruction

K80.46 Calculus of bile duct with acute and chronic cholecystitis without obstruction

K80.47 Calculus of bile duct with acute and chronic cholecystitis with obstruction

✓5ᵗʰ **K80.5** Calculus of bile duct without cholangitis or cholecystitis
Choledocholithiasis (without cholangitis or cholecystitis)
Gallstone (impacted) of bile duct NOS (without cholangitis or cholecystitis)
Gallstone (impacted) of common duct (without cholangitis or cholecystitis)
Gallstone (impacted) of hepatic duct (without cholangitis or cholecystitis)
Hepatic cholelithiasis (without cholangitis or cholecystitis)
Hepatic colic (recurrent) (without cholangitis or cholecystitis)
DEF: Cholangitis: Inflammation of the bile ducts.

K80.50 Calculus of bile duct without cholangitis or cholecystitis without obstruction

K80.51 Calculus of bile duct without cholangitis or cholecystitis with obstruction

✓5ᵗʰ **K80.6** Calculus of gallbladder and bile duct with cholecystitis
Use additional code if applicable for associated gangrene of gallbladder (K82.A1), or perforation of gallbladder (K82.A2)

K80.60 Calculus of gallbladder and bile duct with cholecystitis, unspecified, without obstruction

K80.61 Calculus of gallbladder and bile duct with cholecystitis, unspecified, with obstruction

K80.62 Calculus of gallbladder and bile duct with acute cholecystitis without obstruction

K80.63 Calculus of gallbladder and bile duct with acute cholecystitis with obstruction

K80.64 Calculus of gallbladder and bile duct with chronic cholecystitis without obstruction

K80.65 Calculus of gallbladder and bile duct with chronic cholecystitis with obstruction

K80.66 Calculus of gallbladder and bile duct with acute and chronic cholecystitis without obstruction

K80.67 Calculus of gallbladder and bile duct with acute and chronic cholecystitis with obstruction

✓5ᵗʰ **K80.7** Calculus of gallbladder and bile duct without cholecystitis

K80.70 Calculus of gallbladder and bile duct without cholecystitis without obstruction

K80.71 Calculus of gallbladder and bile duct without cholecystitis with obstruction

✓5ᵗʰ **K80.8** Other cholelithiasis

K80.80 Other cholelithiasis without obstruction

K80.81 Other cholelithiasis with obstruction

✓4ᵗʰ **K81** Cholecystitis
Use additional code if applicable for associated gangrene of gallbladder (K82.A1), or perforation of gallbladder (K82.A2)
EXCLUDES 1 cholecystitis with cholelithiasis (K80.-)
AHA: 2018,4Q,20

K81.0 Acute cholecystitis
Abscess of gallbladder
Angiocholecystitis
Emphysematous (acute) cholecystitis
Empyema of gallbladder
Gangrene of gallbladder
Gangrenous cholecystitis
Suppurative cholecystitis

K81.1 Chronic cholecystitis

K81.2 Acute cholecystitis with chronic cholecystitis

K81.9 Cholecystitis, unspecified

✓4ᵗʰ **K82** Other diseases of gallbladder
EXCLUDES 1 nonvisualization of gallbladder (R93.2)
postcholecystectomy syndrome (K91.5)

K82.0 Obstruction of gallbladder
Occlusion of cystic duct or gallbladder without cholelithiasis
Stenosis of cystic duct or gallbladder without cholelithiasis
Stricture of cystic duct or gallbladder without cholelithiasis
EXCLUDES 1 obstruction of gallbladder with cholelithiasis (K80.-)

K82.1 Hydrops of gallbladder
Mucocele of gallbladder

K82.2 Perforation of gallbladder
Rupture of cystic duct or gallbladder
EXCLUDES 1 perforation of gallbladder in cholecystitis (K82.A2)

K82.3 Fistula of gallbladder
Cholecystocolic fistula
Cholecystoduodenal fistula

K82.4 Cholesterolosis of gallbladder
Strawberry gallbladder
EXCLUDES 1 cholesterolosis of gallbladder with cholecystitis (K81.-)
cholesterolosis of gallbladder with cholelithiasis (K80.-)

K82.8 Other specified diseases of gallbladder
Adhesions of cystic duct or gallbladder
Atrophy of cystic duct or gallbladder
Cyst of cystic duct or gallbladder
Dyskinesia of cystic duct or gallbladder
Hypertrophy of cystic duct or gallbladder
Nonfunctioning of cystic duct or gallbladder
Ulcer of cystic duct or gallbladder

K82.9 Disease of gallbladder, unspecified

✓5ᵗʰ **K82.A** Disorders of gallbladder in diseases classified elsewhere
Code first the type of cholecystitis (K81.-), or cholelithiasis with cholecystitis (K80.00-K80.19, K80.40-K80.47, K80.60-K80.67)
AHA: 2018,4Q,19-20

K82.A1 Gangrene of gallbladder in cholecystitis

K82.A2 Perforation of gallbladder in cholecystitis

✓4ᵗʰ **K83** Other diseases of biliary tract
EXCLUDES 1 postcholecystectomy syndrome (K91.5)
EXCLUDES 2 conditions involving the gallbladder (K81-K82)
conditions involving the cystic duct (K81-K82)

✓5ᵗʰ **K83.0** Cholangitis
EXCLUDES 1 cholangitic liver abscess (K75.0)
cholangitis with choledocholithiasis (K80.3-, K80.4-)
EXCLUDES 2 chronic nonsuppurative destructive cholangitis (K74.3)
primary biliary cholangitis (K74.3)
primary biliary cirrhosis (K74.3)
AHA: 2018,4Q,20

K83.01 Primary sclerosing cholangitis

K83.09   **Other cholangitis**
Ascending cholangitis
Cholangitis NOS
Primary cholangitis
Recurrent cholangitis
Sclerosing cholangitis
Secondary cholangitis
Stenosing cholangitis
Suppurative cholangitis

K83.1   **Obstruction of bile duct**
Occlusion of bile duct without cholelithiasis
Stenosis of bile duct without cholelithiasis
Stricture of bile duct without cholelithiasis
   EXCLUDES 1   *congenital obstruction of bile duct (Q44.3)*
       obstruction of bile duct with cholelithiasis (K80.-)
   AHA: 2016,1Q,18

K83.2   **Perforation of bile duct**
Rupture of bile duct

K83.3   **Fistula of bile duct**
Choledochoduodenal fistula
   AHA: 2019,1Q,17

K83.4   **Spasm of sphincter of Oddi**

K83.5   **Biliary cyst**

K83.8   **Other specified diseases of biliary tract**
Adhesions of biliary tract
Atrophy of biliary tract
Hypertrophy of biliary tract
Ulcer of biliary tract

K83.9   **Disease of biliary tract, unspecified**

✓4ᵗʰ **K85**   **Acute pancreatitis**
   INCLUDES   acute (recurrent) pancreatitis
       subacute pancreatitis
   AHA: 2016,4Q,34

✓5ᵗʰ **K85.0**   **Idiopathic acute pancreatitis**
   K85.00   **Idiopathic acute pancreatitis** without necrosis or infection   COM
   K85.01   **Idiopathic acute pancreatitis** with uninfected necrosis   COM
   K85.02   **Idiopathic acute pancreatitis** with infected necrosis   COM

✓5ᵗʰ **K85.1**   **Biliary acute pancreatitis**
Gallstone pancreatitis
   K85.10   **Biliary acute pancreatitis** without necrosis or infection   COM
   K85.11   **Biliary acute pancreatitis** with uninfected necrosis   COM
   K85.12   **Biliary acute pancreatitis** with infected necrosis   COM

✓5ᵗʰ **K85.2**   **Alcohol induced acute pancreatitis**
   EXCLUDES 2   *alcohol induced chronic pancreatitis (K86.0)*
   K85.20   **Alcohol induced acute pancreatitis** without necrosis or infection   COM
       AHA: 2020,1Q,9
   K85.21   **Alcohol induced acute pancreatitis** with uninfected necrosis   COM
   K85.22   **Alcohol induced acute pancreatitis** with infected necrosis   COM

✓5ᵗʰ **K85.3**   **Drug induced acute pancreatitis**
Use additional code for adverse effect, if applicable, to identify drug (T36-T50 with fifth or sixth character 5)
Use additional code to identify drug abuse and dependence (F11.- F17.-)
   K85.30   **Drug induced acute pancreatitis** without necrosis or infection   COM
   K85.31   **Drug induced acute pancreatitis** with uninfected necrosis   COM
   K85.32   **Drug induced acute pancreatitis** with infected necrosis   COM

✓5ᵗʰ **K85.8**   **Other acute pancreatitis**
   K85.80   **Other acute pancreatitis** without necrosis or infection   COM
   K85.81   **Other acute pancreatitis** with uninfected necrosis   COM
   K85.82   **Other acute pancreatitis** with infected necrosis   COM

✓5ᵗʰ **K85.9**   **Acute pancreatitis, unspecified**
Pancreatitis NOS
   K85.90   **Acute pancreatitis** without necrosis or infection, unspecified   COM
   K85.91   **Acute pancreatitis** with uninfected necrosis, unspecified   COM
   K85.92   **Acute pancreatitis** with infected necrosis, unspecified   COM

✓4ᵗʰ **K86**   **Other diseases of pancreas**
   EXCLUDES 2   *fibrocystic disease of pancreas (E84.-)*
       islet cell tumor (of pancreas) (D13.7)
       pancreatic steatorrhea (K90.3)

K86.0   **Alcohol-induced chronic pancreatitis**   HCC Rx ESR COM
Use additional code to identify:
   alcohol abuse and dependence (F10.-)
Code also exocrine pancreatic insufficiency (K86.81)
   EXCLUDES 2   *alcohol induced acute pancreatitis (K85.2-)*

K86.1   **Other chronic pancreatitis**   HCC Rx ESR COM
Chronic pancreatitis NOS
Infectious chronic pancreatitis
Recurrent chronic pancreatitis
Relapsing chronic pancreatitis
Code also exocrine pancreatic insufficiency (K86.81)

K86.2   **Cyst of pancreas**   Rx

K86.3   **Pseudocyst of pancreas**   Rx

✓5ᵗʰ **K86.8**   **Other specified diseases of pancreas**
   AHA: 2016,4Q,34-35
   K86.81   **Exocrine pancreatic insufficiency**   Rx
   K86.89   **Other specified diseases of pancreas**   Rx
       Aseptic pancreatic necrosis, unrelated to acute pancreatitis
       Atrophy of pancreas
       Calculus of pancreas
       Cirrhosis of pancreas
       Fibrosis of pancreas
       Pancreatic fat necrosis, unrelated to acute pancreatitis
       Pancreatic infantilism
       Pancreatic necrosis NOS, unrelated to acute pancreatitis

K86.9   **Disease of pancreas, unspecified**   Rx

K87   ***Disorders of gallbladder, biliary tract and pancreas in diseases classified elsewhere***   Rx
Code first underlying disease
   EXCLUDES 1   *cytomegaloviral pancreatitis (B25.2)*
       mumps pancreatitis (B26.3)
       syphilitic gallbladder (A52.74)
       syphilitic pancreas (A52.74)
       tuberculosis of gallbladder (A18.83)
       tuberculosis of pancreas (A18.83)

Other diseases of the digestive system (K90-K95)

✓4ᵗʰ **K90**   **Intestinal malabsorption**
   EXCLUDES 1   *intestinal malabsorption following gastrointestinal surgery (K91.2)*
   AHA: 2017,4Q,108

K90.0   **Celiac disease**   Rx
Celiac disease with steatorrhea
Celiac gluten-sensitive enteropathy
Nontropical sprue
Use additional code for associated disorders including:
   dermatitis herpetiformis (L13.0)
   gluten ataxia (G32.81)
Code also exocrine pancreatic insufficiency (K86.81)
DEF: Malabsorption syndrome due to gluten consumption. Symptoms include fetid, bulky, frothy, oily stools; a distended abdomen; gas; asthenia; electrolyte depletion; and vitamin B, D, and K deficiency.

K90.1   **Tropical sprue**   Rx
Sprue NOS
Tropical steatorrhea

K90.2   **Blind loop syndrome, not elsewhere classified**   Rx
Blind loop syndrome NOS
   EXCLUDES 1   *congenital blind loop syndrome (Q43.8)*
       postsurgical blind loop syndrome (K91.2)

K90.3   **Pancreatic steatorrhea**   Rx

✅ Additional Character Required   ✓x7ᵗʰ Placeholder Alert   Manifestation   Unspecified Dx   Q QPP   UPD Unacceptable PDx

Chapter 11. Diseases of the Digestive System

✓5ᵗʰ K90.4 Other malabsorption due to intolerance
> EXCLUDES 2   celiac gluten-sensitive enteropathy (K90.0)
>   lactose intolerance (E73.-)

     AHA: 2016,4Q,35-36

     K90.41 Non-celiac gluten sensitivity
         Gluten sensitivity NOS
         Non-celiac gluten sensitive enteropathy

     K90.49 Malabsorption due to intolerance, not elsewhere classified   Rx
         Malabsorption due to intolerance to carbohydrate
         Malabsorption due to intolerance to fat
         Malabsorption due to intolerance to protein
         Malabsorption due to intolerance to starch

✓5ᵗʰ K90.8 Other intestinal malabsorption

     K90.81 Whipple's disease   Rx

     K90.89 Other intestinal malabsorption   Rx

K90.9 Intestinal malabsorption, unspecified   Rx

✓4ᵗʰ K91 Intraoperative and postprocedural complications and disorders of digestive system, not elsewhere classified
> EXCLUDES 2   complications of artificial opening of digestive system (K94.-)
>   complications of bariatric procedures (K95.-)
>   gastrojejunal ulcer (K28.-)
>   postprocedural (radiation) retroperitoneal abscess (K68.11)
>   radiation colitis (K52.0)
>   radiation gastroenteritis (K52.0)
>   radiation proctitis (K62.7)

     AHA: 2016,4Q,9-10

K91.0 Vomiting following gastrointestinal surgery

K91.1 Postgastric surgery syndromes
     Dumping syndrome
     Postgastrectomy syndrome
     Postvagotomy syndrome

K91.2 Postsurgical malabsorption, not elsewhere classified   Rx
     Postsurgical blind loop syndrome
> EXCLUDES 1   malabsorption osteomalacia in adults (M83.2)
>   malabsorption osteoporosis, postsurgical (M80.8-, M81.8)

✓5ᵗʰ K91.3 Postprocedural intestinal obstruction
     AHA: 2017,4Q,16-17; 2017,1Q,40

     K91.30 Postprocedural intestinal obstruction, unspecified as to partial versus complete
         Postprocedural intestinal obstruction NOS

     K91.31 Postprocedural partial intestinal obstruction
         Postprocedural incomplete intestinal obstruction

     K91.32 Postprocedural complete intestinal obstruction

K91.5 Postcholecystectomy syndrome

✓5ᵗʰ K91.6 Intraoperative hemorrhage and hematoma of a digestive system organ or structure complicating a procedure
> EXCLUDES 1   intraoperative hemorrhage and hematoma of a digestive system organ or structure due to accidental puncture and laceration during a procedure (K91.7-)

     K91.61 Intraoperative hemorrhage and hematoma of a digestive system organ or structure complicating a digestive system procedure
         AHA: 2020,1Q,19

     K91.62 Intraoperative hemorrhage and hematoma of a digestive system organ or structure complicating other procedure

✓5ᵗʰ K91.7 Accidental puncture and laceration of a digestive system organ or structure during a procedure
     AHA: 2022,1Q,51

     K91.71 Accidental puncture and laceration of a digestive system organ or structure during a digestive system procedure
         AHA: 2021,2Q,11

     K91.72 Accidental puncture and laceration of a digestive system organ or structure during other procedure
         AHA: 2019,2Q,23

✓5ᵗʰ K91.8 Other intraoperative and postprocedural complications and disorders of digestive system

     K91.81 Other intraoperative complications of digestive system

     K91.82 Postprocedural hepatic failure

     K91.83 Postprocedural hepatorenal syndrome

✓6ᵗʰ K91.84 Postprocedural hemorrhage of a digestive system organ or structure following a procedure

     K91.840 Postprocedural hemorrhage of a digestive system organ or structure following a digestive system procedure
         AHA: 2016,1Q,15

     K91.841 Postprocedural hemorrhage of a digestive system organ or structure following other procedure

✓6ᵗʰ K91.85 Complications of intestinal pouch

     K91.850 Pouchitis   HCC ESR COM
         Inflammation of internal ileoanal pouch
         DEF: Inflammatory complication of an existing surgically created ileoanal pouch, resulting in multiple GI complaints, including diarrhea, abdominal pain, rectal bleeding, fecal urgency, or incontinence.

     K91.858 Other complications of intestinal pouch   HCC ESR COM
         AHA: 2019,2Q,13

K91.86 Retained cholelithiasis following cholecystectomy

✓6ᵗʰ K91.87 Postprocedural hematoma and seroma of a digestive system organ or structure following a procedure

     K91.870 Postprocedural hematoma of a digestive system organ or structure following a digestive system procedure
         AHA: 2022,1Q,24

     K91.871 Postprocedural hematoma of a digestive system organ or structure following other procedure

     K91.872 Postprocedural seroma of a digestive system organ or structure following a digestive system procedure

     K91.873 Postprocedural seroma of a digestive system organ or structure following other procedure

     K91.89 Other postprocedural complications and disorders of digestive system
         Use additional code, if applicable, to further specify disorder
> EXCLUDES 2   postprocedural retroperitoneal abscess (K68.11)

         AHA: 2020,2Q,22; 2017,1Q,40

✓4ᵗʰ K92 Other diseases of digestive system
> EXCLUDES 1   neonatal gastrointestinal hemorrhage (P54.0-P54.3)

K92.0 Hematemesis

K92.1 Melena
> EXCLUDES 1   occult blood in feces (R19.5)

K92.2 Gastrointestinal hemorrhage, unspecified
     Gastric hemorrhage NOS
     Intestinal hemorrhage NOS
> EXCLUDES 1   acute hemorrhagic gastritis (K29.01)
>   hemorrhage of anus and rectum (K62.5)
>   angiodysplasia of stomach with hemorrhage (K31.811)
>   diverticular disease with hemorrhage (K57.-)
>   gastritis and duodenitis with hemorrhage (K29.-)
>   peptic ulcer with hemorrhage (K25-K28)

     AHA: 2021,1Q,11

✓6ᵗʰ K92.8 Other specified diseases of the digestive system

     K92.81 Gastrointestinal mucositis (ulcerative)
         Code also type of associated therapy, such as:
         antineoplastic and immunosuppressive drugs (T45.1X-)
         radiological procedure and radiotherapy (Y84.2)
> EXCLUDES 2   mucositis (ulcerative) of vagina and vulva (N76.81)
>   nasal mucositis (ulcerative) (J34.81)
>   oral mucositis (ulcerative) (K12.3-)

     K92.89 Other specified diseases of the digestive system

K92.9 Disease of digestive system, unspecified

✓4ᵗʰ K94 Complications of artificial openings of the digestive system

✓5ᵗʰ K94.0 Colostomy complications

     K94.00 Colostomy complication, unspecified   HCC ESR COM

     K94.01 Colostomy hemorrhage   HCC ESR COM

K94.02   **Colostomy** infection   `HCC` `ESR` `COM`
Use additional code to specify type of infection, such as:
cellulitis of abdominal wall (L03.311)
sepsis (A40.-, A41.-)

K94.03   **Colostomy** malfunction   `HCC` `ESR` `COM`
Mechanical complication of colostomy

K94.09   **Other complications of colostomy**   `HCC` `ESR` `COM`

✓5ᵗʰ   **K94.1**   **Enterostomy** complications

K94.10   **Enterostomy complication, unspecified**   `HCC` `ESR` `COM`

K94.11   **Enterostomy** hemorrhage   `HCC` `ESR` `COM`

K94.12   **Enterostomy** infection   `HCC` `ESR` `COM`
Use additional code to specify type of infection, such as:
cellulitis of abdominal wall (L03.311)
sepsis (A40.-, A41.-)

K94.13   **Enterostomy** malfunction   `HCC` `ESR` `COM`
Mechanical complication of enterostomy

K94.19   **Other complications of enterostomy**   `HCC` `ESR` `COM`

✓5ᵗʰ   **K94.2**   **Gastrostomy** complications

K94.20   **Gastrostomy complication, unspecified**   `HCC` `ESR` `COM`

K94.21   **Gastrostomy** hemorrhage   `HCC` `ESR` `COM`

K94.22   **Gastrostomy** infection   `HCC` `ESR` `COM`
Use additional code to specify type of infection, such as:
cellulitis of abdominal wall (L03.311)
sepsis (A40.-, A41.-)

K94.23   **Gastrostomy** malfunction   `HCC` `ESR` `COM`
Mechanical complication of gastrostomy
AHA: 2019,1Q,26

K94.29   **Other complications of gastrostomy**   `HCC` `ESR` `COM`

✓5ᵗʰ   **K94.3**   **Esophagostomy** complications

K94.30   **Esophagostomy complications, unspecified**   `HCC` `ESR` `COM`

K94.31   **Esophagostomy** hemorrhage   `HCC` `ESR` `COM`

K94.32   **Esophagostomy** infection   `HCC` `ESR` `COM`
Use additional code to identify the infection

K94.33   **Esophagostomy** malfunction   `HCC` `ESR` `COM`
Mechanical complication of esophagostomy

K94.39   **Other complications of esophagostomy**   `HCC` `ESR` `COM`

✓4ᵗʰ   **K95**   **Complications of bariatric procedures**

✓5ᵗʰ   **K95.0**   **Complications of** gastric band procedure

K95.01   **Infection** due to gastric band procedure
Use additional code to specify type of infection or organism, such as:
bacterial and viral infectious agents (B95.-, B96.-)
cellulitis of abdominal wall (L03.311)
sepsis (A40.-, A41.-)

K95.09   **Other complications of gastric band procedure**
Use additional code, if applicable, to further specify complication

✓5ᵗʰ   **K95.8**   **Complications of other bariatric procedure**

EXCLUDES 1   complications of gastric band surgery (K95.0-)

K95.81   **Infection** due to other bariatric procedure
Use additional code to specify type of infection or organism, such as:
bacterial and viral infectious agents (B95.-, B96.-)
cellulitis of abdominal wall (L03.311)
sepsis (A40.-, A41.-)

K95.89   **Other complications of other bariatric procedure**
Use additional code, if applicable, to further specify complication

---

☑ Additional Character Required   ✓x7ᵗʰ Placeholder Alert   Manifestation   Unspecified Dx   Q QPP   UPD Unacceptable PDx

Chapter 12. Diseases of the Skin and Subcutaneous Tissue (L00–L99)

Chapter-specific Guidelines with Coding Examples

The chapter-specific guidelines from the ICD-10-CM Official Guidelines for Coding and Reporting have been provided below. Along with these guidelines are coding examples, contained in the shaded boxes, that have been developed to help illustrate the coding and/or sequencing guidance found in these guidelines.

a. Pressure ulcer stage codes

1) Pressure ulcer stages

Codes in category L89, Pressure ulcer, identify the site and stage of the pressure ulcer.

The ICD-10-CM classifies pressure ulcer stages based on severity, which is designated by stages 1-4, deep tissue pressure injury, unspecified stage, and unstageable.

Assign as many codes from category L89 as needed to identify all the pressure ulcers the patient has, if applicable.

See Section I.B.14. for pressure ulcer stage documentation by clinicians other than patient's provider.

> Stage 3 pressure ulcer left ankle, 6 x 7 cm that invades the fascia; stage 2 pressure ulcer of left hip
>
> **L89.523   Pressure ulcer of left ankle, stage 3**
>
> **L89.222   Pressure ulcer of left hip, stage 2**
>
> *Explanation:* Patient has a left ankle pressure ulcer documented as stage 3 and a left hip pressure ulcer documented as stage 2. Combination codes from category L89 Pressure ulcer, identify the site of the pressure ulcer as well as the stage. Assign as many codes from category L89 as needed to identify all the pressure ulcers the patient has.

2) Unstageable pressure ulcers

Assignment of the code for unstageable pressure ulcer (L89.--0) should be based on the clinical documentation. These codes are used for pressure ulcers whose stage cannot be clinically determined (e.g., the ulcer is covered by eschar or has been treated with a skin or muscle graft). This code should not be confused with the codes for unspecified stage (L89.--9). When there is no documentation regarding the stage of the pressure ulcer, assign the appropriate code for unspecified stage (L89.--9).

> Pressure ulcer of the right lower back documented as unstageable due to the presence of thick eschar covering the ulcer
>
> **L89.130   Pressure ulcer of right lower back, unstageable**
>
> *Explanation:* Codes for unstageable pressure ulcers are assigned when the stage cannot be clinically determined (e.g., the ulcer is covered by eschar or has been treated with a skin or muscle graft).

If during an encounter, the stage of an unstageable pressure ulcer is revealed after debridement, assign only the code for the stage revealed following debridement.

3) Documented pressure ulcer stage

Assignment of the pressure ulcer stage code should be guided by clinical documentation of the stage or documentation of the terms found in the Alphabetic Index. For clinical terms describing the stage that are not found in the Alphabetic Index, and there is no documentation of the stage, the provider should be queried.

> Left heel pressure ulcer with partial thickness skin loss involving the dermis
>
> **L89.622   Pressure ulcer of left heel, stage 2**
>
> *Explanation:* Code assignment for the pressure ulcer stage should be guided by either the clinical documentation of the stage or the documentation of terms found in the Alphabetic Index. The clinical documentation describing the left heel pressure ulcer "partial thickness skin loss involving the dermis" matches the ICD-10-CM index parenthetical description for stage 2 "(abrasion, blister, partial thickness skin loss involving epidermis and/or dermis)."

4) Patients admitted with pressure ulcers documented as healed

No code is assigned if the documentation states that the pressure ulcer is completely healed at the time of admission.

> Patient receiving follow-up examination of a completely healed pressure ulcer of the foot
>
> **Z09   Encounter for follow-up examination after completed treatment for conditions other than malignant neoplasm**
>
> **Z87.2   Personal history of diseases of the skin and subcutaneous tissue**
>
> *Explanation:* Assign only codes for the reason for the encounter and the personal history of the pressure ulcer. Personal history code Z87.2 includes conditions classifiable to L00–L99 such as pressure ulcer. No code is assigned for a pressure ulcer documented as completely healed.

5) Pressure ulcers documented as healing

Pressure ulcers described as healing should be assigned the appropriate pressure ulcer stage code based on the documentation in the medical record. If the documentation does not provide information about the stage of the healing pressure ulcer, assign the appropriate code for unspecified stage.

If the documentation is unclear as to whether the patient has a current (new) pressure ulcer or if the patient is being treated for a healing pressure ulcer, query the provider.

For ulcers that were present on admission but healed at the time of discharge, assign the code for the site and stage of the pressure ulcer at the time of admission.

6) Patient admitted with pressure ulcer evolving into another stage during the admission

If a patient is admitted to an inpatient hospital with a pressure ulcer at one stage and it progresses to a higher stage, two separate codes should be assigned: one code for the site and stage of the ulcer on admission and a second code for the same ulcer site and the highest stage reported during the stay.

7) Pressure-induced deep tissue damage

For pressure-induced deep tissue damage or deep tissue pressure injury, assign only the appropriate code for pressure-induced deep tissue damage (L89.--6).

b. Non-pressure chronic ulcers

1) Patients admitted with non-pressure ulcers documented as healed

No code is assigned if the documentation states that the non-pressure ulcer is completely healed at the time of admission.

2) Non-pressure ulcers documented as healing

Non-pressure ulcers described as healing should be assigned the appropriate non-pressure ulcer code based on the documentation in the medical record. If the documentation does not provide information about the severity of the healing non-pressure ulcer, assign the appropriate code for unspecified severity.

If the documentation is unclear as to whether the patient has a current (new) non-pressure ulcer or if the patient is being treated for a healing non-pressure ulcer, query the provider.

For ulcers that were present on admission but healed at the time of discharge, assign the code for the site and severity of the non-pressure ulcer at the time of admission.

3) Patient admitted with non-pressure ulcer that progresses to another severity level during the admission

If a patient is admitted to an inpatient hospital with a non-pressure ulcer at one severity level and it progresses to a higher severity level, two separate codes should be assigned: one code for the site and severity level of the ulcer on admission and a second code for the same ulcer site and the highest severity level reported during the stay.

See Section I.B.14. for pressure ulcer stage documentation by clinicians other than patient's provider.

Chapter 12. Diseases of the Skin and Subcutaneous Tissue (L00-L99)

EXCLUDES 2   *certain conditions originating in the perinatal period (P04-P96)*
certain infectious and parasitic diseases (A00-B99)
complications of pregnancy, childbirth and the puerperium (O00-O9A)
congenital malformations, deformations, and chromosomal abnormalities (Q00-Q99)
endocrine, nutritional and metabolic diseases (E00-E88)
lipomelanotic reticulosis (I89.8)
neoplasms (C00-D49)
symptoms, signs and abnormal clinical and laboratory findings, not elsewhere classified (R00-R94)
systemic connective tissue disorders (M30-M36)
viral warts (B07.-)

AHA: 2022,2Q,7

This chapter contains the following blocks:

L00-L08   Infections of the skin and subcutaneous tissue
L10-L14   Bullous disorders
L20-L30   Dermatitis and eczema
L40-L45   Papulosquamous disorders
L49-L54   Urticaria and erythema
L55-L59   Radiation-related disorders of the skin and subcutaneous tissue
L60-L75   Disorders of skin appendages
L76   Intraoperative and postprocedural complications of skin and subcutaneous tissue
L80-L99   Other disorders of the skin and subcutaneous tissue

Infections of the skin and subcutaneous tissue (L00-L08)

Use additional code (B95-B97) to identify infectious agent
EXCLUDES 2   *hordeolum (H00.0)*
infective dermatitis (L30.3)
local infections of skin classified in Chapter 1
lupus panniculitis (L93.2)
panniculitis NOS (M79.3)
panniculitis of neck and back (M54.0-)
perlèche NOS (K13.0)
perlèche due to candidiasis (B37.0)
perlèche due to riboflavin deficiency (E53.0)
pyogenic granuloma (L98.0)
relapsing panniculitis [Weber-Christian] (M35.6)
viral warts (B07.-)
zoster (B02.-)

L00   **Staphylococcal scalded skin syndrome**   COM
Ritter's disease
Use additional code to identify percentage of skin exfoliation (L49.-)
EXCLUDES 1   *bullous impetigo (L01.03)*
pemphigus neonatorum (L01.03)
toxic epidermal necrolysis [Lyell] (L51.2)
DEF: Infectious skin disease of children younger than 5 years marked by eruptions ranging from a few localized blisters to widespread, easily ruptured, fine vesicles and bullae affecting almost the entire body. It results in exfoliation of large planes of skin and leaves raw areas.

✓4th L01   **Impetigo**
EXCLUDES 1   *impetigo herpetiformis (L40.1)*
DEF: Acute, superficial, highly contagious skin infection commonly occurring in children. Skin lesions usually appear on the face and consist of vesicles and bullae that burst and form yellow crusts.

✓5th L01.0   **Impetigo**
Impetigo contagiosa
Impetigo vulgaris
    L01.00   **Impetigo, unspecified**
       Impetigo NOS
    L01.01   **Non-bullous impetigo**
    L01.02   **Bockhart's impetigo**
       Impetigo follicularis
       Perifolliculitis NOS
       Superficial pustular perifolliculitis
       DEF: Superficial inflammation of the hair follicles commonly caused by *Staphylococcus aureus* that manifests as rounded, sphere-shaped, pustular eruptions in the areas of the scalp, beard, underarms, extremities, and buttocks.
    L01.03   **Bullous impetigo**
       Impetigo neonatorum
       Pemphigus neonatorum
    L01.09   **Other impetigo**
       Ulcerative impetigo
    L01.1   **Impetiginization of other dermatoses**

✓4th L02   **Cutaneous abscess, furuncle and carbuncle**
Use additional code to identify organism (B95-B96)
EXCLUDES 2   *abscess of anus and rectal regions (K61.-)*
abscess of female genital organs (external) (N76.4)
abscess of male genital organs (external) (N48.2, N49.-)
DEF: Carbuncle: Infection of the skin that arises from a collection of interconnected infected boils or furuncles, usually from hair follicles infected by *Staphylococcus.* This condition can produce pus and form drainage cavities.
DEF: Furuncle: Inflamed, painful abscess, cyst, or nodule on the skin caused by bacteria, often *Staphylococcus,* entering along the hair follicle.

✓5th L02.0   **Cutaneous abscess, furuncle and carbuncle of face**
    EXCLUDES 2   *abscess of ear, external (H60.0)*
       abscess of eyelid (H00.0)
       abscess of head [any part, except face] (L02.8)
       abscess of lacrimal gland (H04.0)
       abscess of lacrimal passages (H04.3)
       abscess of mouth (K12.2)
       abscess of nose (J34.0)
       abscess of orbit (H05.0)
       submandibular abscess (K12.2)
    L02.01   **Cutaneous abscess of face**
    L02.02   **Furuncle of face**
       Boil of face
       Folliculitis of face
    L02.03   **Carbuncle of face**

✓5th L02.1   **Cutaneous abscess, furuncle and carbuncle of neck**
    L02.11   **Cutaneous abscess of neck**
    L02.12   **Furuncle of neck**
       Boil of neck
       Folliculitis of neck
    L02.13   **Carbuncle of neck**

✓5th L02.2   **Cutaneous abscess, furuncle and carbuncle of trunk**
    EXCLUDES 1   *non-newborn omphalitis (L08.82)*
       omphalitis of newborn (P38.-)
    EXCLUDES 2   *abscess of breast (N61.1)*
       abscess of buttocks (L02.3)
       abscess of female external genital organs (N76.4)
       abscess of hip (L02.4)
       abscess of male external genital organs (N48.2, N49.-)
    ✓6th L02.21   **Cutaneous abscess of trunk**
       L02.211   **Cutaneous abscess of abdominal wall**
       L02.212   **Cutaneous abscess of back [any part, except buttock]**
       L02.213   **Cutaneous abscess of chest wall**
       L02.214   **Cutaneous abscess of groin**
       L02.215   **Cutaneous abscess of perineum**
       L02.216   **Cutaneous abscess of umbilicus**
       L02.219   **Cutaneous abscess of trunk, unspecified**
    ✓6th L02.22   **Furuncle of trunk**
       Boil of trunk
       Folliculitis of trunk
       L02.221   **Furuncle of abdominal wall**
       L02.222   **Furuncle of back [any part, except buttock]**
       L02.223   **Furuncle of chest wall**
       L02.224   **Furuncle of groin**
       L02.225   **Furuncle of perineum**
       L02.226   **Furuncle of umbilicus**
       L02.229   **Furuncle of trunk, unspecified**
    ✓6th L02.23   **Carbuncle of trunk**
       L02.231   **Carbuncle of abdominal wall**
       L02.232   **Carbuncle of back [any part, except buttock]**
       L02.233   **Carbuncle of chest wall**
       L02.234   **Carbuncle of groin**
       L02.235   **Carbuncle of perineum**
       L02.236   **Carbuncle of umbilicus**
       L02.239   **Carbuncle of trunk, unspecified**

✓5th L02.3   **Cutaneous abscess, furuncle and carbuncle of buttock**
    EXCLUDES 1   *pilonidal cyst with abscess (L05.01)*
    L02.31   **Cutaneous abscess of buttock**
       Cutaneous abscess of gluteal region

L02.32 **Furuncle of buttock**
Boil of buttock
Folliculitis of buttock
Furuncle of gluteal region

L02.33 **Carbuncle of buttock**
Carbuncle of gluteal region

✓5th L02.4 **Cutaneous abscess, furuncle and carbuncle of limb**
EXCLUDES 2   cutaneous abscess, furuncle and carbuncle of groin (L02.214, L02.224, L02.234)
cutaneous abscess, furuncle and carbuncle of hand (L02.5-)
cutaneous abscess, furuncle and carbuncle of foot (L02.6-)

✓6th L02.41 **Cutaneous abscess of limb**
L02.411 **Cutaneous abscess of right axilla**
L02.412 **Cutaneous abscess of left axilla**
L02.413 **Cutaneous abscess of right upper limb**
L02.414 **Cutaneous abscess of left upper limb**
L02.415 **Cutaneous abscess of right lower limb**
L02.416 **Cutaneous abscess of left lower limb**
L02.419 **Cutaneous abscess of limb, unspecified**

✓6th L02.42 **Furuncle of limb**
Boil of limb
Folliculitis of limb
L02.421 **Furuncle of right axilla**
L02.422 **Furuncle of left axilla**
L02.423 **Furuncle of right upper limb**
L02.424 **Furuncle of left upper limb**
L02.425 **Furuncle of right lower limb**
L02.426 **Furuncle of left lower limb**
L02.429 **Furuncle of limb, unspecified**

✓6th L02.43 **Carbuncle of limb**
L02.431 **Carbuncle of right axilla**
L02.432 **Carbuncle of left axilla**
L02.433 **Carbuncle of right upper limb**
L02.434 **Carbuncle of left upper limb**
L02.435 **Carbuncle of right lower limb**
L02.436 **Carbuncle of left lower limb**
L02.439 **Carbuncle of limb, unspecified**

✓5th L02.5 **Cutaneous abscess, furuncle and carbuncle of hand**
✓6th L02.51 **Cutaneous abscess of hand**
L02.511 **Cutaneous abscess of right hand**
L02.512 **Cutaneous abscess of left hand**
L02.519 **Cutaneous abscess of unspecified hand**

✓6th L02.52 **Furuncle hand**
Boil of hand
Folliculitis of hand
L02.521 **Furuncle right hand**
L02.522 **Furuncle left hand**
L02.529 **Furuncle unspecified hand**

✓6th L02.53 **Carbuncle of hand**
L02.531 **Carbuncle of right hand**
L02.532 **Carbuncle of left hand**
L02.539 **Carbuncle of unspecified hand**

✓5th L02.6 **Cutaneous abscess, furuncle and carbuncle of foot**
✓6th L02.61 **Cutaneous abscess of foot**
L02.611 **Cutaneous abscess of right foot**
L02.612 **Cutaneous abscess of left foot**
L02.619 **Cutaneous abscess of unspecified foot**

✓6th L02.62 **Furuncle of foot**
Boil of foot
Folliculitis of foot
L02.621 **Furuncle of right foot**
L02.622 **Furuncle of left foot**
L02.629 **Furuncle of unspecified foot**

✓6th L02.63 **Carbuncle of foot**
L02.631 **Carbuncle of right foot**
L02.632 **Carbuncle of left foot**
L02.639 **Carbuncle of unspecified foot**

✓5th L02.8 **Cutaneous abscess, furuncle and carbuncle of other sites**
✓6th L02.81 **Cutaneous abscess of other sites**
L02.811 **Cutaneous abscess of head [any part, except face]**
L02.818 **Cutaneous abscess of other sites**

✓6th L02.82 **Furuncle of other sites**
Boil of other sites
Folliculitis of other sites
L02.821 **Furuncle of head [any part, except face]**
L02.828 **Furuncle of other sites**

✓6th L02.83 **Carbuncle of other sites**
L02.831 **Carbuncle of head [any part, except face]**
L02.838 **Carbuncle of other sites**

✓5th L02.9 **Cutaneous abscess, furuncle and carbuncle, unspecified**
L02.91 **Cutaneous abscess, unspecified**
L02.92 **Furuncle, unspecified**
Boil NOS
Furunculosis NOS
L02.93 **Carbuncle, unspecified**

✓4th L03 **Cellulitis and acute lymphangitis**
EXCLUDES 2   cellulitis of anal and rectal region (K61.-)
cellulitis of external auditory canal (H60.1)
cellulitis of eyelid (H00.0)
cellulitis of female external genital organs (N76.4)
cellulitis of lacrimal apparatus (H04.3)
cellulitis of male external genital organs (N48.2, N49.-)
cellulitis of mouth (K12.2)
cellulitis of nose (J34.0)
eosinophilic cellulitis [Wells] (L98.3)
febrile neutrophilic dermatosis [Sweet] (L98.2)
lymphangitis (chronic) (subacute) (I89.1)
AHA: 2017,4Q,100
DEF: Cellulitis: Infection of the skin and subcutaneous tissues, most often caused by *Staphylococcus* or *Streptococcus* bacteria secondary to a cutaneous lesion. Progression of the inflammation may lead to abscess and tissue death, or even systemic infection-like bacteremia.
DEF: Lymphangitis: Inflammation of the lymph channels most often caused by *Streptococcus*.

✓5th L03.0 **Cellulitis and acute lymphangitis of finger and toe**
Infection of nail
Onychia
Paronychia
Perionychia

✓6th L03.01 **Cellulitis of finger**
Felon
Whitlow
EXCLUDES 1   herpetic whitlow (B00.89)
DEF: Felon: Superficial bacterial skin infection at the tip of the finger.
L03.011 **Cellulitis of right finger**
L03.012 **Cellulitis of left finger**
L03.019 **Cellulitis of unspecified finger**

✓6th L03.02 **Acute lymphangitis of finger**
Hangnail with lymphangitis of finger
L03.021 **Acute lymphangitis of right finger**
L03.022 **Acute lymphangitis of left finger**
L03.029 **Acute lymphangitis of unspecified finger**

✓6th L03.03 **Cellulitis of toe**
L03.031 **Cellulitis of right toe**
L03.032 **Cellulitis of left toe**
L03.039 **Cellulitis of unspecified toe**

✓6th L03.04 **Acute lymphangitis of toe**
Hangnail with lymphangitis of toe
L03.041 **Acute lymphangitis of right toe**
L03.042 **Acute lymphangitis of left toe**
L03.049 **Acute lymphangitis of unspecified toe**

✓5th L03.1 **Cellulitis and acute lymphangitis of other parts of limb**
✓6th L03.11 **Cellulitis of other parts of limb**
EXCLUDES 2   cellulitis of fingers (L03.01-)
cellulitis of toes (L03.03-)
groin (L03.314)
L03.111 **Cellulitis of right axilla**
L03.112 **Cellulitis of left axilla**
L03.113 **Cellulitis of right upper limb**
L03.114 **Cellulitis of left upper limb**
L03.115 **Cellulitis of right lower limb**
L03.116 **Cellulitis of left lower limb**
L03.119 **Cellulitis of unspecified part of limb**

√6ᵗʰ **L03.12   Acute lymphangitis of other parts of limb**
  EXCLUDES 2   *acute lymphangitis of fingers (L03.2-)*
               acute lymphangitis of groin (L03.324)
               acute lymphangitis of toes (L03.04-)
  L03.121   Acute lymphangitis of right axilla
  L03.122   Acute lymphangitis of left axilla
  L03.123   Acute lymphangitis of right upper limb
  L03.124   Acute lymphangitis of left upper limb
  L03.125   Acute lymphangitis of right lower limb
  L03.126   Acute lymphangitis of left lower limb
  L03.129   Acute lymphangitis of unspecified part of limb

√5ᵗʰ **L03.2   Cellulitis and acute lymphangitis of face and neck**
  √6ᵗʰ **L03.21   Cellulitis and acute lymphangitis of face**
    L03.211   Cellulitis of face
      EXCLUDES 2   *abscess of orbit (H05.01-)*
                   cellulitis of ear (H60.1-)
                   cellulitis of eyelid (H00.0-)
                   cellulitis of head (L03.81)
                   cellulitis of lacrimal apparatus (H04.3)
                   cellulitis of lip (K13.0)
                   cellulitis of mouth (K12.2)
                   cellulitis of nose (internal) (J34.0)
                   cellulitis of orbit (H05.01-)
                   cellulitis of scalp (L03.81)
      AHA: 2013,4Q,123
    L03.212   Acute lymphangitis of face
    L03.213   Periorbital cellulitis
      Preseptal cellulitis
      AHA: 2016,4Q,36
  √6ᵗʰ **L03.22   Cellulitis and acute lymphangitis of neck**
    L03.221   Cellulitis of neck
    L03.222   Acute lymphangitis of neck

√5ᵗʰ **L03.3   Cellulitis and acute lymphangitis of trunk**
  √6ᵗʰ **L03.31   Cellulitis of trunk**
    EXCLUDES 2   *cellulitis of anal and rectal regions (K61.-)*
                 cellulitis of breast NOS (N61.0)
                 cellulitis of female external genital organs (N76.4)
                 cellulitis of male external genital organs (N48.2, N49.-)
                 omphalitis of newborn (P38.-)
                 puerperal cellulitis of breast (O91.2)
    L03.311   Cellulitis of abdominal wall
      EXCLUDES 2   *cellulitis of umbilicus (L03.316)*
                   cellulitis of groin (L03.314)
    L03.312   Cellulitis of back [any part except buttock]
    L03.313   Cellulitis of chest wall
    L03.314   Cellulitis of groin
    L03.315   Cellulitis of perineum
    L03.316   Cellulitis of umbilicus
    L03.317   Cellulitis of buttock
    L03.319   Cellulitis of trunk, unspecified
  √6ᵗʰ **L03.32   Acute lymphangitis of trunk**
    L03.321   Acute lymphangitis of abdominal wall
    L03.322   Acute lymphangitis of back [any part except buttock]
    L03.323   Acute lymphangitis of chest wall
    L03.324   Acute lymphangitis of groin
    L03.325   Acute lymphangitis of perineum
    L03.326   Acute lymphangitis of umbilicus
    L03.327   Acute lymphangitis of buttock
    L03.329   Acute lymphangitis of trunk, unspecified

√5ᵗʰ **L03.8   Cellulitis and acute lymphangitis of other sites**
  √6ᵗʰ **L03.81   Cellulitis of other sites**
    L03.811   Cellulitis of head [any part, except face]
      Cellulitis of scalp
      EXCLUDES 2   *cellulitis of face (L03.211)*
    L03.818   Cellulitis of other sites
  √6ᵗʰ **L03.89   Acute lymphangitis of other sites**
    L03.891   Acute lymphangitis of head [any part, except face]

L03.898   Acute lymphangitis of other sites
√5ᵗʰ **L03.9   Cellulitis and acute lymphangitis, unspecified**
  L03.90   Cellulitis, unspecified
  L03.91   Acute lymphangitis, unspecified
    EXCLUDES 1   *lymphangitis NOS (I89.1)*

√4ᵗʰ **L04   Acute lymphadenitis**
  INCLUDES   abscess (acute) of lymph nodes, except mesenteric
             acute lymphadenitis, except mesenteric
  EXCLUDES 1   *chronic or subacute lymphadenitis, except mesenteric (I88.1)*
               enlarged lymph nodes (R59.-)
               human immunodeficiency virus [HIV] disease resulting in generalized lymphadenopathy (B20)
               lymphadenitis NOS (I88.9)
               nonspecific mesenteric lymphadenitis (I88.0)
  DEF: Inflammation or enlargement of the lymph nodes.
  L04.0   Acute lymphadenitis of face, head and neck
  L04.1   Acute lymphadenitis of trunk
  L04.2   Acute lymphadenitis of upper limb
    Acute lymphadenitis of axilla
    Acute lymphadenitis of shoulder
  L04.3   Acute lymphadenitis of lower limb
    Acute lymphadenitis of hip
    EXCLUDES 2   *acute lymphadenitis of groin (L04.1)*
  L04.8   Acute lymphadenitis of other sites
  L04.9   Acute lymphadenitis, unspecified

√4ᵗʰ **L05   Pilonidal cyst and sinus**
  DEF: Pilonidal cyst: Sac or sinus cavity of trapped epithelial tissues in the sacrococcygeal region, usually associated with ingrown hair.
  DEF: Pilonidal sinus: Fistula, tract, or channel that extends from an infected area of ingrown hair to another site within the skin or out to the skin surface.

Pilonidal Cyst

Skin
Fistula
Pilonidal cyst
Fat
Bone

√5ᵗʰ **L05.0   Pilonidal cyst and sinus with abscess**
  L05.01   Pilonidal cyst with abscess
    Pilonidal abscess
    Pilonidal dimple with abscess
    Postanal dimple with abscess
    EXCLUDES 2   *congenital sacral dimple (Q82.6)*
                 parasacral dimple (Q82.6)
  L05.02   Pilonidal sinus with abscess
    Coccygeal fistula with abscess
    Coccygeal sinus with abscess
    Pilonidal fistula with abscess
√5ᵗʰ **L05.9   Pilonidal cyst and sinus without abscess**
  L05.91   Pilonidal cyst without abscess
    Pilonidal dimple
    Postanal dimple
    Pilonidal cyst NOS
    EXCLUDES 2   *congenital sacral dimple (Q82.6)*
                 parasacral dimple (Q82.6)
  L05.92   Pilonidal sinus without abscess
    Coccygeal fistula
    Coccygeal sinus without abscess
    Pilonidal fistula

☑️4ᵗʰ **L08 Other local infections of skin and subcutaneous tissue**

     L08.0 Pyoderma
         Dermatitis gangrenosa
         Purulent dermatitis
         Septic dermatitis
         Suppurative dermatitis
         EXCLUDES 1   *pyoderma gangrenosum (L88)*
                  pyoderma vegetans (L08.81)
         DEF: Any superficial skin disease commonly characterized by the discharging of pus not attributed to another condition.

     L08.1 Erythrasma
         DEF: Chronic, superficial skin infection of brown scaly patches, commonly found in skin folds most prevalent in the overweight or diabetic population.

     ☑️5ᵗʰ **L08.8 Other specified local infections of the skin and subcutaneous tissue**

         L08.81 Pyoderma vegetans
               EXCLUDES 1   *pyoderma gangrenosum (L88)*
                          pyoderma NOS (L08.0)

         L08.82 Omphalitis not of newborn
               EXCLUDES 1   *omphalitis of newborn (P38.-)*

         L08.89 Other specified local infections of the skin and subcutaneous tissue

     L08.9 Local infection of the skin and subcutaneous tissue, unspecified

Bullous disorders (L10-L14)

EXCLUDES 1   *benign familial pemphigus [Hailey-Hailey] (Q82.8)*
              staphylococcal scalded skin syndrome (L00)
              toxic epidermal necrolysis [Lyell] (L51.2)

☑️4ᵗʰ **L10 Pemphigus**

     EXCLUDES 1   *pemphigus neonatorum (L01.03)*

     L10.0 Pemphigus vulgaris   Rx COM
     L10.1 Pemphigus vegetans   Rx COM
     L10.2 Pemphigus foliaceous   Rx COM
     L10.3 Brazilian pemphigus [fogo selvagem]   Rx COM
     L10.4 Pemphigus erythematosus   Rx COM
         Senear-Usher syndrome
     L10.5 Drug-induced pemphigus   Rx COM
         Use additional code for adverse effect, if applicable, to identify drug (T36-T50 with fifth or sixth character 5)

     ☑️5ᵗʰ **L10.8 Other pemphigus**
         L10.81 Paraneoplastic pemphigus   Rx COM
         L10.89 Other pemphigus   Rx COM
     L10.9 Pemphigus, unspecified   Rx COM

☑️4ᵗʰ **L11 Other acantholytic disorders**

     L11.0 Acquired keratosis follicularis
         EXCLUDES 1   *keratosis follicularis (congenital) [Darier-White] (Q82.8)*
         AHA: 2021,3Q,10

     L11.1 Transient acantholytic dermatosis [Grover]
     L11.8 Other specified acantholytic disorders
     L11.9 Acantholytic disorder, unspecified

☑️4ᵗʰ **L12 Pemphigoid**

     EXCLUDES 1   *herpes gestationis (O26.4-)*
              impetigo herpetiformis (L40.1)

     L12.0 Bullous pemphigoid   Rx COM
     L12.1 Cicatricial pemphigoid   Rx COM
         Benign mucous membrane pemphigoid
         DEF: Chronic autoimmune disease characterized by subepidermal blistering lesions of the mucosa, including the conjunctiva. It is seen predominantly in the elderly and produces adhesions and scarring.

     L12.2 Chronic bullous disease of childhood   Rx P
         Juvenile dermatitis herpetiformis

     ☑️5ᵗʰ **L12.3 Acquired epidermolysis bullosa**
         EXCLUDES 1   *epidermolysis bullosa (congenital) (Q81.-)*
         L12.30 Acquired epidermolysis bullosa, unspecified   HCC ESR COM
         L12.31 Epidermolysis bullosa due to drug   HCC ESR COM
              Use additional code for adverse effect, if applicable, to identify drug (T36-T50 with fifth or sixth character 5)
         L12.35 Other acquired epidermolysis bullosa   HCC ESR COM

     L12.8 Other pemphigoid   Rx COM
     L12.9 Pemphigoid, unspecified   Rx COM

☑️4ᵗʰ **L13 Other bullous disorders**

     L13.0 Dermatitis herpetiformis   Rx
         Duhring's disease
         Hydroa herpetiformis
         EXCLUDES 1   *juvenile dermatitis herpetiformis (L12.2)*
                  senile dermatitis herpetiformis (L12.0)
         DEF: Skin disease to which people are genetically predisposed resulting from an immunological response to gluten. Dermatitis herpetiformis is an extremely pruritic eruption of various lesions that frequently heal, leaving hyperpigmentation or hypopigmentation and occasionally scarring. It is usually associated with asymptomatic gluten-sensitive enteropathy.

     L13.1 Subcorneal pustular dermatitis   Rx
         Sneddon-Wilkinson disease

     L13.8 Other specified bullous disorders   Rx
     L13.9 Bullous disorder, unspecified   Rx

L14 *Bullous disorders in diseases classified elsewhere*   Rx
     Code first underlying disease

Dermatitis and eczema (L20-L30)

NOTE   In this block the terms dermatitis and eczema are used synonymously and interchangeably.

EXCLUDES 2   *chronic (childhood) granulomatous disease (D71)*
              dermatitis gangrenosa (L08.0)
              dermatitis herpetiformis (L13.0)
              dry skin dermatitis (L85.3)
              factitial dermatitis (L98.1)
              perioral dermatitis (L71.0)
              radiation-related disorders of the skin and subcutaneous tissue (L55-L59)
              stasis dermatitis (I87.2)

☑️4ᵗʰ **L20 Atopic dermatitis**

     L20.0 Besnier's prurigo

     ☑️5ᵗʰ **L20.8 Other atopic dermatitis**
         EXCLUDES 2   *circumscribed neurodermatitis (L28.0)*
         L20.81 Atopic neurodermatitis
              Diffuse neurodermatitis
         L20.82 Flexural eczema
         L20.83 Infantile (acute) (chronic) eczema   P
         L20.84 Intrinsic (allergic) eczema
         L20.89 Other atopic dermatitis
     L20.9 Atopic dermatitis, unspecified

☑️4ᵗʰ **L21 Seborrheic dermatitis**

     EXCLUDES 2   *infective dermatitis (L30.3)*
              seborrheic keratosis (L82.-)

     L21.0 Seborrhea capitis
         Cradle cap
         AHA: 2018,1Q,6
         TIP: Assign for dandruff in an adult patient.

     L21.1 Seborrheic infantile dermatitis   P
     L21.8 Other seborrheic dermatitis
     L21.9 Seborrheic dermatitis, unspecified
         Seborrhea NOS

L22 Diaper dermatitis
     Diaper erythema
     Diaper rash
     Psoriasiform diaper rash
     AHA: 2021,4Q,18

☑️ Additional Character Required   ✓x7ᵗʰ Placeholder Alert   Manifestation   Unspecified Dx   Q QPP   UPD Unacceptable PDx

✓4th L23 Allergic contact dermatitis

> EXCLUDES 1   allergy NOS (T78.40)
> contact dermatitis NOS (L25.9)
> dermatitis NOS (L30.9)
>
> EXCLUDES 2   dermatitis due to substances taken internally (L27.-)
> dermatitis of eyelid (H01.1-)
> diaper dermatitis (L22)
> eczema of external ear (H60.5-)
> irritant contact dermatitis (L24.-)
> perioral dermatitis (L71.0)
> radiation-related disorders of the skin and subcutaneous
> tissue (L55-L59)

L23.0 Allergic contact dermatitis due to metals
Allergic contact dermatitis due to chromium
Allergic contact dermatitis due to nickel

L23.1 Allergic contact dermatitis due to adhesives

L23.2 Allergic contact dermatitis due to cosmetics

L23.3 Allergic contact dermatitis due to drugs in contact with skin
Use additional code for adverse effect, if applicable, to identify
drug (T36-T50 with fifth or sixth character 5)
> EXCLUDES 2   dermatitis due to ingested drugs and medicaments
> (L27.0-L27.1)

L23.4 Allergic contact dermatitis due to dyes

L23.5 Allergic contact dermatitis due to other chemical products
Allergic contact dermatitis due to cement
Allergic contact dermatitis due to insecticide
Allergic contact dermatitis due to plastic
Allergic contact dermatitis due to rubber

L23.6 Allergic contact dermatitis due to food in contact with the skin
> EXCLUDES 2   dermatitis due to ingested food (L27.2)

L23.7 Allergic contact dermatitis due to plants, except food
> EXCLUDES 2   allergy NOS due to pollen (J30.1)

✓5th L23.8 Allergic contact dermatitis due to other agents

L23.81 Allergic contact dermatitis due to animal (cat) (dog) dander
Allergic contact dermatitis due to animal (cat) (dog)
hair

L23.89 Allergic contact dermatitis due to other agents

L23.9 Allergic contact dermatitis, unspecified cause
Allergic contact eczema NOS

✓4th L24 Irritant contact dermatitis

> EXCLUDES 1   allergy NOS (T78.40)
> contact dermatitis NOS (L25.9)
> dermatitis NOS (L30.9)
>
> EXCLUDES 2   allergic contact dermatitis (L23.-)
> dermatitis due to substances taken internally (L27.-)
> dermatitis of eyelid (H01.1-)
> diaper dermatitis (L22)
> eczema of external ear (H60.5-)
> perioral dermatitis (L71.0)
> radiation-related disorders of the skin and subcutaneous
> tissue (L55-L59)

L24.0 Irritant contact dermatitis due to detergents

L24.1 Irritant contact dermatitis due to oils and greases

L24.2 Irritant contact dermatitis due to solvents
Irritant contact dermatitis due to chlorocompound
Irritant contact dermatitis due to cyclohexane
Irritant contact dermatitis due to ester
Irritant contact dermatitis due to glycol
Irritant contact dermatitis due to hydrocarbon
Irritant contact dermatitis due to ketone

L24.3 Irritant contact dermatitis due to cosmetics

L24.4 Irritant contact dermatitis due to drugs in contact with skin
Use additional code for adverse effect, if applicable, to identify
drug (T36-T50 with fifth or sixth character 5)

L24.5 Irritant contact dermatitis due to other chemical products
Irritant contact dermatitis due to cement
Irritant contact dermatitis due to insecticide
Irritant contact dermatitis due to plastic
Irritant contact dermatitis due to rubber

L24.6 Irritant contact dermatitis due to food in contact with skin
> EXCLUDES 2   dermatitis due to ingested food (L27.2)

L24.7 Irritant contact dermatitis due to plants, except food
> EXCLUDES 2   allergy NOS to pollen (J30.1)

✓5th L24.8 Irritant contact dermatitis due to other agents

L24.81 Irritant contact dermatitis due to metals
Irritant contact dermatitis due to chromium
Irritant contact dermatitis due to nickel

L24.89 Irritant contact dermatitis due to other agents
Irritant contact dermatitis due to dyes

L24.9 Irritant contact dermatitis, unspecified cause
Irritant contact eczema NOS

✓5th L24.A Irritant contact dermatitis due to friction or contact with body fluids
> EXCLUDES 1   irritant contact dermatitis related to stoma or fistula
> (L24.B-)
> EXCLUDES 2   erythema intertrigo (L30.4)
>
> AHA: 2021,4Q,16-18

L24.A0 Irritant contact dermatitis due to friction or contact with body fluids, unspecified

L24.A1 Irritant contact dermatitis due to saliva

L24.A2 Irritant contact dermatitis due to fecal, urinary or dual incontinence
> EXCLUDES 1   diaper dermatitis (L22)

L24.A9 Irritant contact dermatitis due friction or contact with other specified body fluids
Irritant contact dermatitis related to endotracheal
tube
Wound fluids, exudate

✓5th L24.B Irritant contact dermatitis related to stoma or fistula
Use additional code to identify any artificial opening status
(Z93.-), if applicable, for contact dermatitis related to stoma
secretions
> AHA: 2021,4Q,16-18

L24.B0 Irritant contact dermatitis related to unspecified stoma or fistula
Irritant contact dermatitis related to fistula NOS
Irritant contact dermatitis related to stoma NOS

L24.B1 Irritant contact dermatitis related to digestive stoma or fistula
Irritant contact dermatitis related to gastrostomy
Irritant contact dermatitis related to jejunostomy
Irritant contact dermatitis related to saliva or spit
fistula

L24.B2 Irritant contact dermatitis related to respiratory stoma or fistula
Irritant contact dermatitis related to tracheostomy

L24.B3 Irritant contact dermatitis related to fecal or urinary stoma or fistula
Irritant contact dermatitis related to colostomy
Irritant contact dermatitis related to enterocutaneous
fistula
Irritant contact dermatitis related to ileostomy

✓4th L25 Unspecified contact dermatitis

> EXCLUDES 1   allergic contact dermatitis (L23.-)
> allergy NOS (T78.40)
> dermatitis NOS (L30.9)
> irritant contact dermatitis (L24.-)
>
> EXCLUDES 2   dermatitis due to ingested substances (L27.-)
> dermatitis of eyelid (H01.1-)
> eczema of external ear (H60.5-)
> perioral dermatitis (L71.0)
> radiation-related disorders of the skin and subcutaneous
> tissue (L55-L59)

L25.0 Unspecified contact dermatitis due to cosmetics

L25.1 Unspecified contact dermatitis due to drugs in contact with skin
Use additional code for adverse effect, if applicable, to identify
drug (T36-T50 with fifth or sixth character 5)
> EXCLUDES 2   dermatitis due to ingested drugs and medicaments
> (L27.0-L27.1)

L25.2 Unspecified contact dermatitis due to dyes

L25.3 Unspecified contact dermatitis due to other chemical products
Unspecified contact dermatitis due to cement
Unspecified contact dermatitis due to insecticide

L25.4 Unspecified contact dermatitis due to **food in contact with skin**
> EXCLUDES 2   *dermatitis due to ingested food (L27.2)*

L25.5 Unspecified contact dermatitis due to **plants, except food**
> EXCLUDES 1   *nettle rash (L50.9)*
> EXCLUDES 2   *allergy NOS due to pollen (J30.1)*

L25.8 Unspecified contact dermatitis due to **other agents**

L25.9 Unspecified contact dermatitis, **unspecified cause**
> Contact dermatitis (occupational) NOS
> Contact eczema (occupational) NOS

L26 **Exfoliative dermatitis**
> Hebra's pityriasis
> EXCLUDES 1   *Ritter's disease (L00)*

✓4ᵗʰ **L27** **Dermatitis due to substances taken internally**
> EXCLUDES 1   *allergy NOS (T78.40)*
> EXCLUDES 2   *adverse food reaction, except dermatitis (T78.0-T78.1)*
>   *contact dermatitis (L23-L25)*
>   *drug photoallergic response (L56.1)*
>   *drug phototoxic response (L56.0)*
>   *urticaria (L50.-)*

L27.0 Generalized **skin eruption due to drugs and medicaments taken internally**
> Use additional code for adverse effect, if applicable, to identify drug (T36-T50 with fifth or sixth character 5)

L27.1 Localized **skin eruption due to drugs and medicaments taken internally**
> Use additional code for adverse effect, if applicable, to identify drug (T36-T50 with fifth or sixth character 5)

L27.2 Dermatitis **due to ingested food**
> EXCLUDES 2   *dermatitis due to food in contact with skin (L23.6, L24.6, L25.4)*

L27.8 Dermatitis due to other substances taken internally

L27.9 Dermatitis due to unspecified substance taken internally

✓4ᵗʰ **L28** **Lichen simplex chronicus and prurigo**

L28.0 **Lichen simplex chronicus**
> Circumscribed neurodermatitis
> Lichen NOS

L28.1 **Prurigo nodularis**

L28.2 **Other prurigo**
> Prurigo NOS
> Prurigo Hebra
> Prurigo mitis
> Urticaria papulosa

✓4ᵗʰ **L29** **Pruritus**
> EXCLUDES 1   *neurotic excoriation (L98.1)*
>   *psychogenic pruritus (F45.8)*

L29.0 **Pruritus ani**

L29.1 **Pruritus scroti**   ♂

L29.2 **Pruritus vulvae**   ♀

L29.3 **Anogenital pruritus, unspecified**

L29.8 **Other pruritus**

L29.9 **Pruritus, unspecified**
> Itch NOS

✓4ᵗʰ **L30** **Other and unspecified dermatitis**
> EXCLUDES 2   *contact dermatitis (L23-L25)*
>   *dry skin dermatitis (L85.3)*
>   *small plaque parapsoriasis (L41.3)*
>   *stasis dermatitis (I87.2)*

L30.0 **Nummular dermatitis**

L30.1 **Dyshidrosis [pompholyx]**

L30.2 **Cutaneous autosensitization**
> Candidid [levurid]
> Dermatophytid
> Eczematid

L30.3 **Infective dermatitis**
> Infectious eczematoid dermatitis

L30.4 **Erythema intertrigo**

L30.5 **Pityriasis alba**
> AHA: 2018,1Q,6

L30.8 **Other specified dermatitis**

L30.9 **Dermatitis, unspecified**
> Eczema NOS

Papulosquamous disorders (L40-L45)

✓4ᵗʰ **L40** **Psoriasis**
> **DEF:** Chronic autoimmune condition that speeds up skin cell growth, causing excessive immature skin cells to form raised, rounded erythematous lesions covered by dry, silvery scaling patches. Most commonly found on the scalp, elbows, knees, hands, feet, and genitals, it can also affect the joints with stiffness and swelling.

L40.0 **Psoriasis vulgaris**   Rx
> Nummular psoriasis
> Plaque psoriasis

L40.1 **Generalized pustular psoriasis**   Rx
> Impetigo herpetiformis
> Von Zumbusch's disease

L40.2 **Acrodermatitis continua**   Rx

L40.3 **Pustulosis palmaris et plantaris**   Rx

L40.4 **Guttate psoriasis**   Rx

✓5ᵗʰ **L40.5** **Arthropathic psoriasis**

L40.50 **Arthropathic psoriasis, unspecified**   HCC Rx ESR COM

L40.51 **Distal interphalangeal psoriatic arthropathy**   HCC Rx ESR COM

L40.52 **Psoriatic arthritis mutilans**   HCC Rx ESR COM

L40.53 **Psoriatic spondylitis**   HCC Rx ESR COM

L40.54 **Psoriatic juvenile arthropathy**   HCC Rx ESR COM

L40.59 **Other psoriatic arthropathy**   HCC Rx ESR COM

L40.8 **Other psoriasis**   Rx
> Flexural psoriasis

L40.9 **Psoriasis, unspecified**   Rx

✓4ᵗʰ **L41** **Parapsoriasis**
> EXCLUDES 1   *poikiloderma vasculare atrophicans (L94.5)*

L41.0 **Pityriasis lichenoides et varioliformis acuta**   Rx
> Mucha-Habermann disease

L41.1 **Pityriasis lichenoides chronica**   Rx

L41.3 **Small plaque parapsoriasis**   Rx

L41.4 **Large plaque parapsoriasis**   Rx

L41.5 **Retiform parapsoriasis**   Rx

L41.8 **Other parapsoriasis**   Rx

L41.9 **Parapsoriasis, unspecified**   Rx

L42 **Pityriasis rosea**

✓4ᵗʰ **L43** **Lichen planus**
> EXCLUDES 1   *lichen planopilaris (L66.1)*

L43.0 **Hypertrophic lichen planus**

L43.1 **Bullous lichen planus**

L43.2 **Lichenoid drug reaction**
> Use additional code for adverse effect, if applicable, to identify drug (T36-T50 with fifth or sixth character 5)

L43.3 **Subacute (active) lichen planus**
> Lichen planus tropicus

L43.8 **Other lichen planus**

L43.9 **Lichen planus, unspecified**

✓4ᵗʰ **L44** **Other papulosquamous disorders**

L44.0 **Pityriasis rubra pilaris**

L44.1 **Lichen nitidus**
> **DEF:** Chronic, inflammatory, asymptomatic skin disorder, characterized by numerous glistening, flat-topped, discrete, skin-colored micropapules, most often on the penis, lower abdomen, inner thighs, wrists, forearms, breasts, and buttocks.

L44.2 **Lichen striatus**

L44.3 **Lichen ruber moniliformis**

L44.4 **Infantile papular acrodermatitis [Gianotti-Crosti]**   P

L44.8 **Other specified papulosquamous disorders**

L44.9 **Papulosquamous disorder, unspecified**

L45 *Papulosquamous disorders in diseases classified elsewhere*
> Code first underlying disease

✔ Additional Character Required   ✓x7ᵗʰ Placeholder Alert   Manifestation   Unspecified Dx   Q QPP   UPD Unacceptable PDx

Urticaria and erythema (L49-L54)

EXCLUDES 1   *Lyme disease (A69.2-)*
       rosacea (L71.-)

✓4ᵗʰ **L49 Exfoliation due to erythematous conditions according to extent of body surface involved**

Code first erythematous condition causing exfoliation, such as:
Ritter's disease (L00)
(Staphylococcal) scalded skin syndrome (L00)
Stevens-Johnson syndrome (L51.1)
Stevens-Johnson syndrome-toxic epidermal necrolysis overlap syndrome (L51.3)
toxic epidermal necrolysis (L51.2)
DEF: Exfoliation: Falling or sloughing off skin in layers.

L49.0 Exfoliation due to erythematous condition involving less than 10 percent of body surface   UPD
     Exfoliation due to erythematous condition NOS

L49.1 Exfoliation due to erythematous condition involving 10-19 percent of body surface   COM   UPD

L49.2 Exfoliation due to erythematous condition involving 20-29 percent of body surface   COM   UPD

L49.3 Exfoliation due to erythematous condition involving 30-39 percent of body surface   COM   UPD

L49.4 Exfoliation due to erythematous condition involving 40-49 percent of body surface   COM   UPD

L49.5 Exfoliation due to erythematous condition involving 50-59 percent of body surface   COM   UPD

L49.6 Exfoliation due to erythematous condition involving 60-69 percent of body surface   COM   UPD

L49.7 Exfoliation due to erythematous condition involving 70-79 percent of body surface   COM   UPD

L49.8 Exfoliation due to erythematous condition involving 80-89 percent of body surface   COM   UPD

L49.9 Exfoliation due to erythematous condition involving 90 or more percent of body surface   COM   UPD

✓4ᵗʰ **L50 Urticaria**

EXCLUDES 1   *allergic contact dermatitis (L23.-)*
       angioneurotic edema (T78.3)
       giant urticaria (T78.3)
       hereditary angio-edema (D84.1)
       Quincke's edema (T78.3)
       serum urticaria (T80.6-)
       solar urticaria (L56.3)
       urticaria neonatorum (P83.8)
       urticaria papulosa (L28.2)
       urticaria pigmentosa (D47.01)

DEF: Eruption of itching edema of the skin. **Synonym(s):** *hives.*

L50.0 Allergic urticaria
L50.1 Idiopathic urticaria
L50.2 Urticaria due to cold and heat
     EXCLUDES 2   *familial cold urticaria (M04.2)*
L50.3 Dermatographic urticaria
L50.4 Vibratory urticaria
L50.5 Cholinergic urticaria
L50.6 Contact urticaria
L50.8 Other urticaria
     Chronic urticaria
     Recurrent periodic urticaria
L50.9 Urticaria, unspecified

✓4ᵗʰ **L51 Erythema multiforme**

Use additional code for adverse effect, if applicable, to identify drug (T36-T50 with fifth or sixth character 5)
Use additional code to identify associated manifestations, such as:
arthropathy associated with dermatological disorders (M14.8-)
conjunctival edema (H11.42)
conjunctivitis (H10.22-)
corneal scars and opacities (H17.-)
corneal ulcer (H16.0-)
edema of eyelid (H02.84-)
inflammation of eyelid (H01.8)
keratoconjunctivitis sicca (H16.22-)
mechanical lagophthalmos (H02.22-)
stomatitis (K12.-)
symblepharon (H11.23-)
Use additional code to identify percentage of skin exfoliation (L49.-)
EXCLUDES 1   *staphylococcal scalded skin syndrome (L00)*
       Ritter's disease (L00)

DEF: Acute complex of symptoms with a varied pattern of skin eruptions, such as macular, bullous, papular, nodose, or vesicular lesions on the neck, face, and legs. Erythema (redness of skin and mucous membranes) multiforme (multiple forms) is a hypersensitivity (allergic) reaction that can occur at any age but primarily affects children or young adults.

L51.0 Nonbullous erythema multiforme
L51.1 Stevens-Johnson syndrome   HCC   ESR   COM
L51.2 Toxic epidermal necrolysis [Lyell]   HCC   ESR   COM
L51.3 Stevens-Johnson syndrome-toxic epidermal necrolysis overlap syndrome   HCC   ESR   COM
     SJS-TEN overlap syndrome
L51.8 Other erythema multiforme
L51.9 Erythema multiforme, unspecified
     Erythema iris
     Erythema multiforme major NOS
     Erythema multiforme minor NOS
     Herpes iris

L52 Erythema nodosum

EXCLUDES 1   *tuberculous erythema nodosum (A18.4)*

DEF: Form of panniculitis (inflammation of the fat layer beneath the skin) most often occurring in women. Commonly seen as a hypersensitivity reaction to infections, drugs, sarcoidosis, and specific enteropathies. The acute stage is associated with fever, malaise, and arthralgia. The lesions are pink to blue in color as tender nodules and are found on the front of the legs below the knees.

✓4ᵗʰ **L53 Other erythematous conditions**

EXCLUDES 1   *erythema ab igne (L59.0)*
       erythema due to external agents in contact with skin (L23-L25)
       erythema intertrigo (L30.4)

L53.0 Toxic erythema
     Code first poisoning due to drug or toxin, if applicable (T36-T65 with fifth or sixth character 1-4 or 6)
     Use additional code for adverse effect, if applicable, to identify drug (T36-T50 with fifth or sixth character 5)
     EXCLUDES 1   *neonatal erythema toxicum (P83.1)*
L53.1 Erythema annulare centrifugum
L53.2 Erythema marginatum
L53.3 Other chronic figurate erythema
L53.8 Other specified erythematous conditions
L53.9 Erythematous condition, unspecified
     Erythema NOS
     Erythroderma NOS

L54 Erythema in diseases classified elsewhere
     Code first underlying disease

Radiation-related disorders of the skin and subcutaneous tissue (L55-L59)

✓4ᵗʰ **L55 Sunburn**

L55.0 Sunburn of first degree
L55.1 Sunburn of second degree
L55.2 Sunburn of third degree   COM
L55.9 Sunburn, unspecified

✓5ᵗʰ **M05.2** **Rheumatoid** vasculitis with rheumatoid arthritis

     M05.20 Rheumatoid vasculitis with rheumatoid arthritis of unspecified site   `HCC` `Rx` `ESR` `COM`

     ✓6ᵗʰ **M05.21** **Rheumatoid vasculitis with rheumatoid arthritis of** shoulder

         M05.211 Rheumatoid vasculitis with rheumatoid arthritis of right shoulder   `HCC` `Rx` `ESR` `COM`

         M05.212 Rheumatoid vasculitis with rheumatoid arthritis of left shoulder   `HCC` `Rx` `ESR` `COM`

         M05.219 Rheumatoid vasculitis with rheumatoid arthritis of unspecified shoulder   `HCC` `Rx` `ESR` `COM`

     ✓6ᵗʰ **M05.22** **Rheumatoid vasculitis with rheumatoid arthritis of** elbow

         M05.221 Rheumatoid vasculitis with rheumatoid arthritis of right elbow   `HCC` `Rx` `ESR` `COM`

         M05.222 Rheumatoid vasculitis with rheumatoid arthritis of left elbow   `HCC` `Rx` `ESR` `COM`

         M05.229 Rheumatoid vasculitis with rheumatoid arthritis of unspecified elbow   `HCC` `Rx` `ESR` `COM`

     ✓6ᵗʰ **M05.23** **Rheumatoid vasculitis with rheumatoid arthritis of** wrist

         Rheumatoid vasculitis with rheumatoid arthritis, carpal bones

         M05.231 Rheumatoid vasculitis with rheumatoid arthritis of right wrist   `HCC` `Rx` `ESR` `COM`

         M05.232 Rheumatoid vasculitis with rheumatoid arthritis of left wrist   `HCC` `Rx` `ESR` `COM`

         M05.239 Rheumatoid vasculitis with rheumatoid arthritis of unspecified wrist   `HCC` `Rx` `ESR` `COM`

     ✓6ᵗʰ **M05.24** **Rheumatoid vasculitis with rheumatoid arthritis of** hand

         Rheumatoid vasculitis with rheumatoid arthritis, metacarpus and phalanges

         M05.241 Rheumatoid vasculitis with rheumatoid arthritis of right hand   `HCC` `Rx` `ESR` `COM`

         M05.242 Rheumatoid vasculitis with rheumatoid arthritis of left hand   `HCC` `Rx` `ESR` `COM`

         M05.249 Rheumatoid vasculitis with rheumatoid arthritis of unspecified hand   `HCC` `Rx` `ESR` `COM`

     ✓6ᵗʰ **M05.25** **Rheumatoid vasculitis with rheumatoid arthritis of** hip

         M05.251 Rheumatoid vasculitis with rheumatoid arthritis of right hip   `HCC` `Rx` `ESR` `COM`

         M05.252 Rheumatoid vasculitis with rheumatoid arthritis of left hip   `HCC` `Rx` `ESR` `COM`

         M05.259 Rheumatoid vasculitis with rheumatoid arthritis of unspecified hip   `HCC` `Rx` `ESR` `COM`

     ✓6ᵗʰ **M05.26** **Rheumatoid vasculitis with rheumatoid arthritis of** knee

         M05.261 Rheumatoid vasculitis with rheumatoid arthritis of right knee   `HCC` `Rx` `ESR` `COM`

         M05.262 Rheumatoid vasculitis with rheumatoid arthritis of left knee   `HCC` `Rx` `ESR` `COM`

         M05.269 Rheumatoid vasculitis with rheumatoid arthritis of unspecified knee   `HCC` `Rx` `ESR` `COM`

     ✓6ᵗʰ **M05.27** **Rheumatoid vasculitis with rheumatoid arthritis of** ankle and foot

         Rheumatoid vasculitis with rheumatoid arthritis, tarsus, metatarsus and phalanges

         M05.271 Rheumatoid vasculitis with rheumatoid arthritis of right ankle and foot   `HCC` `Rx` `ESR` `COM`

         M05.272 Rheumatoid vasculitis with rheumatoid arthritis of left ankle and foot   `HCC` `Rx` `ESR` `COM`

         M05.279 Rheumatoid vasculitis with rheumatoid arthritis of unspecified ankle and foot   `HCC` `Rx` `ESR` `COM`

     M05.29 Rheumatoid vasculitis with rheumatoid arthritis of multiple sites   `HCC` `Rx` `ESR` `COM`

✓5ᵗʰ **M05.3** **Rheumatoid** heart disease with rheumatoid arthritis

     Rheumatoid carditis

     Rheumatoid endocarditis

     Rheumatoid myocarditis

     Rheumatoid pericarditis

     M05.30 Rheumatoid heart disease with rheumatoid arthritis of unspecified site   `HCC` `Rx` `ESR` `COM`

     ✓6ᵗʰ **M05.31** **Rheumatoid heart disease with rheumatoid arthritis of** shoulder

         M05.311 Rheumatoid heart disease with rheumatoid arthritis of right shoulder   `HCC` `Rx` `ESR` `COM`

         M05.312 Rheumatoid heart disease with rheumatoid arthritis of left shoulder   `HCC` `Rx` `ESR` `COM`

         M05.319 Rheumatoid heart disease with rheumatoid arthritis of unspecified shoulder   `HCC` `Rx` `ESR` `COM`

     ✓6ᵗʰ **M05.32** **Rheumatoid heart disease with rheumatoid arthritis of** elbow

         M05.321 Rheumatoid heart disease with rheumatoid arthritis of right elbow   `HCC` `Rx` `ESR` `COM`

         M05.322 Rheumatoid heart disease with rheumatoid arthritis of left elbow   `HCC` `Rx` `ESR` `COM`

         M05.329 Rheumatoid heart disease with rheumatoid arthritis of unspecified elbow   `HCC` `Rx` `ESR` `COM`

     ✓6ᵗʰ **M05.33** **Rheumatoid heart disease with rheumatoid arthritis of** wrist

         Rheumatoid heart disease with rheumatoid arthritis, carpal bones

         M05.331 Rheumatoid heart disease with rheumatoid arthritis of right wrist   `HCC` `Rx` `ESR` `COM`

         M05.332 Rheumatoid heart disease with rheumatoid arthritis of left wrist   `HCC` `Rx` `ESR` `COM`

         M05.339 Rheumatoid heart disease with rheumatoid arthritis of unspecified wrist   `HCC` `Rx` `ESR` `COM`

     ✓6ᵗʰ **M05.34** **Rheumatoid heart disease with rheumatoid arthritis of** hand

         Rheumatoid heart disease with rheumatoid arthritis, metacarpus and phalanges

         M05.341 Rheumatoid heart disease with rheumatoid arthritis of right hand   `HCC` `Rx` `ESR` `COM`

         M05.342 Rheumatoid heart disease with rheumatoid arthritis of left hand   `HCC` `Rx` `ESR` `COM`

         M05.349 Rheumatoid heart disease with rheumatoid arthritis of unspecified hand   `HCC` `Rx` `ESR` `COM`

     ✓6ᵗʰ **M05.35** **Rheumatoid heart disease with rheumatoid arthritis of** hip

         M05.351 Rheumatoid heart disease with rheumatoid arthritis of right hip   `HCC` `Rx` `ESR` `COM`

         M05.352 Rheumatoid heart disease with rheumatoid arthritis of left hip   `HCC` `Rx` `ESR` `COM`

         M05.359 Rheumatoid heart disease with rheumatoid arthritis of unspecified hip   `HCC` `Rx` `ESR` `COM`

     ✓6ᵗʰ **M05.36** **Rheumatoid heart disease with rheumatoid arthritis of** knee

         M05.361 Rheumatoid heart disease with rheumatoid arthritis of right knee   `HCC` `Rx` `ESR` `COM`

         M05.362 Rheumatoid heart disease with rheumatoid arthritis of left knee   `HCC` `Rx` `ESR` `COM`

         M05.369 Rheumatoid heart disease with rheumatoid arthritis of unspecified knee   `HCC` `Rx` `ESR` `COM`

✔ Additional Character Required   ✓x7ᵗʰ Placeholder Alert   Manifestation   Unspecified Dx   🄠 QPP   `UPD` Unacceptable PDx

√6ᵗʰ **M05.37** **Rheumatoid heart disease with rheumatoid arthritis of** ankle and foot
Rheumatoid heart disease with rheumatoid arthritis, tarsus, metatarsus and phalanges

M05.371 Rheumatoid heart disease with rheumatoid arthritis of right ankle and foot `HCC` `Rx` `ESR` `COM`

M05.372 Rheumatoid heart disease with rheumatoid arthritis of left ankle and foot `HCC` `Rx` `ESR` `COM`

M05.379 Rheumatoid heart disease with rheumatoid arthritis of unspecified ankle and foot `HCC` `Rx` `ESR` `COM`

M05.39 **Rheumatoid heart disease with rheumatoid arthritis of** multiple sites `HCC` `Rx` `ESR` `COM`

√5ᵗʰ **M05.4** **Rheumatoid** myopathy with rheumatoid arthritis

M05.40 **Rheumatoid myopathy with rheumatoid arthritis of unspecified site** `HCC` `Rx` `ESR` `COM`

√6ᵗʰ **M05.41** **Rheumatoid myopathy with rheumatoid arthritis of** shoulder

M05.411 Rheumatoid myopathy with rheumatoid arthritis of right shoulder `HCC` `Rx` `ESR` `COM`

M05.412 Rheumatoid myopathy with rheumatoid arthritis of left shoulder `HCC` `Rx` `ESR` `COM`

M05.419 Rheumatoid myopathy with rheumatoid arthritis of unspecified shoulder `HCC` `Rx` `ESR` `COM`

√6ᵗʰ **M05.42** **Rheumatoid myopathy with rheumatoid arthritis of** elbow

M05.421 Rheumatoid myopathy with rheumatoid arthritis of right elbow `HCC` `Rx` `ESR` `COM`

M05.422 Rheumatoid myopathy with rheumatoid arthritis of left elbow `HCC` `Rx` `ESR` `COM`

M05.429 Rheumatoid myopathy with rheumatoid arthritis of unspecified elbow `HCC` `Rx` `ESR` `COM`

√6ᵗʰ **M05.43** **Rheumatoid myopathy with rheumatoid arthritis of** wrist
Rheumatoid myopathy with rheumatoid arthritis, carpal bones

M05.431 Rheumatoid myopathy with rheumatoid arthritis of right wrist `HCC` `Rx` `ESR` `COM`

M05.432 Rheumatoid myopathy with rheumatoid arthritis of left wrist `HCC` `Rx` `ESR` `COM`

M05.439 Rheumatoid myopathy with rheumatoid arthritis of unspecified wrist `HCC` `Rx` `ESR` `COM`

√6ᵗʰ **M05.44** **Rheumatoid myopathy with rheumatoid arthritis of** hand
Rheumatoid myopathy with rheumatoid arthritis, metacarpus and phalanges

M05.441 Rheumatoid myopathy with rheumatoid arthritis of right hand `HCC` `Rx` `ESR` `COM`

M05.442 Rheumatoid myopathy with rheumatoid arthritis of left hand `HCC` `Rx` `ESR` `COM`

M05.449 Rheumatoid myopathy with rheumatoid arthritis of unspecified hand `HCC` `Rx` `ESR` `COM`

√6ᵗʰ **M05.45** **Rheumatoid myopathy with rheumatoid arthritis of** hip

M05.451 Rheumatoid myopathy with rheumatoid arthritis of right hip `HCC` `Rx` `ESR` `COM`

M05.452 Rheumatoid myopathy with rheumatoid arthritis of left hip `HCC` `Rx` `ESR` `COM`

M05.459 Rheumatoid myopathy with rheumatoid arthritis of unspecified hip `HCC` `Rx` `ESR` `COM`

√6ᵗʰ **M05.46** **Rheumatoid myopathy with rheumatoid arthritis of** knee

M05.461 Rheumatoid myopathy with rheumatoid arthritis of right knee `HCC` `Rx` `ESR` `COM`

M05.462 Rheumatoid myopathy with rheumatoid arthritis of left knee `HCC` `Rx` `ESR` `COM`

M05.469 Rheumatoid myopathy with rheumatoid arthritis of unspecified knee `HCC` `Rx` `ESR` `COM`

√6ᵗʰ **M05.47** **Rheumatoid myopathy with rheumatoid arthritis of** ankle and foot
Rheumatoid myopathy with rheumatoid arthritis, tarsus, metatarsus and phalanges

M05.471 Rheumatoid myopathy with rheumatoid arthritis of right ankle and foot `HCC` `Rx` `ESR` `COM`

M05.472 Rheumatoid myopathy with rheumatoid arthritis of left ankle and foot `HCC` `Rx` `ESR` `COM`

M05.479 Rheumatoid myopathy with rheumatoid arthritis of unspecified ankle and foot `HCC` `Rx` `ESR` `COM`

M05.49 **Rheumatoid myopathy with rheumatoid arthritis of** multiple sites `HCC` `Rx` `ESR` `COM`

√5ᵗʰ **M05.5** **Rheumatoid** polyneuropathy with rheumatoid arthritis

M05.50 **Rheumatoid polyneuropathy with rheumatoid arthritis of unspecified site** `HCC` `Rx` `ESR` `COM`

√6ᵗʰ **M05.51** **Rheumatoid polyneuropathy with rheumatoid arthritis of** shoulder

M05.511 Rheumatoid polyneuropathy with rheumatoid arthritis of right shoulder `HCC` `Rx` `ESR` `COM`

M05.512 Rheumatoid polyneuropathy with rheumatoid arthritis of left shoulder `HCC` `Rx` `ESR` `COM`

M05.519 Rheumatoid polyneuropathy with rheumatoid arthritis of unspecified shoulder `HCC` `Rx` `ESR` `COM`

√6ᵗʰ **M05.52** **Rheumatoid polyneuropathy with rheumatoid arthritis of** elbow

M05.521 Rheumatoid polyneuropathy with rheumatoid arthritis of right elbow `HCC` `Rx` `ESR` `COM`

M05.522 Rheumatoid polyneuropathy with rheumatoid arthritis of left elbow `HCC` `Rx` `ESR` `COM`

M05.529 Rheumatoid polyneuropathy with rheumatoid arthritis of unspecified elbow `HCC` `Rx` `ESR` `COM`

√6ᵗʰ **M05.53** **Rheumatoid polyneuropathy with rheumatoid arthritis of** wrist
Rheumatoid polyneuropathy with rheumatoid arthritis, carpal bones

M05.531 Rheumatoid polyneuropathy with rheumatoid arthritis of right wrist `HCC` `Rx` `ESR` `COM`

M05.532 Rheumatoid polyneuropathy with rheumatoid arthritis of left wrist `HCC` `Rx` `ESR` `COM`

M05.539 Rheumatoid polyneuropathy with rheumatoid arthritis of unspecified wrist `HCC` `Rx` `ESR` `COM`

√6ᵗʰ **M05.54** **Rheumatoid polyneuropathy with rheumatoid arthritis of** hand
Rheumatoid polyneuropathy with rheumatoid arthritis, metacarpus and phalanges

M05.541 Rheumatoid polyneuropathy with rheumatoid arthritis of right hand `HCC` `Rx` `ESR` `COM`

M05.542 Rheumatoid polyneuropathy with rheumatoid arthritis of left hand `HCC` `Rx` `ESR` `COM`

M05.549 Rheumatoid polyneuropathy with rheumatoid arthritis of unspecified hand `HCC` `Rx` `ESR` `COM`

√6ᵗʰ **M05.55** **Rheumatoid polyneuropathy with rheumatoid arthritis of** hip

M05.551 Rheumatoid polyneuropathy with rheumatoid arthritis of right hip `HCC` `Rx` `ESR` `COM`

M05.552 Rheumatoid polyneuropathy with rheumatoid arthritis of left hip `HCC` `Rx` `ESR` `COM`

M05.559 Rheumatoid polyneuropathy with rheumatoid arthritis of unspecified hip `HCC` `Rx` `ESR` `COM`

√6ᵗʰ **M05.56** **Rheumatoid polyneuropathy with rheumatoid arthritis of** knee

M05.561 Rheumatoid polyneuropathy with rheumatoid arthritis of right knee `HCC` `Rx` `ESR` `COM`

M05.562 **Rheumatoid polyneuropathy with rheumatoid arthritis of left knee** `HCC` `Rx` `ESR` `COM`

M05.569 **Rheumatoid polyneuropathy with rheumatoid arthritis of unspecified knee** `HCC` `Rx` `ESR` `COM`

☑6ᵗʰ M05.57 **Rheumatoid polyneuropathy with rheumatoid arthritis of ankle and foot**
Rheumatoid polyneuropathy with rheumatoid arthritis, tarsus, metatarsus and phalanges

M05.571 **Rheumatoid polyneuropathy with rheumatoid arthritis of right ankle and foot** `HCC` `Rx` `ESR` `COM`

M05.572 **Rheumatoid polyneuropathy with rheumatoid arthritis of left ankle and foot** `HCC` `Rx` `ESR` `COM`

M05.579 **Rheumatoid polyneuropathy with rheumatoid arthritis of unspecified ankle and foot** `HCC` `Rx` `ESR` `COM`

M05.59 **Rheumatoid polyneuropathy with rheumatoid arthritis of multiple sites** `HCC` `Rx` `ESR` `COM`

☑5ᵗʰ M05.6 **Rheumatoid arthritis with involvement of other organs and systems**

M05.60 **Rheumatoid arthritis of unspecified site with involvement of other organs and systems** `HCC` `Rx` `ESR` `COM`

☑6ᵗʰ M05.61 **Rheumatoid arthritis of shoulder with involvement of other organs and systems**

M05.611 **Rheumatoid arthritis of right shoulder with involvement of other organs and systems** `HCC` `Rx` `ESR` `COM`

M05.612 **Rheumatoid arthritis of left shoulder with involvement of other organs and systems** `HCC` `Rx` `ESR` `COM`

M05.619 **Rheumatoid arthritis of unspecified shoulder with involvement of other organs and systems** `HCC` `Rx` `ESR` `COM`

☑6ᵗʰ M05.62 **Rheumatoid arthritis of elbow with involvement of other organs and systems**

M05.621 **Rheumatoid arthritis of right elbow with involvement of other organs and systems** `HCC` `Rx` `ESR` `COM`

M05.622 **Rheumatoid arthritis of left elbow with involvement of other organs and systems** `HCC` `Rx` `ESR` `COM`

M05.629 **Rheumatoid arthritis of unspecified elbow with involvement of other organs and systems** `HCC` `Rx` `ESR` `COM`

☑6ᵗʰ M05.63 **Rheumatoid arthritis of wrist with involvement of other organs and systems**
Rheumatoid arthritis of carpal bones with involvement of other organs and systems

M05.631 **Rheumatoid arthritis of right wrist with involvement of other organs and systems** `HCC` `Rx` `ESR` `COM`

M05.632 **Rheumatoid arthritis of left wrist with involvement of other organs and systems** `HCC` `Rx` `ESR` `COM`

M05.639 **Rheumatoid arthritis of unspecified wrist with involvement of other organs and systems** `HCC` `Rx` `ESR` `COM`

☑6ᵗʰ M05.64 **Rheumatoid arthritis of hand with involvement of other organs and systems**
Rheumatoid arthritis of metacarpus and phalanges with involvement of other organs and systems

M05.641 **Rheumatoid arthritis of right hand with involvement of other organs and systems** `HCC` `Rx` `ESR` `COM`

M05.642 **Rheumatoid arthritis of left hand with involvement of other organs and systems** `HCC` `Rx` `ESR` `COM`

M05.649 **Rheumatoid arthritis of unspecified hand with involvement of other organs and systems** `HCC` `Rx` `ESR` `COM`

☑6ᵗʰ M05.65 **Rheumatoid arthritis of hip with involvement of other organs and systems**

M05.651 **Rheumatoid arthritis of right hip with involvement of other organs and systems** `HCC` `Rx` `ESR` `COM`

M05.652 **Rheumatoid arthritis of left hip with involvement of other organs and systems**

M05.659 **Rheumatoid arthritis of unspecified hip with involvement of other organs and systems** `HCC` `Rx` `ESR` `COM`

☑6ᵗʰ M05.66 **Rheumatoid arthritis of knee with involvement of other organs and systems**

M05.661 **Rheumatoid arthritis of right knee with involvement of other organs and systems** `HCC` `Rx` `ESR` `COM`

M05.662 **Rheumatoid arthritis of left knee with involvement of other organs and systems** `HCC` `Rx` `ESR` `COM`

M05.669 **Rheumatoid arthritis of unspecified knee with involvement of other organs and systems** `HCC` `Rx` `ESR` `COM`

☑6ᵗʰ M05.67 **Rheumatoid arthritis of ankle and foot with involvement of other organs and systems**
Rheumatoid arthritis of tarsus, metatarsus and phalanges with involvement of other organs and systems

M05.671 **Rheumatoid arthritis of right ankle and foot with involvement of other organs and systems** `HCC` `Rx` `ESR` `COM`

M05.672 **Rheumatoid arthritis of left ankle and foot with involvement of other organs and systems** `HCC` `Rx` `ESR` `COM`

M05.679 **Rheumatoid arthritis of unspecified ankle and foot with involvement of other organs and systems** `HCC` `Rx` `ESR` `COM`

M05.69 **Rheumatoid arthritis of multiple sites with involvement of other organs and systems**

☑5ᵗʰ M05.7 **Rheumatoid arthritis with rheumatoid factor without organ or systems involvement**

M05.70 **Rheumatoid arthritis with rheumatoid factor of unspecified site without organ or systems involvement** `HCC` `Rx` `ESR` `COM`

☑6ᵗʰ M05.71 **Rheumatoid arthritis with rheumatoid factor of shoulder without organ or systems involvement**

M05.711 **Rheumatoid arthritis with rheumatoid factor of right shoulder without organ or systems involvement** `HCC` `Rx` `ESR` `COM`

M05.712 **Rheumatoid arthritis with rheumatoid factor of left shoulder without organ or systems involvement** `HCC` `Rx` `ESR` `COM`

M05.719 **Rheumatoid arthritis with rheumatoid factor of unspecified shoulder without organ or systems involvement** `HCC` `Rx` `ESR` `COM`

☑6ᵗʰ M05.72 **Rheumatoid arthritis with rheumatoid factor of elbow without organ or systems involvement**

M05.721 **Rheumatoid arthritis with rheumatoid factor of right elbow without organ or systems involvement** `HCC` `Rx` `ESR` `COM`

M05.722 **Rheumatoid arthritis with rheumatoid factor of left elbow without organ or systems involvement** `HCC` `Rx` `ESR` `COM`

M05.729 **Rheumatoid arthritis with rheumatoid factor of unspecified elbow without organ or systems involvement** `HCC` `Rx` `ESR` `COM`

☑6ᵗʰ M05.73 **Rheumatoid arthritis with rheumatoid factor of wrist without organ or systems involvement**

M05.731 **Rheumatoid arthritis with rheumatoid factor of right wrist without organ or systems involvement** `HCC` `Rx` `ESR` `COM`

M05.732 **Rheumatoid arthritis with rheumatoid factor of left wrist without organ or systems involvement** `HCC` `Rx` `ESR` `COM`

M05.739 **Rheumatoid arthritis with rheumatoid factor of unspecified wrist without organ or systems involvement** `HCC` `Rx` `ESR` `COM`

☑6ᵗʰ M05.74 **Rheumatoid arthritis with rheumatoid factor of hand without organ or systems involvement**

M05.741 **Rheumatoid arthritis with rheumatoid factor of right hand without organ or systems involvement** `HCC` `Rx` `ESR` `COM`

M05.742 **Rheumatoid arthritis with rheumatoid factor of left hand without organ or systems involvement** `HCC` `Rx` `ESR` `COM`

M05.749 Rheumatoid arthritis with rheumatoid factor of unspecified hand without organ or systems involvement `HCC` `Rx` `ESR` `COM`

√6ᵗʰ M05.75 Rheumatoid arthritis with rheumatoid factor of hip without organ or systems involvement

M05.751 Rheumatoid arthritis with rheumatoid factor of right hip without organ or systems involvement `HCC` `Rx` `ESR` `COM`

M05.752 Rheumatoid arthritis with rheumatoid factor of left hip without organ or systems involvement `HCC` `Rx` `ESR` `COM`

M05.759 Rheumatoid arthritis with rheumatoid factor of unspecified hip without organ or systems involvement `HCC` `Rx` `ESR` `COM`

√6ᵗʰ M05.76 Rheumatoid arthritis with rheumatoid factor of knee without organ or systems involvement

M05.761 Rheumatoid arthritis with rheumatoid factor of right knee without organ or systems involvement `HCC` `Rx` `ESR` `COM`

M05.762 Rheumatoid arthritis with rheumatoid factor of left knee without organ or systems involvement `HCC` `Rx` `ESR` `COM`

M05.769 Rheumatoid arthritis with rheumatoid factor of unspecified knee without organ or systems involvement `HCC` `Rx` `ESR` `COM`

√6ᵗʰ M05.77 Rheumatoid arthritis with rheumatoid factor of ankle and foot without organ or systems involvement

M05.771 Rheumatoid arthritis with rheumatoid factor of right ankle and foot without organ or systems involvement `HCC` `Rx` `ESR` `COM`

M05.772 Rheumatoid arthritis with rheumatoid factor of left ankle and foot without organ or systems involvement `HCC` `Rx` `ESR` `COM`

M05.779 Rheumatoid arthritis with rheumatoid factor of unspecified ankle and foot without organ or systems involvement `HCC` `Rx` `ESR` `COM`

M05.79 Rheumatoid arthritis with rheumatoid factor of multiple sites without organ or systems involvement `HCC` `Rx` `ESR` `COM`

M05.7A Rheumatoid arthritis with rheumatoid factor of other specified site without organ or systems involvement `HCC` `Rx` `ESR` `COM`

√5ᵗʰ M05.8 Other rheumatoid arthritis with rheumatoid factor

M05.80 Other rheumatoid arthritis with rheumatoid factor of unspecified site `HCC` `Rx` `ESR` `COM`

√6ᵗʰ M05.81 Other rheumatoid arthritis with rheumatoid factor of shoulder

M05.811 Other rheumatoid arthritis with rheumatoid factor of right shoulder `HCC` `Rx` `ESR` `COM`

M05.812 Other rheumatoid arthritis with rheumatoid factor of left shoulder `HCC` `Rx` `ESR` `COM`

M05.819 Other rheumatoid arthritis with rheumatoid factor of unspecified shoulder `HCC` `Rx` `ESR` `COM`

√6ᵗʰ M05.82 Other rheumatoid arthritis with rheumatoid factor of elbow

M05.821 Other rheumatoid arthritis with rheumatoid factor of right elbow `HCC` `Rx` `ESR` `COM`

M05.822 Other rheumatoid arthritis with rheumatoid factor of left elbow `HCC` `Rx` `ESR` `COM`

M05.829 Other rheumatoid arthritis with rheumatoid factor of unspecified elbow `HCC` `Rx` `ESR` `COM`

√6ᵗʰ M05.83 Other rheumatoid arthritis with rheumatoid factor of wrist

M05.831 Other rheumatoid arthritis with rheumatoid factor of right wrist `HCC` `Rx` `ESR` `COM`

M05.832 Other rheumatoid arthritis with rheumatoid factor of left wrist `HCC` `Rx` `ESR` `COM`

M05.839 Other rheumatoid arthritis with rheumatoid factor of unspecified wrist `HCC` `Rx` `ESR` `COM`

√6ᵗʰ M05.84 Other rheumatoid arthritis with rheumatoid factor of hand

M05.841 Other rheumatoid arthritis with rheumatoid factor of right hand `HCC` `Rx` `ESR` `COM`

M05.842 Other rheumatoid arthritis with rheumatoid factor of left hand `HCC` `Rx` `ESR` `COM`

M05.849 Other rheumatoid arthritis with rheumatoid factor of unspecified hand `HCC` `Rx` `ESR` `COM`

√6ᵗʰ M05.85 Other rheumatoid arthritis with rheumatoid factor of hip

M05.851 Other rheumatoid arthritis with rheumatoid factor of right hip `HCC` `Rx` `ESR` `COM`

M05.852 Other rheumatoid arthritis with rheumatoid factor of left hip `HCC` `Rx` `ESR` `COM`

M05.859 Other rheumatoid arthritis with rheumatoid factor of unspecified hip `HCC` `Rx` `ESR` `COM`

√6ᵗʰ M05.86 Other rheumatoid arthritis with rheumatoid factor of knee

M05.861 Other rheumatoid arthritis with rheumatoid factor of right knee `HCC` `Rx` `ESR` `COM`

M05.862 Other rheumatoid arthritis with rheumatoid factor of left knee `HCC` `Rx` `ESR` `COM`

M05.869 Other rheumatoid arthritis with rheumatoid factor of unspecified knee `HCC` `Rx` `ESR` `COM`

√6ᵗʰ M05.87 Other rheumatoid arthritis with rheumatoid factor of ankle and foot

M05.871 Other rheumatoid arthritis with rheumatoid factor of right ankle and foot `HCC` `Rx` `ESR` `COM`

M05.872 Other rheumatoid arthritis with rheumatoid factor of left ankle and foot `HCC` `Rx` `ESR` `COM`

M05.879 Other rheumatoid arthritis with rheumatoid factor of unspecified ankle and foot `HCC` `Rx` `ESR` `COM`

M05.89 Other rheumatoid arthritis with rheumatoid factor of multiple sites `HCC` `Rx` `ESR` `COM`

M05.8A Other rheumatoid arthritis with rheumatoid factor of other specified site `HCC` `Rx` `ESR` `COM`

M05.9 Rheumatoid arthritis with rheumatoid factor, unspecified `HCC` `Rx` `ESR` `COM`

√4ᵗʰ **M06 Other rheumatoid arthritis**

AHA: 2020,4Q,31-32

DEF: Rheumatoid arthritis: Autoimmune systemic disease that causes chronic inflammation of the joints and other areas of the body, manifested by inflammatory changes in articular structures and synovial membranes, atrophy, and loss in bone density.

√5ᵗʰ M06.0 Rheumatoid arthritis without rheumatoid factor

M06.00 Rheumatoid arthritis without rheumatoid factor, unspecified site `HCC` `Rx` `ESR` `COM`

√6ᵗʰ M06.01 Rheumatoid arthritis without rheumatoid factor, shoulder

M06.011 Rheumatoid arthritis without rheumatoid factor, right shoulder `HCC` `Rx` `ESR` `COM`

M06.012 Rheumatoid arthritis without rheumatoid factor, left shoulder `HCC` `Rx` `ESR` `COM`

M06.019 Rheumatoid arthritis without rheumatoid factor, unspecified shoulder `HCC` `Rx` `ESR` `COM`

√6ᵗʰ M06.02 Rheumatoid arthritis without rheumatoid factor, elbow

M06.021 Rheumatoid arthritis without rheumatoid factor, right elbow `HCC` `Rx` `ESR` `COM`

M06.022 Rheumatoid arthritis without rheumatoid factor, left elbow `HCC` `Rx` `ESR` `COM`

M06.029 Rheumatoid arthritis without rheumatoid factor, unspecified elbow `HCC` `Rx` `ESR` `COM`

`HCC` CMS-HCC · `Rx` Rx HCC · `ESR` ESRD HCC · `COM` Commercial HCC · `N` Newborn: 0 · `P` Pediatric: 0-17 · `M` Maternity: 9-64 · `A` Adult: 15-124

786 ICD-10-CM 2023

√6ᵗʰ **M06.03** Rheumatoid arthritis without rheumatoid factor, wrist

     M06.031 Rheumatoid arthritis without rheumatoid factor, right wrist `HCC` `Rx` `ESR` `COM`

     M06.032 Rheumatoid arthritis without rheumatoid factor, left wrist `HCC` `Rx` `ESR` `COM`

     M06.039 Rheumatoid arthritis without rheumatoid factor, unspecified wrist

√6ᵗʰ **M06.04** Rheumatoid arthritis without rheumatoid factor, hand

     M06.041 Rheumatoid arthritis without rheumatoid factor, right hand `HCC` `Rx` `ESR` `COM`

     M06.042 Rheumatoid arthritis without rheumatoid factor, left hand `HCC` `Rx` `ESR` `COM`

     M06.049 Rheumatoid arthritis without rheumatoid factor, unspecified hand `HCC` `Rx` `ESR` `COM`

√6ᵗʰ **M06.05** Rheumatoid arthritis without rheumatoid factor, hip

     M06.051 Rheumatoid arthritis without rheumatoid factor, right hip `HCC` `Rx` `ESR` `COM`

     M06.052 Rheumatoid arthritis without rheumatoid factor, left hip `HCC` `Rx` `ESR` `COM`

     M06.059 Rheumatoid arthritis without rheumatoid factor, unspecified hip `HCC` `Rx` `ESR` `COM`

√6ᵗʰ **M06.06** Rheumatoid arthritis without rheumatoid factor, knee

     M06.061 Rheumatoid arthritis without rheumatoid factor, right knee `HCC` `Rx` `ESR` `COM`

     M06.062 Rheumatoid arthritis without rheumatoid factor, left knee `HCC` `Rx` `ESR` `COM`

     M06.069 Rheumatoid arthritis without rheumatoid factor, unspecified knee `HCC` `Rx` `ESR` `COM`

√6ᵗʰ **M06.07** Rheumatoid arthritis without rheumatoid factor, ankle and foot

     M06.071 Rheumatoid arthritis without rheumatoid factor, right ankle and foot `HCC` `Rx` `ESR` `COM`

     M06.072 Rheumatoid arthritis without rheumatoid factor, left ankle and foot `HCC` `Rx` `ESR` `COM`

     M06.079 Rheumatoid arthritis without rheumatoid factor, unspecified ankle and foot `HCC` `Rx` `ESR` `COM`

     M06.08 Rheumatoid arthritis without rheumatoid factor, vertebrae `HCC` `Rx` `ESR` `COM`

     M06.09 Rheumatoid arthritis without rheumatoid factor, multiple sites `HCC` `Rx` `ESR` `COM`

     M06.0A Rheumatoid arthritis without rheumatoid factor, other specified site `HCC` `Rx` `ESR` `COM`

M06.1 Adult-onset Still's disease `HCC` `Rx` `ESR` `COM` `A`

     EXCLUDES 1   Still's disease NOS (M08.2-)

     DEF: Type of systemic arthritis characterized by a transient rash and spiking fevers. This condition may resolve or develop into a chronic condition and may affect internal organs, as well as joints.

     Synonym(s): AOSD

√5ᵗʰ **M06.2** Rheumatoid bursitis

     M06.20 Rheumatoid bursitis, unspecified site `HCC` `Rx` `ESR` `COM`

√6ᵗʰ **M06.21** Rheumatoid bursitis, shoulder

     M06.211 Rheumatoid bursitis, right shoulder `HCC` `Rx` `ESR` `COM`

     M06.212 Rheumatoid bursitis, left shoulder `HCC` `Rx` `ESR` `COM`

     M06.219 Rheumatoid bursitis, unspecified shoulder `HCC` `Rx` `ESR` `COM`

√6ᵗʰ **M06.22** Rheumatoid bursitis, elbow

     M06.221 Rheumatoid bursitis, right elbow `HCC` `Rx` `ESR` `COM`

     M06.222 Rheumatoid bursitis, left elbow `HCC` `Rx` `ESR` `COM`

     M06.229 Rheumatoid bursitis, unspecified elbow `HCC` `Rx` `ESR` `COM`

√6ᵗʰ **M06.23** Rheumatoid bursitis, wrist

     M06.231 Rheumatoid bursitis, right wrist `HCC` `Rx` `ESR` `COM`

     M06.232 Rheumatoid bursitis, left wrist `HCC` `Rx` `ESR` `COM`

     M06.239 Rheumatoid bursitis, unspecified wrist `HCC` `Rx` `ESR` `COM`

√6ᵗʰ **M06.24** Rheumatoid bursitis, hand

     M06.241 Rheumatoid bursitis, right hand `HCC` `Rx` `ESR` `COM`

     M06.242 Rheumatoid bursitis, left hand `HCC` `Rx` `ESR` `COM`

     M06.249 Rheumatoid bursitis, unspecified hand `HCC` `Rx` `ESR` `COM`

√6ᵗʰ **M06.25** Rheumatoid bursitis, hip

     M06.251 Rheumatoid bursitis, right hip `HCC` `Rx` `ESR` `COM`

     M06.252 Rheumatoid bursitis, left hip `HCC` `Rx` `ESR` `COM`

     M06.259 Rheumatoid bursitis, unspecified hip `HCC` `Rx` `ESR` `COM`

√6ᵗʰ **M06.26** Rheumatoid bursitis, knee

     M06.261 Rheumatoid bursitis, right knee `HCC` `Rx` `ESR` `COM`

     M06.262 Rheumatoid bursitis, left knee `HCC` `Rx` `ESR` `COM`

     M06.269 Rheumatoid bursitis, unspecified knee `HCC` `Rx` `ESR` `COM`

√6ᵗʰ **M06.27** Rheumatoid bursitis, ankle and foot

     M06.271 Rheumatoid bursitis, right ankle and foot `HCC` `Rx` `ESR` `COM`

     M06.272 Rheumatoid bursitis, left ankle and foot `HCC` `Rx` `ESR` `COM`

     M06.279 Rheumatoid bursitis, unspecified ankle and foot `HCC` `Rx` `ESR` `COM`

     M06.28 Rheumatoid bursitis, vertebrae `HCC` `Rx` `ESR` `COM`

     M06.29 Rheumatoid bursitis, multiple sites `HCC` `Rx` `ESR` `COM`

√5ᵗʰ **M06.3** Rheumatoid nodule

     M06.30 Rheumatoid nodule, unspecified site `HCC` `Rx` `ESR` `COM`

√6ᵗʰ **M06.31** Rheumatoid nodule, shoulder

     M06.311 Rheumatoid nodule, right shoulder `HCC` `Rx` `ESR` `COM`

     M06.312 Rheumatoid nodule, left shoulder `HCC` `Rx` `ESR` `COM`

     M06.319 Rheumatoid nodule, unspecified shoulder `HCC` `Rx` `ESR` `COM`

√6ᵗʰ **M06.32** Rheumatoid nodule, elbow

     M06.321 Rheumatoid nodule, right elbow `HCC` `Rx` `ESR` `COM`

     M06.322 Rheumatoid nodule, left elbow `HCC` `Rx` `ESR` `COM`

     M06.329 Rheumatoid nodule, unspecified elbow `HCC` `Rx` `ESR` `COM`

√6ᵗʰ **M06.33** Rheumatoid nodule, wrist

     M06.331 Rheumatoid nodule, right wrist `HCC` `Rx` `ESR` `COM`

     M06.332 Rheumatoid nodule, left wrist `HCC` `Rx` `ESR` `COM`

     M06.339 Rheumatoid nodule, unspecified wrist `HCC` `Rx` `ESR` `COM`

√6ᵗʰ **M06.34** Rheumatoid nodule, hand

     M06.341 Rheumatoid nodule, right hand `HCC` `Rx` `ESR` `COM`

     M06.342 Rheumatoid nodule, left hand `HCC` `Rx` `ESR` `COM`

     M06.349 Rheumatoid nodule, unspecified hand `HCC` `Rx` `ESR` `COM`

√6ᵗʰ **M06.35** Rheumatoid nodule, hip

     M06.351 Rheumatoid nodule, right hip `HCC` `Rx` `ESR` `COM`

     M06.352 Rheumatoid nodule, left hip `HCC` `Rx` `ESR` `COM`

     M06.359 Rheumatoid nodule, unspecified hip `HCC` `Rx` `ESR` `COM`

√6ᵗʰ **M06.36** Rheumatoid nodule, knee

     M06.361 Rheumatoid nodule, right knee `HCC` `Rx` `ESR` `COM`

     M06.362 Rheumatoid nodule, left knee `HCC` `Rx` `ESR` `COM`

☑ Additional Character Required   √x7ᵗʰ Placeholder Alert   Manifestation   Unspecified Dx   `Q` QPP   `UPD` Unacceptable PDx

        M06.369 Rheumatoid nodule, unspecified knee `HCC` `Rx` `ESR` `COM`

    ✓6ᵗʰ M06.37 **Rheumatoid nodule,** ankle and foot

        M06.371 **Rheumatoid nodule,** right ankle and foot

        M06.372 **Rheumatoid nodule,** left ankle and foot `HCC` `Rx` `ESR` `COM`

        M06.379 **Rheumatoid nodule,** unspecified ankle and foot `HCC` `Rx` `ESR` `COM`

    M06.38 **Rheumatoid nodule,** vertebrae `HCC` `Rx` `ESR` `COM`

    M06.39 **Rheumatoid nodule,** multiple sites `HCC` `Rx` `ESR` `COM`

  M06.4 **Inflammatory polyarthropathy**
    EXCLUDES 1   polyarthritis NOS (M13.0)

✓5ᵗʰ M06.8 **Other specified rheumatoid arthritis**

    M06.80 **Other specified rheumatoid arthritis, unspecified site** `HCC` `Rx` `ESR` `COM`

    ✓6ᵗʰ M06.81 **Other specified rheumatoid arthritis,** shoulder

        M06.811 **Other specified rheumatoid arthritis,** right shoulder `HCC` `Rx` `ESR` `COM`

        M06.812 **Other specified rheumatoid arthritis,** left shoulder `HCC` `Rx` `ESR` `COM`

        M06.819 **Other specified rheumatoid arthritis, unspecified shoulder** `HCC` `Rx` `ESR` `COM`

    ✓6ᵗʰ M06.82 **Other specified rheumatoid arthritis,** elbow

        M06.821 **Other specified rheumatoid arthritis,** right elbow `HCC` `Rx` `ESR` `COM`

        M06.822 **Other specified rheumatoid arthritis,** left elbow `HCC` `Rx` `ESR` `COM`

        M06.829 **Other specified rheumatoid arthritis, unspecified elbow**

    ✓6ᵗʰ M06.83 **Other specified rheumatoid arthritis,** wrist

        M06.831 **Other specified rheumatoid arthritis,** right wrist `HCC` `Rx` `ESR` `COM`

        M06.832 **Other specified rheumatoid arthritis,** left wrist `HCC` `Rx` `ESR` `COM`

        M06.839 **Other specified rheumatoid arthritis, unspecified wrist** `HCC` `Rx` `ESR` `COM`

    ✓6ᵗʰ M06.84 **Other specified rheumatoid arthritis,** hand

        M06.841 **Other specified rheumatoid arthritis,** right hand `HCC` `Rx` `ESR` `COM`

        M06.842 **Other specified rheumatoid arthritis,** left hand `HCC` `Rx` `ESR` `COM`

        M06.849 **Other specified rheumatoid arthritis, unspecified hand** `HCC` `Rx` `ESR` `COM`

    ✓6ᵗʰ M06.85 **Other specified rheumatoid arthritis,** hip

        M06.851 **Other specified rheumatoid arthritis,** right hip `HCC` `Rx` `ESR` `COM`

        M06.852 **Other specified rheumatoid arthritis,** left hip `HCC` `Rx` `ESR` `COM`

        M06.859 **Other specified rheumatoid arthritis, unspecified hip** `HCC` `Rx` `ESR` `COM`

    ✓6ᵗʰ M06.86 **Other specified rheumatoid arthritis,** knee

        M06.861 **Other specified rheumatoid arthritis,** right knee `HCC` `Rx` `ESR` `COM`

        M06.862 **Other specified rheumatoid arthritis,** left knee `HCC` `Rx` `ESR` `COM`

        M06.869 **Other specified rheumatoid arthritis, unspecified knee** `HCC` `Rx` `ESR` `COM`

    ✓6ᵗʰ M06.87 **Other specified rheumatoid arthritis,** ankle and foot

        M06.871 **Other specified rheumatoid arthritis,** right ankle and foot `HCC` `Rx` `ESR` `COM`

        M06.872 **Other specified rheumatoid arthritis,** left ankle and foot `HCC` `Rx` `ESR` `COM`

        M06.879 **Other specified rheumatoid arthritis, unspecified ankle and foot** `HCC` `Rx` `ESR` `COM`

    M06.88 **Other specified rheumatoid arthritis,** vertebrae `HCC` `Rx` `ESR` `COM`

    M06.89 **Other specified rheumatoid arthritis,** multiple sites `HCC` `Rx` `ESR` `COM`

    M06.8A **Other specified rheumatoid arthritis,** other specified site `HCC` `Rx` `ESR` `COM`

  M06.9 **Rheumatoid arthritis, unspecified** `HCC` `Rx` `ESR` `COM`

✓4ᵗʰ **M07 Enteropathic arthropathies**
    Code also associated enteropathy, such as:
      regional enteritis [Crohn's disease] (K50.-)
      ulcerative colitis (K51.-)
    EXCLUDES 1   psoriatic arthropathies (L40.5-)

   ✓5ᵗʰ M07.6 **Enteropathic arthropathies**

    M07.60 **Enteropathic arthropathies, unspecified site**

    ✓6ᵗʰ M07.61 **Enteropathic arthropathies,** shoulder

        M07.611 **Enteropathic arthropathies,** right shoulder

        M07.612 **Enteropathic arthropathies,** left shoulder

        M07.619 **Enteropathic arthropathies, unspecified shoulder**

    ✓6ᵗʰ M07.62 **Enteropathic arthropathies,** elbow

        M07.621 **Enteropathic arthropathies,** right elbow

        M07.622 **Enteropathic arthropathies,** left elbow

        M07.629 **Enteropathic arthropathies, unspecified elbow**

    ✓6ᵗʰ M07.63 **Enteropathic arthropathies,** wrist

        M07.631 **Enteropathic arthropathies,** right wrist

        M07.632 **Enteropathic arthropathies,** left wrist

        M07.639 **Enteropathic arthropathies, unspecified wrist**

    ✓6ᵗʰ M07.64 **Enteropathic arthropathies,** hand

        M07.641 **Enteropathic arthropathies,** right hand

        M07.642 **Enteropathic arthropathies,** left hand

        M07.649 **Enteropathic arthropathies, unspecified hand**

    ✓6ᵗʰ M07.65 **Enteropathic arthropathies,** hip

        M07.651 **Enteropathic arthropathies,** right hip

        M07.652 **Enteropathic arthropathies,** left hip

        M07.659 **Enteropathic arthropathies, unspecified hip**

    ✓6ᵗʰ M07.66 **Enteropathic arthropathies,** knee

        M07.661 **Enteropathic arthropathies,** right knee

        M07.662 **Enteropathic arthropathies,** left knee

        M07.669 **Enteropathic arthropathies, unspecified knee**

    ✓6ᵗʰ M07.67 **Enteropathic arthropathies,** ankle and foot

        M07.671 **Enteropathic arthropathies,** right ankle and foot

        M07.672 **Enteropathic arthropathies,** left ankle and foot

        M07.679 **Enteropathic arthropathies, unspecified ankle and foot**

    M07.68 **Enteropathic arthropathies,** vertebrae

    M07.69 **Enteropathic arthropathies,** multiple sites

✓4ᵗʰ **M08 Juvenile arthritis**
    Code also any associated underlying condition, such as:
      regional enteritis [Crohn's disease] (K50.-)
      ulcerative colitis (K51.-)
    EXCLUDES 1   arthropathy in Whipple's disease (M14.8)
                 Felty's syndrome (M05.0)
                 juvenile dermatomyositis (M33.0-)
                 psoriatic juvenile arthropathy (L40.54)
    AHA: 2020,4Q,31-32

   ✓5ᵗʰ M08.0 **Unspecified juvenile rheumatoid arthritis**
      Juvenile rheumatoid arthritis with or without rheumatoid factor

    M08.00 **Unspecified juvenile rheumatoid arthritis of unspecified site** `HCC` `Rx` `ESR` `COM`

    ✓6ᵗʰ M08.01 **Unspecified juvenile rheumatoid arthritis,** shoulder

        M08.011 **Unspecified juvenile rheumatoid arthritis,** right shoulder `HCC` `Rx` `ESR` `COM`

        M08.012 **Unspecified juvenile rheumatoid arthritis,** left shoulder `HCC` `Rx` `ESR` `COM`

        M08.019 **Unspecified juvenile rheumatoid arthritis, unspecified shoulder** `HCC` `Rx` `ESR` `COM`

    ✓6ᵗʰ M08.02 **Unspecified juvenile rheumatoid arthritis of** elbow

        M08.021 **Unspecified juvenile rheumatoid arthritis,** right elbow `HCC` `Rx` `ESR` `COM`

        M08.022 **Unspecified juvenile rheumatoid arthritis,** left elbow `HCC` `Rx` `ESR` `COM`

        M08.029 **Unspecified juvenile rheumatoid arthritis, unspecified elbow** `HCC` `Rx` `ESR` `COM`

`HCC` CMS-HCC   `Rx` Rx HCC   `ESR` ESRD HCC   `COM` Commercial HCC   `N` Newborn: 0   `P` Pediatric: 0-17   `M` Maternity: 9-64   `A` Adult: 15-124

788   ICD-10-CM 2023

✓6ᵗʰ **M08.03** Unspecified juvenile rheumatoid arthritis, wrist
- **M08.031** Unspecified juvenile rheumatoid arthritis, right wrist `HCC` `Rx` `ESR` `COM`
- **M08.032** Unspecified juvenile rheumatoid arthritis, left wrist `HCC` `Rx` `ESR` `COM`
- **M08.039** Unspecified juvenile rheumatoid arthritis, unspecified wrist `HCC` `Rx` `ESR` `COM`

✓6ᵗʰ **M08.04** Unspecified juvenile rheumatoid arthritis, hand
- **M08.041** Unspecified juvenile rheumatoid arthritis, right hand `HCC` `Rx` `ESR` `COM`
- **M08.042** Unspecified juvenile rheumatoid arthritis, left hand `HCC` `Rx` `ESR` `COM`
- **M08.049** Unspecified juvenile rheumatoid arthritis, unspecified hand `HCC` `Rx` `ESR` `COM`

✓6ᵗʰ **M08.05** Unspecified juvenile rheumatoid arthritis, hip
- **M08.051** Unspecified juvenile rheumatoid arthritis, right hip `HCC` `Rx` `ESR` `COM`
- **M08.052** Unspecified juvenile rheumatoid arthritis, left hip `HCC` `Rx` `ESR` `COM`
- **M08.059** Unspecified juvenile rheumatoid arthritis, unspecified hip `HCC` `Rx` `ESR` `COM`

✓6ᵗʰ **M08.06** Unspecified juvenile rheumatoid arthritis, knee
- **M08.061** Unspecified juvenile rheumatoid arthritis, right knee `HCC` `Rx` `ESR` `COM`
- **M08.062** Unspecified juvenile rheumatoid arthritis, left knee `HCC` `Rx` `ESR` `COM`
- **M08.069** Unspecified juvenile rheumatoid arthritis, unspecified knee `HCC` `Rx` `ESR` `COM`

✓6ᵗʰ **M08.07** Unspecified juvenile rheumatoid arthritis, ankle and foot
- **M08.071** Unspecified juvenile rheumatoid arthritis, right ankle and foot `HCC` `Rx` `ESR` `COM`
- **M08.072** Unspecified juvenile rheumatoid arthritis, left ankle and foot `HCC` `Rx` `ESR` `COM`
- **M08.079** Unspecified juvenile rheumatoid arthritis, unspecified ankle and foot `HCC` `Rx` `ESR` `COM`

M08.08 Unspecified juvenile rheumatoid arthritis, vertebrae `HCC` `Rx` `ESR` `COM`

M08.09 Unspecified juvenile rheumatoid arthritis, multiple sites `HCC` `Rx` `ESR` `COM`

M08.0A Unspecified juvenile rheumatoid arthritis, other specified site `HCC` `Rx` `ESR` `COM`

M08.1 Juvenile ankylosing spondylitis `HCC` `Rx` `ESR` `COM`
- EXCLUDES 1   ankylosing spondylitis in adults (M45.0-)

✓5ᵗʰ **M08.2** Juvenile rheumatoid arthritis with systemic onset
- Still's disease NOS
- EXCLUDES 1   adult-onset Still's disease (M06.1-)
- **DEF:** Systemic juvenile rheumatoid arthritis characterized by a transient rash and spiking fevers that may affect internal organs, as well as joints.
- **M08.20** Juvenile rheumatoid arthritis with systemic onset, unspecified site `HCC` `Rx` `ESR` `COM`

✓6ᵗʰ **M08.21** Juvenile rheumatoid arthritis with systemic onset, shoulder
- **M08.211** Juvenile rheumatoid arthritis with systemic onset, right shoulder `HCC` `Rx` `ESR` `COM`
- **M08.212** Juvenile rheumatoid arthritis with systemic onset, left shoulder `HCC` `Rx` `ESR` `COM`
- **M08.219** Juvenile rheumatoid arthritis with systemic onset, unspecified shoulder `HCC` `Rx` `ESR` `COM`

✓6ᵗʰ **M08.22** Juvenile rheumatoid arthritis with systemic onset, elbow
- **M08.221** Juvenile rheumatoid arthritis with systemic onset, right elbow `HCC` `Rx` `ESR` `COM`
- **M08.222** Juvenile rheumatoid arthritis with systemic onset, left elbow `HCC` `Rx` `ESR` `COM`
- **M08.229** Juvenile rheumatoid arthritis with systemic onset, unspecified elbow `HCC` `Rx` `ESR` `COM`

✓6ᵗʰ **M08.23** Juvenile rheumatoid arthritis with systemic onset, wrist
- **M08.231** Juvenile rheumatoid arthritis with systemic onset, right wrist `HCC` `Rx` `ESR` `COM`
- **M08.232** Juvenile rheumatoid arthritis with systemic onset, left wrist `HCC` `Rx` `ESR` `COM`
- **M08.239** Juvenile rheumatoid arthritis with systemic onset, unspecified wrist `HCC` `Rx` `ESR` `COM`

✓6ᵗʰ **M08.24** Juvenile rheumatoid arthritis with systemic onset, hand
- **M08.241** Juvenile rheumatoid arthritis with systemic onset, right hand `HCC` `Rx` `ESR` `COM`
- **M08.242** Juvenile rheumatoid arthritis with systemic onset, left hand `HCC` `Rx` `ESR` `COM`
- **M08.249** Juvenile rheumatoid arthritis with systemic onset, unspecified hand `HCC` `Rx` `ESR` `COM`

✓6ᵗʰ **M08.25** Juvenile rheumatoid arthritis with systemic onset, hip
- **M08.251** Juvenile rheumatoid arthritis with systemic onset, right hip `HCC` `Rx` `ESR` `COM`
- **M08.252** Juvenile rheumatoid arthritis with systemic onset, left hip `HCC` `Rx` `ESR` `COM`
- **M08.259** Juvenile rheumatoid arthritis with systemic onset, unspecified hip `HCC` `Rx` `ESR` `COM`

✓6ᵗʰ **M08.26** Juvenile rheumatoid arthritis with systemic onset, knee
- **M08.261** Juvenile rheumatoid arthritis with systemic onset, right knee `HCC` `Rx` `ESR` `COM`
- **M08.262** Juvenile rheumatoid arthritis with systemic onset, left knee `HCC` `Rx` `ESR` `COM`
- **M08.269** Juvenile rheumatoid arthritis with systemic onset, unspecified knee `HCC` `Rx` `ESR` `COM`

✓6ᵗʰ **M08.27** Juvenile rheumatoid arthritis with systemic onset, ankle and foot
- **M08.271** Juvenile rheumatoid arthritis with systemic onset, right ankle and foot `HCC` `Rx` `ESR` `COM`
- **M08.272** Juvenile rheumatoid arthritis with systemic onset, left ankle and foot `HCC` `Rx` `ESR` `COM`
- **M08.279** Juvenile rheumatoid arthritis with systemic onset, unspecified ankle and foot `HCC` `Rx` `ESR` `COM`

M08.28 Juvenile rheumatoid arthritis with systemic onset, vertebrae `HCC` `Rx` `ESR` `COM`

M08.29 Juvenile rheumatoid arthritis with systemic onset, multiple sites `HCC` `Rx` `ESR` `COM`

M08.2A Juvenile rheumatoid arthritis with systemic onset, other specified site `HCC` `Rx` `ESR` `COM`

M08.3 Juvenile rheumatoid polyarthritis (seronegative) `HCC` `Rx` `ESR` `COM`

✓5ᵗʰ **M08.4** Pauciarticular juvenile rheumatoid arthritis
- **M08.40** Pauciarticular juvenile rheumatoid arthritis, unspecified site `HCC` `Rx` `ESR` `COM`

✓6ᵗʰ **M08.41** Pauciarticular juvenile rheumatoid arthritis, shoulder
- **M08.411** Pauciarticular juvenile rheumatoid arthritis, right shoulder `HCC` `Rx` `ESR` `COM`
- **M08.412** Pauciarticular juvenile rheumatoid arthritis, left shoulder `HCC` `Rx` `ESR` `COM`
- **M08.419** Pauciarticular juvenile rheumatoid arthritis, unspecified shoulder `HCC` `Rx` `ESR` `COM`

✓6ᵗʰ **M08.42** Pauciarticular juvenile rheumatoid arthritis, elbow
- **M08.421** Pauciarticular juvenile rheumatoid arthritis, right elbow `HCC` `Rx` `ESR` `COM`
- **M08.422** Pauciarticular juvenile rheumatoid arthritis, left elbow `HCC` `Rx` `ESR` `COM`
- **M08.429** Pauciarticular juvenile rheumatoid arthritis, unspecified elbow `HCC` `Rx` `ESR` `COM`

✓6ᵗʰ **M08.43** Pauciarticular juvenile rheumatoid arthritis, wrist
- **M08.431** Pauciarticular juvenile rheumatoid arthritis, right wrist `HCC` `Rx` `ESR` `COM`

M08.432   Pauciarticular juvenile rheumatoid arthritis, left wrist   `HCC` `Rx` `ESR` `COM`

M08.439   Pauciarticular juvenile rheumatoid arthritis, unspecified wrist   `HCC` `Rx` `ESR` `COM`

√6ᵗʰ M08.44   Pauciarticular juvenile rheumatoid arthritis, hand

    M08.441   Pauciarticular juvenile rheumatoid arthritis, right hand   `HCC` `Rx` `ESR` `COM`

    M08.442   Pauciarticular juvenile rheumatoid arthritis, left hand   `HCC` `Rx` `ESR` `COM`

    M08.449   Pauciarticular juvenile rheumatoid arthritis, unspecified hand   `HCC` `Rx` `ESR` `COM`

√6ᵗʰ M08.45   Pauciarticular juvenile rheumatoid arthritis, hip

    M08.451   Pauciarticular juvenile rheumatoid arthritis, right hip   `HCC` `Rx` `ESR` `COM`

    M08.452   Pauciarticular juvenile rheumatoid arthritis, left hip   `HCC` `Rx` `ESR` `COM`

    M08.459   Pauciarticular juvenile rheumatoid arthritis, unspecified hip   `HCC` `Rx` `ESR` `COM`

√6ᵗʰ M08.46   Pauciarticular juvenile rheumatoid arthritis, knee

    M08.461   Pauciarticular juvenile rheumatoid arthritis, right knee   `HCC` `Rx` `ESR` `COM`

    M08.462   Pauciarticular juvenile rheumatoid arthritis, left knee   `HCC` `Rx` `ESR` `COM`

    M08.469   Pauciarticular juvenile rheumatoid arthritis, unspecified knee   `HCC` `Rx` `ESR` `COM`

√6ᵗʰ M08.47   Pauciarticular juvenile rheumatoid arthritis, ankle and foot

    M08.471   Pauciarticular juvenile rheumatoid arthritis, right ankle and foot   `HCC` `Rx` `ESR` `COM`

    M08.472   Pauciarticular juvenile rheumatoid arthritis, left ankle and foot   `HCC` `Rx` `ESR` `COM`

    M08.479   Pauciarticular juvenile rheumatoid arthritis, unspecified ankle and foot   `HCC` `Rx` `ESR` `COM`

    M08.48   Pauciarticular juvenile rheumatoid arthritis, vertebrae   `HCC` `Rx` `ESR` `COM`

    M08.4A   Pauciarticular juvenile rheumatoid arthritis, other specified site   `HCC` `Rx` `ESR` `COM`

√5ᵗʰ M08.8   Other juvenile arthritis

    M08.80   Other juvenile arthritis, unspecified site   `HCC` `Rx` `ESR` `COM`

√6ᵗʰ M08.81   Other juvenile arthritis, shoulder

    M08.811   Other juvenile arthritis, right shoulder   `HCC` `Rx` `ESR` `COM`

    M08.812   Other juvenile arthritis, left shoulder   `HCC` `Rx` `ESR` `COM`

    M08.819   Other juvenile arthritis, unspecified shoulder   `HCC` `Rx` `ESR` `COM`

√6ᵗʰ M08.82   Other juvenile arthritis, elbow

    M08.821   Other juvenile arthritis, right elbow   `HCC` `Rx` `ESR` `COM`

    M08.822   Other juvenile arthritis, left elbow   `HCC` `Rx` `ESR` `COM`

    M08.829   Other juvenile arthritis, unspecified elbow   `HCC` `Rx` `ESR` `COM`

√6ᵗʰ M08.83   Other juvenile arthritis, wrist

    M08.831   Other juvenile arthritis, right wrist   `HCC` `Rx` `ESR` `COM`

    M08.832   Other juvenile arthritis, left wrist   `HCC` `Rx` `ESR` `COM`

    M08.839   Other juvenile arthritis, unspecified wrist   `HCC` `Rx` `ESR` `COM`

√6ᵗʰ M08.84   Other juvenile arthritis, hand

    M08.841   Other juvenile arthritis, right hand   `HCC` `Rx` `ESR` `COM`

    M08.842   Other juvenile arthritis, left hand   `HCC` `Rx` `ESR` `COM`

    M08.849   Other juvenile arthritis, unspecified hand   `HCC` `Rx` `ESR` `COM`

√6ᵗʰ M08.85   Other juvenile arthritis, hip

    M08.851   Other juvenile arthritis, right hip   `HCC` `Rx` `ESR` `COM`

    M08.852   Other juvenile arthritis, left hip   `HCC` `Rx` `ESR` `COM`

    M08.859   Other juvenile arthritis, unspecified hip   `HCC` `Rx` `ESR` `COM`

√6ᵗʰ M08.86   Other juvenile arthritis, knee

    M08.861   Other juvenile arthritis, right knee   `HCC` `Rx` `ESR` `COM`

    M08.862   Other juvenile arthritis, left knee   `HCC` `Rx` `ESR` `COM`

    M08.869   Other juvenile arthritis, unspecified knee   `HCC` `Rx` `ESR` `COM`

√6ᵗʰ M08.87   Other juvenile arthritis, ankle and foot

    M08.871   Other juvenile arthritis, right ankle and foot   `HCC` `Rx` `ESR` `COM`

    M08.872   Other juvenile arthritis, left ankle and foot   `HCC` `Rx` `ESR` `COM`

    M08.879   Other juvenile arthritis, unspecified ankle and foot   `HCC` `Rx` `ESR` `COM`

    M08.88   Other juvenile arthritis, other specified site

       Other juvenile arthritis, vertebrae

    M08.89   Other juvenile arthritis, multiple sites   `HCC` `Rx` `ESR` `COM`

√5ᵗʰ M08.9   Juvenile arthritis, unspecified

    EXCLUDES 1   *juvenile rheumatoid arthritis, unspecified (M08.0-)*

    M08.90   Juvenile arthritis, unspecified, unspecified site   `HCC` `Rx` `ESR` `COM`

√6ᵗʰ M08.91   Juvenile arthritis, unspecified, shoulder

    M08.911   Juvenile arthritis, unspecified, right shoulder   `HCC` `Rx` `ESR` `COM`

    M08.912   Juvenile arthritis, unspecified, left shoulder   `HCC` `Rx` `ESR` `COM`

    M08.919   Juvenile arthritis, unspecified, unspecified shoulder   `HCC` `Rx` `ESR` `COM`

√6ᵗʰ M08.92   Juvenile arthritis, unspecified, elbow

    M08.921   Juvenile arthritis, unspecified, right elbow   `HCC` `Rx` `ESR` `COM`

    M08.922   Juvenile arthritis, unspecified, left elbow   `HCC` `Rx` `ESR` `COM`

    M08.929   Juvenile arthritis, unspecified, unspecified elbow   `HCC` `Rx` `ESR` `COM`

√6ᵗʰ M08.93   Juvenile arthritis, unspecified, wrist

    M08.931   Juvenile arthritis, unspecified, right wrist   `HCC` `Rx` `ESR` `COM`

    M08.932   Juvenile arthritis, unspecified, left wrist   `HCC` `Rx` `ESR` `COM`

    M08.939   Juvenile arthritis, unspecified, unspecified wrist   `HCC` `Rx` `ESR` `COM`

√6ᵗʰ M08.94   Juvenile arthritis, unspecified, hand

    M08.941   Juvenile arthritis, unspecified, right hand   `HCC` `Rx` `ESR` `COM`

    M08.942   Juvenile arthritis, unspecified, left hand   `HCC` `Rx` `ESR` `COM`

    M08.949   Juvenile arthritis, unspecified, unspecified hand   `HCC` `Rx` `ESR` `COM`

√6ᵗʰ M08.95   Juvenile arthritis, unspecified, hip

    M08.951   Juvenile arthritis, unspecified, right hip   `HCC` `Rx` `ESR` `COM`

    M08.952   Juvenile arthritis, unspecified, left hip   `HCC` `Rx` `ESR` `COM`

    M08.959   Juvenile arthritis, unspecified, unspecified hip   `HCC` `Rx` `ESR` `COM`

√6ᵗʰ M08.96   Juvenile arthritis, unspecified, knee

    M08.961   Juvenile arthritis, unspecified, right knee   `HCC` `Rx` `ESR` `COM`

    M08.962   Juvenile arthritis, unspecified, left knee   `HCC` `Rx` `ESR` `COM`

    M08.969   Juvenile arthritis, unspecified, unspecified knee   `HCC` `Rx` `ESR` `COM`

√6ᵗʰ M08.97   Juvenile arthritis, unspecified, ankle and foot

    M08.971   Juvenile arthritis, unspecified, right ankle and foot   `HCC` `Rx` `ESR` `COM`

    M08.972   Juvenile arthritis, unspecified, left ankle and foot   `HCC` `Rx` `ESR` `COM`

    M08.979   Juvenile arthritis, unspecified, unspecified ankle and foot   `HCC` `Rx` `ESR` `COM`

`HCC` CMS-HCC   `Rx` Rx HCC   `ESR` ESRD HCC   `COM` Commercial HCC   N Newborn: 0   P Pediatric: 0-17   M Maternity: 9-64   A Adult: 15-124

790   ICD-10-CM 2023

      M08.98   Juvenile arthritis, unspecified, vertebrae   `HCC` `Rx` `ESR` `COM`

      M08.99   Juvenile arthritis, unspecified, multiple sites   `HCC` `Rx` `ESR` `COM`

      M08.9A   Juvenile arthritis, unspecified, other specified site   `HCC` `Rx` `ESR` `COM`

√4ᵗʰ M1A   **Chronic gout**

     Use additional code to identify:

       autonomic neuropathy in diseases classified elsewhere (G99.Ø)

       calculus of urinary tract in diseases classified elsewhere (N22)

       cardiomyopathy in diseases classified elsewhere (I43)

       disorders of external ear in diseases classified elsewhere (H61.1-, H62.8-)

       disorders of iris and ciliary body in diseases classified elsewhere (H22)

       glomerular disorders in diseases classified elsewhere (NØ8)

     EXCLUDES 1   *gout NOS (M1Ø.-)*

     EXCLUDES 2   *acute gout (M1Ø.-)*

> The appropriate 7th character is to be added to each code from category M1A.
> Ø   without tophus (tophi)
> 1   with tophus (tophi)

√6ᵗʰ M1A.Ø   Idiopathic chronic gout

     Chronic gouty bursitis

     Primary chronic gout

     √x7ᵗʰ M1A.ØØ   Idiopathic chronic gout, unspecified site

     √6ᵗʰ M1A.Ø1   Idiopathic chronic gout, shoulder

         √7ᵗʰ M1A.Ø11   Idiopathic chronic gout, right shoulder

         √7ᵗʰ M1A.Ø12   Idiopathic chronic gout, left shoulder

         √7ᵗʰ M1A.Ø19   Idiopathic chronic gout, unspecified shoulder

     √6ᵗʰ M1A.Ø2   Idiopathic chronic gout, elbow

         √7ᵗʰ M1A.Ø21   Idiopathic chronic gout, right elbow

         √7ᵗʰ M1A.Ø22   Idiopathic chronic gout, left elbow

         √7ᵗʰ M1A.Ø29   Idiopathic chronic gout, unspecified elbow

     √6ᵗʰ M1A.Ø3   Idiopathic chronic gout, wrist

         √7ᵗʰ M1A.Ø31   Idiopathic chronic gout, right wrist

         √7ᵗʰ M1A.Ø32   Idiopathic chronic gout, left wrist

         √7ᵗʰ M1A.Ø39   Idiopathic chronic gout, unspecified wrist

     √6ᵗʰ M1A.Ø4   Idiopathic chronic gout, hand

         √7ᵗʰ M1A.Ø41   Idiopathic chronic gout, right hand

         √7ᵗʰ M1A.Ø42   Idiopathic chronic gout, left hand

         √7ᵗʰ M1A.Ø49   Idiopathic chronic gout, unspecified hand

     √6ᵗʰ M1A.Ø5   Idiopathic chronic gout, hip

         √7ᵗʰ M1A.Ø51   Idiopathic chronic gout, right hip

         √7ᵗʰ M1A.Ø52   Idiopathic chronic gout, left hip

         √7ᵗʰ M1A.Ø59   Idiopathic chronic gout, unspecified hip

     √6ᵗʰ M1A.Ø6   Idiopathic chronic gout, knee

         √7ᵗʰ M1A.Ø61   Idiopathic chronic gout, right knee

         √7ᵗʰ M1A.Ø62   Idiopathic chronic gout, left knee

         √7ᵗʰ M1A.Ø69   Idiopathic chronic gout, unspecified knee

     √6ᵗʰ M1A.Ø7   Idiopathic chronic gout, ankle and foot

         √7ᵗʰ M1A.Ø71   Idiopathic chronic gout, right ankle and foot

         √7ᵗʰ M1A.Ø72   Idiopathic chronic gout, left ankle and foot

         √7ᵗʰ M1A.Ø79   Idiopathic chronic gout, unspecified ankle and foot

     √x7ᵗʰ M1A.Ø8   Idiopathic chronic gout, vertebrae

     √x7ᵗʰ M1A.Ø9   Idiopathic chronic gout, multiple sites

√5ᵗʰ M1A.1   Lead-induced chronic gout

     Code first toxic effects of lead and its compounds (T56.Ø-)

     √x7ᵗʰ M1A.1Ø   Lead-induced chronic gout, unspecified site

     √6ᵗʰ M1A.11   Lead-induced chronic gout, shoulder

         √7ᵗʰ M1A.111   Lead-induced chronic gout, right shoulder

         √7ᵗʰ M1A.112   Lead-induced chronic gout, left shoulder

         √7ᵗʰ M1A.119   Lead-induced chronic gout, unspecified shoulder

     √6ᵗʰ M1A.12   Lead-induced chronic gout, elbow

         √7ᵗʰ M1A.121   Lead-induced chronic gout, right elbow

         √7ᵗʰ M1A.122   Lead-induced chronic gout, left elbow

         √7ᵗʰ M1A.129   Lead-induced chronic gout, unspecified elbow

     √6ᵗʰ M1A.13   Lead-induced chronic gout, wrist

         √7ᵗʰ M1A.131   Lead-induced chronic gout, right wrist

         √7ᵗʰ M1A.132   Lead-induced chronic gout, left wrist

         √7ᵗʰ M1A.139   Lead-induced chronic gout, unspecified wrist

     √6ᵗʰ M1A.14   Lead-induced chronic gout, hand

         √7ᵗʰ M1A.141   Lead-induced chronic gout, right hand

         √7ᵗʰ M1A.142   Lead-induced chronic gout, left hand

         √7ᵗʰ M1A.149   Lead-induced chronic gout, unspecified hand

     √6ᵗʰ M1A.15   Lead-induced chronic gout, hip

         √7ᵗʰ M1A.151   Lead-induced chronic gout, right hip

         √7ᵗʰ M1A.152   Lead-induced chronic gout, left hip

         √7ᵗʰ M1A.159   Lead-induced chronic gout, unspecified hip

     √6ᵗʰ M1A.16   Lead-induced chronic gout, knee

         √7ᵗʰ M1A.161   Lead-induced chronic gout, right knee

         √7ᵗʰ M1A.162   Lead-induced chronic gout, left knee

         √7ᵗʰ M1A.169   Lead-induced chronic gout, unspecified knee

     √6ᵗʰ M1A.17   Lead-induced chronic gout, ankle and foot

         √7ᵗʰ M1A.171   Lead-induced chronic gout, right ankle and foot

         √7ᵗʰ M1A.172   Lead-induced chronic gout, left ankle and foot

         √7ᵗʰ M1A.179   Lead-induced chronic gout, unspecified ankle and foot

     √x7ᵗʰ M1A.18   Lead-induced chronic gout, vertebrae

     √x7ᵗʰ M1A.19   Lead-induced chronic gout, multiple sites

√5ᵗʰ M1A.2   Drug-induced chronic gout

     Use additional code for adverse effect, if applicable, to identify drug (T36-T5Ø with fifth or sixth character 5)

     √x7ᵗʰ M1A.2Ø   Drug-induced chronic gout, unspecified site

     √6ᵗʰ M1A.21   Drug-induced chronic gout, shoulder

         √7ᵗʰ M1A.211   Drug-induced chronic gout, right shoulder

         √7ᵗʰ M1A.212   Drug-induced chronic gout, left shoulder

         √7ᵗʰ M1A.219   Drug-induced chronic gout, unspecified shoulder

     √6ᵗʰ M1A.22   Drug-induced chronic gout, elbow

         √7ᵗʰ M1A.221   Drug-induced chronic gout, right elbow

         √7ᵗʰ M1A.222   Drug-induced chronic gout, left elbow

         √7ᵗʰ M1A.229   Drug-induced chronic gout, unspecified elbow

     √6ᵗʰ M1A.23   Drug-induced chronic gout, wrist

         √7ᵗʰ M1A.231   Drug-induced chronic gout, right wrist

         √7ᵗʰ M1A.232   Drug-induced chronic gout, left wrist

         √7ᵗʰ M1A.239   Drug-induced chronic gout, unspecified wrist

     √6ᵗʰ M1A.24   Drug-induced chronic gout, hand

         √7ᵗʰ M1A.241   Drug-induced chronic gout, right hand

         √7ᵗʰ M1A.242   Drug-induced chronic gout, left hand

         √7ᵗʰ M1A.249   Drug-induced chronic gout, unspecified hand

     √6ᵗʰ M1A.25   Drug-induced chronic gout, hip

         √7ᵗʰ M1A.251   Drug-induced chronic gout, right hip

         √7ᵗʰ M1A.252   Drug-induced chronic gout, left hip

         √7ᵗʰ M1A.259   Drug-induced chronic gout, unspecified hip

     √6ᵗʰ M1A.26   Drug-induced chronic gout, knee

         √7ᵗʰ M1A.261   Drug-induced chronic gout, right knee

         √7ᵗʰ M1A.262   Drug-induced chronic gout, left knee

         √7ᵗʰ M1A.269   Drug-induced chronic gout, unspecified knee

     √6ᵗʰ M1A.27   Drug-induced chronic gout, ankle and foot

         √7ᵗʰ M1A.271   Drug-induced chronic gout, right ankle and foot

         √7ᵗʰ M1A.272   Drug-induced chronic gout, left ankle and foot

✓7ᵗʰ **M1A.279** Drug-induced chronic gout, unspecified ankle and foot

✓x 7ᵗʰ **M1A.28** Drug-induced chronic gout, vertebrae

✓x 7ᵗʰ **M1A.29** Drug-induced chronic gout, multiple sites

✓5ᵗʰ **M1A.3** Chronic gout due to renal impairment
Code first associated renal disease

✓x 7ᵗʰ **M1A.30** Chronic gout due to renal impairment, unspecified site

✓6ᵗʰ **M1A.31** Chronic gout due to renal impairment, shoulder

✓7ᵗʰ **M1A.311** Chronic gout due to renal impairment, right shoulder

✓7ᵗʰ **M1A.312** Chronic gout due to renal impairment, left shoulder

✓7ᵗʰ **M1A.319** Chronic gout due to renal impairment, unspecified shoulder

✓6ᵗʰ **M1A.32** Chronic gout due to renal impairment, elbow

✓7ᵗʰ **M1A.321** Chronic gout due to renal impairment, right elbow

✓7ᵗʰ **M1A.322** Chronic gout due to renal impairment, left elbow

✓7ᵗʰ **M1A.329** Chronic gout due to renal impairment, unspecified elbow

✓6ᵗʰ **M1A.33** Chronic gout due to renal impairment, wrist

✓7ᵗʰ **M1A.331** Chronic gout due to renal impairment, right wrist

✓7ᵗʰ **M1A.332** Chronic gout due to renal impairment, left wrist

✓7ᵗʰ **M1A.339** Chronic gout due to renal impairment, unspecified wrist

✓6ᵗʰ **M1A.34** Chronic gout due to renal impairment, hand

✓7ᵗʰ **M1A.341** Chronic gout due to renal impairment, right hand

✓7ᵗʰ **M1A.342** Chronic gout due to renal impairment, left hand

✓7ᵗʰ **M1A.349** Chronic gout due to renal impairment, unspecified hand

✓6ᵗʰ **M1A.35** Chronic gout due to renal impairment, hip

✓7ᵗʰ **M1A.351** Chronic gout due to renal impairment, right hip

✓7ᵗʰ **M1A.352** Chronic gout due to renal impairment, left hip

✓7ᵗʰ **M1A.359** Chronic gout due to renal impairment, unspecified hip

✓6ᵗʰ **M1A.36** Chronic gout due to renal impairment, knee

✓7ᵗʰ **M1A.361** Chronic gout due to renal impairment, right knee

✓7ᵗʰ **M1A.362** Chronic gout due to renal impairment, left knee

✓7ᵗʰ **M1A.369** Chronic gout due to renal impairment, unspecified knee

✓6ᵗʰ **M1A.37** Chronic gout due to renal impairment, ankle and foot

✓7ᵗʰ **M1A.371** Chronic gout due to renal impairment, right ankle and foot

✓7ᵗʰ **M1A.372** Chronic gout due to renal impairment, left ankle and foot

✓7ᵗʰ **M1A.379** Chronic gout due to renal impairment, unspecified ankle and foot

✓x 7ᵗʰ **M1A.38** Chronic gout due to renal impairment, vertebrae

✓x 7ᵗʰ **M1A.39** Chronic gout due to renal impairment, multiple sites

✓5ᵗʰ **M1A.4** Other secondary chronic gout
Code first associated condition

✓x 7ᵗʰ **M1A.40** Other secondary chronic gout, unspecified site

✓6ᵗʰ **M1A.41** Other secondary chronic gout, shoulder

✓7ᵗʰ **M1A.411** Other secondary chronic gout, right shoulder

✓7ᵗʰ **M1A.412** Other secondary chronic gout, left shoulder

✓7ᵗʰ **M1A.419** Other secondary chronic gout, unspecified shoulder

✓6ᵗʰ **M1A.42** Other secondary chronic gout, elbow

✓7ᵗʰ **M1A.421** Other secondary chronic gout, right elbow

✓7ᵗʰ **M1A.422** Other secondary chronic gout, left elbow

✓7ᵗʰ **M1A.429** Other secondary chronic gout, unspecified elbow

✓6ᵗʰ **M1A.43** Other secondary chronic gout, wrist

✓7ᵗʰ **M1A.431** Other secondary chronic gout, right wrist

✓7ᵗʰ **M1A.432** Other secondary chronic gout, left wrist

✓7ᵗʰ **M1A.439** Other secondary chronic gout, unspecified wrist

✓6ᵗʰ **M1A.44** Other secondary chronic gout, hand

✓7ᵗʰ **M1A.441** Other secondary chronic gout, right hand

✓7ᵗʰ **M1A.442** Other secondary chronic gout, left hand

✓7ᵗʰ **M1A.449** Other secondary chronic gout, unspecified hand

✓6ᵗʰ **M1A.45** Other secondary chronic gout, hip

✓7ᵗʰ **M1A.451** Other secondary chronic gout, right hip

✓7ᵗʰ **M1A.452** Other secondary chronic gout, left hip

✓7ᵗʰ **M1A.459** Other secondary chronic gout, unspecified hip

✓6ᵗʰ **M1A.46** Other secondary chronic gout, knee

✓7ᵗʰ **M1A.461** Other secondary chronic gout, right knee

✓7ᵗʰ **M1A.462** Other secondary chronic gout, left knee

✓7ᵗʰ **M1A.469** Other secondary chronic gout, unspecified knee

✓6ᵗʰ **M1A.47** Other secondary chronic gout, ankle and foot

✓7ᵗʰ **M1A.471** Other secondary chronic gout, right ankle and foot

✓7ᵗʰ **M1A.472** Other secondary chronic gout, left ankle and foot

✓7ᵗʰ **M1A.479** Other secondary chronic gout, unspecified ankle and foot

✓x 7ᵗʰ **M1A.48** Other secondary chronic gout, vertebrae

✓x 7ᵗʰ **M1A.49** Other secondary chronic gout, multiple sites

✓x 7ᵗʰ **M1A.9** Chronic gout, unspecified

✓4ᵗʰ **M10** Gout
Acute gout
Gout attack
Gout flare
Podagra
Use additional code to identify:
autonomic neuropathy in diseases classified elsewhere (G99.0)
calculus of urinary tract in diseases classified elsewhere (N22)
cardiomyopathy in diseases classified elsewhere (I43)
disorders of external ear in diseases classified elsewhere (H61.1-, H62.8-)
disorders of iris and ciliary body in diseases classified elsewhere (H22)
glomerular disorders in diseases classified elsewhere (N08)
EXCLUDES 2   chronic gout (M1A.-)
DEF: Purine and pyrimidine metabolic disorders, manifested by hyperuricemia and recurrent acute inflammatory arthritis. Monosodium urate or monohydrate crystals may be deposited in and around the joints, leading to joint destruction and severe crippling.

✓5ᵗʰ **M10.0** Idiopathic gout
Gouty bursitis
Primary gout

M10.00 Idiopathic gout, unspecified site

✓6ᵗʰ **M10.01** Idiopathic gout, shoulder

M10.011 Idiopathic gout, right shoulder
M10.012 Idiopathic gout, left shoulder
M10.019 Idiopathic gout, unspecified shoulder

✓6ᵗʰ **M10.02** Idiopathic gout, elbow

M10.021 Idiopathic gout, right elbow
M10.022 Idiopathic gout, left elbow
M10.029 Idiopathic gout, unspecified elbow

✓6ᵗʰ **M10.03** Idiopathic gout, wrist

M10.031 Idiopathic gout, right wrist
M10.032 Idiopathic gout, left wrist
M10.039 Idiopathic gout, unspecified wrist

✓6ᵗʰ **M10.04** Idiopathic gout, hand

M10.041 Idiopathic gout, right hand
M10.042 Idiopathic gout, left hand
M10.049 Idiopathic gout, unspecified hand

✓6ᵗʰ **M10.05** Idiopathic gout, hip

M10.051 Idiopathic gout, right hip
M10.052 Idiopathic gout, left hip
M10.059 Idiopathic gout, unspecified hip

✓6ᵗʰ **M10.06** Idiopathic gout, knee

M10.061 Idiopathic gout, right knee

M10.062 Idiopathic gout, left knee
M10.069 Idiopathic gout, unspecified knee
√6th M10.07 Idiopathic gout, ankle and foot
M10.071 Idiopathic gout, right ankle and foot
M10.072 Idiopathic gout, left ankle and foot
M10.079 Idiopathic gout, unspecified ankle and foot
M10.08 Idiopathic gout, vertebrae
M10.09 Idiopathic gout, multiple sites
√5th M10.1 Lead-induced gout
Code first toxic effects of lead and its compounds (T56.0-)
M10.10 Lead-induced gout, unspecified site
√6th M10.11 Lead-induced gout, shoulder
M10.111 Lead-induced gout, right shoulder
M10.112 Lead-induced gout, left shoulder
M10.119 Lead-induced gout, unspecified shoulder
√6th M10.12 Lead-induced gout, elbow
M10.121 Lead-induced gout, right elbow
M10.122 Lead-induced gout, left elbow
M10.129 Lead-induced gout, unspecified elbow
√6th M10.13 Lead-induced gout, wrist
M10.131 Lead-induced gout, right wrist
M10.132 Lead-induced gout, left wrist
M10.139 Lead-induced gout, unspecified wrist
√6th M10.14 Lead-induced gout, hand
M10.141 Lead-induced gout, right hand
M10.142 Lead-induced gout, left hand
M10.149 Lead-induced gout, unspecified hand
√6th M10.15 Lead-induced gout, hip
M10.151 Lead-induced gout, right hip
M10.152 Lead-induced gout, left hip
M10.159 Lead-induced gout, unspecified hip
√6th M10.16 Lead-induced gout, knee
M10.161 Lead-induced gout, right knee
M10.162 Lead-induced gout, left knee
M10.169 Lead-induced gout, unspecified knee
√6th M10.17 Lead-induced gout, ankle and foot
M10.171 Lead-induced gout, right ankle and foot
M10.172 Lead-induced gout, left ankle and foot
M10.179 Lead-induced gout, unspecified ankle and foot
M10.18 Lead-induced gout, vertebrae
M10.19 Lead-induced gout, multiple sites
√6th M10.2 Drug-induced gout
Use additional code for adverse effect, if applicable, to identify drug (T36-T50 with fifth or sixth character 5)
M10.20 Drug-induced gout, unspecified site
√6th M10.21 Drug-induced gout, shoulder
M10.211 Drug-induced gout, right shoulder
M10.212 Drug-induced gout, left shoulder
M10.219 Drug-induced gout, unspecified shoulder
√6th M10.22 Drug-induced gout, elbow
M10.221 Drug-induced gout, right elbow
M10.222 Drug-induced gout, left elbow
M10.229 Drug-induced gout, unspecified elbow
√6th M10.23 Drug-induced gout, wrist
M10.231 Drug-induced gout, right wrist
M10.232 Drug-induced gout, left wrist
M10.239 Drug-induced gout, unspecified wrist
√6th M10.24 Drug-induced gout, hand
M10.241 Drug-induced gout, right hand
M10.242 Drug-induced gout, left hand
M10.249 Drug-induced gout, unspecified hand
√6th M10.25 Drug-induced gout, hip
M10.251 Drug-induced gout, right hip
M10.252 Drug-induced gout, left hip
M10.259 Drug-induced gout, unspecified hip
√6th M10.26 Drug-induced gout, knee
M10.261 Drug-induced gout, right knee
M10.262 Drug-induced gout, left knee
M10.269 Drug-induced gout, unspecified knee
√6th M10.27 Drug-induced gout, ankle and foot
M10.271 Drug-induced gout, right ankle and foot
M10.272 Drug-induced gout, left ankle and foot

M10.279 Drug-induced gout, unspecified ankle and foot
M10.28 Drug-induced gout, vertebrae
M10.29 Drug-induced gout, multiple sites
√5th M10.3 Gout due to renal impairment
Code first associated renal disease
M10.30 Gout due to renal impairment, unspecified site
√6th M10.31 Gout due to renal impairment, shoulder
M10.311 Gout due to renal impairment, right shoulder
M10.312 Gout due to renal impairment, left shoulder
M10.319 Gout due to renal impairment, unspecified shoulder
√6th M10.32 Gout due to renal impairment, elbow
M10.321 Gout due to renal impairment, right elbow
M10.322 Gout due to renal impairment, left elbow
M10.329 Gout due to renal impairment, unspecified elbow
√6th M10.33 Gout due to renal impairment, wrist
M10.331 Gout due to renal impairment, right wrist
M10.332 Gout due to renal impairment, left wrist
M10.339 Gout due to renal impairment, unspecified wrist
√6th M10.34 Gout due to renal impairment, hand
M10.341 Gout due to renal impairment, right hand
M10.342 Gout due to renal impairment, left hand
M10.349 Gout due to renal impairment, unspecified hand
√6th M10.35 Gout due to renal impairment, hip
M10.351 Gout due to renal impairment, right hip
M10.352 Gout due to renal impairment, left hip
M10.359 Gout due to renal impairment, unspecified hip
√6th M10.36 Gout due to renal impairment, knee
M10.361 Gout due to renal impairment, right knee
M10.362 Gout due to renal impairment, left knee
M10.369 Gout due to renal impairment, unspecified knee
√6th M10.37 Gout due to renal impairment, ankle and foot
M10.371 Gout due to renal impairment, right ankle and foot
M10.372 Gout due to renal impairment, left ankle and foot
M10.379 Gout due to renal impairment, unspecified ankle and foot
M10.38 Gout due to renal impairment, vertebrae
M10.39 Gout due to renal impairment, multiple sites
√5th M10.4 Other secondary gout
Code first associated condition
M10.40 Other secondary gout, unspecified site
√6th M10.41 Other secondary gout, shoulder
M10.411 Other secondary gout, right shoulder
M10.412 Other secondary gout, left shoulder
M10.419 Other secondary gout, unspecified shoulder
√6th M10.42 Other secondary gout, elbow
M10.421 Other secondary gout, right elbow
M10.422 Other secondary gout, left elbow
M10.429 Other secondary gout, unspecified elbow
√6th M10.43 Other secondary gout, wrist
M10.431 Other secondary gout, right wrist
M10.432 Other secondary gout, left wrist
M10.439 Other secondary gout, unspecified wrist
√6th M10.44 Other secondary gout, hand
M10.441 Other secondary gout, right hand
M10.442 Other secondary gout, left hand
M10.449 Other secondary gout, unspecified hand
√6th M10.45 Other secondary gout, hip
M10.451 Other secondary gout, right hip
M10.452 Other secondary gout, left hip
M10.459 Other secondary gout, unspecified hip
√6th M10.46 Other secondary gout, knee
M10.461 Other secondary gout, right knee
M10.462 Other secondary gout, left knee
M10.469 Other secondary gout, unspecified knee

√6ᵗʰ **M10.47** Other secondary gout, ankle and foot

     M10.471 Other secondary gout, right ankle and foot

     M10.472 Other secondary gout, left ankle and foot

     M10.479 Other secondary gout, unspecified ankle and foot

   M10.48 Other secondary gout, vertebrae

   M10.49 Other secondary gout, multiple sites

M10.9 Gout, unspecified
     Gout NOS

√4ᵗʰ **M11** Other crystal arthropathies

√5ᵗʰ **M11.0** Hydroxyapatite deposition disease

     DEF: Disease caused by deposits of calcium phosphate crystals in the soft tissues close to the joint (especially tendons) or in the joints. These calcifications can be mono or polyarticular and can cause destruction of the joint involved.

   M11.00 Hydroxyapatite deposition disease, unspecified site

√6ᵗʰ **M11.01** Hydroxyapatite deposition disease, shoulder

     M11.011 Hydroxyapatite deposition disease, right shoulder

     M11.012 Hydroxyapatite deposition disease, left shoulder

     M11.019 Hydroxyapatite deposition disease, unspecified shoulder

√6ᵗʰ **M11.02** Hydroxyapatite deposition disease, elbow

     M11.021 Hydroxyapatite deposition disease, right elbow

     M11.022 Hydroxyapatite deposition disease, left elbow

     M11.029 Hydroxyapatite deposition disease, unspecified elbow

√6ᵗʰ **M11.03** Hydroxyapatite deposition disease, wrist

     M11.031 Hydroxyapatite deposition disease, right wrist

     M11.032 Hydroxyapatite deposition disease, left wrist

     M11.039 Hydroxyapatite deposition disease, unspecified wrist

√6ᵗʰ **M11.04** Hydroxyapatite deposition disease, hand

     M11.041 Hydroxyapatite deposition disease, right hand

     M11.042 Hydroxyapatite deposition disease, left hand

     M11.049 Hydroxyapatite deposition disease, unspecified hand

√6ᵗʰ **M11.05** Hydroxyapatite deposition disease, hip

     M11.051 Hydroxyapatite deposition disease, right hip

     M11.052 Hydroxyapatite deposition disease, left hip

     M11.059 Hydroxyapatite deposition disease, unspecified hip

√6ᵗʰ **M11.06** Hydroxyapatite deposition disease, knee

     M11.061 Hydroxyapatite deposition disease, right knee

     M11.062 Hydroxyapatite deposition disease, left knee

     M11.069 Hydroxyapatite deposition disease, unspecified knee

√6ᵗʰ **M11.07** Hydroxyapatite deposition disease, ankle and foot

     M11.071 Hydroxyapatite deposition disease, right ankle and foot

     M11.072 Hydroxyapatite deposition disease, left ankle and foot

     M11.079 Hydroxyapatite deposition disease, unspecified ankle and foot

   M11.08 Hydroxyapatite deposition disease, vertebrae

   M11.09 Hydroxyapatite deposition disease, multiple sites

√5ᵗʰ **M11.1** Familial chondrocalcinosis

   M11.10 Familial chondrocalcinosis, unspecified site

√6ᵗʰ **M11.11** Familial chondrocalcinosis, shoulder

     M11.111 Familial chondrocalcinosis, right shoulder

     M11.112 Familial chondrocalcinosis, left shoulder

     M11.119 Familial chondrocalcinosis, unspecified shoulder

√6ᵗʰ **M11.12** Familial chondrocalcinosis, elbow

     M11.121 Familial chondrocalcinosis, right elbow

     M11.122 Familial chondrocalcinosis, left elbow

     M11.129 Familial chondrocalcinosis, unspecified elbow

√6ᵗʰ **M11.13** Familial chondrocalcinosis, wrist

     M11.131 Familial chondrocalcinosis, right wrist

     M11.132 Familial chondrocalcinosis, left wrist

     M11.139 Familial chondrocalcinosis, unspecified wrist

√6ᵗʰ **M11.14** Familial chondrocalcinosis, hand

     M11.141 Familial chondrocalcinosis, right hand

     M11.142 Familial chondrocalcinosis, left hand

     M11.149 Familial chondrocalcinosis, unspecified hand

√6ᵗʰ **M11.15** Familial chondrocalcinosis, hip

     M11.151 Familial chondrocalcinosis, right hip

     M11.152 Familial chondrocalcinosis, left hip

     M11.159 Familial chondrocalcinosis, unspecified hip

√6ᵗʰ **M11.16** Familial chondrocalcinosis, knee

     M11.161 Familial chondrocalcinosis, right knee

     M11.162 Familial chondrocalcinosis, left knee

     M11.169 Familial chondrocalcinosis, unspecified knee

√6ᵗʰ **M11.17** Familial chondrocalcinosis, ankle and foot

     M11.171 Familial chondrocalcinosis, right ankle and foot

     M11.172 Familial chondrocalcinosis, left ankle and foot

     M11.179 Familial chondrocalcinosis, unspecified ankle and foot

   M11.18 Familial chondrocalcinosis, vertebrae

   M11.19 Familial chondrocalcinosis, multiple sites

√5ᵗʰ **M11.2** Other chondrocalcinosis

     Chondrocalcinosis NOS

     AHA: 2018,3Q,20

     TIP: Pseudogout is captured with codes in this subcategory.

   M11.20 Other chondrocalcinosis, unspecified site

√6ᵗʰ **M11.21** Other chondrocalcinosis, shoulder

     M11.211 Other chondrocalcinosis, right shoulder

     M11.212 Other chondrocalcinosis, left shoulder

     M11.219 Other chondrocalcinosis, unspecified shoulder

√6ᵗʰ **M11.22** Other chondrocalcinosis, elbow

     M11.221 Other chondrocalcinosis, right elbow

     M11.222 Other chondrocalcinosis, left elbow

     M11.229 Other chondrocalcinosis, unspecified elbow

√6ᵗʰ **M11.23** Other chondrocalcinosis, wrist

     M11.231 Other chondrocalcinosis, right wrist

     M11.232 Other chondrocalcinosis, left wrist

     M11.239 Other chondrocalcinosis, unspecified wrist

√6ᵗʰ **M11.24** Other chondrocalcinosis, hand

     M11.241 Other chondrocalcinosis, right hand

     M11.242 Other chondrocalcinosis, left hand

     M11.249 Other chondrocalcinosis, unspecified hand

√6ᵗʰ **M11.25** Other chondrocalcinosis, hip

     M11.251 Other chondrocalcinosis, right hip

     M11.252 Other chondrocalcinosis, left hip

     M11.259 Other chondrocalcinosis, unspecified hip

√6ᵗʰ **M11.26** Other chondrocalcinosis, knee

     M11.261 Other chondrocalcinosis, right knee

     M11.262 Other chondrocalcinosis, left knee

     M11.269 Other chondrocalcinosis, unspecified knee

√6ᵗʰ **M11.27** Other chondrocalcinosis, ankle and foot

     M11.271 Other chondrocalcinosis, right ankle and foot

     M11.272 Other chondrocalcinosis, left ankle and foot

     M11.279 Other chondrocalcinosis, unspecified ankle and foot

   M11.28 Other chondrocalcinosis, vertebrae

   M11.29 Other chondrocalcinosis, multiple sites

√5ᵗʰ **M11.8** Other specified crystal arthropathies

   M11.80 Other specified crystal arthropathies, unspecified site

HCC CMS-HCC   **Rx** Rx HCC   **ESR** ESRD HCC   **COM** Commercial HCC   **N** Newborn: 0   **P** Pediatric: 0-17   **M** Maternity: 9-64   **A** Adult: 15-124

794   ICD-10-CM 2023

✓6ᵗʰ **M11.81 Other specified crystal arthropathies, shoulder**

    M11.811 Other specified crystal arthropathies, right shoulder

    M11.812 Other specified crystal arthropathies, left shoulder

    M11.819 Other specified crystal arthropathies, unspecified shoulder

✓6ᵗʰ **M11.82 Other specified crystal arthropathies, elbow**

    M11.821 Other specified crystal arthropathies, right elbow

    M11.822 Other specified crystal arthropathies, left elbow

    M11.829 Other specified crystal arthropathies, unspecified elbow

✓6ᵗʰ **M11.83 Other specified crystal arthropathies, wrist**

    M11.831 Other specified crystal arthropathies, right wrist

    M11.832 Other specified crystal arthropathies, left wrist

    M11.839 Other specified crystal arthropathies, unspecified wrist

✓6ᵗʰ **M11.84 Other specified crystal arthropathies, hand**

    M11.841 Other specified crystal arthropathies, right hand

    M11.842 Other specified crystal arthropathies, left hand

    M11.849 Other specified crystal arthropathies, unspecified hand

✓6ᵗʰ **M11.85 Other specified crystal arthropathies, hip**

    M11.851 Other specified crystal arthropathies, right hip

    M11.852 Other specified crystal arthropathies, left hip

    M11.859 Other specified crystal arthropathies, unspecified hip

✓6ᵗʰ **M11.86 Other specified crystal arthropathies, knee**

    M11.861 Other specified crystal arthropathies, right knee

    M11.862 Other specified crystal arthropathies, left knee

    M11.869 Other specified crystal arthropathies, unspecified knee

✓6ᵗʰ **M11.87 Other specified crystal arthropathies, ankle and foot**

    M11.871 Other specified crystal arthropathies, right ankle and foot

    M11.872 Other specified crystal arthropathies, left ankle and foot

    M11.879 Other specified crystal arthropathies, unspecified ankle and foot

    M11.88 Other specified crystal arthropathies, vertebrae

    M11.89 Other specified crystal arthropathies, multiple sites

M11.9 Crystal arthropathy, unspecified

✓4ᵗʰ **M12 Other and unspecified arthropathy**

    EXCLUDES 1   arthrosis (M15-M19)

          cricoarytenoid arthropathy (J38.7)

✓5ᵗʰ **M12.0 Chronic postrheumatic arthropathy [Jaccoud]**

    M12.00 Chronic postrheumatic arthropathy [Jaccoud], unspecified site   HCC Rx ESR COM

✓6ᵗʰ **M12.01 Chronic postrheumatic arthropathy [Jaccoud], shoulder**

    M12.011 Chronic postrheumatic arthropathy [Jaccoud], right shoulder   HCC Rx ESR COM

    M12.012 Chronic postrheumatic arthropathy [Jaccoud], left shoulder   HCC Rx ESR COM

    M12.019 Chronic postrheumatic arthropathy [Jaccoud], unspecified shoulder   HCC Rx ESR COM

✓6ᵗʰ **M12.02 Chronic postrheumatic arthropathy [Jaccoud], elbow**

    M12.021 Chronic postrheumatic arthropathy [Jaccoud], right elbow   HCC Rx ESR COM

    M12.022 Chronic postrheumatic arthropathy [Jaccoud], left elbow   HCC Rx ESR COM

    M12.029 Chronic postrheumatic arthropathy [Jaccoud], unspecified elbow   HCC Rx ESR COM

✓6ᵗʰ **M12.03 Chronic postrheumatic arthropathy [Jaccoud], wrist**

    M12.031 Chronic postrheumatic arthropathy [Jaccoud], right wrist   HCC Rx ESR COM

    M12.032 Chronic postrheumatic arthropathy [Jaccoud], left wrist   HCC Rx ESR COM

    M12.039 Chronic postrheumatic arthropathy [Jaccoud], unspecified wrist   HCC Rx ESR COM

✓6ᵗʰ **M12.04 Chronic postrheumatic arthropathy [Jaccoud], hand**

    M12.041 Chronic postrheumatic arthropathy [Jaccoud], right hand   HCC Rx ESR COM

    M12.042 Chronic postrheumatic arthropathy [Jaccoud], left hand   HCC Rx ESR COM

    M12.049 Chronic postrheumatic arthropathy [Jaccoud], unspecified hand   HCC Rx ESR COM

✓6ᵗʰ **M12.05 Chronic postrheumatic arthropathy [Jaccoud], hip**

    M12.051 Chronic postrheumatic arthropathy [Jaccoud], right hip   HCC Rx ESR COM

    M12.052 Chronic postrheumatic arthropathy [Jaccoud], left hip   HCC Rx ESR COM

    M12.059 Chronic postrheumatic arthropathy [Jaccoud], unspecified hip   HCC Rx ESR COM

✓6ᵗʰ **M12.06 Chronic postrheumatic arthropathy [Jaccoud], knee**

    M12.061 Chronic postrheumatic arthropathy [Jaccoud], right knee   HCC Rx ESR COM

    M12.062 Chronic postrheumatic arthropathy [Jaccoud], left knee   HCC Rx ESR COM

    M12.069 Chronic postrheumatic arthropathy [Jaccoud], unspecified knee   HCC Rx ESR COM

✓6ᵗʰ **M12.07 Chronic postrheumatic arthropathy [Jaccoud], ankle and foot**

    M12.071 Chronic postrheumatic arthropathy [Jaccoud], right ankle and foot   HCC Rx ESR COM

    M12.072 Chronic postrheumatic arthropathy [Jaccoud], left ankle and foot   HCC Rx ESR COM

    M12.079 Chronic postrheumatic arthropathy [Jaccoud], unspecified ankle and foot   HCC Rx ESR COM

    M12.08 Chronic postrheumatic arthropathy [Jaccoud], other specified site   HCC Rx ESR COM

      Chronic postrheumatic arthropathy [Jaccoud], vertebrae

    M12.09 Chronic postrheumatic arthropathy [Jaccoud], multiple sites   HCC Rx ESR COM

✓5ᵗʰ **M12.1 Kaschin-Beck disease**

      Osteochondroarthrosis deformans endemica

    M12.10 Kaschin-Beck disease, unspecified site

✓6ᵗʰ **M12.11 Kaschin-Beck disease, shoulder**

    M12.111 Kaschin-Beck disease, right shoulder

    M12.112 Kaschin-Beck disease, left shoulder

    M12.119 Kaschin-Beck disease, unspecified shoulder

✓6ᵗʰ **M12.12 Kaschin-Beck disease, elbow**

    M12.121 Kaschin-Beck disease, right elbow

    M12.122 Kaschin-Beck disease, left elbow

    M12.129 Kaschin-Beck disease, unspecified elbow

✓6ᵗʰ **M12.13 Kaschin-Beck disease, wrist**

    M12.131 Kaschin-Beck disease, right wrist

    M12.132 Kaschin-Beck disease, left wrist

    M12.139 Kaschin-Beck disease, unspecified wrist

✓6ᵗʰ **M12.14 Kaschin-Beck disease, hand**

    M12.141 Kaschin-Beck disease, right hand

    M12.142 Kaschin-Beck disease, left hand

    M12.149 Kaschin-Beck disease, unspecified hand

✓6ᵗʰ **M12.15 Kaschin-Beck disease, hip**

    M12.151 Kaschin-Beck disease, right hip

    M12.152 Kaschin-Beck disease, left hip

    M12.159 Kaschin-Beck disease, unspecified hip

✓6ᵗʰ **M12.16 Kaschin-Beck disease, knee**

    M12.161 Kaschin-Beck disease, right knee

    M12.162 Kaschin-Beck disease, left knee

    M12.169 Kaschin-Beck disease, unspecified knee

✓6ᵗʰ M12.17   **Kaschin-Beck disease, ankle and foot**
   M12.171   Kaschin-Beck disease, right ankle and foot
   M12.172   Kaschin-Beck disease, left ankle and foot
   M12.179   Kaschin-Beck disease, unspecified ankle and foot
  M12.18   **Kaschin-Beck disease, vertebrae**
  M12.19   **Kaschin-Beck disease, multiple sites**

✓5ᵗʰ M12.2   **Villonodular synovitis (pigmented)**
   M12.20   Villonodular synovitis (pigmented), unspecified site
  ✓6ᵗʰ M12.21   **Villonodular synovitis (pigmented), shoulder**
   M12.211   Villonodular synovitis (pigmented), right shoulder
   M12.212   Villonodular synovitis (pigmented), left shoulder
   M12.219   Villonodular synovitis (pigmented), unspecified shoulder
  ✓6ᵗʰ M12.22   **Villonodular synovitis (pigmented), elbow**
   M12.221   Villonodular synovitis (pigmented), right elbow
   M12.222   Villonodular synovitis (pigmented), left elbow
   M12.229   Villonodular synovitis (pigmented), unspecified elbow
  ✓6ᵗʰ M12.23   **Villonodular synovitis (pigmented), wrist**
   M12.231   Villonodular synovitis (pigmented), right wrist
   M12.232   Villonodular synovitis (pigmented), left wrist
   M12.239   Villonodular synovitis (pigmented), unspecified wrist
  ✓6ᵗʰ M12.24   **Villonodular synovitis (pigmented), hand**
   M12.241   Villonodular synovitis (pigmented), right hand
   M12.242   Villonodular synovitis (pigmented), left hand
   M12.249   Villonodular synovitis (pigmented), unspecified hand
  ✓6ᵗʰ M12.25   **Villonodular synovitis (pigmented), hip**
   M12.251   Villonodular synovitis (pigmented), right hip
   M12.252   Villonodular synovitis (pigmented), left hip
   M12.259   Villonodular synovitis (pigmented), unspecified hip
  ✓6ᵗʰ M12.26   **Villonodular synovitis (pigmented), knee**
   M12.261   Villonodular synovitis (pigmented), right knee
   M12.262   Villonodular synovitis (pigmented), left knee
   M12.269   Villonodular synovitis (pigmented), unspecified knee
  ✓6ᵗʰ M12.27   **Villonodular synovitis (pigmented), ankle and foot**
   M12.271   Villonodular synovitis (pigmented), right ankle and foot
   M12.272   Villonodular synovitis (pigmented), left ankle and foot
   M12.279   Villonodular synovitis (pigmented), unspecified ankle and foot
  M12.28   **Villonodular synovitis (pigmented), other specified site**
    Villonodular synovitis (pigmented), vertebrae
  M12.29   **Villonodular synovitis (pigmented), multiple sites**

✓5ᵗʰ M12.3   **Palindromic rheumatism**
   DEF: Sudden and recurring attacks of moderate to severe joint pain and swelling generally occurring in the hands or feet of unknown etiology. After the attack subsides, the joints appear normal again.
   M12.30   Palindromic rheumatism, unspecified site
  ✓6ᵗʰ M12.31   **Palindromic rheumatism, shoulder**
   M12.311   Palindromic rheumatism, right shoulder
   M12.312   Palindromic rheumatism, left shoulder
   M12.319   Palindromic rheumatism, unspecified shoulder
  ✓6ᵗʰ M12.32   **Palindromic rheumatism, elbow**
   M12.321   Palindromic rheumatism, right elbow
   M12.322   Palindromic rheumatism, left elbow

   M12.329   Palindromic rheumatism, unspecified elbow
  ✓6ᵗʰ M12.33   **Palindromic rheumatism, wrist**
   M12.331   Palindromic rheumatism, right wrist
   M12.332   Palindromic rheumatism, left wrist
   M12.339   Palindromic rheumatism, unspecified wrist
  ✓6ᵗʰ M12.34   **Palindromic rheumatism, hand**
   M12.341   Palindromic rheumatism, right hand
   M12.342   Palindromic rheumatism, left hand
   M12.349   Palindromic rheumatism, unspecified hand
  ✓6ᵗʰ M12.35   **Palindromic rheumatism, hip**
   M12.351   Palindromic rheumatism, right hip
   M12.352   Palindromic rheumatism, left hip
   M12.359   Palindromic rheumatism, unspecified hip
  ✓6ᵗʰ M12.36   **Palindromic rheumatism, knee**
   M12.361   Palindromic rheumatism, right knee
   M12.362   Palindromic rheumatism, left knee
   M12.369   Palindromic rheumatism, unspecified knee
  ✓6ᵗʰ M12.37   **Palindromic rheumatism, ankle and foot**
   M12.371   Palindromic rheumatism, right ankle and foot
   M12.372   Palindromic rheumatism, left ankle and foot
   M12.379   Palindromic rheumatism, unspecified ankle and foot
  M12.38   **Palindromic rheumatism, other specified site**
    Palindromic rheumatism, vertebrae
  M12.39   **Palindromic rheumatism, multiple sites**

✓5ᵗʰ M12.4   **Intermittent hydrarthrosis**
   M12.40   Intermittent hydrarthrosis, unspecified site
  ✓6ᵗʰ M12.41   **Intermittent hydrarthrosis, shoulder**
   M12.411   Intermittent hydrarthrosis, right shoulder
   M12.412   Intermittent hydrarthrosis, left shoulder
   M12.419   Intermittent hydrarthrosis, unspecified shoulder
  ✓6ᵗʰ M12.42   **Intermittent hydrarthrosis, elbow**
   M12.421   Intermittent hydrarthrosis, right elbow
   M12.422   Intermittent hydrarthrosis, left elbow
   M12.429   Intermittent hydrarthrosis, unspecified elbow
  ✓6ᵗʰ M12.43   **Intermittent hydrarthrosis, wrist**
   M12.431   Intermittent hydrarthrosis, right wrist
   M12.432   Intermittent hydrarthrosis, left wrist
   M12.439   Intermittent hydrarthrosis, unspecified wrist
  ✓6ᵗʰ M12.44   **Intermittent hydrarthrosis, hand**
   M12.441   Intermittent hydrarthrosis, right hand
   M12.442   Intermittent hydrarthrosis, left hand
   M12.449   Intermittent hydrarthrosis, unspecified hand
  ✓6ᵗʰ M12.45   **Intermittent hydrarthrosis, hip**
   M12.451   Intermittent hydrarthrosis, right hip
   M12.452   Intermittent hydrarthrosis, left hip
   M12.459   Intermittent hydrarthrosis, unspecified hip
  ✓6ᵗʰ M12.46   **Intermittent hydrarthrosis, knee**
   M12.461   Intermittent hydrarthrosis, right knee
   M12.462   Intermittent hydrarthrosis, left knee
   M12.469   Intermittent hydrarthrosis, unspecified knee
  ✓6ᵗʰ M12.47   **Intermittent hydrarthrosis, ankle and foot**
   M12.471   Intermittent hydrarthrosis, right ankle and foot
   M12.472   Intermittent hydrarthrosis, left ankle and foot
   M12.479   Intermittent hydrarthrosis, unspecified ankle and foot
  M12.48   **Intermittent hydrarthrosis, other site**
  M12.49   **Intermittent hydrarthrosis, multiple sites**

√5ᵗʰ **M12.5 Traumatic arthropathy**

> EXCLUDES 1   *current injury–see Alphabetic Index*
> *post-traumatic osteoarthritis of first carpometacarpal joint (M18.2-M18.3)*
> *post-traumatic osteoarthritis of hip (M16.4-M16.5)*
> *post-traumatic osteoarthritis of knee (M17.2-M17.3)*
> *post-traumatic osteoarthritis NOS (M19.1-)*
> *post-traumatic osteoarthritis of other single joints (M19.1-)*

> **AHA:** 2015,1Q,17

     M12.50   Traumatic arthropathy, unspecified site

√6ᵗʰ   **M12.51**   Traumatic arthropathy, shoulder
     M12.511   Traumatic arthropathy, right shoulder
     M12.512   Traumatic arthropathy, left shoulder
     M12.519   Traumatic arthropathy, unspecified shoulder

√6ᵗʰ   **M12.52**   Traumatic arthropathy, elbow
     M12.521   Traumatic arthropathy, right elbow
     M12.522   Traumatic arthropathy, left elbow
     M12.529   Traumatic arthropathy, unspecified elbow

√6ᵗʰ   **M12.53**   Traumatic arthropathy, wrist
     M12.531   Traumatic arthropathy, right wrist
     M12.532   Traumatic arthropathy, left wrist
     M12.539   Traumatic arthropathy, unspecified wrist

√6ᵗʰ   **M12.54**   Traumatic arthropathy, hand
     M12.541   Traumatic arthropathy, right hand
     M12.542   Traumatic arthropathy, left hand
     M12.549   Traumatic arthropathy, unspecified hand

√6ᵗʰ   **M12.55**   Traumatic arthropathy, hip
     M12.551   Traumatic arthropathy, right hip
     M12.552   Traumatic arthropathy, left hip
     M12.559   Traumatic arthropathy, unspecified hip

√6ᵗʰ   **M12.56**   Traumatic arthropathy, knee
     M12.561   Traumatic arthropathy, right knee
     M12.562   Traumatic arthropathy, left knee
     M12.569   Traumatic arthropathy, unspecified knee

√6ᵗʰ   **M12.57**   Traumatic arthropathy, ankle and foot
     M12.571   Traumatic arthropathy, right ankle and foot
     M12.572   Traumatic arthropathy, left ankle and foot
     M12.579   Traumatic arthropathy, unspecified ankle and foot

     M12.58   Traumatic arthropathy, other specified site
         Traumatic arthropathy, vertebrae

     M12.59   Traumatic arthropathy, multiple sites

√5ᵗʰ **M12.8 Other specific arthropathies, not elsewhere classified**
     Transient arthropathy

     M12.80   Other specific arthropathies, not elsewhere classified, unspecified site

√6ᵗʰ   **M12.81**   Other specific arthropathies, not elsewhere classified, shoulder
     M12.811   Other specific arthropathies, not elsewhere classified, right shoulder
     M12.812   Other specific arthropathies, not elsewhere classified, left shoulder
     M12.819   Other specific arthropathies, not elsewhere classified, unspecified shoulder

√6ᵗʰ   **M12.82**   Other specific arthropathies, not elsewhere classified, elbow
     M12.821   Other specific arthropathies, not elsewhere classified, right elbow
     M12.822   Other specific arthropathies, not elsewhere classified, left elbow
     M12.829   Other specific arthropathies, not elsewhere classified, unspecified elbow

√6ᵗʰ   **M12.83**   Other specific arthropathies, not elsewhere classified, wrist
     M12.831   Other specific arthropathies, not elsewhere classified, right wrist
     M12.832   Other specific arthropathies, not elsewhere classified, left wrist
     M12.839   Other specific arthropathies, not elsewhere classified, unspecified wrist

√6ᵗʰ   **M12.84**   Other specific arthropathies, not elsewhere classified, hand
     M12.841   Other specific arthropathies, not elsewhere classified, right hand
     M12.842   Other specific arthropathies, not elsewhere classified, left hand
     M12.849   Other specific arthropathies, not elsewhere classified, unspecified hand

√6ᵗʰ   **M12.85**   Other specific arthropathies, not elsewhere classified, hip
     M12.851   Other specific arthropathies, not elsewhere classified, right hip
     M12.852   Other specific arthropathies, not elsewhere classified, left hip
     M12.859   Other specific arthropathies, not elsewhere classified, unspecified hip

√6ᵗʰ   **M12.86**   Other specific arthropathies, not elsewhere classified, knee
     M12.861   Other specific arthropathies, not elsewhere classified, right knee
     M12.862   Other specific arthropathies, not elsewhere classified, left knee
     M12.869   Other specific arthropathies, not elsewhere classified, unspecified knee

√6ᵗʰ   **M12.87**   Other specific arthropathies, not elsewhere classified, ankle and foot
     M12.871   Other specific arthropathies, not elsewhere classified, right ankle and foot
     M12.872   Other specific arthropathies, not elsewhere classified, left ankle and foot
     M12.879   Other specific arthropathies, not elsewhere classified, unspecified ankle and foot

     M12.88   Other specific arthropathies, not elsewhere classified, other specified site
         Other specific arthropathies, not elsewhere classified, vertebrae

     M12.89   Other specific arthropathies, not elsewhere classified, multiple sites

M12.9 Arthropathy, unspecified

√4ᵗʰ **M13 Other arthritis**

> EXCLUDES 1   *arthrosis (M15-M19)*
> *osteoarthritis (M15-M19)*

M13.0 Polyarthritis, unspecified

√5ᵗʰ **M13.1 Monoarthritis, not elsewhere classified**

     M13.10   Monoarthritis, not elsewhere classified, unspecified site

√6ᵗʰ   **M13.11**   Monoarthritis, not elsewhere classified, shoulder
     M13.111   Monoarthritis, not elsewhere classified, right shoulder
     M13.112   Monoarthritis, not elsewhere classified, left shoulder
     M13.119   Monoarthritis, not elsewhere classified, unspecified shoulder

√6ᵗʰ   **M13.12**   Monoarthritis, not elsewhere classified, elbow
     M13.121   Monoarthritis, not elsewhere classified, right elbow
     M13.122   Monoarthritis, not elsewhere classified, left elbow
     M13.129   Monoarthritis, not elsewhere classified, unspecified elbow

√6ᵗʰ   **M13.13**   Monoarthritis, not elsewhere classified, wrist
     M13.131   Monoarthritis, not elsewhere classified, right wrist
     M13.132   Monoarthritis, not elsewhere classified, left wrist
     M13.139   Monoarthritis, not elsewhere classified, unspecified wrist

√6ᵗʰ   **M13.14**   Monoarthritis, not elsewhere classified, hand
     M13.141   Monoarthritis, not elsewhere classified, right hand
     M13.142   Monoarthritis, not elsewhere classified, left hand
     M13.149   Monoarthritis, not elsewhere classified, unspecified hand

√6ᵗʰ   **M13.15**   Monoarthritis, not elsewhere classified, hip
     M13.151   Monoarthritis, not elsewhere classified, right hip
     M13.152   Monoarthritis, not elsewhere classified, left hip

Chapter 13. Diseases of the Musculoskeletal System and Connective Tissue

M13.159   Monoarthritis, not elsewhere classified, unspecified hip

√6ᵗʰ   M13.16   Monoarthritis, not elsewhere classified, knee

M13.161   Monoarthritis, not elsewhere classified, right knee

M13.162   Monoarthritis, not elsewhere classified, left knee

M13.169   Monoarthritis, not elsewhere classified, unspecified knee

√6ᵗʰ   M13.17   Monoarthritis, not elsewhere classified, ankle and foot

M13.171   Monoarthritis, not elsewhere classified, right ankle and foot

M13.172   Monoarthritis, not elsewhere classified, left ankle and foot

M13.179   Monoarthritis, not elsewhere classified, unspecified ankle and foot

√5ᵗʰ   **M13.8   Other specified arthritis**

Allergic arthritis

EXCLUDES 1   osteoarthritis (M15-M19)

M13.80   Other specified arthritis, unspecified site

√6ᵗʰ   M13.81   Other specified arthritis, shoulder

M13.811   Other specified arthritis, right shoulder

M13.812   Other specified arthritis, left shoulder

M13.819   Other specified arthritis, unspecified shoulder

√6ᵗʰ   M13.82   Other specified arthritis, elbow

M13.821   Other specified arthritis, right elbow

M13.822   Other specified arthritis, left elbow

M13.829   Other specified arthritis, unspecified elbow

√6ᵗʰ   M13.83   Other specified arthritis, wrist

M13.831   Other specified arthritis, right wrist

M13.832   Other specified arthritis, left wrist

M13.839   Other specified arthritis, unspecified wrist

√6ᵗʰ   M13.84   Other specified arthritis, hand

M13.841   Other specified arthritis, right hand

M13.842   Other specified arthritis, left hand

M13.849   Other specified arthritis, unspecified hand

√6ᵗʰ   M13.85   Other specified arthritis, hip

M13.851   Other specified arthritis, right hip

M13.852   Other specified arthritis, left hip

M13.859   Other specified arthritis, unspecified hip

√6ᵗʰ   M13.86   Other specified arthritis, knee

M13.861   Other specified arthritis, right knee

M13.862   Other specified arthritis, left knee

M13.869   Other specified arthritis, unspecified knee

√6ᵗʰ   M13.87   Other specified arthritis, ankle and foot

M13.871   Other specified arthritis, right ankle and foot

M13.872   Other specified arthritis, left ankle and foot

M13.879   Other specified arthritis, unspecified ankle and foot

M13.88   Other specified arthritis, other site

M13.89   Other specified arthritis, multiple sites

√4ᵗʰ   **M14   Arthropathies in other diseases classified elsewhere**

EXCLUDES 1   arthropathy in:

diabetes mellitus (E08-E13 with .61-)

hematological disorders (M36.2-M36.3)

hypersensitivity reactions (M36.4)

neoplastic disease (M36.1)

neurosyphillis (A52.16)

sarcoidosis (D86.86)

enteropathic arthropathies (M07.-)

juvenile psoriatic arthropathy (L40.54)

lipoid dermatoarthritis (E78.81)

√5ᵗʰ   **M14.6   Charcôt's joint**

Neuropathic arthropathy

EXCLUDES 1   Charcôt's joint in diabetes mellitus (E08-E13 with .610)

Charcôt's joint in tabes dorsalis (A52.16)

DEF: Progressive neurologic arthropathy in which chronic degeneration of joints in the weight-bearing areas with peripheral hypertrophy occurs as a complication of a neuropathy disorder. Supporting structures relax from a loss of sensation resulting in chronic joint instability.

M14.60   Charcôt's joint, unspecified site

√6ᵗʰ   M14.61   Charcôt's joint, shoulder

M14.611   Charcôt's joint, right shoulder

M14.612   Charcôt's joint, left shoulder

M14.619   Charcôt's joint, unspecified shoulder

√6ᵗʰ   M14.62   Charcôt's joint, elbow

M14.621   Charcôt's joint, right elbow

M14.622   Charcôt's joint, left elbow

M14.629   Charcôt's joint, unspecified elbow

√6ᵗʰ   M14.63   Charcôt's joint, wrist

M14.631   Charcôt's joint, right wrist

M14.632   Charcôt's joint, left wrist

M14.639   Charcôt's joint, unspecified wrist

√6ᵗʰ   M14.64   Charcôt's joint, hand

M14.641   Charcôt's joint, right hand

M14.642   Charcôt's joint, left hand

M14.649   Charcôt's joint, unspecified hand

√6ᵗʰ   M14.65   Charcôt's joint, hip

M14.651   Charcôt's joint, right hip

M14.652   Charcôt's joint, left hip

M14.659   Charcôt's joint, unspecified hip

√6ᵗʰ   M14.66   Charcôt's joint, knee

M14.661   Charcôt's joint, right knee

M14.662   Charcôt's joint, left knee

M14.669   Charcôt's joint, unspecified knee

√6ᵗʰ   M14.67   Charcôt's joint, ankle and foot

M14.671   Charcôt's joint, right ankle and foot

M14.672   Charcôt's joint, left ankle and foot

M14.679   Charcôt's joint, unspecified ankle and foot

M14.68   Charcôt's joint, vertebrae

M14.69   Charcôt's joint, multiple sites

√5ᵗʰ   **M14.8   Arthropathies in other specified diseases classified elsewhere**

Code first underlying disease, such as:

amyloidosis (E85.-)

erythema multiforme (L51.-)

erythema nodosum (L52)

hemochromatosis (E83.11-)

hyperparathyroidism (E21.-)

hypothyroidism (E00-E03)

sickle-cell disorders (D57.-)

thyrotoxicosis [hyperthyroidism] (E05.-)

Whipple's disease (K90.81)

M14.80   Arthropathies in other specified diseases classified elsewhere, unspecified site

√6ᵗʰ   M14.81   Arthropathies in other specified diseases classified elsewhere, shoulder

M14.811   Arthropathies in other specified diseases classified elsewhere, right shoulder

M14.812   Arthropathies in other specified diseases classified elsewhere, left shoulder

M14.819   Arthropathies in other specified diseases classified elsewhere, unspecified shoulder

---

√6th M14.82 Arthropathies in other specified diseases classified elsewhere, elbow
- *M14.821 Arthropathies in other specified diseases classified elsewhere, right elbow*
- *M14.822 Arthropathies in other specified diseases classified elsewhere, left elbow*
- *M14.829 Arthropathies in other specified diseases classified elsewhere, unspecified elbow*

√6th M14.83 Arthropathies in other specified diseases classified elsewhere, wrist
- *M14.831 Arthropathies in other specified diseases classified elsewhere, right wrist*
- *M14.832 Arthropathies in other specified diseases classified elsewhere, left wrist*
- *M14.839 Arthropathies in other specified diseases classified elsewhere, unspecified wrist*

√6th M14.84 Arthropathies in other specified diseases classified elsewhere, hand
- *M14.841 Arthropathies in other specified diseases classified elsewhere, right hand*
- *M14.842 Arthropathies in other specified diseases classified elsewhere, left hand*
- *M14.849 Arthropathies in other specified diseases classified elsewhere, unspecified hand*

√6th M14.85 Arthropathies in other specified diseases classified elsewhere, hip
- *M14.851 Arthropathies in other specified diseases classified elsewhere, right hip*
- *M14.852 Arthropathies in other specified diseases classified elsewhere, left hip*
- *M14.859 Arthropathies in other specified diseases classified elsewhere, unspecified hip*

√6th M14.86 Arthropathies in other specified diseases classified elsewhere, knee
- *M14.861 Arthropathies in other specified diseases classified elsewhere, right knee*
- *M14.862 Arthropathies in other specified diseases classified elsewhere, left knee*
- *M14.869 Arthropathies in other specified diseases classified elsewhere, unspecified knee*

√6th M14.87 Arthropathies in other specified diseases classified elsewhere, ankle and foot
- *M14.871 Arthropathies in other specified diseases classified elsewhere, right ankle and foot*
- *M14.872 Arthropathies in other specified diseases classified elsewhere, left ankle and foot*
- *M14.879 Arthropathies in other specified diseases classified elsewhere, unspecified ankle and foot*

- *M14.88 Arthropathies in other specified diseases classified elsewhere, vertebrae*
- *M14.89 Arthropathies in other specified diseases classified elsewhere, multiple sites*

Osteoarthritis (M15-M19)

EXCLUDES 2   osteoarthritis of spine (M47.-)
AHA: 2020,2Q,14; 2016,4Q,147
TIP: Assign a primary osteoarthritis code when the site of the osteoarthritis is documented but the type of osteoarthritis — primary, secondary, generalized, or post-traumatic — is not documented. Primary is considered the default.

√4th M15 Polyosteoarthritis
INCLUDES   arthritis of multiple sites
EXCLUDES 1   bilateral involvement of single joint (M16-M19)

M15.Ø Primary generalized (osteo)arthritis

M15.1 Heberden's nodes (with arthropathy)
    Interphalangeal distal osteoarthritis

M15.2 Bouchard's nodes (with arthropathy)
    Juxtaphalangeal distal osteoarthritis

M15.3 Secondary multiple arthritis
    Post-traumatic polyosteoarthritis

M15.4 Erosive (osteo)arthritis

M15.8 Other polyosteoarthritis

M15.9 Polyosteoarthritis, unspecified
    Generalized osteoarthritis NOS

√4th M16 Osteoarthritis of hip
    AHA: 2016,4Q,146

M16.Ø Bilateral primary osteoarthritis of hip
    AHA: 2018,2Q,15

√5th M16.1 Unilateral primary osteoarthritis of hip
    Primary osteoarthritis of hip NOS
    AHA: 2018,2Q,15
- **M16.10 Unilateral primary osteoarthritis, unspecified hip**
- **M16.11 Unilateral primary osteoarthritis, right hip**
- **M16.12 Unilateral primary osteoarthritis, left hip**

M16.2 Bilateral osteoarthritis resulting from hip dysplasia

√5th M16.3 Unilateral osteoarthritis resulting from hip dysplasia
    Dysplastic osteoarthritis of hip NOS
- **M16.30 Unilateral osteoarthritis resulting from hip dysplasia, unspecified hip**
- **M16.31 Unilateral osteoarthritis resulting from hip dysplasia, right hip**
- **M16.32 Unilateral osteoarthritis resulting from hip dysplasia, left hip**

M16.4 Bilateral post-traumatic osteoarthritis of hip

√5th M16.5 Unilateral post-traumatic osteoarthritis of hip
    Post-traumatic osteoarthritis of hip NOS
- **M16.50 Unilateral post-traumatic osteoarthritis, unspecified hip**
- **M16.51 Unilateral post-traumatic osteoarthritis, right hip**
- **M16.52 Unilateral post-traumatic osteoarthritis, left hip**

M16.6 Other bilateral secondary osteoarthritis of hip

M16.7 Other unilateral secondary osteoarthritis of hip
    Secondary osteoarthritis of hip NOS

M16.9 Osteoarthritis of hip, unspecified

√4th M17 Osteoarthritis of knee
    AHA: 2016,4Q,146-147

M17.Ø Bilateral primary osteoarthritis of knee
    AHA: 2018,2Q,15

√5th M17.1 Unilateral primary osteoarthritis of knee
    Primary osteoarthritis of knee NOS
    AHA: 2018,2Q,15
- **M17.10 Unilateral primary osteoarthritis, unspecified knee**
- **M17.11 Unilateral primary osteoarthritis, right knee**
- **M17.12 Unilateral primary osteoarthritis, left knee**

M17.2 Bilateral post-traumatic osteoarthritis of knee

√5th M17.3 Unilateral post-traumatic osteoarthritis of knee
    Post-traumatic osteoarthritis of knee NOS
- **M17.30 Unilateral post-traumatic osteoarthritis, unspecified knee**
- **M17.31 Unilateral post-traumatic osteoarthritis, right knee**
- **M17.32 Unilateral post-traumatic osteoarthritis, left knee**

M17.4 Other bilateral secondary osteoarthritis of knee

M17.5 Other unilateral secondary osteoarthritis of knee
    Secondary osteoarthritis of knee NOS

M17.9 Osteoarthritis of knee, unspecified

√4th M18 Osteoarthritis of first carpometacarpal joint

M18.Ø Bilateral primary osteoarthritis of first carpometacarpal joints

√5th M18.1 Unilateral primary osteoarthritis of first carpometacarpal joint
    Primary osteoarthritis of first carpometacarpal joint NOS
- **M18.10 Unilateral primary osteoarthritis of first carpometacarpal joint, unspecified hand**
- **M18.11 Unilateral primary osteoarthritis of first carpometacarpal joint, right hand**
- **M18.12 Unilateral primary osteoarthritis of first carpometacarpal joint, left hand**

M18.2 Bilateral post-traumatic osteoarthritis of first carpometacarpal joints

√5th M18.3 Unilateral post-traumatic osteoarthritis of first carpometacarpal joint
    Post-traumatic osteoarthritis of first carpometacarpal joint NOS
- **M18.30 Unilateral post-traumatic osteoarthritis of first carpometacarpal joint, unspecified hand**
- **M18.31 Unilateral post-traumatic osteoarthritis of first carpometacarpal joint, right hand**
- **M18.32 Unilateral post-traumatic osteoarthritis of first carpometacarpal joint, left hand**

M18.4 Other bilateral secondary osteoarthritis of first carpometacarpal joints

√5th M18.5 Other unilateral secondary osteoarthritis of first carpometacarpal joint
    Secondary osteoarthritis of first carpometacarpal joint NOS
- **M18.50 Other unilateral secondary osteoarthritis of first carpometacarpal joint, unspecified hand**

M18.51 Other unilateral secondary osteoarthritis of first carpometacarpal joint, **right** hand

M18.52 Other unilateral secondary osteoarthritis of first carpometacarpal joint, **left** hand

M18.9 Osteoarthritis of first carpometacarpal joint, unspecified

✓4ᵗʰ **M19** Other and unspecified osteoarthritis

> *EXCLUDES 1*   polyarthritis (M15.-)
> *EXCLUDES 2*   arthrosis of spine (M47.-)
>   hallux rigidus (M20.2)
>   osteoarthritis of spine (M47.-)
> **AHA:** 2020,4Q,31-32

✓5ᵗʰ **M19.0** Primary osteoarthritis of other joints

> **AHA:** 2018,2Q,15; 2016,4Q,145

✓6ᵗʰ **M19.01** Primary osteoarthritis, **shoulder**

M19.011 Primary osteoarthritis, **right** shoulder
M19.012 Primary osteoarthritis, **left** shoulder
M19.019 Primary osteoarthritis, **unspecified** shoulder

✓6ᵗʰ **M19.02** Primary osteoarthritis, **elbow**

M19.021 Primary osteoarthritis, **right** elbow
M19.022 Primary osteoarthritis, **left** elbow
M19.029 Primary osteoarthritis, **unspecified** elbow

✓6ᵗʰ **M19.03** Primary osteoarthritis, **wrist**

M19.031 Primary osteoarthritis, **right** wrist
M19.032 Primary osteoarthritis, **left** wrist
M19.039 Primary osteoarthritis, **unspecified** wrist

✓6ᵗʰ **M19.04** Primary osteoarthritis, **hand**

> *EXCLUDES 2*   primary osteoarthritis of first carpometacarpal joint (M18.0-, M18.1-)

M19.041 Primary osteoarthritis, **right** hand
M19.042 Primary osteoarthritis, **left** hand
M19.049 Primary osteoarthritis, **unspecified** hand

✓6ᵗʰ **M19.07** Primary osteoarthritis **ankle and foot**

M19.071 Primary osteoarthritis, **right** ankle and foot
M19.072 Primary osteoarthritis, **left** ankle and foot
M19.079 Primary osteoarthritis, **unspecified** ankle and foot

M19.09 Primary osteoarthritis, other specified site

✓5ᵗʰ **M19.1** Post-traumatic osteoarthritis of other joints

✓6ᵗʰ **M19.11** Post-traumatic osteoarthritis, **shoulder**

M19.111 Post-traumatic osteoarthritis, **right** shoulder
M19.112 Post-traumatic osteoarthritis, **left** shoulder
M19.119 Post-traumatic osteoarthritis, **unspecified** shoulder

✓6ᵗʰ **M19.12** Post-traumatic osteoarthritis, **elbow**

M19.121 Post-traumatic osteoarthritis, **right** elbow
M19.122 Post-traumatic osteoarthritis, **left** elbow
M19.129 Post-traumatic osteoarthritis, **unspecified** elbow

✓6ᵗʰ **M19.13** Post-traumatic osteoarthritis, **wrist**

M19.131 Post-traumatic osteoarthritis, **right** wrist
M19.132 Post-traumatic osteoarthritis, **left** wrist
M19.139 Post-traumatic osteoarthritis, **unspecified** wrist

✓6ᵗʰ **M19.14** Post-traumatic osteoarthritis, **hand**

> *EXCLUDES 2*   post-traumatic osteoarthritis of first carpometacarpal joint (M18.2-, M18.3-)

M19.141 Post-traumatic osteoarthritis, **right** hand
M19.142 Post-traumatic osteoarthritis, **left** hand
M19.149 Post-traumatic osteoarthritis, **unspecified** hand

✓6ᵗʰ **M19.17** Post-traumatic osteoarthritis, **ankle and foot**

M19.171 Post-traumatic osteoarthritis, **right** ankle and foot
M19.172 Post-traumatic osteoarthritis, **left** ankle and foot
M19.179 Post-traumatic osteoarthritis, **unspecified** ankle and foot

M19.19 Post-traumatic osteoarthritis, other specified site

✓5ᵗʰ **M19.2** Secondary osteoarthritis of other joints

✓6ᵗʰ **M19.21** Secondary osteoarthritis, **shoulder**

M19.211 Secondary osteoarthritis, **right** shoulder
M19.212 Secondary osteoarthritis, **left** shoulder
M19.219 Secondary osteoarthritis, **unspecified** shoulder

✓6ᵗʰ **M19.22** Secondary osteoarthritis, **elbow**

M19.221 Secondary osteoarthritis, **right** elbow
M19.222 Secondary osteoarthritis, **left** elbow
M19.229 Secondary osteoarthritis, **unspecified** elbow

✓6ᵗʰ **M19.23** Secondary osteoarthritis, **wrist**

M19.231 Secondary osteoarthritis, **right** wrist
M19.232 Secondary osteoarthritis, **left** wrist
M19.239 Secondary osteoarthritis, **unspecified** wrist

✓6ᵗʰ **M19.24** Secondary osteoarthritis, **hand**

M19.241 Secondary osteoarthritis, **right** hand
M19.242 Secondary osteoarthritis, **left** hand
M19.249 Secondary osteoarthritis, **unspecified** hand

✓6ᵗʰ **M19.27** Secondary osteoarthritis, **ankle and foot**

M19.271 Secondary osteoarthritis, **right** ankle and foot
M19.272 Secondary osteoarthritis, **left** ankle and foot
M19.279 Secondary osteoarthritis, **unspecified** ankle and foot

M19.29 Secondary osteoarthritis, other specified site

✓5ᵗʰ **M19.9** Osteoarthritis, unspecified site

> **TIP:** Assign M19.90 when neither the site nor the type of osteoarthritis — primary, secondary, or post-traumatic — is documented.

M19.90 Unspecified osteoarthritis, unspecified site
Arthrosis NOS
Arthritis NOS
Osteoarthritis NOS
AHA: 2016,4Q,145-147

M19.91 Primary osteoarthritis, unspecified site
Primary osteoarthritis NOS

M19.92 Post-traumatic osteoarthritis, unspecified site
Post-traumatic osteoarthritis NOS

M19.93 Secondary osteoarthritis, unspecified site
Secondary osteoarthritis NOS

Other joint disorders (M20-M25)

> *EXCLUDES 2*   joints of the spine (M40-M54)

✓4ᵗʰ **M20** Acquired deformities of fingers and toes

> *EXCLUDES 1*   acquired absence of fingers and toes (Z89.-)
>   congenital absence of fingers and toes (Q71.3-, Q72.3-)
>   congenital deformities and malformations of fingers and toes (Q66.-, Q68-Q70, Q74.-)

✓5ᵗʰ **M20.0** Deformity of finger(s)

> *EXCLUDES 1*   clubbing of fingers (R68.3)
>   palmar fascial fibromatosis [Dupuytren] (M72.0)
>   trigger finger (M65.3)

✓6ᵗʰ **M20.00** Unspecified deformity of finger(s)

M20.001 Unspecified deformity of **right** finger(s)
M20.002 Unspecified deformity of **left** finger(s)
M20.009 Unspecified deformity of **unspecified** finger(s)

✓6ᵗʰ **M20.01** Mallet finger

M20.011 Mallet finger of **right** finger(s)
M20.012 Mallet finger of **left** finger(s)
M20.019 Mallet finger of unspecified finger(s)

✓6ᵗʰ **M20.02** Boutonnière deformity

> **DEF:** Deformity of the finger caused by flexion of the proximal interphalangeal joint and hyperextension of the distal joint. The deformity results from rheumatoid arthritis, osteoarthritis, or injury.

M20.021 Boutonnière deformity of **right** finger(s)
M20.022 Boutonnière deformity of **left** finger(s)
M20.029 Boutonnière deformity of **unspecified** finger(s)

√6ᵗʰ **M20.03   Swan-neck deformity**

DEF: Flexed distal and hyperextended proximal interphalangeal joint most commonly caused by rheumatoid arthritis.

M20.031   Swan-neck deformity of **right** finger(s)

M20.032   Swan-neck deformity of **left** finger(s)

M20.039   Swan-neck deformity of **unspecified** finger(s)

√6ᵗʰ **M20.09   Other deformity of finger(s)**

M20.091   Other deformity of **right** finger(s)

M20.092   Other deformity of **left** finger(s)

M20.099   Other deformity of finger(s), **unspecified** finger(s)

√5ᵗʰ **M20.1   Hallux valgus (acquired)**

EXCLUDES 2   bunion (M21.6-)

AHA: 2016,4Q,38

DEF: Deformity in which the great toe deviates toward the other toes and may even be positioned over or under the second toe.

Hallux Valgus

Hallux valgus

Medial eminence of metatarsal bone

Right foot

M20.10   Hallux valgus (acquired), **unspecified** foot

M20.11   Hallux valgus (acquired), **right** foot

M20.12   Hallux valgus (acquired), **left** foot

√5ᵗʰ **M20.2   Hallux rigidus**

M20.20   Hallux rigidus, **unspecified** foot

M20.21   Hallux rigidus, **right** foot

M20.22   Hallux rigidus, **left** foot

√5ᵗʰ **M20.3   Hallux varus (acquired)**

DEF: Deformity in which the great toe deviates away from the other toes.

M20.30   Hallux varus (acquired), **unspecified** foot

M20.31   Hallux varus (acquired), **right** foot

M20.32   Hallux varus (acquired), **left** foot

√5ᵗʰ **M20.4   Other hammer toe(s) (acquired)**

M20.40   Other hammer toe(s) (acquired), **unspecified** foot

M20.41   Other hammer toe(s) (acquired), **right** foot

M20.42   Other hammer toe(s) (acquired), **left** foot

√5ᵗʰ **M20.5   Other deformities of toe(s) (acquired)**

√6ᵗʰ **M20.5X   Other deformities of toe(s) (acquired)**

M20.5X1   Other deformities of toe(s) (acquired), **right** foot

M20.5X2   Other deformities of toe(s) (acquired), **left** foot

M20.5X9   Other deformities of toe(s) (acquired), **unspecified** foot

√5ᵗʰ **M20.6   Acquired deformities of toe(s), unspecified**

M20.60   Acquired deformities of toe(s), unspecified, **unspecified** foot

M20.61   Acquired deformities of toe(s), unspecified, **right** foot

M20.62   Acquired deformities of toe(s), unspecified, **left** foot

√4ᵗʰ **M21   Other acquired deformities of limbs**

EXCLUDES 1   acquired absence of limb (Z89.-)

congenital absence of limbs (Q71-Q73)

congenital deformities and malformations of limbs (Q65-Q66, Q68-Q74)

EXCLUDES 2   acquired deformities of fingers or toes (M20.-)

coxa plana (M91.2)

√5ᵗʰ **M21.0   Valgus deformity, not elsewhere classified**

EXCLUDES 1   metatarsus valgus (Q66.6)

talipes calcaneovalgus (Q66.4-)

M21.00   Valgus deformity, not elsewhere classified, **unspecified** site

√6ᵗʰ **M21.02   Valgus deformity, not elsewhere classified, elbow**

Cubitus valgus

M21.021   Valgus deformity, not elsewhere classified, **right** elbow

M21.022   Valgus deformity, not elsewhere classified, **left** elbow

M21.029   Valgus deformity, not elsewhere classified, **unspecified** elbow

√6ᵗʰ **M21.05   Valgus deformity, not elsewhere classified, hip**

M21.051   Valgus deformity, not elsewhere classified, **right** hip

M21.052   Valgus deformity, not elsewhere classified, **left** hip

M21.059   Valgus deformity, not elsewhere classified, **unspecified** hip

√6ᵗʰ **M21.06   Valgus deformity, not elsewhere classified, knee**

Genu valgum

Knock knee

DEF: Genu valga/valgum: Condition in which the thighs slant inward, causing the knees to be angled abnormally close together, leaving the space between the ankles wider than normal.

Genu Valga (knock-knee)

M21.061   Valgus deformity, not elsewhere classified, **right** knee

M21.062   Valgus deformity, not elsewhere classified, **left** knee

M21.069   Valgus deformity, not elsewhere classified, **unspecified** knee

√6ᵗʰ **M21.07   Valgus deformity, not elsewhere classified, ankle**

M21.071   Valgus deformity, not elsewhere classified, **right** ankle

M21.072   Valgus deformity, not elsewhere classified, **left** ankle

M21.079   Valgus deformity, not elsewhere classified, **unspecified** ankle

√5ᵗʰ **M21.1   Varus deformity, not elsewhere classified**

EXCLUDES 1   metatarsus varus (Q66.22-)

tibia vara (M92.51-)

M21.10   Varus deformity, not elsewhere classified, **unspecified** site

√6ᵗʰ **M21.12 Varus deformity, not elsewhere classified,** elbow
Cubitus varus, elbow

M21.121 Varus deformity, not elsewhere classified, right **elbow**

M21.122 Varus deformity, not elsewhere classified, left **elbow**

M21.129 Varus deformity, not elsewhere classified, unspecified elbow

√6ᵗʰ **M21.15 Varus deformity, not elsewhere classified,** hip

M21.151 Varus deformity, not elsewhere classified, right **hip**

M21.152 Varus deformity, not elsewhere classified, left **hip**

M21.159 Varus deformity, not elsewhere classified, unspecified

√6ᵗʰ **M21.16 Varus deformity, not elsewhere classified,** knee
Bow leg
Genu varum
DEF: Genu varus/varum: Condition in which the thighs and/or legs are bowed in an outward curve with an abnormally increased space between the knees.

Genu Varus (bowleg)

M21.161 Varus deformity, not elsewhere classified, right **knee**

M21.162 Varus deformity, not elsewhere classified, left **knee**

M21.169 Varus deformity, not elsewhere classified, unspecified knee

√6ᵗʰ **M21.17 Varus deformity, not elsewhere classified,** ankle

M21.171 Varus deformity, not elsewhere classified, right **ankle**

M21.172 Varus deformity, not elsewhere classified, left **ankle**

M21.179 Varus deformity, not elsewhere classified, unspecified ankle

√5ᵗʰ **M21.2 Flexion deformity**

M21.20 Flexion deformity, unspecified site

√6ᵗʰ **M21.21 Flexion deformity,** shoulder

M21.211 Flexion deformity, right **shoulder**

M21.212 Flexion deformity, left **shoulder**

M21.219 Flexion deformity, unspecified shoulder

√6ᵗʰ **M21.22 Flexion deformity,** elbow

M21.221 Flexion deformity, right **elbow**

M21.222 Flexion deformity, left **elbow**

M21.229 Flexion deformity, unspecified elbow

√6ᵗʰ **M21.23 Flexion deformity,** wrist

M21.231 Flexion deformity, right **wrist**

M21.232 Flexion deformity, left **wrist**

M21.239 Flexion deformity, unspecified wrist

√6ᵗʰ **M21.24 Flexion deformity,** finger joints

M21.241 Flexion deformity, right **finger joints**

M21.242 Flexion deformity, left **finger joints**

M21.249 Flexion deformity, unspecified finger joints

√6ᵗʰ **M21.25 Flexion deformity,** hip

M21.251 Flexion deformity, right **hip**

M21.252 Flexion deformity, left **hip**

M21.259 Flexion deformity, unspecified hip

√6ᵗʰ **M21.26 Flexion deformity,** knee

M21.261 Flexion deformity, right **knee**

M21.262 Flexion deformity, left **knee**

M21.269 Flexion deformity, unspecified knee

√6ᵗʰ **M21.27 Flexion deformity,** ankle and toes

M21.271 Flexion deformity, right **ankle and toes**

M21.272 Flexion deformity, left **ankle and toes**

M21.279 Flexion deformity, unspecified ankle and toes

√5ᵗʰ **M21.3 Wrist or foot drop (acquired)**

√6ᵗʰ **M21.33 Wrist drop (acquired)**

M21.331 Wrist drop, right **wrist**

M21.332 Wrist drop, left **wrist**

M21.339 Wrist drop, unspecified wrist

√6ᵗʰ **M21.37 Foot drop (acquired)**

M21.371 Foot drop, right **foot**

M21.372 Foot drop, left **foot**

M21.379 Foot drop, unspecified foot

√5ᵗʰ **M21.4 Flat foot [pes planus] (acquired)**

  EXCLUDES 1   congenital pes planus (Q66.5-)

M21.40 Flat foot [pes planus] (acquired), unspecified foot

M21.41 Flat foot [pes planus] (acquired), right **foot**

M21.42 Flat foot [pes planus] (acquired), left **foot**

√5ᵗʰ **M21.5 Acquired** clawhand, clubhand, clawfoot and clubfoot

  EXCLUDES 1   clubfoot, not specified as acquired (Q66.89)

√6ᵗʰ **M21.51 Acquired** clawhand

M21.511 Acquired clawhand, right **hand**

M21.512 Acquired clawhand, left **hand**

M21.519 Acquired clawhand, unspecified hand

√6ᵗʰ **M21.52 Acquired** clubhand

M21.521 Acquired clubhand, right **hand**

M21.522 Acquired clubhand, left **hand**

M21.529 Acquired clubhand, unspecified hand

√6ᵗʰ **M21.53 Acquired** clawfoot

DEF: High foot arch with hyperextended toes at the metatarsophalangeal joint and flexed toes at the distal joints.

M21.531 Acquired clawfoot, right **foot**

M21.532 Acquired clawfoot, left **foot**

M21.539 Acquired clawfoot, unspecified foot

√6ᵗʰ **M21.54 Acquired** clubfoot

DEF: Acquired anomaly of the foot with the heel elevated and rotated outward and the toes pointing inward.

M21.541 Acquired clubfoot, right **foot**

M21.542 Acquired clubfoot, left **foot**

M21.549 Acquired clubfoot, unspecified foot

√5ᵗʰ **M21.6 Other acquired deformities of foot**

  EXCLUDES 2   deformities of toe (acquired) (M20.1-M20.6-)

AHA: 2016,4Q,38

√6ᵗʰ **M21.61 Bunion**

M21.611 Bunion of right **foot**

M21.612 Bunion of left **foot**

M21.619 Bunion of unspecified foot

√6ᵗʰ **M21.62 Bunionette**

M21.621 Bunionette of right **foot**

M21.622 Bunionette of left **foot**

M21.629 Bunionette of unspecified foot

√6ᵗʰ **M21.6X Other acquired deformities of** foot

M21.6X1 Other acquired deformities of right **foot**

M21.6X2 Other acquired deformities of left **foot**

M21.6X9 Other acquired deformities of unspecified foot

√5ᵗʰ **M21.7 Unequal limb length (acquired)**

  NOTE   The site used should correspond to the shorter limb

M21.70 Unequal limb length (acquired), unspecified site

√6ᵗʰ **M21.72 Unequal limb length (acquired),** humerus

M21.721 Unequal limb length (acquired), right **humerus**

HCC CMS-HCC   **Rx** Rx HCC   **ESR** ESRD HCC   **COM** Commercial HCC   **N** Newborn: 0   **P** Pediatric: 0-17   **M** Maternity: 9-64   **A** Adult: 15-124

802   ICD-10-CM 2023

M21.722 Unequal limb length (acquired), left humerus

M21.729 Unequal limb length (acquired), unspecified humerus

√6ᵗʰ M21.73 Unequal limb length (acquired), ulna and radius

M21.731 Unequal limb length (acquired), right ulna

M21.732 Unequal limb length (acquired), left ulna

M21.733 Unequal limb length (acquired), right radius

M21.734 Unequal limb length (acquired), left radius

M21.739 Unequal limb length (acquired), unspecified ulna and radius

√6ᵗʰ M21.75 Unequal limb length (acquired), femur

M21.751 Unequal limb length (acquired), right femur

M21.752 Unequal limb length (acquired), left femur

M21.759 Unequal limb length (acquired), unspecified femur

√6ᵗʰ M21.76 Unequal limb length (acquired), tibia and fibula

M21.761 Unequal limb length (acquired), right tibia

M21.762 Unequal limb length (acquired), left tibia

M21.763 Unequal limb length (acquired), right fibula

M21.764 Unequal limb length (acquired), left fibula

M21.769 Unequal limb length (acquired), unspecified tibia and fibula

√5ᵗʰ M21.8 Other specified acquired deformities of limbs

EXCLUDES 2   coxa plana (M91.2)

M21.80 Other specified acquired deformities of unspecified limb

√6ᵗʰ M21.82 Other specified acquired deformities of upper arm

M21.821 Other specified acquired deformities of right upper arm

M21.822 Other specified acquired deformities of left upper arm

M21.829 Other specified acquired deformities of unspecified upper arm

√6ᵗʰ M21.83 Other specified acquired deformities of forearm

M21.831 Other specified acquired deformities of right forearm

M21.832 Other specified acquired deformities of left forearm

M21.839 Other specified acquired deformities of unspecified forearm

√6ᵗʰ M21.85 Other specified acquired deformities of thigh

M21.851 Other specified acquired deformities of right thigh

M21.852 Other specified acquired deformities of left thigh

M21.859 Other specified acquired deformities of unspecified thigh

√6ᵗʰ M21.86 Other specified acquired deformities of lower leg

M21.861 Other specified acquired deformities of right lower leg

M21.862 Other specified acquired deformities of left lower leg

M21.869 Other specified acquired deformities of unspecified lower leg

√5ᵗʰ M21.9 Unspecified acquired deformity of limb and hand

M21.90 Unspecified acquired deformity of unspecified limb

√6ᵗʰ M21.92 Unspecified acquired deformity of upper arm

M21.921 Unspecified acquired deformity of right upper arm

M21.922 Unspecified acquired deformity of left upper arm

M21.929 Unspecified acquired deformity of unspecified upper arm

√6ᵗʰ M21.93 Unspecified acquired deformity of forearm

M21.931 Unspecified acquired deformity of right forearm

M21.932 Unspecified acquired deformity of left forearm

M21.939 Unspecified acquired deformity of unspecified forearm

√6ᵗʰ M21.94 Unspecified acquired deformity of hand

M21.941 Unspecified acquired deformity of hand, right hand

M21.942 Unspecified acquired deformity of hand, left hand

M21.949 Unspecified acquired deformity of hand, unspecified hand

√6ᵗʰ M21.95 Unspecified acquired deformity of thigh

M21.951 Unspecified acquired deformity of right thigh

M21.952 Unspecified acquired deformity of left thigh

M21.959 Unspecified acquired deformity of unspecified thigh

√6ᵗʰ M21.96 Unspecified acquired deformity of lower leg

M21.961 Unspecified acquired deformity of right lower leg

M21.962 Unspecified acquired deformity of left lower leg

M21.969 Unspecified acquired deformity of unspecified lower leg

√4ᵗʰ **M22 Disorder of patella**

EXCLUDES 2   traumatic dislocation of patella (S83.0-)

√5ᵗʰ M22.0 Recurrent dislocation of patella

M22.00 Recurrent dislocation of patella, unspecified knee

M22.01 Recurrent dislocation of patella, right knee

M22.02 Recurrent dislocation of patella, left knee

√5ᵗʰ M22.1 Recurrent subluxation of patella

Incomplete dislocation of patella

M22.10 Recurrent subluxation of patella, unspecified knee

M22.11 Recurrent subluxation of patella, right knee

M22.12 Recurrent subluxation of patella, left knee

√5ᵗʰ M22.2 Patellofemoral disorders

√6ᵗʰ M22.2X Patellofemoral disorders

M22.2X1 Patellofemoral disorders, right knee

M22.2X2 Patellofemoral disorders, left knee

M22.2X9 Patellofemoral disorders, unspecified knee

√5ᵗʰ M22.3 Other derangements of patella

√6ᵗʰ M22.3X Other derangements of patella

M22.3X1 Other derangements of patella, right knee

M22.3X2 Other derangements of patella, left knee

M22.3X9 Other derangements of patella, unspecified knee

√5ᵗʰ M22.4 Chondromalacia patellae

M22.40 Chondromalacia patellae, unspecified knee

M22.41 Chondromalacia patellae, right knee

M22.42 Chondromalacia patellae, left knee

√5ᵗʰ M22.8 Other disorders of patella

√6ᵗʰ M22.8X Other disorders of patella

M22.8X1 Other disorders of patella, right knee

M22.8X2 Other disorders of patella, left knee

M22.8X9 Other disorders of patella, unspecified knee

√5ᵗʰ M22.9 Unspecified disorder of patella

M22.90 Unspecified disorder of patella, unspecified knee

M22.91 Unspecified disorder of patella, right knee

M22.92 Unspecified disorder of patella, left knee

√4ᵗʰ **M23 Internal derangement of knee**

EXCLUDES 1   ankylosis (M24.66)

deformity of knee (M21.-)

osteochondritis dissecans (M93.2)

EXCLUDES 2   current injury - see injury of knee and lower leg (S80-S89)

recurrent dislocation or subluxation of joints (M24.4)

recurrent dislocation or subluxation of patella (M22.0-M22.1)

√5ᵗʰ M23.0 Cystic meniscus

√6ᵗʰ M23.00 Cystic meniscus, unspecified meniscus

Cystic meniscus, unspecified lateral meniscus

Cystic meniscus, unspecified medial meniscus

M23.000 Cystic meniscus, unspecified lateral meniscus, right knee

M23.001 Cystic meniscus, unspecified lateral meniscus, left knee

M23.002 Cystic meniscus, unspecified lateral meniscus, unspecified knee

M23.003 Cystic meniscus, unspecified medial meniscus, right knee

M23.004 Cystic meniscus, unspecified medial meniscus, left knee

M23.005 Cystic meniscus, unspecified medial meniscus, unspecified knee

M23.006 Cystic meniscus, unspecified meniscus, right knee

M23.007 Cystic meniscus, unspecified meniscus, left knee

M23.009 Cystic meniscus, unspecified meniscus, unspecified knee

✓6ᵗʰ M23.01 Cystic meniscus, anterior horn of medial meniscus

M23.011 Cystic meniscus, anterior horn of medial meniscus, right knee

M23.012 Cystic meniscus, anterior horn of medial meniscus, left knee

M23.019 Cystic meniscus, anterior horn of medial meniscus, unspecified knee

✓6ᵗʰ M23.02 Cystic meniscus, posterior horn of medial meniscus

M23.021 Cystic meniscus, posterior horn of medial meniscus, right knee

M23.022 Cystic meniscus, posterior horn of medial meniscus, left knee

M23.029 Cystic meniscus, posterior horn of medial meniscus, unspecified knee

✓6ᵗʰ M23.03 Cystic meniscus, other medial meniscus

M23.031 Cystic meniscus, other medial meniscus, right knee

M23.032 Cystic meniscus, other medial meniscus, left knee

M23.039 Cystic meniscus, other medial meniscus, unspecified knee

✓6ᵗʰ M23.04 Cystic meniscus, anterior horn of lateral meniscus

M23.041 Cystic meniscus, anterior horn of lateral meniscus, right knee

M23.042 Cystic meniscus, anterior horn of lateral meniscus, left knee

M23.049 Cystic meniscus, anterior horn of lateral meniscus, unspecified knee

✓6ᵗʰ M23.05 Cystic meniscus, posterior horn of lateral meniscus

M23.051 Cystic meniscus, posterior horn of lateral meniscus, right knee

M23.052 Cystic meniscus, posterior horn of lateral meniscus, left knee

M23.059 Cystic meniscus, posterior horn of lateral meniscus, unspecified knee

✓6ᵗʰ M23.06 Cystic meniscus, other lateral meniscus

M23.061 Cystic meniscus, other lateral meniscus, right knee

M23.062 Cystic meniscus, other lateral meniscus, left knee

M23.069 Cystic meniscus, other lateral meniscus, unspecified knee

✓5ᵗʰ M23.2 Derangement of meniscus due to old tear or injury

Old bucket-handle tear

AHA: 2019,2Q,26

Derangement of Meniscus

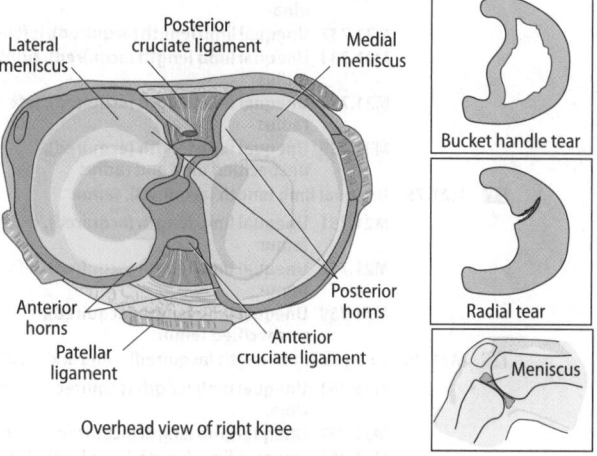

Overhead view of right knee

Bucket handle tear

Radial tear

Meniscus

✓6ᵗʰ M23.20 Derangement of unspecified meniscus due to old tear or injury

Derangement of unspecified lateral meniscus due to old tear or injury

Derangement of unspecified medial meniscus due to old tear or injury

M23.200 Derangement of unspecified lateral meniscus due to old tear or injury, right knee

M23.201 Derangement of unspecified lateral meniscus due to old tear or injury, left knee

M23.202 Derangement of unspecified lateral meniscus due to old tear or injury, unspecified knee

M23.203 Derangement of unspecified medial meniscus due to old tear or injury, right knee

M23.204 Derangement of unspecified medial meniscus due to old tear or injury, left knee

M23.205 Derangement of unspecified medial meniscus due to old tear or injury, unspecified knee

M23.206 Derangement of unspecified meniscus due to old tear or injury, right knee

M23.207 Derangement of unspecified meniscus due to old tear or injury, left knee

M23.209 Derangement of unspecified meniscus due to old tear or injury, unspecified knee

✓6ᵗʰ M23.21 Derangement of anterior horn of medial meniscus due to old tear or injury

M23.211 Derangement of anterior horn of medial meniscus due to old tear or injury, right knee

M23.212 Derangement of anterior horn of medial meniscus due to old tear or injury, left knee

M23.219 Derangement of anterior horn of medial meniscus due to old tear or injury, unspecified knee

✓6ᵗʰ M23.22 Derangement of posterior horn of medial meniscus due to old tear or injury

M23.221 Derangement of posterior horn of medial meniscus due to old tear or injury, right knee

M23.222 Derangement of posterior horn of medial meniscus due to old tear or injury, left knee

M23.229 Derangement of posterior horn of medial meniscus due to old tear or injury, unspecified knee

✓6ᵗʰ M23.23 Derangement of other medial meniscus due to old tear or injury

M23.231 Derangement of other medial meniscus due to old tear or injury, right knee

M23.232   Derangement of other medial meniscus due to old tear or injury, **left** knee

M23.239   Derangement of other medial meniscus due to old tear or injury, unspecified knee

√6ᵗʰ **M23.24** Derangement of **anterior horn of lateral** meniscus due to old tear or injury

M23.241   Derangement of anterior horn of lateral meniscus due to old tear or injury, **right** knee

M23.242   Derangement of anterior horn of lateral meniscus due to old tear or injury, **left** knee

M23.249   Derangement of anterior horn of lateral meniscus due to old tear or injury, unspecified knee

√6ᵗʰ **M23.25** Derangement of **posterior horn of lateral** meniscus due to old tear or injury

M23.251   Derangement of posterior horn of lateral meniscus due to old tear or injury, **right** knee

M23.252   Derangement of posterior horn of lateral meniscus due to old tear or injury, **left** knee

M23.259   Derangement of posterior horn of lateral meniscus due to old tear or injury, unspecified knee

√6ᵗʰ **M23.26** Derangement of **other lateral** meniscus due to old tear or injury

M23.261   Derangement of other lateral meniscus due to old tear or injury, **right** knee

M23.262   Derangement of other lateral meniscus due to old tear or injury, **left** knee

M23.269   Derangement of other lateral meniscus due to old tear or injury, unspecified knee

√5ᵗʰ **M23.3**   **Other meniscus derangements**

Degenerate meniscus
Detached meniscus
Retained meniscus

√6ᵗʰ **M23.30** Other meniscus derangements, unspecified meniscus

Other meniscus derangements, unspecified lateral meniscus

Other meniscus derangements, unspecified medial meniscus

M23.300   Other meniscus derangements, unspecified **lateral** meniscus, **right** knee

M23.301   Other meniscus derangements, unspecified **lateral** meniscus, **left** knee

M23.302   Other meniscus derangements, unspecified **lateral** meniscus, unspecified knee

M23.303   Other meniscus derangements, unspecified **medial** meniscus, **right** knee

M23.304   Other meniscus derangements, unspecified **medial** meniscus, **left** knee

M23.305   Other meniscus derangements, unspecified **medial** meniscus, unspecified knee

M23.306   Other meniscus derangements, unspecified meniscus, **right** knee

M23.307   Other meniscus derangements, unspecified meniscus, **left** knee

M23.309   Other meniscus derangements, unspecified meniscus, unspecified knee

√6ᵗʰ **M23.31** Other meniscus derangements, **anterior horn of medial** meniscus

M23.311   Other meniscus derangements, anterior horn of medial meniscus, **right** knee

M23.312   Other meniscus derangements, anterior horn of medial meniscus, **left** knee

M23.319   Other meniscus derangements, anterior horn of medial meniscus, unspecified knee

√6ᵗʰ **M23.32** Other meniscus derangements, **posterior horn of medial** meniscus

M23.321   Other meniscus derangements, posterior horn of medial meniscus, **right** knee

M23.322   Other meniscus derangements, posterior horn of medial meniscus, **left** knee

M23.329   Other meniscus derangements, posterior horn of medial meniscus, unspecified knee

√6ᵗʰ **M23.33** Other meniscus derangements, **other medial** meniscus

M23.331   Other meniscus derangements, other medial meniscus, **right** knee

M23.332   Other meniscus derangements, other medial meniscus, **left** knee

M23.339   Other meniscus derangements, other medial meniscus, unspecified knee

√6ᵗʰ **M23.34** Other meniscus derangements, **anterior horn of lateral** meniscus

M23.341   Other meniscus derangements, anterior horn of lateral meniscus, **right** knee

M23.342   Other meniscus derangements, anterior horn of lateral meniscus, **left** knee

M23.349   Other meniscus derangements, anterior horn of lateral meniscus, unspecified knee

√6ᵗʰ **M23.35** Other meniscus derangements, **posterior horn of lateral** meniscus

M23.351   Other meniscus derangements, posterior horn of lateral meniscus, **right** knee

M23.352   Other meniscus derangements, posterior horn of lateral meniscus, **left** knee

M23.359   Other meniscus derangements, posterior horn of lateral meniscus, unspecified knee

√6ᵗʰ **M23.36** Other meniscus derangements, **other lateral** meniscus

M23.361   Other meniscus derangements, other lateral meniscus, **right** knee

M23.362   Other meniscus derangements, other lateral meniscus, **left** knee

M23.369   Other meniscus derangements, other lateral meniscus, unspecified knee

√5ᵗʰ **M23.4**   **Loose body in knee**

M23.40   Loose body in knee, unspecified knee

M23.41   Loose body in knee, **right** knee

M23.42   Loose body in knee, **left** knee

√5ᵗʰ **M23.5**   **Chronic instability of knee**

M23.50   Chronic instability of knee, unspecified knee

M23.51   Chronic instability of knee, **right** knee

M23.52   Chronic instability of knee, **left** knee

√5ᵗʰ **M23.6**   **Other spontaneous disruption of ligament(s) of knee**

√6ᵗʰ **M23.60** Other spontaneous disruption of unspecified ligament of knee

M23.601   Other spontaneous disruption of unspecified ligament of **right** knee

M23.602   Other spontaneous disruption of unspecified ligament of **left** knee

M23.609   Other spontaneous disruption of unspecified ligament of unspecified knee

√6ᵗʰ **M23.61** Other spontaneous disruption of **anterior cruciate** ligament of knee

M23.611   Other spontaneous disruption of anterior cruciate ligament of **right** knee

M23.612   Other spontaneous disruption of anterior cruciate ligament of **left** knee

M23.619   Other spontaneous disruption of anterior cruciate ligament of unspecified knee

√6ᵗʰ **M23.62** Other spontaneous disruption of **posterior cruciate** ligament of knee

M23.621   Other spontaneous disruption of posterior cruciate ligament of **right** knee

M23.622   Other spontaneous disruption of posterior cruciate ligament of **left** knee

M23.629   Other spontaneous disruption of posterior cruciate ligament of unspecified knee

√6ᵗʰ **M23.63** Other spontaneous disruption of **medial collateral** ligament of knee

M23.631   Other spontaneous disruption of medial collateral ligament of **right** knee

M23.632   Other spontaneous disruption of medial collateral ligament of **left** knee

M23.639   Other spontaneous disruption of medial collateral ligament of unspecified knee

√6ᵗʰ **M23.64** Other spontaneous disruption of **lateral collateral** ligament of knee

M23.641   Other spontaneous disruption of lateral collateral ligament of **right** knee

M23.642   Other spontaneous disruption of lateral collateral ligament of **left** knee

---

☑ Additional Character Required   √x7ᵗʰ Placeholder Alert   Manifestation   Unspecified Dx   ℚ QPP   ᵁᴾᴰ Unacceptable PDx

M23.649 Other spontaneous disruption of lateral collateral ligament of unspecified knee

✓6ᵗʰ **M23.67** Other spontaneous disruption of capsular ligament of knee

M23.671 Other spontaneous disruption of capsular ligament of right knee

M23.672 Other spontaneous disruption of capsular ligament of left knee

M23.679 Other spontaneous disruption of capsular ligament of unspecified knee

✓5ᵗʰ **M23.8** Other internal derangements of knee

Laxity of ligament of knee
Snapping knee

✓6ᵗʰ **M23.8X** Other internal derangements of knee

M23.8X1 Other internal derangements of right knee

M23.8X2 Other internal derangements of left knee

M23.8X9 Other internal derangements of unspecified knee

✓5ᵗʰ **M23.9** Unspecified internal derangement of knee

M23.90 Unspecified internal derangement of unspecified knee

M23.91 Unspecified internal derangement of right knee

M23.92 Unspecified internal derangement of left knee

✓4ᵗʰ **M24** **Other specific joint derangements**

> **EXCLUDES 1**   *current injury - see injury of joint by body region*
> **EXCLUDES 2**   *ganglion (M67.4)*
> *snapping knee (M23.8-)*
> *temporomandibular joint disorders (M26.6-)*

AHA: 2020,4Q,31-32

✓5ᵗʰ **M24.0** Loose body in joint

> **EXCLUDES 2**   *loose body in knee (M23.4)*

M24.00 Loose body in unspecified joint

✓6ᵗʰ **M24.01** Loose body in shoulder

M24.011 Loose body in right shoulder
M24.012 Loose body in left shoulder
M24.019 Loose body in unspecified shoulder

✓6ᵗʰ **M24.02** Loose body in elbow

M24.021 Loose body in right elbow
M24.022 Loose body in left elbow
M24.029 Loose body in unspecified elbow

✓6ᵗʰ **M24.03** Loose body in wrist

M24.031 Loose body in right wrist
M24.032 Loose body in left wrist
M24.039 Loose body in unspecified wrist

✓6ᵗʰ **M24.04** Loose body in finger joints

M24.041 Loose body in right finger joint(s)
M24.042 Loose body in left finger joint(s)
M24.049 Loose body in unspecified finger joint(s)

✓6ᵗʰ **M24.05** Loose body in hip

M24.051 Loose body in right hip
M24.052 Loose body in left hip
M24.059 Loose body in unspecified hip

✓6ᵗʰ **M24.07** Loose body in ankle and toe joints

M24.071 Loose body in right ankle
M24.072 Loose body in left ankle
M24.073 Loose body in unspecified ankle
M24.074 Loose body in right toe joint(s)
M24.075 Loose body in left toe joint(s)
M24.076 Loose body in unspecified toe joints

M24.08 Loose body, other site

✓5ᵗʰ **M24.1** Other articular cartilage disorders

> **EXCLUDES 2**   *chondrocalcinosis (M11.1, M11.2-)*
> *internal derangement of knee (M23.-)*
> *metastatic calcification (E83.5)*
> *ochronosis (E70.2)*

M24.10 Other articular cartilage disorders, unspecified site

✓6ᵗʰ **M24.11** Other articular cartilage disorders, shoulder

M24.111 Other articular cartilage disorders, right shoulder

M24.112 Other articular cartilage disorders, left shoulder

M24.119 Other articular cartilage disorders, unspecified shoulder

✓6ᵗʰ **M24.12** Other articular cartilage disorders, elbow

M24.121 Other articular cartilage disorders, right elbow

M24.122 Other articular cartilage disorders, left elbow

M24.129 Other articular cartilage disorders, unspecified elbow

✓6ᵗʰ **M24.13** Other articular cartilage disorders, wrist

M24.131 Other articular cartilage disorders, right wrist

M24.132 Other articular cartilage disorders, left wrist

M24.139 Other articular cartilage disorders, unspecified wrist

✓6ᵗʰ **M24.14** Other articular cartilage disorders, hand

M24.141 Other articular cartilage disorders, right hand

M24.142 Other articular cartilage disorders, left hand

M24.149 Other articular cartilage disorders, unspecified hand

✓6ᵗʰ **M24.15** Other articular cartilage disorders, hip

M24.151 Other articular cartilage disorders, right hip

M24.152 Other articular cartilage disorders, left hip

M24.159 Other articular cartilage disorders, unspecified hip

✓6ᵗʰ **M24.17** Other articular cartilage disorders, ankle and foot

M24.171 Other articular cartilage disorders, right ankle

M24.172 Other articular cartilage disorders, left ankle

M24.173 Other articular cartilage disorders, unspecified ankle

M24.174 Other articular cartilage disorders, right foot

M24.175 Other articular cartilage disorders, left foot

M24.176 Other articular cartilage disorders, unspecified foot

M24.19 Other articular cartilage disorders, other specified site

✓5ᵗʰ **M24.2** Disorder of ligament

Instability secondary to old ligament injury
Ligamentous laxity NOS

> **EXCLUDES 1**   *familial ligamentous laxity (M35.7)*
> **EXCLUDES 2**   *internal derangement of knee (M23.5-M23.8X9)*

M24.20 Disorder of ligament, unspecified site

✓6ᵗʰ **M24.21** Disorder of ligament, shoulder

M24.211 Disorder of ligament, right shoulder
M24.212 Disorder of ligament, left shoulder
M24.219 Disorder of ligament, unspecified shoulder

✓6ᵗʰ **M24.22** Disorder of ligament, elbow

M24.221 Disorder of ligament, right elbow
M24.222 Disorder of ligament, left elbow
M24.229 Disorder of ligament, unspecified elbow

✓6ᵗʰ **M24.23** Disorder of ligament, wrist

M24.231 Disorder of ligament, right wrist
M24.232 Disorder of ligament, left wrist
M24.239 Disorder of ligament, unspecified wrist

✓6ᵗʰ **M24.24** Disorder of ligament, hand

M24.241 Disorder of ligament, right hand
M24.242 Disorder of ligament, left hand
M24.249 Disorder of ligament, unspecified hand

✓6ᵗʰ **M24.25** Disorder of ligament, hip

M24.251 Disorder of ligament, right hip
M24.252 Disorder of ligament, left hip
M24.259 Disorder of ligament, unspecified hip

✓6ᵗʰ **M24.27** Disorder of ligament, ankle and foot

M24.271 Disorder of ligament, right ankle
M24.272 Disorder of ligament, left ankle
M24.273 Disorder of ligament, unspecified ankle
M24.274 Disorder of ligament, right foot
M24.275 Disorder of ligament, left foot
M24.276 Disorder of ligament, unspecified foot

M24.28 Disorder of ligament, vertebrae

M24.29   Disorder of ligament, other specified site

☑5ᵗʰ **M24.3**   **Pathological dislocation of joint, not elsewhere classified**

> EXCLUDES 1   *congenital dislocation or displacement of joint - see congenital malformations and deformations of the musculoskeletal system (Q65-Q79)*
> *current injury - see injury of joints and ligaments by body region*
> *recurrent dislocation of joint (M24.4-)*

    M24.30   Pathological dislocation of unspecified joint, not elsewhere classified

   ☑6ᵗʰ **M24.31**   Pathological dislocation of shoulder, not elsewhere classified

     M24.311   Pathological dislocation of right shoulder, not elsewhere classified

     M24.312   Pathological dislocation of left shoulder, not elsewhere classified

     M24.319   Pathological dislocation of unspecified shoulder, not elsewhere classified

   ☑6ᵗʰ **M24.32**   Pathological dislocation of elbow, not elsewhere classified

     M24.321   Pathological dislocation of right elbow, not elsewhere classified

     M24.322   Pathological dislocation of left elbow, not elsewhere classified

     M24.329   Pathological dislocation of unspecified elbow, not elsewhere classified

   ☑6ᵗʰ **M24.33**   Pathological dislocation of wrist, not elsewhere classified

     M24.331   Pathological dislocation of right wrist, not elsewhere classified

     M24.332   Pathological dislocation of left wrist, not elsewhere classified

     M24.339   Pathological dislocation of unspecified wrist, not elsewhere classified

   ☑6ᵗʰ **M24.34**   Pathological dislocation of hand, not elsewhere classified

     M24.341   Pathological dislocation of right hand, not elsewhere classified

     M24.342   Pathological dislocation of left hand, not elsewhere classified

     M24.349   Pathological dislocation of unspecified hand, not elsewhere classified

   ☑6ᵗʰ **M24.35**   Pathological dislocation of hip, not elsewhere classified

     AHA: 2022,1Q,32

     M24.351   Pathological dislocation of right hip, not elsewhere classified

     M24.352   Pathological dislocation of left hip, not elsewhere classified

     M24.359   Pathological dislocation of unspecified hip, not elsewhere classified

   ☑6ᵗʰ **M24.36**   Pathological dislocation of knee, not elsewhere classified

     M24.361   Pathological dislocation of right knee, not elsewhere classified

     M24.362   Pathological dislocation of left knee, not elsewhere classified

     M24.369   Pathological dislocation of unspecified knee, not elsewhere classified

   ☑6ᵗʰ **M24.37**   Pathological dislocation of ankle and foot, not elsewhere classified

     M24.371   Pathological dislocation of right ankle, not elsewhere classified

     M24.372   Pathological dislocation of left ankle, not elsewhere classified

     M24.373   Pathological dislocation of unspecified ankle, not elsewhere classified

     M24.374   Pathological dislocation of right foot, not elsewhere classified

     M24.375   Pathological dislocation of left foot, not elsewhere classified

     M24.376   Pathological dislocation of unspecified foot, not elsewhere classified

    M24.39   Pathological dislocation of other specified joint, not elsewhere classified

☑5ᵗʰ **M24.4**   **Recurrent dislocation of joint**

    Recurrent subluxation of joint

> EXCLUDES 2   *recurrent dislocation of patella (M22.0-M22.1)*
> *recurrent vertebral dislocation (M43.3-, M43.4, M43.5-)*

    M24.40   Recurrent dislocation, unspecified joint

   ☑6ᵗʰ **M24.41**   Recurrent dislocation, shoulder

     M24.411   Recurrent dislocation, right shoulder
     M24.412   Recurrent dislocation, left shoulder
     M24.419   Recurrent dislocation, unspecified shoulder

   ☑6ᵗʰ **M24.42**   Recurrent dislocation, elbow

     M24.421   Recurrent dislocation, right elbow
     M24.422   Recurrent dislocation, left elbow
     M24.429   Recurrent dislocation, unspecified elbow

   ☑6ᵗʰ **M24.43**   Recurrent dislocation, wrist

     M24.431   Recurrent dislocation, right wrist
     M24.432   Recurrent dislocation, left wrist
     M24.439   Recurrent dislocation, unspecified wrist

   ☑6ᵗʰ **M24.44**   Recurrent dislocation, hand and finger(s)

     M24.441   Recurrent dislocation, right hand
     M24.442   Recurrent dislocation, left hand
     M24.443   Recurrent dislocation, unspecified hand
     M24.444   Recurrent dislocation, right finger
     M24.445   Recurrent dislocation, left finger
     M24.446   Recurrent dislocation, unspecified finger

   ☑6ᵗʰ **M24.45**   Recurrent dislocation, hip

     M24.451   Recurrent dislocation, right hip
     M24.452   Recurrent dislocation, left hip
     M24.459   Recurrent dislocation, unspecified hip

   ☑6ᵗʰ **M24.46**   Recurrent dislocation, knee

     M24.461   Recurrent dislocation, right knee
     M24.462   Recurrent dislocation, left knee
     M24.469   Recurrent dislocation, unspecified knee

   ☑6ᵗʰ **M24.47**   Recurrent dislocation, ankle, foot and toes

     M24.471   Recurrent dislocation, right ankle
     M24.472   Recurrent dislocation, left ankle
     M24.473   Recurrent dislocation, unspecified ankle
     M24.474   Recurrent dislocation, right foot
     M24.475   Recurrent dislocation, left foot
     M24.476   Recurrent dislocation, unspecified foot
     M24.477   Recurrent dislocation, right toe(s)
     M24.478   Recurrent dislocation, left toe(s)
     M24.479   Recurrent dislocation, unspecified toe(s)

    M24.49   Recurrent dislocation, other specified joint

☑5ᵗʰ **M24.5**   **Contracture of joint**

> EXCLUDES 1   *contracture of muscle without contracture of joint (M62.4-)*
> *contracture of tendon (sheath) without contracture of joint (M62.4-)*
> *Dupuytren's contracture (M72.0)*
>
> EXCLUDES 2   *acquired deformities of limbs (M20-M21)*

    AHA: 2016,2Q,6

    M24.50   Contracture, unspecified joint

   ☑6ᵗʰ **M24.51**   Contracture, shoulder

     M24.511   Contracture, right shoulder
     M24.512   Contracture, left shoulder
     M24.519   Contracture, unspecified shoulder

   ☑6ᵗʰ **M24.52**   Contracture, elbow

     M24.521   Contracture, right elbow
     M24.522   Contracture, left elbow
     M24.529   Contracture, unspecified elbow

   ☑6ᵗʰ **M24.53**   Contracture, wrist

     M24.531   Contracture, right wrist
     M24.532   Contracture, left wrist
     M24.539   Contracture, unspecified wrist

   ☑6ᵗʰ **M24.54**   Contracture, hand

     M24.541   Contracture, right hand
     M24.542   Contracture, left hand
     M24.549   Contracture, unspecified hand

   ☑6ᵗʰ **M24.55**   Contracture, hip

     M24.551   Contracture, right hip
     M24.552   Contracture, left hip
     M24.559   Contracture, unspecified hip

   ☑6ᵗʰ **M24.56**   Contracture, knee

     M24.561   Contracture, right knee
     M24.562   Contracture, left knee
     M24.569   Contracture, unspecified knee

   ☑6ᵗʰ **M24.57**   Contracture, ankle and foot

     M24.571   Contracture, right ankle
     M24.572   Contracture, left ankle

M24.573 Contracture, unspecified ankle
M24.574 Contracture, right foot
M24.575 Contracture, left foot
M24.576 Contracture, unspecified foot
M24.59 Contracture, other specified joint

√5ᵗʰ **M24.6 Ankylosis of joint**

EXCLUDES 1   stiffness of joint without ankylosis (M25.6-)
EXCLUDES 2   spine (M43.2-)
DEF: Ankylosis: Abnormal union or fusion of bones in a joint, which is normally moveable.

M24.60 Ankylosis, unspecified joint

√6ᵗʰ **M24.61** Ankylosis, shoulder
M24.611 Ankylosis, right shoulder
M24.612 Ankylosis, left shoulder
M24.619 Ankylosis, unspecified shoulder

√6ᵗʰ **M24.62** Ankylosis, elbow
M24.621 Ankylosis, right elbow
M24.622 Ankylosis, left elbow
M24.629 Ankylosis, unspecified elbow

√6ᵗʰ **M24.63** Ankylosis, wrist
M24.631 Ankylosis, right wrist
M24.632 Ankylosis, left wrist
M24.639 Ankylosis, unspecified wrist

√6ᵗʰ **M24.64** Ankylosis, hand
M24.641 Ankylosis, right hand
M24.642 Ankylosis, left hand
M24.649 Ankylosis, unspecified hand

√6ᵗʰ **M24.65** Ankylosis, hip
M24.651 Ankylosis, right hip
M24.652 Ankylosis, left hip
M24.659 Ankylosis, unspecified hip

√6ᵗʰ **M24.66** Ankylosis, knee
M24.661 Ankylosis, right knee
M24.662 Ankylosis, left knee
M24.669 Ankylosis, unspecified knee

√6ᵗʰ **M24.67** Ankylosis, ankle and foot
M24.671 Ankylosis, right ankle
M24.672 Ankylosis, left ankle
M24.673 Ankylosis, unspecified ankle
M24.674 Ankylosis, right foot
M24.675 Ankylosis, left foot
M24.676 Ankylosis, unspecified foot
M24.69 Ankylosis, other specified joint

M24.7 Protrusio acetabuli
DEF: Intrapelvic protrusion of the acetabulum characterized by the sinking of the floor of the acetabulum, causing the femoral head to protrude. It limits hip movement and is of unknown etiology. *Synonym(s):* Otto's pelvis.

√5ᵗʰ **M24.8 Other specific joint derangements, not elsewhere classified**
EXCLUDES 2   iliotibial band syndrome (M76.3)

M24.80 Other specific joint derangements of unspecified joint, not elsewhere classified

√6ᵗʰ **M24.81** Other specific joint derangements of shoulder, not elsewhere classified
M24.811 Other specific joint derangements of right shoulder, not elsewhere classified
M24.812 Other specific joint derangements of left shoulder, not elsewhere classified
M24.819 Other specific joint derangements of unspecified shoulder, not elsewhere classified

√6ᵗʰ **M24.82** Other specific joint derangements of elbow, not elsewhere classified
M24.821 Other specific joint derangements of right elbow, not elsewhere classified
M24.822 Other specific joint derangements of left elbow, not elsewhere classified
M24.829 Other specific joint derangements of unspecified elbow, not elsewhere classified

√6ᵗʰ **M24.83** Other specific joint derangements of wrist, not elsewhere classified
M24.831 Other specific joint derangements of right wrist, not elsewhere classified
M24.832 Other specific joint derangements of left wrist, not elsewhere classified
M24.839 Other specific joint derangements of unspecified wrist, not elsewhere classified

√6ᵗʰ **M24.84** Other specific joint derangements of hand, not elsewhere classified
M24.841 Other specific joint derangements of right hand, not elsewhere classified
M24.842 Other specific joint derangements of left hand, not elsewhere classified
M24.849 Other specific joint derangements of unspecified hand, not elsewhere classified

√6ᵗʰ **M24.85** Other specific joint derangements of hip, not elsewhere classified
Irritable hip
M24.851 Other specific joint derangements of right hip, not elsewhere classified
M24.852 Other specific joint derangements of left hip, not elsewhere classified
M24.859 Other specific joint derangements of unspecified hip, not elsewhere classified

√6ᵗʰ **M24.87** Other specific joint derangements of ankle and foot, not elsewhere classified
M24.871 Other specific joint derangements of right ankle, not elsewhere classified
M24.872 Other specific joint derangements of left ankle, not elsewhere classified
M24.873 Other specific joint derangements of unspecified ankle, not elsewhere classified
M24.874 Other specific joint derangements of right foot, not elsewhere classified
M24.875 Other specific joint derangements left foot, not elsewhere classified
M24.876 Other specific joint derangements of unspecified foot, not elsewhere classified
M24.89 Other specific joint derangement of other specified joint, not elsewhere classified

M24.9 Joint derangement, unspecified

√4ᵗʰ **M25 Other joint disorder, not elsewhere classified**
EXCLUDES 2   abnormality of gait and mobility (R26.-)
acquired deformities of limb (M20-M21)
calcification of bursa (M71.4-)
calcification of shoulder (joint) (M75.3)
calcification of tendon (M65.2-)
difficulty in walking (R26.2)
temporomandibular joint disorder (M26.6-)
AHA: 2020,4Q,31-32

√5ᵗʰ **M25.0 Hemarthrosis**
EXCLUDES 1   current injury - see injury of joint by body region
hemophilic arthropathy (M36.2)

M25.00 Hemarthrosis, unspecified joint

√6ᵗʰ **M25.01** Hemarthrosis, shoulder
M25.011 Hemarthrosis, right shoulder
M25.012 Hemarthrosis, left shoulder
M25.019 Hemarthrosis, unspecified shoulder

√6ᵗʰ **M25.02** Hemarthrosis, elbow
M25.021 Hemarthrosis, right elbow
M25.022 Hemarthrosis, left elbow
M25.029 Hemarthrosis, unspecified elbow

√6ᵗʰ **M25.03** Hemarthrosis, wrist
M25.031 Hemarthrosis, right wrist
M25.032 Hemarthrosis, left wrist
M25.039 Hemarthrosis, unspecified wrist

√6ᵗʰ **M25.04** Hemarthrosis, hand
M25.041 Hemarthrosis, right hand
M25.042 Hemarthrosis, left hand
M25.049 Hemarthrosis, unspecified hand

√6ᵗʰ **M25.05** Hemarthrosis, hip
M25.051 Hemarthrosis, right hip
M25.052 Hemarthrosis, left hip
M25.059 Hemarthrosis, unspecified hip

√6ᵗʰ **M25.06** Hemarthrosis, knee
M25.061 Hemarthrosis, right knee
M25.062 Hemarthrosis, left knee
M25.069 Hemarthrosis, unspecified knee

√6ᵗʰ **M25.07** Hemarthrosis, ankle and foot
M25.071 Hemarthrosis, right ankle
M25.072 Hemarthrosis, left ankle
M25.073 Hemarthrosis, unspecified ankle
M25.074 Hemarthrosis, right foot

M25.075 Hemarthrosis, **left foot**
M25.076 Hemarthrosis, **unspecified foot**
M25.08 Hemarthrosis, **other specified site**
    Hemarthrosis, vertebrae

√5ᵗʰ M25.1 **Fistula of joint**

M25.10 Fistula, **unspecified joint**
√6ᵗʰ M25.11 Fistula, **shoulder**

M25.111 Fistula, **right shoulder**
M25.112 Fistula, **left shoulder**
M25.119 Fistula, **unspecified shoulder**

√6ᵗʰ M25.12 Fistula, **elbow**

M25.121 Fistula, **right elbow**
M25.122 Fistula, **left elbow**
M25.129 Fistula, **unspecified elbow**

√6ᵗʰ M25.13 Fistula, **wrist**

M25.131 Fistula, **right wrist**
M25.132 Fistula, **left wrist**
M25.139 Fistula, **unspecified wrist**

√6ᵗʰ M25.14 Fistula, **hand**

M25.141 Fistula, **right hand**
M25.142 Fistula, **left hand**
M25.149 Fistula, **unspecified hand**

√6ᵗʰ M25.15 Fistula, **hip**

M25.151 Fistula, **right hip**
M25.152 Fistula, **left hip**
M25.159 Fistula, **unspecified hip**

√6ᵗʰ M25.16 Fistula, **knee**

M25.161 Fistula, **right knee**
M25.162 Fistula, **left knee**
M25.169 Fistula, **unspecified knee**

√6ᵗʰ M25.17 Fistula, **ankle and foot**

M25.171 Fistula, **right ankle**
M25.172 Fistula, **left ankle**
M25.173 Fistula, **unspecified ankle**
M25.174 Fistula, **right foot**
M25.175 Fistula, **left foot**
M25.176 Fistula, **unspecified foot**

M25.18 Fistula, **other specified site**
    Fistula, vertebrae

√5ᵗʰ M25.2 **Flail joint**

DEF: Hinged joint that exhibits an abnormal or excessive degree of range and mobility.

M25.20 Flail joint, **unspecified joint**
√6ᵗʰ M25.21 Flail joint, **shoulder**

M25.211 Flail joint, **right shoulder**
M25.212 Flail joint, **left shoulder**
M25.219 Flail joint, **unspecified shoulder**

√6ᵗʰ M25.22 Flail joint, **elbow**

M25.221 Flail joint, **right elbow**
M25.222 Flail joint, **left elbow**
M25.229 Flail joint, **unspecified elbow**

√6ᵗʰ M25.23 Flail joint, **wrist**

M25.231 Flail joint, **right wrist**
M25.232 Flail joint, **left wrist**
M25.239 Flail joint, **unspecified wrist**

√6ᵗʰ M25.24 Flail joint, **hand**

M25.241 Flail joint, **right hand**
M25.242 Flail joint, **left hand**
M25.249 Flail joint, **unspecified hand**

√6ᵗʰ M25.25 Flail joint, **hip**

M25.251 Flail joint, **right hip**
M25.252 Flail joint, **left hip**
M25.259 Flail joint, **unspecified hip**

√6ᵗʰ M25.26 Flail joint, **knee**

M25.261 Flail joint, **right knee**
M25.262 Flail joint, **left knee**
M25.269 Flail joint, **unspecified knee**

√6ᵗʰ M25.27 Flail joint, **ankle and foot**

M25.271 Flail joint, **right ankle and foot**
M25.272 Flail joint, **left ankle and foot**
M25.279 Flail joint, **unspecified ankle and foot**

M25.28 Flail joint, **other site**

√5ᵗʰ M25.3 **Other instability of joint**

EXCLUDES 1   instability of joint secondary to old ligament injury (M24.2-)
    instability of joint secondary to removal of joint prosthesis (M96.8-)
EXCLUDES 2   spinal instabilities (M53.2-)

M25.30 Other instability, **unspecified joint**
√6ᵗʰ M25.31 Other instability, **shoulder**

M25.311 Other instability, **right shoulder**
M25.312 Other instability, **left shoulder**
M25.319 Other instability, **unspecified shoulder**

√6ᵗʰ M25.32 Other instability, **elbow**

M25.321 Other instability, **right elbow**
M25.322 Other instability, **left elbow**
M25.329 Other instability, **unspecified elbow**

√6ᵗʰ M25.33 Other instability, **wrist**

M25.331 Other instability, **right wrist**
M25.332 Other instability, **left wrist**
M25.339 Other instability, **unspecified wrist**

√6ᵗʰ M25.34 Other instability, **hand**

M25.341 Other instability, **right hand**
M25.342 Other instability, **left hand**
M25.349 Other instability, **unspecified hand**

√6ᵗʰ M25.35 Other instability, **hip**

M25.351 Other instability, **right hip**
M25.352 Other instability, **left hip**
M25.359 Other instability, **unspecified hip**

√6ᵗʰ M25.36 Other instability, **knee**

M25.361 Other instability, **right knee**
M25.362 Other instability, **left knee**
M25.369 Other instability, **unspecified knee**

√6ᵗʰ M25.37 Other instability, **ankle and foot**

M25.371 Other instability, **right ankle**
M25.372 Other instability, **left ankle**
M25.373 Other instability, **unspecified ankle**
M25.374 Other instability, **right foot**
M25.375 Other instability, **left foot**
M25.376 Other instability, **unspecified foot**

M25.39 Other instability, **other specified joint**

√5ᵗʰ M25.4 **Effusion of joint**

EXCLUDES 1   hydrarthrosis in yaws (A66.6)
    intermittent hydrarthrosis (M12.4-)
    other infective (teno)synovitis (M65.1-)

M25.40 Effusion, **unspecified joint**
√6ᵗʰ M25.41 Effusion, **shoulder**

M25.411 Effusion, **right shoulder**
M25.412 Effusion, **left shoulder**
M25.419 Effusion, **unspecified shoulder**

√6ᵗʰ M25.42 Effusion, **elbow**

M25.421 Effusion, **right elbow**
M25.422 Effusion, **left elbow**
M25.429 Effusion, **unspecified elbow**

√6ᵗʰ M25.43 Effusion, **wrist**

M25.431 Effusion, **right wrist**
M25.432 Effusion, **left wrist**
M25.439 Effusion, **unspecified wrist**

√6ᵗʰ M25.44 Effusion, **hand**

M25.441 Effusion, **right hand**
M25.442 Effusion, **left hand**
M25.449 Effusion, **unspecified hand**

√6ᵗʰ M25.45 Effusion, **hip**

M25.451 Effusion, **right hip**
M25.452 Effusion, **left hip**
M25.459 Effusion, **unspecified hip**

√6ᵗʰ M25.46 Effusion, **knee**

M25.461 Effusion, **right knee**
M25.462 Effusion, **left knee**
M25.469 Effusion, **unspecified knee**

√6ᵗʰ M25.47 Effusion, **ankle and foot**

M25.471 Effusion, **right ankle**
M25.472 Effusion, **left ankle**
M25.473 Effusion, **unspecified ankle**
M25.474 Effusion, **right foot**
M25.475 Effusion, **left foot**
M25.476 Effusion, **unspecified foot**

☑ Additional Character Required   √x7ᵗʰ Placeholder Alert   Manifestation   Unspecified Dx   ℚ QPP   UPD Unacceptable PDx

Chapter 13. Diseases of the Musculoskeletal System and Connective Tissue

M25.48   **Effusion, other site**

✓5ᵗʰ **M25.5**   **Pain in joint**

> EXCLUDES 2   *pain in hand (M79.64-)*
> *pain in fingers (M79.64-)*
> *pain in foot (M79.67-)*
> *pain in limb (M79.6-)*
> *pain in toes (M79.67-)*

   M25.50   **Pain in unspecified joint**

✓6ᵗʰ **M25.51**   **Pain in shoulder**

   M25.511   Pain in right shoulder
   M25.512   Pain in left shoulder
   M25.519   Pain in unspecified shoulder

✓6ᵗʰ **M25.52**   **Pain in elbow**

   M25.521   Pain in right elbow
   M25.522   Pain in left elbow
   M25.529   Pain in unspecified elbow

✓6ᵗʰ **M25.53**   **Pain in wrist**

   M25.531   Pain in right wrist
   M25.532   Pain in left wrist
   M25.539   Pain in unspecified wrist

✓6ᵗʰ **M25.54**   **Pain in joints of hand**

   AHA: 2016,4Q,38
   M25.541   Pain in joints of right hand
   M25.542   Pain in joints of left hand
   M25.549   Pain in joints of unspecified hand
     Pain in joints of hand NOS

✓6ᵗʰ **M25.55**   **Pain in hip**

   M25.551   Pain in right hip
   M25.552   Pain in left hip
   M25.559   Pain in unspecified hip

✓6ᵗʰ **M25.56**   **Pain in knee**

   M25.561   Pain in right knee
   M25.562   Pain in left knee
   M25.569   Pain in unspecified knee

✓6ᵗʰ **M25.57**   **Pain in ankle and joints of foot**

   M25.571   Pain in right ankle and joints of right foot
   M25.572   Pain in left ankle and joints of left foot
   M25.579   Pain in unspecified ankle and joints of unspecified foot

   M25.59   **Pain in other specified joint**

✓5ᵗʰ **M25.6**   **Stiffness of joint, not elsewhere classified**

> EXCLUDES 1   *ankylosis of joint (M24.6-)*
> *contracture of joint (M24.5-)*

   M25.60   **Stiffness of unspecified joint, not elsewhere classified**

✓6ᵗʰ **M25.61**   **Stiffness of shoulder, not elsewhere classified**

   M25.611   Stiffness of right shoulder, not elsewhere classified
   M25.612   Stiffness of left shoulder, not elsewhere classified
   M25.619   Stiffness of unspecified shoulder, not elsewhere classified

✓6ᵗʰ **M25.62**   **Stiffness of elbow, not elsewhere classified**

   M25.621   Stiffness of right elbow, not elsewhere classified
   M25.622   Stiffness of left elbow, not elsewhere classified
   M25.629   Stiffness of unspecified elbow, not elsewhere classified

✓6ᵗʰ **M25.63**   **Stiffness of wrist, not elsewhere classified**

   M25.631   Stiffness of right wrist, not elsewhere classified
   M25.632   Stiffness of left wrist, not elsewhere classified
   M25.639   Stiffness of unspecified wrist, not elsewhere classified

✓6ᵗʰ **M25.64**   **Stiffness of hand, not elsewhere classified**

   M25.641   Stiffness of right hand, not elsewhere classified
   M25.642   Stiffness of left hand, not elsewhere classified
   M25.649   Stiffness of unspecified hand, not elsewhere classified

✓6ᵗʰ **M25.65**   **Stiffness of hip, not elsewhere classified**

   M25.651   Stiffness of right hip, not elsewhere classified

   M25.652   Stiffness of left hip, not elsewhere classified
   M25.659   Stiffness of unspecified hip, not elsewhere classified

✓6ᵗʰ **M25.66**   **Stiffness of knee, not elsewhere classified**

   M25.661   Stiffness of right knee, not elsewhere classified
   M25.662   Stiffness of left knee, not elsewhere classified
   M25.669   Stiffness of unspecified knee, not elsewhere classified

✓6ᵗʰ **M25.67**   **Stiffness of ankle and foot, not elsewhere classified**

   M25.671   Stiffness of right ankle, not elsewhere classified
   M25.672   Stiffness of left ankle, not elsewhere classified
   M25.673   Stiffness of unspecified ankle, not elsewhere classified
   M25.674   Stiffness of right foot, not elsewhere classified
   M25.675   Stiffness of left foot, not elsewhere classified
   M25.676   Stiffness of unspecified foot, not elsewhere classified

   M25.69   **Stiffness of other specified joint, not elsewhere classified**

✓5ᵗʰ **M25.7**   **Osteophyte**

   M25.70   **Osteophyte, unspecified joint**

✓6ᵗʰ **M25.71**   **Osteophyte, shoulder**

   M25.711   Osteophyte, right shoulder
   M25.712   Osteophyte, left shoulder
   M25.719   Osteophyte, unspecified shoulder

✓6ᵗʰ **M25.72**   **Osteophyte, elbow**

   M25.721   Osteophyte, right elbow
   M25.722   Osteophyte, left elbow
   M25.729   Osteophyte, unspecified elbow

✓6ᵗʰ **M25.73**   **Osteophyte, wrist**

   M25.731   Osteophyte, right wrist
   M25.732   Osteophyte, left wrist
   M25.739   Osteophyte, unspecified wrist

✓6ᵗʰ **M25.74**   **Osteophyte, hand**

   M25.741   Osteophyte, right hand
   M25.742   Osteophyte, left hand
   M25.749   Osteophyte, unspecified hand

✓6ᵗʰ **M25.75**   **Osteophyte, hip**

   M25.751   Osteophyte, right hip
   M25.752   Osteophyte, left hip
   M25.759   Osteophyte, unspecified hip

✓6ᵗʰ **M25.76**   **Osteophyte, knee**

   M25.761   Osteophyte, right knee
   M25.762   Osteophyte, left knee
   M25.769   Osteophyte, unspecified knee

✓6ᵗʰ **M25.77**   **Osteophyte, ankle and foot**

   M25.771   Osteophyte, right ankle
   M25.772   Osteophyte, left ankle
   M25.773   Osteophyte, unspecified ankle
   M25.774   Osteophyte, right foot
   M25.775   Osteophyte, left foot
   M25.776   Osteophyte, unspecified foot

   M25.78   **Osteophyte, vertebrae**

✓5ᵗʰ **M25.8**   **Other specified joint disorders**

   M25.80   **Other specified joint disorders, unspecified joint**

✓6ᵗʰ **M25.81**   **Other specified joint disorders, shoulder**

   M25.811   Other specified joint disorders, right shoulder
   M25.812   Other specified joint disorders, left shoulder
   M25.819   Other specified joint disorders, unspecified shoulder

✓6ᵗʰ **M25.82**   **Other specified joint disorders, elbow**

   M25.821   Other specified joint disorders, right elbow
   M25.822   Other specified joint disorders, left elbow
   M25.829   Other specified joint disorders, unspecified elbow

✓6ᵗʰ **M25.83**   **Other specified joint disorders, wrist**

   M25.831   Other specified joint disorders, right wrist

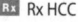

M25.832   Other specified joint disorders, left wrist
M25.839   Other specified joint disorders, unspecified wrist

✓6ᵗʰ   **M25.84**   **Other specified joint disorders, hand**

M25.841   Other specified joint disorders, right hand
M25.842   Other specified joint disorders, left hand
M25.849   Other specified joint disorders, unspecified hand

✓6ᵗʰ   **M25.85**   **Other specified joint disorders, hip**

AHA: 2014,4Q,25

M25.851   Other specified joint disorders, right hip
M25.852   Other specified joint disorders, left hip
M25.859   Other specified joint disorders, unspecified hip

✓6ᵗʰ   **M25.86**   **Other specified joint disorders, knee**

M25.861   Other specified joint disorders, right knee
M25.862   Other specified joint disorders, left knee
M25.869   Other specified joint disorders, unspecified knee

✓6ᵗʰ   **M25.87**   **Other specified joint disorders, ankle and foot**

M25.871   Other specified joint disorders, right ankle and foot
M25.872   Other specified joint disorders, left ankle and foot
M25.879   Other specified joint disorders, unspecified ankle and foot

M25.9   Joint disorder, unspecified

Dentofacial anomalies [including malocclusion] and other disorders of jaw (M26-M27)

EXCLUDES 1   hemifacial atrophy or hypertrophy (Q67.4)
unilateral condylar hyperplasia or hypoplasia (M27.8)

✓4ᵗʰ   **M26**   **Dentofacial anomalies [including malocclusion]**

✓5ᵗʰ   **M26.0**   **Major anomalies of jaw size**

EXCLUDES 1   acromegaly (E22.0)
Robin's syndrome (Q87.0)

M26.00   Unspecified anomaly of jaw size
M26.01   Maxillary hyperplasia
M26.02   Maxillary hypoplasia
AHA: 2014,3Q,23
M26.03   Mandibular hyperplasia
M26.04   Mandibular hypoplasia
M26.05   Macrogenia
M26.06   Microgenia
M26.07   Excessive tuberosity of jaw
Entire maxillary tuberosity
M26.09   Other specified anomalies of jaw size

✓5ᵗʰ   **M26.1**   **Anomalies of jaw-cranial base relationship**

M26.10   Unspecified anomaly of jaw-cranial base relationship
M26.11   Maxillary asymmetry
M26.12   Other jaw asymmetry
M26.19   Other specified anomalies of jaw-cranial base relationship
AHA: 2020,1Q,21

✓5ᵗʰ   **M26.2**   **Anomalies of dental arch relationship**

M26.20   Unspecified anomaly of dental arch relationship

✓6ᵗʰ   **M26.21**   **Malocclusion, Angle's class**

M26.211   Malocclusion, Angle's class I
Neutro-occlusion
M26.212   Malocclusion, Angle's class II
Disto-occlusion Division I
Disto-occlusion Division II
M26.213   Malocclusion, Angle's class III
Mesio-occlusion
M26.219   Malocclusion, Angle's class, unspecified

✓6ᵗʰ   **M26.22**   **Open occlusal relationship**

M26.220   Open anterior occlusal relationship
Anterior open bite
M26.221   Open posterior occlusal relationship
Posterior open bite
M26.23   Excessive horizontal overlap
Excessive horizontal overjet
M26.24   Reverse articulation
Crossbite (anterior) (posterior)
M26.25   Anomalies of interarch distance

M26.29   Other anomalies of dental arch relationship
Midline deviation of dental arch
Overbite (excessive) deep
Overbite (excessive) horizontal
Overbite (excessive) vertical
Posterior lingual occlusion of mandibular teeth

✓5ᵗʰ   **M26.3**   **Anomalies of tooth position of fully erupted tooth or teeth**

EXCLUDES 2   embedded and impacted teeth (K01.-)

M26.30   Unspecified anomaly of tooth position of fully erupted tooth or teeth
Abnormal spacing of fully erupted tooth or teeth NOS
Displacement of fully erupted tooth or teeth NOS
Transposition of fully erupted tooth or teeth NOS
M26.31   Crowding of fully erupted teeth
M26.32   Excessive spacing of fully erupted teeth
Diastema of fully erupted tooth or teeth NOS
M26.33   Horizontal displacement of fully erupted tooth or teeth
Tipped tooth or teeth
Tipping of fully erupted tooth
M26.34   Vertical displacement of fully erupted tooth or teeth
Extruded tooth
Infraeruption of tooth or teeth
Supraeruption of tooth or teeth
M26.35   Rotation of fully erupted tooth or teeth
M26.36   Insufficient interocclusal distance of fully erupted teeth (ridge)
Lack of adequate intermaxillary vertical dimension of fully erupted teeth
M26.37   Excessive interocclusal distance of fully erupted teeth
Excessive intermaxillary vertical dimension of fully erupted teeth
Loss of occlusal vertical dimension of fully erupted teeth
M26.39   Other anomalies of tooth position of fully erupted tooth or teeth

M26.4   Malocclusion, unspecified

✓5ᵗʰ   **M26.5**   **Dentofacial functional abnormalities**

EXCLUDES 1   bruxism (F45.8)
teeth-grinding NOS (F45.8)

M26.50   Dentofacial functional abnormalities, unspecified
M26.51   Abnormal jaw closure
M26.52   Limited mandibular range of motion
M26.53   Deviation in opening and closing of the mandible
M26.54   Insufficient anterior guidance
Insufficient anterior occlusal guidance
M26.55   Centric occlusion maximum intercuspation discrepancy
EXCLUDES 1   centric occlusion NOS (M26.59)
M26.56   Non-working side interference
Balancing side interference
M26.57   Lack of posterior occlusal support
M26.59   Other dentofacial functional abnormalities
Centric occlusion (of teeth) NOS
Malocclusion due to abnormal swallowing
Malocclusion due to mouth breathing
Malocclusion due to tongue, lip or finger habits

√5ᵗʰ M26.6 Temporomandibular joint disorders

> *EXCLUDES 2* *current temporomandibular joint dislocation (S03.0)*
> *current temporomandibular joint sprain (S03.4)*

AHA: 2016,4Q,38-39

Temporomandibular Joint

Cutaway detail

Upper joint space

Articular disc (meniscus)

Lower joint space

Condyle

Mandible

Cutaway view of temporomandibular joint (TMJ)

√6ᵗʰ M26.60 Temporomandibular joint disorder, unspecified

M26.601 Right temporomandibular joint disorder, unspecified

M26.602 Left temporomandibular joint disorder, unspecified

M26.603 Bilateral temporomandibular joint disorder, unspecified

M26.609 Unspecified temporomandibular joint disorder, unspecified side
Temporomandibular joint disorder NOS

√6ᵗʰ M26.61 Adhesions and ankylosis of temporomandibular joint

M26.611 Adhesions and ankylosis of right temporomandibular joint

M26.612 Adhesions and ankylosis of left temporomandibular joint

M26.613 Adhesions and ankylosis of bilateral temporomandibular joint

M26.619 Adhesions and ankylosis of temporomandibular joint, unspecified side

√6ᵗʰ M26.62 Arthralgia of temporomandibular joint

M26.621 Arthralgia of right temporomandibular joint

M26.622 Arthralgia of left temporomandibular joint

M26.623 Arthralgia of bilateral temporomandibular joint

M26.629 Arthralgia of temporomandibular joint, unspecified side

√6ᵗʰ M26.63 Articular disc disorder of temporomandibular joint

M26.631 Articular disc disorder of right temporomandibular joint

M26.632 Articular disc disorder of left temporomandibular joint

M26.633 Articular disc disorder of bilateral temporomandibular joint

M26.639 Articular disc disorder of temporomandibular joint, unspecified side

√6ᵗʰ M26.64 Arthritis of temporomandibular joint

AHA: 2020,4Q,32

M26.641 Arthritis of right temporomandibular joint

M26.642 Arthritis of left temporomandibular joint

M26.643 Arthritis of bilateral temporomandibular joint

M26.649 Arthritis of unspecified temporomandibular joint

√6ᵗʰ M26.65 Arthropathy of temporomandibular joint

AHA: 2020,4Q,32

M26.651 Arthropathy of right temporomandibular joint

M26.652 Arthropathy of left temporomandibular joint

M26.653 Arthropathy of bilateral temporomandibular joint

M26.659 Arthropathy of unspecified temporomandibular joint

M26.69 Other specified disorders of temporomandibular joint

√5ᵗʰ M26.7 Dental alveolar anomalies

M26.70 Unspecified alveolar anomaly

M26.71 Alveolar maxillary hyperplasia

M26.72 Alveolar mandibular hyperplasia

M26.73 Alveolar maxillary hypoplasia

M26.74 Alveolar mandibular hypoplasia

M26.79 Other specified alveolar anomalies

√6ᵗʰ M26.8 Other dentofacial anomalies

M26.81 Anterior soft tissue impingement
Anterior soft tissue impingement on teeth

M26.82 Posterior soft tissue impingement
Posterior soft tissue impingement on teeth

M26.89 Other dentofacial anomalies

M26.9 Dentofacial anomaly, unspecified

√4ᵗʰ M27 Other diseases of jaws

M27.0 Developmental disorders of jaws
Latent bone cyst of jaw
Stafne's cyst
Torus mandibularis
Torus palatinus

M27.1 Giant cell granuloma, central
Giant cell granuloma NOS

> *EXCLUDES 1* *peripheral giant cell granuloma (K06.8)*

M27.2 Inflammatory conditions of jaws
Osteitis of jaw(s)
Osteomyelitis (neonatal) jaw(s)
Osteoradionecrosis jaw(s)
Periostitis jaw(s)
Sequestrum of jaw bone
Use additional code (W88-W90, X39.0) to identify radiation, if radiation-induced

> *EXCLUDES 2* *osteonecrosis of jaw due to drug (M87.180)*

M27.3 Alveolitis of jaws
Alveolar osteitis
Dry socket

√5ᵗʰ M27.4 Other and unspecified cysts of jaw

> *EXCLUDES 1* *cysts of oral region (K09.-)*
> *latent bone cyst of jaw (M27.0)*
> *Stafne's cyst (M27.0)*

M27.40 Unspecified cyst of jaw
Cyst of jaw NOS

M27.49 Other cysts of jaw
Aneurysmal cyst of jaw
Hemorrhagic cyst of jaw
Traumatic cyst of jaw

√5ᵗʰ M27.5 Periradicular pathology associated with previous endodontic treatment

M27.51 Perforation of root canal space due to endodontic treatment

M27.52 Endodontic overfill

M27.53 Endodontic underfill

M27.59 Other periradicular pathology associated with previous endodontic treatment

√5ᵗʰ M27.6 Endosseous dental implant failure

M27.61 Osseointegration failure of dental implant
Hemorrhagic complications of dental implant placement
Iatrogenic osseointegration failure of dental implant
Osseointegration failure of dental implant due to complications of systemic disease
Osseointegration failure of dental implant due to poor bone quality
Pre-integration failure of dental implant NOS
Pre-osseointegration failure of dental implant

HCC CMS-HCC   **Rx** Rx HCC   **ESR** ESRD HCC   **COM** Commercial HCC   **N** Newborn: 0   **P** Pediatric: 0-17   **M** Maternity: 9-64   **A** Adult: 15-124

812   ICD-10-CM 2023

M27.62 Post-osseointegration biological failure of dental implant
Failure of dental implant due to lack of attached gingiva
Failure of dental implant due to occlusal trauma (caused by poor prosthetic design)
Failure of dental implant due to parafunctional habits
Failure of dental implant due to periodontal infection (peri-implantitis)
Failure of dental implant due to poor oral hygiene
Iatrogenic post-osseointegration failure of dental implant
Post-osseointegration failure of dental implant due to complications of systemic disease

M27.63 Post-osseointegration mechanical failure of dental implant
Failure of dental prosthesis causing loss of dental implant
Fracture of dental implant
EXCLUDES 2 cracked tooth (K03.81)
fractured dental restorative material with loss of material (K08.531)
fractured dental restorative material without loss of material (K08.530)
fractured tooth (S02.5)

M27.69 Other endosseous dental implant failure
Dental implant failure NOS

M27.8 Other specified diseases of jaws
Cherubism
Exostosis
Fibrous dysplasia
Unilateral condylar hyperplasia
Unilateral condylar hypoplasia
EXCLUDES 1 jaw pain (R68.84)

M27.9 Disease of jaws, unspecified

Systemic connective tissue disorders (M30-M36)

INCLUDES autoimmune disease NOS
collagen (vascular) disease NOS
systemic autoimmune disease
systemic collagen (vascular) disease
EXCLUDES 1 autoimmune disease, single organ or single cell-type-code to relevant condition category

✓4ᵗʰ **M30 Polyarteritis nodosa and related conditions**
EXCLUDES 1 microscopic polyarteritis (M31.7)

M30.0 Polyarteritis nodosa `HCC` `Rx` `ESR` `COM`

M30.1 Polyarteritis with lung involvement [Churg-Strauss] `HCC` `Rx` `ESR` `COM`
Allergic granulomatous angiitis
Eosinophilic granulomatosis with polyangiitis [EGPA]
AHA: 2021,1Q,23

M30.2 Juvenile polyarteritis `HCC` `Rx` `ESR` `COM`

M30.3 Mucocutaneous lymph node syndrome [Kawasaki] `HCC` `Rx` `ESR` `COM`

M30.8 Other conditions related to polyarteritis nodosa `HCC` `Rx` `ESR` `COM`
Polyangiitis overlap syndrome

✓4ᵗʰ **M31 Other necrotizing vasculopathies**

M31.0 Hypersensitivity angiitis `HCC` `Rx` `ESR` `COM`
Goodpasture's syndrome

✓5ᵗʰ **M31.1 Thrombotic microangiopathy**
AHA: 2021,4Q,19

M31.10 Thrombotic microangiopathy, unspecified `HCC` `Rx` `ESR` `COM`

M31.11 Hematopoietic stem cell transplantation-associated thrombotic microangiopathy [HSCT-TMA] `HCC` `Rx` `ESR` `COM`
Transplant-associated thrombotic microangiopathy [TA-TMA]
Code first if applicable:
complications of bone marrow transplant (T86.0-)
complications of stem cell transplant (T86.5)
Use additional code to identify specific organ dysfunction, such as:
acute kidney failure (N17.-)
acute respiratory distress syndrome (J80)
capillary leak syndrome (I78.8)
diffuse alveolar hemorrhage (R04.89)
encephalopathy (metabolic) (septic) (G93.41)
fluid overload, unspecified (E87.70)
graft versus host disease (D89.81-)
hemolytic uremic syndrome ▶(D59.3-)◀
hepatic failure (K72.-)
hepatic veno-occlusive disease (K76.5)
idiopathic interstitial pneumonia (J84.11-)
sinusoidal obstruction syndrome (K76.5)

M31.19 Other thrombotic microangiopathy `HCC` `Rx` `ESR` `COM`
Thrombotic thrombocytopenic purpura

M31.2 Lethal midline granuloma `HCC` `Rx` `ESR` `COM`

✓5ᵗʰ **M31.3 Wegener's granulomatosis**
Granulomatosis with polyangiitis
Necrotizing respiratory granulomatosis
AHA: 2021,1Q,23

M31.30 Wegener's granulomatosis without renal involvement `HCC` `Rx` `ESR` `COM`
Wegener's granulomatosis NOS
AHA: 2021,2Q,10

M31.31 Wegener's granulomatosis with renal involvement `HCC` `Rx` `ESR` `COM`

M31.4 Aortic arch syndrome [Takayasu] `HCC` `Rx` `ESR` `COM`

M31.5 Giant cell arteritis with polymyalgia rheumatica `HCC` `Rx` `ESR` `COM`

M31.6 Other giant cell arteritis `HCC` `Rx` `ESR` `COM`

M31.7 Microscopic polyangiitis `HCC` `Rx` `ESR` `COM`
Microscopic polyarteritis
EXCLUDES 1 polyarteritis nodosa (M30.0)
AHA: 2021,1Q,23

M31.8 Other specified necrotizing vasculopathies `HCC` `ESR`
Hypocomplementemic vasculitis
Septic vasculitis

M31.9 Necrotizing vasculopathy, unspecified `HCC` `ESR`

✓4ᵗʰ **M32 Systemic lupus erythematosus (SLE)**
EXCLUDES 1 lupus erythematosus (discoid) (NOS) (L93.0)
AHA: 2020,4Q,11; 2018,3Q,14
TIP: There is no default code for "lupus NOS." Query the provider for the specific type of lupus in order to assign the appropriate code.

M32.0 Drug-induced systemic lupus erythematosus `HCC` `Rx` `ESR` `COM`
Use additional code for adverse effect, if applicable, to identify drug (T36-T50 with fifth or sixth character 5)

✓5ᵗʰ **M32.1 Systemic lupus erythematosus with organ or system involvement**

M32.10 Systemic lupus erythematosus, organ or system involvement unspecified `HCC` `Rx` `ESR` `COM`

M32.11 Endocarditis in systemic lupus erythematosus `HCC` `Rx` `ESR` `COM`
Libman-Sacks disease

M32.12 Pericarditis in systemic lupus erythematosus `HCC` `Rx` `ESR` `COM`
Lupus pericarditis

M32.13 Lung involvement in systemic lupus erythematosus `HCC` `Rx` `ESR` `COM`
Pleural effusion due to systemic lupus erythematosus

M32.14 Glomerular disease in systemic lupus erythematosus `HCC` `Rx` `ESR` `COM`
Lupus renal disease NOS
AHA: 2013,4Q,125

M32.15 Tubulo-interstitial nephropathy in systemic lupus erythematosus `HCC` `Rx` `ESR` `COM`

M32.19   **Other organ or system involvement in systemic lupus erythematosus** `HCC` `Rx` `ESR` `COM`

M32.8   **Other forms of systemic lupus erythematosus** `HCC` `Rx` `ESR` `COM`

M32.9   **Systemic lupus erythematosus, unspecified** `HCC` `Rx` `ESR` `COM`
SLE NOS
Systemic lupus erythematosus NOS
Systemic lupus erythematosus without organ involvement

☑4ᵗʰ **M33**   **Dermatopolymyositis**
AHA: 2017,4Q,18

☑5ᵗʰ **M33.0**   **Juvenile dermatomyositis**

M33.00   **Juvenile dermatomyositis, organ involvement unspecified** `HCC` `Rx` `ESR` `COM`

M33.01   **Juvenile dermatomyositis with respiratory involvement** `HCC` `Rx` `ESR` `COM`

M33.02   **Juvenile dermatomyositis with myopathy** `HCC` `Rx` `ESR` `COM`

M33.03   **Juvenile dermatomyositis without myopathy** `HCC` `Rx` `ESR` `COM`

M33.09   **Juvenile dermatomyositis with other organ involvement** `HCC` `Rx` `ESR` `COM`

☑5ᵗʰ **M33.1**   **Other dermatomyositis**
Adult dermatomyositis

M33.10   **Other dermatomyositis, organ involvement unspecified** `HCC` `Rx` `ESR` `COM`

M33.11   **Other dermatomyositis with respiratory involvement** `HCC` `Rx` `ESR` `COM`

M33.12   **Other dermatomyositis with myopathy** `HCC` `Rx` `ESR` `COM`

M33.13   **Other dermatomyositis without myopathy** `HCC` `Rx` `ESR` `COM`
Dermatomyositis NOS

M33.19   **Other dermatomyositis with other organ involvement** `HCC` `Rx` `ESR` `COM`

☑5ᵗʰ **M33.2**   **Polymyositis**

M33.20   **Polymyositis, organ involvement unspecified** `HCC` `Rx` `ESR` `COM`

M33.21   **Polymyositis with respiratory involvement** `HCC` `Rx` `ESR` `COM`

M33.22   **Polymyositis with myopathy** `HCC` `Rx` `ESR` `COM`

M33.29   **Polymyositis with other organ involvement** `HCC` `Rx` `ESR` `COM`

☑5ᵗʰ **M33.9**   **Dermatopolymyositis, unspecified**

M33.90   **Dermatopolymyositis, unspecified, organ involvement unspecified** `HCC` `Rx` `ESR` `COM`

M33.91   **Dermatopolymyositis, unspecified with respiratory involvement** `HCC` `Rx` `ESR` `COM`

M33.92   **Dermatopolymyositis, unspecified with myopathy** `HCC` `Rx` `ESR` `COM`

M33.93   **Dermatopolymyositis, unspecified without myopathy** `HCC` `Rx` `ESR` `COM`

M33.99   **Dermatopolymyositis, unspecified with other organ involvement** `HCC` `Rx` `ESR` `COM`

☑4ᵗʰ **M34**   **Systemic sclerosis [scleroderma]**
`EXCLUDES 1`   *circumscribed scleroderma (L94.0)*
neonatal scleroderma (P83.88)

M34.0   **Progressive systemic sclerosis** `HCC` `Rx` `ESR` `COM`

M34.1   **CR(E)ST syndrome** `HCC` `Rx` `ESR` `COM`
Combination of calcinosis, Raynaud's phenomenon, esophageal dysfunction, sclerodactyly, telangiectasia

M34.2   **Systemic sclerosis induced by drug and chemical** `HCC` `Rx` `ESR` `COM`
Code first poisoning due to drug or toxin, if applicable (T36-T65 with fifth or sixth character 1-4 or 6)
Use additional code for adverse effect, if applicable, to identify drug (T36-T50 with fifth or sixth character 5)

☑5ᵗʰ **M34.8**   **Other forms of systemic sclerosis**

M34.81   **Systemic sclerosis with lung involvement** `HCC` `Rx` `ESR` `COM`
Code also if applicable:
  other interstitial pulmonary diseases (J84.89)
  secondary pulmonary arterial hypertension (I27.21)

M34.82   **Systemic sclerosis with myopathy** `HCC` `Rx` `ESR` `COM`

M34.83   **Systemic sclerosis with polyneuropathy** `HCC` `Rx` `ESR` `COM`

M34.89   **Other systemic sclerosis** `HCC` `Rx` `ESR` `COM`

M34.9   **Systemic sclerosis, unspecified** `HCC` `Rx` `ESR` `COM`

☑4ᵗʰ **M35**   **Other systemic involvement of connective tissue**
`EXCLUDES 1`   *reactive perforating collagenosis (L87.1)*

☑5ᵗʰ **M35.0**   **Sjögren syndrome**
Sicca syndrome
Use additional code to identify associated manifestations
`EXCLUDES 1`   *dry mouth, unspecified (R68.2)*
AHA: 2021,4Q,20
DEF: Autoimmune disease associated with keratoconjunctivitis, laryngopharyngitis, rhinitis, dry mouth, enlarged parotid gland, and chronic polyarthritis.

M35.00   **Sjögren syndrome, unspecified** `HCC` `Rx` `ESR` `COM`

M35.01   **Sjögren syndrome with keratoconjunctivitis** `HCC` `Rx` `ESR` `COM`

M35.02   **Sjögren syndrome with lung involvement** `HCC` `Rx` `ESR` `COM`

M35.03   **Sjögren syndrome with myopathy** `HCC` `Rx` `ESR` `COM`

M35.04   **Sjögren syndrome with tubulo-interstitial nephropathy** `HCC` `Rx` `ESR` `COM`
Renal tubular acidosis in sicca syndrome

M35.05   **Sjögren syndrome with inflammatory arthritis** `HCC` `Rx` `ESR` `COM`

M35.06   **Sjögren syndrome with peripheral nervous system involvement** `HCC` `Rx` `ESR` `COM`

M35.07   **Sjögren syndrome with central nervous system involvement** `HCC` `Rx` `ESR` `COM`

M35.08   **Sjögren syndrome with gastrointestinal involvement** `HCC` `Rx` `ESR` `COM`

M35.0A   **Sjögren syndrome with glomerular disease** `HCC` `Rx` `ESR` `COM`

M35.0B   **Sjögren syndrome with vasculitis** `HCC` `Rx` `ESR` `COM`

M35.0C   **Sjögren syndrome with dental involvement** `HCC` `Rx` `ESR` `COM`

M35.09   **Sjögren syndrome with other organ involvement** `HCC` `Rx` `ESR` `COM`

M35.1   **Other overlap syndromes** `HCC` `Rx` `ESR` `COM`
Mixed connective tissue disease
`EXCLUDES 1`   *polyangiitis overlap syndrome (M30.8)*

M35.2   **Behçet's disease** `HCC` `ESR` `COM`

M35.3   **Polymyalgia rheumatica** `HCC` `ESR` `COM`
`EXCLUDES 1`   *polymyalgia rheumatica with giant cell arteritis (M31.5)*

M35.4   **Diffuse (eosinophilic) fasciitis**

M35.5   **Multifocal fibrosclerosis** `HCC` `Rx` `ESR` `COM`

M35.6   **Relapsing panniculitis [Weber-Christian]**
`EXCLUDES 1`   *lupus panniculitis (L93.2)*
panniculitis NOS (M79.3-)

M35.7   **Hypermobility syndrome**
Familial ligamentous laxity
`EXCLUDES 1`   *ligamentous laxity, NOS (M24.2-)*
`EXCLUDES 2`   *Ehlers-Danlos syndromes (Q79.6-)*

✓5ᵗʰ **M35.8 Other specified systemic involvement of connective tissue**
    AHA: 2021,1Q,36; 2020,3Q,13-14

  M35.81 Multisystem inflammatory syndrome   HCC ESR COM
    MIS-A
    MIS-C
    Multisystem inflammatory syndrome in adults
    Multisystem inflammatory syndrome in children
    Pediatric inflammatory multisystem syndrome
    PIMS
    Code first, if applicable, COVID-19 (U07.1)
    Code also any associated complications such as:
      acute hepatic failure (K72.0-)
      acute kidney failure (N17.-)
      acute myocarditis (I40.-)
      acute respiratory distress syndrome (J80)
      cardiac arrhythmia (I47-I49.-)
      pneumonia due to COVID-19 (J12.82)
      severe sepsis (R65.2-)
      viral cardiomyopathy (B33.24)
      viral pericarditis (B33.23)
    Use additional code, if applicable, for:
      exposure to COVID-19 or SARS-CoV-2 infection (Z20.822)
      personal history of COVID-19 (Z86.16)
      post COVID-19 condition (U09.9)
    AHA: 2021,4Q,102; 2021,1Q,29,36,41
    DEF: Hyperinflammatory condition that seems to be largely associated with past or present coronavirus disease 2019 (COVID-19) infection. Predominantly occurring in children, with less frequent occurrences in adults, symptoms often include fever, laboratory evidence of inflammation, and evidence of clinically severe illness requiring hospitalization with multisystem (two or more) organ involvement. ***Synonym(s):*** MIS, MIS-C.

  M35.89 Other specified systemic involvement of connective tissue   HCC Rx ESR COM

M35.9 Systemic involvement of connective tissue, unspecified   HCC Rx ESR COM
    Autoimmune disease (systemic) NOS
    Collagen (vascular) disease NOS

✓4ᵗʰ **M36 Systemic disorders of connective tissue in diseases classified elsewhere**
    EXCLUDES 2   *arthropathies in diseases classified elsewhere (M14.-)*

  M36.0 *Dermato(poly)myositis in neoplastic disease*   HCC Rx ESR COM
    Code first underlying neoplasm (C00-D49)

  M36.1 *Arthropathy in neoplastic disease*
    Code first underlying neoplasm, such as:
      leukemia (C91-C95)
      malignant histiocytosis (C96.A)
      multiple myeloma (C90.0)

  M36.2 *Hemophilic arthropathy*
    Hemarthrosis in hemophilic arthropathy
    Code first underlying disease, such as:
      factor VIII deficiency (D66)
        with vascular defect ▶(D68.0-)◀
      factor IX deficiency (D67)
      hemophilia (classical) (D66)
      hemophilia B (D67)
      hemophilia C (D68.1)

  M36.3 *Arthropathy in other blood disorders*

  M36.4 *Arthropathy in hypersensitivity reactions classified elsewhere*
    Code first underlying disease, such as:
      Henoch (-Schönlein) purpura (D69.0)
      serum sickness (T80.6-)

  M36.8 *Systemic disorders of connective tissue in other diseases classified elsewhere*   HCC Rx ESR COM
    Code first underlying disease, such as:
      alkaptonuria (E70.2)
      hypogammaglobulinemia (D80.-)
      ochronosis (E70.2)

DORSOPATHIES (M40-M54)

Deforming dorsopathies (M40-M43)

✓4ᵗʰ **M40 Kyphosis and lordosis**
    Code first underlying disease
    EXCLUDES 1   *congenital kyphosis and lordosis (Q76.4)*
                 kyphoscoliosis (M41.-)
                 postprocedural kyphosis and lordosis (M96.-)

Kyphosis and Lordosis

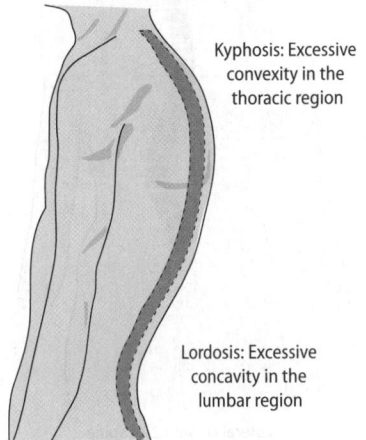

Kyphosis: Excessive convexity in the thoracic region

Lordosis: Excessive concavity in the lumbar region

✓5ᵗʰ **M40.0 Postural kyphosis**
    EXCLUDES 1   *osteochondrosis of spine (M42.-)*
  M40.00 Postural kyphosis, site unspecified
  M40.03 Postural kyphosis, cervicothoracic region
  M40.04 Postural kyphosis, thoracic region
  M40.05 Postural kyphosis, thoracolumbar region

✓5ᵗʰ **M40.1 Other secondary kyphosis**
  M40.10 Other secondary kyphosis, site unspecified   UPD
  M40.12 Other secondary kyphosis, cervical region   UPD
  M40.13 Other secondary kyphosis, cervicothoracic region   UPD
  M40.14 Other secondary kyphosis, thoracic region   UPD
  M40.15 Other secondary kyphosis, thoracolumbar region   UPD

✓5ᵗʰ **M40.2 Other and unspecified kyphosis**
  ✓6ᵗʰ **M40.20 Unspecified kyphosis**
    M40.202 Unspecified kyphosis, cervical region
    M40.203 Unspecified kyphosis, cervicothoracic region
    M40.204 Unspecified kyphosis, thoracic region
    M40.205 Unspecified kyphosis, thoracolumbar region
    M40.209 Unspecified kyphosis, site unspecified
  ✓6ᵗʰ **M40.29 Other kyphosis**
    M40.292 Other kyphosis, cervical region
    M40.293 Other kyphosis, cervicothoracic region
    M40.294 Other kyphosis, thoracic region
    M40.295 Other kyphosis, thoracolumbar region
    M40.299 Other kyphosis, site unspecified

✓5ᵗʰ **M40.3 Flatback syndrome**
  M40.30 Flatback syndrome, site unspecified
  M40.35 Flatback syndrome, thoracolumbar region
  M40.36 Flatback syndrome, lumbar region
  M40.37 Flatback syndrome, lumbosacral region

✓5ᵗʰ **M40.4 Postural lordosis**
    Acquired lordosis
  M40.40 Postural lordosis, site unspecified
  M40.45 Postural lordosis, thoracolumbar region
  M40.46 Postural lordosis, lumbar region
  M40.47 Postural lordosis, lumbosacral region

✓5ᵗʰ **M40.5 Lordosis, unspecified**
  M40.50 Lordosis, unspecified, site unspecified
  M40.55 Lordosis, unspecified, thoracolumbar region
  M40.56 Lordosis, unspecified, lumbar region
  M40.57 Lordosis, unspecified, lumbosacral region

✓4th **M41 Scoliosis**

INCLUDES   kyphoscoliosis
EXCLUDES 1   *congenital scoliosis due to bony malformation (Q76.3)*
congenital scoliosis NOS (Q67.5)
kyphoscoliotic heart disease (I27.1)
postural congenital scoliosis (Q67.5)
EXCLUDES 2   *postprocedural scoliosis (M96.-)*
AHA: 2022,1Q,30

Scoliosis

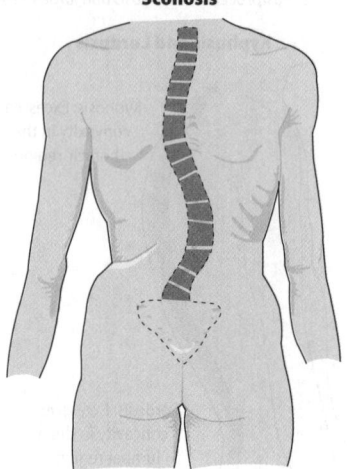

Lateral curvature of spine

✓5th **M41.0 Infantile idiopathic scoliosis**
AHA: 2014,4Q,26

M41.00 Infantile idiopathic scoliosis, site unspecified
M41.02 Infantile idiopathic scoliosis, cervical region
M41.03 Infantile idiopathic scoliosis, cervicothoracic region
M41.04 Infantile idiopathic scoliosis, thoracic region
M41.05 Infantile idiopathic scoliosis, thoracolumbar region
M41.06 Infantile idiopathic scoliosis, lumbar region
M41.07 Infantile idiopathic scoliosis, lumbosacral region
M41.08 Infantile idiopathic scoliosis, sacral and sacrococcygeal region

✓5th **M41.1 Juvenile and adolescent idiopathic scoliosis**

✓6th **M41.11 Juvenile idiopathic scoliosis**
AHA: 2014,4Q,28

M41.112 Juvenile idiopathic scoliosis, cervical region
M41.113 Juvenile idiopathic scoliosis, cervicothoracic region
M41.114 Juvenile idiopathic scoliosis, thoracic region
M41.115 Juvenile idiopathic scoliosis, thoracolumbar region
M41.116 Juvenile idiopathic scoliosis, lumbar region
M41.117 Juvenile idiopathic scoliosis, lumbosacral region
M41.119 Juvenile idiopathic scoliosis, site unspecified

✓6th **M41.12 Adolescent scoliosis**

M41.122 Adolescent idiopathic scoliosis, cervical region
M41.123 Adolescent idiopathic scoliosis, cervicothoracic region
M41.124 Adolescent idiopathic scoliosis, thoracic region
M41.125 Adolescent idiopathic scoliosis, thoracolumbar region
M41.126 Adolescent idiopathic scoliosis, lumbar region
M41.127 Adolescent idiopathic scoliosis, lumbosacral region
M41.129 Adolescent idiopathic scoliosis, site unspecified

✓5th **M41.2 Other idiopathic scoliosis**
M41.20 Other idiopathic scoliosis, site unspecified
M41.22 Other idiopathic scoliosis, cervical region
M41.23 Other idiopathic scoliosis, cervicothoracic region

M41.24 Other idiopathic scoliosis, thoracic region
M41.25 Other idiopathic scoliosis, thoracolumbar region
M41.26 Other idiopathic scoliosis, lumbar region
M41.27 Other idiopathic scoliosis, lumbosacral region

✓6th **M41.3 Thoracogenic scoliosis**
M41.30 Thoracogenic scoliosis, site unspecified
M41.34 Thoracogenic scoliosis, thoracic region
M41.35 Thoracogenic scoliosis, thoracolumbar region

✓6th **M41.4 Neuromuscular scoliosis**

Scoliosis secondary to cerebral palsy, Friedreich's ataxia, poliomyelitis and other neuromuscular disorders
Code also underlying condition
AHA: 2014,4Q,27

M41.40 Neuromuscular scoliosis, site unspecified
M41.41 Neuromuscular scoliosis, occipito-atlanto-axial region
M41.42 Neuromuscular scoliosis, cervical region
M41.43 Neuromuscular scoliosis, cervicothoracic region
M41.44 Neuromuscular scoliosis, thoracic region
M41.45 Neuromuscular scoliosis, thoracolumbar region
M41.46 Neuromuscular scoliosis, lumbar region
M41.47 Neuromuscular scoliosis, lumbosacral region

✓5th **M41.5 Other secondary scoliosis**

Code first underlying disease
AHA: 2019,1Q,19

M41.50 Other secondary scoliosis, site unspecified   UPD
M41.52 Other secondary scoliosis, cervical region   UPD
M41.53 Other secondary scoliosis, cervicothoracic region   UPD
M41.54 Other secondary scoliosis, thoracic region   UPD
M41.55 Other secondary scoliosis, thoracolumbar region   UPD
M41.56 Other secondary scoliosis, lumbar region   UPD
M41.57 Other secondary scoliosis, lumbosacral region   UPD

✓6th **M41.8 Other forms of scoliosis**
AHA: 2022,1Q,30

M41.80 Other forms of scoliosis, site unspecified
M41.82 Other forms of scoliosis, cervical region
M41.83 Other forms of scoliosis, cervicothoracic region
M41.84 Other forms of scoliosis, thoracic region
M41.85 Other forms of scoliosis, thoracolumbar region
M41.86 Other forms of scoliosis, lumbar region
M41.87 Other forms of scoliosis, lumbosacral region

M41.9 Scoliosis, unspecified
AHA: 2022,1Q,30

✓4th **M42 Spinal osteochondrosis**

✓5th **M42.0 Juvenile osteochondrosis of spine**

Calvé's disease
Scheuermann's disease
EXCLUDES 1   *postural kyphosis (M40.0)*

M42.00 Juvenile osteochondrosis of spine, site unspecified   COM
M42.01 Juvenile osteochondrosis of spine, occipito-atlanto-axial region   COM
M42.02 Juvenile osteochondrosis of spine, cervical region   COM
M42.03 Juvenile osteochondrosis of spine, cervicothoracic region   COM
M42.04 Juvenile osteochondrosis of spine, thoracic region   COM
M42.05 Juvenile osteochondrosis of spine, thoracolumbar region   COM
M42.06 Juvenile osteochondrosis of spine, lumbar region   COM
M42.07 Juvenile osteochondrosis of spine, lumbosacral region   COM
M42.08 Juvenile osteochondrosis of spine, sacral and sacrococcygeal region   COM
M42.09 Juvenile osteochondrosis of spine, multiple sites in spine   COM

✓6th **M42.1 Adult osteochondrosis of spine**

M42.10 Adult osteochondrosis of spine, site unspecified   A
M42.11 Adult osteochondrosis of spine, occipito-atlanto-axial region   A

M42.12 Adult osteochondrosis of spine, cervical region   A

M42.13 Adult osteochondrosis of spine, cervicothoracic region   A

M42.14 Adult osteochondrosis of spine, thoracic region   A

M42.15 Adult osteochondrosis of spine, thoracolumbar region   A

M42.16 Adult osteochondrosis of spine, lumbar region   A

M42.17 Adult osteochondrosis of spine, lumbosacral region   A

M42.18 Adult osteochondrosis of spine, sacral and sacrococcygeal region   A

M42.19 Adult osteochondrosis of spine, multiple sites in spine   A

M42.9 Spinal osteochondrosis, unspecified

✓4ᵗʰ **M43** Other deforming dorsopathies

> *EXCLUDES 1*   congenital spondylolysis and spondylolisthesis (Q76.2)
> hemivertebra (Q76.3-Q76.4)
> Klippel-Feil syndrome (Q76.1)
> lumbarization and sacralization (Q76.4)
> platyspondylisis (Q76.4)
> spina bifida occulta (Q76.0)
> spinal curvature in osteoporosis (M80.-)
> spinal curvature in Paget's disease of bone [osteitis deformans] (M88.-)

✓5ᵗʰ **M43.0** Spondylolysis

> *EXCLUDES 1*   congenital spondylolysis (Q76.2)
> spondylolisthesis (M43.1)

M43.00 Spondylolysis, site unspecified

M43.01 Spondylolysis, occipito-atlanto-axial region

M43.02 Spondylolysis, cervical region

M43.03 Spondylolysis, cervicothoracic region

M43.04 Spondylolysis, thoracic region

M43.05 Spondylolysis, thoracolumbar region

M43.06 Spondylolysis, lumbar region

M43.07 Spondylolysis, lumbosacral region

M43.08 Spondylolysis, sacral and sacrococcygeal region

M43.09 Spondylolysis, multiple sites in spine

✓5ᵗʰ **M43.1** Spondylolisthesis

> *EXCLUDES 1*   acute traumatic of lumbosacral region (S33.1)
> acute traumatic of sites other than lumbosacral - code to Fracture, vertebra, by region
> congenital spondylolisthesis (Q76.2)

AHA: 2020,2Q,21; 2018,3Q,18

TIP: Code also any associated radiculopathy (M54.1-) and/or myelopathy (G99.2).

M43.10 Spondylolisthesis, site unspecified

M43.11 Spondylolisthesis, occipito-atlanto-axial region

M43.12 Spondylolisthesis, cervical region

M43.13 Spondylolisthesis, cervicothoracic region

M43.14 Spondylolisthesis, thoracic region

M43.15 Spondylolisthesis, thoracolumbar region

M43.16 Spondylolisthesis, lumbar region

M43.17 Spondylolisthesis, lumbosacral region

M43.18 Spondylolisthesis, sacral and sacrococcygeal region

M43.19 Spondylolisthesis, multiple sites in spine

✓5ᵗʰ **M43.2** Fusion of spine

> Ankylosis of spinal joint
>
> *EXCLUDES 1*   ankylosing spondylitis (M45.0-)
> congenital fusion of spine (Q76.4)
>
> *EXCLUDES 2*   arthrodesis status (Z98.1)
> pseudoarthrosis after fusion or arthrodesis (M96.0)

M43.20 Fusion of spine, site unspecified

M43.21 Fusion of spine, occipito-atlanto-axial region

M43.22 Fusion of spine, cervical region

M43.23 Fusion of spine, cervicothoracic region

M43.24 Fusion of spine, thoracic region

M43.25 Fusion of spine, thoracolumbar region

M43.26 Fusion of spine, lumbar region

M43.27 Fusion of spine, lumbosacral region

M43.28 Fusion of spine, sacral and sacrococcygeal region

M43.3 Recurrent atlantoaxial dislocation with myelopathy

M43.4 Other recurrent atlantoaxial dislocation

✓5ᵗʰ **M43.5** Other recurrent vertebral dislocation

> *EXCLUDES 1*   biomechanical lesions NEC (M99.-)

✓6ᵗʰ **M43.5X** Other recurrent vertebral dislocation

M43.5X2 Other recurrent vertebral dislocation, cervical region

M43.5X3 Other recurrent vertebral dislocation, cervicothoracic region

M43.5X4 Other recurrent vertebral dislocation, thoracic region

M43.5X5 Other recurrent vertebral dislocation, thoracolumbar region

M43.5X6 Other recurrent vertebral dislocation, lumbar region

M43.5X7 Other recurrent vertebral dislocation, lumbosacral region

M43.5X8 Other recurrent vertebral dislocation, sacral and sacrococcygeal region

M43.5X9 Other recurrent vertebral dislocation, site unspecified

M43.6 Torticollis

> *EXCLUDES 1*   congenital (sternomastoid) torticollis (Q68.0)
> current injury - see Injury, of spine, by body region
> ocular torticollis (R29.891)
> psychogenic torticollis (F45.8)
> spasmodic torticollis (G24.3)
> torticollis due to birth injury (P15.2)

DEF: Twisted, unnatural position of the neck due to contracted cervical muscles that pull the head to one side.

✓5ᵗʰ **M43.8** Other specified deforming dorsopathies

> *EXCLUDES 2*   kyphosis and lordosis (M40.-)
> scoliosis (M41.-)

✓6ᵗʰ **M43.8X** Other specified deforming dorsopathies

M43.8X1 Other specified deforming dorsopathies, occipito-atlanto-axial region

M43.8X2 Other specified deforming dorsopathies, cervical region

M43.8X3 Other specified deforming dorsopathies, cervicothoracic region

M43.8X4 Other specified deforming dorsopathies, thoracic region

M43.8X5 Other specified deforming dorsopathies, thoracolumbar region

M43.8X6 Other specified deforming dorsopathies, lumbar region

M43.8X7 Other specified deforming dorsopathies, lumbosacral region

M43.8X8 Other specified deforming dorsopathies, sacral and sacrococcygeal region

M43.8X9 Other specified deforming dorsopathies, site unspecified

M43.9 Deforming dorsopathy, unspecified

> Curvature of spine NOS

Spondylopathies (M45-M49)

✓4ᵗʰ **M45** Ankylosing spondylitis

> Rheumatoid arthritis of spine
>
> *EXCLUDES 1*   arthropathy in Reiter's disease (M02.3-)
> juvenile (ankylosing) spondylitis (M08.1)
>
> *EXCLUDES 2*   Behçet's disease (M35.2)

M45.0 Ankylosing spondylitis of multiple sites in spine   HCC Rx ESR COM

M45.1 Ankylosing spondylitis of occipito-atlanto-axial region   HCC Rx ESR COM

M45.2 Ankylosing spondylitis of cervical region   HCC Rx ESR COM

M45.3 Ankylosing spondylitis of cervicothoracic region   HCC Rx ESR COM

M45.4 Ankylosing spondylitis of thoracic region   HCC Rx ESR COM

M45.5 Ankylosing spondylitis of thoracolumbar region   HCC Rx ESR COM

M45.6 Ankylosing spondylitis lumbar region   HCC Rx ESR COM

M45.7 Ankylosing spondylitis of lumbosacral region   HCC Rx ESR COM

M45.8 Ankylosing spondylitis sacral and sacrococcygeal region   HCC Rx ESR COM

M45.9 Ankylosing spondylitis of unspecified sites in spine   HCC Rx ESR COM

✓5ᵗʰ **M45.A Non-radiographic axial spondyloarthritis**
AHA: 2021,4Q,21-22

M45.A0 Non-radiographic axial spondyloarthritis of unspecified sites in spine HCC Rx ESR COM

M45.A1 Non-radiographic axial spondyloarthritis of occipito-atlanto-axial region HCC Rx ESR COM

M45.A2 Non-radiographic axial spondyloarthritis of cervical region HCC Rx ESR COM

M45.A3 Non-radiographic axial spondyloarthritis of cervicothoracic region HCC Rx ESR COM

M45.A4 Non-radiographic axial spondyloarthritis of thoracic region HCC Rx ESR COM

M45.A5 Non-radiographic axial spondyloarthritis of thoracolumbar region HCC Rx ESR COM

M45.A6 Non-radiographic axial spondyloarthritis of lumbar region HCC Rx ESR COM

M45.A7 Non-radiographic axial spondyloarthritis of lumbosacral region HCC Rx ESR COM

M45.A8 Non-radiographic axial spondyloarthritis of sacral and sacrococcygeal region HCC Rx ESR COM

M45.AB Non-radiographic axial spondyloarthritis of multiple sites in spine HCC Rx ESR COM

✓4ᵗʰ **M46 Other inflammatory spondylopathies**

✓5ᵗʰ **M46.0 Spinal enthesopathy**
Disorder of ligamentous or muscular attachments of spine

M46.00 Spinal enthesopathy, site unspecified HCC ESR

M46.01 Spinal enthesopathy, occipito-atlanto-axial region HCC ESR

M46.02 Spinal enthesopathy, cervical region HCC ESR

M46.03 Spinal enthesopathy, cervicothoracic region HCC ESR

M46.04 Spinal enthesopathy, thoracic region HCC ESR

M46.05 Spinal enthesopathy, thoracolumbar region HCC ESR

M46.06 Spinal enthesopathy, lumbar region HCC ESR

M46.07 Spinal enthesopathy, lumbosacral region HCC ESR

M46.08 Spinal enthesopathy, sacral and sacrococcygeal region HCC ESR

M46.09 Spinal enthesopathy, multiple sites in spine HCC ESR

M46.1 Sacroiliitis, not elsewhere classified HCC ESR
AHA: 2020,2Q,14
DEF: Inflammation of the sacroiliac joint (situated at the juncture of the sacrum and hip). Symptoms include pain in the buttocks or lower back that can extend down one or both legs.

✓5ᵗʰ **M46.2 Osteomyelitis of vertebra**

M46.20 Osteomyelitis of vertebra, site unspecified HCC ESR COM

M46.21 Osteomyelitis of vertebra, occipito-atlanto-axial region HCC ESR COM

M46.22 Osteomyelitis of vertebra, cervical region HCC ESR COM

M46.23 Osteomyelitis of vertebra, cervicothoracic region HCC ESR COM

M46.24 Osteomyelitis of vertebra, thoracic region HCC ESR COM

M46.25 Osteomyelitis of vertebra, thoracolumbar region HCC ESR COM

M46.26 Osteomyelitis of vertebra, lumbar region HCC ESR COM

M46.27 Osteomyelitis of vertebra, lumbosacral region HCC ESR COM

M46.28 Osteomyelitis of vertebra, sacral and sacrococcygeal region HCC ESR COM

✓5ᵗʰ **M46.3 Infection of intervertebral disc (pyogenic)**
Use additional code (B95-B97) to identify infectious agent

M46.30 Infection of intervertebral disc (pyogenic), site unspecified HCC ESR COM

M46.31 Infection of intervertebral disc (pyogenic), occipito-atlanto-axial region HCC ESR COM

M46.32 Infection of intervertebral disc (pyogenic), cervical region HCC ESR COM

M46.33 Infection of intervertebral disc (pyogenic), cervicothoracic region HCC ESR COM

M46.34 Infection of intervertebral disc (pyogenic), thoracic region HCC ESR COM

M46.35 Infection of intervertebral disc (pyogenic), thoracolumbar region HCC ESR COM

M46.36 Infection of intervertebral disc (pyogenic), lumbar region HCC ESR COM

M46.37 Infection of intervertebral disc (pyogenic), lumbosacral region HCC ESR COM

M46.38 Infection of intervertebral disc (pyogenic), sacral and sacrococcygeal region HCC ESR COM

M46.39 Infection of intervertebral disc (pyogenic), multiple sites in spine HCC ESR COM

✓5ᵗʰ **M46.4 Discitis, unspecified**

M46.40 Discitis, unspecified, site unspecified

M46.41 Discitis, unspecified, occipito-atlanto-axial region

M46.42 Discitis, unspecified, cervical region

M46.43 Discitis, unspecified, cervicothoracic region

M46.44 Discitis, unspecified, thoracic region

M46.45 Discitis, unspecified, thoracolumbar region

M46.46 Discitis, unspecified, lumbar region

M46.47 Discitis, unspecified, lumbosacral region

M46.48 Discitis, unspecified, sacral and sacrococcygeal region

M46.49 Discitis, unspecified, multiple sites in spine

✓5ᵗʰ **M46.5 Other infective spondylopathies**

M46.50 Other infective spondylopathies, site unspecified HCC ESR

M46.51 Other infective spondylopathies, occipito-atlanto-axial region HCC ESR

M46.52 Other infective spondylopathies, cervical region HCC ESR

M46.53 Other infective spondylopathies, cervicothoracic region HCC ESR

M46.54 Other infective spondylopathies, thoracic region HCC ESR

M46.55 Other infective spondylopathies, thoracolumbar region HCC ESR

M46.56 Other infective spondylopathies, lumbar region HCC ESR

M46.57 Other infective spondylopathies, lumbosacral region HCC ESR

M46.58 Other infective spondylopathies, sacral and sacrococcygeal region HCC ESR

M46.59 Other infective spondylopathies, multiple sites in spine HCC ESR

✓5ᵗʰ **M46.8 Other specified inflammatory spondylopathies**

M46.80 Other specified inflammatory spondylopathies, site unspecified HCC ESR

M46.81 Other specified inflammatory spondylopathies, occipito-atlanto-axial region HCC ESR

M46.82 Other specified inflammatory spondylopathies, cervical region HCC ESR

M46.83 Other specified inflammatory spondylopathies, cervicothoracic region HCC ESR

M46.84 Other specified inflammatory spondylopathies, thoracic region HCC ESR

M46.85 Other specified inflammatory spondylopathies, thoracolumbar region HCC ESR

M46.86 Other specified inflammatory spondylopathies, lumbar region HCC ESR

M46.87 Other specified inflammatory spondylopathies, lumbosacral region HCC ESR

M46.88 Other specified inflammatory spondylopathies, sacral and sacrococcygeal region HCC ESR

M46.89 Other specified inflammatory spondylopathies, multiple sites in spine HCC ESR

✓5ᵗʰ **M46.9 Unspecified inflammatory spondylopathy**

M46.90 Unspecified inflammatory spondylopathy, site unspecified HCC ESR

M46.91 Unspecified inflammatory spondylopathy, occipito-atlanto-axial region HCC ESR

M46.92 Unspecified inflammatory spondylopathy, cervical region HCC ESR
AHA: 2019,3Q,10

M46.93 Unspecified inflammatory spondylopathy, cervicothoracic region HCC ESR

M46.94 Unspecified inflammatory spondylopathy, thoracic region HCC ESR

M46.95 Unspecified inflammatory spondylopathy, thoracolumbar region HCC ESR

M46.96   Unspecified inflammatory spondylopathy, **lumbar region** `HCC` `ESR`

M46.97   Unspecified inflammatory spondylopathy, **lumbosacral region** `HCC` `ESR`

M46.98   Unspecified inflammatory spondylopathy, **sacral and sacrococcygeal region** `HCC` `ESR`

M46.99   Unspecified inflammatory spondylopathy, **multiple sites in spine** `HCC` `ESR`

☑4ᵗʰ **M47   Spondylosis**

> INCLUDES   arthrosis or osteoarthritis of spine
> degeneration of facet joints
> **AHA:** 2020,1Q,17; 2019,3Q,10-11; 2016,4Q,147

☑5ᵗʰ **M47.0   Anterior spinal and vertebral artery compression syndromes**

   ☑6ᵗʰ **M47.01   Anterior spinal artery compression syndromes**

     M47.011   Anterior spinal artery compression syndromes, **occipito-atlanto-axial region**

     M47.012   Anterior spinal artery compression syndromes, **cervical region**

     M47.013   Anterior spinal artery compression syndromes, **cervicothoracic region**

     M47.014   Anterior spinal artery compression syndromes, **thoracic region**

     M47.015   Anterior spinal artery compression syndromes, **thoracolumbar region**

     M47.016   Anterior spinal artery compression syndromes, **lumbar region**

     M47.019   Anterior spinal artery compression syndromes, **site unspecified**

   ☑6ᵗʰ **M47.02   Vertebral artery compression syndromes**

     M47.021   Vertebral artery compression syndromes, **occipito-atlanto-axial region**

     M47.022   Vertebral artery compression syndromes, **cervical region**

     M47.029   Vertebral artery compression syndromes, **site unspecified**

☑5ᵗʰ **M47.1   Other spondylosis with myelopathy**

> Spondylogenic compression of spinal cord
> EXCLUDES 1   *vertebral subluxation (M43.3-M43.5X9)*
> **AHA:** 2020,1Q,17

   M47.10   **Other spondylosis with myelopathy, site unspecified**

   M47.11   Other spondylosis with myelopathy, **occipito-atlanto-axial region**

   M47.12   Other spondylosis with myelopathy, **cervical region**

   M47.13   Other spondylosis with myelopathy, **cervicothoracic region**

   M47.14   Other spondylosis with myelopathy, **thoracic region**

   M47.15   Other spondylosis with myelopathy, **thoracolumbar region**

   M47.16   Other spondylosis with myelopathy, **lumbar region**

☑5ᵗʰ **M47.2   Other spondylosis with radiculopathy**

> **AHA:** 2020,1Q,17

   M47.20   **Other spondylosis with radiculopathy, site unspecified**

   M47.21   Other spondylosis with radiculopathy, **occipito-atlanto-axial region**

   M47.22   Other spondylosis with radiculopathy, **cervical region**

   M47.23   Other spondylosis with radiculopathy, **cervicothoracic region**

   M47.24   Other spondylosis with radiculopathy, **thoracic region**

   M47.25   Other spondylosis with radiculopathy, **thoracolumbar region**

   M47.26   Other spondylosis with radiculopathy, **lumbar region**

   M47.27   Other spondylosis with radiculopathy, **lumbosacral region**

   M47.28   Other spondylosis with radiculopathy, **sacral and sacrococcygeal region**

☑5ᵗʰ **M47.8   Other spondylosis**

   ☑6ᵗʰ **M47.81   Spondylosis without myelopathy or radiculopathy**

> **AHA:** 2019,3Q,10-11; 2018,2Q,14

     M47.811   Spondylosis without myelopathy or radiculopathy, **occipito-atlanto-axial region**

     M47.812   Spondylosis without myelopathy or radiculopathy, **cervical region**

     M47.813   Spondylosis without myelopathy or radiculopathy, **cervicothoracic region**

     M47.814   Spondylosis without myelopathy or radiculopathy, **thoracic region**

     M47.815   Spondylosis without myelopathy or radiculopathy, **thoracolumbar region**

     M47.816   Spondylosis without myelopathy or radiculopathy, **lumbar region**

     M47.817   Spondylosis without myelopathy or radiculopathy, **lumbosacral region**

     M47.818   Spondylosis without myelopathy or radiculopathy, **sacral and sacrococcygeal region**

     M47.819   Spondylosis without myelopathy or radiculopathy, **site unspecified**

   ☑6ᵗʰ **M47.89   Other spondylosis**

     M47.891   Other spondylosis, **occipito-atlanto-axial region**

     M47.892   Other spondylosis, **cervical region**

     M47.893   Other spondylosis, **cervicothoracic region**

     M47.894   Other spondylosis, **thoracic region**

     M47.895   Other spondylosis, **thoracolumbar region**

     M47.896   Other spondylosis, **lumbar region**

     M47.897   Other spondylosis, **lumbosacral region**

     M47.898   Other spondylosis, **sacral and sacrococcygeal region**

     M47.899   **Other spondylosis, site unspecified**

   M47.9   Spondylosis, unspecified

☑4ᵗʰ **M48   Other spondylopathies**

☑5ᵗʰ **M48.0   Spinal stenosis**

> Caudal stenosis
> **AHA:** 2020,1Q,17; 2018,3Q,18-19
> **TIP:** Code also any associated radiculopathy (M54.1-) and/or myelopathy (G99.2).

   M48.00   **Spinal stenosis, site unspecified**

   M48.01   **Spinal stenosis, occipito-atlanto-axial region**

   M48.02   **Spinal stenosis, cervical region**

   M48.03   **Spinal stenosis, cervicothoracic region**

   M48.04   **Spinal stenosis, thoracic region**

   M48.05   **Spinal stenosis, thoracolumbar region**

   ☑6ᵗʰ **M48.06   Spinal stenosis, lumbar region**

> **AHA:** 2018,3Q,19; 2017,4Q,18-19

     M48.061   **Spinal stenosis, lumbar region without neurogenic claudication**
> Spinal stenosis, lumbar region NOS

     M48.062   **Spinal stenosis, lumbar region with neurogenic claudication**

   M48.07   **Spinal stenosis, lumbosacral region**

   M48.08   **Spinal stenosis, sacral and sacrococcygeal region**

☑5ᵗʰ **M48.1   Ankylosing hyperostosis [Forestier]**

> Diffuse idiopathic skeletal hyperostosis [DISH]

   M48.10   **Ankylosing hyperostosis [Forestier], site unspecified**

   M48.11   Ankylosing hyperostosis [Forestier], **occipito-atlanto-axial region**

   M48.12   Ankylosing hyperostosis [Forestier], **cervical region**

   M48.13   Ankylosing hyperostosis [Forestier], **cervicothoracic region**

   M48.14   Ankylosing hyperostosis [Forestier], **thoracic region**

   M48.15   Ankylosing hyperostosis [Forestier], **thoracolumbar region**

   M48.16   Ankylosing hyperostosis [Forestier], **lumbar region**

   M48.17   Ankylosing hyperostosis [Forestier], **lumbosacral region**

   M48.18   Ankylosing hyperostosis [Forestier], **sacral and sacrococcygeal region**

   M48.19   Ankylosing hyperostosis [Forestier], **multiple sites in spine**

☑5ᵗʰ **M48.2   Kissing spine**

   M48.20   **Kissing spine, site unspecified**

   M48.21   Kissing spine, **occipito-atlanto-axial region**

   M48.22   Kissing spine, **cervical region**

   M48.23   Kissing spine, **cervicothoracic region**

   M48.24   Kissing spine, **thoracic region**

   M48.25   Kissing spine, **thoracolumbar region**

   M48.26   Kissing spine, **lumbar region**

   M48.27   Kissing spine, **lumbosacral region**

√5th **M48.3 Traumatic spondylopathy**

     M48.30 Traumatic spondylopathy, site unspecified

     M48.31 Traumatic spondylopathy, occipito-atlanto-axial region

     M48.32 Traumatic spondylopathy, cervical region

     M48.33 Traumatic spondylopathy, cervicothoracic region

     M48.34 Traumatic spondylopathy, thoracic region

     M48.35 Traumatic spondylopathy, thoracolumbar region

     M48.36 Traumatic spondylopathy, lumbar region

     M48.37 Traumatic spondylopathy, lumbosacral region

     M48.38 Traumatic spondylopathy, sacral and sacrococcygeal region

√5th **M48.4 Fatigue fracture of vertebra**

     Stress fracture of vertebra

     EXCLUDES 1   *pathological fracture NOS (M84.4-)*

          pathological fracture of vertebra due to neoplasm (M84.58)

          pathological fracture of vertebra due to osteoporosis (M80.-)

          pathological fracture of vertebra due to other diagnosis (M84.68)

          traumatic fracture of vertebrae (S12.0-S12.3-, S22.0-, S32.0-)

> The appropriate 7th character is to be added to each code from subcategory M48.4.
> A   initial encounter for fracture
> D   subsequent encounter for fracture with routine healing
> G   subsequent encounter for fracture with delayed healing
> S   sequela of fracture

√x7th **M48.40 Fatigue fracture of vertebra, site unspecified**   Q

√x7th **M48.41 Fatigue fracture of vertebra, occipito-atlanto-axial region**   Q

√x7th **M48.42 Fatigue fracture of vertebra, cervical region**   Q

√x7th **M48.43 Fatigue fracture of vertebra, cervicothoracic region**   Q

√x7th **M48.44 Fatigue fracture of vertebra, thoracic region**   Q

√x7th **M48.45 Fatigue fracture of vertebra, thoracolumbar region**   Q

√x7th **M48.46 Fatigue fracture of vertebra, lumbar region**   Q

√x7th **M48.47 Fatigue fracture of vertebra, lumbosacral region**   Q

√x7th **M48.48 Fatigue fracture of vertebra, sacral and sacrococcygeal region**   Q

√5th **M48.5 Collapsed vertebra, not elsewhere classified**

     Collapsed vertebra NOS

     Compression fracture of vertebra NOS

     Wedging of vertebra NOS

     EXCLUDES 1   *current injury - see Injury of spine, by body region*

          fatigue fracture of vertebra (M48.4)

          pathological fracture NOS (M84.4-)

          pathological fracture of vertebra due to neoplasm (M84.58)

          pathological fracture of vertebra due to osteoporosis (M80.-)

          pathological fracture of vertebra due to other diagnosis (M84.68)

          stress fracture of vertebra (M48.4-)

          traumatic fracture of vertebra (S12.-, S22.-, S32.-)

> The appropriate 7th character is to be added to each code from subcategory M48.5.
> A   initial encounter for fracture
> D   subsequent encounter for fracture with routine healing
> G   subsequent encounter for fracture with delayed healing
> S   sequela of fracture

1   √x7th **M48.50 Collapsed vertebra, not elsewhere classified, site unspecified**   HCC Rx ESR COM

1   √x7th **M48.51 Collapsed vertebra, not elsewhere classified, occipito-atlanto-axial region**   HCC Rx ESR COM

1   √x7th **M48.52 Collapsed vertebra, not elsewhere classified, cervical region**   HCC Rx ESR COM

1   √x7th **M48.53 Collapsed vertebra, not elsewhere classified, cervicothoracic region**   HCC Rx ESR COM

1   √x7th **M48.54 Collapsed vertebra, not elsewhere classified, thoracic region**   HCC Rx ESR COM

1   √x7th **M48.55 Collapsed vertebra, not elsewhere classified, thoracolumbar region**   HCC Rx ESR COM

1   √x7th **M48.56 Collapsed vertebra, not elsewhere classified, lumbar region**   HCC Rx ESR COM

1   √x7th **M48.57 Collapsed vertebra, not elsewhere classified, lumbosacral region**   HCC Rx ESR COM

1   √x7th **M48.58 Collapsed vertebra, not elsewhere classified, sacral and sacrococcygeal region**   HCC Rx ESR COM

√5th **M48.8 Other specified spondylopathies**

     Ossification of posterior longitudinal ligament

     √6th **M48.8X Other specified spondylopathies**

         M48.8X1 Other specified spondylopathies, occipito-atlanto-axial region   HCC Rx ESR COM

         M48.8X2 Other specified spondylopathies, cervical region   HCC Rx ESR COM

         M48.8X3 Other specified spondylopathies, cervicothoracic region   HCC Rx ESR COM

         M48.8X4 Other specified spondylopathies, thoracic region   HCC Rx ESR COM

         M48.8X5 Other specified spondylopathies, thoracolumbar region   HCC Rx ESR COM

         M48.8X6 Other specified spondylopathies, lumbar region   HCC Rx ESR COM

         M48.8X7 Other specified spondylopathies, lumbosacral region   HCC Rx ESR COM

         M48.8X8 Other specified spondylopathies, sacral and sacrococcygeal region   HCC Rx ESR COM

         M48.8X9 Other specified spondylopathies, site unspecified   HCC Rx ESR COM

     M48.9 Spondylopathy, unspecified

√4th **M49 Spondylopathies in diseases classified elsewhere**

     INCLUDES   curvature of spine in diseases classified elsewhere

          deformity of spine in diseases classified elsewhere

          kyphosis in diseases classified elsewhere

          scoliosis in diseases classified elsewhere

          spondylopathy in diseases classified elsewhere

     Code first underlying disease, such as:

       brucellosis (A23.-)

       Charcôt-Marie-Tooth disease (G60.0)

       enterobacterial infections (A01-A04)

       osteitis fibrosa cystica (E21.0)

     EXCLUDES 1   *curvature of spine in tuberculosis [Pott's] (A18.01)*

          enteropathic arthropathies (M07.-)

          gonococcal spondylitis (A54.41)

          neuropathic spondylopathy in syringomyelia (G95.0)

          neuropathic spondylopathy in tabes dorsalis (A52.11)

          neuropathic [tabes dorsalis] spondylitis (A52.11)

          nonsyphilitic neuropathic spondylopathy NEC (G98.0)

          spondylitis in syphilis (acquired) (A52.77)

          tuberculous spondylitis (A18.01)

          typhoid fever spondylitis (A01.05)

√5th **M49.8 Spondylopathy in diseases classified elsewhere**

     M49.80 Spondylopathy in diseases classified elsewhere, site unspecified   HCC ESR

     M49.81 Spondylopathy in diseases classified elsewhere, occipito-atlanto-axial region   HCC ESR

     M49.82 Spondylopathy in diseases classified elsewhere, cervical region   HCC ESR

     M49.83 Spondylopathy in diseases classified elsewhere, cervicothoracic region   HCC ESR

     M49.84 Spondylopathy in diseases classified elsewhere, thoracic region   HCC ESR

     M49.85 Spondylopathy in diseases classified elsewhere, thoracolumbar region   HCC ESR

     M49.86 Spondylopathy in diseases classified elsewhere, lumbar region   HCC ESR

     M49.87 Spondylopathy in diseases classified elsewhere, lumbosacral region   HCC ESR

     M49.88 Spondylopathy in diseases classified elsewhere, sacral and sacrococcygeal region   HCC ESR

     M49.89 Spondylopathy in diseases classified elsewhere, multiple sites in spine   HCC ESR

Other dorsopathies (M50-M54)

EXCLUDES 1   current injury - see injury of spine by body region
discitis NOS (M46.4-)

✓4th **M50 Cervical disc disorders**

> NOTE   ~~Code to the most superior level of disorder~~
>
> INCLUDES   cervicothoracic disc disorders
> cervicothoracic disc disorders with cervicalgia
>
> AHA: 2016,4Q,39-40; 2016,1Q,17

✓5th **M50.0 Cervical disc disorder with myelopathy**

> AHA: 2018,3Q,19

M50.00   **Cervical disc disorder with myelopathy, unspecified cervical region**

M50.01   **Cervical disc disorder with myelopathy, high cervical region**
> C2-C3 disc disorder with myelopathy
> C3-C4 disc disorder with myelopathy

✓6th **M50.02**   **Cervical disc disorder with myelopathy, mid-cervical region**

> **M50.020**   **Cervical disc disorder with myelopathy, mid-cervical region, unspecified level**
>
> M50.021   **Cervical disc disorder at C4-C5 level with myelopathy**
> > C4-C5 disc disorder with myelopathy
>
> M50.022   **Cervical disc disorder at C5-C6 level with myelopathy**
> > C5-C6 disc disorder with myelopathy
>
> M50.023   **Cervical disc disorder at C6-C7 level with myelopathy**
> > C6-C7 disc disorder with myelopathy

M50.03   **Cervical disc disorder with myelopathy, cervicothoracic region**
> C7-T1 disc disorder with myelopathy

✓5th **M50.1 Cervical disc disorder with radiculopathy**

> EXCLUDES 2   brachial radiculitis NOS (M54.13)
>
> AHA: 2018,3Q,19

M50.10   **Cervical disc disorder with radiculopathy, unspecified cervical region**

M50.11   **Cervical disc disorder with radiculopathy, high cervical region**
> C2-C3 disc disorder with radiculopathy
> C3 radiculopathy due to disc disorder
> C3-C4 disc disorder with radiculopathy
> C4 radiculopathy due to disc disorder

✓6th **M50.12**   **Cervical disc disorder with radiculopathy, mid-cervical region**

> **M50.120**   **Mid-cervical disc disorder, unspecified level**
>
> M50.121   **Cervical disc disorder at C4-C5 level with radiculopathy**
> > C4-C5 disc disorder with radiculopathy
> > C5 radiculopathy due to disc disorder
>
> M50.122   **Cervical disc disorder at C5-C6 level with radiculopathy**
> > C5-C6 disc disorder with radiculopathy
> > C6 radiculopathy due to disc disorder
>
> M50.123   **Cervical disc disorder at C6-C7 level with radiculopathy**
> > C6-C7 disc disorder with radiculopathy
> > C7 radiculopathy due to disc disorder

M50.13   **Cervical disc disorder with radiculopathy, cervicothoracic region**
> C7-T1 disc disorder with radiculopathy
> C8 radiculopathy due to disc disorder

✓5th **M50.2 Other cervical disc displacement**

M50.20   **Other cervical disc displacement, unspecified cervical region**

M50.21   **Other cervical disc displacement, high cervical region**
> Other C2-C3 cervical disc displacement
> Other C3-C4 cervical disc displacement

✓6th **M50.22**   **Other cervical disc displacement, mid-cervical region**

> **M50.220**   **Other cervical disc displacement, mid-cervical region, unspecified level**
>
> M50.221   **Other cervical disc displacement at C4-C5 level**
> > Other C4-C5 cervical disc displacement

> M50.222   **Other cervical disc displacement at C5-C6 level**
> > Other C5-C6 cervical disc displacement
>
> M50.223   **Other cervical disc displacement at C6-C7 level**
> > Other C6-C7 cervical disc displacement

M50.23   **Other cervical disc displacement, cervicothoracic region**
> Other C7-T1 cervical disc displacement

✓5th **M50.3 Other cervical disc degeneration**

M50.30   **Other cervical disc degeneration, unspecified cervical region**

M50.31   **Other cervical disc degeneration, high cervical region**
> Other C2-C3 cervical disc degeneration
> Other C3-C4 cervical disc degeneration

✓6th **M50.32**   **Other cervical disc degeneration, mid-cervical region**

> **M50.320**   **Other cervical disc degeneration, mid-cervical region, unspecified level**
>
> M50.321   **Other cervical disc degeneration at C4-C5 level**
> > Other C4-C5 cervical disc degeneration
>
> M50.322   **Other cervical disc degeneration at C5-C6 level**
> > Other C5-C6 cervical disc degeneration
>
> M50.323   **Other cervical disc degeneration at C6-C7 level**
> > Other C6-C7 cervical disc degeneration

M50.33   **Other cervical disc degeneration, cervicothoracic region**
> Other C7-T1 cervical disc degeneration

✓5th **M50.8 Other cervical disc disorders**

M50.80   **Other cervical disc disorders, unspecified cervical region**

M50.81   **Other cervical disc disorders, high cervical region**
> Other C2-C3 cervical disc disorders
> Other C3-C4 cervical disc disorders

✓6th **M50.82**   **Other cervical disc disorders, mid-cervical region**

> **M50.820**   **Other cervical disc disorders, mid-cervical region, unspecified level**
>
> M50.821   **Other cervical disc disorders at C4-C5 level**
> > Other C4-C5 cervical disc disorders
>
> M50.822   **Other cervical disc disorders at C5-C6 level**
> > Other C5-C6 cervical disc disorders
>
> M50.823   **Other cervical disc disorders at C6-C7 level**
> > Other C6-C7 cervical disc disorders

M50.83   **Other cervical disc disorders, cervicothoracic region**
> Other C7-T1 cervical disc disorders

✓5th **M50.9 Cervical disc disorder, unspecified**

M50.90   **Cervical disc disorder, unspecified, unspecified cervical region**

M50.91   **Cervical disc disorder, unspecified, high cervical region**
> C2-C3 cervical disc disorder, unspecified
> C3-C4 cervical disc disorder, unspecified

✓6th **M50.92**   **Cervical disc disorder, unspecified, mid-cervical region**

> **M50.920**   **Unspecified cervical disc disorder, mid-cervical region, unspecified level**
>
> **M50.921**   **Unspecified cervical disc disorder at C4-C5 level**
> > Unspecified C4-C5 cervical disc disorder
>
> **M50.922**   **Unspecified cervical disc disorder at C5-C6 level**
> > Unspecified C5-C6 cervical disc disorder
>
> **M50.923**   **Unspecified cervical disc disorder at C6-C7 level**
> > Unspecified C6-C7 cervical disc disorder

M50.93   **Cervical disc disorder, unspecified, cervicothoracic region**
> C7-T1 cervical disc disorder, unspecified

✓4th M51 Thoracic, thoracolumbar, and lumbosacral intervertebral disc disorders

EXCLUDES 2   *cervical and cervicothoracic disc disorders (M50.-)*
sacral and sacrococcygeal disorders (M53.3)

✓5th M51.0 Thoracic, thoracolumbar and lumbosacral intervertebral disc disorders with myelopathy

M51.04 Intervertebral disc disorders with myelopathy, thoracic region

M51.05 Intervertebral disc disorders with myelopathy, thoracolumbar region

M51.06 Intervertebral disc disorders with myelopathy, lumbar region

✓5th M51.1 Thoracic, thoracolumbar and lumbosacral intervertebral disc disorders with radiculopathy

Sciatica due to intervertebral disc disorder

EXCLUDES 1   *lumbar radiculitis NOS (M54.16)*
sciatica NOS (M54.3)

AHA: 2018,3Q,18

M51.14 Intervertebral disc disorders with radiculopathy, thoracic region

M51.15 Intervertebral disc disorders with radiculopathy, thoracolumbar region

M51.16 Intervertebral disc disorders with radiculopathy, lumbar region

M51.17 Intervertebral disc disorders with radiculopathy, lumbosacral region

✓5th M51.2 Other thoracic, thoracolumbar and lumbosacral intervertebral disc displacement

Lumbago due to displacement of intervertebral disc

AHA: 2022,1Q,26

Displacement Intervertebral Disc

Nucleus pulposus — Lamina — Ligamentum flavum — Disc annulus — Nucleus pulposus — Spinal cord — Herniates through annulus — Spinal nerve

Normal Top View   Herniated Top View

M51.24 Other intervertebral disc displacement, thoracic region

M51.25 Other intervertebral disc displacement, thoracolumbar region

M51.26 Other intervertebral disc displacement, lumbar region

M51.27 Other intervertebral disc displacement, lumbosacral region

✓5th M51.3 Other thoracic, thoracolumbar and lumbosacral intervertebral disc degeneration

AHA: 2022,1Q,26; 2018,2Q,15; 2013,3Q,22

M51.34 Other intervertebral disc degeneration, thoracic region

M51.35 Other intervertebral disc degeneration, thoracolumbar region

M51.36 Other intervertebral disc degeneration, lumbar region

M51.37 Other intervertebral disc degeneration, lumbosacral region

✓5th M51.4 Schmorl's nodes

DEF: Irregular bone defect in the margin of the vertebral body that causes herniation into the end plate of the vertebral body.

M51.44 Schmorl's nodes, thoracic region

M51.45 Schmorl's nodes, thoracolumbar region

M51.46 Schmorl's nodes, lumbar region

M51.47 Schmorl's nodes, lumbosacral region

✓5th M51.8 Other thoracic, thoracolumbar and lumbosacral intervertebral disc disorders

M51.84 Other intervertebral disc disorders, thoracic region

M51.85 Other intervertebral disc disorders, thoracolumbar region

M51.86 Other intervertebral disc disorders, lumbar region

M51.87 Other intervertebral disc disorders, lumbosacral region

M51.9 Unspecified thoracic, thoracolumbar and lumbosacral intervertebral disc disorder

✓5th M51.A Other lumbar and lumbosacral annulus fibrosus disc defects

M51.A0 Intervertebral annulus fibrosus defect, lumbar region, unspecified size

Code first, if applicable, lumbar disc herniation (M51.06, M51.16, M51.26)

M51.A1 Intervertebral annulus fibrosus defect, small, lumbar region

Code first, if applicable, lumbar disc herniation (M51.06, M51.16, M51.26)

M51.A2 Intervertebral annulus fibrosus defect, large, lumbar region

Code first, if applicable, lumbar disc herniation (M51.06, M51.16, M51.26)

M51.A3 Intervertebral annulus fibrosus defect, lumbosacral region, unspecified size

Code first, if applicable, lumbosacral disc herniation (M51.17, M51.27)

M51.A4 Intervertebral annulus fibrosus defect, small, lumbosacral region

Code first, if applicable, lumbosacral disc herniation (M51.17, M51.27)

M51.A5 Intervertebral annulus fibrosus defect, large, lumbosacral region

Code first, if applicable, lumbosacral disc herniation (M51.17, M51.27)

✓4th M53 Other and unspecified dorsopathies, not elsewhere classified

M53.0 Cervicocranial syndrome

Posterior cervical sympathetic syndrome

M53.1 Cervicobrachial syndrome

EXCLUDES 2   *cervical disc disorder (M50.-)*
thoracic outlet syndrome (G54.0)

✓5th M53.2 Spinal instabilities

✓6th M53.2X Spinal instabilities

M53.2X1 Spinal instabilities, occipito-atlanto-axial region

M53.2X2 Spinal instabilities, cervical region

M53.2X3 Spinal instabilities, cervicothoracic region

M53.2X4 Spinal instabilities, thoracic region

M53.2X5 Spinal instabilities, thoracolumbar region

M53.2X6 Spinal instabilities, lumbar region

M53.2X7 Spinal instabilities, lumbosacral region

M53.2X8 Spinal instabilities, sacral and sacrococcygeal region

M53.2X9 Spinal instabilities, site unspecified

M53.3 Sacrococcygeal disorders, not elsewhere classified

Coccygodynia

✓5th M53.8 Other specified dorsopathies

M53.80 Other specified dorsopathies, site unspecified

M53.81 Other specified dorsopathies, occipito-atlanto-axial region

M53.82 Other specified dorsopathies, cervical region

M53.83 Other specified dorsopathies, cervicothoracic region

M53.84 Other specified dorsopathies, thoracic region

M53.85 Other specified dorsopathies, thoracolumbar region

M53.86 Other specified dorsopathies, lumbar region

M53.87 Other specified dorsopathies, lumbosacral region

M53.88 Other specified dorsopathies, sacral and sacrococcygeal region

M53.9 Dorsopathy, unspecified

✓4th M54 Dorsalgia

EXCLUDES 1   *psychogenic dorsalgia (F45.41)*

✓5th M54.0 Panniculitis affecting regions of neck and back

EXCLUDES 1   *lupus panniculitis (L93.2)*
panniculitis NOS (M79.3)
relapsing [Weber-Christian] panniculitis (M35.6)

M54.00 Panniculitis affecting regions of neck and back, site unspecified

M54.01 Panniculitis affecting regions of neck and back, occipito-atlanto-axial region

M54.02 Panniculitis affecting regions of neck and back, cervical region

Chapter 13. Diseases of the Musculoskeletal System and Connective Tissue

M54.Ø3 **Panniculitis affecting regions of neck and back, cervicothoracic region**

M54.Ø4 **Panniculitis affecting regions of neck and back, thoracic region**

M54.Ø5 **Panniculitis affecting regions of neck and back, thoracolumbar region**

M54.Ø6 **Panniculitis affecting regions of neck and back, lumbar region**

M54.Ø7 **Panniculitis affecting regions of neck and back, lumbosacral region**

M54.Ø8 **Panniculitis affecting regions of neck and back, sacral and sacrococcygeal region**

M54.Ø9 **Panniculitis affecting regions, neck and back, multiple sites in spine**

☑5ᵗʰ M54.1 **Radiculopathy**

Brachial neuritis or radiculitis NOS
Lumbar neuritis or radiculitis NOS
Lumbosacral neuritis or radiculitis NOS
Thoracic neuritis or radiculitis NOS
Radiculitis NOS

EXCLUDES 1 *neuralgia and neuritis NOS (M79.2)*
radiculopathy with cervical disc disorder (M50.1)
radiculopathy with lumbar and other intervertebral disc disorder (M51.1-)
radiculopathy with spondylosis (M47.2-)

AHA: 2018,3Q,18
TIP: A code from this subcategory can be used in addition to a spondylolisthesis code (M43.1-) or a spinal stenosis code (M48.0-) when either condition is documented as the cause of the radiculopathy.

M54.1Ø **Radiculopathy, site unspecified**
M54.11 **Radiculopathy, occipito-atlanto-axial region**
M54.12 **Radiculopathy, cervical region**
M54.13 **Radiculopathy, cervicothoracic region**
M54.14 **Radiculopathy, thoracic region**
M54.15 **Radiculopathy, thoracolumbar region**
M54.16 **Radiculopathy, lumbar region**
M54.17 **Radiculopathy, lumbosacral region**
M54.18 **Radiculopathy, sacral and sacrococcygeal region**

M54.2 **Cervicalgia**
EXCLUDES 1 *cervicalgia due to intervertebral cervical disc disorder (M50.-)*

☑5ᵗʰ M54.3 **Sciatica**
EXCLUDES 1 *lesion of sciatic nerve (G57.Ø)*
sciatica due to intervertebral disc disorder (M51.1-)
sciatica with lumbago (M54.4-)

M54.3Ø **Sciatica, unspecified side**
M54.31 **Sciatica, right side**
M54.32 **Sciatica, left side**

☑5ᵗʰ M54.4 **Lumbago with sciatica**
EXCLUDES 1 *lumbago with sciatica due to intervertebral disc disorder (M51.1-)*

AHA: 2016,2Q,7
M54.4Ø **Lumbago with sciatica, unspecified side**
M54.41 **Lumbago with sciatica, right side**
M54.42 **Lumbago with sciatica, left side**

☑5ᵗʰ M54.5 **Low back pain**
EXCLUDES 1 *low back strain (S39.Ø12)*
lumbago due to intervertebral disc displacement (M51.2-)
lumbago with sciatica (M54.4-)

AHA: 2021,4Q,22
M54.5Ø **Low back pain, unspecified**
Loin pain
Lumbago NOS
M54.51 **Vertebrogenic low back pain**
Low back vertebral endplate pain
M54.59 **Other low back pain**

M54.6 **Pain in thoracic spine**
EXCLUDES 1 *pain in thoracic spine due to intervertebral disc disorder (M51.-)*

☑5ᵗʰ M54.8 **Other dorsalgia**
EXCLUDES 1 *dorsalgia in thoracic region (M54.6)*
low back pain (M54.5-)

M54.81 **Occipital neuralgia**
M54.89 **Other dorsalgia**

M54.9 **Dorsalgia, unspecified**
Backache NOS
Back pain NOS

SOFT TISSUE DISORDERS (M60-M79)

Disorders of muscles (M6Ø-M63)

EXCLUDES 1 *dermatopolymyositis (M33.-)*
muscular dystrophies and myopathies (G71-G72)
myopathy in amyloidosis (E85.-)
myopathy in polyarteritis nodosa (M30.Ø)
myopathy in rheumatoid arthritis (MØ5.32)
myopathy in scleroderma (M34.-)
myopathy in Sjögren's syndrome (M35.Ø3)
myopathy in systemic lupus erythematosus (M32.-)

EXCLUDES 2 ▶*muscular dystrophies and myopathies (G71-G72)*◀

☑4ᵗʰ **M6Ø Myositis**
EXCLUDES 2 *inclusion body myositis [IBM] (G72.41)*

☑5ᵗʰ M6Ø.Ø **Infective myositis**
Tropical pyomyositis
Use additional code (B95-B97) to identify infectious agent

☑6ᵗʰ M6Ø.ØØ **Infective myositis, unspecified site**
M6Ø.ØØØ **Infective myositis, unspecified right arm**
Infective myositis, right upper limb NOS
M6Ø.ØØ1 **Infective myositis, unspecified left arm**
Infective myositis, left upper limb NOS
M6Ø.ØØ2 **Infective myositis, unspecified arm**
Infective myositis, upper limb NOS
M6Ø.ØØ3 **Infective myositis, unspecified right leg**
Infective myositis, right lower limb NOS
M6Ø.ØØ4 **Infective myositis, unspecified left leg**
Infective myositis, left lower limb NOS
M6Ø.ØØ5 **Infective myositis, unspecified leg**
Infective myositis, lower limb NOS
M6Ø.ØØ9 **Infective myositis, unspecified site**

☑6ᵗʰ M6Ø.Ø1 **Infective myositis, shoulder**
M6Ø.Ø11 **Infective myositis, right shoulder**
M6Ø.Ø12 **Infective myositis, left shoulder**
M6Ø.Ø19 **Infective myositis, unspecified shoulder**

☑6ᵗʰ M6Ø.Ø2 **Infective myositis, upper arm**
M6Ø.Ø21 **Infective myositis, right upper arm**
M6Ø.Ø22 **Infective myositis, left upper arm**
M6Ø.Ø29 **Infective myositis, unspecified upper arm**

☑6ᵗʰ M6Ø.Ø3 **Infective myositis, forearm**
M6Ø.Ø31 **Infective myositis, right forearm**
M6Ø.Ø32 **Infective myositis, left forearm**
M6Ø.Ø39 **Infective myositis, unspecified forearm**

☑6ᵗʰ M6Ø.Ø4 **Infective myositis, hand and fingers**
M6Ø.Ø41 **Infective myositis, right hand**
M6Ø.Ø42 **Infective myositis, left hand**
M6Ø.Ø43 **Infective myositis, unspecified hand**
M6Ø.Ø44 **Infective myositis, right finger(s)**
M6Ø.Ø45 **Infective myositis, left finger(s)**
M6Ø.Ø46 **Infective myositis, unspecified finger(s)**

☑6ᵗʰ M6Ø.Ø5 **Infective myositis, thigh**
M6Ø.Ø51 **Infective myositis, right thigh**
M6Ø.Ø52 **Infective myositis, left thigh**
M6Ø.Ø59 **Infective myositis, unspecified thigh**

☑6ᵗʰ M6Ø.Ø6 **Infective myositis, lower leg**
M6Ø.Ø61 **Infective myositis, right lower leg**
M6Ø.Ø62 **Infective myositis, left lower leg**
M6Ø.Ø69 **Infective myositis, unspecified lower leg**

☑6ᵗʰ M6Ø.Ø7 **Infective myositis, ankle, foot and toes**
M6Ø.Ø7Ø **Infective myositis, right ankle**
M6Ø.Ø71 **Infective myositis, left ankle**
M6Ø.Ø72 **Infective myositis, unspecified ankle**
M6Ø.Ø73 **Infective myositis, right foot**
M6Ø.Ø74 **Infective myositis, left foot**
M6Ø.Ø75 **Infective myositis, unspecified foot**
M6Ø.Ø76 **Infective myositis, right toe(s)**
M6Ø.Ø77 **Infective myositis, left toe(s)**
M6Ø.Ø78 **Infective myositis, unspecified toe(s)**

M6Ø.Ø8 **Infective myositis, other site**
M6Ø.Ø9 **Infective myositis, multiple sites**

☑5ᵗʰ M6Ø.1 **Interstitial myositis**
M6Ø.1Ø **Interstitial myositis of unspecified site**

√6ᵗʰ **M60.11** Interstitial myositis, shoulder

  M60.111 Interstitial myositis, right shoulder
  M60.112 Interstitial myositis, left shoulder
  M60.119 Interstitial myositis, unspecified shoulder

√6ᵗʰ **M60.12** Interstitial myositis, upper arm

  M60.121 Interstitial myositis, right upper arm
  M60.122 Interstitial myositis, left upper arm
  M60.129 Interstitial myositis, unspecified upper arm

√6ᵗʰ **M60.13** Interstitial myositis, forearm

  M60.131 Interstitial myositis, right forearm
  M60.132 Interstitial myositis, left forearm
  M60.139 Interstitial myositis, unspecified forearm

√6ᵗʰ **M60.14** Interstitial myositis, hand

  M60.141 Interstitial myositis, right hand
  M60.142 Interstitial myositis, left hand
  M60.149 Interstitial myositis, unspecified hand

√6ᵗʰ **M60.15** Interstitial myositis, thigh

  M60.151 Interstitial myositis, right thigh
  M60.152 Interstitial myositis, left thigh
  M60.159 Interstitial myositis, unspecified thigh

√6ᵗʰ **M60.16** Interstitial myositis, lower leg

  M60.161 Interstitial myositis, right lower leg
  M60.162 Interstitial myositis, left lower leg
  M60.169 Interstitial myositis, unspecified lower leg

√6ᵗʰ **M60.17** Interstitial myositis, ankle and foot

  M60.171 Interstitial myositis, right ankle and foot
  M60.172 Interstitial myositis, left ankle and foot
  M60.179 Interstitial myositis, unspecified ankle and foot

M60.18 Interstitial myositis, other site
M60.19 Interstitial myositis, multiple sites

√5ᵗʰ **M60.2** Foreign body granuloma of soft tissue, not elsewhere classified

  Use additional code to identify the type of retained foreign body (Z18.-)

   EXCLUDES 1   foreign body granuloma of skin and subcutaneous tissue (L92.3)

  M60.20 Foreign body granuloma of soft tissue, not elsewhere classified, unspecified site

√6ᵗʰ **M60.21** Foreign body granuloma of soft tissue, not elsewhere classified, shoulder

  M60.211 Foreign body granuloma of soft tissue, not elsewhere classified, right shoulder
  M60.212 Foreign body granuloma of soft tissue, not elsewhere classified, left shoulder
  M60.219 Foreign body granuloma of soft tissue, not elsewhere classified, unspecified shoulder

√6ᵗʰ **M60.22** Foreign body granuloma of soft tissue, not elsewhere classified, upper arm

  M60.221 Foreign body granuloma of soft tissue, not elsewhere classified, right upper arm
  M60.222 Foreign body granuloma of soft tissue, not elsewhere classified, left upper arm
  M60.229 Foreign body granuloma of soft tissue, not elsewhere classified, unspecified upper arm

√6ᵗʰ **M60.23** Foreign body granuloma of soft tissue, not elsewhere classified, forearm

  M60.231 Foreign body granuloma of soft tissue, not elsewhere classified, right forearm
  M60.232 Foreign body granuloma of soft tissue, not elsewhere classified, left forearm
  M60.239 Foreign body granuloma of soft tissue, not elsewhere classified, unspecified forearm

√6ᵗʰ **M60.24** Foreign body granuloma of soft tissue, not elsewhere classified, hand

  M60.241 Foreign body granuloma of soft tissue, not elsewhere classified, right hand
  M60.242 Foreign body granuloma of soft tissue, not elsewhere classified, left hand
  M60.249 Foreign body granuloma of soft tissue, not elsewhere classified, unspecified hand

√6ᵗʰ **M60.25** Foreign body granuloma of soft tissue, not elsewhere classified, thigh

  M60.251 Foreign body granuloma of soft tissue, not elsewhere classified, right thigh
  M60.252 Foreign body granuloma of soft tissue, not elsewhere classified, left thigh
  M60.259 Foreign body granuloma of soft tissue, not elsewhere classified, unspecified thigh

√6ᵗʰ **M60.26** Foreign body granuloma of soft tissue, not elsewhere classified, lower leg

  M60.261 Foreign body granuloma of soft tissue, not elsewhere classified, right lower leg
  M60.262 Foreign body granuloma of soft tissue, not elsewhere classified, left lower leg
  M60.269 Foreign body granuloma of soft tissue, not elsewhere classified, unspecified lower leg

√6ᵗʰ **M60.27** Foreign body granuloma of soft tissue, not elsewhere classified, ankle and foot

  M60.271 Foreign body granuloma of soft tissue, not elsewhere classified, right ankle and foot
  M60.272 Foreign body granuloma of soft tissue, not elsewhere classified, left ankle and foot
  M60.279 Foreign body granuloma of soft tissue, not elsewhere classified, unspecified ankle and foot

M60.28 Foreign body granuloma of soft tissue, not elsewhere classified, other site

√5ᵗʰ **M60.8** Other myositis

  M60.80 Other myositis, unspecified site

√6ᵗʰ **M60.81** Other myositis shoulder

  M60.811 Other myositis, right shoulder
  M60.812 Other myositis, left shoulder
  M60.819 Other myositis, unspecified shoulder

√6ᵗʰ **M60.82** Other myositis, upper arm

  M60.821 Other myositis, right upper arm
  M60.822 Other myositis, left upper arm
  M60.829 Other myositis, unspecified upper arm

√6ᵗʰ **M60.83** Other myositis, forearm

  M60.831 Other myositis, right forearm
  M60.832 Other myositis, left forearm
  M60.839 Other myositis, unspecified forearm

√6ᵗʰ **M60.84** Other myositis, hand

  M60.841 Other myositis, right hand
  M60.842 Other myositis, left hand
  M60.849 Other myositis, unspecified hand

√6ᵗʰ **M60.85** Other myositis, thigh

  M60.851 Other myositis, right thigh
  M60.852 Other myositis, left thigh
  M60.859 Other myositis, unspecified thigh

√6ᵗʰ **M60.86** Other myositis, lower leg

  M60.861 Other myositis, right lower leg
  M60.862 Other myositis, left lower leg
  M60.869 Other myositis, unspecified lower leg

√6ᵗʰ **M60.87** Other myositis, ankle and foot

  M60.871 Other myositis, right ankle and foot
  M60.872 Other myositis, left ankle and foot
  M60.879 Other myositis, unspecified ankle and foot

M60.88 Other myositis, other site
M60.89 Other myositis, multiple sites

M60.9 Myositis, unspecified

√4ᵗʰ **M61** Calcification and ossification of muscle

√5ᵗʰ **M61.0** Myositis ossificans traumatica

  M61.00 Myositis ossificans traumatica, unspecified site

√6ᵗʰ **M61.01** Myositis ossificans traumatica, shoulder

  M61.011 Myositis ossificans traumatica, right shoulder
  M61.012 Myositis ossificans traumatica, left shoulder
  M61.019 Myositis ossificans traumatica, unspecified shoulder

√6ᵗʰ **M61.02** Myositis ossificans traumatica, upper arm

  M61.021 Myositis ossificans traumatica, right upper arm

M61.022 Myositis ossificans traumatica, left upper arm

M61.029 Myositis ossificans traumatica, unspecified upper arm

√6th **M61.03** Myositis ossificans traumatica, forearm

M61.031 Myositis ossificans traumatica, right forearm

M61.032 Myositis ossificans traumatica, left forearm

M61.039 Myositis ossificans traumatica, unspecified forearm

√6th **M61.04** Myositis ossificans traumatica, hand

M61.041 Myositis ossificans traumatica, right hand

M61.042 Myositis ossificans traumatica, left hand

M61.049 Myositis ossificans traumatica, unspecified hand

√6th **M61.05** Myositis ossificans traumatica, thigh

M61.051 Myositis ossificans traumatica, right thigh

M61.052 Myositis ossificans traumatica, left thigh

M61.059 Myositis ossificans traumatica, unspecified thigh

√6th **M61.06** Myositis ossificans traumatica, lower leg

M61.061 Myositis ossificans traumatica, right lower leg

M61.062 Myositis ossificans traumatica, left lower leg

M61.069 Myositis ossificans traumatica, unspecified lower leg

√6th **M61.07** Myositis ossificans traumatica, ankle and foot

M61.071 Myositis ossificans traumatica, right ankle and foot

M61.072 Myositis ossificans traumatica, left ankle and foot

M61.079 Myositis ossificans traumatica, unspecified ankle and foot

M61.08 Myositis ossificans traumatica, other site

M61.09 Myositis ossificans traumatica, multiple sites

√5th **M61.1** Myositis ossificans progressiva

Fibrodysplasia ossificans progressiva

M61.10 Myositis ossificans progressiva, unspecified site

√6th **M61.11** Myositis ossificans progressiva, shoulder

M61.111 Myositis ossificans progressiva, right shoulder

M61.112 Myositis ossificans progressiva, left shoulder

M61.119 Myositis ossificans progressiva, unspecified shoulder

√6th **M61.12** Myositis ossificans progressiva, upper arm

M61.121 Myositis ossificans progressiva, right upper arm

M61.122 Myositis ossificans progressiva, left upper arm

M61.129 Myositis ossificans progressiva, unspecified arm

√6th **M61.13** Myositis ossificans progressiva, forearm

M61.131 Myositis ossificans progressiva, right forearm

M61.132 Myositis ossificans progressiva, left forearm

M61.139 Myositis ossificans progressiva, unspecified forearm

√6th **M61.14** Myositis ossificans progressiva, hand and finger(s)

M61.141 Myositis ossificans progressiva, right hand

M61.142 Myositis ossificans progressiva, left hand

M61.143 Myositis ossificans progressiva, unspecified hand

M61.144 Myositis ossificans progressiva, right finger(s)

M61.145 Myositis ossificans progressiva, left finger(s)

M61.146 Myositis ossificans progressiva, unspecified finger(s)

√6th **M61.15** Myositis ossificans progressiva, thigh

M61.151 Myositis ossificans progressiva, right thigh

M61.152 Myositis ossificans progressiva, left thigh

M61.159 Myositis ossificans progressiva, unspecified thigh

√6th **M61.16** Myositis ossificans progressiva, lower leg

M61.161 Myositis ossificans progressiva, right lower leg

M61.162 Myositis ossificans progressiva, left lower leg

M61.169 Myositis ossificans progressiva, unspecified lower leg

√6th **M61.17** Myositis ossificans progressiva, ankle, foot and toe(s)

M61.171 Myositis ossificans progressiva, right ankle

M61.172 Myositis ossificans progressiva, left ankle

M61.173 Myositis ossificans progressiva, unspecified ankle

M61.174 Myositis ossificans progressiva, right foot

M61.175 Myositis ossificans progressiva, left foot

M61.176 Myositis ossificans progressiva, unspecified foot

M61.177 Myositis ossificans progressiva, right toe(s)

M61.178 Myositis ossificans progressiva, left toe(s)

M61.179 Myositis ossificans progressiva, unspecified toe(s)

M61.18 Myositis ossificans progressiva, other site

M61.19 Myositis ossificans progressiva, multiple sites

√5th **M61.2** Paralytic calcification and ossification of muscle

Myositis ossificans associated with quadriplegia or paraplegia

M61.20 Paralytic calcification and ossification of muscle, unspecified site

√6th **M61.21** Paralytic calcification and ossification of muscle, shoulder

M61.211 Paralytic calcification and ossification of muscle, right shoulder

M61.212 Paralytic calcification and ossification of muscle, left shoulder

M61.219 Paralytic calcification and ossification of muscle, unspecified shoulder

√6th **M61.22** Paralytic calcification and ossification of muscle, upper arm

M61.221 Paralytic calcification and ossification of muscle, right upper arm

M61.222 Paralytic calcification and ossification of muscle, left upper arm

M61.229 Paralytic calcification and ossification of muscle, unspecified upper arm

√6th **M61.23** Paralytic calcification and ossification of muscle, forearm

M61.231 Paralytic calcification and ossification of muscle, right forearm

M61.232 Paralytic calcification and ossification of muscle, left forearm

M61.239 Paralytic calcification and ossification of muscle, unspecified forearm

√6th **M61.24** Paralytic calcification and ossification of muscle, hand

M61.241 Paralytic calcification and ossification of muscle, right hand

M61.242 Paralytic calcification and ossification of muscle, left hand

M61.249 Paralytic calcification and ossification of muscle, unspecified hand

√6th **M61.25** Paralytic calcification and ossification of muscle, thigh

M61.251 Paralytic calcification and ossification of muscle, right thigh

M61.252 Paralytic calcification and ossification of muscle, left thigh

M61.259 Paralytic calcification and ossification of muscle, unspecified thigh

√6th **M61.26** Paralytic calcification and ossification of muscle, lower leg

M61.261 Paralytic calcification and ossification of muscle, right lower leg

M61.262 Paralytic calcification and ossification of muscle, left lower leg

M61.269 Paralytic calcification and ossification of muscle, unspecified lower leg

√6th **M61.27** Paralytic calcification and ossification of muscle, ankle and foot

M61.271 Paralytic calcification and ossification of muscle, right ankle and foot

Chapter 13. Diseases of the Musculoskeletal System and Connective Tissue

M61.272–M61.559

M61.272 Paralytic calcification and ossification of muscle, left ankle and foot

M61.279 Paralytic calcification and ossification of muscle, unspecified ankle and foot

M61.28 Paralytic calcification and ossification of muscle, other site

M61.29 Paralytic calcification and ossification of muscle, multiple sites

✓5ᵗʰ M61.3 Calcification and ossification of muscles associated with burns
   Myositis ossificans associated with burns

M61.30 Calcification and ossification of muscles associated with burns, unspecified site

✓6ᵗʰ M61.31 Calcification and ossification of muscles associated with burns, shoulder

M61.311 Calcification and ossification of muscles associated with burns, right shoulder

M61.312 Calcification and ossification of muscles associated with burns, left shoulder

M61.319 Calcification and ossification of muscles associated with burns, unspecified shoulder

✓6ᵗʰ M61.32 Calcification and ossification of muscles associated with burns, upper arm

M61.321 Calcification and ossification of muscles associated with burns, right upper arm

M61.322 Calcification and ossification of muscles associated with burns, left upper arm

M61.329 Calcification and ossification of muscles associated with burns, unspecified upper arm

✓6ᵗʰ M61.33 Calcification and ossification of muscles associated with burns, forearm

M61.331 Calcification and ossification of muscles associated with burns, right forearm

M61.332 Calcification and ossification of muscles associated with burns, left forearm

M61.339 Calcification and ossification of muscles associated with burns, unspecified forearm

✓6ᵗʰ M61.34 Calcification and ossification of muscles associated with burns, hand

M61.341 Calcification and ossification of muscles associated with burns, right hand

M61.342 Calcification and ossification of muscles associated with burns, left hand

M61.349 Calcification and ossification of muscles associated with burns, unspecified hand

✓6ᵗʰ M61.35 Calcification and ossification of muscles associated with burns, thigh

M61.351 Calcification and ossification of muscles associated with burns, right thigh

M61.352 Calcification and ossification of muscles associated with burns, left thigh

M61.359 Calcification and ossification of muscles associated with burns, unspecified thigh

✓6ᵗʰ M61.36 Calcification and ossification of muscles associated with burns, lower leg

M61.361 Calcification and ossification of muscles associated with burns, right lower leg

M61.362 Calcification and ossification of muscles associated with burns, left lower leg

M61.369 Calcification and ossification of muscles associated with burns, unspecified lower leg

✓6ᵗʰ M61.37 Calcification and ossification of muscles associated with burns, ankle and foot

M61.371 Calcification and ossification of muscles associated with burns, right ankle and foot

M61.372 Calcification and ossification of muscles associated with burns, left ankle and foot

M61.379 Calcification and ossification of muscles associated with burns, unspecified ankle and foot

M61.38 Calcification and ossification of muscles associated with burns, other site

M61.39 Calcification and ossification of muscles associated with burns, multiple sites

✓5ᵗʰ M61.4 Other calcification of muscle

EXCLUDES 1 calcific tendinitis NOS (M65.2-)
   calcific tendinitis of shoulder (M75.3)

M61.40 Other calcification of muscle, unspecified site

✓6ᵗʰ M61.41 Other calcification of muscle, shoulder

M61.411 Other calcification of muscle, right shoulder

M61.412 Other calcification of muscle, left shoulder

M61.419 Other calcification of muscle, unspecified shoulder

✓6ᵗʰ M61.42 Other calcification of muscle, upper arm

M61.421 Other calcification of muscle, right upper arm

M61.422 Other calcification of muscle, left upper arm

M61.429 Other calcification of muscle, unspecified upper arm

✓6ᵗʰ M61.43 Other calcification of muscle, forearm

M61.431 Other calcification of muscle, right forearm

M61.432 Other calcification of muscle, left forearm

M61.439 Other calcification of muscle, unspecified forearm

✓6ᵗʰ M61.44 Other calcification of muscle, hand

M61.441 Other calcification of muscle, right hand

M61.442 Other calcification of muscle, left hand

M61.449 Other calcification of muscle, unspecified hand

✓6ᵗʰ M61.45 Other calcification of muscle, thigh

M61.451 Other calcification of muscle, right thigh

M61.452 Other calcification of muscle, left thigh

M61.459 Other calcification of muscle, unspecified thigh

✓6ᵗʰ M61.46 Other calcification of muscle, lower leg

M61.461 Other calcification of muscle, right lower leg

M61.462 Other calcification of muscle, left lower leg

M61.469 Other calcification of muscle, unspecified lower leg

✓6ᵗʰ M61.47 Other calcification of muscle, ankle and foot

M61.471 Other calcification of muscle, right ankle and foot

M61.472 Other calcification of muscle, left ankle and foot

M61.479 Other calcification of muscle, unspecified ankle and foot

M61.48 Other calcification of muscle, other site

M61.49 Other calcification of muscle, multiple sites

✓5ᵗʰ M61.5 Other ossification of muscle

M61.50 Other ossification of muscle, unspecified site

✓6ᵗʰ M61.51 Other ossification of muscle, shoulder

M61.511 Other ossification of muscle, right shoulder

M61.512 Other ossification of muscle, left shoulder

M61.519 Other ossification of muscle, unspecified shoulder

✓6ᵗʰ M61.52 Other ossification of muscle, upper arm

M61.521 Other ossification of muscle, right upper arm

M61.522 Other ossification of muscle, left upper arm

M61.529 Other ossification of muscle, unspecified upper arm

✓6ᵗʰ M61.53 Other ossification of muscle, forearm

M61.531 Other ossification of muscle, right forearm

M61.532 Other ossification of muscle, left forearm

M61.539 Other ossification of muscle, unspecified forearm

✓6ᵗʰ M61.54 Other ossification of muscle, hand

M61.541 Other ossification of muscle, right hand

M61.542 Other ossification of muscle, left hand

M61.549 Other ossification of muscle, unspecified hand

✓6ᵗʰ M61.55 Other ossification of muscle, thigh

M61.551 Other ossification of muscle, right thigh

M61.552 Other ossification of muscle, left thigh

M61.559 Other ossification of muscle, unspecified thigh

✓6ᵗʰ **M61.56** **Other ossification of muscle,** lower leg

     M61.561 **Other ossification of muscle,** right lower leg

     M61.562 **Other ossification of muscle,** left lower leg

     M61.569 **Other ossification of muscle, unspecified** lower leg

✓6ᵗʰ **M61.57** **Other ossification of muscle,** ankle and foot

     M61.571 **Other ossification of muscle,** right ankle and foot

     M61.572 **Other ossification of muscle,** left ankle and foot

     M61.579 **Other ossification of muscle, unspecified ankle and foot**

M61.58 **Other ossification of muscle, other site**

M61.59 **Other ossification of muscle,** multiple sites

M61.9 **Calcification and ossification of muscle, unspecified**

✓4ᵗʰ **M62** **Other disorders of muscle**

     EXCLUDES 1   *alcoholic myopathy (G72.1)*

                cramp and spasm (R25.2)

                drug-induced myopathy (G72.0)

                myalgia (M79.1-)

                stiff-man syndrome (G25.82)

     EXCLUDES 2   *nontraumatic hematoma of muscle (M79.81)*

✓5ᵗʰ **M62.0** **Separation of muscle (nontraumatic)**

     Diastasis of muscle

         EXCLUDES 1   *diastasis recti complicating pregnancy, labor and delivery (O71.8)*

                   traumatic separation of muscle - see strain of muscle by body region

     M62.00 **Separation of muscle (nontraumatic), unspecified site**

✓6ᵗʰ **M62.01** **Separation of muscle (nontraumatic),** shoulder

     M62.011 **Separation of muscle (nontraumatic),** right shoulder

     M62.012 **Separation of muscle (nontraumatic),** left shoulder

     M62.019 **Separation of muscle (nontraumatic), unspecified shoulder**

✓6ᵗʰ **M62.02** **Separation of muscle (nontraumatic),** upper arm

     M62.021 **Separation of muscle (nontraumatic),** right upper arm

     M62.022 **Separation of muscle (nontraumatic),** left upper arm

     M62.029 **Separation of muscle (nontraumatic), unspecified upper arm**

✓6ᵗʰ **M62.03** **Separation of muscle (nontraumatic),** forearm

     M62.031 **Separation of muscle (nontraumatic),** right forearm

     M62.032 **Separation of muscle (nontraumatic),** left forearm

     M62.039 **Separation of muscle (nontraumatic), unspecified forearm**

✓6ᵗʰ **M62.04** **Separation of muscle (nontraumatic),** hand

     M62.041 **Separation of muscle (nontraumatic),** right hand

     M62.042 **Separation of muscle (nontraumatic),** left hand

     M62.049 **Separation of muscle (nontraumatic), unspecified hand**

✓6ᵗʰ **M62.05** **Separation of muscle (nontraumatic),** thigh

     M62.051 **Separation of muscle (nontraumatic),** right thigh

     M62.052 **Separation of muscle (nontraumatic),** left thigh

     M62.059 **Separation of muscle (nontraumatic), unspecified thigh**

✓6ᵗʰ **M62.06** **Separation of muscle (nontraumatic),** lower leg

     M62.061 **Separation of muscle (nontraumatic),** right lower leg

     M62.062 **Separation of muscle (nontraumatic),** left lower leg

     M62.069 **Separation of muscle (nontraumatic), unspecified lower leg**

✓6ᵗʰ **M62.07** **Separation of muscle (nontraumatic),** ankle and foot

     M62.071 **Separation of muscle (nontraumatic),** right ankle and foot

---

     M62.072 **Separation of muscle (nontraumatic),** left ankle and foot

     M62.079 **Separation of muscle (nontraumatic), unspecified ankle and foot**

     M62.08 **Separation of muscle (nontraumatic), other site**

✓5ᵗʰ **M62.1** **Other rupture of muscle (nontraumatic)**

     EXCLUDES 1   *traumatic rupture of muscle - see strain of muscle by body region*

     EXCLUDES 2   *rupture of tendon (M66.-)*

     M62.10 **Other rupture of muscle (nontraumatic), unspecified site**

✓6ᵗʰ **M62.11** **Other rupture of muscle (nontraumatic),** shoulder

     M62.111 **Other rupture of muscle (nontraumatic),** right shoulder

     M62.112 **Other rupture of muscle (nontraumatic),** left shoulder

     M62.119 **Other rupture of muscle (nontraumatic), unspecified shoulder**

✓6ᵗʰ **M62.12** **Other rupture of muscle (nontraumatic),** upper arm

     M62.121 **Other rupture of muscle (nontraumatic),** right upper arm

     M62.122 **Other rupture of muscle (nontraumatic),** left upper arm

     M62.129 **Other rupture of muscle (nontraumatic), unspecified upper arm**

✓6ᵗʰ **M62.13** **Other rupture of muscle (nontraumatic),** forearm

     M62.131 **Other rupture of muscle (nontraumatic),** right forearm

     M62.132 **Other rupture of muscle (nontraumatic),** left forearm

     M62.139 **Other rupture of muscle (nontraumatic), unspecified forearm**

✓6ᵗʰ **M62.14** **Other rupture of muscle (nontraumatic),** hand

     M62.141 **Other rupture of muscle (nontraumatic),** right hand

     M62.142 **Other rupture of muscle (nontraumatic),** left hand

     M62.149 **Other rupture of muscle (nontraumatic), unspecified hand**

✓6ᵗʰ **M62.15** **Other rupture of muscle (nontraumatic),** thigh

     M62.151 **Other rupture of muscle (nontraumatic),** right thigh

     M62.152 **Other rupture of muscle (nontraumatic),** left thigh

     M62.159 **Other rupture of muscle (nontraumatic), unspecified thigh**

✓6ᵗʰ **M62.16** **Other rupture of muscle (nontraumatic),** lower leg

     M62.161 **Other rupture of muscle (nontraumatic),** right lower leg

     M62.162 **Other rupture of muscle (nontraumatic),** left lower leg

     M62.169 **Other rupture of muscle (nontraumatic), unspecified lower leg**

✓6ᵗʰ **M62.17** **Other rupture of muscle (nontraumatic),** ankle and foot

     M62.171 **Other rupture of muscle (nontraumatic),** right ankle and foot

     M62.172 **Other rupture of muscle (nontraumatic),** left ankle and foot

     M62.179 **Other rupture of muscle (nontraumatic), unspecified ankle and foot**

     M62.18 **Other rupture of muscle (nontraumatic), other site**

✓5ᵗʰ **M62.2** **Nontraumatic ischemic infarction of muscle**

     EXCLUDES 1   *compartment syndrome (traumatic) (T79.A-)*

                nontraumatic compartment syndrome (M79.A-)

                rhabdomyolysis (M62.82)

                traumatic ischemia of muscle (T79.6)

                Volkmann's ischemic contracture (T79.6)

     M62.20 **Nontraumatic ischemic infarction of muscle, unspecified site**

✓6ᵗʰ **M62.21** **Nontraumatic ischemic infarction of muscle,** shoulder

     M62.211 **Nontraumatic ischemic infarction of muscle,** right shoulder

     M62.212 **Nontraumatic ischemic infarction of muscle,** left shoulder

     M62.219 **Nontraumatic ischemic infarction of muscle, unspecified shoulder**

√6ᵗʰ **M62.22** **Nontraumatic ischemic infarction of muscle,** upper arm

    M62.221 **Nontraumatic ischemic infarction of muscle,** right **upper arm**

    M62.222 **Nontraumatic ischemic infarction of muscle,** left **upper arm**

    M62.229 **Nontraumatic ischemic infarction of muscle, unspecified upper arm**

√6ᵗʰ **M62.23** **Nontraumatic ischemic infarction of muscle,** forearm

    M62.231 **Nontraumatic ischemic infarction of muscle,** right **forearm**

    M62.232 **Nontraumatic ischemic infarction of muscle,** left **forearm**

    M62.239 **Nontraumatic ischemic infarction of muscle, unspecified forearm**

√6ᵗʰ **M62.24** **Nontraumatic ischemic infarction of muscle,** hand

    M62.241 **Nontraumatic ischemic infarction of muscle,** right **hand**

    M62.242 **Nontraumatic ischemic infarction of muscle,** left **hand**

    M62.249 **Nontraumatic ischemic infarction of muscle, unspecified hand**

√6ᵗʰ **M62.25** **Nontraumatic ischemic infarction of muscle,** thigh

    M62.251 **Nontraumatic ischemic infarction of muscle,** right **thigh**

    M62.252 **Nontraumatic ischemic infarction of muscle,** left **thigh**

    M62.259 **Nontraumatic ischemic infarction of muscle, unspecified thigh**

√6ᵗʰ **M62.26** **Nontraumatic ischemic infarction of muscle,** lower leg

    M62.261 **Nontraumatic ischemic infarction of muscle,** right **lower leg**

    M62.262 **Nontraumatic ischemic infarction of muscle,** left **lower leg**

    M62.269 **Nontraumatic ischemic infarction of muscle, unspecified lower leg**

√6ᵗʰ **M62.27** **Nontraumatic ischemic infarction of muscle,** ankle and foot

    M62.271 **Nontraumatic ischemic infarction of muscle,** right **ankle and foot**

    M62.272 **Nontraumatic ischemic infarction of muscle,** left **ankle and foot**

    M62.279 **Nontraumatic ischemic infarction of muscle, unspecified ankle and foot**

    M62.28 **Nontraumatic ischemic infarction of muscle, other site**

    M62.3 **Immobility syndrome (paraplegic)**

√5ᵗʰ **M62.4** **Contracture of muscle**

    Contracture of tendon (sheath)

    EXCLUDES 1   *contracture of joint (M24.5-)*

    M62.40 **Contracture of muscle, unspecified site**

√6ᵗʰ **M62.41** **Contracture of muscle,** shoulder

    M62.411 **Contracture of muscle,** right **shoulder**

    M62.412 **Contracture of muscle,** left **shoulder**

    M62.419 **Contracture of muscle, unspecified shoulder**

√6ᵗʰ **M62.42** **Contracture of muscle,** upper arm

    M62.421 **Contracture of muscle,** right **upper arm**

    M62.422 **Contracture of muscle,** left **upper arm**

    M62.429 **Contracture of muscle, unspecified upper arm**

√6ᵗʰ **M62.43** **Contracture of muscle,** forearm

    M62.431 **Contracture of muscle,** right **forearm**

    M62.432 **Contracture of muscle,** left **forearm**

    M62.439 **Contracture of muscle, unspecified forearm**

√6ᵗʰ **M62.44** **Contracture of muscle,** hand

    M62.441 **Contracture of muscle,** right **hand**

    M62.442 **Contracture of muscle,** left **hand**

    M62.449 **Contracture of muscle, unspecified hand**

√6ᵗʰ **M62.45** **Contracture of muscle,** thigh

    M62.451 **Contracture of muscle,** right **thigh**

    M62.452 **Contracture of muscle,** left **thigh**

    M62.459 **Contracture of muscle, unspecified thigh**

√6ᵗʰ **M62.46** **Contracture of muscle,** lower leg

    M62.461 **Contracture of muscle,** right **lower leg**

    M62.462 **Contracture of muscle,** left **lower leg**

    M62.469 **Contracture of muscle, unspecified lower leg**

√6ᵗʰ **M62.47** **Contracture of muscle,** ankle and foot

    M62.471 **Contracture of muscle,** right **ankle and foot**

    M62.472 **Contracture of muscle,** left **ankle and foot**

    M62.479 **Contracture of muscle, unspecified ankle and foot**

    M62.48 **Contracture of muscle, other site**

    M62.49 **Contracture of muscle,** multiple sites

√5ᵗʰ **M62.5** **Muscle wasting and atrophy, not elsewhere classified**

    Disuse atrophy NEC

    EXCLUDES 1   *neuralgic amyotrophy (G54.5)*

        progressive muscular atrophy (G12.21)

        sarcopenia (M62.84)

    EXCLUDES 2   *pelvic muscle wasting (N81.84)*

    M62.50 **Muscle wasting and atrophy, not elsewhere classified, unspecified site**

√6ᵗʰ **M62.51** **Muscle wasting and atrophy, not elsewhere classified,** shoulder

    M62.511 **Muscle wasting and atrophy, not elsewhere classified,** right **shoulder**

    M62.512 **Muscle wasting and atrophy, not elsewhere classified,** left **shoulder**

    M62.519 **Muscle wasting and atrophy, not elsewhere classified, unspecified shoulder**

√6ᵗʰ **M62.52** **Muscle wasting and atrophy, not elsewhere classified,** upper arm

    M62.521 **Muscle wasting and atrophy, not elsewhere classified,** right **upper arm**

    M62.522 **Muscle wasting and atrophy, not elsewhere classified,** left **upper arm**

    M62.529 **Muscle wasting and atrophy, not elsewhere classified, unspecified upper arm**

√6ᵗʰ **M62.53** **Muscle wasting and atrophy, not elsewhere classified,** forearm

    M62.531 **Muscle wasting and atrophy, not elsewhere classified,** right **forearm**

    M62.532 **Muscle wasting and atrophy, not elsewhere classified,** left **forearm**

    M62.539 **Muscle wasting and atrophy, not elsewhere classified, unspecified forearm**

√6ᵗʰ **M62.54** **Muscle wasting and atrophy, not elsewhere classified,** hand

    M62.541 **Muscle wasting and atrophy, not elsewhere classified,** right **hand**

    M62.542 **Muscle wasting and atrophy, not elsewhere classified,** left **hand**

    M62.549 **Muscle wasting and atrophy, not elsewhere classified, unspecified hand**

√6ᵗʰ **M62.55** **Muscle wasting and atrophy, not elsewhere classified,** thigh

    M62.551 **Muscle wasting and atrophy, not elsewhere classified,** right **thigh**

    M62.552 **Muscle wasting and atrophy, not elsewhere classified,** left **thigh**

    M62.559 **Muscle wasting and atrophy, not elsewhere classified, unspecified thigh**

√6ᵗʰ **M62.56** **Muscle wasting and atrophy, not elsewhere classified,** lower leg

    M62.561 **Muscle wasting and atrophy, not elsewhere classified,** right **lower leg**

    M62.562 **Muscle wasting and atrophy, not elsewhere classified,** left **lower leg**

    M62.569 **Muscle wasting and atrophy, not elsewhere classified, unspecified lower leg**

√6ᵗʰ **M62.57** **Muscle wasting and atrophy, not elsewhere classified,** ankle and foot

    M62.571 **Muscle wasting and atrophy, not elsewhere classified,** right **ankle and foot**

    M62.572 **Muscle wasting and atrophy, not elsewhere classified,** left **ankle and foot**

    M62.579 **Muscle wasting and atrophy, not elsewhere classified, unspecified ankle and foot**

    M62.58 **Muscle wasting and atrophy, not elsewhere classified, other site**

    M62.59 **Muscle wasting and atrophy, not elsewhere classified,** multiple sites

HCC CMS-HCC   **Rx** Rx HCC   **ESR** ESRD HCC   **COM** Commercial HCC   **N** Newborn: 0   **P** Pediatric: 0-17   **M** Maternity: 9-64   **A** Adult: 15-124

828   ICD-10-CM 2023

- ☑6ᵗʰ **M62.5A** **Muscle wasting and atrophy, not elsewhere classified, back**
- **M62.5A0** **Muscle wasting and atrophy, not elsewhere classified, back, cervical**
- **M62.5A1** **Muscle wasting and atrophy, not elsewhere classified, back, thoracic**
- **M62.5A2** **Muscle wasting and atrophy, not elsewhere classified, back, lumbosacral**
- **M62.5A9** **Muscle wasting and atrophy, not elsewhere classified, back, unspecified level**

☑5ᵗʰ **M62.8** **Other specified disorders of muscle**

EXCLUDES 2   nontraumatic hematoma of muscle (M79.81)

M62.81 **Muscle weakness (generalized)**

EXCLUDES 1   muscle weakness in sarcopenia (M62.84)

M62.82 **Rhabdomyolysis**

EXCLUDES 1   traumatic rhabdomyolysis (T79.6)

AHA: 2019,2Q,12

DEF: Rapid disintegration or destruction of skeletal muscle caused by direct or indirect injury, resulting in the excretion of muscle protein myoglobin into the urine.

☑6ᵗʰ **M62.83** **Muscle spasm**

M62.830 **Muscle spasm of back**

M62.831 **Muscle spasm of calf**
Charley-horse

M62.838 **Other muscle spasm**

M62.84 **Sarcopenia**
Age-related sarcopenia
Code first underlying disease, if applicable, such as:
disorders of myoneural junction and muscle disease in diseases classified elsewhere (G73.-)
other and unspecified myopathies (G72.-)
primary disorders of muscles (G71.-)
AHA: 2016,4Q,41

M62.89 **Other specified disorders of muscle**
Muscle (sheath) hernia

M62.9 **Disorder of muscle, unspecified**

☑4ᵗʰ **M63** **Disorders of muscle in diseases classified elsewhere**

Code first underlying disease, such as:
leprosy (A30.-)
neoplasm (C49.-, C79.89, D21.-, D48.1)
schistosomiasis (B65.-)
trichinellosis (B75)

EXCLUDES 1   myopathy in cysticercosis (B69.81)
myopathy in endocrine diseases (G73.7)
myopathy in metabolic diseases (G73.7)
myopathy in sarcoidosis (D86.87)
myopathy in secondary syphilis (A51.49)
myopathy in syphilis (late) (A52.78)
myopathy in toxoplasmosis (B58.82)
myopathy in tuberculosis (A18.09)

☑5ᵗʰ **M63.8** **Disorders of muscle in diseases classified elsewhere**

M63.80 *Disorders of muscle in diseases classified elsewhere, unspecified site*

☑6ᵗʰ **M63.81** **Disorders of muscle in diseases classified elsewhere, shoulder**

M63.811 *Disorders of muscle in diseases classified elsewhere, right shoulder*

M63.812 *Disorders of muscle in diseases classified elsewhere, left shoulder*

M63.819 *Disorders of muscle in diseases classified elsewhere, unspecified shoulder*

☑6ᵗʰ **M63.82** **Disorders of muscle in diseases classified elsewhere, upper arm**

M63.821 *Disorders of muscle in diseases classified elsewhere, right upper arm*

M63.822 *Disorders of muscle in diseases classified elsewhere, left upper arm*

M63.829 *Disorders of muscle in diseases classified elsewhere, unspecified upper arm*

☑6ᵗʰ **M63.83** **Disorders of muscle in diseases classified elsewhere, forearm**

M63.831 *Disorders of muscle in diseases classified elsewhere, right forearm*

M63.832 *Disorders of muscle in diseases classified elsewhere, left forearm*

M63.839 *Disorders of muscle in diseases classified elsewhere, unspecified forearm*

☑6ᵗʰ **M63.84** **Disorders of muscle in diseases classified elsewhere, hand**

M63.841 *Disorders of muscle in diseases classified elsewhere, right hand*

M63.842 *Disorders of muscle in diseases classified elsewhere, left hand*

M63.849 *Disorders of muscle in diseases classified elsewhere, unspecified hand*

☑6ᵗʰ **M63.85** **Disorders of muscle in diseases classified elsewhere, thigh**

M63.851 *Disorders of muscle in diseases classified elsewhere, right thigh*

M63.852 *Disorders of muscle in diseases classified elsewhere, left thigh*

M63.859 *Disorders of muscle in diseases classified elsewhere, unspecified thigh*

☑6ᵗʰ **M63.86** **Disorders of muscle in diseases classified elsewhere, lower leg**

M63.861 *Disorders of muscle in diseases classified elsewhere, right lower leg*

M63.862 *Disorders of muscle in diseases classified elsewhere, left lower leg*

M63.869 *Disorders of muscle in diseases classified elsewhere, unspecified lower leg*

☑6ᵗʰ **M63.87** **Disorders of muscle in diseases classified elsewhere, ankle and foot**

M63.871 *Disorders of muscle in diseases classified elsewhere, right ankle and foot*

M63.872 *Disorders of muscle in diseases classified elsewhere, left ankle and foot*

M63.879 *Disorders of muscle in diseases classified elsewhere, unspecified ankle and foot*

M63.88 *Disorders of muscle in diseases classified elsewhere, other site*

M63.89 *Disorders of muscle in diseases classified elsewhere, multiple sites*

Disorders of synovium and tendon (M65-M67)

☑4ᵗʰ **M65** **Synovitis and tenosynovitis**

EXCLUDES 1   chronic crepitant synovitis of hand and wrist (M70.0-)
current injury - see injury of ligament or tendon by body region
soft tissue disorders related to use, overuse and pressure (M70.-)

☑5ᵗʰ **M65.0** **Abscess of tendon sheath**
Use additional code (B95-B96) to identify bacterial agent.

M65.00 **Abscess of tendon sheath, unspecified site**

☑6ᵗʰ **M65.01** **Abscess of tendon sheath, shoulder**

M65.011 **Abscess of tendon sheath, right shoulder**

M65.012 **Abscess of tendon sheath, left shoulder**

M65.019 **Abscess of tendon sheath, unspecified shoulder**

☑6ᵗʰ **M65.02** **Abscess of tendon sheath, upper arm**

M65.021 **Abscess of tendon sheath, right upper arm**

M65.022 **Abscess of tendon sheath, left upper arm**

M65.029 **Abscess of tendon sheath, unspecified upper arm**

☑6ᵗʰ **M65.03** **Abscess of tendon sheath, forearm**

M65.031 **Abscess of tendon sheath, right forearm**

M65.032 **Abscess of tendon sheath, left forearm**

M65.039 **Abscess of tendon sheath, unspecified forearm**

☑6ᵗʰ **M65.04** **Abscess of tendon sheath, hand**

M65.041 **Abscess of tendon sheath, right hand**

M65.042 **Abscess of tendon sheath, left hand**

M65.049 **Abscess of tendon sheath, unspecified hand**

☑6ᵗʰ **M65.05** **Abscess of tendon sheath, thigh**

M65.051 **Abscess of tendon sheath, right thigh**

M65.052 **Abscess of tendon sheath, left thigh**

M65.059 **Abscess of tendon sheath, unspecified thigh**

☑6ᵗʰ **M65.06** **Abscess of tendon sheath, lower leg**

M65.061 **Abscess of tendon sheath, right lower leg**

M65.062 **Abscess of tendon sheath, left lower leg**

M65.069 **Abscess of tendon sheath, unspecified lower leg**

☑6ᵗʰ **M65.Ø7** **Abscess of tendon sheath,** ankle and foot

    M65.Ø71 **Abscess of tendon sheath,** right ankle and foot

    M65.Ø72 **Abscess of tendon sheath,** left ankle and foot

    M65.Ø79 **Abscess of tendon sheath, unspecified ankle and foot**

  M65.Ø8 **Abscess of tendon sheath, other site**

☑5ᵗʰ **M65.1** **Other infective (teno)synovitis**

  M65.1Ø **Other infective (teno)synovitis, unspecified site**

☑6ᵗʰ **M65.11** **Other infective (teno)synovitis,** shoulder

    M65.111 **Other infective (teno)synovitis,** right shoulder

    M65.112 **Other infective (teno)synovitis,** left shoulder

    M65.119 **Other infective (teno)synovitis, unspecified shoulder**

☑6ᵗʰ **M65.12** **Other infective (teno)synovitis,** elbow

    M65.121 **Other infective (teno)synovitis,** right elbow

    M65.122 **Other infective (teno)synovitis,** left elbow

    M65.129 **Other infective (teno)synovitis, unspecified elbow**

☑6ᵗʰ **M65.13** **Other infective (teno)synovitis,** wrist

    M65.131 **Other infective (teno)synovitis,** right wrist

    M65.132 **Other infective (teno)synovitis,** left wrist

    M65.139 **Other infective (teno)synovitis, unspecified wrist**

☑6ᵗʰ **M65.14** **Other infective (teno)synovitis,** hand

    M65.141 **Other infective (teno)synovitis,** right hand

    M65.142 **Other infective (teno)synovitis,** left hand

    M65.149 **Other infective (teno)synovitis, unspecified hand**

☑6ᵗʰ **M65.15** **Other infective (teno)synovitis,** hip

    M65.151 **Other infective (teno)synovitis,** right hip

    M65.152 **Other infective (teno)synovitis,** left hip

    M65.159 **Other infective (teno)synovitis, unspecified hip**

☑6ᵗʰ **M65.16** **Other infective (teno)synovitis,** knee

    M65.161 **Other infective (teno)synovitis,** right knee

    M65.162 **Other infective (teno)synovitis,** left knee

    M65.169 **Other infective (teno)synovitis, unspecified knee**

☑6ᵗʰ **M65.17** **Other infective (teno)synovitis,** ankle and foot

    M65.171 **Other infective (teno)synovitis,** right ankle and foot

    M65.172 **Other infective (teno)synovitis,** left ankle and foot

    M65.179 **Other infective (teno)synovitis, unspecified ankle and foot**

  M65.18 **Other infective (teno)synovitis, other site**

  M65.19 **Other infective (teno)synovitis,** multiple sites

☑5ᵗʰ **M65.2** **Calcific tendinitis**

    EXCLUDES 1   *tendinitis as classified in M75-M77*

                calcified tendinitis of shoulder (M75.3)

  M65.2Ø **Calcific tendinitis, unspecified site**

☑6ᵗʰ **M65.22** **Calcific tendinitis,** upper arm

    M65.221 **Calcific tendinitis,** right upper arm

    M65.222 **Calcific tendinitis,** left upper arm

    M65.229 **Calcific tendinitis, unspecified upper arm**

☑6ᵗʰ **M65.23** **Calcific tendinitis,** forearm

    M65.231 **Calcific tendinitis,** right forearm

    M65.232 **Calcific tendinitis,** left forearm

    M65.239 **Calcific tendinitis, unspecified forearm**

☑6ᵗʰ **M65.24** **Calcific tendinitis,** hand

    M65.241 **Calcific tendinitis,** right hand

    M65.242 **Calcific tendinitis,** left hand

    M65.249 **Calcific tendinitis, unspecified hand**

☑6ᵗʰ **M65.25** **Calcific tendinitis,** thigh

    M65.251 **Calcific tendinitis,** right thigh

    M65.252 **Calcific tendinitis,** left thigh

    M65.259 **Calcific tendinitis, unspecified thigh**

☑6ᵗʰ **M65.26** **Calcific tendinitis,** lower leg

    M65.261 **Calcific tendinitis,** right lower leg

    M65.262 **Calcific tendinitis,** left lower leg

    M65.269 **Calcific tendinitis, unspecified lower leg**

☑6ᵗʰ **M65.27** **Calcific tendinitis,** ankle and foot

    M65.271 **Calcific tendinitis,** right ankle and foot

    M65.272 **Calcific tendinitis,** left ankle and foot

    M65.279 **Calcific tendinitis, unspecified ankle and foot**

  M65.28 **Calcific tendinitis, other site**

  M65.29 **Calcific tendinitis,** multiple sites

☑5ᵗʰ **M65.3** **Trigger finger**

    Nodular tendinous disease

  M65.3Ø **Trigger finger, unspecified finger**

☑6ᵗʰ **M65.31** **Trigger** thumb

    M65.311 **Trigger thumb,** right thumb

    M65.312 **Trigger thumb,** left thumb

    M65.319 **Trigger thumb, unspecified thumb**

☑6ᵗʰ **M65.32** **Trigger finger,** index finger

    M65.321 **Trigger finger,** right index finger

    M65.322 **Trigger finger,** left index finger

    M65.329 **Trigger finger, unspecified index finger**

☑6ᵗʰ **M65.33** **Trigger finger,** middle finger

    M65.331 **Trigger finger,** right middle finger

    M65.332 **Trigger finger,** left middle finger

    M65.339 **Trigger finger, unspecified middle finger**

☑6ᵗʰ **M65.34** **Trigger finger,** ring finger

    M65.341 **Trigger finger,** right ring finger

    M65.342 **Trigger finger,** left ring finger

    M65.349 **Trigger finger, unspecified ring finger**

☑6ᵗʰ **M65.35** **Trigger finger,** little finger

    M65.351 **Trigger finger,** right little finger

    M65.352 **Trigger finger,** left little finger

    M65.359 **Trigger finger, unspecified little finger**

  M65.4 **Radial styloid tenosynovitis [de Quervain]**

☑5ᵗʰ **M65.8** **Other synovitis and tenosynovitis**

  M65.8Ø **Other synovitis and tenosynovitis, unspecified site**

☑6ᵗʰ **M65.81** **Other synovitis and tenosynovitis,** shoulder

    M65.811 **Other synovitis and tenosynovitis,** right shoulder

    M65.812 **Other synovitis and tenosynovitis,** left shoulder

    M65.819 **Other synovitis and tenosynovitis, unspecified shoulder**

☑6ᵗʰ **M65.82** **Other synovitis and tenosynovitis,** upper arm

    M65.821 **Other synovitis and tenosynovitis,** right upper arm

    M65.822 **Other synovitis and tenosynovitis,** left upper arm

    M65.829 **Other synovitis and tenosynovitis, unspecified upper arm**

☑6ᵗʰ **M65.83** **Other synovitis and tenosynovitis,** forearm

    M65.831 **Other synovitis and tenosynovitis,** right forearm

    M65.832 **Other synovitis and tenosynovitis,** left forearm

    M65.839 **Other synovitis and tenosynovitis, unspecified forearm**

☑6ᵗʰ **M65.84** **Other synovitis and tenosynovitis,** hand

    M65.841 **Other synovitis and tenosynovitis,** right hand

    M65.842 **Other synovitis and tenosynovitis,** left hand

    M65.849 **Other synovitis and tenosynovitis, unspecified hand**

☑6ᵗʰ **M65.85** **Other synovitis and tenosynovitis,** thigh

    M65.851 **Other synovitis and tenosynovitis,** right thigh

    M65.852 **Other synovitis and tenosynovitis,** left thigh

    M65.859 **Other synovitis and tenosynovitis, unspecified thigh**

☑6ᵗʰ **M65.86** **Other synovitis and tenosynovitis,** lower leg

    M65.861 **Other synovitis and tenosynovitis,** right lower leg

    M65.862 **Other synovitis and tenosynovitis,** left lower leg

    M65.869 **Other synovitis and tenosynovitis, unspecified lower leg**

☑6ᵗʰ **M65.87** **Other synovitis and tenosynovitis,** ankle and foot

    M65.871 **Other synovitis and tenosynovitis,** right ankle and foot

M65.872 Other synovitis and tenosynovitis, left ankle and foot

M65.879 Other synovitis and tenosynovitis, unspecified ankle and foot

M65.88 Other synovitis and tenosynovitis, other site

M65.89 Other synovitis and tenosynovitis, multiple sites

M65.9 Synovitis and tenosynovitis, unspecified

✅4ᵗʰ M66 Spontaneous rupture of synovium and tendon

INCLUDES rupture that occurs when a normal force is applied to tissues that are inferred to have less than normal strength

EXCLUDES 2 rotator cuff syndrome (M75.1-)

rupture where an abnormal force is applied to normal tissue - see injury of tendon by body region

M66.0 Rupture of popliteal cyst

✅5ᵗʰ M66.1 Rupture of synovium

Rupture of synovial cyst

EXCLUDES 2 rupture of popliteal cyst (M66.0)

M66.10 Rupture of synovium, unspecified joint

✅6ᵗʰ M66.11 Rupture of synovium, shoulder

M66.111 Rupture of synovium, right shoulder

M66.112 Rupture of synovium, left shoulder

M66.119 Rupture of synovium, unspecified shoulder

✅6ᵗʰ M66.12 Rupture of synovium, elbow

M66.121 Rupture of synovium, right elbow

M66.122 Rupture of synovium, left elbow

M66.129 Rupture of synovium, unspecified elbow

✅6ᵗʰ M66.13 Rupture of synovium, wrist

M66.131 Rupture of synovium, right wrist

M66.132 Rupture of synovium, left wrist

M66.139 Rupture of synovium, unspecified wrist

✅6ᵗʰ M66.14 Rupture of synovium, hand and fingers

M66.141 Rupture of synovium, right hand

M66.142 Rupture of synovium, left hand

M66.143 Rupture of synovium, unspecified hand

M66.144 Rupture of synovium, right finger(s)

M66.145 Rupture of synovium, left finger(s)

M66.146 Rupture of synovium, unspecified finger(s)

✅6ᵗʰ M66.15 Rupture of synovium, hip

M66.151 Rupture of synovium, right hip

M66.152 Rupture of synovium, left hip

M66.159 Rupture of synovium, unspecified hip

✅6ᵗʰ M66.17 Rupture of synovium, ankle, foot and toes

M66.171 Rupture of synovium, right ankle

M66.172 Rupture of synovium, left ankle

M66.173 Rupture of synovium, unspecified ankle

M66.174 Rupture of synovium, right foot

M66.175 Rupture of synovium, left foot

M66.176 Rupture of synovium, unspecified foot

M66.177 Rupture of synovium, right toe(s)

M66.178 Rupture of synovium, left toe(s)

M66.179 Rupture of synovium, unspecified toe(s)

M66.18 Rupture of synovium, other site

✅5ᵗʰ M66.2 Spontaneous rupture of extensor tendons

TIP: Refer to the Muscle/Tendon table at the beginning of this chapter.

M66.20 Spontaneous rupture of extensor tendons, unspecified site

✅6ᵗʰ M66.21 Spontaneous rupture of extensor tendons, shoulder

M66.211 Spontaneous rupture of extensor tendons, right shoulder

M66.212 Spontaneous rupture of extensor tendons, left shoulder

M66.219 Spontaneous rupture of extensor tendons, unspecified shoulder

✅6ᵗʰ M66.22 Spontaneous rupture of extensor tendons, upper arm

M66.221 Spontaneous rupture of extensor tendons, right upper arm

M66.222 Spontaneous rupture of extensor tendons, left upper arm

M66.229 Spontaneous rupture of extensor tendons, unspecified upper arm

✅6ᵗʰ M66.23 Spontaneous rupture of extensor tendons, forearm

M66.231 Spontaneous rupture of extensor tendons, right forearm

M66.232 Spontaneous rupture of extensor tendons, left forearm

M66.239 Spontaneous rupture of extensor tendons, unspecified forearm

✅6ᵗʰ M66.24 Spontaneous rupture of extensor tendons, hand

M66.241 Spontaneous rupture of extensor tendons, right hand

M66.242 Spontaneous rupture of extensor tendons, left hand

M66.249 Spontaneous rupture of extensor tendons, unspecified hand

✅6ᵗʰ M66.25 Spontaneous rupture of extensor tendons, thigh

M66.251 Spontaneous rupture of extensor tendons, right thigh

M66.252 Spontaneous rupture of extensor tendons, left thigh

M66.259 Spontaneous rupture of extensor tendons, unspecified thigh

✅6ᵗʰ M66.26 Spontaneous rupture of extensor tendons, lower leg

M66.261 Spontaneous rupture of extensor tendons, right lower leg

M66.262 Spontaneous rupture of extensor tendons, left lower leg

M66.269 Spontaneous rupture of extensor tendons, unspecified lower leg

✅6ᵗʰ M66.27 Spontaneous rupture of extensor tendons, ankle and foot

M66.271 Spontaneous rupture of extensor tendons, right ankle and foot

M66.272 Spontaneous rupture of extensor tendons, left ankle and foot

M66.279 Spontaneous rupture of extensor tendons, unspecified ankle and foot

M66.28 Spontaneous rupture of extensor tendons, other site

M66.29 Spontaneous rupture of extensor tendons, multiple sites

✅5ᵗʰ M66.3 Spontaneous rupture of flexor tendons

TIP: Refer to the Muscle/Tendon table at the beginning of this chapter.

M66.30 Spontaneous rupture of flexor tendons, unspecified site

✅6ᵗʰ M66.31 Spontaneous rupture of flexor tendons, shoulder

M66.311 Spontaneous rupture of flexor tendons, right shoulder

M66.312 Spontaneous rupture of flexor tendons, left shoulder

M66.319 Spontaneous rupture of flexor tendons, unspecified shoulder

✅6ᵗʰ M66.32 Spontaneous rupture of flexor tendons, upper arm

M66.321 Spontaneous rupture of flexor tendons, right upper arm

M66.322 Spontaneous rupture of flexor tendons, left upper arm

M66.329 Spontaneous rupture of flexor tendons, unspecified upper arm

✅6ᵗʰ M66.33 Spontaneous rupture of flexor tendons, forearm

M66.331 Spontaneous rupture of flexor tendons, right forearm

M66.332 Spontaneous rupture of flexor tendons, left forearm

M66.339 Spontaneous rupture of flexor tendons, unspecified forearm

✅6ᵗʰ M66.34 Spontaneous rupture of flexor tendons, hand

M66.341 Spontaneous rupture of flexor tendons, right hand

M66.342 Spontaneous rupture of flexor tendons, left hand

M66.349 Spontaneous rupture of flexor tendons, unspecified hand

✅6ᵗʰ M66.35 Spontaneous rupture of flexor tendons, thigh

M66.351 Spontaneous rupture of flexor tendons, right thigh

M66.352 Spontaneous rupture of flexor tendons, left thigh

M66.359 Spontaneous rupture of flexor tendons, unspecified thigh

✓6ᵗʰ **M66.36** Spontaneous rupture of flexor tendons, lower leg
- **M66.361** Spontaneous rupture of flexor tendons, right lower leg
- **M66.362** Spontaneous rupture of flexor tendons, left lower leg
- **M66.369** Spontaneous rupture of flexor tendons, unspecified lower leg

✓6ᵗʰ **M66.37** Spontaneous rupture of flexor tendons, ankle and foot
- **M66.371** Spontaneous rupture of flexor tendons, right ankle and foot
- **M66.372** Spontaneous rupture of flexor tendons, left ankle and foot
- **M66.379** Spontaneous rupture of flexor tendons, unspecified ankle and foot

M66.38 Spontaneous rupture of flexor tendons, other site

M66.39 Spontaneous rupture of flexor tendons, multiple sites

✓5ᵗʰ **M66.8** Spontaneous rupture of other tendons

TIP: Refer to the Muscle/Tendon table at the beginning of this chapter.

M66.80 Spontaneous rupture of other tendons, unspecified site

✓6ᵗʰ **M66.81** Spontaneous rupture of other tendons, shoulder
- **M66.811** Spontaneous rupture of other tendons, right shoulder
- **M66.812** Spontaneous rupture of other tendons, left shoulder
- **M66.819** Spontaneous rupture of other tendons, unspecified shoulder

✓6ᵗʰ **M66.82** Spontaneous rupture of other tendons, upper arm
- **M66.821** Spontaneous rupture of other tendons, right upper arm
- **M66.822** Spontaneous rupture of other tendons, left upper arm
- **M66.829** Spontaneous rupture of other tendons, unspecified upper arm

✓6ᵗʰ **M66.83** Spontaneous rupture of other tendons, forearm
- **M66.831** Spontaneous rupture of other tendons, right forearm
- **M66.832** Spontaneous rupture of other tendons, left forearm
- **M66.839** Spontaneous rupture of other tendons, unspecified forearm

✓6ᵗʰ **M66.84** Spontaneous rupture of other tendons, hand
- **M66.841** Spontaneous rupture of other tendons, right hand
- **M66.842** Spontaneous rupture of other tendons, left hand
- **M66.849** Spontaneous rupture of other tendons, unspecified hand

✓6ᵗʰ **M66.85** Spontaneous rupture of other tendons, thigh
- **M66.851** Spontaneous rupture of other tendons, right thigh
- **M66.852** Spontaneous rupture of other tendons, left thigh
- **M66.859** Spontaneous rupture of other tendons, unspecified thigh

✓6ᵗʰ **M66.86** Spontaneous rupture of other tendons, lower leg
- **M66.861** Spontaneous rupture of other tendons, right lower leg
- **M66.862** Spontaneous rupture of other tendons, left lower leg
- **M66.869** Spontaneous rupture of other tendons, unspecified lower leg

✓6ᵗʰ **M66.87** Spontaneous rupture of other tendons, ankle and foot
- **M66.871** Spontaneous rupture of other tendons, right ankle and foot
- **M66.872** Spontaneous rupture of other tendons, left ankle and foot
- **M66.879** Spontaneous rupture of other tendons, unspecified ankle and foot

M66.88 Spontaneous rupture of other tendons, other sites

M66.89 Spontaneous rupture of other tendons, multiple sites

M66.9 Spontaneous rupture of unspecified tendon
Rupture at musculotendinous junction, nontraumatic

✓4ᵗʰ **M67** **Other disorders of synovium and tendon**

EXCLUDES 1   *palmar fascial fibromatosis [Dupuytren] (M72.0)*
tendinitis NOS (M77.9-)
xanthomatosis localized to tendons (E78.2)

✓5ᵗʰ **M67.0** Short Achilles tendon (acquired)
- **M67.00** Short Achilles tendon (acquired), unspecified ankle
- **M67.01** Short Achilles tendon (acquired), right ankle
- **M67.02** Short Achilles tendon (acquired), left ankle

✓5ᵗʰ **M67.2** Synovial hypertrophy, not elsewhere classified

EXCLUDES 1   *villonodular synovitis (pigmented) (M12.2-)*

M67.20 Synovial hypertrophy, not elsewhere classified, unspecified site

✓6ᵗʰ **M67.21** Synovial hypertrophy, not elsewhere classified, shoulder
- **M67.211** Synovial hypertrophy, not elsewhere classified, right shoulder
- **M67.212** Synovial hypertrophy, not elsewhere classified, left shoulder
- **M67.219** Synovial hypertrophy, not elsewhere classified, unspecified shoulder

✓6ᵗʰ **M67.22** Synovial hypertrophy, not elsewhere classified, upper arm
- **M67.221** Synovial hypertrophy, not elsewhere classified, right upper arm
- **M67.222** Synovial hypertrophy, not elsewhere classified, left upper arm
- **M67.229** Synovial hypertrophy, not elsewhere classified, unspecified upper arm

✓6ᵗʰ **M67.23** Synovial hypertrophy, not elsewhere classified, forearm
- **M67.231** Synovial hypertrophy, not elsewhere classified, right forearm
- **M67.232** Synovial hypertrophy, not elsewhere classified, left forearm
- **M67.239** Synovial hypertrophy, not elsewhere classified, unspecified forearm

✓6ᵗʰ **M67.24** Synovial hypertrophy, not elsewhere classified, hand
- **M67.241** Synovial hypertrophy, not elsewhere classified, right hand
- **M67.242** Synovial hypertrophy, not elsewhere classified, left hand
- **M67.249** Synovial hypertrophy, not elsewhere classified, unspecified hand

✓6ᵗʰ **M67.25** Synovial hypertrophy, not elsewhere classified, thigh
- **M67.251** Synovial hypertrophy, not elsewhere classified, right thigh
- **M67.252** Synovial hypertrophy, not elsewhere classified, left thigh
- **M67.259** Synovial hypertrophy, not elsewhere classified, unspecified thigh

✓6ᵗʰ **M67.26** Synovial hypertrophy, not elsewhere classified, lower leg
- **M67.261** Synovial hypertrophy, not elsewhere classified, right lower leg
- **M67.262** Synovial hypertrophy, not elsewhere classified, left lower leg
- **M67.269** Synovial hypertrophy, not elsewhere classified, unspecified lower leg

✓6ᵗʰ **M67.27** Synovial hypertrophy, not elsewhere classified, ankle and foot
- **M67.271** Synovial hypertrophy, not elsewhere classified, right ankle and foot
- **M67.272** Synovial hypertrophy, not elsewhere classified, left ankle and foot
- **M67.279** Synovial hypertrophy, not elsewhere classified, unspecified ankle and foot

M67.28 Synovial hypertrophy, not elsewhere classified, other site

M67.29 Synovial hypertrophy, not elsewhere classified, multiple sites

✓5ᵗʰ **M67.3** Transient synovitis
Toxic synovitis
EXCLUDES 1   *palindromic rheumatism (M12.3-)*

M67.30 Transient synovitis, unspecified site

✓6ᵗʰ **M67.31** Transient synovitis, shoulder
- **M67.311** Transient synovitis, right shoulder
- **M67.312** Transient synovitis, left shoulder
- **M67.319** Transient synovitis, unspecified shoulder

✓6ᵗʰ M67.32 Transient synovitis, elbow

    M67.321 Transient synovitis, right elbow
    M67.322 Transient synovitis, left elbow
    M67.329 Transient synovitis, unspecified elbow

✓6ᵗʰ M67.33 Transient synovitis, wrist

    M67.331 Transient synovitis, right wrist
    M67.332 Transient synovitis, left wrist
    M67.339 Transient synovitis, unspecified wrist

✓6ᵗʰ M67.34 Transient synovitis, hand

    M67.341 Transient synovitis, right hand
    M67.342 Transient synovitis, left hand
    M67.349 Transient synovitis, unspecified hand

✓6ᵗʰ M67.35 Transient synovitis, hip

    M67.351 Transient synovitis, right hip
    M67.352 Transient synovitis, left hip
    M67.359 Transient synovitis, unspecified hip

✓6ᵗʰ M67.36 Transient synovitis, knee

    M67.361 Transient synovitis, right knee
    M67.362 Transient synovitis, left knee
    M67.369 Transient synovitis, unspecified knee

✓6ᵗʰ M67.37 Transient synovitis, ankle and foot

    M67.371 Transient synovitis, right ankle and foot
    M67.372 Transient synovitis, left ankle and foot
    M67.379 Transient synovitis, unspecified ankle and foot

    M67.38 Transient synovitis, other site
    M67.39 Transient synovitis, multiple sites

✓5ᵗʰ M67.4 Ganglion

    Ganglion of joint or tendon (sheath)

    EXCLUDES 1 *ganglion in yaws (A66.6)*

    EXCLUDES 2 *cyst of bursa (M71.2-M71.3)*
                   cyst of synovium (M71.2-M71.3)

    DEF: Fluid-filled, benign cyst appearing on a tendon sheath or aponeurosis, frequently connecting to an underlying joint.

    M67.40 Ganglion, unspecified site

✓6ᵗʰ M67.41 Ganglion, shoulder

    M67.411 Ganglion, right shoulder
    M67.412 Ganglion, left shoulder
    M67.419 Ganglion, unspecified shoulder

✓6ᵗʰ M67.42 Ganglion, elbow

    M67.421 Ganglion, right elbow
    M67.422 Ganglion, left elbow
    M67.429 Ganglion, unspecified elbow

✓6ᵗʰ M67.43 Ganglion, wrist

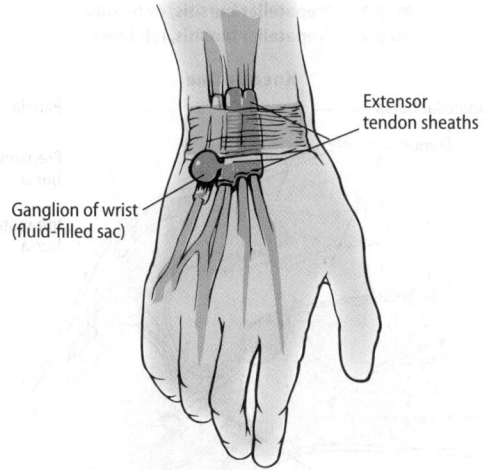

Ganglion of Wrist

Extensor tendon sheaths

Ganglion of wrist (fluid-filled sac)

    M67.431 Ganglion, right wrist
    M67.432 Ganglion, left wrist
    M67.439 Ganglion, unspecified wrist

✓6ᵗʰ M67.44 Ganglion, hand

    M67.441 Ganglion, right hand
    M67.442 Ganglion, left hand
    M67.449 Ganglion, unspecified hand

✓6ᵗʰ M67.45 Ganglion, hip

    M67.451 Ganglion, right hip

    M67.452 Ganglion, left hip
    M67.459 Ganglion, unspecified hip

✓6ᵗʰ M67.46 Ganglion, knee

    M67.461 Ganglion, right knee
    M67.462 Ganglion, left knee
    M67.469 Ganglion, unspecified knee

✓6ᵗʰ M67.47 Ganglion, ankle and foot

    M67.471 Ganglion, right ankle and foot
    M67.472 Ganglion, left ankle and foot
    M67.479 Ganglion, unspecified ankle and foot

    M67.48 Ganglion, other site
    M67.49 Ganglion, multiple sites

✓5ᵗʰ M67.5 Plica syndrome

    Plica knee

    M67.50 Plica syndrome, unspecified knee
    M67.51 Plica syndrome, right knee
    M67.52 Plica syndrome, left knee

✓5ᵗʰ M67.8 Other specified disorders of synovium and tendon

    M67.80 Other specified disorders of synovium and tendon, unspecified site

✓6ᵗʰ M67.81 Other specified disorders of synovium and tendon, shoulder

    M67.811 Other specified disorders of synovium, right shoulder
    M67.812 Other specified disorders of synovium, left shoulder
    M67.813 Other specified disorders of tendon, right shoulder
    M67.814 Other specified disorders of tendon, left shoulder
    M67.819 Other specified disorders of synovium and tendon, unspecified shoulder

✓6ᵗʰ M67.82 Other specified disorders of synovium and tendon, elbow

    M67.821 Other specified disorders of synovium, right elbow
    M67.822 Other specified disorders of synovium, left elbow
    M67.823 Other specified disorders of tendon, right elbow
    M67.824 Other specified disorders of tendon, left elbow
    M67.829 Other specified disorders of synovium and tendon, unspecified elbow

✓6ᵗʰ M67.83 Other specified disorders of synovium and tendon, wrist

    M67.831 Other specified disorders of synovium, right wrist
    M67.832 Other specified disorders of synovium, left wrist
    M67.833 Other specified disorders of tendon, right wrist
    M67.834 Other specified disorders of tendon, left wrist
    M67.839 Other specified disorders of synovium and tendon, unspecified wrist

✓6ᵗʰ M67.84 Other specified disorders of synovium and tendon, hand

    M67.841 Other specified disorders of synovium, right hand
    M67.842 Other specified disorders of synovium, left hand
    M67.843 Other specified disorders of tendon, right hand
    M67.844 Other specified disorders of tendon, left hand
    M67.849 Other specified disorders of synovium and tendon, unspecified hand

✓6ᵗʰ M67.85 Other specified disorders of synovium and tendon, hip

    M67.851 Other specified disorders of synovium, right hip
    M67.852 Other specified disorders of synovium, left hip
    M67.853 Other specified disorders of tendon, right hip
    M67.854 Other specified disorders of tendon, left hip
    M67.859 Other specified disorders of synovium and tendon, unspecified hip

✓6ᵗʰ **M67.86** Other specified disorders of synovium and tendon, knee
    M67.861 Other specified disorders of synovium, right knee
    M67.862 Other specified disorders of synovium, left knee
    M67.863 Other specified disorders of tendon, right knee
    M67.864 Other specified disorders of tendon, left knee
    M67.869 Other specified disorders of synovium and tendon, unspecified knee

✓6ᵗʰ **M67.87** Other specified disorders of synovium and tendon, ankle and foot
    M67.871 Other specified disorders of synovium, right ankle and foot
    M67.872 Other specified disorders of synovium, left ankle and foot
    M67.873 Other specified disorders of tendon, right ankle and foot
    M67.874 Other specified disorders of tendon, left ankle and foot
    M67.879 Other specified disorders of synovium and tendon, unspecified ankle and foot

M67.88 Other specified disorders of synovium and tendon, other site

M67.89 Other specified disorders of synovium and tendon, multiple sites

✓5ᵗʰ **M67.9** Unspecified disorder of synovium and tendon

    M67.90 Unspecified disorder of synovium and tendon, unspecified site

✓6ᵗʰ **M67.91** Unspecified disorder of synovium and tendon, shoulder
    M67.911 Unspecified disorder of synovium and tendon, right shoulder
    M67.912 Unspecified disorder of synovium and tendon, left shoulder
    M67.919 Unspecified disorder of synovium and tendon, unspecified shoulder

✓6ᵗʰ **M67.92** Unspecified disorder of synovium and tendon, upper arm
    M67.921 Unspecified disorder of synovium and tendon, right upper arm
    M67.922 Unspecified disorder of synovium and tendon, left upper arm
    M67.929 Unspecified disorder of synovium and tendon, unspecified upper arm

✓6ᵗʰ **M67.93** Unspecified disorder of synovium and tendon, forearm
    M67.931 Unspecified disorder of synovium and tendon, right forearm
    M67.932 Unspecified disorder of synovium and tendon, left forearm
    M67.939 Unspecified disorder of synovium and tendon, unspecified forearm

✓6ᵗʰ **M67.94** Unspecified disorder of synovium and tendon, hand
    M67.941 Unspecified disorder of synovium and tendon, right hand
    M67.942 Unspecified disorder of synovium and tendon, left hand
    M67.949 Unspecified disorder of synovium and tendon, unspecified hand

✓6ᵗʰ **M67.95** Unspecified disorder of synovium and tendon, thigh
    M67.951 Unspecified disorder of synovium and tendon, right thigh
    M67.952 Unspecified disorder of synovium and tendon, left thigh
    M67.959 Unspecified disorder of synovium and tendon, unspecified thigh

✓6ᵗʰ **M67.96** Unspecified disorder of synovium and tendon, lower leg
    M67.961 Unspecified disorder of synovium and tendon, right lower leg
    M67.962 Unspecified disorder of synovium and tendon, left lower leg
    M67.969 Unspecified disorder of synovium and tendon, unspecified lower leg

✓6ᵗʰ **M67.97** Unspecified disorder of synovium and tendon, ankle and foot
    M67.971 Unspecified disorder of synovium and tendon, right ankle and foot

    M67.972 Unspecified disorder of synovium and tendon, left ankle and foot
    M67.979 Unspecified disorder of synovium and tendon, unspecified ankle and foot

M67.98 Unspecified disorder of synovium and tendon, other site

M67.99 Unspecified disorder of synovium and tendon, multiple sites

Other soft tissue disorders (M70-M79)

✓4ᵗʰ **M70** Soft tissue disorders related to use, overuse and pressure

    INCLUDES soft tissue disorders of occupational origin

    Use additional external cause code to identify activity causing disorder (Y93.-)

    EXCLUDES 1 bursitis NOS (M71.9-)

    EXCLUDES 2 bursitis of shoulder (M75.5)
             enthesopathies (M76-M77)
             pressure ulcer (pressure area) (L89.-)

✓5ᵗʰ **M70.0** Crepitant synovitis (acute) (chronic) of hand and wrist

    ✓6ᵗʰ **M70.03** Crepitant synovitis (acute) (chronic), wrist
       M70.031 Crepitant synovitis (acute) (chronic), right wrist
       M70.032 Crepitant synovitis (acute) (chronic), left wrist
       M70.039 Crepitant synovitis (acute) (chronic), unspecified wrist

    ✓6ᵗʰ **M70.04** Crepitant synovitis (acute) (chronic), hand
       M70.041 Crepitant synovitis (acute) (chronic), right hand
       M70.042 Crepitant synovitis (acute) (chronic), left hand
       M70.049 Crepitant synovitis (acute) (chronic), unspecified hand

✓5ᵗʰ **M70.1** Bursitis of hand

    M70.10 Bursitis, unspecified hand
    M70.11 Bursitis, right hand
    M70.12 Bursitis, left hand

✓5ᵗʰ **M70.2** Olecranon bursitis

    M70.20 Olecranon bursitis, unspecified elbow
    M70.21 Olecranon bursitis, right elbow
    M70.22 Olecranon bursitis, left elbow

✓5ᵗʰ **M70.3** Other bursitis of elbow

    M70.30 Other bursitis of elbow, unspecified elbow
    M70.31 Other bursitis of elbow, right elbow
    M70.32 Other bursitis of elbow, left elbow

✓5ᵗʰ **M70.4** Prepatellar bursitis

    M70.40 Prepatellar bursitis, unspecified knee
    M70.41 Prepatellar bursitis, right knee
    M70.42 Prepatellar bursitis, left knee

Knee Bursae

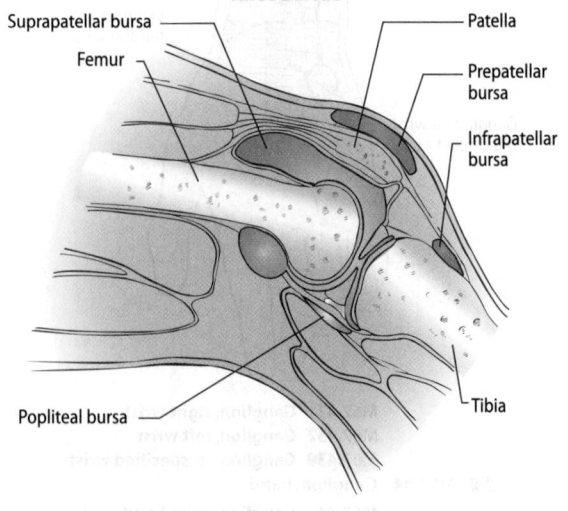

Suprapatellar bursa · Femur · Patella · Prepatellar bursa · Infrapatellar bursa · Popliteal bursa · Tibia

✓5ᵗʰ **M70.5** Other bursitis of knee

    M70.50 Other bursitis of knee, unspecified knee
    M70.51 Other bursitis of knee, right knee
    M70.52 Other bursitis of knee, left knee

HCC CMS-HCC   **Rx** Rx HCC   **ESR** ESRD HCC   **COM** Commercial HCC   **N** Newborn: 0   **P** Pediatric: 0-17   **M** Maternity: 9-64   **A** Adult: 15-124

834   ICD-10-CM 2023

☑5ᵗʰ **M70.6** Trochanteric bursitis
     Trochanteric tendinitis

     M70.60 Trochanteric bursitis, unspecified hip
     M70.61 Trochanteric bursitis, right hip
     M70.62 Trochanteric bursitis, left hip

☑5ᵗʰ **M70.7** Other bursitis of hip
     Ischial bursitis

     M70.70 Other bursitis of hip, unspecified hip
     M70.71 Other bursitis of hip, right hip
     M70.72 Other bursitis of hip, left hip

☑5ᵗʰ **M70.8** Other soft tissue disorders related to use, overuse and pressure

     M70.80 Other soft tissue disorders related to use, overuse and pressure of unspecified site

☑6ᵗʰ   **M70.81** Other soft tissue disorders related to use, overuse and pressure of shoulder
     M70.811 Other soft tissue disorders related to use, overuse and pressure, right shoulder
     M70.812 Other soft tissue disorders related to use, overuse and pressure, left shoulder
     M70.819 Other soft tissue disorders related to use, overuse and pressure, unspecified shoulder

☑6ᵗʰ   **M70.82** Other soft tissue disorders related to use, overuse and pressure of upper arm
     M70.821 Other soft tissue disorders related to use, overuse and pressure, right upper arm
     M70.822 Other soft tissue disorders related to use, overuse and pressure, left upper arm
     M70.829 Other soft tissue disorders related to use, overuse and pressure, unspecified upper arms

☑6ᵗʰ   **M70.83** Other soft tissue disorders related to use, overuse and pressure of forearm
     M70.831 Other soft tissue disorders related to use, overuse and pressure, right forearm
     M70.832 Other soft tissue disorders related to use, overuse and pressure, left forearm
     M70.839 Other soft tissue disorders related to use, overuse and pressure, unspecified forearm

☑6ᵗʰ   **M70.84** Other soft tissue disorders related to use, overuse and pressure of hand
     M70.841 Other soft tissue disorders related to use, overuse and pressure, right hand
     M70.842 Other soft tissue disorders related to use, overuse and pressure, left hand
     M70.849 Other soft tissue disorders related to use, overuse and pressure, unspecified hand

☑6ᵗʰ   **M70.85** Other soft tissue disorders related to use, overuse and pressure of thigh
     M70.851 Other soft tissue disorders related to use, overuse and pressure, right thigh
     M70.852 Other soft tissue disorders related to use, overuse and pressure, left thigh
     M70.859 Other soft tissue disorders related to use, overuse and pressure, unspecified thigh

☑6ᵗʰ   **M70.86** Other soft tissue disorders related to use, overuse and pressure lower leg
     M70.861 Other soft tissue disorders related to use, overuse and pressure, right lower leg
     M70.862 Other soft tissue disorders related to use, overuse and pressure, left lower leg
     M70.869 Other soft tissue disorders related to use, overuse and pressure, unspecified leg

☑6ᵗʰ   **M70.87** Other soft tissue disorders related to use, overuse and pressure of ankle and foot
     M70.871 Other soft tissue disorders related to use, overuse and pressure, right ankle and foot
     M70.872 Other soft tissue disorders related to use, overuse and pressure, left ankle and foot
     M70.879 Other soft tissue disorders related to use, overuse and pressure, unspecified ankle and foot

     M70.88 Other soft tissue disorders related to use, overuse and pressure other site

     M70.89 Other soft tissue disorders related to use, overuse and pressure multiple sites

☑5ᵗʰ **M70.9** Unspecified soft tissue disorder related to use, overuse and pressure

     M70.90 Unspecified soft tissue disorder related to use, overuse and pressure of unspecified site

☑6ᵗʰ   **M70.91** Unspecified soft tissue disorder related to use, overuse and pressure of shoulder
     M70.911 Unspecified soft tissue disorder related to use, overuse and pressure, right shoulder
     M70.912 Unspecified soft tissue disorder related to use, overuse and pressure, left shoulder
     M70.919 Unspecified soft tissue disorder related to use, overuse and pressure, unspecified shoulder

☑6ᵗʰ   **M70.92** Unspecified soft tissue disorder related to use, overuse and pressure of upper arm
     M70.921 Unspecified soft tissue disorder related to use, overuse and pressure, right upper arm
     M70.922 Unspecified soft tissue disorder related to use, overuse and pressure, left upper arm
     M70.929 Unspecified soft tissue disorder related to use, overuse and pressure, unspecified upper arm

☑6ᵗʰ   **M70.93** Unspecified soft tissue disorder related to use, overuse and pressure of forearm
     M70.931 Unspecified soft tissue disorder related to use, overuse and pressure, right forearm
     M70.932 Unspecified soft tissue disorder related to use, overuse and pressure, left forearm
     M70.939 Unspecified soft tissue disorder related to use, overuse and pressure, unspecified forearm

☑6ᵗʰ   **M70.94** Unspecified soft tissue disorder related to use, overuse and pressure of hand
     M70.941 Unspecified soft tissue disorder related to use, overuse and pressure, right hand
     M70.942 Unspecified soft tissue disorder related to use, overuse and pressure, left hand
     M70.949 Unspecified soft tissue disorder related to use, overuse and pressure, unspecified hand

☑6ᵗʰ   **M70.95** Unspecified soft tissue disorder related to use, overuse and pressure of thigh
     M70.951 Unspecified soft tissue disorder related to use, overuse and pressure, right thigh
     M70.952 Unspecified soft tissue disorder related to use, overuse and pressure, left thigh
     M70.959 Unspecified soft tissue disorder related to use, overuse and pressure, unspecified thigh

☑6ᵗʰ   **M70.96** Unspecified soft tissue disorder related to use, overuse and pressure lower leg
     M70.961 Unspecified soft tissue disorder related to use, overuse and pressure, right lower leg
     M70.962 Unspecified soft tissue disorder related to use, overuse and pressure, left lower leg
     M70.969 Unspecified soft tissue disorder related to use, overuse and pressure, unspecified lower leg

☑6ᵗʰ   **M70.97** Unspecified soft tissue disorder related to use, overuse and pressure of ankle and foot
     M70.971 Unspecified soft tissue disorder related to use, overuse and pressure, right ankle and foot
     M70.972 Unspecified soft tissue disorder related to use, overuse and pressure, left ankle and foot
     M70.979 Unspecified soft tissue disorder related to use, overuse and pressure, unspecified ankle and foot

     M70.98 Unspecified soft tissue disorder related to use, overuse and pressure other

     M70.99 Unspecified soft tissue disorder related to use, overuse and pressure multiple sites

✓4ᵗʰ M71 Other bursopathies

> EXCLUDES 1   *bunion (M20.1)*
> *bursitis related to use, overuse or pressure (M70.-)*
> *enthesopathies (M76-M77)*

✓5ᵗʰ M71.0 Abscess of bursa

> Use additional code (B95.-, B96.-) to identify causative organism

M71.00 Abscess of bursa, unspecified site

✓6ᵗʰ M71.01 Abscess of bursa, shoulder

M71.011 Abscess of bursa, right shoulder
M71.012 Abscess of bursa, left shoulder
M71.019 Abscess of bursa, unspecified shoulder

✓6ᵗʰ M71.02 Abscess of bursa, elbow

M71.021 Abscess of bursa, right elbow
M71.022 Abscess of bursa, left elbow
M71.029 Abscess of bursa, unspecified elbow

✓6ᵗʰ M71.03 Abscess of bursa, wrist

M71.031 Abscess of bursa, right wrist
M71.032 Abscess of bursa, left wrist
M71.039 Abscess of bursa, unspecified wrist

✓6ᵗʰ M71.04 Abscess of bursa, hand

M71.041 Abscess of bursa, right hand
M71.042 Abscess of bursa, left hand
M71.049 Abscess of bursa, unspecified hand

✓6ᵗʰ M71.05 Abscess of bursa, hip

M71.051 Abscess of bursa, right hip
M71.052 Abscess of bursa, left hip
M71.059 Abscess of bursa, unspecified hip

✓6ᵗʰ M71.06 Abscess of bursa, knee

M71.061 Abscess of bursa, right knee
M71.062 Abscess of bursa, left knee
M71.069 Abscess of bursa, unspecified knee

✓6ᵗʰ M71.07 Abscess of bursa, ankle and foot

M71.071 Abscess of bursa, right ankle and foot
M71.072 Abscess of bursa, left ankle and foot
M71.079 Abscess of bursa, unspecified ankle and foot

M71.08 Abscess of bursa, other site

M71.09 Abscess of bursa, multiple sites

✓5ᵗʰ M71.1 Other infective bursitis

> Use additional code (B95.-, B96.-) to identify causative organism

M71.10 Other infective bursitis, unspecified site

✓6ᵗʰ M71.11 Other infective bursitis, shoulder

M71.111 Other infective bursitis, right shoulder
M71.112 Other infective bursitis, left shoulder
M71.119 Other infective bursitis, unspecified shoulder

✓6ᵗʰ M71.12 Other infective bursitis, elbow

M71.121 Other infective bursitis, right elbow
M71.122 Other infective bursitis, left elbow
M71.129 Other infective bursitis, unspecified elbow

✓6ᵗʰ M71.13 Other infective bursitis, wrist

M71.131 Other infective bursitis, right wrist
M71.132 Other infective bursitis, left wrist
M71.139 Other infective bursitis, unspecified wrist

✓6ᵗʰ M71.14 Other infective bursitis, hand

M71.141 Other infective bursitis, right hand
M71.142 Other infective bursitis, left hand
M71.149 Other infective bursitis, unspecified hand

✓6ᵗʰ M71.15 Other infective bursitis, hip

M71.151 Other infective bursitis, right hip
M71.152 Other infective bursitis, left hip
M71.159 Other infective bursitis, unspecified hip

✓6ᵗʰ M71.16 Other infective bursitis, knee

M71.161 Other infective bursitis, right knee
M71.162 Other infective bursitis, left knee
M71.169 Other infective bursitis, unspecified knee

✓6ᵗʰ M71.17 Other infective bursitis, ankle and foot

M71.171 Other infective bursitis, right ankle and foot
M71.172 Other infective bursitis, left ankle and foot
M71.179 Other infective bursitis, unspecified ankle and foot

M71.18 Other infective bursitis, other site

M71.19 Other infective bursitis, multiple sites

✓5ᵗʰ M71.2 Synovial cyst of popliteal space [Baker]

> EXCLUDES 1   *synovial cyst of popliteal space with rupture (M66.0)*
> **DEF:** Sac filled with clear synovial fluid in adults, usually secondary to disease inside the joint, located on the back of the knee in the popliteal fossa area. In children, the cyst usually represents a ganglion of one of the tendons in the knee.

Baker's Cyst

Baker's cyst connected to knee joint synovial cavity

M71.20 Synovial cyst of popliteal space [Baker], unspecified knee

M71.21 Synovial cyst of popliteal space [Baker], right knee

M71.22 Synovial cyst of popliteal space [Baker], left knee

✓5ᵗʰ M71.3 Other bursal cyst

> Synovial cyst NOS
> EXCLUDES 1   *synovial cyst with rupture (M66.1-)*

M71.30 Other bursal cyst, unspecified site

✓6ᵗʰ M71.31 Other bursal cyst, shoulder

M71.311 Other bursal cyst, right shoulder
M71.312 Other bursal cyst, left shoulder
M71.319 Other bursal cyst, unspecified shoulder

✓6ᵗʰ M71.32 Other bursal cyst, elbow

M71.321 Other bursal cyst, right elbow
M71.322 Other bursal cyst, left elbow
M71.329 Other bursal cyst, unspecified elbow

✓6ᵗʰ M71.33 Other bursal cyst, wrist

M71.331 Other bursal cyst, right wrist
M71.332 Other bursal cyst, left wrist
M71.339 Other bursal cyst, unspecified wrist

✓6ᵗʰ M71.34 Other bursal cyst, hand

M71.341 Other bursal cyst, right hand
M71.342 Other bursal cyst, left hand
M71.349 Other bursal cyst, unspecified hand

✓6ᵗʰ M71.35 Other bursal cyst, hip

M71.351 Other bursal cyst, right hip
M71.352 Other bursal cyst, left hip
M71.359 Other bursal cyst, unspecified hip

✓6ᵗʰ M71.37 Other bursal cyst, ankle and foot

M71.371 Other bursal cyst, right ankle and foot
M71.372 Other bursal cyst, left ankle and foot
M71.379 Other bursal cyst, unspecified ankle and foot

M71.38 Other bursal cyst, other site

M71.39 Other bursal cyst, multiple sites

✓5ᵗʰ M71.4 Calcium deposit in bursa

> EXCLUDES 2   *calcium deposit in bursa of shoulder (M75.3)*

M71.40 Calcium deposit in bursa, unspecified site

✓6ᵗʰ M71.42 Calcium deposit in bursa, elbow

M71.421 Calcium deposit in bursa, right elbow
M71.422 Calcium deposit in bursa, left elbow
M71.429 Calcium deposit in bursa, unspecified elbow

✓6ᵗʰ M71.43 Calcium deposit in bursa, wrist

M71.431 Calcium deposit in bursa, right wrist
M71.432 Calcium deposit in bursa, left wrist

M71.439 **Calcium deposit in bursa, unspecified wrist**

√6ᵗʰ **M71.44 Calcium deposit in bursa, hand**

    M71.441 **Calcium deposit in bursa, right hand**
    M71.442 **Calcium deposit in bursa, left hand**
    M71.449 **Calcium deposit in bursa, unspecified hand**

√6ᵗʰ **M71.45 Calcium deposit in bursa, hip**

    M71.451 **Calcium deposit in bursa, right hip**
    M71.452 **Calcium deposit in bursa, left hip**
    M71.459 **Calcium deposit in bursa, unspecified hip**

√6ᵗʰ **M71.46 Calcium deposit in bursa, knee**

    M71.461 **Calcium deposit in bursa, right knee**
    M71.462 **Calcium deposit in bursa, left knee**
    M71.469 **Calcium deposit in bursa, unspecified knee**

√6ᵗʰ **M71.47 Calcium deposit in bursa, ankle and foot**

    M71.471 **Calcium deposit in bursa, right ankle and foot**
    M71.472 **Calcium deposit in bursa, left ankle and foot**
    M71.479 **Calcium deposit in bursa, unspecified ankle and foot**

    M71.48 **Calcium deposit in bursa, other site**
    M71.49 **Calcium deposit in bursa, multiple sites**

√5ᵗʰ **M71.5 Other bursitis, not elsewhere classified**

    EXCLUDES 1   *bursitis NOS (M71.9-)*
    EXCLUDES 2   *bursitis of shoulder (M75.5)*
              bursitis of tibial collateral [Pellegrini-Stieda] (M76.4-)

    M71.50 **Other bursitis, not elsewhere classified, unspecified site**

√6ᵗʰ **M71.52 Other bursitis, not elsewhere classified, elbow**

    M71.521 **Other bursitis, not elsewhere classified, right elbow**
    M71.522 **Other bursitis, not elsewhere classified, left elbow**
    M71.529 **Other bursitis, not elsewhere classified, unspecified elbow**

√6ᵗʰ **M71.53 Other bursitis, not elsewhere classified, wrist**

    M71.531 **Other bursitis, not elsewhere classified, right wrist**
    M71.532 **Other bursitis, not elsewhere classified, left wrist**
    M71.539 **Other bursitis, not elsewhere classified, unspecified wrist**

√6ᵗʰ **M71.54 Other bursitis, not elsewhere classified, hand**

    M71.541 **Other bursitis, not elsewhere classified, right hand**
    M71.542 **Other bursitis, not elsewhere classified, left hand**
    M71.549 **Other bursitis, not elsewhere classified, unspecified hand**

√6ᵗʰ **M71.55 Other bursitis, not elsewhere classified, hip**

    M71.551 **Other bursitis, not elsewhere classified, right hip**
    M71.552 **Other bursitis, not elsewhere classified, left hip**
    M71.559 **Other bursitis, not elsewhere classified, unspecified hip**

√6ᵗʰ **M71.56 Other bursitis, not elsewhere classified, knee**

    M71.561 **Other bursitis, not elsewhere classified, right knee**
    M71.562 **Other bursitis, not elsewhere classified, left knee**
    M71.569 **Other bursitis, not elsewhere classified, unspecified knee**

√6ᵗʰ **M71.57 Other bursitis, not elsewhere classified, ankle and foot**

    M71.571 **Other bursitis, not elsewhere classified, right ankle and foot**
    M71.572 **Other bursitis, not elsewhere classified, left ankle and foot**
    M71.579 **Other bursitis, not elsewhere classified, unspecified ankle and foot**

    M71.58 **Other bursitis, not elsewhere classified, other site**

√5ᵗʰ **M71.8 Other specified bursopathies**

    M71.80 **Other specified bursopathies, unspecified site**

√6ᵗʰ **M71.81 Other specified bursopathies, shoulder**

    M71.811 **Other specified bursopathies, right shoulder**
    M71.812 **Other specified bursopathies, left shoulder**
    M71.819 **Other specified bursopathies, unspecified shoulder**

√6ᵗʰ **M71.82 Other specified bursopathies, elbow**

    M71.821 **Other specified bursopathies, right elbow**
    M71.822 **Other specified bursopathies, left elbow**
    M71.829 **Other specified bursopathies, unspecified elbow**

√6ᵗʰ **M71.83 Other specified bursopathies, wrist**

    M71.831 **Other specified bursopathies, right wrist**
    M71.832 **Other specified bursopathies, left wrist**
    M71.839 **Other specified bursopathies, unspecified wrist**

√6ᵗʰ **M71.84 Other specified bursopathies, hand**

    M71.841 **Other specified bursopathies, right hand**
    M71.842 **Other specified bursopathies, left hand**
    M71.849 **Other specified bursopathies, unspecified hand**

√6ᵗʰ **M71.85 Other specified bursopathies, hip**

    M71.851 **Other specified bursopathies, right hip**
    M71.852 **Other specified bursopathies, left hip**
    M71.859 **Other specified bursopathies, unspecified hip**

√6ᵗʰ **M71.86 Other specified bursopathies, knee**

    M71.861 **Other specified bursopathies, right knee**
    M71.862 **Other specified bursopathies, left knee**
    M71.869 **Other specified bursopathies, unspecified knee**

√6ᵗʰ **M71.87 Other specified bursopathies, ankle and foot**

    M71.871 **Other specified bursopathies, right ankle and foot**
    M71.872 **Other specified bursopathies, left ankle and foot**
    M71.879 **Other specified bursopathies, unspecified ankle and foot**

    M71.88 **Other specified bursopathies, other site**
    M71.89 **Other specified bursopathies, multiple sites**

M71.9 Bursopathy, unspecified
    Bursitis NOS

√4ᵗʰ **M72 Fibroblastic disorders**

    EXCLUDES 2   *retroperitoneal fibromatosis (D48.3)*

    M72.0 **Palmar fascial fibromatosis [Dupuytren]**   **A**
       DEF: Dupuytren's contracture: Flexion deformity of a finger, due to shortened, thickened fibrosing of palmar fascia. The cause is unknown, but it is associated with long-standing epilepsy.

    M72.1 **Knuckle pads**

    M72.2 **Plantar fascial fibromatosis**
       Plantar fasciitis
       DEF: Rapid-growing and multiplanar nodular swellings and pain in the foot that is not associated with contractures.

    M72.4 **Pseudosarcomatous fibromatosis**
       Nodular fasciitis

    M72.6 **Necrotizing fasciitis**   **HCC** **ESR** **COM**
       Use additional code (B95.-, B96.-) to identify causative organism

    M72.8 **Other fibroblastic disorders**
       Abscess of fascia
       Fasciitis NEC
       Other infective fasciitis
       Use additional code to (B95.-, B96.-) identify causative organism
       EXCLUDES 1   *diffuse (eosinophilic) fasciitis (M35.4)*
                  necrotizing fasciitis (M72.6)
                  nodular fasciitis (M72.4)
                  perirenal fasciitis NOS (N13.5)
                  perirenal fasciitis with infection (N13.6)
                  plantar fasciitis (M72.2)

    M72.9 **Fibroblastic disorder, unspecified**
       Fasciitis NOS
       Fibromatosis NOS

✓4ᵗʰ **M75** **Shoulder lesions**

     EXCLUDES 2   *shoulder-hand syndrome (M89.0-)*

   ✓5ᵗʰ **M75.0** **Adhesive capsulitis of shoulder**

     Frozen shoulder

     Periarthritis of shoulder

     AHA: 2015,2Q,23

     M75.00   **Adhesive capsulitis of unspecified shoulder**

     M75.01   **Adhesive capsulitis of right shoulder**

     M75.02   **Adhesive capsulitis of left shoulder**

   ✓5ᵗʰ **M75.1** **Rotator cuff tear or rupture, not specified as traumatic**

     Rotator cuff syndrome

     Supraspinatus syndrome

     Supraspinatus tear or rupture, not specified as traumatic

     EXCLUDES 1   *tear of rotator cuff, traumatic (S46.01-)*

     ✓6ᵗʰ **M75.10** **Unspecified rotator cuff tear or rupture, not specified as traumatic**

       M75.100   **Unspecified rotator cuff tear or rupture of unspecified shoulder, not specified as traumatic**

       M75.101   **Unspecified rotator cuff tear or rupture of right shoulder, not specified as traumatic**

       M75.102   **Unspecified rotator cuff tear or rupture of left shoulder, not specified as traumatic**

     ✓6ᵗʰ **M75.11** **Incomplete rotator cuff tear or rupture not specified as traumatic**

       M75.110   **Incomplete rotator cuff tear or rupture of unspecified shoulder, not specified as traumatic**

       M75.111   **Incomplete rotator cuff tear or rupture of right shoulder, not specified as traumatic**

       M75.112   **Incomplete rotator cuff tear or rupture of left shoulder, not specified as traumatic**

     ✓6ᵗʰ **M75.12** **Complete rotator cuff tear or rupture not specified as traumatic**

       M75.120   **Complete rotator cuff tear or rupture of unspecified shoulder, not specified as traumatic**

       M75.121   **Complete rotator cuff tear or rupture of right shoulder, not specified as traumatic**

       M75.122   **Complete rotator cuff tear or rupture of left shoulder, not specified as traumatic**

   ✓5ᵗʰ **M75.2** **Bicipital tendinitis**

     M75.20   **Bicipital tendinitis, unspecified shoulder**

     M75.21   **Bicipital tendinitis, right shoulder**

     M75.22   **Bicipital tendinitis, left shoulder**

   ✓5ᵗʰ **M75.3** **Calcific tendinitis of shoulder**

     Calcified bursa of shoulder

     M75.30   **Calcific tendinitis of unspecified shoulder**

     M75.31   **Calcific tendinitis of right shoulder**

     M75.32   **Calcific tendinitis of left shoulder**

   ✓5ᵗʰ **M75.4** **Impingement syndrome of shoulder**

     M75.40   **Impingement syndrome of unspecified shoulder**

     M75.41   **Impingement syndrome of right shoulder**

     M75.42   **Impingement syndrome of left shoulder**

   ✓5ᵗʰ **M75.5** **Bursitis of shoulder**

     M75.50   **Bursitis of unspecified shoulder**

     M75.51   **Bursitis of right shoulder**

     M75.52   **Bursitis of left shoulder**

   ✓5ᵗʰ **M75.8** **Other shoulder lesions**

     M75.80   **Other shoulder lesions, unspecified shoulder**

     M75.81   **Other shoulder lesions, right shoulder**

     M75.82   **Other shoulder lesions, left shoulder**

   ✓5ᵗʰ **M75.9** **Shoulder lesion, unspecified**

     M75.90   **Shoulder lesion, unspecified, unspecified shoulder**

     M75.91   **Shoulder lesion, unspecified, right shoulder**

     M75.92   **Shoulder lesion, unspecified, left shoulder**

✓4ᵗʰ **M76** **Enthesopathies, lower limb, excluding foot**

     EXCLUDES 2   *bursitis due to use, overuse and pressure (M70.-)*

             enthesopathies of ankle and foot (M77.5-)

   ✓6ᵗʰ **M76.0** **Gluteal tendinitis**

     M76.00   **Gluteal tendinitis, unspecified hip**

     M76.01   **Gluteal tendinitis, right hip**

     M76.02   **Gluteal tendinitis, left hip**

   ✓5ᵗʰ **M76.1** **Psoas tendinitis**

     M76.10   **Psoas tendinitis, unspecified hip**

     M76.11   **Psoas tendinitis, right hip**

     M76.12   **Psoas tendinitis, left hip**

   ✓5ᵗʰ **M76.2** **Iliac crest spur**

     M76.20   **Iliac crest spur, unspecified hip**

     M76.21   **Iliac crest spur, right hip**

     M76.22   **Iliac crest spur, left hip**

   ✓5ᵗʰ **M76.3** **Iliotibial band syndrome**

     M76.30   **Iliotibial band syndrome, unspecified leg**

     M76.31   **Iliotibial band syndrome, right leg**

     M76.32   **Iliotibial band syndrome, left leg**

   ✓5ᵗʰ **M76.4** **Tibial collateral bursitis [Pellegrini-Stieda]**

     M76.40   **Tibial collateral bursitis [Pellegrini-Stieda], unspecified leg**

     M76.41   **Tibial collateral bursitis [Pellegrini-Stieda], right leg**

     M76.42   **Tibial collateral bursitis [Pellegrini-Stieda], left leg**

   ✓5ᵗʰ **M76.5** **Patellar tendinitis**

     M76.50   **Patellar tendinitis, unspecified knee**

     M76.51   **Patellar tendinitis, right knee**

     M76.52   **Patellar tendinitis, left knee**

   ✓5ᵗʰ **M76.6** **Achilles tendinitis**

     Achilles bursitis

     M76.60   **Achilles tendinitis, unspecified leg**

     M76.61   **Achilles tendinitis, right leg**

     M76.62   **Achilles tendinitis, left leg**

   ✓5ᵗʰ **M76.7** **Peroneal tendinitis**

     M76.70   **Peroneal tendinitis, unspecified leg**

     M76.71   **Peroneal tendinitis, right leg**

     M76.72   **Peroneal tendinitis, left leg**

   ✓5ᵗʰ **M76.8** **Other specified enthesopathies of lower limb, excluding foot**

     ✓6ᵗʰ **M76.81** **Anterior tibial syndrome**

       M76.811   **Anterior tibial syndrome, right leg**

       M76.812   **Anterior tibial syndrome, left leg**

       M76.819   **Anterior tibial syndrome, unspecified leg**

     ✓6ᵗʰ **M76.82** **Posterior tibial tendinitis**

       M76.821   **Posterior tibial tendinitis, right leg**

       M76.822   **Posterior tibial tendinitis, left leg**

       M76.829   **Posterior tibial tendinitis, unspecified leg**

     ✓6ᵗʰ **M76.89** **Other specified enthesopathies of lower limb, excluding foot**

       M76.891   **Other specified enthesopathies of right lower limb, excluding foot**

       M76.892   **Other specified enthesopathies of left lower limb, excluding foot**

       M76.899   **Other specified enthesopathies of unspecified lower limb, excluding foot**

     M76.9   **Unspecified enthesopathy, lower limb, excluding foot**

✓4ᵗʰ **M77** **Other enthesopathies**

     EXCLUDES 1   *bursitis NOS (M71.9-)*

     EXCLUDES 2   *bursitis due to use, overuse and pressure (M70.-)*

             osteophyte (M25.7)

             spinal enthesopathy (M46.0-)

   ✓5ᵗʰ **M77.0** **Medial epicondylitis**

     M77.00   **Medial epicondylitis, unspecified elbow**

     M77.01   **Medial epicondylitis, right elbow**

     M77.02   **Medial epicondylitis, left elbow**

   ✓5ᵗʰ **M77.1** **Lateral epicondylitis**

     Tennis elbow

     M77.10   **Lateral epicondylitis, unspecified elbow**

     M77.11   **Lateral epicondylitis, right elbow**

     M77.12   **Lateral epicondylitis, left elbow**

   ✓5ᵗʰ **M77.2** **Periarthritis of wrist**

     M77.20   **Periarthritis, unspecified wrist**

     M77.21   **Periarthritis, right wrist**

     M77.22   **Periarthritis, left wrist**

   ✓5ᵗʰ **M77.3** **Calcaneal spur**

     DEF: Overgrowth of calcaneus bone on the underside of the heel that causes pain on walking. Calcaneal spur is due to a chronic avulsion injury of the plantar fascia from the calcaneus.

     M77.30   **Calcaneal spur, unspecified foot**

     M77.31   **Calcaneal spur, right foot**

     M77.32   **Calcaneal spur, left foot**

☑️5ᵗʰ **M77.4** **Metatarsalgia**
- EXCLUDES 1   *Morton's metatarsalgia (G57.6)*
  - **M77.40** **Metatarsalgia, unspecified foot**
  - **M77.41** **Metatarsalgia, right foot**
  - **M77.42** **Metatarsalgia, left foot**

☑️5ᵗʰ **M77.5** **Other enthesopathy of foot and ankle**
  - **M77.50** **Other enthesopathy of unspecified foot and ankle**
  - **M77.51** **Other enthesopathy of right foot and ankle**
  - **M77.52** **Other enthesopathy of left foot and ankle**

M77.8 **Other enthesopathies, not elsewhere classified**

M77.9 **Enthesopathy, unspecified**
- Bone spur NOS
- Capsulitis NOS
- Periarthritis NOS
- Tendinitis NOS

☑️4ᵗʰ **M79** **Other and unspecified soft tissue disorders, not elsewhere classified**
- EXCLUDES 1   *psychogenic rheumatism (F45.8)*
  - *soft tissue pain, psychogenic (F45.41)*

M79.0 **Rheumatism, unspecified**
- EXCLUDES 1   *fibromyalgia (M79.7)*
  - *palindromic rheumatism (M12.3-)*

☑️5ᵗʰ **M79.1** **Myalgia**
- Myofascial pain syndrome
- EXCLUDES 1   *fibromyalgia (M79.7)*
  - *myositis (M60.-)*
- **AHA:** 2018,4Q,21
  - **M79.10** **Myalgia, unspecified site**
  - **M79.11** **Myalgia of mastication muscle**
  - **M79.12** **Myalgia of auxiliary muscles, head and neck**
  - **M79.18** **Myalgia, other site**

M79.2 **Neuralgia and neuritis, unspecified**
- EXCLUDES 1   *brachial radiculitis NOS (M54.1)*
  - *lumbosacral radiculitis NOS (M54.1)*
  - *mononeuropathies (G56-G58)*
  - *radiculitis NOS (M54.1)*
  - *sciatica (M54.3-M54.4)*
- **TIP:** Assign for documented neuropathic pain.

M79.3 **Panniculitis, unspecified**
- EXCLUDES 1   *lupus panniculitis (L93.2)*
  - *neck and back panniculitis (M54.0-)*
  - *relapsing [Weber-Christian] panniculitis (M35.6)*

M79.4 **Hypertrophy of (infrapatellar) fat pad**

M79.5 **Residual foreign body in soft tissue**
- EXCLUDES 1   *foreign body granuloma of skin and subcutaneous tissue (L92.3)*
  - *foreign body granuloma of soft tissue (M60.2-)*

☑️5ᵗʰ **M79.6** **Pain in limb, hand, foot, fingers and toes**
- EXCLUDES 2   *pain in joint (M25.5-)*
  - ☑️6ᵗʰ **M79.60** **Pain in limb, unspecified**
    - **M79.601** **Pain in right arm**
      - Pain in right upper limb NOS
    - **M79.602** **Pain in left arm**
      - Pain in left upper limb NOS
    - **M79.603** **Pain in arm, unspecified**
      - Pain in upper limb NOS
    - **M79.604** **Pain in right leg**
      - Pain in right lower limb NOS
    - **M79.605** **Pain in left leg**
      - Pain in left lower limb NOS
    - **M79.606** **Pain in leg, unspecified**
      - Pain in lower limb NOS
    - **M79.609** **Pain in unspecified limb**
      - Pain in limb NOS
  - ☑️6ᵗʰ **M79.62** **Pain in upper arm**
    - Pain in axillary region
    - **M79.621** **Pain in right upper arm**
    - **M79.622** **Pain in left upper arm**
    - **M79.629** **Pain in unspecified upper arm**
  - ☑️6ᵗʰ **M79.63** **Pain in forearm**
    - **M79.631** **Pain in right forearm**
    - **M79.632** **Pain in left forearm**
    - **M79.639** **Pain in unspecified forearm**
  - ☑️6ᵗʰ **M79.64** **Pain in hand and fingers**
    - **M79.641** **Pain in right hand**

- **M79.642** **Pain in left hand**
- **M79.643** **Pain in unspecified hand**
- **M79.644** **Pain in right finger(s)**
- **M79.645** **Pain in left finger(s)**
- **M79.646** **Pain in unspecified finger(s)**
  - ☑️6ᵗʰ **M79.65** **Pain in thigh**
    - **M79.651** **Pain in right thigh**
    - **M79.652** **Pain in left thigh**
    - **M79.659** **Pain in unspecified thigh**
  - ☑️6ᵗʰ **M79.66** **Pain in lower leg**
    - **M79.661** **Pain in right lower leg**
    - **M79.662** **Pain in left lower leg**
    - **M79.669** **Pain in unspecified lower leg**
  - ☑️6ᵗʰ **M79.67** **Pain in foot and toes**
    - **M79.671** **Pain in right foot**
    - **M79.672** **Pain in left foot**
    - **M79.673** **Pain in unspecified foot**
    - **M79.674** **Pain in right toe(s)**
    - **M79.675** **Pain in left toe(s)**
    - **M79.676** **Pain in unspecified toe(s)**

M79.7 **Fibromyalgia**
- Fibromyositis
- Fibrositis
- Myofibrositis

☑️5ᵗʰ **M79.A** **Nontraumatic compartment syndrome**
- Code first, if applicable, associated postprocedural complication
- EXCLUDES 1   *compartment syndrome NOS (T79.A-)*
  - *fibromyalgia (M79.7)*
  - *nontraumatic ischemic infarction of muscle (M62.2-)*
  - *traumatic compartment syndrome (T79.A-)*
- ☑️6ᵗʰ **M79.A1** **Nontraumatic compartment syndrome of upper extremity**
  - Nontraumatic compartment syndrome of shoulder, arm, forearm, wrist, hand, and fingers
  - **M79.A11** **Nontraumatic compartment syndrome of right upper extremity**
  - **M79.A12** **Nontraumatic compartment syndrome of left upper extremity**
  - **M79.A19** **Nontraumatic compartment syndrome of unspecified upper extremity**
- ☑️6ᵗʰ **M79.A2** **Nontraumatic compartment syndrome of lower extremity**
  - Nontraumatic compartment syndrome of hip, buttock, thigh, leg, foot, and toes
  - **M79.A21** **Nontraumatic compartment syndrome of right lower extremity**
  - **M79.A22** **Nontraumatic compartment syndrome of left lower extremity**
  - **M79.A29** **Nontraumatic compartment syndrome of unspecified lower extremity**
- **M79.A3** **Nontraumatic compartment syndrome of abdomen**
- **M79.A9** **Nontraumatic compartment syndrome of other sites**

☑️5ᵗʰ **M79.8** **Other specified soft tissue disorders**
- **M79.81** **Nontraumatic hematoma of soft tissue**
  - Nontraumatic hematoma of muscle
  - Nontraumatic seroma of muscle and soft tissue
- **M79.89** **Other specified soft tissue disorders**
  - Polyalgia

M79.9 **Soft tissue disorder, unspecified**

| ☑️ Additional Character Required | ⚠️7ᵗʰ Placeholder Alert | Manifestation | Unspecified Dx | ℚ QPP | ⓊⓅⒹ Unacceptable PDx |

OSTEOPATHIES AND CHONDROPATHIES (M80-M94)

Disorders of bone density and structure (M80-M85)

√4ᵗʰ M80 Osteoporosis with current pathological fracture

     INCLUDES osteoporosis with current fragility fracture

     Use additional code to identify major osseous defect, if applicable (M89.7-)

     EXCLUDES 1 collapsed vertebra NOS (M48.5)
           pathological fracture NOS (M84.4)
           wedging of vertebra NOS (M48.5)

     EXCLUDES 2 personal history of (healed) osteoporosis fracture (Z87.310)

     AHA: 2018,2Q,12

     TIP: The site codes in this category identify the site of the fracture, not the site of the osteoporosis.

> The appropriate 7th character is to be added to each code from category M80:
> A   initial encounter for fracture
> D   subsequent encounter for fracture with routine healing
> G   subsequent encounter for fracture with delayed healing
> K   subsequent encounter for fracture with nonunion
> P   subsequent encounter for fracture with malunion
> S   sequela

√5ᵗʰ M80.0 Age-related osteoporosis with current pathological fracture

     Involutional osteoporosis with current pathological fracture
     Osteoporosis NOS with current pathological fracture
     Postmenopausal osteoporosis with current pathological fracture
     Senile osteoporosis with current pathological fracture

     √x7ᵗʰ M80.00 Age-related osteoporosis with current pathological fracture, unspecified site   Rx Q A

     √6ᵗʰ M80.01 Age-related osteoporosis with current pathological fracture, **shoulder**

         √7ᵗʰ M80.011 Age-related osteoporosis with current pathological fracture, **right shoulder**   Rx Q A

         √7ᵗʰ M80.012 Age-related osteoporosis with current pathological fracture, **left shoulder**   Rx Q A

         √7ᵗʰ M80.019 Age-related osteoporosis with current pathological fracture, unspecified shoulder   Rx Q A

     √6ᵗʰ M80.02 Age-related osteoporosis with current pathological fracture, **humerus**

         √7ᵗʰ M80.021 Age-related osteoporosis with current pathological fracture, **right humerus**   Rx Q A

         √7ᵗʰ M80.022 Age-related osteoporosis with current pathological fracture, **left humerus**   Rx Q A

         √7ᵗʰ M80.029 Age-related osteoporosis with current pathological fracture, unspecified humerus   Rx Q A

     √6ᵗʰ M80.03 Age-related osteoporosis with current pathological fracture, **forearm**

         Age-related osteoporosis with current pathological fracture of wrist

         √7ᵗʰ M80.031 Age-related osteoporosis with current pathological fracture, **right forearm**   Rx Q A

         √7ᵗʰ M80.032 Age-related osteoporosis with current pathological fracture, **left forearm**   Rx Q A

         √7ᵗʰ M80.039 Age-related osteoporosis with current pathological fracture, unspecified forearm   Rx Q A

     √6ᵗʰ M80.04 Age-related osteoporosis with current pathological fracture, **hand**

         √7ᵗʰ M80.041 Age-related osteoporosis with current pathological fracture, **right hand**   Rx Q A

         √7ᵗʰ M80.042 Age-related osteoporosis with current pathological fracture, **left hand**   Rx Q A

         √7ᵗʰ M80.049 Age-related osteoporosis with current pathological fracture, unspecified hand   Rx Q A

     √6ᵗʰ M80.05 Age-related osteoporosis with current pathological fracture, **femur**

         Age-related osteoporosis with current pathological fracture of hip

         ¹ **√7ᵗʰ M80.051** Age-related osteoporosis with current pathological fracture, **right femur**   HCC Rx ESR COM Q A

         ¹ **√7ᵗʰ M80.052** Age-related osteoporosis with current pathological fracture, **left femur**   HCC Rx ESR COM Q A

         ¹ **√7ᵗʰ M80.059** Age-related osteoporosis with current pathological fracture, unspecified femur   HCC Rx ESR COM Q A

     √6ᵗʰ M80.06 Age-related osteoporosis with current pathological fracture, **lower leg**

         √7ᵗʰ M80.061 Age-related osteoporosis with current pathological fracture, **right lower leg**   Rx Q A

         √7ᵗʰ M80.062 Age-related osteoporosis with current pathological fracture, **left lower leg**   Rx Q A

         √7ᵗʰ M80.069 Age-related osteoporosis with current pathological fracture, unspecified lower leg   Rx Q A

     √6ᵗʰ M80.07 Age-related osteoporosis with current pathological fracture, **ankle and foot**

         √7ᵗʰ M80.071 Age-related osteoporosis with current pathological fracture, **right ankle and foot**   Rx Q A

         √7ᵗʰ M80.072 Age-related osteoporosis with current pathological fracture, **left ankle and foot**   Rx Q A

         √7ᵗʰ M80.079 Age-related osteoporosis with current pathological fracture, unspecified ankle and foot   Rx Q A

     ¹ **√x7ᵗʰ M80.08** Age-related osteoporosis with current pathological fracture, **vertebra(e)**   HCC Rx ESR COM Q A

     √x7ᵗʰ M80.0A Age-related osteoporosis with current pathological fracture, **other site**   Rx Q A

         AHA: 2020,4Q,32-33

√5ᵗʰ M80.8 Other osteoporosis with current pathological fracture

     Drug-induced osteoporosis with current pathological fracture
     Idiopathic osteoporosis with current pathological fracture
     Osteoporosis of disuse with current pathological fracture
     Postoophorectomy osteoporosis with current pathological fracture
     Postsurgical malabsorption osteoporosis with current pathological fracture
     Post-traumatic osteoporosis with current pathological fracture
     Use additional code for adverse effect, if applicable, to identify drug (T36-T50 with fifth or sixth character 5)

     √x7ᵗʰ M80.80 Other osteoporosis with current pathological fracture, unspecified site   Rx Q

     √6ᵗʰ M80.81 Other osteoporosis with pathological fracture, **shoulder**

         √7ᵗʰ M80.811 Other osteoporosis with current pathological fracture, **right shoulder**   Rx Q

         √7ᵗʰ M80.812 Other osteoporosis with current pathological fracture, **left shoulder**   Rx Q

         √7ᵗʰ M80.819 Other osteoporosis with current pathological fracture, unspecified shoulder   Rx Q

     √6ᵗʰ M80.82 Other osteoporosis with current pathological fracture, **humerus**

         √7ᵗʰ M80.821 Other osteoporosis with current pathological fracture, **right humerus**   Rx Q

         √7ᵗʰ M80.822 Other osteoporosis with current pathological fracture, **left humerus**   Rx Q

         √7ᵗʰ M80.829 Other osteoporosis with current pathological fracture, unspecified humerus   Rx Q

√6th M80.83 Other osteoporosis with current pathological fracture, forearm
Other osteoporosis with current pathological fracture of wrist

    √7th M80.831 Other osteoporosis with current pathological fracture, right forearm Rx Q

    √7th M80.832 Other osteoporosis with current pathological fracture, left forearm Rx Q

    √7th M80.839 Other osteoporosis with current pathological fracture, unspecified forearm Rx Q

√6th M80.84 Other osteoporosis with current pathological fracture, hand

    √7th M80.841 Other osteoporosis with current pathological fracture, right hand Rx Q

    √7th M80.842 Other osteoporosis with current pathological fracture, left hand Rx Q

    √7th M80.849 Other osteoporosis with current pathological fracture, unspecified hand

√6th M80.85 Other osteoporosis with current pathological fracture, femur
Other osteoporosis with current pathological fracture of hip

    1 **√7th M80.851 Other osteoporosis with current pathological fracture, right femur** HCC Rx ESR COM Q

    1 **√7th M80.852 Other osteoporosis with current pathological fracture, left femur** HCC Rx ESR COM Q

    1 **√7th M80.859 Other osteoporosis with current pathological fracture, unspecified femur** HCC Rx ESR COM Q

√6th M80.86 Other osteoporosis with current pathological fracture, lower leg

    √7th M80.861 Other osteoporosis with current pathological fracture, right lower leg Rx Q

    √7th M80.862 Other osteoporosis with current pathological fracture, left lower leg Rx Q

    √7th M80.869 Other osteoporosis with current pathological fracture, unspecified lower leg Rx Q

√6th M80.87 Other osteoporosis with current pathological fracture, ankle and foot

    √7th M80.871 Other osteoporosis with current pathological fracture, right ankle and foot Rx Q

    √7th M80.872 Other osteoporosis with current pathological fracture, left ankle and foot Rx Q

    √7th M80.879 Other osteoporosis with current pathological fracture, unspecified ankle and foot Rx Q

   1 **√x7th M80.88 Other osteoporosis with current pathological fracture, vertebra(e)** HCC Rx ESR COM Q

   √x7th M80.8A Other osteoporosis with current pathological fracture, other site Rx Q
AHA: 2020,4Q,32

√4th M81 Osteoporosis without current pathological fracture
Use additional code to identify:
major osseous defect, if applicable (M89.7-)
personal history of (healed) osteoporosis fracture, if applicable (Z87.310)
EXCLUDES 1   osteoporosis with current pathological fracture (M80.-)
      Sudeck's atrophy (M89.0)

M81.0 Age-related osteoporosis without current pathological fracture Rx Q A
Involutional osteoporosis without current pathological fracture
Osteoporosis NOS
Postmenopausal osteoporosis without current pathological fracture
Senile osteoporosis without current pathological fracture

M81.6 Localized osteoporosis [Lequesne] Rx Q
EXCLUDES 1   Sudeck's atrophy (M89.0)

M81.8 Other osteoporosis without current pathological fracture Rx Q
Drug-induced osteoporosis without current pathological fracture
Idiopathic osteoporosis without current pathological fracture
Osteoporosis of disuse without current pathological fracture
Postoophorectomy osteoporosis without current pathological fracture
Postsurgical malabsorption osteoporosis without current pathological fracture
Post-traumatic osteoporosis without current pathological fracture
Use additional code for adverse effect, if applicable, to identify drug (T36-T50 with fifth or sixth character 5)

√4th M83 Adult osteomalacia
EXCLUDES 1   infantile and juvenile osteomalacia (E55.0)
      renal osteodystrophy (N25.0)
      rickets (active) (E55.0)
      rickets (active) sequelae (E64.3)
      vitamin D-resistant osteomalacia (E83.3)
      vitamin D-resistant rickets (active) (E83.3)

M83.0 Puerperal osteomalacia Rx M ♀

M83.1 Senile osteomalacia Rx A

M83.2 Adult osteomalacia due to malabsorption Rx A
Postsurgical malabsorption osteomalacia in adults

M83.3 Adult osteomalacia due to malnutrition Rx A

M83.4 Aluminum bone disease Rx

M83.5 Other drug-induced osteomalacia in adults Rx A
Use additional code for adverse effect, if applicable, to identify drug (T36-T50 with fifth or sixth character 5)

M83.8 Other adult osteomalacia Rx A

M83.9 Adult osteomalacia, unspecified Rx A

√4th M84 Disorder of continuity of bone
EXCLUDES 2   traumatic fracture of bone-see fracture, by site

√5th M84.3 Stress fracture
Fatigue fracture
March fracture
Stress fracture NOS
Stress reaction
Use additional external cause code(s) to identify the cause of the stress fracture
EXCLUDES 1   pathological fracture due to osteoporosis (M80.-)
      pathological fracture NOS (M84.4.-)
      traumatic fracture (S12.-, S22.-, S32.-, S42.-, S52.-, S62.-, S72.-, S82.-, S92.-)
EXCLUDES 2   personal history of (healed) stress (fatigue) fracture (Z87.312)
      stress fracture of vertebra (M48.4-)

> The appropriate 7th character is to be added to each code from subcategory M84.3.
> A   initial encounter for fracture
> D   subsequent encounter for fracture with routine healing
> G   subsequent encounter for fracture with delayed healing
> K   subsequent encounter for fracture with nonunion
> P   subsequent encounter for fracture with malunion
> S   sequela

√x7th M84.30 Stress fracture, unspecified site

√6th M84.31 Stress fracture, shoulder

    √7th M84.311 Stress fracture, right shoulder Q

    √7th M84.312 Stress fracture, left shoulder Q

    √7th M84.319 Stress fracture, unspecified shoulder Q

√6th M84.32 Stress fracture, humerus

    √7th M84.321 Stress fracture, right humerus Q

    √7th M84.322 Stress fracture, left humerus Q

    √7th M84.329 Stress fracture, unspecified humerus Q

√6th M84.33 Stress fracture, ulna and radius

    √7th M84.331 Stress fracture, right ulna Q

    √7th M84.332 Stress fracture, left ulna Q

    √7th M84.333 Stress fracture, right radius Q

    √7th M84.334 Stress fracture, left radius Q

Chapter 13. Diseases of the Musculoskeletal System and Connective Tissue

M84.339–M84.522

√7ᵗʰ **M84.339** Stress fracture, unspecified ulna and radius   Q

√6ᵗʰ **M84.34** Stress fracture, hand and fingers

  √7ᵗʰ **M84.341** Stress fracture, right hand   Q
  √7ᵗʰ **M84.342** Stress fracture, left hand   Q
  √7ᵗʰ **M84.343** Stress fracture, unspecified hand   Q
  √7ᵗʰ **M84.344** Stress fracture, right finger(s)
  √7ᵗʰ **M84.345** Stress fracture, left finger(s)
  √7ᵗʰ **M84.346** Stress fracture, unspecified finger(s)

√6ᵗʰ **M84.35** Stress fracture, pelvis and femur
  Stress fracture, hip

  √7ᵗʰ **M84.350** Stress fracture, pelvis   Q
  √7ᵗʰ **M84.351** Stress fracture, right femur   Q
  √7ᵗʰ **M84.352** Stress fracture, left femur   Q
  √7ᵗʰ **M84.353** Stress fracture, unspecified femur   Q
  √7ᵗʰ **M84.359** Stress fracture, hip, unspecified   Q

√6ᵗʰ **M84.36** Stress fracture, tibia and fibula

  √7ᵗʰ **M84.361** Stress fracture, right tibia   Q
  √7ᵗʰ **M84.362** Stress fracture, left tibia   Q
  √7ᵗʰ **M84.363** Stress fracture, right fibula   Q
  √7ᵗʰ **M84.364** Stress fracture, left fibula   Q
  √7ᵗʰ **M84.369** Stress fracture, unspecified tibia and fibula   Q

√6ᵗʰ **M84.37** Stress fracture, ankle, foot and toes

  √7ᵗʰ **M84.371** Stress fracture, right ankle   Q
  √7ᵗʰ **M84.372** Stress fracture, left ankle   Q
  √7ᵗʰ **M84.373** Stress fracture, unspecified ankle   Q
  √7ᵗʰ **M84.374** Stress fracture, right foot   Q
  √7ᵗʰ **M84.375** Stress fracture, left foot   Q
  √7ᵗʰ **M84.376** Stress fracture, unspecified foot   Q
  √7ᵗʰ **M84.377** Stress fracture, right toe(s)
  √7ᵗʰ **M84.378** Stress fracture, left toe(s)
  √7ᵗʰ **M84.379** Stress fracture, unspecified toe(s)

√x7ᵗʰ **M84.38** Stress fracture, other site   Q
    EXCLUDES 2   stress fracture of vertebra (M48.4-)

√5ᵗʰ **M84.4** Pathological fracture, not elsewhere classified
  Chronic fracture
  Pathological fracture NOS
  EXCLUDES 1   collapsed vertebra NEC (M48.5)
       pathological fracture in neoplastic disease (M84.5-)
       pathological fracture in osteoporosis (M80.-)
       pathological fracture in other disease (M84.6-)
       stress fracture (M84.3-)
       traumatic fracture (S12.-, S22.-, S32.-, S42.-, S52.-, S62.-, S72.-, S82.-, S92.-)
  EXCLUDES 2   personal history of (healed) pathological fracture (Z87.311)

  The appropriate 7th character is to be added to each code from subcategory M84.4.
  A   initial encounter for fracture
  D   subsequent encounter for fracture with routine healing
  G   subsequent encounter for fracture with delayed healing
  K   subsequent encounter for fracture with nonunion
  P   subsequent encounter for fracture with malunion
  S   sequela

√x7ᵗʰ **M84.40** Pathological fracture, unspecified site   Rx

√6ᵗʰ **M84.41** Pathological fracture, shoulder

  √7ᵗʰ **M84.411** Pathological fracture, right shoulder   Rx
  √7ᵗʰ **M84.412** Pathological fracture, left shoulder   Rx
  √7ᵗʰ **M84.419** Pathological fracture, unspecified shoulder   Rx

√6ᵗʰ **M84.42** Pathological fracture, humerus

  √7ᵗʰ **M84.421** Pathological fracture, right humerus   Rx
  √7ᵗʰ **M84.422** Pathological fracture, left humerus   Rx
  √7ᵗʰ **M84.429** Pathological fracture, unspecified humerus   Rx

√6ᵗʰ **M84.43** Pathological fracture, ulna and radius

  √7ᵗʰ **M84.431** Pathological fracture, right ulna   Rx

  √7ᵗʰ **M84.432** Pathological fracture, left ulna   Rx
  √7ᵗʰ **M84.433** Pathological fracture, right radius   Rx
  √7ᵗʰ **M84.434** Pathological fracture, left radius   Rx
  √7ᵗʰ **M84.439** Pathological fracture, unspecified ulna and radius   Rx

√6ᵗʰ **M84.44** Pathological fracture, hand and fingers

  √7ᵗʰ **M84.441** Pathological fracture, right hand   Rx
  √7ᵗʰ **M84.442** Pathological fracture, left hand   Rx
  √7ᵗʰ **M84.443** Pathological fracture, unspecified hand   Rx
  √7ᵗʰ **M84.444** Pathological fracture, right finger(s)
  √7ᵗʰ **M84.445** Pathological fracture, left finger(s)   Rx
  √7ᵗʰ **M84.446** Pathological fracture, unspecified finger(s)   Rx

√6ᵗʰ **M84.45** Pathological fracture, femur and pelvis
  AHA: 2016,4Q,43

  ¹ √7ᵗʰ **M84.451** Pathological fracture, right femur   HCC Rx ESR COM
  ¹ √7ᵗʰ **M84.452** Pathological fracture, left femur   HCC Rx ESR COM
  ¹ √7ᵗʰ **M84.453** Pathological fracture, unspecified femur   HCC Rx ESR COM
  √7ᵗʰ **M84.454** Pathological fracture, pelvis   Rx
  ¹ √7ᵗʰ **M84.459** Pathological fracture, hip, unspecified   HCC Rx ESR COM

√6ᵗʰ **M84.46** Pathological fracture, tibia and fibula

  √7ᵗʰ **M84.461** Pathological fracture, right tibia   Rx
  √7ᵗʰ **M84.462** Pathological fracture, left tibia   Rx
  √7ᵗʰ **M84.463** Pathological fracture, right fibula   Rx
  √7ᵗʰ **M84.464** Pathological fracture, left fibula   Rx
  √7ᵗʰ **M84.469** Pathological fracture, unspecified tibia and fibula   Rx

√6ᵗʰ **M84.47** Pathological fracture, ankle, foot and toes

  √7ᵗʰ **M84.471** Pathological fracture, right ankle   Rx
  √7ᵗʰ **M84.472** Pathological fracture, left ankle   Rx
  √7ᵗʰ **M84.473** Pathological fracture, unspecified ankle   Rx
  √7ᵗʰ **M84.474** Pathological fracture, right foot   Rx
  √7ᵗʰ **M84.475** Pathological fracture, left foot   Rx
  √7ᵗʰ **M84.476** Pathological fracture, unspecified foot   Rx
  √7ᵗʰ **M84.477** Pathological fracture, right toe(s)   Rx
  √7ᵗʰ **M84.478** Pathological fracture, left toe(s)   Rx
  √7ᵗʰ **M84.479** Pathological fracture, unspecified toe(s)   Rx

√x7ᵗʰ **M84.48** Pathological fracture, other site   Rx

√5ᵗʰ **M84.5** Pathological fracture in neoplastic disease
  Code also underlying neoplasm

  The appropriate 7th character is to be added to each code from subcategory M84.5.
  A   initial encounter for fracture
  D   subsequent encounter for fracture with routine healing
  G   subsequent encounter for fracture with delayed healing
  K   subsequent encounter for fracture with nonunion
  P   subsequent encounter for fracture with malunion
  S   sequela

√x7ᵗʰ **M84.50** Pathological fracture in neoplastic disease, unspecified site   Rx

√6ᵗʰ **M84.51** Pathological fracture in neoplastic disease, shoulder

  √7ᵗʰ **M84.511** Pathological fracture in neoplastic disease, right shoulder   Rx
  √7ᵗʰ **M84.512** Pathological fracture in neoplastic disease, left shoulder   Rx
  √7ᵗʰ **M84.519** Pathological fracture in neoplastic disease, unspecified shoulder   Rx

√6ᵗʰ **M84.52** Pathological fracture in neoplastic disease, humerus

  √7ᵗʰ **M84.521** Pathological fracture in neoplastic disease, right humerus   Rx
  √7ᵗʰ **M84.522** Pathological fracture in neoplastic disease, left humerus   Rx

√6ᵗʰ **M84.529** Pathological fracture in neoplastic disease, unspecified humerus `Rx`

√6ᵗʰ **M84.53** Pathological fracture in neoplastic disease, ulna and radius

  √7ᵗʰ **M84.531** Pathological fracture in neoplastic disease, right ulna `Rx`

  √7ᵗʰ **M84.532** Pathological fracture in neoplastic disease, left ulna `Rx`

  √7ᵗʰ **M84.533** Pathological fracture in neoplastic disease, right radius `Rx`

  √7ᵗʰ **M84.534** Pathological fracture in neoplastic disease, left radius `Rx`

  √7ᵗʰ **M84.539** Pathological fracture in neoplastic disease, unspecified ulna and radius `Rx`

√6ᵗʰ **M84.54** Pathological fracture in neoplastic disease, hand

  √7ᵗʰ **M84.541** Pathological fracture in neoplastic disease, right hand `Rx`

  √7ᵗʰ **M84.542** Pathological fracture in neoplastic disease, left hand `Rx`

  √7ᵗʰ **M84.549** Pathological fracture in neoplastic disease, unspecified hand `Rx`

√6ᵗʰ **M84.55** Pathological fracture in neoplastic disease, pelvis and femur

  √7ᵗʰ **M84.550** Pathological fracture in neoplastic disease, pelvis `Rx`

  1 √7ᵗʰ **M84.551** Pathological fracture in neoplastic disease, right femur `HCC` `Rx` `ESR` `COM`

  1 √7ᵗʰ **M84.552** Pathological fracture in neoplastic disease, left femur `HCC` `Rx` `ESR` `COM`

  1 √7ᵗʰ **M84.553** Pathological fracture in neoplastic disease, unspecified femur `HCC` `Rx` `ESR` `COM`

  1 √7ᵗʰ **M84.559** Pathological fracture in neoplastic disease, hip, unspecified `HCC` `Rx` `ESR` `COM`

√6ᵗʰ **M84.56** Pathological fracture in neoplastic disease, tibia and fibula

  √7ᵗʰ **M84.561** Pathological fracture in neoplastic disease, right tibia `Rx`

  √7ᵗʰ **M84.562** Pathological fracture in neoplastic disease, left tibia `Rx`

  √7ᵗʰ **M84.563** Pathological fracture in neoplastic disease, right fibula `Rx`

  √7ᵗʰ **M84.564** Pathological fracture in neoplastic disease, left fibula `Rx`

  √7ᵗʰ **M84.569** Pathological fracture in neoplastic disease, unspecified tibia and fibula `Rx`

√6ᵗʰ **M84.57** Pathological fracture in neoplastic disease, ankle and foot

  √7ᵗʰ **M84.571** Pathological fracture in neoplastic disease, right ankle `Rx`

  √7ᵗʰ **M84.572** Pathological fracture in neoplastic disease, left ankle `Rx`

  √7ᵗʰ **M84.573** Pathological fracture in neoplastic disease, unspecified ankle `Rx`

  √7ᵗʰ **M84.574** Pathological fracture in neoplastic disease, right foot `Rx`

  √7ᵗʰ **M84.575** Pathological fracture in neoplastic disease, left foot `Rx`

  √7ᵗʰ **M84.576** Pathological fracture in neoplastic disease, unspecified foot `Rx`

√x7ᵗʰ **M84.58** Pathological fracture in neoplastic disease, other specified site `Rx`

    Pathological fracture in neoplastic disease, vertebrae

√5ᵗʰ **M84.6** Pathological fracture in other disease

  Code also underlying condition

    EXCLUDES 1 *pathological fracture in osteoporosis (M80.-)*

    The appropriate 7th character is to be added to each code from subcategory M84.6.
    A   initial encounter for fracture
    D   subsequent encounter for fracture with routine healing
    G   subsequent encounter for fracture with delayed healing
    K   subsequent encounter for fracture with nonunion
    P   subsequent encounter for fracture with malunion
    S   sequela

√x7ᵗʰ **M84.60** Pathological fracture in other disease, unspecified site `Rx`

√6ᵗʰ **M84.61** Pathological fracture in other disease, shoulder

  √7ᵗʰ **M84.611** Pathological fracture in other disease, right shoulder `Rx`

  √7ᵗʰ **M84.612** Pathological fracture in other disease, left shoulder `Rx`

  √7ᵗʰ **M84.619** Pathological fracture in other disease, unspecified shoulder `Rx`

√6ᵗʰ **M84.62** Pathological fracture in other disease, humerus

  √7ᵗʰ **M84.621** Pathological fracture in other disease, right humerus `Rx`

  √7ᵗʰ **M84.622** Pathological fracture in other disease, left humerus `Rx`

  √7ᵗʰ **M84.629** Pathological fracture in other disease, unspecified humerus `Rx`

√6ᵗʰ **M84.63** Pathological fracture in other disease, ulna and radius

  √7ᵗʰ **M84.631** Pathological fracture in other disease, right ulna `Rx`

  √7ᵗʰ **M84.632** Pathological fracture in other disease, left ulna `Rx`

  √7ᵗʰ **M84.633** Pathological fracture in other disease, right radius `Rx`

  √7ᵗʰ **M84.634** Pathological fracture in other disease, left radius `Rx`

  √7ᵗʰ **M84.639** Pathological fracture in other disease, unspecified ulna and radius `Rx`

√6ᵗʰ **M84.64** Pathological fracture in other disease, hand

  √7ᵗʰ **M84.641** Pathological fracture in other disease, right hand `Rx`

  √7ᵗʰ **M84.642** Pathological fracture in other disease, left hand `Rx`

  √7ᵗʰ **M84.649** Pathological fracture in other disease, unspecified hand `Rx`

√6ᵗʰ **M84.65** Pathological fracture in other disease, pelvis and femur

  √7ᵗʰ **M84.650** Pathological fracture in other disease, pelvis `Rx`

  1 √7ᵗʰ **M84.651** Pathological fracture in other disease, right femur `HCC` `Rx` `ESR` `COM`

  1 √7ᵗʰ **M84.652** Pathological fracture in other disease, left femur `HCC` `Rx` `ESR` `COM`

  1 √7ᵗʰ **M84.653** Pathological fracture in other disease, unspecified femur `HCC` `Rx` `ESR` `COM`

  1 √7ᵗʰ **M84.659** Pathological fracture in other disease, hip, unspecified `HCC` `Rx` `ESR` `COM`

√6ᵗʰ **M84.66** Pathological fracture in other disease, tibia and fibula

  √7ᵗʰ **M84.661** Pathological fracture in other disease, right tibia `Rx`

  √7ᵗʰ **M84.662** Pathological fracture in other disease, left tibia `Rx`

  √7ᵗʰ **M84.663** Pathological fracture in other disease, right fibula `Rx`

  √7ᵗʰ **M84.664** Pathological fracture in other disease, left fibula `Rx`

  √7ᵗʰ **M84.669** Pathological fracture in other disease, unspecified tibia and fibula `Rx`

√6ᵗʰ **M84.67** Pathological fracture in other disease, ankle and foot

  √7ᵗʰ **M84.671** Pathological fracture in other disease, right ankle `Rx`

  √7ᵗʰ **M84.672** Pathological fracture in other disease, left ankle `Rx`

  √7ᵗʰ **M84.673** Pathological fracture in other disease, unspecified ankle `Rx`

  √7ᵗʰ **M84.674** Pathological fracture in other disease, right foot `Rx`

  √7ᵗʰ **M84.675** Pathological fracture in other disease, left foot `Rx`

  √7ᵗʰ **M84.676** Pathological fracture in other disease, unspecified foot `Rx`

√x7ᵗʰ **M84.68** Pathological fracture in other disease, other site `Rx`

☑ Additional Character Required   √x7ᵗʰ Placeholder Alert   Manifestation   Unspecified Dx   🔟 QPP   UPD Unacceptable PDx

√5th **M84.7** **Nontraumatic fracture, not elsewhere classified**

√6th **M84.75** **Atypical** femoral fracture

AHA: 2016,4Q,41-42

> The appropriate 7th character is to be added to each code from M84.75.
> A   initial encounter for fracture
> D   subsequent encounter for fracture with routine healing
> G   subsequent encounter for fracture with delayed healing
> K   subsequent encounter for fracture with nonunion
> P   subsequent encounter for fracture with malunion
> S   sequela

√7th **M84.750** **Atypical femoral fracture, unspecified**   Q

√7th **M84.751** **Incomplete atypical femoral fracture, right leg**   Q

√7th **M84.752** **Incomplete atypical femoral fracture, left leg**   Q

√7th **M84.753** **Incomplete atypical femoral fracture, unspecified leg**   Q

1 √7th **M84.754** **Complete transverse atypical femoral fracture, right leg**   HCC ESR COM Q

1 √7th **M84.755** **Complete transverse atypical femoral fracture, left leg**   HCC ESR COM Q

1 √7th **M84.756** **Complete transverse atypical femoral fracture, unspecified leg**   HCC ESR COM Q

1 √7th **M84.757** **Complete oblique atypical femoral fracture, right leg**   HCC ESR COM Q

1 √7th **M84.758** **Complete oblique atypical femoral fracture, left leg**   HCC ESR COM

1 √7th **M84.759** **Complete oblique atypical femoral fracture, unspecified leg**   HCC ESR COM Q

√5th **M84.8** **Other disorders of continuity of bone**

M84.80 **Other disorders of continuity of bone, unspecified site**

√6th **M84.81** **Other disorders of continuity of bone, shoulder**

M84.811 **Other disorders of continuity of bone, right shoulder**

M84.812 **Other disorders of continuity of bone, left shoulder**

M84.819 **Other disorders of continuity of bone, unspecified shoulder**

√6th **M84.82** **Other disorders of continuity of bone, humerus**

M84.821 **Other disorders of continuity of bone, right humerus**

M84.822 **Other disorders of continuity of bone, left humerus**

M84.829 **Other disorders of continuity of bone, unspecified humerus**

√6th **M84.83** **Other disorders of continuity of bone, ulna and radius**

M84.831 **Other disorders of continuity of bone, right ulna**

M84.832 **Other disorders of continuity of bone, left ulna**

M84.833 **Other disorders of continuity of bone, right radius**

M84.834 **Other disorders of continuity of bone, left radius**

M84.839 **Other disorders of continuity of bone, unspecified ulna and radius**

√6th **M84.84** **Other disorders of continuity of bone, hand**

M84.841 **Other disorders of continuity of bone, right hand**

M84.842 **Other disorders of continuity of bone, left hand**

M84.849 **Other disorders of continuity of bone, unspecified hand**

√6th **M84.85** **Other disorders of continuity of bone, pelvic region and thigh**

M84.851 **Other disorders of continuity of bone, right pelvic region and thigh**

M84.852 **Other disorders of continuity of bone, left pelvic region and thigh**

M84.859 **Other disorders of continuity of bone, unspecified pelvic region and thigh**

√6th **M84.86** **Other disorders of continuity of bone, tibia and fibula**

M84.861 **Other disorders of continuity of bone, right tibia**

M84.862 **Other disorders of continuity of bone, left tibia**

M84.863 **Other disorders of continuity of bone, right fibula**

M84.864 **Other disorders of continuity of bone, left fibula**

M84.869 **Other disorders of continuity of bone, unspecified tibia and fibula**

√6th **M84.87** **Other disorders of continuity of bone, ankle and foot**

M84.871 **Other disorders of continuity of bone, right ankle and foot**

M84.872 **Other disorders of continuity of bone, left ankle and foot**

M84.879 **Other disorders of continuity of bone, unspecified ankle and foot**

M84.88 **Other disorders of continuity of bone, other site**

M84.9 **Disorder of continuity of bone, unspecified**

√4th **M85** **Other disorders of bone density and structure**

EXCLUDES 1   osteogenesis imperfecta (Q78.0)
       osteopetrosis (Q78.2)
       osteopoikilosis (Q78.8)
       polyostotic fibrous dysplasia (Q78.1)

√5th **M85.0** **Fibrous dysplasia (monostotic)**

EXCLUDES 2   fibrous dysplasia of jaw (M27.8)

M85.00 **Fibrous dysplasia (monostotic), unspecified site**

√6th **M85.01** **Fibrous dysplasia (monostotic), shoulder**

M85.011 **Fibrous dysplasia (monostotic), right shoulder**

M85.012 **Fibrous dysplasia (monostotic), left shoulder**

M85.019 **Fibrous dysplasia (monostotic), unspecified shoulder**

√6th **M85.02** **Fibrous dysplasia (monostotic), upper arm**

M85.021 **Fibrous dysplasia (monostotic), right upper arm**

M85.022 **Fibrous dysplasia (monostotic), left upper arm**

M85.029 **Fibrous dysplasia (monostotic), unspecified upper arm**

√6th **M85.03** **Fibrous dysplasia (monostotic), forearm**

M85.031 **Fibrous dysplasia (monostotic), right forearm**

M85.032 **Fibrous dysplasia (monostotic), left forearm**

M85.039 **Fibrous dysplasia (monostotic), unspecified forearm**

√6th **M85.04** **Fibrous dysplasia (monostotic), hand**

M85.041 **Fibrous dysplasia (monostotic), right hand**

M85.042 **Fibrous dysplasia (monostotic), left hand**

M85.049 **Fibrous dysplasia (monostotic), unspecified hand**

√6th **M85.05** **Fibrous dysplasia (monostotic), thigh**

M85.051 **Fibrous dysplasia (monostotic), right thigh**

M85.052 **Fibrous dysplasia (monostotic), left thigh**

M85.059 **Fibrous dysplasia (monostotic), unspecified thigh**

√6th **M85.06** **Fibrous dysplasia (monostotic), lower leg**

M85.061 **Fibrous dysplasia (monostotic), right lower leg**

M85.062 **Fibrous dysplasia (monostotic), left lower leg**

M85.069 **Fibrous dysplasia (monostotic), unspecified lower leg**

√6th **M85.07** **Fibrous dysplasia (monostotic), ankle and foot**

M85.071 **Fibrous dysplasia (monostotic), right ankle and foot**

M85.072 **Fibrous dysplasia (monostotic), left ankle and foot**

M85.079 **Fibrous dysplasia (monostotic), unspecified ankle and foot**

M85.Ø8   **Fibrous dysplasia (monostotic), other site**

M85.Ø9   **Fibrous dysplasia (monostotic),** multiple sites

☑5ᵗʰ **M85.1**   **Skeletal fluorosis**

   M85.1Ø   **Skeletal fluorosis, unspecified site**

   ☑6ᵗʰ **M85.11**   **Skeletal fluorosis,** shoulder

     M85.111   **Skeletal fluorosis,** right **shoulder**

     M85.112   **Skeletal fluorosis,** left **shoulder**

     M85.119   **Skeletal fluorosis, unspecified shoulder**

   ☑6ᵗʰ **M85.12**   **Skeletal fluorosis,** upper arm

     M85.121   **Skeletal fluorosis,** right **upper arm**

     M85.122   **Skeletal fluorosis,** left **upper arm**

     M85.129   **Skeletal fluorosis, unspecified upper arm**

   ☑6ᵗʰ **M85.13**   **Skeletal fluorosis,** forearm

     M85.131   **Skeletal fluorosis,** right **forearm**

     M85.132   **Skeletal fluorosis,** left **forearm**

     M85.139   **Skeletal fluorosis, unspecified forearm**

   ☑6ᵗʰ **M85.14**   **Skeletal fluorosis,** hand

     M85.141   **Skeletal fluorosis,** right **hand**

     M85.142   **Skeletal fluorosis,** left **hand**

     M85.149   **Skeletal fluorosis, unspecified hand**

   ☑6ᵗʰ **M85.15**   **Skeletal fluorosis,** thigh

     M85.151   **Skeletal fluorosis,** right **thigh**

     M85.152   **Skeletal fluorosis,** left **thigh**

     M85.159   **Skeletal fluorosis, unspecified thigh**

   ☑6ᵗʰ **M85.16**   **Skeletal fluorosis,** lower leg

     M85.161   **Skeletal fluorosis,** right **lower leg**

     M85.162   **Skeletal fluorosis,** left **lower leg**

     M85.169   **Skeletal fluorosis, unspecified lower leg**

   ☑6ᵗʰ **M85.17**   **Skeletal fluorosis,** ankle and foot

     M85.171   **Skeletal fluorosis,** right **ankle and foot**

     M85.172   **Skeletal fluorosis,** left **ankle and foot**

     M85.179   **Skeletal fluorosis, unspecified ankle and foot**

   M85.18   **Skeletal fluorosis, other site**

   M85.19   **Skeletal fluorosis,** multiple sites

M85.2   **Hyperostosis of skull**

   DEF: Abnormal bone growth on the inner aspect of the cranial bones.

☑5ᵗʰ **M85.3**   **Osteitis condensans**

   M85.3Ø   **Osteitis condensans, unspecified site**

   ☑6ᵗʰ **M85.31**   **Osteitis condensans,** shoulder

     M85.311   **Osteitis condensans,** right **shoulder**

     M85.312   **Osteitis condensans,** left **shoulder**

     M85.319   **Osteitis condensans, unspecified shoulder**

   ☑6ᵗʰ **M85.32**   **Osteitis condensans,** upper arm

     M85.321   **Osteitis condensans,** right **upper arm**

     M85.322   **Osteitis condensans,** left **upper arm**

     M85.329   **Osteitis condensans, unspecified upper arm**

   ☑6ᵗʰ **M85.33**   **Osteitis condensans,** forearm

     M85.331   **Osteitis condensans,** right **forearm**

     M85.332   **Osteitis condensans,** left **forearm**

     M85.339   **Osteitis condensans, unspecified forearm**

   ☑6ᵗʰ **M85.34**   **Osteitis condensans,** hand

     M85.341   **Osteitis condensans,** right **hand**

     M85.342   **Osteitis condensans,** left **hand**

     M85.349   **Osteitis condensans, unspecified hand**

   ☑6ᵗʰ **M85.35**   **Osteitis condensans,** thigh

     M85.351   **Osteitis condensans,** right **thigh**

     M85.352   **Osteitis condensans,** left **thigh**

     M85.359   **Osteitis condensans, unspecified thigh**

   ☑6ᵗʰ **M85.36**   **Osteitis condensans,** lower leg

     M85.361   **Osteitis condensans,** right **lower leg**

     M85.362   **Osteitis condensans,** left **lower leg**

     M85.369   **Osteitis condensans, unspecified lower leg**

   ☑6ᵗʰ **M85.37**   **Osteitis condensans,** ankle and foot

     M85.371   **Osteitis condensans,** right **ankle and foot**

     M85.372   **Osteitis condensans,** left **ankle and foot**

     M85.379   **Osteitis condensans, unspecified ankle and foot**

   M85.38   **Osteitis condensans, other site**

   M85.39   **Osteitis condensans,** multiple sites

☑5ᵗʰ **M85.4**   **Solitary bone cyst**

   EXCLUDES 2   *solitary cyst of jaw (M27.4)*

   M85.4Ø   **Solitary bone cyst, unspecified site**

   ☑6ᵗʰ **M85.41**   **Solitary bone cyst,** shoulder

     M85.411   **Solitary bone cyst,** right **shoulder**

     M85.412   **Solitary bone cyst,** left **shoulder**

     M85.419   **Solitary bone cyst, unspecified shoulder**

   ☑6ᵗʰ **M85.42**   **Solitary bone cyst,** humerus

     M85.421   **Solitary bone cyst,** right **humerus**

     M85.422   **Solitary bone cyst,** left **humerus**

     M85.429   **Solitary bone cyst, unspecified humerus**

   ☑6ᵗʰ **M85.43**   **Solitary bone cyst,** ulna and radius

     M85.431   **Solitary bone cyst,** right **ulna and radius**

     M85.432   **Solitary bone cyst,** left **ulna and radius**

     M85.439   **Solitary bone cyst, unspecified ulna and radius**

   ☑6ᵗʰ **M85.44**   **Solitary bone cyst,** hand

     M85.441   **Solitary bone cyst,** right **hand**

     M85.442   **Solitary bone cyst,** left **hand**

     M85.449   **Solitary bone cyst, unspecified hand**

   ☑6ᵗʰ **M85.45**   **Solitary bone cyst,** pelvis

     M85.451   **Solitary bone cyst,** right **pelvis**

     M85.452   **Solitary bone cyst,** left **pelvis**

     M85.459   **Solitary bone cyst, unspecified pelvis**

   ☑6ᵗʰ **M85.46**   **Solitary bone cyst,** tibia and fibula

     M85.461   **Solitary bone cyst,** right **tibia and fibula**

     M85.462   **Solitary bone cyst,** left **tibia and fibula**

     M85.469   **Solitary bone cyst, unspecified tibia and fibula**

   ☑6ᵗʰ **M85.47**   **Solitary bone cyst,** ankle and foot

     M85.471   **Solitary bone cyst,** right **ankle and foot**

     M85.472   **Solitary bone cyst,** left **ankle and foot**

     M85.479   **Solitary bone cyst, unspecified ankle and foot**

   M85.48   **Solitary bone cyst, other site**

☑5ᵗʰ **M85.5**   **Aneurysmal bone cyst**

   EXCLUDES 2   *aneurysmal cyst of jaw (M27.4)*

   DEF: Solitary bone lesion that bulges into the periosteum and is marked by a calcified rim.

   M85.5Ø   **Aneurysmal bone cyst, unspecified site**

   ☑6ᵗʰ **M85.51**   **Aneurysmal bone cyst,** shoulder

     M85.511   **Aneurysmal bone cyst,** right **shoulder**

     M85.512   **Aneurysmal bone cyst,** left **shoulder**

     M85.519   **Aneurysmal bone cyst, unspecified shoulder**

   ☑6ᵗʰ **M85.52**   **Aneurysmal bone cyst,** upper arm

     M85.521   **Aneurysmal bone cyst,** right **upper arm**

     M85.522   **Aneurysmal bone cyst,** left **upper arm**

     M85.529   **Aneurysmal bone cyst, unspecified upper arm**

   ☑6ᵗʰ **M85.53**   **Aneurysmal bone cyst,** forearm

     M85.531   **Aneurysmal bone cyst,** right **forearm**

     M85.532   **Aneurysmal bone cyst,** left **forearm**

     M85.539   **Aneurysmal bone cyst, unspecified forearm**

   ☑6ᵗʰ **M85.54**   **Aneurysmal bone cyst,** hand

     M85.541   **Aneurysmal bone cyst,** right **hand**

     M85.542   **Aneurysmal bone cyst,** left **hand**

     M85.549   **Aneurysmal bone cyst, unspecified hand**

   ☑6ᵗʰ **M85.55**   **Aneurysmal bone cyst,** thigh

     M85.551   **Aneurysmal bone cyst,** right **thigh**

     M85.552   **Aneurysmal bone cyst,** left **thigh**

     M85.559   **Aneurysmal bone cyst, unspecified thigh**

   ☑6ᵗʰ **M85.56**   **Aneurysmal bone cyst,** lower leg

     M85.561   **Aneurysmal bone cyst,** right **lower leg**

     M85.562   **Aneurysmal bone cyst,** left **lower leg**

     M85.569   **Aneurysmal bone cyst, unspecified lower leg**

   ☑6ᵗʰ **M85.57**   **Aneurysmal bone cyst,** ankle and foot

     M85.571   **Aneurysmal bone cyst,** right **ankle and foot**

     M85.572   **Aneurysmal bone cyst,** left **ankle and foot**

     M85.579   **Aneurysmal bone cyst, unspecified ankle and foot**

   M85.58   **Aneurysmal bone cyst, other site**

   M85.59   **Aneurysmal bone cyst,** multiple sites

√5ᵗʰ M85.6 Other cyst of bone

> EXCLUDES 1   cyst of jaw NEC (M27.4)
>
> osteitis fibrosa cystica generalisata [von Recklinghausen's disease of bone] (E21.0)

M85.60 Other cyst of bone, unspecified site

√6ᵗʰ M85.61 Other cyst of bone, shoulder

     M85.611 Other cyst of bone, right shoulder
     M85.612 Other cyst of bone, left shoulder
     M85.619 Other cyst of bone, unspecified shoulder

√6ᵗʰ M85.62 Other cyst of bone, upper arm

     M85.621 Other cyst of bone, right upper arm
     M85.622 Other cyst of bone, left upper arm
     M85.629 Other cyst of bone, unspecified upper arm

√6ᵗʰ M85.63 Other cyst of bone, forearm

     M85.631 Other cyst of bone, right forearm
     M85.632 Other cyst of bone, left forearm
     M85.639 Other cyst of bone, unspecified forearm

√6ᵗʰ M85.64 Other cyst of bone, hand

     M85.641 Other cyst of bone, right hand
     M85.642 Other cyst of bone, left hand
     M85.649 Other cyst of bone, unspecified hand

√6ᵗʰ M85.65 Other cyst of bone, thigh

     M85.651 Other cyst of bone, right thigh
     M85.652 Other cyst of bone, left thigh
     M85.659 Other cyst of bone, unspecified thigh

√6ᵗʰ M85.66 Other cyst of bone, lower leg

     M85.661 Other cyst of bone, right lower leg
     M85.662 Other cyst of bone, left lower leg
     M85.669 Other cyst of bone, unspecified lower leg

√6ᵗʰ M85.67 Other cyst of bone, ankle and foot

     M85.671 Other cyst of bone, right ankle and foot
     M85.672 Other cyst of bone, left ankle and foot
     M85.679 Other cyst of bone, unspecified ankle and foot

M85.68 Other cyst of bone, other site

M85.69 Other cyst of bone, multiple sites

√5ᵗʰ M85.8 Other specified disorders of bone density and structure

> Hyperostosis of bones, except skull
> Osteosclerosis, acquired
>
> EXCLUDES 1   diffuse idiopathic skeletal hyperostosis [DISH] (M48.1)
> osteosclerosis congenita (Q77.4)
> osteosclerosis fragilitas (generalista) (Q78.2)
> osteosclerosis myelofibrosis (D75.81)

M85.80 Other specified disorders of bone density and structure, unspecified site

√6ᵗʰ M85.81 Other specified disorders of bone density and structure, shoulder

     M85.811 Other specified disorders of bone density and structure, right shoulder
     M85.812 Other specified disorders of bone density and structure, left shoulder
     M85.819 Other specified disorders of bone density and structure, unspecified shoulder

√6ᵗʰ M85.82 Other specified disorders of bone density and structure, upper arm

     M85.821 Other specified disorders of bone density and structure, right upper arm
     M85.822 Other specified disorders of bone density and structure, left upper arm
     M85.829 Other specified disorders of bone density and structure, unspecified upper arm

√6ᵗʰ M85.83 Other specified disorders of bone density and structure, forearm

     M85.831 Other specified disorders of bone density and structure, right forearm
     M85.832 Other specified disorders of bone density and structure, left forearm
     M85.839 Other specified disorders of bone density and structure, unspecified forearm

√6ᵗʰ M85.84 Other specified disorders of bone density and structure, hand

     M85.841 Other specified disorders of bone density and structure, right hand
     M85.842 Other specified disorders of bone density and structure, left hand
     M85.849 Other specified disorders of bone density and structure, unspecified hand

√6ᵗʰ M85.85 Other specified disorders of bone density and structure, thigh

     M85.851 Other specified disorders of bone density and structure, right thigh
     M85.852 Other specified disorders of bone density and structure, left thigh
     M85.859 Other specified disorders of bone density and structure, unspecified thigh

√6ᵗʰ M85.86 Other specified disorders of bone density and structure, lower leg

     M85.861 Other specified disorders of bone density and structure, right lower leg
     M85.862 Other specified disorders of bone density and structure, left lower leg
     M85.869 Other specified disorders of bone density and structure, unspecified lower leg

√6ᵗʰ M85.87 Other specified disorders of bone density and structure, ankle and foot

     M85.871 Other specified disorders of bone density and structure, right ankle and foot
     M85.872 Other specified disorders of bone density and structure, left ankle and foot
     M85.879 Other specified disorders of bone density and structure, unspecified ankle and foot

M85.88 Other specified disorders of bone density and structure, other site

M85.89 Other specified disorders of bone density and structure, multiple sites

M85.9 Disorder of bone density and structure, unspecified

AHA: 2021,3Q,11

Other osteopathies (M86-M90)

EXCLUDES 1   postprocedural osteopathies (M96.-)

√4ᵗʰ M86 Osteomyelitis

> Use additional code (B95-B97) to identify infectious agent
> Use additional code to identify major osseous defect, if applicable (M89.7-)
>
> EXCLUDES 1   osteomyelitis due to:
> echinococcus (B67.2)
> gonococcus (A54.43)
> salmonella (A02.24)
>
> EXCLUDES 2   ostemyelitis of:
> orbit (H05.0-)
> petrous bone (H70.2-)
> vertebra (M46.2-)

√5ᵗʰ M86.0 Acute hematogenous osteomyelitis

M86.00 Acute hematogenous osteomyelitis, unspecified site HCC ESR COM

√6ᵗʰ M86.01 Acute hematogenous osteomyelitis, shoulder

     M86.011 Acute hematogenous osteomyelitis, right shoulder HCC ESR COM
     M86.012 Acute hematogenous osteomyelitis, left shoulder HCC ESR COM
     M86.019 Acute hematogenous osteomyelitis, unspecified shoulder HCC ESR COM

√6ᵗʰ M86.02 Acute hematogenous osteomyelitis, humerus

     M86.021 Acute hematogenous osteomyelitis, right humerus HCC ESR COM
     M86.022 Acute hematogenous osteomyelitis, left humerus HCC ESR COM
     M86.029 Acute hematogenous osteomyelitis, unspecified humerus HCC ESR COM

√6ᵗʰ M86.03 Acute hematogenous osteomyelitis, radius and ulna

     M86.031 Acute hematogenous osteomyelitis, right radius and ulna HCC ESR COM
     M86.032 Acute hematogenous osteomyelitis, left radius and ulna HCC ESR COM
     M86.039 Acute hematogenous osteomyelitis, unspecified radius and ulna HCC ESR COM

√6ᵗʰ M86.04 Acute hematogenous osteomyelitis, hand

     M86.041 Acute hematogenous osteomyelitis, right hand HCC ESR COM
     M86.042 Acute hematogenous osteomyelitis, left hand HCC ESR COM
     M86.049 Acute hematogenous osteomyelitis, unspecified hand HCC ESR COM

√6ᵗʰ **M86.05** Acute hematogenous osteomyelitis, femur

     M86.051 Acute hematogenous osteomyelitis, right femur `HCC` `ESR` `COM`

     M86.052 Acute hematogenous osteomyelitis, left femur `HCC` `ESR` `COM`

     M86.059 Acute hematogenous osteomyelitis, unspecified femur `HCC` `ESR` `COM`

√6ᵗʰ **M86.06** Acute hematogenous osteomyelitis, tibia and fibula

     M86.061 Acute hematogenous osteomyelitis, right tibia and fibula `HCC` `ESR` `COM`

     M86.062 Acute hematogenous osteomyelitis, left tibia and fibula `HCC` `ESR` `COM`

     M86.069 Acute hematogenous osteomyelitis, unspecified tibia and fibula `HCC` `ESR` `COM`

√6ᵗʰ **M86.07** Acute hematogenous osteomyelitis, ankle and foot

     M86.071 Acute hematogenous osteomyelitis, right ankle and foot `HCC` `ESR` `COM`

     M86.072 Acute hematogenous osteomyelitis, left ankle and foot `HCC` `ESR` `COM`

     M86.079 Acute hematogenous osteomyelitis, unspecified ankle and foot `HCC` `ESR` `COM`

M86.08 Acute hematogenous osteomyelitis, other sites `HCC` `ESR` `COM`

M86.09 Acute hematogenous osteomyelitis, multiple sites `HCC` `ESR` `COM`

√5ᵗʰ **M86.1** Other acute osteomyelitis

     M86.10 Other acute osteomyelitis, unspecified site `HCC` `ESR` `COM`

√6ᵗʰ **M86.11** Other acute osteomyelitis, shoulder

     M86.111 Other acute osteomyelitis, right shoulder

     M86.112 Other acute osteomyelitis, left shoulder

     M86.119 Other acute osteomyelitis, unspecified shoulder `HCC` `ESR` `COM`

√6ᵗʰ **M86.12** Other acute osteomyelitis, humerus

     M86.121 Other acute osteomyelitis, right humerus `HCC` `ESR` `COM`

     M86.122 Other acute osteomyelitis, left humerus `HCC` `ESR` `COM`

     M86.129 Other acute osteomyelitis, unspecified humerus `HCC` `ESR` `COM`

√6ᵗʰ **M86.13** Other acute osteomyelitis, radius and ulna

     M86.131 Other acute osteomyelitis, right radius and ulna `HCC` `ESR` `COM`

     M86.132 Other acute osteomyelitis, left radius and ulna `HCC` `ESR` `COM`

     M86.139 Other acute osteomyelitis, unspecified radius and ulna `HCC` `ESR` `COM`

√6ᵗʰ **M86.14** Other acute osteomyelitis, hand

     M86.141 Other acute osteomyelitis, right hand `HCC` `ESR` `COM`

     M86.142 Other acute osteomyelitis, left hand `HCC` `ESR` `COM`

     M86.149 Other acute osteomyelitis, unspecified hand `HCC` `ESR` `COM`

√6ᵗʰ **M86.15** Other acute osteomyelitis, femur

     M86.151 Other acute osteomyelitis, right femur `HCC` `ESR` `COM`

     M86.152 Other acute osteomyelitis, left femur `HCC` `ESR` `COM`

     M86.159 Other acute osteomyelitis, unspecified femur `HCC` `ESR` `COM`

√6ᵗʰ **M86.16** Other acute osteomyelitis, tibia and fibula

     M86.161 Other acute osteomyelitis, right tibia and fibula `HCC` `ESR` `COM`

     M86.162 Other acute osteomyelitis, left tibia and fibula `HCC` `ESR` `COM`

     M86.169 Other acute osteomyelitis, unspecified tibia and fibula `HCC` `ESR` `COM`

√6ᵗʰ **M86.17** Other acute osteomyelitis, ankle and foot

     AHA: 2020,1Q,12

     M86.171 Other acute osteomyelitis, right ankle and foot `HCC` `ESR` `COM`

     M86.172 Other acute osteomyelitis, left ankle and foot `HCC` `ESR` `COM`

     M86.179 Other acute osteomyelitis, unspecified ankle and foot `HCC` `ESR` `COM`

M86.18 Other acute osteomyelitis, other site `HCC` `ESR` `COM`

M86.19 Other acute osteomyelitis, multiple sites `HCC` `ESR` `COM`

√5ᵗʰ **M86.2** Subacute osteomyelitis

     M86.20 Subacute osteomyelitis, unspecified site `HCC` `ESR` `COM`

√6ᵗʰ **M86.21** Subacute osteomyelitis, shoulder

     M86.211 Subacute osteomyelitis, right shoulder `HCC` `ESR` `COM`

     M86.212 Subacute osteomyelitis, left shoulder `HCC` `ESR` `COM`

     M86.219 Subacute osteomyelitis, unspecified shoulder `HCC` `ESR` `COM`

√6ᵗʰ **M86.22** Subacute osteomyelitis, humerus

     M86.221 Subacute osteomyelitis, right humerus `HCC` `ESR` `COM`

     M86.222 Subacute osteomyelitis, left humerus `HCC` `ESR` `COM`

     M86.229 Subacute osteomyelitis, unspecified humerus `HCC` `ESR` `COM`

√6ᵗʰ **M86.23** Subacute osteomyelitis, radius and ulna

     M86.231 Subacute osteomyelitis, right radius and ulna `HCC` `ESR` `COM`

     M86.232 Subacute osteomyelitis, left radius and ulna `HCC` `ESR` `COM`

     M86.239 Subacute osteomyelitis, unspecified radius and ulna `HCC` `ESR` `COM`

√6ᵗʰ **M86.24** Subacute osteomyelitis, hand

     M86.241 Subacute osteomyelitis, right hand `HCC` `ESR` `COM`

     M86.242 Subacute osteomyelitis, left hand `HCC` `ESR` `COM`

     M86.249 Subacute osteomyelitis, unspecified hand `HCC` `ESR` `COM`

√6ᵗʰ **M86.25** Subacute osteomyelitis, femur

     M86.251 Subacute osteomyelitis, right femur `HCC` `ESR` `COM`

     M86.252 Subacute osteomyelitis, left femur `HCC` `ESR` `COM`

     M86.259 Subacute osteomyelitis, unspecified femur `HCC` `ESR` `COM`

√6ᵗʰ **M86.26** Subacute osteomyelitis, tibia and fibula

     M86.261 Subacute osteomyelitis, right tibia and fibula `HCC` `ESR` `COM`

     M86.262 Subacute osteomyelitis, left tibia and fibula `HCC` `ESR` `COM`

     M86.269 Subacute osteomyelitis, unspecified tibia and fibula `HCC` `ESR` `COM`

√6ᵗʰ **M86.27** Subacute osteomyelitis, ankle and foot

     M86.271 Subacute osteomyelitis, right ankle and foot `HCC` `ESR` `COM`

     M86.272 Subacute osteomyelitis, left ankle and foot `HCC` `ESR` `COM`

     M86.279 Subacute osteomyelitis, unspecified ankle and foot `HCC` `ESR` `COM`

M86.28 Subacute osteomyelitis, other site `HCC` `ESR` `COM`

M86.29 Subacute osteomyelitis, multiple sites `HCC` `ESR` `COM`

√5ᵗʰ **M86.3** Chronic multifocal osteomyelitis

     M86.30 Chronic multifocal osteomyelitis, unspecified site `HCC` `ESR` `COM`

√6ᵗʰ **M86.31** Chronic multifocal osteomyelitis, shoulder

     M86.311 Chronic multifocal osteomyelitis, right shoulder `HCC` `ESR` `COM`

     M86.312 Chronic multifocal osteomyelitis, left shoulder `HCC` `ESR` `COM`

     M86.319 Chronic multifocal osteomyelitis, unspecified shoulder `HCC` `ESR` `COM`

√6ᵗʰ **M86.32** Chronic multifocal osteomyelitis, humerus

     M86.321 Chronic multifocal osteomyelitis, right humerus `HCC` `ESR` `COM`

     M86.322 Chronic multifocal osteomyelitis, left humerus `HCC` `ESR` `COM`

M86.329 Chronic multifocal osteomyelitis, unspecified humerus `HCC` `ESR` `COM`

✓6ᵗʰ M86.33 Chronic multifocal osteomyelitis, radius and ulna

M86.331 Chronic multifocal osteomyelitis, right radius and ulna `HCC` `ESR` `COM`

M86.332 Chronic multifocal osteomyelitis, left radius and ulna `HCC` `ESR` `COM`

M86.339 Chronic multifocal osteomyelitis, unspecified radius and ulna `HCC` `ESR` `COM`

✓6ᵗʰ M86.34 Chronic multifocal osteomyelitis, hand

M86.341 Chronic multifocal osteomyelitis, right hand `HCC` `ESR` `COM`

M86.342 Chronic multifocal osteomyelitis, left hand `HCC` `ESR` `COM`

M86.349 Chronic multifocal osteomyelitis, unspecified hand `HCC` `ESR` `COM`

✓6ᵗʰ M86.35 Chronic multifocal osteomyelitis, femur

M86.351 Chronic multifocal osteomyelitis, right femur `HCC` `ESR` `COM`

M86.352 Chronic multifocal osteomyelitis, left femur `HCC` `ESR` `COM`

M86.359 Chronic multifocal osteomyelitis, unspecified femur `HCC` `ESR` `COM`

✓6ᵗʰ M86.36 Chronic multifocal osteomyelitis, tibia and fibula

M86.361 Chronic multifocal osteomyelitis, right tibia and fibula `HCC` `ESR` `COM`

M86.362 Chronic multifocal osteomyelitis, left tibia and fibula `HCC` `ESR` `COM`

M86.369 Chronic multifocal osteomyelitis, unspecified tibia and fibula `HCC` `ESR` `COM`

✓6ᵗʰ M86.37 Chronic multifocal osteomyelitis, ankle and foot

M86.371 Chronic multifocal osteomyelitis, right ankle and foot `HCC` `ESR` `COM`

M86.372 Chronic multifocal osteomyelitis, left ankle and foot `HCC` `ESR` `COM`

M86.379 Chronic multifocal osteomyelitis, unspecified ankle and foot `HCC` `ESR` `COM`

M86.38 Chronic multifocal osteomyelitis, other site `HCC` `ESR` `COM`

M86.39 Chronic multifocal osteomyelitis, multiple sites `HCC` `ESR` `COM`

✓5ᵗʰ M86.4 Chronic osteomyelitis with draining sinus

M86.40 Chronic osteomyelitis with draining sinus, unspecified site `HCC` `ESR` `COM`

✓6ᵗʰ M86.41 Chronic osteomyelitis with draining sinus, shoulder

M86.411 Chronic osteomyelitis with draining sinus, right shoulder `HCC` `ESR` `COM`

M86.412 Chronic osteomyelitis with draining sinus, left shoulder `HCC` `ESR` `COM`

M86.419 Chronic osteomyelitis with draining sinus, unspecified shoulder `HCC` `ESR` `COM`

✓6ᵗʰ M86.42 Chronic osteomyelitis with draining sinus, humerus

M86.421 Chronic osteomyelitis with draining sinus, right humerus `HCC` `ESR` `COM`

M86.422 Chronic osteomyelitis with draining sinus, left humerus `HCC` `ESR` `COM`

M86.429 Chronic osteomyelitis with draining sinus, unspecified humerus `HCC` `ESR` `COM`

✓6ᵗʰ M86.43 Chronic osteomyelitis with draining sinus, radius and ulna

M86.431 Chronic osteomyelitis with draining sinus, right radius and ulna `HCC` `ESR` `COM`

M86.432 Chronic osteomyelitis with draining sinus, left radius and ulna `HCC` `ESR` `COM`

M86.439 Chronic osteomyelitis with draining sinus, unspecified radius and ulna `HCC` `ESR` `COM`

✓6ᵗʰ M86.44 Chronic osteomyelitis with draining sinus, hand

M86.441 Chronic osteomyelitis with draining sinus, right hand `HCC` `ESR` `COM`

M86.442 Chronic osteomyelitis with draining sinus, left hand `HCC` `ESR` `COM`

M86.449 Chronic osteomyelitis with draining sinus, unspecified hand `HCC` `ESR` `COM`

✓6ᵗʰ M86.45 Chronic osteomyelitis with draining sinus, femur

M86.451 Chronic osteomyelitis with draining sinus, right femur `HCC` `ESR` `COM`

M86.452 Chronic osteomyelitis with draining sinus, left femur `HCC` `ESR` `COM`

M86.459 Chronic osteomyelitis with draining sinus, unspecified femur `HCC` `ESR` `COM`

✓6ᵗʰ M86.46 Chronic osteomyelitis with draining sinus, tibia and fibula

M86.461 Chronic osteomyelitis with draining sinus, right tibia and fibula `HCC` `ESR` `COM`

M86.462 Chronic osteomyelitis with draining sinus, left tibia and fibula `HCC` `ESR` `COM`

M86.469 Chronic osteomyelitis with draining sinus, unspecified tibia and fibula `HCC` `ESR` `COM`

✓6ᵗʰ M86.47 Chronic osteomyelitis with draining sinus, ankle and foot

M86.471 Chronic osteomyelitis with draining sinus, right ankle and foot `HCC` `ESR` `COM`

M86.472 Chronic osteomyelitis with draining sinus, left ankle and foot `HCC` `ESR` `COM`

M86.479 Chronic osteomyelitis with draining sinus, unspecified ankle and foot `HCC` `ESR` `COM`

M86.48 Chronic osteomyelitis with draining sinus, other site `HCC` `ESR` `COM`

M86.49 Chronic osteomyelitis with draining sinus, multiple sites `HCC` `ESR` `COM`

✓5ᵗʰ M86.5 Other chronic hematogenous osteomyelitis

M86.50 Other chronic hematogenous osteomyelitis, unspecified site `HCC` `ESR` `COM`

✓6ᵗʰ M86.51 Other chronic hematogenous osteomyelitis, shoulder

M86.511 Other chronic hematogenous osteomyelitis, right shoulder `HCC` `ESR` `COM`

M86.512 Other chronic hematogenous osteomyelitis, left shoulder `HCC` `ESR` `COM`

M86.519 Other chronic hematogenous osteomyelitis, unspecified shoulder `HCC` `ESR` `COM`

✓6ᵗʰ M86.52 Other chronic hematogenous osteomyelitis, humerus

M86.521 Other chronic hematogenous osteomyelitis, right humerus `HCC` `ESR` `COM`

M86.522 Other chronic hematogenous osteomyelitis, left humerus `HCC` `ESR` `COM`

M86.529 Other chronic hematogenous osteomyelitis, unspecified humerus `HCC` `ESR` `COM`

✓6ᵗʰ M86.53 Other chronic hematogenous osteomyelitis, radius and ulna

M86.531 Other chronic hematogenous osteomyelitis, right radius and ulna `HCC` `ESR` `COM`

M86.532 Other chronic hematogenous osteomyelitis, left radius and ulna `HCC` `ESR` `COM`

M86.539 Other chronic hematogenous osteomyelitis, unspecified radius and ulna `HCC` `ESR` `COM`

✓6ᵗʰ M86.54 Other chronic hematogenous osteomyelitis, hand

M86.541 Other chronic hematogenous osteomyelitis, right hand `HCC` `ESR` `COM`

M86.542 Other chronic hematogenous osteomyelitis, left hand `HCC` `ESR` `COM`

M86.549 Other chronic hematogenous osteomyelitis, unspecified hand `HCC` `ESR` `COM`

✓6ᵗʰ M86.55 Other chronic hematogenous osteomyelitis, femur

M86.551 Other chronic hematogenous osteomyelitis, right femur `HCC` `ESR` `COM`

M86.552 Other chronic hematogenous osteomyelitis, left femur `HCC` `ESR` `COM`

M86.559 Other chronic hematogenous osteomyelitis, unspecified femur `HCC` `ESR` `COM`

✓6ᵗʰ **M86.56** Other chronic hematogenous osteomyelitis, tibia and fibula

    M86.561 Other chronic hematogenous osteomyelitis, right tibia and fibula `HCC` `ESR` `COM`

    M86.562 Other chronic hematogenous osteomyelitis, left tibia and fibula `HCC` `ESR` `COM`

    M86.569 Other chronic hematogenous osteomyelitis, unspecified tibia and fibula `HCC` `ESR` `COM`

✓6ᵗʰ **M86.57** Other chronic hematogenous osteomyelitis, ankle and foot

    M86.571 Other chronic hematogenous osteomyelitis, right ankle and foot `HCC` `ESR` `COM`

    M86.572 Other chronic hematogenous osteomyelitis, left ankle and foot `HCC` `ESR` `COM`

    M86.579 Other chronic hematogenous osteomyelitis, unspecified ankle and foot `HCC` `ESR` `COM`

  M86.58 Other chronic hematogenous osteomyelitis, other site `HCC` `ESR` `COM`

  M86.59 Other chronic hematogenous osteomyelitis, multiple sites `HCC` `ESR` `COM`

✓5ᵗʰ **M86.6** Other chronic osteomyelitis

  M86.60 Other chronic osteomyelitis, unspecified site `HCC` `ESR` `COM`

✓6ᵗʰ **M86.61** Other chronic osteomyelitis, shoulder

    M86.611 Other chronic osteomyelitis, right shoulder `HCC` `ESR` `COM`

    M86.612 Other chronic osteomyelitis, left shoulder `HCC` `ESR` `COM`

    M86.619 Other chronic osteomyelitis, unspecified shoulder `HCC` `ESR` `COM`

✓6ᵗʰ **M86.62** Other chronic osteomyelitis, humerus

    M86.621 Other chronic osteomyelitis, right humerus `HCC` `ESR` `COM`

    M86.622 Other chronic osteomyelitis, left humerus `HCC` `ESR` `COM`

    M86.629 Other chronic osteomyelitis, unspecified humerus `HCC` `ESR` `COM`

✓6ᵗʰ **M86.63** Other chronic osteomyelitis, radius and ulna

    M86.631 Other chronic osteomyelitis, right radius and ulna `HCC` `ESR` `COM`

    M86.632 Other chronic osteomyelitis, left radius and ulna `HCC` `ESR` `COM`

    M86.639 Other chronic osteomyelitis, unspecified radius and ulna `HCC` `ESR` `COM`

✓6ᵗʰ **M86.64** Other chronic osteomyelitis, hand

    M86.641 Other chronic osteomyelitis, right hand `HCC` `ESR` `COM`

    M86.642 Other chronic osteomyelitis, left hand `HCC` `ESR` `COM`

    M86.649 Other chronic osteomyelitis, unspecified hand `HCC` `ESR` `COM`

✓6ᵗʰ **M86.65** Other chronic osteomyelitis, thigh

    M86.651 Other chronic osteomyelitis, right thigh `HCC` `ESR` `COM`

    M86.652 Other chronic osteomyelitis, left thigh `HCC` `ESR` `COM`

    M86.659 Other chronic osteomyelitis, unspecified thigh `HCC` `ESR` `COM`

✓6ᵗʰ **M86.66** Other chronic osteomyelitis, tibia and fibula

    M86.661 Other chronic osteomyelitis, right tibia and fibula `HCC` `ESR` `COM`

    M86.662 Other chronic osteomyelitis, left tibia and fibula `HCC` `ESR` `COM`

    M86.669 Other chronic osteomyelitis, unspecified tibia and fibula `HCC` `ESR` `COM`

✓6ᵗʰ **M86.67** Other chronic osteomyelitis, ankle and foot

    M86.671 Other chronic osteomyelitis, right ankle and foot `HCC` `ESR` `COM`

      AHA: 2016,1Q,13

    M86.672 Other chronic osteomyelitis, left ankle and foot `HCC` `ESR` `COM`

    M86.679 Other chronic osteomyelitis, unspecified ankle and foot `HCC` `ESR` `COM`

  M86.68 Other chronic osteomyelitis, other site `HCC` `ESR` `COM`

  M86.69 Other chronic osteomyelitis, multiple sites `HCC` `ESR` `COM`

✓5ᵗʰ **M86.8** Other osteomyelitis

  Brodie's abscess

  AHA: 2022,1Q,31

✓6ᵗʰ **M86.8X** Other osteomyelitis

    M86.8X0 Other osteomyelitis, multiple sites `HCC` `ESR` `COM`

    M86.8X1 Other osteomyelitis, shoulder `HCC` `ESR` `COM`

    M86.8X2 Other osteomyelitis, upper arm `HCC` `ESR` `COM`

    M86.8X3 Other osteomyelitis, forearm `HCC` `ESR` `COM`

    M86.8X4 Other osteomyelitis, hand `HCC` `ESR` `COM`

    M86.8X5 Other osteomyelitis, thigh `HCC` `ESR` `COM`

    M86.8X6 Other osteomyelitis, lower leg `HCC` `ESR` `COM`

    M86.8X7 Other osteomyelitis, ankle and foot `HCC` `ESR` `COM`

    M86.8X8 Other osteomyelitis, other site `HCC` `ESR` `COM`

    M86.8X9 Other osteomyelitis, unspecified sites `HCC` `ESR` `COM`

  M86.9 Osteomyelitis, unspecified `HCC` `ESR` `COM`

    Infection of bone NOS

    Periostitis without osteomyelitis

✓4ᵗʰ **M87** Osteonecrosis

  `INCLUDES` avascular necrosis of bone

  Use additional code to identify major osseous defect, if applicable (M89.7-)

  `EXCLUDES 1` juvenile osteonecrosis (M91-M92)

    osteochondropathies (M90-M93)

✓5ᵗʰ **M87.0** Idiopathic aseptic necrosis of bone

  M87.00 Idiopathic aseptic necrosis of unspecified bone `HCC` `Rx` `ESR` `COM`

✓6ᵗʰ **M87.01** Idiopathic aseptic necrosis of shoulder

    Idiopathic aseptic necrosis of clavicle and scapula

    M87.011 Idiopathic aseptic necrosis of right shoulder `HCC` `Rx` `ESR` `COM`

    M87.012 Idiopathic aseptic necrosis of left shoulder `HCC` `Rx` `ESR` `COM`

    M87.019 Idiopathic aseptic necrosis of unspecified shoulder `HCC` `Rx` `ESR` `COM`

✓6ᵗʰ **M87.02** Idiopathic aseptic necrosis of humerus

    M87.021 Idiopathic aseptic necrosis of right humerus `HCC` `Rx` `ESR` `COM`

    M87.022 Idiopathic aseptic necrosis of left humerus `HCC` `Rx` `ESR` `COM`

    M87.029 Idiopathic aseptic necrosis of unspecified humerus `HCC` `Rx` `ESR` `COM`

✓6ᵗʰ **M87.03** Idiopathic aseptic necrosis of radius, ulna and carpus

    M87.031 Idiopathic aseptic necrosis of right radius `HCC` `Rx` `ESR` `COM`

    M87.032 Idiopathic aseptic necrosis of left radius `HCC` `Rx` `ESR` `COM`

    M87.033 Idiopathic aseptic necrosis of unspecified radius `HCC` `Rx` `ESR` `COM`

    M87.034 Idiopathic aseptic necrosis of right ulna `HCC` `Rx` `ESR` `COM`

    M87.035 Idiopathic aseptic necrosis of left ulna `HCC` `Rx` `ESR` `COM`

    M87.036 Idiopathic aseptic necrosis of unspecified ulna `HCC` `Rx` `ESR` `COM`

    M87.037 Idiopathic aseptic necrosis of right carpus `HCC` `Rx` `ESR` `COM`

    M87.038 Idiopathic aseptic necrosis of left carpus `HCC` `Rx` `ESR` `COM`

    M87.039 Idiopathic aseptic necrosis of unspecified carpus `HCC` `Rx` `ESR` `COM`

☑ Additional Character Required   ✓x7ᵗʰ Placeholder Alert   Manifestation   Unspecified Dx   ⓠ QPP   `UPD` Unacceptable PDx

Chapter 13. Diseases of the Musculoskeletal System and Connective Tissue

M87.04–M87.179

√6ᵗʰ **M87.04 Idiopathic aseptic necrosis of** hand and fingers
Idiopathic aseptic necrosis of metacarpals and phalanges of hands

M87.041 Idiopathic aseptic necrosis of right hand `HCC` `Rx` `ESR` `COM`

M87.042 Idiopathic aseptic necrosis of left hand `HCC` `Rx` `ESR` `COM`

M87.043 Idiopathic aseptic necrosis of unspecified hand `HCC` `Rx` `ESR` `COM`

M87.044 Idiopathic aseptic necrosis of right finger(s) `HCC` `Rx` `ESR` `COM`

M87.045 Idiopathic aseptic necrosis of left finger(s) `HCC` `Rx` `ESR` `COM`

M87.046 Idiopathic aseptic necrosis of unspecified finger(s) `HCC` `Rx` `ESR` `COM`

√6ᵗʰ **M87.05 Idiopathic aseptic necrosis of** pelvis and femur

M87.050 Idiopathic aseptic necrosis of pelvis `HCC` `Rx` `ESR` `COM`

M87.051 Idiopathic aseptic necrosis of right femur `HCC` `Rx` `ESR` `COM`

M87.052 Idiopathic aseptic necrosis of left femur `HCC` `Rx` `ESR` `COM`

M87.059 Idiopathic aseptic necrosis of unspecified femur `HCC` `Rx` `ESR` `COM`

√6ᵗʰ **M87.06 Idiopathic aseptic necrosis of** tibia and fibula

M87.061 Idiopathic aseptic necrosis of right tibia `HCC` `Rx` `ESR` `COM`

M87.062 Idiopathic aseptic necrosis of left tibia `HCC` `Rx` `ESR` `COM`

M87.063 Idiopathic aseptic necrosis of unspecified tibia `HCC` `Rx` `ESR` `COM`

M87.064 Idiopathic aseptic necrosis of right fibula `HCC` `Rx` `ESR` `COM`

M87.065 Idiopathic aseptic necrosis of left fibula `HCC` `Rx` `ESR` `COM`

M87.066 Idiopathic aseptic necrosis of unspecified fibula `HCC` `Rx` `ESR` `COM`

√6ᵗʰ **M87.07 Idiopathic aseptic necrosis of** ankle, foot and toes
Idiopathic aseptic necrosis of metatarsus, tarsus, and phalanges of toes

M87.071 Idiopathic aseptic necrosis of right ankle `HCC` `Rx` `ESR` `COM`

M87.072 Idiopathic aseptic necrosis of left ankle `HCC` `Rx` `ESR` `COM`

M87.073 Idiopathic aseptic necrosis of unspecified ankle `HCC` `Rx` `ESR` `COM`

M87.074 Idiopathic aseptic necrosis of right foot `HCC` `Rx` `ESR` `COM`

M87.075 Idiopathic aseptic necrosis of left foot `HCC` `Rx` `ESR` `COM`

M87.076 Idiopathic aseptic necrosis of unspecified foot `HCC` `Rx` `ESR` `COM`

M87.077 Idiopathic aseptic necrosis of right toe(s) `HCC` `Rx` `ESR` `COM`

M87.078 Idiopathic aseptic necrosis of left toe(s) `HCC` `Rx` `ESR` `COM`

M87.079 Idiopathic aseptic necrosis of unspecified toe(s) `HCC` `Rx` `ESR` `COM`

M87.08 Idiopathic aseptic necrosis of bone, other site

M87.09 Idiopathic aseptic necrosis of bone, multiple sites `HCC` `Rx` `ESR` `COM`

√5ᵗʰ **M87.1 Osteonecrosis** due to drugs
Use additional code for adverse effect, if applicable, to identify drug (T36-T50 with fifth or sixth character 5)

M87.10 Osteonecrosis due to drugs, unspecified bone `HCC` `Rx` `ESR` `COM`

√6ᵗʰ **M87.11 Osteonecrosis due to drugs,** shoulder

M87.111 Osteonecrosis due to drugs, right shoulder `HCC` `Rx` `ESR` `COM`

M87.112 Osteonecrosis due to drugs, left shoulder `HCC` `Rx` `ESR` `COM`

M87.119 Osteonecrosis due to drugs, unspecified shoulder `HCC` `Rx` `ESR` `COM`

√6ᵗʰ **M87.12 Osteonecrosis due to drugs,** humerus

M87.121 Osteonecrosis due to drugs, right humerus `HCC` `Rx` `ESR` `COM`

M87.122 Osteonecrosis due to drugs, left humerus `HCC` `Rx` `ESR` `COM`

M87.129 Osteonecrosis due to drugs, unspecified humerus `HCC` `Rx` `ESR` `COM`

√6ᵗʰ **M87.13 Osteonecrosis due to drugs of** radius, ulna and carpus

M87.131 Osteonecrosis due to drugs of right radius `HCC` `Rx` `ESR` `COM`

M87.132 Osteonecrosis due to drugs of left radius `HCC` `Rx` `ESR` `COM`

M87.133 Osteonecrosis due to drugs of unspecified radius `HCC` `Rx` `ESR` `COM`

M87.134 Osteonecrosis due to drugs of right ulna `HCC` `Rx` `ESR` `COM`

M87.135 Osteonecrosis due to drugs of left ulna `HCC` `Rx` `ESR` `COM`

M87.136 Osteonecrosis due to drugs of unspecified ulna `HCC` `Rx` `ESR` `COM`

M87.137 Osteonecrosis due to drugs of right carpus `HCC` `Rx` `ESR` `COM`

M87.138 Osteonecrosis due to drugs of left carpus `HCC` `Rx` `ESR` `COM`

M87.139 Osteonecrosis due to drugs of unspecified carpus `HCC` `Rx` `ESR` `COM`

√6ᵗʰ **M87.14 Osteonecrosis due to drugs,** hand and fingers

M87.141 Osteonecrosis due to drugs, right hand `HCC` `Rx` `ESR` `COM`

M87.142 Osteonecrosis due to drugs, left hand `HCC` `Rx` `ESR` `COM`

M87.143 Osteonecrosis due to drugs, unspecified hand `HCC` `Rx` `ESR` `COM`

M87.144 Osteonecrosis due to drugs, right finger(s) `HCC` `Rx` `ESR` `COM`

M87.145 Osteonecrosis due to drugs, left finger(s) `HCC` `Rx` `ESR` `COM`

M87.146 Osteonecrosis due to drugs, unspecified finger(s) `HCC` `Rx` `ESR` `COM`

√6ᵗʰ **M87.15 Osteonecrosis due to drugs,** pelvis and femur

M87.150 Osteonecrosis due to drugs, pelvis `HCC` `Rx` `ESR` `COM`

M87.151 Osteonecrosis due to drugs, right femur `HCC` `Rx` `ESR` `COM`

M87.152 Osteonecrosis due to drugs, left femur `HCC` `Rx` `ESR` `COM`

M87.159 Osteonecrosis due to drugs, unspecified femur `HCC` `Rx` `ESR` `COM`

√6ᵗʰ **M87.16 Osteonecrosis due to drugs,** tibia and fibula

M87.161 Osteonecrosis due to drugs, right tibia `HCC` `Rx` `ESR` `COM`

M87.162 Osteonecrosis due to drugs, left tibia `HCC` `Rx` `ESR` `COM`

M87.163 Osteonecrosis due to drugs, unspecified tibia `HCC` `Rx` `ESR` `COM`

M87.164 Osteonecrosis due to drugs, right fibula `HCC` `Rx` `ESR` `COM`

M87.165 Osteonecrosis due to drugs, left fibula `HCC` `Rx` `ESR` `COM`

M87.166 Osteonecrosis due to drugs, unspecified fibula `HCC` `Rx` `ESR` `COM`

√6ᵗʰ **M87.17 Osteonecrosis due to drugs,** ankle, foot and toes

M87.171 Osteonecrosis due to drugs, right ankle `HCC` `Rx` `ESR` `COM`

M87.172 Osteonecrosis due to drugs, left ankle `HCC` `Rx` `ESR` `COM`

M87.173 Osteonecrosis due to drugs, unspecified ankle `HCC` `Rx` `ESR` `COM`

M87.174 Osteonecrosis due to drugs, right foot `HCC` `Rx` `ESR` `COM`

M87.175 Osteonecrosis due to drugs, left foot `HCC` `Rx` `ESR` `COM`

M87.176 Osteonecrosis due to drugs, unspecified foot `HCC` `Rx` `ESR` `COM`

M87.177 Osteonecrosis due to drugs, right toe(s) `HCC` `Rx` `ESR` `COM`

M87.178 Osteonecrosis due to drugs, left toe(s) `HCC` `Rx` `ESR` `COM`

M87.179 Osteonecrosis due to drugs, unspecified toe(s) `HCC` `Rx` `ESR` `COM`

`HCC` CMS-HCC   `Rx` Rx HCC   `ESR` ESRD HCC   `COM` Commercial HCC   N Newborn: 0   P Pediatric: 0-17   M Maternity: 9-64   A Adult: 15-124

850   ICD-10-CM 2023

✓6ᵗʰ **M87.18** Osteonecrosis due to drugs, other site

    M87.180 Osteonecrosis due to drugs, jaw `HCC` `Rx` `ESR` `COM`

    M87.188 Osteonecrosis due to drugs, other site `HCC` `Rx` `ESR` `COM`

  M87.19 Osteonecrosis due to drugs, multiple sites `HCC` `Rx` `ESR` `COM`

✓5ᵗʰ **M87.2** Osteonecrosis due to previous trauma

  M87.20 Osteonecrosis due to previous trauma, unspecified bone `HCC` `Rx` `ESR` `COM`

✓6ᵗʰ **M87.21** Osteonecrosis due to previous trauma, shoulder

    M87.211 Osteonecrosis due to previous trauma, right shoulder `HCC` `Rx` `ESR` `COM`

    M87.212 Osteonecrosis due to previous trauma, left shoulder `HCC` `Rx` `ESR` `COM`

    M87.219 Osteonecrosis due to previous trauma, unspecified shoulder `HCC` `Rx` `ESR` `COM`

✓6ᵗʰ **M87.22** Osteonecrosis due to previous trauma, humerus

    M87.221 Osteonecrosis due to previous trauma, right humerus `HCC` `Rx` `ESR` `COM`

    M87.222 Osteonecrosis due to previous trauma, left humerus `HCC` `Rx` `ESR` `COM`

    M87.229 Osteonecrosis due to previous trauma, unspecified humerus `HCC` `Rx` `ESR` `COM`

✓6ᵗʰ **M87.23** Osteonecrosis due to previous trauma of radius, ulna and carpus

    M87.231 Osteonecrosis due to previous trauma of right radius `HCC` `Rx` `ESR` `COM`

    M87.232 Osteonecrosis due to previous trauma of left radius `HCC` `Rx` `ESR` `COM`

    M87.233 Osteonecrosis due to previous trauma of unspecified radius `HCC` `Rx` `ESR` `COM`

    M87.234 Osteonecrosis due to previous trauma of right ulna `HCC` `Rx` `ESR` `COM`

    M87.235 Osteonecrosis due to previous trauma of left ulna `HCC` `Rx` `ESR` `COM`

    M87.236 Osteonecrosis due to previous trauma of unspecified ulna `HCC` `Rx` `ESR` `COM`

    M87.237 Osteonecrosis due to previous trauma of right carpus `HCC` `Rx` `ESR` `COM`

    M87.238 Osteonecrosis due to previous trauma of left carpus `HCC` `Rx` `ESR` `COM`

    M87.239 Osteonecrosis due to previous trauma of unspecified carpus `HCC` `Rx` `ESR` `COM`

✓6ᵗʰ **M87.24** Osteonecrosis due to previous trauma, hand and fingers

    M87.241 Osteonecrosis due to previous trauma, right hand `HCC` `Rx` `ESR` `COM`

    M87.242 Osteonecrosis due to previous trauma, left hand `HCC` `Rx` `ESR` `COM`

    M87.243 Osteonecrosis due to previous trauma, unspecified hand `HCC` `Rx` `ESR` `COM`

    M87.244 Osteonecrosis due to previous trauma, right finger(s) `HCC` `Rx` `ESR` `COM`

    M87.245 Osteonecrosis due to previous trauma, left finger(s) `HCC` `Rx` `ESR` `COM`

    M87.246 Osteonecrosis due to previous trauma, unspecified finger(s) `HCC` `Rx` `ESR` `COM`

✓6ᵗʰ **M87.25** Osteonecrosis due to previous trauma, pelvis and femur

    M87.250 Osteonecrosis due to previous trauma, pelvis `HCC` `Rx` `ESR` `COM`

    M87.251 Osteonecrosis due to previous trauma, right femur `HCC` `Rx` `ESR` `COM`

    M87.252 Osteonecrosis due to previous trauma, left femur `HCC` `Rx` `ESR` `COM`

    M87.256 Osteonecrosis due to previous trauma, unspecified femur `HCC` `Rx` `ESR` `COM`

✓6ᵗʰ **M87.26** Osteonecrosis due to previous trauma, tibia and fibula

    M87.261 Osteonecrosis due to previous trauma, right tibia `HCC` `Rx` `ESR` `COM`

    M87.262 Osteonecrosis due to previous trauma, left tibia `HCC` `Rx` `ESR` `COM`

    M87.263 Osteonecrosis due to previous trauma, unspecified tibia `HCC` `Rx` `ESR` `COM`

    M87.264 Osteonecrosis due to previous trauma, right fibula `HCC` `Rx` `ESR` `COM`

    M87.265 Osteonecrosis due to previous trauma, left fibula `HCC` `Rx` `ESR` `COM`

    M87.266 Osteonecrosis due to previous trauma, unspecified fibula `HCC` `Rx` `ESR` `COM`

✓6ᵗʰ **M87.27** Osteonecrosis due to previous trauma, ankle, foot and toes

    M87.271 Osteonecrosis due to previous trauma, right ankle `HCC` `Rx` `ESR` `COM`

    M87.272 Osteonecrosis due to previous trauma, left ankle `HCC` `Rx` `ESR` `COM`

    M87.273 Osteonecrosis due to previous trauma, unspecified ankle `HCC` `Rx` `ESR` `COM`

    M87.274 Osteonecrosis due to previous trauma, right foot `HCC` `Rx` `ESR` `COM`

    M87.275 Osteonecrosis due to previous trauma, left foot `HCC` `Rx` `ESR` `COM`

    M87.276 Osteonecrosis due to previous trauma, unspecified foot `HCC` `Rx` `ESR` `COM`

    M87.277 Osteonecrosis due to previous trauma, right toe(s) `HCC` `Rx` `ESR` `COM`

    M87.278 Osteonecrosis due to previous trauma, left toe(s) `HCC` `Rx` `ESR` `COM`

    M87.279 Osteonecrosis due to previous trauma, unspecified toe(s) `HCC` `Rx` `ESR` `COM`

  M87.28 Osteonecrosis due to previous trauma, other site `HCC` `Rx` `ESR` `COM`

  M87.29 Osteonecrosis due to previous trauma, multiple sites `HCC` `Rx` `ESR` `COM`

✓5ᵗʰ **M87.3** Other secondary osteonecrosis

  M87.30 Other secondary osteonecrosis, unspecified bone `HCC` `Rx` `ESR` `COM`

✓6ᵗʰ **M87.31** Other secondary osteonecrosis, shoulder

    M87.311 Other secondary osteonecrosis, right shoulder `HCC` `Rx` `ESR` `COM`

    M87.312 Other secondary osteonecrosis, left shoulder `HCC` `Rx` `ESR` `COM`

    M87.319 Other secondary osteonecrosis, unspecified shoulder `HCC` `Rx` `ESR` `COM`

✓6ᵗʰ **M87.32** Other secondary osteonecrosis, humerus

    M87.321 Other secondary osteonecrosis, right humerus `HCC` `Rx` `ESR` `COM`

    M87.322 Other secondary osteonecrosis, left humerus `HCC` `Rx` `ESR` `COM`

    M87.329 Other secondary osteonecrosis, unspecified humerus `HCC` `Rx` `ESR` `COM`

✓6ᵗʰ **M87.33** Other secondary osteonecrosis of radius, ulna and carpus

    M87.331 Other secondary osteonecrosis of right radius `HCC` `Rx` `ESR` `COM`

    M87.332 Other secondary osteonecrosis of left radius `HCC` `Rx` `ESR` `COM`

    M87.333 Other secondary osteonecrosis of unspecified radius `HCC` `Rx` `ESR` `COM`

    M87.334 Other secondary osteonecrosis of right ulna `HCC` `Rx` `ESR` `COM`

    M87.335 Other secondary osteonecrosis of left ulna `HCC` `Rx` `ESR` `COM`

    M87.336 Other secondary osteonecrosis of unspecified ulna `HCC` `Rx` `ESR` `COM`

    M87.337 Other secondary osteonecrosis of right carpus `HCC` `Rx` `ESR` `COM`

    M87.338 Other secondary osteonecrosis of left carpus `HCC` `Rx` `ESR` `COM`

    M87.339 Other secondary osteonecrosis of unspecified carpus `HCC` `Rx` `ESR` `COM`

✓6ᵗʰ **M87.34** Other secondary osteonecrosis, hand and fingers

    M87.341 Other secondary osteonecrosis, right hand `HCC` `Rx` `ESR` `COM`

    M87.342 Other secondary osteonecrosis, left hand `HCC` `Rx` `ESR` `COM`

    M87.343 Other secondary osteonecrosis, unspecified hand `HCC` `Rx` `ESR` `COM`

    M87.344 Other secondary osteonecrosis, right finger(s) `HCC` `Rx` `ESR` `COM`

    M87.345 Other secondary osteonecrosis, left finger(s) `HCC` `Rx` `ESR` `COM`

    M87.346 Other secondary osteonecrosis, unspecified finger(s) `HCC` `Rx` `ESR` `COM`

☑ Additional Character Required   ✓x7ᵗʰ Placeholder Alert   Manifestation   Unspecified Dx   🄌 QPP   `UPD` Unacceptable PDx

✓6ᵗʰ **M87.35** Other secondary osteonecrosis, **pelvis and femur**
- **M87.350** Other secondary osteonecrosis, **pelvis** `HCC` `Rx` `ESR` `COM`
- **M87.351** Other secondary osteonecrosis, **right femur** `HCC` `Rx` `ESR` `COM`
- **M87.352** Other secondary osteonecrosis, **left femur** `HCC` `Rx` `ESR` `COM`
- **M87.353** Other secondary osteonecrosis, **unspecified femur** `HCC` `Rx` `ESR` `COM`

✓6ᵗʰ **M87.36** Other secondary osteonecrosis, **tibia and fibula**
- **M87.361** Other secondary osteonecrosis, **right tibia** `HCC` `Rx` `ESR` `COM`
- **M87.362** Other secondary osteonecrosis, **left tibia** `HCC` `Rx` `ESR` `COM`
- **M87.363** Other secondary osteonecrosis, **unspecified tibia** `HCC` `Rx` `ESR` `COM`
- **M87.364** Other secondary osteonecrosis, **right fibula** `HCC` `Rx` `ESR` `COM`
- **M87.365** Other secondary osteonecrosis, **left fibula** `HCC` `Rx` `ESR` `COM`
- **M87.366** Other secondary osteonecrosis, **unspecified fibula** `HCC` `Rx` `ESR` `COM`

✓6ᵗʰ **M87.37** Other secondary osteonecrosis, **ankle and foot**
- **M87.371** Other secondary osteonecrosis, **right ankle** `HCC` `Rx` `ESR` `COM`
- **M87.372** Other secondary osteonecrosis, **left ankle** `HCC` `Rx` `ESR` `COM`
- **M87.373** Other secondary osteonecrosis, **unspecified ankle** `HCC` `Rx` `ESR` `COM`
- **M87.374** Other secondary osteonecrosis, **right foot** `HCC` `Rx` `ESR` `COM`
- **M87.375** Other secondary osteonecrosis, **left foot** `HCC` `Rx` `ESR` `COM`
- **M87.376** Other secondary osteonecrosis, **unspecified foot** `HCC` `Rx` `ESR` `COM`
- **M87.377** Other secondary osteonecrosis, **right toe(s)** `HCC` `Rx` `ESR` `COM`
- **M87.378** Other secondary osteonecrosis, **left toe(s)** `HCC` `Rx` `ESR` `COM`
- **M87.379** Other secondary osteonecrosis, **unspecified toe(s)** `HCC` `Rx` `ESR` `COM`

M87.38 Other secondary osteonecrosis, other site `HCC` `Rx` `ESR` `COM`

M87.39 Other secondary osteonecrosis, **multiple sites** `HCC` `Rx` `ESR` `COM`

✓5ᵗʰ **M87.8** Other osteonecrosis
- **M87.80** Other osteonecrosis, unspecified bone `HCC` `Rx` `ESR` `COM`

✓6ᵗʰ **M87.81** Other osteonecrosis, **shoulder**
- **M87.811** Other osteonecrosis, **right shoulder** `HCC` `Rx` `ESR` `COM`
- **M87.812** Other osteonecrosis, **left shoulder** `HCC` `Rx` `ESR` `COM`
- **M87.819** Other osteonecrosis, unspecified shoulder `HCC` `Rx` `ESR` `COM`

✓6ᵗʰ **M87.82** Other osteonecrosis, **humerus**
- **M87.821** Other osteonecrosis, **right humerus** `HCC` `Rx` `ESR` `COM`
- **M87.822** Other osteonecrosis, **left humerus** `HCC` `Rx` `ESR` `COM`
- **M87.829** Other osteonecrosis, unspecified humerus `HCC` `Rx` `ESR` `COM`

✓6ᵗʰ **M87.83** Other osteonecrosis of **radius, ulna and carpus**
- **M87.831** Other osteonecrosis of **right radius** `HCC` `Rx` `ESR` `COM`
- **M87.832** Other osteonecrosis of **left radius** `HCC` `Rx` `ESR` `COM`
- **M87.833** Other osteonecrosis of unspecified radius `HCC` `Rx` `ESR` `COM`
- **M87.834** Other osteonecrosis of **right ulna** `HCC` `Rx` `ESR` `COM`
- **M87.835** Other osteonecrosis of **left ulna** `HCC` `Rx` `ESR` `COM`
- **M87.836** Other osteonecrosis of unspecified ulna `HCC` `Rx` `ESR` `COM`
- **M87.837** Other osteonecrosis of **right carpus** `HCC` `Rx` `ESR` `COM`
- **M87.838** Other osteonecrosis of **left carpus** `HCC` `Rx` `ESR` `COM`
- **M87.839** Other osteonecrosis of unspecified carpus `HCC` `Rx` `ESR` `COM`

✓6ᵗʰ **M87.84** Other osteonecrosis, **hand and fingers**
- **M87.841** Other osteonecrosis, **right hand** `HCC` `Rx` `ESR` `COM`
- **M87.842** Other osteonecrosis, **left hand** `HCC` `Rx` `ESR` `COM`
- **M87.843** Other osteonecrosis, unspecified hand `HCC` `Rx` `ESR` `COM`
- **M87.844** Other osteonecrosis, **right finger(s)** `HCC` `Rx` `ESR` `COM`
- **M87.845** Other osteonecrosis, **left finger(s)** `HCC` `Rx` `ESR` `COM`
- **M87.849** Other osteonecrosis, unspecified finger(s) `HCC` `Rx` `ESR` `COM`

✓6ᵗʰ **M87.85** Other osteonecrosis, **pelvis and femur**
- **M87.850** Other osteonecrosis, **pelvis** `HCC` `Rx` `ESR` `COM`
- **M87.851** Other osteonecrosis, **right femur** `HCC` `Rx` `ESR` `COM`
- **M87.852** Other osteonecrosis, **left femur** `HCC` `Rx` `ESR` `COM`
- **M87.859** Other osteonecrosis, unspecified femur `HCC` `Rx` `ESR` `COM`

✓6ᵗʰ **M87.86** Other osteonecrosis, **tibia and fibula**
- **M87.861** Other osteonecrosis, **right tibia** `HCC` `Rx` `ESR` `COM`
- **M87.862** Other osteonecrosis, **left tibia** `HCC` `Rx` `ESR` `COM`
- **M87.863** Other osteonecrosis, unspecified tibia `HCC` `Rx` `ESR` `COM`
- **M87.864** Other osteonecrosis, **right fibula** `HCC` `Rx` `ESR` `COM`
- **M87.865** Other osteonecrosis, **left fibula** `HCC` `Rx` `ESR` `COM`
- **M87.869** Other osteonecrosis, unspecified fibula `HCC` `Rx` `ESR` `COM`

✓6ᵗʰ **M87.87** Other osteonecrosis, **ankle, foot and toes**
- **M87.871** Other osteonecrosis, **right ankle** `HCC` `Rx` `ESR` `COM`
- **M87.872** Other osteonecrosis, **left ankle** `HCC` `Rx` `ESR` `COM`
- **M87.873** Other osteonecrosis, unspecified ankle `HCC` `Rx` `ESR` `COM`
- **M87.874** Other osteonecrosis, **right foot** `HCC` `Rx` `ESR` `COM`
- **M87.875** Other osteonecrosis, **left foot** `HCC` `Rx` `ESR` `COM`
- **M87.876** Other osteonecrosis, unspecified foot `HCC` `Rx` `ESR` `COM`
- **M87.877** Other osteonecrosis, **right toe(s)** `HCC` `Rx` `ESR` `COM`
- **M87.878** Other osteonecrosis, **left toe(s)** `HCC` `Rx` `ESR` `COM`
- **M87.879** Other osteonecrosis, unspecified toe(s) `HCC` `Rx` `ESR` `COM`

M87.88 Other osteonecrosis, other site `HCC` `Rx` `ESR` `COM`

M87.89 Other osteonecrosis, **multiple sites** `HCC` `Rx` `ESR` `COM`

M87.9 Osteonecrosis, unspecified `HCC` `Rx` `ESR` `COM`
Necrosis of bone NOS

✓4ᵗʰ **M88** Osteitis deformans [Paget's disease of bone]
EXCLUDES 1   osteitis deformans in neoplastic disease (M90.6)

DEF: Bone disease characterized by numerous cycles of bone resorption by the body. Resorption is followed by accelerated repair attempts, causing bone deformities and bowing, with associated fractures and pain.

M88.0 Osteitis deformans of **skull**

M88.1 Osteitis deformans of **vertebrae**

✓5ᵗʰ **M88.8** Osteitis deformans of other bones
✓6ᵗʰ **M88.81** Osteitis deformans of **shoulder**
- **M88.811** Osteitis deformans of **right shoulder**
- **M88.812** Osteitis deformans of **left shoulder**
- **M88.819** Osteitis deformans of unspecified shoulder

`HCC` CMS-HCC   `Rx` Rx HCC   `ESR` ESRD HCC   `COM` Commercial HCC   `N` Newborn: 0   `P` Pediatric: 0-17   `M` Maternity: 9-64   `A` Adult: 15-124

852   ICD-10-CM 2023

✓6ᵗʰ M88.82 Osteitis deformans of upper arm

M88.821 Osteitis deformans of right upper arm
M88.822 Osteitis deformans of left upper arm
M88.829 Osteitis deformans of unspecified upper arm

✓6ᵗʰ M88.83 Osteitis deformans of forearm

M88.831 Osteitis deformans of right forearm
M88.832 Osteitis deformans of left forearm
M88.839 Osteitis deformans of unspecified forearm

✓6ᵗʰ M88.84 Osteitis deformans of hand

M88.841 Osteitis deformans of right hand
M88.842 Osteitis deformans of left hand
M88.849 Osteitis deformans of unspecified hand

✓6ᵗʰ M88.85 Osteitis deformans of thigh

M88.851 Osteitis deformans of right thigh
M88.852 Osteitis deformans of left thigh
M88.859 Osteitis deformans of unspecified thigh

✓6ᵗʰ M88.86 Osteitis deformans of lower leg

M88.861 Osteitis deformans of right lower leg
M88.862 Osteitis deformans of left lower leg
M88.869 Osteitis deformans of unspecified lower leg

✓6ᵗʰ M88.87 Osteitis deformans of ankle and foot

M88.871 Osteitis deformans of right ankle and foot
M88.872 Osteitis deformans of left ankle and foot
M88.879 Osteitis deformans of unspecified ankle and foot

M88.88 Osteitis deformans of other bones

EXCLUDES 2 *osteitis deformans of skull (M88.0)*
osteitis deformans of vertebrae (M88.1)

M88.89 Osteitis deformans of multiple sites

M88.9 Osteitis deformans of unspecified bone

✓4ᵗʰ **M89 Other disorders of bone**

✓5ᵗʰ M89.0 Algoneurodystrophy

Shoulder-hand syndrome
Sudeck's atrophy

EXCLUDES 1 *causalgia, lower limb (G57.7-)*
causalgia, upper limb (G56.4-)
complex regional pain syndrome II, lower limb (G57.7-)
complex regional pain syndrome II, upper limb (G56.4-)
reflex sympathetic dystrophy (G90.5-)

M89.00 Algoneurodystrophy, unspecified site

✓6ᵗʰ M89.01 Algoneurodystrophy, shoulder

M89.011 Algoneurodystrophy, right shoulder
M89.012 Algoneurodystrophy, left shoulder
M89.019 Algoneurodystrophy, unspecified shoulder

✓6ᵗʰ M89.02 Algoneurodystrophy, upper arm

M89.021 Algoneurodystrophy, right upper arm
M89.022 Algoneurodystrophy, left upper arm
M89.029 Algoneurodystrophy, unspecified upper arm

✓6ᵗʰ M89.03 Algoneurodystrophy, forearm

M89.031 Algoneurodystrophy, right forearm
M89.032 Algoneurodystrophy, left forearm
M89.039 Algoneurodystrophy, unspecified forearm

✓6ᵗʰ M89.04 Algoneurodystrophy, hand

M89.041 Algoneurodystrophy, right hand
M89.042 Algoneurodystrophy, left hand
M89.049 Algoneurodystrophy, unspecified hand

✓6ᵗʰ M89.05 Algoneurodystrophy, thigh

M89.051 Algoneurodystrophy, right thigh
M89.052 Algoneurodystrophy, left thigh
M89.059 Algoneurodystrophy, unspecified thigh

✓6ᵗʰ M89.06 Algoneurodystrophy, lower leg

M89.061 Algoneurodystrophy, right lower leg
M89.062 Algoneurodystrophy, left lower leg
M89.069 Algoneurodystrophy, unspecified lower leg

✓6ᵗʰ M89.07 Algoneurodystrophy, ankle and foot

M89.071 Algoneurodystrophy, right ankle and foot
M89.072 Algoneurodystrophy, left ankle and foot

M89.079 Algoneurodystrophy, unspecified ankle and foot

M89.08 Algoneurodystrophy, other site
M89.09 Algoneurodystrophy, multiple sites

✓5ᵗʰ M89.1 Physeal arrest

Arrest of growth plate
Epiphyseal arrest
Growth plate arrest

✓6ᵗʰ M89.12 Physeal arrest, humerus

M89.121 Complete physeal arrest, right proximal humerus
M89.122 Complete physeal arrest, left proximal humerus
M89.123 Partial physeal arrest, right proximal humerus
M89.124 Partial physeal arrest, left proximal humerus
M89.125 Complete physeal arrest, right distal humerus
M89.126 Complete physeal arrest, left distal humerus
M89.127 Partial physeal arrest, right distal humerus
M89.128 Partial physeal arrest, left distal humerus
M89.129 Physeal arrest, humerus, unspecified

✓6ᵗʰ M89.13 Physeal arrest, forearm

M89.131 Complete physeal arrest, right distal radius
M89.132 Complete physeal arrest, left distal radius
M89.133 Partial physeal arrest, right distal radius
M89.134 Partial physeal arrest, left distal radius
M89.138 Other physeal arrest of forearm
M89.139 Physeal arrest, forearm, unspecified

✓6ᵗʰ M89.15 Physeal arrest, femur

M89.151 Complete physeal arrest, right proximal femur
M89.152 Complete physeal arrest, left proximal femur
M89.153 Partial physeal arrest, right proximal femur
M89.154 Partial physeal arrest, left proximal femur
M89.155 Complete physeal arrest, right distal femur
M89.156 Complete physeal arrest, left distal femur
M89.157 Partial physeal arrest, right distal femur
M89.158 Partial physeal arrest, left distal femur
M89.159 Physeal arrest, femur, unspecified

✓6ᵗʰ M89.16 Physeal arrest, lower leg

M89.160 Complete physeal arrest, right proximal tibia
M89.161 Complete physeal arrest, left proximal tibia
M89.162 Partial physeal arrest, right proximal tibia
M89.163 Partial physeal arrest, left proximal tibia
M89.164 Complete physeal arrest, right distal tibia
M89.165 Complete physeal arrest, left distal tibia
M89.166 Partial physeal arrest, right distal tibia
M89.167 Partial physeal arrest, left distal tibia
M89.168 Other physeal arrest of lower leg
M89.169 Physeal arrest, lower leg, unspecified

M89.18 Physeal arrest, other site

✓5ᵗʰ M89.2 Other disorders of bone development and growth

M89.20 Other disorders of bone development and growth, unspecified site

✓6ᵗʰ M89.21 Other disorders of bone development and growth, shoulder

M89.211 Other disorders of bone development and growth, right shoulder
M89.212 Other disorders of bone development and growth, left shoulder
M89.219 Other disorders of bone development and growth, unspecified shoulder

✓6ᵗʰ M89.22 Other disorders of bone development and growth, humerus

M89.221 Other disorders of bone development and growth, right humerus
M89.222 Other disorders of bone development and growth, left humerus
M89.229 Other disorders of bone development and growth, unspecified humerus

√6ᵗʰ **M89.23** **Other disorders of bone development and growth, ulna and radius**

     M89.231 Other disorders of bone development and growth, **right ulna**

     M89.232 Other disorders of bone development and growth, **left ulna**

     M89.233 Other disorders of bone development and growth, **right radius**

     M89.234 Other disorders of bone development and growth, **left radius**

     M89.239 Other disorders of bone development and growth, **unspecified ulna and radius**

√6ᵗʰ **M89.24** **Other disorders of bone development and growth, hand**

     M89.241 Other disorders of bone development and growth, **right hand**

     M89.242 Other disorders of bone development and growth, **left hand**

     M89.249 Other disorders of bone development and growth, **unspecified hand**

√6ᵗʰ **M89.25** **Other disorders of bone development and growth, femur**

     M89.251 Other disorders of bone development and growth, **right femur**

     M89.252 Other disorders of bone development and growth, **left femur**

     M89.259 Other disorders of bone development and growth, **unspecified femur**

√6ᵗʰ **M89.26** **Other disorders of bone development and growth, tibia and fibula**

     M89.261 Other disorders of bone development and growth, **right tibia**

     M89.262 Other disorders of bone development and growth, **left tibia**

     M89.263 Other disorders of bone development and growth, **right fibula**

     M89.264 Other disorders of bone development and growth, **left fibula**

     M89.269 Other disorders of bone development and growth, **unspecified lower leg**

√6ᵗʰ **M89.27** **Other disorders of bone development and growth, ankle and foot**

     M89.271 Other disorders of bone development and growth, **right ankle and foot**

     M89.272 Other disorders of bone development and growth, **left ankle and foot**

     M89.279 Other disorders of bone development and growth, **unspecified ankle and foot**

     M89.28 Other disorders of bone development and growth, **other site**

     M89.29 Other disorders of bone development and growth, **multiple sites**

√5ᵗʰ **M89.3** **Hypertrophy of bone**

     M89.30 Hypertrophy of bone, **unspecified site**

√6ᵗʰ **M89.31** **Hypertrophy of bone, shoulder**

     M89.311 Hypertrophy of bone, **right shoulder**

     M89.312 Hypertrophy of bone, **left shoulder**

     M89.319 Hypertrophy of bone, **unspecified shoulder**

√6ᵗʰ **M89.32** **Hypertrophy of bone, humerus**

     M89.321 Hypertrophy of bone, **right humerus**

     M89.322 Hypertrophy of bone, **left humerus**

     M89.329 Hypertrophy of bone, **unspecified humerus**

√6ᵗʰ **M89.33** **Hypertrophy of bone, ulna and radius**

     M89.331 Hypertrophy of bone, **right ulna**

     M89.332 Hypertrophy of bone, **left ulna**

     M89.333 Hypertrophy of bone, **right radius**

     M89.334 Hypertrophy of bone, **left radius**

     M89.339 Hypertrophy of bone, **unspecified ulna and radius**

√6ᵗʰ **M89.34** **Hypertrophy of bone, hand**

     M89.341 Hypertrophy of bone, **right hand**

     M89.342 Hypertrophy of bone, **left hand**

     M89.349 Hypertrophy of bone, **unspecified hand**

√6ᵗʰ **M89.35** **Hypertrophy of bone, femur**

     M89.351 Hypertrophy of bone, **right femur**

     M89.352 Hypatrophy of bone, **left femur**

     M89.359 Hypertrophy of bone, **unspecified femur**

√6ᵗʰ **M89.36** **Hypertrophy of bone, tibia and fibula**

     M89.361 Hypertrophy of bone, **right tibia**

     M89.362 Hypertrophy of bone, **left tibia**

     M89.363 Hypertrophy of bone, **right fibula**

     M89.364 Hypertrophy of bone, **left fibula**

     M89.369 Hypertrophy of bone, **unspecified tibia and fibula**

√6ᵗʰ **M89.37** **Hypertrophy of bone, ankle and foot**

     M89.371 Hypertrophy of bone, **right ankle and foot**

     M89.372 Hypertrophy of bone, **left ankle and foot**

     M89.379 Hypertrophy of bone, **unspecified ankle and foot**

     M89.38 Hypertrophy of bone, **other site**

     M89.39 Hypertrophy of bone, **multiple sites**

√5ᵗʰ **M89.4** **Other hypertrophic osteoarthropathy**

     Marie-Bamberger disease

     Pachydermoperiostosis

     M89.40 **Other hypertrophic osteoarthropathy, unspecified site**

√6ᵗʰ **M89.41** **Other hypertrophic osteoarthropathy, shoulder**

     M89.411 Other hypertrophic osteoarthropathy, **right shoulder**

     M89.412 Other hypertrophic osteoarthropathy, **left shoulder**

     M89.419 Other hypertrophic osteoarthropathy, **unspecified shoulder**

√6ᵗʰ **M89.42** **Other hypertrophic osteoarthropathy, upper arm**

     M89.421 Other hypertrophic osteoarthropathy, **right upper arm**

     M89.422 Other hypertrophic osteoarthropathy, **left upper arm**

     M89.429 Other hypertrophic osteoarthropathy, **unspecified upper arm**

√6ᵗʰ **M89.43** **Other hypertrophic osteoarthropathy, forearm**

     M89.431 Other hypertrophic osteoarthropathy, **right forearm**

     M89.432 Other hypertrophic osteoarthropathy, **left forearm**

     M89.439 Other hypertrophic osteoarthropathy, **unspecified forearm**

√6ᵗʰ **M89.44** **Other hypertrophic osteoarthropathy, hand**

     M89.441 Other hypertrophic osteoarthropathy, **right hand**

     M89.442 Other hypertrophic osteoarthropathy, **left hand**

     M89.449 Other hypertrophic osteoarthropathy, **unspecified hand**

√6ᵗʰ **M89.45** **Other hypertrophic osteoarthropathy, thigh**

     M89.451 Other hypertrophic osteoarthropathy, **right thigh**

     M89.452 Other hypertrophic osteoarthropathy, **left thigh**

     M89.459 Other hypertrophic osteoarthropathy, **unspecified thigh**

√6ᵗʰ **M89.46** **Other hypertrophic osteoarthropathy, lower leg**

     M89.461 Other hypertrophic osteoarthropathy, **right lower leg**

     M89.462 Other hypertrophic osteoarthropathy, **left lower leg**

     M89.469 Other hypertrophic osteoarthropathy, **unspecified lower leg**

√6ᵗʰ **M89.47** **Other hypertrophic osteoarthropathy, ankle and foot**

     M89.471 Other hypertrophic osteoarthropathy, **right ankle and foot**

     M89.472 Other hypertrophic osteoarthropathy, **left ankle and foot**

     M89.479 Other hypertrophic osteoarthropathy, **unspecified ankle and foot**

     M89.48 Other hypertrophic osteoarthropathy, **other site**

     M89.49 Other hypertrophic osteoarthropathy, **multiple sites**

√5ᵗʰ **M89.5** **Osteolysis**

     Use additional code to identify major osseous defect, if applicable (M89.7-)

     EXCLUDES 2   periprosthetic osteolysis of internal prosthetic joint (T84.05-)

     M89.50 **Osteolysis, unspecified site**

✓6ᵗʰ **M89.51** Osteolysis, shoulder

　　　M89.511 Osteolysis, right shoulder
　　　M89.512 Osteolysis, left shoulder
　　　M89.519 Osteolysis, unspecified shoulder

✓6ᵗʰ **M89.52** Osteolysis, upper arm

　　　M89.521 Osteolysis, right upper arm
　　　M89.522 Osteolysis, left upper arm
　　　M89.529 Osteolysis, unspecified upper arm

✓6ᵗʰ **M89.53** Osteolysis, forearm

　　　M89.531 Osteolysis, right forearm
　　　M89.532 Osteolysis, left forearm
　　　M89.539 Osteolysis, unspecified forearm

✓6ᵗʰ **M89.54** Osteolysis, hand

　　　M89.541 Osteolysis, right hand
　　　M89.542 Osteolysis, left hand
　　　M89.549 Osteolysis, unspecified hand

✓6ᵗʰ **M89.55** Osteolysis, thigh

　　　M89.551 Osteolysis, right thigh
　　　M89.552 Osteolysis, left thigh
　　　M89.559 Osteolysis, unspecified thigh

✓6ᵗʰ **M89.56** Osteolysis, lower leg

　　　M89.561 Osteolysis, right lower leg
　　　M89.562 Osteolysis, left lower leg
　　　M89.569 Osteolysis, unspecified lower leg

✓6ᵗʰ **M89.57** Osteolysis, ankle and foot

　　　M89.571 Osteolysis, right ankle and foot
　　　M89.572 Osteolysis, left ankle and foot
　　　M89.579 Osteolysis, unspecified ankle and foot

　　M89.58 Osteolysis, other site
　　M89.59 Osteolysis, multiple sites

✓5ᵗʰ **M89.6** Osteopathy after poliomyelitis

　　　Use additional code (B91) to identify previous poliomyelitis
　　　EXCLUDES 1 *postpolio syndrome (G14)*

　　M89.60 Osteopathy after poliomyelitis, unspecified
　　　　site　　HCC ESR COM

✓6ᵗʰ **M89.61** Osteopathy after poliomyelitis, shoulder

　　　M89.611 Osteopathy after poliomyelitis, right
　　　　　shoulder　　HCC ESR COM
　　　M89.612 Osteopathy after poliomyelitis, left
　　　　　shoulder　　HCC ESR COM
　　　M89.619 Osteopathy after poliomyelitis,
　　　　　unspecified shoulder　　HCC ESR COM

✓6ᵗʰ **M89.62** Osteopathy after poliomyelitis, upper arm

　　　M89.621 Osteopathy after poliomyelitis, right
　　　　　upper arm　　HCC ESR COM
　　　M89.622 Osteopathy after poliomyelitis, left upper
　　　　　arm　　HCC ESR COM
　　　M89.629 Osteopathy after poliomyelitis,
　　　　　unspecified upper arm　　HCC ESR COM

✓6ᵗʰ **M89.63** Osteopathy after poliomyelitis, forearm

　　　M89.631 Osteopathy after poliomyelitis, right
　　　　　forearm　　HCC ESR COM
　　　M89.632 Osteopathy after poliomyelitis, left
　　　　　forearm　　HCC ESR COM
　　　M89.639 Osteopathy after poliomyelitis,
　　　　　unspecified forearm　　HCC ESR COM

✓6ᵗʰ **M89.64** Osteopathy after poliomyelitis, hand

　　　M89.641 Osteopathy after poliomyelitis, right
　　　　　hand　　HCC ESR COM
　　　M89.642 Osteopathy after poliomyelitis, left
　　　　　hand　　HCC ESR COM
　　　M89.649 Osteopathy after poliomyelitis,
　　　　　unspecified hand　　HCC ESR COM

✓6ᵗʰ **M89.65** Osteopathy after poliomyelitis, thigh

　　　M89.651 Osteopathy after poliomyelitis, right
　　　　　thigh　　HCC ESR COM
　　　M89.652 Osteopathy after poliomyelitis, left
　　　　　thigh　　HCC ESR COM
　　　M89.659 Osteopathy after poliomyelitis,
　　　　　unspecified thigh　　HCC ESR COM

✓6ᵗʰ **M89.66** Osteopathy after poliomyelitis, lower leg

　　　M89.661 Osteopathy after poliomyelitis, right
　　　　　lower leg　　HCC ESR COM
　　　M89.662 Osteopathy after poliomyelitis, left lower
　　　　　leg　　HCC ESR COM

　　　M89.669 Osteopathy after poliomyelitis,
　　　　　unspecified lower leg　　HCC ESR COM

✓6ᵗʰ **M89.67** Osteopathy after poliomyelitis, ankle and foot

　　　M89.671 Osteopathy after poliomyelitis, right
　　　　　ankle and foot　　HCC ESR COM
　　　M89.672 Osteopathy after poliomyelitis, left ankle
　　　　　and foot　　HCC ESR COM
　　　M89.679 Osteopathy after poliomyelitis,
　　　　　unspecified ankle and
　　　　　foot　　HCC ESR COM

　　M89.68 Osteopathy after poliomyelitis, other
　　　　site　　HCC ESR COM
　　M89.69 Osteopathy after poliomyelitis, multiple
　　　　sites　　HCC ESR COM

✓5ᵗʰ **M89.7** Major osseous defect

　　　Code first underlying disease, if known, such as:
　　　　aseptic necrosis of bone (M87.-)
　　　　malignant neoplasm of bone (C40.-)
　　　　osteolysis (M89.5)
　　　　osteomyelitis (M86.-)
　　　　osteonecrosis (M87.-)
　　　　osteoporosis (M80.-, M81.-)
　　　　periprosthetic osteolysis (T84.05-)

　　M89.70 Major osseous defect, unspecified site

✓6ᵗʰ **M89.71** Major osseous defect, shoulder region

　　　　Major osseous defect clavicle or scapula

　　　M89.711 Major osseous defect, right shoulder
　　　　　region
　　　M89.712 Major osseous defect, left shoulder region
　　　M89.719 Major osseous defect, unspecified
　　　　　shoulder region

✓6ᵗʰ **M89.72** Major osseous defect, humerus

　　　M89.721 Major osseous defect, right humerus
　　　M89.722 Major osseous defect, left humerus
　　　M89.729 Major osseous defect, unspecified
　　　　　humerus

✓6ᵗʰ **M89.73** Major osseous defect, forearm

　　　　Major osseous defect of radius and ulna

　　　M89.731 Major osseous defect, right forearm
　　　M89.732 Major osseous defect, left forearm
　　　M89.739 Major osseous defect, unspecified
　　　　　forearm

✓6ᵗʰ **M89.74** Major osseous defect, hand

　　　　Major osseous defect of carpus, fingers, metacarpus

　　　M89.741 Major osseous defect, right hand
　　　M89.742 Major osseous defect, left hand
　　　M89.749 Major osseous defect, unspecified hand

✓6ᵗʰ **M89.75** Major osseous defect, pelvic region and thigh

　　　　Major osseous defect of femur and pelvis

　　　M89.751 Major osseous defect, right pelvic region
　　　　　and thigh
　　　M89.752 Major osseous defect, left pelvic region
　　　　　and thigh
　　　M89.759 Major osseous defect, unspecified pelvic
　　　　　region and thigh

✓6ᵗʰ **M89.76** Major osseous defect, lower leg

　　　　Major osseous defect of fibula and tibia

　　　M89.761 Major osseous defect, right lower leg
　　　M89.762 Major osseous defect, left lower leg
　　　M89.769 Major osseous defect, unspecified lower
　　　　　leg

✓6ᵗʰ **M89.77** Major osseous defect, ankle and foot

　　　　Major osseous defect of metatarsus, tarsus, toes

　　　M89.771 Major osseous defect, right ankle and
　　　　　foot
　　　M89.772 Major osseous defect, left ankle and foot
　　　M89.779 Major osseous defect, unspecified ankle
　　　　　and foot

　　M89.78 Major osseous defect, other site
　　M89.79 Major osseous defect, multiple sites

✓5ᵗʰ **M89.8** Other specified disorders of bone

　　　Infantile cortical hyperostoses
　　　Post-traumatic subperiosteal ossification
　　　AHA: 2022,2Q,10

✓6ᵗʰ **M89.8X** Other specified disorders of bone

　　　M89.8X0 Other specified disorders of bone,
　　　　　multiple sites

M89.8X1 **Other specified disorders of bone,** shoulder

M89.8X2 **Other specified disorders of bone,** upper arm

M89.8X3 **Other specified disorders of bone,** forearm
   AHA: 2019,3Q,9

M89.8X4 **Other specified disorders of bone,** hand

M89.8X5 **Other specified disorders of bone,** thigh

M89.8X6 **Other specified disorders of bone,** lower leg

M89.8X7 **Other specified disorders of bone,** ankle and foot

M89.8X8 **Other specified disorders of bone,** other site

M89.8X9 **Other specified disorders of bone,** unspecified site

M89.9 Disorder of bone, unspecified

☑4ᵗʰ **M90 Osteopathies in diseases classified elsewhere**

   EXCLUDES 1 *osteochondritis, osteomyelitis, and osteopathy (in):*
      cryptococcosis (B45.3)
      diabetes mellitus (E08-E13 with .69-)
      gonococcal (A54.43)
      neurogenic syphilis (A52.11)
      renal osteodystrophy (N25.0)
      salmonellosis (A02.24)
      secondary syphilis (A51.46)
      syphilis (late) (A52.77)

☑5ᵗʰ **M90.5 Osteonecrosis in diseases classified elsewhere**

   Code first underlying disease, such as:
   caisson disease (T70.3)
   hemoglobinopathy (D50-D64)

   M90.50 *Osteonecrosis in diseases classified elsewhere, unspecified site* HCC Rx ESR COM

☑6ᵗʰ **M90.51 Osteonecrosis in diseases classified elsewhere,** shoulder

   M90.511 *Osteonecrosis in diseases classified elsewhere, right shoulder* HCC Rx ESR COM

   M90.512 *Osteonecrosis in diseases classified elsewhere, left shoulder* HCC Rx ESR COM

   M90.519 *Osteonecrosis in diseases classified elsewhere, unspecified shoulder* HCC Rx ESR COM

☑6ᵗʰ **M90.52 Osteonecrosis in diseases classified elsewhere,** upper arm

   M90.521 *Osteonecrosis in diseases classified elsewhere, right upper arm* HCC Rx ESR COM

   M90.522 *Osteonecrosis in diseases classified elsewhere, left upper arm* HCC Rx ESR COM

   M90.529 *Osteonecrosis in diseases classified elsewhere, unspecified upper arm* HCC Rx ESR COM

☑6ᵗʰ **M90.53 Osteonecrosis in diseases classified elsewhere,** forearm

   M90.531 *Osteonecrosis in diseases classified elsewhere, right forearm* HCC Rx ESR COM

   M90.532 *Osteonecrosis in diseases classified elsewhere, left forearm* HCC Rx ESR COM

   M90.539 *Osteonecrosis in diseases classified elsewhere, unspecified forearm* HCC Rx ESR COM

☑6ᵗʰ **M90.54 Osteonecrosis in diseases classified elsewhere,** hand

   M90.541 *Osteonecrosis in diseases classified elsewhere, right hand* HCC Rx ESR COM

   M90.542 *Osteonecrosis in diseases classified elsewhere, left hand* HCC Rx ESR COM

   M90.549 *Osteonecrosis in diseases classified elsewhere, unspecified hand* HCC Rx ESR COM

☑6ᵗʰ **M90.55 Osteonecrosis in diseases classified elsewhere,** thigh

   M90.551 *Osteonecrosis in diseases classified elsewhere, right thigh* HCC Rx ESR COM

   M90.552 *Osteonecrosis in diseases classified elsewhere, left thigh* HCC Rx ESR COM

   M90.559 *Osteonecrosis in diseases classified elsewhere, unspecified thigh* HCC Rx ESR COM

☑6ᵗʰ **M90.56 Osteonecrosis in diseases classified elsewhere,** lower leg

   M90.561 *Osteonecrosis in diseases classified elsewhere, right lower leg* HCC Rx ESR COM

   M90.562 *Osteonecrosis in diseases classified elsewhere, left lower leg* HCC Rx ESR COM

   M90.569 *Osteonecrosis in diseases classified elsewhere, unspecified lower leg* HCC Rx ESR COM

☑6ᵗʰ **M90.57 Osteonecrosis in diseases classified elsewhere,** ankle and foot

   M90.571 *Osteonecrosis in diseases classified elsewhere, right ankle and foot* HCC Rx ESR COM

   M90.572 *Osteonecrosis in diseases classified elsewhere, left ankle and foot* HCC Rx ESR COM

   M90.579 *Osteonecrosis in diseases classified elsewhere, unspecified ankle and foot* HCC Rx ESR COM

   M90.58 **Osteonecrosis in diseases classified elsewhere, other site** HCC Rx ESR COM

   M90.59 **Osteonecrosis in diseases classified elsewhere,** multiple sites HCC Rx ESR COM

☑5ᵗʰ **M90.6 Osteitis deformans in neoplastic diseases**

   Osteitis deformans in malignant neoplasm of bone
   Code first the neoplasm (C40.-, C41.-)

   EXCLUDES 1 *osteitis deformans [Paget's disease of bone] (M88.-)*

   M90.60 *Osteitis deformans in neoplastic diseases, unspecified site*

☑6ᵗʰ **M90.61 Osteitis deformans in neoplastic diseases,** shoulder

   M90.611 *Osteitis deformans in neoplastic diseases, right shoulder*

   M90.612 *Osteitis deformans in neoplastic diseases, left shoulder*

   M90.619 *Osteitis deformans in neoplastic diseases, unspecified shoulder*

☑6ᵗʰ **M90.62 Osteitis deformans in neoplastic diseases,** upper arm

   M90.621 *Osteitis deformans in neoplastic diseases, right upper arm*

   M90.622 *Osteitis deformans in neoplastic diseases, left upper arm*

   M90.629 *Osteitis deformans in neoplastic diseases, unspecified upper arm*

☑6ᵗʰ **M90.63 Osteitis deformans in neoplastic diseases,** forearm

   M90.631 *Osteitis deformans in neoplastic diseases, right forearm*

   M90.632 *Osteitis deformans in neoplastic diseases, left forearm*

   M90.639 *Osteitis deformans in neoplastic diseases, unspecified forearm*

☑6ᵗʰ **M90.64 Osteitis deformans in neoplastic diseases,** hand

   M90.641 *Osteitis deformans in neoplastic diseases, right hand*

   M90.642 *Osteitis deformans in neoplastic diseases, left hand*

   M90.649 *Osteitis deformans in neoplastic diseases, unspecified hand*

☑6ᵗʰ **M90.65 Osteitis deformans in neoplastic diseases,** thigh

   M90.651 *Osteitis deformans in neoplastic diseases, right thigh*

   M90.652 *Osteitis deformans in neoplastic diseases, left thigh*

   M90.659 *Osteitis deformans in neoplastic diseases, unspecified thigh*

☑6ᵗʰ **M90.66 Osteitis deformans in neoplastic diseases,** lower leg

   M90.661 *Osteitis deformans in neoplastic diseases, right lower leg*

   M90.662 *Osteitis deformans in neoplastic diseases, left lower leg*

   M90.669 *Osteitis deformans in neoplastic diseases, unspecified lower leg*

✓6ᵗʰ **M90.67** Osteitis deformans in neoplastic diseases, ankle and foot

    M90.671 *Osteitis deformans in neoplastic diseases, right ankle and foot*

    M90.672 *Osteitis deformans in neoplastic diseases, left ankle and foot*

    M90.679 *Osteitis deformans in neoplastic diseases, unspecified ankle and foot*

    M90.68 Osteitis deformans in neoplastic diseases, other site

    M90.69 Osteitis deformans in neoplastic diseases, multiple sites

✓5ᵗʰ **M90.8** Osteopathy in diseases classified elsewhere

    Code first underlying disease, such as:
      rickets (E55.0)
      vitamin-D-resistant rickets (E83.3)

    M90.80 *Osteopathy in diseases classified elsewhere, unspecified site*

✓6ᵗʰ **M90.81** Osteopathy in diseases classified elsewhere, shoulder

    M90.811 *Osteopathy in diseases classified elsewhere, right shoulder*

    M90.812 *Osteopathy in diseases classified elsewhere, left shoulder*

    M90.819 *Osteopathy in diseases classified elsewhere, unspecified shoulder*

✓6ᵗʰ **M90.82** Osteopathy in diseases classified elsewhere, upper arm

    M90.821 *Osteopathy in diseases classified elsewhere, right upper arm*

    M90.822 *Osteopathy in diseases classified elsewhere, left upper arm*

    M90.829 *Osteopathy in diseases classified elsewhere, unspecified upper arm*

✓6ᵗʰ **M90.83** Osteopathy in diseases classified elsewhere, forearm

    M90.831 *Osteopathy in diseases classified elsewhere, right forearm*

    M90.832 *Osteopathy in diseases classified elsewhere, left forearm*

    M90.839 *Osteopathy in diseases classified elsewhere, unspecified forearm*

✓6ᵗʰ **M90.84** Osteopathy in diseases classified elsewhere, hand

    M90.841 *Osteopathy in diseases classified elsewhere, right hand*

    M90.842 *Osteopathy in diseases classified elsewhere, left hand*

    M90.849 *Osteopathy in diseases classified elsewhere, unspecified hand*

✓6ᵗʰ **M90.85** Osteopathy in diseases classified elsewhere, thigh

    M90.851 *Osteopathy in diseases classified elsewhere, right thigh*

    M90.852 *Osteopathy in diseases classified elsewhere, left thigh*

    M90.859 *Osteopathy in diseases classified elsewhere, unspecified thigh*

✓6ᵗʰ **M90.86** Osteopathy in diseases classified elsewhere, lower leg

    M90.861 *Osteopathy in diseases classified elsewhere, right lower leg*

    M90.862 *Osteopathy in diseases classified elsewhere, left lower leg*

    M90.869 *Osteopathy in diseases classified elsewhere, unspecified lower leg*

✓6ᵗʰ **M90.87** Osteopathy in diseases classified elsewhere, ankle and foot

    M90.871 *Osteopathy in diseases classified elsewhere, right ankle and foot*

    M90.872 *Osteopathy in diseases classified elsewhere, left ankle and foot*

    M90.879 *Osteopathy in diseases classified elsewhere, unspecified ankle and foot*

    M90.88 Osteopathy in diseases classified elsewhere, other site

    M90.89 Osteopathy in diseases classified elsewhere, multiple sites

Chondropathies (M91-M94)

EXCLUDES 1   *postprocedural chondropathies (M96.-)*

✓4ᵗʰ **M91** Juvenile osteochondrosis of hip and pelvis

    EXCLUDES 1   *slipped upper femoral epiphysis (nontraumatic) ▶(M93.0-)◀*

    M91.0 Juvenile osteochondrosis of pelvis COM

      Osteochondrosis (juvenile) of acetabulum
      Osteochondrosis (juvenile) of iliac crest [Buchanan]
      Osteochondrosis (juvenile) of ischiopubic synchondrosis [van Neck]
      Osteochondrosis (juvenile) of symphysis pubis [Pierson]

✓5ᵗʰ **M91.1** Juvenile osteochondrosis of head of femur [Legg-Calvé-Perthes]

    M91.10 Juvenile osteochondrosis of head of femur [Legg-Calvé-Perthes], unspecified leg COM

    M91.11 Juvenile osteochondrosis of head of femur [Legg-Calvé-Perthes], right leg COM

    M91.12 Juvenile osteochondrosis of head of femur [Legg-Calvé-Perthes], left leg COM

✓5ᵗʰ **M91.2** Coxa plana

    Hip deformity due to previous juvenile osteochondrosis

    M91.20 Coxa plana, unspecified hip COM

    M91.21 Coxa plana, right hip COM

    M91.22 Coxa plana, left hip COM

✓5ᵗʰ **M91.3** Pseudocoxalgia

    M91.30 Pseudocoxalgia, unspecified hip COM

    M91.31 Pseudocoxalgia, right hip COM

    M91.32 Pseudocoxalgia, left hip COM

✓5ᵗʰ **M91.4** Coxa magna

    M91.40 Coxa magna, unspecified hip COM

    M91.41 Coxa magna, right hip COM

    M91.42 Coxa magna, left hip COM

✓5ᵗʰ **M91.8** Other juvenile osteochondrosis of hip and pelvis

    Juvenile osteochondrosis after reduction of congenital dislocation of hip

    M91.80 Other juvenile osteochondrosis of hip and pelvis, unspecified leg COM

    M91.81 Other juvenile osteochondrosis of hip and pelvis, right leg COM

    M91.82 Other juvenile osteochondrosis of hip and pelvis, left leg COM

✓5ᵗʰ **M91.9** Juvenile osteochondrosis of hip and pelvis, unspecified

    M91.90 Juvenile osteochondrosis of hip and pelvis, unspecified, unspecified leg COM

    M91.91 Juvenile osteochondrosis of hip and pelvis, unspecified, right leg COM

    M91.92 Juvenile osteochondrosis of hip and pelvis, unspecified, left leg COM

✓4ᵗʰ **M92** Other juvenile osteochondrosis

✓5ᵗʰ **M92.0** Juvenile osteochondrosis of humerus

    Osteochondrosis (juvenile) of capitulum of humerus [Panner]
    Osteochondrosis (juvenile) of head of humerus [Haas]

    M92.00 Juvenile osteochondrosis of humerus, unspecified arm

    M92.01 Juvenile osteochondrosis of humerus, right arm

    M92.02 Juvenile osteochondrosis of humerus, left arm

✓5ᵗʰ **M92.1** Juvenile osteochondrosis of radius and ulna

    Osteochondrosis (juvenile) of lower ulna [Burns]
    Osteochondrosis (juvenile) of radial head [Brailsford]

    M92.10 Juvenile osteochondrosis of radius and ulna, unspecified arm

    M92.11 Juvenile osteochondrosis of radius and ulna, right arm

    M92.12 Juvenile osteochondrosis of radius and ulna, left arm

✓5ᵗʰ **M92.2** Juvenile osteochondrosis, hand

✓6ᵗʰ **M92.20** Unspecified juvenile osteochondrosis, hand

    M92.201 Unspecified juvenile osteochondrosis, right hand

    M92.202 Unspecified juvenile osteochondrosis, left hand

    M92.209 Unspecified juvenile osteochondrosis, unspecified hand

☑6ᵗʰ **M92.21** **Osteochondrosis (juvenile) of** carpal lunate [Kienböck]

     M92.211 **Osteochondrosis (juvenile) of carpal lunate [Kienböck],** right **hand**

     M92.212 **Osteochondrosis (juvenile) of carpal lunate [Kienböck],** left **hand**

     M92.219 **Osteochondrosis (juvenile) of carpal lunate [Kienböck], unspecified hand**

☑6ᵗʰ **M92.22** **Osteochondrosis (juvenile) of** metacarpal heads [Mauclaire]

     M92.221 **Osteochondrosis (juvenile) of metacarpal heads [Mauclaire],** right **hand**

     M92.222 **Osteochondrosis (juvenile) of metacarpal heads [Mauclaire],** left **hand**

     M92.229 **Osteochondrosis (juvenile) of metacarpal heads [Mauclaire], unspecified hand**

☑6ᵗʰ **M92.29** **Other juvenile osteochondrosis,** hand

     M92.291 **Other juvenile osteochondrosis,** right **hand**

     M92.292 **Other juvenile osteochondrosis,** left **hand**

     M92.299 **Other juvenile osteochondrosis, unspecified hand**

☑5ᵗʰ **M92.3** **Other juvenile osteochondrosis,** upper limb

     M92.30 **Other juvenile osteochondrosis, unspecified upper limb**

     M92.31 **Other juvenile osteochondrosis,** right **upper limb**

     M92.32 **Other juvenile osteochondrosis,** left **upper limb**

☑5ᵗʰ **M92.4** **Juvenile osteochondrosis of** patella

Osteochondrosis (juvenile) of primary patellar center [Köhler]

Osteochondrosis (juvenile) of secondary patellar centre [Sinding Larsen]

     M92.40 **Juvenile osteochondrosis of patella, unspecified knee**

     M92.41 **Juvenile osteochondrosis of patella,** right **knee**

     M92.42 **Juvenile osteochondrosis of patella,** left **knee**

☑5ᵗʰ **M92.5** **Juvenile osteochondrosis of** tibia and fibula

AHA: 2020,4Q,33-34

☑6ᵗʰ **M92.50** **Unspecified juvenile osteochondrosis of tibia and fibula**

     M92.501 **Unspecified juvenile osteochondrosis,** right **leg**

     M92.502 **Unspecified juvenile osteochondrosis,** left **leg**

     M92.503 **Unspecified juvenile osteochondrosis,** bilateral **leg**

     M92.509 **Unspecified juvenile osteochondrosis, unspecified leg**

☑6ᵗʰ **M92.51** **Juvenile osteochondrosis of** proximal tibia

Blount disease

Tibia vara

     M92.511 **Juvenile osteochondrosis of proximal tibia,** right **leg**

     M92.512 **Juvenile osteochondrosis of proximal tibia,** left **leg**

     M92.513 **Juvenile osteochondrosis of proximal tibia,** bilateral

     M92.519 **Juvenile osteochondrosis of proximal tibia, unspecified leg**

☑6ᵗʰ **M92.52** **Juvenile osteochondrosis of** tibia tubercle

Osgood-Schlatter disease

     M92.521 **Juvenile osteochondrosis of tibia tubercle,** right **leg**

     M92.522 **Juvenile osteochondrosis of tibia tubercle,** left **leg**

     M92.523 **Juvenile osteochondrosis of tibia tubercle,** bilateral

     M92.529 **Juvenile osteochondrosis of tibia tubercle, unspecified leg**

☑6ᵗʰ **M92.59** **Other juvenile osteochondrosis of tibia and fibula**

     M92.591 **Other juvenile osteochondrosis of tibia and fibula,** right **leg**

     M92.592 **Other juvenile osteochondrosis of tibia and fibula,** left **leg**

     M92.593 **Other juvenile osteochondrosis of tibia and fibula,** bilateral

     M92.599 **Other juvenile osteochondrosis of tibia and fibula, unspecified leg**

☑6ᵗʰ **M92.6** **Juvenile osteochondrosis of** tarsus

Osteochondrosis (juvenile) of calcaneum [Sever]

Osteochondrosis (juvenile) of os tibiale externum [Haglund]

Osteochondrosis (juvenile) of talus [Diaz]

Osteochondrosis (juvenile) of tarsal navicular [Köhler]

     M92.60 **Juvenile osteochondrosis of tarsus, unspecified ankle**

     M92.61 **Juvenile osteochondrosis of tarsus,** right **ankle**

     M92.62 **Juvenile osteochondrosis of tarsus,** left **ankle**

☑6ᵗʰ **M92.7** **Juvenile osteochondrosis of** metatarsus

Osteochondrosis (juvenile) of fifth metatarsus [Iselin]

Osteochondrosis (juvenile) of second metatarsus [Freiberg]

     M92.70 **Juvenile osteochondrosis of metatarsus, unspecified foot**

     M92.71 **Juvenile osteochondrosis of metatarsus,** right **foot**

     M92.72 **Juvenile osteochondrosis of metatarsus,** left **foot**

M92.8 **Other specified juvenile osteochondrosis**

Calcaneal apophysitis

DEF: Calcaneal apophysitis: Inflammation of the calcaneus at the point of Achilles tendon insertion usually occurring in boys ages 8 to 14. Pain, tenderness, and localized swelling are present.

M92.9 **Juvenile osteochondrosis, unspecified**

Juvenile apophysitis NOS

Juvenile epiphysitis NOS

Juvenile osteochondritis NOS

Juvenile osteochondrosis NOS

☑4ᵗʰ **M93** **Other osteochondropathies**

     EXCLUDES 2   *osteochondrosis of spine (M42.-)*

☑5ᵗʰ **M93.0** **Slipped upper femoral epiphysis (nontraumatic)**

     ▶Slipped capital femoral epiphysis (SCFE)◀

     ▶Slipped upper femoral epiphysis (SUFE)◀

     Use additional code for associated chondrolysis (M94.3)

☑6ᵗʰ **M93.00** **Unspecified slipped upper femoral epiphysis (nontraumatic)**

     M93.001 **Unspecified slipped upper femoral epiphysis (nontraumatic),** right **hip** COM

     M93.002 **Unspecified slipped upper femoral epiphysis (nontraumatic),** left **hip** COM

     M93.003 **Unspecified slipped upper femoral epiphysis (nontraumatic), unspecified hip** COM

●   **M93.004** **Unspecified slipped upper femoral epiphysis (nontraumatic),** bilateral **hips**

▲ ☑6ᵗʰ **M93.01** **Acute slipped upper femoral epiphysis,** stable **(nontraumatic)**

▲   **M93.011** **Acute slipped upper femoral epiphysis, stable (nontraumatic),** right **hip** COM

▲   **M93.012** **Acute slipped upper femoral epiphysis, stable (nontraumatic),** left **hip** COM

▲   **M93.013** **Acute slipped upper femoral epiphysis, stable (nontraumatic), unspecified hip** COM

●   **M93.014** **Acute slipped upper femoral epiphysis, stable (nontraumatic),** bilateral **hips**

▲ ☑6ᵗʰ **M93.02** **Chronic slipped upper femoral epiphysis,** stable **(nontraumatic)**

▲   **M93.021** **Chronic slipped upper femoral epiphysis, stable (nontraumatic),** right **hip** COM

▲   **M93.022** **Chronic slipped upper femoral epiphysis, stable (nontraumatic),** left **hip** COM

▲   **M93.023** **Chronic slipped upper femoral epiphysis, stable (nontraumatic), unspecified hip** COM

●   **M93.024** **Chronic slipped upper femoral epiphysis, stable (nontraumatic),** bilateral **hips**

▲ ☑6ᵗʰ **M93.03** **Acute on chronic slipped upper femoral epiphysis,** stable **(nontraumatic)**

▲   **M93.031** **Acute on chronic slipped upper femoral epiphysis, stable (nontraumatic),** right **hip** COM

▲   **M93.032** **Acute on chronic slipped upper femoral epiphysis, stable (nontraumatic),** left **hip** COM

▲   **M93.033** **Acute on chronic slipped upper femoral epiphysis, stable (nontraumatic), unspecified hip** COM

●   **M93.034** **Acute on chronic slipped upper femoral epiphysis, stable (nontraumatic),** bilateral **hips**

● ✓6ᵗʰ **M93.04** Acute slipped upper femoral epiphysis, unstable (nontraumatic)

●   **M93.041** Acute slipped upper femoral epiphysis, unstable (nontraumatic), right hip

●   **M93.042** Acute slipped upper femoral epiphysis, unstable (nontraumatic), left hip

●   **M93.043** Acute slipped upper femoral epiphysis, unstable (nontraumatic), unspecified hip

●   **M93.044** Acute slipped upper femoral epiphysis, unstable (nontraumatic), bilateral hips

● ✓6ᵗʰ **M93.05** Acute on chronic slipped upper femoral epiphysis, unstable (nontraumatic)

●   **M93.051** Acute on chronic slipped upper femoral epiphysis, unstable (nontraumatic), right hip

●   **M93.052** Acute on chronic slipped upper femoral epiphysis, unstable (nontraumatic), left hip

●   **M93.053** Acute on chronic slipped upper femoral epiphysis, unstable (nontraumatic), unspecified hip

●   **M93.054** Acute on chronic slipped upper femoral epiphysis, unstable (nontraumatic), bilateral hips

● ✓6ᵗʰ **M93.06** Acute slipped upper femoral epiphysis, unspecified stability (nontraumatic)

●   **M93.061** Acute slipped upper femoral epiphysis, unspecified stability (nontraumatic), right hip

●   **M93.062** Acute slipped upper femoral epiphysis, unspecified stability (nontraumatic), left hip

●   **M93.063** Acute slipped upper femoral epiphysis, unspecified stability (nontraumatic), unspecified hip

●   **M93.064** Acute slipped upper femoral epiphysis, unspecified stability (nontraumatic), bilateral hips

● ✓6ᵗʰ **M93.07** Acute on chronic slipped upper femoral epiphysis, unspecified stability (nontraumatic)

●   **M93.071** Acute on chronic slipped upper femoral epiphysis, unspecified stability (nontraumatic), right hip

●   **M93.072** Acute on chronic slipped upper femoral epiphysis, unspecified stability (nontraumatic), left hip

●   **M93.073** Acute on chronic slipped upper femoral epiphysis, unspecified stability (nontraumatic), unspecified hip

●   **M93.074** Acute on chronic slipped upper femoral epiphysis, unspecified stability (nontraumatic), bilateral hips

      M93.1 Kienböck's disease of adults   🄰
        Adult osteochondrosis of carpal lunates

✓5ᵗʰ **M93.2** Osteochondritis dissecans

      DEF: Avascular necrosis caused by lack of blood flow to the bone and cartilage of a joint causing the bone to die. This can result in splinters or pieces of cartilage breaking off in the joint.

      M93.20 Osteochondritis dissecans of unspecified site

✓6ᵗʰ **M93.21** Osteochondritis dissecans of shoulder

      M93.211 Osteochondritis dissecans, right shoulder
      M93.212 Osteochondritis dissecans, left shoulder
      M93.219 Osteochondritis dissecans, unspecified shoulder

✓6ᵗʰ **M93.22** Osteochondritis dissecans of elbow

      M93.221 Osteochondritis dissecans, right elbow
      M93.222 Osteochondritis dissecans, left elbow
      M93.229 Osteochondritis dissecans, unspecified elbow

✓6ᵗʰ **M93.23** Osteochondritis dissecans of wrist

      M93.231 Osteochondritis dissecans, right wrist
      M93.232 Osteochondritis dissecans, left wrist
      M93.239 Osteochondritis dissecans, unspecified wrist

✓6ᵗʰ **M93.24** Osteochondritis dissecans of joints of hand

      M93.241 Osteochondritis dissecans, joints of right hand
      M93.242 Osteochondritis dissecans, joints of left hand
      M93.249 Osteochondritis dissecans, joints of unspecified hand

✓6ᵗʰ **M93.25** Osteochondritis dissecans of hip

      M93.251 Osteochondritis dissecans, right hip
      M93.252 Osteochondritis dissecans, left hip
      M93.259 Osteochondritis dissecans, unspecified hip

✓6ᵗʰ **M93.26** Osteochondritis dissecans knee

      M93.261 Osteochondritis dissecans, right knee
      M93.262 Osteochondritis dissecans, left knee
      M93.269 Osteochondritis dissecans, unspecified knee

✓6ᵗʰ **M93.27** Osteochondritis dissecans of ankle and joints of foot

      M93.271 Osteochondritis dissecans, right ankle and joints of right foot
      M93.272 Osteochondritis dissecans, left ankle and joints of left foot
      M93.279 Osteochondritis dissecans, unspecified ankle and joints of foot

      M93.28 Osteochondritis dissecans other site
      M93.29 Osteochondritis dissecans multiple sites

✓5ᵗʰ **M93.8** Other specified osteochondropathies

      M93.80 Other specified osteochondropathies of unspecified site

✓6ᵗʰ **M93.81** Other specified osteochondropathies of shoulder

      M93.811 Other specified osteochondropathies, right shoulder
      M93.812 Other specified osteochondropathies, left shoulder
      M93.819 Other specified osteochondropathies, unspecified shoulder

✓6ᵗʰ **M93.82** Other specified osteochondropathies of upper arm

      M93.821 Other specified osteochondropathies, right upper arm
      M93.822 Other specified osteochondropathies, left upper arm
      M93.829 Other specified osteochondropathies, unspecified upper arm

✓6ᵗʰ **M93.83** Other specified osteochondropathies of forearm

      M93.831 Other specified osteochondropathies, right forearm
      M93.832 Other specified osteochondropathies, left forearm
      M93.839 Other specified osteochondropathies, unspecified forearm

✓6ᵗʰ **M93.84** Other specified osteochondropathies of hand

      M93.841 Other specified osteochondropathies, right hand
      M93.842 Other specified osteochondropathies, left hand
      M93.849 Other specified osteochondropathies, unspecified hand

✓6ᵗʰ **M93.85** Other specified osteochondropathies of thigh

      M93.851 Other specified osteochondropathies, right thigh
      M93.852 Other specified osteochondropathies, left thigh
      M93.859 Other specified osteochondropathies, unspecified thigh

✓6ᵗʰ **M93.86** Other specified osteochondropathies lower leg

      M93.861 Other specified osteochondropathies, right lower leg
      M93.862 Other specified osteochondropathies, left lower leg
      M93.869 Other specified osteochondropathies, unspecified lower leg

✓6ᵗʰ **M93.87** Other specified osteochondropathies of ankle and foot

      M93.871 Other specified osteochondropathies, right ankle and foot
      M93.872 Other specified osteochondropathies, left ankle and foot
      M93.879 Other specified osteochondropathies, unspecified ankle and foot

      M93.88 Other specified osteochondropathies other site
      M93.89 Other specified osteochondropathies multiple sites

✓6ᵗʰ **M93.9** **Osteochondropathy, unspecified**
    Apophysitis NOS
    Epiphysitis NOS
    Osteochondritis NOS
    Osteochondrosis NOS

    M93.90 **Osteochondropathy, unspecified of unspecified site**

    ✓6ᵗʰ **M93.91** **Osteochondropathy, unspecified of shoulder**
      M93.911 **Osteochondropathy, unspecified, right shoulder**
      M93.912 **Osteochondropathy, unspecified, left shoulder**
      M93.919 **Osteochondropathy, unspecified, unspecified shoulder**

    ✓6ᵗʰ **M93.92** **Osteochondropathy, unspecified of upper arm**
      M93.921 **Osteochondropathy, unspecified, right upper arm**
      M93.922 **Osteochondropathy, unspecified, left upper arm**
      M93.929 **Osteochondropathy, unspecified, unspecified upper arm**

    ✓6ᵗʰ **M93.93** **Osteochondropathy, unspecified of forearm**
      M93.931 **Osteochondropathy, unspecified, right forearm**
      M93.932 **Osteochondropathy, unspecified, left forearm**
      M93.939 **Osteochondropathy, unspecified, unspecified forearm**

    ✓6ᵗʰ **M93.94** **Osteochondropathy, unspecified of hand**
      M93.941 **Osteochondropathy, unspecified, right hand**
      M93.942 **Osteochondropathy, unspecified, left hand**
      M93.949 **Osteochondropathy, unspecified, unspecified hand**

    ✓6ᵗʰ **M93.95** **Osteochondropathy, unspecified of thigh**
      M93.951 **Osteochondropathy, unspecified, right thigh**
      M93.952 **Osteochondropathy, unspecified, left thigh**
      M93.959 **Osteochondropathy, unspecified, unspecified thigh**

    ✓6ᵗʰ **M93.96** **Osteochondropathy, unspecified lower leg**
      M93.961 **Osteochondropathy, unspecified, right lower leg**
      M93.962 **Osteochondropathy, unspecified, left lower leg**
      M93.969 **Osteochondropathy, unspecified, unspecified lower leg**

    ✓6ᵗʰ **M93.97** **Osteochondropathy, unspecified of ankle and foot**
      M93.971 **Osteochondropathy, unspecified, right ankle and foot**
      M93.972 **Osteochondropathy, unspecified, left ankle and foot**
      M93.979 **Osteochondropathy, unspecified, unspecified ankle and foot**

    M93.98 **Osteochondropathy, unspecified other site**
    M93.99 **Osteochondropathy, unspecified multiple sites**

✓4ᵗʰ **M94** **Other disorders of cartilage**

    M94.0 **Chondrocostal junction syndrome [Tietze]**
      Costochondritis

    M94.1 **Relapsing polychondritis**

    ✓5ᵗʰ **M94.2** **Chondromalacia**
      EXCLUDES 1   *chondromalacia patellae (M22.4)*

      M94.20 **Chondromalacia, unspecified site**

      ✓6ᵗʰ **M94.21** **Chondromalacia, shoulder**
        M94.211 **Chondromalacia, right shoulder**
        M94.212 **Chondromalacia, left shoulder**
        M94.219 **Chondromalacia, unspecified shoulder**

      ✓6ᵗʰ **M94.22** **Chondromalacia, elbow**
        M94.221 **Chondromalacia, right elbow**
        M94.222 **Chondromalacia, left elbow**
        M94.229 **Chondromalacia, unspecified elbow**

      ✓6ᵗʰ **M94.23** **Chondromalacia, wrist**
        M94.231 **Chondromalacia, right wrist**
        M94.232 **Chondromalacia, left wrist**
        M94.239 **Chondromalacia, unspecified wrist**

      ✓6ᵗʰ **M94.24** **Chondromalacia, joints of hand**
        M94.241 **Chondromalacia, joints of right hand**
        M94.242 **Chondromalacia, joints of left hand**
        M94.249 **Chondromalacia, joints of unspecified hand**

      ✓6ᵗʰ **M94.25** **Chondromalacia, hip**
        M94.251 **Chondromalacia, right hip**
        M94.252 **Chondromalacia, left hip**
        M94.259 **Chondromalacia, unspecified hip**

      ✓6ᵗʰ **M94.26** **Chondromalacia, knee**
        M94.261 **Chondromalacia, right knee**
        M94.262 **Chondromalacia, left knee**
        M94.269 **Chondromalacia, unspecified knee**

      ✓6ᵗʰ **M94.27** **Chondromalacia, ankle and joints of foot**
        M94.271 **Chondromalacia, right ankle and joints of right foot**
        M94.272 **Chondromalacia, left ankle and joints of left foot**
        M94.279 **Chondromalacia, unspecified ankle and joints of foot**

      M94.28 **Chondromalacia, other site**
      M94.29 **Chondromalacia, multiple sites**

    ✓5ᵗʰ **M94.3** **Chondrolysis**
      Code first any associated slipped upper femoral epiphysis (nontraumatic) (M93.0-)

      ✓6ᵗʰ **M94.35** **Chondrolysis, hip**
        M94.351 **Chondrolysis, right hip**
        M94.352 **Chondrolysis, left hip**
        M94.359 **Chondrolysis, unspecified hip**

    ✓5ᵗʰ **M94.8** **Other specified disorders of cartilage**
      ✓6ᵗʰ **M94.8X** **Other specified disorders of cartilage**
        M94.8X0 **Other specified disorders of cartilage, multiple sites**
        M94.8X1 **Other specified disorders of cartilage, shoulder**
        M94.8X2 **Other specified disorders of cartilage, upper arm**
        M94.8X3 **Other specified disorders of cartilage, forearm**
        M94.8X4 **Other specified disorders of cartilage, hand**
        M94.8X5 **Other specified disorders of cartilage, thigh**
        M94.8X6 **Other specified disorders of cartilage, lower leg**
        M94.8X7 **Other specified disorders of cartilage, ankle and foot**
        M94.8X8 **Other specified disorders of cartilage, other site**
        M94.8X9 **Other specified disorders of cartilage, unspecified sites**

    M94.9 **Disorder of cartilage, unspecified**

Other disorders of the musculoskeletal system and connective tissue (M95)

✓4ᵗʰ **M95** **Other acquired deformities of musculoskeletal system and connective tissue**
    EXCLUDES 2   *acquired absence of limbs and organs (Z89-Z90)*
        acquired deformities of limbs (M20-M21)
        congenital malformations and deformations of the musculoskeletal system (Q65-Q79)
        deforming dorsopathies (M40-M43)
        dentofacial anomalies [including malocclusion] (M26.-)
        postprocedural musculoskeletal disorders (M96.-)

    M95.0 **Acquired deformity of nose**
      EXCLUDES 2   *deviated nasal septum (J34.2)*

    ✓5ᵗʰ **M95.1** **Cauliflower ear**
      EXCLUDES 2   *other acquired deformities of ear (H61.1)*
      DEF: Acquired deformity of the external ear due to injury or subsequent perichondritis.

      M95.10 **Cauliflower ear, unspecified ear**
      M95.11 **Cauliflower ear, right ear**
      M95.12 **Cauliflower ear, left ear**

    M95.2 **Other acquired deformity of head**
      AHA: 2022, 1Q, 34

    M95.3 **Acquired deformity of neck**

M95.4 **Acquired** deformity of chest and rib
    AHA: 2022,2Q,14; 2014,4Q,26-27

M95.5 **Acquired** deformity of pelvis
    EXCLUDES 1   *maternal care for known or suspected disproportion (O33.-)*

M95.8 **Other specified acquired deformities of musculoskeletal system**

M95.9 **Acquired deformity of musculoskeletal system, unspecified**

Intraoperative and postprocedural complications and disorders of musculoskeletal system, not elsewhere classified (M96)

✓4ᵗʰ M96 **Intraoperative and postprocedural complications and disorders of musculoskeletal system, not elsewhere classified**
    EXCLUDES 2   *arthropathy following intestinal bypass (M02.0-)*
        complications of internal orthopedic prosthetic devices, implants and grafts (T84.-)
        disorders associated with osteoporosis (M80)
        periprosthetic fracture around internal prosthetic joint (M97.-)
        presence of functional implants and other devices (Z96-Z97)

M96.0 **Pseudarthrosis after fusion or arthrodesis**

M96.1 **Postlaminectomy syndrome, not elsewhere classified**

M96.2 **Postradiation kyphosis**

M96.3 **Postlaminectomy kyphosis**

M96.4 **Postsurgical lordosis**

M96.5 **Postradiation scoliosis**

✓5ᵗʰ M96.6 **Fracture of bone following insertion of orthopedic implant, joint prosthesis, or bone plate**
    Intraoperative fracture of bone during insertion of orthopedic implant, joint prosthesis, or bone plate
    EXCLUDES 2   *complication of internal orthopedic devices, implants or grafts (T84.-)*

  ✓6ᵗʰ M96.62 **Fracture of** humerus **following insertion of orthopedic implant, joint prosthesis, or bone plate**
     M96.621 **Fracture of humerus following insertion of orthopedic implant, joint prosthesis, or bone plate,** right **arm** `HCC` `ESR`
     M96.622 **Fracture of humerus following insertion of orthopedic implant, joint prosthesis, or bone plate,** left **arm** `HCC` `ESR`
     M96.629 **Fracture of humerus following insertion of orthopedic implant, joint prosthesis, or bone plate, unspecified arm** `HCC` `ESR`

  ✓6ᵗʰ M96.63 **Fracture of** radius or ulna **following insertion of orthopedic implant, joint prosthesis, or bone plate**
     M96.631 **Fracture of radius or ulna following insertion of orthopedic implant, joint prosthesis, or bone plate,** right **arm** `HCC` `ESR`
     M96.632 **Fracture of radius or ulna following insertion of orthopedic implant, joint prosthesis, or bone plate,** left **arm** `HCC` `ESR`
     M96.639 **Fracture of radius or ulna following insertion of orthopedic implant, joint prosthesis, or bone plate, unspecified arm** `HCC` `ESR`

  M96.65 **Fracture of** pelvis **following insertion of orthopedic implant, joint prosthesis, or bone plate** `HCC` `ESR`

  ✓6ᵗʰ M96.66 **Fracture of** femur **following insertion of orthopedic implant, joint prosthesis, or bone plate**
     M96.661 **Fracture of femur following insertion of orthopedic implant, joint prosthesis, or bone plate,** right **leg** `HCC` `ESR`
     M96.662 **Fracture of femur following insertion of orthopedic implant, joint prosthesis, or bone plate,** left **leg** `HCC` `ESR`
     M96.669 **Fracture of femur following insertion of orthopedic implant, joint prosthesis, or bone plate, unspecified leg** `HCC` `ESR`

  ✓6ᵗʰ M96.67 **Fracture of** tibia or fibula **following insertion of orthopedic implant, joint prosthesis, or bone plate**
     M96.671 **Fracture of tibia or fibula following insertion of orthopedic implant, joint prosthesis, or bone plate,** right **leg** `HCC` `ESR`

M96.672 **Fracture of tibia or fibula following insertion of orthopedic implant, joint prosthesis, or bone plate,** left **leg** `HCC` `ESR`

M96.679 **Fracture of tibia or fibula following insertion of orthopedic implant, joint prosthesis, or bone plate, unspecified leg** `HCC` `ESR`

M96.69 **Fracture of other bone following insertion of orthopedic implant, joint prosthesis, or bone plate** `HCC` `ESR`

✓5ᵗʰ M96.8 **Other intraoperative and postprocedural complications and disorders of musculoskeletal system, not elsewhere classified**
    AHA: 2016,4Q,9-10

  ✓6ᵗʰ M96.81 Intraoperative hemorrhage and hematoma **of a musculoskeletal structure complicating a procedure**
    EXCLUDES 1   *intraoperative hemorrhage and hematoma of a musculoskeletal structure due to accidental puncture and laceration during a procedure (M96.82-)*
     M96.810 **Intraoperative hemorrhage and hematoma of a musculoskeletal structure complicating a** musculoskeletal system procedure
     M96.811 **Intraoperative hemorrhage and hematoma of a musculoskeletal structure complicating** other procedure

  ✓6ᵗʰ M96.82 Accidental puncture and laceration **of a musculoskeletal structure during a procedure**
     M96.820 **Accidental puncture and laceration of a musculoskeletal structure during a** musculoskeletal system procedure
     M96.821 **Accidental puncture and laceration of a musculoskeletal structure during** other procedure

  ✓6ᵗʰ M96.83 Postprocedural hemorrhage **of a musculoskeletal structure following a procedure**
     M96.830 **Postprocedural hemorrhage of a musculoskeletal structure following a** musculoskeletal system procedure
     M96.831 **Postprocedural hemorrhage of a musculoskeletal structure following** other procedure

  ✓6ᵗʰ M96.84 Postprocedural hematoma and seroma **of a musculoskeletal structure following a procedure**
     M96.840 **Postprocedural** hematoma **of a musculoskeletal structure following a** musculoskeletal system procedure
     M96.841 **Postprocedural** hematoma **of a musculoskeletal structure following** other procedure
       AHA: 2016,4Q,10
     M96.842 **Postprocedural** seroma **of a musculoskeletal structure following a** musculoskeletal system procedure
     M96.843 **Postprocedural** seroma **of a musculoskeletal structure following** other procedure
       AHA: 2018,3Q,6

  M96.89 **Other intraoperative and postprocedural complications and disorders of the musculoskeletal system**
    Instability of joint secondary to removal of joint prosthesis
    Use additional code, if applicable, to further specify disorder
    AHA: 2022,2Q,14; 2021,1Q,5

● **✓5ᵗʰ M96.A** **Fracture of ribs, sternum and thorax** associated with compression of the chest and cardiopulmonary resuscitation

● **M96.A1** **Fracture of sternum** associated with chest compression and cardiopulmonary resuscitation
    Fracture of xiphoid process associated with chest compression and cardiopulmonary resuscitation

● **M96.A2** **Fracture of one rib** associated with chest compression and cardiopulmonary resuscitation

● **M96.A3** **Multiple fractures of ribs** associated with chest compression and cardiopulmonary resuscitation

● **M96.A4** **Flail chest** associated with chest compression and cardiopulmonary resuscitation

● **M96.A9** **Other fracture** associated with chest compression and cardiopulmonary resuscitation

---

✅ Additional Character Required   ✓x7ᵗʰ Placeholder Alert   Manifestation   Unspecified Dx   🅠 QPP   🆄🅿🅳 Unacceptable PDx

Periprosthetic fractures around internal prosthetic joint (M97)

✓4ᵗʰ M97 Periprosthetic fracture around internal prosthetic joint

EXCLUDES 2   breakage (fracture) of prosthetic joint (T84.01-)
fracture of bone following insertion of orthopedic implant, joint prosthesis or bone plate (M96.6-)

AHA: 2016,4Q,42-43

> The appropriate 7th character is to be added to each code from category M97.
> A initial encounter
> D subsequent encounter
> S sequela

✓5ᵗʰ M97.0 Periprosthetic fracture around internal prosthetic hip joint
AHA: 2018,1Q,21; 2016,4Q,42

¹ **✓x7ᵗʰ M97.01 Periprosthetic fracture around internal prosthetic right hip joint**   HCC ESR Q

¹ **✓x7ᵗʰ M97.02 Periprosthetic fracture around internal prosthetic left hip joint**   HCC ESR Q

✓5ᵗʰ M97.1 Periprosthetic fracture around internal prosthetic knee joint

✓x7ᵗʰ M97.11 Periprosthetic fracture around internal prosthetic right knee joint   Q

✓x7ᵗʰ M97.12 Periprosthetic fracture around internal prosthetic left knee joint   Q

✓5ᵗʰ M97.2 Periprosthetic fracture around internal prosthetic ankle joint

✓x7ᵗʰ M97.21 Periprosthetic fracture around internal prosthetic right ankle joint   Q

✓x7ᵗʰ M97.22 Periprosthetic fracture around internal prosthetic left ankle joint   Q

✓5ᵗʰ M97.3 Periprosthetic fracture around internal prosthetic shoulder joint

✓x7ᵗʰ M97.31 Periprosthetic fracture around internal prosthetic right shoulder joint   Q

✓x7ᵗʰ M97.32 Periprosthetic fracture around internal prosthetic left shoulder joint   Q

✓5ᵗʰ M97.4 Periprosthetic fracture around internal prosthetic elbow joint

✓x7ᵗʰ M97.41 Periprosthetic fracture around internal prosthetic right elbow joint   Q

✓x7ᵗʰ M97.42 Periprosthetic fracture around internal prosthetic left elbow joint   Q

✓x7ᵗʰ M97.8 Periprosthetic fracture around other internal prosthetic joint
Periprosthetic fracture around internal prosthetic finger joint
Periprosthetic fracture around internal prosthetic spinal joint
Periprosthetic fracture around internal prosthetic toe joint
Periprosthetic fracture around internal prosthetic wrist joint
Use additional code to identify the joint (Z96.6-)

✓x7ᵗʰ M97.9 Periprosthetic fracture around unspecified internal prosthetic joint

Biomechanical lesions, not elsewhere classified (M99)

✓4ᵗʰ M99 Biomechanical lesions, not elsewhere classified

NOTE   This category should not be used if the condition can be classified elsewhere.

DEF: Biomechanical lesion: Term used by osteopathic and chiropractic physicians to describe musculoskeletal conditions treated that are not more appropriately classified elsewhere.

✓6ᵗʰ M99.0 Segmental and somatic dysfunction
M99.00 Segmental and somatic dysfunction of head region
M99.01 Segmental and somatic dysfunction of cervical region
M99.02 Segmental and somatic dysfunction of thoracic region
M99.03 Segmental and somatic dysfunction of lumbar region
M99.04 Segmental and somatic dysfunction of sacral region
M99.05 Segmental and somatic dysfunction of pelvic region
M99.06 Segmental and somatic dysfunction of lower extremity
M99.07 Segmental and somatic dysfunction of upper extremity
M99.08 Segmental and somatic dysfunction of rib cage
M99.09 Segmental and somatic dysfunction of abdomen and other regions

✓5ᵗʰ M99.1 Subluxation complex (vertebral)
M99.10 Subluxation complex (vertebral) of head region

M99.11 Subluxation complex (vertebral) of cervical region
M99.12 Subluxation complex (vertebral) of thoracic region
M99.13 Subluxation complex (vertebral) of lumbar region
M99.14 Subluxation complex (vertebral) of sacral region
M99.15 Subluxation complex (vertebral) of pelvic region
M99.16 Subluxation complex (vertebral) of lower extremity
M99.17 Subluxation complex (vertebral) of upper extremity
M99.18 Subluxation complex (vertebral) of rib cage
M99.19 Subluxation complex (vertebral) of abdomen and other regions

✓5ᵗʰ M99.2 Subluxation stenosis of neural canal
M99.20 Subluxation stenosis of neural canal of head region
M99.21 Subluxation stenosis of neural canal of cervical region
M99.22 Subluxation stenosis of neural canal of thoracic region
M99.23 Subluxation stenosis of neural canal of lumbar region
M99.24 Subluxation stenosis of neural canal of sacral region
M99.25 Subluxation stenosis of neural canal of pelvic region
M99.26 Subluxation stenosis of neural canal of lower extremity
M99.27 Subluxation stenosis of neural canal of upper extremity
M99.28 Subluxation stenosis of neural canal of rib cage
M99.29 Subluxation stenosis of neural canal of abdomen and other regions

✓5ᵗʰ M99.3 Osseous stenosis of neural canal
M99.30 Osseous stenosis of neural canal of head region
M99.31 Osseous stenosis of neural canal of cervical region
M99.32 Osseous stenosis of neural canal of thoracic region
M99.33 Osseous stenosis of neural canal of lumbar region
M99.34 Osseous stenosis of neural canal of sacral region
M99.35 Osseous stenosis of neural canal of pelvic region
M99.36 Osseous stenosis of neural canal of lower extremity
M99.37 Osseous stenosis of neural canal of upper extremity
M99.38 Osseous stenosis of neural canal of rib cage
M99.39 Osseous stenosis of neural canal of abdomen and other regions

✓5ᵗʰ M99.4 Connective tissue stenosis of neural canal
M99.40 Connective tissue stenosis of neural canal of head region
M99.41 Connective tissue stenosis of neural canal of cervical region
M99.42 Connective tissue stenosis of neural canal of thoracic region
M99.43 Connective tissue stenosis of neural canal of lumbar region
M99.44 Connective tissue stenosis of neural canal of sacral region
M99.45 Connective tissue stenosis of neural canal of pelvic region
M99.46 Connective tissue stenosis of neural canal of lower extremity
M99.47 Connective tissue stenosis of neural canal of upper extremity
M99.48 Connective tissue stenosis of neural canal of rib cage
M99.49 Connective tissue stenosis of neural canal of abdomen and other regions

✓5ᵗʰ M99.5 Intervertebral disc stenosis of neural canal
M99.50 Intervertebral disc stenosis of neural canal of head region
M99.51 Intervertebral disc stenosis of neural canal of cervical region
M99.52 Intervertebral disc stenosis of neural canal of thoracic region
M99.53 Intervertebral disc stenosis of neural canal of lumbar region
M99.54 Intervertebral disc stenosis of neural canal of sacral region
M99.55 Intervertebral disc stenosis of neural canal of pelvic region
M99.56 Intervertebral disc stenosis of neural canal of lower extremity
M99.57 Intervertebral disc stenosis of neural canal of upper extremity
M99.58 Intervertebral disc stenosis of neural canal of rib cage

M99.59   **Intervertebral disc stenosis of neural canal of** abdomen and other **regions**

✓5ᵗʰ **M99.6   Osseous and subluxation stenosis of intervertebral foramina**

M99.60   **Osseous and subluxation stenosis of intervertebral foramina of** head **region**

M99.61   **Osseous and subluxation stenosis of intervertebral foramina of** cervical **region**

M99.62   **Osseous and subluxation stenosis of intervertebral foramina of** thoracic **region**

M99.63   **Osseous and subluxation stenosis of intervertebral foramina of** lumbar **region**

M99.64   **Osseous and subluxation stenosis of intervertebral foramina of** sacral **region**

M99.65   **Osseous and subluxation stenosis of intervertebral foramina of** pelvic **region**

M99.66   **Osseous and subluxation stenosis of intervertebral foramina of** lower extremity

M99.67   **Osseous and subluxation stenosis of intervertebral foramina of** upper extremity

M99.68   **Osseous and subluxation stenosis of intervertebral foramina of** rib cage

M99.69   **Osseous and subluxation stenosis of intervertebral foramina of** abdomen and other **regions**

✓5ᵗʰ **M99.7   Connective tissue and disc stenosis of intervertebral foramina**

M99.70   **Connective tissue and disc stenosis of intervertebral foramina of** head **region**

M99.71   **Connective tissue and disc stenosis of intervertebral foramina of** cervical **region**

M99.72   **Connective tissue and disc stenosis of intervertebral foramina of** thoracic **region**

M99.73   **Connective tissue and disc stenosis of intervertebral foramina of** lumbar **region**

M99.74   **Connective tissue and disc stenosis of intervertebral foramina of** sacral **region**

M99.75   **Connective tissue and disc stenosis of intervertebral foramina of** pelvic **region**

M99.76   **Connective tissue and disc stenosis of intervertebral foramina of** lower extremity

M99.77   **Connective tissue and disc stenosis of intervertebral foramina of** upper extremity

M99.78   **Connective tissue and disc stenosis of intervertebral foramina of** rib cage

M99.79   **Connective tissue and disc stenosis of intervertebral foramina of** abdomen and other **regions**

✓5ᵗʰ **M99.8   Other biomechanical lesions**

M99.80   **Other biomechanical lesions of** head region

M99.81   **Other biomechanical lesions of** cervical **region**

M99.82   **Other biomechanical lesions of** thoracic **region**

M99.83   **Other biomechanical lesions of** lumbar **region**

M99.84   **Other biomechanical lesions of** sacral **region**

M99.85   **Other biomechanical lesions of** pelvic **region**

M99.86   **Other biomechanical lesions of** lower extremity

M99.87   **Other biomechanical lesions of** upper extremity

M99.88   **Other biomechanical lesions of** rib cage

M99.89   **Other biomechanical lesions of** abdomen and other **regions**

M99.9   Biomechanical lesion, unspecified

☑ Additional Character Required   ✓x7ᵗʰ Placeholder Alert   Manifestation   Unspecified Dx   ᐤ QPP   UPD Unacceptable PDx

Chapter 14. Diseases of Genitourinary System (N00–N99)

Chapter-specific Guidelines with Coding Examples

The chapter-specific guidelines from the ICD-10-CM Official Guidelines for Coding and Reporting have been provided below. Along with these guidelines are coding examples, contained in the shaded boxes, that have been developed to help illustrate the coding and/or sequencing guidance found in these guidelines.

a. Chronic kidney disease

1) Stages of chronic kidney disease (CKD)

The ICD-10-CM classifies CKD based on severity. The severity of CKD is designated by stages 1-5. Stage 2, code N18.2, equates to mild CKD; stage 3, codes N18.30-N18.32, equate to moderate CKD; and stage 4, code N18.4, equates to severe CKD. Code N18.6, End stage renal disease (ESRD), is assigned when the provider has documented end-stage renal disease (ESRD).

If both a stage of CKD and ESRD are documented, assign code N18.6 only.

Stage 5 chronic kidney disease with ESRD requiring chronic dialysis

N18.6   **End stage renal disease**

Z99.2   **Dependence on renal dialysis**

Explanation: The diagnostic statement indicates the patient has chronic kidney disease, documented both as stage 5 and as ESRD requiring chronic dialysis. Code N18.6 End stage renal disease (ESRD), is assigned when the provider has documented end-stage-renal disease (ESRD). If both a stage of CKD and ESRD are documented, assign code N18.6 only.

2) Chronic kidney disease and kidney transplant status

Patients who have undergone kidney transplant may still have some form of chronic kidney disease (CKD) because the kidney transplant may not fully restore kidney function. Therefore, the presence of CKD alone does not constitute a transplant complication. Assign the appropriate N18 code for the patient's stage of CKD and code Z94.0, Kidney transplant status. If a transplant complication such as failure or rejection or other transplant complication is documented, see section I.C.19.g for information on coding complications of a kidney transplant. If the documentation is unclear as to whether the patient has a complication of the transplant, query the provider.

Patient with residual chronic kidney disease stage 1 after kidney transplant

N18.1   **Chronic kidney disease, stage 1**

Z94.0   **Kidney transplant status**

Explanation: Patients who have undergone kidney transplant may still have some form of chronic kidney disease (CKD) because the kidney transplant may not fully restore kidney function. The presence of CKD alone does not constitute a transplant complication. Assign the appropriate N18 code for the patient's stage of CKD and code Z94.0 Kidney transplant status.

3) Chronic kidney disease with other conditions

Patients with CKD may also suffer from other serious conditions, most commonly diabetes mellitus and hypertension. The sequencing of the CKD code in relationship to codes for other contributing conditions is based on the conventions in the Tabular List.

See I.C.9. Hypertensive chronic kidney disease.

See I.C.19. Chronic kidney disease and kidney transplant complications.

Type 1 diabetic chronic kidney disease, stage 2

E10.22   **Type 1 diabetes mellitus with diabetic chronic kidney disease**

N18.2   **Chronic kidney disease, stage 2 (mild)**

Explanation: Patients with CKD may also suffer from other serious conditions such as diabetes mellitus. The sequencing of the CKD code in relationship to codes for other contributing conditions is based on the conventions in the Tabular List. Diabetic CKD code E10.22 includes an instructional note to "Use additional code to identify stage of chronic kidney disease (N18.1–N18.6)," thus providing sequencing direction.

Chapter 14. Diseases of the Genitourinary System (N00-N99)

EXCLUDES 2
certain conditions originating in the perinatal period (P04-P96)
certain infectious and parasitic diseases (A00-B99)
complications of pregnancy, childbirth and the puerperium (O00-O9A)
congenital malformations, deformations and chromosomal abnormalities (Q00-Q99)
endocrine, nutritional and metabolic diseases (E00-E88)
injury, poisoning and certain other consequences of external causes (S00-T88)
neoplasms (C00-D49)
symptoms, signs and abnormal clinical and laboratory findings, not elsewhere classified (R00-R94)

This chapter contains the following blocks:

N00-N08   Glomerular diseases
N10-N16   Renal tubulo-interstitial diseases
N17-N19   Acute kidney failure and chronic kidney disease
N20-N23   Urolithiasis
N25-N29   Other disorders of kidney and ureter
N30-N39   Other diseases of the urinary system
N40-N53   Diseases of male genital organs
N60-N65   Disorders of breast
N70-N77   Inflammatory diseases of female pelvic organs
N80-N98   Noninflammatory disorders of female genital tract
N99   Intraoperative and postprocedural complications and disorders of genitourinary system, not elsewhere classified

Glomerular diseases (N00-N08)

Code also any associated kidney failure (N17-N19).
EXCLUDES 1   hypertensive chronic kidney disease (I12.-)
AHA: 2020,4Q,34-35
DEF: Glomeruli: Clusters of microscopic blood vessels located within the kidneys containing small pores through which waste products are filtered from the blood and urine is formed.
DEF: Glomerulonephritis: Disease of the kidney with diffuse inflammation of the capillary loops of the glomeruli.

✓4ᵗʰ N00   Acute nephritic syndrome

INCLUDES   acute glomerular disease
acute glomerulonephritis
acute nephritis
EXCLUDES 1   acute tubulo-interstitial nephritis (N10)
nephritic syndrome NOS (N05.-)

AHA: 2021,1Q,23

N00.0   Acute nephritic syndrome with minor glomerular abnormality
Acute nephritic syndrome with minimal change lesion

N00.1   Acute nephritic syndrome with focal and segmental glomerular lesions
Acute nephritic syndrome with focal and segmental hyalinosis
Acute nephritic syndrome with focal and segmental sclerosis
Acute nephritic syndrome with focal glomerulonephritis

N00.2   Acute nephritic syndrome with diffuse membranous glomerulonephritis

N00.3   Acute nephritic syndrome with diffuse mesangial proliferative glomerulonephritis

N00.4   Acute nephritic syndrome with diffuse endocapillary proliferative glomerulonephritis

N00.5   Acute nephritic syndrome with diffuse mesangiocapillary glomerulonephritis
Acute nephritic syndrome with membranoproliferative glomerulonephritis, types 1 and 3, or NOS
EXCLUDES 1   acute nephritic syndrome with C3 glomerulonephritis (N00.A)
acute nephritic syndrome with C3 glomerulopathy (N00.A)

N00.6   Acute nephritic syndrome with dense deposit disease
Acute nephritic syndrome with C3 glomerulopathy with dense deposit disease
Acute nephritic syndrome with membranoproliferative glomerulonephritis, type 2

N00.7   Acute nephritic syndrome with diffuse crescentic glomerulonephritis
Acute nephritic syndrome with extracapillary glomerulonephritis

N00.8   Acute nephritic syndrome with other morphologic changes
Acute nephritic syndrome with proliferative glomerulonephritis NOS

N00.9   Acute nephritic syndrome with unspecified morphologic changes

N00.A   Acute nephritic syndrome with C3 glomerulonephritis
Acute nephritic syndrome with C3 glomerulopathy, NOS
EXCLUDES 1   acute nephritic syndrome (with C3 glomerulopathy) with dense deposit disease (N00.6)

✓4ᵗʰ N01   Rapidly progressive nephritic syndrome

INCLUDES   rapidly progressive glomerular disease
rapidly progressive glomerulonephritis
rapidly progressive nephritis
EXCLUDES 1   nephritic syndrome NOS (N05.-)

AHA: 2021,1Q,23

N01.0   Rapidly progressive nephritic syndrome with minor glomerular abnormality
Rapidly progressive nephritic syndrome with minimal change lesion

N01.1   Rapidly progressive nephritic syndrome with focal and segmental glomerular lesions
Rapidly progressive nephritic syndrome with focal and segmental hyalinosis
Rapidly progressive nephritic syndrome with focal and segmental sclerosis
Rapidly progressive nephritic syndrome with focal glomerulonephritis

N01.2   Rapidly progressive nephritic syndrome with diffuse membranous glomerulonephritis

N01.3   Rapidly progressive nephritic syndrome with diffuse mesangial proliferative glomerulonephritis

N01.4   Rapidly progressive nephritic syndrome with diffuse endocapillary proliferative glomerulonephritis

N01.5   Rapidly progressive nephritic syndrome with diffuse mesangiocapillary glomerulonephritis
Rapidly progressive nephritic syndrome with membranoproliferative glomerulonephritis, types 1 and 3, or NOS
EXCLUDES 1   rapidly progressive nephritic syndrome with C3 glomerulonephritis (N01.A)
rapidly progressive nephritic syndrome with C3 glomerulopathy (N01.A)

N01.6   Rapidly progressive nephritic syndrome with dense deposit disease
Rapidly progressive nephritic syndrome with C3 glomerulopathy with dense deposit disease
Rapidly progressive nephritic syndrome with membranoproliferative glomerulonephritis, type 2

N01.7   Rapidly progressive nephritic syndrome with diffuse crescentic glomerulonephritis
Rapidly progressive nephritic syndrome with extracapillary glomerulonephritis

N01.8   Rapidly progressive nephritic syndrome with other morphologic changes
Rapidly progressive nephritic syndrome with proliferative glomerulonephritis NOS

N01.9   Rapidly progressive nephritic syndrome with unspecified morphologic changes

N01.A   Rapidly progressive nephritic syndrome with C3 glomerulonephritis
Rapidly progressive nephritic syndrome with C3 glomerulopathy, NOS
EXCLUDES 1   rapidly progressive nephritic syndrome (with C3 glomerulopathy) with dense deposit disease (N01.6)

✓4ᵗʰ N02   Recurrent and persistent hematuria

EXCLUDES 1   acute cystitis with hematuria (N30.01)
hematuria NOS (R31.9)
hematuria not associated with specified morphologic lesions (R31.-)

N02.0   Recurrent and persistent hematuria with minor glomerular abnormality
Recurrent and persistent hematuria with minimal change lesion

N02.1   Recurrent and persistent hematuria with focal and segmental glomerular lesions
Recurrent and persistent hematuria with focal and segmental hyalinosis
Recurrent and persistent hematuria with focal and segmental sclerosis
Recurrent and persistent hematuria with focal glomerulonephritis

N02.2   Recurrent and persistent hematuria with diffuse membranous glomerulonephritis

N02.3 Recurrent and persistent hematuria with diffuse mesangial proliferative glomerulonephritis

N02.4 Recurrent and persistent hematuria with diffuse endocapillary proliferative glomerulonephritis

N02.5 Recurrent and persistent hematuria with diffuse mesangiocapillary glomerulonephritis

Recurrent and persistent hematuria with membranoproliferative glomerulonephritis, types 1 and 3, or NOS

EXCLUDES 1   *recurrent and persistent hematuria with C3 glomerulonephritis (N02.A)*
recurrent and persistent hematuria with C3 glomerulopathy (N02.A)

N02.6 Recurrent and persistent hematuria with dense deposit disease

Recurrent and persistent hematuria with C3 glomerulopathy with dense deposit disease
Recurrent and persistent hematuria with membranoproliferative glomerulonephritis, type 2

N02.7 Recurrent and persistent hematuria with diffuse crescentic glomerulonephritis

Recurrent and persistent hematuria with extracapillary glomerulonephritis

N02.8 Recurrent and persistent hematuria with other morphologic changes

Recurrent and persistent hematuria with proliferative glomerulonephritis NOS

N02.9 Recurrent and persistent hematuria with unspecified morphologic changes

AHA: 2017,2Q,5

N02.A Recurrent and persistent hematuria with C3 glomerulonephritis

Recurrent and persistent hematuria with C3 glomerulopathy

EXCLUDES 1   *recurrent and persistent hematuria (with C3 glomerulopathy) with dense deposit disease (N02.6)*

☑4ᵗʰ N03 Chronic nephritic syndrome

INCLUDES   chronic glomerular disease
chronic glomerulonephritis
chronic nephritis

EXCLUDES 1   *chronic tubulo-interstitial nephritis (N11.-)*
diffuse sclerosing glomerulonephritis (N05.8-)
nephritic syndrome NOS (N05.-)

AHA: 2021,1Q,23

DEF: Slow, progressive type of nephritis characterized by inflammation of the capillary loops in the glomeruli of the kidney, which leads to renal failure.

N03.0 Chronic nephritic syndrome with minor glomerular abnormality

Chronic nephritic syndrome with minimal change lesion

N03.1 Chronic nephritic syndrome with focal and segmental glomerular lesions

Chronic nephritic syndrome with focal and segmental hyalinosis
Chronic nephritic syndrome with focal and segmental sclerosis
Chronic nephritic syndrome with focal glomerulonephritis

N03.2 Chronic nephritic syndrome with diffuse membranous glomerulonephritis

N03.3 Chronic nephritic syndrome with diffuse mesangial proliferative glomerulonephritis

N03.4 Chronic nephritic syndrome with diffuse endocapillary proliferative glomerulonephritis

N03.5 Chronic nephritic syndrome with diffuse mesangiocapillary glomerulonephritis

Chronic nephritic syndrome with membranoproliferative glomerulonephritis, types 1 and 3, or NOS

EXCLUDES 1   *chronic nephritic syndrome with C3 glomerulonephritis (N03.A)*
chronic nephritic syndrome with C3 glomerulopathy (N03.A)

N03.6 Chronic nephritic syndrome with dense deposit disease

Chronic nephritic syndrome with C3 glomerulopathy with dense deposit disease
Chronic nephritic syndrome with membranoproliferative glomerulonephritis, type 2

N03.7 Chronic nephritic syndrome with diffuse crescentic glomerulonephritis

Chronic nephritic syndrome with extracapillary glomerulonephritis

N03.8 Chronic nephritic syndrome with other morphologic changes

Chronic nephritic syndrome with proliferative glomerulonephritis NOS

N03.9 Chronic nephritic syndrome with unspecified morphologic changes

N03.A Chronic nephritic syndrome with C3 glomerulonephritis

Chronic nephritic syndrome with C3 glomerulopathy

EXCLUDES 1   *chronic nephritic syndrome (with C3 glomerulopathy) with dense deposit disease (N03.6)*

☑4ᵗʰ N04 Nephrotic syndrome

INCLUDES   congenital nephrotic syndrome
lipoid nephrosis

N04.0 Nephrotic syndrome with minor glomerular abnormality

Nephrotic syndrome with minimal change lesion

N04.1 Nephrotic syndrome with focal and segmental glomerular lesions

Nephrotic syndrome with focal and segmental hyalinosis
Nephrotic syndrome with focal and segmental sclerosis
Nephrotic syndrome with focal glomerulonephritis

N04.2 Nephrotic syndrome with diffuse membranous glomerulonephritis

N04.3 Nephrotic syndrome with diffuse mesangial proliferative glomerulonephritis

N04.4 Nephrotic syndrome with diffuse endocapillary proliferative glomerulonephritis

N04.5 Nephrotic syndrome with diffuse mesangiocapillary glomerulonephritis

Nephrotic syndrome with membranoproliferative glomerulonephritis, types 1 and 3, or NOS

EXCLUDES 1   *nephrotic syndrome with C3 glomerulonephritis (N04.A)*
nephrotic syndrome with C3 glomerulopathy (N04.A)

N04.6 Nephrotic syndrome with dense deposit disease

Nephrotic syndrome with C3 glomerulopathy with dense deposit disease
Nephrotic syndrome with membranoproliferative glomerulonephritis, type 2

N04.7 Nephrotic syndrome with diffuse crescentic glomerulonephritis

Nephrotic syndrome with extracapillary glomerulonephritis

N04.8 Nephrotic syndrome with other morphologic changes

Nephrotic syndrome with proliferative glomerulonephritis NOS

N04.9 Nephrotic syndrome with unspecified morphologic changes

N04.A Nephrotic syndrome with C3 glomerulonephritis

Nephrotic syndrome with C3 glomerulopathy

EXCLUDES 1   *nephrotic syndrome (with C3 glomerulopathy) with dense deposit disease (N04.6)*

☑4ᵗʰ N05 Unspecified nephritic syndrome

INCLUDES   glomerular disease NOS
glomerulonephritis NOS
nephritis NOS
nephropathy NOS and renal disease NOS with morphological lesion specified in .0-.8

EXCLUDES 1   *nephropathy NOS with no stated morphological lesion (N28.9)*
renal disease NOS with no stated morphological lesion (N28.9)
tubulo-interstitial nephritis NOS (N12)

N05.0 Unspecified nephritic syndrome with minor glomerular abnormality

Unspecified nephritic syndrome with minimal change lesion

N05.1 Unspecified nephritic syndrome with focal and segmental glomerular lesions

Unspecified nephritic syndrome with focal and segmental hyalinosis
Unspecified nephritic syndrome with focal and segmental sclerosis
Unspecified nephritic syndrome with focal glomerulonephritis

N05.2 Unspecified nephritic syndrome with diffuse membranous glomerulonephritis

N05.3 Unspecified nephritic syndrome with diffuse mesangial proliferative glomerulonephritis

N05.4 Unspecified nephritic syndrome with diffuse endocapillary proliferative glomerulonephritis

N05.5 **Unspecified nephritic syndrome with** diffuse mesangiocapillary glomerulonephritis

Unspecified nephritic syndrome with membranoproliferative glomerulonephritis, types 1 and 3, or NOS

> *EXCLUDES 1*   *unspecified nephritic syndrome with C3 glomerulonephritis (N05.A)*
> *unspecified nephritic syndrome with C3 glomerulopathy (N05.A)*

N05.6 **Unspecified nephritic syndrome with** dense deposit disease

Unspecified nephritic syndrome with C3 glomerulopathy with dense deposit disease

Unspecified nephritic syndrome with membranoproliferative glomerulonephritis, type 2

N05.7 **Unspecified nephritic syndrome with** diffuse crescentic glomerulonephritis

Unspecified nephritic syndrome with extracapillary glomerulonephritis

N05.8 **Unspecified nephritic syndrome with other morphologic changes**

Unspecified nephritic syndrome with proliferative glomerulonephritis NOS

N05.9 **Unspecified nephritic syndrome with unspecified morphologic changes**

N05.A **Unspecified nephritic syndrome with** C3 glomerulonephritis

Unspecified nephritic syndrome with C3 glomerulopathy

> *EXCLUDES 1*   *unspecified nephritic syndrome (with C3 glomerulopathy) with dense deposit disease (N05.6)*

✓4ᵗʰ **N06** **Isolated proteinuria with specified morphological lesion**

> *EXCLUDES 1*   *proteinuria not associated with specific morphologic lesions (R80.0)*

N06.0 **Isolated proteinuria with** minor glomerular abnormality

Isolated proteinuria with minimal change lesion

N06.1 **Isolated proteinuria with** focal and segmental glomerular lesions

Isolated proteinuria with focal and segmental hyalinosis

Isolated proteinuria with focal and segmental sclerosis

Isolated proteinuria with focal glomerulonephritis

N06.2 **Isolated proteinuria with** diffuse membranous glomerulonephritis

N06.3 **Isolated proteinuria with** diffuse mesangial proliferative glomerulonephritis

N06.4 **Isolated proteinuria with** diffuse endocapillary proliferative glomerulonephritis

N06.5 **Isolated proteinuria with** diffuse mesangiocapillary glomerulonephritis

Isolated proteinuria with membranoproliferative glomerulonephritis, types 1 and 3, or NOS

> *EXCLUDES 1*   *isolated proteinuria with C3 glomerulonephritis (N06.A)*
> *isolated proteinuria with C3 glomerulopathy (N06.A)*

N06.6 **Isolated proteinuria with** dense deposit disease

Isolated proteinuria with C3 glomerulopathy with dense deposit disease

Isolated proteinuria with membranoproliferative glomerulonephritis, type 2

N06.7 **Isolated proteinuria with** diffuse crescentic glomerulonephritis

Isolated proteinuria with extracapillary glomerulonephritis

N06.8 **Isolated proteinuria with other morphologic lesion**

Isolated proteinuria with proliferative glomerulonephritis NOS

N06.9 **Isolated proteinuria with unspecified morphologic lesion**

N06.A **Isolated proteinuria with** C3 glomerulonephritis

Isolated proteinuria with C3 glomerulopathy

> *EXCLUDES 1*   *isolated proteinuria (with C3 glomerulopathy) with dense deposit disease (N06.6)*

✓4ᵗʰ **N07** **Hereditary nephropathy, not elsewhere classified**

> *EXCLUDES 2*   *Alport's syndrome (Q87.81-)*
> *hereditary amyloid nephropathy (E85.-)*
> *nail patella syndrome (Q87.2)*
> *non-neuropathic heredofamilial amyloidosis (E85.-)*

N07.0 **Hereditary nephropathy, not elsewhere classified with** minor glomerular abnormality

Hereditary nephropathy, not elsewhere classified with minimal change lesion

N07.1 **Hereditary nephropathy, not elsewhere classified with** focal and segmental glomerular lesions

Hereditary nephropathy, not elsewhere classified with focal and segmental hyalinosis

Hereditary nephropathy, not elsewhere classified with focal and segmental sclerosis

Hereditary nephropathy, not elsewhere classified with focal glomerulonephritis

N07.2 **Hereditary nephropathy, not elsewhere classified with diffuse membranous glomerulonephritis**

N07.3 **Hereditary nephropathy, not elsewhere classified with diffuse mesangial proliferative glomerulonephritis**

N07.4 **Hereditary nephropathy, not elsewhere classified with diffuse endocapillary proliferative glomerulonephritis**

N07.5 **Hereditary nephropathy, not elsewhere classified with diffuse mesangiocapillary glomerulonephritis**

Hereditary nephropathy, not elsewhere classified with membranoproliferative glomerulonephritis, types 1 and 3, or NOS

> *EXCLUDES 1*   *hereditary nephropathy, not elsewhere classified with C3 glomerulonephritis (N07.A)*
> *hereditary nephropathy, not elsewhere classified with C3 glomerulopathy (N07.A)*

N07.6 **Hereditary nephropathy, not elsewhere classified with** dense deposit disease

Hereditary nephropathy, not elsewhere classified with C3 glomerulopathy with dense deposit disease

Hereditary nephropathy, not elsewhere classified with membranoproliferative glomerulonephritis, type 2

N07.7 **Hereditary nephropathy, not elsewhere classified with diffuse crescentic glomerulonephritis**

Hereditary nephropathy, not elsewhere classified with extracapillary glomerulonephritis

N07.8 **Hereditary nephropathy, not elsewhere classified with other morphologic lesions**

Hereditary nephropathy, not elsewhere classified with proliferative glomerulonephritis NOS

N07.9 **Hereditary nephropathy, not elsewhere classified with unspecified morphologic lesions**

N07.A **Hereditary nephropathy, not elsewhere classified with** C3 glomerulonephritis

Hereditary nephropathy, not elsewhere classified with C3 glomerulopathy

> *EXCLUDES 1*   *hereditary nephropathy, not elsewhere classified (with C3 glomerulopathy) with dense deposit disease (N07.6)*

N08 *Glomerular disorders in diseases classified elsewhere*

Glomerulonephritis
Nephritis
Nephropathy

Code first underlying disease, such as:
amyloidosis (E85.-)
congenital syphilis (A50.5)
cryoglobulinemia (D89.1)
disseminated intravascular coagulation (D65)
gout (M1A.-, M10.-)
microscopic polyangiitis (M31.7)
multiple myeloma (C90.0-)
sepsis (A40.0-A41.9)
sickle-cell disease (D57.0-D57.8)

> *EXCLUDES 1*   *glomerulonephritis, nephritis and nephropathy (in):*
> *antiglomerular basement membrane disease (M31.0)*
> *diabetes (E08-E13 with .21)*
> *gonococcal (A54.21)*
> *Goodpasture's syndrome (M31.0)*
> *hemolytic-uremic syndrome ▶(D59.3-)◀*
> *lupus (M32.14)*
> *mumps (B26.83)*
> *syphilis (A52.75)*
> *systemic lupus erythematosus (M32.14)*
> *Wegener's granulomatosis (M31.31)*
> *pyelonephritis in diseases classified elsewhere (N16)*
> *renal tubulo-interstitial disorders classified elsewhere (N16)*

Renal tubulo-interstitial diseases (N10-N16)

INCLUDES   pyelonephritis

EXCLUDES 1   pyeloureteritis cystica (N28.85)

N10   Acute pyelonephritis

     Acute infectious interstitial nephritis

     Acute pyelitis

     Acute tubulo-interstitial nephritis

     Hemoglobin nephrosis

     Myoglobin nephrosis

     Use additional code (B95-B97), to identify infectious agent

     AHA: 2020,3Q,25; 2019,3Q,13

☑4ᵗʰ   N11   Chronic tubulo-interstitial nephritis

     INCLUDES   chronic infectious interstitial nephritis

                 chronic pyelitis

                 chronic pyelonephritis

     Use additional code (B95-B97), to identify infectious agent

     N11.0   Nonobstructive reflux-associated chronic pyelonephritis

         Pyelonephritis (chronic) associated with (vesicoureteral) reflux

         EXCLUDES 1   vesicoureteral reflux NOS (N13.70)

     N11.1   Chronic obstructive pyelonephritis

         Pyelonephritis (chronic) associated with anomaly of pelviureteric junction

         Pyelonephritis (chronic) associated with anomaly of pyeloureteric junction

         Pyelonephritis (chronic) associated with crossing of vessel

         Pyelonephritis (chronic) associated with kinking of ureter

         Pyelonephritis (chronic) associated with obstruction of ureter

         Pyelonephritis (chronic) associated with stricture of pelviureteric junction

         Pyelonephritis (chronic) associated with stricture of ureter

         EXCLUDES 1   calculous pyelonephritis (N20.9)

                       obstructive uropathy (N13.-)

     N11.8   Other chronic tubulo-interstitial nephritis

         Nonobstructive chronic pyelonephritis NOS

     N11.9   Chronic tubulo-interstitial nephritis, unspecified

         Chronic interstitial nephritis NOS

         Chronic pyelitis NOS

         Chronic pyelonephritis NOS

N12   Tubulo-interstitial nephritis, not specified as acute or chronic

     Interstitial nephritis NOS

     Pyelitis NOS

     Pyelonephritis NOS

     EXCLUDES 1   calculous pyelonephritis (N20.9)

☑4ᵗʰ   N13   Obstructive and reflux uropathy

     EXCLUDES 2   calculus of kidney and ureter without hydronephrosis (N20.-)

                 congenital obstructive defects of renal pelvis and ureter (Q62.0-Q62.3)

                 hydronephrosis with ureteropelvic junction obstruction (Q62.11)

                 obstructive pyelonephritis (N11.1)

     DEF: Hydronephrosis: Distension of the kidney caused by an accumulation of urine that cannot flow out due to an obstruction that may be caused by conditions such as kidney stones or vesicoureteral reflux.

     N13.0   Hydronephrosis with ureteropelvic junction obstruction

         Hydronephrosis due to acquired occlusion of ureteropelvic junction

         EXCLUDES 2   hydronephrosis with ureteropelvic junction obstruction due to calculus (N13.2)

         AHA: 2016,4Q,43

Hydronephrosis/UPJ Obstruction

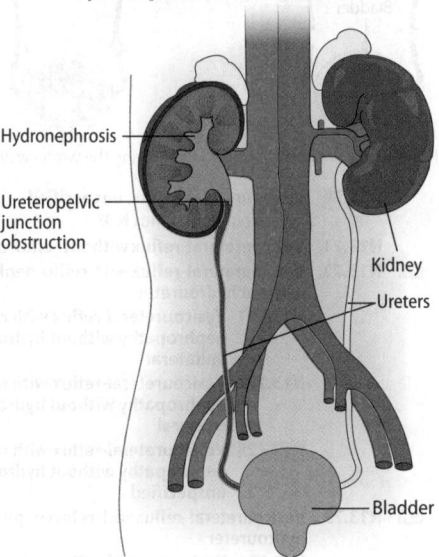

Hydronephrosis

Ureteropelvic junction obstruction

Kidney

Ureters

Bladder

     N13.1   Hydronephrosis with ureteral stricture, not elsewhere classified

         EXCLUDES 1   hydronephrosis with ureteral stricture with infection (N13.6)

     N13.2   Hydronephrosis with renal and ureteral calculous obstruction

         EXCLUDES 1   hydronephrosis with renal and ureteral calculous obstruction with infection (N13.6)

     ☑5ᵗʰ   N13.3   Other and unspecified hydronephrosis

         EXCLUDES 1   hydronephrosis with infection (N13.6)

         N13.30   Unspecified hydronephrosis

         N13.39   Other hydronephrosis

     N13.4   Hydroureter

         EXCLUDES 1   congenital hydroureter (Q62.3-)

                 hydroureter with infection (N13.6)

                 vesicoureteral-reflux with hydroureter (N13.73-)

         DEF: Abnormal enlargement or distension of the ureter with water or urine caused by an obstruction.

     N13.5   Crossing vessel and stricture of ureter without hydronephrosis

         Kinking and stricture of ureter without hydronephrosis

         EXCLUDES 1   crossing vessel and stricture of ureter without hydronephrosis with infection (N13.6)

     N13.6   Pyonephrosis

         Conditions in N13.0-N13.5 with infection

         Obstructive uropathy with infection

         Use additional code (B95-B97), to identify infectious agent

         AHA: 2018,2Q,21

☑6ᵗʰ N13.7 Vesicoureteral-reflux
> *EXCLUDES 1*   reflux-associated pyelonephritis (N11.0)
>
> **DEF:** Urine passage from the bladder flows backward up into the ureter and kidneys that can lead to bacterial infection and an increase in hydrostatic pressure, causing kidney damage.

Vesicoureteral Reflux

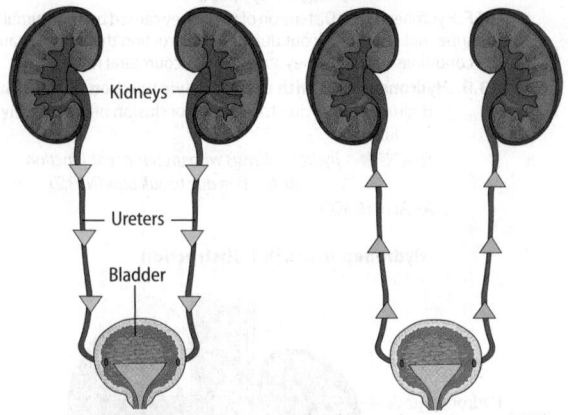

Kidneys — Ureters — Bladder

Normal flow of urine   Urine flowing the wrong way (VUR)

    N13.70 Vesicoureteral-reflux, unspecified
      Vesicoureteral-reflux NOS
    N13.71 Vesicoureteral-reflux without reflux nephropathy
☑6ᵗʰ N13.72 Vesicoureteral-reflux with reflux nephropathy without hydroureter
      N13.721 Vesicoureteral-reflux with reflux nephropathy without hydroureter, unilateral
      N13.722 Vesicoureteral-reflux with reflux nephropathy without hydroureter, bilateral
      N13.729 Vesicoureteral-reflux with reflux nephropathy without hydroureter, unspecified
☑6ᵗʰ N13.73 Vesicoureteral-reflux with reflux nephropathy with hydroureter
      N13.731 Vesicoureteral-reflux with reflux nephropathy with hydroureter, unilateral
      N13.732 Vesicoureteral-reflux with reflux nephropathy with hydroureter, bilateral
      N13.739 Vesicoureteral-reflux with reflux nephropathy with hydroureter, unspecified
    N13.8 Other obstructive and reflux uropathy
      Urinary tract obstruction due to specified cause
      Code first, if applicable, any causal condition, such as:
        enlarged prostate (N40.1)
    N13.9 Obstructive and reflux uropathy, unspecified
      Urinary tract obstruction NOS

▲ ☑4ᵗʰ N14 Drug- and heavy-metal-induced tubulo-interstitial and tubular conditions
    Code first poisoning due to drug or toxin, if applicable (T36-T65 with fifth or sixth character 1-4 or 6)
    Use additional code for adverse effect, if applicable, to identify drug (T36-T50 with fifth or sixth character 5)
    N14.0 Analgesic nephropathy
▲ ☑5ᵗʰ N14.1 Nephropathy induced by other drugs, medicaments and biological substances
      AHA: 2021,3Q,9-10
  ●   **N14.11 Contrast-induced** nephropathy
        Contrast medium, radiography nephropathy
        EXCLUDES 2   acute kidney failure (N17.-)
  ●   **N14.19 Nephropathy induced by other drugs, medicaments and biological substances**
    N14.2 Nephropathy induced by unspecified drug, medicament or biological substance
    N14.3 Nephropathy induced by heavy metals
    N14.4 Toxic nephropathy, not elsewhere classified

☑4ᵗʰ N15 Other renal tubulo-interstitial diseases
    N15.0 Balkan nephropathy
      Balkan endemic nephropathy
    N15.1 Renal and perinephric abscess
    N15.8 Other specified renal tubulo-interstitial diseases

    N15.9 Renal tubulo-interstitial disease, unspecified
      Infection of kidney NOS
      EXCLUDES 1   urinary tract infection NOS (N39.0)

N16   *Renal tubulo-interstitial disorders in diseases classified elsewhere*
    Pyelonephritis
    Tubulo-interstitial nephritis
    Code first underlying disease, such as:
      brucellosis (A23.0-A23.9)
      cryoglobulinemia (D89.1)
      glycogen storage disease (E74.0)
      leukemia (C91-C95)
      lymphoma (C81.0-C85.9, C96.0-C96.9)
      multiple myeloma (C90.0-)
      sepsis (A40.0-A41.9)
      Wilson's disease (E83.0)
    EXCLUDES 1   diphtheritic pyelonephritis and tubulo-interstitial nephritis (A36.84)
      pyelonephritis and tubulo-interstitial nephritis in candidiasis (B37.49)
      pyelonephritis and tubulo-interstitial nephritis in cystinosis (E72.04)
      pyelonephritis and tubulo-interstitial nephritis in salmonella infection (A02.25)
      pyelonephritis and tubulo-interstitial nephritis in sarcoidosis (D86.84)
      pyelonephritis and tubulo-interstitial nephritis in Sjögren syndrome (M35.04)
      pyelonephritis and tubulo-interstitial nephritis in systemic lupus erythematosus (M32.15)
      pyelonephritis and tubulo-interstitial nephritis in toxoplasmosis (B58.83)
      renal tubular degeneration in diabetes (E08-E13 with .29)
      syphilitic pyelonephritis and tubulo-interstitial nephritis (A52.75)

Acute kidney failure and chronic kidney disease (N17-N19)

> *EXCLUDES 2*   congenital renal failure (P96.0)
> drug- and heavy-metal-induced tubulo-interstitial and tubular conditions (N14.-)
> extrarenal uremia (R39.2)
> hemolytic-uremic syndrome ▶(D59.3-)◀
> hepatorenal syndrome (K76.7)
> postpartum hepatorenal syndrome (O90.4)
> posttraumatic renal failure (T79.5)
> prerenal uremia (R39.2)
> renal failure complicating abortion or ectopic or molar pregnancy (O00-O07, O08.4)
> renal failure following labor and delivery (O90.4)
> renal failure postprocedural (N99.0)

☑4ᵗʰ N17   Acute kidney failure
    Code also associated underlying condition
    EXCLUDES 1   posttraumatic renal failure (T79.5)
    AHA: 2020,3Q,22; 2019,2Q,7; 2019,1Q,12; 2013,4Q,124

    N17.0 Acute kidney failure with tubular necrosis   HCC ESR
      Acute tubular necrosis
      Renal tubular necrosis
      Tubular necrosis NOS
      AHA: 2021,3Q,10

    N17.1 Acute kidney failure with acute cortical necrosis   HCC ESR
      Acute cortical necrosis
      Cortical necrosis NOS
      Renal cortical necrosis

    N17.2 Acute kidney failure with medullary necrosis   HCC ESR
      Medullary [papillary] necrosis NOS
      Acute medullary [papillary] necrosis
      Renal medullary [papillary] necrosis

    N17.8 Other acute kidney failure   HCC ESR

    N17.9 Acute kidney failure, unspecified   HCC ESR
      Acute kidney injury (nontraumatic)
      EXCLUDES 2   traumatic kidney injury (S37.0-)

✓4ᵗʰ **N18 Chronic kidney disease (CKD)**
   Code first any associated:
   diabetic chronic kidney disease (E08.22, E09.22, E10.22, E11.22, E13.22)
   hypertensive chronic kidney disease (I12.-, I13.-)
   Use additional code to identify kidney transplant status, if applicable, (Z94.0)
   AHA: 2019,3Q,3; 2018,4Q,88; 2013,1Q,24
   TIP: CKD/ESRD occurring in an individual with a history of kidney transplant should not be assumed to be a transplant complication unless specifically indicated as such by provider documentation.

   N18.1 Chronic kidney disease, stage 1
   N18.2 Chronic kidney disease, stage 2 (mild)
✓5ᵗʰ **N18.3 Chronic kidney disease, stage 3 (moderate)**
   AHA: 2020,4Q,35
   N18.30 Chronic kidney disease, stage 3 unspecified HCC ESR
   N18.31 Chronic kidney disease, stage 3a HCC ESR
   N18.32 Chronic kidney disease, stage 3b HCC ESR
   N18.4 Chronic kidney disease, stage 4 (severe) HCC Rx ESR COM
   N18.5 Chronic kidney disease, stage 5 HCC ESR COM
   EXCLUDES 1 chronic kidney disease, stage 5 requiring chronic dialysis (N18.6)
   DEF: End-stage renal disease (ESRD) with a GFR value of 15 ml/min or less not yet requiring chronic dialysis.
   TIP: When both ESRD and CKD 5 are documented, code only for ESRD.
   N18.6 End stage renal disease HCC Rx ESR COM
   Chronic kidney disease requiring chronic dialysis
   Use additional code to identify dialysis status (Z99.2)
   AHA: 2016,3Q,22; 2016,1Q,12; 2013,4Q,124-125
   TIP: When both ESRD and CKD 5 are documented, code only for ESRD.
   N18.9 Chronic kidney disease, unspecified
   Chronic renal disease
   Chronic renal failure NOS
   Chronic renal insufficiency
   Chronic uremia NOS
   Diffuse sclerosing glomerulonephritis NOS

N19 Unspecified kidney failure
   Uremia NOS
   EXCLUDES 1 acute kidney failure (N17.-)
   chronic kidney disease (N18.-)
   chronic uremia (N18.9)
   extrarenal uremia (R39.2)
   prerenal uremia (R39.2)
   renal insufficiency (acute) (N28.9)
   uremia of newborn (P96.0)

Urolithiasis (N20-N23)

AHA: 2017,1Q,5; 2015,2Q,8
TIP: Codes from this code block can be assigned based on the diagnosis listed in a radiology report when authenticated by a radiologist and available at the time of code assignment.

✓4ᵗʰ **N20 Calculus of kidney and ureter**
   Calculous pyelonephritis
   EXCLUDES 1 nephrocalcinosis (E83.5)
   that with hydronephrosis (N13.2)
   AHA: 2019,3Q,13
   N20.0 Calculus of kidney
   Nephrolithiasis NOS
   Renal calculus
   Renal stone
   Staghorn calculus
   Stone in kidney
   AHA: 2019,3Q,13
   N20.1 Calculus of ureter
   Calculus of the ureteropelvic junction
   Ureteric stone
   AHA: 2016,3Q,22
   N20.2 Calculus of kidney with calculus of ureter
   N20.9 Urinary calculus, unspecified

✓4ᵗʰ **N21 Calculus of lower urinary tract**
   INCLUDES calculus of lower urinary tract with cystitis and urethritis
   N21.0 Calculus in bladder
   Calculus in diverticulum of bladder
   Urinary bladder stone
   EXCLUDES 2 staghorn calculus (N20.0)
   N21.1 Calculus in urethra
   EXCLUDES 2 calculus of prostate (N42.0)
   N21.8 Other lower urinary tract calculus
   N21.9 Calculus of lower urinary tract, unspecified
   EXCLUDES 1 calculus of urinary tract NOS (N20.9)

N22 Calculus of urinary tract in diseases classified elsewhere
   Code first underlying disease, such as:
   gout (M1A.-, M10.-)
   schistosomiasis (B65.0-B65.9)

N23 Unspecified renal colic

Other disorders of kidney and ureter (N25-N29)

   EXCLUDES 2 disorders of kidney and ureter with urolithiasis (N20-N23)

✓4ᵗʰ **N25 Disorders resulting from impaired renal tubular function**
   N25.0 Renal osteodystrophy Rx
   Azotemic osteodystrophy
   Phosphate-losing tubular disorders
   Renal rickets
   Renal short stature
   EXCLUDES 2 metabolic disorders classifiable to E70-E88
   DEF: Various bone diseases occurring when kidney function is impaired or fails. Abnormal levels of phosphorous and calcium can lead to osteomalacia, osteoporosis, or osteosclerosis.
   N25.1 Nephrogenic diabetes insipidus HCC Rx ESR COM
   EXCLUDES 1 diabetes insipidus NOS (E23.2)
   DEF: Type of diabetes due to the inability of renal tubules to reabsorb water back into the body. It is not responsive to vasopressin (antidiuretic hormone) and it is characterized by excessive thirst and excessive urine production. It may develop into chronic renal insufficiency.
✓5ᵗʰ **N25.8 Other disorders resulting from impaired renal tubular function**
   N25.81 Secondary hyperparathyroidism of renal origin HCC Rx ESR COM
   EXCLUDES 1 secondary hyperparathyroidism, non-renal (E21.1)
   EXCLUDES 2 metabolic disorders classifiable to E70-E88
   DEF: Parathyroid dysfunction caused by chronic renal failure. Phosphate clearance and vitamin D production is impaired resulting in lowered calcium blood levels and an excessive production of parathyroid hormone.
   N25.89 Other disorders resulting from impaired renal tubular function
   Hypokalemic nephropathy
   Lightwood-Albright syndrome
   Renal tubular acidosis NOS
   N25.9 Disorder resulting from impaired renal tubular function, unspecified

✓4ᵗʰ **N26 Unspecified contracted kidney**
   EXCLUDES 1 contracted kidney due to hypertension (I12.-)
   diffuse sclerosing glomerulonephritis (N05.8.-)
   hypertensive nephrosclerosis (arteriolar) (arteriosclerotic) (I12.-)
   small kidney of unknown cause (N27.-)
   N26.1 Atrophy of kidney (terminal)
   N26.2 Page kidney Rx
   N26.9 Renal sclerosis, unspecified

✓4ᵗʰ **N27 Small kidney of unknown cause**
   INCLUDES oligonephronia
   N27.0 Small kidney, unilateral
   N27.1 Small kidney, bilateral
   N27.9 Small kidney, unspecified

✓ Additional Character Required   ✓x7ᵗʰ Placeholder Alert   Manifestation   Unspecified Dx   Q QPP   UPD Unacceptable PDx
ICD-10-CM 2023   871

N18–N27.9

Chapter 14. Diseases of the Genitourinary System

✓4th **N28** **Other disorders of kidney and ureter, not elsewhere classified**

    N28.0 **Ischemia and infarction of kidney** `HCC` `ESR` `COM`
        Renal artery embolism
        Renal artery obstruction
        Renal artery occlusion
        Renal artery thrombosis
        Renal infarct
        EXCLUDES 1   *atherosclerosis of renal artery (extrarenal part) (I70.1)*
                    congenital stenosis of renal artery (Q27.1)
                    Goldblatt's kidney (I70.1)

    N28.1 **Cyst of kidney, acquired**
        Cyst (multiple) (solitary) of kidney (acquired)
        EXCLUDES 1   *cystic kidney disease (congenital) (Q61.-)*

  ✓5th **N28.8** **Other specified disorders of kidney and ureter**
        EXCLUDES 1   *hydroureter (N13.4)*
                    ureteric stricture with hydronephrosis (N13.1)
                    ureteric stricture without hydronephrosis (N13.5)

        N28.81 **Hypertrophy of kidney**
        N28.82 **Megaloureter**
        N28.83 **Nephroptosis**
        N28.84 **Pyelitis cystica**
        N28.85 **Pyeloureteritis cystica**
        N28.86 **Ureteritis cystica**
        N28.89 **Other specified disorders of kidney and ureter**

    N28.9 **Disorder of kidney and ureter, unspecified**
        Nephropathy NOS
        Renal disease (acute) NOS
        Renal insufficiency (acute)
        EXCLUDES 1   *chronic renal insufficiency (N18.9)*
                    unspecified nephritic syndrome (N05.-)
        AHA: 2016,1Q,13

N29 *Other disorders of kidney and ureter in diseases classified elsewhere*
    Code first underlying disease, such as:
      amyloidosis (E85.-)
      nephrocalcinosis (E83.5)
      schistosomiasis (B65.0-B65.9)
    EXCLUDES 1   *disorders of kidney and ureter in:*
                cystinosis (E72.0)
                gonorrhea (A54.21)
                syphilis (A52.75)
                tuberculosis (A18.11)

Other diseases of the urinary system (N30-N39)

EXCLUDES 2   *urinary infection (complicating):*
        abortion or ectopic or molar pregnancy (O00-O07, O08.8)
        pregnancy, childbirth and the puerperium (O23.-, O75.3, O86.2-)

✓4th **N30** **Cystitis**
    Use additional code to identify infectious agent (B95-B97)
    EXCLUDES 1   *prostatocystitis (N41.3)*
    AHA: 2017,1Q,6
    DEF: Inflammation of the urinary bladder. Symptoms include dysuria, frequency of urination, urgency, and hematuria.

  ✓5th **N30.0** **Acute cystitis**
        EXCLUDES 1   *irradiation cystitis (N30.4-)*
                    trigonitis (N30.3-)
        N30.00 **Acute cystitis without hematuria**
        N30.01 **Acute cystitis with hematuria**

  ✓5th **N30.1** **Interstitial cystitis (chronic)**
        N30.10 **Interstitial cystitis (chronic) without hematuria**
        N30.11 **Interstitial cystitis (chronic) with hematuria**

  ✓5th **N30.2** **Other chronic cystitis**
        N30.20 **Other chronic cystitis without hematuria**
        N30.21 **Other chronic cystitis with hematuria**

  ✓5th **N30.3** **Trigonitis**
        Urethrotrigonitis
        N30.30 **Trigonitis without hematuria**
        N30.31 **Trigonitis with hematuria**

  ✓5th **N30.4** **Irradiation cystitis**
        N30.40 **Irradiation cystitis without hematuria**
        N30.41 **Irradiation cystitis with hematuria**

  ✓5th **N30.8** **Other cystitis**
        Abscess of bladder
        N30.80 **Other cystitis without hematuria**
        N30.81 **Other cystitis with hematuria**

  ✓5th **N30.9** **Cystitis, unspecified**
        N30.90 **Cystitis, unspecified without hematuria**
        N30.91 **Cystitis, unspecified with hematuria**

✓4th **N31** **Neuromuscular dysfunction of bladder, not elsewhere classified**
    Use additional code to identify any associated urinary incontinence (N39.3-N39.4-)
    EXCLUDES 1   *cord bladder NOS (G95.89)*
                neurogenic bladder due to cauda equina syndrome (G83.4)
                neuromuscular dysfunction due to spinal cord lesion (G95.89)

    N31.0 **Uninhibited neuropathic bladder, not elsewhere classified**
    N31.1 **Reflex neuropathic bladder, not elsewhere classified**
    N31.2 **Flaccid neuropathic bladder, not elsewhere classified**
        Atonic (motor) (sensory) neuropathic bladder
        Autonomous neuropathic bladder
        Nonreflex neuropathic bladder

    N31.8 **Other neuromuscular dysfunction of bladder**
    N31.9 **Neuromuscular dysfunction of bladder, unspecified**
        Neurogenic bladder dysfunction NOS

✓4th **N32** **Other disorders of bladder**
    EXCLUDES 2   *calculus of bladder (N21.0)*
                cystocele (N81.1-)
                hernia or prolapse of bladder, female (N81.1-)

    N32.0 **Bladder-neck obstruction**
        Bladder-neck stenosis (acquired)
        EXCLUDES 1   *congenital bladder-neck obstruction (Q64.3-)*
        DEF: Bladder outlet and vesicourethral obstruction that occurs as a consequence of benign prostatic hypertrophy or prostatic cancer. It may also occur in either sex due to strictures, radiation, cystoscopy, catheterization, injury, infection, blood clots, bladder cancer, impaction, or other disease that compresses the bladder neck.

    N32.1 **Vesicointestinal fistula**
        Vesicorectal fistula

    N32.2 **Vesical fistula, not elsewhere classified**
        EXCLUDES 1   *fistula between bladder and female genital tract (N82.0-N82.1)*

    N32.3 **Diverticulum of bladder**
        EXCLUDES 1   *congenital diverticulum of bladder (Q64.6)*
                diverticulitis of bladder (N30.8-)

  ✓5th **N32.8** **Other specified disorders of bladder**
        N32.81 **Overactive bladder**
            Detrusor muscle hyperactivity
            EXCLUDES 1   *frequent urination due to specified bladder condition — code to condition*
            DEF: Sudden involuntary contractions of the muscular wall of the bladder that results in a sudden, strong urge to urinate.

        N32.89 **Other specified disorders of bladder**
            Bladder hemorrhage
            Bladder hypertrophy
            Calcified bladder
            Contracted bladder

    N32.9 **Bladder disorder, unspecified**

N33 *Bladder disorders in diseases classified elsewhere*
    Code first underlying disease, such as:
      schistosomiasis (B65.0-B65.9)
    EXCLUDES 1   *bladder disorder in syphilis (A52.76)*
                bladder disorder in tuberculosis (A18.12)
                candidal cystitis (B37.41)
                chlamydial cystitis (A56.01)
                cystitis in gonorrhea (A54.01)
                cystitis in neurogenic bladder (N31.-)
                diphtheritic cystitis (A36.85)
                neurogenic bladder (N31.-)
                syphilitic cystitis (A52.76)
                trichomonal cystitis (A59.03)

Chapter 14. Diseases of the Genitourinary System

✓4ᵗʰ **N34** **Urethritis and urethral syndrome**
Use additional code (B95-B97), to identify infectious agent
> EXCLUDES 2   Reiter's disease (M02.3-)
> urethritis in diseases with a predominantly sexual mode of transmission (A50-A64)
> urethrotrigonitis (N30.3-)

AHA: 2017,1Q,6

N34.0 **Urethral abscess**
Abscess (of) Cowper's gland
Abscess (of) Littré's gland
Abscess (of) urethral (gland)
Periurethral abscess
> EXCLUDES 1   urethral caruncle (N36.2)

N34.1 **Nonspecific urethritis**
Nongonococcal urethritis
Nonvenereal urethritis

N34.2 **Other urethritis**
Meatitis, urethral
Postmenopausal urethritis
Ulcer of urethra (meatus)
Urethritis NOS

N34.3 **Urethral syndrome, unspecified**

✓4ᵗʰ **N35** **Urethral stricture**
> EXCLUDES 1   congenital urethral stricture (Q64.3-)
> postprocedural urethral stricture (N99.1-)

AHA: 2018,4Q,21-22

✓5ᵗʰ **N35.0** **Post-traumatic urethral stricture**
Urethral stricture due to injury
> EXCLUDES 1   postprocedural urethral stricture (N99.1-)

✓6ᵗʰ **N35.01** **Post-traumatic urethral stricture, male**

N35.010 **Post-traumatic urethral stricture, male, meatal** ♂

N35.011 **Post-traumatic bulbous urethral stricture** ♂

N35.012 **Post-traumatic membranous urethral stricture** ♂

N35.013 **Post-traumatic anterior urethral stricture** ♂

N35.014 **Post-traumatic urethral stricture, male, unspecified** ♂

N35.016 **Post-traumatic urethral stricture, male, overlapping sites** ♂

✓6ᵗʰ **N35.02** **Post-traumatic urethral stricture, female**

N35.021 **Urethral stricture due to childbirth** ♀

N35.028 **Other post-traumatic urethral stricture, female** ♀

✓5ᵗʰ **N35.1** **Postinfective urethral stricture, not elsewhere classified**
> EXCLUDES 1   gonococcal urethral stricture (A54.01)
> syphilitic urethral stricture (A52.76)
> urethral stricture associated with schistosomiasis (B65.-, N29)

✓6ᵗʰ **N35.11** **Postinfective urethral stricture, not elsewhere classified, male**

N35.111 **Postinfective urethral stricture, not elsewhere classified, male, meatal** ♂

N35.112 **Postinfective bulbous urethral stricture, not elsewhere classified, male** ♂

N35.113 **Postinfective membranous urethral stricture, not elsewhere classified, male** ♂

N35.114 **Postinfective anterior urethral stricture, not elsewhere classified, male** ♂

N35.116 **Postinfective urethral stricture, not elsewhere classified, male, overlapping sites** ♂

N35.119 **Postinfective urethral stricture, not elsewhere classified, male, unspecified** ♂

N35.12 **Postinfective urethral stricture, not elsewhere classified, female** ♀

✓5ᵗʰ **N35.8** **Other urethral stricture**
> EXCLUDES 1   postprocedural urethral stricture (N99.1-)

✓6ᵗʰ **N35.81** **Other urethral stricture, male**

N35.811 **Other urethral stricture, male, meatal** ♂

N35.812 **Other urethral bulbous stricture, male** ♂

N35.813 **Other membranous urethral stricture, male** ♂

N35.814 **Other anterior urethral stricture, male** ♂

N35.816 **Other urethral stricture, male, overlapping sites** ♂

N35.819 **Other urethral stricture, male, unspecified site** ♂

N35.82 **Other urethral stricture, female** ♀

✓5ᵗʰ **N35.9** **Urethral stricture, unspecified**

✓6ᵗʰ **N35.91** **Urethral stricture, unspecified, male**

N35.911 **Unspecified urethral stricture, male, meatal** ♂

N35.912 **Unspecified bulbous urethral stricture, male** ♂

N35.913 **Unspecified membranous urethral stricture, male** ♂

N35.914 **Unspecified anterior urethral stricture, male** ♂

N35.916 **Unspecified urethral stricture, male, overlapping sites** ♂

N35.919 **Unspecified urethral stricture, male, unspecified site** ♂
Pinhole meatus NOS
Urethral stricture NOS

N35.92 **Unspecified urethral stricture, female** ♀

✓4ᵗʰ **N36** **Other disorders of urethra**

N36.0 **Urethral fistula**
Urethroperineal fistula
Urethrorectal fistula
Urinary fistula NOS
> EXCLUDES 1   urethroscrotal fistula (N50.89)
> urethrovaginal fistula (N82.1)
> urethrovesicovaginal fistula (N82.1)

N36.1 **Urethral diverticulum**

N36.2 **Urethral caruncle**

✓5ᵗʰ **N36.4** **Urethral functional and muscular disorders**
Use additional code to identify associated urinary stress incontinence (N39.3)

N36.41 **Hypermobility of urethra**

N36.42 **Intrinsic sphincter deficiency (ISD)**

N36.43 **Combined hypermobility of urethra and intrinsic sphincter deficiency**

N36.44 **Muscular disorders of urethra**
Bladder sphincter dyssynergy

N36.5 **Urethral false passage**

N36.8 **Other specified disorders of urethra**
> EXCLUDES 1   congenital urethrocele (Q64.7)
> female urethrocele (N81.0)

AHA: 2022,2Q,7

N36.9 **Urethral disorder, unspecified**

N37 **Urethral disorders in diseases classified elsewhere**
Code first underlying disease
> EXCLUDES 1   urethritis (in):
> candidal infection (B37.41)
> chlamydial (A56.01)
> gonorrhea (A54.01)
> syphilis (A52.76)
> trichomonal infection (A59.03)
> tuberculosis (A18.13)

N39 Other disorders of urinary system

> EXCLUDES 2   hematuria NOS (R31.-)
>
> recurrent or persistent hematuria (N02.-)
>
> recurrent or persistent hematuria with specified morphological lesion (N02.-)
>
> proteinuria NOS (R80.-)

N39.0 Urinary tract infection, site not specified

> Use additional code (B95-B97), to identify infectious agent
>
> EXCLUDES 1   candidiasis of urinary tract (B37.4-)
>
> neonatal urinary tract infection (P39.3)
>
> pyuria (R82.81)
>
> urinary tract infection of specified site, such as:
>
> cystitis (N30.-)
>
> urethritis (N34.-)
>
> **AHA:** 2019,3Q,17; 2018,2Q,21,22; 2018,1Q,16; 2017,1Q,6; 2012,4Q,94

N39.3 Stress incontinence (female) (male)

> Code also any associated overactive bladder (N32.81)
>
> EXCLUDES 1   mixed incontinence (N39.46)

N39.4 Other specified urinary incontinence

> Code also any associated overactive bladder (N32.81)
>
> EXCLUDES 1   enuresis NOS (R32)
>
> functional urinary incontinence (R39.81)
>
> urinary incontinence associated with cognitive impairment (R39.81)
>
> urinary incontinence NOS (R32)
>
> urinary incontinence of nonorganic origin (F98.0)

N39.41 Urge incontinence

> EXCLUDES 1   mixed incontinence (N39.46)

N39.42 Incontinence without sensory awareness

> Insensible (urinary) incontinence

N39.43 Post-void dribbling

N39.44 Nocturnal enuresis

> EXCLUDES 2   nocturnal polyuria (R35.81)

N39.45 Continuous leakage

N39.46 Mixed incontinence

> Urge and stress incontinence

N39.49 Other specified urinary incontinence

> **AHA:** 2016,4Q,44

N39.490 Overflow incontinence
N39.491 Coital incontinence
N39.492 Postural (urinary) incontinence
N39.498 Other specified urinary incontinence
> Reflex incontinence
>
> Total incontinence

N39.8 Other specified disorders of urinary system

N39.9 Disorder of urinary system, unspecified

Diseases of male genital organs (N40-N53)

N40 Benign prostatic hyperplasia

> INCLUDES   adenofibromatous hypertrophy of prostate
>
> benign hypertrophy of the prostate
>
> benign prostatic hypertrophy
>
> BPH
>
> enlarged prostate
>
> nodular prostate
>
> polyp of prostate
>
> EXCLUDES 1   benign neoplasms of prostate (adenoma, benign) (fibroadenoma) (fibroma) (myoma) (D29.1)
>
> EXCLUDES 2   malignant neoplasm of prostate (C61)
>
> **DEF:** Enlargement of the prostate gland due to an abnormal proliferation of fibrostromal tissue in the paraurethral glands. This condition causes impingement of the urethra resulting in obstructed urinary flow.

N40.0 Benign prostatic hyperplasia without lower urinary tract symptoms   A ♂

> Enlarged prostate NOS
>
> Enlarged prostate without LUTS

N40.1 Benign prostatic hyperplasia with lower urinary tract symptoms   A ♂

> Enlarged prostate with LUTS
>
> Use additional code for associated symptoms, when specified:
>
> incomplete bladder emptying (R39.14)
>
> nocturia (R35.1)
>
> straining on urination (R39.16)
>
> urinary frequency (R35.0)
>
> urinary hesitancy (R39.11)
>
> urinary incontinence (N39.4-)
>
> urinary obstruction (N13.8)
>
> urinary retention (R33.8)
>
> urinary urgency (R39.15)
>
> weak urinary stream (R39.12)
>
> **AHA:** 2018,4Q,55

N40.2 Nodular prostate without lower urinary tract symptoms   A ♂

> Nodular prostate without LUTS

N40.3 Nodular prostate with lower urinary tract symptoms   A ♂

> Use additional code for associated symptoms, when specified:
>
> incomplete bladder emptying (R39.14)
>
> nocturia (R35.1)
>
> straining on urination (R39.16)
>
> urinary frequency (R35.0)
>
> urinary hesitancy (R39.11)
>
> urinary incontinence (N39.4-)
>
> urinary obstruction (N13.8)
>
> urinary retention (R33.8)
>
> urinary urgency (R39.15)
>
> weak urinary stream (R39.12)

N41 Inflammatory diseases of prostate

> Use additional code (B95-B97), to identify infectious agent

N41.0 Acute prostatitis   A ♂
N41.1 Chronic prostatitis   A ♂
N41.2 Abscess of prostate   A ♂
N41.3 Prostatocystitis   A ♂
N41.4 Granulomatous prostatitis   A ♂
N41.8 Other inflammatory diseases of prostate   A ♂
N41.9 Inflammatory disease of prostate, unspecified   A ♂
> Prostatitis NOS

N42 Other and unspecified disorders of prostate

N42.0 Calculus of prostate   A ♂

> Prostatic stone
>
> **DEF:** Formation of a small, solid stone often composed of calcium carbonate or calcium phosphate in the prostate gland.

N42.1 Congestion and hemorrhage of prostate   A ♂

> EXCLUDES 1   enlarged prostate (N40.-)
>
> hematuria (R31.-)
>
> hyperplasia of prostate (N40.-)
>
> inflammatory diseases of prostate (N41.-)

N42.3 Dysplasia of prostate

> **AHA:** 2016,4Q,44

N42.30 Unspecified dysplasia of prostate   ♂

N42.31 Prostatic intraepithelial neoplasia   ♂

> PIN
>
> Prostatic intraepithelial neoplasia I (PIN I)
>
> Prostatic intraepithelial neoplasia II (PIN II)
>
> EXCLUDES 1   prostatic intraepithelial neoplasia III (PIN III) (D07.5)
>
> **DEF:** Abnormality of shape and size of the intraepithelial tissues of the prostate. It is a premalignant condition characterized by stalks and absence of a basilar cell layer.

N42.32 Atypical small acinar proliferation of prostate   ♂
N42.39 Other dysplasia of prostate   ♂

N42.8 Other specified disorders of prostate

N42.81 Prostatodynia syndrome   A ♂
> Painful prostate syndrome

N42.82 Prostatosis syndrome   A ♂
N42.83 Cyst of prostate   A ♂
N42.89 Other specified disorders of prostate   A ♂

N42.9 Disorder of prostate, unspecified   A ♂

N43 Hydrocele and spermatocele

INCLUDES hydrocele of spermatic cord, testis or tunica vaginalis
EXCLUDES 1 congenital hydrocele (P83.5)
DEF: Hydrocele: Serous fluid that collects in the tunica vaginalis of the scrotum along the spermatic cord in males.

N43.0 Encysted hydrocele ♂
N43.1 Infected hydrocele
     Use additional code (B95-B97), to identify infectious agent
N43.2 Other hydrocele ♂

Hydrocele

Testicle
Scrotum

Normal   Noncommunicating   Communicating   Hydrocele
hydrocele   hydrocele   of the cord

N43.3 Hydrocele, unspecified ♂
N43.4 Spermatocele of epididymis
     Spermatic cyst
     DEF: Spermatocele: Noncancerous accumulation of fluid and dead sperm cells normally located at the head of the epididymis that exhibits itself as a hard, smooth scrotal mass and do not normally require treatment unless they become enlarged or cause pain.

     N43.40 Spermatocele of epididymis, unspecified ♂
     N43.41 Spermatocele of epididymis, single ♂
     N43.42 Spermatocele of epididymis, multiple ♂

N44 Noninflammatory disorders of testis

N44.0 Torsion of testis
     N44.00 Torsion of testis, unspecified ♂
     N44.01 Extravaginal torsion of spermatic cord ♂
        DEF: Torsion of the spermatic cord just below the tunica vaginalis attachments.
     N44.02 Intravaginal torsion of spermatic cord ♂
        Torsion of spermatic cord NOS
     N44.03 Torsion of appendix testis ♂
     N44.04 Torsion of appendix epididymis ♂
N44.1 Cyst of tunica albuginea testis ♂
N44.2 Benign cyst of testis ♂
N44.8 Other noninflammatory disorders of the testis ♂

N45 Orchitis and epididymitis

     Use additional code (B95-B97), to identify infectious agent
N45.1 Epididymitis ♂
N45.2 Orchitis ♂
N45.3 Epididymo-orchitis ♂
N45.4 Abscess of epididymis or testis ♂

N46 Male infertility

EXCLUDES 1 vasectomy status (Z98.52)
N46.0 Azoospermia
     Absolute male infertility
     Male infertility due to germinal (cell) aplasia
     Male infertility due to spermatogenic arrest (complete)
     DEF: Failure of the development of sperm or the absence of sperm in semen.
     N46.01 Organic azoospermia A ♂
        Azoospermia NOS
     N46.02 Azoospermia due to extratesticular causes
        Code also associated cause
        N46.021 Azoospermia due to drug therapy A ♂
        N46.022 Azoospermia due to infection A ♂
        N46.023 Azoospermia due to obstruction of efferent ducts A ♂
        N46.024 Azoospermia due to radiation A ♂

        N46.025 Azoospermia due to systemic disease A ♂
        N46.029 Azoospermia due to other extratesticular causes A ♂
N46.1 Oligospermia
     Male infertility due to germinal cell desquamation
     Male infertility due to hypospermatogenesis
     Male infertility due to incomplete spermatogenic arrest
     DEF: Insufficient production of sperm in semen.
     N46.11 Organic oligospermia A ♂
        Oligospermia NOS
     N46.12 Oligospermia due to extratesticular causes
        Code also associated cause
        N46.121 Oligospermia due to drug therapy A ♂
        N46.122 Oligospermia due to infection A ♂
        N46.123 Oligospermia due to obstruction of efferent ducts A ♂
        N46.124 Oligospermia due to radiation A ♂
        N46.125 Oligospermia due to systemic disease A ♂
        N46.129 Oligospermia due to other extratesticular causes A ♂
N46.8 Other male infertility A ♂
N46.9 Male infertility, unspecified A ♂

N47 Disorders of prepuce

N47.0 Adherent prepuce, newborn N ♂
N47.1 Phimosis ♂
     DEF: Condition in which the foreskin is contracted and cannot be drawn back behind the glans penis.
N47.2 Paraphimosis ♂
N47.3 Deficient foreskin ♂
N47.4 Benign cyst of prepuce ♂
N47.5 Adhesions of prepuce and glans penis ♂
N47.6 Balanoposthitis ♂
     Use additional code (B95-B97), to identify infectious agent
     EXCLUDES 1 balanitis (N48.1)
N47.7 Other inflammatory diseases of prepuce ♂
     Use additional code (B95-B97), to identify infectious agent
N47.8 Other disorders of prepuce ♂

N48 Other disorders of penis

N48.0 Leukoplakia of penis ♂
     Balanitis xerotica obliterans
     Kraurosis of penis
     Lichen sclerosus of external male genital organs
     EXCLUDES 1 carcinoma in situ of penis (D07.4)
N48.1 Balanitis ♂
     Use additional code (B95-B97), to identify infectious agent
     EXCLUDES 1 amebic balanitis (A06.8)
        balanitis xerotica obliterans (N48.0)
        candidal balanitis (B37.42)
        gonococcal balanitis (A54.23)
        herpesviral [herpes simplex] balanitis (A60.01)
     DEF: Inflammation of the glans penis, most often affecting uncircumcised males.
N48.2 Other inflammatory disorders of penis
     Use additional code (B95-B97), to identify infectious agent
     EXCLUDES 1 balanitis (N48.1)
        balanitis xerotica obliterans (N48.0)
        balanoposthitis (N47.6)
     N48.21 Abscess of corpus cavernosum and penis ♂
     N48.22 Cellulitis of corpus cavernosum and penis ♂
     N48.29 Other inflammatory disorders of penis ♂
N48.3 Priapism
     Painful erection
     Code first underlying cause
     N48.30 Priapism, unspecified ♂
     N48.31 Priapism due to trauma ♂
     N48.32 Priapism due to disease classified elsewhere ♂
     N48.33 Priapism, drug-induced ♂
     N48.39 Other priapism ♂
N48.5 Ulcer of penis

N48.6   **Induration penis plastica**   ♂
       Peyronie's disease
       Plastic induration of penis

✓5ᵗʰ **N48.8**   **Other specified disorders of penis**

     N48.81   **Thrombosis of superficial vein of penis**   ♂

     N48.82   **Acquired torsion of penis**   ♂
         Acquired torsion of penis NOS
         EXCLUDES 1   *congenital torsion of penis (Q55.63)*

     N48.83   **Acquired buried penis**   ♂
         EXCLUDES 1   *congenital hidden penis (Q55.64)*

     N48.89   **Other specified disorders of penis**   ♂

N48.9   **Disorder of penis, unspecified**   ♂

✓4ᵗʰ **N49**   **Inflammatory disorders of male genital organs, not elsewhere classified**
      Use additional code (B95-B97), to identify infectious agent
       EXCLUDES 1   *inflammation of penis (N48.1, N48.2-)*
                orchitis and epididymitis (N45.-)

N49.0   **Inflammatory disorders of** seminal vesicle   ♂
       Vesiculitis NOS

N49.1   **Inflammatory disorders of** spermatic cord, tunica vaginalis **and vas deferens**   ♂
       Vasitis

N49.2   **Inflammatory disorders of** scrotum   ♂

N49.3   **Fournier gangrene**   ♂
       AHA: 2020,2Q,18

N49.8   **Inflammatory disorders of other specified male genital organs**   ♂
       Inflammation of multiple sites in male genital organs

N49.9   **Inflammatory disorder of unspecified male genital organ**   ♂
       Abscess of unspecified male genital organ
       Boil of unspecified male genital organ
       Carbuncle of unspecified male genital organ
       Cellulitis of unspecified male genital organ

✓4ᵗʰ **N50**   **Other and unspecified disorders of male genital organs**
       EXCLUDES 2   *torsion of testis (N44.0-)*

N50.0   **Atrophy of testis**   ♂

N50.1   **Vascular disorders of male genital organs**   ♂
       Hematocele, NOS, of male genital organs
       Hemorrhage of male genital organs
       Thrombosis of male genital organs

N50.3   **Cyst of epididymis**   ♂

✓5ᵗʰ **N50.8**   **Other specified disorders of male genital organs**
       AHA: 2016,4Q,45

     ✓6ᵗʰ **N50.81**   **Testicular pain**

         N50.811   **Right** testicular pain   ♂
         N50.812   **Left** testicular pain   ♂
         N50.819   **Testicular pain, unspecified**   ♂

     N50.82   **Scrotal pain**   ♂

     N50.89   **Other specified disorders of the male genital organs**   ♂
         Atrophy of scrotum, seminal vesicle, spermatic cord, tunica vaginalis and vas deferens
         Chylocele, tunica vaginalis (nonfilarial) NOS
         Edema of scrotum, seminal vesicle, spermatic cord, tunica vaginalis and vas deferens
         Hypertrophy of scrotum, seminal vesicle, spermatic cord, tunica vaginalis and vas deferens
         Stricture of spermatic cord, tunica vaginalis, and vas deferens
         Ulcer of scrotum, seminal vesicle, spermatic cord, testis, tunica vaginalis and vas deferens
         Urethroscrotal fistula

N50.9   **Disorder of male genital organs, unspecified**   ♂

N51   *Disorders of male genital organs in diseases classified elsewhere*   ♂
       Code first underlying disease, such as:
         filariasis (B74.0-B74.9)
       EXCLUDES 1   *amebic balanitis (A06.8)*
                candidal balanitis (B37.42)
                gonococcal balanitis (A54.23)
                gonococcal prostatitis (A54.22)
                herpesviral [herpes simplex] balanitis (A60.01)
                trichomonal prostatitis (A59.02)
                tuberculous prostatitis (A18.14)

✓4ᵗʰ **N52**   **Male erectile dysfunction**
       EXCLUDES 1   *psychogenic impotence (F52.21)*

✓5ᵗʰ **N52.0**   **Vasculogenic** erectile dysfunction

     N52.01   **Erectile dysfunction due to** arterial insufficiency   A ♂

     N52.02   **Corporo-venous occlusive** erectile dysfunction   A ♂

     N52.03   **Combined arterial insufficiency and corporo-venous occlusive** erectile dysfunction   A ♂

N52.1   *Erectile dysfunction due to diseases classified elsewhere*   A ♂
       Code first underlying disease

N52.2   **Drug-induced** erectile dysfunction   A ♂

✓5ᵗʰ **N52.3**   **Postprocedural** erectile dysfunction
       AHA: 2016,4Q,45

     N52.31   **Erectile dysfunction following** radical prostatectomy   A ♂

     N52.32   **Erectile dysfunction following** radical cystectomy   A ♂

     N52.33   **Erectile dysfunction following** urethral surgery   A ♂

     N52.34   **Erectile dysfunction following** simple prostatectomy   A ♂

     N52.35   **Erectile dysfunction following** radiation therapy   A ♂

     N52.36   **Erectile dysfunction following** interstitial seed therapy   A ♂

     N52.37   **Erectile dysfunction following** prostate ablative therapy   A ♂
         Erectile dysfunction following cryotherapy
         Erectile dysfunction following other prostate ablative therapies
         Erectile dysfunction following ultrasound ablative therapies

     N52.39   **Other and unspecified postprocedural erectile dysfunction**   A ♂

N52.8   **Other male erectile dysfunction**   A ♂

N52.9   **Male erectile dysfunction, unspecified**   A ♂
       Impotence NOS

✓4ᵗʰ **N53**   **Other male sexual dysfunction**
       EXCLUDES 1   *psychogenic sexual dysfunction (F52.-)*

✓5ᵗʰ **N53.1**   **Ejaculatory dysfunction**
       EXCLUDES 1   *premature ejaculation (F52.4)*

     N53.11   **Retarded** ejaculation   ♂
     N53.12   **Painful** ejaculation   ♂
     N53.13   **Anejaculatory** orgasm   ♂
     N53.14   **Retrograde** ejaculation   ♂
         DEF: Form of male sexual dysfunction in which the semen enters the bladder instead of going out through the urethra during ejaculation.

     N53.19   **Other ejaculatory dysfunction**   ♂
         Ejaculatory dysfunction NOS

N53.8   **Other male sexual dysfunction**   ♂

N53.9   **Unspecified male sexual dysfunction**   ♂

Disorders of breast (N60-N65)

       EXCLUDES 1   *disorders of breast associated with childbirth (O91-O92)*

✓4ᵗʰ **N60**   **Benign mammary dysplasia**
       INCLUDES   fibrocystic mastopathy

✓5ᵗʰ **N60.0**   **Solitary cyst of breast**
       Cyst of breast

     N60.01   **Solitary cyst of** right **breast**
     N60.02   **Solitary cyst of** left **breast**
     N60.09   **Solitary cyst of unspecified breast**

✓5ᵗʰ **N60.1 Diffuse cystic mastopathy**
    Cystic breast
    Fibrocystic disease of breast
    EXCLUDES 1   *diffuse cystic mastopathy with epithelial proliferation (N60.3-)*

    N60.11 Diffuse cystic mastopathy of right breast   Ⓐ
    N60.12 Diffuse cystic mastopathy of left breast   Ⓐ
    N60.19 Diffuse cystic mastopathy of unspecified breast   Ⓐ

✓5ᵗʰ **N60.2 Fibroadenosis of breast**
    Adenofibrosis of breast
    EXCLUDES 2   *fibroadenoma of breast (D24.-)*

    N60.21 Fibroadenosis of right breast
    N60.22 Fibroadenosis of left breast
    N60.29 Fibroadenosis of unspecified breast

✓5ᵗʰ **N60.3 Fibrosclerosis of breast**
    Cystic mastopathy with epithelial proliferation
    N60.31 Fibrosclerosis of right breast
    N60.32 Fibrosclerosis of left breast
    N60.39 Fibrosclerosis of unspecified breast

✓5ᵗʰ **N60.4 Mammary duct ectasia**
    N60.41 Mammary duct ectasia of right breast
    N60.42 Mammary duct ectasia of left breast
    N60.49 Mammary duct ectasia of unspecified breast

✓5ᵗʰ **N60.8 Other benign mammary dysplasias**
    N60.81 Other benign mammary dysplasias of right breast
    N60.82 Other benign mammary dysplasias of left breast
    N60.89 Other benign mammary dysplasias of unspecified breast

✓5ᵗʰ **N60.9 Unspecified benign mammary dysplasia**
    N60.91 Unspecified benign mammary dysplasia of right breast
    N60.92 Unspecified benign mammary dysplasia of left breast
    N60.99 Unspecified benign mammary dysplasia of unspecified breast

✓4ᵗʰ **N61 Inflammatory disorders of breast**
    EXCLUDES 1   *inflammatory carcinoma of breast (C50.9)*
        inflammatory disorder of breast associated with childbirth (O91.-)
        neonatal infective mastitis (P39.0)
        thrombophlebitis of breast [Mondor's disease] (I80.8)

    N61.0 Mastitis without abscess
    Infective mastitis (acute) (nonpuerperal) (subacute)
    Mastitis (acute) (nonpuerperal) (subacute) NOS
    Cellulitis (acute) (nonpuerperal) (subacute) of breast NOS
    Cellulitis (acute) (nonpuerperal) (subacute) of nipple NOS

    N61.1 Abscess of the breast and nipple
    Abscess (acute) (chronic) (nonpuerperal) of areola
    Abscess (acute) (chronic) (nonpuerperal) of breast
    Carbuncle of breast
    Mastitis with abscess

✓5ᵗʰ **N61.2 Granulomatous mastitis**
    AHA: 2020,4Q,35
    N61.20 Granulomatous mastitis, unspecified breast
    N61.21 Granulomatous mastitis, right breast
    N61.22 Granulomatous mastitis, left breast
    N61.23 Granulomatous mastitis, bilateral breast

N62 Hypertrophy of breast
    Gynecomastia
    Hypertrophy of breast NOS
    Massive pubertal hypertrophy of breast
    EXCLUDES 1   *breast engorgement of newborn (P83.4)*
        disproportion of reconstructed breast (N65.1)

✓4ᵗʰ **N63 Unspecified lump in breast**
    Nodule(s) NOS in breast
    AHA: 2019,4Q,12; 2017,4Q,19
    N63.0 Unspecified lump in unspecified breast
✓5ᵗʰ   **N63.1 Unspecified lump in the right breast**
    N63.10 Unspecified lump in the right breast, unspecified quadrant
    N63.11 Unspecified lump in the right breast, upper outer quadrant
    N63.12 Unspecified lump in the right breast, upper inner quadrant

N63.13 Unspecified lump in the right breast, lower outer quadrant
N63.14 Unspecified lump in the right breast, lower inner quadrant
N63.15 Unspecified lump in the right breast, overlapping quadrants

✓5ᵗʰ **N63.2 Unspecified lump in the left breast**
    N63.20 Unspecified lump in the left breast, unspecified quadrant
    N63.21 Unspecified lump in the left breast, upper outer quadrant
    N63.22 Unspecified lump in the left breast, upper inner quadrant
    N63.23 Unspecified lump in the left breast, lower outer quadrant
    N63.24 Unspecified lump in the left breast, lower inner quadrant
    N63.25 Unspecified lump in the left breast, overlapping quadrants

✓5ᵗʰ **N63.3 Unspecified lump in axillary tail**
    N63.31 Unspecified lump in axillary tail of the right breast
    N63.32 Unspecified lump in axillary tail of the left breast

✓5ᵗʰ **N63.4 Unspecified lump in breast, subareolar**
    N63.41 Unspecified lump in right breast, subareolar
    N63.42 Unspecified lump in left breast, subareolar

✓4ᵗʰ **N64 Other disorders of breast**
    EXCLUDES 2   *mechanical complication of breast prosthesis and implant (T85.4-)*

    N64.0 Fissure and fistula of nipple
    N64.1 Fat necrosis of breast
    Fat necrosis (segmental) of breast
    Code first breast necrosis due to breast graft (T85.898)

    N64.2 Atrophy of breast
    N64.3 Galactorrhea not associated with childbirth
    N64.4 Mastodynia
✓5ᵗʰ   **N64.5 Other signs and symptoms in breast**
    EXCLUDES 2   *abnormal findings on diagnostic imaging of breast (R92.-)*
    N64.51 Induration of breast
    N64.52 Nipple discharge
    EXCLUDES 1   *abnormal findings in nipple discharge (R89.-)*
    N64.53 Retraction of nipple
    N64.59 Other signs and symptoms in breast
✓5ᵗʰ   **N64.8 Other specified disorders of breast**
    N64.81 Ptosis of breast   Ⓐ
    EXCLUDES 1   *ptosis of native breast in relation to reconstructed breast (N65.1)*
    N64.82 Hypoplasia of breast   Ⓐ
    Micromastia
    EXCLUDES 1   *congenital absence of breast (Q83.0)*
        hypoplasia of native breast in relation to reconstructed breast (N65.1)
    N64.89 Other specified disorders of breast
    Galactocele
    Subinvolution of breast (postlactational)
    AHA: 2019,1Q,32; 2018,1Q,3
    N64.9 Disorder of breast, unspecified

✓4ᵗʰ **N65 Deformity and disproportion of reconstructed breast**
    N65.0 Deformity of reconstructed breast   Ⓐ
    Contour irregularity in reconstructed breast
    Excess tissue in reconstructed breast
    Misshapen reconstructed breast

    N65.1 Disproportion of reconstructed breast   Ⓐ
    Breast asymmetry between native breast and reconstructed breast
    Disproportion between native breast and reconstructed breast

Chapter 14. Diseases of the Genitourinary System

Inflammatory diseases of female pelvic organs (N70-N77)

EXCLUDES 1   inflammatory diseases of female pelvic organs complicating:
abortion or ectopic or molar pregnancy (O00-O07, O08.0)
pregnancy, childbirth and the puerperium (O23.-, O75.3, O85, O86.-)

✓4ᵗʰ N70   Salpingitis and oophoritis

INCLUDES   abscess (of) fallopian tube
abscess (of) ovary
pyosalpinx
salpingo-oophoritis
tubo-ovarian abscess
tubo-ovarian inflammatory disease

Use additional code (B95-B97), to identify infectious agent

EXCLUDES 1   gonococcal infection (A54.24)
tuberculous infection (A18.17)

✓5ᵗʰ **N70.0**   Acute **salpingitis and oophoritis**

N70.01   Acute **salpingitis** ♀
N70.02   Acute **oophoritis** ♀
N70.03   Acute **salpingitis and oophoritis** ♀

✓5ᵗʰ **N70.1**   Chronic **salpingitis and oophoritis**

Hydrosalpinx

N70.11   Chronic **salpingitis** ♀
N70.12   Chronic **oophoritis** ♀
N70.13   Chronic **salpingitis and oophoritis** ♀

✓5ᵗʰ **N70.9**   Salpingitis and oophoritis, unspecified

N70.91   Salpingitis, unspecified ♀
N70.92   Oophoritis, unspecified ♀
N70.93   Salpingitis and oophoritis, **unspecified** ♀

✓4ᵗʰ N71   Inflammatory disease of uterus, except cervix

INCLUDES   endo (myo) metritis
metritis
myometritis
pyometra
uterine abscess

Use additional code (B95-B97), to identify infectious agent

EXCLUDES 1   hyperplastic endometritis (N85.0-)
infection of uterus following delivery (O85, O86.-)

N71.0   Acute **inflammatory disease of uterus** ♀
N71.1   Chronic **inflammatory disease of uterus** ♀
N71.9   Inflammatory disease of uterus, unspecified ♀

N72   Inflammatory disease of cervix uteri ♀

INCLUDES   cervicitis (with or without erosion or ectropion)
endocervicitis (with or without erosion or ectropion)
exocervicitis (with or without erosion or ectropion)

Use additional code (B95-B97), to identify infectious agent

EXCLUDES 1   erosion and ectropion of cervix without cervicitis (N86)

✓4ᵗʰ N73   Other female pelvic inflammatory diseases

Use additional code (B95-B97), to identify infectious agent

N73.0   Acute **parametritis and pelvic cellulitis** ♀
Abscess of broad ligament
Abscess of parametrium
Pelvic cellulitis, female
DEF: Parametritis: Inflammation of the parametrium.

N73.1   Chronic **parametritis and pelvic cellulitis** ♀
Any condition in N73.0 specified as chronic
EXCLUDES 1   tuberculous parametritis and pelvic cellulitis (A18.17)

N73.2   Unspecified **parametritis and pelvic cellulitis** ♀
Any condition in N73.0 unspecified whether acute or chronic

N73.3   Female acute **pelvic peritonitis** ♀
N73.4   Female chronic **pelvic peritonitis** ♀
EXCLUDES 1   tuberculous pelvic (female) peritonitis (A18.17)

N73.5   Female pelvic peritonitis, unspecified ♀

N73.6   Female pelvic **peritoneal adhesions (postinfective)** ♀
EXCLUDES 2   postprocedural pelvic peritoneal adhesions (N99.4)
AHA: 2014,1Q,6

N73.8   Other specified **female pelvic inflammatory diseases** ♀

N73.9   Female pelvic inflammatory disease, unspecified ♀
Female pelvic infection or inflammation NOS

N74   *Female pelvic inflammatory disorders in diseases classified elsewhere* ♀

Code first underlying disease

EXCLUDES 1   chlamydial cervicitis (A56.02)
chlamydial pelvic inflammatory disease (A56.11)
gonococcal cervicitis (A54.03)
gonococcal pelvic inflammatory disease (A54.24)
herpesviral [herpes simplex] cervicitis (A60.03)
herpesviral [herpes simplex] pelvic inflammatory disease (A60.09)
syphilitic cervicitis (A52.76)
syphilitic pelvic inflammatory disease (A52.76)
trichomonal cervicitis (A59.09)
tuberculous cervicitis (A18.16)
tuberculous pelvic inflammatory disease (A18.17)

✓4ᵗʰ N75   Diseases of Bartholin's gland

DEF: Bartholin's gland: Mucous-producing gland found in the vestibular bulbs on either side of the vaginal orifice and connected to the mucosal membrane at the opening by a duct.

N75.0   Cyst **of Bartholin's gland** ♀
N75.1   Abscess **of Bartholin's gland** ♀
N75.8   Other diseases of Bartholin's gland ♀
Bartholinitis
N75.9   Disease of Bartholin's gland, unspecified ♀

✓4ᵗʰ N76   Other inflammation of vagina and vulva

Use additional code (B95-B97), to identify infectious agent

EXCLUDES 2   senile (atrophic) vaginitis (N95.2)
vulvar vestibulitis (N94.810)

N76.0   Acute **vaginitis** ♀
Acute vulvovaginitis
Vaginitis NOS
Vulvovaginitis NOS

N76.1   Subacute and chronic **vaginitis** ♀
Chronic vulvovaginitis
Subacute vulvovaginitis

N76.2   Acute **vulvitis** ♀
Vulvitis NOS

N76.3   Subacute and chronic **vulvitis** ♀
N76.4   Abscess **of vulva** ♀
Furuncle of vulva

N76.5   Ulceration **of vagina** ♀
N76.6   Ulceration **of vulva** ♀

✓5ᵗʰ **N76.8**   Other specified **inflammation of vagina and vulva**

N76.81   Mucositis (ulcerative) of vagina and vulva ♀
Code also type of associated therapy, such as:
antineoplastic and immunosuppressive drugs (T45.1X-)
radiological procedure and radiotherapy (Y84.2)
EXCLUDES 2   gastrointestinal mucositis (ulcerative) (K92.81)
nasal mucositis (ulcerative) (J34.81)
oral mucositis (ulcerative) (K12.3-)

N76.82   Fournier disease **of vagina and vulva**
Fournier gangrene of vagina and vulva
Code also, if applicable, diabetes mellitus (E08-E13 with .9)
EXCLUDES 1   gangrene in diabetes mellitus (E08-E13 with .52)

N76.89   Other specified **inflammation of vagina and vulva** ♀

✓4ᵗʰ N77   Vulvovaginal ulceration and inflammation in diseases classified elsewhere

N77.0   *Ulceration of vulva in diseases classified elsewhere* ♀
Code first underlying disease, such as:
Behçet's disease (M35.2)
EXCLUDES 1   ulceration of vulva in gonococcal infection (A54.02)
ulceration of vulva in herpesviral [herpes simplex] infection (A60.04)
ulceration of vulva in syphilis (A51.0)
ulceration of vulva in tuberculosis (A18.18)

HCC CMS-HCC   **Rx** Rx HCC   **ESR** ESRD HCC   **COM** Commercial HCC   **N** Newborn: 0   **P** Pediatric: 0-17   **M** Maternity: 9-64   **A** Adult: 15-124

878

ICD-10-CM 2023

N77.1   *Vaginitis, vulvitis and vulvovaginitis in diseases classified elsewhere* ♀

Code first underlying disease, such as:
pinworm (B80)

EXCLUDES 1   *candidal vulvovaginitis ▶(B37.3-)◀*
chlamydial vulvovaginitis (A56.02)
gonococcal vulvovaginitis (A54.02)
herpesviral [herpes simplex] vulvovaginitis (A60.04)
trichomonal vulvovaginitis (A59.01)
tuberculous vulvovaginitis (A18.18)
vulvovaginitis in early syphilis (A51.0)
vulvovaginitis in late syphilis (A52.76)

Noninflammatory disorders of female genital tract (N80-N98)

✓4ᵗʰ **N80**   **Endometriosis**

DEF: Aberrant uterine mucosal tissue appearing in areas of the pelvic cavity outside of its normal location, lining the uterus, and inflaming surrounding tissues often resulting in infertility or spontaneous abortion.

▲   ✓5ᵗʰ **N80.0**   **Endometriosis of** uterus

~~Adenomyosis~~
▶Endometriosis of the cervix◀

EXCLUDES 1   *stromal endometriosis (D39.0)*

- **N80.00**   **Endometriosis of the uterus, unspecified**
- **N80.01**   **Superficial endometriosis of the uterus**
- **N80.02**   **Deep endometriosis of the uterus**
  Deep retrocervical endometriosis
- **N80.03**   **Adenomyosis of the uterus**
  Adenomyosis NOS

▲   ✓5ᵗʰ **N80.1**   **Endometriosis of** ovary

- ✓6ᵗʰ **N80.10**   **Endometriosis of ovary, unspecified depth**
  - **N80.101**   **Endometriosis of** right **ovary, unspecified depth**
  - **N80.102**   **Endometriosis of** left **ovary, unspecified depth**
  - **N80.103**   **Endometriosis of** bilateral **ovaries, unspecified depth**
  - **N80.109**   **Endometriosis of ovary, unspecified side, unspecified depth**
    Endometriosis of ovary NOS
- ✓6ᵗʰ **N80.11**   **Superficial endometriosis of the ovary**
  - **N80.111**   **Superficial endometriosis of** right **ovary**
  - **N80.112**   **Superficial endometriosis of** left **ovary**
  - **N80.113**   **Superficial endometriosis of** bilateral **ovaries**
  - **N80.119**   **Superficial endometriosis of ovary, unspecified ovary**
- ✓6ᵗʰ **N80.12**   **Deep endometriosis of ovary**
  Deep ovarian endometriosis
  Endometrioma
  - **N80.121**   **Deep endometriosis of** right **ovary**
  - **N80.122**   **Deep endometriosis of** left **ovary**
  - **N80.123**   **Deep endometriosis of** bilateral **ovaries**
  - **N80.129**   **Deep endometriosis of ovary, unspecified ovary**

▲   ✓5ᵗʰ **N80.2**   **Endometriosis of** fallopian tube

- ✓6ᵗʰ **N80.20**   **Endometriosis of fallopian tube, unspecified depth**
  - **N80.201**   **Endometriosis of** right **fallopian tube, unspecified depth**
  - **N80.202**   **Endometriosis of** left **fallopian tube, unspecified depth**
  - **N80.203**   **Endometriosis of** bilateral **fallopian tubes, unspecified depth**
  - **N80.209**   **Endometriosis of unspecified fallopian tube, unspecified depth**
    Endometriosis fallopian tube NOS
- ✓6ᵗʰ **N80.21**   **Superficial endometriosis of fallopian tube**
  - **N80.211**   **Superficial endometriosis of** right **fallopian tube**
  - **N80.212**   **Superficial endometriosis of** left **fallopian tube**
  - **N80.213**   **Superficial endometriosis of** bilateral **fallopian tubes**
  - **N80.219**   **Superficial endometriosis of unspecified fallopian tube**

- ✓6ᵗʰ **N80.22**   **Deep endometriosis of the fallopian tube**
  Deep endometriosis involving muscular wall of fallopian tube
  - **N80.221**   **Deep endometriosis of** right **fallopian tube**
  - **N80.222**   **Deep endometriosis of** left **fallopian tube**
  - **N80.223**   **Deep endometriosis of** bilateral **fallopian tubes**
  - **N80.229**   **Deep endometriosis of unspecified fallopian tube**

▲   ✓5ᵗʰ **N80.3**   **Endometriosis of** pelvic peritoneum

- **N80.30**   **Endometriosis of pelvic peritoneum, unspecified**
  Endometriosis of the retroperitoneum NOS
- ✓6ᵗʰ **N80.31**   **Endometriosis of the** anterior cul-de-sac
  - **N80.311**   **Superficial endometriosis of the anterior cul-de-sac**
  - **N80.312**   **Deep endometriosis of the anterior cul-de-sac**
  - **N80.319**   **Endometriosis of the anterior cul-de-sac, unspecified depth**
    Endometriosis of the anterior cul-de-sac NOS
- ✓6ᵗʰ **N80.32**   **Endometriosis of the** posterior cul-de-sac
  - **N80.321**   **Superficial endometriosis of the posterior cul-de-sac**
  - **N80.322**   **Deep endometriosis of the posterior cul-de-sac**
  - **N80.329**   **Endometriosis of the posterior cul-de-sac, unspecified depth**
    Endometriosis of the posterior cul-de-sac NOS
- ✓6ᵗʰ **N80.33**   **Superficial endometriosis of the** pelvic sidewall
  - **N80.331**   **Superficial endometriosis of the** right **pelvic sidewall**
  - **N80.332**   **Superficial endometriosis of the** left **pelvic sidewall**
  - **N80.333**   **Superficial endometriosis of** bilateral **pelvic sidewall**
  - **N80.339**   **Superficial endometriosis of pelvic sidewall, unspecified side**
- ✓6ᵗʰ **N80.34**   **Deep endometriosis of the** pelvic sidewall
  - **N80.341**   **Deep endometriosis of the** right **pelvic sidewall**
  - **N80.342**   **Deep endometriosis of the** left **pelvic sidewall**
  - **N80.343**   **Deep endometriosis of the** bilateral **pelvic sidewall**
  - **N80.349**   **Deep endometriosis of the pelvic sidewall, unspecified side**
- ✓6ᵗʰ **N80.35**   **Endometriosis of the pelvic sidewall, unspecified depth**
  - **N80.351**   **Endometriosis of the** right **pelvic sidewall, unspecified depth**
  - **N80.352**   **Endometriosis of the** left **pelvic sidewall, unspecified depth**
  - **N80.353**   **Endometriosis of** bilateral **pelvic sidewall, unspecified depth**
  - **N80.359**   **Endometriosis of pelvic sidewall, unspecified side, unspecified depth**
    Endometriosis of the pelvic sidewall NOS
- ✓6ᵗʰ **N80.36**   **Superficial endometriosis of the** pelvic brim
  - **N80.361**   **Superficial endometriosis of the** right **pelvic brim**
  - **N80.362**   **Superficial endometriosis of the** left **pelvic brim**
  - **N80.363**   **Superficial endometriosis of** bilateral **pelvic brim**
  - **N80.369**   **Superficial endometriosis of the pelvic brim, unspecified side**
- ✓6ᵗʰ **N80.37**   **Deep endometriosis of the** pelvic brim
  - **N80.371**   **Deep endometriosis of the** right **pelvic brim**
  - **N80.372**   **Deep endometriosis of the** left **pelvic brim**
  - **N80.373**   **Deep endometriosis of** bilateral **pelvic brim**
  - **N80.379**   **Deep endometriosis of the pelvic brim, unspecified side**
- ✓6ᵗʰ **N80.38**   **Endometriosis of the pelvic brim, unspecified depth**
  - **N80.381**   **Endometriosis of the** right **pelvic brim, unspecified depth**

☑ Additional Character Required   ✓x7ᵗʰ Placeholder Alert   Manifestation   Unspecified Dx   Q QPP   UPD Unacceptable PDx

N80.382 Endometriosis of the left pelvic brim, unspecified depth

N80.383 Endometriosis of bilateral pelvic brim, unspecified depth

N80.389 Endometriosis of the pelvic brim, unspecified side, unspecified depth
Endometriosis of the pelvic brim NOS

✓6ᵗʰ N80.3A Superficial endometriosis of the uterosacral ligament(s)

N80.3A1 Superficial endometriosis of the right uterosacral ligament

N80.3A2 Superficial endometriosis of the left uterosacral ligament

N80.3A3 Superficial endometriosis of the bilateral uterosacral ligament(s)

N80.3A9 Superficial endometriosis of the uterosacral ligament(s), unspecified side

✓6ᵗʰ N80.3B Deep endometriosis of the uterosacral ligament(s)

N80.3B1 Deep endometriosis of the right uterosacral ligament

N80.3B2 Deep endometriosis of the left uterosacral ligament

N80.3B3 Deep endometriosis of bilateral uterosacral ligament(s)

N80.3B9 Deep endometriosis of the uterosacral ligament(s), unspecified side

✓6ᵗʰ N80.3C Endometriosis of the uterosacral ligament(s), unspecified depth

N80.3C1 Endometriosis of the right uterosacral ligament, unspecified depth

N80.3C2 Endometriosis of the left uterosacral ligament, unspecified depth

N80.3C3 Endometriosis of bilateral uterosacral ligament(s), unspecified depth

N80.3C9 Endometriosis of the uterosacral ligament(s), unspecified side, unspecified depth
Endometriosis of the uterosacral ligament(s) NOS

✓6ᵗʰ N80.39 Endometriosis of other pelvic peritoneum

N80.391 Superficial endometriosis of the pelvic peritoneum, other specified sites

N80.392 Deep endometriosis of the pelvic peritoneum, other specified sites

N80.399 Endometriosis of the pelvic peritoneum, other specified sites, unspecified depth

▲ ✓5ᵗʰ N80.4 Endometriosis of rectovaginal septum and vagina

N80.40 Endometriosis of rectovaginal septum, unspecified involvement of vagina
Endometriosis of the rectovaginal septum, NOS

N80.41 Endometriosis of rectovaginal septum without involvement of vagina

N80.42 Endometriosis of rectovaginal septum with involvement of vagina

▲ ✓5ᵗʰ N80.5 Endometriosis of intestine

N80.50 Endometriosis of intestine, unspecified

✓6ᵗʰ N80.51 Endometriosis of the rectum

N80.511 Superficial endometriosis of the rectum

N80.512 Deep endometriosis of the rectum
Deep endometriosis of the rectum, multifocal

N80.519 Endometriosis of the rectum, unspecified depth
Endometriosis of the rectum NOS

✓6ᵗʰ N80.52 Endometriosis of the sigmoid colon

N80.521 Superficial endometriosis of the sigmoid colon

N80.522 Deep endometriosis of the sigmoid colon

N80.529 Endometriosis of the sigmoid colon, unspecified depth
Endometriosis of the sigmoid colon NOS

✓6ᵗʰ N80.53 Endometriosis of the cecum

N80.531 Superficial endometriosis of the cecum

N80.532 Deep endometriosis of the cecum

N80.539 Endometriosis of the cecum, unspecified depth
Endometriosis of the cecum NOS

✓6ᵗʰ N80.54 Endometriosis of the appendix

N80.541 Superficial endometriosis of the appendix

N80.542 Deep endometriosis of the appendix

N80.549 Endometriosis of the appendix, unspecified depth
Endometriosis of the appendix NOS

✓6ᵗʰ N80.55 Endometriosis of other parts of the colon
Endometriosis of descending colon
Endometriosis of transverse colon

N80.551 Superficial endometriosis of other parts of the colon

N80.552 Deep endometriosis of other parts of the colon

N80.559 Endometriosis of other parts of the colon, unspecified depth
Endometriosis of colon NOS

✓6ᵗʰ N80.56 Endometriosis of the small intestine

N80.561 Superficial endometriosis of the small intestine

N80.562 Deep endometriosis of the small intestine
Deep endometriosis of the small intestine, multifocal

N80.569 Endometriosis of the small intestine, unspecified depth
Endometriosis of the small intestine NOS

N80.6 Endometriosis in cutaneous scar   ♀

✓5ᵗʰ N80.A Endometriosis of bladder and ureters

N80.A0 Endometriosis of bladder, unspecified depth
Endometriosis of bladder NOS

N80.A1 Superficial endometriosis of bladder

N80.A2 Deep endometriosis of bladder

✓6ᵗʰ N80.A4 Superficial endometriosis of ureter
Extrinsic endometriosis of ureter
Code also, if applicable, obstructive and reflux uropathy (N13.-)

N80.A41 Superficial endometriosis of right ureter

N80.A42 Superficial endometriosis of left ureter

N80.A43 Superficial endometriosis of bilateral ureters

N80.A49 Superficial endometriosis of unspecified ureter

✓6ᵗʰ N80.A5 Deep endometriosis of ureter
Intrinsic endometriosis of ureter
Code also, if applicable, obstructive and reflux uropathy (N13.-)

N80.A51 Deep endometriosis of right ureter

N80.A52 Deep endometriosis of left ureter

N80.A53 Deep endometriosis of bilateral ureters

N80.A59 Deep endometriosis of unspecified ureter

✓6ᵗʰ N80.A6 Endometriosis of ureter, unspecified depth
Code also, if applicable, obstructive and reflux uropathy (N13.-)

N80.A61 Endometriosis of right ureter, unspecified depth

N80.A62 Endometriosis of left ureter, unspecified depth

N80.A63 Endometriosis of bilateral ureters, unspecified depth

N80.A69 Endometriosis of unspecified ureter, unspecified depth

✓5ᵗʰ N80.B Endometriosis of cardiothoracic space
Endometriosis of thorax
Code also, if applicable:
catamenial hemothorax (J94.2)
catamenial pneumothorax (J93.12)

N80.B1 Endometriosis of pleura

N80.B2 Endometriosis of lung

✓6ᵗʰ N80.B3 Endometriosis of diaphragm

N80.B31 Superficial endometriosis of diaphragm

N80.B32 Deep endometriosis of diaphragm

N80.B39 Endometriosis of diaphragm, unspecified depth
Endometriosis of the diaphragm NOS

N80.B4 Endometriosis of the pericardial space

N80.B5 Endometriosis of the mediastinal space

N80.B6 Endometriosis of cardiothoracic space

- ✓5ᵗʰ **N80.C** **Endometriosis of the** abdomen
-     **N80.C0** **Endometriosis of the abdomen, unspecified**
  - Endometriosis of the abdomen NOS
-     ✓6ᵗʰ **N80.C1** **Endometriosis of the** anterior **abdominal wall**
  - **N80.C10** **Endometriosis of the anterior abdominal wall,** subcutaneous tissue
  - **N80.C11** **Endometriosis of the anterior abdominal wall,** fascia and muscular layers
  - **N80.C19** **Endometriosis of the anterior abdominal wall, unspecified depth**
    - Endometriosis of the anterior abdominal wall NOS
-     **N80.C2** **Endometriosis of the** umbilicus
-     **N80.C3** **Endometriosis of the** inguinal canal
-     **N80.C4** **Endometriosis of** extra-pelvic abdominal peritoneum
-     **N80.C9** **Endometriosis of other site of abdomen**
- ✓5ᵗʰ **N80.D** **Endometriosis of the** pelvic nerves
  - Endometriosis of the nerves of the retroperitoneum
-     **N80.D0** **Endometriosis of the pelvic nerves, unspecified**
  - Endometriosis of nerve of the retroperitoneum, NOS
-     **N80.D1** **Endometriosis of the** sacral splanchnic nerves
  - Endometriosis of the pelvic splanchnic nerves
-     **N80.D2** **Endometriosis of the** sacral nerve roots
-     **N80.D3** **Endometriosis of the** obturator nerve
-     **N80.D4** **Endometriosis of the** sciatic nerve
-     **N80.D5** **Endometriosis of the** pudendal nerve
-     **N80.D6** **Endometriosis of the** femoral nerve
-     **N80.D9** **Endometriosis of other pelvic nerve**
  - Endometriosis of the other nerves of the retroperitoneum
-     **N80.8** **Other endometriosis**   ♀
  - ▶Endometriosis of other site◀
-     **N80.9** **Endometriosis, unspecified**   ♀

✓4ᵗʰ **N81** **Female genital prolapse**
> EXCLUDES 1   genital prolapse complicating pregnancy, labor or delivery (O34.5-)
> prolapse and hernia of ovary and fallopian tube (N83.4-)
> prolapse of vaginal vault after hysterectomy (N99.3)

Types of Pelvic Organ Prolapse

Urethrocele

Cystocele

Rectocele

Enterocele

- **N81.0** **Urethrocele**   ♀
  > EXCLUDES 1   urethrocele with cystocele (N81.1-)
  > urethrocele with prolapse of uterus (N81.2-N81.4)
- ✓5ᵗʰ **N81.1** **Cystocele**
  - Cystocele with urethrocele
  - Cystourethrocele
  > EXCLUDES 1   cystocele with prolapse of uterus (N81.2-N81.4)
  - **N81.10** **Cystocele, unspecified**   Q ♀
    - Prolapse of (anterior) vaginal wall NOS
  - **N81.11** **Cystocele,** midline   Q ♀

-   **N81.12** **Cystocele,** lateral   Q ♀
  - Paravaginal cystocele
  - **DEF:** Detachment of the lateral support connections of the vagina at the arcus tendineus fasciae pelvis (ATFP) that results in bladder drop. The bladder herniates into the vagina laterally.
- **N81.2** **Incomplete uterovaginal prolapse**   Q ♀
  - First degree uterine prolapse
  - Prolapse of cervix NOS
  - Second degree uterine prolapse
  > EXCLUDES 1   cervical stump prolapse (N81.85)
- **N81.3** **Complete uterovaginal prolapse**   Q ♀
  - Procidentia (uteri) NOS
  - Third degree uterine prolapse
- **N81.4** **Uterovaginal prolapse, unspecified**   Q ♀
  - Prolapse of uterus NOS
- **N81.5** **Vaginal enterocele**   ♀
  > EXCLUDES 1   enterocele with prolapse of uterus (N81.2-N81.4)
- **N81.6** **Rectocele**   ♀
  - Prolapse of posterior vaginal wall
  - Use additional code for any associated fecal incontinence, if applicable (R15.-)
  > EXCLUDES 2   perineocele (N81.81)
  > rectal prolapse (K62.3)
  > rectocele with prolapse of uterus (N81.2-N81.4)
- ✓5ᵗʰ **N81.8** **Other female genital prolapse**
  - **N81.81** **Perineocele**   ♀
  - **N81.82** **Incompetence or weakening of** pubocervical tissue   ♀
  - **N81.83** **Incompetence or weakening of** rectovaginal tissue   ♀
  - **N81.84** **Pelvic muscle wasting**   ♀
    - Disuse atrophy of pelvic muscles and anal sphincter
  - **N81.85** **Cervical stump prolapse**   ♀
  - **N81.89** **Other female genital prolapse**   Q ♀
    - Deficient perineum
    - Old laceration of muscles of pelvic floor
- **N81.9** **Female genital prolapse, unspecified**   Q ♀

✓4ᵗʰ **N82** **Fistulae involving female genital tract**
> EXCLUDES 1   vesicointestinal fistulae (N32.1)

- **N82.0** **Vesicovaginal fistula**   ♀
- **N82.1** **Other female urinary-genital tract fistulae**   ♀
  - Cervicovesical fistula
  - Ureterovaginal fistula
  - Urethrovaginal fistula
  - Uteroureteric fistula
  - Uterovesical fistula
  - **AHA:** 2017,3Q,3
- **N82.2** **Fistula of vagina to** small **intestine**   ♀
- **N82.3** **Fistula of vagina to** large **intestine**   ♀
  - Rectovaginal fistula
- **N82.4** **Other female intestinal-genital tract fistulae**   ♀
  - Intestinouterine fistula
- **N82.5** **Female** genital tract-skin **fistulae**   ♀
  - Uterus to abdominal wall fistula
  - Vaginoperineal fistula
- **N82.8** **Other female genital tract fistulae**   ♀
- **N82.9** **Female genital tract fistula, unspecified**   ♀

✓4ᵗʰ **N83** **Noninflammatory disorders of ovary, fallopian tube and broad ligament**
> EXCLUDES 2   hydrosalpinx (N70.1-)
> **AHA:** 2016,4Q,46

- ✓5ᵗʰ **N83.0** **Follicular cyst of ovary**
  - Cyst of graafian follicle
  - Hemorrhagic follicular cyst (of ovary)
  - **N83.00** **Follicular cyst of ovary, unspecified side**   ♀
  - **N83.01** **Follicular cyst of** right **ovary**   ♀
  - **N83.02** **Follicular cyst of** left **ovary**   ♀
- ✓5ᵗʰ **N83.1** **Corpus luteum cyst**
  - Hemorrhagic corpus luteum cyst
  - **AHA:** 2022,1Q,23
  - **N83.10** **Corpus luteum cyst of ovary, unspecified side**   ♀
  - **N83.11** **Corpus luteum cyst of** right **ovary**   ♀
  - **N83.12** **Corpus luteum cyst of** left **ovary**   ♀

✓5ᵗʰ N83.2 Other and unspecified ovarian cysts

EXCLUDES 1   *developmental ovarian cyst (Q50.1)*
     neoplastic ovarian cyst (D27.-)
     polycystic ovarian syndrome (E28.2)
     Stein-Leventhal syndrome (E28.2)

AHA: 2022,1Q,23

     ✓6ᵗʰ N83.20 Unspecified ovarian cysts

        N83.201 Unspecified ovarian cyst, right side ♀
        N83.202 Unspecified ovarian cyst, left side ♀
        N83.209 Unspecified ovarian cyst, unspecified side ♀
          Ovarian cyst, NOS

     ✓6ᵗʰ N83.29 Other ovarian cysts

        Retention cyst of ovary
        Simple cyst of ovary
        N83.291 Other ovarian cyst, right side ♀
        N83.292 Other ovarian cyst, left side ♀
        N83.299 Other ovarian cyst, unspecified side ♀

✓5ᵗʰ N83.3 Acquired atrophy of ovary and fallopian tube

     ✓6ᵗʰ N83.31 Acquired atrophy of ovary

        N83.311 Acquired atrophy of right ovary ♀
        N83.312 Acquired atrophy of left ovary ♀
        N83.319 Acquired atrophy of ovary, unspecified side ♀
          Acquired atrophy of ovary, NOS

     ✓6ᵗʰ N83.32 Acquired atrophy of fallopian tube

        N83.321 Acquired atrophy of right fallopian tube ♀
        N83.322 Acquired atrophy of left fallopian tube ♀
        N83.329 Acquired atrophy of fallopian tube, unspecified side ♀
          Acquired atrophy of fallopian tube, NOS

     ✓6ᵗʰ N83.33 Acquired atrophy of ovary and fallopian tube

        N83.331 Acquired atrophy of right ovary and fallopian tube ♀
        N83.332 Acquired atrophy of left ovary and fallopian tube ♀
        N83.339 Acquired atrophy of ovary and fallopian tube, unspecified side ♀
          Acquired atrophy of ovary and fallopian tube, NOS

✓5ᵗʰ N83.4 Prolapse and hernia of ovary and fallopian tube

     N83.40 Prolapse and hernia of ovary and fallopian tube, unspecified side ♀
        Prolapse and hernia of ovary and fallopian tube, NOS
     N83.41 Prolapse and hernia of right ovary and fallopian tube ♀
     N83.42 Prolapse and hernia of left ovary and fallopian tube ♀

✓5ᵗʰ N83.5 Torsion of ovary, ovarian pedicle and fallopian tube

     Torsion of accessory tube

     ✓6ᵗʰ N83.51 Torsion of ovary and ovarian pedicle

        N83.511 Torsion of right ovary and ovarian pedicle ♀
        N83.512 Torsion of left ovary and ovarian pedicle ♀
        N83.519 Torsion of ovary and ovarian pedicle, unspecified side ♀
          Torsion of ovary and ovarian pedicle, NOS

     ✓6ᵗʰ N83.52 Torsion of fallopian tube

        Torsion of hydatid of Morgagni
        N83.521 Torsion of right fallopian tube ♀
        N83.522 Torsion of left fallopian tube ♀
        N83.529 Torsion of fallopian tube, unspecified side ♀
          Torsion of fallopian tube, NOS

     N83.53 Torsion of ovary, ovarian pedicle and fallopian tube ♀

N83.6 Hematosalpinx ♀

EXCLUDES 1   *hematosalpinx (with) (in):*
     hematocolpos (N89.7)
     hematometra (N85.7)
     tubal pregnancy (O00.1-)

N83.7 Hematoma of broad ligament ♀

N83.8 Other noninflammatory disorders of ovary, fallopian tube and broad ligament ♀

     Broad ligament laceration syndrome [Allen-Masters]

N83.9 Noninflammatory disorder of ovary, fallopian tube and broad ligament, unspecified ♀

✓4ᵗʰ N84 Polyp of female genital tract

EXCLUDES 1   *adenomatous polyp (D28.-)*
     placental polyp (O90.89)

N84.0 Polyp of corpus uteri ♀
     Polyp of endometrium
     Polyp of uterus NOS
     EXCLUDES 1   *polypoid endometrial hyperplasia (N85.0-)*

N84.1 Polyp of cervix uteri ♀
     Mucous polyp of cervix

N84.2 Polyp of vagina ♀

N84.3 Polyp of vulva ♀
     Polyp of labia

N84.8 Polyp of other parts of female genital tract ♀

N84.9 Polyp of female genital tract, unspecified ♀

✓4ᵗʰ N85 Other noninflammatory disorders of uterus, except cervix

EXCLUDES 1   *endometriosis (N80.-)*
     inflammatory diseases of uterus (N71.-)
     noninflammatory disorders of cervix, except malposition (N86-N88)
     polyp of corpus uteri (N84.0)
     uterine prolapse (N81.-)

✓5ᵗʰ N85.0 Endometrial hyperplasia

     N85.00 Endometrial hyperplasia, unspecified ♀
        Hyperplasia (adenomatous) (cystic) (glandular) of endometrium
        Hyperplastic endometritis

     N85.01 Benign endometrial hyperplasia ♀
        Endometrial hyperplasia (complex) (simple) without atypia

     N85.02 Endometrial intraepithelial neoplasia [EIN] ♀
        Endometrial hyperplasia with atypia
        EXCLUDES 1   *malignant neoplasm of endometrium (with endometrial intraepithelial neoplasia [EIN]) (C54.1)*

N85.2 Hypertrophy of uterus ♀
     Bulky or enlarged uterus
     EXCLUDES 1   *puerperal hypertrophy of uterus (O90.89)*

N85.3 Subinvolution of uterus ♀
     EXCLUDES 1   *puerperal subinvolution of uterus (O90.89)*

N85.4 Malposition of uterus ♀
     Anteversion of uterus
     Retroflexion of uterus
     Retroversion of uterus
     EXCLUDES 1   *malposition of uterus complicating pregnancy, labor or delivery (O34.5-, O65.5)*

N85.5 Inversion of uterus ♀
     EXCLUDES 1   *current obstetric trauma (O71.2)*
        postpartum inversion of uterus (O71.2)
     DEF: Abnormality in which the uterus turns inside out.

Inversion of Uterus

Uterus

N85.6 Intrauterine synechiae ♀

HCC CMS-HCC   Rx Rx HCC   ESR ESRD HCC   COM Commercial HCC   N Newborn: 0   P Pediatric: 0-17   M Maternity: 9-64   A Adult: 15-124

N85.7 **Hematometra** ♀
    Hematosalpinx with hematometra
        EXCLUDES 1   *hematometra with hematocolpos (N89.7)*
        DEF: Accumulation of blood within the uterus.

N85.8 **Other specified noninflammatory disorders of uterus** ♀
    Atrophy of uterus, acquired
    Fibrosis of uterus NOS

N85.9 **Noninflammatory disorder of uterus, unspecified** ♀
    Disorder of uterus NOS

● **N85.A** **Isthmocele**
    Isthmocele (non-pregnant state)
    Code also any associated conditions such as:
       abnormal uterine and vaginal bleeding, unspecified (N93.9)
       female infertility of uterine origin (N97.2)
       pelvic and perineal pain (R10.2)
        EXCLUDES 1   *maternal care for cesarean scar defect (isthmocele)*
            (O34.22)

N86 **Erosion and ectropion of cervix uteri** ♀
    Decubitus (trophic) ulcer of cervix
    Eversion of cervix
        EXCLUDES 1   *erosion and ectropion of cervix with cervicitis (N72)*

☑4ᵗʰ **N87** **Dysplasia of cervix uteri**
        EXCLUDES 1   *abnormal results from cervical cytologic examination without*
            histologic confirmation (R87.61-)
            carcinoma in situ of cervix uteri (D06.-)
            cervical intraepithelial neoplasia III [CIN III] (D06.-)
            HGSIL of cervix (R87.613)
            severe dysplasia of cervix uteri (D06.-)

N87.0 **Mild cervical dysplasia** ♀
    Cervical intraepithelial neoplasia I [CIN I]

N87.1 **Moderate cervical dysplasia** ♀
    Cervical intraepithelial neoplasia II [CIN II]

N87.9 **Dysplasia of cervix uteri, unspecified** ♀
    Anaplasia of cervix
    Cervical atypism
    Cervical dysplasia NOS

☑4ᵗʰ **N88** **Other noninflammatory disorders of cervix uteri**
        EXCLUDES 2   *inflammatory disease of cervix (N72)*
            polyp of cervix (N84.1)

N88.0 **Leukoplakia of cervix uteri** ♀

N88.1 **Old laceration of cervix uteri** ♀
    Adhesions of cervix
        EXCLUDES 1   *current obstetric trauma (O71.3)*

N88.2 **Stricture and stenosis of cervix uteri** ♀
        EXCLUDES 1   *stricture and stenosis of cervix uteri complicating*
            labor (O65.5)

N88.3 **Incompetence of cervix uteri** ♀
    Investigation and management of (suspected) cervical
       incompetence in a nonpregnant woman
        EXCLUDES 1   *cervical incompetence complicating pregnancy*
            (O34.3-)
        DEF: Inadequate functioning of the cervix marked by abnormal
       widening during pregnancy and causing premature birth or
       miscarriage.

N88.4 **Hypertrophic elongation of cervix uteri** ♀

N88.8 **Other specified noninflammatory disorders of cervix uteri** ♀
        EXCLUDES 1   *current obstetric trauma (O71.3)*

N88.9 **Noninflammatory disorder of cervix uteri, unspecified** ♀

☑4ᵗʰ **N89** **Other noninflammatory disorders of vagina**
        EXCLUDES 1   *abnormal results from vaginal cytologic examination without*
            histologic confirmation (R87.62-)
            carcinoma in situ of vagina (D07.2)
            HGSIL of vagina (R87.623)
            inflammation of vagina (N76.-)
            senile (atrophic) vaginitis (N95.2)
            severe dysplasia of vagina (D07.2)
            trichomonal leukorrhea (A59.00)
            vaginal intraepithelial neoplasia [VAIN], grade III (D07.2)

N89.0 **Mild vaginal dysplasia** ♀
    Vaginal intraepithelial neoplasia [VAIN], grade I

N89.1 **Moderate vaginal dysplasia** ♀
    Vaginal intraepithelial neoplasia [VAIN], grade II

N89.3 **Dysplasia of vagina, unspecified** ♀

N89.4 **Leukoplakia of vagina** ♀

N89.5 **Stricture and atresia of vagina** ♀
    Vaginal adhesions
    Vaginal stenosis
        EXCLUDES 1   *congenital atresia or stricture (Q52.4)*
            postprocedural adhesions of vagina (N99.2)

N89.6 **Tight hymenal ring** ♀
    Rigid hymen
    Tight introitus
        EXCLUDES 1   *imperforate hymen (Q52.3)*

N89.7 **Hematocolpos** ♀
    Hematocolpos with hematometra or hematosalpinx
    AHA: 2016,4Q,58

N89.8 **Other specified noninflammatory disorders of vagina** ♀
    Leukorrhea NOS
    Old vaginal laceration
    Pessary ulcer of vagina
        EXCLUDES 1   *current obstetric trauma (O70.-, O71.4, O71.7-O71.8)*
            old laceration involving muscles of pelvic floor
            (N81.8)

N89.9 **Noninflammatory disorder of vagina, unspecified** ♀

☑4ᵗʰ **N90** **Other noninflammatory disorders of vulva and perineum**
        EXCLUDES 1   *anogenital (venereal) warts (A63.0)*
            carcinoma in situ of vulva (D07.1)
            condyloma acuminatum (A63.0)
            current obstetric trauma (O70.-, O71.7-O71.8)
            inflammation of vulva (N76.-)
            severe dysplasia of vulva (D07.1)
            vulvar intraepithelial neoplasm III [VIN III] (D07.1)

N90.0 **Mild vulvar dysplasia** ♀
    Vulvar intraepithelial neoplasia [VIN], grade I

N90.1 **Moderate vulvar dysplasia** ♀
    Vulvar intraepithelial neoplasia [VIN], grade II

N90.3 **Dysplasia of vulva, unspecified** ♀

N90.4 **Leukoplakia of vulva** ♀
    Dystrophy of vulva
    Kraurosis of vulva
    Lichen sclerosus of external female genital organs

N90.5 **Atrophy of vulva** ♀
    Stenosis of vulva

☑5ᵗʰ **N90.6** **Hypertrophy of vulva**
    AHA: 2016,4Q,46

N90.60 **Unspecified hypertrophy of vulva** ♀
    Unspecified hypertrophy of labia

N90.61 **Childhood asymmetric labium majus enlargement** ♀
    CALME

N90.69 **Other specified hypertrophy of vulva** ♀
    Other specified hypertrophy of labia

N90.7 **Vulvar cyst** ♀

☑5ᵗʰ **N90.8** **Other specified noninflammatory disorders of vulva and perineum**

   ☑6ᵗʰ **N90.81** **Female genital mutilation status**
    Female genital cutting status

      N90.810 **Female genital mutilation status, unspecified** ♀
      Female genital cutting status, unspecified
      Female genital mutilation status NOS

      N90.811 **Female genital mutilation Type I status** ♀
      Clitorectomy status
      Female genital cutting Type I status

      N90.812 **Female genital mutilation Type II status** ♀
      Clitorectomy with excision of labia minora status
      Female genital cutting Type II status

      N90.813 **Female genital mutilation Type III status** ♀
      Female genital cutting Type III status
      Infibulation status

N90.818 Other female genital mutilation status ♀
Female genital cutting Type IV status
Female genital mutilation Type IV status
Other female genital cutting status

N90.89 Other specified noninflammatory disorders of vulva and perineum ♀
Adhesions of vulva
Hypertrophy of clitoris

N90.9 Noninflammatory disorder of vulva and perineum, unspecified ♀

✓4ᵗʰ **N91 Absent, scanty and rare menstruation**
EXCLUDES 1   *ovarian dysfunction (E28.-)*

N91.0 Primary amenorrhea ♀
N91.1 Secondary amenorrhea ♀
N91.2 Amenorrhea, unspecified ♀
N91.3 Primary oligomenorrhea ♀
N91.4 Secondary oligomenorrhea ♀
N91.5 Oligomenorrhea, unspecified ♀
Hypomenorrhea NOS

✓4ᵗʰ **N92 Excessive, frequent and irregular menstruation**
EXCLUDES 1   *postmenopausal bleeding (N95.0)*
precocious puberty (menstruation) (E30.1)

N92.0 Excessive and frequent menstruation with regular cycle ♀
Heavy periods NOS
Menorrhagia NOS
Polymenorrhea

N92.1 Excessive and frequent menstruation with irregular cycle ♀
Irregular intermenstrual bleeding
Irregular, shortened intervals between menstrual bleeding
Menometrorrhagia
Metrorrhagia

N92.2 Excessive menstruation at puberty P ♀
Excessive bleeding associated with onset of menstrual periods
Pubertal menorrhagia
Puberty bleeding

N92.3 Ovulation bleeding ♀
Regular intermenstrual bleeding

N92.4 Excessive bleeding in the premenopausal period ♀
Climacteric menorrhagia or metrorrhagia
Menopausal menorrhagia or metrorrhagia
Perimenopausal bleeding
Perimenopausal menorrhagia or metrorrhagia
Preclimacteric menorrhagia or metrorrhagia
Premenopausal menorrhagia or metrorrhagia

N92.5 Other specified irregular menstruation ♀
N92.6 Irregular menstruation, unspecified ♀
Irregular bleeding NOS
Irregular periods NOS
EXCLUDES 1   *irregular menstruation with:*
lengthened intervals or scanty bleeding (N91.3-N91.5)
shortened intervals or excessive bleeding (N92.1)

✓4ᵗʰ **N93 Other abnormal uterine and vaginal bleeding**
EXCLUDES 1   *neonatal vaginal hemorrhage (P54.6)*
precocious puberty (menstruation) (E30.1)
pseudomenses (P54.6)

N93.0 Postcoital and contact bleeding ♀
N93.1 Pre-pubertal vaginal bleeding ♀
AHA: 2016,4Q,47

N93.8 Other specified abnormal uterine and vaginal bleeding ♀
Dysfunctional or functional uterine or vaginal bleeding NOS

N93.9 Abnormal uterine and vaginal bleeding, unspecified ♀

✓4ᵗʰ **N94 Pain and other conditions associated with female genital organs and menstrual cycle**

N94.0 Mittelschmerz ♀
DEF: One-sided, lower abdominal pain occurring between menstrual periods that is associated with ovulation.

✓5ᵗʰ **N94.1 Dyspareunia**
EXCLUDES 1   *psychogenic dyspareunia (F52.6)*
AHA: 2016,4Q,47

N94.10 Unspecified dyspareunia ♀
N94.11 Superficial (introital) dyspareunia ♀

N94.12 Deep dyspareunia ♀
N94.19 Other specified dyspareunia ♀

N94.2 Vaginismus ♀
EXCLUDES 1   *psychogenic vaginismus (F52.5)*
DEF: Spontaneous contractions of the muscles surrounding the vagina, causing it to constrict or close.

N94.3 Premenstrual tension syndrome ♀
Code also associated menstrual migraine (G43.82-, G43.83-)
EXCLUDES 1   *premenstrual dysphoric disorder (F32.81)*

N94.4 Primary dysmenorrhea ♀
N94.5 Secondary dysmenorrhea ♀
N94.6 Dysmenorrhea, unspecified ♀
EXCLUDES 1   *psychogenic dysmenorrhea (F45.8)*

✓5ᵗʰ **N94.8 Other specified conditions associated with female genital organs and menstrual cycle**

✓6ᵗʰ **N94.81 Vulvodynia**

N94.810 Vulvar vestibulitis ♀
N94.818 Other vulvodynia ♀
N94.819 Vulvodynia, unspecified ♀
Vulvodynia NOS

N94.89 Other specified conditions associated with female genital organs and menstrual cycle ♀
DEF: Hydrocele: Serous fluid that collects in the canal of Nuck in females.

N94.9 Unspecified condition associated with female genital organs and menstrual cycle ♀

✓4ᵗʰ **N95 Menopausal and other perimenopausal disorders**
Menopausal and other perimenopausal disorders due to naturally occurring (age-related) menopause and perimenopause
EXCLUDES 1   *excessive bleeding in the premenopausal period (N92.4)*
menopausal and perimenopausal disorders due to artificial or premature menopause (E89.4-, E28.31-)
premature menopause (E28.31-)
EXCLUDES 2   *postmenopausal osteoporosis (M81.0-)*
postmenopausal osteoporosis with current pathological fracture (M80.0-)
postmenopausal urethritis (N34.2)

N95.0 Postmenopausal bleeding ♀
N95.1 Menopausal and female climacteric states ♀
Symptoms such as flushing, sleeplessness, headache, lack of concentration, associated with natural (age-related) menopause
Use additional code for associated symptoms
EXCLUDES 1   *asymptomatic menopausal state (Z78.0)*
symptoms associated with artificial menopause (E89.41)
symptoms associated with premature menopause (E28.310)

N95.2 Postmenopausal atrophic vaginitis ♀
Senile (atrophic) vaginitis

N95.8 Other specified menopausal and perimenopausal disorders ♀

N95.9 Unspecified menopausal and perimenopausal disorder ♀

N96 Recurrent pregnancy loss ♀
Investigation or care in a nonpregnant woman with history of recurrent pregnancy loss
EXCLUDES 1   *recurrent pregnancy loss with current pregnancy (O26.2-)*

✓4ᵗʰ **N97 Female infertility**
INCLUDES   inability to achieve a pregnancy
sterility, female NOS
EXCLUDES 2   *female infertility associated with:*
hypopituitarism (E23.0)
Stein-Leventhal syndrome (E28.2)
incompetence of cervix uteri (N88.3)
DEF: Infertility: Inability to conceive for at least one year with regular intercourse.
DEF: Primary infertility: Infertility occurring in patients who have never conceived.
DEF: Secondary infertility: Infertility occurring in patients who have previously conceived.

N97.0 Female infertility associated with anovulation ♀
AHA: 2022,2Q,16

N97.1 **Female infertility of** tubal origin ♀
     Female infertility associated with congenital anomaly of tube
     Female infertility due to tubal block
     Female infertility due to tubal occlusion
     Female infertility due to tubal stenosis

N97.2 **Female infertility of** uterine origin ♀
     Female infertility associated with congenital anomaly of uterus
     Female infertility due to nonimplantation of ovum

N97.8 **Female infertility of other origin** ♀
     AHA: 2022,2Q,15

N97.9 **Female infertility, unspecified** ♀

✓4ᵗʰ **N98** **Complications associated with artificial fertilization**

N98.0 Infection **associated with artificial insemination** ♀

N98.1 Hyperstimulation of ovaries ♀
     Hyperstimulation of ovaries NOS
     Hyperstimulation of ovaries associated with induced ovulation

N98.2 **Complications of attempted** introduction of fertilized ovum **following in vitro fertilization** ♀

N98.3 **Complications of attempted** introduction of embryo in **embryo transfer** ♀

N98.8 **Other complications associated with artificial fertilization** ♀

N98.9 **Complication associated with artificial fertilization, unspecified** ♀

Intraoperative and postprocedural complications and disorders of genitourinary system, not elsewhere classified (N99)

✓4ᵗʰ **N99** **Intraoperative and postprocedural complications and disorders of genitourinary system, not elsewhere classified**
     EXCLUDES 2   irradiation cystitis (N30.4-)
            postoophorectomy osteoporosis with current pathological fracture (M80.8-)
            postoophorectomy osteoporosis without current pathological fracture (M81.8)

N99.0 **Postprocedural (acute) (chronic)** kidney failure
     Use additional code to type of kidney disease

✓5ᵗʰ **N99.1** **Postprocedural** urethral stricture
     Postcatheterization urethral stricture

     ✓6ᵗʰ **N99.11** **Postprocedural urethral stricture,** male
         AHA: 2016,4Q,47-48
         N99.110 **Postprocedural urethral stricture, male, meatal** ♂
         N99.111 **Postprocedural** bulbous **urethral stricture, male** ♂
         N99.112 **Postprocedural** membranous **urethral stricture, male** ♂
         N99.113 **Postprocedural** anterior bulbous **urethral stricture, male** ♂
         N99.114 **Postprocedural urethral stricture, male, unspecified** ♂
         N99.115 **Postprocedural** fossa navicularis **urethral stricture** ♂
         N99.116 **Postprocedural urethral stricture, male, overlapping sites** ♂

     N99.12 **Postprocedural urethral stricture,** female ♀

N99.2 **Postprocedural** adhesions of vagina ♀

N99.3 Prolapse of vaginal vault **after hysterectomy** ♀

N99.4 **Postprocedural** pelvic peritoneal adhesions
     EXCLUDES 2   pelvic peritoneal adhesions NOS (N73.6)
            postinfective pelvic peritoneal adhesions (N73.6)

✓5ᵗʰ **N99.5** **Complications of stoma of urinary tract**
     EXCLUDES 2   mechanical complication of urinary catheter (T83.0-)
     AHA: 2016,4Q,48

     ✓6ᵗʰ **N99.51** **Complication of** cystostomy
         N99.510 **Cystostomy** hemorrhage   HCC ESR
         N99.511 **Cystostomy** infection   HCC ESR
         N99.512 **Cystostomy** malfunction   HCC ESR
         N99.518 **Other cystostomy complication**   HCC ESR

     ✓6ᵗʰ **N99.52** **Complication of** incontinent external stoma **of urinary tract**
         N99.520 Hemorrhage **of incontinent external stoma of urinary tract**   HCC ESR
         N99.521 Infection **of incontinent external stoma of urinary tract**   HCC ESR

         N99.522 Malfunction **of incontinent external stoma of urinary tract**   HCC ESR
         N99.523 Herniation **of incontinent stoma of urinary tract**   HCC ESR
         N99.524 Stenosis **of incontinent stoma of urinary tract**   HCC ESR
         N99.528 **Other complication of incontinent external stoma of urinary tract**   HCC ESR

     ✓6ᵗʰ **N99.53** **Complication of** continent stoma **of urinary tract**
         N99.530 Hemorrhage **of continent stoma of urinary tract**   HCC ESR
         N99.531 Infection **of continent stoma of urinary tract**   HCC ESR
         N99.532 Malfunction **of continent stoma of urinary tract**   HCC ESR
         N99.533 Herniation **of continent stoma of urinary tract**   HCC ESR
         N99.534 Stenosis **of continent stoma of urinary tract**   HCC ESR
         N99.538 **Other complication of continent stoma of urinary tract**   HCC ESR

✓5ᵗʰ **N99.6** Intraoperative hemorrhage and hematoma **of a genitourinary system organ or structure complicating a procedure**
     EXCLUDES 1   intraoperative hemorrhage and hematoma of a genitourinary system organ or structure due to accidental puncture or laceration during a procedure (N99.7-)

     N99.61 **Intraoperative hemorrhage and hematoma of a genitourinary system organ or structure complicating a** genitourinary system procedure
     N99.62 **Intraoperative hemorrhage and hematoma of a genitourinary system organ or structure complicating** other procedure

✓5ᵗʰ **N99.7** Accidental puncture and laceration **of a genitourinary system organ or structure during a procedure**
     N99.71 **Accidental puncture and laceration of a genitourinary system organ or structure during a** genitourinary system procedure
     N99.72 **Accidental puncture and laceration of a genitourinary system organ or structure during** other procedure

✓5ᵗʰ **N99.8** **Other intraoperative and postprocedural complications and disorders of genitourinary system**
     AHA: 2016,4Q,9-10
     N99.81 **Other** intraoperative complications **of genitourinary system**

     ✓6ᵗʰ **N99.82** Postprocedural hemorrhage **of a genitourinary system organ or structure following a procedure**
         N99.820 **Postprocedural hemorrhage of a genitourinary system organ or structure following a** genitourinary system procedure
         N99.821 **Postprocedural hemorrhage of a genitourinary system organ or structure following** other procedure

     N99.83 Residual ovary syndrome ♀

     ✓6ᵗʰ **N99.84** Postprocedural hematoma and seroma **of a genitourinary system organ or structure following a procedure**
         N99.840 **Postprocedural** hematoma **of a genitourinary system organ or structure following a** genitourinary system procedure
         N99.841 **Postprocedural** hematoma **of a genitourinary system organ or structure following** other procedure
         N99.842 **Postprocedural** seroma **of a genitourinary system organ or structure following a** genitourinary system procedure
         N99.843 **Postprocedural** seroma **of a genitourinary system organ or structure following** other procedure

     N99.85 Post endometrial ablation syndrome ♀
         AHA: 2019,4Q,12

     N99.89 **Other postprocedural complications and disorders of genitourinary system**

✓ Additional Character Required   ✓x7ᵗʰ Placeholder Alert   Manifestation   Unspecified Dx   Q QPP   UPD Unacceptable PDx

Chapter 15. Pregnancy, Childbirth, and the Puerperium (O00–O9A)

Chapter-specific Guidelines with Coding Examples

The chapter-specific guidelines from the ICD-10-CM Official Guidelines for Coding and Reporting have been provided below. Along with these guidelines are coding examples, contained in the shaded boxes, that have been developed to help illustrate the coding and/or sequencing guidance found in these guidelines.

a. General rules for obstetric cases

1) Codes from Chapter 15 and sequencing priority

Obstetric cases require codes from chapter 15, codes in the range O00-O9A, Pregnancy, Childbirth, and the Puerperium. Chapter 15 codes have sequencing priority over codes from other chapters. Additional codes from other chapters may be used in conjunction with chapter 15 codes to further specify conditions. Should the provider document that the pregnancy is incidental to the encounter, then code Z33.1, Pregnant state, incidental, should be used in place of any chapter 15 codes. It is the provider's responsibility to state that the condition being treated is not affecting the pregnancy.

> Bladder abscess in pregnant patient at 25 weeks' gestation
>
> **O23.12**   **Infections of bladder in pregnancy, second trimester**
>
> **N30.80**   **Other cystitis without hematuria**
>
> **Z3A.25**   **25 weeks gestation of pregnancy**
>
> *Explanation:* The documentation does not indicate that the pregnancy is incidental or in any way unaffected by the bladder abscess; therefore, an obstetrics code should be sequenced first. An additional code was provided to identify the specific bladder condition as this information is not called out specifically in the obstetrics code.

2) Chapter 15 codes used only on the maternal record

Chapter 15 codes are to be used only on the maternal record, never on the record of the newborn.

3) Final character for trimester

The majority of codes in Chapter 15 have a final character indicating the trimester of pregnancy. The timeframes for the trimesters are indicated at the beginning of the chapter. If trimester is not a component of a code, it is because the condition always occurs in a specific trimester, or the concept of trimester of pregnancy is not applicable. Certain codes have characters for only certain trimesters because the condition does not occur in all trimesters, but it may occur in more than just one. Assignment of the final character for trimester should be based on the provider's documentation of the trimester (or number of weeks) for the current admission/encounter. This applies to the assignment of trimester for pre-existing conditions as well as those that develop during or are due to the pregnancy. The provider's documentation of the number of weeks may be used to assign the appropriate code identifying the trimester.

> Pregnant patient at 21 weeks' gestation admitted with excessive vomiting
>
> **O21.2**   **Late vomiting of pregnancy**
>
> **Z3A.21**   **21 weeks gestation of pregnancy**
>
> *Explanation:* Category O21 classifies vomiting in pregnancy. Although code selection is based on whether the vomiting is before or after 20 completed weeks, these codes are not further classified by trimester. If vomiting only in the second trimester was documented, the provider should be queried for the specific week of gestation, as this will affect code selection.

Whenever delivery occurs during the current admission, and there is an "in childbirth" option for the obstetric complication being coded, the "in childbirth" code should be assigned. When the classification does not provide an obstetric code with an "in childbirth" option, it is appropriate to assign a code describing the current trimester.

4) Selection of trimester for inpatient admissions that encompass more than one trimester

In instances when a patient is admitted to a hospital for complications of pregnancy during one trimester and remains in the hospital into a subsequent trimester, the trimester character for the antepartum complication code should be assigned on the basis of the trimester when the complication developed, not the trimester of the discharge. If the condition developed prior to the current admission/encounter or

represents a pre-existing condition, the trimester character for the trimester at the time of the admission/encounter should be assigned.

5) Unspecified trimester

Each category that includes codes for trimester has a code for "unspecified trimester." The "unspecified trimester" code should rarely be used, such as when the documentation in the record is insufficient to determine the trimester and it is not possible to obtain clarification.

6) 7th character for fetus identification

Where applicable, a 7th character is to be assigned for certain categories (O31, O32, O33.3 - O33.6, O35, O36, O40, O41, O60.1, O60.2, O64, and O69) to identify the fetus for which the complication code applies.

Assign 7th character "0":

- For single gestations.
- When the documentation in the record is insufficient to determine the fetus affected and it is not possible to obtain clarification.
- When it is not possible to clinically determine which fetus is affected.

> Maternal patient with twin gestations is seen after ultrasound identifies fetus B to be in breech presentation
>
> **O32.1XX2**   **Maternal care for breech presentation, fetus 2**
>
> *Explanation:* The documentation indicates that although there are two fetuses, only one fetus is determined to be in breech presentation. Whether fetus 2 or fetus B is used, the coder can assign the seventh character of 2 to identify the second fetus as the one in breech.

7) Completed weeks of gestation

In ICD-10-CM, "completed" weeks of gestation refers to full weeks. For example, if the provider documents gestation at 39 weeks and 6 days, the code for 39 weeks of gestation should be assigned, as the patient has not yet reached 40 completed weeks.

b. Selection of OB principal or first-listed diagnosis

1) Routine outpatient prenatal visits

For routine outpatient prenatal visits when no complications are present, a code from category Z34, Encounter for supervision of normal pregnancy, should be used as the first-listed diagnosis. These codes should not be used in conjunction with chapter 15 codes.

2) Supervision of high-risk pregnancy

Codes from category O09, Supervision of high-risk pregnancy, are intended for use only during the prenatal period. For complications during the labor or delivery episode as a result of a high-risk pregnancy, assign the applicable complication codes from Chapter 15. If there are no complications during the labor or delivery episode, assign code O80, Encounter for full-term uncomplicated delivery.

For routine prenatal outpatient visits for patients with high-risk pregnancies, a code from category O09, Supervision of high-risk pregnancy, should be used as the first-listed diagnosis. Secondary chapter 15 codes may be used in conjunction with these codes if appropriate.

> 36-year-old seen in labor with second child at 39 weeks' gestation, delivered a healthy baby, delivery complicated by tear of fourchette that was repaired
>
> **O70.0**   **First degree perineal laceration during delivery**
>
> **Z3A.39**   **39 weeks gestation of pregnancy**
>
> **Z37.0**   **Single live birth**
>
> Explanation: Although this patient is over 35 and having her second child (elderly multigravida), do not append a code from subcategory O09.5-. A code describing the tear of the fourchette, which complicated the delivery, should be used in addition to the applicable Z codes.

3) Episodes when no delivery occurs

In episodes when no delivery occurs, the principal diagnosis should correspond to the principal complication of the pregnancy which necessitated the encounter. Should more than one complication exist, all of which are treated or monitored, any of the complication codes may be sequenced first.

4) When a delivery occurs

When an obstetric patient is admitted and delivers during that admission, the condition that prompted the admission should be sequenced as the principal diagnosis. If multiple conditions prompted the admission, sequence the one most related to the delivery as the principal diagnosis. A code for any complication of the delivery should be assigned as an additional diagnosis. In cases of cesarean delivery, if the patient was admitted with a condition that resulted in the performance of a cesarean procedure, that condition should be selected as the principal diagnosis. If the reason for the admission was unrelated to the condition resulting in the cesarean delivery, the condition related to the reason for the admission should be selected as the principal diagnosis.

Maternal patient with diet-controlled gestational diabetes was seen at 38 weeks' gestation in obstructed labor due to footling presentation; cesarean performed for the malpresentation

Code	Description
O64.8XX0	Obstructed labor due to other malposition and malpresentation, not applicable or unspecified
O24.420	Gestational diabetes mellitus in childbirth, diet controlled
Z3A.38	38 weeks gestation of pregnancy
Z37.0	Single live birth

Explanation: The obstructed labor necessitated the cesarean procedure.

5) Outcome of delivery

A code from category Z37, Outcome of delivery, should be included on every maternal record when a delivery has occurred. These codes are not to be used on subsequent records or on the newborn record.

c. Pre-existing conditions versus conditions due to the pregnancy

Certain categories in Chapter 15 distinguish between conditions of the mother that existed prior to pregnancy (pre-existing) and those that are a direct result of pregnancy. When assigning codes from Chapter 15, it is important to assess if a condition was pre-existing prior to pregnancy or developed during or due to the pregnancy in order to assign the correct code.

Categories that do not distinguish between pre-existing and pregnancy-related conditions may be used for either. It is acceptable to use codes specifically for the puerperium with codes complicating pregnancy and childbirth if a condition arises postpartum during the delivery encounter.

Type 2 diabetic patient presents at 19 weeks gestation for glucose check. Patient has been taking oral metformin for several years and currently is experiencing no diabetic complications.

Code	Description
O24.112	Pre-existing type 2 diabetes mellitus, in pregnancy, second trimester
E11.9	Type 2 diabetes mellitus without complications
Z79.84	Long term (current) use of oral hypoglycemic drugs

Explanation: The documentation states that the patient has been on a diabetic medication (oral metformin) for several years, indicating the patient was diabetic prior to becoming pregnant. Reporting pre-existing Type 2 diabetes in a pregnant patient requires two codes to capture the condition, a code from category O24 and a code from category E11. A note at E11 indicates that the code for long-term use of oral hypoglycemic drugs should also be reported.

d. Pre-existing hypertension in pregnancy

Category O10, Pre-existing hypertension complicating pregnancy, childbirth and the puerperium, includes codes for hypertensive heart and hypertensive chronic kidney disease. When assigning one of the O10 codes that includes hypertensive heart disease or hypertensive chronic kidney disease, it is necessary to add a secondary code from the appropriate hypertension category to specify the type of heart failure or chronic kidney disease.
See Section I.C.9. Hypertension.

e. Fetal conditions affecting the management of the mother

1) Codes from categories O35 and O36

Codes from categories O35, Maternal care for known or suspected fetal abnormality and damage, and O36, Maternal care for other fetal problems, are assigned only when the fetal condition is actually responsible for modifying the management of the mother, i.e., by requiring diagnostic studies, additional observation, special care, or termination of pregnancy. The fact that the fetal condition exists does not justify assigning a code from this series to the mother's record.

A patient with twin gestation is seen for spotting 15 weeks into her pregnancy; the doctors also suspect fetal hydrocephalus. Patient is instructed to return in one week for additional diagnostic testing, sooner if the problem worsens.

Code	Description
O35.00X0	Maternal care for (suspected) central nervous system malformation or damage in fetus, unspecified, not applicable or unspecified
O26.852	Spotting complicating pregnancy, second trimester
Z3A.15	15 weeks gestation of pregnancy

Explanation: Whether the fetal hydrocephalus was suspected or confirmed, an additional code is warranted for this condition since documentation indicates the patient is to return sooner than her routine visit for further testing.

2) In utero surgery

In cases when surgery is performed on the fetus, a diagnosis code from category O35, Maternal care for known or suspected fetal abnormality and damage, should be assigned identifying the fetal condition. Assign the appropriate procedure code for the procedure performed.

No code from Chapter 16, the perinatal codes, should be used on the mother's record to identify fetal conditions. Surgery performed in utero on a fetus is still to be coded as an obstetric encounter.

f. HIV infection in pregnancy, childbirth and the puerperium

During pregnancy, childbirth or the puerperium, a patient admitted because of an HIV-related illness should receive a principal diagnosis from subcategory O98.7-, Human immunodeficiency [HIV] disease complicating pregnancy, childbirth and the puerperium, followed by the code(s) for the HIV-related illness(es).

Patients with asymptomatic HIV infection status admitted during pregnancy, childbirth, or the puerperium should receive codes of O98.7- and Z21, Asymptomatic human immunodeficiency virus [HIV] infection status.

A previously asymptomatic HIV patient who is 13 weeks pregnant is evaluated for HIV-related candidal bronchitis

Code	Description
O98.711	Human immunodeficiency virus [HIV] disease complicating pregnancy, first trimester
B20	Human immunodeficiency virus [HIV] disease
B37.1	Pulmonary candidiasis
Z3A.13	13 weeks gestation of pregnancy

Explanation: Because candidal bronchitis is an AIDS-related condition, this patient is now considered to have HIV disease. An obstetrics code indicating that HIV is complicating the pregnancy is coded first, followed by B20 for HIV disease as well as a code for the candidal bronchitis.

g. Diabetes mellitus in pregnancy

Diabetes mellitus is a significant complicating factor in pregnancy. Pregnant patients who are diabetic should be assigned a code from category O24, Diabetes mellitus in pregnancy, childbirth, and the puerperium, first, followed by the appropriate diabetes code(s) (E08-E13) from Chapter 4.

h. Long term use of insulin and oral hypoglycemics

See section I.C.4.a.3 for information on the long term-use of insulin and oral hypoglycemics.

i. Gestational (pregnancy induced) diabetes

Gestational (pregnancy induced) diabetes can occur during the second and third trimester of pregnancy in patients who were not diabetic prior to pregnancy. Gestational diabetes can cause complications in the pregnancy similar to those of pre-existing diabetes mellitus. It also puts the patient at greater risk of developing diabetes after the pregnancy.

Codes for gestational diabetes are in subcategory O24.4, Gestational diabetes mellitus. No other code from category O24, Diabetes mellitus in pregnancy, childbirth, and the puerperium, should be used with a code from O24.4.

The codes under subcategory O24.4 include diet controlled, insulin controlled, and controlled by oral hypoglycemic drugs. If a patient with gestational diabetes is treated with both diet and insulin, only the code for insulin-controlled is required. If a patient with gestational diabetes is treated with both diet and oral hypoglycemic medications, only the code for "controlled by oral hypoglycemic drugs" is required. Codes Z79.4, Long-term (current) use of insulin, Z79.84, Long-term (current) use of oral hypoglycemic drugs, **and Z79.85, Long-term (current) use of injectable non-insulin antidiabetic drugs,** should not be assigned with codes from subcategory O24.4.

An abnormal glucose tolerance in pregnancy is assigned a code from subcategory O99.81, Abnormal glucose complicating pregnancy, childbirth, and the puerperium.

j. Sepsis and septic shock complicating abortion, pregnancy, childbirth and the puerperium

When assigning a chapter 15 code for sepsis complicating abortion, pregnancy, childbirth, and the puerperium, a code for the specific type of infection should be assigned as an additional diagnosis. If severe sepsis is present, a code from subcategory R65.2, Severe sepsis, and code(s) for associated organ dysfunction(s) should also be assigned as additional diagnoses.

Patient is seen several days after a miscarriage with sepsis; cultures return MSSA

O03.87   **Sepsis following complete or unspecified spontaneous abortion**

B95.61   **Methicillin susceptible Staphylococcus aureus infection as the cause of diseases classified elsewhere**

Explanation: The type of infection that caused this patient to become septic was methicillin susceptible *Staphylococcus aureus* (MSSA), which as a secondary code helps capture all aspects related to this patient's septic condition.

k. Puerperal sepsis

Code O85, Puerperal sepsis, should be assigned with a secondary code to identify the causal organism (e.g., for a bacterial infection, assign a code from category B95-B96, Bacterial infections in conditions classified elsewhere). A code from category A40, Streptococcal sepsis, or A41, Other sepsis, should not be used for puerperal sepsis. If applicable, use additional codes to identify severe sepsis (R65.2-) and any associated acute organ dysfunction.

Code O85 should not be assigned for sepsis following an obstetrical procedure (See Section I.C.1.d.5.b., Sepsis due to a postprocedural infection).

l. Alcohol, tobacco and drug use during pregnancy, childbirth and the puerperium

1) Alcohol use during pregnancy, childbirth and the puerperium

Codes under subcategory O99.31, Alcohol use complicating pregnancy, childbirth, and the puerperium, should be assigned for any pregnancy case when a patient uses alcohol during the pregnancy or postpartum. A secondary code from category F10, Alcohol related disorders, should also be assigned to identify manifestations of the alcohol use.

2) Tobacco use during pregnancy, childbirth and the puerperium

Codes under subcategory O99.33, Smoking (tobacco) complicating pregnancy, childbirth, and the puerperium, should be assigned for any pregnancy case when a patient uses any type of tobacco product during the pregnancy or postpartum.

A secondary code from category F17, Nicotine dependence, should also be assigned to identify the type of nicotine dependence.

3) Drug use during pregnancy, childbirth and the puerperium

Codes under subcategory O99.32, Drug use complicating pregnancy, childbirth, and the puerperium, should be assigned for any pregnancy case when a patient uses drugs during the pregnancy or postpartum. This can involve illegal drugs, or inappropriate use or abuse of prescription drugs. Secondary code(s) from categories F11-F16 and F18-F19 should also be assigned to identify manifestations of the drug use.

m. Poisoning, toxic effects, adverse effects and underdosing in a pregnant patient

A code from subcategory O9A.2, Injury, poisoning and certain other consequences of external causes complicating pregnancy, childbirth, and the puerperium, should be sequenced first, followed by the appropriate injury, poisoning, toxic effect, adverse effect or underdosing code, and then the additional code(s) that specifies the condition caused by the poisoning, toxic effect, adverse effect or underdosing.

See Section I.C.19. Adverse effects, poisoning, underdosing and toxic effects.

Patient treated for accidental carbon monoxide poisoning from a gas heating implement; the patient is 18 weeks' pregnant

O9A.212   **Injury, poisoning and certain other consequences of external causes complicating pregnancy, second trimester**

T58.11XA   **Toxic effect of carbon monoxide from utility gas, accidental (unintentional), initial encounter**

Z3A.18   **18 weeks gestation of pregnancy**

Explanation: Although the carbon monoxide poisoning is the reason for the encounter, a code from the obstetrics chapter must be sequenced first. Chapter 15 codes have sequencing priority over codes from other chapters.

n. Normal delivery, code O80

1) Encounter for full term uncomplicated delivery

Code O80 should be assigned when a patient is admitted for a full-term normal delivery and delivers a single, healthy infant without any complications antepartum, during the delivery, or postpartum during the delivery episode. Code O80 is always a principal diagnosis. It is not to be used if any other code from chapter 15 is needed to describe a current complication of the antenatal, delivery, or postnatal period. Additional codes from other chapters may be used with code O80 if they are not related to or are in any way complicating the pregnancy.

2) Uncomplicated delivery with resolved antepartum complication

Code O80 may be used if the patient had a complication at some point during the pregnancy, but the complication is not present at the time of the admission for delivery.

Patient presents in labor at 39 weeks' gestation and delivers a healthy newborn; patient had abnormal glucose levels in her first trimester, which have since resolved

O80   **Encounter for full-term uncomplicated delivery**

Z37.0   **Single live birth**

Explanation: The abnormal glucose levels during the first trimester cannot be coded if they are not affecting the patient's current trimester. Without additional complications associated with the pregnancy, fetus, or mother, code O80 is appropriate.

3) Outcome of delivery for O80

Z37.0, Single live birth, is the only outcome of delivery code appropriate for use with O80.

o. The peripartum and postpartum periods

1) Peripartum and postpartum periods

The postpartum period begins immediately after delivery and continues for six weeks following delivery. The peripartum period is defined as the last month of pregnancy to five months postpartum.

2) Peripartum and postpartum complication

A postpartum complication is any complication occurring within the six-week period.

3) Pregnancy-related complications after 6-week period

Chapter 15 codes may also be used to describe pregnancy-related complications after the peripartum or postpartum period if the provider documents that a condition is pregnancy related.

Patient referred for varicose veins. She had a baby boy three months ago; the varicose veins started to appear one month ago. The doctor attributes the patient's pregnancy as the cause of the varicose veins, which continue to be painful and bother the patient. She is seeking surgical relief.

O87.4   **Varicose veins of the lower extremity in the puerperium**

Explanation: Although the varicose veins occurred several months after the delivery of the newborn, the doctor attributed the varicose veins to pregnancy and therefore a code from chapter 15 is appropriate.

4) Admission for routine postpartum care following delivery outside hospital

When the mother delivers outside the hospital prior to admission and is admitted for routine postpartum care and no complications are noted, code Z39.0, Encounter for care and examination of mother immediately after delivery, should be assigned as the principal diagnosis.

5) Pregnancy associated cardiomyopathy

Pregnancy associated cardiomyopathy, code O90.3, is unique in that it may be diagnosed in the third trimester of pregnancy but may continue to progress months after delivery. For this reason, it is referred to as peripartum cardiomyopathy. Code O90.3 is only for use when the cardiomyopathy develops as a result of pregnancy in a patient who did not have pre-existing heart disease.

p. Code O94, Sequelae of complication of pregnancy, childbirth, and the puerperium

1) Code O94

Code O94, Sequelae of complication of pregnancy, childbirth, and the puerperium, is for use in those cases when an initial complication of a pregnancy develops a sequela or sequelae requiring care or treatment at a future date.

2) After the initial postpartum period

This code may be used at any time after the initial postpartum period.

3) Sequencing of code O94

This code, like all sequela codes, is to be sequenced following the code describing the sequelae of the complication.

q. Termination of pregnancy and spontaneous abortions

1) Abortion with Liveborn Fetus

When an attempted termination of pregnancy results in a liveborn fetus, assign code Z33.2, Encounter for elective termination of pregnancy and a code from category Z37, Outcome of Delivery.

2) Retained Products of Conception following an abortion

Subsequent encounters for retained products of conception following a spontaneous abortion or elective termination of pregnancy, without complications are assigned O03.4, Incomplete spontaneous abortion without complication, or code O07.4, Failed attempted termination of pregnancy without complication. This advice is appropriate even when the patient was discharged previously with a discharge diagnosis of complete abortion. If the patient has a specific complication associated with the spontaneous abortion or elective termination of pregnancy in addition to retained products of conception, assign the appropriate complication code (e.g., O03.-, O04.-, O07.-) instead of code O03.4 or O07.4.

Patient was seen two days ago for complete spontaneous abortion but returns today for urinary tract infection (UTI) with ultrasound showing retained products of conception

O03.38   **Urinary tract infection following incomplete spontaneous abortion**

Explanation: Although the diagnosis from the patient's previous stay indicated that the patient had a complete abortion, it is now determined that there were actually retained products of conception (POC). An abortion with retained POC is considered incomplete and in this case resulted in the patient developing a UTI.

3) Complications leading to abortion

Codes from Chapter 15 may be used as additional codes to identify any documented complications of the pregnancy in conjunction with codes in categories in O04, O07 and O08.

4) Hemorrhage following elective abortion

For hemorrhage post elective abortion, assign code O04.6, Delayed or excessive hemorrhage following (induced) termination of pregnancy. Do not assign code O72.1, Other immediate postpartum hemorrhage, as this code should not be assigned for post abortion conditions. Do not assign code Z33.2, Encounter for elective termination of pregnancy, when the patient experiences a complication post elective abortion.

r. Abuse in a pregnant patient

For suspected or confirmed cases of abuse of a pregnant patient, a code(s) from subcategories O9A.3, Physical abuse complicating pregnancy, childbirth, and the puerperium, O9A.4, Sexual abuse complicating pregnancy, childbirth, and the puerperium, and O9A.5, Psychological abuse complicating pregnancy, childbirth, and the puerperium, should be sequenced first, followed by the appropriate codes (if applicable) to identify any associated current injury due to physical abuse, sexual abuse, and the perpetrator of abuse.

See Section I.C.19. Adult and child abuse, neglect and other maltreatment.

s. COVID-19 infection in pregnancy, childbirth, and the puerperium

During pregnancy, childbirth or the puerperium, when COVID-19 is the reason for admission/encounter, code O98.5-, Other viral diseases complicating pregnancy, childbirth and the puerperium, should be sequenced as the principal/first-listed diagnosis, and code U07.1, COVID-19, and the appropriate codes for associated manifestation(s) should be assigned as additional diagnoses. Codes from Chapter 15 always take sequencing priority.

If the reason for admission/encounter is unrelated to COVID-19 but the patient tests positive for COVID-19 during the admission/encounter, the appropriate code for the reason for admission/encounter should be sequenced as the principal/first-listed diagnosis, and codes O98.5-and U07.1, as well as the appropriate codes for associated COVID-19 manifestations, should be assigned as additional diagnoses.

Chapter 15. Pregnancy, Childbirth and the Puerperium (O00-O9A)

NOTE   CODES FROM THIS CHAPTER ARE FOR USE ONLY ON MATERNAL RECORDS, NEVER ON NEWBORN RECORDS

Codes from this chapter are for use for conditions related to or aggravated by the pregnancy, childbirth, or by the puerperium (maternal causes or obstetric causes)

NOTE   Trimesters are counted from the first day of the last menstrual period. They are defined as follows:

1st trimester- less than 14 weeks 0 days

2nd trimester- 14 weeks 0 days to less than 28 weeks 0 days

3rd trimester- 28 weeks 0 days until delivery

Use additional code from category Z3A, Weeks of gestation, to identify the specific week of the pregnancy, if known.

EXCLUDES 1   supervision of normal pregnancy (Z34.-)

EXCLUDES 2   mental and behavioral disorders associated with the puerperium (F53.-)
obstetrical tetanus (A34)
postpartum necrosis of pituitary gland (E23.0)
puerperal osteomalacia (M83.0)

AHA: 2016,1Q,3-5; 2014,3Q,17

This chapter contains the following blocks:

O00-O08   Pregnancy with abortive outcome
O09   Supervision of high risk pregnancy
O10-O16   Edema, proteinuria and hypertensive disorders in pregnancy, childbirth and the puerperium
O20-O29   Other maternal disorders predominantly related to pregnancy
O30-O48   Maternal care related to the fetus and amniotic cavity and possible delivery problems
O60-O77   Complications of labor and delivery
O80-O82   Encounter for delivery
O85-O92   Complications predominantly related to the puerperium
O94-O9A   Other obstetric conditions, not elsewhere classified

Pregnancy with abortive outcome (O00-O08)

EXCLUDES 1   continuing pregnancy in multiple gestation after abortion of one fetus or more (O31.1-, O31.3-)

TIP: Do not assign a code from category Z3A with codes in this code block.

✓4ᵗʰ **O00 Ectopic pregnancy**

INCLUDES   ruptured ectopic pregnancy

Use additional code from category O08 to identify any associated complication

AHA: 2016,4Q,48-50; 2014,3Q,17

DEF: Implantation of a fertilized egg outside the uterus, usually in the fallopian tube or abdomen that requires emergency treatment.

  ✓5ᵗʰ **O00.0 Abdominal pregnancy**

EXCLUDES 1   maternal care for viable fetus in abdominal pregnancy (O36.7-)

    O00.00 Abdominal pregnancy without intrauterine pregnancy COM M ♀
Abdominal pregnancy NOS

    O00.01 Abdominal pregnancy with intrauterine pregnancy COM M ♀

  ✓5ᵗʰ **O00.1 Tubal pregnancy**
Fallopian pregnancy
Rupture of (fallopian) tube due to pregnancy
Tubal abortion

AHA: 2017,4Q,20

    ✓6ᵗʰ **O00.10 Tubal pregnancy without intrauterine pregnancy**
Tubal pregnancy NOS

      O00.101 Right tubal pregnancy without intrauterine pregnancy COM M ♀

      O00.102 Left tubal pregnancy without intrauterine pregnancy COM M ♀

      O00.109 Unspecified tubal pregnancy without intrauterine pregnancy COM M ♀

    ✓6ᵗʰ **O00.11 Tubal pregnancy with intrauterine pregnancy**

      O00.111 Right tubal pregnancy with intrauterine pregnancy COM M ♀

      O00.112 Left tubal pregnancy with intrauterine pregnancy COM M ♀

      O00.119 Unspecified tubal pregnancy with intrauterine pregnancy COM M ♀

  ✓5ᵗʰ **O00.2 Ovarian pregnancy**

AHA: 2017,4Q,20

    ✓6ᵗʰ **O00.20 Ovarian pregnancy without intrauterine pregnancy**
Ovarian pregnancy NOS

      O00.201 Right ovarian pregnancy without intrauterine pregnancy COM M ♀

      O00.202 Left ovarian pregnancy without intrauterine pregnancy COM M ♀

      O00.209 Unspecified ovarian pregnancy without intrauterine pregnancy COM M ♀

    ✓6ᵗʰ **O00.21 Ovarian pregnancy with intrauterine pregnancy**

      O00.211 Right ovarian pregnancy with intrauterine pregnancy COM M ♀

      O00.212 Left ovarian pregnancy with intrauterine pregnancy COM M ♀

      O00.219 Unspecified ovarian pregnancy with intrauterine pregnancy COM M ♀

  ✓5ᵗʰ **O00.8 Other ectopic pregnancy**
Cervical pregnancy
Cornual pregnancy
Intraligamentous pregnancy
Mural pregnancy

    O00.80 Other ectopic pregnancy without intrauterine pregnancy COM M ♀
Other ectopic pregnancy NOS

    O00.81 Other ectopic pregnancy with intrauterine pregnancy COM M ♀

  ✓5ᵗʰ **O00.9 Ectopic pregnancy, unspecified**

    O00.90 Unspecified ectopic pregnancy without intrauterine pregnancy COM M ♀
Ectopic pregnancy NOS

    O00.91 Unspecified ectopic pregnancy with intrauterine pregnancy COM M ♀

✓4ᵗʰ **O01 Hydatidiform mole**

Use additional code from category O08 to identify any associated complication

EXCLUDES 1   chorioadenoma (destruens) (D39.2)
malignant hydatidiform mole (D39.2)

AHA: 2014,3Q,17

DEF: Abnormal product of pregnancy, marked by a mass of cysts resembling a bunch of grapes due to chorionic villi proliferation and dissolution. It must be surgically removed.

  O01.0 Classical hydatidiform mole COM M ♀
Complete hydatidiform mole

  O01.1 Incomplete and partial hydatidiform mole COM M ♀

  O01.9 Hydatidiform mole, unspecified COM M ♀
Trophoblastic disease NOS
Vesicular mole NOS

✓4ᵗʰ **O02 Other abnormal products of conception**

Use additional code from category O08 to identify any associated complication

EXCLUDES 1   papyraceous fetus (O31.0-)

AHA: 2014,3Q,17

  O02.0 Blighted ovum and nonhydatidiform mole COM M ♀
Carneous mole
Fleshy mole
Intrauterine mole NOS
Molar pregnancy NEC
Pathological ovum

  O02.1 Missed abortion COM M ♀
Early fetal death, before completion of 20 weeks of gestation, with retention of dead fetus

EXCLUDES 1   failed induced abortion (O07.-)
fetal death (intrauterine) (late) (O36.4)
missed abortion with blighted ovum (O02.0)
missed abortion with hydatidiform mole (O01.-)
missed abortion with nonhydatidiform (O02.0)
missed abortion with other abnormal products of conception (O02.8-)
missed delivery (O36.4)
stillbirth (P95)

AHA: 2022,2Q,3; 2019,3Q,11

Chapter 15. Pregnancy, Childbirth and the Puerperium

✓5ᵗʰ **O02.8 Other specified abnormal products of conception**

EXCLUDES 1   *abnormal products of conception with blighted ovum (O02.0)*
abnormal products of conception with hydatidiform mole (O01.-)
abnormal products of conception with nonhydatidiform mole (O02.0)

O02.81 Inappropriate change in quantitative human chorionic gonadotropin (hCG) in early pregnancy COM M ♀
Biochemical pregnancy
Chemical pregnancy
Inappropriate level of quantitative human chorionic gonadotropin (hCG) for gestational age in early pregnancy

O02.89 Other abnormal products of conception COM M ♀

O02.9 Abnormal product of conception, unspecified COM M ♀

✓4ᵗʰ **O03 Spontaneous abortion**

NOTE   Incomplete abortion includes retained products of conception following spontaneous abortion

INCLUDES   miscarriage

O03.0 Genital tract and pelvic infection following incomplete spontaneous abortion COM M ♀
Endometritis following incomplete spontaneous abortion
Oophoritis following incomplete spontaneous abortion
Parametritis following incomplete spontaneous abortion
Pelvic peritonitis following incomplete spontaneous abortion
Salpingitis following incomplete spontaneous abortion
Salpingo-oophoritis following incomplete spontaneous abortion

EXCLUDES 1   *sepsis following incomplete spontaneous abortion (O03.37)*
urinary tract infection following incomplete spontaneous abortion (O03.38)

O03.1 Delayed or excessive hemorrhage following incomplete spontaneous abortion COM M ♀
Afibrinogenemia following incomplete spontaneous abortion
Defibrination syndrome following incomplete spontaneous abortion
Hemolysis following incomplete spontaneous abortion
Intravascular coagulation following incomplete spontaneous abortion

AHA: 2022,1Q,19

O03.2 Embolism following incomplete spontaneous abortion COM M ♀
Air embolism following incomplete spontaneous abortion
Amniotic fluid embolism following incomplete spontaneous abortion
Blood-clot embolism following incomplete spontaneous abortion
Embolism NOS following incomplete spontaneous abortion
Fat embolism following incomplete spontaneous abortion
Pulmonary embolism following incomplete spontaneous abortion
Pyemic embolism following incomplete spontaneous abortion
Septic or septicopyemic embolism following incomplete spontaneous abortion
Soap embolism following incomplete spontaneous abortion

✓5ᵗʰ **O03.3 Other and unspecified complications following incomplete spontaneous abortion**

O03.30 Unspecified complication following incomplete spontaneous abortion COM M ♀

O03.31 Shock following incomplete spontaneous abortion COM M ♀
Circulatory collapse following incomplete spontaneous abortion
Shock (postprocedural) following incomplete spontaneous abortion

EXCLUDES 1   *shock due to infection following incomplete spontaneous abortion (O03.37)*

O03.32 Renal failure following incomplete spontaneous abortion COM M ♀
Kidney failure (acute) following incomplete spontaneous abortion
Oliguria following incomplete spontaneous abortion
Renal shutdown following incomplete spontaneous abortion
Renal tubular necrosis following incomplete spontaneous abortion
Uremia following incomplete spontaneous abortion

O03.33 Metabolic disorder following incomplete spontaneous abortion COM M ♀

O03.34 Damage to pelvic organs following incomplete spontaneous abortion COM M ♀
Laceration, perforation, tear or chemical damage of bladder following incomplete spontaneous abortion
Laceration, perforation, tear or chemical damage of bowel following incomplete spontaneous abortion
Laceration, perforation, tear or chemical damage of broad ligament following incomplete spontaneous abortion
Laceration, perforation, tear or chemical damage of cervix following incomplete spontaneous abortion
Laceration, perforation, tear or chemical damage of periurethral tissue following incomplete spontaneous abortion
Laceration, perforation, tear or chemical damage of uterus following incomplete spontaneous abortion
Laceration, perforation, tear or chemical damage of vagina following incomplete spontaneous abortion

O03.35 Other venous complications following incomplete spontaneous abortion COM M ♀

O03.36 Cardiac arrest following incomplete spontaneous abortion COM M ♀

O03.37 Sepsis following incomplete spontaneous abortion COM M ♀
Use additional code to identify infectious agent (B95-B97)
Use additional code to identify severe sepsis, if applicable (R65.2-)

EXCLUDES 1   *septic or septicopyemic embolism following incomplete spontaneous abortion (O03.2)*

O03.38 Urinary tract infection following incomplete spontaneous abortion COM M ♀
Cystitis following incomplete spontaneous abortion

O03.39 Incomplete spontaneous abortion with other complications COM M ♀

O03.4 Incomplete spontaneous abortion without complication COM M ♀

O03.5 Genital tract and pelvic infection following complete or unspecified spontaneous abortion COM M ♀
Endometritis following complete or unspecified spontaneous abortion
Oophoritis following complete or unspecified spontaneous abortion
Parametritis following complete or unspecified spontaneous abortion
Pelvic peritonitis following complete or unspecified spontaneous abortion
Salpingitis following complete or unspecified spontaneous abortion
Salpingo-oophoritis following complete or unspecified spontaneous abortion

EXCLUDES 1   *sepsis following complete or unspecified spontaneous abortion (O03.87)*
urinary tract infection following complete or unspecified spontaneous abortion (O03.88)

O03.6 **Delayed or excessive hemorrhage following** complete or unspecified **spontaneous abortion** `COM` `M` ♀

Afibrinogenemia following complete or unspecified spontaneous abortion

Defibrination syndrome following complete or unspecified spontaneous abortion

Hemolysis following complete or unspecified spontaneous abortion

Intravascular coagulation following complete or unspecified spontaneous abortion

AHA: 2022,1Q,19

O03.7 **Embolism following** complete or unspecified **spontaneous abortion** `COM` `M` ♀

Air embolism following complete or unspecified spontaneous abortion

Amniotic fluid embolism following complete or unspecified spontaneous abortion

Blood-clot embolism following complete or unspecified spontaneous abortion

Embolism NOS following complete or unspecified spontaneous abortion

Fat embolism following complete or unspecified spontaneous abortion

Pulmonary embolism following complete or unspecified spontaneous abortion

Pyemic embolism following complete or unspecified spontaneous abortion

Septic or septicopyemic embolism following complete or unspecified spontaneous abortion

Soap embolism following complete or unspecified spontaneous abortion

✓6ᵗʰ **O03.8** **Other and unspecified complications following complete or unspecified spontaneous abortion**

  O03.80 **Unspecified complication following** complete or unspecified **spontaneous abortion** `COM` `M` ♀

  O03.81 **Shock following** complete or unspecified **spontaneous abortion** `COM` `M` ♀

Circulatory collapse following complete or unspecified spontaneous abortion

Shock (postprocedural) following complete or unspecified spontaneous abortion

EXCLUDES 1   *shock due to infection following complete or unspecified spontaneous abortion (O03.87)*

  O03.82 **Renal failure following** complete or unspecified **spontaneous abortion** `COM` `M` ♀

Kidney failure (acute) following complete or unspecified spontaneous abortion

Oliguria following complete or unspecified spontaneous abortion

Renal shutdown following complete or unspecified spontaneous abortion

Renal tubular necrosis following complete or unspecified spontaneous abortion

Uremia following complete or unspecified spontaneous abortion

  O03.83 **Metabolic disorder following** complete or unspecified **spontaneous abortion** `COM` `M` ♀

O03.84 **Damage to pelvic organs following** complete or unspecified **spontaneous abortion** `COM` `M` ♀

Laceration, perforation, tear or chemical damage of bladder following complete or unspecified spontaneous abortion

Laceration, perforation, tear or chemical damage of bowel following complete or unspecified spontaneous abortion

Laceration, perforation, tear or chemical damage of broad ligament following complete or unspecified spontaneous abortion

Laceration, perforation, tear or chemical damage of cervix following complete or unspecified spontaneous abortion

Laceration, perforation, tear or chemical damage of periurethral tissue following complete or unspecified spontaneous abortion

Laceration, perforation, tear or chemical damage of uterus following complete or unspecified spontaneous abortion

Laceration, perforation, tear or chemical damage of vagina following complete or unspecified spontaneous abortion

O03.85 **Other** venous **complications following** complete or unspecified **spontaneous abortion** `COM` `M` ♀

O03.86 **Cardiac arrest following** complete or unspecified **spontaneous abortion** `COM` `M` ♀

O03.87 **Sepsis following** complete or unspecified **spontaneous abortion** `COM` `M` ♀

Use additional code to identify infectious agent (B95-B97)

Use additional code to identify severe sepsis, if applicable (R65.2-)

EXCLUDES 1   *septic or septicopyemic embolism following complete or unspecified spontaneous abortion (O03.7)*

O03.88 **Urinary tract infection following** complete or unspecified **spontaneous abortion** `COM` `M` ♀

Cystitis following complete or unspecified spontaneous abortion

O03.89 **Complete or unspecified spontaneous abortion with other complications** `COM` `M` ♀

O03.9 **Complete or unspecified spontaneous abortion without complication** `COM` `M` ♀

Miscarriage NOS

Spontaneous abortion NOS

✓4ᵗʰ **O04** **Complications following (induced) termination of pregnancy**

  INCLUDES   complications following (induced) termination of pregnancy

  EXCLUDES 1   *encounter for elective termination of pregnancy, uncomplicated (Z33.2)*

    failed attempted termination of pregnancy (O07.-)

O04.5 **Genital tract and pelvic infection following (induced) termination of pregnancy** `M` ♀

Endometritis following (induced) termination of pregnancy

Oophoritis following (induced) termination of pregnancy

Parametritis following (induced) termination of pregnancy

Pelvic peritonitis following (induced) termination of pregnancy

Salpingitis following (induced) termination of pregnancy

Salpingo-oophoritis following (induced) termination of pregnancy

EXCLUDES 1   *sepsis following (induced) termination of pregnancy (O04.87)*

  urinary tract infection following (induced) termination of pregnancy (O04.88)

O04.6 **Delayed or excessive hemorrhage following (induced) termination of pregnancy** `M` ♀

Afibrinogenemia following (induced) termination of pregnancy

Defibrination syndrome following (induced) termination of pregnancy

Hemolysis following (induced) termination of pregnancy

Intravascular coagulation following (induced) termination of pregnancy

AHA: 2019,3Q,11

O04.7 Embolism following (induced) termination of **pregnancy**   M ♀

     Air embolism following (induced) termination of pregnancy

     Amniotic fluid embolism following (induced) termination of pregnancy

     Blood-clot embolism following (induced) termination of pregnancy

     Embolism NOS following (induced) termination of pregnancy

     Fat embolism following (induced) termination of pregnancy

     Pulmonary embolism following (induced) termination of pregnancy

     Pyemic embolism following (induced) termination of pregnancy

     Septic or septicopyemic embolism following (induced) termination of pregnancy

     Soap embolism following (induced) termination of pregnancy

✓5ᵗʰ **O04.8 (Induced) termination of pregnancy with other and unspecified complications**

     O04.80 (Induced) termination of pregnancy with unspecified complications   M ♀

     O04.81 Shock following (induced) termination of **pregnancy**   M ♀

         Circulatory collapse following (induced) termination of pregnancy

         Shock (postprocedural) following (induced) termination of pregnancy

         EXCLUDES 1   *shock due to infection following (induced) termination of pregnancy (O04.87)*

     O04.82 Renal failure following (induced) termination of **pregnancy**   M ♀

         Kidney failure (acute) following (induced) termination of pregnancy

         Oliguria following (induced) termination of pregnancy

         Renal shutdown following (induced) termination of pregnancy

         Renal tubular necrosis following (induced) termination of pregnancy

         Uremia following (induced) termination of pregnancy

     O04.83 Metabolic disorder following (induced) termination **of pregnancy**   M ♀

     O04.84 Damage to pelvic organs following (induced) **termination of pregnancy**   M ♀

         Laceration, perforation, tear or chemical damage of bladder following (induced) termination of pregnancy

         Laceration, perforation, tear or chemical damage of bowel following (induced) termination of pregnancy

         Laceration, perforation, tear or chemical damage of broad ligament following (induced) termination of pregnancy

         Laceration, perforation, tear or chemical damage of cervix following (induced) termination of pregnancy

         Laceration, perforation, tear or chemical damage of periurethral tissue following (induced) termination of pregnancy

         Laceration, perforation, tear or chemical damage of uterus following (induced) termination of pregnancy

         Laceration, perforation, tear or chemical damage of vagina following (induced) termination of pregnancy

     O04.85 Other venous complications following (induced) termination of pregnancy   M ♀

     O04.86 Cardiac arrest following (induced) termination of **pregnancy**   M ♀

     O04.87 Sepsis following (induced) termination of **pregnancy**   M ♀

         Use additional code to identify infectious agent (B95-B97)

         Use additional code to identify severe sepsis, if applicable (R65.2-)

         EXCLUDES 1   *septic or septicopyemic embolism following (induced) termination of pregnancy (O04.7)*

     O04.88 Urinary tract infection following (induced) **termination of pregnancy**   M ♀

         Cystitis following (induced) termination of pregnancy

O04.89 (Induced) termination of pregnancy with other complications   M ♀

✓4ᵗʰ **O07 Failed attempted termination of pregnancy**

     INCLUDES   failure of attempted induction of termination of pregnancy

                 incomplete elective abortion

     EXCLUDES 1   *incomplete spontaneous abortion (O03.0-)*

O07.0 Genital tract and pelvic infection following **failed attempted termination of pregnancy**   M ♀

     Endometritis following failed attempted termination of pregnancy

     Oophoritis following failed attempted termination of pregnancy

     Parametritis following failed attempted termination of pregnancy

     Pelvic peritonitis following failed attempted termination of pregnancy

     Salpingitis following failed attempted termination of pregnancy

     Salpingo-oophoritis following failed attempted termination of pregnancy

     EXCLUDES 1   *sepsis following failed attempted termination of pregnancy (O07.37)*

              urinary tract infection following failed attempted termination of pregnancy (O07.38)

O07.1 Delayed or excessive hemorrhage following **failed attempted termination of pregnancy**   M ♀

     Afibrinogenemia following failed attempted termination of pregnancy

     Defibrination syndrome following failed attempted termination of pregnancy

     Hemolysis following failed attempted termination of pregnancy

     Intravascular coagulation following failed attempted termination of pregnancy

O07.2 Embolism following **failed attempted termination of pregnancy**   M ♀

     Air embolism following failed attempted termination of pregnancy

     Amniotic fluid embolism following failed attempted termination of pregnancy

     Blood-clot embolism following failed attempted termination of pregnancy

     Embolism NOS following failed attempted termination of pregnancy

     Fat embolism following failed attempted termination of pregnancy

     Pulmonary embolism following failed attempted termination of pregnancy

     Pyemic embolism following failed attempted termination of pregnancy

     Septic or septicopyemic embolism following failed attempted termination of pregnancy

     Soap embolism following failed attempted termination of pregnancy

✓5ᵗʰ **O07.3 Failed attempted termination of pregnancy with other and unspecified complications**

     O07.30 Failed attempted termination of pregnancy with unspecified complications   M ♀

     O07.31 Shock following **failed attempted termination of pregnancy**   M ♀

         Circulatory collapse following failed attempted termination of pregnancy

         Shock (postprocedural) following failed attempted termination of pregnancy

         EXCLUDES 1   *shock due to infection following failed attempted termination of pregnancy (O07.37)*

     O07.32 Renal failure following **failed attempted termination of pregnancy**   M ♀

         Kidney failure (acute) following failed attempted termination of pregnancy

         Oliguria following failed attempted termination of pregnancy

         Renal shutdown following failed attempted termination of pregnancy

         Renal tubular necrosis following failed attempted termination of pregnancy

         Uremia following failed attempted termination of pregnancy

     O07.33 Metabolic disorder following **failed attempted termination of pregnancy**   M ♀

O07.34 **Damage to pelvic organs following failed attempted termination of pregnancy** Ⓜ ♀

Laceration, perforation, tear or chemical damage of bladder following failed attempted termination of pregnancy

Laceration, perforation, tear or chemical damage of bowel following failed attempted termination of pregnancy

Laceration, perforation, tear or chemical damage of broad ligament following failed attempted termination of pregnancy

Laceration, perforation, tear or chemical damage of cervix following failed attempted termination of pregnancy

Laceration, perforation, tear or chemical damage of periurethral tissue following failed attempted termination of pregnancy

Laceration, perforation, tear or chemical damage of uterus following failed attempted termination of pregnancy

Laceration, perforation, tear or chemical damage of vagina following failed attempted termination of pregnancy

O07.35 **Other venous complications following failed attempted termination of pregnancy** Ⓜ ♀

O07.36 **Cardiac arrest following failed attempted termination of pregnancy** Ⓜ ♀

O07.37 **Sepsis following failed attempted termination of pregnancy** Ⓜ ♀

Use additional code (B95-B97), to identify infectious agent

Use additional code (R65.2-) to identify severe sepsis, if applicable

> *EXCLUDES 1*   *septic or septicopyemic embolism following failed attempted termination of pregnancy (O07.2)*

O07.38 **Urinary tract infection following failed attempted termination of pregnancy** Ⓜ ♀

Cystitis following failed attempted termination of pregnancy

O07.39 **Failed attempted termination of pregnancy with other complications** Ⓜ ♀

O07.4 **Failed attempted termination of pregnancy without complication** Ⓜ ♀

☑4ᵗʰ **O08** **Complications following ectopic and molar pregnancy**

This category is for use with categories O00-O02 to identify any associated complications

O08.0 **Genital tract and pelvic infection following ectopic and molar pregnancy** COM Ⓜ ♀

Endometritis following ectopic and molar pregnancy
Oophoritis following ectopic and molar pregnancy
Parametritis following ectopic and molar pregnancy
Pelvic peritonitis following ectopic and molar pregnancy
Salpingitis following ectopic and molar pregnancy
Salpingo-oophoritis following ectopic and molar pregnancy

> *EXCLUDES 1*   *sepsis following ectopic and molar pregnancy (O08.82)*
> *urinary tract infection (O08.83)*

O08.1 **Delayed or excessive hemorrhage following ectopic and molar pregnancy** COM Ⓜ ♀

Afibrinogenemia following ectopic and molar pregnancy
Defibrination syndrome following ectopic and molar pregnancy
Hemolysis following ectopic and molar pregnancy
Intravascular coagulation following ectopic and molar pregnancy

> *EXCLUDES 1*   *delayed or excessive hemorrhage due to incomplete abortion (O03.1)*

O08.2 **Embolism following ectopic and molar pregnancy** COM ♀

Air embolism following ectopic and molar pregnancy
Amniotic fluid embolism following ectopic and molar pregnancy
Blood-clot embolism following ectopic and molar pregnancy
Embolism NOS following ectopic and molar pregnancy
Fat embolism following ectopic and molar pregnancy
Pulmonary embolism following ectopic and molar pregnancy
Pyemic embolism following ectopic and molar pregnancy
Septic or septicopyemic embolism following ectopic and molar pregnancy
Soap embolism following ectopic and molar pregnancy

O08.3 **Shock following ectopic and molar pregnancy** COM Ⓜ ♀

Circulatory collapse following ectopic and molar pregnancy
Shock (postprocedural) following ectopic and molar pregnancy

> *EXCLUDES 1*   *shock due to infection following ectopic and molar pregnancy (O08.82)*

O08.4 **Renal failure following ectopic and molar pregnancy** COM Ⓜ ♀

Kidney failure (acute) following ectopic and molar pregnancy
Oliguria following ectopic and molar pregnancy
Renal shutdown following ectopic and molar pregnancy
Renal tubular necrosis following ectopic and molar pregnancy
Uremia following ectopic and molar pregnancy

O08.5 **Metabolic disorders following an ectopic and molar pregnancy** COM Ⓜ ♀

O08.6 **Damage to pelvic organs and tissues following an ectopic and molar pregnancy** COM Ⓜ ♀

Laceration, perforation, tear or chemical damage of bladder following an ectopic and molar pregnancy

Laceration, perforation, tear or chemical damage of bowel following an ectopic and molar pregnancy

Laceration, perforation, tear or chemical damage of broad ligament following an ectopic and molar pregnancy

Laceration, perforation, tear or chemical damage of cervix following an ectopic and molar pregnancy

Laceration, perforation, tear or chemical damage of periurethral tissue following an ectopic and molar pregnancy

Laceration, perforation, tear or chemical damage of uterus following an ectopic and molar pregnancy

Laceration, perforation, tear or chemical damage of vagina following an ectopic and molar pregnancy

O08.7 **Other venous complications following an ectopic and molar pregnancy** COM Ⓜ ♀

☑5ᵗʰ **O08.8** **Other complications following an ectopic and molar pregnancy**

O08.81 **Cardiac arrest following an ectopic and molar pregnancy** COM Ⓜ ♀

O08.82 **Sepsis following an ectopic and molar pregnancy** COM Ⓜ ♀

Use additional code (B95-B97), to identify infectious agent

Use additional code (R65.2-) to identify severe sepsis, if applicable

> *EXCLUDES 1*   *septic or septicopyemic embolism following ectopic and molar pregnancy (O08.2)*

O08.83 **Urinary tract infection following an ectopic and molar pregnancy** COM Ⓜ ♀

Cystitis following an ectopic and molar pregnancy

O08.89 **Other complications following an ectopic and molar pregnancy** COM ♀

O08.9 **Unspecified complication following an ectopic and molar pregnancy** COM Ⓜ ♀

Supervision of high risk pregnancy (O09)

☑4ᵗʰ **O09** **Supervision of high risk pregnancy**

AHA: 2019,3Q,5; 2016,4Q,48-50,150

☑5ᵗʰ **O09.0** **Supervision of pregnancy with history of infertility**

O09.00 **Supervision of pregnancy with history of infertility, unspecified trimester** COM ♀

O09.01 **Supervision of pregnancy with history of infertility, first trimester** COM ♀

O09.02 **Supervision of pregnancy with history of infertility, second trimester** COM ♀

O09.03 **Supervision of pregnancy with history of infertility, third trimester** COM ♀

✓5ᵗʰ O09.1 Supervision of pregnancy with history of ectopic **pregnancy**

O09.10 Supervision of pregnancy with history of ectopic pregnancy, unspecified trimester ᶜᵒᵐ Ⓜ ♀

O09.11 Supervision of pregnancy with history of ectopic pregnancy, first trimester ᶜᵒᵐ Ⓜ ♀

O09.12 Supervision of pregnancy with history of ectopic pregnancy, second trimester ᶜᵒᵐ Ⓜ ♀

O09.13 Supervision of pregnancy with history of ectopic pregnancy, third trimester ᶜᵒᵐ Ⓜ ♀

✓5ᵗʰ O09.A Supervision of pregnancy with history of molar **pregnancy**

DEF: Molar pregnancy: Trophoblastic neoplasm that mimics pregnancy by proliferating from a pathologic ovum and resulting only in a mass of cysts resembling grapes, 80 percent of which are benign, but require surgical removal.

O09.A0 Supervision of pregnancy with history of molar pregnancy, unspecified trimester ᶜᵒᵐ Ⓜ ♀

O09.A1 Supervision of pregnancy with history of molar pregnancy, first trimester ᶜᵒᵐ Ⓜ ♀

O09.A2 Supervision of pregnancy with history of molar pregnancy, second trimester ᶜᵒᵐ Ⓜ ♀

O09.A3 Supervision of pregnancy with history of molar pregnancy, third trimester ᶜᵒᵐ Ⓜ ♀

✓5ᵗʰ O09.2 Supervision of pregnancy with other poor reproductive or obstetric history

EXCLUDES 2   *pregnancy care for patient with history of recurrent pregnancy loss (O26.2-)*

✓6ᵗʰ O09.21 Supervision of pregnancy with history of pre-term labor

O09.211 Supervision of pregnancy with history of pre-term labor, first trimester ᶜᵒᵐ Ⓜ ♀

O09.212 Supervision of pregnancy with history of pre-term labor, second trimester ᶜᵒᵐ Ⓜ ♀

O09.213 Supervision of pregnancy with history of pre-term labor, third trimester ᶜᵒᵐ Ⓜ ♀

O09.219 Supervision of pregnancy with history of pre-term labor, unspecified trimester ᶜᵒᵐ Ⓜ ♀

✓6ᵗʰ O09.29 Supervision of pregnancy with other poor reproductive or obstetric history

Supervision of pregnancy with history of neonatal death

Supervision of pregnancy with history of stillbirth

O09.291 Supervision of pregnancy with other poor reproductive or obstetric history, first trimester ᶜᵒᵐ Ⓜ ♀

O09.292 Supervision of pregnancy with other poor reproductive or obstetric history, second trimester ᶜᵒᵐ Ⓜ ♀

O09.293 Supervision of pregnancy with other poor reproductive or obstetric history, third trimester ᶜᵒᵐ Ⓜ ♀

O09.299 Supervision of pregnancy with other poor reproductive or obstetric history, unspecified trimester ᶜᵒᵐ Ⓜ ♀

✓5ᵗʰ O09.3 Supervision of pregnancy with insufficient antenatal care

Supervision of concealed pregnancy

Supervision of hidden pregnancy

O09.30 Supervision of pregnancy with insufficient antenatal care, unspecified trimester ᶜᵒᵐ Ⓜ ♀

O09.31 Supervision of pregnancy with insufficient antenatal care, first trimester ᶜᵒᵐ Ⓜ ♀

O09.32 Supervision of pregnancy with insufficient antenatal care, second trimester ᶜᵒᵐ Ⓜ ♀

O09.33 Supervision of pregnancy with insufficient antenatal care, third trimester ᶜᵒᵐ Ⓜ ♀

✓5ᵗʰ O09.4 Supervision of pregnancy with grand multiparity

O09.40 Supervision of pregnancy with grand multiparity, unspecified trimester ᶜᵒᵐ Ⓜ ♀

O09.41 Supervision of pregnancy with grand multiparity, first trimester ᶜᵒᵐ Ⓜ ♀

O09.42 Supervision of pregnancy with grand multiparity, second trimester ᶜᵒᵐ Ⓜ ♀

O09.43 Supervision of pregnancy with grand multiparity, third trimester ᶜᵒᵐ Ⓜ ♀

✓5ᵗʰ O09.5 Supervision of elderly primigravida and multigravida

Pregnancy for a female 35 years and older at expected date of delivery

✓6ᵗʰ O09.51 Supervision of elderly primigravida

O09.511 Supervision of elderly primigravida, first trimester ᶜᵒᵐ ♀

O09.512 Supervision of elderly primigravida, second trimester ᶜᵒᵐ ♀

O09.513 Supervision of elderly primigravida, third trimester ᶜᵒᵐ ♀

O09.519 Supervision of elderly primigravida, unspecified trimester ᶜᵒᵐ ♀

✓6ᵗʰ O09.52 Supervision of elderly multigravida

O09.521 Supervision of elderly multigravida, first trimester ᶜᵒᵐ ♀

O09.522 Supervision of elderly multigravida, second trimester ᶜᵒᵐ ♀

O09.523 Supervision of elderly multigravida, third trimester ᶜᵒᵐ ♀

O09.529 Supervision of elderly multigravida, unspecified trimester ᶜᵒᵐ ♀

✓5ᵗʰ O09.6 Supervision of young primigravida and multigravida

Supervision of pregnancy for a female less than 16 years old at expected date of delivery

✓6ᵗʰ O09.61 Supervision of young primigravida

O09.611 Supervision of young primigravida, first trimester ᶜᵒᵐ ♀

O09.612 Supervision of young primigravida, second trimester ᶜᵒᵐ ♀

O09.613 Supervision of young primigravida, third trimester ᶜᵒᵐ ♀

O09.619 Supervision of young primigravida, unspecified trimester ᶜᵒᵐ ♀

✓6ᵗʰ O09.62 Supervision of young multigravida

O09.621 Supervision of young multigravida, first trimester ᶜᵒᵐ ♀

O09.622 Supervision of young multigravida, second trimester ᶜᵒᵐ ♀

O09.623 Supervision of young multigravida, third trimester ᶜᵒᵐ ♀

O09.629 Supervision of young multigravida, unspecified trimester ᶜᵒᵐ ♀

✓5ᵗʰ O09.7 Supervision of high risk pregnancy due to social problems

O09.70 Supervision of high risk pregnancy due to social problems, unspecified trimester ᶜᵒᵐ Ⓜ ♀

O09.71 Supervision of high risk pregnancy due to social problems, first trimester ᶜᵒᵐ Ⓜ ♀

O09.72 Supervision of high risk pregnancy due to social problems, second trimester ᶜᵒᵐ Ⓜ ♀

O09.73 Supervision of high risk pregnancy due to social problems, third trimester ᶜᵒᵐ Ⓜ ♀

✓5ᵗʰ O09.8 Supervision of other high risk pregnancies

✓6ᵗʰ O09.81 Supervision of pregnancy resulting from assisted reproductive technology

Supervision of pregnancy resulting from in-vitro fertilization

EXCLUDES 2   *gestational carrier status (Z33.3)*

O09.811 Supervision of pregnancy resulting from assisted reproductive technology, first trimester ᶜᵒᵐ Ⓜ ♀

O09.812 Supervision of pregnancy resulting from assisted reproductive technology, second trimester ᶜᵒᵐ Ⓜ ♀

O09.813 Supervision of pregnancy resulting from assisted reproductive technology, third trimester ᶜᵒᵐ Ⓜ ♀

O09.819 Supervision of pregnancy resulting from assisted reproductive technology, unspecified trimester ᶜᵒᵐ Ⓜ ♀

✓6ᵗʰ O09.82 Supervision of pregnancy with history of in utero procedure during previous pregnancy

O09.821 Supervision of pregnancy with history of in utero procedure during previous pregnancy, first trimester ᶜᵒᵐ Ⓜ ♀

O09.822 Supervision of pregnancy with history of in utero procedure during previous pregnancy, second trimester ᶜᵒᵐ Ⓜ ♀

O09.823 Supervision of pregnancy with history of in utero procedure during previous pregnancy, third trimester `COM` `M` ♀

O09.829 Supervision of pregnancy with history of in utero procedure during previous pregnancy, unspecified trimester `COM` `M` ♀

　　　EXCLUDES 1　supervision of pregnancy affected by in utero procedure during current pregnancy (O35.7)

✓6th **O09.89** Supervision of other high risk pregnancies

O09.891 Supervision of other high risk pregnancies, first trimester `COM` `M` ♀

O09.892 Supervision of other high risk pregnancies, second trimester `COM` `M` ♀

O09.893 Supervision of other high risk pregnancies, third trimester `COM` `M` ♀

O09.899 Supervision of other high risk pregnancies, unspecified trimester `COM` `M` ♀

✓5th **O09.9** Supervision of high risk pregnancy, unspecified

O09.90 Supervision of high risk pregnancy, unspecified, unspecified trimester `COM` `M` ♀

O09.91 Supervision of high risk pregnancy, unspecified, first trimester `COM` `M` ♀

O09.92 Supervision of high risk pregnancy, unspecified, second trimester `COM` `M` ♀

O09.93 Supervision of high risk pregnancy, unspecified, third trimester `COM` `M` ♀

Edema, proteinuria and hypertensive disorders in pregnancy, childbirth and the puerperium (O10-O16)

AHA: 2016,4Q,50

✓4th **O10** Pre-existing hypertension complicating pregnancy, childbirth and the puerperium

　　　INCLUDES　pre-existing hypertension with pre-existing proteinuria complicating pregnancy, childbirth and the puerperium

　　　EXCLUDES 2　pre-existing hypertension with superimposed pre-eclampsia complicating pregnancy, childbirth and the puerperium (O11.-)

✓5th **O10.0** Pre-existing essential hypertension complicating pregnancy, childbirth and the puerperium

　　　Any condition in I10 specified as a reason for obstetric care during pregnancy, childbirth or the puerperium

✓6th **O10.01** Pre-existing essential hypertension complicating pregnancy

O10.011 Pre-existing essential hypertension complicating pregnancy, first trimester `COM` `M` ♀

O10.012 Pre-existing essential hypertension complicating pregnancy, second trimester `COM` `M` ♀

O10.013 Pre-existing essential hypertension complicating pregnancy, third trimester `COM` `M` ♀

O10.019 Pre-existing essential hypertension complicating pregnancy, unspecified trimester `COM` `M` ♀

O10.02 Pre-existing essential hypertension complicating childbirth `COM` `M` ♀

O10.03 Pre-existing essential hypertension complicating the puerperium `COM` `M` ♀

✓5th **O10.1** Pre-existing hypertensive heart disease complicating pregnancy, childbirth and the puerperium

　　　Any condition in I11 specified as a reason for obstetric care during pregnancy, childbirth or the puerperium

　　　Use additional code from I11 to identify the type of hypertensive heart disease

✓6th **O10.11** Pre-existing hypertensive heart disease complicating pregnancy

O10.111 Pre-existing hypertensive heart disease complicating pregnancy, first trimester `COM` `M` ♀

O10.112 Pre-existing hypertensive heart disease complicating pregnancy, second trimester `COM` `M` ♀

O10.113 Pre-existing hypertensive heart disease complicating pregnancy, third trimester `COM` `M` ♀

O10.119 Pre-existing hypertensive heart disease complicating pregnancy, unspecified trimester `COM` `M` ♀

O10.12 Pre-existing hypertensive heart disease complicating childbirth `COM` `M` ♀

O10.13 Pre-existing hypertensive heart disease complicating the puerperium `COM` `M` ♀

✓5th **O10.2** Pre-existing hypertensive chronic kidney disease complicating pregnancy, childbirth and the puerperium

　　　Any condition in I12 specified as a reason for obstetric care during pregnancy, childbirth or the puerperium

　　　Use additional code from I12 to identify the type of hypertensive chronic kidney disease

✓6th **O10.21** Pre-existing hypertensive chronic kidney disease complicating pregnancy

O10.211 Pre-existing hypertensive chronic kidney disease complicating pregnancy, first trimester `COM` `M` ♀

O10.212 Pre-existing hypertensive chronic kidney disease complicating pregnancy, second trimester `COM` `M` ♀

O10.213 Pre-existing hypertensive chronic kidney disease complicating pregnancy, third trimester `COM` `M` ♀

O10.219 Pre-existing hypertensive chronic kidney disease complicating pregnancy, unspecified trimester `COM` `M` ♀

O10.22 Pre-existing hypertensive chronic kidney disease complicating childbirth `COM` `M` ♀

O10.23 Pre-existing hypertensive chronic kidney disease complicating the puerperium `COM` `M` ♀

✓5th **O10.3** Pre-existing hypertensive heart and chronic kidney disease complicating pregnancy, childbirth and the puerperium

　　　Any condition in I13 specified as a reason for obstetric care during pregnancy, childbirth or the puerperium

　　　Use additional code from I13 to identify the type of hypertensive heart and chronic kidney disease

✓6th **O10.31** Pre-existing hypertensive heart and chronic kidney disease complicating pregnancy

O10.311 Pre-existing hypertensive heart and chronic kidney disease complicating pregnancy, first trimester `COM` `M` ♀

O10.312 Pre-existing hypertensive heart and chronic kidney disease complicating pregnancy, second trimester `COM` `M` ♀

O10.313 Pre-existing hypertensive heart and chronic kidney disease complicating pregnancy, third trimester `COM` `M` ♀

O10.319 Pre-existing hypertensive heart and chronic kidney disease complicating pregnancy, unspecified trimester `COM` `M` ♀

O10.32 Pre-existing hypertensive heart and chronic kidney disease complicating childbirth `COM` `M` ♀

O10.33 Pre-existing hypertensive heart and chronic kidney disease complicating the puerperium `COM` `M` ♀

✓5th **O10.4** Pre-existing secondary hypertension complicating pregnancy, childbirth and the puerperium

　　　Any condition in I15 specified as a reason for obstetric care during pregnancy, childbirth or the puerperium

　　　Use additional code from I15 to identify the type of secondary hypertension

✓6th **O10.41** Pre-existing secondary hypertension complicating pregnancy

O10.411 Pre-existing secondary hypertension complicating pregnancy, first trimester `COM` `M` ♀

O10.412 Pre-existing secondary hypertension complicating pregnancy, second trimester `COM` `M` ♀

O10.413 Pre-existing secondary hypertension complicating pregnancy, third trimester `COM` `M` ♀

O10.419 Pre-existing secondary hypertension complicating pregnancy, unspecified trimester `COM` `M` ♀

O10.42 Pre-existing secondary hypertension complicating childbirth `COM` `M` ♀

Chapter 15. Pregnancy, Childbirth and the Puerperium

    O10.43   Pre-existing secondary hypertension complicating the puerperium   COM M ♀

✓5th **O10.9**   Unspecified pre-existing hypertension complicating pregnancy, childbirth and the puerperium

    ✓6th **O10.91**   Unspecified pre-existing hypertension complicating pregnancy

       O10.911   Unspecified pre-existing hypertension complicating pregnancy, first trimester   COM M ♀

       O10.912   Unspecified pre-existing hypertension complicating pregnancy, second trimester   COM M ♀

       O10.913   Unspecified pre-existing hypertension complicating pregnancy, third trimester   COM M ♀

       O10.919   Unspecified pre-existing hypertension complicating pregnancy, unspecified trimester   COM M ♀

    O10.92   Unspecified pre-existing hypertension complicating childbirth   COM M ♀

    O10.93   Unspecified pre-existing hypertension complicating the puerperium   COM M ♀

✓4th **O11**   Pre-existing hypertension with pre-eclampsia

    INCLUDES   conditions in O10 complicated by pre-eclampsia

         pre-eclampsia superimposed pre-existing in hypertension

Use additional code from O10 to identify the type of hypertension

DEF: Complication of pregnancy manifesting in the development of borderline hypertension, protein in the urine, and unresponsive swelling between the 20th week of pregnancy and the end of the first week following birth in mild to moderate cases. Severe preeclampsia presents with hypertension, associated with marked swelling, proteinuria, abdominal pain, and/or visual changes.

    O11.1   Pre-existing hypertension with pre-eclampsia, first trimester   COM M ♀

    O11.2   Pre-existing hypertension with pre-eclampsia, second trimester   COM M ♀

    O11.3   Pre-existing hypertension with pre-eclampsia, third trimester   COM M ♀

    O11.4   Pre-existing hypertension with pre-eclampsia, complicating childbirth   COM M ♀

    O11.5   Pre-existing hypertension with pre-eclampsia, complicating the puerperium   COM M ♀

    O11.9   Pre-existing hypertension with pre-eclampsia, unspecified trimester   COM M ♀

✓4th **O12**   Gestational [pregnancy-induced] edema and proteinuria without hypertension

    ✓5th **O12.0**   Gestational edema

      O12.00   Gestational edema, unspecified trimester   COM M ♀

      O12.01   Gestational edema, first trimester   COM M ♀

      O12.02   Gestational edema, second trimester   COM M ♀

      O12.03   Gestational edema, third trimester   COM M ♀

      O12.04   Gestational edema, complicating childbirth   COM M ♀

      O12.05   Gestational edema, complicating the puerperium   COM M ♀

    ✓5th **O12.1**   Gestational proteinuria

      O12.10   Gestational proteinuria, unspecified trimester   COM M ♀

      O12.11   Gestational proteinuria, first trimester   COM M ♀

      O12.12   Gestational proteinuria, second trimester   COM M ♀

      O12.13   Gestational proteinuria, third trimester   COM M ♀

      O12.14   Gestational proteinuria, complicating childbirth   COM M ♀

      O12.15   Gestational proteinuria, complicating the puerperium   COM M ♀

    ✓5th **O12.2**   Gestational edema with proteinuria

      O12.20   Gestational edema with proteinuria, unspecified trimester   COM M ♀

      O12.21   Gestational edema with proteinuria, first trimester   COM M ♀

      O12.22   Gestational edema with proteinuria, second trimester   COM M ♀

      O12.23   Gestational edema with proteinuria, third trimester   COM M ♀

      O12.24   Gestational edema with proteinuria, complicating childbirth   COM M ♀

      O12.25   Gestational edema with proteinuria, complicating the puerperium   COM M ♀

✓4th **O13**   Gestational [pregnancy-induced] hypertension without significant proteinuria

    INCLUDES   gestational hypertension NOS

         transient hypertension of pregnancy

    AHA: 2016,1Q,5

    O13.1   Gestational [pregnancy-induced] hypertension without significant proteinuria, first trimester   COM M ♀

    O13.2   Gestational [pregnancy-induced] hypertension without significant proteinuria, second trimester   COM M ♀

    O13.3   Gestational [pregnancy-induced] hypertension without significant proteinuria, third trimester   COM M ♀

    O13.4   Gestational [pregnancy-induced] hypertension without significant proteinuria, complicating childbirth   COM M ♀

    O13.5   Gestational [pregnancy-induced] hypertension without significant proteinuria, complicating the puerperium   COM M ♀

    O13.9   Gestational [pregnancy-induced] hypertension without significant proteinuria, unspecified trimester   COM M ♀

✓4th **O14**   Pre-eclampsia

    EXCLUDES 1   pre-existing hypertension with pre-eclampsia (O11)

    DEF: Complication of pregnancy manifesting in the development of borderline hypertension, protein in the urine, and unresponsive swelling between the 20th week of pregnancy and the end of the first week following birth in mild to moderate cases. Severe preeclampsia presents with hypertension, associated with marked swelling, proteinuria, abdominal pain, and/or visual changes.

    ✓5th **O14.0**   Mild to moderate pre-eclampsia

    AHA: 2019,3Q,12; 2019,2Q,8

      O14.00   Mild to moderate pre-eclampsia, unspecified trimester   COM M ♀

      O14.02   Mild to moderate pre-eclampsia, second trimester   COM M ♀

      O14.03   Mild to moderate pre-eclampsia, third trimester   COM M ♀

      O14.04   Mild to moderate pre-eclampsia, complicating childbirth   COM M ♀

         AHA: 2019,2Q,8

      O14.05   Mild to moderate pre-eclampsia, complicating the puerperium   COM M ♀

    ✓5th **O14.1**   Severe pre-eclampsia

    EXCLUDES 1   HELLP syndrome (O14.2-)

    AHA: 2019,3Q,12

      O14.10   Severe pre-eclampsia, unspecified trimester   COM M ♀

      O14.12   Severe pre-eclampsia, second trimester   COM M ♀

      O14.13   Severe pre-eclampsia, third trimester   COM M ♀

      O14.14   Severe pre-eclampsia complicating childbirth   COM M ♀

      O14.15   Severe pre-eclampsia, complicating the puerperium   COM M ♀

    ✓5th **O14.2**   HELLP syndrome

         Severe pre-eclampsia with hemolysis, elevated liver enzymes and low platelet count (HELLP)

    AHA: 2019,3Q,12

      O14.20   HELLP syndrome (HELLP), unspecified trimester   COM M ♀

      O14.22   HELLP syndrome (HELLP), second trimester   COM M ♀

      O14.23   HELLP syndrome (HELLP), third trimester   COM M ♀

      O14.24   HELLP syndrome, complicating childbirth   COM M ♀

      O14.25   HELLP syndrome, complicating the puerperium   COM M ♀

    ✓5th **O14.9**   Unspecified pre-eclampsia

      O14.90   Unspecified pre-eclampsia, unspecified trimester   COM M ♀

      O14.92   Unspecified pre-eclampsia, second trimester   COM M ♀

      O14.93   Unspecified pre-eclampsia, third trimester   COM M ♀

      O14.94   Unspecified pre-eclampsia, complicating childbirth   COM M ♀

      O14.95   Unspecified pre-eclampsia, complicating the puerperium   COM M ♀

✓4ᵗʰ O15 Eclampsia

> **INCLUDES**   convulsions following conditions in O10-O14 and O16
>
> **DEF:** Tetany and toxemia producing seizure activity or coma in a pregnant patient who most often has presented with prior preeclampsia (i.e., hypertension, albuminuria, and edema).

> **✓5ᵗʰ O15.0 Eclampsia complicating pregnancy**
>
> > **O15.00**   **Eclampsia complicating pregnancy, unspecified trimester**   COM M ♀
> >
> > **O15.02**   **Eclampsia complicating pregnancy, second trimester**   COM M ♀
> >
> > **O15.03**   **Eclampsia complicating pregnancy, third trimester**   COM M ♀
>
> **O15.1**   **Eclampsia complicating labor**   COM M ♀
>
> **O15.2**   **Eclampsia complicating the puerperium**   COM M ♀
>
> **O15.9**   **Eclampsia, unspecified as to time period**   COM M ♀
> > Eclampsia NOS

✓4ᵗʰ O16 Unspecified maternal hypertension

> **O16.1**   **Unspecified maternal hypertension, first trimester**   COM M ♀
>
> **O16.2**   **Unspecified maternal hypertension, second trimester**   COM M ♀
>
> **O16.3**   **Unspecified maternal hypertension, third trimester**   COM M ♀
>
> **O16.4**   **Unspecified maternal hypertension, complicating childbirth**   COM M ♀
>
> **O16.5**   **Unspecified maternal hypertension, complicating the puerperium**   COM M ♀
>
> **O16.9**   **Unspecified maternal hypertension, unspecified trimester**   COM M ♀

Other maternal disorders predominantly related to pregnancy (O20-O29)

> **EXCLUDES 2**   maternal care related to the fetus and amniotic cavity and possible delivery problems (O30-O48)
> maternal diseases classifiable elsewhere but complicating pregnancy, labor and delivery, and the puerperium (O98-O99)

✓4ᵗʰ O20 Hemorrhage in early pregnancy

> **INCLUDES**   hemorrhage before completion of 20 weeks gestation
>
> **EXCLUDES 1**   pregnancy with abortive outcome (O00-O08)

> **O20.0**   **Threatened abortion**   COM M ♀
> > Hemorrhage specified as due to threatened abortion
> > **DEF:** Bloody discharge during pregnancy. The cervix may be dilated and pregnancy threatened, but the pregnancy is not terminated.
>
> **O20.8**   **Other hemorrhage in early pregnancy**   COM M ♀
>
> **O20.9**   **Hemorrhage in early pregnancy, unspecified**   COM M ♀

✓4ᵗʰ O21 Excessive vomiting in pregnancy

> **O21.0**   **Mild hyperemesis gravidarum**   COM M ♀
> > Hyperemesis gravidarum, mild or unspecified, starting before the end of the 20th week of gestation
>
> **O21.1**   **Hyperemesis gravidarum with metabolic disturbance**   COM M ♀
> > Hyperemesis gravidarum, starting before the end of the 20th week of gestation, with metabolic disturbance such as carbohydrate depletion
> > Hyperemesis gravidarum, starting before the end of the 20th week of gestation, with metabolic disturbance such as dehydration
> > Hyperemesis gravidarum, starting before the end of the 20th week of gestation, with metabolic disturbance such as electrolyte imbalance
>
> **O21.2**   **Late vomiting of pregnancy**   COM M ♀
> > Excessive vomiting starting after 20 completed weeks of gestation
>
> **O21.8**   **Other vomiting complicating pregnancy**   COM M ♀
> > Vomiting due to diseases classified elsewhere, complicating pregnancy
> > Use additional code, to identify cause
>
> **O21.9**   **Vomiting of pregnancy, unspecified**   COM M ♀

✓4ᵗʰ O22 Venous complications and hemorrhoids in pregnancy

> **EXCLUDES 1**   venous complications of:
> > abortion NOS (O03.9)
> > ectopic or molar pregnancy (O08.7)
> > failed attempted abortion (O07.35)
> > induced abortion (O04.85)
> > spontaneous abortion (O03.89)
>
> **EXCLUDES 2**   obstetric pulmonary embolism (O88.-)
> > venous complications and hemorrhoids of childbirth and the puerperium (O87.-)

> **✓5ᵗʰ O22.0 Varicose veins of lower extremity in pregnancy**
> > Varicose veins NOS in pregnancy
> > **DEF:** Distended, tortuous veins of the lower extremities associated with pregnancy.
> >
> > **O22.00**   **Varicose veins of lower extremity in pregnancy, unspecified trimester**   COM M ♀
> >
> > **O22.01**   **Varicose veins of lower extremity in pregnancy, first trimester**   COM M ♀
> >
> > **O22.02**   **Varicose veins of lower extremity in pregnancy, second trimester**   COM M ♀
> >
> > **O22.03**   **Varicose veins of lower extremity in pregnancy, third trimester**   COM M ♀

> **✓5ᵗʰ O22.1 Genital varices in pregnancy**
> > Perineal varices in pregnancy
> > Vaginal varices in pregnancy
> > Vulval varices in pregnancy
> >
> > **O22.10**   **Genital varices in pregnancy, unspecified trimester**   COM M ♀
> >
> > **O22.11**   **Genital varices in pregnancy, first trimester**   COM M ♀
> >
> > **O22.12**   **Genital varices in pregnancy, second trimester**   COM M ♀
> >
> > **O22.13**   **Genital varices in pregnancy, third trimester**   COM M ♀

> **✓5ᵗʰ O22.2 Superficial thrombophlebitis in pregnancy**
> > Phlebitis in pregnancy NOS
> > Thrombophlebitis of legs in pregnancy
> > Thrombosis in pregnancy NOS
> > Use additional code to identify the superficial thrombophlebitis (I80.0-)
> >
> > **O22.20**   **Superficial thrombophlebitis in pregnancy, unspecified trimester**   COM M ♀
> >
> > **O22.21**   **Superficial thrombophlebitis in pregnancy, first trimester**   COM M ♀
> >
> > **O22.22**   **Superficial thrombophlebitis in pregnancy, second trimester**   COM M ♀
> >
> > **O22.23**   **Superficial thrombophlebitis in pregnancy, third trimester**   COM M ♀

> **✓5ᵗʰ O22.3 Deep phlebothrombosis in pregnancy**
> > Deep vein thrombosis, antepartum
> > Use additional code to identify the deep vein thrombosis (I82.4-, I82.5-, I82.62-, I82.72-)
> > Use additional code, if applicable, for associated long-term (current) use of anticoagulants (Z79.01)
> >
> > **O22.30**   **Deep phlebothrombosis in pregnancy, unspecified trimester**   COM M ♀
> >
> > **O22.31**   **Deep phlebothrombosis in pregnancy, first trimester**   COM M ♀
> >
> > **O22.32**   **Deep phlebothrombosis in pregnancy, second trimester**   COM M ♀
> >
> > **O22.33**   **Deep phlebothrombosis in pregnancy, third trimester**   COM M ♀

> **✓5ᵗʰ O22.4 Hemorrhoids in pregnancy**
> > **O22.40**   **Hemorrhoids in pregnancy, unspecified trimester**   COM M ♀
> >
> > **O22.41**   **Hemorrhoids in pregnancy, first trimester**   COM M ♀
> >
> > **O22.42**   **Hemorrhoids in pregnancy, second trimester**   COM M ♀
> >
> > **O22.43**   **Hemorrhoids in pregnancy, third trimester**   COM M ♀

> **✓5ᵗʰ O22.5 Cerebral venous thrombosis in pregnancy**
> > Cerebrovenous sinus thrombosis in pregnancy
> >
> > **O22.50**   **Cerebral venous thrombosis in pregnancy, unspecified trimester**   COM M ♀
> >
> > **O22.51**   **Cerebral venous thrombosis in pregnancy, first trimester**   COM M ♀

✔ Additional Character Required   ✔x7ᵗʰ Placeholder Alert   Manifestation   Unspecified Dx   Q QPP   UPD Unacceptable PDx

Chapter 15. Pregnancy, Childbirth and the Puerperium

O22.52　Cerebral venous thrombosis in pregnancy, second trimester `COM` `M` ♀

O22.53　Cerebral venous thrombosis in pregnancy, third trimester `COM` `M` ♀

✓5th **O22.8**　Other venous complications in pregnancy

　✓6th **O22.8X**　Other venous complications in pregnancy

　　O22.8X1　Other venous complications in pregnancy, first trimester `COM` `M` ♀

　　O22.8X2　Other venous complications in pregnancy, second trimester `COM` `M` ♀

　　O22.8X3　Other venous complications in pregnancy, third trimester `COM` `M` ♀

　　O22.8X9　Other venous complications in pregnancy, unspecified trimester `COM` `M` ♀

✓5th **O22.9**　Venous complication in pregnancy, unspecified

　　Gestational phlebitis NOS
　　Gestational phlebopathy NOS
　　Gestational thrombosis NOS

　　O22.90　Venous complication in pregnancy, unspecified, unspecified trimester `COM` `M` ♀

　　O22.91　Venous complication in pregnancy, unspecified, first trimester `COM` `M` ♀

　　O22.92　Venous complication in pregnancy, unspecified, second trimester `COM` `M` ♀

　　O22.93　Venous complication in pregnancy, unspecified, third trimester `COM` `M` ♀

✓4th **O23**　Infections of genitourinary tract in pregnancy

　　Use additional code to identify organism (B95.-, B96.-)

　　EXCLUDES 2　*gonococcal infections complicating pregnancy, childbirth and the puerperium (O98.2)*

　　infections with a predominantly sexual mode of transmission NOS complicating pregnancy, childbirth and the puerperium (O98.3)

　　syphilis complicating pregnancy, childbirth and the puerperium (O98.1)

　　tuberculosis of genitourinary system complicating pregnancy, childbirth and the puerperium (O98.0)

　　venereal disease NOS complicating pregnancy, childbirth and the puerperium (O98.3)

　　AHA: 2018,2Q,20

✓5th **O23.0**　Infections of kidney in pregnancy

　　Pyelonephritis in pregnancy

　　O23.00　Infections of kidney in pregnancy, unspecified trimester `COM` `M` ♀

　　O23.01　Infections of kidney in pregnancy, first trimester `COM` `M` ♀

　　O23.02　Infections of kidney in pregnancy, second trimester `COM` `M` ♀

　　O23.03　Infections of kidney in pregnancy, third trimester `COM` `M` ♀

✓5th **O23.1**　Infections of bladder in pregnancy

　　O23.10　Infections of bladder in pregnancy, unspecified trimester `COM` `M` ♀

　　O23.11　Infections of bladder in pregnancy, first trimester `COM` `M` ♀

　　O23.12　Infections of bladder in pregnancy, second trimester `COM` `M` ♀

　　O23.13　Infections of bladder in pregnancy, third trimester `COM` `M` ♀

✓5th **O23.2**　Infections of urethra in pregnancy

　　O23.20　Infections of urethra in pregnancy, unspecified trimester `COM` `M` ♀

　　O23.21　Infections of urethra in pregnancy, first trimester `COM` `M` ♀

　　O23.22　Infections of urethra in pregnancy, second trimester `COM` `M` ♀

　　O23.23　Infections of urethra in pregnancy, third trimester `COM` `M` ♀

✓5th **O23.3**　Infections of other parts of urinary tract in pregnancy

　　O23.30　Infections of other parts of urinary tract in pregnancy, unspecified trimester `COM` `M` ♀

　　O23.31　Infections of other parts of urinary tract in pregnancy, first trimester `COM` `M` ♀

　　O23.32　Infections of other parts of urinary tract in pregnancy, second trimester `COM` `M` ♀

O23.33　Infections of other parts of urinary tract in pregnancy, third trimester `COM` `M` ♀

✓5th **O23.4**　Unspecified infection of urinary tract in pregnancy

　　O23.40　Unspecified infection of urinary tract in pregnancy, unspecified trimester `COM` `M` ♀

　　O23.41　Unspecified infection of urinary tract in pregnancy, first trimester `COM` `M` ♀

　　O23.42　Unspecified infection of urinary tract in pregnancy, second trimester `COM` `M` ♀

　　O23.43　Unspecified infection of urinary tract in pregnancy, third trimester `COM` `M` ♀

✓5th **O23.5**　Infections of the genital tract in pregnancy

　✓6th **O23.51**　Infection of cervix in pregnancy

　　O23.511　Infections of cervix in pregnancy, first trimester `COM` `M` ♀

　　O23.512　Infections of cervix in pregnancy, second trimester `COM` `M` ♀

　　O23.513　Infections of cervix in pregnancy, third trimester `COM` `M` ♀

　　O23.519　Infections of cervix in pregnancy, unspecified trimester `COM` `M` ♀

　✓6th **O23.52**　Salpingo-oophoritis in pregnancy

　　Oophoritis in pregnancy
　　Salpingitis in pregnancy

　　O23.521　Salpingo-oophoritis in pregnancy, first trimester `COM` `M` ♀

　　O23.522　Salpingo-oophoritis in pregnancy, second trimester `COM` `M` ♀

　　O23.523　Salpingo-oophoritis in pregnancy, third trimester `COM` `M` ♀

　　O23.529　Salpingo-oophoritis in pregnancy, unspecified trimester `COM` `M` ♀

　✓6th **O23.59**　Infection of other part of genital tract in pregnancy

　　AHA: 2022,1Q,20

　　O23.591　Infection of other part of genital tract in pregnancy, first trimester `COM` `M` ♀

　　O23.592　Infection of other part of genital tract in pregnancy, second trimester `COM` `M` ♀

　　O23.593　Infection of other part of genital tract in pregnancy, third trimester `COM` `M` ♀

　　O23.599　Infection of other part of genital tract in pregnancy, unspecified trimester `COM` `M` ♀

✓5th **O23.9**　Unspecified genitourinary tract infection in pregnancy

　　Genitourinary tract infection in pregnancy NOS

　　O23.90　Unspecified genitourinary tract infection in pregnancy, unspecified trimester `COM` `M` ♀

　　O23.91　Unspecified genitourinary tract infection in pregnancy, first trimester `COM` `M` ♀

　　O23.92　Unspecified genitourinary tract infection in pregnancy, second trimester `COM` `M` ♀

　　O23.93　Unspecified genitourinary tract infection in pregnancy, third trimester `COM` `M` ♀

✓4th **O24**　Diabetes mellitus in pregnancy, childbirth and the puerperium

　✓5th **O24.0**　Pre-existing type 1 diabetes mellitus, in pregnancy, childbirth and the puerperium

　　Juvenile onset diabetes mellitus, in pregnancy, childbirth and the puerperium

　　Ketosis-prone diabetes mellitus in pregnancy, childbirth and the puerperium

　　Use additional code from category E10 to further identify any manifestations

　✓6th **O24.01**　Pre-existing type 1 diabetes mellitus, in pregnancy

　　O24.011　Pre-existing type 1 diabetes mellitus, in pregnancy, first trimester `COM` `Q` `M` ♀

　　O24.012　Pre-existing type 1 diabetes mellitus, in pregnancy, second trimester `COM` `Q` `M` ♀

　　O24.013　Pre-existing type 1 diabetes mellitus, in pregnancy, third trimester `COM` `Q` `M` ♀

　　O24.019　Pre-existing type 1 diabetes mellitus, in pregnancy, unspecified trimester `COM` `Q` `M` ♀

　　O24.02　Pre-existing type 1 diabetes mellitus, in childbirth `COM` `Q` `M` ♀

　　O24.03　Pre-existing type 1 diabetes mellitus, in the puerperium `COM` `Q` `M` ♀

√5th **O24.1 Pre-existing type 2 diabetes mellitus, in pregnancy, childbirth and the puerperium**
    Insulin-resistant diabetes mellitus in pregnancy, childbirth and the puerperium
    Use additional code (for):
      from category E11 to further identify any manifestations
      long-term (current) use of insulin (Z79.4)

  √6th **O24.11 Pre-existing type 2 diabetes mellitus, in** pregnancy

     O24.111 Pre-existing type 2 diabetes mellitus, in pregnancy, first trimester COM Q M ♀
     O24.112 Pre-existing type 2 diabetes mellitus, in pregnancy, second trimester COM Q M ♀
     O24.113 Pre-existing type 2 diabetes mellitus, in pregnancy, third trimester COM Q M ♀
     O24.119 Pre-existing type 2 diabetes mellitus, in pregnancy, unspecified trimester COM Q M ♀

  O24.12 Pre-existing type 2 diabetes mellitus, in childbirth COM Q M ♀
  O24.13 Pre-existing type 2 diabetes mellitus, in the puerperium COM Q M ♀

√5th **O24.3 Unspecified pre-existing diabetes mellitus in pregnancy, childbirth and the puerperium**
    Use additional code (for):
      from category E11 to further identify any manifestation
      long-term (current) use of insulin (Z79.4)

  √6th **O24.31 Unspecified pre-existing diabetes mellitus in** pregnancy

     O24.311 Unspecified pre-existing diabetes mellitus in pregnancy, first trimester COM Q M ♀
     O24.312 Unspecified pre-existing diabetes mellitus in pregnancy, second trimester COM Q M ♀
     O24.313 Unspecified pre-existing diabetes mellitus in pregnancy, third trimester COM Q M ♀
     O24.319 Unspecified pre-existing diabetes mellitus in pregnancy, unspecified trimester COM Q M ♀

  O24.32 Unspecified pre-existing diabetes mellitus in childbirth COM Q M ♀
  O24.33 Unspecified pre-existing diabetes mellitus in the puerperium COM Q M ♀

√5th **O24.4 Gestational diabetes mellitus**
    Diabetes mellitus arising in pregnancy
    Gestational diabetes mellitus NOS
    AHA: 2020,3Q,30; 2016,4Q,50; 2015,4Q,34

  √6th **O24.41 Gestational diabetes mellitus in** pregnancy

     O24.410 Gestational diabetes mellitus in pregnancy, diet controlled COM M ♀
     O24.414 Gestational diabetes mellitus in pregnancy, insulin controlled COM M ♀
     O24.415 Gestational diabetes mellitus in pregnancy, controlled by oral hypoglycemic drugs COM M ♀
       Gestational diabetes mellitus in pregnancy, controlled by oral antidiabetic drugs
     O24.419 Gestational diabetes mellitus in pregnancy, unspecified control COM M ♀

  √6th **O24.42 Gestational diabetes mellitus in** childbirth
    AHA: 2016,1Q,5

     O24.420 Gestational diabetes mellitus in childbirth, diet controlled COM M ♀
     O24.424 Gestational diabetes mellitus in childbirth, insulin controlled COM M ♀
     O24.425 Gestational diabetes mellitus in childbirth, controlled by oral hypoglycemic drugs COM M ♀
       Gestational diabetes mellitus in childbirth, controlled by oral antidiabetic drugs
     O24.429 Gestational diabetes mellitus in childbirth, unspecified control COM M ♀

  √6th **O24.43 Gestational diabetes mellitus in the** puerperium

     O24.430 Gestational diabetes mellitus in the puerperium, diet controlled COM M ♀

     O24.434 Gestational diabetes mellitus in the puerperium, insulin controlled COM M ♀
     O24.435 Gestational diabetes mellitus in puerperium, controlled by oral hypoglycemic drugs COM M ♀
       Gestational diabetes mellitus in puerperium, controlled by oral antidiabetic drugs
     O24.439 Gestational diabetes mellitus in the puerperium, unspecified control COM M ♀

√5th **O24.8 Other pre-existing diabetes mellitus in pregnancy, childbirth, and the puerperium**
    Use additional code (for):
      from categories E08, E09 and E13 to further identify any manifestation
      long-term (current) use of insulin (Z79.4)

  √6th **O24.81 Other pre-existing diabetes mellitus in** pregnancy

     O24.811 Other pre-existing diabetes mellitus in pregnancy, first trimester COM Q M ♀
     O24.812 Other pre-existing diabetes mellitus in pregnancy, second trimester COM Q M ♀
     O24.813 Other pre-existing diabetes mellitus in pregnancy, third trimester COM Q M ♀
     O24.819 Other pre-existing diabetes mellitus in pregnancy, unspecified trimester COM Q M ♀

  O24.82 Other pre-existing diabetes mellitus in childbirth COM Q M ♀
  O24.83 Other pre-existing diabetes mellitus in the puerperium COM Q M ♀

√5th **O24.9 Unspecified diabetes mellitus in pregnancy, childbirth and the puerperium**
    Use additional code for long-term (current) use of insulin (Z79.4)

  √6th **O24.91 Unspecified diabetes mellitus in** pregnancy

     O24.911 Unspecified diabetes mellitus in pregnancy, first trimester COM M ♀
     O24.912 Unspecified diabetes mellitus in pregnancy, second trimester COM M ♀
     O24.913 Unspecified diabetes mellitus in pregnancy, third trimester COM M ♀
     O24.919 Unspecified diabetes mellitus in pregnancy, unspecified trimester COM M ♀

  O24.92 Unspecified diabetes mellitus in childbirth COM M ♀
  O24.93 Unspecified diabetes mellitus in the puerperium COM M ♀

√4th **O25 Malnutrition in pregnancy, childbirth and the puerperium**

  √5th **O25.1 Malnutrition in** pregnancy

    O25.10 Malnutrition in pregnancy, unspecified trimester COM M ♀
    O25.11 Malnutrition in pregnancy, first trimester COM M ♀
    O25.12 Malnutrition in pregnancy, second trimester COM M ♀
    O25.13 Malnutrition in pregnancy, third trimester COM M ♀

  O25.2 Malnutrition in childbirth COM M ♀
  O25.3 Malnutrition in the puerperium COM M ♀

√4th **O26 Maternal care for other conditions predominantly related to pregnancy**

  √5th **O26.0 Excessive weight gain in pregnancy**
    EXCLUDES 2 *gestational edema (O12.0, O12.2)*

    O26.00 Excessive weight gain in pregnancy, unspecified trimester COM M ♀
    O26.01 Excessive weight gain in pregnancy, first trimester COM M ♀
    O26.02 Excessive weight gain in pregnancy, second trimester COM M ♀
    O26.03 Excessive weight gain in pregnancy, third trimester COM M ♀

  √5th **O26.1 Low weight gain in pregnancy**

    O26.10 Low weight gain in pregnancy, unspecified trimester COM M ♀

☑ Additional Character Required   √x7th Placeholder Alert   Manifestation   Unspecified Dx   Q QPP   UPD Unacceptable PDx

O26.11 Low weight gain in pregnancy, first trimester COM M ♀

O26.12 Low weight gain in pregnancy, second trimester COM M ♀

O26.13 Low weight gain in pregnancy, third trimester COM M ♀

✓5th **O26.2** Pregnancy care for patient with recurrent pregnancy loss

O26.20 Pregnancy care for patient with recurrent pregnancy loss, unspecified trimester COM M ♀

O26.21 Pregnancy care for patient with recurrent pregnancy loss, first trimester COM M ♀

O26.22 Pregnancy care for patient with recurrent pregnancy loss, second trimester COM M ♀

O26.23 Pregnancy care for patient with recurrent pregnancy loss, third trimester COM M ♀

✓5th **O26.3** Retained intrauterine contraceptive device in pregnancy

O26.30 Retained intrauterine contraceptive device in pregnancy, unspecified trimester COM M ♀

O26.31 Retained intrauterine contraceptive device in pregnancy, first trimester COM M ♀

O26.32 Retained intrauterine contraceptive device in pregnancy, second trimester COM M ♀

O26.33 Retained intrauterine contraceptive device in pregnancy, third trimester COM M ♀

✓5th **O26.4** Herpes gestationis

DEF: Rare skin disorder of unknown origin that appears on the abdomen in the second and third trimester as intensely itchy blisters that spread to other sites.

O26.40 Herpes gestationis, unspecified trimester COM M ♀

O26.41 Herpes gestationis, first trimester COM M ♀

O26.42 Herpes gestationis, second trimester COM M ♀

O26.43 Herpes gestationis, third trimester COM M ♀

✓5th **O26.5** Maternal hypotension syndrome

Supine hypotensive syndrome

O26.50 Maternal hypotension syndrome, unspecified trimester COM M ♀

O26.51 Maternal hypotension syndrome, first trimester COM M ♀

O26.52 Maternal hypotension syndrome, second trimester COM M ♀

O26.53 Maternal hypotension syndrome, third trimester COM M ♀

✓5th **O26.6** Liver and biliary tract disorders in pregnancy, childbirth and the puerperium

Use additional code to identify the specific disorder

EXCLUDES 2 hepatorenal syndrome following labor and delivery (O90.4)

✓6th **O26.61** Liver and biliary tract disorders in pregnancy

O26.611 Liver and biliary tract disorders in pregnancy, first trimester COM M ♀

O26.612 Liver and biliary tract disorders in pregnancy, second trimester COM M ♀

O26.613 Liver and biliary tract disorders in pregnancy, third trimester COM M ♀

O26.619 Liver and biliary tract disorders in pregnancy, unspecified trimester COM M ♀

O26.62 Liver and biliary tract disorders in childbirth COM M ♀

O26.63 Liver and biliary tract disorders in the puerperium COM M ♀

✓5th **O26.7** Subluxation of symphysis (pubis) in pregnancy, childbirth and the puerperium

EXCLUDES 1 traumatic separation of symphysis (pubis) during childbirth (O71.6)

✓6th **O26.71** Subluxation of symphysis (pubis) in pregnancy

O26.711 Subluxation of symphysis (pubis) in pregnancy, first trimester COM M ♀

O26.712 Subluxation of symphysis (pubis) in pregnancy, second trimester COM M ♀

O26.713 Subluxation of symphysis (pubis) in pregnancy, third trimester COM M ♀

O26.719 Subluxation of symphysis (pubis) in pregnancy, unspecified trimester COM M ♀

O26.72 Subluxation of symphysis (pubis) in childbirth COM M ♀

O26.73 Subluxation of symphysis (pubis) in the puerperium COM M ♀

✓5th **O26.8** Other specified pregnancy related conditions

✓6th **O26.81** Pregnancy related exhaustion and fatigue

O26.811 Pregnancy related exhaustion and fatigue, first trimester COM M ♀

O26.812 Pregnancy related exhaustion and fatigue, second trimester COM M ♀

O26.813 Pregnancy related exhaustion and fatigue, third trimester COM M ♀

O26.819 Pregnancy related exhaustion and fatigue, unspecified trimester COM M ♀

✓6th **O26.82** Pregnancy related peripheral neuritis

O26.821 Pregnancy related peripheral neuritis, first trimester COM M ♀

O26.822 Pregnancy related peripheral neuritis, second trimester COM M ♀

O26.823 Pregnancy related peripheral neuritis, third trimester COM M ♀

O26.829 Pregnancy related peripheral neuritis, unspecified trimester COM M ♀

✓6th **O26.83** Pregnancy related renal disease

Use additional code to identify the specific disorder

O26.831 Pregnancy related renal disease, first trimester COM M ♀

O26.832 Pregnancy related renal disease, second trimester COM M ♀

O26.833 Pregnancy related renal disease, third trimester COM M ♀

O26.839 Pregnancy related renal disease, unspecified trimester COM M ♀

✓6th **O26.84** Uterine size-date discrepancy complicating pregnancy

EXCLUDES 1 encounter for suspected problem with fetal growth ruled out (Z03.74)

O26.841 Uterine size-date discrepancy, first trimester COM M ♀

O26.842 Uterine size-date discrepancy, second trimester COM M ♀

O26.843 Uterine size-date discrepancy, third trimester COM M ♀

O26.849 Uterine size-date discrepancy, unspecified trimester COM M ♀

✓6th **O26.85** Spotting complicating pregnancy

O26.851 Spotting complicating pregnancy, first trimester COM M ♀

O26.852 Spotting complicating pregnancy, second trimester COM M ♀

O26.853 Spotting complicating pregnancy, third trimester COM M ♀

O26.859 Spotting complicating pregnancy, unspecified trimester COM M ♀

O26.86 Pruritic urticarial papules and plaques of pregnancy (PUPPP) COM M ♀

Polymorphic eruption of pregnancy

✓6th **O26.87** Cervical shortening

EXCLUDES 1 encounter for suspected cervical shortening ruled out (Z03.75)

DEF: Cervix that has shortened to less than 25 mm before the 24th week of pregnancy. A shortened cervix is a warning sign for impending premature delivery and is treated by cervical cerclage placement or progesterone.

O26.872 Cervical shortening, second trimester COM M ♀

O26.873 Cervical shortening, third trimester COM M ♀

O26.879 Cervical shortening, unspecified trimester COM M ♀

✓6th **O26.89** Other specified pregnancy related conditions

AHA: 2015,3Q,40

O26.891 Other specified pregnancy related conditions, first trimester COM M ♀

O26.892 Other specified pregnancy related conditions, second trimester COM M ♀

O26.893 Other specified pregnancy related conditions, third trimester COM M ♀

O26.899   Other specified pregnancy related conditions, unspecified trimester   COM M ♀

✓5th O26.9   **Pregnancy related conditions, unspecified**

O26.90   Pregnancy related conditions, unspecified, unspecified trimester   COM M ♀

O26.91   Pregnancy related conditions, unspecified, first trimester   COM M ♀

O26.92   Pregnancy related conditions, unspecified, second trimester   COM M ♀

O26.93   Pregnancy related conditions, unspecified, third trimester   COM M ♀

✓4th **O28**   **Abnormal findings on antenatal screening of mother**

    EXCLUDES 1   *diagnostic findings classified elsewhere - see Alphabetical Index*

O28.0   Abnormal hematological finding on antenatal screening of mother   M ♀

O28.1   Abnormal biochemical finding on antenatal screening of mother   M ♀

O28.2   Abnormal cytological finding on antenatal screening of mother   M ♀

O28.3   Abnormal ultrasonic finding on antenatal screening of mother   M ♀

O28.4   Abnormal radiological finding on antenatal screening of mother   M ♀

O28.5   Abnormal chromosomal and genetic finding on antenatal screening of mother   M ♀

O28.8   Other abnormal findings on antenatal screening of mother   M ♀

O28.9   Unspecified abnormal findings on antenatal screening of mother   M ♀

✓4th **O29**   **Complications of anesthesia during pregnancy**

    INCLUDES   maternal complications arising from the administration of a general, regional or local anesthetic, analgesic or other sedation during pregnancy

    Use additional code, if necessary, to identify the complication

    EXCLUDES 2   *complications of anesthesia during labor and delivery (O74.-)*
             complications of anesthesia during the puerperium (O89.-)

✓5th O29.0   **Pulmonary complications of anesthesia during pregnancy**

✓6th O29.01   Aspiration pneumonitis due to anesthesia during pregnancy

     Inhalation of stomach contents or secretions NOS due to anesthesia during pregnancy

     Mendelson's syndrome due to anesthesia during pregnancy

O29.011   Aspiration pneumonitis due to anesthesia during pregnancy, first trimester   COM M ♀

O29.012   Aspiration pneumonitis due to anesthesia during pregnancy, second trimester   COM M ♀

O29.013   Aspiration pneumonitis due to anesthesia during pregnancy, third trimester   COM M ♀

O29.019   Aspiration pneumonitis due to anesthesia during pregnancy, unspecified trimester   COM M ♀

✓6th O29.02   Pressure collapse of lung due to anesthesia during pregnancy

O29.021   Pressure collapse of lung due to anesthesia during pregnancy, first trimester   COM M ♀

O29.022   Pressure collapse of lung due to anesthesia during pregnancy, second trimester   COM M ♀

O29.023   Pressure collapse of lung due to anesthesia during pregnancy, third trimester   COM M ♀

O29.029   Pressure collapse of lung due to anesthesia during pregnancy, unspecified trimester   COM M ♀

✓6th O29.09   Other pulmonary complications of anesthesia during pregnancy

O29.091   Other pulmonary complications of anesthesia during pregnancy, first trimester   COM M ♀

O29.092   Other pulmonary complications of anesthesia during pregnancy, second trimester   COM M ♀

O29.093   Other pulmonary complications of anesthesia during pregnancy, third trimester   COM M ♀

O29.099   Other pulmonary complications of anesthesia during pregnancy, unspecified trimester   COM M ♀

✓5th O29.1   **Cardiac complications of anesthesia during pregnancy**

✓6th O29.11   Cardiac arrest due to anesthesia during pregnancy

O29.111   Cardiac arrest due to anesthesia during pregnancy, first trimester   COM M ♀

O29.112   Cardiac arrest due to anesthesia during pregnancy, second trimester   COM M ♀

O29.113   Cardiac arrest due to anesthesia during pregnancy, third trimester   COM M ♀

O29.119   Cardiac arrest due to anesthesia during pregnancy, unspecified trimester   COM M ♀

✓6th O29.12   Cardiac failure due to anesthesia during pregnancy

O29.121   Cardiac failure due to anesthesia during pregnancy, first trimester   COM M ♀

O29.122   Cardiac failure due to anesthesia during pregnancy, second trimester   COM M ♀

O29.123   Cardiac failure due to anesthesia during pregnancy, third trimester   COM M ♀

O29.129   Cardiac failure due to anesthesia during pregnancy, unspecified trimester   COM M ♀

✓6th O29.19   Other cardiac complications of anesthesia during pregnancy

O29.191   Other cardiac complications of anesthesia during pregnancy, first trimester   COM M ♀

O29.192   Other cardiac complications of anesthesia during pregnancy, second trimester   COM M ♀

O29.193   Other cardiac complications of anesthesia during pregnancy, third trimester   COM M ♀

O29.199   Other cardiac complications of anesthesia during pregnancy, unspecified trimester   COM M ♀

✓5th O29.2   **Central nervous system complications of anesthesia during pregnancy**

✓6th O29.21   Cerebral anoxia due to anesthesia during pregnancy

O29.211   Cerebral anoxia due to anesthesia during pregnancy, first trimester   COM M ♀

O29.212   Cerebral anoxia due to anesthesia during pregnancy, second trimester   COM M ♀

O29.213   Cerebral anoxia due to anesthesia during pregnancy, third trimester   COM M ♀

O29.219   Cerebral anoxia due to anesthesia during pregnancy, unspecified trimester   COM M ♀

✓6th O29.29   Other central nervous system complications of anesthesia during pregnancy

O29.291   Other central nervous system complications of anesthesia during pregnancy, first trimester   COM M ♀

O29.292   Other central nervous system complications of anesthesia during pregnancy, second trimester   COM M ♀

O29.293   Other central nervous system complications of anesthesia during pregnancy, third trimester   COM M ♀

O29.299   Other central nervous system complications of anesthesia during pregnancy, unspecified trimester   COM M ♀

✓5th O29.3   **Toxic reaction to local anesthesia during pregnancy**

✓6th O29.3X   Toxic reaction to local anesthesia during pregnancy

O29.3X1   Toxic reaction to local anesthesia during pregnancy, first trimester   COM M ♀

O29.3X2   Toxic reaction to local anesthesia during pregnancy, second trimester   COM M ♀

O29.3X3   Toxic reaction to local anesthesia during pregnancy, third trimester   COM M ♀

O29.3X9   Toxic reaction to local anesthesia during pregnancy, unspecified trimester   COM M ♀

✓ Additional Character Required   ✓x7th Placeholder Alert   Manifestation   Unspecified Dx   Q QPP   UPD Unacceptable PDx

√5ᵗʰ **O29.4** Spinal and epidural anesthesia induced headache **during pregnancy**

     O29.40 Spinal and epidural anesthesia induced headache during pregnancy, unspecified trimester   COM M ♀

     O29.41 Spinal and epidural anesthesia induced headache during pregnancy, first trimester   COM M ♀

     O29.42 Spinal and epidural anesthesia induced headache during pregnancy, second trimester   COM M ♀

     O29.43 Spinal and epidural anesthesia induced headache during pregnancy, third trimester   COM M ♀

√5ᵗʰ **O29.5** Other complications of spinal and epidural anesthesia **during pregnancy**

   √6ᵗʰ **O29.5X** Other complications of spinal and epidural anesthesia during pregnancy

     O29.5X1 Other complications of spinal and epidural anesthesia during pregnancy, first trimester   COM M ♀

     O29.5X2 Other complications of spinal and epidural anesthesia during pregnancy, second trimester   COM M ♀

     O29.5X3 Other complications of spinal and epidural anesthesia during pregnancy, third trimester   COM M ♀

     O29.5X9 Other complications of spinal and epidural anesthesia during pregnancy, unspecified trimester   COM M ♀

√5ᵗʰ **O29.6** Failed or difficult intubation for anesthesia during pregnancy

     O29.60 Failed or difficult intubation for anesthesia during pregnancy, unspecified trimester   COM M ♀

     O29.61 Failed or difficult intubation for anesthesia during pregnancy, first trimester   COM M ♀

     O29.62 Failed or difficult intubation for anesthesia during pregnancy, second trimester   COM M ♀

     O29.63 Failed or difficult intubation for anesthesia during pregnancy, third trimester   COM M ♀

√5ᵗʰ **O29.8** Other complications of anesthesia during pregnancy

   √6ᵗʰ **O29.8X** Other complications of anesthesia during pregnancy

     O29.8X1 Other complications of anesthesia during pregnancy, first trimester   COM M ♀

     O29.8X2 Other complications of anesthesia during pregnancy, second trimester   COM M ♀

     O29.8X3 Other complications of anesthesia during pregnancy, third trimester   COM M ♀

     O29.8X9 Other complications of anesthesia during pregnancy, unspecified trimester   COM M ♀

√5ᵗʰ **O29.9** Unspecified complication of anesthesia during pregnancy

     O29.90 Unspecified complication of anesthesia during pregnancy, unspecified trimester   COM M ♀

     O29.91 Unspecified complication of anesthesia during pregnancy, first trimester   COM M ♀

     O29.92 Unspecified complication of anesthesia during pregnancy, second trimester   COM M ♀

     O29.93 Unspecified complication of anesthesia during pregnancy, third trimester   COM M ♀

Maternal care related to the fetus and amniotic cavity and possible delivery problems (O30-O48)

√4ᵗʰ **O30** **Multiple gestation**

   Code also any complications specific to multiple gestation

   AHA: 2016,4Q,51

√5ᵗʰ **O30.0** Twin pregnancy

   √6ᵗʰ **O30.00** Twin pregnancy, unspecified number of placenta and unspecified number of amniotic sacs

     O30.001 Twin pregnancy, unspecified number of placenta and unspecified number of amniotic sacs, first trimester   COM M ♀

     O30.002 Twin pregnancy, unspecified number of placenta and unspecified number of amniotic sacs, second trimester   COM M ♀

     O30.003 Twin pregnancy, unspecified number of placenta and unspecified number of amniotic sacs, third trimester   COM M ♀

     O30.009 Twin pregnancy, unspecified number of placenta and unspecified number of amniotic sacs, unspecified trimester   COM M ♀

   √6ᵗʰ **O30.01** Twin pregnancy, monochorionic/monoamniotic

     Twin pregnancy, one placenta, one amniotic sac

     EXCLUDES 1   conjoined twins (O30.02-)

     O30.011 Twin pregnancy, monochorionic/monoamniotic, first trimester   COM M ♀

     O30.012 Twin pregnancy, monochorionic/monoamniotic, second trimester   COM M ♀

     O30.013 Twin pregnancy, monochorionic/monoamniotic, third trimester   COM M ♀

     O30.019 Twin pregnancy, monochorionic/monoamniotic, unspecified trimester   COM M ♀

   √6ᵗʰ **O30.02** Conjoined twin pregnancy

     O30.021 Conjoined twin pregnancy, first trimester   COM M ♀

     O30.022 Conjoined twin pregnancy, second trimester   COM M ♀

     O30.023 Conjoined twin pregnancy, third trimester   COM M ♀

     O30.029 Conjoined twin pregnancy, unspecified trimester   COM M ♀

   √6ᵗʰ **O30.03** Twin pregnancy, monochorionic/diamniotic

     Twin pregnancy, one placenta, two amniotic sacs

     O30.031 Twin pregnancy, monochorionic/diamniotic, first trimester   COM M ♀

     O30.032 Twin pregnancy, monochorionic/diamniotic, second trimester   COM M ♀

     O30.033 Twin pregnancy, monochorionic/diamniotic, third trimester   COM M ♀

     O30.039 Twin pregnancy, monochorionic/diamniotic, unspecified trimester   COM M ♀

   √6ᵗʰ **O30.04** Twin pregnancy, dichorionic/diamniotic

     Twin pregnancy, two placentae, two amniotic sacs

     O30.041 Twin pregnancy, dichorionic/diamniotic, first trimester   COM M ♀

     O30.042 Twin pregnancy, dichorionic/diamniotic, second trimester   COM M ♀

     O30.043 Twin pregnancy, dichorionic/diamniotic, third trimester   COM M ♀

     O30.049 Twin pregnancy, dichorionic/diamniotic, unspecified trimester   COM M ♀

   √6ᵗʰ **O30.09** Twin pregnancy, unable to determine number of placenta and number of amniotic sacs

     O30.091 Twin pregnancy, unable to determine number of placenta and number of amniotic sacs, first trimester   COM M ♀

     O30.092 Twin pregnancy, unable to determine number of placenta and number of amniotic sacs, second trimester   COM M ♀

     O30.093 Twin pregnancy, unable to determine number of placenta and number of amniotic sacs, third trimester   COM M ♀

     O30.099 Twin pregnancy, unable to determine number of placenta and number of amniotic sacs, unspecified trimester   COM M ♀

√5ᵗʰ **O30.1** Triplet pregnancy

   √6ᵗʰ **O30.10** Triplet pregnancy, unspecified number of placenta and unspecified number of amniotic sacs

     AHA: 2016,2Q,8

     O30.101 Triplet pregnancy, unspecified number of placenta and unspecified number of amniotic sacs, first trimester   COM M ♀

     O30.102 Triplet pregnancy, unspecified number of placenta and unspecified number of amniotic sacs, second trimester   COM M ♀

O30.103 Triplet pregnancy, unspecified number of placenta and unspecified number of amniotic sacs, third trimester   COM M ♀

O30.109 Triplet pregnancy, unspecified number of placenta and unspecified number of amniotic sacs, unspecified trimester   COM M ♀

✓6ᵗʰ **O30.11** Triplet pregnancy with two or more monochorionic fetuses

  O30.111 Triplet pregnancy with two or more monochorionic fetuses, first trimester   COM M ♀

  O30.112 Triplet pregnancy with two or more monochorionic fetuses, second trimester   COM M ♀

  O30.113 Triplet pregnancy with two or more monochorionic fetuses, third trimester   COM M ♀

  O30.119 Triplet pregnancy with two or more monochorionic fetuses, unspecified trimester   COM M ♀

✓6ᵗʰ **O30.12** Triplet pregnancy with two or more monoamniotic fetuses

  O30.121 Triplet pregnancy with two or more monoamniotic fetuses, first trimester   COM M ♀

  O30.122 Triplet pregnancy with two or more monoamniotic fetuses, second trimester   COM M ♀

  O30.123 Triplet pregnancy with two or more monoamniotic fetuses, third trimester   COM M ♀

  O30.129 Triplet pregnancy with two or more monoamniotic fetuses, unspecified trimester   COM M ♀

✓6ᵗʰ **O30.13** Triplet pregnancy, trichorionic/triamniotic

    AHA: 2018,4Q,22

  O30.131 Triplet pregnancy, trichorionic/triamniotic, first trimester   COM M ♀

  O30.132 Triplet pregnancy, trichorionic/triamniotic, second trimester   COM M ♀

  O30.133 Triplet pregnancy, trichorionic/triamniotic, third trimester   COM M ♀

  O30.139 Triplet pregnancy, trichorionic/triamniotic, unspecified trimester   COM M ♀

✓6ᵗʰ **O30.19** Triplet pregnancy, unable to determine number of placenta and number of amniotic sacs

  O30.191 Triplet pregnancy, unable to determine number of placenta and number of amniotic sacs, first trimester   COM M ♀

  O30.192 Triplet pregnancy, unable to determine number of placenta and number of amniotic sacs, second trimester   COM M ♀

  O30.193 Triplet pregnancy, unable to determine number of placenta and number of amniotic sacs, third trimester   COM M ♀

  O30.199 Triplet pregnancy, unable to determine number of placenta and number of amniotic sacs, unspecified trimester   COM M ♀

✓5ᵗʰ **O30.2** Quadruplet pregnancy

✓6ᵗʰ **O30.20** Quadruplet pregnancy, unspecified number of placenta and unspecified number of amniotic sacs

  O30.201 Quadruplet pregnancy, unspecified number of placenta and unspecified number of amniotic sacs, first trimester   COM M ♀

  O30.202 Quadruplet pregnancy, unspecified number of placenta and unspecified number of amniotic sacs, second trimester   COM M ♀

  O30.203 Quadruplet pregnancy, unspecified number of placenta and unspecified number of amniotic sacs, third trimester   COM M ♀

O30.209 Quadruplet pregnancy, unspecified number of placenta and unspecified number of amniotic sacs, unspecified trimester   COM M ♀

✓6ᵗʰ **O30.21** Quadruplet pregnancy with two or more monochorionic fetuses

  O30.211 Quadruplet pregnancy with two or more monochorionic fetuses, first trimester   COM M ♀

  O30.212 Quadruplet pregnancy with two or more monochorionic fetuses, second trimester   COM M ♀

  O30.213 Quadruplet pregnancy with two or more monochorionic fetuses, third trimester   COM M ♀

  O30.219 Quadruplet pregnancy with two or more monochorionic fetuses, unspecified trimester   COM M ♀

✓6ᵗʰ **O30.22** Quadruplet pregnancy with two or more monoamniotic fetuses

  O30.221 Quadruplet pregnancy with two or more monoamniotic fetuses, first trimester   COM M ♀

  O30.222 Quadruplet pregnancy with two or more monoamniotic fetuses, second trimester   COM M ♀

  O30.223 Quadruplet pregnancy with two or more monoamniotic fetuses, third trimester   COM M ♀

  O30.229 Quadruplet pregnancy with two or more monoamniotic fetuses, unspecified trimester   COM M ♀

✓6ᵗʰ **O30.23** Quadruplet pregnancy, quadrachorionic/quadra-amniotic

    AHA: 2018,4Q,22

  O30.231 Quadruplet pregnancy, quadrachorionic/quadra-amniotic, first trimester   COM M ♀

  O30.232 Quadruplet pregnancy, quadrachorionic/quadra-amniotic, second trimester   COM M ♀

  O30.233 Quadruplet pregnancy, quadrachorionic/quadra-amniotic, third trimester   COM M ♀

  O30.239 Quadruplet pregnancy, quadrachorionic/quadra-amniotic, unspecified trimester   COM M ♀

✓6ᵗʰ **O30.29** Quadruplet pregnancy, unable to determine number of placenta and number of amniotic sacs

  O30.291 Quadruplet pregnancy, unable to determine number of placenta and number of amniotic sacs, first trimester   COM M ♀

  O30.292 Quadruplet pregnancy, unable to determine number of placenta and number of amniotic sacs, second trimester   COM M ♀

  O30.293 Quadruplet pregnancy, unable to determine number of placenta and number of amniotic sacs, third trimester   COM M ♀

  O30.299 Quadruplet pregnancy, unable to determine number of placenta and number of amniotic sacs, unspecified trimester   COM M ♀

✓5ᵗʰ **O30.8** Other specified multiple gestation

    Multiple gestation pregnancy greater then quadruplets

✓6ᵗʰ **O30.80** Other specified multiple gestation, unspecified number of placenta and unspecified number of amniotic sacs

  O30.801 Other specified multiple gestation, unspecified number of placenta and unspecified number of amniotic sacs, first trimester   COM M ♀

  O30.802 Other specified multiple gestation, unspecified number of placenta and unspecified number of amniotic sacs, second trimester   COM M ♀

  O30.803 Other specified multiple gestation, unspecified number of placenta and unspecified number of amniotic sacs, third trimester   COM M ♀

Chapter 15. Pregnancy, Childbirth and the Puerperium

O30.809 Other specified multiple gestation, unspecified number of placenta and unspecified number of amniotic sacs, unspecified trimester   COM M ♀

✓6ᵗʰ **O30.81** Other specified multiple gestation with two or more monochorionic fetuses

O30.811 Other specified multiple gestation with two or more monochorionic fetuses, first trimester   COM M ♀

O30.812 Other specified multiple gestation with two or more monochorionic fetuses, second trimester   COM M ♀

O30.813 Other specified multiple gestation with two or more monochorionic fetuses, third trimester   COM M ♀

O30.819 Other specified multiple gestation with two or more monochorionic fetuses, unspecified trimester   COM M ♀

✓6ᵗʰ **O30.82** Other specified multiple gestation with two or more monoamniotic fetuses

O30.821 Other specified multiple gestation with two or more monoamniotic fetuses, first trimester   COM M ♀

O30.822 Other specified multiple gestation with two or more monoamniotic fetuses, second trimester   COM M ♀

O30.823 Other specified multiple gestation with two or more monoamniotic fetuses, third trimester   COM M ♀

O30.829 Other specified multiple gestation with two or more monoamniotic fetuses, unspecified trimester   COM M ♀

✓6ᵗʰ **O30.83** Other specified multiple gestation, number of chorions and amnions are both equal to the number of fetuses

Pentachorionic, penta-amniotic pregnancy (quintuplets)

Hexachorionic, hexa-amniotic pregnancy (sextuplets)

Heptachorionic, hepta-amniotic pregnancy (septuplets)

AHA: 2018,4Q,22

O30.831 Other specified multiple gestation, number of chorions and amnions are both equal to the number of fetuses, first trimester   COM M ♀

O30.832 Other specified multiple gestation, number of chorions and amnions are both equal to the number of fetuses, second trimester   COM M ♀

O30.833 Other specified multiple gestation, number of chorions and amnions are both equal to the number of fetuses, third trimester   COM M ♀

O30.839 Other specified multiple gestation, number of chorions and amnions are both equal to the number of fetuses, unspecified trimester   COM M ♀

✓6ᵗʰ **O30.89** Other specified multiple gestation, unable to determine number of placenta and number of amniotic sacs

O30.891 Other specified multiple gestation, unable to determine number of placenta and number of amniotic sacs, first trimester   COM M ♀

O30.892 Other specified multiple gestation, unable to determine number of placenta and number of amniotic sacs, second trimester   COM M ♀

O30.893 Other specified multiple gestation, unable to determine number of placenta and number of amniotic sacs, third trimester   COM M ♀

O30.899 Other specified multiple gestation, unable to determine number of placenta and number of amniotic sacs, unspecified trimester   COM M ♀

✓5ᵗʰ **O30.9** Multiple gestation, unspecified

Multiple pregnancy NOS

O30.90 Multiple gestation, unspecified, unspecified trimester   COM M ♀

O30.91 Multiple gestation, unspecified, first trimester   COM M ♀

O30.92 Multiple gestation, unspecified, second trimester   COM M ♀

O30.93 Multiple gestation, unspecified, third trimester   COM M ♀

✓4ᵗʰ **O31 Complications specific to multiple gestation**

EXCLUDES 2   delayed delivery of second twin, triplet, etc. (O63.2)

malpresentation of one fetus or more (O32.9)

placental transfusion syndromes (O43.0-)

AHA: 2012,4Q,107

One of the following 7th characters is to be assigned to each code under category O31. 7th character 0 is for single gestations and multiple gestations where the fetus is unspecified. 7th characters 1 through 9 are for cases of multiple gestations to identify the fetus for which the code applies. The appropriate code from category O30, Multiple gestation, must also be assigned when assigning a code from category O31 that has a 7th character of 1 through 9.

0   not applicable or unspecified
1   fetus 1
2   fetus 2
3   fetus 3
4   fetus 4
5   fetus 5
9   other fetus

✓5ᵗʰ **O31.0 Papyraceous fetus**

Fetus compressus

DEF: Fetus that has died, but remains in utero for weeks before delivery, becoming compacted and mummified in appearance, with skin resembling parchment. Occurs most commonly in multigestational pregnancies. *Synonym(s):* paper doll fetus.

✓x7ᵗʰ **O31.00** Papyraceous fetus, unspecified trimester   COM M ♀

✓x7ᵗʰ **O31.01** Papyraceous fetus, first trimester   COM M ♀

✓x7ᵗʰ **O31.02** Papyraceous fetus, second trimester   COM M ♀

✓x7ᵗʰ **O31.03** Papyraceous fetus, third trimester   COM M ♀

✓5ᵗʰ **O31.1 Continuing pregnancy after spontaneous abortion of one fetus or more**

✓x7ᵗʰ **O31.10** Continuing pregnancy after spontaneous abortion of one fetus or more, unspecified trimester   COM M ♀

✓x7ᵗʰ **O31.11** Continuing pregnancy after spontaneous abortion of one fetus or more, first trimester   COM M ♀

✓x7ᵗʰ **O31.12** Continuing pregnancy after spontaneous abortion of one fetus or more, second trimester   COM M ♀

✓x7ᵗʰ **O31.13** Continuing pregnancy after spontaneous abortion of one fetus or more, third trimester   COM M ♀

✓5ᵗʰ **O31.2 Continuing pregnancy after intrauterine death of one fetus or more**

✓x7ᵗʰ **O31.20** Continuing pregnancy after intrauterine death of one fetus or more, unspecified trimester   COM M ♀

✓x7ᵗʰ **O31.21** Continuing pregnancy after intrauterine death of one fetus or more, first trimester   COM M ♀

✓x7ᵗʰ **O31.22** Continuing pregnancy after intrauterine death of one fetus or more, second trimester   COM M ♀

✓x7ᵗʰ **O31.23** Continuing pregnancy after intrauterine death of one fetus or more, third trimester   COM M ♀

✓5ᵗʰ **O31.3 Continuing pregnancy after elective fetal reduction of one fetus or more**

Continuing pregnancy after selective termination of one fetus or more

✓x7ᵗʰ **O31.30** Continuing pregnancy after elective fetal reduction of one fetus or more, unspecified trimester   COM M ♀

✓x7ᵗʰ **O31.31** Continuing pregnancy after elective fetal reduction of one fetus or more, first trimester   COM M ♀

✓x7ᵗʰ **O31.32** Continuing pregnancy after elective fetal reduction of one fetus or more, second trimester   COM M ♀

✓x7ᵗʰ **O31.33** Continuing pregnancy after elective fetal reduction of one fetus or more, third trimester   COM M ♀

✓5ᵗʰ **O31.8 Other complications specific to multiple gestation**   COM

✓6ᵗʰ **O31.8X** Other complications specific to multiple gestation

✓7ᵗʰ **O31.8X1** Other complications specific to multiple gestation, first trimester   M ♀

✓7ᵗʰ **O31.8X2** Other complications specific to multiple gestation, second trimester   M ♀

✓7ᵗʰ **O31.8X3** Other complications specific to multiple gestation, third trimester   COM M ♀

✓7ᵗʰ **O31.8X9** Other complications specific to multiple
gestation, unspecified trimester   Ⓜ ♀

✓4ᵗʰ **O32** **Maternal care for malpresentation of fetus**

     INCLUDES   the listed conditions as a reason for observation,
hospitalization or other obstetric care of the mother,
or for cesarean delivery before onset of labor

     EXCLUDES 1   *malpresentation of fetus with obstructed labor (O64.-)*

     AHA: 2012,4Q,107

One of the following 7th characters is to be assigned to each code
under category O32. 7th character Ø is for single gestations and
multiple gestations where the fetus is unspecified. 7th characters 1
through 9 are for cases of multiple gestations to identify the fetus for
which the code applies. The appropriate code from category O3Ø,
Multiple gestation, must also be assigned when assigning a code
from category O32 that has a 7th character of 1 through 9.

   Ø   not applicable or unspecified
   1   fetus 1
   2   fetus 2
   3   fetus 3
   4   fetus 4
   5   fetus 5
   9   other fetus

Fetal Malpresentation

Breech — Mother's pelvis

Shoulder (arm prolapse)

Compound (extremity together with head)

Face (mentum)

Oblique

✓x7ᵗʰ **O32.0** **Maternal care for** unstable lie   COM Ⓜ ♀

✓x7ᵗʰ **O32.1** **Maternal care for** breech presentation   COM Ⓜ ♀

     Maternal care for buttocks presentation
     Maternal care for complete breech
     Maternal care for frank breech

     EXCLUDES 1   *footling presentation (O32.8)*
               incomplete breech (O32.8)

     DEF: Fetus presentation in a longitudinal lie with the buttocks or
feet closest to birth canal that may require external cephalic
version or cesarean delivery.

✓x7ᵗʰ **O32.2** **Maternal care for** transverse and oblique lie   COM Ⓜ ♀

     Maternal care for oblique presentation
     Maternal care for transverse presentation

✓x7ᵗʰ **O32.3** **Maternal care for** face, brow and chin
presentation   COM Ⓜ ♀

✓x7ᵗʰ **O32.4** **Maternal care for** high head at term   COM Ⓜ ♀

     Maternal care for failure of head to enter pelvic brim

✓x7ᵗʰ **O32.6** **Maternal care for** compound presentation   COM Ⓜ ♀

✓x7ᵗʰ **O32.8** **Maternal care for** other malpresentation of fetus   COM Ⓜ ♀

     Maternal care for footling presentation
     Maternal care for incomplete breech

✓x7ᵗʰ **O32.9** **Maternal care for** malpresentation of fetus,
unspecified   COM Ⓜ ♀

✓4ᵗʰ **O33** **Maternal care for disproportion**

     INCLUDES   the listed conditions as a reason for observation,
hospitalization or other obstetric care of the mother,
or for cesarean delivery before onset of labor

     EXCLUDES 1   *disproportion with obstructed labor (O65-O66)*

O33.0 **Maternal care for disproportion due to** deformity of maternal
pelvic bones   COM Ⓜ ♀

     Maternal care for disproportion due to pelvic deformity causing
disproportion NOS

O33.1 **Maternal care for disproportion due to** generally contracted
pelvis   COM Ⓜ ♀

     Maternal care for disproportion due to contracted pelvis NOS
causing disproportion

O33.2 **Maternal care for disproportion due to** inlet contraction of
pelvis   COM Ⓜ ♀

     Maternal care for disproportion due to inlet contraction (pelvis)
causing disproportion

✓x7ᵗʰ **O33.3** **Maternal care for disproportion due to** outlet contraction of
pelvis   COM Ⓜ ♀

     Maternal care for disproportion due to mid-cavity contraction
(pelvis)

     Maternal care for disproportion due to outlet contraction (pelvis)

One of the following 7th characters is to be assigned to code
O33.3. 7th character Ø is for single gestations and multiple
gestations where the fetus is unspecified. 7th characters 1
through 9 are for cases of multiple gestations to identify the
fetus for which the code applies. The appropriate code from
category O3Ø, Multiple gestation, must also be assigned when
assigning code O33.3 with a 7th character of 1 through 9.

   Ø   not applicable or unspecified
   1   fetus 1
   2   fetus 2
   3   fetus 3
   4   fetus 4
   5   fetus 5
   9   other fetus

✓x7ᵗʰ **O33.4** **Maternal care for disproportion of mixed maternal and fetal
origin**   COM Ⓜ ♀

One of the following 7th characters is to be assigned to code
O33.4. 7th character Ø is for single gestations and multiple
gestations where the fetus is unspecified. 7th characters 1
through 9 are for cases of multiple gestations to identify the
fetus for which the code applies. The appropriate code from
category O3Ø, Multiple gestation, must also be assigned when
assigning code O33.4 with a 7th character of 1 through 9.

   Ø   not applicable or unspecified
   1   fetus 1
   2   fetus 2
   3   fetus 3
   4   fetus 4
   5   fetus 5
   9   other fetus

✓x7ᵗʰ **O33.5** **Maternal care for disproportion due to** unusually large
fetus   COM Ⓜ ♀

     Maternal care for disproportion due to disproportion of fetal
origin with normally formed fetus

     Maternal care for disproportion due to fetal disproportion NOS

One of the following 7th characters is to be assigned to code
O33.5. 7th character Ø is for single gestations and multiple
gestations where the fetus is unspecified. 7th characters 1
through 9 are for cases of multiple gestations to identify the
fetus for which the code applies. The appropriate code from
category O3Ø, Multiple gestation, must also be assigned when
assigning code O33.5 with a 7th character of 1 through 9.

   Ø   not applicable or unspecified
   1   fetus 1
   2   fetus 2
   3   fetus 3
   4   fetus 4
   5   fetus 5
   9   other fetus

√x7ᵗʰ **O33.6 Maternal care for disproportion due to hydrocephalic fetus** COM M ♀

> One of the following 7th characters is to be assigned to code O33.6. 7th character Ø is for single gestations and multiple gestations where the fetus is unspecified. 7th characters 1 through 9 are for cases of multiple gestations to identify the fetus for which the code applies. The appropriate code from category O3Ø, Multiple gestation, must also be assigned when assigning code O33.6 with a 7th character of 1 through 9.
> Ø   not applicable or unspecified
> 1   fetus 1
> 2   fetus 2
> 3   fetus 3
> 4   fetus 4
> 5   fetus 5
> 9   other fetus

√x7ᵗʰ **O33.7 Maternal care for disproportion due to other fetal deformities** COM M ♀

> Maternal care for disproportion due to fetal ascites
> Maternal care for disproportion due to fetal hydrops
> Maternal care for disproportion due to fetal meningomyelocele
> Maternal care for disproportion due to fetal sacral teratoma
> Maternal care for disproportion due to fetal tumor
>
> EXCLUDES 1   *obstructed labor due to other fetal deformities (O66.3)*
>
> **AHA:** 2016,4Q,51

> One of the following 7th characters is to be assigned to code O33.7. 7th character Ø is for single gestations and multiple gestations where the fetus is unspecified. 7th characters 1 through 9 are for cases of multiple gestations to identify the fetus for which the code applies. The appropriate code from category O3Ø, Multiple gestation, must also be assigned when assigning code O33.7 with a 7th character of 1 through 9.
> Ø   not applicable or unspecified
> 1   fetus 1
> 2   fetus 2
> 3   fetus 3
> 4   fetus 4
> 5   fetus 5
> 9   other fetus

O33.8 Maternal care for disproportion of other origin COM M ♀

O33.9 Maternal care for disproportion, unspecified COM M ♀
> Maternal care for disproportion due to cephalopelvic disproportion NOS
> Maternal care for disproportion due to fetopelvic disproportion NOS

√4ᵗʰ **O34 Maternal care for abnormality of pelvic organs**

> INCLUDES   the listed conditions as a reason for hospitalization or other obstetric care of the mother, or for cesarean delivery before onset of labor

> Code first any associated obstructed labor (O65.5)
> Use additional code for specific condition

√5ᵗʰ **O34.Ø Maternal care for congenital malformation of uterus**
> Maternal care for double uterus
> Maternal care for uterus bicornis

O34.ØØ Maternal care for unspecified congenital malformation of uterus, unspecified trimester COM M ♀

O34.Ø1 Maternal care for unspecified congenital malformation of uterus, first trimester COM M ♀

O34.Ø2 Maternal care for unspecified congenital malformation of uterus, second trimester COM M ♀

O34.Ø3 Maternal care for unspecified congenital malformation of uterus, third trimester COM M ♀

√5ᵗʰ **O34.1 Maternal care for benign tumor of corpus uteri**
> EXCLUDES 2   *maternal care for benign tumor of cervix (O34.4-)*
> *maternal care for malignant neoplasm of uterus (O9A.1-)*

O34.1Ø Maternal care for benign tumor of corpus uteri, unspecified trimester COM M ♀

O34.11 Maternal care for benign tumor of corpus uteri, first trimester COM M ♀

O34.12 Maternal care for benign tumor of corpus uteri, second trimester COM M ♀

O34.13 Maternal care for benign tumor of corpus uteri, third trimester COM M ♀

√5ᵗʰ **O34.2 Maternal care due to** uterine scar from previous surgery
> **AHA:** 2020,4Q,36; 2016,4Q,76

√6ᵗʰ **O34.21 Maternal care for scar** from previous cesarean delivery
> **AHA:** 2018,3Q,23; 2016,4Q,51-52

O34.211 Maternal care for low transverse scar **from previous cesarean delivery** COM M ♀

O34.212 Maternal care for vertical scar from **previous cesarean delivery** COM M ♀
> Maternal care for classical scar from previous cesarean delivery

O34.218 Maternal care for other type scar from previous cesarean delivery COM M ♀
> Mid-transverse T incision

O34.219 Maternal care for unspecified type scar from previous cesarean delivery COM M ♀

O34.22 Maternal care for cesarean scar defect **(isthmocele)** COM M ♀

O34.29 Maternal care due to uterine scar from other previous surgery COM M ♀
> Maternal care due to uterine scar from other transmural uterine incision

√5ᵗʰ **O34.3 Maternal care for** cervical incompetence
> Maternal care for cerclage with or without cervical incompetence
> Maternal care for Shirodkar suture with or without cervical incompetence
> **DEF:** Inadequate functioning of the cervix marked by abnormal widening during pregnancy and causing premature birth or miscarriage.

O34.3Ø Maternal care for cervical incompetence, unspecified trimester COM M ♀

O34.31 Maternal care for cervical incompetence, first trimester COM M ♀

O34.32 Maternal care for cervical incompetence, second trimester COM M ♀

O34.33 Maternal care for cervical incompetence, third trimester COM M ♀

√5ᵗʰ **O34.4 Maternal care for** other abnormalities of cervix

O34.4Ø Maternal care for other abnormalities of cervix, unspecified trimester COM M ♀

O34.41 Maternal care for other abnormalities of cervix, first trimester COM M ♀

O34.42 Maternal care for other abnormalities of cervix, second trimester COM M ♀

O34.43 Maternal care for other abnormalities of cervix, third trimester COM M ♀

√5ᵗʰ **O34.5 Maternal care for** other abnormalities of gravid uterus

√6ᵗʰ **O34.51 Maternal care for** incarceration of gravid uterus

O34.511 Maternal care for incarceration of gravid uterus, first trimester COM M ♀

O34.512 Maternal care for incarceration of gravid uterus, second trimester COM M ♀

O34.513 Maternal care for incarceration of gravid uterus, third trimester COM M ♀

O34.519 Maternal care for incarceration of gravid uterus, unspecified trimester COM M ♀

√6ᵗʰ **O34.52 Maternal care for** prolapse of gravid uterus

O34.521 Maternal care for prolapse of gravid uterus, first trimester COM M ♀

O34.522 Maternal care for prolapse of gravid uterus, second trimester COM M ♀

O34.523 Maternal care for prolapse of gravid uterus, third trimester COM M ♀

O34.529 Maternal care for prolapse of gravid uterus, unspecified trimester COM M ♀

√6ᵗʰ **O34.53 Maternal care for** retroversion of gravid uterus

O34.531 Maternal care for retroversion of gravid uterus, first trimester COM M ♀

O34.532 Maternal care for retroversion of gravid uterus, second trimester COM M ♀

O34.533 Maternal care for retroversion of gravid uterus, third trimester COM M ♀

O34.539 Maternal care for retroversion of gravid uterus, unspecified trimester COM M ♀

☑6ᵗʰ **O34.59 Maternal care for other abnormalities of gravid uterus**

     O34.591 Maternal care for other abnormalities of gravid uterus, first trimester COM M ♀

     O34.592 Maternal care for other abnormalities of gravid uterus, second trimester COM M ♀

     O34.593 Maternal care for other abnormalities of gravid uterus, third trimester COM M ♀

     O34.599 Maternal care for other abnormalities of gravid uterus, unspecified trimester COM M ♀

☑5ᵗʰ **O34.6 Maternal care for abnormality of vagina**

     EXCLUDES 2   *maternal care for vaginal varices in pregnancy (O22.1-)*

     O34.60 Maternal care for abnormality of vagina, unspecified trimester COM M ♀

     O34.61 Maternal care for abnormality of vagina, first trimester COM M ♀

     O34.62 Maternal care for abnormality of vagina, second trimester COM M ♀

     O34.63 Maternal care for abnormality of vagina, third trimester COM M ♀

☑5ᵗʰ **O34.7 Maternal care for abnormality of vulva and perineum**

     EXCLUDES 2   *maternal care for perineal and vulval varices in pregnancy (O22.1-)*

     O34.70 Maternal care for abnormality of vulva and perineum, unspecified trimester COM M ♀

     O34.71 Maternal care for abnormality of vulva and perineum, first trimester COM M ♀

     O34.72 Maternal care for abnormality of vulva and perineum, second trimester COM M ♀

     O34.73 Maternal care for abnormality of vulva and perineum, third trimester COM M ♀

☑5ᵗʰ **O34.8 Maternal care for other abnormalities of pelvic organs**

     O34.80 Maternal care for other abnormalities of pelvic organs, unspecified trimester COM M ♀

     O34.81 Maternal care for other abnormalities of pelvic organs, first trimester COM M ♀

     O34.82 Maternal care for other abnormalities of pelvic organs, second trimester COM M ♀

     O34.83 Maternal care for other abnormalities of pelvic organs, third trimester COM M ♀

☑5ᵗʰ **O34.9 Maternal care for abnormality of pelvic organ, unspecified**

     O34.90 Maternal care for abnormality of pelvic organ, unspecified, unspecified trimester COM M ♀

     O34.91 Maternal care for abnormality of pelvic organ, unspecified, first trimester COM M ♀

     O34.92 Maternal care for abnormality of pelvic organ, unspecified, second trimester COM M ♀

     O34.93 Maternal care for abnormality of pelvic organ, unspecified, third trimester COM M ♀

☑4ᵗʰ **O35 Maternal care for known or suspected fetal abnormality and damage**

     INCLUDES   the listed conditions in the fetus as a reason for hospitalization or other obstetric care to the mother, or for termination of pregnancy

     Code also any associated maternal condition

     EXCLUDES 1   *encounter for suspected maternal and fetal conditions ruled out (Z03.7-)*

     One of the following 7th characters is to be assigned to each code under category O35. 7th character Ø is for single gestations and multiple gestations where the fetus is unspecified. 7th characters 1 through 9 are for cases of multiple gestations to identify the fetus for which the code applies. The appropriate code from category O30, Multiple gestation, must also be assigned when assigning a code from category O35 that has a 7th character of 1 through 9.

     Ø   not applicable or unspecified
     1   fetus 1
     2   fetus 2
     3   fetus 3
     4   fetus 4
     5   fetus 5
     9   other fetus

☑5ᵗʰ **O35.0 Maternal care for (suspected) central nervous system malformation in fetus**

     ~~Maternal care for fetal anencephaly~~
     ~~Maternal care for fetal hydrocephalus~~
     ~~Maternal care for fetal spina bifida~~

     EXCLUDES 2   *chromosomal abnormality in fetus ▶(O35.1-)◀*

● ✓x7ᵗʰ **O35.00 Maternal care for (suspected) central nervous system malformation or damage in fetus, unspecified**

● ✓x7ᵗʰ **O35.01 Maternal care for (suspected) central nervous system malformation or damage in fetus, agenesis of the corpus callosum**

● ✓x7ᵗʰ **O35.02 Maternal care for (suspected) central nervous system malformation or damage in fetus, anencephaly**

● ✓x7ᵗʰ **O35.03 Maternal care for (suspected) central nervous system malformation or damage in fetus, choroid plexus cysts**

● ✓x7ᵗʰ **O35.04 Maternal care for (suspected) central nervous system malformation or damage in fetus, encephalocele**

● ✓x7ᵗʰ **O35.05 Maternal care for (suspected) central nervous system malformation or damage in fetus, holoprosencephaly**

● ✓x7ᵗʰ **O35.06 Maternal care for (suspected) central nervous system malformation or damage in fetus, hydrocephaly**
     Maternal care for fetal hydrocephalus

● ✓x7ᵗʰ **O35.07 Maternal care for (suspected) central nervous system malformation or damage in fetus, microcephaly**

● ✓x7ᵗʰ **O35.08 Maternal care for (suspected) central nervous system malformation or damage in fetus, spina bifida**

● ✓x7ᵗʰ **O35.09 Maternal care for (suspected) other central nervous system malformation or damage in fetus**

☑5ᵗʰ **O35.1 Maternal care for (suspected) chromosomal abnormality in fetus**

● ✓x7ᵗʰ **O35.10 Maternal care for (suspected) chromosomal abnormality in fetus, unspecified**

● ✓x7ᵗʰ **O35.11 Maternal care for (suspected) chromosomal abnormality in fetus, Trisomy 13**

● ✓x7ᵗʰ **O35.12 Maternal care for (suspected) chromosomal abnormality in fetus, Trisomy 18**

● ✓x7ᵗʰ **O35.13 Maternal care for (suspected) chromosomal abnormality in fetus, Trisomy 21**

● ✓x7ᵗʰ **O35.14 Maternal care for (suspected) chromosomal abnormality in fetus, Turner Syndrome**

● ✓x7ᵗʰ **O35.15 Maternal care for (suspected) chromosomal abnormality in fetus, sex chromosome abnormality**

● ✓x7ᵗʰ **O35.19 Maternal care for (suspected) chromosomal abnormality in fetus, other chromosomal abnormality**

● ✓x7ᵗʰ **O35.A Maternal care for other (suspected) fetal abnormality and damage, fetal facial anomalies**

● ✓x7ᵗʰ **O35.B Maternal care for other (suspected) fetal abnormality and damage, fetal cardiac anomalies**

● ✓x7ᵗʰ **O35.C Maternal care for other (suspected) fetal abnormality and damage, fetal pulmonary anomalies**

- √x 7th **O35.D** **Maternal care for other (suspected) fetal abnormality and damage,** fetal gastrointestinal anomalies
- √x 7th **O35.E** **Maternal care for other (suspected) fetal abnormality and damage,** fetal genitourinary anomalies
- √x 7th **O35.F** **Maternal care for other (suspected) fetal abnormality and damage,** fetal musculoskeletal anomalies of trunk

  > **EXCLUDES 2**   maternal care for other (suspected) fetal abnormality and damage, fetal lower extremities anomalies (O35.H)
  > maternal care for other (suspected) fetal abnormality and damage, fetal upper extremities anomalies (O35.G)

- √x 7th **O35.G** **Maternal care for other (suspected) fetal abnormality and damage,** fetal upper extremities anomalies
- √x 7th **O35.H** **Maternal care for other (suspected) fetal abnormality and damage,** fetal lower extremities anomalies

√x 7th **O35.2** **Maternal care for (suspected)** hereditary disease in fetus   COM M ♀

  > **EXCLUDES 2**   chromosomal abnormality in fetus ▶(O35.1-)◀

√x 7th **O35.3** **Maternal care for (suspected)** damage to fetus from viral disease in mother   COM M ♀

  Maternal care for damage to fetus from maternal cytomegalovirus infection
  Maternal care for damage to fetus from maternal rubella

√x 7th **O35.4** **Maternal care for (suspected)** damage to fetus from alcohol   COM M ♀

√x 7th **O35.5** **Maternal care for (suspected)** damage to fetus by drugs   COM M ♀

  Maternal care for damage to fetus from drug addiction

√x 7th **O35.6** **Maternal care for (suspected)** damage to fetus by radiation   COM M ♀

√x 7th **O35.7** **Maternal care for (suspected)** damage to fetus by other medical procedures   COM M ♀

  Maternal care for damage to fetus by amniocentesis
  Maternal care for damage to fetus by biopsy procedures
  Maternal care for damage to fetus by hematological investigation
  Maternal care for damage to fetus by intrauterine contraceptive device
  Maternal care for damage to fetus by intrauterine surgery

√x 7th **O35.8** **Maternal care for other (suspected) fetal abnormality and damage**   COM M ♀

  Maternal care for damage to fetus from maternal listeriosis
  Maternal care for damage to fetus from maternal toxoplasmosis

√x 7th **O35.9** **Maternal care for (suspected) fetal abnormality and damage, unspecified**   COM M ♀

√4th **O36** **Maternal care for other fetal problems**

  > **INCLUDES**   the listed conditions in the fetus as a reason for hospitalization or other obstetric care of the mother, or for termination of pregnancy
  > **EXCLUDES 1**   encounter for suspected maternal and fetal conditions ruled out (Z03.7-)
  > placental transfusion syndromes (O43.0-)
  > **EXCLUDES 2**   labor and delivery complicated by fetal stress (O77.-)

  AHA: 2015,3Q,40

  > One of the following 7th characters is to be assigned to each code under category O36. 7th character Ø is for single gestations and multiple gestations where the fetus is unspecified. 7th characters 1 through 9 are for cases of multiple gestations to identify the fetus for which the code applies. The appropriate code from category O30, Multiple gestation, must also be assigned when assigning a code from category O36 that has a 7th character of 1 through 9.
  > Ø   not applicable or unspecified
  > 1   fetus 1
  > 2   fetus 2
  > 3   fetus 3
  > 4   fetus 4
  > 5   fetus 5
  > 9   other fetus

√5th **O36.0** **Maternal care for rhesus isoimmunization**

  Maternal care for Rh incompatibility (with hydrops fetalis)

  √6th **O36.01** **Maternal care for** anti-D [Rh] antibodies

    AHA: 2014,4Q,17

    √7th **O36.011** **Maternal care for anti-D [Rh] antibodies, first trimester**   COM M ♀

    √7th **O36.012** **Maternal care for anti-D [Rh] antibodies, second trimester**   COM M ♀

    √7th **O36.013** **Maternal care for anti-D [Rh] antibodies, third trimester**   COM M ♀

    √7th **O36.019** **Maternal care for anti-D [Rh] antibodies, unspecified trimester**   COM M ♀

  √6th **O36.09** **Maternal care for other rhesus isoimmunization**

    √7th **O36.091** **Maternal care for other rhesus isoimmunization,** first trimester   COM M ♀

    √7th **O36.092** **Maternal care for other rhesus isoimmunization,** second trimester   COM M ♀

    √7th **O36.093** **Maternal care for other rhesus isoimmunization,** third trimester   COM M ♀

    √7th **O36.099** **Maternal care for other rhesus isoimmunization, unspecified** trimester   COM M ♀

√5th **O36.1** **Maternal care for other isoimmunization**

  Maternal care for ABO isoimmunization

  √6th **O36.11** **Maternal care for** Anti-A sensitization

    Maternal care for isoimmunization NOS (with hydrops fetalis)

    √7th **O36.111** **Maternal care for Anti-A sensitization, first trimester**   COM M ♀

    √7th **O36.112** **Maternal care for Anti-A sensitization, second trimester**   COM M ♀

    √7th **O36.113** **Maternal care for Anti-A sensitization, third trimester**   COM M ♀

    √7th **O36.119** **Maternal care for Anti-A sensitization, unspecified trimester**   COM M ♀

  √6th **O36.19** **Maternal care for other isoimmunization**

    Maternal care for Anti-B sensitization

    √7th **O36.191** **Maternal care for other isoimmunization, first trimester**   COM M ♀

    √7th **O36.192** **Maternal care for other isoimmunization, second trimester**   COM M ♀

    √7th **O36.193** **Maternal care for other isoimmunization, third trimester**   COM M ♀

    √7th **O36.199** **Maternal care for other isoimmunization, unspecified trimester**   COM M ♀

√5th **O36.2** **Maternal care for hydrops fetalis**

  Maternal care for hydrops fetalis NOS
  Maternal care for hydrops fetalis not associated with isoimmunization

  > **EXCLUDES 1**   hydrops fetalis associated with ABO isoimmunization (O36.1-)
  > hydrops fetalis associated with rhesus isoimmunization (O36.0-)

  DEF: Hydrops fetalis: Abnormal fluid buildup in at least two of the following fetal organ spaces: the skin (edema), abdomen (ascites), around the heart (pericardia effusion), and around the lung (pleural effusion). Fluid accumulation may also occur in the mother as polyhydramnios and edema of the placenta.

  √x 7th **O36.20** **Maternal care for hydrops fetalis, unspecified trimester**   COM M ♀

  √x 7th **O36.21** **Maternal care for hydrops fetalis, first** trimester   COM M ♀

  √x 7th **O36.22** **Maternal care for hydrops fetalis, second** trimester   COM M ♀

  √x 7th **O36.23** **Maternal care for hydrops fetalis, third** trimester   COM M ♀

√x 7th **O36.4** **Maternal care for intrauterine death**   COM M ♀

  Maternal care for intrauterine fetal death NOS
  Maternal care for intrauterine fetal death after completion of 20 weeks of gestation
  Maternal care for late fetal death
  Maternal care for missed delivery

  > **EXCLUDES 1**   missed abortion (O02.1)
  > stillbirth (P95)

  AHA: 2022,2Q,3

√5th **O36.5** **Maternal care for known or suspected poor fetal growth**

  √6th **O36.51** **Maternal care for known or suspected placental insufficiency**

    √7th **O36.511** **Maternal care for known or suspected placental insufficiency, first** trimester   COM M ♀

☑7ᵗʰ O36.512 Maternal care for known or suspected placental insufficiency, second trimester   COM M ♀

☑7ᵗʰ O36.513 Maternal care for known or suspected placental insufficiency, third trimester   COM M ♀

☑7ᵗʰ O36.519 Maternal care for known or suspected placental insufficiency, unspecified trimester   COM M ♀

☑6ᵗʰ O36.59 Maternal care for other known or suspected poor fetal growth

Maternal care for known or suspected light-for-dates NOS

Maternal care for known or suspected small-for-dates NOS

☑7ᵗʰ O36.591 Maternal care for other known or suspected poor fetal growth, first trimester   COM M ♀

☑7ᵗʰ O36.592 Maternal care for other known or suspected poor fetal growth, second trimester   COM M ♀

☑7ᵗʰ O36.593 Maternal care for other known or suspected poor fetal growth, third trimester   COM M ♀

☑7ᵗʰ O36.599 Maternal care for other known or suspected poor fetal growth, unspecified trimester   COM M ♀

☑5ᵗʰ O36.6 Maternal care for excessive fetal growth

Maternal care for known or suspected large-for-dates

☑x7ᵗʰ O36.60 Maternal care for excessive fetal growth, unspecified trimester   COM M ♀

☑x7ᵗʰ O36.61 Maternal care for excessive fetal growth, first trimester   COM M ♀

☑x7ᵗʰ O36.62 Maternal care for excessive fetal growth, second trimester   COM M ♀

☑x7ᵗʰ O36.63 Maternal care for excessive fetal growth, third trimester   COM M ♀

☑5ᵗʰ O36.7 Maternal care for viable fetus in abdominal pregnancy

☑x7ᵗʰ O36.70 Maternal care for viable fetus in abdominal pregnancy, unspecified trimester   COM M ♀

☑x7ᵗʰ O36.71 Maternal care for viable fetus in abdominal pregnancy, first trimester   COM M ♀

☑x7ᵗʰ O36.72 Maternal care for viable fetus in abdominal pregnancy, second trimester   COM M ♀

☑x7ᵗʰ O36.73 Maternal care for viable fetus in abdominal pregnancy, third trimester   COM M ♀

☑5ᵗʰ O36.8 Maternal care for other specified fetal problems

☑x7ᵗʰ O36.80 Pregnancy with inconclusive fetal viability   COM M ♀

Encounter to determine fetal viability of pregnancy

AHA: 2019,2Q,29

☑6ᵗʰ O36.81 Decreased fetal movements

☑7ᵗʰ O36.812 Decreased fetal movements, second trimester   COM M ♀

☑7ᵗʰ O36.813 Decreased fetal movements, third trimester   COM M ♀

☑7ᵗʰ O36.819 Decreased fetal movements, unspecified trimester   COM M ♀

☑6ᵗʰ O36.82 Fetal anemia and thrombocytopenia

☑7ᵗʰ O36.821 Fetal anemia and thrombocytopenia, first trimester   COM M ♀

☑7ᵗʰ O36.822 Fetal anemia and thrombocytopenia, second trimester   COM M ♀

☑7ᵗʰ O36.823 Fetal anemia and thrombocytopenia, third trimester   COM M ♀

☑7ᵗʰ O36.829 Fetal anemia and thrombocytopenia, unspecified trimester   COM M ♀

☑6ᵗʰ O36.83 Maternal care for abnormalities of the fetal heart rate or rhythm

Maternal care for depressed fetal heart rate tones

Maternal care for fetal bradycardia

Maternal care for fetal heart rate abnormal variability

Maternal care for fetal heart rate decelerations

Maternal care for fetal heart rate irregularity

Maternal care for fetal tachycardia

Maternal care for non-reassuring fetal heart rate or rhythm

AHA: 2017,4Q,20

TIP: Assign for documented fetal tachycardia, bradycardia, decelerations, or loss of variability detected during antenatal testing.

☑7ᵗʰ O36.831 Maternal care for abnormalities of the fetal heart rate or rhythm, first trimester   COM M ♀

☑7ᵗʰ O36.832 Maternal care for abnormalities of the fetal heart rate or rhythm, second trimester   COM M ♀

☑7ᵗʰ O36.833 Maternal care for abnormalities of the fetal heart rate or rhythm, third trimester   COM M ♀

☑7ᵗʰ O36.839 Maternal care for abnormalities of the fetal heart rate or rhythm, unspecified trimester   COM M ♀

☑6ᵗʰ O36.89 Maternal care for other specified fetal problems

☑7ᵗʰ O36.891 Maternal care for other specified fetal problems, first trimester   COM M ♀

☑7ᵗʰ O36.892 Maternal care for other specified fetal problems, second trimester   COM M ♀

☑7ᵗʰ O36.893 Maternal care for other specified fetal problems, third trimester   COM M ♀

☑7ᵗʰ O36.899 Maternal care for other specified fetal problems, unspecified trimester   COM M ♀

☑5ᵗʰ O36.9 Maternal care for fetal problem, unspecified

☑x7ᵗʰ O36.90 Maternal care for fetal problem, unspecified, unspecified trimester   COM M ♀

☑x7ᵗʰ O36.91 Maternal care for fetal problem, unspecified, first trimester   COM M ♀

☑x7ᵗʰ O36.92 Maternal care for fetal problem, unspecified, second trimester   COM M ♀

☑x7ᵗʰ O36.93 Maternal care for fetal problem, unspecified, third trimester   COM M ♀

☑4ᵗʰ O40 Polyhydramnios

INCLUDES hydramnios

EXCLUDES 1 encounter for suspected maternal and fetal conditions ruled out (Z03.7-)

AHA: 2016,1Q,4

DEF: Excess amniotic fluid surrounding the fetus, typically defined as a total fluid volume of greater than 24 cm.

One of the following 7th characters is to be assigned to each code under category O40. 7th character 0 is for single gestations and multiple gestations where the fetus is unspecified. 7th characters 1 through 9 are for cases of multiple gestations to identify the fetus for which the code applies. The appropriate code from category O30, Multiple gestation, must also be assigned when assigning a code from category O40 that has a 7th character of 1 through 9.

0   not applicable or unspecified

1   fetus 1

2   fetus 2

3   fetus 3

4   fetus 4

5   fetus 5

9   other fetus

☑x7ᵗʰ O40.1 Polyhydramnios, first trimester   COM M ♀

☑x7ᵗʰ O40.2 Polyhydramnios, second trimester   COM M ♀

☑x7ᵗʰ O40.3 Polyhydramnios, third trimester   COM M ♀

☑x7ᵗʰ O40.9 Polyhydramnios, unspecified trimester   COM M ♀

Chapter 15. Pregnancy, Childbirth and the Puerperium

O36.512–O40.9

✓4ᵗʰ O41 Other disorders of amniotic fluid and membranes

> EXCLUDES 1   encounter for suspected maternal and fetal conditions ruled out (Z03.7-)

> One of the following 7th characters is to be assigned to each code under category O41. 7th character Ø is for single gestations and multiple gestations where the fetus is unspecified. 7th characters 1 through 9 are for cases of multiple gestations to identify the fetus for which the code applies. The appropriate code from category O30, Multiple gestation, must also be assigned when assigning a code from category O41 that has a 7th character of 1 through 9.
> Ø   not applicable or unspecified
> 1   fetus 1
> 2   fetus 2
> 3   fetus 3
> 4   fetus 4
> 5   fetus 5
> 9   other fetus

✓5ᵗʰ O41.Ø Oligohydramnios

Oligohydramnios without rupture of membranes
DEF: Low amniotic fluid, occurring most frequently in the last trimester.

- ✓x7ᵗʰ **O41.ØØ Oligohydramnios, unspecified trimester** COM M ♀
- ✓x7ᵗʰ **O41.Ø1 Oligohydramnios, first trimester** COM M ♀
- ✓x7ᵗʰ **O41.Ø2 Oligohydramnios, second trimester** COM M ♀
- ✓x7ᵗʰ **O41.Ø3 Oligohydramnios, third trimester** COM M ♀

✓5ᵗʰ O41.1 Infection of amniotic sac and membranes

- ✓6ᵗʰ **O41.1Ø Infection of amniotic sac and membranes, unspecified**
  - ✓7ᵗʰ **O41.1Ø1 Infection of amniotic sac and membranes, unspecified, first trimester** COM M ♀
  - ✓7ᵗʰ **O41.1Ø2 Infection of amniotic sac and membranes, unspecified, second trimester** COM M ♀
  - ✓7ᵗʰ **O41.1Ø3 Infection of amniotic sac and membranes, unspecified, third trimester** COM M ♀
  - ✓7ᵗʰ **O41.1Ø9 Infection of amniotic sac and membranes, unspecified, unspecified trimester** COM M ♀

- ✓6ᵗʰ **O41.12 Chorioamnionitis**
  AHA: 2019,2Q,34
  - ✓7ᵗʰ **O41.121 Chorioamnionitis, first trimester** COM M ♀
  - ✓7ᵗʰ **O41.122 Chorioamnionitis, second trimester** COM M ♀
  - ✓7ᵗʰ **O41.123 Chorioamnionitis, third trimester** COM M ♀
  - ✓7ᵗʰ **O41.129 Chorioamnionitis, unspecified trimester** COM M ♀

- ✓6ᵗʰ **O41.14 Placentitis**
  - ✓7ᵗʰ **O41.141 Placentitis, first trimester** COM M ♀
  - ✓7ᵗʰ **O41.142 Placentitis, second trimester** COM M ♀
  - ✓7ᵗʰ **O41.143 Placentitis, third trimester** COM M ♀
  - ✓7ᵗʰ **O41.149 Placentitis, unspecified trimester** COM M ♀

✓5ᵗʰ O41.8 Other specified disorders of amniotic fluid and membranes

- ✓6ᵗʰ **O41.8X Other specified disorders of amniotic fluid and membranes**
  - ✓7ᵗʰ **O41.8X1 Other specified disorders of amniotic fluid and membranes, first trimester** COM M ♀
  - ✓7ᵗʰ **O41.8X2 Other specified disorders of amniotic fluid and membranes, second trimester** COM M ♀
  - ✓7ᵗʰ **O41.8X3 Other specified disorders of amniotic fluid and membranes, third trimester** COM M ♀
  - ✓7ᵗʰ **O41.8X9 Other specified disorders of amniotic fluid and membranes, unspecified trimester** COM M ♀

✓5ᵗʰ O41.9 Disorder of amniotic fluid and membranes, unspecified

- ✓x7ᵗʰ **O41.9Ø Disorder of amniotic fluid and membranes, unspecified, unspecified trimester** COM M ♀
- ✓x7ᵗʰ **O41.91 Disorder of amniotic fluid and membranes, unspecified, first trimester** COM M ♀
- ✓x7ᵗʰ **O41.92 Disorder of amniotic fluid and membranes, unspecified, second trimester** COM M ♀

- ✓x7ᵗʰ **O41.93 Disorder of amniotic fluid and membranes, unspecified, third trimester** COM M ♀

✓4ᵗʰ O42 Premature rupture of membranes
AHA: 2016,1Q,3

✓5ᵗʰ O42.Ø Premature rupture of membranes, onset of labor within 24 hours of rupture

- **O42.ØØ Premature rupture of membranes, onset of labor within 24 hours of rupture, unspecified weeks of gestation** COM M ♀
- ✓6ᵗʰ **O42.Ø1 Preterm premature rupture of membranes, onset of labor within 24 hours of rupture**
  Premature rupture of membranes before 37 completed weeks of gestation
  - **O42.Ø11 Preterm premature rupture of membranes, onset of labor within 24 hours of rupture, first trimester** COM M ♀
  - **O42.Ø12 Preterm premature rupture of membranes, onset of labor within 24 hours of rupture, second trimester** COM M ♀
  - **O42.Ø13 Preterm premature rupture of membranes, onset of labor within 24 hours of rupture, third trimester** COM M ♀
  - **O42.Ø19 Preterm premature rupture of membranes, onset of labor within 24 hours of rupture, unspecified trimester** COM M ♀
- **O42.Ø2 Full-term premature rupture of membranes, onset of labor within 24 hours of rupture** COM M ♀
  Premature rupture of membranes at or after 37 completed weeks of gestation, onset of labor within 24 hours of rupture

✓5ᵗʰ O42.1 Premature rupture of membranes, onset of labor more than 24 hours following rupture
AHA: 2016,1Q,5

- **O42.1Ø Premature rupture of membranes, onset of labor more than 24 hours following rupture, unspecified weeks of gestation** COM M ♀
- ✓6ᵗʰ **O42.11 Preterm premature rupture of membranes, onset of labor more than 24 hours following rupture**
  Premature rupture of membranes before 37 completed weeks of gestation
  - **O42.111 Preterm premature rupture of membranes, onset of labor more than 24 hours following rupture, first trimester** COM M ♀
  - **O42.112 Preterm premature rupture of membranes, onset of labor more than 24 hours following rupture, second trimester** COM M ♀
  - **O42.113 Preterm premature rupture of membranes, onset of labor more than 24 hours following rupture, third trimester** COM M ♀
  - **O42.119 Preterm premature rupture of membranes, onset of labor more than 24 hours following rupture, unspecified trimester** COM M ♀
- **O42.12 Full-term premature rupture of membranes, onset of labor more than 24 hours following rupture** COM M ♀
  Premature rupture of membranes at or after 37 completed weeks of gestation, onset of labor more than 24 hours following rupture

✓5ᵗʰ O42.9 Premature rupture of membranes, unspecified as to length of time between rupture and onset of labor

- **O42.9Ø Premature rupture of membranes, unspecified as to length of time between rupture and onset of labor, unspecified weeks of gestation** COM M ♀
- ✓6ᵗʰ **O42.91 Preterm premature rupture of membranes, unspecified as to length of time between rupture and onset of labor**
  Premature rupture of membranes before 37 completed weeks of gestation
  - **O42.911 Preterm premature rupture of membranes, unspecified as to length of time between rupture and onset of labor, first trimester** COM M ♀

O42.912 **Preterm premature rupture of membranes, unspecified as to length of time between rupture and onset of labor, second trimester** `COM` `M` ♀

O42.913 **Preterm premature rupture of membranes, unspecified as to length of time between rupture and onset of labor, third trimester** `COM` `M` ♀

O42.919 **Preterm premature rupture of membranes, unspecified as to length of time between rupture and onset of labor, unspecified trimester** `COM` `M` ♀

O42.92 **Full-term premature rupture of membranes, unspecified as to length of time between rupture and onset of labor** `COM` `M` ♀

Premature rupture of membranes at or after 37 completed weeks of gestation, unspecified as to length of time between rupture and onset of labor

✓4ᵗʰ **O43** **Placental disorders**

EXCLUDES 2   *maternal care for poor fetal growth due to placental insufficiency (O36.5-)*
placenta previa (O44.-)
placental polyp (O90.89)
placentitis (O41.14-)
premature separation of placenta [abruptio placentae] (O45.-)

✓5ᵗʰ **O43.0** **Placental transfusion syndromes**

✓6ᵗʰ **O43.01** **Fetomaternal placental transfusion syndrome**
Maternofetal placental transfusion syndrome

O43.011 **Fetomaternal placental transfusion syndrome, first trimester** `COM` `M` ♀

O43.012 **Fetomaternal placental transfusion syndrome, second trimester** `COM` `M` ♀

O43.013 **Fetomaternal placental transfusion syndrome, third trimester** `COM` `M` ♀

O43.019 **Fetomaternal placental transfusion syndrome, unspecified trimester** `COM` `M` ♀

✓6ᵗʰ **O43.02** **Fetus-to-fetus placental transfusion syndrome**
DEF: Condition in which an imbalance in amniotic fluid occurs due to uneven blood flow between twins sharing a placenta.

Twin to Twin Transfusion Syndrome (TTTS)

Healthy twins   Twins with TTTS

O43.021 **Fetus-to-fetus placental transfusion syndrome, first trimester** `COM` `M` ♀

O43.022 **Fetus-to-fetus placental transfusion syndrome, second trimester** `COM` `M` ♀

O43.023 **Fetus-to-fetus placental transfusion syndrome, third trimester** `COM` `M` ♀

O43.029 **Fetus-to-fetus placental transfusion syndrome, unspecified trimester** `COM` `M` ♀

✓5ᵗʰ **O43.1** **Malformation of placenta**

✓6ᵗʰ **O43.10** **Malformation of placenta, unspecified**
Abnormal placenta NOS

O43.101 **Malformation of placenta, unspecified, first trimester** `COM` `M` ♀

O43.102 **Malformation of placenta, unspecified, second trimester** `COM` `M` ♀

O43.103 **Malformation of placenta, unspecified, third trimester** `COM` `M` ♀

O43.109 **Malformation of placenta, unspecified, unspecified trimester** `COM` `M` ♀

✓6ᵗʰ **O43.11** **Circumvallate placenta**

O43.111 **Circumvallate placenta, first trimester** `COM` `M` ♀

O43.112 **Circumvallate placenta, second trimester** `COM` `M` ♀

O43.113 **Circumvallate placenta, third trimester** `COM` `M` ♀

O43.119 **Circumvallate placenta, unspecified trimester** `COM` `M` ♀

✓6ᵗʰ **O43.12** **Velamentous insertion of umbilical cord**

O43.121 **Velamentous insertion of umbilical cord, first trimester** `COM` `M` ♀

O43.122 **Velamentous insertion of umbilical cord, second trimester** `COM` `M` ♀

O43.123 **Velamentous insertion of umbilical cord, third trimester** `COM` `M` ♀

O43.129 **Velamentous insertion of umbilical cord, unspecified trimester** `COM` `M` ♀

✓6ᵗʰ **O43.19** **Other malformation of placenta**

O43.191 **Other malformation of placenta, first trimester** `COM` `M` ♀

O43.192 **Other malformation of placenta, second trimester** `COM` `M` ♀

O43.193 **Other malformation of placenta, third trimester** `COM` `M` ♀

O43.199 **Other malformation of placenta, unspecified trimester** `COM` `M` ♀

✓5ᵗʰ **O43.2** **Morbidly adherent placenta**
Code also associated third stage postpartum hemorrhage, if applicable (O72.0)
EXCLUDES 1   *retained placenta (O73.-)*

✓6ᵗʰ **O43.21** **Placenta accreta**
DEF: Condition where the placenta adheres too deeply to the uterine wall; often associated with placenta previa.

O43.211 **Placenta accreta, first trimester** `COM` `M` ♀

O43.212 **Placenta accreta, second trimester** `COM` `M` ♀

O43.213 **Placenta accreta, third trimester** `COM` `M` ♀

O43.219 **Placenta accreta, unspecified trimester** `COM` `M` ♀

✓6ᵗʰ **O43.22** **Placenta increta**
AHA: 2022,1Q,20
DEF: Condition where the placenta adheres too deeply to the uterine wall and penetrates the muscle; often associated with placenta previa.

O43.221 **Placenta increta, first trimester** `COM` `M` ♀

O43.222 **Placenta increta, second trimester** `COM` `M` ♀

O43.223 **Placenta increta, third trimester** `COM` `M` ♀

O43.229 **Placenta increta, unspecified trimester** `COM` `M` ♀

✓6ᵗʰ **O43.23** **Placenta percreta**
DEF: Condition where the placenta attaches through the uterine muscle and may invade other organs, resulting in antenatal complications, premature delivery, retention of all or a portion of the placenta, or postpartum bleeding.

O43.231 **Placenta percreta, first trimester** `COM` `M` ♀

O43.232 **Placenta percreta, second trimester** `COM` `M` ♀

O43.233 **Placenta percreta, third trimester** `COM` `M` ♀

O43.239 **Placenta percreta, unspecified trimester** `COM` `M` ♀

✓5ᵗʰ **O43.8** **Other placental disorders**

✓6ᵗʰ **O43.81** **Placental infarction**

O43.811 **Placental infarction, first trimester** `COM` `M` ♀

O43.812 **Placental infarction, second trimester** `COM` `M` ♀

    O43.813 **Placental infarction, third trimester** COM M ♀

    O43.819 **Placental infarction, unspecified trimester** HCC COM M ♀

√6ᵗʰ **O43.89 Other placental disorders**

    Placental dysfunction

    O43.891 **Other placental disorders, first trimester** COM M ♀

    O43.892 **Other placental disorders, second trimester** COM M ♀

    O43.893 **Other placental disorders, third trimester** COM M ♀

    O43.899 **Other placental disorders, unspecified trimester** COM M ♀

√5ᵗʰ **O43.9 Unspecified placental disorder**

    O43.90 **Unspecified placental disorder, unspecified trimester** COM M ♀

    O43.91 **Unspecified placental disorder, first trimester** COM M ♀

    O43.92 **Unspecified placental disorder, second trimester** COM M ♀

    O43.93 **Unspecified placental disorder, third trimester** COM M ♀

√4ᵗʰ **O44 Placenta previa**

    AHA: 2016,4Q,52-53

    DEF: Placenta implanted in the lower segment of the uterus, which commonly causes hemorrhage in the last trimester of pregnancy.

√5ᵗʰ **O44.0 Complete placenta previa NOS or without hemorrhage**

    Placenta previa NOS

    O44.00 **Complete placenta previa NOS or without hemorrhage, unspecified trimester** COM M ♀

    O44.01 **Complete placenta previa NOS or without hemorrhage, first trimester** COM M ♀

    O44.02 **Complete placenta previa NOS or without hemorrhage, second trimester** COM M ♀

    O44.03 **Complete placenta previa NOS or without hemorrhage, third trimester** COM M ♀

√5ᵗʰ **O44.1 Complete placenta previa with hemorrhage**

    EXCLUDES 1   *labor and delivery complicated by hemorrhage from vasa previa (O69.4)*

    O44.10 **Complete placenta previa with hemorrhage, unspecified trimester** COM M ♀

    O44.11 **Complete placenta previa with hemorrhage, first trimester** COM M ♀

    O44.12 **Complete placenta previa with hemorrhage, second trimester** COM M ♀

    O44.13 **Complete placenta previa with hemorrhage, third trimester** COM M ♀

√5ᵗʰ **O44.2 Partial placenta previa without hemorrhage**

    Marginal placenta previa, NOS or without hemorrhage

    O44.20 **Partial placenta previa NOS or without hemorrhage, unspecified trimester** COM M ♀

    O44.21 **Partial placenta previa NOS or without hemorrhage, first trimester** COM M ♀

    O44.22 **Partial placenta previa NOS or without hemorrhage, second trimester** COM M ♀

    O44.23 **Partial placenta previa NOS or without hemorrhage, third trimester** COM M ♀

√5ᵗʰ **O44.3 Partial placenta previa with hemorrhage**

    Marginal placenta previa with hemorrhage

    O44.30 **Partial placenta previa with hemorrhage, unspecified trimester** COM M ♀

    O44.31 **Partial placenta previa with hemorrhage, first trimester** COM M ♀

    O44.32 **Partial placenta previa with hemorrhage, second trimester** COM M ♀

    O44.33 **Partial placenta previa with hemorrhage, third trimester** COM M ♀

√5ᵗʰ **O44.4 Low lying placenta NOS or without hemorrhage**

    Low implantation of placenta NOS or without hemorrhage

    O44.40 **Low lying placenta NOS or without hemorrhage, unspecified trimester** COM M ♀

    O44.41 **Low lying placenta NOS or without hemorrhage, first trimester** COM M ♀

    O44.42 **Low lying placenta NOS or without hemorrhage, second trimester** COM M ♀

    O44.43 **Low lying placenta NOS or without hemorrhage, third trimester** COM M ♀

√5ᵗʰ **O44.5 Low lying placenta with hemorrhage**

    Low implantation of placenta with hemorrhage

    O44.50 **Low lying placenta with hemorrhage, unspecified trimester** COM M ♀

    O44.51 **Low lying placenta with hemorrhage, first trimester** COM M ♀

    O44.52 **Low lying placenta with hemorrhage, second trimester** COM M ♀

    O44.53 **Low lying placenta with hemorrhage, third trimester** COM M ♀

√4ᵗʰ **O45 Premature separation of placenta [abruptio placentae]**

√5ᵗʰ **O45.0 Premature separation of placenta with coagulation defect**

√6ᵗʰ **O45.00 Premature separation of placenta with coagulation defect, unspecified**

    O45.001 **Premature separation of placenta with coagulation defect, unspecified, first trimester** COM M ♀

    O45.002 **Premature separation of placenta with coagulation defect, unspecified, second trimester** COM M ♀

    O45.003 **Premature separation of placenta with coagulation defect, unspecified, third trimester** COM M ♀

    O45.009 **Premature separation of placenta with coagulation defect, unspecified, unspecified trimester** COM M ♀

√6ᵗʰ **O45.01 Premature separation of placenta with afibrinogenemia**

    Premature separation of placenta with hypofibrinogenemia

    O45.011 **Premature separation of placenta with afibrinogenemia, first trimester** COM M ♀

    O45.012 **Premature separation of placenta with afibrinogenemia, second trimester** COM M ♀

    O45.013 **Premature separation of placenta with afibrinogenemia, third trimester** COM M ♀

    O45.019 **Premature separation of placenta with afibrinogenemia, unspecified trimester** COM M ♀

√6ᵗʰ **O45.02 Premature separation of placenta with disseminated intravascular coagulation**

    O45.021 **Premature separation of placenta with disseminated intravascular coagulation, first trimester** COM M ♀

    O45.022 **Premature separation of placenta with disseminated intravascular coagulation, second trimester** COM M ♀

    O45.023 **Premature separation of placenta with disseminated intravascular coagulation, third trimester** COM M ♀

    O45.029 **Premature separation of placenta with disseminated intravascular coagulation, unspecified trimester** COM M ♀

√6ᵗʰ **O45.09 Premature separation of placenta with other coagulation defect**

    O45.091 **Premature separation of placenta with other coagulation defect, first trimester** COM M ♀

    O45.092 **Premature separation of placenta with other coagulation defect, second trimester** COM M ♀

    O45.093 **Premature separation of placenta with other coagulation defect, third trimester** COM M ♀

    O45.099 **Premature separation of placenta with other coagulation defect, unspecified trimester** COM M ♀

√5ᵗʰ **O45.8 Other premature separation of placenta**

√6ᵗʰ **O45.8X Other premature separation of placenta**

    O45.8X1 **Other premature separation of placenta, first trimester** COM M ♀

    O45.8X2 **Other premature separation of placenta, second trimester** COM M ♀

    O45.8X3 **Other premature separation of placenta, third trimester** COM M ♀

     O45.8X9 **Other premature separation of placenta, unspecified trimester** COM M ♀

☑5th **O45.9 Premature separation of placenta, unspecified**
    Abruptio placentae NOS
    O45.90 **Premature separation of placenta, unspecified, unspecified trimester** COM M ♀
    O45.91 **Premature separation of placenta, unspecified, first trimester** COM M ♀
    O45.92 **Premature separation of placenta, unspecified, second trimester** COM M ♀
    O45.93 **Premature separation of placenta, unspecified, third trimester** COM M ♀

☑4th **O46 Antepartum hemorrhage, not elsewhere classified**
    EXCLUDES1 *hemorrhage in early pregnancy (O20.-)*
       intrapartum hemorrhage NEC (O67.-)
       placenta previa (O44.-)
       premature separation of placenta [abruptio placentae] (O45.-)
    DEF: Uterine hemorrhage prior to delivery that is not related to placenta previa or abruptio placentae.

☑5th **O46.0 Antepartum hemorrhage** with coagulation defect
  ☑6th **O46.00 Antepartum hemorrhage with coagulation defect, unspecified**
    O46.001 **Antepartum hemorrhage with coagulation defect, unspecified, first trimester** COM M ♀
    O46.002 **Antepartum hemorrhage with coagulation defect, unspecified, second trimester** COM M ♀
    O46.003 **Antepartum hemorrhage with coagulation defect, unspecified, third trimester** COM M ♀
    O46.009 **Antepartum hemorrhage with coagulation defect, unspecified, unspecified trimester** COM M ♀
  ☑6th **O46.01 Antepartum hemorrhage** with afibrinogenemia
    Antepartum hemorrhage with hypofibrinogenemia
    O46.011 **Antepartum hemorrhage with afibrinogenemia, first trimester** COM M ♀
    O46.012 **Antepartum hemorrhage with afibrinogenemia, second trimester** COM M ♀
    O46.013 **Antepartum hemorrhage with afibrinogenemia, third trimester** COM M ♀
    O46.019 **Antepartum hemorrhage with afibrinogenemia, unspecified trimester** COM M ♀
  ☑6th **O46.02 Antepartum hemorrhage** with disseminated intravascular coagulation
    O46.021 **Antepartum hemorrhage with disseminated intravascular coagulation, first trimester** COM M ♀
    O46.022 **Antepartum hemorrhage with disseminated intravascular coagulation, second trimester** COM M ♀
    O46.023 **Antepartum hemorrhage with disseminated intravascular coagulation, third trimester** COM M ♀
    O46.029 **Antepartum hemorrhage with disseminated intravascular coagulation, unspecified trimester** COM M ♀
  ☑6th **O46.09 Antepartum hemorrhage** with other coagulation defect
    O46.091 **Antepartum hemorrhage with other coagulation defect, first trimester** COM M ♀
    O46.092 **Antepartum hemorrhage with other coagulation defect, second trimester** COM M ♀
    O46.093 **Antepartum hemorrhage with other coagulation defect, third trimester** COM M ♀
    O46.099 **Antepartum hemorrhage with other coagulation defect, unspecified trimester** COM M ♀

☑5th **O46.8 Other antepartum hemorrhage**
  ☑6th **O46.8X Other antepartum hemorrhage**
    O46.8X1 **Other antepartum hemorrhage, first trimester** COM M ♀
    O46.8X2 **Other antepartum hemorrhage, second trimester** COM M ♀
    O46.8X3 **Other antepartum hemorrhage, third trimester** COM M ♀
    O46.8X9 **Other antepartum hemorrhage, unspecified trimester** COM M ♀

☑5th **O46.9 Antepartum hemorrhage, unspecified**
    O46.90 **Antepartum hemorrhage, unspecified, unspecified trimester** COM M ♀
    O46.91 **Antepartum hemorrhage, unspecified, first trimester** COM M ♀
    O46.92 **Antepartum hemorrhage, unspecified, second trimester** COM M ♀
    O46.93 **Antepartum hemorrhage, unspecified, third trimester** COM M ♀

☑4th **O47 False labor**
    INCLUDES Braxton Hicks contractions
       threatened labor
    EXCLUDES1 *preterm labor (O60.-)*
    AHA: 2021,1Q,10

☑5th **O47.0 False labor** before 37 completed weeks of gestation
    O47.00 **False labor before 37 completed weeks of gestation, unspecified trimester** COM M ♀
    O47.02 **False labor before 37 completed weeks of gestation, second trimester** COM M ♀
    O47.03 **False labor before 37 completed weeks of gestation, third trimester** COM M ♀
  O47.1 **False labor** at or after 37 completed weeks of gestation COM M ♀
  O47.9 **False labor, unspecified** COM M ♀

☑4th **O48 Late pregnancy**
    AHA: 2022,2Q,3
  O48.0 **Post-term pregnancy** COM M ♀
    Pregnancy over 40 completed weeks to 42 completed weeks gestation
  O48.1 **Prolonged pregnancy** COM M ♀
    Pregnancy which has advanced beyond 42 completed weeks gestation
    AHA: 2016,1Q,5

Complications of labor and delivery (O60-O77)

☑4th **O60 Preterm labor**
    INCLUDES onset (spontaneous) of labor before 37 completed weeks of gestation
    EXCLUDES1 *false labor (O47.0-)*
       threatened labor NOS (O47.0-)

☑5th **O60.0 Preterm labor** without delivery
    O60.00 **Preterm labor without delivery, unspecified trimester** COM M ♀
    O60.02 **Preterm labor without delivery, second trimester** COM M ♀
    O60.03 **Preterm labor without delivery, third trimester** COM M ♀

☑5th **O60.1 Preterm labor** with preterm delivery
    AHA: 2016,2Q,10

    One of the following 7th characters is to be assigned to each code under subcategory O60.1. 7th character 0 is for single gestations and multiple gestations where the fetus is unspecified. 7th characters 1 through 9 are for cases of multiple gestations to identify the fetus for which the code applies. The appropriate code from category O30, Multiple gestation, must also be assigned when assigning a code from subcategory O60.1 that has a 7th character of 1 through 9.
    0 not applicable or unspecified
    1 fetus 1
    2 fetus 2
    3 fetus 3
    4 fetus 4
    5 fetus 5
    9 other fetus

    √x7th **O60.10 Preterm labor with preterm delivery, unspecified trimester** COM M ♀
       Preterm labor with delivery NOS
    √x7th **O60.12 Preterm labor** second trimester **with preterm delivery** second trimester COM M ♀

✓x7ᵗʰ **O60.13** Preterm labor second trimester with preterm delivery third trimester COM M ♀

✓x7ᵗʰ **O60.14** Preterm labor third trimester with preterm delivery third trimester COM M ♀

✓5ᵗʰ **O60.2** Term delivery with preterm labor

> One of the following 7th characters is to be assigned to each code under subcategory O60.2. 7th character 0 is for single gestations and multiple gestations where the fetus is unspecified. 7th characters 1 through 9 are for cases of multiple gestations to identify the fetus for which the code applies. The appropriate code from category O30, Multiple gestation, must also be assigned when assigning a code from subcategory O60.2 that has a 7th character of 1 through 9.
> 0 not applicable or unspecified
> 1 fetus 1
> 2 fetus 2
> 3 fetus 3
> 4 fetus 4
> 5 fetus 5
> 9 other fetus

✓x7ᵗʰ **O60.20** Term delivery with preterm labor, unspecified trimester COM M ♀

✓x7ᵗʰ **O60.22** Term delivery with preterm labor, second trimester COM M ♀

✓x7ᵗʰ **O60.23** Term delivery with preterm labor, third trimester COM M ♀

✓4ᵗʰ **O61** Failed induction of labor

O61.0 Failed medical induction of labor COM M ♀
Failed induction (of labor) by oxytocin
Failed induction (of labor) by prostaglandins

O61.1 Failed instrumental induction of labor COM M ♀
Failed mechanical induction (of labor)
Failed surgical induction (of labor)

O61.8 Other failed induction of labor COM M ♀

O61.9 Failed induction of labor, unspecified COM M ♀

✓4ᵗʰ **O62** Abnormalities of forces of labor

DEF: Uterine inertia: Weak or poorly coordinated contractions of the uterus during labor.

O62.0 Primary inadequate contractions COM M ♀
Failure of cervical dilatation
Primary hypotonic uterine dysfunction
Uterine inertia during latent phase of labor

O62.1 Secondary uterine inertia COM M ♀
Arrested active phase of labor
Secondary hypotonic uterine dysfunction

O62.2 Other uterine inertia COM M ♀
Atony of uterus without hemorrhage
Atony of uterus NOS
Desultory labor
Hypotonic uterine dysfunction NOS
Irregular labor
Poor contractions
Slow slope active phase of labor
Uterine inertia NOS
> EXCLUDES 1 atony of uterus with hemorrhage (postpartum) (O72.1)
> postpartum atony of uterus without hemorrhage (O75.89)

DEF: Uterine atony: Failure of the uterine muscles to contract after the fetus and placenta are delivered.

O62.3 Precipitate labor COM M ♀
DEF: Rapid labor with delivery occurring in three hours or less from the onset of contractions.

O62.4 Hypertonic, incoordinate, and prolonged uterine contractions COM M ♀
Cervical spasm
Contraction ring dystocia
Dyscoordinate labor
Hour-glass contraction of uterus
Hypertonic uterine dysfunction
Incoordinate uterine action
Tetanic contractions
Uterine dystocia NOS
Uterine spasm
> EXCLUDES 1 dystocia (fetal) (maternal) NOS (O66.9)

O62.8 Other abnormalities of forces of labor COM M ♀

O62.9 Abnormality of forces of labor, unspecified COM M ♀

✓4ᵗʰ **O63** Long labor

O63.0 Prolonged first stage (of labor) COM M ♀

O63.1 Prolonged second stage (of labor) COM M ♀

O63.2 Delayed delivery of second twin, triplet, etc. COM M ♀

O63.9 Long labor, unspecified COM M ♀
Prolonged labor NOS

✓4ᵗʰ **O64** Obstructed labor due to malposition and malpresentation of fetus

> One of the following 7th characters is to be assigned to each code under category O64. 7th character 0 is for single gestations and multiple gestations where the fetus is unspecified. 7th characters 1 through 9 are for cases of multiple gestations to identify the fetus for which the code applies. The appropriate code from category O30, Multiple gestation, must also be assigned when assigning a code from category O64 that has a 7th character of 1 through 9.
> 0 not applicable or unspecified
> 1 fetus 1
> 2 fetus 2
> 3 fetus 3
> 4 fetus 4
> 5 fetus 5
> 9 other fetus

Fetal Malposition

Breech
Mother's pelvis
Shoulder (arm prolapse)
Face (mentum)
Oblique
Compound (extremity together with head)

✓x7ᵗʰ **O64.0** Obstructed labor due to incomplete rotation of fetal head COM M ♀
Deep transverse arrest
Obstructed labor due to persistent occipitoiliac (position)
Obstructed labor due to persistent occipitoposterior (position)
Obstructed labor due to persistent occipitosacral (position)
Obstructed labor due to persistent occipitotransverse (position)

✓x7ᵗʰ **O64.1** Obstructed labor due to breech presentation COM M ♀
Obstructed labor due to buttocks presentation
Obstructed labor due to complete breech presentation
Obstructed labor due to frank breech presentation

✓x7ᵗʰ **O64.2** Obstructed labor due to face presentation COM M ♀
Obstructed labor due to chin presentation

✓x7ᵗʰ **O64.3** Obstructed labor due to brow presentation COM M ♀

✓x7ᵗʰ **O64.4** Obstructed labor due to shoulder presentation COM M ♀
Prolapsed arm
> EXCLUDES 1 impacted shoulders (O66.0)
> shoulder dystocia (O66.0)

✓x7ᵗʰ **O64.5** Obstructed labor due to compound presentation COM M ♀

✓x7ᵗʰ **O64.8** Obstructed labor due to other malposition and malpresentation COM M ♀
Obstructed labor due to footling presentation
Obstructed labor due to incomplete breech presentation

✓x7ᵗʰ **O64.9** Obstructed labor due to malposition and malpresentation, unspecified COM M ♀

✓4ᵗʰ **O65** Obstructed labor due to maternal pelvic abnormality

O65.0 Obstructed labor due to deformed pelvis COM M ♀

O65.1 Obstructed labor due to generally contracted pelvis COM M ♀

O65.2 Obstructed labor due to pelvic inlet contraction COM M ♀

O65.3 Obstructed labor due to pelvic outlet and mid-cavity contraction COM M ♀

HCC CMS-HCC | Rx Rx HCC | ESR ESRD HCC | COM Commercial HCC | N Newborn: 0 | P Pediatric: 0-17 | M Maternity: 9-64 | A Adult: 15-124

916 | ICD-10-CM 2023

O65.4 **Obstructed labor due to** fetopelvic disproportion, unspecified   COM M ♀
     EXCLUDES 1   *dystocia due to abnormality of fetus (O66.2-O66.3)*

O65.5 **Obstructed labor due to** abnormality of maternal pelvic organs   COM M ♀
     Obstructed labor due to conditions listed in O34.-
     Use additional code to identify abnormality of pelvic organs O34.-

O65.8 **Obstructed labor due to other maternal pelvic abnormalities**   COM M ♀

O65.9 **Obstructed labor due to maternal pelvic abnormality, unspecified**   COM M ♀

✓4ᵗʰ **O66** **Other obstructed labor**

O66.0 **Obstructed labor due to** shoulder dystocia   COM M ♀
     Impacted shoulders
     DEF: Obstructed labor due to impacted fetal shoulders. It is an emergency condition that may require cesarean section, forceps delivery, vacuum extraction, or symphysiotomy.

O66.1 **Obstructed labor due to** locked twins   COM M ♀

O66.2 **Obstructed labor due to** unusually large fetus   COM M ♀

O66.3 **Obstructed labor due to other abnormalities of fetus**   COM M ♀
     Dystocia due to fetal ascites
     Dystocia due to fetal hydrops
     Dystocia due to fetal meningomyelocele
     Dystocia due to fetal sacral teratoma
     Dystocia due to fetal tumor
     Dystocia due to hydrocephalic fetus
     Use additional code to identify cause of obstruction

✓5ᵗʰ **O66.4** **Failed trial of labor**

     O66.40 **Failed trial of labor, unspecified**   COM M ♀

     O66.41 **Failed** attempted vaginal birth after previous cesarean delivery   COM M ♀
         Code first rupture of uterus, if applicable (O71.0-, O71.1)

O66.5 **Attempted application of** vacuum extractor and forceps   COM M ♀
     Attempted application of vacuum or forceps, with subsequent delivery by forceps or cesarean delivery

O66.6 **Obstructed labor due to other multiple fetuses**   COM M ♀

O66.8 **Other specified obstructed labor**   COM M ♀
     Use additional code to identify cause of obstruction

O66.9 **Obstructed labor, unspecified**   COM M ♀
     Dystocia NOS
     Fetal dystocia NOS
     Maternal dystocia NOS

✓4ᵗʰ **O67** **Labor and delivery complicated by intrapartum hemorrhage, not elsewhere classified**
     EXCLUDES 1   *antepartum hemorrhage NEC (O46.-)*
         placenta previa (O44.-)
         premature separation of placenta [abruptio placentae] (O45.-)
     EXCLUDES 2   *postpartum hemorrhage (O72.-)*

O67.0 **Intrapartum hemorrhage with coagulation defect**   COM M ♀
     Intrapartum hemorrhage (excessive) associated with afibrinogenemia
     Intrapartum hemorrhage (excessive) associated with disseminated intravascular coagulation
     Intrapartum hemorrhage (excessive) associated with hyperfibrinolysis
     Intrapartum hemorrhage (excessive) associated with hypofibrinogenemia

O67.8 **Other intrapartum hemorrhage**   COM M ♀
     Excessive intrapartum hemorrhage

O67.9 **Intrapartum hemorrhage, unspecified**   COM M ♀

O68 **Labor and delivery complicated by abnormality of fetal acid-base balance**   COM M ♀
     Fetal acidemia complicating labor and delivery
     Fetal acidosis complicating labor and delivery
     Fetal alkalosis complicating labor and delivery
     Fetal metabolic acidemia complicating labor and delivery
     EXCLUDES 1   *fetal stress NOS (O77.9)*
         labor and delivery complicated by electrocardiographic evidence of fetal stress (O77.8)
         labor and delivery complicated by ultrasonic evidence of fetal stress (O77.8)
     EXCLUDES 2   *abnormality in fetal heart rate or rhythm (O76)*
         labor and delivery complicated by meconium in amniotic fluid (O77.0)

✓4ᵗʰ **O69** **Labor and delivery complicated by umbilical cord complications**
     AHA: 2016,1Q,5

     One of the following 7th characters is to be assigned to each code under category O69. 7th character Ø is for single gestations and multiple gestations where the fetus is unspecified. 7th characters 1 through 9 are for cases of multiple gestations to identify the fetus for which the code applies. The appropriate code from category O3Ø, Multiple gestation, must also be assigned when assigning a code from category O69 that has a 7th character of 1 through 9.
     Ø   not applicable or unspecified
     1   fetus 1
     2   fetus 2
     3   fetus 3
     4   fetus 4
     5   fetus 5
     9   other fetus

✓x7ᵗʰ **O69.0** **Labor and delivery complicated by** prolapse of cord   COM M ♀
     DEF: Abnormal presentation of the fetus marked by a protruding umbilical cord during labor. It can cause fetal death.

✓x7ᵗʰ **O69.1** **Labor and delivery complicated by** cord around neck, with compression   COM M ♀
     EXCLUDES 1   *labor and delivery complicated by cord around neck, without compression (O69.81)*

✓x7ᵗʰ **O69.2** **Labor and delivery complicated by** other cord entanglement, with compression   COM M ♀
     Labor and delivery complicated by compression of cord NOS
     Labor and delivery complicated by entanglement of cords of twins in monoamniotic sac
     Labor and delivery complicated by knot in cord
     EXCLUDES 1   *labor and delivery complicated by other cord entanglement, without compression (O69.82)*

✓x7ᵗʰ **O69.3** **Labor and delivery complicated by** short cord   COM M ♀

✓x7ᵗʰ **O69.4** **Labor and delivery complicated by** vasa previa   COM M ♀
     Labor and delivery complicated by hemorrhage from vasa previa

✓x7ᵗʰ **O69.5** **Labor and delivery complicated by** vascular lesion of cord   COM M ♀
     Labor and delivery complicated by cord bruising
     Labor and delivery complicated by cord hematoma
     Labor and delivery complicated by thrombosis of umbilical vessels

✓5ᵗʰ **O69.8** **Labor and delivery complicated by other cord complications**

     ✓x7ᵗʰ **O69.81** **Labor and delivery complicated by** cord around neck, without compression   COM M ♀
         AHA: 2016,1Q,5

     ✓x7ᵗʰ **O69.82** **Labor and delivery complicated by** other cord entanglement, without compression   COM M ♀

     ✓x7ᵗʰ **O69.89** **Labor and delivery complicated by** other cord complications   COM M ♀

✓x7ᵗʰ **O69.9** **Labor and delivery complicated by cord complication, unspecified**   COM M ♀

Chapter 15. Pregnancy, Childbirth and the Puerperium

O7Ø–O73.1

☑4ᵗʰ **O7Ø Perineal laceration during delivery**

INCLUDES   episiotomy extended by laceration

EXCLUDES 1   *obstetric high vaginal laceration alone (O71.4)*

AHA: 2016,2Q,34; 2016,1Q,3-4,5

O7Ø.Ø First degree **perineal laceration during delivery**   COM M ♀

Perineal laceration, rupture or tear involving fourchette during delivery

Perineal laceration, rupture or tear involving labia during delivery

Perineal laceration, rupture or tear involving skin during delivery

Perineal laceration, rupture or tear involving vagina during delivery

Perineal laceration, rupture or tear involving vulva during delivery

Slight perineal laceration, rupture or tear during delivery

O7Ø.1 Second degree **perineal laceration during delivery**   COM M ♀

Perineal laceration, rupture or tear during delivery as in O7Ø.Ø, also involving pelvic floor

Perineal laceration, rupture or tear during delivery as in O7Ø.Ø, also involving perineal muscles

Perineal laceration, rupture or tear during delivery as in O7Ø.Ø, also involving vaginal muscles

EXCLUDES 1   *perineal laceration involving anal sphincter (O7Ø.2)*

☑5ᵗʰ **O7Ø.2** Third degree **perineal laceration during delivery**

Perineal laceration, rupture or tear during delivery as in O7Ø.1, also involving anal sphincter

Perineal laceration, rupture or tear during delivery as in O7Ø.1, also involving rectovaginal septum

Perineal laceration, rupture or tear during delivery as in O7Ø.1, also involving sphincter NOS

EXCLUDES 1   *anal sphincter tear during delivery without third degree perineal laceration (O7Ø.4)*

perineal laceration involving anal or rectal mucosa (O7Ø.3)

AHA: 2016,4Q,53-54

O7Ø.2Ø Third degree perineal laceration during delivery, unspecified   COM M ♀

O7Ø.21 Third degree perineal laceration during delivery, IIIa   COM M ♀

Third degree perineal laceration during delivery with less than 50% of external anal sphincter (EAS) thickness torn

O7Ø.22 Third degree perineal laceration during delivery, IIIb   COM M ♀

Third degree perineal laceration during delivery with more than 50% external anal sphincter (EAS) thickness torn

O7Ø.23 Third degree perineal laceration during delivery, IIIc   COM M ♀

Third degree perineal laceration during delivery with both external anal sphincter (EAS) and internal anal sphincter (IAS) torn

O7Ø.3 Fourth degree **perineal laceration during delivery**   COM M ♀

Perineal laceration, rupture or tear during delivery as in O7Ø.2, also involving anal mucosa

Perineal laceration, rupture or tear during delivery as in O7Ø.2, also involving rectal mucosa

O7Ø.4 Anal sphincter tear **complicating delivery, not associated with third degree laceration**   COM M ♀

EXCLUDES 1   *anal sphincter tear with third degree perineal laceration (O7Ø.2)*

O7Ø.9 Perineal laceration during delivery, unspecified   COM M ♀

☑4ᵗʰ **O71 Other obstetric trauma**

INCLUDES   obstetric damage from instruments

☑5ᵗʰ **O71.Ø** **Rupture of uterus (spontaneous)** before onset of labor

EXCLUDES 1   *disruption of (current) cesarean delivery wound (O9Ø.Ø)*

laceration of uterus, NEC (O71.81)

O71.ØØ Rupture of uterus before onset of labor, unspecified trimester   COM M ♀

O71.Ø2 Rupture of uterus before onset of labor, second trimester   COM M ♀

O71.Ø3 Rupture of uterus before onset of labor, third trimester   COM M ♀

O71.1 **Rupture of uterus** during labor   COM M ♀

Rupture of uterus not stated as occurring before onset of labor

EXCLUDES 1   *disruption of cesarean delivery wound (O9Ø.Ø)*

laceration of uterus, NEC (O71.81)

O71.2 **Postpartum** inversion of uterus   COM M ♀

O71.3 **Obstetric** laceration of cervix   COM M ♀

Annular detachment of cervix

O71.4 **Obstetric** high vaginal laceration **alone**   COM M ♀

Laceration of vaginal wall without perineal laceration

EXCLUDES 1   *obstetric high vaginal laceration with perineal laceration (O7Ø.-)*

AHA: 2016,1Q,5

O71.5 **Other obstetric injury to pelvic organs**   COM M ♀

Obstetric injury to bladder

Obstetric injury to urethra

EXCLUDES 2   *obstetric periurethral trauma (O71.82)*

AHA: 2014,4Q,18

O71.6 **Obstetric damage to** pelvic joints and ligaments   COM M ♀

Obstetric avulsion of inner symphyseal cartilage

Obstetric damage to coccyx

Obstetric traumatic separation of symphysis (pubis)

O71.7 **Obstetric** hematoma of pelvis   COM M ♀

Obstetric hematoma of perineum

Obstetric hematoma of vagina

Obstetric hematoma of vulva

☑6ᵗʰ **O71.8** **Other specified obstetric trauma**

O71.81 Laceration of uterus, not elsewhere classified   COM M ♀

O71.82 Other specified trauma to perineum and vulva   COM M ♀

Obstetric periurethral trauma

AHA: 2016,1Q,4; 2014,4Q,18

O71.89 Other specified obstetric trauma   COM M ♀

O71.9 Obstetric trauma, unspecified   COM M ♀

☑4ᵗʰ **O72 Postpartum hemorrhage**

INCLUDES   hemorrhage after delivery of fetus or infant

O72.Ø Third-stage **hemorrhage**   COM M ♀

Hemorrhage associated with retained, trapped or adherent placenta

Retained placenta NOS

Code also type of adherent placenta (O43.2-)

AHA: 2019,3Q,11

O72.1 **Other** immediate **postpartum hemorrhage**   COM M ♀

Hemorrhage following delivery of placenta

Postpartum hemorrhage (atonic) NOS

Uterine atony with hemorrhage

EXCLUDES 1   *uterine atony NOS (O62.2)*

uterine atony without hemorrhage (O62.2)

postpartum atony of uterus without hemorrhage (O75.89)

AHA: 2016,1Q,4

DEF: Uterine atony: Failure of the uterine muscles to contract after the fetus and placenta are delivered.

O72.2 Delayed and secondary **postpartum hemorrhage**   COM M ♀

Hemorrhage associated with retained portions of placenta or membranes after the first 24 hours following delivery of placenta

Retained products of conception NOS, following delivery

O72.3 **Postpartum** coagulation defects   COM M ♀

Postpartum afibrinogenemia

Postpartum fibrinolysis

☑4ᵗʰ **O73 Retained placenta and membranes, without hemorrhage**

EXCLUDES 1   *placenta accreta (O43.21-)*

placenta increta (O43.22-)

placenta percreta (O43.23-)

DEF: Postpartum condition resulting from failure to expel placental membrane tissues due to failed contractions of the uterine wall.

O73.Ø **Retained** placenta **without hemorrhage**   COM M ♀

Adherent placenta, without hemorrhage

Trapped placenta without hemorrhage

O73.1 **Retained** portions of placenta and membranes, **without hemorrhage**   COM M ♀

Retained products of conception following delivery, without hemorrhage

Chapter 15. Pregnancy, Childbirth and the Puerperium

☑️4th **O74 Complications of anesthesia during labor and delivery**

    INCLUDES   maternal complications arising from the administration of a general, regional or local anesthetic, analgesic or other sedation during labor and delivery

    Use additional code, if applicable, to identify specific complication

  O74.0 Aspiration pneumonitis due to anesthesia during labor and delivery COM M ♀

    Inhalation of stomach contents or secretions NOS due to anesthesia during labor and delivery

    Mendelson's syndrome due to anesthesia during labor and delivery

  O74.1 Other pulmonary complications of anesthesia during labor and delivery COM M ♀

  O74.2 Cardiac complications of anesthesia during labor and delivery COM M ♀

  O74.3 Central nervous system complications of anesthesia during labor and delivery COM M ♀

  O74.4 Toxic reaction to local anesthesia during labor and delivery COM M ♀

  O74.5 Spinal and epidural anesthesia-induced headache during labor and delivery COM M ♀

  O74.6 Other complications of spinal and epidural anesthesia during labor and delivery COM M ♀

  O74.7 Failed or difficult intubation for anesthesia during labor and delivery COM M ♀

  O74.8 Other complications of anesthesia during labor and delivery COM M ♀

  O74.9 Complication of anesthesia during labor and delivery, unspecified COM M ♀

☑️4th **O75 Other complications of labor and delivery, not elsewhere classified**

    EXCLUDES 2   puerperal (postpartum) infection (O86.-)

                puerperal (postpartum) sepsis (O85)

  O75.0 Maternal distress during labor and delivery COM M ♀

  O75.1 Shock during or following labor and delivery COM M ♀

    Obstetric shock following labor and delivery

  O75.2 Pyrexia during labor, not elsewhere classified COM M ♀

  O75.3 Other infection during labor COM M ♀

    Sepsis during labor

    Use additional code (B95-B97), to identify infectious agent

  O75.4 Other complications of obstetric surgery and procedures COM M ♀

    Cardiac arrest following obstetric surgery or procedures

    Cardiac failure following obstetric surgery or procedures

    Cerebral anoxia following obstetric surgery or procedures

    Pulmonary edema following obstetric surgery or procedures

    Use additional code to identify specific complication

    EXCLUDES 2   complications of anesthesia during labor and delivery (O74.-)

                disruption of obstetrical (surgical) wound (O90.0-O90.1)

                hematoma of obstetrical (surgical) wound (O90.2)

                infection of obstetrical (surgical) wound (O86.0-)

  O75.5 Delayed delivery after artificial rupture of membranes COM M ♀

☑️5th **O75.8 Other specified complications of labor and delivery**

    O75.81 Maternal exhaustion complicating labor and delivery COM M ♀

    O75.82 Onset (spontaneous) of labor after 37 completed weeks of gestation but before 39 completed weeks gestation, with delivery by (planned) cesarean section COM M ♀

      Delivery by (planned) cesarean section occurring after 37 completed weeks of gestation but before 39 completed weeks gestation due to (spontaneous) onset of labor

      Code first to specify reason for planned cesarean section such as:

      cephalopelvic disproportion (normally formed fetus) (O33.9)

      previous cesarean delivery (O34.21)

      AHA: 2022,2Q,3

    O75.89 Other specified complications of labor and delivery COM M ♀

  O75.9 Complication of labor and delivery, unspecified COM M ♀

O76 Abnormality in fetal heart rate and rhythm complicating labor and delivery COM M ♀

  Depressed fetal heart rate tones complicating labor and delivery

  Fetal bradycardia complicating labor and delivery

  Fetal heart rate decelerations complicating labor and delivery

  Fetal heart rate irregularity complicating labor and delivery

  Fetal heart rate abnormal variability complicating labor and delivery

  Fetal tachycardia complicating labor and delivery

  Non-reassuring fetal heart rate or rhythm complicating labor and delivery

    EXCLUDES 1   fetal stress NOS (O77.9)

                labor and delivery complicated by electrocardiographic evidence of fetal stress (O77.8)

                labor and delivery complicated by ultrasonic evidence of fetal stress (O77.8)

    EXCLUDES 2   fetal metabolic acidemia (O68)

                other fetal stress (O77.0-O77.1)

  AHA: 2013,4Q,118

☑️4th **O77 Other fetal stress complicating labor and delivery**

  O77.0 Labor and delivery complicated by meconium in amniotic fluid COM M ♀

    AHA: 2022,2Q,16; 2013,4Q,117-118

  O77.1 Fetal stress in labor or delivery due to drug administration COM M ♀

  O77.8 Labor and delivery complicated by other evidence of fetal stress COM M ♀

    Labor and delivery complicated by electrocardiographic evidence of fetal stress

    Labor and delivery complicated by ultrasonic evidence of fetal stress

    EXCLUDES 1   abnormality of fetal acid-base balance (O68)

                abnormality in fetal heart rate or rhythm (O76)

                fetal metabolic acidemia (O68)

  O77.9 Labor and delivery complicated by fetal stress, unspecified COM M ♀

    EXCLUDES 1   abnormality of fetal acid-base balance (O68)

                abnormality in fetal heart rate or rhythm (O76)

                fetal metabolic acidemia (O68)

Encounter for delivery (O80-O82)

O80 Encounter for full-term uncomplicated delivery COM M ♀

    NOTE   Delivery requiring minimal or no assistance, with or without episiotomy, without fetal manipulation [e.g., rotation version] or instrumentation [forceps] of a spontaneous, cephalic, vaginal, full-term, single, live-born infant. This code is for use as a single diagnosis code and is not to be used with any other code from chapter 15.

  Use additional code to indicate outcome of delivery (Z37.0)

  AHA: 2016,4Q,150; 2014,2Q,9

O82 Encounter for cesarean delivery without indication COM M ♀

  Use additional code to indicate outcome of delivery (Z37.0)

Complications predominantly related to the puerperium (O85-O92)

    EXCLUDES 2   mental and behavioral disorders associated with the puerperium (F53.-)

                obstetrical tetanus (A34)

                puerperal osteomalacia (M83.0)

O85 Puerperal sepsis COM M ♀

  Postpartum sepsis

  Puerperal peritonitis

  Puerperal pyemia

  Use additional code (B95-B97), to identify infectious agent

  Use additional code (R65.2-) to identify severe sepsis, if applicable

    EXCLUDES 1   fever of unknown origin following delivery (O86.4)

                genital tract infection following delivery (O86.1-)

                obstetric pyemic and septic embolism (O88.3-)

                puerperal septic thrombophlebitis (O86.81)

                urinary tract infection following delivery (O86.2-)

    EXCLUDES 2   sepsis during labor (O75.3)

  AHA: 2022,2Q,5; 2020,2Q,32; 2019,2Q,39; 2018,4Q,23

☑️ Additional Character Required   ✓x7th Placeholder Alert   Manifestation   Unspecified Dx   🅀 QPP   UPD Unacceptable PDx

Chapter 15. Pregnancy, Childbirth and the Puerperium

✓4ᵗʰ O86 Other puerperal infections

Use additional code (B95-B97), to identify infectious agent

EXCLUDES 2   *infection during labor (O75.3)*

           obstetrical tetanus (A34)

✓5ᵗʰ O86.0 Infection of obstetric surgical wound

Infected cesarean delivery wound following delivery

Infected perineal repair following delivery

EXCLUDES 1   *complications of procedures, not elsewhere classified (T81.4-)*

           postprocedural fever NOS (R50.82)

           postprocedural retroperitoneal abscess (K68.11)

AHA: 2020,2Q,32; 2018,4Q,22-23,62

O86.00 Infection of obstetric surgical wound, unspecified   COM M ♀

O86.01 Infection of obstetric surgical wound, superficial incisional site   COM M ♀

Subcutaneous abscess following an obstetrical procedure

Stitch abscess following an obstetrical procedure

O86.02 Infection of obstetric surgical wound, deep incisional site   COM M ♀

Intramuscular abscess following an obstetrical procedure

Sub-fascial abscess following an obstetrical procedure

AHA: 2020,2Q,32

O86.03 Infection of obstetric surgical wound, organ and space site   COM M ♀

Intraabdominal abscess following an obstetrical procedure

Subphrenic abscess following an obstetrical procedure

O86.04 Sepsis following an obstetrical procedure   COM M ♀

Use additional code to identify the sepsis

AHA: 2020,2Q,32; 2019,2Q,39

O86.09 Infection of obstetric surgical wound, other surgical site   COM M ♀

✓5ᵗʰ O86.1 Other infection of genital tract following delivery

O86.11 Cervicitis following delivery   COM M ♀

O86.12 Endometritis following delivery   COM M ♀

O86.13 Vaginitis following delivery   COM M ♀

O86.19 Other infection of genital tract following delivery   COM M ♀

✓5ᵗʰ O86.2 Urinary tract infection following delivery

O86.20 Urinary tract infection following delivery, unspecified   COM M ♀

Puerperal urinary tract infection NOS

AHA: 2022,2Q,5

O86.21 Infection of kidney following delivery   COM M ♀

O86.22 Infection of bladder following delivery   COM M ♀

Infection of urethra following delivery

O86.29 Other urinary tract infection following delivery   COM M ♀

O86.4 Pyrexia of unknown origin following delivery   COM M ♀

Puerperal infection NOS following delivery

Puerperal pyrexia NOS following delivery

EXCLUDES 2   *pyrexia during labor (O75.2)*

DEF: Fever of unknown origin experienced by the mother after childbirth.

✓5ᵗʰ O86.8 Other specified puerperal infections

O86.81 Puerperal septic thrombophlebitis   COM M ♀

O86.89 Other specified puerperal infections   COM M ♀

✓4ᵗʰ O87 Venous complications and hemorrhoids in the puerperium

INCLUDES   venous complications in labor, delivery and the puerperium

EXCLUDES 2   *obstetric embolism (O88.-)*

           puerperal septic thrombophlebitis (O86.81)

           venous complications in pregnancy (O22.-)

O87.0 Superficial thrombophlebitis in the puerperium   COM M ♀

Puerperal phlebitis NOS

Puerperal thrombosis NOS

O87.1 Deep phlebothrombosis in the puerperium   COM M ♀

Deep vein thrombosis, postpartum

Pelvic thrombophlebitis, postpartum

Use additional code to identify the deep vein thrombosis (I82.4-, I82.5-, I82.62-, I82.72-)

Use additional code, if applicable, for associated long-term (current) use of anticoagulants (Z79.01)

O87.2 Hemorrhoids in the puerperium   COM M ♀

O87.3 Cerebral venous thrombosis in the puerperium   COM M ♀

Cerebrovenous sinus thrombosis in the puerperium

O87.4 Varicose veins of lower extremity in the puerperium   COM M ♀

O87.8 Other venous complications in the puerperium   COM M ♀

Genital varices in the puerperium

O87.9 Venous complication in the puerperium, unspecified   COM M ♀

Puerperal phlebopathy NOS

✓4ᵗʰ O88 Obstetric embolism

EXCLUDES 1   *embolism complicating abortion NOS (O03.2)*

           embolism complicating ectopic or molar pregnancy (O08.2)

           embolism complicating failed attempted abortion (O07.2)

           embolism complicating induced abortion (O04.7)

           embolism complicating spontaneous abortion (O03.2, O03.7)

✓5ᵗʰ O88.0 Obstetric air embolism

DEF: Sudden blocking of the pulmonary artery or right ventricle with air or nitrogen bubbles.

✓6ᵗʰ O88.01 Obstetric air embolism in pregnancy

O88.011 Air embolism in pregnancy, first trimester   COM M ♀

O88.012 Air embolism in pregnancy, second trimester   COM M ♀

O88.013 Air embolism in pregnancy, third trimester   COM M ♀

O88.019 Air embolism in pregnancy, unspecified trimester   COM M ♀

O88.02 Air embolism in childbirth   COM M ♀

O88.03 Air embolism in the puerperium   COM M ♀

✓5ᵗʰ O88.1 Amniotic fluid embolism

Anaphylactoid syndrome in pregnancy

✓6ᵗʰ O88.11 Amniotic fluid embolism in pregnancy

O88.111 Amniotic fluid embolism in pregnancy, first trimester   COM M ♀

O88.112 Amniotic fluid embolism in pregnancy, second trimester   COM M ♀

O88.113 Amniotic fluid embolism in pregnancy, third trimester   COM M ♀

O88.119 Amniotic fluid embolism in pregnancy, unspecified trimester   COM M ♀

O88.12 Amniotic fluid embolism in childbirth   COM M ♀

O88.13 Amniotic fluid embolism in the puerperium   COM M ♀

✓5ᵗʰ O88.2 Obstetric thromboembolism

✓6ᵗʰ O88.21 Thromboembolism in pregnancy

Obstetric (pulmonary) embolism NOS

O88.211 Thromboembolism in pregnancy, first trimester   COM M ♀

O88.212 Thromboembolism in pregnancy, second trimester   COM M ♀

O88.213 Thromboembolism in pregnancy, third trimester   COM M ♀

O88.219 Thromboembolism in pregnancy, unspecified trimester   COM M ♀

O88.22 Thromboembolism in childbirth   COM M ♀

O88.23 Thromboembolism in the puerperium   COM M ♀

Puerperal (pulmonary) embolism NOS

✓5ᵗʰ O88.3 Obstetric pyemic and septic embolism

✓6ᵗʰ O88.31 Pyemic and septic embolism in pregnancy

O88.311 Pyemic and septic embolism in pregnancy, first trimester   COM M ♀

O88.312 Pyemic and septic embolism in pregnancy, second trimester   COM M ♀

O88.313 Pyemic and septic embolism in pregnancy, third trimester   COM M ♀

O88.319 Pyemic and septic embolism in pregnancy, unspecified trimester   COM M ♀

O88.32   **Pyemic and septic embolism in childbirth**   COM M ♀

O88.33   **Pyemic and septic embolism in the puerperium**   COM M ♀

✓5ᵗʰ **O88.8**   **Other obstetric embolism**
Obstetric fat embolism

✓6ᵗʰ **O88.81**   **Other embolism in** pregnancy

O88.811   **Other embolism in pregnancy, first trimester**   COM M ♀

O88.812   **Other embolism in pregnancy, second trimester**   COM M ♀

O88.813   **Other embolism in pregnancy, third trimester**   COM M ♀

O88.819   **Other embolism in pregnancy, unspecified trimester**   COM M ♀

O88.82   **Other embolism in** childbirth   COM M ♀

O88.83   **Other embolism in the** puerperium   COM M ♀

✓4ᵗʰ **O89**   **Complications of anesthesia during the puerperium**

INCLUDES   maternal complications arising from the administration of a general, regional or local anesthetic, analgesic or other sedation during the puerperium

Use additional code, if applicable, to identify specific complication

✓5ᵗʰ **O89.0**   **Pulmonary complications of anesthesia during the puerperium**

O89.01   **Aspiration pneumonitis due to anesthesia during the puerperium**   COM M ♀
Inhalation of stomach contents or secretions NOS due to anesthesia during the puerperium
Mendelson's syndrome due to anesthesia during the puerperium

O89.09   **Other pulmonary complications of anesthesia during the puerperium**   COM M ♀

O89.1   **Cardiac complications of anesthesia during the puerperium**   COM M ♀

O89.2   **Central nervous system complications of anesthesia during the puerperium**   COM M ♀

O89.3   **Toxic reaction to local anesthesia during the puerperium**   COM M ♀

O89.4   **Spinal and epidural anesthesia-induced headache during the puerperium**   COM M ♀

O89.5   **Other complications of spinal and epidural anesthesia during the puerperium**   COM M ♀

O89.6   **Failed or difficult intubation for anesthesia during the puerperium**   COM M ♀

O89.8   **Other complications of anesthesia during the puerperium**   COM M ♀

O89.9   **Complication of anesthesia during the puerperium, unspecified**   COM M ♀

✓4ᵗʰ **O90**   **Complications of the puerperium, not elsewhere classified**

O90.0   **Disruption of cesarean delivery wound**   COM M ♀
Dehiscence of cesarean delivery wound
EXCLUDES 1   rupture of uterus (spontaneous) before onset of labor (O71.0-)
rupture of uterus during labor (O71.1)

O90.1   **Disruption of perineal obstetric wound**   COM M ♀
Disruption of wound of episiotomy
Disruption of wound of perineal laceration
Secondary perineal tear

O90.2   **Hematoma of obstetric wound**   COM M ♀

O90.3   **Peripartum cardiomyopathy**   COM M ♀
Conditions in I42- arising during pregnancy and the puerperium
EXCLUDES 1   pre-existing heart disease complicating pregnancy and the puerperium (O99.4-)
DEF: Any structural or functional abnormality of the ventricular myocardium. It is a noninflammatory disease of obscure or unknown etiology with onset during the postpartum period.

O90.4   **Postpartum acute kidney failure**   COM M ♀
Hepatorenal syndrome following labor and delivery

O90.5   **Postpartum thyroiditis**   COM M ♀

O90.6   **Postpartum mood disturbance**   COM Q M ♀
Postpartum blues
Postpartum dysphoria
Postpartum sadness
EXCLUDES 1   postpartum depression (F53.0)
puerperal psychosis (F53.1)

✓5ᵗʰ **O90.8**   **Other complications of the puerperium, not elsewhere classified**

O90.81   **Anemia of the puerperium**   COM M ♀
Postpartum anemia NOS
EXCLUDES 1   pre-existing anemia complicating the puerperium (O99.03)
AHA: 2019,3Q,11

O90.89   **Other complications of the puerperium, not elsewhere classified**   COM M ♀
Placental polyp

O90.9   **Complication of the puerperium, unspecified**   COM M ♀

✓4ᵗʰ **O91**   **Infections of breast associated with pregnancy, the puerperium and lactation**
Use additional code to identify infection

✓5ᵗʰ **O91.0**   **Infection of nipple associated with pregnancy, the puerperium and lactation**

✓6ᵗʰ **O91.01**   **Infection of nipple associated with** pregnancy
Gestational abscess of nipple

O91.011   **Infection of nipple associated with pregnancy, first trimester**   COM M ♀

O91.012   **Infection of nipple associated with pregnancy, second trimester**   COM M ♀

O91.013   **Infection of nipple associated with pregnancy, third trimester**   COM M ♀

O91.019   **Infection of nipple associated with pregnancy, unspecified trimester**   COM M ♀

O91.02   **Infection of nipple associated with the puerperium**   M ♀
Puerperal abscess of nipple

O91.03   **Infection of nipple associated with** lactation   M ♀
Abscess of nipple associated with lactation

✓5ᵗʰ **O91.1**   **Abscess of breast associated with pregnancy, the puerperium and lactation**

✓6ᵗʰ **O91.11**   **Abscess of breast associated with** pregnancy
Gestational mammary abscess
Gestational purulent mastitis
Gestational subareolar abscess

O91.111   **Abscess of breast associated with pregnancy, first trimester**   COM M ♀

O91.112   **Abscess of breast associated with pregnancy, second trimester**   COM M ♀

O91.113   **Abscess of breast associated with pregnancy, third trimester**   COM M ♀

O91.119   **Abscess of breast associated with pregnancy, unspecified trimester**   COM M ♀

O91.12   **Abscess of breast associated with the puerperium**   M ♀
Puerperal mammary abscess
Puerperal purulent mastitis
Puerperal subareolar abscess

O91.13   **Abscess of breast associated with** lactation   M ♀
Mammary abscess associated with lactation
Purulent mastitis associated with lactation
Subareolar abscess associated with lactation

✓5ᵗʰ **O91.2**   **Nonpurulent mastitis associated with pregnancy, the puerperium and lactation**

✓6ᵗʰ **O91.21**   **Nonpurulent mastitis associated with** pregnancy
Gestational interstitial mastitis
Gestational lymphangitis of breast
Gestational mastitis NOS
Gestational parenchymatous mastitis

O91.211   **Nonpurulent mastitis associated with pregnancy, first trimester**   COM M ♀

O91.212   **Nonpurulent mastitis associated with pregnancy, second trimester**   COM M ♀

O91.213   **Nonpurulent mastitis associated with pregnancy, third trimester**   COM M ♀

O91.219   **Nonpurulent mastitis associated with pregnancy, unspecified trimester**   COM M ♀

O91.22   **Nonpurulent mastitis associated with the puerperium**   M ♀
- Puerperal interstitial mastitis
- Puerperal lymphangitis of breast
- Puerperal mastitis NOS
- Puerperal parenchymatous mastitis

O91.23   **Nonpurulent mastitis associated with lactation**   M ♀
- Interstitial mastitis associated with lactation
- Lymphangitis of breast associated with lactation
- Mastitis NOS associated with lactation
- Parenchymatous mastitis associated with lactation

✓4ᵗʰ **O92**   **Other disorders of breast and disorders of lactation associated with pregnancy and the puerperium**

✓5ᵗʰ **O92.0**   **Retracted nipple associated with pregnancy, the puerperium, and lactation**

   ✓6ᵗʰ **O92.01**   **Retracted nipple associated with pregnancy**

     O92.011   **Retracted nipple associated with pregnancy, first trimester**   COM M ♀

     O92.012   **Retracted nipple associated with pregnancy, second trimester**   COM M ♀

     O92.013   **Retracted nipple associated with pregnancy, third trimester**   COM M ♀

     O92.019   **Retracted nipple associated with pregnancy, unspecified trimester**   COM M ♀

   O92.02   **Retracted nipple associated with the puerperium**   M ♀

   O92.03   **Retracted nipple associated with lactation**   M ♀

✓5ᵗʰ **O92.1**   **Cracked nipple associated with pregnancy, the puerperium, and lactation**
- Fissure of nipple, gestational or puerperal

   ✓6ᵗʰ **O92.11**   **Cracked nipple associated with pregnancy**

     O92.111   **Cracked nipple associated with pregnancy, first trimester**   COM M ♀

     O92.112   **Cracked nipple associated with pregnancy, second trimester**   COM M ♀

     O92.113   **Cracked nipple associated with pregnancy, third trimester**   COM M ♀

     O92.119   **Cracked nipple associated with pregnancy, unspecified trimester**   COM M ♀

   O92.12   **Cracked nipple associated with the puerperium**   M ♀

   O92.13   **Cracked nipple associated with lactation**   M ♀

✓5ᵗʰ **O92.2**   **Other and unspecified disorders of breast associated with pregnancy and the puerperium**

   O92.20   **Unspecified disorder of breast associated with pregnancy and the puerperium**   M ♀

   O92.29   **Other disorders of breast associated with pregnancy and the puerperium**   M ♀

O92.3   **Agalactia**   M ♀
- Primary agalactia

   EXCLUDES 1   elective agalactia (O92.5)
     secondary agalactia (O92.5)
     therapeutic agalactia (O92.5)

   DEF: Absence of milk secretion in a female after delivery.

O92.4   **Hypogalactia**   M ♀

O92.5   **Suppressed lactation**   M ♀
- Elective agalactia
- Secondary agalactia
- Therapeutic agalactia

   EXCLUDES 1   primary agalactia (O92.3)

O92.6   **Galactorrhea**   M ♀

   DEF: Excessive or persistent milk secretion by the breast that may occur in the absence of nursing.

✓5ᵗʰ **O92.7**   **Other and unspecified disorders of lactation**

   O92.70   **Unspecified disorders of lactation**   M ♀

   O92.79   **Other disorders of lactation**   M ♀
- Puerperal galactocele

Other obstetric conditions, not elsewhere classified (O94-O9A)

O94   **Sequelae of complication of pregnancy, childbirth, and the puerperium**   UPD M ♀

   NOTE   This category is to be used to indicate conditions in O00-O77.-, O85-O94 and O98-O9A.- as the cause of late effects. The sequelae include conditions specified as such, or as late effects, which may occur at any time after the puerperium

   Code first condition resulting from (sequela) of complication of pregnancy, childbirth, and the puerperium

✓4ᵗʰ **O98**   **Maternal infectious and parasitic diseases classifiable elsewhere but complicating pregnancy, childbirth and the puerperium**

   INCLUDES   the listed conditions when complicating the pregnant state, when aggravated by the pregnancy, or as a reason for obstetric care

   Use additional code (Chapter 1), to identify specific infectious or parasitic disease

   EXCLUDES 2   herpes gestationis (O26.4-)
     infectious carrier state (O99.82-, O99.83-)
     obstetrical tetanus (A34)
     puerperal infection (O86.-)
     puerperal sepsis (O85)
     when the reason for maternal care is that the disease is known or suspected to have affected the fetus (O35-O36)

✓5ᵗʰ **O98.0**   **Tuberculosis complicating pregnancy, childbirth and the puerperium**
- Conditions in A15-A19

   ✓6ᵗʰ **O98.01**   **Tuberculosis complicating pregnancy**

     O98.011   **Tuberculosis complicating pregnancy, first trimester**   COM M ♀

     O98.012   **Tuberculosis complicating pregnancy, second trimester**   COM M ♀

     O98.013   **Tuberculosis complicating pregnancy, third trimester**   COM M ♀

     O98.019   **Tuberculosis complicating pregnancy, unspecified trimester**   COM M ♀

   O98.02   **Tuberculosis complicating childbirth**   COM M ♀

   O98.03   **Tuberculosis complicating the puerperium**   COM M ♀

✓5ᵗʰ **O98.1**   **Syphilis complicating pregnancy, childbirth and the puerperium**
- Conditions in A50-A53

   ✓6ᵗʰ **O98.11**   **Syphilis complicating pregnancy**

     O98.111   **Syphilis complicating pregnancy, first trimester**   COM M ♀

     O98.112   **Syphilis complicating pregnancy, second trimester**   COM M ♀

     O98.113   **Syphilis complicating pregnancy, third trimester**   COM M ♀

     O98.119   **Syphilis complicating pregnancy, unspecified trimester**   COM M ♀

   O98.12   **Syphilis complicating childbirth**   COM M ♀

   O98.13   **Syphilis complicating the puerperium**   COM M ♀

✓5ᵗʰ **O98.2**   **Gonorrhea complicating pregnancy, childbirth and the puerperium**
- Conditions in A54.-

   ✓6ᵗʰ **O98.21**   **Gonorrhea complicating pregnancy**

     O98.211   **Gonorrhea complicating pregnancy, first trimester**   COM M ♀

     O98.212   **Gonorrhea complicating pregnancy, second trimester**   COM M ♀

     O98.213   **Gonorrhea complicating pregnancy, third trimester**   COM M ♀

     O98.219   **Gonorrhea complicating pregnancy, unspecified trimester**   COM M ♀

   O98.22   **Gonorrhea complicating childbirth**   COM M ♀

   O98.23   **Gonorrhea complicating the puerperium**   COM M ♀

✓5ᵗʰ **O98.3** **Other infections with a predominantly sexual mode of transmission complicating pregnancy, childbirth and the puerperium**
Conditions in A55-A64
AHA: 2020,1Q,20

✓6ᵗʰ **O98.31** **Other infections with a predominantly sexual mode of transmission complicating** pregnancy

O98.311 **Other infections with a predominantly sexual mode of transmission complicating pregnancy,** first trimester ᴄᴏᴹ Ⓜ ♀

O98.312 **Other infections with a predominantly sexual mode of transmission complicating pregnancy,** second trimester ᴄᴏᴹ Ⓜ ♀

O98.313 **Other infections with a predominantly sexual mode of transmission complicating pregnancy,** third trimester ᴄᴏᴹ Ⓜ ♀

O98.319 **Other infections with a predominantly sexual mode of transmission complicating pregnancy, unspecified trimester** ᴄᴏᴹ Ⓜ ♀

O98.32 **Other infections with a predominantly sexual mode of transmission complicating** childbirth ᴄᴏᴹ Ⓜ ♀

O98.33 **Other infections with a predominantly sexual mode of transmission complicating the** puerperium ᴄᴏᴹ Ⓜ ♀

✓5ᵗʰ **O98.4** **Viral hepatitis complicating pregnancy, childbirth and the puerperium**
Conditions in B15-B19

✓6ᵗʰ **O98.41** **Viral hepatitis complicating** pregnancy

O98.411 **Viral hepatitis complicating pregnancy,** first trimester ᴄᴏᴹ Ⓜ ♀

O98.412 **Viral hepatitis complicating pregnancy,** second trimester ᴄᴏᴹ Ⓜ ♀

O98.413 **Viral hepatitis complicating pregnancy,** third trimester ᴄᴏᴹ Ⓜ ♀

O98.419 **Viral hepatitis complicating pregnancy, unspecified trimester** ᴄᴏᴹ Ⓜ ♀

O98.42 **Viral hepatitis complicating** childbirth ᴄᴏᴹ Ⓜ ♀

O98.43 **Viral hepatitis complicating the** puerperium ᴄᴏᴹ Ⓜ ♀

✓5ᵗʰ **O98.5** **Other viral diseases complicating pregnancy, childbirth and the puerperium**
Conditions in A80-B09, B25-B34, R87.81-, R87.82-
EXCLUDES 1 *human immunodeficiency virus [HIV] disease complicating pregnancy, childbirth and the puerperium (O98.7-)*
TIP: Assign a code from this subcategory as the principal or first-listed diagnosis for a patient admitted/presenting during pregnancy, childbirth, or the puerperium because of COVID-19; assign U07.1 and codes for associated manifestations as secondary codes.

✓6ᵗʰ **O98.51** **Other viral diseases complicating** pregnancy

O98.511 **Other viral diseases complicating pregnancy,** first trimester ᴄᴏᴹ Ⓜ ♀

O98.512 **Other viral diseases complicating pregnancy,** second trimester ᴄᴏᴹ Ⓜ ♀

O98.513 **Other viral diseases complicating pregnancy,** third trimester ᴄᴏᴹ Ⓜ ♀

O98.519 **Other viral diseases complicating pregnancy, unspecified trimester** ᴄᴏᴹ Ⓜ ♀

O98.52 **Other viral diseases complicating** childbirth ᴄᴏᴹ Ⓜ ♀

O98.53 **Other viral diseases complicating the** puerperium ᴄᴏᴹ Ⓜ ♀

✓5ᵗʰ **O98.6** **Protozoal diseases complicating pregnancy, childbirth and the puerperium**
Conditions in B50-B64

✓6ᵗʰ **O98.61** **Protozoal diseases complicating** pregnancy

O98.611 **Protozoal diseases complicating pregnancy,** first trimester ᴄᴏᴹ Ⓜ ♀

O98.612 **Protozoal diseases complicating pregnancy,** second trimester ᴄᴏᴹ Ⓜ ♀

O98.613 **Protozoal diseases complicating pregnancy,** third trimester ᴄᴏᴹ Ⓜ ♀

O98.619 **Protozoal diseases complicating pregnancy, unspecified trimester** ᴄᴏᴹ Ⓜ ♀

O98.62 **Protozoal diseases complicating** childbirth ᴄᴏᴹ Ⓜ ♀

O98.63 **Protozoal diseases complicating the** puerperium ᴄᴏᴹ Ⓜ ♀

✓5ᵗʰ **O98.7** **Human immunodeficiency virus [HIV] disease complicating pregnancy, childbirth and the puerperium**
Use additional code to identify the type of HIV disease:
acquired immune deficiency syndrome (AIDS) (B20)
asymptomatic HIV status (Z21)
HIV positive NOS (Z21)
symptomatic HIV disease (B20)

✓6ᵗʰ **O98.71** **Human immunodeficiency virus [HIV] disease complicating** pregnancy

O98.711 **Human immunodeficiency virus [HIV] disease complicating pregnancy,** first trimester ᴄᴏᴹ Ⓜ ♀

O98.712 **Human immunodeficiency virus [HIV] disease complicating pregnancy,** second trimester ᴄᴏᴹ Ⓜ ♀

O98.713 **Human immunodeficiency virus [HIV] disease complicating pregnancy,** third trimester ᴄᴏᴹ Ⓜ ♀

O98.719 **Human immunodeficiency virus [HIV] disease complicating pregnancy, unspecified trimester** ᴄᴏᴹ Ⓜ ♀

O98.72 **Human immunodeficiency virus [HIV] disease complicating** childbirth ᴄᴏᴹ Ⓜ ♀

O98.73 **Human immunodeficiency virus [HIV] disease complicating the** puerperium ᴄᴏᴹ Ⓜ ♀

✓5ᵗʰ **O98.8** **Other maternal infectious and parasitic diseases complicating pregnancy, childbirth and the puerperium**
AHA: 2020,1Q,10

✓6ᵗʰ **O98.81** **Other maternal infectious and parasitic diseases complicating** pregnancy

O98.811 **Other maternal infectious and parasitic diseases complicating pregnancy,** first trimester ᴄᴏᴹ Ⓜ ♀

O98.812 **Other maternal infectious and parasitic diseases complicating pregnancy,** second trimester ᴄᴏᴹ Ⓜ ♀

O98.813 **Other maternal infectious and parasitic diseases complicating pregnancy,** third trimester ᴄᴏᴹ Ⓜ ♀

O98.819 **Other maternal infectious and parasitic diseases complicating pregnancy, unspecified trimester** ᴄᴏᴹ Ⓜ ♀

O98.82 **Other maternal infectious and parasitic diseases complicating** childbirth ᴄᴏᴹ Ⓜ ♀

O98.83 **Other maternal infectious and parasitic diseases complicating the** puerperium ᴄᴏᴹ Ⓜ ♀
AHA: 2022,2Q,5

✓5ᵗʰ **O98.9** **Unspecified maternal infectious and parasitic disease complicating pregnancy, childbirth and the puerperium**

✓6ᵗʰ **O98.91** **Unspecified maternal infectious and parasitic disease complicating** pregnancy

O98.911 **Unspecified maternal infectious and parasitic disease complicating pregnancy,** first trimester ᴄᴏᴹ Ⓜ ♀

O98.912 **Unspecified maternal infectious and parasitic disease complicating pregnancy,** second trimester ᴄᴏᴹ Ⓜ ♀

O98.913 **Unspecified maternal infectious and parasitic disease complicating pregnancy,** third trimester ᴄᴏᴹ Ⓜ ♀

O98.919 **Unspecified maternal infectious and parasitic disease complicating pregnancy, unspecified trimester** ᴄᴏᴹ Ⓜ ♀

O98.92 **Unspecified maternal infectious and parasitic disease complicating** childbirth ᴄᴏᴹ Ⓜ ♀

O98.93 **Unspecified maternal infectious and parasitic disease complicating the** puerperium ᴄᴏᴹ Ⓜ ♀

Chapter 15. Pregnancy, Childbirth and the Puerperium

O99–O99.325

✓4ᵗʰ **O99** **Other maternal diseases classifiable elsewhere but complicating pregnancy, childbirth and the puerperium**
> INCLUDES   conditions which complicate the pregnant state, are aggravated by the pregnancy or are a main reason for obstetric care
> Use additional code to identify specific condition
> EXCLUDES 2   *when the reason for maternal care is that the condition is known or suspected to have affected the fetus (O35-O36)*

✓5ᵗʰ **O99.0** **Anemia complicating pregnancy, childbirth and the puerperium**
> Conditions in D50-D64
> EXCLUDES 1   *anemia arising in the puerperium (O90.81)*
> *postpartum anemia NOS (O90.81)*
> AHA: 2019,3Q,11

     ✓6ᵗʰ **O99.01** **Anemia complicating pregnancy**
>   AHA: 2016,1Q,4

         O99.011 **Anemia complicating pregnancy, first trimester** COM M ♀

         O99.012 **Anemia complicating pregnancy, second trimester** COM M ♀

         O99.013 **Anemia complicating pregnancy, third trimester** COM M ♀

         O99.019 **Anemia complicating pregnancy, unspecified trimester** COM M ♀

     O99.02 **Anemia complicating childbirth** COM M ♀

     O99.03 **Anemia complicating the puerperium** COM M ♀
>   EXCLUDES 1   *postpartum anemia not pre-existing prior to delivery (O90.81)*

✓5ᵗʰ **O99.1** **Other diseases of the blood and blood-forming organs and certain disorders involving the immune mechanism complicating pregnancy, childbirth and the puerperium**
> Conditions in D65-D89
> EXCLUDES 1   *hemorrhage with coagulation defects (O45.-, O46.0-, O67.0, O72.3)*

     ✓6ᵗʰ **O99.11** **Other diseases of the blood and blood-forming organs and certain disorders involving the immune mechanism complicating pregnancy**

         O99.111 **Other diseases of the blood and blood-forming organs and certain disorders involving the immune mechanism complicating pregnancy, first trimester** COM M ♀

         O99.112 **Other diseases of the blood and blood-forming organs and certain disorders involving the immune mechanism complicating pregnancy, second trimester** COM M ♀

         O99.113 **Other diseases of the blood and blood-forming organs and certain disorders involving the immune mechanism complicating pregnancy, third trimester** COM M ♀

         O99.119 **Other diseases of the blood and blood-forming organs and certain disorders involving the immune mechanism complicating pregnancy, unspecified trimester** COM M ♀

     O99.12 **Other diseases of the blood and blood-forming organs and certain disorders involving the immune mechanism complicating childbirth** COM M ♀

     O99.13 **Other diseases of the blood and blood-forming organs and certain disorders involving the immune mechanism complicating the puerperium** COM M ♀

✓5ᵗʰ **O99.2** **Endocrine, nutritional and metabolic diseases complicating pregnancy, childbirth and the puerperium**
> Conditions in E00-E89
> EXCLUDES 2   *diabetes mellitus (O24.-)*
> *malnutrition (O25.-)*
> *postpartum thyroiditis (O90.5)*

     ✓6ᵗʰ **O99.21** **Obesity complicating pregnancy, childbirth, and the puerperium**
>   Use additional code to identify the type of obesity (E66.-)
>   AHA: 2021,2Q,10; 2018,4Q,80
>   TIP: Do not assign a BMI code (Z68.-) for obese or overweight patients who are pregnant.

         O99.210 **Obesity complicating pregnancy, unspecified trimester** COM M ♀

         O99.211 **Obesity complicating pregnancy, first trimester** COM M ♀

         O99.212 **Obesity complicating pregnancy, second trimester** COM M ♀

         O99.213 **Obesity complicating pregnancy, third trimester** COM M ♀

         O99.214 **Obesity complicating childbirth** COM M ♀

         O99.215 **Obesity complicating the puerperium** COM M ♀

     ✓6ᵗʰ **O99.28** **Other endocrine, nutritional and metabolic diseases complicating pregnancy, childbirth and the puerperium**
>   AHA: 2021,1Q,8

         O99.280 **Endocrine, nutritional and metabolic diseases complicating pregnancy, unspecified trimester** COM M ♀

         O99.281 **Endocrine, nutritional and metabolic diseases complicating pregnancy, first trimester** COM M ♀

         O99.282 **Endocrine, nutritional and metabolic diseases complicating pregnancy, second trimester** COM M ♀

         O99.283 **Endocrine, nutritional and metabolic diseases complicating pregnancy, third trimester** COM M ♀

         O99.284 **Endocrine, nutritional and metabolic diseases complicating childbirth** COM M ♀

         O99.285 **Endocrine, nutritional and metabolic diseases complicating the puerperium** COM M ♀

✓5ᵗʰ **O99.3** **Mental disorders and diseases of the nervous system complicating pregnancy, childbirth and the puerperium**

     ✓6ᵗʰ **O99.31** **Alcohol use complicating pregnancy, childbirth, and the puerperium**
>   Use additional code(s) from F10 to identify manifestations of the alcohol use

         O99.310 **Alcohol use complicating pregnancy, unspecified trimester** COM M ♀

         O99.311 **Alcohol use complicating pregnancy, first trimester** COM M ♀

         O99.312 **Alcohol use complicating pregnancy, second trimester** COM M ♀

         O99.313 **Alcohol use complicating pregnancy, third trimester** COM M ♀

         O99.314 **Alcohol use complicating childbirth** COM M ♀

         O99.315 **Alcohol use complicating the puerperium** COM M ♀

     ✓6ᵗʰ **O99.32** **Drug use complicating pregnancy, childbirth, and the puerperium**
>   Use additional code(s) from F11-F16 and F18-F19 to identify manifestations of the drug use
>   AHA: 2018,4Q,69-70; 2018,2Q,10
>   TIP: When drug use is documented during pregnancy, assign first a code from this subcategory followed by an additional code from F11-F16 and F18-F19 identifying the specific drug use even if not documented as associated with a physical, mental, or behavioral disorder. According to chapter 15 guidelines, it is the provider's responsibility to state that the condition being treated is *not* affecting the pregnancy.

         O99.320 **Drug use complicating pregnancy, unspecified trimester** COM M ♀

         O99.321 **Drug use complicating pregnancy, first trimester** COM M ♀

         O99.322 **Drug use complicating pregnancy, second trimester** COM M ♀

         O99.323 **Drug use complicating pregnancy, third trimester** COM M ♀

         O99.324 **Drug use complicating childbirth** COM M ♀

         O99.325 **Drug use complicating the puerperium** COM M ♀

Chapter 15. Pregnancy, Childbirth and the Puerperium

✓6ᵗʰ **O99.33 Tobacco use disorder complicating pregnancy, childbirth, and the puerperium**
Smoking complicating pregnancy, childbirth, and the puerperium
Use additional code from category F17 to identify type of tobacco nicotine dependence

- **O99.330 Smoking (tobacco) complicating pregnancy, unspecified trimester** COM M ♀
- **O99.331 Smoking (tobacco) complicating pregnancy, first trimester** COM M ♀
- **O99.332 Smoking (tobacco) complicating pregnancy, second trimester** COM M ♀
- **O99.333 Smoking (tobacco) complicating pregnancy, third trimester** COM M ♀
- **O99.334 Smoking (tobacco) complicating childbirth** COM M ♀
- **O99.335 Smoking (tobacco) complicating the puerperium** COM M ♀

✓6ᵗʰ **O99.34 Other mental disorders complicating pregnancy, childbirth, and the puerperium**
Conditions in F01-F09, F20-F52 and F54-F99
EXCLUDES 2 postpartum mood disturbance (O90.6)
postnatal psychosis (F53.1)
puerperal psychosis (F53.1)

- **O99.340 Other mental disorders complicating pregnancy, unspecified trimester** COM Q M ♀
- **O99.341 Other mental disorders complicating pregnancy, first trimester** COM Q M ♀
- **O99.342 Other mental disorders complicating pregnancy, second trimester** COM Q M ♀
- **O99.343 Other mental disorders complicating pregnancy, third trimester** COM Q M ♀
- **O99.344 Other mental disorders complicating childbirth** COM M ♀
- **O99.345 Other mental disorders complicating the puerperium** COM Q M ♀
  AHA: 2018,4Q,8

✓6ᵗʰ **O99.35 Diseases of the nervous system complicating pregnancy, childbirth, and the puerperium**
Conditions in G00-G99
EXCLUDES 2 pregnancy related peripheral neuritis (O26.8-)

- **O99.350 Diseases of the nervous system complicating pregnancy, unspecified trimester** COM M ♀
- **O99.351 Diseases of the nervous system complicating pregnancy, first trimester** COM M ♀
- **O99.352 Diseases of the nervous system complicating pregnancy, second trimester** COM M ♀
- **O99.353 Diseases of the nervous system complicating pregnancy, third trimester** COM M ♀
- **O99.354 Diseases of the nervous system complicating childbirth** COM M ♀
- **O99.355 Diseases of the nervous system complicating the puerperium** COM M ♀

✓5ᵗʰ **O99.4 Diseases of the circulatory system complicating pregnancy, childbirth and the puerperium**
Conditions in I00-I99
EXCLUDES 1 peripartum cardiomyopathy (O90.3)
EXCLUDES 2 hypertensive disorders (O10-O16)
obstetric embolism (O88.-)
venous complications and cerebrovenous sinus thrombosis in labor, childbirth and the puerperium (O87.-)
venous complications and cerebrovenous sinus thrombosis in pregnancy (O22.-)
AHA: 2016,2Q,8

✓6ᵗʰ **O99.41 Diseases of the circulatory system complicating pregnancy**
- **O99.411 Diseases of the circulatory system complicating pregnancy, first trimester** COM M ♀
- **O99.412 Diseases of the circulatory system complicating pregnancy, second trimester** COM M ♀
- **O99.413 Diseases of the circulatory system complicating pregnancy, third trimester** COM M ♀
- **O99.419 Diseases of the circulatory system complicating pregnancy, unspecified trimester** COM M ♀

O99.42 Diseases of the circulatory system complicating childbirth COM M ♀
O99.43 Diseases of the circulatory system complicating the puerperium COM M ♀

✓5ᵗʰ **O99.5 Diseases of the respiratory system complicating pregnancy, childbirth and the puerperium**
Conditions in J00-J99

✓6ᵗʰ **O99.51 Diseases of the respiratory system complicating pregnancy**
- **O99.511 Diseases of the respiratory system complicating pregnancy, first trimester** COM M ♀
- **O99.512 Diseases of the respiratory system complicating pregnancy, second trimester** COM M ♀
- **O99.513 Diseases of the respiratory system complicating pregnancy, third trimester** COM M ♀
- **O99.519 Diseases of the respiratory system complicating pregnancy, unspecified trimester** COM M ♀

O99.52 Diseases of the respiratory system complicating childbirth COM M ♀
O99.53 Diseases of the respiratory system complicating the puerperium COM M ♀

✓5ᵗʰ **O99.6 Diseases of the digestive system complicating pregnancy, childbirth and the puerperium**
Conditions in K00-K93
EXCLUDES 2 hemorrhoids in pregnancy (O22.4-)
liver and biliary tract disorders in pregnancy, childbirth and the puerperium (O26.6-)

✓6ᵗʰ **O99.61 Diseases of the digestive system complicating pregnancy**
AHA: 2016,1Q,4
- **O99.611 Diseases of the digestive system complicating pregnancy, first trimester** COM M ♀
- **O99.612 Diseases of the digestive system complicating pregnancy, second trimester** COM M ♀
- **O99.613 Diseases of the digestive system complicating pregnancy, third trimester** COM M ♀
- **O99.619 Diseases of the digestive system complicating pregnancy, unspecified trimester** COM M ♀

O99.62 Diseases of the digestive system complicating childbirth COM M ♀
O99.63 Diseases of the digestive system complicating the puerperium COM M ♀

✓5ᵗʰ **O99.7 Diseases of the skin and subcutaneous tissue complicating pregnancy, childbirth and the puerperium**
Conditions in L00-L99
EXCLUDES 2 herpes gestationis (O26.4)
pruritic urticarial papules and plaques of pregnancy (PUPPP) (O26.86)

✓6ᵗʰ **O99.71 Diseases of the skin and subcutaneous tissue complicating pregnancy**
- **O99.711 Diseases of the skin and subcutaneous tissue complicating pregnancy, first trimester** COM M ♀
- **O99.712 Diseases of the skin and subcutaneous tissue complicating pregnancy, second trimester** COM M ♀
- **O99.713 Diseases of the skin and subcutaneous tissue complicating pregnancy, third trimester** COM M ♀
- **O99.719 Diseases of the skin and subcutaneous tissue complicating pregnancy, unspecified trimester** COM M ♀

O99.72 Diseases of the skin and subcutaneous tissue complicating childbirth COM M ♀

O99.73 **Diseases of the skin and subcutaneous tissue complicating the** puerperium   COM M ♀

√5ᵗʰ O99.8 **Other specified diseases and conditions complicating pregnancy, childbirth and the puerperium**
Conditions in D00-D48, H00-H95, M00-N99, and Q00-Q99
Use additional code to identify condition
EXCLUDES 2   *genitourinary infections in pregnancy (O23.-)*
infection of genitourinary tract following delivery (O86.1-O86.4)
malignant neoplasm complicating pregnancy, childbirth and the puerperium (O9A.1-)
maternal care for known or suspected abnormality of maternal pelvic organs (O34.-)
postpartum acute kidney failure (O90.4)
traumatic injuries in pregnancy (O9A.2-)

√6ᵗʰ O99.81 **Abnormal glucose complicating pregnancy, childbirth and the puerperium**
EXCLUDES 1   *gestational diabetes (O24.4-)*

    O99.810 **Abnormal glucose complicating pregnancy**   COM M ♀
    O99.814 **Abnormal glucose complicating childbirth**   COM M ♀
    O99.815 **Abnormal glucose complicating the puerperium**   COM M ♀

√6ᵗʰ O99.82 **Streptococcus B carrier state complicating pregnancy, childbirth and the puerperium**
EXCLUDES 1   *carrier of streptococcus group B (GBS) in a nonpregnant woman (Z22.330)*
DEF: *Streptococcus* group B colonization: Bacteria normally found in the vagina or lower intestine of many healthy adult women that may infect the fetus during childbirth, causing mental or physical handicaps or death. Women who test positive for *Streptococcus* group B during pregnancy are considered a "colonized" status and are treated with IV antibiotics at the time of delivery and may also be treated with oral antibiotics during the pregnancy.

    O99.820 **Streptococcus B carrier state complicating pregnancy**   COM M ♀
    O99.824 **Streptococcus B carrier state complicating childbirth**   COM M ♀
      AHA: 2019,2Q,8
    O99.825 **Streptococcus B carrier state complicating the** puerperium   COM M ♀

√6ᵗʰ O99.83 **Other infection carrier state complicating pregnancy, childbirth and the puerperium**
Use additional code to identify the carrier state (Z22.-)

    O99.830 **Other infection carrier state complicating pregnancy**   COM M ♀
    O99.834 **Other infection carrier state complicating childbirth**   COM M ♀
    O99.835 **Other infection carrier state complicating the** puerperium   COM M ♀

√6ᵗʰ O99.84 **Bariatric surgery status complicating pregnancy, childbirth and the puerperium**
Gastric banding status complicating pregnancy, childbirth and the puerperium
Gastric bypass status for obesity complicating pregnancy, childbirth and the puerperium
Obesity surgery status complicating pregnancy, childbirth and the puerperium

    O99.840 **Bariatric surgery status complicating pregnancy, unspecified trimester**   COM M ♀
    O99.841 **Bariatric surgery status complicating pregnancy, first trimester**   COM M ♀
    O99.842 **Bariatric surgery status complicating pregnancy, second trimester**   COM M ♀
    O99.843 **Bariatric surgery status complicating pregnancy, third trimester**   COM M ♀
    O99.844 **Bariatric surgery status complicating childbirth**   COM M ♀
    O99.845 **Bariatric surgery status complicating the** puerperium   COM M ♀

√6ᵗʰ O99.89 **Other specified diseases and conditions complicating pregnancy, childbirth and the puerperium**
AHA: 2020,4Q,36-37

    O99.891 **Other specified diseases and conditions complicating** pregnancy   COM M ♀
    O99.892 **Other specified diseases and conditions complicating** childbirth   COM M ♀
    O99.893 **Other specified diseases and conditions complicating** puerperium   COM M ♀

√4ᵗʰ O9A **Maternal malignant neoplasms, traumatic injuries and abuse classifiable elsewhere but complicating pregnancy, childbirth and the puerperium**

√5ᵗʰ O9A.1 Malignant neoplasm **complicating pregnancy, childbirth and the puerperium**
Conditions in C00-C96
Use additional code to identify neoplasm
EXCLUDES 2   *maternal care for benign tumor of corpus uteri (O34.1-)*
maternal care for benign tumor of cervix (O34.4-)
AHA: 2015,3Q,19

√6ᵗʰ O9A.11 **Malignant neoplasm complicating** pregnancy

    O9A.111 **Malignant neoplasm complicating pregnancy, first trimester**   COM M ♀
    O9A.112 **Malignant neoplasm complicating pregnancy, second trimester**   COM M ♀
    O9A.113 **Malignant neoplasm complicating pregnancy, third trimester**   COM M ♀
    O9A.119 **Malignant neoplasm complicating pregnancy, unspecified trimester**   COM M ♀

   O9A.12 **Malignant neoplasm complicating** childbirth   COM M ♀
   O9A.13 **Malignant neoplasm complicating the** puerperium   COM M ♀

√5ᵗʰ O9A.2 Injury, poisoning and **certain other consequences of** external causes **complicating pregnancy, childbirth and the puerperium**
Conditions in S00-T88, except T74 and T76
Use additional code(s) to identify the injury or poisoning
EXCLUDES 2   *physical, sexual and psychological abuse complicating pregnancy, childbirth and the puerperium (O9A.3-, O9A.4-, O9A.5-)*

√6ᵗʰ O9A.21 **Injury, poisoning and certain other consequences of external causes complicating** pregnancy

    O9A.211 **Injury, poisoning and certain other consequences of external causes complicating pregnancy, first trimester**   COM M ♀
    O9A.212 **Injury, poisoning and certain other consequences of external causes complicating pregnancy, second trimester**   COM M ♀
    O9A.213 **Injury, poisoning and certain other consequences of external causes complicating pregnancy, third trimester**   COM M ♀
    O9A.219 **Injury, poisoning and certain other consequences of external causes complicating pregnancy, unspecified trimester**   COM M ♀

   O9A.22 **Injury, poisoning and certain other consequences of external causes complicating** childbirth   COM M ♀
   O9A.23 **Injury, poisoning and certain other consequences of external causes complicating the** puerperium   COM M ♀

√5ᵗʰ O9A.3 Physical abuse **complicating pregnancy, childbirth and the puerperium**
Conditions in T74.11 or T76.11
Use additional code (if applicable):
to identify any associated current injury due to physical abuse
to identify the perpetrator of abuse (Y07.-)
EXCLUDES 2   *sexual abuse complicating pregnancy, childbirth and the puerperium (O9A.4)*

√6ᵗʰ O9A.31 **Physical abuse complicating** pregnancy

    O9A.311 **Physical abuse complicating pregnancy, first trimester**   COM M ♀
    O9A.312 **Physical abuse complicating pregnancy, second trimester**   COM M ♀
    O9A.313 **Physical abuse complicating pregnancy, third trimester**   COM M ♀
    O9A.319 **Physical abuse complicating pregnancy, unspecified trimester**   COM M ♀

   O9A.32 **Physical abuse complicating** childbirth   COM M ♀

O9A.33   **Physical abuse complicating the**
             puerperium   COM M ♀

√5ᵗʰ **O9A.4**   Sexual abuse **complicating pregnancy, childbirth and the**
             puerperium
             Conditions in T74.21 or T76.21
             Use additional code (if applicable):
                to identify any associated current injury due to sexual abuse
                to identify the perpetrator of abuse (Y07.-)

√6ᵗʰ **O9A.41**   **Sexual abuse complicating** pregnancy

   O9A.411   **Sexual abuse complicating pregnancy,**
                first trimester   COM M ♀
   O9A.412   **Sexual abuse complicating pregnancy,**
                second trimester   COM M ♀
   O9A.413   **Sexual abuse complicating pregnancy,**
                third trimester   COM M ♀
   O9A.419   **Sexual abuse complicating pregnancy,**
                unspecified trimester   COM M ♀

O9A.42   **Sexual abuse complicating** childbirth   COM M ♀
O9A.43   **Sexual abuse complicating the**
             puerperium   COM M ♀

√5ᵗʰ **O9A.5**   Psychological abuse **complicating pregnancy, childbirth and**
             the puerperium
             Conditions in T74.31 or T76.31
             Use additional code to identify the perpetrator of abuse (Y07.-)

√6ᵗʰ **O9A.51**   **Psychological abuse complicating** pregnancy

   O9A.511   **Psychological abuse complicating**
                pregnancy, first trimester   COM M ♀
   O9A.512   **Psychological abuse complicating**
                pregnancy, second trimester   COM M ♀
   O9A.513   **Psychological abuse complicating**
                pregnancy, third trimester   COM M ♀
   O9A.519   **Psychological abuse complicating**
                pregnancy, unspecified
                trimester   COM M ♀

O9A.52   **Psychological abuse complicating**
             childbirth   COM M ♀
O9A.53   **Psychological abuse complicating the**
             puerperium   COM M ♀

✔ Additional Character Required   √x7ᵗʰ Placeholder Alert   Manifestation   Unspecified Dx   Ⅱ QPP   UPD Unacceptable PDx

Chapter 16. Certain Conditions Originating in the Perinatal Period (PØØ–P96)

Chapter-specific Guidelines with Coding Examples

The chapter-specific guidelines from the ICD-10-CM Official Guidelines for Coding and Reporting have been provided below. Along with these guidelines are coding examples, contained in the shaded boxes, that have been developed to help illustrate the coding and/or sequencing guidance found in these guidelines.

For coding and reporting purposes the perinatal period is defined as before birth through the 28th day following birth. The following guidelines are provided for reporting purposes

a. General perinatal rules

1) Use of Chapter 16 codes

Codes in this chapter are <u>never</u> for use on the maternal record. Codes from Chapter 15, the obstetric chapter, are never permitted on the newborn record. Chapter 16 codes may be used throughout the life of the patient if the condition is still present.

2) Principal diagnosis for birth record

When coding the birth episode in a newborn record, assign a code from category Z38, Liveborn infants according to place of birth and type of delivery, as the principal diagnosis. A code from category Z38 is assigned only once, to a newborn at the time of birth. If a newborn is transferred to another institution, a code from category Z38 should not be used at the receiving hospital.

A code from category Z38 is used only on the newborn record, not on the mother's record.

3) Use of codes from other chapters with codes from Chapter 16

Codes from other chapters may be used with codes from chapter 16 if the codes from the other chapters provide more specific detail. Codes for signs and symptoms may be assigned when a definitive diagnosis has not been established. If the reason for the encounter is a perinatal condition, the code from chapter 16 should be sequenced first.

4) Use of Chapter 16 codes after the perinatal period

Should a condition originate in the perinatal period, and continue throughout the life of the patient, the perinatal code should continue to be used regardless of the patient's age.

> A 7-year-old patient with history of birth injury that resulted in Erb's palsy is seen for subscapularis release
>
> **P14.Ø**   **Erb's paralysis due to birth injury**
>
> *Explanation:* Although in this instance Erb's palsy is specifically related to a birth injury, it has not resolved and continues to be a health concern. A perinatal code is appropriate even though this patient is beyond the perinatal period.

5) Birth process or community acquired conditions

If a newborn has a condition that may be either due to the birth process or community acquired and the documentation does not indicate which it is, the default is due to the birth process and the code from Chapter 16 should be used. If the condition is community-acquired, a code from Chapter 16 should not be assigned.

For COVID-19 infection in a newborn, see guideline I.C.16.h.

6) Code all clinically significant conditions

All clinically significant conditions noted on routine newborn examination should be coded. A condition is clinically significant if it requires:

clinical evaluation; or

therapeutic treatment; or

diagnostic procedures; or

extended length of hospital stay; or

increased nursing care and/or monitoring; or

has implications for future health care needs

Note: The perinatal guidelines listed above are the same as the general coding guidelines for "additional diagnoses", except for the final point regarding implications for future health care needs. Codes should be assigned for conditions that have been specified by the provider as having implications for future health care needs.

b. Observation and evaluation of newborns for suspected conditions not found

1) Use of Z05 codes

Assign a code from category Z05, Observation and evaluation of newborn for suspected **diseases and** conditions ruled out, to identify those instances when a healthy newborn is evaluated for a suspected condition/**disease** that is determined after study not to be present. Do not use a code from category Z05 when the patient **is documented to have** signs or symptoms of a suspected problem; in such cases code the sign or symptom.

2) Z05 on other than the birth record

A code from category Z05 may also be assigned as a principal or first-listed code for readmissions or encounters when the code from category Z38 code no longer applies. Codes from category Z05 are for use only for healthy newborns and infants for which no condition after study is found to be present.

3) Z05 on a birth record

A code from category Z05 is to be used as a secondary code after the code from category Z38, Liveborn infants according to place of birth and type of delivery.

> Newborn delivered via vaginal delivery; previous ultrasounds showed what appeared to be an abnormality of the right kidney. Kidney function tests were performed and ultrasounds taken and any genitourinary conditions ruled out.
>
> **Z38.ØØ**   **Single liveborn infant, delivered vaginally**
>
> **Z05.6**   **Observation and evaluation of newborn for suspected genitourinary condition ruled out**
>
> *Explanation:* The newborn had no signs or symptoms of kidney or other genitourinary condition but was evaluated after delivery due to the abnormal prenatal ultrasound findings. A Z code describing the type and place of birth should be coded first, followed by a Z05 category code for the work performed to rule out a suspected genitourinary condition.

c. Coding additional perinatal diagnoses

1) Assigning codes for conditions that require treatment

Assign codes for conditions that require treatment or further investigation, prolong the length of stay, or require resource utilization.

2) Codes for conditions specified as having implications for future health care needs

Assign codes for conditions that have been specified by the provider as having implications for future health care needs.

Note: This guideline should not be used for adult patients.

> An abnormal noise was heard in the left hip of a post-term newborn during a physical examination. The pediatrician would like to follow the patient after discharge as a hip click can be an early sign of hip dysplasia. The newborn was delivered via cesarean at 41 weeks.
>
> **Z38.Ø1**   **Single liveborn infant, delivered by cesarean**
>
> **PØ8.21**   **Post-term newborn**
>
> **R29.4**   **Clicking hip**
>
> *Explanation:* The abnormal hip noise or click is appended as a secondary diagnosis not only because it is an abnormal finding upon examination, but also due to its potential to be part of a bigger health issue. The hip dysplasia has not yet been diagnosed and does not warrant a code at this time.

d. Prematurity and fetal growth retardation

Providers utilize different criteria in determining prematurity. A code for prematurity should not be assigned unless it is documented. Assignment of codes in categories P05, Disorders of newborn related to slow fetal growth and fetal malnutrition, and P07, Disorders of newborn related to short gestation and low birth weight, not elsewhere classified, should be based on the recorded birth weight and estimated gestational age.

When both birth weight and gestational age are available, two codes from category P07 should be assigned, with the code for birth weight sequenced before the code for gestational age.

e. Low birth weight and immaturity status

Codes from category P07, Disorders of newborn related to short gestation and low birth weight, not elsewhere classified, are for use for a child or adult who was premature or had a low birth weight as a newborn and this is affecting the patient's current health status.

See Section I.C.21. Factors influencing health status and contact with health services, Status.

A 35-year-old patient, who weighed 659 grams at birth, is seen for heart disease documented as being a consequence of the low birth weight

I51.9   Heart disease, unspecified

P07.02   Extremely low birth weight newborn, 500–749 grams

Explanation: A code from subcategories P07.0- and P07.1- is appropriate, regardless of the age of the patient, as long as the documentation provides a clear link between the patient's current illness and the low birth weight.

f. Bacterial sepsis of newborn

Category P36, Bacterial sepsis of newborn, includes congenital sepsis. If a perinate is documented as having sepsis without documentation of congenital or community acquired, the default is congenital and a code from category P36 should be assigned. If the P36 code includes the causal organism, an additional code from category B95, Streptococcus, Staphylococcus, and Enterococcus as the cause of diseases classified elsewhere, or B96, Other bacterial agents as the cause of diseases classified elsewhere, should not be assigned. If the P36 code does not include the causal organism, assign an additional code from category B96. If applicable, use additional codes to identify severe sepsis (R65.2-) and any associated acute organ dysfunction.

A full-term infant develops severe sepsis 24 hours after discharge from the hospital and is readmitted; cultures identified *E. coli* as the infective agent

P36.4   Sepsis of newborn due to Escherichia coli

R65.20   Severe sepsis without septic shock

Explanation: Even though this newborn was discharged and could have acquired *E. coli* from his/her external environment, due to the lack of documentation specifying specifically how this pathogen was acquired, the default is to code the *E. coli* sepsis as congenital. A code from chapter 1, "Certain Infectious and Parasitic Diseases," is not required because the perinatal sepsis code identifies both the sepsis and the bacteria causing the sepsis.

g. Stillbirth

Code P95, Stillbirth, is only for use in institutions that maintain separate records for stillbirths. No other code should be used with P95. Code P95 should not be used on the mother's record.

h. COVID-19 infection in newborn

For a newborn that tests positive for COVID-19, assign code U07.1, COVID-19, and the appropriate codes for associated manifestation(s) in neonates/newborns in the absence of documentation indicating a specific type of transmission. For a newborn that tests positive for COVID-19 and the provider documents the condition was contracted in utero or during the birth process, assign codes P35.8, Other congenital viral diseases, and U07.1, COVID-19. When coding the birth episode in a newborn record, the appropriate code from category Z38, Liveborn infants according to place of birth and type of delivery, should be assigned as the principal diagnosis.

Chapter 16. Certain Conditions Originating in the Perinatal Period (P00-P96)

NOTE Codes from this chapter are for use on newborn records only, never on maternal records

INCLUDES conditions that have their origin in the fetal or perinatal period (before birth through the first 28 days after birth) even if morbidity occurs later

EXCLUDES 2 congenital malformations, deformations and chromosomal abnormalities (Q00-Q99)

endocrine, nutritional and metabolic diseases (E00-E88)

injury, poisoning and certain other consequences of external causes (S00-T88)

neoplasms (C00-D49)

tetanus neonatorum (A33)

This chapter contains the following blocks:

P00-P04   Newborn affected by maternal factors and by complications of pregnancy, labor, and delivery
P05-P08   Disorders of newborn related to length of gestation and fetal growth
P09   Abnormal findings on neonatal screening
P10-P15   Birth trauma
P19-P29   Respiratory and cardiovascular disorders specific to the perinatal period
P35-P39   Infections specific to the perinatal period
P50-P61   Hemorrhagic and hematological disorders of newborn
P70-P74   Transitory endocrine and metabolic disorders specific to newborn
P76-P78   Digestive system disorders of newborn
P80-P83   Conditions involving the integument and temperature regulation of newborn
P84   Other problems with newborn
P90-P96   Other disorders originating in the perinatal period

Newborn affected by maternal factors and by complications of pregnancy, labor, and delivery (P00-P04)

NOTE These codes are for use when the listed maternal conditions are specified as the cause of confirmed morbidity or potential morbidity which have their origin in the perinatal period (before birth through the first 28 days after birth).

AHA: 2016,4Q,54-55

☑4ᵗʰ **P00 Newborn affected by maternal conditions that may be unrelated to present pregnancy**

Code first any current condition in newborn

EXCLUDES 2 encounter for observation of newborn for suspected diseases and conditions ruled out (Z05.-)

newborn affected by maternal complications of pregnancy (P01.-)

newborn affected by maternal endocrine and metabolic disorders (P70-P74)

newborn affected by noxious substances transmitted via placenta or breast milk (P04.-)

P00.0 Newborn affected by maternal hypertensive disorders

Newborn affected by maternal conditions classifiable to O10-O11, O13-O16

P00.1 Newborn affected by maternal renal and urinary tract diseases

Newborn affected by maternal conditions classifiable to N00-N39

P00.2 Newborn affected by maternal infectious and parasitic diseases

Newborn affected by maternal infectious disease classifiable to A00-B99, J09 and J10

EXCLUDES 1 maternal genital tract or other localized infections (P00.8)

EXCLUDES 2 infections specific to the perinatal period (P35-P39)

newborn affected by (positive) maternal group B streptococcus (GBS) colonization (P00.82)

AHA: 2019,2Q,10; 2015,3Q,20

P00.3 Newborn affected by other maternal circulatory and respiratory diseases

Newborn affected by maternal conditions classifiable to I00-I99, J00-J99, Q20-Q34 and not included in P00.0, P00.2

P00.4 Newborn affected by maternal nutritional disorders

Newborn affected by maternal disorders classifiable to E40-E64

Maternal malnutrition NOS

P00.5 Newborn affected by maternal injury

Newborn affected by maternal conditions classifiable to O9A.2-

P00.6 Newborn affected by surgical procedure on mother

Newborn affected by amniocentesis

EXCLUDES 1 Cesarean delivery for present delivery (P03.4)

damage to placenta from amniocentesis, Cesarean delivery or surgical induction (P02.1)

previous surgery to uterus or pelvic organs (P03.89)

EXCLUDES 2 newborn affected by complication of (fetal) intrauterine procedure (P96.5)

P00.7 Newborn affected by other medical procedures on mother, not elsewhere classified

Newborn affected by radiation to mother

EXCLUDES 1 damage to placenta from amniocentesis, cesarean delivery or surgical induction (P02.1)

newborn affected by other complications of labor and delivery (P03.-)

☑5ᵗʰ **P00.8 Newborn affected by other maternal conditions**

P00.81 Newborn affected by periodontal disease in mother

P00.82 Newborn affected by (positive) maternal group B streptococcus (GBS) colonization

Contact with positive maternal group B streptococcus

AHA: 2021,4Q,23

P00.89 Newborn affected by other maternal conditions

Newborn affected by conditions classifiable to T80-T88

Newborn affected by maternal genital tract or other localized infections

Newborn affected by maternal systemic lupus erythematosus

Use additional code to identify infectious agent, if known

EXCLUDES 2 newborn affected by positive maternal group B streptococcus (GBS) colonization (P00.82)

AHA: 2019,2Q,9

P00.9 Newborn affected by unspecified maternal condition

☑4ᵗʰ **P01 Newborn affected by maternal complications of pregnancy**

Code first any current condition in newborn

EXCLUDES 2 encounter for observation of newborn for suspected diseases and conditions ruled out (Z05.-)

P01.0 Newborn affected by incompetent cervix

P01.1 Newborn affected by premature rupture of membranes

P01.2 Newborn affected by oligohydramnios

EXCLUDES 1 oligohydramnios due to premature rupture of membranes (P01.1)

DEF: Low amniotic fluid level, resulting in underdeveloped organs in the fetus.

P01.3 Newborn affected by polyhydramnios

Newborn affected by hydramnios

DEF: Excess amniotic fluid surrounding the fetus, typically defined as a total fluid volume of greater than 24 cm.

P01.4 Newborn affected by ectopic pregnancy

Newborn affected by abdominal pregnancy

P01.5 Newborn affected by multiple pregnancy

Newborn affected by triplet (pregnancy)

Newborn affected by twin (pregnancy)

P01.6 Newborn affected by maternal death

P01.7 Newborn affected by malpresentation before labor

Newborn affected by breech presentation before labor

Newborn affected by external version before labor

Newborn affected by face presentation before labor

Newborn affected by transverse lie before labor

Newborn affected by unstable lie before labor

P01.8 Newborn affected by other maternal complications of pregnancy

P01.9 Newborn affected by maternal complication of pregnancy, unspecified

☑4ᵗʰ **P02 Newborn affected by complications of placenta, cord and membranes**

Code first any current condition in newborn

EXCLUDES 2 encounter for observation of newborn for suspected diseases and conditions ruled out (Z05.-)

P02.0 Newborn affected by placenta previa

DEF: Placenta developed in the lower segment of the uterus that can cause hemorrhaging leading to preterm delivery.

Chapter 16. Certain Conditions Originating in the Perinatal Period

P02.1   **Newborn affected by other forms of placental separation and hemorrhage**
Newborn affected by abruptio placenta
Newborn affected by accidental hemorrhage
Newborn affected by antepartum hemorrhage
Newborn affected by damage to placenta from amniocentesis, cesarean delivery or surgical induction
Newborn affected by maternal blood loss
Newborn affected by premature separation of placenta

✓5ᵗʰ **P02.2**   **Newborn affected by other and unspecified morphological and functional abnormalities of placenta**

    P02.20   **Newborn affected by unspecified morphological and functional abnormalities of placenta**

    P02.29   **Newborn affected by other morphological and functional abnormalities of placenta**
Newborn affected by placental dysfunction
Newborn affected by placental infarction
Newborn affected by placental insufficiency

P02.3   **Newborn affected by placental transfusion syndromes**
Newborn affected by placental and cord abnormalities resulting in twin-to-twin or other transplacental transfusion

P02.4   **Newborn affected by prolapsed cord**

P02.5   **Newborn affected by other compression of umbilical cord**
Newborn affected by umbilical cord (tightly) around neck
Newborn affected by entanglement of umbilical cord
Newborn affected by knot in umbilical cord
AHA: 2022,1Q,22

✓5ᵗʰ **P02.6**   **Newborn affected by other and unspecified conditions of umbilical cord**

    P02.60   **Newborn affected by unspecified conditions of umbilical cord**

    P02.69   **Newborn affected by other conditions of umbilical cord**
Newborn affected by short umbilical cord
Newborn affected by vasa previa
EXCLUDES 1   *newborn affected by single umbilical artery (Q27.0)*

✓5ᵗʰ **P02.7**   **Newborn affected by chorioamnionitis**
AHA: 2018,4Q,23-24
DEF: Inflammation of the fetal membranes due to maternal infection characterized by fetal tachycardia, respiratory distress, apnea, weak cries, and poor sucking.

    P02.70   **Newborn affected by fetal inflammatory response syndrome**   HCC ESR COM
Newborn affected by FIRS

    P02.78   **Newborn affected by other conditions from chorioamnionitis**
Newborn affected by amnionitis
Newborn affected by membranitis
Newborn affected by placentitis

P02.8   **Newborn affected by other abnormalities of membranes**

P02.9   **Newborn affected by abnormality of membranes, unspecified**

✓4ᵗʰ **P03**   **Newborn affected by other complications of labor and delivery**
Code first any current condition in newborn
EXCLUDES 2   *encounter for observation of newborn for suspected diseases and conditions ruled out (Z05.-)*

P03.0   **Newborn affected by breech delivery and extraction**

P03.1   **Newborn affected by other malpresentation, malposition and disproportion during labor and delivery**
Newborn affected by contracted pelvis
Newborn affected by conditions classifiable to O64-O66
Newborn affected by persistent occipitoposterior
Newborn affected by transverse lie

P03.2   **Newborn affected by forceps delivery**

Forceps Assisted Birth

Forceps extractor

P03.3   **Newborn affected by delivery by vacuum extractor [ventouse]**

Vacuum Assisted Birth

Vacuum extractor

P03.4   **Newborn affected by Cesarean delivery**

P03.5   **Newborn affected by precipitate delivery**
Newborn affected by rapid second stage

P03.6   **Newborn affected by abnormal uterine contractions**
Newborn affected by conditions classifiable to O62.-, except O62.3
Newborn affected by hypertonic labor
Newborn affected by uterine inertia

✓5ᵗʰ **P03.8**   **Newborn affected by other specified complications of labor and delivery**

    ✓6ᵗʰ **P03.81**   **Newborn affected by abnormality in fetal (intrauterine) heart rate or rhythm**
EXCLUDES 1   *neonatal cardiac dysrhythmia (P29.1-)*

      P03.810   **Newborn affected by abnormality in fetal (intrauterine) heart rate or rhythm before the onset of labor**

      P03.811   **Newborn affected by abnormality in fetal (intrauterine) heart rate or rhythm during labor**

      P03.819   **Newborn affected by abnormality in fetal (intrauterine) heart rate or rhythm, unspecified as to time of onset**

    P03.82   **Meconium passage during delivery**
EXCLUDES 1   *meconium aspiration (P24.00, P24.01)*
meconium staining (P96.83)
DEF: Fetal intestinal activity that increases in response to a fetomaternal distressed state during delivery. The anal sphincter relaxes and meconium is passed into the amniotic fluid.

    P03.89   **Newborn affected by other specified complications of labor and delivery**
Newborn affected by abnormality of maternal soft tissues
Newborn affected by conditions classifiable to O60-O75 and by procedures used in labor and delivery not included in P02.- and P03.0-P03.6
Newborn affected by induction of labor

P03.9   **Newborn affected by complication of labor and delivery, unspecified**

✓4ᵗʰ **P04**   **Newborn affected by noxious substances transmitted via placenta or breast milk**
INCLUDES   nonteratogenic effects of substances transmitted via placenta
Code first any current condition in newborn, if applicable
EXCLUDES 2   *congenital malformations (Q00-Q99)*
encounter for observation of newborn for suspected diseases and conditions ruled out (Z05.-)
neonatal jaundice from excessive hemolysis due to drugs or toxins transmitted from mother (P58.4)
newborn in contact with and (suspected) exposures hazardous to health not transmitted via placenta or breast milk (Z77.-)

P04.0   **Newborn affected by maternal anesthesia and analgesia in pregnancy, labor and delivery**   COM
Newborn affected by reactions and intoxications from maternal opiates and tranquilizers administered for procedures during pregnancy or labor and delivery
EXCLUDES 2   *newborn affected by other maternal medication (P04.1-)*

✓5ᵗʰ **P04.1 Newborn affected by other maternal medication**
Code first withdrawal symptoms from maternal use of drugs of addiction, if applicable (P96.1)

    EXCLUDES 1   *dysmorphism due to warfarin (Q86.2)*
                 fetal hydantoin syndrome (Q86.1)
    EXCLUDES 2   *maternal anesthesia and analgesia in pregnancy, labor and delivery (P04.0)*
                 maternal use of drugs of addiction (P04.4-)

    AHA: 2018,4Q,24-25

    P04.11 Newborn affected by maternal antineoplastic **chemotherapy** COM
    P04.12 Newborn affected by maternal cytotoxic **drugs** COM
    P04.13 Newborn affected by maternal use of anticonvulsants COM
    P04.14 Newborn affected by maternal use of opiates COM
    P04.15 Newborn affected by maternal use of antidepressants COM
    P04.16 Newborn affected by maternal use of amphetamines COM
    P04.17 Newborn affected by maternal use of sedative-hypnotics COM
    P04.1A Newborn affected by maternal use of anxiolytics COM
    P04.18 Newborn affected by other maternal medication COM
    P04.19 Newborn affected by maternal use of unspecified medication COM

P04.2 Newborn affected by maternal use of tobacco COM
Newborn affected by exposure in utero to tobacco smoke
    EXCLUDES 2   *newborn exposure to environmental tobacco smoke (P96.81)*

P04.3 Newborn affected by maternal use of alcohol COM
    EXCLUDES 1   *fetal alcohol syndrome (Q86.0)*

✓5ᵗʰ **P04.4 Newborn affected by maternal use of** drugs of addiction
    AHA: 2018,4Q,25

    P04.40 Newborn affected by maternal use of unspecified drugs of addiction COM
    P04.41 Newborn affected by maternal use of cocaine COM
    P04.42 Newborn affected by maternal use of hallucinogens COM
        EXCLUDES 2   *newborn affected by other maternal medication (P04.1-)*
    P04.49 Newborn affected by maternal use of other drugs of addiction
        EXCLUDES 2   *newborn affected by maternal anesthesia and analgesia (P04.0)*
                 withdrawal symptoms from maternal use of drugs of addiction (P96.1)

P04.5 Newborn affected by maternal use of nutritional chemical substances COM

P04.6 Newborn affected by maternal exposure to environmental chemical substances COM

✓5ᵗʰ **P04.8 Newborn affected by other maternal** noxious substances
    AHA: 2018,4Q,25

    P04.81 Newborn affected by maternal use of cannabis COM
    P04.89 Newborn affected by other maternal noxious substances COM

P04.9 Newborn affected by maternal noxious substance, unspecified COM

Disorders of newborn related to length of gestation and fetal growth (P05-P08)

✓4ᵗʰ **P05 Disorders of newborn related to slow fetal growth and fetal malnutrition**
    AHA: 2016,4Q,55-56

✓5ᵗʰ **P05.0 Newborn light for gestational age**
Newborn light-for-dates
Weight below but length above 10th percentile for gestational age

    P05.00 Newborn light for gestational age, unspecified weight COM
    P05.01 Newborn light for gestational age, less than 500 grams COM

P05.02 Newborn light for gestational age, 500-749 grams COM
P05.03 Newborn light for gestational age, 750-999 grams COM
P05.04 Newborn light for gestational age, 1000-1249 grams COM
P05.05 Newborn light for gestational age, 1250-1499 grams COM
P05.06 Newborn light for gestational age, 1500-1749 grams COM
P05.07 Newborn light for gestational age, 1750-1999 grams COM
P05.08 Newborn light for gestational age, 2000-2499 grams COM
P05.09 Newborn light for gestational age, 2500 grams and over COM
Newborn light for gestational age, other

✓5ᵗʰ **P05.1 Newborn small for gestational age**
Newborn small-and-light-for-dates
Newborn small-for-dates
Weight and length below 10th percentile for gestational age

    P05.10 Newborn small for gestational age, unspecified weight COM
    P05.11 Newborn small for gestational age, less than 500 grams COM
    P05.12 Newborn small for gestational age, 500-749 grams COM
    P05.13 Newborn small for gestational age, 750-999 grams COM
    P05.14 Newborn small for gestational age, 1000-1249 grams COM
    P05.15 Newborn small for gestational age, 1250-1499 grams COM
    P05.16 Newborn small for gestational age, 1500-1749 grams COM
    P05.17 Newborn small for gestational age, 1750-1999 grams COM
    P05.18 Newborn small for gestational age, 2000-2499 grams COM
    P05.19 Newborn small for gestational age, other COM
    Newborn small for gestational age, 2500 grams and over

P05.2 Newborn affected by fetal (intrauterine) malnutrition **not light or small for gestational age** COM
Infant, not light or small for gestational age, showing signs of fetal malnutrition, such as dry, peeling skin and loss of subcutaneous tissue
    EXCLUDES 1   *newborn affected by fetal malnutrition with light for gestational age (P05.0-)*
                 newborn affected by fetal malnutrition with small for gestational age (P05.1-)

P05.9 Newborn affected by slow intrauterine growth, unspecified COM
Newborn affected by fetal growth retardation NOS

✓4ᵗʰ **P07 Disorders of newborn related to short gestation and low birth weight, not elsewhere classified**

    NOTE   When both birth weight and gestational age of the newborn are available, both should be coded with birth weight sequenced before gestational age

    INCLUDES   the listed conditions, without further specification, as the cause of morbidity or additional care, in newborn

✓5ᵗʰ **P07.0 Extremely low birth weight newborn**
Newborn birth weight 999 g. or less
    EXCLUDES 1   *low birth weight due to slow fetal growth and fetal malnutrition (P05.-)*

    P07.00 Extremely low birth weight newborn, unspecified weight COM
    P07.01 Extremely low birth weight newborn, less than 500 grams COM
    P07.02 Extremely low birth weight newborn, 500-749 grams COM
    P07.03 Extremely low birth weight newborn, 750-999 grams COM

Chapter 16. Certain Conditions Originating in the Perinatal Period

P07.1–P09.8

✓5ᵗʰ **P07.1 Other low birth weight newborn**
Newborn birth weight 1000-2499 g.
   EXCLUDES 1   *low birth weight due to slow fetal growth and fetal malnutrition (P05.-)*

  P07.10 **Other low birth weight newborn, unspecified weight** `COM`

  P07.14 **Other low birth weight newborn, 1000-1249 grams** `COM`

  P07.15 **Other low birth weight newborn, 1250-1499 grams** `COM`

  P07.16 **Other low birth weight newborn, 1500-1749 grams** `COM`

  P07.17 **Other low birth weight newborn, 1750-1999 grams** `COM`

  P07.18 **Other low birth weight newborn, 2000-2499 grams** `COM`

✓5ᵗʰ **P07.2 Extreme immaturity of newborn**
Less than 28 completed weeks (less than 196 completed days) of gestation.

  P07.20 **Extreme immaturity of newborn, unspecified weeks of gestation** `COM`
Gestational age less than 28 completed weeks NOS

  P07.21 **Extreme immaturity of newborn, gestational age less than 23 completed weeks** `COM`
Extreme immaturity of newborn, gestational age less than 23 weeks, 0 days

  P07.22 **Extreme immaturity of newborn, gestational age 23 completed weeks** `COM`
Extreme immaturity of newborn, gestational age 23 weeks, 0 days through 23 weeks, 6 days

  P07.23 **Extreme immaturity of newborn, gestational age 24 completed weeks** `COM`
Extreme immaturity of newborn, gestational age 24 weeks, 0 days through 24 weeks, 6 days

  P07.24 **Extreme immaturity of newborn, gestational age 25 completed weeks** `COM`
Extreme immaturity of newborn, gestational age 25 weeks, 0 days through 25 weeks, 6 days

  P07.25 **Extreme immaturity of newborn, gestational age 26 completed weeks** `COM`
Extreme immaturity of newborn, gestational age 26 weeks, 0 days through 26 weeks, 6 days

  P07.26 **Extreme immaturity of newborn, gestational age 27 completed weeks** `COM`
Extreme immaturity of newborn, gestational age 27 weeks, 0 days through 27 weeks, 6 days

✓5ᵗʰ **P07.3 Preterm [premature] newborn [other]**
28 completed weeks or more but less than 37 completed weeks (196 completed days but less than 259 completed days) of gestation
Prematurity NOS
AHA: 2017,3Q,26

  P07.30 **Preterm newborn, unspecified weeks of gestation** `COM`

  P07.31 **Preterm newborn, gestational age 28 completed weeks** `COM`
Preterm newborn, gestational age 28 weeks, 0 days through 28 weeks, 6 days

  P07.32 **Preterm newborn, gestational age 29 completed weeks** `COM`
Preterm newborn, gestational age 29 weeks, 0 days through 29 weeks, 6 days

  P07.33 **Preterm newborn, gestational age 30 completed weeks** `COM`
Preterm newborn, gestational age 30 weeks, 0 days through 30 weeks, 6 days

  P07.34 **Preterm newborn, gestational age 31 completed weeks** `COM`
Preterm newborn, gestational age 31 weeks, 0 days through 31 weeks, 6 days

  P07.35 **Preterm newborn, gestational age 32 completed weeks** `COM`
Preterm newborn, gestational age 32 weeks, 0 days through 32 weeks, 6 days

  P07.36 **Preterm newborn, gestational age 33 completed weeks** `COM`
Preterm newborn, gestational age 33 weeks, 0 days through 33 weeks, 6 days

  P07.37 **Preterm newborn, gestational age 34 completed weeks** `COM`
Preterm newborn, gestational age 34 weeks, 0 days through 34 weeks, 6 days

  P07.38 **Preterm newborn, gestational age 35 completed weeks** `COM`
Preterm newborn, gestational age 35 weeks, 0 days through 35 weeks, 6 days

  P07.39 **Preterm newborn, gestational age 36 completed weeks** `COM`
Preterm newborn, gestational age 36 weeks, 0 days through 36 weeks, 6 days

✓4ᵗʰ **P08 Disorders of newborn related to long gestation and high birth weight**
  NOTE   When both birth weight and gestational age of the newborn are available, priority of assignment should be given to birth weight
  INCLUDES   the listed conditions, without further specification, as causes of morbidity or additional care, in newborn

  P08.0 **Exceptionally large newborn baby** `COM`
Usually implies a birth weight of 4500 g. or more
   EXCLUDES 1   *syndrome of infant of diabetic mother (P70.1)*
       syndrome of infant of mother with gestational diabetes (P70.0)

  P08.1 **Other heavy for gestational age newborn** `COM`
Other newborn heavy- or large-for-dates regardless of period of gestation
Usually implies a birth weight of 4000 g. to 4499 g.
   EXCLUDES 1   *newborn with a birth weight of 4500 or more (P08.0)*
       syndrome of infant of diabetic mother (P70.1)
       syndrome of infant of mother with gestational diabetes (P70.0)

✓5ᵗʰ **P08.2 Late newborn, not heavy for gestational age**
AHA: 2014,1Q,14

  P08.21 **Post-term newborn** `COM`
Newborn with gestation period over 40 completed weeks to 42 completed weeks

  P08.22 **Prolonged gestation of newborn** `COM`
Newborn with gestation period over 42 completed weeks (294 days or more), not heavy- or large-for-dates.
Postmaturity NOS

Abnormal findings on neonatal screening (P09)

✓4ᵗʰ **P09 Abnormal findings on neonatal screening**
  INCLUDES   abnormal findings on state mandated newborn screens
       failed newborn screening
  EXCLUDES 2   *nonspecific serologic evidence of human immunodeficiency virus [HIV] (R75)*
  AHA: 2021,4Q,24

  P09.1 **Abnormal findings on neonatal screening for inborn errors of metabolism**

  P09.2 **Abnormal findings on neonatal screening for congenital endocrine disease**
Abnormal findings on neonatal screening for congenital adrenal hyperplasia
Abnormal findings on neonatal screening for hypothyroidism screen

  P09.3 **Abnormal findings on neonatal screening for congenital hematologic disorders**
Abnormal findings for hemoglobinothies screen
Abnormal findings on red cell membrane defects screen
Abnormal findings on sickle cell screen

  P09.4 **Abnormal findings on neonatal screening for cystic fibrosis**

  P09.5 **Abnormal findings on neonatal screening for critical congenital heart disease**
Neonatal congenital heart disease screening failure

  P09.6 **Abnormal findings on neonatal screening for neonatal hearing loss**
   EXCLUDES 2   *encounter for hearing examination following failed hearing screening (Z01.110)*

  P09.8 **Other abnormal findings on neonatal screening**

P09.9   Abnormal findings on neonatal screening, unspecified

Birth trauma (P10-P15)

✓4ᵗʰ **P10**   **Intracranial laceration and hemorrhage** due to birth injury
> *EXCLUDES 1*   intracranial hemorrhage of newborn NOS (P52.9)
> intracranial hemorrhage of newborn due to anoxia or hypoxia (P52.-)
> nontraumatic intracranial hemorrhage of newborn (P52.-)

   P10.0   **Subdural** hemorrhage due to birth injury   COM
     Subdural hematoma (localized) due to birth injury
> *EXCLUDES 1*   subdural hemorrhage accompanying tentorial tear (P10.4)

   P10.1   **Cerebral** hemorrhage due to birth injury   COM
   P10.2   **Intraventricular** hemorrhage due to birth injury   COM
   P10.3   **Subarachnoid** hemorrhage due to birth injury   COM
   P10.4   **Tentorial tear** due to birth injury   COM
   P10.8   **Other intracranial lacerations and hemorrhages due to birth injury**   COM
   P10.9   **Unspecified intracranial laceration and hemorrhage due to birth injury**   COM

✓4ᵗʰ **P11**   **Other birth injuries to central nervous system**
   P11.0   **Cerebral edema** due to birth injury   COM
   P11.1   **Other specified brain damage** due to birth injury   COM
   P11.2   **Unspecified brain damage** due to birth injury   COM
   P11.3   **Birth injury to facial nerve**
     Facial palsy due to birth injury
   P11.4   **Birth injury to other cranial nerves**
   P11.5   **Birth injury to spine and spinal cord**   COM
     Fracture of spine due to birth injury
   P11.9   **Birth injury to central nervous system, unspecified**

✓4ᵗʰ **P12**   **Birth injury to scalp**

Birth Injuries to Scalp

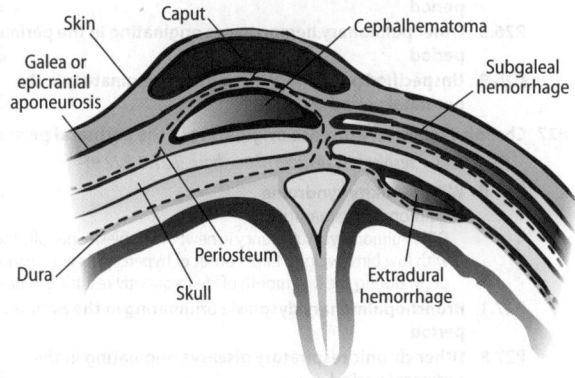

   P12.0   **Cephalhematoma** due to birth injury
> **DEF:** Condition that occurs in a neonate when blood vessels between the skull and periosteum rupture and blood collects in the subperiosteal space (below the periosteum). It is typically caused by prolonged labor or trauma due to instrument-assisted delivery (e.g., forceps, vacuum extraction), although in rare circumstances, it may indicate a linear skull fracture with intracranial hemorrhage.

   P12.1   **Chignon (from vacuum extraction)** due to birth injury
> **DEF:** Artificial swelling of the scalp that occurs when a collection of interstitial fluid and blood forms in the area of the scalp where the suction cup was applied during a vacuum-assisted delivery.

   P12.2   **Epicranial subaponeurotic hemorrhage** due to birth injury
     Subgaleal hemorrhage

   P12.3   **Bruising of scalp** due to birth injury

   P12.4   **Injury of scalp of newborn due to monitoring equipment**
     Sampling incision of scalp of newborn
     Scalp clip (electrode) injury of newborn

✓5ᵗʰ **P12.8**   **Other birth injuries to scalp**
     P12.81   **Caput succedaneum**
> **DEF:** Swelling of the scalp as a result of pressure being exerted on the head from the vaginal walls, uterus, or instrumentation used in assisting a delivery (e.g., vacuum).

     P12.89   **Other birth injuries to scalp**
   P12.9   **Birth injury to scalp, unspecified**

✓4ᵗʰ **P13**   **Birth injury to skeleton**
> *EXCLUDES 2*   birth injury to spine (P11.5)

   P13.0   **Fracture of skull** due to birth injury
   P13.1   **Other birth injuries to skull**
> *EXCLUDES 1*   cephalhematoma (P12.0)

   P13.2   **Birth injury to femur**
   P13.3   **Birth injury to other long bones**
   P13.4   **Fracture of clavicle** due to birth injury
   P13.8   **Birth injuries to other parts of skeleton**
   P13.9   **Birth injury to skeleton, unspecified**

✓4ᵗʰ **P14**   **Birth injury to peripheral nervous system**
   P14.0   **Erb's paralysis** due to birth injury
> **DEF:** Erb's paralysis: Most common type of brachial plexus (peripheral nerve) injury in a neonate that involves nerve damage at the level of C5-C6. *Synonym(s): Erb's palsy*

   P14.1   **Klumpke's paralysis** due to birth injury
   P14.2   **Phrenic nerve paralysis** due to birth injury
   P14.3   **Other brachial plexus birth injuries**
   P14.8   **Birth injuries to other parts of peripheral nervous system**
   P14.9   **Birth injury to peripheral nervous system, unspecified**

✓4ᵗʰ **P15**   **Other birth injuries**
   P15.0   **Birth injury to liver**
     Rupture of liver due to birth injury
   P15.1   **Birth injury to spleen**
     Rupture of spleen due to birth injury
   P15.2   **Sternomastoid** injury due to birth injury
   P15.3   **Birth injury to eye**
     Subconjunctival hemorrhage due to birth injury
     Traumatic glaucoma due to birth injury
   P15.4   **Birth injury to face**
     Facial congestion due to birth injury
   P15.5   **Birth injury to external genitalia**
   P15.6   **Subcutaneous fat necrosis** due to birth injury
   P15.8   **Other specified birth injuries**
   P15.9   **Birth injury, unspecified**

Respiratory and cardiovascular disorders specific to the perinatal period (P19-P29)

✓4ᵗʰ **P19**   **Metabolic acidemia in newborn**
> *INCLUDES*   metabolic acidemia in newborn

   P19.0   **Metabolic acidemia in newborn first noted** before onset of labor
   P19.1   **Metabolic acidemia in newborn first noted** during labor
   P19.2   **Metabolic acidemia noted** at birth
   P19.9   **Metabolic acidemia, unspecified**

✓4ᵗʰ **P22**   **Respiratory distress of newborn**
> **AHA:** 2019,2Q,29

   P22.0   **Respiratory distress syndrome of newborn**   COM
     Cardiorespiratory distress syndrome of newborn
     Hyaline membrane disease
     Idiopathic respiratory distress syndrome [IRDS or RDS] of newborn
     Pulmonary hypoperfusion syndrome
     Respiratory distress syndrome, type I
> *EXCLUDES 2*   respiratory arrest of newborn (P28.81)
> respiratory failure of newborn NOS (P28.5)
> **AHA:** 2019,2Q,29
> **DEF:** Severe chest contractions upon air intake and expiratory grunting. The infant appears blue due to oxygen deficiency and has a rapid respiratory rate, formerly called hyaline membrane disease.

   P22.1   **Transient tachypnea of newborn**
     Idiopathic tachypnea of newborn
     Respiratory distress syndrome, type II
     Wet lung syndrome
> **DEF:** Rapid, labored breathing of a newborn. It is a short-term problem that begins after birth and lasts about three days.

   P22.8   **Other respiratory distress of newborn**
> *EXCLUDES 1*   respiratory arrest of newborn (P28.81)
> respiratory failure of newborn NOS (P28.5)

   P22.9   **Respiratory distress of newborn, unspecified**
> *EXCLUDES 1*   respiratory arrest of newborn (P28.81)
> respiratory failure of newborn NOS (P28.5)

✓4ᵗʰ P23 Congenital pneumonia

> **INCLUDES** infective pneumonia acquired in utero or during birth
> **EXCLUDES 1** *neonatal pneumonia resulting from aspiration (P24.-)*

P23.0 Congenital pneumonia due to viral agent [COM]
> Use additional code (B97) to identify organism
> **EXCLUDES 1** *congenital rubella pneumonitis (P35.0)*

P23.1 Congenital pneumonia due to Chlamydia [COM]

P23.2 Congenital pneumonia due to staphylococcus [COM]

P23.3 Congenital pneumonia due to streptococcus, group B [COM]

P23.4 Congenital pneumonia due to Escherichia coli [COM]

P23.5 Congenital pneumonia due to Pseudomonas [COM]

P23.6 Congenital pneumonia due to other bacterial agents [COM]
> Congenital pneumonia due to Hemophilus influenzae
> Congenital pneumonia due to Klebsiella pneumoniae
> Congenital pneumonia due to Mycoplasma
> Congenital pneumonia due to Streptococcus, except group B
> Use additional code (B95-B96) to identify organism

P23.8 Congenital pneumonia due to other organisms [COM]

P23.9 Congenital pneumonia, unspecified [COM]

✓4ᵗʰ P24 Neonatal aspiration

> **INCLUDES** aspiration in utero and during delivery

✓5ᵗʰ P24.0 Meconium aspiration

> **EXCLUDES 1** *meconium passage (without aspiration) during delivery (P03.82)*
> *meconium staining (P96.83)*
> **DEF:** Meconium in the trachea or seen on chest x-ray after birth.

P24.00 Meconium aspiration without respiratory symptoms
> Meconium aspiration NOS

P24.01 Meconium aspiration with respiratory symptoms [COM]
> Meconium aspiration pneumonia
> Meconium aspiration pneumonitis
> Meconium aspiration syndrome NOS
> Use additional code to identify any secondary pulmonary hypertension, if applicable (I27.2-)
> **DEF:** Aspiration of fetal intestinal material during or prior to delivery. It is usually a complication of placental insufficiency, causing pneumonitis and bronchial obstruction (inflammatory reaction of lungs).

✓5ᵗʰ P24.1 Neonatal aspiration of (clear) amniotic fluid and mucus
> Neonatal aspiration of liquor (amnii)

P24.10 Neonatal aspiration of (clear) amniotic fluid and mucus without respiratory symptoms
> Neonatal aspiration of amniotic fluid and mucus NOS

P24.11 Neonatal aspiration of (clear) amniotic fluid and mucus with respiratory symptoms [COM]
> Neonatal aspiration of amniotic fluid and mucus with pneumonia
> Neonatal aspiration of amniotic fluid and mucus with pneumonitis
> Use additional code to identify any secondary pulmonary hypertension, if applicable (I27.2-)

✓5ᵗʰ P24.2 Neonatal aspiration of blood

P24.20 Neonatal aspiration of blood without respiratory symptoms
> Neonatal aspiration of blood NOS

P24.21 Neonatal aspiration of blood with respiratory symptoms [COM]
> Neonatal aspiration of blood with pneumonia
> Neonatal aspiration of blood with pneumonitis
> Use additional code to identify any secondary pulmonary hypertension, if applicable (I27.2-)

✓5ᵗʰ P24.3 Neonatal aspiration of milk and regurgitated food
> Neonatal aspiration of stomach contents

P24.30 Neonatal aspiration of milk and regurgitated food without respiratory symptoms
> Neonatal aspiration of milk and regurgitated food NOS

P24.31 Neonatal aspiration of milk and regurgitated food with respiratory symptoms [COM]
> Neonatal aspiration of milk and regurgitated food with pneumonia
> Neonatal aspiration of milk and regurgitated food with pneumonitis
> Use additional code to identify any secondary pulmonary hypertension, if applicable (I27.2-)

✓5ᵗʰ P24.8 Other neonatal aspiration

P24.80 Other neonatal aspiration without respiratory symptoms
> Neonatal aspiration NEC

P24.81 Other neonatal aspiration with respiratory symptoms [COM]
> Neonatal aspiration pneumonia NEC
> Neonatal aspiration with pneumonitis NEC
> Neonatal aspiration with pneumonia NOS
> Neonatal aspiration with pneumonitis NOS
> Use additional code to identify any secondary pulmonary hypertension, if applicable (I27.2-)

P24.9 Neonatal aspiration, unspecified

✓4ᵗʰ P25 Interstitial emphysema and related conditions originating in the perinatal period

P25.0 Interstitial emphysema originating in the perinatal period

P25.1 Pneumothorax originating in the perinatal period

P25.2 Pneumomediastinum originating in the perinatal period

P25.3 Pneumopericardium originating in the perinatal period

P25.8 Other conditions related to interstitial emphysema originating in the perinatal period

✓4ᵗʰ P26 Pulmonary hemorrhage originating in the perinatal period

> **EXCLUDES 1** *acute idiopathic hemorrhage in infants over 28 days old (R04.81)*

P26.0 Tracheobronchial hemorrhage originating in the perinatal period [COM]

P26.1 Massive pulmonary hemorrhage originating in the perinatal period [COM]

P26.8 Other pulmonary hemorrhages originating in the perinatal period [COM]

P26.9 Unspecified pulmonary hemorrhage originating in the perinatal period [COM]

✓4ᵗʰ P27 Chronic respiratory disease originating in the perinatal period

> **EXCLUDES 2** *respiratory distress of newborn (P22.0-P22.9)*

P27.0 Wilson-Mikity syndrome [COM]
> Pulmonary dysmaturity
> **DEF:** Pulmonary insufficiency in newborn babies, especially those with low birth weight. Rapid onset of hypercapnia and cyanosis occur during the first month of life frequently resulting in death.

P27.1 Bronchopulmonary dysplasia originating in the perinatal period [COM]

P27.8 Other chronic respiratory diseases originating in the perinatal period [COM]
> Congenital pulmonary fibrosis
> Ventilator lung in newborn

P27.9 Unspecified chronic respiratory disease originating in the perinatal period [COM]

✓4ᵗʰ P28 Other respiratory conditions originating in the perinatal period

> ▶Code also, if applicable, congenital malformations of the respiratory system (Q30-Q34)◀
> **EXCLUDES 1** *congenital malformations of the respiratory system (Q30-Q34)*

P28.0 Primary atelectasis of newborn [COM]
> Primary failure to expand terminal respiratory units
> Pulmonary hypoplasia associated with short gestation
> Pulmonary immaturity NOS

✓5ᵗʰ P28.1 Other and unspecified atelectasis of newborn

P28.10 Unspecified atelectasis of newborn [COM]
> Atelectasis of newborn NOS

P28.11 Resorption atelectasis without respiratory distress syndrome [COM]
> **EXCLUDES 1** *resorption atelectasis with respiratory distress syndrome (P22.0)*

P28.19 Other atelectasis of newborn [COM]
> Partial atelectasis of newborn
> Secondary atelectasis of newborn

P28.2 Cyanotic attacks of newborn
> **EXCLUDES 1** *apnea of newborn ▶(P28.3- - P28.4-)◀*

[HCC] CMS-HCC   [Rx] Rx HCC   [ESR] ESRD HCC   [COM] Commercial HCC   [N] Newborn: 0   [P] Pediatric: 0-17   [M] Maternity: 9-64   [A] Adult: 15-124

936   ICD-10-CM 2023

▲   √5ᵗʰ   **P28.3**   Primary **sleep apnea of newborn**
     ~~Central sleep apnea of newborn~~
     ~~Obstructive sleep apnea of newborn~~
     Sleep apnea of newborn NOS
     EXCLUDES 2   ▶*other apnea of newborn (P28.4-)*◀
     DEF: Unexplained cessation of breathing when a neonate makes no respiratory effort for 20 seconds or longer or when a neonate's breathing cessation is accompanied by cyanosis, bradycardia, or hypotonia.

●   **P28.30**   **Primary sleep apnea of newborn, unspecified**
         Transient oxygen desaturation spells of newborn during sleep

●   **P28.31**   **Primary** central **sleep apnea of newborn**
●   **P28.32**   **Primary** obstructive **sleep apnea of newborn**
●   **P28.33**   **Primary** mixed **sleep apnea of newborn**
●   **P28.39**   **Other primary sleep apnea of newborn**

▲   √5ᵗʰ   **P28.4**   **Other apnea of newborn**
     ~~Apnea of prematurity~~
     ~~Obstructive apnea of newborn~~
     EXCLUDES 1   *obstructive sleep apnea of newborn (P28.3)*
     EXCLUDES 2   ▶*primary sleep apnea of newborn (P28.3-)*◀

●   **P28.40**   **Unspecified apnea of newborn**
         Apnea of newborn, NOS
         Transient oxygen desaturation spells of newborn

●   **P28.41**   Central **neonatal apnea of newborn**
●   **P28.42**   Obstructive **apnea of newborn**
●   **P28.43**   Mixed **neonatal apnea of newborn**
●   **P28.49**   **Other apnea of newborn**
         Apnea of prematurity

    P28.5   **Respiratory failure of newborn**   COM
     EXCLUDES 1   *respiratory arrest of newborn (P28.81)*
                 respiratory distress of newborn (P22.0-)
     AHA: 2019,2Q,29

√5ᵗʰ   **P28.8**   **Other specified respiratory conditions of newborn**
    P28.81   **Respiratory arrest of newborn**   COM
    P28.89   **Other specified respiratory conditions of newborn**
         Congenital laryngeal stridor
         Sniffles in newborn
         Snuffles in newborn
         EXCLUDES 1   *early congenital syphilitic rhinitis (A50.05)*

    P28.9   **Respiratory condition of newborn, unspecified**
     Respiratory depression in newborn

√4ᵗʰ   **P29**   **Cardiovascular disorders originating in the perinatal period**
     EXCLUDES 2   *congenital malformations of the circulatory system (Q20-Q28)*

    P29.0   **Neonatal cardiac failure**   COM
√5ᵗʰ   **P29.1**   **Neonatal cardiac dysrhythmia**
    P29.11   **Neonatal** tachycardia
    P29.12   **Neonatal** bradycardia
    P29.2   **Neonatal hypertension**
√5ᵗʰ   **P29.3**   **Persistent fetal circulation**
     AHA: 2017,4Q,20-21
    P29.30   **Pulmonary hypertension of newborn**   COM
         Persistent pulmonary hypertension of newborn
         DEF: Condition that occurs when pressure within the pulmonary artery is elevated and vascular resistance is observed in the lungs.
    P29.38   **Other persistent fetal circulation**   COM
         Delayed closure of ductus arteriosus
    P29.4   **Transient myocardial ischemia in newborn**
√5ᵗʰ   **P29.8**   **Other cardiovascular disorders originating in the perinatal period**
    P29.81   **Cardiac arrest of newborn**   COM
    P29.89   **Other cardiovascular disorders originating in the perinatal period**
         AHA: 2014,4Q,23
    P29.9   **Cardiovascular disorder originating in the perinatal period, unspecified**

Infections specific to the perinatal period (P35-P39)

Infections acquired in utero, during birth via the umbilicus, or during the first 28 days after birth
    EXCLUDES 2   *asymptomatic human immunodeficiency virus [HIV] infection status (Z21)*
                 congenital gonococcal infection (A54.-)
                 congenital pneumonia (P23.-)
                 congenital syphilis (A50.-)
                 human immunodeficiency virus [HIV] disease (B20)
                 infant botulism (A48.51)
                 infectious diseases not specific to the perinatal period (A00-B99, J09, J10.-)
                 intestinal infectious disease (A00-A09)
                 laboratory evidence of human immunodeficiency virus [HIV] (R75)
                 tetanus neonatorum (A33)

√4ᵗʰ   **P35**   **Congenital viral diseases**
    INCLUDES   infections acquired in utero or during birth
    P35.0   **Congenital** rubella **syndrome**
         Congenital rubella pneumonitis
    P35.1   **Congenital** cytomegalovirus **infection**   COM
    P35.2   **Congenital** herpesviral [herpes simplex] **infection**
    P35.3   **Congenital** viral hepatitis
    P35.4   **Congenital** Zika virus **disease**
         Use additional code to identify manifestations of congenital Zika virus disease
         AHA: 2018,4Q,25-26
    P35.8   **Other congenital viral diseases**
         Congenital varicella [chickenpox]
         AHA: 2020,2Q,13
    P35.9   **Congenital viral disease, unspecified**

√4ᵗʰ   **P36**   **Bacterial sepsis of newborn**
    INCLUDES   congenital sepsis
    Use additional code(s), if applicable, to identify severe sepsis (R65.2-) and associated acute organ dysfunction(s)
    P36.0   **Sepsis of newborn due to** streptococcus, group B   HCC ESR COM
√5ᵗʰ   **P36.1**   **Sepsis of newborn due to other and unspecified** streptococci
    P36.10   **Sepsis of newborn due to unspecified streptococci**   HCC ESR COM
    P36.19   **Sepsis of newborn due to other streptococci**   HCC ESR COM
    P36.2   **Sepsis of newborn due to** Staphylococcus aureus   HCC ESR COM
√5ᵗʰ   **P36.3**   **Sepsis of newborn due to other and unspecified** staphylococci
    P36.30   **Sepsis of newborn due to unspecified staphylococci**   HCC ESR COM
    P36.39   **Sepsis of newborn due to other staphylococci**   HCC ESR COM
    P36.4   **Sepsis of newborn due to** Escherichia coli   HCC ESR COM
    P36.5   **Sepsis of newborn due to** anaerobes   HCC ESR COM
    P36.8   **Other** bacterial sepsis **of newborn**   HCC ESR COM
         Use additional code from category B96 to identify organism
    P36.9   **Bacterial sepsis of newborn, unspecified**   HCC ESR COM

√4ᵗʰ   **P37**   **Other congenital infectious and parasitic diseases**
    EXCLUDES 2   *congenital syphilis (A50.-)*
                 infectious neonatal diarrhea (A00-A09)
                 necrotizing enterocolitis in newborn (P77.-)
                 noninfectious neonatal diarrhea (P78.3)
                 ophthalmia neonatorum due to gonococcus (A54.31)
                 tetanus neonatorum (A33)
    P37.0   **Congenital** tuberculosis
    P37.1   **Congenital** toxoplasmosis
         Hydrocephalus due to congenital toxoplasmosis
    P37.2   **Neonatal (disseminated)** listeriosis
    P37.3   **Congenital** falciparum malaria
    P37.4   **Other congenital** malaria
    P37.5   **Neonatal** candidiasis
    P37.8   **Other specified congenital infectious and parasitic diseases**
    P37.9   **Congenital infectious or parasitic disease, unspecified**

✓4ᵗʰ **P38 Omphalitis of newborn**

> EXCLUDES 1   *omphalitis not of newborn (L08.82)*
> *tetanus omphalitis (A33)*
> *umbilical hemorrhage of newborn (P51.-)*

DEF: Omphalitis: Infection and inflammation of the umbilical stump, often due to bacteria that can spread beyond the umbilical stump to the fascia, muscle, or even the umbilical vessels.

P38.1   Omphalitis with mild hemorrhage

P38.9   Omphalitis without hemorrhage
Omphalitis of newborn NOS

✓4ᵗʰ **P39 Other infections specific to the perinatal period**

Use additional code to identify organism or specific infection

P39.0   Neonatal infective mastitis

> EXCLUDES 1   *breast engorgement of newborn (P83.4)*
> *noninfective mastitis of newborn (P83.4)*

P39.1   Neonatal conjunctivitis and dacryocystitis
Neonatal chlamydial conjunctivitis
Ophthalmia neonatorum NOS

> EXCLUDES 1   *gonococcal conjunctivitis (A54.31)*

P39.2   Intra-amniotic infection affecting newborn, not elsewhere classified

P39.3   Neonatal urinary tract infection

P39.4   Neonatal skin infection
Neonatal pyoderma

> EXCLUDES 1   *pemphigus neonatorum (L00)*
> *staphylococcal scalded skin syndrome (L00)*

P39.8   Other specified infections specific to the perinatal period

P39.9   Infection specific to the perinatal period, unspecified

Hemorrhagic and hematological disorders of newborn (P50-P61)

> EXCLUDES 1   *congenital stenosis and stricture of bile ducts (Q44.3)*
> *Crigler-Najjar syndrome (E80.5)*
> *Dubin-Johnson syndrome (E80.6)*
> *Gilbert syndrome (E80.4)*
> *hereditary hemolytic anemias (D55-D58)*

✓4ᵗʰ **P50 Newborn affected by intrauterine (fetal) blood loss**

> EXCLUDES 1   *congenital anemia from intrauterine (fetal) blood loss (P61.3)*

P50.0   Newborn affected by intrauterine (fetal) blood loss from vasa previa

P50.1   Newborn affected by intrauterine (fetal) blood loss from ruptured cord

P50.2   Newborn affected by intrauterine (fetal) blood loss from placenta

P50.3   Newborn affected by hemorrhage into co-twin

P50.4   Newborn affected by hemorrhage into maternal circulation

P50.5   Newborn affected by intrauterine (fetal) blood loss from cut end of co-twin's cord

P50.8   Newborn affected by other intrauterine (fetal) blood loss

P50.9   Newborn affected by intrauterine (fetal) blood loss, unspecified
Newborn affected by fetal hemorrhage NOS

✓4ᵗʰ **P51 Umbilical hemorrhage of newborn**

> EXCLUDES 1   *omphalitis with mild hemorrhage (P38.1)*
> *umbilical hemorrhage from cut end of co-twins cord (P50.5)*

P51.0   Massive umbilical hemorrhage of newborn

P51.8   Other umbilical hemorrhages of newborn
Slipped umbilical ligature NOS

P51.9   Umbilical hemorrhage of newborn, unspecified

✓4ᵗʰ **P52 Intracranial nontraumatic hemorrhage of newborn**

> INCLUDES   intracranial hemorrhage due to anoxia or hypoxia
> EXCLUDES 1   *intracranial hemorrhage due to birth injury (P10.-)*
> *intracranial hemorrhage due to other injury (S06.-)*

P52.0   Intraventricular (nontraumatic) hemorrhage, grade 1, of newborn   COM
Subependymal hemorrhage (without intraventricular extension)
Bleeding into germinal matrix

P52.1   Intraventricular (nontraumatic) hemorrhage, grade 2, of newborn   COM
Subependymal hemorrhage with intraventricular extension
Bleeding into ventricle

✓5ᵗʰ **P52.2   Intraventricular (nontraumatic) hemorrhage, grade 3 and grade 4, of newborn**

P52.21   Intraventricular (nontraumatic) hemorrhage, grade 3, of newborn   COM
Subependymal hemorrhage with intraventricular extension with enlargement of ventricle

P52.22   Intraventricular (nontraumatic) hemorrhage, grade 4, of newborn   COM
Bleeding into cerebral cortex
Subependymal hemorrhage with intracerebral extension

P52.3   Unspecified intraventricular (nontraumatic) hemorrhage of newborn   COM

P52.4   Intracerebral (nontraumatic) hemorrhage of newborn   COM

P52.5   Subarachnoid (nontraumatic) hemorrhage of newborn   COM

P52.6   Cerebellar (nontraumatic) and posterior fossa hemorrhage of newborn   COM

P52.8   Other intracranial (nontraumatic) hemorrhages of newborn   COM

P52.9   Intracranial (nontraumatic) hemorrhage of newborn, unspecified   COM

P53   Hemorrhagic disease of newborn   COM
Vitamin K deficiency of newborn

✓4ᵗʰ **P54 Other neonatal hemorrhages**

> EXCLUDES 1   *newborn affected by (intrauterine) blood loss (P50.-)*
> *pulmonary hemorrhage originating in the perinatal period (P26.-)*

P54.0   Neonatal hematemesis

> EXCLUDES 1   *neonatal hematemesis due to swallowed maternal blood (P78.2)*

P54.1   Neonatal melena

> EXCLUDES 1   *neonatal melena due to swallowed maternal blood (P78.2)*

P54.2   Neonatal rectal hemorrhage

P54.3   Other neonatal gastrointestinal hemorrhage

P54.4   Neonatal adrenal hemorrhage

P54.5   Neonatal cutaneous hemorrhage
Neonatal bruising
Neonatal ecchymoses
Neonatal petechiae
Neonatal superficial hematomata

> EXCLUDES 2   *bruising of scalp due to birth injury (P12.3)*
> *cephalhematoma due to birth injury (P12.0)*

P54.6   Neonatal vaginal hemorrhage   ♀
Neonatal pseudomenses

P54.8   Other specified neonatal hemorrhages

P54.9   Neonatal hemorrhage, unspecified

✓4ᵗʰ **P55 Hemolytic disease of newborn**

P55.0   Rh isoimmunization of newborn   COM
DEF: Incompatible Rh fetal-maternal blood grouping that prematurely destroys red blood cells. Symptoms include jaundice, asphyxia, pulmonary hypertension, edema, respiratory distress, kernicterus, and coagulopathies. It is detected by a Coombs test.
TIP: A positive Coombs test without documentation of associated Rh isoimmunization should be coded to R79.89 Other specified abnormal findings of blood chemistry.

P55.1   ABO isoimmunization of newborn   COM
AHA: 2015,3Q,20

P55.8   Other hemolytic diseases of newborn   COM
AHA: 2018,3Q,24

P55.9   Hemolytic disease of newborn, unspecified   COM

✓4ᵗʰ **P56 Hydrops fetalis due to hemolytic disease**

> EXCLUDES 1   *hydrops fetalis NOS (P83.2)*

P56.0   Hydrops fetalis due to isoimmunization   COM

✓5ᵗʰ **P56.9   Hydrops fetalis due to other and unspecified hemolytic disease**

P56.90   Hydrops fetalis due to unspecified hemolytic disease   COM

P56.99   Hydrops fetalis due to other hemolytic disease   COM

✓4ᵗʰ P57 Kernicterus

P57.0 Kernicterus due to isoimmunization `COM`
DEF: Complication of erythroblastosis fetalis associated with severe neural symptoms, high blood bilirubin levels, and nerve cell destruction. It results in bilirubin-pigmented gray matter of the central nervous system.

P57.8 Other specified kernicterus `COM`
EXCLUDES 1 *Crigler-Najjar syndrome (E80.5)*

P57.9 Kernicterus, unspecified `COM`

✓4ᵗʰ P58 Neonatal jaundice due to other excessive hemolysis
EXCLUDES 1 *jaundice due to isoimmunization (P55-P57)*

P58.0 Neonatal jaundice due to bruising
P58.1 Neonatal jaundice due to bleeding
P58.2 Neonatal jaundice due to infection
P58.3 Neonatal jaundice due to polycythemia

✓5ᵗʰ P58.4 Neonatal jaundice due to drugs or toxins transmitted from mother or given to newborn
Code first poisoning due to drug or toxin, if applicable (T36-T65 with fifth or sixth character 1-4 or 6)
Use additional code for adverse effect, if applicable, to identify drug (T36-T50 with fifth or sixth character 5)

P58.41 Neonatal jaundice due to drugs or toxins transmitted from mother
P58.42 Neonatal jaundice due to drugs or toxins given to newborn

P58.5 Neonatal jaundice due to swallowed maternal blood
P58.8 Neonatal jaundice due to other specified excessive hemolysis
P58.9 Neonatal jaundice due to excessive hemolysis, unspecified

✓4ᵗʰ P59 Neonatal jaundice from other and unspecified causes
EXCLUDES 1 *jaundice due to inborn errors of metabolism (E70-E88)*
kernicterus (P57.-)

P59.0 Neonatal jaundice associated with preterm delivery
Hyperbilirubinemia of prematurity
Jaundice due to delayed conjugation associated with preterm delivery

P59.1 Inspissated bile syndrome `COM`
DEF: Biliary obstruction in newborn resulting from obstruction of outflow tract.

✓5ᵗʰ P59.2 Neonatal jaundice from other and unspecified hepatocellular damage
EXCLUDES 1 *congenital viral hepatitis (P35.3)*

P59.20 Neonatal jaundice from unspecified hepatocellular damage `COM`
P59.29 Neonatal jaundice from other hepatocellular damage `COM`
Neonatal giant cell hepatitis
Neonatal (idiopathic) hepatitis

P59.3 Neonatal jaundice from breast milk inhibitor
P59.8 Neonatal jaundice from other specified causes
P59.9 Neonatal jaundice, unspecified
Neonatal physiological jaundice (intense)(prolonged) NOS
AHA: 2015,3Q,20

P60 Disseminated intravascular coagulation of newborn `COM`
Defibrination syndrome of newborn

✓4ᵗʰ P61 Other perinatal hematological disorders
EXCLUDES 1 *transient hypogammaglobulinemia of infancy (D80.7)*

P61.0 Transient neonatal thrombocytopenia `COM`
Neonatal thrombocytopenia due to exchange transfusion
Neonatal thrombocytopenia due to idiopathic maternal thrombocytopenia
Neonatal thrombocytopenia due to isoimmunization
DEF: Temporary decrease in blood platelets of a newborn that is secondary to placental insufficiency.

P61.1 Polycythemia neonatorum
DEF: Abnormal increase of total red blood cells of a newborn that results in hyperviscosity, which slows the flow of blood through small blood vessels.

P61.2 Anemia of prematurity
P61.3 Congenital anemia from fetal blood loss
P61.4 Other congenital anemias, not elsewhere classified
Congenital anemia NOS

P61.5 Transient neonatal neutropenia `COM`
EXCLUDES 1 *congenital neutropenia (nontransient) (D70.0)*
DEF: Low blood neutrophil counts of newborn that occurs due to maternal hypertension, sepsis, twin-twin transfusion, alloimmunization, and hemolytic disease.

P61.6 Other transient neonatal disorders of coagulation `COM`
P61.8 Other specified perinatal hematological disorders
P61.9 Perinatal hematological disorder, unspecified

Transitory endocrine and metabolic disorders specific to newborn (P70-P74)

INCLUDES transitory endocrine and metabolic disturbances caused by the infant's response to maternal endocrine and metabolic factors, or its adjustment to extrauterine environment
AHA: 2018,2Q,6

✓4ᵗʰ P70 Transitory disorders of carbohydrate metabolism specific to newborn

P70.0 Syndrome of infant of mother with gestational diabetes
Newborn (with hypoglycemia) affected by maternal gestational diabetes
EXCLUDES 1 *newborn (with hypoglycemia) affected by maternal (pre-existing) diabetes mellitus (P70.1)*
syndrome of infant of a diabetic mother (P70.1)

P70.1 Syndrome of infant of a diabetic mother
Newborn (with hypoglycemia) affected by maternal (pre-existing) diabetes mellitus
EXCLUDES 1 *newborn (with hypoglycemia) affected by maternal gestational diabetes (P70.0)*
syndrome of infant of mother with gestational diabetes (P70.0)

P70.2 Neonatal diabetes mellitus
P70.3 Iatrogenic neonatal hypoglycemia
P70.4 Other neonatal hypoglycemia
Transitory neonatal hypoglycemia
P70.8 Other transitory disorders of carbohydrate metabolism of newborn
P70.9 Transitory disorder of carbohydrate metabolism of newborn, unspecified

✓4ᵗʰ P71 Transitory neonatal disorders of calcium and magnesium metabolism
P71.0 Cow's milk hypocalcemia in newborn
P71.1 Other neonatal hypocalcemia
EXCLUDES 1 *neonatal hypoparathyroidism (P71.4)*
P71.2 Neonatal hypomagnesemia
P71.3 Neonatal tetany without calcium or magnesium deficiency
Neonatal tetany NOS
P71.4 Transitory neonatal hypoparathyroidism
P71.8 Other transitory neonatal disorders of calcium and magnesium metabolism
AHA: 2016,4Q,54
P71.9 Transitory neonatal disorder of calcium and magnesium metabolism, unspecified

✓4ᵗʰ P72 Other transitory neonatal endocrine disorders
EXCLUDES 1 *congenital hypothyroidism with or without goiter (E03.0-E03.1)*
dyshormogenetic goiter (E07.1)
Pendred's syndrome (E07.1)

P72.0 Neonatal goiter, not elsewhere classified
Transitory congenital goiter with normal functioning
P72.1 Transitory neonatal hyperthyroidism
Neonatal thyrotoxicosis
P72.2 Other transitory neonatal disorders of thyroid function, not elsewhere classified
Transitory neonatal hypothyroidism
P72.8 Other specified transitory neonatal endocrine disorders
P72.9 Transitory neonatal endocrine disorder, unspecified

✓4ᵗʰ P74 Other transitory neonatal electrolyte and metabolic disturbances
AHA: 2018,4Q,26-27
P74.0 Late metabolic acidosis of newborn
EXCLUDES 1 *(fetal) metabolic acidosis of newborn (P19)*
P74.1 Dehydration of newborn
✓5ᵗʰ P74.2 Disturbances of sodium balance of newborn
P74.21 Hypernatremia of newborn
P74.22 Hyponatremia of newborn
✓5ᵗʰ P74.3 Disturbances of potassium balance of newborn
P74.31 Hyperkalemia of newborn

P74.32   **Hypokalemia** of newborn

√5ᵗʰ P74.4   **Other transitory electrolyte disturbances of newborn**

   P74.41   **Alkalosis** of newborn
     Hyperbicarbonatemia

√6ᵗʰ P74.42   **Disturbances of chlorine balance of newborn**

     P74.421   **Hyperchloremia** of newborn
       Hyperchloremic metabolic acidosis
       EXCLUDES 2   *late metabolic acidosis of the newborn (P74.0)*

     P74.422   **Hypochloremia** of newborn

   P74.49   **Other transitory electrolyte disturbance of newborn**

P74.5   **Transitory tyrosinemia of newborn**

P74.6   **Transitory hyperammonemia of newborn**

P74.8   **Other transitory metabolic disturbances of newborn**
   Amino-acid metabolic disorders described as transitory

P74.9   **Transitory metabolic disturbance of newborn, unspecified**

Digestive system disorders of newborn (P76-P78)

√4ᵗʰ **P76**   **Other intestinal obstruction of newborn**

P76.0   **Meconium plug syndrome**
   Meconium ileus NOS
   EXCLUDES 1   *meconium ileus in cystic fibrosis (E84.11)*
   DEF: Meconium obstruction of a newborn's intestines, resulting from unusually thick or hard meconium.

P76.1   **Transitory ileus of newborn**
   EXCLUDES 1   *Hirschsprung's disease (Q43.1)*

P76.2   **Intestinal obstruction due to inspissated milk**

P76.8   **Other specified intestinal obstruction of newborn**
   EXCLUDES 1   *intestinal obstruction classifiable to K56.-*

P76.9   **Intestinal obstruction of newborn, unspecified**

√4ᵗʰ **P77**   **Necrotizing enterocolitis of newborn**
   DEF: Serious intestinal infection and inflammation in preterm infants. Severity is measured by stages and may progress to life-threatening perforation or peritonitis. Resection surgical treatment may be necessary.

P77.1   **Stage 1 necrotizing enterocolitis in newborn**   COM
   Necrotizing enterocolitis without pneumatosis, without perforation
   DEF: Broad-spectrum symptoms with nonspecific signs, including feeding intolerance, abdominal distention, bradycardia, and metabolic abnormalities.

P77.2   **Stage 2 necrotizing enterocolitis in newborn**   COM
   Necrotizing enterocolitis with pneumatosis, without perforation
   DEF: Radiographic confirmation of necrotizing enterocolitis showing intestinal dilatation, fixed loops of bowels, pneumatosis intestinalis, metabolic acidosis, and thrombocytopenia.

P77.3   **Stage 3 necrotizing enterocolitis in newborn**   COM
   Necrotizing enterocolitis with perforation
   Necrotizing enterocolitis with pneumatosis and perforation
   DEF: Advanced stage in which an infant demonstrates signs of bowel perforation, septic shock, metabolic acidosis, ascites, disseminated intravascular coagulopathy, and neutropenia.

P77.9   **Necrotizing enterocolitis in newborn, unspecified**   COM
   Necrotizing enterocolitis in newborn, NOS

√4ᵗʰ **P78**   **Other perinatal digestive system disorders**
   EXCLUDES 1   *cystic fibrosis (E84.0-E84.9)*
       neonatal gastrointestinal hemorrhages (P54.0-P54.3)

P78.0   **Perinatal intestinal perforation**   COM
   Meconium peritonitis

P78.1   **Other neonatal peritonitis**
   Neonatal peritonitis NOS

P78.2   **Neonatal hematemesis and melena due to swallowed maternal blood**

P78.3   **Noninfective neonatal diarrhea**
   Neonatal diarrhea NOS

√5ᵗʰ P78.8   **Other specified perinatal digestive system disorders**

   P78.81   **Congenital cirrhosis (of liver)**

   P78.82   **Peptic ulcer of newborn**

   P78.83   **Newborn esophageal reflux**
     Neonatal esophageal reflux

   P78.84   **Gestational alloimmune liver disease**   COM
     GALD
     Neonatal hemochromatosis
     EXCLUDES 1   *hemochromatosis (E83.11-)*
     AHA: 2017,4Q,21
     DEF: Severe hepatic injury with onset during fetal development with manifestations beginning during fetal life. It is due to maternal antibodies to fetal hepatic cells (hepatocytes) that cross the placenta into the fetal circulation, causing hepatic cell necrosis.

   P78.89   **Other specified perinatal digestive system disorders**

P78.9   **Perinatal digestive system disorder, unspecified**

Conditions involving the integument and temperature regulation of newborn (P80-P83)

√4ᵗʰ **P80**   **Hypothermia of newborn**
   DEF: Decrease in newborn body temperature due to their larger ratio of surface area to body weight, thin skin with blood vessels close to the surface, and a limited amount of subcutaneous fat.

P80.0   **Cold injury syndrome**
   Severe and usually chronic hypothermia associated with a pink flushed appearance, edema and neurological and biochemical abnormalities.
   EXCLUDES 1   *mild hypothermia of newborn (P80.8)*

P80.8   **Other hypothermia of newborn**
   Mild hypothermia of newborn

P80.9   **Hypothermia of newborn, unspecified**

√4ᵗʰ **P81**   **Other disturbances of temperature regulation of newborn**

P81.0   **Environmental hyperthermia of newborn**

P81.8   **Other specified disturbances of temperature regulation of newborn**

P81.9   **Disturbance of temperature regulation of newborn, unspecified**
   Fever of newborn NOS

√4ᵗʰ **P83**   **Other conditions of integument specific to newborn**
   EXCLUDES 1   *congenital malformations of skin and integument (Q80-Q84)*
       hydrops fetalis due to hemolytic disease (P56.-)
       neonatal skin infection (P39.4)
       staphylococcal scalded skin syndrome (L00)
   EXCLUDES 2   *cradle cap (L21.0)*
       diaper [napkin] dermatitis (L22)

P83.0   **Sclerema neonatorum**
   DEF: Diffuse, rapidly progressing white, waxy, nonpitting hardening of tissue, usually of legs and feet that is life-threatening. It is found in preterm or debilitated infants. Etiology is unknown.

P83.1   **Neonatal erythema toxicum**

P83.2   **Hydrops fetalis not due to hemolytic disease**
   Hydrops fetalis NOS
   DEF: Severe, life-threatening problem of a newborn characterized by severe edema of the entire body. It is unrelated to immune response.

√5ᵗʰ P83.3   **Other and unspecified edema specific to newborn**

   P83.30   **Unspecified edema specific to newborn**

   P83.39   **Other edema specific to newborn**

P83.4   **Breast engorgement of newborn**
   Noninfective mastitis of newborn

P83.5   **Congenital hydrocele**   ♂
   DEF: Hydrocele: Serous fluid that collects in the tunica vaginalis of the scrotum along the spermatic cord in males.

P83.6   **Umbilical polyp of newborn**

√5ᵗʰ P83.8   **Other specified conditions of integument specific to newborn**
   AHA: 2017,4Q,21-22

   P83.81   **Umbilical granuloma**
     EXCLUDES 2   *granulomatous disorder of the skin and subcutaneous tissue, unspecified (L92.9)*

   P83.88   **Other specified conditions of integument specific to newborn**
     Bronze baby syndrome
     Neonatal scleroderma
     Urticaria neonatorum

P83.9   **Condition of the integument specific to newborn, unspecified**

Other problems with newborn (P84)

P84 Other problems with newborn
Acidemia of newborn
Acidosis of newborn
Anoxia of newborn NOS
Asphyxia of newborn NOS
Hypercapnia of newborn
Hypoxemia of newborn
Hypoxia of newborn NOS
Mixed metabolic and respiratory acidosis of newborn
  EXCLUDES 1   intracranial hemorrhage due to anoxia or hypoxia (P52.-)
        hypoxic ischemic encephalopathy [HIE] (P91.6-)
        late metabolic acidosis of newborn (P74.0)

Other disorders originating in the perinatal period (P90-P96)

P90 Convulsions of newborn   COM
  EXCLUDES 1   benign myoclonic epilepsy in infancy (G40.3-)
        benign neonatal convulsions (familial) (G40.3-)

✓4ᵗʰ **P91 Other disturbances of cerebral status of newborn**

  P91.0 Neonatal cerebral ischemia   COM
      EXCLUDES 1   neonatal cerebral infarction (P91.82-)

  P91.1 Acquired periventricular cysts of newborn   COM

  P91.2 Neonatal cerebral leukomalacia   COM
      Periventricular leukomalacia

  P91.3 Neonatal cerebral irritability   COM

  P91.4 Neonatal cerebral depression   COM

  P91.5 Neonatal coma   COM

  ✓5ᵗʰ **P91.6 Hypoxic ischemic encephalopathy [HIE]**
      EXCLUDES 1   neonatal cerebral depression (P91.4)
            neonatal cerebral irritability (P91.3)
            neonatal coma (P91.5)
      AHA: 2017,4Q,22

    P91.60 Hypoxic ischemic encephalopathy [HIE], unspecified   COM

    P91.61 Mild hypoxic ischemic encephalopathy [HIE]   COM

    P91.62 Moderate hypoxic ischemic encephalopathy [HIE]   COM

    P91.63 Severe hypoxic ischemic encephalopathy [HIE]   COM

  ✓5ᵗʰ **P91.8 Other specified disturbances of cerebral status of newborn**
      AHA: 2017,4Q,22

    ✓6ᵗʰ **P91.81 Neonatal encephalopathy**

      P91.811 Neonatal encephalopathy in diseases classified elsewhere   COM
            Code first underlying condition, if known, such as:
            congenital cirrhosis (of liver) (P78.81)
            intracranial nontraumatic hemorrhage of newborn (P52.-)
            kernicterus (P57.-)

      P91.819 Neonatal encephalopathy, unspecified   COM

    ✓6ᵗʰ **P91.82 Neonatal cerebral infarction**
          Neonatal stroke
          Perinatal arterial ischemic stroke
          Perinatal cerebral infarction
          EXCLUDES 1   cerebral infarction (I63.-)
          EXCLUDES 2   intracranial hemorrhage of newborn (P52.-)
          AHA: 2020,4Q,37-38

      P91.821 Neonatal cerebral infarction, right side of brain   HCC ESR COM

      P91.822 Neonatal cerebral infarction, left side of brain   HCC ESR COM

      P91.823 Neonatal cerebral infarction, bilateral   HCC ESR COM

      P91.829 Neonatal cerebral infarction, unspecified side   HCC ESR COM

    P91.88 Other specified disturbances of cerebral status of newborn   COM

  P91.9 Disturbance of cerebral status of newborn, unspecified   COM

✓4ᵗʰ **P92 Feeding problems of newborn**
    EXCLUDES 1   eating disorders (F50.-)
    EXCLUDES 2   feeding problems in child over 28 days old (R63.3)
    AHA: 2016,3Q,19

  ✓5ᵗʰ **P92.0 Vomiting of newborn**
      EXCLUDES 1   vomiting of child over 28 days old (R11.-)

    P92.01 Bilious vomiting of newborn
        EXCLUDES 1   bilious vomiting in child over 28 days old (R11.14)

    P92.09 Other vomiting of newborn
        EXCLUDES 1   regurgitation of food in newborn (P92.1)

  P92.1 Regurgitation and rumination of newborn

  P92.2 Slow feeding of newborn

  P92.3 Underfeeding of newborn

  P92.4 Overfeeding of newborn

  P92.5 Neonatal difficulty in feeding at breast
      AHA: 2017,1Q,28

  P92.6 Failure to thrive in newborn
      EXCLUDES 1   failure to thrive in child over 28 days old (R62.51)

  P92.8 Other feeding problems of newborn

  P92.9 Feeding problem of newborn, unspecified

✓4ᵗʰ **P93 Reactions and intoxications due to drugs administered to newborn**
    INCLUDES   reactions and intoxications due to drugs administered to fetus affecting newborn
    EXCLUDES 1   jaundice due to drugs or toxins transmitted from mother or given to newborn (P58.4-)
          reactions and intoxications from maternal opiates, tranquilizers and other medication (P04.0-P04.1, P04.4-)
          withdrawal symptoms from maternal use of drugs of addiction (P96.1)
          withdrawal symptoms from therapeutic use of drugs in newborn (P96.2)

  P93.0 Grey baby syndrome   COM
      Grey syndrome from chloramphenicol administration in newborn

  P93.8 Other reactions and intoxications due to drugs administered to newborn   COM
      Use additional code for adverse effect, if applicable, to identify drug (T36-T50 with fifth or sixth character 5)

✓4ᵗʰ **P94 Disorders of muscle tone of newborn**

  P94.0 Transient neonatal myasthenia gravis
      EXCLUDES 1   myasthenia gravis (G70.0)

  P94.1 Congenital hypertonia

  P94.2 Congenital hypotonia
      Floppy baby syndrome, unspecified

  P94.8 Other disorders of muscle tone of newborn

  P94.9 Disorder of muscle tone of newborn, unspecified

P95 Stillbirth
    Deadborn fetus NOS
    Fetal death of unspecified cause
    Stillbirth NOS
    EXCLUDES 1   maternal care for intrauterine death (O36.4)
          missed abortion (O02.1)
          outcome of delivery, stillbirth (Z37.1, Z37.3, Z37.4, Z37.7)

✓4ᵗʰ **P96 Other conditions originating in the perinatal period**

  P96.0 Congenital renal failure
      Uremia of newborn

  P96.1 Neonatal withdrawal symptoms from maternal use of drugs of addiction   COM
      Drug withdrawal syndrome in infant of dependent mother
      Neonatal abstinence syndrome
      EXCLUDES 1   reactions and intoxications from maternal opiates and tranquilizers administered during labor and delivery (P04.0)
      AHA: 2018,4Q,24-25

  P96.2 Withdrawal symptoms from therapeutic use of drugs in newborn   COM

  P96.3 Wide cranial sutures of newborn
      Neonatal craniotabes

  P96.5 Complication to newborn due to (fetal) intrauterine procedure
      EXCLUDES 2   newborn affected by amniocentesis (P00.6)

✓5ᵗʰ **P96.8 Other specified conditions originating in the perinatal period**

    P96.81 Exposure to (parental) (environmental) tobacco smoke in the perinatal period

        EXCLUDES 2   *newborn affected by in utero exposure to tobacco (P04.2)*

                        exposure to environmental tobacco smoke after the perinatal period (Z77.22)

    P96.82 Delayed separation of umbilical cord

    P96.83 Meconium staining

        EXCLUDES 1   *meconium aspiration (P24.00, P24.01)*

                        meconium passage during delivery (P03.82)

        DEF: Meconium passed in utero causing discoloration on the fetal skin and nails or on the umbilicus. This staining may be incidental or may be an indicator of significant fetal stress that could affect outcomes.

    P96.89 Other specified conditions originating in the perinatal period

        Use additional code to specify condition

P96.9 Condition originating in the perinatal period, unspecified

    Congenital debility NOS

Chapter 17. Congenital Malformations, Deformations, and Chromosomal Abnormalities (Q00–Q99)

Chapter-specific Guidelines with Coding Examples

The chapter-specific guidelines from the ICD-10-CM Official Guidelines for Coding and Reporting have been provided below. Along with these guidelines are coding examples, contained in the shaded boxes, that have been developed to help illustrate the coding and/or sequencing guidance found in these guidelines.

Assign an appropriate code(s) from categories Q00-Q99, Congenital malformations, deformations, and chromosomal abnormalities when a malformation/deformation or chromosomal abnormality is documented. A malformation/deformation/or chromosomal abnormality may be the principal/first-listed diagnosis on a record or a secondary diagnosis.

When a malformation/deformation/or chromosomal abnormality does not have a unique code assignment, assign additional code(s) for any manifestations that may be present.

When the code assignment specifically identifies the malformation/deformation/or chromosomal abnormality, manifestations that are an inherent component of the anomaly should not be coded separately. Additional codes should be assigned for manifestations that are not an inherent component.

8-day-old infant with tetralogy of Fallot and pulmonary stenosis

Q21.3   **Tetralogy of Fallot**

Explanation: Pulmonary stenosis is inherent in the disease process of tetralogy of Fallot. When the code assignment specifically identifies the malformation/deformation/or chromosomal abnormality, manifestations that are inherent components of the anomaly should not be coded separately.

7-month-old infant with Down syndrome and common atrioventricular canal

Q90.9   **Down syndrome, unspecified**

Q21.23   **Complete atrioventricular septal defect**

Explanation: While a common atrioventricular canal is often associated with patients with Down syndrome, this manifestation is not an inherent component and may be reported separately. When the code assignment specifically identifies the anomaly, manifestations that are inherent components of the condition should not be coded separately. Additional codes should be assigned for manifestations that are not inherent components.

Codes from Chapter 17 may be used throughout the life of the patient. If a congenital malformation or deformity has been corrected, a personal history code should be used to identify the history of the malformation or deformity. Although present at birth, a malformation/deformation/or chromosomal abnormality may not be identified until later in life. Whenever the condition is diagnosed by the provider, it is appropriate to assign a code from codes Q00-Q99. For the birth admission, the appropriate code from category Z38, Liveborn infants, according to place of birth and type of delivery, should be sequenced as the principal diagnosis, followed by any congenital anomaly codes, Q00- Q99.

Three-year-old with history of corrected ventricular septal defect

Z87.74   **Personal history of (corrected) congenital malformations of heart and circulatory system**

Explanation: If a congenital malformation or deformity has been corrected, a personal history code should be used to identify the history of the malformation or deformity.

Forty-year-old man with headaches diagnosed with congenital arteriovenous malformation of cerebral vessels by brain scan

Q28.2   **Arteriovenous malformation of cerebral vessels**

Explanation: Although present at birth, malformations may not be identified until later in life. Whenever a congenital condition is diagnosed by the physician, it is appropriate to assign a code from the range Q00–Q99.

Chapter 17. Congenital Malformations, Deformations and Chromosomal Abnormalities (Q00-Q99)

NOTE Codes from this chapter are not for use on maternal records

EXCLUDES 2 *inborn errors of metabolism (E70-E88)*

This chapter contains the following blocks:

Q00-Q07 Congenital malformations of the nervous system
Q10-Q18 Congenital malformations of eye, ear, face and neck
Q20-Q28 Congenital malformations of the circulatory system
Q30-Q34 Congenital malformations of the respiratory system
Q35-Q37 Cleft lip and cleft palate
Q38-Q45 Other congenital malformations of the digestive system
Q50-Q56 Congenital malformations of genital organs
Q60-Q64 Congenital malformations of the urinary system
Q65-Q79 Congenital malformations and deformations of the musculoskeletal system
Q80-Q89 Other congenital malformations
Q90-Q99 Chromosomal abnormalities, not elsewhere classified

Congenital malformations of the nervous system (Q00-Q07)

☑4ᵗʰ **Q00 Anencephaly and similar malformations**

Q00.0 Anencephaly HCC Rx ESR COM
Acephaly
Acrania
Amyelencephaly
Hemianencephaly
Hemicephaly

Q00.1 Craniorachischisis HCC Rx ESR COM

Q00.2 Iniencephaly HCC Rx ESR COM

☑4ᵗʰ **Q01 Encephalocele**

INCLUDES Arnold-Chiari syndrome, type III
encephalocystocele
encephalomyelocele
hydroencephalocele
hydromeningocele, cranial
meningocele, cerebral
meningoencephalocele

EXCLUDES 1 *Meckel-Gruber syndrome (Q61.9)*

DEF: Congenital protrusion of brain tissue through a defect in the skull.

Q01.0 Frontal encephalocele HCC Rx ESR COM

Q01.1 Nasofrontal encephalocele HCC Rx ESR COM

Q01.2 Occipital encephalocele HCC Rx ESR COM

Q01.8 Encephalocele of other sites HCC Rx ESR COM

Q01.9 Encephalocele, unspecified HCC Rx ESR COM

Q02 Microcephaly HCC Rx ESR COM

INCLUDES hydromicrocephaly
micrencephalon

Code first, if applicable, congenital Zika virus disease

EXCLUDES 1 *Meckel-Gruber syndrome (Q61.9)*

AHA: 2018,4Q,26

DEF: Congenital disorder in which the head circumference is more than two standard deviations below the mean for age, sex, race, and gestation and associated with a decreased life expectancy.

☑4ᵗʰ **Q03 Congenital hydrocephalus**

INCLUDES hydrocephalus in newborn

EXCLUDES 1 *Arnold-Chiari syndrome, type II (Q07.0-)*
acquired hydrocephalus (G91.-)
hydrocephalus due to congenital toxoplasmosis (P37.1)
hydrocephalus with spina bifida (Q05.0-Q05.4)

DEF: Hydrocephalus: Abnormal buildup of cerebrospinal fluid in the brain causing dilation of the ventricles.

Congenital Hydrocephalus

Pressure

Normal ventricles   Hydrocephalic ventricles

Q03.0 Malformations of aqueduct of Sylvius HCC Rx ESR COM
Anomaly of aqueduct of Sylvius
Obstruction of aqueduct of Sylvius, congenital
Stenosis of aqueduct of Sylvius

Q03.1 Atresia of foramina of Magendie and Luschka HCC Rx ESR COM
Dandy-Walker syndrome

Q03.8 Other congenital hydrocephalus HCC Rx ESR COM

Q03.9 Congenital hydrocephalus, unspecified HCC Rx ESR COM

☑4ᵗʰ **Q04 Other congenital malformations of brain**

EXCLUDES 1 *cyclopia (Q87.0)*
macrocephaly (Q75.3)

Q04.0 Congenital malformations of corpus callosum HCC Rx ESR COM
Agenesis of corpus callosum

Q04.1 Arhinencephaly HCC Rx ESR COM

Q04.2 Holoprosencephaly HCC Rx ESR COM

Q04.3 Other reduction deformities of brain HCC Rx ESR COM
Absence of part of brain
Agenesis of part of brain
Agyria
Aplasia of part of brain
Hydranencephaly
Hypoplasia of part of brain
Lissencephaly
Microgyria
Pachygyria

EXCLUDES 1 *congenital malformations of corpus callosum (Q04.0)*

Q04.4 Septo-optic dysplasia of brain HCC Rx ESR COM

Q04.5 Megalencephaly HCC Rx ESR COM

Q04.6 Congenital cerebral cysts HCC Rx ESR COM
Porencephaly
Schizencephaly

EXCLUDES 1 *acquired porencephalic cyst (G93.0)*

Q04.8 Other specified congenital malformations of brain HCC Rx ESR COM
Arnold-Chiari syndrome, type IV
Macrogyria

Q04.9 Congenital malformation of brain, unspecified HCC Rx ESR COM
Congenital anomaly NOS of brain
Congenital deformity NOS of brain
Congenital disease or lesion NOS of brain
Multiple anomalies NOS of brain, congenital

✓4th Q05 Spina bifida

INCLUDES   hydromeningocele (spinal)
    meningocele (spinal)
    meningomyelocele
    myelocele
    myelomeningocele
    rachischisis
    spina bifida (aperta)(cystica)
    syringomyelocele

Use additional code for any associated paraplegia (paraparesis) (G82.2-)

EXCLUDES 1   Arnold-Chiari syndrome, type II (Q07.0-)
    spina bifida occulta (Q76.0)

DEF: Lack of closure in the vertebral column with protrusion of the spinal cord through the defect, often in the lumbosacral area. This condition can be recognized by the presence of alpha-fetoproteins in the amniotic fluid.

Spina Bifida

Spina bifida occulta   Meningocele   Myelomeningocele

Q05.0 **Cervical spina bifida with hydrocephalus**   HCC Rx ESR COM

Q05.1 **Thoracic spina bifida with hydrocephalus**   HCC Rx ESR COM
    Dorsal spina bifida with hydrocephalus
    Thoracolumbar spina bifida with hydrocephalus

Q05.2 **Lumbar spina bifida with hydrocephalus**   HCC Rx ESR COM
    Lumbosacral spina bifida with hydrocephalus

Q05.3 **Sacral spina bifida with hydrocephalus**   HCC Rx ESR COM

Q05.4 **Unspecified spina bifida with hydrocephalus**   HCC Rx ESR COM

Q05.5 **Cervical spina bifida without hydrocephalus**   HCC Rx ESR COM

Q05.6 **Thoracic spina bifida without hydrocephalus**   HCC Rx ESR COM
    Dorsal spina bifida NOS
    Thoracolumbar spina bifida NOS

Q05.7 **Lumbar spina bifida without hydrocephalus**   HCC Rx ESR COM
    Lumbosacral spina bifida NOS

Q05.8 **Sacral spina bifida without hydrocephalus**   HCC Rx ESR COM

Q05.9 **Spina bifida, unspecified**   HCC Rx ESR COM

✓4th Q06 Other congenital malformations of spinal cord

Q06.0 **Amyelia**   HCC Rx ESR COM

Q06.1 **Hypoplasia and dysplasia of spinal cord**   HCC Rx ESR COM
    Atelomyelia
    Myelatelia
    Myelodysplasia of spinal cord

Q06.2 **Diastematomyelia**   HCC Rx ESR COM
    DEF: Rare congenital anomaly often associated with spina bifida. The spinal cord is separated into longitudinal halves by a bony, cartilaginous or fibrous septum, each half surrounded by a dural sac.

Q06.3 **Other congenital cauda equina malformations**   HCC Rx ESR COM

Q06.4 **Hydromyelia**   HCC Rx ESR COM
    Hydrorachis

Q06.8 **Other specified congenital malformations of spinal cord**   HCC Rx ESR COM

Q06.9 **Congenital malformation of spinal cord, unspecified**   HCC Rx ESR COM
    Congenital anomaly NOS of spinal cord
    Congenital deformity NOS of spinal cord
    Congenital disease or lesion NOS of spinal cord

✓4th Q07 Other congenital malformations of nervous system

EXCLUDES 2   congenital central alveolar hypoventilation syndrome (G47.35)
    familial dysautonomia [Riley-Day] (G90.1)
    neurofibromatosis (nonmalignant) (Q85.0-)

✓5th Q07.0 Arnold-Chiari syndrome

Arnold-Chiari syndrome, type II

EXCLUDES 1   Arnold-Chiari syndrome, type III (Q01.-)
    Arnold-Chiari syndrome, type IV (Q04.8)

DEF: Congenital malformation of the brain in which the cerebellum protrudes through the foramen magnum into the spinal canal.

Q07.00 **Arnold-Chiari syndrome** without spina bifida or hydrocephalus   HCC Rx ESR COM

Q07.01 **Arnold-Chiari syndrome** with spina bifida   HCC Rx ESR COM

Q07.02 **Arnold-Chiari syndrome** with hydrocephalus   HCC Rx ESR COM

Q07.03 **Arnold-Chiari syndrome** with spina bifida and hydrocephalus   HCC Rx ESR COM

Q07.8 **Other specified congenital malformations of nervous system**   HCC Rx ESR COM
    Agenesis of nerve
    Displacement of brachial plexus
    Jaw-winking syndrome
    Marcus Gunn's syndrome

Q07.9 **Congenital malformation of nervous system, unspecified**   HCC Rx ESR COM
    Congenital anomaly NOS of nervous system
    Congenital deformity NOS of nervous system
    Congenital disease or lesion NOS of nervous system

Congenital malformations of eye, ear, face and neck (Q10-Q18)

EXCLUDES 2   cleft lip and cleft palate (Q35-Q37)
    congenital malformation of cervical spine (Q05.0, Q05.5, Q67.5, Q76.0-Q76.4)
    congenital malformation of larynx (Q31.-)
    congenital malformation of lip NEC (Q38.0)
    congenital malformation of nose (Q30.-)
    congenital malformation of parathyroid gland (Q89.2)
    congenital malformation of thyroid gland (Q89.2)

✓4th Q10 Congenital malformations of eyelid, lacrimal apparatus and orbit

EXCLUDES 1   cryptophthalmos NOS (Q11.2)
    cryptophthalmos syndrome (Q87.0)

Q10.0 **Congenital ptosis**
    DEF: Congenital drooping of the eyelid. Ptosis is mostly idiopathic, but may occur genetically.

Q10.1 **Congenital ectropion**

Q10.2 **Congenital entropion**

Q10.3 **Other congenital malformations of eyelid**
    Ablepharon
    Blepharophimosis, congenital
    Coloboma of eyelid
    Congenital absence or agenesis of cilia
    Congenital absence or agenesis of eyelid
    Congenital accessory eyelid
    Congenital accessory eye muscle
    Congenital malformation of eyelid NOS

Q10.4 **Absence and agenesis of lacrimal apparatus**
    Congenital absence of punctum lacrimale

Q10.5 **Congenital stenosis and stricture of lacrimal duct**

Q10.6 **Other congenital malformations of lacrimal apparatus**
    Congenital malformation of lacrimal apparatus NOS

Q10.7 **Congenital malformation of orbit**

✓4th Q11 Anophthalmos, microphthalmos and macrophthalmos

Q11.0 **Cystic eyeball**

Q11.1 **Other anophthalmos**
    Anophthalmos NOS
    Agenesis of eye
    Aplasia of eye

Q11.2 **Microphthalmos**
    Cryptophthalmos NOS
    Dysplasia of eye
    Hypoplasia of eye
    Rudimentary eye

EXCLUDES 1   cryptophthalmos syndrome (Q87.0)

✓ Additional Character Required   ✓x7th Placeholder Alert   Manifestation   Unspecified Dx   Q QPP   UPD Unacceptable PDx

Q11.3 Macrophthalmos
> EXCLUDES 1   *macrophthalmos in congenital glaucoma (Q15.0)*

✓4ᵗʰ **Q12 Congenital lens malformations**

Q12.0 Congenital cataract

Q12.1 Congenital displaced lens

Q12.2 Coloboma of lens

Coloboma of Lens

Coloboma

Q12.3 Congenital aphakia

Q12.4 Spherophakia

Q12.8 Other congenital lens malformations
Microphakia

Q12.9 Congenital lens malformation, unspecified

✓4ᵗʰ **Q13 Congenital malformations of anterior segment of eye**

Q13.0 Coloboma of iris
Coloboma NOS
DEF: Defective or absent section of ocular tissue that may present as mild cupping or a small pit in the ocular disc due to extensive defects in the iris, ciliary body, choroids, and retina.

Q13.1 Absence of iris
Aniridia
Use additional code for associated glaucoma (H42)
DEF: Incompletely formed or absent iris. It affects both eyes and is a dominant trait.

Q13.2 Other congenital malformations of iris
Anisocoria, congenital
Atresia of pupil
Congenital malformation of iris NOS
Corectopia

Q13.3 Congenital corneal opacity

Q13.4 Other congenital corneal malformations
Congenital malformation of cornea NOS
Microcornea
Peter's anomaly

Q13.5 Blue sclera

✓5ᵗʰ **Q13.8 Other congenital malformations of anterior segment of eye**

    Q13.81 Rieger's anomaly
        Use additional code for associated glaucoma (H42)

    Q13.89 Other congenital malformations of anterior segment of eye

Q13.9 Congenital malformation of anterior segment of eye, unspecified

✓4ᵗʰ **Q14 Congenital malformations of posterior segment of eye**
> EXCLUDES 2   *optic nerve hypoplasia (H47.03-)*

Q14.0 Congenital malformation of vitreous humor
Congenital vitreous opacity

Q14.1 Congenital malformation of retina
Congenital retinal aneurysm

Q14.2 Congenital malformation of optic disc
Coloboma of optic disc

Q14.3 Congenital malformation of choroid

Q14.8 Other congenital malformations of posterior segment of eye
Coloboma of the fundus

Q14.9 Congenital malformation of posterior segment of eye, unspecified

✓4ᵗʰ **Q15 Other congenital malformations of eye**
> EXCLUDES 1   *congenital nystagmus (H55.01)*
> *ocular albinism (E70.31-)*
> *optic nerve hypoplasia (H47.03-)*
> *retinitis pigmentosa (H35.52)*

Q15.0 Congenital glaucoma
Axenfeld's anomaly
Buphthalmos
Glaucoma of childhood
Glaucoma of newborn
Hydrophthalmos
Keratoglobus, congenital, with glaucoma
Macrocornea with glaucoma
Macrophthalmos in congenital glaucoma
Megalocornea with glaucoma

Q15.8 Other specified congenital malformations of eye

Q15.9 Congenital malformation of eye, unspecified
Congenital anomaly of eye
Congenital deformity of eye

✓4ᵗʰ **Q16 Congenital malformations of ear causing impairment of hearing**
> EXCLUDES 1   *congenital deafness (H90.-)*

Q16.0 Congenital absence of (ear) auricle

Q16.1 Congenital absence, atresia and stricture of auditory canal (external)
Congenital atresia or stricture of osseous meatus

Q16.2 Absence of eustachian tube

Q16.3 Congenital malformation of ear ossicles
Congenital fusion of ear ossicles

Q16.4 Other congenital malformations of middle ear
Congenital malformation of middle ear NOS

Q16.5 Congenital malformation of inner ear
Congenital anomaly of membranous labyrinth
Congenital anomaly of organ of Corti

Q16.9 Congenital malformation of ear causing impairment of hearing, unspecified
Congenital absence of ear NOS

✓4ᵗʰ **Q17 Other congenital malformations of ear**
> EXCLUDES 1   *congenital malformations of ear with impairment of hearing (Q16.0-Q16.9)*
> *preauricular sinus (Q18.1)*

Q17.0 Accessory auricle
Accessory tragus
Polyotia
Preauricular appendage or tag
Supernumerary ear
Supernumerary lobule

Q17.1 Macrotia
DEF: Birth defect characterized by abnormal enlargement of the pinna of the ear.

Q17.2 Microtia

Q17.3 Other misshapen ear
Pointed ear

Q17.4 Misplaced ear
Low-set ears
> EXCLUDES 1   *cervical auricle (Q18.2)*

Q17.5 Prominent ear
Bat ear

Q17.8 Other specified congenital malformations of ear
Congenital absence of lobe of ear

Q17.9 Congenital malformation of ear, unspecified
Congenital anomaly of ear NOS

✓4ᵗʰ **Q18 Other congenital malformations of face and neck**
> EXCLUDES 1   *cleft lip and cleft palate (Q35-Q37)*
> *conditions classified to Q67.0-Q67.4*
> *congenital malformations of skull and face bones (Q75.-)*
> *cyclopia (Q87.0)*
> *dentofacial anomalies [including malocclusion] (M26.-)*
> *malformation syndromes affecting facial appearance (Q87.0)*
> *persistent thyroglossal duct (Q89.2)*

Q18.0 Sinus, fistula and cyst of branchial cleft
Branchial vestige

Q18.1 Preauricular sinus and cyst
Fistula of auricle, congenital
Cervicoaural fistula

Q18.2　Other branchial cleft malformations
Branchial cleft malformation NOS
Cervical auricle
Otocephaly

Q18.3　Webbing of neck
Pterygium colli
DEF: Congenital malformation characterized by a thick, triangular skinfold that stretches from the lateral side of the neck across the shoulder. It is associated with genetic conditions such as Turner's and Noonan's syndromes.

Q18.4　Macrostomia
DEF: Rare congenital craniofacial bilateral or unilateral anomaly of the mouth due to malformed maxillary and mandibular processes. It results in an abnormally large mouth extending toward the ear.

Q18.5　Microstomia

Q18.6　Macrocheilia
Hypertrophy of lip, congenital

Q18.7　Microcheilia

Q18.8　Other specified congenital malformations of face and neck
Medial cyst of face and neck
Medial fistula of face and neck
Medial sinus of face and neck

Q18.9　Congenital malformation of face and neck, unspecified
Congenital anomaly NOS of face and neck

Congenital malformations of the circulatory system (Q20-Q28)

✓4ᵗʰ　Q20　Congenital malformations of cardiac chambers and connections
　　EXCLUDES 1　dextrocardia with situs inversus (Q89.3)
　　　　　　mirror-image atrial arrangement with situs inversus (Q89.3)

Q20.0　Common arterial trunk　　Rx COM
Persistent truncus arteriosus
　EXCLUDES 1　aortic septal defect (Q21.4)

Q20.1　Double outlet right ventricle　　Rx COM
Taussig-Bing syndrome

Q20.2　Double outlet left ventricle　　Rx COM

Q20.3　Discordant ventriculoarterial connection　　Rx COM
Dextrotransposition of aorta
Transposition of great vessels (complete)

Q20.4　Double inlet ventricle　　Rx COM
Common ventricle
Cor triloculare biatriatum
Single ventricle

Q20.5　Discordant atrioventricular connection　　Rx COM
Corrected transposition
Levotransposition
Ventricular inversion

Q20.6　Isomerism of atrial appendages　　COM
Isomerism of atrial appendages with asplenia or polysplenia

Q20.8　Other congenital malformations of cardiac chambers and connections　　Rx COM
Cor binoculare

Q20.9　Congenital malformation of cardiac chambers and connections, unspecified　　COM

✓4ᵗʰ　Q21　Congenital malformations of cardiac septa
　　EXCLUDES 1　acquired cardiac septal defect (I51.0)

Q21.0　Ventricular septal defect　　Rx COM
Roger's disease

Ventricular Septal Defect

✓5ᵗʰ　Q21.1　Atrial septal defect ▲
~~Coronary sinus defect~~
~~Patent or persistent foramen ovale~~
~~Patent or persistent ostium secundum defect (type II)~~
~~Patent or persistent sinus venosus defect~~
　EXCLUDES 2　▶ostium primum atrial septal defect (type I) (Q21.20)◀

Atrial Septal Defect

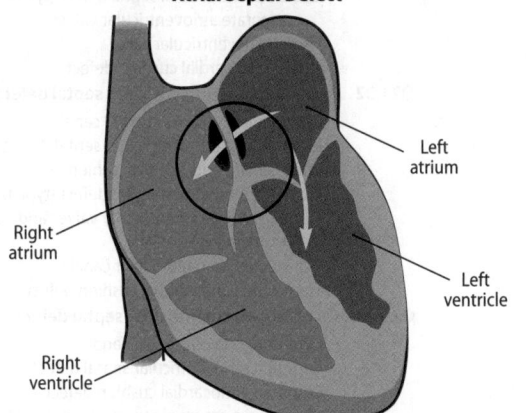

Left atrium
Right atrium
Left ventricle
Right ventricle

● **Q21.10　Atrial septal defect, unspecified**

● **Q21.11　Secundum atrial septal defect**
Fenestrated atrial septum
Patent or persistent ostium secundum defect (type II)

● **Q21.12　Patent foramen ovale**
Persistent foramen ovale

● **Q21.13　Coronary sinus atrial septal defect**
Coronary sinus defect
Unroofed coronary sinus

● **Q21.14　Superior sinus venosus atrial septal defect**
Superior vena cava type atrial septal defect

● **Q21.15　Inferior sinus venosus atrial septal defect**
Inferior vena cava type atrial septal defect

● **Q21.16　Sinus venosus atrial septal defect, unspecified**
Sinus venosus defect, NOS

● **Q21.19　Other specified atrial septal defect**
Common atrium
Other specified atrial septal abnormality

Chapter 17. Congenital Malformations, Deformations and Chromosomal Abnormalities

Q18.2–Q21.19

Chapter 17. Congenital Malformations, Deformations and Chromosomal Abnormalities

Q21.2–Q25.0

▲ ☑5ᵗʰ **Q21.2** Atrioventricular septal defect
> ►Atrioventricular canal defect◄
> ~~Common atrioventricular canal~~
> Endocardial cushion defect
> Ostium primum atrial septal defect (type I)

Atrioventricular Septal Defect

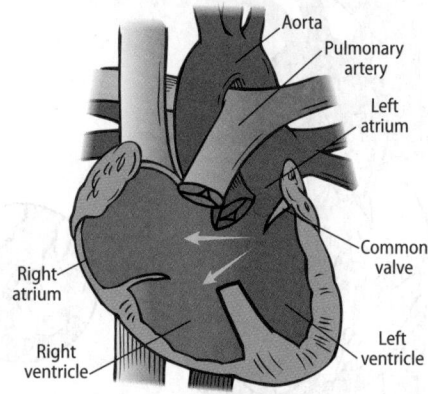

- **Q21.20** Atrioventricular septal defect, unspecified as to partial or complete
  Atrioventricular canal, NOS
  Endocardial cushion defect NOS
  Ostium primum atrial septal defect (type I) NOS

- **Q21.21** Partial atrioventricular septal defect
  Incomplete atrioventricular canal
  Incomplete atrioventricular septal defect
  Incomplete endocardial cushion defect
  Ostium primum atrial septal defect (type I) with separate atrioventricular valves
  Partial atrioventricular canal
  Partial endocardial cushion defect

- **Q21.22** Transitional atrioventricular septal defect
  Intermediate atrioventricular canal
  Intermediate atrioventricular septal defect
  Intermediate endocardial cushion defect
  Ostium primum atrial septal defect (type I) with separate atrioventricular valves and a small or restrictive inlet VSD
  Transitional atrioventricular canal
  Transitional endocardial cushion defect

- **Q21.23** Complete atrioventricular septal defect
  Common atrioventricular canal
  Common atrioventricular septal defect
  Common endocardial cushion defect
  Ostium primum atrial septal defect (type I) with common atrioventricular valve and a moderate or larger inlet VSD

Q21.3 Tetralogy of Fallot `Rx` `COM`
> Ventricular septal defect with pulmonary stenosis or atresia, dextroposition of aorta and hypertrophy of right ventricle.
> **AHA:** 2014,3Q,16

Q21.4 Aortopulmonary septal defect `COM`
> Aortic septal defect
> Aortopulmonary window

Q21.8 Other congenital malformations of cardiac septa `COM`
> Eisenmenger's defect
> Pentalogy of Fallot
> Code also, if applicable:
>> Eisenmenger's complex (I27.83)
>> Eisenmenger's syndrome (I27.83)

Q21.9 Congenital malformation of cardiac septum, unspecified `COM`
> Septal (heart) defect NOS

☑4ᵗʰ **Q22** Congenital malformations of pulmonary and tricuspid valves

Q22.0 Pulmonary valve atresia `Rx` `COM`

Q22.1 Congenital pulmonary valve stenosis `COM`

Q22.2 Congenital pulmonary valve insufficiency `COM`
> Congenital pulmonary valve regurgitation

Q22.3 Other congenital malformations of pulmonary valve `COM`
> Congenital malformation of pulmonary valve NOS
> Supernumerary cusps of pulmonary valve

Q22.4 Congenital tricuspid stenosis `COM`
> Congenital tricuspid atresia

Q22.5 Ebstein's anomaly `COM`
> **DEF:** Malformation of the tricuspid valve characterized by septal and posterior leaflets attaching to the wall of the right ventricle. Ebstein's anomaly causes the right ventricle to fuse with the atrium into a large right atrium and a small ventricle and leads to heart failure and abnormal cardiac rhythm.

Q22.6 Hypoplastic right heart syndrome `COM`

Q22.8 Other congenital malformations of tricuspid valve `COM`

Q22.9 Congenital malformation of tricuspid valve, unspecified `COM`

☑4ᵗʰ **Q23** Congenital malformations of aortic and mitral valves

Q23.0 Congenital stenosis of aortic valve `COM`
> Congenital aortic atresia
> Congenital aortic stenosis NOS
> *EXCLUDES 1*   congenital stenosis of aortic valve in hypoplastic left heart syndrome (Q23.4)
>   congenital subaortic stenosis (Q24.4)
>   supravalvular aortic stenosis (congenital) (Q25.3)

Q23.1 Congenital insufficiency of aortic valve `COM`
> Bicuspid aortic valve
> Congenital aortic insufficiency

Q23.2 Congenital mitral stenosis `COM`
> Congenital mitral atresia

Q23.3 Congenital mitral insufficiency `COM`

Q23.4 Hypoplastic left heart syndrome `Rx` `COM`

Q23.8 Other congenital malformations of aortic and mitral valves `COM`

Q23.9 Congenital malformation of aortic and mitral valves, unspecified `COM`

☑4ᵗʰ **Q24** Other congenital malformations of heart
> *EXCLUDES 1*   endocardial fibroelastosis (I42.4)

Q24.0 Dextrocardia `COM`
> *EXCLUDES 1*   dextrocardia with situs inversus (Q89.3)
>   isomerism of atrial appendages (with asplenia or polysplenia) (Q20.6)
>   mirror-image atrial arrangement with situs inversus (Q89.3)
> **DEF:** Congenital condition in which the heart is located on the right side of the chest rather than in its normal position on the left.

Q24.1 Levocardia `COM`

Q24.2 Cor triatriatum `COM`

Q24.3 Pulmonary infundibular stenosis `COM`
> Subvalvular pulmonic stenosis

Q24.4 Congenital subaortic stenosis `COM`
> **DEF:** Congenital heart defect characterized by stenosis of the left ventricular outflow tract due to a fibrous tissue ring or septal hypertrophy below the aortic valve.

Q24.5 Malformation of coronary vessels `Rx` `COM`
> Congenital coronary (artery) aneurysm

Q24.6 Congenital heart block `COM`

Q24.8 Other specified congenital malformations of heart `COM`
> Congenital diverticulum of left ventricle
> Congenital malformation of myocardium
> Congenital malformation of pericardium
> Malposition of heart
> Uhl's disease

Q24.9 Congenital malformation of heart, unspecified `COM`
> Congenital anomaly of heart
> Congenital disease of heart

☑4ᵗʰ **Q25** Congenital malformations of great arteries

Q25.0 Patent ductus arteriosus `Rx` `COM`
> Patent ductus Botallo
> Persistent ductus arteriosus
> **DEF:** Condition in which the normal channel between the pulmonary artery and the aorta fails to close at birth, causing arterial blood to recirculate in the lungs and inhibiting the blood supply to the aorta. **Synonym(s):** PDA.

Q25.1   Coarctation of aorta   `COM`
Coarctation of aorta (preductal) (postductal)
Stenosis of aorta
AHA: 2016,4Q,56-57

✓5ᵗʰ **Q25.2**   Atresia of aorta
AHA: 2016,4Q,56-57

    Q25.21   Interruption of aortic arch   `COM`
Atresia of aortic arch

    Q25.29   Other atresia of aorta   `COM`
Atresia of aorta

Q25.3   Supravalvular aortic stenosis   `COM`
`EXCLUDES 1`   congenital aortic stenosis NOS (Q23.0)
congenital stenosis of aortic valve (Q23.0)

✓5ᵗʰ **Q25.4**   Other congenital malformations of aorta
`EXCLUDES 1`   hypoplasia of aorta in hypoplastic left heart syndrome (Q23.4)
AHA: 2016,4Q,57

    Q25.40   Congenital malformation of aorta unspecified   `COM`

    Q25.41   Absence and aplasia of aorta   `COM`

    Q25.42   Hypoplasia of aorta   `COM`

    Q25.43   Congenital aneurysm of aorta   `COM`
Congenital aneurysm of aortic root
Congenital aneurysm of aortic sinus

    Q25.44   Congenital dilation of aorta   `COM`

    Q25.45   Double aortic arch   `COM`
Vascular ring of aorta

Aortic Arch Anomalies

Normal aortic arch

Double aortic arch   Right aortic arch

    Q25.46   Tortuous aortic arch   `COM`
Persistent convolutions of aortic arch

    Q25.47   Right aortic arch   `COM`
Persistent right aortic arch

    Q25.48   Anomalous origin of subclavian artery   `COM`

    Q25.49   Other congenital malformations of aorta   `COM`
Aortic arch
Bovine arch

Q25.5   Atresia of pulmonary artery   `Rx` `COM`

Q25.6   Stenosis of pulmonary artery   `COM`
Supravalvular pulmonary stenosis

✓5ᵗʰ **Q25.7**   Other congenital malformations of pulmonary artery

    Q25.71   Coarctation of pulmonary artery   `Rx` `COM`

    Q25.72   Congenital pulmonary arteriovenous malformation   `COM`
Congenital pulmonary arteriovenous aneurysm

    Q25.79   Other congenital malformations of pulmonary artery   `COM`
Aberrant pulmonary artery
Agenesis of pulmonary artery
Congenital aneurysm of pulmonary artery
Congenital anomaly of pulmonary artery
Hypoplasia of pulmonary artery

Q25.8   Other congenital malformations of other great arteries   `COM`

Q25.9   Congenital malformation of great arteries, unspecified   `COM`

✓4ᵗʰ **Q26**   Congenital malformations of great veins

Q26.0   Congenital stenosis of vena cava   `Rx` `COM`
Congenital stenosis of vena cava (inferior)(superior)

Q26.1   Persistent left superior vena cava   `Rx` `COM`

Q26.2   Total anomalous pulmonary venous connection   `Rx` `COM`
Total anomalous pulmonary venous return [TAPVR], subdiaphragmatic
Total anomalous pulmonary venous return [TAPVR], supradiaphragmatic

Q26.3   Partial anomalous pulmonary venous connection   `Rx` `COM`
Partial anomalous pulmonary venous return

Q26.4   Anomalous pulmonary venous connection, unspecified   `Rx` `COM`

Q26.5   Anomalous portal venous connection   `COM`

Q26.6   Portal vein-hepatic artery fistula   `COM`

Q26.8   Other congenital malformations of great veins   `Rx` `COM`
Absence of vena cava (inferior) (superior)
Azygos continuation of inferior vena cava
Persistent left posterior cardinal vein
Scimitar syndrome

Q26.9   Congenital malformation of great vein, unspecified   `Rx` `COM`
Congenital anomaly of vena cava (inferior) (superior) NOS

✓4ᵗʰ **Q27**   Other congenital malformations of peripheral vascular system
`EXCLUDES 2`   anomalies of cerebral and precerebral vessels (Q28.0-Q28.3)
anomalies of coronary vessels (Q24.5)
anomalies of pulmonary artery (Q25.5-Q25.7)
congenital retinal aneurysm (Q14.1)
hemangioma and lymphangioma (D18.-)

Q27.0   Congenital absence and hypoplasia of umbilical artery   `COM`
Single umbilical artery

Q27.1   Congenital renal artery stenosis   `COM`

Q27.2   Other congenital malformations of renal artery   `COM`
Congenital malformation of renal artery NOS
Multiple renal arteries

✓5ᵗʰ **Q27.3**   Arteriovenous malformation (peripheral)
Arteriovenous aneurysm
`EXCLUDES 1`   acquired arteriovenous aneurysm (I77.0)
`EXCLUDES 2`   arteriovenous malformation of cerebral vessels (Q28.2)
arteriovenous malformation of precerebral vessels (Q28.0)
DEF: Arteriovenous malformation: Connecting passage between an artery and a vein.

    Q27.30   Arteriovenous malformation, site unspecified   `COM`

    Q27.31   Arteriovenous malformation of vessel of upper limb   `COM`

    Q27.32   Arteriovenous malformation of vessel of lower limb   `COM`

    Q27.33   Arteriovenous malformation of digestive system vessel   `COM`
AHA: 2018,3Q,21

    Q27.34   Arteriovenous malformation of renal vessel   `COM`

    Q27.39   Arteriovenous malformation, other site   `COM`

Q27.4   Congenital phlebectasia   `COM`

Chapter 17. Congenital Malformations, Deformations and Chromosomal Abnormalities

Q27.8   **Other specified congenital malformations of peripheral vascular system**   COM
   Absence of peripheral vascular system
   Atresia of peripheral vascular system
   Congenital aneurysm (peripheral)
   Congenital stricture, artery
   Congenital varix
   EXCLUDES 1   *arteriovenous malformation (Q27.3-)*

Q27.9   **Congenital malformation of peripheral vascular system, unspecified**   COM
   Anomaly of artery or vein NOS

✓4th **Q28**   **Other congenital malformations of circulatory system**
   EXCLUDES 1   *congenital aneurysm NOS (Q27.8)*
   congenital coronary aneurysm (Q24.5)
   ruptured cerebral arteriovenous malformation (I60.8)
   ruptured malformation of precerebral vessels (I72.0)
   EXCLUDES 2   *congenital peripheral aneurysm (Q27.8)*
   congenital pulmonary aneurysm (Q25.79)
   congenital retinal aneurysm (Q14.1)

Q28.0   **Arteriovenous malformation of precerebral vessels**   COM
   Congenital arteriovenous precerebral aneurysm (nonruptured)

Q28.1   **Other malformations of precerebral vessels**   COM
   Congenital malformation of precerebral vessels NOS
   Congenital precerebral aneurysm (nonruptured)

Q28.2   **Arteriovenous malformation of cerebral vessels**   COM
   Arteriovenous malformation of brain NOS
   Congenital arteriovenous cerebral aneurysm (nonruptured)

Q28.3   **Other malformations of cerebral vessels**   COM
   Congenital cerebral aneurysm (nonruptured)
   Congenital malformation of cerebral vessels NOS
   Developmental venous anomaly

Q28.8   **Other specified congenital malformations of circulatory system**   COM
   Congenital aneurysm, specified site NEC
   Spinal vessel anomaly

Q28.9   **Congenital malformation of circulatory system, unspecified**   COM

Congenital malformations of the respiratory system (Q30-Q34)

✓4th **Q30**   **Congenital malformations of nose**
   EXCLUDES 1   *congenital deviation of nasal septum (Q67.4)*

Q30.0   **Choanal atresia**
   Atresia of nares (anterior) (posterior)
   Congenital stenosis of nares (anterior) (posterior)

Q30.1   **Agenesis and underdevelopment of nose**
   Congenital absent of nose

Q30.2   **Fissured, notched and cleft nose**

Q30.3   **Congenital perforated nasal septum**

Q30.8   **Other congenital malformations of nose**
   Accessory nose
   Congenital anomaly of nasal sinus wall
   AHA: 2022,2Q,17

Q30.9   **Congenital malformation of nose, unspecified**

✓4th **Q31**   **Congenital malformations of larynx**
   EXCLUDES 1   *congenital laryngeal stridor NOS (P28.89)*

Q31.0   **Web of larynx**
   Glottic web of larynx
   Subglottic web of larynx
   Web of larynx NOS
   DEF: Congenital malformation of the larynx marked by thin, translucent, or thick fibrotic membrane-like structure between the vocal folds. It is characterized by shortness of breath and stridor.

Q31.1   **Congenital subglottic stenosis**

Q31.2   **Laryngeal hypoplasia**

Q31.3   **Laryngocele**

Q31.5   **Congenital laryngomalacia**

Q31.8   **Other congenital malformations of larynx**
   Absence of larynx
   Agenesis of larynx
   Atresia of larynx
   Congenital cleft thyroid cartilage
   Congenital fissure of epiglottis
   Congenital stenosis of larynx NEC
   Posterior cleft of cricoid cartilage

Q31.9   **Congenital malformation of larynx, unspecified**

✓4th **Q32**   **Congenital malformations of trachea and bronchus**
   EXCLUDES 1   *congenital bronchiectasis (Q33.4)*

Q32.0   **Congenital tracheomalacia**

Q32.1   **Other congenital malformations of trachea**
   Atresia of trachea
   Congenital anomaly of tracheal cartilage
   Congenital dilatation of trachea
   Congenital malformation of trachea
   Congenital stenosis of trachea
   Congenital tracheocele

Q32.2   **Congenital bronchomalacia**

Q32.3   **Congenital stenosis of bronchus**

Q32.4   **Other congenital malformations of bronchus**
   Absence of bronchus
   Agenesis of bronchus
   Atresia of bronchus
   Congenital diverticulum of bronchus
   Congenital malformation of bronchus NOS

✓4th **Q33**   **Congenital malformations of lung**

Q33.0   **Congenital cystic lung**
   Congenital cystic lung disease
   Congenital honeycomb lung
   Congenital polycystic lung disease
   EXCLUDES 1   *cystic fibrosis (E84.0)*
   cystic lung disease, acquired or unspecified (J98.4)

Q33.1   **Accessory lobe of lung**
   Azygos lobe (fissured), lung

Q33.2   **Sequestration of lung**

Q33.3   **Agenesis of lung**
   Congenital absence of lung (lobe)

Q33.4   **Congenital bronchiectasis**

Q33.5   **Ectopic tissue in lung**

Q33.6   **Congenital hypoplasia and dysplasia of lung**
   EXCLUDES 1   *pulmonary hypoplasia associated with short gestation (P28.0)*

Q33.8   **Other congenital malformations of lung**

Q33.9   **Congenital malformation of lung, unspecified**

✓4th **Q34**   **Other congenital malformations of respiratory system**
   EXCLUDES 2   *congenital central alveolar hypoventilation syndrome (G47.35)*

Q34.0   **Anomaly of pleura**

Q34.1   **Congenital cyst of mediastinum**

Q34.8   **Other specified congenital malformations of respiratory system**
   Atresia of nasopharynx

Q34.9   **Congenital malformation of respiratory system, unspecified**
   Congenital absence of respiratory system
   Congenital anomaly of respiratory system NOS

Cleft lip and cleft palate (Q35-Q37)

Use additional code to identify associated malformation of the nose (Q30.2)

EXCLUDES 2   *Robin's syndrome (Q87.0)*

☑4ᵗʰ **Q35 Cleft palate**

    INCLUDES   fissure of palate
                palatoschisis

    EXCLUDES 1   *cleft palate with cleft lip (Q37.-)*

    DEF: Congenital fissure or defect of the roof of the mouth opening to the nasal cavity due to failure of embryonic cells to fuse completely.

Cleft Palate

Cleft in soft palate   Cleft in hard and soft palate

Hard palate —   Soft palate —   Cleft   Cleft

    Q35.1 Cleft hard palate   `COM`
    Q35.3 Cleft soft palate   `COM`
    Q35.5 Cleft hard palate with cleft soft palate   `COM`
    Q35.7 Cleft uvula   `COM`
    Q35.9 Cleft palate, unspecified   `COM`
        Cleft palate NOS

☑4ᵗʰ **Q36 Cleft lip**

    INCLUDES   cheiloschisis
                congenital fissure of lip
                harelip
                labium leporinum

    EXCLUDES 1   *cleft lip with cleft palate (Q37.-)*

    DEF: Congenital fissure or opening in the upper lip due to failure of embryonic cells to fuse completely.

Cleft Lip

Unilateral incomplete   Unilateral complete   Bilateral complete

    Q36.0 Cleft lip, bilateral   `COM`
    Q36.1 Cleft lip, median   `COM`
    Q36.9 Cleft lip, unilateral   `COM`
        Cleft lip NOS

☑4ᵗʰ **Q37 Cleft palate with cleft lip**

    INCLUDES   cheilopalatoschisis

    Q37.0 Cleft hard palate with bilateral cleft lip   `COM`
    Q37.1 Cleft hard palate with unilateral cleft lip   `COM`
        Cleft hard palate with cleft lip NOS
    Q37.2 Cleft soft palate with bilateral cleft lip   `COM`
    Q37.3 Cleft soft palate with unilateral cleft lip   `COM`
        Cleft soft palate with cleft lip NOS
    Q37.4 Cleft hard and soft palate with bilateral cleft lip   `COM`
    Q37.5 Cleft hard and soft palate with unilateral cleft lip   `COM`
        Cleft hard and soft palate with cleft lip NOS
    Q37.8 Unspecified cleft palate with bilateral cleft lip   `COM`
    Q37.9 Unspecified cleft palate with unilateral cleft lip   `COM`
        Cleft palate with cleft lip NOS

Other congenital malformations of the digestive system (Q38-Q45)

☑4ᵗʰ **Q38 Other congenital malformations of tongue, mouth and pharynx**

    EXCLUDES 1   *dentofacial anomalies (M26.-)*
                  macrostomia (Q18.4)
                  microstomia (Q18.5)

    Q38.0 Congenital malformations of lips, not elsewhere classified
        Congenital fistula of lip
        Congenital malformation of lip NOS
        Van der Woude's syndrome
      EXCLUDES 1   *cleft lip (Q36.-)*
                cleft lip with cleft palate (Q37.-)
                macrocheilia (Q18.6)
                microcheilia (Q18.7)

    Q38.1 Ankyloglossia
        Tongue tie

    Q38.2 Macroglossia
        Congenital hypertrophy of tongue

    Q38.3 Other congenital malformations of tongue
        Aglossia
        Bifid tongue
        Congenital adhesion of tongue
        Congenital fissure of tongue
        Congenital malformation of tongue NOS
        Double tongue
        Hypoglossia
        Hypoplasia of tongue
        Microglossia

    Q38.4 Congenital malformations of salivary glands and ducts
        Atresia of salivary glands and ducts
        Congenital absence of salivary glands and ducts
        Congenital accessory salivary glands and ducts
        Congenital fistula of salivary gland

    Q38.5 Congenital malformations of palate, not elsewhere classified
        Congenital absence of uvula
        Congenital malformation of palate NOS
        Congenital high arched palate
      EXCLUDES 1   *cleft palate (Q35.-)*
                cleft palate with cleft lip (Q37.-)

    Q38.6 Other congenital malformations of mouth
        Congenital malformation of mouth NOS

    Q38.7 Congenital pharyngeal pouch
        Congenital diverticulum of pharynx
      EXCLUDES 1   *pharyngeal pouch syndrome (D82.1)*

    Q38.8 Other congenital malformations of pharynx
        Congenital malformation of pharynx NOS
        Imperforate pharynx

☑4ᵗʰ **Q39 Congenital malformations of esophagus**

    Q39.0 Atresia of esophagus without fistula   `COM`
        Atresia of esophagus NOS
    Q39.1 Atresia of esophagus with tracheo-esophageal fistula   `COM`
        Atresia of esophagus with broncho-esophageal fistula
    Q39.2 Congenital tracheo-esophageal fistula without atresia   `COM`
        Congenital tracheo-esophageal fistula NOS
    Q39.3 Congenital stenosis and stricture of esophagus   `COM`
    Q39.4 Esophageal web   `COM`
    Q39.5 Congenital dilatation of esophagus
        Congenital cardiospasm
    Q39.6 Congenital diverticulum of esophagus
        Congenital esophageal pouch
    Q39.8 Other congenital malformations of esophagus
        Congenital absence of esophagus
        Congenital displacement of esophagus
        Congenital duplication of esophagus
    Q39.9 Congenital malformation of esophagus, unspecified

☑4ᵗʰ **Q40 Other congenital malformations of upper alimentary tract**

    Q40.0 Congenital hypertrophic pyloric stenosis   `COM`
        Congenital or infantile constriction
        Congenital or infantile hypertrophy
        Congenital or infantile spasm
        Congenital or infantile stenosis
        Congenital or infantile stricture

Q40.1　Congenital hiatus hernia
Congenital displacement of cardia through esophageal hiatus
EXCLUDES 1　*congenital diaphragmatic hernia (Q79.0)*

Q40.2　Other specified congenital malformations of stomach
Congenital displacement of stomach
Congenital diverticulum of stomach
Congenital hourglass stomach
Congenital duplication of stomach
Megalogastria
Microgastria

Q40.3　Congenital malformation of stomach, unspecified

Q40.8　Other specified congenital malformations of upper alimentary tract

Q40.9　Congenital malformation of upper alimentary tract, unspecified
Congenital anomaly of upper alimentary tract
Congenital deformity of upper alimentary tract

✓4ᵗʰ Q41　Congenital absence, atresia and stenosis of small intestine
INCLUDES　congenital obstruction, occlusion or stricture of small intestine or intestine NOS
EXCLUDES 1　*cystic fibrosis with intestinal manifestation (E84.11)*
meconium ileus NOS (without cystic fibrosis) (P76.0)

Q41.0　Congenital absence, atresia and stenosis of duodenum COM

Q41.1　Congenital absence, atresia and stenosis of jejunum COM
Apple peel syndrome
Imperforate jejunum

Q41.2　Congenital absence, atresia and stenosis of ileum COM

Q41.8　Congenital absence, atresia and stenosis of other specified parts of small intestine COM

Q41.9　Congenital absence, atresia and stenosis of small intestine, part unspecified COM
Congenital absence, atresia and stenosis of intestine NOS

✓4ᵗʰ Q42　Congenital absence, atresia and stenosis of large intestine
INCLUDES　congenital obstruction, occlusion and stricture of large intestine

Q42.0　Congenital absence, atresia and stenosis of rectum with fistula COM

Q42.1　Congenital absence, atresia and stenosis of rectum without fistula COM
Imperforate rectum

Q42.2　Congenital absence, atresia and stenosis of anus with fistula COM

Q42.3　Congenital absence, atresia and stenosis of anus without fistula COM
Imperforate anus

Q42.8　Congenital absence, atresia and stenosis of other parts of large intestine COM

Q42.9　Congenital absence, atresia and stenosis of large intestine, part unspecified COM

✓4ᵗʰ Q43　Other congenital malformations of intestine

Q43.0　Meckel's diverticulum (displaced) (hypertrophic)
Persistent omphalomesenteric duct
Persistent vitelline duct
DEF: Congenital, abnormal remnant of embryonic digestive system development that leaves a sacculation or outpouching from the wall of the small intestine near the terminal part of the ileum made of acid-secreting tissue as in the stomach.

Q43.1　Hirschsprung's disease COM
Aganglionosis
Congenital (aganglionic) megacolon
DEF: Congenital enlargement or dilation of the colon, with the absence of nerve cells in a segment of colon distally that causes the inability to defecate.

Q43.2　Other congenital functional disorders of colon COM
Congenital dilatation of colon

Q43.3　Congenital malformations of intestinal fixation COM
Congenital omental, anomalous adhesions [bands]
Congenital peritoneal adhesions [bands]
Incomplete rotation of cecum and colon
Insufficient rotation of cecum and colon
Jackson's membrane
Malrotation of colon
Rotation failure of cecum and colon
Universal mesentery

Q43.4　Duplication of intestine
Q43.5　Ectopic anus

Q43.6　Congenital fistula of rectum and anus
EXCLUDES 1　*congenital fistula of anus with absence, atresia and stenosis (Q42.2)*
congenital fistula of rectum with absence, atresia and stenosis (Q42.0)
congenital rectovaginal fistula (Q52.2)
congenital urethrorectal fistula (Q64.73)
pilonidal fistula or sinus (L05.-)

Q43.7　Persistent cloaca
Cloaca NOS

Q43.8　Other specified congenital malformations of intestine
Congenital blind loop syndrome
Congenital diverticulitis, colon
Congenital diverticulum, intestine
Dolichocolon
Megaloappendix
Megaloduodenum
Microcolon
Transposition of appendix
Transposition of colon
Transposition of intestine
AHA: 2013,2Q,31

Q43.9　Congenital malformation of intestine, unspecified

✓4ᵗʰ Q44　Congenital malformations of gallbladder, bile ducts and liver

Q44.0　Agenesis, aplasia and hypoplasia of gallbladder
Congenital absence of gallbladder

Q44.1　Other congenital malformations of gallbladder
Congenital malformation of gallbladder NOS
Intrahepatic gallbladder

Q44.2　Atresia of bile ducts
Q44.3　Congenital stenosis and stricture of bile ducts
Q44.4　Choledochal cyst
Q44.5　Other congenital malformations of bile ducts
Accessory hepatic duct
Biliary duct duplication
Congenital malformation of bile duct NOS
Cystic duct duplication

Q44.6　Cystic disease of liver
Fibrocystic disease of liver

Q44.7　Other congenital malformations of liver
Accessory liver
Alagille's syndrome
Congenital absence of liver
Congenital hepatomegaly
Congenital malformation of liver NOS

✓4ᵗʰ Q45　Other congenital malformations of digestive system
EXCLUDES 2　*congenital diaphragmatic hernia (Q79.0)*
congenital hiatus hernia (Q40.1)

Q45.0　Agenesis, aplasia and hypoplasia of pancreas
Congenital absence of pancreas

Q45.1　Annular pancreas
Q45.2　Congenital pancreatic cyst
Q45.3　Other congenital malformations of pancreas and pancreatic duct
Accessory pancreas
Congenital malformation of pancreas or pancreatic duct NOS
EXCLUDES 1　*congenital diabetes mellitus (E10.-)*
cystic fibrosis (E84.0-E84.9)
fibrocystic disease of pancreas (E84.-)
neonatal diabetes mellitus (P70.2)

Q45.8　Other specified congenital malformations of digestive system
Absence (complete) (partial) of alimentary tract NOS
Duplication of digestive system
Malposition, congenital of digestive system

Q45.9　Congenital malformation of digestive system, unspecified
Congenital anomaly of digestive system
Congenital deformity of digestive system

Congenital malformations of genital organs (Q50-Q56)

EXCLUDES 1 *androgen insensitivity syndrome (E34.5-)*
syndromes associated with anomalies in the number and form of chromosomes (Q90-Q99)

√4ᵗʰ **Q50 Congenital malformations of ovaries, fallopian tubes and broad ligaments**

√5ᵗʰ **Q50.0 Congenital absence of ovary**

EXCLUDES 1 *Turner's syndrome (Q96.-)*

Q50.01 Congenital absence of ovary, unilateral ♀
Q50.02 Congenital absence of ovary, bilateral ♀

Q50.1 Developmental ovarian cyst ♀
Q50.2 Congenital torsion of ovary ♀

√5ᵗʰ **Q50.3 Other congenital malformations of ovary**

Q50.31 Accessory ovary ♀
Q50.32 Ovarian streak ♀
46, XX with streak gonads
Q50.39 Other congenital malformation of ovary ♀
Congenital malformation of ovary NOS

Q50.4 Embryonic cyst of fallopian tube ♀
Fimbrial cyst
Q50.5 Embryonic cyst of broad ligament ♀
Epoophoron cyst
Parovarian cyst
Q50.6 Other congenital malformations of fallopian tube and broad ligament ♀
Absence of fallopian tube and broad ligament
Accessory fallopian tube and broad ligament
Atresia of fallopian tube and broad ligament
Congenital malformation of fallopian tube or broad ligament NOS

√4ᵗʰ **Q51 Congenital malformations of uterus and cervix**

Q51.0 Agenesis and aplasia of uterus ♀
Congenital absence of uterus

√5ᵗʰ **Q51.1 Doubling of uterus with doubling of cervix and vagina**

Q51.10 Doubling of uterus with doubling of cervix and vagina without obstruction ♀
Doubling of uterus with doubling of cervix and vagina NOS
Q51.11 Doubling of uterus with doubling of cervix and vagina with obstruction ♀

√5ᵗʰ **Q51.2 Other doubling of uterus**
Doubling of uterus NOS
Septate uterus
AHA: 2018,4Q,27
Q51.21 Complete doubling of uterus ♀
Complete septate uterus
Q51.22 Partial doubling of uterus ♀
Partial septate uterus
Q51.28 Other and unspecified doubling of uterus ♀
Septate uterus NOS

Q51.3 Bicornate uterus ♀
Bicornate uterus, complete or partial
Q51.4 Unicornate uterus ♀
Unicornate uterus with or without a separate uterine horn
Uterus with only one functioning horn
Q51.5 Agenesis and aplasia of cervix ♀
Congenital absence of cervix
Q51.6 Embryonic cyst of cervix ♀
Q51.7 Congenital fistulae between uterus and digestive and urinary tracts ♀

√6ᵗʰ **Q51.8 Other congenital malformations of uterus and cervix**

√6ᵗʰ **Q51.81 Other congenital malformations of uterus**
Q51.810 Arcuate uterus ♀
Arcuatus uterus
Q51.811 Hypoplasia of uterus ♀
Q51.818 Other congenital malformations of uterus ♀
Müllerian anomaly of uterus NEC

√6ᵗʰ **Q51.82 Other congenital malformations of cervix**
Q51.820 Cervical duplication ♀
Q51.821 Hypoplasia of cervix ♀
Q51.828 Other congenital malformations of cervix ♀

Q51.9 Congenital malformation of uterus and cervix, unspecified ♀

√4ᵗʰ **Q52 Other congenital malformations of female genitalia**

Q52.0 Congenital absence of vagina ♀
Vaginal agenesis, total or partial

√5ᵗʰ **Q52.1 Doubling of vagina**

EXCLUDES 1 *doubling of vagina with doubling of uterus and cervix (Q51.1-)*

Q52.10 Doubling of vagina, unspecified ♀
Septate vagina NOS
Q52.11 Transverse vaginal septum ♀

√6ᵗʰ **Q52.12 Longitudinal vaginal septum**
AHA: 2016,4Q,58-59
Q52.120 Longitudinal vaginal septum, nonobstructing ♀
Q52.121 Longitudinal vaginal septum, obstructing, right side ♀
Q52.122 Longitudinal vaginal septum, obstructing, left side ♀
Q52.123 Longitudinal vaginal septum, microperforate, right side ♀
Q52.124 Longitudinal vaginal septum, microperforate, left side ♀
Q52.129 Other and unspecified longitudinal vaginal septum ♀

Q52.2 Congenital rectovaginal fistula ♀
EXCLUDES 1 *cloaca (Q43.7)*
Q52.3 Imperforate hymen ♀
DEF: Obstructive anomaly of vagina, characterized by complete closure of the membranous fold around the external opening of the vagina, obstructing the vaginal introitus.
Q52.4 Other congenital malformations of vagina ♀
Canal of Nuck cyst, congenital
Congenital malformation of vagina NOS
Embryonic vaginal cyst
Gartner's duct cyst
AHA: 2022,2Q,15
Q52.5 Fusion of labia ♀
Q52.6 Congenital malformation of clitoris ♀

√5ᵗʰ **Q52.7 Other and unspecified congenital malformations of vulva**

Q52.70 Unspecified congenital malformations of vulva ♀
Congenital malformation of vulva NOS
Q52.71 Congenital absence of vulva ♀
Q52.79 Other congenital malformations of vulva ♀
Congenital cyst of vulva

Q52.8 Other specified congenital malformations of female genitalia ♀
Q52.9 Congenital malformation of female genitalia, unspecified ♀

√4ᵗʰ **Q53 Undescended and ectopic testicle**

√5ᵗʰ **Q53.0 Ectopic testis**

Q53.00 Ectopic testis, unspecified ♂
Q53.01 Ectopic testis, unilateral ♂
Q53.02 Ectopic testes, bilateral ♂

√5ᵗʰ **Q53.1 Undescended testicle, unilateral**
AHA: 2017,4Q,22-23
Q53.10 Unspecified undescended testicle, unilateral ♂

√6ᵗʰ **Q53.11 Abdominal testis, unilateral**
Q53.111 Unilateral intraabdominal testis ♂
Q53.112 Unilateral inguinal testis ♂
Q53.12 Ectopic perineal testis, unilateral ♂
Q53.13 Unilateral high scrotal testis ♂

√5ᵗʰ **Q53.2 Undescended testicle, bilateral**
AHA: 2017,4Q,22-23
Q53.20 Undescended testicle, unspecified, bilateral ♂

√6ᵗʰ **Q53.21 Abdominal testis, bilateral**
Q53.211 Bilateral intraabdominal testes ♂
Q53.212 Bilateral inguinal testes ♂
Q53.22 Ectopic perineal testis, bilateral ♂
Q53.23 Bilateral high scrotal testes ♂

Q53.9 Undescended testicle, unspecified ♂
Cryptorchism NOS

☑ Additional Character Required   √x7ᵗʰ Placeholder Alert   Manifestation   Unspecified Dx   Q QPP   UPD Unacceptable PDx

✓4ᵗʰ **Q54 Hypospadias**

> **EXCLUDES 1** epispadias (Q64.0)

DEF: Abnormal opening of the urethra on the ventral (underside) surface of the penis.

Hypospadias

- Balanic (glanular, coronal) hypospadias
- Subcoronal hypospadias
- Penile hypospadias
- Penile raphe
- Scrotal hypospadias
- Penoscrotal hypospadias
- Scrotum
- Scrotal raphe
- Perineal hypospadias

Hypospadias (ventral view)

Q54.0 Hypospadias, balanic ♂
Hypospadias, coronal
Hypospadias, glandular

Q54.1 Hypospadias, penile ♂

Q54.2 Hypospadias, penoscrotal ♂

Q54.3 Hypospadias, perineal ♂

Q54.4 Congenital chordee ♂
Chordee without hypospadias

Q54.8 Other hypospadias ♂
Hypospadias with intersex state

Q54.9 Hypospadias, unspecified ♂

✓4ᵗʰ **Q55 Other congenital malformations of male genital organs**

> **EXCLUDES 1** congenital hydrocele (P83.5)
> hypospadias (Q54.-)

Q55.0 Absence and aplasia of testis ♂
Monorchism

Q55.1 Hypoplasia of testis and scrotum ♂
Fusion of testes

✓5ᵗʰ **Q55.2 Other and unspecified congenital malformations of testis and scrotum**

Q55.20 Unspecified congenital malformations of testis and scrotum ♂
Congenital malformation of testis or scrotum NOS

Q55.21 Polyorchism ♂
DEF: Congenital anomaly in which there are more than two testes.

Q55.22 Retractile testis ♂

Q55.23 Scrotal transposition ♂

Q55.29 Other congenital malformations of testis and scrotum ♂

Q55.3 Atresia of vas deferens ♂
Code first any associated cystic fibrosis (E84.-)

Q55.4 Other congenital malformations of vas deferens, epididymis, seminal vesicles and prostate ♂
Absence or aplasia of prostate
Absence or aplasia of spermatic cord
Congenital malformation of vas deferens, epididymis, seminal vesicles or prostate NOS

Q55.5 Congenital absence and aplasia of penis ♂

✓5ᵗʰ **Q55.6 Other congenital malformations of penis**

Q55.61 Curvature of penis (lateral) ♂

Q55.62 Hypoplasia of penis ♂
Micropenis

Q55.63 Congenital torsion of penis ♂
> **EXCLUDES 1** acquired torsion of penis (N48.82)

Q55.64 Hidden penis ♂
Buried penis
Concealed penis
> **EXCLUDES 1** acquired buried penis (N48.83)

Q55.69 Other congenital malformation of penis ♂
Congenital malformation of penis NOS

Q55.7 Congenital vasocutaneous fistula ♂

Q55.8 Other specified congenital malformations of male genital organs ♂

Q55.9 Congenital malformation of male genital organ, unspecified ♂
Congenital anomaly of male genital organ
Congenital deformity of male genital organ

✓4ᵗʰ **Q56 Indeterminate sex and pseudohermaphroditism**

> **EXCLUDES 1** 46, XX true hermaphrodite (Q99.1)
> androgen insensitivity syndrome (E34.5-)
> chimera 46, XX/46, XY true hermaphrodite (Q99.0)
> female pseudohermaphroditism with adrenocortical disorder (E25.-)
> pseudohermaphroditism with specified chromosomal anomaly (Q96-Q99)
> pure gonadal dysgenesis (Q99.1)

DEF: Indeterminate sex: External genitalia that is nondescript, lacking the physical appearance specific to either sex.
DEF: Pseudohermaphroditism: Presence of gonads of one sex and external genitalia of another sex.

Q56.0 Hermaphroditism, not elsewhere classified
Ovotestis

Q56.1 Male pseudohermaphroditism, not elsewhere classified ♂
46, XY with streak gonads
Male pseudohermaphroditism NOS

Q56.2 Female pseudohermaphroditism, not elsewhere classified ♀
Female pseudohermaphroditism NOS

Q56.3 Pseudohermaphroditism, unspecified

Q56.4 Indeterminate sex, unspecified
Ambiguous genitalia

Congenital malformations of the urinary system (Q60-Q64)

✓4ᵗʰ **Q60 Renal agenesis and other reduction defects of kidney**

> **INCLUDES** congenital absence of kidney
> congenital atrophy of kidney
> infantile atrophy of kidney

Q60.0 Renal agenesis, unilateral

Q60.1 Renal agenesis, bilateral

Q60.2 Renal agenesis, unspecified

Q60.3 Renal hypoplasia, unilateral

Q60.4 Renal hypoplasia, bilateral

Q60.5 Renal hypoplasia, unspecified

Q60.6 Potter's syndrome

✓4ᵗʰ **Q61 Cystic kidney disease**

> **EXCLUDES 1** acquired cyst of kidney (N28.1)
> Potter's syndrome (Q60.6)

✓5ᵗʰ **Q61.0 Congenital renal cyst**

Q61.00 Congenital renal cyst, unspecified
Cyst of kidney NOS (congenital)

Q61.01 Congenital single renal cyst

Q61.02 Congenital multiple renal cysts

✓5ᵗʰ **Q61.1 Polycystic kidney, infantile type**
Polycystic kidney, autosomal recessive

Q61.11 Cystic dilatation of collecting ducts `COM`

Q61.19 Other polycystic kidney, infantile type `COM`

Q61.2 Polycystic kidney, adult type
Polycystic kidney, autosomal dominant

Q61.3 Polycystic kidney, unspecified
AHA: 2016,3Q,22

Q61.4 Renal dysplasia
Multicystic dysplastic kidney
Multicystic kidney (development)
Multicystic kidney disease
Multicystic renal dysplasia
> **EXCLUDES 1** polycystic kidney disease (Q61.11-Q61.3)

Q61.5 Medullary cystic kidney
Nephronophthisis
Sponge kidney NOS
DEF: Sponge kidney: Dilated collecting tubules that are usually asymptomatic. Calcinosis in tubules may cause renal insufficiency.

Q61.8 Other cystic kidney diseases
Fibrocystic kidney
Fibrocystic renal degeneration or disease

Q61.9 Cystic kidney disease, unspecified
Meckel-Gruber syndrome

☑4ᵗʰ **Q62 Congenital obstructive defects of renal pelvis and congenital malformations of ureter**

    Q62.0 Congenital hydronephrosis

☑5ᵗʰ **Q62.1 Congenital occlusion of ureter**
        Atresia and stenosis of ureter

        Q62.10 Congenital occlusion of ureter, unspecified

        Q62.11 Congenital occlusion of ureteropelvic junction

        Q62.12 Congenital occlusion of ureterovesical orifice

    Q62.2 Congenital megaureter
        Congenital dilatation of ureter

☑5ᵗʰ **Q62.3 Other obstructive defects of renal pelvis and ureter**

        Q62.31 Congenital ureterocele, orthotopic

        Q62.32 Cecoureterocele
          Ectopic ureterocele

        Q62.39 Other obstructive defects of renal pelvis and ureter
          Ureteropelvic junction obstruction NOS

    Q62.4 Agenesis of ureter
        Congenital absence ureter

    Q62.5 Duplication of ureter
        Accessory ureter
        Double ureter

☑5ᵗʰ **Q62.6 Malposition of ureter**

        Q62.60 Malposition of ureter, unspecified

        Q62.61 Deviation of ureter

        Q62.62 Displacement of ureter

        Q62.63 Anomalous implantation of ureter
          Ectopia of ureter
          Ectopic ureter

        Q62.69 Other malposition of ureter

    Q62.7 Congenital vesico-uretero-renal reflux

    Q62.8 Other congenital malformations of ureter
        Anomaly of ureter NOS

☑4ᵗʰ **Q63 Other congenital malformations of kidney**

    EXCLUDES 1   congenital nephrotic syndrome (N04.-)

    Q63.0 Accessory kidney

    Q63.1 Lobulated, fused and horseshoe kidney

    Q63.2 Ectopic kidney
        Congenital displaced kidney
        Malrotation of kidney

    Q63.3 Hyperplastic and giant kidney
        Compensatory hypertrophy of kidney

    Q63.8 Other specified congenital malformations of kidney
        Congenital renal calculi

    Q63.9 Congenital malformation of kidney, unspecified

☑4ᵗʰ **Q64 Other congenital malformations of urinary system**

    Q64.0 Epispadias

        EXCLUDES 1   hypospadias (Q54.-)

Epispadias

Normal external urethral orifice

Glans penis

Foreskin (retracted)

Epispadias

Epispadias (dorsal view)

☑5ᵗʰ **Q64.1 Exstrophy of urinary bladder**

        Q64.10 Exstrophy of urinary bladder, unspecified COM
          Ectopia vesicae

        Q64.11 Supravesical fissure of urinary bladder COM

        Q64.12 Cloacal exstrophy of urinary bladder COM

        Q64.19 Other exstrophy of urinary bladder COM
          Extroversion of bladder

    Q64.2 Congenital posterior urethral valves

☑5ᵗʰ **Q64.3 Other atresia and stenosis of urethra and bladder neck**

        Q64.31 Congenital bladder neck obstruction
          Congenital obstruction of vesicourethral orifice

        Q64.32 Congenital stricture of urethra

        Q64.33 Congenital stricture of urinary meatus

        Q64.39 Other atresia and stenosis of urethra and bladder neck
          Atresia and stenosis of urethra and bladder neck NOS

    Q64.4 Malformation of urachus
        Cyst of urachus
        Patent urachus
        Prolapse of urachus

    Q64.5 Congenital absence of bladder and urethra

    Q64.6 Congenital diverticulum of bladder

☑6ᵗʰ **Q64.7 Other and unspecified congenital malformations of bladder and urethra**

        EXCLUDES 1   congenital prolapse of bladder (mucosa) (Q79.4)

        Q64.70 Unspecified congenital malformation of bladder and urethra
          Malformation of bladder or urethra NOS

        Q64.71 Congenital prolapse of urethra

        Q64.72 Congenital prolapse of urinary meatus

        Q64.73 Congenital urethrorectal fistula

        Q64.74 Double urethra

        Q64.75 Double urinary meatus

        Q64.79 Other congenital malformations of bladder and urethra

    Q64.8 Other specified congenital malformations of urinary system

    Q64.9 Congenital malformation of urinary system, unspecified
        Congenital anomaly NOS of urinary system
        Congenital deformity NOS of urinary system

Congenital malformations and deformations of the musculoskeletal system (Q65-Q79)

☑4ᵗʰ **Q65 Congenital deformities of hip**

    EXCLUDES 1   clicking hip (R29.4)

☑5ᵗʰ **Q65.0 Congenital dislocation of hip, unilateral**

        Q65.00 Congenital dislocation of unspecified hip, unilateral COM

        Q65.01 Congenital dislocation of right hip, unilateral COM

        Q65.02 Congenital dislocation of left hip, unilateral COM

    Q65.1 Congenital dislocation of hip, bilateral COM

    Q65.2 Congenital dislocation of hip, unspecified COM

☑5ᵗʰ **Q65.3 Congenital partial dislocation of hip, unilateral**

        Q65.30 Congenital partial dislocation of unspecified hip, unilateral COM

        Q65.31 Congenital partial dislocation of right hip, unilateral COM

        Q65.32 Congenital partial dislocation of left hip, unilateral COM

    Q65.4 Congenital partial dislocation of hip, bilateral COM

    Q65.5 Congenital partial dislocation of hip, unspecified COM

    Q65.6 Congenital unstable hip COM
        Congenital dislocatable hip

☑5ᵗʰ **Q65.8 Other congenital deformities of hip**

        Q65.81 Congenital coxa valga COM

        Q65.82 Congenital coxa vara COM

        Q65.89 Other specified congenital deformities of hip COM
          Anteversion of femoral neck
          Congenital acetabular dysplasia

    Q65.9 Congenital deformity of hip, unspecified COM

☑4ᵗʰ **Q66 Congenital deformities of feet**

    EXCLUDES 1   reduction defects of feet (Q72.-)
          valgus deformities (acquired) (M21.0-)
          varus deformities (acquired) (M21.1-)

    AHA: 2019,4Q,13

☑5ᵗʰ **Q66.0 Congenital talipes equinovarus**

        Q66.00 Congenital talipes equinovarus, unspecified foot

        Q66.01 Congenital talipes equinovarus, right foot

        Q66.02 Congenital talipes equinovarus, left foot

☑5ᵗʰ **Q66.1 Congenital talipes calcaneovarus**

        Q66.10 Congenital talipes calcaneovarus, unspecified foot

        Q66.11 Congenital talipes calcaneovarus, right foot

        Q66.12 Congenital talipes calcaneovarus, left foot

✓5th **Q66.2 Congenital metatarsus (primus) varus**
   AHA: 2016,4Q,59
   ✓6th **Q66.21   Congenital metatarsus primus varus**
      Q66.211 Congenital metatarsus primus varus, right foot
      Q66.212 Congenital metatarsus primus varus, left foot
      Q66.219 Congenital metatarsus primus varus, unspecified foot
   ✓6th **Q66.22   Congenital metatarsus adductus**
      Congenital metatarsus varus
      Q66.221 Congenital metatarsus adductus, right foot
      Q66.222 Congenital metatarsus adductus, left foot
      Q66.229 Congenital metatarsus adductus, unspecified foot
✓5th **Q66.3 Other congenital varus deformities of feet**
   Hallux varus, congenital
   Q66.30   Other congenital varus deformities of feet, unspecified foot
   Q66.31   Other congenital varus deformities of feet, right foot
   Q66.32   Other congenital varus deformities of feet, left foot
✓5th **Q66.4 Congenital talipes calcaneovalgus**
   Q66.40   Congenital talipes calcaneovalgus, unspecified foot
   Q66.41   Congenital talipes calcaneovalgus, right foot
   Q66.42   Congenital talipes calcaneovalgus, left foot
✓5th **Q66.5 Congenital pes planus**
   Congenital flat foot
   Congenital rigid flat foot
   Congenital spastic (everted) flat foot
   EXCLUDES 1   *pes planus, acquired (M21.4)*
   Q66.50   Congenital pes planus, unspecified foot
   Q66.51   Congenital pes planus, right foot
   Q66.52   Congenital pes planus, left foot
Q66.6 Other congenital valgus deformities of feet
   Congenital metatarsus valgus
✓5th **Q66.7 Congenital pes cavus**
   Q66.70   Congenital pes cavus, unspecified foot
   Q66.71   Congenital pes cavus, right foot
   Q66.72   Congenital pes cavus, left foot
✓5th **Q66.8 Other congenital deformities of feet**
   Q66.80   Congenital vertical talus deformity, unspecified foot
   Q66.81   Congenital vertical talus deformity, right foot
   Q66.82   Congenital vertical talus deformity, left foot
   Q66.89   Other specified congenital deformities of feet
      Congenital asymmetric talipes
      Congenital clubfoot NOS
      Congenital talipes NOS
      Congenital tarsal coalition
      Hammer toe, congenital
      DEF: Clubfoot: Congenital anomaly of the foot with the heel elevated and rotated outward and the toes pointing inward.
✓5th **Q66.9 Congenital deformity of feet, unspecified**
   Q66.90   Congenital deformity of feet, unspecified, unspecified foot
   Q66.91   Congenital deformity of feet, unspecified, right foot
   Q66.92   Congenital deformity of feet, unspecified, left foot
✓4th **Q67 Congenital musculoskeletal deformities of head, face, spine and chest**
   EXCLUDES 1   *congenital malformation syndromes classified to Q87.- Potter's syndrome (Q60.6)*
   Q67.0 Congenital facial asymmetry
   Q67.1 Congenital compression facies
   Q67.2 Dolichocephaly
   Q67.3 Plagiocephaly

Q67.4 Other congenital deformities of skull, face and jaw
   Congenital depressions in skull
   Congenital hemifacial atrophy or hypertrophy
   Deviation of nasal septum, congenital
   Squashed or bent nose, congenital
   EXCLUDES 1   *dentofacial anomalies [including malocclusion] (M26.-)*
      syphilitic saddle nose (A50.5)
   DEF: Deviated septum: Condition in which the nasal septum, a thin wall composed of cartilage and bone that separates the two nostrils, is crooked or displaced from the midline.
Q67.5 Congenital deformity of spine
   Congenital postural scoliosis
   Congenital scoliosis NOS
   EXCLUDES 1   *infantile idiopathic scoliosis (M41.0)*
      scoliosis due to congenital bony malformation (Q76.3)
   AHA: 2014,4Q,26
Q67.6 Pectus excavatum
   Congenital funnel chest
Q67.7 Pectus carinatum
   Congenital pigeon chest
Q67.8 Other congenital deformities of chest
   Congenital deformity of chest wall NOS
✓4th **Q68 Other congenital musculoskeletal deformities**
   EXCLUDES 1   *reduction defects of limb(s) (Q71-Q73)*
   EXCLUDES 2   *congenital myotonic chondrodystrophy (G71.13)*
   Q68.0 Congenital deformity of sternocleidomastoid muscle
      Congenital contracture of sternocleidomastoid (muscle)
      Congenital (sternomastoid) torticollis
      Sternomastoid tumor (congenital)
   Q68.1 Congenital deformity of finger(s) and hand
      Congenital clubfinger
      Spade-like hand (congenital)
   Q68.2 Congenital deformity of knee
      Congenital dislocation of knee
      Congenital genu recurvatum
   Q68.3 Congenital bowing of femur
      EXCLUDES 1   *anteversion of femur (neck) (Q65.89)*
   Q68.4 Congenital bowing of tibia and fibula
   Q68.5 Congenital bowing of long bones of leg, unspecified
   Q68.6 Discoid meniscus
   Q68.8 Other specified congenital musculoskeletal deformities
      Congenital deformity of clavicle
      Congenital deformity of elbow
      Congenital deformity of forearm
      Congenital deformity of scapula
      Congenital deformity of wrist
      Congenital dislocation of elbow
      Congenital dislocation of shoulder
      Congenital dislocation of wrist
✓4th **Q69 Polydactyly**
   Q69.0 Accessory finger(s)
   Q69.1 Accessory thumb(s)
   Q69.2 Accessory toe(s)
      Accessory hallux
   Q69.9 Polydactyly, unspecified
      Supernumerary digit(s) NOS
✓4th **Q70 Syndactyly**
   ✓5th **Q70.0 Fused fingers**
      Complex syndactyly of fingers with synostosis
      Q70.00   Fused fingers, unspecified hand
      Q70.01   Fused fingers, right hand
      Q70.02   Fused fingers, left hand
      Q70.03   Fused fingers, bilateral
   ✓5th **Q70.1 Webbed fingers**
      Simple syndactyly of fingers without synostosis
      Q70.10   Webbed fingers, unspecified hand
      Q70.11   Webbed fingers, right hand
      Q70.12   Webbed fingers, left hand
      Q70.13   Webbed fingers, bilateral
   ✓5th **Q70.2 Fused toes**
      Complex syndactyly of toes with synostosis
      Q70.20   Fused toes, unspecified foot
      Q70.21   Fused toes, right foot

Q70.22   **Fused toes,** left **foot**

Q70.23   **Fused toes,** bilateral

√5ᵗʰ **Q70.3   Webbed toes**

    Simple syndactyly of toes without synostosis

Q70.30   **Webbed toes, unspecified foot**

Q70.31   **Webbed toes,** right **foot**

Q70.32   **Webbed toes,** left **foot**

Q70.33   **Webbed toes,** bilateral

Q70.4   Polysyndactyly, unspecified

    EXCLUDES 1   *specified syndactyly of hand and feet - code to specified conditions (Q70.0-Q70.3-)*

Q70.9   Syndactyly, unspecified

    Symphalangy NOS

√4ᵗʰ **Q71   Reduction defects of** upper limb

√5ᵗʰ **Q71.0   Congenital** complete absence **of upper limb**

Q71.00   **Congenital complete absence of unspecified upper limb**

Q71.01   **Congenital complete absence of** right **upper limb**

Q71.02   **Congenital complete absence of** left **upper limb**

Q71.03   **Congenital complete absence of upper limb,** bilateral

√5ᵗʰ **Q71.1   Congenital** absence of upper arm and forearm with hand present

Q71.10   **Congenital absence of unspecified upper arm and forearm with hand present**

Q71.11   **Congenital absence of** right **upper arm and forearm with hand present**

Q71.12   **Congenital absence of** left **upper arm and forearm with hand present**

Q71.13   **Congenital absence of upper arm and forearm with hand present,** bilateral

√5ᵗʰ **Q71.2   Congenital** absence of both forearm and hand

Q71.20   **Congenital absence of both forearm and hand, unspecified upper limb**

Q71.21   **Congenital absence of both forearm and hand,** right **upper limb**

Q71.22   **Congenital absence of both forearm and hand,** left **upper limb**

Q71.23   **Congenital absence of both forearm and hand,** bilateral

√5ᵗʰ **Q71.3   Congenital** absence of hand and finger

Q71.30   **Congenital absence of unspecified hand and finger**

Q71.31   **Congenital absence of** right **hand and finger**

Q71.32   **Congenital absence of** left **hand and finger**

Q71.33   **Congenital absence of hand and finger,** bilateral

√5ᵗʰ **Q71.4   Longitudinal reduction defect of** radius

    Clubhand (congenital)

    Radial clubhand

Q71.40   **Longitudinal reduction defect of unspecified radius**

Q71.41   **Longitudinal reduction defect of** right **radius**

Q71.42   **Longitudinal reduction defect of** left **radius**

Q71.43   **Longitudinal reduction defect of radius,** bilateral

√5ᵗʰ **Q71.5   Longitudinal reduction defect of** ulna

Q71.50   **Longitudinal reduction defect of unspecified ulna**

Q71.51   **Longitudinal reduction defect of** right **ulna**

Q71.52   **Longitudinal reduction defect of** left **ulna**

Q71.53   **Longitudinal reduction defect of ulna,** bilateral

√5ᵗʰ **Q71.6   Lobster-claw hand**

Q71.60   **Lobster-claw hand, unspecified hand**

Q71.61   **Lobster-claw** right **hand**

Q71.62   **Lobster-claw** left **hand**

Q71.63   **Lobster-claw hand,** bilateral

√5ᵗʰ **Q71.8   Other reduction defects of** upper limb

√6ᵗʰ Q71.81   **Congenital** shortening **of upper limb**

Q71.811   **Congenital shortening of** right **upper limb**

Q71.812   **Congenital shortening of** left **upper limb**

Q71.813   **Congenital shortening of upper limb,** bilateral

Q71.819   **Congenital shortening of unspecified upper limb**

√6ᵗʰ Q71.89   **Other reduction defects of upper limb**

Q71.891   **Other reduction defects of** right **upper limb**

Q71.892   **Other reduction defects of** left **upper limb**

Q71.893   **Other reduction defects of upper limb,** bilateral

Q71.899   **Other reduction defects of unspecified upper limb**

√5ᵗʰ **Q71.9   Unspecified reduction defect of upper limb**

Q71.90   **Unspecified reduction defect of unspecified upper limb**

Q71.91   **Unspecified reduction defect of** right **upper limb**

Q71.92   **Unspecified reduction defect of** left **upper limb**

Q71.93   **Unspecified reduction defect of upper limb,** bilateral

√4ᵗʰ **Q72   Reduction defects of** lower limb

√5ᵗʰ **Q72.0   Congenital** complete absence **of lower limb**

Q72.00   **Congenital complete absence of unspecified lower limb**

Q72.01   **Congenital complete absence of** right **lower limb**

Q72.02   **Congenital complete absence of** left **lower limb**

Q72.03   **Congenital complete absence of lower limb,** bilateral

√5ᵗʰ **Q72.1   Congenital** absence of thigh and lower leg with foot present

Q72.10   **Congenital absence of unspecified thigh and lower leg with foot present**

Q72.11   **Congenital absence of** right **thigh and lower leg with foot present**

Q72.12   **Congenital absence of** left **thigh and lower leg with foot present**

Q72.13   **Congenital absence of thigh and lower leg with foot present,** bilateral

√5ᵗʰ **Q72.2   Congenital** absence of both lower leg and foot

Q72.20   **Congenital absence of both lower leg and foot, unspecified lower limb**

Q72.21   **Congenital absence of both lower leg and foot,** right **lower limb**

Q72.22   **Congenital absence of both lower leg and foot,** left **lower limb**

Q72.23   **Congenital absence of both lower leg and foot,** bilateral

√5ᵗʰ **Q72.3   Congenital** absence of foot and toe(s)

Q72.30   **Congenital absence of unspecified foot and toe(s)**

Q72.31   **Congenital absence of** right **foot and toe(s)**

Q72.32   **Congenital absence of** left **foot and toe(s)**

Q72.33   **Congenital absence of foot and toe(s),** bilateral

√5ᵗʰ **Q72.4   Longitudinal reduction defect of** femur

    Proximal femoral focal deficiency

Q72.40   **Longitudinal reduction defect of unspecified femur**

Q72.41   **Longitudinal reduction defect of** right **femur**

Q72.42   **Longitudinal reduction defect of** left **femur**

Q72.43   **Longitudinal reduction defect of femur,** bilateral

√5ᵗʰ **Q72.5   Longitudinal reduction defect of** tibia

Q72.50   **Longitudinal reduction defect of unspecified tibia**

Q72.51   **Longitudinal reduction defect of** right **tibia**

Q72.52   **Longitudinal reduction defect of** left **tibia**

Q72.53   **Longitudinal reduction defect of tibia,** bilateral

√5ᵗʰ **Q72.6   Longitudinal reduction defect of** fibula

Q72.60   **Longitudinal reduction defect of unspecified fibula**

Q72.61   **Longitudinal reduction defect of** right **fibula**

Q72.62   **Longitudinal reduction defect of** left **fibula**

Q72.63   **Longitudinal reduction defect of fibula,** bilateral

√5ᵗʰ **Q72.7   Split foot**

Q72.70   **Split foot, unspecified lower limb**

Q72.71   **Split foot,** right **lower limb**

Q72.72   **Split foot,** left **lower limb**

Q72.73   **Split foot,** bilateral

√5ᵗʰ **Q72.8   Other reduction defects of lower limb**

√6ᵗʰ Q72.81   **Congenital** shortening **of lower limb**

Q72.811   **Congenital shortening of** right **lower limb**

Q72.812   **Congenital shortening of** left **lower limb**

Q72.813   **Congenital shortening of lower limb,** bilateral

Q72.819   **Congenital shortening of unspecified lower limb**

√6ᵗʰ Q72.89   **Other reduction defects of lower limb**

Q72.891   **Other reduction defects of** right **lower limb**

Q72.892   **Other reduction defects of** left **lower limb**

Q72.893   **Other reduction defects of lower limb,** bilateral

Q72.899 Other reduction defects of unspecified lower limb

✓5ᵗʰ Q72.9 Unspecified reduction defect of lower limb

Q72.90 Unspecified reduction defect of unspecified lower limb

Q72.91 Unspecified reduction defect of right lower limb

Q72.92 Unspecified reduction defect of left lower limb

Q72.93 Unspecified reduction defect of lower limb, bilateral

✓4ᵗʰ Q73 Reduction defects of unspecified limb

Q73.0 Congenital absence of unspecified limb(s)
Amelia NOS

Q73.1 Phocomelia, unspecified limb(s)
Phocomelia NOS

Q73.8 Other reduction defects of unspecified limb(s)
Longitudinal reduction deformity of unspecified limb(s)
Ectromelia of limb NOS
Hemimelia of limb NOS
Reduction defect of limb NOS

✓4ᵗʰ Q74 Other congenital malformations of limb(s)
EXCLUDES 1   polydactyly (Q69.-)
reduction defect of limb (Q71-Q73)
syndactyly (Q70.-)

Q74.0 Other congenital malformations of upper limb(s), including shoulder girdle
Accessory carpal bones
Cleidocranial dysostosis
Congenital pseudarthrosis of clavicle
Macrodactylia (fingers)
Madelung's deformity
Radioulnar synostosis
Sprengel's deformity
Triphalangeal thumb

Q74.1 Congenital malformation of knee
Congenital absence of patella
Congenital dislocation of patella
Congenital genu valgum
Congenital genu varum
Rudimentary patella
EXCLUDES 1   congenital dislocation of knee (Q68.2)
congenital genu recurvatum (Q68.2)
nail patella syndrome (Q87.2)

Q74.2 Other congenital malformations of lower limb(s), including pelvic girdle
Congenital fusion of sacroiliac joint
Congenital malformation of ankle joint
Congenital malformation of sacroiliac joint
EXCLUDES 1   anteversion of femur (neck) (Q65.89)

Q74.3 Arthrogryposis multiplex congenita

Q74.8 Other specified congenital malformations of limb(s)

Q74.9 Unspecified congenital malformation of limb(s)
Congenital anomaly of limb(s) NOS

✓4ᵗʰ Q75 Other congenital malformations of skull and face bones
EXCLUDES 1   congenital malformation of face NOS (Q18.-)
congenital malformation syndromes classified to Q87.-
dentofacial anomalies [including malocclusion] (M26.-)
musculoskeletal deformities of head and face (Q67.0-Q67.4)
skull defects associated with congenital anomalies of brain such as:
anencephaly (Q00.0)
encephalocele (Q01.-)
hydrocephalus (Q03.-)
microcephaly (Q02)

Q75.0 Craniosynostosis
Acrocephaly
Imperfect fusion of skull
Oxycephaly
Trigonocephaly
DEF: Congenital condition in which one or more of the cranial sutures fuse prematurely, creating a deformed or aberrant head shape.

Q75.1 Craniofacial dysostosis
Crouzon's disease

Q75.2 Hypertelorism

Q75.3 Macrocephaly

Q75.4 Mandibulofacial dysostosis
Franceschetti syndrome
Treacher Collins syndrome

Q75.5 Oculomandibular dysostosis

Q75.8 Other specified congenital malformations of skull and face bones
Absence of skull bone, congenital
Congenital deformity of forehead
Platybasia

Q75.9 Congenital malformation of skull and face bones, unspecified
Congenital anomaly of face bones NOS
Congenital anomaly of skull NOS

✓4ᵗʰ Q76 Congenital malformations of spine and bony thorax
EXCLUDES 1   congenital musculoskeletal deformities of spine and chest (Q67.5-Q67.8)

Q76.0 Spina bifida occulta
EXCLUDES 1   meningocele (spinal) (Q05.-)
spina bifida (aperta) (cystica) (Q05.-)

Q76.1 Klippel-Feil syndrome
Cervical fusion syndrome

Q76.2 Congenital spondylolisthesis
Congenital spondylolysis
EXCLUDES 1   spondylolisthesis (acquired) (M43.1-)
spondylolysis (acquired) (M43.0-)

Q76.3 Congenital scoliosis due to congenital bony malformation
Hemivertebra fusion or failure of segmentation with scoliosis

✓5ᵗʰ Q76.4 Other congenital malformations of spine, not associated with scoliosis

✓6ᵗʰ Q76.41 Congenital kyphosis

Q76.411 Congenital kyphosis, occipito-atlanto-axial region
Q76.412 Congenital kyphosis, cervical region
Q76.413 Congenital kyphosis, cervicothoracic region
Q76.414 Congenital kyphosis, thoracic region
Q76.415 Congenital kyphosis, thoracolumbar region
Q76.419 Congenital kyphosis, unspecified region

✓6ᵗʰ Q76.42 Congenital lordosis

Q76.425 Congenital lordosis, thoracolumbar region
Q76.426 Congenital lordosis, lumbar region
Q76.427 Congenital lordosis, lumbosacral region
Q76.428 Congenital lordosis, sacral and sacrococcygeal region
Q76.429 Congenital lordosis, unspecified region

Q76.49 Other congenital malformations of spine, not associated with scoliosis
Congenital absence of vertebra NOS
Congenital fusion of spine NOS
Congenital malformation of lumbosacral (joint) (region) NOS
Congenital malformation of spine NOS
Hemivertebra NOS
Malformation of spine NOS
Platyspondylisis NOS
Supernumerary vertebra NOS

Q76.5 Cervical rib
Supernumerary rib in cervical region

Q76.6 Other congenital malformations of ribs
Accessory rib
Congenital absence of rib
Congenital fusion of ribs
Congenital malformation of ribs NOS
EXCLUDES 1   short rib syndrome (Q77.2)

Q76.7 Congenital malformation of sternum
Congenital absence of sternum
Sternum bifidum

Q76.8 Other congenital malformations of bony thorax

Q76.9 Congenital malformation of bony thorax, unspecified

✓4ᵗʰ Q77 Osteochondrodysplasia with defects of growth of tubular bones and spine
EXCLUDES 1   mucopolysaccharidosis (E76.0-E76.3)
EXCLUDES 2   congenital myotonic chondrodystrophy (G71.13)

Q77.0 Achondrogenesis COM
Hypochondrogenesis

Q77.1 Thanatophoric short stature COM

Q77.2 Short rib syndrome `COM`
Asphyxiating thoracic dysplasia [Jeune]

Q77.3 Chondrodysplasia punctata `COM`
EXCLUDES 1   *Rhizomelic chondrodysplasia punctata (E71.43)*

Q77.4 Achondroplasia `COM`
Hypochondroplasia
Osteosclerosis congenita

Q77.5 Diastrophic dysplasia `COM`

Q77.6 Chondroectodermal dysplasia `COM`
Ellis-van Creveld syndrome

Q77.7 Spondyloepiphyseal dysplasia `COM`

Q77.8 Other osteochondrodysplasia with defects of growth of tubular bones and spine `COM`

Q77.9 Osteochondrodysplasia with defects of growth of tubular bones and spine, unspecified `COM`

☑4ᵗʰ **Q78 Other osteochondrodysplasias**
EXCLUDES 2   *congenital myotonic chondrodystrophy (G71.13)*

Q78.0 Osteogenesis imperfecta `COM`
Fragilitas ossium
Osteopsathyrosis

Q78.1 Polyostotic fibrous dysplasia `COM`
Albright(-McCune)(-Sternberg) syndrome

Q78.2 Osteopetrosis `COM`
Albers-Schönberg syndrome
Osteosclerosis NOS
DEF: Rare congenital condition in which the bones are excessively dense, resulting from a discrepancy in the formation and breakdown of bone.

Q78.3 Progressive diaphyseal dysplasia `COM`
Camurati-Engelmann syndrome

Q78.4 Enchondromatosis `COM`
Maffucci's syndrome
Ollier's disease

Q78.5 Metaphyseal dysplasia `COM`
Pyle's syndrome

Q78.6 Multiple congenital exostoses `COM`
Diaphyseal aclasis

Q78.8 Other specified osteochondrodysplasias `COM`
Osteopoikilosis

Q78.9 Osteochondrodysplasia, unspecified `COM`
Chondrodystrophy NOS
Osteodystrophy NOS

☑4ᵗʰ **Q79 Congenital malformations of musculoskeletal system, not elsewhere classified**
EXCLUDES 2   *congenital (sternomastoid) torticollis (Q68.0)*

Q79.0 Congenital diaphragmatic hernia `COM`
EXCLUDES 1   *congenital hiatus hernia (Q40.1)*

Q79.1 Other congenital malformations of diaphragm `COM`
Absence of diaphragm
Congenital malformation of diaphragm NOS
Eventration of diaphragm

Q79.2 Exomphalos `COM`
Omphalocele
EXCLUDES 1   *umbilical hernia (K42.-)*

Q79.3 Gastroschisis `COM`

Gastroschisis

Herniated small bowel (gastroschisis)

Rectus abdominus m.

Umbilicus

skin

distal

proximal

Defect

Q79.4 Prune belly syndrome `COM`
Congenital prolapse of bladder mucosa
Eagle-Barrett syndrome

☑5ᵗʰ **Q79.5 Other congenital malformations of abdominal wall**
EXCLUDES 1   *umbilical hernia (K42.-)*

Q79.51 Congenital hernia of bladder `COM`
Q79.59 Other congenital malformations of abdominal wall

☑5ᵗʰ **Q79.6 Ehlers-Danlos syndromes**
AHA: 2019,4Q,13-14
DEF: Connective tissue disorder that causes hyperextended skin and joints and results in fragile blood vessels with bleeding, poor wound healing, and subcutaneous pseudotumors.

Q79.60 Ehlers-Danlos syndrome, unspecified `Rx` `COM`
Q79.61 Classical Ehlers-Danlos syndrome `Rx` `COM`
Classical EDS (cEDS)
Q79.62 Hypermobile Ehlers-Danlos syndrome `Rx` `COM`
Hypermobile EDS (hEDS)
Q79.63 Vascular Ehlers-Danlos syndrome `Rx` `COM`
Vascular EDS (vEDS)
Q79.69 Other Ehlers-Danlos syndromes `Rx` `COM`

Q79.8 Other congenital malformations of musculoskeletal system
Absence of muscle
Absence of tendon
Accessory muscle
Amyotrophia congenita
Congenital constricting bands
Congenital shortening of tendon
Poland syndrome

Q79.9 Congenital malformation of musculoskeletal system, unspecified
Congenital anomaly of musculoskeletal system NOS
Congenital deformity of musculoskeletal system NOS

Other congenital malformations (Q80-Q89)

☑4ᵗʰ **Q80 Congenital ichthyosis**
EXCLUDES 1   *Refsum's disease (G60.1)*
DEF: Excessive production of skin cells resulting in red, dry, scaly skin.

Q80.0 Ichthyosis vulgaris
Q80.1 X-linked ichthyosis
Q80.2 Lamellar ichthyosis
Collodion baby
Q80.3 Congenital bullous ichthyosiform erythroderma
Q80.4 Harlequin fetus
Q80.8 Other congenital ichthyosis
Q80.9 Congenital ichthyosis, unspecified

☑4ᵗʰ **Q81 Epidermolysis bullosa**

Q81.0 Epidermolysis bullosa simplex `COM`
EXCLUDES 1   *Cockayne's syndrome (Q87.19)*

Q81.1 Epidermolysis bullosa letalis `COM`
Herlitz' syndrome

Q81.2 Epidermolysis bullosa dystrophica `COM`
Q81.8 Other epidermolysis bullosa `COM`
Q81.9 Epidermolysis bullosa, unspecified `COM`

☑4ᵗʰ **Q82 Other congenital malformations of skin**
EXCLUDES 1   *acrodermatitis enteropathica (E83.2)*
congenital erythropoietic porphyria (E80.0)
pilonidal cyst or sinus (L05.-)
Sturge-Weber (-Dimitri) syndrome ▶(Q85.89)◀

Q82.0 Hereditary lymphedema
Q82.1 Xeroderma pigmentosum
Q82.2 Congenital cutaneous mastocytosis
Congenital diffuse cutaneous mastocytosis
Congenital maculopapular cutaneous mastocytosis
Congenital urticaria pigmentosa
EXCLUDES 1   *cutaneous mastocytosis NOS (D47.01)*
diffuse cutaneous mastocytosis (with onset after newborn period) (D47.01)
malignant mastocytosis (C96.2-)
systemic mastocytosis (D47.02)
urticaria pigmentosa (non-congenital) (with onset after newborn period) (D47.01)
AHA: 2017,4Q,5

Q82.3 Incontinentia pigmenti
Q82.4 Ectodermal dysplasia (anhidrotic)
EXCLUDES 1   *Ellis-van Creveld syndrome (Q77.6)*

☑ Additional Character Required   ☑x7ᵗʰ Placeholder Alert   Manifestation   Unspecified Dx   ◘ QPP   `UPD` Unacceptable PDx

Q82.5 Congenital non-neoplastic nevus
Birthmark NOS
Flammeus Nevus
Portwine Nevus
Sanguineous Nevus
Strawberry Nevus
Vascular Nevus NOS
Verrucous Nevus
EXCLUDES 2   *araneus nevus (I78.1)*
Café au lait spots (L81.3)
lentigo (L81.4)
melanocytic nevus (D22.-)
nevus NOS (D22.-)
pigmented nevus (D22.-)
spider nevus (I78.1)
stellar nevus (I78.1)

Q82.6 Congenital sacral dimple
Parasacral dimple
EXCLUDES 2   *pilonidal cyst with abscess (L05.01)*
pilonidal cyst without abscess (L05.91)
AHA: 2016,4Q,60

Q82.8 Other specified congenital malformations of skin
Abnormal palmar creases
Accessory skin tags
Benign familial pemphigus [Hailey-Hailey]
Congenital poikiloderma
Cutis laxa (hyperelastica)
Dermatoglyphic anomalies
Inherited keratosis palmaris et plantaris
Keratosis follicularis [Darier-White]
EXCLUDES 1   *Ehlers-Danlos syndromes (Q79.6-)*
AHA: 2021,3Q,10; 2016,1Q,17

Q82.9 Congenital malformation of skin, unspecified

✓4th **Q83 Congenital malformations of breast**
EXCLUDES 2   *absence of pectoral muscle (Q79.8)*
hypoplasia of breast (N64.82)
micromastia (N64.82)

Q83.0 Congenital absence of breast with absent nipple

Q83.1 Accessory breast
Supernumerary breast

Q83.2 Absent nipple

Q83.3 Accessory nipple
Supernumerary nipple

Q83.8 Other congenital malformations of breast

Q83.9 Congenital malformation of breast, unspecified

✓4th **Q84 Other congenital malformations of integument**

Q84.0 Congenital alopecia
Congenital atrichosis

Q84.1 Congenital morphological disturbances of hair, not elsewhere classified
Beaded hair
Monilethrix
Pili annulati
EXCLUDES 1   *Menkes' kinky hair syndrome (E83.0)*

Q84.2 Other congenital malformations of hair
Congenital hypertrichosis
Congenital malformation of hair NOS
Persistent lanugo

Q84.3 Anonychia
EXCLUDES 1   *nail patella syndrome (Q87.2)*

Q84.4 Congenital leukonychia

Q84.5 Enlarged and hypertrophic nails
Congenital onychauxis
Pachyonychia

Q84.6 Other congenital malformations of nails
Congenital clubnail
Congenital koilonychia
Congenital malformation of nail NOS

Q84.8 Other specified congenital malformations of integument
Aplasia cutis congenita

Q84.9 Congenital malformation of integument, unspecified
Congenital anomaly of integument NOS
Congenital deformity of integument NOS

✓4th **Q85 Phakomatoses, not elsewhere classified**
EXCLUDES 1   *ataxia telangiectasia [Louis-Bar] (G11.3)*
familial dysautonomia [Riley-Day] (G90.1)

✓6th **Q85.0 Neurofibromatosis (nonmalignant)**

Q85.00 Neurofibromatosis, unspecified   HCC ESR COM

Q85.01 Neurofibromatosis, type 1   HCC ESR COM
Von Recklinghausen disease

Q85.02 Neurofibromatosis, type 2   HCC ESR COM
Acoustic neurofibromatosis
DEF: Inherited condition with cutaneous lesions, benign tumors of peripheral nerves, and bilateral 8th nerve masses.

Q85.03 Schwannomatosis   HCC ESR COM
DEF: Genetic mutation (SMARCB1/INI1) causing multiple benign tumors along the nerve pathways, except on the 8th cranial (vestibular) nerve.

Q85.09 Other neurofibromatosis   HCC ESR COM

Q85.1 Tuberous sclerosis   HCC Rx ESR COM
Bourneville's disease
Epiloia

▲ ✓5th **Q85.8 Other phakomatoses, not elsewhere classified**
~~Peutz-Jeghers Syndrome~~
~~Sturge-Weber(-Dimitri) syndrome~~
~~von Hippel-Lindau syndrome~~
EXCLUDES 1   *Meckel-Gruber syndrome (Q61.9)*
AHA: 2021,3Q,12

● **Q85.81 PTEN tumor syndrome**
PHTS
PTEN hamartoma tumor syndrome
PTEN related Cowden syndrome
Code also, if applicable, genetic susceptibility to malignant neoplasm (Z15.0-)

● **Q85.82 Other Cowden syndrome**

● **Q85.83 Von Hippel-Lindau syndrome**
Code also manifestations

● **Q85.89 Other phakomatoses, not elsewhere classified**
Peutz-Jeghers syndrome
Sturge-Weber(-Dimitri) syndrome

Q85.9 Phakomatosis, unspecified   HCC Rx ESR COM
Hamartosis NOS

✓4th **Q86 Congenital malformation syndromes due to known exogenous causes, not elsewhere classified**
EXCLUDES 2   *iodine-deficiency-related hypothyroidism (E00-E02)*
nonteratogenic effects of substances transmitted via placenta or breast milk (P04.-)

Q86.0 Fetal alcohol syndrome (dysmorphic)   COM

Q86.1 Fetal hydantoin syndrome   COM
Meadow's syndrome

Q86.2 Dysmorphism due to warfarin   COM

Q86.8 Other congenital malformation syndromes due to known exogenous causes   COM

✓4th **Q87 Other specified congenital malformation syndromes affecting multiple systems**
Use additional code(s) to identify all associated manifestations

Q87.0 Congenital malformation syndromes predominantly affecting facial appearance
Acrocephalopolysyndactyly
Acrocephalosyndactyly [Apert]
Cryptophthalmos syndrome
Cyclopia
Goldenhar syndrome
Moebius syndrome
Oro-facial-digital syndrome
Robin syndrome
Whistling face

✓5th **Q87.1 Congenital malformation syndromes predominantly associated with short stature**
EXCLUDES 1   *Ellis-van Creveld syndrome (Q77.6)*
Smith-Lemli-Opitz syndrome (E78.72)
AHA: 2019,4Q,14-15

Q87.11 Prader-Willi syndrome   Rx COM

Q87.19   **Other congenital malformation syndromes predominantly associated with short stature** `COM`
- Aarskog syndrome
- Cockayne syndrome
- De Lange syndrome
- Dubowitz syndrome
- Noonan syndrome
- Robinow-Silverman-Smith syndrome
- Russell-Silver syndrome
- Seckel syndrome

Q87.2   **Congenital malformation syndromes predominantly involving limbs** `COM`
- Holt-Oram syndrome
- Klippel-Trenaunay-Weber syndrome
- Nail patella syndrome
- Rubinstein-Taybi syndrome
- Sirenomelia syndrome
- Thrombocytopenia with absent radius [TAR] syndrome
- VATER syndrome

Q87.3   **Congenital malformation syndromes involving early overgrowth** `COM`
- Beckwith-Wiedemann syndrome
- Sotos syndrome
- Weaver syndrome

✅5ᵗʰ **Q87.4**   **Marfan's syndrome**
> **DEF:** Disorder that affects the connective tissue of multiple systems, including disproportionally long or abnormal bone structure and eye and cardiovascular complications.

   Q87.40   **Marfan's syndrome, unspecified** `Rx` `COM`

✅6ᵗʰ **Q87.41**   **Marfan's syndrome with cardiovascular manifestations**

     Q87.410   **Marfan's syndrome with aortic dilation** `Rx` `COM`

     Q87.418   **Marfan's syndrome with other cardiovascular manifestations** `Rx` `COM`

   Q87.42   **Marfan's syndrome with ocular manifestations** `Rx` `COM`

   Q87.43   **Marfan's syndrome with skeletal manifestation** `Rx` `COM`

Q87.5   **Other congenital malformation syndromes with other skeletal changes** `COM`

✅5ᵗʰ **Q87.8**   **Other specified congenital malformation syndromes, not elsewhere classified**
> `EXCLUDES 1`   *Zellweger syndrome (E71.510)*

   Q87.81   **Alport syndrome** `COM`
> Use additional code to identify stage of chronic kidney disease (N18.1-N18.6)

   Q87.82   **Arterial tortuosity syndrome** `Rx` `COM`
> **AHA:** 2016,4Q,60-61

   Q87.89   **Other specified congenital malformation syndromes, not elsewhere classified** `COM`
> Laurence-Moon (-Bardet)-Biedl syndrome

✅4ᵗʰ **Q89**   **Other congenital malformations, not elsewhere classified**

✅5ᵗʰ **Q89.0**   **Congenital absence and malformations of spleen**
> `EXCLUDES 1`   *isomerism of atrial appendages (with asplenia or polysplenia) (Q20.6)*

   Q89.01   **Asplenia (congenital)**

   Q89.09   **Congenital malformations of spleen**
> Congenital splenomegaly

Q89.1   **Congenital malformations of adrenal gland**
> `EXCLUDES 1`   *adrenogenital disorders (E25.-)*
>   *congenital adrenal hyperplasia (E25.0)*

Q89.2   **Congenital malformations of other endocrine glands**
> Congenital malformation of parathyroid or thyroid gland
> Persistent thyroglossal duct
> Thyroglossal cyst
> `EXCLUDES 1`   *congenital goiter (E03.0)*
>   *congenital hypothyroidism (E03.1)*

Q89.3   **Situs inversus** `COM`
- Dextrocardia with situs inversus
- Mirror-image atrial arrangement with situs inversus
- Situs inversus or transversus abdominalis
- Situs inversus or transversus thoracis
- Transposition of abdominal viscera
- Transposition of thoracic viscera
> `EXCLUDES 1`   *dextrocardia NOS (Q24.0)*
> **DEF:** Congenital anomaly in which the internal thoracic and abdominal organs are transposed laterally and found on the opposite side from the normal position.

Q89.4   **Conjoined twins** `COM`
- Craniopagus
- Dicephaly
- Pygopagus
- Thoracopagus

Q89.7   **Multiple congenital malformations, not elsewhere classified**
- Multiple congenital anomalies NOS
- Multiple congenital deformities NOS
> `EXCLUDES 1`   *congenital malformation syndromes affecting multiple systems (Q87.-)*

Q89.8   **Other specified congenital malformations** `COM`
> Use additional code(s) to identify all associated manifestations
> **AHA:** 2021,3Q,12

Q89.9   **Congenital malformation, unspecified**
- Congenital anomaly NOS
- Congenital deformity NOS

Chromosomal abnormalities, not elsewhere classified (Q90-Q99)

> `EXCLUDES 2`   *mitochondrial metabolic disorders (E88.4-)*

✅4ᵗʰ **Q90**   **Down syndrome**
> Use additional code(s) to identify any associated physical conditions and degree of intellectual disabilities (F70-F79)

   Q90.0   **Trisomy 21, nonmosaicism (meiotic nondisjunction)** `COM`

   Q90.1   **Trisomy 21, mosaicism (mitotic nondisjunction)** `COM`

   Q90.2   **Trisomy 21, translocation** `COM`

   Q90.9   **Down syndrome, unspecified** `COM`
> Trisomy 21 NOS

✅4ᵗʰ **Q91**   **Trisomy 18 and Trisomy 13**

   Q91.0   **Trisomy 18, nonmosaicism (meiotic nondisjunction)** `Rx` `COM`

   Q91.1   **Trisomy 18, mosaicism (mitotic nondisjunction)** `Rx` `COM`

   Q91.2   **Trisomy 18, translocation** `Rx` `COM`

   Q91.3   **Trisomy 18, unspecified** `Rx` `COM`

   Q91.4   **Trisomy 13, nonmosaicism (meiotic nondisjunction)** `Rx` `COM`

   Q91.5   **Trisomy 13, mosaicism (mitotic nondisjunction)** `Rx` `COM`

   Q91.6   **Trisomy 13, translocation** `Rx` `COM`

   Q91.7   **Trisomy 13, unspecified** `Rx` `COM`

✅4ᵗʰ **Q92**   **Other trisomies and partial trisomies of the autosomes, not elsewhere classified**
> `INCLUDES`   unbalanced translocations and insertions
> `EXCLUDES 1`   *trisomies of chromosomes 13, 18, 21 (Q90-Q91)*

   Q92.0   **Whole chromosome trisomy, nonmosaicism (meiotic nondisjunction)** `Rx` `COM`

   Q92.1   **Whole chromosome trisomy, mosaicism (mitotic nondisjunction)** `Rx` `COM`

   Q92.2   **Partial trisomy** `Rx` `COM`
- Less than whole arm duplicated
- Whole arm or more duplicated
> `EXCLUDES 1`   *partial trisomy due to unbalanced translocation (Q92.5)*

   Q92.5   **Duplications with other complex rearrangements** `Rx` `COM`
> Partial trisomy due to unbalanced translocations
> Code also any associated deletions due to unbalanced translocations, inversions and insertions (Q93.7)

✅5ᵗʰ **Q92.6**   **Marker chromosomes**
- Trisomies due to dicentrics
- Trisomies due to extra rings
- Trisomies due to isochromosomes
- Individual with marker heterochromatin

   Q92.61   **Marker chromosomes in normal individual** `Rx` `COM`

Q92.62   **Marker chromosomes in abnormal individual** `Rx` `COM`

Q92.7   **Triploidy and polyploidy** `Rx` `COM`

Q92.8   **Other specified trisomies and partial trisomies of autosomes** `Rx` `COM`
Duplications identified by fluorescence in situ hybridization (FISH)
Duplications identified by in situ hybridization (ISH)
Duplications seen only at prometaphase

Q92.9   **Trisomy and partial trisomy of autosomes, unspecified** `Rx` `COM`

✓4ᵗʰ **Q93** **Monosomies and deletions from the autosomes, not elsewhere classified**

Q93.0   **Whole chromosome monosomy, nonmosaicism (meiotic nondisjunction)** `Rx` `COM`

Q93.1   **Whole chromosome monosomy, mosaicism (mitotic nondisjunction)** `Rx` `COM`

Q93.2   **Chromosome replaced with ring, dicentric or isochromosome** `Rx` `COM`

Q93.3   **Deletion of short arm of chromosome 4** `Rx` `COM`
Wolff-Hirschorn syndrome

Q93.4   **Deletion of short arm of chromosome 5** `Rx` `COM`
Cri-du-chat syndrome

✓5ᵗʰ **Q93.5**   **Other deletions of part of a chromosome**
AHA: 2018,4Q,28

Q93.51   **Angelman syndrome** `Rx` `COM`

Q93.59   **Other deletions of part of a chromosome** `Rx` `COM`

Q93.7   **Deletions with other complex rearrangements** `Rx` `COM`
Deletions due to unbalanced translocations, inversions and insertions
Code also any associated duplications due to unbalanced translocations, inversions and insertions (Q92.5)

✓5ᵗʰ **Q93.8**   **Other deletions from the autosomes**

Q93.81   **Velo-cardio-facial syndrome** `Rx` `COM`
Deletion 22q11.2
AHA: 2019,3Q,14
DEF: Microdeletion syndrome affecting multiple organs characterized by a cleft palate, heart defects, an elongated face with almond-shaped eyes, wide nose, small ears, weak immune system, weak musculature, hypothyroidism, short stature, and scoliosis. The deletion occurs at q11.2 on the long arm of the chromosome 22.

Q93.82   **Williams syndrome** `Rx` `COM`
AHA: 2018,4Q,28-29

Q93.88   **Other microdeletions** `Rx` `COM`
Miller-Dieker syndrome
Smith-Magenis syndrome

Q93.89   **Other deletions from the autosomes** `Rx` `COM`
Deletions identified by fluorescence in situ hybridization (FISH)
Deletions identified by in situ hybridization (ISH)
Deletions seen only at prometaphase

Q93.9   **Deletion from autosomes, unspecified** `Rx` `COM`

✓4ᵗʰ **Q95** **Balanced rearrangements and structural markers, not elsewhere classified**
INCLUDES   Robertsonian and balanced reciprocal translocations and insertions

Q95.0   **Balanced translocation and insertion in normal individual**

Q95.1   **Chromosome inversion in normal individual**

Q95.2   **Balanced autosomal rearrangement in abnormal individual** `Rx` `COM`

Q95.3   **Balanced sex/autosomal rearrangement in abnormal individual** `Rx` `COM`

Q95.5   **Individual with autosomal fragile site**

Q95.8   **Other balanced rearrangements and structural markers**

Q95.9   **Balanced rearrangement and structural marker, unspecified**

✓4ᵗʰ **Q96** **Turner's syndrome**
EXCLUDES 1   Noonan syndrome (Q87.19)

Q96.0   **Karyotype 45, X** `COM` ♀

Q96.1   **Karyotype 46, X iso (Xq)** `COM` ♀
Karyotype 46, isochromosome Xq

Q96.2   **Karyotype 46, X with abnormal sex chromosome, except iso (Xq)** `COM` ♀
Karyotype 46, X with abnormal sex chromosome, except isochromosome Xq

Q96.3   **Mosaicism, 45, X/46, XX or XY** `COM` ♀

Q96.4   **Mosaicism, 45, X/other cell line(s) with abnormal sex chromosome** `COM` ♀

Q96.8   **Other variants of Turner's syndrome** `COM` ♀

Q96.9   **Turner's syndrome, unspecified** `COM` ♀

✓4ᵗʰ **Q97** **Other sex chromosome abnormalities, female phenotype, not elsewhere classified**
EXCLUDES 1   Turner's syndrome (Q96.-)

Q97.0   **Karyotype 47, XXX** `COM` ♀

Q97.1   **Female with more than three X chromosomes** `COM` ♀

Q97.2   **Mosaicism, lines with various numbers of X chromosomes** `COM` ♀

Q97.3   **Female with 46, XY karyotype** `COM` ♀

Q97.8   **Other specified sex chromosome abnormalities, female phenotype** `COM` ♀

Q97.9   **Sex chromosome abnormality, female phenotype, unspecified** `COM` ♀

✓4ᵗʰ **Q98** **Other sex chromosome abnormalities, male phenotype, not elsewhere classified**

Q98.0   **Klinefelter syndrome karyotype 47, XXY** `COM` ♂

Q98.1   **Klinefelter syndrome, male with more than two X chromosomes** `COM` ♂

Q98.3   **Other male with 46, XX karyotype** `COM` ♂

Q98.4   **Klinefelter syndrome, unspecified** `COM` ♂

Q98.5   **Karyotype 47, XYY** `COM`

Q98.6   **Male with structurally abnormal sex chromosome** `COM` ♂

Q98.7   **Male with sex chromosome mosaicism** `COM` ♂

Q98.8   **Other specified sex chromosome abnormalities, male phenotype** `COM` ♂

Q98.9   **Sex chromosome abnormality, male phenotype, unspecified** `COM` ♂

✓4ᵗʰ **Q99** **Other chromosome abnormalities, not elsewhere classified**

Q99.0   **Chimera 46, XX/46, XY** `COM`
Chimera 46, XX/46, XY true hermaphrodite

Q99.1   **46, XX true hermaphrodite** `COM`
46, XX with streak gonads
46, XY with streak gonads
Pure gonadal dysgenesis

Q99.2   **Fragile X chromosome** `Rx` `COM`
Fragile X syndrome

Q99.8   **Other specified chromosome abnormalities** `COM`

Q99.9   **Chromosomal abnormality, unspecified** `COM`

Chapter 18. Symptoms, Signs and Abnormal Clinical and Laboratory Findings (R00–R99)

Chapter-specific Guidelines with Coding Examples

The chapter-specific guidelines from the ICD-10-CM Official Guidelines for Coding and Reporting have been provided below. Along with these guidelines are coding examples, contained in the shaded boxes, that have been developed to help illustrate the coding and/or sequencing guidance found in these guidelines.

Chapter 18 includes symptoms, signs, abnormal results of clinical or other investigative procedures, and ill-defined conditions regarding which no diagnosis classifiable elsewhere is recorded. Signs and symptoms that point to a specific diagnosis have been assigned to a category in other chapters of the classification.

a. Use of symptom codes

Codes that describe symptoms and signs are acceptable for reporting purposes when a related definitive diagnosis has not been established (confirmed) by the provider.

> Tenderness and localized pain in the right upper quadrant; based on presentation, probable gallstones
>
> **R10.11**   **Right upper quadrant pain**
>
> **R10.811**   **Right upper quadrant abdominal tenderness**
>
> *Explanation:* Codes that describe symptoms such as abdominal pain are acceptable for reporting purposes when the provider has not established (confirmed) a definitive diagnosis.

b. Use of a symptom code with a definitive diagnosis code

Codes for signs and symptoms may be reported in addition to a related definitive diagnosis when the sign or symptom is not routinely associated with that diagnosis, such as the various signs and symptoms associated with complex syndromes. The definitive diagnosis code should be sequenced before the symptom code.

Signs or symptoms that are associated routinely with a disease process should not be assigned as additional codes, unless otherwise instructed by the classification.

> Pneumonia with hemoptysis
>
> **J18.9**   **Pneumonia, unspecified organism**
>
> **R04.2**   **Hemoptysis**
>
> *Explanation:* Codes for signs and symptoms may be reported in addition to a related definitive diagnosis when the sign or symptom is not routinely associated with that diagnosis.

> Abdominal pain due to acute appendicitis
>
> **K35.80**   **Unspecified acute appendicitis**
>
> *Explanation:* Codes for signs or symptoms routinely associated with a disease process should not be assigned unless the classification instructs otherwise.

c. Combination codes that include symptoms

ICD-10-CM contains a number of combination codes that identify both the definitive diagnosis and common symptoms of that diagnosis. When using one of these combination codes, an additional code should not be assigned for the symptom.

> IBS with diarrhea
>
> **K58.0**   **Irritable bowel syndrome with diarrhea**
>
> *Explanation:* When a combination code identifies both the definitive diagnosis and the symptom, an additional code should not be assigned for the symptom.

d. Repeated falls

Code R29.6, Repeated falls, is for use for encounters when a patient has recently fallen and the reason for the fall is being investigated.

Code Z91.81, History of falling, is for use when a patient has fallen in the past and is at risk for future falls. When appropriate, both codes R29.6 and Z91.81 may be assigned together.

e. Coma

Code R40.20, Unspecified coma, may be assigned in conjunction with codes for any medical condition.

Do not report codes for unspecified coma, individual or total Glasgow coma scale scores for a patient with a medically induced coma or a sedated patient.

1) Coma scale

The coma scale codes (R40.21- to R40.24-) can be used in conjunction with traumatic brain injury codes. These codes are primarily for use by trauma registries, but they may be used in any setting where this information is collected. The coma scale codes should be sequenced after the diagnosis code(s).

These codes, one from each subcategory, are needed to complete the scale. The 7th character indicates when the scale was recorded. The 7th character should match for all three codes.

At a minimum, report the initial score documented on presentation at your facility. This may be a score from the emergency medicine technician (EMT) or in the emergency department. If desired, a facility may choose to capture multiple coma scale scores.

Assign code R40.24-, Glasgow coma scale, total score, when only the total score is documented in the medical record and not the individual score(s).

If multiple coma scores are captured within the first 24 hours after hospital admission, assign only the code for the score at the time of admission. ICD-10-CM does not classify coma scores that are reported after admission but less than 24 hours later.

See Section I.B.14. for coma scale documentation by clinicians other than patient's provider

> 36-year-old man found down after unknown injury with skull fracture and with concussion and loss of consciousness of unknown duration. Upon hospital admission, the patient was evaluated with the following Glasgow coma scores:
>
> Eye-opening response—3: eyes open to speech
>
> Verbal response—3: random speech with no conversational exchange
>
> Motor response—4: pulls limb away from painful stimulus
>
> **S02.0XXA**   **Fracture of vault of skull, initial encounter for closed fracture**
>
> **S06.0X9A**   **Concussion with loss of consciousness of unspecified duration, initial encounter**
>
> **R40.2133**   **Coma scale, eyes open, to sound, at hospital admission**
>
> **R40.2233**   **Coma scale, best verbal response, inappropriate words, at hospital admission**
>
> **R40.2343**   **Coma scale, best motor response, flexion withdrawal, at hospital admission**
>
> *Explanation:* When individual scores for the Glasgow coma scale are documented, one code from each category is needed to complete the scale. The seventh character indicates when the scale was recorded and should match for all three codes. Assign a code from subcategory R40.24- Glasgow coma scale, total score, when only the total and not the individual score(s) is documented.

f. Functional quadriplegia

GUIDELINE HAS BEEN DELETED EFFECTIVE OCTOBER 1, 2017

g. SIRS due to non-infectious process

The systemic inflammatory response syndrome (SIRS) can develop as a result of certain non-infectious disease processes, such as trauma, malignant neoplasm, or pancreatitis. When SIRS is documented with a noninfectious condition, and no subsequent infection is documented, the code for the underlying condition, such as an injury, should be assigned, followed by code R65.10, Systemic inflammatory response syndrome (SIRS) of non-infectious origin without acute organ dysfunction, or code R65.11, Systemic inflammatory response syndrome (SIRS) of non-infectious origin with acute organ dysfunction. If an associated acute organ dysfunction is documented, the appropriate code(s) for the specific type of organ dysfunction(s) should be assigned in addition to code R65.11. If acute organ dysfunction is documented, but it cannot be determined if the acute organ dysfunction is associated with SIRS or due to another condition (e.g., directly due to the trauma), the provider should be queried.

> Systemic inflammatory response syndrome (SIRS) due to acute gallstone pancreatitis
>
> **K85.10   Biliary acute pancreatitis without necrosis or infection**
>
> **R65.10   Systemic inflammatory response syndrome [SIRS] of non-infectious origin without acute organ dysfunction**
>
> *Explanation:* When SIRS is documented with a non-infectious condition without subsequent infection documented, the code for the underlying condition such as pancreatitis should be assigned followed by the appropriate code for SIRS of noninfectious origin, either with or without associated organ dysfunction.

h. Death NOS

Code R99, Ill-defined and unknown cause of mortality, is only for use in the very limited circumstance when a patient who has already died is brought into an emergency department or other healthcare facility and is pronounced dead upon arrival. It does not represent the discharge disposition of death.

i. NIHSS stroke scale

The NIH stroke scale (NIHSS) codes (R29.7- -) can be used in conjunction with acute stroke codes (I63) to identify the patient's neurological status and the severity of the stroke. The stroke scale codes should be sequenced after the acute stroke diagnosis code(s).

At a minimum, report the initial score documented. If desired, a facility may choose to capture multiple stroke scale scores.

See Section I.B.14. for NIHSS stroke scale documentation by clinicians other than patient's provider

Chapter 18. Symptoms, Signs and Abnormal Clinical and Laboratory Findings, Not Elsewhere Classified (R00-R99)

NOTE   This chapter includes symptoms, signs, abnormal results of clinical or other investigative procedures, and ill-defined conditions regarding which no diagnosis classifiable elsewhere is recorded.

Signs and symptoms that point rather definitely to a given diagnosis have been assigned to a category in other chapters of the classification. In general, categories in this chapter include the less well-defined conditions and symptoms that, without the necessary study of the case to establish a final diagnosis, point perhaps equally to two or more diseases or to two or more systems of the body. Practically all categories in the chapter could be designated 'not otherwise specified', 'unknown etiology' or 'transient'. The Alphabetical Index should be consulted to determine which symptoms and signs are to be allocated here and which to other chapters. The residual subcategories, numbered .8, are generally provided for other relevant symptoms that cannot be allocated elsewhere in the classification.

The conditions and signs or symptoms included in categories R00-R94 consist of:

(a)   cases for which no more specific diagnosis can be made even after all the facts bearing on the case have been investigated;

(b)   signs or symptoms existing at the time of initial encounter that proved to be transient and whose causes could not be determined;

(c)   provisional diagnosis in a patient who failed to return for further investigation or care;

(d)   cases referred elsewhere for investigation or treatment before the diagnosis was made;

(e)   cases in which a more precise diagnosis was not available for any other reason;

(f)   certain symptoms, for which supplementary information is provided, that represent important problems in medical care in their own right.

EXCLUDES 2   *abnormal findings on antenatal screening of mother (O28.-)*
certain conditions originating in the perinatal period (P04-P96)
signs and symptoms classified in the body system chapters
signs and symptoms of breast (N63, N64.5)

AHA: 2017,1Q,6,7

This chapter contains the following blocks:

R00-R09   Symptoms and signs involving the circulatory and respiratory systems
R10-R19   Symptoms and signs involving the digestive system and abdomen
R20-R23   Symptoms and signs involving the skin and subcutaneous tissue
R25-R29   Symptoms and signs involving the nervous and musculoskeletal systems
R30-R39   Symptoms and signs involving the genitourinary system
R40-R46   Symptoms and signs involving cognition, perception, emotional state and behavior
R47-R49   Symptoms and signs involving speech and voice
R50-R69   General symptoms and signs
R70-R79   Abnormal findings on examination of blood, without diagnosis
R80-R82   Abnormal findings on examination of urine, without diagnosis
R83-R89   Abnormal findings on examination of other body fluids, substances and tissues, without diagnosis
R90-R94   Abnormal findings on diagnostic imaging and in function studies, without diagnosis
R97   Abnormal tumor markers
R99   Ill-defined and unknown cause of mortality

Symptoms and signs involving the circulatory and respiratory systems (R00-R09)

✓4ᵗʰ R00   Abnormalities of heart beat
    EXCLUDES 1   *abnormalities originating in the perinatal period (P29.1-)*
    EXCLUDES 2   *specified arrhythmias (I47-I49)*

   R00.0   Tachycardia, unspecified
     Rapid heart beat
     Sinoauricular tachycardia NOS
     Sinus [sinusal] tachycardia NOS
     EXCLUDES 1   *neonatal tachycardia (P29.11)*
                 paroxysmal tachycardia (I47.-)
     DEF: Excessively rapid heart rate of more than 100 beats per minute.

R00.1   Bradycardia, unspecified
    Sinoatrial bradycardia
    Sinus bradycardia
    Slow heart beat
    Vagal bradycardia
    Use additional code for adverse effect, if applicable, to identify drug (T36-T50 with fifth or sixth character 5)
    EXCLUDES 1   *neonatal bradycardia (P29.12)*
    AHA: 2020,2Q,23
    DEF: Slowed heartbeat, usually defined as a rate fewer than 60 beats per minute. Heart rhythm may be slow as a result of a congenital defect or an acquired problem.

R00.2   Palpitations
    Awareness of heart beat

R00.8   Other abnormalities of heart beat

R00.9   Unspecified abnormalities of heart beat

✓4ᵗʰ R01   Cardiac murmurs and other cardiac sounds
    EXCLUDES 1   *cardiac murmurs and sounds originating in the perinatal period (P29.8)*

   R01.0   Benign and innocent cardiac murmurs
     Functional cardiac murmur

   R01.1   Cardiac murmur, unspecified
     Cardiac bruit NOS
     Heart murmur NOS
     Systolic murmur NOS

   R01.2   Other cardiac sounds
     Cardiac dullness, increased or decreased
     Precordial friction

✓4ᵗʰ R03   Abnormal blood-pressure reading, without diagnosis

   R03.0   Elevated blood-pressure reading, without diagnosis of hypertension
     NOTE   This category is to be used to record an episode of elevated blood pressure in a patient in whom no formal diagnosis of hypertension has been made, or as an isolated incidental finding.

   R03.1   Nonspecific low blood-pressure reading
     EXCLUDES 1   *hypotension (I95.-)*
                 maternal hypotension syndrome (O26.5-)
                 neurogenic orthostatic hypotension (G90.3)

✓4ᵗʰ R04   Hemorrhage from respiratory passages

   R04.0   Epistaxis
     Hemorrhage from nose
     Nosebleed

   R04.1   Hemorrhage from throat
     EXCLUDES 2   *hemoptysis (R04.2)*

   R04.2   Hemoptysis
     Blood-stained sputum
     Cough with hemorrhage
     AHA: 2013,4Q,118

   ✓5ᵗʰ R04.8   Hemorrhage from other sites in respiratory passages

     R04.81   Acute idiopathic pulmonary hemorrhage in infants   **P**
        AIPHI
        Acute idiopathic hemorrhage in infants over 28 days old
        EXCLUDES 1   *perinatal pulmonary hemorrhage (P26.-)*
                    ▶*von Willebrand disease (D68.0-)*◀

     R04.89   Hemorrhage from other sites in respiratory passages
        Pulmonary hemorrhage NOS

   R04.9   Hemorrhage from respiratory passages, unspecified

✓4ᵗʰ R05   Cough
    EXCLUDES 1   *paroxysmal cough due to Bordetella pertussis (A37.0-)*
                 smoker's cough (J41.0)
    EXCLUDES 2   *cough with hemorrhage (R04.2)*
    AHA: 2021,4Q,24-25; 2016,2Q,33

   R05.1   Acute cough

   R05.2   Subacute cough

   R05.3   Chronic cough
     Persistent cough
     Refractory cough
     Unexplained cough

   R05.4   Cough syncope   **UPD**
     Code first syncope and collapse (R55)

   R05.8   Other specified cough

Chapter 18. Symptoms, Signs and Abnormal Clinical and Laboratory Findings

R05.9 **Cough, unspecified**

✓4th **R06 Abnormalities of breathing**
- EXCLUDES 1   *acute respiratory distress syndrome (J80)*
  - *respiratory arrest (R09.2)*
  - *respiratory arrest of newborn (P28.81)*
  - *respiratory distress syndrome of newborn (P22.-)*
  - *respiratory failure (J96.-)*
  - *respiratory failure of newborn (P28.5)*

✓5th **R06.0 Dyspnea**
- EXCLUDES 1   *tachypnea NOS (R06.82)*
  - *transient tachypnea of newborn (P22.1)*

  R06.00 **Dyspnea, unspecified**
  - **AHA:** 2017,1Q,26
  R06.01 **Orthopnea**
  R06.02 **Shortness of breath**
  R06.03 **Acute respiratory distress**
  - **AHA:** 2017,4Q,23
  R06.09 **Other forms of dyspnea**

R06.1 Stridor
- EXCLUDES 1   *congenital laryngeal stridor (P28.89)*
  - *laryngismus (stridulus) (J38.5)*
- **DEF:** Certain type of wheezing described as a loud, constant, musical sound produced when breathing with an obstructed airway, like the inspiratory sound heard when laryngeal or esophageal obstruction is present.

R06.2 Wheezing
- EXCLUDES 1   *asthma (J45.-)*
- **AHA:** 2016,2Q,33
- **DEF:** High-pitched whistling sound during breathing due to stenosis of the respiratory passageway. Wheezing is associated with asthma, sleep apnea, bronchiectasis, bronchiolitis, COPD, and pleural effusion.

R06.3 Periodic breathing
- Cheyne-Stokes breathing

R06.4 Hyperventilation
- EXCLUDES 1   *psychogenic hyperventilation (F45.8)*

R06.5 Mouth breathing
- EXCLUDES 2   *dry mouth NOS (R68.2)*

R06.6 Hiccough
- EXCLUDES 1   *psychogenic hiccough (F45.8)*

R06.7 Sneezing

✓5th **R06.8 Other abnormalities of breathing**
  R06.81 **Apnea, not elsewhere classified**
  - Apnea NOS
    - EXCLUDES 1   *apnea (of) newborn ▶(P28.4-)◀*
      - *sleep apnea (G47.3-)*
      - *sleep apnea of newborn (primary)*
        - ▶(P28.3-)◀
  R06.82 **Tachypnea, not elsewhere classified**
  - Tachypnea NOS
    - EXCLUDES 1   *transitory tachypnea of newborn (P22.1)*
  R06.83 **Snoring**
  R06.89 **Other abnormalities of breathing**
  - Breath-holding (spells)
  - Sighing

  R06.9 **Unspecified abnormalities of breathing**

✓4th **R07 Pain in throat and chest**
- EXCLUDES 1   *epidemic myalgia (B33.0)*
- EXCLUDES 2   *jaw pain R68.84*
  - *pain in breast (N64.4)*

R07.0 Pain in throat
- EXCLUDES 1   *chronic sore throat (J31.2)*
  - *sore throat (acute) NOS (J02.9)*
- EXCLUDES 2   *dysphagia (R13.1-)*
  - *pain in neck (M54.2)*

R07.1 Chest pain on breathing
- Painful respiration

R07.2 Precordial pain
- **DEF:** Pain felt in the anterior (front) chest wall over the region of the heart. This type of pain is generally felt slightly to the left of the sternum, but may also extend into the surrounding chest wall region.

✓5th **R07.8 Other chest pain**
  R07.81 **Pleurodynia**
  - Pleurodynia NOS
    - EXCLUDES 1   *epidemic pleurodynia (B33.0)*
  R07.82 **Intercostal pain**
  R07.89 **Other chest pain**
  - Anterior chest-wall pain NOS
  - **AHA:** 2021,1Q,42

  R07.9 **Chest pain, unspecified**

✓4th **R09 Other symptoms and signs involving the circulatory and respiratory system**
- EXCLUDES 1   *acute respiratory distress syndrome (J80)*
  - *respiratory arrest of newborn (P28.81)*
  - *respiratory distress syndrome of newborn (P22.0)*
  - *respiratory failure (J96.-)*
  - *respiratory failure of newborn (P28.5)*

✓5th **R09.0 Asphyxia and hypoxemia**
- EXCLUDES 1   *asphyxia due to carbon monoxide (T58.-)*
  - *asphyxia due to foreign body in respiratory tract (T17.-)*
  - *birth (intrauterine) asphyxia (P84)*
  - *hyperventilation (R06.4)*
  - *traumatic asphyxia (T71.-)*
- EXCLUDES 2   *hypercapnia (R06.89)*

  R09.01 **Asphyxia**
  - **DEF:** Interference of oxygen intake due to obstruction or injury of airways resulting in a lack of oxygen perfusion to the tissues or excessive carbon dioxide in the blood. Can cause unconsciousness or death.
  R09.02 **Hypoxemia**
  - **AHA:** 2019,3Q,15
  - **DEF:** Insufficient oxygen in the arterial blood resulting in inadequate delivery of oxygen to the body tissues.

R09.1 Pleurisy
- EXCLUDES 1   *pleurisy with effusion (J90)*

R09.2 Respiratory arrest   HCC ESR COM
- Cardiorespiratory failure
  - EXCLUDES 1   *cardiac arrest (I46.-)*
    - *respiratory arrest of newborn (P28.81)*
    - *respiratory distress of newborn (P22.0)*
    - *respiratory failure (J96.-)*
    - *respiratory failure of newborn (P28.5)*
    - *respiratory insufficiency (R06.89)*
    - *respiratory insufficiency of newborn (P28.5)*

R09.3 Abnormal sputum
- Abnormal amount of sputum
- Abnormal color of sputum
- Abnormal odor of sputum
- Excessive sputum
  - EXCLUDES 1   *blood-stained sputum (R04.2)*

✓5th **R09.8 Other specified symptoms and signs involving the circulatory and respiratory systems**
  R09.81 **Nasal congestion**
  R09.82 **Postnasal drip**
  R09.89 **Other specified symptoms and signs involving the circulatory and respiratory systems**
  - Abnormal chest percussion
  - Bruit (arterial)
  - Chest tympany
  - Choking sensation
  - Feeling of foreign body in throat
  - Friction sounds in chest
  - Rales
  - Weak pulse
    - EXCLUDES 2   *foreign body in throat (T17.2-)*
      - *wheezing (R06.2)*
  - **AHA:** 2021,1Q,42

Symptoms and signs involving the digestive system and abdomen (R10-R19)

> EXCLUDES 2   *congenital or infantile pylorospasm (Q40.0)*
> *gastrointestinal hemorrhage (K92.0-K92.2)*
> *intestinal obstruction (K56.-)*
> *newborn gastrointestinal hemorrhage (P54.0-P54.3)*
> *newborn intestinal obstruction (P76.-)*
> *pylorospasm (K31.3)*
> *signs and symptoms involving the urinary system (R30-R39)*
> *symptoms referable to female genital organs (N94.-)*
> *symptoms referable to male genital organs (N48-N50)*

☑️4ᵗʰ **R10** **Abdominal and pelvic pain**
> EXCLUDES 1   *renal colic (N23)*
> EXCLUDES 2   *dorsalgia (M54.-)*
>   *flatulence and related conditions (R14.-)*

   R10.0 **Acute abdomen**
         Severe abdominal pain (generalized) (with abdominal rigidity)
> EXCLUDES 1   *abdominal rigidity NOS (R19.3)*
>   *generalized abdominal pain NOS (R10.84)*
>   *localized abdominal pain (R10.1-R10.3-)*

☑️5ᵗʰ **R10.1** **Pain localized to upper abdomen**
       R10.10 **Upper abdominal pain, unspecified**
       R10.11 **Right upper quadrant pain**
       R10.12 **Left upper quadrant pain**
       R10.13 **Epigastric pain**
             Dyspepsia
>   EXCLUDES 1   *functional dyspepsia (K30)*

Abdominal Pain

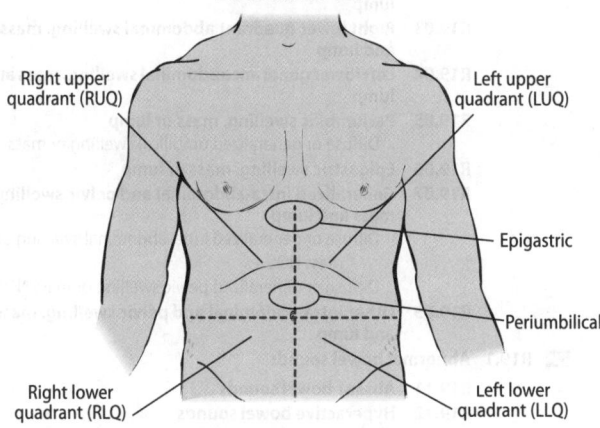

Right upper quadrant (RUQ)

Left upper quadrant (LUQ)

Epigastric

Periumbilical

Right lower quadrant (RLQ)

Left lower quadrant (LLQ)

   R10.2 **Pelvic and perineal pain**
>   EXCLUDES 1   *vulvodynia (N94.81)*

☑️5ᵗʰ **R10.3** **Pain localized to other parts of lower abdomen**
       R10.30 **Lower abdominal pain, unspecified**
       R10.31 **Right lower quadrant pain**
       R10.32 **Left lower quadrant pain**
       R10.33 **Periumbilical pain**

☑️5ᵗʰ **R10.8** **Other abdominal pain**
   ☑️6ᵗʰ **R10.81** **Abdominal tenderness**
          Abdominal tenderness NOS
          R10.811 **Right upper quadrant abdominal tenderness**
          R10.812 **Left upper quadrant abdominal tenderness**
          R10.813 **Right lower quadrant abdominal tenderness**
          R10.814 **Left lower quadrant abdominal tenderness**
          R10.815 **Periumbilic abdominal tenderness**
          R10.816 **Epigastric abdominal tenderness**
          R10.817 **Generalized abdominal tenderness**
          R10.819 **Abdominal tenderness, unspecified site**
   ☑️6ᵗʰ **R10.82** **Rebound abdominal tenderness**
          R10.821 **Right upper quadrant rebound abdominal tenderness**
          R10.822 **Left upper quadrant rebound abdominal tenderness**
          R10.823 **Right lower quadrant rebound abdominal tenderness**

          R10.824 **Left lower quadrant rebound abdominal tenderness**
          R10.825 **Periumbilic rebound abdominal tenderness**
          R10.826 **Epigastric rebound abdominal tenderness**
          R10.827 **Generalized rebound abdominal tenderness**
          R10.829 **Rebound abdominal tenderness, unspecified site**
       R10.83 **Colic**   P
          Colic NOS
          Infantile colic
>   EXCLUDES 1   *colic in adult and child over 12 months old (R10.84)*

          DEF: Inconsolable crying in an otherwise well-fed and healthy infant for more than three hours a day, three days a week, for more than three weeks.
       R10.84 **Generalized abdominal pain**
>   EXCLUDES 1   *generalized abdominal pain associated with acute abdomen (R10.0)*

   R10.9 **Unspecified abdominal pain**

☑️4ᵗʰ **R11** **Nausea and vomiting**
> EXCLUDES 1   *cyclical vomiting associated with migraine (G43.A-)*
> *excessive vomiting in pregnancy (O21.-)*
> *hematemesis (K92.0)*
> *neonatal hematemesis (P54.0)*
> *newborn vomiting (P92.0-)*
> *psychogenic vomiting (F50.89)*
> *vomiting associated with bulimia nervosa (F50.2)*
> *vomiting following gastrointestinal surgery (K91.0)*

   AHA: 2017,1Q,28
   R11.0 **Nausea**
         Nausea NOS
         Nausea without vomiting
☑️5ᵗʰ **R11.1** **Vomiting**
       R11.10 **Vomiting, unspecified**
          Vomiting NOS
       R11.11 **Vomiting without nausea**
       R11.12 **Projectile vomiting**
       R11.13 **Vomiting of fecal matter**
       R11.14 **Bilious vomiting**
          Bilious emesis
       R11.15 **Cyclical vomiting syndrome unrelated to migraine**
          Cyclic vomiting syndrome NOS
          Persistent vomiting
>   EXCLUDES 1   *cyclical vomiting in migraine (G43.A-)*
>   EXCLUDES 2   *bulimia nervosa (F50.2)*
>   *diabetes mellitus due to underlying condition (E08.-)*

          AHA: 2019,4Q,15
   R11.2 **Nausea with vomiting, unspecified**
         Persistent nausea with vomiting NOS
         AHA: 2020,1Q,8

R12 **Heartburn**
> EXCLUDES 1   *dyspepsia NOS (R10.13)*
>   *functional dyspepsia (K30)*

☑️4ᵗʰ **R13** **Aphagia and dysphagia**
   R13.0 **Aphagia**
         Inability to swallow
>   EXCLUDES 1   *psychogenic aphagia (F50.9)*

Chapter 18. Symptoms, Signs and Abnormal Clinical and Laboratory Findings

R13.1–R19.4

✓5ᵗʰ **R13.1 Dysphagia**

Code first, if applicable, dysphagia following cerebrovascular disease (I69. with final characters -91)

EXCLUDES 1   *psychogenic dysphagia (F45.8)*

Swallowing Function

Oral phase

Oropharyngeal phase

Pharyngeal phase

Pharyngoesophageal phase

R13.10 Dysphagia, unspecified
Difficulty in swallowing NOS

R13.11 Dysphagia, oral phase

R13.12 Dysphagia, oropharyngeal phase

R13.13 Dysphagia, pharyngeal phase

R13.14 Dysphagia, pharyngoesophageal phase

R13.19 Other dysphagia
Cervical dysphagia
Neurogenic dysphagia

✓4ᵗʰ **R14 Flatulence and related conditions**

EXCLUDES 1   *psychogenic aerophagy (F45.8)*

R14.0 Abdominal distension (gaseous)
Bloating
Tympanites (abdominal) (intestinal)

R14.1 Gas pain

R14.2 Eructation

R14.3 Flatulence

✓4ᵗʰ **R15 Fecal incontinence**

INCLUDES   encopresis NOS

EXCLUDES 1   *fecal incontinence of nonorganic origin (F98.1)*

R15.0 Incomplete defecation
EXCLUDES 1   *constipation (K59.0-)*
             fecal impaction (K56.41)

R15.1 Fecal smearing
Fecal soiling

R15.2 Fecal urgency

R15.9 Full incontinence of feces
Fecal incontinence NOS

✓4ᵗʰ **R16 Hepatomegaly and splenomegaly, not elsewhere classified**

R16.0 Hepatomegaly, not elsewhere classified
Hepatomegaly NOS

R16.1 Splenomegaly, not elsewhere classified
Splenomegaly NOS

R16.2 Hepatomegaly with splenomegaly, not elsewhere classified
Hepatosplenomegaly NOS

R17 Unspecified jaundice
EXCLUDES 1   *neonatal jaundice (P55, P57-P59)*

✓4ᵗʰ **R18 Ascites**

INCLUDES   fluid in peritoneal cavity

EXCLUDES 1   *ascites in alcoholic cirrhosis (K70.31)*
             ascites in alcoholic hepatitis (K70.11)
             ascites in toxic liver disease with chronic active hepatitis (K71.51)

DEF: Abnormal accumulation of free fluid in the abdominal cavity, causing distention and tightness in addition to shortness of breath as the fluid accumulates. Ascites is usually an underlying disorder and can be a manifestation of any number of diseases.

R18.0 Malignant ascites   UPD
Code first malignancy, such as:
malignant neoplasm of ovary (C56.-)
secondary malignant neoplasm of retroperitoneum and peritoneum (C78.6)

R18.8 Other ascites
Ascites NOS
Peritoneal effusion (chronic)
AHA: 2018,1Q,4

✓4ᵗʰ **R19 Other symptoms and signs involving the digestive system and abdomen**

EXCLUDES 1   *acute abdomen (R10.0)*

✓5ᵗʰ **R19.0 Intra-abdominal and pelvic swelling, mass and lump**

EXCLUDES 1   *abdominal distension (gaseous) (R14.-)*
             ascites (R18.-)

R19.00 Intra-abdominal and pelvic swelling, mass and lump, unspecified site

R19.01 Right upper quadrant abdominal swelling, mass and lump

R19.02 Left upper quadrant abdominal swelling, mass and lump

R19.03 Right lower quadrant abdominal swelling, mass and lump

R19.04 Left lower quadrant abdominal swelling, mass and lump

R19.05 Periumbilic swelling, mass or lump
Diffuse or generalized umbilical swelling or mass

R19.06 Epigastric swelling, mass or lump

R19.07 Generalized intra-abdominal and pelvic swelling, mass and lump
Diffuse or generalized intra-abdominal swelling or mass NOS
Diffuse or generalized pelvic swelling or mass NOS

R19.09 Other intra-abdominal and pelvic swelling, mass and lump

✓6ᵗʰ **R19.1 Abnormal bowel sounds**

R19.11 Absent bowel sounds

R19.12 Hyperactive bowel sounds

R19.15 Other abnormal bowel sounds
Abnormal bowel sounds NOS

R19.2 Visible peristalsis
Hyperperistalsis
DEF: Visible movements of muscular attempts to move food through the digestive tract due to pyloric obstruction, stomach obstruction, or intestinal obstruction.

✓5ᵗʰ **R19.3 Abdominal rigidity**

EXCLUDES 1   *abdominal rigidity with severe abdominal pain (R10.0)*

R19.30 Abdominal rigidity, unspecified site

R19.31 Right upper quadrant abdominal rigidity

R19.32 Left upper quadrant abdominal rigidity

R19.33 Right lower quadrant abdominal rigidity

R19.34 Left lower quadrant abdominal rigidity

R19.35 Periumbilic abdominal rigidity

R19.36 Epigastric abdominal rigidity

R19.37 Generalized abdominal rigidity

R19.4 Change in bowel habit
EXCLUDES 1   *constipation (K59.0-)*
             functional diarrhea (K59.1)

R19.5 **Other fecal abnormalities**
Abnormal stool color
Bulky stools
Mucus in stools
Occult blood in feces
Occult blood in stools
EXCLUDES 1   *melena (K92.1)*
neonatal melena (P54.1)
AHA: 2021,1Q,9; 2019,1Q,32

R19.6 **Halitosis**
R19.7 **Diarrhea, unspecified**
Diarrhea NOS
EXCLUDES 1   *functional diarrhea (K59.1)*
neonatal diarrhea (P78.3)
psychogenic diarrhea (F45.8)
AHA: 2021,3Q,3

R19.8 **Other specified symptoms and signs involving the digestive system and abdomen**

Symptoms and signs involving the skin and subcutaneous tissue (R20-R23)

EXCLUDES 2   *symptoms relating to breast (N64.4-N64.5)*

✓4th **R20** **Disturbances of skin sensation**
EXCLUDES 1   *dissociative anesthesia and sensory loss (F44.6)*
psychogenic disturbances (F45.8)
R20.0 **Anesthesia of skin**
R20.1 **Hypoesthesia of skin**
R20.2 **Paresthesia of skin**
Formication
Pins and needles
Tingling skin
EXCLUDES 1   *acroparesthesia (I73.8)*
R20.3 **Hyperesthesia**
R20.8 **Other disturbances of skin sensation**
R20.9 **Unspecified disturbances of skin sensation**

R21 **Rash and other nonspecific skin eruption**
INCLUDES   rash NOS
EXCLUDES 1   *specified type of rash - code to condition*
vesicular eruption (R23.8)

✓4th **R22** **Localized swelling, mass and lump of skin and subcutaneous tissue**
INCLUDES   subcutaneous nodules (localized)(superficial)
EXCLUDES 1   *abnormal findings on diagnostic imaging (R90-R93)*
edema (R60.-)
enlarged lymph nodes (R59.-)
localized adiposity (E65)
swelling of joint (M25.4-)
R22.0 **Localized swelling, mass and lump, head**
R22.1 **Localized swelling, mass and lump, neck**
R22.2 **Localized swelling, mass and lump, trunk**
EXCLUDES 1   *intra-abdominal or pelvic mass and lump (R19.0-)*
intra-abdominal or pelvic swelling (R19.0-)
EXCLUDES 2   *breast mass and lump (N63)*
✓5th **R22.3** **Localized swelling, mass and lump, upper limb**
R22.30 Localized swelling, mass and lump, unspecified upper limb
R22.31 Localized swelling, mass and lump, right upper limb
R22.32 Localized swelling, mass and lump, left upper limb
R22.33 Localized swelling, mass and lump, upper limb, bilateral
✓5th **R22.4** **Localized swelling, mass and lump, lower limb**
R22.40 Localized swelling, mass and lump, unspecified lower limb
R22.41 Localized swelling, mass and lump, right lower limb
R22.42 Localized swelling, mass and lump, left lower limb
R22.43 Localized swelling, mass and lump, lower limb, bilateral
R22.9 **Localized swelling, mass and lump, unspecified**

✓4th **R23** **Other skin changes**
R23.0 **Cyanosis**
EXCLUDES 1   *acrocyanosis (I73.8)*
cyanotic attacks of newborn (P28.2)
DEF: Bluish or purplish discoloration of the skin due to an inadequate oxygen blood level.

R23.1 **Pallor**
Clammy skin
R23.2 **Flushing**
Excessive blushing
Code first, if applicable, menopausal and female climacteric states (N95.1)
R23.3 **Spontaneous ecchymoses**
Petechiae
EXCLUDES 1   *ecchymoses of newborn (P54.5)*
purpura (D69.-)
R23.4 **Changes in skin texture**
Desquamation of skin
Induration of skin
Scaling of skin
EXCLUDES 1   *epidermal thickening NOS (L85.9)*
R23.8 **Other skin changes**
R23.9 **Unspecified skin changes**

Symptoms and signs involving the nervous and musculoskeletal systems (R25-R29)

✓4th **R25** **Abnormal involuntary movements**
EXCLUDES 1   *specific movement disorders (G20-G26)*
stereotyped movement disorders (F98.4)
tic disorders (F95.-)
R25.0 **Abnormal head movements**
R25.1 **Tremor, unspecified**
EXCLUDES 1   *chorea NOS (G25.5)*
essential tremor (G25.0)
hysterical tremor (F44.4)
intention tremor (G25.2)
R25.2 **Cramp and spasm**
EXCLUDES 2   *carpopedal spasm (R29.0)*
charley-horse (M62.831)
infantile spasms (G40.4-)
muscle spasm of back (M62.830)
muscle spasm of calf (M62.831)
R25.3 **Fasciculation**
Twitching NOS
R25.8 **Other abnormal involuntary movements**
R25.9 **Unspecified abnormal involuntary movements**

✓4th **R26** **Abnormalities of gait and mobility**
EXCLUDES 1   *ataxia NOS (R27.0)*
hereditary ataxia (G11.-)
locomotor (syphilitic) ataxia (A52.11)
immobility syndrome (paraplegic) (M62.3)
R26.0 **Ataxic gait**
Staggering gait
AHA: 2022,2Q,12
R26.1 **Paralytic gait**
Spastic gait
R26.2 **Difficulty in walking, not elsewhere classified**
EXCLUDES 1   *falling (R29.6)*
unsteadiness on feet (R26.81)
AHA: 2016,2Q,7
✓5th **R26.8** **Other abnormalities of gait and mobility**
R26.81 Unsteadiness on feet
R26.89 Other abnormalities of gait and mobility
AHA: 2020,2Q,29
R26.9 **Unspecified abnormalities of gait and mobility**

✓4th **R27** **Other lack of coordination**
EXCLUDES 1   *ataxic gait (R26.0)*
hereditary ataxia (G11.-)
vertigo NOS (R42)
R27.0 **Ataxia, unspecified**
EXCLUDES 1   *ataxia following cerebrovascular disease (I69. with final characters -93)*
R27.8 **Other lack of coordination**
R27.9 **Unspecified lack of coordination**

Chapter 18. Symptoms, Signs and Abnormal Clinical and Laboratory Findings

R29–R31.9

✓4th **R29** **Other symptoms and signs involving the nervous and musculoskeletal systems**

R29.0 **Tetany**
Carpopedal spasm
  EXCLUDES 1   hysterical tetany (F44.5)
             neonatal tetany (P71.3)
             parathyroid tetany (E20.9)
             post-thyroidectomy tetany (E89.2)
DEF: Calcium or other mineral imbalance causing voluntary muscles such as hands, feet, or larynx to spasm rhythmically.

R29.1 **Meningismus**

R29.2 **Abnormal reflex**
  EXCLUDES 2   abnormal pupillary reflex (H57.0)
             hyperactive gag reflex (J39.2)
             vasovagal reaction or syncope (R55)

R29.3 **Abnormal posture**

R29.4 **Clicking hip**
  EXCLUDES 1   congenital deformities of hip (Q65.-)

R29.5 **Transient paralysis**
Code first any associated spinal cord injury (S14.0, S14.1-, S24.0, S24.1-, S34.0-, S34.1-)
  EXCLUDES 1   transient ischemic attack (G45.9)

R29.6 **Repeated falls**
Falling
Tendency to fall
  EXCLUDES 2   at risk for falling (Z91.81)
             history of falling (Z91.81)
AHA: 2016,2Q,6
TIP: Code in addition to Parkinson's disease (G20), when documented.

✓5th **R29.7** **National Institutes of Health Stroke Scale (NIHSS) score**
Code first the type of cerebral infarction (I63.-)
AHA: 2016,4Q,61-62
TIP: Codes from this subcategory may be assigned based on medical record documentation from clinicians who are not the patient's provider.

✓6th **R29.70** **NIHSS score 0-9**
  R29.700   NIHSS score 0   UPD
  R29.701   NIHSS score 1   UPD
  R29.702   NIHSS score 2   UPD
  R29.703   NIHSS score 3   UPD
  R29.704   NIHSS score 4   UPD
  R29.705   NIHSS score 5   UPD
  R29.706   NIHSS score 6   UPD
  R29.707   NIHSS score 7   UPD
  R29.708   NIHSS score 8   UPD
  R29.709   NIHSS score 9   UPD

✓6th **R29.71** **NIHSS score 10-19**
  R29.710   NIHSS score 10   UPD
  R29.711   NIHSS score 11   UPD
  R29.712   NIHSS score 12   UPD
  R29.713   NIHSS score 13   UPD
  R29.714   NIHSS score 14   UPD
  R29.715   NIHSS score 15   UPD
  R29.716   NIHSS score 16   UPD
  R29.717   NIHSS score 17   UPD
  R29.718   NIHSS score 18   UPD
  R29.719   NIHSS score 19   UPD

✓6th **R29.72** **NIHSS score 20-29**
  R29.720   NIHSS score 20   UPD
  R29.721   NIHSS score 21   UPD
  R29.722   NIHSS score 22   UPD
  R29.723   NIHSS score 23   UPD
  R29.724   NIHSS score 24   UPD
  R29.725   NIHSS score 25   UPD
  R29.726   NIHSS score 26   UPD
  R29.727   NIHSS score 27   UPD
  R29.728   NIHSS score 28   UPD
  R29.729   NIHSS score 29   UPD

✓6th **R29.73** **NIHSS score 30-39**
  R29.730   NIHSS score 30   UPD
  R29.731   NIHSS score 31   UPD
  R29.732   NIHSS score 32   UPD
  R29.733   NIHSS score 33   UPD
  R29.734   NIHSS score 34   UPD

  R29.735   NIHSS score 35   UPD
  R29.736   NIHSS score 36   UPD
  R29.737   NIHSS score 37   UPD
  R29.738   NIHSS score 38   UPD
  R29.739   NIHSS score 39   UPD

✓6th **R29.74** **NIHSS score 40-42**
  R29.740   NIHSS score 40   UPD
  R29.741   NIHSS score 41   UPD
  R29.742   NIHSS score 42   UPD

✓5th **R29.8** **Other symptoms and signs involving the nervous and musculoskeletal systems**

✓6th **R29.81** **Other symptoms and signs involving the nervous system**
R29.810 **Facial weakness**
Facial droop
  EXCLUDES 1   Bell's palsy (G51.0)
             facial weakness following cerebrovascular disease (I69. with final characters -92)
R29.818 **Other symptoms and signs involving the nervous system**

✓6th **R29.89** **Other symptoms and signs involving the musculoskeletal system**
  EXCLUDES 2   pain in limb (M79.6-)
R29.890 **Loss of height**
  EXCLUDES 1   osteoporosis (M80-M81)
R29.891 **Ocular torticollis**
  EXCLUDES 1   congenital (sternomastoid) torticollis Q68.0
             psychogenic torticollis (F45.8)
             spasmodic torticollis (G24.3)
             torticollis due to birth injury (P15.8)
             torticollis NOS M43.6
DEF: Abnormal head posture as a result of a contracted state of cervical muscles to correct a visual disturbance, either double vision or a visual field defect.
R29.898 **Other symptoms and signs involving the musculoskeletal system**

✓5th **R29.9** **Unspecified symptoms and signs involving the nervous and musculoskeletal systems**
R29.90 **Unspecified symptoms and signs involving the nervous system**
R29.91 **Unspecified symptoms and signs involving the musculoskeletal system**

Symptoms and signs involving the genitourinary system (R30-R39)

✓4th **R30** **Pain associated with micturition**
  EXCLUDES 1   psychogenic pain associated with micturition (F45.8)
R30.0 **Dysuria**
Strangury
R30.1 **Vesical tenesmus**
DEF: Feeling of a full bladder even when there is little or no urine in the bladder.
R30.9 **Painful micturition, unspecified**
Painful urination NOS

✓4th **R31** **Hematuria**
  EXCLUDES 1   hematuria included with underlying conditions, such as:
             acute cystitis with hematuria (N30.01)
             recurrent and persistent hematuria in glomerular diseases (N02.-)
AHA: 2017,1Q,17
R31.0 **Gross hematuria**
R31.1 **Benign essential microscopic hematuria**
✓5th **R31.2** **Other microscopic hematuria**
AHA: 2016,4Q,62
R31.21 **Asymptomatic microscopic hematuria**
AMH
R31.29 **Other microscopic hematuria**
R31.9 **Hematuria, unspecified**

R32 **Unspecified urinary incontinence**
Enuresis NOS
> *EXCLUDES 1*   *functional urinary incontinence (R39.81)*
> *nonorganic enuresis (F98.0)*
> *stress incontinence and other specified urinary incontinence (N39.3-N39.4-)*
> *urinary incontinence associated with cognitive impairment (R39.81)*

✓4ᵗʰ R33 **Retention of urine**
> *EXCLUDES 1*   *psychogenic retention of urine (F45.8)*

   R33.0   Drug induced **retention of urine**
       Use additional code for adverse effect, if applicable, to identify drug (T36-T50 with fifth or sixth character 5)

   R33.8   **Other retention of urine**
       Code first, if applicable, any causal condition, such as:
       enlarged prostate (N40.1)
       AHA: 2018,4Q,55

   R33.9   **Retention of urine, unspecified**

R34 **Anuria and oliguria**
> *EXCLUDES 1*   *anuria and oliguria complicating abortion or ectopic or molar pregnancy (O00-O07, O08.4)*
> *anuria and oliguria complicating pregnancy (O26.83-)*
> *anuria and oliguria complicating the puerperium (O90.4)*

✓4ᵗʰ R35 **Polyuria**
       Code first, if applicable, any causal condition, such as:
       enlarged prostate (N40.1)
> *EXCLUDES 1*   *psychogenic polyuria (F45.8)*

   R35.0   **Frequency of micturition**
   R35.1   **Nocturia**
✓5ᵗʰ **R35.8**   **Other polyuria**
       AHA: 2021,4Q,26
       R35.81   Nocturnal **polyuria**
          EXCLUDES 2   *nocturnal enuresis (N39.44)*
       R35.89   **Other polyuria**
          Polyuria NOS

✓4ᵗʰ R36 **Urethral discharge**
   R36.0   **Urethral discharge without blood**
   R36.1   **Hematospermia**   ♂
   R36.9   **Urethral discharge, unspecified**
       Penile discharge NOS
       Urethrorrhea

R37 **Sexual dysfunction, unspecified**

✓4ᵗʰ R39 **Other and unspecified symptoms and signs involving the genitourinary system**
   R39.0   **Extravasation of urine**
✓5ᵗʰ **R39.1**   **Other difficulties with micturition**
       Code first, if applicable, any causal condition, such as:
       enlarged prostate (N40.1)
       R39.11   **Hesitancy of micturition**
       R39.12   **Poor urinary stream**
          Weak urinary steam
       R39.13   **Splitting of urinary stream**
       R39.14   **Feeling of incomplete bladder emptying**
       R39.15   **Urgency of urination**
          EXCLUDES 1   *urge incontinence (N39.41, N39.46)*
       R39.16   **Straining to void**
✓6ᵗʰ   **R39.19**   **Other difficulties with micturition**
          AHA: 2016,4Q,63
          R39.191   **Need to immediately re-void**
          R39.192   **Position dependent micturition**
          R39.198   **Other difficulties with micturition**
   R39.2   **Extrarenal uremia**
       Prerenal uremia
       EXCLUDES 1   *uremia NOS (N19)*
✓5ᵗʰ **R39.8**   **Other symptoms and signs involving the genitourinary system**
       AHA: 2017,4Q,22-23
       R39.81   **Functional urinary incontinence**
          Urinary incontinence due to cognitive impairment, or severe physical disability or immobility
          EXCLUDES 1   *stress incontinence and other specified urinary incontinence (N39.3-N39.4-)*
             urinary incontinence NOS (R32)

   R39.82   **Chronic bladder pain**
       AHA: 2016,4Q,64
   R39.83   **Unilateral non-palpable testicle**   ♂
   R39.84   **Bilateral non-palpable testicles**   ♂
   R39.89   **Other symptoms and signs involving the genitourinary system**
   R39.9   **Unspecified symptoms and signs involving the genitourinary system**

Symptoms and signs involving cognition, perception, emotional state and behavior (R40-R46)

> *EXCLUDES 2*   *symptoms and signs constituting part of a pattern of mental disorder (F01-F99)*

✓4ᵗʰ R40 **Somnolence, stupor and coma**
> *EXCLUDES 1*   *neonatal coma (P91.5)*
> *somnolence, stupor and coma in diabetes (E08-E13)*
> *somnolence, stupor and coma in hepatic failure (K72.-)*
> *somnolence, stupor and coma in hypoglycemia (nondiabetic) (E15)*

   R40.0   **Somnolence**
       Drowsiness
       EXCLUDES 1   *coma (R40.2-)*

   R40.1   **Stupor**
       Catatonic stupor
       Semicoma
       EXCLUDES 1   *catatonic schizophrenia (F20.2)*
             coma (R40.2-)
             depressive stupor (F31-F33)
             dissociative stupor (F44.2)
             manic stupor (F30.2)

✓5ᵗʰ **R40.2**   **Coma**
       Code first any associated:
       fracture of skull (S02.-)
       intracranial injury (S06.-)
       NOTE   One code from each subcategory, R40.21-R40.23, is required to complete the coma scale
       AHA: 2020,3Q,46; 2019,2Q,12; 2018,4Q,70; 2017,4Q,23-25,95; 2015,2Q,17; 2014,1Q,19
       TIP: Codes for individual (R40.21-, R40.22-, R40.23-) or total (R40.24-) coma scale scores may be assigned based on medical record documentation from clinicians who are not the patient's provider.
       TIP: It is not appropriate to assign individual (R40.21-, R40.22-, R40.23-) or total (R40.24-) coma scale score codes for patients who are sedated or in medically induced comas.

   R40.20   **Unspecified coma**   HCC   ESR   COM
       Coma NOS
       Unconsciousness NOS
       AHA: 2021,4Q,112-113; 2021,2Q,5

✓6ᵗʰ   **R40.21**   **Coma scale,** eyes open

> The following appropriate 7th character is to be added to subcategory R40.21-, R40.22-, R40.23-, and R40.24-.
> 0   unspecified time
> 1   in the field [EMT or ambulance]
> 2   at arrival to emergency department
> 3   at hospital admission
> 4   24 hours or more after hospital admission

✓7ᵗʰ   **R40.211**   **Coma scale, eyes open, never**   HCC   ESR   COM   UPD
          Coma scale eye opening score of 1
✓7ᵗʰ   **R40.212**   **Coma scale, eyes open, to pain**   HCC   ESR   COM   UPD
          Coma scale eye opening score of 2
✓7ᵗʰ   **R40.213**   **Coma scale, eyes open, to sound**   UPD
          Coma scale eye opening score of 3
✓7ᵗʰ   **R40.214**   **Coma scale, eyes open, spontaneous**   UPD
          Coma scale eye opening score of 4
✓6ᵗʰ   **R40.22**   **Coma scale,** best verbal response
✓7ᵗʰ   **R40.221**   **Coma scale, best verbal response, none**   HCC   ESR   COM   UPD
          Coma scale verbal score of 1

Chapter 18. Symptoms, Signs and Abnormal Clinical and Laboratory Findings

R40.222–R43.2

√7ᵗʰ **R40.222 Coma scale, best verbal response, incomprehensible words** `HCC` `ESR` `COM` `UPD`
Coma scale verbal score of 2
Incomprehensible sounds (2-5 years of age)
Moans/grunts to pain; restless (< 2 years old)

√7ᵗʰ **R40.223 Coma scale, best verbal response, inappropriate words** `UPD`
Coma scale verbal score of 3
Inappropriate crying or screaming (< 2 years of age)
Screaming (2-5 years of age)

√7ᵗʰ **R40.224 Coma scale, best verbal response, confused conversation** `UPD`
Coma scale verbal score of 4
Inappropriate words (2-5 years of age)
Irritable cries (< 2 years of age)

√7ᵗʰ **R40.225 Coma scale, best verbal response, oriented** `UPD`
Coma scale verbal score of 5
Cooing or babbling or crying appropriately (< 2 years of age)
Uses appropriate words (2-5 years of age)

√6ᵗʰ **R40.23 Coma scale, best motor response**

√7ᵗʰ **R40.231 Coma scale, best motor response, none** `HCC` `ESR` `COM` `UPD`
Coma scale motor score of 1

√7ᵗʰ **R40.232 Coma scale, best motor response, extension** `HCC` `ESR` `COM` `UPD`
Abnormal extensor posturing to pain or noxious stimuli (< 2 years of age)
Coma scale motor score of 2
Extensor posturing to pain or noxious stimuli (2-5 years of age)

√7ᵗʰ **R40.233 Coma scale, best motor response, abnormal flexion** `UPD`
Abnormal flexure posturing to pain or noxious stimuli (2-5 years of age)
Coma scale motor score of 3
Flexion/decorticate posturing (< 2 years of age)

√7ᵗʰ **R40.234 Coma scale, best motor response, flexion withdrawal** `HCC` `ESR` `COM` `UPD`
Coma scale motor score of 4
Withdraws from pain or noxious stimuli (2-5 years of age)

√7ᵗʰ **R40.235 Coma scale, best motor response, localizes pain** `UPD`
Coma scale motor score of 5
Localizes pain (2-5 years of age)
Withdraws to touch (< 2 years of age)

√7ᵗʰ **R40.236 Coma scale, best motor response, obeys commands** `UPD`
Coma scale motor score of 6
Normal or spontaneous movement (< 2 years of age)
Obeys commands (2-5 years of age)

√6ᵗʰ **R40.24 Glasgow coma scale, total score**

NOTE Assign a code from subcategory R40.24, when only the total coma score is documented

AHA: 2021,2Q,4; 2016,4Q,64-65

√7ᵗʰ **R40.241 Glasgow coma scale score 13-15** `UPD`

√7ᵗʰ **R40.242 Glasgow coma scale score 9-12** `UPD`

√7ᵗʰ **R40.243 Glasgow coma scale score 3-8** `HCC` `ESR` `COM` `UPD`

√7ᵗʰ **R40.244 Other coma, without documented Glasgow coma scale score, or with partial score reported** `HCC` `ESR` `COM`

R40.3 Persistent vegetative state `HCC` `ESR` `COM`
DEF: Persistent wakefulness without consciousness due to a nonfunctioning cerebral cortex.

R40.4 Transient alteration of awareness
AHA: 2020,2Q,24

√4ᵗʰ **R41 Other symptoms and signs involving cognitive functions and awareness**
EXCLUDES 1   *dissociative [conversion] disorders (F44.-)*
mild cognitive impairment, so stated (G31.84)

R41.0 Disorientation, unspecified
Confusion NOS
Delirium NOS
AHA: 2022,2Q,11; 2019,2Q,34

R41.1 Anterograde amnesia

R41.2 Retrograde amnesia

R41.3 Other amnesia
Amnesia NOS
Memory loss NOS
EXCLUDES 1   *amnestic disorder due to known physiologic condition (F04)*
amnestic syndrome due to psychoactive substance use (F10-F19 with 5th character .6)
mild memory disturbance due to known physiological condition (F06.8)
transient global amnesia (G45.4)

R41.4 Neurologic neglect syndrome
Asomatognosia
Hemi-akinesia
Hemi-inattention
Hemispatial neglect
Left-sided neglect
Sensory neglect
Visuospatial neglect
EXCLUDES 1   *visuospatial deficit (R41.842)*

√5ᵗʰ **R41.8 Other symptoms and signs involving cognitive functions and awareness**

R41.81 Age-related cognitive decline `A`
Senility NOS

R41.82 Altered mental status, unspecified
Change in mental status NOS
EXCLUDES 1   *altered level of consciousness (R40.-)*
altered mental status due to known condition - code to condition
delirium NOS (R41.0)
AHA: 2012,4Q,97

R41.83 Borderline intellectual functioning
IQ level 71 to 84
EXCLUDES 1   *intellectual disabilities (F70-F79)*

√6ᵗʰ **R41.84 Other specified cognitive deficit**
EXCLUDES 1   *cognitive deficits as sequelae of cerebrovascular disease (I69.01-, I69.11-, I69.21-, I69.31-, I69.81-, I69.91-)*

R41.840 Attention and concentration deficit
EXCLUDES 1   *attention-deficit hyperactivity disorders (F90.-)*

R41.841 Cognitive communication deficit
R41.842 Visuospatial deficit
R41.843 Psychomotor deficit
R41.844 Frontal lobe and executive function deficit

R41.89 Other symptoms and signs involving cognitive functions and awareness
Anosognosia

R41.9 Unspecified symptoms and signs involving cognitive functions and awareness
Unspecified neurocognitive disorder

R42 Dizziness and giddiness `Q`
Light-headedness
Vertigo NOS
EXCLUDES 1   *vertiginous syndromes (H81.-)*
vertigo from infrasound (T75.23)

√4ᵗʰ **R43 Disturbances of smell and taste**

R43.0 Anosmia
DEF: Permanent or transient absence of smell that may be congenital or acquired.

R43.1 Parosmia
DEF: Abnormal perception of smell usually triggered by environmental odors.

R43.2 Parageusia
DEF: Abnormal perception of taste.

`HCC` CMS-HCC   `Rx` Rx HCC   `ESR` ESRD HCC   `COM` Commercial HCC   `N` Newborn: 0   `P` Pediatric: 0-17   `M` Maternity: 9-64   `A` Adult: 15-124

972   ICD-10-CM 2023

R43.8　Other disturbances of smell and taste
　　　Mixed disturbance of smell and taste

R43.9　Unspecified disturbances of smell and taste

✓4ᵗʰ **R44　Other symptoms and signs involving general sensations and perceptions**
　　EXCLUDES 1　alcoholic hallucinations (F10.151, F10.251, F10.951)
　　　　hallucinations in drug psychosis (F11-F19 with fifth to sixth characters 51)
　　　　hallucinations in mood disorders with psychotic symptoms (F30.2, F31.5, F32.3, F33.3)
　　　　hallucinations in schizophrenia, schizotypal and delusional disorders (F20-F29)
　　EXCLUDES 2　disturbances of skin sensation (R20.-)

R44.0　Auditory hallucinations
R44.1　Visual hallucinations
R44.2　Other hallucinations
R44.3　Hallucinations, unspecified
　　　AHA: 2022,2Q,11
R44.8　Other symptoms and signs involving general sensations and perceptions
R44.9　Unspecified symptoms and signs involving general sensations and perceptions

✓4ᵗʰ **R45　Symptoms and signs involving emotional state**

R45.0　Nervousness
　　　Nervous tension
R45.1　Restlessness and agitation
R45.2　Unhappiness
R45.3　Demoralization and apathy
　　EXCLUDES 1　anhedonia (R45.84)
R45.4　Irritability and anger
R45.5　Hostility
R45.6　Violent behavior
R45.7　State of emotional shock and stress, unspecified
R45.8　Other symptoms and signs involving emotional state

✓5ᵗʰ 　**R45.81　Low self-esteem**
　　R45.82　Worries
　　R45.83　Excessive crying of child, adolescent or adult
　　　EXCLUDES 1　excessive crying of infant (baby) R68.11
　　R45.84　Anhedonia
　✓6ᵗʰ **R45.85　Homicidal and suicidal ideations**
　　　EXCLUDES 1　suicide attempt (T14.91)
　　　R45.850　Homicidal ideations
　　　R45.851　Suicidal ideations
　　　　AHA: 2022,1Q,29
　　　　DEF: Thoughts of committing suicide but no actual attempt of suicide has been made.
　　R45.86　Emotional lability
　　R45.87　Impulsiveness
　　R45.88　Nonsuicidal self-harm　HCC　Rx　ESR　COM
　　　Nonsuicidal self-injury
　　　Nonsuicidal self-mutilation
　　　Self-inflicted injury without suicidal intent
　　　Code also injury, if known
　　　AHA: 2021,4Q,26-27
　　R45.89　Other symptoms and signs involving emotional state

✓4ᵗʰ **R46　Symptoms and signs involving appearance and behavior**
　　EXCLUDES 1　appearance and behavior in schizophrenia, schizotypal and delusional disorders (F20-F29)
　　　　mental and behavioral disorders (F01-F99)
R46.0　Very low level of personal hygiene
R46.1　Bizarre personal appearance
R46.2　Strange and inexplicable behavior
R46.3　Overactivity
R46.4　Slowness and poor responsiveness
　　EXCLUDES 1　stupor (R40.1)
R46.5　Suspiciousness and marked evasiveness
R46.6　Undue concern and preoccupation with stressful events
R46.7　Verbosity and circumstantial detail obscuring reason for contact
✓5ᵗʰ **R46.8　Other symptoms and signs involving appearance and behavior**
　　R46.81　Obsessive-compulsive behavior
　　　EXCLUDES 1　obsessive-compulsive disorder (F42.-)

R46.89　Other symptoms and signs involving appearance and behavior

Symptoms and signs involving speech and voice (R47-R49)

✓4ᵗʰ **R47　Speech disturbances, not elsewhere classified**
　　EXCLUDES 1　autism (F84.0)
　　　　cluttering (F80.81)
　　　　specific developmental disorders of speech and language (F80.-)
　　　　stuttering (F80.81)

✓5ᵗʰ **R47.0　Dysphasia and aphasia**
　　R47.01　Aphasia
　　　EXCLUDES 1　aphasia following cerebrovascular disease (I69. with final characters -20)
　　　　progressive isolated aphasia (G31.01)
　　R47.02　Dysphasia
　　　EXCLUDES 1　dysphasia following cerebrovascular disease (I69. with final characters -21)
R47.1　Dysarthria and anarthria
　　EXCLUDES 1　dysarthria following cerebrovascular disease (I69. with final characters -22)
✓5ᵗʰ **R47.8　Other speech disturbances**
　　EXCLUDES 1　dysarthria following cerebrovascular disease (I69. with final characters -28)
　　R47.81　Slurred speech
　　R47.82　Fluency disorder in conditions classified elsewhere
　　　Stuttering in conditions classified elsewhere
　　　Code first underlying disease or condition, such as:
　　　Parkinson's disease (G20)
　　　EXCLUDES 1　adult onset fluency disorder (F98.5)
　　　　childhood onset fluency disorder (F80.81)
　　　　fluency disorder (stuttering) following cerebrovascular disease (I69. with final characters -23)
　　R47.89　Other speech disturbances
R47.9　Unspecified speech disturbances

✓4ᵗʰ **R48　Dyslexia and other symbolic dysfunctions, not elsewhere classified**
　　EXCLUDES 1　specific developmental disorders of scholastic skills (F81.-)
R48.0　Dyslexia and alexia
R48.1　Agnosia
　　Astereognosia (astereognosis)
　　Autotopagnosia
　　EXCLUDES 1　visual object agnosia (R48.3)
　　DEF: Inability to recognize common things such as faces, objects, smells, or voices.
R48.2　Apraxia
　　EXCLUDES 1　apraxia following cerebrovascular disease (I69. with final characters -90)
R48.3　Visual agnosia
　　Prosopagnosia
　　Simultanagnosia (asimultagnosia)
R48.8　Other symbolic dysfunctions
　　Acalculia
　　Agraphia
　　AHA: 2017,1Q,27
R48.9　Unspecified symbolic dysfunctions

✓4ᵗʰ **R49　Voice and resonance disorders**
　　EXCLUDES 1　psychogenic voice and resonance disorders (F44.4)
R49.0　Dysphonia
　　Hoarseness
R49.1　Aphonia
　　Loss of voice
✓5ᵗʰ **R49.2　Hypernasality and hyponasality**
　　R49.21　Hypernasality
　　R49.22　Hyponasality
R49.8　Other voice and resonance disorders
R49.9　Unspecified voice and resonance disorder
　　Change in voice NOS
　　Resonance disorder NOS

Chapter 18. Symptoms, Signs and Abnormal Clinical and Laboratory Findings

General symptoms and signs (R50-R69)

✓4ᵗʰ R50   Fever of other and unknown origin
EXCLUDES 1   *chills without fever (R68.83)*
febrile convulsions (R56.0-)
fever of unknown origin during labor (O75.2)
fever of unknown origin in newborn (P81.9)
hypothermia due to illness (R68.0)
malignant hyperthermia due to anesthesia (T88.3)
puerperal pyrexia NOS (O86.4)

R50.2   Drug induced **fever**
Use additional code for adverse effect, if applicable, to identify drug (T36-T50 with fifth or sixth character 5)
EXCLUDES 1   *postvaccination (postimmunization) fever (R50.83)*

✓5ᵗʰ R50.8   Other specified fever

R50.81   *Fever presenting with conditions classified elsewhere*
Code first underlying condition when associated fever is present, such as with:
leukemia (C91-C95)
neutropenia (D70.-)
sickle-cell disease (D57.-)
AHA: 2020,3Q,22; 2014,4Q,22

R50.82   Postprocedural **fever**
EXCLUDES 1   *postprocedural infection (T81.4-)*
posttransfusion fever (R50.84)
postvaccination (postimmunization) fever (R50.83)

R50.83   Postvaccination **fever**
Postimmunization fever

R50.84   Febrile nonhemolytic transfusion reaction
FNHTR
Posttransfusion fever

R50.9   Fever, unspecified
Fever NOS
Fever of unknown origin [FUO]
Fever with chills
Fever with rigors
Hyperpyrexia NOS
Persistent fever
Pyrexia NOS

✓4ᵗʰ R51   Headache
EXCLUDES 2   *atypical face pain (G50.1)*
migraine and other headache syndromes (G43-G44)
trigeminal neuralgia (G50.0)
AHA: 2020,4Q,38-39

R51.0   Headache with orthostatic component, not elsewhere classified
Headache with positional component, not elsewhere classified

R51.9   Headache, unspecified
Facial pain NOS

R52   Pain, unspecified
Acute pain NOS
Generalized pain NOS
Pain NOS
EXCLUDES 1   *acute and chronic pain, not elsewhere classified (G89.-)*
localized pain, unspecified type - code to pain by site, such as:
abdomen pain (R10.-)
back pain (M54.9)
breast pain (N64.4)
chest pain (R07.1-R07.9)
ear pain (H92.0-)
eye pain (H57.1)
headache (R51.9)
joint pain (M25.5-)
limb pain (M79.6-)
lumbar region pain (M54.5-)
pelvic and perineal pain (R10.2)
renal colic (N23)
shoulder pain (M25.51-)
spine pain (M54.-)
throat pain (R07.0)
tongue pain (K14.6)
tooth pain (K08.8)
pain disorders exclusively related to psychological factors (F45.41)

✓4ᵗʰ R53   Malaise and fatigue

R53.0   Neoplastic (malignant) related fatigue
Code first associated neoplasm

R53.1   Weakness
Asthenia NOS
EXCLUDES 1   *age-related weakness (R54)*
muscle weakness (generalized) (M62.81)
sarcopenia (M62.84)
senile asthenia (R54)
AHA: 2017,1Q,7; 2015,1Q,25

R53.2   Functional quadriplegia   HCC ESR COM
Complete immobility due to severe physical disability or frailty
EXCLUDES 1   *frailty NOS (R54)*
hysterical paralysis (F44.4)
immobility syndrome (M62.3)
neurologic quadriplegia (G82.5-)
quadriplegia (G82.50)
AHA: 2016,2Q,6
DEF: Inability to move due to a nonphysiological condition, such as dementia. The patient has no mental ability to move independently.

✓5ᵗʰ R53.8   Other malaise and fatigue
EXCLUDES 1   *combat exhaustion and fatigue (F43.0)*
congenital debility (P96.9)
exhaustion and fatigue due to excessive exertion (T73.3)
exhaustion and fatigue due to exposure (T73.2)
exhaustion and fatigue due to heat (T67.-)
exhaustion and fatigue due to pregnancy (O26.8-)
exhaustion and fatigue due to recurrent depressive episode (F33)
exhaustion and fatigue due to senile debility (R54)

R53.81   Other malaise
Chronic debility
Debility NOS
General physical deterioration
Malaise NOS
Nervous debility
EXCLUDES 1   *age-related physical debility (R54)*
AHA: 2021,1Q,43

R53.82   Chronic fatigue, unspecified
~~Chronic fatigue syndrome NOS~~
EXCLUDES 1   ►*chronic fatigue syndrome (G93.32)*◄
►*myalgic encephalomyelitis (G93.32)*◄
►*post infection and related fatigue syndromes (G93.39)*◄
postviral fatigue syndrome ►*(G93.31)*◄

R53.83 Other fatigue
Fatigue NOS
Lack of energy
Lethargy
Tiredness
EXCLUDES 2 exhaustion and fatigue due to depressive episode (F32.-)

R54 Age-related physical debility   A
Frailty
Old age
Senescence
Senile asthenia
Senile debility
EXCLUDES 1 age-related cognitive decline (R41.81)
sarcopenia (M62.84)
senile psychosis (F03)
senility NOS (R41.81)

R55 Syncope and collapse
Blackout
Fainting
Vasovagal attack
EXCLUDES 1 cardiogenic shock (R57.0)
carotid sinus syncope (G90.01)
heat syncope (T67.1)
neurocirculatory asthenia (F45.8)
neurogenic orthostatic hypotension (G90.3)
orthostatic hypotension (I95.1)
postprocedural shock (T81.1-)
psychogenic syncope (F48.8)
shock NOS (R57.9)
shock complicating or following abortion or ectopic or molar pregnancy (O00-O07, O08.3)
shock complicating or following labor and delivery (O75.1)
Stokes-Adams attack (I45.9)
unconsciousness NOS (R40.2-)

✓4ᵗʰ R56 Convulsions, not elsewhere classified
EXCLUDES 1 dissociative convulsions and seizures (F44.5)
epileptic convulsions and seizures (G40.-)
newborn convulsions and seizures (P90)

✓5ᵗʰ R56.0 Febrile convulsions

R56.00 Simple febrile convulsions   HCC ESR COM
Febrile convulsion NOS
Febrile seizure NOS

R56.01 Complex febrile convulsions   HCC ESR COM
Atypical febrile seizure
Complex febrile seizure
Complicated febrile seizure
EXCLUDES 1 status epilepticus (G40.901)

R56.1 Post traumatic seizures   HCC ESR COM
EXCLUDES 1 post traumatic epilepsy (G40.-)

R56.9 Unspecified convulsions   HCC ESR COM
Convulsion disorder
Fit NOS
Recurrent convulsions
Seizure(s) (convulsive) NOS
AHA: 2021,1Q,3; 2019,1Q,19

✓4ᵗʰ R57 Shock, not elsewhere classified
EXCLUDES 1 anaphylactic shock NOS (T78.2)
anaphylactic reaction or shock due to adverse food reaction (T78.0-)
anaphylactic shock due to adverse effect of correct drug or medicament properly administered (T88.6)
anaphylactic shock due to serum (T80.5-)
electric shock (T75.4)
obstetric shock (O75.1)
postprocedural shock (T81.1-)
psychic shock (F43.0)
shock complicating or following ectopic or molar pregnancy (O00-O07, O08.3)
shock due to anesthesia (T88.2)
shock due to lightning (T75.01)
toxic shock syndrome (A48.3)
traumatic shock (T79.4)

R57.0 Cardiogenic shock   HCC ESR COM
EXCLUDES 2 septic shock (R65.21)
AHA: 2020,3Q,26
DEF: Associated with myocardial infarction, cardiac tamponade, and massive pulmonary embolism. Symptoms include mental confusion, reduced blood pressure, tachycardia, pallor, and cold, clammy skin.

R57.1 Hypovolemic shock   HCC ESR COM
AHA: 2019,2Q,7

R57.8 Other shock   HCC ESR COM

R57.9 Shock, unspecified   HCC ESR COM
Failure of peripheral circulation NOS

R58 Hemorrhage, not elsewhere classified
Hemorrhage NOS
EXCLUDES 1 hemorrhage included with underlying conditions, such as:
acute duodenal ulcer with hemorrhage (K26.0)
acute gastritis with bleeding (K29.01)
ulcerative enterocolitis with rectal bleeding (K51.01)

✓4ᵗʰ R59 Enlarged lymph nodes
INCLUDES swollen glands
EXCLUDES 1 acute lymphadenitis (L04.-)
chronic lymphadenitis (I88.1)
lymphadenitis NOS (I88.9)
mesenteric (acute) (chronic) lymphadenitis (I88.0)

R59.0 Localized enlarged lymph nodes

R59.1 Generalized enlarged lymph nodes
Lymphadenopathy NOS

R59.9 Enlarged lymph nodes, unspecified

✓4ᵗʰ R60 Edema, not elsewhere classified
EXCLUDES 1 angioneurotic edema (T78.3)
ascites (R18.-)
cerebral edema (G93.6)
cerebral edema due to birth injury (P11.0)
edema of larynx (J38.4)
edema of nasopharynx (J39.2)
edema of pharynx (J39.2)
gestational edema (O12.0-)
hereditary edema (Q82.0)
hydrops fetalis NOS (P83.2)
hydrothorax (J94.8)
newborn edema (P83.3)
pulmonary edema (J81.-)

R60.0 Localized edema

R60.1 Generalized edema
EXCLUDES 2 nutritional edema (E40-E46)

R60.9 Edema, unspecified
Fluid retention NOS

R61 Generalized hyperhidrosis
Excessive sweating
Night sweats
Secondary hyperhidrosis
Code first, if applicable, menopausal and female climacteric states (N95.1)
EXCLUDES 1 focal (primary) (secondary) hyperhidrosis (L74.5-)
Frey's syndrome (L74.52)
localized (primary) (secondary) hyperhidrosis (L74.5-)

Chapter 18. Symptoms, Signs and Abnormal Clinical and Laboratory Findings

R62–R65.11

✓4ᵗʰ **R62 Lack of expected normal physiological development in childhood and adults**
> EXCLUDES 1   *delayed puberty (E30.0)*
> *gonadal dysgenesis (Q99.1)*
> *hypopituitarism (E23.0)*

R62.0 Delayed milestone in childhood   P
> Delayed attainment of expected physiological developmental stage
> Late talker
> Late walker

✓5ᵗʰ **R62.5 Other and unspecified lack of expected normal physiological development in childhood**
> EXCLUDES 1   *HIV disease resulting in failure to thrive (B20)*
> *physical retardation due to malnutrition (E45)*

R62.50 Unspecified lack of expected normal physiological development in childhood
> Infantilism NOS

R62.51 Failure to thrive (child)   P
> Failure to gain weight
> EXCLUDES 1   *failure to thrive in child under 28 days old (P92.6)*
>
> **AHA:** 2018,4Q,82
> **DEF:** Organic failure to thrive (FTT): Acute or chronic illness that interferes with nutritional intake, absorption, metabolism excretion, and energy requirements.
> **DEF:** Nonorganic failure to thrive (FTT): Symptom of neglect or abuse.

R62.52 Short stature (child)
> Lack of growth
> Physical retardation
> Short stature NOS
> EXCLUDES 1   *short stature due to endocrine disorder*
> ▶*(E34.3-)*◄

R62.59 Other lack of expected normal physiological development in childhood

R62.7 Adult failure to thrive   A

✓4ᵗʰ **R63 Symptoms and signs concerning food and fluid intake**
> EXCLUDES 1   *bulimia NOS (F50.2)*

R63.0 Anorexia
> Loss of appetite
> EXCLUDES 1   *anorexia nervosa (F50.0-)*
> *loss of appetite of nonorganic origin (F50.89)*
>
> **AHA:** 2018,4Q,82
> **TIP:** Assign an additional code from category Z68 when BMI is documented. BMI can be based on documentation from clinicians who are not the patient's provider.

R63.1 Polydipsia
> Excessive thirst

R63.2 Polyphagia
> Excessive eating
> Hyperalimentation NOS

✓5ᵗʰ **R63.3 Feeding difficulties**
> EXCLUDES 2   *eating disorders (F50.-)*
> *feeding problems of newborn (P92.-)*
> *infant feeding disorder of nonorganic origin (F98.2-)*
>
> **AHA:** 2021,4Q,27-28; 2017,1Q,28; 2016,3Q,19

R63.30 Feeding difficulties, unspecified

R63.31 Pediatric feeding disorder, acute   P
> Pediatric feeding dysfunction, acute
> Code also, if applicable, associated conditions such as:
> aspiration pneumonia (J69.0)
> dysphagia (R13.1-)
> gastro-esophageal reflux disease (K21.-)
> malnutrition (E40-E46)

R63.32 Pediatric feeding disorder, chronic   P
> Pediatric feeding dysfunction, chronic
> Code also, if applicable, associated conditions such as:
> aspiration pneumonia (J69.0)
> dysphagia (R13.1-)
> gastro-esophageal reflux disease (K21.-)
> malnutrition (E40-E46)

R63.39 Other feeding difficulties
> Feeding problem (elderly) (infant) NOS
> Picky eater

R63.4 Abnormal weight loss
> **AHA:** 2018,4Q,82
> **TIP:** Assign an additional code from category Z68 when BMI is documented. BMI can be based on documentation from clinicians who are not the patient's provider.

R63.5 Abnormal weight gain
> EXCLUDES 1   *excessive weight gain in pregnancy (O26.0-)*
> *obesity (E66.-)*
>
> **AHA:** 2018,4Q,82
> **TIP:** Assign an additional code from category Z68 when BMI is documented. BMI can be based on documentation from clinicians who are not the patient's provider.

R63.6 Underweight
> Use additional code to identify body mass index (BMI), if known (Z68.-)
> EXCLUDES 1   *abnormal weight loss (R63.4)*
> *anorexia nervosa (F50.0-)*
> *malnutrition (E40-E46)*
>
> **AHA:** 2018,4Q,82

R63.8 Other symptoms and signs concerning food and fluid intake

R64 Cachexia   HCC ESR COM
> Wasting syndrome
> Code first underlying condition, if known
> EXCLUDES 1   *abnormal weight loss (R63.4)*
> *nutritional marasmus (E41)*
>
> **AHA:** 2018,4Q,82; 2017,3Q,24
> **TIP:** Assign code E43 when emaciated or emaciation is documented in relation to malnutrition.

✓4ᵗʰ **R65 Symptoms and signs specifically associated with systemic inflammation and infection**
> **AHA:** 2019,2Q,38
> **TIP:** When documentation states SIRS with an infection, assign only a code for the infection. ICD-10-CM does not offer a code for SIRS due to infectious process. If sepsis is suspected, query the provider.

✓5ᵗʰ **R65.1 Systemic inflammatory response syndrome [SIRS] of non-infectious origin**
> Code first underlying condition, such as:
> heatstroke (T67.0-)
> injury and trauma (S00-T88)
> EXCLUDES 1   *sepsis - code to infection*
> *severe sepsis (R65.2)*

R65.10 Systemic inflammatory response syndrome [SIRS] of non-infectious origin without acute organ dysfunction   HCC ESR COM UPD
> Systemic inflammatory response syndrome (SIRS) NOS
> **AHA:** 2019,2Q,24

R65.11 Systemic inflammatory response syndrome [SIRS] of non-infectious origin with acute organ dysfunction   HCC ESR COM UPD
> Use additional code to identify specific acute organ dysfunction, such as:
> acute kidney failure (N17.-)
> acute respiratory failure (J96.0-)
> critical illness myopathy (G72.81)
> critical illness polyneuropathy (G62.81)
> disseminated intravascular coagulopathy [DIC] (D65)
> encephalopathy (metabolic) (septic) (G93.41)
> hepatic failure (K72.0-)

✓5ᵗʰ **R65.2** Severe sepsis

    Infection with associated acute organ dysfunction

    Sepsis with acute organ dysfunction

    Sepsis with multiple organ dysfunction

    Systemic inflammatory response syndrome due to infectious process with acute organ dysfunction

    Code first underlying infection, such as:

      infection following a procedure (T81.4-)

      infections following infusion, transfusion and therapeutic injection (T80.2-)

      puerperal sepsis (O85)

      sepsis following complete or unspecified spontaneous abortion (O03.87)

      sepsis following ectopic and molar pregnancy (O08.82)

      sepsis following incomplete spontaneous abortion (O03.37)

      sepsis following (induced) termination of pregnancy (O04.87)

      sepsis NOS (A41.9)

    Use additional code to identify specific acute organ dysfunction, such as:

      acute kidney failure (N17.-)

      acute respiratory failure (J96.0-)

      critical illness myopathy (G72.81)

      critical illness polyneuropathy (G62.81)

      disseminated intravascular coagulopathy [DIC] (D65)

      encephalopathy (metabolic) (septic) (G93.41)

      hepatic failure (K72.0-)

    AHA: 2020,2Q,17; 2018,4Q,62-63; 2017,4Q,98-99; 2016,3Q,8

    R65.20 **Severe sepsis** without septic shock   HCC ESR COM UPD

      Severe sepsis NOS

      AHA: 2020,2Q,17; 2016,3Q,14; 2013,4Q,119

    R65.21 **Severe sepsis** with septic shock   HCC ESR COM UPD

      AHA: 2018,4Q,63

✓4ᵗʰ **R68** Other general symptoms and signs

    R68.0 **Hypothermia, not associated with low environmental temperature**

      EXCLUDES 1   hypothermia NOS (accidental) (T68)

               hypothermia due to anesthesia (T88.51)

               hypothermia due to low environmental temperature (T68)

               newborn hypothermia (P80.-)

    ✓5ᵗʰ **R68.1** **Nonspecific symptoms peculiar to infancy**

      EXCLUDES 1   colic, infantile (R10.83)

               neonatal cerebral irritability (P91.3)

               teething syndrome (K00.7)

      R68.11 **Excessive crying of infant (baby)**   P

          EXCLUDES 1   excessive crying of child, adolescent, or adult (R45.83)

      R68.12 **Fussy infant (baby)**   P

          Irritable infant

      R68.13 **Apparent life threatening event in infant (ALTE)**   P

          Apparent life threatening event in newborn

          Brief resolved unexplained event (BRUE)

          Code first confirmed diagnosis, if known

          Use additional code(s) for associated signs and symptoms if no confirmed diagnosis established, or if signs and symptoms are not associated routinely with confirmed diagnosis, or provide additional information for cause of ALTE

      R68.19 **Other nonspecific symptoms peculiar to infancy**   P

    R68.2 **Dry mouth, unspecified**

      EXCLUDES 1   dry mouth due to dehydration (E86.0)

               dry mouth due to Sjögren syndrome (M35.0-)

               salivary gland hyposecretion (K11.7)

    R68.3 **Clubbing of fingers**

      Clubbing of nails

      EXCLUDES 1   congenital clubfinger (Q68.1)

      DEF: Enlarged soft tissue of the distal fingers that usually occurs in heart and lung diseases.

    ✓5ᵗʰ **R68.8** **Other general symptoms and signs**

      R68.81 **Early satiety**

          DEF: Premature feeling of being full after eating only a small amount of food. The mechanism of satiety is multifactorial.

      R68.82 **Decreased libido**   A

          Decreased sexual desire

      R68.83 **Chills (without fever)**

          Chills NOS

          EXCLUDES 1   chills with fever (R50.9)

      R68.84 **Jaw pain**

          Mandibular pain

          Maxilla pain

          EXCLUDES 1   temporomandibular joint arthralgia (M26.62-)

      R68.89 **Other general symptoms and signs**

R69 **Illness, unspecified**

    Unknown and unspecified cases of morbidity

Abnormal findings on examination of blood, without diagnosis (R70-R79)

    EXCLUDES 2   abnormal findings on antenatal screening of mother (O28.-)

               abnormalities of lipids (E78.-)

               abnormalities of platelets and thrombocytes (D69.-)

               abnormalities of white blood cells classified elsewhere (D70-D72)

               coagulation hemorrhagic disorders (D65-D68)

               diagnostic abnormal findings classified elsewhere - see Alphabetical Index

               hemorrhagic and hematological disorders of newborn (P50-P61)

✓4ᵗʰ **R70** Elevated erythrocyte sedimentation rate and abnormality of plasma viscosity

    R70.0 **Elevated erythrocyte sedimentation rate**

    R70.1 **Abnormal plasma viscosity**

✓4ᵗʰ **R71** Abnormality of red blood cells

    EXCLUDES 1   anemias (D50-D64)

               anemia of premature infant (P61.2)

               benign (familial) polycythemia (D75.0)

               congenital anemias (P61.2-P61.4)

               newborn anemia due to isoimmunization (P55.-)

               polycythemia neonatorum (P61.1)

               polycythemia NOS (D75.1)

               polycythemia vera (D45)

               secondary polycythemia (D75.1)

    R71.0 **Precipitous drop in hematocrit**

      Drop (precipitous) in hemoglobin

      Drop in hematocrit

    R71.8 **Other abnormality of red blood cells**

      Abnormal red-cell morphology NOS

      Abnormal red-cell volume NOS

      Anisocytosis

      Poikilocytosis

✓4ᵗʰ **R73** Elevated blood glucose level

    EXCLUDES 1   diabetes mellitus (E08-E13)

               diabetes mellitus in pregnancy, childbirth and the puerperium (O24.-)

               neonatal disorders (P70.0-P70.2)

               postsurgical hypoinsulinemia (E89.1)

    ✓5ᵗʰ **R73.0** **Abnormal glucose**

      EXCLUDES 1   abnormal glucose in pregnancy (O99.81-)

               diabetes mellitus (E08-E13)

               dysmetabolic syndrome X (E88.81)

               gestational diabetes (O24.4-)

               glycosuria (R81)

               hypoglycemia (E16.2)

      R73.01 **Impaired fasting glucose**

          Elevated fasting glucose

      R73.02 **Impaired glucose tolerance (oral)**

          Elevated glucose tolerance

      R73.03 **Prediabetes**

          Latent diabetes

          AHA: 2016,4Q,65

      R73.09 **Other abnormal glucose**

          Abnormal glucose NOS

          Abnormal non-fasting glucose tolerance

    R73.9 **Hyperglycemia, unspecified**

☑4ᵗʰ **R74 Abnormal serum enzyme levels**

☑5ᵗʰ **R74.0 Nonspecific elevation of levels of transaminase and lactic acid dehydrogenase [LDH]**
AHA: 2020,4Q,39

R74.01 Elevation of levels of liver transaminase levels
Elevation of levels of alanine transaminase (ALT)
Elevation of levels of aspartate transaminase (AST)

R74.02 Elevation of levels of lactic acid dehydrogenase [LDH]

R74.8 Abnormal levels of other serum enzymes
Abnormal level of acid phosphatase
Abnormal level of alkaline phosphatase
Abnormal level of amylase
Abnormal level of lipase [triacylglycerol lipase]
AHA: 2019,2Q,6

R74.9 Abnormal serum enzyme level, unspecified

R75 Inconclusive laboratory evidence of human immunodeficiency virus [HIV]
Nonconclusive HIV-test finding in infants
EXCLUDES 1 asymptomatic human immunodeficiency virus [HIV] infection status (Z21)
human immunodeficiency virus [HIV] disease (B20)

☑4ᵗʰ **R76 Other abnormal immunological findings in serum**

R76.0 Raised antibody titer
EXCLUDES 1 isoimmunization in pregnancy (O36.0-O36.1)
isoimmunization affecting newborn (P55.-)
AHA: 2021,1Q,6

☑5ᵗʰ **R76.1 Nonspecific reaction to test for tuberculosis**

R76.11 Nonspecific reaction to tuberculin skin test without active tuberculosis
Abnormal result of Mantoux test
PPD positive
Tuberculin (skin test) positive
Tuberculin (skin test) reactor
EXCLUDES 1 nonspecific reaction to cell mediated immunity measurement of gamma interferon antigen response without active tuberculosis (R76.12)

R76.12 Nonspecific reaction to cell mediated immunity measurement of gamma interferon antigen response without active tuberculosis
Nonspecific reaction to QuantiFERON-TB test (QFT) without active tuberculosis
EXCLUDES 1 nonspecific reaction to tuberculin skin test without active tuberculosis (R76.11)
positive tuberculin skin test (R76.11)

R76.8 Other specified abnormal immunological findings in serum
Raised level of immunoglobulins NOS
AHA: 2021,1Q,6

R76.9 Abnormal immunological finding in serum, unspecified

☑4ᵗʰ **R77 Other abnormalities of plasma proteins**
EXCLUDES 1 disorders of plasma-protein metabolism (E88.0-)

R77.0 Abnormality of albumin

R77.1 Abnormality of globulin
Hyperglobulinemia NOS

R77.2 Abnormality of alphafetoprotein

R77.8 Other specified abnormalities of plasma proteins

R77.9 Abnormality of plasma protein, unspecified
AHA: 2019,2Q,6

☑4ᵗʰ **R78 Findings of drugs and other substances, not normally found in blood**
Use additional code to identify the any retained foreign body, if applicable (Z18.-)
EXCLUDES 1 mental or behavioral disorders due to psychoactive substance use (F10-F19)

R78.0 Finding of alcohol in blood
Use additional external cause code (Y90.-), for detail regarding alcohol level

R78.1 Finding of opiate drug in blood

R78.2 Finding of cocaine in blood

R78.3 Finding of hallucinogen in blood

R78.4 Finding of other drugs of addictive potential in blood

R78.5 Finding of other psychotropic drug in blood

R78.6 Finding of steroid agent in blood

☑5ᵗʰ **R78.7 Finding of abnormal level of heavy metals in blood**

R78.71 Abnormal lead level in blood
EXCLUDES 1 lead poisoning (T56.0-)

R78.79 Finding of abnormal level of heavy metals in blood

☑5ᵗʰ **R78.8 Finding of other specified substances, not normally found in blood**

R78.81 Bacteremia
EXCLUDES 1 sepsis — code to specified infection
DEF: Laboratory finding of bacteria in the blood in the absence of two or more signs of sepsis. Transient in nature, it can progress to septicemia with a severe infectious process.

R78.89 Finding of other specified substances, not normally found in blood
Finding of abnormal level of lithium in blood

R78.9 Finding of unspecified substance, not normally found in blood

☑4ᵗʰ **R79 Other abnormal findings of blood chemistry**
Use additional code to identify any retained foreign body, if applicable (Z18.-)
EXCLUDES 1 asymptomatic hyperuricemia (E79.0)
hyperglycemia NOS (R73.9)
hypoglycemia NOS (E16.2)
neonatal hypoglycemia (P70.3-P70.4)
specific findings indicating disorder of amino-acid metabolism (E70-E72)
specific findings indicating disorder of carbohydrate metabolism (E73-E74)
specific findings indicating disorder of lipid metabolism (E75.-)

R79.0 Abnormal level of blood mineral
Abnormal blood level of cobalt
Abnormal blood level of copper
Abnormal blood level of iron
Abnormal blood level of magnesium
Abnormal blood level of mineral NEC
Abnormal blood level of zinc
EXCLUDES 1 abnormal level of lithium (R78.89)
disorders of mineral metabolism (E83.-)
neonatal hypomagnesemia (P71.2)
nutritional mineral deficiency (E58-E61)

R79.1 Abnormal coagulation profile
Abnormal or prolonged bleeding time
Abnormal or prolonged coagulation time
Abnormal or prolonged partial thromboplastin time [PTT]
Abnormal or prolonged prothrombin time [PT]
▶Low von Willebrand factor◀
EXCLUDES 1 coagulation defects (D68.-)
EXCLUDES 2 abnormality of fluid, electrolyte or acid-base balance (E86-E87)

☑5ᵗʰ **R79.8 Other specified abnormal findings of blood chemistry**

R79.81 Abnormal blood-gas level

R79.82 Elevated C-reactive protein [CRP]

R79.83 Abnormal findings of blood amino-acid level
Homocysteinemia
EXCLUDES 1 disorders of amino-acid metabolism (E70-E72)
AHA: 2021,4Q,28

R79.89 Other specified abnormal findings of blood chemistry
AHA: 2019,2Q,6
TIP: Assign for positive Coombs test when not further clarified in the documentation.

R79.9 Abnormal finding of blood chemistry, unspecified

Abnormal findings on examination of urine, without diagnosis (R80-R82)

EXCLUDES 1   *abnormal findings on antenatal screening of mother (O28.-)*
diagnostic abnormal findings classified elsewhere - see Alphabetical Index
specific findings indicating disorder of amino-acid metabolism (E70-E72)
specific findings indicating disorder of carbohydrate metabolism (E73-E74)

✓4ᵗʰ **R80   Proteinuria**
  EXCLUDES 1   *gestational proteinuria (O12.1-)*

R80.0   Isolated proteinuria
  Idiopathic proteinuria
  EXCLUDES 1   *isolated proteinuria with specific morphological lesion (N06.-)*

R80.1   Persistent proteinuria, unspecified
R80.2   Orthostatic proteinuria, unspecified
  Postural proteinuria
R80.3   Bence Jones proteinuria
R80.8   Other proteinuria
R80.9   Proteinuria, unspecified
  Albuminuria NOS

R81   Glycosuria
  EXCLUDES 1   *renal glycosuria (E74.818)*

✓4ᵗʰ **R82   Other and unspecified abnormal findings in urine**
  INCLUDES   chromoabnormalities in urine
  Use additional code to identify any retained foreign body, if applicable (Z18.-)
  EXCLUDES 2   *hematuria (R31.-)*

R82.0   Chyluria
  EXCLUDES 1   *filarial chyluria (B74.-)*

R82.1   Myoglobinuria
R82.2   Biliuria
R82.3   Hemoglobinuria
  EXCLUDES 1   *hemoglobinuria due to hemolysis from external causes NEC (D59.6)*
  hemoglobinuria due to paroxysmal nocturnal [Marchiafava-Micheli] (D59.5)
  DEF: Free hemoglobin in blood due to rapid hemolysis of red blood cells. Causes include burns, crushed injury, sickle cell anemia, thalassemia, parasitic infections, or kidney infections.

R82.4   Acetonuria
  Ketonuria
  DEF: Excessive excretion of acetone in urine that commonly occurs in diabetic acidosis.

R82.5   Elevated urine levels of drugs, medicaments and biological substances
  Elevated urine levels of catecholamines
  Elevated urine levels of indoleacetic acid
  Elevated urine levels of 17-ketosteroids
  Elevated urine levels of steroids

R82.6   Abnormal urine levels of substances chiefly nonmedicinal as to source
  Abnormal urine level of heavy metals

✓5ᵗʰ **R82.7   Abnormal findings on microbiological examination of urine**
  EXCLUDES 1   *colonization status (Z22.-)*
  AHA: 2016,4Q,65
  R82.71   Bacteriuria
  R82.79   Other abnormal findings on microbiological examination of urine
    Positive culture findings of urine

✓5ᵗʰ **R82.8   Abnormal findings on cytological and histological examination of urine**
  AHA: 2019,4Q,16
  R82.81   Pyuria
    Sterile pyuria
  R82.89   Other abnormal findings on cytological and histological examination of urine

✓5ᵗʰ **R82.9   Other and unspecified abnormal findings in urine**

  R82.90   Unspecified abnormal findings in urine

  R82.91   Other chromoabnormalities of urine
    Chromoconversion (dipstick)
    Idiopathic dipstick converts positive for blood with no cellular forms in sediment
    EXCLUDES 1   *hemoglobinuria (R82.3)*
    myoglobinuria (R82.1)

✓6ᵗʰ **R82.99   Other abnormal findings in urine**
    AHA: 2018,4Q,29-30
    R82.991   Hypocitraturia
    R82.992   Hyperoxaluria
      EXCLUDES 1   *primary hyperoxaluria (E72.53)*
    R82.993   Hyperuricosuria
    R82.994   Hypercalciuria
      Idiopathic hypercalciuria
    R82.998   Other abnormal findings in urine
      Cells and casts in urine
      Crystalluria
      Melanuria

Abnormal findings on examination of other body fluids, substances and tissues, without diagnosis (R83-R89)

EXCLUDES 1   *abnormal findings on antenatal screening of mother (O28.-)*
diagnostic abnormal findings classified elsewhere - see Alphabetical Index

EXCLUDES 2   *abnormal findings on examination of blood, without diagnosis (R70-R79)*
abnormal findings on examination of urine, without diagnosis (R80-R82)
abnormal tumor markers (R97.-)

✓4ᵗʰ **R83   Abnormal findings in cerebrospinal fluid**

R83.0   Abnormal level of enzymes in cerebrospinal fluid
R83.1   Abnormal level of hormones in cerebrospinal fluid
R83.2   Abnormal level of other drugs, medicaments and biological substances in cerebrospinal fluid
R83.3   Abnormal level of substances chiefly nonmedicinal as to source in cerebrospinal fluid
R83.4   Abnormal immunological findings in cerebrospinal fluid
R83.5   Abnormal microbiological findings in cerebrospinal fluid
  Positive culture findings in cerebrospinal fluid
  EXCLUDES 1   *colonization status (Z22.-)*
R83.6   Abnormal cytological findings in cerebrospinal fluid
R83.8   Other abnormal findings in cerebrospinal fluid
  Abnormal chromosomal findings in cerebrospinal fluid
R83.9   Unspecified abnormal finding in cerebrospinal fluid

✓4ᵗʰ **R84   Abnormal findings in specimens from respiratory organs and thorax**
  INCLUDES   abnormal findings in bronchial washings
    abnormal findings in nasal secretions
    abnormal findings in pleural fluid
    abnormal findings in sputum
    abnormal findings in throat scrapings
  EXCLUDES 1   *blood-stained sputum (R04.2)*

R84.0   Abnormal level of enzymes in specimens from respiratory organs and thorax
R84.1   Abnormal level of hormones in specimens from respiratory organs and thorax
R84.2   Abnormal level of other drugs, medicaments and biological substances in specimens from respiratory organs and thorax
R84.3   Abnormal level of substances chiefly nonmedicinal as to source in specimens from respiratory organs and thorax
R84.4   Abnormal immunological findings in specimens from respiratory organs and thorax
R84.5   Abnormal microbiological findings in specimens from respiratory organs and thorax
  Positive culture findings in specimens from respiratory organs and thorax
  EXCLUDES 1   *colonization status (Z22.-)*
R84.6   Abnormal cytological findings in specimens from respiratory organs and thorax
R84.7   Abnormal histological findings in specimens from respiratory organs and thorax
R84.8   Other abnormal findings in specimens from respiratory organs and thorax
  Abnormal chromosomal findings in specimens from respiratory organs and thorax
R84.9   Unspecified abnormal finding in specimens from respiratory organs and thorax

☑4ᵗʰ **R85** **Abnormal findings in specimens from digestive organs and abdominal cavity**
INCLUDES   abnormal findings in peritoneal fluid
     abnormal findings in saliva
EXCLUDES 1   cloudy peritoneal dialysis effluent (R88.0)
     fecal abnormalities (R19.5)

R85.0 **Abnormal level of enzymes in specimens from digestive organs and abdominal cavity**

R85.1 **Abnormal level of hormones in specimens from digestive organs and abdominal cavity**

R85.2 **Abnormal level of other drugs, medicaments and biological substances in specimens from digestive organs and abdominal cavity**

R85.3 **Abnormal level of substances chiefly nonmedicinal as to source in specimens from digestive organs and abdominal cavity**

R85.4 **Abnormal immunological findings in specimens from digestive organs and abdominal cavity**

R85.5 **Abnormal microbiological findings in specimens from digestive organs and abdominal cavity**
     Positive culture findings in specimens from digestive organs and abdominal cavity
     EXCLUDES 1   colonization status (Z22.-)

☑5ᵗʰ **R85.6** **Abnormal cytological findings in specimens from digestive organs and abdominal cavity**

     ☑6ᵗʰ **R85.61** **Abnormal cytologic smear of anus**
       EXCLUDES 1   abnormal cytological findings in specimens from other digestive organs and abdominal cavity (R85.69)
       anal intraepithelial neoplasia I [AIN I] (K62.82)
       anal intraepithelial neoplasia II [AIN II] (K62.82)
       anal intraepithelial neoplasia III [AIN III] (D01.3)
       carcinoma in situ of anus (histologically confirmed) (D01.3)
       dysplasia (mild) (moderate) of anus (histologically confirmed) (K62.82)
       severe dysplasia of anus (histologically confirmed) (D01.3)
       EXCLUDES 2   anal high risk human papillomavirus (HPV) DNA test positive (R85.81)
       anal low risk human papillomavirus (HPV) DNA test positive (R85.82)

       R85.610 **Atypical squamous cells of undetermined significance on cytologic smear of anus [ASC-US]**

       R85.611 **Atypical squamous cells cannot exclude high grade squamous intraepithelial lesion on cytologic smear of anus [ASC-H]**

       R85.612 **Low grade squamous intraepithelial lesion on cytologic smear of anus [LGSIL]**

       R85.613 **High grade squamous intraepithelial lesion on cytologic smear of anus [HGSIL]**

       R85.614 **Cytologic evidence of malignancy on smear of anus**

       R85.615 **Unsatisfactory cytologic smear of anus**
         Inadequate sample of cytologic smear of anus

       R85.616 **Satisfactory anal smear but lacking transformation zone**

       R85.618 **Other abnormal cytological findings on specimens from anus**

       R85.619 **Unspecified abnormal cytological findings in specimens from anus**
         Abnormal anal cytology NOS
         Atypical glandular cells of anus NOS

     R85.69 **Abnormal cytological findings in specimens from other digestive organs and abdominal cavity**

R85.7 **Abnormal histological findings in specimens from digestive organs and abdominal cavity**

☑5ᵗʰ **R85.8** **Other abnormal findings in specimens from digestive organs and abdominal cavity**

     R85.81 **Anal high risk human papillomavirus [HPV] DNA test positive**
       EXCLUDES 1   anogenital warts due to human papillomavirus (HPV) (A63.0)
       condyloma acuminatum (A63.0)

     R85.82 **Anal low risk human papillomavirus [HPV] DNA test positive**
       Use additional code for associated human papillomavirus (B97.7)

     R85.89 **Other abnormal findings in specimens from digestive organs and abdominal cavity**
       Abnormal chromosomal findings in specimens from digestive organs and abdominal cavity

R85.9 **Unspecified abnormal finding in specimens from digestive organs and abdominal cavity**

☑4ᵗʰ **R86** **Abnormal findings in specimens from male genital organs**
INCLUDES   abnormal findings in prostatic secretions
     abnormal findings in semen, seminal fluid
     abnormal spermatozoa
EXCLUDES 1   azoospermia (N46.0-)
     oligospermia (N46.1-)

R86.0 **Abnormal level of enzymes in specimens from male genital organs** ♂

R86.1 **Abnormal level of hormones in specimens from male genital organs** ♂

R86.2 **Abnormal level of other drugs, medicaments and biological substances in specimens from male genital organs** ♂

R86.3 **Abnormal level of substances chiefly nonmedicinal as to source in specimens from male genital organs** ♂

R86.4 **Abnormal immunological findings in specimens from male genital organs** ♂

R86.5 **Abnormal microbiological findings in specimens from male genital organs** ♂
     Positive culture findings in specimens from male genital organs
     EXCLUDES 1   colonization status (Z22.-)

R86.6 **Abnormal cytological findings in specimens from male genital organs** ♂

R86.7 **Abnormal histological findings in specimens from male genital organs** ♂

R86.8 **Other abnormal findings in specimens from male genital organs** ♂
     Abnormal chromosomal findings in specimens from male genital organs

R86.9 **Unspecified abnormal finding in specimens from male genital organs** ♂

☑4ᵗʰ **R87** **Abnormal findings in specimens from female genital organs**
INCLUDES   abnormal findings in secretion and smears from cervix uteri
     abnormal findings in secretion and smears from vagina
     abnormal findings in secretion and smears from vulva

R87.0 **Abnormal level of enzymes in specimens from female genital organs** ♀

R87.1 **Abnormal level of hormones in specimens from female genital organs** ♀

R87.2 **Abnormal level of other drugs, medicaments and biological substances in specimens from female genital organs** ♀

R87.3 **Abnormal level of substances chiefly nonmedicinal as to source in specimens from female genital organs** ♀

R87.4 **Abnormal immunological findings in specimens from female genital organs** ♀

R87.5 **Abnormal microbiological findings in specimens from female genital organs** ♀
     Positive culture findings in specimens from female genital organs
     EXCLUDES 1   colonization status (Z22.-)

✓5ᵗʰ **R87.6** **Abnormal cytological findings in specimens from female genital organs**

✓6ᵗʰ **R87.61** **Abnormal cytological findings in specimens from cervix uteri**

> EXCLUDES 1   *abnormal cytological findings in specimens from other female genital organs (R87.69)*
> *abnormal cytological findings in specimens from vagina (R87.62-)*
> *carcinoma in situ of cervix uteri (histologically confirmed) (D06.-)*
> *cervical intraepithelial neoplasia I [CIN I] (N87.0)*
> *cervical intraepithelial neoplasia II [CIN II] (N87.1)*
> *cervical intraepithelial neoplasia III [CIN III] (D06.-)*
> *dysplasia (mild) (moderate) of cervix uteri (histologically confirmed) (N87.-)*
> *severe dysplasia of cervix uteri (histologically confirmed) (D06.-)*

> EXCLUDES 2   *cervical high risk human papillomavirus (HPV) DNA test positive (R87.810)*
> *cervical low risk human papillomavirus (HPV) DNA test positive (R87.820)*

R87.610 **Atypical squamous cells of undetermined significance on cytologic smear of cervix [ASC-US]**

R87.611 **Atypical squamous cells cannot exclude high grade squamous intraepithelial lesion on cytologic smear of cervix [ASC-H]** ♀

R87.612 **Low grade squamous intraepithelial lesion on cytologic smear of cervix [LGSIL]** ♀

R87.613 **High grade squamous intraepithelial lesion on cytologic smear of cervix [HGSIL]** ♀

R87.614 **Cytologic evidence of malignancy on smear of cervix** ♀

R87.615 **Unsatisfactory cytologic smear of cervix** ♀
> Inadequate sample of cytologic smear of cervix

R87.616 **Satisfactory cervical smear but lacking transformation zone** ♀

R87.618 **Other abnormal cytological findings on specimens from cervix uteri** ♀

R87.619 **Unspecified abnormal cytological findings in specimens from cervix uteri** ♀
> Abnormal cervical cytology NOS
> Abnormal Papanicolaou smear of cervix NOS
> Abnormal thin preparation smear of cervix NOS
> Atypical endocervial cells of cervix NOS
> Atypical endometrial cells of cervix NOS
> Atypical glandular cells of cervix NOS

✓6ᵗʰ **R87.62** **Abnormal cytological findings in specimens from vagina**

> Use additional code to identify acquired absence of uterus and cervix, if applicable (Z90.71-)

> EXCLUDES 1   *abnormal cytological findings in specimens from cervix uteri (R87.61-)*
> *abnormal cytological findings in specimens from other female genital organs (R87.69)*
> *carcinoma in situ of vagina (histologically confirmed) (D07.2)*
> *dysplasia (mild) (moderate) of vagina (histologically confirmed) (N89.-)*
> *severe dysplasia of vagina (histologically confirmed) (D07.2)*
> *vaginal intraepithelial neoplasia I [VAIN I] (N89.0)*
> *vaginal intraepithelial neoplasia II [VAIN II] (N89.1)*
> *vaginal intraepithelial neoplasia III [VAIN III] (D07.2)*

> EXCLUDES 2   *vaginal high risk human papillomavirus (HPV) DNA test positive (R87.811)*
> *vaginal low risk human papillomavirus (HPV) DNA test positive (R87.821)*

R87.620 **Atypical squamous cells of undetermined significance on cytologic smear of vagina [ASC-US]**

R87.621 **Atypical squamous cells cannot exclude high grade squamous intraepithelial lesion on cytologic smear of vagina [ASC-H]** ♀

R87.622 **Low grade squamous intraepithelial lesion on cytologic smear of vagina [LGSIL]** ♀

R87.623 **High grade squamous intraepithelial lesion on cytologic smear of vagina [HGSIL]** ♀

R87.624 **Cytologic evidence of malignancy on smear of vagina** ♀

R87.625 **Unsatisfactory cytologic smear of vagina** ♀
> Inadequate sample of cytologic smear of vagina

R87.628 **Other abnormal cytological findings on specimens from vagina** ♀

R87.629 **Unspecified abnormal cytological findings in specimens from vagina** ♀
> Abnormal Papanicolaou smear of vagina NOS
> Abnormal thin preparation smear of vagina NOS
> Abnormal vaginal cytology NOS
> Atypical endocervical cells of vagina NOS
> Atypical endometrial cells of vagina NOS
> Atypical glandular cells of vagina NOS

R87.69 **Abnormal cytological findings in specimens from other female genital organs** ♀
> Abnormal cytological findings in specimens from female genital organs NOS

> EXCLUDES 1   *dysplasia of vulva (histologically confirmed) (N90.0-N90.3)*

R87.7 **Abnormal histological findings in specimens from female genital organs** ♀

> EXCLUDES 1   *carcinoma in situ (histologically confirmed) of female genital organs (D06-D07.3)*
> *cervical intraepithelial neoplasia I [CIN I] (N87.0)*
> *cervical intraepithelial neoplasia II [CIN II] (N87.1)*
> *cervical intraepithelial neoplasia III [CIN III] (D06.-)*
> *dysplasia (mild) (moderate) of cervix uteri (histologically confirmed) (N87.-)*
> *dysplasia (mild) (moderate) of vagina (histologically confirmed) (N89.-)*
> *severe dysplasia of cervix uteri (histologically confirmed) (D06.-)*
> *severe dysplasia of vagina (histologically confirmed) (D07.2)*
> *vaginal intraepithelial neoplasia I [VAIN I] (N89.0)*
> *vaginal intraepithelial neoplasia II [VAIN II] (N89.1)*
> *vaginal intraepithelial neoplasia III [VAIN III] (D07.2)*

✓5ᵗʰ **R87.8** **Other abnormal findings in specimens from female genital organs**

     ✓6ᵗʰ **R87.81** **High risk human papillomavirus [HPV] DNA test positive from female genital organs**

>   EXCLUDES 1   *anogenital warts due to human papillomavirus (HPV) (A63.0)*
> *condyloma acuminatum (A63.0)*

         R87.810 **Cervical high risk human papillomavirus [HPV] DNA test positive** ♀

         R87.811 **Vaginal high risk human papillomavirus [HPV] DNA test positive** ♀

     ✓6ᵗʰ **R87.82** **Low risk human papillomavirus [HPV] DNA test positive from female genital organs**

         Use additional code for associated human papillomavirus (B97.7)

         R87.820 **Cervical low risk human papillomavirus [HPV] DNA test positive** ♀

         R87.821 **Vaginal low risk human papillomavirus [HPV] DNA test positive** ♀

     R87.89 **Other abnormal findings in specimens from female genital organs** ♀

         Abnormal chromosomal findings in specimens from female genital organs

R87.9 **Unspecified abnormal finding in specimens from female genital organs** ♀

✓4ᵗʰ **R88** **Abnormal findings in other body fluids and substances**

     R88.0 **Cloudy (hemodialysis) (peritoneal) dialysis effluent**

     R88.8 **Abnormal findings in other body fluids and substances**

✓4ᵗʰ **R89** **Abnormal findings in specimens from other organs, systems and tissues**

> INCLUDES   abnormal findings in nipple discharge
> abnormal findings in synovial fluid
> abnormal findings in wound secretions

     R89.0 **Abnormal level of enzymes in specimens from other organs, systems and tissues**

     R89.1 **Abnormal level of hormones in specimens from other organs, systems and tissues**

     R89.2 **Abnormal level of other drugs, medicaments and biological substances in specimens from other organs, systems and tissues**

     R89.3 **Abnormal level of substances chiefly nonmedicinal as to source in specimens from other organs, systems and tissues**

     R89.4 **Abnormal immunological findings in specimens from other organs, systems and tissues**

     R89.5 **Abnormal microbiological findings in specimens from other organs, systems and tissues**

         Positive culture findings in specimens from other organs, systems and tissues

>   EXCLUDES 1   *colonization status (Z22.-)*

     R89.6 **Abnormal cytological findings in specimens from other organs, systems and tissues**

     R89.7 **Abnormal histological findings in specimens from other organs, systems and tissues**

     R89.8 **Other abnormal findings in specimens from other organs, systems and tissues**

         Abnormal chromosomal findings in specimens from other organs, systems and tissues

     R89.9 **Unspecified abnormal finding in specimens from other organs, systems and tissues**

Abnormal findings on diagnostic imaging and in function studies, without diagnosis (R90-R94)

> INCLUDES   nonspecific abnormal findings on diagnostic imaging by computerized axial tomography [CAT scan]
> nonspecific abnormal findings on diagnostic imaging by magnetic resonance imaging [MRI][NMR]
> nonspecific abnormal findings on diagnostic imaging by positron emission tomography [PET scan]
> nonspecific abnormal findings on diagnostic imaging by thermography
> nonspecific abnormal findings on diagnostic imaging by ultrasound [echogram]
> nonspecific abnormal findings on diagnostic imaging by X-ray examination

> EXCLUDES 1   *abnormal findings on antenatal screening of mother (O28.-)*
> *diagnostic abnormal findings classified elsewhere - see Alphabetical Index*

✓4ᵗʰ **R90** **Abnormal findings on diagnostic imaging of central nervous system**

     R90.0 **Intracranial space-occupying lesion found on diagnostic imaging of central nervous system**

     ✓5ᵗʰ **R90.8** **Other abnormal findings on diagnostic imaging of central nervous system**

         R90.81 **Abnormal echoencephalogram**

         R90.82 **White matter disease, unspecified**

         R90.89 **Other abnormal findings on diagnostic imaging of central nervous system**

             Other cerebrovascular abnormality found on diagnostic imaging of central nervous system

✓4ᵗʰ **R91** **Abnormal findings on diagnostic imaging of lung**

     R91.1 **Solitary pulmonary nodule**

         Coin lesion lung

         Solitary pulmonary nodule, subsegmental branch of the bronchial tree

     R91.8 **Other nonspecific abnormal finding of lung field**

         Lung mass NOS found on diagnostic imaging of lung

         Pulmonary infiltrate NOS

         Shadow, lung

✓4ᵗʰ **R92** **Abnormal and inconclusive findings on diagnostic imaging of breast**

     R92.0 **Mammographic microcalcification found on diagnostic imaging of breast**

>   EXCLUDES 2   *mammographic calcification (calculus) found on diagnostic imaging of breast (R92.1)*

         DEF: Calcium and cellular debris deposits in the breast that cannot be felt but can be detected on a mammogram. The deposits can be a sign of cancer, benign conditions, or changes in the breast tissue as a result of inflammation, injury, or an obstructed duct.

     R92.1 **Mammographic calcification found on diagnostic imaging of breast**

         Mammographic calculus found on diagnostic imaging of breast

     R92.2 **Inconclusive mammogram**

         Dense breasts NOS

         Inconclusive mammogram NEC

         Inconclusive mammography due to dense breasts

         Inconclusive mammography NEC

         AHA: 2015,1Q,24

     R92.8 **Other abnormal and inconclusive findings on diagnostic imaging of breast**

✓4ᵗʰ **R93** **Abnormal findings on diagnostic imaging of other body structures**

     R93.0 **Abnormal findings on diagnostic imaging of skull and head, not elsewhere classified**

>   EXCLUDES 1   *intracranial space-occupying lesion found on diagnostic imaging (R90.0)*

     R93.1 **Abnormal findings on diagnostic imaging of heart and coronary circulation**

         Abnormal echocardiogram NOS

         Abnormal heart shadow

     R93.2 **Abnormal findings on diagnostic imaging of liver and biliary tract**

         Nonvisualization of gallbladder

     R93.3 **Abnormal findings on diagnostic imaging of other parts of digestive tract**

✓5ᵗʰ **R93.4** **Abnormal findings on diagnostic imaging of urinary organs**
> EXCLUDES 2   hypertrophy of kidney (N28.81)

     AHA: 2016,4Q,66

     R93.41 **Abnormal radiologic findings on diagnostic imaging of renal pelvis, ureter, or bladder**
> Filling defect of bladder found on diagnostic imaging
> Filling defect of renal pelvis found on diagnostic imaging
> Filling defect of ureter found on diagnostic imaging

✓6ᵗʰ   **R93.42** **Abnormal radiologic findings on diagnostic imaging of kidney**
     R93.421 **Abnormal radiologic findings on diagnostic imaging of right kidney**
     R93.422 **Abnormal radiologic findings on diagnostic imaging of left kidney**
     R93.429 **Abnormal radiologic findings on diagnostic imaging of unspecified kidney**
     R93.49 **Abnormal radiologic findings on diagnostic imaging of other urinary organs**

R93.5 **Abnormal findings on diagnostic imaging of other abdominal regions, including retroperitoneum**

R93.6 **Abnormal findings on diagnostic imaging of limbs**
> EXCLUDES 2   abnormal finding in skin and subcutaneous tissue (R93.8-)

     AHA: 2020,1Q,14

R93.7 **Abnormal findings on diagnostic imaging of other parts of musculoskeletal system**
> EXCLUDES 2   abnormal findings on diagnostic imaging of skull (R93.0)

✓5ᵗʰ **R93.8** **Abnormal findings on diagnostic imaging of other specified body structures**
     AHA: 2018,4Q,30

✓6ᵗʰ   **R93.81** **Abnormal radiologic findings on diagnostic imaging of testis**
     R93.811 **Abnormal radiologic findings on diagnostic imaging of right testicle** ♂
     R93.812 **Abnormal radiologic findings on diagnostic imaging of left testicle** ♂
     R93.813 **Abnormal radiologic findings on diagnostic imaging of testicles, bilateral** ♂
     R93.819 **Abnormal radiologic findings on diagnostic imaging of unspecified testicle** ♂

     R93.89 **Abnormal findings on diagnostic imaging of other specified body structures**
> Abnormal finding by radioisotope localization of placenta
> Abnormal radiological finding in skin and subcutaneous tissue
> Mediastinal shift

R93.9 **Diagnostic imaging inconclusive due to excess body fat of patient**

✓4ᵗʰ **R94** **Abnormal results of function studies**
> INCLUDES   abnormal results of radionuclide [radioisotope] uptake studies
> abnormal results of scintigraphy

✓5ᵗʰ **R94.0** **Abnormal results of function studies of central nervous system**
     R94.01 **Abnormal electroencephalogram [EEG]**
     R94.02 **Abnormal brain scan**
     R94.09 **Abnormal results of other function studies of central nervous system**

✓5ᵗʰ **R94.1** **Abnormal results of function studies of peripheral nervous system and special senses**
✓6ᵗʰ   **R94.11** **Abnormal results of function studies of eye**
     R94.110 **Abnormal electro-oculogram [EOG]**
     R94.111 **Abnormal electroretinogram [ERG]**
> Abnormal retinal function study

     R94.112 **Abnormal visually evoked potential [VEP]**
     R94.113 **Abnormal oculomotor study**
     R94.118 **Abnormal results of other function studies of eye**

✓6ᵗʰ   **R94.12** **Abnormal results of function studies of ear and other special senses**
     AHA: 2016,3Q,17
     R94.120 **Abnormal auditory function study**
     R94.121 **Abnormal vestibular function study**
     R94.128 **Abnormal results of other function studies of ear and other special senses**

✓6ᵗʰ   **R94.13** **Abnormal results of function studies of peripheral nervous system**
     R94.130 **Abnormal response to nerve stimulation, unspecified**
     R94.131 **Abnormal electromyogram [EMG]**
> EXCLUDES 1   electromyogram of eye (R94.113)

     R94.138 **Abnormal results of other function studies of peripheral nervous system**

R94.2 **Abnormal results of pulmonary function studies**
> Reduced ventilatory capacity
> Reduced vital capacity

✓5ᵗʰ **R94.3** **Abnormal results of cardiovascular function studies**
     R94.30 **Abnormal result of cardiovascular function study, unspecified**
     R94.31 **Abnormal electrocardiogram [ECG] [EKG]**
> EXCLUDES 1   long QT syndrome (I45.81)

     R94.39 **Abnormal result of other cardiovascular function study**
> Abnormal electrophysiological intracardiac studies
> Abnormal phonocardiogram
> Abnormal vectorcardiogram

R94.4 **Abnormal results of kidney function studies**
> Abnormal renal function test

R94.5 **Abnormal results of liver function studies**

R94.6 **Abnormal results of thyroid function studies**

R94.7 **Abnormal results of other endocrine function studies**
> EXCLUDES 2   abnormal glucose (R73.0-)

R94.8 **Abnormal results of function studies of other organs and systems**
> Abnormal basal metabolic rate [BMR]
> Abnormal bladder function test
> Abnormal splenic function test

Abnormal tumor markers (R97)

✓4ᵗʰ **R97** **Abnormal tumor markers**
> Elevated tumor associated antigens [TAA]
> Elevated tumor specific antigens [TSA]

R97.0 **Elevated carcinoembryonic antigen [CEA]**

R97.1 **Elevated cancer antigen 125 [CA 125]**

✓5ᵗʰ **R97.2** **Elevated prostate specific antigen [PSA]**
     AHA: 2016,4Q,66
     R97.20 **Elevated prostate specific antigen [PSA]** 🄰♂
     R97.21 **Rising PSA following treatment for malignant neoplasm of prostate** 🄰♂

R97.8 **Other abnormal tumor markers**

Ill-defined and unknown cause of mortality (R99)

R99 **Ill-defined and unknown cause of mortality**
> Death (unexplained) NOS
> Unspecified cause of mortality

Chapter 19. Injury, Poisoning, and Certain Other Consequences of External Causes (S00–T88)

Chapter-specific Guidelines with Coding Examples

The chapter-specific guidelines from the ICD-10-CM Official Guidelines for Coding and Reporting have been provided below. Along with these guidelines are coding examples, contained in the shaded boxes, that have been developed to help illustrate the coding and/or sequencing guidance found in these guidelines.

a. Application of 7th characters in Chapter 19

Most categories in chapter 19 have a 7th character requirement for each applicable code. Most categories in this chapter have three 7th character values (with the exception of fractures): A, initial encounter, D, subsequent encounter and S, sequela. Categories for traumatic fractures have additional 7th character values. While the patient may be seen by a new or different provider over the course of treatment for an injury, assignment of the 7th character is based on whether the patient is undergoing active treatment and not whether the provider is seeing the patient for the first time.

For complication codes, active treatment refers to treatment for the condition described by the code, even though it may be related to an earlier precipitating problem. For example, code T84.50XA, Infection and inflammatory reaction due to unspecified internal joint prosthesis, initial encounter, is used when active treatment is provided for the infection, even though the condition relates to the prosthetic device, implant or graft that was placed at a previous encounter.

7th character "A", initial encounter is used for each encounter where the patient is receiving active treatment for the condition.

> Patient evaluated after fall from a skateboard onto the sidewalk, x-rays identify a nondisplaced fracture to the distal pole of the right scaphoid bone. The patient is placed in a cast.
>
> **S62.014A**   **Nondisplaced fracture of distal pole of navicular [scaphoid] bone of right wrist, initial encounter for closed fracture**
>
> **V00.131A**   **Fall from skateboard, initial encounter**
>
> **Y93.51**   **Activity, roller skating (inline) and skateboarding**
>
> **Y92.480**   **Sidewalk as the place of occurrence of the external cause**
>
> **Y99.8**   **Other external cause status**
>
> *Explanation:* This fracture would be coded with a seventh character A for initial encounter because the patient received x-rays to identify the site of the fracture and treatment was rendered; this would be considered active treatment.

7th character "D" subsequent encounter is used for encounters after the patient has completed active treatment of the condition and is receiving routine care for the condition during the healing or recovery phase.

> Patient seen in follow-up after fall from a skateboard onto the sidewalk resulted in casting of the right arm. X-rays are taken to evaluate how well the nondisplaced fracture to the distal pole of the right scaphoid bone is healing. The physician feels the fracture is healing appropriately; no adjustments to the cast are made.
>
> **S62.014D**   **Nondisplaced fracture of distal pole of navicular [scaphoid] bone of right wrist, subsequent encounter for fracture with routine healing**
>
> **V00.131D**   **Fall from skateboard, subsequent encounter**
>
> *Explanation:* This fracture would be coded with a seventh character D for subsequent encounter, whether the same physician who provided the initial cast application or a different physician is now seeing the patient. Although the patient received x-rays, the intent of the x-rays was to assess how the fracture was healing. There was no active treatment rendered and the visit is therefore considered a subsequent encounter.

The aftercare Z codes should not be used for aftercare for conditions such as injuries or poisonings, where 7th characters are provided to identify subsequent care. For example, for aftercare of an injury, assign the acute injury code with the 7th character "D" (subsequent encounter).

7th character "S", sequela, is for use for complications or conditions that arise as a direct result of a condition, such as scar formation after a burn. The scars are sequelae of the burn. When using 7th character "S", it is necessary to use both the injury code that precipitated the sequela and the code for the sequela itself. The "S" is added only to the injury code, not the sequela code. The 7th character "S" identifies the injury responsible for the sequela. The

specific type of sequela (e.g. scar) is sequenced first, followed by the injury code.

See Section I.B.10. Sequelae, (Late Effects)

> Patient with a history of a nondisplaced fracture to the distal pole of the right scaphoid bone due to a fall from a skateboard is seen for evaluation of arthritis to the right wrist that has developed as a consequence of the traumatic fracture.
>
> **M12.531**   **Traumatic arthropathy, right wrist**
>
> **S62.014S**   **Nondisplaced fracture of distal pole of navicular [scaphoid] bone of right wrist, sequela**
>
> **V00.131S**   **Fall from skateboard, sequela**
>
> *Explanation:* The code identifying the specific sequela condition (traumatic arthritis) should be coded first followed by the injury that instigated the development of the sequela (fracture). The scaphoid fracture injury code is given a 7th character S for sequela to represent its role as the inciting injury. The fracture has healed and is not being managed or treated on this admit and therefore is not applicable as a first listed or principal diagnosis. However, it is directly related to the development of the arthritis and should be appended as a secondary code to signify this cause and effect relationship.

b. Coding of injuries

When coding injuries, assign separate codes for each injury unless a combination code is provided, in which case the combination code is assigned. Codes from category T07, Unspecified multiple injuries should not be assigned in the inpatient setting unless information for a more specific code is not available. Traumatic injury codes (S00–T14.9) are not to be used for normal, healing surgical wounds or to identify complications of surgical wounds.

> 11-year-old girl fell from her horse, resulting in a laceration to her right forearm with several large pieces of wooden fragments embedded in the wound as well as abrasions to her right ear; in addition, her right shoulder was dislocated.
>
> **S43.004A**   **Unspecified dislocation of right shoulder joint, initial encounter**
>
> **S51.821A**   **Laceration with foreign body of right forearm, initial encounter**
>
> **S00.411A**   **Abrasion of right ear, initial encounter**
>
> **V80.010A**   **Animal-rider injured by fall from or being thrown from horse in noncollision accident, initial encounter**
>
> **Y93.52**   **Activity, horseback riding**
>
> *Explanation:* Each separate injury should be reported. The patient's injury to the forearm is reported with one combination code that captures both the laceration and the foreign body.

The code for the most serious injury, as determined by the provider and the focus of treatment, is sequenced first.

1) Superficial injuries

Superficial injuries such as abrasions or contusions are not coded when associated with more severe injuries of the same site.

2) Primary injury with damage to nerves/blood vessels

When a primary injury results in minor damage to peripheral nerves or blood vessels, the primary injury is sequenced first with additional code(s) for injuries to nerves and spinal cord (such as category S04), and/or injury to blood vessels (such as category S15). When the primary injury is to the blood vessels or nerves, that injury should be sequenced first.

3) Iatrogenic injuries

Injury codes from Chapter 19 should not be assigned for injuries that occur during, or as a result of, a medical intervention. Assign the appropriate complication code(s).

c. Coding of traumatic fractures

The principles of multiple coding of injuries should be followed in coding fractures. Fractures of specified sites are coded individually by site in accordance with both the provisions within categories S02, S12, S22, S32, S42, S49, S52, S59, S62, S72, S79, S82, S89, S92 and the level of detail furnished by medical record content.

A fracture not indicated as open or closed should be coded to closed. A fracture not indicated whether displaced or not displaced should be coded to displaced.

More specific guidelines are as follows:

1) Initial vs. subsequent encounter for fractures

Traumatic fractures are coded using the appropriate 7th character for initial encounter (A, B, C) for each encounter where the patient is receiving active treatment for the fracture. The appropriate 7th character for initial encounter should also be assigned for a patient who delayed seeking treatment for the fracture or nonunion.

Fractures are coded using the appropriate 7th character for subsequent care for encounters after the patient has completed active treatment of the fracture and is receiving routine care for the fracture during the healing or recovery phase.

Care for complications of surgical treatment for fracture repairs during the healing or recovery phase should be coded with the appropriate complication codes.

Care of complications of fractures, such as malunion and nonunion, should be reported with the appropriate 7th character for subsequent care with nonunion (K, M, N,) or subsequent care with malunion (P, Q, R).

Malunion/nonunion: The appropriate 7th character for initial encounter should also be assigned for a patient who delayed seeking treatment for the fracture or nonunion.

> Female patient fell during a forest hiking excursion almost six months ago and until recently did not feel she needed to seek medical attention for her left ankle pain; x-rays show nonunion of lateral malleolus and surgery has been scheduled
>
> | S82.62XA | Displaced fracture of lateral malleolus of left fibula, initial encounter for closed fracture |
> |---|---|
> | W01.0XXA | Fall on same level from slipping, tripping and stumbling without subsequent striking against object, initial encounter |
> | Y92.821 | Forest as place of occurrence of the external cause |
> | Y93.01 | Activity, walking, marching and hiking |
> | Y99.8 | Other external cause status |
>
> *Explanation:* A seventh character of A is used for the lateral malleolus nonunion fracture to signify that the fracture is receiving active treatment. The delayed care for the fracture has resulted in a nonunion, but capturing the nonunion in the seventh character is trumped by the provision of active care.

The open fracture designations in the assignment of the 7th character for fractures of the forearm, femur and lower leg, including ankle are based on the Gustilo open fracture classification. When the Gustilo classification type is not specified for an open fracture, the 7th character for open fracture type I or II should be assigned (B, E, H, M, Q).

A code from category M80, not a traumatic fracture code, should be used for any patient with known osteoporosis who suffers a fracture, even if the patient had a minor fall or trauma, if that fall or trauma would not usually break a normal, healthy bone.

See Section I.C.13. Osteoporosis.

The aftercare Z codes should not be used for aftercare for traumatic fractures. For aftercare of a traumatic fracture, assign the acute fracture code with the appropriate 7th character.

2) Multiple fractures sequencing

Multiple fractures are sequenced in accordance with the severity of the fracture.

3) Physeal fractures

For physeal fractures, assign only the code identifying the type of physeal fracture. Do not assign a separate code to identify the specific bone that is fractured.

d. Coding of burns and corrosions

The ICD-10-CM makes a distinction between burns and corrosions. The burn codes are for thermal burns, except sunburns, that come from a heat source, such as a fire or hot appliance. The burn codes are also for burns resulting from electricity and radiation. Corrosions are burns due to chemicals. The guidelines are the same for burns and corrosions.

Current burns (T20-T25) are classified by depth, extent and by agent (X code). Burns are classified by depth as first degree (erythema), second degree (blistering), and third degree (full-thickness involvement). Burns of the eye and internal organs (T26-T28) are classified by site, but not by degree.

1) Sequencing of burn and related condition codes

Sequence first the code that reflects the highest degree of burn when more than one burn is present.

a. When the reason for the admission or encounter is for treatment of external multiple burns, sequence first the code that reflects the burn of the highest degree.

b. When a patient has both internal and external burns, the circumstances of admission govern the selection of the principal diagnosis or first-listed diagnosis.

c. When a patient is admitted for burn injuries and other related conditions such as smoke inhalation and/or respiratory failure, the circumstances of admission govern the selection of the principal or first-listed diagnosis.

> Patient referred for minor first-degree burns to multiple sites of her right and left hands as well as severe smoke inhalation. While she was sleeping at home, a candle on her dresser lit the bedroom curtains on fire.
>
> | T59.811A | Toxic effect of smoke, accidental (unintentional), initial encounter |
> |---|---|
> | J70.5 | Respiratory conditions due to smoke inhalation |
> | T23.191A | Burn of first degree of multiple sites of right wrist and hand, initial encounter |
> | T23.192A | Burn of first degree of multiple sites of left wrist and hand, initial encounter |
> | X08.8XXA | Exposure to other specified smoke, fire and flames, initial encounter |
> | Y99.8 | Other external cause status |
> | Y92.003 | Bedroom of unspecified non-institutional (private) residence as the place of occurrence of the external cause |
> | Y93.84 | Activity, sleeping |
>
> *Explanation:* Based on the documentation, the inhalation injury is more severe than the first-degree burns and is sequenced first. The burns to the hands are appended as secondary diagnoses.

2) Burns of the same anatomic site

Classify burns of the same anatomic site and on the same side but of different degrees to the subcategory identifying the highest degree recorded in the diagnosis (e.g., for second and third degree burns of right thigh, assign only code T24.311-).

3) Non-healing burns

Non-healing burns are coded as acute burns.

Necrosis of burned skin should be coded as a non-healed burn.

4) Infected burn

For any documented infected burn site, use an additional code for the infection.

5) Assign separate codes for each burn site

When coding burns, assign separate codes for each burn site. Category T30, Burn and corrosion, body region unspecified is extremely vague and should rarely be used.

Codes for burns of "multiple sites" should only be assigned when the medical record documentation does not specify the individual sites.

6) Burns and corrosions classified according to extent of body surface involved

Assign codes from category T31, Burns classified according to extent of body surface involved, or T32, Corrosions classified according to extent of body surface involved, for acute burns or corrosions when the site of the burn or corrosion is not specified or when there is a need for additional data. It is advisable to use category T31 as additional coding when needed to provide data for evaluating burn mortality, such as that needed by burn units. It is also advisable to use category T31 as an additional code for reporting purposes when there is mention of a third- degree burn involving 20 percent or more of the body surface. Codes from categories T31 and T32 should not be used for sequelae of burns or corrosions.

Categories T31 and T32 are based on the classic "rule of nines" in estimating body surface involved: head and neck are assigned nine percent, each arm nine percent, each leg 18 percent, the anterior trunk 18 percent, posterior trunk 18 percent, and genitalia one percent. Providers may change these percentage assignments where necessary to accommodate infants and children who have proportionately larger heads than adults, and patients who have large buttocks, thighs, or abdomen that involve burns.

ICD-10-CM 2023   Chapter 19. Injury, Poisoning, and Certain Other Consequences of External Causes   **Guidelines and Examples**

Chapter 19. Injury, Poisoning, and Certain Other Consequences of External Causes

Patient seen for dressing change after he accidentally spilled acetic acid on himself two days ago. The second-degree burns to his right thigh, covering about 3 percent of his body surface, are healing appropriately.

T54.2X1D	Toxic effect of corrosive acids and acid-like substances, accidental (unintentional), subsequent encounter
T24.611D	Corrosion of second degree of right thigh, subsequent encounter
T32.0	Corrosions involving less than 10% of body surface

Explanation: Code T32.0 provides additional information as to how much of the patient's body was affected by the corrosive substance.

7) Encounters for treatment of sequela of burns

Encounters for the treatment of the late effects of burns or corrosions (i.e., scars or joint contractures) should be coded with a burn or corrosion code with the 7th character "S" for sequela.

8) Sequelae with a late effect code and current burn

When appropriate, both a code for a current burn or corrosion with 7th character "A" or "D" and a burn or corrosion code with 7th character "S" may be assigned on the same record (when both a current burn and sequelae of an old burn exist). Burns and corrosions do not heal at the same rate and a current healing wound may still exist with sequela of a healed burn or corrosion.

See Section I.B.10. Sequela (Late Effects)

Female patient seen for second-degree burn to the left ear; she also has significant scarring on her left elbow from a third-degree burn from childhood

T20.212A	Burn of second degree of left ear [any part, except ear drum], initial encounter
L90.5	Scar conditions and fibrosis of skin
T22.322S	Burn of third degree of left elbow, sequela

Explanation: The patient is being seen for management of a current second-degree burn, which is reflected in the code by appending the seventh character of A, indicating active treatment or management of this burn. The elbow scarring is a sequela of a previous third-degree burn. The sequela condition precedes the original burn injury, which is appended with a seventh character of S.

9) Use of an external cause code with burns and corrosions

An external cause code should be used with burns and corrosions to identify the source and intent of the burn, as well as the place where it occurred.

e. Adverse effects, poisoning, underdosing and toxic effects

Codes in categories T36-T65 are combination codes that include the substance that was taken as well as the intent. No additional external cause code is required for poisonings, toxic effects, adverse effects and underdosing codes.

1) Do not code directly from the Table of Drugs

Do not code directly from the Table of Drugs and Chemicals. Always refer back to the Tabular List.

2) Use as many codes as necessary to describe

Use as many codes as necessary to describe completely all drugs, medicinal or biological substances.

3) If the same code would describe the causative agent

If the same code would describe the causative agent for more than one adverse reaction, poisoning, toxic effect or underdosing, assign the code only once.

4) If two or more drugs, medicinal or biological substances

If two or more drugs, medicinal or biological substances are taken, code each individually unless a combination code is listed in the Table of Drugs and Chemicals.

If multiple unspecified drugs, medicinal or biological substances were taken, assign the appropriate code from subcategory T50.91, Poisoning by, adverse effect of and underdosing of multiple unspecified drugs, medicaments and biological substances.

5) The occurrence of drug toxicity is classified in ICD-10-CM as follows:

(a) Adverse effect

When coding an adverse effect of a drug that has been correctly prescribed and properly administered, assign the appropriate code for the nature of the adverse effect followed by the appropriate code for the adverse effect of the drug (T36-T50). The code for the drug should have a 5th or 6th character "5" (for example T36.0X5-) Examples of the

nature of an adverse effect are tachycardia, delirium, gastrointestinal hemorrhaging, vomiting, hypokalemia, hepatitis, renal failure, or respiratory failure.

(b) Poisoning

When coding a poisoning or reaction to the improper use of a medication (e.g., overdose, wrong substance given or taken in error, wrong route of administration), first assign the appropriate code from categories T36-T50. The poisoning codes have an associated intent as their 5th or 6th character (accidental, intentional self-harm, assault and undetermined). If the intent of the poisoning is unknown or unspecified, code the intent as accidental intent. The undetermined intent is only for use if the documentation in the record specifies that the intent cannot be determined. Use additional code(s) for all manifestations of poisonings.

If there is also a diagnosis of abuse or dependence of the substance, the abuse or dependence is assigned as an additional code.

Examples of poisoning include:

(i) Error was made in drug prescription
Errors made in drug prescription or in the administration of the drug by provider, nurse, patient, or other person.

(ii) Overdose of a drug intentionally taken
If an overdose of a drug was intentionally taken or administered and resulted in drug toxicity, it would be coded as a poisoning.

(iii) Nonprescribed drug taken with correctly prescribed and properly administered drug
If a nonprescribed drug or medicinal agent was taken in combination with a correctly prescribed and properly administered drug, any drug toxicity or other reaction resulting from the interaction of the two drugs would be classified as a poisoning.

(iv) Interaction of drug(s) and alcohol
When a reaction results from the interaction of a drug(s) and alcohol, this would be classified as poisoning.
See Section I.C.4. if poisoning is the result of insulin pump malfunctions.

(c) Underdosing

Underdosing refers to taking less of a medication than is prescribed by a provider or a manufacturer's instruction. Discontinuing the use of a prescribed medication on the patient's own initiative (not directed by the patient's provider) is also classified as an underdosing. For underdosing, assign the code from categories T36-T50 (fifth or sixth character "6"). **Documentation of a change in the patient's condition is not required in order to assign an underdosing code. Documentation that the patient is taking less of a medication than is prescribed or discontinued the prescribed medication is sufficient for code assignment.**

Codes for underdosing should never be assigned as principal or first-listed codes. If a patient has a relapse or exacerbation of the medical condition for which the drug is prescribed because of the reduction in dose, then the medical condition itself should be coded.

Noncompliance (Z91.12-, Z91.13- and Z91.14-) or complication of care (Y63.6-Y63.9) codes are to be used with an underdosing code to indicate intent, if known.

Patient referred for atrial fibrillation with history of chronic atrial fibrillation for which she is prescribed amiodarone. Financial concerns have left the patient unable to pay for her prescriptions and she has been skipping her amiodarone dose every other day to offset the cost.

I48.20	Chronic atrial fibrillation, unspecified
T46.2X6A	Underdosing of other antidysrhythmic drugs, initial encounter
Z91.120	Patient's intentional underdosing of medication regimen due to financial hardship

Explanation: By skipping her amiodarone pill every other day, the patient's atrial fibrillation returned. The condition for which the drug was being taken is reported first, followed by an underdosing code to show that the patient was not adhering to her prescription regiment. The Z code helps elaborate on the patient's social and/or economic circumstances that led to the patient taking less then what she was prescribed.

(d) Toxic effects

When a harmful substance is ingested or comes in contact with a person, this is classified as a toxic effect. The toxic effect codes are in categories T51-T65.

Toxic effect codes have an associated intent: accidental, intentional self-harm, assault and undetermined.

f. Adult and child abuse, neglect and other maltreatment

Sequence first the appropriate code from categories T74, Adult and child abuse, neglect and other maltreatment, confirmed, or T76, Adult and child abuse, neglect and other maltreatment, suspected, for abuse, neglect and other maltreatment, followed by any accompanying mental health or injury code(s).

If the documentation in the medical record states abuse or neglect, it is coded as confirmed (T74.-). It is coded as suspected if it is documented as suspected (T76.-).

For cases of confirmed abuse or neglect an external cause code from the assault section (X92-Y09) should be added to identify the cause of any physical injuries. A perpetrator code (Y07) should be added when the perpetrator of the abuse is known. For suspected cases of abuse or neglect, do not report external cause or perpetrator code.

If a suspected case of abuse, neglect or mistreatment is ruled out during an encounter code Z04.71, Encounter for examination and observation following alleged physical adult abuse, ruled out, or code Z04.72, Encounter for examination and observation following alleged child physical abuse, ruled out, should be used, not a code from T76.

If a suspected case of alleged rape or sexual abuse is ruled out during an encounter code Z04.41, Encounter for examination and observation following alleged adult rape or code Z04.42, Encounter for examination and observation following alleged child rape, should be used, not a code from T76.

If a suspected case of forced sexual exploitation or forced labor exploitation is ruled out during an encounter, code Z04.81, Encounter for examination and observation of victim following forced sexual exploitation, or code Z04.82, Encounter for examination and observation of victim following forced labor exploitation, should be used, not a code from T76.

See Section I.C.15. Abuse in a pregnant patient.

g. Complications of care

1) General guidelines for complications of care

(a) Documentation of complications of care

See Section I.B.16. for information on documentation of complications of care.

2) Pain due to medical devices

Pain associated with devices, implants or grafts left in a surgical site (for example painful hip prosthesis) is assigned to the appropriate code(s) found in Chapter 19, Injury, poisoning, and certain other consequences of external causes. Specific codes for pain due to medical devices are found in the T code section of the ICD-10-CM. Use additional code(s) from category G89 to identify acute or chronic pain due to presence of the device, implant or graft (G89.18 or G89.28).

Chronic left breast pain secondary to breast implant	
T85.848A	Pain due to other internal prosthetic devices, implants and grafts, initial encounter
N64.4	Mastodynia
G89.28	Other chronic postprocedural pain

Explanation: As the pain is a complication related to the breast implant, the complication code is sequenced first. The T code does not describe the site or type of pain, so additional codes may be appended to indicate that the patient is experiencing chronic pain in the breast.

3) Transplant complications

(a) Transplant complications other than kidney

Codes under category T86, Complications of transplanted organs and tissues, are for use for both complications and rejection of transplanted organs. A transplant complication code is only assigned if the complication affects the function of the transplanted organ. Two codes are required to fully describe a transplant complication: the appropriate code from category T86 and a secondary code that identifies the complication.

Pre-existing conditions or conditions that develop after the transplant are not coded as complications unless they affect the function of the transplanted organs.

See I.C.21. for transplant organ removal status

See I.C.2. for malignant neoplasm associated with transplanted organ.

(b) Kidney transplant complications

Patients who have undergone kidney transplant may still have some form of chronic kidney disease (CKD) because the kidney transplant may not fully restore kidney function. Code T86.1- should be assigned for documented complications of a kidney transplant, such as transplant failure or rejection or other transplant complication. Code T86.1- should not be assigned for post kidney transplant patients who have chronic kidney (CKD) unless a transplant complication such as transplant failure or rejection is documented. If the documentation is unclear as to whether the patient has a complication of the transplant, query the provider.

Conditions that affect the function of the transplanted kidney, other than CKD, should be assigned a code from subcategory T86.1, Complications of transplanted organ, Kidney, and a secondary code that identifies the complication.

For patients with CKD following a kidney transplant, but who do not have a complication such as failure or rejection, *see section I.C.14. Chronic kidney disease and kidney transplant status.*

Patient seen for chronic kidney disease stage 2; history of successful kidney transplant with no complications identified	
N18.2	Chronic kidney disease, stage 2 (mild)
Z94.0	Kidney transplant status

Explanation: This patient's stage 2 CKD is not indicated as being due to the transplanted kidney but instead is just the residual disease the patient had prior to the transplant.

4) Complication codes that include the external cause

As with certain other T codes, some of the complications of care codes have the external cause included in the code. The code includes the nature of the complication as well as the type of procedure that caused the complication. No external cause code indicating the type of procedure is necessary for these codes.

5) Complications of care codes within the body system chapters

Intraoperative and postprocedural complication codes are found within the body system chapters with codes specific to the organs and structures of that body system. These codes should be sequenced first, followed by a code(s) for the specific complication, if applicable.

Postprocedural ischemic infarction of the left middle cerebral artery due to cardiac surgery	
I97.820	Postprocedural cerebrovascular infarction following cardiac surgery
I63.512	Cerebral infarction due to unspecified occlusion or stenosis of left middle cerebral artery

Explanation: The infarction was caused by the cardiac procedure and is coded as a postprocedural complication. The postprocedural cerebrovascular infarction is the first-listed diagnosis, followed by the code for the infarction itself.

Complication codes from the body system chapters should be assigned for intraoperative and postprocedural complications (e.g., the appropriate complication code from chapter 9 would be assigned for a vascular intraoperative or postprocedural complication) unless the complication is specifically indexed to a T code in chapter 19.

Muscle/Tendon Table

ICD-10-CM categorizes certain muscles and tendons in the upper and lower extremities by their action (e.g., extension, flexion), their anatomical location (e.g., posterior, anterior), and/or whether they are intrinsic or extrinsic to a certain anatomical area. The Muscle/Tendon Table is provided at the beginning of chapters 13 and 19 as a resource to help users when code selection depends on one or more of these characteristics. A **TIP** has been placed at those categories and/or subcategories that relate to this table. Please note that this table is not all-inclusive, and proper code assignment should be based on the provider's documentation.

Body Region	Muscle	Extensor Tendon	Flexor Tendon	Other Tendon
Shoulder				
	Deltoid	Posterior deltoid	Anterior deltoid	
	Rotator cuff			
	Infraspinatus			Infraspinatus
	Subscapularis			Subscapularis
	Supraspinatus			Supraspinatus
	Teres minor			Teres minor
	Teres major	Teres major		
Upper arm				
	Anterior muscles			
	Biceps brachii — long head		Biceps brachii — long head	
	Biceps brachii — short head		Biceps brachii — short head	
	Brachialis		Brachialis	
	Coracobrachialis		Coracobrachialis	
	Posterior muscles			
	Triceps brachii	Triceps brachii		
Forearm				
	Anterior muscles			
	Flexors			
	Deep			
	Flexor digitorum profundus		Flexor digitorum profundus	
	Flexor pollicis longus		Flexor pollicis longus	
	Intermediate			
	Flexor digitorum superficialis		Flexor digitorum superficialis	
	Superficial			
	Flexor carpi radialis		Flexor carpi radialis	
	Flexor carpi ulnaris		Flexor carpi ulnaris	
	Palmaris longus		Palmaris longus	
	Pronators			
	Pronator quadratus			Pronator quadratus
	Pronator teres			Pronator teres
	Posterior muscles			
	Extensors			
	Deep			
	Abductor pollicis longus			Abductor pollicis longus
	Extensor indicis	Extensor indicis		
	Extensor pollicis brevis	Extensor pollicis brevis		
	Extensor pollicis longus	Extensor pollicis longus		
	Superficial			
	Brachioradialis			Brachioradialis
	Extensor carpi radialis brevis	Extensor carpi radialis brevis		
	Extensor carpi radialis longus	Extensor carpi radialis longus		
	Extensor carpi ulnaris	Extensor carpi ulnaris		
	Extensor digiti minimi	Extensor digiti minimi		
	Extensor digitorum	Extensor digitorum		
	Anconeus	Anconeus		
	Supinator			Supinator

Body Region	Muscle	Extensor Tendon	Flexor Tendon	Other Tendon
Hand				
Extrinsic — attach to a site in the forearm as well as a site in the hand with action related to hand movement at the wrist				
	Extensor carpi radialis brevis	Extensor carpi radialis brevis		
	Extensor carpi radialis longus	Extensor carpi radialis longus		
	Extensor carpi ulnaris	Extensor carpi ulnaris		
	Flexor carpi radialis		Flexor carpi radialis	
	Flexor carpi ulnaris		Flexor carpi ulnaris	
	Flexor digitorum superficialis		Flexor digitorum superficialis	
	Palmaris longus		Palmaris longus	
Extrinsic — attach to a site in the forearm as well as a site in the hand with action in the hand related to finger movement				
	Adductor pollicis longus			Adductor pollicis longus
	Extensor digiti minimi	Extensor digiti minimi		
	Extensor digitorum	Extensor digitorum		
	Extensor indicis	Extensor indicis		
	Flexor digitorum profundus		Flexor digitorum profundus	
	Flexor digitorum superficialis		Flexor digitorum superficialis	
Extrinsic — attach to a site in the forearm as well as a site in the hand with action in the hand related to thumb movement				
	Extensor pollicis brevis	Extensor pollicis brevis		
	Extensor pollicis longus	Extensor pollicis longus		
	Flexor pollicis longus		Flexor pollicis longus	
Intrinsic — found within the hand only				
	Adductor pollicis			Adductor pollicis
	Dorsal interossei	Dorsal interossei	Dorsal interossei	
	Lumbricals	Lumbricals	Lumbricals	
	Palmaris brevis			Palmaris brevis
	Palmar interossei	Palmar interossei	Palmar interossei	
	Hypothenar muscles			
	Abductor digiti minimi			Abductor digiti minimi
	Flexor digiti minimi brevis		Flexor digiti minimi brevis	
	Opponens digiti minimi		Opponens digiti minimi	
	Thenar muscles			
	Abductor pollicis brevis			Abductor pollicis brevis
	Flexor pollicis brevis		Flexor pollicis brevis	
	Opponens pollicis		Opponens pollicis	
Thigh				
	Anterior muscles			
	Iliopsoas		Iliopsoas	
	Pectineus		Pectineus	
	Quadriceps	Quadriceps		
	Rectus femoris	Rectus femoris — Extends knee	Rectus femoris — Flexes hip	
	Vastus intermedius	Vastus intermedius		
	Vastus lateralis	Vastus lateralis		
	Vastus medialis	Vastus medialis		
	Sartorius		Sartorius	
	Medial muscles			
	Adductor brevis			Adductor brevis
	Adductor longus			Adductor longus
	Adductor magnus			Adductor magnus
	Gracilis			Gracilis
	Obturator externus			Obturator externus
	Posterior muscles			
	Hamstring	Hamstring — Extends hip	Hamstring — Flexes knee	
	Biceps femoris	Biceps femoris	Biceps femoris	
	Semimembranosus	Semimembranosus	Semimembranosus	
	Semitendinosus	Semitendinosus	Semitendinosus	

Body Region	Muscle	Extensor Tendon	Flexor Tendon	Other Tendon
Lower leg				
	Anterior muscles			
	Extensor digitorum longus	Extensor digitorum longus		
	Extensor hallucis longus	Extensor hallucis longus		
	Fibularis (peroneus) tertius	Fibularis (peroneus) tertius		
	Tibialis anterior	Tibialis anterior		Tibialis anterior
	Lateral muscles			
	Fibularis (peroneus) brevis		Fibularis (peroneus) brevis	
	Fibularis (peroneus) longus		Fibularis (peroneus) longus	
	Posterior muscles			
	Deep			
	Flexor digitorum longus		Flexor digitorum longus	
	Flexor hallucis longus		Flexor hallucis longus	
	Popliteus		Popliteus	
	Tibialis posterior		Tibialis posterior	
	Superficial			
	Gastrocnemius		Gastrocnemius	
	Plantaris		Plantaris	
	Soleus		Soleus	
				Calcaneal (Achilles)
Ankle/Foot				
Extrinsic — attach to a site in the lower leg as well as a site in the foot with action related to foot movement at the ankle				
	Plantaris		Plantaris	
	Soleus		Soleus	
	Tibialis anterior	Tibialis anterior		
	Tibialis posterior		Tibialis posterior	
Extrinsic — attach to a site in the lower leg as well as a site in the foot with action in the foot related to toe movement				
	Extensor digitorum longus	Extensor digitorum longus		
	Extensor hallucis longus	Extensor hallucis longus		
	Flexor digitorum longus		Flexor digitorum longus	
	Flexor hallucis longus		Flexor hallucis longus	
Intrinsic — found within the ankle/foot only				
	Dorsal muscles			
	Extensor digitorum brevis	Extensor digitorum brevis		
	Extensor hallucis brevis	Extensor hallucis brevis		
	Plantar muscles			
	Abductor digiti minimi		Abductor digiti minimi	
	Abductor hallucis		Abductor hallucis	
	Dorsal interossei	Dorsal interossei	Dorsal interossei	
	Flexor digiti minimi brevis		Flexor digiti minimi brevis	
	Flexor digitorum brevis		Flexor digitorum brevis	
	Flexor hallucis brevis		Flexor hallucis brevis	
	Lumbricals	Lumbricals	Lumbricals	
	Quadratus plantae		Quadratus plantae	
	Plantar interossei	Plantar interossei	Plantar interossei	

Chapter 19. Injury, Poisoning and Certain Other Consequences of External Causes (S00-T88)

NOTE Use secondary code(s) from Chapter 20, External causes of morbidity, to indicate cause of injury. Codes within the T section that include the external cause do not require an additional external cause code.

Use additional code to identify any retained foreign body, if applicable (Z18.-)

EXCLUDES 1   birth trauma (P10-P15)
           obstetric trauma (O70-O71)

NOTE The chapter uses the S-section for coding different types of injuries related to single body regions and the T-section to cover injuries to unspecified body regions as well as poisoning and certain other consequences of external causes.

AHA: 2016,2Q,3-7; 2015,4Q,35-38; 2015,3Q,37-39,40; 2015,2Q,6; 2015,1Q,3-21

TIP: The specific site of an injury can be determined from the radiology report when authenticated by a radiologist and available at the time of code assignment.

This chapter contains the following blocks:

S00-S09	Injuries to the head
S10-S19	Injuries to the neck
S20-S29	Injuries to the thorax
S30-S39	Injuries to the abdomen, lower back, lumbar spine, pelvis and external genitals
S40-S49	Injuries to the shoulder and upper arm
S50-S59	Injuries to the elbow and forearm
S60-S69	Injuries to the wrist, hand and fingers
S70-S79	Injuries to the hip and thigh
S80-S89	Injuries to the knee and lower leg
S90-S99	Injuries to the ankle and foot
T07	Injuries involving multiple body regions
T14	Injury of unspecified body region
T15-T19	Effects of foreign body entering through natural orifice
T20-T25	Burns and corrosions of external body surface, specified by site
T26-T28	Burns and corrosions confined to eye and internal organs
T30-T32	Burns and corrosions of multiple and unspecified body regions
T33-T34	Frostbite
T36-T50	Poisoning by, adverse effect of and underdosing of drugs, medicaments and biological substances
T51-T65	Toxic effects of substances chiefly nonmedicinal as to source
T66-T78	Other and unspecified effects of external causes
T79	Certain early complications of trauma
T80-T88	Complications of surgical and medical care, not elsewhere classified

Injuries to the head (S00-S09)

INCLUDES injuries of ear
         injuries of eye
         injuries of face [any part]
         injuries of gum
         injuries of jaw
         injuries of oral cavity
         injuries of palate
         injuries of periocular area
         injuries of scalp
         injuries of temporomandibular joint area
         injuries of tongue
         injuries of tooth

Code also for any associated infection

EXCLUDES 2   burns and corrosions (T20-T32)
           effects of foreign body in ear (T16)
           effects of foreign body in larynx (T17.3)
           effects of foreign body in mouth NOS (T18.0)
           effects of foreign body in nose (T17.0-T17.1)
           effects of foreign body in pharynx (T17.2)
           effects of foreign body on external eye (T15.-)
           frostbite (T33-T34)
           insect bite or sting, venomous (T63.4)

√4ᵗʰ **S00   Superficial injury of head**

    EXCLUDES 1   diffuse cerebral contusion (S06.2-)
             focal cerebral contusion (S06.3-)
             injury of eye and orbit (S05.-)
             open wound of head (S01.-)

> The appropriate 7th character is to be added to each code from category S00.
> A   initial encounter
> D   subsequent encounter
> S   sequela

   √5ᵗʰ **S00.0   Superficial injury of scalp**

      √x7ᵗʰ   **S00.00   Unspecified superficial injury of scalp**

      √x7ᵗʰ   **S00.01   Abrasion of scalp**

      √x7ᵗʰ   **S00.02   Blister (nonthermal) of scalp**

√x7ᵗʰ   **S00.03   Contusion of scalp**   🄠
          Bruise of scalp
          Hematoma of scalp

√x7ᵗʰ   **S00.04   External constriction of part of scalp**

√x7ᵗʰ   **S00.05   Superficial foreign body of scalp**
          Splinter in the scalp

√x7ᵗʰ   **S00.06   Insect bite (nonvenomous) of scalp**

√x7ᵗʰ   **S00.07   Other superficial bite of scalp**
       EXCLUDES 1   open bite of scalp (S01.05)

√5ᵗʰ   **S00.1   Contusion of eyelid and periocular area**
      Black eye
      EXCLUDES 2   contusion of eyeball and orbital tissues (S05.1-)

   √x7ᵗʰ   **S00.10   Contusion of unspecified eyelid and periocular area**

   √x7ᵗʰ   **S00.11   Contusion of right eyelid and periocular area**

   √x7ᵗʰ   **S00.12   Contusion of left eyelid and periocular area**

√5ᵗʰ   **S00.2   Other and unspecified superficial injuries of eyelid and periocular area**
      EXCLUDES 2   superficial injury of conjunctiva and cornea (S05.0-)

   √6ᵗʰ   **S00.20   Unspecified superficial injury of eyelid and periocular area**

      √7ᵗʰ   **S00.201   Unspecified superficial injury of right eyelid and periocular area**

      √7ᵗʰ   **S00.202   Unspecified superficial injury of left eyelid and periocular area**

      √7ᵗʰ   **S00.209   Unspecified superficial injury of unspecified eyelid and periocular area**

   √6ᵗʰ   **S00.21   Abrasion of eyelid and periocular area**

      √7ᵗʰ   **S00.211   Abrasion of right eyelid and periocular area**

      √7ᵗʰ   **S00.212   Abrasion of left eyelid and periocular area**

      √7ᵗʰ   **S00.219   Abrasion of unspecified eyelid and periocular area**

   √6ᵗʰ   **S00.22   Blister (nonthermal) of eyelid and periocular area**

      √7ᵗʰ   **S00.221   Blister (nonthermal) of right eyelid and periocular area**

      √7ᵗʰ   **S00.222   Blister (nonthermal) of left eyelid and periocular area**

      √7ᵗʰ   **S00.229   Blister (nonthermal) of unspecified eyelid and periocular area**

   √6ᵗʰ   **S00.24   External constriction of eyelid and periocular area**

      √7ᵗʰ   **S00.241   External constriction of right eyelid and periocular area**

      √7ᵗʰ   **S00.242   External constriction of left eyelid and periocular area**

      √7ᵗʰ   **S00.249   External constriction of unspecified eyelid and periocular area**

   √6ᵗʰ   **S00.25   Superficial foreign body of eyelid and periocular area**
      Splinter of eyelid and periocular area
      EXCLUDES 2   retained foreign body in eyelid (H02.81-)

      √7ᵗʰ   **S00.251   Superficial foreign body of right eyelid and periocular area**

      √7ᵗʰ   **S00.252   Superficial foreign body of left eyelid and periocular area**

      √7ᵗʰ   **S00.259   Superficial foreign body of unspecified eyelid and periocular area**

   √6ᵗʰ   **S00.26   Insect bite (nonvenomous) of eyelid and periocular area**

      √7ᵗʰ   **S00.261   Insect bite (nonvenomous) of right eyelid and periocular area**

      √7ᵗʰ   **S00.262   Insect bite (nonvenomous) of left eyelid and periocular area**

      √7ᵗʰ   **S00.269   Insect bite (nonvenomous) of unspecified eyelid and periocular area**

   √6ᵗʰ   **S00.27   Other superficial bite of eyelid and periocular area**
      EXCLUDES 1   open bite of eyelid and periocular area (S01.15)

      √7ᵗʰ   **S00.271   Other superficial bite of right eyelid and periocular area**

      √7ᵗʰ   **S00.272   Other superficial bite of left eyelid and periocular area**

      √7ᵗʰ   **S00.279   Other superficial bite of unspecified eyelid and periocular area**

√5ᵗʰ   **S00.3   Superficial injury of nose**

   √x7ᵗʰ   **S00.30   Unspecified superficial injury of nose**

   √x7ᵗʰ   **S00.31   Abrasion of nose**

   √x7ᵗʰ   **S00.32   Blister (nonthermal) of nose**

√x7ᵗʰ **S00.33** **Contusion** of nose Q
Bruise of nose
Hematoma of nose

√x7ᵗʰ **S00.34** **External constriction** of nose

√x7ᵗʰ **S00.35** **Superficial** foreign body of nose
Splinter in the nose

√x7ᵗʰ **S00.36** **Insect bite** (nonvenomous) of nose

√x7ᵗʰ **S00.37** **Other superficial** bite of nose
EXCLUDES 1   *open bite of nose (S01.25)*

√5ᵗʰ **S00.4** **Superficial injury** of ear

√6ᵗʰ **S00.40** **Unspecified superficial injury** of ear

√7ᵗʰ **S00.401** **Unspecified superficial injury** of **right** ear

√7ᵗʰ **S00.402** **Unspecified superficial injury** of **left** ear

√7ᵗʰ **S00.409** **Unspecified superficial injury** of unspecified ear

√6ᵗʰ **S00.41** **Abrasion** of ear

√7ᵗʰ **S00.411** **Abrasion** of **right** ear

√7ᵗʰ **S00.412** **Abrasion** of **left** ear

√7ᵗʰ **S00.419** **Abrasion** of unspecified ear

√6ᵗʰ **S00.42** **Blister** (nonthermal) of ear

√7ᵗʰ **S00.421** **Blister** (nonthermal) of **right** ear

√7ᵗʰ **S00.422** **Blister** (nonthermal) of **left** ear

√7ᵗʰ **S00.429** **Blister** (nonthermal) of unspecified ear

√6ᵗʰ **S00.43** **Contusion** of ear
Bruise of ear
Hematoma of ear

√7ᵗʰ **S00.431** **Contusion** of **right** ear Q

√7ᵗʰ **S00.432** **Contusion** of **left** ear Q

√7ᵗʰ **S00.439** **Contusion** of unspecified ear Q

√6ᵗʰ **S00.44** **External constriction** of ear

√7ᵗʰ **S00.441** **External constriction** of **right** ear

√7ᵗʰ **S00.442** **External constriction** of **left** ear

√7ᵗʰ **S00.449** **External constriction** of unspecified ear

√6ᵗʰ **S00.45** **Superficial** foreign body of ear
Splinter in the ear

√7ᵗʰ **S00.451** **Superficial foreign body** of **right** ear

√7ᵗʰ **S00.452** **Superficial foreign body** of **left** ear

√7ᵗʰ **S00.459** **Superficial foreign body** of unspecified ear

√6ᵗʰ **S00.46** **Insect bite** (nonvenomous) of ear

√7ᵗʰ **S00.461** **Insect bite** (nonvenomous) of **right** ear

√7ᵗʰ **S00.462** **Insect bite** (nonvenomous) of **left** ear

√7ᵗʰ **S00.469** **Insect bite** (nonvenomous) of unspecified ear

√6ᵗʰ **S00.47** **Other superficial** bite of ear
EXCLUDES 1   *open bite of ear (S01.35)*

√7ᵗʰ **S00.471** **Other superficial** bite of **right** ear

√7ᵗʰ **S00.472** **Other superficial** bite of **left** ear

√7ᵗʰ **S00.479** **Other superficial** bite of unspecified ear

√5ᵗʰ **S00.5** **Superficial injury** of lip and oral cavity

√6ᵗʰ **S00.50** **Unspecified superficial injury** of lip and oral cavity

√7ᵗʰ **S00.501** **Unspecified superficial injury** of lip

√7ᵗʰ **S00.502** **Unspecified superficial injury** of oral cavity

√6ᵗʰ **S00.51** **Abrasion** of lip and oral cavity

√7ᵗʰ **S00.511** **Abrasion** of lip

√7ᵗʰ **S00.512** **Abrasion** of oral cavity

√6ᵗʰ **S00.52** **Blister** (nonthermal) of lip and oral cavity

√7ᵗʰ **S00.521** **Blister** (nonthermal) of lip

√7ᵗʰ **S00.522** **Blister** (nonthermal) of oral cavity

√6ᵗʰ **S00.53** **Contusion** of lip and oral cavity

√7ᵗʰ **S00.531** **Contusion** of lip Q
Bruise of lip
Hematoma of lip

√7ᵗʰ **S00.532** **Contusion** of oral cavity Q
Bruise of oral cavity
Hematoma of oral cavity

√6ᵗʰ **S00.54** **External constriction** of lip and oral cavity

√7ᵗʰ **S00.541** **External constriction** of lip

√7ᵗʰ **S00.542** **External constriction** of oral cavity

√6ᵗʰ **S00.55** **Superficial** foreign body of lip and oral cavity

√7ᵗʰ **S00.551** **Superficial foreign body** of lip
Splinter of lip and oral cavity

√7ᵗʰ **S00.552** **Superficial foreign body** of oral cavity
Splinter of lip and oral cavity

√6ᵗʰ **S00.56** **Insect bite** (nonvenomous) of lip and oral cavity

√7ᵗʰ **S00.561** **Insect bite** (nonvenomous) of lip

√7ᵗʰ **S00.562** **Insect bite** (nonvenomous) of oral cavity

√6ᵗʰ **S00.57** **Other superficial** bite of lip and oral cavity

√7ᵗʰ **S00.571** **Other superficial bite** of lip
EXCLUDES 1   *open bite of lip (S01.551)*

√7ᵗʰ **S00.572** **Other superficial bite** of oral cavity
EXCLUDES 1   *open bite of oral cavity (S01.552)*

√5ᵗʰ **S00.8** **Superficial injury** of other parts of head
Superficial injuries of face [any part]

√x7ᵗʰ **S00.80** **Unspecified superficial injury** of other part of head

√x7ᵗʰ **S00.81** **Abrasion** of other part of head

√x7ᵗʰ **S00.82** **Blister** (nonthermal) of other part of head

√x7ᵗʰ **S00.83** **Contusion** of other part of head Q
Bruise of other part of head
Hematoma of other part of head

√x7ᵗʰ **S00.84** **External constriction** of other part of head

√x7ᵗʰ **S00.85** **Superficial** foreign body of other part of head
Splinter in other part of head

√x7ᵗʰ **S00.86** **Insect bite** (nonvenomous) of other part of head

√x7ᵗʰ **S00.87** **Other superficial** bite of other part of head
EXCLUDES 1   *open bite of other part of head (S01.85)*

√5ᵗʰ **S00.9** **Superficial injury** of unspecified part of head

√x7ᵗʰ **S00.90** **Unspecified superficial injury** of unspecified part of head

√x7ᵗʰ **S00.91** **Abrasion** of unspecified part of head

√x7ᵗʰ **S00.92** **Blister** (nonthermal) of unspecified part of head

√x7ᵗʰ **S00.93** **Contusion** of unspecified part of head Q
Bruise of head
Hematoma of head

√x7ᵗʰ **S00.94** **External constriction** of unspecified part of head

√x7ᵗʰ **S00.95** **Superficial** foreign body of unspecified part of head
Splinter of head

√x7ᵗʰ **S00.96** **Insect bite** (nonvenomous) of unspecified part of head

√x7ᵗʰ **S00.97** **Other superficial** bite of unspecified part of head
EXCLUDES 1   *open bite of head (S01.95)*

√4ᵗʰ **S01** **Open wound of head**
Code also any associated:
injury of cranial nerve (S04.-)
injury of muscle and tendon of head (S09.1-)
intracranial injury (S06.-)
wound infection
EXCLUDES 1   *open skull fracture (S02.- with 7th character B)*
EXCLUDES 2   *injury of eye and orbit (S05.-)*
traumatic amputation of part of head (S08.-)

The appropriate 7th character is to be added to each code from category S01.
A   initial encounter
D   subsequent encounter
S   sequela

√5ᵗʰ **S01.0** **Open wound of scalp**
EXCLUDES 1   *avulsion of scalp (S08.0-)*

√x7ᵗʰ **S01.00** **Unspecified open wound** of scalp

√x7ᵗʰ **S01.01** **Laceration without foreign body** of scalp

√x7ᵗʰ **S01.02** **Laceration with foreign body** of scalp

√x7ᵗʰ **S01.03** **Puncture wound without foreign body** of scalp

√x7ᵗʰ **S01.04** **Puncture wound with foreign body** of scalp

√x7ᵗʰ **S01.05** **Open bite** of scalp
Bite of scalp NOS
EXCLUDES 1   *superficial bite of scalp (S00.06, S00.07-)*

√5ᵗʰ **S01.1** Open wound of eyelid and periocular area

Open wound of eyelid and periocular area with or without involvement of lacrimal passages

√6ᵗʰ **S01.10** Unspecified open wound of eyelid and periocular area

√7ᵗʰ **S01.101** Unspecified open wound of right eyelid and periocular area

√7ᵗʰ **S01.102** Unspecified open wound of left eyelid and periocular area

√7ᵗʰ **S01.109** Unspecified open wound of unspecified eyelid and periocular area

√6ᵗʰ **S01.11** Laceration without foreign body of eyelid and periocular area

√7ᵗʰ **S01.111** Laceration without foreign body of right eyelid and periocular area

√7ᵗʰ **S01.112** Laceration without foreign body of left eyelid and periocular area

√7ᵗʰ **S01.119** Laceration without foreign body of unspecified eyelid and periocular area

√6ᵗʰ **S01.12** Laceration with foreign body of eyelid and periocular area

√7ᵗʰ **S01.121** Laceration with foreign body of right eyelid and periocular area

√7ᵗʰ **S01.122** Laceration with foreign body of left eyelid and periocular area

√7ᵗʰ **S01.129** Laceration with foreign body of unspecified eyelid and periocular area

√6ᵗʰ **S01.13** Puncture wound without foreign body of eyelid and periocular area

√7ᵗʰ **S01.131** Puncture wound without foreign body of right eyelid and periocular area

√7ᵗʰ **S01.132** Puncture wound without foreign body of left eyelid and periocular area

√7ᵗʰ **S01.139** Puncture wound without foreign body of unspecified eyelid and periocular area

√6ᵗʰ **S01.14** Puncture wound with foreign body of eyelid and periocular area

√7ᵗʰ **S01.141** Puncture wound with foreign body of right eyelid and periocular area

√7ᵗʰ **S01.142** Puncture wound with foreign body of left eyelid and periocular area

√7ᵗʰ **S01.149** Puncture wound with foreign body of unspecified eyelid and periocular area

√6ᵗʰ **S01.15** Open bite of eyelid and periocular area

Bite of eyelid and periocular area NOS

EXCLUDES 1   superficial bite of eyelid and periocular area (S00.26, S00.27)

√7ᵗʰ **S01.151** Open bite of right eyelid and periocular area

√7ᵗʰ **S01.152** Open bite of left eyelid and periocular area

√7ᵗʰ **S01.159** Open bite of unspecified eyelid and periocular area

√5ᵗʰ **S01.2** Open wound of nose

√x7ᵗʰ **S01.20** Unspecified open wound of nose

√x7ᵗʰ **S01.21** Laceration without foreign body of nose

√x7ᵗʰ **S01.22** Laceration with foreign body of nose

√x7ᵗʰ **S01.23** Puncture wound without foreign body of nose

√x7ᵗʰ **S01.24** Puncture wound with foreign body of nose

√x7ᵗʰ **S01.25** Open bite of nose

Bite of nose NOS

EXCLUDES 1   superficial bite of nose (S00.36, S00.37)

√5ᵗʰ **S01.3** Open wound of ear

√6ᵗʰ **S01.30** Unspecified open wound of ear

√7ᵗʰ **S01.301** Unspecified open wound of right ear

√7ᵗʰ **S01.302** Unspecified open wound of left ear

√7ᵗʰ **S01.309** Unspecified open wound of unspecified ear

√6ᵗʰ **S01.31** Laceration without foreign body of ear

√7ᵗʰ **S01.311** Laceration without foreign body of right ear

√7ᵗʰ **S01.312** Laceration without foreign body of left ear

√7ᵗʰ **S01.319** Laceration without foreign body of unspecified ear

√6ᵗʰ **S01.32** Laceration with foreign body of ear

√7ᵗʰ **S01.321** Laceration with foreign body of right ear

√7ᵗʰ **S01.322** Laceration with foreign body of left ear

√7ᵗʰ **S01.329** Laceration with foreign body of unspecified ear

√6ᵗʰ **S01.33** Puncture wound without foreign body of ear

√7ᵗʰ **S01.331** Puncture wound without foreign body of right ear

√7ᵗʰ **S01.332** Puncture wound without foreign body of left ear

√7ᵗʰ **S01.339** Puncture wound without foreign body of unspecified ear

√6ᵗʰ **S01.34** Puncture wound with foreign body of ear

√7ᵗʰ **S01.341** Puncture wound with foreign body of right ear

√7ᵗʰ **S01.342** Puncture wound with foreign body of left ear

√7ᵗʰ **S01.349** Puncture wound with foreign body of unspecified ear

√6ᵗʰ **S01.35** Open bite of ear

Bite of ear NOS

EXCLUDES 1   superficial bite of ear (S00.46, S00.47)

√7ᵗʰ **S01.351** Open bite of right ear

√7ᵗʰ **S01.352** Open bite of left ear

√7ᵗʰ **S01.359** Open bite of unspecified ear

√5ᵗʰ **S01.4** Open wound of cheek and temporomandibular area

√6ᵗʰ **S01.40** Unspecified open wound of cheek and temporomandibular area

√7ᵗʰ **S01.401** Unspecified open wound of right cheek and temporomandibular area

√7ᵗʰ **S01.402** Unspecified open wound of left cheek and temporomandibular area

√7ᵗʰ **S01.409** Unspecified open wound of unspecified cheek and temporomandibular area

√6ᵗʰ **S01.41** Laceration without foreign body of cheek and temporomandibular area

√7ᵗʰ **S01.411** Laceration without foreign body of right cheek and temporomandibular area

√7ᵗʰ **S01.412** Laceration without foreign body of left cheek and temporomandibular area

√7ᵗʰ **S01.419** Laceration without foreign body of unspecified cheek and temporomandibular area

√6ᵗʰ **S01.42** Laceration with foreign body of cheek and temporomandibular area

√7ᵗʰ **S01.421** Laceration with foreign body of right cheek and temporomandibular area

√7ᵗʰ **S01.422** Laceration with foreign body of left cheek and temporomandibular area

√7ᵗʰ **S01.429** Laceration with foreign body of unspecified cheek and temporomandibular area

√6ᵗʰ **S01.43** Puncture wound without foreign body of cheek and temporomandibular area

√7ᵗʰ **S01.431** Puncture wound without foreign body of right cheek and temporomandibular area

√7ᵗʰ **S01.432** Puncture wound without foreign body of left cheek and temporomandibular area

√7ᵗʰ **S01.439** Puncture wound without foreign body of unspecified cheek and temporomandibular area

√6ᵗʰ **S01.44** Puncture wound with foreign body of cheek and temporomandibular area

√7ᵗʰ **S01.441** Puncture wound with foreign body of right cheek and temporomandibular area

√7ᵗʰ **S01.442** Puncture wound with foreign body of left cheek and temporomandibular area

√7ᵗʰ **S01.449** Puncture wound with foreign body of unspecified cheek and temporomandibular area

√6ᵗʰ **S01.45** Open bite of cheek and temporomandibular area

Bite of cheek and temporomandibular area NOS

EXCLUDES 2   superficial bite of cheek and temporomandibular area (S00.86, S00.87)

√7ᵗʰ **S01.451** Open bite of right cheek and temporomandibular area

√7ᵗʰ **S01.452** Open bite of left cheek and temporomandibular area

√7ᵗʰ **S01.459** Open bite of unspecified cheek and temporomandibular area

√5ᵗʰ S01.5   Open wound of lip and oral cavity

> *EXCLUDES 2*   tooth dislocation (S03.2)
> tooth fracture (S02.5)

√6ᵗʰ S01.50   Unspecified open wound of lip and oral cavity

> **√7ᵗʰ S01.501**   Unspecified open wound of lip
>
> **√7ᵗʰ S01.502**   Unspecified open wound of oral cavity

√6ᵗʰ S01.51   Laceration of lip and oral cavity without foreign body

> **√7ᵗʰ S01.511**   Laceration without foreign body of lip
>
> **√7ᵗʰ S01.512**   Laceration without foreign body of oral cavity

√6ᵗʰ S01.52   Laceration of lip and oral cavity with foreign body

> **√7ᵗʰ S01.521**   Laceration with foreign body of lip
>
> **√7ᵗʰ S01.522**   Laceration with foreign body of oral cavity

√6ᵗʰ S01.53   Puncture wound of lip and oral cavity without foreign body

> **√7ᵗʰ S01.531**   Puncture wound without foreign body of lip
>
> **√7ᵗʰ S01.532**   Puncture wound without foreign body of oral cavity

√6ᵗʰ S01.54   Puncture wound of lip and oral cavity with foreign body

> **√7ᵗʰ S01.541**   Puncture wound with foreign body of lip
>
> **√7ᵗʰ S01.542**   Puncture wound with foreign body of oral cavity

√6ᵗʰ S01.55   Open bite of lip and oral cavity

> **√7ᵗʰ S01.551**   Open bite of lip
>
> Bite of lip NOS
> *EXCLUDES 1*   superficial bite of lip (S00.571)
>
> **√7ᵗʰ S01.552**   Open bite of oral cavity
>
> Bite of oral cavity NOS
> *EXCLUDES 1*   superficial bite of oral cavity (S00.572)

√5ᵗʰ S01.8   Open wound of other parts of head

> **√x7ᵗʰ S01.80**   Unspecified open wound of other part of head
>
> **√x7ᵗʰ S01.81**   Laceration without foreign body of other part of head
>
> **√x7ᵗʰ S01.82**   Laceration with foreign body of other part of head
>
> **√x7ᵗʰ S01.83**   Puncture wound without foreign body of other part of head
>
> **√x7ᵗʰ S01.84**   Puncture wound with foreign body of other part of head
>
> **√x7ᵗʰ S01.85**   Open bite of other part of head
>
> Bite of other part of head NOS
> *EXCLUDES 1*   superficial bite of other part of head (S00.87)

√5ᵗʰ S01.9   Open wound of unspecified part of head

> **√x7ᵗʰ S01.90**   Unspecified open wound of unspecified part of head
>
> **√x7ᵗʰ S01.91**   Laceration without foreign body of unspecified part of head
>
> **√x7ᵗʰ S01.92**   Laceration with foreign body of unspecified part of head
>
> **√x7ᵗʰ S01.93**   Puncture wound without foreign body of unspecified part of head
>
> **√x7ᵗʰ S01.94**   Puncture wound with foreign body of unspecified part of head
>
> **√x7ᵗʰ S01.95**   Open bite of unspecified part of head
>
> Bite of head NOS
> *EXCLUDES 1*   superficial bite of head NOS (S00.97)

√4ᵗʰ S02   Fracture of skull and facial bones

> **NOTE**   A fracture not indicated as open or closed should be coded to closed.

Code also any associated intracranial injury (S06.-)
AHA: 2021,1Q,6; 2017,1Q,42; 2016,4Q,66-67

> The appropriate 7th character is to be added to each code from category S02.
> A   initial encounter for closed fracture
> B   initial encounter for open fracture
> D   subsequent encounter for fracture with routine healing
> G   subsequent encounter for fracture with delayed healing
> K   subsequent encounter for fracture with nonunion
> S   sequela

² **√x7ᵗʰ S02.0**   Fracture of vault of skull   HCC ESR

> Fracture of frontal bone
> Fracture of parietal bone

√5ᵗʰ S02.1   Fracture of base of skull

> *EXCLUDES 2*   lateral orbital wall (S02.84-)
> medial orbital wall (S02.83-)
> orbital floor (S02.3-)
>
> **AHA:** 2019,4Q,16-17

√6ᵗʰ S02.10   Unspecified fracture of base of skull

> ² **√7ᵗʰ S02.101**   Fracture of base of skull, right side   HCC ESR
>
> ² **√7ᵗʰ S02.102**   Fracture of base of skull, left side   HCC ESR
>
> ² **√7ᵗʰ S02.109**   Fracture of base of skull, unspecified side   HCC ESR

√6ᵗʰ S02.11   Fracture of occiput

> ² **√7ᵗʰ S02.110**   Type I occipital condyle fracture, unspecified side   HCC ESR
>
> ² **√7ᵗʰ S02.111**   Type II occipital condyle fracture, unspecified side   HCC ESR
>
> ² **√7ᵗʰ S02.112**   Type III occipital condyle fracture, unspecified side   HCC ESR
>
> ² **√7ᵗʰ S02.113**   Unspecified occipital condyle fracture   HCC ESR
>
> ² **√7ᵗʰ S02.118**   Other fracture of occiput, unspecified side   HCC ESR
>
> ² **√7ᵗʰ S02.119**   Unspecified fracture of occiput   HCC ESR
>
> ² **√7ᵗʰ S02.11A**   Type I occipital condyle fracture, right side   HCC ESR
>
> ² **√7ᵗʰ S02.11B**   Type I occipital condyle fracture, left side   HCC ESR
>
> ² **√7ᵗʰ S02.11C**   Type II occipital condyle fracture, right side   HCC ESR
>
> ² **√7ᵗʰ S02.11D**   Type II occipital condyle fracture, left side   HCC ESR
>
> ² **√7ᵗʰ S02.11E**   Type III occipital condyle fracture, right side   HCC ESR
>
> ² **√7ᵗʰ S02.11F**   Type III occipital condyle fracture, left side   HCC ESR
>
> ² **√7ᵗʰ S02.11G**   Other fracture of occiput, right side   HCC ESR
>
> ² **√7ᵗʰ S02.11H**   Other fracture of occiput, left side   HCC ESR

√6ᵗʰ S02.12   Fracture of orbital roof

> **AHA:** 2019,4Q,16-17
>
> ² **√7ᵗʰ S02.121**   Fracture of orbital roof, right side   HCC ESR
>
> ² **√7ᵗʰ S02.122**   Fracture of orbital roof, left side   HCC ESR
>
> ² **√7ᵗʰ S02.129**   Fracture of orbital roof, unspecified side   HCC ESR

² **√x7ᵗʰ S02.19**   Other fracture of base of skull   HCC ESR

> Fracture of anterior fossa of base of skull
> Fracture of ethmoid sinus
> Fracture of frontal sinus
> Fracture of middle fossa of base of skull
> Fracture of posterior fossa of base of skull
> Fracture of sphenoid
> Fracture of temporal bone

√x7ᵗʰ S02.2   Fracture of nasal bones

Chapter 19. Injury, Poisoning and Certain Other Consequences of External Causes

S02.3–S02.849

√5th **S02.3** **Fracture of orbital floor**
Fracture of inferior orbital wall
EXCLUDES 1   orbit NOS (S02.85)
EXCLUDES 2   lateral orbital wall (S02.84-)
             medial orbital wall (S02.83-)
             orbital roof (S02.1-)

   2 √x7th **S02.30** **Fracture of orbital floor, unspecified side** HCC ESR
   2 √x7th **S02.31** **Fracture of orbital floor, right side** HCC ESR
   2 √x7th **S02.32** **Fracture of orbital floor, left side** HCC ESR

√5th **S02.4** **Fracture of malar, maxillary and zygoma bones**
Fracture of superior maxilla
Fracture of upper jaw (bone)
Fracture of zygomatic process of temporal bone

   √6th **S02.40** **Fracture of malar, maxillary and zygoma bones, unspecified**
     2 √7th **S02.400** **Malar fracture, unspecified side** HCC ESR
     2 √7th **S02.401** **Maxillary fracture, unspecified side** HCC ESR
     2 √7th **S02.402** **Zygomatic fracture, unspecified side** HCC ESR
     2 √7th **S02.40A** **Malar fracture, right side** HCC ESR
     2 √7th **S02.40B** **Malar fracture, left side** HCC ESR
     2 √7th **S02.40C** **Maxillary fracture, right side** HCC ESR
     2 √7th **S02.40D** **Maxillary fracture, left side** HCC ESR
     2 √7th **S02.40E** **Zygomatic fracture, right side** HCC ESR
     2 √7th **S02.40F** **Zygomatic fracture, left side** HCC ESR

   √6th **S02.41** **LeFort fracture**
DEF: Named for Rene Le Fort, these fractures describe different combinations of multiple fractures that occur from significant force to the midface. A common denominator in all three types of LeFort fractures is fracture of the pterygoid processes, which are two bony plates resembling wings that extend downward from the sphenoid bone.

LeFort Fracture Types

Frontal bone
Type III
Nasal bone
Orbital floor
Type II
Type I
Maxilla
Zygomatic bone (malar) and arch

     2 √7th **S02.411** **LeFort I fracture** HCC ESR
     2 √7th **S02.412** **LeFort II fracture** HCC ESR
     2 √7th **S02.413** **LeFort III fracture** HCC ESR
   2 √x7th **S02.42** **Fracture of alveolus of maxilla** HCC ESR

√x7th **S02.5** **Fracture of tooth (traumatic)**
Broken tooth
EXCLUDES 1   cracked tooth (nontraumatic) (K03.81)

√5th **S02.6** **Fracture of mandible**
Fracture of lower jaw (bone)
   √6th **S02.60** **Fracture of mandible, unspecified**
     2 √7th **S02.600** **Fracture of unspecified part of body of mandible, unspecified side** HCC ESR
     2 √7th **S02.601** **Fracture of unspecified part of body of right mandible** HCC ESR
     2 √7th **S02.602** **Fracture of unspecified part of body of left mandible** HCC ESR

   2 √7th **S02.609** **Fracture of mandible, unspecified** HCC ESR

   √6th **S02.61** **Fracture of condylar process of mandible**
     2 √7th **S02.610** **Fracture of condylar process of mandible, unspecified side** HCC ESR
     2 √7th **S02.611** **Fracture of condylar process of right mandible** HCC ESR
     2 √7th **S02.612** **Fracture of condylar process of left mandible** HCC ESR

   √6th **S02.62** **Fracture of subcondylar process of mandible**
     2 √7th **S02.620** **Fracture of subcondylar process of mandible, unspecified side** HCC ESR
     2 √7th **S02.621** **Fracture of subcondylar process of right mandible** HCC ESR
     2 √7th **S02.622** **Fracture of subcondylar process of left mandible** HCC ESR

   √6th **S02.63** **Fracture of coronoid process of mandible**
     2 √7th **S02.630** **Fracture of coronoid process of mandible, unspecified side** HCC ESR
     2 √7th **S02.631** **Fracture of coronoid process of right mandible** HCC ESR
     2 √7th **S02.632** **Fracture of coronoid process of left mandible** HCC ESR

   √6th **S02.64** **Fracture of ramus of mandible**
     2 √7th **S02.640** **Fracture of ramus of mandible, unspecified side** HCC ESR
     2 √7th **S02.641** **Fracture of ramus of right mandible** HCC ESR
     2 √7th **S02.642** **Fracture of ramus of left mandible** HCC ESR

   √6th **S02.65** **Fracture of angle of mandible**
     2 √7th **S02.650** **Fracture of angle of mandible, unspecified side** HCC ESR
     2 √7th **S02.651** **Fracture of angle of right mandible** HCC ESR
     2 √7th **S02.652** **Fracture of angle of left mandible** HCC ESR

   2 √x7th **S02.66** **Fracture of symphysis of mandible** HCC ESR

   √6th **S02.67** **Fracture of alveolus of mandible**
     2 √7th **S02.670** **Fracture of alveolus of mandible, unspecified side** HCC ESR
     2 √7th **S02.671** **Fracture of alveolus of right mandible** HCC ESR
     2 √7th **S02.672** **Fracture of alveolus of left mandible** HCC ESR

   2 √x7th **S02.69** **Fracture of mandible of other specified site** HCC ESR

√5th **S02.8** **Fractures of other specified skull and facial bones**
Fracture of palate
EXCLUDES 2   fracture of orbital floor (S02.3-)
             fracture of orbital roof (S02.12-)

   2 √x7th **S02.80** **Fracture of other specified skull and facial bones, unspecified side** HCC ESR
   2 √x7th **S02.81** **Fracture of other specified skull and facial bones, right side** HCC ESR
   2 √x7th **S02.82** **Fracture of other specified skull and facial bones, left side** HCC ESR

   √6th **S02.83** **Fracture of medial orbital wall**
EXCLUDES 2   orbital floor (S02.3-)
             orbital roof (S02.12-)
AHA: 2019,4Q,16-17
     2 √7th **S02.831** **Fracture of medial orbital wall, right side** HCC ESR
     2 √7th **S02.832** **Fracture of medial orbital wall, left side** HCC ESR
     2 √7th **S02.839** **Fracture of medial orbital wall, unspecified side** HCC ESR

   √6th **S02.84** **Fracture of lateral orbital wall**
EXCLUDES 2   orbital floor (S02.3-)
             orbital roof (S02.12-)
AHA: 2019,4Q,16-17
     2 √7th **S02.841** **Fracture of lateral orbital wall, right side** HCC ESR
     2 √7th **S02.842** **Fracture of lateral orbital wall, left side** HCC ESR
     2 √7th **S02.849** **Fracture of lateral orbital wall, unspecified side** HCC ESR

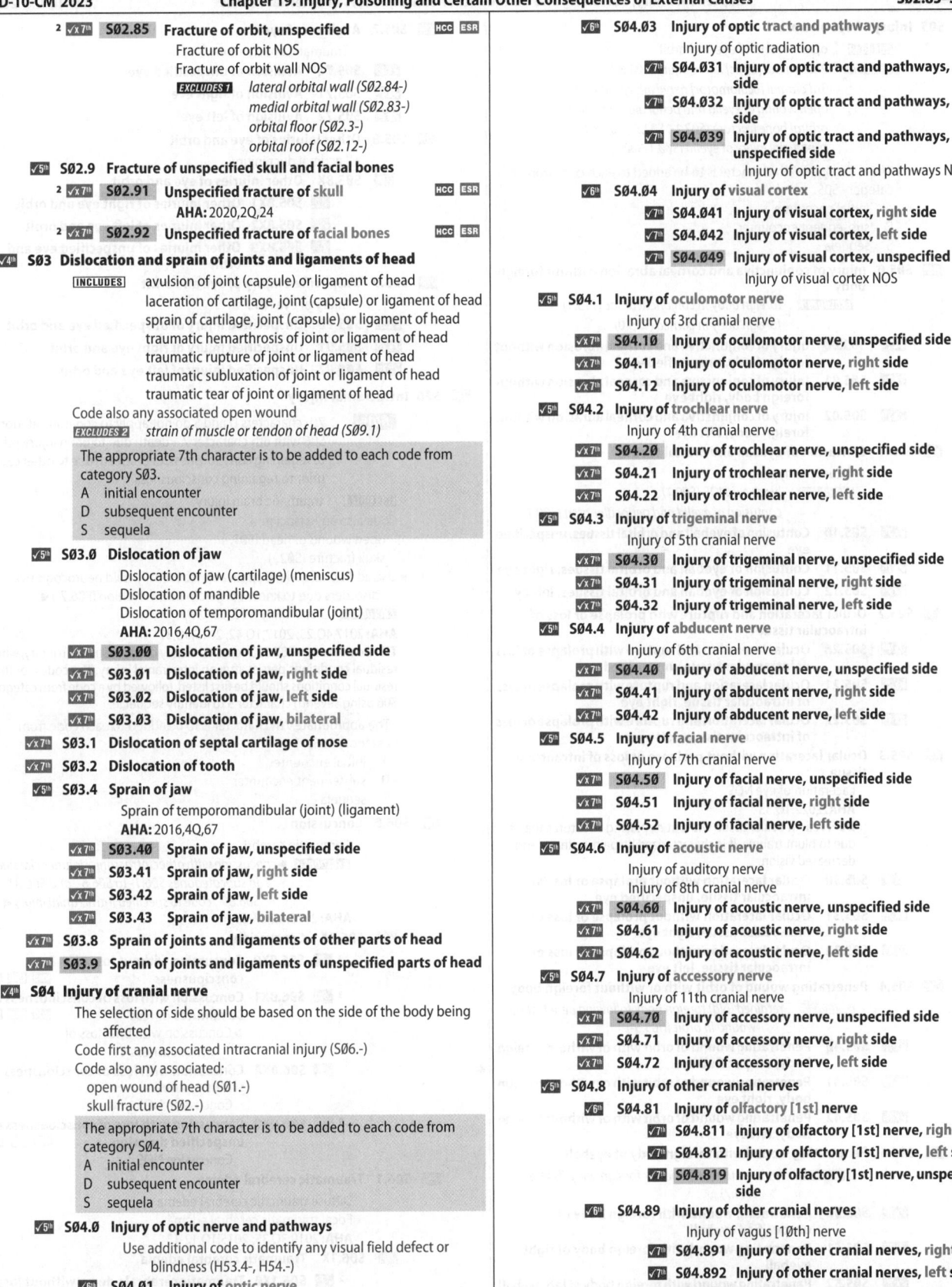

² √x7ᵗʰ **S02.85** **Fracture of orbit, unspecified** `HCC` `ESR`
Fracture of orbit NOS
Fracture of orbit wall NOS
EXCLUDES 1   *lateral orbital wall (S02.84-)*
medial orbital wall (S02.83-)
orbital floor (S02.3-)
orbital roof (S02.12-)

√5ᵗʰ **S02.9** **Fracture of unspecified skull and facial bones**

² √x7ᵗʰ **S02.91** **Unspecified fracture of skull** `HCC` `ESR`
AHA: 2020,2Q,24

² √x7ᵗʰ **S02.92** **Unspecified fracture of facial bones** `HCC` `ESR`

√4ᵗʰ **S03** **Dislocation and sprain of joints and ligaments of head**
INCLUDES   avulsion of joint (capsule) or ligament of head
laceration of cartilage, joint (capsule) or ligament of head
sprain of cartilage, joint (capsule) or ligament of head
traumatic hemarthrosis of joint or ligament of head
traumatic rupture of joint or ligament of head
traumatic subluxation of joint or ligament of head
traumatic tear of joint or ligament of head
Code also any associated open wound
EXCLUDES 2   *strain of muscle or tendon of head (S09.1)*

The appropriate 7th character is to be added to each code from
category S03.
A   initial encounter
D   subsequent encounter
S   sequela

√5ᵗʰ **S03.0** **Dislocation of jaw**
Dislocation of jaw (cartilage) (meniscus)
Dislocation of mandible
Dislocation of temporomandibular (joint)
AHA: 2016,4Q,67

√x7ᵗʰ **S03.00** **Dislocation of jaw, unspecified side**

√x7ᵗʰ **S03.01** **Dislocation of jaw, right side**

√x7ᵗʰ **S03.02** **Dislocation of jaw, left side**

√x7ᵗʰ **S03.03** **Dislocation of jaw, bilateral**

√x7ᵗʰ **S03.1** **Dislocation of septal cartilage of nose**

√x7ᵗʰ **S03.2** **Dislocation of tooth**

√5ᵗʰ **S03.4** **Sprain of jaw**
Sprain of temporomandibular (joint) (ligament)
AHA: 2016,4Q,67

√x7ᵗʰ **S03.40** **Sprain of jaw, unspecified side**

√x7ᵗʰ **S03.41** **Sprain of jaw, right side**

√x7ᵗʰ **S03.42** **Sprain of jaw, left side**

√x7ᵗʰ **S03.43** **Sprain of jaw, bilateral**

√x7ᵗʰ **S03.8** **Sprain of joints and ligaments of other parts of head**

√x7ᵗʰ **S03.9** **Sprain of joints and ligaments of unspecified parts of head**

√4ᵗʰ **S04** **Injury of cranial nerve**
The selection of side should be based on the side of the body being
affected
Code first any associated intracranial injury (S06.-)
Code also any associated:
open wound of head (S01.-)
skull fracture (S02.-)

The appropriate 7th character is to be added to each code from
category S04.
A   initial encounter
D   subsequent encounter
S   sequela

√5ᵗʰ **S04.0** **Injury of optic nerve and pathways**
Use additional code to identify any visual field defect or
blindness (H53.4-, H54.-)

√6ᵗʰ **S04.01** **Injury of optic nerve**
Injury of 2nd cranial nerve

√7ᵗʰ **S04.011** **Injury of optic nerve, right eye**

√7ᵗʰ **S04.012** **Injury of optic nerve, left eye**

√7ᵗʰ **S04.019** **Injury of optic nerve, unspecified eye**
Injury of optic nerve NOS

√x7ᵗʰ **S04.02** **Injury of optic chiasm**

√6ᵗʰ **S04.03** **Injury of optic tract and pathways**
Injury of optic radiation

√7ᵗʰ **S04.031** **Injury of optic tract and pathways, right
side**

√7ᵗʰ **S04.032** **Injury of optic tract and pathways, left
side**

√7ᵗʰ **S04.039** **Injury of optic tract and pathways,
unspecified side**
Injury of optic tract and pathways NOS

√6ᵗʰ **S04.04** **Injury of visual cortex**

√7ᵗʰ **S04.041** **Injury of visual cortex, right side**

√7ᵗʰ **S04.042** **Injury of visual cortex, left side**

√7ᵗʰ **S04.049** **Injury of visual cortex, unspecified side**
Injury of visual cortex NOS

√5ᵗʰ **S04.1** **Injury of oculomotor nerve**
Injury of 3rd cranial nerve

√x7ᵗʰ **S04.10** **Injury of oculomotor nerve, unspecified side**

√x7ᵗʰ **S04.11** **Injury of oculomotor nerve, right side**

√x7ᵗʰ **S04.12** **Injury of oculomotor nerve, left side**

√5ᵗʰ **S04.2** **Injury of trochlear nerve**
Injury of 4th cranial nerve

√x7ᵗʰ **S04.20** **Injury of trochlear nerve, unspecified side**

√x7ᵗʰ **S04.21** **Injury of trochlear nerve, right side**

√x7ᵗʰ **S04.22** **Injury of trochlear nerve, left side**

√5ᵗʰ **S04.3** **Injury of trigeminal nerve**
Injury of 5th cranial nerve

√x7ᵗʰ **S04.30** **Injury of trigeminal nerve, unspecified side**

√x7ᵗʰ **S04.31** **Injury of trigeminal nerve, right side**

√x7ᵗʰ **S04.32** **Injury of trigeminal nerve, left side**

√5ᵗʰ **S04.4** **Injury of abducent nerve**
Injury of 6th cranial nerve

√x7ᵗʰ **S04.40** **Injury of abducent nerve, unspecified side**

√x7ᵗʰ **S04.41** **Injury of abducent nerve, right side**

√x7ᵗʰ **S04.42** **Injury of abducent nerve, left side**

√5ᵗʰ **S04.5** **Injury of facial nerve**
Injury of 7th cranial nerve

√x7ᵗʰ **S04.50** **Injury of facial nerve, unspecified side**

√x7ᵗʰ **S04.51** **Injury of facial nerve, right side**

√x7ᵗʰ **S04.52** **Injury of facial nerve, left side**

√5ᵗʰ **S04.6** **Injury of acoustic nerve**
Injury of auditory nerve
Injury of 8th cranial nerve

√x7ᵗʰ **S04.60** **Injury of acoustic nerve, unspecified side**

√x7ᵗʰ **S04.61** **Injury of acoustic nerve, right side**

√x7ᵗʰ **S04.62** **Injury of acoustic nerve, left side**

√5ᵗʰ **S04.7** **Injury of accessory nerve**
Injury of 11th cranial nerve

√x7ᵗʰ **S04.70** **Injury of accessory nerve, unspecified side**

√x7ᵗʰ **S04.71** **Injury of accessory nerve, right side**

√x7ᵗʰ **S04.72** **Injury of accessory nerve, left side**

√5ᵗʰ **S04.8** **Injury of other cranial nerves**

√6ᵗʰ **S04.81** **Injury of olfactory [1st] nerve**

√7ᵗʰ **S04.811** **Injury of olfactory [1st] nerve, right side**

√7ᵗʰ **S04.812** **Injury of olfactory [1st] nerve, left side**

√7ᵗʰ **S04.819** **Injury of olfactory [1st] nerve, unspecified
side**

√6ᵗʰ **S04.89** **Injury of other cranial nerves**
Injury of vagus [10th] nerve

√7ᵗʰ **S04.891** **Injury of other cranial nerves, right side**

√7ᵗʰ **S04.892** **Injury of other cranial nerves, left side**

√7ᵗʰ **S04.899** **Injury of other cranial nerves, unspecified
side**

√x7ᵗʰ **S04.9** **Injury of unspecified cranial nerve**

☑ Additional Character Required   √x7ᵗʰ Placeholder Alert   Manifestation   Unspecified Dx   Q QPP   UPD Unacceptable PDx

✓4ᵗʰ S05 Injury of eye and orbit

INCLUDES   open wound of eye and orbit

EXCLUDES 2   *2nd cranial [optic] nerve injury (S04.0-)*
3rd cranial [oculomotor] nerve injury (S04.1-)
open wound of eyelid and periocular area (S01.1-)
orbital bone fracture (S02.1-, S02.3-, S02.8-)
superficial injury of eyelid (S00.1-S00.2)

The appropriate 7th character is to be added to each code from category S05.
A   initial encounter
D   subsequent encounter
S   sequela

✓5ᵗʰ S05.0 Injury of conjunctiva and corneal abrasion without foreign body

EXCLUDES 1   *foreign body in conjunctival sac (T15.1)*
foreign body in cornea (T15.0)

✓x7ᵗʰ **S05.00**   Injury of conjunctiva and corneal abrasion without foreign body, unspecified eye

✓x7ᵗʰ **S05.01**   Injury of conjunctiva and corneal abrasion without foreign body, right eye

✓x7ᵗʰ **S05.02**   Injury of conjunctiva and corneal abrasion without foreign body, left eye

✓5ᵗʰ S05.1 Contusion of eyeball and orbital tissues

Traumatic hyphema

EXCLUDES 2   *black eye NOS (S00.1)*
contusion of eyelid and periocular area (S00.1)

✓x7ᵗʰ **S05.10**   Contusion of eyeball and orbital tissues, unspecified eye

✓x7ᵗʰ **S05.11**   Contusion of eyeball and orbital tissues, right eye

✓x7ᵗʰ **S05.12**   Contusion of eyeball and orbital tissues, left eye

✓5ᵗʰ S05.2 Ocular laceration and rupture with prolapse or loss of intraocular tissue

✓x7ᵗʰ **S05.20**   Ocular laceration and rupture with prolapse or loss of intraocular tissue, unspecified eye

✓x7ᵗʰ **S05.21**   Ocular laceration and rupture with prolapse or loss of intraocular tissue, right eye

✓x7ᵗʰ **S05.22**   Ocular laceration and rupture with prolapse or loss of intraocular tissue, left eye

✓5ᵗʰ S05.3 Ocular laceration without prolapse or loss of intraocular tissue

Laceration of eye NOS
AHA: 2022,1Q,33
DEF: Tear in ocular tissue without displacing structures that is due to blunt trauma. It is characterized by pain, redness, and decreased vision.

✓x7ᵗʰ **S05.30**   Ocular laceration without prolapse or loss of intraocular tissue, unspecified eye

✓x7ᵗʰ **S05.31**   Ocular laceration without prolapse or loss of intraocular tissue, right eye

✓x7ᵗʰ **S05.32**   Ocular laceration without prolapse or loss of intraocular tissue, left eye

✓5ᵗʰ S05.4 Penetrating wound of orbit with or without foreign body

EXCLUDES 2   *retained (old) foreign body following penetrating wound in orbit (H05.5-)*

✓x7ᵗʰ **S05.40**   Penetrating wound of orbit with or without foreign body, unspecified eye

✓x7ᵗʰ **S05.41**   Penetrating wound of orbit with or without foreign body, right eye

✓x7ᵗʰ **S05.42**   Penetrating wound of orbit with or without foreign body, left eye

✓5ᵗʰ S05.5 Penetrating wound with foreign body of eyeball

EXCLUDES 2   *retained (old) intraocular foreign body (H44.6-, H44.7)*

✓x7ᵗʰ **S05.50**   Penetrating wound with foreign body of unspecified eyeball

✓x7ᵗʰ **S05.51**   Penetrating wound with foreign body of right eyeball

✓x7ᵗʰ **S05.52**   Penetrating wound with foreign body of left eyeball

✓5ᵗʰ S05.6 Penetrating wound without foreign body of eyeball

Ocular penetration NOS

✓x7ᵗʰ **S05.60**   Penetrating wound without foreign body of unspecified eyeball

✓x7ᵗʰ **S05.61**   Penetrating wound without foreign body of right eyeball

✓x7ᵗʰ **S05.62**   Penetrating wound without foreign body of left eyeball

✓5ᵗʰ S05.7 Avulsion of eye

Traumatic enucleation

✓x7ᵗʰ **S05.70**   Avulsion of unspecified eye

✓x7ᵗʰ **S05.71**   Avulsion of right eye

✓x7ᵗʰ **S05.72**   Avulsion of left eye

✓5ᵗʰ S05.8 Other injuries of eye and orbit

Lacrimal duct injury

✓6ᵗʰ **S05.8X**   Other injuries of eye and orbit

✓7ᵗʰ **S05.8X1**   Other injuries of right eye and orbit

✓7ᵗʰ **S05.8X2**   Other injuries of left eye and orbit

✓7ᵗʰ **S05.8X9**   Other injuries of unspecified eye and orbit

✓5ᵗʰ S05.9 Unspecified injury of eye and orbit

Injury of eye NOS

✓x7ᵗʰ **S05.90**   Unspecified injury of unspecified eye and orbit

✓x7ᵗʰ **S05.91**   Unspecified injury of right eye and orbit

✓x7ᵗʰ **S05.92**   Unspecified injury of left eye and orbit

✓4ᵗʰ S06 Intracranial injury

NOTE   7th characters D and S do not apply to codes in category S06 with 6th character 7 – death due to brain injury prior to regaining consciousness, or 8 – death due to other cause prior to regaining consciousness.

INCLUDES   traumatic brain injury

Code also any associated:
open wound of head (S01.-)
skull fracture (S02.-)

▶Use additional code, if applicable, to identify mild neurocognitive disorders due to known physiological condition (F06.7-)◀

EXCLUDES 1   *head injury NOS (S09.90)*

AHA: 2017,4Q,25; 2017,1Q,42; 2015,3Q,37

TIP: Do not assign Z87.820 Personal history of traumatic brain injury, when residual conditions persist after an intracranial injury. The codes for the residual conditions should be first listed, followed by a code from category S06 using seventh character S to identify sequelae.

The appropriate 7th character is to be added to each code from category S06.
A   initial encounter
D   subsequent encounter
S   sequela

✓5ᵗʰ S06.0 Concussion

Commotio cerebri

EXCLUDES 1   ▶*concussion with other intracranial injuries classified in subcategories S06.1- to S06.6-, and S06.81- to S06.89-, code to specified intracranial injury*◀

AHA: 2016,4Q,67-68

✓6ᵗʰ **S06.0X**   Concussion

³ ✓7ᵗʰ **S06.0X0**   Concussion without loss of consciousness   HCC ESR Q

³ ✓7ᵗʰ **S06.0X1**   Concussion with loss of consciousness of 30 minutes or less   HCC ESR Q
▶Concussion with brief loss of consciousness◀

✓7ᵗʰ **S06.0XA**   Concussion with loss of consciousness status unknown
Concussion NOS

³ ✓7ᵗʰ **S06.0X9**   Concussion with loss of consciousness of unspecified duration   HCC ESR Q
~~Concussion NOS~~

✓5ᵗʰ S06.1 Traumatic cerebral edema

Diffuse traumatic cerebral edema
Focal traumatic cerebral edema
AHA: 2019,3Q,35; 2015,1Q,12-13

✓6ᵗʰ **S06.1X**   Traumatic cerebral edema

² ✓7ᵗʰ **S06.1X0**   Traumatic cerebral edema without loss of consciousness   HCC ESR Q

² ✓7ᵗʰ **S06.1X1**   Traumatic cerebral edema with loss of consciousness of 30 minutes or less   HCC ESR Q
▶Traumatic cerebral edema with brief loss of consciousness◀

² ✓7ᵗʰ **S06.1X2**   Traumatic cerebral edema with loss of consciousness of 31 minutes to 59 minutes   HCC ESR Q

² √7ᵗʰ **S06.1X3**   **Traumatic cerebral edema with loss of consciousness of** 1 hour to 5 hours 59 minutes   HCC ESR COM Q

² √7ᵗʰ **S06.1X4**   **Traumatic cerebral edema with loss of consciousness of** 6 hours to 24 hours   HCC ESR COM Q

² √7ᵗʰ **S06.1X5**   **Traumatic cerebral edema with loss of consciousness** greater than 24 hours with return to pre-existing conscious level   HCC ESR COM

² √7ᵗʰ **S06.1X6**   **Traumatic cerebral edema with loss of consciousness** greater than 24 hours without return to pre-existing conscious level with patient surviving   HCC ESR COM

√7ᵗʰ **S06.1X7**   **Traumatic cerebral edema with loss of consciousness of** any duration with death due to brain injury prior to regaining consciousness

√7ᵗʰ **S06.1X8**   **Traumatic cerebral edema with loss of consciousness of** any duration with death due to **other** cause prior to regaining consciousness

√7ᵗʰ **S06.1XA**   **Traumatic cerebral edema with loss of consciousness** status unknown
Traumatic cerebral edema NOS

² √7ᵗʰ **S06.1X9**   **Traumatic cerebral edema with loss of consciousness of unspecified duration**   HCC ESR Q
~~Traumatic cerebral edema NOS~~

√5ᵗʰ **S06.2**   **Diffuse traumatic brain injury**
Diffuse axonal brain injury
Use additional code, if applicable, for traumatic brain compression or herniation (S06.A-)
EXCLUDES 1   *traumatic diffuse cerebral edema (S06.1X-)*
AHA: 2020,3Q,46

√6ᵗʰ **S06.2X**   **Diffuse traumatic brain injury**

² √7ᵗʰ **S06.2X0**   **Diffuse traumatic brain injury** without loss of consciousness   HCC ESR Q

² √7ᵗʰ **S06.2X1**   **Diffuse traumatic brain injury with loss of consciousness of** 30 minutes or less   HCC ESR Q
▶Diffuse traumatic brain injury with brief loss of consciousness◀

² √7ᵗʰ **S06.2X2**   **Diffuse traumatic brain injury with loss of consciousness of** 31 minutes to 59 minutes   HCC ESR Q

² √7ᵗʰ **S06.2X3**   **Diffuse traumatic brain injury with loss of consciousness of** 1 hour to 5 hours 59 minutes   HCC ESR Q

² √7ᵗʰ **S06.2X4**   **Diffuse traumatic brain injury with loss of consciousness of** 6 hours to 24 hours   HCC ESR COM Q

² √7ᵗʰ **S06.2X5**   **Diffuse traumatic brain injury with loss of consciousness** greater than 24 hours with return to pre-existing conscious levels   HCC ESR COM

² √7ᵗʰ **S06.2X6**   **Diffuse traumatic brain injury with loss of consciousness** greater than 24 hours without return to pre-existing conscious level with patient surviving   HCC ESR COM

√7ᵗʰ **S06.2X7**   **Diffuse traumatic brain injury with loss of consciousness of** any duration with death due to brain injury prior to regaining consciousness

√7ᵗʰ **S06.2X8**   **Diffuse traumatic brain injury with loss of consciousness of** any duration with death due to **other** cause prior to regaining consciousness

√7ᵗʰ **S06.2XA**   **Diffuse traumatic brain injury with loss of consciousness** status unknown
Diffuse traumatic brain injury NOS

² √7ᵗʰ **S06.2X9**   **Diffuse traumatic brain injury with loss of consciousness of unspecified duration**   HCC ESR Q
~~Diffuse traumatic brain injury NOS~~

√5ᵗʰ **S06.3**   **Focal traumatic brain injury**
Use additional code, if applicable, for traumatic brain compression or herniation (S06.A-)
EXCLUDES 1   *any condition classifiable to S06.4-S06.6*
EXCLUDES 2   *focal cerebral edema (S06.1)*
AHA: 2020,3Q,46; 2019,3Q,35; 2015,1Q,12-13

√6ᵗʰ **S06.30**   **Unspecified focal traumatic brain injury**

² √7ᵗʰ **S06.300**   **Unspecified focal traumatic brain injury** without loss of consciousness   HCC ESR Q

² √7ᵗʰ **S06.301**   **Unspecified focal traumatic brain injury with loss of consciousness of** 30 minutes or less   HCC ESR Q
▶Unspecified focal traumatic brain injury with brief loss of consciousness◀

² √7ᵗʰ **S06.302**   **Unspecified focal traumatic brain injury with loss of consciousness of** 31 minutes to 59 minutes   HCC ESR Q

² √7ᵗʰ **S06.303**   **Unspecified focal traumatic brain injury with loss of consciousness of** 1 hour to 5 hours 59 minutes   HCC ESR COM Q

² √7ᵗʰ **S06.304**   **Unspecified focal traumatic brain injury with loss of consciousness of** 6 hours to 24 hours   HCC ESR COM Q

² √7ᵗʰ **S06.305**   **Unspecified focal traumatic brain injury with loss of consciousness** greater than 24 hours with return to pre-existing conscious level   HCC ESR COM

² √7ᵗʰ **S06.306**   **Unspecified focal traumatic brain injury with loss of consciousness** greater than 24 hours without return to pre-existing conscious level with patient surviving   HCC ESR COM

√7ᵗʰ **S06.307**   **Unspecified focal traumatic brain injury with loss of consciousness of** any duration with death due to brain injury prior to regaining consciousness

√7ᵗʰ **S06.308**   **Unspecified focal traumatic brain injury with loss of consciousness of** any duration with death due to **other** cause prior to regaining consciousness

√7ᵗʰ **S06.30A**   **Unspecified focal traumatic brain injury with loss of consciousness** status unknown
Unspecified focal traumatic brain injury NOS

² √7ᵗʰ **S06.309**   **Unspecified focal traumatic brain injury with loss of consciousness of unspecified duration**   HCC ESR Q
~~Unspecified focal traumatic brain injury NOS~~

√6ᵗʰ **S06.31**   **Contusion and laceration of right cerebrum**

² √7ᵗʰ **S06.310**   **Contusion and laceration of right cerebrum** without loss of consciousness   HCC ESR

² √7ᵗʰ **S06.311**   **Contusion and laceration of right cerebrum with loss of consciousness of** 30 minutes or less   HCC ESR
▶Contusion and laceration of right cerebrum with brief loss of consciousness◀

² √7ᵗʰ **S06.312**   **Contusion and laceration of right cerebrum with loss of consciousness of** 31 minutes to 59 minutes   HCC ESR

² √7ᵗʰ **S06.313**   **Contusion and laceration of right cerebrum with loss of consciousness of** 1 hour to 5 hours 59 minutes   HCC ESR COM

² √7ᵗʰ **S06.314**   **Contusion and laceration of right cerebrum with loss of consciousness of** 6 hours to 24 hours   HCC ESR COM

² √7ᵗʰ **S06.315**   **Contusion and laceration of right cerebrum with loss of consciousness** greater than 24 hours with return to pre-existing conscious level   HCC ESR COM

² √7ᵗʰ **S06.316**   **Contusion and laceration of right cerebrum with loss of consciousness** greater than 24 hours without return to pre-existing conscious level with patient surviving   HCC ESR COM

Chapter 19. Injury, Poisoning and Certain Other Consequences of External Causes

S06.317–S06.350

√7ᵗʰ **S06.317 Contusion and laceration of right cerebrum with loss of consciousness of any duration with death due to brain injury prior to regaining consciousness**

√7ᵗʰ **S06.318 Contusion and laceration of right cerebrum with loss of consciousness of any duration with death due to other cause prior to regaining consciousness**

√7ᵗʰ **S06.31A Contusion and laceration of right cerebrum with loss of consciousness status unknown**

    Contusion and laceration of right cerebrum NOS

2 √7ᵗʰ **S06.319 Contusion and laceration of right cerebrum with loss of consciousness of unspecified duration** HCC ESR

    ~~Contusion and laceration of right cerebrum NOS~~

√6ᵗʰ **S06.32 Contusion and laceration of left cerebrum**

2 √7ᵗʰ **S06.320 Contusion and laceration of left cerebrum without loss of consciousness** HCC ESR

2 √7ᵗʰ **S06.321 Contusion and laceration of left cerebrum with loss of consciousness of 30 minutes or less**

    ►Contusion and laceration of left cerebrum with brief loss of consciousness◄

2 √7ᵗʰ **S06.322 Contusion and laceration of left cerebrum with loss of consciousness of 31 minutes to 59 minutes** HCC ESR

2 √7ᵗʰ **S06.323 Contusion and laceration of left cerebrum with loss of consciousness of 1 hour to 5 hours 59 minutes** HCC ESR COM

2 √7ᵗʰ **S06.324 Contusion and laceration of left cerebrum with loss of consciousness of 6 hours to 24 hours** HCC ESR COM

2 √7ᵗʰ **S06.325 Contusion and laceration of left cerebrum with loss of consciousness greater than 24 hours with return to pre-existing conscious level** HCC ESR COM

2 √7ᵗʰ **S06.326 Contusion and laceration of left cerebrum with loss of consciousness greater than 24 hours without return to pre-existing conscious level with patient surviving** HCC ESR COM

√7ᵗʰ **S06.327 Contusion and laceration of left cerebrum with loss of consciousness of any duration with death due to brain injury prior to regaining consciousness**

√7ᵗʰ **S06.328 Contusion and laceration of left cerebrum with loss of consciousness of any duration with death due to other cause prior to regaining consciousness**

√7ᵗʰ **S06.32A Contusion and laceration of left cerebrum with loss of consciousness status unknown**

    Contusion and laceration of left cerebrum NOS

2 √7ᵗʰ **S06.329 Contusion and laceration of left cerebrum with loss of consciousness of unspecified duration** HCC ESR

    ~~Contusion and laceration of left cerebrum NOS~~

√6ᵗʰ **S06.33 Contusion and laceration of cerebrum, unspecified**

2 √7ᵗʰ **S06.330 Contusion and laceration of cerebrum, unspecified, without loss of consciousness** HCC ESR

2 √7ᵗʰ **S06.331 Contusion and laceration of cerebrum, unspecified, with loss of consciousness of 30 minutes or less** HCC ESR

    ►Contusion and laceration of cerebrum, unspecified, with brief loss of consciousness◄

2 √7ᵗʰ **S06.332 Contusion and laceration of cerebrum, unspecified, with loss of consciousness of 31 minutes to 59 minutes** HCC ESR

2 √7ᵗʰ **S06.333 Contusion and laceration of cerebrum, unspecified, with loss of consciousness of 1 hour to 5 hours 59 minutes** HCC ESR COM

2 √7ᵗʰ **S06.334 Contusion and laceration of cerebrum, unspecified, with loss of consciousness of 6 hours to 24 hours** HCC ESR COM

2 √7ᵗʰ **S06.335 Contusion and laceration of cerebrum, unspecified, with loss of consciousness greater than 24 hours with return to pre-existing conscious level** HCC ESR COM

2 √7ᵗʰ **S06.336 Contusion and laceration of cerebrum, unspecified, with loss of consciousness greater than 24 hours without return to pre-existing conscious level with patient surviving** HCC ESR COM

√7ᵗʰ **S06.337 Contusion and laceration of cerebrum, unspecified, with loss of consciousness of any duration with death due to brain injury prior to regaining consciousness**

√7ᵗʰ **S06.338 Contusion and laceration of cerebrum, unspecified, with loss of consciousness of any duration with death due to other cause prior to regaining consciousness**

√7ᵗʰ **S06.33A Contusion and laceration of cerebrum, unspecified, with loss of consciousness status unknown**

    Contusion and laceration of cerebrum NOS

2 √7ᵗʰ **S06.339 Contusion and laceration of cerebrum, unspecified, with loss of consciousness of unspecified duration** HCC ESR

    ~~Contusion and laceration of cerebrum NOS~~

√6ᵗʰ **S06.34 Traumatic hemorrhage of right cerebrum**

    Traumatic intracerebral hemorrhage and hematoma of right cerebrum

2 √7ᵗʰ **S06.340 Traumatic hemorrhage of right cerebrum without loss of consciousness** HCC ESR Q

2 √7ᵗʰ **S06.341 Traumatic hemorrhage of right cerebrum with loss of consciousness of 30 minutes or less** HCC ESR Q

    ►Traumatic hemorrhage of right cerebrum with loss of consciousness◄

2 √7ᵗʰ **S06.342 Traumatic hemorrhage of right cerebrum with loss of consciousness of 31 minutes to 59 minutes** HCC ESR Q

2 √7ᵗʰ **S06.343 Traumatic hemorrhage of right cerebrum with loss of consciousness of 1 hours to 5 hours 59 minutes** HCC ESR COM Q

2 √7ᵗʰ **S06.344 Traumatic hemorrhage of right cerebrum with loss of consciousness of 6 hours to 24 hours** HCC ESR COM Q

2 √7ᵗʰ **S06.345 Traumatic hemorrhage of right cerebrum with loss of consciousness greater than 24 hours with return to pre-existing conscious level** HCC ESR COM

2 √7ᵗʰ **S06.346 Traumatic hemorrhage of right cerebrum with loss of consciousness greater than 24 hours without return to pre-existing conscious level with patient surviving** HCC ESR COM

√7ᵗʰ **S06.347 Traumatic hemorrhage of right cerebrum with loss of consciousness of any duration with death due to brain injury prior to regaining consciousness**

√7ᵗʰ **S06.348 Traumatic hemorrhage of right cerebrum with loss of consciousness of any duration with death due to other cause prior to regaining consciousness**

√7ᵗʰ **S06.34A Traumatic hemorrhage of right cerebrum with loss of consciousness status unknown**

    Traumatic hemorrhage of right cerebrum NOS

2 √7ᵗʰ **S06.349 Traumatic hemorrhage of right cerebrum with loss of consciousness of unspecified duration** HCC ESR Q

    ~~Traumatic hemorrhage of right cerebrum NOS~~

√6ᵗʰ **S06.35 Traumatic hemorrhage of left cerebrum**

    Traumatic intracerebral hemorrhage and hematoma of left cerebrum

2 √7ᵗʰ **S06.350 Traumatic hemorrhage of left cerebrum without loss of consciousness** HCC ESR Q

² √7ᵗʰ **S06.351 Traumatic hemorrhage of left cerebrum with loss of consciousness of** 30 minutes or less   HCC ESR Q
▶Traumatic hemorrhage of left cerebrum with brief loss of consciousness◀

² √7ᵗʰ **S06.352 Traumatic hemorrhage of left cerebrum with loss of consciousness of** 31 minutes to 59 minutes   HCC ESR Q

² √7ᵗʰ **S06.353 Traumatic hemorrhage of left cerebrum with loss of consciousness of** 1 hours to 5 hours 59 minutes   HCC ESR COM Q

² √7ᵗʰ **S06.354 Traumatic hemorrhage of left cerebrum with loss of consciousness of** 6 hours to 24 hours   HCC ESR COM Q

² √7ᵗʰ **S06.355 Traumatic hemorrhage of left cerebrum with loss of consciousness** greater than 24 hours with return to pre-existing conscious level   HCC ESR COM

² √7ᵗʰ **S06.356 Traumatic hemorrhage of left cerebrum with loss of consciousness** greater than 24 hours without return to pre-existing conscious level with patient surviving   HCC ESR COM

√7ᵗʰ **S06.357 Traumatic hemorrhage of left cerebrum with loss of consciousness of** any duration with death due to brain injury prior to regaining consciousness

√7ᵗʰ **S06.358 Traumatic hemorrhage of left cerebrum with loss of consciousness of** any duration with death due to **other** cause prior to regaining consciousness

● √7ᵗʰ **S06.35A Traumatic hemorrhage of left cerebrum with loss of consciousness** status unknown
Traumatic hemorrhage of left cerebrum NOS

² √7ᵗʰ **S06.359 Traumatic hemorrhage of left cerebrum with loss of consciousness of unspecified duration**   HCC ESR Q
~~Traumatic hemorrhage of left cerebrum NOS~~

√6ᵗʰ **S06.36 Traumatic hemorrhage of cerebrum, unspecified**
Traumatic intracerebral hemorrhage and hematoma, unspecified

² √7ᵗʰ **S06.360 Traumatic hemorrhage of cerebrum, unspecified,** without loss of consciousness   HCC ESR Q

² √7ᵗʰ **S06.361 Traumatic hemorrhage of cerebrum, unspecified, with loss of consciousness of** 30 minutes or less   HCC ESR Q
▶Traumatic hemorrhage of cerebrum, unspecified, with brief loss of consciousness◀

² √7ᵗʰ **S06.362 Traumatic hemorrhage of cerebrum, unspecified, with loss of consciousness of** 31 minutes to 59 minutes   HCC ESR Q

² √7ᵗʰ **S06.363 Traumatic hemorrhage of cerebrum, unspecified, with loss of consciousness of** 1 hours to 5 hours 59 minutes   HCC ESR COM Q

² √7ᵗʰ **S06.364 Traumatic hemorrhage of cerebrum, unspecified, with loss of consciousness of** 6 hours to 24 hours   HCC ESR COM Q

² √7ᵗʰ **S06.365 Traumatic hemorrhage of cerebrum, unspecified, with loss of consciousness** greater than 24 hours with return to pre-existing conscious level   HCC ESR COM

² √7ᵗʰ **S06.366 Traumatic hemorrhage of cerebrum, unspecified, with loss of consciousness** greater than 24 hours without return to pre-existing conscious level with patient surviving   HCC ESR COM

√7ᵗʰ **S06.367 Traumatic hemorrhage of cerebrum, unspecified, with loss of consciousness of** any duration with death due to brain injury prior to regaining consciousness

√7ᵗʰ **S06.368 Traumatic hemorrhage of cerebrum, unspecified, with loss of consciousness of** any duration with death due to **other** cause prior to regaining consciousness

● √7ᵗʰ **S06.36A Traumatic hemorrhage of cerebrum, unspecified, with loss of consciousness** status unknown
Traumatic hemorrhage of cerebrum NOS

² √7ᵗʰ **S06.369 Traumatic hemorrhage of cerebrum, unspecified, with loss of consciousness of unspecified duration**   HCC ESR Q
~~Traumatic hemorrhage of cerebrum NOS~~

√6ᵗʰ **S06.37 Contusion, laceration, and hemorrhage of cerebellum**

² √7ᵗʰ **S06.370 Contusion, laceration, and hemorrhage of cerebellum** without loss of consciousness   HCC ESR

² √7ᵗʰ **S06.371 Contusion, laceration, and hemorrhage of cerebellum with loss of consciousness of** 30 minutes or less   HCC ESR
▶Contusion, laceration, and hemorrhage of cerebellum with brief loss of consciousness◀

² √7ᵗʰ **S06.372 Contusion, laceration, and hemorrhage of cerebellum with loss of consciousness of** 31 minutes to 59 minutes   HCC ESR

² √7ᵗʰ **S06.373 Contusion, laceration, and hemorrhage of cerebellum with loss of consciousness of** 1 hour to 5 hours 59 minutes   HCC ESR COM

² √7ᵗʰ **S06.374 Contusion, laceration, and hemorrhage of cerebellum with loss of consciousness of** 6 hours to 24 hours   HCC ESR COM

² √7ᵗʰ **S06.375 Contusion, laceration, and hemorrhage of cerebellum with loss of consciousness** greater than 24 hours with return to pre-existing conscious level   HCC ESR COM

² √7ᵗʰ **S06.376 Contusion, laceration, and hemorrhage of cerebellum with loss of consciousness** greater than 24 hours without return to pre-existing conscious level with patient surviving   HCC ESR COM

√7ᵗʰ **S06.377 Contusion, laceration, and hemorrhage of cerebellum with loss of consciousness of** any duration with death due to brain injury prior to regaining consciousness

√7ᵗʰ **S06.378 Contusion, laceration, and hemorrhage of cerebellum with loss of consciousness of** any duration with death due to **other** cause prior to regaining consciousness

● √7ᵗʰ **S06.37A Contusion, laceration, and hemorrhage of cerebellum with loss of consciousness** status unknown
Contusion, laceration, and hemorrhage of cerebellum NOS

² √7ᵗʰ **S06.379 Contusion, laceration, and hemorrhage of cerebellum with loss of consciousness of unspecified duration**   HCC ESR
~~Contusion, laceration, and hemorrhage of cerebellum NOS~~

√6ᵗʰ **S06.38 Contusion, laceration, and hemorrhage of brainstem**

² √7ᵗʰ **S06.380 Contusion, laceration, and hemorrhage of brainstem** without loss of consciousness   HCC ESR

² √7ᵗʰ **S06.381 Contusion, laceration, and hemorrhage of brainstem with loss of consciousness of** 30 minutes or less   HCC ESR
▶Contusion, laceration, and hemorrhage of brainstem with brief loss of consciousness◀

² √7ᵗʰ **S06.382 Contusion, laceration, and hemorrhage of brainstem with loss of consciousness of** 31 minutes to 59 minutes   HCC ESR

² √7ᵗʰ **S06.383 Contusion, laceration, and hemorrhage of brainstem with loss of consciousness of** 1 hour to 5 hours 59 minutes   HCC ESR COM

² √7ᵗʰ **S06.384 Contusion, laceration, and hemorrhage of brainstem with loss of consciousness of** 6 hours to 24 hours   HCC ESR COM

² √7ᵗʰ **S06.385 Contusion, laceration, and hemorrhage of brainstem with loss of consciousness** greater than 24 hours with return to pre-existing conscious level   HCC ESR COM

2 √7ᵗʰ **S06.386 Contusion, laceration, and hemorrhage of brainstem with loss of consciousness greater than 24 hours without return to pre-existing conscious level with patient surviving** HCC ESR COM

√7ᵗʰ **S06.387 Contusion, laceration, and hemorrhage of brainstem with loss of consciousness of any duration with death due to brain injury prior to regaining consciousness**

√7ᵗʰ **S06.388 Contusion, laceration, and hemorrhage of brainstem with loss of consciousness of any duration with death due to other cause prior to regaining consciousness**

√7ᵗʰ **S06.38A Contusion, laceration, and hemorrhage of brainstem with loss of consciousness status unknown**
Contusion, laceration, and hemorrhage of brainstem NOS

2 √7ᵗʰ **S06.389 Contusion, laceration, and hemorrhage of brainstem with loss of consciousness of unspecified duration** HCC ESR
~~Contusion, laceration, and hemorrhage of brainstem NOS~~

√5ᵗʰ **S06.4 Epidural hemorrhage**
Extradural hemorrhage NOS
Extradural hemorrhage (traumatic)
DEF: Epidural space: Space between the endosteum of the cranium (skull) and the dura mater, the outermost layer of a three-layer membrane that covers the brain.

√6ᵗʰ **S06.4X Epidural hemorrhage**

2 √7ᵗʰ **S06.4X0 Epidural hemorrhage without loss of consciousness** HCC ESR Q

2 √7ᵗʰ **S06.4X1 Epidural hemorrhage with loss of consciousness of 30 minutes or less** HCC ESR Q
▶Epidural hemorrhage with brief loss of consciousness◀

2 √7ᵗʰ **S06.4X2 Epidural hemorrhage with loss of consciousness of 31 minutes to 59 minutes** HCC ESR Q

2 √7ᵗʰ **S06.4X3 Epidural hemorrhage with loss of consciousness of 1 hour to 5 hours 59 minutes** HCC ESR COM Q

2 √7ᵗʰ **S06.4X4 Epidural hemorrhage with loss of consciousness of 6 hours to 24 hours** HCC ESR COM Q

2 √7ᵗʰ **S06.4X5 Epidural hemorrhage with loss of consciousness greater than 24 hours with return to pre-existing conscious level** HCC ESR COM

2 √7ᵗʰ **S06.4X6 Epidural hemorrhage with loss of consciousness greater than 24 hours without return to pre-existing conscious level with patient surviving** HCC ESR COM

√7ᵗʰ **S06.4X7 Epidural hemorrhage with loss of consciousness of any duration with death due to brain injury prior to regaining consciousness**

√7ᵗʰ **S06.4X8 Epidural hemorrhage with loss of consciousness of any duration with death due to other causes prior to regaining consciousness**

√7ᵗʰ **S06.4XA Epidural hemorrhage with loss of consciousness status unknown**
Epidural hemorrhage NOS

2 √7ᵗʰ **S06.4X9 Epidural hemorrhage with loss of consciousness of unspecified duration** HCC ESR Q
~~Epidural hemorrhage NOS~~

√5ᵗʰ **S06.5 Traumatic subdural hemorrhage**
Use additional code, if applicable, for traumatic brain compression or herniation (S06.A-)
AHA: 2021,2Q,5; 2021,1Q,4
DEF: Subdural: Potential space between the dura mater and arachnoid membrane around the brain.

√6ᵗʰ **S06.5X Traumatic subdural hemorrhage**

2 √7ᵗʰ **S06.5X0 Traumatic subdural hemorrhage without loss of consciousness** HCC ESR Q

2 √7ᵗʰ **S06.5X1 Traumatic subdural hemorrhage with loss of consciousness of 30 minutes or less** HCC ESR Q
▶Traumatic subdural hemorrhage with brief loss of consciousness◀

2 √7ᵗʰ **S06.5X2 Traumatic subdural hemorrhage with loss of consciousness of 31 minutes to 59 minutes** HCC ESR Q

2 √7ᵗʰ **S06.5X3 Traumatic subdural hemorrhage with loss of consciousness of 1 hour to 5 hours 59 minutes** HCC ESR COM Q

2 √7ᵗʰ **S06.5X4 Traumatic subdural hemorrhage with loss of consciousness of 6 hours to 24 hours** HCC ESR COM Q

2 √7ᵗʰ **S06.5X5 Traumatic subdural hemorrhage with loss of consciousness greater than 24 hours with return to pre-existing conscious level** HCC ESR COM

2 √7ᵗʰ **S06.5X6 Traumatic subdural hemorrhage with loss of consciousness greater than 24 hours without return to pre-existing conscious level with patient surviving** HCC ESR COM

√7ᵗʰ **S06.5X7 Traumatic subdural hemorrhage with loss of consciousness of any duration with death due to brain injury before regaining consciousness**

√7ᵗʰ **S06.5X8 Traumatic subdural hemorrhage with loss of consciousness of any duration with death due to other cause before regaining consciousness**

√7ᵗʰ **S06.5XA Traumatic subdural hemorrhage with loss of consciousness status unknown**
Traumatic subdural hemorrhage NOS

2 √7ᵗʰ **S06.5X9 Traumatic subdural hemorrhage with loss of consciousness of unspecified duration** HCC ESR Q
~~Traumatic subdural hemorrhage NOS~~

√5ᵗʰ **S06.6 Traumatic subarachnoid hemorrhage**
Use additional code, if applicable, for traumatic brain compression or herniation (S06.A-)
AHA: 2021,2Q,5; 2021,1Q,4
DEF: Subarachnoid: Space located between the arachnoid membrane and the pia mater that contains cerebrospinal fluid.

√6ᵗʰ **S06.6X Traumatic subarachnoid hemorrhage**

2 √7ᵗʰ **S06.6X0 Traumatic subarachnoid hemorrhage without loss of consciousness** HCC ESR Q

2 √7ᵗʰ **S06.6X1 Traumatic subarachnoid hemorrhage with loss of consciousness of 30 minutes or less** HCC ESR Q
▶Traumatic subarachnoid hemorrhage with brief loss of consciousness◀

2 √7ᵗʰ **S06.6X2 Traumatic subarachnoid hemorrhage with loss of consciousness of 31 minutes to 59 minutes** HCC ESR Q

2 √7ᵗʰ **S06.6X3 Traumatic subarachnoid hemorrhage with loss of consciousness of 1 hour to 5 hours 59 minutes** HCC ESR COM Q

2 √7ᵗʰ **S06.6X4 Traumatic subarachnoid hemorrhage with loss of consciousness of 6 hours to 24 hours** HCC ESR COM Q

2 √7ᵗʰ **S06.6X5 Traumatic subarachnoid hemorrhage with loss of consciousness greater than 24 hours with return to pre-existing conscious level** HCC ESR COM

2 √7ᵗʰ **S06.6X6 Traumatic subarachnoid hemorrhage with loss of consciousness greater than 24 hours without return to pre-existing conscious level with patient surviving** HCC ESR COM

√7ᵗʰ **S06.6X7 Traumatic subarachnoid hemorrhage with loss of consciousness of any duration with death due to brain injury prior to regaining consciousness**

√7ᵗʰ **S06.6X8 Traumatic subarachnoid hemorrhage with loss of consciousness of any duration with death due to other cause prior to regaining consciousness**

✓7ᵗʰ S06.6XA Traumatic subarachnoid hemorrhage with loss of consciousness status unknown

　Traumatic subarachnoid hemorrhage NOS

² **✓7ᵗʰ S06.6X9 Traumatic subarachnoid hemorrhage with loss of consciousness of unspecified duration** HCC ESR Q

　~~Traumatic subarachnoid hemorrhage NOS~~

✓5ᵗʰ S06.8 Other specified intracranial injuries

✓6ᵗʰ S06.81 Injury of right internal carotid artery, intracranial **portion, not elsewhere classified**

² **✓7ᵗʰ S06.810 Injury of right internal carotid artery, intracranial portion, not elsewhere classified** without loss of **consciousness** HCC ESR Q

² **✓7ᵗʰ S06.811 Injury of right internal carotid artery, intracranial portion, not elsewhere classified** with loss of consciousness of 30 **minutes or less** HCC ESR Q

　▶Injury of right internal carotid artery, intracranial portion, not elsewhere classified with brief loss of consciousness◀

² **✓7ᵗʰ S06.812 Injury of right internal carotid artery, intracranial portion, not elsewhere classified** with loss of consciousness of 31 **minutes to 59 minutes** HCC ESR Q

² **✓7ᵗʰ S06.813 Injury of right internal carotid artery, intracranial portion, not elsewhere classified** with loss of consciousness of 1 **hour to 5 hours 59 minutes** HCC ESR COM Q

² **✓7ᵗʰ S06.814 Injury of right internal carotid artery, intracranial portion, not elsewhere classified** with loss of consciousness of 6 **hours to 24 hours** HCC ESR COM Q

² **✓7ᵗʰ S06.815 Injury of right internal carotid artery, intracranial portion, not elsewhere classified** with loss of consciousness greater than 24 hours with return to pre-existing conscious **level** HCC ESR COM

² **✓7ᵗʰ S06.816 Injury of right internal carotid artery, intracranial portion, not elsewhere classified** with loss of consciousness greater than 24 hours without return to pre-existing conscious level with patient **surviving** HCC ESR COM

✓7ᵗʰ S06.817 Injury of right internal carotid artery, intracranial portion, not elsewhere classified with loss of consciousness of any duration with death due to brain injury prior to regaining consciousness

✓7ᵗʰ S06.818 Injury of right internal carotid artery, intracranial portion, not elsewhere classified with loss of consciousness of any duration with death due to **other** cause prior to regaining consciousness

✓7ᵗʰ S06.81A Injury of right internal carotid artery, intracranial portion, not elsewhere classified with loss of consciousness status unknown

　Injury of right internal carotid artery, intracranial portion, not elsewhere classified NOS

² **✓7ᵗʰ S06.819 Injury of right internal carotid artery, intracranial portion, not elsewhere classified** with loss of consciousness of unspecified **duration** HCC ESR Q

　~~Injury of right internal carotid artery, intracranial portion, not elsewhere classified NOS~~

✓6ᵗʰ S06.82 Injury of left internal carotid artery, intracranial **portion, not elsewhere classified**

² **✓7ᵗʰ S06.820 Injury of left internal carotid artery, intracranial portion, not elsewhere classified** without loss of **consciousness** HCC ESR Q

² **✓7ᵗʰ S06.821 Injury of left internal carotid artery, intracranial portion, not elsewhere classified** with loss of consciousness of 30 **minutes or less** HCC ESR Q

　▶Injury of left internal carotid artery, intracranial portion, not elsewhere classified with brief loss of consciousness◀

² **✓7ᵗʰ S06.822 Injury of left internal carotid artery, intracranial portion, not elsewhere classified** with loss of consciousness of 31 **minutes to 59 minutes** HCC ESR Q

² **✓7ᵗʰ S06.823 Injury of left internal carotid artery, intracranial portion, not elsewhere classified** with loss of consciousness of 1 **hour to 5 hours 59 minutes** HCC ESR COM Q

² **✓7ᵗʰ S06.824 Injury of left internal carotid artery, intracranial portion, not elsewhere classified** with loss of consciousness of 6 **hours to 24 hours** HCC ESR COM Q

² **✓7ᵗʰ S06.825 Injury of left internal carotid artery, intracranial portion, not elsewhere classified** with loss of consciousness greater than 24 hours with return to pre-existing conscious **level** HCC ESR COM

² **✓7ᵗʰ S06.826 Injury of left internal carotid artery, intracranial portion, not elsewhere classified** with loss of consciousness greater than 24 hours without return to pre-existing conscious level with patient **surviving** HCC ESR COM

✓7ᵗʰ S06.827 Injury of left internal carotid artery, intracranial portion, not elsewhere classified with loss of consciousness of any duration with death due to brain injury prior to regaining consciousness

✓7ᵗʰ S06.828 Injury of left internal carotid artery, intracranial portion, not elsewhere classified with loss of consciousness of any duration with death due to **other** cause prior to regaining consciousness

✓7ᵗʰ S06.82A Injury of left internal carotid artery, intracranial portion, not elsewhere classified with loss of consciousness status unknown

　Injury of left internal carotid artery, intracranial portion, not elsewhere classified NOS

² **✓7ᵗʰ S06.829 Injury of left internal carotid artery, intracranial portion, not elsewhere classified** with loss of consciousness of unspecified **duration** HCC ESR Q

　~~Injury of left internal carotid artery, intracranial portion, not elsewhere classified NOS~~

✓6ᵗʰ S06.8A Primary blast injury of brain, not elsewhere classified

　Code also, if applicable, focal traumatic brain injury (S06.3-)

　EXCLUDES 2 traumatic cerebral edema (S06.1)

✓7ᵗʰ S06.8A0 Primary blast injury of brain, not elsewhere classified without loss of consciousness

✓7ᵗʰ S06.8A1 Primary blast injury of brain, not elsewhere classified with loss of consciousness of 30 minutes or less

　Primary blast injury of brain, not elsewhere classified with brief loss of consciousness

✓7ᵗʰ S06.8A2 Primary blast injury of brain, not elsewhere classified with loss of consciousness of 31 minutes to 59 minutes

✓7ᵗʰ S06.8A3 Primary blast injury of brain, not elsewhere classified with loss of consciousness of 1 hour to 5 hours 59 minutes

✓7ᵗʰ S06.8A4 Primary blast injury of brain, not elsewhere classified with loss of consciousness of 6 hours to 24 hours

- √7ᵗʰ **S06.8A5** **Primary blast injury of brain, not elsewhere classified with loss of consciousness greater than 24 hours with return to pre-existing conscious level**
- √7ᵗʰ **S06.8A6** **Primary blast injury of brain, not elsewhere classified with loss of consciousness greater than 24 hours without return to pre-existing conscious level with patient surviving**
- √7ᵗʰ **S06.8A7** **Primary blast injury of brain, not elsewhere classified with loss of consciousness of any duration with death due to brain injury prior to regaining consciousness**
- √7ᵗʰ **S06.8A8** **Primary blast injury of brain, not elsewhere classified with loss of consciousness of any duration with death due to other cause prior to regaining consciousness**
- √7ᵗʰ **S06.8AA** **Primary blast injury of brain, not elsewhere classified with loss of consciousness status unknown**
    Primary blast injury of brain NOS
- √7ᵗʰ **S06.8A9** **Primary blast injury of brain, not elsewhere classified with loss of consciousness of unspecified duration**

√6ᵗʰ **S06.89** **Other specified intracranial injury**
     EXCLUDES 1 concussion (S06.0X-)

- 2 √7ᵗʰ **S06.890** **Other specified intracranial injury without loss of consciousness** HCC ESR Q
- 2 √7ᵗʰ **S06.891** **Other specified intracranial injury with loss of consciousness of 30 minutes or less** HCC ESR Q
    ▶Other specified intracranial injury with brief loss of consciousness◀
- 2 √7ᵗʰ **S06.892** **Other specified intracranial injury with loss of consciousness of 31 minutes to 59 minutes** HCC ESR Q
- 2 √7ᵗʰ **S06.893** **Other specified intracranial injury with loss of consciousness of 1 hour to 5 hours 59 minutes** HCC ESR COM Q
- 2 √7ᵗʰ **S06.894** **Other specified intracranial injury with loss of consciousness of 6 hours to 24 hours** HCC ESR COM Q
- 2 √7ᵗʰ **S06.895** **Other specified intracranial injury with loss of consciousness greater than 24 hours with return to pre-existing conscious level** HCC ESR COM
- 2 √7ᵗʰ **S06.896** **Other specified intracranial injury with loss of consciousness greater than 24 hours without return to pre-existing conscious level with patient surviving** HCC ESR COM
- √7ᵗʰ **S06.897** **Other specified intracranial injury with loss of consciousness of any duration with death due to brain injury prior to regaining consciousness**
- √7ᵗʰ **S06.898** **Other specified intracranial injury with loss of consciousness of any duration with death due to other cause prior to regaining consciousness**
- √7ᵗʰ **S06.89A** **Other specified intracranial injury with loss of consciousness status unknown**
- 2 √7ᵗʰ **S06.899** **Other specified intracranial injury with loss of consciousness of unspecified duration** HCC ESR

√5ᵗʰ **S06.9** **Unspecified intracranial injury**
     Brain injury NOS
     Head injury NOS with loss of consciousness
     Traumatic brain injury NOS
     EXCLUDES 1 conditions classifiable to S06.0- to S06.8- code to specified intracranial injury
         head injury NOS (S09.90)
     AHA: 2020,3Q,46; 2020,2Q,31

√6ᵗʰ **S06.9X** **Unspecified intracranial injury**
- 2 √7ᵗʰ **S06.9X0** **Unspecified intracranial injury without loss of consciousness** HCC ESR Q

- 2 √7ᵗʰ **S06.9X1** **Unspecified intracranial injury with loss of consciousness of 30 minutes or less** HCC ESR Q
    ▶Unspecified intracranial injury with brief loss of consciousness◀
- 2 √7ᵗʰ **S06.9X2** **Unspecified intracranial injury with loss of consciousness of 31 minutes to 59 minutes** HCC ESR Q
- 2 √7ᵗʰ **S06.9X3** **Unspecified intracranial injury with loss of consciousness of 1 hour to 5 hours 59 minutes** HCC ESR COM Q
- 2 √7ᵗʰ **S06.9X4** **Unspecified intracranial injury with loss of consciousness of 6 hours to 24 hours** HCC ESR COM Q
- 2 √7ᵗʰ **S06.9X5** **Unspecified intracranial injury with loss of consciousness greater than 24 hours with return to pre-existing conscious level** HCC ESR COM
- 2 √7ᵗʰ **S06.9X6** **Unspecified intracranial injury with loss of consciousness greater than 24 hours without return to pre-existing conscious level with patient surviving** HCC ESR COM
- √7ᵗʰ **S06.9X7** **Unspecified intracranial injury with loss of consciousness of any duration with death due to brain injury prior to regaining consciousness**
- √7ᵗʰ **S06.9X8** **Unspecified intracranial injury with loss of consciousness of any duration with death due to other cause prior to regaining consciousness**
- √7ᵗʰ **S06.9XA** **Unspecified intracranial injury with loss of consciousness status unknown**
- 2 √7ᵗʰ **S06.9X9** **Unspecified intracranial injury with loss of consciousness of unspecified duration** HCC ESR Q

√5ᵗʰ **S06.A** **Traumatic brain compression and herniation**
     Traumatic cerebral compression
     Code first the underlying traumatic brain injury, such as:
         diffuse traumatic brain injury (S06.2-)
         focal traumatic brain injury (S06.3-)
         traumatic subdural hemorrhage (S06.5-)
         traumatic subarachnoid hemorrhage (S06.6-)
     AHA: 2021,4Q,29

√x7ᵗʰ **S06.A0** **Traumatic brain compression without herniation** HCC ESR UPD
     Traumatic brain compression NOS
     Traumatic cerebral compression NOS

√x7ᵗʰ **S06.A1** **Traumatic brain compression with herniation** HCC ESR UPD
     Traumatic brain herniation
     Traumatic brainstem compression with herniation
     Traumatic cerebellar compression with herniation
     Traumatic cerebral compression with herniation

√4ᵗʰ **S07** **Crushing injury of head**
     Use additional code for all associated injuries, such as:
         intracranial injuries (S06.-)
         skull fractures (S02.-)

     The appropriate 7th character is to be added to each code from category S07.
     A   initial encounter
     D   subsequent encounter
     S   sequela

√x7ᵗʰ **S07.0** **Crushing injury of face**

√x7ᵗʰ **S07.1** **Crushing injury of skull**

√x7ᵗʰ **S07.8** **Crushing injury of other parts of head**

√x7ᵗʰ **S07.9** **Crushing injury of head, part unspecified**

√4ᵗʰ **S08** **Avulsion and traumatic amputation of part of head**
     An amputation not identified as partial or complete should be coded to complete

     The appropriate 7th character is to be added to each code from category S08.
     A   initial encounter
     D   subsequent encounter
     S   sequela

√x7ᵗʰ **S08.0** **Avulsion of scalp**

√5ᵗʰ **S08.1 Traumatic amputation of** ear
   √6ᵗʰ **S08.11 Complete** traumatic amputation of ear
      √7ᵗʰ **S08.111 Complete** traumatic amputation of **right** ear
      √7ᵗʰ **S08.112 Complete** traumatic amputation of **left** ear
      √7ᵗʰ **S08.119 Complete** traumatic amputation of **unspecified** ear
   √6ᵗʰ **S08.12 Partial** traumatic amputation of ear
      √7ᵗʰ **S08.121 Partial** traumatic amputation of **right** ear
      √7ᵗʰ **S08.122 Partial** traumatic amputation of **left** ear
      √7ᵗʰ **S08.129 Partial** traumatic amputation of **unspecified** ear
√5ᵗʰ **S08.8 Traumatic amputation of other parts of head**
   √6ᵗʰ **S08.81 Traumatic amputation of** nose
      √7ᵗʰ **S08.811 Complete** traumatic amputation of nose
      √7ᵗʰ **S08.812 Partial** traumatic amputation of nose
   √x7ᵗʰ **S08.89 Traumatic amputation of other parts of head**

√4ᵗʰ **S09 Other and unspecified injuries of head**

> The appropriate 7th character is to be added to each code from category S09.
> A   initial encounter
> D   subsequent encounter
> S   sequela

   √x7ᵗʰ **S09.0 Injury of** blood vessels **of head, not elsewhere classified**
      EXCLUDES 1   *injury of cerebral blood vessels (S06.-)*
                   injury of precerebral blood vessels (S15.-)
   √5ᵗʰ **S09.1 Injury of** muscle and tendon **of head**
      Code also any associated open wound (S01.-)
      EXCLUDES 2   *sprain to joints and ligament of head (S03.9)*
      √x7ᵗʰ **S09.10 Unspecified injury of muscle and tendon of head**
         Injury of muscle and tendon of head NOS
      √x7ᵗʰ **S09.11 Strain of muscle and tendon of head**   Q
      √x7ᵗʰ **S09.12 Laceration of muscle and tendon of head**
      √x7ᵗʰ **S09.19 Other specified injury of muscle and tendon of head**   Q
   √5ᵗʰ **S09.2 Traumatic rupture of** ear drum
      EXCLUDES 1   *traumatic rupture of ear drum due to blast injury (S09.31-)*
      √x7ᵗʰ **S09.20 Traumatic rupture of unspecified ear drum**
      √x7ᵗʰ **S09.21 Traumatic rupture of right ear drum**
      √x7ᵗʰ **S09.22 Traumatic rupture of left ear drum**
   √5ᵗʰ **S09.3 Other specified and unspecified injury of middle and inner ear**
      EXCLUDES 1   *injury to ear NOS (S09.91-)*
      EXCLUDES 2   *injury to external ear (S00.4-, S01.3-, S08.1-)*
      √6ᵗʰ **S09.30 Unspecified injury of** middle and inner ear
         √7ᵗʰ **S09.301 Unspecified injury of right** middle and inner ear
         √7ᵗʰ **S09.302 Unspecified injury of left** middle and inner ear
         √7ᵗʰ **S09.309 Unspecified injury of unspecified middle and inner ear**
      √6ᵗʰ **S09.31 Primary** blast injury **of ear**
         Blast injury of ear NOS
         √7ᵗʰ **S09.311 Primary blast injury of right** ear
         √7ᵗʰ **S09.312 Primary blast injury of left** ear
         √7ᵗʰ **S09.313 Primary blast injury of ear, bilateral**
         √7ᵗʰ **S09.319 Primary blast injury of unspecified** ear
      √6ᵗʰ **S09.39 Other specified injury of middle and inner ear**
         Secondary blast injury to ear
         √7ᵗʰ **S09.391 Other specified injury of right** middle and inner ear
         √7ᵗʰ **S09.392 Other specified injury of left** middle and inner ear
         √7ᵗʰ **S09.399 Other specified injury of unspecified middle and inner ear**
   √x7ᵗʰ **S09.8 Other specified injuries of head**   Q

√5ᵗʰ **S09.9 Unspecified injury of face and head**
   √x7ᵗʰ **S09.90 Unspecified injury of** head
      Head injury NOS
      EXCLUDES 1   *brain injury NOS (S06.9-)*
                   head injury NOS with loss of consciousness (S06.9-)
                   intracranial injury NOS (S06.9-)
   √x7ᵗʰ **S09.91 Unspecified injury of** ear
      Injury of ear NOS
   √x7ᵗʰ **S09.92 Unspecified injury of** nose
      Injury of nose NOS
   √x7ᵗʰ **S09.93 Unspecified injury of** face
      Injury of face NOS
      AHA: 2019,2Q,23

Injuries to the neck (S10-S19)

INCLUDES   injuries of nape
           injuries of supraclavicular region
           injuries of throat
EXCLUDES 2   *burns and corrosions (T20-T32)*
             effects of foreign body in esophagus (T18.1)
             effects of foreign body in larynx (T17.3)
             effects of foreign body in pharynx (T17.2)
             effects of foreign body in trachea (T17.4)
             frostbite (T33-T34)
             insect bite or sting, venomous (T63.4)

√4ᵗʰ **S10 Superficial injury of neck**

> The appropriate 7th character is to be added to each code from category S10.
> A   initial encounter
> D   subsequent encounter
> S   sequela

   √x7ᵗʰ **S10.0 Contusion of throat**
      Contusion of cervical esophagus
      Contusion of larynx
      Contusion of pharynx
      Contusion of trachea
   √5ᵗʰ **S10.1 Other and unspecified superficial injuries of throat**
      √7ᵗʰ **S10.10 Unspecified superficial injuries of throat**
      √7ᵗʰ **S10.11 Abrasion of throat**
      √7ᵗʰ **S10.12 Blister (nonthermal) of throat**
      √7ᵗʰ **S10.14 External constriction of part of throat**
      √7ᵗʰ **S10.15 Superficial foreign body of throat**
         Splinter in the throat
      √7ᵗʰ **S10.16 Insect bite (nonvenomous) of throat**
      √7ᵗʰ **S10.17 Other superficial bite of throat**
         EXCLUDES 1   *open bite of throat (S11.85)*
   √5ᵗʰ **S10.8 Superficial injury of other specified parts of neck**
      √x7ᵗʰ **S10.80 Unspecified superficial injury of other specified part of neck**
      √x7ᵗʰ **S10.81 Abrasion of other specified part of neck**
      √x7ᵗʰ **S10.82 Blister (nonthermal) of other specified part of neck**
      √x7ᵗʰ **S10.83 Contusion of other specified part of neck**
      √x7ᵗʰ **S10.84 External constriction of other specified part of neck**
      √x7ᵗʰ **S10.85 Superficial foreign body of other specified part of neck**
         Splinter in other specified part of neck
      √x7ᵗʰ **S10.86 Insect bite of other specified part of neck**
      √x7ᵗʰ **S10.87 Other superficial bite of other specified part of neck**
         EXCLUDES 1   *open bite of other specified parts of neck (S11.85)*
   √5ᵗʰ **S10.9 Superficial injury of unspecified part of neck**
      √x7ᵗʰ **S10.90 Unspecified superficial injury of unspecified part of neck**
      √x7ᵗʰ **S10.91 Abrasion of unspecified part of neck**
      √x7ᵗʰ **S10.92 Blister (nonthermal) of unspecified part of neck**
      √x7ᵗʰ **S10.93 Contusion of unspecified part of neck**
      √x7ᵗʰ **S10.94 External constriction of unspecified part of neck**
      √x7ᵗʰ **S10.95 Superficial foreign body of unspecified part of neck**
      √x7ᵗʰ **S10.96 Insect bite of unspecified part of neck**
      √x7ᵗʰ **S10.97 Other superficial bite of unspecified part of neck**

☑4ᵗʰ S11 Open wound of neck

Code also any associated:
spinal cord injury (S14.0, S14.1-)
wound infection

EXCLUDES 2   open fracture of vertebra (S12.- with 7th character B)

The appropriate 7th character is to be added to each code from category S11.
A   initial encounter
D   subsequent encounter
S   sequela

☑5ᵗʰ S11.0 Open wound of larynx and trachea

☑6ᵗʰ S11.01 Open wound of larynx

EXCLUDES 2   open wound of vocal cord (S11.03)

- ☑7ᵗʰ **S11.011** Laceration without foreign body of larynx
- ☑7ᵗʰ **S11.012** Laceration with foreign body of larynx
- ☑7ᵗʰ **S11.013** Puncture wound without foreign body of larynx
- ☑7ᵗʰ **S11.014** Puncture wound with foreign body of larynx
- ☑7ᵗʰ **S11.015** Open bite of larynx
  Bite of larynx NOS
- ☑7ᵗʰ **S11.019** Unspecified open wound of larynx

☑6ᵗʰ S11.02 Open wound of trachea

Open wound of cervical trachea
Open wound of trachea NOS

EXCLUDES 2   open wound of thoracic trachea (S27.5-)

- ☑7ᵗʰ **S11.021** Laceration without foreign body of trachea
- ☑7ᵗʰ **S11.022** Laceration with foreign body of trachea
- ☑7ᵗʰ **S11.023** Puncture wound without foreign body of trachea
- ☑7ᵗʰ **S11.024** Puncture wound with foreign body of trachea
- ☑7ᵗʰ **S11.025** Open bite of trachea
  Bite of trachea NOS
- ☑7ᵗʰ **S11.029** Unspecified open wound of trachea

☑6ᵗʰ S11.03 Open wound of vocal cord

- ☑7ᵗʰ **S11.031** Laceration without foreign body of vocal cord
- ☑7ᵗʰ **S11.032** Laceration with foreign body of vocal cord
- ☑7ᵗʰ **S11.033** Puncture wound without foreign body of vocal cord
- ☑7ᵗʰ **S11.034** Puncture wound with foreign body of vocal cord
- ☑7ᵗʰ **S11.035** Open bite of vocal cord
  Bite of vocal cord NOS
- ☑7ᵗʰ **S11.039** Unspecified open wound of vocal cord

☑5ᵗʰ S11.1 Open wound of thyroid gland

- ☑x7ᵗʰ **S11.10** Unspecified open wound of thyroid gland
- ☑x7ᵗʰ **S11.11** Laceration without foreign body of thyroid gland
- ☑x7ᵗʰ **S11.12** Laceration with foreign body of thyroid gland
- ☑x7ᵗʰ **S11.13** Puncture wound without foreign body of thyroid gland
- ☑x7ᵗʰ **S11.14** Puncture wound with foreign body of thyroid gland
- ☑x7ᵗʰ **S11.15** Open bite of thyroid gland
  Bite of thyroid gland NOS

☑5ᵗʰ S11.2 Open wound of pharynx and cervical esophagus

EXCLUDES 1   open wound of esophagus NOS (S27.8-)

- ☑x7ᵗʰ **S11.20** Unspecified open wound of pharynx and cervical esophagus
- ☑x7ᵗʰ **S11.21** Laceration without foreign body of pharynx and cervical esophagus
- ☑x7ᵗʰ **S11.22** Laceration with foreign body of pharynx and cervical esophagus
- ☑x7ᵗʰ **S11.23** Puncture wound without foreign body of pharynx and cervical esophagus
- ☑x7ᵗʰ **S11.24** Puncture wound with foreign body of pharynx and cervical esophagus
- ☑x7ᵗʰ **S11.25** Open bite of pharynx and cervical esophagus
  Bite of pharynx and cervical esophagus NOS

☑5ᵗʰ S11.8 Open wound of other specified parts of neck

- ☑x7ᵗʰ **S11.80** Unspecified open wound of other specified part of neck

- ☑x7ᵗʰ **S11.81** Laceration without foreign body of other specified part of neck
- ☑x7ᵗʰ **S11.82** Laceration with foreign body of other specified part of neck
- ☑x7ᵗʰ **S11.83** Puncture wound without foreign body of other specified part of neck
- ☑x7ᵗʰ **S11.84** Puncture wound with foreign body of other specified part of neck
- ☑x7ᵗʰ **S11.85** Open bite of other specified part of neck
  Bite of other specified part of neck NOS
  EXCLUDES 1   superficial bite of other specified part of neck (S10.87)
- ☑x7ᵗʰ **S11.89** Other open wound of other specified part of neck

☑5ᵗʰ S11.9 Open wound of unspecified part of neck

- ☑x7ᵗʰ **S11.90** Unspecified open wound of unspecified part of neck
- ☑x7ᵗʰ **S11.91** Laceration without foreign body of unspecified part of neck
- ☑x7ᵗʰ **S11.92** Laceration with foreign body of unspecified part of neck
- ☑x7ᵗʰ **S11.93** Puncture wound without foreign body of unspecified part of neck
- ☑x7ᵗʰ **S11.94** Puncture wound with foreign body of unspecified part of neck
- ☑x7ᵗʰ **S11.95** Open bite of unspecified part of neck
  Bite of neck NOS
  EXCLUDES 1   superficial bite of neck (S10.97)

☑4ᵗʰ S12 Fracture of cervical vertebra and other parts of neck

NOTE   A fracture not indicated as displaced or nondisplaced should be coded to displaced.

A fracture not indicated as open or closed should be coded to closed.

INCLUDES   fracture of cervical neural arch
fracture of cervical spine
fracture of cervical spinous process
fracture of cervical transverse process
fracture of cervical vertebral arch
fracture of neck

Code first any associated cervical spinal cord injury (S14.0, S14.1-)
AHA: 2021,1Q,6; 2018,2Q,12; 2015,3Q,37-39

The appropriate 7th character is to be added to all codes from subcategories S12.0-S12.6.
A   initial encounter for closed fracture
B   initial encounter for open fracture
D   subsequent encounter for fracture with routine healing
G   subsequent encounter for fracture with delayed healing
K   subsequent encounter for fracture with nonunion
S   sequela

☑5ᵗʰ S12.0 Fracture of first cervical vertebra

Atlas

☑6ᵗʰ S12.00 Unspecified fracture of first cervical vertebra

- ¹ ☑7ᵗʰ **S12.000** Unspecified displaced fracture of first cervical vertebra   HCC ESR COM Q
- ¹ ☑7ᵗʰ **S12.001** Unspecified nondisplaced fracture of first cervical vertebra   HCC ESR COM Q

- ¹ ☑x7ᵗʰ **S12.01** Stable burst fracture of first cervical vertebra   HCC ESR COM Q
- ¹ ☑x7ᵗʰ **S12.02** Unstable burst fracture of first cervical vertebra   HCC ESR COM Q

☑6ᵗʰ S12.03 Posterior arch fracture of first cervical vertebra

- ¹ ☑7ᵗʰ **S12.030** Displaced posterior arch fracture of first cervical vertebra   HCC ESR COM Q
- ¹ ☑7ᵗʰ **S12.031** Nondisplaced posterior arch fracture of first cervical vertebra   HCC ESR COM Q

☑6ᵗʰ S12.04 Lateral mass fracture of first cervical vertebra

- ¹ ☑7ᵗʰ **S12.040** Displaced lateral mass fracture of first cervical vertebra   HCC ESR COM Q
- ¹ ☑7ᵗʰ **S12.041** Nondisplaced lateral mass fracture of first cervical vertebra   HCC ESR COM Q

☑6ᵗʰ S12.09 Other fracture of first cervical vertebra

- ¹ ☑7ᵗʰ **S12.090** Other displaced fracture of first cervical vertebra   HCC ESR COM Q
- ¹ ☑7ᵗʰ **S12.091** Other nondisplaced fracture of first cervical vertebra   HCC ESR COM Q

√5ᵗʰ **S12.1** **Fracture of** second **cervical vertebra**
　　Axis
　√6ᵗʰ **S12.10** **Unspecified fracture of second cervical vertebra**
　　1 √7ᵗʰ **S12.100** Unspecified displaced fracture of second cervical vertebra   HCC ESR COM Q
　　1 √7ᵗʰ **S12.101** Unspecified nondisplaced fracture of second vertebra   HCC ESR COM Q
　√6ᵗʰ **S12.11** Type II dens **fracture**
　　1 √7ᵗʰ **S12.110** Anterior displaced Type II dens fracture   HCC ESR COM Q
　　1 √7ᵗʰ **S12.111** Posterior displaced Type II dens fracture   HCC ESR COM Q
　　1 √7ᵗʰ **S12.112** Nondisplaced Type II dens fracture   HCC ESR COM Q
　√6ᵗʰ **S12.12** **Other dens fracture**
　　1 √7ᵗʰ **S12.120** Other displaced dens fracture   HCC ESR COM Q
　　1 √7ᵗʰ **S12.121** Other nondisplaced dens fracture   HCC ESR COM Q
　√6ᵗʰ **S12.13** **Unspecified traumatic** spondylolisthesis **of second cervical vertebra**
　　1 √7ᵗʰ **S12.130** Unspecified traumatic displaced spondylolisthesis of second cervical vertebra   HCC ESR COM Q
　　1 √7ᵗʰ **S12.131** Unspecified traumatic nondisplaced spondylolisthesis of second cervical vertebra   HCC ESR COM Q
　1 √x7ᵗʰ **S12.14** Type III traumatic spondylolisthesis **of second cervical vertebra**   HCC ESR COM Q
　√6ᵗʰ **S12.15** **Other traumatic** spondylolisthesis **of second cervical vertebra**
　　1 √7ᵗʰ **S12.150** Other traumatic displaced spondylolisthesis of second cervical vertebra   HCC ESR COM Q
　　1 √7ᵗʰ **S12.151** Other traumatic nondisplaced spondylolisthesis of second cervical vertebra   HCC ESR COM Q
　√6ᵗʰ **S12.19** **Other fracture of second cervical vertebra**
　　1 √7ᵗʰ **S12.190** Other displaced fracture of second cervical vertebra   HCC ESR COM Q
　　1 √7ᵗʰ **S12.191** Other nondisplaced fracture of second cervical vertebra   HCC ESR COM Q
√5ᵗʰ **S12.2** **Fracture of** third **cervical vertebra**
　√6ᵗʰ **S12.20** **Unspecified fracture of third cervical vertebra**
　　1 √7ᵗʰ **S12.200** Unspecified displaced fracture of third cervical vertebra   HCC ESR COM Q
　　1 √7ᵗʰ **S12.201** Unspecified nondisplaced fracture of third cervical vertebra   HCC ESR COM Q
　√6ᵗʰ **S12.23** **Unspecified traumatic** spondylolisthesis **of third cervical vertebra**
　　1 √7ᵗʰ **S12.230** Unspecified traumatic displaced spondylolisthesis of third cervical vertebra   HCC ESR COM Q
　　1 √7ᵗʰ **S12.231** Unspecified traumatic nondisplaced spondylolisthesis of third cervical vertebra   HCC ESR COM Q
　1 √x7ᵗʰ **S12.24** Type III traumatic spondylolisthesis **of third cervical vertebra**   HCC ESR COM Q
　√6ᵗʰ **S12.25** **Other traumatic spondylolisthesis of third cervical vertebra**
　　1 √7ᵗʰ **S12.250** Other traumatic displaced spondylolisthesis of third cervical vertebra   HCC ESR COM Q
　　1 √7ᵗʰ **S12.251** Other traumatic nondisplaced spondylolisthesis of third cervical vertebra   HCC ESR COM Q
　√6ᵗʰ **S12.29** **Other fracture of third cervical vertebra**
　　1 √7ᵗʰ **S12.290** Other displaced fracture of third cervical vertebra   HCC ESR COM Q
　　1 √7ᵗʰ **S12.291** Other nondisplaced fracture of third cervical vertebra   HCC ESR COM Q
√5ᵗʰ **S12.3** **Fracture of** fourth **cervical vertebra**
　√6ᵗʰ **S12.30** **Unspecified fracture of fourth cervical vertebra**
　　1 √7ᵗʰ **S12.300** Unspecified displaced fracture of fourth cervical vertebra   HCC ESR COM Q
　　1 √7ᵗʰ **S12.301** Unspecified nondisplaced fracture of fourth cervical vertebra   HCC ESR COM Q

√6ᵗʰ **S12.33** **Unspecified traumatic** spondylolisthesis **of fourth cervical vertebra**
　1 √7ᵗʰ **S12.330** Unspecified traumatic displaced spondylolisthesis of fourth cervical vertebra   HCC ESR COM Q
　1 √7ᵗʰ **S12.331** Unspecified traumatic nondisplaced spondylolisthesis of fourth cervical vertebra   HCC ESR COM Q
1 √x7ᵗʰ **S12.34** Type III traumatic spondylolisthesis **of fourth cervical vertebra**
√6ᵗʰ **S12.35** **Other traumatic** spondylolisthesis **of fourth cervical vertebra**
　1 √7ᵗʰ **S12.350** Other traumatic displaced spondylolisthesis of fourth cervical vertebra   HCC ESR COM Q
　1 √7ᵗʰ **S12.351** Other traumatic nondisplaced spondylolisthesis of fourth cervical vertebra   HCC ESR COM Q
√6ᵗʰ **S12.39** **Other fracture of fourth cervical vertebra**
　1 √7ᵗʰ **S12.390** Other displaced fracture of fourth cervical vertebra   HCC ESR COM Q
　1 √7ᵗʰ **S12.391** Other nondisplaced fracture of fourth cervical vertebra   HCC ESR COM Q
√5ᵗʰ **S12.4** **Fracture of** fifth **cervical vertebra**
　√6ᵗʰ **S12.40** **Unspecified fracture of fifth cervical vertebra**
　　1 √7ᵗʰ **S12.400** Unspecified displaced fracture of fifth cervical vertebra   HCC ESR COM Q
　　1 √7ᵗʰ **S12.401** Unspecified nondisplaced fracture of fifth cervical vertebra   HCC ESR COM Q
　√6ᵗʰ **S12.43** **Unspecified traumatic** spondylolisthesis **of fifth cervical vertebra**
　　1 √7ᵗʰ **S12.430** Unspecified traumatic displaced spondylolisthesis of fifth cervical vertebra   HCC ESR COM Q
　　1 √7ᵗʰ **S12.431** Unspecified traumatic nondisplaced spondylolisthesis of fifth cervical vertebra   HCC ESR COM Q
　1 √x7ᵗʰ **S12.44** Type III traumatic spondylolisthesis **of fifth cervical vertebra**   HCC ESR COM Q
　√6ᵗʰ **S12.45** **Other traumatic** spondylolisthesis **of fifth cervical vertebra**
　　1 √7ᵗʰ **S12.450** Other traumatic displaced spondylolisthesis of fifth cervical vertebra   HCC ESR COM Q
　　1 √7ᵗʰ **S12.451** Other traumatic nondisplaced spondylolisthesis of fifth cervical vertebra   HCC ESR COM Q
　√6ᵗʰ **S12.49** **Other fracture of fifth cervical vertebra**
　　1 √7ᵗʰ **S12.490** Other displaced fracture of fifth cervical vertebra   HCC ESR COM Q
　　1 √7ᵗʰ **S12.491** Other nondisplaced fracture of fifth cervical vertebra   HCC ESR COM Q
√5ᵗʰ **S12.5** **Fracture of** sixth **cervical vertebra**
　√6ᵗʰ **S12.50** **Unspecified fracture of sixth cervical vertebra**
　　1 √7ᵗʰ **S12.500** Unspecified displaced fracture of sixth cervical vertebra   HCC ESR COM Q
　　1 √7ᵗʰ **S12.501** Unspecified nondisplaced fracture of sixth cervical vertebra   HCC ESR COM Q
　√6ᵗʰ **S12.53** **Unspecified traumatic** spondylolisthesis **of sixth cervical vertebra**
　　1 √7ᵗʰ **S12.530** Unspecified traumatic displaced spondylolisthesis of sixth cervical vertebra   HCC ESR COM Q
　　1 √7ᵗʰ **S12.531** Unspecified traumatic nondisplaced spondylolisthesis of sixth cervical vertebra   HCC ESR COM Q
　1 √x7ᵗʰ **S12.54** Type III traumatic spondylolisthesis **of sixth cervical vertebra**   HCC ESR COM Q
　√6ᵗʰ **S12.55** **Other traumatic** spondylolisthesis **of sixth cervical vertebra**
　　1 √7ᵗʰ **S12.550** Other traumatic displaced spondylolisthesis of sixth cervical vertebra   HCC ESR COM Q
　　1 √7ᵗʰ **S12.551** Other traumatic nondisplaced spondylolisthesis of sixth cervical vertebra   HCC ESR COM Q
　√6ᵗʰ **S12.59** **Other fracture of sixth cervical vertebra**
　　1 √7ᵗʰ **S12.590** Other displaced fracture of sixth cervical vertebra   HCC ESR COM Q

¹ ✓7ᵗʰ **S12.591** Other nondisplaced fracture of sixth cervical vertebra   HCC ESR COM Q

✓5ᵗʰ **S12.6** Fracture of seventh cervical vertebra

  ✓6ᵗʰ **S12.60** Unspecified fracture of seventh cervical vertebra

    ¹ ✓7ᵗʰ **S12.600** Unspecified displaced fracture of seventh cervical vertebra

    ¹ ✓7ᵗʰ **S12.601** Unspecified nondisplaced fracture of seventh cervical vertebra   HCC ESR COM Q

  ✓6ᵗʰ **S12.63** Unspecified traumatic spondylolisthesis of seventh cervical vertebra

    ¹ ✓7ᵗʰ **S12.630** Unspecified traumatic displaced spondylolisthesis of seventh cervical vertebra   HCC ESR COM Q

    ¹ ✓7ᵗʰ **S12.631** Unspecified traumatic nondisplaced spondylolisthesis of seventh cervical vertebra   HCC ESR COM Q

  ¹ ✓x7ᵗʰ **S12.64** Type III traumatic spondylolisthesis of seventh cervical vertebra   HCC ESR COM Q

  ✓6ᵗʰ **S12.65** Other traumatic spondylolisthesis of seventh cervical vertebra

    ¹ ✓7ᵗʰ **S12.650** Other traumatic displaced spondylolisthesis of seventh cervical vertebra   HCC ESR COM Q

    ¹ ✓7ᵗʰ **S12.651** Other traumatic nondisplaced spondylolisthesis of seventh cervical vertebra   HCC ESR COM Q

  ✓6ᵗʰ **S12.69** Other fracture of seventh cervical vertebra

    ¹ ✓7ᵗʰ **S12.690** Other displaced fracture of seventh cervical vertebra   HCC ESR COM Q

    ¹ ✓7ᵗʰ **S12.691** Other nondisplaced fracture of seventh cervical vertebra   HCC ESR COM Q

¹ ✓x7ᵗʰ **S12.8** Fracture of other parts of neck   HCC ESR COM Q

    Hyoid bone
    Larynx
    Thyroid cartilage
    Trachea

    The appropriate 7th character is to be added to code S12.8.
    A initial encounter
    D subsequent encounter
    S sequela

¹ ✓x7ᵗʰ **S12.9** Fracture of neck, unspecified   HCC ESR COM Q

    Fracture of neck NOS
    Fracture of cervical spine NOS
    Fracture of cervical vertebra NOS

    The appropriate 7th character is to be added to code S12.9.
    A initial encounter
    D subsequent encounter
    S sequela

✓4ᵗʰ **S13** Dislocation and sprain of joints and ligaments at neck level

  INCLUDES   avulsion of joint or ligament at neck level
    laceration of cartilage, joint or ligament at neck level
    sprain of cartilage, joint or ligament at neck level
    traumatic hemarthrosis of joint or ligament at neck level
    traumatic rupture of joint or ligament at neck level
    traumatic subluxation of joint or ligament at neck level
    traumatic tear of joint or ligament at neck level

  Code also any associated open wound
  EXCLUDES 2   strain of muscle or tendon at neck level (S16.1)

    The appropriate 7th character is to be added to each code from category S13.
    A initial encounter
    D subsequent encounter
    S sequela

  ✓x7ᵗʰ **S13.0** Traumatic rupture of cervical intervertebral disc

    EXCLUDES 1   rupture or displacement (nontraumatic) of cervical intervertebral disc NOS (M50.-)

  ✓5ᵗʰ **S13.1** Subluxation and dislocation of cervical vertebrae

    Code also any associated:
      open wound of neck (S11.-)
      spinal cord injury (S14.1-)
    EXCLUDES 2   fracture of cervical vertebrae (S12.0-S12.3-)

    ✓6ᵗʰ **S13.10** Subluxation and dislocation of unspecified cervical vertebrae

      ✓7ᵗʰ **S13.100** Subluxation of unspecified cervical vertebrae

      ✓7ᵗʰ **S13.101** Dislocation of unspecified cervical vertebrae

    ✓6ᵗʰ **S13.11** Subluxation and dislocation of C0/C1 cervical vertebrae

      Subluxation and dislocation of atlantooccipital joint
      Subluxation and dislocation of atloidooccipital joint
      Subluxation and dislocation of occipitoatloid joint

      ✓7ᵗʰ **S13.110** Subluxation of C0/C1 cervical vertebrae

      ✓7ᵗʰ **S13.111** Dislocation of C0/C1 cervical vertebrae

    ✓6ᵗʰ **S13.12** Subluxation and dislocation of C1/C2 cervical vertebrae

      Subluxation and dislocation of atlantoaxial joint

      ✓7ᵗʰ **S13.120** Subluxation of C1/C2 cervical vertebrae

      ✓7ᵗʰ **S13.121** Dislocation of C1/C2 cervical vertebrae

    ✓6ᵗʰ **S13.13** Subluxation and dislocation of C2/C3 cervical vertebrae

      ✓7ᵗʰ **S13.130** Subluxation of C2/C3 cervical vertebrae

      ✓7ᵗʰ **S13.131** Dislocation of C2/C3 cervical vertebrae

    ✓6ᵗʰ **S13.14** Subluxation and dislocation of C3/C4 cervical vertebrae

      ✓7ᵗʰ **S13.140** Subluxation of C3/C4 cervical vertebrae

      ✓7ᵗʰ **S13.141** Dislocation of C3/C4 cervical vertebrae

    ✓6ᵗʰ **S13.15** Subluxation and dislocation of C4/C5 cervical vertebrae

      ✓7ᵗʰ **S13.150** Subluxation of C4/C5 cervical vertebrae

      ✓7ᵗʰ **S13.151** Dislocation of C4/C5 cervical vertebrae

    ✓6ᵗʰ **S13.16** Subluxation and dislocation of C5/C6 cervical vertebrae

      ✓7ᵗʰ **S13.160** Subluxation of C5/C6 cervical vertebrae

      ✓7ᵗʰ **S13.161** Dislocation of C5/C6 cervical vertebrae

    ✓6ᵗʰ **S13.17** Subluxation and dislocation of C6/C7 cervical vertebrae

      ✓7ᵗʰ **S13.170** Subluxation of C6/C7 cervical vertebrae

      ✓7ᵗʰ **S13.171** Dislocation of C6/C7 cervical vertebrae

    ✓6ᵗʰ **S13.18** Subluxation and dislocation of C7/T1 cervical vertebrae

      ✓7ᵗʰ **S13.180** Subluxation of C7/T1 cervical vertebrae

      ✓7ᵗʰ **S13.181** Dislocation of C7/T1 cervical vertebrae

  ✓5ᵗʰ **S13.2** Dislocation of other and unspecified parts of neck

    ✓x7ᵗʰ **S13.20** Dislocation of unspecified parts of neck

    ✓x7ᵗʰ **S13.29** Dislocation of other parts of neck

  ✓x7ᵗʰ **S13.4** Sprain of ligaments of cervical spine

    Sprain of anterior longitudinal (ligament), cervical
    Sprain of atlanto-axial (joints)
    Sprain of atlanto-occipital (joints)
    Whiplash injury of cervical spine

  ✓x7ᵗʰ **S13.5** Sprain of thyroid region

    Sprain of cricoarytenoid (joint) (ligament)
    Sprain of cricothyroid (joint) (ligament)
    Sprain of thyroid cartilage

  ✓x7ᵗʰ **S13.8** Sprain of joints and ligaments of other parts of neck

  ✓x7ᵗʰ **S13.9** Sprain of joints and ligaments of unspecified parts of neck

✓4ᵗʰ **S14** Injury of nerves and spinal cord at neck level

  NOTE   Code to highest level of cervical cord injury

  Code also any associated:
    fracture of cervical vertebra (S12.0- — S12.6.-)
    open wound of neck (S11.-)
    transient paralysis (R29.5)

    The appropriate 7th character is to be added to each code from category S14.
    A initial encounter
    D subsequent encounter
    S sequela

  ✓x7ᵗʰ **S14.0** Concussion and edema of cervical spinal cord   HCC ESR COM

  ✓5ᵗʰ **S14.1** Other and unspecified injuries of cervical spinal cord

    ✓6ᵗʰ **S14.10** Unspecified injury of cervical spinal cord

      ✓7ᵗʰ **S14.101** Unspecified injury at C1 level of cervical spinal cord   HCC ESR COM

      ✓7ᵗʰ **S14.102** Unspecified injury at C2 level of cervical spinal cord   HCC ESR COM

      ✓7ᵗʰ **S14.103** Unspecified injury at C3 level of cervical spinal cord   HCC ESR COM

√7ᵗʰ **S14.104** Unspecified injury at C4 level of cervical spinal cord `HCC` `ESR` `COM`

√7ᵗʰ **S14.105** Unspecified injury at C5 level of cervical spinal cord `HCC` `ESR` `COM`

√7ᵗʰ **S14.106** Unspecified injury at C6 level of cervical spinal cord `HCC` `ESR` `COM`

√7ᵗʰ **S14.107** Unspecified injury at C7 level of cervical spinal cord `HCC` `ESR` `COM`

√7ᵗʰ **S14.108** Unspecified injury at C8 level of cervical spinal cord `HCC` `ESR` `COM`

√7ᵗʰ **S14.109** Unspecified injury at unspecified level of cervical spinal cord `HCC` `ESR` `COM`

     Injury of cervical spinal cord NOS

√6ᵗʰ **S14.11** Complete lesion of cervical spinal cord

√7ᵗʰ **S14.111** Complete lesion at C1 level of cervical spinal cord `HCC` `ESR` `COM`

√7ᵗʰ **S14.112** Complete lesion at C2 level of cervical spinal cord `HCC` `ESR` `COM`

√7ᵗʰ **S14.113** Complete lesion at C3 level of cervical spinal cord `HCC` `ESR` `COM`

√7ᵗʰ **S14.114** Complete lesion at C4 level of cervical spinal cord `HCC` `ESR` `COM`

√7ᵗʰ **S14.115** Complete lesion at C5 level of cervical spinal cord `HCC` `ESR` `COM`

√7ᵗʰ **S14.116** Complete lesion at C6 level of cervical spinal cord `HCC` `ESR` `COM`

√7ᵗʰ **S14.117** Complete lesion at C7 level of cervical spinal cord `HCC` `ESR` `COM`

√7ᵗʰ **S14.118** Complete lesion at C8 level of cervical spinal cord `HCC` `ESR` `COM`

√7ᵗʰ **S14.119** Complete lesion at unspecified level of cervical spinal cord `HCC` `ESR` `COM`

√6ᵗʰ **S14.12** Central cord syndrome of cervical spinal cord

√7ᵗʰ **S14.121** Central cord syndrome at C1 level of cervical spinal cord `HCC` `ESR` `COM`

√7ᵗʰ **S14.122** Central cord syndrome at C2 level of cervical spinal cord `HCC` `ESR` `COM`

√7ᵗʰ **S14.123** Central cord syndrome at C3 level of cervical spinal cord `HCC` `ESR` `COM`

√7ᵗʰ **S14.124** Central cord syndrome at C4 level of cervical spinal cord `HCC` `ESR` `COM`

√7ᵗʰ **S14.125** Central cord syndrome at C5 level of cervical spinal cord `HCC` `ESR` `COM`

√7ᵗʰ **S14.126** Central cord syndrome at C6 level of cervical spinal cord `HCC` `ESR` `COM`

√7ᵗʰ **S14.127** Central cord syndrome at C7 level of cervical spinal cord `HCC` `ESR` `COM`

√7ᵗʰ **S14.128** Central cord syndrome at C8 level of cervical spinal cord `HCC` `ESR` `COM`

√7ᵗʰ **S14.129** Central cord syndrome at unspecified level of cervical spinal cord `HCC` `ESR` `COM`

√6ᵗʰ **S14.13** Anterior cord syndrome of cervical spinal cord

√7ᵗʰ **S14.131** Anterior cord syndrome at C1 level of cervical spinal cord `HCC` `ESR` `COM`

√7ᵗʰ **S14.132** Anterior cord syndrome at C2 level of cervical spinal cord `HCC` `ESR` `COM`

√7ᵗʰ **S14.133** Anterior cord syndrome at C3 level of cervical spinal cord `HCC` `ESR` `COM`

√7ᵗʰ **S14.134** Anterior cord syndrome at C4 level of cervical spinal cord `HCC` `ESR` `COM`

√7ᵗʰ **S14.135** Anterior cord syndrome at C5 level of cervical spinal cord `HCC` `ESR` `COM`

√7ᵗʰ **S14.136** Anterior cord syndrome at C6 level of cervical spinal cord `HCC` `ESR` `COM`

√7ᵗʰ **S14.137** Anterior cord syndrome at C7 level of cervical spinal cord `HCC` `ESR` `COM`

√7ᵗʰ **S14.138** Anterior cord syndrome at C8 level of cervical spinal cord `HCC` `ESR` `COM`

√7ᵗʰ **S14.139** Anterior cord syndrome at unspecified level of cervical spinal cord `HCC` `ESR` `COM`

√6ᵗʰ **S14.14** Brown-Séquard syndrome of cervical spinal cord

√7ᵗʰ **S14.141** Brown-Séquard syndrome at C1 level of cervical spinal cord `HCC` `ESR` `COM`

√7ᵗʰ **S14.142** Brown-Séquard syndrome at C2 level of cervical spinal cord `HCC` `ESR` `COM`

√7ᵗʰ **S14.143** Brown-Séquard syndrome at C3 level of cervical spinal cord `HCC` `ESR` `COM`

√7ᵗʰ **S14.144** Brown-Séquard syndrome at C4 level of cervical spinal cord `HCC` `ESR` `COM`

√7ᵗʰ **S14.145** Brown-Séquard syndrome at C5 level of cervical spinal cord `HCC` `ESR` `COM`

√7ᵗʰ **S14.146** Brown-Séquard syndrome at C6 level of cervical spinal cord `HCC` `ESR` `COM`

√7ᵗʰ **S14.147** Brown-Séquard syndrome at C7 level of cervical spinal cord `HCC` `ESR` `COM`

√7ᵗʰ **S14.148** Brown-Séquard syndrome at C8 level of cervical spinal cord `HCC` `ESR` `COM`

√7ᵗʰ **S14.149** Brown-Séquard syndrome at unspecified level of cervical spinal cord `HCC` `ESR` `COM`

√6ᵗʰ **S14.15** Other incomplete lesions of cervical spinal cord

     Incomplete lesion of cervical spinal cord NOS
     Posterior cord syndrome of cervical spinal cord

√7ᵗʰ **S14.151** Other incomplete lesion at C1 level of cervical spinal cord `HCC` `ESR` `COM`

√7ᵗʰ **S14.152** Other incomplete lesion at C2 level of cervical spinal cord `HCC` `ESR` `COM`

√7ᵗʰ **S14.153** Other incomplete lesion at C3 level of cervical spinal cord `HCC` `ESR` `COM`

√7ᵗʰ **S14.154** Other incomplete lesion at C4 level of cervical spinal cord `HCC` `ESR` `COM`

√7ᵗʰ **S14.155** Other incomplete lesion at C5 level of cervical spinal cord `HCC` `ESR` `COM`

√7ᵗʰ **S14.156** Other incomplete lesion at C6 level of cervical spinal cord `HCC` `ESR` `COM`

√7ᵗʰ **S14.157** Other incomplete lesion at C7 level of cervical spinal cord `HCC` `ESR` `COM`

√7ᵗʰ **S14.158** Other incomplete lesion at C8 level of cervical spinal cord `HCC` `ESR` `COM`

√7ᵗʰ **S14.159** Other incomplete lesion at unspecified level of cervical spinal cord `HCC` `ESR` `COM`

√x7ᵗʰ **S14.2** Injury of nerve root of cervical spine

√x7ᵗʰ **S14.3** Injury of brachial plexus

√x7ᵗʰ **S14.4** Injury of peripheral nerves of neck

√x7ᵗʰ **S14.5** Injury of cervical sympathetic nerves

√x7ᵗʰ **S14.8** Injury of other specified nerves of neck

√x7ᵗʰ **S14.9** Injury of unspecified nerves of neck

√4ᵗʰ **S15** Injury of blood vessels at neck level

     Code also any associated open wound (S11.-)

> The appropriate 7th character is to be added to each code from category S15.
> A   initial encounter
> D   subsequent encounter
> S   sequela

√5ᵗʰ **S15.0** Injury of carotid artery of neck

     Injury of carotid artery (common) (external) (internal, extracranial portion)
     Injury of carotid artery NOS
     EXCLUDES 1   *injury of internal carotid artery, intracranial portion (S06.8)*

√6ᵗʰ **S15.00** Unspecified injury of carotid artery

√7ᵗʰ **S15.001** Unspecified injury of right carotid artery

√7ᵗʰ **S15.002** Unspecified injury of left carotid artery

√7ᵗʰ **S15.009** Unspecified injury of unspecified carotid artery

√6ᵗʰ **S15.01** Minor laceration of carotid artery

     Incomplete transection of carotid artery
     Laceration of carotid artery NOS
     Superficial laceration of carotid artery

√7ᵗʰ **S15.011** Minor laceration of right carotid artery

√7ᵗʰ **S15.012** Minor laceration of left carotid artery

√7ᵗʰ **S15.019** Minor laceration of unspecified carotid artery

√6ᵗʰ **S15.02** Major laceration of carotid artery

     Complete transection of carotid artery
     Traumatic rupture of carotid artery

√7ᵗʰ **S15.021** Major laceration of right carotid artery

√7ᵗʰ **S15.022** Major laceration of left carotid artery

√7ᵗʰ **S15.029** Major laceration of unspecified carotid artery

Chapter 19. Injury, Poisoning and Certain Other Consequences of External Causes

S15.09–S19.85

√6ᵗʰ **S15.09** **Other specified injury of carotid artery**
- √7ᵗʰ **S15.091** **Other specified injury of right carotid artery**
- √7ᵗʰ **S15.092** **Other specified injury of left carotid artery**
- √7ᵗʰ **S15.099** **Other specified injury of unspecified carotid artery**

√5ᵗʰ **S15.1** **Injury of vertebral artery**
- √6ᵗʰ **S15.10** **Unspecified injury of vertebral artery**
  - √7ᵗʰ **S15.101** **Unspecified injury of right vertebral artery**
  - √7ᵗʰ **S15.102** **Unspecified injury of left vertebral artery**
  - √7ᵗʰ **S15.109** **Unspecified injury of unspecified vertebral artery**
- √6ᵗʰ **S15.11** **Minor laceration of vertebral artery**
  - Incomplete transection of vertebral artery
  - Laceration of vertebral artery NOS
  - Superficial laceration of vertebral artery
  - √7ᵗʰ **S15.111** **Minor laceration of right vertebral artery**
  - √7ᵗʰ **S15.112** **Minor laceration of left vertebral artery**
  - √7ᵗʰ **S15.119** **Minor laceration of unspecified vertebral artery**
- √6ᵗʰ **S15.12** **Major laceration of vertebral artery**
  - Complete transection of vertebral artery
  - Traumatic rupture of vertebral artery
  - √7ᵗʰ **S15.121** **Major laceration of right vertebral artery**
  - √7ᵗʰ **S15.122** **Major laceration of left vertebral artery**
  - √7ᵗʰ **S15.129** **Major laceration of unspecified vertebral artery**
- √6ᵗʰ **S15.19** **Other specified injury of vertebral artery**
  - √7ᵗʰ **S15.191** **Other specified injury of right vertebral artery**
  - √7ᵗʰ **S15.192** **Other specified injury of left vertebral artery**
  - √7ᵗʰ **S15.199** **Other specified injury of unspecified vertebral artery**

√5ᵗʰ **S15.2** **Injury of external jugular vein**
- √6ᵗʰ **S15.20** **Unspecified injury of external jugular vein**
  - √7ᵗʰ **S15.201** **Unspecified injury of right external jugular vein**
  - √7ᵗʰ **S15.202** **Unspecified injury of left external jugular vein**
  - √7ᵗʰ **S15.209** **Unspecified injury of unspecified external jugular vein**
- √6ᵗʰ **S15.21** **Minor laceration of external jugular vein**
  - Incomplete transection of external jugular vein
  - Laceration of external jugular vein NOS
  - Superficial laceration of external jugular vein
  - √7ᵗʰ **S15.211** **Minor laceration of right external jugular vein**
  - √7ᵗʰ **S15.212** **Minor laceration of left external jugular vein**
  - √7ᵗʰ **S15.219** **Minor laceration of unspecified external jugular vein**
- √6ᵗʰ **S15.22** **Major laceration of external jugular vein**
  - Complete transection of external jugular vein
  - Traumatic rupture of external jugular vein
  - √7ᵗʰ **S15.221** **Major laceration of right external jugular vein**
  - √7ᵗʰ **S15.222** **Major laceration of left external jugular vein**
  - √7ᵗʰ **S15.229** **Major laceration of unspecified external jugular vein**
- √6ᵗʰ **S15.29** **Other specified injury of external jugular vein**
  - √7ᵗʰ **S15.291** **Other specified injury of right external jugular vein**
  - √7ᵗʰ **S15.292** **Other specified injury of left external jugular vein**
  - √7ᵗʰ **S15.299** **Other specified injury of unspecified external jugular vein**

√5ᵗʰ **S15.3** **Injury of internal jugular vein**
- √6ᵗʰ **S15.30** **Unspecified injury of internal jugular vein**
  - √7ᵗʰ **S15.301** **Unspecified injury of right internal jugular vein**
  - √7ᵗʰ **S15.302** **Unspecified injury of left internal jugular vein**
  - √7ᵗʰ **S15.309** **Unspecified injury of unspecified internal jugular vein**

√6ᵗʰ **S15.31** **Minor laceration of internal jugular vein**
- Incomplete transection of internal jugular vein
- Laceration of internal jugular vein NOS
- Superficial laceration of internal jugular vein
- √7ᵗʰ **S15.311** **Minor laceration of right internal jugular vein**
- √7ᵗʰ **S15.312** **Minor laceration of left internal jugular vein**
- √7ᵗʰ **S15.319** **Minor laceration of unspecified internal jugular vein**

√6ᵗʰ **S15.32** **Major laceration of internal jugular vein**
- Complete transection of internal jugular vein
- Traumatic rupture of internal jugular vein
- √7ᵗʰ **S15.321** **Major laceration of right internal jugular vein**
- √7ᵗʰ **S15.322** **Major laceration of left internal jugular vein**
- √7ᵗʰ **S15.329** **Major laceration of unspecified internal jugular vein**

√6ᵗʰ **S15.39** **Other specified injury of internal jugular vein**
- √7ᵗʰ **S15.391** **Other specified injury of right internal jugular vein**
- √7ᵗʰ **S15.392** **Other specified injury of left internal jugular vein**
- √7ᵗʰ **S15.399** **Other specified injury of unspecified internal jugular vein**

√x7ᵗʰ **S15.8** **Injury of other specified blood vessels at neck level**

√x7ᵗʰ **S15.9** **Injury of unspecified blood vessel at neck level**

√4ᵗʰ **S16** **Injury of muscle, fascia and tendon at neck level**
- Code also any associated open wound (S11.-)
- *EXCLUDES 2*   sprain of joint or ligament at neck level (S13.9)

> The appropriate 7th character is to be added to each code from category S16.
> A   initial encounter
> D   subsequent encounter
> S   sequela

√x7ᵗʰ **S16.1** **Strain of muscle, fascia and tendon at neck level**

√x7ᵗʰ **S16.2** **Laceration of muscle, fascia and tendon at neck level**

√x7ᵗʰ **S16.8** **Other specified injury of muscle, fascia and tendon at neck level**

√x7ᵗʰ **S16.9** **Unspecified injury of muscle, fascia and tendon at neck level**

√4ᵗʰ **S17** **Crushing injury of neck**
- Use additional code for all associated injuries, such as:
  - injury of blood vessels (S15.-)
  - open wound of neck (S11.-)
  - spinal cord injury (S14.0, S14.1-)
  - vertebral fracture (S12.0- — S12.3-)

> The appropriate 7th character is to be added to each code from category S17.
> A   initial encounter
> D   subsequent encounter
> S   sequela

√x7ᵗʰ **S17.0** **Crushing injury of larynx and trachea**

√x7ᵗʰ **S17.8** **Crushing injury of other specified parts of neck**

√x7ᵗʰ **S17.9** **Crushing injury of neck, part unspecified**

√4ᵗʰ **S19** **Other specified and unspecified injuries of neck**

> The appropriate 7th character is to be added to each code from category S19.
> A   initial encounter
> D   subsequent encounter
> S   sequela

√5ᵗʰ **S19.8** **Other specified injuries of neck**
- √x7ᵗʰ **S19.80** **Other specified injuries of unspecified part of neck**
- √x7ᵗʰ **S19.81** **Other specified injuries of larynx**
- √x7ᵗʰ **S19.82** **Other specified injuries of cervical trachea**
  - *EXCLUDES 2*   other specified injury of thoracic trachea (S27.5-)
- √x7ᵗʰ **S19.83** **Other specified injuries of vocal cord**
- √x7ᵗʰ **S19.84** **Other specified injuries of thyroid gland**
- √x7ᵗʰ **S19.85** **Other specified injuries of pharynx and cervical esophagus**
  - **AHA:** 2022,1Q,27

√x 7ᵗʰ **S19.89** Other specified injuries of other specified part of neck

√x 7ᵗʰ **S19.9** Unspecified injury of neck

Injuries to the thorax (S20-S29)

INCLUDES injuries of breast
injuries of chest (wall)
injuries of interscapular area
EXCLUDES 2 *burns and corrosions (T20-T32)*
effects of foreign body in bronchus (T17.5)
effects of foreign body in esophagus (T18.1)
effects of foreign body in lung (T17.8)
effects of foreign body in trachea (T17.4)
frostbite (T33-T34)
injuries of axilla
injuries of clavicle
injuries of scapular region
injuries of shoulder
insect bite or sting, venomous (T63.4)

√4ᵗʰ **S20** **Superficial injury of thorax**

AHA: 2020,4Q,39

The appropriate 7th character is to be added to each code from category S20.
A   initial encounter
D   subsequent encounter
S   sequela

√5ᵗʰ **S20.0** **Contusion of breast**

√x 7ᵗʰ **S20.00** Contusion of breast, unspecified breast

√x 7ᵗʰ **S20.01** Contusion of right breast

√x 7ᵗʰ **S20.02** Contusion of left breast

√5ᵗʰ **S20.1** Other and unspecified superficial injuries of breast

√6ᵗʰ **S20.10** Unspecified superficial injuries of breast

√7ᵗʰ **S20.101** Unspecified superficial injuries of breast, right breast

√7ᵗʰ **S20.102** Unspecified superficial injuries of breast, left breast

√7ᵗʰ **S20.109** Unspecified superficial injuries of breast, unspecified breast

√6ᵗʰ **S20.11** Abrasion of breast

√7ᵗʰ **S20.111** Abrasion of breast, right breast

√7ᵗʰ **S20.112** Abrasion of breast, left breast

√7ᵗʰ **S20.119** Abrasion of breast, unspecified breast

√6ᵗʰ **S20.12** Blister (nonthermal) of breast

√7ᵗʰ **S20.121** Blister (nonthermal) of breast, right breast

√7ᵗʰ **S20.122** Blister (nonthermal) of breast, left breast

√7ᵗʰ **S20.129** Blister (nonthermal) of breast, unspecified breast

√6ᵗʰ **S20.14** External constriction of part of breast

√7ᵗʰ **S20.141** External constriction of part of breast, right breast

√7ᵗʰ **S20.142** External constriction of part of breast, left breast

√7ᵗʰ **S20.149** External constriction of part of breast, unspecified breast

√6ᵗʰ **S20.15** Superficial foreign body of breast

Splinter in the breast

√7ᵗʰ **S20.151** Superficial foreign body of breast, right breast

√7ᵗʰ **S20.152** Superficial foreign body of breast, left breast

√7ᵗʰ **S20.159** Superficial foreign body of breast, unspecified breast

√6ᵗʰ **S20.16** Insect bite (nonvenomous) of breast

√7ᵗʰ **S20.161** Insect bite (nonvenomous) of breast, right breast

√7ᵗʰ **S20.162** Insect bite (nonvenomous) of breast, left breast

√7ᵗʰ **S20.169** Insect bite (nonvenomous) of breast, unspecified breast

√6ᵗʰ **S20.17** Other superficial bite of breast

EXCLUDES 1 *open bite of breast (S21.05-)*

√7ᵗʰ **S20.171** Other superficial bite of breast, right breast

√7ᵗʰ **S20.172** Other superficial bite of breast, left breast

√7ᵗʰ **S20.179** Other superficial bite of breast, unspecified breast

√5ᵗʰ **S20.2** **Contusion of thorax**

√x 7ᵗʰ **S20.20** Contusion of thorax, unspecified

√6ᵗʰ **S20.21** Contusion of front wall of thorax

√7ᵗʰ **S20.211** Contusion of right front wall of thorax

√7ᵗʰ **S20.212** Contusion of left front wall of thorax

√7ᵗʰ **S20.213** Contusion of bilateral front wall of thorax

√7ᵗʰ **S20.214** Contusion of middle front wall of thorax

√7ᵗʰ **S20.219** Contusion of unspecified front wall of thorax

√6ᵗʰ **S20.22** Contusion of back wall of thorax

√7ᵗʰ **S20.221** Contusion of right back wall of thorax

√7ᵗʰ **S20.222** Contusion of left back wall of thorax

√7ᵗʰ **S20.223** Contusion of bilateral back wall of thorax

√7ᵗʰ **S20.224** Contusion of middle back wall of thorax

√7ᵗʰ **S20.229** Contusion of unspecified back wall of thorax

√5ᵗʰ **S20.3** **Other and unspecified superficial injuries of front wall of thorax**

√6ᵗʰ **S20.30** Unspecified superficial injuries of front wall of thorax

√7ᵗʰ **S20.301** Unspecified superficial injuries of right front wall of thorax

√7ᵗʰ **S20.302** Unspecified superficial injuries of left front wall of thorax

√7ᵗʰ **S20.303** Unspecified superficial injuries of bilateral front wall of thorax

√7ᵗʰ **S20.304** Unspecified superficial injuries of middle front wall of thorax

√7ᵗʰ **S20.309** Unspecified superficial injuries of unspecified front wall of thorax

√6ᵗʰ **S20.31** Abrasion of front wall of thorax

√7ᵗʰ **S20.311** Abrasion of right front wall of thorax

√7ᵗʰ **S20.312** Abrasion of left front wall of thorax

√7ᵗʰ **S20.313** Abrasion of bilateral front wall of thorax

√7ᵗʰ **S20.314** Abrasion of middle front wall of thorax

√7ᵗʰ **S20.319** Abrasion of unspecified front wall of thorax

√6ᵗʰ **S20.32** Blister (nonthermal) of front wall of thorax

√7ᵗʰ **S20.321** Blister (nonthermal) of right front wall of thorax

√7ᵗʰ **S20.322** Blister (nonthermal) of left front wall of thorax

√7ᵗʰ **S20.323** Blister (nonthermal) of bilateral front wall of thorax

√7ᵗʰ **S20.324** Blister (nonthermal) of middle front wall of thorax

√7ᵗʰ **S20.329** Blister (nonthermal) of unspecified front wall of thorax

√6ᵗʰ **S20.34** External constriction of front wall of thorax

√7ᵗʰ **S20.341** External constriction of right front wall of thorax

√7ᵗʰ **S20.342** External constriction of left front wall of thorax

√7ᵗʰ **S20.343** External constriction of bilateral front wall of thorax

√7ᵗʰ **S20.344** External constriction of middle front wall of thorax

√7ᵗʰ **S20.349** External constriction of unspecified front wall of thorax

√6ᵗʰ **S20.35** Superficial foreign body of front wall of thorax

Splinter in front wall of thorax

√7ᵗʰ **S20.351** Superficial foreign body of right front wall of thorax

√7ᵗʰ **S20.352** Superficial foreign body of left front wall of thorax

√7ᵗʰ **S20.353** Superficial foreign body of bilateral front wall of thorax

√7ᵗʰ **S20.354** Superficial foreign body of middle front wall of thorax

√7ᵗʰ **S20.359** Superficial foreign body of unspecified front wall of thorax

√6ᵗʰ **S20.36** Insect bite (nonvenomous) of front wall of thorax

√7ᵗʰ **S20.361** Insect bite (nonvenomous) of right front wall of thorax

√7ᵗʰ **S20.362　Insect bite (nonvenomous) of** left **front wall of thorax**

√7ᵗʰ **S20.363　Insect bite (nonvenomous) of** bilateral **front wall of thorax**

√7ᵗʰ **S20.364　Insect bite (nonvenomous) of** middle **front wall of thorax**

√7ᵗʰ **S20.369　Insect bite (nonvenomous) of unspecified front wall of thorax**

√6ᵗʰ **S20.37　Other superficial** bite **of front wall of thorax**
> EXCLUDES 1　*open bite of front wall of thorax (S21.15)*

√7ᵗʰ **S20.371　Other superficial bite of** right **front wall of thorax**

√7ᵗʰ **S20.372　Other superficial bite of** left **front wall of thorax**

√7ᵗʰ **S20.373　Other superficial bite of** bilateral **front wall of thorax**

√7ᵗʰ **S20.374　Other superficial bite of** middle **front wall of thorax**

√7ᵗʰ **S20.379　Other superficial bite of unspecified front wall of thorax**

√5ᵗʰ **S20.4　Other and unspecified superficial injuries of** back wall of thorax

√6ᵗʰ **S20.40　Unspecified superficial injuries of back wall of thorax**

√7ᵗʰ **S20.401　Unspecified superficial injuries of** right **back wall of thorax**

√7ᵗʰ **S20.402　Unspecified superficial injuries of** left **back wall of thorax**

√7ᵗʰ **S20.409　Unspecified superficial injuries of unspecified back wall of thorax**

√6ᵗʰ **S20.41　Abrasion of back wall of thorax**

√7ᵗʰ **S20.411　Abrasion of** right **back wall of thorax**

√7ᵗʰ **S20.412　Abrasion of** left **back wall of thorax**

√7ᵗʰ **S20.419　Abrasion of unspecified back wall of thorax**

√6ᵗʰ **S20.42　Blister (nonthermal) of back wall of thorax**

√7ᵗʰ **S20.421　Blister (nonthermal) of** right **back wall of thorax**

√7ᵗʰ **S20.422　Blister (nonthermal) of** left **back wall of thorax**

√7ᵗʰ **S20.429　Blister (nonthermal) of unspecified back wall of thorax**

√6ᵗʰ **S20.44　External constriction of back wall of thorax**

√7ᵗʰ **S20.441　External constriction of** right **back wall of thorax**

√7ᵗʰ **S20.442　External constriction of** left **back wall of thorax**

√7ᵗʰ **S20.449　External constriction of unspecified back wall of thorax**

√6ᵗʰ **S20.45　Superficial** foreign body **of back wall of thorax**
> Splinter of back wall of thorax

√7ᵗʰ **S20.451　Superficial foreign body of** right **back wall of thorax**

√7ᵗʰ **S20.452　Superficial foreign body of** left **back wall of thorax**

√7ᵗʰ **S20.459　Superficial foreign body of unspecified back wall of thorax**

√6ᵗʰ **S20.46　Insect bite (nonvenomous) of back wall of thorax**

√7ᵗʰ **S20.461　Insect bite (nonvenomous) of** right **back wall of thorax**

√7ᵗʰ **S20.462　Insect bite (nonvenomous) of** left **back wall of thorax**

√7ᵗʰ **S20.469　Insect bite (nonvenomous) of unspecified back wall of thorax**

√6ᵗʰ **S20.47　Other superficial** bite **of back wall of thorax**
> EXCLUDES 1　*open bite of back wall of thorax (S21.25)*

√7ᵗʰ **S20.471　Other superficial bite of** right **back wall of thorax**

√7ᵗʰ **S20.472　Other superficial bite of** left **back wall of thorax**

√7ᵗʰ **S20.479　Other superficial bite of unspecified back wall of thorax**

√5ᵗʰ **S20.9　Superficial injury of unspecified parts of thorax**
> EXCLUDES 1　*contusion of thorax NOS (S20.20)*

√×7ᵗʰ **S20.90　Unspecified superficial injury of unspecified parts of thorax**
> Superficial injury of thoracic wall NOS

√×7ᵗʰ **S20.91　Abrasion of unspecified parts of thorax**

√×7ᵗʰ **S20.92　Blister (nonthermal) of unspecified parts of thorax**

√×7ᵗʰ **S20.94　External constriction of unspecified parts of thorax**

√×7ᵗʰ **S20.95　Superficial foreign body of unspecified parts of thorax**
> Splinter in thorax NOS

√×7ᵗʰ **S20.96　Insect bite (nonvenomous) of unspecified parts of thorax**

√×7ᵗʰ **S20.97　Other superficial bite of unspecified parts of thorax**
> EXCLUDES 1　*open bite of thorax NOS (S21.95)*

√4ᵗʰ **S21　Open wound of thorax**
> Code also any associated injury, such as:
> injury of heart (S26.-)
> injury of intrathoracic organs (S27.-)
> rib fracture (S22.3-, S22.4-)
> spinal cord injury (S24.0-, S24.1-)
> traumatic hemopneumothorax (S27.3)
> traumatic hemothorax (S27.1)
> traumatic pneumothorax (S27.0)
> wound infection
> EXCLUDES 1　*traumatic amputation (partial) of thorax (S28.1)*

> The appropriate 7th character is to be added to each code from category S21.
> A　initial encounter
> D　subsequent encounter
> S　sequela

√5ᵗʰ **S21.0　Open wound of** breast

√6ᵗʰ **S21.00　Unspecified open wound of breast**

√7ᵗʰ **S21.001　Unspecified open wound of** right **breast**

√7ᵗʰ **S21.002　Unspecified open wound of** left **breast**

√7ᵗʰ **S21.009　Unspecified open wound of unspecified breast**

√6ᵗʰ **S21.01　Laceration without foreign body of breast**

√7ᵗʰ **S21.011　Laceration without foreign body of** right **breast**

√7ᵗʰ **S21.012　Laceration without foreign body of** left **breast**

√7ᵗʰ **S21.019　Laceration without foreign body of unspecified breast**

√6ᵗʰ **S21.02　Laceration with foreign body of breast**

√7ᵗʰ **S21.021　Laceration with foreign body of** right **breast**

√7ᵗʰ **S21.022　Laceration with foreign body of** left **breast**

√7ᵗʰ **S21.029　Laceration with foreign body of unspecified breast**

√6ᵗʰ **S21.03　Puncture wound without foreign body of breast**

√7ᵗʰ **S21.031　Puncture wound without foreign body of** right **breast**

√7ᵗʰ **S21.032　Puncture wound without foreign body of** left **breast**

√7ᵗʰ **S21.039　Puncture wound without foreign body of unspecified breast**

√6ᵗʰ **S21.04　Puncture wound with foreign body of breast**

√7ᵗʰ **S21.041　Puncture wound with foreign body of** right **breast**

√7ᵗʰ **S21.042　Puncture wound with foreign body of** left **breast**

√7ᵗʰ **S21.049　Puncture wound with foreign body of unspecified breast**

√6ᵗʰ **S21.05　Open bite of breast**
> Bite of breast NOS
> EXCLUDES 1　*superficial bite of breast (S20.17)*

√7ᵗʰ **S21.051　Open bite of** right **breast**

√7ᵗʰ **S21.052　Open bite of** left **breast**

√7ᵗʰ **S21.059　Open bite of unspecified breast**

√5ᵗʰ **S21.1　Open wound of** front wall of thorax without penetration into thoracic cavity
> Open wound of chest without penetration into thoracic cavity

√6ᵗʰ **S21.10　Unspecified open wound of front wall of thorax without penetration into thoracic cavity**

√7ᵗʰ **S21.101　Unspecified open wound of** right **front wall of thorax without penetration into thoracic cavity**

√7ᵗʰ **S21.102　Unspecified open wound of** left **front wall of thorax without penetration into thoracic cavity**

√7ᵗʰ **S21.109** Unspecified open wound of unspecified front wall of thorax without penetration into thoracic cavity

√6ᵗʰ **S21.11** Laceration without foreign body of front wall of thorax without penetration into thoracic cavity

√7ᵗʰ **S21.111** Laceration without foreign body of right front wall of thorax without penetration into thoracic cavity

√7ᵗʰ **S21.112** Laceration without foreign body of left front wall of thorax without penetration into thoracic cavity

√7ᵗʰ **S21.119** Laceration without foreign body of unspecified front wall of thorax without penetration into thoracic cavity

√6ᵗʰ **S21.12** Laceration with foreign body of front wall of thorax without penetration into thoracic cavity

√7ᵗʰ **S21.121** Laceration with foreign body of right front wall of thorax without penetration into thoracic cavity

√7ᵗʰ **S21.122** Laceration with foreign body of left front wall of thorax without penetration into thoracic cavity

√7ᵗʰ **S21.129** Laceration with foreign body of unspecified front wall of thorax without penetration into thoracic cavity

√6ᵗʰ **S21.13** Puncture wound without foreign body of front wall of thorax without penetration into thoracic cavity

√7ᵗʰ **S21.131** Puncture wound without foreign body of right front wall of thorax without penetration into thoracic cavity

√7ᵗʰ **S21.132** Puncture wound without foreign body of left front wall of thorax without penetration into thoracic cavity

√7ᵗʰ **S21.139** Puncture wound without foreign body of unspecified front wall of thorax without penetration into thoracic cavity

√6ᵗʰ **S21.14** Puncture wound with foreign body of front wall of thorax without penetration into thoracic cavity

√7ᵗʰ **S21.141** Puncture wound with foreign body of right front wall of thorax without penetration into thoracic cavity

√7ᵗʰ **S21.142** Puncture wound with foreign body of left front wall of thorax without penetration into thoracic cavity

√7ᵗʰ **S21.149** Puncture wound with foreign body of unspecified front wall of thorax without penetration into thoracic cavity

√6ᵗʰ **S21.15** Open bite of front wall of thorax without penetration into thoracic cavity
Bite of front wall of thorax NOS
EXCLUDES 1   superficial bite of front wall of thorax (S20.37)

√7ᵗʰ **S21.151** Open bite of right front wall of thorax without penetration into thoracic cavity

√7ᵗʰ **S21.152** Open bite of left front wall of thorax without penetration into thoracic cavity

√7ᵗʰ **S21.159** Open bite of unspecified front wall of thorax without penetration into thoracic cavity

√5ᵗʰ **S21.2** Open wound of back wall of thorax without penetration into thoracic cavity

√6ᵗʰ **S21.20** Unspecified open wound of back wall of thorax without penetration into thoracic cavity

√7ᵗʰ **S21.201** Unspecified open wound of right back wall of thorax without penetration into thoracic cavity

√7ᵗʰ **S21.202** Unspecified open wound of left back wall of thorax without penetration into thoracic cavity

√7ᵗʰ **S21.209** Unspecified open wound of unspecified back wall of thorax without penetration into thoracic cavity

√6ᵗʰ **S21.21** Laceration without foreign body of back wall of thorax without penetration into thoracic cavity

√7ᵗʰ **S21.211** Laceration without foreign body of right back wall of thorax without penetration into thoracic cavity

√7ᵗʰ **S21.212** Laceration without foreign body of left back wall of thorax without penetration into thoracic cavity

√7ᵗʰ **S21.219** Laceration without foreign body of unspecified back wall of thorax without penetration into thoracic cavity

√6ᵗʰ **S21.22** Laceration with foreign body of back wall of thorax without penetration into thoracic cavity

√7ᵗʰ **S21.221** Laceration with foreign body of right back wall of thorax without penetration into thoracic cavity

√7ᵗʰ **S21.222** Laceration with foreign body of left back wall of thorax without penetration into thoracic cavity

√7ᵗʰ **S21.229** Laceration with foreign body of unspecified back wall of thorax without penetration into thoracic cavity

√6ᵗʰ **S21.23** Puncture wound without foreign body of back wall of thorax without penetration into thoracic cavity

√7ᵗʰ **S21.231** Puncture wound without foreign body of right back wall of thorax without penetration into thoracic cavity

√7ᵗʰ **S21.232** Puncture wound without foreign body of left back wall of thorax without penetration into thoracic cavity

√7ᵗʰ **S21.239** Puncture wound without foreign body of unspecified back wall of thorax without penetration into thoracic cavity

√6ᵗʰ **S21.24** Puncture wound with foreign body of back wall of thorax without penetration into thoracic cavity

√7ᵗʰ **S21.241** Puncture wound with foreign body of right back wall of thorax without penetration into thoracic cavity

√7ᵗʰ **S21.242** Puncture wound with foreign body of left back wall of thorax without penetration into thoracic cavity

√7ᵗʰ **S21.249** Puncture wound with foreign body of unspecified back wall of thorax without penetration into thoracic cavity

√6ᵗʰ **S21.25** Open bite of back wall of thorax without penetration into thoracic cavity
Bite of back wall of thorax NOS
EXCLUDES 1   superficial bite of back wall of thorax (S20.47)

√7ᵗʰ **S21.251** Open bite of right back wall of thorax without penetration into thoracic cavity

√7ᵗʰ **S21.252** Open bite of left back wall of thorax without penetration into thoracic cavity

√7ᵗʰ **S21.259** Open bite of unspecified back wall of thorax without penetration into thoracic cavity

√5ᵗʰ **S21.3** Open wound of front wall of thorax with penetration into thoracic cavity
Open wound of chest with penetration into thoracic cavity

√6ᵗʰ **S21.30** Unspecified open wound of front wall of thorax with penetration into thoracic cavity

√7ᵗʰ **S21.301** Unspecified open wound of right front wall of thorax with penetration into thoracic cavity

√7ᵗʰ **S21.302** Unspecified open wound of left front wall of thorax with penetration into thoracic cavity

√7ᵗʰ **S21.309** Unspecified open wound of unspecified front wall of thorax with penetration into thoracic cavity

√6ᵗʰ **S21.31** Laceration without foreign body of front wall of thorax with penetration into thoracic cavity

√7ᵗʰ **S21.311** Laceration without foreign body of right front wall of thorax with penetration into thoracic cavity

√7ᵗʰ **S21.312** Laceration without foreign body of left front wall of thorax with penetration into thoracic cavity

√7ᵗʰ **S21.319** Laceration without foreign body of unspecified front wall of thorax with penetration into thoracic cavity

√6ᵗʰ **S21.32** Laceration with foreign body of front wall of thorax with penetration into thoracic cavity

√7ᵗʰ **S21.321** Laceration with foreign body of right front wall of thorax with penetration into thoracic cavity

√7ᵗʰ **S21.322** Laceration with foreign body of left front wall of thorax with penetration into thoracic cavity

√7ᵗʰ **S21.329** Laceration with foreign body of unspecified front wall of thorax with penetration into thoracic cavity

✓6ᵗʰ **S21.33** Puncture wound without foreign body of front wall of thorax with penetration into thoracic cavity

     ✓7ᵗʰ **S21.331** Puncture wound without foreign body of right front wall of thorax with penetration into thoracic cavity

     ✓7ᵗʰ **S21.332** Puncture wound without foreign body of left front wall of thorax with penetration into thoracic cavity

     ✓7ᵗʰ **S21.339** Puncture wound without foreign body of unspecified front wall of thorax with penetration into thoracic cavity

✓6ᵗʰ **S21.34** Puncture wound with foreign body of front wall of thorax with penetration into thoracic cavity

     ✓7ᵗʰ **S21.341** Puncture wound with foreign body of right front wall of thorax with penetration into thoracic cavity

     ✓7ᵗʰ **S21.342** Puncture wound with foreign body of left front wall of thorax with penetration into thoracic cavity

     ✓7ᵗʰ **S21.349** Puncture wound with foreign body of unspecified front wall of thorax with penetration into thoracic cavity

✓6ᵗʰ **S21.35** Open bite of front wall of thorax with penetration into thoracic cavity

     EXCLUDES 1 superficial bite of front wall of thorax (S20.37)

     ✓7ᵗʰ **S21.351** Open bite of right front wall of thorax with penetration into thoracic cavity

     ✓7ᵗʰ **S21.352** Open bite of left front wall of thorax with penetration into thoracic cavity

     ✓7ᵗʰ **S21.359** Open bite of unspecified front wall of thorax with penetration into thoracic cavity

✓5ᵗʰ **S21.4** Open wound of back wall of thorax with penetration into thoracic cavity

     ✓6ᵗʰ **S21.40** Unspecified open wound of back wall of thorax with penetration into thoracic cavity

     ✓7ᵗʰ **S21.401** Unspecified open wound of right back wall of thorax with penetration into thoracic cavity

     ✓7ᵗʰ **S21.402** Unspecified open wound of left back wall of thorax with penetration into thoracic cavity

     ✓7ᵗʰ **S21.409** Unspecified open wound of unspecified back wall of thorax with penetration into thoracic cavity

✓6ᵗʰ **S21.41** Laceration without foreign body of back wall of thorax with penetration into thoracic cavity

     ✓7ᵗʰ **S21.411** Laceration without foreign body of right back wall of thorax with penetration into thoracic cavity

     ✓7ᵗʰ **S21.412** Laceration without foreign body of left back wall of thorax with penetration into thoracic cavity

     ✓7ᵗʰ **S21.419** Laceration without foreign body of unspecified back wall of thorax with penetration into thoracic cavity

✓6ᵗʰ **S21.42** Laceration with foreign body of back wall of thorax with penetration into thoracic cavity

     ✓7ᵗʰ **S21.421** Laceration with foreign body of right back wall of thorax with penetration into thoracic cavity

     ✓7ᵗʰ **S21.422** Laceration with foreign body of left back wall of thorax with penetration into thoracic cavity

     ✓7ᵗʰ **S21.429** Laceration with foreign body of unspecified back wall of thorax with penetration into thoracic cavity

✓6ᵗʰ **S21.43** Puncture wound without foreign body of back wall of thorax with penetration into thoracic cavity

     ✓7ᵗʰ **S21.431** Puncture wound without foreign body of right back wall of thorax with penetration into thoracic cavity

     ✓7ᵗʰ **S21.432** Puncture wound without foreign body of left back wall of thorax with penetration into thoracic cavity

     ✓7ᵗʰ **S21.439** Puncture wound without foreign body of unspecified back wall of thorax with penetration into thoracic cavity

✓6ᵗʰ **S21.44** Puncture wound with foreign body of back wall of thorax with penetration into thoracic cavity

     ✓7ᵗʰ **S21.441** Puncture wound with foreign body of right back wall of thorax with penetration into thoracic cavity

     ✓7ᵗʰ **S21.442** Puncture wound with foreign body of left back wall of thorax with penetration into thoracic cavity

     ✓7ᵗʰ **S21.449** Puncture wound with foreign body of unspecified back wall of thorax with penetration into thoracic cavity

✓6ᵗʰ **S21.45** Open bite of back wall of thorax with penetration into thoracic cavity

     Bite of back wall of thorax NOS

     EXCLUDES 1 superficial bite of back wall of thorax (S20.47)

     ✓7ᵗʰ **S21.451** Open bite of right back wall of thorax with penetration into thoracic cavity

     ✓7ᵗʰ **S21.452** Open bite of left back wall of thorax with penetration into thoracic cavity

     ✓7ᵗʰ **S21.459** Open bite of unspecified back wall of thorax with penetration into thoracic cavity

✓5ᵗʰ **S21.9** Open wound of unspecified part of thorax

     Open wound of thoracic wall NOS

     ✓x7ᵗʰ **S21.90** Unspecified open wound of unspecified part of thorax

     ✓x7ᵗʰ **S21.91** Laceration without foreign body of unspecified part of thorax

     ✓x7ᵗʰ **S21.92** Laceration with foreign body of unspecified part of thorax

     ✓x7ᵗʰ **S21.93** Puncture wound without foreign body of unspecified part of thorax

     ✓x7ᵗʰ **S21.94** Puncture wound with foreign body of unspecified part of thorax

     ✓x7ᵗʰ **S21.95** Open bite of unspecified part of thorax

     EXCLUDES 1 superficial bite of thorax (S20.97)

✓4ᵗʰ **S22** **Fracture of rib(s), sternum and thoracic spine**

     NOTE A fracture not indicated as displaced or nondisplaced should be coded to displaced

     A fracture not indicated as open or closed should be coded to closed

     INCLUDES fracture of thoracic neural arch

     fracture of thoracic spinous process

     fracture of thoracic transverse process

     fracture of thoracic vertebra

     fracture of thoracic vertebral arch

     Code first any associated:

     injury of intrathoracic organ (S27.-)

     spinal cord injury (S24.0-, S24.1-)

     EXCLUDES 1 transection of thorax (S28.1)

     EXCLUDES 2 fracture of clavicle (S42.0-)

     fracture of scapula (S42.1-)

     AHA: 2021,1Q,6; 2018,2Q,12; 2015,3Q,37-39

     The appropriate 7th character is to be added to each code from category S22.

     A   initial encounter for closed fracture

     B   initial encounter for open fracture

     D   subsequent encounter for fracture with routine healing

     G   subsequent encounter for fracture with delayed healing

     K   subsequent encounter for fracture with nonunion

     S   sequela

✓5ᵗʰ **S22.0** **Fracture of thoracic vertebra**

     ✓6ᵗʰ **S22.00** Fracture of unspecified thoracic vertebra

     ¹ ✓7ᵗʰ **S22.000** Wedge compression fracture of unspecified thoracic vertebra   HCC ESR COM Q

     ¹ ✓7ᵗʰ **S22.001** Stable burst fracture of unspecified thoracic vertebra   HCC ESR COM Q

     ¹ ✓7ᵗʰ **S22.002** Unstable burst fracture of unspecified thoracic vertebra   HCC ESR COM Q

     ¹ ✓7ᵗʰ **S22.008** Other fracture of unspecified thoracic vertebra   HCC ESR COM Q

     ¹ ✓7ᵗʰ **S22.009** Unspecified fracture of unspecified thoracic vertebra   HCC ESR COM Q

     ✓6ᵗʰ **S22.01** Fracture of first thoracic vertebra

     ¹ ✓7ᵗʰ **S22.010** Wedge compression fracture of first thoracic vertebra   HCC ESR COM Q

     ¹ ✓7ᵗʰ **S22.011** Stable burst fracture of first thoracic vertebra   HCC ESR COM Q

     ¹ ✓7ᵗʰ **S22.012** Unstable burst fracture of first thoracic vertebra   HCC ESR COM Q

HCC CMS-HCC   **Rx** Rx HCC   **ESR** ESRD HCC   **COM** Commercial HCC   **N** Newborn: 0   **P** Pediatric: 0-17   **M** Maternity: 9-64   **A** Adult: 15-124

1014   ICD-10-CM 2023

¹ √7ᵗʰ **S22.018** Other fracture of first thoracic vertebra `HCC` `ESR` `COM` `Q`

¹ √7ᵗʰ **S22.019** Unspecified fracture of first thoracic vertebra `HCC` `ESR` `COM` `Q`

√6ᵗʰ **S22.02** Fracture of second thoracic vertebra

  ¹ √7ᵗʰ **S22.020** Wedge compression fracture of second thoracic vertebra `HCC` `ESR` `COM`

  ¹ √7ᵗʰ **S22.021** Stable burst fracture of second thoracic vertebra `HCC` `ESR` `COM`

  ¹ √7ᵗʰ **S22.022** Unstable burst fracture of second thoracic vertebra `HCC` `ESR` `COM`

  ¹ √7ᵗʰ **S22.028** Other fracture of second thoracic vertebra `HCC` `ESR` `COM`

  ¹ √7ᵗʰ **S22.029** Unspecified fracture of second thoracic vertebra `HCC` `ESR` `COM`

√6ᵗʰ **S22.03** Fracture of third thoracic vertebra

  ¹ √7ᵗʰ **S22.030** Wedge compression fracture of third thoracic vertebra `HCC` `ESR` `COM`

  ¹ √7ᵗʰ **S22.031** Stable burst fracture of third thoracic vertebra `HCC` `ESR` `COM`

  ¹ √7ᵗʰ **S22.032** Unstable burst fracture of third thoracic vertebra `HCC` `ESR` `COM`

  ¹ √7ᵗʰ **S22.038** Other fracture of third thoracic vertebra `HCC` `ESR` `COM`

  ¹ √7ᵗʰ **S22.039** Unspecified fracture of third thoracic vertebra `HCC` `ESR` `COM`

√6ᵗʰ **S22.04** Fracture of fourth thoracic vertebra

  ¹ √7ᵗʰ **S22.040** Wedge compression fracture of fourth thoracic vertebra `HCC` `ESR` `COM`

  ¹ √7ᵗʰ **S22.041** Stable burst fracture of fourth thoracic vertebra `HCC` `ESR` `COM`

  ¹ √7ᵗʰ **S22.042** Unstable burst fracture of fourth thoracic vertebra `HCC` `ESR` `COM`

  ¹ √7ᵗʰ **S22.048** Other fracture of fourth thoracic vertebra `HCC` `ESR` `COM`

  ¹ √7ᵗʰ **S22.049** Unspecified fracture of fourth thoracic vertebra `HCC` `ESR` `COM`

√6ᵗʰ **S22.05** Fracture of T5-T6 vertebra

  ¹ √7ᵗʰ **S22.050** Wedge compression fracture of T5-T6 vertebra `HCC` `ESR` `COM`

  ¹ √7ᵗʰ **S22.051** Stable burst fracture of T5-T6 vertebra `HCC` `ESR` `COM`

  ¹ √7ᵗʰ **S22.052** Unstable burst fracture of T5-T6 vertebra `HCC` `ESR` `COM`

  ¹ √7ᵗʰ **S22.058** Other fracture of T5-T6 vertebra `HCC` `ESR` `COM`

  ¹ √7ᵗʰ **S22.059** Unspecified fracture of T5-T6 vertebra `HCC` `ESR` `COM`

√6ᵗʰ **S22.06** Fracture of T7-T8 vertebra

  ¹ √7ᵗʰ **S22.060** Wedge compression fracture of T7-T8 vertebra `HCC` `ESR` `COM`

  ¹ √7ᵗʰ **S22.061** Stable burst fracture of T7-T8 vertebra `HCC` `ESR` `COM`

  ¹ √7ᵗʰ **S22.062** Unstable burst fracture of T7-T8 vertebra `HCC` `ESR` `COM`

  ¹ √7ᵗʰ **S22.068** Other fracture of T7-T8 thoracic vertebra `HCC` `ESR` `COM`

  ¹ √7ᵗʰ **S22.069** Unspecified fracture of T7-T8 vertebra `HCC` `ESR` `COM`

√6ᵗʰ **S22.07** Fracture of T9-T10 vertebra

  ¹ √7ᵗʰ **S22.070** Wedge compression fracture of T9-T10 vertebra `HCC` `ESR` `COM`

  ¹ √7ᵗʰ **S22.071** Stable burst fracture of T9-T10 vertebra `HCC` `ESR` `COM`

  ¹ √7ᵗʰ **S22.072** Unstable burst fracture of T9-T10 vertebra `HCC` `ESR` `COM`

  ¹ √7ᵗʰ **S22.078** Other fracture of T9-T10 vertebra `HCC` `ESR` `COM`

  ¹ √7ᵗʰ **S22.079** Unspecified fracture of T9-T10 vertebra `HCC` `ESR` `COM`

√6ᵗʰ **S22.08** Fracture of T11-T12 vertebra

  ¹ √7ᵗʰ **S22.080** Wedge compression fracture of T11-T12 vertebra `HCC` `ESR` `COM`

  ¹ √7ᵗʰ **S22.081** Stable burst fracture of T11-T12 vertebra `HCC` `ESR` `COM`

  ¹ √7ᵗʰ **S22.082** Unstable burst fracture of T11-T12 vertebra `HCC` `ESR` `COM`

---

¹ √7ᵗʰ **S22.088** Other fracture of T11-T12 vertebra `HCC` `ESR` `COM` `Q`

¹ √7ᵗʰ **S22.089** Unspecified fracture of T11-T12 vertebra `HCC` `ESR` `COM` `Q`

√5ᵗʰ **S22.2** Fracture of sternum

  DEF: Break in flat bone (breast bone) in the anterior thorax caused by blunt trauma to the anterior chest.

√x7ᵗʰ **S22.20** Unspecified fracture of sternum `Q`

√x7ᵗʰ **S22.21** Fracture of manubrium `Q`

√x7ᵗʰ **S22.22** Fracture of body of sternum `Q`

√x7ᵗʰ **S22.23** Sternal manubrial dissociation `Q`

√x7ᵗʰ **S22.24** Fracture of xiphoid process `Q`

√5ᵗʰ **S22.3** Fracture of one rib

  AHA: 2021,1Q,5

√x7ᵗʰ **S22.31** Fracture of one rib, right side `Q`

√x7ᵗʰ **S22.32** Fracture of one rib, left side `Q`

√x7ᵗʰ **S22.39** Fracture of one rib, unspecified side `Q`

√5ᵗʰ **S22.4** Multiple fractures of ribs

  Fractures of two or more ribs

  `EXCLUDES 1`   flail chest (S22.5-)

  AHA: 2021,1Q,5

√x7ᵗʰ **S22.41** Multiple fractures of ribs, right side `Q`

√x7ᵗʰ **S22.42** Multiple fractures of ribs, left side `Q`

√x7ᵗʰ **S22.43** Multiple fractures of ribs, bilateral `Q`

√x7ᵗʰ **S22.49** Multiple fractures of ribs, unspecified side `Q`

√x7ᵗʰ **S22.5** Flail chest `Q`

√x7ᵗʰ **S22.9** Fracture of bony thorax, part unspecified `Q`

√4ᵗʰ **S23** Dislocation and sprain of joints and ligaments of thorax

  `INCLUDES`   avulsion of joint or ligament of thorax

      laceration of cartilage, joint or ligament of thorax

      sprain of cartilage, joint or ligament of thorax

      traumatic hemarthrosis of joint or ligament of thorax

      traumatic rupture of joint or ligament of thorax

      traumatic subluxation of joint or ligament of thorax

      traumatic tear of joint or ligament of thorax

  Code also any associated open wound

  `EXCLUDES 2`   dislocation, sprain of sternoclavicular joint (S43.2, S43.6)

      strain of muscle or tendon of thorax (S29.01-)

> The appropriate 7th character is to be added to each code from category S23.
> A   initial encounter
> D   subsequent encounter
> S   sequela

√x7ᵗʰ **S23.0** Traumatic rupture of thoracic intervertebral disc

  `EXCLUDES 1`   rupture or displacement (nontraumatic) of thoracic intervertebral disc NOS (M51.- with fifth character 4)

√5ᵗʰ **S23.1** Subluxation and dislocation of thoracic vertebra

  Code also any associated:

     open wound of thorax (S21.-)

     spinal cord injury (S24.0-, S24.1-)

  `EXCLUDES 2`   fracture of thoracic vertebrae (S22.0-)

√6ᵗʰ **S23.10** Subluxation and dislocation of unspecified thoracic vertebra

  √7ᵗʰ **S23.100** Subluxation of unspecified thoracic vertebra

  √7ᵗʰ **S23.101** Dislocation of unspecified thoracic vertebra

√6ᵗʰ **S23.11** Subluxation and dislocation of T1/T2 thoracic vertebra

  √7ᵗʰ **S23.110** Subluxation of T1/T2 thoracic vertebra

  √7ᵗʰ **S23.111** Dislocation of T1/T2 thoracic vertebra

√6ᵗʰ **S23.12** Subluxation and dislocation of T2/T3-T3/T4 thoracic vertebra

  √7ᵗʰ **S23.120** Subluxation of T2/T3 thoracic vertebra

  √7ᵗʰ **S23.121** Dislocation of T2/T3 thoracic vertebra

  √7ᵗʰ **S23.122** Subluxation of T3/T4 thoracic vertebra

  √7ᵗʰ **S23.123** Dislocation of T3/T4 thoracic vertebra

√6ᵗʰ **S23.13** Subluxation and dislocation of T4/T5-T5/T6 thoracic vertebra

  √7ᵗʰ **S23.130** Subluxation of T4/T5 thoracic vertebra

  √7ᵗʰ **S23.131** Dislocation of T4/T5 thoracic vertebra

        √7ᵗʰ **S23.132** Subluxation of T5/T6 thoracic vertebra

        √7ᵗʰ **S23.133** Dislocation of T5/T6 thoracic vertebra

    √6ᵗʰ **S23.14** **Subluxation and dislocation of** T6/T7-T7/T8 **thoracic vertebra**

        √7ᵗʰ **S23.140** Subluxation of T6/T7 thoracic vertebra

        √7ᵗʰ **S23.141** Dislocation of T6/T7 thoracic vertebra

        √7ᵗʰ **S23.142** Subluxation of T7/T8 thoracic vertebra

        √7ᵗʰ **S23.143** Dislocation of T7/T8 thoracic vertebra

    √6ᵗʰ **S23.15** **Subluxation and dislocation of** T8/T9-T9/T10 **thoracic vertebra**

        √7ᵗʰ **S23.150** Subluxation of T8/T9 thoracic vertebra

        √7ᵗʰ **S23.151** Dislocation of T8/T9 thoracic vertebra

        √7ᵗʰ **S23.152** Subluxation of T9/T10 thoracic vertebra

        √7ᵗʰ **S23.153** Dislocation of T9/T10 thoracic vertebra

    √6ᵗʰ **S23.16** **Subluxation and dislocation of** T10/T11-T11/T12 **thoracic vertebra**

        √7ᵗʰ **S23.160** Subluxation of T10/T11 thoracic vertebra

        √7ᵗʰ **S23.161** Dislocation of T10/T11 thoracic vertebra

        √7ᵗʰ **S23.162** Subluxation of T11/T12 thoracic vertebra

        √7ᵗʰ **S23.163** Dislocation of T11/T12 thoracic vertebra

    √6ᵗʰ **S23.17** **Subluxation and dislocation of** T12/L1 **thoracic vertebra**

        √7ᵗʰ **S23.170** Subluxation of T12/L1 thoracic vertebra

        √7ᵗʰ **S23.171** Dislocation of T12/L1 thoracic vertebra

  √5ᵗʰ **S23.2** **Dislocation of other and unspecified parts of thorax**

    √x7ᵗʰ **S23.20** **Dislocation of unspecified part of thorax**

    √x7ᵗʰ **S23.29** **Dislocation of other parts of thorax**

  √x7ᵗʰ **S23.3** **Sprain of ligaments of thoracic spine**

  √5ᵗʰ **S23.4** **Sprain of ribs and sternum**

    √x7ᵗʰ **S23.41** **Sprain of ribs**

    √6ᵗʰ **S23.42** **Sprain of sternum**

        √7ᵗʰ **S23.420** Sprain of sternoclavicular (joint) (ligament)

        √7ᵗʰ **S23.421** Sprain of chondrosternal joint

        √7ᵗʰ **S23.428** Other sprain of sternum

        √7ᵗʰ **S23.429** Unspecified sprain of sternum

  √x7ᵗʰ **S23.8** **Sprain of other specified parts of thorax**

  √x7ᵗʰ **S23.9** **Sprain of unspecified parts of thorax**

√4ᵗʰ **S24** **Injury of nerves and spinal cord at thorax level**

> **NOTE**   Code to highest level of thoracic spinal cord injury.
>
> Injuries to the spinal cord (S24.0 and S24.1) refer to the cord level and not bone level injury, and can affect nerve roots at and below the level given.

Code also any associated:
   fracture of thoracic vertebra (S22.0-)
   open wound of thorax (S21.-)
   transient paralysis (R29.5)

EXCLUDES 2   *injury of brachial plexus (S14.3)*

> The appropriate 7th character is to be added to each code from category S24.
> A   initial encounter
> D   subsequent encounter
> S   sequela

  √x7ᵗʰ **S24.0** **Concussion and edema of thoracic spinal cord** HCC ESR COM

  √5ᵗʰ **S24.1** **Other and unspecified injuries of thoracic spinal cord**

    √6ᵗʰ **S24.10** **Unspecified injury of thoracic spinal cord**

        √7ᵗʰ **S24.101** Unspecified injury at T1 level of thoracic spinal cord HCC ESR COM

        √7ᵗʰ **S24.102** Unspecified injury at T2-T6 level of thoracic spinal cord HCC ESR COM

        √7ᵗʰ **S24.103** Unspecified injury at T7-T10 level of thoracic spinal cord HCC ESR COM

        √7ᵗʰ **S24.104** Unspecified injury at T11-T12 level of thoracic spinal cord HCC ESR COM

        √7ᵗʰ **S24.109** Unspecified injury at unspecified level of thoracic spinal cord HCC ESR COM

            Injury of thoracic spinal cord NOS

    √6ᵗʰ **S24.11** **Complete lesion of thoracic spinal cord**

        √7ᵗʰ **S24.111** Complete lesion at T1 level of thoracic spinal cord HCC ESR COM

        √7ᵗʰ **S24.112** Complete lesion at T2-T6 level of thoracic spinal cord HCC ESR COM

        √7ᵗʰ **S24.113** Complete lesion at T7-T10 level of thoracic spinal cord HCC ESR COM

        √7ᵗʰ **S24.114** Complete lesion at T11-T12 level of thoracic spinal cord HCC ESR COM

        √7ᵗʰ **S24.119** Complete lesion at unspecified level of thoracic spinal cord HCC ESR COM

    √6ᵗʰ **S24.13** **Anterior cord syndrome of thoracic spinal cord**

        √7ᵗʰ **S24.131** Anterior cord syndrome at T1 level of thoracic spinal cord HCC ESR COM

        √7ᵗʰ **S24.132** Anterior cord syndrome at T2-T6 level of thoracic spinal cord HCC ESR COM

        √7ᵗʰ **S24.133** Anterior cord syndrome at T7-T10 level of thoracic spinal cord HCC ESR COM

        √7ᵗʰ **S24.134** Anterior cord syndrome at T11-T12 level of thoracic spinal cord HCC ESR COM

        √7ᵗʰ **S24.139** Anterior cord syndrome at unspecified level of thoracic spinal cord HCC ESR COM

    √6ᵗʰ **S24.14** **Brown-Séquard syndrome of thoracic spinal cord**

        √7ᵗʰ **S24.141** Brown-Séquard syndrome at T1 level of thoracic spinal cord HCC ESR COM

        √7ᵗʰ **S24.142** Brown-Séquard syndrome at T2-T6 level of thoracic spinal cord HCC ESR COM

        √7ᵗʰ **S24.143** Brown-Séquard syndrome at T7-T10 level of thoracic spinal cord HCC ESR COM

        √7ᵗʰ **S24.144** Brown-Séquard syndrome at T11-T12 level of thoracic spinal cord HCC ESR COM

        √7ᵗʰ **S24.149** Brown-Séquard syndrome at unspecified level of thoracic spinal cord HCC ESR COM

    √6ᵗʰ **S24.15** **Other incomplete lesions of thoracic spinal cord**

        Incomplete lesion of thoracic spinal cord NOS
        Posterior cord syndrome of thoracic spinal cord

        √7ᵗʰ **S24.151** Other incomplete lesion at T1 level of thoracic spinal cord HCC ESR COM

        √7ᵗʰ **S24.152** Other incomplete lesion at T2-T6 level of thoracic spinal cord HCC ESR COM

        √7ᵗʰ **S24.153** Other incomplete lesion at T7-T10 level of thoracic spinal cord HCC ESR COM

        √7ᵗʰ **S24.154** Other incomplete lesion at T11-T12 level of thoracic spinal cord HCC ESR COM

        √7ᵗʰ **S24.159** Other incomplete lesion at unspecified level of thoracic spinal cord HCC ESR COM

  √x7ᵗʰ **S24.2** **Injury of nerve root of thoracic spine**

  √x7ᵗʰ **S24.3** **Injury of peripheral nerves of thorax**

  √x7ᵗʰ **S24.4** **Injury of thoracic sympathetic nervous system**

        Injury of cardiac plexus
        Injury of esophageal plexus
        Injury of pulmonary plexus
        Injury of stellate ganglion
        Injury of thoracic sympathetic ganglion

  √x7ᵗʰ **S24.8** **Injury of other specified nerves of thorax**

  √x7ᵗʰ **S24.9** **Injury of unspecified nerve of thorax**

√4ᵗʰ **S25** **Injury of blood vessels of thorax**

    Code also any associated open wound (S21.-)

> The appropriate 7th character is to be added to each code from category S25.
> A   initial encounter
> D   subsequent encounter
> S   sequela

  √5ᵗʰ **S25.0** **Injury of thoracic aorta**

    Injury of aorta NOS

    √x7ᵗʰ **S25.00** **Unspecified injury of thoracic aorta**

    √x7ᵗʰ **S25.01** **Minor laceration of thoracic aorta**

        Incomplete transection of thoracic aorta
        Laceration of thoracic aorta NOS
        Superficial laceration of thoracic aorta

    √x7ᵗʰ **S25.02** **Major laceration of thoracic aorta**

        Complete transection of thoracic aorta
        Traumatic rupture of thoracic aorta

    √x7ᵗʰ **S25.09** **Other specified injury of thoracic aorta**

√5ᵗʰ **S25.1 Injury of innominate or subclavian artery**

  √6ᵗʰ **S25.10 Unspecified injury of innominate or subclavian artery**

    √7ᵗʰ **S25.101 Unspecified injury of right innominate or subclavian artery**

    √7ᵗʰ **S25.102 Unspecified injury of left innominate or subclavian artery**

    √7ᵗʰ **S25.109 Unspecified injury of unspecified innominate or subclavian artery**

  √6ᵗʰ **S25.11 Minor laceration of innominate or subclavian artery**

    Incomplete transection of innominate or subclavian artery

    Laceration of innominate or subclavian artery NOS

    Superficial laceration of innominate or subclavian artery

    √7ᵗʰ **S25.111 Minor laceration of right innominate or subclavian artery**

    √7ᵗʰ **S25.112 Minor laceration of left innominate or subclavian artery**

    √7ᵗʰ **S25.119 Minor laceration of unspecified innominate or subclavian artery**

  √6ᵗʰ **S25.12 Major laceration of innominate or subclavian artery**

    Complete transection of innominate or subclavian artery

    Traumatic rupture of innominate or subclavian artery

    √7ᵗʰ **S25.121 Major laceration of right innominate or subclavian artery**

    √7ᵗʰ **S25.122 Major laceration of left innominate or subclavian artery**

    √7ᵗʰ **S25.129 Major laceration of unspecified innominate or subclavian artery**

  √6ᵗʰ **S25.19 Other specified injury of innominate or subclavian artery**

    √7ᵗʰ **S25.191 Other specified injury of right innominate or subclavian artery**

    √7ᵗʰ **S25.192 Other specified injury of left innominate or subclavian artery**

    √7ᵗʰ **S25.199 Other specified injury of unspecified innominate or subclavian artery**

√5ᵗʰ **S25.2 Injury of superior vena cava**

  Injury of vena cava NOS

  √x7ᵗʰ **S25.20 Unspecified injury of superior vena cava**

  √x7ᵗʰ **S25.21 Minor laceration of superior vena cava**

    Incomplete transection of superior vena cava

    Laceration of superior vena cava NOS

    Superficial laceration of superior vena cava

  √x7ᵗʰ **S25.22 Major laceration of superior vena cava**

    Complete transection of superior vena cava

    Traumatic rupture of superior vena cava

  √x7ᵗʰ **S25.29 Other specified injury of superior vena cava**

√5ᵗʰ **S25.3 Injury of innominate or subclavian vein**

  √6ᵗʰ **S25.30 Unspecified injury of innominate or subclavian vein**

    √7ᵗʰ **S25.301 Unspecified injury of right innominate or subclavian vein**

    √7ᵗʰ **S25.302 Unspecified injury of left innominate or subclavian vein**

    √7ᵗʰ **S25.309 Unspecified injury of unspecified innominate or subclavian vein**

  √6ᵗʰ **S25.31 Minor laceration of innominate or subclavian vein**

    Incomplete transection of innominate or subclavian vein

    Laceration of innominate or subclavian vein NOS

    Superficial laceration of innominate or subclavian vein

    √7ᵗʰ **S25.311 Minor laceration of right innominate or subclavian vein**

    √7ᵗʰ **S25.312 Minor laceration of left innominate or subclavian vein**

    √7ᵗʰ **S25.319 Minor laceration of unspecified innominate or subclavian vein**

  √6ᵗʰ **S25.32 Major laceration of innominate or subclavian vein**

    Complete transection of innominate or subclavian vein

    Traumatic rupture of innominate or subclavian vein

    √7ᵗʰ **S25.321 Major laceration of right innominate or subclavian vein**

    √7ᵗʰ **S25.322 Major laceration of left innominate or subclavian vein**

    √7ᵗʰ **S25.329 Major laceration of unspecified innominate or subclavian vein**

  √6ᵗʰ **S25.39 Other specified injury of innominate or subclavian vein**

    √7ᵗʰ **S25.391 Other specified injury of right innominate or subclavian vein**

    √7ᵗʰ **S25.392 Other specified injury of left innominate or subclavian vein**

    √7ᵗʰ **S25.399 Other specified injury of unspecified innominate or subclavian vein**

√5ᵗʰ **S25.4 Injury of pulmonary blood vessels**

  √6ᵗʰ **S25.40 Unspecified injury of pulmonary blood vessels**

    √7ᵗʰ **S25.401 Unspecified injury of right pulmonary blood vessels**

    √7ᵗʰ **S25.402 Unspecified injury of left pulmonary blood vessels**

    √7ᵗʰ **S25.409 Unspecified injury of unspecified pulmonary blood vessels**

  √6ᵗʰ **S25.41 Minor laceration of pulmonary blood vessels**

    Incomplete transection of pulmonary blood vessels

    Laceration of pulmonary blood vessels NOS

    Superficial laceration of pulmonary blood vessels

    √7ᵗʰ **S25.411 Minor laceration of right pulmonary blood vessels**

    √7ᵗʰ **S25.412 Minor laceration of left pulmonary blood vessels**

    √7ᵗʰ **S25.419 Minor laceration of unspecified pulmonary blood vessels**

  √6ᵗʰ **S25.42 Major laceration of pulmonary blood vessels**

    Complete transection of pulmonary blood vessels

    Traumatic rupture of pulmonary blood vessels

    √7ᵗʰ **S25.421 Major laceration of right pulmonary blood vessels**

    √7ᵗʰ **S25.422 Major laceration of left pulmonary blood vessels**

    √7ᵗʰ **S25.429 Major laceration of unspecified pulmonary blood vessels**

  √6ᵗʰ **S25.49 Other specified injury of pulmonary blood vessels**

    √7ᵗʰ **S25.491 Other specified injury of right pulmonary blood vessels**

    √7ᵗʰ **S25.492 Other specified injury of left pulmonary blood vessels**

    √7ᵗʰ **S25.499 Other specified injury of unspecified pulmonary blood vessels**

√5ᵗʰ **S25.5 Injury of intercostal blood vessels**

  √6ᵗʰ **S25.50 Unspecified injury of intercostal blood vessels**

    √7ᵗʰ **S25.501 Unspecified injury of intercostal blood vessels, right side**

    √7ᵗʰ **S25.502 Unspecified injury of intercostal blood vessels, left side**

    √7ᵗʰ **S25.509 Unspecified injury of intercostal blood vessels, unspecified side**

  √6ᵗʰ **S25.51 Laceration of intercostal blood vessels**

    √7ᵗʰ **S25.511 Laceration of intercostal blood vessels, right side**

    √7ᵗʰ **S25.512 Laceration of intercostal blood vessels, left side**

    √7ᵗʰ **S25.519 Laceration of intercostal blood vessels, unspecified side**

  √6ᵗʰ **S25.59 Other specified injury of intercostal blood vessels**

    √7ᵗʰ **S25.591 Other specified injury of intercostal blood vessels, right side**

    √7ᵗʰ **S25.592 Other specified injury of intercostal blood vessels, left side**

    √7ᵗʰ **S25.599 Other specified injury of intercostal blood vessels, unspecified side**

√5ᵗʰ **S25.8 Injury of other blood vessels of thorax**

  Injury of azygos vein

  Injury of mammary artery or vein

  √6ᵗʰ **S25.80 Unspecified injury of other blood vessels of thorax**

    √7ᵗʰ **S25.801 Unspecified injury of other blood vessels of thorax, right side**

    √7ᵗʰ **S25.802 Unspecified injury of other blood vessels of thorax, left side**

    √7ᵗʰ **S25.809 Unspecified injury of other blood vessels of thorax, unspecified side**

  √6ᵗʰ **S25.81 Laceration of other blood vessels of thorax**

    √7ᵗʰ **S25.811 Laceration of other blood vessels of thorax, right side**

        ✓7ᵗʰ **S25.812**   Laceration of other blood vessels of thorax, **left** side

        ✓7ᵗʰ **S25.819**   Laceration of other blood vessels of thorax, unspecified side

       ✓6ᵗʰ **S25.89**   Other specified injury of other blood vessels of thorax

        ✓7ᵗʰ **S25.891**   Other specified injury of other blood vessels of thorax, **right** side

        ✓7ᵗʰ **S25.892**   Other specified injury of other blood vessels of thorax, **left** side

        ✓7ᵗʰ **S25.899**   Other specified injury of other blood vessels of thorax, unspecified side

      ✓5ᵗʰ **S25.9**   Injury of unspecified blood vessel of thorax

       ✓×7ᵗʰ **S25.90**   Unspecified injury of unspecified blood vessel of thorax

       ✓×7ᵗʰ **S25.91**   Laceration of unspecified blood vessel of thorax

       ✓×7ᵗʰ **S25.99**   Other specified injury of unspecified blood vessel of thorax

✓4ᵗʰ **S26**   **Injury of heart**

Code also any associated:
open wound of thorax (S21.-)
traumatic hemopneumothorax (S27.2)
traumatic hemothorax (S27.1)
traumatic pneumothorax (S27.0)

> The appropriate 7th character is to be added to each code from category S26.
> A   initial encounter
> D   subsequent encounter
> S   sequela

      ✓5ᵗʰ **S26.0**   Injury of heart with hemopericardium

       ✓×7ᵗʰ **S26.00**   Unspecified injury of heart with hemopericardium

       ✓×7ᵗʰ **S26.01**   Contusion of heart with hemopericardium

       ✓6ᵗʰ **S26.02**   Laceration of heart with hemopericardium

        ✓7ᵗʰ **S26.020**   **Mild** laceration of heart with hemopericardium

         Laceration of heart without penetration of heart chamber

        ✓7ᵗʰ **S26.021**   **Moderate** laceration of heart with hemopericardium

         Laceration of heart with penetration of heart chamber

        ✓7ᵗʰ **S26.022**   **Major** laceration of heart with hemopericardium

         Laceration of heart with penetration of multiple heart chambers

       ✓×7ᵗʰ **S26.09**   Other injury of heart with hemopericardium

      ✓5ᵗʰ **S26.1**   Injury of heart without hemopericardium

       ✓×7ᵗʰ **S26.10**   Unspecified injury of heart without hemopericardium

       ✓×7ᵗʰ **S26.11**   Contusion of heart without hemopericardium

       ✓×7ᵗʰ **S26.12**   Laceration of heart without hemopericardium

       ✓×7ᵗʰ **S26.19**   Other injury of heart without hemopericardium

      ✓5ᵗʰ **S26.9**   Injury of heart, unspecified with or without hemopericardium

       ✓×7ᵗʰ **S26.90**   Unspecified injury of heart, unspecified with or without hemopericardium

       ✓×7ᵗʰ **S26.91**   Contusion of heart, unspecified with or without hemopericardium

        DEF: Bruising within the heart muscle, with no mention of an open wound, usually caused by blunt chest trauma in motor vehicle accidents, falling from great heights, or receiving CPR.

       ✓×7ᵗʰ **S26.92**   Laceration of heart, unspecified with or without hemopericardium

        Laceration of heart NOS

        AHA: 2019,2Q,24

       ✓×7ᵗʰ **S26.99**   Other injury of heart, unspecified with or without hemopericardium

✓4ᵗʰ **S27**   **Injury of other and unspecified intrathoracic organs**

Code also any associated open wound of thorax (S21.-)

EXCLUDES 2   injury of cervical esophagus (S10-S19)
               injury of trachea (cervical) (S10-S19)

> The appropriate 7th character is to be added to each code from category S27.
> A   initial encounter
> D   subsequent encounter
> S   sequela

      ✓7ᵗʰ **S27.0**   **Traumatic pneumothorax**

        EXCLUDES 1   spontaneous pneumothorax (J93.-)

      ✓7ᵗʰ **S27.1**   **Traumatic hemothorax**

      ✓7ᵗʰ **S27.2**   **Traumatic hemopneumothorax**

      ✓5ᵗʰ **S27.3**   **Other and unspecified injuries of lung**

       ✓6ᵗʰ **S27.30**   Unspecified injury of lung

        ✓7ᵗʰ **S27.301**   Unspecified injury of lung, unilateral

        ✓7ᵗʰ **S27.302**   Unspecified injury of lung, bilateral

        ✓7ᵗʰ **S27.309**   Unspecified injury of lung, unspecified

       ✓6ᵗʰ **S27.31**   Primary blast injury of lung

        Blast injury of lung NOS

        ✓7ᵗʰ **S27.311**   Primary blast injury of lung, unilateral

        ✓7ᵗʰ **S27.312**   Primary blast injury of lung, bilateral

        ✓7ᵗʰ **S27.319**   Primary blast injury of lung, unspecified

       ✓6ᵗʰ **S27.32**   Contusion of lung

        DEF: Bruising of the lung without mention of an open wound.

        ✓7ᵗʰ **S27.321**   Contusion of lung, unilateral

        ✓7ᵗʰ **S27.322**   Contusion of lung, bilateral

        ✓7ᵗʰ **S27.329**   Contusion of lung, unspecified

       ✓6ᵗʰ **S27.33**   Laceration of lung

        ✓7ᵗʰ **S27.331**   Laceration of lung, unilateral

        ✓7ᵗʰ **S27.332**   Laceration of lung, bilateral

        ✓7ᵗʰ **S27.339**   Laceration of lung, unspecified

       ✓6ᵗʰ **S27.39**   Other injuries of lung

        Secondary blast injury of lung

        ✓7ᵗʰ **S27.391**   Other injuries of lung, unilateral

        ✓7ᵗʰ **S27.392**   Other injuries of lung, bilateral

        ✓7ᵗʰ **S27.399**   Other injuries of lung, unspecified

      ✓5ᵗʰ **S27.4**   **Injury of bronchus**

       ✓6ᵗʰ **S27.40**   Unspecified injury of bronchus

        ✓7ᵗʰ **S27.401**   Unspecified injury of bronchus, unilateral

        ✓7ᵗʰ **S27.402**   Unspecified injury of bronchus, bilateral

        ✓7ᵗʰ **S27.409**   Unspecified injury of bronchus, unspecified

       ✓6ᵗʰ **S27.41**   Primary blast injury of bronchus

        Blast injury of bronchus NOS

        ✓7ᵗʰ **S27.411**   Primary blast injury of bronchus, unilateral

        ✓7ᵗʰ **S27.412**   Primary blast injury of bronchus, bilateral

        ✓7ᵗʰ **S27.419**   Primary blast injury of bronchus, unspecified

       ✓6ᵗʰ **S27.42**   Contusion of bronchus

        ✓7ᵗʰ **S27.421**   Contusion of bronchus, unilateral

        ✓7ᵗʰ **S27.422**   Contusion of bronchus, bilateral

        ✓7ᵗʰ **S27.429**   Contusion of bronchus, unspecified

       ✓6ᵗʰ **S27.43**   Laceration of bronchus

        ✓7ᵗʰ **S27.431**   Laceration of bronchus, unilateral

        ✓7ᵗʰ **S27.432**   Laceration of bronchus, bilateral

        ✓7ᵗʰ **S27.439**   Laceration of bronchus, unspecified

       ✓6ᵗʰ **S27.49**   Other injury of bronchus

        Secondary blast injury of bronchus

        ✓7ᵗʰ **S27.491**   Other injury of bronchus, unilateral

        ✓7ᵗʰ **S27.492**   Other injury of bronchus, bilateral

        ✓7ᵗʰ **S27.499**   Other injury of bronchus, unspecified

      ✓5ᵗʰ **S27.5**   **Injury of thoracic trachea**

       ✓×7ᵗʰ **S27.50**   Unspecified injury of thoracic trachea

       ✓×7ᵗʰ **S27.51**   Primary blast injury of thoracic trachea

        Blast injury of thoracic trachea NOS

       ✓×7ᵗʰ **S27.52**   Contusion of thoracic trachea

    √x 7ᵗʰ   **S27.53**   Laceration of thoracic trachea

    √x 7ᵗʰ   **S27.59**   **Other injury of thoracic trachea**

       Secondary blast injury of thoracic trachea

√5ᵗʰ   **S27.6**   **Injury of** pleura

    √x 7ᵗʰ   **S27.60**   **Unspecified injury of pleura**

    √x 7ᵗʰ   **S27.63**   Laceration of pleura

    √x 7ᵗʰ   **S27.69**   **Other injury of pleura**

√5ᵗʰ   **S27.8**   **Injury of other specified intrathoracic organs**

    √6ᵗʰ   **S27.80**   **Injury of** diaphragm

       √7ᵗʰ   **S27.802**   **Contusion of diaphragm**

       √7ᵗʰ   **S27.803**   Laceration of diaphragm

       √7ᵗʰ   **S27.808**   **Other injury of diaphragm**

       √7ᵗʰ   **S27.809**   **Unspecified injury of diaphragm**

    √6ᵗʰ   **S27.81**   **Injury of** esophagus (thoracic part)

       √7ᵗʰ   **S27.812**   **Contusion of esophagus (thoracic part)**

       √7ᵗʰ   **S27.813**   Laceration of esophagus (thoracic part)

       √7ᵗʰ   **S27.818**   **Other injury of esophagus (thoracic part)**

       √7ᵗʰ   **S27.819**   **Unspecified injury of esophagus (thoracic part)**

    √6ᵗʰ   **S27.89**   **Injury of other specified intrathoracic organs**

       Injury of lymphatic thoracic duct

       Injury of thymus gland

       √7ᵗʰ   **S27.892**   **Contusion of other specified intrathoracic organs**

       √7ᵗʰ   **S27.893**   Laceration of other specified intrathoracic organs

       √7ᵗʰ   **S27.898**   **Other injury of other specified intrathoracic organs**

       √7ᵗʰ   **S27.899**   **Unspecified injury of other specified intrathoracic organs**

√x 7ᵗʰ   **S27.9**   **Injury of unspecified intrathoracic organ**

√4ᵗʰ   **S28**   **Crushing injury of thorax, and traumatic amputation of part of thorax**

> The appropriate 7th character is to be added to each code from category S28.
> A   initial encounter
> D   subsequent encounter
> S   sequela

√x 7ᵗʰ   **S28.0**   **Crushed chest**

       Use additional code for all associated injuries

       EXCLUDES 1   flail chest (S22.5)

√x 7ᵗʰ   **S28.1**   **Traumatic amputation (partial) of** part of thorax, except breast

√5ᵗʰ   **S28.2**   **Traumatic amputation of** breast

    √6ᵗʰ   **S28.21**   **Complete traumatic amputation of breast**

       Traumatic amputation of breast NOS

       √7ᵗʰ   **S28.211**   **Complete traumatic amputation of** right **breast**

       √7ᵗʰ   **S28.212**   **Complete traumatic amputation of** left **breast**

       √7ᵗʰ   **S28.219**   **Complete traumatic amputation of unspecified breast**

    √6ᵗʰ   **S28.22**   Partial **traumatic amputation of breast**

       √7ᵗʰ   **S28.221**   **Partial traumatic amputation of** right **breast**

       √7ᵗʰ   **S28.222**   **Partial traumatic amputation of** left **breast**

       √7ᵗʰ   **S28.229**   **Partial traumatic amputation of unspecified breast**

√4ᵗʰ   **S29**   **Other and unspecified injuries of thorax**

       Code also any associated open wound (S21.-)

> The appropriate 7th character is to be added to each code from category S29.
> A   initial encounter
> D   subsequent encounter
> S   sequela

√5ᵗʰ   **S29.0**   **Injury of muscle and tendon at thorax level**

    √6ᵗʰ   **S29.00**   **Unspecified injury of muscle and tendon of thorax**

       √7ᵗʰ   **S29.001**   **Unspecified injury of muscle and tendon of** front **wall of thorax**

       √7ᵗʰ   **S29.002**   **Unspecified injury of muscle and tendon of** back **wall of thorax**

       √7ᵗʰ   **S29.009**   **Unspecified injury of muscle and tendon of unspecified wall of thorax**

    √6ᵗʰ   **S29.01**   **Strain** of muscle and tendon of thorax

       √7ᵗʰ   **S29.011**   **Strain of muscle and tendon of** front **wall of thorax**

       √7ᵗʰ   **S29.012**   **Strain of muscle and tendon of** back **wall of thorax**

       √7ᵗʰ   **S29.019**   **Strain of muscle and tendon of unspecified wall of thorax**

    √6ᵗʰ   **S29.02**   Laceration of muscle and tendon of thorax

       √7ᵗʰ   **S29.021**   Laceration of muscle and tendon of front wall of thorax

       √7ᵗʰ   **S29.022**   Laceration of muscle and tendon of back wall of thorax

       √7ᵗʰ   **S29.029**   Laceration of muscle and tendon of unspecified wall of thorax

    √6ᵗʰ   **S29.09**   **Other injury of muscle and tendon of thorax**

       √7ᵗʰ   **S29.091**   **Other injury of muscle and tendon of** front **wall of thorax**

       √7ᵗʰ   **S29.092**   **Other injury of muscle and tendon of** back **wall of thorax**

       √7ᵗʰ   **S29.099**   **Other injury of muscle and tendon of unspecified wall of thorax**

√x 7ᵗʰ   **S29.8**   **Other specified injuries of thorax**

√x 7ᵗʰ   **S29.9**   **Unspecified injury of thorax**

Injuries to the abdomen, lower back, lumbar spine, pelvis and external genitals (S30-S39)

INCLUDES   injuries to the abdominal wall
       injuries to the anus
       injuries to the buttock
       injuries to the external genitalia
       injuries to the flank
       injuries to the groin

EXCLUDES 2   burns and corrosions (T20-T32)
       effects of foreign body in anus and rectum (T18.5)
       effects of foreign body in genitourinary tract (T19.-)
       effects of foreign body in stomach, small intestine and colon (T18.2-T18.4)
       frostbite (T33-T34)
       insect bite or sting, venomous (T63.4)

√4ᵗʰ   **S30**   **Superficial injury of abdomen, lower back, pelvis and external genitals**

       EXCLUDES 2   superficial injury of hip (S70.-)

> The appropriate 7th character is to be added to each code from category S30.
> A   initial encounter
> D   subsequent encounter
> S   sequela

√x 7ᵗʰ   **S30.0**   **Contusion of lower back and pelvis**

       Contusion of buttock

√x 7ᵗʰ   **S30.1**   **Contusion of abdominal wall**

       Contusion of flank

       Contusion of groin

√5ᵗʰ   **S30.2**   **Contusion of** external genital organs

    √6ᵗʰ   **S30.20**   **Contusion of unspecified external genital organ**

       √7ᵗʰ   **S30.201**   **Contusion of unspecified external genital organ,** male   ♂

       √7ᵗʰ   **S30.202**   **Contusion of unspecified external genital organ,** female   ♀

    √x 7ᵗʰ   **S30.21**   **Contusion of** penis   ♂

    √x 7ᵗʰ   **S30.22**   **Contusion of** scrotum and testes   ♂

    √x 7ᵗʰ   **S30.23**   **Contusion of** vagina and vulva   ♀

√x 7ᵗʰ   **S30.3**   **Contusion of anus**

√5ᵗʰ   **S30.8**   **Other superficial injuries of abdomen, lower back, pelvis and external genitals**

    √6ᵗʰ   **S30.81**   Abrasion **of abdomen, lower back, pelvis and external genitals**

       √7ᵗʰ   **S30.810**   **Abrasion of** lower back and pelvis

       √7ᵗʰ   **S30.811**   **Abrasion of** abdominal wall

       √7ᵗʰ   **S30.812**   **Abrasion of** penis   ♂

       √7ᵗʰ   **S30.813**   **Abrasion of** scrotum and testes   ♂

       √7ᵗʰ   **S30.814**   **Abrasion of** vagina and vulva   ♀

       √7ᵗʰ   **S30.815**   **Abrasion of unspecified** external genital **organs, male**   ♂

√7ᵗʰ **S30.816** **Abrasion of unspecified** external genital organs, female ♀

√7ᵗʰ **S30.817** **Abrasion of** anus

√6ᵗʰ **S30.82** **Blister** (nonthermal) of abdomen, lower back, pelvis and external genitals

   √7ᵗʰ **S30.820** **Blister (nonthermal) of** lower back and pelvis

   √7ᵗʰ **S30.821** **Blister (nonthermal) of** abdominal wall

   √7ᵗʰ **S30.822** **Blister (nonthermal) of** penis ♂

   √7ᵗʰ **S30.823** **Blister (nonthermal) of** scrotum and testes ♂

   √7ᵗʰ **S30.824** **Blister (nonthermal) of** vagina and vulva ♀

   √7ᵗʰ **S30.825** **Blister (nonthermal) of unspecified** external genital organs, male ♂

   √7ᵗʰ **S30.826** **Blister (nonthermal) of unspecified** external genital organs, female ♀

   √7ᵗʰ **S30.827** **Blister (nonthermal) of** anus

√6ᵗʰ **S30.84** **External constriction of** abdomen, lower back, pelvis and external genitals

   √7ᵗʰ **S30.840** **External constriction of** lower back and pelvis

   √7ᵗʰ **S30.841** **External constriction of** abdominal wall

   √7ᵗʰ **S30.842** **External constriction of** penis ♂

       Hair tourniquet syndrome of penis
       Use additional cause code to identify the constricting item (W49.0-)

   √7ᵗʰ **S30.843** **External constriction of** scrotum and testes ♂

   √7ᵗʰ **S30.844** **External constriction of** vagina and vulva ♀

   √7ᵗʰ **S30.845** **External constriction of unspecified** external genital organs, male ♂

   √7ᵗʰ **S30.846** **External constriction of unspecified** external genital organs, female ♀

√6ᵗʰ **S30.85** **Superficial** foreign body of abdomen, lower back, pelvis and external genitals

       Splinter in the abdomen, lower back, pelvis and external genitals

   √7ᵗʰ **S30.850** **Superficial foreign body of** lower back and pelvis

   √7ᵗʰ **S30.851** **Superficial foreign body of** abdominal wall

   √7ᵗʰ **S30.852** **Superficial foreign body of** penis ♂

   √7ᵗʰ **S30.853** **Superficial foreign body of** scrotum and testes ♂

   √7ᵗʰ **S30.854** **Superficial foreign body of** vagina and vulva ♀

   √7ᵗʰ **S30.855** **Superficial foreign body of unspecified** external genital organs, male ♂

   √7ᵗʰ **S30.856** **Superficial foreign body of unspecified** external genital organs, female ♀

   √7ᵗʰ **S30.857** **Superficial foreign body of** anus

√6ᵗʰ **S30.86** **Insect bite** (nonvenomous) of abdomen, lower back, pelvis and external genitals

   √7ᵗʰ **S30.860** **Insect bite (nonvenomous) of** lower back and pelvis

   √7ᵗʰ **S30.861** **Insect bite (nonvenomous) of** abdominal wall

   √7ᵗʰ **S30.862** **Insect bite (nonvenomous) of** penis ♂

   √7ᵗʰ **S30.863** **Insect bite (nonvenomous) of** scrotum and testes ♂

   √7ᵗʰ **S30.864** **Insect bite (nonvenomous) of** vagina and vulva ♀

   √7ᵗʰ **S30.865** **Insect bite (nonvenomous) of unspecified** external genital organs, male ♂

   √7ᵗʰ **S30.866** **Insect bite (nonvenomous) of unspecified** external genital organs, female ♀

   √7ᵗʰ **S30.867** **Insect bite (nonvenomous) of** anus

√6ᵗʰ **S30.87** **Other superficial** bite of abdomen, lower back, pelvis and external genitals

    EXCLUDES 1   *open bite of abdomen, lower back, pelvis and external genitals (S31.05, S31.15, S31.25, S31.35, S31.45, S31.55)*

   √7ᵗʰ **S30.870** **Other superficial bite of** lower back and pelvis

   √7ᵗʰ **S30.871** **Other superficial bite of** abdominal wall

   √7ᵗʰ **S30.872** **Other superficial bite of** penis ♂

√7ᵗʰ **S30.873** **Other superficial bite of** scrotum and testes ♂

√7ᵗʰ **S30.874** **Other superficial bite of** vagina and vulva ♀

√7ᵗʰ **S30.875** **Other superficial bite of unspecified** external genital organs, male ♂

√7ᵗʰ **S30.876** **Other superficial bite of unspecified** external genital organs, female ♀

√7ᵗʰ **S30.877** **Other superficial bite of** anus

√5ᵗʰ **S30.9** **Unspecified superficial injury of abdomen, lower back, pelvis and external genitals**

   √x7ᵗʰ **S30.91** **Unspecified superficial injury of** lower back and pelvis

   √x7ᵗʰ **S30.92** **Unspecified superficial injury of** abdominal wall

   √x7ᵗʰ **S30.93** **Unspecified superficial injury of** penis ♂

   √x7ᵗʰ **S30.94** **Unspecified superficial injury of** scrotum and testes ♂

   √x7ᵗʰ **S30.95** **Unspecified superficial injury of** vagina and vulva ♀

   √x7ᵗʰ **S30.96** **Unspecified superficial injury of unspecified** external genital organs, male ♂

   √x7ᵗʰ **S30.97** **Unspecified superficial injury of unspecified** external genital organs, female ♀

   √x7ᵗʰ **S30.98** **Unspecified superficial injury of** anus

√4ᵗʰ **S31** **Open wound of abdomen, lower back, pelvis and external genitals**

   Code also any associated:
      spinal cord injury (S24.0, S24.1-, S34.0-, S34.1-)
      wound infection

   EXCLUDES 1   *traumatic amputation of part of abdomen, lower back and pelvis (S38.2-, S38.3)*

   EXCLUDES 2   *open wound of hip (S71.00-S71.02)*
              open fracture of pelvis (S32.1-- S32.9 with 7th character B)

   The appropriate 7th character is to be added to each code from category S31.
   A   initial encounter
   D   subsequent encounter
   S   sequela

√5ᵗʰ **S31.0** **Open wound of** lower back and pelvis

   √6ᵗʰ **S31.00** **Unspecified open wound of lower back and pelvis**

      √7ᵗʰ **S31.000** **Unspecified open wound of lower back and pelvis** without penetration into retroperitoneum
         Unspecified open wound of lower back and pelvis NOS

      √7ᵗʰ **S31.001** **Unspecified open wound of lower back and pelvis** with penetration into retroperitoneum

   √6ᵗʰ **S31.01** **Laceration** without foreign body **of lower back and pelvis**

      √7ᵗʰ **S31.010** **Laceration without foreign body of lower back and pelvis** without penetration into retroperitoneum
         Laceration without foreign body of lower back and pelvis NOS

      √7ᵗʰ **S31.011** **Laceration without foreign body of lower back and pelvis** with penetration into retroperitoneum

   √6ᵗʰ **S31.02** **Laceration with foreign body of lower back and pelvis**

      √7ᵗʰ **S31.020** **Laceration with foreign body of lower back and pelvis** without penetration into retroperitoneum
         Laceration with foreign body of lower back and pelvis NOS

      √7ᵗʰ **S31.021** **Laceration with foreign body of lower back and pelvis** with penetration into retroperitoneum

   √6ᵗʰ **S31.03** **Puncture wound without foreign body of lower back and pelvis**

      √7ᵗʰ **S31.030** **Puncture wound without foreign body of lower back and pelvis** without penetration into retroperitoneum
         Puncture wound without foreign body of lower back and pelvis NOS

      √7ᵗʰ **S31.031** **Puncture wound without foreign body of lower back and pelvis** with penetration into retroperitoneum

√6ᵗʰ **S31.04** Puncture wound with foreign body of lower back and pelvis

     √7ᵗʰ **S31.040** Puncture wound with foreign body of lower back and pelvis without penetration into retroperitoneum

       Puncture wound with foreign body of lower back and pelvis NOS

     √7ᵗʰ **S31.041** Puncture wound with foreign body of lower back and pelvis with penetration into retroperitoneum

√6ᵗʰ **S31.05** Open bite of lower back and pelvis

     Bite of lower back and pelvis NOS

     EXCLUDES 1   superficial bite of lower back and pelvis (S30.860, S30.870)

     √7ᵗʰ **S31.050** Open bite of lower back and pelvis without penetration into retroperitoneum

       Open bite of lower back and pelvis NOS

     √7ᵗʰ **S31.051** Open bite of lower back and pelvis with penetration into retroperitoneum

√5ᵗʰ **S31.1** Open wound of abdominal wall without penetration into peritoneal cavity

     Open wound of abdominal wall NOS

     EXCLUDES 2   open wound of abdominal wall with penetration into peritoneal cavity (S31.6-)

√6ᵗʰ **S31.10** Unspecified open wound of abdominal wall without penetration into peritoneal cavity

     √7ᵗʰ **S31.100** Unspecified open wound of abdominal wall, right upper quadrant without penetration into peritoneal cavity

     √7ᵗʰ **S31.101** Unspecified open wound of abdominal wall, left upper quadrant without penetration into peritoneal cavity

     √7ᵗʰ **S31.102** Unspecified open wound of abdominal wall, epigastric region without penetration into peritoneal cavity

     √7ᵗʰ **S31.103** Unspecified open wound of abdominal wall, right lower quadrant without penetration into peritoneal cavity

     √7ᵗʰ **S31.104** Unspecified open wound of abdominal wall, left lower quadrant without penetration into peritoneal cavity

     √7ᵗʰ **S31.105** Unspecified open wound of abdominal wall, periumbilic region without penetration into peritoneal cavity

     √7ᵗʰ **S31.109** Unspecified open wound of abdominal wall, unspecified quadrant without penetration into peritoneal cavity

       Unspecified open wound of abdominal wall NOS

√6ᵗʰ **S31.11** Laceration without foreign body of abdominal wall without penetration into peritoneal cavity

     √7ᵗʰ **S31.110** Laceration without foreign body of abdominal wall, right upper quadrant without penetration into peritoneal cavity

     √7ᵗʰ **S31.111** Laceration without foreign body of abdominal wall, left upper quadrant without penetration into peritoneal cavity

     √7ᵗʰ **S31.112** Laceration without foreign body of abdominal wall, epigastric region without penetration into peritoneal cavity

     √7ᵗʰ **S31.113** Laceration without foreign body of abdominal wall, right lower quadrant without penetration into peritoneal cavity

     √7ᵗʰ **S31.114** Laceration without foreign body of abdominal wall, left lower quadrant without penetration into peritoneal cavity

     √7ᵗʰ **S31.115** Laceration without foreign body of abdominal wall, periumbilic region without penetration into peritoneal cavity

     √7ᵗʰ **S31.119** Laceration without foreign body of abdominal wall, unspecified quadrant without penetration into peritoneal cavity

√6ᵗʰ **S31.12** Laceration with foreign body of abdominal wall without penetration into peritoneal cavity

     √7ᵗʰ **S31.120** Laceration of abdominal wall with foreign body, right upper quadrant without penetration into peritoneal cavity

     √7ᵗʰ **S31.121** Laceration of abdominal wall with foreign body, left upper quadrant without penetration into peritoneal cavity

     √7ᵗʰ **S31.122** Laceration of abdominal wall with foreign body, epigastric region without penetration into peritoneal cavity

     √7ᵗʰ **S31.123** Laceration of abdominal wall with foreign body, right lower quadrant without penetration into peritoneal cavity

     √7ᵗʰ **S31.124** Laceration of abdominal wall with foreign body, left lower quadrant without penetration into peritoneal cavity

     √7ᵗʰ **S31.125** Laceration of abdominal wall with foreign body, periumbilic region without penetration into peritoneal cavity

     √7ᵗʰ **S31.129** Laceration of abdominal wall with foreign body, unspecified quadrant without penetration into peritoneal cavity

√6ᵗʰ **S31.13** Puncture wound of abdominal wall without foreign body without penetration into peritoneal cavity

     √7ᵗʰ **S31.130** Puncture wound of abdominal wall without foreign body, right upper quadrant without penetration into peritoneal cavity

     √7ᵗʰ **S31.131** Puncture wound of abdominal wall without foreign body, left upper quadrant without penetration into peritoneal cavity

     √7ᵗʰ **S31.132** Puncture wound of abdominal wall without foreign body, epigastric region without penetration into peritoneal cavity

     √7ᵗʰ **S31.133** Puncture wound of abdominal wall without foreign body, right lower quadrant without penetration into peritoneal cavity

     √7ᵗʰ **S31.134** Puncture wound of abdominal wall without foreign body, left lower quadrant without penetration into peritoneal cavity

     √7ᵗʰ **S31.135** Puncture wound of abdominal wall without foreign body, periumbilic region without penetration into peritoneal cavity

     √7ᵗʰ **S31.139** Puncture wound of abdominal wall without foreign body, unspecified quadrant without penetration into peritoneal cavity

√6ᵗʰ **S31.14** Puncture wound of abdominal wall with foreign body without penetration into peritoneal cavity

     √7ᵗʰ **S31.140** Puncture wound of abdominal wall with foreign body, right upper quadrant without penetration into peritoneal cavity

     √7ᵗʰ **S31.141** Puncture wound of abdominal wall with foreign body, left upper quadrant without penetration into peritoneal cavity

     √7ᵗʰ **S31.142** Puncture wound of abdominal wall with foreign body, epigastric region without penetration into peritoneal cavity

     √7ᵗʰ **S31.143** Puncture wound of abdominal wall with foreign body, right lower quadrant without penetration into peritoneal cavity

     √7ᵗʰ **S31.144** Puncture wound of abdominal wall with foreign body, left lower quadrant without penetration into peritoneal cavity

     √7ᵗʰ **S31.145** Puncture wound of abdominal wall with foreign body, periumbilic region without penetration into peritoneal cavity

     √7ᵗʰ **S31.149** Puncture wound of abdominal wall with foreign body, unspecified quadrant without penetration into peritoneal cavity

√6ᵗʰ **S31.15** Open bite of abdominal wall without penetration into peritoneal cavity

     Bite of abdominal wall NOS

     EXCLUDES 1   superficial bite of abdominal wall (S30.871)

     √7ᵗʰ **S31.150** Open bite of abdominal wall, right upper quadrant without penetration into peritoneal cavity

√7ᵗʰ **S31.151** Open bite of abdominal wall, *left upper quadrant* without penetration into peritoneal cavity

√7ᵗʰ **S31.152** Open bite of abdominal wall, *epigastric region* without penetration into peritoneal cavity

√7ᵗʰ **S31.153** Open bite of abdominal wall, *right lower quadrant* without penetration into peritoneal cavity

√7ᵗʰ **S31.154** Open bite of abdominal wall, *left lower quadrant* without penetration into peritoneal cavity

√7ᵗʰ **S31.155** Open bite of abdominal wall, *periumbilic region* without penetration into peritoneal cavity

√7ᵗʰ **S31.159** Open bite of abdominal wall, unspecified quadrant without penetration into peritoneal cavity

√5ᵗʰ **S31.2** Open wound of penis

√x7ᵗʰ **S31.20** Unspecified open wound of penis ♂

√x7ᵗʰ **S31.21** Laceration without foreign body of penis ♂

√x7ᵗʰ **S31.22** Laceration with foreign body of penis ♂

√x7ᵗʰ **S31.23** Puncture wound without foreign body of penis ♂

√x7ᵗʰ **S31.24** Puncture wound with foreign body of penis ♂

√x7ᵗʰ **S31.25** Open bite of penis ♂
Bite of penis NOS
EXCLUDES 1   *superficial bite of penis (S30.862, S30.872)*

√5ᵗʰ **S31.3** Open wound of scrotum and testes

√x7ᵗʰ **S31.30** Unspecified open wound of scrotum and testes ♂

√x7ᵗʰ **S31.31** Laceration without foreign body of scrotum and testes ♂

√x7ᵗʰ **S31.32** Laceration with foreign body of scrotum and testes ♂

√x7ᵗʰ **S31.33** Puncture wound without foreign body of scrotum and testes ♂

√x7ᵗʰ **S31.34** Puncture wound with foreign body of scrotum and testes ♂

√x7ᵗʰ **S31.35** Open bite of scrotum and testes ♂
Bite of scrotum and testes NOS
EXCLUDES 1   *superficial bite of scrotum and testes (S30.863, S30.873)*

√5ᵗʰ **S31.4** Open wound of vagina and vulva
EXCLUDES 1   *injury to vagina and vulva during delivery (O70.-, O71.4)*

√x7ᵗʰ **S31.40** Unspecified open wound of vagina and vulva ♀

√x7ᵗʰ **S31.41** Laceration without foreign body of vagina and vulva ♀

√x7ᵗʰ **S31.42** Laceration with foreign body of vagina and vulva ♀

√x7ᵗʰ **S31.43** Puncture wound without foreign body of vagina and vulva ♀

√x7ᵗʰ **S31.44** Puncture wound with foreign body of vagina and vulva ♀

√x7ᵗʰ **S31.45** Open bite of vagina and vulva ♀
Bite of vagina and vulva NOS
EXCLUDES 1   *superficial bite of vagina and vulva (S30.864, S30.874)*

√5ᵗʰ **S31.5** Open wound of unspecified external genital organs
EXCLUDES 1   *traumatic amputation of external genital organs (S38.21, S38.22)*

√6ᵗʰ **S31.50** Unspecified open wound of unspecified external genital organs

√7ᵗʰ **S31.501** Unspecified open wound of unspecified external genital organs, male ♂

√7ᵗʰ **S31.502** Unspecified open wound of unspecified external genital organs, female ♀

√6ᵗʰ **S31.51** Laceration without foreign body of unspecified external genital organs

√7ᵗʰ **S31.511** Laceration without foreign body of unspecified external genital organs, male ♂

√7ᵗʰ **S31.512** Laceration without foreign body of unspecified external genital organs, female ♀

√6ᵗʰ **S31.52** Laceration with foreign body of unspecified external genital organs

√7ᵗʰ **S31.521** Laceration with foreign body of unspecified external genital organs, male ♂

√7ᵗʰ **S31.522** Laceration with foreign body of unspecified external genital organs, female ♀

√6ᵗʰ **S31.53** Puncture wound without foreign body of unspecified external genital organs

√7ᵗʰ **S31.531** Puncture wound without foreign body of unspecified external genital organs, male ♂

√7ᵗʰ **S31.532** Puncture wound without foreign body of unspecified external genital organs, female ♀

√6ᵗʰ **S31.54** Puncture wound with foreign body of unspecified external genital organs

√7ᵗʰ **S31.541** Puncture wound with foreign body of unspecified external genital organs, male ♂

√7ᵗʰ **S31.542** Puncture wound with foreign body of unspecified external genital organs, female ♀

√6ᵗʰ **S31.55** Open bite of unspecified external genital organs
Bite of unspecified external genital organs NOS
EXCLUDES 1   *superficial bite of unspecified external genital organs (S30.865, S30.866, S30.875, S30.876)*

√7ᵗʰ **S31.551** Open bite of unspecified external genital organs, male ♂

√7ᵗʰ **S31.552** Open bite of unspecified external genital organs, female ♀

√5ᵗʰ **S31.6** Open wound of abdominal wall with penetration into peritoneal cavity

√6ᵗʰ **S31.60** Unspecified open wound of abdominal wall with penetration into peritoneal cavity

√7ᵗʰ **S31.600** Unspecified open wound of abdominal wall, *right upper quadrant* with penetration into peritoneal cavity

√7ᵗʰ **S31.601** Unspecified open wound of abdominal wall, *left upper quadrant* with penetration into peritoneal cavity

√7ᵗʰ **S31.602** Unspecified open wound of abdominal wall, *epigastric region* with penetration into peritoneal cavity

√7ᵗʰ **S31.603** Unspecified open wound of abdominal wall, *right lower quadrant* with penetration into peritoneal cavity

√7ᵗʰ **S31.604** Unspecified open wound of abdominal wall, *left lower quadrant* with penetration into peritoneal cavity

√7ᵗʰ **S31.605** Unspecified open wound of abdominal wall, *periumbilic region* with penetration into peritoneal cavity

√7ᵗʰ **S31.609** Unspecified open wound of abdominal wall, unspecified quadrant with penetration into peritoneal cavity

√6ᵗʰ **S31.61** Laceration without foreign body of abdominal wall with penetration into peritoneal cavity

√7ᵗʰ **S31.610** Laceration without foreign body of abdominal wall, *right upper quadrant* with penetration into peritoneal cavity

√7ᵗʰ **S31.611** Laceration without foreign body of abdominal wall, *left upper quadrant* with penetration into peritoneal cavity

√7ᵗʰ **S31.612** Laceration without foreign body of abdominal wall, *epigastric region* with penetration into peritoneal cavity

√7ᵗʰ **S31.613** Laceration without foreign body of abdominal wall, *right lower quadrant* with penetration into peritoneal cavity

√7ᵗʰ **S31.614** Laceration without foreign body of abdominal wall, *left lower quadrant* with penetration into peritoneal cavity

√7ᵗʰ **S31.615** Laceration without foreign body of abdominal wall, *periumbilic region* with penetration into peritoneal cavity

√7ᵗʰ **S31.619** Laceration without foreign body of abdominal wall, unspecified quadrant with penetration into peritoneal cavity

✓6ᵗʰ **S31.62** Laceration with foreign body of abdominal wall with penetration into peritoneal cavity

   ✓7ᵗʰ **S31.620** Laceration with foreign body of abdominal wall, right upper quadrant with penetration into peritoneal cavity

   ✓7ᵗʰ **S31.621** Laceration with foreign body of abdominal wall, left upper quadrant with penetration into peritoneal cavity

   ✓7ᵗʰ **S31.622** Laceration with foreign body of abdominal wall, epigastric region with penetration into peritoneal cavity

   ✓7ᵗʰ **S31.623** Laceration with foreign body of abdominal wall, right lower quadrant with penetration into peritoneal cavity

   ✓7ᵗʰ **S31.624** Laceration with foreign body of abdominal wall, left lower quadrant with penetration into peritoneal cavity

   ✓7ᵗʰ **S31.625** Laceration with foreign body of abdominal wall, periumbilic region with penetration into peritoneal cavity

   ✓7ᵗʰ **S31.629** Laceration with foreign body of abdominal wall, unspecified quadrant with penetration into peritoneal cavity

✓6ᵗʰ **S31.63** Puncture wound without foreign body of abdominal wall with penetration into peritoneal cavity

   ✓7ᵗʰ **S31.630** Puncture wound without foreign body of abdominal wall, right upper quadrant with penetration into peritoneal cavity

   ✓7ᵗʰ **S31.631** Puncture wound without foreign body of abdominal wall, left upper quadrant with penetration into peritoneal cavity

   ✓7ᵗʰ **S31.632** Puncture wound without foreign body of abdominal wall, epigastric region with penetration into peritoneal cavity

   ✓7ᵗʰ **S31.633** Puncture wound without foreign body of abdominal wall, right lower quadrant with penetration into peritoneal cavity

   ✓7ᵗʰ **S31.634** Puncture wound without foreign body of abdominal wall, left lower quadrant with penetration into peritoneal cavity

   ✓7ᵗʰ **S31.635** Puncture wound without foreign body of abdominal wall, periumbilic region with penetration into peritoneal cavity

   ✓7ᵗʰ **S31.639** Puncture wound without foreign body of abdominal wall, unspecified quadrant with penetration into peritoneal cavity

✓6ᵗʰ **S31.64** Puncture wound with foreign body of abdominal wall with penetration into peritoneal cavity

   ✓7ᵗʰ **S31.640** Puncture wound with foreign body of abdominal wall, right upper quadrant with penetration into peritoneal cavity

   ✓7ᵗʰ **S31.641** Puncture wound with foreign body of abdominal wall, left upper quadrant with penetration into peritoneal cavity

   ✓7ᵗʰ **S31.642** Puncture wound with foreign body of abdominal wall, epigastric region with penetration into peritoneal cavity

   ✓7ᵗʰ **S31.643** Puncture wound with foreign body of abdominal wall, right lower quadrant with penetration into peritoneal cavity

   ✓7ᵗʰ **S31.644** Puncture wound with foreign body of abdominal wall, left lower quadrant with penetration into peritoneal cavity

   ✓7ᵗʰ **S31.645** Puncture wound with foreign body of abdominal wall, periumbilic region with penetration into peritoneal cavity

   ✓7ᵗʰ **S31.649** Puncture wound with foreign body of abdominal wall, unspecified quadrant with penetration into peritoneal cavity

✓6ᵗʰ **S31.65** Open bite of abdominal wall with penetration into peritoneal cavity

   EXCLUDES 1   superficial bite of abdominal wall (S30.861, S30.871)

   ✓7ᵗʰ **S31.650** Open bite of abdominal wall, right upper quadrant with penetration into peritoneal cavity

   ✓7ᵗʰ **S31.651** Open bite of abdominal wall, left upper quadrant with penetration into peritoneal cavity

   ✓7ᵗʰ **S31.652** Open bite of abdominal wall, epigastric region with penetration into peritoneal cavity

   ✓7ᵗʰ **S31.653** Open bite of abdominal wall, right lower quadrant with penetration into peritoneal cavity

   ✓7ᵗʰ **S31.654** Open bite of abdominal wall, left lower quadrant with penetration into peritoneal cavity

   ✓7ᵗʰ **S31.655** Open bite of abdominal wall, periumbilic region with penetration into peritoneal cavity

   ✓7ᵗʰ **S31.659** Open bite of abdominal wall, unspecified quadrant with penetration into peritoneal cavity

✓5ᵗʰ **S31.8** Open wound of other parts of abdomen, lower back and pelvis

✓6ᵗʰ **S31.80** Open wound of unspecified buttock

   ✓7ᵗʰ **S31.801** Laceration without foreign body of unspecified buttock

   ✓7ᵗʰ **S31.802** Laceration with foreign body of unspecified buttock

   ✓7ᵗʰ **S31.803** Puncture wound without foreign body of unspecified buttock

   ✓7ᵗʰ **S31.804** Puncture wound with foreign body of unspecified buttock

   ✓7ᵗʰ **S31.805** Open bite of unspecified buttock

     Bite of buttock NOS

     EXCLUDES 1   superficial bite of buttock (S30.870)

   ✓7ᵗʰ **S31.809** Unspecified open wound of unspecified buttock

✓6ᵗʰ **S31.81** Open wound of right buttock

   ✓7ᵗʰ **S31.811** Laceration without foreign body of right buttock

   ✓7ᵗʰ **S31.812** Laceration with foreign body of right buttock

   ✓7ᵗʰ **S31.813** Puncture wound without foreign body of right buttock

   ✓7ᵗʰ **S31.814** Puncture wound with foreign body of right buttock

   ✓7ᵗʰ **S31.815** Open bite of right buttock

     Bite of right buttock NOS

     EXCLUDES 1   superficial bite of buttock (S30.870)

   ✓7ᵗʰ **S31.819** Unspecified open wound of right buttock

✓6ᵗʰ **S31.82** Open wound of left buttock

   ✓7ᵗʰ **S31.821** Laceration without foreign body of left buttock

   ✓7ᵗʰ **S31.822** Laceration with foreign body of left buttock

   ✓7ᵗʰ **S31.823** Puncture wound without foreign body of left buttock

   ✓7ᵗʰ **S31.824** Puncture wound with foreign body of left buttock

   ✓7ᵗʰ **S31.825** Open bite of left buttock

     Bite of left buttock NOS

     EXCLUDES 1   superficial bite of buttock (S30.870)

   ✓7ᵗʰ **S31.829** Unspecified open wound of left buttock

✓6ᵗʰ **S31.83** Open wound of anus

   ✓7ᵗʰ **S31.831** Laceration without foreign body of anus

   ✓7ᵗʰ **S31.832** Laceration with foreign body of anus

   ✓7ᵗʰ **S31.833** Puncture wound without foreign body of anus

   ✓7ᵗʰ **S31.834** Puncture wound with foreign body of anus

   ✓7ᵗʰ **S31.835** Open bite of anus

     Bite of anus NOS

     EXCLUDES 1   superficial bite of anus (S30.877)

   ✓7ᵗʰ **S31.839** Unspecified open wound of anus

☑ Additional Character Required   ✓x7ᵗʰ Placeholder Alert   Manifestation   Unspecified Dx   ◻ QPP   UPD Unacceptable PDx

☑4ᵗʰ **S32   Fracture of lumbar spine and pelvis**

> **NOTE**   A fracture not indicated as displaced or nondisplaced should be coded to displaced.
>
> A fracture not indicated as opened or closed should be coded to closed.

> **INCLUDES**   fracture of lumbosacral neural arch
> fracture of lumbosacral spinous process
> fracture of lumbosacral transverse process
> fracture of lumbosacral vertebra
> fracture of lumbosacral vertebral arch

Code first any associated spinal cord and spinal nerve injury (S34.-)

EXCLUDES 1   *transection of abdomen (S38.3)*

EXCLUDES 2   *fracture of hip NOS (S72.0-)*

AHA: 2021,1Q,6; 2018,2Q,12; 2015,3Q,37-39; 2012,4Q,93

> The appropriate 7th character is to be added to each code from category S32.
> A   initial encounter for closed fracture
> B   initial encounter for open fracture
> D   subsequent encounter for fracture with routine healing
> G   subsequent encounter for fracture with delayed healing
> K   subsequent encounter for fracture with nonunion
> S   sequela

☑5ᵗʰ **S32.0   Fracture of lumbar vertebra**

Fracture of lumbar spine NOS

☑6ᵗʰ **S32.00   Fracture of unspecified lumbar vertebra**

¹ ☑7ᵗʰ **S32.000   Wedge compression fracture of unspecified lumbar vertebra** HCC ESR COM Q

¹ ☑7ᵗʰ **S32.001   Stable burst fracture of unspecified lumbar vertebra** HCC ESR COM Q

¹ ☑7ᵗʰ **S32.002   Unstable burst fracture of unspecified lumbar vertebra** HCC ESR COM Q

¹ ☑7ᵗʰ **S32.008   Other fracture of unspecified lumbar vertebra** HCC ESR COM Q

¹ ☑7ᵗʰ **S32.009   Unspecified fracture of unspecified lumbar vertebra** HCC ESR COM Q

☑6ᵗʰ **S32.01   Fracture of first lumbar vertebra**

¹ ☑7ᵗʰ **S32.010   Wedge compression fracture of first lumbar vertebra** HCC ESR COM Q

¹ ☑7ᵗʰ **S32.011   Stable burst fracture of first lumbar vertebra** HCC ESR COM Q

¹ ☑7ᵗʰ **S32.012   Unstable burst fracture of first lumbar vertebra** HCC ESR COM Q

¹ ☑7ᵗʰ **S32.018   Other fracture of first lumbar vertebra** HCC ESR COM Q

¹ ☑7ᵗʰ **S32.019   Unspecified fracture of first lumbar vertebra** HCC ESR COM Q

☑6ᵗʰ **S32.02   Fracture of second lumbar vertebra**

¹ ☑7ᵗʰ **S32.020   Wedge compression fracture of second lumbar vertebra** HCC ESR COM Q

¹ ☑7ᵗʰ **S32.021   Stable burst fracture of second lumbar vertebra** HCC ESR COM Q

¹ ☑7ᵗʰ **S32.022   Unstable burst fracture of second lumbar vertebra** HCC ESR COM Q

¹ ☑7ᵗʰ **S32.028   Other fracture of second lumbar vertebra** HCC ESR COM Q

¹ ☑7ᵗʰ **S32.029   Unspecified fracture of second lumbar vertebra** HCC ESR COM Q

☑6ᵗʰ **S32.03   Fracture of third lumbar vertebra**

¹ ☑7ᵗʰ **S32.030   Wedge compression fracture of third lumbar vertebra** HCC ESR COM Q

¹ ☑7ᵗʰ **S32.031   Stable burst fracture of third lumbar vertebra** HCC ESR COM Q

¹ ☑7ᵗʰ **S32.032   Unstable burst fracture of third lumbar vertebra** HCC ESR COM Q

¹ ☑7ᵗʰ **S32.038   Other fracture of third lumbar vertebra** HCC ESR COM Q

¹ ☑7ᵗʰ **S32.039   Unspecified fracture of third lumbar vertebra** HCC ESR COM Q

☑6ᵗʰ **S32.04   Fracture of fourth lumbar vertebra**

¹ ☑7ᵗʰ **S32.040   Wedge compression fracture of fourth lumbar vertebra** HCC ESR COM Q

¹ ☑7ᵗʰ **S32.041   Stable burst fracture of fourth lumbar vertebra** HCC ESR COM Q

¹ ☑7ᵗʰ **S32.042   Unstable burst fracture of fourth lumbar vertebra** HCC ESR COM Q

¹ ☑7ᵗʰ **S32.048   Other fracture of fourth lumbar vertebra** HCC ESR COM Q

¹ ☑7ᵗʰ **S32.049   Unspecified fracture of fourth lumbar vertebra** HCC ESR COM Q

☑6ᵗʰ **S32.05   Fracture of fifth lumbar vertebra**

¹ ☑7ᵗʰ **S32.050   Wedge compression fracture of fifth lumbar vertebra** HCC ESR COM Q

¹ ☑7ᵗʰ **S32.051   Stable burst fracture of fifth lumbar vertebra** HCC ESR COM Q

¹ ☑7ᵗʰ **S32.052   Unstable burst fracture of fifth lumbar vertebra** HCC ESR COM Q

¹ ☑7ᵗʰ **S32.058   Other fracture of fifth lumbar vertebra** HCC ESR COM Q

¹ ☑7ᵗʰ **S32.059   Unspecified fracture of fifth lumbar vertebra** HCC ESR COM Q

☑5ᵗʰ **S32.1   Fracture of sacrum**

> **NOTE**   For vertical fractures, code to most medial fracture extension
>
> Use two codes if both a vertical and transverse fracture are present

Code also any associated fracture of pelvic ring (S32.8-)

¹ ☑x7ᵗʰ **S32.10   Unspecified fracture of sacrum** HCC ESR COM Q

☑6ᵗʰ **S32.11   Zone I fracture of sacrum**

Vertical sacral ala fracture of sacrum

Vertical Sacral Fracture Zones

Zones: ① ② ③

¹ ☑7ᵗʰ **S32.110   Nondisplaced Zone I fracture of sacrum** HCC ESR COM Q

¹ ☑7ᵗʰ **S32.111   Minimally displaced Zone I fracture of sacrum** HCC ESR COM Q

¹ ☑7ᵗʰ **S32.112   Severely displaced Zone I fracture of sacrum** HCC ESR COM Q

¹ ☑7ᵗʰ **S32.119   Unspecified Zone I fracture of sacrum** HCC ESR COM Q

☑6ᵗʰ **S32.12   Zone II fracture of sacrum**

Vertical foraminal region fracture of sacrum

¹ ☑7ᵗʰ **S32.120   Nondisplaced Zone II fracture of sacrum** HCC ESR COM Q

¹ ☑7ᵗʰ **S32.121   Minimally displaced Zone II fracture of sacrum** HCC ESR COM Q

¹ ☑7ᵗʰ **S32.122   Severely displaced Zone II fracture of sacrum** HCC ESR COM Q

¹ ☑7ᵗʰ **S32.129   Unspecified Zone II fracture of sacrum** HCC ESR COM Q

☑6ᵗʰ **S32.13   Zone III fracture of sacrum**

Vertical fracture into spinal canal region of sacrum

¹ ☑7ᵗʰ **S32.130   Nondisplaced Zone III fracture of sacrum** HCC ESR COM Q

¹ ☑7ᵗʰ **S32.131   Minimally displaced Zone III fracture of sacrum** HCC ESR COM Q

¹ ☑7ᵗʰ **S32.132   Severely displaced Zone III fracture of sacrum** HCC ESR COM Q

¹ √7ᵗʰ **S32.139** Unspecified Zone III fracture of sacrum   HCC ESR COM Q

Transverse Sacral Fracture Types

Type 1   Type 2   Type 3   Type 4

¹ √x7ᵗʰ **S32.14** Type 1 fracture of sacrum   HCC ESR COM Q
  Transverse flexion fracture of sacrum without displacement

¹ √x7ᵗʰ **S32.15** Type 2 fracture of sacrum   HCC ESR COM Q
  Transverse flexion fracture of sacrum with posterior displacement

¹ √x7ᵗʰ **S32.16** Type 3 fracture of sacrum   HCC ESR COM Q
  Transverse extension fracture of sacrum with anterior displacement

¹ √x7ᵗʰ **S32.17** Type 4 fracture of sacrum   HCC ESR COM Q
  Transverse segmental comminution of upper sacrum

¹ √x7ᵗʰ **S32.19** Other fracture of sacrum   HCC ESR COM Q

¹ √x7ᵗʰ **S32.2** Fracture of coccyx   HCC ESR COM Q

√5ᵗʰ **S32.3** Fracture of ilium

  EXCLUDES 1   fracture of ilium with associated disruption of pelvic ring (S32.8-)

√6ᵗʰ **S32.30** Unspecified fracture of ilium

¹ √7ᵗʰ **S32.301** Unspecified fracture of right ilium   HCC ESR COM Q

¹ √7ᵗʰ **S32.302** Unspecified fracture of left ilium   HCC ESR COM Q

¹ √7ᵗʰ **S32.309** Unspecified fracture of unspecified ilium   HCC ESR COM Q

√6ᵗʰ **S32.31** Avulsion fracture of ilium

¹ √7ᵗʰ **S32.311** Displaced avulsion fracture of right ilium   HCC ESR COM Q

¹ √7ᵗʰ **S32.312** Displaced avulsion fracture of left ilium   HCC ESR COM Q

¹ √7ᵗʰ **S32.313** Displaced avulsion fracture of unspecified ilium   HCC ESR COM Q

¹ √7ᵗʰ **S32.314** Nondisplaced avulsion fracture of right ilium   HCC ESR COM Q

¹ √7ᵗʰ **S32.315** Nondisplaced avulsion fracture of left ilium   HCC ESR COM Q

¹ √7ᵗʰ **S32.316** Nondisplaced avulsion fracture of unspecified ilium   HCC ESR COM Q

√6ᵗʰ **S32.39** Other fracture of ilium

¹ √7ᵗʰ **S32.391** Other fracture of right ilium   HCC ESR COM Q

¹ √7ᵗʰ **S32.392** Other fracture of left ilium   HCC ESR COM Q

¹ √7ᵗʰ **S32.399** Other fracture of unspecified ilium   HCC ESR COM Q

√5ᵗʰ **S32.4** Fracture of acetabulum
  Code also any associated fracture of pelvic ring (S32.8-)
  AHA: 2016,3Q,16

√6ᵗʰ **S32.40** Unspecified fracture of acetabulum

¹ √7ᵗʰ **S32.401** Unspecified fracture of right acetabulum   HCC ESR COM Q

¹ √7ᵗʰ **S32.402** Unspecified fracture of left acetabulum   HCC ESR COM Q

¹ √7ᵗʰ **S32.409** Unspecified fracture of unspecified acetabulum   HCC ESR COM Q

√6ᵗʰ **S32.41** Fracture of anterior wall of acetabulum

¹ √7ᵗʰ **S32.411** Displaced fracture of anterior wall of right acetabulum   HCC ESR COM Q

¹ √7ᵗʰ **S32.412** Displaced fracture of anterior wall of left acetabulum   HCC ESR COM Q

¹ √7ᵗʰ **S32.413** Displaced fracture of anterior wall of unspecified acetabulum   HCC ESR COM Q

¹ √7ᵗʰ **S32.414** Nondisplaced fracture of anterior wall of right acetabulum   HCC ESR COM Q

¹ √7ᵗʰ **S32.415** Nondisplaced fracture of anterior wall of left acetabulum   HCC ESR COM Q

¹ √7ᵗʰ **S32.416** Nondisplaced fracture of anterior wall of unspecified acetabulum   HCC ESR COM Q

√6ᵗʰ **S32.42** Fracture of posterior wall of acetabulum

¹ √7ᵗʰ **S32.421** Displaced fracture of posterior wall of right acetabulum   HCC ESR COM Q

¹ √7ᵗʰ **S32.422** Displaced fracture of posterior wall of left acetabulum   HCC ESR COM Q

¹ √7ᵗʰ **S32.423** Displaced fracture of posterior wall of unspecified acetabulum   HCC ESR COM Q

¹ √7ᵗʰ **S32.424** Nondisplaced fracture of posterior wall of right acetabulum   HCC ESR COM Q

¹ √7ᵗʰ **S32.425** Nondisplaced fracture of posterior wall of left acetabulum   HCC ESR COM Q

¹ √7ᵗʰ **S32.426** Nondisplaced fracture of posterior wall of unspecified acetabulum   HCC ESR COM Q

√6ᵗʰ **S32.43** Fracture of anterior column [iliopubic] of acetabulum

¹ √7ᵗʰ **S32.431** Displaced fracture of anterior column [iliopubic] of right acetabulum   HCC ESR COM Q

¹ √7ᵗʰ **S32.432** Displaced fracture of anterior column [iliopubic] of left acetabulum   HCC ESR COM Q

¹ √7ᵗʰ **S32.433** Displaced fracture of anterior column [iliopubic] of unspecified acetabulum   HCC ESR COM Q

¹ √7ᵗʰ **S32.434** Nondisplaced fracture of anterior column [iliopubic] of right acetabulum   HCC ESR COM Q

¹ √7ᵗʰ **S32.435** Nondisplaced fracture of anterior column [iliopubic] of left acetabulum   HCC ESR COM Q

¹ √7ᵗʰ **S32.436** Nondisplaced fracture of anterior column [iliopubic] of unspecified acetabulum   HCC ESR COM Q

√6ᵗʰ **S32.44** Fracture of posterior column [ilioischial] of acetabulum

¹ √7ᵗʰ **S32.441** Displaced fracture of posterior column [ilioischial] of right acetabulum   HCC ESR COM Q

¹ √7ᵗʰ **S32.442** Displaced fracture of posterior column [ilioischial] of left acetabulum   HCC ESR COM Q

¹ √7ᵗʰ **S32.443** Displaced fracture of posterior column [ilioischial] of unspecified acetabulum   HCC ESR COM Q

¹ √7ᵗʰ **S32.444** Nondisplaced fracture of posterior column [ilioischial] of right acetabulum   HCC ESR COM Q

¹ √7ᵗʰ **S32.445** Nondisplaced fracture of posterior column [ilioischial] of left acetabulum   HCC ESR COM Q

¹ √7ᵗʰ **S32.446** Nondisplaced fracture of posterior column [ilioischial] of unspecified acetabulum   HCC ESR COM Q

√6ᵗʰ **S32.45** Transverse fracture of acetabulum

¹ √7ᵗʰ **S32.451** Displaced transverse fracture of right acetabulum   HCC ESR COM Q

¹ √7ᵗʰ **S32.452** Displaced transverse fracture of left acetabulum   HCC ESR COM Q

¹ √7ᵗʰ **S32.453** Displaced transverse fracture of unspecified acetabulum   HCC ESR COM Q

¹ √7ᵗʰ **S32.454** Nondisplaced transverse fracture of right acetabulum   HCC ESR COM Q

¹ √7ᵗʰ **S32.455** Nondisplaced transverse fracture of left acetabulum   HCC ESR COM Q

¹ √7ᵗʰ **S32.456** Nondisplaced transverse fracture of unspecified acetabulum   HCC ESR COM Q

√6ᵗʰ **S32.46** Associated transverse-posterior fracture of acetabulum

- ¹ √7ᵗʰ **S32.461** Displaced associated transverse-posterior fracture of right acetabulum `HCC` `ESR` `COM` `Q`
- ¹ √7ᵗʰ **S32.462** Displaced associated transverse-posterior fracture of left acetabulum `HCC` `ESR` `COM` `Q`
- ¹ √7ᵗʰ **S32.463** Displaced associated transverse-posterior fracture of unspecified acetabulum `HCC` `ESR` `COM` `Q`
- ¹ √7ᵗʰ **S32.464** Nondisplaced associated transverse-posterior fracture of right acetabulum `HCC` `ESR` `COM` `Q`
- ¹ √7ᵗʰ **S32.465** Nondisplaced associated transverse-posterior fracture of left acetabulum `HCC` `ESR` `COM` `Q`
- ¹ √7ᵗʰ **S32.466** Nondisplaced associated transverse-posterior fracture of unspecified acetabulum `HCC` `ESR` `COM` `Q`

√6ᵗʰ **S32.47** Fracture of medial wall of acetabulum

- ¹ √7ᵗʰ **S32.471** Displaced fracture of medial wall of right acetabulum `HCC` `ESR` `COM` `Q`
- ¹ √7ᵗʰ **S32.472** Displaced fracture of medial wall of left acetabulum `HCC` `ESR` `COM` `Q`
- ¹ √7ᵗʰ **S32.473** Displaced fracture of medial wall of unspecified acetabulum `HCC` `ESR` `COM` `Q`
- ¹ √7ᵗʰ **S32.474** Nondisplaced fracture of medial wall of right acetabulum `HCC` `ESR` `COM` `Q`
- ¹ √7ᵗʰ **S32.475** Nondisplaced fracture of medial wall of left acetabulum `HCC` `ESR` `COM` `Q`
- ¹ √7ᵗʰ **S32.476** Nondisplaced fracture of medial wall of unspecified acetabulum `HCC` `ESR` `COM` `Q`

√6ᵗʰ **S32.48** Dome fracture of acetabulum

- ¹ √7ᵗʰ **S32.481** Displaced dome fracture of right acetabulum `HCC` `ESR` `COM` `Q`
- ¹ √7ᵗʰ **S32.482** Displaced dome fracture of left acetabulum `HCC` `ESR` `COM` `Q`
- ¹ √7ᵗʰ **S32.483** Displaced dome fracture of unspecified acetabulum `HCC` `ESR` `COM` `Q`
- ¹ √7ᵗʰ **S32.484** Nondisplaced dome fracture of right acetabulum `HCC` `ESR` `COM` `Q`
- ¹ √7ᵗʰ **S32.485** Nondisplaced dome fracture of left acetabulum `HCC` `ESR` `COM` `Q`
- ¹ √7ᵗʰ **S32.486** Nondisplaced dome fracture of unspecified acetabulum `HCC` `ESR` `COM` `Q`

√6ᵗʰ **S32.49** Other specified fracture of acetabulum

- ¹ √7ᵗʰ **S32.491** Other specified fracture of right acetabulum `HCC` `ESR` `COM` `Q`
- ¹ √7ᵗʰ **S32.492** Other specified fracture of left acetabulum `HCC` `ESR` `COM` `Q`
- ¹ √7ᵗʰ **S32.499** Other specified fracture of unspecified acetabulum `HCC` `ESR` `COM` `Q`

√5ᵗʰ **S32.5** Fracture of pubis

EXCLUDES 1 *fracture of pubis with associated disruption of pelvic ring (S32.8-)*

√6ᵗʰ **S32.50** Unspecified fracture of pubis

- ¹ √7ᵗʰ **S32.501** Unspecified fracture of right pubis `HCC` `ESR` `COM` `Q`
- ¹ √7ᵗʰ **S32.502** Unspecified fracture of left pubis `HCC` `ESR` `COM` `Q`
- ¹ √7ᵗʰ **S32.509** Unspecified fracture of unspecified pubis `HCC` `ESR` `COM` `Q`

√6ᵗʰ **S32.51** Fracture of superior rim of pubis

- ¹ √7ᵗʰ **S32.511** Fracture of superior rim of right pubis `HCC` `ESR` `COM` `Q`
- ¹ √7ᵗʰ **S32.512** Fracture of superior rim of left pubis `HCC` `ESR` `COM` `Q`
- ¹ √7ᵗʰ **S32.519** Fracture of superior rim of unspecified pubis `HCC` `ESR` `COM` `Q`

√6ᵗʰ **S32.59** Other specified fracture of pubis

- ¹ √7ᵗʰ **S32.591** Other specified fracture of right pubis `HCC` `ESR` `COM` `Q`
- ¹ √7ᵗʰ **S32.592** Other specified fracture of left pubis `HCC` `ESR` `COM` `Q`

- ¹ √7ᵗʰ **S32.599** Other specified fracture of unspecified pubis `HCC` `ESR` `COM` `Q`

√5ᵗʰ **S32.6** Fracture of ischium

EXCLUDES 1 *fracture of ischium with associated disruption of pelvic ring (S32.8-)*

√6ᵗʰ **S32.60** Unspecified fracture of ischium

- ¹ √7ᵗʰ **S32.601** Unspecified fracture of right ischium `HCC` `ESR` `COM` `Q`
- ¹ √7ᵗʰ **S32.602** Unspecified fracture of left ischium `HCC` `ESR` `COM` `Q`
- ¹ √7ᵗʰ **S32.609** Unspecified fracture of unspecified ischium `HCC` `ESR` `COM` `Q`

√6ᵗʰ **S32.61** Avulsion fracture of ischium

- ¹ √7ᵗʰ **S32.611** Displaced avulsion fracture of right ischium `HCC` `ESR` `COM` `Q`
- ¹ √7ᵗʰ **S32.612** Displaced avulsion fracture of left ischium `HCC` `ESR` `COM` `Q`
- ¹ √7ᵗʰ **S32.613** Displaced avulsion fracture of unspecified ischium `HCC` `ESR` `COM` `Q`
- ¹ √7ᵗʰ **S32.614** Nondisplaced avulsion fracture of right ischium `HCC` `ESR` `COM` `Q`
- ¹ √7ᵗʰ **S32.615** Nondisplaced avulsion fracture of left ischium `HCC` `ESR` `COM` `Q`
- ¹ √7ᵗʰ **S32.616** Nondisplaced avulsion fracture of unspecified ischium `HCC` `ESR` `COM` `Q`

√6ᵗʰ **S32.69** Other specified fracture of ischium

- ¹ √7ᵗʰ **S32.691** Other specified fracture of right ischium `HCC` `ESR` `COM` `Q`
- ¹ √7ᵗʰ **S32.692** Other specified fracture of left ischium `HCC` `ESR` `COM` `Q`
- ¹ √7ᵗʰ **S32.699** Other specified fracture of unspecified ischium `HCC` `ESR` `COM` `Q`

√5ᵗʰ **S32.8** Fracture of other parts of pelvis

Code also any associated:
  fracture of acetabulum (S32.4-)
  sacral fracture (S32.1-)

Fractures Disrupting Pelvic Circle

Pelvic circle — Stable

Unstable (two-place fracture)

Iliac crest
Anterior superior iliac spine
Ischial spine
Acetabulum
Femur
Ilium
L5
Sacrum
Coccyx
Pubis
Ischium
Pubic symphysis
Pelvic Bones

√6ᵗʰ **S32.81** Multiple fractures of pelvis with disruption of pelvic ring

Multiple pelvic fractures with disruption of pelvic circle

- ¹ √7ᵗʰ **S32.810** Multiple fractures of pelvis with stable disruption of pelvic ring `HCC` `ESR` `COM` `Q`
- ¹ √7ᵗʰ **S32.811** Multiple fractures of pelvis with unstable disruption of pelvic ring `HCC` `ESR` `COM` `Q`

¹ √x7ᵗʰ **S32.82** Multiple fractures of pelvis without disruption of pelvic ring `HCC` `ESR` `COM` `Q`

Multiple pelvic fractures without disruption of pelvic circle

¹ √x7ᵗʰ **S32.89** Fracture of other parts of pelvis `HCC` `ESR` `COM` `Q`

¹ √x7ᵗʰ **S32.9** Fracture of unspecified parts of lumbosacral spine and pelvis `HCC` `ESR` `COM` `Q`

Fracture of lumbosacral spine NOS
Fracture of pelvis NOS
AHA: 2012,4Q,93

`HCC` CMS-HCC   `Rx` Rx HCC   `ESR` ESRD HCC   `COM` Commercial HCC   `N` Newborn: 0   `P` Pediatric: 0-17   `M` Maternity: 9-64   `A` Adult: 15-124

1026
ICD-10-CM 2023

☑4ᵗʰ **S33 Dislocation and sprain of joints and ligaments of lumbar spine and pelvis**

INCLUDES   avulsion of joint or ligament of lumbar spine and pelvis

laceration of cartilage, joint or ligament of lumbar spine and pelvis

sprain of cartilage, joint or ligament of lumbar spine and pelvis

traumatic hemarthrosis of joint or ligament of lumbar spine and pelvis

traumatic rupture of joint or ligament of lumbar spine and pelvis

traumatic subluxation of joint or ligament of lumbar spine and pelvis

traumatic tear of joint or ligament of lumbar spine and pelvis

Code also any associated open wound

EXCLUDES 1   *nontraumatic rupture or displacement of lumbar intervertebral disc NOS (M51.-)*

obstetric damage to pelvic joints and ligaments (O71.6)

EXCLUDES 2   *dislocation and sprain of joints and ligaments of hip (S73.-)*

strain of muscle of lower back and pelvis (S39.01-)

The appropriate 7th character is to be added to each code from category S33.
A   initial encounter
D   subsequent encounter
S   sequela

☑x7ᵗʰ **S33.0 Traumatic rupture of lumbar intervertebral disc**

EXCLUDES 1   *rupture or displacement (nontraumatic) of lumbar intervertebral disc NOS (M51.- with fifth character 6)*

☑5ᵗʰ **S33.1 Subluxation and dislocation of lumbar vertebra**

Code also any associated:

open wound of abdomen, lower back and pelvis (S31)

spinal cord injury (S24.0, S24.1-, S34.0-, S34.1-)

EXCLUDES 2   *fracture of lumbar vertebrae (S32.0-)*

☑6ᵗʰ **S33.10 Subluxation and dislocation of unspecified lumbar vertebra**

☑7ᵗʰ **S33.100 Subluxation** of unspecified lumbar vertebra

☑7ᵗʰ **S33.101 Dislocation** of unspecified lumbar vertebra

☑6ᵗʰ **S33.11 Subluxation and dislocation of L1/L2 lumbar vertebra**

☑7ᵗʰ **S33.110 Subluxation** of L1/L2 lumbar vertebra

☑7ᵗʰ **S33.111 Dislocation** of L1/L2 lumbar vertebra

☑6ᵗʰ **S33.12 Subluxation and dislocation of L2/L3 lumbar vertebra**

☑7ᵗʰ **S33.120 Subluxation** of L2/L3 lumbar vertebra

☑7ᵗʰ **S33.121 Dislocation** of L2/L3 lumbar vertebra

☑6ᵗʰ **S33.13 Subluxation and dislocation of L3/L4 lumbar vertebra**

☑7ᵗʰ **S33.130 Subluxation** of L3/L4 lumbar vertebra

☑7ᵗʰ **S33.131 Dislocation** of L3/L4 lumbar vertebra

☑6ᵗʰ **S33.14 Subluxation and dislocation of L4/L5 lumbar vertebra**

☑7ᵗʰ **S33.140 Subluxation** of L4/L5 lumbar vertebra

☑7ᵗʰ **S33.141 Dislocation** of L4/L5 lumbar vertebra

☑x7ᵗʰ **S33.2 Dislocation of sacroiliac and sacrococcygeal joint**

☑5ᵗʰ **S33.3 Dislocation of other and unspecified parts of lumbar spine and pelvis**

☑x7ᵗʰ **S33.30 Dislocation of unspecified parts of lumbar spine and pelvis**

☑x7ᵗʰ **S33.39 Dislocation of other parts of lumbar spine and pelvis**

☑x7ᵗʰ **S33.4 Traumatic rupture of symphysis pubis**

☑x7ᵗʰ **S33.5 Sprain of ligaments of lumbar spine**

☑x7ᵗʰ **S33.6 Sprain of sacroiliac joint**

☑x7ᵗʰ **S33.8 Sprain of other parts of lumbar spine and pelvis**

☑x7ᵗʰ **S33.9 Sprain of unspecified parts of lumbar spine and pelvis**

☑4ᵗʰ **S34 Injury of lumbar and sacral spinal cord and nerves at abdomen, lower back and pelvis level**

NOTE   Code to highest level of lumbar cord injury.

Injuries to the spinal cord (S34.0 and S34.1) refer to the cord level and not bone level injury, and can affect nerve roots at and below the level given.

Code also any associated:

fracture of vertebra (S22.0-, S32.0-)

open wound of abdomen, lower back and pelvis (S31.-)

transient paralysis (R29.5)

The appropriate 7th character is to be added to each code from category S34.
A   initial encounter
D   subsequent encounter
S   sequela

☑5ᵗʰ **S34.0 Concussion and edema of lumbar and sacral spinal cord**

☑x7ᵗʰ **S34.01 Concussion and edema of lumbar spinal cord** HCC ESR COM

☑x7ᵗʰ **S34.02 Concussion and edema of sacral spinal cord** HCC ESR COM

Concussion and edema of conus medullaris

☑5ᵗʰ **S34.1 Other and unspecified injury of lumbar and sacral spinal cord**

☑6ᵗʰ **S34.10 Unspecified injury to lumbar spinal cord**

☑7ᵗʰ **S34.101 Unspecified injury to L1 level of lumbar spinal cord** HCC ESR COM

Unspecified injury to lumbar spinal cord level 1

☑7ᵗʰ **S34.102 Unspecified injury to L2 level of lumbar spinal cord** HCC ESR COM

Unspecified injury to lumbar spinal cord level 2

☑7ᵗʰ **S34.103 Unspecified injury to L3 level of lumbar spinal cord** HCC ESR COM

Unspecified injury to lumbar spinal cord level 3

☑7ᵗʰ **S34.104 Unspecified injury to L4 level of lumbar spinal cord** HCC ESR COM

Unspecified injury to lumbar spinal cord level 4

☑7ᵗʰ **S34.105 Unspecified injury to L5 level of lumbar spinal cord** HCC ESR COM

Unspecified injury to lumbar spinal cord level 5

☑7ᵗʰ **S34.109 Unspecified injury to unspecified level of lumbar spinal cord** HCC ESR COM

☑6ᵗʰ **S34.11 Complete lesion of lumbar spinal cord**

☑7ᵗʰ **S34.111 Complete lesion of L1 level of lumbar spinal cord** HCC ESR COM

Complete lesion of lumbar spinal cord level 1

☑7ᵗʰ **S34.112 Complete lesion of L2 level of lumbar spinal cord** HCC ESR COM

Complete lesion of lumbar spinal cord level 2

☑7ᵗʰ **S34.113 Complete lesion of L3 level of lumbar spinal cord** HCC ESR COM

Complete lesion of lumbar spinal cord level 3

☑7ᵗʰ **S34.114 Complete lesion of L4 level of lumbar spinal cord** HCC ESR COM

Complete lesion of lumbar spinal cord level 4

☑7ᵗʰ **S34.115 Complete lesion of L5 level of lumbar spinal cord** HCC ESR COM

Complete lesion of lumbar spinal cord level 5

☑7ᵗʰ **S34.119 Complete lesion of unspecified level of lumbar spinal cord** HCC ESR COM

☑6ᵗʰ **S34.12 Incomplete lesion of lumbar spinal cord**

☑7ᵗʰ **S34.121 Incomplete lesion of L1 level of lumbar spinal cord** HCC ESR COM

Incomplete lesion of lumbar spinal cord level 1

√7ᵗʰ **S34.122 Incomplete lesion of L2 level of lumbar spinal cord** HCC ESR COM
     Incomplete lesion of lumbar spinal cord level 2

√7ᵗʰ **S34.123 Incomplete lesion of L3 level of lumbar spinal cord** HCC ESR COM
     Incomplete lesion of lumbar spinal cord level 3

√7ᵗʰ **S34.124 Incomplete lesion of L4 level of lumbar spinal cord** HCC ESR COM
     Incomplete lesion of lumbar spinal cord level 4

√7ᵗʰ **S34.125 Incomplete lesion of L5 level of lumbar spinal cord** HCC ESR COM
     Incomplete lesion of lumbar spinal cord level 5

√7ᵗʰ **S34.129 Incomplete lesion of unspecified level of lumbar spinal cord** HCC ESR COM

√6ᵗʰ **S34.13 Other and unspecified injury to sacral spinal cord**
     Other injury to conus medullaris

√7ᵗʰ **S34.131 Complete lesion of sacral spinal cord** HCC ESR COM
     Complete lesion of conus medullaris

√7ᵗʰ **S34.132 Incomplete lesion of sacral spinal cord** HCC ESR COM
     Incomplete lesion of conus medullaris

√7ᵗʰ **S34.139 Unspecified injury to sacral spinal cord** HCC ESR COM
     Unspecified injury of conus medullaris

√5ᵗʰ **S34.2 Injury of nerve root of lumbar and sacral spine**

√x7ᵗʰ **S34.21 Injury of nerve root of lumbar spine**

√x7ᵗʰ **S34.22 Injury of nerve root of sacral spine**

¹ √x7ᵗʰ **S34.3 Injury of cauda equina** HCC ESR COM

√x7ᵗʰ **S34.4 Injury of lumbosacral plexus**

√x7ᵗʰ **S34.5 Injury of lumbar, sacral and pelvic sympathetic nerves**
     Injury of celiac ganglion or plexus
     Injury of hypogastric plexus
     Injury of mesenteric plexus (inferior) (superior)
     Injury of splanchnic nerve

√x7ᵗʰ **S34.6 Injury of peripheral nerve(s) at abdomen, lower back and pelvis level**

√x7ᵗʰ **S34.8 Injury of other nerves at abdomen, lower back and pelvis level**

√x7ᵗʰ **S34.9 Injury of unspecified nerves at abdomen, lower back and pelvis level**

√4ᵗʰ **S35 Injury of blood vessels at abdomen, lower back and pelvis level**
     Code also any associated open wound (S31.-)

     The appropriate 7th character is to be added to each code from category S35.
     A   initial encounter
     D   subsequent encounter
     S   sequela

√5ᵗʰ **S35.0 Injury of abdominal aorta**
     EXCLUDES 1   injury of aorta NOS (S25.0)

√x7ᵗʰ **S35.00 Unspecified injury of abdominal aorta**

√x7ᵗʰ **S35.01 Minor laceration of abdominal aorta**
     Incomplete transection of abdominal aorta
     Laceration of abdominal aorta NOS
     Superficial laceration of abdominal aorta

√x7ᵗʰ **S35.02 Major laceration of abdominal aorta**
     Complete transection of abdominal aorta
     Traumatic rupture of abdominal aorta

√x7ᵗʰ **S35.09 Other injury of abdominal aorta**

√5ᵗʰ **S35.1 Injury of inferior vena cava**
     Injury of hepatic vein
     EXCLUDES 1   injury of vena cava NOS (S25.2)

√x7ᵗʰ **S35.10 Unspecified injury of inferior vena cava**

√x7ᵗʰ **S35.11 Minor laceration of inferior vena cava**
     Incomplete transection of inferior vena cava
     Laceration of inferior vena cava NOS
     Superficial laceration of inferior vena cava

√x7ᵗʰ **S35.12 Major laceration of inferior vena cava**
     Complete transection of inferior vena cava
     Traumatic rupture of inferior vena cava

√x7ᵗʰ **S35.19 Other injury of inferior vena cava**

√5ᵗʰ **S35.2 Injury of celiac or mesenteric artery and branches**

√6ᵗʰ **S35.21 Injury of celiac artery**

√7ᵗʰ **S35.211 Minor laceration of celiac artery**
     Incomplete transection of celiac artery
     Laceration of celiac artery NOS
     Superficial laceration of celiac artery

√7ᵗʰ **S35.212 Major laceration of celiac artery**
     Complete transection of celiac artery
     Traumatic rupture of celiac artery

√7ᵗʰ **S35.218 Other injury of celiac artery**

√7ᵗʰ **S35.219 Unspecified injury of celiac artery**

√6ᵗʰ **S35.22 Injury of superior mesenteric artery**

√7ᵗʰ **S35.221 Minor laceration of superior mesenteric artery**
     Incomplete transection of superior mesenteric artery
     Laceration of superior mesenteric artery NOS
     Superficial laceration of superior mesenteric artery

√7ᵗʰ **S35.222 Major laceration of superior mesenteric artery**
     Complete transection of superior mesenteric artery
     Traumatic rupture of superior mesenteric artery

√7ᵗʰ **S35.228 Other injury of superior mesenteric artery**

√7ᵗʰ **S35.229 Unspecified injury of superior mesenteric artery**

√6ᵗʰ **S35.23 Injury of inferior mesenteric artery**

√7ᵗʰ **S35.231 Minor laceration of inferior mesenteric artery**
     Incomplete transection of inferior mesenteric artery
     Laceration of inferior mesenteric artery NOS
     Superficial laceration of inferior mesenteric artery

√7ᵗʰ **S35.232 Major laceration of inferior mesenteric artery**
     Complete transection of inferior mesenteric artery
     Traumatic rupture of inferior mesenteric artery

√7ᵗʰ **S35.238 Other injury of inferior mesenteric artery**

√7ᵗʰ **S35.239 Unspecified injury of inferior mesenteric artery**

√6ᵗʰ **S35.29 Injury of branches of celiac and mesenteric artery**
     Injury of gastric artery
     Injury of gastroduodenal artery
     Injury of hepatic artery
     Injury of splenic artery

√7ᵗʰ **S35.291 Minor laceration of branches of celiac and mesenteric artery**
     Incomplete transection of branches of celiac and mesenteric artery
     Laceration of branches of celiac and mesenteric artery NOS
     Superficial laceration of branches of celiac and mesenteric artery

√7ᵗʰ **S35.292 Major laceration of branches of celiac and mesenteric artery**
     Complete transection of branches of celiac and mesenteric artery
     Traumatic rupture of branches of celiac and mesenteric artery

√7ᵗʰ **S35.298 Other injury of branches of celiac and mesenteric artery**

√7ᵗʰ **S35.299 Unspecified injury of branches of celiac and mesenteric artery**

√5ᵗʰ **S35.3** **Injury of portal or splenic vein and branches**

  √6ᵗʰ **S35.31** **Injury of** portal vein

    √7ᵗʰ **S35.311** Laceration of portal vein

    √7ᵗʰ **S35.318** **Other specified injury of portal vein**

    √7ᵗʰ **S35.319** **Unspecified injury of portal vein**

  √6ᵗʰ **S35.32** **Injury of** splenic vein

    √7ᵗʰ **S35.321** Laceration of splenic vein

    √7ᵗʰ **S35.328** **Other specified injury of splenic vein**

    √7ᵗʰ **S35.329** **Unspecified injury of splenic vein**

  √6ᵗʰ **S35.33** **Injury of** superior mesenteric vein

    √7ᵗʰ **S35.331** Laceration of superior mesenteric vein

    √7ᵗʰ **S35.338** **Other specified injury of superior mesenteric vein**

    √7ᵗʰ **S35.339** **Unspecified injury of superior mesenteric vein**

  √6ᵗʰ **S35.34** **Injury of** inferior mesenteric vein

    √7ᵗʰ **S35.341** Laceration of inferior mesenteric vein

    √7ᵗʰ **S35.348** **Other specified injury of inferior mesenteric vein**

    √7ᵗʰ **S35.349** **Unspecified injury of inferior mesenteric vein**

√5ᵗʰ **S35.4** **Injury of** renal blood vessels

  √6ᵗʰ **S35.40** **Unspecified injury of renal blood vessel**

    √7ᵗʰ **S35.401** **Unspecified injury of** right renal artery

    √7ᵗʰ **S35.402** **Unspecified injury of** left renal artery

    √7ᵗʰ **S35.403** **Unspecified injury of unspecified renal artery**

    √7ᵗʰ **S35.404** **Unspecified injury of** right renal vein

    √7ᵗʰ **S35.405** **Unspecified injury of** left renal vein

    √7ᵗʰ **S35.406** **Unspecified injury of unspecified renal vein**

  √6ᵗʰ **S35.41** Laceration of renal blood vessel

    √7ᵗʰ **S35.411** Laceration of right renal artery

    √7ᵗʰ **S35.412** Laceration of left renal artery

    √7ᵗʰ **S35.413** Laceration of unspecified renal artery

    √7ᵗʰ **S35.414** Laceration of right renal vein

    √7ᵗʰ **S35.415** Laceration of left renal vein

    √7ᵗʰ **S35.416** Laceration of unspecified renal vein

  √6ᵗʰ **S35.49** **Other specified injury of renal blood vessel**

    √7ᵗʰ **S35.491** **Other specified injury of** right renal artery

    √7ᵗʰ **S35.492** **Other specified injury of** left renal artery

    √7ᵗʰ **S35.493** **Other specified injury of unspecified renal artery**

    √7ᵗʰ **S35.494** **Other specified injury of** right renal vein

    √7ᵗʰ **S35.495** **Other specified injury of** left renal vein

    √7ᵗʰ **S35.496** **Other specified injury of unspecified renal vein**

√5ᵗʰ **S35.5** **Injury of** iliac blood vessels

  √ₓ7ᵗʰ **S35.50** **Injury of unspecified iliac blood vessel(s)**

  √6ᵗʰ **S35.51** **Injury of** iliac artery or vein

    Injury of hypogastric artery or vein

    √7ᵗʰ **S35.511** **Injury of** right iliac artery

    √7ᵗʰ **S35.512** **Injury of** left iliac artery

    √7ᵗʰ **S35.513** **Injury of unspecified iliac artery**

    √7ᵗʰ **S35.514** **Injury of** right iliac vein

    √7ᵗʰ **S35.515** **Injury of** left iliac vein

    √7ᵗʰ **S35.516** **Injury of unspecified iliac vein**

  √6ᵗʰ **S35.53** **Injury of** uterine artery or vein

    √7ᵗʰ **S35.531** **Injury of** right uterine artery ♀

    √7ᵗʰ **S35.532** **Injury of** left uterine artery ♀

    √7ᵗʰ **S35.533** **Injury of unspecified uterine artery** ♀

    √7ᵗʰ **S35.534** **Injury of** right uterine vein ♀

    √7ᵗʰ **S35.535** **Injury of** left uterine vein ♀

    √7ᵗʰ **S35.536** **Injury of unspecified uterine vein** ♀

  √ₓ7ᵗʰ **S35.59** **Injury of other iliac blood vessels**

√5ᵗʰ **S35.8** **Injury of other blood vessels at abdomen, lower back and pelvis level**

  Injury of ovarian artery or vein

  √6ᵗʰ **S35.8X** **Injury of other blood vessels at abdomen, lower back and pelvis level**

    √7ᵗʰ **S35.8X1** Laceration of other blood vessels at abdomen, lower back and pelvis level

    √7ᵗʰ **S35.8X8** **Other specified injury of other blood vessels at abdomen, lower back and pelvis level**

    √7ᵗʰ **S35.8X9** **Unspecified injury of other blood vessels at abdomen, lower back and pelvis level**

√5ᵗʰ **S35.9** **Injury of unspecified blood vessel at abdomen, lower back and pelvis level**

  √ₓ7ᵗʰ **S35.90** **Unspecified injury of unspecified blood vessel at abdomen, lower back and pelvis level**

  √ₓ7ᵗʰ **S35.91** Laceration of unspecified blood vessel at abdomen, lower back and pelvis level

  √ₓ7ᵗʰ **S35.99** **Other specified injury of unspecified blood vessel at abdomen, lower back and pelvis level**

√4ᵗʰ **S36** **Injury of intra-abdominal organs**

  Code also any associated open wound (S31.-)

  The appropriate 7th character is to be added to each code from category S36.
  A   initial encounter
  D   subsequent encounter
  S   sequela

√5ᵗʰ **S36.0** **Injury of** spleen

  AHA: 2015,2Q,36; 2015,1Q,10

  √ₓ7ᵗʰ **S36.00** **Unspecified injury of spleen**

  √6ᵗʰ **S36.02** **Contusion of spleen**

    √7ᵗʰ **S36.020** **Minor contusion of spleen**

      Contusion of spleen less than 2 cm

    √7ᵗʰ **S36.021** **Major contusion of spleen**

      Contusion of spleen greater than 2 cm

    √7ᵗʰ **S36.029** **Unspecified contusion of spleen**

  √6ᵗʰ **S36.03** **Laceration of spleen**

    √7ᵗʰ **S36.030** **Superficial (capsular) laceration of spleen**

      Laceration of spleen less than 1 cm
      Minor laceration of spleen

    √7ᵗʰ **S36.031** **Moderate laceration of spleen**

      Laceration of spleen 1 to 3 cm

    √7ᵗʰ **S36.032** **Major laceration of spleen**

      Avulsion of spleen
      Laceration of spleen greater than 3 cm
      Massive laceration of spleen
      Multiple moderate lacerations of spleen
      Stellate laceration of spleen

    √7ᵗʰ **S36.039** **Unspecified laceration of spleen**

  √ₓ7ᵗʰ **S36.09** **Other injury of spleen**

√5ᵗʰ **S36.1** **Injury of liver and gallbladder and bile duct**

  √6ᵗʰ **S36.11** **Injury of liver**

    √7ᵗʰ **S36.112** **Contusion of liver**

    √7ᵗʰ **S36.113** Laceration of liver, unspecified degree

    √7ᵗʰ **S36.114** **Minor laceration of liver**

      Laceration involving capsule only, or, without significant involvement of hepatic parenchyma [i.e., less than 1 cm deep]

    √7ᵗʰ **S36.115** **Moderate laceration of liver**

      Laceration involving parenchyma but without major disruption of parenchyma [i.e., less than 10 cm long and less than 3 cm deep]

    √7ᵗʰ **S36.116** **Major laceration of liver**

      Laceration with significant disruption of hepatic parenchyma [i.e., greater than 10 cm long and 3 cm deep]
      Multiple moderate lacerations, with or without hematoma
      Stellate laceration of liver

    √7ᵗʰ **S36.118** **Other injury of liver**

    √7ᵗʰ **S36.119** **Unspecified injury of liver**

S36.12 Injury of gallbladder
- **S36.122 Contusion** of gallbladder
- **S36.123 Laceration** of gallbladder
- **S36.128 Other injury** of gallbladder
- **S36.129 Unspecified injury** of gallbladder

S36.13 Injury of bile duct

S36.2 Injury of pancreas

S36.20 Unspecified injury of pancreas
- **S36.200 Unspecified injury of** head of pancreas
- **S36.201 Unspecified injury of** body of pancreas
- **S36.202 Unspecified injury of** tail of pancreas
- **S36.209 Unspecified injury of** unspecified part of pancreas

S36.22 Contusion of pancreas
- **S36.220 Contusion of** head of pancreas
- **S36.221 Contusion of** body of pancreas
- **S36.222 Contusion of** tail of pancreas
- **S36.229 Contusion of** unspecified part of pancreas

S36.23 Laceration of pancreas, unspecified degree
- **S36.230 Laceration of** head of pancreas, unspecified degree
- **S36.231 Laceration of** body of pancreas, unspecified degree
- **S36.232 Laceration of** tail of pancreas, unspecified degree
- **S36.239 Laceration of** unspecified part of pancreas, unspecified degree

S36.24 Minor laceration of pancreas
- **S36.240 Minor laceration of** head of pancreas
- **S36.241 Minor laceration of** body of pancreas
- **S36.242 Minor laceration of** tail of pancreas
- **S36.249 Minor laceration of** unspecified part of pancreas

S36.25 Moderate laceration of pancreas
- **S36.250 Moderate laceration of** head of pancreas
- **S36.251 Moderate laceration of** body of pancreas
- **S36.252 Moderate laceration of** tail of pancreas
- **S36.259 Moderate laceration of** unspecified part of pancreas

S36.26 Major laceration of pancreas
- **S36.260 Major laceration of** head of pancreas
- **S36.261 Major laceration of** body of pancreas
- **S36.262 Major laceration of** tail of pancreas
- **S36.269 Major laceration of** unspecified part of pancreas

S36.29 Other injury of pancreas
- **S36.290 Other injury of** head of pancreas
- **S36.291 Other injury of** body of pancreas
- **S36.292 Other injury of** tail of pancreas
- **S36.299 Other injury of** unspecified part of pancreas

S36.3 Injury of stomach
- **S36.30 Unspecified injury of stomach**
- **S36.32 Contusion of stomach**
- **S36.33 Laceration of stomach**
- **S36.39 Other injury of stomach**

S36.4 Injury of small intestine

S36.40 Unspecified injury of small intestine
- **S36.400 Unspecified injury of** duodenum
- **S36.408 Unspecified injury of** other part of small intestine
- **S36.409 Unspecified injury of** unspecified part of small intestine

S36.41 Primary blast injury of small intestine

Blast injury of small intestine NOS
- **S36.410 Primary blast injury of** duodenum
- **S36.418 Primary blast injury of** other part of small intestine
- **S36.419 Primary blast injury of** unspecified part of small intestine

S36.42 Contusion of small intestine
- **S36.420 Contusion of** duodenum
- **S36.428 Contusion of other part of small intestine**
- **S36.429 Contusion of unspecified part of small intestine**

S36.43 Laceration of small intestine
- **S36.430 Laceration of** duodenum
- **S36.438 Laceration of other part of small intestine**
- **S36.439 Laceration of unspecified part of small intestine**

S36.49 Other injury of small intestine
- **S36.490 Other injury of** duodenum
- **S36.498 Other injury of other part of small intestine**
- **S36.499 Other injury of unspecified part of small intestine**

S36.5 Injury of colon

> EXCLUDES 2   injury of rectum (S36.6-)

S36.50 Unspecified injury of colon
- **S36.500 Unspecified injury of** ascending [right] colon
- **S36.501 Unspecified injury of** transverse colon
- **S36.502 Unspecified injury of** descending [left] colon
- **S36.503 Unspecified injury of** sigmoid colon
- **S36.508 Unspecified injury of other part of colon**
- **S36.509 Unspecified injury of unspecified part of colon**

S36.51 Primary blast injury of colon

Blast injury of colon NOS
- **S36.510 Primary blast injury of** ascending [right] colon
- **S36.511 Primary blast injury of** transverse colon
- **S36.512 Primary blast injury of** descending [left] colon
- **S36.513 Primary blast injury of** sigmoid colon
- **S36.518 Primary blast injury of other part of colon**
- **S36.519 Primary blast injury of unspecified part of colon**

S36.52 Contusion of colon
- **S36.520 Contusion of** ascending [right] colon
- **S36.521 Contusion of** transverse colon
- **S36.522 Contusion of** descending [left] colon
- **S36.523 Contusion of** sigmoid colon
- **S36.528 Contusion of other part of colon**
- **S36.529 Contusion of unspecified part of colon**

S36.53 Laceration of colon
- **S36.530 Laceration of** ascending [right] colon
- **S36.531 Laceration of** transverse colon
- **S36.532 Laceration of** descending [left] colon
- **S36.533 Laceration of** sigmoid colon
- **S36.538 Laceration of other part of colon**
- **S36.539 Laceration of unspecified part of colon**

S36.59 Other injury of colon

Secondary blast injury of colon
- **S36.590 Other injury of** ascending [right] colon
- **S36.591 Other injury of** transverse colon
- **S36.592 Other injury of** descending [left] colon
- **S36.593 Other injury of** sigmoid colon
- **S36.598 Other injury of other part of colon**
- **S36.599 Other injury of unspecified part of colon**

S36.6 Injury of rectum
- **S36.60 Unspecified injury of rectum**
- **S36.61 Primary blast injury of rectum**

Blast injury of rectum NOS
- **S36.62 Contusion of rectum**
- **S36.63 Laceration of rectum**
- **S36.69 Other injury of rectum**

Secondary blast injury of rectum

√5ᵗʰ **S36.8** **Injury of other intra-abdominal organs**

    √x7ᵗʰ **S36.81** **Injury of** peritoneum

    √6ᵗʰ **S36.89** **Injury of other intra-abdominal organs**

       Injury of retroperitoneum

       √7ᵗʰ **S36.892** **Contusion of other intra-abdominal organs**

       √7ᵗʰ **S36.893** **Laceration of other intra-abdominal organs**

       √7ᵗʰ **S36.898** **Other injury of other intra-abdominal organs**

       √7ᵗʰ **S36.899** **Unspecified injury of other intra-abdominal organs**

√5ᵗʰ **S36.9** **Injury of unspecified intra-abdominal organ**

    √x7ᵗʰ **S36.90** **Unspecified injury of unspecified intra-abdominal organ**

    √x7ᵗʰ **S36.92** **Contusion of unspecified intra-abdominal organ**

    √x7ᵗʰ **S36.93** **Laceration of unspecified intra-abdominal organ**

    √x7ᵗʰ **S36.99** **Other injury of unspecified intra-abdominal organ**

√4ᵗʰ **S37** **Injury of urinary and pelvic organs**

    Code also any associated open wound (S31.-)

    EXCLUDES 1   obstetric trauma to pelvic organs (O71.-)

    EXCLUDES 2   injury of peritoneum (S36.81)

            injury of retroperitoneum (S36.89-)

    The appropriate 7th character is to be added to each code from category S37.
    A   initial encounter
    D   subsequent encounter
    S   sequela

√5ᵗʰ **S37.0** **Injury of** kidney

      EXCLUDES 2   acute kidney injury (nontraumatic) (N17.9)

    √6ᵗʰ **S37.00** **Unspecified injury of kidney**

       √7ᵗʰ **S37.001** **Unspecified injury of** right **kidney**

       √7ᵗʰ **S37.002** **Unspecified injury of** left **kidney**

       √7ᵗʰ **S37.009** **Unspecified injury of unspecified kidney**

    √6ᵗʰ **S37.01** **Minor contusion of kidney**

       Contusion of kidney less than 2 cm
       Contusion of kidney NOS

       √7ᵗʰ **S37.011** **Minor contusion of** right **kidney**

       √7ᵗʰ **S37.012** **Minor contusion of** left **kidney**

       √7ᵗʰ **S37.019** **Minor contusion of unspecified kidney**

    √6ᵗʰ **S37.02** **Major contusion of kidney**

       Contusion of kidney greater than 2 cm

       √7ᵗʰ **S37.021** **Major contusion of** right **kidney**

       √7ᵗʰ **S37.022** **Major contusion of** left **kidney**

       √7ᵗʰ **S37.029** **Major contusion of unspecified kidney**

    √6ᵗʰ **S37.03** **Laceration of kidney, unspecified degree**

       √7ᵗʰ **S37.031** **Laceration of** right **kidney, unspecified degree**

       √7ᵗʰ **S37.032** **Laceration of** left **kidney, unspecified degree**

       √7ᵗʰ **S37.039** **Laceration of unspecified kidney, unspecified degree**

    √6ᵗʰ **S37.04** **Minor laceration of kidney**

       Laceration of kidney less than 1 cm

       √7ᵗʰ **S37.041** **Minor laceration of** right **kidney**

       √7ᵗʰ **S37.042** **Minor laceration of** left **kidney**

       √7ᵗʰ **S37.049** **Minor laceration of unspecified kidney**

    √6ᵗʰ **S37.05** **Moderate laceration of kidney**

       Laceration of kidney 1 to 3 cm

       √7ᵗʰ **S37.051** **Moderate laceration of** right **kidney**

       √7ᵗʰ **S37.052** **Moderate laceration of** left **kidney**

       √7ᵗʰ **S37.059** **Moderate laceration of unspecified kidney**

    √6ᵗʰ **S37.06** **Major laceration of kidney**

       Avulsion of kidney
       Laceration of kidney greater than 3 cm
       Massive laceration of kidney
       Multiple moderate lacerations of kidney
       Stellate laceration of kidney

       √7ᵗʰ **S37.061** **Major laceration of** right **kidney**

       √7ᵗʰ **S37.062** **Major laceration of** left **kidney**

       √7ᵗʰ **S37.069** **Major laceration of unspecified kidney**

    √6ᵗʰ **S37.09** **Other injury of kidney**

       √7ᵗʰ **S37.091** **Other injury of** right **kidney**

       √7ᵗʰ **S37.092** **Other injury of** left **kidney**

       √7ᵗʰ **S37.099** **Other injury of unspecified kidney**

√5ᵗʰ **S37.1** **Injury of** ureter

    √x7ᵗʰ **S37.10** **Unspecified injury of ureter**

    √x7ᵗʰ **S37.12** **Contusion of ureter**

    √x7ᵗʰ **S37.13** **Laceration of ureter**

    √x7ᵗʰ **S37.19** **Other injury of ureter**

√5ᵗʰ **S37.2** **Injury of** bladder

    √x7ᵗʰ **S37.20** **Unspecified injury of bladder**

    √x7ᵗʰ **S37.22** **Contusion of bladder**

    √x7ᵗʰ **S37.23** **Laceration of bladder**

    √x7ᵗʰ **S37.29** **Other injury of bladder**

√5ᵗʰ **S37.3** **Injury of** urethra

    √x7ᵗʰ **S37.30** **Unspecified injury of urethra**

    √x7ᵗʰ **S37.32** **Contusion of urethra**

    √x7ᵗʰ **S37.33** **Laceration of urethra**

    √x7ᵗʰ **S37.39** **Other injury of urethra**

√5ᵗʰ **S37.4** **Injury of** ovary

    √6ᵗʰ **S37.40** **Unspecified injury of ovary**

       √7ᵗʰ **S37.401** **Unspecified injury of ovary, unilateral** ♀

       √7ᵗʰ **S37.402** **Unspecified injury of ovary, bilateral** ♀

       √7ᵗʰ **S37.409** **Unspecified injury of ovary, unspecified** ♀

    √6ᵗʰ **S37.42** **Contusion of ovary**

       √7ᵗʰ **S37.421** **Contusion of ovary,** unilateral ♀

       √7ᵗʰ **S37.422** **Contusion of ovary,** bilateral ♀

       √7ᵗʰ **S37.429** **Contusion of ovary, unspecified** ♀

    √6ᵗʰ **S37.43** **Laceration of ovary**

       √7ᵗʰ **S37.431** **Laceration of ovary,** unilateral ♀

       √7ᵗʰ **S37.432** **Laceration of ovary,** bilateral ♀

       √7ᵗʰ **S37.439** **Laceration of ovary, unspecified** ♀

    √6ᵗʰ **S37.49** **Other injury of ovary**

       √7ᵗʰ **S37.491** **Other injury of ovary,** unilateral ♀

       √7ᵗʰ **S37.492** **Other injury of ovary,** bilateral ♀

       √7ᵗʰ **S37.499** **Other injury of ovary, unspecified** ♀

√5ᵗʰ **S37.5** **Injury of** fallopian tube

    √6ᵗʰ **S37.50** **Unspecified injury of fallopian tube**

       √7ᵗʰ **S37.501** **Unspecified injury of fallopian tube, unilateral** ♀

       √7ᵗʰ **S37.502** **Unspecified injury of fallopian tube, bilateral** ♀

       √7ᵗʰ **S37.509** **Unspecified injury of fallopian tube, unspecified** ♀

    √6ᵗʰ **S37.51** **Primary blast injury of fallopian tube**

       Blast injury of fallopian tube NOS

       √7ᵗʰ **S37.511** **Primary blast injury of fallopian tube, unilateral** ♀

       √7ᵗʰ **S37.512** **Primary blast injury of fallopian tube, bilateral** ♀

       √7ᵗʰ **S37.519** **Primary blast injury of fallopian tube, unspecified** ♀

    √6ᵗʰ **S37.52** **Contusion of fallopian tube**

       √7ᵗʰ **S37.521** **Contusion of fallopian tube, unilateral** ♀

       √7ᵗʰ **S37.522** **Contusion of fallopian tube, bilateral** ♀

       √7ᵗʰ **S37.529** **Contusion of fallopian tube, unspecified** ♀

    √6ᵗʰ **S37.53** **Laceration of fallopian tube**

       √7ᵗʰ **S37.531** **Laceration of fallopian tube, unilateral** ♀

       √7ᵗʰ **S37.532** **Laceration of fallopian tube, bilateral** ♀

       √7ᵗʰ **S37.539** **Laceration of fallopian tube, unspecified** ♀

✓ Additional Character Required   √x7ᵗʰ Placeholder Alert   Manifestation   Unspecified Dx   Q QPP   UPD Unacceptable PDx

√6ᵗʰ **S37.59** **Other injury of fallopian tube**

Secondary blast injury of fallopian tube

√7ᵗʰ **S37.591** **Other injury of fallopian tube, unilateral** ♀

√7ᵗʰ **S37.592** **Other injury of fallopian tube, bilateral** ♀

√7ᵗʰ **S37.599** **Other injury of fallopian tube, unspecified** ♀

√5ᵗʰ **S37.6** **Injury of** uterus

EXCLUDES 1   *injury to gravid uterus (O9A.2-)*
               injury to uterus during delivery (O71.-)

√x7ᵗʰ **S37.60** **Unspecified injury of uterus** ♀

√x7ᵗʰ **S37.62** **Contusion of uterus** ♀

√x7ᵗʰ **S37.63** **Laceration of uterus** ♀

√x7ᵗʰ **S37.69** **Other injury of uterus** ♀

√5ᵗʰ **S37.8** **Injury of other urinary and pelvic organs**

√6ᵗʰ **S37.81** **Injury of** adrenal gland

√7ᵗʰ **S37.812** **Contusion of adrenal gland**

√7ᵗʰ **S37.813** **Laceration of adrenal gland**

√7ᵗʰ **S37.818** **Other injury of adrenal gland**

√7ᵗʰ **S37.819** **Unspecified injury of adrenal gland**

√6ᵗʰ **S37.82** **Injury of** prostate

√7ᵗʰ **S37.822** **Contusion of prostate** ♂

√7ᵗʰ **S37.823** **Laceration of prostate** ♂

√7ᵗʰ **S37.828** **Other injury of prostate** ♂

√7ᵗʰ **S37.829** **Unspecified injury of prostate** ♂

√6ᵗʰ **S37.89** **Injury of other urinary and pelvic organ**

√7ᵗʰ **S37.892** **Contusion of other urinary and pelvic organ**

√7ᵗʰ **S37.893** **Laceration of other urinary and pelvic organ**

√7ᵗʰ **S37.898** **Other injury of other urinary and pelvic organ**

√7ᵗʰ **S37.899** **Unspecified injury of other urinary and pelvic organ**

√5ᵗʰ **S37.9** **Injury of unspecified urinary and pelvic organ**

√x7ᵗʰ **S37.90** **Unspecified injury of unspecified urinary and pelvic organ**

√x7ᵗʰ **S37.92** **Contusion of unspecified urinary and pelvic organ**

√x7ᵗʰ **S37.93** **Laceration of unspecified urinary and pelvic organ**

√x7ᵗʰ **S37.99** **Other injury of unspecified urinary and pelvic organ**

√4ᵗʰ **S38** **Crushing injury and traumatic amputation of abdomen, lower back, pelvis and external genitals**

NOTE   An amputation not identified as partial or complete should be coded to complete

The appropriate 7th character is to be added to each code from category S38.
A   initial encounter
D   subsequent encounter
S   sequela

√5ᵗʰ **S38.0** **Crushing injury of** external genital organs

Use additional code for any associated injuries

√6ᵗʰ **S38.00** **Crushing injury of unspecified external genital organs**

√7ᵗʰ **S38.001** **Crushing injury of unspecified external genital organs, male** ♂

√7ᵗʰ **S38.002** **Crushing injury of unspecified external genital organs, female** ♀

√x7ᵗʰ **S38.01** **Crushing injury of** penis ♂

√x7ᵗʰ **S38.02** **Crushing injury of** scrotum and testis ♂

√x7ᵗʰ **S38.03** **Crushing injury of** vulva ♀

√x7ᵗʰ **S38.1** **Crushing injury of abdomen, lower back, and pelvis**

Use additional code for all associated injuries, such as:
  fracture of thoracic or lumbar spine and pelvis (S22.0-, S32.-)
  injury to intra-abdominal organs (S36.-)
  injury to urinary and pelvic organs (S37.-)
  open wound of abdominal wall (S31.-)
  spinal cord injury (S34.0, S34.1-)

EXCLUDES 2   *crushing injury of external genital organs (S38.0-)*

√5ᵗʰ **S38.2** **Traumatic amputation of external genital organs**

√6ᵗʰ **S38.21** **Traumatic amputation of** female **external genital organs**

Traumatic amputation of clitoris
Traumatic amputation of labium (majus) (minus)
Traumatic amputation of vulva

√7ᵗʰ **S38.211** **Complete traumatic amputation of female external genital organs** ♀

√7ᵗʰ **S38.212** **Partial traumatic amputation of female external genital organs** ♀

√6ᵗʰ **S38.22** **Traumatic amputation of** penis

√7ᵗʰ **S38.221** **Complete traumatic amputation of penis** ♂

√7ᵗʰ **S38.222** **Partial traumatic amputation of penis** ♂

√6ᵗʰ **S38.23** **Traumatic amputation of** scrotum and testis

√7ᵗʰ **S38.231** **Complete traumatic amputation of scrotum and testis** ♂

√7ᵗʰ **S38.232** **Partial traumatic amputation of scrotum and testis** ♂

√x7ᵗʰ **S38.3** **Transection (partial) of abdomen**

√4ᵗʰ **S39** **Other and unspecified injuries of abdomen, lower back, pelvis and external genitals**

Code also any associated open wound (S31.-)

EXCLUDES 2   *sprain of joints and ligaments of lumbar spine and pelvis (S33.-)*

The appropriate 7th character is to be added to each code from category S39.
A   initial encounter
D   subsequent encounter
S   sequela

√5ᵗʰ **S39.0** **Injury of muscle, fascia and tendon of abdomen, lower back and pelvis**

√6ᵗʰ **S39.00** **Unspecified injury of muscle, fascia and tendon of abdomen, lower back and pelvis**

√7ᵗʰ **S39.001** **Unspecified injury of muscle, fascia and tendon of** abdomen

√7ᵗʰ **S39.002** **Unspecified injury of muscle, fascia and tendon of** lower back

√7ᵗʰ **S39.003** **Unspecified injury of muscle, fascia and tendon of** pelvis

√6ᵗʰ **S39.01** **Strain of muscle, fascia and tendon of abdomen, lower back and pelvis**

√7ᵗʰ **S39.011** **Strain of muscle, fascia and tendon of** abdomen

√7ᵗʰ **S39.012** **Strain of muscle, fascia and tendon of** lower back

√7ᵗʰ **S39.013** **Strain of muscle, fascia and tendon of** pelvis

√6ᵗʰ **S39.02** **Laceration of muscle, fascia and tendon of abdomen, lower back and pelvis**

√7ᵗʰ **S39.021** **Laceration of muscle, fascia and tendon of** abdomen

√7ᵗʰ **S39.022** **Laceration of muscle, fascia and tendon of** lower back

√7ᵗʰ **S39.023** **Laceration of muscle, fascia and tendon of** pelvis

√6ᵗʰ **S39.09** **Other injury of muscle, fascia and tendon of abdomen, lower back and pelvis**

√7ᵗʰ **S39.091** **Other injury of muscle, fascia and tendon of** abdomen

√7ᵗʰ **S39.092** **Other injury of muscle, fascia and tendon of** lower back

√7ᵗʰ **S39.093** **Other injury of muscle, fascia and tendon of** pelvis

√5ᵗʰ **S39.8** **Other specified injuries of abdomen, lower back, pelvis and external genitals**

√x7ᵗʰ **S39.81** **Other specified injuries of** abdomen

√x7ᵗʰ **S39.82** **Other specified injuries of** lower back

√x7ᵗʰ **S39.83** **Other specified injuries of** pelvis

√6ᵗʰ **S39.84** **Other specified injuries of** external genitals

√7ᵗʰ **S39.840** **Fracture of** corpus cavernosum penis ♂

√7ᵗʰ **S39.848** **Other specified injuries of external genitals**

√5ᵗʰ **S39.9** **Unspecified injury of abdomen, lower back, pelvis and external genitals**

√x7ᵗʰ **S39.91** **Unspecified injury of** abdomen

√x7ᵗʰ **S39.92** Unspecified injury of lower back

√x7ᵗʰ **S39.93** Unspecified injury of pelvis

√x7ᵗʰ **S39.94** Unspecified injury of external genitals

Injuries to the shoulder and upper arm (S40-S49)

INCLUDES   injuries of axilla
       injuries of scapular region
EXCLUDES 2   burns and corrosions (T20-T32)
       frostbite (T33-T34)
       injuries of elbow (S50-S59)
       insect bite or sting, venomous (T63.4)

√4ᵗʰ **S40** **Superficial injury of shoulder and upper arm**

> The appropriate 7th character is to be added to each code from category S40.
> A   initial encounter
> D   subsequent encounter
> S   sequela

√5ᵗʰ **S40.0** **Contusion of shoulder and upper arm**

√6ᵗʰ **S40.01** **Contusion of** shoulder

√7ᵗʰ **S40.011** **Contusion of** right **shoulder**

√7ᵗʰ **S40.012** **Contusion of** left **shoulder**

√7ᵗʰ **S40.019** **Contusion of unspecified shoulder**

√6ᵗʰ **S40.02** **Contusion of** upper arm

√7ᵗʰ **S40.021** **Contusion of** right **upper arm**

√7ᵗʰ **S40.022** **Contusion of** left **upper arm**

√7ᵗʰ **S40.029** **Contusion of unspecified upper arm**

√5ᵗʰ **S40.2** **Other superficial injuries of** shoulder

√6ᵗʰ **S40.21** **Abrasion of** shoulder

√7ᵗʰ **S40.211** **Abrasion of** right **shoulder**

√7ᵗʰ **S40.212** **Abrasion of** left **shoulder**

√7ᵗʰ **S40.219** **Abrasion of unspecified shoulder**

√6ᵗʰ **S40.22** **Blister (nonthermal) of shoulder**

√7ᵗʰ **S40.221** **Blister (nonthermal) of** right **shoulder**

√7ᵗʰ **S40.222** **Blister (nonthermal) of** left **shoulder**

√7ᵗʰ **S40.229** **Blister (nonthermal) of unspecified shoulder**

√6ᵗʰ **S40.24** **External constriction of shoulder**

√7ᵗʰ **S40.241** **External constriction of** right **shoulder**

√7ᵗʰ **S40.242** **External constriction of** left **shoulder**

√7ᵗʰ **S40.249** **External constriction of unspecified shoulder**

√6ᵗʰ **S40.25** **Superficial** foreign body **of shoulder**

     Splinter in the shoulder

√7ᵗʰ **S40.251** **Superficial foreign body of** right **shoulder**

√7ᵗʰ **S40.252** **Superficial foreign body of** left **shoulder**

√7ᵗʰ **S40.259** **Superficial foreign body of unspecified shoulder**

√6ᵗʰ **S40.26** **Insect bite** (nonvenomous) **of shoulder**

√7ᵗʰ **S40.261** **Insect bite (nonvenomous) of** right **shoulder**

√7ᵗʰ **S40.262** **Insect bite (nonvenomous) of** left **shoulder**

√7ᵗʰ **S40.269** **Insect bite (nonvenomous) of unspecified shoulder**

√6ᵗʰ **S40.27** **Other superficial** bite **of shoulder**

EXCLUDES 1   open bite of shoulder (S41.05)

√7ᵗʰ **S40.271** **Other superficial bite of** right **shoulder**

√7ᵗʰ **S40.272** **Other superficial bite of** left **shoulder**

√7ᵗʰ **S40.279** **Other superficial bite of unspecified shoulder**

√5ᵗʰ **S40.8** **Other superficial injuries of** upper arm

√6ᵗʰ **S40.81** **Abrasion of** upper arm

√7ᵗʰ **S40.811** **Abrasion of** right **upper arm**

√7ᵗʰ **S40.812** **Abrasion of** left **upper arm**

√7ᵗʰ **S40.819** **Abrasion of unspecified upper arm**

√6ᵗʰ **S40.82** **Blister (nonthermal) of** upper arm

√7ᵗʰ **S40.821** **Blister (nonthermal) of** right **upper arm**

√7ᵗʰ **S40.822** **Blister (nonthermal) of** left **upper arm**

√7ᵗʰ **S40.829** **Blister (nonthermal) of unspecified upper arm**

√6ᵗʰ **S40.84** **External constriction of upper arm**

√7ᵗʰ **S40.841** **External constriction of** right **upper arm**

√7ᵗʰ **S40.842** **External constriction of** left **upper arm**

√7ᵗʰ **S40.849** **External constriction of unspecified upper arm**

√6ᵗʰ **S40.85** **Superficial** foreign body **of upper arm**

     Splinter in the upper arm

√7ᵗʰ **S40.851** **Superficial foreign body of** right **upper arm**

√7ᵗʰ **S40.852** **Superficial foreign body of** left **upper arm**

√7ᵗʰ **S40.859** **Superficial foreign body of unspecified upper arm**

√6ᵗʰ **S40.86** **Insect bite** (nonvenomous) **of upper arm**

√7ᵗʰ **S40.861** **Insect bite (nonvenomous) of** right **upper arm**

√7ᵗʰ **S40.862** **Insect bite (nonvenomous) of** left **upper arm**

√7ᵗʰ **S40.869** **Insect bite (nonvenomous) of unspecified upper arm**

√6ᵗʰ **S40.87** **Other superficial** bite **of upper arm**

EXCLUDES 1   open bite of upper arm (S41.14)
EXCLUDES 2   other superficial bite of shoulder (S40.27-)

√7ᵗʰ **S40.871** **Other superficial bite of** right **upper arm**

√7ᵗʰ **S40.872** **Other superficial bite of** left **upper arm**

√7ᵗʰ **S40.879** **Other superficial bite of unspecified upper arm**

√5ᵗʰ **S40.9** **Unspecified superficial injury of shoulder and upper arm**

√6ᵗʰ **S40.91** **Unspecified superficial injury of** shoulder

√7ᵗʰ **S40.911** **Unspecified superficial injury of** right **shoulder**

√7ᵗʰ **S40.912** **Unspecified superficial injury of** left **shoulder**

√7ᵗʰ **S40.919** **Unspecified superficial injury of unspecified shoulder**

√6ᵗʰ **S40.92** **Unspecified superficial injury of** upper arm

√7ᵗʰ **S40.921** **Unspecified superficial injury of** right **upper arm**

√7ᵗʰ **S40.922** **Unspecified superficial injury of** left **upper arm**

√7ᵗʰ **S40.929** **Unspecified superficial injury of unspecified upper arm**

√4ᵗʰ **S41** **Open wound of shoulder and upper arm**

Code also any associated wound infection
EXCLUDES 1   traumatic amputation of shoulder and upper arm (S48.-)
EXCLUDES 2   open fracture of shoulder and upper arm (S42.- with 7th character B or C)

> The appropriate 7th character is to be added to each code from category S41.
> A   initial encounter
> D   subsequent encounter
> S   sequela

√5ᵗʰ **S41.0** **Open wound of** shoulder

√6ᵗʰ **S41.00** **Unspecified open wound of shoulder**

√7ᵗʰ **S41.001** **Unspecified open wound of** right **shoulder**

√7ᵗʰ **S41.002** **Unspecified open wound of** left **shoulder**

√7ᵗʰ **S41.009** **Unspecified open wound of unspecified shoulder**

√6ᵗʰ **S41.01** **Laceration without foreign body of shoulder**

√7ᵗʰ **S41.011** **Laceration without foreign body of** right **shoulder**

√7ᵗʰ **S41.012** **Laceration without foreign body of** left **shoulder**

√7ᵗʰ **S41.019** **Laceration without foreign body of unspecified shoulder**

√6ᵗʰ **S41.02** **Laceration with foreign body of shoulder**

√7ᵗʰ **S41.021** **Laceration with foreign body of** right **shoulder**

√7ᵗʰ **S41.022** **Laceration with foreign body of** left **shoulder**

√7ᵗʰ **S41.029** **Laceration with foreign body of unspecified shoulder**

√6ᵗʰ **S41.03** **Puncture wound without foreign body of shoulder**

√7ᵗʰ **S41.031** **Puncture wound without foreign body of** right **shoulder**

✓7ᵗʰ **S41.032** Puncture wound without foreign body of left shoulder

✓7ᵗʰ **S41.039** Puncture wound without foreign body of unspecified shoulder

✓6ᵗʰ **S41.04** Puncture wound with foreign body of shoulder

✓7ᵗʰ **S41.041** Puncture wound with foreign body of right shoulder

✓7ᵗʰ **S41.042** Puncture wound with foreign body of left shoulder

✓7ᵗʰ **S41.049** Puncture wound with foreign body of unspecified shoulder

✓6ᵗʰ **S41.05** Open bite of shoulder

Bite of shoulder NOS

EXCLUDES 1   *superficial bite of shoulder (S40.27)*

✓7ᵗʰ **S41.051** Open bite of right shoulder

✓7ᵗʰ **S41.052** Open bite of left shoulder

✓7ᵗʰ **S41.059** Open bite of unspecified shoulder

✓5ᵗʰ **S41.1** Open wound of upper arm

✓6ᵗʰ **S41.10** Unspecified open wound of upper arm

AHA: 2016,3Q,24

✓7ᵗʰ **S41.101** Unspecified open wound of right upper arm

✓7ᵗʰ **S41.102** Unspecified open wound of left upper arm

✓7ᵗʰ **S41.109** Unspecified open wound of unspecified upper arm

✓6ᵗʰ **S41.11** Laceration without foreign body of upper arm

✓7ᵗʰ **S41.111** Laceration without foreign body of right upper arm

✓7ᵗʰ **S41.112** Laceration without foreign body of left upper arm

✓7ᵗʰ **S41.119** Laceration without foreign body of unspecified upper arm

✓6ᵗʰ **S41.12** Laceration with foreign body of upper arm

✓7ᵗʰ **S41.121** Laceration with foreign body of right upper arm

✓7ᵗʰ **S41.122** Laceration with foreign body of left upper arm

✓7ᵗʰ **S41.129** Laceration with foreign body of unspecified upper arm

✓6ᵗʰ **S41.13** Puncture wound without foreign body of upper arm

AHA: 2016,3Q,24

✓7ᵗʰ **S41.131** Puncture wound without foreign body of right upper arm

✓7ᵗʰ **S41.132** Puncture wound without foreign body of left upper arm

✓7ᵗʰ **S41.139** Puncture wound without foreign body of unspecified upper arm

✓6ᵗʰ **S41.14** Puncture wound with foreign body of upper arm

AHA: 2016,3Q,24

✓7ᵗʰ **S41.141** Puncture wound with foreign body of right upper arm

✓7ᵗʰ **S41.142** Puncture wound with foreign body of left upper arm

✓7ᵗʰ **S41.149** Puncture wound with foreign body of unspecified upper arm

✓6ᵗʰ **S41.15** Open bite of upper arm

Bite of upper arm NOS

EXCLUDES 1   *superficial bite of upper arm (S40.87)*

✓7ᵗʰ **S41.151** Open bite of right upper arm

✓7ᵗʰ **S41.152** Open bite of left upper arm

✓7ᵗʰ **S41.159** Open bite of unspecified upper arm

✓4ᵗʰ **S42** Fracture of shoulder and upper arm

NOTE   A fracture not indicated as displaced or nondisplaced should be coded to displaced

A fracture not indicated as open or closed should be coded to closed

EXCLUDES 1   *traumatic amputation of shoulder and upper arm (S48.-)*

AHA: 2018,2Q,12; 2015,3Q,37-39

DEF: Diaphysis: Central shaft of a long bone.

DEF: Epiphysis: Proximal and distal rounded ends of a long bone, communicates with the joint.

DEF: Metaphysis: Section of a long bone located between the epiphysis and diaphysis at the proximal and distal ends.

DEF: Physis (growth plate): Narrow zone of cartilaginous tissue between the epiphysis and metaphysis at each end of a long bone. In childhood, proliferation of cells in this zone lengthens the bone. As the bone matures, this area thins, ossification eventually fusing into solid bone and growth stops. *Synonym(s): Epiphyseal plate.*

The appropriate 7th character is to be added to all codes from category S42 [unless otherwise indicated].

A   initial encounter for closed fracture
B   initial encounter for open fracture
D   subsequent encounter for fracture with routine healing
G   subsequent encounter for fracture with delayed healing
K   subsequent encounter for fracture with nonunion
P   subsequent encounter for fracture with malunion
S   sequela

✓5ᵗʰ **S42.0** Fracture of clavicle

✓6ᵗʰ **S42.00** Fracture of unspecified part of clavicle

✓7ᵗʰ **S42.001** Fracture of unspecified part of right clavicle ⓪

✓7ᵗʰ **S42.002** Fracture of unspecified part of left clavicle ⓪

✓7ᵗʰ **S42.009** Fracture of unspecified part of unspecified clavicle ⓪

AHA: 2012,4Q,93

✓6ᵗʰ **S42.01** Fracture of sternal end of clavicle

✓7ᵗʰ **S42.011** Anterior displaced fracture of sternal end of right clavicle ⓪

✓7ᵗʰ **S42.012** Anterior displaced fracture of sternal end of left clavicle ⓪

✓7ᵗʰ **S42.013** Anterior displaced fracture of sternal end of unspecified clavicle ⓪

Displaced fracture of sternal end of clavicle NOS

✓7ᵗʰ **S42.014** Posterior displaced fracture of sternal end of right clavicle ⓪

✓7ᵗʰ **S42.015** Posterior displaced fracture of sternal end of left clavicle ⓪

✓7ᵗʰ **S42.016** Posterior displaced fracture of sternal end of unspecified clavicle ⓪

✓7ᵗʰ **S42.017** Nondisplaced fracture of sternal end of right clavicle ⓪

✓7ᵗʰ **S42.018** Nondisplaced fracture of sternal end of left clavicle ⓪

✓7ᵗʰ **S42.019** Nondisplaced fracture of sternal end of unspecified clavicle ⓪

✓6ᵗʰ **S42.02** Fracture of shaft of clavicle

✓7ᵗʰ **S42.021** Displaced fracture of shaft of right clavicle ⓪

✓7ᵗʰ **S42.022** Displaced fracture of shaft of left clavicle ⓪

✓7ᵗʰ **S42.023** Displaced fracture of shaft of unspecified clavicle ⓪

✓7ᵗʰ **S42.024** Nondisplaced fracture of shaft of right clavicle ⓪

✓7ᵗʰ **S42.025** Nondisplaced fracture of shaft of left clavicle ⓪

✓7ᵗʰ **S42.026** Nondisplaced fracture of shaft of unspecified clavicle ⓪

✓6ᵗʰ **S42.03** Fracture of lateral end of clavicle

Fracture of acromial end of clavicle

✓7ᵗʰ **S42.031** Displaced fracture of lateral end of right clavicle ⓪

✓7ᵗʰ **S42.032** Displaced fracture of lateral end of left clavicle ⓪

✓7ᵗʰ **S42.033** Displaced fracture of lateral end of unspecified clavicle ⓪

| HCC CMS-HCC | Rx Rx HCC | ESR ESRD HCC | COM Commercial HCC | N Newborn: 0 | P Pediatric: 0-17 | M Maternity: 9-64 | A Adult: 15-124 |

1034

ICD-10-CM 2023

√7ᵗʰ **S42.034** Nondisplaced fracture of lateral end of right clavicle ◘

√7ᵗʰ **S42.035** Nondisplaced fracture of lateral end of left clavicle ◘

√7ᵗʰ **S42.036** Nondisplaced fracture of lateral end of unspecified clavicle ◘

√5ᵗʰ **S42.1** Fracture of scapula

√6ᵗʰ **S42.10** Fracture of unspecified part of scapula

√7ᵗʰ **S42.101** Fracture of unspecified part of scapula, right shoulder ◘

√7ᵗʰ **S42.102** Fracture of unspecified part of scapula, left shoulder ◘

√7ᵗʰ **S42.109** Fracture of unspecified part of scapula, unspecified shoulder ◘

√6ᵗʰ **S42.11** Fracture of body of scapula

√7ᵗʰ **S42.111** Displaced fracture of body of scapula, right shoulder ◘

√7ᵗʰ **S42.112** Displaced fracture of body of scapula, left shoulder ◘

√7ᵗʰ **S42.113** Displaced fracture of body of scapula, unspecified shoulder ◘

√7ᵗʰ **S42.114** Nondisplaced fracture of body of scapula, right shoulder ◘

√7ᵗʰ **S42.115** Nondisplaced fracture of body of scapula, left shoulder ◘

√7ᵗʰ **S42.116** Nondisplaced fracture of body of scapula, unspecified shoulder ◘

√6ᵗʰ **S42.12** Fracture of acromial process

√7ᵗʰ **S42.121** Displaced fracture of acromial process, right shoulder ◘

√7ᵗʰ **S42.122** Displaced fracture of acromial process, left shoulder ◘

√7ᵗʰ **S42.123** Displaced fracture of acromial process, unspecified shoulder ◘

√7ᵗʰ **S42.124** Nondisplaced fracture of acromial process, right shoulder ◘

√7ᵗʰ **S42.125** Nondisplaced fracture of acromial process, left shoulder ◘

√7ᵗʰ **S42.126** Nondisplaced fracture of acromial process, unspecified shoulder ◘

√6ᵗʰ **S42.13** Fracture of coracoid process

√7ᵗʰ **S42.131** Displaced fracture of coracoid process, right shoulder ◘

√7ᵗʰ **S42.132** Displaced fracture of coracoid process, left shoulder ◘

√7ᵗʰ **S42.133** Displaced fracture of coracoid process, unspecified shoulder ◘

√7ᵗʰ **S42.134** Nondisplaced fracture of coracoid process, right shoulder ◘

√7ᵗʰ **S42.135** Nondisplaced fracture of coracoid process, left shoulder ◘

√7ᵗʰ **S42.136** Nondisplaced fracture of coracoid process, unspecified shoulder ◘

√6ᵗʰ **S42.14** Fracture of glenoid cavity of scapula

√7ᵗʰ **S42.141** Displaced fracture of glenoid cavity of scapula, right shoulder ◘

√7ᵗʰ **S42.142** Displaced fracture of glenoid cavity of scapula, left shoulder ◘

√7ᵗʰ **S42.143** Displaced fracture of glenoid cavity of scapula, unspecified shoulder ◘

√7ᵗʰ **S42.144** Nondisplaced fracture of glenoid cavity of scapula, right shoulder ◘

√7ᵗʰ **S42.145** Nondisplaced fracture of glenoid cavity of scapula, left shoulder ◘

√7ᵗʰ **S42.146** Nondisplaced fracture of glenoid cavity of scapula, unspecified shoulder ◘

√6ᵗʰ **S42.15** Fracture of neck of scapula

√7ᵗʰ **S42.151** Displaced fracture of neck of scapula, right shoulder ◘

√7ᵗʰ **S42.152** Displaced fracture of neck of scapula, left shoulder ◘

√7ᵗʰ **S42.153** Displaced fracture of neck of scapula, unspecified shoulder ◘

√7ᵗʰ **S42.154** Nondisplaced fracture of neck of scapula, right shoulder ◘

√7ᵗʰ **S42.155** Nondisplaced fracture of neck of scapula, left shoulder ◘

√7ᵗʰ **S42.156** Nondisplaced fracture of neck of scapula, unspecified shoulder ◘

√6ᵗʰ **S42.19** Fracture of other part of scapula

√7ᵗʰ **S42.191** Fracture of other part of scapula, right shoulder ◘

√7ᵗʰ **S42.192** Fracture of other part of scapula, left shoulder ◘

√7ᵗʰ **S42.199** Fracture of other part of scapula, unspecified shoulder ◘

√5ᵗʰ **S42.2** Fracture of upper end of humerus

Fracture of proximal end of humerus

EXCLUDES 2   *fracture of shaft of humerus (S42.3-)*

physeal fracture of upper end of humerus (S49.0-)

√6ᵗʰ **S42.20** Unspecified fracture of upper end of humerus

√7ᵗʰ **S42.201** Unspecified fracture of upper end of right humerus ◘

√7ᵗʰ **S42.202** Unspecified fracture of upper end of left humerus ◘

√7ᵗʰ **S42.209** Unspecified fracture of upper end of unspecified humerus ◘

√6ᵗʰ **S42.21** Unspecified fracture of surgical neck of humerus

Fracture of neck of humerus NOS

√7ᵗʰ **S42.211** Unspecified displaced fracture of surgical neck of right humerus ◘

√7ᵗʰ **S42.212** Unspecified displaced fracture of surgical neck of left humerus ◘

√7ᵗʰ **S42.213** Unspecified displaced fracture of surgical neck of unspecified humerus ◘

√7ᵗʰ **S42.214** Unspecified nondisplaced fracture of surgical neck of right humerus ◘

√7ᵗʰ **S42.215** Unspecified nondisplaced fracture of surgical neck of left humerus ◘

√7ᵗʰ **S42.216** Unspecified nondisplaced fracture of surgical neck of unspecified humerus ◘

√6ᵗʰ **S42.22** 2-part fracture of surgical neck of humerus

√7ᵗʰ **S42.221** 2-part displaced fracture of surgical neck of right humerus ◘

√7ᵗʰ **S42.222** 2-part displaced fracture of surgical neck of left humerus ◘

√7ᵗʰ **S42.223** 2-part displaced fracture of surgical neck of unspecified humerus ◘

√7ᵗʰ **S42.224** 2-part nondisplaced fracture of surgical neck of right humerus ◘

√7ᵗʰ **S42.225** 2-part nondisplaced fracture of surgical neck of left humerus ◘

√7ᵗʰ **S42.226** 2-part nondisplaced fracture of surgical neck of unspecified humerus ◘

√6ᵗʰ **S42.23** 3-part fracture of surgical neck of humerus

√7ᵗʰ **S42.231** 3-part fracture of surgical neck of right humerus ◘

√7ᵗʰ **S42.232** 3-part fracture of surgical neck of left humerus ◘

√7ᵗʰ **S42.239** 3-part fracture of surgical neck of unspecified humerus ◘

√6ᵗʰ **S42.24** 4-part fracture of surgical neck of humerus

√7ᵗʰ **S42.241** 4-part fracture of surgical neck of right humerus ◘

√7ᵗʰ **S42.242** 4-part fracture of surgical neck of left humerus ◘

√7ᵗʰ **S42.249** 4-part fracture of surgical neck of unspecified humerus ◘

√6ᵗʰ **S42.25** Fracture of greater tuberosity of humerus

√7ᵗʰ **S42.251** Displaced fracture of greater tuberosity of right humerus ◘

√7ᵗʰ **S42.252** Displaced fracture of greater tuberosity of left humerus ◘

√7ᵗʰ **S42.253** Displaced fracture of greater tuberosity of unspecified humerus ◘

√7ᵗʰ **S42.254** Nondisplaced fracture of greater tuberosity of right humerus ◘

√7ᵗʰ **S42.255** Nondisplaced fracture of greater tuberosity of left humerus ◘

√7ᵗʰ **S42.256** Nondisplaced fracture of greater tuberosity of unspecified humerus ◘

√6ᵗʰ **S42.26** Fracture of lesser tuberosity of humerus

√7ᵗʰ **S42.261** Displaced fracture of lesser tuberosity of right humerus ◘

√7ᵗʰ **S42.262** Displaced fracture of lesser tuberosity of left humerus ◘

√7ᵗʰ **S42.263** Displaced fracture of lesser tuberosity of unspecified humerus

√7ᵗʰ **S42.264** Nondisplaced fracture of lesser tuberosity of right humerus

√7ᵗʰ **S42.265** Nondisplaced fracture of lesser tuberosity of left humerus

√7ᵗʰ **S42.266** Nondisplaced fracture of lesser tuberosity of unspecified humerus

√6ᵗʰ **S42.27** Torus fracture of upper end of humerus

The appropriate 7th character is to be added to all codes in subcategory S42.27
A initial encounter for closed fracture
D subsequent encounter for fracture with routine healing
G subsequent encounter for fracture with delayed healing
K subsequent encounter for fracture with nonunion
P subsequent encounter for fracture with malunion
S sequela

√7ᵗʰ **S42.271** Torus fracture of upper end of right humerus

√7ᵗʰ **S42.272** Torus fracture of upper end of left humerus

√7ᵗʰ **S42.279** Torus fracture of upper end of unspecified humerus

√6ᵗʰ **S42.29** Other fracture of upper end of humerus
Fracture of anatomical neck of humerus
Fracture of articular head of humerus
AHA: 2019,1Q,18

√7ᵗʰ **S42.291** Other displaced fracture of upper end of right humerus

√7ᵗʰ **S42.292** Other displaced fracture of upper end of left humerus

√7ᵗʰ **S42.293** Other displaced fracture of upper end of unspecified humerus

√7ᵗʰ **S42.294** Other nondisplaced fracture of upper end of right humerus

√7ᵗʰ **S42.295** Other nondisplaced fracture of upper end of left humerus

√7ᵗʰ **S42.296** Other nondisplaced fracture of upper end of unspecified humerus

√5ᵗʰ **S42.3** Fracture of shaft of humerus
Fracture of humerus NOS
Fracture of upper arm NOS
EXCLUDES 2 physeal fractures of upper end of humerus (S49.0-)
physeal fractures of lower end of humerus (S49.1-)

√6ᵗʰ **S42.30** Unspecified fracture of shaft of humerus

√7ᵗʰ **S42.301** Unspecified fracture of shaft of humerus, right arm

√7ᵗʰ **S42.302** Unspecified fracture of shaft of humerus, left arm

√7ᵗʰ **S42.309** Unspecified fracture of shaft of humerus, unspecified arm

√6ᵗʰ **S42.31** Greenstick fracture of shaft of humerus

The appropriate 7th character is to be added to all codes in subcategory S42.31
A initial encounter for closed fracture
D subsequent encounter for fracture with routine healing
G subsequent encounter for fracture with delayed healing
K subsequent encounter for fracture with nonunion
P subsequent encounter for fracture with malunion
S sequela

√7ᵗʰ **S42.311** Greenstick fracture of shaft of humerus, right arm

√7ᵗʰ **S42.312** Greenstick fracture of shaft of humerus, left arm

√7ᵗʰ **S42.319** Greenstick fracture of shaft of humerus, unspecified arm

√6ᵗʰ **S42.32** Transverse fracture of shaft of humerus

√7ᵗʰ **S42.321** Displaced transverse fracture of shaft of humerus, right arm

√7ᵗʰ **S42.322** Displaced transverse fracture of shaft of humerus, left arm

√7ᵗʰ **S42.323** Displaced transverse fracture of shaft of humerus, unspecified arm

√7ᵗʰ **S42.324** Nondisplaced transverse fracture of shaft of humerus, right arm

√7ᵗʰ **S42.325** Nondisplaced transverse fracture of shaft of humerus, left arm

√7ᵗʰ **S42.326** Nondisplaced transverse fracture of shaft of humerus, unspecified arm

√6ᵗʰ **S42.33** Oblique fracture of shaft of humerus

√7ᵗʰ **S42.331** Displaced oblique fracture of shaft of humerus, right arm

√7ᵗʰ **S42.332** Displaced oblique fracture of shaft of humerus, left arm

√7ᵗʰ **S42.333** Displaced oblique fracture of shaft of humerus, unspecified arm

√7ᵗʰ **S42.334** Nondisplaced oblique fracture of shaft of humerus, right arm

√7ᵗʰ **S42.335** Nondisplaced oblique fracture of shaft of humerus, left arm

√7ᵗʰ **S42.336** Nondisplaced oblique fracture of shaft of humerus, unspecified arm

√6ᵗʰ **S42.34** Spiral fracture of shaft of humerus

√7ᵗʰ **S42.341** Displaced spiral fracture of shaft of humerus, right arm

√7ᵗʰ **S42.342** Displaced spiral fracture of shaft of humerus, left arm

√7ᵗʰ **S42.343** Displaced spiral fracture of shaft of humerus, unspecified arm

√7ᵗʰ **S42.344** Nondisplaced spiral fracture of shaft of humerus, right arm

√7ᵗʰ **S42.345** Nondisplaced spiral fracture of shaft of humerus, left arm

√7ᵗʰ **S42.346** Nondisplaced spiral fracture of shaft of humerus, unspecified arm

√6ᵗʰ **S42.35** Comminuted fracture of shaft of humerus

√7ᵗʰ **S42.351** Displaced comminuted fracture of shaft of humerus, right arm

√7ᵗʰ **S42.352** Displaced comminuted fracture of shaft of humerus, left arm

√7ᵗʰ **S42.353** Displaced comminuted fracture of shaft of humerus, unspecified arm

√7ᵗʰ **S42.354** Nondisplaced comminuted fracture of shaft of humerus, right arm

√7ᵗʰ **S42.355** Nondisplaced comminuted fracture of shaft of humerus, left arm

√7ᵗʰ **S42.356** Nondisplaced comminuted fracture of shaft of humerus, unspecified arm

√6ᵗʰ **S42.36** Segmental fracture of shaft of humerus

√7ᵗʰ **S42.361** Displaced segmental fracture of shaft of humerus, right arm

√7ᵗʰ **S42.362** Displaced segmental fracture of shaft of humerus, left arm

√7ᵗʰ **S42.363** Displaced segmental fracture of shaft of humerus, unspecified arm

√7ᵗʰ **S42.364** Nondisplaced segmental fracture of shaft of humerus, right arm

√7ᵗʰ **S42.365** Nondisplaced segmental fracture of shaft of humerus, left arm

√7ᵗʰ **S42.366** Nondisplaced segmental fracture of shaft of humerus, unspecified arm

√6ᵗʰ **S42.39** Other fracture of shaft of humerus

√7ᵗʰ **S42.391** Other fracture of shaft of right humerus

√7ᵗʰ **S42.392** Other fracture of shaft of left humerus

√7ᵗʰ **S42.399** Other fracture of shaft of unspecified humerus

√5ᵗʰ **S42.4** Fracture of lower end of humerus
Fracture of distal end of humerus
EXCLUDES 2 fracture of shaft of humerus (S42.3-)
physeal fracture of lower end of humerus (S49.1-)

√6ᵗʰ **S42.40** Unspecified fracture of lower end of humerus
Fracture of elbow NOS

√7ᵗʰ **S42.401** Unspecified fracture of lower end of right humerus

√7ᵗʰ **S42.402** Unspecified fracture of lower end of left humerus

√7ᵗʰ **S42.409** Unspecified fracture of lower end of unspecified humerus Ⓠ

√6ᵗʰ **S42.41** Simple supracondylar fracture without intercondylar fracture of humerus

√7ᵗʰ **S42.411** Displaced simple supracondylar fracture without intercondylar fracture of right humerus Ⓠ

√7ᵗʰ **S42.412** Displaced simple supracondylar fracture without intercondylar fracture of left humerus Ⓠ

√7ᵗʰ **S42.413** Displaced simple supracondylar fracture without intercondylar fracture of unspecified humerus Ⓠ

√7ᵗʰ **S42.414** Nondisplaced simple supracondylar fracture without intercondylar fracture of right humerus Ⓠ

√7ᵗʰ **S42.415** Nondisplaced simple supracondylar fracture without intercondylar fracture of left humerus Ⓠ

√7ᵗʰ **S42.416** Nondisplaced simple supracondylar fracture without intercondylar fracture of unspecified humerus Ⓠ

√6ᵗʰ **S42.42** Comminuted supracondylar fracture without intercondylar fracture of humerus

√7ᵗʰ **S42.421** Displaced comminuted supracondylar fracture without intercondylar fracture of right humerus Ⓠ

√7ᵗʰ **S42.422** Displaced comminuted supracondylar fracture without intercondylar fracture of left humerus Ⓠ

√7ᵗʰ **S42.423** Displaced comminuted supracondylar fracture without intercondylar fracture of unspecified humerus Ⓠ

√7ᵗʰ **S42.424** Nondisplaced comminuted supracondylar fracture without intercondylar fracture of right humerus Ⓠ

√7ᵗʰ **S42.425** Nondisplaced comminuted supracondylar fracture without intercondylar fracture of left humerus Ⓠ

√7ᵗʰ **S42.426** Nondisplaced comminuted supracondylar fracture without intercondylar fracture of unspecified humerus Ⓠ

√6ᵗʰ **S42.43** Fracture (avulsion) of lateral epicondyle of humerus

√7ᵗʰ **S42.431** Displaced fracture (avulsion) of lateral epicondyle of right humerus Ⓠ

√7ᵗʰ **S42.432** Displaced fracture (avulsion) of lateral epicondyle of left humerus Ⓠ

√7ᵗʰ **S42.433** Displaced fracture (avulsion) of lateral epicondyle of unspecified humerus Ⓠ

√7ᵗʰ **S42.434** Nondisplaced fracture (avulsion) of lateral epicondyle of right humerus Ⓠ

√7ᵗʰ **S42.435** Nondisplaced fracture (avulsion) of lateral epicondyle of left humerus Ⓠ

√7ᵗʰ **S42.436** Nondisplaced fracture (avulsion) of lateral epicondyle of unspecified humerus Ⓠ

√6ᵗʰ **S42.44** Fracture (avulsion) of medial epicondyle of humerus

√7ᵗʰ **S42.441** Displaced fracture (avulsion) of medial epicondyle of right humerus Ⓠ

√7ᵗʰ **S42.442** Displaced fracture (avulsion) of medial epicondyle of left humerus Ⓠ

√7ᵗʰ **S42.443** Displaced fracture (avulsion) of medial epicondyle of unspecified humerus Ⓠ

√7ᵗʰ **S42.444** Nondisplaced fracture (avulsion) of medial epicondyle of right humerus Ⓠ

√7ᵗʰ **S42.445** Nondisplaced fracture (avulsion) of medial epicondyle of left humerus Ⓠ

√7ᵗʰ **S42.446** Nondisplaced fracture (avulsion) of medial epicondyle of unspecified humerus Ⓠ

√7ᵗʰ **S42.447** Incarcerated fracture (avulsion) of medial epicondyle of right humerus Ⓠ

√7ᵗʰ **S42.448** Incarcerated fracture (avulsion) of medial epicondyle of left humerus Ⓠ

√7ᵗʰ **S42.449** Incarcerated fracture (avulsion) of medial epicondyle of unspecified humerus Ⓠ

√6ᵗʰ **S42.45** Fracture of lateral condyle of humerus
Fracture of capitellum of humerus

√7ᵗʰ **S42.451** Displaced fracture of lateral condyle of right humerus Ⓠ

√7ᵗʰ **S42.452** Displaced fracture of lateral condyle of left humerus Ⓠ

√7ᵗʰ **S42.453** Displaced fracture of lateral condyle of unspecified humerus Ⓠ

√7ᵗʰ **S42.454** Nondisplaced fracture of lateral condyle of right humerus Ⓠ

√7ᵗʰ **S42.455** Nondisplaced fracture of lateral condyle of left humerus Ⓠ

√7ᵗʰ **S42.456** Nondisplaced fracture of lateral condyle of unspecified humerus Ⓠ

√6ᵗʰ **S42.46** Fracture of medial condyle of humerus
Trochlea fracture of humerus

√7ᵗʰ **S42.461** Displaced fracture of medial condyle of right humerus Ⓠ

√7ᵗʰ **S42.462** Displaced fracture of medial condyle of left humerus Ⓠ

√7ᵗʰ **S42.463** Displaced fracture of medial condyle of unspecified humerus Ⓠ

√7ᵗʰ **S42.464** Nondisplaced fracture of medial condyle of right humerus Ⓠ

√7ᵗʰ **S42.465** Nondisplaced fracture of medial condyle of left humerus Ⓠ

√7ᵗʰ **S42.466** Nondisplaced fracture of medial condyle of unspecified humerus Ⓠ

√6ᵗʰ **S42.47** Transcondylar fracture of humerus

√7ᵗʰ **S42.471** Displaced transcondylar fracture of right humerus Ⓠ

√7ᵗʰ **S42.472** Displaced transcondylar fracture of left humerus Ⓠ

√7ᵗʰ **S42.473** Displaced transcondylar fracture of unspecified humerus Ⓠ

√7ᵗʰ **S42.474** Nondisplaced transcondylar fracture of right humerus Ⓠ

√7ᵗʰ **S42.475** Nondisplaced transcondylar fracture of left humerus Ⓠ

√7ᵗʰ **S42.476** Nondisplaced transcondylar fracture of unspecified humerus Ⓠ

√6ᵗʰ **S42.48** Torus fracture of lower end of humerus

> The appropriate 7th character is to be added to all codes in subcategory S42.48.
> A   initial encounter for closed fracture
> D   subsequent encounter for fracture with routine healing
> G   subsequent encounter for fracture with delayed healing
> K   subsequent encounter for fracture with nonunion
> P   subsequent encounter for fracture with malunion
> S   sequela

√7ᵗʰ **S42.481** Torus fracture of lower end of right humerus Ⓠ

√7ᵗʰ **S42.482** Torus fracture of lower end of left humerus Ⓠ

√7ᵗʰ **S42.489** Torus fracture of lower end of unspecified humerus Ⓠ

√6ᵗʰ **S42.49** Other fracture of lower end of humerus

√7ᵗʰ **S42.491** Other displaced fracture of lower end of right humerus Ⓠ

√7ᵗʰ **S42.492** Other displaced fracture of lower end of left humerus Ⓠ

√7ᵗʰ **S42.493** Other displaced fracture of lower end of unspecified humerus Ⓠ

√7ᵗʰ **S42.494** Other nondisplaced fracture of lower end of right humerus Ⓠ

√7ᵗʰ **S42.495** Other nondisplaced fracture of lower end of left humerus Ⓠ

√7ᵗʰ **S42.496** Other nondisplaced fracture of lower end of unspecified humerus Ⓠ

√5ᵗʰ **S42.9** Fracture of shoulder girdle, part unspecified
Fracture of shoulder NOS

√x7ᵗʰ **S42.90** Fracture of unspecified shoulder girdle, part unspecified Ⓠ

√x7ᵗʰ **S42.91** Fracture of right shoulder girdle, part unspecified Ⓠ

√x7ᵗʰ **S42.92** Fracture of left shoulder girdle, part unspecified Ⓠ

√4ᵗʰ **S43   Dislocation and sprain of joints and ligaments of shoulder girdle**

INCLUDES   avulsion of joint or ligament of shoulder girdle
laceration of cartilage, joint or ligament of shoulder girdle
sprain of cartilage, joint or ligament of shoulder girdle
traumatic hemarthrosis of joint or ligament of shoulder girdle
traumatic rupture of joint or ligament of shoulder girdle
traumatic subluxation of joint or ligament of shoulder girdle
traumatic tear of joint or ligament of shoulder girdle

Code also any associated open wound

EXCLUDES 2   strain of muscle, fascia and tendon of shoulder and upper arm (S46.-)

The appropriate 7th character is to be added to each code from category S43.
A   initial encounter
D   subsequent encounter
S   sequela

√5ᵗʰ **S43.0   Subluxation and dislocation of shoulder joint**

Dislocation of glenohumeral joint
Subluxation of glenohumeral joint

√6ᵗʰ **S43.00   Unspecified subluxation and dislocation of shoulder joint**

Dislocation of humerus NOS
Subluxation of humerus NOS

√7ᵗʰ **S43.001   Unspecified subluxation of right shoulder joint**

√7ᵗʰ **S43.002   Unspecified subluxation of left shoulder joint**

√7ᵗʰ **S43.003   Unspecified subluxation of unspecified shoulder joint**

√7ᵗʰ **S43.004   Unspecified dislocation of right shoulder joint**

√7ᵗʰ **S43.005   Unspecified dislocation of left shoulder joint**

√7ᵗʰ **S43.006   Unspecified dislocation of unspecified shoulder joint**

√6ᵗʰ **S43.01   Anterior subluxation and dislocation of humerus**

√7ᵗʰ **S43.011   Anterior subluxation of right humerus**

√7ᵗʰ **S43.012   Anterior subluxation of left humerus**

√7ᵗʰ **S43.013   Anterior subluxation of unspecified humerus**

√7ᵗʰ **S43.014   Anterior dislocation of right humerus**

√7ᵗʰ **S43.015   Anterior dislocation of left humerus**

√7ᵗʰ **S43.016   Anterior dislocation of unspecified humerus**

√6ᵗʰ **S43.02   Posterior subluxation and dislocation of humerus**

√7ᵗʰ **S43.021   Posterior subluxation of right humerus**

√7ᵗʰ **S43.022   Posterior subluxation of left humerus**

√7ᵗʰ **S43.023   Posterior subluxation of unspecified humerus**

√7ᵗʰ **S43.024   Posterior dislocation of right humerus**

√7ᵗʰ **S43.025   Posterior dislocation of left humerus**

√7ᵗʰ **S43.026   Posterior dislocation of unspecified humerus**

√6ᵗʰ **S43.03   Inferior subluxation and dislocation of humerus**

√7ᵗʰ **S43.031   Inferior subluxation of right humerus**

√7ᵗʰ **S43.032   Inferior subluxation of left humerus**

√7ᵗʰ **S43.033   Inferior subluxation of unspecified humerus**

√7ᵗʰ **S43.034   Inferior dislocation of right humerus**

√7ᵗʰ **S43.035   Inferior dislocation of left humerus**

√7ᵗʰ **S43.036   Inferior dislocation of unspecified humerus**

√6ᵗʰ **S43.08   Other subluxation and dislocation of shoulder joint**

√7ᵗʰ **S43.081   Other subluxation of right shoulder joint**

√7ᵗʰ **S43.082   Other subluxation of left shoulder joint**

√7ᵗʰ **S43.083   Other subluxation of unspecified shoulder joint**

√7ᵗʰ **S43.084   Other dislocation of right shoulder joint**

√7ᵗʰ **S43.085   Other dislocation of left shoulder joint**

√7ᵗʰ **S43.086   Other dislocation of unspecified shoulder joint**

√5ᵗʰ **S43.1   Subluxation and dislocation of acromioclavicular joint**

√6ᵗʰ **S43.10   Unspecified dislocation of acromioclavicular joint**

√7ᵗʰ **S43.101   Unspecified dislocation of right acromioclavicular joint**

√7ᵗʰ **S43.102   Unspecified dislocation of left acromioclavicular joint**

√7ᵗʰ **S43.109   Unspecified dislocation of unspecified acromioclavicular joint**

√6ᵗʰ **S43.11   Subluxation of acromioclavicular joint**

√7ᵗʰ **S43.111   Subluxation of right acromioclavicular joint**

√7ᵗʰ **S43.112   Subluxation of left acromioclavicular joint**

√7ᵗʰ **S43.119   Subluxation of unspecified acromioclavicular joint**

√6ᵗʰ **S43.12   Dislocation of acromioclavicular joint, 100%-200% displacement**

√7ᵗʰ **S43.121   Dislocation of right acromioclavicular joint, 100%-200% displacement**

√7ᵗʰ **S43.122   Dislocation of left acromioclavicular joint, 100%-200% displacement**

√7ᵗʰ **S43.129   Dislocation of unspecified acromioclavicular joint, 100%-200% displacement**

√6ᵗʰ **S43.13   Dislocation of acromioclavicular joint, greater than 200% displacement**

√7ᵗʰ **S43.131   Dislocation of right acromioclavicular joint, greater than 200% displacement**

√7ᵗʰ **S43.132   Dislocation of left acromioclavicular joint, greater than 200% displacement**

√7ᵗʰ **S43.139   Dislocation of unspecified acromioclavicular joint, greater than 200% displacement**

√6ᵗʰ **S43.14   Inferior dislocation of acromioclavicular joint**

√7ᵗʰ **S43.141   Inferior dislocation of right acromioclavicular joint**

√7ᵗʰ **S43.142   Inferior dislocation of left acromioclavicular joint**

√7ᵗʰ **S43.149   Inferior dislocation of unspecified acromioclavicular joint**

√6ᵗʰ **S43.15   Posterior dislocation of acromioclavicular joint**

√7ᵗʰ **S43.151   Posterior dislocation of right acromioclavicular joint**

√7ᵗʰ **S43.152   Posterior dislocation of left acromioclavicular joint**

√7ᵗʰ **S43.159   Posterior dislocation of unspecified acromioclavicular joint**

√5ᵗʰ **S43.2   Subluxation and dislocation of sternoclavicular joint**

√6ᵗʰ **S43.20   Unspecified subluxation and dislocation of sternoclavicular joint**

√7ᵗʰ **S43.201   Unspecified subluxation of right sternoclavicular joint**

√7ᵗʰ **S43.202   Unspecified subluxation of left sternoclavicular joint**

√7ᵗʰ **S43.203   Unspecified subluxation of unspecified sternoclavicular joint**

√7ᵗʰ **S43.204   Unspecified dislocation of right sternoclavicular joint**

√7ᵗʰ **S43.205   Unspecified dislocation of left sternoclavicular joint**

√7ᵗʰ **S43.206   Unspecified dislocation of unspecified sternoclavicular joint**

√6ᵗʰ **S43.21   Anterior subluxation and dislocation of sternoclavicular joint**

√7ᵗʰ **S43.211   Anterior subluxation of right sternoclavicular joint**

√7ᵗʰ **S43.212   Anterior subluxation of left sternoclavicular joint**

√7ᵗʰ **S43.213   Anterior subluxation of unspecified sternoclavicular joint**

√7ᵗʰ **S43.214   Anterior dislocation of right sternoclavicular joint**

√7ᵗʰ **S43.215   Anterior dislocation of left sternoclavicular joint**

√7ᵗʰ **S43.216   Anterior dislocation of unspecified sternoclavicular joint**

√6ᵗʰ **S43.22   Posterior subluxation and dislocation of sternoclavicular joint**

√7ᵗʰ **S43.221   Posterior subluxation of right sternoclavicular joint**

√7ᵗʰ **S43.222   Posterior subluxation of left sternoclavicular joint**

√7ᵗʰ **S43.223** Posterior subluxation of unspecified sternoclavicular joint

√7ᵗʰ **S43.224** Posterior dislocation of right sternoclavicular joint

√7ᵗʰ **S43.225** Posterior dislocation of left sternoclavicular joint

√7ᵗʰ **S43.226** Posterior dislocation of unspecified sternoclavicular joint

√5ᵗʰ **S43.3** Subluxation and dislocation of other and unspecified parts of shoulder girdle

√6ᵗʰ **S43.30** Subluxation and dislocation of unspecified parts of shoulder girdle

Dislocation of shoulder girdle NOS

Subluxation of shoulder girdle NOS

√7ᵗʰ **S43.301** Subluxation of unspecified parts of right shoulder girdle

√7ᵗʰ **S43.302** Subluxation of unspecified parts of left shoulder girdle

√7ᵗʰ **S43.303** Subluxation of unspecified parts of unspecified shoulder girdle

√7ᵗʰ **S43.304** Dislocation of unspecified parts of right shoulder girdle

√7ᵗʰ **S43.305** Dislocation of unspecified parts of left shoulder girdle

√7ᵗʰ **S43.306** Dislocation of unspecified parts of unspecified shoulder girdle

√6ᵗʰ **S43.31** Subluxation and dislocation of scapula

√7ᵗʰ **S43.311** Subluxation of right scapula

√7ᵗʰ **S43.312** Subluxation of left scapula

√7ᵗʰ **S43.313** Subluxation of unspecified scapula

√7ᵗʰ **S43.314** Dislocation of right scapula

√7ᵗʰ **S43.315** Dislocation of left scapula

√7ᵗʰ **S43.316** Dislocation of unspecified scapula

√6ᵗʰ **S43.39** Subluxation and dislocation of other parts of shoulder girdle

√7ᵗʰ **S43.391** Subluxation of other parts of right shoulder girdle

√7ᵗʰ **S43.392** Subluxation of other parts of left shoulder girdle

√7ᵗʰ **S43.393** Subluxation of other parts of unspecified shoulder girdle

√7ᵗʰ **S43.394** Dislocation of other parts of right shoulder girdle

√7ᵗʰ **S43.395** Dislocation of other parts of left shoulder girdle

√7ᵗʰ **S43.396** Dislocation of other parts of unspecified shoulder girdle

√5ᵗʰ **S43.4** Sprain of shoulder joint

√6ᵗʰ **S43.40** Unspecified sprain of shoulder joint

√7ᵗʰ **S43.401** Unspecified sprain of right shoulder joint

√7ᵗʰ **S43.402** Unspecified sprain of left shoulder joint

√7ᵗʰ **S43.409** Unspecified sprain of unspecified shoulder joint

√6ᵗʰ **S43.41** Sprain of coracohumeral (ligament)

√7ᵗʰ **S43.411** Sprain of right coracohumeral (ligament)

√7ᵗʰ **S43.412** Sprain of left coracohumeral (ligament)

√7ᵗʰ **S43.419** Sprain of unspecified coracohumeral (ligament)

√6ᵗʰ **S43.42** Sprain of rotator cuff capsule

EXCLUDES 1   rotator cuff syndrome (complete) (incomplete), not specified as traumatic (M75.1-)

EXCLUDES 2   injury of tendon of rotator cuff (S46.0-)

√7ᵗʰ **S43.421** Sprain of right rotator cuff capsule

√7ᵗʰ **S43.422** Sprain of left rotator cuff capsule

√7ᵗʰ **S43.429** Sprain of unspecified rotator cuff capsule

√6ᵗʰ **S43.43** Superior glenoid labrum lesion

SLAP lesion

AHA: 2019,2Q,26

DEF: Detachment injury of the superior aspect of the glenoid labrum, which is the ring of fibrocartilage attached to the rim of the glenoid cavity of the scapula.

√7ᵗʰ **S43.431** Superior glenoid labrum lesion of right shoulder

√7ᵗʰ **S43.432** Superior glenoid labrum lesion of left shoulder

√7ᵗʰ **S43.439** Superior glenoid labrum lesion of unspecified shoulder

√6ᵗʰ **S43.49** Other sprain of shoulder joint

√7ᵗʰ **S43.491** Other sprain of right shoulder joint

√7ᵗʰ **S43.492** Other sprain of left shoulder joint

√7ᵗʰ **S43.499** Other sprain of unspecified shoulder joint

√5ᵗʰ **S43.5** Sprain of acromioclavicular joint

Sprain of acromioclavicular ligament

√x7ᵗʰ **S43.50** Sprain of unspecified acromioclavicular joint

√x7ᵗʰ **S43.51** Sprain of right acromioclavicular joint

√x7ᵗʰ **S43.52** Sprain of left acromioclavicular joint

√5ᵗʰ **S43.6** Sprain of sternoclavicular joint

√x7ᵗʰ **S43.60** Sprain of unspecified sternoclavicular joint

√x7ᵗʰ **S43.61** Sprain of right sternoclavicular joint

√x7ᵗʰ **S43.62** Sprain of left sternoclavicular joint

√5ᵗʰ **S43.8** Sprain of other specified parts of shoulder girdle

√x7ᵗʰ **S43.80** Sprain of other specified parts of unspecified shoulder girdle

√x7ᵗʰ **S43.81** Sprain of other specified parts of right shoulder girdle

√x7ᵗʰ **S43.82** Sprain of other specified parts of left shoulder girdle

√5ᵗʰ **S43.9** Sprain of unspecified parts of shoulder girdle

√x7ᵗʰ **S43.90** Sprain of unspecified parts of unspecified shoulder girdle

Sprain of shoulder girdle NOS

√x7ᵗʰ **S43.91** Sprain of unspecified parts of right shoulder girdle

√x7ᵗʰ **S43.92** Sprain of unspecified parts of left shoulder girdle

√4ᵗʰ **S44** Injury of nerves at shoulder and upper arm level

Code also any associated open wound (S41.-)

EXCLUDES 2   injury of brachial plexus (S14.3-)

The appropriate 7th character is to be added to each code from category S44.

A   initial encounter

D   subsequent encounter

S   sequela

√5ᵗʰ **S44.0** Injury of ulnar nerve at upper arm level

EXCLUDES 1   ulnar nerve NOS (S54.0)

√x7ᵗʰ **S44.00** Injury of ulnar nerve at upper arm level, unspecified arm

√x7ᵗʰ **S44.01** Injury of ulnar nerve at upper arm level, right arm

√x7ᵗʰ **S44.02** Injury of ulnar nerve at upper arm level, left arm

√5ᵗʰ **S44.1** Injury of median nerve at upper arm level

EXCLUDES 1   median nerve NOS (S54.1)

√x7ᵗʰ **S44.10** Injury of median nerve at upper arm level, unspecified arm

√x7ᵗʰ **S44.11** Injury of median nerve at upper arm level, right arm

√x7ᵗʰ **S44.12** Injury of median nerve at upper arm level, left arm

√5ᵗʰ **S44.2** Injury of radial nerve at upper arm level

EXCLUDES 1   radial nerve NOS (S54.2)

√x7ᵗʰ **S44.20** Injury of radial nerve at upper arm level, unspecified arm

√x7ᵗʰ **S44.21** Injury of radial nerve at upper arm level, right arm

√x7ᵗʰ **S44.22** Injury of radial nerve at upper arm level, left arm

√5ᵗʰ **S44.3** Injury of axillary nerve

√x7ᵗʰ **S44.30** Injury of axillary nerve, unspecified arm

√x7ᵗʰ **S44.31** Injury of axillary nerve, right arm

√x7ᵗʰ **S44.32** Injury of axillary nerve, left arm

√5ᵗʰ **S44.4** Injury of musculocutaneous nerve

√x7ᵗʰ **S44.40** Injury of musculocutaneous nerve, unspecified arm

√x7ᵗʰ **S44.41** Injury of musculocutaneous nerve, right arm

√x7ᵗʰ **S44.42** Injury of musculocutaneous nerve, left arm

√5ᵗʰ **S44.5** Injury of cutaneous sensory nerve at shoulder and upper arm level

√x7ᵗʰ **S44.50** Injury of cutaneous sensory nerve at shoulder and upper arm level, unspecified arm

√x7ᵗʰ **S44.51** Injury of cutaneous sensory nerve at shoulder and upper arm level, right arm

√x7ᵗʰ **S44.52** Injury of cutaneous sensory nerve at shoulder and upper arm level, left arm

√5ᵗʰ **S44.8** Injury of other nerves at shoulder and upper arm level

     √6ᵗʰ **S44.8X** Injury of other nerves at shoulder and upper arm level

         √7ᵗʰ **S44.8X1** Injury of other nerves at shoulder and upper arm level, right arm

         √7ᵗʰ **S44.8X2** Injury of other nerves at shoulder and upper arm level, left arm

         √7ᵗʰ **S44.8X9** Injury of other nerves at shoulder and upper arm level, unspecified arm

√5ᵗʰ **S44.9** Injury of unspecified nerve at shoulder and upper arm level

     √x7ᵗʰ **S44.90** Injury of unspecified nerve at shoulder and upper arm level, unspecified arm

     √x7ᵗʰ **S44.91** Injury of unspecified nerve at shoulder and upper arm level, right arm

     √x7ᵗʰ **S44.92** Injury of unspecified nerve at shoulder and upper arm level, left arm

√4ᵗʰ **S45 Injury of blood vessels at shoulder and upper arm level**

     Code also any associated open wound (S41.-)

     EXCLUDES 2   injury of subclavian artery (S25.1)

                  injury of subclavian vein (S25.3)

     The appropriate 7th character is to be added to each code from category S45.

     A   initial encounter

     D   subsequent encounter

     S   sequela

     √5ᵗʰ **S45.0** Injury of axillary artery

         √6ᵗʰ **S45.00** Unspecified injury of axillary artery

             √7ᵗʰ **S45.001** Unspecified injury of axillary artery, right side

             √7ᵗʰ **S45.002** Unspecified injury of axillary artery, left side

             √7ᵗʰ **S45.009** Unspecified injury of axillary artery, unspecified side

         √6ᵗʰ **S45.01** Laceration of axillary artery

             √7ᵗʰ **S45.011** Laceration of axillary artery, right side

             √7ᵗʰ **S45.012** Laceration of axillary artery, left side

             √7ᵗʰ **S45.019** Laceration of axillary artery, unspecified side

         √6ᵗʰ **S45.09** Other specified injury of axillary artery

             √7ᵗʰ **S45.091** Other specified injury of axillary artery, right side

             √7ᵗʰ **S45.092** Other specified injury of axillary artery, left side

             √7ᵗʰ **S45.099** Other specified injury of axillary artery, unspecified side

     √5ᵗʰ **S45.1** Injury of brachial artery

         √6ᵗʰ **S45.10** Unspecified injury of brachial artery

             √7ᵗʰ **S45.101** Unspecified injury of brachial artery, right side

             √7ᵗʰ **S45.102** Unspecified injury of brachial artery, left side

             √7ᵗʰ **S45.109** Unspecified injury of brachial artery, unspecified side

         √6ᵗʰ **S45.11** Laceration of brachial artery

             √7ᵗʰ **S45.111** Laceration of brachial artery, right side

             √7ᵗʰ **S45.112** Laceration of brachial artery, left side

             √7ᵗʰ **S45.119** Laceration of brachial artery, unspecified side

         √6ᵗʰ **S45.19** Other specified injury of brachial artery

             √7ᵗʰ **S45.191** Other specified injury of brachial artery, right side

             √7ᵗʰ **S45.192** Other specified injury of brachial artery, left side

             √7ᵗʰ **S45.199** Other specified injury of brachial artery, unspecified side

     √5ᵗʰ **S45.2** Injury of axillary or brachial vein

         √6ᵗʰ **S45.20** Unspecified injury of axillary or brachial vein

             √7ᵗʰ **S45.201** Unspecified injury of axillary or brachial vein, right side

             √7ᵗʰ **S45.202** Unspecified injury of axillary or brachial vein, left side

             √7ᵗʰ **S45.209** Unspecified injury of axillary or brachial vein, unspecified side

         √6ᵗʰ **S45.21** Laceration of axillary or brachial vein

             √7ᵗʰ **S45.211** Laceration of axillary or brachial vein, right side

             √7ᵗʰ **S45.212** Laceration of axillary or brachial vein, left side

             √7ᵗʰ **S45.219** Laceration of axillary or brachial vein, unspecified side

         √6ᵗʰ **S45.29** Other specified injury of axillary or brachial vein

             √7ᵗʰ **S45.291** Other specified injury of axillary or brachial vein, right side

             √7ᵗʰ **S45.292** Other specified injury of axillary or brachial vein, left side

             √7ᵗʰ **S45.299** Other specified injury of axillary or brachial vein, unspecified side

     √5ᵗʰ **S45.3** Injury of superficial vein at shoulder and upper arm level

         √6ᵗʰ **S45.30** Unspecified injury of superficial vein at shoulder and upper arm level

             √7ᵗʰ **S45.301** Unspecified injury of superficial vein at shoulder and upper arm level, right arm

             √7ᵗʰ **S45.302** Unspecified injury of superficial vein at shoulder and upper arm level, left arm

             √7ᵗʰ **S45.309** Unspecified injury of superficial vein at shoulder and upper arm level, unspecified arm

         √6ᵗʰ **S45.31** Laceration of superficial vein at shoulder and upper arm level

             √7ᵗʰ **S45.311** Laceration of superficial vein at shoulder and upper arm level, right arm

             √7ᵗʰ **S45.312** Laceration of superficial vein at shoulder and upper arm level, left arm

             √7ᵗʰ **S45.319** Laceration of superficial vein at shoulder and upper arm level, unspecified arm

         √6ᵗʰ **S45.39** Other specified injury of superficial vein at shoulder and upper arm level

             √7ᵗʰ **S45.391** Other specified injury of superficial vein at shoulder and upper arm level, right arm

             √7ᵗʰ **S45.392** Other specified injury of superficial vein at shoulder and upper arm level, left arm

             √7ᵗʰ **S45.399** Other specified injury of superficial vein at shoulder and upper arm level, unspecified arm

     √5ᵗʰ **S45.8** Injury of other specified blood vessels at shoulder and upper arm level

         √6ᵗʰ **S45.80** Unspecified injury of other specified blood vessels at shoulder and upper arm level

             √7ᵗʰ **S45.801** Unspecified injury of other specified blood vessels at shoulder and upper arm level, right arm

             √7ᵗʰ **S45.802** Unspecified injury of other specified blood vessels at shoulder and upper arm level, left arm

             √7ᵗʰ **S45.809** Unspecified injury of other specified blood vessels at shoulder and upper arm level, unspecified arm

         √6ᵗʰ **S45.81** Laceration of other specified blood vessels at shoulder and upper arm level

             √7ᵗʰ **S45.811** Laceration of other specified blood vessels at shoulder and upper arm level, right arm

             √7ᵗʰ **S45.812** Laceration of other specified blood vessels at shoulder and upper arm level, left arm

             √7ᵗʰ **S45.819** Laceration of other specified blood vessels at shoulder and upper arm level, unspecified arm

         √6ᵗʰ **S45.89** Other specified injury of other specified blood vessels at shoulder and upper arm level

             √7ᵗʰ **S45.891** Other specified injury of other specified blood vessels at shoulder and upper arm level, right arm

             √7ᵗʰ **S45.892** Other specified injury of other specified blood vessels at shoulder and upper arm level, left arm

             √7ᵗʰ **S45.899** Other specified injury of other specified blood vessels at shoulder and upper arm level, unspecified arm

     √5ᵗʰ **S45.9** Injury of unspecified blood vessel at shoulder and upper arm level

         √6ᵗʰ **S45.90** Unspecified injury of unspecified blood vessel at shoulder and upper arm level

             √7ᵗʰ **S45.901** Unspecified injury of unspecified blood vessel at shoulder and upper arm level, right arm

√7ʰ **S45.902** Unspecified injury of unspecified blood vessel at shoulder and upper arm level, **left** arm

√7ʰ **S45.909** Unspecified injury of unspecified blood vessel at shoulder and upper arm level, unspecified arm

√6ʰ **S45.91** Laceration of unspecified blood vessel at shoulder and upper arm level

√7ʰ **S45.911** Laceration of unspecified blood vessel at shoulder and upper arm level, **right** arm

√7ʰ **S45.912** Laceration of unspecified blood vessel at shoulder and upper arm level, **left** arm

√7ʰ **S45.919** Laceration of unspecified blood vessel at shoulder and upper arm level, unspecified arm

√6ʰ **S45.99** Other specified injury of unspecified blood vessel at shoulder and upper arm level

√7ʰ **S45.991** Other specified injury of unspecified blood vessel at shoulder and upper arm level, **right** arm

√7ʰ **S45.992** Other specified injury of unspecified blood vessel at shoulder and upper arm level, **left** arm

√7ʰ **S45.999** Other specified injury of unspecified blood vessel at shoulder and upper arm level, unspecified arm

√4ʰ **S46** **Injury of muscle, fascia and tendon at shoulder and upper arm level**

Code also any associated open wound (S41.-)

EXCLUDES 2 injury of muscle, fascia and tendon at elbow (S56.-)
sprain of joints and ligaments of shoulder girdle (S43.9)

TIP: Refer to the Muscle/Tendon table at the beginning of this chapter.

The appropriate 7th character is to be added to each code from category S46.
A initial encounter
D subsequent encounter
S sequela

√5ʰ **S46.0** Injury of muscle(s) and tendon(s) of the rotator cuff of shoulder

√6ʰ **S46.00** Unspecified injury of muscle(s) and tendon(s) of the rotator cuff of shoulder

√7ʰ **S46.001** Unspecified injury of muscle(s) and tendon(s) of the rotator cuff of **right** shoulder

√7ʰ **S46.002** Unspecified injury of muscle(s) and tendon(s) of the rotator cuff of **left** shoulder

√7ʰ **S46.009** Unspecified injury of muscle(s) and tendon(s) of the rotator cuff of unspecified shoulder

√6ʰ **S46.01** Strain of muscle(s) and tendon(s) of the rotator cuff of shoulder

√7ʰ **S46.011** Strain of muscle(s) and tendon(s) of the rotator cuff of **right** shoulder

√7ʰ **S46.012** Strain of muscle(s) and tendon(s) of the rotator cuff of **left** shoulder

√7ʰ **S46.019** Strain of muscle(s) and tendon(s) of the rotator cuff of unspecified shoulder

√6ʰ **S46.02** Laceration of muscle(s) and tendon(s) of the rotator cuff of shoulder

√7ʰ **S46.021** Laceration of muscle(s) and tendon(s) of the rotator cuff of **right** shoulder

√7ʰ **S46.022** Laceration of muscle(s) and tendon(s) of the rotator cuff of **left** shoulder

√7ʰ **S46.029** Laceration of muscle(s) and tendon(s) of the rotator cuff of unspecified shoulder

√6ʰ **S46.09** Other injury of muscle(s) and tendon(s) of the rotator cuff of shoulder

√7ʰ **S46.091** Other injury of muscle(s) and tendon(s) of the rotator cuff of **right** shoulder

√7ʰ **S46.092** Other injury of muscle(s) and tendon(s) of the rotator cuff of **left** shoulder

√7ʰ **S46.099** Other injury of muscle(s) and tendon(s) of the rotator cuff of unspecified shoulder

√5ʰ **S46.1** Injury of muscle, fascia and tendon of long head of biceps

√6ʰ **S46.10** Unspecified injury of muscle, fascia and tendon of long head of biceps

√7ʰ **S46.101** Unspecified injury of muscle, fascia and tendon of long head of biceps, **right** arm

√7ʰ **S46.102** Unspecified injury of muscle, fascia and tendon of long head of biceps, **left** arm

√7ʰ **S46.109** Unspecified injury of muscle, fascia and tendon of long head of biceps, unspecified arm

√6ʰ **S46.11** Strain of muscle, fascia and tendon of long head of biceps

AHA: 2020,1Q,38; 2019,2Q,27

√7ʰ **S46.111** Strain of muscle, fascia and tendon of long head of biceps, **right** arm

√7ʰ **S46.112** Strain of muscle, fascia and tendon of long head of biceps, **left** arm

√7ʰ **S46.119** Strain of muscle, fascia and tendon of long head of biceps, unspecified arm

√6ʰ **S46.12** Laceration of muscle, fascia and tendon of long head of biceps

√7ʰ **S46.121** Laceration of muscle, fascia and tendon of long head of biceps, **right** arm

√7ʰ **S46.122** Laceration of muscle, fascia and tendon of long head of biceps, **left** arm

√7ʰ **S46.129** Laceration of muscle, fascia and tendon of long head of biceps, unspecified arm

√6ʰ **S46.19** Other injury of muscle, fascia and tendon of long head of biceps

√7ʰ **S46.191** Other injury of muscle, fascia and tendon of long head of biceps, **right** arm

√7ʰ **S46.192** Other injury of muscle, fascia and tendon of long head of biceps, **left** arm

√7ʰ **S46.199** Other injury of muscle, fascia and tendon of long head of biceps, unspecified arm

√5ʰ **S46.2** Injury of muscle, fascia and tendon of other parts of biceps

√6ʰ **S46.20** Unspecified injury of muscle, fascia and tendon of other parts of biceps

√7ʰ **S46.201** Unspecified injury of muscle, fascia and tendon of other parts of biceps, **right** arm

√7ʰ **S46.202** Unspecified injury of muscle, fascia and tendon of other parts of biceps, **left** arm

√7ʰ **S46.209** Unspecified injury of muscle, fascia and tendon of other parts of biceps, unspecified arm

√6ʰ **S46.21** Strain of muscle, fascia and tendon of other parts of biceps

√7ʰ **S46.211** Strain of muscle, fascia and tendon of other parts of biceps, **right** arm

√7ʰ **S46.212** Strain of muscle, fascia and tendon of other parts of biceps, **left** arm

√7ʰ **S46.219** Strain of muscle, fascia and tendon of other parts of biceps, unspecified arm

√6ʰ **S46.22** Laceration of muscle, fascia and tendon of other parts of biceps

√7ʰ **S46.221** Laceration of muscle, fascia and tendon of other parts of biceps, **right** arm

√7ʰ **S46.222** Laceration of muscle, fascia and tendon of other parts of biceps, **left** arm

√7ʰ **S46.229** Laceration of muscle, fascia and tendon of other parts of biceps, unspecified arm

√6ʰ **S46.29** Other injury of muscle, fascia and tendon of other parts of biceps

√7ʰ **S46.291** Other injury of muscle, fascia and tendon of other parts of biceps, **right** arm

√7ʰ **S46.292** Other injury of muscle, fascia and tendon of other parts of biceps, **left** arm

√7ʰ **S46.299** Other injury of muscle, fascia and tendon of other parts of biceps, unspecified arm

√5ʰ **S46.3** Injury of muscle, fascia and tendon of triceps

√6ʰ **S46.30** Unspecified injury of muscle, fascia and tendon of triceps

√7ʰ **S46.301** Unspecified injury of muscle, fascia and tendon of triceps, **right** arm

√7ʰ **S46.302** Unspecified injury of muscle, fascia and tendon of triceps, **left** arm

√7ʰ **S46.309** Unspecified injury of muscle, fascia and tendon of triceps, unspecified arm

√6ʰ **S46.31** Strain of muscle, fascia and tendon of triceps

√7ʰ **S46.311** Strain of muscle, fascia and tendon of triceps, **right** arm

√7ʰ **S46.312** Strain of muscle, fascia and tendon of triceps, **left** arm

√7ʰ **S46.319** Strain of muscle, fascia and tendon of triceps, unspecified arm

√6ʰ **S46.32** Laceration of muscle, fascia and tendon of triceps

√7ʰ **S46.321** Laceration of muscle, fascia and tendon of triceps, **right** arm

√7ᵗʰ **S46.322** Laceration of muscle, fascia and tendon of triceps, left arm

√7ᵗʰ **S46.329** Laceration of muscle, fascia and tendon of triceps, unspecified arm

√6ᵗʰ **S46.39** Other injury of muscle, fascia and tendon of triceps

√7ᵗʰ **S46.391** Other injury of muscle, fascia and tendon of triceps, right arm

√7ᵗʰ **S46.392** Other injury of muscle, fascia and tendon of triceps, left arm

√7ᵗʰ **S46.399** Other injury of muscle, fascia and tendon of triceps, unspecified arm

√5ᵗʰ **S46.8** Injury of other muscles, fascia and tendons at shoulder and upper arm level

√6ᵗʰ **S46.80** Unspecified injury of other muscles, fascia and tendons at shoulder and upper arm level

√7ᵗʰ **S46.801** Unspecified injury of other muscles, fascia and tendons at shoulder and upper arm level, right arm

√7ᵗʰ **S46.802** Unspecified injury of other muscles, fascia and tendons at shoulder and upper arm level, left arm

√7ᵗʰ **S46.809** Unspecified injury of other muscles, fascia and tendons at shoulder and upper arm level, unspecified arm

√6ᵗʰ **S46.81** Strain of other muscles, fascia and tendons at shoulder and upper arm level

√7ᵗʰ **S46.811** Strain of other muscles, fascia and tendons at shoulder and upper arm level, right arm

√7ᵗʰ **S46.812** Strain of other muscles, fascia and tendons at shoulder and upper arm level, left arm

√7ᵗʰ **S46.819** Strain of other muscles, fascia and tendons at shoulder and upper arm level, unspecified arm

√6ᵗʰ **S46.82** Laceration of other muscles, fascia and tendons at shoulder and upper arm level

√7ᵗʰ **S46.821** Laceration of other muscles, fascia and tendons at shoulder and upper arm level, right arm

√7ᵗʰ **S46.822** Laceration of other muscles, fascia and tendons at shoulder and upper arm level, left arm

√7ᵗʰ **S46.829** Laceration of other muscles, fascia and tendons at shoulder and upper arm level, unspecified arm

√6ᵗʰ **S46.89** Other injury of other muscles, fascia and tendons at shoulder and upper arm level

√7ᵗʰ **S46.891** Other injury of other muscles, fascia and tendons at shoulder and upper arm level, right arm

√7ᵗʰ **S46.892** Other injury of other muscles, fascia and tendons at shoulder and upper arm level, left arm

√7ᵗʰ **S46.899** Other injury of other muscles, fascia and tendons at shoulder and upper arm level, unspecified arm

√5ᵗʰ **S46.9** Injury of unspecified muscle, fascia and tendon at shoulder and upper arm level

√6ᵗʰ **S46.90** Unspecified injury of unspecified muscle, fascia and tendon at shoulder and upper arm level

√7ᵗʰ **S46.901** Unspecified injury of unspecified muscle, fascia and tendon at shoulder and upper arm level, right arm

√7ᵗʰ **S46.902** Unspecified injury of unspecified muscle, fascia and tendon at shoulder and upper arm level, left arm

√7ᵗʰ **S46.909** Unspecified injury of unspecified muscle, fascia and tendon at shoulder and upper arm level, unspecified arm

√6ᵗʰ **S46.91** Strain of unspecified muscle, fascia and tendon at shoulder and upper arm level

√7ᵗʰ **S46.911** Strain of unspecified muscle, fascia and tendon at shoulder and upper arm level, right arm

√7ᵗʰ **S46.912** Strain of unspecified muscle, fascia and tendon at shoulder and upper arm level, left arm

√7ᵗʰ **S46.919** Strain of unspecified muscle, fascia and tendon at shoulder and upper arm level, unspecified arm

√6ᵗʰ **S46.92** Laceration of unspecified muscle, fascia and tendon at shoulder and upper arm level

√7ᵗʰ **S46.921** Laceration of unspecified muscle, fascia and tendon at shoulder and upper arm level, right arm

√7ᵗʰ **S46.922** Laceration of unspecified muscle, fascia and tendon at shoulder and upper arm level, left arm

√7ᵗʰ **S46.929** Laceration of unspecified muscle, fascia and tendon at shoulder and upper arm level, unspecified arm

√6ᵗʰ **S46.99** Other injury of unspecified muscle, fascia and tendon at shoulder and upper arm level

√7ᵗʰ **S46.991** Other injury of unspecified muscle, fascia and tendon at shoulder and upper arm level, right arm

√7ᵗʰ **S46.992** Other injury of unspecified muscle, fascia and tendon at shoulder and upper arm level, left arm

√7ᵗʰ **S46.999** Other injury of unspecified muscle, fascia and tendon at shoulder and upper arm level, unspecified arm

√4ᵗʰ **S47** Crushing injury of shoulder and upper arm

Use additional code for all associated injuries

EXCLUDES 2   crushing injury of elbow (S57.0-)

> The appropriate 7th character is to be added to each code from category S47.
> A   initial encounter
> D   subsequent encounter
> S   sequela

√x7ᵗʰ **S47.1** Crushing injury of right shoulder and upper arm

√x7ᵗʰ **S47.2** Crushing injury of left shoulder and upper arm

√x7ᵗʰ **S47.9** Crushing injury of shoulder and upper arm, unspecified arm

√4ᵗʰ **S48** Traumatic amputation of shoulder and upper arm

An amputation not identified as partial or complete should be coded to complete

EXCLUDES 1   traumatic amputation at elbow level (S58.0)

> The appropriate 7th character is to be added to each code from category S48.
> A   initial encounter
> D   subsequent encounter
> S   sequela

√5ᵗʰ **S48.0** Traumatic amputation at shoulder joint

√6ᵗʰ **S48.01** Complete traumatic amputation at shoulder joint

² √7ᵗʰ **S48.011** Complete traumatic amputation at right shoulder joint   HCC ESR COM

² √7ᵗʰ **S48.012** Complete traumatic amputation at left shoulder joint   HCC ESR COM

² √7ᵗʰ **S48.019** Complete traumatic amputation at unspecified shoulder joint   HCC ESR COM

√6ᵗʰ **S48.02** Partial traumatic amputation at shoulder joint

² √7ᵗʰ **S48.021** Partial traumatic amputation at right shoulder joint   HCC ESR COM

² √7ᵗʰ **S48.022** Partial traumatic amputation at left shoulder joint   HCC ESR COM

² √7ᵗʰ **S48.029** Partial traumatic amputation at unspecified shoulder joint   HCC ESR COM

√5ᵗʰ **S48.1** Traumatic amputation at level between shoulder and elbow

√6ᵗʰ **S48.11** Complete traumatic amputation at level between shoulder and elbow

² √7ᵗʰ **S48.111** Complete traumatic amputation at level between right shoulder and elbow   HCC ESR COM

² √7ᵗʰ **S48.112** Complete traumatic amputation at level between left shoulder and elbow   HCC ESR COM

² √7ᵗʰ **S48.119** Complete traumatic amputation at level between unspecified shoulder and elbow   HCC ESR COM

√6ᵗʰ **S48.12** Partial traumatic amputation at level between shoulder and elbow

² √7ᵗʰ **S48.121** Partial traumatic amputation at level between right shoulder and elbow   HCC ESR COM

² √7ᵗʰ **S48.122** Partial traumatic amputation at level between left shoulder and elbow   HCC ESR COM

✓4ᵗʰ **S72 Fracture of femur**

> **NOTE**   A fracture not indicated as displaced or nondisplaced should be coded to displaced.
>
> A fracture not indicated as open or closed should be coded to closed.
>
> The open fracture designations are based on the Gustilo open fracture classification.

   EXCLUDES 1   traumatic amputation of hip and thigh (S78.-)

   EXCLUDES 2   fracture of lower leg and ankle (S82.-)

           fracture of foot (S92.-)

           periprosthetic fracture of prosthetic implant of hip (M97.0-)

AHA: 2018,2Q,12; 2016,1Q,33; 2015,3Q,37-39; 2015,1Q,17; 2013,4Q,128

DEF: Diaphysis: Central shaft of a long bone.

DEF: Epiphysis: Proximal and distal rounded ends of a long bone communicates with the joint.

DEF: Metaphysis: Section of a long bone located between the epiphysis and diaphysis at the proximal and distal ends.

DEF: Physis (growth plate): Narrow zone of cartilaginous tissue between the epiphysis and metaphysis at each end of a long bone. In childhood, proliferation of cells in this zone lengthens the bone. As the bone matures, this area thins, ossification eventually fusing into solid bone and growth stops. ***Synonym(s):*** *Epiphyseal plate.*

> The appropriate 7th character is to be added to all codes from category S72 [unless otherwise indicated].
>
> A   initial encounter for closed fracture
> B   initial encounter for open fracture type I or II
>   initial encounter for open fracture NOS
> C   initial encounter for open fracture type IIIA, IIIB, or IIIC
> D   subsequent encounter for closed fracture with routine healing
> E   subsequent encounter for open fracture type I or II with routine healing
> F   subsequent encounter for open fracture type IIIA, IIIB, or IIIC with routine healing
> G   subsequent encounter for closed fracture with delayed healing
> H   subsequent encounter for open fracture type I or II with delayed healing
> J   subsequent encounter for open fracture type IIIA, IIIB, or IIIC with delayed healing
> K   subsequent encounter for closed fracture with nonunion
> M   subsequent encounter for open fracture type I or II with nonunion
> N   subsequent encounter for open fracture type IIIA, IIIB, or IIIC with nonunion
> P   subsequent encounter for closed fracture with malunion
> Q   subsequent encounter for open fracture type I or II with malunion
> R   subsequent encounter for open fracture type IIIA, IIIB, or IIIC with malunion
> S   sequela

✓5ᵗʰ **S72.0 Fracture of head and neck of femur**

   EXCLUDES 2   physeal fracture of upper end of femur (S79.0-)

   AHA: 2016,3Q,16

✓6ᵗʰ **S72.00 Fracture of unspecified part of neck of femur**

     Fracture of hip NOS

     Fracture of neck of femur NOS

   1 ✓7ᵗʰ **S72.001 Fracture of unspecified part of neck of right femur** HCC ESR COM Q

   1 ✓7ᵗʰ **S72.002 Fracture of unspecified part of neck of left femur** HCC ESR COM Q

   1 ✓7ᵗʰ **S72.009 Fracture of unspecified part of neck of unspecified femur** HCC ESR COM Q

✓6ᵗʰ **S72.01 Unspecified intracapsular fracture of femur**

     Subcapital fracture of femur

   1 ✓7ᵗʰ **S72.011 Unspecified intracapsular fracture of right femur** HCC ESR COM Q

   1 ✓7ᵗʰ **S72.012 Unspecified intracapsular fracture of left femur** HCC ESR COM Q

   1 ✓7ᵗʰ **S72.019 Unspecified intracapsular fracture of unspecified femur** HCC ESR COM Q

✓6ᵗʰ **S72.02 Fracture of epiphysis (separation) (upper) of femur**

     Transepiphyseal fracture of femur

   EXCLUDES 1   capital femoral epiphyseal fracture (pediatric) of femur (S79.01-)

           Salter-Harris Type I physeal fracture of upper end of femur (S79.01-)

   1 ✓7ᵗʰ **S72.021 Displaced fracture of epiphysis (separation) (upper) of right femur** HCC ESR COM Q

   1 ✓7ᵗʰ **S72.022 Displaced fracture of epiphysis (separation) (upper) of left femur** HCC ESR COM Q

   1 ✓7ᵗʰ **S72.023 Displaced fracture of epiphysis (separation) (upper) of unspecified femur** HCC ESR COM Q

   1 ✓7ᵗʰ **S72.024 Nondisplaced fracture of epiphysis (separation) (upper) of right femur** HCC ESR COM Q

   1 ✓7ᵗʰ **S72.025 Nondisplaced fracture of epiphysis (separation) (upper) of left femur** HCC ESR COM Q

   1 ✓7ᵗʰ **S72.026 Nondisplaced fracture of epiphysis (separation) (upper) of unspecified femur** HCC ESR COM Q

✓6ᵗʰ **S72.03 Midcervical fracture of femur**

     Transcervical fracture of femur NOS

   1 ✓7ᵗʰ **S72.031 Displaced midcervical fracture of right femur** HCC ESR COM Q

   1 ✓7ᵗʰ **S72.032 Displaced midcervical fracture of left femur** HCC ESR COM Q

   1 ✓7ᵗʰ **S72.033 Displaced midcervical fracture of unspecified femur** HCC ESR COM Q

   1 ✓7ᵗʰ **S72.034 Nondisplaced midcervical fracture of right femur** HCC ESR COM Q

   1 ✓7ᵗʰ **S72.035 Nondisplaced midcervical fracture of left femur** HCC ESR COM Q

   1 ✓7ᵗʰ **S72.036 Nondisplaced midcervical fracture of unspecified femur** HCC ESR COM Q

✓6ᵗʰ **S72.04 Fracture of base of neck of femur**

     Cervicotrochanteric fracture of femur

   1 ✓7ᵗʰ **S72.041 Displaced fracture of base of neck of right femur** HCC ESR COM Q

   1 ✓7ᵗʰ **S72.042 Displaced fracture of base of neck of left femur** HCC ESR COM Q

   1 ✓7ᵗʰ **S72.043 Displaced fracture of base of neck of unspecified femur** HCC ESR COM Q

   1 ✓7ᵗʰ **S72.044 Nondisplaced fracture of base of neck of right femur** HCC ESR COM Q

   1 ✓7ᵗʰ **S72.045 Nondisplaced fracture of base of neck of left femur** HCC ESR COM Q

   1 ✓7ᵗʰ **S72.046 Nondisplaced fracture of base of neck of unspecified femur** HCC ESR COM Q

✓6ᵗʰ **S72.05 Unspecified fracture of head of femur**

     Fracture of head of femur NOS

   1 ✓7ᵗʰ **S72.051 Unspecified fracture of head of right femur** HCC ESR COM Q

   1 ✓7ᵗʰ **S72.052 Unspecified fracture of head of left femur** HCC ESR COM Q

   1 ✓7ᵗʰ **S72.059 Unspecified fracture of head of unspecified femur** HCC ESR COM Q

✓6ᵗʰ **S72.06 Articular fracture of head of femur**

   1 ✓7ᵗʰ **S72.061 Displaced articular fracture of head of right femur** HCC ESR COM Q

   1 ✓7ᵗʰ **S72.062 Displaced articular fracture of head of left femur** HCC ESR COM Q

   1 ✓7ᵗʰ **S72.063 Displaced articular fracture of head of unspecified femur** HCC ESR COM Q

   1 ✓7ᵗʰ **S72.064 Nondisplaced articular fracture of head of right femur** HCC ESR COM Q

   1 ✓7ᵗʰ **S72.065 Nondisplaced articular fracture of head of left femur** HCC ESR COM Q

   1 ✓7ᵗʰ **S72.066 Nondisplaced articular fracture of head of unspecified femur** HCC ESR COM Q

✓6ᵗʰ **S72.09 Other fracture of head and neck of femur**

   1 ✓7ᵗʰ **S72.091 Other fracture of head and neck of right femur** HCC ESR COM Q

   1 ✓7ᵗʰ **S72.092 Other fracture of head and neck of left femur** HCC ESR COM Q

   1 ✓7ᵗʰ **S72.099 Other fracture of head and neck of unspecified femur** HCC ESR COM Q

✓5ᵗʰ **S72.1 Pertrochanteric fracture**

   AHA: 2016,3Q,16

✓6ᵗʰ **S72.10 Unspecified trochanteric fracture of femur**

     Fracture of trochanter NOS

   1 ✓7ᵗʰ **S72.101 Unspecified trochanteric fracture of right femur** HCC ESR COM Q

   1 ✓7ᵗʰ **S72.102 Unspecified trochanteric fracture of left femur** HCC ESR COM Q

✓ Additional Character Required   ✓×7ᵗʰ Placeholder Alert   Manifestation   Unspecified Dx   Q QPP   UPD Unacceptable PDx

Chapter 19. Injury, Poisoning and Certain Other Consequences of External Causes

S72.109–S72.399

¹ ✓7ᵗʰ **S72.109** Unspecified trochanteric fracture of unspecified femur `HCC` `ESR` `COM` `Q`

✓6ᵗʰ **S72.11** Fracture of greater trochanter of femur

¹ ✓7ᵗʰ **S72.111** Displaced fracture of greater trochanter of right femur `HCC` `ESR` `COM` `Q`

¹ ✓7ᵗʰ **S72.112** Displaced fracture of greater trochanter of left femur `HCC` `ESR` `COM` `Q`

¹ ✓7ᵗʰ **S72.113** Displaced fracture of greater trochanter of unspecified femur `HCC` `ESR` `COM` `Q`

¹ ✓7ᵗʰ **S72.114** Nondisplaced fracture of greater trochanter of right femur `HCC` `ESR` `COM` `Q`

¹ ✓7ᵗʰ **S72.115** Nondisplaced fracture of greater trochanter of left femur `HCC` `ESR` `COM` `Q`

¹ ✓7ᵗʰ **S72.116** Nondisplaced fracture of greater trochanter of unspecified femur `HCC` `ESR` `COM` `Q`

✓6ᵗʰ **S72.12** Fracture of lesser trochanter of femur

¹ ✓7ᵗʰ **S72.121** Displaced fracture of lesser trochanter of right femur `HCC` `ESR` `COM` `Q`

¹ ✓7ᵗʰ **S72.122** Displaced fracture of lesser trochanter of left femur `HCC` `ESR` `COM` `Q`

¹ ✓7ᵗʰ **S72.123** Displaced fracture of lesser trochanter of unspecified femur `HCC` `ESR` `COM` `Q`

¹ ✓7ᵗʰ **S72.124** Nondisplaced fracture of lesser trochanter of right femur `HCC` `ESR` `COM` `Q`

¹ ✓7ᵗʰ **S72.125** Nondisplaced fracture of lesser trochanter of left femur `HCC` `ESR` `COM` `Q`

¹ ✓7ᵗʰ **S72.126** Nondisplaced fracture of lesser trochanter of unspecified femur `HCC` `ESR` `COM` `Q`

✓6ᵗʰ **S72.13** Apophyseal fracture of femur

> **EXCLUDES 1**   chronic (nontraumatic) slipped upper femoral epiphysis (M93.0-)

¹ ✓7ᵗʰ **S72.131** Displaced apophyseal fracture of right femur `HCC` `ESR` `COM` `Q`

¹ ✓7ᵗʰ **S72.132** Displaced apophyseal fracture of left femur `HCC` `ESR` `COM` `Q`

¹ ✓7ᵗʰ **S72.133** Displaced apophyseal fracture of unspecified femur `HCC` `ESR` `COM` `Q`

¹ ✓7ᵗʰ **S72.134** Nondisplaced apophyseal fracture of right femur `HCC` `ESR` `COM` `Q`

¹ ✓7ᵗʰ **S72.135** Nondisplaced apophyseal fracture of left femur `HCC` `ESR` `COM` `Q`

¹ ✓7ᵗʰ **S72.136** Nondisplaced apophyseal fracture of unspecified femur `HCC` `ESR` `COM` `Q`

✓6ᵗʰ **S72.14** Intertrochanteric fracture of femur

¹ ✓7ᵗʰ **S72.141** Displaced intertrochanteric fracture of right femur `HCC` `ESR` `COM` `Q`

¹ ✓7ᵗʰ **S72.142** Displaced intertrochanteric fracture of left femur `HCC` `ESR` `COM` `Q`

¹ ✓7ᵗʰ **S72.143** Displaced intertrochanteric fracture of unspecified femur `HCC` `ESR` `COM` `Q`

¹ ✓7ᵗʰ **S72.144** Nondisplaced intertrochanteric fracture of right femur `HCC` `ESR` `COM` `Q`

¹ ✓7ᵗʰ **S72.145** Nondisplaced intertrochanteric fracture of left femur `HCC` `ESR` `COM` `Q`

¹ ✓7ᵗʰ **S72.146** Nondisplaced intertrochanteric fracture of unspecified femur `HCC` `ESR` `COM` `Q`

✓5ᵗʰ **S72.2** Subtrochanteric fracture of femur

¹ ✓x7ᵗʰ **S72.21** Displaced subtrochanteric fracture of right femur `HCC` `ESR` `COM` `Q`

¹ ✓x7ᵗʰ **S72.22** Displaced subtrochanteric fracture of left femur `HCC` `ESR` `COM` `Q`

¹ ✓x7ᵗʰ **S72.23** Displaced subtrochanteric fracture of unspecified femur `HCC` `ESR` `COM` `Q`

¹ ✓x7ᵗʰ **S72.24** Nondisplaced subtrochanteric fracture of right femur `HCC` `ESR` `COM` `Q`

¹ ✓x7ᵗʰ **S72.25** Nondisplaced subtrochanteric fracture of left femur `HCC` `ESR` `COM` `Q`

¹ ✓x7ᵗʰ **S72.26** Nondisplaced subtrochanteric fracture of unspecified femur `HCC` `ESR` `COM` `Q`

✓5ᵗʰ **S72.3** Fracture of shaft of femur

✓6ᵗʰ **S72.30** Unspecified fracture of shaft of femur

¹ ✓7ᵗʰ **S72.301** Unspecified fracture of shaft of right femur `HCC` `ESR` `Q`

¹ ✓7ᵗʰ **S72.302** Unspecified fracture of shaft of left femur `HCC` `ESR` `Q`

¹ ✓7ᵗʰ **S72.309** Unspecified fracture of shaft of unspecified femur `HCC` `ESR` `Q`

✓6ᵗʰ **S72.32** Transverse fracture of shaft of femur

¹ ✓7ᵗʰ **S72.321** Displaced transverse fracture of shaft of right femur `HCC` `ESR` `Q`

¹ ✓7ᵗʰ **S72.322** Displaced transverse fracture of shaft of left femur `HCC` `ESR` `Q`

¹ ✓7ᵗʰ **S72.323** Displaced transverse fracture of shaft of unspecified femur `HCC` `ESR` `Q`

¹ ✓7ᵗʰ **S72.324** Nondisplaced transverse fracture of shaft of right femur `HCC` `ESR` `Q`

¹ ✓7ᵗʰ **S72.325** Nondisplaced transverse fracture of shaft of left femur `HCC` `ESR` `Q`

¹ ✓7ᵗʰ **S72.326** Nondisplaced transverse fracture of shaft of unspecified femur `HCC` `ESR` `Q`

✓6ᵗʰ **S72.33** Oblique fracture of shaft of femur

¹ ✓7ᵗʰ **S72.331** Displaced oblique fracture of shaft of right femur `HCC` `ESR` `Q`

¹ ✓7ᵗʰ **S72.332** Displaced oblique fracture of shaft of left femur `HCC` `ESR` `Q`

¹ ✓7ᵗʰ **S72.333** Displaced oblique fracture of shaft of unspecified femur `HCC` `ESR` `Q`

¹ ✓7ᵗʰ **S72.334** Nondisplaced oblique fracture of shaft of right femur `HCC` `ESR` `Q`

¹ ✓7ᵗʰ **S72.335** Nondisplaced oblique fracture of shaft of left femur `HCC` `ESR` `Q`

¹ ✓7ᵗʰ **S72.336** Nondisplaced oblique fracture of shaft of unspecified femur `HCC` `ESR` `Q`

✓6ᵗʰ **S72.34** Spiral fracture of shaft of femur

¹ ✓7ᵗʰ **S72.341** Displaced spiral fracture of shaft of right femur `HCC` `ESR` `Q`

¹ ✓7ᵗʰ **S72.342** Displaced spiral fracture of shaft of left femur `HCC` `ESR` `Q`

¹ ✓7ᵗʰ **S72.343** Displaced spiral fracture of shaft of unspecified femur `HCC` `ESR` `Q`

¹ ✓7ᵗʰ **S72.344** Nondisplaced spiral fracture of shaft of right femur `HCC` `ESR` `Q`

¹ ✓7ᵗʰ **S72.345** Nondisplaced spiral fracture of shaft of left femur `HCC` `ESR` `Q`

¹ ✓7ᵗʰ **S72.346** Nondisplaced spiral fracture of shaft of unspecified femur `HCC` `ESR` `Q`

✓6ᵗʰ **S72.35** Comminuted fracture of shaft of femur

¹ ✓7ᵗʰ **S72.351** Displaced comminuted fracture of shaft of right femur `HCC` `ESR` `Q`

¹ ✓7ᵗʰ **S72.352** Displaced comminuted fracture of shaft of left femur `HCC` `ESR` `Q`

¹ ✓7ᵗʰ **S72.353** Displaced comminuted fracture of shaft of unspecified femur `HCC` `ESR` `Q`

¹ ✓7ᵗʰ **S72.354** Nondisplaced comminuted fracture of shaft of right femur `HCC` `ESR` `Q`

¹ ✓7ᵗʰ **S72.355** Nondisplaced comminuted fracture of shaft of left femur `HCC` `ESR` `Q`

¹ ✓7ᵗʰ **S72.356** Nondisplaced comminuted fracture of shaft of unspecified femur `HCC` `ESR` `Q`

✓6ᵗʰ **S72.36** Segmental fracture of shaft of femur

¹ ✓7ᵗʰ **S72.361** Displaced segmental fracture of shaft of right femur `HCC` `ESR` `Q`

¹ ✓7ᵗʰ **S72.362** Displaced segmental fracture of shaft of left femur `HCC` `ESR` `Q`

¹ ✓7ᵗʰ **S72.363** Displaced segmental fracture of shaft of unspecified femur `HCC` `ESR` `Q`

¹ ✓7ᵗʰ **S72.364** Nondisplaced segmental fracture of shaft of right femur `HCC` `ESR` `Q`

¹ ✓7ᵗʰ **S72.365** Nondisplaced segmental fracture of shaft of left femur `HCC` `ESR` `Q`

¹ ✓7ᵗʰ **S72.366** Nondisplaced segmental fracture of shaft of unspecified femur `HCC` `ESR` `Q`

✓6ᵗʰ **S72.39** Other fracture of shaft of femur

¹ ✓7ᵗʰ **S72.391** Other fracture of shaft of right femur `HCC` `ESR` `Q`

¹ ✓7ᵗʰ **S72.392** Other fracture of shaft of left femur `HCC` `ESR` `Q`

¹ ✓7ᵗʰ **S72.399** Other fracture of shaft of unspecified femur `HCC` `ESR` `Q`

`HCC` CMS-HCC   `Rx` Rx HCC   `ESR` ESRD HCC   `COM` Commercial HCC   `N` Newborn: 0   `P` Pediatric: 0-17   `M` Maternity: 9-64   `A` Adult: 15-124

1082

ICD-10-CM 2023

√5ᵗʰ **S72.4** **Fracture of lower end of femur**
Fracture of distal end of femur
EXCLUDES 2   *fracture of shaft of femur (S72.3-)*
physeal fracture of lower end of femur (S79.1-)
AHA: 2016,4Q,42

√6ᵗʰ **S72.40** **Unspecified fracture of lower end of femur**
AHA: 2018,1Q,21; 2016,4Q,42
¹ √7ᵗʰ **S72.401** Unspecified fracture of lower end of **right** femur ᴴᶜᶜ ᴱˢᴿ ◻
¹ √7ᵗʰ **S72.402** Unspecified fracture of lower end of **left** femur ᴴᶜᶜ ᴱˢᴿ ◻
¹ √7ᵗʰ **S72.409** Unspecified fracture of lower end of **unspecified** femur ᴴᶜᶜ ᴱˢᴿ ◻

√6ᵗʰ **S72.41** **Unspecified condyle fracture of lower end of femur**
Condyle fracture of femur NOS
¹ √7ᵗʰ **S72.411** Displaced unspecified condyle fracture of lower end of **right** femur ᴴᶜᶜ ᴱˢᴿ ◻
¹ √7ᵗʰ **S72.412** Displaced unspecified condyle fracture of lower end of **left** femur ᴴᶜᶜ ᴱˢᴿ ◻
¹ √7ᵗʰ **S72.413** Displaced unspecified condyle fracture of lower end of unspecified femur ᴴᶜᶜ ᴱˢᴿ ◻
¹ √7ᵗʰ **S72.414** Nondisplaced unspecified condyle fracture of lower end of **right** femur ᴴᶜᶜ ᴱˢᴿ ◻
¹ √7ᵗʰ **S72.415** Nondisplaced unspecified condyle fracture of lower end of **left** femur ᴴᶜᶜ ᴱˢᴿ ◻
¹ √7ᵗʰ **S72.416** Nondisplaced unspecified condyle fracture of lower end of unspecified femur ᴴᶜᶜ ᴱˢᴿ ◻

√6ᵗʰ **S72.42** **Fracture of lateral condyle of femur**
¹ √7ᵗʰ **S72.421** Displaced fracture of lateral condyle of **right** femur ᴴᶜᶜ ᴱˢᴿ ◻
¹ √7ᵗʰ **S72.422** Displaced fracture of lateral condyle of **left** femur ᴴᶜᶜ ᴱˢᴿ ◻
¹ √7ᵗʰ **S72.423** Displaced fracture of lateral condyle of unspecified femur ᴴᶜᶜ ᴱˢᴿ ◻
¹ √7ᵗʰ **S72.424** Nondisplaced fracture of lateral condyle of **right** femur ᴴᶜᶜ ᴱˢᴿ ◻
¹ √7ᵗʰ **S72.425** Nondisplaced fracture of lateral condyle of **left** femur ᴴᶜᶜ ᴱˢᴿ ◻
¹ √7ᵗʰ **S72.426** Nondisplaced fracture of lateral condyle of unspecified femur ᴴᶜᶜ ᴱˢᴿ ◻

√6ᵗʰ **S72.43** **Fracture of medial condyle of femur**
¹ √7ᵗʰ **S72.431** Displaced fracture of medial condyle of **right** femur ᴴᶜᶜ ᴱˢᴿ ◻
¹ √7ᵗʰ **S72.432** Displaced fracture of medial condyle of **left** femur ᴴᶜᶜ ᴱˢᴿ ◻
¹ √7ᵗʰ **S72.433** Displaced fracture of medial condyle of unspecified femur ᴴᶜᶜ ᴱˢᴿ ◻
¹ √7ᵗʰ **S72.434** Nondisplaced fracture of medial condyle of **right** femur ᴴᶜᶜ ᴱˢᴿ ◻
¹ √7ᵗʰ **S72.435** Nondisplaced fracture of medial condyle of **left** femur ᴴᶜᶜ ᴱˢᴿ ◻
¹ √7ᵗʰ **S72.436** Nondisplaced fracture of medial condyle of unspecified femur ᴴᶜᶜ ᴱˢᴿ ◻

√6ᵗʰ **S72.44** **Fracture of lower epiphysis (separation) of femur**
EXCLUDES 1   *Salter-Harris Type I physeal fracture of lower end of femur (S79.11-)*
¹ √7ᵗʰ **S72.441** Displaced fracture of lower epiphysis (separation) of **right** femur ᴴᶜᶜ ᴱˢᴿ ◻
¹ √7ᵗʰ **S72.442** Displaced fracture of lower epiphysis (separation) of **left** femur ᴴᶜᶜ ᴱˢᴿ ◻
¹ √7ᵗʰ **S72.443** Displaced fracture of lower epiphysis (separation) of unspecified femur ᴴᶜᶜ ᴱˢᴿ ◻
¹ √7ᵗʰ **S72.444** Nondisplaced fracture of lower epiphysis (separation) of **right** femur ᴴᶜᶜ ᴱˢᴿ ◻
¹ √7ᵗʰ **S72.445** Nondisplaced fracture of lower epiphysis (separation) of **left** femur ᴴᶜᶜ ᴱˢᴿ ◻
¹ √7ᵗʰ **S72.446** Nondisplaced fracture of lower epiphysis (separation) of unspecified femur ᴴᶜᶜ ᴱˢᴿ ◻

√6ᵗʰ **S72.45** **Supracondylar fracture without intracondylar extension of lower end of femur**
Supracondylar fracture of lower end of femur NOS
EXCLUDES 1   *supracondylar fracture with intracondylar extension of lower end of femur (S72.46-)*
¹ √7ᵗʰ **S72.451** Displaced supracondylar fracture without intracondylar extension of lower end of **right** femur ᴴᶜᶜ ᴱˢᴿ ◻
¹ √7ᵗʰ **S72.452** Displaced supracondylar fracture without intracondylar extension of lower end of **left** femur ᴴᶜᶜ ᴱˢᴿ ◻
¹ √7ᵗʰ **S72.453** Displaced supracondylar fracture without intracondylar extension of lower end of unspecified femur ᴴᶜᶜ ᴱˢᴿ ◻
¹ √7ᵗʰ **S72.454** Nondisplaced supracondylar fracture without intracondylar extension of lower end of **right** femur ᴴᶜᶜ ᴱˢᴿ ◻
¹ √7ᵗʰ **S72.455** Nondisplaced supracondylar fracture without intracondylar extension of lower end of **left** femur ᴴᶜᶜ ᴱˢᴿ ◻
¹ √7ᵗʰ **S72.456** Nondisplaced supracondylar fracture without intracondylar extension of lower end of unspecified femur ᴴᶜᶜ ᴱˢᴿ ◻

√6ᵗʰ **S72.46** **Supracondylar fracture with intracondylar extension of lower end of femur**
EXCLUDES 1   *supracondylar fracture without intracondylar extension of lower end of femur (S72.45-)*
¹ √7ᵗʰ **S72.461** Displaced supracondylar fracture with intracondylar extension of lower end of **right** femur ᴴᶜᶜ ᴱˢᴿ ◻
¹ √7ᵗʰ **S72.462** Displaced supracondylar fracture with intracondylar extension of lower end of **left** femur ᴴᶜᶜ ᴱˢᴿ ◻
¹ √7ᵗʰ **S72.463** Displaced supracondylar fracture with intracondylar extension of lower end of unspecified femur ᴴᶜᶜ ᴱˢᴿ ◻
¹ √7ᵗʰ **S72.464** Nondisplaced supracondylar fracture with intracondylar extension of lower end of **right** femur ᴴᶜᶜ ᴱˢᴿ ◻
¹ √7ᵗʰ **S72.465** Nondisplaced supracondylar fracture with intracondylar extension of lower end of **left** femur ᴴᶜᶜ ᴱˢᴿ ◻
¹ √7ᵗʰ **S72.466** Nondisplaced supracondylar fracture with intracondylar extension of lower end of unspecified femur ᴴᶜᶜ ᴱˢᴿ ◻

√6ᵗʰ **S72.47** **Torus fracture of lower end of femur**

The appropriate 7th character is to be added to all codes in subcategory S72.47.
A   initial encounter for closed fracture
D   subsequent encounter for fracture with routine healing
G   subsequent encounter for fracture with delayed healing
K   subsequent encounter for fracture with nonunion
P   subsequent encounter for fracture with malunion
S   sequela

¹ √7ᵗʰ **S72.471** Torus fracture of lower end of **right** femur ᴴᶜᶜ ᴱˢᴿ ◻
¹ √7ᵗʰ **S72.472** Torus fracture of lower end of **left** femur ᴴᶜᶜ ᴱˢᴿ ◻
¹ √7ᵗʰ **S72.479** Torus fracture of lower end of unspecified femur ᴴᶜᶜ ᴱˢᴿ ◻

√6ᵗʰ **S72.49** **Other fracture of lower end of femur**
¹ √7ᵗʰ **S72.491** Other fracture of lower end of **right** femur ᴴᶜᶜ ᴱˢᴿ ◻
¹ √7ᵗʰ **S72.492** Other fracture of lower end of **left** femur ᴴᶜᶜ ᴱˢᴿ ◻
¹ √7ᵗʰ **S72.499** Other fracture of lower end of unspecified femur ᴴᶜᶜ ᴱˢᴿ ◻

√5ᵗʰ **S72.8** **Other fracture of femur**
√6ᵗʰ **S72.8X** **Other fracture of femur**
¹ √7ᵗʰ **S72.8X1** Other fracture of **right** femur ᴴᶜᶜ ᴱˢᴿ ◻
¹ √7ᵗʰ **S72.8X2** Other fracture of **left** femur ᴴᶜᶜ ᴱˢᴿ ◻

¹ ✓7ᵗʰ **S72.8X9** **Other fracture of unspecified femur** `HCC` `ESR` `Q`

✓5ᵗʰ **S72.9** **Unspecified fracture of femur**
Fracture of thigh NOS
Fracture of upper leg NOS
   EXCLUDES 1   *fracture of hip NOS (S72.00-, S72.01-)*

¹ ✓x7ᵗʰ **S72.90** **Unspecified fracture of unspecified femur** `HCC` `ESR` `Q`
   AHA: 2012,4Q,93

¹ ✓x7ᵗʰ **S72.91** **Unspecified fracture of right femur** `HCC` `ESR` `Q`

¹ ✓x7ᵗʰ **S72.92** **Unspecified fracture of left femur** `HCC` `ESR` `Q`

✓4ᵗʰ **S73** **Dislocation and sprain of joint and ligaments of hip**
   INCLUDES   avulsion of joint or ligament of hip
           laceration of cartilage, joint or ligament of hip
           sprain of cartilage, joint or ligament of hip
           traumatic hemarthrosis of joint or ligament of hip
           traumatic rupture of joint or ligament of hip
           traumatic subluxation of joint or ligament of hip
           traumatic tear of joint or ligament of hip
Code also any associated open wound
   EXCLUDES 2   *strain of muscle, fascia and tendon of hip and thigh (S76.-)*

The appropriate 7th character is to be added to each code from category S73.
A   initial encounter
D   subsequent encounter
S   sequela

✓5ᵗʰ **S73.0** **Subluxation and dislocation of hip**
   EXCLUDES 2   *dislocation and subluxation of hip prosthesis (T84.020, T84.021)*

✓6ᵗʰ **S73.00** **Unspecified subluxation and dislocation of hip**
Dislocation of hip NOS
Subluxation of hip NOS

¹ ✓7ᵗʰ **S73.001** **Unspecified subluxation of right hip** `HCC` `ESR`

¹ ✓7ᵗʰ **S73.002** **Unspecified subluxation of left hip** `HCC` `ESR`

¹ ✓7ᵗʰ **S73.003** **Unspecified subluxation of unspecified hip** `HCC` `ESR`

¹ ✓7ᵗʰ **S73.004** **Unspecified dislocation of right hip** `HCC` `ESR`

¹ ✓7ᵗʰ **S73.005** **Unspecified dislocation of left hip** `HCC` `ESR`

¹ ✓7ᵗʰ **S73.006** **Unspecified dislocation of unspecified hip** `HCC` `ESR`

✓6ᵗʰ **S73.01** **Posterior subluxation and dislocation of hip**

¹ ✓7ᵗʰ **S73.011** **Posterior subluxation of right hip** `HCC` `ESR`

¹ ✓7ᵗʰ **S73.012** **Posterior subluxation of left hip** `HCC` `ESR`

¹ ✓7ᵗʰ **S73.013** **Posterior subluxation of unspecified hip** `HCC` `ESR`

¹ ✓7ᵗʰ **S73.014** **Posterior dislocation of right hip** `HCC` `ESR`

¹ ✓7ᵗʰ **S73.015** **Posterior dislocation of left hip** `HCC` `ESR`

¹ ✓7ᵗʰ **S73.016** **Posterior dislocation of unspecified hip** `HCC` `ESR`

✓6ᵗʰ **S73.02** **Obturator subluxation and dislocation of hip**

¹ ✓7ᵗʰ **S73.021** **Obturator subluxation of right hip** `HCC` `ESR`

¹ ✓7ᵗʰ **S73.022** **Obturator subluxation of left hip** `HCC` `ESR`

¹ ✓7ᵗʰ **S73.023** **Obturator subluxation of unspecified hip** `HCC` `ESR`

¹ ✓7ᵗʰ **S73.024** **Obturator dislocation of right hip** `HCC` `ESR`

¹ ✓7ᵗʰ **S73.025** **Obturator dislocation of left hip** `HCC` `ESR`

¹ ✓7ᵗʰ **S73.026** **Obturator dislocation of unspecified hip** `HCC` `ESR`

✓6ᵗʰ **S73.03** **Other anterior subluxation and dislocation of hip**

¹ ✓7ᵗʰ **S73.031** **Other anterior subluxation of right hip** `HCC` `ESR`

¹ ✓7ᵗʰ **S73.032** **Other anterior subluxation of left hip** `HCC` `ESR`

¹ ✓7ᵗʰ **S73.033** **Other anterior subluxation of unspecified hip** `HCC` `ESR`

¹ ✓7ᵗʰ **S73.034** **Other anterior dislocation of right hip** `HCC` `ESR`

¹ ✓7ᵗʰ **S73.035** **Other anterior dislocation of left hip** `HCC` `ESR`

¹ ✓7ᵗʰ **S73.036** **Other anterior dislocation of unspecified hip** `HCC` `ESR`

✓6ᵗʰ **S73.04** **Central subluxation and dislocation of hip**

¹ ✓7ᵗʰ **S73.041** **Central subluxation of right hip** `HCC` `ESR`

¹ ✓7ᵗʰ **S73.042** **Central subluxation of left hip** `HCC` `ESR`

¹ ✓7ᵗʰ **S73.043** **Central subluxation of unspecified hip** `HCC` `ESR`

¹ ✓7ᵗʰ **S73.044** **Central dislocation of right hip** `HCC` `ESR`

¹ ✓7ᵗʰ **S73.045** **Central dislocation of left hip** `HCC` `ESR`

¹ ✓7ᵗʰ **S73.046** **Central dislocation of unspecified hip** `HCC` `ESR`

✓5ᵗʰ **S73.1** **Sprain of hip**
   AHA: 2014,4Q,25

✓6ᵗʰ **S73.10** **Unspecified sprain of hip**

✓7ᵗʰ **S73.101** **Unspecified sprain of right hip**

✓7ᵗʰ **S73.102** **Unspecified sprain of left hip**

✓7ᵗʰ **S73.109** **Unspecified sprain of unspecified hip**

✓6ᵗʰ **S73.11** **Iliofemoral ligament sprain of hip**

✓7ᵗʰ **S73.111** **Iliofemoral ligament sprain of right hip**

✓7ᵗʰ **S73.112** **Iliofemoral ligament sprain of left hip**

✓7ᵗʰ **S73.119** **Iliofemoral ligament sprain of unspecified hip**

✓6ᵗʰ **S73.12** **Ischiocapsular (ligament) sprain of hip**

✓7ᵗʰ **S73.121** **Ischiocapsular ligament sprain of right hip**

✓7ᵗʰ **S73.122** **Ischiocapsular ligament sprain of left hip**

✓7ᵗʰ **S73.129** **Ischiocapsular ligament sprain of unspecified hip**

✓6ᵗʰ **S73.19** **Other sprain of hip**

✓7ᵗʰ **S73.191** **Other sprain of right hip**

✓7ᵗʰ **S73.192** **Other sprain of left hip**

✓7ᵗʰ **S73.199** **Other sprain of unspecified hip**

✓4ᵗʰ **S74** **Injury of nerves at hip and thigh level**
Code also any associated open wound (S71.-)
   EXCLUDES 2   *injury of nerves at ankle and foot level (S94.-)*
                    injury of nerves at lower leg level (S84.-)

The appropriate 7th character is to be added to each code from category S74.
A   initial encounter
D   subsequent encounter
S   sequela

✓5ᵗʰ **S74.0** **Injury of sciatic nerve at hip and thigh level**

✓x7ᵗʰ **S74.00** **Injury of sciatic nerve at hip and thigh level, unspecified leg**

✓x7ᵗʰ **S74.01** **Injury of sciatic nerve at hip and thigh level, right leg**

✓x7ᵗʰ **S74.02** **Injury of sciatic nerve at hip and thigh level, left leg**

✓5ᵗʰ **S74.1** **Injury of femoral nerve at hip and thigh level**

✓x7ᵗʰ **S74.10** **Injury of femoral nerve at hip and thigh level, unspecified leg**

✓x7ᵗʰ **S74.11** **Injury of femoral nerve at hip and thigh level, right leg**

✓x7ᵗʰ **S74.12** **Injury of femoral nerve at hip and thigh level, left leg**

✓5ᵗʰ **S74.2** **Injury of cutaneous sensory nerve at hip and thigh level**

✓x7ᵗʰ **S74.20** **Injury of cutaneous sensory nerve at hip and thigh level, unspecified leg**

✓x7ᵗʰ **S74.21** **Injury of cutaneous sensory nerve at hip and high level, right leg**

✓x7ᵗʰ **S74.22** **Injury of cutaneous sensory nerve at hip and thigh level, left leg**

✓5ᵗʰ **S74.8** **Injury of other nerves at hip and thigh level**

✓6ᵗʰ **S74.8X** **Injury of other nerves at hip and thigh level**

✓7ᵗʰ **S74.8X1** **Injury of other nerves at hip and thigh level, right leg**

`HCC` CMS-HCC   `Rx` Rx HCC   `ESR` ESRD HCC   `COM` Commercial HCC   `N` Newborn: 0   `P` Pediatric: 0-17   `M` Maternity: 9-64   `A` Adult: 15-124

1084   ICD-10-CM 2023

√7ᵗʰ **S74.8X2** Injury of other nerves at hip and thigh level, left leg

√7ᵗʰ **S74.8X9** Injury of other nerves at hip and thigh level, unspecified leg

√5ᵗʰ **S74.9** Injury of unspecified nerve at hip and thigh level

√×7ᵗʰ **S74.90** Injury of unspecified nerve at hip and thigh level, unspecified leg

√×7ᵗʰ **S74.91** Injury of unspecified nerve at hip and thigh level, right leg

√×7ᵗʰ **S74.92** Injury of unspecified nerve at hip and thigh level, left leg

√4ᵗʰ **S75** **Injury of blood vessels at hip and thigh level**

Code also any associated open wound (S71.-)

EXCLUDES 2   *injury of blood vessels at lower leg level (S85.-)*
            injury of popliteal artery (S85.0)

The appropriate 7th character is to be added to each code from category S75.
A   initial encounter
D   subsequent encounter
S   sequela

√5ᵗʰ **S75.0** Injury of femoral artery

√6ᵗʰ **S75.00** Unspecified injury of femoral artery

√7ᵗʰ **S75.001** Unspecified injury of femoral artery, right leg

√7ᵗʰ **S75.002** Unspecified injury of femoral artery, left leg

√7ᵗʰ **S75.009** Unspecified injury of femoral artery, unspecified leg

√6ᵗʰ **S75.01** Minor laceration of femoral artery

Incomplete transection of femoral artery
Laceration of femoral artery NOS
Superficial laceration of femoral artery

√7ᵗʰ **S75.011** Minor laceration of femoral artery, right leg

√7ᵗʰ **S75.012** Minor laceration of femoral artery, left leg

√7ᵗʰ **S75.019** Minor laceration of femoral artery, unspecified leg

√6ᵗʰ **S75.02** Major laceration of femoral artery

Complete transection of femoral artery
Traumatic rupture of femoral artery

√7ᵗʰ **S75.021** Major laceration of femoral artery, right leg

√7ᵗʰ **S75.022** Major laceration of femoral artery, left leg

√7ᵗʰ **S75.029** Major laceration of femoral artery, unspecified leg

√6ᵗʰ **S75.09** Other specified injury of femoral artery

√7ᵗʰ **S75.091** Other specified injury of femoral artery, right leg

√7ᵗʰ **S75.092** Other specified injury of femoral artery, left leg

√7ᵗʰ **S75.099** Other specified injury of femoral artery, unspecified leg

√5ᵗʰ **S75.1** Injury of femoral vein at hip and thigh level

√6ᵗʰ **S75.10** Unspecified injury of femoral vein at hip and thigh level

√7ᵗʰ **S75.101** Unspecified injury of femoral vein at hip and thigh level, right leg

√7ᵗʰ **S75.102** Unspecified injury of femoral vein at hip and thigh level, left leg

√7ᵗʰ **S75.109** Unspecified injury of femoral vein at hip and thigh level, unspecified leg

√6ᵗʰ **S75.11** Minor laceration of femoral vein at hip and thigh level

Incomplete transection of femoral vein at hip and thigh level
Laceration of femoral vein at hip and thigh level NOS
Superficial laceration of femoral vein at hip and thigh level

√7ᵗʰ **S75.111** Minor laceration of femoral vein at hip and thigh level, right leg

√7ᵗʰ **S75.112** Minor laceration of femoral vein at hip and thigh level, left leg

√7ᵗʰ **S75.119** Minor laceration of femoral vein at hip and thigh level, unspecified leg

√6ᵗʰ **S75.12** Major laceration of femoral vein at hip and thigh level

Complete transection of femoral vein at hip and thigh level
Traumatic rupture of femoral vein at hip and thigh level

√7ᵗʰ **S75.121** Major laceration of femoral vein at hip and thigh level, right leg

√7ᵗʰ **S75.122** Major laceration of femoral vein at hip and thigh level, left leg

√7ᵗʰ **S75.129** Major laceration of femoral vein at hip and thigh level, unspecified leg

√6ᵗʰ **S75.19** Other specified injury of femoral vein at hip and thigh level

√7ᵗʰ **S75.191** Other specified injury of femoral vein at hip and thigh level, right leg

√7ᵗʰ **S75.192** Other specified injury of femoral vein at hip and thigh level, left leg

√7ᵗʰ **S75.199** Other specified injury of femoral vein at hip and thigh level, unspecified leg

√5ᵗʰ **S75.2** Injury of greater saphenous vein at hip and thigh level

EXCLUDES 1   *greater saphenous vein NOS (S85.3)*

√6ᵗʰ **S75.20** Unspecified injury of greater saphenous vein at hip and thigh level

√7ᵗʰ **S75.201** Unspecified injury of greater saphenous vein at hip and thigh level, right leg

√7ᵗʰ **S75.202** Unspecified injury of greater saphenous vein at hip and thigh level, left leg

√7ᵗʰ **S75.209** Unspecified injury of greater saphenous vein at hip and thigh level, unspecified leg

√6ᵗʰ **S75.21** Minor laceration of greater saphenous vein at hip and thigh level

Incomplete transection of greater saphenous vein at hip and thigh level
Laceration of greater saphenous vein at hip and thigh level NOS
Superficial laceration of greater saphenous vein at hip and thigh level

√7ᵗʰ **S75.211** Minor laceration of greater saphenous vein at hip and thigh level, right leg

√7ᵗʰ **S75.212** Minor laceration of greater saphenous vein at hip and thigh level, left leg

√7ᵗʰ **S75.219** Minor laceration of greater saphenous vein at hip and thigh level, unspecified leg

√6ᵗʰ **S75.22** Major laceration of greater saphenous vein at hip and thigh level

Complete transection of greater saphenous vein at hip and thigh level
Traumatic rupture of greater saphenous vein at hip and thigh level

√7ᵗʰ **S75.221** Major laceration of greater saphenous vein at hip and thigh level, right leg

√7ᵗʰ **S75.222** Major laceration of greater saphenous vein at hip and thigh level, left leg

√7ᵗʰ **S75.229** Major laceration of greater saphenous vein at hip and thigh level, unspecified leg

√6ᵗʰ **S75.29** Other specified injury of greater saphenous vein at hip and thigh level

√7ᵗʰ **S75.291** Other specified injury of greater saphenous vein at hip and thigh level, right leg

√7ᵗʰ **S75.292** Other specified injury of greater saphenous vein at hip and thigh level, left leg

√7ᵗʰ **S75.299** Other specified injury of greater saphenous vein at hip and thigh level, unspecified leg

√5ᵗʰ **S75.8** Injury of other blood vessels at hip and thigh level

√6ᵗʰ **S75.80** Unspecified injury of other blood vessels at hip and thigh level

√7ᵗʰ **S75.801** Unspecified injury of other blood vessels at hip and thigh level, right leg

√7ᵗʰ **S75.802** Unspecified injury of other blood vessels at hip and thigh level, left leg

√7ᵗʰ **S75.809** Unspecified injury of other blood vessels at hip and thigh level, unspecified leg

√6ᵗʰ **S75.81** Laceration of other blood vessels at hip and thigh level

  √7ᵗʰ **S75.811** Laceration of other blood vessels at hip and thigh level, right leg

  √7ᵗʰ **S75.812** Laceration of other blood vessels at hip and thigh level, left leg

  √7ᵗʰ **S75.819** Laceration of other blood vessels at hip and thigh level, unspecified leg

√6ᵗʰ **S75.89** Other specified injury of other blood vessels at hip and thigh level

  √7ᵗʰ **S75.891** Other specified injury of other blood vessels at hip and thigh level, right leg

  √7ᵗʰ **S75.892** Other specified injury of other blood vessels at hip and thigh level, left leg

  √7ᵗʰ **S75.899** Other specified injury of other blood vessels at hip and thigh level, unspecified leg

√5ᵗʰ **S75.9** Injury of unspecified blood vessel at hip and thigh level

√6ᵗʰ **S75.90** Unspecified injury of unspecified blood vessel at hip and thigh level

  √7ᵗʰ **S75.901** Unspecified injury of unspecified blood vessel at hip and thigh level, right leg

  √7ᵗʰ **S75.902** Unspecified injury of unspecified blood vessel at hip and thigh level, left leg

  √7ᵗʰ **S75.909** Unspecified injury of unspecified blood vessel at hip and thigh level, unspecified leg

√6ᵗʰ **S75.91** Laceration of unspecified blood vessel at hip and thigh level

  √7ᵗʰ **S75.911** Laceration of unspecified blood vessel at hip and thigh level, right leg

  √7ᵗʰ **S75.912** Laceration of unspecified blood vessel at hip and thigh level, left leg

  √7ᵗʰ **S75.919** Laceration of unspecified blood vessel at hip and thigh level, unspecified leg

√6ᵗʰ **S75.99** Other specified injury of unspecified blood vessel at hip and thigh level

  √7ᵗʰ **S75.991** Other specified injury of unspecified blood vessel at hip and thigh level, right leg

  √7ᵗʰ **S75.992** Other specified injury of unspecified blood vessel at hip and thigh level, left leg

  √7ᵗʰ **S75.999** Other specified injury of unspecified blood vessel at hip and thigh level, unspecified leg

√4ᵗʰ **S76 Injury of muscle, fascia and tendon at hip and thigh level**

Code also any associated open wound (S71.-)

EXCLUDES 2   injury of muscle, fascia and tendon at lower leg level (S86)
         sprain of joint and ligament of hip (S73.1)

TIP: Refer to the Muscle/Tendon table at the beginning of this chapter.

The appropriate 7th character is to be added to each code from category S76.
A   initial encounter
D   subsequent encounter
S   sequela

√5ᵗʰ **S76.0** Injury of muscle, fascia and tendon of hip

√6ᵗʰ **S76.00** Unspecified injury of muscle, fascia and tendon of hip

  √7ᵗʰ **S76.001** Unspecified injury of muscle, fascia and tendon of right hip

  √7ᵗʰ **S76.002** Unspecified injury of muscle, fascia and tendon of left hip

  √7ᵗʰ **S76.009** Unspecified injury of muscle, fascia and tendon of unspecified hip

√6ᵗʰ **S76.01** Strain of muscle, fascia and tendon of hip

  √7ᵗʰ **S76.011** Strain of muscle, fascia and tendon of right hip

  √7ᵗʰ **S76.012** Strain of muscle, fascia and tendon of left hip

  √7ᵗʰ **S76.019** Strain of muscle, fascia and tendon of unspecified hip

√6ᵗʰ **S76.02** Laceration of muscle, fascia and tendon of hip

  √7ᵗʰ **S76.021** Laceration of muscle, fascia and tendon of right hip

  √7ᵗʰ **S76.022** Laceration of muscle, fascia and tendon of left hip

  √7ᵗʰ **S76.029** Laceration of muscle, fascia and tendon of unspecified hip

√6ᵗʰ **S76.09** Other specified injury of muscle, fascia and tendon of hip

  √7ᵗʰ **S76.091** Other specified injury of muscle, fascia and tendon of right hip

  √7ᵗʰ **S76.092** Other specified injury of muscle, fascia and tendon of left hip

  √7ᵗʰ **S76.099** Other specified injury of muscle, fascia and tendon of unspecified hip

√5ᵗʰ **S76.1** Injury of quadriceps muscle, fascia and tendon

Injury of patellar ligament (tendon)

√6ᵗʰ **S76.10** Unspecified injury of quadriceps muscle, fascia and tendon

  √7ᵗʰ **S76.101** Unspecified injury of right quadriceps muscle, fascia and tendon

  √7ᵗʰ **S76.102** Unspecified injury of left quadriceps muscle, fascia and tendon

  √7ᵗʰ **S76.109** Unspecified injury of unspecified quadriceps muscle, fascia and tendon

√6ᵗʰ **S76.11** Strain of quadriceps muscle, fascia and tendon

  √7ᵗʰ **S76.111** Strain of right quadriceps muscle, fascia and tendon

  √7ᵗʰ **S76.112** Strain of left quadriceps muscle, fascia and tendon

  √7ᵗʰ **S76.119** Strain of unspecified quadriceps muscle, fascia and tendon

√6ᵗʰ **S76.12** Laceration of quadriceps muscle, fascia and tendon

  √7ᵗʰ **S76.121** Laceration of right quadriceps muscle, fascia and tendon

  √7ᵗʰ **S76.122** Laceration of left quadriceps muscle, fascia and tendon

  √7ᵗʰ **S76.129** Laceration of unspecified quadriceps muscle, fascia and tendon

√6ᵗʰ **S76.19** Other specified injury of quadriceps muscle, fascia and tendon

  √7ᵗʰ **S76.191** Other specified injury of right quadriceps muscle, fascia and tendon

  √7ᵗʰ **S76.192** Other specified injury of left quadriceps muscle, fascia and tendon

  √7ᵗʰ **S76.199** Other specified injury of unspecified quadriceps muscle, fascia and tendon

√5ᵗʰ **S76.2** Injury of adductor muscle, fascia and tendon of thigh

√6ᵗʰ **S76.20** Unspecified injury of adductor muscle, fascia and tendon of thigh

  √7ᵗʰ **S76.201** Unspecified injury of adductor muscle, fascia and tendon of right thigh

  √7ᵗʰ **S76.202** Unspecified injury of adductor muscle, fascia and tendon of left thigh

  √7ᵗʰ **S76.209** Unspecified injury of adductor muscle, fascia and tendon of unspecified thigh

√6ᵗʰ **S76.21** Strain of adductor muscle, fascia and tendon of thigh

  √7ᵗʰ **S76.211** Strain of adductor muscle, fascia and tendon of right thigh

  √7ᵗʰ **S76.212** Strain of adductor muscle, fascia and tendon of left thigh

  √7ᵗʰ **S76.219** Strain of adductor muscle, fascia and tendon of unspecified thigh

√6ᵗʰ **S76.22** Laceration of adductor muscle, fascia and tendon of thigh

  √7ᵗʰ **S76.221** Laceration of adductor muscle, fascia and tendon of right thigh

  √7ᵗʰ **S76.222** Laceration of adductor muscle, fascia and tendon of left thigh

  √7ᵗʰ **S76.229** Laceration of adductor muscle, fascia and tendon of unspecified thigh

√6ᵗʰ **S76.29** Other injury of adductor muscle, fascia and tendon of thigh

  √7ᵗʰ **S76.291** Other injury of adductor muscle, fascia and tendon of right thigh

  √7ᵗʰ **S76.292** Other injury of adductor muscle, fascia and tendon of left thigh

  √7ᵗʰ **S76.299** Other injury of adductor muscle, fascia and tendon of unspecified thigh

√5ᵗʰ **S76.3** Injury of muscle, fascia and tendon of the posterior muscle group at thigh level

√6ᵗʰ **S76.30** Unspecified injury of muscle, fascia and tendon of the posterior muscle group at thigh level

  √7ᵗʰ **S76.301** Unspecified injury of muscle, fascia and tendon of the posterior muscle group at thigh level, right thigh

☑6ᵗʰ **S76.302** Unspecified injury of muscle, fascia and tendon of the posterior muscle group at thigh level, left thigh

☑7ᵗʰ **S76.309** Unspecified injury of muscle, fascia and tendon of the posterior muscle group at thigh level, unspecified thigh

☑6ᵗʰ **S76.31** Strain of muscle, fascia and tendon of the posterior muscle group at thigh level

☑7ᵗʰ **S76.311** Strain of muscle, fascia and tendon of the posterior muscle group at thigh level, right thigh

☑7ᵗʰ **S76.312** Strain of muscle, fascia and tendon of the posterior muscle group at thigh level, left thigh

☑7ᵗʰ **S76.319** Strain of muscle, fascia and tendon of the posterior muscle group at thigh level, unspecified thigh

☑6ᵗʰ **S76.32** Laceration of muscle, fascia and tendon of the posterior muscle group at thigh level

☑7ᵗʰ **S76.321** Laceration of muscle, fascia and tendon of the posterior muscle group at thigh level, right thigh

☑7ᵗʰ **S76.322** Laceration of muscle, fascia and tendon of the posterior muscle group at thigh level, left thigh

☑7ᵗʰ **S76.329** Laceration of muscle, fascia and tendon of the posterior muscle group at thigh level, unspecified thigh

☑6ᵗʰ **S76.39** Other specified injury of muscle, fascia and tendon of the posterior muscle group at thigh level

☑7ᵗʰ **S76.391** Other specified injury of muscle, fascia and tendon of the posterior muscle group at thigh level, right thigh

☑7ᵗʰ **S76.392** Other specified injury of muscle, fascia and tendon of the posterior muscle group at thigh level, left thigh

☑7ᵗʰ **S76.399** Other specified injury of muscle, fascia and tendon of the posterior muscle group at thigh level, unspecified thigh

☑5ᵗʰ **S76.8** Injury of other specified muscles, fascia and tendons at thigh level

☑6ᵗʰ **S76.80** Unspecified injury of other specified muscles, fascia and tendons at thigh level

☑7ᵗʰ **S76.801** Unspecified injury of other specified muscles, fascia and tendons at thigh level, right thigh

☑7ᵗʰ **S76.802** Unspecified injury of other specified muscles, fascia and tendons at thigh level, left thigh

☑7ᵗʰ **S76.809** Unspecified injury of other specified muscles, fascia and tendons at thigh level, unspecified thigh

☑6ᵗʰ **S76.81** Strain of other specified muscles, fascia and tendons at thigh level

☑7ᵗʰ **S76.811** Strain of other specified muscles, fascia and tendons at thigh level, right thigh

☑7ᵗʰ **S76.812** Strain of other specified muscles, fascia and tendons at thigh level, left thigh

☑7ᵗʰ **S76.819** Strain of other specified muscles, fascia and tendons at thigh level, unspecified thigh

☑6ᵗʰ **S76.82** Laceration of other specified muscles, fascia and tendons at thigh level

☑7ᵗʰ **S76.821** Laceration of other specified muscles, fascia and tendons at thigh level, right thigh

☑7ᵗʰ **S76.822** Laceration of other specified muscles, fascia and tendons at thigh level, left thigh

☑7ᵗʰ **S76.829** Laceration of other specified muscles, fascia and tendons at thigh level, unspecified thigh

☑6ᵗʰ **S76.89** Other injury of other specified muscles, fascia and tendons at thigh level

☑7ᵗʰ **S76.891** Other injury of other specified muscles, fascia and tendons at thigh level, right thigh

☑7ᵗʰ **S76.892** Other injury of other specified muscles, fascia and tendons at thigh level, left thigh

☑7ᵗʰ **S76.899** Other injury of other specified muscles, fascia and tendons at thigh level, unspecified thigh

☑5ᵗʰ **S76.9** Injury of unspecified muscles, fascia and tendons at thigh level

☑6ᵗʰ **S76.90** Unspecified injury of unspecified muscles, fascia and tendons at thigh level

☑7ᵗʰ **S76.901** Unspecified injury of unspecified muscles, fascia and tendons at thigh level, right thigh

☑7ᵗʰ **S76.902** Unspecified injury of unspecified muscles, fascia and tendons at thigh level, left thigh

☑7ᵗʰ **S76.909** Unspecified injury of unspecified muscles, fascia and tendons at thigh level, unspecified thigh

☑6ᵗʰ **S76.91** Strain of unspecified muscles, fascia and tendons at thigh level

☑7ᵗʰ **S76.911** Strain of unspecified muscles, fascia and tendons at thigh level, right thigh

☑7ᵗʰ **S76.912** Strain of unspecified muscles, fascia and tendons at thigh level, left thigh

☑7ᵗʰ **S76.919** Strain of unspecified muscles, fascia and tendons at thigh level, unspecified thigh

☑6ᵗʰ **S76.92** Laceration of unspecified muscles, fascia and tendons at thigh level

☑7ᵗʰ **S76.921** Laceration of unspecified muscles, fascia and tendons at thigh level, right thigh

☑7ᵗʰ **S76.922** Laceration of unspecified muscles, fascia and tendons at thigh level, left thigh

☑7ᵗʰ **S76.929** Laceration of unspecified muscles, fascia and tendons at thigh level, unspecified thigh

☑6ᵗʰ **S76.99** Other specified injury of unspecified muscles, fascia and tendons at thigh level

☑7ᵗʰ **S76.991** Other specified injury of unspecified muscles, fascia and tendons at thigh level, right thigh

☑7ᵗʰ **S76.992** Other specified injury of unspecified muscles, fascia and tendons at thigh level, left thigh

☑7ᵗʰ **S76.999** Other specified injury of unspecified muscles, fascia and tendons at thigh level, unspecified thigh

☑4ᵗʰ **S77** Crushing injury of hip and thigh

Use additional code(s) for all associated injuries

EXCLUDES 2   crushing injury of ankle and foot (S97.-)
               crushing injury of lower leg (S87.-)

The appropriate 7th character is to be added to each code from category S77.
A   initial encounter
D   subsequent encounter
S   sequela

☑5ᵗʰ **S77.0** Crushing injury of hip

☑x7ᵗʰ **S77.00** Crushing injury of unspecified hip

☑x7ᵗʰ **S77.01** Crushing injury of right hip

☑x7ᵗʰ **S77.02** Crushing injury of left hip

☑5ᵗʰ **S77.1** Crushing injury of thigh

☑x7ᵗʰ **S77.10** Crushing injury of unspecified thigh

☑x7ᵗʰ **S77.11** Crushing injury of right thigh

☑x7ᵗʰ **S77.12** Crushing injury of left thigh

☑5ᵗʰ **S77.2** Crushing injury of hip with thigh

☑x7ᵗʰ **S77.20** Crushing injury of unspecified hip with thigh

☑x7ᵗʰ **S77.21** Crushing injury of right hip with thigh

☑x7ᵗʰ **S77.22** Crushing injury of left hip with thigh

☑4ᵗʰ **S78** Traumatic amputation of hip and thigh

An amputation not identified as partial or complete should be coded to complete

EXCLUDES 1   traumatic amputation of knee (S88.0-)

The appropriate 7th character is to be added to each code from category S78.
A   initial encounter
D   subsequent encounter
S   sequela

☑5ᵗʰ **S78.0** Traumatic amputation at hip joint

☑6ᵗʰ **S78.01** Complete traumatic amputation at hip joint

☑7ᵗʰ **S78.011** Complete traumatic amputation at right hip joint   HCC ESR COM

√7th **S78.012** Complete traumatic amputation at left hip joint `HCC` `ESR` `COM`

√7th **S78.019** Complete traumatic amputation at unspecified hip joint `HCC` `ESR` `COM`

√6th **S78.02** Partial traumatic amputation at hip joint

√7th **S78.021** Partial traumatic amputation at right hip joint `HCC` `ESR` `COM`

√7th **S78.022** Partial traumatic amputation at left hip joint `HCC` `ESR` `COM`

√7th **S78.029** Partial traumatic amputation at unspecified hip joint `HCC` `ESR` `COM`

√5th **S78.1** Traumatic amputation at level between hip and knee

EXCLUDES 1   *traumatic amputation of knee (S88.0-)*

√6th **S78.11** Complete traumatic amputation at level between hip and knee

√7th **S78.111** Complete traumatic amputation at level between right hip and knee `HCC` `ESR` `COM`

√7th **S78.112** Complete traumatic amputation at level between left hip and knee `HCC` `ESR` `COM`

√7th **S78.119** Complete traumatic amputation at level between unspecified hip and knee `HCC` `ESR` `COM`

√6th **S78.12** Partial traumatic amputation at level between hip and knee

√7th **S78.121** Partial traumatic amputation at level between right hip and knee `HCC` `ESR` `COM`

√7th **S78.122** Partial traumatic amputation at level between left hip and knee `HCC` `ESR` `COM`

√7th **S78.129** Partial traumatic amputation at level between unspecified hip and knee `HCC` `ESR` `COM`

√5th **S78.9** Traumatic amputation of hip and thigh, level unspecified

√6th **S78.91** Complete traumatic amputation of hip and thigh, level unspecified

√7th **S78.911** Complete traumatic amputation of right hip and thigh, level unspecified `HCC` `ESR` `COM`

√7th **S78.912** Complete traumatic amputation of left hip and thigh, level unspecified `HCC` `ESR` `COM`

√7th **S78.919** Complete traumatic amputation of unspecified hip and thigh, level unspecified `HCC` `ESR` `COM`

√6th **S78.92** Partial traumatic amputation of hip and thigh, level unspecified

√7th **S78.921** Partial traumatic amputation of right hip and thigh, level unspecified `HCC` `ESR` `COM`

√7th **S78.922** Partial traumatic amputation of left hip and thigh, level unspecified `HCC` `ESR` `COM`

√7th **S78.929** Partial traumatic amputation of unspecified hip and thigh, level unspecified `HCC` `ESR` `COM`

√4th **S79 Other and unspecified injuries of hip and thigh**

NOTE   A fracture not indicated as open or closed should be coded to closed

AHA: 2018,2Q,12; 2018,1Q,3; 2015,3Q,37-39

The appropriate 7th character is to be added to each code from subcategories S79.0 and S79.1.
A   initial encounter for closed fracture
D   subsequent encounter for fracture with routine healing
G   subsequent encounter for fracture with delayed healing
K   subsequent encounter for fracture with nonunion
P   subsequent encounter for fracture with malunion
S   sequela

√5th **S79.0** Physeal fracture of upper end of femur

EXCLUDES 1   *apophyseal fracture of upper end of femur (S72.13-)*
nontraumatic slipped upper femoral epiphysis (M93.0-)

AHA: 2019,4Q,56

√6th **S79.00** Unspecified physeal fracture of upper end of femur

1 √7th **S79.001** Unspecified physeal fracture of upper end of right femur `HCC` `ESR` `COM` `Q`

1 √7th **S79.002** Unspecified physeal fracture of upper end of left femur `HCC` `ESR` `COM` `Q`

1 √7th **S79.009** Unspecified physeal fracture of upper end of unspecified femur `HCC` `ESR` `COM` `Q`

√6th **S79.01** Salter-Harris Type I physeal fracture of upper end of femur

Acute on chronic slipped capital femoral epiphysis (traumatic)
Acute slipped capital femoral epiphysis (traumatic)
Capital femoral epiphyseal fracture

EXCLUDES 1   *chronic slipped upper femoral epiphysis (nontraumatic) (M93.02-)*

1 √7th **S79.011** Salter-Harris Type I physeal fracture of upper end of right femur `HCC` `ESR` `COM` `Q`

1 √7th **S79.012** Salter-Harris Type I physeal fracture of upper end of left femur `HCC` `ESR` `COM` `Q`

1 √7th **S79.019** Salter-Harris Type I physeal fracture of upper end of unspecified femur `HCC` `ESR` `COM` `Q`

√6th **S79.09** Other physeal fracture of upper end of femur

1 √7th **S79.091** Other physeal fracture of upper end of right femur `HCC` `ESR` `COM` `Q`

1 √7th **S79.092** Other physeal fracture of upper end of left femur `HCC` `ESR` `COM` `Q`

1 √7th **S79.099** Other physeal fracture of upper end of unspecified femur `HCC` `ESR` `COM` `Q`

√5th **S79.1** Physeal fracture of lower end of femur

AHA: 2019,4Q,56

√6th **S79.10** Unspecified physeal fracture of lower end of femur

1 √7th **S79.101** Unspecified physeal fracture of lower end of right femur `HCC` `ESR` `Q`

1 √7th **S79.102** Unspecified physeal fracture of lower end of left femur `HCC` `ESR` `Q`

1 √7th **S79.109** Unspecified physeal fracture of lower end of unspecified femur `HCC` `ESR` `Q`

√6th **S79.11** Salter-Harris Type I physeal fracture of lower end of femur

1 √7th **S79.111** Salter-Harris Type I physeal fracture of lower end of right femur `HCC` `ESR` `Q`

1 √7th **S79.112** Salter-Harris Type I physeal fracture of lower end of left femur `HCC` `ESR` `Q`

1 √7th **S79.119** Salter-Harris Type I physeal fracture of lower end of unspecified femur `HCC` `ESR` `Q`

√6th **S79.12** Salter-Harris Type II physeal fracture of lower end of femur

1 √7th **S79.121** Salter-Harris Type II physeal fracture of lower end of right femur `HCC` `ESR` `Q`

1 √7th **S79.122** Salter-Harris Type II physeal fracture of lower end of left femur `HCC` `ESR` `Q`

1 √7th **S79.129** Salter-Harris Type II physeal fracture of lower end of unspecified femur `HCC` `ESR` `Q`

√6th **S79.13** Salter-Harris Type III physeal fracture of lower end of femur

1 √7th **S79.131** Salter-Harris Type III physeal fracture of lower end of right femur `HCC` `ESR` `Q`

1 √7th **S79.132** Salter-Harris Type III physeal fracture of lower end of left femur `HCC` `ESR` `Q`

1 √7th **S79.139** Salter-Harris Type III physeal fracture of lower end of unspecified femur `HCC` `ESR` `Q`

√6th **S79.14** Salter-Harris Type IV physeal fracture of lower end of femur

1 √7th **S79.141** Salter-Harris Type IV physeal fracture of lower end of right femur `HCC` `ESR` `Q`

1 √7th **S79.142** Salter-Harris Type IV physeal fracture of lower end of left femur `HCC` `ESR` `Q`

1 √7th **S79.149** Salter-Harris Type IV physeal fracture of lower end of unspecified femur `HCC` `ESR` `Q`

√6th **S79.19** Other physeal fracture of lower end of femur

1 √7th **S79.191** Other physeal fracture of lower end of right femur `HCC` `ESR` `Q`

1 √7th **S79.192** Other physeal fracture of lower end of left femur `HCC` `ESR` `Q`

1 √7th **S79.199** Other physeal fracture of lower end of unspecified femur `HCC` `ESR` `Q`

✓5ᵗʰ **S79.8 Other specified injuries of hip and thigh**

> The appropriate 7th character is to be added to each code in subcategory S79.8.
> A   initial encounter
> D   subsequent encounter
> S   sequela

  ✓6ᵗʰ **S79.81 Other specified injuries of hip**
    ✓7ᵗʰ **S79.811 Other specified injuries of right hip**
    ✓7ᵗʰ **S79.812 Other specified injuries of left hip**
    ✓7ᵗʰ **S79.819 Other specified injuries of unspecified hip**
  ✓6ᵗʰ **S79.82 Other specified injuries of thigh**
    ✓7ᵗʰ **S79.821 Other specified injuries of right thigh**
    ✓7ᵗʰ **S79.822 Other specified injuries of left thigh**
    ✓7ᵗʰ **S79.829 Other specified injuries of unspecified thigh**

✓5ᵗʰ **S79.9 Unspecified injury of hip and thigh**

> The appropriate 7th character is to be added to each code in subcategory S79.9.
> A   initial encounter
> D   subsequent encounter
> S   sequela

  ✓6ᵗʰ **S79.91 Unspecified injury of hip**
    ✓7ᵗʰ **S79.911 Unspecified injury of right hip**
    ✓7ᵗʰ **S79.912 Unspecified injury of left hip**
    ✓7ᵗʰ **S79.919 Unspecified injury of unspecified hip**
  ✓6ᵗʰ **S79.92 Unspecified injury of thigh**
    ✓7ᵗʰ **S79.921 Unspecified injury of right thigh**
    ✓7ᵗʰ **S79.922 Unspecified injury of left thigh**
    ✓7ᵗʰ **S79.929 Unspecified injury of unspecified thigh**

Injuries to the knee and lower leg (S80-S89)

EXCLUDES 2   *burns and corrosions (T20-T32)*
    frostbite (T33-T34)
    injuries of ankle and foot, except fracture of ankle and malleolus (S90-S99)
    insect bite or sting, venomous (T63.4)

✓4ᵗʰ **S80 Superficial injury of knee and lower leg**
  EXCLUDES 2   *superficial injury of ankle and foot (S90.-)*

> The appropriate 7th character is to be added to each code from category S80.
> A   initial encounter
> D   subsequent encounter
> S   sequela

✓5ᵗʰ **S80.0 Contusion of knee**
  ✓x7ᵗʰ **S80.00 Contusion of unspecified knee**
  ✓x7ᵗʰ **S80.01 Contusion of right knee**
  ✓x7ᵗʰ **S80.02 Contusion of left knee**
✓5ᵗʰ **S80.1 Contusion of lower leg**
  ✓x7ᵗʰ **S80.10 Contusion of unspecified lower leg**
  ✓x7ᵗʰ **S80.11 Contusion of right lower leg**
  ✓x7ᵗʰ **S80.12 Contusion of left lower leg**
✓5ᵗʰ **S80.2 Other superficial injuries of knee**
  ✓6ᵗʰ **S80.21 Abrasion of knee**
    ✓7ᵗʰ **S80.211 Abrasion, right knee**
    ✓7ᵗʰ **S80.212 Abrasion, left knee**
    ✓7ᵗʰ **S80.219 Abrasion, unspecified knee**
  ✓6ᵗʰ **S80.22 Blister (nonthermal) of knee**
    ✓7ᵗʰ **S80.221 Blister (nonthermal), right knee**
    ✓7ᵗʰ **S80.222 Blister (nonthermal), left knee**
    ✓7ᵗʰ **S80.229 Blister (nonthermal), unspecified knee**
  ✓6ᵗʰ **S80.24 External constriction of knee**
    ✓7ᵗʰ **S80.241 External constriction, right knee**
    ✓7ᵗʰ **S80.242 External constriction, left knee**
    ✓7ᵗʰ **S80.249 External constriction, unspecified knee**
  ✓6ᵗʰ **S80.25 Superficial foreign body of knee**
    Splinter in the knee
    ✓7ᵗʰ **S80.251 Superficial foreign body, right knee**
    ✓7ᵗʰ **S80.252 Superficial foreign body, left knee**

    ✓7ᵗʰ **S80.259 Superficial foreign body, unspecified knee**
  ✓6ᵗʰ **S80.26 Insect bite (nonvenomous) of knee**
    ✓7ᵗʰ **S80.261 Insect bite (nonvenomous), right knee**
    ✓7ᵗʰ **S80.262 Insect bite (nonvenomous), left knee**
    ✓7ᵗʰ **S80.269 Insect bite (nonvenomous), unspecified knee**
  ✓6ᵗʰ **S80.27 Other superficial bite of knee**
    EXCLUDES 1   *open bite of knee (S81.05-)*
    ✓7ᵗʰ **S80.271 Other superficial bite of right knee**
    ✓7ᵗʰ **S80.272 Other superficial bite of left knee**
    ✓7ᵗʰ **S80.279 Other superficial bite of unspecified knee**
✓5ᵗʰ **S80.8 Other superficial injuries of lower leg**
  ✓6ᵗʰ **S80.81 Abrasion of lower leg**
    ✓7ᵗʰ **S80.811 Abrasion, right lower leg**
    ✓7ᵗʰ **S80.812 Abrasion, left lower leg**
    ✓7ᵗʰ **S80.819 Abrasion, unspecified lower leg**
  ✓6ᵗʰ **S80.82 Blister (nonthermal) of lower leg**
    ✓7ᵗʰ **S80.821 Blister (nonthermal), right lower leg**
    ✓7ᵗʰ **S80.822 Blister (nonthermal), left lower leg**
    ✓7ᵗʰ **S80.829 Blister (nonthermal), unspecified lower leg**
  ✓6ᵗʰ **S80.84 External constriction of lower leg**
    ✓7ᵗʰ **S80.841 External constriction, right lower leg**
    ✓7ᵗʰ **S80.842 External constriction, left lower leg**
    ✓7ᵗʰ **S80.849 External constriction, unspecified lower leg**
  ✓6ᵗʰ **S80.85 Superficial foreign body of lower leg**
    Splinter in the lower leg
    ✓7ᵗʰ **S80.851 Superficial foreign body, right lower leg**
    ✓7ᵗʰ **S80.852 Superficial foreign body, left lower leg**
    ✓7ᵗʰ **S80.859 Superficial foreign body, unspecified lower leg**
  ✓6ᵗʰ **S80.86 Insect bite (nonvenomous) of lower leg**
    ✓7ᵗʰ **S80.861 Insect bite (nonvenomous), right lower leg**
    ✓7ᵗʰ **S80.862 Insect bite (nonvenomous), left lower leg**
    ✓7ᵗʰ **S80.869 Insect bite (nonvenomous), unspecified lower leg**
  ✓6ᵗʰ **S80.87 Other superficial bite of lower leg**
    EXCLUDES 1   *open bite of lower leg (S81.85-)*
    ✓7ᵗʰ **S80.871 Other superficial bite, right lower leg**
    ✓7ᵗʰ **S80.872 Other superficial bite, left lower leg**
    ✓7ᵗʰ **S80.879 Other superficial bite, unspecified lower leg**
✓5ᵗʰ **S80.9 Unspecified superficial injury of knee and lower leg**
  ✓6ᵗʰ **S80.91 Unspecified superficial injury of knee**
    ✓7ᵗʰ **S80.911 Unspecified superficial injury of right knee**
    ✓7ᵗʰ **S80.912 Unspecified superficial injury of left knee**
    ✓7ᵗʰ **S80.919 Unspecified superficial injury of unspecified knee**
  ✓6ᵗʰ **S80.92 Unspecified superficial injury of lower leg**
    ✓7ᵗʰ **S80.921 Unspecified superficial injury of right lower leg**
    ✓7ᵗʰ **S80.922 Unspecified superficial injury of left lower leg**
    ✓7ᵗʰ **S80.929 Unspecified superficial injury of unspecified lower leg**

✓4ᵗʰ **S81 Open wound of knee and lower leg**
  Code also any associated wound infection
  EXCLUDES 1   *open fracture of knee and lower leg (S82.-)*
    traumatic amputation of lower leg (S88.-)
  EXCLUDES 2   *open wound of ankle and foot (S91.-)*

> The appropriate 7th character is to be added to each code from category S81.
> A   initial encounter
> D   subsequent encounter
> S   sequela

✓5ᵗʰ **S81.0 Open wound of knee**
  ✓6ᵗʰ **S81.00 Unspecified open wound of knee**
    ✓7ᵗʰ **S81.001 Unspecified open wound, right knee**

✓7ᵗʰ **S81.002** Unspecified open wound, left knee

✓7ᵗʰ **S81.009** Unspecified open wound, unspecified knee

✓6ᵗʰ **S81.01** Laceration without foreign body of knee

    ✓7ᵗʰ **S81.011** Laceration without foreign body, right knee

    ✓7ᵗʰ **S81.012** Laceration without foreign body, left knee

    ✓7ᵗʰ **S81.019** Laceration without foreign body, unspecified knee

✓6ᵗʰ **S81.02** Laceration with foreign body of knee

    ✓7ᵗʰ **S81.021** Laceration with foreign body, right knee

    ✓7ᵗʰ **S81.022** Laceration with foreign body, left knee

    ✓7ᵗʰ **S81.029** Laceration with foreign body, unspecified knee

✓6ᵗʰ **S81.03** Puncture wound without foreign body of knee

    ✓7ᵗʰ **S81.031** Puncture wound without foreign body, right knee

    ✓7ᵗʰ **S81.032** Puncture wound without foreign body, left knee

    ✓7ᵗʰ **S81.039** Puncture wound without foreign body, unspecified knee

✓6ᵗʰ **S81.04** Puncture wound with foreign body of knee

    ✓7ᵗʰ **S81.041** Puncture wound with foreign body, right knee

    ✓7ᵗʰ **S81.042** Puncture wound with foreign body, left knee

    ✓7ᵗʰ **S81.049** Puncture wound with foreign body, unspecified knee

✓6ᵗʰ **S81.05** Open bite of knee

    Bite of knee NOS

    EXCLUDES 1   *superficial bite of knee (S80.27-)*

    ✓7ᵗʰ **S81.051** Open bite, right knee

    ✓7ᵗʰ **S81.052** Open bite, left knee

    ✓7ᵗʰ **S81.059** Open bite, unspecified knee

✓5ᵗʰ **S81.8** Open wound of lower leg

  ✓6ᵗʰ **S81.80** Unspecified open wound of lower leg

    AHA: 2016,3Q,24

    ✓7ᵗʰ **S81.801** Unspecified open wound, right lower leg

    ✓7ᵗʰ **S81.802** Unspecified open wound, left lower leg

    ✓7ᵗʰ **S81.809** Unspecified open wound, unspecified lower leg

  ✓6ᵗʰ **S81.81** Laceration without foreign body of lower leg

    ✓7ᵗʰ **S81.811** Laceration without foreign body, right lower leg

    ✓7ᵗʰ **S81.812** Laceration without foreign body, left lower leg

    ✓7ᵗʰ **S81.819** Laceration without foreign body, unspecified lower leg

  ✓6ᵗʰ **S81.82** Laceration with foreign body of lower leg

    ✓7ᵗʰ **S81.821** Laceration with foreign body, right lower leg

    ✓7ᵗʰ **S81.822** Laceration with foreign body, left lower leg

    ✓7ᵗʰ **S81.829** Laceration with foreign body, unspecified lower leg

  ✓6ᵗʰ **S81.83** Puncture wound without foreign body of lower leg

    AHA: 2016,3Q,24

    ✓7ᵗʰ **S81.831** Puncture wound without foreign body, right lower leg

    ✓7ᵗʰ **S81.832** Puncture wound without foreign body, left lower leg

    ✓7ᵗʰ **S81.839** Puncture wound without foreign body, unspecified lower leg

  ✓6ᵗʰ **S81.84** Puncture wound with foreign body of lower leg

    AHA: 2016,3Q,24

    ✓7ᵗʰ **S81.841** Puncture wound with foreign body, right lower leg

    ✓7ᵗʰ **S81.842** Puncture wound with foreign body, left lower leg

    ✓7ᵗʰ **S81.849** Puncture wound with foreign body, unspecified lower leg

  ✓6ᵗʰ **S81.85** Open bite of lower leg

    Bite of lower leg NOS

    EXCLUDES 1   *superficial bite of lower leg (S80.86-, S80.87-)*

    ✓7ᵗʰ **S81.851** Open bite, right lower leg

✓7ᵗʰ **S81.852** Open bite, left lower leg

✓7ᵗʰ **S81.859** Open bite, unspecified lower leg

✓4ᵗʰ **S82** Fracture of lower leg, including ankle

NOTE   A fracture not indicated as displaced or nondisplaced should be coded to displaced

     A fracture not indicated as open or closed should be coded to closed

     The open fracture designations are based on the Gustilo open fracture classification.

INCLUDES   fracture of malleolus

EXCLUDES 1   *traumatic amputation of lower leg (S88.-)*

EXCLUDES 2   *fracture of foot, except ankle (S92.-)*

     periprosthetic fracture around internal prosthetic implant of knee joint (M97.1-)

AHA: 2018,2Q,12; 2016,1Q,33; 2015,3Q,37-39

DEF: Diaphysis: Central shaft of a long bone.

DEF: Epiphysis: Proximal and distal rounded ends of a long bone, communicates with the joint.

DEF: Metaphysis: Section of a long bone located between the epiphysis and diaphysis at the proximal and distal ends.

DEF: Physis (growth plate): Narrow zone of cartilaginous tissue between the epiphysis and metaphysis at each end of a long bone. In childhood, proliferation of cells in this zone lengthens the bone. As the bone matures, this area thins, ossification eventually fusing into solid bone and growth stops. **Synonym(s):** *Epiphyseal plate.*

The appropriate 7th character is to be added to all codes from category S82 [unless otherwise indicated].

A   initial encounter for closed fracture

B   initial encounter for open fracture type I or II
     initial encounter for open fracture NOS

C   initial encounter for open fracture type IIIA, IIIB, or IIIC

D   subsequent encounter for closed fracture with routine healing

E   subsequent encounter for open fracture type I or II with routine healing

F   subsequent encounter for open fracture type IIIA, IIIB, or IIIC with routine healing

G   subsequent encounter for closed fracture with delayed healing

H   subsequent encounter for open fracture type I or II with delayed healing

J   subsequent encounter for open fracture type IIIA, IIIB, or IIIC with delayed healing

K   subsequent encounter for closed fracture with nonunion

M   subsequent encounter for open fracture type I or II with nonunion

N   subsequent encounter for open fracture type IIIA, IIIB, or IIIC with nonunion

P   subsequent encounter for closed fracture with malunion

Q   subsequent encounter for open fracture type I or II with malunion

R   subsequent encounter for open fracture type IIIA, IIIB, or IIIC with malunion

S   sequela

✓5ᵗʰ **S82.0** Fracture of patella

  Knee cap

  ✓6ᵗʰ **S82.00** Unspecified fracture of patella

    ✓7ᵗʰ **S82.001** Unspecified fracture of right patella 🅾

    ✓7ᵗʰ **S82.002** Unspecified fracture of left patella 🅾

    ✓7ᵗʰ **S82.009** Unspecified fracture of unspecified patella 🅾

  ✓6ᵗʰ **S82.01** Osteochondral fracture of patella

    ✓7ᵗʰ **S82.011** Displaced osteochondral fracture of right patella 🅾

    ✓7ᵗʰ **S82.012** Displaced osteochondral fracture of left patella 🅾

    ✓7ᵗʰ **S82.013** Displaced osteochondral fracture of unspecified patella 🅾

    ✓7ᵗʰ **S82.014** Nondisplaced osteochondral fracture of right patella 🅾

    ✓7ᵗʰ **S82.015** Nondisplaced osteochondral fracture of left patella 🅾

    ✓7ᵗʰ **S82.016** Nondisplaced osteochondral fracture of unspecified patella 🅾

  ✓6ᵗʰ **S82.02** Longitudinal fracture of patella

    ✓7ᵗʰ **S82.021** Displaced longitudinal fracture of right patella 🅾

    ✓7ᵗʰ **S82.022** Displaced longitudinal fracture of left patella 🅾

HCC CMS-HCC   **Rx** Rx HCC   **ESR** ESRD HCC   **COM** Commercial HCC   **N** Newborn: 0   **P** Pediatric: 0-17   **M** Maternity: 9-64   **A** Adult: 15-124

1090   ICD-10-CM 2023

√7ᵗʰ **S82.023** Displaced longitudinal fracture of unspecified patella [Q]

√7ᵗʰ **S82.024** Nondisplaced longitudinal fracture of right patella [Q]

√7ᵗʰ **S82.025** Nondisplaced longitudinal fracture of left patella [Q]

√7ᵗʰ **S82.026** Nondisplaced longitudinal fracture of unspecified patella [Q]

√6ᵗʰ **S82.03** Transverse fracture of patella

√7ᵗʰ **S82.031** Displaced transverse fracture of right patella [Q]

√7ᵗʰ **S82.032** Displaced transverse fracture of left patella [Q]

√7ᵗʰ **S82.033** Displaced transverse fracture of unspecified patella [Q]

√7ᵗʰ **S82.034** Nondisplaced transverse fracture of right patella [Q]

√7ᵗʰ **S82.035** Nondisplaced transverse fracture of left patella [Q]

√7ᵗʰ **S82.036** Nondisplaced transverse fracture of unspecified patella [Q]

√6ᵗʰ **S82.04** Comminuted fracture of patella

√7ᵗʰ **S82.041** Displaced comminuted fracture of right patella [Q]

√7ᵗʰ **S82.042** Displaced comminuted fracture of left patella [Q]

√7ᵗʰ **S82.043** Displaced comminuted fracture of unspecified patella [Q]

√7ᵗʰ **S82.044** Nondisplaced comminuted fracture of right patella [Q]

√7ᵗʰ **S82.045** Nondisplaced comminuted fracture of left patella [Q]

√7ᵗʰ **S82.046** Nondisplaced comminuted fracture of unspecified patella [Q]

√6ᵗʰ **S82.09** Other fracture of patella

√7ᵗʰ **S82.091** Other fracture of right patella [Q]

√7ᵗʰ **S82.092** Other fracture of left patella [Q]

√7ᵗʰ **S82.099** Other fracture of unspecified patella [Q]

√5ᵗʰ **S82.1** Fracture of upper end of tibia

Fracture of proximal end of tibia

EXCLUDES 2 *fracture of shaft of tibia (S82.2-)*
physeal fracture of upper end of tibia (S89.0-)

√6ᵗʰ **S82.10** Unspecified fracture of upper end of tibia

√7ᵗʰ **S82.101** Unspecified fracture of upper end of right tibia [Q]

√7ᵗʰ **S82.102** Unspecified fracture of upper end of left tibia [Q]

√7ᵗʰ **S82.109** Unspecified fracture of upper end of unspecified tibia [Q]

√6ᵗʰ **S82.11** Fracture of tibial spine

√7ᵗʰ **S82.111** Displaced fracture of right tibial spine [Q]

√7ᵗʰ **S82.112** Displaced fracture of left tibial spine [Q]

√7ᵗʰ **S82.113** Displaced fracture of unspecified tibial spine [Q]

√7ᵗʰ **S82.114** Nondisplaced fracture of right tibial spine [Q]

√7ᵗʰ **S82.115** Nondisplaced fracture of left tibial spine [Q]

√7ᵗʰ **S82.116** Nondisplaced fracture of unspecified tibial spine [Q]

√6ᵗʰ **S82.12** Fracture of lateral condyle of tibia

√7ᵗʰ **S82.121** Displaced fracture of lateral condyle of right tibia [Q]

√7ᵗʰ **S82.122** Displaced fracture of lateral condyle of left tibia [Q]

√7ᵗʰ **S82.123** Displaced fracture of lateral condyle of unspecified tibia [Q]

√7ᵗʰ **S82.124** Nondisplaced fracture of lateral condyle of right tibia [Q]

√7ᵗʰ **S82.125** Nondisplaced fracture of lateral condyle of left tibia [Q]

√7ᵗʰ **S82.126** Nondisplaced fracture of lateral condyle of unspecified tibia [Q]

√6ᵗʰ **S82.13** Fracture of medial condyle of tibia

√7ᵗʰ **S82.131** Displaced fracture of medial condyle of right tibia [Q]

√7ᵗʰ **S82.132** Displaced fracture of medial condyle of left tibia [Q]

√7ᵗʰ **S82.133** Displaced fracture of medial condyle of unspecified tibia [Q]

√7ᵗʰ **S82.134** Nondisplaced fracture of medial condyle of right tibia [Q]

√7ᵗʰ **S82.135** Nondisplaced fracture of medial condyle of left tibia [Q]

√7ᵗʰ **S82.136** Nondisplaced fracture of medial condyle of unspecified tibia [Q]

√6ᵗʰ **S82.14** Bicondylar fracture of tibia

Fracture of tibial plateau NOS

√7ᵗʰ **S82.141** Displaced bicondylar fracture of right tibia [Q]

√7ᵗʰ **S82.142** Displaced bicondylar fracture of left tibia [Q]

√7ᵗʰ **S82.143** Displaced bicondylar fracture of unspecified tibia [Q]

√7ᵗʰ **S82.144** Nondisplaced bicondylar fracture of right tibia [Q]

√7ᵗʰ **S82.145** Nondisplaced bicondylar fracture of left tibia [Q]

√7ᵗʰ **S82.146** Nondisplaced bicondylar fracture of unspecified tibia [Q]

√6ᵗʰ **S82.15** Fracture of tibial tuberosity

√7ᵗʰ **S82.151** Displaced fracture of right tibial tuberosity [Q]

√7ᵗʰ **S82.152** Displaced fracture of left tibial tuberosity [Q]

√7ᵗʰ **S82.153** Displaced fracture of unspecified tibial tuberosity [Q]

√7ᵗʰ **S82.154** Nondisplaced fracture of right tibial tuberosity [Q]

√7ᵗʰ **S82.155** Nondisplaced fracture of left tibial tuberosity [Q]

√7ᵗʰ **S82.156** Nondisplaced fracture of unspecified tibial tuberosity [Q]

√6ᵗʰ **S82.16** Torus fracture of upper end of tibia

The appropriate 7th character is to be added to all codes in subcategory S82.16.
A   initial encounter for closed fracture
D   subsequent encounter for fracture with routine healing
G   subsequent encounter for fracture with delayed healing
K   subsequent encounter for fracture with nonunion
P   subsequent encounter for fracture with malunion
S   sequela

√7ᵗʰ **S82.161** Torus fracture of upper end of right tibia [Q]

√7ᵗʰ **S82.162** Torus fracture of upper end of left tibia [Q]

√7ᵗʰ **S82.169** Torus fracture of upper end of unspecified tibia [Q]

√6ᵗʰ **S82.19** Other fracture of upper end of tibia

√7ᵗʰ **S82.191** Other fracture of upper end of right tibia [Q]

√7ᵗʰ **S82.192** Other fracture of upper end of left tibia [Q]

√7ᵗʰ **S82.199** Other fracture of upper end of unspecified tibia [Q]

√5ᵗʰ **S82.2** Fracture of shaft of tibia

√6ᵗʰ **S82.20** Unspecified fracture of shaft of tibia

Fracture of tibia NOS

√7ᵗʰ **S82.201** Unspecified fracture of shaft of right tibia [Q]

√7ᵗʰ **S82.202** Unspecified fracture of shaft of left tibia [Q]

√7ᵗʰ **S82.209** Unspecified fracture of shaft of unspecified tibia [Q]

√6ᵗʰ **S82.22** Transverse fracture of shaft of tibia

√7ᵗʰ **S82.221** Displaced transverse fracture of shaft of right tibia [Q]

Chapter 19. Injury, Poisoning and Certain Other Consequences of External Causes

√7ᵗʰ **S82.222** Displaced **transverse fracture of shaft of** left tibia ◘

√7ᵗʰ **S82.223** Displaced **transverse fracture of shaft of** unspecified tibia ◘

√7ᵗʰ **S82.224** Nondisplaced **transverse fracture of shaft of** right tibia ◘

√7ᵗʰ **S82.225** Nondisplaced **transverse fracture of shaft of** left tibia ◘

√7ᵗʰ **S82.226** Nondisplaced **transverse fracture of shaft of** unspecified tibia ◘

√6ᵗʰ **S82.23** Oblique **fracture of shaft of tibia**

√7ᵗʰ **S82.231** Displaced **oblique fracture of shaft of** right tibia ◘

√7ᵗʰ **S82.232** Displaced **oblique fracture of shaft of** left tibia ◘

√7ᵗʰ **S82.233** Displaced **oblique fracture of shaft of** unspecified tibia ◘

√7ᵗʰ **S82.234** Nondisplaced **oblique fracture of shaft of** right tibia ◘

√7ᵗʰ **S82.235** Nondisplaced **oblique fracture of shaft of** left tibia ◘

√7ᵗʰ **S82.236** Nondisplaced **oblique fracture of shaft of** unspecified tibia ◘

√6ᵗʰ **S82.24** Spiral **fracture of shaft of tibia**

Toddler fracture

√7ᵗʰ **S82.241** Displaced **spiral fracture of shaft of** right tibia ◘

√7ᵗʰ **S82.242** Displaced **spiral fracture of shaft of** left tibia ◘

√7ᵗʰ **S82.243** Displaced **spiral fracture of shaft of** unspecified tibia ◘

√7ᵗʰ **S82.244** Nondisplaced **spiral fracture of shaft of** right tibia ◘

√7ᵗʰ **S82.245** Nondisplaced **spiral fracture of shaft of** left tibia ◘

√7ᵗʰ **S82.246** Nondisplaced **spiral fracture of shaft of** unspecified tibia ◘

√6ᵗʰ **S82.25** Comminuted **fracture of shaft of tibia**

√7ᵗʰ **S82.251** Displaced **comminuted fracture of shaft of** right tibia ◘

√7ᵗʰ **S82.252** Displaced **comminuted fracture of shaft of** left tibia ◘

√7ᵗʰ **S82.253** Displaced **comminuted fracture of shaft of** unspecified tibia ◘

√7ᵗʰ **S82.254** Nondisplaced **comminuted fracture of shaft of** right tibia ◘

√7ᵗʰ **S82.255** Nondisplaced **comminuted fracture of shaft of** left tibia ◘

√7ᵗʰ **S82.256** Nondisplaced **comminuted fracture of shaft of** unspecified tibia ◘

√6ᵗʰ **S82.26** Segmental **fracture of shaft of tibia**

√7ᵗʰ **S82.261** Displaced **segmental fracture of shaft of** right tibia ◘

√7ᵗʰ **S82.262** Displaced **segmental fracture of shaft of** left tibia ◘

√7ᵗʰ **S82.263** Displaced **segmental fracture of shaft of** unspecified tibia ◘

√7ᵗʰ **S82.264** Nondisplaced **segmental fracture of shaft of** right tibia ◘

√7ᵗʰ **S82.265** Nondisplaced **segmental fracture of shaft of** left tibia ◘

√7ᵗʰ **S82.266** Nondisplaced **segmental fracture of shaft of** unspecified tibia ◘

√6ᵗʰ **S82.29** Other **fracture of shaft of tibia**

√7ᵗʰ **S82.291** Other **fracture of shaft of** right tibia ◘

√7ᵗʰ **S82.292** Other **fracture of shaft of** left tibia ◘

√7ᵗʰ **S82.299** Other **fracture of shaft of** unspecified tibia ◘

√5ᵗʰ **S82.3** Fracture of lower end of tibia

EXCLUDES 1   bimalleolar fracture of lower leg (S82.84-)

fracture of medial malleolus alone (S82.5-)

Maisonneuve's fracture (S82.86-)

pilon fracture of distal tibia (S82.87-)

trimalleolar fractures of lower leg (S82.85-)

√6ᵗʰ **S82.30** Unspecified **fracture of lower end of tibia**

√7ᵗʰ **S82.301** Unspecified **fracture of lower end of** right tibia ◘

√7ᵗʰ **S82.302** Unspecified **fracture of lower end of** left tibia ◘

√7ᵗʰ **S82.309** Unspecified **fracture of lower end of** unspecified tibia ◘

√6ᵗʰ **S82.31** Torus **fracture of lower end of tibia**

The appropriate 7th character is to be added to all codes in subcategory S82.31.
A   initial encounter for closed fracture
D   subsequent encounter for fracture with routine healing
G   subsequent encounter for fracture with delayed healing
K   subsequent encounter for fracture with nonunion
P   subsequent encounter for fracture with malunion
S   sequela

√7ᵗʰ **S82.311** Torus **fracture of lower end of** right tibia ◘

√7ᵗʰ **S82.312** Torus **fracture of lower end of** left tibia ◘

√7ᵗʰ **S82.319** Torus **fracture of lower end of** unspecified tibia ◘

√6ᵗʰ **S82.39** Other **fracture of lower end of tibia**

AHA: 2015,1Q,25

√7ᵗʰ **S82.391** Other **fracture of lower end of** right tibia ◘

√7ᵗʰ **S82.392** Other **fracture of lower end of** left tibia ◘

√7ᵗʰ **S82.399** Other **fracture of lower end of** unspecified tibia ◘

√5ᵗʰ **S82.4** Fracture of shaft of fibula

EXCLUDES 2   fracture of lateral malleolus alone (S82.6-)

√6ᵗʰ **S82.40** Unspecified **fracture of shaft of fibula**

√7ᵗʰ **S82.401** Unspecified **fracture of shaft of** right fibula ◘

√7ᵗʰ **S82.402** Unspecified **fracture of shaft of** left fibula ◘

√7ᵗʰ **S82.409** Unspecified **fracture of shaft of** unspecified fibula ◘

√6ᵗʰ **S82.42** Transverse **fracture of shaft of fibula**

√7ᵗʰ **S82.421** Displaced **transverse fracture of shaft of** right fibula ◘

√7ᵗʰ **S82.422** Displaced **transverse fracture of shaft of** left fibula ◘

√7ᵗʰ **S82.423** Displaced **transverse fracture of shaft of** unspecified fibula ◘

√7ᵗʰ **S82.424** Nondisplaced **transverse fracture of shaft of** right fibula ◘

√7ᵗʰ **S82.425** Nondisplaced **transverse fracture of shaft of** left fibula ◘

√7ᵗʰ **S82.426** Nondisplaced **transverse fracture of shaft of** unspecified fibula ◘

√6ᵗʰ **S82.43** Oblique **fracture of shaft of fibula**

√7ᵗʰ **S82.431** Displaced **oblique fracture of shaft of** right fibula ◘

√7ᵗʰ **S82.432** Displaced **oblique fracture of shaft of** left fibula ◘

√7ᵗʰ **S82.433** Displaced **oblique fracture of shaft of** unspecified fibula ◘

√7ᵗʰ **S82.434** Nondisplaced **oblique fracture of shaft of** right fibula ◘

√7ᵗʰ **S82.435** Nondisplaced **oblique fracture of shaft of** left fibula ◘

√7ᵗʰ **S82.436** Nondisplaced **oblique fracture of shaft of** unspecified fibula ◘

√6ᵗʰ **S82.44** Spiral **fracture of shaft of fibula**

√7ᵗʰ **S82.441** Displaced **spiral fracture of shaft of** right fibula ◘

√7ᵗʰ **S82.442** Displaced **spiral fracture of shaft of** left fibula ◘

√7ᵗʰ **S82.443** Displaced **spiral fracture of shaft of** unspecified fibula ◘

√7ᵗʰ **S82.444** Nondisplaced **spiral fracture of shaft of** right fibula ◘

√7ᵗʰ **S82.445** Nondisplaced **spiral fracture of shaft of** left fibula ◘

HCC CMS-HCC   **Rx** Rx HCC   **ESR** ESRD HCC   **COM** Commercial HCC   **N** Newborn: 0   **P** Pediatric: 0-17   **M** Maternity: 9-64   **A** Adult: 15-124

1092   ICD-10-CM 2023

√7ʰ **S82.446** Nondisplaced spiral fracture of shaft of unspecified fibula   Q

√6ʰ **S82.45** Comminuted fracture of shaft of fibula

√7ʰ **S82.451** Displaced comminuted fracture of shaft of right fibula

√7ʰ **S82.452** Displaced comminuted fracture of shaft of left fibula   Q

√7ʰ **S82.453** Displaced comminuted fracture of shaft of unspecified fibula   Q

√7ʰ **S82.454** Nondisplaced comminuted fracture of shaft of right fibula

√7ʰ **S82.455** Nondisplaced comminuted fracture of shaft of left fibula   Q

√7ʰ **S82.456** Nondisplaced comminuted fracture of shaft of unspecified fibula   Q

√6ʰ **S82.46** Segmental fracture of shaft of fibula

√7ʰ **S82.461** Displaced segmental fracture of shaft of right fibula

√7ʰ **S82.462** Displaced segmental fracture of shaft of left fibula   Q

√7ʰ **S82.463** Displaced segmental fracture of shaft of unspecified fibula   Q

√7ʰ **S82.464** Nondisplaced segmental fracture of shaft of right fibula

√7ʰ **S82.465** Nondisplaced segmental fracture of shaft of left fibula   Q

√7ʰ **S82.466** Nondisplaced segmental fracture of shaft of unspecified fibula   Q

√6ʰ **S82.49** Other fracture of shaft of fibula

√7ʰ **S82.491** Other fracture of shaft of right fibula   Q

√7ʰ **S82.492** Other fracture of shaft of left fibula   Q

√7ʰ **S82.499** Other fracture of shaft of unspecified fibula   Q

√5ʰ **S82.5** Fracture of medial malleolus

     EXCLUDES 1   pilon fracture of distal tibia (S82.87-)
                 Salter-Harris type III of lower end of tibia (S89.13-)
                 Salter-Harris type IV of lower end of tibia (S89.14-)

√x7ʰ **S82.51** Displaced fracture of medial malleolus of right tibia   Q

√x7ʰ **S82.52** Displaced fracture of medial malleolus of left tibia   Q

√x7ʰ **S82.53** Displaced fracture of medial malleolus of unspecified tibia   Q

√x7ʰ **S82.54** Nondisplaced fracture of medial malleolus of right tibia   Q

√x7ʰ **S82.55** Nondisplaced fracture of medial malleolus of left tibia   Q

√x7ʰ **S82.56** Nondisplaced fracture of medial malleolus of unspecified tibia   Q

√5ʰ **S82.6** Fracture of lateral malleolus

     EXCLUDES 1   pilon fracture of distal tibia (S82.87-)

√x7ʰ **S82.61** Displaced fracture of lateral malleolus of right fibula   Q

√x7ʰ **S82.62** Displaced fracture of lateral malleolus of left fibula   Q

√x7ʰ **S82.63** Displaced fracture of lateral malleolus of unspecified fibula   Q

√x7ʰ **S82.64** Nondisplaced fracture of lateral malleolus of right fibula   Q

√x7ʰ **S82.65** Nondisplaced fracture of lateral malleolus of left fibula   Q

√x7ʰ **S82.66** Nondisplaced fracture of lateral malleolus of unspecified fibula   Q

√5ʰ **S82.8** Other fractures of lower leg

√6ʰ **S82.81** Torus fracture of upper end of fibula

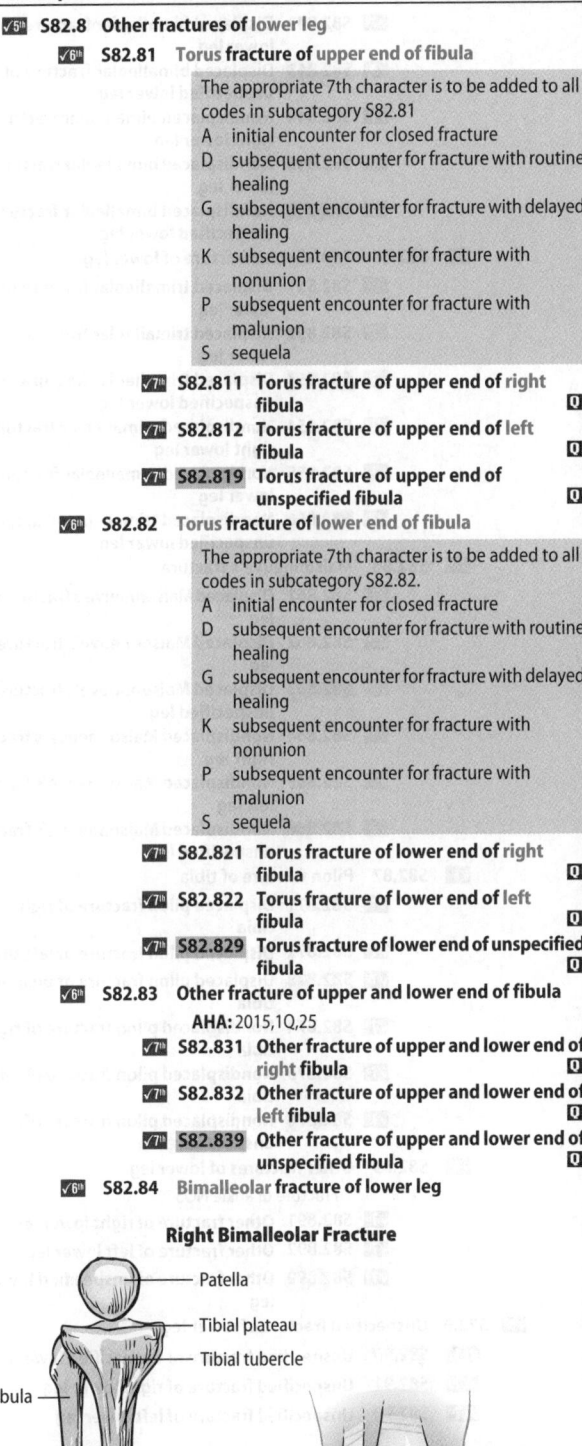

The appropriate 7th character is to be added to all codes in subcategory S82.81
A   initial encounter for closed fracture
D   subsequent encounter for fracture with routine healing
G   subsequent encounter for fracture with delayed healing
K   subsequent encounter for fracture with nonunion
P   subsequent encounter for fracture with malunion
S   sequela

√7ʰ **S82.811** Torus fracture of upper end of right fibula   Q

√7ʰ **S82.812** Torus fracture of upper end of left fibula   Q

√7ʰ **S82.819** Torus fracture of upper end of unspecified fibula   Q

√6ʰ **S82.82** Torus fracture of lower end of fibula

The appropriate 7th character is to be added to all codes in subcategory S82.82
A   initial encounter for closed fracture
D   subsequent encounter for fracture with routine healing
G   subsequent encounter for fracture with delayed healing
K   subsequent encounter for fracture with nonunion
P   subsequent encounter for fracture with malunion
S   sequela

√7ʰ **S82.821** Torus fracture of lower end of right fibula   Q

√7ʰ **S82.822** Torus fracture of lower end of left fibula   Q

√7ʰ **S82.829** Torus fracture of lower end of unspecified fibula   Q

√6ʰ **S82.83** Other fracture of upper and lower end of fibula

     AHA: 2015,1Q,25

√7ʰ **S82.831** Other fracture of upper and lower end of right fibula   Q

√7ʰ **S82.832** Other fracture of upper and lower end of left fibula   Q

√7ʰ **S82.839** Other fracture of upper and lower end of unspecified fibula   Q

√6ʰ **S82.84** Bimalleolar fracture of lower leg

Right Bimalleolar Fracture

Patella
Tibial plateau
Tibial tubercle
Fibula
Tibia
Fracture medial malleolus
Fracture lateral malleolus
Talus
Medial (tibial) malleolus
Lateral (fibular) malleolus

√7ʰ **S82.841** Displaced bimalleolar fracture of right lower leg   Q

√7ᵗʰ S82.842　Displaced bimalleolar fracture of left lower leg　◻

√7ᵗʰ **S82.843**　Displaced bimalleolar fracture of unspecified lower leg　◻

√7ᵗʰ S82.844　Nondisplaced bimalleolar fracture of right lower leg　◻

√7ᵗʰ S82.845　Nondisplaced bimalleolar fracture of left lower leg　◻

√7ᵗʰ **S82.846**　Nondisplaced bimalleolar fracture of unspecified lower leg　◻

√6ᵗʰ S82.85　Trimalleolar fracture of lower leg

√7ᵗʰ S82.851　Displaced trimalleolar fracture of right lower leg　◻

√7ᵗʰ S82.852　Displaced trimalleolar fracture of left lower leg　◻

√7ᵗʰ **S82.853**　Displaced trimalleolar fracture of unspecified lower leg　◻

√7ᵗʰ S82.854　Nondisplaced trimalleolar fracture of right lower leg　◻

√7ᵗʰ S82.855　Nondisplaced trimalleolar fracture of left lower leg　◻

√7ᵗʰ **S82.856**　Nondisplaced trimalleolar fracture of unspecified lower leg　◻

√6ᵗʰ S82.86　Maisonneuve's fracture

√7ᵗʰ S82.861　Displaced Maisonneuve's fracture of right leg　◻

√7ᵗʰ S82.862　Displaced Maisonneuve's fracture of left leg　◻

√7ᵗʰ **S82.863**　Displaced Maisonneuve's fracture of unspecified leg　◻

√7ᵗʰ S82.864　Nondisplaced Maisonneuve's fracture of right leg　◻

√7ᵗʰ S82.865　Nondisplaced Maisonneuve's fracture of left leg　◻

√7ᵗʰ **S82.866**　Nondisplaced Maisonneuve's fracture of unspecified leg　◻

√6ᵗʰ S82.87　Pilon fracture of tibia

√7ᵗʰ S82.871　Displaced pilon fracture of right tibia　◻

√7ᵗʰ S82.872　Displaced pilon fracture of left tibia　◻

√7ᵗʰ **S82.873**　Displaced pilon fracture of unspecified tibia　◻

√7ᵗʰ S82.874　Nondisplaced pilon fracture of right tibia　◻

√7ᵗʰ S82.875　Nondisplaced pilon fracture of left tibia　◻

√7ᵗʰ **S82.876**　Nondisplaced pilon fracture of unspecified tibia　◻

√6ᵗʰ S82.89　Other fractures of lower leg
　　　　Fracture of ankle NOS

√7ᵗʰ S82.891　Other fracture of right lower leg　◻

√7ᵗʰ S82.892　Other fracture of left lower leg　◻

√7ᵗʰ **S82.899**　Other fracture of unspecified lower leg　◻

√5ᵗʰ S82.9　Unspecified fracture of lower leg

√x7ᵗʰ **S82.90**　Unspecified fracture of unspecified lower leg　◻

√x7ᵗʰ **S82.91**　Unspecified fracture of right lower leg　◻

√x7ᵗʰ **S82.92**　Unspecified fracture of left lower leg　◻

√4ᵗʰ **S83**　**Dislocation and sprain of joints and ligaments of knee**

INCLUDES　avulsion of joint or ligament of knee
　　　　laceration of cartilage, joint or ligament of knee
　　　　sprain of cartilage, joint or ligament of knee
　　　　traumatic hemarthrosis of joint or ligament of knee
　　　　traumatic rupture of joint or ligament of knee
　　　　traumatic subluxation of joint or ligament of knee
　　　　traumatic tear of joint or ligament of knee

Code also any associated open wound

EXCLUDES 2　*derangement of patella (M22.0-M22.3)*
　　　　injury of patellar ligament (tendon) (S76.1-)
　　　　internal derangement of knee (M23.-)
　　　　old dislocation of knee (M24.36)
　　　　pathological dislocation of knee (M24.36)
　　　　recurrent dislocation of knee (M22.0)
　　　　strain of muscle, fascia and tendon of lower leg (S86.-)

> The appropriate 7th character is to be added to each code from category S83.
> A　initial encounter
> D　subsequent encounter
> S　sequela

√5ᵗʰ **S83.0**　**Subluxation and dislocation of patella**

√6ᵗʰ S83.00　Unspecified subluxation and dislocation of patella

√7ᵗʰ S83.001　Unspecified subluxation of right patella

√7ᵗʰ S83.002　Unspecified subluxation of left patella

√7ᵗʰ **S83.003**　Unspecified subluxation of unspecified patella

√7ᵗʰ S83.004　Unspecified dislocation of right patella

√7ᵗʰ S83.005　Unspecified dislocation of left patella

√7ᵗʰ **S83.006**　Unspecified dislocation of unspecified patella

√6ᵗʰ S83.01　Lateral subluxation and dislocation of patella

√7ᵗʰ S83.011　Lateral subluxation of right patella

√7ᵗʰ S83.012　Lateral subluxation of left patella

√7ᵗʰ S83.013　Lateral subluxation of unspecified patella

√7ᵗʰ S83.014　Lateral dislocation of right patella

√7ᵗʰ S83.015　Lateral dislocation of left patella

√7ᵗʰ **S83.016**　Lateral dislocation of unspecified patella

√6ᵗʰ S83.09　Other subluxation and dislocation of patella

√7ᵗʰ S83.091　Other subluxation of right patella

√7ᵗʰ S83.092　Other subluxation of left patella

√7ᵗʰ **S83.093**　Other subluxation of unspecified patella

√7ᵗʰ S83.094　Other dislocation of right patella

√7ᵗʰ S83.095　Other dislocation of left patella

√7ᵗʰ **S83.096**　Other dislocation of unspecified patella

√5ᵗʰ **S83.1**　**Subluxation and dislocation of knee**

EXCLUDES 2　*instability of knee prosthesis (T84.022, T84.023)*

√6ᵗʰ S83.10　Unspecified subluxation and dislocation of knee

√7ᵗʰ **S83.101**　Unspecified subluxation of right knee

√7ᵗʰ **S83.102**　Unspecified subluxation of left knee

√7ᵗʰ **S83.103**　Unspecified subluxation of unspecified knee

√7ᵗʰ **S83.104**　Unspecified dislocation of right knee

√7ᵗʰ **S83.105**　Unspecified dislocation of left knee

√7ᵗʰ **S83.106**　Unspecified dislocation of unspecified knee

√6ᵗʰ S83.11　Anterior subluxation and dislocation of proximal end of tibia
　　　　Posterior subluxation and dislocation of distal end of femur

√7ᵗʰ S83.111　Anterior subluxation of proximal end of tibia, right knee

√7ᵗʰ S83.112　Anterior subluxation of proximal end of tibia, left knee

√7ᵗʰ **S83.113**　Anterior subluxation of proximal end of tibia, unspecified knee

√7ᵗʰ S83.114　Anterior dislocation of proximal end of tibia, right knee

√7ᵗʰ S83.115　Anterior dislocation of proximal end of tibia, left knee

√7ᵗʰ **S83.116**　Anterior dislocation of proximal end of tibia, unspecified knee

√6ᵗʰ **S83.12** Posterior subluxation and dislocation of proximal end of tibia

     Anterior dislocation of distal end of femur

     √7ᵗʰ **S83.121** Posterior subluxation of proximal end of tibia, right knee

     √7ᵗʰ **S83.122** Posterior subluxation of proximal end of tibia, left knee

     √7ᵗʰ **S83.123** Posterior subluxation of proximal end of tibia, unspecified knee

     √7ᵗʰ **S83.124** Posterior dislocation of proximal end of tibia, right knee

     √7ᵗʰ **S83.125** Posterior dislocation of proximal end of tibia, left knee

     √7ᵗʰ **S83.126** Posterior dislocation of proximal end of tibia, unspecified knee

√6ᵗʰ **S83.13** Medial subluxation and dislocation of proximal end of tibia

     √7ᵗʰ **S83.131** Medial subluxation of proximal end of tibia, right knee

     √7ᵗʰ **S83.132** Medial subluxation of proximal end of tibia, left knee

     √7ᵗʰ **S83.133** Medial subluxation of proximal end of tibia, unspecified knee

     √7ᵗʰ **S83.134** Medial dislocation of proximal end of tibia, right knee

     √7ᵗʰ **S83.135** Medial dislocation of proximal end of tibia, left knee

     √7ᵗʰ **S83.136** Medial dislocation of proximal end of tibia, unspecified knee

√6ᵗʰ **S83.14** Lateral subluxation and dislocation of proximal end of tibia

     √7ᵗʰ **S83.141** Lateral subluxation of proximal end of tibia, right knee

     √7ᵗʰ **S83.142** Lateral subluxation of proximal end of tibia, left knee

     √7ᵗʰ **S83.143** Lateral subluxation of proximal end of tibia, unspecified knee

     √7ᵗʰ **S83.144** Lateral dislocation of proximal end of tibia, right knee

     √7ᵗʰ **S83.145** Lateral dislocation of proximal end of tibia, left knee

     √7ᵗʰ **S83.146** Lateral dislocation of proximal end of tibia, unspecified knee

√6ᵗʰ **S83.19** Other subluxation and dislocation of knee

     √7ᵗʰ **S83.191** Other subluxation of right knee

     √7ᵗʰ **S83.192** Other subluxation of left knee

     √7ᵗʰ **S83.193** Other subluxation of unspecified knee

     √7ᵗʰ **S83.194** Other dislocation of right knee

     √7ᵗʰ **S83.195** Other dislocation of left knee

     √7ᵗʰ **S83.196** Other dislocation of unspecified knee

√5ᵗʰ **S83.2** Tear of meniscus, current injury

     EXCLUDES 1   old bucket-handle tear (M23.2)

     AHA: 2019,2Q,26

√6ᵗʰ **S83.20** Tear of unspecified meniscus, current injury

     Tear of meniscus of knee NOS

     √7ᵗʰ **S83.200** Bucket-handle tear of unspecified meniscus, current injury, right knee

     √7ᵗʰ **S83.201** Bucket-handle tear of unspecified meniscus, current injury, left knee

     √7ᵗʰ **S83.202** Bucket-handle tear of unspecified meniscus, current injury, unspecified knee

     √7ᵗʰ **S83.203** Other tear of unspecified meniscus, current injury, right knee

     √7ᵗʰ **S83.204** Other tear of unspecified meniscus, current injury, left knee

     √7ᵗʰ **S83.205** Other tear of unspecified meniscus, current injury, unspecified knee

     √7ᵗʰ **S83.206** Unspecified tear of unspecified meniscus, current injury, right knee

     √7ᵗʰ **S83.207** Unspecified tear of unspecified meniscus, current injury, left knee

     √7ᵗʰ **S83.209** Unspecified tear of unspecified meniscus, current injury, unspecified knee

√6ᵗʰ **S83.21** Bucket-handle tear of medial meniscus, current injury

     √7ᵗʰ **S83.211** Bucket-handle tear of medial meniscus, current injury, right knee

     √7ᵗʰ **S83.212** Bucket-handle tear of medial meniscus, current injury, left knee

√7ᵗʰ **S83.219** Bucket-handle tear of medial meniscus, current injury, unspecified knee

√6ᵗʰ **S83.22** Peripheral tear of medial meniscus, current injury

     √7ᵗʰ **S83.221** Peripheral tear of medial meniscus, current injury, right knee

     √7ᵗʰ **S83.222** Peripheral tear of medial meniscus, current injury, left knee

     √7ᵗʰ **S83.229** Peripheral tear of medial meniscus, current injury, unspecified knee

√6ᵗʰ **S83.23** Complex tear of medial meniscus, current injury

     √7ᵗʰ **S83.231** Complex tear of medial meniscus, current injury, right knee

     √7ᵗʰ **S83.232** Complex tear of medial meniscus, current injury, left knee

     √7ᵗʰ **S83.239** Complex tear of medial meniscus, current injury, unspecified knee

√6ᵗʰ **S83.24** Other tear of medial meniscus, current injury

     √7ᵗʰ **S83.241** Other tear of medial meniscus, current injury, right knee

     √7ᵗʰ **S83.242** Other tear of medial meniscus, current injury, left knee

     √7ᵗʰ **S83.249** Other tear of medial meniscus, current injury, unspecified knee

√6ᵗʰ **S83.25** Bucket-handle tear of lateral meniscus, current injury

     √7ᵗʰ **S83.251** Bucket-handle tear of lateral meniscus, current injury, right knee

     √7ᵗʰ **S83.252** Bucket-handle tear of lateral meniscus, current injury, left knee

     √7ᵗʰ **S83.259** Bucket-handle tear of lateral meniscus, current injury, unspecified knee

√6ᵗʰ **S83.26** Peripheral tear of lateral meniscus, current injury

     √7ᵗʰ **S83.261** Peripheral tear of lateral meniscus, current injury, right knee

     √7ᵗʰ **S83.262** Peripheral tear of lateral meniscus, current injury, left knee

     √7ᵗʰ **S83.269** Peripheral tear of lateral meniscus, current injury, unspecified knee

√6ᵗʰ **S83.27** Complex tear of lateral meniscus, current injury

     √7ᵗʰ **S83.271** Complex tear of lateral meniscus, current injury, right knee

     √7ᵗʰ **S83.272** Complex tear of lateral meniscus, current injury, left knee

     √7ᵗʰ **S83.279** Complex tear of lateral meniscus, current injury, unspecified knee

√6ᵗʰ **S83.28** Other tear of lateral meniscus, current injury

     √7ᵗʰ **S83.281** Other tear of lateral meniscus, current injury, right knee

     √7ᵗʰ **S83.282** Other tear of lateral meniscus, current injury, left knee

     √7ᵗʰ **S83.289** Other tear of lateral meniscus, current injury, unspecified knee

√5ᵗʰ **S83.3** Tear of articular cartilage of knee, current

     √x7ᵗʰ **S83.30** Tear of articular cartilage of unspecified knee, current

     √x7ᵗʰ **S83.31** Tear of articular cartilage of right knee, current

     √x7ᵗʰ **S83.32** Tear of articular cartilage of left knee, current

√5ᵗʰ **S83.4** Sprain of collateral ligament of knee

     √6ᵗʰ **S83.40** Sprain of unspecified collateral ligament of knee

       √7ᵗʰ **S83.401** Sprain of unspecified collateral ligament of right knee

       √7ᵗʰ **S83.402** Sprain of unspecified collateral ligament of left knee

       √7ᵗʰ **S83.409** Sprain of unspecified collateral ligament of unspecified knee

     √6ᵗʰ **S83.41** Sprain of medial collateral ligament of knee

       Sprain of tibial collateral ligament

       √7ᵗʰ **S83.411** Sprain of medial collateral ligament of right knee

       √7ᵗʰ **S83.412** Sprain of medial collateral ligament of left knee

       √7ᵗʰ **S83.419** Sprain of medial collateral ligament of unspecified knee

     √6ᵗʰ **S83.42** Sprain of lateral collateral ligament of knee

       Sprain of fibular collateral ligament

       √7ᵗʰ **S83.421** Sprain of lateral collateral ligament of right knee

       √7ᵗʰ **S83.422** Sprain of lateral collateral ligament of left knee

√7ᵗʰ **S83.429** Sprain of lateral collateral ligament of unspecified knee

√5ᵗʰ **S83.5** Sprain of cruciate ligament of knee

     AHA: 2016,2Q,3

√6ᵗʰ   **S83.50** Sprain of unspecified cruciate ligament of knee

√7ᵗʰ **S83.501** Sprain of unspecified cruciate ligament of right knee

√7ᵗʰ **S83.502** Sprain of unspecified cruciate ligament of left knee

√7ᵗʰ **S83.509** Sprain of unspecified cruciate ligament of unspecified knee

√6ᵗʰ   **S83.51** Sprain of anterior cruciate ligament of knee

√7ᵗʰ **S83.511** Sprain of anterior cruciate ligament of right knee

√7ᵗʰ **S83.512** Sprain of anterior cruciate ligament of left knee

√7ᵗʰ **S83.519** Sprain of anterior cruciate ligament of unspecified knee

√6ᵗʰ   **S83.52** Sprain of posterior cruciate ligament of knee

√7ᵗʰ **S83.521** Sprain of posterior cruciate ligament of right knee

√7ᵗʰ **S83.522** Sprain of posterior cruciate ligament of left knee

√7ᵗʰ **S83.529** Sprain of posterior cruciate ligament of unspecified knee

√5ᵗʰ **S83.6** Sprain of the superior tibiofibular joint and ligament

√x7ᵗʰ **S83.60** Sprain of the superior tibiofibular joint and ligament, unspecified knee

√x7ᵗʰ **S83.61** Sprain of the superior tibiofibular joint and ligament, right knee

√x7ᵗʰ **S83.62** Sprain of the superior tibiofibular joint and ligament, left knee

√5ᵗʰ **S83.8** Sprain of other specified parts of knee

√6ᵗʰ   **S83.8X** Sprain of other specified parts of knee

√7ᵗʰ **S83.8X1** Sprain of other specified parts of right knee

√7ᵗʰ **S83.8X2** Sprain of other specified parts of left knee

√7ᵗʰ **S83.8X9** Sprain of other specified parts of unspecified knee

√5ᵗʰ **S83.9** Sprain of unspecified site of knee

√x7ᵗʰ **S83.90** Sprain of unspecified site of unspecified knee

√x7ᵗʰ **S83.91** Sprain of unspecified site of right knee

√x7ᵗʰ **S83.92** Sprain of unspecified site of left knee

√4ᵗʰ **S84** Injury of nerves at lower leg level

     Code also any associated open wound (S81.-)

     EXCLUDES 2   injury of nerves at ankle and foot level (S94.-)

> The appropriate 7th character is to be added to each code from category S84.
> A   initial encounter
> D   subsequent encounter
> S   sequela

√5ᵗʰ **S84.0** Injury of tibial nerve at lower leg level

√x7ᵗʰ **S84.00** Injury of tibial nerve at lower leg level, unspecified leg

√x7ᵗʰ **S84.01** Injury of tibial nerve at lower leg level, right leg

√x7ᵗʰ **S84.02** Injury of tibial nerve at lower leg level, left leg

√5ᵗʰ **S84.1** Injury of peroneal nerve at lower leg level

√x7ᵗʰ **S84.10** Injury of peroneal nerve at lower leg level, unspecified leg

√x7ᵗʰ **S84.11** Injury of peroneal nerve at lower leg level, right leg

√x7ᵗʰ **S84.12** Injury of peroneal nerve at lower leg level, left leg

√5ᵗʰ **S84.2** Injury of cutaneous sensory nerve at lower leg level

√x7ᵗʰ **S84.20** Injury of cutaneous sensory nerve at lower leg level, unspecified leg

√x7ᵗʰ **S84.21** Injury of cutaneous sensory nerve at lower leg level, right leg

√x7ᵗʰ **S84.22** Injury of cutaneous sensory nerve at lower leg level, left leg

√5ᵗʰ **S84.8** Injury of other nerves at lower leg level

√6ᵗʰ   **S84.80** Injury of other nerves at lower leg level

√7ᵗʰ **S84.801** Injury of other nerves at lower leg level, right leg

√7ᵗʰ **S84.802** Injury of other nerves at lower leg level, left leg

√7ᵗʰ **S84.809** Injury of other nerves at lower leg level, unspecified leg

√6ᵗʰ   **S84.9** Injury of unspecified nerve at lower leg level

√x7ᵗʰ **S84.90** Injury of unspecified nerve at lower leg level, unspecified leg

√x7ᵗʰ **S84.91** Injury of unspecified nerve at lower leg level, right leg

√x7ᵗʰ **S84.92** Injury of unspecified nerve at lower leg level, left leg

√4ᵗʰ **S85** Injury of blood vessels at lower leg level

     Code also any associated open wound (S81.-)

     EXCLUDES 2   injury of blood vessels at ankle and foot level (S95.-)

> The appropriate 7th character is to be added to each code from category S85.
> A   initial encounter
> D   subsequent encounter
> S   sequela

√5ᵗʰ **S85.0** Injury of popliteal artery

√6ᵗʰ   **S85.00** Unspecified injury of popliteal artery

√7ᵗʰ **S85.001** Unspecified injury of popliteal artery, right leg

√7ᵗʰ **S85.002** Unspecified injury of popliteal artery, left leg

√7ᵗʰ **S85.009** Unspecified injury of popliteal artery, unspecified leg

√6ᵗʰ   **S85.01** Laceration of popliteal artery

√7ᵗʰ **S85.011** Laceration of popliteal artery, right leg

√7ᵗʰ **S85.012** Laceration of popliteal artery, left leg

√7ᵗʰ **S85.019** Laceration of popliteal artery, unspecified leg

√6ᵗʰ   **S85.09** Other specified injury of popliteal artery

√7ᵗʰ **S85.091** Other specified injury of popliteal artery, right leg

√7ᵗʰ **S85.092** Other specified injury of popliteal artery, left leg

√7ᵗʰ **S85.099** Other specified injury of popliteal artery, unspecified leg

√5ᵗʰ **S85.1** Injury of tibial artery

√6ᵗʰ   **S85.10** Unspecified injury of unspecified tibial artery

     Injury of tibial artery NOS

√7ᵗʰ **S85.101** Unspecified injury of unspecified tibial artery, right leg

√7ᵗʰ **S85.102** Unspecified injury of unspecified tibial artery, left leg

√7ᵗʰ **S85.109** Unspecified injury of unspecified tibial artery, unspecified leg

√6ᵗʰ   **S85.11** Laceration of unspecified tibial artery

√7ᵗʰ **S85.111** Laceration of unspecified tibial artery, right leg

√7ᵗʰ **S85.112** Laceration of unspecified tibial artery, left leg

√7ᵗʰ **S85.119** Laceration of unspecified tibial artery, unspecified leg

√6ᵗʰ   **S85.12** Other specified injury of unspecified tibial artery

√7ᵗʰ **S85.121** Other specified injury of unspecified tibial artery, right leg

√7ᵗʰ **S85.122** Other specified injury of unspecified tibial artery, left leg

√7ᵗʰ **S85.129** Other specified injury of unspecified tibial artery, unspecified leg

√6ᵗʰ   **S85.13** Unspecified injury of anterior tibial artery

√7ᵗʰ **S85.131** Unspecified injury of anterior tibial artery, right leg

√7ᵗʰ **S85.132** Unspecified injury of anterior tibial artery, left leg

√7ᵗʰ **S85.139** Unspecified injury of anterior tibial artery, unspecified leg

√6ᵗʰ   **S85.14** Laceration of anterior tibial artery

√7ᵗʰ **S85.141** Laceration of anterior tibial artery, right leg

√7ᵗʰ **S85.142** Laceration of anterior tibial artery, left leg

√7ᵗʰ **S85.149** Laceration of anterior tibial artery, unspecified leg

√6ᵗʰ   **S85.15** Other specified injury of anterior tibial artery

√7ᵗʰ **S85.151** Other specified injury of anterior tibial artery, right leg

HCC CMS-HCC   **Rx** Rx HCC   **ESR** ESRD HCC   **COM** Commercial HCC   **N** Newborn: 0   **P** Pediatric: 0-17   **M** Maternity: 9-64   **A** Adult: 15-124

1096

ICD-10-CM 2023

√7ᵗʰ **S85.152** Other specified injury of anterior tibial artery, left leg

√7ᵗʰ **S85.159** Other specified injury of anterior tibial artery, unspecified leg

√6ᵗʰ **S85.16** Unspecified injury of posterior tibial artery

√7ᵗʰ **S85.161** Unspecified injury of posterior tibial artery, right leg

√7ᵗʰ **S85.162** Unspecified injury of posterior tibial artery, left leg

√7ᵗʰ **S85.169** Unspecified injury of posterior tibial artery, unspecified leg

√6ᵗʰ **S85.17** Laceration of posterior tibial artery

√7ᵗʰ **S85.171** Laceration of posterior tibial artery, right leg

√7ᵗʰ **S85.172** Laceration of posterior tibial artery, left leg

√7ᵗʰ **S85.179** Laceration of posterior tibial artery, unspecified leg

√6ᵗʰ **S85.18** Other specified injury of posterior tibial artery

√7ᵗʰ **S85.181** Other specified injury of posterior tibial artery, right leg

√7ᵗʰ **S85.182** Other specified injury of posterior tibial artery, left leg

√7ᵗʰ **S85.189** Other specified injury of posterior tibial artery, unspecified leg

√5ᵗʰ **S85.2** Injury of peroneal artery

√6ᵗʰ **S85.20** Unspecified injury of peroneal artery

√7ᵗʰ **S85.201** Unspecified injury of peroneal artery, right leg

√7ᵗʰ **S85.202** Unspecified injury of peroneal artery, left leg

√7ᵗʰ **S85.209** Unspecified injury of peroneal artery, unspecified leg

√6ᵗʰ **S85.21** Laceration of peroneal artery

√7ᵗʰ **S85.211** Laceration of peroneal artery, right leg

√7ᵗʰ **S85.212** Laceration of peroneal artery, left leg

√7ᵗʰ **S85.219** Laceration of peroneal artery, unspecified leg

√6ᵗʰ **S85.29** Other specified injury of peroneal artery

√7ᵗʰ **S85.291** Other specified injury of peroneal artery, right leg

√7ᵗʰ **S85.292** Other specified injury of peroneal artery, left leg

√7ᵗʰ **S85.299** Other specified injury of peroneal artery, unspecified leg

√5ᵗʰ **S85.3** Injury of greater saphenous vein at lower leg level

Injury of greater saphenous vein NOS
Injury of saphenous vein NOS

√6ᵗʰ **S85.30** Unspecified injury of greater saphenous vein at lower leg level

√7ᵗʰ **S85.301** Unspecified injury of greater saphenous vein at lower leg level, right leg

√7ᵗʰ **S85.302** Unspecified injury of greater saphenous vein at lower leg level, left leg

√7ᵗʰ **S85.309** Unspecified injury of greater saphenous vein at lower leg level, unspecified leg

√6ᵗʰ **S85.31** Laceration of greater saphenous vein at lower leg level

√7ᵗʰ **S85.311** Laceration of greater saphenous vein at lower leg level, right leg

√7ᵗʰ **S85.312** Laceration of greater saphenous vein at lower leg level, left leg

√7ᵗʰ **S85.319** Laceration of greater saphenous vein at lower leg level, unspecified leg

√6ᵗʰ **S85.39** Other specified injury of greater saphenous vein at lower leg level

√7ᵗʰ **S85.391** Other specified injury of greater saphenous vein at lower leg level, right leg

√7ᵗʰ **S85.392** Other specified injury of greater saphenous vein at lower leg level, left leg

√7ᵗʰ **S85.399** Other specified injury of greater saphenous vein at lower leg level, unspecified leg

√5ᵗʰ **S85.4** Injury of lesser saphenous vein at lower leg level

√6ᵗʰ **S85.40** Unspecified injury of lesser saphenous vein at lower leg level

√7ᵗʰ **S85.401** Unspecified injury of lesser saphenous vein at lower leg level, right leg

√7ᵗʰ **S85.402** Unspecified injury of lesser saphenous vein at lower leg level, left leg

√7ᵗʰ **S85.409** Unspecified injury of lesser saphenous vein at lower leg level, unspecified leg

√6ᵗʰ **S85.41** Laceration of lesser saphenous vein at lower leg level

√7ᵗʰ **S85.411** Laceration of lesser saphenous vein at lower leg level, right leg

√7ᵗʰ **S85.412** Laceration of lesser saphenous vein at lower leg level, left leg

√7ᵗʰ **S85.419** Laceration of lesser saphenous vein at lower leg level, unspecified leg

√6ᵗʰ **S85.49** Other specified injury of lesser saphenous vein at lower leg level

√7ᵗʰ **S85.491** Other specified injury of lesser saphenous vein at lower leg level, right leg

√7ᵗʰ **S85.492** Other specified injury of lesser saphenous vein at lower leg level, left leg

√7ᵗʰ **S85.499** Other specified injury of lesser saphenous vein at lower leg level, unspecified leg

√5ᵗʰ **S85.5** Injury of popliteal vein

√6ᵗʰ **S85.50** Unspecified injury of popliteal vein

√7ᵗʰ **S85.501** Unspecified injury of popliteal vein, right leg

√7ᵗʰ **S85.502** Unspecified injury of popliteal vein, left leg

√7ᵗʰ **S85.509** Unspecified injury of popliteal vein, unspecified leg

√6ᵗʰ **S85.51** Laceration of popliteal vein

√7ᵗʰ **S85.511** Laceration of popliteal vein, right leg

√7ᵗʰ **S85.512** Laceration of popliteal vein, left leg

√7ᵗʰ **S85.519** Laceration of popliteal vein, unspecified leg

√6ᵗʰ **S85.59** Other specified injury of popliteal vein

√7ᵗʰ **S85.591** Other specified injury of popliteal vein, right leg

√7ᵗʰ **S85.592** Other specified injury of popliteal vein, left leg

√7ᵗʰ **S85.599** Other specified injury of popliteal vein, unspecified leg

√5ᵗʰ **S85.8** Injury of other blood vessels at lower leg level

√6ᵗʰ **S85.80** Unspecified injury of other blood vessels at lower leg level

√7ᵗʰ **S85.801** Unspecified injury of other blood vessels at lower leg level, right leg

√7ᵗʰ **S85.802** Unspecified injury of other blood vessels at lower leg level, left leg

√7ᵗʰ **S85.809** Unspecified injury of other blood vessels at lower leg level, unspecified leg

√6ᵗʰ **S85.81** Laceration of other blood vessels at lower leg level

√7ᵗʰ **S85.811** Laceration of other blood vessels at lower leg level, right leg

√7ᵗʰ **S85.812** Laceration of other blood vessels at lower leg level, left leg

√7ᵗʰ **S85.819** Laceration of other blood vessels at lower leg level, unspecified leg

√6ᵗʰ **S85.89** Other specified injury of other blood vessels at lower leg level

√7ᵗʰ **S85.891** Other specified injury of other blood vessels at lower leg level, right leg

√7ᵗʰ **S85.892** Other specified injury of other blood vessels at lower leg level, left leg

√7ᵗʰ **S85.899** Other specified injury of other blood vessels at lower leg level, unspecified leg

√5ᵗʰ **S85.9** Injury of unspecified blood vessel at lower leg level

√6ᵗʰ **S85.90** Unspecified injury of unspecified blood vessel at lower leg level

√7ᵗʰ **S85.901** Unspecified injury of unspecified blood vessel at lower leg level, right leg

√7ᵗʰ **S85.902** Unspecified injury of unspecified blood vessel at lower leg level, left leg

√7ᵗʰ **S85.909** Unspecified injury of unspecified blood vessel at lower leg level, unspecified leg

√6ᵗʰ **S85.91** Laceration of unspecified blood vessel at lower leg level

√7ᵗʰ **S85.911** Laceration of unspecified blood vessel at lower leg level, right leg

√7ᵗʰ **S85.912** Laceration of unspecified blood vessel at lower leg level, left leg

√7ᵗʰ **S85.919** Laceration of unspecified blood vessel at lower leg level, unspecified leg

√6ᵗʰ **S85.99** **Other specified injury of unspecified blood vessel at lower leg level**

- √7ᵗʰ **S85.991** Other specified injury of unspecified blood vessel at lower leg level, right leg
- √7ᵗʰ **S85.992** Other specified injury of unspecified blood vessel at lower leg level, left leg
- √7ᵗʰ **S85.999** Other specified injury of unspecified blood vessel at lower leg level, unspecified leg

√4ᵗʰ **S86** **Injury of muscle, fascia and tendon at lower leg level**

Code also any associated open wound (S81.-)

EXCLUDES 2   injury of muscle, fascia and tendon at ankle (S96.-)
        injury of patellar ligament (tendon) (S76.1-)
        sprain of joints and ligaments of knee (S83.-)

TIP: Refer to the Muscle/Tendon table at the beginning of this chapter.

The appropriate 7th character is to be added to each code from category S86.
A   initial encounter
D   subsequent encounter
S   sequela

√5ᵗʰ **S86.0** **Injury of Achilles tendon**

√6ᵗʰ **S86.00** **Unspecified injury of Achilles tendon**

- √7ᵗʰ **S86.001** Unspecified injury of right Achilles tendon
- √7ᵗʰ **S86.002** Unspecified injury of left Achilles tendon
- √7ᵗʰ **S86.009** Unspecified injury of unspecified Achilles tendon

√6ᵗʰ **S86.01** **Strain of Achilles tendon**

- √7ᵗʰ **S86.011** Strain of right Achilles tendon
- √7ᵗʰ **S86.012** Strain of left Achilles tendon
- √7ᵗʰ **S86.019** Strain of unspecified Achilles tendon

√6ᵗʰ **S86.02** **Laceration of Achilles tendon**

- √7ᵗʰ **S86.021** Laceration of right Achilles tendon
- √7ᵗʰ **S86.022** Laceration of left Achilles tendon
- √7ᵗʰ **S86.029** Laceration of unspecified Achilles tendon

√6ᵗʰ **S86.09** **Other specified injury of Achilles tendon**

- √7ᵗʰ **S86.091** Other specified injury of right Achilles tendon
- √7ᵗʰ **S86.092** Other specified injury of left Achilles tendon
- √7ᵗʰ **S86.099** Other specified injury of unspecified Achilles tendon

√5ᵗʰ **S86.1** **Injury of other muscle(s) and tendon(s) of posterior muscle group at lower leg level**

√6ᵗʰ **S86.10** **Unspecified injury of other muscle(s) and tendon(s) of posterior muscle group at lower leg level**

- √7ᵗʰ **S86.101** Unspecified injury of other muscle(s) and tendon(s) of posterior muscle group at lower leg level, right leg
- √7ᵗʰ **S86.102** Unspecified injury of other muscle(s) and tendon(s) of posterior muscle group at lower leg level, left leg
- √7ᵗʰ **S86.109** Unspecified injury of other muscle(s) and tendon(s) of posterior muscle group at lower leg level, unspecified leg

√6ᵗʰ **S86.11** **Strain of other muscle(s) and tendon(s) of posterior muscle group at lower leg level**

- √7ᵗʰ **S86.111** Strain of other muscle(s) and tendon(s) of posterior muscle group at lower leg level, right leg
- √7ᵗʰ **S86.112** Strain of other muscle(s) and tendon(s) of posterior muscle group at lower leg level, left leg
- √7ᵗʰ **S86.119** Strain of other muscle(s) and tendon(s) of posterior muscle group at lower leg level, unspecified leg

√6ᵗʰ **S86.12** **Laceration of other muscle(s) and tendon(s) of posterior muscle group at lower leg level**

- √7ᵗʰ **S86.121** Laceration of other muscle(s) and tendon(s) of posterior muscle group at lower leg level, right leg
- √7ᵗʰ **S86.122** Laceration of other muscle(s) and tendon(s) of posterior muscle group at lower leg level, left leg
- √7ᵗʰ **S86.129** Laceration of other muscle(s) and tendon(s) of posterior muscle group at lower leg level, unspecified leg

√6ᵗʰ **S86.19** **Other injury of other muscle(s) and tendon(s) of posterior muscle group at lower leg level**

- √7ᵗʰ **S86.191** Other injury of other muscle(s) and tendon(s) of posterior muscle group at lower leg level, right leg
- √7ᵗʰ **S86.192** Other injury of other muscle(s) and tendon(s) of posterior muscle group at lower leg level, left leg
- √7ᵗʰ **S86.199** Other injury of other muscle(s) and tendon(s) of posterior muscle group at lower leg level, unspecified leg

√5ᵗʰ **S86.2** **Injury of muscle(s) and tendon(s) of anterior muscle group at lower leg level**

√6ᵗʰ **S86.20** **Unspecified injury of muscle(s) and tendon(s) of anterior muscle group at lower leg level**

- √7ᵗʰ **S86.201** Unspecified injury of muscle(s) and tendon(s) of anterior muscle group at lower leg level, right leg
- √7ᵗʰ **S86.202** Unspecified injury of muscle(s) and tendon(s) of anterior muscle group at lower leg level, left leg
- √7ᵗʰ **S86.209** Unspecified injury of muscle(s) and tendon(s) of anterior muscle group at lower leg level, unspecified leg

√6ᵗʰ **S86.21** **Strain of muscle(s) and tendon(s) of anterior muscle group at lower leg level**

- √7ᵗʰ **S86.211** Strain of muscle(s) and tendon(s) of anterior muscle group at lower leg level, right leg
- √7ᵗʰ **S86.212** Strain of muscle(s) and tendon(s) of anterior muscle group at lower leg level, left leg
- √7ᵗʰ **S86.219** Strain of muscle(s) and tendon(s) of anterior muscle group at lower leg level, unspecified leg

√6ᵗʰ **S86.22** **Laceration of muscle(s) and tendon(s) of anterior muscle group at lower leg level**

- √7ᵗʰ **S86.221** Laceration of muscle(s) and tendon(s) of anterior muscle group at lower leg level, right leg
- √7ᵗʰ **S86.222** Laceration of muscle(s) and tendon(s) of anterior muscle group at lower leg level, left leg
- √7ᵗʰ **S86.229** Laceration of muscle(s) and tendon(s) of anterior muscle group at lower leg level, unspecified leg

√6ᵗʰ **S86.29** **Other injury of muscle(s) and tendon(s) of anterior muscle group at lower leg level**

- √7ᵗʰ **S86.291** Other injury of muscle(s) and tendon(s) of anterior muscle group at lower leg level, right leg
- √7ᵗʰ **S86.292** Other injury of muscle(s) and tendon(s) of anterior muscle group at lower leg level, left leg
- √7ᵗʰ **S86.299** Other injury of muscle(s) and tendon(s) of anterior muscle group at lower leg level, unspecified leg

√5ᵗʰ **S86.3** **Injury of muscle(s) and tendon(s) of peroneal muscle group at lower leg level**

√6ᵗʰ **S86.30** **Unspecified injury of muscle(s) and tendon(s) of peroneal muscle group at lower leg level**

- √7ᵗʰ **S86.301** Unspecified injury of muscle(s) and tendon(s) of peroneal muscle group at lower leg level, right leg
- √7ᵗʰ **S86.302** Unspecified injury of muscle(s) and tendon(s) of peroneal muscle group at lower leg level, left leg
- √7ᵗʰ **S86.309** Unspecified injury of muscle(s) and tendon(s) of peroneal muscle group at lower leg level, unspecified leg

√6ᵗʰ **S86.31** **Strain of muscle(s) and tendon(s) of peroneal muscle group at lower leg level**

- √7ᵗʰ **S86.311** Strain of muscle(s) and tendon(s) of peroneal muscle group at lower leg level, right leg
- √7ᵗʰ **S86.312** Strain of muscle(s) and tendon(s) of peroneal muscle group at lower leg level, left leg
- √7ᵗʰ **S86.319** Strain of muscle(s) and tendon(s) of peroneal muscle group at lower leg level, unspecified leg

√6ᵗʰ **S86.32** Laceration of muscle(s) and tendon(s) of peroneal muscle group at lower leg level
  √7ᵗʰ **S86.321** Laceration of muscle(s) and tendon(s) of peroneal muscle group at lower leg level, right leg
  √7ᵗʰ **S86.322** Laceration of muscle(s) and tendon(s) of peroneal muscle group at lower leg level, left leg
  √7ᵗʰ **S86.329** Laceration of muscle(s) and tendon(s) of peroneal muscle group at lower leg level, unspecified leg
√6ᵗʰ **S86.39** Other injury of muscle(s) and tendon(s) of peroneal muscle group at lower leg level
  √7ᵗʰ **S86.391** Other injury of muscle(s) and tendon(s) of peroneal muscle group at lower leg level, right leg
  √7ᵗʰ **S86.392** Other injury of muscle(s) and tendon(s) of peroneal muscle group at lower leg level, left leg
  √7ᵗʰ **S86.399** Other injury of muscle(s) and tendon(s) of peroneal muscle group at lower leg level, unspecified leg

√5ᵗʰ **S86.8** Injury of other muscles and tendons at lower leg level
√6ᵗʰ **S86.80** Unspecified injury of other muscles and tendons at lower leg level
  √7ᵗʰ **S86.801** Unspecified injury of other muscle(s) and tendon(s) at lower leg level, right leg
  √7ᵗʰ **S86.802** Unspecified injury of other muscle(s) and tendon(s) at lower leg level, left leg
  √7ᵗʰ **S86.809** Unspecified injury of other muscle(s) and tendon(s) at lower leg level, unspecified leg
√6ᵗʰ **S86.81** Strain of other muscles and tendons at lower leg level
  √7ᵗʰ **S86.811** Strain of other muscle(s) and tendon(s) at lower leg level, right leg
  √7ᵗʰ **S86.812** Strain of other muscle(s) and tendon(s) at lower leg level, left leg
  √7ᵗʰ **S86.819** Strain of other muscle(s) and tendon(s) at lower leg level, unspecified leg
√6ᵗʰ **S86.82** Laceration of other muscles and tendons at lower leg level
  √7ᵗʰ **S86.821** Laceration of other muscle(s) and tendon(s) at lower leg level, right leg
  √7ᵗʰ **S86.822** Laceration of other muscle(s) and tendon(s) at lower leg level, left leg
  √7ᵗʰ **S86.829** Laceration of other muscle(s) and tendon(s) at lower leg level, unspecified leg
√6ᵗʰ **S86.89** Other injury of other muscles and tendons at lower leg level
  √7ᵗʰ **S86.891** Other injury of other muscle(s) and tendon(s) at lower leg level, right leg
  √7ᵗʰ **S86.892** Other injury of other muscle(s) and tendon(s) at lower leg level, left leg
  √7ᵗʰ **S86.899** Other injury of other muscle(s) and tendon(s) at lower leg level, unspecified leg

√5ᵗʰ **S86.9** Injury of unspecified muscle and tendon at lower leg level
√6ᵗʰ **S86.90** Unspecified injury of unspecified muscle and tendon at lower leg level
  √7ᵗʰ **S86.901** Unspecified injury of unspecified muscle(s) and tendon(s) at lower leg level, right leg
  √7ᵗʰ **S86.902** Unspecified injury of unspecified muscle(s) and tendon(s) at lower leg level, left leg
  √7ᵗʰ **S86.909** Unspecified injury of unspecified muscle(s) and tendon(s) at lower leg level, unspecified leg
√6ᵗʰ **S86.91** Strain of unspecified muscle and tendon at lower leg level
  √7ᵗʰ **S86.911** Strain of unspecified muscle(s) and tendon(s) at lower leg level, right leg
  √7ᵗʰ **S86.912** Strain of unspecified muscle(s) and tendon(s) at lower leg level, left leg
  √7ᵗʰ **S86.919** Strain of unspecified muscle(s) and tendon(s) at lower leg level, unspecified leg
√6ᵗʰ **S86.92** Laceration of unspecified muscle and tendon at lower leg level
  √7ᵗʰ **S86.921** Laceration of unspecified muscle(s) and tendon(s) at lower leg level, right leg

  √7ᵗʰ **S86.922** Laceration of unspecified muscle(s) and tendon(s) at lower leg level, left leg
  √7ᵗʰ **S86.929** Laceration of unspecified muscle(s) and tendon(s) at lower leg level, unspecified leg
√6ᵗʰ **S86.99** Other injury of unspecified muscle and tendon at lower leg level
  √7ᵗʰ **S86.991** Other injury of unspecified muscle(s) and tendon(s) at lower leg level, right leg
  √7ᵗʰ **S86.992** Other injury of unspecified muscle(s) and tendon(s) at lower leg level, left leg
  √7ᵗʰ **S86.999** Other injury of unspecified muscle(s) and tendon(s) at lower leg level, unspecified leg

√4ᵗʰ **S87 Crushing injury of lower leg**
Use additional code(s) for all associated injuries
EXCLUDES 2   crushing injury of ankle and foot (S97.-)

The appropriate 7th character is to be added to each code from category S87.
A   initial encounter
D   subsequent encounter
S   sequela

√5ᵗʰ **S87.0** Crushing injury of knee
  √x7ᵗʰ **S87.00** Crushing injury of unspecified knee
  √x7ᵗʰ **S87.01** Crushing injury of right knee
  √x7ᵗʰ **S87.02** Crushing injury of left knee
√5ᵗʰ **S87.8** Crushing injury of lower leg
  √x7ᵗʰ **S87.80** Crushing injury of unspecified lower leg
  √x7ᵗʰ **S87.81** Crushing injury of right lower leg
  √x7ᵗʰ **S87.82** Crushing injury of left lower leg

√4ᵗʰ **S88 Traumatic amputation of lower leg**
An amputation not identified as partial or complete should be coded to complete
EXCLUDES 1   traumatic amputation of ankle and foot (S98.-)

The appropriate 7th character is to be added to each code from category S88.
A   initial encounter
D   subsequent encounter
S   sequela

√5ᵗʰ **S88.0** Traumatic amputation at knee level
√6ᵗʰ **S88.01** Complete traumatic amputation at knee level
  √7ᵗʰ **S88.011** Complete traumatic amputation at knee level, right lower leg   HCC ESR COM
  √7ᵗʰ **S88.012** Complete traumatic amputation at knee level, left lower leg   HCC ESR COM
  √7ᵗʰ **S88.019** Complete traumatic amputation at knee level, unspecified lower leg   HCC ESR COM
√6ᵗʰ **S88.02** Partial traumatic amputation at knee level
  √7ᵗʰ **S88.021** Partial traumatic amputation at knee level, right lower leg   HCC ESR COM
  √7ᵗʰ **S88.022** Partial traumatic amputation at knee level, left lower leg   HCC ESR COM
  √7ᵗʰ **S88.029** Partial traumatic amputation at knee level, unspecified lower leg   HCC ESR COM
√5ᵗʰ **S88.1** Traumatic amputation at level between knee and ankle
√6ᵗʰ **S88.11** Complete traumatic amputation at level between knee and ankle
  √7ᵗʰ **S88.111** Complete traumatic amputation at level between knee and ankle, right lower leg   HCC ESR COM
  √7ᵗʰ **S88.112** Complete traumatic amputation at level between knee and ankle, left lower leg   HCC ESR COM
  √7ᵗʰ **S88.119** Complete traumatic amputation at level between knee and ankle, unspecified lower leg   HCC ESR COM
√6ᵗʰ **S88.12** Partial traumatic amputation at level between knee and ankle
  √7ᵗʰ **S88.121** Partial traumatic amputation at level between knee and ankle, right lower leg   HCC ESR COM
  √7ᵗʰ **S88.122** Partial traumatic amputation at level between knee and ankle, left lower leg   HCC ESR COM

√7ᵗʰ **S88.129** Partial traumatic amputation at level between knee and ankle, unspecified lower leg   HCC ESR COM

√5ᵗʰ **S88.9** Traumatic amputation of lower leg, level unspecified

√6ᵗʰ **S88.91** Complete traumatic amputation of lower leg, level unspecified

√7ᵗʰ **S88.911** Complete traumatic amputation of right lower leg, level unspecified   HCC ESR COM

√7ᵗʰ **S88.912** Complete traumatic amputation of left lower leg, level unspecified   HCC ESR COM

√7ᵗʰ **S88.919** Complete traumatic amputation of unspecified lower leg, level unspecified   HCC ESR COM

√6ᵗʰ **S88.92** Partial traumatic amputation of lower leg, level unspecified

√7ᵗʰ **S88.921** Partial traumatic amputation of right lower leg, level unspecified   HCC ESR COM

√7ᵗʰ **S88.922** Partial traumatic amputation of left lower leg, level unspecified   HCC ESR COM

√7ᵗʰ **S88.929** Partial traumatic amputation of unspecified lower leg, level unspecified   HCC ESR COM

√4ᵗʰ **S89** Other and unspecified injuries of lower leg

> **NOTE** A fracture not indicated as open or closed should be coded to closed.

> **EXCLUDES 2** other and unspecified injuries of ankle and foot (S99.-)

AHA: 2018,2Q,12; 2018,1Q,3; 2015,3Q,37-39

> The appropriate 7th character is to be added to each code from subcategories S89.0, S89.1, S89.2, and S89.3.
> A   initial encounter for closed fracture
> D   subsequent encounter for fracture with routine healing
> G   subsequent encounter for fracture with delayed healing
> K   subsequent encounter for fracture with nonunion
> P   subsequent encounter for fracture with malunion
> S   sequela

√5ᵗʰ **S89.0** Physeal fracture of upper end of tibia

AHA: 2019,4Q,56

√6ᵗʰ **S89.00** Unspecified physeal fracture of upper end of tibia

√7ᵗʰ **S89.001** Unspecified physeal fracture of upper end of right tibia   Q

√7ᵗʰ **S89.002** Unspecified physeal fracture of upper end of left tibia   Q

√7ᵗʰ **S89.009** Unspecified physeal fracture of upper end of unspecified tibia   Q

√6ᵗʰ **S89.01** Salter-Harris Type I physeal fracture of upper end of tibia

√7ᵗʰ **S89.011** Salter-Harris Type I physeal fracture of upper end of right tibia   Q

√7ᵗʰ **S89.012** Salter-Harris Type I physeal fracture of upper end of left tibia   Q

√7ᵗʰ **S89.019** Salter-Harris Type I physeal fracture of upper end of unspecified tibia   Q

√6ᵗʰ **S89.02** Salter-Harris Type II physeal fracture of upper end of tibia

√7ᵗʰ **S89.021** Salter-Harris Type II physeal fracture of upper end of right tibia   Q

√7ᵗʰ **S89.022** Salter-Harris Type II physeal fracture of upper end of left tibia   Q

√7ᵗʰ **S89.029** Salter-Harris Type II physeal fracture of upper end of unspecified tibia   Q

√6ᵗʰ **S89.03** Salter-Harris Type III physeal fracture of upper end of tibia

√7ᵗʰ **S89.031** Salter-Harris Type III physeal fracture of upper end of right tibia   Q

√7ᵗʰ **S89.032** Salter-Harris Type III physeal fracture of upper end of left tibia   Q

√7ᵗʰ **S89.039** Salter-Harris Type III physeal fracture of upper end of unspecified tibia   Q

√6ᵗʰ **S89.04** Salter-Harris Type IV physeal fracture of upper end of tibia

√7ᵗʰ **S89.041** Salter-Harris Type IV physeal fracture of upper end of right tibia   Q

√7ᵗʰ **S89.042** Salter-Harris Type IV physeal fracture of upper end of left tibia   Q

√7ᵗʰ **S89.049** Salter-Harris Type IV physeal fracture of upper end of unspecified tibia   Q

√6ᵗʰ **S89.09** Other physeal fracture of upper end of tibia

√7ᵗʰ **S89.091** Other physeal fracture of upper end of right tibia   Q

√7ᵗʰ **S89.092** Other physeal fracture of upper end of left tibia   Q

√7ᵗʰ **S89.099** Other physeal fracture of upper end of unspecified tibia   Q

√5ᵗʰ **S89.1** Physeal fracture of lower end of tibia

AHA: 2019,4Q,56

√6ᵗʰ **S89.10** Unspecified physeal fracture of lower end of tibia

√7ᵗʰ **S89.101** Unspecified physeal fracture of lower end of right tibia   Q

√7ᵗʰ **S89.102** Unspecified physeal fracture of lower end of left tibia   Q

√7ᵗʰ **S89.109** Unspecified physeal fracture of lower end of unspecified tibia   Q

√6ᵗʰ **S89.11** Salter-Harris Type I physeal fracture of lower end of tibia

√7ᵗʰ **S89.111** Salter-Harris Type I physeal fracture of lower end of right tibia   Q

√7ᵗʰ **S89.112** Salter-Harris Type I physeal fracture of lower end of left tibia   Q

√7ᵗʰ **S89.119** Salter-Harris Type I physeal fracture of lower end of unspecified tibia   Q

√6ᵗʰ **S89.12** Salter-Harris Type II physeal fracture of lower end of tibia

√7ᵗʰ **S89.121** Salter-Harris Type II physeal fracture of lower end of right tibia   Q

√7ᵗʰ **S89.122** Salter-Harris Type II physeal fracture of lower end of left tibia   Q

√7ᵗʰ **S89.129** Salter-Harris Type II physeal fracture of lower end of unspecified tibia   Q

√6ᵗʰ **S89.13** Salter-Harris Type III physeal fracture of lower end of tibia

> **EXCLUDES 1** fracture of medial malleolus (adult) (S82.5-)

√7ᵗʰ **S89.131** Salter-Harris Type III physeal fracture of lower end of right tibia   Q

√7ᵗʰ **S89.132** Salter-Harris Type III physeal fracture of lower end of left tibia   Q

√7ᵗʰ **S89.139** Salter-Harris Type III physeal fracture of lower end of unspecified tibia   Q

√6ᵗʰ **S89.14** Salter-Harris Type IV physeal fracture of lower end of tibia

> **EXCLUDES 1** fracture of medial malleolus (adult) (S82.5-)

√7ᵗʰ **S89.141** Salter-Harris Type IV physeal fracture of lower end of right tibia   Q

√7ᵗʰ **S89.142** Salter-Harris Type IV physeal fracture of lower end of left tibia   Q

√7ᵗʰ **S89.149** Salter-Harris Type IV physeal fracture of lower end of unspecified tibia   Q

√6ᵗʰ **S89.19** Other physeal fracture of lower end of tibia

√7ᵗʰ **S89.191** Other physeal fracture of lower end of right tibia   Q

√7ᵗʰ **S89.192** Other physeal fracture of lower end of left tibia   Q

√7ᵗʰ **S89.199** Other physeal fracture of lower end of unspecified tibia   Q

√5ᵗʰ **S89.2** Physeal fracture of upper end of fibula

AHA: 2019,4Q,56

√6ᵗʰ **S89.20** Unspecified physeal fracture of upper end of fibula

√7ᵗʰ **S89.201** Unspecified physeal fracture of upper end of right fibula   Q

√7ᵗʰ **S89.202** Unspecified physeal fracture of upper end of left fibula   Q

√7ᵗʰ **S89.209** Unspecified physeal fracture of upper end of unspecified fibula   Q

√6ᵗʰ **S89.21** Salter-Harris Type I physeal fracture of upper end of fibula

√7ᵗʰ **S89.211** Salter-Harris Type I physeal fracture of upper end of right fibula   Q

√7ᵗʰ **S89.212** Salter-Harris Type I physeal fracture of upper end of left fibula   Q

√7ᵗʰ **S89.219** Salter-Harris Type I physeal fracture of upper end of unspecified fibula   Q

√6ᵗʰ **S89.22** Salter-Harris Type II physeal fracture of upper end of fibula

√7ᵗʰ **S89.221** Salter-Harris Type II physeal fracture of upper end of right fibula   Q

√7ᵗʰ **S89.222** Salter-Harris Type II physeal fracture of upper end of left fibula   ◻

√7ᵗʰ **S89.229** Salter-Harris Type II physeal fracture of upper end of unspecified fibula   ◻

√6ᵗʰ **S89.29** Other physeal fracture of upper end of fibula

√7ᵗʰ **S89.291** Other physeal fracture of upper end of right fibula   ◻

√7ᵗʰ **S89.292** Other physeal fracture of upper end of left fibula   ◻

√7ᵗʰ **S89.299** Other physeal fracture of upper end of unspecified fibula   ◻

√5ᵗʰ **S89.3** Physeal fracture of lower end of fibula

     AHA: 2019,4Q,56

√6ᵗʰ **S89.30** Unspecified physeal fracture of lower end of fibula

√7ᵗʰ **S89.301** Unspecified physeal fracture of lower end of right fibula   ◻

√7ᵗʰ **S89.302** Unspecified physeal fracture of lower end of left fibula   ◻

√7ᵗʰ **S89.309** Unspecified physeal fracture of lower end of unspecified fibula   ◻

√6ᵗʰ **S89.31** Salter-Harris Type I physeal fracture of lower end of fibula

√7ᵗʰ **S89.311** Salter-Harris Type I physeal fracture of lower end of right fibula   ◻

√7ᵗʰ **S89.312** Salter-Harris Type I physeal fracture of lower end of left fibula   ◻

√7ᵗʰ **S89.319** Salter-Harris Type I physeal fracture of lower end of unspecified fibula   ◻

√6ᵗʰ **S89.32** Salter-Harris Type II physeal fracture of lower end of fibula

√7ᵗʰ **S89.321** Salter-Harris Type II physeal fracture of lower end of right fibula   ◻

√7ᵗʰ **S89.322** Salter-Harris Type II physeal fracture of lower end of left fibula   ◻

√7ᵗʰ **S89.329** Salter-Harris Type II physeal fracture of lower end of unspecified fibula   ◻

√6ᵗʰ **S89.39** Other physeal fracture of lower end of fibula

√7ᵗʰ **S89.391** Other physeal fracture of lower end of right fibula   ◻

√7ᵗʰ **S89.392** Other physeal fracture of lower end of left fibula   ◻

√7ᵗʰ **S89.399** Other physeal fracture of lower end of unspecified fibula   ◻

√5ᵗʰ **S89.8** Other specified injuries of lower leg

> The appropriate 7th character is to be added to each code in subcategory S89.8.
> A   initial encounter
> D   subsequent encounter
> S   sequela

√x7ᵗʰ **S89.80** Other specified injuries of unspecified lower leg

√x7ᵗʰ **S89.81** Other specified injuries of right lower leg

√x7ᵗʰ **S89.82** Other specified injuries of left lower leg

√6ᵗʰ **S89.9** Unspecified injury of lower leg

> The appropriate 7th character is to be added to each code in subcategory S89.9.
> A   initial encounter
> D   subsequent encounter
> S   sequela

√x7ᵗʰ **S89.90** Unspecified injury of unspecified lower leg

√x7ᵗʰ **S89.91** Unspecified injury of right lower leg

√x7ᵗʰ **S89.92** Unspecified injury of left lower leg

Injuries to the ankle and foot (S90-S99)

EXCLUDES 2   burns and corrosions (T20-T32)
     fracture of ankle and malleolus (S82.-)
     frostbite (T33-T34)
     insect bite or sting, venomous (T63.4)

√4ᵗʰ **S90** Superficial injury of ankle, foot and toes

> The appropriate 7th character is to be added to each code from category S90.
> A   initial encounter
> D   subsequent encounter
> S   sequela

√6ᵗʰ **S90.0** Contusion of ankle

√x7ᵗʰ **S90.00** Contusion of unspecified ankle

√x7ᵗʰ **S90.01** Contusion of right ankle

√x7ᵗʰ **S90.02** Contusion of left ankle

√5ᵗʰ **S90.1** Contusion of toe without damage to nail

√6ᵗʰ **S90.11** Contusion of great toe without damage to nail

√7ᵗʰ **S90.111** Contusion of right great toe without damage to nail

√7ᵗʰ **S90.112** Contusion of left great toe without damage to nail

√7ᵗʰ **S90.119** Contusion of unspecified great toe without damage to nail

√6ᵗʰ **S90.12** Contusion of lesser toe without damage to nail

√7ᵗʰ **S90.121** Contusion of right lesser toe(s) without damage to nail

√7ᵗʰ **S90.122** Contusion of left lesser toe(s) without damage to nail

√7ᵗʰ **S90.129** Contusion of unspecified lesser toe(s) without damage to nail
     Contusion of toe NOS

√5ᵗʰ **S90.2** Contusion of toe with damage to nail

√6ᵗʰ **S90.21** Contusion of great toe with damage to nail

√7ᵗʰ **S90.211** Contusion of right great toe with damage to nail

√7ᵗʰ **S90.212** Contusion of left great toe with damage to nail

√7ᵗʰ **S90.219** Contusion of unspecified great toe with damage to nail

√6ᵗʰ **S90.22** Contusion of lesser toe with damage to nail

√7ᵗʰ **S90.221** Contusion of right lesser toe(s) with damage to nail

√7ᵗʰ **S90.222** Contusion of left lesser toe(s) with damage to nail

√7ᵗʰ **S90.229** Contusion of unspecified lesser toe(s) with damage to nail

√5ᵗʰ **S90.3** Contusion of foot

EXCLUDES 2   contusion of toes (S90.1-, S90.2-)

√x7ᵗʰ **S90.30** Contusion of unspecified foot
     Contusion of foot NOS

√x7ᵗʰ **S90.31** Contusion of right foot

√x7ᵗʰ **S90.32** Contusion of left foot

√5ᵗʰ **S90.4** Other superficial injuries of toe

√6ᵗʰ **S90.41** Abrasion of toe

√7ᵗʰ **S90.411** Abrasion, right great toe

√7ᵗʰ **S90.412** Abrasion, left great toe

√7ᵗʰ **S90.413** Abrasion, unspecified great toe

√7ᵗʰ **S90.414** Abrasion, right lesser toe(s)

√7ᵗʰ **S90.415** Abrasion, left lesser toe(s)

√7ᵗʰ **S90.416** Abrasion, unspecified lesser toe(s)

√6ᵗʰ **S90.42** Blister (nonthermal) of toe

√7ᵗʰ **S90.421** Blister (nonthermal), right great toe

√7ᵗʰ **S90.422** Blister (nonthermal), left great toe

√7ᵗʰ **S90.423** Blister (nonthermal), unspecified great toe

√7ᵗʰ **S90.424** Blister (nonthermal), right lesser toe(s)

√7ᵗʰ **S90.425** Blister (nonthermal), left lesser toe(s)

√7ᵗʰ **S90.426** Blister (nonthermal), unspecified lesser toe(s)

√6ᵗʰ **S90.44** External constriction of toe
     Hair tourniquet syndrome of toe

√7ᵗʰ **S90.441** External constriction, right great toe

√7ᵗʰ **S90.442** External constriction, left great toe

√7ᵗʰ **S90.443** External constriction, unspecified great toe

√7ᵗʰ **S90.444** External constriction, right lesser toe(s)

√7ᵗʰ **S90.445** External constriction, left lesser toe(s)

√7ᵗʰ **S90.446** External constriction, unspecified lesser toe(s)

√6ᵗʰ **S90.45** Superficial foreign body of toe
     Splinter in the toe

√7ᵗʰ **S90.451** Superficial foreign body, right great toe

√7ᵗʰ **S90.452** Superficial foreign body, left great toe

√7ᵗʰ **S90.453** Superficial foreign body, unspecified great toe

√7ᵗʰ **S90.454** Superficial foreign body, right lesser toe(s)

Chapter 19. Injury, Poisoning and Certain Other Consequences of External Causes

✓7ᵗʰ **S90.455** Superficial foreign body, left lesser toe(s)

✓7ᵗʰ **S90.456** Superficial foreign body, unspecified lesser toe(s)

✓6ᵗʰ **S90.46** Insect bite (nonvenomous) of toe

  ✓7ᵗʰ **S90.461** Insect bite (nonvenomous), right great toe

  ✓7ᵗʰ **S90.462** Insect bite (nonvenomous), left great toe

  ✓7ᵗʰ **S90.463** Insect bite (nonvenomous), unspecified great toe

  ✓7ᵗʰ **S90.464** Insect bite (nonvenomous), right lesser toe(s)

  ✓7ᵗʰ **S90.465** Insect bite (nonvenomous), left lesser toe(s)

  ✓7ᵗʰ **S90.466** Insect bite (nonvenomous), unspecified lesser toe(s)

✓5ᵗʰ **S90.47** Other superficial bite of toe

  EXCLUDES 1   *open bite of toe (S91.15-, S91.25-)*

  ✓7ᵗʰ **S90.471** Other superficial bite of right great toe

  ✓7ᵗʰ **S90.472** Other superficial bite of left great toe

  ✓7ᵗʰ **S90.473** Other superficial bite of unspecified great toe

  ✓7ᵗʰ **S90.474** Other superficial bite of right lesser toe(s)

  ✓7ᵗʰ **S90.475** Other superficial bite of left lesser toe(s)

  ✓7ᵗʰ **S90.476** Other superficial bite of unspecified lesser toe(s)

✓5ᵗʰ **S90.5** Other superficial injuries of ankle

  ✓6ᵗʰ **S90.51** Abrasion of ankle

    ✓7ᵗʰ **S90.511** Abrasion, right ankle

    ✓7ᵗʰ **S90.512** Abrasion, left ankle

    ✓7ᵗʰ **S90.519** Abrasion, unspecified ankle

  ✓6ᵗʰ **S90.52** Blister (nonthermal) of ankle

    ✓7ᵗʰ **S90.521** Blister (nonthermal), right ankle

    ✓7ᵗʰ **S90.522** Blister (nonthermal), left ankle

    ✓7ᵗʰ **S90.529** Blister (nonthermal), unspecified ankle

  ✓6ᵗʰ **S90.54** External constriction of ankle

    ✓7ᵗʰ **S90.541** External constriction, right ankle

    ✓7ᵗʰ **S90.542** External constriction, left ankle

    ✓7ᵗʰ **S90.549** External constriction, unspecified ankle

  ✓6ᵗʰ **S90.55** Superficial foreign body of ankle

    Splinter in the ankle

    ✓7ᵗʰ **S90.551** Superficial foreign body, right ankle

    ✓7ᵗʰ **S90.552** Superficial foreign body, left ankle

    ✓7ᵗʰ **S90.559** Superficial foreign body, unspecified ankle

  ✓6ᵗʰ **S90.56** Insect bite (nonvenomous) of ankle

    ✓7ᵗʰ **S90.561** Insect bite (nonvenomous), right ankle

    ✓7ᵗʰ **S90.562** Insect bite (nonvenomous), left ankle

    ✓7ᵗʰ **S90.569** Insect bite (nonvenomous), unspecified ankle

  ✓6ᵗʰ **S90.57** Other superficial bite of ankle

    EXCLUDES 1   *open bite of ankle (S91.05-)*

    ✓7ᵗʰ **S90.571** Other superficial bite of ankle, right ankle

    ✓7ᵗʰ **S90.572** Other superficial bite of ankle, left ankle

    ✓7ᵗʰ **S90.579** Other superficial bite of ankle, unspecified ankle

✓5ᵗʰ **S90.8** Other superficial injuries of foot

  ✓6ᵗʰ **S90.81** Abrasion of foot

    ✓7ᵗʰ **S90.811** Abrasion, right foot

    ✓7ᵗʰ **S90.812** Abrasion, left foot

    ✓7ᵗʰ **S90.819** Abrasion, unspecified foot

  ✓6ᵗʰ **S90.82** Blister (nonthermal) of foot

    ✓7ᵗʰ **S90.821** Blister (nonthermal), right foot

    ✓7ᵗʰ **S90.822** Blister (nonthermal), left foot

    ✓7ᵗʰ **S90.829** Blister (nonthermal), unspecified foot

  ✓6ᵗʰ **S90.84** External constriction of foot

    ✓7ᵗʰ **S90.841** External constriction, right foot

    ✓7ᵗʰ **S90.842** External constriction, left foot

    ✓7ᵗʰ **S90.849** External constriction, unspecified foot

  ✓6ᵗʰ **S90.85** Superficial foreign body of foot

    Splinter in the foot

    ✓7ᵗʰ **S90.851** Superficial foreign body, right foot

✓7ᵗʰ **S90.852** Superficial foreign body, left foot

✓7ᵗʰ **S90.859** Superficial foreign body, unspecified foot

✓6ᵗʰ **S90.86** Insect bite (nonvenomous) of foot

  ✓7ᵗʰ **S90.861** Insect bite (nonvenomous), right foot

  ✓7ᵗʰ **S90.862** Insect bite (nonvenomous), left foot

  ✓7ᵗʰ **S90.869** Insect bite (nonvenomous), unspecified foot

✓6ᵗʰ **S90.87** Other superficial bite of foot

  EXCLUDES 1   *open bite of foot (S91.35-)*

  ✓7ᵗʰ **S90.871** Other superficial bite of right foot

  ✓7ᵗʰ **S90.872** Other superficial bite of left foot

  ✓7ᵗʰ **S90.879** Other superficial bite of unspecified foot

✓5ᵗʰ **S90.9** Unspecified superficial injury of ankle, foot and toe

  ✓6ᵗʰ **S90.91** Unspecified superficial injury of ankle

    ✓7ᵗʰ **S90.911** Unspecified superficial injury of right ankle

    ✓7ᵗʰ **S90.912** Unspecified superficial injury of left ankle

    ✓7ᵗʰ **S90.919** Unspecified superficial injury of unspecified ankle

  ✓6ᵗʰ **S90.92** Unspecified superficial injury of foot

    ✓7ᵗʰ **S90.921** Unspecified superficial injury of right foot

    ✓7ᵗʰ **S90.922** Unspecified superficial injury of left foot

    ✓7ᵗʰ **S90.929** Unspecified superficial injury of unspecified foot

  ✓6ᵗʰ **S90.93** Unspecified superficial injury of toes

    ✓7ᵗʰ **S90.931** Unspecified superficial injury of right great toe

    ✓7ᵗʰ **S90.932** Unspecified superficial injury of left great toe

    ✓7ᵗʰ **S90.933** Unspecified superficial injury of unspecified great toe

    ✓7ᵗʰ **S90.934** Unspecified superficial injury of right lesser toe(s)

    ✓7ᵗʰ **S90.935** Unspecified superficial injury of left lesser toe(s)

    ✓7ᵗʰ **S90.936** Unspecified superficial injury of unspecified lesser toe(s)

✓4ᵗʰ **S91** **Open wound of ankle, foot and toes**

  Code also any associated wound infection

  EXCLUDES 1   *open fracture of ankle, foot and toes (S92.- with 7th character B)*

  traumatic amputation of ankle and foot (S98.-)

  AHA: 2021,1Q,7

  The appropriate 7th character is to be added to each code from category S91.
  A   initial encounter
  D   subsequent encounter
  S   sequela

✓5ᵗʰ **S91.0** Open wound of ankle

  ✓6ᵗʰ **S91.00** Unspecified open wound of ankle

    ✓7ᵗʰ **S91.001** Unspecified open wound, right ankle

    ✓7ᵗʰ **S91.002** Unspecified open wound, left ankle

    ✓7ᵗʰ **S91.009** Unspecified open wound, unspecified ankle

  ✓6ᵗʰ **S91.01** Laceration without foreign body of ankle

    ✓7ᵗʰ **S91.011** Laceration without foreign body, right ankle

    ✓7ᵗʰ **S91.012** Laceration without foreign body, left ankle

    ✓7ᵗʰ **S91.019** Laceration without foreign body, unspecified ankle

  ✓6ᵗʰ **S91.02** Laceration with foreign body of ankle

    ✓7ᵗʰ **S91.021** Laceration with foreign body, right ankle

    ✓7ᵗʰ **S91.022** Laceration with foreign body, left ankle

    ✓7ᵗʰ **S91.029** Laceration with foreign body, unspecified ankle

  ✓6ᵗʰ **S91.03** Puncture wound without foreign body of ankle

    ✓7ᵗʰ **S91.031** Puncture wound without foreign body, right ankle

    ✓7ᵗʰ **S91.032** Puncture wound without foreign body, left ankle

    ✓7ᵗʰ **S91.039** Puncture wound without foreign body, unspecified ankle

√6ᵗʰ **S91.04** Puncture wound with foreign body of ankle

     √7ᵗʰ **S91.041** Puncture wound with foreign body, right ankle

     √7ᵗʰ **S91.042** Puncture wound with foreign body, left ankle

     √7ᵗʰ **S91.049** Puncture wound with foreign body, unspecified ankle

√6ᵗʰ **S91.05** Open bite of ankle

     EXCLUDES 1   superficial bite of ankle (S90.56-, S90.57-)

     √7ᵗʰ **S91.051** Open bite, right ankle

     √7ᵗʰ **S91.052** Open bite, left ankle

     √7ᵗʰ **S91.059** Open bite, unspecified ankle

√5ᵗʰ **S91.1** Open wound of toe without damage to nail

√6ᵗʰ **S91.10** Unspecified open wound of toe without damage to nail

     √7ᵗʰ **S91.101** Unspecified open wound of right great toe without damage to nail

     √7ᵗʰ **S91.102** Unspecified open wound of left great toe without damage to nail

     √7ᵗʰ **S91.103** Unspecified open wound of unspecified great toe without damage to nail

     √7ᵗʰ **S91.104** Unspecified open wound of right lesser toe(s) without damage to nail

     √7ᵗʰ **S91.105** Unspecified open wound of left lesser toe(s) without damage to nail

     √7ᵗʰ **S91.106** Unspecified open wound of unspecified lesser toe(s) without damage to nail

     √7ᵗʰ **S91.109** Unspecified open wound of unspecified toe(s) without damage to nail

√6ᵗʰ **S91.11** Laceration without foreign body of toe without damage to nail

     √7ᵗʰ **S91.111** Laceration without foreign body right great toe without damage to nail

     √7ᵗʰ **S91.112** Laceration without foreign body of left great toe without damage to nail

     √7ᵗʰ **S91.113** Laceration without foreign body of unspecified great toe without damage to nail

     √7ᵗʰ **S91.114** Laceration without foreign body of right lesser toe(s) without damage to nail

     √7ᵗʰ **S91.115** Laceration without foreign body of left lesser toe(s) without damage to nail

     √7ᵗʰ **S91.116** Laceration without foreign body of unspecified lesser toe(s) without damage to nail

     √7ᵗʰ **S91.119** Laceration without foreign body of unspecified toe without damage to nail

√6ᵗʰ **S91.12** Laceration with foreign body of toe without damage to nail

     √7ᵗʰ **S91.121** Laceration with foreign body of right great toe without damage to nail

     √7ᵗʰ **S91.122** Laceration with foreign body of left great toe without damage to nail

     √7ᵗʰ **S91.123** Laceration with foreign body of unspecified great toe without damage to nail

     √7ᵗʰ **S91.124** Laceration with foreign body of right lesser toe(s) without damage to nail

     √7ᵗʰ **S91.125** Laceration with foreign body of left lesser toe(s) without damage to nail

     √7ᵗʰ **S91.126** Laceration with foreign body of unspecified lesser toe(s) without damage to nail

     √7ᵗʰ **S91.129** Laceration with foreign body of unspecified toe(s) without damage to nail

√6ᵗʰ **S91.13** Puncture wound without foreign body of toe without damage to nail

     √7ᵗʰ **S91.131** Puncture wound without foreign body of right great toe without damage to nail

     √7ᵗʰ **S91.132** Puncture wound without foreign body of left great toe without damage to nail

     √7ᵗʰ **S91.133** Puncture wound without foreign body of unspecified great toe without damage to nail

     √7ᵗʰ **S91.134** Puncture wound without foreign body of right lesser toe(s) without damage to nail

     √7ᵗʰ **S91.135** Puncture wound without foreign body of left lesser toe(s) without damage to nail

     √7ᵗʰ **S91.136** Puncture wound without foreign body of unspecified lesser toe(s) without damage to nail

     √7ᵗʰ **S91.139** Puncture wound without foreign body of unspecified toe(s) without damage to nail

√6ᵗʰ **S91.14** Puncture wound with foreign body of toe without damage to nail

     √7ᵗʰ **S91.141** Puncture wound with foreign body of right great toe without damage to nail

     √7ᵗʰ **S91.142** Puncture wound with foreign body of left great toe without damage to nail

     √7ᵗʰ **S91.143** Puncture wound with foreign body of unspecified great toe without damage to nail

     √7ᵗʰ **S91.144** Puncture wound with foreign body of right lesser toe(s) without damage to nail

     √7ᵗʰ **S91.145** Puncture wound with foreign body of left lesser toe(s) without damage to nail

     √7ᵗʰ **S91.146** Puncture wound with foreign body of unspecified lesser toe(s) without damage to nail

     √7ᵗʰ **S91.149** Puncture wound with foreign body of unspecified toe(s) without damage to nail

√6ᵗʰ **S91.15** Open bite of toe without damage to nail

     Bite of toe NOS

     EXCLUDES 1   superficial bite of toe (S90.46-, S90.47-)

     √7ᵗʰ **S91.151** Open bite of right great toe without damage to nail

     √7ᵗʰ **S91.152** Open bite of left great toe without damage to nail

     √7ᵗʰ **S91.153** Open bite of unspecified great toe without damage to nail

     √7ᵗʰ **S91.154** Open bite of right lesser toe(s) without damage to nail

     √7ᵗʰ **S91.155** Open bite of left lesser toe(s) without damage to nail

     √7ᵗʰ **S91.156** Open bite of unspecified lesser toe(s) without damage to nail

     √7ᵗʰ **S91.159** Open bite of unspecified toe(s) without damage to nail

√5ᵗʰ **S91.2** Open wound of toe with damage to nail

√6ᵗʰ **S91.20** Unspecified open wound of toe with damage to nail

     √7ᵗʰ **S91.201** Unspecified open wound of right great toe with damage to nail

     √7ᵗʰ **S91.202** Unspecified open wound of left great toe with damage to nail

     √7ᵗʰ **S91.203** Unspecified open wound of unspecified great toe with damage to nail

     √7ᵗʰ **S91.204** Unspecified open wound of right lesser toe(s) with damage to nail

     √7ᵗʰ **S91.205** Unspecified open wound of left lesser toe(s) with damage to nail

     √7ᵗʰ **S91.206** Unspecified open wound of unspecified lesser toe(s) with damage to nail

     √7ᵗʰ **S91.209** Unspecified open wound of unspecified toe(s) with damage to nail

√6ᵗʰ **S91.21** Laceration without foreign body of toe with damage to nail

     √7ᵗʰ **S91.211** Laceration without foreign body of right great toe with damage to nail

     √7ᵗʰ **S91.212** Laceration without foreign body of left great toe with damage to nail

     √7ᵗʰ **S91.213** Laceration without foreign body of unspecified great toe with damage to nail

     √7ᵗʰ **S91.214** Laceration without foreign body of right lesser toe(s) with damage to nail

     √7ᵗʰ **S91.215** Laceration without foreign body of left lesser toe(s) with damage to nail

     √7ᵗʰ **S91.216** Laceration without foreign body of unspecified lesser toe(s) with damage to nail

     √7ᵗʰ **S91.219** Laceration without foreign body of unspecified toe(s) with damage to nail

√6ᵗʰ **S91.22** Laceration with foreign body of toe with damage to nail

     √7ᵗʰ **S91.221** Laceration with foreign body of right great toe with damage to nail

     √7ᵗʰ **S91.222** Laceration with foreign body of left great toe with damage to nail

     √7ᵗʰ **S91.223** Laceration with foreign body of unspecified great toe with damage to nail

     √7ᵗʰ **S91.224** Laceration with foreign body of right lesser toe(s) with damage to nail

     √7ᵗʰ **S91.225** Laceration with foreign body of left lesser toe(s) with damage to nail

---

√7ᵗʰ **S91.226** **Laceration with foreign body of unspecified lesser toe(s) with damage to nail**

√7ᵗʰ **S91.229** **Laceration with foreign body of unspecified toe(s) with damage to nail**

√6ᵗʰ **S91.23** **Puncture wound without foreign body of toe with damage to nail**

√7ᵗʰ **S91.231** **Puncture wound without foreign body of right great toe with damage to nail**

√7ᵗʰ **S91.232** **Puncture wound without foreign body of left great toe with damage to nail**

√7ᵗʰ **S91.233** **Puncture wound without foreign body of unspecified great toe with damage to nail**

√7ᵗʰ **S91.234** **Puncture wound without foreign body of right lesser toe(s) with damage to nail**

√7ᵗʰ **S91.235** **Puncture wound without foreign body of left lesser toe(s) with damage to nail**

√7ᵗʰ **S91.236** **Puncture wound without foreign body of unspecified lesser toe(s) with damage to nail**

√7ᵗʰ **S91.239** **Puncture wound without foreign body of unspecified toe(s) with damage to nail**

√6ᵗʰ **S91.24** **Puncture wound with foreign body of toe with damage to nail**

√7ᵗʰ **S91.241** **Puncture wound with foreign body of right great toe with damage to nail**

√7ᵗʰ **S91.242** **Puncture wound with foreign body of left great toe with damage to nail**

√7ᵗʰ **S91.243** **Puncture wound with foreign body of unspecified great toe with damage to nail**

√7ᵗʰ **S91.244** **Puncture wound with foreign body of right lesser toe(s) with damage to nail**

√7ᵗʰ **S91.245** **Puncture wound with foreign body of left lesser toe(s) with damage to nail**

√7ᵗʰ **S91.246** **Puncture wound with foreign body of unspecified lesser toe(s) with damage to nail**

√7ᵗʰ **S91.249** **Puncture wound with foreign body of unspecified toe(s) with damage to nail**

√6ᵗʰ **S91.25** **Open bite of toe with damage to nail**

Bite of toe with damage to nail NOS

EXCLUDES 1   *superficial bite of toe (S90.46-, S90.47-)*

√7ᵗʰ **S91.251** **Open bite of right great toe with damage to nail**

√7ᵗʰ **S91.252** **Open bite of left great toe with damage to nail**

√7ᵗʰ **S91.253** **Open bite of unspecified great toe with damage to nail**

√7ᵗʰ **S91.254** **Open bite of right lesser toe(s) with damage to nail**

√7ᵗʰ **S91.255** **Open bite of left lesser toe(s) with damage to nail**

√7ᵗʰ **S91.256** **Open bite of unspecified lesser toe(s) with damage to nail**

√7ᵗʰ **S91.259** **Open bite of unspecified toe(s) with damage to nail**

√5ᵗʰ **S91.3** **Open wound of foot**

√6ᵗʰ **S91.30** **Unspecified open wound of foot**

√7ᵗʰ **S91.301** **Unspecified open wound, right foot**

√7ᵗʰ **S91.302** **Unspecified open wound, left foot**

√7ᵗʰ **S91.309** **Unspecified open wound, unspecified foot**

√6ᵗʰ **S91.31** **Laceration without foreign body of foot**

√7ᵗʰ **S91.311** **Laceration without foreign body, right foot**

√7ᵗʰ **S91.312** **Laceration without foreign body, left foot**

√7ᵗʰ **S91.319** **Laceration without foreign body, unspecified foot**

√6ᵗʰ **S91.32** **Laceration with foreign body of foot**

√7ᵗʰ **S91.321** **Laceration with foreign body, right foot**

√7ᵗʰ **S91.322** **Laceration with foreign body, left foot**

√7ᵗʰ **S91.329** **Laceration with foreign body, unspecified foot**

√6ᵗʰ **S91.33** **Puncture wound without foreign body of foot**

√7ᵗʰ **S91.331** **Puncture wound without foreign body, right foot**

√7ᵗʰ **S91.332** **Puncture wound without foreign body, left foot**

√7ᵗʰ **S91.339** **Puncture wound without foreign body, unspecified foot**

√6ᵗʰ **S91.34** **Puncture wound with foreign body of foot**

√7ᵗʰ **S91.341** **Puncture wound with foreign body, right foot**

√7ᵗʰ **S91.342** **Puncture wound with foreign body, left foot**

√7ᵗʰ **S91.349** **Puncture wound with foreign body, unspecified foot**

√6ᵗʰ **S91.35** **Open bite of foot**

EXCLUDES 1   *superficial bite of foot (S90.86-, S90.87-)*

√7ᵗʰ **S91.351** **Open bite, right foot**

√7ᵗʰ **S91.352** **Open bite, left foot**

√7ᵗʰ **S91.359** **Open bite, unspecified foot**

√4ᵗʰ **S92** **Fracture of foot and toe, except ankle**

NOTE   A fracture not indicated as displaced or nondisplaced should be coded to displaced

A fracture not indicated as open or closed should be coded to closed.

EXCLUDES 2   *fracture of ankle (S82.-)*
fracture of malleolus (S82.-)
traumatic amputation of ankle and foot (S98.-)

AHA: 2018,2Q,12; 2015,3Q,37-39

The appropriate 7th character is to be added to each code from category S92.
A   initial encounter for closed fracture
B   initial encounter for open fracture
D   subsequent encounter for fracture with routine healing
G   subsequent encounter for fracture with delayed healing
K   subsequent encounter for fracture with nonunion
P   subsequent encounter for fracture with malunion
S   sequela

√5ᵗʰ **S92.0** **Fracture of calcaneus**

Heel bone
Os calcis

EXCLUDES 2   *physeal fracture of calcaneus (S99.0-)*

√6ᵗʰ **S92.00** **Unspecified fracture of calcaneus**

√7ᵗʰ **S92.001** **Unspecified fracture of right calcaneus**   🔟

√7ᵗʰ **S92.002** **Unspecified fracture of left calcaneus**   🔟

√7ᵗʰ **S92.009** **Unspecified fracture of unspecified calcaneus**   🔟

√6ᵗʰ **S92.01** **Fracture of body of calcaneus**

√7ᵗʰ **S92.011** **Displaced fracture of body of right calcaneus**   🔟

√7ᵗʰ **S92.012** **Displaced fracture of body of left calcaneus**   🔟

√7ᵗʰ **S92.013** **Displaced fracture of body of unspecified calcaneus**   🔟

√7ᵗʰ **S92.014** **Nondisplaced fracture of body of right calcaneus**   🔟

√7ᵗʰ **S92.015** **Nondisplaced fracture of body of left calcaneus**   🔟

√7ᵗʰ **S92.016** **Nondisplaced fracture of body of unspecified calcaneus**   🔟

√6ᵗʰ **S92.02** **Fracture of anterior process of calcaneus**

√7ᵗʰ **S92.021** **Displaced fracture of anterior process of right calcaneus**   🔟

√7ᵗʰ **S92.022** **Displaced fracture of anterior process of left calcaneus**   🔟

√7ᵗʰ **S92.023** **Displaced fracture of anterior process of unspecified calcaneus**   🔟

√7ᵗʰ **S92.024** **Nondisplaced fracture of anterior process of right calcaneus**   🔟

√7ᵗʰ **S92.025** **Nondisplaced fracture of anterior process of left calcaneus**   🔟

√7ᵗʰ **S92.026** **Nondisplaced fracture of anterior process of unspecified calcaneus**   🔟

√6ᵗʰ **S92.03** **Avulsion fracture of tuberosity of calcaneus**

√7ᵗʰ **S92.031** **Displaced avulsion fracture of tuberosity of right calcaneus**   🔟

√7ᵗʰ **S92.032** **Displaced avulsion fracture of tuberosity of left calcaneus**   🔟

√7ᵗʰ **S92.033** **Displaced avulsion fracture of tuberosity of unspecified calcaneus**   🔟

√7ᵗʰ **S92.034** **Nondisplaced avulsion fracture of tuberosity of right calcaneus**   🔟

√7ᵗʰ **S92.035** Nondisplaced avulsion fracture of tuberosity of left calcaneus 🄀

√7ᵗʰ **S92.036** Nondisplaced avulsion fracture of tuberosity of unspecified calcaneus 🄀

√6ᵗʰ **S92.04** Other fracture of tuberosity of calcaneus

√7ᵗʰ **S92.041** Displaced other fracture of tuberosity of right calcaneus 🄀

√7ᵗʰ **S92.042** Displaced other fracture of tuberosity of left calcaneus 🄀

√7ᵗʰ **S92.043** Displaced other fracture of tuberosity of unspecified calcaneus 🄀

√7ᵗʰ **S92.044** Nondisplaced other fracture of tuberosity of right calcaneus 🄀

√7ᵗʰ **S92.045** Nondisplaced other fracture of tuberosity of left calcaneus 🄀

√7ᵗʰ **S92.046** Nondisplaced other fracture of tuberosity of unspecified calcaneus 🄀

√6ᵗʰ **S92.05** Other extraarticular fracture of calcaneus

√7ᵗʰ **S92.051** Displaced other extraarticular fracture of right calcaneus 🄀

√7ᵗʰ **S92.052** Displaced other extraarticular fracture of left calcaneus 🄀

√7ᵗʰ **S92.053** Displaced other extraarticular fracture of unspecified calcaneus 🄀

√7ᵗʰ **S92.054** Nondisplaced other extraarticular fracture of right calcaneus 🄀

√7ᵗʰ **S92.055** Nondisplaced other extraarticular fracture of left calcaneus 🄀

√7ᵗʰ **S92.056** Nondisplaced other extraarticular fracture of unspecified calcaneus 🄀

√6ᵗʰ **S92.06** Intraarticular fracture of calcaneus

√7ᵗʰ **S92.061** Displaced intraarticular fracture of right calcaneus 🄀

√7ᵗʰ **S92.062** Displaced intraarticular fracture of left calcaneus 🄀

√7ᵗʰ **S92.063** Displaced intraarticular fracture of unspecified calcaneus 🄀

√7ᵗʰ **S92.064** Nondisplaced intraarticular fracture of right calcaneus 🄀

√7ᵗʰ **S92.065** Nondisplaced intraarticular fracture of left calcaneus 🄀

√7ᵗʰ **S92.066** Nondisplaced intraarticular fracture of unspecified calcaneus 🄀

√5ᵗʰ **S92.1** Fracture of talus

Astragalus

√6ᵗʰ **S92.10** Unspecified fracture of talus

√7ᵗʰ **S92.101** Unspecified fracture of right talus 🄀

√7ᵗʰ **S92.102** Unspecified fracture of left talus 🄀

√7ᵗʰ **S92.109** Unspecified fracture of unspecified talus 🄀

√6ᵗʰ **S92.11** Fracture of neck of talus

√7ᵗʰ **S92.111** Displaced fracture of neck of right talus 🄀

√7ᵗʰ **S92.112** Displaced fracture of neck of left talus 🄀

√7ᵗʰ **S92.113** Displaced fracture of neck of unspecified talus 🄀

√7ᵗʰ **S92.114** Nondisplaced fracture of neck of right talus 🄀

√7ᵗʰ **S92.115** Nondisplaced fracture of neck of left talus 🄀

√7ᵗʰ **S92.116** Nondisplaced fracture of neck of unspecified talus 🄀

√6ᵗʰ **S92.12** Fracture of body of talus

√7ᵗʰ **S92.121** Displaced fracture of body of right talus 🄀

√7ᵗʰ **S92.122** Displaced fracture of body of left talus 🄀

√7ᵗʰ **S92.123** Displaced fracture of body of unspecified talus 🄀

√7ᵗʰ **S92.124** Nondisplaced fracture of body of right talus 🄀

√7ᵗʰ **S92.125** Nondisplaced fracture of body of left talus 🄀

√7ᵗʰ **S92.126** Nondisplaced fracture of body of unspecified talus 🄀

√6ᵗʰ **S92.13** Fracture of posterior process of talus

√7ᵗʰ **S92.131** Displaced fracture of posterior process of right talus 🄀

√7ᵗʰ **S92.132** Displaced fracture of posterior process of left talus 🄀

√7ᵗʰ **S92.133** Displaced fracture of posterior process of unspecified talus 🄀

√7ᵗʰ **S92.134** Nondisplaced fracture of posterior process of right talus 🄀

√7ᵗʰ **S92.135** Nondisplaced fracture of posterior process of left talus 🄀

√7ᵗʰ **S92.136** Nondisplaced fracture of posterior process of unspecified talus 🄀

√6ᵗʰ **S92.14** Dome fracture of talus

EXCLUDES 1   osteochondritis dissecans (M93.2)

√7ᵗʰ **S92.141** Displaced dome fracture of right talus 🄀

√7ᵗʰ **S92.142** Displaced dome fracture of left talus 🄀

√7ᵗʰ **S92.143** Displaced dome fracture of unspecified talus 🄀

√7ᵗʰ **S92.144** Nondisplaced dome fracture of right talus 🄀

√7ᵗʰ **S92.145** Nondisplaced dome fracture of left talus 🄀

√7ᵗʰ **S92.146** Nondisplaced dome fracture of unspecified talus 🄀

√6ᵗʰ **S92.15** Avulsion fracture (chip fracture) of talus

√7ᵗʰ **S92.151** Displaced avulsion fracture (chip fracture) of right talus 🄀

√7ᵗʰ **S92.152** Displaced avulsion fracture (chip fracture) of left talus 🄀

√7ᵗʰ **S92.153** Displaced avulsion fracture (chip fracture) of unspecified talus 🄀

√7ᵗʰ **S92.154** Nondisplaced avulsion fracture (chip fracture) of right talus 🄀

√7ᵗʰ **S92.155** Nondisplaced avulsion fracture (chip fracture) of left talus 🄀

√7ᵗʰ **S92.156** Nondisplaced avulsion fracture (chip fracture) of unspecified talus 🄀

√6ᵗʰ **S92.19** Other fracture of talus

√7ᵗʰ **S92.191** Other fracture of right talus 🄀

√7ᵗʰ **S92.192** Other fracture of left talus 🄀

√7ᵗʰ **S92.199** Other fracture of unspecified talus 🄀

√5ᵗʰ **S92.2** Fracture of other and unspecified tarsal bone(s)

√6ᵗʰ **S92.20** Fracture of unspecified tarsal bone(s)

√7ᵗʰ **S92.201** Fracture of unspecified tarsal bone(s) of right foot 🄀

√7ᵗʰ **S92.202** Fracture of unspecified tarsal bone(s) of left foot 🄀

√7ᵗʰ **S92.209** Fracture of unspecified tarsal bone(s) of unspecified foot 🄀

√6ᵗʰ **S92.21** Fracture of cuboid bone

√7ᵗʰ **S92.211** Displaced fracture of cuboid bone of right foot 🄀

√7ᵗʰ **S92.212** Displaced fracture of cuboid bone of left foot 🄀

√7ᵗʰ **S92.213** Displaced fracture of cuboid bone of unspecified foot 🄀

√7ᵗʰ **S92.214** Nondisplaced fracture of cuboid bone of right foot 🄀

√7ᵗʰ **S92.215** Nondisplaced fracture of cuboid bone of left foot 🄀

√7ᵗʰ **S92.216** Nondisplaced fracture of cuboid bone of unspecified foot 🄀

√6ᵗʰ **S92.22** Fracture of lateral cuneiform

√7ᵗʰ **S92.221** Displaced fracture of lateral cuneiform of right foot 🄀

√7ᵗʰ **S92.222** Displaced fracture of lateral cuneiform of left foot 🄀

√7ᵗʰ **S92.223** Displaced fracture of lateral cuneiform of unspecified foot 🄀

√7ᵗʰ **S92.224** Nondisplaced fracture of lateral cuneiform of right foot 🄀

√7ᵗʰ **S92.225** Nondisplaced fracture of lateral cuneiform of left foot 🄀

√7ᵗʰ **S92.226** Nondisplaced fracture of lateral cuneiform of unspecified foot 🄀

√6ᵗʰ **S92.23** Fracture of intermediate cuneiform

√7ᵗʰ **S92.231** Displaced fracture of intermediate cuneiform of right foot 🄀

√7ᵗʰ **S92.232** Displaced **fracture of intermediate cuneiform of** left **foot** 🄞

√7ᵗʰ **S92.233** Displaced **fracture of intermediate cuneiform of unspecified foot** 🄞

√7ᵗʰ **S92.234** Nondisplaced **fracture of intermediate cuneiform of** right **foot** 🄞

√7ᵗʰ **S92.235** Nondisplaced **fracture of intermediate cuneiform of** left **foot** 🄞

√7ᵗʰ **S92.236** Nondisplaced **fracture of intermediate cuneiform of unspecified foot** 🄞

√6ᵗʰ **S92.24** Fracture of medial cuneiform

√7ᵗʰ **S92.241** Displaced **fracture of medial cuneiform of right foot** 🄞

√7ᵗʰ **S92.242** Displaced **fracture of medial cuneiform of** left **foot** 🄞

√7ᵗʰ **S92.243** Displaced **fracture of medial cuneiform of unspecified foot** 🄞

√7ᵗʰ **S92.244** Nondisplaced **fracture of medial cuneiform of** right **foot** 🄞

√7ᵗʰ **S92.245** Nondisplaced **fracture of medial cuneiform of** left **foot** 🄞

√7ᵗʰ **S92.246** Nondisplaced **fracture of medial cuneiform of unspecified foot** 🄞

√6ᵗʰ **S92.25** Fracture of navicular [scaphoid] of foot

√7ᵗʰ **S92.251** Displaced **fracture of navicular [scaphoid] of right foot** 🄞

√7ᵗʰ **S92.252** Displaced **fracture of navicular [scaphoid] of** left **foot** 🄞

√7ᵗʰ **S92.253** Displaced **fracture of navicular [scaphoid] of unspecified foot** 🄞

√7ᵗʰ **S92.254** Nondisplaced **fracture of navicular [scaphoid] of** right **foot** 🄞

√7ᵗʰ **S92.255** Nondisplaced **fracture of navicular [scaphoid] of** left **foot** 🄞

√7ᵗʰ **S92.256** Nondisplaced **fracture of navicular [scaphoid] of unspecified foot** 🄞

√5ᵗʰ **S92.3** Fracture of metatarsal bone(s)

EXCLUDES 2   *physeal fracture of metatarsal (S99.1-)*

AHA: 2018,1Q,3

√6ᵗʰ **S92.30** Fracture of unspecified metatarsal bone(s)

√7ᵗʰ **S92.301** Fracture of unspecified metatarsal bone(s), right **foot** 🄞

√7ᵗʰ **S92.302** Fracture of unspecified metatarsal bone(s), left **foot** 🄞

√7ᵗʰ **S92.309** Fracture of unspecified metatarsal bone(s), unspecified **foot** 🄞

√6ᵗʰ **S92.31** Fracture of first metatarsal bone

√7ᵗʰ **S92.311** Displaced **fracture of first metatarsal bone,** right **foot** 🄞

√7ᵗʰ **S92.312** Displaced **fracture of first metatarsal bone,** left **foot** 🄞

√7ᵗʰ **S92.313** Displaced **fracture of first metatarsal bone, unspecified foot** 🄞

√7ᵗʰ **S92.314** Nondisplaced **fracture of first metatarsal bone,** right **foot** 🄞

√7ᵗʰ **S92.315** Nondisplaced **fracture of first metatarsal bone,** left **foot** 🄞

√7ᵗʰ **S92.316** Nondisplaced **fracture of first metatarsal bone, unspecified foot** 🄞

√6ᵗʰ **S92.32** Fracture of second metatarsal bone

√7ᵗʰ **S92.321** Displaced **fracture of second metatarsal bone,** right **foot** 🄞

√7ᵗʰ **S92.322** Displaced **fracture of second metatarsal bone,** left **foot** 🄞

√7ᵗʰ **S92.323** Displaced **fracture of second metatarsal bone, unspecified foot** 🄞

√7ᵗʰ **S92.324** Nondisplaced **fracture of second metatarsal bone,** right **foot** 🄞

√7ᵗʰ **S92.325** Nondisplaced **fracture of second metatarsal bone,** left **foot** 🄞

√7ᵗʰ **S92.326** Nondisplaced **fracture of second metatarsal bone, unspecified foot** 🄞

√6ᵗʰ **S92.33** Fracture of third metatarsal bone

√7ᵗʰ **S92.331** Displaced **fracture of third metatarsal bone,** right **foot** 🄞

√7ᵗʰ **S92.332** Displaced **fracture of third metatarsal bone,** left **foot** 🄞

√7ᵗʰ **S92.333** Displaced **fracture of third metatarsal bone, unspecified foot** 🄞

√7ᵗʰ **S92.334** Nondisplaced **fracture of third metatarsal bone,** right **foot** 🄞

√7ᵗʰ **S92.335** Nondisplaced **fracture of third metatarsal bone,** left **foot** 🄞

√7ᵗʰ **S92.336** Nondisplaced **fracture of third metatarsal bone, unspecified foot** 🄞

√6ᵗʰ **S92.34** Fracture of fourth metatarsal bone

√7ᵗʰ **S92.341** Displaced **fracture of fourth metatarsal bone,** right **foot** 🄞

√7ᵗʰ **S92.342** Displaced **fracture of fourth metatarsal bone,** left **foot** 🄞

√7ᵗʰ **S92.343** Displaced **fracture of fourth metatarsal bone, unspecified foot** 🄞

√7ᵗʰ **S92.344** Nondisplaced **fracture of fourth metatarsal bone,** right **foot** 🄞

√7ᵗʰ **S92.345** Nondisplaced **fracture of fourth metatarsal bone,** left **foot** 🄞

√7ᵗʰ **S92.346** Nondisplaced **fracture of fourth metatarsal bone, unspecified foot** 🄞

√6ᵗʰ **S92.35** Fracture of fifth metatarsal bone

√7ᵗʰ **S92.351** Displaced **fracture of fifth metatarsal bone,** right **foot** 🄞

√7ᵗʰ **S92.352** Displaced **fracture of fifth metatarsal bone,** left **foot** 🄞

√7ᵗʰ **S92.353** Displaced **fracture of fifth metatarsal bone, unspecified foot** 🄞

√7ᵗʰ **S92.354** Nondisplaced **fracture of fifth metatarsal bone,** right **foot** 🄞

√7ᵗʰ **S92.355** Nondisplaced **fracture of fifth metatarsal bone,** left **foot** 🄞

√7ᵗʰ **S92.356** Nondisplaced **fracture of fifth metatarsal bone, unspecified foot** 🄞

√5ᵗʰ **S92.4** Fracture of great toe

EXCLUDES 2   *physeal fracture of phalanx of toe (S99.2-)*

√6ᵗʰ **S92.40** Unspecified fracture of great toe

√7ᵗʰ **S92.401** Displaced **unspecified fracture of** right **great toe**

√7ᵗʰ **S92.402** Displaced **unspecified fracture of** left **great toe**

√7ᵗʰ **S92.403** Displaced **unspecified fracture of unspecified great toe**

√7ᵗʰ **S92.404** Nondisplaced **unspecified fracture of** right **great toe**

√7ᵗʰ **S92.405** Nondisplaced **unspecified fracture of** left **great toe**

√7ᵗʰ **S92.406** Nondisplaced **unspecified fracture of unspecified great toe**

√6ᵗʰ **S92.41** Fracture of proximal phalanx of great toe

√7ᵗʰ **S92.411** Displaced **fracture of proximal phalanx of** right **great toe**

√7ᵗʰ **S92.412** Displaced **fracture of proximal phalanx of** left **great toe**

√7ᵗʰ **S92.413** Displaced **fracture of proximal phalanx of unspecified great toe**

√7ᵗʰ **S92.414** Nondisplaced **fracture of proximal phalanx of** right **great toe**

√7ᵗʰ **S92.415** Nondisplaced **fracture of proximal phalanx of** left **great toe**

√7ᵗʰ **S92.416** Nondisplaced **fracture of proximal phalanx of unspecified great toe**

√6ᵗʰ **S92.42** Fracture of distal phalanx of great toe

√7ᵗʰ **S92.421** Displaced **fracture of distal phalanx of** right **great toe**

√7ᵗʰ **S92.422** Displaced **fracture of distal phalanx of** left **great toe**

√7ᵗʰ **S92.423** Displaced **fracture of distal phalanx of unspecified great toe**

√7ᵗʰ **S92.424** Nondisplaced **fracture of distal phalanx of** right **great toe**

√7ᵗʰ **S92.425** Nondisplaced **fracture of distal phalanx of** left **great toe**

√7ᵗʰ **S92.426** Nondisplaced **fracture of distal phalanx of unspecified great toe**

√6ᵗʰ **S92.49** Other fracture of great toe

√7ᵗʰ **S92.491** Other fracture of right **great toe**

√7ᵗʰ **S92.492** Other fracture of left **great toe**

√7ᵗʰ **S92.499** Other fracture of unspecified **great toe**

HCC CMS-HCC   **Rx** Rx HCC   **ESR** ESRD HCC   **COM** Commercial HCC   **N** Newborn: 0   **P** Pediatric: 0-17   **M** Maternity: 9-64   **A** Adult: 15-124

1106   ICD-10-CM 2023

☑5ᵗʰ **S92.5** Fracture of lesser toe(s)

EXCLUDES 2 *physeal fracture of phalanx of toe (S99.2-)*

☑6ᵗʰ **S92.50** Unspecified fracture of lesser toe(s)

☑7ᵗʰ **S92.501** Displaced unspecified fracture of right lesser toe(s)

☑7ᵗʰ **S92.502** Displaced unspecified fracture of left lesser toe(s)

☑7ᵗʰ **S92.503** Displaced unspecified fracture of unspecified lesser toe(s)

☑7ᵗʰ **S92.504** Nondisplaced unspecified fracture of right lesser toe(s)

☑7ᵗʰ **S92.505** Nondisplaced unspecified fracture of left lesser toe(s)

☑7ᵗʰ **S92.506** Nondisplaced unspecified fracture of unspecified lesser toe(s)

☑6ᵗʰ **S92.51** Fracture of proximal phalanx of lesser toe(s)

☑7ᵗʰ **S92.511** Displaced fracture of proximal phalanx of right lesser toe(s)

☑7ᵗʰ **S92.512** Displaced fracture of proximal phalanx of left lesser toe(s)

☑7ᵗʰ **S92.513** Displaced fracture of proximal phalanx of unspecified lesser toe(s)

☑7ᵗʰ **S92.514** Nondisplaced fracture of proximal phalanx of right lesser toe(s)

☑7ᵗʰ **S92.515** Nondisplaced fracture of proximal phalanx of left lesser toe(s)

☑7ᵗʰ **S92.516** Nondisplaced fracture of proximal phalanx of unspecified lesser toe(s)

☑6ᵗʰ **S92.52** Fracture of middle phalanx of lesser toe(s)

☑7ᵗʰ **S92.521** Displaced fracture of middle phalanx of right lesser toe(s)

☑7ᵗʰ **S92.522** Displaced fracture of middle phalanx of left lesser toe(s)

☑7ᵗʰ **S92.523** Displaced fracture of middle phalanx of unspecified lesser toe(s)

☑7ᵗʰ **S92.524** Nondisplaced fracture of middle phalanx of right lesser toe(s)

☑7ᵗʰ **S92.525** Nondisplaced fracture of middle phalanx of left lesser toe(s)

☑7ᵗʰ **S92.526** Nondisplaced fracture of middle phalanx of unspecified lesser toe(s)

☑6ᵗʰ **S92.53** Fracture of distal phalanx of lesser toe(s)

☑7ᵗʰ **S92.531** Displaced fracture of distal phalanx of right lesser toe(s)

☑7ᵗʰ **S92.532** Displaced fracture of distal phalanx of left lesser toe(s)

☑7ᵗʰ **S92.533** Displaced fracture of distal phalanx of unspecified lesser toe(s)

☑7ᵗʰ **S92.534** Nondisplaced fracture of distal phalanx of right lesser toe(s)

☑7ᵗʰ **S92.535** Nondisplaced fracture of distal phalanx of left lesser toe(s)

☑7ᵗʰ **S92.536** Nondisplaced fracture of distal phalanx of unspecified lesser toe(s)

☑6ᵗʰ **S92.59** Other fracture of lesser toe(s)

☑7ᵗʰ **S92.591** Other fracture of right lesser toe(s)

☑7ᵗʰ **S92.592** Other fracture of left lesser toe(s)

☑7ᵗʰ **S92.599** Other fracture of unspecified lesser toe(s)

☑5ᵗʰ **S92.8** Other fracture of foot, except ankle

☑6ᵗʰ **S92.81** Other fracture of foot

Sesamoid fracture of foot

AHA: 2016,4Q,68

☑7ᵗʰ **S92.811** Other fracture of right foot ▣

☑7ᵗʰ **S92.812** Other fracture of left foot ▣

☑7ᵗʰ **S92.819** Other fracture of unspecified foot ▣

☑5ᵗʰ **S92.9** Unspecified fracture of foot and toe

☑6ᵗʰ **S92.90** Unspecified fracture of foot

☑7ᵗʰ **S92.901** Unspecified fracture of right foot ▣

☑7ᵗʰ **S92.902** Unspecified fracture of left foot ▣

☑7ᵗʰ **S92.909** Unspecified fracture of unspecified foot ▣

☑6ᵗʰ **S92.91** Unspecified fracture of toe

☑7ᵗʰ **S92.911** Unspecified fracture of right toe(s)

☑7ᵗʰ **S92.912** Unspecified fracture of left toe(s)

☑7ᵗʰ **S92.919** Unspecified fracture of unspecified toe(s)

☑4ᵗʰ **S93** Dislocation and sprain of joints and ligaments at ankle, foot and toe level

INCLUDES avulsion of joint or ligament of ankle, foot and toe
laceration of cartilage, joint or ligament of ankle, foot and toe
sprain of cartilage, joint or ligament of ankle, foot and toe
traumatic hemarthrosis of joint or ligament of ankle, foot and toe
traumatic rupture of joint or ligament of ankle, foot and toe
traumatic subluxation of joint or ligament of ankle, foot and toe
traumatic tear of joint or ligament of ankle, foot and toe

Code also any associated open wound

EXCLUDES 2 *strain of muscle and tendon of ankle and foot (S96.-)*

The appropriate 7th character is to be added to each code from category S93.
A initial encounter
D subsequent encounter
S sequela

☑5ᵗʰ **S93.0** Subluxation and dislocation of ankle joint

Subluxation and dislocation of astragalus
Subluxation and dislocation of fibula, lower end
Subluxation and dislocation of talus
Subluxation and dislocation of tibia, lower end

☑x7ᵗʰ **S93.01** Subluxation of right ankle joint

☑x7ᵗʰ **S93.02** Subluxation of left ankle joint

☑x7ᵗʰ **S93.03** Subluxation of unspecified ankle joint

☑x7ᵗʰ **S93.04** Dislocation of right ankle joint

☑x7ᵗʰ **S93.05** Dislocation of left ankle joint

☑x7ᵗʰ **S93.06** Dislocation of unspecified ankle joint

☑5ᵗʰ **S93.1** Subluxation and dislocation of toe

☑6ᵗʰ **S93.10** Unspecified subluxation and dislocation of toe

Dislocation of toe NOS
Subluxation of toe NOS

☑7ᵗʰ **S93.101** Unspecified subluxation of right toe(s)

☑7ᵗʰ **S93.102** Unspecified subluxation of left toe(s)

☑7ᵗʰ **S93.103** Unspecified subluxation of unspecified toe(s)

☑7ᵗʰ **S93.104** Unspecified dislocation of right toe(s)

☑7ᵗʰ **S93.105** Unspecified dislocation of left toe(s)

☑7ᵗʰ **S93.106** Unspecified dislocation of unspecified toe(s)

☑6ᵗʰ **S93.11** Dislocation of interphalangeal joint

☑7ᵗʰ **S93.111** Dislocation of interphalangeal joint of right great toe

☑7ᵗʰ **S93.112** Dislocation of interphalangeal joint of left great toe

☑7ᵗʰ **S93.113** Dislocation of interphalangeal joint of unspecified great toe

☑7ᵗʰ **S93.114** Dislocation of interphalangeal joint of right lesser toe(s)

☑7ᵗʰ **S93.115** Dislocation of interphalangeal joint of left lesser toe(s)

☑7ᵗʰ **S93.116** Dislocation of interphalangeal joint of unspecified lesser toe(s)

☑7ᵗʰ **S93.119** Dislocation of interphalangeal joint of unspecified toe(s)

☑6ᵗʰ **S93.12** Dislocation of metatarsophalangeal joint

☑7ᵗʰ **S93.121** Dislocation of metatarsophalangeal joint of right great toe

☑7ᵗʰ **S93.122** Dislocation of metatarsophalangeal joint of left great toe

☑7ᵗʰ **S93.123** Dislocation of metatarsophalangeal joint of unspecified great toe

☑7ᵗʰ **S93.124** Dislocation of metatarsophalangeal joint of right lesser toe(s)

☑7ᵗʰ **S93.125** Dislocation of metatarsophalangeal joint of left lesser toe(s)

☑7ᵗʰ **S93.126** Dislocation of metatarsophalangeal joint of unspecified lesser toe(s)

☑7ᵗʰ **S93.129** Dislocation of metatarsophalangeal joint of unspecified toe(s)

☑6ᵗʰ **S93.13** Subluxation of interphalangeal joint

☑7ᵗʰ **S93.131** Subluxation of interphalangeal joint of right great toe

☑ Additional Character Required   ☑x7ᵗʰ Placeholder Alert   Manifestation   Unspecified Dx   ▣ QPP   UPD Unacceptable PDx

√7ᵗʰ **S93.132** Subluxation of interphalangeal joint of left great toe

√7ᵗʰ **S93.133** Subluxation of interphalangeal joint of unspecified great toe

√7ᵗʰ **S93.134** Subluxation of interphalangeal joint of right lesser toe(s)

√7ᵗʰ **S93.135** Subluxation of interphalangeal joint of left lesser toe(s)

√7ᵗʰ **S93.136** Subluxation of interphalangeal joint of unspecified lesser toe(s)

√7ᵗʰ **S93.139** Subluxation of interphalangeal joint of unspecified toe(s)

√6ᵗʰ **S93.14** Subluxation of metatarsophalangeal joint

√7ᵗʰ **S93.141** Subluxation of metatarsophalangeal joint of right great toe

√7ᵗʰ **S93.142** Subluxation of metatarsophalangeal joint of left great toe

√7ᵗʰ **S93.143** Subluxation of metatarsophalangeal joint of unspecified great toe

√7ᵗʰ **S93.144** Subluxation of metatarsophalangeal joint of right lesser toe(s)

√7ᵗʰ **S93.145** Subluxation of metatarsophalangeal joint of left lesser toe(s)

√7ᵗʰ **S93.146** Subluxation of metatarsophalangeal joint of unspecified lesser toe(s)

√7ᵗʰ **S93.149** Subluxation of metatarsophalangeal joint of unspecified toe(s)

√5ᵗʰ **S93.3** Subluxation and dislocation of foot

     EXCLUDES 2   *dislocation of toe (S93.1-)*

√6ᵗʰ **S93.30** Unspecified subluxation and dislocation of foot

     Dislocation of foot NOS
     Subluxation of foot NOS

√7ᵗʰ **S93.301** Unspecified subluxation of right foot

√7ᵗʰ **S93.302** Unspecified subluxation of left foot

√7ᵗʰ **S93.303** Unspecified subluxation of unspecified foot

√7ᵗʰ **S93.304** Unspecified dislocation of right foot

√7ᵗʰ **S93.305** Unspecified dislocation of left foot

√7ᵗʰ **S93.306** Unspecified dislocation of unspecified foot

√6ᵗʰ **S93.31** Subluxation and dislocation of tarsal joint

√7ᵗʰ **S93.311** Subluxation of tarsal joint of right foot

√7ᵗʰ **S93.312** Subluxation of tarsal joint of left foot

√7ᵗʰ **S93.313** Subluxation of tarsal joint of unspecified foot

√7ᵗʰ **S93.314** Dislocation of tarsal joint of right foot

√7ᵗʰ **S93.315** Dislocation of tarsal joint of left foot

√7ᵗʰ **S93.316** Dislocation of tarsal joint of unspecified foot

√6ᵗʰ **S93.32** Subluxation and dislocation of tarsometatarsal joint

√7ᵗʰ **S93.321** Subluxation of tarsometatarsal joint of right foot

√7ᵗʰ **S93.322** Subluxation of tarsometatarsal joint of left foot

√7ᵗʰ **S93.323** Subluxation of tarsometatarsal joint of unspecified foot

√7ᵗʰ **S93.324** Dislocation of tarsometatarsal joint of right foot

√7ᵗʰ **S93.325** Dislocation of tarsometatarsal joint of left foot

√7ᵗʰ **S93.326** Dislocation of tarsometatarsal joint of unspecified foot

√6ᵗʰ **S93.33** Other subluxation and dislocation of foot

√7ᵗʰ **S93.331** Other subluxation of right foot

√7ᵗʰ **S93.332** Other subluxation of left foot

√7ᵗʰ **S93.333** Other subluxation of unspecified foot

√7ᵗʰ **S93.334** Other dislocation of right foot

√7ᵗʰ **S93.335** Other dislocation of left foot

√7ᵗʰ **S93.336** Other dislocation of unspecified foot

√5ᵗʰ **S93.4** Sprain of ankle

     EXCLUDES 2   *injury of Achilles tendon (S86.0-)*

√6ᵗʰ **S93.40** Sprain of unspecified ligament of ankle

     Sprain of ankle NOS
     Sprained ankle NOS

√7ᵗʰ **S93.401** Sprain of unspecified ligament of right ankle

√7ᵗʰ **S93.402** Sprain of unspecified ligament of left ankle

√7ᵗʰ **S93.409** Sprain of unspecified ligament of unspecified ankle

√6ᵗʰ **S93.41** Sprain of calcaneofibular ligament

√7ᵗʰ **S93.411** Sprain of calcaneofibular ligament of right ankle

√7ᵗʰ **S93.412** Sprain of calcaneofibular ligament of left ankle

√7ᵗʰ **S93.419** Sprain of calcaneofibular ligament of unspecified ankle

√6ᵗʰ **S93.42** Sprain of deltoid ligament

√7ᵗʰ **S93.421** Sprain of deltoid ligament of right ankle

√7ᵗʰ **S93.422** Sprain of deltoid ligament of left ankle

√7ᵗʰ **S93.429** Sprain of deltoid ligament of unspecified ankle

√6ᵗʰ **S93.43** Sprain of tibiofibular ligament

√7ᵗʰ **S93.431** Sprain of tibiofibular ligament of right ankle

√7ᵗʰ **S93.432** Sprain of tibiofibular ligament of left ankle

√7ᵗʰ **S93.439** Sprain of tibiofibular ligament of unspecified ankle

√6ᵗʰ **S93.49** Sprain of other ligament of ankle

     Sprain of internal collateral ligament
     Sprain of talofibular ligament

√7ᵗʰ **S93.491** Sprain of other ligament of right ankle

√7ᵗʰ **S93.492** Sprain of other ligament of left ankle

√7ᵗʰ **S93.499** Sprain of other ligament of unspecified ankle

√5ᵗʰ **S93.5** Sprain of toe

√6ᵗʰ **S93.50** Unspecified sprain of toe

√7ᵗʰ **S93.501** Unspecified sprain of right great toe

√7ᵗʰ **S93.502** Unspecified sprain of left great toe

√7ᵗʰ **S93.503** Unspecified sprain of unspecified great toe

√7ᵗʰ **S93.504** Unspecified sprain of right lesser toe(s)

√7ᵗʰ **S93.505** Unspecified sprain of left lesser toe(s)

√7ᵗʰ **S93.506** Unspecified sprain of unspecified lesser toe(s)

√7ᵗʰ **S93.509** Unspecified sprain of unspecified toe(s)

√6ᵗʰ **S93.51** Sprain of interphalangeal joint of toe

√7ᵗʰ **S93.511** Sprain of interphalangeal joint of right great toe

√7ᵗʰ **S93.512** Sprain of interphalangeal joint of left great toe

√7ᵗʰ **S93.513** Sprain of interphalangeal joint of unspecified great toe

√7ᵗʰ **S93.514** Sprain of interphalangeal joint of right lesser toe(s)

√7ᵗʰ **S93.515** Sprain of interphalangeal joint of left lesser toe(s)

√7ᵗʰ **S93.516** Sprain of interphalangeal joint of unspecified lesser toe(s)

√7ᵗʰ **S93.519** Sprain of interphalangeal joint of unspecified toe(s)

√6ᵗʰ **S93.52** Sprain of metatarsophalangeal joint of toe

√7ᵗʰ **S93.521** Sprain of metatarsophalangeal joint of right great toe

√7ᵗʰ **S93.522** Sprain of metatarsophalangeal joint of left great toe

√7ᵗʰ **S93.523** Sprain of metatarsophalangeal joint of unspecified great toe

√7ᵗʰ **S93.524** Sprain of metatarsophalangeal joint of right lesser toe(s)

√7ᵗʰ **S93.525** Sprain of metatarsophalangeal joint of left lesser toe(s)

√7ᵗʰ **S93.526** Sprain of metatarsophalangeal joint of unspecified lesser toe(s)

√7ᵗʰ **S93.529** Sprain of metatarsophalangeal joint of unspecified toe(s)

√5ᵗʰ **S93.6** Sprain of foot

     EXCLUDES 2   *sprain of metatarsophalangeal joint of toe (S93.52-)*
                sprain of toe (S93.5-)

√6ᵗʰ **S93.60** Unspecified sprain of foot

√7ᵗʰ **S93.601** Unspecified sprain of right foot

√7ᵗʰ **S93.602** Unspecified sprain of left foot

√7ᵗʰ **S93.609** Unspecified sprain of unspecified foot

√6ᵗʰ **S93.61** Sprain of tarsal ligament of foot

     √7ᵗʰ **S93.611** Sprain of tarsal ligament of right foot

     √7ᵗʰ **S93.612** Sprain of tarsal ligament of left foot

     √7ᵗʰ **S93.619** Sprain of tarsal ligament of unspecified foot

√6ᵗʰ **S93.62** Sprain of tarsometatarsal ligament of foot

     √7ᵗʰ **S93.621** Sprain of tarsometatarsal ligament of right foot

     √7ᵗʰ **S93.622** Sprain of tarsometatarsal ligament of left foot

     √7ᵗʰ **S93.629** Sprain of tarsometatarsal ligament of unspecified foot

√6ᵗʰ **S93.69** Other sprain of foot

     √7ᵗʰ **S93.691** Other sprain of right foot

     √7ᵗʰ **S93.692** Other sprain of left foot

     √7ᵗʰ **S93.699** Other sprain of unspecified foot

√4ᵗʰ **S94 Injury of nerves at ankle and foot level**

Code also any associated open wound (S91.-)

> The appropriate 7th character is to be added to each code from category S94.
> A initial encounter
> D subsequent encounter
> S sequela

√5ᵗʰ **S94.0** Injury of lateral plantar nerve

   √x7ᵗʰ **S94.00** Injury of lateral plantar nerve, unspecified leg

   √x7ᵗʰ **S94.01** Injury of lateral plantar nerve, right leg

   √x7ᵗʰ **S94.02** Injury of lateral plantar nerve, left leg

√5ᵗʰ **S94.1** Injury of medial plantar nerve

   √x7ᵗʰ **S94.10** Injury of medial plantar nerve, unspecified leg

   √x7ᵗʰ **S94.11** Injury of medial plantar nerve, right leg

   √x7ᵗʰ **S94.12** Injury of medial plantar nerve, left leg

√5ᵗʰ **S94.2** Injury of deep peroneal nerve at ankle and foot level

Injury of terminal, lateral branch of deep peroneal nerve

   √x7ᵗʰ **S94.20** Injury of deep peroneal nerve at ankle and foot level, unspecified leg

   √x7ᵗʰ **S94.21** Injury of deep peroneal nerve at ankle and foot level, right leg

   √x7ᵗʰ **S94.22** Injury of deep peroneal nerve at ankle and foot level, left leg

√5ᵗʰ **S94.3** Injury of cutaneous sensory nerve at ankle and foot level

   √x7ᵗʰ **S94.30** Injury of cutaneous sensory nerve at ankle and foot level, unspecified leg

   √x7ᵗʰ **S94.31** Injury of cutaneous sensory nerve at ankle and foot level, right leg

   √x7ᵗʰ **S94.32** Injury of cutaneous sensory nerve at ankle and foot level, left leg

√5ᵗʰ **S94.8** Injury of other nerves at ankle and foot level

   √6ᵗʰ **S94.8X** Injury of other nerves at ankle and foot level

     √7ᵗʰ **S94.8X1** Injury of other nerves at ankle and foot level, right leg

     √7ᵗʰ **S94.8X2** Injury of other nerves at ankle and foot level, left leg

     √7ᵗʰ **S94.8X9** Injury of other nerves at ankle and foot level, unspecified leg

√5ᵗʰ **S94.9** Injury of unspecified nerve at ankle and foot level

   √x7ᵗʰ **S94.90** Injury of unspecified nerve at ankle and foot level, unspecified leg

   √x7ᵗʰ **S94.91** Injury of unspecified nerve at ankle and foot level, right leg

   √x7ᵗʰ **S94.92** Injury of unspecified nerve at ankle and foot level, left leg

√4ᵗʰ **S95 Injury of blood vessels at ankle and foot level**

Code also any associated open wound (S91.-)

EXCLUDES 2   *injury of posterior tibial artery and vein (S85.1-, S85.8-)*

> The appropriate 7th character is to be added to each code from category S95.
> A initial encounter
> D subsequent encounter
> S sequela

√5ᵗʰ **S95.0** Injury of dorsal artery of foot

   √6ᵗʰ **S95.00** Unspecified injury of dorsal artery of foot

     √7ᵗʰ **S95.001** Unspecified injury of dorsal artery of right foot

     √7ᵗʰ **S95.002** Unspecified injury of dorsal artery of left foot

     √7ᵗʰ **S95.009** Unspecified injury of dorsal artery of unspecified foot

   √6ᵗʰ **S95.01** Laceration of dorsal artery of foot

     √7ᵗʰ **S95.011** Laceration of dorsal artery of right foot

     √7ᵗʰ **S95.012** Laceration of dorsal artery of left foot

     √7ᵗʰ **S95.019** Laceration of dorsal artery of unspecified foot

   √6ᵗʰ **S95.09** Other specified injury of dorsal artery of foot

     √7ᵗʰ **S95.091** Other specified injury of dorsal artery of right foot

     √7ᵗʰ **S95.092** Other specified injury of dorsal artery of left foot

     √7ᵗʰ **S95.099** Other specified injury of dorsal artery of unspecified foot

√5ᵗʰ **S95.1** Injury of plantar artery of foot

   √6ᵗʰ **S95.10** Unspecified injury of plantar artery of foot

     √7ᵗʰ **S95.101** Unspecified injury of plantar artery of right foot

     √7ᵗʰ **S95.102** Unspecified injury of plantar artery of left foot

     √7ᵗʰ **S95.109** Unspecified injury of plantar artery of unspecified foot

   √6ᵗʰ **S95.11** Laceration of plantar artery of foot

     √7ᵗʰ **S95.111** Laceration of plantar artery of right foot

     √7ᵗʰ **S95.112** Laceration of plantar artery of left foot

     √7ᵗʰ **S95.119** Laceration of plantar artery of unspecified foot

   √6ᵗʰ **S95.19** Other specified injury of plantar artery of foot

     √7ᵗʰ **S95.191** Other specified injury of plantar artery of right foot

     √7ᵗʰ **S95.192** Other specified injury of plantar artery of left foot

     √7ᵗʰ **S95.199** Other specified injury of plantar artery of unspecified foot

√5ᵗʰ **S95.2** Injury of dorsal vein of foot

   √6ᵗʰ **S95.20** Unspecified injury of dorsal vein of foot

     √7ᵗʰ **S95.201** Unspecified injury of dorsal vein of right foot

     √7ᵗʰ **S95.202** Unspecified injury of dorsal vein of left foot

     √7ᵗʰ **S95.209** Unspecified injury of dorsal vein of unspecified foot

   √6ᵗʰ **S95.21** Laceration of dorsal vein of foot

     √7ᵗʰ **S95.211** Laceration of dorsal vein of right foot

     √7ᵗʰ **S95.212** Laceration of dorsal vein of left foot

     √7ᵗʰ **S95.219** Laceration of dorsal vein of unspecified foot

   √6ᵗʰ **S95.29** Other specified injury of dorsal vein of foot

     √7ᵗʰ **S95.291** Other specified injury of dorsal vein of right foot

     √7ᵗʰ **S95.292** Other specified injury of dorsal vein of left foot

     √7ᵗʰ **S95.299** Other specified injury of dorsal vein of unspecified foot

√5ᵗʰ **S95.8** Injury of other blood vessels at ankle and foot level

   √6ᵗʰ **S95.80** Unspecified injury of other blood vessels at ankle and foot level

     √7ᵗʰ **S95.801** Unspecified injury of other blood vessels at ankle and foot level, right leg

     √7ᵗʰ **S95.802** Unspecified injury of other blood vessels at ankle and foot level, left leg

     √7ᵗʰ **S95.809** Unspecified injury of other blood vessels at ankle and foot level, unspecified leg

☑6ᵗʰ **S95.81** Laceration of other blood vessels at ankle and foot level

     ☑7ᵗʰ **S95.811** Laceration of other blood vessels at ankle and foot level, right leg

     ☑7ᵗʰ **S95.812** Laceration of other blood vessels at ankle and foot level, left leg

     ☑7ᵗʰ **S95.819** Laceration of other blood vessels at ankle and foot level, unspecified leg

☑6ᵗʰ **S95.89** Other specified injury of other blood vessels at ankle and foot level

     ☑7ᵗʰ **S95.891** Other specified injury of other blood vessels at ankle and foot level, right leg

     ☑7ᵗʰ **S95.892** Other specified injury of other blood vessels at ankle and foot level, left leg

     ☑7ᵗʰ **S95.899** Other specified injury of other blood vessels at ankle and foot level, unspecified leg

☑5ᵗʰ **S95.9** Injury of unspecified blood vessel at ankle and foot level

   ☑6ᵗʰ **S95.90** Unspecified injury of unspecified blood vessel at ankle and foot level

     ☑7ᵗʰ **S95.901** Unspecified injury of unspecified blood vessel at ankle and foot level, right leg

     ☑7ᵗʰ **S95.902** Unspecified injury of unspecified blood vessel at ankle and foot level, left leg

     ☑7ᵗʰ **S95.909** Unspecified injury of unspecified blood vessel at ankle and foot level, unspecified leg

   ☑6ᵗʰ **S95.91** Laceration of unspecified blood vessel at ankle and foot level

     ☑7ᵗʰ **S95.911** Laceration of unspecified blood vessel at ankle and foot level, right leg

     ☑7ᵗʰ **S95.912** Laceration of unspecified blood vessel at ankle and foot level, left leg

     ☑7ᵗʰ **S95.919** Laceration of unspecified blood vessel at ankle and foot level, unspecified leg

   ☑6ᵗʰ **S95.99** Other specified injury of unspecified blood vessel at ankle and foot level

     ☑7ᵗʰ **S95.991** Other specified injury of unspecified blood vessel at ankle and foot level, right leg

     ☑7ᵗʰ **S95.992** Other specified injury of unspecified blood vessel at ankle and foot level, left leg

     ☑7ᵗʰ **S95.999** Other specified injury of unspecified blood vessel at ankle and foot level, unspecified leg

☑4ᵗʰ **S96 Injury of muscle and tendon at ankle and foot level**

   Code also any associated open wound (S91.-)

   EXCLUDES 2   injury of Achilles tendon (S86.0-)

            sprain of joints and ligaments of ankle and foot (S93.-)

   TIP: Refer to the Muscle/Tendon table at the beginning of this chapter,

   The appropriate 7th character is to be added to each code from category S96.
   A   initial encounter
   D   subsequent encounter
   S   sequela

☑5ᵗʰ **S96.0** Injury of muscle and tendon of long flexor muscle of toe at ankle and foot level

   ☑6ᵗʰ **S96.00** Unspecified injury of muscle and tendon of long flexor muscle of toe at ankle and foot level

     ☑7ᵗʰ **S96.001** Unspecified injury of muscle and tendon of long flexor muscle of toe at ankle and foot level, right foot

     ☑7ᵗʰ **S96.002** Unspecified injury of muscle and tendon of long flexor muscle of toe at ankle and foot level, left foot

     ☑7ᵗʰ **S96.009** Unspecified injury of muscle and tendon of long flexor muscle of toe at ankle and foot level, unspecified foot

   ☑6ᵗʰ **S96.01** Strain of muscle and tendon of long flexor muscle of toe at ankle and foot level

     ☑7ᵗʰ **S96.011** Strain of muscle and tendon of long flexor muscle of toe at ankle and foot level, right foot

     ☑7ᵗʰ **S96.012** Strain of muscle and tendon of long flexor muscle of toe at ankle and foot level, left foot

     ☑7ᵗʰ **S96.019** Strain of muscle and tendon of long flexor muscle of toe at ankle and foot level, unspecified foot

☑6ᵗʰ **S96.02** Laceration of muscle and tendon of long flexor muscle of toe at ankle and foot level

     ☑7ᵗʰ **S96.021** Laceration of muscle and tendon of long flexor muscle of toe at ankle and foot level, right foot

     ☑7ᵗʰ **S96.022** Laceration of muscle and tendon of long flexor muscle of toe at ankle and foot level, left foot

     ☑7ᵗʰ **S96.029** Laceration of muscle and tendon of long flexor muscle of toe at ankle and foot level, unspecified foot

☑6ᵗʰ **S96.09** Other injury of muscle and tendon of long flexor muscle of toe at ankle and foot level

     ☑7ᵗʰ **S96.091** Other injury of muscle and tendon of long flexor muscle of toe at ankle and foot level, right foot

     ☑7ᵗʰ **S96.092** Other injury of muscle and tendon of long flexor muscle of toe at ankle and foot level, left foot

     ☑7ᵗʰ **S96.099** Other injury of muscle and tendon of long flexor muscle of toe at ankle and foot level, unspecified foot

☑5ᵗʰ **S96.1** Injury of muscle and tendon of long extensor muscle of toe at ankle and foot level

   ☑6ᵗʰ **S96.10** Unspecified injury of muscle and tendon of long extensor muscle of toe at ankle and foot level

     ☑7ᵗʰ **S96.101** Unspecified injury of muscle and tendon of long extensor muscle of toe at ankle and foot level, right foot

     ☑7ᵗʰ **S96.102** Unspecified injury of muscle and tendon of long extensor muscle of toe at ankle and foot level, left foot

     ☑7ᵗʰ **S96.109** Unspecified injury of muscle and tendon of long extensor muscle of toe at ankle and foot level, unspecified foot

   ☑6ᵗʰ **S96.11** Strain of muscle and tendon of long extensor muscle of toe at ankle and foot level

     ☑7ᵗʰ **S96.111** Strain of muscle and tendon of long extensor muscle of toe at ankle and foot level, right foot

     ☑7ᵗʰ **S96.112** Strain of muscle and tendon of long extensor muscle of toe at ankle and foot level, left foot

     ☑7ᵗʰ **S96.119** Strain of muscle and tendon of long extensor muscle of toe at ankle and foot level, unspecified foot

   ☑6ᵗʰ **S96.12** Laceration of muscle and tendon of long extensor muscle of toe at ankle and foot level

     ☑7ᵗʰ **S96.121** Laceration of muscle and tendon of long extensor muscle of toe at ankle and foot level, right foot

     ☑7ᵗʰ **S96.122** Laceration of muscle and tendon of long extensor muscle of toe at ankle and foot level, left foot

     ☑7ᵗʰ **S96.129** Laceration of muscle and tendon of long extensor muscle of toe at ankle and foot level, unspecified foot

   ☑6ᵗʰ **S96.19** Other specified injury of muscle and tendon of long extensor muscle of toe at ankle and foot level

     ☑7ᵗʰ **S96.191** Other specified injury of muscle and tendon of long extensor muscle of toe at ankle and foot level, right foot

     ☑7ᵗʰ **S96.192** Other specified injury of muscle and tendon of long extensor muscle of toe at ankle and foot level, left foot

     ☑7ᵗʰ **S96.199** Other specified injury of muscle and tendon of long extensor muscle of toe at ankle and foot level, unspecified foot

☑5ᵗʰ **S96.2** Injury of intrinsic muscle and tendon at ankle and foot level

   ☑6ᵗʰ **S96.20** Unspecified injury of intrinsic muscle and tendon at ankle and foot level

     ☑7ᵗʰ **S96.201** Unspecified injury of intrinsic muscle and tendon at ankle and foot level, right foot

     ☑7ᵗʰ **S96.202** Unspecified injury of intrinsic muscle and tendon at ankle and foot level, left foot

     ☑7ᵗʰ **S96.209** Unspecified injury of intrinsic muscle and tendon at ankle and foot level, unspecified foot

   ☑6ᵗʰ **S96.21** Strain of intrinsic muscle and tendon at ankle and foot level

     ☑7ᵗʰ **S96.211** Strain of intrinsic muscle and tendon at ankle and foot level, right foot

     ☑7ᵗʰ **S96.212** Strain of intrinsic muscle and tendon at ankle and foot level, left foot

√7ᵗʰ **S96.219** Strain of intrinsic muscle and tendon at ankle and foot level, unspecified foot

√6ᵗʰ **S96.22** Laceration of intrinsic muscle and tendon at ankle and foot level

√7ᵗʰ **S96.221** Laceration of intrinsic muscle and tendon at ankle and foot level, right foot

√7ᵗʰ **S96.222** Laceration of intrinsic muscle and tendon at ankle and foot level, left foot

√7ᵗʰ **S96.229** Laceration of intrinsic muscle and tendon at ankle and foot level, unspecified foot

√6ᵗʰ **S96.29** Other specified injury of intrinsic muscle and tendon at ankle and foot level

√7ᵗʰ **S96.291** Other specified injury of intrinsic muscle and tendon at ankle and foot level, right foot

√7ᵗʰ **S96.292** Other specified injury of intrinsic muscle and tendon at ankle and foot level, left foot

√7ᵗʰ **S96.299** Other specified injury of intrinsic muscle and tendon at ankle and foot level, unspecified foot

√5ᵗʰ **S96.8** Injury of other specified muscles and tendons at ankle and foot level

√6ᵗʰ **S96.80** Unspecified injury of other specified muscles and tendons at ankle and foot level

√7ᵗʰ **S96.801** Unspecified injury of other specified muscles and tendons at ankle and foot level, right foot

√7ᵗʰ **S96.802** Unspecified injury of other specified muscles and tendons at ankle and foot level, left foot

√7ᵗʰ **S96.809** Unspecified injury of other specified muscles and tendons at ankle and foot level, unspecified foot

√6ᵗʰ **S96.81** Strain of other specified muscles and tendons at ankle and foot level

√7ᵗʰ **S96.811** Strain of other specified muscles and tendons at ankle and foot level, right foot

√7ᵗʰ **S96.812** Strain of other specified muscles and tendons at ankle and foot level, left foot

√7ᵗʰ **S96.819** Strain of other specified muscles and tendons at ankle and foot level, unspecified foot

√6ᵗʰ **S96.82** Laceration of other specified muscles and tendons at ankle and foot level

√7ᵗʰ **S96.821** Laceration of other specified muscles and tendons at ankle and foot level, right foot

√7ᵗʰ **S96.822** Laceration of other specified muscles and tendons at ankle and foot level, left foot

√7ᵗʰ **S96.829** Laceration of other specified muscles and tendons at ankle and foot level, unspecified foot

√6ᵗʰ **S96.89** Other specified injury of other specified muscles and tendons at ankle and foot level

√7ᵗʰ **S96.891** Other specified injury of other specified muscles and tendons at ankle and foot level, right foot

√7ᵗʰ **S96.892** Other specified injury of other specified muscles and tendons at ankle and foot level, left foot

√7ᵗʰ **S96.899** Other specified injury of other specified muscles and tendons at ankle and foot level, unspecified foot

√5ᵗʰ **S96.9** Injury of unspecified muscle and tendon at ankle and foot level

√6ᵗʰ **S96.90** Unspecified injury of unspecified muscle and tendon at ankle and foot level

√7ᵗʰ **S96.901** Unspecified injury of unspecified muscle and tendon at ankle and foot level, right foot

√7ᵗʰ **S96.902** Unspecified injury of unspecified muscle and tendon at ankle and foot level, left foot

√7ᵗʰ **S96.909** Unspecified injury of unspecified muscle and tendon at ankle and foot level, unspecified foot

√6ᵗʰ **S96.91** Strain of unspecified muscle and tendon at ankle and foot level

√7ᵗʰ **S96.911** Strain of unspecified muscle and tendon at ankle and foot level, right foot

√7ᵗʰ **S96.912** Strain of unspecified muscle and tendon at ankle and foot level, left foot

√7ᵗʰ **S96.919** Strain of unspecified muscle and tendon at ankle and foot level, unspecified foot

√6ᵗʰ **S96.92** Laceration of unspecified muscle and tendon at ankle and foot level

√7ᵗʰ **S96.921** Laceration of unspecified muscle and tendon at ankle and foot level, right foot

√7ᵗʰ **S96.922** Laceration of unspecified muscle and tendon at ankle and foot level, left foot

√7ᵗʰ **S96.929** Laceration of unspecified muscle and tendon at ankle and foot level, unspecified foot

√6ᵗʰ **S96.99** Other specified injury of unspecified muscle and tendon at ankle and foot level

√7ᵗʰ **S96.991** Other specified injury of unspecified muscle and tendon at ankle and foot level, right foot

√7ᵗʰ **S96.992** Other specified injury of unspecified muscle and tendon at ankle and foot level, left foot

√7ᵗʰ **S96.999** Other specified injury of unspecified muscle and tendon at ankle and foot level, unspecified foot

√4ᵗʰ **S97** **Crushing injury of ankle and foot**

Use additional code(s) for all associated injuries

The appropriate 7th character is to be added to each code from category S97.
A   initial encounter
D   subsequent encounter
S   sequela

√5ᵗʰ **S97.0** Crushing injury of ankle

√x7ᵗʰ **S97.00** Crushing injury of unspecified ankle

√x7ᵗʰ **S97.01** Crushing injury of right ankle

√x7ᵗʰ **S97.02** Crushing injury of left ankle

√5ᵗʰ **S97.1** Crushing injury of toe

√6ᵗʰ **S97.10** Crushing injury of unspecified toe(s)

√7ᵗʰ **S97.101** Crushing injury of unspecified right toe(s)

√7ᵗʰ **S97.102** Crushing injury of unspecified left toe(s)

√7ᵗʰ **S97.109** Crushing injury of unspecified toe(s)

Crushing injury of toe NOS

√6ᵗʰ **S97.11** Crushing injury of great toe

√7ᵗʰ **S97.111** Crushing injury of right great toe

√7ᵗʰ **S97.112** Crushing injury of left great toe

√7ᵗʰ **S97.119** Crushing injury of unspecified great toe

√6ᵗʰ **S97.12** Crushing injury of lesser toe(s)

√7ᵗʰ **S97.121** Crushing injury of right lesser toe(s)

√7ᵗʰ **S97.122** Crushing injury of left lesser toe(s)

√7ᵗʰ **S97.129** Crushing injury of unspecified lesser toe(s)

√5ᵗʰ **S97.8** Crushing injury of foot

√x7ᵗʰ **S97.80** Crushing injury of unspecified foot

Crushing injury of foot NOS

√x7ᵗʰ **S97.81** Crushing injury of right foot

√x7ᵗʰ **S97.82** Crushing injury of left foot

√4ᵗʰ **S98** **Traumatic amputation of ankle and foot**

An amputation not identified as partial or complete should be coded to complete

The appropriate 7th character is to be added to each code from category S98.
A   initial encounter
D   subsequent encounter
S   sequela

√5ᵗʰ **S98.0** Traumatic amputation of foot at ankle level

√6ᵗʰ **S98.01** Complete traumatic amputation of foot at ankle level

√7ᵗʰ **S98.011** Complete traumatic amputation of right foot at ankle level   HCC ESR COM

√7ᵗʰ **S98.012** Complete traumatic amputation of left foot at ankle level   HCC ESR COM

√7ᵗʰ **S98.019** Complete traumatic amputation of unspecified foot at ankle level   HCC ESR COM

√6ᵗʰ **S98.02** Partial traumatic amputation of foot at ankle level

√7ᵗʰ **S98.021** Partial traumatic amputation of right foot at ankle level   HCC ESR COM

√7ᵗʰ **S98.022** Partial traumatic amputation of left foot at ankle level   HCC ESR COM

√7ᵗʰ **S98.029** Partial traumatic amputation of unspecified foot at ankle level `HCC` `ESR` `COM`

√5ᵗʰ **S98.1** Traumatic amputation of one toe

  √6ᵗʰ **S98.11** Complete traumatic amputation of great toe

    √7ᵗʰ **S98.111** Complete traumatic amputation of right great toe `HCC` `ESR`

    √7ᵗʰ **S98.112** Complete traumatic amputation of left great toe `HCC` `ESR`

    √7ᵗʰ **S98.119** Complete traumatic amputation of unspecified great toe `HCC` `ESR`

  √6ᵗʰ **S98.12** Partial traumatic amputation of great toe

    √7ᵗʰ **S98.121** Partial traumatic amputation of right great toe `HCC` `ESR`

    √7ᵗʰ **S98.122** Partial traumatic amputation of left great toe `HCC` `ESR`

    √7ᵗʰ **S98.129** Partial traumatic amputation of unspecified great toe `HCC` `ESR`

  √6ᵗʰ **S98.13** Complete traumatic amputation of one lesser toe

    Traumatic amputation of toe NOS

    √7ᵗʰ **S98.131** Complete traumatic amputation of one right lesser toe `HCC` `ESR`

    √7ᵗʰ **S98.132** Complete traumatic amputation of one left lesser toe `HCC` `ESR`

    √7ᵗʰ **S98.139** Complete traumatic amputation of one unspecified lesser toe `HCC` `ESR`

  √6ᵗʰ **S98.14** Partial traumatic amputation of one lesser toe

    √7ᵗʰ **S98.141** Partial traumatic amputation of one right lesser toe `HCC` `ESR`

    √7ᵗʰ **S98.142** Partial traumatic amputation of one left lesser toe `HCC` `ESR`

    √7ᵗʰ **S98.149** Partial traumatic amputation of one unspecified lesser toe `HCC` `ESR`

√5ᵗʰ **S98.2** Traumatic amputation of two or more lesser toes

  √6ᵗʰ **S98.21** Complete traumatic amputation of two or more lesser toes

    √7ᵗʰ **S98.211** Complete traumatic amputation of two or more right lesser toes `HCC` `ESR`

    √7ᵗʰ **S98.212** Complete traumatic amputation of two or more left lesser toes `HCC` `ESR`

    √7ᵗʰ **S98.219** Complete traumatic amputation of two or more unspecified lesser toes `HCC` `ESR`

  √6ᵗʰ **S98.22** Partial traumatic amputation of two or more lesser toes

    √7ᵗʰ **S98.221** Partial traumatic amputation of two or more right lesser toes `HCC` `ESR`

    √7ᵗʰ **S98.222** Partial traumatic amputation of two or more left lesser toes `HCC` `ESR`

    √7ᵗʰ **S98.229** Partial traumatic amputation of two or more unspecified lesser toes `HCC` `ESR`

√5ᵗʰ **S98.3** Traumatic amputation of midfoot

  √6ᵗʰ **S98.31** Complete traumatic amputation of midfoot

    √7ᵗʰ **S98.311** Complete traumatic amputation of right midfoot `HCC` `ESR` `COM`

    √7ᵗʰ **S98.312** Complete traumatic amputation of left midfoot `HCC` `ESR` `COM`

    √7ᵗʰ **S98.319** Complete traumatic amputation of unspecified midfoot `HCC` `ESR` `COM`

  √6ᵗʰ **S98.32** Partial traumatic amputation of midfoot

    √7ᵗʰ **S98.321** Partial traumatic amputation of right midfoot `HCC` `ESR` `COM`

    √7ᵗʰ **S98.322** Partial traumatic amputation of left midfoot `HCC` `ESR` `COM`

    √7ᵗʰ **S98.329** Partial traumatic amputation of unspecified midfoot `HCC` `ESR` `COM`

√5ᵗʰ **S98.9** Traumatic amputation of foot, level unspecified

  √6ᵗʰ **S98.91** Complete traumatic amputation of foot, level unspecified

    √7ᵗʰ **S98.911** Complete traumatic amputation of right foot, level unspecified `HCC` `ESR` `COM`

    √7ᵗʰ **S98.912** Complete traumatic amputation of left foot, level unspecified `HCC` `ESR` `COM`

    √7ᵗʰ **S98.919** Complete traumatic amputation of unspecified foot, level unspecified `HCC` `ESR` `COM`

  √6ᵗʰ **S98.92** Partial traumatic amputation of foot, level unspecified

    √7ᵗʰ **S98.921** Partial traumatic amputation of right foot, level unspecified `HCC` `ESR` `COM`

    √7ᵗʰ **S98.922** Partial traumatic amputation of left foot, level unspecified `HCC` `ESR` `COM`

    √7ᵗʰ **S98.929** Partial traumatic amputation of unspecified foot, level unspecified `HCC` `ESR` `COM`

√4ᵗʰ **S99** Other and unspecified injuries of ankle and foot

  AHA: 2018,2Q,12; 2018,1Q,3; 2016,4Q,68-69

√5ᵗʰ **S99.0** Physeal fracture of calcaneus

  AHA: 2019,4Q,56

> The appropriate 7th character is to be added to each code from subcategory S99.0.
> A   initial encounter for closed fracture
> B   initial encounter for open fracture
> D   subsequent encounter for fracture with routine healing
> G   subsequent encounter for fracture with delayed healing
> K   subsequent encounter for fracture with nonunion
> P   subsequent encounter for fracture with malunion
> S   sequela

  √6ᵗʰ **S99.00** Unspecified physeal fracture of calcaneus

    √7ᵗʰ **S99.001** Unspecified physeal fracture of right calcaneus `Q`

    √7ᵗʰ **S99.002** Unspecified physeal fracture of left calcaneus `Q`

    √7ᵗʰ **S99.009** Unspecified physeal fracture of unspecified calcaneus `Q`

  √6ᵗʰ **S99.01** Salter-Harris Type I physeal fracture of calcaneus

    √7ᵗʰ **S99.011** Salter-Harris Type I physeal fracture of right calcaneus `Q`

    √7ᵗʰ **S99.012** Salter-Harris Type I physeal fracture of left calcaneus `Q`

    √7ᵗʰ **S99.019** Salter-Harris Type I physeal fracture of unspecified calcaneus `Q`

  √6ᵗʰ **S99.02** Salter-Harris Type II physeal fracture of calcaneus

    √7ᵗʰ **S99.021** Salter-Harris Type II physeal fracture of right calcaneus `Q`

    √7ᵗʰ **S99.022** Salter-Harris Type II physeal fracture of left calcaneus `Q`

    √7ᵗʰ **S99.029** Salter-Harris Type II physeal fracture of unspecified calcaneus `Q`

  √6ᵗʰ **S99.03** Salter-Harris Type III physeal fracture of calcaneus

    √7ᵗʰ **S99.031** Salter-Harris Type III physeal fracture of right calcaneus `Q`

    √7ᵗʰ **S99.032** Salter-Harris Type III physeal fracture of left calcaneus `Q`

    √7ᵗʰ **S99.039** Salter-Harris Type III physeal fracture of unspecified calcaneus `Q`

  √6ᵗʰ **S99.04** Salter-Harris Type IV physeal fracture of calcaneus

    √7ᵗʰ **S99.041** Salter-Harris Type IV physeal fracture of right calcaneus `Q`

    √7ᵗʰ **S99.042** Salter-Harris Type IV physeal fracture of left calcaneus `Q`

    √7ᵗʰ **S99.049** Salter-Harris Type IV physeal fracture of unspecified calcaneus `Q`

  √6ᵗʰ **S99.09** Other physeal fracture of calcaneus

    √7ᵗʰ **S99.091** Other physeal fracture of right calcaneus `Q`

    √7ᵗʰ **S99.092** Other physeal fracture of left calcaneus `Q`

    √7ᵗʰ **S99.099** Other physeal fracture of unspecified calcaneus `Q`

`HCC` CMS-HCC   `Rx` Rx HCC   `ESR` ESRD HCC   `COM` Commercial HCC   `N` Newborn: 0   `P` Pediatric: 0-17   `M` Maternity: 9-64   `A` Adult: 15-124

1112   ICD-10-CM 2023

√5ᵗʰ **S99.1 Physeal fracture of metatarsal**

AHA: 2019,4Q,56

The appropriate 7th character is to be added to each code from subcategory S99.1
- A initial encounter for closed fracture
- B initial encounter for open fracture
- D subsequent encounter for fracture with routine healing
- G subsequent encounter for fracture with delayed healing
- K subsequent encounter for fracture with nonunion
- P subsequent encounter for fracture with malunion
- S sequela

√6ᵗʰ **S99.10   Unspecified physeal fracture of metatarsal**

√7ᵗʰ **S99.101   Unspecified physeal fracture of right metatarsal** Q

√7ᵗʰ **S99.102   Unspecified physeal fracture of left metatarsal** Q

√7ᵗʰ **S99.109   Unspecified physeal fracture of unspecified metatarsal** Q

√6ᵗʰ **S99.11   Salter-Harris Type I physeal fracture of metatarsal**

√7ᵗʰ **S99.111   Salter-Harris Type I physeal fracture of right metatarsal** Q

√7ᵗʰ **S99.112   Salter-Harris Type I physeal fracture of left metatarsal** Q

√7ᵗʰ **S99.119   Salter-Harris Type I physeal fracture of unspecified metatarsal** Q

√6ᵗʰ **S99.12   Salter-Harris Type II physeal fracture of metatarsal**

√7ᵗʰ **S99.121   Salter-Harris Type II physeal fracture of right metatarsal** Q

√7ᵗʰ **S99.122   Salter-Harris Type II physeal fracture of left metatarsal** Q

√7ᵗʰ **S99.129   Salter-Harris Type II physeal fracture of unspecified metatarsal** Q

√6ᵗʰ **S99.13   Salter-Harris Type III physeal fracture of metatarsal**

√7ᵗʰ **S99.131   Salter-Harris Type III physeal fracture of right metatarsal** Q

√7ᵗʰ **S99.132   Salter-Harris Type III physeal fracture of left metatarsal** Q

√7ᵗʰ **S99.139   Salter-Harris Type III physeal fracture of unspecified metatarsal** Q

√6ᵗʰ **S99.14   Salter-Harris Type IV physeal fracture of metatarsal**

√7ᵗʰ **S99.141   Salter-Harris Type IV physeal fracture of right metatarsal** Q

√7ᵗʰ **S99.142   Salter-Harris Type IV physeal fracture of left metatarsal** Q

√7ᵗʰ **S99.149   Salter-Harris Type IV physeal fracture of unspecified metatarsal** Q

√6ᵗʰ **S99.19   Other physeal fracture of metatarsal**

√7ᵗʰ **S99.191   Other physeal fracture of right metatarsal** Q

√7ᵗʰ **S99.192   Other physeal fracture of left metatarsal** Q

√7ᵗʰ **S99.199   Other physeal fracture of unspecified metatarsal** Q

√5ᵗʰ **S99.2 Physeal fracture of phalanx of toe**

AHA: 2019,4Q,56

The appropriate 7th character is to be added to each code from subcategories S99.2.
- A initial encounter for closed fracture
- B initial encounter for open fracture
- D subsequent encounter for fracture with routine healing
- G subsequent encounter for fracture with delayed healing
- K subsequent encounter for fracture with nonunion
- P subsequent encounter for fracture with malunion
- S sequela

√6ᵗʰ **S99.20   Unspecified physeal fracture of phalanx of toe**

√7ᵗʰ **S99.201   Unspecified physeal fracture of phalanx of right toe**

√7ᵗʰ **S99.202   Unspecified physeal fracture of phalanx of left toe**

√7ᵗʰ **S99.209   Unspecified physeal fracture of phalanx of unspecified toe**

√6ᵗʰ **S99.21   Salter-Harris Type I physeal fracture of phalanx of toe**

√7ᵗʰ **S99.211   Salter-Harris Type I physeal fracture of phalanx of right toe**

√7ᵗʰ **S99.212   Salter-Harris Type I physeal fracture of phalanx of left toe**

√7ᵗʰ **S99.219   Salter-Harris Type I physeal fracture of phalanx of unspecified toe**

√6ᵗʰ **S99.22   Salter-Harris Type II physeal fracture of phalanx of toe**

√7ᵗʰ **S99.221   Salter-Harris Type II physeal fracture of phalanx of right toe**

√7ᵗʰ **S99.222   Salter-Harris Type II physeal fracture of phalanx of left toe**

√7ᵗʰ **S99.229   Salter-Harris Type II physeal fracture of phalanx of unspecified toe**

√6ᵗʰ **S99.23   Salter-Harris Type III physeal fracture of phalanx of toe**

√7ᵗʰ **S99.231   Salter-Harris Type III physeal fracture of phalanx of right toe**

√7ᵗʰ **S99.232   Salter-Harris Type III physeal fracture of phalanx of left toe**

√7ᵗʰ **S99.239   Salter-Harris Type III physeal fracture of phalanx of unspecified toe**

√6ᵗʰ **S99.24   Salter-Harris Type IV physeal fracture of phalanx of toe**

√7ᵗʰ **S99.241   Salter-Harris Type IV physeal fracture of phalanx of right toe**

√7ᵗʰ **S99.242   Salter-Harris Type IV physeal fracture of phalanx of left toe**

√7ᵗʰ **S99.249   Salter-Harris Type IV physeal fracture of phalanx of unspecified toe**

√6ᵗʰ **S99.29   Other physeal fracture of phalanx of toe**

√7ᵗʰ **S99.291   Other physeal fracture of phalanx of right toe**

√7ᵗʰ **S99.292   Other physeal fracture of phalanx of left toe**

√7ᵗʰ **S99.299   Other physeal fracture of phalanx of unspecified toe**

√5ᵗʰ **S99.8 Other specified injuries of ankle and foot**

The appropriate 7th character is to be added to each code from subcategory S99.8.
- A initial encounter
- D subsequent encounter
- S sequela

√6ᵗʰ **S99.81   Other specified injuries of ankle**

√7ᵗʰ **S99.811   Other specified injuries of right ankle**

√7ᵗʰ **S99.812   Other specified injuries of left ankle**

√7ᵗʰ **S99.819   Other specified injuries of unspecified ankle**

√6ᵗʰ **S99.82   Other specified injuries of foot**

√7ᵗʰ **S99.821   Other specified injuries of right foot**

√7ᵗʰ **S99.822   Other specified injuries of left foot**

√7ᵗʰ **S99.829   Other specified injuries of unspecified foot**

√5ᵗʰ **S99.9 Unspecified injury of ankle and foot**

The appropriate 7th character is to be added to each code from subcategory S99.9.
- A initial encounter
- D subsequent encounter
- S sequela

√6ᵗʰ **S99.91   Unspecified injury of ankle**

√7ᵗʰ **S99.911   Unspecified injury of right ankle**

√7ᵗʰ **S99.912   Unspecified injury of left ankle**

√7ᵗʰ **S99.919   Unspecified injury of unspecified ankle**

√6ᵗʰ **S99.92   Unspecified injury of foot**

√7ᵗʰ **S99.921   Unspecified injury of right foot**

√7ᵗʰ **S99.922   Unspecified injury of left foot**

√7ᵗʰ **S99.929   Unspecified injury of unspecified foot**

INJURY, POISONING AND CERTAIN OTHER CONSEQUENCES OF EXTERNAL CAUSES (T07-T88)

Injuries involving multiple body regions (T07)

EXCLUDES 1   burns and corrosions (T20-T32)
frostbite (T33-T34)
insect bite or sting, venomous (T63.4)
sunburn (L55.-)

✓x7th **T07** **Unspecified multiple injuries**

     EXCLUDES 1   injury NOS (T14.90)

     AHA: 2017,4Q,26

The appropriate 7th character is to be added to code T07.
A   initial encounter
D   subsequent encounter
S   sequela

Injury of unspecified body region (T14)

✓4th **T14** **Injury of unspecified body region**

     EXCLUDES 1   multiple unspecified injuries (T07)

     AHA: 2017,4Q,26

The appropriate 7th character is to be added to each code from category T14.
A   initial encounter
D   subsequent encounter
S   sequela

✓x7th **T14.8**   **Other injury of unspecified body region**
     Abrasion NOS
     Contusion NOS
     Crush injury NOS
     Fracture NOS
     Skin injury NOS
     Vascular injury NOS
     Wound NOS

✓5th **T14.9**   **Unspecified injury**

     ✓x7th **T14.90**   **Injury, unspecified**
         Injury NOS

     ✓x7th **T14.91**   **Suicide attempt**   HCC Rx ESR COM
         Attempted suicide NOS

Effects of foreign body entering through natural orifice (T15-T19)

EXCLUDES 2   foreign body accidentally left in operation wound (T81.5-)
foreign body in penetrating wound - see open wound by body region
residual foreign body in soft tissue (M79.5)
splinter, without open wound - see superficial injury by body region

✓4th **T15** **Foreign body on external eye**

     EXCLUDES 2   foreign body in penetrating wound of orbit and eye ball
         (S05.4-, S05.5-)
         open wound of eyelid and periocular area (S01.1-)
         retained foreign body in eyelid (H02.8-)
         retained (old) foreign body in penetrating wound of orbit and
         eye ball (H05.5-, H44.6-, H44.7-)
         superficial foreign body of eyelid and periocular area (S00.25-)

The appropriate 7th character is to be added to each code from category T15.
A   initial encounter
D   subsequent encounter
S   sequela

✓6th **T15.0**   **Foreign body in cornea**
     ✓x7th **T15.00**   **Foreign body in cornea, unspecified eye**
     ✓x7th **T15.01**   **Foreign body in cornea, right eye**
     ✓x7th **T15.02**   **Foreign body in cornea, left eye**

✓5th **T15.1**   **Foreign body in conjunctival sac**
     ✓x7th **T15.10**   **Foreign body in conjunctival sac, unspecified eye**
     ✓x7th **T15.11**   **Foreign body in conjunctival sac, right eye**
     ✓x7th **T15.12**   **Foreign body in conjunctival sac, left eye**

✓6th **T15.8**   **Foreign body in other and multiple parts of external eye**
     Foreign body in lacrimal punctum
     ✓x7th **T15.80**   **Foreign body in other and multiple parts of external eye, unspecified eye**

     ✓x7th **T15.81**   **Foreign body in other and multiple parts of external eye, right eye**
     ✓x7th **T15.82**   **Foreign body in other and multiple parts of external eye, left eye**

✓5th **T15.9**   **Foreign body on external eye, part unspecified**
     ✓x7th **T15.90**   **Foreign body on external eye, part unspecified, unspecified eye**
     ✓x7th **T15.91**   **Foreign body on external eye, part unspecified, right eye**
     ✓x7th **T15.92**   **Foreign body on external eye, part unspecified, left eye**

✓4th **T16** **Foreign body in ear**

     INCLUDES   foreign body in auditory canal

The appropriate 7th character is to be added to each code from category T16.
A   initial encounter
D   subsequent encounter
S   sequela

✓x7th **T16.1**   **Foreign body in right ear**
✓x7th **T16.2**   **Foreign body in left ear**
✓x7th **T16.9**   **Foreign body in ear, unspecified ear**

✓4th **T17** **Foreign body in respiratory tract**

The appropriate 7th character is to be added to each code from category T17.
A   initial encounter
D   subsequent encounter
S   sequela

✓x7th **T17.0**   **Foreign body in nasal sinus**

✓x7th **T17.1**   **Foreign body in nostril**
     Foreign body in nose NOS

✓5th **T17.2**   **Foreign body in pharynx**
     Foreign body in nasopharynx
     Foreign body in throat NOS
     ✓6th **T17.20**   **Unspecified foreign body in pharynx**
         ✓7th **T17.200**   **Unspecified foreign body in pharynx causing asphyxiation**
         ✓7th **T17.208**   **Unspecified foreign body in pharynx causing other injury**
     ✓6th **T17.21**   **Gastric contents in pharynx**
         Aspiration of gastric contents into pharynx
         Vomitus in pharynx
         ✓7th **T17.210**   **Gastric contents in pharynx causing asphyxiation**
         ✓7th **T17.218**   **Gastric contents in pharynx causing other injury**
     ✓6th **T17.22**   **Food in pharynx**
         Bones in pharynx
         Seeds in pharynx
         ✓7th **T17.220**   **Food in pharynx causing asphyxiation**
         ✓7th **T17.228**   **Food in pharynx causing other injury**
     ✓6th **T17.29**   **Other foreign object in pharynx**
         ✓7th **T17.290**   **Other foreign object in pharynx causing asphyxiation**
         ✓7th **T17.298**   **Other foreign object in pharynx causing other injury**

✓5th **T17.3**   **Foreign body in larynx**
     ✓6th **T17.30**   **Unspecified foreign body in larynx**
         ✓7th **T17.300**   **Unspecified foreign body in larynx causing asphyxiation**
         ✓7th **T17.308**   **Unspecified foreign body in larynx causing other injury**
     ✓6th **T17.31**   **Gastric contents in larynx**
         Aspiration of gastric contents into larynx
         Vomitus in larynx
         ✓7th **T17.310**   **Gastric contents in larynx causing asphyxiation**
         ✓7th **T17.318**   **Gastric contents in larynx causing other injury**
     ✓6th **T17.32**   **Food in larynx**
         Bones in larynx
         Seeds in larynx
         ✓7th **T17.320**   **Food in larynx causing asphyxiation**
         ✓7th **T17.328**   **Food in larynx causing other injury**

☑6ᵗʰ   **T17.39**   **Other foreign object in larynx**

    ☑7ᵗʰ   **T17.390**   **Other foreign object in larynx** causing asphyxiation

    ☑7ᵗʰ   **T17.398**   **Other foreign object in larynx** causing other injury

☑5ᵗʰ   **T17.4**   **Foreign body in** trachea

   ☑6ᵗʰ   **T17.40**   **Unspecified foreign body in trachea**

    ☑7ᵗʰ   **T17.400**   **Unspecified foreign body in trachea causing asphyxiation**

    ☑7ᵗʰ   **T17.408**   **Unspecified foreign body in trachea causing other injury**

   ☑6ᵗʰ   **T17.41**   **Gastric contents in trachea**

     Aspiration of gastric contents into trachea
     Vomitus in trachea

    ☑7ᵗʰ   **T17.410**   **Gastric contents in trachea** causing asphyxiation

    ☑7ᵗʰ   **T17.418**   **Gastric contents in trachea** causing other injury

   ☑6ᵗʰ   **T17.42**   **Food in trachea**

     Bones in trachea
     Seeds in trachea

    ☑7ᵗʰ   **T17.420**   **Food in trachea** causing asphyxiation

    ☑7ᵗʰ   **T17.428**   **Food in trachea** causing other injury

   ☑6ᵗʰ   **T17.49**   **Other foreign object in trachea**

    ☑7ᵗʰ   **T17.490**   **Other foreign object in trachea** causing asphyxiation

    ☑7ᵗʰ   **T17.498**   **Other foreign object in trachea** causing other injury

☑5ᵗʰ   **T17.5**   **Foreign body in** bronchus

   ☑6ᵗʰ   **T17.50**   **Unspecified foreign body in bronchus**

    ☑7ᵗʰ   **T17.500**   **Unspecified foreign body in bronchus causing asphyxiation**

    ☑7ᵗʰ   **T17.508**   **Unspecified foreign body in bronchus causing other injury**

   ☑6ᵗʰ   **T17.51**   **Gastric contents in bronchus**

     Aspiration of gastric contents into bronchus
     Vomitus in bronchus

    ☑7ᵗʰ   **T17.510**   **Gastric contents in bronchus** causing asphyxiation

    ☑7ᵗʰ   **T17.518**   **Gastric contents in bronchus** causing other injury

   ☑6ᵗʰ   **T17.52**   **Food in bronchus**

     Bones in bronchus
     Seeds in bronchus

    ☑7ᵗʰ   **T17.520**   **Food in bronchus** causing asphyxiation

    ☑7ᵗʰ   **T17.528**   **Food in bronchus** causing other injury

   ☑6ᵗʰ   **T17.59**   **Other foreign object in bronchus**

    ☑7ᵗʰ   **T17.590**   **Other foreign object in bronchus** causing asphyxiation

    ☑7ᵗʰ   **T17.598**   **Other foreign object in bronchus** causing other injury

☑5ᵗʰ   **T17.8**   **Foreign body in other parts of respiratory tract**

     Foreign body in bronchioles
     Foreign body in lung

   ☑6ᵗʰ   **T17.80**   **Unspecified foreign body in other parts of respiratory tract**

    ☑7ᵗʰ   **T17.800**   **Unspecified foreign body in other parts of respiratory tract** causing asphyxiation

    ☑7ᵗʰ   **T17.808**   **Unspecified foreign body in other parts of respiratory tract** causing other injury

   ☑6ᵗʰ   **T17.81**   **Gastric contents in other parts of respiratory tract**

     Aspiration of gastric contents into other parts of respiratory tract
     Vomitus in other parts of respiratory tract

    ☑7ᵗʰ   **T17.810**   **Gastric contents in other parts of respiratory tract** causing asphyxiation

    ☑7ᵗʰ   **T17.818**   **Gastric contents in other parts of respiratory tract** causing other injury

   ☑6ᵗʰ   **T17.82**   **Food in other parts of respiratory tract**

     Bones in other parts of respiratory tract
     Seeds in other parts of respiratory tract

    ☑7ᵗʰ   **T17.820**   **Food in other parts of respiratory tract causing asphyxiation**

    ☑7ᵗʰ   **T17.828**   **Food in other parts of respiratory tract causing other injury**

☑6ᵗʰ   **T17.89**   **Other foreign object in other parts of respiratory tract**

    ☑7ᵗʰ   **T17.890**   **Other foreign object in other parts of respiratory tract** causing asphyxiation

    ☑7ᵗʰ   **T17.898**   **Other foreign object in other parts of respiratory tract** causing other injury

☑5ᵗʰ   **T17.9**   **Foreign body in respiratory tract, part unspecified**

   ☑6ᵗʰ   **T17.90**   **Unspecified foreign body in respiratory tract, part unspecified**

    ☑7ᵗʰ   **T17.900**   **Unspecified foreign body in respiratory tract, part unspecified** causing asphyxiation

    ☑7ᵗʰ   **T17.908**   **Unspecified foreign body in respiratory tract, part unspecified** causing other injury

   ☑6ᵗʰ   **T17.91**   **Gastric contents in respiratory tract, part unspecified**

     Aspiration of gastric contents into respiratory tract, part unspecified
     Vomitus in trachea respiratory tract, part unspecified

    ☑7ᵗʰ   **T17.910**   **Gastric contents in respiratory tract, part unspecified** causing asphyxiation

    ☑7ᵗʰ   **T17.918**   **Gastric contents in respiratory tract, part unspecified** causing other injury

   ☑6ᵗʰ   **T17.92**   **Food in respiratory tract, part unspecified**

     Bones in respiratory tract, part unspecified
     Seeds in respiratory tract, part unspecified

    ☑7ᵗʰ   **T17.920**   **Food in respiratory tract, part unspecified** causing asphyxiation

    ☑7ᵗʰ   **T17.928**   **Food in respiratory tract, part unspecified** causing other injury

   ☑6ᵗʰ   **T17.99**   **Other foreign object in respiratory tract, part unspecified**

    ☑7ᵗʰ   **T17.990**   **Other foreign object in respiratory tract, part unspecified in** causing asphyxiation
      AHA: 2019,3Q,15

    ☑7ᵗʰ   **T17.998**   **Other foreign object in respiratory tract, part unspecified** causing other injury

☑4ᵗʰ   **T18**   **Foreign body in alimentary tract**

   EXCLUDES 2   *foreign body in pharynx (T17.2-)*

    The appropriate 7th character is to be added to each code from category T18.
    A   initial encounter
    D   subsequent encounter
    S   sequela

☑x7ᵗʰ   **T18.0**   **Foreign body in** mouth

☑5ᵗʰ   **T18.1**   **Foreign body in** esophagus

   EXCLUDES 2   *foreign body in respiratory tract (T17.-)*

   ☑6ᵗʰ   **T18.10**   **Unspecified foreign body in esophagus**

    ☑7ᵗʰ   **T18.100**   **Unspecified foreign body in esophagus causing compression of trachea**
      Unspecified foreign body in esophagus causing obstruction of respiration

    ☑7ᵗʰ   **T18.108**   **Unspecified foreign body in esophagus causing other injury**

   ☑6ᵗʰ   **T18.11**   **Gastric contents in esophagus**

     Vomitus in esophagus

    ☑7ᵗʰ   **T18.110**   **Gastric contents in esophagus** causing compression of trachea
      Gastric contents in esophagus causing obstruction of respiration

    ☑7ᵗʰ   **T18.118**   **Gastric contents in esophagus** causing other injury

   ☑6ᵗʰ   **T18.12**   **Food in esophagus**

     Bones in esophagus
     Seeds in esophagus

    ☑7ᵗʰ   **T18.120**   **Food in esophagus** causing compression of trachea
      Food in esophagus causing obstruction of respiration

    ☑7ᵗʰ   **T18.128**   **Food in esophagus** causing other injury

✓6ᵗʰ T18.19 Other foreign object in esophagus
> AHA: 2022,1Q,27; 2015,1Q,23

> **✓7ᵗʰ T18.190 Other foreign object in esophagus causing compression of trachea**
>> Other foreign body in esophagus causing obstruction of respiration
>> **TIP:** Any foreign object lodged in the esophagus requires immediate treatment and is considered an injury. Assign this code when there is respiratory compromise or compression. If no respiratory compromise or compression is documented, assign code T18.198-.

> **✓7ᵗʰ T18.198 Other foreign object in esophagus causing other injury**
>> **TIP:** Any foreign object lodged in the esophagus requires immediate treatment and is considered an injury. Assign this code when there is no respiratory compromise or compression. If respiratory compromise or compression is documented, assign code T18.190-.

✓x7ᵗʰ T18.2 Foreign body in stomach

✓x7ᵗʰ T18.3 Foreign body in small intestine

✓x7ᵗʰ T18.4 Foreign body in colon

✓x7ᵗʰ T18.5 Foreign body in anus and rectum
> Foreign body in rectosigmoid (junction)

✓x7ᵗʰ T18.8 Foreign body in other parts of alimentary tract

✓x7ᵗʰ T18.9 Foreign body of alimentary tract, part unspecified
> Foreign body in digestive system NOS
> Swallowed foreign body NOS

✓4ᵗʰ T19 Foreign body in genitourinary tract
> *EXCLUDES 2*   *complications due to implanted mesh (T83.7-)*
> *mechanical complications of contraceptive device (intrauterine) (vaginal) (T83.3-)*
> *presence of contraceptive device (intrauterine) (vaginal) (Z97.5)*

> The appropriate 7th character is to be added to each code from category T19.
> A   initial encounter
> D   subsequent encounter
> S   sequela

✓x7ᵗʰ T19.0 Foreign body in urethra

✓x7ᵗʰ T19.1 Foreign body in bladder

✓x7ᵗʰ T19.2 Foreign body in vulva and vagina   ♀

✓x7ᵗʰ T19.3 Foreign body in uterus   ♀

✓x7ᵗʰ T19.4 Foreign body in penis   ♂

✓x7ᵗʰ T19.8 Foreign body in other parts of genitourinary tract

✓x7ᵗʰ T19.9 Foreign body in genitourinary tract, part unspecified

BURNS AND CORROSIONS (T20-T32)

INCLUDES   burns (thermal) from electrical heating appliances
burns (thermal) from electricity
burns (thermal) from flame
burns (thermal) from friction
burns (thermal) from hot air and hot gases
burns (thermal) from hot objects
burns (thermal) from lightning
burns (thermal) from radiation
chemical burn [corrosion] (external) (internal)
scalds

EXCLUDES 2   *erythema [dermatitis] ab igne (L59.0)*
radiation-related disorders of the skin and subcutaneous tissue (L55-L59)
sunburn (L55.-)

AHA: 2016,2Q,4

Burns and corrosions of external body surface, specified by site (T20-T25)

INCLUDES   burns and corrosions of first degree [erythema]
burns and corrosions of second degree [blisters] [epidermal loss]
burns and corrosions of third degree [deep necrosis of underlying tissue] [full-thickness skin loss]

Use additional code from category T31 or T32 to identify extent of body surface involved

✓4ᵗʰ T20 Burn and corrosion of head, face, and neck
> *EXCLUDES 2*   *burn and corrosion of ear drum (T28.41, T28.91)*
> *burn and corrosion of eye and adnexa (T26.-)*
> *burn and corrosion of mouth and pharynx (T28.0)*

> **AHA:** 2015,1Q,18-19

> The appropriate 7th character is to be added to each code from category T20.
> A   initial encounter
> D   subsequent encounter
> S   sequela

✓5ᵗʰ T20.0 Burn of unspecified degree of head, face, and neck
> Use additional external cause code to identify the source, place and intent of the burn (X00-X19, X75-X77, X96-X98, Y92)

> **✓x7ᵗʰ T20.00 Burn of unspecified degree of head, face, and neck, unspecified site**

> **✓6ᵗʰ T20.01 Burn of unspecified degree of ear [any part, except ear drum]**
>> *EXCLUDES 2*   *burn of ear drum (T28.41-)*
>> **✓7ᵗʰ T20.011 Burn of unspecified degree of right ear [any part, except ear drum]**
>> **✓7ᵗʰ T20.012 Burn of unspecified degree of left ear [any part, except ear drum]**
>> **✓7ᵗʰ T20.019 Burn of unspecified degree of unspecified ear [any part, except ear drum]**

> **✓x7ᵗʰ T20.02 Burn of unspecified degree of lip(s)**

> **✓x7ᵗʰ T20.03 Burn of unspecified degree of chin**

> **✓x7ᵗʰ T20.04 Burn of unspecified degree of nose (septum)**

> **✓x7ᵗʰ T20.05 Burn of unspecified degree of scalp [any part]**

> **✓x7ᵗʰ T20.06 Burn of unspecified degree of forehead and cheek**

> **✓x7ᵗʰ T20.07 Burn of unspecified degree of neck**

> **✓x7ᵗʰ T20.09 Burn of unspecified degree of multiple sites of head, face, and neck**

✓5ᵗʰ T20.1 Burn of first degree of head, face, and neck
> Use additional external cause code to identify the source, place and intent of the burn (X00-X19, X75-X77, X96-X98, Y92)

> **✓x7ᵗʰ T20.10 Burn of first degree of head, face, and neck, unspecified site**

> **✓6ᵗʰ T20.11 Burn of first degree of ear [any part, except ear drum]**
>> *EXCLUDES 2*   *burn of ear drum (T28.41-)*
>> **✓7ᵗʰ T20.111 Burn of first degree of right ear [any part, except ear drum]**
>> **✓7ᵗʰ T20.112 Burn of first degree of left ear [any part, except ear drum]**
>> **✓7ᵗʰ T20.119 Burn of first degree of unspecified ear [any part, except ear drum]**

> **✓x7ᵗʰ T20.12 Burn of first degree of lip(s)**

> **✓x7ᵗʰ T20.13 Burn of first degree of chin**

> **✓x7ᵗʰ T20.14 Burn of first degree of nose (septum)**

> **✓x7ᵗʰ T20.15 Burn of first degree of scalp [any part]**

> **✓x7ᵗʰ T20.16 Burn of first degree of forehead and cheek**

| **HCC** CMS-HCC | **Rx** Rx HCC | **ESR** ESRD HCC | **COM** Commercial HCC | **N** Newborn: 0 | **P** Pediatric: 0-17 | **M** Maternity: 9-64 | **A** Adult: 15-124 |

1116   ICD-10-CM 2023

✓x7ᵗʰ **T20.17** **Burn of first degree of neck**

✓x7ᵗʰ **T20.19** **Burn of first degree of multiple sites of head, face, and neck**

Degree of Burns

Normal   First Degree Burn

Second Degree Burn   Third Degree Burn

Epidermis
Dermis
Subcutaneous

✓5ᵗʰ **T20.2** **Burn of second degree of head, face, and neck**

Use additional external cause code to identify the source, place and intent of the burn (X00-X19, X75-X77, X96-X98, Y92)

✓x7ᵗʰ **T20.20** **Burn of second degree of head, face, and neck, unspecified site**

✓6ᵗʰ **T20.21** **Burn of second degree of ear [any part, except ear drum]**

EXCLUDES 2   *burn of ear drum (T28.41-)*

✓7ᵗʰ **T20.211** **Burn of second degree of right ear [any part, except ear drum]**

✓7ᵗʰ **T20.212** **Burn of second degree of left ear [any part, except ear drum]**

✓7ᵗʰ **T20.219** **Burn of second degree of unspecified ear [any part, except ear drum]**

✓x7ᵗʰ **T20.22** **Burn of second degree of lip(s)**

✓x7ᵗʰ **T20.23** **Burn of second degree of chin**

✓x7ᵗʰ **T20.24** **Burn of second degree of nose (septum)**

✓x7ᵗʰ **T20.25** **Burn of second degree of scalp [any part]**

✓x7ᵗʰ **T20.26** **Burn of second degree of forehead and cheek**

✓x7ᵗʰ **T20.27** **Burn of second degree of neck**

✓x7ᵗʰ **T20.29** **Burn of second degree of multiple sites of head, face, and neck**

✓5ᵗʰ **T20.3** **Burn of third degree of head, face, and neck**

Use additional external cause code to identify the source, place and intent of the burn (X00-X19, X75-X77, X96-X98, Y92)

✓x7ᵗʰ **T20.30** **Burn of third degree of head, face, and neck, unspecified site** COM

✓6ᵗʰ **T20.31** **Burn of third degree of ear [any part, except ear drum]**

EXCLUDES 2   *burn of ear drum (T28.41-)*

AHA: 2015,1Q,18

✓7ᵗʰ **T20.311** **Burn of third degree of right ear [any part, except ear drum]** COM

✓7ᵗʰ **T20.312** **Burn of third degree of left ear [any part, except ear drum]** COM

✓7ᵗʰ **T20.319** **Burn of third degree of unspecified ear [any part, except ear drum]** COM

✓x7ᵗʰ **T20.32** **Burn of third degree of lip(s)** COM

✓x7ᵗʰ **T20.33** **Burn of third degree of chin** COM

✓x7ᵗʰ **T20.34** **Burn of third degree of nose (septum)** COM

✓x7ᵗʰ **T20.35** **Burn of third degree of scalp [any part]** COM

✓x7ᵗʰ **T20.36** **Burn of third degree of forehead and cheek** COM

✓x7ᵗʰ **T20.37** **Burn of third degree of neck** COM

✓x7ᵗʰ **T20.39** **Burn of third degree of multiple sites of head, face, and neck** COM

✓5ᵗʰ **T20.4** **Corrosion of unspecified degree of head, face, and neck**

Code first (T51-T65) to identify chemical and intent
Use additional external cause code to identify place (Y92)

✓x7ᵗʰ **T20.40** **Corrosion of unspecified degree of head, face, and neck, unspecified site**

✓6ᵗʰ **T20.41** **Corrosion of unspecified degree of ear [any part, except ear drum]**

EXCLUDES 2   *corrosion of ear drum (T28.91-)*

✓7ᵗʰ **T20.411** **Corrosion of unspecified degree of right ear [any part, except ear drum]**

✓7ᵗʰ **T20.412** **Corrosion of unspecified degree of left ear [any part, except ear drum]**

✓7ᵗʰ **T20.419** **Corrosion of unspecified degree of unspecified ear [any part, except ear drum]**

✓x7ᵗʰ **T20.42** **Corrosion of unspecified degree of lip(s)**

✓x7ᵗʰ **T20.43** **Corrosion of unspecified degree of chin**

✓x7ᵗʰ **T20.44** **Corrosion of unspecified degree of nose (septum)**

✓x7ᵗʰ **T20.45** **Corrosion of unspecified degree of scalp [any part]**

✓x7ᵗʰ **T20.46** **Corrosion of unspecified degree of forehead and cheek**

✓x7ᵗʰ **T20.47** **Corrosion of unspecified degree of neck**

✓x7ᵗʰ **T20.49** **Corrosion of unspecified degree of multiple sites of head, face, and neck**

✓5ᵗʰ **T20.5** **Corrosion of first degree of head, face, and neck**

Code first (T51-T65) to identify chemical and intent
Use additional external cause code to identify place (Y92)

✓x7ᵗʰ **T20.50** **Corrosion of first degree of head, face, and neck, unspecified site**

✓6ᵗʰ **T20.51** **Corrosion of first degree of ear [any part, except ear drum]**

EXCLUDES 2   *corrosion of ear drum (T28.91-)*

✓7ᵗʰ **T20.511** **Corrosion of first degree of right ear [any part, except ear drum]**

✓7ᵗʰ **T20.512** **Corrosion of first degree of left ear [any part, except ear drum]**

✓7ᵗʰ **T20.519** **Corrosion of first degree of unspecified ear [any part, except ear drum]**

✓x7ᵗʰ **T20.52** **Corrosion of first degree of lip(s)**

✓x7ᵗʰ **T20.53** **Corrosion of first degree of chin**

✓x7ᵗʰ **T20.54** **Corrosion of first degree of nose (septum)**

✓x7ᵗʰ **T20.55** **Corrosion of first degree of scalp [any part]**

✓x7ᵗʰ **T20.56** **Corrosion of first degree of forehead and cheek**

✓x7ᵗʰ **T20.57** **Corrosion of first degree of neck**

✓x7ᵗʰ **T20.59** **Corrosion of first degree of multiple sites of head, face, and neck**

✓5ᵗʰ **T20.6** **Corrosion of second degree of head, face, and neck**

Code first (T51-T65) to identify chemical and intent
Use additional external cause code to identify place (Y92)

✓x7ᵗʰ **T20.60** **Corrosion of second degree of head, face, and neck, unspecified site**

✓6ᵗʰ **T20.61** **Corrosion of second degree of ear [any part, except ear drum]**

EXCLUDES 2   *corrosion of ear drum (T28.91-)*

✓7ᵗʰ **T20.611** **Corrosion of second degree of right ear [any part, except ear drum]**

✓7ᵗʰ **T20.612** **Corrosion of second degree of left ear [any part, except ear drum]**

✓7ᵗʰ **T20.619** **Corrosion of second degree of unspecified ear [any part, except ear drum]**

✓x7ᵗʰ **T20.62** **Corrosion of second degree of lip(s)**

✓x7ᵗʰ **T20.63** **Corrosion of second degree of chin**

✓x7ᵗʰ **T20.64** **Corrosion of second degree of nose (septum)**

✓x7ᵗʰ **T20.65** **Corrosion of second degree of scalp [any part]**

✓x7ᵗʰ **T20.66** **Corrosion of second degree of forehead and cheek**

✓x7ᵗʰ **T20.67** **Corrosion of second degree of neck**

✓x7ᵗʰ **T20.69** **Corrosion of second degree of multiple sites of head, face, and neck**

✓6ᵗʰ **T20.7** **Corrosion of third degree of head, face, and neck**

Code first (T51-T65) to identify chemical and intent
Use additional external cause code to identify place (Y92)

✓x7ᵗʰ **T20.70** **Corrosion of third degree of head, face, and neck, unspecified site** COM

✔ Additional Character Required   ✓x7ᵗʰ Placeholder Alert   Manifestation   Unspecified Dx   🄠 QPP   UPD Unacceptable PDx

√6ᵗʰ **T20.71 Corrosion of third degree of ear [any part, except ear drum]**
> *EXCLUDES 2*   corrosion of ear drum (T28.91-)

√7ᵗʰ **T20.711 Corrosion of third degree of right ear [any part, except ear drum]** `COM`

√7ᵗʰ **T20.712 Corrosion of third degree of left ear [any part, except ear drum]** `COM`

√7ᵗʰ **T20.719 Corrosion of third degree of unspecified ear [any part, except ear drum]** `COM`

√x7ᵗʰ **T20.72 Corrosion of third degree of lip(s)** `COM`

√x7ᵗʰ **T20.73 Corrosion of third degree of chin** `COM`

√x7ᵗʰ **T20.74 Corrosion of third degree of nose (septum)** `COM`

√x7ᵗʰ **T20.75 Corrosion of third degree of scalp [any part]** `COM`

√x7ᵗʰ **T20.76 Corrosion of third degree of forehead and cheek** `COM`

√x7ᵗʰ **T20.77 Corrosion of third degree of neck** `COM`

√x7ᵗʰ **T20.79 Corrosion of third degree of multiple sites of head, face, and neck** `COM`

√4ᵗʰ **T21 Burn and corrosion of trunk**
> **INCLUDES**   burns and corrosion of hip region
> *EXCLUDES 2*   burns and corrosion of axilla (T22.- with fifth character 4)
> burns and corrosion of scapular region (T22.- with fifth character 6)
> burns and corrosion of shoulder (T22.- with fifth character 5)

> The appropriate 7th character is to be added to each code from category T21.
> A   initial encounter
> D   subsequent encounter
> S   sequela

√5ᵗʰ **T21.0 Burn of unspecified degree of trunk**
> Use additional external cause code to identify the source, place and intent of the burn (X00-X19, X75-X77, X96-X98, Y92)

√7ᵗʰ **T21.00 Burn of unspecified degree of trunk, unspecified site**

√7ᵗʰ **T21.01 Burn of unspecified degree of chest wall**
> Burn of unspecified degree of breast

√7ᵗʰ **T21.02 Burn of unspecified degree of abdominal wall**
> Burn of unspecified degree of flank
> Burn of unspecified degree of groin

√7ᵗʰ **T21.03 Burn of unspecified degree of upper back**
> Burn of unspecified degree of interscapular region

√7ᵗʰ **T21.04 Burn of unspecified degree of lower back**

√7ᵗʰ **T21.05 Burn of unspecified degree of buttock**
> Burn of unspecified degree of anus

√7ᵗʰ **T21.06 Burn of unspecified degree of male genital region** ♂
> Burn of unspecified degree of penis
> Burn of unspecified degree of scrotum
> Burn of unspecified degree of testis

√7ᵗʰ **T21.07 Burn of unspecified degree of female genital region** ♀
> Burn of unspecified degree of labium (majus) (minus)
> Burn of unspecified degree of perineum
> Burn of unspecified degree of vulva
> *EXCLUDES 2*   burn of vagina (T28.3)

√7ᵗʰ **T21.09 Burn of unspecified degree of other site of trunk**

√5ᵗʰ **T21.1 Burn of first degree of trunk**
> Use additional external cause code to identify the source, place and intent of the burn (X00-X19, X75-X77, X96-X98, Y92)

√7ᵗʰ **T21.10 Burn of first degree of trunk, unspecified site**

√7ᵗʰ **T21.11 Burn of first degree of chest wall**
> Burn of first degree of breast

√7ᵗʰ **T21.12 Burn of first degree of abdominal wall**
> Burn of first degree of flank
> Burn of first degree of groin

√7ᵗʰ **T21.13 Burn of first degree of upper back**
> Burn of first degree of interscapular region

√7ᵗʰ **T21.14 Burn of first degree of lower back**

√7ᵗʰ **T21.15 Burn of first degree of buttock**
> Burn of first degree of anus

√x7ᵗʰ **T21.16 Burn of first degree of male genital region** ♂
> Burn of first degree of penis
> Burn of first degree of scrotum
> Burn of first degree of testis

√x7ᵗʰ **T21.17 Burn of first degree of female genital region** ♀
> Burn of first degree of labium (majus) (minus)
> Burn of first degree of perineum
> Burn of first degree of vulva
> *EXCLUDES 2*   burn of vagina (T28.3)

√x7ᵗʰ **T21.19 Burn of first degree of other site of trunk**

√5ᵗʰ **T21.2 Burn of second degree of trunk**
> Use additional external cause code to identify the source, place and intent of the burn (X00-X19, X75-X77, X96-X98, Y92)

√x7ᵗʰ **T21.20 Burn of second degree of trunk, unspecified site**

√x7ᵗʰ **T21.21 Burn of second degree of chest wall**
> Burn of second degree of breast

√x7ᵗʰ **T21.22 Burn of second degree of abdominal wall**
> Burn of second degree of flank
> Burn of second degree of groin

√x7ᵗʰ **T21.23 Burn of second degree of upper back**
> Burn of second degree of interscapular region

√x7ᵗʰ **T21.24 Burn of second degree of lower back**

√x7ᵗʰ **T21.25 Burn of second degree of buttock**
> Burn of second degree of anus

√x7ᵗʰ **T21.26 Burn of second degree of male genital region** ♂
> Burn of second degree of penis
> Burn of second degree of scrotum
> Burn of second degree of testis

√x7ᵗʰ **T21.27 Burn of second degree of female genital region** ♀
> Burn of second degree of labium (majus) (minus)
> Burn of second degree of perineum
> Burn of second degree of vulva
> *EXCLUDES 2*   burn of vagina (T28.3)

√x7ᵗʰ **T21.29 Burn of second degree of other site of trunk**

√5ᵗʰ **T21.3 Burn of third degree of trunk**
> Use additional external cause code to identify the source, place and intent of the burn (X00-X19, X75-X77, X96-X98, Y92)

√x7ᵗʰ **T21.30 Burn of third degree of trunk, unspecified site** `COM`

√x7ᵗʰ **T21.31 Burn of third degree of chest wall** `COM`
> Burn of third degree of breast
> **AHA:** 2016,2Q,5

√x7ᵗʰ **T21.32 Burn of third degree of abdominal wall** `COM`
> Burn of third degree of flank
> Burn of third degree of groin

√x7ᵗʰ **T21.33 Burn of third degree of upper back** `COM`
> Burn of third degree of interscapular region

√x7ᵗʰ **T21.34 Burn of third degree of lower back** `COM`

√x7ᵗʰ **T21.35 Burn of third degree of buttock** `COM`
> Burn of third degree of anus

√x7ᵗʰ **T21.36 Burn of third degree of male genital region** `COM` ♂
> Burn of third degree of penis
> Burn of third degree of scrotum
> Burn of third degree of testis

√x7ᵗʰ **T21.37 Burn of third degree of female genital region** `COM` ♀
> Burn of third degree of labium (majus) (minus)
> Burn of third degree of perineum
> Burn of third degree of vulva
> *EXCLUDES 2*   burn of vagina (T28.3)

√x7ᵗʰ **T21.39 Burn of third degree of other site of trunk** `COM`

√5ᵗʰ **T21.4 Corrosion of unspecified degree of trunk**
> Code first (T51-T65) to identify chemical and intent
> Use additional external cause code to identify place (Y92)

√x7ᵗʰ **T21.40 Corrosion of unspecified degree of trunk, unspecified site**

√x7ᵗʰ **T21.41 Corrosion of unspecified degree of chest wall**
> Corrosion of unspecified degree of breast

`HCC` CMS-HCC   `Rx` Rx HCC   `ESR` ESRD HCC   `COM` Commercial HCC   `N` Newborn: 0   `P` Pediatric: 0-17   `M` Maternity: 9-64   `A` Adult: 15-124

1118   ICD-10-CM 2023

✓x7ᵗʰ **T21.42** **Corrosion of unspecified degree of abdominal wall**
     Corrosion of unspecified degree of flank
     Corrosion of unspecified degree of groin

✓x7ᵗʰ **T21.43** **Corrosion of unspecified degree of upper back**
     Corrosion of unspecified degree of interscapular region

✓x7ᵗʰ **T21.44** **Corrosion of unspecified degree of lower back**

✓x7ᵗʰ **T21.45** **Corrosion of unspecified degree of buttock**
     Corrosion of unspecified degree of anus

✓x7ᵗʰ **T21.46** **Corrosion of unspecified degree of male genital region** ♂
     Corrosion of unspecified degree of penis
     Corrosion of unspecified degree of scrotum
     Corrosion of unspecified degree of testis

✓x7ᵗʰ **T21.47** **Corrosion of unspecified degree of female genital region** ♀
     Corrosion of unspecified degree of labium (majus) (minus)
     Corrosion of unspecified degree of perineum
     Corrosion of unspecified degree of vulva
     EXCLUDES 2   *corrosion of vagina (T28.8)*

✓x7ᵗʰ **T21.49** **Corrosion of unspecified degree of other site of trunk**

✓5ᵗʰ **T21.5** **Corrosion of first degree of trunk**
     Code first (T51-T65) to identify chemical and intent
     Use additional external cause code to identify place (Y92)

✓x7ᵗʰ **T21.50** **Corrosion of first degree of trunk, unspecified site**

✓x7ᵗʰ **T21.51** **Corrosion of first degree of chest wall**
     Corrosion of first degree of breast

✓x7ᵗʰ **T21.52** **Corrosion of first degree of abdominal wall**
     Corrosion of first degree of flank
     Corrosion of first degree of groin

✓x7ᵗʰ **T21.53** **Corrosion of first degree of upper back**
     Corrosion of first degree of interscapular region

✓x7ᵗʰ **T21.54** **Corrosion of first degree of lower back**

✓x7ᵗʰ **T21.55** **Corrosion of first degree of buttock**
     Corrosion of first degree of anus

✓x7ᵗʰ **T21.56** **Corrosion of first degree of male genital region** ♂
     Corrosion of first degree of penis
     Corrosion of first degree of scrotum
     Corrosion of first degree of testis

✓x7ᵗʰ **T21.57** **Corrosion of first degree of female genital region** ♀
     Corrosion of first degree of labium (majus) (minus)
     Corrosion of first degree of perineum
     Corrosion of first degree of vulva
     EXCLUDES 2   *corrosion of vagina (T28.8)*

✓x7ᵗʰ **T21.59** **Corrosion of first degree of other site of trunk**

✓5ᵗʰ **T21.6** **Corrosion of second degree of trunk**
     Code first (T51-T65) to identify chemical and intent
     Use additional external cause code to identify place (Y92)

✓x7ᵗʰ **T21.60** **Corrosion of second degree of trunk, unspecified site**

✓x7ᵗʰ **T21.61** **Corrosion of second degree of chest wall**
     Corrosion of second degree of breast

✓x7ᵗʰ **T21.62** **Corrosion of second degree of abdominal wall**
     Corrosion of second degree of flank
     Corrosion of second degree of groin

✓x7ᵗʰ **T21.63** **Corrosion of second degree of upper back**
     Corrosion of second degree of interscapular region

✓x7ᵗʰ **T21.64** **Corrosion of second degree of lower back**

✓x7ᵗʰ **T21.65** **Corrosion of second degree of buttock**
     Corrosion of second degree of anus

✓x7ᵗʰ **T21.66** **Corrosion of second degree of male genital region** ♂
     Corrosion of second degree of penis
     Corrosion of second degree of scrotum
     Corrosion of second degree of testis

✓x7ᵗʰ **T21.67** **Corrosion of second degree of female genital region** ♀
     Corrosion of second degree of labium (majus) (minus)
     Corrosion of second degree of perineum
     Corrosion of second degree of vulva
     EXCLUDES 2   *corrosion of vagina (T28.8)*

✓x7ᵗʰ **T21.69** **Corrosion of second degree of other site of trunk**

✓5ᵗʰ **T21.7** **Corrosion of third degree of trunk**
     Code first (T51-T65) to identify chemical and intent
     Use additional external cause code to identify place (Y92)

✓x7ᵗʰ **T21.70** **Corrosion of third degree of trunk, unspecified site** COM

✓x7ᵗʰ **T21.71** **Corrosion of third degree of chest wall** COM
     Corrosion of third degree of breast

✓x7ᵗʰ **T21.72** **Corrosion of third degree of abdominal wall** COM
     Corrosion of third degree of flank
     Corrosion of third degree of groin

✓x7ᵗʰ **T21.73** **Corrosion of third degree of upper back** COM
     Corrosion of third degree of interscapular region

✓x7ᵗʰ **T21.74** **Corrosion of third degree of lower back** COM

✓x7ᵗʰ **T21.75** **Corrosion of third degree of buttock** COM
     Corrosion of third degree of anus

✓x7ᵗʰ **T21.76** **Corrosion of third degree of male genital region** COM ♂
     Corrosion of third degree of penis
     Corrosion of third degree of scrotum
     Corrosion of third degree of testis

✓x7ᵗʰ **T21.77** **Corrosion of third degree of female genital region** COM ♀
     Corrosion of third degree of labium (majus) (minus)
     Corrosion of third degree of perineum
     Corrosion of third degree of vulva
     EXCLUDES 2   *corrosion of vagina (T28.8)*

✓x7ᵗʰ **T21.79** **Corrosion of third degree of other site of trunk** COM

✓4ᵗʰ **T22** **Burn and corrosion of shoulder and upper limb, except wrist and hand**
     EXCLUDES 2   *burn and corrosion of interscapular region (T21.-)*
                  burn and corrosion of wrist and hand (T23.-)

The appropriate 7th character is to be added to each code from category T22.
A   initial encounter
D   subsequent encounter
S   sequela

✓5ᵗʰ **T22.0** **Burn of unspecified degree of shoulder and upper limb, except wrist and hand**
     Use additional external cause code to identify the source, place and intent of the burn (X00-X19, X75-X77, X96-X98, Y92)

✓x7ᵗʰ **T22.00** **Burn of unspecified degree of shoulder and upper limb, except wrist and hand, unspecified site**

✓6ᵗʰ **T22.01** **Burn of unspecified degree of forearm**

✓7ᵗʰ **T22.011** **Burn of unspecified degree of right forearm**

✓7ᵗʰ **T22.012** **Burn of unspecified degree of left forearm**

✓7ᵗʰ **T22.019** **Burn of unspecified degree of unspecified forearm**

✓6ᵗʰ **T22.02** **Burn of unspecified degree of elbow**

✓7ᵗʰ **T22.021** **Burn of unspecified degree of right elbow**

✓7ᵗʰ **T22.022** **Burn of unspecified degree of left elbow**

✓7ᵗʰ **T22.029** **Burn of unspecified degree of unspecified elbow**

✓6ᵗʰ **T22.03** **Burn of unspecified degree of upper arm**

✓7ᵗʰ **T22.031** **Burn of unspecified degree of right upper arm**

✓7ᵗʰ **T22.032** **Burn of unspecified degree of left upper arm**

✓7ᵗʰ **T22.039** **Burn of unspecified degree of unspecified upper arm**

✓6ᵗʰ **T22.04** **Burn of unspecified degree of axilla**

✓7ᵗʰ **T22.041** **Burn of unspecified degree of right axilla**

✓7ᵗʰ **T22.042** **Burn of unspecified degree of left axilla**

✓7ᵗʰ **T22.049** **Burn of unspecified degree of unspecified axilla**

✓6ᵗʰ **T22.05** **Burn of unspecified degree of** shoulder
　　✓7ᵗʰ **T22.051** **Burn of unspecified degree of** right shoulder
　　✓7ᵗʰ **T22.052** **Burn of unspecified degree of** left shoulder
　　✓7ᵗʰ **T22.059** **Burn of unspecified degree of unspecified shoulder**

✓6ᵗʰ **T22.06** **Burn of unspecified degree of** scapular region
　　✓7ᵗʰ **T22.061** **Burn of unspecified degree of** right scapular region
　　✓7ᵗʰ **T22.062** **Burn of unspecified degree of** left scapular region
　　✓7ᵗʰ **T22.069** **Burn of unspecified degree of unspecified scapular region**

✓6ᵗʰ **T22.09** **Burn of unspecified degree of** multiple sites **of shoulder and upper limb, except wrist and hand**
　　✓7ᵗʰ **T22.091** **Burn of unspecified degree of multiple sites of** right **shoulder and upper limb, except wrist and hand**
　　✓7ᵗʰ **T22.092** **Burn of unspecified degree of multiple sites of** left **shoulder and upper limb, except wrist and hand**
　　✓7ᵗʰ **T22.099** **Burn of unspecified degree of multiple sites of unspecified shoulder and upper limb, except wrist and hand**

✓5ᵗʰ **T22.1** **Burn of** first degree **of shoulder and upper limb, except wrist and hand**
　　Use additional external cause code to identify the source, place and intent of the burn (X00-X19, X75-X77, X96-X98, Y92)
　✓x7ᵗʰ **T22.10** **Burn of first degree of shoulder and upper limb, except wrist and hand, unspecified site**

✓6ᵗʰ **T22.11** **Burn of first degree of** forearm
　　✓7ᵗʰ **T22.111** **Burn of first degree of** right **forearm**
　　✓7ᵗʰ **T22.112** **Burn of first degree of** left **forearm**
　　✓7ᵗʰ **T22.119** **Burn of first degree of unspecified forearm**

✓6ᵗʰ **T22.12** **Burn of first degree of** elbow
　　✓7ᵗʰ **T22.121** **Burn of first degree of** right **elbow**
　　✓7ᵗʰ **T22.122** **Burn of first degree of** left **elbow**
　　✓7ᵗʰ **T22.129** **Burn of first degree of unspecified elbow**

✓6ᵗʰ **T22.13** **Burn of first degree of** upper arm
　　✓7ᵗʰ **T22.131** **Burn of first degree of** right **upper arm**
　　✓7ᵗʰ **T22.132** **Burn of first degree of** left **upper arm**
　　✓7ᵗʰ **T22.139** **Burn of first degree of unspecified upper arm**

✓6ᵗʰ **T22.14** **Burn of first degree of** axilla
　　✓7ᵗʰ **T22.141** **Burn of first degree of** right **axilla**
　　✓7ᵗʰ **T22.142** **Burn of first degree of** left **axilla**
　　✓7ᵗʰ **T22.149** **Burn of first degree of unspecified axilla**

✓6ᵗʰ **T22.15** **Burn of first degree of** shoulder
　　✓7ᵗʰ **T22.151** **Burn of first degree of** right **shoulder**
　　✓7ᵗʰ **T22.152** **Burn of first degree of** left **shoulder**
　　✓7ᵗʰ **T22.159** **Burn of first degree of unspecified shoulder**

✓6ᵗʰ **T22.16** **Burn of first degree of** scapular region
　　✓7ᵗʰ **T22.161** **Burn of first degree of** right **scapular region**
　　✓7ᵗʰ **T22.162** **Burn of first degree of** left **scapular region**
　　✓7ᵗʰ **T22.169** **Burn of first degree of unspecified scapular region**

✓6ᵗʰ **T22.19** **Burn of first degree of** multiple sites **of shoulder and upper limb, except wrist and hand**
　　✓7ᵗʰ **T22.191** **Burn of first degree of multiple sites of** right **shoulder and upper limb, except wrist and hand**
　　✓7ᵗʰ **T22.192** **Burn of first degree of multiple sites of** left **shoulder and upper limb, except wrist and hand**
　　✓7ᵗʰ **T22.199** **Burn of first degree of multiple sites of unspecified shoulder and upper limb, except wrist and hand**

✓5ᵗʰ **T22.2** **Burn of** second degree **of shoulder and upper limb, except wrist and hand**
　　Use additional external cause code to identify the source, place and intent of the burn (X00-X19, X75-X77, X96-X98, Y92)
　✓x7ᵗʰ **T22.20** **Burn of second degree of shoulder and upper limb, except wrist and hand, unspecified site**

✓6ᵗʰ **T22.21** **Burn of second degree of** forearm
　　✓7ᵗʰ **T22.211** **Burn of second degree of** right **forearm**
　　✓7ᵗʰ **T22.212** **Burn of second degree of** left **forearm**
　　✓7ᵗʰ **T22.219** **Burn of second degree of unspecified forearm**

✓6ᵗʰ **T22.22** **Burn of second degree of** elbow
　　✓7ᵗʰ **T22.221** **Burn of second degree of** right **elbow**
　　✓7ᵗʰ **T22.222** **Burn of second degree of** left **elbow**
　　✓7ᵗʰ **T22.229** **Burn of second degree of unspecified elbow**

✓6ᵗʰ **T22.23** **Burn of second degree of** upper arm
　　✓7ᵗʰ **T22.231** **Burn of second degree of** right **upper arm**
　　✓7ᵗʰ **T22.232** **Burn of second degree of** left **upper arm**
　　✓7ᵗʰ **T22.239** **Burn of second degree of unspecified upper arm**

✓6ᵗʰ **T22.24** **Burn of second degree of** axilla
　　✓7ᵗʰ **T22.241** **Burn of second degree of** right **axilla**
　　✓7ᵗʰ **T22.242** **Burn of second degree of** left **axilla**
　　✓7ᵗʰ **T22.249** **Burn of second degree of unspecified axilla**

✓6ᵗʰ **T22.25** **Burn of second degree of** shoulder
　　✓7ᵗʰ **T22.251** **Burn of second degree of** right **shoulder**
　　✓7ᵗʰ **T22.252** **Burn of second degree of** left **shoulder**
　　✓7ᵗʰ **T22.259** **Burn of second degree of unspecified shoulder**

✓6ᵗʰ **T22.26** **Burn of second degree of** scapular region
　　✓7ᵗʰ **T22.261** **Burn of second degree of** right **scapular region**
　　✓7ᵗʰ **T22.262** **Burn of second degree of** left **scapular region**
　　✓7ᵗʰ **T22.269** **Burn of second degree of unspecified scapular region**

✓6ᵗʰ **T22.29** **Burn of second degree of** multiple sites **of shoulder and upper limb, except wrist and hand**
　　✓7ᵗʰ **T22.291** **Burn of second degree of multiple sites of** right **shoulder and upper limb, except wrist and hand**
　　✓7ᵗʰ **T22.292** **Burn of second degree of multiple sites of** left **shoulder and upper limb, except wrist and hand**
　　✓7ᵗʰ **T22.299** **Burn of second degree of multiple sites of unspecified shoulder and upper limb, except wrist and hand**

✓5ᵗʰ **T22.3** **Burn of** third degree **of shoulder and upper limb, except wrist and hand**
　　Use additional external cause code to identify the source, place and intent of the burn (X00-X19, X75-X77, X96-X98, Y92)
　✓x7ᵗʰ **T22.30** **Burn of third degree of shoulder and upper limb, except wrist and hand, unspecified site** COM

✓6ᵗʰ **T22.31** **Burn of third degree of** forearm
　　✓7ᵗʰ **T22.311** **Burn of third degree of** right **forearm** COM
　　✓7ᵗʰ **T22.312** **Burn of third degree of** left **forearm** COM
　　✓7ᵗʰ **T22.319** **Burn of third degree of unspecified forearm** COM

✓6ᵗʰ **T22.32** **Burn of third degree of** elbow
　　✓7ᵗʰ **T22.321** **Burn of third degree of** right **elbow** COM
　　✓7ᵗʰ **T22.322** **Burn of third degree of** left **elbow** COM
　　✓7ᵗʰ **T22.329** **Burn of third degree of unspecified elbow** COM

✓6ᵗʰ **T22.33** **Burn of third degree of** upper arm
　　✓7ᵗʰ **T22.331** **Burn of third degree of** right **upper arm** COM
　　✓7ᵗʰ **T22.332** **Burn of third degree of** left **upper arm** COM
　　✓7ᵗʰ **T22.339** **Burn of third degree of unspecified upper arm** COM

✓6ᵗʰ **T22.34** **Burn of third degree of** axilla
　　✓7ᵗʰ **T22.341** **Burn of third degree of** right **axilla** COM
　　✓7ᵗʰ **T22.342** **Burn of third degree of** left **axilla** COM
　　✓7ᵗʰ **T22.349** **Burn of third degree of unspecified axilla** COM

√6ᵗʰ **T22.35** Burn of third degree of shoulder

    √7ᵗʰ **T22.351** Burn of third degree of right shoulder `COM`

    √7ᵗʰ **T22.352** Burn of third degree of left shoulder `COM`

    √7ᵗʰ **T22.359** Burn of third degree of unspecified shoulder `COM`

√6ᵗʰ **T22.36** Burn of third degree of scapular region

    √7ᵗʰ **T22.361** Burn of third degree of right scapular region `COM`

    √7ᵗʰ **T22.362** Burn of third degree of left scapular region `COM`

    √7ᵗʰ **T22.369** Burn of third degree of unspecified scapular region `COM`

√6ᵗʰ **T22.39** Burn of third degree of multiple sites of shoulder and upper limb, except wrist and hand

    √7ᵗʰ **T22.391** Burn of third degree of multiple sites of right shoulder and upper limb, except wrist and hand `COM`

    √7ᵗʰ **T22.392** Burn of third degree of multiple sites of left shoulder and upper limb, except wrist and hand `COM`

    √7ᵗʰ **T22.399** Burn of third degree of multiple sites of unspecified shoulder and upper limb, except wrist and hand `COM`

√5ᵗʰ **T22.4** Corrosion of unspecified degree of shoulder and upper limb, except wrist and hand

    Code first (T51-T65) to identify chemical and intent

    Use additional external cause code to identify place (Y92)

√x7ᵗʰ **T22.40** Corrosion of unspecified degree of shoulder and upper limb, except wrist and hand, unspecified site

√6ᵗʰ **T22.41** Corrosion of unspecified degree of forearm

    √7ᵗʰ **T22.411** Corrosion of unspecified degree of right forearm

    √7ᵗʰ **T22.412** Corrosion of unspecified degree of left forearm

    √7ᵗʰ **T22.419** Corrosion of unspecified degree of unspecified forearm

√6ᵗʰ **T22.42** Corrosion of unspecified degree of elbow

    √7ᵗʰ **T22.421** Corrosion of unspecified degree of right elbow

    √7ᵗʰ **T22.422** Corrosion of unspecified degree of left elbow

    √7ᵗʰ **T22.429** Corrosion of unspecified degree of unspecified elbow

√6ᵗʰ **T22.43** Corrosion of unspecified degree of upper arm

    √7ᵗʰ **T22.431** Corrosion of unspecified degree of right upper arm

    √7ᵗʰ **T22.432** Corrosion of unspecified degree of left upper arm

    √7ᵗʰ **T22.439** Corrosion of unspecified degree of unspecified upper arm

√6ᵗʰ **T22.44** Corrosion of unspecified degree of axilla

    √7ᵗʰ **T22.441** Corrosion of unspecified degree of right axilla

    √7ᵗʰ **T22.442** Corrosion of unspecified degree of left axilla

    √7ᵗʰ **T22.449** Corrosion of unspecified degree of unspecified axilla

√6ᵗʰ **T22.45** Corrosion of unspecified degree of shoulder

    √7ᵗʰ **T22.451** Corrosion of unspecified degree of right shoulder

    √7ᵗʰ **T22.452** Corrosion of unspecified degree of left shoulder

    √7ᵗʰ **T22.459** Corrosion of unspecified degree of unspecified shoulder

√6ᵗʰ **T22.46** Corrosion of unspecified degree of scapular region

    √7ᵗʰ **T22.461** Corrosion of unspecified degree of right scapular region

    √7ᵗʰ **T22.462** Corrosion of unspecified degree of left scapular region

    √7ᵗʰ **T22.469** Corrosion of unspecified degree of unspecified scapular region

√6ᵗʰ **T22.49** Corrosion of unspecified degree of multiple sites of shoulder and upper limb, except wrist and hand

    √7ᵗʰ **T22.491** Corrosion of unspecified degree of multiple sites of right shoulder and upper limb, except wrist and hand

    √7ᵗʰ **T22.492** Corrosion of unspecified degree of multiple sites of left shoulder and upper limb, except wrist and hand

    √7ᵗʰ **T22.499** Corrosion of unspecified degree of multiple sites of unspecified shoulder and upper limb, except wrist and hand

√5ᵗʰ **T22.5** Corrosion of first degree of shoulder and upper limb, except wrist and hand

    Code first (T51-T65) to identify chemical and intent

    Use additional external cause code to identify place (Y92)

√x7ᵗʰ **T22.50** Corrosion of first degree of shoulder and upper limb, except wrist and hand unspecified site

√6ᵗʰ **T22.51** Corrosion of first degree of forearm

    √7ᵗʰ **T22.511** Corrosion of first degree of right forearm

    √7ᵗʰ **T22.512** Corrosion of first degree of left forearm

    √7ᵗʰ **T22.519** Corrosion of first degree of unspecified forearm

√6ᵗʰ **T22.52** Corrosion of first degree of elbow

    √7ᵗʰ **T22.521** Corrosion of first degree of right elbow

    √7ᵗʰ **T22.522** Corrosion of first degree of left elbow

    √7ᵗʰ **T22.529** Corrosion of first degree of unspecified elbow

√6ᵗʰ **T22.53** Corrosion of first degree of upper arm

    √7ᵗʰ **T22.531** Corrosion of first degree of right upper arm

    √7ᵗʰ **T22.532** Corrosion of first degree of left upper arm

    √7ᵗʰ **T22.539** Corrosion of first degree of unspecified upper arm

√6ᵗʰ **T22.54** Corrosion of first degree of axilla

    √7ᵗʰ **T22.541** Corrosion of first degree of right axilla

    √7ᵗʰ **T22.542** Corrosion of first degree of left axilla

    √7ᵗʰ **T22.549** Corrosion of first degree of unspecified axilla

√6ᵗʰ **T22.55** Corrosion of first degree of shoulder

    √7ᵗʰ **T22.551** Corrosion of first degree of right shoulder

    √7ᵗʰ **T22.552** Corrosion of first degree of left shoulder

    √7ᵗʰ **T22.559** Corrosion of first degree of unspecified shoulder

√6ᵗʰ **T22.56** Corrosion of first degree of scapular region

    √7ᵗʰ **T22.561** Corrosion of first degree of right scapular region

    √7ᵗʰ **T22.562** Corrosion of first degree of left scapular region

    √7ᵗʰ **T22.569** Corrosion of first degree of unspecified scapular region

√6ᵗʰ **T22.59** Corrosion of first degree of multiple sites of shoulder and upper limb, except wrist and hand

    √7ᵗʰ **T22.591** Corrosion of first degree of multiple sites of right shoulder and upper limb, except wrist and hand

    √7ᵗʰ **T22.592** Corrosion of first degree of multiple sites of left shoulder and upper limb, except wrist and hand

    √7ᵗʰ **T22.599** Corrosion of first degree of multiple sites of unspecified shoulder and upper limb, except wrist and hand

√5ᵗʰ **T22.6** Corrosion of second degree of shoulder and upper limb, except wrist and hand

    Code first (T51-T65) to identify chemical and intent

    Use additional external cause code to identify place (Y92)

√x7ᵗʰ **T22.60** Corrosion of second degree of shoulder and upper limb, except wrist and hand, unspecified site

√6ᵗʰ **T22.61** Corrosion of second degree of forearm

    √7ᵗʰ **T22.611** Corrosion of second degree of right forearm

    √7ᵗʰ **T22.612** Corrosion of second degree of left forearm

    √7ᵗʰ **T22.619** Corrosion of second degree of unspecified forearm

√6ᵗʰ **T22.62** Corrosion of second degree of elbow

    √7ᵗʰ **T22.621** Corrosion of second degree of right elbow

    √7ᵗʰ **T22.622** Corrosion of second degree of left elbow

    √7ᵗʰ **T22.629** Corrosion of second degree of unspecified elbow

√6ᵗʰ **T22.63** Corrosion of second degree of upper arm

    √7ᵗʰ **T22.631** Corrosion of second degree of right upper arm

√7ᵗʰ **T22.632** Corrosion of second degree of left upper arm

√7ᵗʰ **T22.639** Corrosion of second degree of unspecified upper arm

√6ᵗʰ **T22.64** Corrosion of second degree of axilla

√7ᵗʰ **T22.641** Corrosion of second degree of right axilla

√7ᵗʰ **T22.642** Corrosion of second degree of left axilla

√7ᵗʰ **T22.649** Corrosion of second degree of unspecified axilla

√6ᵗʰ **T22.65** Corrosion of second degree of shoulder

√7ᵗʰ **T22.651** Corrosion of second degree of right shoulder

√7ᵗʰ **T22.652** Corrosion of second degree of left shoulder

√7ᵗʰ **T22.659** Corrosion of second degree of unspecified shoulder

√6ᵗʰ **T22.66** Corrosion of second degree of scapular region

√7ᵗʰ **T22.661** Corrosion of second degree of right scapular region

√7ᵗʰ **T22.662** Corrosion of second degree of left scapular region

√7ᵗʰ **T22.669** Corrosion of second degree of unspecified scapular region

√6ᵗʰ **T22.69** Corrosion of second degree of multiple sites of shoulder and upper limb, except wrist and hand

√7ᵗʰ **T22.691** Corrosion of second degree of multiple sites of right shoulder and upper limb, except wrist and hand

√7ᵗʰ **T22.692** Corrosion of second degree of multiple sites of left shoulder and upper limb, except wrist and hand

√7ᵗʰ **T22.699** Corrosion of second degree of multiple sites of unspecified shoulder and upper limb, except wrist and hand

√5ᵗʰ **T22.7** Corrosion of third degree of shoulder and upper limb, except wrist and hand

Code first (T51-T65) to identify chemical and intent
Use additional external cause code to identify place (Y92)

√x7ᵗʰ **T22.70** Corrosion of third degree of shoulder and upper limb, except wrist and hand, unspecified site   `COM`

√6ᵗʰ **T22.71** Corrosion of third degree of forearm

√7ᵗʰ **T22.711** Corrosion of third degree of right forearm   `COM`

√7ᵗʰ **T22.712** Corrosion of third degree of left forearm   `COM`

√7ᵗʰ **T22.719** Corrosion of third degree of unspecified forearm   `COM`

√6ᵗʰ **T22.72** Corrosion of third degree of elbow

√7ᵗʰ **T22.721** Corrosion of third degree of right elbow   `COM`

√7ᵗʰ **T22.722** Corrosion of third degree of left elbow   `COM`

√7ᵗʰ **T22.729** Corrosion of third degree of unspecified elbow   `COM`

√6ᵗʰ **T22.73** Corrosion of third degree of upper arm

√7ᵗʰ **T22.731** Corrosion of third degree of right upper arm   `COM`

√7ᵗʰ **T22.732** Corrosion of third degree of left upper arm   `COM`

√7ᵗʰ **T22.739** Corrosion of third degree of unspecified upper arm   `COM`

√6ᵗʰ **T22.74** Corrosion of third degree of axilla

√7ᵗʰ **T22.741** Corrosion of third degree of right axilla   `COM`

√7ᵗʰ **T22.742** Corrosion of third degree of left axilla   `COM`

√7ᵗʰ **T22.749** Corrosion of third degree of unspecified axilla   `COM`

√6ᵗʰ **T22.75** Corrosion of third degree of shoulder

√7ᵗʰ **T22.751** Corrosion of third degree of right shoulder   `COM`

√7ᵗʰ **T22.752** Corrosion of third degree of left shoulder   `COM`

√7ᵗʰ **T22.759** Corrosion of third degree of unspecified shoulder   `COM`

√6ᵗʰ **T22.76** Corrosion of third degree of scapular region

√7ᵗʰ **T22.761** Corrosion of third degree of right scapular region   `COM`

√7ᵗʰ **T22.762** Corrosion of third degree of left scapular region   `COM`

√7ᵗʰ **T22.769** Corrosion of third degree of unspecified scapular region   `COM`

√6ᵗʰ **T22.79** Corrosion of third degree of multiple sites of shoulder and upper limb, except wrist and hand

√7ᵗʰ **T22.791** Corrosion of third degree of multiple sites of right shoulder and upper limb, except wrist and hand   `COM`

√7ᵗʰ **T22.792** Corrosion of third degree of multiple sites of left shoulder and upper limb, except wrist and hand   `COM`

√7ᵗʰ **T22.799** Corrosion of third degree of multiple sites of unspecified shoulder and upper limb, except wrist and hand   `COM`

√4ᵗʰ **T23** Burn and corrosion of wrist and hand

AHA: 2015,1Q,19

The appropriate 7th character is to be added to each code from category T23.
A   initial encounter
D   subsequent encounter
S   sequela

√5ᵗʰ **T23.0** Burn of unspecified degree of wrist and hand

Use additional external cause code to identify the source, place and intent of the burn (X00-X19, X75-X77, X96-X98, Y92)

√6ᵗʰ **T23.00** Burn of unspecified degree of hand, unspecified site

√7ᵗʰ **T23.001** Burn of unspecified degree of right hand, unspecified site

√7ᵗʰ **T23.002** Burn of unspecified degree of left hand, unspecified site

√7ᵗʰ **T23.009** Burn of unspecified degree of unspecified hand, unspecified site

√6ᵗʰ **T23.01** Burn of unspecified degree of thumb (nail)

√7ᵗʰ **T23.011** Burn of unspecified degree of right thumb (nail)

√7ᵗʰ **T23.012** Burn of unspecified degree of left thumb (nail)

√7ᵗʰ **T23.019** Burn of unspecified degree of unspecified thumb (nail)

√6ᵗʰ **T23.02** Burn of unspecified degree of single finger (nail) except thumb

√7ᵗʰ **T23.021** Burn of unspecified degree of single right finger (nail) except thumb

√7ᵗʰ **T23.022** Burn of unspecified degree of single left finger (nail) except thumb

√7ᵗʰ **T23.029** Burn of unspecified degree of unspecified single finger (nail) except thumb

√6ᵗʰ **T23.03** Burn of unspecified degree of multiple fingers (nail), not including thumb

√7ᵗʰ **T23.031** Burn of unspecified degree of multiple right fingers (nail), not including thumb

√7ᵗʰ **T23.032** Burn of unspecified degree of multiple left fingers (nail), not including thumb

√7ᵗʰ **T23.039** Burn of unspecified degree of unspecified multiple fingers (nail), not including thumb

√6ᵗʰ **T23.04** Burn of unspecified degree of multiple fingers (nail), including thumb

√7ᵗʰ **T23.041** Burn of unspecified degree of multiple right fingers (nail), including thumb

√7ᵗʰ **T23.042** Burn of unspecified degree of multiple left fingers (nail), including thumb

√7ᵗʰ **T23.049** Burn of unspecified degree of unspecified multiple fingers (nail), including thumb

√6ᵗʰ **T23.05** Burn of unspecified degree of palm

√7ᵗʰ **T23.051** Burn of unspecified degree of right palm

√7ᵗʰ **T23.052** Burn of unspecified degree of left palm

√7ᵗʰ **T23.059** Burn of unspecified degree of unspecified palm

√6ᵗʰ **T23.06** Burn of unspecified degree of back of hand

√7ᵗʰ **T23.061** Burn of unspecified degree of back of right hand

√7ᵗʰ **T23.062** Burn of unspecified degree of back of left hand

√7ᵗʰ **T23.069** Burn of unspecified degree of back of unspecified hand

√6ᵗʰ **T23.07** Burn of unspecified degree of wrist

√7ᵗʰ **T23.071** Burn of unspecified degree of right wrist

✓7ᵗʰ **T23.072** Burn of unspecified degree of left wrist

✓7ᵗʰ **T23.079** Burn of unspecified degree of unspecified wrist

✓6ᵗʰ **T23.09** Burn of unspecified degree of multiple sites of wrist and hand

✓7ᵗʰ **T23.091** Burn of unspecified degree of multiple sites of right wrist and hand

✓7ᵗʰ **T23.092** Burn of unspecified degree of multiple sites of left wrist and hand

✓7ᵗʰ **T23.099** Burn of unspecified degree of multiple sites of unspecified wrist and hand

✓5ᵗʰ **T23.1** Burn of first degree of wrist and hand

Use additional external cause code to identify the source, place and intent of the burn (X00-X19, X75-X77, X96-X98, Y92)

✓6ᵗʰ **T23.10** Burn of first degree of hand, unspecified site

✓7ᵗʰ **T23.101** Burn of first degree of right hand, unspecified site

✓7ᵗʰ **T23.102** Burn of first degree of left hand, unspecified site

✓7ᵗʰ **T23.109** Burn of first degree of unspecified hand, unspecified site

✓6ᵗʰ **T23.11** Burn of first degree of thumb (nail)

✓7ᵗʰ **T23.111** Burn of first degree of right thumb (nail)

✓7ᵗʰ **T23.112** Burn of first degree of left thumb (nail)

✓7ᵗʰ **T23.119** Burn of first degree of unspecified thumb (nail)

✓6ᵗʰ **T23.12** Burn of first degree of single finger (nail) except thumb

✓7ᵗʰ **T23.121** Burn of first degree of single right finger (nail) except thumb

✓7ᵗʰ **T23.122** Burn of first degree of single left finger (nail) except thumb

✓7ᵗʰ **T23.129** Burn of first degree of unspecified single finger (nail) except thumb

✓6ᵗʰ **T23.13** Burn of first degree of multiple fingers (nail), not including thumb

✓7ᵗʰ **T23.131** Burn of first degree of multiple right fingers (nail), not including thumb

✓7ᵗʰ **T23.132** Burn of first degree of multiple left fingers (nail), not including thumb

✓7ᵗʰ **T23.139** Burn of first degree of unspecified multiple fingers (nail), not including thumb

✓6ᵗʰ **T23.14** Burn of first degree of multiple fingers (nail), including thumb

✓7ᵗʰ **T23.141** Burn of first degree of multiple right fingers (nail), including thumb

✓7ᵗʰ **T23.142** Burn of first degree of multiple left fingers (nail), including thumb

✓7ᵗʰ **T23.149** Burn of first degree of unspecified multiple fingers (nail), including thumb

✓6ᵗʰ **T23.15** Burn of first degree of palm

✓7ᵗʰ **T23.151** Burn of first degree of right palm

✓7ᵗʰ **T23.152** Burn of first degree of left palm

✓7ᵗʰ **T23.159** Burn of first degree of unspecified palm

✓6ᵗʰ **T23.16** Burn of first degree of back of hand

✓7ᵗʰ **T23.161** Burn of first degree of back of right hand

✓7ᵗʰ **T23.162** Burn of first degree of back of left hand

✓7ᵗʰ **T23.169** Burn of first degree of back of unspecified hand

✓6ᵗʰ **T23.17** Burn of first degree of wrist

✓7ᵗʰ **T23.171** Burn of first degree of right wrist

✓7ᵗʰ **T23.172** Burn of first degree of left wrist

✓7ᵗʰ **T23.179** Burn of first degree of unspecified wrist

✓6ᵗʰ **T23.19** Burn of first degree of multiple sites of wrist and hand

✓7ᵗʰ **T23.191** Burn of first degree of multiple sites of right wrist and hand

✓7ᵗʰ **T23.192** Burn of first degree of multiple sites of left wrist and hand

✓7ᵗʰ **T23.199** Burn of first degree of multiple sites of unspecified wrist and hand

✓5ᵗʰ **T23.2** Burn of second degree of wrist and hand

Use additional external cause code to identify the source, place and intent of the burn (X00-X19, X75-X77, X96-X98, Y92)

✓6ᵗʰ **T23.20** Burn of second degree of hand, unspecified site

✓7ᵗʰ **T23.201** Burn of second degree of right hand, unspecified site

✓7ᵗʰ **T23.202** Burn of second degree of left hand, unspecified site

✓7ᵗʰ **T23.209** Burn of second degree of unspecified hand, unspecified site

✓6ᵗʰ **T23.21** Burn of second degree of thumb (nail)

✓7ᵗʰ **T23.211** Burn of second degree of right thumb (nail)

✓7ᵗʰ **T23.212** Burn of second degree of left thumb (nail)

✓7ᵗʰ **T23.219** Burn of second degree of unspecified thumb (nail)

✓6ᵗʰ **T23.22** Burn of second degree of single finger (nail) except thumb

✓7ᵗʰ **T23.221** Burn of second degree of single right finger (nail) except thumb

✓7ᵗʰ **T23.222** Burn of second degree of single left finger (nail) except thumb

✓7ᵗʰ **T23.229** Burn of second degree of unspecified single finger (nail) except thumb

✓6ᵗʰ **T23.23** Burn of second degree of multiple fingers (nail), not including thumb

✓7ᵗʰ **T23.231** Burn of second degree of multiple right fingers (nail), not including thumb

✓7ᵗʰ **T23.232** Burn of second degree of multiple left fingers (nail), not including thumb

✓7ᵗʰ **T23.239** Burn of second degree of unspecified multiple fingers (nail), not including thumb

✓6ᵗʰ **T23.24** Burn of second degree of multiple fingers (nail), including thumb

✓7ᵗʰ **T23.241** Burn of second degree of multiple right fingers (nail), including thumb

✓7ᵗʰ **T23.242** Burn of second degree of multiple left fingers (nail), including thumb

✓7ᵗʰ **T23.249** Burn of second degree of unspecified multiple fingers (nail), including thumb

✓6ᵗʰ **T23.25** Burn of second degree of palm

✓7ᵗʰ **T23.251** Burn of second degree of right palm

✓7ᵗʰ **T23.252** Burn of second degree of left palm

✓7ᵗʰ **T23.259** Burn of second degree of unspecified palm

✓6ᵗʰ **T23.26** Burn of second degree of back of hand

✓7ᵗʰ **T23.261** Burn of second degree of back of right hand

✓7ᵗʰ **T23.262** Burn of second degree of back of left hand

✓7ᵗʰ **T23.269** Burn of second degree of back of unspecified hand

✓6ᵗʰ **T23.27** Burn of second degree of wrist

✓7ᵗʰ **T23.271** Burn of second degree of right wrist

✓7ᵗʰ **T23.272** Burn of second degree of left wrist

✓7ᵗʰ **T23.279** Burn of second degree of unspecified wrist

✓6ᵗʰ **T23.29** Burn of second degree of multiple sites of wrist and hand

✓7ᵗʰ **T23.291** Burn of second degree of multiple sites of right wrist and hand

✓7ᵗʰ **T23.292** Burn of second degree of multiple sites of left wrist and hand

✓7ᵗʰ **T23.299** Burn of second degree of multiple sites of unspecified wrist and hand

✓5ᵗʰ **T23.3** Burn of third degree of wrist and hand

Use additional external cause code to identify the source, place and intent of the burn (X00-X19, X75-X77, X96-X98, Y92)

✓6ᵗʰ **T23.30** Burn of third degree of hand, unspecified site

AHA: 2016,2Q,5

✓7ᵗʰ **T23.301** Burn of third degree of right hand, unspecified site   COM

✓7ᵗʰ **T23.302** Burn of third degree of left hand, unspecified site   COM

✓7ᵗʰ **T23.309** Burn of third degree of unspecified hand, unspecified site   COM

✓6ᵗʰ **T23.31** Burn of third degree of thumb (nail)

✓7ᵗʰ **T23.311** Burn of third degree of right thumb (nail)   COM

✓7ᵗʰ **T23.312** Burn of third degree of left thumb (nail)   COM

✓7ᵗʰ **T23.319** Burn of third degree of unspecified thumb (nail)   COM

✓6ᵗʰ **T23.32** **Burn of third degree of** single finger (nail) except thumb

     ✓7ᵗʰ **T23.321** **Burn of third degree of single** right **finger (nail) except thumb** `COM`

     ✓7ᵗʰ **T23.322** **Burn of third degree of single** left **finger (nail) except thumb** `COM`

     ✓7ᵗʰ **T23.329** **Burn of third degree of unspecified single finger (nail) except thumb** `COM`

✓6ᵗʰ **T23.33** **Burn of third degree of** multiple fingers (nail), not including thumb

     ✓7ᵗʰ **T23.331** **Burn of third degree of multiple** right **fingers (nail), not including thumb** `COM`

     ✓7ᵗʰ **T23.332** **Burn of third degree of multiple** left **fingers (nail), not including thumb** `COM`

     ✓7ᵗʰ **T23.339** **Burn of third degree of unspecified multiple fingers (nail), not including thumb** `COM`

✓6ᵗʰ **T23.34** **Burn of third degree of** multiple fingers (nail), including thumb

     ✓7ᵗʰ **T23.341** **Burn of third degree of multiple** right **fingers (nail), including thumb** `COM`

     ✓7ᵗʰ **T23.342** **Burn of third degree of multiple** left **fingers (nail), including thumb** `COM`

     ✓7ᵗʰ **T23.349** **Burn of third degree of unspecified multiple fingers (nail), including thumb** `COM`

✓6ᵗʰ **T23.35** **Burn of third degree of** palm

     ✓7ᵗʰ **T23.351** **Burn of third degree of** right **palm** `COM`

     ✓7ᵗʰ **T23.352** **Burn of third degree of** left **palm** `COM`

     ✓7ᵗʰ **T23.359** **Burn of third degree of unspecified palm** `COM`

✓6ᵗʰ **T23.36** **Burn of third degree of** back of hand

     ✓7ᵗʰ **T23.361** **Burn of third degree of back of** right **hand** `COM`

     ✓7ᵗʰ **T23.362** **Burn of third degree of back of** left **hand** `COM`

     ✓7ᵗʰ **T23.369** **Burn of third degree of back of unspecified hand** `COM`

✓6ᵗʰ **T23.37** **Burn of third degree of** wrist

     ✓7ᵗʰ **T23.371** **Burn of third degree of** right **wrist** `COM`

     ✓7ᵗʰ **T23.372** **Burn of third degree of** left **wrist** `COM`

     ✓7ᵗʰ **T23.379** **Burn of third degree of unspecified wrist** `COM`

✓6ᵗʰ **T23.39** **Burn of third degree of** multiple sites of wrist and hand

     ✓7ᵗʰ **T23.391** **Burn of third degree of multiple sites of** right **wrist and hand** `COM`

     ✓7ᵗʰ **T23.392** **Burn of third degree of multiple sites of** left **wrist and hand** `COM`

     ✓7ᵗʰ **T23.399** **Burn of third degree of multiple sites of unspecified wrist and hand** `COM`

✓5ᵗʰ **T23.4** **Corrosion of unspecified degree of wrist and hand**

     Code first (T51-T65) to identify chemical and intent
     Use additional external cause code to identify place (Y92)

     ✓6ᵗʰ **T23.40** **Corrosion of unspecified degree of hand, unspecified site**

       ✓7ᵗʰ **T23.401** **Corrosion of unspecified degree of** right **hand, unspecified site**

       ✓7ᵗʰ **T23.402** **Corrosion of unspecified degree of** left **hand, unspecified site**

       ✓7ᵗʰ **T23.409** **Corrosion of unspecified degree of unspecified hand, unspecified site**

     ✓6ᵗʰ **T23.41** **Corrosion of unspecified degree of** thumb (nail)

       ✓7ᵗʰ **T23.411** **Corrosion of unspecified degree of** right **thumb (nail)**

       ✓7ᵗʰ **T23.412** **Corrosion of unspecified degree of** left **thumb (nail)**

       ✓7ᵗʰ **T23.419** **Corrosion of unspecified degree of unspecified thumb (nail)**

     ✓6ᵗʰ **T23.42** **Corrosion of unspecified degree of** single finger (nail) except thumb

       ✓7ᵗʰ **T23.421** **Corrosion of unspecified degree of single** right **finger (nail) except thumb**

       ✓7ᵗʰ **T23.422** **Corrosion of unspecified degree of single** left **finger (nail) except thumb**

       ✓7ᵗʰ **T23.429** **Corrosion of unspecified degree of unspecified single finger (nail) except thumb**

✓6ᵗʰ **T23.43** **Corrosion of unspecified degree of** multiple fingers (nail), not including thumb

     ✓7ᵗʰ **T23.431** **Corrosion of unspecified degree of multiple** right **fingers (nail), not including thumb**

     ✓7ᵗʰ **T23.432** **Corrosion of unspecified degree of multiple** left **fingers (nail), not including thumb**

     ✓7ᵗʰ **T23.439** **Corrosion of unspecified degree of unspecified multiple fingers (nail), not including thumb**

✓6ᵗʰ **T23.44** **Corrosion of unspecified degree of** multiple fingers (nail), including thumb

     ✓7ᵗʰ **T23.441** **Corrosion of unspecified degree of multiple** right **fingers (nail), including thumb**

     ✓7ᵗʰ **T23.442** **Corrosion of unspecified degree of multiple** left **fingers (nail), including thumb**

     ✓7ᵗʰ **T23.449** **Corrosion of unspecified degree of unspecified multiple fingers (nail), including thumb**

✓6ᵗʰ **T23.45** **Corrosion of unspecified degree of** palm

     ✓7ᵗʰ **T23.451** **Corrosion of unspecified degree of** right **palm**

     ✓7ᵗʰ **T23.452** **Corrosion of unspecified degree of** left **palm**

     ✓7ᵗʰ **T23.459** **Corrosion of unspecified degree of unspecified palm**

✓6ᵗʰ **T23.46** **Corrosion of unspecified degree of** back of hand

     ✓7ᵗʰ **T23.461** **Corrosion of unspecified degree of back of** right **hand**

     ✓7ᵗʰ **T23.462** **Corrosion of unspecified degree of back of** left **hand**

     ✓7ᵗʰ **T23.469** **Corrosion of unspecified degree of back of unspecified hand**

✓6ᵗʰ **T23.47** **Corrosion of unspecified degree of** wrist

     ✓7ᵗʰ **T23.471** **Corrosion of unspecified degree of** right **wrist**

     ✓7ᵗʰ **T23.472** **Corrosion of unspecified degree of** left **wrist**

     ✓7ᵗʰ **T23.479** **Corrosion of unspecified degree of unspecified wrist**

✓6ᵗʰ **T23.49** **Corrosion of unspecified degree of** multiple sites of wrist and hand

     ✓7ᵗʰ **T23.491** **Corrosion of unspecified degree of multiple sites of** right **wrist and hand**

     ✓7ᵗʰ **T23.492** **Corrosion of unspecified degree of multiple sites of** left **wrist and hand**

     ✓7ᵗʰ **T23.499** **Corrosion of unspecified degree of multiple sites of unspecified wrist and hand**

✓5ᵗʰ **T23.5** **Corrosion of** first degree of wrist and hand

     Code first (T51-T65) to identify chemical and intent
     Use additional external cause code to identify place (Y92)

     ✓6ᵗʰ **T23.50** **Corrosion of first degree of hand, unspecified site**

       ✓7ᵗʰ **T23.501** **Corrosion of first degree of** right **hand, unspecified site**

       ✓7ᵗʰ **T23.502** **Corrosion of first degree of** left **hand, unspecified site**

       ✓7ᵗʰ **T23.509** **Corrosion of first degree of unspecified hand, unspecified site**

     ✓6ᵗʰ **T23.51** **Corrosion of first degree of** thumb (nail)

       ✓7ᵗʰ **T23.511** **Corrosion of first degree of** right **thumb (nail)**

       ✓7ᵗʰ **T23.512** **Corrosion of first degree of** left **thumb (nail)**

       ✓7ᵗʰ **T23.519** **Corrosion of first degree of unspecified thumb (nail)**

     ✓6ᵗʰ **T23.52** **Corrosion of first degree of** single finger (nail) except thumb

       ✓7ᵗʰ **T23.521** **Corrosion of first degree of single** right **finger (nail) except thumb**

       ✓7ᵗʰ **T23.522** **Corrosion of first degree of single** left **finger (nail) except thumb**

       ✓7ᵗʰ **T23.529** **Corrosion of first degree of unspecified single finger (nail) except thumb**

     ✓6ᵗʰ **T23.53** **Corrosion of first degree of** multiple fingers (nail), not including thumb

       ✓7ᵗʰ **T23.531** **Corrosion of first degree of multiple** right **fingers (nail), not including thumb**

`HCC` CMS-HCC   `Rx` Rx HCC   `ESR` ESRD HCC   `COM` Commercial HCC   `N` Newborn: 0   `P` Pediatric: 0-17   `M` Maternity: 9-64   `A` Adult: 15-124

1124   ICD-10-CM 2023

√7ᵗʰ **T23.532** Corrosion of first degree of multiple left fingers (nail), not including thumb

√7ᵗʰ **T23.539** Corrosion of first degree of unspecified multiple fingers (nail), not including thumb

√6ᵗʰ **T23.54** Corrosion of first degree of multiple fingers (nail), including thumb

√7ᵗʰ **T23.541** Corrosion of first degree of multiple right fingers (nail), including thumb

√7ᵗʰ **T23.542** Corrosion of first degree of multiple left fingers (nail), including thumb

√7ᵗʰ **T23.549** Corrosion of first degree of unspecified multiple fingers (nail), including thumb

√6ᵗʰ **T23.55** Corrosion of first degree of palm

√7ᵗʰ **T23.551** Corrosion of first degree of right palm

√7ᵗʰ **T23.552** Corrosion of first degree of left palm

√7ᵗʰ **T23.559** Corrosion of first degree of unspecified palm

√6ᵗʰ **T23.56** Corrosion of first degree of back of hand

√7ᵗʰ **T23.561** Corrosion of first degree of back of right hand

√7ᵗʰ **T23.562** Corrosion of first degree of back of left hand

√7ᵗʰ **T23.569** Corrosion of first degree of back of unspecified hand

√6ᵗʰ **T23.57** Corrosion of first degree of wrist

√7ᵗʰ **T23.571** Corrosion of first degree of right wrist

√7ᵗʰ **T23.572** Corrosion of first degree of left wrist

√7ᵗʰ **T23.579** Corrosion of first degree of unspecified wrist

√6ᵗʰ **T23.59** Corrosion of first degree of multiple sites of wrist and hand

√7ᵗʰ **T23.591** Corrosion of first degree of multiple sites of right wrist and hand

√7ᵗʰ **T23.592** Corrosion of first degree of multiple sites of left wrist and hand

√7ᵗʰ **T23.599** Corrosion of first degree of multiple sites of unspecified wrist and hand

√5ᵗʰ **T23.6** Corrosion of second degree of wrist and hand

Code first (T51-T65) to identify chemical and intent

Use additional external cause code to identify place (Y92)

√6ᵗʰ **T23.60** Corrosion of second degree of hand, unspecified site

√7ᵗʰ **T23.601** Corrosion of second degree of right hand, unspecified site

√7ᵗʰ **T23.602** Corrosion of second degree of left hand, unspecified site

√7ᵗʰ **T23.609** Corrosion of second degree of unspecified hand, unspecified site

√6ᵗʰ **T23.61** Corrosion of second degree of thumb (nail)

√7ᵗʰ **T23.611** Corrosion of second degree of right thumb (nail)

√7ᵗʰ **T23.612** Corrosion of second degree of left thumb (nail)

√7ᵗʰ **T23.619** Corrosion of second degree of unspecified thumb (nail)

√6ᵗʰ **T23.62** Corrosion of second degree of single finger (nail) except thumb

√7ᵗʰ **T23.621** Corrosion of second degree of single right finger (nail) except thumb

√7ᵗʰ **T23.622** Corrosion of second degree of single left finger (nail) except thumb

√7ᵗʰ **T23.629** Corrosion of second degree of unspecified single finger (nail) except thumb

√6ᵗʰ **T23.63** Corrosion of second degree of multiple fingers (nail), not including thumb

√7ᵗʰ **T23.631** Corrosion of second degree of multiple right fingers (nail), not including thumb

√7ᵗʰ **T23.632** Corrosion of second degree of multiple left fingers (nail), not including thumb

√7ᵗʰ **T23.639** Corrosion of second degree of unspecified multiple fingers (nail), not including thumb

√6ᵗʰ **T23.64** Corrosion of second degree of multiple fingers (nail), including thumb

√7ᵗʰ **T23.641** Corrosion of second degree of multiple right fingers (nail), including thumb

√7ᵗʰ **T23.642** Corrosion of second degree of multiple left fingers (nail), including thumb

√7ᵗʰ **T23.649** Corrosion of second degree of unspecified multiple fingers (nail), including thumb

√6ᵗʰ **T23.65** Corrosion of second degree of palm

√7ᵗʰ **T23.651** Corrosion of second degree of right palm

√7ᵗʰ **T23.652** Corrosion of second degree of left palm

√7ᵗʰ **T23.659** Corrosion of second degree of unspecified palm

√6ᵗʰ **T23.66** Corrosion of second degree of back of hand

√7ᵗʰ **T23.661** Corrosion of second degree back of right hand

√7ᵗʰ **T23.662** Corrosion of second degree back of left hand

√7ᵗʰ **T23.669** Corrosion of second degree back of unspecified hand

√6ᵗʰ **T23.67** Corrosion of second degree of wrist

√7ᵗʰ **T23.671** Corrosion of second degree of right wrist

√7ᵗʰ **T23.672** Corrosion of second degree of left wrist

√7ᵗʰ **T23.679** Corrosion of second degree of unspecified wrist

√6ᵗʰ **T23.69** Corrosion of second degree of multiple sites of wrist and hand

√7ᵗʰ **T23.691** Corrosion of second degree of multiple sites of right wrist and hand

√7ᵗʰ **T23.692** Corrosion of second degree of multiple sites of left wrist and hand

√7ᵗʰ **T23.699** Corrosion of second degree of multiple sites of unspecified wrist and hand

√5ᵗʰ **T23.7** Corrosion of third degree of wrist and hand

Code first (T51-T65) to identify chemical and intent

Use additional external cause code to identify place (Y92)

√6ᵗʰ **T23.70** Corrosion of third degree of hand, unspecified site

√7ᵗʰ **T23.701** Corrosion of third degree of right hand, unspecified site   `COM`

√7ᵗʰ **T23.702** Corrosion of third degree of left hand, unspecified site   `COM`

√7ᵗʰ **T23.709** Corrosion of third degree of unspecified hand, unspecified site   `COM`

√6ᵗʰ **T23.71** Corrosion of third degree of thumb (nail)

√7ᵗʰ **T23.711** Corrosion of third degree of right thumb (nail)   `COM`

√7ᵗʰ **T23.712** Corrosion of third degree of left thumb (nail)   `COM`

√7ᵗʰ **T23.719** Corrosion of third degree of unspecified thumb (nail)   `COM`

√6ᵗʰ **T23.72** Corrosion of third degree of single finger (nail) except thumb

√7ᵗʰ **T23.721** Corrosion of third degree of single right finger (nail) except thumb   `COM`

√7ᵗʰ **T23.722** Corrosion of third degree of single left finger (nail) except thumb   `COM`

√7ᵗʰ **T23.729** Corrosion of third degree of unspecified single finger (nail) except thumb   `COM`

√6ᵗʰ **T23.73** Corrosion of third degree of multiple fingers (nail), not including thumb

√7ᵗʰ **T23.731** Corrosion of third degree of multiple right fingers (nail), not including thumb   `COM`

√7ᵗʰ **T23.732** Corrosion of third degree of multiple left fingers (nail), not including thumb   `COM`

√7ᵗʰ **T23.739** Corrosion of third degree of unspecified multiple fingers (nail), not including thumb   `COM`

√6ᵗʰ **T23.74** Corrosion of third degree of multiple fingers (nail), including thumb

√7ᵗʰ **T23.741** Corrosion of third degree of multiple right fingers (nail), including thumb   `COM`

√7ᵗʰ **T23.742** Corrosion of third degree of multiple left fingers (nail), including thumb   `COM`

√7ᵗʰ **T23.749** Corrosion of third degree of unspecified multiple fingers (nail), including thumb   `COM`

√6ᵗʰ **T23.75** Corrosion of third degree of palm

√7ᵗʰ **T23.751** Corrosion of third degree of right palm   `COM`

√7ᵗʰ **T23.752** Corrosion of third degree of left palm   `COM`

√7ᵗʰ **T23.759** Corrosion of third degree of unspecified palm   `COM`

☑6ᵗʰ **T23.76 Corrosion of third degree of** back of hand

    ☑7ᵗʰ **T23.761 Corrosion of third degree of back of** right **hand** `COM`

    ☑7ᵗʰ **T23.762 Corrosion of third degree of back of** left **hand** `COM`

    ☑7ᵗʰ **T23.769 Corrosion of third degree back of unspecified hand** `COM`

☑6ᵗʰ **T23.77 Corrosion of third degree of** wrist

    ☑7ᵗʰ **T23.771 Corrosion of third degree of** right **wrist** `COM`

    ☑7ᵗʰ **T23.772 Corrosion of third degree of** left **wrist** `COM`

    ☑7ᵗʰ **T23.779 Corrosion of third degree of unspecified wrist** `COM`

☑6ᵗʰ **T23.79 Corrosion of third degree of** multiple sites **of wrist and hand**

    ☑7ᵗʰ **T23.791 Corrosion of third degree of multiple sites of** right **wrist and hand** `COM`

    ☑7ᵗʰ **T23.792 Corrosion of third degree of multiple sites of** left **wrist and hand** `COM`

    ☑7ᵗʰ **T23.799 Corrosion of third degree of multiple sites of unspecified wrist and hand** `COM`

☑4ᵗʰ **T24 Burn and corrosion of lower limb, except ankle and foot**

    `EXCLUDES 2` *burn and corrosion of ankle and foot (T25.-)*
    burn and corrosion of hip region (T21.-)

    The appropriate 7th character is to be added to each code from category T24.
    A   initial encounter
    D   subsequent encounter
    S   sequela

☑5ᵗʰ **T24.0 Burn of unspecified degree of lower limb, except ankle and foot**

    Use additional external cause code to identify the source, place and intent of the burn (X00-X19, X75-X77, X96-X98, Y92)

    ☑6ᵗʰ **T24.00 Burn of unspecified degree of unspecified site of lower limb, except ankle and foot**

        ☑7ᵗʰ **T24.001 Burn of unspecified degree of unspecified site of** right **lower limb, except ankle and foot**

        ☑7ᵗʰ **T24.002 Burn of unspecified degree of unspecified site of** left **lower limb, except ankle and foot**

        ☑7ᵗʰ **T24.009 Burn of unspecified degree of unspecified site of unspecified lower limb, except ankle and foot**

    ☑6ᵗʰ **T24.01 Burn of unspecified degree of** thigh

        ☑7ᵗʰ **T24.011 Burn of unspecified degree of** right **thigh**

        ☑7ᵗʰ **T24.012 Burn of unspecified degree of** left **thigh**

        ☑7ᵗʰ **T24.019 Burn of unspecified degree of unspecified thigh**

    ☑6ᵗʰ **T24.02 Burn of unspecified degree of** knee

        ☑7ᵗʰ **T24.021 Burn of unspecified degree of** right **knee**

        ☑7ᵗʰ **T24.022 Burn of unspecified degree of** left **knee**

        ☑7ᵗʰ **T24.029 Burn of unspecified degree of unspecified knee**

    ☑6ᵗʰ **T24.03 Burn of unspecified degree of** lower leg

        ☑7ᵗʰ **T24.031 Burn of unspecified degree of** right **lower leg**

        ☑7ᵗʰ **T24.032 Burn of unspecified degree of** left **lower leg**

        ☑7ᵗʰ **T24.039 Burn of unspecified degree of unspecified lower leg**

    ☑6ᵗʰ **T24.09 Burn of unspecified degree of** multiple sites **of lower limb, except ankle and foot**

        ☑7ᵗʰ **T24.091 Burn of unspecified degree of multiple sites of** right **lower limb, except ankle and foot**

        ☑7ᵗʰ **T24.092 Burn of unspecified degree of multiple sites of** left **lower limb, except ankle and foot**

        ☑7ᵗʰ **T24.099 Burn of unspecified degree of multiple sites of unspecified lower limb, except ankle and foot**

☑5ᵗʰ **T24.1 Burn of** first degree **of lower limb, except ankle and foot**

    Use additional external cause code to identify the source, place and intent of the burn (X00-X19, X75-X77, X96-X98, Y92)

    ☑6ᵗʰ **T24.10 Burn of first degree of unspecified site of lower limb, except ankle and foot**

        ☑7ᵗʰ **T24.101 Burn of first degree of unspecified site of** right **lower limb, except ankle and foot**

        ☑7ᵗʰ **T24.102 Burn of first degree of unspecified site of** left **lower limb, except ankle and foot**

        ☑7ᵗʰ **T24.109 Burn of first degree of unspecified site of unspecified lower limb, except ankle and foot**

    ☑6ᵗʰ **T24.11 Burn of first degree of** thigh

        ☑7ᵗʰ **T24.111 Burn of first degree of** right **thigh**

        ☑7ᵗʰ **T24.112 Burn of first degree of** left **thigh**

        ☑7ᵗʰ **T24.119 Burn of first degree of unspecified thigh**

    ☑6ᵗʰ **T24.12 Burn of first degree of** knee

        ☑7ᵗʰ **T24.121 Burn of first degree of** right **knee**

        ☑7ᵗʰ **T24.122 Burn of first degree of** left **knee**

        ☑7ᵗʰ **T24.129 Burn of first degree of unspecified knee**

    ☑6ᵗʰ **T24.13 Burn of first degree of** lower leg

        ☑7ᵗʰ **T24.131 Burn of first degree of** right **lower leg**

        ☑7ᵗʰ **T24.132 Burn of first degree of** left **lower leg**

        ☑7ᵗʰ **T24.139 Burn of first degree of unspecified lower leg**

    ☑6ᵗʰ **T24.19 Burn of first degree of** multiple sites **of lower limb, except ankle and foot**

        ☑7ᵗʰ **T24.191 Burn of first degree of multiple sites of** right **lower limb, except ankle and foot**

        ☑7ᵗʰ **T24.192 Burn of first degree of multiple sites of** left **lower limb, except ankle and foot**

        ☑7ᵗʰ **T24.199 Burn of first degree of multiple sites of unspecified lower limb, except ankle and foot**

☑5ᵗʰ **T24.2 Burn of** second degree **of lower limb, except ankle and foot**

    Use additional external cause code to identify the source, place and intent of the burn (X00-X19, X75-X77, X96-X98, Y92)

    ☑6ᵗʰ **T24.20 Burn of second degree of unspecified site of lower limb, except ankle and foot**

        ☑7ᵗʰ **T24.201 Burn of second degree of unspecified site of** right **lower limb, except ankle and foot**

        ☑7ᵗʰ **T24.202 Burn of second degree of unspecified site of** left **lower limb, except ankle and foot**

        ☑7ᵗʰ **T24.209 Burn of second degree of unspecified site of unspecified lower limb, except ankle and foot**

    ☑6ᵗʰ **T24.21 Burn of second degree of** thigh

        ☑7ᵗʰ **T24.211 Burn of second degree of** right **thigh**

        ☑7ᵗʰ **T24.212 Burn of second degree of** left **thigh**

        ☑7ᵗʰ **T24.219 Burn of second degree of unspecified thigh**

    ☑6ᵗʰ **T24.22 Burn of second degree of** knee

        ☑7ᵗʰ **T24.221 Burn of second degree of** right **knee**

        ☑7ᵗʰ **T24.222 Burn of second degree of** left **knee**

        ☑7ᵗʰ **T24.229 Burn of second degree of unspecified knee**

    ☑6ᵗʰ **T24.23 Burn of second degree of** lower leg

        ☑7ᵗʰ **T24.231 Burn of second degree of** right **lower leg**

        ☑7ᵗʰ **T24.232 Burn of second degree of** left **lower leg**

        ☑7ᵗʰ **T24.239 Burn of second degree of unspecified lower leg**

    ☑6ᵗʰ **T24.29 Burn of second degree of** multiple sites **of lower limb, except ankle and foot**

        ☑7ᵗʰ **T24.291 Burn of second degree of multiple sites of** right **lower limb, except ankle and foot**

        ☑7ᵗʰ **T24.292 Burn of second degree of multiple sites of** left **lower limb, except ankle and foot**

        ☑7ᵗʰ **T24.299 Burn of second degree of multiple sites of unspecified lower limb, except ankle and foot**

✓5ᵗʰ **T24.3**   **Burn of third degree of lower limb, except ankle and foot**
Use additional external cause code to identify the source, place and intent of the burn (X00-X19, X75-X77, X96-X98, Y92)

   ✓6ᵗʰ **T24.30**   **Burn of third degree of unspecified site of lower limb, except ankle and foot**

     ✓7ᵗʰ **T24.301**   Burn of third degree of unspecified site of right lower limb, except ankle and foot   `COM`

     ✓7ᵗʰ **T24.302**   Burn of third degree of unspecified site of left lower limb, except ankle and foot   `COM`

     ✓7ᵗʰ **T24.309**   Burn of third degree of unspecified site of unspecified lower limb, except ankle and foot   `COM`

   ✓6ᵗʰ **T24.31**   **Burn of third degree of thigh**

     ✓7ᵗʰ **T24.311**   Burn of third degree of right thigh   `COM`

     ✓7ᵗʰ **T24.312**   Burn of third degree of left thigh   `COM`

     ✓7ᵗʰ **T24.319**   Burn of third degree of unspecified thigh   `COM`

   ✓6ᵗʰ **T24.32**   **Burn of third degree of knee**

     ✓7ᵗʰ **T24.321**   Burn of third degree of right knee   `COM`

     ✓7ᵗʰ **T24.322**   Burn of third degree of left knee   `COM`

     ✓7ᵗʰ **T24.329**   Burn of third degree of unspecified knee   `COM`

   ✓6ᵗʰ **T24.33**   **Burn of third degree of lower leg**

     ✓7ᵗʰ **T24.331**   Burn of third degree of right lower leg   `COM`

     ✓7ᵗʰ **T24.332**   Burn of third degree of left lower leg   `COM`

     ✓7ᵗʰ **T24.339**   Burn of third degree of unspecified lower leg   `COM`

   ✓6ᵗʰ **T24.39**   **Burn of third degree of multiple sites of lower limb, except ankle and foot**
     AHA: 2016,2Q,4

     ✓7ᵗʰ **T24.391**   Burn of third degree of multiple sites of right lower limb, except ankle and foot   `COM`

     ✓7ᵗʰ **T24.392**   Burn of third degree of multiple sites of left lower limb, except ankle and foot   `COM`

     ✓7ᵗʰ **T24.399**   Burn of third degree of multiple sites of unspecified lower limb, except ankle and foot   `COM`

✓5ᵗʰ **T24.4**   **Corrosion of unspecified degree of lower limb, except ankle and foot**
Code first (T51-T65) to identify chemical and intent
Use additional external cause code to identify place (Y92)

   ✓6ᵗʰ **T24.40**   **Corrosion of unspecified degree of unspecified site of lower limb, except ankle and foot**

     ✓7ᵗʰ **T24.401**   Corrosion of unspecified degree of unspecified site of right lower limb, except ankle and foot

     ✓7ᵗʰ **T24.402**   Corrosion of unspecified degree of unspecified site of left lower limb, except ankle and foot

     ✓7ᵗʰ **T24.409**   Corrosion of unspecified degree of unspecified site of unspecified lower limb, except ankle and foot

   ✓6ᵗʰ **T24.41**   **Corrosion of unspecified degree of thigh**

     ✓7ᵗʰ **T24.411**   Corrosion of unspecified degree of right thigh

     ✓7ᵗʰ **T24.412**   Corrosion of unspecified degree of left thigh

     ✓7ᵗʰ **T24.419**   Corrosion of unspecified degree of unspecified thigh

   ✓6ᵗʰ **T24.42**   **Corrosion of unspecified degree of knee**

     ✓7ᵗʰ **T24.421**   Corrosion of unspecified degree of right knee

     ✓7ᵗʰ **T24.422**   Corrosion of unspecified degree of left knee

     ✓7ᵗʰ **T24.429**   Corrosion of unspecified degree of unspecified knee

   ✓6ᵗʰ **T24.43**   **Corrosion of unspecified degree of lower leg**

     ✓7ᵗʰ **T24.431**   Corrosion of unspecified degree of right lower leg

     ✓7ᵗʰ **T24.432**   Corrosion of unspecified degree of left lower leg

     ✓7ᵗʰ **T24.439**   Corrosion of unspecified degree of unspecified lower leg

   ✓6ᵗʰ **T24.49**   **Corrosion of unspecified degree of multiple sites of lower limb, except ankle and foot**

     ✓7ᵗʰ **T24.491**   Corrosion of unspecified degree of multiple sites of right lower limb, except ankle and foot

     ✓7ᵗʰ **T24.492**   Corrosion of unspecified degree of multiple sites of left lower limb, except ankle and foot

     ✓7ᵗʰ **T24.499**   Corrosion of unspecified degree of multiple sites of unspecified lower limb, except ankle and foot

✓5ᵗʰ **T24.5**   **Corrosion of first degree of lower limb, except ankle and foot**
Code first (T51-T65) to identify chemical and intent
Use additional external cause code to identify place (Y92)

   ✓6ᵗʰ **T24.50**   **Corrosion of first degree of unspecified site of lower limb, except ankle and foot**

     ✓7ᵗʰ **T24.501**   Corrosion of first degree of unspecified site of right lower limb, except ankle and foot

     ✓7ᵗʰ **T24.502**   Corrosion of first degree of unspecified site of left lower limb, except ankle and foot

     ✓7ᵗʰ **T24.509**   Corrosion of first degree of unspecified site of unspecified lower limb, except ankle and foot

   ✓6ᵗʰ **T24.51**   **Corrosion of first degree of thigh**

     ✓7ᵗʰ **T24.511**   Corrosion of first degree of right thigh

     ✓7ᵗʰ **T24.512**   Corrosion of first degree of left thigh

     ✓7ᵗʰ **T24.519**   Corrosion of first degree of unspecified thigh

   ✓6ᵗʰ **T24.52**   **Corrosion of first degree of knee**

     ✓7ᵗʰ **T24.521**   Corrosion of first degree of right knee

     ✓7ᵗʰ **T24.522**   Corrosion of first degree of left knee

     ✓7ᵗʰ **T24.529**   Corrosion of first degree of unspecified knee

   ✓6ᵗʰ **T24.53**   **Corrosion of first degree of lower leg**

     ✓7ᵗʰ **T24.531**   Corrosion of first degree of right lower leg

     ✓7ᵗʰ **T24.532**   Corrosion of first degree of left lower leg

     ✓7ᵗʰ **T24.539**   Corrosion of first degree of unspecified lower leg

   ✓6ᵗʰ **T24.59**   **Corrosion of first degree of multiple sites of lower limb, except ankle and foot**

     ✓7ᵗʰ **T24.591**   Corrosion of first degree of multiple sites of right lower limb, except ankle and foot

     ✓7ᵗʰ **T24.592**   Corrosion of first degree of multiple sites of left lower limb, except ankle and foot

     ✓7ᵗʰ **T24.599**   Corrosion of first degree of multiple sites of unspecified lower limb, except ankle and foot

✓5ᵗʰ **T24.6**   **Corrosion of second degree of lower limb, except ankle and foot**
Code first (T51-T65) to identify chemical and intent
Use additional external cause code to identify place (Y92)

   ✓6ᵗʰ **T24.60**   **Corrosion of second degree of unspecified site of lower limb, except ankle and foot**

     ✓7ᵗʰ **T24.601**   Corrosion of second degree of unspecified site of right lower limb, except ankle and foot

     ✓7ᵗʰ **T24.602**   Corrosion of second degree of unspecified site of left lower limb, except ankle and foot

     ✓7ᵗʰ **T24.609**   Corrosion of second degree of unspecified site of unspecified lower limb, except ankle and foot

   ✓6ᵗʰ **T24.61**   **Corrosion of second degree of thigh**

     ✓7ᵗʰ **T24.611**   Corrosion of second degree of right thigh

     ✓7ᵗʰ **T24.612**   Corrosion of second degree of left thigh

     ✓7ᵗʰ **T24.619**   Corrosion of second degree of unspecified thigh

   ✓6ᵗʰ **T24.62**   **Corrosion of second degree of knee**

     ✓7ᵗʰ **T24.621**   Corrosion of second degree of right knee

     ✓7ᵗʰ **T24.622**   Corrosion of second degree of left knee

     ✓7ᵗʰ **T24.629**   Corrosion of second degree of unspecified knee

   ✓6ᵗʰ **T24.63**   **Corrosion of second degree of lower leg**

     ✓7ᵗʰ **T24.631**   Corrosion of second degree of right lower leg

---

✓ Additional Character Required   ✓×7ᵗʰ Placeholder Alert   Manifestation   Unspecified Dx   **Q** QPP   **UPD** Unacceptable PDx

✓7ᵗʰ **T24.632** Corrosion of second degree of left lower leg

✓7ᵗʰ **T24.639** Corrosion of second degree of unspecified lower leg

✓6ᵗʰ **T24.69** Corrosion of second degree of multiple sites of lower limb, except ankle and foot

✓7ᵗʰ **T24.691** Corrosion of second degree of multiple sites of right lower limb, except ankle and foot

✓7ᵗʰ **T24.692** Corrosion of second degree of multiple sites of left lower limb, except ankle and foot

✓7ᵗʰ **T24.699** Corrosion of second degree of multiple sites of unspecified lower limb, except ankle and foot

✓5ᵗʰ **T24.7** Corrosion of third degree of lower limb, except ankle and foot

Code first (T51-T65) to identify chemical and intent
Use additional external cause code to identify place (Y92)

✓6ᵗʰ **T24.70** Corrosion of third degree of unspecified site of lower limb, except ankle and foot

✓7ᵗʰ **T24.701** Corrosion of third degree of unspecified site of right lower limb, except ankle and foot   COM

✓7ᵗʰ **T24.702** Corrosion of third degree of unspecified site of left lower limb, except ankle and foot   COM

✓7ᵗʰ **T24.709** Corrosion of third degree of unspecified site of unspecified lower limb, except ankle and foot   COM

✓6ᵗʰ **T24.71** Corrosion of third degree of thigh

✓7ᵗʰ **T24.711** Corrosion of third degree of right thigh   COM

✓7ᵗʰ **T24.712** Corrosion of third degree of left thigh   COM

✓7ᵗʰ **T24.719** Corrosion of third degree of unspecified thigh   COM

✓6ᵗʰ **T24.72** Corrosion of third degree of knee

✓7ᵗʰ **T24.721** Corrosion of third degree of right knee   COM

✓7ᵗʰ **T24.722** Corrosion of third degree of left knee   COM

✓7ᵗʰ **T24.729** Corrosion of third degree of unspecified knee   COM

✓6ᵗʰ **T24.73** Corrosion of third degree of lower leg

✓7ᵗʰ **T24.731** Corrosion of third degree of right lower leg   COM

✓7ᵗʰ **T24.732** Corrosion of third degree of left lower leg   COM

✓7ᵗʰ **T24.739** Corrosion of third degree of unspecified lower leg   COM

✓6ᵗʰ **T24.79** Corrosion of third degree of multiple sites of lower limb, except ankle and foot

✓7ᵗʰ **T24.791** Corrosion of third degree of multiple sites of right lower limb, except ankle and foot   COM

✓7ᵗʰ **T24.792** Corrosion of third degree of multiple sites of left lower limb, except ankle and foot   COM

✓7ᵗʰ **T24.799** Corrosion of third degree of multiple sites of unspecified lower limb, except ankle and foot   COM

✓4ᵗʰ **T25** Burn and corrosion of ankle and foot

The appropriate 7th character is to be added to each code from category T25.
A   initial encounter
D   subsequent encounter
S   sequela

✓5ᵗʰ **T25.0** Burn of unspecified degree of ankle and foot

Use additional external cause code to identify the source, place and intent of the burn (X00-X19, X75-X77, X96-X98, Y92)

✓6ᵗʰ **T25.01** Burn of unspecified degree of ankle

✓7ᵗʰ **T25.011** Burn of unspecified degree of right ankle

✓7ᵗʰ **T25.012** Burn of unspecified degree of left ankle

✓7ᵗʰ **T25.019** Burn of unspecified degree of unspecified ankle

✓6ᵗʰ **T25.02** Burn of unspecified degree of foot

EXCLUDES 2   burn of unspecified degree of toe(s) (nail) (T25.03-)

✓7ᵗʰ **T25.021** Burn of unspecified degree of right foot

✓7ᵗʰ **T25.022** Burn of unspecified degree of left foot

✓7ᵗʰ **T25.029** Burn of unspecified degree of unspecified foot

✓6ᵗʰ **T25.03** Burn of unspecified degree of toe(s) (nail)

✓7ᵗʰ **T25.031** Burn of unspecified degree of right toe(s) (nail)

✓7ᵗʰ **T25.032** Burn of unspecified degree of left toe(s) (nail)

✓7ᵗʰ **T25.039** Burn of unspecified degree of unspecified toe(s) (nail)

✓6ᵗʰ **T25.09** Burn of unspecified degree of multiple sites of ankle and foot

✓7ᵗʰ **T25.091** Burn of unspecified degree of multiple sites of right ankle and foot

✓7ᵗʰ **T25.092** Burn of unspecified degree of multiple sites of left ankle and foot

✓7ᵗʰ **T25.099** Burn of unspecified degree of multiple sites of unspecified ankle and foot

✓5ᵗʰ **T25.1** Burn of first degree of ankle and foot

Use additional external cause code to identify the source, place and intent of the burn (X00-X19, X75-X77, X96-X98, Y92)

✓6ᵗʰ **T25.11** Burn of first degree of ankle

✓7ᵗʰ **T25.111** Burn of first degree of right ankle

✓7ᵗʰ **T25.112** Burn of first degree of left ankle

✓7ᵗʰ **T25.119** Burn of first degree of unspecified ankle

✓6ᵗʰ **T25.12** Burn of first degree of foot

EXCLUDES 2   burn of first degree of toe(s) (nail) (T25.13-)

✓7ᵗʰ **T25.121** Burn of first degree of right foot

✓7ᵗʰ **T25.122** Burn of first degree of left foot

✓7ᵗʰ **T25.129** Burn of first degree of unspecified foot

✓6ᵗʰ **T25.13** Burn of first degree of toe(s) (nail)

✓7ᵗʰ **T25.131** Burn of first degree of right toe(s) (nail)

✓7ᵗʰ **T25.132** Burn of first degree of left toe(s) (nail)

✓7ᵗʰ **T25.139** Burn of first degree of unspecified toe(s) (nail)

✓6ᵗʰ **T25.19** Burn of first degree of multiple sites of ankle and foot

✓7ᵗʰ **T25.191** Burn of first degree of multiple sites of right ankle and foot

✓7ᵗʰ **T25.192** Burn of first degree of multiple sites of left ankle and foot

✓7ᵗʰ **T25.199** Burn of first degree of multiple sites of unspecified ankle and foot

✓5ᵗʰ **T25.2** Burn of second degree of ankle and foot

Use additional external cause code to identify the source, place and intent of the burn (X00-X19, X75-X77, X96-X98, Y92)

✓6ᵗʰ **T25.21** Burn of second degree of ankle

✓7ᵗʰ **T25.211** Burn of second degree of right ankle

✓7ᵗʰ **T25.212** Burn of second degree of left ankle

✓7ᵗʰ **T25.219** Burn of second degree of unspecified ankle

✓6ᵗʰ **T25.22** Burn of second degree of foot

EXCLUDES 2   burn of second degree of toe(s) (nail) (T25.23-)

✓7ᵗʰ **T25.221** Burn of second degree of right foot

✓7ᵗʰ **T25.222** Burn of second degree of left foot

✓7ᵗʰ **T25.229** Burn of second degree of unspecified foot

✓6ᵗʰ **T25.23** Burn of second degree of toe(s) (nail)

✓7ᵗʰ **T25.231** Burn of second degree of right toe(s) (nail)

✓7ᵗʰ **T25.232** Burn of second degree of left toe(s) (nail)

✓7ᵗʰ **T25.239** Burn of second degree of unspecified toe(s) (nail)

✓6ᵗʰ **T25.29** Burn of second degree of multiple sites of ankle and foot

✓7ᵗʰ **T25.291** Burn of second degree of multiple sites of right ankle and foot

✓7ᵗʰ **T25.292** Burn of second degree of multiple sites of left ankle and foot

✓7ᵗʰ **T25.299** Burn of second degree of multiple sites of unspecified ankle and foot

✓5ᵗʰ **T25.3 Burn of third degree of ankle and foot**
> Use additional external cause code to identify the source, place and intent of the burn (X00-X19, X75-X77, X96-X98, Y92)

  ✓6ᵗʰ **T25.31 Burn of third degree of ankle**
    ✓7ᵗʰ **T25.311 Burn of third degree of right ankle** COM
    ✓7ᵗʰ **T25.312 Burn of third degree of left ankle** COM
    ✓7ᵗʰ **T25.319 Burn of third degree of unspecified ankle** COM

  ✓6ᵗʰ **T25.32 Burn of third degree of foot**
> EXCLUDES 2   burn of third degree of toe(s) (nail) (T25.33-)

    ✓7ᵗʰ **T25.321 Burn of third degree of right foot** COM
    ✓7ᵗʰ **T25.322 Burn of third degree of left foot** COM
    ✓7ᵗʰ **T25.329 Burn of third degree of unspecified foot** COM

  ✓6ᵗʰ **T25.33 Burn of third degree of toe(s) (nail)**
    ✓7ᵗʰ **T25.331 Burn of third degree of right toe(s) (nail)** COM
    ✓7ᵗʰ **T25.332 Burn of third degree of left toe(s) (nail)** COM
    ✓7ᵗʰ **T25.339 Burn of third degree of unspecified toe(s) (nail)** COM

  ✓6ᵗʰ **T25.39 Burn of third degree of multiple sites of ankle and foot**
    ✓7ᵗʰ **T25.391 Burn of third degree of multiple sites of right ankle and foot** COM
    ✓7ᵗʰ **T25.392 Burn of third degree of multiple sites of left ankle and foot** COM
    ✓7ᵗʰ **T25.399 Burn of third degree of multiple sites of unspecified ankle and foot** COM

✓5ᵗʰ **T25.4 Corrosion of unspecified degree of ankle and foot**
> Code first (T51-T65) to identify chemical and intent
> Use additional external cause code to identify place (Y92)

  ✓6ᵗʰ **T25.41 Corrosion of unspecified degree of ankle**
    ✓7ᵗʰ **T25.411 Corrosion of unspecified degree of right ankle**
    ✓7ᵗʰ **T25.412 Corrosion of unspecified degree of left ankle**
    ✓7ᵗʰ **T25.419 Corrosion of unspecified degree of unspecified ankle**

  ✓6ᵗʰ **T25.42 Corrosion of unspecified degree of foot**
> EXCLUDES 2   corrosion of unspecified degree of toe(s) (nail) (T25.43-)

    ✓7ᵗʰ **T25.421 Corrosion of unspecified degree of right foot**
    ✓7ᵗʰ **T25.422 Corrosion of unspecified degree of left foot**
    ✓7ᵗʰ **T25.429 Corrosion of unspecified degree of unspecified foot**

  ✓6ᵗʰ **T25.43 Corrosion of unspecified degree of toe(s) (nail)**
    ✓7ᵗʰ **T25.431 Corrosion of unspecified degree of right toe(s) (nail)**
    ✓7ᵗʰ **T25.432 Corrosion of unspecified degree of left toe(s) (nail)**
    ✓7ᵗʰ **T25.439 Corrosion of unspecified degree of unspecified toe(s) (nail)**

  ✓6ᵗʰ **T25.49 Corrosion of unspecified degree of multiple sites of ankle and foot**
    ✓7ᵗʰ **T25.491 Corrosion of unspecified degree of multiple sites of right ankle and foot**
    ✓7ᵗʰ **T25.492 Corrosion of unspecified degree of multiple sites of left ankle and foot**
    ✓7ᵗʰ **T25.499 Corrosion of unspecified degree of multiple sites of unspecified ankle and foot**

✓5ᵗʰ **T25.5 Corrosion of first degree of ankle and foot**
> Code first (T51-T65) to identify chemical and intent
> Use additional external cause code to identify place (Y92)

  ✓6ᵗʰ **T25.51 Corrosion of first degree of ankle**
    ✓7ᵗʰ **T25.511 Corrosion of first degree of right ankle**
    ✓7ᵗʰ **T25.512 Corrosion of first degree of left ankle**
    ✓7ᵗʰ **T25.519 Corrosion of first degree of unspecified ankle**

  ✓6ᵗʰ **T25.52 Corrosion of first degree of foot**
> EXCLUDES 2   corrosion of first degree of toe(s) (nail) (T25.53-)

    ✓7ᵗʰ **T25.521 Corrosion of first degree of right foot**
    ✓7ᵗʰ **T25.522 Corrosion of first degree of left foot**
    ✓7ᵗʰ **T25.529 Corrosion of first degree of unspecified foot**

  ✓6ᵗʰ **T25.53 Corrosion of first degree of toe(s) (nail)**
    ✓7ᵗʰ **T25.531 Corrosion of first degree of right toe(s) (nail)**
    ✓7ᵗʰ **T25.532 Corrosion of first degree of left toe(s) (nail)**
    ✓7ᵗʰ **T25.539 Corrosion of first degree of unspecified toe(s) (nail)**

  ✓6ᵗʰ **T25.59 Corrosion of first degree of multiple sites of ankle and foot**
    ✓7ᵗʰ **T25.591 Corrosion of first degree of multiple sites of right ankle and foot**
    ✓7ᵗʰ **T25.592 Corrosion of first degree of multiple sites of left ankle and foot**
    ✓7ᵗʰ **T25.599 Corrosion of first degree of multiple sites of unspecified ankle and foot**

✓5ᵗʰ **T25.6 Corrosion of second degree of ankle and foot**
> Code first (T51-T65) to identify chemical and intent
> Use additional external cause code to identify place (Y92)

  ✓6ᵗʰ **T25.61 Corrosion of second degree of ankle**
    ✓7ᵗʰ **T25.611 Corrosion of second degree of right ankle**
    ✓7ᵗʰ **T25.612 Corrosion of second degree of left ankle**
    ✓7ᵗʰ **T25.619 Corrosion of second degree of unspecified ankle**

  ✓6ᵗʰ **T25.62 Corrosion of second degree of foot**
> EXCLUDES 2   corrosion of second degree of toe(s) (nail) (T25.63-)

    ✓7ᵗʰ **T25.621 Corrosion of second degree of right foot**
    ✓7ᵗʰ **T25.622 Corrosion of second degree of left foot**
    ✓7ᵗʰ **T25.629 Corrosion of second degree of unspecified foot**

  ✓6ᵗʰ **T25.63 Corrosion of second degree of toe(s) (nail)**
    ✓7ᵗʰ **T25.631 Corrosion of second degree of right toe(s) (nail)**
    ✓7ᵗʰ **T25.632 Corrosion of second degree of left toe(s) (nail)**
    ✓7ᵗʰ **T25.639 Corrosion of second degree of unspecified toe(s) (nail)**

  ✓6ᵗʰ **T25.69 Corrosion of second degree of multiple sites of ankle and foot**
    ✓7ᵗʰ **T25.691 Corrosion of second degree of right ankle and foot**
    ✓7ᵗʰ **T25.692 Corrosion of second degree of left ankle and foot**
    ✓7ᵗʰ **T25.699 Corrosion of second degree of unspecified ankle and foot**

✓5ᵗʰ **T25.7 Corrosion of third degree of ankle and foot**
> Code first (T51-T65) to identify chemical and intent
> Use additional external cause code to identify place (Y92)

  ✓6ᵗʰ **T25.71 Corrosion of third degree of ankle**
    ✓7ᵗʰ **T25.711 Corrosion of third degree of right ankle** COM
    ✓7ᵗʰ **T25.712 Corrosion of third degree of left ankle** COM
    ✓7ᵗʰ **T25.719 Corrosion of third degree of unspecified ankle** COM

  ✓6ᵗʰ **T25.72 Corrosion of third degree of foot**
> EXCLUDES 2   corrosion of third degree of toe(s) (nail) (T25.73-)

    ✓7ᵗʰ **T25.721 Corrosion of third degree of right foot** COM
    ✓7ᵗʰ **T25.722 Corrosion of third degree of left foot** COM
    ✓7ᵗʰ **T25.729 Corrosion of third degree of unspecified foot** COM

  ✓6ᵗʰ **T25.73 Corrosion of third degree of toe(s) (nail)**
    ✓7ᵗʰ **T25.731 Corrosion of third degree of right toe(s) (nail)** COM
    ✓7ᵗʰ **T25.732 Corrosion of third degree of left toe(s) (nail)** COM
    ✓7ᵗʰ **T25.739 Corrosion of third degree of unspecified toe(s) (nail)**

  ✓6ᵗʰ **T25.79 Corrosion of third degree of multiple sites of ankle and foot**
    ✓7ᵗʰ **T25.791 Corrosion of third degree of multiple sites of right ankle and foot** COM

✓ Additional Character Required   ✗7ᵗʰ Placeholder Alert   Manifestation   Unspecified Dx   Ⓠ QPP   UPD Unacceptable PDx

☑7ᵗʰ **T25.792** Corrosion of third degree of multiple sites of **left** ankle and foot   `COM`

☑7ᵗʰ **T25.799** Corrosion of third degree of multiple sites of unspecified ankle and foot   `COM`

Burns and corrosions confined to eye and internal organs (T26-T28)

☑4ᵗʰ **T26** **Burn and corrosion confined to eye and adnexa**

> The appropriate 7th character is to be added to each code from category T26.
> A   initial encounter
> D   subsequent encounter
> S   sequela

☑5ᵗʰ **T26.0** **Burn of** eyelid and periocular area

> Use additional external cause code to identify the source, place and intent of the burn (X00-X19, X75-X77, X96-X98, Y92)

☑x7ᵗʰ **T26.00** **Burn of unspecified eyelid and periocular area**

☑x7ᵗʰ **T26.01** **Burn of** right **eyelid and periocular area**

☑x7ᵗʰ **T26.02** **Burn of** left **eyelid and periocular area**

☑5ᵗʰ **T26.1** **Burn of** cornea and conjunctival sac

> Use additional external cause code to identify the source, place and intent of the burn (X00-X19, X75-X77, X96-X98, Y92)

☑x7ᵗʰ **T26.10** **Burn of cornea and conjunctival sac, unspecified eye**

☑x7ᵗʰ **T26.11** **Burn of cornea and conjunctival sac,** right **eye**

☑x7ᵗʰ **T26.12** **Burn of cornea and conjunctival sac,** left **eye**

☑5ᵗʰ **T26.2** **Burn with resulting** rupture and destruction of eyeball

> Use additional external cause code to identify the source, place and intent of the burn (X00-X19, X75-X77, X96-X98, Y92)

☑x7ᵗʰ **T26.20** **Burn with resulting rupture and destruction of unspecified eyeball**

☑x7ᵗʰ **T26.21** **Burn with resulting rupture and destruction of** right **eyeball**

☑x7ᵗʰ **T26.22** **Burn with resulting rupture and destruction of** left **eyeball**

☑5ᵗʰ **T26.3** **Burns of other specified parts of eye and adnexa**

> Use additional external cause code to identify the source, place and intent of the burn (X00-X19, X75-X77, X96-X98, Y92)

☑x7ᵗʰ **T26.30** **Burns of other specified parts of unspecified eye and adnexa**

☑x7ᵗʰ **T26.31** **Burns of other specified parts of** right **eye and adnexa**

☑x7ᵗʰ **T26.32** **Burns of other specified parts of** left **eye and adnexa**

☑5ᵗʰ **T26.4** **Burn of eye and adnexa, part unspecified**

> Use additional external cause code to identify the source, place and intent of the burn (X00-X19, X75-X77, X96-X98, Y92)

☑x7ᵗʰ **T26.40** **Burn of unspecified eye and adnexa, part unspecified**

☑x7ᵗʰ **T26.41** **Burn of** right **eye and adnexa, part unspecified**

☑x7ᵗʰ **T26.42** **Burn of** left **eye and adnexa, part unspecified**

☑5ᵗʰ **T26.5** **Corrosion of** eyelid and periocular area

> Code first (T51-T65) to identify chemical and intent
> Use additional external cause code to identify place (Y92)

☑x7ᵗʰ **T26.50** **Corrosion of unspecified eyelid and periocular area**

☑x7ᵗʰ **T26.51** **Corrosion of** right **eyelid and periocular area**

☑x7ᵗʰ **T26.52** **Corrosion of** left **eyelid and periocular area**

☑5ᵗʰ **T26.6** **Corrosion of** cornea and conjunctival sac

> Code first (T51-T65) to identify chemical and intent
> Use additional external cause code to identify place (Y92)

☑x7ᵗʰ **T26.60** **Corrosion of cornea and conjunctival sac, unspecified eye**

☑x7ᵗʰ **T26.61** **Corrosion of cornea and conjunctival sac,** right **eye**

☑x7ᵗʰ **T26.62** **Corrosion of cornea and conjunctival sac,** left **eye**

☑5ᵗʰ **T26.7** **Corrosion with resulting** rupture and destruction of eyeball

> Code first (T51-T65) to identify chemical and intent
> Use additional external cause code to identify place (Y92)

☑x7ᵗʰ **T26.70** **Corrosion with resulting rupture and destruction of unspecified eyeball**

☑x7ᵗʰ **T26.71** **Corrosion with resulting rupture and destruction of** right **eyeball**

☑x7ᵗʰ **T26.72** **Corrosion with resulting rupture and destruction of** left **eyeball**

☑5ᵗʰ **T26.8** **Corrosions of other specified parts of eye and adnexa**

> Code first (T51-T65) to identify chemical and intent
> Use additional external cause code to identify place (Y92)

☑x7ᵗʰ **T26.80** **Corrosions of other specified parts of unspecified eye and adnexa**

☑x7ᵗʰ **T26.81** **Corrosions of other specified parts of** right **eye and adnexa**

☑x7ᵗʰ **T26.82** **Corrosions of other specified parts of** left **eye and adnexa**

☑5ᵗʰ **T26.9** **Corrosion of eye and adnexa, part unspecified**

> Code first (T51-T65) to identify chemical and intent
> Use additional external cause code to identify place (Y92)

☑x7ᵗʰ **T26.90** **Corrosion of unspecified eye and adnexa, part unspecified**

☑x7ᵗʰ **T26.91** **Corrosion of** right **eye and adnexa, part unspecified**

☑x7ᵗʰ **T26.92** **Corrosion of** left **eye and adnexa, part unspecified**

☑4ᵗʰ **T27** **Burn and corrosion of respiratory tract**

> Use additional external cause code to identify the source and intent of the burn (X00-X19, X75-X77, X96-X98)
> Use additional external cause code to identify place (Y92)

> The appropriate 7th character is to be added to each code from category T27.
> A   initial encounter
> D   subsequent encounter
> S   sequela

☑x7ᵗʰ **T27.0** **Burn of** larynx and trachea

☑x7ᵗʰ **T27.1** **Burn involving** larynx and trachea with lung

☑x7ᵗʰ **T27.2** **Burn of other parts of respiratory tract**

> Burn of thoracic cavity

☑x7ᵗʰ **T27.3** **Burn of respiratory tract, part unspecified**

☑x7ᵗʰ **T27.4** **Corrosion of** larynx and trachea

> Code first (T51-T65) to identify chemical and intent

☑x7ᵗʰ **T27.5** **Corrosion involving** larynx and trachea with lung

> Code first (T51-T65) to identify chemical and intent

☑x7ᵗʰ **T27.6** **Corrosion of other parts of respiratory tract**

> Code first (T51-T65) to identify chemical and intent

☑x7ᵗʰ **T27.7** **Corrosion of respiratory tract, part unspecified**

> Code first (T51-T65) to identify chemical and intent

☑4ᵗʰ **T28** **Burn and corrosion of other internal organs**

> Use additional external cause code to identify the source and intent of the burn (X00-X19, X75-X77, X96-X98)
> Use additional external cause code to identify place (Y92)

> The appropriate 7th character is to be added to each code from category T28.
> A   initial encounter
> D   subsequent encounter
> S   sequela

☑x7ᵗʰ **T28.0** **Burn of** mouth and pharynx

☑x7ᵗʰ **T28.1** **Burn of** esophagus

☑x7ᵗʰ **T28.2** **Burn of** other parts of alimentary tract

☑x7ᵗʰ **T28.3** **Burn of** internal genitourinary organs

☑5ᵗʰ **T28.4** **Burns of other and unspecified internal organs**

☑x7ᵗʰ **T28.40** **Burn of** unspecified internal organ

☑6ᵗʰ **T28.41** **Burn of** ear drum

☑7ᵗʰ **T28.411** **Burn of** right **ear drum**

☑7ᵗʰ **T28.412** **Burn of** left **ear drum**

☑7ᵗʰ **T28.419** **Burn of** unspecified ear drum

☑x7ᵗʰ **T28.49** **Burn of** other internal organ

☑x7ᵗʰ **T28.5** **Corrosion of** mouth and pharynx

> Code first (T51-T65) to identify chemical and intent

☑x7ᵗʰ **T28.6** **Corrosion of** esophagus

> Code first (T51-T65) to identify chemical and intent

☑x7ᵗʰ **T28.7** **Corrosion of** other parts of alimentary tract

> Code first (T51-T65) to identify chemical and intent

☑x7ᵗʰ **T28.8** **Corrosion of** internal genitourinary organs

> Code first (T51-T65) to identify chemical and intent

☑5ᵗʰ **T28.9** **Corrosions of other and unspecified internal organs**

> Code first (T51-T65) to identify chemical and intent

☑x7ᵗʰ **T28.90** **Corrosions of** unspecified internal organs

`HCC` CMS-HCC   `Rx` Rx HCC   `ESR` ESRD HCC   `COM` Commercial HCC   `N` Newborn: 0   `P` Pediatric: 0-17   `M` Maternity: 9-64   `A` Adult: 15-124

1130   ICD-10-CM 2023

✓6ᵗʰ **T28.91 Corrosions of ear drum**
    ✓7ᵗʰ **T28.911 Corrosions of right ear drum**
    ✓7ᵗʰ **T28.912 Corrosions of left ear drum**
    ✓7ᵗʰ **T28.919 Corrosions of unspecified ear drum**
✓×7ᵗʰ **T28.99 Corrosions of other internal organs**

Burns and corrosions of multiple and unspecified body regions (T30-T32)

✓4ᵗʰ **T30 Burn and corrosion, body region unspecified**

T30.0 Burn of unspecified body region, unspecified degree
This code is not for inpatient use. Code to specified site and degree of burns
Burn NOS
Multiple burns NOS

T30.4 Corrosion of unspecified body region, unspecified degree
This code is not for inpatient use. Code to specified site and degree of corrosion
Corrosion NOS
Multiple corrosion NOS

✓4ᵗʰ **T31 Burns classified according to extent of body surface involved**

NOTE   This category is to be used as the primary code only when the site of the burn is unspecified. It should be used as a supplementary code with categories T20-T25 when the site is specified.

T31.0 Burns involving less than 10% of body surface
✓5ᵗʰ **T31.1 Burns involving 10-19% of body surface**

T31.10 Burns involving 10-19% of body surface with 0% to 9% third degree burns `COM`
Burns involving 10-19% of body surface NOS
T31.11 Burns involving 10-19% of body surface with 10-19% third degree burns `HCC` `ESR` `COM`

✓5ᵗʰ **T31.2 Burns involving 20-29% of body surface**

T31.20 Burns involving 20-29% of body surface with 0% to 9% third degree burns `COM`
Burns involving 20-29% of body surface NOS
T31.21 Burns involving 20-29% of body surface with 10-19% third degree burns `HCC` `ESR` `COM`
T31.22 Burns involving 20-29% of body surface with 20-29% third degree burns `HCC` `ESR` `COM`

✓5ᵗʰ **T31.3 Burns involving 30-39% of body surface**

T31.30 Burns involving 30-39% of body surface with 0% to 9% third degree burns `COM`
Burns involving 30-39% of body surface NOS
T31.31 Burns involving 30-39% of body surface with 10-19% third degree burns `HCC` `ESR` `COM`
T31.32 Burns involving 30-39% of body surface with 20-29% third degree burns `HCC` `ESR` `COM`
T31.33 Burns involving 30-39% of body surface with 30-39% third degree burns `HCC` `ESR` `COM`

✓5ᵗʰ **T31.4 Burns involving 40-49% of body surface**

T31.40 Burns involving 40-49% of body surface with 0% to 9% third degree burns `COM`
Burns involving 40-49% of body surface NOS
T31.41 Burns involving 40-49% of body surface with 10-19% third degree burns `HCC` `ESR` `COM`
T31.42 Burns involving 40-49% of body surface with 20-29% third degree burns `HCC` `ESR` `COM`
T31.43 Burns involving 40-49% of body surface with 30-39% third degree burns `HCC` `ESR` `COM`
T31.44 Burns involving 40-49% of body surface with 40-49% third degree burns `HCC` `ESR` `COM`

✓5ᵗʰ **T31.5 Burns involving 50-59% of body surface**

T31.50 Burns involving 50-59% of body surface with 0% to 9% third degree burns `COM`
Burns involving 50-59% of body surface NOS
T31.51 Burns involving 50-59% of body surface with 10-19% third degree burns `HCC` `ESR` `COM`
T31.52 Burns involving 50-59% of body surface with 20-29% third degree burns `HCC` `ESR` `COM`
T31.53 Burns involving 50-59% of body surface with 30-39% third degree burns `HCC` `ESR` `COM`
T31.54 Burns involving 50-59% of body surface with 40-49% third degree burns `HCC` `ESR` `COM`
T31.55 Burns involving 50-59% of body surface with 50-59% third degree burns `HCC` `ESR` `COM`

✓5ᵗʰ **T31.6 Burns involving 60-69% of body surface**

T31.60 Burns involving 60-69% of body surface with 0% to 9% third degree burns `COM`
Burns involving 60-69% of body surface NOS
T31.61 Burns involving 60-69% of body surface with 10-19% third degree burns `HCC` `ESR` `COM`
T31.62 Burns involving 60-69% of body surface with 20-29% third degree burns `HCC` `ESR` `COM`
T31.63 Burns involving 60-69% of body surface with 30-39% third degree burns `HCC` `ESR` `COM`
T31.64 Burns involving 60-69% of body surface with 40-49% third degree burns `HCC` `ESR` `COM`
T31.65 Burns involving 60-69% of body surface with 50-59% third degree burns `HCC` `ESR` `COM`
T31.66 Burns involving 60-69% of body surface with 60-69% third degree burns `HCC` `ESR` `COM`

✓5ᵗʰ **T31.7 Burns involving 70-79% of body surface**

T31.70 Burns involving 70-79% of body surface with 0% to 9% third degree burns `COM`
Burns involving 70-79% of body surface NOS
T31.71 Burns involving 70-79% of body surface with 10-19% third degree burns `HCC` `ESR` `COM`
T31.72 Burns involving 70-79% of body surface with 20-29% third degree burns `HCC` `ESR` `COM`
T31.73 Burns involving 70-79% of body surface with 30-39% third degree burns `HCC` `ESR` `COM`
T31.74 Burns involving 70-79% of body surface with 40-49% third degree burns `HCC` `ESR` `COM`
T31.75 Burns involving 70-79% of body surface with 50-59% third degree burns `HCC` `ESR` `COM`
T31.76 Burns involving 70-79% of body surface with 60-69% third degree burns `HCC` `ESR` `COM`
T31.77 Burns involving 70-79% of body surface with 70-79% third degree burns `HCC` `ESR` `COM`

✓5ᵗʰ **T31.8 Burns involving 80-89% of body surface**

T31.80 Burns involving 80-89% of body surface with 0% to 9% third degree burns `COM`
Burns involving 80-89% of body surface NOS
T31.81 Burns involving 80-89% of body surface with 10-19% third degree burns `HCC` `ESR` `COM`
T31.82 Burns involving 80-89% of body surface with 20-29% third degree burns `HCC` `ESR` `COM`
T31.83 Burns involving 80-89% of body surface with 30-39% third degree burns `HCC` `ESR` `COM`
T31.84 Burns involving 80-89% of body surface with 40-49% third degree burns `HCC` `ESR` `COM`
T31.85 Burns involving 80-89% of body surface with 50-59% third degree burns `HCC` `ESR` `COM`
T31.86 Burns involving 80-89% of body surface with 60-69% third degree burns `HCC` `ESR` `COM`
T31.87 Burns involving 80-89% of body surface with 70-79% third degree burns `HCC` `ESR` `COM`
T31.88 Burns involving 80-89% of body surface with 80-89% third degree burns `HCC` `ESR` `COM`

✓5ᵗʰ **T31.9 Burns involving 90% or more of body surface**

T31.90 Burns involving 90% or more of body surface with 0% to 9% third degree burns `COM`
Burns involving 90% or more of body surface NOS
T31.91 Burns involving 90% or more of body surface with 10-19% third degree burns `HCC` `ESR` `COM`
T31.92 Burns involving 90% or more of body surface with 20-29% third degree burns `HCC` `ESR`
T31.93 Burns involving 90% or more of body surface with 30-39% third degree burns `HCC` `ESR` `COM`
T31.94 Burns involving 90% or more of body surface with 40-49% third degree burns `HCC` `ESR` `COM`
T31.95 Burns involving 90% or more of body surface with 50-59% third degree burns `HCC` `ESR` `COM`
T31.96 Burns involving 90% or more of body surface with 60-69% third degree burns `HCC` `ESR` `COM`
T31.97 Burns involving 90% or more of body surface with 70-79% third degree burns `HCC` `ESR` `COM`
T31.98 Burns involving 90% or more of body surface with 80-89% third degree burns `HCC` `ESR` `COM`

✔ Additional Character Required   ✓×7ᵗʰ Placeholder Alert   Manifestation   Unspecified Dx   **Q** QPP   **UPD** Unacceptable PDx

T31.99   **Burns involving 90% or more of body surface with 90% or more third degree burns** `HCC` `ESR` `COM`

Rule of Nines Estimation of Total Body Surface Burned

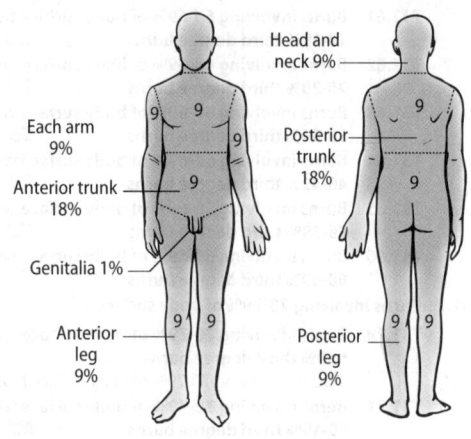

- Head and neck 9%
- Each arm 9%
- Posterior trunk 18%
- Anterior trunk 18%
- Genitalia 1%
- Anterior leg 9%
- Posterior leg 9%

`√4ᵗʰ` **T32**   Corrosions **classified** according to extent of body surface involved

> **NOTE**   This category is to be used as the primary code only when the site of the corrosion is unspecified. It may be used as a supplementary code with categories T20-T25 when the site is specified.

T32.0   Corrosions involving less than 10% of body surface

`√5ᵗʰ` **T32.1**   Corrosions involving 10-19% of body surface

     T32.10   **Corrosions involving 10-19% of body surface with 0% to 9% third degree corrosion** `COM`
             Corrosions involving 10-19% of body surface NOS

     T32.11   **Corrosions involving 10-19% of body surface with 10-19% third degree corrosion** `HCC` `ESR` `COM`

`√5ᵗʰ` **T32.2**   Corrosions involving 20-29% of body surface

     T32.20   **Corrosions involving 20-29% of body surface with 0% to 9% third degree corrosion** `COM`

     T32.21   **Corrosions involving 20-29% of body surface with 10-19% third degree corrosion** `HCC` `ESR` `COM`

     T32.22   **Corrosions involving 20-29% of body surface with 20-29% third degree corrosion** `HCC` `ESR` `COM`

`√5ᵗʰ` **T32.3**   Corrosions involving 30-39% of body surface

     T32.30   **Corrosions involving 30-39% of body surface with 0% to 9% third degree corrosion** `COM`

     T32.31   **Corrosions involving 30-39% of body surface with 10-19% third degree corrosion** `HCC` `ESR` `COM`

     T32.32   **Corrosions involving 30-39% of body surface with 20-29% third degree corrosion** `HCC` `ESR` `COM`

     T32.33   **Corrosions involving 30-39% of body surface with 30-39% third degree corrosion** `HCC` `ESR` `COM`

`√5ᵗʰ` **T32.4**   Corrosions involving 40-49% of body surface

     T32.40   **Corrosions involving 40-49% of body surface with 0% to 9% third degree corrosion** `COM`

     T32.41   **Corrosions involving 40-49% of body surface with 10-19% third degree corrosion** `HCC` `ESR` `COM`

     T32.42   **Corrosions involving 40-49% of body surface with 20-29% third degree corrosion** `HCC` `ESR` `COM`

     T32.43   **Corrosions involving 40-49% of body surface with 30-39% third degree corrosion** `HCC` `ESR` `COM`

     T32.44   **Corrosions involving 40-49% of body surface with 40-49% third degree corrosion** `HCC` `ESR` `COM`

`√5ᵗʰ` **T32.5**   Corrosions involving 50-59% of body surface

     T32.50   **Corrosions involving 50-59% of body surface with 0% to 9% third degree corrosion** `COM`

     T32.51   **Corrosions involving 50-59% of body surface with 10-19% third degree corrosion** `HCC` `ESR` `COM`

     T32.52   **Corrosions involving 50-59% of body surface with 20-29% third degree corrosion** `HCC` `ESR` `COM`

     T32.53   **Corrosions involving 50-59% of body surface with 30-39% third degree corrosion** `HCC` `ESR` `COM`

     T32.54   **Corrosions involving 50-59% of body surface with 40-49% third degree corrosion** `HCC` `ESR` `COM`

     T32.55   **Corrosions involving 50-59% of body surface with 50-59% third degree corrosion** `HCC` `ESR` `COM`

`√5ᵗʰ` **T32.6**   Corrosions involving 60-69% of body surface

     T32.60   **Corrosions involving 60-69% of body surface with 0% to 9% third degree corrosion** `COM`

     T32.61   **Corrosions involving 60-69% of body surface with 10-19% third degree corrosion** `HCC` `ESR` `COM`

     T32.62   **Corrosions involving 60-69% of body surface with 20-29% third degree corrosion** `HCC` `ESR` `COM`

     T32.63   **Corrosions involving 60-69% of body surface with 30-39% third degree corrosion** `HCC` `ESR` `COM`

     T32.64   **Corrosions involving 60-69% of body surface with 40-49% third degree corrosion** `HCC` `ESR` `COM`

     T32.65   **Corrosions involving 60-69% of body surface with 50-59% third degree corrosion** `HCC` `ESR` `COM`

     T32.66   **Corrosions involving 60-69% of body surface with 60-69% third degree corrosion** `HCC` `ESR` `COM`

`√5ᵗʰ` **T32.7**   Corrosions involving 70-79% of body surface

     T32.70   **Corrosions involving 70-79% of body surface with 0% to 9% third degree corrosion** `COM`

     T32.71   **Corrosions involving 70-79% of body surface with 10-19% third degree corrosion** `HCC` `ESR` `COM`

     T32.72   **Corrosions involving 70-79% of body surface with 20-29% third degree corrosion** `HCC` `ESR` `COM`

     T32.73   **Corrosions involving 70-79% of body surface with 30-39% third degree corrosion** `HCC` `ESR` `COM`

     T32.74   **Corrosions involving 70-79% of body surface with 40-49% third degree corrosion** `HCC` `ESR` `COM`

     T32.75   **Corrosions involving 70-79% of body surface with 50-59% third degree corrosion** `HCC` `ESR` `COM`

     T32.76   **Corrosions involving 70-79% of body surface with 60-69% third degree corrosion** `HCC` `ESR` `COM`

     T32.77   **Corrosions involving 70-79% of body surface with 70-79% third degree corrosion** `HCC` `ESR` `COM`

`√5ᵗʰ` **T32.8**   Corrosions involving 80-89% of body surface

     T32.80   **Corrosions involving 80-89% of body surface with 0% to 9% third degree corrosion** `COM`

     T32.81   **Corrosions involving 80-89% of body surface with 10-19% third degree corrosion** `HCC` `ESR` `COM`

     T32.82   **Corrosions involving 80-89% of body surface with 20-29% third degree corrosion** `HCC` `ESR` `COM`

     T32.83   **Corrosions involving 80-89% of body surface with 30-39% third degree corrosion** `HCC` `ESR` `COM`

     T32.84   **Corrosions involving 80-89% of body surface with 40-49% third degree corrosion** `HCC` `ESR` `COM`

     T32.85   **Corrosions involving 80-89% of body surface with 50-59% third degree corrosion** `HCC` `ESR` `COM`

     T32.86   **Corrosions involving 80-89% of body surface with 60-69% third degree corrosion** `HCC` `ESR` `COM`

     T32.87   **Corrosions involving 80-89% of body surface with 70-79% third degree corrosion** `HCC` `ESR` `COM`

     T32.88   **Corrosions involving 80-89% of body surface with 80-89% third degree corrosion** `HCC` `ESR` `COM`

`√5ᵗʰ` **T32.9**   Corrosions involving 90% or more of body surface

     T32.90   **Corrosions involving 90% or more of body surface with 0% to 9% third degree corrosion** `COM`

     T32.91   **Corrosions involving 90% or more of body surface with 10-19% third degree corrosion** `HCC` `ESR` `COM`

     T32.92   **Corrosions involving 90% or more of body surface with 20-29% third degree corrosion** `HCC` `ESR` `COM`

     T32.93   **Corrosions involving 90% or more of body surface with 30-39% third degree corrosion** `HCC` `ESR` `COM`

     T32.94   **Corrosions involving 90% or more of body surface with 40-49% third degree corrosion** `HCC` `ESR` `COM`

     T32.95   **Corrosions involving 90% or more of body surface with 50-59% third degree corrosion** `HCC` `ESR` `COM`

     T32.96   **Corrosions involving 90% or more of body surface with 60-69% third degree corrosion** `HCC` `ESR` `COM`

     T32.97   **Corrosions involving 90% or more of body surface with 70-79% third degree corrosion** `HCC` `ESR` `COM`

     T32.98   **Corrosions involving 90% or more of body surface with 80-89% third degree corrosion** `HCC` `ESR` `COM`

     T32.99   **Corrosions involving 90% or more of body surface with 90% or more third degree corrosion** `HCC` `ESR` `COM`

`HCC` CMS-HCC   `Rx` Rx HCC   `ESR` ESRD HCC   `COM` Commercial HCC   `N` Newborn: 0   `P` Pediatric: 0-17   `M` Maternity: 9-64   `A` Adult: 15-124

1132   ICD-10-CM 2023

Frostbite (T33-T34)

EXCLUDES 2   *hypothermia and other effects of reduced temperature (T68, T69.-)*

☑4ᵗʰ **T33** **Superficial frostbite**

INCLUDES   frostbite with partial thickness skin loss

> The appropriate 7th character is to be added to each code from category T33.
> A   initial encounter
> D   subsequent encounter
> S   sequela

☑5ᵗʰ **T33.0** **Superficial frostbite of** head

   ☑6ᵗʰ **T33.01** **Superficial frostbite of** ear

     7ᵗʰ **T33.011** **Superficial frostbite of** right ear

     7ᵗʰ **T33.012** **Superficial frostbite of** left ear

     7ᵗʰ **T33.019** **Superficial frostbite of** unspecified ear

   ✓x7ᵗʰ **T33.02** **Superficial frostbite of** nose

   ✓x7ᵗʰ **T33.09** **Superficial frostbite of** other part of head

✓x7ᵗʰ **T33.1** **Superficial frostbite of** neck

✓x7ᵗʰ **T33.2** **Superficial frostbite of** thorax

✓x7ᵗʰ **T33.3** **Superficial frostbite of** abdominal wall, lower back and pelvis

☑5ᵗʰ **T33.4** **Superficial frostbite of** arm

   EXCLUDES 2   *superficial frostbite of wrist and hand (T33.5-)*

   ✓x7ᵗʰ **T33.40** **Superficial frostbite of** unspecified arm

   ✓x7ᵗʰ **T33.41** **Superficial frostbite of** right arm

   ✓x7ᵗʰ **T33.42** **Superficial frostbite of** left arm

☑5ᵗʰ **T33.5** **Superficial frostbite of** wrist, hand, and fingers

   ☑6ᵗʰ **T33.51** **Superficial frostbite of** wrist

     7ᵗʰ **T33.511** **Superficial frostbite of** right wrist

     7ᵗʰ **T33.512** **Superficial frostbite of** left wrist

     7ᵗʰ **T33.519** **Superficial frostbite of** unspecified wrist

   ☑6ᵗʰ **T33.52** **Superficial frostbite of** hand

     EXCLUDES 2   *superficial frostbite of fingers (T33.53-)*

     7ᵗʰ **T33.521** **Superficial frostbite of** right hand

     7ᵗʰ **T33.522** **Superficial frostbite of** left hand

     7ᵗʰ **T33.529** **Superficial frostbite of** unspecified hand

   ☑6ᵗʰ **T33.53** **Superficial frostbite of** finger(s)

     7ᵗʰ **T33.531** **Superficial frostbite of** right finger(s)

     7ᵗʰ **T33.532** **Superficial frostbite of** left finger(s)

     7ᵗʰ **T33.539** **Superficial frostbite of** unspecified finger(s)

☑5ᵗʰ **T33.6** **Superficial frostbite of** hip and thigh

   ✓x7ᵗʰ **T33.60** **Superficial frostbite of** unspecified hip and thigh

   ✓x7ᵗʰ **T33.61** **Superficial frostbite of** right hip and thigh

   ✓x7ᵗʰ **T33.62** **Superficial frostbite of** left hip and thigh

☑5ᵗʰ **T33.7** **Superficial frostbite of** knee and lower leg

   EXCLUDES 2   *superficial frostbite of ankle and foot (T33.8-)*

   ✓x7ᵗʰ **T33.70** **Superficial frostbite of** unspecified knee and lower leg

   ✓x7ᵗʰ **T33.71** **Superficial frostbite of** right knee and lower leg

   ✓x7ᵗʰ **T33.72** **Superficial frostbite of** left knee and lower leg

☑5ᵗʰ **T33.8** **Superficial frostbite of** ankle, foot, and toe(s)

   ☑6ᵗʰ **T33.81** **Superficial frostbite of** ankle

     7ᵗʰ **T33.811** **Superficial frostbite of** right ankle

     7ᵗʰ **T33.812** **Superficial frostbite of** left ankle

     7ᵗʰ **T33.819** **Superficial frostbite of** unspecified ankle

   ☑6ᵗʰ **T33.82** **Superficial frostbite of** foot

     7ᵗʰ **T33.821** **Superficial frostbite of** right foot

     7ᵗʰ **T33.822** **Superficial frostbite of** left foot

     7ᵗʰ **T33.829** **Superficial frostbite of** unspecified foot

   ☑6ᵗʰ **T33.83** **Superficial frostbite of** toe(s)

     7ᵗʰ **T33.831** **Superficial frostbite of** right toe(s)

     7ᵗʰ **T33.832** **Superficial frostbite of** left toe(s)

     7ᵗʰ **T33.839** **Superficial frostbite of** unspecified toe(s)

☑5ᵗʰ **T33.9** **Superficial frostbite of** other and unspecified sites

   ✓x7ᵗʰ **T33.90** **Superficial frostbite of** unspecified sites

     Superficial frostbite NOS

   ✓x7ᵗʰ **T33.99** **Superficial frostbite of** other sites

     Superficial frostbite of leg NOS
     Superficial frostbite of trunk NOS

☑4ᵗʰ **T34** **Frostbite with tissue necrosis**

> The appropriate 7th character is to be added to each code from category T34.
> A   initial encounter
> D   subsequent encounter
> S   sequela

☑5ᵗʰ **T34.0** **Frostbite with tissue necrosis of** head

   ☑6ᵗʰ **T34.01** **Frostbite with tissue necrosis of** ear

     7ᵗʰ **T34.011** **Frostbite with tissue necrosis of** right ear   COM

     7ᵗʰ **T34.012** **Frostbite with tissue necrosis of** left ear   COM

     7ᵗʰ **T34.019** **Frostbite with tissue necrosis of** unspecified ear   COM

   ✓x7ᵗʰ **T34.02** **Frostbite with tissue necrosis of** nose   COM

   ✓x7ᵗʰ **T34.09** **Frostbite with tissue necrosis of** other part of head   COM

✓x7ᵗʰ **T34.1** **Frostbite with tissue necrosis of** neck   COM

✓x7ᵗʰ **T34.2** **Frostbite with tissue necrosis of** thorax   COM

✓x7ᵗʰ **T34.3** **Frostbite with tissue necrosis of** abdominal wall, lower back and pelvis   COM

☑5ᵗʰ **T34.4** **Frostbite with tissue necrosis of** arm

   EXCLUDES 2   *frostbite with tissue necrosis of wrist and hand (T34.5-)*

   ✓x7ᵗʰ **T34.40** **Frostbite with tissue necrosis of** unspecified arm   COM

   ✓x7ᵗʰ **T34.41** **Frostbite with tissue necrosis of** right arm   COM

   ✓x7ᵗʰ **T34.42** **Frostbite with tissue necrosis of** left arm   COM

☑5ᵗʰ **T34.5** **Frostbite with tissue necrosis of** wrist, hand, and finger(s)

   ☑6ᵗʰ **T34.51** **Frostbite with tissue necrosis of** wrist

     7ᵗʰ **T34.511** **Frostbite with tissue necrosis of** right wrist   COM

     7ᵗʰ **T34.512** **Frostbite with tissue necrosis of** left wrist   COM

     7ᵗʰ **T34.519** **Frostbite with tissue necrosis of** unspecified wrist   COM

   ☑6ᵗʰ **T34.52** **Frostbite with tissue necrosis of** hand

     EXCLUDES 2   *frostbite with tissue necrosis of finger(s) (T34.53-)*

     7ᵗʰ **T34.521** **Frostbite with tissue necrosis of** right hand   COM

     7ᵗʰ **T34.522** **Frostbite with tissue necrosis of** left hand   COM

     7ᵗʰ **T34.529** **Frostbite with tissue necrosis of** unspecified hand   COM

   ☑6ᵗʰ **T34.53** **Frostbite with tissue necrosis of** finger(s)

     7ᵗʰ **T34.531** **Frostbite with tissue necrosis of** right finger(s)   COM

     7ᵗʰ **T34.532** **Frostbite with tissue necrosis of** left finger(s)   COM

     7ᵗʰ **T34.539** **Frostbite with tissue necrosis of** unspecified finger(s)   COM

☑5ᵗʰ **T34.6** **Frostbite with tissue necrosis of** hip and thigh

   ✓x7ᵗʰ **T34.60** **Frostbite with tissue necrosis of** unspecified hip and thigh

   ✓x7ᵗʰ **T34.61** **Frostbite with tissue necrosis of** right hip and thigh

   ✓x7ᵗʰ **T34.62** **Frostbite with tissue necrosis of** left hip and thigh   COM

☑5ᵗʰ **T34.7** **Frostbite with tissue necrosis of** knee and lower leg

   EXCLUDES 2   *frostbite with tissue necrosis of ankle and foot (T34.8-)*

   ✓x7ᵗʰ **T34.70** **Frostbite with tissue necrosis of** unspecified knee and lower leg   COM

   ✓x7ᵗʰ **T34.71** **Frostbite with tissue necrosis of** right knee and lower leg   COM

   ✓x7ᵗʰ **T34.72** **Frostbite with tissue necrosis of** left knee and lower leg   COM

☑5ᵗʰ **T34.8** **Frostbite with tissue necrosis of** ankle, foot, and toe(s)

   ☑6ᵗʰ **T34.81** **Frostbite with tissue necrosis of** ankle

     7ᵗʰ **T34.811** **Frostbite with tissue necrosis of** right ankle   COM

√7ᵗʰ **T34.812** **Frostbite with tissue necrosis of** left **ankle** `COM`

√7ᵗʰ **T34.819** **Frostbite with tissue necrosis of unspecified ankle** `COM`

√6ᵗʰ **T34.82** **Frostbite with tissue necrosis of** foot

√7ᵗʰ **T34.821** **Frostbite with tissue necrosis of** right **foot**

√7ᵗʰ **T34.822** **Frostbite with tissue necrosis of** left **foot**

√7ᵗʰ **T34.829** **Frostbite with tissue necrosis of unspecified foot**

√6ᵗʰ **T34.83** **Frostbite with tissue necrosis of** toe(s)

√7ᵗʰ **T34.831** **Frostbite with tissue necrosis of** right **toe(s)**

√7ᵗʰ **T34.832** **Frostbite with tissue necrosis of** left **toe(s)**

√7ᵗʰ **T34.839** **Frostbite with tissue necrosis of unspecified toe(s)**

√5ᵗʰ **T34.9** **Frostbite with tissue necrosis of other and unspecified sites**

√x7ᵗʰ **T34.90** **Frostbite with tissue necrosis of unspecified sites**
Frostbite with tissue necrosis NOS

√x7ᵗʰ **T34.99** **Frostbite with tissue necrosis of other sites**
Frostbite with tissue necrosis of leg NOS
Frostbite with tissue necrosis of trunk NOS

Poisoning by, adverse effects of and underdosing of drugs, medicaments and biological substances (T36-T50)

`INCLUDES` adverse effect of correct substance properly administered
poisoning by overdose of substance
poisoning by wrong substance given or taken in error
underdosing by (inadvertently) (deliberately) taking less substance than prescribed or instructed
Code first, for adverse effects, the nature of the adverse effect, such as:
adverse effect NOS (T88.7)
aspirin gastritis (K29.-)
blood disorders (D56-D76)
contact dermatitis (L23-L25)
dermatitis due to substances taken internally (L27.-)
nephropathy (N14.0-N14.2)

`NOTE` The drug giving rise to the adverse effect should be identified by use of codes from categories T36-T50 with fifth or sixth character 5.

Use additional code(s) to specify:
manifestations of poisoning
underdosing or failure in dosage during medical and surgical care (Y63.6, Y63.8-Y63.9)
underdosing of medication regimen (Z91.12-, Z91.13-)
`EXCLUDES 1` toxic reaction to local anesthesia in pregnancy (O29.3-)
`EXCLUDES 2` abuse and dependence of psychoactive substances (F10-F19)
abuse of non-dependence-producing substances (F55.-)
drug reaction and poisoning affecting newborn (P00-P96)
immunodeficiency due to drugs (D84.821)
pathological drug intoxication (inebriation) (F10-F19)
AHA: 2018,4Q,71; 2016,2Q,8; 2015,3Q,22

√4ᵗʰ **T36** **Poisoning by, adverse effect of and underdosing of systemic antibiotics**
`EXCLUDES 1` antineoplastic antibiotics (T45.1-)
locally applied antibiotic NEC (T49.0)
topically used antibiotic for ear, nose and throat (T49.6)
topically used antibiotic for eye (T49.5)

The appropriate 7th character is to be added to each code from category T36.
A   initial encounter
D   subsequent encounter
S   sequela

√5ᵗʰ **T36.0** **Poisoning by, adverse effect of and underdosing of penicillins**

√6ᵗʰ **T36.0X** **Poisoning by, adverse effect of and underdosing of** penicillins

√7ᵗʰ **T36.0X1** **Poisoning by penicillins,** accidental **(unintentional)**
Poisoning by penicillins NOS

² √7ᵗʰ **T36.0X2** **Poisoning by penicillins,** intentional **self-harm** `HCC` `Rx` `ESR` `COM`

√7ᵗʰ **T36.0X3** **Poisoning by penicillins,** assault

√7ᵗʰ **T36.0X4** **Poisoning by penicillins,** undetermined

√7ᵗʰ **T36.0X5** **Adverse effect** of penicillins `UPD`

√7ᵗʰ **T36.0X6** **Underdosing** of penicillins `UPD`

√5ᵗʰ **T36.1** **Poisoning by, adverse effect of and underdosing of cephalosporins and other beta-lactam antibiotics**

√6ᵗʰ **T36.1X** **Poisoning by, adverse effect of and underdosing of** cephalosporins and other beta-lactam antibiotics

√7ᵗʰ **T36.1X1** **Poisoning by cephalosporins and other beta-lactam antibiotics,** accidental **(unintentional)**
Poisoning by cephalosporins and other beta-lactam antibiotics NOS

² √7ᵗʰ **T36.1X2** **Poisoning by cephalosporins and other beta-lactam antibiotics,** intentional **self-harm** `HCC` `Rx` `ESR` `COM`

√7ᵗʰ **T36.1X3** **Poisoning by cephalosporins and other beta-lactam antibiotics,** assault

√7ᵗʰ **T36.1X4** **Poisoning by cephalosporins and other beta-lactam antibiotics,** undetermined

√7ᵗʰ **T36.1X5** **Adverse effect** of cephalosporins and other beta-lactam antibiotics `UPD`

√7ᵗʰ **T36.1X6** **Underdosing** of cephalosporins and other beta-lactam antibiotics `UPD`

√5ᵗʰ **T36.2** **Poisoning by, adverse effect of and underdosing of chloramphenicol group**

√6ᵗʰ **T36.2X** **Poisoning by, adverse effect of and underdosing of** chloramphenicol group

√7ᵗʰ **T36.2X1** **Poisoning by chloramphenicol group,** accidental **(unintentional)**
Poisoning by chloramphenicol group NOS

² √7ᵗʰ **T36.2X2** **Poisoning by chloramphenicol group,** intentional self-harm `HCC` `Rx` `ESR` `COM`

√7ᵗʰ **T36.2X3** **Poisoning by chloramphenicol group,** assault

√7ᵗʰ **T36.2X4** **Poisoning by chloramphenicol group,** undetermined

√7ᵗʰ **T36.2X5** **Adverse effect** of chloramphenicol group `UPD`

√7ᵗʰ **T36.2X6** **Underdosing** of chloramphenicol group `UPD`

√5ᵗʰ **T36.3** **Poisoning by, adverse effect of and underdosing of macrolides**

√6ᵗʰ **T36.3X** **Poisoning by, adverse effect of and underdosing of** macrolides

√7ᵗʰ **T36.3X1** **Poisoning by macrolides,** accidental **(unintentional)**
Poisoning by macrolides NOS

² √7ᵗʰ **T36.3X2** **Poisoning by macrolides,** intentional **self-harm** `HCC` `Rx` `ESR` `COM`

√7ᵗʰ **T36.3X3** **Poisoning by macrolides,** assault

√7ᵗʰ **T36.3X4** **Poisoning by macrolides,** undetermined

√7ᵗʰ **T36.3X5** **Adverse effect** of macrolides `UPD`

√7ᵗʰ **T36.3X6** **Underdosing** of macrolides `UPD`

√5ᵗʰ **T36.4** **Poisoning by, adverse effect of and underdosing of tetracyclines**

√6ᵗʰ **T36.4X** **Poisoning by, adverse effect of and underdosing of** tetracyclines

√7ᵗʰ **T36.4X1** **Poisoning by tetracyclines,** accidental **(unintentional)**
Poisoning by tetracyclines NOS

² √7ᵗʰ **T36.4X2** **Poisoning by tetracyclines,** intentional **self-harm** `HCC` `Rx` `ESR` `COM`

√7ᵗʰ **T36.4X3** **Poisoning by tetracyclines,** assault

√7ᵗʰ **T36.4X4** **Poisoning by tetracyclines,** undetermined

√7ᵗʰ **T36.4X5** **Adverse effect** of tetracyclines `UPD`

√7ᵗʰ **T36.4X6** **Underdosing** of tetracyclines `UPD`

√5ᵗʰ **T36.5** **Poisoning by, adverse effect of and underdosing of aminoglycosides**
Poisoning by, adverse effect of and underdosing of streptomycin

√6ᵗʰ **T36.5X** **Poisoning by, adverse effect of and underdosing of** aminoglycosides

√7ᵗʰ **T36.5X1** **Poisoning by aminoglycosides,** accidental **(unintentional)**
Poisoning by aminoglycosides NOS

² √7ᵗʰ **T36.5X2** **Poisoning by aminoglycosides,** intentional self-harm `HCC` `Rx` `ESR` `COM`

√7ᵗʰ **T36.5X3** **Poisoning by aminoglycosides,** assault

√7ᵗʰ **T36.5X4** **Poisoning by aminoglycosides,** undetermined

√7ᵗʰ **T36.5X5** **Adverse effect** of aminoglycosides `UPD`

√7ᵗʰ **T36.5X6** **Underdosing** of aminoglycosides `UPD`

`HCC` CMS-HCC   `Rx` Rx HCC   `ESR` ESRD HCC   `COM` Commercial HCC   `N` Newborn: 0   `P` Pediatric: 0-17   `M` Maternity: 9-64   `A` Adult: 15-124

1134
ICD-10-CM 2023

✓5ᵗʰ T36.6 Poisoning by, adverse effect of and underdosing of rifampicins

    ✓6ᵗʰ T36.6X Poisoning by, adverse effect of and underdosing of rifampicins

        ✓7ᵗʰ T36.6X1 Poisoning by rifampicins, accidental (unintentional)
            Poisoning by rifampicins NOS

        ² **✓7ᵗʰ T36.6X2 Poisoning by rifampicins, intentional self-harm** HCC Rx ESR COM

        ✓7ᵗʰ T36.6X3 Poisoning by rifampicins, assault

        ✓7ᵗʰ T36.6X4 Poisoning by rifampicins, undetermined

        ✓7ᵗʰ T36.6X5 Adverse effect of rifampicins UPD

        ✓7ᵗʰ T36.6X6 Underdosing of rifampicins UPD

✓5ᵗʰ T36.7 Poisoning by, adverse effect of and underdosing of antifungal antibiotics, systemically used

    ✓6ᵗʰ T36.7X Poisoning by, adverse effect of and underdosing of antifungal antibiotics, systemically used

        ✓7ᵗʰ T36.7X1 Poisoning by antifungal antibiotics, systemically used, accidental (unintentional)
            Poisoning by antifungal antibiotics, systemically used NOS

        ² **✓7ᵗʰ T36.7X2 Poisoning by antifungal antibiotics, systemically used, intentional self-harm** HCC Rx ESR COM

        ✓7ᵗʰ T36.7X3 Poisoning by antifungal antibiotics, systemically used, assault

        ✓7ᵗʰ T36.7X4 Poisoning by antifungal antibiotics, systemically used, undetermined

        ✓7ᵗʰ T36.7X5 Adverse effect of antifungal antibiotics, systemically used UPD

        ✓7ᵗʰ T36.7X6 Underdosing of antifungal antibiotics, systemically used UPD

✓5ᵗʰ T36.8 Poisoning by, adverse effect of and underdosing of other systemic antibiotics

    ✓6ᵗʰ T36.8X Poisoning by, adverse effect of and underdosing of other systemic antibiotics
        AHA: 2017, 1Q, 39

        ✓7ᵗʰ T36.8X1 Poisoning by other systemic antibiotics, accidental (unintentional)
            Poisoning by other systemic antibiotics NOS

        ² **✓7ᵗʰ T36.8X2 Poisoning by other systemic antibiotics, intentional self-harm** HCC Rx ESR COM

        ✓7ᵗʰ T36.8X3 Poisoning by other systemic antibiotics, assault

        ✓7ᵗʰ T36.8X4 Poisoning by other systemic antibiotics, undetermined

        ✓7ᵗʰ T36.8X5 Adverse effect of other systemic antibiotics UPD

        ✓7ᵗʰ T36.8X6 Underdosing of other systemic antibiotics UPD

✓5ᵗʰ T36.9 Poisoning by, adverse effect of and underdosing of unspecified systemic antibiotic

    ✓×7ᵗʰ T36.91 Poisoning by unspecified systemic antibiotic, accidental (unintentional)
        Poisoning by systemic antibiotic NOS

    ² **✓×7ᵗʰ T36.92 Poisoning by unspecified systemic antibiotic, intentional self-harm** HCC Rx ESR COM

    ✓×7ᵗʰ T36.93 Poisoning by unspecified systemic antibiotic, assault

    ✓×7ᵗʰ T36.94 Poisoning by unspecified systemic antibiotic, undetermined

    ✓×7ᵗʰ T36.95 Adverse effect of unspecified systemic antibiotic UPD

    ✓×7ᵗʰ T36.96 Underdosing of unspecified systemic antibiotic UPD

✓4ᵗʰ T37 Poisoning by, adverse effect of and underdosing of other systemic anti-infectives and antiparasitics

    EXCLUDES 1   *anti-infectives topically used for ear, nose and throat (T49.6-)*
            anti-infectives topically used for eye (T49.5-)
            locally applied anti-infectives NEC (T49.0-)

> The appropriate 7th character is to be added to each code from category T37.
> A   initial encounter
> D   subsequent encounter
> S   sequela

✓5ᵗʰ T37.0 Poisoning by, adverse effect of and underdosing of sulfonamides

    ✓6ᵗʰ T37.0X Poisoning by, adverse effect of and underdosing of sulfonamides

        ✓7ᵗʰ T37.0X1 Poisoning by sulfonamides, accidental (unintentional)
            Poisoning by sulfonamides NOS

        ² **✓7ᵗʰ T37.0X2 Poisoning by sulfonamides, intentional self-harm** HCC Rx ESR COM

        ✓7ᵗʰ T37.0X3 Poisoning by sulfonamides, assault

        ✓7ᵗʰ T37.0X4 Poisoning by sulfonamides, undetermined

        ✓7ᵗʰ T37.0X5 Adverse effect of sulfonamides UPD

        ✓7ᵗʰ T37.0X6 Underdosing of sulfonamides UPD

✓5ᵗʰ T37.1 Poisoning by, adverse effect of and underdosing of antimycobacterial drugs

    EXCLUDES 1   *rifampicins (T36.6-)*
            streptomycin (T36.5-)

    ✓6ᵗʰ T37.1X Poisoning by, adverse effect of and underdosing of antimycobacterial drugs

        ✓7ᵗʰ T37.1X1 Poisoning by antimycobacterial drugs, accidental (unintentional)
            Poisoning by antimycobacterial drugs NOS

        ² **✓7ᵗʰ T37.1X2 Poisoning by antimycobacterial drugs, intentional self-harm** HCC Rx ESR COM

        ✓7ᵗʰ T37.1X3 Poisoning by antimycobacterial drugs, assault

        ✓7ᵗʰ T37.1X4 Poisoning by antimycobacterial drugs, undetermined

        ✓7ᵗʰ T37.1X5 Adverse effect of antimycobacterial drugs UPD

        ✓7ᵗʰ T37.1X6 Underdosing of antimycobacterial drugs UPD

✓5ᵗʰ T37.2 Poisoning by, adverse effect of and underdosing of antimalarials and drugs acting on other blood protozoa

    EXCLUDES 1   *hydroxyquinoline derivatives (T37.8-)*

    ✓6ᵗʰ T37.2X Poisoning by, adverse effect of and underdosing of antimalarials and drugs acting on other blood protozoa

        ✓7ᵗʰ T37.2X1 Poisoning by antimalarials and drugs acting on other blood protozoa, accidental (unintentional)
            Poisoning by antimalarials and drugs acting on other blood protozoa NOS

        ² **✓7ᵗʰ T37.2X2 Poisoning by antimalarials and drugs acting on other blood protozoa, intentional self-harm** HCC Rx ESR COM

        ✓7ᵗʰ T37.2X3 Poisoning by antimalarials and drugs acting on other blood protozoa, assault

        ✓7ᵗʰ T37.2X4 Poisoning by antimalarials and drugs acting on other blood protozoa, undetermined

        ✓7ᵗʰ T37.2X5 Adverse effect of antimalarials and drugs acting on other blood protozoa UPD

        ✓7ᵗʰ T37.2X6 Underdosing of antimalarials and drugs acting on other blood protozoa UPD

✓5ᵗʰ T37.3 Poisoning by, adverse effect of and underdosing of other antiprotozoal drugs

    ✓6ᵗʰ T37.3X Poisoning by, adverse effect of and underdosing of other antiprotozoal drugs

        ✓7ᵗʰ T37.3X1 Poisoning by other antiprotozoal drugs, accidental (unintentional)
            Poisoning by other antiprotozoal drugs NOS

        ² **✓7ᵗʰ T37.3X2 Poisoning by other antiprotozoal drugs, intentional self-harm** HCC Rx ESR COM

        ✓7ᵗʰ T37.3X3 Poisoning by other antiprotozoal drugs, assault

        ✓7ᵗʰ T37.3X4 Poisoning by other antiprotozoal drugs, undetermined

Chapter 19. Injury, Poisoning and Certain Other Consequences of External Causes

T37.3X5–T38.3X2

✓7ᵗʰ **T37.3X5** Adverse effect of other antiprotozoal drugs   UPD

✓7ᵗʰ **T37.3X6** Underdosing of other antiprotozoal drugs   UPD

✓5ᵗʰ **T37.4** Poisoning by, adverse effect of and underdosing of anthelminthics

  ✓6ᵗʰ **T37.4X** Poisoning by, adverse effect of and underdosing of anthelminthics

    ✓7ᵗʰ **T37.4X1** Poisoning by anthelminthics, accidental (unintentional)

       Poisoning by anthelminthics NOS

    ² ✓7ᵗʰ **T37.4X2** Poisoning by anthelminthics, intentional self-harm   HCC Rx ESR COM

    ✓7ᵗʰ **T37.4X3** Poisoning by anthelminthics, assault

    ✓7ᵗʰ **T37.4X4** Poisoning by anthelminthics, undetermined

    ✓7ᵗʰ **T37.4X5** Adverse effect of anthelminthics   UPD

    ✓7ᵗʰ **T37.4X6** Underdosing of anthelminthics   UPD

✓5ᵗʰ **T37.5** Poisoning by, adverse effect of and underdosing of antiviral drugs

    EXCLUDES 1   amantadine (T42.8-)

              cytarabine (T45.1-)

  ✓6ᵗʰ **T37.5X** Poisoning by, adverse effect of and underdosing of antiviral drugs

    ✓7ᵗʰ **T37.5X1** Poisoning by antiviral drugs, accidental (unintentional)

       Poisoning by antiviral drugs NOS

    ² ✓7ᵗʰ **T37.5X2** Poisoning by antiviral drugs, intentional self-harm   HCC Rx ESR COM

    ✓7ᵗʰ **T37.5X3** Poisoning by antiviral drugs, assault

    ✓7ᵗʰ **T37.5X4** Poisoning by antiviral drugs, undetermined

    ✓7ᵗʰ **T37.5X5** Adverse effect of antiviral drugs   UPD

    ✓7ᵗʰ **T37.5X6** Underdosing of antiviral drugs   UPD

✓5ᵗʰ **T37.8** Poisoning by, adverse effect of and underdosing of other specified systemic anti-infectives and antiparasitics

     Poisoning by, adverse effect of and underdosing of hydroxyquinoline derivatives

    EXCLUDES 1   antimalarial drugs (T37.2-)

  ✓6ᵗʰ **T37.8X** Poisoning by, adverse effect of and underdosing of other specified systemic anti-infectives and antiparasitics

    ✓7ᵗʰ **T37.8X1** Poisoning by other specified systemic anti-infectives and antiparasitics, accidental (unintentional)

       Poisoning by other specified systemic anti-infectives and antiparasitics NOS

    ² ✓7ᵗʰ **T37.8X2** Poisoning by other specified systemic anti-infectives and antiparasitics, intentional self-harm   HCC Rx ESR COM

    ✓7ᵗʰ **T37.8X3** Poisoning by other specified systemic anti-infectives and antiparasitics, assault

    ✓7ᵗʰ **T37.8X4** Poisoning by other specified systemic anti-infectives and antiparasitics, undetermined

    ✓7ᵗʰ **T37.8X5** Adverse effect of other specified systemic anti-infectives and antiparasitics   UPD

    ✓7ᵗʰ **T37.8X6** Underdosing of other specified systemic anti-infectives and antiparasitics   UPD

✓5ᵗʰ **T37.9** Poisoning by, adverse effect of and underdosing of unspecified systemic anti-infective and antiparasitics

  ✓x7ᵗʰ **T37.91** Poisoning by unspecified systemic anti-infective and antiparasitics, accidental (unintentional)

     Poisoning by, adverse effect of and underdosing of systemic anti-infective and antiparasitics NOS

  ² ✓x7ᵗʰ **T37.92** Poisoning by unspecified systemic anti-infective and antiparasitics, intentional self-harm   HCC Rx ESR COM

  ✓x7ᵗʰ **T37.93** Poisoning by unspecified systemic anti-infective and antiparasitics, assault

  ✓x7ᵗʰ **T37.94** Poisoning by unspecified systemic anti-infective and antiparasitics, undetermined

  ✓x7ᵗʰ **T37.95** Adverse effect of unspecified systemic anti-infective and antiparasitic   UPD

  ✓x7ᵗʰ **T37.96** Underdosing of unspecified systemic anti-infectives and antiparasitics   UPD

✓4ᵗʰ **T38** Poisoning by, adverse effect of and underdosing of hormones and their synthetic substitutes and antagonists, not elsewhere classified

    EXCLUDES 1   mineralocorticoids and their antagonists (T50.0-)

              oxytocic hormones (T48.0-)

              parathyroid hormones and derivatives (T50.9-)

> The appropriate 7th character is to be added to each code from category T38.
> A   initial encounter
> D   subsequent encounter
> S   sequela

✓5ᵗʰ **T38.0** Poisoning by, adverse effect of and underdosing of glucocorticoids and synthetic analogues

    EXCLUDES 1   glucocorticoids, topically used (T49.-)

  ✓6ᵗʰ **T38.0X** Poisoning by, adverse effect of and underdosing of glucocorticoids and synthetic analogues

    ✓7ᵗʰ **T38.0X1** Poisoning by glucocorticoids and synthetic analogues, accidental (unintentional)

       Poisoning by glucocorticoids and synthetic analogues NOS

    ² ✓7ᵗʰ **T38.0X2** Poisoning by glucocorticoids and synthetic analogues, intentional self-harm   HCC Rx ESR COM

    ✓7ᵗʰ **T38.0X3** Poisoning by glucocorticoids and synthetic analogues, assault

    ✓7ᵗʰ **T38.0X4** Poisoning by glucocorticoids and synthetic analogues, undetermined

    ✓7ᵗʰ **T38.0X5** Adverse effect of glucocorticoids and synthetic analogues   UPD

    ✓7ᵗʰ **T38.0X6** Underdosing of glucocorticoids and synthetic analogues   UPD

✓5ᵗʰ **T38.1** Poisoning by, adverse effect of and underdosing of thyroid hormones and substitutes

  ✓6ᵗʰ **T38.1X** Poisoning by, adverse effect of and underdosing of thyroid hormones and substitutes

    ✓7ᵗʰ **T38.1X1** Poisoning by thyroid hormones and substitutes, accidental (unintentional)

       Poisoning by thyroid hormones and substitutes NOS

    ² ✓7ᵗʰ **T38.1X2** Poisoning by thyroid hormones and substitutes, intentional self-harm   HCC Rx ESR COM

    ✓7ᵗʰ **T38.1X3** Poisoning by thyroid hormones and substitutes, assault

    ✓7ᵗʰ **T38.1X4** Poisoning by thyroid hormones and substitutes, undetermined

    ✓7ᵗʰ **T38.1X5** Adverse effect of thyroid hormones and substitutes   UPD

    ✓7ᵗʰ **T38.1X6** Underdosing of thyroid hormones and substitutes   UPD

✓5ᵗʰ **T38.2** Poisoning by, adverse effect of and underdosing of antithyroid drugs

  ✓6ᵗʰ **T38.2X** Poisoning by, adverse effect of and underdosing of antithyroid drugs

    ✓7ᵗʰ **T38.2X1** Poisoning by antithyroid drugs, accidental (unintentional)

       Poisoning by antithyroid drugs NOS

    ² ✓7ᵗʰ **T38.2X2** Poisoning by antithyroid drugs, intentional self-harm   HCC Rx ESR COM

    ✓7ᵗʰ **T38.2X3** Poisoning by antithyroid drugs, assault

    ✓7ᵗʰ **T38.2X4** Poisoning by antithyroid drugs, undetermined

    ✓7ᵗʰ **T38.2X5** Adverse effect of antithyroid drugs   UPD

    ✓7ᵗʰ **T38.2X6** Underdosing of antithyroid drugs   UPD

✓5ᵗʰ **T38.3** Poisoning by, adverse effect of and underdosing of insulin and oral hypoglycemic [antidiabetic] drugs

  ✓6ᵗʰ **T38.3X** Poisoning by, adverse effect of and underdosing of insulin and oral hypoglycemic [antidiabetic] drugs

    ✓7ᵗʰ **T38.3X1** Poisoning by insulin and oral hypoglycemic [antidiabetic] drugs, accidental (unintentional)

       Poisoning by insulin and oral hypoglycemic [antidiabetic] drugs NOS

    ² ✓7ᵗʰ **T38.3X2** Poisoning by insulin and oral hypoglycemic [antidiabetic] drugs, intentional self-harm   HCC Rx ESR COM

✓7ᵗʰ **T38.3X3** **Poisoning** by insulin and oral hypoglycemic [antidiabetic] drugs, **assault**

✓7ᵗʰ **T38.3X4** **Poisoning** by insulin and oral hypoglycemic [antidiabetic] drugs, **undetermined**

✓7ᵗʰ **T38.3X5** **Adverse effect** of insulin and oral hypoglycemic [antidiabetic] drugs **UPD**

✓7ᵗʰ **T38.3X6** **Underdosing** of insulin and oral hypoglycemic [antidiabetic] drugs **UPD**

✓5ᵗʰ **T38.4** **Poisoning by, adverse effect of and underdosing of oral contraceptives**
    Poisoning by, adverse effect of and underdosing of multiple- and single-ingredient oral contraceptive preparations

✓6ᵗʰ **T38.4X** **Poisoning by, adverse effect of and underdosing of oral contraceptives**

✓7ᵗʰ **T38.4X1** **Poisoning** by oral contraceptives, **accidental (unintentional)**
    Poisoning by oral contraceptives NOS

² ✓7ᵗʰ **T38.4X2** **Poisoning** by oral contraceptives, **intentional self-harm** HCC Rx ESR COM

✓7ᵗʰ **T38.4X3** **Poisoning** by oral contraceptives, **assault**

✓7ᵗʰ **T38.4X4** **Poisoning** by oral contraceptives, **undetermined**

✓7ᵗʰ **T38.4X5** **Adverse effect** of oral contraceptives **UPD**

✓7ᵗʰ **T38.4X6** **Underdosing** of oral contraceptives **UPD**

✓5ᵗʰ **T38.5** **Poisoning by, adverse effect of and underdosing of other estrogens and progestogens**
    Poisoning by, adverse effect of and underdosing of estrogens and progestogens mixtures and substitutes

✓6ᵗʰ **T38.5X** **Poisoning by, adverse effect of and underdosing of other estrogens and progestogens**

✓7ᵗʰ **T38.5X1** **Poisoning** by other estrogens and progestogens, **accidental (unintentional)**
    Poisoning by other estrogens and progestogens NOS

² ✓7ᵗʰ **T38.5X2** **Poisoning** by other estrogens and progestogens, **intentional self-harm** HCC Rx ESR COM

✓7ᵗʰ **T38.5X3** **Poisoning** by other estrogens and progestogens, **assault**

✓7ᵗʰ **T38.5X4** **Poisoning** by other estrogens and progestogens, **undetermined**

✓7ᵗʰ **T38.5X5** **Adverse effect** of other estrogens and progestogens **UPD**

✓7ᵗʰ **T38.5X6** **Underdosing** of other estrogens and progestogens **UPD**

✓5ᵗʰ **T38.6** **Poisoning by, adverse effect of and underdosing of antigonadotrophins, antiestrogens, antiandrogens, not elsewhere classified**
    Poisoning by, adverse effect of and underdosing of tamoxifen

✓6ᵗʰ **T38.6X** **Poisoning by, adverse effect of and underdosing of antigonadotrophins, antiestrogens, antiandrogens, not elsewhere classified**

✓7ᵗʰ **T38.6X1** **Poisoning** by antigonadotrophins, antiestrogens, antiandrogens, not elsewhere classified, **accidental (unintentional)**
    Poisoning by antigonadotrophins, antiestrogens, antiandrogens, not elsewhere classified NOS

² ✓7ᵗʰ **T38.6X2** **Poisoning** by antigonadotrophins, antiestrogens, antiandrogens, not elsewhere classified, **intentional self-harm** HCC Rx ESR COM

✓7ᵗʰ **T38.6X3** **Poisoning** by antigonadotrophins, antiestrogens, antiandrogens, not elsewhere classified, **assault**

✓7ᵗʰ **T38.6X4** **Poisoning** by antigonadotrophins, antiestrogens, antiandrogens, not elsewhere classified, **undetermined**

✓7ᵗʰ **T38.6X5** **Adverse effect** of antigonadotrophins, antiestrogens, antiandrogens, not elsewhere classified **UPD**

✓7ᵗʰ **T38.6X6** **Underdosing** of antigonadotrophins, antiestrogens, antiandrogens, not elsewhere classified **UPD**

✓5ᵗʰ **T38.7** **Poisoning by, adverse effect of and underdosing of androgens and anabolic congeners**

✓6ᵗʰ **T38.7X** **Poisoning by, adverse effect of and underdosing of androgens and anabolic congeners**

✓7ᵗʰ **T38.7X1** **Poisoning** by androgens and anabolic congeners, **accidental (unintentional)**
    Poisoning by androgens and anabolic congeners NOS

² ✓7ᵗʰ **T38.7X2** **Poisoning** by androgens and anabolic congeners, **intentional self-harm** HCC Rx ESR COM

✓7ᵗʰ **T38.7X3** **Poisoning** by androgens and anabolic congeners, **assault**

✓7ᵗʰ **T38.7X4** **Poisoning** by androgens and anabolic congeners, **undetermined**

✓7ᵗʰ **T38.7X5** **Adverse effect** of androgens and anabolic congeners **UPD**

✓7ᵗʰ **T38.7X6** **Underdosing** of androgens and anabolic congeners **UPD**

✓5ᵗʰ **T38.8** **Poisoning by, adverse effect of and underdosing of other and unspecified hormones and synthetic substitutes**

✓6ᵗʰ **T38.80** **Poisoning by, adverse effect of and underdosing of unspecified hormones and synthetic substitutes**

✓7ᵗʰ **T38.801** **Poisoning** by unspecified hormones and synthetic substitutes, **accidental (unintentional)**
    Poisoning by unspecified hormones and synthetic substitutes NOS

² ✓7ᵗʰ **T38.802** **Poisoning** by unspecified hormones and synthetic substitutes, **intentional self-harm** HCC Rx ESR COM

✓7ᵗʰ **T38.803** **Poisoning** by unspecified hormones and synthetic substitutes, **assault**

✓7ᵗʰ **T38.804** **Poisoning** by unspecified hormones and synthetic substitutes, **undetermined**

✓7ᵗʰ **T38.805** **Adverse effect** of unspecified hormones and synthetic substitutes **UPD**

✓7ᵗʰ **T38.806** **Underdosing** of unspecified hormones and synthetic substitutes **UPD**

✓6ᵗʰ **T38.81** **Poisoning by, adverse effect of and underdosing of anterior pituitary [adenohypophyseal] hormones**

✓7ᵗʰ **T38.811** **Poisoning** by anterior pituitary [adenohypophyseal] hormones, **accidental (unintentional)**
    Poisoning by anterior pituitary [adenohypophyseal] hormones NOS

² ✓7ᵗʰ **T38.812** **Poisoning** by anterior pituitary [adenohypophyseal] hormones, **intentional self-harm** HCC Rx ESR COM

✓7ᵗʰ **T38.813** **Poisoning** by anterior pituitary [adenohypophyseal] hormones, **assault**

✓7ᵗʰ **T38.814** **Poisoning** by anterior pituitary [adenohypophyseal] hormones, **undetermined**

✓7ᵗʰ **T38.815** **Adverse effect** of anterior pituitary [adenohypophyseal] hormones **UPD**

✓7ᵗʰ **T38.816** **Underdosing** of anterior pituitary [adenohypophyseal] hormones **UPD**

✓6ᵗʰ **T38.89** **Poisoning by, adverse effect of and underdosing of other hormones and synthetic substitutes**

✓7ᵗʰ **T38.891** **Poisoning** by other hormones and synthetic substitutes, **accidental (unintentional)**
    Poisoning by other hormones and synthetic substitutes NOS

² ✓7ᵗʰ **T38.892** **Poisoning** by other hormones and synthetic substitutes, **intentional self-harm** HCC Rx ESR COM

✓7ᵗʰ **T38.893** **Poisoning** by other hormones and synthetic substitutes, **assault**

✓7ᵗʰ **T38.894** **Poisoning** by other hormones and synthetic substitutes, **undetermined**

✓7ᵗʰ **T38.895** **Adverse effect** of other hormones and synthetic substitutes **UPD**

✓7ᵗʰ **T38.896** **Underdosing** of other hormones and synthetic substitutes **UPD**

Chapter 19. Injury, Poisoning and Certain Other Consequences of External Causes

T38.9–T39.396

✓5ᵗʰ **T38.9 Poisoning by, adverse effect of and underdosing of other and unspecified hormone antagonists**

  ✓6ᵗʰ **T38.90 Poisoning by, adverse effect of and underdosing of unspecified hormone antagonists**

    ✓7ᵗʰ **T38.901 Poisoning by unspecified hormone antagonists, accidental (unintentional)**
      Poisoning by unspecified hormone antagonists NOS

    ² ✓7ᵗʰ **T38.902 Poisoning by unspecified hormone antagonists, intentional self-harm** `HCC` `Rx` `ESR` `COM`

    ✓7ᵗʰ **T38.903 Poisoning by unspecified hormone antagonists, assault**

    ✓7ᵗʰ **T38.904 Poisoning by unspecified hormone antagonists, undetermined**

    ✓7ᵗʰ **T38.905 Adverse effect of unspecified hormone antagonists** `UPD`

    ✓7ᵗʰ **T38.906 Underdosing of unspecified hormone antagonists** `UPD`

  ✓6ᵗʰ **T38.99 Poisoning by, adverse effect of and underdosing of other hormone antagonists**

    ✓7ᵗʰ **T38.991 Poisoning by other hormone antagonists, accidental (unintentional)**
      Poisoning by other hormone antagonists NOS

    ² ✓7ᵗʰ **T38.992 Poisoning by other hormone antagonists, intentional self-harm** `HCC` `Rx` `ESR` `COM`

    ✓7ᵗʰ **T38.993 Poisoning by other hormone antagonists, assault**

    ✓7ᵗʰ **T38.994 Poisoning by other hormone antagonists, undetermined**

    ✓7ᵗʰ **T38.995 Adverse effect of other hormone antagonists** `UPD`

    ✓7ᵗʰ **T38.996 Underdosing of other hormone antagonists** `UPD`

✓4ᵗʰ **T39 Poisoning by, adverse effect of and underdosing of nonopioid analgesics, antipyretics and antirheumatics**

> The appropriate 7th character is to be added to each code from category T39.
> A   initial encounter
> D   subsequent encounter
> S   sequela

✓5ᵗʰ **T39.0 Poisoning by, adverse effect of and underdosing of salicylates**

  ✓6ᵗʰ **T39.01 Poisoning by, adverse effect of and underdosing of aspirin**
    Poisoning by, adverse effect of and underdosing of acetylsalicylic acid

    ✓7ᵗʰ **T39.011 Poisoning by aspirin, accidental (unintentional)**

    ² ✓7ᵗʰ **T39.012 Poisoning by aspirin, intentional self-harm** `HCC` `Rx` `ESR` `COM`

    ✓7ᵗʰ **T39.013 Poisoning by aspirin, assault**

    ✓7ᵗʰ **T39.014 Poisoning by aspirin, undetermined**

    ✓7ᵗʰ **T39.015 Adverse effect of aspirin** `UPD`
      AHA: 2016,1Q,15

    ✓7ᵗʰ **T39.016 Underdosing of aspirin** `UPD`

  ✓6ᵗʰ **T39.09 Poisoning by, adverse effect of and underdosing of other salicylates**

    ✓7ᵗʰ **T39.091 Poisoning by salicylates, accidental (unintentional)**
      Poisoning by salicylates NOS

    ² ✓7ᵗʰ **T39.092 Poisoning by salicylates, intentional self-harm** `HCC` `Rx` `ESR` `COM`

    ✓7ᵗʰ **T39.093 Poisoning by salicylates, assault**

    ✓7ᵗʰ **T39.094 Poisoning by salicylates, undetermined**

    ✓7ᵗʰ **T39.095 Adverse effect of salicylates** `UPD`

    ✓7ᵗʰ **T39.096 Underdosing of salicylates** `UPD`

✓5ᵗʰ **T39.1 Poisoning by, adverse effect of and underdosing of 4-Aminophenol derivatives**

  ✓6ᵗʰ **T39.1X Poisoning by, adverse effect of and underdosing of 4-Aminophenol derivatives**

    ✓7ᵗʰ **T39.1X1 Poisoning by 4-Aminophenol derivatives, accidental (unintentional)**
      Poisoning by 4-Aminophenol derivatives NOS

    ² ✓7ᵗʰ **T39.1X2 Poisoning by 4-Aminophenol derivatives, intentional self-harm** `HCC` `Rx` `ESR` `COM`

    ✓7ᵗʰ **T39.1X3 Poisoning by 4-Aminophenol derivatives, assault**

    ✓7ᵗʰ **T39.1X4 Poisoning by 4-Aminophenol derivatives, undetermined**

    ✓7ᵗʰ **T39.1X5 Adverse effect of 4-Aminophenol derivatives** `UPD`

    ✓7ᵗʰ **T39.1X6 Underdosing of 4-Aminophenol derivatives** `UPD`

✓5ᵗʰ **T39.2 Poisoning by, adverse effect of and underdosing of pyrazolone derivatives**

  ✓6ᵗʰ **T39.2X Poisoning by, adverse effect of and underdosing of pyrazolone derivatives**

    ✓7ᵗʰ **T39.2X1 Poisoning by pyrazolone derivatives, accidental (unintentional)**
      Poisoning by pyrazolone derivatives NOS

    ² ✓7ᵗʰ **T39.2X2 Poisoning by pyrazolone derivatives, intentional self-harm** `HCC` `Rx` `ESR` `COM`

    ✓7ᵗʰ **T39.2X3 Poisoning by pyrazolone derivatives, assault**

    ✓7ᵗʰ **T39.2X4 Poisoning by pyrazolone derivatives, undetermined**

    ✓7ᵗʰ **T39.2X5 Adverse effect of pyrazolone derivatives** `UPD`

    ✓7ᵗʰ **T39.2X6 Underdosing of pyrazolone derivatives** `UPD`

✓5ᵗʰ **T39.3 Poisoning by, adverse effect of and underdosing of other nonsteroidal anti-inflammatory drugs [NSAID]**

  ✓6ᵗʰ **T39.31 Poisoning by, adverse effect of and underdosing of propionic acid derivatives**
    Poisoning by, adverse effect of and underdosing of fenoprofen
    Poisoning by, adverse effect of and underdosing of flurbiprofen
    Poisoning by, adverse effect of and underdosing of ibuprofen
    Poisoning by, adverse effect of and underdosing of ketoprofen
    Poisoning by, adverse effect of and underdosing of naproxen
    Poisoning by, adverse effect of and underdosing of oxaprozin

    ✓7ᵗʰ **T39.311 Poisoning by propionic acid derivatives, accidental (unintentional)**

    ² ✓7ᵗʰ **T39.312 Poisoning by propionic acid derivatives, intentional self-harm** `HCC` `Rx` `ESR` `COM`

    ✓7ᵗʰ **T39.313 Poisoning by propionic acid derivatives, assault**

    ✓7ᵗʰ **T39.314 Poisoning by propionic acid derivatives, undetermined**

    ✓7ᵗʰ **T39.315 Adverse effect of propionic acid derivatives** `UPD`

    ✓7ᵗʰ **T39.316 Underdosing of propionic acid derivatives** `UPD`

  ✓6ᵗʰ **T39.39 Poisoning by, adverse effect of and underdosing of other nonsteroidal anti-inflammatory drugs [NSAID]**

    ✓7ᵗʰ **T39.391 Poisoning by other nonsteroidal anti-inflammatory drugs [NSAID], accidental (unintentional)**
      Poisoning by other nonsteroidal anti-inflammatory drugs NOS

    ² ✓7ᵗʰ **T39.392 Poisoning by other nonsteroidal anti-inflammatory drugs [NSAID], intentional self-harm** `HCC` `Rx` `ESR` `COM`

    ✓7ᵗʰ **T39.393 Poisoning by other nonsteroidal anti-inflammatory drugs [NSAID], assault**

    ✓7ᵗʰ **T39.394 Poisoning by other nonsteroidal anti-inflammatory drugs [NSAID], undetermined**

    ✓7ᵗʰ **T39.395 Adverse effect of other nonsteroidal anti-inflammatory drugs [NSAID]** `UPD`

    ✓7ᵗʰ **T39.396 Underdosing of other nonsteroidal anti-inflammatory drugs [NSAID]** `UPD`

☑5ᵗʰ **T39.4** **Poisoning by, adverse effect of and underdosing of antirheumatics, not elsewhere classified**

    EXCLUDES 1   *poisoning by, adverse effect of and underdosing of glucocorticoids (T38.0-)*

              poisoning by, adverse effect of and underdosing of salicylates (T39.0-)

  ☑6ᵗʰ **T39.4X** **Poisoning by, adverse effect of and underdosing of antirheumatics, not elsewhere classified**

    ☑7ᵗʰ **T39.4X1** **Poisoning by antirheumatics, not elsewhere classified, accidental (unintentional)**
        Poisoning by antirheumatics, not elsewhere classified NOS

    ² ☑7ᵗʰ **T39.4X2** **Poisoning by antirheumatics, not elsewhere classified, intentional self-harm** HCC Rx ESR COM

    ☑7ᵗʰ **T39.4X3** **Poisoning by antirheumatics, not elsewhere classified, assault**

    ☑7ᵗʰ **T39.4X4** **Poisoning by antirheumatics, not elsewhere classified, undetermined**

    ☑7ᵗʰ **T39.4X5** **Adverse effect of antirheumatics, not elsewhere classified** UPD

    ☑7ᵗʰ **T39.4X6** **Underdosing of antirheumatics, not elsewhere classified** UPD

☑5ᵗʰ **T39.8** **Poisoning by, adverse effect of and underdosing of other nonopioid analgesics and antipyretics, not elsewhere classified**

  ☑6ᵗʰ **T39.8X** **Poisoning by, adverse effect of and underdosing of other nonopioid analgesics and antipyretics, not elsewhere classified**

    ☑7ᵗʰ **T39.8X1** **Poisoning by other nonopioid analgesics and antipyretics, not elsewhere classified, accidental (unintentional)**
        Poisoning by other nonopioid analgesics and antipyretics, not elsewhere classified NOS

    ² ☑7ᵗʰ **T39.8X2** **Poisoning by other nonopioid analgesics and antipyretics, not elsewhere classified, intentional self-harm** HCC Rx ESR COM

    ☑7ᵗʰ **T39.8X3** **Poisoning by other nonopioid analgesics and antipyretics, not elsewhere classified, assault**

    ☑7ᵗʰ **T39.8X4** **Poisoning by other nonopioid analgesics and antipyretics, not elsewhere classified, undetermined**

    ☑7ᵗʰ **T39.8X5** **Adverse effect of other nonopioid analgesics and antipyretics, not elsewhere classified** UPD

    ☑7ᵗʰ **T39.8X6** **Underdosing of other nonopioid analgesics and antipyretics, not elsewhere classified** UPD

☑5ᵗʰ **T39.9** **Poisoning by, adverse effect of and underdosing of unspecified nonopioid analgesic, antipyretic and antirheumatic**

  ☑✗7ᵗʰ **T39.91** **Poisoning by unspecified nonopioid analgesic, antipyretic and antirheumatic, accidental (unintentional)**
    Poisoning by nonopioid analgesic, antipyretic and antirheumatic NOS

  ² ☑✗7ᵗʰ **T39.92** **Poisoning by unspecified nonopioid analgesic, antipyretic and antirheumatic, intentional self-harm** HCC Rx ESR COM

  ☑✗7ᵗʰ **T39.93** **Poisoning by unspecified nonopioid analgesic, antipyretic and antirheumatic, assault**

  ☑✗7ᵗʰ **T39.94** **Poisoning by unspecified nonopioid analgesic, antipyretic and antirheumatic, undetermined**

  ☑✗7ᵗʰ **T39.95** **Adverse effect of unspecified nonopioid analgesic, antipyretic and antirheumatic** UPD

  ☑✗7ᵗʰ **T39.96** **Underdosing of unspecified nonopioid analgesic, antipyretic and antirheumatic** UPD

☑4ᵗʰ **T40** **Poisoning by, adverse effect of and underdosing of narcotics and psychodysleptics [hallucinogens]**

    EXCLUDES 2   *drug dependence and related mental and behavioral disorders due to psychoactive substance use (F10.-F19.-)*

  The appropriate 7th character is to be added to each code from category T40.
  A initial encounter
  D subsequent encounter
  S sequela

  ☑5ᵗʰ **T40.0** **Poisoning by, adverse effect of and underdosing of opium**

    ☑6ᵗʰ **T40.0X** **Poisoning by, adverse effect of and underdosing of opium**

      ¹ ☑7ᵗʰ **T40.0X1** **Poisoning by opium, accidental (unintentional)** HCC ESR COM
          Poisoning by opium NOS

      ² ☑7ᵗʰ **T40.0X2** **Poisoning by opium, intentional self-harm** HCC Rx ESR COM

      ☑7ᵗʰ **T40.0X3** **Poisoning by opium, assault**

      ¹ ☑7ᵗʰ **T40.0X4** **Poisoning by opium, undetermined** HCC ESR COM

      ☑7ᵗʰ **T40.0X5** **Adverse effect of opium** UPD

      ☑7ᵗʰ **T40.0X6** **Underdosing of opium** UPD

  ☑5ᵗʰ **T40.1** **Poisoning by and adverse effect of heroin**

    ☑6ᵗʰ **T40.1X** **Poisoning by and adverse effect of heroin**

      ¹ ☑7ᵗʰ **T40.1X1** **Poisoning by heroin, accidental (unintentional)** HCC ESR COM
          Poisoning by heroin NOS

      ² ☑7ᵗʰ **T40.1X2** **Poisoning by heroin, intentional self-harm** HCC Rx ESR COM

      ☑7ᵗʰ **T40.1X3** **Poisoning by heroin, assault**

      ¹ ☑7ᵗʰ **T40.1X4** **Poisoning by heroin, undetermined** HCC ESR COM

  ☑5ᵗʰ **T40.2** **Poisoning by, adverse effect of and underdosing of other opioids**

    ☑6ᵗʰ **T40.2X** **Poisoning by, adverse effect of and underdosing of other opioids**

      ¹ ☑7ᵗʰ **T40.2X1** **Poisoning by other opioids, accidental (unintentional)** HCC ESR COM
          Poisoning by other opioids NOS

      ² ☑7ᵗʰ **T40.2X2** **Poisoning by other opioids, intentional self-harm** HCC Rx ESR COM

      ☑7ᵗʰ **T40.2X3** **Poisoning by other opioids, assault**

      ¹ ☑7ᵗʰ **T40.2X4** **Poisoning by other opioids, undetermined** HCC ESR COM

      ☑7ᵗʰ **T40.2X5** **Adverse effect of other opioids** UPD
          AHA: 2020,2Q,24

      ☑7ᵗʰ **T40.2X6** **Underdosing of other opioids** UPD

  ☑5ᵗʰ **T40.3** **Poisoning by, adverse effect of and underdosing of methadone**

    ☑6ᵗʰ **T40.3X** **Poisoning by, adverse effect of and underdosing of methadone**

      ¹ ☑7ᵗʰ **T40.3X1** **Poisoning by methadone, accidental (unintentional)** HCC ESR COM
          Poisoning by methadone NOS

      ² ☑7ᵗʰ **T40.3X2** **Poisoning by methadone, intentional self-harm** HCC Rx ESR COM

      ☑7ᵗʰ **T40.3X3** **Poisoning by methadone, assault**

      ☑7ᵗʰ **T40.3X4** **Poisoning by methadone, undetermined** HCC ESR COM

      ☑7ᵗʰ **T40.3X5** **Adverse effect of methadone** UPD

      ☑7ᵗʰ **T40.3X6** **Underdosing of methadone** UPD

  ☑5ᵗʰ **T40.4** **Poisoning by, adverse effect of and underdosing of other synthetic narcotics**
    AHA: 2020,4Q,40

    ☑6ᵗʰ **T40.41** **Poisoning by, adverse effect of and underdosing of fentanyl or fentanyl analogs**

      ☑7ᵗʰ **T40.411** **Poisoning by fentanyl or fentanyl analogs, accidental (unintentional)** HCC ESR COM

      ☑7ᵗʰ **T40.412** **Poisoning by fentanyl or fentanyl analogs, intentional self-harm** HCC Rx ESR COM

      ☑7ᵗʰ **T40.413** **Poisoning by fentanyl or fentanyl analogs, assault**

      ☑7ᵗʰ **T40.414** **Poisoning by fentanyl or fentanyl analogs, undetermined** HCC ESR COM

✓7ᵗʰ **T40.415** Adverse effect of fentanyl or fentanyl analogs **UPD**

✓7ᵗʰ **T40.416** Underdosing of fentanyl or fentanyl analogs **UPD**

✓6ᵗʰ **T40.42** Poisoning by, adverse effect of and underdosing of tramadol

✓7ᵗʰ **T40.421** Poisoning by tramadol, accidental (unintentional) **HCC ESR COM**

✓7ᵗʰ **T40.422** Poisoning by tramadol, intentional self-harm **HCC Rx COM**

✓7ᵗʰ **T40.423** Poisoning by tramadol, assault

✓7ᵗʰ **T40.424** Poisoning by tramadol, undetermined **HCC ESR COM**

✓7ᵗʰ **T40.425** Adverse effect of tramadol **UPD**

✓7ᵗʰ **T40.426** Underdosing of tramadol **UPD**

✓6ᵗʰ **T40.49** Poisoning by, adverse effect of and underdosing of other synthetic narcotics

✓7ᵗʰ **T40.491** Poisoning by other synthetic narcotics, accidental (unintentional) **HCC ESR COM**

✓7ᵗʰ **T40.492** Poisoning by other synthetic narcotics, intentional self-harm **HCC Rx ESR COM**

✓7ᵗʰ **T40.493** Poisoning by other synthetic narcotics, assault

✓7ᵗʰ **T40.494** Poisoning by other synthetic narcotics, undetermined **HCC ESR COM**

✓7ᵗʰ **T40.495** Adverse effect of other synthetic narcotics **UPD**

✓7ᵗʰ **T40.496** Underdosing of other synthetic narcotics **UPD**

✓5ᵗʰ **T40.5** Poisoning by, adverse effect of and underdosing of cocaine

✓6ᵗʰ **T40.5X** Poisoning by, adverse effect of and underdosing of cocaine

¹ ✓7ᵗʰ **T40.5X1** Poisoning by cocaine, accidental (unintentional) **HCC ESR COM**
Poisoning by cocaine NOS
AHA: 2016,2Q,8

² ✓7ᵗʰ **T40.5X2** Poisoning by cocaine, intentional self-harm **HCC Rx ESR COM**

✓7ᵗʰ **T40.5X3** Poisoning by cocaine, assault

¹ ✓7ᵗʰ **T40.5X4** Poisoning by cocaine, undetermined **HCC ESR COM**

✓7ᵗʰ **T40.5X5** Adverse effect of cocaine **UPD**

✓7ᵗʰ **T40.5X6** Underdosing of cocaine **UPD**

✓5ᵗʰ **T40.6** Poisoning by, adverse effect of and underdosing of other and unspecified narcotics

✓6ᵗʰ **T40.60** Poisoning by, adverse effect of and underdosing of unspecified narcotics

¹ ✓7ᵗʰ **T40.601** Poisoning by unspecified narcotics, accidental (unintentional) **HCC ESR COM**
Poisoning by narcotics NOS

² ✓7ᵗʰ **T40.602** Poisoning by unspecified narcotics, intentional self-harm **HCC Rx ESR COM**

✓7ᵗʰ **T40.603** Poisoning by unspecified narcotics, assault

¹ ✓7ᵗʰ **T40.604** Poisoning by unspecified narcotics, undetermined **HCC ESR COM**

✓7ᵗʰ **T40.605** Adverse effect of unspecified narcotics **UPD**

✓7ᵗʰ **T40.606** Underdosing of unspecified narcotics **UPD**

✓6ᵗʰ **T40.69** Poisoning by, adverse effect of and underdosing of other narcotics

¹ ✓7ᵗʰ **T40.691** Poisoning by other narcotics, accidental (unintentional) **HCC ESR COM**
Poisoning by other narcotics NOS

² ✓7ᵗʰ **T40.692** Poisoning by other narcotics, intentional self-harm **HCC Rx ESR COM**

✓7ᵗʰ **T40.693** Poisoning by other narcotics, assault

¹ ✓7ᵗʰ **T40.694** Poisoning by other narcotics, undetermined **HCC ESR COM**

✓7ᵗʰ **T40.695** Adverse effect of other narcotics **UPD**

✓7ᵗʰ **T40.696** Underdosing of other narcotics **UPD**

✓5ᵗʰ **T40.7** Poisoning by, adverse effect of and underdosing of cannabis (derivatives)

✓6ᵗʰ **T40.71** Poisoning by, adverse effect of and underdosing of cannabis (derivatives)
AHA: 2021,4Q,30

✓7ᵗʰ **T40.711** Poisoning by cannabis, accidental (unintentional)

✓7ᵗʰ **T40.712** Poisoning by cannabis, intentional self-harm **HCC Rx ESR COM**

✓7ᵗʰ **T40.713** Poisoning by cannabis, assault

✓7ᵗʰ **T40.714** Poisoning by cannabis, undetermined

✓7ᵗʰ **T40.715** Adverse effect of cannabis **UPD**

✓7ᵗʰ **T40.716** Underdosing of cannabis **UPD**

✓6ᵗʰ **T40.72** Poisoning by, adverse effect of and underdosing of synthetic cannabinoids
AHA: 2021,4Q,30

✓7ᵗʰ **T40.721** Poisoning by synthetic cannabinoids, accidental (unintentional)

✓7ᵗʰ **T40.722** Poisoning by synthetic cannabinoids, intentional self-harm **HCC Rx ESR COM**

✓7ᵗʰ **T40.723** Poisoning by synthetic cannabinoids, assault

✓7ᵗʰ **T40.724** Poisoning by synthetic cannabinoids, undetermined

✓7ᵗʰ **T40.725** Adverse effect of synthetic cannabinoids **UPD**

✓7ᵗʰ **T40.726** Underdosing of synthetic cannabinoids **UPD**

✓5ᵗʰ **T40.8** Poisoning by and adverse effect of lysergide [LSD]

✓6ᵗʰ **T40.8X** Poisoning by and adverse effect of lysergide [LSD]

¹ ✓7ᵗʰ **T40.8X1** Poisoning by lysergide [LSD], accidental (unintentional) **HCC ESR COM**
Poisoning by lysergide [LSD] NOS

² ✓7ᵗʰ **T40.8X2** Poisoning by lysergide [LSD], intentional self-harm **HCC Rx ESR COM**

✓7ᵗʰ **T40.8X3** Poisoning by lysergide [LSD], assault

¹ ✓7ᵗʰ **T40.8X4** Poisoning by lysergide [LSD], undetermined **HCC ESR COM**

✓5ᵗʰ **T40.9** Poisoning by, adverse effect of and underdosing of other and unspecified psychodysleptics [hallucinogens]

✓6ᵗʰ **T40.90** Poisoning by, adverse effect of and underdosing of unspecified psychodysleptics [hallucinogens]

¹ ✓7ᵗʰ **T40.901** Poisoning by unspecified psychodysleptics [hallucinogens], accidental (unintentional) **HCC ESR COM**

² ✓7ᵗʰ **T40.902** Poisoning by unspecified psychodysleptics [hallucinogens], intentional self-harm **HCC Rx ESR COM**

✓7ᵗʰ **T40.903** Poisoning by unspecified psychodysleptics [hallucinogens], assault

¹ ✓7ᵗʰ **T40.904** Poisoning by unspecified psychodysleptics [hallucinogens], undetermined **HCC ESR COM**

✓7ᵗʰ **T40.905** Adverse effect of unspecified psychodysleptics [hallucinogens] **UPD**

✓7ᵗʰ **T40.906** Underdosing of unspecified psychodysleptics [hallucinogens] **UPD**

✓6ᵗʰ **T40.99** Poisoning by, adverse effect of and underdosing of other psychodysleptics [hallucinogens]

¹ ✓7ᵗʰ **T40.991** Poisoning by other psychodysleptics [hallucinogens], accidental (unintentional) **HCC ESR COM**
Poisoning by other psychodysleptics [hallucinogens] NOS

² ✓7ᵗʰ **T40.992** Poisoning by other psychodysleptics [hallucinogens], intentional self-harm **HCC Rx ESR COM**

✓7ᵗʰ **T40.993** Poisoning by other psychodysleptics [hallucinogens], assault

¹ ✓7ᵗʰ **T40.994** Poisoning by other psychodysleptics [hallucinogens], undetermined **HCC ESR COM**

✓7ᵗʰ **T40.995** Adverse effect of other psychodysleptics [hallucinogens] **UPD**

✓7ᵗʰ **T40.996** Underdosing of other psychodysleptics [hallucinogens] **UPD**

☑4ᵗʰ **T41** **Poisoning by, adverse effect of and underdosing of anesthetics and therapeutic gases**

   EXCLUDES 1   *benzodiazepines (T42.4-)*
             cocaine (T40.5-)
             complications of anesthesia during labor and delivery (O74.-)
             complications of anesthesia during pregnancy (O29.-)
             complications of anesthesia during the puerperium (O89.-)
             opioids (T40.0-T40.2-)

> The appropriate 7th character is to be added to each code from category T41.
> A   initial encounter
> D   subsequent encounter
> S   sequela

   ☑5ᵗʰ **T41.0** **Poisoning by, adverse effect of and underdosing of inhaled anesthetics**
      EXCLUDES 1   *oxygen (T41.5-)*

     ☑6ᵗʰ **T41.0X** **Poisoning by, adverse effect of and underdosing of inhaled anesthetics**
       ☑7ᵗʰ **T41.0X1** **Poisoning by inhaled anesthetics, accidental (unintentional)**
          Poisoning by inhaled anesthetics NOS
       ² ☑7ᵗʰ **T41.0X2** **Poisoning by inhaled anesthetics, intentional self-harm** HCC Rx ESR COM
       ☑7ᵗʰ **T41.0X3** **Poisoning by inhaled anesthetics, assault**
       ☑7ᵗʰ **T41.0X4** **Poisoning by inhaled anesthetics, undetermined**
       ☑7ᵗʰ **T41.0X5** **Adverse effect of inhaled anesthetics** UPD
       ☑7ᵗʰ **T41.0X6** **Underdosing of inhaled anesthetics** UPD

   ☑5ᵗʰ **T41.1** **Poisoning by, adverse effect of and underdosing of intravenous anesthetics**
      Poisoning by, adverse effect of and underdosing of thiobarbiturates

     ☑6ᵗʰ **T41.1X** **Poisoning by, adverse effect of and underdosing of intravenous anesthetics**
       ☑7ᵗʰ **T41.1X1** **Poisoning by intravenous anesthetics, accidental (unintentional)**
          Poisoning by intravenous anesthetics NOS
       ² ☑7ᵗʰ **T41.1X2** **Poisoning by intravenous anesthetics, intentional self-harm** HCC Rx ESR COM
       ☑7ᵗʰ **T41.1X3** **Poisoning by intravenous anesthetics, assault**
       ☑7ᵗʰ **T41.1X4** **Poisoning by intravenous anesthetics, undetermined**
       ☑7ᵗʰ **T41.1X5** **Adverse effect of intravenous anesthetics** UPD
       ☑7ᵗʰ **T41.1X6** **Underdosing of intravenous anesthetics** UPD

   ☑5ᵗʰ **T41.2** **Poisoning by, adverse effect of and underdosing of other and unspecified general anesthetics**
     ☑6ᵗʰ **T41.20** **Poisoning by, adverse effect of and underdosing of unspecified general anesthetics**
       ☑7ᵗʰ **T41.201** **Poisoning by unspecified general anesthetics, accidental (unintentional)**
          Poisoning by general anesthetics NOS
       ² ☑7ᵗʰ **T41.202** **Poisoning by unspecified general anesthetics, intentional self-harm** HCC Rx ESR COM
       ☑7ᵗʰ **T41.203** **Poisoning by unspecified general anesthetics, assault**
       ☑7ᵗʰ **T41.204** **Poisoning by unspecified general anesthetics, undetermined**
       ☑7ᵗʰ **T41.205** **Adverse effect of unspecified general anesthetics** UPD
          AHA: 2016,4Q,73
       ☑7ᵗʰ **T41.206** **Underdosing of unspecified general anesthetics** UPD

     ☑6ᵗʰ **T41.29** **Poisoning by, adverse effect of and underdosing of other general anesthetics**
       ☑7ᵗʰ **T41.291** **Poisoning by other general anesthetics, accidental (unintentional)**
          Poisoning by other general anesthetics NOS
       ² ☑7ᵗʰ **T41.292** **Poisoning by other general anesthetics, intentional self-harm** HCC Rx ESR COM
       ☑7ᵗʰ **T41.293** **Poisoning by other general anesthetics, assault**
       ☑7ᵗʰ **T41.294** **Poisoning by other general anesthetics, undetermined**

       ☑7ᵗʰ **T41.295** **Adverse effect of other general anesthetics** UPD
       ☑7ᵗʰ **T41.296** **Underdosing of other general anesthetics** UPD

   ☑5ᵗʰ **T41.3** **Poisoning by, adverse effect of and underdosing of local anesthetics**
      Cocaine (topical)
      EXCLUDES 2   *poisoning by cocaine used as a central nervous system stimulant (T40.5X1-T40.5X4)*

     ☑6ᵗʰ **T41.3X** **Poisoning by, adverse effect of and underdosing of local anesthetics**
       ☑7ᵗʰ **T41.3X1** **Poisoning by local anesthetics, accidental (unintentional)**
          Poisoning by local anesthetics NOS
       ² ☑7ᵗʰ **T41.3X2** **Poisoning by local anesthetics, intentional self-harm** HCC Rx ESR COM
       ☑7ᵗʰ **T41.3X3** **Poisoning by local anesthetics, assault**
       ☑7ᵗʰ **T41.3X4** **Poisoning by local anesthetics, undetermined**
       ☑7ᵗʰ **T41.3X5** **Adverse effect of local anesthetics** UPD
       ☑7ᵗʰ **T41.3X6** **Underdosing of local anesthetics** UPD

   ☑5ᵗʰ **T41.4** **Poisoning by, adverse effect of and underdosing of unspecified anesthetic**
     ☑x7ᵗʰ **T41.41** **Poisoning by unspecified anesthetic, accidental (unintentional)**
       Poisoning by anesthetic NOS
     ² ☑x7ᵗʰ **T41.42** **Poisoning by unspecified anesthetic, intentional self-harm** HCC Rx ESR COM
     ☑x7ᵗʰ **T41.43** **Poisoning by unspecified anesthetic, assault**
     ☑x7ᵗʰ **T41.44** **Poisoning by unspecified anesthetic, undetermined**
     ☑x7ᵗʰ **T41.45** **Adverse effect of unspecified anesthetic** UPD
     ☑x7ᵗʰ **T41.46** **Underdosing of unspecified anesthetics** UPD

   ☑5ᵗʰ **T41.5** **Poisoning by, adverse effect of and underdosing of therapeutic gases**
     ☑6ᵗʰ **T41.5X** **Poisoning by, adverse effect of and underdosing of therapeutic gases**
       ☑7ᵗʰ **T41.5X1** **Poisoning by therapeutic gases, accidental (unintentional)**
          Poisoning by therapeutic gases NOS
       ² ☑7ᵗʰ **T41.5X2** **Poisoning by therapeutic gases, intentional self-harm** HCC Rx ESR COM
       ☑7ᵗʰ **T41.5X3** **Poisoning by therapeutic gases, assault**
       ☑7ᵗʰ **T41.5X4** **Poisoning by therapeutic gases, undetermined**
       ☑7ᵗʰ **T41.5X5** **Adverse effect of therapeutic gases** UPD
       ☑7ᵗʰ **T41.5X6** **Underdosing of therapeutic gases** UPD

☑4ᵗʰ **T42** **Poisoning by, adverse effect of and underdosing of antiepileptic, sedative- hypnotic and antiparkinsonism drugs**
   EXCLUDES 2   *drug dependence and related mental and behavioral disorders due to psychoactive substance use (F10.-- F19.-)*

> The appropriate 7th character is to be added to each code from category T42.
> A   initial encounter
> D   subsequent encounter
> S   sequela

   ☑5ᵗʰ **T42.0** **Poisoning by, adverse effect of and underdosing of hydantoin derivatives**
     ☑6ᵗʰ **T42.0X** **Poisoning by, adverse effect of and underdosing of hydantoin derivatives**
       ☑7ᵗʰ **T42.0X1** **Poisoning by hydantoin derivatives, accidental (unintentional)**
          Poisoning by hydantoin derivatives NOS
       ² ☑7ᵗʰ **T42.0X2** **Poisoning by hydantoin derivatives, intentional self-harm** HCC Rx ESR COM
       ☑7ᵗʰ **T42.0X3** **Poisoning by hydantoin derivatives, assault**
       ☑7ᵗʰ **T42.0X4** **Poisoning by hydantoin derivatives, undetermined**
       ☑7ᵗʰ **T42.0X5** **Adverse effect of hydantoin derivatives** UPD
       ☑7ᵗʰ **T42.0X6** **Underdosing of hydantoin derivatives** UPD

☑ Additional Character Required   ☑x7ᵗʰ Placeholder Alert   Manifestation   Unspecified Dx   ☑ QPP   UPD Unacceptable PDx

√5th **T42.1** **Poisoning by, adverse effect of and underdosing of iminostilbenes**

Poisoning by, adverse effect of and underdosing of carbamazepine

√6th **T42.1X** **Poisoning by, adverse effect of and underdosing of** iminostilbenes

√7th **T42.1X1** **Poisoning by iminostilbenes, accidental (unintentional)**

Poisoning by iminostilbenes NOS

2 √7th **T42.1X2** **Poisoning by iminostilbenes, intentional self-harm** HCC Rx ESR COM

√7th **T42.1X3** **Poisoning by iminostilbenes, assault**

√7th **T42.1X4** **Poisoning by iminostilbenes, undetermined**

√7th **T42.1X5** **Adverse effect of iminostilbenes** UPD

√7th **T42.1X6** **Underdosing of iminostilbenes** UPD

√5th **T42.2** **Poisoning by, adverse effect of and underdosing of succinimides and oxazolidinediones**

√6th **T42.2X** **Poisoning by, adverse effect of and underdosing of** succinimides and oxazolidinediones

√7th **T42.2X1** **Poisoning by succinimides and oxazolidinediones, accidental (unintentional)**

Poisoning by succinimides and oxazolidinediones NOS

2 √7th **T42.2X2** **Poisoning by succinimides and oxazolidinediones, intentional self-harm** HCC Rx ESR COM

√7th **T42.2X3** **Poisoning by succinimides and oxazolidinediones, assault**

√7th **T42.2X4** **Poisoning by succinimides and oxazolidinediones, undetermined**

√7th **T42.2X5** **Adverse effect of succinimides and oxazolidinediones** UPD

√7th **T42.2X6** **Underdosing of succinimides and oxazolidinediones** UPD

√5th **T42.3** **Poisoning by, adverse effect of and underdosing of barbiturates**

EXCLUDES 1   *poisoning by, adverse effect of and underdosing of thiobarbiturates (T41.1-)*

√6th **T42.3X** **Poisoning by, adverse effect of and underdosing of** barbiturates

√7th **T42.3X1** **Poisoning by barbiturates, accidental (unintentional)**

Poisoning by barbiturates NOS

2 √7th **T42.3X2** **Poisoning by barbiturates, intentional self-harm** HCC Rx ESR COM

√7th **T42.3X3** **Poisoning by barbiturates, assault**

√7th **T42.3X4** **Poisoning by barbiturates, undetermined**

√7th **T42.3X5** **Adverse effect of barbiturates** UPD

√7th **T42.3X6** **Underdosing of barbiturates** UPD

√5th **T42.4** **Poisoning by, adverse effect of and underdosing of benzodiazepines**

√6th **T42.4X** **Poisoning by, adverse effect of and underdosing of** benzodiazepines

√7th **T42.4X1** **Poisoning by benzodiazepines, accidental (unintentional)**

Poisoning by benzodiazepines NOS

2 √7th **T42.4X2** **Poisoning by benzodiazepines, intentional self-harm** HCC Rx ESR COM

√7th **T42.4X3** **Poisoning by benzodiazepines, assault**

√7th **T42.4X4** **Poisoning by benzodiazepines, undetermined**

√7th **T42.4X5** **Adverse effect of benzodiazepines** UPD

√7th **T42.4X6** **Underdosing of benzodiazepines** UPD

√5th **T42.5** **Poisoning by, adverse effect of and underdosing of mixed antiepileptics**

√6th **T42.5X** **Poisoning by, adverse effect of and underdosing of** antiepileptics

√7th **T42.5X1** **Poisoning by mixed antiepileptics, accidental (unintentional)**

Poisoning by mixed antiepileptics NOS

2 √7th **T42.5X2** **Poisoning by mixed antiepileptics, intentional self-harm** HCC Rx ESR COM

√7th **T42.5X3** **Poisoning by mixed antiepileptics, assault**

√7th **T42.5X4** **Poisoning by mixed antiepileptics, undetermined**

√7th **T42.5X5** **Adverse effect of mixed antiepileptics** UPD

√7th **T42.5X6** **Underdosing of mixed antiepileptics** UPD

√5th **T42.6** **Poisoning by, adverse effect of and underdosing of other antiepileptic and sedative-hypnotic drugs**

Poisoning by, adverse effect of and underdosing of methaqualone

Poisoning by, adverse effect of and underdosing of valproic acid

EXCLUDES 1   *poisoning by, adverse effect of and underdosing of carbamazepine (T42.1-)*

√6th **T42.6X** **Poisoning by, adverse effect of and underdosing of other antiepileptic and sedative-hypnotic drugs**

√7th **T42.6X1** **Poisoning by other antiepileptic and sedative-hypnotic drugs, accidental (unintentional)**

Poisoning by other antiepileptic and sedative-hypnotic drugs NOS

2 √7th **T42.6X2** **Poisoning by other antiepileptic and sedative-hypnotic drugs, intentional self-harm** HCC Rx ESR COM

√7th **T42.6X3** **Poisoning by other antiepileptic and sedative-hypnotic drugs, assault**

√7th **T42.6X4** **Poisoning by other antiepileptic and sedative-hypnotic drugs, undetermined**

√7th **T42.6X5** **Adverse effect of other antiepileptic and sedative-hypnotic drugs** UPD

√7th **T42.6X6** **Underdosing of other antiepileptic and sedative-hypnotic drugs** UPD

√6th **T42.7** **Poisoning by, adverse effect of and underdosing of unspecified antiepileptic and sedative-hypnotic drugs**

√x7th **T42.71** **Poisoning by unspecified antiepileptic and sedative-hypnotic drugs, accidental (unintentional)**

Poisoning by antiepileptic and sedative-hypnotic drugs NOS

2 √x7th **T42.72** **Poisoning by unspecified antiepileptic and sedative-hypnotic drugs, intentional self-harm** HCC Rx ESR COM

√x7th **T42.73** **Poisoning by unspecified antiepileptic and sedative-hypnotic drugs, assault**

√x7th **T42.74** **Poisoning by unspecified antiepileptic and sedative-hypnotic drugs, undetermined**

√x7th **T42.75** **Adverse effect of unspecified antiepileptic and sedative-hypnotic drugs** UPD

√x7th **T42.76** **Underdosing of unspecified antiepileptic and sedative-hypnotic drugs** UPD

√5th **T42.8** **Poisoning by, adverse effect of and underdosing of antiparkinsonism drugs and other central muscle-tone depressants**

Poisoning by, adverse effect of and underdosing of amantadine

√6th **T42.8X** **Poisoning by, adverse effect of and underdosing of** antiparkinsonism drugs and other central muscle-tone depressants

√7th **T42.8X1** **Poisoning by antiparkinsonism drugs and other central muscle-tone depressants, accidental (unintentional)**

Poisoning by antiparkinsonism drugs and other central muscle-tone depressants NOS

2 √7th **T42.8X2** **Poisoning by antiparkinsonism drugs and other central muscle-tone depressants, intentional self-harm** HCC Rx ESR COM

√7th **T42.8X3** **Poisoning by antiparkinsonism drugs and other central muscle-tone depressants, assault**

√7th **T42.8X4** **Poisoning by antiparkinsonism drugs and other central muscle-tone depressants, undetermined**

√7th **T42.8X5** **Adverse effect of antiparkinsonism drugs and other central muscle-tone depressants** UPD

√7th **T42.8X6** **Underdosing of antiparkinsonism drugs and other central muscle-tone depressants** UPD

✓4ᵗʰ **T43 Poisoning by, adverse effect of and underdosing of psychotropic drugs, not elsewhere classified**

    EXCLUDES 1   *appetite depressants (T50.5-)*
               barbiturates (T42.3-)
               benzodiazepines (T42.4-)
               methaqualone (T42.6-)
               psychodysleptics [hallucinogens] (T40.7-T40.9-)

    EXCLUDES 2   *drug dependence and related mental and behavioral disorders due to psychoactive substance use (F10.- – F19.-)*

> The appropriate 7th character is to be added to each code from category T43.
> A   initial encounter
> D   subsequent encounter
> S   sequela

✓5ᵗʰ **T43.0 Poisoning by, adverse effect of and underdosing of tricyclic and tetracyclic antidepressants**

    ✓6ᵗʰ **T43.01 Poisoning by, adverse effect of and underdosing of tricyclic antidepressants**

       ✓7ᵗʰ **T43.011 Poisoning by tricyclic antidepressants, accidental (unintentional)**
           Poisoning by tricyclic antidepressants NOS

       2 ✓7ᵗʰ **T43.012 Poisoning by tricyclic antidepressants, intentional self-harm** HCC Rx ESR COM

       ✓7ᵗʰ **T43.013 Poisoning by tricyclic antidepressants, assault**

       ✓7ᵗʰ **T43.014 Poisoning by tricyclic antidepressants, undetermined**

       ✓7ᵗʰ **T43.015 Adverse effect of tricyclic antidepressants** UPD

       ✓7ᵗʰ **T43.016 Underdosing of tricyclic antidepressants** UPD

    ✓6ᵗʰ **T43.02 Poisoning by, adverse effect of and underdosing of tetracyclic antidepressants**

       ✓7ᵗʰ **T43.021 Poisoning by tetracyclic antidepressants, accidental (unintentional)**
           Poisoning by tetracyclic antidepressants NOS

       2 ✓7ᵗʰ **T43.022 Poisoning by tetracyclic antidepressants, intentional self-harm** HCC Rx ESR COM

       ✓7ᵗʰ **T43.023 Poisoning by tetracyclic antidepressants, assault**

       ✓7ᵗʰ **T43.024 Poisoning by tetracyclic antidepressants, undetermined**

       ✓7ᵗʰ **T43.025 Adverse effect of tetracyclic antidepressants** UPD

       ✓7ᵗʰ **T43.026 Underdosing of tetracyclic antidepressants** UPD

✓5ᵗʰ **T43.1 Poisoning by, adverse effect of and underdosing of monoamine-oxidase-inhibitor antidepressants**

    ✓6ᵗʰ **T43.1X Poisoning by, adverse effect of and underdosing of monoamine-oxidase-inhibitor antidepressants**

       ✓7ᵗʰ **T43.1X1 Poisoning by monoamine-oxidase-inhibitor antidepressants, accidental (unintentional)**
           Poisoning by monoamine-oxidase-inhibitor antidepressants NOS

       2 ✓7ᵗʰ **T43.1X2 Poisoning by monoamine-oxidase-inhibitor antidepressants, intentional self-harm** HCC Rx ESR COM

       ✓7ᵗʰ **T43.1X3 Poisoning by monoamine-oxidase-inhibitor antidepressants, assault**

       ✓7ᵗʰ **T43.1X4 Poisoning by monoamine-oxidase-inhibitor antidepressants, undetermined**

       ✓7ᵗʰ **T43.1X5 Adverse effect of monoamine-oxidase-inhibitor antidepressants** UPD

       ✓7ᵗʰ **T43.1X6 Underdosing of monoamine-oxidase-inhibitor antidepressants** UPD

✓5ᵗʰ **T43.2 Poisoning by, adverse effect of and underdosing of other and unspecified antidepressants**

    ✓6ᵗʰ **T43.20 Poisoning by, adverse effect of and underdosing of unspecified antidepressants**

       ✓7ᵗʰ **T43.201 Poisoning by unspecified antidepressants, accidental (unintentional)**
           Poisoning by antidepressants NOS

       2 ✓7ᵗʰ **T43.202 Poisoning by unspecified antidepressants, intentional self-harm** HCC Rx ESR COM

       ✓7ᵗʰ **T43.203 Poisoning by unspecified antidepressants, assault**

       ✓7ᵗʰ **T43.204 Poisoning by unspecified antidepressants, undetermined**

       ✓7ᵗʰ **T43.205 Adverse effect of unspecified antidepressants** UPD
           Antidepressant discontinuation syndrome

       ✓7ᵗʰ **T43.206 Underdosing of unspecified antidepressants** UPD

    ✓6ᵗʰ **T43.21 Poisoning by, adverse effect of and underdosing of selective serotonin and norepinephrine reuptake inhibitors**
       Poisoning by, adverse effect of and underdosing of SSNRI antidepressants

       ✓7ᵗʰ **T43.211 Poisoning by selective serotonin and norepinephrine reuptake inhibitors, accidental (unintentional)**

       2 ✓7ᵗʰ **T43.212 Poisoning by selective serotonin and norepinephrine reuptake inhibitors, intentional self-harm** HCC Rx ESR COM

       ✓7ᵗʰ **T43.213 Poisoning by selective serotonin and norepinephrine reuptake inhibitors, assault**

       ✓7ᵗʰ **T43.214 Poisoning by selective serotonin and norepinephrine reuptake inhibitors, undetermined**

       ✓7ᵗʰ **T43.215 Adverse effect of selective serotonin and norepinephrine reuptake inhibitors** UPD

       ✓7ᵗʰ **T43.216 Underdosing of selective serotonin and norepinephrine reuptake inhibitors** UPD

    ✓6ᵗʰ **T43.22 Poisoning by, adverse effect of and underdosing of selective serotonin reuptake inhibitors**
       Poisoning by, adverse effect of and underdosing of SSRI antidepressants

       ✓7ᵗʰ **T43.221 Poisoning by selective serotonin reuptake inhibitors, accidental (unintentional)**

       2 ✓7ᵗʰ **T43.222 Poisoning by selective serotonin reuptake inhibitors, intentional self-harm** HCC Rx ESR COM

       ✓7ᵗʰ **T43.223 Poisoning by selective serotonin reuptake inhibitors, assault**

       ✓7ᵗʰ **T43.224 Poisoning by selective serotonin reuptake inhibitors, undetermined**

       ✓7ᵗʰ **T43.225 Adverse effect of selective serotonin reuptake inhibitors** UPD
           AHA: 2022,2Q,11

       ✓7ᵗʰ **T43.226 Underdosing of selective serotonin reuptake inhibitors** UPD

    ✓6ᵗʰ **T43.29 Poisoning by, adverse effect of and underdosing of other antidepressants**

       ✓7ᵗʰ **T43.291 Poisoning by other antidepressants, accidental (unintentional)**
           Poisoning by other antidepressants NOS

       2 ✓7ᵗʰ **T43.292 Poisoning by other antidepressants, intentional self-harm** HCC Rx ESR COM

       ✓7ᵗʰ **T43.293 Poisoning by other antidepressants, assault**

       ✓7ᵗʰ **T43.294 Poisoning by other antidepressants, undetermined**

       ✓7ᵗʰ **T43.295 Adverse effect of other antidepressants** UPD

       ✓7ᵗʰ **T43.296 Underdosing of other antidepressants** UPD

✓5ᵗʰ T43.3   Poisoning by, adverse effect of and underdosing of phenothiazine antipsychotics and neuroleptics

    ✓6ᵗʰ T43.3X   Poisoning by, adverse effect of and underdosing of phenothiazine antipsychotics and neuroleptics

       ✓7ᵗʰ T43.3X1   Poisoning by phenothiazine antipsychotics and neuroleptics, accidental (unintentional)
          Poisoning by phenothiazine antipsychotics and neuroleptics NOS

       ² **✓7ᵗʰ T43.3X2**   Poisoning by phenothiazine antipsychotics and neuroleptics, intentional self-harm   HCC Rx ESR COM

       ✓7ᵗʰ T43.3X3   Poisoning by phenothiazine antipsychotics and neuroleptics, assault

       ✓7ᵗʰ T43.3X4   Poisoning by phenothiazine antipsychotics and neuroleptics, undetermined

       ✓7ᵗʰ T43.3X5   Adverse effect of phenothiazine antipsychotics and neuroleptics   UPD

       ✓7ᵗʰ T43.3X6   Underdosing of phenothiazine antipsychotics and neuroleptics   UPD

✓5ᵗʰ T43.4   Poisoning by, adverse effect of and underdosing of butyrophenone and thiothixene neuroleptics

    ✓6ᵗʰ T43.4X   Poisoning by, adverse effect of and underdosing of butyrophenone and thiothixene neuroleptics

       ✓7ᵗʰ T43.4X1   Poisoning by butyrophenone and thiothixene neuroleptics, accidental (unintentional)
          Poisoning by butyrophenone and thiothixene neuroleptics NOS

       ² **✓7ᵗʰ T43.4X2**   Poisoning by butyrophenone and thiothixene neuroleptics, intentional self-harm   HCC Rx ESR COM

       ✓7ᵗʰ T43.4X3   Poisoning by butyrophenone and thiothixene neuroleptics, assault

       ✓7ᵗʰ T43.4X4   Poisoning by butyrophenone and thiothixene neuroleptics, undetermined

       ✓7ᵗʰ T43.4X5   Adverse effect of butyrophenone and thiothixene neuroleptics   UPD

       ✓7ᵗʰ T43.4X6   Underdosing of butyrophenone and thiothixene neuroleptics   UPD

✓5ᵗʰ T43.5   Poisoning by, adverse effect of and underdosing of other and unspecified antipsychotics and neuroleptics

    EXCLUDES 1   poisoning by, adverse effect of and underdosing of rauwolfia (T46.5-)

    ✓6ᵗʰ T43.50   Poisoning by, adverse effect of and underdosing of unspecified antipsychotics and neuroleptics

       ✓7ᵗʰ T43.501   Poisoning by unspecified antipsychotics and neuroleptics, accidental (unintentional)
          Poisoning by antipsychotics and neuroleptics NOS

       ² **✓7ᵗʰ T43.502**   Poisoning by unspecified antipsychotics and neuroleptics, intentional self-harm   HCC Rx ESR COM

       ✓7ᵗʰ T43.503   Poisoning by unspecified antipsychotics and neuroleptics, assault

       ✓7ᵗʰ T43.504   Poisoning by unspecified antipsychotics and neuroleptics, undetermined

       ✓7ᵗʰ T43.505   Adverse effect of unspecified antipsychotics and neuroleptics   UPD

       ✓7ᵗʰ T43.506   Underdosing of unspecified antipsychotics and neuroleptics   UPD

    ✓6ᵗʰ T43.59   Poisoning by, adverse effect of and underdosing of other antipsychotics and neuroleptics
      AHA: 2017,1Q,40

       ✓7ᵗʰ T43.591   Poisoning by other antipsychotics and neuroleptics, accidental (unintentional)
          Poisoning by other antipsychotics and neuroleptics NOS

       ² **✓7ᵗʰ T43.592**   Poisoning by other antipsychotics and neuroleptics, intentional self-harm   HCC Rx ESR COM

       ✓7ᵗʰ T43.593   Poisoning by other antipsychotics and neuroleptics, assault

       ✓7ᵗʰ T43.594   Poisoning by other antipsychotics and neuroleptics, undetermined

       ✓7ᵗʰ T43.595   Adverse effect of other antipsychotics and neuroleptics   UPD
      AHA: 2022,2Q,11

       ✓7ᵗʰ T43.596   Underdosing of other antipsychotics and neuroleptics   UPD

✓5ᵗʰ T43.6   Poisoning by, adverse effect of and underdosing of psychostimulants
    EXCLUDES 1   poisoning by, adverse effect of and underdosing of cocaine (T40.5-)

    ✓6ᵗʰ T43.60   Poisoning by, adverse effect of and underdosing of unspecified psychostimulant

       ¹ **✓7ᵗʰ T43.601**   Poisoning by unspecified psychostimulants, accidental (unintentional)   HCC ESR COM
          Poisoning by psychostimulants NOS

       ² **✓7ᵗʰ T43.602**   Poisoning by unspecified psychostimulants, intentional self-harm   HCC Rx ESR COM

       ✓7ᵗʰ T43.603   Poisoning by unspecified psychostimulants, assault

       ¹ **✓7ᵗʰ T43.604**   Poisoning by unspecified psychostimulants, undetermined   HCC ESR COM

       ✓7ᵗʰ T43.605   Adverse effect of unspecified psychostimulants   UPD

       ✓7ᵗʰ T43.606   Underdosing of unspecified psychostimulants   UPD

    ✓6ᵗʰ T43.61   Poisoning by, adverse effect of and underdosing of caffeine

       ¹ **✓7ᵗʰ T43.611**   Poisoning by caffeine, accidental (unintentional)   HCC ESR COM
          Poisoning by caffeine NOS

       ² **✓7ᵗʰ T43.612**   Poisoning by caffeine, intentional self-harm   HCC Rx ESR COM

       ✓7ᵗʰ T43.613   Poisoning by caffeine, assault

       ¹ **✓7ᵗʰ T43.614**   Poisoning by caffeine, undetermined   HCC ESR COM

       ✓7ᵗʰ T43.615   Adverse effect of caffeine   UPD

       ✓7ᵗʰ T43.616   Underdosing of caffeine   UPD

    ✓6ᵗʰ T43.62   Poisoning by, adverse effect of and underdosing of amphetamines
      Poisoning by, adverse effect of and underdosing of methamphetamines

       ¹ **✓7ᵗʰ T43.621**   Poisoning by amphetamines, accidental (unintentional)   HCC ESR COM
          Poisoning by amphetamines NOS
          AHA: 2021,3Q,8

       ² **✓7ᵗʰ T43.622**   Poisoning by amphetamines, intentional self-harm   HCC Rx ESR COM

       ✓7ᵗʰ T43.623   Poisoning by amphetamines, assault

       ¹ **✓7ᵗʰ T43.624**   Poisoning by amphetamines, undetermined   HCC ESR COM

       ✓7ᵗʰ T43.625   Adverse effect of amphetamines   UPD

       ✓7ᵗʰ T43.626   Underdosing of amphetamines   UPD

    ✓6ᵗʰ T43.63   Poisoning by, adverse effect of and underdosing of methylphenidate

       ¹ **✓7ᵗʰ T43.631**   Poisoning by methylphenidate, accidental (unintentional)   HCC ESR COM
          Poisoning by methylphenidate NOS

       ² **✓7ᵗʰ T43.632**   Poisoning by methylphenidate, intentional self-harm   HCC Rx ESR COM

       ✓7ᵗʰ T43.633   Poisoning by methylphenidate, assault

       ¹ **✓7ᵗʰ T43.634**   Poisoning by methylphenidate, undetermined   HCC ESR COM

       ✓7ᵗʰ T43.635   Adverse effect of methylphenidate   UPD

       ✓7ᵗʰ T43.636   Underdosing of methylphenidate   UPD

    ✓6ᵗʰ T43.64   Poisoning by ecstasy
      Poisoning by MDMA
      Poisoning by 3,4-methylenedioxymethamphetamine
      AHA: 2018,4Q,30-31

       ¹ **✓7ᵗʰ T43.641**   Poisoning by ecstasy, accidental (unintentional)   HCC ESR COM
          Poisoning by ecstasy NOS

       ² **✓7ᵗʰ T43.642**   Poisoning by ecstasy, intentional self-harm   HCC Rx ESR COM

       ✓7ᵗʰ T43.643   Poisoning by ecstasy, assault

       ¹ **✓7ᵗʰ T43.644**   Poisoning by ecstasy, undetermined   HCC ESR COM

● ✓6ᵗʰ **T43.65 Poisoning by, adverse effect of and underdosing of** methamphetamines

●   ✓7ᵗʰ **T43.651 Poisoning by methamphetamines accidental (unintentional)**
         Poisoning by methamphetamines NOS

●   ✓7ᵗʰ **T43.652 Poisoning by methamphetamines intentional self-harm**

●   ✓7ᵗʰ **T43.653 Poisoning by methamphetamines, assault**

●   ✓7ᵗʰ **T43.654 Poisoning by methamphetamines, undetermined**

●   ✓7ᵗʰ **T43.655 Adverse effect of methamphetamines**

●   ✓7ᵗʰ **T43.656 Underdosing of methamphetamines**

✓6ᵗʰ **T43.69 Poisoning by, adverse effect of and underdosing of other psychostimulants**

¹ ✓7ᵗʰ **T43.691 Poisoning by other psychostimulants, accidental (unintentional)** HCC Rx ESR COM
         Poisoning by other psychostimulants NOS

² ✓7ᵗʰ **T43.692 Poisoning by other psychostimulants, intentional self-harm** HCC Rx ESR COM

✓7ᵗʰ **T43.693 Poisoning by other psychostimulants, assault**

¹ ✓7ᵗʰ **T43.694 Poisoning by other psychostimulants, undetermined** HCC ESR COM

✓7ᵗʰ **T43.695 Adverse effect of other psychostimulants** UPD

✓7ᵗʰ **T43.696 Underdosing of other psychostimulants** UPD

✓5ᵗʰ **T43.8 Poisoning by, adverse effect of and underdosing of other psychotropic drugs**

✓6ᵗʰ **T43.8X Poisoning by, adverse effect of and underdosing of other psychotropic drugs**

✓7ᵗʰ **T43.8X1 Poisoning by other psychotropic drugs, accidental (unintentional)**
         Poisoning by other psychotropic drugs NOS

² ✓7ᵗʰ **T43.8X2 Poisoning by other psychotropic drugs, intentional self-harm** HCC Rx ESR COM

✓7ᵗʰ **T43.8X3 Poisoning by other psychotropic drugs, assault**

✓7ᵗʰ **T43.8X4 Poisoning by other psychotropic drugs, undetermined**

✓7ᵗʰ **T43.8X5 Adverse effect of other psychotropic drugs** UPD

✓7ᵗʰ **T43.8X6 Underdosing of other psychotropic drugs** UPD

✓5ᵗʰ **T43.9 Poisoning by, adverse effect of and underdosing of unspecified psychotropic drug**

✓x7ᵗʰ **T43.91 Poisoning by unspecified psychotropic drug, accidental (unintentional)**
         Poisoning by psychotropic drug NOS

² ✓x7ᵗʰ **T43.92 Poisoning by unspecified psychotropic drug, intentional self-harm** HCC Rx ESR COM

✓x7ᵗʰ **T43.93 Poisoning by unspecified psychotropic drug, assault**

✓x7ᵗʰ **T43.94 Poisoning by unspecified psychotropic drug, undetermined**

✓x7ᵗʰ **T43.95 Adverse effect of unspecified psychotropic drug** UPD

✓x7ᵗʰ **T43.96 Underdosing of unspecified psychotropic drug** UPD

✓4ᵗʰ **T44 Poisoning by, adverse effect of and underdosing of drugs primarily affecting the autonomic nervous system**

> The appropriate 7th character is to be added to each code from category T44.
> A   initial encounter
> D   subsequent encounter
> S   sequela

✓5ᵗʰ **T44.0 Poisoning by, adverse effect of and underdosing of anticholinesterase agents**

✓6ᵗʰ **T44.0X Poisoning by, adverse effect of and underdosing of anticholinesterase agents**

✓7ᵗʰ **T44.0X1 Poisoning by anticholinesterase agents, accidental (unintentional)**
         Poisoning by anticholinesterase agents NOS

² ✓7ᵗʰ **T44.0X2 Poisoning by anticholinesterase agents, intentional self-harm** HCC Rx ESR COM

✓7ᵗʰ **T44.0X3 Poisoning by anticholinesterase agents, assault**

✓7ᵗʰ **T44.0X4 Poisoning by anticholinesterase agents, undetermined**

✓7ᵗʰ **T44.0X5 Adverse effect of anticholinesterase agents** UPD

✓7ᵗʰ **T44.0X6 Underdosing of anticholinesterase agents** UPD

✓5ᵗʰ **T44.1 Poisoning by, adverse effect of and underdosing of other parasympathomimetics [cholinergics]**

✓6ᵗʰ **T44.1X Poisoning by, adverse effect of and underdosing of other parasympathomimetics [cholinergics]**

✓7ᵗʰ **T44.1X1 Poisoning by other parasympathomimetics [cholinergics], accidental (unintentional)**
         Poisoning by other parasympathomimetics [cholinergics] NOS

² ✓7ᵗʰ **T44.1X2 Poisoning by other parasympathomimetics [cholinergics], intentional self-harm** HCC Rx ESR COM

✓7ᵗʰ **T44.1X3 Poisoning by other parasympathomimetics [cholinergics], assault**

✓7ᵗʰ **T44.1X4 Poisoning by other parasympathomimetics [cholinergics], undetermined**

✓7ᵗʰ **T44.1X5 Adverse effect of other parasympathomimetics [cholinergics]** UPD

✓7ᵗʰ **T44.1X6 Underdosing of other parasympathomimetics [cholinergics]** UPD

✓5ᵗʰ **T44.2 Poisoning by, adverse effect of and underdosing of ganglionic blocking drugs**

✓6ᵗʰ **T44.2X Poisoning by, adverse effect of and underdosing of ganglionic blocking drugs**

✓7ᵗʰ **T44.2X1 Poisoning by ganglionic blocking drugs, accidental (unintentional)**
         Poisoning by ganglionic blocking drugs NOS

² ✓7ᵗʰ **T44.2X2 Poisoning by ganglionic blocking drugs, intentional self-harm** HCC Rx ESR COM

✓7ᵗʰ **T44.2X3 Poisoning by ganglionic blocking drugs, assault**

✓7ᵗʰ **T44.2X4 Poisoning by ganglionic blocking drugs, undetermined**

✓7ᵗʰ **T44.2X5 Adverse effect of ganglionic blocking drugs** UPD

✓7ᵗʰ **T44.2X6 Underdosing of ganglionic blocking drugs** UPD

✓5ᵗʰ **T44.3 Poisoning by, adverse effect of and underdosing of other parasympatholytics [anticholinergics and antimuscarinics] and spasmolytics**
     Poisoning by, adverse effect of and underdosing of papaverine

✓6ᵗʰ **T44.3X Poisoning by, adverse effect of and underdosing of other parasympatholytics [anticholinergics and antimuscarinics] and spasmolytics**

✓7ᵗʰ **T44.3X1 Poisoning by other parasympatholytics [anticholinergics and antimuscarinics] and spasmolytics, accidental (unintentional)**
         Poisoning by other parasympatholytics [anticholinergics and antimuscarinics] and spasmolytics NOS

² ✓7ᵗʰ **T44.3X2 Poisoning by other parasympatholytics [anticholinergics and antimuscarinics] and spasmolytics, intentional self-harm** HCC Rx ESR COM

✓7ᵗʰ **T44.3X3 Poisoning by other parasympatholytics [anticholinergics and antimuscarinics] and spasmolytics, assault**

✓7ᵗʰ **T44.3X4 Poisoning by other parasympatholytics [anticholinergics and antimuscarinics] and spasmolytics, undetermined**

✓7ᵗʰ **T44.3X5 Adverse effect of other parasympatholytics [anticholinergics and antimuscarinics] and spasmolytics** UPD

✓7ᵗʰ **T44.3X6 Underdosing of other parasympatholytics [anticholinergics and antimuscarinics] and spasmolytics** UPD

✓5th T44.4 Poisoning by, adverse effect of and underdosing of predominantly alpha-adrenoreceptor agonists
Poisoning by, adverse effect of and underdosing of metaraminol

✓6th T44.4X Poisoning by, adverse effect of and underdosing of predominantly alpha-adrenoreceptor agonists

    ✓7th T44.4X1 Poisoning by predominantly alpha-adrenoreceptor agonists, accidental (unintentional)
        Poisoning by predominantly alpha-adrenoreceptor agonists NOS

    2 ✓7th T44.4X2 Poisoning by predominantly alpha-adrenoreceptor agonists, intentional self-harm HCC Rx ESR COM

    ✓7th T44.4X3 Poisoning by predominantly alpha-adrenoreceptor agonists, assault

    ✓7th T44.4X4 Poisoning by predominantly alpha-adrenoreceptor agonists, undetermined

    ✓7th T44.4X5 Adverse effect of predominantly alpha-adrenoreceptor agonists UPD

    ✓7th T44.4X6 Underdosing of predominantly alpha-adrenoreceptor agonists UPD

✓5th T44.5 Poisoning by, adverse effect of and underdosing of predominantly beta-adrenoreceptor agonists
EXCLUDES 1 poisoning by, adverse effect of and underdosing of beta-adrenoreceptor agonists used in asthma therapy (T48.6-)

✓6th T44.5X Poisoning by, adverse effect of and underdosing of predominantly beta-adrenoreceptor agonists

    ✓7th T44.5X1 Poisoning by predominantly beta-adrenoreceptor agonists, accidental (unintentional)
        Poisoning by predominantly beta-adrenoreceptor agonists NOS

    2 ✓7th T44.5X2 Poisoning by predominantly beta-adrenoreceptor agonists, intentional self-harm HCC Rx ESR COM

    ✓7th T44.5X3 Poisoning by predominantly beta-adrenoreceptor agonists, assault

    ✓7th T44.5X4 Poisoning by predominantly beta-adrenoreceptor agonists, undetermined

    ✓7th T44.5X5 Adverse effect of predominantly beta-adrenoreceptor agonists UPD

    ✓7th T44.5X6 Underdosing of predominantly beta-adrenoreceptor agonists UPD

✓5th T44.6 Poisoning by, adverse effect of and underdosing of alpha-adrenoreceptor antagonists
EXCLUDES 1 poisoning by, adverse effect of and underdosing of ergot alkaloids (T48.0)

✓6th T44.6X Poisoning by, adverse effect of and underdosing of alpha-adrenoreceptor antagonists

    ✓7th T44.6X1 Poisoning by alpha-adrenoreceptor antagonists, accidental (unintentional)
        Poisoning by alpha-adrenoreceptor antagonists NOS

    2 ✓7th T44.6X2 Poisoning by alpha-adrenoreceptor antagonists, intentional self-harm HCC Rx ESR COM

    ✓7th T44.6X3 Poisoning by alpha-adrenoreceptor antagonists, assault

    ✓7th T44.6X4 Poisoning by alpha-adrenoreceptor antagonists, undetermined

    ✓7th T44.6X5 Adverse effect of alpha-adrenoreceptor antagonists UPD

    ✓7th T44.6X6 Underdosing of alpha-adrenoreceptor antagonists UPD

✓5th T44.7 Poisoning by, adverse effect of and underdosing of beta-adrenoreceptor antagonists

✓6th T44.7X Poisoning by, adverse effect of and underdosing of beta-adrenoreceptor antagonists

    ✓7th T44.7X1 Poisoning by beta-adrenoreceptor antagonists, accidental (unintentional)
        Poisoning by beta-adrenoreceptor antagonists NOS

    2 ✓7th T44.7X2 Poisoning by beta-adrenoreceptor antagonists, intentional self-harm HCC Rx ESR COM

    ✓7th T44.7X3 Poisoning by beta-adrenoreceptor antagonists, assault

    ✓7th T44.7X4 Poisoning by beta-adrenoreceptor antagonists, undetermined

    ✓7th T44.7X5 Adverse effect of beta-adrenoreceptor antagonists UPD

    ✓7th T44.7X6 Underdosing of beta-adrenoreceptor antagonists UPD

✓5th T44.8 Poisoning by, adverse effect of and underdosing of centrally-acting and adrenergic-neuron- blocking agents
EXCLUDES 2 poisoning by, adverse effect of and underdosing of clonidine (T46.5)
poisoning by, adverse effect of and underdosing of guanethidine (T46.5)

✓6th T44.8X Poisoning by, adverse effect of and underdosing of centrally-acting and adrenergic- neuron-blocking agents

    ✓7th T44.8X1 Poisoning by centrally-acting and adrenergic-neuron-blocking agents, accidental (unintentional)
        Poisoning by centrally-acting and adrenergic-neuron-blocking agents NOS

    2 ✓7th T44.8X2 Poisoning by centrally-acting and adrenergic-neuron-blocking agents, intentional self-harm HCC Rx ESR COM

    ✓7th T44.8X3 Poisoning by centrally-acting and adrenergic-neuron-blocking agents, assault

    ✓7th T44.8X4 Poisoning by centrally-acting and adrenergic-neuron-blocking agents, undetermined

    ✓7th T44.8X5 Adverse effect of centrally-acting and adrenergic-neuron-blocking agents UPD

    ✓7th T44.8X6 Underdosing of centrally-acting and adrenergic-neuron-blocking agents UPD

✓5th T44.9 Poisoning by, adverse effect of and underdosing of other and unspecified drugs primarily affecting the autonomic nervous system
Poisoning by, adverse effect of and underdosing of drug stimulating both alpha and beta-adrenoreceptors

✓6th T44.90 Poisoning by, adverse effect of and underdosing of unspecified drugs primarily affecting the autonomic nervous system

    ✓7th T44.901 Poisoning by unspecified drugs primarily affecting the autonomic nervous system, accidental (unintentional)
        Poisoning by unspecified drugs primarily affecting the autonomic nervous system NOS

    2 ✓7th T44.902 Poisoning by unspecified drugs primarily affecting the autonomic nervous system, intentional self-harm HCC Rx ESR COM

    ✓7th T44.903 Poisoning by unspecified drugs primarily affecting the autonomic nervous system, assault

    ✓7th T44.904 Poisoning by unspecified drugs primarily affecting the autonomic nervous system, undetermined

    ✓7th T44.905 Adverse effect of unspecified drugs primarily affecting the autonomic nervous system UPD

    ✓7th T44.906 Underdosing of unspecified drugs primarily affecting the autonomic nervous system UPD

✓6th T44.99 Poisoning by, adverse effect of and underdosing of other drugs primarily affecting the autonomic nervous system

    ✓7th T44.991 Poisoning by other drug primarily affecting the autonomic nervous system, accidental (unintentional)
        Poisoning by other drugs primarily affecting the autonomic nervous system NOS

    2 ✓7th T44.992 Poisoning by other drug primarily affecting the autonomic nervous system, intentional self-harm HCC Rx ESR COM

    ✓7th T44.993 Poisoning by other drug primarily affecting the autonomic nervous system, assault

    ✓7th T44.994 Poisoning by other drug primarily affecting the autonomic nervous system, undetermined

√7ᵗʰ **T44.995** Adverse effect of other drug primarily affecting the autonomic nervous system **UPD**

√7ᵗʰ **T44.996** Underdosing of other drug primarily affecting the autonomic nervous system **UPD**

√4ᵗʰ **T45** **Poisoning by, adverse effect of and underdosing of primarily systemic and hematological agents, not elsewhere classified**

> The appropriate 7th character is to be added to each code from category T45.
> A initial encounter
> D subsequent encounter
> S sequela

√5ᵗʰ **T45.Ø** **Poisoning by, adverse effect of and underdosing of antiallergic and antiemetic drugs**

> **EXCLUDES 1**   poisoning by, adverse effect of and underdosing of phenothiazine-based neuroleptics (T43.3)

√6ᵗʰ **T45.ØX** **Poisoning by, adverse effect of and underdosing of antiallergic and antiemetic drugs**

√7ᵗʰ **T45.ØX1** **Poisoning by antiallergic and antiemetic drugs, accidental (unintentional)**
Poisoning by antiallergic and antiemetic drugs NOS

² √7ᵗʰ **T45.ØX2** **Poisoning by antiallergic and antiemetic drugs, intentional self-harm** **HCC Rx ESR COM**

√7ᵗʰ **T45.ØX3** **Poisoning by antiallergic and antiemetic drugs, assault**

√7ᵗʰ **T45.ØX4** **Poisoning by antiallergic and antiemetic drugs, undetermined**

√7ᵗʰ **T45.ØX5** Adverse effect of antiallergic and antiemetic drugs **UPD**

√7ᵗʰ **T45.ØX6** Underdosing of antiallergic and antiemetic drugs **UPD**

√5ᵗʰ **T45.1** **Poisoning by, adverse effect of and underdosing of antineoplastic and immunosuppressive drugs**

> **EXCLUDES 1**   poisoning by, adverse effect of and underdosing of tamoxifen (T38.6)

AHA: 2019,1Q,17,20; 2014,4Q,22

√6ᵗʰ **T45.1X** **Poisoning by, adverse effect of and underdosing of antineoplastic and immunosuppressive drugs**

√7ᵗʰ **T45.1X1** **Poisoning by antineoplastic and immunosuppressive drugs, accidental (unintentional)**
Poisoning by antineoplastic and immunosuppressive drugs NOS

² √7ᵗʰ **T45.1X2** **Poisoning by antineoplastic and immunosuppressive drugs, intentional self-harm** **HCC Rx ESR COM**

√7ᵗʰ **T45.1X3** **Poisoning by antineoplastic and immunosuppressive drugs, assault**

√7ᵗʰ **T45.1X4** **Poisoning by antineoplastic and immunosuppressive drugs, undetermined**

√7ᵗʰ **T45.1X5** Adverse effect of antineoplastic and immunosuppressive drugs **UPD**
AHA: 2021,3Q,4; 2020,4Q,11; 2020,3Q,22; 2019,2Q,24,28

√7ᵗʰ **T45.1X6** Underdosing of antineoplastic and immunosuppressive drugs **UPD**

√5ᵗʰ **T45.2** **Poisoning by, adverse effect of and underdosing of vitamins**

> **EXCLUDES 2**   poisoning by, adverse effect of and underdosing of iron (T45.4)
> poisoning by, adverse effect of and underdosing of nicotinic acid (derivatives) (T46.7)
> poisoning by, adverse effect of and underdosing of vitamin K (T45.7)

√6ᵗʰ **T45.2X** **Poisoning by, adverse effect of and underdosing of vitamins**

√7ᵗʰ **T45.2X1** **Poisoning by vitamins, accidental (unintentional)**
Poisoning by vitamins NOS

² √7ᵗʰ **T45.2X2** **Poisoning by vitamins, intentional self-harm** **HCC Rx ESR COM**

√7ᵗʰ **T45.2X3** **Poisoning by vitamins, assault**

√7ᵗʰ **T45.2X4** **Poisoning by vitamins, undetermined**

√7ᵗʰ **T45.2X5** Adverse effect of vitamins **UPD**

√7ᵗʰ **T45.2X6** Underdosing of vitamins **UPD**
> **EXCLUDES 1**   vitamin deficiencies (E5Ø-E56)

√5ᵗʰ **T45.3** **Poisoning by, adverse effect of and underdosing of enzymes**

√6ᵗʰ **T45.3X** **Poisoning by, adverse effect of and underdosing of enzymes**

√7ᵗʰ **T45.3X1** **Poisoning by enzymes, accidental (unintentional)**
Poisoning by enzymes NOS

² √7ᵗʰ **T45.3X2** **Poisoning by enzymes, intentional self-harm** **HCC Rx ESR COM**

√7ᵗʰ **T45.3X3** **Poisoning by enzymes, assault**

√7ᵗʰ **T45.3X4** **Poisoning by enzymes, undetermined**

√7ᵗʰ **T45.3X5** Adverse effect of enzymes **UPD**

√7ᵗʰ **T45.3X6** Underdosing of enzymes **UPD**

√5ᵗʰ **T45.4** **Poisoning by, adverse effect of and underdosing of iron and its compounds**

√6ᵗʰ **T45.4X** **Poisoning by, adverse effect of and underdosing of iron and its compounds**

√7ᵗʰ **T45.4X1** **Poisoning by iron and its compounds, accidental (unintentional)**
Poisoning by iron and its compounds NOS

² √7ᵗʰ **T45.4X2** **Poisoning by iron and its compounds, intentional self-harm** **HCC Rx ESR COM**

√7ᵗʰ **T45.4X3** **Poisoning by iron and its compounds, assault**

√7ᵗʰ **T45.4X4** **Poisoning by iron and its compounds, undetermined**

√7ᵗʰ **T45.4X5** Adverse effect of iron and its compounds **UPD**

√7ᵗʰ **T45.4X6** Underdosing of iron and its compounds **UPD**
> **EXCLUDES 1**   iron deficiency (E61.1)

√5ᵗʰ **T45.5** **Poisoning by, adverse effect of and underdosing of anticoagulants and antithrombotic drugs**

√6ᵗʰ **T45.51** **Poisoning by, adverse effect of and underdosing of anticoagulants**

√7ᵗʰ **T45.511** **Poisoning by anticoagulants, accidental (unintentional)**
Poisoning by anticoagulants NOS

² √7ᵗʰ **T45.512** **Poisoning by anticoagulants, intentional self-harm** **HCC Rx ESR COM**

√7ᵗʰ **T45.513** **Poisoning by anticoagulants, assault**

√7ᵗʰ **T45.514** **Poisoning by anticoagulants, undetermined**

√7ᵗʰ **T45.515** Adverse effect of anticoagulants **UPD**
AHA: 2021,1Q,4; 2016,1Q,14; 2013,2Q,34

√7ᵗʰ **T45.516** Underdosing of anticoagulants **UPD**

√6ᵗʰ **T45.52** **Poisoning by, adverse effect of and underdosing of antithrombotic drugs**
Poisoning by, adverse effect of and underdosing of antiplatelet drugs

> **EXCLUDES 2**   poisoning by, adverse effect of and underdosing of aspirin (T39.Ø1-)
> poisoning by, adverse effect of and underdosing of acetylsalicylic acid (T39.Ø1-)

√7ᵗʰ **T45.521** **Poisoning by antithrombotic drugs, accidental (unintentional)**
Poisoning by antithrombotic drug NOS

² √7ᵗʰ **T45.522** **Poisoning by antithrombotic drugs, intentional self-harm** **HCC Rx ESR COM**

√7ᵗʰ **T45.523** **Poisoning by antithrombotic drugs, assault**

√7ᵗʰ **T45.524** **Poisoning by antithrombotic drugs, undetermined**

√7ᵗʰ **T45.525** Adverse effect of antithrombotic drugs **UPD**
AHA: 2016,1Q,15

√7ᵗʰ **T45.526** Underdosing of antithrombotic drugs **UPD**

✓5ᵗʰ T45.6 Poisoning by, adverse effect of and underdosing of fibrinolysis-affecting drugs

    ✓6ᵗʰ T45.60 Poisoning by, adverse effect of and underdosing of unspecified fibrinolysis-affecting drugs

        ✓7ᵗʰ T45.601 Poisoning by unspecified fibrinolysis-affecting drugs, accidental (unintentional)
             Poisoning by fibrinolysis-affecting drug NOS

        ² **✓7ᵗʰ T45.602 Poisoning by unspecified fibrinolysis-affecting drugs, intentional self-harm** HCC Rx ESR COM

        ✓7ᵗʰ T45.603 Poisoning by unspecified fibrinolysis-affecting drugs, assault

        ✓7ᵗʰ T45.604 Poisoning by unspecified fibrinolysis-affecting drugs, undetermined

        ✓7ᵗʰ T45.605 Adverse effect of unspecified fibrinolysis-affecting drugs UPD

        ✓7ᵗʰ T45.606 Underdosing of unspecified fibrinolysis-affecting drugs UPD

    ✓6ᵗʰ T45.61 Poisoning by, adverse effect of and underdosing of thrombolytic drugs

        ✓7ᵗʰ T45.611 Poisoning by thrombolytic drug, accidental (unintentional)
             Poisoning by thrombolytic drug NOS

        ² **✓7ᵗʰ T45.612 Poisoning by thrombolytic drug, intentional self-harm** HCC Rx ESR COM

        ✓7ᵗʰ T45.613 Poisoning by thrombolytic drug, assault

        ✓7ᵗʰ T45.614 Poisoning by thrombolytic drug, undetermined

        ✓7ᵗʰ T45.615 Adverse effect of thrombolytic drugs UPD
             AHA: 2017,2Q,9

        ✓7ᵗʰ T45.616 Underdosing of thrombolytic drugs UPD

    ✓6ᵗʰ T45.62 Poisoning by, adverse effect of and underdosing of hemostatic drugs

        ✓7ᵗʰ T45.621 Poisoning by hemostatic drug, accidental (unintentional)
             Poisoning by hemostatic drug NOS

        ² **✓7ᵗʰ T45.622 Poisoning by hemostatic drug, intentional self-harm** HCC Rx ESR COM

        ✓7ᵗʰ T45.623 Poisoning by hemostatic drug, assault

        ✓7ᵗʰ T45.624 Poisoning by hemostatic drug, undetermined

        ✓7ᵗʰ T45.625 Adverse effect of hemostatic drug UPD

        ✓7ᵗʰ T45.626 Underdosing of hemostatic drugs UPD

    ✓6ᵗʰ T45.69 Poisoning by, adverse effect of and underdosing of other fibrinolysis-affecting drugs

        ✓7ᵗʰ T45.691 Poisoning by other fibrinolysis-affecting drugs, accidental (unintentional)
             Poisoning by other fibrinolysis-affecting drug NOS

        ² **✓7ᵗʰ T45.692 Poisoning by other fibrinolysis-affecting drugs, intentional self-harm** HCC Rx ESR COM

        ✓7ᵗʰ T45.693 Poisoning by other fibrinolysis-affecting drugs, assault

        ✓7ᵗʰ T45.694 Poisoning by other fibrinolysis-affecting drugs, undetermined

        ✓7ᵗʰ T45.695 Adverse effect of other fibrinolysis-affecting drugs UPD

        ✓7ᵗʰ T45.696 Underdosing of other fibrinolysis-affecting drugs UPD

✓5ᵗʰ T45.7 Poisoning by, adverse effect of and underdosing of anticoagulant antagonists, vitamin K and other coagulants

    ✓6ᵗʰ T45.7X Poisoning by, adverse effect of and underdosing of anticoagulant antagonists, vitamin K and other coagulants

        ✓7ᵗʰ T45.7X1 Poisoning by anticoagulant antagonists, vitamin K and other coagulants, accidental (unintentional)
             Poisoning by anticoagulant antagonists, vitamin K and other coagulants NOS

        ² **✓7ᵗʰ T45.7X2 Poisoning by anticoagulant antagonists, vitamin K and other coagulants, intentional self-harm** HCC Rx ESR COM

        ✓7ᵗʰ T45.7X3 Poisoning by anticoagulant antagonists, vitamin K and other coagulants, assault

        ✓7ᵗʰ T45.7X4 Poisoning by anticoagulant antagonists, vitamin K and other coagulants, undetermined

        ✓7ᵗʰ T45.7X5 Adverse effect of anticoagulant antagonists, vitamin K and other coagulants UPD

        ✓7ᵗʰ T45.7X6 Underdosing of anticoagulant antagonist, vitamin K and other coagulants UPD
             EXCLUDES 1 *vitamin K deficiency (E56.1)*

✓5ᵗʰ T45.8 Poisoning by, adverse effect of and underdosing of other primarily systemic and hematological agents
     Poisoning by, adverse effect of and underdosing of liver preparations and other antianemic agents
     Poisoning by, adverse effect of and underdosing of natural blood and blood products
     Poisoning by, adverse effect of and underdosing of plasma substitute
    EXCLUDES 2 *poisoning by, adverse effect of and underdosing of immunoglobulin (T50.Z1)*
           poisoning by, adverse effect of and underdosing of iron (T45.4)
           transfusion reactions (T80.-)

    ✓6ᵗʰ T45.8X Poisoning by, adverse effect of and underdosing of other primarily systemic and hematological agents

        ✓7ᵗʰ T45.8X1 Poisoning by other primarily systemic and hematological agents, accidental (unintentional)
             Poisoning by other primarily systemic and hematological agents NOS

        ² **✓7ᵗʰ T45.8X2 Poisoning by other primarily systemic and hematological agents, intentional self-harm** HCC Rx ESR COM

        ✓7ᵗʰ T45.8X3 Poisoning by other primarily systemic and hematological agents, assault

        ✓7ᵗʰ T45.8X4 Poisoning by other primarily systemic and hematological agents, undetermined

        ✓7ᵗʰ T45.8X5 Adverse effect of other primarily systemic and hematological agents UPD
             AHA: 2016,4Q,42

        ✓7ᵗʰ T45.8X6 Underdosing of other primarily systemic and hematological agents UPD

✓5ᵗʰ T45.9 Poisoning by, adverse effect of and underdosing of unspecified primarily systemic and hematological agent

    ✓x7ᵗʰ T45.91 Poisoning by unspecified primarily systemic and hematological agent, accidental (unintentional)
          Poisoning by primarily systemic and hematological agent NOS

    ² **✓x7ᵗʰ T45.92 Poisoning by unspecified primarily systemic and hematological agent, intentional self-harm** HCC Rx ESR COM

    ✓x7ᵗʰ T45.93 Poisoning by unspecified primarily systemic and hematological agent, assault

    ✓x7ᵗʰ T45.94 Poisoning by unspecified primarily systemic and hematological agent, undetermined

    ✓x7ᵗʰ T45.95 Adverse effect of unspecified primarily systemic and hematological agent UPD

    ✓x7ᵗʰ T45.96 Underdosing of unspecified primarily systemic and hematological agent UPD

✓4ᵗʰ T46 Poisoning by, adverse effect of and underdosing of agents primarily affecting the cardiovascular system
    EXCLUDES 1 *poisoning by, adverse effect of and underdosing of metaraminol (T44.4)*

> The appropriate 7th character is to be added to each code from category T46.
> A   initial encounter
> D   subsequent encounter
> S   sequela

✓5ᵗʰ T46.0 Poisoning by, adverse effect of and underdosing of cardiac-stimulant glycosides and drugs of similar action

    ✓6ᵗʰ T46.0X Poisoning by, adverse effect of and underdosing of cardiac-stimulant glycosides and drugs of similar action

        ✓7ᵗʰ T46.0X1 Poisoning by cardiac-stimulant glycosides and drugs of similar action, accidental (unintentional)
             Poisoning by cardiac-stimulant glycosides and drugs of similar action NOS

² ✓7ᵗʰ **T46.0X2** **Poisoning by cardiac-stimulant glycosides and drugs of similar action, intentional self-harm** `HCC` `Rx` `ESR` `COM`

✓7ᵗʰ **T46.0X3** **Poisoning by cardiac-stimulant glycosides and drugs of similar action, assault**

✓7ᵗʰ **T46.0X4** **Poisoning by cardiac-stimulant glycosides and drugs of similar action, undetermined**

✓7ᵗʰ **T46.0X5** **Adverse effect of cardiac-stimulant glycosides and drugs of similar action** `UPD`

✓7ᵗʰ **T46.0X6** **Underdosing of cardiac-stimulant glycosides and drugs of similar action** `UPD`

✓5ᵗʰ **T46.1** **Poisoning by, adverse effect of and underdosing of calcium-channel blockers**

  ✓6ᵗʰ **T46.1X** **Poisoning by, adverse effect of and underdosing of calcium-channel blockers**

    ✓7ᵗʰ **T46.1X1** **Poisoning by calcium-channel blockers, accidental (unintentional)**
      Poisoning by calcium-channel blockers NOS

    ² ✓7ᵗʰ **T46.1X2** **Poisoning by calcium-channel blockers, intentional self-harm** `HCC` `Rx` `ESR` `COM`

    ✓7ᵗʰ **T46.1X3** **Poisoning by calcium-channel blockers, assault**

    ✓7ᵗʰ **T46.1X4** **Poisoning by calcium-channel blockers, undetermined**

    ✓7ᵗʰ **T46.1X5** **Adverse effect of calcium-channel blockers** `UPD`

    ✓7ᵗʰ **T46.1X6** **Underdosing of calcium-channel blockers** `UPD`

✓5ᵗʰ **T46.2** **Poisoning by, adverse effect of and underdosing of other antidysrhythmic drugs, not elsewhere classified**
    EXCLUDES 1   *poisoning by, adverse effect of and underdosing of beta-adrenoreceptor antagonists (T44.7-)*

  ✓6ᵗʰ **T46.2X** **Poisoning by, adverse effect of and underdosing of other antidysrhythmic drugs**

    ✓7ᵗʰ **T46.2X1** **Poisoning by other antidysrhythmic drugs, accidental (unintentional)**
      Poisoning by other antidysrhythmic drugs NOS

    ² ✓7ᵗʰ **T46.2X2** **Poisoning by other antidysrhythmic drugs, intentional self-harm** `HCC` `Rx` `ESR` `COM`

    ✓7ᵗʰ **T46.2X3** **Poisoning by other antidysrhythmic drugs, assault**

    ✓7ᵗʰ **T46.2X4** **Poisoning by other antidysrhythmic drugs, undetermined**

    ✓7ᵗʰ **T46.2X5** **Adverse effect of other antidysrhythmic drugs** `UPD`

    ✓7ᵗʰ **T46.2X6** **Underdosing of other antidysrhythmic drugs** `UPD`

✓5ᵗʰ **T46.3** **Poisoning by, adverse effect of and underdosing of coronary vasodilators**
    Poisoning by, adverse effect of and underdosing of dipyridamole
    EXCLUDES 1   *poisoning by, adverse effect of and underdosing of calcium-channel blockers (T46.1)*

  ✓6ᵗʰ **T46.3X** **Poisoning by, adverse effect of and underdosing of coronary vasodilators**

    ✓7ᵗʰ **T46.3X1** **Poisoning by coronary vasodilators, accidental (unintentional)**
      Poisoning by coronary vasodilators NOS

    ² ✓7ᵗʰ **T46.3X2** **Poisoning by coronary vasodilators, intentional self-harm** `HCC` `Rx` `ESR` `COM`

    ✓7ᵗʰ **T46.3X3** **Poisoning by coronary vasodilators, assault**

    ✓7ᵗʰ **T46.3X4** **Poisoning by coronary vasodilators, undetermined**

    ✓7ᵗʰ **T46.3X5** **Adverse effect of coronary vasodilators** `UPD`

    ✓7ᵗʰ **T46.3X6** **Underdosing of coronary vasodilators** `UPD`

✓5ᵗʰ **T46.4** **Poisoning by, adverse effect of and underdosing of angiotensin-converting-enzyme inhibitors**

  ✓6ᵗʰ **T46.4X** **Poisoning by, adverse effect of and underdosing of angiotensin-converting-enzyme inhibitors**

    ✓7ᵗʰ **T46.4X1** **Poisoning by angiotensin-converting-enzyme inhibitors, accidental (unintentional)**
      Poisoning by angiotensin-converting-enzyme inhibitors NOS

    ² ✓7ᵗʰ **T46.4X2** **Poisoning by angiotensin-converting-enzyme inhibitors, intentional self-harm** `HCC` `Rx` `ESR` `COM`

    ✓7ᵗʰ **T46.4X3** **Poisoning by angiotensin-converting-enzyme inhibitors, assault**

    ✓7ᵗʰ **T46.4X4** **Poisoning by angiotensin-converting-enzyme inhibitors, undetermined**

    ✓7ᵗʰ **T46.4X5** **Adverse effect of angiotensin-converting-enzyme inhibitors** `UPD`

    ✓7ᵗʰ **T46.4X6** **Underdosing of angiotensin-converting-enzyme inhibitors** `UPD`

✓5ᵗʰ **T46.5** **Poisoning by, adverse effect of and underdosing of other antihypertensive drugs**
    EXCLUDES 2   *poisoning by, adverse effect of and underdosing of beta-adrenoreceptor antagonists (T44.7)*
      poisoning by, adverse effect of and underdosing of calcium-channel blockers (T46.1)
      poisoning by, adverse effect of and underdosing of diuretics (T50.0-T50.2)

  ✓6ᵗʰ **T46.5X** **Poisoning by, adverse effect of and underdosing of other antihypertensive drugs**

    ✓7ᵗʰ **T46.5X1** **Poisoning by other antihypertensive drugs, accidental (unintentional)**
      Poisoning by other antihypertensive drugs NOS

    ² ✓7ᵗʰ **T46.5X2** **Poisoning by other antihypertensive drugs, intentional self-harm** `HCC` `Rx` `ESR` `COM`

    ✓7ᵗʰ **T46.5X3** **Poisoning by other antihypertensive drugs, assault**

    ✓7ᵗʰ **T46.5X4** **Poisoning by other antihypertensive drugs, undetermined**

    ✓7ᵗʰ **T46.5X5** **Adverse effect of other antihypertensive drugs** `UPD`

    ✓7ᵗʰ **T46.5X6** **Underdosing of other antihypertensive drugs** `UPD`
      AHA: 2022,1Q,36

✓5ᵗʰ **T46.6** **Poisoning by, adverse effect of and underdosing of antihyperlipidemic and antiarteriosclerotic drugs**

  ✓6ᵗʰ **T46.6X** **Poisoning by, adverse effect of and underdosing of antihyperlipidemic and antiarteriosclerotic drugs**

    ✓7ᵗʰ **T46.6X1** **Poisoning by antihyperlipidemic and antiarteriosclerotic drugs, accidental (unintentional)**
      Poisoning by antihyperlipidemic and antiarteriosclerotic drugs NOS

    ² ✓7ᵗʰ **T46.6X2** **Poisoning by antihyperlipidemic and antiarteriosclerotic drugs, intentional self-harm** `HCC` `Rx` `ESR` `COM`

    ✓7ᵗʰ **T46.6X3** **Poisoning by antihyperlipidemic and antiarteriosclerotic drugs, assault**

    ✓7ᵗʰ **T46.6X4** **Poisoning by antihyperlipidemic and antiarteriosclerotic drugs, undetermined**

    ✓7ᵗʰ **T46.6X5** **Adverse effect of antihyperlipidemic and antiarteriosclerotic drugs** `UPD`

    ✓7ᵗʰ **T46.6X6** **Underdosing of antihyperlipidemic and antiarteriosclerotic drugs** `UPD`

Chapter 19. Injury, Poisoning and Certain Other Consequences of External Causes

T46.7–T47.3X2

√5ᵗʰ **T46.7** **Poisoning by, adverse effect of and underdosing of peripheral vasodilators**
  Poisoning by, adverse effect of and underdosing of nicotinic acid (derivatives)
  EXCLUDES 1   *poisoning by, adverse effect of and underdosing of papaverine (T44.3)*

√6ᵗʰ **T46.7X** **Poisoning by, adverse effect of and underdosing of** peripheral vasodilators

√7ᵗʰ **T46.7X1** **Poisoning by peripheral vasodilators, accidental (unintentional)**
  Poisoning by peripheral vasodilators NOS

² √7ᵗʰ **T46.7X2** **Poisoning by peripheral vasodilators, intentional self-harm** HCC Rx ESR COM

√7ᵗʰ **T46.7X3** **Poisoning by peripheral vasodilators, assault**

√7ᵗʰ **T46.7X4** **Poisoning by peripheral vasodilators, undetermined**

√7ᵗʰ **T46.7X5** **Adverse effect of peripheral vasodilators** UPD

√7ᵗʰ **T46.7X6** **Underdosing of peripheral vasodilators** UPD

√5ᵗʰ **T46.8** **Poisoning by, adverse effect of and underdosing of antivaricose drugs, including sclerosing agents**

√6ᵗʰ **T46.8X** **Poisoning by, adverse effect of and underdosing of** antivaricose drugs, including sclerosing agents

√7ᵗʰ **T46.8X1** **Poisoning by antivaricose drugs, including sclerosing agents, accidental (unintentional)**
  Poisoning by antivaricose drugs, including sclerosing agents NOS

² √7ᵗʰ **T46.8X2** **Poisoning by antivaricose drugs, including sclerosing agents, intentional self-harm** HCC Rx ESR COM

√7ᵗʰ **T46.8X3** **Poisoning by antivaricose drugs, including sclerosing agents, assault**

√7ᵗʰ **T46.8X4** **Poisoning by antivaricose drugs, including sclerosing agents, undetermined**

√7ᵗʰ **T46.8X5** **Adverse effect of antivaricose drugs, including sclerosing agents** UPD

√7ᵗʰ **T46.8X6** **Underdosing of antivaricose drugs, including sclerosing agents** UPD

√5ᵗʰ **T46.9** **Poisoning by, adverse effect of and underdosing of other and unspecified agents primarily affecting the cardiovascular system**

√6ᵗʰ **T46.90** **Poisoning by, adverse effect of and underdosing of unspecified agents primarily affecting the cardiovascular system**

√7ᵗʰ **T46.901** **Poisoning by unspecified agents primarily affecting the cardiovascular system, accidental (unintentional)**

² √7ᵗʰ **T46.902** **Poisoning by unspecified agents primarily affecting the cardiovascular system, intentional self-harm** HCC Rx ESR COM

√7ᵗʰ **T46.903** **Poisoning by unspecified agents primarily affecting the cardiovascular system, assault**

√7ᵗʰ **T46.904** **Poisoning by unspecified agents primarily affecting the cardiovascular system, undetermined**

√7ᵗʰ **T46.905** **Adverse effect of unspecified agents primarily affecting the cardiovascular system** UPD

√7ᵗʰ **T46.906** **Underdosing of unspecified agents primarily affecting the cardiovascular system** UPD

√6ᵗʰ **T46.99** **Poisoning by, adverse effect of and underdosing of other agents primarily affecting the cardiovascular system**

√7ᵗʰ **T46.991** **Poisoning by other agents primarily affecting the cardiovascular system, accidental (unintentional)**

² √7ᵗʰ **T46.992** **Poisoning by other agents primarily affecting the cardiovascular system, intentional self-harm** HCC Rx ESR COM

√7ᵗʰ **T46.993** **Poisoning by other agents primarily affecting the cardiovascular system, assault**

√7ᵗʰ **T46.994** **Poisoning by other agents primarily affecting the cardiovascular system, undetermined**

√7ᵗʰ **T46.995** **Adverse effect of other agents primarily affecting the cardiovascular system** UPD

√7ᵗʰ **T46.996** **Underdosing of other agents primarily affecting the cardiovascular system** UPD

√4ᵗʰ **T47** **Poisoning by, adverse effect of and underdosing of agents primarily affecting the gastrointestinal system**

The appropriate 7th character is to be added to each code from category T47.
A   initial encounter
D   subsequent encounter
S   sequela

√5ᵗʰ **T47.0** **Poisoning by, adverse effect of and underdosing of histamine H2-receptor blockers**

√6ᵗʰ **T47.0X** **Poisoning by, adverse effect of and underdosing of** histamine H2-receptor blockers

√7ᵗʰ **T47.0X1** **Poisoning by histamine H2-receptor blockers, accidental (unintentional)**
  Poisoning by histamine H2-receptor blockers NOS

² √7ᵗʰ **T47.0X2** **Poisoning by histamine H2-receptor blockers, intentional self-harm** HCC Rx ESR COM

√7ᵗʰ **T47.0X3** **Poisoning by histamine H2-receptor blockers, assault**

√7ᵗʰ **T47.0X4** **Poisoning by histamine H2-receptor blockers, undetermined**

√7ᵗʰ **T47.0X5** **Adverse effect of histamine H2-receptor blockers** UPD

√7ᵗʰ **T47.0X6** **Underdosing of histamine H2-receptor blockers** UPD

√5ᵗʰ **T47.1** **Poisoning by, adverse effect of and underdosing of other antacids and anti-gastric-secretion drugs**

√6ᵗʰ **T47.1X** **Poisoning by, adverse effect of and underdosing of other antacids and anti-gastric-secretion drugs**

√7ᵗʰ **T47.1X1** **Poisoning by other antacids and anti-gastric-secretion drugs, accidental (unintentional)**
  Poisoning by other antacids and anti-gastric-secretion drugs NOS

² √7ᵗʰ **T47.1X2** **Poisoning by other antacids and anti-gastric-secretion drugs, intentional self-harm** HCC Rx ESR COM

√7ᵗʰ **T47.1X3** **Poisoning by other antacids and anti-gastric-secretion drugs, assault**

√7ᵗʰ **T47.1X4** **Poisoning by other antacids and anti-gastric-secretion drugs, undetermined**

√7ᵗʰ **T47.1X5** **Adverse effect of other antacids and anti-gastric-secretion drugs** UPD

√7ᵗʰ **T47.1X6** **Underdosing of other antacids and anti-gastric-secretion drugs** UPD

√5ᵗʰ **T47.2** **Poisoning by, adverse effect of and underdosing of stimulant laxatives**

√6ᵗʰ **T47.2X** **Poisoning by, adverse effect of and underdosing of** stimulant laxatives

√7ᵗʰ **T47.2X1** **Poisoning by stimulant laxatives, accidental (unintentional)**
  Poisoning by stimulant laxatives NOS

² √7ᵗʰ **T47.2X2** **Poisoning by stimulant laxatives, intentional self-harm** HCC Rx ESR COM

√7ᵗʰ **T47.2X3** **Poisoning by stimulant laxatives, assault**

√7ᵗʰ **T47.2X4** **Poisoning by stimulant laxatives, undetermined**

√7ᵗʰ **T47.2X5** **Adverse effect of stimulant laxatives** UPD

√7ᵗʰ **T47.2X6** **Underdosing of stimulant laxatives** UPD

√5ᵗʰ **T47.3** **Poisoning by, adverse effect of and underdosing of saline and osmotic laxatives**

√6ᵗʰ **T47.3X** **Poisoning by and adverse effect of** saline and osmotic laxatives

√7ᵗʰ **T47.3X1** **Poisoning by saline and osmotic laxatives, accidental (unintentional)**
  Poisoning by saline and osmotic laxatives NOS

² √7ᵗʰ **T47.3X2** **Poisoning by saline and osmotic laxatives, intentional self-harm** HCC Rx ESR COM

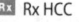

✓7ᵗʰ **T47.3X3** **Poisoning by saline and osmotic laxatives,** assault

✓7ᵗʰ **T47.3X4** **Poisoning by saline and osmotic laxatives,** undetermined

✓7ᵗʰ **T47.3X5** **Adverse effect** of saline and osmotic laxatives   UPD

✓7ᵗʰ **T47.3X6** **Underdosing** of saline and osmotic laxatives   UPD

✓5ᵗʰ **T47.4** **Poisoning by, adverse effect of and underdosing of other laxatives**

✓6ᵗʰ **T47.4X** **Poisoning by, adverse effect of and underdosing of other laxatives**

✓7ᵗʰ **T47.4X1** **Poisoning by other laxatives,** accidental (unintentional)
Poisoning by other laxatives NOS

² ✓7ᵗʰ **T47.4X2** **Poisoning by other laxatives,** intentional self-harm   HCC Rx ESR COM

✓7ᵗʰ **T47.4X3** **Poisoning by other laxatives,** assault

✓7ᵗʰ **T47.4X4** **Poisoning by other laxatives,** undetermined

✓7ᵗʰ **T47.4X5** **Adverse effect** of other laxatives   UPD

✓7ᵗʰ **T47.4X6** **Underdosing** of other laxatives   UPD

✓5ᵗʰ **T47.5** **Poisoning by, adverse effect of and underdosing of digestants**

✓6ᵗʰ **T47.5X** **Poisoning by, adverse effect of and underdosing of digestants**

✓7ᵗʰ **T47.5X1** **Poisoning by digestants,** accidental (unintentional)
Poisoning by digestants NOS

² ✓7ᵗʰ **T47.5X2** **Poisoning by digestants,** intentional self-harm   HCC Rx ESR COM

✓7ᵗʰ **T47.5X3** **Poisoning by digestants,** assault

✓7ᵗʰ **T47.5X4** **Poisoning by digestants,** undetermined

✓7ᵗʰ **T47.5X5** **Adverse effect** of digestants   UPD

✓7ᵗʰ **T47.5X6** **Underdosing** of digestants   UPD

✓5ᵗʰ **T47.6** **Poisoning by, adverse effect of and underdosing of antidiarrheal drugs**

EXCLUDES 2   poisoning by, adverse effect of and underdosing of systemic antibiotics and other anti-infectives (T36-T37)

✓6ᵗʰ **T47.6X** **Poisoning by, adverse effect of and underdosing of antidiarrheal drugs**

✓7ᵗʰ **T47.6X1** **Poisoning by antidiarrheal drugs,** accidental (unintentional)
Poisoning by antidiarrheal drugs NOS

² ✓7ᵗʰ **T47.6X2** **Poisoning by antidiarrheal drugs,** intentional self-harm   HCC Rx ESR COM

✓7ᵗʰ **T47.6X3** **Poisoning by antidiarrheal drugs,** assault

✓7ᵗʰ **T47.6X4** **Poisoning by antidiarrheal drugs,** undetermined

✓7ᵗʰ **T47.6X5** **Adverse effect** of antidiarrheal drugs   UPD

✓7ᵗʰ **T47.6X6** **Underdosing** of antidiarrheal drugs   UPD

✓5ᵗʰ **T47.7** **Poisoning by, adverse effect of and underdosing of emetics**

✓6ᵗʰ **T47.7X** **Poisoning by, adverse effect of and underdosing of emetics**

✓7ᵗʰ **T47.7X1** **Poisoning by emetics,** accidental (unintentional)
Poisoning by emetics NOS

² ✓7ᵗʰ **T47.7X2** **Poisoning by emetics,** intentional self-harm   HCC Rx ESR COM

✓7ᵗʰ **T47.7X3** **Poisoning by emetics,** assault

✓7ᵗʰ **T47.7X4** **Poisoning by emetics,** undetermined

✓7ᵗʰ **T47.7X5** **Adverse effect** of emetics   UPD

✓7ᵗʰ **T47.7X6** **Underdosing** of emetics   UPD

✓5ᵗʰ **T47.8** **Poisoning by, adverse effect of and underdosing of other agents primarily affecting gastrointestinal system**

✓6ᵗʰ **T47.8X** **Poisoning by, adverse effect of and underdosing of other agents primarily affecting gastrointestinal system**

✓7ᵗʰ **T47.8X1** **Poisoning by other agents primarily affecting gastrointestinal system,** accidental (unintentional)
Poisoning by other agents primarily affecting gastrointestinal system NOS

² ✓7ᵗʰ **T47.8X2** **Poisoning by other agents primarily affecting gastrointestinal system,** intentional self-harm   HCC Rx ESR COM

✓7ᵗʰ **T47.8X3** **Poisoning by other agents primarily affecting gastrointestinal system,** assault

✓7ᵗʰ **T47.8X4** **Poisoning by other agents primarily affecting gastrointestinal system,** undetermined

✓7ᵗʰ **T47.8X5** **Adverse effect** of other agents primarily affecting gastrointestinal system   UPD

✓7ᵗʰ **T47.8X6** **Underdosing** of other agents primarily affecting gastrointestinal system   UPD

✓5ᵗʰ **T47.9** **Poisoning by, adverse effect of and underdosing of unspecified agents primarily affecting the gastrointestinal system**

✓x7ᵗʰ **T47.91** **Poisoning by unspecified agents primarily affecting the gastrointestinal system,** accidental (unintentional)
Poisoning by agents primarily affecting the gastrointestinal system NOS

² ✓x7ᵗʰ **T47.92** **Poisoning by unspecified agents primarily affecting the gastrointestinal system,** intentional self-harm   HCC Rx ESR COM

✓x7ᵗʰ **T47.93** **Poisoning by unspecified agents primarily affecting the gastrointestinal system,** assault

✓x7ᵗʰ **T47.94** **Poisoning by unspecified agents primarily affecting the gastrointestinal system,** undetermined

✓x7ᵗʰ **T47.95** **Adverse effect** of unspecified agents primarily affecting the gastrointestinal system   UPD

✓x7ᵗʰ **T47.96** **Underdosing** of unspecified agents primarily affecting the gastrointestinal system   UPD

✓4ᵗʰ **T48** **Poisoning by, adverse effect of and underdosing of agents primarily acting on smooth and skeletal muscles and the respiratory system**

The appropriate 7th character is to be added to each code from category T48.
A   initial encounter
D   subsequent encounter
S   sequela

✓5ᵗʰ **T48.0** **Poisoning by, adverse effect of and underdosing of oxytocic drugs**

EXCLUDES 1   poisoning by, adverse effect of and underdosing of estrogens, progestogens and antagonists (T38.4-T38.6)

✓6ᵗʰ **T48.0X** **Poisoning by, adverse effect of and underdosing of oxytocic drugs**

✓7ᵗʰ **T48.0X1** **Poisoning by oxytocic drugs,** accidental (unintentional)
Poisoning by oxytocic drugs NOS

² ✓7ᵗʰ **T48.0X2** **Poisoning by oxytocic drugs,** intentional self-harm   HCC Rx ESR COM

✓7ᵗʰ **T48.0X3** **Poisoning by oxytocic drugs,** assault

✓7ᵗʰ **T48.0X4** **Poisoning by oxytocic drugs,** undetermined

✓7ᵗʰ **T48.0X5** **Adverse effect** of oxytocic drugs   UPD

✓7ᵗʰ **T48.0X6** **Underdosing** of oxytocic drugs   UPD

✓5ᵗʰ **T48.1** **Poisoning by, adverse effect of and underdosing of skeletal muscle relaxants [neuromuscular blocking agents]**

✓6ᵗʰ **T48.1X** **Poisoning by, adverse effect of and underdosing of skeletal muscle relaxants [neuromuscular blocking agents]**

✓7ᵗʰ **T48.1X1** **Poisoning by skeletal muscle relaxants [neuromuscular blocking agents],** accidental (unintentional)
Poisoning by skeletal muscle relaxants [neuromuscular blocking agents] NOS

² ✓7ᵗʰ **T48.1X2** **Poisoning by skeletal muscle relaxants [neuromuscular blocking agents],** intentional self-harm   HCC Rx ESR COM

✓7ᵗʰ **T48.1X3** **Poisoning by skeletal muscle relaxants [neuromuscular blocking agents],** assault

✓7ᵗʰ **T48.1X4** **Poisoning by skeletal muscle relaxants [neuromuscular blocking agents],** undetermined

✓7ᵗʰ **T48.1X5** **Adverse effect** of skeletal muscle relaxants [neuromuscular blocking agents]   UPD

✓7ᵗʰ **T48.1X6** **Underdosing** of skeletal muscle relaxants [neuromuscular blocking agents]   UPD

✓5ᵗʰ **T48.2** **Poisoning by, adverse effect of and underdosing of other and unspecified drugs acting on muscles**

  ✓6ᵗʰ **T48.20** **Poisoning by, adverse effect of and underdosing of unspecified drugs acting on muscles**

    ✓7ᵗʰ **T48.201** **Poisoning by unspecified drugs acting on muscles, accidental (unintentional)**
Poisoning by unspecified drugs acting on muscles NOS

    ² ✓7ᵗʰ **T48.202** **Poisoning by unspecified drugs acting on muscles, intentional self-harm** `HCC` `Rx` `ESR` `COM`

    ✓7ᵗʰ **T48.203** **Poisoning by unspecified drugs acting on muscles, assault**

    ✓7ᵗʰ **T48.204** **Poisoning by unspecified drugs acting on muscles, undetermined**

    ✓7ᵗʰ **T48.205** **Adverse effect of unspecified drugs acting on muscles** `UPD`

    ✓7ᵗʰ **T48.206** **Underdosing of unspecified drugs acting on muscles** `UPD`

  ✓6ᵗʰ **T48.29** **Poisoning by, adverse effect of and underdosing of other drugs acting on muscles**

    ✓7ᵗʰ **T48.291** **Poisoning by other drugs acting on muscles, accidental (unintentional)**
Poisoning by other drugs acting on muscles NOS

    ² ✓7ᵗʰ **T48.292** **Poisoning by other drugs acting on muscles, intentional self-harm** `HCC` `Rx` `ESR` `COM`

    ✓7ᵗʰ **T48.293** **Poisoning by other drugs acting on muscles, assault**

    ✓7ᵗʰ **T48.294** **Poisoning by other drugs acting on muscles, undetermined**

    ✓7ᵗʰ **T48.295** **Adverse effect of other drugs acting on muscles** `UPD`

    ✓7ᵗʰ **T48.296** **Underdosing of other drugs acting on muscles** `UPD`

✓5ᵗʰ **T48.3** **Poisoning by, adverse effect of and underdosing of antitussives**

  ✓6ᵗʰ **T48.3X** **Poisoning by, adverse effect of and underdosing of antitussives**

    ✓7ᵗʰ **T48.3X1** **Poisoning by antitussives, accidental (unintentional)**
Poisoning by antitussives NOS

    ² ✓7ᵗʰ **T48.3X2** **Poisoning by antitussives, intentional self-harm** `HCC` `Rx` `ESR` `COM`

    ✓7ᵗʰ **T48.3X3** **Poisoning by antitussives, assault**

    ✓7ᵗʰ **T48.3X4** **Poisoning by antitussives, undetermined**

    ✓7ᵗʰ **T48.3X5** **Adverse effect of antitussives** `UPD`

    ✓7ᵗʰ **T48.3X6** **Underdosing of antitussives** `UPD`

✓5ᵗʰ **T48.4** **Poisoning by, adverse effect of and underdosing of expectorants**

  ✓6ᵗʰ **T48.4X** **Poisoning by, adverse effect of and underdosing of expectorants**

    ✓7ᵗʰ **T48.4X1** **Poisoning by expectorants, accidental (unintentional)**
Poisoning by expectorants NOS

    ² ✓7ᵗʰ **T48.4X2** **Poisoning by expectorants, intentional self-harm** `HCC` `Rx` `ESR` `COM`

    ✓7ᵗʰ **T48.4X3** **Poisoning by expectorants, assault**

    ✓7ᵗʰ **T48.4X4** **Poisoning by expectorants, undetermined**

    ✓7ᵗʰ **T48.4X5** **Adverse effect of expectorants** `UPD`

    ✓7ᵗʰ **T48.4X6** **Underdosing of expectorants** `UPD`

✓5ᵗʰ **T48.5** **Poisoning by, adverse effect of and underdosing of other anti-common-cold drugs**
Poisoning by, adverse effect of and underdosing of decongestants

  EXCLUDES 2 *poisoning by, adverse effect of and underdosing of antipyretics, NEC (T39.9-)*
poisoning by, adverse effect of and underdosing of non-steroidal antiinflammatory drugs (T39.3-)
poisoning by, adverse effect of and underdosing of salicylates (T39.0-)

  ✓6ᵗʰ **T48.5X** **Poisoning by, adverse effect of and underdosing of other anti-common-cold drugs**

    ✓7ᵗʰ **T48.5X1** **Poisoning by other anti-common-cold drugs, accidental (unintentional)**
Poisoning by other anti-common-cold drugs NOS

    ² ✓7ᵗʰ **T48.5X2** **Poisoning by other anti-common-cold drugs, intentional self-harm** `HCC` `Rx` `ESR` `COM`

    ✓7ᵗʰ **T48.5X3** **Poisoning by other anti-common-cold drugs, assault**

    ✓7ᵗʰ **T48.5X4** **Poisoning by other anti-common-cold drugs, undetermined**

    ✓7ᵗʰ **T48.5X5** **Adverse effect of other anti-common-cold drugs** `UPD`

    ✓7ᵗʰ **T48.5X6** **Underdosing of other anti-common-cold drugs** `UPD`

✓5ᵗʰ **T48.6** **Poisoning by, adverse effect of and underdosing of antiasthmatics, not elsewhere classified**
Poisoning by, adverse effect of and underdosing of beta-adrenoreceptor agonists used in asthma therapy

  EXCLUDES 1 *poisoning by, adverse effect of and underdosing of anterior pituitary [adenohypophyseal] hormones (T38.8)*
poisoning by, adverse effect of and underdosing of beta-adrenoreceptor agonists not used in asthma therapy (T44.5)

  ✓6ᵗʰ **T48.6X** **Poisoning by, adverse effect of and underdosing of antiasthmatics**

    ✓7ᵗʰ **T48.6X1** **Poisoning by antiasthmatics, accidental (unintentional)**
Poisoning by antiasthmatics NOS

    ² ✓7ᵗʰ **T48.6X2** **Poisoning by antiasthmatics, intentional self-harm** `HCC` `Rx` `ESR` `COM`

    ✓7ᵗʰ **T48.6X3** **Poisoning by antiasthmatics, assault**

    ✓7ᵗʰ **T48.6X4** **Poisoning by antiasthmatics, undetermined**

    ✓7ᵗʰ **T48.6X5** **Adverse effect of antiasthmatics** `UPD`

    ✓7ᵗʰ **T48.6X6** **Underdosing of antiasthmatics** `UPD`

✓5ᵗʰ **T48.9** **Poisoning by, adverse effect of and underdosing of other and unspecified agents primarily acting on the respiratory system**

  ✓6ᵗʰ **T48.90** **Poisoning by, adverse effect of and underdosing of unspecified agents primarily acting on the respiratory system**

    ✓7ᵗʰ **T48.901** **Poisoning by unspecified agents primarily acting on the respiratory system, accidental (unintentional)**

    ² ✓7ᵗʰ **T48.902** **Poisoning by unspecified agents primarily acting on the respiratory system, intentional self-harm** `HCC` `Rx` `ESR` `COM`

    ✓7ᵗʰ **T48.903** **Poisoning by unspecified agents primarily acting on the respiratory system, assault**

    ✓7ᵗʰ **T48.904** **Poisoning by unspecified agents primarily acting on the respiratory system, undetermined**

    ✓7ᵗʰ **T48.905** **Adverse effect of unspecified agents primarily acting on the respiratory system** `UPD`

    ✓7ᵗʰ **T48.906** **Underdosing of unspecified agents primarily acting on the respiratory system** `UPD`

  ✓6ᵗʰ **T48.99** **Poisoning by, adverse effect of and underdosing of other agents primarily acting on the respiratory system**

    ✓7ᵗʰ **T48.991** **Poisoning by other agents primarily acting on the respiratory system, accidental (unintentional)**

    ² ✓7ᵗʰ **T48.992** **Poisoning by other agents primarily acting on the respiratory system, intentional self-harm** `HCC` `Rx` `ESR` `COM`

    ✓7ᵗʰ **T48.993** **Poisoning by other agents primarily acting on the respiratory system, assault**

    ✓7ᵗʰ **T48.994** **Poisoning by other agents primarily acting on the respiratory system, undetermined**

    ✓7ᵗʰ **T48.995** **Adverse effect of other agents primarily acting on the respiratory system** `UPD`

    ✓7ᵗʰ **T48.996** **Underdosing of other agents primarily acting on the respiratory system** `UPD`

`HCC` CMS-HCC `Rx` Rx HCC `ESR` ESRD HCC `COM` Commercial HCC `N` Newborn: 0 `P` Pediatric: 0-17 `M` Maternity: 9-64 `A` Adult: 15-124

1152 ICD-10-CM 2023

☑4ᵗʰ **T49** **Poisoning by, adverse effect of and underdosing of topical agents primarily affecting skin and mucous membrane and by ophthalmological, otorhinolaryngological and dental drugs**

    INCLUDES   poisoning by, adverse effect of and underdosing of glucocorticoids, topically used

The appropriate 7th character is to be added to each code from category T49.
A   initial encounter
D   subsequent encounter
S   sequela

☑5ᵗʰ **T49.0** **Poisoning by, adverse effect of and underdosing of local antifungal, anti-infective and anti-inflammatory drugs**

   ☑6ᵗʰ **T49.0X** **Poisoning by, adverse effect of and underdosing of** local antifungal, anti-infective and anti-inflammatory drugs

     ☑7ᵗʰ **T49.0X1** **Poisoning by local antifungal, anti-infective and anti-inflammatory drugs,** accidental **(unintentional)**
       Poisoning by local antifungal, anti-infective and anti-inflammatory drugs NOS

    ² ☑7ᵗʰ **T49.0X2** **Poisoning by local antifungal, anti-infective and anti-inflammatory drugs,** intentional **self-harm**   HCC Rx ESR COM

     ☑7ᵗʰ **T49.0X3** **Poisoning by local antifungal, anti-infective and anti-inflammatory drugs,** assault

     ☑7ᵗʰ **T49.0X4** **Poisoning by local antifungal, anti-infective and anti-inflammatory drugs,** undetermined

     ☑7ᵗʰ **T49.0X5** **Adverse effect of local antifungal, anti-infective and anti-inflammatory drugs**   UPD

     ☑7ᵗʰ **T49.0X6** **Underdosing of local antifungal, anti-infective and anti-inflammatory drugs**   UPD

☑5ᵗʰ **T49.1** **Poisoning by, adverse effect of and underdosing of antipruritics**

   ☑6ᵗʰ **T49.1X** **Poisoning by, adverse effect of and underdosing of** antipruritics

     ☑7ᵗʰ **T49.1X1** **Poisoning by antipruritics,** accidental **(unintentional)**
       Poisoning by antipruritics NOS

    ² ☑7ᵗʰ **T49.1X2** **Poisoning by antipruritics,** intentional **self-harm**   HCC Rx ESR COM

     ☑7ᵗʰ **T49.1X3** **Poisoning by antipruritics,** assault

     ☑7ᵗʰ **T49.1X4** **Poisoning by antipruritics,** undetermined

     ☑7ᵗʰ **T49.1X5** **Adverse effect of antipruritics**   UPD

     ☑7ᵗʰ **T49.1X6** **Underdosing of antipruritics**   UPD

☑5ᵗʰ **T49.2** **Poisoning by, adverse effect of and underdosing of local astringents and local detergents**

   ☑6ᵗʰ **T49.2X** **Poisoning by, adverse effect of and underdosing of** local astringents and local detergents

     ☑7ᵗʰ **T49.2X1** **Poisoning by local astringents and local detergents,** accidental **(unintentional)**
       Poisoning by local astringents and local detergents NOS

    ² ☑7ᵗʰ **T49.2X2** **Poisoning by local astringents and local detergents,** intentional **self-harm**   HCC Rx ESR COM

     ☑7ᵗʰ **T49.2X3** **Poisoning by local astringents and local detergents,** assault

     ☑7ᵗʰ **T49.2X4** **Poisoning by local astringents and local detergents,** undetermined

     ☑7ᵗʰ **T49.2X5** **Adverse effect of local astringents and local detergents**   UPD

     ☑7ᵗʰ **T49.2X6** **Underdosing of local astringents and local detergents**   UPD

☑5ᵗʰ **T49.3** **Poisoning by, adverse effect of and underdosing of emollients, demulcents and protectants**

   ☑6ᵗʰ **T49.3X** **Poisoning by, adverse effect of and underdosing of** emollients, demulcents and protectants

     ☑7ᵗʰ **T49.3X1** **Poisoning by emollients, demulcents and protectants,** accidental **(unintentional)**
       Poisoning by emollients, demulcents and protectants NOS

    ² ☑7ᵗʰ **T49.3X2** **Poisoning by emollients, demulcents and protectants,** intentional **self-harm**   HCC Rx ESR COM

     ☑7ᵗʰ **T49.3X3** **Poisoning by emollients, demulcents and protectants,** assault

     ☑7ᵗʰ **T49.3X4** **Poisoning by emollients, demulcents and protectants,** undetermined

     ☑7ᵗʰ **T49.3X5** **Adverse effect of emollients, demulcents and protectants**   UPD

     ☑7ᵗʰ **T49.3X6** **Underdosing of emollients, demulcents and protectants**   UPD

☑5ᵗʰ **T49.4** **Poisoning by, adverse effect of and underdosing of keratolytics, keratoplastics, and other hair treatment drugs and preparations**

   ☑6ᵗʰ **T49.4X** **Poisoning by, adverse effect of and underdosing of** keratolytics, keratoplastics, and other hair treatment drugs and preparations

     ☑7ᵗʰ **T49.4X1** **Poisoning by keratolytics, keratoplastics, and other hair treatment drugs and preparations,** accidental **(unintentional)**
       Poisoning by keratolytics, keratoplastics, and other hair treatment drugs and preparations NOS

    ² ☑7ᵗʰ **T49.4X2** **Poisoning by keratolytics, keratoplastics, and other hair treatment drugs and preparations,** intentional **self-harm**   HCC Rx ESR COM

     ☑7ᵗʰ **T49.4X3** **Poisoning by keratolytics, keratoplastics, and other hair treatment drugs and preparations,** assault

     ☑7ᵗʰ **T49.4X4** **Poisoning by keratolytics, keratoplastics, and other hair treatment drugs and preparations,** undetermined

     ☑7ᵗʰ **T49.4X5** **Adverse effect of keratolytics, keratoplastics, and other hair treatment drugs and preparations**   UPD

     ☑7ᵗʰ **T49.4X6** **Underdosing of keratolytics, keratoplastics, and other hair treatment drugs and preparations**   UPD

☑5ᵗʰ **T49.5** **Poisoning by, adverse effect of and underdosing of ophthalmological drugs and preparations**

   ☑6ᵗʰ **T49.5X** **Poisoning by, adverse effect of and underdosing of** ophthalmological drugs and preparations

     ☑7ᵗʰ **T49.5X1** **Poisoning by ophthalmological drugs and preparations,** accidental **(unintentional)**
       Poisoning by ophthalmological drugs and preparations NOS

    ² ☑7ᵗʰ **T49.5X2** **Poisoning by ophthalmological drugs and preparations,** intentional **self-harm**   HCC Rx ESR COM

     ☑7ᵗʰ **T49.5X3** **Poisoning by ophthalmological drugs and preparations,** assault

     ☑7ᵗʰ **T49.5X4** **Poisoning by ophthalmological drugs and preparations,** undetermined

     ☑7ᵗʰ **T49.5X5** **Adverse effect of ophthalmological drugs and preparations**   UPD

     ☑7ᵗʰ **T49.5X6** **Underdosing of ophthalmological drugs and preparations**   UPD

☑5ᵗʰ **T49.6** **Poisoning by, adverse effect of and underdosing of otorhinolaryngological drugs and preparations**

   ☑6ᵗʰ **T49.6X** **Poisoning by, adverse effect of and underdosing of** otorhinolaryngological drugs and preparations

     ☑7ᵗʰ **T49.6X1** **Poisoning by otorhinolaryngological drugs and preparations,** accidental **(unintentional)**
       Poisoning by otorhinolaryngological drugs and preparations NOS

    ² ☑7ᵗʰ **T49.6X2** **Poisoning by otorhinolaryngological drugs and preparations,** intentional **self-harm**   HCC Rx ESR COM

     ☑7ᵗʰ **T49.6X3** **Poisoning by otorhinolaryngological drugs and preparations,** assault

     ☑7ᵗʰ **T49.6X4** **Poisoning by otorhinolaryngological drugs and preparations,** undetermined

     ☑7ᵗʰ **T49.6X5** **Adverse effect of otorhinolaryngological drugs and preparations**   UPD

     ☑7ᵗʰ **T49.6X6** **Underdosing of otorhinolaryngological drugs and preparations**   UPD

☑5ᵗʰ **T49.7** **Poisoning by, adverse effect of and underdosing of dental drugs, topically applied**

   ☑6ᵗʰ **T49.7X** **Poisoning by, adverse effect of and underdosing of** dental drugs, topically applied

     ☑7ᵗʰ **T49.7X1** **Poisoning by dental drugs, topically applied,** accidental **(unintentional)**
       Poisoning by dental drugs, topically applied NOS

☑ Additional Character Required   ☑x7ᵗʰ Placeholder Alert   Manifestation   Unspecified Dx   Q QPP   UPD Unacceptable PDx

² ✓7ᵗʰ **T49.7X2 Poisoning** by dental drugs, topically applied, **intentional self-harm** `HCC` `Rx` `ESR` `COM`

✓7ᵗʰ **T49.7X3 Poisoning** by dental drugs, topically applied, **assault**

✓7ᵗʰ **T49.7X4 Poisoning** by dental drugs, topically applied, **undetermined**

✓7ᵗʰ **T49.7X5 Adverse effect** of dental drugs, topically applied `UPD`

✓7ᵗʰ **T49.7X6 Underdosing** of dental drugs, topically applied `UPD`

✓5ᵗʰ **T49.8 Poisoning by, adverse effect of and underdosing of other topical agents**

Poisoning by, adverse effect of and underdosing of spermicides

✓6ᵗʰ **T49.8X Poisoning by, adverse effect of and underdosing of other topical agents**

✓7ᵗʰ **T49.8X1 Poisoning** by other topical agents, **accidental (unintentional)**

Poisoning by other topical agents NOS

² ✓7ᵗʰ **T49.8X2 Poisoning** by other topical agents, **intentional self-harm** `HCC` `Rx` `ESR` `COM`

✓7ᵗʰ **T49.8X3 Poisoning** by other topical agents, **assault**

✓7ᵗʰ **T49.8X4 Poisoning** by other topical agents, **undetermined**

✓7ᵗʰ **T49.8X5 Adverse effect** of other topical agents `UPD`

✓7ᵗʰ **T49.8X6 Underdosing** of other topical agents `UPD`

✓5ᵗʰ **T49.9 Poisoning by, adverse effect of and underdosing of unspecified topical agent**

✓x7ᵗʰ **T49.91 Poisoning** by unspecified topical agent, **accidental (unintentional)**

² ✓x7ᵗʰ **T49.92 Poisoning** by unspecified topical agent, **intentional self-harm** `HCC` `Rx` `ESR` `COM`

✓x7ᵗʰ **T49.93 Poisoning** by unspecified topical agent, **assault**

✓x7ᵗʰ **T49.94 Poisoning** by unspecified topical agent, **undetermined**

✓x7ᵗʰ **T49.95 Adverse effect** of unspecified topical agent `UPD`

✓x7ᵗʰ **T49.96 Underdosing** of unspecified topical agent `UPD`

✓4ᵗʰ **T50 Poisoning by, adverse effect of and underdosing of diuretics and other and unspecified drugs, medicaments and biological substances**

> The appropriate 7th character is to be added to each code from category T50.
> A   initial encounter
> D   subsequent encounter
> S   sequela

✓5ᵗʰ **T50.0 Poisoning by, adverse effect of and underdosing of mineralocorticoids and their antagonists**

✓6ᵗʰ **T50.0X Poisoning by, adverse effect of and underdosing of mineralocorticoids and their antagonists**

✓7ᵗʰ **T50.0X1 Poisoning** by mineralocorticoids and their antagonists, **accidental (unintentional)**

Poisoning by mineralocorticoids and their antagonists NOS

² ✓7ᵗʰ **T50.0X2 Poisoning** by mineralocorticoids and their antagonists, **intentional self-harm** `HCC` `Rx` `ESR` `COM`

✓7ᵗʰ **T50.0X3 Poisoning** by mineralocorticoids and their antagonists, **assault**

✓7ᵗʰ **T50.0X4 Poisoning** by mineralocorticoids and their antagonists, **undetermined**

✓7ᵗʰ **T50.0X5 Adverse effect** of mineralocorticoids and their antagonists `UPD`

✓7ᵗʰ **T50.0X6 Underdosing** of mineralocorticoids and their antagonists `UPD`

✓5ᵗʰ **T50.1 Poisoning by, adverse effect of and underdosing of loop [high-ceiling] diuretics**

✓6ᵗʰ **T50.1X Poisoning by, adverse effect of and underdosing of loop [high-ceiling] diuretics**

✓7ᵗʰ **T50.1X1 Poisoning** by loop [high-ceiling] diuretics, **accidental (unintentional)**

Poisoning by loop [high-ceiling] diuretics NOS

² ✓7ᵗʰ **T50.1X2 Poisoning** by loop [high-ceiling] diuretics, **intentional self-harm** `HCC` `Rx` `ESR` `COM`

✓7ᵗʰ **T50.1X3 Poisoning** by loop [high-ceiling] diuretics, **assault**

✓7ᵗʰ **T50.1X4 Poisoning** by loop [high-ceiling] diuretics, **undetermined**

✓7ᵗʰ **T50.1X5 Adverse effect** of loop [high-ceiling] diuretics `UPD`

✓7ᵗʰ **T50.1X6 Underdosing** of loop [high-ceiling] diuretics `UPD`

✓5ᵗʰ **T50.2 Poisoning by, adverse effect of and underdosing of carbonic-anhydrase inhibitors, benzothiadiazides and other diuretics**

Poisoning by, adverse effect of and underdosing of acetazolamide

✓6ᵗʰ **T50.2X Poisoning by, adverse effect of and underdosing of carbonic-anhydrase inhibitors, benzothiadiazides and other diuretics**

✓7ᵗʰ **T50.2X1 Poisoning** by carbonic-anhydrase inhibitors, benzothiadiazides and other diuretics, **accidental (unintentional)**

Poisoning by carbonic-anhydrase inhibitors, benzothiadiazides and other diuretics NOS

² ✓7ᵗʰ **T50.2X2 Poisoning** by carbonic-anhydrase inhibitors, benzothiadiazides and other diuretics, **intentional self-harm** `HCC` `Rx` `ESR` `COM`

✓7ᵗʰ **T50.2X3 Poisoning** by carbonic-anhydrase inhibitors, benzothiadiazides and other diuretics, **assault**

✓7ᵗʰ **T50.2X4 Poisoning** by carbonic-anhydrase inhibitors, benzothiadiazides and other diuretics, **undetermined**

✓7ᵗʰ **T50.2X5 Adverse effect** of carbonic-anhydrase inhibitors, benzothiadiazides and other diuretics `UPD`

✓7ᵗʰ **T50.2X6 Underdosing** of carbonic-anhydrase inhibitors, benzothiadiazides and other diuretics `UPD`

✓5ᵗʰ **T50.3 Poisoning by, adverse effect of and underdosing of electrolytic, caloric and water-balance agents**

Poisoning by, adverse effect of and underdosing of oral rehydration salts

✓6ᵗʰ **T50.3X Poisoning by, adverse effect of and underdosing of electrolytic, caloric and water-balance agents**

✓7ᵗʰ **T50.3X1 Poisoning** by electrolytic, caloric and water-balance agents, **accidental (unintentional)**

Poisoning by electrolytic, caloric and water-balance agents NOS

² ✓7ᵗʰ **T50.3X2 Poisoning** by electrolytic, caloric and water-balance agents, **intentional self-harm** `HCC` `Rx` `ESR` `COM`

✓7ᵗʰ **T50.3X3 Poisoning** by electrolytic, caloric and water-balance agents, **assault**

✓7ᵗʰ **T50.3X4 Poisoning** by electrolytic, caloric and water-balance agents, **undetermined**

✓7ᵗʰ **T50.3X5 Adverse effect** of electrolytic, caloric and water-balance agents `UPD`

     AHA: 2022,2Q,10

✓7ᵗʰ **T50.3X6 Underdosing** of electrolytic, caloric and water-balance agents `UPD`

✓5ᵗʰ **T50.4 Poisoning by, adverse effect of and underdosing of drugs affecting uric acid metabolism**

✓6ᵗʰ **T50.4X Poisoning by, adverse effect of and underdosing of drugs affecting uric acid metabolism**

✓7ᵗʰ **T50.4X1 Poisoning** by drugs affecting uric acid metabolism, **accidental (unintentional)**

Poisoning by drugs affecting uric acid metabolism NOS

² ✓7ᵗʰ **T50.4X2 Poisoning** by drugs affecting uric acid metabolism, **intentional self-harm** `HCC` `Rx` `ESR` `COM`

✓7ᵗʰ **T50.4X3 Poisoning** by drugs affecting uric acid metabolism, **assault**

✓7ᵗʰ **T50.4X4 Poisoning** by drugs affecting uric acid metabolism, **undetermined**

✓7ᵗʰ **T50.4X5 Adverse effect** of drugs affecting uric acid metabolism `UPD`

✓7ᵗʰ **T50.4X6 Underdosing** of drugs affecting uric acid metabolism `UPD`

`HCC` CMS-HCC   `Rx` Rx HCC   `ESR` ESRD HCC   `COM` Commercial HCC   `N` Newborn: 0   `P` Pediatric: 0-17   `M` Maternity: 9-64   `A` Adult: 15-124

1154   ICD-10-CM 2023

☑5ᵗʰ **T50.5 Poisoning by, adverse effect of and underdosing of appetite depressants**

    ☑6ᵗʰ **T50.5X Poisoning by, adverse effect of and underdosing of** appetite depressants

       ☑7ᵗʰ **T50.5X1 Poisoning by appetite depressants, accidental (unintentional)**

          Poisoning by appetite depressants NOS

       ² ☑7ᵗʰ **T50.5X2 Poisoning by appetite depressants, intentional self-harm** `HCC` `Rx` `ESR` `COM`

       ☑7ᵗʰ **T50.5X3 Poisoning by appetite depressants, assault**

       ☑7ᵗʰ **T50.5X4 Poisoning by appetite depressants, undetermined**

       ☑7ᵗʰ **T50.5X5 Adverse effect of appetite depressants** `UPD`

       ☑7ᵗʰ **T50.5X6 Underdosing of appetite depressants** `UPD`

☑5ᵗʰ **T50.6 Poisoning by, adverse effect of and underdosing of antidotes and chelating agents**

    Poisoning by, adverse effect of and underdosing of alcohol deterrents

    ☑6ᵗʰ **T50.6X Poisoning by, adverse effect of and underdosing of** antidotes and chelating agents

       ☑7ᵗʰ **T50.6X1 Poisoning by antidotes and chelating agents, accidental (unintentional)**

          Poisoning by antidotes and chelating agents NOS

       ² ☑7ᵗʰ **T50.6X2 Poisoning by antidotes and chelating agents, intentional self-harm** `HCC` `Rx` `ESR` `COM`

       ☑7ᵗʰ **T50.6X3 Poisoning by antidotes and chelating agents, assault**

       ☑7ᵗʰ **T50.6X4 Poisoning by antidotes and chelating agents, undetermined**

       ☑7ᵗʰ **T50.6X5 Adverse effect of antidotes and chelating agents** `UPD`

       ☑7ᵗʰ **T50.6X6 Underdosing of antidotes and chelating agents** `UPD`

☑5ᵗʰ **T50.7 Poisoning by, adverse effect of and underdosing of analeptics and opioid receptor antagonists**

    ☑6ᵗʰ **T50.7X Poisoning by, adverse effect of and underdosing of** analeptics and opioid receptor antagonists

       ☑7ᵗʰ **T50.7X1 Poisoning by analeptics and opioid receptor antagonists, accidental (unintentional)**

          Poisoning by analeptics and opioid receptor antagonists NOS

       ² ☑7ᵗʰ **T50.7X2 Poisoning by analeptics and opioid receptor antagonists, intentional self-harm** `HCC` `Rx` `ESR` `COM`

       ☑7ᵗʰ **T50.7X3 Poisoning by analeptics and opioid receptor antagonists, assault**

       ☑7ᵗʰ **T50.7X4 Poisoning by analeptics and opioid receptor antagonists, undetermined**

       ☑7ᵗʰ **T50.7X5 Adverse effect of analeptics and opioid receptor antagonists** `UPD`

       ☑7ᵗʰ **T50.7X6 Underdosing of analeptics and opioid receptor antagonists** `UPD`

☑5ᵗʰ **T50.8 Poisoning by, adverse effect of and underdosing of diagnostic agents**

    ☑6ᵗʰ **T50.8X Poisoning by, adverse effect of and underdosing of** diagnostic agents

       ☑7ᵗʰ **T50.8X1 Poisoning by diagnostic agents, accidental (unintentional)**

          Poisoning by diagnostic agents NOS

       ² ☑7ᵗʰ **T50.8X2 Poisoning by diagnostic agents, intentional self-harm** `HCC` `Rx` `ESR` `COM`

       ☑7ᵗʰ **T50.8X3 Poisoning by diagnostic agents, assault**

       ☑7ᵗʰ **T50.8X4 Poisoning by diagnostic agents, undetermined**

       ☑7ᵗʰ **T50.8X5 Adverse effect of diagnostic agents** `UPD`

          AHA: 2021,3Q,9-10

       ☑7ᵗʰ **T50.8X6 Underdosing of diagnostic agents** `UPD`

☑5ᵗʰ **T50.A Poisoning by, adverse effect of and underdosing of bacterial vaccines**

    ☑6ᵗʰ **T50.A1 Poisoning by, adverse effect of and underdosing of** pertussis vaccine, including combinations with a pertussis component

       ☑7ᵗʰ **T50.A11 Poisoning by pertussis vaccine, including combinations with a pertussis component, accidental (unintentional)**

       ² ☑7ᵗʰ **T50.A12 Poisoning by pertussis vaccine, including combinations with a pertussis component, intentional self-harm** `HCC` `Rx` `ESR` `COM`

       ☑7ᵗʰ **T50.A13 Poisoning by pertussis vaccine, including combinations with a pertussis component, assault**

       ☑7ᵗʰ **T50.A14 Poisoning by pertussis vaccine, including combinations with a pertussis component, undetermined**

       ☑7ᵗʰ **T50.A15 Adverse effect of pertussis vaccine, including combinations with a pertussis component**

       ☑7ᵗʰ **T50.A16 Underdosing of pertussis vaccine, including combinations with a pertussis component** `UPD`

    ☑6ᵗʰ **T50.A2 Poisoning by, adverse effect of and underdosing of** mixed bacterial vaccines without a pertussis component

       ☑7ᵗʰ **T50.A21 Poisoning by mixed bacterial vaccines without a pertussis component, accidental (unintentional)**

       ² ☑7ᵗʰ **T50.A22 Poisoning by mixed bacterial vaccines without a pertussis component, intentional self-harm** `HCC` `Rx` `ESR` `COM`

       ☑7ᵗʰ **T50.A23 Poisoning by mixed bacterial vaccines without a pertussis component, assault**

       ☑7ᵗʰ **T50.A24 Poisoning by mixed bacterial vaccines without a pertussis component, undetermined**

       ☑7ᵗʰ **T50.A25 Adverse effect of mixed bacterial vaccines without a pertussis component** `UPD`

       ☑7ᵗʰ **T50.A26 Underdosing of mixed bacterial vaccines without a pertussis component** `UPD`

    ☑6ᵗʰ **T50.A9 Poisoning by, adverse effect of and underdosing of** other bacterial vaccines

       ☑7ᵗʰ **T50.A91 Poisoning by other bacterial vaccines, accidental (unintentional)**

       ² ☑7ᵗʰ **T50.A92 Poisoning by other bacterial vaccines, intentional self-harm** `HCC` `Rx` `ESR` `COM`

       ☑7ᵗʰ **T50.A93 Poisoning by other bacterial vaccines, assault**

       ☑7ᵗʰ **T50.A94 Poisoning by other bacterial vaccines, undetermined**

       ☑7ᵗʰ **T50.A95 Adverse effect of other bacterial vaccines** `UPD`

       ☑7ᵗʰ **T50.A96 Underdosing of other bacterial vaccines** `UPD`

☑5ᵗʰ **T50.B Poisoning by, adverse effect of and underdosing of viral vaccines**

    ☑6ᵗʰ **T50.B1 Poisoning by, adverse effect of and underdosing of** smallpox vaccines

       ☑7ᵗʰ **T50.B11 Poisoning by smallpox vaccines, accidental (unintentional)**

       ² ☑7ᵗʰ **T50.B12 Poisoning by smallpox vaccines, intentional self-harm** `HCC` `Rx` `ESR` `COM`

       ☑7ᵗʰ **T50.B13 Poisoning by smallpox vaccines, assault**

       ☑7ᵗʰ **T50.B14 Poisoning by smallpox vaccines, undetermined**

       ☑7ᵗʰ **T50.B15 Adverse effect of smallpox vaccines** `UPD`

       ☑7ᵗʰ **T50.B16 Underdosing of smallpox vaccines** `UPD`

    ☑6ᵗʰ **T50.B9 Poisoning by, adverse effect of and underdosing of** other viral vaccines

       ☑7ᵗʰ **T50.B91 Poisoning by other viral vaccines, accidental (unintentional)**

       ² ☑7ᵗʰ **T50.B92 Poisoning by other viral vaccines, intentional self-harm** `HCC` `Rx` `ESR` `COM`

       ☑7ᵗʰ **T50.B93 Poisoning by other viral vaccines, assault**

       ☑7ᵗʰ **T50.B94 Poisoning by other viral vaccines, undetermined**

       ☑7ᵗʰ **T50.B95 Adverse effect of other viral vaccines** `UPD`

          AHA: 2021,1Q,43

       ☑7ᵗʰ **T50.B96 Underdosing of other viral vaccines** `UPD`

☑5ᵗʰ **T50.Z Poisoning by, adverse effect of and underdosing of other vaccines and biological substances**

    ☑6ᵗʰ **T50.Z1 Poisoning by, adverse effect of and underdosing of** immunoglobulin

       ☑7ᵗʰ **T50.Z11 Poisoning by immunoglobulin, accidental (unintentional)**

Chapter 19. Injury, Poisoning and Certain Other Consequences of External Causes *(left margin vertical)*

T50.Z12–T51.3X4 *(left margin vertical)*

² √7ᵗʰ **T50.Z12** **Poisoning by immunoglobulin,**
intentional self-harm `HCC` `Rx` `ESR` `COM`

√7ᵗʰ **T50.Z13** **Poisoning by immunoglobulin,** assault

√7ᵗʰ **T50.Z14** **Poisoning by immunoglobulin,**
undetermined

√7ᵗʰ **T50.Z15** **Adverse effect of immunoglobulin** `UPD`

√7ᵗʰ **T50.Z16** **Underdosing of immunoglobulin** `UPD`

√6ᵗʰ **T50.Z9** **Poisoning by, adverse effect of and underdosing**
of other vaccines and biological substances

√7ᵗʰ **T50.Z91** **Poisoning by other vaccines and**
biological substances, accidental
(unintentional)

² √7ᵗʰ **T50.Z92** **Poisoning by other vaccines and**
biological substances, intentional
self-harm `HCC` `Rx` `ESR` `COM`

√7ᵗʰ **T50.Z93** **Poisoning by other vaccines and**
biological substances, assault

√7ᵗʰ **T50.Z94** **Poisoning by other vaccines and**
biological substances, undetermined

√7ᵗʰ **T50.Z95** **Adverse effect of other vaccines and**
biological substances `UPD`
AHA: 2020,1Q,18

√7ᵗʰ **T50.Z96** **Underdosing of other vaccines and**
biological substances `UPD`

√5ᵗʰ **T50.9** **Poisoning by, adverse effect of and underdosing of other**
and unspecified drugs, medicaments and biological
substances

√6ᵗʰ **T50.90** **Poisoning by, adverse effect of and underdosing**
of unspecified drugs, medicaments and biological
substances

√7ᵗʰ **T50.901** **Poisoning by unspecified drugs,**
medicaments and biological substances,
accidental (unintentional)

² √7ᵗʰ **T50.902** **Poisoning by unspecified drugs,**
medicaments and biological substances,
intentional self-harm `HCC` `Rx` `ESR` `COM`

√7ᵗʰ **T50.903** **Poisoning by unspecified drugs,**
medicaments and biological substances,
assault

√7ᵗʰ **T50.904** **Poisoning by unspecified drugs,**
medicaments and biological substances,
undetermined

√7ᵗʰ **T50.905** **Adverse effect of unspecified drugs,**
medicaments and biological substances

√7ᵗʰ **T50.906** **Underdosing of unspecified drugs,**
medicaments and biological substances

√6ᵗʰ **T50.91** **Poisoning by, adverse effect of and underdosing**
of multiple unspecified drugs, medicaments and
biological substances
Multiple drug ingestion NOS
Code also any specific drugs, medicaments and
biological substances

√7ᵗʰ **T50.911** **Poisoning by multiple unspecified drugs,**
medicaments and biological substances,
accidental (unintentional)

² √7ᵗʰ **T50.912** **Poisoning by multiple unspecified drugs,**
medicaments and biological substances,
intentional self-harm `HCC` `Rx` `ESR` `COM`

√7ᵗʰ **T50.913** **Poisoning by multiple unspecified drugs,**
medicaments and biological substances,
assault

√7ᵗʰ **T50.914** **Poisoning by multiple unspecified drugs,**
medicaments and biological substances,
undetermined

√7ᵗʰ **T50.915** **Adverse effect of multiple unspecified**
drugs, medicaments and biological
substances `UPD`

√7ᵗʰ **T50.916** **Underdosing of multiple unspecified**
drugs, medicaments and biological
substances `UPD`

√6ᵗʰ **T50.99** **Poisoning by, adverse effect of and underdosing**
of other drugs, medicaments and biological
substances

√7ᵗʰ **T50.991** **Poisoning by other drugs, medicaments**
and biological substances, accidental
(unintentional)

² √7ᵗʰ **T50.992** **Poisoning by other drugs, medicaments**
and biological substances, intentional
self-harm `HCC` `Rx` `ESR` `COM`

√7ᵗʰ **T50.993** **Poisoning by other drugs, medicaments**
and biological substances, assault

√7ᵗʰ **T50.994** **Poisoning by other drugs, medicaments**
and biological substances, undetermined

√7ᵗʰ **T50.995** **Adverse effect of other drugs,**
medicaments and biological substances

√7ᵗʰ **T50.996** **Underdosing of other drugs,**
medicaments and biological substances

Toxic effects of substances chiefly nonmedicinal as to source (T51-T65)

`NOTE`   When no intent is indicated code to accidental. Undetermined intent
is only for use when there is specific documentation in the record
that the intent of the toxic effect cannot be determined.

Use additional code(s) for all associated manifestations of toxic effect, such as:
personal history of foreign body fully removed (Z87.821)
respiratory conditions due to external agents (J60-J70)
to identify any retained foreign body, if applicable (Z18.-)

`EXCLUDES 1`   contact with and (suspected) exposure to toxic substances (Z77.-)
AHA: 2017,1Q,39-40

√4ᵗʰ **T51** **Toxic effect of alcohol**

> The appropriate 7th character is to be added to each code from
> category T51.
> A   initial encounter
> D   subsequent encounter
> S   sequela

√5ᵗʰ **T51.0** **Toxic effect of ethanol**
Toxic effect of ethyl alcohol

`EXCLUDES 2`   acute alcohol intoxication or "hangover" effects
(F10.129, F10.229, F10.929)
drunkenness (F10.129, F10.229, F10.929)
pathological alcohol intoxication (F10.129, F10.229,
F10.929)

√6ᵗʰ **T51.0X** **Toxic effect of** ethanol

¹ √7ᵗʰ **T51.0X1** **Toxic effect of ethanol,** accidental
(unintentional) `HCC` `ESR`
Toxic effect of ethanol NOS

² √7ᵗʰ **T51.0X2** **Toxic effect of ethanol,** intentional
self-harm `HCC` `Rx` `ESR` `COM`

√7ᵗʰ **T51.0X3** **Toxic effect of ethanol,** assault

¹ √7ᵗʰ **T51.0X4** **Toxic effect of ethanol,**
undetermined `HCC` `ESR`

√5ᵗʰ **T51.1** **Toxic effect of methanol**
Toxic effect of methyl alcohol

√6ᵗʰ **T51.1X** **Toxic effect of** methanol

√7ᵗʰ **T51.1X1** **Toxic effect of methanol,** accidental
(unintentional)
Toxic effect of methanol NOS

² √7ᵗʰ **T51.1X2** **Toxic effect of methanol,** intentional
self-harm `HCC` `Rx` `ESR` `COM`

√7ᵗʰ **T51.1X3** **Toxic effect of methanol,** assault

√7ᵗʰ **T51.1X4** **Toxic effect of methanol,** undetermined

√5ᵗʰ **T51.2** **Toxic effect of 2-Propanol**
Toxic effect of isopropyl alcohol

√6ᵗʰ **T51.2X** **Toxic effect of** 2-Propanol

√7ᵗʰ **T51.2X1** **Toxic effect of 2-Propanol,** accidental
(unintentional)
Toxic effect of 2-Propanol NOS

² √7ᵗʰ **T51.2X2** **Toxic effect of 2-Propanol,** intentional
self-harm `HCC` `Rx` `ESR` `COM`

√7ᵗʰ **T51.2X3** **Toxic effect of 2-Propanol,** assault

√7ᵗʰ **T51.2X4** **Toxic effect of 2-Propanol,** undetermined

√5ᵗʰ **T51.3** **Toxic effect of fusel oil**
Toxic effect of amyl alcohol
Toxic effect of butyl [1-butanol] alcohol
Toxic effect of propyl [1-propanol] alcohol

√6ᵗʰ **T51.3X** **Toxic effect of** fusel oil

√7ᵗʰ **T51.3X1** **Toxic effect of fusel oil,** accidental
(unintentional)
Toxic effect of fusel oil NOS

² √7ᵗʰ **T51.3X2** **Toxic effect of fusel oil,** intentional
self-harm `HCC` `Rx` `ESR` `COM`

√7ᵗʰ **T51.3X3** **Toxic effect of fusel oil,** assault

√7ᵗʰ **T51.3X4** **Toxic effect of fusel oil,** undetermined

`HCC` CMS-HCC   `Rx` Rx HCC   `ESR` ESRD HCC   `COM` Commercial HCC   Ⓝ Newborn: 0   Ⓟ Pediatric: 0-17   Ⓜ Maternity: 9-64   Ⓐ Adult: 15-124

1156   ICD-10-CM 2023

√5ᵗʰ **T51.8 Toxic effect of other alcohols**

  √6ᵗʰ **T51.8X Toxic effect of other alcohols**

    √7ᵗʰ **T51.8X1 Toxic effect of other alcohols, accidental (unintentional)**
      Toxic effect of other alcohols NOS

    ² √7ᵗʰ **T51.8X2 Toxic effect of other alcohols, intentional self-harm** HCC Rx ESR COM

    √7ᵗʰ **T51.8X3 Toxic effect of other alcohols, assault**

    √7ᵗʰ **T51.8X4 Toxic effect of other alcohols, undetermined**

√5ᵗʰ **T51.9 Toxic effect of unspecified alcohol**

  √x7ᵗʰ **T51.91 Toxic effect of unspecified alcohol, accidental (unintentional)**

  ² √x7ᵗʰ **T51.92 Toxic effect of unspecified alcohol, intentional self-harm** HCC Rx ESR COM

  √x7ᵗʰ **T51.93 Toxic effect of unspecified alcohol, assault**

  √x7ᵗʰ **T51.94 Toxic effect of unspecified alcohol, undetermined**

√4ᵗʰ **T52 Toxic effect of organic solvents**

  EXCLUDES 1   *halogen derivatives of aliphatic and aromatic hydrocarbons (T53.-)*

  The appropriate 7th character is to be added to each code from category T52.
  A   initial encounter
  D   subsequent encounter
  S   sequela

  √5ᵗʰ **T52.0 Toxic effects of petroleum products**
    Toxic effects of ether petroleum
    Toxic effects of gasoline [petrol]
    Toxic effects of kerosene [paraffin oil]
    Toxic effects of naphtha petroleum
    Toxic effects of paraffin wax
    Toxic effects of spirit petroleum

    √6ᵗʰ **T52.0X Toxic effects of petroleum products**

      √7ᵗʰ **T52.0X1 Toxic effect of petroleum products, accidental (unintentional)**
        Toxic effects of petroleum products NOS

      ² √7ᵗʰ **T52.0X2 Toxic effect of petroleum products, intentional self-harm** HCC Rx ESR COM

      √7ᵗʰ **T52.0X3 Toxic effect of petroleum products, assault**

      √7ᵗʰ **T52.0X4 Toxic effect of petroleum products, undetermined**

  √5ᵗʰ **T52.1 Toxic effects of benzene**

    EXCLUDES 1   *homologues of benzene (T52.2)*
        nitroderivatives and aminoderivatives of benzene and its homologues (T65.3)

    √6ᵗʰ **T52.1X Toxic effects of benzene**

      √7ᵗʰ **T52.1X1 Toxic effect of benzene, accidental (unintentional)**
        Toxic effects of benzene NOS

      ² √7ᵗʰ **T52.1X2 Toxic effect of benzene, intentional self-harm** HCC Rx ESR COM

      √7ᵗʰ **T52.1X3 Toxic effect of benzene, assault**

      √7ᵗʰ **T52.1X4 Toxic effect of benzene, undetermined**

  √5ᵗʰ **T52.2 Toxic effects of homologues of benzene**
    Toxic effects of toluene [methylbenzene]
    Toxic effects of xylene [dimethylbenzene]

    √6ᵗʰ **T52.2X Toxic effects of homologues of benzene**

      √7ᵗʰ **T52.2X1 Toxic effect of homologues of benzene, accidental (unintentional)**
        Toxic effects of homologues of benzene NOS

      ² √7ᵗʰ **T52.2X2 Toxic effect of homologues of benzene, intentional self-harm** HCC Rx ESR COM

      √7ᵗʰ **T52.2X3 Toxic effect of homologues of benzene, assault**

      √7ᵗʰ **T52.2X4 Toxic effect of homologues of benzene, undetermined**

  √5ᵗʰ **T52.3 Toxic effects of glycols**

    √6ᵗʰ **T52.3X Toxic effects of glycols**

      √7ᵗʰ **T52.3X1 Toxic effect of glycols, accidental (unintentional)**
        Toxic effects of glycols NOS

      ² √7ᵗʰ **T52.3X2 Toxic effect of glycols, intentional self-harm** HCC Rx ESR COM

      √7ᵗʰ **T52.3X3 Toxic effect of glycols, assault**

      √7ᵗʰ **T52.3X4 Toxic effect of glycols, undetermined**

√5ᵗʰ **T52.4 Toxic effects of ketones**

  √6ᵗʰ **T52.4X Toxic effects of ketones**

    √7ᵗʰ **T52.4X1 Toxic effect of ketones, accidental (unintentional)**
      Toxic effects of ketones NOS

    ² √7ᵗʰ **T52.4X2 Toxic effect of ketones, intentional self-harm** HCC Rx ESR COM

    √7ᵗʰ **T52.4X3 Toxic effect of ketones, assault**

    √7ᵗʰ **T52.4X4 Toxic effect of ketones, undetermined**

√5ᵗʰ **T52.8 Toxic effects of other organic solvents**

  √6ᵗʰ **T52.8X Toxic effects of other organic solvents**

    √7ᵗʰ **T52.8X1 Toxic effect of other organic solvents, accidental (unintentional)**
      Toxic effects of other organic solvents NOS

    ² √7ᵗʰ **T52.8X2 Toxic effect of other organic solvents, intentional self-harm** HCC Rx ESR COM

    √7ᵗʰ **T52.8X3 Toxic effect of other organic solvents, assault**

    √7ᵗʰ **T52.8X4 Toxic effect of other organic solvents, undetermined**

√5ᵗʰ **T52.9 Toxic effects of unspecified organic solvent**

  √x7ᵗʰ **T52.91 Toxic effect of unspecified organic solvent, accidental (unintentional)**

  ² √x7ᵗʰ **T52.92 Toxic effect of unspecified organic solvent, intentional self-harm** HCC Rx ESR COM

  √x7ᵗʰ **T52.93 Toxic effect of unspecified organic solvent, assault**

  √x7ᵗʰ **T52.94 Toxic effect of unspecified organic solvent, undetermined**

√4ᵗʰ **T53 Toxic effect of halogen derivatives of aliphatic and aromatic hydrocarbons**

  The appropriate 7th character is to be added to each code from category T53.
  A   initial encounter
  D   subsequent encounter
  S   sequela

  √5ᵗʰ **T53.0 Toxic effects of carbon tetrachloride**
    Toxic effects of tetrachloromethane

    √6ᵗʰ **T53.0X Toxic effects of carbon tetrachloride**

      √7ᵗʰ **T53.0X1 Toxic effect of carbon tetrachloride, accidental (unintentional)**
        Toxic effects of carbon tetrachloride NOS

      ² √7ᵗʰ **T53.0X2 Toxic effect of carbon tetrachloride, intentional self-harm** HCC Rx ESR COM

      √7ᵗʰ **T53.0X3 Toxic effect of carbon tetrachloride, assault**

      √7ᵗʰ **T53.0X4 Toxic effect of carbon tetrachloride, undetermined**

  √5ᵗʰ **T53.1 Toxic effects of chloroform**
    Toxic effects of trichloromethane

    √6ᵗʰ **T53.1X Toxic effects of chloroform**

      √7ᵗʰ **T53.1X1 Toxic effect of chloroform, accidental (unintentional)**
        Toxic effects of chloroform NOS

      ² √7ᵗʰ **T53.1X2 Toxic effect of chloroform, intentional self-harm** HCC Rx ESR COM

      √7ᵗʰ **T53.1X3 Toxic effect of chloroform, assault**

      √7ᵗʰ **T53.1X4 Toxic effect of chloroform, undetermined**

  √5ᵗʰ **T53.2 Toxic effects of trichloroethylene**
    Toxic effects of trichloroethene

    √6ᵗʰ **T53.2X Toxic effects of trichloroethylene**

      √7ᵗʰ **T53.2X1 Toxic effect of trichloroethylene, accidental (unintentional)**
        Toxic effects of trichloroethylene NOS

      ² √7ᵗʰ **T53.2X2 Toxic effect of trichloroethylene, intentional self-harm** HCC Rx ESR COM

      √7ᵗʰ **T53.2X3 Toxic effect of trichloroethylene, assault**

      √7ᵗʰ **T53.2X4 Toxic effect of trichloroethylene, undetermined**

√5th **T53.3 Toxic effects of tetrachloroethylene**
Toxic effects of perchloroethylene
Toxic effect of tetrachloroethene

√6th **T53.3X Toxic effects of** tetrachloroethylene

√7th **T53.3X1 Toxic effect of tetrachloroethylene, accidental (unintentional)**
Toxic effects of tetrachloroethylene NOS

2 √7th **T53.3X2 Toxic effect of tetrachloroethylene, intentional self-harm** HCC Rx ESR COM

√7th **T53.3X3 Toxic effect of tetrachloroethylene, assault**

√7th **T53.3X4 Toxic effect of tetrachloroethylene, undetermined**

√5th **T53.4 Toxic effects of dichloromethane**
Toxic effects of methylene chloride

√6th **T53.4X Toxic effects of** dichloromethane

√7th **T53.4X1 Toxic effect of dichloromethane, accidental (unintentional)**
Toxic effects of dichloromethane NOS

2 √7th **T53.4X2 Toxic effect of dichloromethane, intentional self-harm** HCC Rx ESR COM

√7th **T53.4X3 Toxic effect of dichloromethane, assault**

√7th **T53.4X4 Toxic effect of dichloromethane, undetermined**

√5th **T53.5 Toxic effects of chlorofluorocarbons**

√6th **T53.5X Toxic effects of** chlorofluorocarbons

√7th **T53.5X1 Toxic effect of chlorofluorocarbons, accidental (unintentional)**
Toxic effects of chlorofluorocarbons NOS

2 √7th **T53.5X2 Toxic effect of chlorofluorocarbons, intentional self-harm** HCC Rx ESR COM

√7th **T53.5X3 Toxic effect of chlorofluorocarbons, assault**

√7th **T53.5X4 Toxic effect of chlorofluorocarbons, undetermined**

√5th **T53.6 Toxic effects of other halogen derivatives of aliphatic hydrocarbons**

√6th **T53.6X Toxic effects of** other halogen derivatives of aliphatic hydrocarbons

√7th **T53.6X1 Toxic effect of other halogen derivatives of aliphatic hydrocarbons, accidental (unintentional)**
Toxic effects of other halogen derivatives of aliphatic hydrocarbons NOS

2 √7th **T53.6X2 Toxic effect of other halogen derivatives of aliphatic hydrocarbons, intentional self-harm** HCC Rx ESR COM

√7th **T53.6X3 Toxic effect of other halogen derivatives of aliphatic hydrocarbons, assault**

√7th **T53.6X4 Toxic effect of other halogen derivatives of aliphatic hydrocarbons, undetermined**

√5th **T53.7 Toxic effects of other halogen derivatives of aromatic hydrocarbons**

√6th **T53.7X Toxic effects of** other halogen derivatives of aromatic hydrocarbons

√7th **T53.7X1 Toxic effect of other halogen derivatives of aromatic hydrocarbons, accidental (unintentional)**
Toxic effects of other halogen derivatives of aromatic hydrocarbons NOS

2 √7th **T53.7X2 Toxic effect of other halogen derivatives of aromatic hydrocarbons, intentional self-harm** HCC Rx ESR COM

√7th **T53.7X3 Toxic effect of other halogen derivatives of aromatic hydrocarbons, assault**

√7th **T53.7X4 Toxic effect of other halogen derivatives of aromatic hydrocarbons, undetermined**

√5th **T53.9 Toxic effects of unspecified halogen derivatives of aliphatic and aromatic hydrocarbons**

√x7th **T53.91 Toxic effect of unspecified halogen derivatives of aliphatic and aromatic hydrocarbons, accidental (unintentional)**

2 √x7th **T53.92 Toxic effect of unspecified halogen derivatives of aliphatic and aromatic hydrocarbons, intentional self-harm** HCC Rx ESR COM

√x7th **T53.93 Toxic effect of unspecified halogen derivatives of aliphatic and aromatic hydrocarbons, assault**

√x7th **T53.94 Toxic effect of unspecified halogen derivatives of aliphatic and aromatic hydrocarbons, undetermined**

√4th **T54 Toxic effect of corrosive substances**

> The appropriate 7th character is to be added to each code from category T54.
> A   initial encounter
> D   subsequent encounter
> S   sequela

√5th **T54.0 Toxic effects of phenol and phenol homologues**

√6th **T54.0X Toxic effects of** phenol and phenol homologues

√7th **T54.0X1 Toxic effect of phenol and phenol homologues, accidental (unintentional)**
Toxic effects of phenol and phenol homologues NOS

2 √7th **T54.0X2 Toxic effect of phenol and phenol homologues, intentional self-harm** HCC Rx ESR COM

√7th **T54.0X3 Toxic effect of phenol and phenol homologues, assault**

√7th **T54.0X4 Toxic effect of phenol and phenol homologues, undetermined**

√5th **T54.1 Toxic effects of other corrosive organic compounds**

√6th **T54.1X Toxic effects of other corrosive organic compounds**

√7th **T54.1X1 Toxic effect of other corrosive organic compounds, accidental (unintentional)**
Toxic effects of other corrosive organic compounds NOS

2 √7th **T54.1X2 Toxic effect of other corrosive organic compounds, intentional self-harm** HCC Rx ESR COM

√7th **T54.1X3 Toxic effect of other corrosive organic compounds, assault**

√7th **T54.1X4 Toxic effect of other corrosive organic compounds, undetermined**

√5th **T54.2 Toxic effects of corrosive acids and acid-like substances**
Toxic effects of hydrochloric acid
Toxic effects of sulfuric acid

√6th **T54.2X Toxic effects of** corrosive acids and acid-like substances

√7th **T54.2X1 Toxic effect of corrosive acids and acid-like substances, accidental (unintentional)**
Toxic effects of corrosive acids and acid-like substances NOS

2 √7th **T54.2X2 Toxic effect of corrosive acids and acid-like substances, intentional self-harm** HCC Rx ESR COM

√7th **T54.2X3 Toxic effect of corrosive acids and acid-like substances, assault**

√7th **T54.2X4 Toxic effect of corrosive acids and acid-like substances, undetermined**

√5th **T54.3 Toxic effects of corrosive alkalis and alkali-like substances**
Toxic effects of potassium hydroxide
Toxic effects of sodium hydroxide

√6th **T54.3X Toxic effects of** corrosive alkalis and alkali-like substances

√7th **T54.3X1 Toxic effect of corrosive alkalis and alkali-like substances, accidental (unintentional)**
Toxic effects of corrosive alkalis and alkali-like substances NOS

2 √7th **T54.3X2 Toxic effect of corrosive alkalis and alkali-like substances, intentional self-harm** HCC Rx ESR COM

√7th **T54.3X3 Toxic effect of corrosive alkalis and alkali-like substances, assault**

√7th **T54.3X4 Toxic effect of corrosive alkalis and alkali-like substances, undetermined**

√5th **T54.9 Toxic effects of unspecified corrosive substance**

√x7th **T54.91 Toxic effect of unspecified corrosive substance, accidental (unintentional)**

2 √x7th **T54.92 Toxic effect of unspecified corrosive substance, intentional self-harm** HCC Rx ESR COM

√x7th **T54.93 Toxic effect of unspecified corrosive substance, assault**

√x7th **T54.94 Toxic effect of unspecified corrosive substance, undetermined**

✓4ᵗʰ **T55 Toxic effect of soaps and detergents**

> The appropriate 7th character is to be added to each code from category T55.
> A initial encounter
> D subsequent encounter
> S sequela

✓5ᵗʰ **T55.0 Toxic effect of soaps**

✓6ᵗʰ **T55.0X Toxic effect of soaps**

✓7ᵗʰ **T55.0X1 Toxic effect of soaps, accidental (unintentional)**
Toxic effect of soaps NOS

² ✓7ᵗʰ **T55.0X2 Toxic effect of soaps, intentional self-harm** HCC Rx ESR COM

✓7ᵗʰ **T55.0X3 Toxic effect of soaps, assault**

✓7ᵗʰ **T55.0X4 Toxic effect of soaps, undetermined**

✓5ᵗʰ **T55.1 Toxic effect of detergents**

✓6ᵗʰ **T55.1X Toxic effect of detergents**

✓7ᵗʰ **T55.1X1 Toxic effect of detergents, accidental (unintentional)**
Toxic effect of detergents NOS

² ✓7ᵗʰ **T55.1X2 Toxic effect of detergents, intentional self-harm** HCC Rx ESR COM

✓7ᵗʰ **T55.1X3 Toxic effect of detergents, assault**

✓7ᵗʰ **T55.1X4 Toxic effect of detergents, undetermined**

✓4ᵗʰ **T56 Toxic effect of metals**

> INCLUDES   toxic effects of fumes and vapors of metals
> toxic effects of metals from all sources, except medicinal substances
> Use additional code to identify any retained metal foreign body, if applicable (Z18.0-, T18.1-)
> EXCLUDES 1   arsenic and its compounds (T57.0)
> manganese and its compounds (T57.2)

> The appropriate 7th character is to be added to each code from category T56.
> A initial encounter
> D subsequent encounter
> S sequela

✓5ᵗʰ **T56.0 Toxic effects of lead and its compounds**

✓6ᵗʰ **T56.0X Toxic effects of lead and its compounds**

✓7ᵗʰ **T56.0X1 Toxic effect of lead and its compounds, accidental (unintentional)**
Toxic effects of lead and its compounds NOS

² ✓7ᵗʰ **T56.0X2 Toxic effect of lead and its compounds, intentional self-harm** HCC Rx ESR COM

✓7ᵗʰ **T56.0X3 Toxic effect of lead and its compounds, assault**

✓7ᵗʰ **T56.0X4 Toxic effect of lead and its compounds, undetermined**

✓5ᵗʰ **T56.1 Toxic effects of mercury and its compounds**

✓6ᵗʰ **T56.1X Toxic effect of mercury and its compounds**

✓7ᵗʰ **T56.1X1 Toxic effect of mercury and its compounds, accidental (unintentional)**
Toxic effects of mercury and its compounds NOS

² ✓7ᵗʰ **T56.1X2 Toxic effect of mercury and its compounds, intentional self-harm** HCC Rx ESR COM

✓7ᵗʰ **T56.1X3 Toxic effect of mercury and its compounds, assault**

✓7ᵗʰ **T56.1X4 Toxic effect of mercury and its compounds, undetermined**

✓5ᵗʰ **T56.2 Toxic effects of chromium and its compounds**

✓6ᵗʰ **T56.2X Toxic effects of chromium and its compounds**

✓7ᵗʰ **T56.2X1 Toxic effect of chromium and its compounds, accidental (unintentional)**
Toxic effects of chromium and its compounds NOS

² ✓7ᵗʰ **T56.2X2 Toxic effect of chromium and its compounds, intentional self-harm** HCC Rx ESR COM

✓7ᵗʰ **T56.2X3 Toxic effect of chromium and its compounds, assault**

✓7ᵗʰ **T56.2X4 Toxic effect of chromium and its compounds, undetermined**

✓5ᵗʰ **T56.3 Toxic effects of cadmium and its compounds**

✓6ᵗʰ **T56.3X Toxic effects of cadmium and its compounds**

✓7ᵗʰ **T56.3X1 Toxic effect of cadmium and its compounds, accidental (unintentional)**
Toxic effects of cadmium and its compounds NOS

² ✓7ᵗʰ **T56.3X2 Toxic effect of cadmium and its compounds, intentional self-harm** HCC Rx ESR COM

✓7ᵗʰ **T56.3X3 Toxic effect of cadmium and its compounds, assault**

✓7ᵗʰ **T56.3X4 Toxic effect of cadmium and its compounds, undetermined**

✓5ᵗʰ **T56.4 Toxic effects of copper and its compounds**

✓6ᵗʰ **T56.4X Toxic effects of copper and its compounds**

✓7ᵗʰ **T56.4X1 Toxic effect of copper and its compounds, accidental (unintentional)**
Toxic effects of copper and its compounds NOS

² ✓7ᵗʰ **T56.4X2 Toxic effect of copper and its compounds, intentional self-harm** HCC Rx ESR COM

✓7ᵗʰ **T56.4X3 Toxic effect of copper and its compounds, assault**

✓7ᵗʰ **T56.4X4 Toxic effect of copper and its compounds, undetermined**

✓5ᵗʰ **T56.5 Toxic effects of zinc and its compounds**

✓6ᵗʰ **T56.5X Toxic effects of zinc and its compounds**

✓7ᵗʰ **T56.5X1 Toxic effect of zinc and its compounds, accidental (unintentional)**
Toxic effects of zinc and its compounds NOS

² ✓7ᵗʰ **T56.5X2 Toxic effect of zinc and its compounds, intentional self-harm** HCC Rx ESR COM

✓7ᵗʰ **T56.5X3 Toxic effect of zinc and its compounds, assault**

✓7ᵗʰ **T56.5X4 Toxic effect of zinc and its compounds, undetermined**

✓5ᵗʰ **T56.6 Toxic effects of tin and its compounds**

✓6ᵗʰ **T56.6X Toxic effects of tin and its compounds**

✓7ᵗʰ **T56.6X1 Toxic effect of tin and its compounds, accidental (unintentional)**
Toxic effects of tin and its compounds NOS

² ✓7ᵗʰ **T56.6X2 Toxic effect of tin and its compounds, intentional self-harm** HCC Rx ESR COM

✓7ᵗʰ **T56.6X3 Toxic effect of tin and its compounds, assault**

✓7ᵗʰ **T56.6X4 Toxic effect of tin and its compounds, undetermined**

✓5ᵗʰ **T56.7 Toxic effects of beryllium and its compounds**

✓6ᵗʰ **T56.7X Toxic effects of beryllium and its compounds**

✓7ᵗʰ **T56.7X1 Toxic effect of beryllium and its compounds, accidental (unintentional)**
Toxic effects of beryllium and its compounds NOS

² ✓7ᵗʰ **T56.7X2 Toxic effect of beryllium and its compounds, intentional self-harm** HCC Rx ESR COM

✓7ᵗʰ **T56.7X3 Toxic effect of beryllium and its compounds, assault**

✓7ᵗʰ **T56.7X4 Toxic effect of beryllium and its compounds, undetermined**

✓5ᵗʰ **T56.8 Toxic effects of other metals**

✓6ᵗʰ **T56.81 Toxic effect of thallium**

✓7ᵗʰ **T56.811 Toxic effect of thallium, accidental (unintentional)**
Toxic effect of thallium NOS

² ✓7ᵗʰ **T56.812 Toxic effect of thallium, intentional self-harm** HCC Rx ESR COM

✓7ᵗʰ **T56.813 Toxic effect of thallium, assault**

✓7ᵗʰ **T56.814 Toxic effect of thallium, undetermined**

✓6ᵗʰ **T56.89 Toxic effects of other metals**

✓7ᵗʰ **T56.891 Toxic effect of other metals, accidental (unintentional)**
Toxic effect of other metals NOS

² ✓7ᵗʰ **T56.892 Toxic effect of other metals, intentional self-harm** HCC Rx ESR COM

✓7ᵗʰ **T56.893 Toxic effect of other metals, assault**

✓7ᵗʰ **T56.894** Toxic effect of other metals, undetermined

✓5ᵗʰ **T56.9** Toxic effects of unspecified metal

✓x7ᵗʰ **T56.91** Toxic effect of unspecified metal, accidental (unintentional)

² ✓x7ᵗʰ **T56.92** Toxic effect of unspecified metal, intentional self-harm HCC Rx ESR COM

✓x7ᵗʰ **T56.93** Toxic effect of unspecified metal, assault

✓x7ᵗʰ **T56.94** Toxic effect of unspecified metal, undetermined

✓4ᵗʰ **T57** Toxic effect of other inorganic substances

The appropriate 7th character is to be added to each code from category T57.
A   initial encounter
D   subsequent encounter
S   sequela

✓5ᵗʰ **T57.0** Toxic effect of arsenic and its compounds

✓6ᵗʰ **T57.0X** Toxic effect of arsenic and its compounds

✓7ᵗʰ **T57.0X1** Toxic effect of arsenic and its compounds, accidental (unintentional)
Toxic effect of arsenic and its compounds NOS

² ✓7ᵗʰ **T57.0X2** Toxic effect of arsenic and its compounds, intentional self-harm HCC Rx ESR COM

✓7ᵗʰ **T57.0X3** Toxic effect of arsenic and its compounds, assault

✓7ᵗʰ **T57.0X4** Toxic effect of arsenic and its compounds, undetermined

✓5ᵗʰ **T57.1** Toxic effect of phosphorus and its compounds

EXCLUDES 1   organophosphate insecticides (T60.0)

✓6ᵗʰ **T57.1X** Toxic effect of phosphorus and its compounds

✓7ᵗʰ **T57.1X1** Toxic effect of phosphorus and its compounds, accidental (unintentional)
Toxic effect of phosphorus and its compounds NOS

² ✓7ᵗʰ **T57.1X2** Toxic effect of phosphorus and its compounds, intentional self-harm HCC Rx ESR COM

✓7ᵗʰ **T57.1X3** Toxic effect of phosphorus and its compounds, assault

✓7ᵗʰ **T57.1X4** Toxic effect of phosphorus and its compounds, undetermined

✓5ᵗʰ **T57.2** Toxic effect of manganese and its compounds

✓6ᵗʰ **T57.2X** Toxic effect of manganese and its compounds

✓7ᵗʰ **T57.2X1** Toxic effect of manganese and its compounds, accidental (unintentional)
Toxic effect of manganese and its compounds NOS

² ✓7ᵗʰ **T57.2X2** Toxic effect of manganese and its compounds, intentional self-harm HCC Rx ESR COM

✓7ᵗʰ **T57.2X3** Toxic effect of manganese and its compounds, assault

✓7ᵗʰ **T57.2X4** Toxic effect of manganese and its compounds, undetermined

✓5ᵗʰ **T57.3** Toxic effect of hydrogen cyanide

✓6ᵗʰ **T57.3X** Toxic effect of hydrogen cyanide

✓7ᵗʰ **T57.3X1** Toxic effect of hydrogen cyanide, accidental (unintentional)
Toxic effect of hydrogen cyanide NOS

² ✓7ᵗʰ **T57.3X2** Toxic effect of hydrogen cyanide, intentional self-harm HCC Rx ESR COM

✓7ᵗʰ **T57.3X3** Toxic effect of hydrogen cyanide, assault

✓7ᵗʰ **T57.3X4** Toxic effect of hydrogen cyanide, undetermined

✓5ᵗʰ **T57.8** Toxic effect of other specified inorganic substances

✓6ᵗʰ **T57.8X** Toxic effect of other specified inorganic substances

✓7ᵗʰ **T57.8X1** Toxic effect of other specified inorganic substances, accidental (unintentional)
Toxic effect of other specified inorganic substances NOS

² ✓7ᵗʰ **T57.8X2** Toxic effect of other specified inorganic substances, intentional self-harm HCC Rx ESR COM

✓7ᵗʰ **T57.8X3** Toxic effect of other specified inorganic substances, assault

✓7ᵗʰ **T57.8X4** Toxic effect of other specified inorganic substances, undetermined

✓5ᵗʰ **T57.9** Toxic effect of unspecified inorganic substance

✓x7ᵗʰ **T57.91** Toxic effect of unspecified inorganic substance, accidental (unintentional)

² ✓x7ᵗʰ **T57.92** Toxic effect of unspecified inorganic substance, intentional self-harm HCC Rx ESR COM

✓x7ᵗʰ **T57.93** Toxic effect of unspecified inorganic substance, assault

✓x7ᵗʰ **T57.94** Toxic effect of unspecified inorganic substance, undetermined

✓4ᵗʰ **T58** Toxic effect of carbon monoxide

INCLUDES   asphyxiation from carbon monoxide
toxic effect of carbon monoxide from all sources

The appropriate 7th character is to be added to each code from category T58.
A   initial encounter
D   subsequent encounter
S   sequela

✓5ᵗʰ **T58.0** Toxic effect of carbon monoxide from motor vehicle exhaust
Toxic effect of exhaust gas from gas engine
Toxic effect of exhaust gas from motor pump

✓x7ᵗʰ **T58.01** Toxic effect of carbon monoxide from motor vehicle exhaust, accidental (unintentional)

² ✓x7ᵗʰ **T58.02** Toxic effect of carbon monoxide from motor vehicle exhaust, intentional self-harm HCC Rx ESR COM

✓x7ᵗʰ **T58.03** Toxic effect of carbon monoxide from motor vehicle exhaust, assault

✓x7ᵗʰ **T58.04** Toxic effect of carbon monoxide from motor vehicle exhaust, undetermined

✓5ᵗʰ **T58.1** Toxic effect of carbon monoxide from utility gas
Toxic effect of acetylene
Toxic effect of gas NOS used for lighting, heating, cooking
Toxic effect of water gas

✓x7ᵗʰ **T58.11** Toxic effect of carbon monoxide from utility gas, accidental (unintentional)

² ✓x7ᵗʰ **T58.12** Toxic effect of carbon monoxide from utility gas, intentional self-harm HCC Rx ESR COM

✓x7ᵗʰ **T58.13** Toxic effect of carbon monoxide from utility gas, assault

✓x7ᵗʰ **T58.14** Toxic effect of carbon monoxide from utility gas, undetermined

✓5ᵗʰ **T58.2** Toxic effect of carbon monoxide from incomplete combustion of other domestic fuels
Toxic effect of carbon monoxide from incomplete combustion of coal, coke, kerosene, wood

✓6ᵗʰ **T58.2X** Toxic effect of carbon monoxide from incomplete combustion of other domestic fuels

✓7ᵗʰ **T58.2X1** Toxic effect of carbon monoxide from incomplete combustion of other domestic fuels, accidental (unintentional)

² ✓7ᵗʰ **T58.2X2** Toxic effect of carbon monoxide from incomplete combustion of other domestic fuels, intentional self-harm HCC Rx ESR COM

✓7ᵗʰ **T58.2X3** Toxic effect of carbon monoxide from incomplete combustion of other domestic fuels, assault

✓7ᵗʰ **T58.2X4** Toxic effect of carbon monoxide from incomplete combustion of other domestic fuels, undetermined

✓5ᵗʰ **T58.8** Toxic effect of carbon monoxide from other source
Toxic effect of carbon monoxide from blast furnace gas
Toxic effect of carbon monoxide from fuels in industrial use
Toxic effect of carbon monoxide from kiln vapor

✓6ᵗʰ **T58.8X** Toxic effect of carbon monoxide from other source

✓7ᵗʰ **T58.8X1** Toxic effect of carbon monoxide from other source, accidental (unintentional)

² ✓7ᵗʰ **T58.8X2** Toxic effect of carbon monoxide from other source, intentional self-harm HCC Rx ESR COM

✓7ᵗʰ **T58.8X3** Toxic effect of carbon monoxide from other source, assault

✓7ᵗʰ **T58.8X4** Toxic effect of carbon monoxide from other source, undetermined

✓5ᵗʰ **T58.9** Toxic effect of carbon monoxide from unspecified source

✓x7ᵗʰ **T58.91** Toxic effect of carbon monoxide from unspecified source, accidental (unintentional)

² ✓x7ᵗʰ **T58.92** Toxic effect of carbon monoxide from unspecified source, intentional self-harm HCC Rx ESR COM

√x7ᵗʰ **T58.93** **Toxic effect of carbon monoxide from unspecified source,** assault

√x7ᵗʰ **T58.94** **Toxic effect of carbon monoxide from unspecified source,** undetermined

√4ᵗʰ **T59** **Toxic effect of other gases, fumes and vapors**

    INCLUDES   aerosol propellants

    EXCLUDES 1   *chlorofluorocarbons (T53.5)*

> The appropriate 7th character is to be added to each code from category T59.
> A   initial encounter
> D   subsequent encounter
> S   sequela

√5ᵗʰ **T59.0** **Toxic effect of nitrogen oxides**

   √6ᵗʰ **T59.0X** **Toxic effect of** nitrogen oxides

     √7ᵗʰ **T59.0X1** **Toxic effect of nitrogen oxides,** accidental (unintentional)

       Toxic effect of nitrogen oxides NOS

    ² √7ᵗʰ **T59.0X2** **Toxic effect of nitrogen oxides, intentional self-harm** HCC Rx ESR COM

     √7ᵗʰ **T59.0X3** **Toxic effect of nitrogen oxides,** assault

     √7ᵗʰ **T59.0X4** **Toxic effect of nitrogen oxides,** undetermined

√5ᵗʰ **T59.1** **Toxic effect of sulfur dioxide**

   √6ᵗʰ **T59.1X** **Toxic effect of** sulfur dioxide

     √7ᵗʰ **T59.1X1** **Toxic effect of sulfur dioxide,** accidental (unintentional)

       Toxic effect of sulfur dioxide NOS

    ² √7ᵗʰ **T59.1X2** **Toxic effect of sulfur dioxide, intentional self-harm** HCC Rx ESR COM

     √7ᵗʰ **T59.1X3** **Toxic effect of sulfur dioxide,** assault

     √7ᵗʰ **T59.1X4** **Toxic effect of sulfur dioxide,** undetermined

√5ᵗʰ **T59.2** **Toxic effect of formaldehyde**

   √6ᵗʰ **T59.2X** **Toxic effect of** formaldehyde

     √7ᵗʰ **T59.2X1** **Toxic effect of formaldehyde,** accidental (unintentional)

       Toxic effect of formaldehyde NOS

    ² √7ᵗʰ **T59.2X2** **Toxic effect of formaldehyde, intentional self-harm** HCC Rx ESR COM

     √7ᵗʰ **T59.2X3** **Toxic effect of formaldehyde,** assault

     √7ᵗʰ **T59.2X4** **Toxic effect of formaldehyde,** undetermined

√5ᵗʰ **T59.3** **Toxic effect of lacrimogenic gas**

   Toxic effect of tear gas

   √6ᵗʰ **T59.3X** **Toxic effect of** lacrimogenic gas

     √7ᵗʰ **T59.3X1** **Toxic effect of lacrimogenic gas,** accidental (unintentional)

       Toxic effect of lacrimogenic gas NOS

    ² √7ᵗʰ **T59.3X2** **Toxic effect of lacrimogenic gas, intentional self-harm** HCC Rx ESR COM

     √7ᵗʰ **T59.3X3** **Toxic effect of lacrimogenic gas,** assault

     √7ᵗʰ **T59.3X4** **Toxic effect of lacrimogenic gas,** undetermined

√5ᵗʰ **T59.4** **Toxic effect of chlorine gas**

   √6ᵗʰ **T59.4X** **Toxic effect of** chlorine gas

     √7ᵗʰ **T59.4X1** **Toxic effect of chlorine gas,** accidental (unintentional)

       Toxic effect of chlorine gas NOS

    ² √7ᵗʰ **T59.4X2** **Toxic effect of chlorine gas, intentional self-harm** HCC Rx ESR COM

     √7ᵗʰ **T59.4X3** **Toxic effect of chlorine gas,** assault

     √7ᵗʰ **T59.4X4** **Toxic effect of chlorine gas,** undetermined

√5ᵗʰ **T59.5** **Toxic effect of fluorine gas and hydrogen fluoride**

   √6ᵗʰ **T59.5X** **Toxic effect of** fluorine gas and hydrogen fluoride

     √7ᵗʰ **T59.5X1** **Toxic effect of fluorine gas and hydrogen fluoride,** accidental (unintentional)

       Toxic effect of fluorine gas and hydrogen fluoride NOS

    ² √7ᵗʰ **T59.5X2** **Toxic effect of fluorine gas and hydrogen fluoride, intentional self-harm** HCC Rx ESR COM

     √7ᵗʰ **T59.5X3** **Toxic effect of fluorine gas and hydrogen fluoride,** assault

     √7ᵗʰ **T59.5X4** **Toxic effect of fluorine gas and hydrogen fluoride,** undetermined

√5ᵗʰ **T59.6** **Toxic effect of hydrogen sulfide**

   √6ᵗʰ **T59.6X** **Toxic effect of** hydrogen sulfide

     √7ᵗʰ **T59.6X1** **Toxic effect of hydrogen sulfide,** accidental (unintentional)

       Toxic effect of hydrogen sulfide NOS

    ² √7ᵗʰ **T59.6X2** **Toxic effect of hydrogen sulfide, intentional self-harm** HCC Rx ESR COM

     √7ᵗʰ **T59.6X3** **Toxic effect of hydrogen sulfide,** assault

     √7ᵗʰ **T59.6X4** **Toxic effect of hydrogen sulfide,** undetermined

√5ᵗʰ **T59.7** **Toxic effect of carbon dioxide**

   √6ᵗʰ **T59.7X** **Toxic effect of** carbon dioxide

     √7ᵗʰ **T59.7X1** **Toxic effect of carbon dioxide,** accidental (unintentional)

       Toxic effect of carbon dioxide NOS

    ² √7ᵗʰ **T59.7X2** **Toxic effect of carbon dioxide, intentional self-harm** HCC Rx ESR COM

     √7ᵗʰ **T59.7X3** **Toxic effect of carbon dioxide,** assault

     √7ᵗʰ **T59.7X4** **Toxic effect of carbon dioxide,** undetermined

√5ᵗʰ **T59.8** **Toxic effect of other specified gases, fumes and vapors**

   √6ᵗʰ **T59.81** **Toxic effect of** smoke

     Smoke inhalation

     EXCLUDES 2   *toxic effect of cigarette (tobacco) smoke (T65.22-)*

     √7ᵗʰ **T59.811** **Toxic effect of smoke,** accidental (unintentional)

       Toxic effect of smoke NOS

       AHA: 2013,4Q,121

    ² √7ᵗʰ **T59.812** **Toxic effect of smoke, intentional self-harm** HCC Rx ESR COM

     √7ᵗʰ **T59.813** **Toxic effect of smoke,** assault

     √7ᵗʰ **T59.814** **Toxic effect of smoke,** undetermined

   √6ᵗʰ **T59.89** **Toxic effect of other specified gases, fumes and vapors**

     √7ᵗʰ **T59.891** **Toxic effect of other specified gases, fumes and vapors,** accidental (unintentional)

    ² √7ᵗʰ **T59.892** **Toxic effect of other specified gases, fumes and vapors, intentional self-harm** HCC Rx ESR COM

     √7ᵗʰ **T59.893** **Toxic effect of other specified gases, fumes and vapors,** assault

     √7ᵗʰ **T59.894** **Toxic effect of other specified gases, fumes and vapors,** undetermined

√5ᵗʰ **T59.9** **Toxic effect of unspecified gases, fumes and vapors**

   √x7ᵗʰ **T59.91** **Toxic effect of unspecified gases, fumes and vapors, accidental (unintentional)**

   ² √x7ᵗʰ **T59.92** **Toxic effect of unspecified gases, fumes and vapors, intentional self-harm** HCC Rx ESR COM

   √x7ᵗʰ **T59.93** **Toxic effect of unspecified gases, fumes and vapors, assault**

   √x7ᵗʰ **T59.94** **Toxic effect of unspecified gases, fumes and vapors, undetermined**

√4ᵗʰ **T60** **Toxic effect of pesticides**

    INCLUDES   toxic effect of wood preservatives

> The appropriate 7th character is to be added to each code from category T60.
> A   initial encounter
> D   subsequent encounter
> S   sequela

√5ᵗʰ **T60.0** **Toxic effect of organophosphate and carbamate insecticides**

   √6ᵗʰ **T60.0X** **Toxic effect of** organophosphate and carbamate insecticides

     √7ᵗʰ **T60.0X1** **Toxic effect of organophosphate and carbamate insecticides,** accidental (unintentional)

       Toxic effect of organophosphate and carbamate insecticides NOS

    ² √7ᵗʰ **T60.0X2** **Toxic effect of organophosphate and carbamate insecticides, intentional self-harm** HCC Rx ESR COM

     √7ᵗʰ **T60.0X3** **Toxic effect of organophosphate and carbamate insecticides,** assault

     √7ᵗʰ **T60.0X4** **Toxic effect of organophosphate and carbamate insecticides,** undetermined

---

✔ Additional Character Required   √x7ᵗʰ Placeholder Alert   Manifestation   Unspecified Dx   Q QPP   UPD Unacceptable PDx

✓5ᵗʰ **T60.1 Toxic effect of halogenated insecticides**
    EXCLUDES 1   *chlorinated hydrocarbon (T53.-)*

  ✓6ᵗʰ **T60.1X Toxic effect of** halogenated insecticides

    ✓7ᵗʰ **T60.1X1 Toxic effect of halogenated insecticides,** accidental **(unintentional)**
         Toxic effect of halogenated insecticides NOS

    ² ✓7ᵗʰ **T60.1X2 Toxic effect of halogenated insecticides,** intentional self-harm   HCC Rx ESR COM

    ✓7ᵗʰ **T60.1X3 Toxic effect of halogenated insecticides,** assault

    ✓7ᵗʰ **T60.1X4 Toxic effect of halogenated insecticides,** undetermined

✓5ᵗʰ **T60.2 Toxic effect of other insecticides**

  ✓6ᵗʰ **T60.2X Toxic effect of** other insecticides

    ✓7ᵗʰ **T60.2X1 Toxic effect of other insecticides,** accidental **(unintentional)**
         Toxic effect of other insecticides NOS

    ² ✓7ᵗʰ **T60.2X2 Toxic effect of other insecticides,** intentional self-harm   HCC Rx ESR COM

    ✓7ᵗʰ **T60.2X3 Toxic effect of other insecticides,** assault

    ✓7ᵗʰ **T60.2X4 Toxic effect of other insecticides,** undetermined

✓5ᵗʰ **T60.3 Toxic effect of herbicides and fungicides**

  ✓6ᵗʰ **T60.3X Toxic effect of** herbicides and fungicides

    ✓7ᵗʰ **T60.3X1 Toxic effect of herbicides and fungicides,** accidental **(unintentional)**
         Toxic effect of herbicides and fungicides NOS

    ² ✓7ᵗʰ **T60.3X2 Toxic effect of herbicides and fungicides,** intentional self-harm   HCC Rx ESR COM

    ✓7ᵗʰ **T60.3X3 Toxic effect of herbicides and fungicides,** assault

    ✓7ᵗʰ **T60.3X4 Toxic effect of herbicides and fungicides,** undetermined

✓5ᵗʰ **T60.4 Toxic effect of rodenticides**
    EXCLUDES 1   *strychnine and its salts (T65.1)*
                thallium (T56.81-)

  ✓6ᵗʰ **T60.4X Toxic effect of** rodenticides

    ✓7ᵗʰ **T60.4X1 Toxic effect of rodenticides,** accidental **(unintentional)**
         Toxic effect of rodenticides NOS

    ² ✓7ᵗʰ **T60.4X2 Toxic effect of rodenticides,** intentional self-harm   HCC Rx ESR COM

    ✓7ᵗʰ **T60.4X3 Toxic effect of rodenticides,** assault

    ✓7ᵗʰ **T60.4X4 Toxic effect of rodenticides,** undetermined

✓5ᵗʰ **T60.8 Toxic effect of other pesticides**

  ✓6ᵗʰ **T60.8X Toxic effect of** other pesticides

    ✓7ᵗʰ **T60.8X1 Toxic effect of other pesticides,** accidental **(unintentional)**
         Toxic effect of other pesticides NOS

    ² ✓7ᵗʰ **T60.8X2 Toxic effect of other pesticides,** intentional self-harm   HCC Rx ESR COM

    ✓7ᵗʰ **T60.8X3 Toxic effect of other pesticides,** assault

    ✓7ᵗʰ **T60.8X4 Toxic effect of other pesticides,** undetermined

✓5ᵗʰ **T60.9 Toxic effect of unspecified pesticide**

  ✓x7ᵗʰ **T60.91 Toxic effect of unspecified pesticide,** accidental **(unintentional)**

  ² ✓x7ᵗʰ **T60.92 Toxic effect of unspecified pesticide,** intentional self-harm   HCC Rx ESR COM

  ✓x7ᵗʰ **T60.93 Toxic effect of unspecified pesticide,** assault

  ✓x7ᵗʰ **T60.94 Toxic effect of unspecified pesticide,** undetermined

---

✓4ᵗʰ **T61 Toxic effect of noxious substances eaten as seafood**
    EXCLUDES 1   *allergic reaction to food, such as:*
         anaphylactic reaction or shock due to adverse food reaction (T78.0-)
         bacterial foodborne intoxications (A05.-)
         dermatitis (L23.6, L25.4, L27.2)
         food protein-induced enterocolitis syndrome (K52.21)
         food protein-induced enteropathy (K52.22)
         gastroenteritis (noninfective) (K52.29)
       toxic effect of aflatoxin and other mycotoxins (T64)
       toxic effect of cyanides (T65.0-)
       toxic effect of harmful algae bloom (T65.82-)
       toxic effect of hydrogen cyanide (T57.3-)
       toxic effect of mercury (T56.1-)
       toxic effect of red tide (T65.82-)

> The appropriate 7th character is to be added to each code from category T61.
> A   initial encounter
> D   subsequent encounter
> S   sequela

✓5ᵗʰ **T61.0 Ciguatera fish poisoning**

  ✓x7ᵗʰ **T61.01 Ciguatera fish poisoning,** accidental **(unintentional)**

  ² ✓x7ᵗʰ **T61.02 Ciguatera fish poisoning,** intentional self-harm   HCC Rx ESR COM

  ✓x7ᵗʰ **T61.03 Ciguatera fish poisoning,** assault

  ✓x7ᵗʰ **T61.04 Ciguatera fish poisoning,** undetermined

✓5ᵗʰ **T61.1 Scombroid fish poisoning**
     Histamine-like syndrome

  ✓x7ᵗʰ **T61.11 Scombroid fish poisoning,** accidental **(unintentional)**

  ² ✓x7ᵗʰ **T61.12 Scombroid fish poisoning,** intentional self-harm   HCC Rx ESR COM

  ✓x7ᵗʰ **T61.13 Scombroid fish poisoning,** assault

  ✓x7ᵗʰ **T61.14 Scombroid fish poisoning,** undetermined

✓5ᵗʰ **T61.7 Other fish and shellfish poisoning**

  ✓6ᵗʰ **T61.77 Other** fish **poisoning**

    ✓7ᵗʰ **T61.771 Other fish poisoning,** accidental **(unintentional)**

    ² ✓7ᵗʰ **T61.772 Other fish poisoning,** intentional self-harm   HCC Rx ESR COM

    ✓7ᵗʰ **T61.773 Other fish poisoning,** assault

    ✓7ᵗʰ **T61.774 Other fish poisoning,** undetermined

  ✓6ᵗʰ **T61.78 Other** shellfish **poisoning**

    ✓7ᵗʰ **T61.781 Other shellfish poisoning,** accidental **(unintentional)**

    ² ✓7ᵗʰ **T61.782 Other shellfish poisoning,** intentional self-harm   HCC Rx ESR COM

    ✓7ᵗʰ **T61.783 Other shellfish poisoning,** assault

    ✓7ᵗʰ **T61.784 Other shellfish poisoning,** undetermined

✓5ᵗʰ **T61.8 Toxic effect of other seafood**

  ✓6ᵗʰ **T61.8X Toxic effect of other seafood**

    ✓7ᵗʰ **T61.8X1 Toxic effect of other seafood,** accidental **(unintentional)**

    ² ✓7ᵗʰ **T61.8X2 Toxic effect of other seafood,** intentional self-harm   HCC Rx ESR COM

    ✓7ᵗʰ **T61.8X3 Toxic effect of other seafood,** assault

    ✓7ᵗʰ **T61.8X4 Toxic effect of other seafood,** undetermined

✓5ᵗʰ **T61.9 Toxic effect of unspecified seafood**

  ✓x7ᵗʰ **T61.91 Toxic effect of unspecified seafood,** accidental **(unintentional)**

  ² ✓x7ᵗʰ **T61.92 Toxic effect of unspecified seafood,** intentional self-harm   HCC Rx ESR COM

  ✓x7ᵗʰ **T61.93 Toxic effect of unspecified seafood,** assault

  ✓x7ᵗʰ **T61.94 Toxic effect of unspecified seafood,** undetermined

✓4ᵗʰ **T62 Toxic effect of other noxious substances eaten as food**

    EXCLUDES 1   allergic reaction to food, such as:
              anaphylactic shock (reaction) due to adverse food reaction (T78.0-)
              bacterial food borne intoxications (A05.-)
              dermatitis (L23.6, L25.4, L27.2)
              food protein-induced enterocolitis syndrome (K52.21)
              food protein-induced enteropathy (K52.22)
              gastroenteritis (noninfective) (K52.29)
              toxic effect of aflatoxin and other mycotoxins (T64)
              toxic effect of cyanides (T65.0-)
              toxic effect of hydrogen cyanide (T57.3-)
              toxic effect of mercury (T56.1-)

> The appropriate 7th character is to be added to each code from category T62.
> A   initial encounter
> D   subsequent encounter
> S   sequela

✓5ᵗʰ **T62.0 Toxic effect of ingested mushrooms**

    ✓6ᵗʰ **T62.0X Toxic effect of** ingested mushrooms

       ✓7ᵗʰ **T62.0X1 Toxic effect of ingested mushrooms, accidental (unintentional)**
          Toxic effect of ingested mushrooms NOS

       2 ✓7ᵗʰ **T62.0X2 Toxic effect of ingested mushrooms, intentional self-harm** HCC Rx ESR COM

       ✓7ᵗʰ **T62.0X3 Toxic effect of ingested mushrooms, assault**

       ✓7ᵗʰ **T62.0X4 Toxic effect of ingested mushrooms, undetermined**

✓5ᵗʰ **T62.1 Toxic effect of ingested berries**

    ✓6ᵗʰ **T62.1X Toxic effect of** ingested berries

       ✓7ᵗʰ **T62.1X1 Toxic effect of ingested berries, accidental (unintentional)**
          Toxic effect of ingested berries NOS

       2 ✓7ᵗʰ **T62.1X2 Toxic effect of ingested berries, intentional self-harm** HCC Rx ESR COM

       ✓7ᵗʰ **T62.1X3 Toxic effect of ingested berries, assault**

       ✓7ᵗʰ **T62.1X4 Toxic effect of ingested berries, undetermined**

✓5ᵗʰ **T62.2 Toxic effect of other ingested (parts of) plant(s)**

    ✓6ᵗʰ **T62.2X Toxic effect of** other ingested (parts of) plant(s)

       ✓7ᵗʰ **T62.2X1 Toxic effect of other ingested (parts of) plant(s), accidental (unintentional)**
          Toxic effect of other ingested (parts of) plant(s) NOS

       2 ✓7ᵗʰ **T62.2X2 Toxic effect of other ingested (parts of) plant(s), intentional self-harm** HCC Rx ESR COM

       ✓7ᵗʰ **T62.2X3 Toxic effect of other ingested (parts of) plant(s), assault**

       ✓7ᵗʰ **T62.2X4 Toxic effect of other ingested (parts of) plant(s), undetermined**

✓5ᵗʰ **T62.8 Toxic effect of other specified noxious substances eaten as food**

    ✓6ᵗʰ **T62.8X Toxic effect of other specified noxious substances eaten as food**

       ✓7ᵗʰ **T62.8X1 Toxic effect of other specified noxious substances eaten as food, accidental (unintentional)**
          Toxic effect of other specified noxious substances eaten as food NOS

       2 ✓7ᵗʰ **T62.8X2 Toxic effect of other specified noxious substances eaten as food, intentional self-harm** HCC Rx ESR COM

       ✓7ᵗʰ **T62.8X3 Toxic effect of other specified noxious substances eaten as food, assault**

       ✓7ᵗʰ **T62.8X4 Toxic effect of other specified noxious substances eaten as food, undetermined**

✓5ᵗʰ **T62.9 Toxic effect of unspecified noxious substance eaten as food**

    ✓x7ᵗʰ **T62.91 Toxic effect of unspecified noxious substance eaten as food, accidental (unintentional)**
       Toxic effect of unspecified noxious substance eaten as food NOS

    2 ✓x7ᵗʰ **T62.92 Toxic effect of unspecified noxious substance eaten as food, intentional self-harm** HCC Rx ESR COM

    ✓x7ᵗʰ **T62.93 Toxic effect of unspecified noxious substance eaten as food, assault**

    ✓x7ᵗʰ **T62.94 Toxic effect of unspecified noxious substance eaten as food, undetermined**

✓4ᵗʰ **T63 Toxic effect of contact with venomous animals and plants**

    INCLUDES   bite or touch of venomous animal
            pricked or stuck by thorn or leaf
    EXCLUDES 2   ingestion of toxic animal or plant (T61.-, T62.-)

> The appropriate 7th character is to be added to each code from category T63.
> A   initial encounter
> D   subsequent encounter
> S   sequela

✓5ᵗʰ **T63.0 Toxic effect of** snake venom

    ✓6ᵗʰ **T63.00 Toxic effect of unspecified snake venom**

       ✓7ᵗʰ **T63.001 Toxic effect of unspecified snake venom, accidental (unintentional)**
          Toxic effect of unspecified snake venom NOS

       2 ✓7ᵗʰ **T63.002 Toxic effect of unspecified snake venom, intentional self-harm** HCC Rx ESR COM

       ✓7ᵗʰ **T63.003 Toxic effect of unspecified snake venom, assault**

       ✓7ᵗʰ **T63.004 Toxic effect of unspecified snake venom, undetermined**

    ✓6ᵗʰ **T63.01 Toxic effect of** rattlesnake venom

       ✓7ᵗʰ **T63.011 Toxic effect of rattlesnake venom, accidental (unintentional)**
          Toxic effect of rattlesnake venom NOS

       2 ✓7ᵗʰ **T63.012 Toxic effect of rattlesnake venom, intentional self-harm** HCC Rx ESR COM

       ✓7ᵗʰ **T63.013 Toxic effect of rattlesnake venom,** assault

       ✓7ᵗʰ **T63.014 Toxic effect of rattlesnake venom, undetermined**

    ✓6ᵗʰ **T63.02 Toxic effect of** coral snake venom

       ✓7ᵗʰ **T63.021 Toxic effect of coral snake venom, accidental (unintentional)**
          Toxic effect of coral snake venom NOS

       2 ✓7ᵗʰ **T63.022 Toxic effect of coral snake venom, intentional self-harm** HCC Rx ESR COM

       ✓7ᵗʰ **T63.023 Toxic effect of coral snake venom,** assault

       ✓7ᵗʰ **T63.024 Toxic effect of coral snake venom, undetermined**

    ✓6ᵗʰ **T63.03 Toxic effect of** taipan venom

       ✓7ᵗʰ **T63.031 Toxic effect of taipan venom, accidental (unintentional)**
          Toxic effect of taipan venom NOS

       2 ✓7ᵗʰ **T63.032 Toxic effect of taipan venom, intentional self-harm** HCC Rx ESR COM

       ✓7ᵗʰ **T63.033 Toxic effect of taipan venom, assault**

       ✓7ᵗʰ **T63.034 Toxic effect of taipan venom, undetermined**

    ✓6ᵗʰ **T63.04 Toxic effect of** cobra venom

       ✓7ᵗʰ **T63.041 Toxic effect of cobra venom, accidental (unintentional)**
          Toxic effect of cobra venom NOS

       2 ✓7ᵗʰ **T63.042 Toxic effect of cobra venom, intentional self-harm** HCC Rx ESR COM

       ✓7ᵗʰ **T63.043 Toxic effect of cobra venom, assault**

       ✓7ᵗʰ **T63.044 Toxic effect of cobra venom, undetermined**

    ✓6ᵗʰ **T63.06 Toxic effect of venom of** other North and South American snake

       ✓7ᵗʰ **T63.061 Toxic effect of venom of other North and South American snake, accidental (unintentional)**
          Toxic effect of venom of other North and South American snake NOS

       2 ✓7ᵗʰ **T63.062 Toxic effect of venom of other North and South American snake, intentional self-harm** HCC Rx ESR COM

       ✓7ᵗʰ **T63.063 Toxic effect of venom of other North and South American snake, assault**

       ✓7ᵗʰ **T63.064 Toxic effect of venom of other North and South American snake, undetermined**

√6ᵗʰ **T63.07** Toxic effect of venom of other Australian snake

    √7ᵗʰ **T63.071** Toxic effect of venom of other Australian snake, **accidental (unintentional)**
       Toxic effect of venom of other Australian snake NOS

    ² √7ᵗʰ **T63.072** Toxic effect of venom of other Australian snake, **intentional self-harm**   HCC Rx ESR COM

    √7ᵗʰ **T63.073** Toxic effect of venom of other Australian snake, **assault**

    √7ᵗʰ **T63.074** Toxic effect of venom of other Australian snake, **undetermined**

√6ᵗʰ **T63.08** Toxic effect of venom of other African and Asian snake

    √7ᵗʰ **T63.081** Toxic effect of venom of other African and Asian snake, **accidental (unintentional)**
       Toxic effect of venom of other African and Asian snake NOS

    ² √7ᵗʰ **T63.082** Toxic effect of venom of other African and Asian snake, **intentional self-harm**   HCC Rx ESR COM

    √7ᵗʰ **T63.083** Toxic effect of venom of other African and Asian snake, **assault**

    √7ᵗʰ **T63.084** Toxic effect of venom of other African and Asian snake, **undetermined**

√6ᵗʰ **T63.09** Toxic effect of venom of other snake

    √7ᵗʰ **T63.091** Toxic effect of venom of other snake, **accidental (unintentional)**
       Toxic effect of venom of other snake NOS

    ² √7ᵗʰ **T63.092** Toxic effect of venom of other snake, **intentional self-harm**   HCC Rx ESR COM

    √7ᵗʰ **T63.093** Toxic effect of venom of other snake, **assault**

    √7ᵗʰ **T63.094** Toxic effect of venom of other snake, **undetermined**

√5ᵗʰ **T63.1** Toxic effect of venom of other reptiles

   √6ᵗʰ **T63.11** Toxic effect of venom of gila monster

    √7ᵗʰ **T63.111** Toxic effect of venom of gila monster, **accidental (unintentional)**
       Toxic effect of venom of gila monster NOS

    ² √7ᵗʰ **T63.112** Toxic effect of venom of gila monster, **intentional self-harm**   HCC Rx ESR COM

    √7ᵗʰ **T63.113** Toxic effect of venom of gila monster, **assault**

    √7ᵗʰ **T63.114** Toxic effect of venom of gila monster, **undetermined**

   √6ᵗʰ **T63.12** Toxic effect of venom of other venomous lizard

    √7ᵗʰ **T63.121** Toxic effect of venom of other venomous lizard, **accidental (unintentional)**
       Toxic effect of venom of other venomous lizard NOS

    ² √7ᵗʰ **T63.122** Toxic effect of venom of other venomous lizard, **intentional self-harm**   HCC Rx ESR COM

    √7ᵗʰ **T63.123** Toxic effect of venom of other venomous lizard, **assault**

    √7ᵗʰ **T63.124** Toxic effect of venom of other venomous lizard, **undetermined**

   √6ᵗʰ **T63.19** Toxic effect of venom of other reptiles

    √7ᵗʰ **T63.191** Toxic effect of venom of other reptiles, **accidental (unintentional)**
       Toxic effect of venom of other reptiles NOS

    ² √7ᵗʰ **T63.192** Toxic effect of venom of other reptiles, **intentional self-harm**   HCC Rx ESR COM

    √7ᵗʰ **T63.193** Toxic effect of venom of other reptiles, **assault**

    √7ᵗʰ **T63.194** Toxic effect of venom of other reptiles, **undetermined**

√5ᵗʰ **T63.2** Toxic effect of venom of scorpion

   √6ᵗʰ **T63.2X** Toxic effect of venom of scorpion

    √7ᵗʰ **T63.2X1** Toxic effect of venom of scorpion, **accidental (unintentional)**
       Toxic effect of venom of scorpion NOS

    ² √7ᵗʰ **T63.2X2** Toxic effect of venom of scorpion, **intentional self-harm**   HCC Rx ESR COM

    √7ᵗʰ **T63.2X3** Toxic effect of venom of scorpion, **assault**

    √7ᵗʰ **T63.2X4** Toxic effect of venom of scorpion, **undetermined**

√5ᵗʰ **T63.3** Toxic effect of venom of spider

   √6ᵗʰ **T63.30** Toxic effect of unspecified spider venom

    √7ᵗʰ **T63.301** Toxic effect of unspecified spider venom, **accidental (unintentional)**

    ² √7ᵗʰ **T63.302** Toxic effect of unspecified spider venom, **intentional self-harm**   HCC Rx ESR COM

    √7ᵗʰ **T63.303** Toxic effect of unspecified spider venom, **assault**

    √7ᵗʰ **T63.304** Toxic effect of unspecified spider venom, **undetermined**

   √6ᵗʰ **T63.31** Toxic effect of venom of black widow spider

    √7ᵗʰ **T63.311** Toxic effect of venom of black widow spider, **accidental (unintentional)**

    ² √7ᵗʰ **T63.312** Toxic effect of venom of black widow spider, **intentional self-harm**   HCC Rx ESR COM

    √7ᵗʰ **T63.313** Toxic effect of venom of black widow spider, **assault**

    √7ᵗʰ **T63.314** Toxic effect of venom of black widow spider, **undetermined**

   √6ᵗʰ **T63.32** Toxic effect of venom of tarantula

    √7ᵗʰ **T63.321** Toxic effect of venom of tarantula, **accidental (unintentional)**

    ² √7ᵗʰ **T63.322** Toxic effect of venom of tarantula, **intentional self-harm**   HCC Rx ESR COM

    √7ᵗʰ **T63.323** Toxic effect of venom of tarantula, **assault**

    √7ᵗʰ **T63.324** Toxic effect of venom of tarantula, **undetermined**

   √6ᵗʰ **T63.33** Toxic effect of venom of brown recluse spider

    √7ᵗʰ **T63.331** Toxic effect of venom of brown recluse spider, **accidental (unintentional)**

    ² √7ᵗʰ **T63.332** Toxic effect of venom of brown recluse spider, **intentional self-harm**   HCC Rx ESR COM

    √7ᵗʰ **T63.333** Toxic effect of venom of brown recluse spider, **assault**

    √7ᵗʰ **T63.334** Toxic effect of venom of brown recluse spider, **undetermined**

   √6ᵗʰ **T63.39** Toxic effect of venom of other spider

    √7ᵗʰ **T63.391** Toxic effect of venom of other spider, **accidental (unintentional)**

    ² √7ᵗʰ **T63.392** Toxic effect of venom of other spider, **intentional self-harm**   HCC Rx ESR COM

    √7ᵗʰ **T63.393** Toxic effect of venom of other spider, **assault**

    √7ᵗʰ **T63.394** Toxic effect of venom of other spider, **undetermined**

√5ᵗʰ **T63.4** Toxic effect of venom of other arthropods

   √6ᵗʰ **T63.41** Toxic effect of venom of centipedes and venomous millipedes

    √7ᵗʰ **T63.411** Toxic effect of venom of centipedes and venomous millipedes, **accidental (unintentional)**

    ² √7ᵗʰ **T63.412** Toxic effect of venom of centipedes and venomous millipedes, **intentional self-harm**   HCC Rx ESR COM

    √7ᵗʰ **T63.413** Toxic effect of venom of centipedes and venomous millipedes, **assault**

    √7ᵗʰ **T63.414** Toxic effect of venom of centipedes and venomous millipedes, **undetermined**

   √6ᵗʰ **T63.42** Toxic effect of venom of ants

    √7ᵗʰ **T63.421** Toxic effect of venom of ants, **accidental (unintentional)**

    ² √7ᵗʰ **T63.422** Toxic effect of venom of ants, **intentional self-harm**   HCC Rx ESR COM

    √7ᵗʰ **T63.423** Toxic effect of venom of ants, **assault**

    √7ᵗʰ **T63.424** Toxic effect of venom of ants, **undetermined**

   √6ᵗʰ **T63.43** Toxic effect of venom of caterpillars

    √7ᵗʰ **T63.431** Toxic effect of venom of caterpillars, **accidental (unintentional)**

    ² √7ᵗʰ **T63.432** Toxic effect of venom of caterpillars, **intentional self-harm**   HCC Rx ESR COM

    √7ᵗʰ **T63.433** Toxic effect of venom of caterpillars, **assault**

    √7ᵗʰ **T63.434** Toxic effect of venom of caterpillars, **undetermined**

   √6ᵗʰ **T63.44** Toxic effect of venom of bees

    √7ᵗʰ **T63.441** Toxic effect of venom of bees, **accidental (unintentional)**

² √7ᵗʰ **T63.442** Toxic effect of venom of bees, intentional self-harm `HCC` `Rx` `ESR` `COM`

√7ᵗʰ **T63.443** Toxic effect of venom of bees, assault

√7ᵗʰ **T63.444** Toxic effect of venom of bees, undetermined

√6ᵗʰ **T63.45** Toxic effect of venom of hornets

√7ᵗʰ **T63.451** Toxic effect of venom of hornets, accidental (unintentional)

² √7ᵗʰ **T63.452** Toxic effect of venom of hornets, intentional self-harm `HCC` `Rx` `ESR` `COM`

√7ᵗʰ **T63.453** Toxic effect of venom of hornets, assault

√7ᵗʰ **T63.454** Toxic effect of venom of hornets, undetermined

√6ᵗʰ **T63.46** Toxic effect of venom of wasps

     Toxic effect of yellow jacket

√7ᵗʰ **T63.461** Toxic effect of venom of wasps, accidental (unintentional)

² √7ᵗʰ **T63.462** Toxic effect of venom of wasps, intentional self-harm `HCC` `Rx` `ESR` `COM`

√7ᵗʰ **T63.463** Toxic effect of venom of wasps, assault

√7ᵗʰ **T63.464** Toxic effect of venom of wasps, undetermined

√6ᵗʰ **T63.48** Toxic effect of venom of other arthropod

√7ᵗʰ **T63.481** Toxic effect of venom of other arthropod, accidental (unintentional)

² √7ᵗʰ **T63.482** Toxic effect of venom of other arthropod, intentional self-harm `HCC` `Rx` `ESR` `COM`

√7ᵗʰ **T63.483** Toxic effect of venom of other arthropod, assault

√7ᵗʰ **T63.484** Toxic effect of venom of other arthropod, undetermined

√5ᵗʰ **T63.5** Toxic effect of contact with venomous fish

     `EXCLUDES 2`   poisoning by ingestion of fish (T61.-)

√6ᵗʰ **T63.51** Toxic effect of contact with stingray

√7ᵗʰ **T63.511** Toxic effect of contact with stingray, accidental (unintentional)

² √7ᵗʰ **T63.512** Toxic effect of contact with stingray, intentional self-harm `HCC` `Rx` `ESR` `COM`

√7ᵗʰ **T63.513** Toxic effect of contact with stingray, assault

√7ᵗʰ **T63.514** Toxic effect of contact with stingray, undetermined

√6ᵗʰ **T63.59** Toxic effect of contact with other venomous fish

√7ᵗʰ **T63.591** Toxic effect of contact with other venomous fish, accidental (unintentional)

² √7ᵗʰ **T63.592** Toxic effect of contact with other venomous fish, intentional self-harm `HCC` `Rx` `ESR` `COM`

√7ᵗʰ **T63.593** Toxic effect of contact with other venomous fish, assault

√7ᵗʰ **T63.594** Toxic effect of contact with other venomous fish, undetermined

√5ᵗʰ **T63.6** Toxic effect of contact with other venomous marine animals

     `EXCLUDES 1`   sea-snake venom (T63.09)

     `EXCLUDES 2`   poisoning by ingestion of shellfish (T61.78-)

√6ᵗʰ **T63.61** Toxic effect of contact with Portuguese Man-o-war

     Toxic effect of contact with bluebottle

√7ᵗʰ **T63.611** Toxic effect of contact with Portuguese Man-o-war, accidental (unintentional)

² √7ᵗʰ **T63.612** Toxic effect of contact with Portuguese Man-o-war, intentional self-harm `HCC` `Rx` `ESR` `COM`

√7ᵗʰ **T63.613** Toxic effect of contact with Portuguese Man-o-war, assault

√7ᵗʰ **T63.614** Toxic effect of contact with Portuguese Man-o-war, undetermined

√6ᵗʰ **T63.62** Toxic effect of contact with other jellyfish

√7ᵗʰ **T63.621** Toxic effect of contact with other jellyfish, accidental (unintentional)

² √7ᵗʰ **T63.622** Toxic effect of contact with other jellyfish, intentional self-harm `HCC` `Rx` `ESR` `COM`

√7ᵗʰ **T63.623** Toxic effect of contact with other jellyfish, assault

√7ᵗʰ **T63.624** Toxic effect of contact with other jellyfish, undetermined

√6ᵗʰ **T63.63** Toxic effect of contact with sea anemone

√7ᵗʰ **T63.631** Toxic effect of contact with sea anemone, accidental (unintentional)

² √7ᵗʰ **T63.632** Toxic effect of contact with sea anemone, intentional self-harm `HCC` `Rx` `ESR` `COM`

√7ᵗʰ **T63.633** Toxic effect of contact with sea anemone, assault

√7ᵗʰ **T63.634** Toxic effect of contact with sea anemone, undetermined

√6ᵗʰ **T63.69** Toxic effect of contact with other venomous marine animals

√7ᵗʰ **T63.691** Toxic effect of contact with other venomous marine animals, accidental (unintentional)

² √7ᵗʰ **T63.692** Toxic effect of contact with other venomous marine animals, intentional self-harm `HCC` `Rx` `ESR` `COM`

√7ᵗʰ **T63.693** Toxic effect of contact with other venomous marine animals, assault

√7ᵗʰ **T63.694** Toxic effect of contact with other venomous marine animals, undetermined

√5ᵗʰ **T63.7** Toxic effect of contact with venomous plant

√6ᵗʰ **T63.71** Toxic effect of contact with venomous marine plant

√7ᵗʰ **T63.711** Toxic effect of contact with venomous marine plant, accidental (unintentional)

² √7ᵗʰ **T63.712** Toxic effect of contact with venomous marine plant, intentional self-harm `HCC` `Rx` `ESR` `COM`

√7ᵗʰ **T63.713** Toxic effect of contact with venomous marine plant, assault

√7ᵗʰ **T63.714** Toxic effect of contact with venomous marine plant, undetermined

√6ᵗʰ **T63.79** Toxic effect of contact with other venomous plant

√7ᵗʰ **T63.791** Toxic effect of contact with other venomous plant, accidental (unintentional)

² √7ᵗʰ **T63.792** Toxic effect of contact with other venomous plant, intentional self-harm `HCC` `Rx` `ESR` `COM`

√7ᵗʰ **T63.793** Toxic effect of contact with other venomous plant, assault

√7ᵗʰ **T63.794** Toxic effect of contact with other venomous plant, undetermined

√5ᵗʰ **T63.8** Toxic effect of contact with other venomous animals

√6ᵗʰ **T63.81** Toxic effect of contact with venomous frog

     `EXCLUDES 1`   contact with nonvenomous frog (W62.0)

√7ᵗʰ **T63.811** Toxic effect of contact with venomous frog, accidental (unintentional)

² √7ᵗʰ **T63.812** Toxic effect of contact with venomous frog, intentional self-harm `HCC` `Rx` `ESR` `COM`

√7ᵗʰ **T63.813** Toxic effect of contact with venomous frog, assault

√7ᵗʰ **T63.814** Toxic effect of contact with venomous frog, undetermined

√6ᵗʰ **T63.82** Toxic effect of contact with venomous toad

     `EXCLUDES 1`   contact with nonvenomous toad (W62.1)

√7ᵗʰ **T63.821** Toxic effect of contact with venomous toad, accidental (unintentional)

² √7ᵗʰ **T63.822** Toxic effect of contact with venomous toad, intentional self-harm `HCC` `Rx` `ESR` `COM`

√7ᵗʰ **T63.823** Toxic effect of contact with venomous toad, assault

√7ᵗʰ **T63.824** Toxic effect of contact with venomous toad, undetermined

√6ᵗʰ **T63.83** Toxic effect of contact with other venomous amphibian

     `EXCLUDES 1`   contact with nonvenomous amphibian (W62.9)

√7ᵗʰ **T63.831** Toxic effect of contact with other venomous amphibian, accidental (unintentional)

² √7ᵗʰ **T63.832** Toxic effect of contact with other venomous amphibian, intentional self-harm `HCC` `Rx` `ESR` `COM`

√7ᵗʰ **T63.833** Toxic effect of contact with other venomous amphibian, assault

√7ᵗʰ **T63.834** Toxic effect of contact with other venomous amphibian, undetermined

√6ᵗʰ **T63.89** Toxic effect of contact with other venomous animals

√7ᵗʰ **T63.891** Toxic effect of contact with other venomous animals, accidental (unintentional)

² ✓7ᵗʰ **T63.892** **Toxic effect of contact with other venomous animals, intentional self-harm** `HCC` `Rx` `ESR` `COM`

✓7ᵗʰ **T63.893** **Toxic effect of contact with other venomous animals, assault**

✓7ᵗʰ **T63.894** **Toxic effect of contact with other venomous animals, undetermined**

✓5ᵗʰ **T63.9** **Toxic effect of contact with unspecified venomous animal**

✓x7ᵗʰ **T63.91** **Toxic effect of contact with unspecified venomous animal, accidental (unintentional)**

² ✓x7ᵗʰ **T63.92** **Toxic effect of contact with unspecified venomous animal, intentional self-harm** `HCC` `Rx` `ESR` `COM`

✓x7ᵗʰ **T63.93** **Toxic effect of contact with unspecified venomous animal, assault**

✓x7ᵗʰ **T63.94** **Toxic effect of contact with unspecified venomous animal, undetermined**

✓4ᵗʰ **T64** **Toxic effect of aflatoxin and other mycotoxin food contaminants**

> The appropriate 7th character is to be added to each code from category T64.
> A   initial encounter
> D   subsequent encounter
> S   sequela

✓5ᵗʰ **T64.0** **Toxic effect of aflatoxin**

✓x7ᵗʰ **T64.01** **Toxic effect of aflatoxin, accidental (unintentional)**

² ✓x7ᵗʰ **T64.02** **Toxic effect of aflatoxin, intentional self-harm** `HCC` `Rx` `ESR` `COM`

✓x7ᵗʰ **T64.03** **Toxic effect of aflatoxin, assault**

✓x7ᵗʰ **T64.04** **Toxic effect of aflatoxin, undetermined**

✓5ᵗʰ **T64.8** **Toxic effect of other mycotoxin food contaminants**

✓x7ᵗʰ **T64.81** **Toxic effect of other mycotoxin food contaminants, accidental (unintentional)**

² ✓x7ᵗʰ **T64.82** **Toxic effect of other mycotoxin food contaminants, intentional self-harm** `HCC` `Rx` `ESR` `COM`

✓x7ᵗʰ **T64.83** **Toxic effect of other mycotoxin food contaminants, assault**

✓x7ᵗʰ **T64.84** **Toxic effect of other mycotoxin food contaminants, undetermined**

✓4ᵗʰ **T65** **Toxic effect of other and unspecified substances**

> The appropriate 7th character is to be added to each code from category T65.
> A   initial encounter
> D   subsequent encounter
> S   sequela

✓5ᵗʰ **T65.0** **Toxic effect of cyanides**

> `EXCLUDES 1`   *hydrogen cyanide (T57.3-)*

✓6ᵗʰ **T65.0X** **Toxic effect of cyanides**

✓7ᵗʰ **T65.0X1** **Toxic effect of cyanides, accidental (unintentional)**
Toxic effect of cyanides NOS

² ✓7ᵗʰ **T65.0X2** **Toxic effect of cyanides, intentional self-harm** `HCC` `Rx` `ESR` `COM`

✓7ᵗʰ **T65.0X3** **Toxic effect of cyanides, assault**

✓7ᵗʰ **T65.0X4** **Toxic effect of cyanides, undetermined**

✓5ᵗʰ **T65.1** **Toxic effect of strychnine and its salts**

✓6ᵗʰ **T65.1X** **Toxic effect of strychnine and its salts**

✓7ᵗʰ **T65.1X1** **Toxic effect of strychnine and its salts, accidental (unintentional)**
Toxic effect of strychnine and its salts NOS

² ✓7ᵗʰ **T65.1X2** **Toxic effect of strychnine and its salts, intentional self-harm** `HCC` `Rx` `ESR` `COM`

✓7ᵗʰ **T65.1X3** **Toxic effect of strychnine and its salts, assault**

✓7ᵗʰ **T65.1X4** **Toxic effect of strychnine and its salts, undetermined**

✓5ᵗʰ **T65.2** **Toxic effect of tobacco and nicotine**

> `EXCLUDES 2`   *nicotine dependence (F17.-)*

✓6ᵗʰ **T65.21** **Toxic effect of chewing tobacco**

✓7ᵗʰ **T65.211** **Toxic effect of chewing tobacco, accidental (unintentional)**
Toxic effect of chewing tobacco NOS

² ✓7ᵗʰ **T65.212** **Toxic effect of chewing tobacco, intentional self-harm** `HCC` `Rx` `ESR` `COM`

✓7ᵗʰ **T65.213** **Toxic effect of chewing tobacco, assault**

✓7ᵗʰ **T65.214** **Toxic effect of chewing tobacco, undetermined**

✓6ᵗʰ **T65.22** **Toxic effect of tobacco cigarettes**
Toxic effect of tobacco smoke
Use additional code for exposure to second hand tobacco smoke (Z57.31, Z77.22)

✓7ᵗʰ **T65.221** **Toxic effect of tobacco cigarettes, accidental (unintentional)**
Toxic effect of tobacco cigarettes NOS

² ✓7ᵗʰ **T65.222** **Toxic effect of tobacco cigarettes, intentional self-harm** `HCC` `Rx` `ESR` `COM`

✓7ᵗʰ **T65.223** **Toxic effect of tobacco cigarettes, assault**

✓7ᵗʰ **T65.224** **Toxic effect of tobacco cigarettes, undetermined**

✓6ᵗʰ **T65.29** **Toxic effect of other tobacco and nicotine**

✓7ᵗʰ **T65.291** **Toxic effect of other tobacco and nicotine, accidental (unintentional)**
Toxic effect of other tobacco and nicotine NOS

² ✓7ᵗʰ **T65.292** **Toxic effect of other tobacco and nicotine, intentional self-harm** `HCC` `Rx` `ESR` `COM`

✓7ᵗʰ **T65.293** **Toxic effect of other tobacco and nicotine, assault**

✓7ᵗʰ **T65.294** **Toxic effect of other tobacco and nicotine, undetermined**

✓5ᵗʰ **T65.3** **Toxic effect of nitroderivatives and aminoderivatives of benzene and its homologues**
Toxic effect of anilin [benzenamine]
Toxic effect of nitrobenzene
Toxic effect of trinitrotoluene

✓6ᵗʰ **T65.3X** **Toxic effect of nitroderivatives and aminoderivatives of benzene and its homologues**

✓7ᵗʰ **T65.3X1** **Toxic effect of nitroderivatives and aminoderivatives of benzene and its homologues, accidental (unintentional)**
Toxic effect of nitroderivatives and aminoderivatives of benzene and its homologues NOS

² ✓7ᵗʰ **T65.3X2** **Toxic effect of nitroderivatives and aminoderivatives of benzene and its homologues, intentional self-harm** `HCC` `Rx` `ESR` `COM`

✓7ᵗʰ **T65.3X3** **Toxic effect of nitroderivatives and aminoderivatives of benzene and its homologues, assault**

✓7ᵗʰ **T65.3X4** **Toxic effect of nitroderivatives and aminoderivatives of benzene and its homologues, undetermined**

✓5ᵗʰ **T65.4** **Toxic effect of carbon disulfide**

✓6ᵗʰ **T65.4X** **Toxic effect of carbon disulfide**

✓7ᵗʰ **T65.4X1** **Toxic effect of carbon disulfide, accidental (unintentional)**
Toxic effect of carbon disulfide NOS

² ✓7ᵗʰ **T65.4X2** **Toxic effect of carbon disulfide, intentional self-harm** `HCC` `Rx` `ESR` `COM`

✓7ᵗʰ **T65.4X3** **Toxic effect of carbon disulfide, assault**

✓7ᵗʰ **T65.4X4** **Toxic effect of carbon disulfide, undetermined**

✓5ᵗʰ **T65.5** **Toxic effect of nitroglycerin and other nitric acids and esters**
Toxic effect of 1,2,3-Propanetriol trinitrate

✓6ᵗʰ **T65.5X** **Toxic effect of nitroglycerin and other nitric acids and esters**

✓7ᵗʰ **T65.5X1** **Toxic effect of nitroglycerin and other nitric acids and esters, accidental (unintentional)**
Toxic effect of nitroglycerin and other nitric acids and esters NOS

² ✓7ᵗʰ **T65.5X2** **Toxic effect of nitroglycerin and other nitric acids and esters, intentional self-harm** `HCC` `Rx` `ESR` `COM`

✓7ᵗʰ **T65.5X3** **Toxic effect of nitroglycerin and other nitric acids and esters, assault**

✓7ᵗʰ **T65.5X4** **Toxic effect of nitroglycerin and other nitric acids and esters, undetermined**

✓5ᵗʰ **T65.6** **Toxic effect of paints and dyes, not elsewhere classified**

✓6ᵗʰ **T65.6X** **Toxic effect of paints and dyes, not elsewhere classified**

✓7ᵗʰ **T65.6X1** **Toxic effect of paints and dyes, not elsewhere classified, accidental (unintentional)**
Toxic effect of paints and dyes NOS

`HCC` CMS-HCC   `Rx` Rx HCC   `ESR` ESRD HCC   `COM` Commercial HCC   `N` Newborn: 0   `P` Pediatric: 0-17   `M` Maternity: 9-64   `A` Adult: 15-124

1166   ICD-10-CM 2023

² √7ᵗʰ T65.6X2 Toxic effect of paints and dyes, not elsewhere classified, **intentional self-harm** `HCC` `Rx` `ESR` `COM`

√7ᵗʰ T65.6X3 Toxic effect of paints and dyes, not elsewhere classified, **assault**

√7ᵗʰ T65.6X4 Toxic effect of paints and dyes, not elsewhere classified, **undetermined**

√5ᵗʰ T65.8 Toxic effect of other specified substances

√6ᵗʰ T65.81 Toxic effect of **latex**

√7ᵗʰ T65.811 Toxic effect of latex, **accidental (unintentional)**
Toxic effect of latex NOS

² √7ᵗʰ T65.812 Toxic effect of latex, **intentional self-harm** `HCC` `Rx` `ESR` `COM`

√7ᵗʰ T65.813 Toxic effect of latex, **assault**

√7ᵗʰ T65.814 Toxic effect of latex, **undetermined**

√6ᵗʰ T65.82 Toxic effect of harmful **algae and algae toxins**
Toxic effect of (harmful) algae bloom NOS
Toxic effect of blue-green algae bloom
Toxic effect of brown tide
Toxic effect of cyanobacteria bloom
Toxic effect of Florida red tide
Toxic effect of pfiesteria piscicida
Toxic effect of red tide

√7ᵗʰ T65.821 Toxic effect of harmful algae and algae toxins, **accidental (unintentional)**
Toxic effect of harmful algae and algae toxins NOS

² √7ᵗʰ T65.822 Toxic effect of harmful algae and algae toxins, **intentional self-harm** `HCC` `Rx` `ESR` `COM`

√7ᵗʰ T65.823 Toxic effect of harmful algae and algae toxins, **assault**

√7ᵗʰ T65.824 Toxic effect of harmful algae and algae toxins, **undetermined**

√6ᵗʰ T65.83 Toxic effect of **fiberglass**

√7ᵗʰ T65.831 Toxic effect of fiberglass, **accidental (unintentional)**
Toxic effect of fiberglass NOS

² √7ᵗʰ T65.832 Toxic effect of fiberglass, **intentional self-harm** `HCC` `Rx` `ESR` `COM`

√7ᵗʰ T65.833 Toxic effect of fiberglass, **assault**

√7ᵗʰ T65.834 Toxic effect of fiberglass, **undetermined**

√6ᵗʰ T65.89 Toxic effect of **other specified substances**

√7ᵗʰ T65.891 Toxic effect of other specified substances, **accidental (unintentional)**
Toxic effect of other specified substances NOS
AHA: 2018,1Q,5

² √7ᵗʰ T65.892 Toxic effect of other specified substances, **intentional self-harm** `HCC` `Rx` `ESR` `COM`

√7ᵗʰ T65.893 Toxic effect of other specified substances, **assault**

√7ᵗʰ T65.894 Toxic effect of other specified substances, **undetermined**

√5ᵗʰ T65.9 Toxic effect of unspecified substance

√7ᵗʰ T65.91 Toxic effect of unspecified substance, **accidental (unintentional)**
Poisoning NOS

² √7ᵗʰ T65.92 Toxic effect of unspecified substance, **intentional self-harm** `HCC` `Rx` `ESR` `COM`

√7ᵗʰ T65.93 Toxic effect of unspecified substance, **assault**

√7ᵗʰ T65.94 Toxic effect of unspecified substance, **undetermined**

Other and unspecified effects of external causes (T66-T78)

√x7ᵗʰ T66 **Radiation sickness, unspecified**

`EXCLUDES 1`   *specified adverse effects of radiation, such as:*
    burns (T20-T31)
    leukemia (C91-C95)
    radiation gastroenteritis and colitis (K52.0)
    radiation pneumonitis (J70.0)
    radiation related disorders of the skin and subcutaneous tissue (L55-L59)
    radiation sunburn (L55.-)

The appropriate 7th character is to be added to code T66.
A   initial encounter
D   subsequent encounter
S   sequela

√4ᵗʰ T67 **Effects of heat and light**

`EXCLUDES 1`   *erythema [dermatitis] ab igne (L59.0)*
    malignant hyperpyrexia due to anesthesia (T88.3)
    radiation-related disorders of the skin and subcutaneous tissue (L55-L59)

`EXCLUDES 2`   *burns (T20-T31)*
    sunburn (L55.-)
    sweat disorder due to heat (L74-L75)

The appropriate 7th character is to be added to each code from category T67.
A   initial encounter
D   subsequent encounter
S   sequela

√5ᵗʰ T67.0 **Heatstroke and sunstroke**
Use additional code(s) to identify any associated complications of heatstroke, such as:
    coma and stupor (R40.-)
    rhabdomyolysis (M62.82)
    systemic inflammatory response syndrome (R65.1-)
AHA: 2019,4Q,17-18
DEF: Headache, vertigo, cramps, and elevated body temperature due to prolonged exposure to high environmental temperatures that requires emergency intervention.

√x7ᵗʰ T67.01 **Heatstroke and sunstroke**
Heat apoplexy
Heat pyrexia
Siriasis
Thermoplegia

√x7ᵗʰ T67.02 **Exertional heatstroke**

√x7ᵗʰ T67.09 **Other heatstroke and sunstroke**

√x7ᵗʰ T67.1 **Heat syncope**
Heat collapse

√x7ᵗʰ T67.2 **Heat cramp**

√x7ᵗʰ T67.3 **Heat exhaustion, anhydrotic**
Heat prostration due to water depletion
`EXCLUDES 1`   *heat exhaustion due to salt depletion (T67.4)*

√x7ᵗʰ T67.4 **Heat exhaustion due to salt depletion**
Heat prostration due to salt (and water) depletion

√x7ᵗʰ T67.5 **Heat exhaustion, unspecified**
Heat prostration NOS

√x7ᵗʰ T67.6 **Heat fatigue, transient**

√x7ᵗʰ T67.7 **Heat edema**

√x7ᵗʰ T67.8 **Other effects of heat and light**

√x7ᵗʰ T67.9 **Effect of heat and light, unspecified**

√x7th **T68 Hypothermia**

Accidental hypothermia

Hypothermia NOS

Use additional code to identify source of exposure:

exposure to excessive cold of man-made origin (W93)

exposure to excessive cold of natural origin (X31)

EXCLUDES 1   *hypothermia following anesthesia (T88.51)*

hypothermia not associated with low environmental temperature (R68.0)

hypothermia of newborn (P80.-)

EXCLUDES 2   *frostbite (T33-T34)*

The appropriate 7th character is to be added to code T68.

A   initial encounter

D   subsequent encounter

S   sequela

√4th **T69 Other effects of reduced temperature**

Use additional code to identify source of exposure:

exposure to excessive cold of man-made origin (W93)

exposure to excessive cold of natural origin (X31)

EXCLUDES 2   *frostbite (T33-T34)*

The appropriate 7th character is to be added to each code from category T69.

A   initial encounter

D   subsequent encounter

S   sequela

√5th **T69.0 Immersion hand and foot**

√6th **T69.01 Immersion hand**

√7th **T69.011 Immersion hand, right hand**

√7th **T69.012 Immersion hand, left hand**

√7th **T69.019 Immersion hand, unspecified hand**

√6th **T69.02 Immersion foot**

Trench foot

√7th **T69.021 Immersion foot, right foot**

√7th **T69.022 Immersion foot, left foot**

√7th **T69.029 Immersion foot, unspecified foot**

√x7th **T69.1 Chilblains**

DEF: Red, swollen, itchy skin primarily affecting the fingers and toes, nose and ears, and legs. Chilblains follows damp-cold exposure, and can also be associated with pruritus and a burning feeling.

√x7th **T69.8 Other specified effects of reduced temperature**

√x7th **T69.9 Effect of reduced temperature, unspecified**

√4th **T70 Effects of air pressure and water pressure**

The appropriate 7th character is to be added to each code from category T70.

A   initial encounter

D   subsequent encounter

S   sequela

√x7th **T70.0 Otitic barotrauma**

Aero-otitis media

Effects of change in ambient atmospheric pressure or water pressure on ears

√x7th **T70.1 Sinus barotrauma**

Aerosinusitis

Effects of change in ambient atmospheric pressure on sinuses

√5th **T70.2 Other and unspecified effects of high altitude**

EXCLUDES 2   *polycythemia due to high altitude (D75.1)*

√x7th **T70.20 Unspecified effects of high altitude**

√x7th **T70.29 Other effects of high altitude**

Alpine sickness

Anoxia due to high altitude

Barotrauma NOS

Hypobaropathy

Mountain sickness

√x7th **T70.3 Caisson disease [decompression sickness]**

Compressed-air disease

Diver's palsy or paralysis

DEF: Rapid reduction in air pressure while breathing compressed air. Symptoms include skin lesions, joint pains, and respiratory and neurological problems.

√x7th **T70.4 Effects of high-pressure fluids**

Hydraulic jet injection (industrial)

Pneumatic jet injection (industrial)

Traumatic jet injection (industrial)

√x7th **T70.8 Other effects of air pressure and water pressure**

√x7th **T70.9 Effect of air pressure and water pressure, unspecified**

√4th **T71 Asphyxiation**

Mechanical suffocation

Traumatic suffocation

EXCLUDES 1   *acute respiratory distress (syndrome) (J80)*

anoxia due to high altitude (T70.2)

asphyxia NOS (R09.01)

asphyxia from carbon monoxide (T58.-)

asphyxia from inhalation of food or foreign body (T17.-)

asphyxia from other gases, fumes and vapors (T59.-)

respiratory distress (syndrome) in newborn (P22.-)

The appropriate 7th character is to be added to each code from category T71.

A   initial encounter

D   subsequent encounter

S   sequela

√5th **T71.1 Asphyxiation due to mechanical threat to breathing**

Suffocation due to mechanical threat to breathing

√6th **T71.11 Asphyxiation due to smothering under pillow**

√7th **T71.111 Asphyxiation due to smothering under pillow, accidental**

Asphyxiation due to smothering under pillow NOS

2 √7th **T71.112 Asphyxiation due to smothering under pillow, intentional self-harm** HCC Rx ESR COM

√7th **T71.113 Asphyxiation due to smothering under pillow, assault**

√7th **T71.114 Asphyxiation due to smothering under pillow, undetermined**

√6th **T71.12 Asphyxiation due to plastic bag**

√7th **T71.121 Asphyxiation due to plastic bag, accidental**

Asphyxiation due to plastic bag NOS

2 √7th **T71.122 Asphyxiation due to plastic bag, intentional self-harm** HCC Rx ESR COM

√7th **T71.123 Asphyxiation due to plastic bag, assault**

√7th **T71.124 Asphyxiation due to plastic bag, undetermined**

√6th **T71.13 Asphyxiation due to being trapped in bed linens**

√7th **T71.131 Asphyxiation due to being trapped in bed linens, accidental**

Asphyxiation due to being trapped in bed linens NOS

2 √7th **T71.132 Asphyxiation due to being trapped in bed linens, intentional self-harm** HCC Rx ESR COM

√7th **T71.133 Asphyxiation due to being trapped in bed linens, assault**

√7th **T71.134 Asphyxiation due to being trapped in bed linens, undetermined**

√6th **T71.14 Asphyxiation due to smothering under another person's body (in bed)**

√7th **T71.141 Asphyxiation due to smothering under another person's body (in bed), accidental**

Asphyxiation due to smothering under another person's body (in bed) NOS

√7th **T71.143 Asphyxiation due to smothering under another person's body (in bed), assault**

√7th **T71.144 Asphyxiation due to smothering under another person's body (in bed), undetermined**

√6th **T71.15 Asphyxiation due to smothering in furniture**

√7th **T71.151 Asphyxiation due to smothering in furniture, accidental**

Asphyxiation due to smothering in furniture NOS

2 √7th **T71.152 Asphyxiation due to smothering in furniture, intentional self-harm** HCC Rx ESR COM

√7th **T71.153 Asphyxiation due to smothering in furniture, assault**

✓7ᵗʰ **T71.154 Asphyxiation due to smothering in furniture,** undetermined

✓6ᵗʰ **T71.16 Asphyxiation due to** hanging

    Hanging by window shade cord
    Use additional code for any associated injuries, such as:
        crushing injury of neck (S17.-)
        fracture of cervical vertebrae (S12.0-S12.2-)
        open wound of neck (S11.-)

    ✓7ᵗʰ **T71.161 Asphyxiation due to hanging,** accidental
        Asphyxiation due to hanging NOS
        Hanging NOS

    ² ✓7ᵗʰ **T71.162 Asphyxiation due to hanging,** intentional self-harm   HCC Rx ESR COM

    ✓7ᵗʰ **T71.163 Asphyxiation due to hanging,** assault

    ✓7ᵗʰ **T71.164 Asphyxiation due to hanging,** undetermined

✓6ᵗʰ **T71.19 Asphyxiation due to mechanical threat to breathing due to other causes**

    ✓7ᵗʰ **T71.191 Asphyxiation due to mechanical threat to breathing due to other causes,** accidental
        Asphyxiation due to other causes NOS

    ² ✓7ᵗʰ **T71.192 Asphyxiation due to mechanical threat to breathing due to other causes,** intentional self-harm   HCC Rx ESR COM

    ✓7ᵗʰ **T71.193 Asphyxiation due to mechanical threat to breathing due to other causes,** assault

    ✓7ᵗʰ **T71.194 Asphyxiation due to mechanical threat to breathing due to other causes,** undetermined

✓5ᵗʰ **T71.2 Asphyxiation due to** systemic oxygen deficiency due to low oxygen content in ambient air

    Suffocation due to systemic oxygen deficiency due to low oxygen content in ambient air

    ✓x7ᵗʰ **T71.20 Asphyxiation due to systemic oxygen deficiency due to low oxygen content in ambient air due to unspecified cause**

    ✓x7ᵗʰ **T71.21 Asphyxiation due to** cave-in or falling earth
        Use additional code for any associated cataclysm (X34-X38)

✓6ᵗʰ **T71.22 Asphyxiation due to** being trapped in a car trunk

    ✓7ᵗʰ **T71.221 Asphyxiation due to being trapped in a car trunk,** accidental

    ² ✓7ᵗʰ **T71.222 Asphyxiation due to being trapped in a car trunk,** intentional self-harm   HCC Rx ESR COM

    ✓7ᵗʰ **T71.223 Asphyxiation due to being trapped in a car trunk,** assault

    ✓7ᵗʰ **T71.224 Asphyxiation due to being trapped in a car trunk,** undetermined

✓6ᵗʰ **T71.23 Asphyxiation due to being** trapped in a (discarded) refrigerator

    ✓7ᵗʰ **T71.231 Asphyxiation due to being trapped in a (discarded) refrigerator,** accidental

    ² ✓7ᵗʰ **T71.232 Asphyxiation due to being trapped in a (discarded) refrigerator,** intentional self-harm   HCC Rx ESR COM

    ✓7ᵗʰ **T71.233 Asphyxiation due to being trapped in a (discarded) refrigerator,** assault

    ✓7ᵗʰ **T71.234 Asphyxiation due to being trapped in a (discarded) refrigerator,** undetermined

✓x7ᵗʰ **T71.29 Asphyxiation due to being trapped in other low oxygen environment**

✓x7ᵗʰ **T71.9 Asphyxiation due to unspecified cause**

    Suffocation (by strangulation) due to unspecified cause
    Suffocation NOS
    Systemic oxygen deficiency due to low oxygen content in ambient air due to unspecified cause
    Systemic oxygen deficiency due to mechanical threat to breathing due to unspecified cause
    Traumatic asphyxia NOS

✓4ᵗʰ **T73 Effects of other deprivation**

    The appropriate 7th character is to be added to each code from category T73.
    A   initial encounter
    D   subsequent encounter
    S   sequela

✓x7ᵗʰ **T73.0 Starvation**
    Deprivation of food

✓x7ᵗʰ **T73.1 Deprivation of water**

✓x7ᵗʰ **T73.2 Exhaustion due to exposure**

✓x7ᵗʰ **T73.3 Exhaustion due to excessive exertion**
    Exhaustion due to overexertion

✓x7ᵗʰ **T73.8 Other effects of deprivation**

✓x7ᵗʰ **T73.9 Effect of deprivation, unspecified**

✓4ᵗʰ **T74 Adult and child abuse, neglect and other maltreatment,** confirmed

    Use additional code, if applicable, to identify any associated current injury
    Use additional external cause code to identify perpetrator, if known (Y07.-)
    EXCLUDES 1   abuse and maltreatment in pregnancy (O9A.3-, O9A.4-, O9A.5-)
                adult and child maltreatment, suspected (T76.-)

    The appropriate 7th character is to be added to each code from category T74.
    A   initial encounter
    D   subsequent encounter
    S   sequela

✓5ᵗʰ **T74.0 Neglect or abandonment, confirmed**

    ✓x7ᵗʰ **T74.01 Adult neglect or abandonment, confirmed**   A

    ✓x7ᵗʰ **T74.02 Child neglect or abandonment, confirmed**   P

✓5ᵗʰ **T74.1 Physical abuse, confirmed**

    EXCLUDES 2   sexual abuse (T74.2-)

    ✓x7ᵗʰ **T74.11 Adult physical abuse, confirmed**   A

    ✓x7ᵗʰ **T74.12 Child physical abuse, confirmed**   P
        EXCLUDES 2   shaken infant syndrome (T74.4)

✓5ᵗʰ **T74.2 Sexual abuse, confirmed**
    Rape, confirmed
    Sexual assault, confirmed

    ✓x7ᵗʰ **T74.21 Adult sexual abuse, confirmed**   A

    ✓x7ᵗʰ **T74.22 Child sexual abuse, confirmed**   P

✓5ᵗʰ **T74.3 Psychological abuse, confirmed**
    Bullying and intimidation, confirmed
    Intimidation through social media, confirmed

    ✓x7ᵗʰ **T74.31 Adult psychological abuse, confirmed**   A

    ✓x7ᵗʰ **T74.32 Child psychological abuse, confirmed**   P

✓x7ᵗʰ **T74.4 Shaken infant syndrome**   P

✓5ᵗʰ **T74.5 Forced sexual exploitation, confirmed**
    AHA: 2018,4Q,32-33,65

    ✓x7ᵗʰ **T74.51 Adult forced sexual exploitation, confirmed**   A

    ✓x7ᵗʰ **T74.52 Child sexual exploitation, confirmed**   P

✓5ᵗʰ **T74.6 Forced labor exploitation, confirmed**
    AHA: 2018,4Q,32-33,65

    ✓x7ᵗʰ **T74.61 Adult forced labor exploitation, confirmed**   A

    ✓x7ᵗʰ **T74.62 Child forced labor exploitation, confirmed**   P

✓5ᵗʰ **T74.9 Unspecified maltreatment, confirmed**

    ✓x7ᵗʰ **T74.91 Unspecified adult maltreatment, confirmed**   A

    ✓x7ᵗʰ **T74.92 Unspecified child maltreatment, confirmed**   P

✓4ᵗʰ **T75** **Other and unspecified effects of other external causes**
> EXCLUDES1   *adverse effects NEC (T78.-)*
> EXCLUDES2   *burns (electric) (T20-T31)*
>
> The appropriate 7th character is to be added to each code from category T75.
> A   initial encounter
> D   subsequent encounter
> S   sequela

✓5ᵗʰ **T75.0** **Effects of lightning**
> Struck by lightning

✓x7ᵗʰ **T75.00** **Unspecified effects of lightning**
> Struck by lightning NOS

✓x7ᵗʰ **T75.01** **Shock due to being struck by lightning**

✓x7ᵗʰ **T75.09** **Other effects of lightning**
> Use additional code for other effects of lightning

✓x7ᵗʰ **T75.1** **Unspecified effects of drowning and nonfatal submersion**
> Immersion
> EXCLUDES1   *specified effects of drowning - code to effects*

✓5ᵗʰ **T75.2** **Effects of vibration**

✓x7ᵗʰ **T75.20** **Unspecified effects of vibration**

✓x7ᵗʰ **T75.21** **Pneumatic hammer syndrome**

✓x7ᵗʰ **T75.22** **Traumatic vasospastic syndrome**

✓x7ᵗʰ **T75.23** **Vertigo from infrasound**
> EXCLUDES1   *vertigo NOS (R42)*

✓x7ᵗʰ **T75.29** **Other effects of vibration**

✓x7ᵗʰ **T75.3** **Motion sickness**
> Airsickness
> Seasickness
> Travel sickness
> Use additional external cause code to identify vehicle or type of motion (Y92.81-, Y93.5-)

✓x7ᵗʰ **T75.4** **Electrocution**
> Shock from electric current
> Shock from electroshock gun (taser)

✓5ᵗʰ **T75.8** **Other specified effects of external causes**

✓x7ᵗʰ **T75.81** **Effects of abnormal gravitation [G] forces**

✓x7ᵗʰ **T75.82** **Effects of weightlessness**

✓x7ᵗʰ **T75.89** **Other specified effects of external causes**

✓4ᵗʰ **T76** **Adult and child abuse, neglect and other maltreatment, suspected**
> Use additional code, if applicable, to identify any associated current injury
> EXCLUDES1   *adult and child maltreatment, confirmed (T74.-)*
>   *suspected abuse and maltreatment in pregnancy (O9A.3-, O9A.4-, O9A.5-)*
>   *suspected adult physical abuse, ruled out (Z04.71)*
>   *suspected adult sexual abuse, ruled out (Z04.41)*
>   *suspected child physical abuse, ruled out (Z04.72)*
>   *suspected child sexual abuse, ruled out (Z04.42)*
>
> AHA: 2018,4Q,72
>
> The appropriate 7th character is to be added to each code from category T76.
> A   initial encounter
> D   subsequent encounter
> S   sequela

✓5ᵗʰ **T76.0** **Neglect or abandonment, suspected**

✓x7ᵗʰ **T76.01** **Adult neglect or abandonment, suspected** 🅰

✓x7ᵗʰ **T76.02** **Child neglect or abandonment, suspected** 🅿

✓5ᵗʰ **T76.1** **Physical abuse, suspected**

✓x7ᵗʰ **T76.11** **Adult physical abuse, suspected** 🅰

✓x7ᵗʰ **T76.12** **Child physical abuse, suspected** 🅿
> AHA: 2019,2Q,12

✓5ᵗʰ **T76.2** **Sexual abuse, suspected**
> Rape, suspected
> EXCLUDES1   *alleged abuse, ruled out (Z04.7)*

✓x7ᵗʰ **T76.21** **Adult sexual abuse, suspected** 🅰

✓x7ᵗʰ **T76.22** **Child sexual abuse, suspected** 🅿

✓5ᵗʰ **T76.3** **Psychological abuse, suspected**
> Bullying and intimidation, suspected
> Intimidation through social media, suspected

✓x7ᵗʰ **T76.31** **Adult psychological abuse, suspected** 🅰

✓x7ᵗʰ **T76.32** **Child psychological abuse, suspected** 🅿

✓5ᵗʰ **T76.5** **Forced sexual exploitation, suspected**
> AHA: 2018,4Q,32-33,65

✓x7ᵗʰ **T76.51** **Adult forced sexual exploitation, suspected** 🅰

✓x7ᵗʰ **T76.52** **Child sexual exploitation, suspected** 🅿

✓5ᵗʰ **T76.6** **Forced labor exploitation, suspected**
> AHA: 2018,4Q,32-33,65

✓x7ᵗʰ **T76.61** **Adult forced labor exploitation, suspected** 🅰

✓x7ᵗʰ **T76.62** **Child forced labor exploitation, suspected** 🅿

✓5ᵗʰ **T76.9** **Unspecified maltreatment, suspected**

✓x7ᵗʰ **T76.91** **Unspecified adult maltreatment, suspected** 🅰

✓x7ᵗʰ **T76.92** **Unspecified child maltreatment, suspected** 🅿

✓4ᵗʰ **T78** **Adverse effects, not elsewhere classified**
> EXCLUDES2   *complications of surgical and medical care NEC (T80-T88)*
>
> The appropriate 7th character is to be added to each code from category T78.
> A   initial encounter
> D   subsequent encounter
> S   sequela

✓5ᵗʰ **T78.0** **Anaphylactic reaction due to food**
> Anaphylactic reaction due to adverse food reaction
> Anaphylactic shock or reaction due to nonpoisonous foods
> Anaphylactoid reaction due to food

✓x7ᵗʰ **T78.00** **Anaphylactic reaction due to unspecified food**

✓x7ᵗʰ **T78.01** **Anaphylactic reaction due to peanuts**

✓x7ᵗʰ **T78.02** **Anaphylactic reaction due to shellfish (crustaceans)**

✓x7ᵗʰ **T78.03** **Anaphylactic reaction due to other fish**

✓x7ᵗʰ **T78.04** **Anaphylactic reaction due to fruits and vegetables**

✓x7ᵗʰ **T78.05** **Anaphylactic reaction due to tree nuts and seeds**
> EXCLUDES2   *anaphylactic reaction due to peanuts (T78.01)*

✓x7ᵗʰ **T78.06** **Anaphylactic reaction due to food additives**

✓x7ᵗʰ **T78.07** **Anaphylactic reaction due to milk and dairy products**

✓x7ᵗʰ **T78.08** **Anaphylactic reaction due to eggs**

✓x7ᵗʰ **T78.09** **Anaphylactic reaction due to other food products**

✓x7ᵗʰ **T78.1** **Other adverse food reactions, not elsewhere classified**
> Use additional code to identify the type of reaction, if applicable
> EXCLUDES1   *anaphylactic reaction or shock due to adverse food reaction (T78.0-)*
>   *anaphylactic reaction due to food (T78.0-)*
>   *bacterial food borne intoxications (A05.-)*
> EXCLUDES2   *allergic and dietetic gastroenteritis and colitis (K52.29)*
>   *allergic rhinitis due to food (J30.5)*
>   *dermatitis due to food in contact with skin (L23.6, L24.6, L25.4)*
>   *dermatitis due to ingested food (L27.2)*
>   *food protein-induced enterocolitis syndrome (K52.21)*
>   *food protein-induced enteropathy (K52.22)*

✓x7ᵗʰ **T78.2** **Anaphylactic shock, unspecified**
> Allergic shock
> Anaphylactic reaction
> Anaphylaxis
> EXCLUDES1   *anaphylactic reaction or shock due to adverse effect of correct medicinal substance properly administered (T88.6)*
>   *anaphylactic reaction or shock due to adverse food reaction (T78.0-)*
>   *anaphylactic reaction or shock due to serum (T80.5-)*

✓x7ᵗʰ **T78.3** **Angioneurotic edema**
> Allergic angioedema
> Giant urticaria
> Quincke's edema
> EXCLUDES1   *serum urticaria (T80.6-)*
>   *urticaria (L50.-)*

✓5ᵗʰ T78.4 Other and unspecified allergy

EXCLUDES 1   specified types of allergic reaction such as:
allergic diarrhea (K52.29)
allergic gastroenteritis and colitis (K52.29)
dermatitis (L23-L25, L27.-)
food protein-induced enterocolitis syndrome (K52.21)
food protein-induced enteropathy (K52.22)
hay fever (J30.1)

✓x7ᵗʰ   **T78.40   Allergy, unspecified**
Allergic reaction NOS
Hypersensitivity NOS

✓x7ᵗʰ   **T78.41   Arthus phenomenon**
Arthus reaction

✓x7ᵗʰ   **T78.49   Other allergy**
AHA: 2021,1Q,42

✓x7ᵗʰ **T78.8   Other adverse effects, not elsewhere classified**

Certain early complications of trauma (T79)

✓4ᵗʰ **T79   Certain early complications of trauma, not elsewhere classified**

EXCLUDES 2   acute respiratory distress syndrome (J80)
complications occurring during or following medical procedures (T80-T88)
complications of surgical and medical care NEC (T80-T88)
newborn respiratory distress syndrome (P22.0)

The appropriate 7th character is to be added to each code from category T79.
A   initial encounter
D   subsequent encounter
S   sequela

¹ ✓x7ᵗʰ **T79.0   Air embolism (traumatic)**   HCC ESR COM

EXCLUDES 1   air embolism complicating abortion or ectopic or molar pregnancy (O00-O07, O08.2)
air embolism complicating pregnancy, childbirth and the puerperium (O88.0)
air embolism following infusion, transfusion, and therapeutic injection (T80.0)
air embolism following procedure NEC (T81.7-)

DEF: Arterial or venous obstruction due to the introduction of air bubbles into the blood vessels following surgery or trauma.

¹ ✓x7ᵗʰ **T79.1   Fat embolism (traumatic)**   HCC ESR COM

EXCLUDES 1   fat embolism complicating:
abortion or ectopic or molar pregnancy (O00-O07, O08.2)
pregnancy, childbirth and the puerperium (O88.8)

DEF: Arterial blockage due to the entrance of fat into the circulatory system after a fracture of the large bones or administration of corticosteroids.

¹ ✓x7ᵗʰ **T79.2   Traumatic secondary and recurrent hemorrhage and seroma**   HCC ESR

¹ ✓x7ᵗʰ **T79.4   Traumatic shock**   HCC ESR COM
Shock (immediate) (delayed) following injury

EXCLUDES 1   anaphylactic shock due to adverse food reaction (T78.0-)
anaphylactic shock due to correct medicinal substance properly administered (T88.6)
anaphylactic shock due to serum (T80.5-)
anaphylactic shock NOS (T78.2)
electric shock (T75.4)
nontraumatic shock NEC (R57.-)
obstetric shock (O75.1)
postprocedural shock (T81.1-)
septic shock (R65.21)
shock complicating abortion or ectopic or molar pregnancy (O00-O07, O08.3)
shock due to anesthesia (T88.2)
shock due to lightning (T75.01)
shock NOS (R57.9)

¹ ✓x7ᵗʰ **T79.5   Traumatic anuria**   HCC ESR
Crush syndrome
Renal failure following crushing

¹ ✓x7ᵗʰ **T79.6   Traumatic ischemia of muscle**   HCC ESR
Traumatic rhabdomyolysis
Volkmann's ischemic contracture

EXCLUDES 2   anterior tibial syndrome (M76.8)
compartment syndrome (traumatic) (T79.A-)
nontraumatic ischemia of muscle (M62.2-)

AHA: 2019,2Q,12

¹ ✓x7ᵗʰ **T79.7   Traumatic subcutaneous emphysema**   HCC ESR

EXCLUDES 2   emphysema NOS (J43)
emphysema (subcutaneous) resulting from a procedure (T81.82)

✓5ᵗʰ T79.A Traumatic compartment syndrome

EXCLUDES 1   fibromyalgia (M79.7)
nontraumatic compartment syndrome (M79.A-)

EXCLUDES 2   traumatic ischemic infarction of muscle (T79.6)

DEF: Compression of nerves and blood vessels within an enclosed muscle space due to previous trauma, which leads to impaired blood flow and muscle and nerve damage.

¹ ✓x7ᵗʰ   **T79.A0   Compartment syndrome, unspecified**   HCC ESR
Compartment syndrome NOS

✓6ᵗʰ   **T79.A1   Traumatic compartment syndrome of upper extremity**
Traumatic compartment syndrome of shoulder, arm, forearm, wrist, hand, and fingers

¹ ✓7ᵗʰ   **T79.A11   Traumatic compartment syndrome of right upper extremity**   HCC ESR

¹ ✓7ᵗʰ   **T79.A12   Traumatic compartment syndrome of left upper extremity**   HCC ESR

¹ ✓7ᵗʰ   **T79.A19   Traumatic compartment syndrome of unspecified upper extremity**   HCC ESR

✓6ᵗʰ   **T79.A2   Traumatic compartment syndrome of lower extremity**
Traumatic compartment syndrome of hip, buttock, thigh, leg, foot, and toes

¹ ✓7ᵗʰ   **T79.A21   Traumatic compartment syndrome of right lower extremity**   HCC ESR

¹ ✓7ᵗʰ   **T79.A22   Traumatic compartment syndrome of left lower extremity**   HCC ESR

¹ ✓7ᵗʰ   **T79.A29   Traumatic compartment syndrome of unspecified lower extremity**   HCC ESR

¹ ✓x7ᵗʰ   **T79.A3   Traumatic compartment syndrome of abdomen**   HCC ESR

¹ ✓x7ᵗʰ   **T79.A9   Traumatic compartment syndrome of other sites**   HCC ESR

¹ ✓x7ᵗʰ **T79.8   Other early complications of trauma**   HCC ESR

¹ ✓x7ᵗʰ **T79.9   Unspecified early complication of trauma**   HCC ESR

Complications of surgical and medical care, not elsewhere classified (T80-T88)

Use additional code for adverse effect, if applicable, to identify drug (T36-T50 with fifth or sixth character 5)

Use additional code(s) to identify the specified condition resulting from the complication

Use additional code to identify devices involved and details of circumstances (Y62-Y82)

EXCLUDES 2   *any encounters with medical care for postprocedural conditions in which no complications are present, such as:*
     artificial opening status (Z93.-)
     closure of external stoma (Z43.-)
     fitting and adjustment of external prosthetic device (Z44.-)
   burns and corrosions from local applications and irradiation (T20-T32)
   complications of surgical procedures during pregnancy, childbirth and the puerperium (O00-O9A)
   mechanical complication of respirator [ventilator] (J95.850)
   poisoning and toxic effects of drugs and chemicals (T36-T65 with fifth or sixth character 1-4 or 6)
   postprocedural fever (R50.82)
   specified complications classified elsewhere, such as:
     cerebrospinal fluid leak from spinal puncture (G97.0)
     colostomy malfunction (K94.0-)
     disorders of fluid and electrolyte imbalance (E86-E87)
     functional disturbances following cardiac surgery (I97.0-I97.1)
     intraoperative and postprocedural complications of specified body systems (D78.-, E36.-, E89.-, G97.3-, G97.4, H59.3-, H59.-, H95.2-, H95.3, I97.4-, I97.5, J95.6-, J95.7, K91.6-, L76.-, M96.-, N99.-)
     ostomy complications (J95.0-, K94.-, N99.5-)
     postgastric surgery syndromes (K91.1)
     postlaminectomy syndrome NEC (M96.1)
     postmastectomy lymphedema syndrome (I97.2)
     postsurgical blind-loop syndrome (K91.2)
     ventilator associated pneumonia (J95.851)

AHA: 2015,1Q,15

✓4ᵗʰ T80   Complications following infusion, transfusion and therapeutic injection

INCLUDES   complications following perfusion

EXCLUDES 2   *bone marrow transplant rejection (T86.01)*
     febrile nonhemolytic transfusion reaction (R50.84)
     fluid overload due to transfusion (E87.71)
     posttransfusion purpura (D69.51)
     transfusion associated circulatory overload (TACO) (E87.71)
     transfusion (red blood cell) associated hemochromatosis (E83.111)
     transfusion related acute lung injury (TRALI) (J95.84)

The appropriate 7th character is to be added to each code from category T80.
- A   initial encounter
- D   subsequent encounter
- S   sequela

✓x7ᵗʰ T80.0   Air embolism following infusion, transfusion and therapeutic injection

✓x7ᵗʰ T80.1   Vascular complications following infusion, transfusion and therapeutic injection

Use additional code to identify the vascular complication

EXCLUDES 2   *extravasation of vesicant agent (T80.81-)*
     infiltration of vesicant agent (T80.81-)
     postprocedural vascular complications (T81.7-)
     vascular complications specified as due to prosthetic devices, implants and grafts (T82.8-, T83.8-, T84.8-, T85.8-)

✓5ᵗʰ T80.2   Infections following infusion, transfusion and therapeutic injection

Use additional code to identify the specific infection, such as: sepsis (A41.9)

Use additional code (R65.2-) to identify severe sepsis, if applicable

EXCLUDES 2   *infections specified as due to prosthetic devices, implants and grafts (T82.6-T82.7, T83.5-T83.6, T84.5-T84.7, T85.7)*
     postprocedural infections (T81.4-)

AHA: 2018,4Q,62

✓6ᵗʰ T80.21   Infection due to central venous catheter

Infection due to pulmonary artery catheter (Swan-Ganz catheter)

AHA: 2019,1Q,13-14

DEF: Central venous catheter: Catheter positioned in the superior vena cava or right atrium and introduced through a large vein, such as the jugular or subclavian, and used to measure venous pressure or administer fluids or medication.

TIP: Code assignment is based on the location of the catheter and not how the catheter is being used; for example, for hemodialysis. Infections resulting from catheters that are not central lines should be coded to T82.7-.

✓7ᵗʰ T80.211   Bloodstream infection due to central venous catheter

Catheter-related bloodstream infection (CRBSI) NOS

Central line-associated bloodstream infection (CLABSI)

Bloodstream infection due to Hickman catheter

Bloodstream infection due to peripherally inserted central catheter (PICC)

Bloodstream infection due to portacath (port-a-cath)

Bloodstream infection due to pulmonary artery catheter

Bloodstream infection due to triple lumen catheter

Bloodstream infection due to umbilical venous catheter

AHA: 2019,1Q,13,14; 2018,4Q,89

✓7ᵗʰ T80.212   Local infection due to central venous catheter

Exit or insertion site infection

Local infection due to Hickman catheter

Local infection due to peripherally inserted central catheter (PICC)

Local infection due to portacath (port-a-cath)

Local infection due to pulmonary artery catheter

Local infection due to triple lumen catheter

Local infection due to umbilical venous catheter

Port or reservoir infection

Tunnel infection

✓7ᵗʰ T80.218   Other infection due to central venous catheter

Other central line-associated infection

Other infection due to Hickman catheter

Other infection due to peripherally inserted central catheter (PICC)

Other infection due to portacath (port-a-cath)

Other infection due to pulmonary artery catheter

Other infection due to triple lumen catheter

Other infection due to umbilical venous catheter

☑7ᵗʰ **T80.219 Unspecified infection due to central venous catheter**
Central line-associated infection NOS
Unspecified infection due to Hickman catheter
Unspecified infection due to peripherally inserted central catheter (PICC)
Unspecified infection due to portacath (port-a-cath)
Unspecified infection due to pulmonary artery catheter
Unspecified infection due to triple lumen catheter
Unspecified infection due to umbilical venous catheter

√x7ᵗʰ **T80.22 Acute infection following transfusion, infusion, or injection of blood and blood products**

√x7ᵗʰ **T80.29 Infection following other infusion, transfusion and therapeutic injection**

√5ᵗʰ **T80.3 ABO incompatibility reaction due to transfusion of blood or blood products**
> EXCLUDES 1   *minor blood group antigens reactions (Duffy) (E) (K) (Kell) (Kidd) (Lewis) (M) (N) (P) (S) (T80.A-)*

√x7ᵗʰ **T80.30 ABO incompatibility reaction due to transfusion of blood or blood products, unspecified**
ABO incompatibility blood transfusion NOS
Reaction to ABO incompatibility from transfusion NOS

√6ᵗʰ **T80.31 ABO incompatibility with hemolytic transfusion reaction**

√7ᵗʰ **T80.310 ABO incompatibility with acute hemolytic transfusion reaction**
ABO incompatibility with hemolytic transfusion reaction less than 24 hours after transfusion
Acute hemolytic transfusion reaction (AHTR) due to ABO incompatibility

√7ᵗʰ **T80.311 ABO incompatibility with delayed hemolytic transfusion reaction**
ABO incompatibility with hemolytic transfusion reaction 24 hours or more after transfusion
Delayed hemolytic transfusion reaction (DHTR) due to ABO incompatibility

√7ᵗʰ **T80.319 ABO incompatibility with hemolytic transfusion reaction, unspecified**
ABO incompatibility with hemolytic transfusion reaction at unspecified time after transfusion
Hemolytic transfusion reaction (HTR) due to ABO incompatibility NOS

√x7ᵗʰ **T80.39 Other ABO incompatibility reaction due to transfusion of blood or blood products**
Delayed serologic transfusion reaction (DSTR) from ABO incompatibility
Other ABO incompatible blood transfusion
Other reaction to ABO incompatible blood transfusion

√5ᵗʰ **T80.4 Rh incompatibility reaction due to transfusion of blood or blood products**
Reaction due to incompatibility of Rh antigens (C) (c) (D) (E) (e)

√x7ᵗʰ **T80.40 Rh incompatibility reaction due to transfusion of blood or blood products, unspecified**
Reaction due to Rh factor in transfusion NOS
Rh incompatible blood transfusion NOS

√6ᵗʰ **T80.41 Rh incompatibility with hemolytic transfusion reaction**

√7ᵗʰ **T80.410 Rh incompatibility with acute hemolytic transfusion reaction**
Acute hemolytic transfusion reaction (AHTR) due to Rh incompatibility
Rh incompatibility with hemolytic transfusion reaction less than 24 hours after transfusion

√7ᵗʰ **T80.411 Rh incompatibility with delayed hemolytic transfusion reaction**
Delayed hemolytic transfusion reaction (DHTR) due to Rh incompatibility
Rh incompatibility with hemolytic transfusion reaction 24 hours or more after transfusion

√7ᵗʰ **T80.419 Rh incompatibility with hemolytic transfusion reaction, unspecified**
Rh incompatibility with hemolytic transfusion reaction at unspecified time after transfusion
Hemolytic transfusion reaction (HTR) due to Rh incompatibility NOS

√x7ᵗʰ **T80.49 Other Rh incompatibility reaction due to transfusion of blood or blood products**
Delayed serologic transfusion reaction (DSTR) from Rh incompatibility
Other reaction to Rh incompatible blood transfusion

√5ᵗʰ **T80.A Non-ABO incompatibility reaction due to transfusion of blood or blood products**
Reaction due to incompatibility of minor antigens (Duffy) (Kell) (Kidd) (Lewis) (M) (N) (P) (S)

√x7ᵗʰ **T80.A0 Non-ABO incompatibility reaction due to transfusion of blood or blood products, unspecified**
Non-ABO antigen incompatibility reaction from transfusion NOS

√6ᵗʰ **T80.A1 Non-ABO incompatibility with hemolytic transfusion reaction**

√7ᵗʰ **T80.A10 Non-ABO incompatibility with acute hemolytic transfusion reaction**
Acute hemolytic transfusion reaction (AHTR) due to non-ABO incompatibility
Non-ABO incompatibility with hemolytic transfusion reaction less than 24 hours after transfusion

√7ᵗʰ **T80.A11 Non-ABO incompatibility with delayed hemolytic transfusion reaction**
Delayed hemolytic transfusion reaction (DHTR) due to non-ABO incompatibility
Non-ABO incompatibility with hemolytic transfusion reaction 24 or more hours after transfusion

√7ᵗʰ **T80.A19 Non-ABO incompatibility with hemolytic transfusion reaction, unspecified**
Hemolytic transfusion reaction (HTR) due to non-ABO incompatibility NOS
Non-ABO incompatibility with hemolytic transfusion reaction at unspecified time after transfusion

√x7ᵗʰ **T80.A9 Other non-ABO incompatibility reaction due to transfusion of blood or blood products**
Delayed serologic transfusion reaction (DSTR) from non-ABO incompatibility
Other reaction to non-ABO incompatible blood transfusion

√5ᵗʰ **T80.5 Anaphylactic reaction due to serum**
Allergic shock due to serum
Anaphylactic shock due to serum
Anaphylactoid reaction due to serum
Anaphylaxis due to serum
> EXCLUDES 1   *ABO incompatibility reaction due to transfusion of blood or blood products (T80.3-)*
> *allergic reaction or shock NOS (T78.2)*
> *anaphylactic reaction or shock NOS (T78.2)*
> *anaphylactic reaction or shock due to adverse effect of correct medicinal substance properly administered (T88.6)*
> *other serum reaction (T80.6-)*

DEF: Life-threatening hypersensitivity to a foreign serum causing respiratory distress, vascular collapse, and shock.

√x7ᵗʰ **T80.51 Anaphylactic reaction due to administration of blood and blood products**

√x7ᵗʰ **T80.52 Anaphylactic reaction due to vaccination**
AHA: 2021,1Q,43

√x7ᵗʰ **T80.59 Anaphylactic reaction due to other serum**

✓5ᵗʰ T80.6 Other serum reactions
     Intoxication by serum
     Protein sickness
     Serum rash
     Serum sickness
     Serum urticaria
     EXCLUDES 2   serum hepatitis (B16-B19)
     DEF: Serum sickness: Hypersensitivity to a foreign serum that causes fever, hives, swelling, and lymphadenopathy.

     ✓x7ᵗʰ T80.61 Other serum reaction due to administration of blood and blood products

     ✓x7ᵗʰ T80.62 Other serum reaction due to vaccination
         AHA: 2021,1Q,42

     ✓x7ᵗʰ T80.69 Other serum reaction due to other serum
         Code also, if applicable, arthropathy in hypersensitivity reactions classified elsewhere (M36.4)

✓5ᵗʰ T80.8 Other complications following infusion, transfusion and therapeutic injection

     ✓6ᵗʰ T80.81 Extravasation of vesicant agent
         Infiltration of vesicant agent

         ✓7ᵗʰ T80.810 Extravasation of vesicant antineoplastic chemotherapy
             Infiltration of vesicant antineoplastic chemotherapy

         ✓7ᵗʰ T80.818 Extravasation of other vesicant agent
             Infiltration of other vesicant agent

     ✓x7ᵗʰ T80.82 Complication of immune effector cellular therapy
         Complication of chimeric antigen receptor (CAR-T) cell therapy
         Complication of IEC therapy
         Use additional code to identify the specific complication, such as:
            cytokine release syndrome (D89.83-)
            immune effector cell-associated neurotoxicity syndrome (G92.0-)
         EXCLUDES 2   complication of bone marrow transplant (T86.0)
                       complication of stem cell transplant (T86.5)
         AHA: 2021,4Q,31

     ✓x7ᵗʰ T80.89 Other complications following infusion, transfusion and therapeutic injection
         Delayed serologic transfusion reaction (DSTR), unspecified incompatibility
         Use additional code to identify graft-versus-host reaction, if applicable, (D89.81-)
         AHA: 2020,4Q,14

✓5ᵗʰ T80.9 Unspecified complication following infusion, transfusion and therapeutic injection

     ✓x7ᵗʰ T80.90 Unspecified complication following infusion and therapeutic injection

     ✓6ᵗʰ T80.91 Hemolytic transfusion reaction, unspecified incompatibility
         EXCLUDES 1   ABO incompatibility with hemolytic transfusion reaction (T80.31-)
                       non-ABO incompatibility with hemolytic transfusion reaction (T80.A1-)
                       Rh incompatibility with hemolytic transfusion reaction (T80.41-)

         ✓7ᵗʰ T80.910 Acute hemolytic transfusion reaction, unspecified incompatibility

         ✓7ᵗʰ T80.911 Delayed hemolytic transfusion reaction, unspecified incompatibility

         ✓7ᵗʰ T80.919 Hemolytic transfusion reaction, unspecified incompatibility, unspecified as acute or delayed
            Hemolytic transfusion reaction NOS

     ✓x7ᵗʰ T80.92 Unspecified transfusion reaction
         Transfusion reaction NOS

✓4ᵗʰ T81 Complications of procedures, not elsewhere classified
     Use additional code for adverse effect, if applicable, to identify drug (T36-T50 with fifth or sixth character 5)
     EXCLUDES 2   complications following immunization (T88.0-T88.1)
                 complications following infusion, transfusion and therapeutic injection (T80.-)
                 complications of transplanted organs and tissue (T86.-)
                 specified complications classified elsewhere, such as:
                     complication of prosthetic devices, implants and grafts (T82-T85)
                     dermatitis due to drugs and medicaments (L23.3, L24.4, L25.1, L27.0-L27.1)
                     endosseous dental implant failure (M27.6-)
                     floppy iris syndrome (IFIS) (intraoperative) (H21.81)
                     intraoperative and postprocedural complications of specific body system (D78.-, E36.-, E89.-, G97.3-, G97.4, H59.-, H59.-, H95.2-, H95.3, I97.4-, I97.5, J95, K91.-, L76.-, M96.-, N99.-)
                     ostomy complications (J95.0-, K94.-, N99.5-)
                     plateau iris syndrome (post-iridectomy) (postprocedural) H21.82
                     poisoning and toxic effects of drugs and chemicals (T36-T65 with fifth or sixth character 1-4 or 6)
     AHA: 2019,2Q,21

     The appropriate 7th character is to be added to each code from category T81.
     A   initial encounter
     D   subsequent encounter
     S   sequela

✓5ᵗʰ T81.1 Postprocedural shock
     Shock during or resulting from a procedure, not elsewhere classified
     EXCLUDES 1   anaphylactic shock due to correct substance properly administered (T88.6)
                 anaphylactic shock due to serum (T80.5-)
                 anaphylactic shock NOS (T78.2)
                 electric shock (T75.4)
                 obstetric shock (O75.1)
                 septic shock (R65.21)
                 shock due to anesthesia (T88.2)
                 shock following abortion or ectopic or molar pregnancy (O00-O07, O08.3)
                 traumatic shock (T79.4)
     AHA: 2021,1Q,13

     ✓x7ᵗʰ T81.10 Postprocedural shock unspecified
         Collapse NOS during or resulting from a procedure, not elsewhere classified
         Postprocedural failure of peripheral circulation
         Postprocedural shock NOS

     ¹ ✓x7ᵗʰ T81.11 Postprocedural cardiogenic shock   `HCC` `ESR`

     ¹ ✓x7ᵗʰ T81.12 Postprocedural septic shock   `HCC` `ESR` `UPD`
         Postprocedural endotoxic shock resulting from a procedure, not elsewhere classified
         Postprocedural gram-negative shock resulting from a procedure, not elsewhere classified
         Code first underlying infection
         Use additional code, to identify any associated acute organ dysfunction, if applicable
         AHA: 2018,4Q,63

     ✓x7ᵗʰ T81.19 Other postprocedural shock
         Postprocedural hypovolemic shock

✓5ᵗʰ T81.3 Disruption of wound, not elsewhere classified
     Disruption of any suture materials or other closure methods
     EXCLUDES 1   breakdown (mechanical) of permanent sutures (T85.612)
                 displacement of permanent sutures (T85.622)
                 disruption of cesarean delivery wound (O90.0)
                 disruption of perineal obstetric wound (O90.1)
                 mechanical complication of permanent sutures NEC (T85.692)
     AHA: 2014,1Q,23

     ✓x7ᵗʰ T81.30 Disruption of wound, unspecified
         Disruption of wound NOS

✓x7ᵗʰ **T81.31** **Disruption of external operation (surgical) wound, not elsewhere classified**
Dehiscence of operation wound NOS
Disruption of operation wound NOS
Disruption or dehiscence of closure of cornea
Disruption or dehiscence of closure of mucosa
Disruption or dehiscence of closure of skin and subcutaneous tissue
Full-thickness skin disruption or dehiscence
Superficial disruption or dehiscence of operation wound
EXCLUDES 1   *dehiscence of amputation stump (T87.81)*

✓x7ᵗʰ **T81.32** **Disruption of internal operation (surgical) wound, not elsewhere classified**
Deep disruption or dehiscence of operation wound NOS
Disruption or dehiscence of closure of internal organ or other internal tissue
Disruption or dehiscence of closure of muscle or muscle flap
Disruption or dehiscence of closure of ribs or rib cage
Disruption or dehiscence of closure of skull or craniotomy
Disruption or dehiscence of closure of sternum or sternotomy
Disruption or dehiscence of closure of tendon or ligament
Disruption or dehiscence of closure of superficial or muscular fascia
AHA: 2020,2Q,22; 2017,3Q,4

✓x7ᵗʰ **T81.33** **Disruption of traumatic injury wound repair**
Disruption or dehiscence of closure of traumatic laceration (external) (internal)

✓5ᵗʰ **T81.4** **Infection following a procedure**
Wound abscess following a procedure
Use additional code to identify infection
Use additional code (R65.2-) to identify severe sepsis, if applicable
EXCLUDES 2   *bleb associated endophthalmitis (H59.4-)*
          infection due to infusion, transfusion and therapeutic injection (T80.2-)
          infection due to prosthetic devices, implants and grafts (T82.6-T82.7, T83.5-T83.6, T84.5-T84.7, T85.7)
          obstetric surgical wound infection (O86.0-)
          postprocedural fever NOS (R50.82)
          postprocedural retroperitoneal abscess (K68.11)
AHA: 2018,4Q,33-34,62; 2014,1Q,23

✓x7ᵗʰ **T81.40** **Infection following a procedure, unspecified**

✓x7ᵗʰ **T81.41** **Infection following a procedure, superficial incisional surgical site**
Subcutaneous abscess following a procedure
Stitch abscess following a procedure

✓x7ᵗʰ **T81.42** **Infection following a procedure, deep incisional surgical site**
Intra-muscular abscess following a procedure

✓x7ᵗʰ **T81.43** **Infection following a procedure, organ and space surgical site**
Intra-abdominal abscess following a procedure
Subphrenic abscess following a procedure

¹ ✓x7ᵗʰ **T81.44** **Sepsis following a procedure**   HCC ESR COM
Use additional code to identify the sepsis

✓x7ᵗʰ **T81.49** **Infection following a procedure, other surgical site**

✓5ᵗʰ **T81.5** **Complications of foreign body accidentally left in body following procedure**
AHA: 2014,4Q,24

✓6ᵗʰ **T81.50** **Unspecified complication of foreign body accidentally left in body following procedure**

✓7ᵗʰ **T81.500** **Unspecified complication of foreign body accidentally left in body following surgical operation**

✓7ᵗʰ **T81.501** **Unspecified complication of foreign body accidentally left in body following infusion or transfusion**

✓7ᵗʰ **T81.502** **Unspecified complication of foreign body accidentally left in body following kidney dialysis**   HCC Rx ESR

✓7ᵗʰ **T81.503** **Unspecified complication of foreign body accidentally left in body following injection or immunization**

✓7ᵗʰ **T81.504** **Unspecified complication of foreign body accidentally left in body following endoscopic examination**

✓7ᵗʰ **T81.505** **Unspecified complication of foreign body accidentally left in body following heart catheterization**

✓7ᵗʰ **T81.506** **Unspecified complication of foreign body accidentally left in body following aspiration, puncture or other catheterization**

✓7ᵗʰ **T81.507** **Unspecified complication of foreign body accidentally left in body following removal of catheter or packing**

✓7ᵗʰ **T81.508** **Unspecified complication of foreign body accidentally left in body following other procedure**

✓7ᵗʰ **T81.509** **Unspecified complication of foreign body accidentally left in body following unspecified procedure**

✓6ᵗʰ **T81.51** **Adhesions due to foreign body accidentally left in body following procedure**

✓7ᵗʰ **T81.510** **Adhesions due to foreign body accidentally left in body following surgical operation**

✓7ᵗʰ **T81.511** **Adhesions due to foreign body accidentally left in body following infusion or transfusion**

✓7ᵗʰ **T81.512** **Adhesions due to foreign body accidentally left in body following kidney dialysis**   HCC Rx ESR

✓7ᵗʰ **T81.513** **Adhesions due to foreign body accidentally left in body following injection or immunization**

✓7ᵗʰ **T81.514** **Adhesions due to foreign body accidentally left in body following endoscopic examination**

✓7ᵗʰ **T81.515** **Adhesions due to foreign body accidentally left in body following heart catheterization**

✓7ᵗʰ **T81.516** **Adhesions due to foreign body accidentally left in body following aspiration, puncture or other catheterization**

✓7ᵗʰ **T81.517** **Adhesions due to foreign body accidentally left in body following removal of catheter or packing**

✓7ᵗʰ **T81.518** **Adhesions due to foreign body accidentally left in body following other procedure**

✓7ᵗʰ **T81.519** **Adhesions due to foreign body accidentally left in body following unspecified procedure**

✓6ᵗʰ **T81.52** **Obstruction due to foreign body accidentally left in body following procedure**

✓7ᵗʰ **T81.520** **Obstruction due to foreign body accidentally left in body following surgical operation**

✓7ᵗʰ **T81.521** **Obstruction due to foreign body accidentally left in body following infusion or transfusion**

✓7ᵗʰ **T81.522** **Obstruction due to foreign body accidentally left in body following kidney dialysis**   HCC Rx ESR

✓7ᵗʰ **T81.523** **Obstruction due to foreign body accidentally left in body following injection or immunization**

✓7ᵗʰ **T81.524** **Obstruction due to foreign body accidentally left in body following endoscopic examination**

✓7ᵗʰ **T81.525** **Obstruction due to foreign body accidentally left in body following heart catheterization**

✓7ᵗʰ **T81.526** **Obstruction due to foreign body accidentally left in body following aspiration, puncture or other catheterization**

✓7ᵗʰ **T81.527** **Obstruction due to foreign body accidentally left in body following removal of catheter or packing**

✓7ᵗʰ **T81.528** **Obstruction due to foreign body accidentally left in body following other procedure**

✓ Additional Character Required   ✓x7ᵗʰ Placeholder Alert   Manifestation   Unspecified Dx   Q QPP   UPD Unacceptable PDx

√7th **T81.529** **Obstruction due to foreign body accidentally left in body following unspecified procedure**

√6th T81.53 Perforation due to foreign body accidentally left in body following procedure

√7th **T81.530** **Perforation due to foreign body accidentally left in body following surgical operation**

√7th **T81.531** **Perforation due to foreign body accidentally left in body following infusion or transfusion**

√7th **T81.532** **Perforation due to foreign body accidentally left in body following kidney dialysis** HCC Rx ESR

√7th **T81.533** **Perforation due to foreign body accidentally left in body following injection or immunization**

√7th **T81.534** **Perforation due to foreign body accidentally left in body following endoscopic examination**

√7th **T81.535** **Perforation due to foreign body accidentally left in body following heart catheterization**

√7th **T81.536** **Perforation due to foreign body accidentally left in body following aspiration, puncture or other catheterization**

√7th **T81.537** **Perforation due to foreign body accidentally left in body following removal of catheter or packing**

√7th **T81.538** **Perforation due to foreign body accidentally left in body following other procedure**

√7th **T81.539** **Perforation due to foreign body accidentally left in body following unspecified procedure**

√6th T81.59 Other complications of foreign body accidentally left in body following procedure

> EXCLUDES 2   *obstruction or perforation due to prosthetic devices and implants intentionally left in body (T82.0-T82.5, T83.0-T83.4, T83.7, T84.0-T84.4, T85.0-T85.6)*

√7th **T81.590** **Other complications of foreign body accidentally left in body following surgical operation**

√7th **T81.591** **Other complications of foreign body accidentally left in body following infusion or transfusion**

√7th **T81.592** **Other complications of foreign body accidentally left in body following kidney dialysis** HCC Rx ESR

√7th **T81.593** **Other complications of foreign body accidentally left in body following injection or immunization**

√7th **T81.594** **Other complications of foreign body accidentally left in body following endoscopic examination**

√7th **T81.595** **Other complications of foreign body accidentally left in body following heart catheterization**

√7th **T81.596** **Other complications of foreign body accidentally left in body following aspiration, puncture or other catheterization**

√7th **T81.597** **Other complications of foreign body accidentally left in body following removal of catheter or packing**

√7th **T81.598** **Other complications of foreign body accidentally left in body following other procedure**

√7th **T81.599** **Other complications of foreign body accidentally left in body following unspecified procedure**

√5th T81.6 Acute reaction to foreign substance accidentally left during a procedure

> EXCLUDES 2   *complications of foreign body accidentally left in body cavity or operation wound following procedure (T81.5-)*

√x7th **T81.60** **Unspecified acute reaction to foreign substance accidentally left during a procedure**

√x7th **T81.61** Aseptic peritonitis due to foreign substance accidentally left during a procedure

Chemical peritonitis

√x7th **T81.69** **Other acute reaction to foreign substance accidentally left during a procedure**

√5th T81.7 Vascular complications following a procedure, not elsewhere classified

Air embolism following procedure NEC

Phlebitis or thrombophlebitis resulting from a procedure

> EXCLUDES 1   *embolism complicating abortion or ectopic or molar pregnancy (O00-O07, O08.2)*
> *embolism complicating pregnancy, childbirth and the puerperium (O88.-)*
> *traumatic embolism (T79.0)*

> EXCLUDES 2   *embolism due to prosthetic devices, implants and grafts (T82.8-, T83.81, T84.8-, T85.81-)*
> *embolism following infusion, transfusion and therapeutic injection (T80.0)*

AHA: 2019,2Q,22

√6th T81.71 Complication of artery following a procedure, not elsewhere classified

√7th **T81.710** **Complication of mesenteric artery following a procedure, not elsewhere classified**

√7th **T81.711** **Complication of renal artery following a procedure, not elsewhere classified**

√7th **T81.718** **Complication of other artery following a procedure, not elsewhere classified**

AHA: 2019,2Q,21-22

√7th **T81.719** **Complication of unspecified artery following a procedure, not elsewhere classified**

√x7th T81.72 Complication of vein following a procedure, not elsewhere classified

√5th T81.8 Other complications of procedures, not elsewhere classified

> EXCLUDES 2   *hypothermia following anesthesia (T88.51)*
> *malignant hyperpyrexia due to anesthesia (T88.3)*

√x7th **T81.81** **Complication of inhalation therapy**

√x7th **T81.82** **Emphysema (subcutaneous) resulting from a procedure**

√x7th **T81.83** **Persistent postprocedural fistula**

AHA: 2017,3Q,3-4

√x7th **T81.89** **Other complications of procedures, not elsewhere classified**

Use additional code to specify complication, such as: postprocedural delirium (F05)

AHA: 2014,1Q,23

√x7th **T81.9** **Unspecified complication of procedure**

√4th T82 Complications of cardiac and vascular prosthetic devices, implants and grafts

> EXCLUDES 2   *failure and rejection of transplanted organs and tissue (T86.-)*

AHA: 2020,3Q,36-37

> The appropriate 7th character is to be added to each code from category T82.
> A   initial encounter
> D   subsequent encounter
> S   sequela

√5th T82.0 Mechanical complication of heart valve prosthesis

Mechanical complication of artificial heart valve

> EXCLUDES 1   *mechanical complication of biological heart valve graft (T82.22-)*

√x7th **T82.01** **Breakdown (mechanical) of heart valve prosthesis**

√x7th **T82.02** **Displacement of heart valve prosthesis**

Malposition of heart valve prosthesis

√x7th **T82.03** **Leakage of heart valve prosthesis**

√x7th **T82.09** **Other mechanical complication of heart valve prosthesis**

Obstruction (mechanical) of heart valve prosthesis

Perforation of heart valve prosthesis

Protrusion of heart valve prosthesis

√5th T82.1 Mechanical complication of cardiac electronic device

√6th T82.11 Breakdown (mechanical) of cardiac electronic device

√7th **T82.110** **Breakdown (mechanical) of cardiac electrode**

√7th **T82.111** **Breakdown (mechanical) of cardiac pulse generator (battery)**

☑7ᵗʰ **T82.118 Breakdown (mechanical) of other cardiac electronic device**

☑7ᵗʰ **T82.119 Breakdown (mechanical) of unspecified cardiac electronic device**

✓6ᵗʰ **T82.12 Displacement of cardiac electronic device**

Malposition of cardiac electronic device

☑7ᵗʰ **T82.120 Displacement of cardiac electrode**

☑7ᵗʰ **T82.121 Displacement of cardiac pulse generator (battery)**

☑7ᵗʰ **T82.128 Displacement of other cardiac electronic device**

☑7ᵗʰ **T82.129 Displacement of unspecified cardiac electronic device**

✓6ᵗʰ **T82.19 Other mechanical complication of cardiac electronic device**

Leakage of cardiac electronic device

Obstruction of cardiac electronic device

Perforation of cardiac electronic device

Protrusion of cardiac electronic device

☑7ᵗʰ **T82.190 Other mechanical complication of cardiac electrode**

☑7ᵗʰ **T82.191 Other mechanical complication of cardiac pulse generator (battery)**

☑7ᵗʰ **T82.198 Other mechanical complication of other cardiac electronic device**

☑7ᵗʰ **T82.199 Other mechanical complication of unspecified cardiac device**

✓5ᵗʰ **T82.2 Mechanical complication of coronary artery bypass graft and biological heart valve graft**

> EXCLUDES 1   mechanical complication of artificial heart valve prosthesis (T82.0-)

✓6ᵗʰ **T82.21 Mechanical complication of coronary artery bypass graft**

☑7ᵗʰ **T82.211 Breakdown (mechanical) of coronary artery bypass graft**

☑7ᵗʰ **T82.212 Displacement of coronary artery bypass graft**

Malposition of coronary artery bypass graft

☑7ᵗʰ **T82.213 Leakage of coronary artery bypass graft**

☑7ᵗʰ **T82.218 Other mechanical complication of coronary artery bypass graft**

Obstruction, mechanical of coronary artery bypass graft

Perforation of coronary artery bypass graft

Protrusion of coronary artery bypass graft

✓6ᵗʰ **T82.22 Mechanical complication of biological heart valve graft**

☑7ᵗʰ **T82.221 Breakdown (mechanical) of biological heart valve graft**

☑7ᵗʰ **T82.222 Displacement of biological heart valve graft**

Malposition of biological heart valve graft

☑7ᵗʰ **T82.223 Leakage of biological heart valve graft**

☑7ᵗʰ **T82.228 Other mechanical complication of biological heart valve graft**

Obstruction of biological heart valve graft

Perforation of biological heart valve graft

Protrusion of biological heart valve graft

✓5ᵗʰ **T82.3 Mechanical complication of other vascular grafts**

✓6ᵗʰ **T82.31 Breakdown (mechanical) of other vascular grafts**

¹ ☑7ᵗʰ **T82.310 Breakdown (mechanical) of aortic (bifurcation) graft (replacement)** HCC ESR

AHA: 2020,3Q,3-8

¹ ☑7ᵗʰ **T82.311 Breakdown (mechanical) of carotid arterial graft (bypass)** HCC ESR

¹ ☑7ᵗʰ **T82.312 Breakdown (mechanical) of femoral arterial graft (bypass)** HCC ESR

¹ ☑7ᵗʰ **T82.318 Breakdown (mechanical) of other vascular grafts** HCC ESR

¹ ☑7ᵗʰ **T82.319 Breakdown (mechanical) of unspecified vascular grafts** HCC ESR

✓6ᵗʰ **T82.32 Displacement of other vascular grafts**

Malposition of other vascular grafts

¹ ☑7ᵗʰ **T82.320 Displacement of aortic (bifurcation) graft (replacement)** HCC ESR

¹ ☑7ᵗʰ **T82.321 Displacement of carotid arterial graft (bypass)** HCC ESR

¹ ☑7ᵗʰ **T82.322 Displacement of femoral arterial graft (bypass)**

¹ ☑7ᵗʰ **T82.328 Displacement of other vascular grafts** HCC ESR

¹ ☑7ᵗʰ **T82.329 Displacement of unspecified vascular grafts** HCC ESR

✓6ᵗʰ **T82.33 Leakage of other vascular grafts**

¹ ☑7ᵗʰ **T82.330 Leakage of aortic (bifurcation) graft (replacement)** HCC ESR

AHA: 2020,3Q,3-8

¹ ☑7ᵗʰ **T82.331 Leakage of carotid arterial graft (bypass)** HCC ESR

¹ ☑7ᵗʰ **T82.332 Leakage of femoral arterial graft (bypass)** HCC ESR

¹ ☑7ᵗʰ **T82.338 Leakage of other vascular grafts** HCC ESR

¹ ☑7ᵗʰ **T82.339 Leakage of unspecified vascular graft** HCC ESR

✓6ᵗʰ **T82.39 Other mechanical complication of other vascular grafts**

Obstruction (mechanical) of other vascular grafts

Perforation of other vascular grafts

Protrusion of other vascular grafts

¹ ☑7ᵗʰ **T82.390 Other mechanical complication of aortic (bifurcation) graft (replacement)** HCC ESR

AHA: 2020,3Q,3-5

¹ ☑7ᵗʰ **T82.391 Other mechanical complication of carotid arterial graft (bypass)** HCC ESR

¹ ☑7ᵗʰ **T82.392 Other mechanical complication of femoral arterial graft (bypass)** HCC ESR

¹ ☑7ᵗʰ **T82.398 Other mechanical complication of other vascular grafts** HCC ESR

¹ ☑7ᵗʰ **T82.399 Other mechanical complication of unspecified vascular grafts** HCC ESR

✓5ᵗʰ **T82.4 Mechanical complication of vascular dialysis catheter**

Mechanical complication of hemodialysis catheter

> EXCLUDES 1   mechanical complication of intraperitoneal dialysis catheter (T85.62)

✓x7ᵗʰ **T82.41 Breakdown (mechanical) of vascular dialysis catheter** HCC Rx ESR

✓x7ᵗʰ **T82.42 Displacement of vascular dialysis catheter** HCC Rx ESR

Malposition of vascular dialysis catheter

✓x7ᵗʰ **T82.43 Leakage of vascular dialysis catheter** HCC Rx ESR

✓x7ᵗʰ **T82.49 Other complication of vascular dialysis catheter** HCC Rx ESR

Obstruction (mechanical) of vascular dialysis catheter

Perforation of vascular dialysis catheter

Protrusion of vascular dialysis catheter

✓5ᵗʰ **T82.5 Mechanical complication of other cardiac and vascular devices and implants**

> EXCLUDES 2   mechanical complication of epidural and subdural infusion catheter (T85.61)

✓6ᵗʰ **T82.51 Breakdown (mechanical) of other cardiac and vascular devices and implants**

¹ ☑7ᵗʰ **T82.510 Breakdown (mechanical) of surgically created arteriovenous fistula** HCC ESR

AHA: 2020,3Q,36

¹ ☑7ᵗʰ **T82.511 Breakdown (mechanical) of surgically created arteriovenous shunt** HCC ESR

AHA: 2020,3Q,37

☑7ᵗʰ **T82.512 Breakdown (mechanical) of artificial heart**

¹ ☑7ᵗʰ **T82.513 Breakdown (mechanical) of balloon (counterpulsation) device** HCC ESR

¹ ☑7ᵗʰ **T82.514 Breakdown (mechanical) of infusion catheter** HCC ESR

¹ ☑7ᵗʰ **T82.515 Breakdown (mechanical) of umbrella device** HCC ESR

¹ ☑7ᵗʰ **T82.518 Breakdown (mechanical) of other cardiac and vascular devices and implants** HCC ESR

☑7ᵗʰ **T82.519 Breakdown (mechanical) of unspecified cardiac and vascular devices and implants**

Chapter 19. Injury, Poisoning and Certain Other Consequences of External Causes

√6ᵗʰ **T82.52** **Displacement** of other cardiac and vascular devices and implants
     Malposition of other cardiac and vascular devices and implants

1 √7ᵗʰ **T82.520** **Displacement of** surgically created arteriovenous fistula   HCC ESR
     AHA: 2020,3Q,36

1 √7ᵗʰ **T82.521** **Displacement of** surgically created arteriovenous shunt   HCC ESR

√7ᵗʰ **T82.522** **Displacement of** artificial heart

1 √7ᵗʰ **T82.523** **Displacement of** balloon (counterpulsation) device   HCC ESR

1 √7ᵗʰ **T82.524** **Displacement of** infusion catheter   HCC ESR
     AHA: 2020,2Q,21; 2019,3Q,15

1 √7ᵗʰ **T82.525** **Displacement of** umbrella device   HCC ESR

1 √7ᵗʰ **T82.528** **Displacement of other cardiac and vascular devices and implants**   HCC ESR

√7ᵗʰ **T82.529** **Displacement of unspecified cardiac and vascular devices and implants**

√6ᵗʰ **T82.53** **Leakage** of other cardiac and vascular devices and implants

1 √7ᵗʰ **T82.530** **Leakage of** surgically created arteriovenous fistula   HCC ESR
     AHA: 2020,3Q,36

1 √7ᵗʰ **T82.531** **Leakage of** surgically created arteriovenous shunt   HCC ESR

√7ᵗʰ **T82.532** **Leakage of** artificial heart

1 √7ᵗʰ **T82.533** **Leakage of** balloon (counterpulsation) device   HCC ESR

1 √7ᵗʰ **T82.534** **Leakage of** infusion catheter   HCC ESR

1 √7ᵗʰ **T82.535** **Leakage of** umbrella device   HCC ESR

1 √7ᵗʰ **T82.538** **Leakage of other cardiac and vascular devices and implants**   HCC ESR

√7ᵗʰ **T82.539** **Leakage of unspecified cardiac and vascular devices and implants**

√6ᵗʰ **T82.59** **Other mechanical complication of other cardiac and vascular devices and implants**
     Obstruction (mechanical) of other cardiac and vascular devices and implants
     Perforation of other cardiac and vascular devices and implants
     Protrusion of other cardiac and vascular devices and implants

1 √7ᵗʰ **T82.590** **Other mechanical complication of** surgically created arteriovenous fistula   HCC ESR
     AHA: 2020,3Q,36

1 √7ᵗʰ **T82.591** **Other mechanical complication of** surgically created arteriovenous shunt   HCC ESR

√7ᵗʰ **T82.592** **Other mechanical complication of** artificial heart

1 √7ᵗʰ **T82.593** **Other mechanical complication of** balloon (counterpulsation) device   HCC ESR

1 √7ᵗʰ **T82.594** **Other mechanical complication of** infusion catheter   HCC ESR

1 √7ᵗʰ **T82.595** **Other mechanical complication of** umbrella device   HCC ESR

1 √7ᵗʰ **T82.598** **Other mechanical complication of other cardiac and vascular devices and implants**   HCC ESR

√7ᵗʰ **T82.599** **Other mechanical complication of unspecified cardiac and vascular devices and implants**

1 √x7ᵗʰ **T82.6** **Infection and inflammatory reaction due to cardiac valve prosthesis**   HCC ESR
     Use additional code to identify infection

1 √x7ᵗʰ **T82.7** **Infection and inflammatory reaction due to other cardiac and vascular devices, implants and grafts**   HCC ESR
     Use additional code to identify infection
     AHA: 2019,1Q,13-14
     DEF: Midline catheter: Long peripheral catheter introduced via the cephalic, basilic, brachial, or median cubital veins in the upper arm and positioned so that the tip is level or near the level of the axilla and distal to the shoulder. Midline catheters are typically used for IV access, fluid replacement, and medication administration.
     TIP: Assign this code for infections and/or cellulitis resulting from catheters that are not centrally placed (e.g., midline catheters).

√5ᵗʰ **T82.8** **Other specified complications of cardiac and vascular prosthetic devices, implants and grafts**
     AHA: 2016,4Q,70

√6ᵗʰ **T82.81** **Embolism** due to cardiac and vascular prosthetic devices, implants and grafts

√7ᵗʰ **T82.817** **Embolism due to** cardiac prosthetic devices, implants and grafts

1 √7ᵗʰ **T82.818** **Embolism due to** vascular prosthetic devices, implants and grafts   HCC ESR

√6ᵗʰ **T82.82** **Fibrosis** due to cardiac and vascular prosthetic devices, implants and grafts

√7ᵗʰ **T82.827** **Fibrosis due to** cardiac prosthetic devices, implants and grafts

1 √7ᵗʰ **T82.828** **Fibrosis due** vascular prosthetic devices, implants and grafts   HCC ESR

√6ᵗʰ **T82.83** **Hemorrhage** due to cardiac and vascular prosthetic devices, implants and grafts

√7ᵗʰ **T82.837** **Hemorrhage due to** cardiac prosthetic devices, implants and grafts

1 √7ᵗʰ **T82.838** **Hemorrhage due to** vascular prosthetic devices, implants and grafts   HCC ESR
     AHA: 2020,3Q,36-37

√6ᵗʰ **T82.84** **Pain** due to cardiac and vascular prosthetic devices, implants and grafts

√7ᵗʰ **T82.847** **Pain due to** cardiac prosthetic devices, implants and grafts

1 √7ᵗʰ **T82.848** **Pain due to** vascular prosthetic devices, implants and grafts   HCC ESR

√6ᵗʰ **T82.85** **Stenosis** due to cardiac and vascular prosthetic devices, implants and grafts

√7ᵗʰ **T82.855** **Stenosis of** coronary artery stent
     In-stent stenosis (restenosis) of coronary artery stent
     Restenosis of coronary artery stent
     AHA: 2021,3Q,6-7

1 √7ᵗʰ **T82.856** **Stenosis of** peripheral vascular stent   HCC ESR
     In-stent stenosis (restenosis) of peripheral vascular stent
     Restenosis of peripheral vascular stent

√7ᵗʰ **T82.857** **Stenosis of other** cardiac prosthetic devices, implants and grafts

1 √7ᵗʰ **T82.858** **Stenosis of other** vascular prosthetic devices, implants and grafts   HCC ESR

√6ᵗʰ **T82.86** **Thrombosis** of cardiac and vascular prosthetic devices, implants and grafts

√7ᵗʰ **T82.867** **Thrombosis due to** cardiac prosthetic devices, implants and grafts

1 √7ᵗʰ **T82.868** **Thrombosis due to** vascular prosthetic devices, implants and grafts   HCC ESR

√6ᵗʰ **T82.89** **Other specified complication of cardiac and vascular prosthetic devices, implants and grafts**

√7ᵗʰ **T82.897** **Other specified complication of** cardiac prosthetic devices, implants and grafts
     AHA: 2019,2Q,33

1 √7ᵗʰ **T82.898** **Other specified complication of** vascular prosthetic devices, implants and grafts   HCC ESR
     AHA: 2020,3Q,3-5

√x7ᵗʰ **T82.9** **Unspecified complication of cardiac and vascular prosthetic device, implant and graft**

✓4ᵗʰ **T83 Complications of genitourinary prosthetic devices, implants and grafts**

> *EXCLUDES 2*   *failure and rejection of transplanted organs and tissue (T86.-)*

AHA: 2016,4Q,70-71

> The appropriate 7th character is to be added to each code from category T83.
> A   initial encounter
> D   subsequent encounter
> S   sequela

✓5ᵗʰ **T83.0 Mechanical complication of urinary catheter**

> *EXCLUDES 2*   *complications of stoma of urinary tract (N99.5-)*

✓6ᵗʰ **T83.01 Breakdown (mechanical) of urinary catheter**

¹ ✓7ᵗʰ **T83.010 Breakdown (mechanical) of cystostomy catheter** HCC ESR

¹ ✓7ᵗʰ **T83.011 Breakdown (mechanical) of indwelling urethral catheter** HCC ESR

¹ ✓7ᵗʰ **T83.012 Breakdown (mechanical) of nephrostomy catheter** HCC ESR

¹ ✓7ᵗʰ **T83.018 Breakdown (mechanical) of other urinary catheter** HCC ESR
> Breakdown (mechanical) of Hopkins catheter
> Breakdown (mechanical) of ileostomy catheter
> Breakdown (mechanical) urostomy catheter

✓6ᵗʰ **T83.02 Displacement of urinary catheter**
> Malposition of urinary catheter

¹ ✓7ᵗʰ **T83.020 Displacement of cystostomy catheter** HCC ESR

¹ ✓7ᵗʰ **T83.021 Displacement of indwelling urethral catheter** HCC ESR

¹ ✓7ᵗʰ **T83.022 Displacement of nephrostomy catheter** HCC ESR

¹ ✓7ᵗʰ **T83.028 Displacement of other urinary catheter** HCC ESR
> Displacement of Hopkins catheter
> Displacement of ileostomy catheter
> Displacement of urostomy catheter

✓6ᵗʰ **T83.03 Leakage of urinary catheter**

¹ ✓7ᵗʰ **T83.030 Leakage of cystostomy catheter** HCC ESR
> **AHA:** 2021,4Q,18

¹ ✓7ᵗʰ **T83.031 Leakage of indwelling urethral catheter** HCC ESR

¹ ✓7ᵗʰ **T83.032 Leakage of nephrostomy catheter** HCC ESR

¹ ✓7ᵗʰ **T83.038 Leakage of other urinary catheter** HCC ESR
> Leakage of Hopkins catheter
> Leakage of ileostomy catheter
> Leakage of urostomy catheter

✓6ᵗʰ **T83.09 Other mechanical complication of urinary catheter**
> Obstruction (mechanical) of urinary catheter
> Perforation of urinary catheter
> Protrusion of urinary catheter

¹ ✓7ᵗʰ **T83.090 Other mechanical complication of cystostomy catheter** HCC ESR

¹ ✓7ᵗʰ **T83.091 Other mechanical complication of indwelling urethral catheter** HCC ESR

¹ ✓7ᵗʰ **T83.092 Other mechanical complication of nephrostomy catheter** HCC ESR

¹ ✓7ᵗʰ **T83.098 Other mechanical complication of other urinary catheter** HCC ESR
> Other mechanical complication of Hopkins catheter
> Other mechanical complication of ileostomy catheter
> Other mechanical complication of urostomy catheter

✓5ᵗʰ **T83.1 Mechanical complication of other urinary devices and implants**

✓6ᵗʰ **T83.11 Breakdown (mechanical) of other urinary devices and implants**

¹ ✓7ᵗʰ **T83.110 Breakdown (mechanical) of urinary electronic stimulator device** HCC ESR
> *EXCLUDES 2*   *breakdown (mechanical) of electrode (lead) for sacral nerve neurostimulator (T85.111)*
> *breakdown (mechanical) of implanted electronic sacral neurostimulator, pulse generator or receiver (T85.113)*

¹ ✓7ᵗʰ **T83.111 Breakdown (mechanical) of implanted urinary sphincter** HCC ESR

¹ ✓7ᵗʰ **T83.112 Breakdown (mechanical) of indwelling ureteral stent** HCC ESR

¹ ✓7ᵗʰ **T83.113 Breakdown (mechanical) of other urinary stents** HCC ESR
> Breakdown (mechanical) of ileal conduit stent
> Breakdown (mechanical) of nephroureteral stent

¹ ✓7ᵗʰ **T83.118 Breakdown (mechanical) of other urinary devices and implants** HCC ESR

✓6ᵗʰ **T83.12 Displacement of other urinary devices and implants**
> Malposition of other urinary devices and implants

¹ ✓7ᵗʰ **T83.120 Displacement of urinary electronic stimulator device** HCC ESR
> *EXCLUDES 2*   *displacement of electrode (lead) for sacral nerve neurostimulator (T85.121)*
> *displacement of implanted electronic sacral neurostimulator, pulse generator or receiver (T85.123)*

¹ ✓7ᵗʰ **T83.121 Displacement of implanted urinary sphincter** HCC ESR

¹ ✓7ᵗʰ **T83.122 Displacement of indwelling ureteral stent** HCC ESR

¹ ✓7ᵗʰ **T83.123 Displacement of other urinary stents** HCC ESR
> Displacement of ileal conduit stent
> Displacement of nephroureteral stent

¹ ✓7ᵗʰ **T83.128 Displacement of other urinary devices and implants** HCC ESR

✓6ᵗʰ **T83.19 Other mechanical complication of other urinary devices and implants**
> Leakage of other urinary devices and implants
> Obstruction (mechanical) of other urinary devices and implants
> Perforation of other urinary devices and implants
> Protrusion of other urinary devices and implants

¹ ✓7ᵗʰ **T83.190 Other mechanical complication of urinary electronic stimulator device** HCC ESR
> *EXCLUDES 2*   *other mechanical complication of electrode (lead) for sacral nerve neurostimulator (T85.191)*
> *other mechanical complication of implanted electronic sacral neurostimulator, pulse generator or receiver (T85.193)*

¹ ✓7ᵗʰ **T83.191 Other mechanical complication of implanted urinary sphincter** HCC ESR

¹ ✓7ᵗʰ **T83.192 Other mechanical complication of indwelling ureteral stent** HCC ESR

¹ ✓7ᵗʰ **T83.193 Other mechanical complication of other urinary stent** HCC ESR
> Other mechanical complication of ileal conduit stent
> Other mechanical complication of nephroureteral stent

¹ ✓7ᵗʰ **T83.198 Other mechanical complication of other urinary devices and implants** HCC ESR

√5ᵗʰ **T83.2** Mechanical complication of graft of urinary organ

¹ √x7ᵗʰ **T83.21** **Breakdown (mechanical) of graft of urinary organ** HCC ESR

¹ √x7ᵗʰ **T83.22** **Displacement of graft of urinary organ** HCC ESR
Malposition of graft of urinary organ

¹ √x7ᵗʰ **T83.23** **Leakage of graft of urinary organ** HCC ESR

¹ √x7ᵗʰ **T83.24** **Erosion of graft of urinary organ** HCC ESR

¹ √x7ᵗʰ **T83.25** **Exposure of graft of urinary organ** HCC ESR

¹ √x7ᵗʰ **T83.29** **Other mechanical complication of graft of urinary organ**
Obstruction (mechanical) of graft of urinary organ
Perforation of graft of urinary organ
Protrusion of graft of urinary organ

√5ᵗʰ **T83.3** Mechanical complication of intrauterine contraceptive device

√x7ᵗʰ **T83.31** **Breakdown (mechanical) of intrauterine contraceptive device** ♀

√x7ᵗʰ **T83.32** **Displacement of intrauterine contraceptive device** ♀
Malposition of intrauterine contraceptive device
Missing string of intrauterine contraceptive device
AHA: 2018,1Q,5

√x7ᵗʰ **T83.39** **Other mechanical complication of intrauterine contraceptive device** ♀
Leakage of intrauterine contraceptive device
Obstruction (mechanical) of intrauterine contraceptive device
Perforation of intrauterine contraceptive device
Protrusion of intrauterine contraceptive device

√5ᵗʰ **T83.4** Mechanical complication of other prosthetic devices, implants and grafts of genital tract

√6ᵗʰ **T83.41** **Breakdown (mechanical) of other prosthetic devices, implants and grafts of genital tract**

¹ √7ᵗʰ **T83.410** **Breakdown (mechanical) of implanted penile prosthesis** HCC ESR ♂
Breakdown (mechanical) of penile prosthesis cylinder
Breakdown (mechanical) of penile prosthesis pump
Breakdown (mechanical) of penile prosthesis reservoir

¹ √7ᵗʰ **T83.411** **Breakdown (mechanical) of implanted testicular prosthesis** HCC ESR

¹ √7ᵗʰ **T83.418** **Breakdown (mechanical) of other prosthetic devices, implants and grafts of genital tract** HCC ESR

√6ᵗʰ **T83.42** **Displacement of other prosthetic devices, implants and grafts of genital tract**
Malposition of other prosthetic devices, implants and grafts of genital tract

¹ √7ᵗʰ **T83.420** **Displacement of implanted penile prosthesis** HCC ESR ♂
Displacement of penile prosthesis cylinder
Displacement of penile prosthesis pump
Displacement of penile prosthesis reservoir

¹ √7ᵗʰ **T83.421** **Displacement of implanted testicular prosthesis** HCC ESR

¹ √7ᵗʰ **T83.428** **Displacement of other prosthetic devices, implants and grafts of genital tract** HCC ESR
AHA: 2018,1Q,5

√6ᵗʰ **T83.49** **Other mechanical complication of other prosthetic devices, implants and grafts of genital tract**
Leakage of other prosthetic devices, implants and grafts of genital tract
Obstruction, mechanical of other prosthetic devices, implants and grafts of genital tract
Perforation of other prosthetic devices, implants and grafts of genital tract
Protrusion of other prosthetic devices, implants and grafts of genital tract

¹ √7ᵗʰ **T83.490** **Other mechanical complication of implanted penile prosthesis** HCC ESR ♂
Other mechanical complication of penile prosthesis cylinder
Other mechanical complication of penile prosthesis pump
Other mechanical complication of penile prosthesis reservoir

¹ √7ᵗʰ **T83.491** **Other mechanical complication of implanted testicular prosthesis** HCC ESR

¹ √7ᵗʰ **T83.498** **Other mechanical complication of other prosthetic devices, implants and grafts of genital tract** HCC ESR

√5ᵗʰ **T83.5** Infection and inflammatory reaction due to prosthetic device, implant and graft in urinary system
Use additional code to identify infection

√6ᵗʰ **T83.51** **Infection and inflammatory reaction due to urinary catheter**
EXCLUDES 2   complications of stoma of urinary tract (N99.5-)
AHA: 2019,3Q,17

¹ √7ᵗʰ **T83.510** **Infection and inflammatory reaction due to cystostomy catheter** HCC ESR

¹ √7ᵗʰ **T83.511** **Infection and inflammatory reaction due to indwelling urethral catheter** HCC ESR
AHA: 2022,2Q,7

¹ √7ᵗʰ **T83.512** **Infection and inflammatory reaction due to nephrostomy catheter** HCC ESR

¹ √7ᵗʰ **T83.518** **Infection and inflammatory reaction due to other urinary catheter** HCC ESR
Infection and inflammatory reaction due to Hopkins catheter
Infection and inflammatory reaction due to ileostomy catheter
Infection and inflammatory reaction due to urostomy catheter

√6ᵗʰ **T83.59** **Infection and inflammatory reaction due to prosthetic device, implant and graft in urinary system**

¹ √7ᵗʰ **T83.590** **Infection and inflammatory reaction due to implanted urinary neurostimulation device** HCC ESR
EXCLUDES 2   infection and inflammatory reaction due to electrode lead of sacral nerve neurostimulator (T85.732)
infection and inflammatory reaction due to pulse generator or receiver of sacral nerve neurostimulator (T85.734)

¹ √7ᵗʰ **T83.591** **Infection and inflammatory reaction due to implanted urinary sphincter** HCC ESR

¹ √7ᵗʰ **T83.592** **Infection and inflammatory reaction due to indwelling ureteral stent** HCC ESR

¹ √7ᵗʰ **T83.593** **Infection and inflammatory reaction due to other urinary stents** HCC ESR
Infection and inflammatory reaction due to ileal conduit stents
Infection and inflammatory reaction due to nephroureteral stent

¹ √7ᵗʰ **T83.598** **Infection and inflammatory reaction due to other prosthetic device, implant and graft in urinary system** HCC ESR
AHA: 2020,3Q,25

√5ᵗʰ **T83.6** **Infection and inflammatory reaction due to prosthetic device, implant and graft in** genital tract
Use additional code to identify infection

1 √x7ᵗʰ **T83.61** **Infection and inflammatory reaction due to implanted penile prosthesis** HCC ESR
Infection and inflammatory reaction due to penile prosthesis cylinder
Infection and inflammatory reaction due to penile prosthesis pump
Infection and inflammatory reaction due to penile prosthesis reservoir

1 √x7ᵗʰ **T83.62** **Infection and inflammatory reaction due to implanted testicular prosthesis** HCC ESR

1 √x7ᵗʰ **T83.69** **Infection and inflammatory reaction due to other prosthetic device, implant and graft in genital tract** HCC ESR

√5ᵗʰ **T83.7** **Complications due to** implanted mesh and other prosthetic materials

√6ᵗʰ **T83.71** **Erosion of implanted mesh and other prosthetic materials**

1 √7ᵗʰ **T83.711** **Erosion of implanted** vaginal **mesh to surrounding organ or tissue** HCC ESR ♀
Erosion of implanted vaginal mesh into pelvic floor muscles

1 √7ᵗʰ **T83.712** **Erosion of implanted** urethral **mesh to surrounding organ or tissue** HCC ESR
Erosion of implanted female urethral sling
Erosion of implanted male urethral sling
Erosion of implanted urethral mesh into pelvic floor muscles

1 √7ᵗʰ **T83.713** **Erosion of implanted** urethral bulking agent **to surrounding organ or tissue** HCC ESR

1 √7ᵗʰ **T83.714** **Erosion of implanted** ureteral bulking agent **to surrounding organ or tissue** HCC ESR

1 √7ᵗʰ **T83.718** **Erosion of other implanted mesh to organ or tissue** HCC ESR

1 √7ᵗʰ **T83.719** **Erosion of other prosthetic materials to surrounding organ or tissue** HCC ESR

√6ᵗʰ **T83.72** **Exposure** of implanted mesh and other prosthetic materials into surrounding organ or tissue
Extrusion of implanted mesh

1 √7ᵗʰ **T83.721** **Exposure of implanted** vaginal mesh **into vagina** HCC ESR ♀
Exposure of implanted vaginal mesh through vaginal wall

1 √7ᵗʰ **T83.722** **Exposure of implanted** urethral mesh **into urethra** HCC ESR
Exposure of implanted female urethral sling
Exposure of implanted male urethral sling
Exposure of implanted urethral mesh through urethral wall

1 √7ᵗʰ **T83.723** **Exposure of implanted** urethral bulking agent **into urethra** HCC ESR

1 √7ᵗʰ **T83.724** **Exposure of implanted** ureteral bulking agent **into ureter** HCC ESR

1 √7ᵗʰ **T83.728** **Exposure of** other implanted mesh **into organ or tissue** HCC ESR

1 √7ᵗʰ **T83.729** **Exposure of** other prosthetic materials **into organ or tissue** HCC ESR

1 √x7ᵗʰ **T83.79** **Other specified complications due to other genitourinary prosthetic materials** HCC ESR

√5ᵗʰ **T83.8** **Other specified complications of** genitourinary prosthetic devices, implants and grafts

1 √x7ᵗʰ **T83.81** **Embolism due to genitourinary prosthetic devices, implants and grafts** HCC ESR

1 √x7ᵗʰ **T83.82** **Fibrosis due to genitourinary prosthetic devices, implants and grafts** HCC ESR

1 √x7ᵗʰ **T83.83** **Hemorrhage due to genitourinary prosthetic devices, implants and grafts** HCC ESR

1 √x7ᵗʰ **T83.84** **Pain due to genitourinary prosthetic devices, implants and grafts** HCC ESR

1 √x7ᵗʰ **T83.85** **Stenosis due to genitourinary prosthetic devices, implants and grafts** HCC ESR

1 √x7ᵗʰ **T83.86** **Thrombosis due to genitourinary prosthetic devices, implants and grafts** HCC ESR

1 √x7ᵗʰ **T83.89** **Other specified complication of genitourinary prosthetic devices, implants and grafts** HCC ESR
AHA: 2016,1Q,19

1 √x7ᵗʰ **T83.9** **Unspecified complication of genitourinary prosthetic device, implant and graft** HCC ESR

√4ᵗʰ **T84** **Complications of internal orthopedic prosthetic devices, implants and grafts**

EXCLUDES 2 *failure and rejection of transplanted organs and tissues (T86.-)*
fracture of bone following insertion of orthopedic implant, joint prosthesis or bone plate (M96.6)

The appropriate 7th character is to be added to each code from category T84.
A   initial encounter
D   subsequent encounter
S   sequela

√5ᵗʰ **T84.0** **Mechanical complication of** internal joint prosthesis

√6ᵗʰ **T84.01** **Broken** internal joint prosthesis
Breakage (fracture) of prosthetic joint
Broken prosthetic joint implant
EXCLUDES 1 *periprosthetic joint implant fracture (M97.-)*
AHA: 2016,4Q,42

1 √7ᵗʰ **T84.010** **Broken internal** right hip **prosthesis** HCC ESR

1 √7ᵗʰ **T84.011** **Broken internal** left hip **prosthesis** HCC ESR

1 √7ᵗʰ **T84.012** **Broken internal** right knee **prosthesis** HCC ESR

1 √7ᵗʰ **T84.013** **Broken internal** left knee **prosthesis** HCC ESR

1 √7ᵗʰ **T84.018** **Broken internal joint prosthesis, other site** HCC ESR
Use additional code to identify the joint (Z96.6-)

1 √7ᵗʰ **T84.019** **Broken internal joint prosthesis, unspecified site** HCC ESR

√6ᵗʰ **T84.02** **Dislocation** of internal joint prosthesis
Instability of internal joint prosthesis
Subluxation of internal joint prosthesis
AHA: 2019,2Q,27

1 √7ᵗʰ **T84.020** **Dislocation of internal** right hip **prosthesis** HCC ESR

1 √7ᵗʰ **T84.021** **Dislocation of internal** left hip **prosthesis** HCC ESR

1 √7ᵗʰ **T84.022** **Instability of internal** right knee **prosthesis** HCC ESR

1 √7ᵗʰ **T84.023** **Instability of internal** left knee **prosthesis** HCC ESR

1 √7ᵗʰ **T84.028** **Dislocation of other internal joint prosthesis** HCC ESR
Use additional code to identify the joint (Z96.6-)

1 √7ᵗʰ **T84.029** **Dislocation of unspecified internal joint prosthesis** HCC ESR

√6ᵗʰ **T84.03** **Mechanical loosening** of internal prosthetic joint
Aseptic loosening of prosthetic joint

1 √7ᵗʰ **T84.030** **Mechanical loosening of internal** right hip **prosthetic joint** HCC ESR

1 √7ᵗʰ **T84.031** **Mechanical loosening of internal** left hip **prosthetic joint** HCC ESR

1 √7ᵗʰ **T84.032** **Mechanical loosening of internal** right knee **prosthetic joint** HCC ESR

1 √7ᵗʰ **T84.033** **Mechanical loosening of internal** left knee **prosthetic joint** HCC ESR

1 √7ᵗʰ **T84.038** **Mechanical loosening of other internal prosthetic joint** HCC ESR
Use additional code to identify the joint (Z96.6-)

1 √7ᵗʰ **T84.039** **Mechanical loosening of unspecified internal prosthetic joint** HCC ESR

√6ᵗʰ **T84.05** **Periprosthetic osteolysis** of internal prosthetic joint
Use additional code to identify major osseous defect, if applicable (M89.7-)

1 √7ᵗʰ **T84.050** **Periprosthetic osteolysis of internal prosthetic** right hip joint HCC ESR

1 √7ᵗʰ **T84.051** **Periprosthetic osteolysis of internal prosthetic** left hip joint HCC ESR

¹ ✓7ᵗʰ **T84.052 Periprosthetic osteolysis of internal prosthetic** right knee joint `HCC` `ESR`

¹ ✓7ᵗʰ **T84.053 Periprosthetic osteolysis of internal prosthetic** left knee joint `HCC` `ESR`

¹ ✓7ᵗʰ **T84.058 Periprosthetic osteolysis of other internal prosthetic joint** `HCC` `ESR`
Use additional code to identify the joint (Z96.6-)

¹ ✓7ᵗʰ **T84.059 Periprosthetic osteolysis of unspecified internal prosthetic joint** `HCC` `ESR`

✓6ᵗʰ **T84.06 Wear of articular bearing surface of internal prosthetic joint**

¹ ✓7ᵗʰ **T84.060 Wear of articular bearing surface of internal prosthetic** right hip joint `HCC` `ESR`

¹ ✓7ᵗʰ **T84.061 Wear of articular bearing surface of internal prosthetic** left hip joint `HCC` `ESR`

¹ ✓7ᵗʰ **T84.062 Wear of articular bearing surface of internal prosthetic** right knee joint `HCC` `ESR`

¹ ✓7ᵗʰ **T84.063 Wear of articular bearing surface of internal prosthetic** left knee joint `HCC` `ESR`

¹ ✓7ᵗʰ **T84.068 Wear of articular bearing surface of other internal prosthetic joint** `HCC` `ESR`
Use additional code to identify the joint (Z96.6-)

¹ ✓7ᵗʰ **T84.069 Wear of articular bearing surface of unspecified internal prosthetic joint** `HCC` `ESR`

✓6ᵗʰ **T84.09 Other mechanical complication of internal joint prosthesis**
Prosthetic joint implant failure NOS
AHA: 2019,1Q,20

¹ ✓7ᵗʰ **T84.090 Other mechanical complication of internal** right hip prosthesis `HCC` `ESR`

¹ ✓7ᵗʰ **T84.091 Other mechanical complication of internal** left hip prosthesis `HCC` `ESR`

¹ ✓7ᵗʰ **T84.092 Other mechanical complication of internal** right knee prosthesis `HCC` `ESR`

¹ ✓7ᵗʰ **T84.093 Other mechanical complication of internal** left knee prosthesis `HCC` `ESR`

¹ ✓7ᵗʰ **T84.098 Other mechanical complication of other internal joint prosthesis** `HCC` `ESR`
Use additional code to identify the joint (Z96.6-)

¹ ✓7ᵗʰ **T84.099 Other mechanical complication of unspecified internal joint prosthesis** `HCC` `ESR`

✓5ᵗʰ **T84.1 Mechanical complication of** internal fixation device **of bones of limb**
EXCLUDES 2 *mechanical complication of internal fixation device of bones of feet (T84.2-)*
mechanical complication of internal fixation device of bones of fingers (T84.2-)
mechanical complication of internal fixation device of bones of hands (T84.2-)
mechanical complication of internal fixation device of bones of toes (T84.2-)

✓6ᵗʰ **T84.11 Breakdown (mechanical) of internal fixation device of bones of limb**

¹ ✓7ᵗʰ **T84.110 Breakdown (mechanical) of internal fixation device of** right humerus `HCC` `ESR`

¹ ✓7ᵗʰ **T84.111 Breakdown (mechanical) of internal fixation device of** left humerus `HCC` `ESR`

¹ ✓7ᵗʰ **T84.112 Breakdown (mechanical) of internal fixation device of bone of** right forearm `HCC` `ESR`

¹ ✓7ᵗʰ **T84.113 Breakdown (mechanical) of internal fixation device of bone of** left forearm `HCC` `ESR`

¹ ✓7ᵗʰ **T84.114 Breakdown (mechanical) of internal fixation device of** right femur `HCC` `ESR`

¹ ✓7ᵗʰ **T84.115 Breakdown (mechanical) of internal fixation device of** left femur `HCC` `ESR`

¹ ✓7ᵗʰ **T84.116 Breakdown (mechanical) of internal fixation device of bone of** right lower leg `HCC` `ESR`

¹ ✓7ᵗʰ **T84.117 Breakdown (mechanical) of internal fixation device of bone of** left lower leg `HCC` `ESR`

¹ ✓7ᵗʰ **T84.119 Breakdown (mechanical) of internal fixation device of unspecified bone of limb** `HCC` `ESR`

✓6ᵗʰ **T84.12 Displacement of internal fixation device of bones of limb**
Malposition of internal fixation device of bones of limb

¹ ✓7ᵗʰ **T84.120 Displacement of internal fixation device of** right humerus `HCC` `ESR`

¹ ✓7ᵗʰ **T84.121 Displacement of internal fixation device of** left humerus `HCC` `ESR`

¹ ✓7ᵗʰ **T84.122 Displacement of internal fixation device of bone of** right forearm `HCC` `ESR`

¹ ✓7ᵗʰ **T84.123 Displacement of internal fixation device of bone of** left forearm `HCC` `ESR`

¹ ✓7ᵗʰ **T84.124 Displacement of internal fixation device of** right femur `HCC` `ESR`

¹ ✓7ᵗʰ **T84.125 Displacement of internal fixation device of** left femur `HCC` `ESR`

¹ ✓7ᵗʰ **T84.126 Displacement of internal fixation device of bone of** right lower leg `HCC` `ESR`

¹ ✓7ᵗʰ **T84.127 Displacement of internal fixation device of bone of** left lower leg `HCC` `ESR`

¹ ✓7ᵗʰ **T84.129 Displacement of internal fixation device of unspecified bone of limb** `HCC` `ESR`

✓6ᵗʰ **T84.19 Other mechanical complication of internal fixation device of bones of limb**
Obstruction (mechanical) of internal fixation device of bones of limb
Perforation of internal fixation device of bones of limb
Protrusion of internal fixation device of bones of limb

¹ ✓7ᵗʰ **T84.190 Other mechanical complication of internal fixation device of** right humerus `HCC` `ESR`

¹ ✓7ᵗʰ **T84.191 Other mechanical complication of internal fixation device of** left humerus `HCC` `ESR`

¹ ✓7ᵗʰ **T84.192 Other mechanical complication of internal fixation device of bone of** right forearm `HCC` `ESR`

¹ ✓7ᵗʰ **T84.193 Other mechanical complication of internal fixation device of bone of** left forearm `HCC` `ESR`

¹ ✓7ᵗʰ **T84.194 Other mechanical complication of internal fixation device of** right femur `HCC` `ESR`

¹ ✓7ᵗʰ **T84.195 Other mechanical complication of internal fixation device of** left femur `HCC` `ESR`

¹ ✓7ᵗʰ **T84.196 Other mechanical complication of internal fixation device of bone of** right lower leg `HCC` `ESR`

¹ ✓7ᵗʰ **T84.197 Other mechanical complication of internal fixation device of bone of** left lower leg `HCC` `ESR`

¹ ✓7ᵗʰ **T84.199 Other mechanical complication of internal fixation device of unspecified bone of limb** `HCC` `ESR`

✓5ᵗʰ **T84.2 Mechanical complication of** internal fixation device **of** other bones

✓6ᵗʰ **T84.21 Breakdown (mechanical) of internal fixation device of other bones**

¹ ✓7ᵗʰ **T84.210 Breakdown (mechanical) of internal fixation device of bones of** hand and fingers `HCC` `ESR`

¹ ✓7ᵗʰ **T84.213 Breakdown (mechanical) of internal fixation device of bones of** foot and toes `HCC` `ESR`

¹ ✓7ᵗʰ **T84.216 Breakdown (mechanical) of internal fixation device of** vertebrae `HCC` `ESR`

¹ ✓7ᵗʰ **T84.218 Breakdown (mechanical) of internal fixation device of other bones** `HCC` `ESR`

✓6ᵗʰ **T84.22 Displacement of internal fixation device of other bones**
Malposition of internal fixation device of other bones

¹ ✓7ᵗʰ **T84.220 Displacement of internal fixation device of bones of** hand and fingers `HCC` `ESR`

¹ ✓7ᵗʰ **T84.223 Displacement of internal fixation device of bones of** foot and toes `HCC` `ESR`

¹ ✓7ᵗʰ **T84.226 Displacement of internal fixation device of** vertebrae `HCC` `ESR`

¹ ✓7ᵗʰ **T84.228 Displacement of internal fixation device of other bones** `HCC` `ESR`

✓6ᵗʰ **T84.29 Other mechanical complication of internal fixation device of other bones**
Obstruction (mechanical) of internal fixation device of other bones
Perforation of internal fixation device of other bones
Protrusion of internal fixation device of other bones

¹ ✓7ᵗʰ **T84.290 Other mechanical complication of internal fixation device of bones of** hand and fingers `HCC` `ESR`

¹ ✓7ᵗʰ **T84.293 Other mechanical complication of internal fixation device of bones of** foot and toes `HCC` `ESR`

¹ ✓7ᵗʰ **T84.296 Other mechanical complication of internal fixation device of** vertebrae `HCC` `ESR`

¹ ✓7ᵗʰ **T84.298 Other mechanical complication of internal fixation device of other bones** `HCC` `ESR`

✓5ᵗʰ **T84.3 Mechanical complication of other bone devices, implants and grafts**
EXCLUDES 2   other complications of bone graft (T86.83-)

✓6ᵗʰ **T84.31 Breakdown (mechanical) of other bone devices, implants and grafts**

¹ ✓7ᵗʰ **T84.310 Breakdown (mechanical) of** electronic bone stimulator `HCC` `ESR`

¹ ✓7ᵗʰ **T84.318 Breakdown (mechanical) of other bone devices, implants and grafts** `HCC` `ESR`

✓6ᵗʰ **T84.32 Displacement of other bone devices, implants and grafts**
Malposition of other bone devices, implants and grafts

¹ ✓7ᵗʰ **T84.320 Displacement of** electronic bone stimulator `HCC` `ESR`

¹ ✓7ᵗʰ **T84.328 Displacement of other bone devices, implants and grafts** `HCC` `ESR`
AHA: 2014,4Q,28

✓6ᵗʰ **T84.39 Other mechanical complication of other bone devices, implants and grafts**
Obstruction (mechanical) of other bone devices, implants and grafts
Perforation of other bone devices, implants and grafts
Protrusion of other bone devices, implants and grafts

¹ ✓7ᵗʰ **T84.390 Other mechanical complication of** electronic bone stimulator `HCC` `ESR`

¹ ✓7ᵗʰ **T84.398 Other mechanical complication of other bone devices, implants and grafts** `HCC` `ESR`

✓5ᵗʰ **T84.4 Mechanical complication of other internal orthopedic devices, implants and grafts**

✓6ᵗʰ **T84.41 Breakdown (mechanical) of other internal orthopedic devices, implants and grafts**

¹ ✓7ᵗʰ **T84.410 Breakdown (mechanical) of** muscle and tendon graft `HCC` `ESR`

¹ ✓7ᵗʰ **T84.418 Breakdown (mechanical) of other internal orthopedic devices, implants and grafts** `HCC` `ESR`

✓6ᵗʰ **T84.42 Displacement of other internal orthopedic devices, implants and grafts**
Malposition of other internal orthopedic devices, implants and grafts

¹ ✓7ᵗʰ **T84.420 Displacement of** muscle and tendon graft `HCC` `ESR`

¹ ✓7ᵗʰ **T84.428 Displacement of other internal orthopedic devices, implants and grafts** `HCC` `ESR`

✓6ᵗʰ **T84.49 Other mechanical complication of other internal orthopedic devices, implants and grafts**
Mechanical complication of other internal orthopedic devices, implants and grafts NOS
Obstruction (mechanical) of other internal orthopedic devices, implants and grafts
Perforation of other internal orthopedic devices, implants and grafts
Protrusion of other internal orthopedic devices, implants and grafts

¹ ✓7ᵗʰ **T84.490 Other mechanical complication of** muscle and tendon graft `HCC` `ESR`

¹ ✓7ᵗʰ **T84.498 Other mechanical complication of other internal orthopedic devices, implants and grafts** `HCC` `ESR`

✓5ᵗʰ **T84.5 Infection and inflammatory reaction due to** internal joint prosthesis
Use additional code to identify infection
AHA: 2019,3Q,16; 2015,1Q,16

¹ ✓x7ᵗʰ **T84.50 Infection and inflammatory reaction due to unspecified internal joint prosthesis** `HCC` `ESR`

¹ ✓x7ᵗʰ **T84.51 Infection and inflammatory reaction due to internal** right hip **prosthesis** `HCC` `ESR`

¹ ✓x7ᵗʰ **T84.52 Infection and inflammatory reaction due to internal** left hip **prosthesis** `HCC` `ESR`

¹ ✓x7ᵗʰ **T84.53 Infection and inflammatory reaction due to internal** right knee **prosthesis** `HCC` `ESR`

¹ ✓x7ᵗʰ **T84.54 Infection and inflammatory reaction due to internal** left knee **prosthesis** `HCC` `ESR`

¹ ✓x7ᵗʰ **T84.59 Infection and inflammatory reaction due to other internal joint prosthesis** `HCC` `ESR`

✓5ᵗʰ **T84.6 Infection and inflammatory reaction due to** internal fixation device
Use additional code to identify infection

¹ ✓x7ᵗʰ **T84.60 Infection and inflammatory reaction due to internal fixation device of unspecified site** `HCC` `ESR`

✓6ᵗʰ **T84.61 Infection and inflammatory reaction due to internal fixation device of** arm

¹ ✓7ᵗʰ **T84.610 Infection and inflammatory reaction due to internal fixation device of** right humerus `HCC` `ESR`

¹ ✓7ᵗʰ **T84.611 Infection and inflammatory reaction due to internal fixation device of** left humerus `HCC` `ESR`

¹ ✓7ᵗʰ **T84.612 Infection and inflammatory reaction due to internal fixation device of** right radius `HCC` `ESR`

¹ ✓7ᵗʰ **T84.613 Infection and inflammatory reaction due to internal fixation device of** left radius `HCC` `ESR`

¹ ✓7ᵗʰ **T84.614 Infection and inflammatory reaction due to internal fixation device of** right ulna `HCC` `ESR`

¹ ✓7ᵗʰ **T84.615 Infection and inflammatory reaction due to internal fixation device of** left ulna `HCC` `ESR`

¹ ✓7ᵗʰ **T84.619 Infection and inflammatory reaction due to internal fixation device of unspecified bone of arm** `HCC` `ESR`

✓6ᵗʰ **T84.62 Infection and inflammatory reaction due to internal fixation device of** leg

¹ ✓7ᵗʰ **T84.620 Infection and inflammatory reaction due to internal fixation device of** right femur `HCC` `ESR`

¹ ✓7ᵗʰ **T84.621 Infection and inflammatory reaction due to internal fixation device of** left femur `HCC` `ESR`

¹ ✓7ᵗʰ **T84.622 Infection and inflammatory reaction due to internal fixation device of** right tibia `HCC` `ESR`

¹ ✓7ᵗʰ **T84.623 Infection and inflammatory reaction due to internal fixation device of** left tibia `HCC` `ESR`

¹ ✓7ᵗʰ **T84.624 Infection and inflammatory reaction due to internal fixation device of** right fibula `HCC` `ESR`

¹ ✓7ᵗʰ **T84.625 Infection and inflammatory reaction due to internal fixation device of** left fibula `HCC` `ESR`

¹ ✓7ᵗʰ **T84.629** **Infection and inflammatory reaction due to internal fixation device of unspecified bone of leg** `HCC` `ESR`

¹ ✓x7ᵗʰ **T84.63** **Infection and inflammatory reaction due to internal fixation device of** spine `HCC` `ESR`

¹ ✓x7ᵗʰ **T84.69** **Infection and inflammatory reaction due to internal fixation device of other site** `HCC` `ESR`

¹ ✓x7ᵗʰ **T84.7** **Infection and inflammatory reaction due to other internal orthopedic prosthetic devices, implants and grafts** `HCC` `ESR`
Use additional code to identify infection

✓5ᵗʰ **T84.8** **Other specified complications of internal orthopedic prosthetic devices, implants and grafts**

¹ ✓x7ᵗʰ **T84.81** **Embolism due to internal orthopedic prosthetic devices, implants and grafts** `HCC` `ESR`

¹ ✓x7ᵗʰ **T84.82** **Fibrosis due to internal orthopedic prosthetic devices, implants and grafts** `HCC` `ESR`

¹ ✓x7ᵗʰ **T84.83** **Hemorrhage due to internal orthopedic prosthetic devices, implants and grafts** `HCC` `ESR`

¹ ✓x7ᵗʰ **T84.84** **Pain due to internal orthopedic prosthetic devices, implants and grafts** `HCC` `ESR`

¹ ✓x7ᵗʰ **T84.85** **Stenosis due to internal orthopedic prosthetic devices, implants and grafts** `HCC` `ESR`

¹ ✓x7ᵗʰ **T84.86** **Thrombosis due to internal orthopedic prosthetic devices, implants and grafts** `HCC` `ESR`

¹ ✓x7ᵗʰ **T84.89** **Other specified complication of internal orthopedic prosthetic devices, implants and grafts** `HCC` `ESR`

¹ ✓x7ᵗʰ **T84.9** **Unspecified complication of internal orthopedic prosthetic device, implant and graft** `HCC` `ESR`

✓4ᵗʰ **T85** **Complications of other internal prosthetic devices, implants and grafts**

EXCLUDES 2   *failure and rejection of transplanted organs and tissue (T86.-)*
AHA: 2016,4Q,71-72

The appropriate 7th character is to be added to each code from category T85.
A   initial encounter
D   subsequent encounter
S   sequela

✓5ᵗʰ **T85.0** **Mechanical complication of** ventricular intracranial (communicating) shunt

¹ ✓x7ᵗʰ **T85.01** **Breakdown (mechanical) of ventricular intracranial (communicating) shunt** `HCC` `ESR`

¹ ✓x7ᵗʰ **T85.02** **Displacement of ventricular intracranial (communicating) shunt** `HCC` `ESR`
Malposition of ventricular intracranial (communicating) shunt

¹ ✓x7ᵗʰ **T85.03** **Leakage of ventricular intracranial (communicating) shunt** `HCC` `ESR`

¹ ✓x7ᵗʰ **T85.09** **Other mechanical complication of ventricular intracranial (communicating) shunt** `HCC` `ESR`
Obstruction (mechanical) of ventricular intracranial (communicating) shunt
Perforation of ventricular intracranial (communicating) shunt
Protrusion of ventricular intracranial (communicating) shunt

✓5ᵗʰ **T85.1** **Mechanical complication of** implanted electronic stimulator of nervous system

✓6ᵗʰ **T85.11** **Breakdown (mechanical) of implanted electronic stimulator of nervous system**

¹ ✓7ᵗʰ **T85.110** **Breakdown (mechanical) of implanted electronic neurostimulator** of brain electrode (lead) `HCC` `ESR`

¹ ✓7ᵗʰ **T85.111** **Breakdown (mechanical) of implanted electronic neurostimulator** of peripheral nerve electrode (lead) `HCC` `ESR`
Breakdown of electrode (lead) for cranial nerve neurostimulators
Breakdown of electrode (lead) for gastric neurostimulator
Breakdown of electrode (lead) for sacral nerve neurostimulator
Breakdown of electrode (lead) for vagal nerve neurostimulators

¹ ✓7ᵗʰ **T85.112** **Breakdown (mechanical) of implanted electronic neurostimulator** of spinal cord electrode (lead) `HCC` `ESR`

¹ ✓7ᵗʰ **T85.113** **Breakdown (mechanical) of implanted electronic neurostimulator, generator** `HCC` `ESR`
Breakdown (mechanical) of implanted electronic neurostimulator generator, brain, peripheral, gastric, spinal
Breakdown (mechanical) of implanted electronic sacral neurostimulator, pulse generator or receiver

¹ ✓7ᵗʰ **T85.118** **Breakdown (mechanical) of other implanted electronic stimulator of** nervous system `HCC` `ESR`

✓6ᵗʰ **T85.12** **Displacement of implanted electronic stimulator of nervous system**
Malposition of implanted electronic stimulator of nervous system

¹ ✓7ᵗʰ **T85.120** **Displacement of implanted electronic neurostimulator** of brain electrode (lead) `HCC` `ESR`

¹ ✓7ᵗʰ **T85.121** **Displacement of implanted electronic neurostimulator** of peripheral nerve electrode (lead) `HCC` `ESR`
Displacement of electrode (lead) for cranial nerve neurostimulators
Displacement of electrode (lead) for gastric neurostimulator
Displacement of electrode (lead) for sacral nerve neurostimulator
Displacement of electrode (lead) for vagal nerve neurostimulators

¹ ✓7ᵗʰ **T85.122** **Displacement of implanted electronic neurostimulator** of spinal cord electrode (lead) `HCC` `ESR`

¹ ✓7ᵗʰ **T85.123** **Displacement of implanted electronic neurostimulator, generator** `HCC` `ESR`
Displacement of implanted electronic neurostimulator generator, brain, peripheral, gastric, spinal
Displacement of implanted electronic sacral neurostimulator, pulse generator or receiver

¹ ✓7ᵗʰ **T85.128** **Displacement of other implanted electronic stimulator of nervous system** `HCC` `ESR`

✓6ᵗʰ **T85.19** **Other mechanical complication of implanted electronic stimulator of nervous system**
Leakage of implanted electronic stimulator of nervous system
Obstruction (mechanical) of implanted electronic stimulator of nervous system
Perforation of implanted electronic stimulator of nervous system
Protrusion of implanted electronic stimulator of nervous system

¹ ✓7ᵗʰ **T85.190** **Other mechanical complication of implanted electronic neurostimulator** of brain electrode (lead) `HCC` `ESR`

¹ ✓7ᵗʰ **T85.191** **Other mechanical complication of implanted electronic neurostimulator** of peripheral nerve electrode (lead) `HCC` `ESR`
Other mechanical complication of electrode (lead) for cranial nerve neurostimulators
Other mechanical complication of electrode (lead) for gastric neurostimulator
Other mechanical complication of electrode (lead) for sacral nerve neurostimulator
Other mechanical complication of electrode (lead) for vagal nerve neurostimulators

¹ ✓7ᵗʰ **T85.192** **Other mechanical complication of implanted electronic neurostimulator** of spinal cord electrode (lead) `HCC` `ESR`

[1] √7th **T85.193 Other mechanical complication of implanted electronic neurostimulator, generator** HCC ESR

    Other mechanical complication of implanted electronic neurostimulator generator, brain, peripheral, gastric, spinal

    Other mechanical complication of implanted electronic sacral neurostimulator, pulse generator or receiver

[1] √7th **T85.199 Other mechanical complication of other implanted electronic stimulator of nervous system** HCC ESR

√5th **T85.2 Mechanical complication of** intraocular lens

  √x7th **T85.21 Breakdown (mechanical) of intraocular lens**

  √x7th **T85.22 Displacement of intraocular lens**

    Malposition of intraocular lens

  √x7th **T85.29 Other mechanical complication of intraocular lens**

    Obstruction (mechanical) of intraocular lens
    Perforation of intraocular lens
    Protrusion of intraocular lens

√5th **T85.3 Mechanical complication of other ocular prosthetic devices, implants and grafts**

    EXCLUDES 2   *other complications of corneal graft (T86.84-)*

  √6th **T85.31 Breakdown (mechanical) of other ocular prosthetic devices, implants and grafts**

    √7th **T85.310 Breakdown (mechanical) of prosthetic orbit of** right eye

    √7th **T85.311 Breakdown (mechanical) of prosthetic orbit of** left eye

    √7th **T85.318 Breakdown (mechanical) of other ocular prosthetic devices, implants and grafts**

  √6th **T85.32 Displacement of other ocular prosthetic devices, implants and grafts**

    Malposition of other ocular prosthetic devices, implants and grafts

    √7th **T85.320 Displacement of prosthetic orbit of** right eye

    √7th **T85.321 Displacement of prosthetic orbit of** left eye

    √7th **T85.328 Displacement of other ocular prosthetic devices, implants and grafts**

  √6th **T85.39 Other mechanical complication of other ocular prosthetic devices, implants and grafts**

    Obstruction (mechanical) of other ocular prosthetic devices, implants and grafts
    Perforation of other ocular prosthetic devices, implants and grafts
    Protrusion of other ocular prosthetic devices, implants and grafts

    √7th **T85.390 Other mechanical complication of prosthetic orbit of** right eye

    √7th **T85.391 Other mechanical complication of prosthetic orbit of** left eye

    √7th **T85.398 Other mechanical complication of other ocular prosthetic devices, implants and grafts**

√5th **T85.4 Mechanical complication of** breast prosthesis and implant

  √x7th **T85.41 Breakdown (mechanical) of breast prosthesis and implant**

  √x7th **T85.42 Displacement of breast prosthesis and implant**

    Malposition of breast prosthesis and implant

  √x7th **T85.43 Leakage of breast prosthesis and implant**

  √x7th **T85.44 Capsular contracture of breast implant**

  √x7th **T85.49 Other mechanical complication of breast prosthesis and implant**

    Obstruction (mechanical) of breast prosthesis and implant
    Perforation of breast prosthesis and implant
    Protrusion of breast prosthesis and implant

√5th **T85.5 Mechanical complication of** gastrointestinal prosthetic devices, implants and grafts

  √6th **T85.51 Breakdown (mechanical) of gastrointestinal prosthetic devices, implants and grafts**

    √7th **T85.510 Breakdown (mechanical) of** bile duct prosthesis

    √7th **T85.511 Breakdown (mechanical) of** esophageal anti-reflux device

    √7th **T85.518 Breakdown (mechanical) of other gastrointestinal prosthetic devices, implants and grafts**

  √6th **T85.52 Displacement of gastrointestinal prosthetic devices, implants and grafts**

    Malposition of gastrointestinal prosthetic devices, implants and grafts

    √7th **T85.520 Displacement of** bile duct prosthesis

    √7th **T85.521 Displacement of** esophageal anti-reflux device

    √7th **T85.528 Displacement of other gastrointestinal prosthetic devices, implants and grafts**

  √6th **T85.59 Other mechanical complication of gastrointestinal prosthetic devices, implants and**

    Obstruction, mechanical of gastrointestinal prosthetic devices, implants and grafts
    Perforation of gastrointestinal prosthetic devices, implants and grafts
    Protrusion of gastrointestinal prosthetic devices, implants and grafts

    √7th **T85.590 Other mechanical complication of** bile duct prosthesis

    √7th **T85.591 Other mechanical complication of** esophageal anti-reflux device

    √7th **T85.598 Other mechanical complication of other gastrointestinal prosthetic devices, implants and grafts**

√5th **T85.6 Mechanical complication of other specified internal and external prosthetic devices, implants and grafts**

  √6th **T85.61 Breakdown (mechanical) of other specified internal prosthetic devices, implants and grafts**

    √7th **T85.610 Breakdown (mechanical) of** cranial or spinal infusion catheter

    Breakdown (mechanical) of epidural infusion catheter
    Breakdown (mechanical) of intrathecal infusion catheter
    Breakdown (mechanical) of subarachnoid infusion catheter
    Breakdown (mechanical) of subdural infusion catheter

    √7th **T85.611 Breakdown (mechanical) of intraperitoneal dialysis catheter** HCC Rx ESR

      EXCLUDES 1   *mechanical complication of vascular dialysis catheter (T82.4-)*

    √7th **T85.612 Breakdown (mechanical) of** permanent sutures

      EXCLUDES 1   *mechanical complication of permanent (wire) suture used in bone repair (T84.1-T84.2)*

    √7th **T85.613 Breakdown (mechanical) of** artificial skin graft and decellularized allodermis

    Failure of artificial skin graft and decellularized allodermis
    Non-adherence of artificial skin graft and decellularized allodermis
    Poor incorporation of artificial skin graft and decellularized allodermis
    Shearing of artificial skin graft and decellularized allodermis

    √7th **T85.614 Breakdown (mechanical) of** insulin pump

[1] √7th **T85.615 Breakdown (mechanical) of other nervous system device, implant or graft** HCC ESR

    Breakdown (mechanical) of intrathecal infusion pump

    √7th **T85.618 Breakdown (mechanical) of other specified internal prosthetic devices, implants and grafts**

√6ᵗʰ **T85.62** **Displacement** of other specified internal prosthetic devices, implants and grafts

Malposition of other specified internal prosthetic devices, implants and grafts

√7ᵗʰ **T85.620** **Displacement of** cranial or spinal infusion catheter

Displacement of epidural infusion catheter
Displacement of intrathecal infusion catheter
Displacement of subarachnoid infusion catheter
Displacement of subdural infusion catheter

√7ᵗʰ **T85.621** **Displacement of** intraperitoneal dialysis catheter   HCC Rx ESR

EXCLUDES 1   mechanical complication of vascular dialysis catheter (T82.4-)

√7ᵗʰ **T85.622** **Displacement of** permanent sutures

EXCLUDES 1   mechanical complication of permanent (wire) suture used in bone repair (T84.1-T84.2)

√7ᵗʰ **T85.623** **Displacement of** artificial skin graft and decellularized allodermis

Dislodgement of artificial skin graft and decellularized allodermis

√7ᵗʰ **T85.624** **Displacement of** insulin pump

¹ √7ᵗʰ **T85.625** **Displacement of other nervous system device, implant or graft**   HCC ESR

Displacement of intrathecal infusion pump

√7ᵗʰ **T85.628** **Displacement of other specified internal prosthetic devices, implants and grafts**

√6ᵗʰ **T85.63** **Leakage** of other specified internal prosthetic devices, implants and grafts

√7ᵗʰ **T85.630** **Leakage of** cranial or spinal infusion catheter

Leakage of epidural infusion catheter
Leakage of intrathecal infusion infusion catheter
Leakage of subdural infusion catheter
Leakage of subarachnoid infusion catheter

√7ᵗʰ **T85.631** **Leakage of** intraperitoneal dialysis catheter   HCC Rx ESR

EXCLUDES 1   mechanical complication of vascular dialysis catheter (T82.4)

√7ᵗʰ **T85.633** **Leakage of** insulin pump

¹ √7ᵗʰ **T85.635** **Leakage of other nervous system device, implant or graft**   HCC ESR

Leakage of intrathecal infusion pump

√7ᵗʰ **T85.638** **Leakage of other specified internal prosthetic devices, implants and grafts**

√6ᵗʰ **T85.69** **Other mechanical complication of other specified internal prosthetic devices, implants and grafts**

Obstruction, mechanical of other specified internal prosthetic devices, implants and grafts
Perforation of other specified internal prosthetic devices, implants and grafts
Protrusion of other specified internal prosthetic devices, implants and grafts

√7ᵗʰ **T85.690** **Other mechanical complication of** cranial or spinal infusion catheter

Other mechanical complication of epidural infusion catheter
Other mechanical complication of intrathecal infusion catheter
Other mechanical complication of subarachnoid infusion catheter
Other mechanical complication of subdural infusion catheter

√7ᵗʰ **T85.691** **Other mechanical complication of** intraperitoneal dialysis catheter   HCC Rx ESR

EXCLUDES 1   mechanical complication of vascular dialysis catheter (T82.4)

√7ᵗʰ **T85.692** **Other mechanical complication of** permanent sutures

EXCLUDES 1   mechanical complication of permanent (wire) suture used in bone repair (T84.1-T84.2)

√7ᵗʰ **T85.693** **Other mechanical complication of** artificial skin graft and decellularized allodermis

√7ᵗʰ **T85.694** **Other mechanical complication of** insulin pump

¹ √7ᵗʰ **T85.695** **Other mechanical complication of other nervous system device, implant or graft**   HCC ESR

Other mechanical complication of intrathecal infusion pump

√7ᵗʰ **T85.698** **Other mechanical complication of other specified internal prosthetic devices, implants and grafts**

Mechanical complication of nonabsorbable surgical material NOS

√5ᵗʰ **T85.7** **Infection and inflammatory reaction** due to other internal prosthetic devices, implants and grafts

Use additional code to identify infection

√7ᵗʰ **T85.71** **Infection and inflammatory reaction due to** peritoneal dialysis catheter   HCC Rx ESR

¹ √x7ᵗʰ **T85.72** **Infection and inflammatory reaction due to** insulin pump   HCC ESR

√6ᵗʰ **T85.73** **Infection and inflammatory reaction due to** nervous system devices, implants and graft

¹ √7ᵗʰ **T85.730** **Infection and inflammatory reaction due to** ventricular intracranial (communicating) shunt   HCC ESR

¹ √7ᵗʰ **T85.731** **Infection and inflammatory reaction due to implanted electronic neurostimulator of** brain, electrode (lead)   HCC ESR

¹ √7ᵗʰ **T85.732** **Infection and inflammatory reaction due to implanted electronic neurostimulator of** peripheral nerve, electrode (lead)   HCC ESR

Infection and inflammatory reaction due to electrode (lead) for cranial nerve neurostimulators
Infection and inflammatory reaction due to electrode (lead) for gastric neurostimulator
Infection and inflammatory reaction due to electrode (lead) for sacral nerve neurostimulator
Infection and inflammatory reaction due to electrode (lead) for vagal nerve neurostimulators

¹ √7ᵗʰ **T85.733** **Infection and inflammatory reaction due to implanted electronic neurostimulator of** spinal cord, electrode (lead)   HCC ESR

¹ √7ᵗʰ **T85.734** **Infection and inflammatory reaction due to implanted electronic neurostimulator, generator**

Generator pocket infection   HCC ESR

¹ √7ᵗʰ **T85.735** **Infection and inflammatory reaction due to** cranial or spinal infusion catheter   HCC ESR

Infection and inflammatory reaction due to epidural catheter
Infection and inflammatory reaction due to intrathecal infusion catheter
Infection and inflammatory reaction due to subarachnoid catheter
Infection and inflammatory reaction due to subdural catheter

¹ √7ᵗʰ **T85.738** **Infection and inflammatory reaction due to other nervous system device, implant or graft**   HCC ESR

Infection and inflammatory reaction due to intrathecal infusion pump

¹ √x7ᵗʰ **T85.79** **Infection and inflammatory reaction due to other internal prosthetic devices, implants and grafts**   HCC ESR

AHA: 2022,2Q,7

√5ᵗʰ **T85.8** **Other specified complications of internal prosthetic devices, implants and grafts, not elsewhere classified**

√6ᵗʰ **T85.81** **Embolism** due to internal prosthetic devices, implants and grafts, not elsewhere classified

¹ √7ᵗʰ **T85.810** **Embolism** due to **nervous system** prosthetic devices, implants and grafts   HCC ESR

√7ᵗʰ **T85.818** **Embolism** due to other internal prosthetic devices, implants and grafts

√6ᵗʰ **T85.82** **Fibrosis** due to internal prosthetic devices, implants and grafts, not elsewhere classified

¹ √7ᵗʰ **T85.820** **Fibrosis** due to **nervous system** prosthetic devices, implants and grafts   HCC ESR

√7ᵗʰ **T85.828** **Fibrosis** due to other internal prosthetic devices, implants and grafts

√6ᵗʰ **T85.83** **Hemorrhage** due to internal prosthetic devices, implants and grafts, not elsewhere classified

¹ √7ᵗʰ **T85.830** **Hemorrhage** due to **nervous system** prosthetic devices, implants and grafts   HCC ESR

√7ᵗʰ **T85.838** **Hemorrhage** due to other internal prosthetic devices, implants and grafts

√6ᵗʰ **T85.84** **Pain** due to internal prosthetic devices, implants and grafts, not elsewhere classified

¹ √7ᵗʰ **T85.840** **Pain** due to **nervous system** prosthetic devices, implants and grafts   HCC ESR

√7ᵗʰ **T85.848** **Pain** due to other internal prosthetic devices, implants and grafts

√6ᵗʰ **T85.85** **Stenosis** due to internal prosthetic devices, implants and grafts, not elsewhere classified

¹ √7ᵗʰ **T85.850** **Stenosis** due to **nervous system** prosthetic devices, implants and grafts   HCC ESR

√7ᵗʰ **T85.858** **Stenosis** due to other internal prosthetic devices, implants and grafts

√6ᵗʰ **T85.86** **Thrombosis** due to internal prosthetic devices, implants and grafts, not elsewhere classified

¹ √7ᵗʰ **T85.860** **Thrombosis** due to **nervous system** prosthetic devices, implants and grafts   HCC ESR

√7ᵗʰ **T85.868** **Thrombosis** due to other internal prosthetic devices, implants and grafts

√6ᵗʰ **T85.89** **Other specified complication of internal prosthetic devices, implants and grafts, not elsewhere classified**

Erosion or breakdown of subcutaneous device pocket

¹ √7ᵗʰ **T85.890** **Other specified complication of nervous system** prosthetic devices, implants and grafts   HCC ESR

√7ᵗʰ **T85.898** **Other specified complication of other internal prosthetic devices, implants and grafts**

√x7ᵗʰ **T85.9** **Unspecified complication of internal prosthetic device, implant and graft**

Complication of internal prosthetic device, implant and graft NOS

√4ᵗʰ **T86** **Complications of transplanted organs and tissue**

Use additional code to identify other transplant complications, such as:
graft-versus-host disease (D89.81-)
malignancy associated with organ transplant (C80.2)
post-transplant lymphoproliferative disorders (PTLD) (D47.Z1)
AHA: 2020,1Q,18

√5ᵗʰ **T86.0** **Complications of bone marrow transplant**

T86.00 **Unspecified complication of bone marrow transplant**   HCC Rx ESR COM

T86.01 **Bone marrow transplant rejection**   HCC Rx ESR COM

T86.02 **Bone marrow transplant failure**   HCC Rx ESR COM

T86.03 **Bone marrow transplant infection**   HCC Rx ESR COM

T86.09 **Other complications of bone marrow transplant**   HCC Rx ESR COM

√5ᵗʰ **T86.1** **Complications of kidney transplant**

T86.10 **Unspecified complication of kidney transplant**   Rx COM

T86.11 **Kidney transplant rejection**   Rx COM

T86.12 **Kidney transplant failure**   Rx COM
AHA: 2013,1Q,24

T86.13 **Kidney transplant infection**   Rx COM
Use additional code to specify infection

T86.19 **Other complication of kidney transplant**   Rx COM
AHA: 2019,2Q,7

√5ᵗʰ **T86.2** **Complications of heart transplant**

EXCLUDES 1   complication of:
artificial heart device (T82.5-)
heart-lung transplant (T86.3-)

T86.20 **Unspecified complication of heart transplant**   HCC Rx ESR COM

T86.21 **Heart transplant rejection**   HCC Rx ESR COM

T86.22 **Heart transplant failure**   HCC Rx ESR COM

T86.23 **Heart transplant infection**   HCC Rx ESR COM
Use additional code to specify infection

√6ᵗʰ **T86.29** **Other complications of heart transplant**

T86.290 **Cardiac allograft vasculopathy**   HCC Rx ESR COM
EXCLUDES 1   atherosclerosis of coronary arteries (I25.75-, I25.76-, I25.81-)

T86.298 **Other complications of heart transplant**   HCC Rx ESR COM

√5ᵗʰ **T86.3** **Complications of heart-lung transplant**

T86.30 **Unspecified complication of heart-lung transplant**   HCC Rx ESR COM

T86.31 **Heart-lung transplant rejection**   HCC Rx ESR COM

T86.32 **Heart-lung transplant failure**   HCC Rx ESR COM

T86.33 **Heart-lung transplant infection**   HCC Rx ESR COM
Use additional code to specify infection

T86.39 **Other complications of heart-lung transplant**   HCC Rx ESR COM

√5ᵗʰ **T86.4** **Complications of liver transplant**

T86.40 **Unspecified complication of liver transplant**   HCC Rx ESR COM

T86.41 **Liver transplant rejection**   HCC Rx ESR COM

T86.42 **Liver transplant failure**   HCC Rx ESR COM

T86.43 **Liver transplant infection**   HCC Rx ESR COM
Use additional code to identify infection, such as:
cytomegalovirus (CMV) infection (B25.-)

T86.49 **Other complications of liver transplant**   HCC Rx ESR COM

T86.5 **Complications of stem cell transplant**   HCC Rx ESR COM
Complications from stem cells from peripheral blood
Complications from stem cells from umbilical cord
AHA: 2020,4Q,14

√5ᵗʰ **T86.8** **Complications of other transplanted organs and tissues**

√6ᵗʰ **T86.81** **Complications of lung transplant**

EXCLUDES 1   complication of heart-lung transplant (T86.3-)

T86.810 **Lung transplant rejection**   HCC Rx ESR COM

T86.811 **Lung transplant failure**   HCC Rx ESR COM

T86.812 **Lung transplant infection**   HCC Rx ESR COM
Use additional code to specify infection

T86.818 **Other complications of lung transplant**   HCC Rx ESR COM
AHA: 2019,2Q,6

T86.819 **Unspecified complication of lung transplant**   HCC Rx ESR COM

√6ᵗʰ **T86.82** **Complications of skin graft (allograft) (autograft)**

EXCLUDES 2   complication of artificial skin graft (T85.693)

T86.820 **Skin graft (allograft) rejection**

T86.821 **Skin graft (allograft) (autograft) failure**

T86.822 **Skin graft (allograft) (autograft) infection**
Use additional code to specify infection

T86.828 **Other complications of skin graft (allograft) (autograft)**

T86.829 **Unspecified complication of skin graft (allograft) (autograft)**

√6ᵗʰ **T86.83** **Complications of bone graft**

EXCLUDES 2   mechanical complications of bone graft (T84.3-)

T86.830 **Bone graft rejection**

T86.831 **Bone graft failure**

Chapter 19. Injury, Poisoning and Certain Other Consequences of External Causes

T86.832   **Bone graft** infection
Use additional code to specify infection

T86.838   **Other complications of bone graft**

T86.839   **Unspecified complication of bone graft**

√6ᵗʰ   **T86.84**   **Complications of** corneal **transplant**

    EXCLUDES 2   *mechanical complications of corneal graft (T85.3-)*

    AHA: 2020,4Q,40

√7ᵗʰ   **T86.840**   **Corneal transplant** rejection

     T86.8401   **Corneal transplant rejection,** right **eye**

     T86.8402   **Corneal transplant rejection,** left **eye**

     T86.8403   **Corneal transplant rejection,** bilateral

     T86.8409   **Corneal transplant rejection, unspecified eye**

√7ᵗʰ   **T86.841**   **Corneal transplant** failure

     T86.8411   **Corneal transplant failure,** right **eye**

     T86.8412   **Corneal transplant failure,** left **eye**

     T86.8413   **Corneal transplant failure,** bilateral

     T86.8419   **Corneal transplant failure, unspecified eye**

√7ᵗʰ   **T86.842**   **Corneal transplant** infection
Use additional code to specify infection

     T86.8421   **Corneal transplant infection,** right **eye**   HCC ESR

     T86.8422   **Corneal transplant infection,** left **eye**   HCC ESR

     T86.8423   **Corneal transplant infection,** bilateral   HCC ESR

     T86.8429   **Corneal transplant infection, unspecified eye**   HCC ESR

√7ᵗʰ   **T86.848**   **Other complications of corneal transplant**

     T86.8481   **Other complications of corneal transplant,** right **eye**

     T86.8482   **Other complications of corneal transplant,** left **eye**

     T86.8483   **Other complications of corneal transplant,** bilateral

     T86.8489   **Other complications of corneal transplant, unspecified eye**

√7ᵗʰ   **T86.849**   **Unspecified complication of corneal transplant**

     T86.8491   **Unspecified complication of corneal transplant,** right **eye**

     T86.8492   **Unspecified complication of corneal transplant,** left **eye**

     T86.8493   **Unspecified complication of corneal transplant,** bilateral

     T86.8499   **Unspecified complication of corneal transplant, unspecified eye**

√6ᵗʰ   **T86.85**   **Complication of** intestine **transplant**

    T86.850   **Intestine transplant** rejection   HCC Rx ESR COM

    T86.851   **Intestine transplant** failure   HCC Rx ESR COM

    T86.852   **Intestine transplant** infection   HCC Rx ESR COM
Use additional code to specify infection

    T86.858   **Other complications of intestine transplant**   HCC Rx ESR COM

    T86.859   **Unspecified complication of intestine transplant**   HCC Rx ESR COM

√6ᵗʰ   **T86.89**   **Complications of other transplanted tissue**
Transplant failure or rejection of pancreas
    AHA: 2020,1Q,18

    T86.890   **Other transplanted tissue** rejection

    T86.891   **Other transplanted tissue** failure

    T86.892   **Other transplanted tissue** infection
Use additional code to specify infection

    T86.898   **Other complications of other transplanted tissue**

    T86.899   **Unspecified complication of other transplanted tissue**

√5ᵗʰ   **T86.9**   **Complication of unspecified transplanted organ and tissue**

    T86.90   **Unspecified complication of unspecified transplanted organ and tissue**

    T86.91   **Unspecified transplanted organ and tissue** rejection

    T86.92   **Unspecified transplanted organ and tissue** failure

    T86.93   **Unspecified transplanted organ and tissue** infection
Use additional code to specify infection

    T86.99   **Other complications of unspecified transplanted organ and tissue**

√4ᵗʰ   **T87**   **Complications peculiar to reattachment and amputation**

√5ᵗʰ   **T87.0**   **Complications of reattached (part of)** upper extremity

√6ᵗʰ   **T87.0X**   **Complications of reattached (part of) upper extremity**

     T87.0X1   **Complications of reattached (part of)** right **upper extremity**   HCC ESR COM

     T87.0X2   **Complications of reattached (part of)** left **upper extremity**   HCC ESR COM

     T87.0X9   **Complications of reattached (part of) unspecified upper extremity**   HCC ESR COM

√5ᵗʰ   **T87.1**   **Complications of reattached (part of)** lower extremity

√6ᵗʰ   **T87.1X**   **Complications of reattached (part of) lower extremity**

     T87.1X1   **Complications of reattached (part of)** right **lower extremity**   HCC ESR COM

     T87.1X2   **Complications of reattached (part of)** left **lower extremity**   HCC ESR COM

     T87.1X9   **Complications of reattached (part of) unspecified lower extremity**   HCC ESR COM

    T87.2   **Complications of other reattached body part**   HCC ESR

√5ᵗʰ   **T87.3**   **Neuroma of amputation stump**

    DEF: Non-neoplastic tumor generated at the proximal end of severed, partially transected, or injured nerve following amputation.

    T87.30   **Neuroma of amputation stump, unspecified extremity**   HCC ESR COM

    T87.31   **Neuroma of amputation stump,** right upper **extremity**   HCC ESR COM

    T87.32   **Neuroma of amputation stump,** left upper **extremity**   HCC ESR COM

    T87.33   **Neuroma of amputation stump,** right lower **extremity**   HCC ESR COM

    T87.34   **Neuroma of amputation stump,** left lower **extremity**   HCC ESR COM

√6ᵗʰ   **T87.4**   **Infection of amputation stump**

    T87.40   **Infection of amputation stump, unspecified extremity**   HCC ESR COM

    T87.41   **Infection of amputation stump,** right upper **extremity**   HCC ESR COM

    T87.42   **Infection of amputation stump,** left upper **extremity**   HCC ESR COM

    T87.43   **Infection of amputation stump,** right lower **extremity**   HCC ESR COM

    T87.44   **Infection of amputation stump,** left lower **extremity**   HCC ESR COM

√5ᵗʰ   **T87.5**   **Necrosis of amputation stump**

    T87.50   **Necrosis of amputation stump, unspecified extremity**   HCC ESR COM

    T87.51   **Necrosis of amputation stump,** right upper **extremity**   HCC ESR COM

    T87.52   **Necrosis of amputation stump,** left upper **extremity**   HCC ESR COM

    T87.53   **Necrosis of amputation stump,** right lower **extremity**   HCC ESR COM

    T87.54   **Necrosis of amputation stump,** left lower **extremity**   HCC ESR COM

√5ᵗʰ   **T87.8**   **Other complications of amputation stump**

    T87.81   **Dehiscence of amputation stump**   HCC ESR COM

T87.89 **Other complications of amputation stump** `HCC` `ESR` `COM`

Amputation stump contracture

Amputation stump contracture of next proximal joint

Amputation stump flexion

Amputation stump edema

Amputation stump hematoma

> `EXCLUDES 2`   *phantom limb syndrome (G54.6-G54.7)*

T87.9 **Unspecified complications of amputation stump** `HCC` `ESR` `COM`

☑4ᵗʰ **T88** **Other complications of surgical and medical care, not elsewhere classified**

> `EXCLUDES 2`   *complication following infusion, transfusion and therapeutic injection (T80.-)*
>
> *complication following procedure NEC (T81.-)*
>
> *complications of anesthesia in labor and delivery (O74.-)*
>
> *complications of anesthesia in pregnancy (O29.-)*
>
> *complications of anesthesia in puerperium (O89.-)*
>
> *complications of devices, implants and grafts (T82-T85)*
>
> *complications of obstetric surgery and procedure (O75.4)*
>
> *dermatitis due to drugs and medicaments (L23.3, L24.4, L25.1, L27.0-L27.1)*
>
> *poisoning and toxic effects of drugs and chemicals (T36-T65 with fifth or sixth character 1-4 or 6)*
>
> *specified complications classified elsewhere*

The appropriate 7th character is to be added to each code from category T88.

A   initial encounter

D   subsequent encounter

S   sequela

√x7ᵗʰ **T88.0** **Infection following immunization**

Sepsis following immunization

AHA: 2018,4Q,62-63

√x7ᵗʰ **T88.1** **Other complications following immunization, not elsewhere classified**

Generalized vaccinia

Rash following immunization

> `EXCLUDES 1`   *vaccinia not from vaccine (B08.011)*
> `EXCLUDES 2`   *anaphylactic shock due to serum (T80.5-)*
>
> *other serum reactions (T80.6-)*
>
> *postimmunization arthropathy (M02.2)*
>
> *postimmunization encephalitis (G04.02)*
>
> *postimmunization fever (R50.83)*

√x7ᵗʰ **T88.2** **Shock due to anesthesia**

Use additional code for adverse effect, if applicable, to identify drug (T41.- with fifth or sixth character 5)

> `EXCLUDES 1`   *complications of anesthesia (in):*
>
> *labor and delivery (O74.-)*
>
> *postprocedural shock NOS (T81.1-)*
>
> *pregnancy (O29.-)*
>
> *puerperium (O89.-)*

√x7ᵗʰ **T88.3** **Malignant hyperthermia due to anesthesia**

Use additional code for adverse effect, if applicable, to identify drug (T41.- with fifth or sixth character 5)

√x7ᵗʰ **T88.4** **Failed or difficult intubation**

☑6ᵗʰ **T88.5** **Other complications of anesthesia**

Use additional code for adverse effect, if applicable, to identify drug (T41.- with fifth or sixth character 5)

√x7ᵗʰ **T88.51** **Hypothermia following anesthesia**

√x7ᵗʰ **T88.52** **Failed moderate sedation during procedure**

Failed conscious sedation during procedure

> `EXCLUDES 2`   *personal history of failed moderate sedation (Z92.83)*

√x7ᵗʰ **T88.53** **Unintended awareness under general anesthesia during procedure**

> `EXCLUDES 2`   *personal history of unintended awareness under general anesthesia (Z92.84)*

AHA: 2016,4Q,72-73

√x7ᵗʰ **T88.59** **Other complications of anesthesia**

√x7ᵗʰ **T88.6** **Anaphylactic reaction due to adverse effect of correct drug or medicament properly administered**

Anaphylactic shock due to adverse effect of correct drug or medicament properly administered

Anaphylactoid reaction NOS

Use additional code for adverse effect, if applicable, to identify drug (T36-T50 with fifth or sixth character 5)

> `EXCLUDES 1`   *anaphylactic reaction due to serum (T80.5-)*
>
> *anaphylactic shock or reaction due to adverse food reaction (T78.0-)*

AHA: 2020,1Q,18

√x7ᵗʰ **T88.7** **Unspecified adverse effect of drug or medicament**

Drug hypersensitivity NOS

Drug reaction NOS

Use additional code for adverse effect, if applicable, to identify drug (T36-T50 with fifth or sixth character 5)

> `EXCLUDES 1`   *specified adverse effects of drugs and medicaments (A00-R94 and T80-T88.6, T88.8)*

√x7ᵗʰ **T88.8** **Other specified complications of surgical and medical care, not elsewhere classified**

Use additional code to identify the complication

AHA: 2022,2Q,7

√x7ᵗʰ **T88.9** **Complication of surgical and medical care, unspecified**

Chapter 20. External Causes of Morbidity (V00–Y99)

Chapter-specific Guidelines with Coding Examples

The chapter-specific guidelines from the ICD-10-CM Official Guidelines for Coding and Reporting have been provided below. Along with these guidelines are coding examples, contained in the shaded boxes, that have been developed to help illustrate the coding and/or sequencing guidance found in these guidelines.

The external causes of morbidity codes should never be sequenced as the first-listed or principal diagnosis.

External cause codes are intended to provide data for injury research and evaluation of injury prevention strategies. These codes capture how the injury or health condition happened (cause), the intent (unintentional or accidental; or intentional, such as suicide or assault), the place where the event occurred the activity of the patient at the time of the event, and the person's status (e.g., civilian, military).

There is no national requirement for mandatory ICD-10-CM external cause code reporting. Unless a provider is subject to a state-based external cause code reporting mandate or these codes are required by a particular payer, reporting of ICD-10-CM codes in Chapter 20, External Causes of Morbidity, is not required. In the absence of a mandatory reporting requirement, providers are encouraged to voluntarily report external cause codes, as they provide valuable data for injury research and evaluation of injury prevention strategies.

a. General external cause coding guidelines

1) Used with any code in the range of A00.0–T88.9, Z00–Z99

An external cause code may be used with any code in the range of A00.0–T88.9, Z00–Z99, classification that represents a health condition due to an external cause. Though they are most applicable to injuries, they are also valid for use with such things as infections or diseases due to an external source, and other health conditions, such as a heart attack that occurs during strenuous physical activity.

> Actinic reticuloid due to tanning bed use
>
> | | |
> |---|---|
> | **L57.1** | **Actinic reticuloid** |
> | **W89.1XXA** | **Exposure to tanning bed, initial encounter** |
>
> *Explanation:* An external cause code may be used with any code in the range of A00.0–T88.9, Z00–Z99, classifications that describe health conditions due to an external cause. Code W89.1 Exposure to tanning bed requires a seventh character of A to report this initial encounter, with a placeholder X for the fifth and sixth characters.

2) External cause code used for length of treatment

Assign the external cause code, with the appropriate 7th character (initial encounter, subsequent encounter or sequela) for each encounter for which the injury or condition is being treated.

Most categories in chapter 20 have a 7th character requirement for each applicable code. Most categories in this chapter have three 7th character values: A, initial encounter, D, subsequent encounter and S, sequela. While the patient may be seen by a new or different provider over the course of treatment for an injury or condition, assignment of the 7th character for external cause should match the 7th character of the code assigned for the associated injury or condition for the encounter.

3) Use the full range of external cause codes

Use the full range of external cause codes to completely describe the cause, the intent, the place of occurrence, and if applicable, the activity of the patient at the time of the event, and the patient's status, for all injuries, and other health conditions due to an external cause.

4) Assign as many external cause codes as necessary

Assign as many external cause codes as necessary to fully explain each cause. If only one external code can be recorded, assign the code most related to the principal diagnosis.

5) The selection of the appropriate external cause code

The selection of the appropriate external cause code is guided by the Alphabetic Index of External Causes and by Inclusion and Exclusion notes in the Tabular List.

6) External cause code can never be a principal diagnosis

An external cause code can never be a principal (first-listed) diagnosis.

7) Combination external cause codes

Certain of the external cause codes are combination codes that identify sequential events that result in an injury, such as a fall which results in striking against an object. The injury may be due to either event or both.

The combination external cause code used should correspond to the sequence of events regardless of which caused the most serious injury.

> Toddler tripped and fell while walking and struck his head on an end table, sustaining a scalp contusion
>
> | | |
> |---|---|
> | **S00.03XA** | **Contusion of scalp, initial encounter** |
> | **W01.190A** | **Fall on same level from slipping, tripping and stumbling with subsequent striking against furniture, initial encounter** |
>
> *Explanation:* Combination external cause codes identify sequential events that result in an injury, such as a fall resulting in striking against an object. The injury may be due to either or both events.

8) No external cause code needed in certain circumstances

No external cause code from Chapter 20 is needed if the external cause and intent are included in a code from another chapter (e.g., T36.0X1-, Poisoning by penicillins, accidental (unintentional)).

b. Place of occurrence guideline

Codes from category Y92, Place of occurrence of the external cause, are secondary codes for use after other external cause codes to identify the location of the patient at the time of injury or other condition.

Generally, a place of occurrence code is assigned only once, at the initial encounter for treatment. However, in the rare instance that a new injury occurs during hospitalization, an additional place of occurrence code may be assigned. No 7th characters are used for Y92.

Do not use place of occurrence code Y92.9 if the place is not stated or is not applicable.

> A farmer was working in his barn and sustained a foot contusion when the horse stepped on his left foot
>
> | | |
> |---|---|
> | **S90.32XA** | **Contusion of left foot, initial encounter** |
> | **W55.19XA** | **Other contact with horse, initial encounter** |
> | **Y92.71** | **Barn as the place of occurrence of the external cause** |
>
> *Explanation:* A place-of-occurrence code from category Y92 is assigned at the initial encounter to identify the location of the patient at the time the injury occurred.

c. Activity code

Assign a code from category Y93, Activity code, to describe the activity of the patient at the time the injury or other health condition occurred.

An activity code is used only once, at the initial encounter for treatment. Only one code from Y93 should be recorded on a medical record.

The activity codes are not applicable to poisonings, adverse effects, misadventures or sequela.

Do not assign Y93.9, Unspecified activity, if the activity is not stated.

A code from category Y93 is appropriate for use with external cause and intent codes if identifying the activity provides additional information about the event.

> Ranch hand who was grooming a horse sustained a foot contusion when the horse stepped on his left foot
>
> | | |
> |---|---|
> | **S90.32XA** | **Contusion of left foot, initial encounter** |
> | **W55.19XA** | **Other contact with horse, initial encounter** |
> | **Y93.K3** | **Activity, grooming and shearing an animal** |
>
> *Explanation:* One activity code from category Y93 is assigned at the initial encounter only to describe the activity of the patient at the time the injury occurred.

d. Place of occurrence, activity, and status codes used with other external cause code

When applicable, place of occurrence, activity, and external cause status codes are sequenced after the main external cause code(s). Regardless of the number of external cause codes assigned, generally there should be only one place of occurrence code, one activity code, and one external cause status code assigned to an encounter. However, in the rare instance that a new injury occurs during hospitalization, an additional place of occurrence code may be assigned.

e. If the reporting format limits the number of external cause codes

If the reporting format limits the number of external cause codes that can be used in reporting clinical data, report the code for the cause/intent most related to the principal diagnosis. If the format permits capture of additional external cause codes, the cause/intent, including medical misadventures, of the additional events should be reported rather than the codes for place, activity, or external status.

f. Multiple external cause coding guidelines

More than one external cause code is required to fully describe the external cause of an illness or injury. The assignment of external cause codes should be sequenced in the following priority:

If two or more events cause separate injuries, an external cause code should be assigned for each cause. The first-listed external cause code will be selected in the following order:

External codes for child and adult abuse take priority over all other external cause codes.

See Section I.C.19., Child and Adult abuse guidelines.

External cause codes for terrorism events take priority over all other external cause codes except child and adult abuse.

External cause codes for cataclysmic events take priority over all other external cause codes except child and adult abuse and terrorism.

External cause codes for transport accidents take priority over all other external cause codes except cataclysmic events, child and adult abuse and terrorism.

Activity and external cause status codes are assigned following all causal (intent) external cause codes.

The first-listed external cause code should correspond to the cause of the most serious diagnosis due to an assault, accident, or self-harm, following the order of hierarchy listed above..

> 30-year-old man accidentally discharged his hunting rifle, sustaining an open gunshot wound, with no retained bullet fragments, to the right thigh, which caused him to fall down the stairs, resulting in closed displaced comminuted fracture of his left radial shaft
>
> **S71.131A**　**Puncture wound without foreign body, right thigh, initial encounter**
>
> **W33.02XA**　**Accidental discharge of hunting rifle, initial encounter**
>
> **S52.352A**　**Displaced comminuted fracture of shaft of radius, left arm, initial encounter for closed fracture**
>
> **W10.9XXA**　**Fall (on) (from) unspecified stairs and steps, initial encounter**
>
> *Explanation:* If two or more events cause separate injuries, an external cause code should be assigned for each cause.

g. Child and adult abuse guideline

Adult and child abuse, neglect and maltreatment are classified as assault. Any of the assault codes may be used to indicate the external cause of any injury resulting from the confirmed abuse.

For confirmed cases of abuse, neglect and maltreatment, when the perpetrator is known, a code from Y07, Perpetrator of maltreatment and neglect, should accompany any other assault codes.

See Section I.C.19. Adult and child abuse, neglect and other maltreatment

h. Unknown or undetermined intent guideline

If the intent (accident, self-harm, assault) of the cause of an injury or other condition is unknown or unspecified, code the intent as accidental intent. All transport accident categories assume accidental intent.

1) Use of undetermined intent

External cause codes for events of undetermined intent are only for use if the documentation in the record specifies that the intent cannot be determined.

i. Sequelae (late effects) of external cause guidelines

1) Sequelae external cause codes

Sequela are reported using the external cause code with the 7th character "S" for sequela. These codes should be used with any report of a late effect or sequela resulting from a previous injury.

See Section I.B.10. Sequela (Late Effects)

2) Sequela external cause code with a related current injury

A sequela external cause code should never be used with a related current nature of injury code.

3) Use of sequela external cause codes for subsequent visits

Use a late effect external cause code for subsequent visits when a late effect of the initial injury is being treated. Do not use a late effect external cause code for subsequent visits for follow-up care (e.g., to assess healing, to receive rehabilitative therapy) of the injury when no late effect of the injury has been documented.

j. Terrorism guidelines

1) Cause of injury identified by the Federal Government (FBI) as terrorism

When the cause of an injury is identified by the Federal Government (FBI) as terrorism, the first-listed external cause code should be a code from category Y38, Terrorism. The definition of terrorism employed by the FBI is found at the inclusion note at the beginning of category Y38. Use additional code for place of occurrence (Y92.-). More than one Y38 code may be assigned if the injury is the result of more than one mechanism of terrorism.

2) Cause of an injury is suspected to be the result of terrorism

When the cause of an injury is suspected to be the result of terrorism a code from category Y38 should not be assigned. Suspected cases should be classified as assault.

3) Code Y38.9, Terrorism, secondary effects

Assign code Y38.9, Terrorism, secondary effects, for conditions occurring subsequent to the terrorist event. This code should not be assigned for conditions that are due to the initial terrorist act.

It is acceptable to assign code Y38.9 with another code from Y38 if there is an injury due to the initial terrorist event and an injury that is a subsequent result of the terrorist event.

k. External cause status

A code from category Y99, External cause status, should be assigned whenever any other external cause code is assigned for an encounter, including an Activity code, except for the events noted below. Assign a code from category Y99, External cause status, to indicate the work status of the person at the time the event occurred. The status code indicates whether the event occurred during military activity, whether a non-military person was at work, whether an individual including a student or volunteer was involved in a non-work activity at the time of the causal event.

A code from Y99, External cause status, should be assigned, when applicable, with other external cause codes, such as transport accidents and falls. The external cause status codes are not applicable to poisonings, adverse effects, misadventures or late effects.

Do not assign a code from category Y99 if no other external cause codes (cause, activity) are applicable for the encounter.

An external cause status code is used only once, at the initial encounter for treatment. Only one code from Y99 should be recorded on a medical record.

Do not assign code Y99.9, Unspecified external cause status, if the status is not stated.

Chapter 20. External Causes of Morbidity (V00-Y99)

NOTE This chapter permits the classification of environmental events and circumstances as the cause of injury, and other adverse effects. Where a code from this section is applicable, it is intended that it shall be used secondary to a code from another chapter of the Classification indicating the nature of the condition. Most often, the condition will be classifiable to Chapter 19, Injury, poisoning and certain other consequences of external causes (S00-T88). Other conditions that may be stated to be due to external causes are classified in Chapters I to XVIII. For these conditions, codes from Chapter 20 should be used to provide additional information as to the cause of the condition.

AHA: 2018,4Q,58-60

This chapter contains the following blocks:

V00-X58	Accidents
V00-V99	Transport accidents
V00-V09	Pedestrian injured in transport accident
V10-V19	Pedal cycle rider injured in transport accident
V20-V29	Motorcycle rider injured in transport accident
V30-V39	Occupant of three-wheeled motor vehicle injured in transport accident
V40-V49	Car occupant injured in transport accident
V50-V59	Occupant of pick-up truck or van injured in transport accident
V60-V69	Occupant of heavy transport vehicle injured in transport accident
V70-V79	Bus occupant injured in transport accident
V80-V89	Other land transport accidents
V90-V94	Water transport accidents
V95-V97	Air and space transport accidents
V98-V99	Other and unspecified transport accidents
W00-X58	Other external causes of accidental injury
W00-W19	Slipping, tripping, stumbling and falls
W20-W49	Exposure to inanimate mechanical forces
W50-W64	Exposure to animate mechanical forces
W65-W74	Accidental non-transport drowning and submersion
W85-W99	Exposure to electric current, radiation and extreme ambient air temperature and pressure
X00-X08	Exposure to smoke, fire and flames
X10-X19	Contact with heat and hot substances
X30-X39	Exposure to forces of nature
X50	Overexertion and strenuous or repetitive movements
X52-X58	Accidental exposure to other specified factors
X71-X83	Intentional self-harm
X92-Y09	Assault
Y21-Y33	Event of undetermined intent
Y35-Y38	Legal intervention, operations of war, military operations, and terrorism
Y62-Y84	Complications of medical and surgical care
Y62-Y69	Misadventures to patients during surgical and medical care
Y70-Y82	Medical devices associated with adverse incidents in diagnostic and therapeutic use
Y83-Y84	Surgical and other medical procedures as the cause of abnormal reaction of the patient, or of later complication, without mention of misadventure at the time of the procedure
Y90-Y99	Supplementary factors related to causes of morbidity classified elsewhere

ACCIDENTS (V00-X58)

AHA: 2018,2Q,7-8

Transport accidents (V00-V99)

NOTE This section is structured in 12 groups. Those relating to land transport accidents (V00-V89) reflect the victim's mode of transport and are subdivided to identify the victim's 'counterpart' or the type of event. The vehicle of which the injured person is an occupant is identified in the first two characters since it is seen as the most important factor to identify for prevention purposes. A transport accident is one in which the vehicle involved must be moving or running or in use for transport purposes at the time of the accident.

Use additional code to identify:
   airbag injury (W22.1)
   type of street or road (Y92.4-)
   use of cellular telephone and other electronic equipment at the time of the transport accident (Y93.C-)

EXCLUDES 1 *agricultural vehicles in stationary use or maintenance (W31.-)*
assault by crashing of motor vehicle (Y03.-)
automobile or motor cycle in stationary use or maintenance - code to type of accident
crashing of motor vehicle, undetermined intent (Y32)
intentional self-harm by crashing of motor vehicle (X82)
EXCLUDES 2 *transport accidents due to cataclysm (X34-X38)*

NOTE Definitions related to transport accidents:

(a) A transport accident (V00-V99) is any accident involving a device designed primarily for, or used at the time primarily for, conveying persons or good from one place to another.

(b) A public highway [trafficway] or street is the entire width between property lines (or other boundary lines) of land open to the public as a matter of right or custom for purposes of moving persons or property from one place to another. A roadway is that part of the public highway designed, improved and customarily used for vehicular traffic.

(c) A traffic accident is any vehicle accident occurring on the public highway [i.e. originating on, terminating on, or involving a vehicle partially on the highway]. A vehicle accident is assumed to have occurred on the public highway unless another place is specified, except in the case of accidents involving only off-road motor vehicles, which are classified as nontraffic accidents unless the contrary is stated.

(d) A nontraffic accident is any vehicle accident that occurs entirely in any place other than a public highway.

(e) A pedestrian is any person involved in an accident who was not at the time of the accident riding in or on a motor vehicle, railway train, streetcar or animal-drawn or other vehicle, or on a pedal cycle or animal. This includes, a person changing a tire, working on a parked car, or a person on foot. It also includes the user of a pedestrian conveyance such as a baby stroller, ice-skates, skis, sled, roller skates, a skateboard, nonmotorized or motorized wheelchair, motorized mobility scooter, or nonmotorized scooter.

(f) A driver is an occupant of a transport vehicle who is operating or intending to operate it.

(g) A passenger is any occupant of a transport vehicle other than the driver, except a person traveling on the outside of the vehicle.

(h) A person on the outside of a vehicle is any person being transported by a vehicle but not occupying the space normally reserved for the driver or passengers, or the space intended for the transport of property. This includes a person travelling on the bodywork, bumper, fender, roof, running board or step of a vehicle, as well as, hanging on the outside of the vehicle.

(i) A pedal cycle is any land transport vehicle operated solely by nonmotorized pedals including a bicycle or tricycle.

(j) A pedal cyclist is any person riding a pedal cycle or in a sidecar or trailer attached to a pedal cycle.

(k) A motorcycle is a two-wheeled motor vehicle with one or two riding saddles and sometimes with a third wheel for the support of a sidecar. The sidecar is considered part of the motorcycle. This includes a moped, motor scooter, or motorized bicycle.

(l) A motorcycle rider is any person riding a motorcycle or in a sidecar or trailer attached to the motorcycle.

(m) A three-wheeled motor vehicle is a motorized tricycle designed primarily for on-road use. This includes a motor-driven tricycle, a motorized rickshaw, or a three-wheeled motor car.

(n) A car [automobile] is a four-wheeled motor vehicle designed primarily for carrying up to 7 persons. A trailer being towed by the car is considered part of the car. It does not include a van or minivan — see definition (o).

(o) A pick-up truck or van is a four or six-wheeled motor vehicle designed for carrying passengers as well as property or cargo weighing less than the local limit for classification as a heavy goods vehicle, and not requiring a special driver's license. This includes a minivan and a sport-utility vehicle (SUV).

(p) A heavy transport vehicle is a motor vehicle designed primarily for carrying property, meeting local criteria for classification as a heavy goods vehicle in terms of weight and requiring a special driver's license.

(q) A bus (coach) is a motor vehicle designed or adapted primarily for carrying more than 10 passengers, and requiring a special driver's license.

(r) A railway train or railway vehicle is any device, with or without freight or passenger cars couple to it, designed for traffic on a railway track. This includes subterranean (subways) or elevated trains.

(s) A streetcar, is a device designed and used primarily for transporting passengers within a municipality, running on rails, usually subject to normal traffic control signals, and operated principally on a right-of-way that forms part of the roadway. This includes a tram or trolley that runs on rails. A trailer being towed by a streetcar is considered part of the streetcar.

(t) A special vehicle mainly used on industrial premises is a motor vehicle designed primarily for use within the buildings and premises of industrial or commercial establishments. This includes battery-powered airport passenger vehicles or baggage/mail trucks, forklifts, coal-cars in a coal mine, logging cars and trucks used in mines or quarries.

(u) A special vehicle mainly used in agriculture is a motor vehicle designed specifically for use in farming and agriculture (horticulture), to work the land, tend and harvest crops and transport materials on the farm. This includes harvesters, farm machinery and tractor and trailers.

(v)   A special construction vehicle is a motor vehicle designed specifically for use on construction and demolition sites. This includes bulldozers, diggers, earth levellers, dump trucks, backhoes, front-end loaders, pavers, and mechanical shovels.

(w)   A special all-terrain vehicle is a motor vehicle of special design to enable it to negotiate over rough or soft terrain, snow or sand. Examples of special design are high construction, special wheels and tires, tracks, and support on a cushion of air. This includes snow mobiles, All-terrain vehicles (ATV), and dune buggies. It does not include passenger vehicle designated as Sport Utility Vehicles. (SUV)

(x)   A watercraft is any device designed for transporting passengers or goods on water. This includes motor or sailboats, ships, and hovercraft.

(y)   An aircraft is any device for transporting passengers or goods in the air. This includes hot-air balloons, gliders, helicopters and airplanes.

(z)   A military vehicle is any motorized vehicle operating on a public roadway owned by the military and being operated by a member of the military.

Pedestrian injured in transport accident (V00-V09)

INCLUDES   person changing tire on transport vehicle
person examining engine of vehicle broken down in (on side of) road

EXCLUDES 1   *fall due to non-transport collision with other person (W03)*
pedestrian on foot falling (slipping) on ice and snow (W00.-)
struck or bumped by another person (W51)

The appropriate 7th character is to be added to each code from categories V00-V09.
A   initial encounter
D   subsequent encounter
S   sequela

✓4ᵗʰ **V00   Pedestrian conveyance accident**
Use additional place of occurrence and activity external cause codes, if known (Y92.-, Y93.-)

EXCLUDES 1   *collision with another person without fall (W51)*
fall due to person on foot colliding with another person on foot (W03)
fall from non-moving wheelchair, nonmotorized scooter and motorized mobility scooter without collision (W05.-)
pedestrian (conveyance) collision with other land transport vehicle (V01-V09)
pedestrian on foot falling (slipping) on ice and snow (W00.-)

✓5ᵗʰ **V00.0   Pedestrian on foot injured in collision with pedestrian conveyance**

    ✓x7ᵗʰ **V00.01   Pedestrian on foot injured in collision with roller-skater**

    ✓x7ᵗʰ **V00.02   Pedestrian on foot injured in collision with skateboarder**

    ✓6ᵗʰ **V00.03   Pedestrian on foot injured in collision with standing micro-mobility pedestrian conveyance**

        ✓7ᵗʰ **V00.031   Pedestrian on foot injured in collision with rider of standing electric scooter**

        ✓7ᵗʰ **V00.038   Pedestrian on foot injured in collision with rider of other standing micro-mobility pedestrian conveyance**
Pedestrian on foot injured in collision with rider of hoverboard
Pedestrian on foot injured in collision with rider of segway

    ✓x7ᵗʰ **V00.09   Pedestrian on foot injured in collision with other pedestrian conveyance**

✓5ᵗʰ **V00.1   Rolling-type pedestrian conveyance accident**

    EXCLUDES 1   *accident with baby stroller (V00.82-)*
accident with motorized mobility scooter (V00.83-)
accident with wheelchair (powered) (V00.81-)

    ✓6ᵗʰ **V00.11   In-line roller-skate accident**

        ✓7ᵗʰ **V00.111   Fall from in-line roller-skates**

        ✓7ᵗʰ **V00.112   In-line roller-skater colliding with stationary object**

        ✓7ᵗʰ **V00.118   Other in-line roller-skate accident**
        EXCLUDES 1   *roller-skater collision with other land transport vehicle (V01-V09 with 5th character 1)*

    ✓6ᵗʰ **V00.12   Non-in-line roller-skate accident**

        ✓7ᵗʰ **V00.121   Fall from non-in-line roller-skates**

        ✓7ᵗʰ **V00.122   Non-in-line roller-skater colliding with stationary object**

        ✓7ᵗʰ **V00.128   Other non-in-line roller-skating accident**
        EXCLUDES 1   *roller-skater collision with other land transport vehicle (V01-V09 with 5th character 1)*

    ✓6ᵗʰ **V00.13   Skateboard accident**

        ✓7ᵗʰ **V00.131   Fall from skateboard**

        ✓7ᵗʰ **V00.132   Skateboarder colliding with stationary object**

        ✓7ᵗʰ **V00.138   Other skateboard accident**
        EXCLUDES 1   *skateboarder collision with other land transport vehicle (V01-V09 with 5th character 2)*

    ✓6ᵗʰ **V00.14   Scooter (nonmotorized) accident**
        EXCLUDES 1   *motor scooter accident (V20-V29)*

        ✓7ᵗʰ **V00.141   Fall from scooter (nonmotorized)**

        ✓7ᵗʰ **V00.142   Scooter (nonmotorized) colliding with stationary object**

        ✓7ᵗʰ **V00.148   Other scooter (nonmotorized) accident**
        EXCLUDES 1   *scooter (nonmotorized) collision with other land transport vehicle (V01-V09 with fifth character 9)*

    ✓6ᵗʰ **V00.15   Heelies accident**
Rolling shoe
Wheeled shoe
Wheelies accident

        ✓7ᵗʰ **V00.151   Fall from heelies**

        ✓7ᵗʰ **V00.152   Heelies colliding with stationary object**

        ✓7ᵗʰ **V00.158   Other heelies accident**

    ✓6ᵗʰ **V00.18   Accident on other rolling-type pedestrian conveyance**

        ✓7ᵗʰ **V00.181   Fall from other rolling-type pedestrian conveyance**

        ✓7ᵗʰ **V00.182   Pedestrian on other rolling-type pedestrian conveyance colliding with stationary object**

        ✓7ᵗʰ **V00.188   Other accident on other rolling-type pedestrian conveyance**

✓5ᵗʰ **V00.2   Gliding-type pedestrian conveyance accident**

    ✓6ᵗʰ **V00.21   Ice-skates accident**

        ✓7ᵗʰ **V00.211   Fall from ice-skates**

        ✓7ᵗʰ **V00.212   Ice-skater colliding with stationary object**

        ✓7ᵗʰ **V00.218   Other ice-skates accident**
        EXCLUDES 1   *ice-skater collision with other land transport vehicle (V01-V09 with 5th character 9)*

    ✓6ᵗʰ **V00.22   Sled accident**

        ✓7ᵗʰ **V00.221   Fall from sled**

        ✓7ᵗʰ **V00.222   Sledder colliding with stationary object**

        ✓7ᵗʰ **V00.228   Other sled accident**
        EXCLUDES 1   *sled collision with other land transport vehicle (V01-V09 with 5th character 9)*

    ✓6ᵗʰ **V00.28   Other gliding-type pedestrian conveyance accident**

        ✓7ᵗʰ **V00.281   Fall from other gliding-type pedestrian conveyance**

        ✓7ᵗʰ **V00.282   Pedestrian on other gliding-type pedestrian conveyance colliding with stationary object**

☑7ᵗʰ **V00.288 Other accident on other gliding-type pedestrian conveyance**
EXCLUDES 1 gliding-type pedestrian conveyance collision with other land transport vehicle (V01–V09 with 5th character 9)

☑5ᵗʰ **V00.3 Flat-bottomed pedestrian conveyance accident**

☑6ᵗʰ **V00.31 Snowboard accident**

☑7ᵗʰ **V00.311 Fall from snowboard**

☑7ᵗʰ **V00.312 Snowboarder colliding with stationary object**

☑7ᵗʰ **V00.318 Other snowboard accident**
EXCLUDES 1 snowboarder collision with other land transport vehicle (V01–V09 with 5th character 9)

☑6ᵗʰ **V00.32 Snow-ski accident**

☑7ᵗʰ **V00.321 Fall from snow-skis**

☑7ᵗʰ **V00.322 Snow-skier colliding with stationary object**

☑7ᵗʰ **V00.328 Other snow-ski accident**
EXCLUDES 1 snow-skier collision with other land transport vehicle (V01–V09 with 5th character 9)

☑6ᵗʰ **V00.38 Other flat-bottomed pedestrian conveyance accident**

☑7ᵗʰ **V00.381 Fall from other flat-bottomed pedestrian conveyance**

☑7ᵗʰ **V00.382 Pedestrian on other flat-bottomed pedestrian conveyance colliding with stationary object**

☑7ᵗʰ **V00.388 Other accident on other flat-bottomed pedestrian conveyance**

☑5ᵗʰ **V00.8 Accident on other pedestrian conveyance**

☑6ᵗʰ **V00.81 Accident with wheelchair (powered)**

☑7ᵗʰ **V00.811 Fall from moving wheelchair (powered)**
EXCLUDES 1 fall from non-moving wheelchair (W05.0)

☑7ᵗʰ **V00.812 Wheelchair (powered) colliding with stationary object**

☑7ᵗʰ **V00.818 Other accident with wheelchair (powered)**

☑6ᵗʰ **V00.82 Accident with baby stroller**

☑7ᵗʰ **V00.821 Fall from baby stroller**

☑7ᵗʰ **V00.822 Baby stroller colliding with stationary object**

☑7ᵗʰ **V00.828 Other accident with baby stroller**

☑6ᵗʰ **V00.83 Accident with motorized mobility scooter**

☑7ᵗʰ **V00.831 Fall from motorized mobility scooter**
EXCLUDES 1 fall from non-moving motorized mobility scooter (W05.2)

☑7ᵗʰ **V00.832 Motorized mobility scooter colliding with stationary object**

☑7ᵗʰ **V00.838 Other accident with motorized mobility scooter**

☑6ᵗʰ **V00.84 Accident with standing micro-mobility pedestrian conveyance**

☑7ᵗʰ **V00.841 Fall from standing electric scooter**

☑7ᵗʰ **V00.842 Pedestrian on standing electric scooter colliding with stationary object**

☑7ᵗʰ **V00.848 Other accident with standing micro-mobility pedestrian conveyance**
Accident with hoverboard
Accident with segway

☑6ᵗʰ **V00.89 Accident on other pedestrian conveyance**

☑7ᵗʰ **V00.891 Fall from other pedestrian conveyance**

☑7ᵗʰ **V00.892 Pedestrian on other pedestrian conveyance colliding with stationary object**

☑7ᵗʰ **V00.898 Other accident on other pedestrian conveyance**
EXCLUDES 1 other pedestrian (conveyance) collision with other land transport vehicle (V01–V09 with 5th character 9)

☑4ᵗʰ **V01 Pedestrian injured in collision with pedal cycle**

☑5ᵗʰ **V01.0 Pedestrian injured in collision with pedal cycle in nontraffic accident**

☑x7ᵗʰ **V01.00 Pedestrian on foot injured in collision with pedal cycle in nontraffic accident**
Pedestrian NOS injured in collision with pedal cycle in nontraffic accident

☑x7ᵗʰ **V01.01 Pedestrian on roller-skates injured in collision with pedal cycle in nontraffic accident**

☑x7ᵗʰ **V01.02 Pedestrian on skateboard injured in collision with pedal cycle in nontraffic accident**

☑6ᵗʰ **V01.03 Pedestrian on standing micro-mobility pedestrian conveyance injured in collision with pedal cycle in nontraffic accident**

☑7ᵗʰ **V01.031 Pedestrian on standing electric scooter injured in collision with pedal cycle in nontraffic accident**

☑7ᵗʰ **V01.038 Pedestrian on other standing micro-mobility pedestrian conveyance injured in collision with pedal cycle in nontraffic accident**
Pedestrian on hoverboard injured in collision with pedal cycle in nontraffic accident
Pedestrian on segway injured in collision with pedal cycle in nontraffic accident

☑x7ᵗʰ **V01.09 Pedestrian with other conveyance injured in collision with pedal cycle in nontraffic accident**
Pedestrian with baby stroller injured in collision with pedal cycle in nontraffic accident
Pedestrian on ice-skates injured in collision with pedal cycle in nontraffic accident
Pedestrian on nonmotorized scooter injured in collision with pedal cycle in nontraffic accident
Pedestrian on sled injured in collision with pedal cycle in nontraffic accident
Pedestrian on snowboard injured in collision with pedal cycle in nontraffic accident
Pedestrian on snow-skis injured in collision with pedal cycle in nontraffic accident
Pedestrian in wheelchair (powered) injured in collision with pedal cycle in nontraffic accident
Pedestrian in motorized mobility scooter injured in collision with pedal cycle in nontraffic accident

☑5ᵗʰ **V01.1 Pedestrian injured in collision with pedal cycle in traffic accident**

☑x7ᵗʰ **V01.10 Pedestrian on foot injured in collision with pedal cycle in traffic accident**
Pedestrian NOS injured in collision with pedal cycle in traffic accident

☑x7ᵗʰ **V01.11 Pedestrian on roller-skates injured in collision with pedal cycle in traffic accident**

☑x7ᵗʰ **V01.12 Pedestrian on skateboard injured in collision with pedal cycle in traffic accident**

☑6ᵗʰ **V01.13 Pedestrian on standing micro-mobility pedestrian conveyance injured in collision with pedal cycle in traffic accident**

☑7ᵗʰ **V01.131 Pedestrian on standing electric scooter injured in collision with pedal cycle in traffic accident**

☑7ᵗʰ **V01.138 Pedestrian on other standing micro-mobility pedestrian conveyance injured in collision with pedal cycle in traffic accident**
Pedestrian on hoverboard injured in collision with pedal cycle in traffic accident
Pedestrian on segway injured in collision with pedal cycle in traffic accident

---

√x 7ᵗʰ **V01.19** **Pedestrian with other conveyance injured in collision with pedal cycle in traffic accident**

Pedestrian with baby stroller injured in collision with pedal cycle in traffic accident

Pedestrian on ice-skates injured in collision with pedal cycle in traffic accident

Pedestrian on nonmotorized scooter injured in collision with pedal cycle in traffic accident

Pedestrian on sled injured in collision with pedal cycle in traffic accident

Pedestrian on snowboard injured in collision with pedal cycle in traffic accident

Pedestrian on snow-skis injured in collision with pedal cycle in traffic accident

Pedestrian in wheelchair (powered) injured in collision with pedal cycle in traffic accident

Pedestrian in motorized mobility scooter injured in collision with pedal cycle in traffic accident

√5ᵗʰ **V01.9** **Pedestrian injured in collision with pedal cycle, unspecified whether traffic or nontraffic accident**

√x 7ᵗʰ **V01.90** **Pedestrian on foot injured in collision with pedal cycle, unspecified whether traffic or nontraffic accident**

Pedestrian NOS injured in collision with pedal cycle, unspecified whether traffic or nontraffic accident

√x 7ᵗʰ **V01.91** **Pedestrian on roller-skates injured in collision with pedal cycle, unspecified whether traffic or nontraffic accident**

√x 7ᵗʰ **V01.92** **Pedestrian on skateboard injured in collision with pedal cycle, unspecified whether traffic or nontraffic accident**

√6ᵗʰ **V01.93** **Pedestrian on standing micro-mobility pedestrian conveyance injured in collision with pedal cycle, unspecified whether traffic or nontraffic accident**

√7ᵗʰ **V01.931** **Pedestrian on standing electric scooter injured in collision with pedal cycle, unspecified whether traffic or nontraffic accident**

√7ᵗʰ **V01.938** **Pedestrian on other standing micro-mobility pedestrian conveyance injured in collision with pedal cycle, unspecified whether traffic or nontraffic accident**

Pedestrian on hoverboard injured in collision with pedal cycle, unspecified whether traffic or nontraffic accident

Pedestrian on segway injured in collision with pedal cycle, unspecified whether traffic or nontraffic accident

√x 7ᵗʰ **V01.99** **Pedestrian with other conveyance injured in collision with pedal cycle, unspecified whether traffic or nontraffic accident**

Pedestrian with baby stroller injured in collision with pedal cycle, unspecified whether traffic or nontraffic accident

Pedestrian on ice-skates injured in collision with pedal cycle unspecified, whether traffic or nontraffic accident

Pedestrian on nonmotorized scooter injured in collision with pedal cycle, unspecified whether traffic or nontraffic accident

Pedestrian on sled injured in collision with pedal cycle unspecified, whether traffic or nontraffic accident

Pedestrian on snowboard injured in collision with pedal cycle, unspecified whether traffic or nontraffic accident

Pedestrian on snow-skis injured in collision with pedal cycle, unspecified whether traffic or nontraffic accident

Pedestrian in wheelchair (powered) injured in collision with pedal cycle, unspecified whether traffic or nontraffic accident

Pedestrian in motorized mobility scooter injured in collision with pedal cycle, unspecified whether traffic or nontraffic accident

√4ᵗʰ **V02** **Pedestrian injured in collision with two- or three-wheeled motor vehicle**

√5ᵗʰ **V02.0** **Pedestrian injured in collision with two- or three-wheeled motor vehicle in nontraffic accident**

√x 7ᵗʰ **V02.00** **Pedestrian on foot injured in collision with two- or three-wheeled motor vehicle in nontraffic accident**

Pedestrian NOS injured in collision with two- or three-wheeled motor vehicle in nontraffic accident

√x 7ᵗʰ **V02.01** **Pedestrian on roller-skates injured in collision with two- or three-wheeled motor vehicle in nontraffic accident**

√x 7ᵗʰ **V02.02** **Pedestrian on skateboard injured in collision with two- or three-wheeled motor vehicle in nontraffic accident**

√6ᵗʰ **V02.03** **Pedestrian on standing micro-mobility pedestrian conveyance injured in collision with two- or three-wheeled motor vehicle in nontraffic accident**

√7ᵗʰ **V02.031** **Pedestrian on standing electric scooter injured in collision with two- or three-wheeled motor vehicle in nontraffic accident**

√7ᵗʰ **V02.038** **Pedestrian on other standing micro-mobility pedestrian conveyance injured in collision with two- or three-wheeled motor vehicle in nontraffic accident**

Pedestrian on hoverboard injured in collision with two-or three wheeled motor vehicle in nontraffic accident

Pedestrian on segway injured in collision with two- or three-wheeled motor vehicle in nontraffic accident

√x 7ᵗʰ **V02.09** **Pedestrian with other conveyance injured in collision with two- or three-wheeled motor vehicle in nontraffic accident**

Pedestrian with baby stroller injured in collision with two- or three-wheeled motor vehicle in nontraffic accident

Pedestrian on ice-skates injured in collision with two- or three-wheeled motor vehicle in nontraffic accident

Pedestrian on nonmotorized scooter injured in collision with two- or three-wheeled motor vehicle in nontraffic accident

Pedestrian on sled injured in collision with two- or three-wheeled motor vehicle in nontraffic accident

Pedestrian on snowboard injured in collision with two- or three-wheeled motor vehicle in nontraffic accident

Pedestrian on snow-skis injured in collision with two- or three-wheeled motor vehicle in nontraffic accident

Pedestrian in wheelchair (powered) injured in collision with two- or three-wheeled motor vehicle in nontraffic accident

Pedestrian in motorized mobility scooter injured in collision with two- or three-wheeled motor vehicle in nontraffic accident

√5ᵗʰ **V02.1** **Pedestrian injured in collision with two- or three-wheeled motor vehicle in traffic accident**

√x 7ᵗʰ **V02.10** **Pedestrian on foot injured in collision with two- or three-wheeled motor vehicle in traffic accident**

Pedestrian NOS injured in collision with two- or three-wheeled motor vehicle in traffic accident

√x 7ᵗʰ **V02.11** **Pedestrian on roller-skates injured in collision with two- or three-wheeled motor vehicle in traffic accident**

√x 7ᵗʰ **V02.12** **Pedestrian on skateboard injured in collision with two- or three-wheeled motor vehicle in traffic accident**

√6ᵗʰ **V02.13** **Pedestrian on standing micro-mobility pedestrian conveyance injured in collision with two- or three-wheeled motor vehicle in traffic accident**

√7ᵗʰ **V02.131** **Pedestrian on standing electric scooter injured in collision with two- or three-wheeled motor vehicle in traffic accident**

HCC CMS-HCC   **Rx** Rx HCC   **ESR** ESRD HCC   **COM** Commercial HCC   **N** Newborn: 0   **P** Pediatric: 0-17   **M** Maternity: 9-64   **A** Adult: 15-124

1196   ICD-10-CM 2023

☑7ᵗʰ **V02.138 Pedestrian on other standing micro-mobility pedestrian conveyance injured in collision with two- or three-wheeled motor vehicle in traffic accident**

> Pedestrian on hoverboard injured in collision with two-or three wheeled motor vehicle in traffic accident
>
> Pedestrian on segway injured in collision with two- or three-wheeled motor vehicle in traffic accident

☑7ᵗʰ **V02.19 Pedestrian with other conveyance injured in collision with two- or three-wheeled motor vehicle in traffic accident**

> Pedestrian with baby stroller injured in collision with two- or three-wheeled motor vehicle in traffic accident
>
> Pedestrian on ice-skates injured in collision with two- or three-wheeled motor vehicle in traffic accident
>
> Pedestrian on nonmotorized scooter injured in collision with two- or three-wheeled motor vehicle in traffic accident
>
> Pedestrian on sled injured in collision with two- or three-wheeled motor vehicle in traffic accident
>
> Pedestrian on snowboard injured in collision with two- or three-wheeled motor vehicle in traffic accident
>
> Pedestrian on snow-skis injured in collision with two- or three-wheeled motor vehicle in traffic accident
>
> Pedestrian in wheelchair (powered) injured in collision with two- or three-wheeled motor vehicle in traffic accident
>
> Pedestrian in motorized mobility scooter injured in collision with two- or three-wheeled motor vehicle in traffic accident

☑5ᵗʰ **V02.9 Pedestrian injured in collision with two- or three-wheeled motor vehicle, unspecified whether traffic or nontraffic accident**

☑7ᵗʰ **V02.90 Pedestrian on foot injured in collision with two- or three-wheeled motor vehicle, unspecified whether traffic or nontraffic accident**

> Pedestrian NOS injured in collision with two- or three-wheeled motor vehicle, unspecified whether traffic or nontraffic accident

☑7ᵗʰ **V02.91 Pedestrian on roller-skates injured in collision with two- or three-wheeled motor vehicle, unspecified whether traffic or nontraffic accident**

☑7ᵗʰ **V02.92 Pedestrian on skateboard injured in collision with two- or three-wheeled motor vehicle, unspecified whether traffic or nontraffic accident**

☑6ᵗʰ **V02.93 Pedestrian on standing micro-mobility pedestrian conveyance injured in collision with two- or three-wheeled motor vehicle, unspecified whether traffic or nontraffic accident**

☑7ᵗʰ **V02.931 Pedestrian on standing electric scooter injured in collision with two- or three wheeled motor vehicle, unspecified whether traffic or nontraffic accident**

☑7ᵗʰ **V02.938 Pedestrian on other standing micro-mobility pedestrian conveyance injured in collision with two- or three wheeled motor vehicle, unspecified whether traffic or nontraffic accident**

> Pedestrian on hoverboard injured in collision with two-three-wheeled motor vehicle, unspecified whether traffic or nontraffic accident
>
> Pedestrian on segway injured in collision with two- or three wheeled motor vehicle, unspecified whether traffic or nontraffic accident

☑×7ᵗʰ **V02.99 Pedestrian with other conveyance injured in collision with two- or three-wheeled motor vehicle, unspecified whether traffic or nontraffic accident**

> Pedestrian with baby stroller injured in collision with two- or three-wheeled motor vehicle, unspecified whether traffic or nontraffic accident
>
> Pedestrian on ice-skates injured in collision with two- or three-wheeled motor vehicle, unspecified whether traffic or nontraffic accident
>
> Pedestrian on nonmotorized scooter injured in collision with two- or three-wheeled motor vehicle, unspecified whether traffic or nontraffic accident
>
> Pedestrian on sled injured in collision with two- or three-wheeled motor vehicle, unspecified whether traffic or nontraffic accident
>
> Pedestrian on snowboard injured in collision with two- or three-wheeled motor vehicle, unspecified whether traffic or nontraffic accident
>
> Pedestrian on snow-skis injured in collision with two- or three-wheeled motor vehicle, unspecified whether traffic or nontraffic accident
>
> Pedestrian in wheelchair (powered) injured in collision with two- or three-wheeled motor vehicle, unspecified whether traffic or nontraffic accident
>
> Pedestrian in motorized mobility scooter injured in collision with two- or three wheeled motor vehicle, unspecified whether traffic or nontraffic accident

☑4ᵗʰ **V03 Pedestrian injured in collision with car, pick-up truck or van**

☑5ᵗʰ **V03.0 Pedestrian injured in collision with car, pick-up truck or van in nontraffic accident**

☑×7ᵗʰ **V03.00 Pedestrian on foot injured in collision with car, pick-up truck or van in nontraffic accident**

> Pedestrian NOS injured in collision with car, pick-up truck or van in nontraffic accident

☑×7ᵗʰ **V03.01 Pedestrian on roller-skates injured in collision with car, pick-up truck or van in nontraffic accident**

☑×7ᵗʰ **V03.02 Pedestrian on skateboard injured in collision with car, pick-up truck or van in nontraffic accident**

☑6ᵗʰ **V03.03 Pedestrian on standing micro-mobility pedestrian conveyance injured in collision with car, pick-up or van in nontraffic accident**

☑7ᵗʰ **V03.031 Pedestrian on standing electric scooter injured in collision with car, pick-up or van in nontraffic accident**

☑7ᵗʰ **V03.038 Pedestrian on other standing micro-mobility pedestrian conveyance injured in collision with car, pick-up or van in nontraffic accident**

> Pedestrian on hoverboard injured in collision with car, pick-up or van in nontraffic accident
>
> Pedestrian on segway injured in collision with car, pick-up or van in nontraffic accident

☑×7ᵗʰ **V03.09 Pedestrian with other conveyance injured in collision with car, pick-up truck or van in nontraffic accident**

> Pedestrian with baby stroller injured in collision with car, pick-up truck or van in nontraffic accident
>
> Pedestrian on ice-skates injured in collision with car, pick-up truck or van in nontraffic accident
>
> Pedestrian on nonmotorized scooter injured in collision with car, pick-up truck or van in nontraffic accident
>
> Pedestrian on sled injured in collision with car, pick-up truck or van in nontraffic accident
>
> Pedestrian on snowboard injured in collision with car, pick-up truck or van in nontraffic accident
>
> Pedestrian on snow-skis injured in collision with car, pick-up truck or van in nontraffic accident
>
> Pedestrian in wheelchair (powered) injured in collision with car, pick-up truck or van in nontraffic accident
>
> Pedestrian in motorized mobility scooter injured in collision with car, pick-up truck or van in nontraffic accident

Chapter 20. External Causes of Morbidity

√5ᵗʰ **V03.1** **Pedestrian injured in collision with car, pick-up truck or van in traffic accident**

√x7ᵗʰ **V03.10** **Pedestrian on foot injured in collision with car, pick-up truck or van in traffic accident**
Pedestrian NOS injured in collision with car, pick-up truck or van in traffic accident

√x7ᵗʰ **V03.11** **Pedestrian on roller-skates injured in collision with car, pick-up truck or van in traffic accident**

√x7ᵗʰ **V03.12** **Pedestrian on skateboard injured in collision with car, pick-up truck or van in traffic accident**

√6ᵗʰ **V03.13** **Pedestrian on standing micro-mobility pedestrian conveyance injured in collision with car, pick-up or van in traffic accident**

√7ᵗʰ **V03.131** **Pedestrian on standing electric scooter injured in collision with car, pick-up or van in traffic accident**

√7ᵗʰ **V03.138** **Pedestrian on other standing micro-mobility pedestrian conveyance injured in collision with car, pick-up or van in traffic accident**
Pedestrian on hoverboard injured in collision with car, pick-up or van in traffic accident
Pedestrian on segway injured in collision with car, pick-up or van in traffic accident

√x7ᵗʰ **V03.19** **Pedestrian with other conveyance injured in collision with car, pick-up truck or van in traffic accident**
Pedestrian with baby stroller injured in collision with car, pick-up truck or van in traffic accident
Pedestrian on ice-skates injured in collision with car, pick-up truck or van in traffic accident
Pedestrian on nonmotorized scooter injured in collision with car, pick-up truck or van in nontraffic accident
Pedestrian on sled injured in collision with car, pick-up truck or van in traffic accident
Pedestrian on snowboard injured in collision with car, pick-up truck or van in traffic accident
Pedestrian on snow-skis injured in collision with car, pick-up truck or van in traffic accident
Pedestrian in wheelchair (powered) injured in collision with car, pick-up truck or van in traffic accident
Pedestrian in motorized mobility scooter injured in collision with car, pick-up truck or van in nontraffic accident

√5ᵗʰ **V03.9** **Pedestrian injured in collision with car, pick-up truck or van, unspecified whether traffic or nontraffic accident**

√x7ᵗʰ **V03.90** **Pedestrian on foot injured in collision with car, pick-up truck or van, unspecified whether traffic or nontraffic accident**
Pedestrian NOS injured in collision with car, pick-up truck or van, unspecified whether traffic or nontraffic accident

√x7ᵗʰ **V03.91** **Pedestrian on roller-skates injured in collision with car, pick-up truck or van, unspecified whether traffic or nontraffic accident**

√x7ᵗʰ **V03.92** **Pedestrian on skateboard injured in collision with car, pick-up truck or van, unspecified whether traffic or nontraffic accident**

√6ᵗʰ **V03.93** **Pedestrian on standing micro-mobility pedestrian conveyance injured in collision with car, pick-up or van, unspecified whether traffic or nontraffic accident**

√7ᵗʰ **V03.931** **Pedestrian on standing electric scooter injured in collision with car, pick-up or van, unspecified whether traffic or nontraffic accident**

√7ᵗʰ **V03.938** **Pedestrian on other standing micro-mobility pedestrian conveyance injured in collision with car, pick-up or van, unspecified whether traffic or nontraffic accident**
Pedestrian on hoverboard injured in collision with car, pick-up or van, unspecified whether traffic or nontraffic accident
Pedestrian on segway injured in collision with car, pick-up or van, unspecified whether traffic or nontraffic accident

√x7ᵗʰ **V03.99** **Pedestrian with other conveyance injured in collision with car, pick-up truck or van, unspecified whether traffic or nontraffic accident**
Pedestrian with baby stroller injured in collision with car, pick-up truck or van, unspecified whether traffic or nontraffic accident
Pedestrian on ice-skates injured in collision with car, pick-up truck or van, unspecified whether traffic or nontraffic accident
Pedestrian on nonmotorized scooter injured in collision with car, pick-up truck or van, unspecified whether traffic or nontraffic accident
Pedestrian on sled injured in collision with car, pick-up truck or van in nontraffic accident
Pedestrian on snowboard injured in collision with car, pick-up truck or van, unspecified whether traffic or nontraffic accident
Pedestrian on snow-skis injured in collision with car, pick-up truck or van, unspecified whether traffic or nontraffic accident
Pedestrian in wheelchair (powered) injured in collision with car, pick-up truck or van, unspecified whether traffic or nontraffic accident
Pedestrian in motorized mobility scooter injured in collision with car, pick-up truck or van, unspecified whether traffic or nontraffic accident

√4ᵗʰ **V04** **Pedestrian injured in collision with heavy transport vehicle or bus**
EXCLUDES 1   *pedestrian injured in collision with military vehicle (V09.01, V09.21)*

√5ᵗʰ **V04.0** **Pedestrian injured in collision with heavy transport vehicle or bus in nontraffic accident**

√x7ᵗʰ **V04.00** **Pedestrian on foot injured in collision with heavy transport vehicle or bus in nontraffic accident**
Pedestrian NOS injured in collision with heavy transport vehicle or bus in nontraffic accident

√x7ᵗʰ **V04.01** **Pedestrian on roller-skates injured in collision with heavy transport vehicle or bus in nontraffic accident**

√x7ᵗʰ **V04.02** **Pedestrian on skateboard injured in collision with heavy transport vehicle or bus in nontraffic accident**

√6ᵗʰ **V04.03** **Pedestrian on standing micro-mobility pedestrian conveyance injured in collision with heavy transport vehicle or bus in nontraffic accident**

√7ᵗʰ **V04.031** **Pedestrian on standing electric scooter injured in collision with heavy transport vehicle or bus in nontraffic accident**

√7ᵗʰ **V04.038** **Pedestrian on other standing micro-mobility pedestrian conveyance injured in collision with heavy transport vehicle or bus in nontraffic accident**
Pedestrian on hoverboard injured in collision with heavy transport vehicle or bus in nontraffic accident
Pedestrian on segway injured in collision with heavy transport vehicle or bus in nontraffic accident

☑x7ᵗʰ **V04.09** **Pedestrian with other conveyance injured in collision with heavy transport vehicle or bus in nontraffic accident**

Pedestrian with baby stroller injured in collision with heavy transport vehicle or bus in nontraffic accident

Pedestrian on ice-skates injured in collision with heavy transport vehicle or bus in nontraffic accident

Pedestrian on nonmotorized scooter injured in collision with heavy transport vehicle or bus in nontraffic accident

Pedestrian on sled injured in collision with heavy transport vehicle or bus in nontraffic accident

Pedestrian on snowboard injured in collision with heavy transport vehicle or bus in nontraffic accident

Pedestrian on snow-skis injured in collision with heavy transport vehicle or bus in nontraffic accident

Pedestrian in wheelchair (powered) injured in collision with heavy transport vehicle or bus in nontraffic accident

Pedestrian in motorized mobility scooter injured in collision with heavy transport vehicle or bus in nontraffic accident

☑5ᵗʰ **V04.1** **Pedestrian injured in collision with heavy transport vehicle or bus in traffic accident**

☑x7ᵗʰ **V04.10** **Pedestrian on foot injured in collision with heavy transport vehicle or bus in traffic accident**

Pedestrian NOS injured in collision with heavy transport vehicle or bus in traffic accident

☑x7ᵗʰ **V04.11** **Pedestrian on roller-skates injured in collision with heavy transport vehicle or bus in traffic accident**

☑x7ᵗʰ **V04.12** **Pedestrian on skateboard injured in collision with heavy transport vehicle or bus in traffic accident**

☑6ᵗʰ **V04.13** **Pedestrian on standing micro-mobility pedestrian conveyance injured in collision with heavy transport vehicle or bus in traffic accident**

☑7ᵗʰ **V04.131** **Pedestrian on standing electric scooter injured in collision with heavy transport vehicle or bus in traffic accident**

☑7ᵗʰ **V04.138** **Pedestrian on other standing micro-mobility pedestrian conveyance injured in collision with heavy transport vehicle or bus in traffic accident**

Pedestrian on hoverboard injured in collision with heavy transport vehicle or bus in traffic accident

Pedestrian on segway injured in collision with heavy transport vehicle or bus in traffic accident

☑x7ᵗʰ **V04.19** **Pedestrian with other conveyance injured in collision with heavy transport vehicle or bus in traffic accident**

Pedestrian with baby stroller injured in collision with heavy transport vehicle or bus in traffic accident

Pedestrian on ice-skates injured in collision with heavy transport vehicle or bus in traffic accident

Pedestrian on nonmotorized scooter injured in collision with heavy transport vehicle or bus in traffic accident

Pedestrian on sled injured in collision with heavy transport vehicle or bus in traffic accident

Pedestrian on snowboard injured in collision with heavy transport vehicle or bus in traffic accident

Pedestrian on snow-skis injured in collision with heavy transport vehicle or bus in traffic accident

Pedestrian in wheelchair (powered) injured in collision with heavy transport vehicle or bus in traffic accident

Pedestrian in motorized mobility scooter injured in collision with heavy transport vehicle or bus in traffic accident

☑5ᵗʰ **V04.9** **Pedestrian injured in collision with heavy transport vehicle or bus, unspecified whether traffic or nontraffic accident**

☑x7ᵗʰ **V04.90** **Pedestrian on foot injured in collision with heavy transport vehicle or bus, unspecified whether traffic or nontraffic accident**

Pedestrian NOS injured in collision with heavy transport vehicle or bus, unspecified whether traffic or nontraffic accident

☑x7ᵗʰ **V04.91** **Pedestrian on roller-skates injured in collision with heavy transport vehicle or bus, unspecified whether traffic or nontraffic accident**

☑x7ᵗʰ **V04.92** **Pedestrian on skateboard injured in collision with heavy transport vehicle or bus, unspecified whether traffic or nontraffic accident**

☑6ᵗʰ **V04.93** **Pedestrian on standing micro-mobility pedestrian conveyance injured in collision with heavy transport vehicle or bus, unspecified whether traffic or nontraffic accident**

☑7ᵗʰ **V04.931** **Pedestrian on standing electric scooter injured in collision with heavy transport vehicle or bus, unspecified whether traffic or nontraffic accident**

☑7ᵗʰ **V04.938** **Pedestrian on other standing micro-mobility pedestrian conveyance injured in collision with heavy transport vehicle or bus, unspecified whether traffic or nontraffic accident**

Pedestrian on hoverboard injured in collision with heavy transport vehicle or bus, unspecified whether traffic or nontraffic accident

Pedestrian on segway injured in collision with heavy transport vehicle or bus, unspecified whether traffic or nontraffic accident

☑x7ᵗʰ **V04.99** **Pedestrian with other conveyance injured in collision with heavy transport vehicle or bus, unspecified whether traffic or nontraffic accident**

Pedestrian with baby stroller injured in collision with heavy transport vehicle or bus, unspecified whether traffic or nontraffic accident

Pedestrian on ice-skates injured in collision with heavy transport vehicle or bus, unspecified whether traffic or nontraffic accident

Pedestrian on nonmotorized scooter injured in collision with heavy transport vehicle or bus, unspecified whether traffic or nontraffic accident

Pedestrian on sled injured in collision with heavy transport vehicle or bus, unspecified whether traffic or nontraffic accident

Pedestrian on snowboard injured in collision with heavy transport vehicle or bus, unspecified whether traffic or nontraffic accident

Pedestrian on snow-skis injured in collision with heavy transport vehicle or bus, unspecified whether traffic or nontraffic accident

Pedestrian in wheelchair (powered) injured in collision with heavy transport vehicle or bus, unspecified whether traffic or nontraffic accident

Pedestrian in motorized mobility scooter injured in collision with heavy transport vehicle or bus, unspecified whether traffic or nontraffic accident

☑4ᵗʰ **V05** **Pedestrian injured in collision with railway train or railway vehicle**

☑5ᵗʰ **V05.0** **Pedestrian injured in collision with railway train or railway vehicle in nontraffic accident**

☑x7ᵗʰ **V05.00** **Pedestrian on foot injured in collision with railway train or railway vehicle in nontraffic accident**

Pedestrian NOS injured in collision with railway train or railway vehicle in nontraffic accident

☑x7ᵗʰ **V05.01** **Pedestrian on roller-skates injured in collision with railway train or railway vehicle in nontraffic accident**

☑x7ᵗʰ **V05.02** **Pedestrian on skateboard injured in collision with railway train or railway vehicle in nontraffic accident**

☑6ᵗʰ **V05.03** **Pedestrian on standing micro-mobility pedestrian conveyance injured in collision with railway train or railway vehicle in nontraffic accident**

☑7ᵗʰ **V05.031** **Pedestrian on standing electric scooter injured in collision with railway train or railway vehicle in nontraffic accident**

✓7ᵗʰ V05.038 Pedestrian on other standing micro-mobility pedestrian conveyance injured in collision with railway train or railway vehicle in nontraffic accident
  Pedestrian on hoverboard injured in collision with railway train or railway vehicle in nontraffic accident
  Pedestrian on segway injured in collision with railway train or railway vehicle in nontraffic accident

✓x7ᵗʰ V05.09 Pedestrian with other conveyance injured in collision with railway train or railway vehicle in nontraffic accident
  Pedestrian with baby stroller injured in collision with railway train or railway vehicle in nontraffic accident
  Pedestrian on ice-skates injured in collision with railway train or railway vehicle in nontraffic accident
  Pedestrian on nonmotorized scooter injured in collision with railway train or railway vehicle in nontraffic accident
  Pedestrian on sled injured in collision with railway train or railway vehicle in nontraffic accident
  Pedestrian on snowboard injured in collision with railway train or railway vehicle in nontraffic accident
  Pedestrian on snow-skis injured in collision with railway train or railway vehicle in nontraffic accident
  Pedestrian in wheelchair (powered) injured in collision with railway train or railway vehicle in nontraffic accident
  Pedestrian in motorized mobility scooter injured in collision with railway train or railway vehicle in nontraffic accident

✓5ᵗʰ V05.1 Pedestrian injured in collision with railway train or railway vehicle in traffic accident

✓x7ᵗʰ V05.10 Pedestrian on foot injured in collision with railway train or railway vehicle in traffic accident
  Pedestrian NOS injured in collision with railway train or railway vehicle in traffic accident

✓x7ᵗʰ V05.11 Pedestrian on roller-skates injured in collision with railway train or railway vehicle in traffic accident

✓x7ᵗʰ V05.12 Pedestrian on skateboard injured in collision with railway train or railway vehicle in traffic accident

✓6ᵗʰ V05.13 Pedestrian on standing micro-mobility pedestrian conveyance injured in collision with railway train or railway vehicle in traffic accident

✓7ᵗʰ V05.131 Pedestrian on standing electric scooter injured in collision with railway train or railway vehicle in traffic accident

✓7ᵗʰ V05.138 Pedestrian on other standing micro-mobility pedestrian conveyance injured in collision with railway train or railway vehicle in traffic accident
  Pedestrian on hoverboard injured in collision with railway train or railway vehicle in traffic accident
  Pedestrian on segway injured in collision with railway train or railway vehicle in traffic accident

✓x7ᵗʰ V05.19 Pedestrian with other conveyance injured in collision with railway train or railway vehicle in traffic accident
  Pedestrian with baby stroller injured in collision with railway train or railway vehicle in traffic accident
  Pedestrian on ice-skates injured in collision with railway train or railway vehicle in traffic accident
  Pedestrian on nonmotorized scooter injured in collision with railway train or railway vehicle in traffic accident
  Pedestrian on sled injured in collision with railway train or railway vehicle in traffic accident
  Pedestrian on snowboard injured in collision with railway train or railway vehicle in traffic accident
  Pedestrian on snow-skis injured in collision with railway train or railway vehicle in traffic accident
  Pedestrian in wheelchair (powered) injured in collision with railway train or railway vehicle in traffic accident
  Pedestrian in motorized mobility scooter injured in collision with railway train or railway vehicle in traffic accident

✓5ᵗʰ V05.9 Pedestrian injured in collision with railway train or railway vehicle, unspecified whether traffic or nontraffic accident

✓x7ᵗʰ V05.90 Pedestrian on foot injured in collision with railway train or railway vehicle, unspecified whether traffic or nontraffic accident
  Pedestrian NOS injured in collision with railway train or railway vehicle, unspecified whether traffic or nontraffic accident

✓x7ᵗʰ V05.91 Pedestrian on roller-skates injured in collision with railway train or railway vehicle, unspecified whether traffic or nontraffic accident

✓x7ᵗʰ V05.92 Pedestrian on skateboard injured in collision with railway train or railway vehicle, unspecified whether traffic or nontraffic accident

✓6ᵗʰ V05.93 Pedestrian on standing micro-mobility pedestrian conveyance injured in collision with railway train or railway vehicle, unspecified whether traffic or nontraffic accident

✓7ᵗʰ V05.931 Pedestrian on standing electric scooter injured in collision with railway train or railway vehicle, unspecified whether traffic or nontraffic accident

✓7ᵗʰ V05.938 Pedestrian on other standing micro-mobility pedestrian conveyance injured in collision with railway train or railway vehicle, unspecified whether traffic or nontraffic accident
  Pedestrian on hoverboard injured in collision with railway train or railway vehicle, unspecified whether traffic or nontraffic accident
  Pedestrian on segway injured in collision with railway train or railway vehicle, unspecified whether traffic or nontraffic accident

HCC CMS-HCC　　**Rx** Rx HCC　　**ESR** ESRD HCC　　**COM** Commercial HCC　　　**N** Newborn: 0　　**P** Pediatric: 0-17　　**M** Maternity: 9-64　　**A** Adult: 15-124

1200

ICD-10-CM 2023

☑7ᵗʰ **V05.99** **Pedestrian with other conveyance injured in collision with railway train or railway vehicle, unspecified whether traffic or nontraffic accident**
Pedestrian with baby stroller injured in collision with railway train or railway vehicle, unspecified whether traffic or nontraffic
Pedestrian on ice-skates injured in collision with railway train or railway vehicle, unspecified whether traffic or nontraffic
Pedestrian on nonmotorized scooter injured in collision with railway train or railway vehicle, unspecified whether traffic or nontraffic
Pedestrian on sled injured in collision with railway train or railway vehicle, unspecified whether traffic or nontraffic
Pedestrian on snowboard injured in collision with railway train or railway vehicle, unspecified whether traffic or nontraffic
Pedestrian on snow-skis injured in collision with railway train or railway vehicle, unspecified whether traffic or nontraffic
Pedestrian in wheelchair (powered) injured in collision with railway train or railway vehicle, unspecified whether traffic or nontraffic
Pedestrian in motorized mobility scooter injured in collision with railway train or railway vehicle, unspecified whether traffic or nontraffic

☑4ᵗʰ **V06** **Pedestrian injured in collision with other nonmotor vehicle**
INCLUDES   collision with animal-drawn vehicle, animal being ridden, nonpowered streetcar
EXCLUDES 1   pedestrian injured in collision with pedestrian conveyance (V00.0-)

☑5ᵗʰ **V06.0** **Pedestrian injured in collision with other nonmotor vehicle in nontraffic accident**

☑7ᵗʰ **V06.00** **Pedestrian on foot injured in collision with other nonmotor vehicle in nontraffic accident**
Pedestrian NOS injured in collision with other nonmotor vehicle in nontraffic accident

☑7ᵗʰ **V06.01** **Pedestrian on roller-skates injured in collision with other nonmotor vehicle in nontraffic accident**

☑7ᵗʰ **V06.02** **Pedestrian on skateboard injured in collision with other nonmotor vehicle in nontraffic accident**

☑6ᵗʰ **V06.03** **Pedestrian on standing micro-mobility pedestrian conveyance injured in collision with other nonmotor vehicle in nontraffic accident**

☑7ᵗʰ **V06.031** **Pedestrian on standing electric scooter injured in collision with other nonmotor vehicle in nontraffic accident**

☑7ᵗʰ **V06.038** **Pedestrian on other standing micro-mobility pedestrian conveyance injured in collision with other nonmotor vehicle in nontraffic accident**
Pedestrian on hoverboard injured in collision with other nonmotor vehicle in nontraffic accident
Pedestrian on segway injured in collision with other nonmotor vehicle in nontraffic accident

☑7ᵗʰ **V06.09** **Pedestrian with other conveyance injured in collision with other nonmotor vehicle in nontraffic accident**
Pedestrian with baby stroller injured in collision with other nonmotor vehicle in nontraffic accident
Pedestrian on ice-skates injured in collision with other nonmotor vehicle in nontraffic accident
Pedestrian on nonmotorized scooter injured in collision with other nonmotor vehicle in nontraffic accident
Pedestrian on sled injured in collision with other nonmotor vehicle in nontraffic accident
Pedestrian on snowboard injured in collision with other nonmotor vehicle in nontraffic accident
Pedestrian on snow-skis injured in collision with other nonmotor vehicle in nontraffic accident
Pedestrian in wheelchair (powered) injured in collision with other nonmotor vehicle in nontraffic accident
Pedestrian in motorized mobility scooter injured in collision with other nonmotor vehicle in nontraffic accident

☑5ᵗʰ **V06.1** **Pedestrian injured in collision with other nonmotor vehicle in traffic accident**

☑7ᵗʰ **V06.10** **Pedestrian on foot injured in collision with other nonmotor vehicle in traffic accident**
Pedestrian NOS injured in collision with other nonmotor vehicle in traffic accident

☑7ᵗʰ **V06.11** **Pedestrian on roller-skates injured in collision with other nonmotor vehicle in traffic accident**

☑7ᵗʰ **V06.12** **Pedestrian on skateboard injured in collision with other nonmotor vehicle in traffic accident**

☑6ᵗʰ **V06.13** **Pedestrian on standing micro-mobility pedestrian conveyance injured in collision with other nonmotor vehicle in traffic accident**

☑7ᵗʰ **V06.131** **Pedestrian on standing electric scooter injured in collision with other nonmotor vehicle in traffic accident**

☑7ᵗʰ **V06.138** **Pedestrian on other standing micro-mobility pedestrian conveyance injured in collision with other nonmotor vehicle in traffic accident**
Pedestrian on hoverboard injured in collision with other nonmotor vehicle in traffic accident
Pedestrian on segway injured in collision with other nonmotor vehicle in traffic accident

☑7ᵗʰ **V06.19** **Pedestrian with other conveyance injured in collision with other nonmotor vehicle in traffic accident**
Pedestrian with baby stroller injured in collision with other nonmotor vehicle in nontraffic accident
Pedestrian on ice-skates injured in collision with other nonmotor vehicle in traffic accident
Pedestrian on nonmotorized scooter injured in collision with other nonmotor vehicle in traffic accident
Pedestrian on sled injured in collision with other nonmotor vehicle in traffic accident
Pedestrian on snowboard injured in collision with other nonmotor vehicle in traffic accident
Pedestrian on snow-skis injured in collision with other nonmotor vehicle in traffic accident
Pedestrian in wheelchair (powered) injured in collision with other nonmotor vehicle in traffic accident
Pedestrian in motorized mobility scooter injured in collision with other nonmotor vehicle in traffic accident

☑5ᵗʰ **V06.9** **Pedestrian injured in collision with other nonmotor vehicle, unspecified whether traffic or nontraffic accident**

☑7ᵗʰ **V06.90** **Pedestrian on foot injured in collision with other nonmotor vehicle, unspecified whether traffic or nontraffic accident**
Pedestrian NOS injured in collision with other nonmotor vehicle, unspecified whether traffic or nontraffic accident

☑7ᵗʰ **V06.91** **Pedestrian on roller-skates injured in collision with other nonmotor vehicle, unspecified whether traffic or nontraffic accident**

√x7ᵗʰ **V06.92 Pedestrian** on skateboard **injured in collision with other nonmotor vehicle, unspecified whether traffic or nontraffic accident**

√6ᵗʰ **V06.93 Pedestrian on standing micro-mobility pedestrian conveyance injured in collision with other nonmotor vehicle, unspecified whether traffic or nontraffic accident**

√7ᵗʰ **V06.931 Pedestrian** on standing electric scooter **injured in collision with other nonmotor vehicle, unspecified whether traffic or nontraffic accident**

√7ᵗʰ **V06.938 Pedestrian on other standing micro-mobility pedestrian conveyance injured in collision with other nonmotor vehicle, unspecified whether traffic or nontraffic accident**

Pedestrian on hoverboard injured in collision with other nonmotor, unspecified whether traffic or nontraffic accident

Pedestrian on segway injured in collision with other nonmotor vehicle, unspecified whether traffic or nontraffic accident

√x7ᵗʰ **V06.99 Pedestrian with other conveyance injured in collision with other nonmotor vehicle, unspecified whether traffic or nontraffic accident**

Pedestrian with baby stroller injured in collision with other nonmotor vehicle, unspecified whether traffic or nontraffic accident

Pedestrian on ice-skates injured in collision with other nonmotor vehicle, unspecified whether traffic or nontraffic accident

Pedestrian on nonmotorized scooter injured in collision with other nonmotor vehicle, unspecified whether traffic or nontraffic accident

Pedestrian on sled injured in collision with other nonmotor vehicle, unspecified whether traffic or nontraffic accident

Pedestrian on snowboard injured in collision with other nonmotor vehicle, unspecified whether traffic or nontraffic accident

Pedestrian on snow-skis injured in collision with other nonmotor vehicle, unspecified whether traffic or nontraffic accident

Pedestrian in wheelchair (powered) injured in collision with other nonmotor vehicle, unspecified whether traffic or nontraffic accident

Pedestrian in motorized mobility scooter injured in collision with other nonmotorized vehicle, unspecified whether traffic or nontraffic accident

√4ᵗʰ **V09 Pedestrian injured in other and unspecified transport accidents**

√5ᵗʰ **V09.0 Pedestrian injured in** nontraffic **accident involving other and unspecified motor vehicles**

√x7ᵗʰ **V09.00 Pedestrian injured in nontraffic accident involving unspecified motor vehicles**

√x7ᵗʰ **V09.01 Pedestrian injured in nontraffic accident involving** military vehicle

√x7ᵗʰ **V09.09 Pedestrian injured in nontraffic accident involving other motor vehicles**

Pedestrian injured in nontraffic accident by special vehicle

√x7ᵗʰ **V09.1 Pedestrian injured in unspecified** nontraffic **accident**

√5ᵗʰ **V09.2 Pedestrian injured in** traffic accident **involving other and unspecified motor vehicles**

√x7ᵗʰ **V09.20 Pedestrian injured in traffic accident involving unspecified motor vehicles**

√x7ᵗʰ **V09.21 Pedestrian injured in traffic accident involving** military vehicle

√x7ᵗʰ **V09.29 Pedestrian injured in traffic accident involving other motor vehicles**

√x7ᵗʰ **V09.3 Pedestrian injured in unspecified** traffic **accident**

√x7ᵗʰ **V09.9 Pedestrian injured in unspecified** transport **accident**

Pedal cycle rider injured in transport accident (V10-V19)

INCLUDES   any non-motorized vehicle, excluding an animal-drawn vehicle, or a sidecar or trailer attached to the pedal cycle

EXCLUDES 2   *rupture of pedal cycle tire (W37.0)*

The appropriate 7th character is to be added to each code from categories V10-V19.
A   initial encounter
D   subsequent encounter
S   sequela

√4ᵗʰ **V10 Pedal cycle rider injured in collision with pedestrian or animal**

EXCLUDES 1   *pedal cycle rider collision with animal-drawn vehicle or animal being ridden (V16.-)*

√x7ᵗʰ **V10.0 Pedal cycle** driver **injured in collision with pedestrian or animal** in nontraffic accident

√x7ᵗʰ **V10.1 Pedal cycle** passenger **injured in collision with pedestrian or animal** in nontraffic accident

√x7ᵗʰ **V10.2 Unspecified pedal cyclist injured in collision with pedestrian or animal** in nontraffic accident

√x7ᵗʰ **V10.3** Person boarding or alighting **a pedal cycle injured in collision with pedestrian or animal**

√x7ᵗʰ **V10.4 Pedal cycle** driver **injured in collision with pedestrian or animal** in traffic accident

√x7ᵗʰ **V10.5 Pedal cycle** passenger **injured in collision with pedestrian or animal** in traffic accident

√x7ᵗʰ **V10.9 Unspecified pedal cyclist injured in collision with pedestrian or animal** in traffic accident

√4ᵗʰ **V11 Pedal cycle rider injured in collision with other pedal cycle**

√x7ᵗʰ **V11.0 Pedal cycle** driver **injured in collision with other pedal cycle** in nontraffic accident

√x7ᵗʰ **V11.1 Pedal cycle** passenger **injured in collision with other pedal cycle** in nontraffic accident

√x7ᵗʰ **V11.2 Unspecified pedal cyclist injured in collision with other pedal cycle** in nontraffic accident

√x7ᵗʰ **V11.3** Person boarding or alighting **a pedal cycle injured in collision with other pedal cycle**

√x7ᵗʰ **V11.4 Pedal cycle** driver **injured in collision with other pedal cycle** in traffic accident

√x7ᵗʰ **V11.5 Pedal cycle** passenger **injured in collision with other pedal cycle** in traffic accident

√x7ᵗʰ **V11.9 Unspecified pedal cyclist injured in collision with other pedal cycle** in traffic accident

√4ᵗʰ **V12 Pedal cycle rider injured in collision with two- or three-wheeled motor vehicle**

√x7ᵗʰ **V12.0 Pedal cycle** driver **injured in collision with two- or three-wheeled motor vehicle** in nontraffic accident

√x7ᵗʰ **V12.1 Pedal cycle** passenger **injured in collision with two- or three-wheeled motor vehicle** in nontraffic accident

√x7ᵗʰ **V12.2 Unspecified pedal cyclist injured in collision with two- or three-wheeled motor vehicle** in nontraffic accident

√x7ᵗʰ **V12.3** Person boarding or alighting **a pedal cycle injured in collision with two- or three-wheeled motor vehicle**

√x7ᵗʰ **V12.4 Pedal cycle** driver **injured in collision with two- or three-wheeled motor vehicle** in traffic accident

√x7ᵗʰ **V12.5 Pedal cycle** passenger **injured in collision with two- or three-wheeled motor vehicle** in traffic accident

√x7ᵗʰ **V12.9 Unspecified pedal cyclist injured in collision with two- or three-wheeled motor vehicle** in traffic accident

√4ᵗʰ **V13 Pedal cycle rider injured in collision with car, pick-up truck or van**

√x7ᵗʰ **V13.0 Pedal cycle** driver **injured in collision with car, pick-up truck or van** in nontraffic accident

√x7ᵗʰ **V13.1 Pedal cycle** passenger **injured in collision with car, pick-up truck or van** in nontraffic accident

√x7ᵗʰ **V13.2 Unspecified pedal cyclist injured in collision with car, pick-up truck or van** in nontraffic accident

√x7ᵗʰ **V13.3** Person boarding or alighting **a pedal cycle injured in collision with car, pick-up truck or van**

√x7ᵗʰ **V13.4 Pedal cycle** driver **injured in collision with car, pick-up truck or van** in traffic accident

√x7ᵗʰ **V13.5 Pedal cycle** passenger **injured in collision with car, pick-up truck or van** in traffic accident

√x7ᵗʰ **V13.9 Unspecified pedal cyclist injured in collision with car, pick-up truck or van** in traffic accident

√4ᵗʰ **V14 Pedal cycle rider injured in collision with heavy transport vehicle or bus**

EXCLUDES 1   *pedal cycle rider injured in collision with military vehicle (V19.81)*

√x7ᵗʰ **V14.0 Pedal cycle** driver **injured in collision with heavy transport vehicle or bus** in nontraffic accident

✓7th **V14.1** Pedal cycle passenger injured in collision with heavy transport vehicle or bus in nontraffic accident

✓7th **V14.2** Unspecified pedal cyclist injured in collision with heavy transport vehicle or bus in nontraffic accident

✓7th **V14.3** Person boarding or alighting a pedal cycle injured in collision with heavy transport vehicle or bus

✓7th **V14.4** Pedal cycle driver injured in collision with heavy transport vehicle or bus in traffic accident

✓7th **V14.5** Pedal cycle passenger injured in collision with heavy transport vehicle or bus in traffic accident

✓7th **V14.9** Unspecified pedal cyclist injured in collision with heavy transport vehicle or bus in traffic accident

✓4th **V15** Pedal cycle rider injured in collision with railway train or railway vehicle

✓7th **V15.0** Pedal cycle driver injured in collision with railway train or railway vehicle in nontraffic accident

✓7th **V15.1** Pedal cycle passenger injured in collision with railway train or railway vehicle in nontraffic accident

✓7th **V15.2** Unspecified pedal cyclist injured in collision with railway train or railway vehicle in nontraffic accident

✓7th **V15.3** Person boarding or alighting a pedal cycle injured in collision with railway train or railway vehicle

✓7th **V15.4** Pedal cycle driver injured in collision with railway train or railway vehicle in traffic accident

✓7th **V15.5** Pedal cycle passenger injured in collision with railway train or railway vehicle in traffic accident

✓7th **V15.9** Unspecified pedal cyclist injured in collision with railway train or railway vehicle in traffic accident

✓4th **V16** Pedal cycle rider injured in collision with other nonmotor vehicle

> INCLUDES   collision with animal-drawn vehicle, animal being ridden, streetcar

✓7th **V16.0** Pedal cycle driver injured in collision with other nonmotor vehicle in nontraffic accident

✓7th **V16.1** Pedal cycle passenger injured in collision with other nonmotor vehicle in nontraffic accident

✓7th **V16.2** Unspecified pedal cyclist injured in collision with other nonmotor vehicle in nontraffic accident

✓7th **V16.3** Person boarding or alighting a pedal cycle injured in collision with other nonmotor vehicle in nontraffic accident

✓7th **V16.4** Pedal cycle driver injured in collision with other nonmotor vehicle in traffic accident

✓7th **V16.5** Pedal cycle passenger injured in collision with other nonmotor vehicle in traffic accident

✓7th **V16.9** Unspecified pedal cyclist injured in collision with other nonmotor vehicle in traffic accident

✓4th **V17** Pedal cycle rider injured in collision with fixed or stationary object

✓7th **V17.0** Pedal cycle driver injured in collision with fixed or stationary object in nontraffic accident

✓7th **V17.1** Pedal cycle passenger injured in collision with fixed or stationary object in nontraffic accident

✓7th **V17.2** Unspecified pedal cyclist injured in collision with fixed or stationary object in nontraffic accident

✓7th **V17.3** Person boarding or alighting a pedal cycle injured in collision with fixed or stationary object

✓7th **V17.4** Pedal cycle driver injured in collision with fixed or stationary object in traffic accident

✓7th **V17.5** Pedal cycle passenger injured in collision with fixed or stationary object in traffic accident

✓7th **V17.9** Unspecified pedal cyclist injured in collision with fixed or stationary object in traffic accident

✓4th **V18** Pedal cycle rider injured in noncollision transport accident

> INCLUDES   fall or thrown from pedal cycle (without antecedent collision)
> overturning pedal cycle NOS
> overturning pedal cycle without collision

✓7th **V18.0** Pedal cycle driver injured in noncollision transport accident in nontraffic accident

✓7th **V18.1** Pedal cycle passenger injured in noncollision transport accident in nontraffic accident

✓7th **V18.2** Unspecified pedal cyclist injured in noncollision transport accident in nontraffic accident

✓7th **V18.3** Person boarding or alighting a pedal cycle injured in noncollision transport accident

✓7th **V18.4** Pedal cycle driver injured in noncollision transport accident in traffic accident

✓7th **V18.5** Pedal cycle passenger injured in noncollision transport accident in traffic accident

✓7th **V18.9** Unspecified pedal cyclist injured in noncollision transport accident in traffic accident

✓4th **V19** Pedal cycle rider injured in other and unspecified transport accidents

✓5th **V19.0** Pedal cycle driver injured in collision with other and unspecified motor vehicles in nontraffic accident

✓7th **V19.00** Pedal cycle driver injured in collision with unspecified motor vehicles in nontraffic accident

✓7th **V19.09** Pedal cycle driver injured in collision with other motor vehicles in nontraffic accident

✓5th **V19.1** Pedal cycle passenger injured in collision with other and unspecified motor vehicles in nontraffic accident

✓7th **V19.10** Pedal cycle passenger injured in collision with unspecified motor vehicles in nontraffic accident

✓7th **V19.19** Pedal cycle passenger injured in collision with other motor vehicles in nontraffic accident

✓5th **V19.2** Unspecified pedal cyclist injured in collision with other and unspecified motor vehicles in nontraffic accident

✓7th **V19.20** Unspecified pedal cyclist injured in collision with unspecified motor vehicles in nontraffic accident
Pedal cycle collision NOS, nontraffic

✓7th **V19.29** Unspecified pedal cyclist injured in collision with other motor vehicles in nontraffic accident

✓7th **V19.3** Pedal cyclist (driver) (passenger) injured in unspecified nontraffic accident
Pedal cycle accident NOS, nontraffic
Pedal cyclist injured in nontraffic accident NOS

✓5th **V19.4** Pedal cycle driver injured in collision with other and unspecified motor vehicles in traffic accident

✓7th **V19.40** Pedal cycle driver injured in collision with unspecified motor vehicles in traffic accident

✓7th **V19.49** Pedal cycle driver injured in collision with other motor vehicles in traffic accident

✓5th **V19.5** Pedal cycle passenger injured in collision with other and unspecified motor vehicles in traffic accident

✓7th **V19.50** Pedal cycle passenger injured in collision with unspecified motor vehicles in traffic accident

✓7th **V19.59** Pedal cycle passenger injured in collision with other motor vehicles in traffic accident

✓5th **V19.6** Unspecified pedal cyclist injured in collision with other and unspecified motor vehicles in traffic accident

✓7th **V19.60** Unspecified pedal cyclist injured in collision with unspecified motor vehicles in traffic accident
Pedal cycle collision NOS (traffic)

✓7th **V19.69** Unspecified pedal cyclist injured in collision with other motor vehicles in traffic accident

✓5th **V19.8** Pedal cyclist (driver) (passenger) injured in other specified transport accidents

✓7th **V19.81** Pedal cyclist (driver) (passenger) injured in transport accident with military vehicle

✓7th **V19.88** Pedal cyclist (driver) (passenger) injured in other specified transport accidents

✓7th **V19.9** Pedal cyclist (driver) (passenger) injured in unspecified traffic accident
Pedal cycle accident NOS

Motorcycle rider injured in transport accident (V20-V29)

> INCLUDES   ▶electric bicycle◄
> ▶e-bike◄
> ▶e-bicycle◄
> moped
> motorcycle with sidecar
> motorized bicycle
> motor scooter
>
> EXCLUDES 1   three-wheeled motor vehicle (V30-V39)

The appropriate 7th character is to be added to each code from categories V20-V29.
A   initial encounter
D   subsequent encounter
S   sequela

✓4th **V20** Motorcycle rider injured in collision with pedestrian or animal

> EXCLUDES 1   motorcycle rider collision with animal-drawn vehicle or animal being ridden (V26.-)

✓5th **V20.0** Motorcycle driver injured in collision with pedestrian or animal in nontraffic accident

● ✓7th **V20.01** Electric (assisted) bicycle driver injured in collision with pedestrian or animal in nontraffic accident

● ✓7th **V20.09** Other motorcycle driver injured in collision with pedestrian or animal in nontraffic accident

---

✓ Additional Character Required   ✓7th Placeholder Alert   Manifestation   Unspecified Dx   Q QPP   UPD Unacceptable PDx

√5ᵗʰ **V20.1** Motorcycle passenger injured in collision with pedestrian or animal in nontraffic accident

- √x7ᵗʰ **V20.11** Electric (assisted) bicycle passenger injured in collision with pedestrian or animal in nontraffic accident
- √x7ᵗʰ **V20.19** Other motorcycle passenger injured in collision with pedestrian or animal in nontraffic accident

√5ᵗʰ **V20.2** Unspecified motorcycle rider injured in collision with pedestrian or animal in nontraffic accident

- √x7ᵗʰ **V20.21** Unspecified electric (assisted) bicycle rider injured in collision with pedestrian or animal in nontraffic accident
- √x7ᵗʰ **V20.29** Unspecified rider of other motorcycle injured in collision with pedestrian or animal in nontraffic accident

√5ᵗʰ **V20.3** Person boarding or alighting a motorcycle injured in collision with pedestrian or animal

- √x7ᵗʰ **V20.31** Person boarding or alighting an electric (assisted) bicycle injured in collision with pedestrian or animal
- √x7ᵗʰ **V20.39** Person boarding or alighting other motorcycle injured in collision with pedestrian or animal

√5ᵗʰ **V20.4** Motorcycle driver injured in collision with pedestrian or animal in traffic accident

- √x7ᵗʰ **V20.41** Electric (assisted) bicycle driver injured in collision with pedestrian or animal in traffic accident
- √x7ᵗʰ **V20.49** Other motorcycle driver injured in collision with pedestrian or animal in traffic accident

√5ᵗʰ **V20.5** Motorcycle passenger injured in collision with pedestrian or animal in traffic accident

- √x7ᵗʰ **V20.51** Electric (assisted) bicycle passenger injured in collision with pedestrian or animal in traffic accident
- √x7ᵗʰ **V20.59** Other motorcycle passenger injured in collision with pedestrian or animal in traffic accident

√5ᵗʰ **V20.9** Unspecified motorcycle rider injured in collision with pedestrian or animal in traffic accident

- √x7ᵗʰ **V20.91** Unspecified electric (assisted) bicycle rider injured in collision with pedestrian or animal in traffic accident
- √x7ᵗʰ **V20.99** Unspecified rider of other motorcycle injured in collision with pedestrian or animal in traffic accident

√4ᵗʰ **V21** Motorcycle rider injured in collision with pedal cycle

√5ᵗʰ **V21.0** Motorcycle driver injured in collision with pedal cycle in nontraffic accident

- √x7ᵗʰ **V21.01** Electric (assisted) bicycle driver injured in collision with pedal cycle in nontraffic accident
- √x7ᵗʰ **V21.09** Other motorcycle driver injured in collision with pedal cycle in nontraffic accident

√5ᵗʰ **V21.1** Motorcycle passenger injured in collision with pedal cycle in nontraffic accident

- √x7ᵗʰ **V21.11** Electric (assisted) bicycle passenger injured in collision with pedal cycle in nontraffic accident
- √x7ᵗʰ **V21.19** Other motorcycle passenger injured in collision with pedal cycle in nontraffic accident

√5ᵗʰ **V21.2** Unspecified motorcycle rider injured in collision with pedal cycle in nontraffic accident

- √x7ᵗʰ **V21.21** Unspecified electric (assisted) bicycle rider injured in collision with pedal cycle in nontraffic accident
- √x7ᵗʰ **V21.29** Unspecified rider of other motorcycle injured in collision with pedal cycle in nontraffic accident

√5ᵗʰ **V21.3** Person boarding or alighting a motorcycle injured in collision with pedal cycle

- √x7ᵗʰ **V21.31** Person boarding or alighting an electric (assisted) bicycle injured in collision with pedal cycle
- √x7ᵗʰ **V21.39** Person boarding or alighting other motorcycle injured in collision with pedal cycle

√5ᵗʰ **V21.4** Motorcycle driver injured in collision with pedal cycle in traffic accident

- √x7ᵗʰ **V21.41** Electric (assisted) bicycle driver injured in collision with pedal cycle in traffic accident
- √x7ᵗʰ **V21.49** Other motorcycle driver injured in collision with pedal cycle in traffic accident

√5ᵗʰ **V21.5** Motorcycle passenger injured in collision with pedal cycle in traffic accident

- √x7ᵗʰ **V21.51** Electric (assisted) bicycle passenger injured in collision with pedal cycle in traffic accident
- √x7ᵗʰ **V21.59** Other motorcycle passenger injured in collision with pedal cycle in traffic accident

√5ᵗʰ **V21.9** Unspecified motorcycle rider injured in collision with pedal cycle in traffic accident

- √x7ᵗʰ **V21.91** Unspecified electric (assisted) bicycle rider injured in collision with pedal cycle in traffic accident
- √x7ᵗʰ **V21.99** Unspecified rider of other motorcycle injured in collision with pedal cycle in traffic accident

√4ᵗʰ **V22** Motorcycle rider injured in collision with two- or three-wheeled motor vehicle

√5ᵗʰ **V22.0** Motorcycle driver injured in collision with two- or three-wheeled motor vehicle in nontraffic accident

- √x7ᵗʰ **V22.01** Electric (assisted) bicycle driver injured in collision with two- or three-wheeled motor vehicle in nontraffic accident
- √x7ᵗʰ **V22.09** Other motorcycle driver injured in collision with two- or three-wheeled motor vehicle in nontraffic accident

√5ᵗʰ **V22.1** Motorcycle passenger injured in collision with two- or three-wheeled motor vehicle in nontraffic accident

- √x7ᵗʰ **V22.11** Electric (assisted) bicycle passenger injured in collision with two- or three-wheeled motor vehicle in nontraffic accident
- √x7ᵗʰ **V22.19** Other motorcycle passenger injured in collision with two- or three-wheeled motor vehicle in nontraffic accident

√5ᵗʰ **V22.2** Unspecified motorcycle rider injured in collision with two- or three-wheeled motor vehicle in nontraffic accident

- √x7ᵗʰ **V22.21** Unspecified electric (assisted) bicycle rider injured in collision with two- or three-wheeled motor vehicle in nontraffic accident
- √x7ᵗʰ **V22.29** Unspecified rider of other motorcycle injured in collision with two- or three-wheeled motor vehicle in nontraffic accident

√5ᵗʰ **V22.3** Person boarding or alighting a motorcycle injured in collision with two- or three-wheeled motor vehicle

- √x7ᵗʰ **V22.31** Person boarding or alighting an electric (assisted) bicycle injured in collision with two- or three-wheeled motor vehicle
- √x7ᵗʰ **V22.39** Person boarding or alighting other motorcycle injured in collision with two- or three-wheeled motor vehicle

√5ᵗʰ **V22.4** Motorcycle driver injured in collision with two- or three-wheeled motor vehicle in traffic accident

- √x7ᵗʰ **V22.41** Electric (assisted) bicycle driver injured in collision with two- or three-wheeled motor vehicle in traffic accident
- √x7ᵗʰ **V22.49** Other motorcycle driver injured in collision with two- or three-wheeled motor vehicle in traffic accident

√5ᵗʰ **V22.5** Motorcycle passenger injured in collision with two- or three-wheeled motor vehicle in traffic accident

- √x7ᵗʰ **V22.51** Electric (assisted) bicycle passenger injured in collision with two- or three-wheeled motor vehicle in traffic accident
- √x7ᵗʰ **V22.59** Other motorcycle passenger injured in collision with two- or three-wheeled motor vehicle in traffic accident

√5ᵗʰ **V22.9** Unspecified motorcycle rider injured in collision with two- or three-wheeled motor vehicle in traffic accident

- √x7ᵗʰ **V22.91** Unspecified electric (assisted) bicycle rider injured in collision with two- or three-wheeled motor vehicle in traffic accident
- √x7ᵗʰ **V22.99** Unspecified rider of other motorcycle injured in collision with two- or three-wheeled motor vehicle in traffic accident

√4ᵗʰ **V23** Motorcycle rider injured in collision with car, pick-up truck or van

√5ᵗʰ **V23.0** Motorcycle driver injured in collision with car, pick-up truck or van in nontraffic accident

- √x7ᵗʰ **V23.01** Electric (assisted) bicycle driver injured in collision with car, pick-up truck or van in nontraffic accident
- √x7ᵗʰ **V23.09** Other motorcycle driver injured in collision with car, pick-up truck or van in nontraffic accident

√5ᵗʰ **V23.1** Motorcycle passenger injured in collision with car, pick-up truck or van in nontraffic accident

- √x7ᵗʰ **V23.11** Electric (assisted) bicycle passenger injured in collision with car, pick-up truck or van in nontraffic accident
- √x7ᵗʰ **V23.19** Other motorcycle passenger injured in collision with car, pick-up truck or van in nontraffic accident

√5ᵗʰ **V23.2** **Unspecified motorcycle rider injured in collision with car, pick-up truck or van** in nontraffic accident

●   √x7ᵗʰ **V23.21** **Unspecified electric (assisted) bicycle rider injured in collision with car, pick-up truck or van in nontraffic accident**

●   √x7ᵗʰ **V23.29** **Unspecified rider of other motorcycle injured in collision with car, pick-up truck or van in nontraffic accident**

√5ᵗʰ **V23.3** **Person boarding or alighting a motorcycle injured in collision with car, pick-up truck or van**

●   √x7ᵗʰ **V23.31** **Person boarding or alighting an electric (assisted) bicycle injured in collision with car, pick-up truck or van**

●   √x7ᵗʰ **V23.39** **Person boarding or alighting other motorcycle injured in collision with car, pick-up truck or van**

√5ᵗʰ **V23.4** **Motorcycle driver injured in collision with car, pick-up truck or van in traffic accident**

●   √x7ᵗʰ **V23.41** **Electric (assisted) bicycle driver injured in collision with car, pick-up truck or van in traffic accident**

●   √x7ᵗʰ **V23.49** **Other motorcycle driver injured in collision with car, pick-up truck or van in traffic accident**

√5ᵗʰ **V23.5** **Motorcycle passenger injured in collision with car, pick-up truck or van in traffic accident**

●   √x7ᵗʰ **V23.51** **Electric (assisted) bicycle passenger injured in collision with car, pick-up truck or van in traffic accident**

●   √x7ᵗʰ **V23.59** **Other motorcycle passenger injured in collision with car, pick-up truck or van in traffic accident**

√5ᵗʰ **V23.9** **Unspecified motorcycle rider injured in collision with car, pick-up truck or van in traffic accident**

●   √x7ᵗʰ **V23.91** **Unspecified electric (assisted) bicycle rider injured in collision with car, pick-up truck or van in traffic accident**

●   √x7ᵗʰ **V23.99** **Unspecified rider of other motorcycle injured in collision with car, pick-up truck or van in traffic accident**

√4ᵗʰ **V24** **Motorcycle rider injured in collision with heavy transport vehicle or bus**

> EXCLUDES 1   motorcycle rider injured in collision with military vehicle ►(V29.818)◄

√5ᵗʰ **V24.0** **Motorcycle driver injured in collision with heavy transport vehicle or bus in nontraffic accident**

●   √x7ᵗʰ **V24.01** **Electric (assisted) bicycle driver injured in collision with heavy transport vehicle or bus in nontraffic accident**

●   √x7ᵗʰ **V24.09** **Other motorcycle driver injured in collision with heavy transport vehicle or bus in nontraffic accident**

√5ᵗʰ **V24.1** **Motorcycle passenger injured in collision with heavy transport vehicle or bus in nontraffic accident**

●   √x7ᵗʰ **V24.11** **Electric (assisted) bicycle passenger injured in collision with heavy transport vehicle or bus in nontraffic accident**

●   √x7ᵗʰ **V24.19** **Other motorcycle passenger injured in collision with heavy transport vehicle or bus in nontraffic accident**

√5ᵗʰ **V24.2** **Unspecified motorcycle rider injured in collision with heavy transport vehicle or bus in nontraffic accident**

●   √x7ᵗʰ **V24.21** **Unspecified electric (assisted) bicycle rider injured in collision with heavy transport vehicle or bus in nontraffic accident**

●   √x7ᵗʰ **V24.29** **Unspecified rider of other motorcycle injured in collision with heavy transport vehicle or bus in nontraffic accident**

√5ᵗʰ **V24.3** **Person boarding or alighting a motorcycle injured in collision with heavy transport vehicle or bus**

●   √x7ᵗʰ **V24.31** **Person boarding or alighting an electric (assisted) bicycle injured in collision with heavy transport vehicle or bus**

●   √x7ᵗʰ **V24.39** **Person boarding or alighting other motorcycle injured in collision with heavy transport vehicle or bus**

√5ᵗʰ **V24.4** **Motorcycle driver injured in collision with heavy transport vehicle or bus in traffic accident**

●   √x7ᵗʰ **V24.41** **Electric (assisted) bicycle driver injured in collision with heavy transport vehicle or bus in traffic accident**

●   √x7ᵗʰ **V24.49** **Other motorcycle driver injured in collision with heavy transport vehicle or bus in traffic accident**

√5ᵗʰ **V24.5** **Motorcycle passenger injured in collision with heavy transport vehicle or bus in traffic accident**

●   √x7ᵗʰ **V24.51** **Electric (assisted) bicycle passenger injured in collision with heavy transport vehicle or bus in traffic accident**

●   √x7ᵗʰ **V24.59** **Other motorcycle passenger injured in collision with heavy transport vehicle or bus in traffic accident**

√5ᵗʰ **V24.9** **Unspecified motorcycle rider injured in collision with heavy transport vehicle or bus in traffic accident**

●   √x7ᵗʰ **V24.91** **Unspecified electric (assisted) bicycle rider injured in collision with heavy transport vehicle or bus in traffic accident**

●   √x7ᵗʰ **V24.99** **Unspecified rider of other motorcycle injured in collision with heavy transport vehicle or bus in traffic accident**

√4ᵗʰ **V25** **Motorcycle rider injured in collision with railway train or railway vehicle**

√5ᵗʰ **V25.0** **Motorcycle driver injured in collision with railway train or railway vehicle in nontraffic accident**

●   √x7ᵗʰ **V25.01** **Electric (assisted) bicycle driver injured in collision with railway train or railway vehicle in nontraffic accident**

●   √x7ᵗʰ **V25.09** **Other motorcycle driver injured in collision with railway train or railway vehicle in nontraffic accident**

√5ᵗʰ **V25.1** **Motorcycle passenger injured in collision with railway train or railway vehicle in nontraffic accident**

●   √x7ᵗʰ **V25.11** **Electric (assisted) bicycle passenger injured in collision with railway train or railway vehicle in nontraffic accident**

●   √x7ᵗʰ **V25.19** **Other motorcycle passenger injured in collision with railway train or railway vehicle in nontraffic accident**

√5ᵗʰ **V25.2** **Unspecified motorcycle rider injured in collision with railway train or railway vehicle in nontraffic accident**

●   √x7ᵗʰ **V25.21** **Unspecified electric (assisted) bicycle rider injured in collision with railway train or railway vehicle in nontraffic accident**

●   √x7ᵗʰ **V25.29** **Unspecified rider of other motorcycle injured in collision with railway train or railway vehicle in nontraffic accident**

√5ᵗʰ **V25.3** **Person boarding or alighting a motorcycle injured in collision with railway train or railway vehicle**

●   √x7ᵗʰ **V25.31** **Person boarding or alighting an electric (assisted) bicycle injured in collision with railway train or railway vehicle**

●   √x7ᵗʰ **V25.39** **Person boarding or alighting other motorcycle injured in collision with railway train or railway vehicle**

√5ᵗʰ **V25.4** **Motorcycle driver injured in collision with railway train or railway vehicle in traffic accident**

●   √x7ᵗʰ **V25.41** **Electric (assisted) bicycle driver injured in collision with railway train or railway vehicle in traffic accident**

●   √x7ᵗʰ **V25.49** **Other motorcycle driver injured in collision with railway train or railway vehicle in traffic accident**

√5ᵗʰ **V25.5** **Motorcycle passenger injured in collision with railway train or railway vehicle in traffic accident**

●   √x7ᵗʰ **V25.51** **Electric (assisted) bicycle passenger injured in collision with railway train or railway vehicle in traffic accident**

●   √x7ᵗʰ **V25.59** **Other motorcycle passenger injured in collision with railway train or railway vehicle in traffic accident**

√5ᵗʰ **V25.9** **Unspecified motorcycle rider injured in collision with railway train or railway vehicle in traffic accident**

●   √x7ᵗʰ **V25.91** **Unspecified electric (assisted) bicycle rider injured in collision with railway train or railway vehicle in traffic accident**

●   √x7ᵗʰ **V25.99** **Unspecified rider of other motorcycle injured in collision with railway train or railway vehicle in traffic accident**

√4ᵗʰ **V26** **Motorcycle rider injured in collision with other nonmotor vehicle**

> INCLUDES   collision with animal-drawn vehicle, animal being ridden, streetcar

√5ᵗʰ **V26.0** **Motorcycle driver injured in collision with other nonmotor vehicle in nontraffic accident**

●   √x7ᵗʰ **V26.01** **Electric (assisted) bicycle driver injured in collision with other nonmotor vehicle in nontraffic accident**

●   √x7ᵗʰ **V26.09** **Other motorcycle driver injured in collision with other nonmotor vehicle in nontraffic accident**

√5ᵗʰ **V26.1** **Motorcycle passenger injured in collision with other nonmotor vehicle in nontraffic accident**

●   √x7ᵗʰ **V26.11** **Electric (assisted) bicycle passenger injured in collision with other nonmotor vehicle in nontraffic accident**

| ✔ Additional Character Required | √x7ᵗʰ Placeholder Alert | Manifestation | Unspecified Dx | Q QPP | UPD Unacceptable PDx |

ICD-10-CM 2023   1205

✓x7th **V26.19** Other motorcycle passenger injured in collision with other nonmotor vehicle in nontraffic accident

✓5th **V26.2** Unspecified motorcycle rider injured in collision with other nonmotor vehicle in nontraffic accident

• ✓x7th **V26.21** Unspecified electric (assisted) bicycle rider injured in collision with other nonmotor vehicle in nontraffic accident

• ✓x7th **V26.29** Unspecified rider of other motorcycle injured in collision with other nonmotor vehicle in nontraffic accident

✓5th **V26.3** Person boarding or alighting a motorcycle injured in collision with other nonmotor vehicle

• ✓x7th **V26.31** Person boarding or alighting an electric (assisted) bicycle injured in collision with other nonmotor vehicle

✓x7th **V26.39** Person boarding or alighting other motorcycle injured in collision with other nonmotor vehicle

✓5th **V26.4** Motorcycle driver injured in collision with other nonmotor vehicle in traffic accident

• ✓x7th **V26.41** Electric (assisted) bicycle driver injured in collision with other nonmotor vehicle in traffic accident

✓x7th **V26.49** Other motorcycle driver injured in collision with other nonmotor vehicle in traffic accident

✓5th **V26.5** Motorcycle passenger injured in collision with other nonmotor vehicle in traffic accident

• ✓x7th **V26.51** Electric (assisted) bicycle passenger injured in collision with other nonmotor vehicle in traffic accident

• ✓x7th **V26.59** Other motorcycle passenger injured in collision with other nonmotor vehicle in traffic accident

✓5th **V26.9** Unspecified motorcycle rider injured in collision with other nonmotor vehicle in traffic accident

• ✓x7th **V26.91** Unspecified electric (assisted) bicycle rider injured in collision with other nonmotor vehicle in traffic accident

• ✓x7th **V26.99** Unspecified rider of other motorcycle injured in collision with other nonmotor vehicle in traffic accident

✓4th **V27** Motorcycle rider injured in collision with fixed or stationary object

✓5th **V27.0** Motorcycle driver injured in collision with fixed or stationary object in nontraffic accident

• ✓x7th **V27.01** Electric (assisted) bicycle driver injured in collision with fixed or stationary object in nontraffic accident

• ✓x7th **V27.09** Other motorcycle driver injured in collision with fixed or stationary object in nontraffic accident

✓5th **V27.1** Motorcycle passenger injured in collision with fixed or stationary object in nontraffic accident

• ✓x7th **V27.11** Electric (assisted) bicycle passenger injured in collision with fixed or stationary object in nontraffic accident

✓x7th **V27.19** Other motorcycle passenger injured in collision with fixed or stationary object in nontraffic accident

✓5th **V27.2** Unspecified motorcycle rider injured in collision with fixed or stationary object in nontraffic accident

• ✓x7th **V27.21** Unspecified electric (assisted) bicycle rider injured in collision with fixed or stationary object in nontraffic accident

• ✓x7th **V27.29** Unspecified rider of other motorcycle injured in collision with fixed or stationary object in nontraffic accident

✓5th **V27.3** Person boarding or alighting a motorcycle injured in collision with fixed or stationary object

• ✓x7th **V27.31** Person boarding or alighting an electric (assisted) bicycle injured in collision with fixed or stationary object

✓x7th **V27.39** Person boarding or alighting other motorcycle injured in collision with fixed or stationary object

✓5th **V27.4** Motorcycle driver injured in collision with fixed or stationary object in traffic accident

• ✓x7th **V27.41** Electric (assisted) bicycle driver injured in collision with fixed or stationary object in traffic accident

✓x7th **V27.49** Other motorcycle driver injured in collision with fixed or stationary object in traffic accident

✓5th **V27.5** Motorcycle passenger injured in collision with fixed or stationary object in traffic accident

• ✓x7th **V27.51** Electric (assisted) bicycle passenger injured in collision with fixed or stationary object in traffic accident

✓x7th **V27.59** Other motorcycle passenger injured in collision with fixed or stationary object in traffic accident

✓5th **V27.9** Unspecified motorcycle rider injured in collision with fixed or stationary object in traffic accident

• ✓x7th **V27.91** Unspecified electric (assisted) bicycle rider injured in collision with fixed or stationary object in traffic accident

• ✓x7th **V27.99** Unspecified rider of other motorcycle injured in collision with fixed or stationary object in traffic accident

✓4th **V28** Motorcycle rider injured in noncollision transport accident

INCLUDES fall or thrown from motorcycle (without antecedent collision)
overturning motorcycle NOS
overturning motorcycle without collision

✓5th **V28.0** Motorcycle driver injured in noncollision transport accident in nontraffic accident

• ✓x7th **V28.01** Electric (assisted) bicycle driver injured in noncollision transport accident in nontraffic accident

✓x7th **V28.09** Other motorcycle driver injured in noncollision transport accident in nontraffic accident

✓5th **V28.1** Motorcycle passenger injured in noncollision transport accident in nontraffic accident

• ✓x7th **V28.11** Electric (assisted) bicycle passenger injured in noncollision transport accident in nontraffic accident

✓x7th **V28.19** Other motorcycle passenger injured in noncollision transport accident in nontraffic accident

✓5th **V28.2** Unspecified motorcycle rider injured in noncollision transport accident in nontraffic accident

• ✓x7th **V28.21** Unspecified electric (assisted) bicycle rider injured in noncollision transport accident in nontraffic accident

• ✓x7th **V28.29** Unspecified rider of other motorcycle injured in noncollision transport accident in nontraffic accident

✓5th **V28.3** Person boarding or alighting a motorcycle injured in noncollision transport accident

• ✓x7th **V28.31** Person boarding or alighting an electric (assisted) bicycle injured in noncollision transport accident

✓x7th **V28.39** Person boarding or alighting other motorcycle injured in noncollision transport accident

✓5th **V28.4** Motorcycle driver injured in noncollision transport accident in traffic accident

• ✓x7th **V28.41** Electric (assisted) bicycle driver injured in noncollision transport accident in traffic accident

✓x7th **V28.49** Other motorcycle driver injured in noncollision transport accident in traffic accident

✓5th **V28.5** Motorcycle passenger injured in noncollision transport accident in traffic accident

• ✓x7th **V28.51** Electric (assisted) bicycle passenger injured in noncollision transport accident in traffic accident

✓x7th **V28.59** Other motorcycle passenger injured in noncollision transport accident in traffic accident

✓5th **V28.9** Unspecified motorcycle rider injured in noncollision transport accident in traffic accident

• ✓x7th **V28.91** Unspecified electric (assisted) bicycle rider injured in noncollision transport accident in traffic accident

• ✓x7th **V28.99** Unspecified rider of other motorcycle injured in noncollision transport accident in traffic accident

✓4th **V29** Motorcycle rider injured in other and unspecified transport accidents

✓5th **V29.0** Motorcycle driver injured in collision with other and unspecified motor vehicles in nontraffic accident

✓6th **V29.00** Motorcycle driver injured in collision with unspecified motor vehicles in nontraffic accident

• ✓7th **V29.001** Electric (assisted) bicycle driver injured in collision with unspecified motor vehicles in nontraffic accident

• ✓7th **V29.008** Other motorcycle driver injured in collision with unspecified motor vehicles in nontraffic accident

✓6th **V29.09** Motorcycle driver injured in collision with other motor vehicles in nontraffic accident

✓7th **V29.091** Electric (assisted) bicycle driver injured in collision with other motor vehicles in nontraffic accident

✓7th **V29.098** Other motorcycle driver injured in collision with other motor vehicles in nontraffic accident

✓5ᵗʰ **V29.1** Motorcycle passenger injured in collision with other and unspecified motor vehicles in nontraffic accident

  ✓6ᵗʰ **V29.10** Motorcycle passenger injured in collision with unspecified motor vehicles in nontraffic accident

●   ✓7ᵗʰ **V29.101** Electric (assisted) bicycle passenger injured in collision with unspecified motor vehicles in nontraffic accident

●   ✓7ᵗʰ **V29.108** Other motorcycle passenger injured in collision with unspecified motor vehicles in nontraffic accident

  ✓6ᵗʰ **V29.19** Motorcycle passenger injured in collision with other motor vehicles in nontraffic accident

●   ✓7ᵗʰ **V29.191** Electric (assisted) bicycle passenger injured in collision with other motor vehicles in nontraffic accident

●   ✓7ᵗʰ **V29.198** Other motorcycle passenger injured in collision with other motor vehicles in nontraffic accident

✓5ᵗʰ **V29.2** Unspecified motorcycle rider injured in collision with other and unspecified motor vehicles in nontraffic accident

  ✓6ᵗʰ **V29.20** Unspecified motorcycle rider injured in collision with unspecified motor vehicles in nontraffic accident
    Motorcycle collision NOS, nontraffic

●   ✓7ᵗʰ **V29.201** Unspecified electric (assisted) bicycle rider injured in collision with unspecified motor vehicles in nontraffic accident

●   ✓7ᵗʰ **V29.208** Unspecified rider of other motorcycle injured in collision with unspecified motor vehicles in nontraffic accident
      Motorcycle collision NOS, nontraffic

  ✓6ᵗʰ **V29.29** Unspecified motorcycle rider injured in collision with other motor vehicles in nontraffic accident

●   ✓7ᵗʰ **V29.291** Unspecified electric (assisted) bicycle rider injured in collision with other motor vehicles in nontraffic accident

●   ✓7ᵗʰ **V29.298** Unspecified rider of other motorcycle injured in collision with other motor vehicles in nontraffic accident

✓5ᵗʰ **V29.3** Motorcycle rider (driver) (passenger) injured in unspecified nontraffic accident
  Motorcycle accident NOS, nontraffic
  Motorcycle rider injured in nontraffic accident NOS

●   ✓x7ᵗʰ **V29.31** Electric (assisted) bicycle (driver) (passenger) injured in unspecified nontraffic accident

●   ✓x7ᵗʰ **V29.39** Other motorcycle (driver) (passenger) injured in unspecified nontraffic accident
    Motorcycle accident NOS, nontraffic
    Motorcycle rider injured in nontraffic accident NOS

✓5ᵗʰ **V29.4** Motorcycle driver injured in collision with other and unspecified motor vehicles in traffic accident

  ✓6ᵗʰ **V29.40** Motorcycle driver injured in collision with unspecified motor vehicles in traffic accident

●   ✓7ᵗʰ **V29.401** Electric (assisted) bicycle driver injured in collision with unspecified motor vehicles in traffic accident

●   ✓7ᵗʰ **V29.408** Other motorcycle driver injured in collision with unspecified motor vehicles in traffic accident

  ✓6ᵗʰ **V29.49** Motorcycle driver injured in collision with other motor vehicles in traffic accident

●   ✓7ᵗʰ **V29.491** Electric (assisted) bicycle driver injured in collision with other motor vehicles in traffic accident

●   ✓7ᵗʰ **V29.498** Other motorcycle driver injured in collision with other motor vehicles in traffic accident

✓5ᵗʰ **V29.5** Motorcycle passenger injured in collision with other and unspecified motor vehicles in traffic accident

  ✓6ᵗʰ **V29.50** Motorcycle passenger injured in collision with unspecified motor vehicles in traffic accident

●   ✓7ᵗʰ **V29.501** Electric (assisted) bicycle passenger injured in collision with unspecified motor vehicles in traffic accident

●   ✓7ᵗʰ **V29.508** Other motorcycle passenger injured in collision with unspecified motor vehicles in traffic accident

  ✓6ᵗʰ **V29.59** Motorcycle passenger injured in collision with other motor vehicles in traffic accident

●   ✓7ᵗʰ **V29.591** Electric (assisted) bicycle passenger injured in collision with other motor vehicles in traffic accident

●   ✓7ᵗʰ **V29.598** Other motorcycle passenger injured in collision with other motor vehicles in traffic accident

✓5ᵗʰ **V29.6** Unspecified motorcycle rider injured in collision with other and unspecified motor vehicles in traffic accident

  ✓6ᵗʰ **V29.60** Unspecified motorcycle rider injured in collision with unspecified motor vehicles in traffic accident
    Motorcycle collision NOS (traffic)

●   ✓7ᵗʰ **V29.601** Unspecified electric (assisted) bicycle rider injured in collision with unspecified motor vehicles in traffic accident

●   ✓7ᵗʰ **V29.608** Unspecified rider of other motorcycle injured in collision with unspecified motor vehicles in traffic accident
      Motorcycle collision NOS (traffic)

  ✓6ᵗʰ **V29.69** Unspecified motorcycle rider injured in collision with other motor vehicles in traffic accident

●   ✓7ᵗʰ **V29.691** Unspecified electric (assisted) bicycle rider injured in collision with other motor vehicles in traffic accident

●   ✓7ᵗʰ **V29.698** Unspecified rider of other motorcycle injured in collision with other motor vehicles in traffic accident

✓5ᵗʰ **V29.8** Motorcycle rider (driver) (passenger) injured in other specified transport accidents

  ✓6ᵗʰ **V29.81** Motorcycle rider (driver) (passenger) injured in transport accident military vehicle

●   ✓7ᵗʰ **V29.811** Electric (assisted) bicycle rider (driver) (passenger) injured in transport accident with military vehicle

●   ✓7ᵗʰ **V29.818** Rider (driver) (passenger) of other motorcycle injured in transport accident with military vehicle

  ✓6ᵗʰ **V29.88** Motorcycle rider (driver) (passenger) injured in other specified transport accidents

●   ✓7ᵗʰ **V29.881** Electric (assisted) bicycle rider (driver) (passenger) injured in other specified transport accidents

●   ✓7ᵗʰ **V29.888** Rider (driver) (passenger) of other motorcycle injured in other specified transport accidents

✓5ᵗʰ **V29.9** Motorcycle rider (driver) (passenger) injured in unspecified traffic accident
  Motorcycle accident NOS

●   ✓x7ᵗʰ **V29.91** Electric (assisted) bicycle rider (driver) (passenger) injured in unspecified traffic accident

●   ✓x7ᵗʰ **V29.99** Rider (driver) (passenger) of other motorcycle injured in unspecified traffic accident
    Motorcycle accident NOS

Occupant of three-wheeled motor vehicle injured in transport accident (V30-V39)

INCLUDES   motorized tricycle
              motorized rickshaw
              three-wheeled motor car

EXCLUDES 1   all-terrain vehicles (V86.-)
              motorcycle with sidecar (V20-V29)
              vehicle designed primarily for off-road use (V86.-)

The appropriate 7th character is to be added to each code from categories V30-V39.
A   initial encounter
D   subsequent encounter
S   sequela

✓4ᵗʰ **V30** Occupant of three-wheeled motor vehicle injured in collision with pedestrian or animal
  EXCLUDES 1   three-wheeled motor vehicle collision with animal-drawn vehicle or animal being ridden (V36.-)

  ✓x7ᵗʰ **V30.0** Driver of three-wheeled motor vehicle injured in collision with pedestrian or animal in nontraffic accident

  ✓x7ᵗʰ **V30.1** Passenger in three-wheeled motor vehicle injured in collision with pedestrian or animal in nontraffic accident

  ✓x7ᵗʰ **V30.2** Person on outside of three-wheeled motor vehicle injured in collision with pedestrian or animal in nontraffic accident

  ✓x7ᵗʰ **V30.3** Unspecified occupant of three-wheeled motor vehicle injured in collision with pedestrian or animal in nontraffic accident

  ✓x7ᵗʰ **V30.4** Person boarding or alighting a three-wheeled motor vehicle injured in collision with pedestrian or animal

  ✓x7ᵗʰ **V30.5** Driver of three-wheeled motor vehicle injured in collision with pedestrian or animal in traffic accident

  ✓x7ᵗʰ **V30.6** Passenger in three-wheeled motor vehicle injured in collision with pedestrian or animal in traffic accident

---

☑ Additional Character Required   ✓x7ᵗʰ Placeholder Alert   Manifestation   Unspecified Dx   Q QPP   UPD Unacceptable PDx

Chapter 20. External Causes of Morbidity

V30.7 ✓x7ᵗʰ **Person on outside** of three-wheeled motor vehicle injured in collision with pedestrian or animal in traffic accident

V30.9 ✓x7ᵗʰ Unspecified occupant of three-wheeled motor vehicle injured in collision with pedestrian or animal in traffic accident

✓4ᵗʰ **V31 Occupant of three-wheeled motor vehicle injured in collision with pedal cycle**

V31.0 ✓x7ᵗʰ **Driver** of three-wheeled motor vehicle injured in collision with pedal cycle in nontraffic accident

V31.1 ✓x7ᵗʰ **Passenger** in three-wheeled motor vehicle injured in collision with pedal cycle in nontraffic accident

V31.2 ✓x7ᵗʰ **Person on outside** of three-wheeled motor vehicle injured in collision with pedal cycle in nontraffic accident

V31.3 ✓x7ᵗʰ Unspecified occupant of three-wheeled motor vehicle injured in collision with pedal cycle in nontraffic accident

V31.4 ✓x7ᵗʰ **Person boarding or alighting** a three-wheeled motor vehicle injured in collision with pedal cycle

V31.5 ✓x7ᵗʰ **Driver** of three-wheeled motor vehicle injured in collision with pedal cycle in traffic accident

V31.6 ✓x7ᵗʰ **Passenger** in three-wheeled motor vehicle injured in collision with pedal cycle in traffic accident

V31.7 ✓x7ᵗʰ **Person on outside** of three-wheeled motor vehicle injured in collision with pedal cycle in traffic accident

V31.9 ✓x7ᵗʰ Unspecified occupant of three-wheeled motor vehicle injured in collision with pedal cycle in traffic accident

✓4ᵗʰ **V32 Occupant of three-wheeled motor vehicle injured in collision with two- or three-wheeled motor vehicle**

V32.0 ✓x7ᵗʰ **Driver** of three-wheeled motor vehicle injured in collision with two- or three-wheeled motor vehicle in nontraffic accident

V32.1 ✓x7ᵗʰ **Passenger** in three-wheeled motor vehicle injured in collision with two- or three-wheeled motor vehicle in nontraffic accident

V32.2 ✓x7ᵗʰ **Person on outside** of three-wheeled motor vehicle injured in collision with two- or three-wheeled motor vehicle in nontraffic accident

V32.3 ✓x7ᵗʰ Unspecified occupant of three-wheeled motor vehicle injured in collision with two- or three-wheeled motor vehicle in nontraffic accident

V32.4 ✓x7ᵗʰ **Person boarding or alighting** a three-wheeled motor vehicle injured in collision with two- or three-wheeled motor vehicle

V32.5 ✓x7ᵗʰ **Driver** of three-wheeled motor vehicle injured in collision with two- or three-wheeled motor vehicle in traffic accident

V32.6 ✓x7ᵗʰ **Passenger** in three-wheeled motor vehicle injured in collision with two- or three-wheeled motor vehicle in traffic accident

V32.7 ✓x7ᵗʰ **Person on outside** of three-wheeled motor vehicle injured in collision with two- or three-wheeled motor vehicle in traffic accident

V32.9 ✓x7ᵗʰ Unspecified occupant of three-wheeled motor vehicle injured in collision with two- or three-wheeled motor vehicle in traffic accident

✓4ᵗʰ **V33 Occupant of three-wheeled motor vehicle injured in collision with car, pick-up truck or van**

V33.0 ✓x7ᵗʰ **Driver** of three-wheeled motor vehicle injured in collision with car, pick-up truck or van in nontraffic accident

V33.1 ✓x7ᵗʰ **Passenger** in three-wheeled motor vehicle injured in collision with car, pick-up truck or van in nontraffic accident

V33.2 ✓x7ᵗʰ **Person on outside** of three-wheeled motor vehicle injured in collision with car, pick-up truck or van in nontraffic accident

V33.3 ✓x7ᵗʰ Unspecified occupant of three-wheeled motor vehicle injured in collision with car, pick-up truck or van in nontraffic accident

V33.4 ✓x7ᵗʰ **Person boarding or alighting** a three-wheeled motor vehicle injured in collision with car, pick-up truck or van

V33.5 ✓x7ᵗʰ **Driver** of three-wheeled motor vehicle injured in collision with car, pick-up truck or van in traffic accident

V33.6 ✓x7ᵗʰ **Passenger** in three-wheeled motor vehicle injured in collision with car, pick-up truck or van in traffic accident

V33.7 ✓x7ᵗʰ **Person on outside** of three-wheeled motor vehicle injured in collision with car, pick-up truck or van in traffic accident

V33.9 ✓x7ᵗʰ Unspecified occupant of three-wheeled motor vehicle injured in collision with car, pick-up truck or van in traffic accident

✓4ᵗʰ **V34 Occupant of three-wheeled motor vehicle injured in collision with heavy transport vehicle or bus**

EXCLUDES 1 *occupant of three-wheeled motor vehicle injured in collision with military vehicle (V39.81)*

V34.0 ✓x7ᵗʰ **Driver** of three-wheeled motor vehicle injured in collision with heavy transport vehicle or bus in nontraffic accident

V34.1 ✓x7ᵗʰ **Passenger** in three-wheeled motor vehicle injured in collision with heavy transport vehicle or bus in nontraffic accident

V34.2 ✓x7ᵗʰ **Person on outside** of three-wheeled motor vehicle injured in collision with heavy transport vehicle or bus in nontraffic accident

V34.3 ✓x7ᵗʰ Unspecified occupant of three-wheeled motor vehicle injured in collision with heavy transport vehicle or bus in nontraffic accident

V34.4 ✓x7ᵗʰ **Person boarding or alighting** a three-wheeled motor vehicle injured in collision with heavy transport vehicle or bus

V34.5 ✓x7ᵗʰ **Driver** of three-wheeled motor vehicle injured in collision with heavy transport vehicle or bus in traffic accident

V34.6 ✓x7ᵗʰ **Passenger** in three-wheeled motor vehicle injured in collision with heavy transport vehicle or bus in traffic accident

V34.7 ✓x7ᵗʰ **Person on outside** of three-wheeled motor vehicle injured in collision with heavy transport vehicle or bus in traffic accident

V34.9 ✓x7ᵗʰ Unspecified occupant of three-wheeled motor vehicle injured in collision with heavy transport vehicle or bus in traffic accident

✓4ᵗʰ **V35 Occupant of three-wheeled motor vehicle injured in collision with railway train or railway vehicle**

V35.0 ✓x7ᵗʰ **Driver** of three-wheeled motor vehicle injured in collision with railway train or railway vehicle in nontraffic accident

V35.1 ✓x7ᵗʰ **Passenger** in three-wheeled motor vehicle injured in collision with railway train or railway vehicle in nontraffic accident

V35.2 ✓x7ᵗʰ **Person on outside** of three-wheeled motor vehicle injured in collision with railway train or railway vehicle in nontraffic accident

V35.3 ✓x7ᵗʰ Unspecified occupant of three-wheeled motor vehicle injured in collision with railway train or railway vehicle in nontraffic accident

V35.4 ✓x7ᵗʰ **Person boarding or alighting** a three-wheeled motor vehicle injured in collision with railway train or railway vehicle

V35.5 ✓x7ᵗʰ **Driver** of three-wheeled motor vehicle injured in collision with railway train or railway vehicle in traffic accident

V35.6 ✓x7ᵗʰ **Passenger** in three-wheeled motor vehicle injured in collision with railway train or railway vehicle in traffic accident

V35.7 ✓x7ᵗʰ **Person on outside** of three-wheeled motor vehicle injured in collision with railway train or railway vehicle in traffic accident

V35.9 ✓x7ᵗʰ Unspecified occupant of three-wheeled motor vehicle injured in collision with railway train or railway vehicle in traffic accident

✓4ᵗʰ **V36 Occupant of three-wheeled motor vehicle injured in collision with other nonmotor vehicle**

INCLUDES collision with animal-drawn vehicle, animal being ridden, streetcar

V36.0 ✓x7ᵗʰ **Driver** of three-wheeled motor vehicle injured in collision with other nonmotor vehicle in nontraffic accident

V36.1 ✓x7ᵗʰ **Passenger** in three-wheeled motor vehicle injured in collision with other nonmotor vehicle in nontraffic accident

V36.2 ✓x7ᵗʰ **Person on outside** of three-wheeled motor vehicle injured in collision with other nonmotor vehicle in nontraffic accident

V36.3 ✓x7ᵗʰ Unspecified occupant of three-wheeled motor vehicle injured in collision with other nonmotor vehicle in nontraffic accident

V36.4 ✓x7ᵗʰ **Person boarding or alighting** a three-wheeled motor vehicle injured in collision with other nonmotor vehicle

V36.5 ✓x7ᵗʰ **Driver** of three-wheeled motor vehicle injured in collision with other nonmotor vehicle in traffic accident

V36.6 ✓x7ᵗʰ **Passenger** in three-wheeled motor vehicle injured in collision with other nonmotor vehicle in traffic accident

V36.7 ✓x7ᵗʰ **Person on outside** of three-wheeled motor vehicle injured in collision with other nonmotor vehicle in traffic accident

V36.9 ✓x7ᵗʰ Unspecified occupant of three-wheeled motor vehicle injured in collision with other nonmotor vehicle in traffic accident

✓4ᵗʰ **V37 Occupant of three-wheeled motor vehicle injured in collision with fixed or stationary object**

V37.0 ✓x7ᵗʰ **Driver** of three-wheeled motor vehicle injured in collision with fixed or stationary object in nontraffic accident

V37.1 ✓x7ᵗʰ **Passenger** in three-wheeled motor vehicle injured in collision with fixed or stationary object in nontraffic accident

V37.2 ✓x7ᵗʰ **Person on outside** of three-wheeled motor vehicle injured in collision with fixed or stationary object in nontraffic accident

V37.3 ✓x7ᵗʰ Unspecified occupant of three-wheeled motor vehicle injured in collision with fixed or stationary object in nontraffic accident

V37.4 ✓x7ᵗʰ **Person boarding or alighting** a three-wheeled motor vehicle injured in collision with fixed or stationary object

V37.5 ✓x7ᵗʰ **Driver** of three-wheeled motor vehicle injured in collision with fixed or stationary object in traffic accident

HCC CMS-HCC   **Rx** Rx HCC   **ESR** ESRD HCC   **COM** Commercial HCC   **N** Newborn: 0   **P** Pediatric: 0-17   **M** Maternity: 9-64   **A** Adult: 15-124

1208   ICD-10-CM 2023

√7ᵗʰ **V37.6** Passenger in three-wheeled motor vehicle injured in collision with fixed or stationary object in traffic accident

√7ᵗʰ **V37.7** Person on outside of three-wheeled motor vehicle injured in collision with fixed or stationary object in traffic accident

√x7ᵗʰ **V37.9** Unspecified occupant of three-wheeled motor vehicle injured in collision with fixed or stationary object in traffic accident

√4ᵗʰ **V38** Occupant of three-wheeled motor vehicle injured in noncollision transport accident

> INCLUDES   fall or thrown from three-wheeled motor vehicle
> overturning of three-wheeled motor vehicle NOS
> overturning of three-wheeled motor vehicle without collision

√7ᵗʰ **V38.0** Driver of three-wheeled motor vehicle injured in noncollision transport accident in nontraffic accident

√7ᵗʰ **V38.1** Passenger in three-wheeled motor vehicle injured in noncollision transport accident in nontraffic accident

√7ᵗʰ **V38.2** Person on outside of three-wheeled motor vehicle injured in noncollision transport accident in nontraffic accident

√x7ᵗʰ **V38.3** Unspecified occupant of three-wheeled motor vehicle injured in noncollision transport accident in nontraffic accident

√7ᵗʰ **V38.4** Person boarding or alighting a three-wheeled motor vehicle injured in noncollision transport accident

√7ᵗʰ **V38.5** Driver of three-wheeled motor vehicle injured in noncollision transport accident in traffic accident

√7ᵗʰ **V38.6** Passenger in three-wheeled motor vehicle injured in noncollision transport accident in traffic accident

√7ᵗʰ **V38.7** Person on outside of three-wheeled motor vehicle injured in noncollision transport accident in traffic accident

√x7ᵗʰ **V38.9** Unspecified occupant of three-wheeled motor vehicle injured in noncollision transport accident in traffic accident

√4ᵗʰ **V39** Occupant of three-wheeled motor vehicle injured in other and unspecified transport accidents

√6ᵗʰ **V39.0** Driver of three-wheeled motor vehicle injured in collision with other and unspecified motor vehicles in nontraffic accident

    √x7ᵗʰ **V39.00** Driver of three-wheeled motor vehicle injured in collision with unspecified motor vehicles in nontraffic accident

    √x7ᵗʰ **V39.09** Driver of three-wheeled motor vehicle injured in collision with other motor vehicles in nontraffic accident

√5ᵗʰ **V39.1** Passenger in three-wheeled motor vehicle injured in collision with other and unspecified motor vehicles in nontraffic accident

    √x7ᵗʰ **V39.10** Passenger in three-wheeled motor vehicle injured in collision with unspecified motor vehicles in nontraffic accident

    √x7ᵗʰ **V39.19** Passenger in three-wheeled motor vehicle injured in collision with other motor vehicles in nontraffic accident

√5ᵗʰ **V39.2** Unspecified occupant of three-wheeled motor vehicle injured in collision with other and unspecified motor vehicles in nontraffic accident

    √x7ᵗʰ **V39.20** Unspecified occupant of three-wheeled motor vehicle injured in collision with unspecified motor vehicles in nontraffic accident
> Collision NOS involving three-wheeled motor vehicle, nontraffic

    √x7ᵗʰ **V39.29** Unspecified occupant of three-wheeled motor vehicle injured in collision with other motor vehicles in nontraffic accident

√x7ᵗʰ **V39.3** Occupant (driver) (passenger) of three-wheeled motor vehicle injured in unspecified nontraffic accident
> Accident NOS involving three-wheeled motor vehicle, nontraffic
> Occupant of three-wheeled motor vehicle injured in nontraffic accident NOS

√5ᵗʰ **V39.4** Driver of three-wheeled motor vehicle injured in collision with other and unspecified motor vehicles in traffic accident

    √x7ᵗʰ **V39.40** Driver of three-wheeled motor vehicle injured in collision with unspecified motor vehicles in traffic accident

    √x7ᵗʰ **V39.49** Driver of three-wheeled motor vehicle injured in collision with other motor vehicles in traffic accident

√5ᵗʰ **V39.5** Passenger in three-wheeled motor vehicle injured in collision with other and unspecified motor vehicles in traffic accident

    √x7ᵗʰ **V39.50** Passenger in three-wheeled motor vehicle injured in collision with unspecified motor vehicles in traffic accident

    √x7ᵗʰ **V39.59** Passenger in three-wheeled motor vehicle injured in collision with other motor vehicles in traffic accident

√5ᵗʰ **V39.6** Unspecified occupant of three-wheeled motor vehicle injured in collision with other and unspecified motor vehicles in traffic accident

    √x7ᵗʰ **V39.60** Unspecified occupant of three-wheeled motor vehicle injured in collision with unspecified motor vehicles in traffic accident
> Collision NOS involving three-wheeled motor vehicle (traffic)

    √x7ᵗʰ **V39.69** Unspecified occupant of three-wheeled motor vehicle injured in collision with other motor vehicles in traffic accident

√5ᵗʰ **V39.8** Occupant (driver) (passenger) of three-wheeled motor vehicle injured in other specified transport accidents

    √x7ᵗʰ **V39.81** Occupant (driver) (passenger) of three-wheeled motor vehicle injured in transport accident with military vehicle

    √x7ᵗʰ **V39.89** Occupant (driver) (passenger) of three-wheeled motor vehicle injured in other specified transport accidents

√x7ᵗʰ **V39.9** Occupant (driver) (passenger) of three-wheeled motor vehicle injured in unspecified traffic accident
> Accident NOS involving three-wheeled motor vehicle

Car occupant injured in transport accident (V40-V49)

> INCLUDES   a four-wheeled motor vehicle designed primarily for carrying passengers
> automobile (pulling a trailer or camper)

> EXCLUDES 1   bus (V50-V59)
> minibus (V50-V59)
> minivan (V50-V59)
> motorcoach (V70-V79)
> pick-up truck (V50-V59)
> sport utility vehicle (SUV) (V50-V59)

> The appropriate 7th character is to be added to each code from categories V40-V49.
> A   initial encounter
> D   subsequent encounter
> S   sequela

√4ᵗʰ **V40** Car occupant injured in collision with pedestrian or animal

> EXCLUDES 1   car collision with animal-drawn vehicle or animal being ridden (V46.-)

√x7ᵗʰ **V40.0** Car driver injured in collision with pedestrian or animal in nontraffic accident

√x7ᵗʰ **V40.1** Car passenger injured in collision with pedestrian or animal in nontraffic accident

√x7ᵗʰ **V40.2** Person on outside of car injured in collision with pedestrian or animal in nontraffic accident

√x7ᵗʰ **V40.3** Unspecified car occupant injured in collision with pedestrian or animal in nontraffic accident

√x7ᵗʰ **V40.4** Person boarding or alighting a car injured in collision with pedestrian or animal

√x7ᵗʰ **V40.5** Car driver injured in collision with pedestrian or animal in traffic accident

√x7ᵗʰ **V40.6** Car passenger injured in collision with pedestrian or animal in traffic accident

√x7ᵗʰ **V40.7** Person on outside of car injured in collision with pedestrian or animal in traffic accident

√x7ᵗʰ **V40.9** Unspecified car occupant injured in collision with pedestrian or animal in traffic accident

√4ᵗʰ **V41** Car occupant injured in collision with pedal cycle

√x7ᵗʰ **V41.0** Car driver injured in collision with pedal cycle in nontraffic accident

√x7ᵗʰ **V41.1** Car passenger injured in collision with pedal cycle in nontraffic accident

√x7ᵗʰ **V41.2** Person on outside of car injured in collision with pedal cycle in nontraffic accident

√x7ᵗʰ **V41.3** Unspecified car occupant injured in collision with pedal cycle in nontraffic accident

√x7ᵗʰ **V41.4** Person boarding or alighting a car injured in collision with pedal cycle

√x7ᵗʰ **V41.5** Car driver injured in collision with pedal cycle in traffic accident

√x7ᵗʰ **V41.6** Car passenger injured in collision with pedal cycle in traffic accident

√x7ᵗʰ **V41.7** Person on outside of car injured in collision with pedal cycle in traffic accident

√x7ᵗʰ **V41.9** Unspecified car occupant injured in collision with pedal cycle in traffic accident

√4th **V42** **Car occupant injured in collision with two- or three-wheeled motor vehicle**

√x7th **V42.0** Car driver injured in collision with two- or three-wheeled motor vehicle in nontraffic accident

√x7th **V42.1** Car passenger injured in collision with two- or three-wheeled motor vehicle in nontraffic accident

√x7th **V42.2** Person on outside of car injured in collision with two- or three-wheeled motor vehicle in nontraffic accident

√x7th **V42.3** Unspecified car occupant injured in collision with two- or three-wheeled motor vehicle in nontraffic accident

√x7th **V42.4** Person boarding or alighting a car injured in collision with two- or three-wheeled motor vehicle

√x7th **V42.5** Car driver injured in collision with two- or three-wheeled motor vehicle in traffic accident

√x7th **V42.6** Car passenger injured in collision with two- or three-wheeled motor vehicle in traffic accident

√x7th **V42.7** Person on outside of car injured in collision with two- or three-wheeled motor vehicle in traffic accident

√x7th **V42.9** Unspecified car occupant injured in collision with two- or three-wheeled motor vehicle in traffic accident

√4th **V43** **Car occupant injured in collision with car, pick-up truck or van**

√5th **V43.0** Car driver injured in collision with car, pick-up truck or van in nontraffic accident

√x7th **V43.01** Car driver injured in collision with sport utility vehicle in nontraffic accident

√x7th **V43.02** Car driver injured in collision with other type car in nontraffic accident

√x7th **V43.03** Car driver injured in collision with pick-up truck in nontraffic accident

√x7th **V43.04** Car driver injured in collision with van in nontraffic accident

√5th **V43.1** Car passenger injured in collision with car, pick-up truck or van in nontraffic accident

√x7th **V43.11** Car passenger injured in collision with sport utility vehicle in nontraffic accident

√x7th **V43.12** Car passenger injured in collision with other type car in nontraffic accident

√x7th **V43.13** Car passenger injured in collision with pick-up truck in nontraffic accident

√x7th **V43.14** Car passenger injured in collision with van in nontraffic accident

√5th **V43.2** Person on outside of car injured in collision with car, pick-up truck or van in nontraffic accident

√x7th **V43.21** Person on outside of car injured in collision with sport utility vehicle in nontraffic accident

√x7th **V43.22** Person on outside of car injured in collision with other type car in nontraffic accident

√x7th **V43.23** Person on outside of car injured in collision with pick-up truck in nontraffic accident

√x7th **V43.24** Person on outside of car injured in collision with van in nontraffic accident

√5th **V43.3** Unspecified car occupant injured in collision with car, pick-up truck or van in nontraffic accident

√x7th **V43.31** Unspecified car occupant injured in collision with sport utility vehicle in nontraffic accident

√x7th **V43.32** Unspecified car occupant injured in collision with other type car in nontraffic accident

√x7th **V43.33** Unspecified car occupant injured in collision with pick-up truck in nontraffic accident

√x7th **V43.34** Unspecified car occupant injured in collision with van in nontraffic accident

√5th **V43.4** Person boarding or alighting a car injured in collision with car, pick-up truck or van

√x7th **V43.41** Person boarding or alighting a car injured in collision with sport utility vehicle

√x7th **V43.42** Person boarding or alighting a car injured in collision with other type car

√x7th **V43.43** Person boarding or alighting a car injured in collision with pick-up truck

√x7th **V43.44** Person boarding or alighting a car injured in collision with van

√6th **V43.5** Car driver injured in collision with car, pick-up truck or van in traffic accident

√x7th **V43.51** Car driver injured in collision with sport utility vehicle in traffic accident

√x7th **V43.52** Car driver injured in collision with other type car in traffic accident

√x7th **V43.53** Car driver injured in collision with pick-up truck in traffic accident

√x7th **V43.54** Car driver injured in collision with van in traffic accident

√5th **V43.6** Car passenger injured in collision with car, pick-up truck or van in traffic accident

√x7th **V43.61** Car passenger injured in collision with sport utility vehicle in traffic accident

√x7th **V43.62** Car passenger injured in collision with other type car in traffic accident

√x7th **V43.63** Car passenger injured in collision with pick-up truck in traffic accident

√x7th **V43.64** Car passenger injured in collision with van in traffic accident

√5th **V43.7** Person on outside of car injured in collision with car, pick-up truck or van in traffic accident

√x7th **V43.71** Person on outside of car injured in collision with sport utility vehicle in traffic accident

√x7th **V43.72** Person on outside of car injured in collision with other type car in traffic accident

√x7th **V43.73** Person on outside of car injured in collision with pick-up truck in traffic accident

√x7th **V43.74** Person on outside of car injured in collision with van in traffic accident

√5th **V43.9** Unspecified car occupant injured in collision with car, pick-up truck or van in traffic accident

√x7th **V43.91** Unspecified car occupant injured in collision with sport utility vehicle in traffic accident

√x7th **V43.92** Unspecified car occupant injured in collision with other type car in traffic accident

√x7th **V43.93** Unspecified car occupant injured in collision with pick-up truck in traffic accident

√x7th **V43.94** Unspecified car occupant injured in collision with van in traffic accident

√4th **V44** **Car occupant injured in collision with heavy transport vehicle or bus**

EXCLUDES 1 *car occupant injured in collision with military vehicle (V49.81)*

√x7th **V44.0** Car driver injured in collision with heavy transport vehicle or bus in nontraffic accident

√x7th **V44.1** Car passenger injured in collision with heavy transport vehicle or bus in nontraffic accident

√x7th **V44.2** Person on outside of car injured in collision with heavy transport vehicle or bus in nontraffic accident

√x7th **V44.3** Unspecified car occupant injured in collision with heavy transport vehicle or bus in nontraffic accident

√x7th **V44.4** Person boarding or alighting a car injured in collision with heavy transport vehicle or bus

√x7th **V44.5** Car driver injured in collision with heavy transport vehicle or bus in traffic accident

√x7th **V44.6** Car passenger injured in collision with heavy transport vehicle or bus in traffic accident

√x7th **V44.7** Person on outside of car injured in collision with heavy transport vehicle or bus in traffic accident

√x7th **V44.9** Unspecified car occupant injured in collision with heavy transport vehicle or bus in traffic accident

√4th **V45** **Car occupant injured in collision with railway train or railway vehicle**

√x7th **V45.0** Car driver injured in collision with railway train or railway vehicle in nontraffic accident

√x7th **V45.1** Car passenger injured in collision with railway train or railway vehicle in nontraffic accident

√x7th **V45.2** Person on outside of car injured in collision with railway train or railway vehicle in nontraffic accident

√x7th **V45.3** Unspecified car occupant injured in collision with railway train or railway vehicle in nontraffic accident

√x7th **V45.4** Person boarding or alighting a car injured in collision with railway train or railway vehicle

√x7th **V45.5** Car driver injured in collision with railway train or railway vehicle in traffic accident

√x7th **V45.6** Car passenger injured in collision with railway train or railway vehicle in traffic accident

√x7th **V45.7** Person on outside of car injured in collision with railway train or railway vehicle in traffic accident

√x7th **V45.9** Unspecified car occupant injured in collision with railway train or railway vehicle in traffic accident

√4th **V46** **Car occupant injured in collision with other nonmotor vehicle**

INCLUDES collision with animal-drawn vehicle, animal being ridden, streetcar

√x7th **V46.0** Car driver injured in collision with other nonmotor vehicle in nontraffic accident

√x7th **V46.1** Car passenger injured in collision with other nonmotor vehicle in nontraffic accident

√x7th **V46.2** Person on outside of car injured in collision with other nonmotor vehicle in nontraffic accident

√x7ᵗʰ **V46.3** Unspecified car occupant injured in collision with other nonmotor vehicle in nontraffic accident

√x7ᵗʰ **V46.4** Person boarding or alighting a car injured in collision with other nonmotor vehicle

√x7ᵗʰ **V46.5** Car driver injured in collision with other nonmotor vehicle in traffic accident

√x7ᵗʰ **V46.6** Car passenger injured in collision with other nonmotor vehicle in traffic accident

√x7ᵗʰ **V46.7** Person on outside of car injured in collision with other nonmotor vehicle in traffic accident

√x7ᵗʰ **V46.9** Unspecified car occupant injured in collision with other nonmotor vehicle in traffic accident

✓4ᵗʰ **V47** Car occupant injured in collision with fixed or stationary object
    AHA: 2016,4Q,73

√x7ᵗʰ **V47.0** Car driver injured in collision with fixed or stationary object in nontraffic accident

√x7ᵗʰ **V47.1** Car passenger injured in collision with fixed or stationary object in nontraffic accident

√x7ᵗʰ **V47.2** Person on outside of car injured in collision with fixed or stationary object in nontraffic accident

√x7ᵗʰ **V47.3** Unspecified car occupant injured in collision with fixed or stationary object in nontraffic accident

√x7ᵗʰ **V47.4** Person boarding or alighting a car injured in collision with fixed or stationary object

√x7ᵗʰ **V47.5** Car driver injured in collision with fixed or stationary object in traffic accident

√x7ᵗʰ **V47.6** Car passenger injured in collision with fixed or stationary object in traffic accident

√x7ᵗʰ **V47.7** Person on outside of car injured in collision with fixed or stationary object in traffic accident

√x7ᵗʰ **V47.9** Unspecified car occupant injured in collision with fixed or stationary object in traffic accident

✓4ᵗʰ **V48** Car occupant injured in noncollision transport accident
    INCLUDES   overturning car NOS
                overturning car without collision

√x7ᵗʰ **V48.0** Car driver injured in noncollision transport accident in nontraffic accident

√x7ᵗʰ **V48.1** Car passenger injured in noncollision transport accident in nontraffic accident

√x7ᵗʰ **V48.2** Person on outside of car injured in noncollision transport accident in nontraffic accident

√x7ᵗʰ **V48.3** Unspecified car occupant injured in noncollision transport accident in nontraffic accident

√x7ᵗʰ **V48.4** Person boarding or alighting a car injured in noncollision transport accident

√x7ᵗʰ **V48.5** Car driver injured in noncollision transport accident in traffic accident

√x7ᵗʰ **V48.6** Car passenger injured in noncollision transport accident in traffic accident

√x7ᵗʰ **V48.7** Person on outside of car injured in noncollision transport accident in traffic accident

√x7ᵗʰ **V48.9** Unspecified car occupant injured in noncollision transport accident in traffic accident

✓4ᵗʰ **V49** Car occupant injured in other and unspecified transport accidents

✓5ᵗʰ **V49.0** Driver injured in collision with other and unspecified motor vehicles in nontraffic accident

  √x7ᵗʰ **V49.00** Driver injured in collision with unspecified motor vehicles in nontraffic accident

  √x7ᵗʰ **V49.09** Driver injured in collision with other motor vehicles in nontraffic accident

✓5ᵗʰ **V49.1** Passenger injured in collision with other and unspecified motor vehicles in nontraffic accident

  √x7ᵗʰ **V49.10** Passenger injured in collision with unspecified motor vehicles in nontraffic accident

  √x7ᵗʰ **V49.19** Passenger injured in collision with other motor vehicles in nontraffic accident

✓5ᵗʰ **V49.2** Unspecified car occupant injured in collision with other and unspecified motor vehicles in nontraffic accident

  √x7ᵗʰ **V49.20** Unspecified car occupant injured in collision with unspecified motor vehicles in nontraffic accident
         Car collision NOS, nontraffic

  √x7ᵗʰ **V49.29** Unspecified car occupant injured in collision with other motor vehicles in nontraffic accident

√x7ᵗʰ **V49.3** Car occupant (driver) (passenger) injured in unspecified nontraffic accident
      Car accident NOS, nontraffic
      Car occupant injured in nontraffic accident NOS

✓5ᵗʰ **V49.4** Driver injured in collision with other and unspecified motor vehicles in traffic accident

  √x7ᵗʰ **V49.40** Driver injured in collision with unspecified motor vehicles in traffic accident

  √x7ᵗʰ **V49.49** Driver injured in collision with other motor vehicles in traffic accident

✓5ᵗʰ **V49.5** Passenger injured in collision with other and unspecified motor vehicles in traffic accident

  √x7ᵗʰ **V49.50** Passenger injured in collision with unspecified motor vehicles in traffic accident

  √x7ᵗʰ **V49.59** Passenger injured in collision with other motor vehicles in traffic accident

✓5ᵗʰ **V49.6** Unspecified car occupant injured in collision with other and unspecified motor vehicles in traffic accident

  √x7ᵗʰ **V49.60** Unspecified car occupant injured in collision with unspecified motor vehicles in traffic accident
         Car collision NOS (traffic)

  √x7ᵗʰ **V49.69** Unspecified car occupant injured in collision with other motor vehicles in traffic accident

✓5ᵗʰ **V49.8** Car occupant (driver) (passenger) injured in other specified transport accidents

  √x7ᵗʰ **V49.81** Car occupant (driver) (passenger) injured in transport accident with military vehicle

  √x7ᵗʰ **V49.88** Car occupant (driver) (passenger) injured in other specified transport accidents

√x7ᵗʰ **V49.9** Car occupant (driver) (passenger) injured in unspecified traffic accident
      Car accident NOS

Occupant of pick-up truck or van injured in transport accident (V50-V59)

   INCLUDES   a four or six wheel motor vehicle designed primarily for carrying passengers and property but weighing less than the local limit for classification as a heavy goods vehicle
                minibus
                minivan
                sport utility vehicle (SUV)
                truck
                van
   EXCLUDES 1   *heavy transport vehicle (V60-V69)*

The appropriate 7th character is to be added to each code from categories V50-V59.
A   initial encounter
D   subsequent encounter
S   sequela

✓4ᵗʰ **V50** Occupant of pick-up truck or van injured in collision with pedestrian or animal
    EXCLUDES 1   *pick-up truck or van collision with animal-drawn vehicle or animal being ridden (V56.-)*

√x7ᵗʰ **V50.0** Driver of pick-up truck or van injured in collision with pedestrian or animal in nontraffic accident

√x7ᵗʰ **V50.1** Passenger in pick-up truck or van injured in collision with pedestrian or animal in nontraffic accident

√x7ᵗʰ **V50.2** Person on outside of pick-up truck or van injured in collision with pedestrian or animal in nontraffic accident

√x7ᵗʰ **V50.3** Unspecified occupant of pick-up truck or van injured in collision with pedestrian or animal in nontraffic accident

√x7ᵗʰ **V50.4** Person boarding or alighting a pick-up truck or van injured in collision with pedestrian or animal

√x7ᵗʰ **V50.5** Driver of pick-up truck or van injured in collision with pedestrian or animal in traffic accident

√x7ᵗʰ **V50.6** Passenger in pick-up truck or van injured in collision with pedestrian or animal in traffic accident

√x7ᵗʰ **V50.7** Person on outside of pick-up truck or van injured in collision with pedestrian or animal in traffic accident

√x7ᵗʰ **V50.9** Unspecified occupant of pick-up truck or van injured in collision with pedestrian or animal in traffic accident

✓4ᵗʰ **V51** Occupant of pick-up truck or van injured in collision with pedal cycle

√x7ᵗʰ **V51.0** Driver of pick-up truck or van injured in collision with pedal cycle in nontraffic accident

√x7ᵗʰ **V51.1** Passenger in pick-up truck or van injured in collision with pedal cycle in nontraffic accident

√x7ᵗʰ **V51.2** Person on outside of pick-up truck or van injured in collision with pedal cycle in nontraffic accident

√x7ᵗʰ **V51.3** Unspecified occupant of pick-up truck or van injured in collision with pedal cycle in nontraffic accident

√x7ᵗʰ **V51.4** Person boarding or alighting a pick-up truck or van injured in collision with pedal cycle

√x7ᵗʰ **V51.5** Driver of pick-up truck or van injured in collision with pedal cycle in traffic accident

√x7th **V51.6** Passenger in pick-up truck or van injured in collision with pedal cycle in traffic accident

√x7th **V51.7** Person on outside of pick-up truck or van injured in collision with pedal cycle in traffic accident

√x7th **V51.9** Unspecified occupant of pick-up truck or van injured in collision with pedal cycle in traffic accident

√4th **V52** Occupant of pick-up truck or van injured in collision with two- or three-wheeled motor vehicle

√x7th **V52.0** Driver of pick-up truck or van injured in collision with two- or three-wheeled motor vehicle in nontraffic accident

√x7th **V52.1** Passenger in pick-up truck or van injured in collision with two- or three-wheeled motor vehicle in nontraffic accident

√x7th **V52.2** Person on outside of pick-up truck or van injured in collision with two- or three-wheeled motor vehicle in nontraffic accident

√x7th **V52.3** Unspecified occupant of pick-up truck or van injured in collision with two- or three-wheeled motor vehicle in nontraffic accident

√x7th **V52.4** Person boarding or alighting a pick-up truck or van injured in collision with two- or three-wheeled motor vehicle

√x7th **V52.5** Driver of pick-up truck or van injured in collision with two- or three-wheeled motor vehicle in traffic accident

√x7th **V52.6** Passenger in pick-up truck or van injured in collision with two- or three-wheeled motor vehicle in traffic accident

√x7th **V52.7** Person on outside of pick-up truck or van injured in collision with two- or three-wheeled motor vehicle in traffic accident

√x7th **V52.9** Unspecified occupant of pick-up truck or van injured in collision with two- or three-wheeled motor vehicle in traffic accident

√4th **V53** Occupant of pick-up truck or van injured in collision with car, pick-up truck or van

√x7th **V53.0** Driver of pick-up truck or van injured in collision with car, pick-up truck or van in nontraffic accident

√x7th **V53.1** Passenger in pick-up truck or van injured in collision with car, pick-up truck or van in nontraffic accident

√x7th **V53.2** Person on outside of pick-up truck or van injured in collision with car, pick-up truck or van in nontraffic accident

√x7th **V53.3** Unspecified occupant of pick-up truck or van injured in collision with car, pick-up truck or van in nontraffic accident

√x7th **V53.4** Person boarding or alighting a pick-up truck or van injured in collision with car, pick-up truck or van

√x7th **V53.5** Driver of pick-up truck or van injured in collision with car, pick-up truck or van in traffic accident

√x7th **V53.6** Passenger in pick-up truck or van injured in collision with car, pick-up truck or van in traffic accident

√x7th **V53.7** Person on outside of pick-up truck or van injured in collision with car, pick-up truck or van in traffic accident

√x7th **V53.9** Unspecified occupant of pick-up truck or van injured in collision with car, pick-up truck or van in traffic accident

√4th **V54** Occupant of pick-up truck or van injured in collision with heavy transport vehicle or bus

EXCLUDES 1   occupant of pick-up truck or van injured in collision with military vehicle (V59.81)

√x7th **V54.0** Driver of pick-up truck or van injured in collision with heavy transport vehicle or bus in nontraffic accident

√x7th **V54.1** Passenger in pick-up truck or van injured in collision with heavy transport vehicle or bus in nontraffic accident

√x7th **V54.2** Person on outside of pick-up truck or van injured in collision with heavy transport vehicle or bus in nontraffic accident

√x7th **V54.3** Unspecified occupant of pick-up truck or van injured in collision with heavy transport vehicle or bus in nontraffic accident

√x7th **V54.4** Person boarding or alighting a pick-up truck or van injured in collision with heavy transport vehicle or bus

√x7th **V54.5** Driver of pick-up truck or van injured in collision with heavy transport vehicle or bus in traffic accident

√x7th **V54.6** Passenger in pick-up truck or van injured in collision with heavy transport vehicle or bus in traffic accident

√x7th **V54.7** Person on outside of pick-up truck or van injured in collision with heavy transport vehicle or bus in traffic accident

√x7th **V54.9** Unspecified occupant of pick-up truck or van injured in collision with heavy transport vehicle or bus in traffic accident

√4th **V55** Occupant of pick-up truck or van injured in collision with railway train or railway vehicle

√x7th **V55.0** Driver of pick-up truck or van injured in collision with railway train or railway vehicle in nontraffic accident

√x7th **V55.1** Passenger in pick-up truck or van injured in collision with railway train or railway vehicle in nontraffic accident

√x7th **V55.2** Person on outside of pick-up truck or van injured in collision with railway train or railway vehicle in nontraffic accident

√x7th **V55.3** Unspecified occupant of pick-up truck or van injured in collision with railway train or railway vehicle in nontraffic accident

√x7th **V55.4** Person boarding or alighting a pick-up truck or van injured in collision with railway train or railway vehicle

√x7th **V55.5** Driver of pick-up truck or van injured in collision with railway train or railway vehicle in traffic accident

√x7th **V55.6** Passenger in pick-up truck or van injured in collision with railway train or railway vehicle in traffic accident

√x7th **V55.7** Person on outside of pick-up truck or van injured in collision with railway train or railway vehicle in traffic accident

√x7th **V55.9** Unspecified occupant of pick-up truck or van injured in collision with railway train or railway vehicle in traffic accident

√4th **V56** Occupant of pick-up truck or van injured in collision with other nonmotor vehicle

INCLUDES   collision with animal-drawn vehicle, animal being ridden, streetcar

√x7th **V56.0** Driver of pick-up truck or van injured in collision with other nonmotor vehicle in nontraffic accident

√x7th **V56.1** Passenger in pick-up truck or van injured in collision with other nonmotor vehicle in nontraffic accident

√x7th **V56.2** Person on outside of pick-up truck or van injured in collision with other nonmotor vehicle in nontraffic accident

√x7th **V56.3** Unspecified occupant of pick-up truck or van injured in collision with other nonmotor vehicle in nontraffic accident

√x7th **V56.4** Person boarding or alighting a pick-up truck or van injured in collision with other nonmotor vehicle

√x7th **V56.5** Driver of pick-up truck or van injured in collision with other nonmotor vehicle in traffic accident

√x7th **V56.6** Passenger in pick-up truck or van injured in collision with other nonmotor vehicle in traffic accident

√x7th **V56.7** Person on outside of pick-up truck or van injured in collision with other nonmotor vehicle in traffic accident

√x7th **V56.9** Unspecified occupant of pick-up truck or van injured in collision with other nonmotor vehicle in traffic accident

√4th **V57** Occupant of pick-up truck or van injured in collision with fixed or stationary object

√x7th **V57.0** Driver of pick-up truck or van injured in collision with fixed or stationary object in nontraffic accident

√x7th **V57.1** Passenger in pick-up truck or van injured in collision with fixed or stationary object in nontraffic accident

√x7th **V57.2** Person on outside of pick-up truck or van injured in collision with fixed or stationary object in nontraffic accident

√x7th **V57.3** Unspecified occupant of pick-up truck or van injured in collision with fixed or stationary object in nontraffic accident

√x7th **V57.4** Person boarding or alighting a pick-up truck or van injured in collision with fixed or stationary object

√x7th **V57.5** Driver of pick-up truck or van injured in collision with fixed or stationary object in traffic accident

√x7th **V57.6** Passenger in pick-up truck or van injured in collision with fixed or stationary object in traffic accident

√x7th **V57.7** Person on outside of pick-up truck or van injured in collision with fixed or stationary object in traffic accident

√x7th **V57.9** Unspecified occupant of pick-up truck or van injured in collision with fixed or stationary object in traffic accident

√4th **V58** Occupant of pick-up truck or van injured in noncollision transport accident

INCLUDES   overturning pick-up truck or van NOS
overturning pick-up truck or van without collision

√x7th **V58.0** Driver of pick-up truck or van injured in noncollision transport accident in nontraffic accident

√x7th **V58.1** Passenger in pick-up truck or van injured in noncollision transport accident in nontraffic accident

√x7th **V58.2** Person on outside of pick-up truck or van injured in noncollision transport accident in nontraffic accident

√x7th **V58.3** Unspecified occupant of pick-up truck or van injured in noncollision transport accident in nontraffic accident

√x7th **V58.4** Person boarding or alighting a pick-up truck or van injured in noncollision transport accident

√x7th **V58.5** Driver of pick-up truck or van injured in noncollision transport accident in traffic accident

√x7th **V58.6** Passenger in pick-up truck or van injured in noncollision transport accident in traffic accident

√x7th **V58.7** Person on outside of pick-up truck or van injured in noncollision transport accident in traffic accident

√x7th **V58.9** Unspecified occupant of pick-up truck or van injured in noncollision transport accident in traffic accident

☑4ᵗʰ **V59 Occupant of pick-up truck or van injured in other and unspecified transport accidents**

    ☑5ᵗʰ **V59.0** Driver of pick-up truck or van injured in collision with other and unspecified motor vehicles in nontraffic accident

       ✓x 7ᵗʰ **V59.00** Driver of pick-up truck or van injured in collision with unspecified motor vehicles in nontraffic accident

       ✓x 7ᵗʰ **V59.09** Driver of pick-up truck or van injured in collision with other motor vehicles in nontraffic accident

    ☑5ᵗʰ **V59.1** Passenger in pick-up truck or van injured in collision with other and unspecified motor vehicles in nontraffic accident

       ✓x 7ᵗʰ **V59.10** Passenger in pick-up truck or van injured in collision with unspecified motor vehicles in nontraffic accident

       ✓x 7ᵗʰ **V59.19** Passenger in pick-up truck or van injured in collision with other motor vehicles in nontraffic accident

    ☑5ᵗʰ **V59.2** Unspecified occupant of pick-up truck or van injured in collision with other and unspecified motor vehicles in nontraffic accident

       ✓x 7ᵗʰ **V59.20** Unspecified occupant of pick-up truck or van injured in collision with unspecified motor vehicles in nontraffic accident

          Collision NOS involving pick-up truck or van, nontraffic

       ✓x 7ᵗʰ **V59.29** Unspecified occupant of pick-up truck or van injured in collision with other motor vehicles in nontraffic accident

    ✓x 7ᵗʰ **V59.3** Occupant (driver) (passenger) of pick-up truck or van injured in unspecified nontraffic accident

       Accident NOS involving pick-up truck or van, nontraffic

       Occupant of pick-up truck or van injured in nontraffic accident NOS

    ☑5ᵗʰ **V59.4** Driver of pick-up truck or van injured in collision with other and unspecified motor vehicles in traffic accident

       ✓x 7ᵗʰ **V59.40** Driver of pick-up truck or van injured in collision with unspecified motor vehicles in traffic accident

       ✓x 7ᵗʰ **V59.49** Driver of pick-up truck or van injured in collision with other motor vehicles in traffic accident

    ☑5ᵗʰ **V59.5** Passenger in pick-up truck or van injured in collision with other and unspecified motor vehicles in traffic accident

       ✓x 7ᵗʰ **V59.50** Passenger in pick-up truck or van injured in collision with unspecified motor vehicles in traffic accident

       ✓x 7ᵗʰ **V59.59** Passenger in pick-up truck or van injured in collision with other motor vehicles in traffic accident

    ☑5ᵗʰ **V59.6** Unspecified occupant of pick-up truck or van injured in collision with other and unspecified motor vehicles in traffic accident

       ✓x 7ᵗʰ **V59.60** Unspecified occupant of pick-up truck or van injured in collision with unspecified motor vehicles in traffic accident

          Collision NOS involving pick-up truck or van (traffic)

       ✓x 7ᵗʰ **V59.69** Unspecified occupant of pick-up truck or van injured in collision with other motor vehicles in traffic accident

    ☑5ᵗʰ **V59.8** Occupant (driver) (passenger) of pick-up truck or van injured in other specified transport accidents

       ✓x 7ᵗʰ **V59.81** Occupant (driver) (passenger) of pick-up truck or van injured in transport accident with military vehicle

       ✓x 7ᵗʰ **V59.88** Occupant (driver) (passenger) of pick-up truck or van injured in other specified transport accidents

    ✓x 7ᵗʰ **V59.9** Occupant (driver) (passenger) of pick-up truck or van injured in unspecified traffic accident

       Accident NOS involving pick-up truck or van

Occupant of heavy transport vehicle injured in transport accident (V60-V69)

INCLUDES	18 wheeler
	armored car
	panel truck
EXCLUDES 1	bus
	motorcoach

The appropriate 7th character is to be added to each code from categories V60-V69.
A   initial encounter
D   subsequent encounter
S   sequela

☑4ᵗʰ **V60 Occupant of heavy transport vehicle injured in collision with pedestrian or animal**

    EXCLUDES 1   *heavy transport vehicle collision with animal-drawn vehicle or animal being ridden (V66.-)*

    ✓x 7ᵗʰ **V60.0** Driver of heavy transport vehicle injured in collision with pedestrian or animal in nontraffic accident

    ✓x 7ᵗʰ **V60.1** Passenger in heavy transport vehicle injured in collision with pedestrian or animal in nontraffic accident

    ✓x 7ᵗʰ **V60.2** Person on outside of heavy transport vehicle injured in collision with pedestrian or animal in nontraffic accident

    ✓x 7ᵗʰ **V60.3** Unspecified occupant of heavy transport vehicle injured in collision with pedestrian or animal in nontraffic accident

    ✓x 7ᵗʰ **V60.4** Person boarding or alighting a heavy transport vehicle injured in collision with pedestrian or animal

    ✓x 7ᵗʰ **V60.5** Driver of heavy transport vehicle injured in collision with pedestrian or animal in traffic accident

    ✓x 7ᵗʰ **V60.6** Passenger in heavy transport vehicle injured in collision with pedestrian or animal in traffic accident

    ✓x 7ᵗʰ **V60.7** Person on outside of heavy transport vehicle injured in collision with pedestrian or animal in traffic accident

    ✓x 7ᵗʰ **V60.9** Unspecified occupant of heavy transport vehicle injured in collision with pedestrian or animal in traffic accident

☑4ᵗʰ **V61 Occupant of heavy transport vehicle injured in collision with pedal cycle**

    ✓x 7ᵗʰ **V61.0** Driver of heavy transport vehicle injured in collision with pedal cycle in nontraffic accident

    ✓x 7ᵗʰ **V61.1** Passenger in heavy transport vehicle injured in collision with pedal cycle in nontraffic accident

    ✓x 7ᵗʰ **V61.2** Person on outside of heavy transport vehicle injured in collision with pedal cycle in nontraffic accident

    ✓x 7ᵗʰ **V61.3** Unspecified occupant of heavy transport vehicle injured in collision with pedal cycle in nontraffic accident

    ✓x 7ᵗʰ **V61.4** Person boarding or alighting a heavy transport vehicle injured in collision with pedal cycle while boarding or alighting

    ✓x 7ᵗʰ **V61.5** Driver of heavy transport vehicle injured in collision with pedal cycle in traffic accident

    ✓x 7ᵗʰ **V61.6** Passenger in heavy transport vehicle injured in collision with pedal cycle in traffic accident

    ✓x 7ᵗʰ **V61.7** Person on outside of heavy transport vehicle injured in collision with pedal cycle in traffic accident

    ✓x 7ᵗʰ **V61.9** Unspecified occupant of heavy transport vehicle injured in collision with pedal cycle in traffic accident

☑4ᵗʰ **V62 Occupant of heavy transport vehicle injured in collision with two- or three-wheeled motor vehicle**

    ✓x 7ᵗʰ **V62.0** Driver of heavy transport vehicle injured in collision with two- or three-wheeled motor vehicle in nontraffic accident

    ✓x 7ᵗʰ **V62.1** Passenger in heavy transport vehicle injured in collision with two- or three-wheeled motor vehicle in nontraffic accident

    ✓x 7ᵗʰ **V62.2** Person on outside of heavy transport vehicle injured in collision with two- or three-wheeled motor vehicle in nontraffic accident

    ✓x 7ᵗʰ **V62.3** Unspecified occupant of heavy transport vehicle injured in collision with two- or three-wheeled motor vehicle in nontraffic accident

    ✓x 7ᵗʰ **V62.4** Person boarding or alighting a heavy transport vehicle injured in collision with two- or three-wheeled motor vehicle

    ✓x 7ᵗʰ **V62.5** Driver of heavy transport vehicle injured in collision with two- or three-wheeled motor vehicle in traffic accident

    ✓x 7ᵗʰ **V62.6** Passenger in heavy transport vehicle injured in collision with two- or three-wheeled motor vehicle in traffic accident

    ✓x 7ᵗʰ **V62.7** Person on outside of heavy transport vehicle injured in collision with two- or three-wheeled motor vehicle in traffic accident

    ✓x 7ᵗʰ **V62.9** Unspecified occupant of heavy transport vehicle injured in collision with two- or three-wheeled motor vehicle in traffic accident

✓4ᵗʰ **V63** Occupant of heavy transport vehicle injured in collision with car, pick-up truck or van

✓x7ᵗʰ **V63.Ø** Driver of heavy transport vehicle injured in collision with car, pick-up truck or van in nontraffic accident

✓x7ᵗʰ **V63.1** Passenger in heavy transport vehicle injured in collision with car, pick-up truck or van in nontraffic accident

✓x7ᵗʰ **V63.2** Person on outside of heavy transport vehicle injured in collision with car, pick-up truck or van in nontraffic accident

✓x7ᵗʰ **V63.3** Unspecified occupant of heavy transport vehicle injured in collision with car, pick-up truck or van in nontraffic accident

✓x7ᵗʰ **V63.4** Person boarding or alighting a heavy transport vehicle injured in collision with car, pick-up truck or van

✓x7ᵗʰ **V63.5** Driver of heavy transport vehicle injured in collision with car, pick-up truck or van in traffic accident

✓x7ᵗʰ **V63.6** Passenger in heavy transport vehicle injured in collision with car, pick-up truck or van in traffic accident

✓x7ᵗʰ **V63.7** Person on outside of heavy transport vehicle injured in collision with car, pick-up truck or van in traffic accident

✓x7ᵗʰ **V63.9** Unspecified occupant of heavy transport vehicle injured in collision with car, pick-up truck or van in traffic accident

✓4ᵗʰ **V64** Occupant of heavy transport vehicle injured in collision with heavy transport vehicle or bus

EXCLUDES 1 occupant of heavy transport vehicle injured in collision with military vehicle (V69.81)

✓x7ᵗʰ **V64.Ø** Driver of heavy transport vehicle injured in collision with heavy transport vehicle or bus in nontraffic accident

✓x7ᵗʰ **V64.1** Passenger in heavy transport vehicle injured in collision with heavy transport vehicle or bus in nontraffic accident

✓x7ᵗʰ **V64.2** Person on outside of heavy transport vehicle injured in collision with heavy transport vehicle or bus in nontraffic accident

✓x7ᵗʰ **V64.3** Unspecified occupant of heavy transport vehicle injured in collision with heavy transport vehicle or bus in nontraffic accident

✓x7ᵗʰ **V64.4** Person boarding or alighting a heavy transport vehicle injured in collision with heavy transport vehicle or bus while boarding or alighting

✓x7ᵗʰ **V64.5** Driver of heavy transport vehicle injured in collision with heavy transport vehicle or bus in traffic accident

✓x7ᵗʰ **V64.6** Passenger in heavy transport vehicle injured in collision with heavy transport vehicle or bus in traffic accident

✓x7ᵗʰ **V64.7** Person on outside of heavy transport vehicle injured in collision with heavy transport vehicle or bus in traffic accident

✓x7ᵗʰ **V64.9** Unspecified occupant of heavy transport vehicle injured in collision with heavy transport vehicle or bus in traffic accident

✓4ᵗʰ **V65** Occupant of heavy transport vehicle injured in collision with railway train or railway vehicle

✓x7ᵗʰ **V65.Ø** Driver of heavy transport vehicle injured in collision with railway train or railway vehicle in nontraffic accident

✓x7ᵗʰ **V65.1** Passenger in heavy transport vehicle injured in collision with railway train or railway vehicle in nontraffic accident

✓x7ᵗʰ **V65.2** Person on outside of heavy transport vehicle injured in collision with railway train or railway vehicle in nontraffic accident

✓x7ᵗʰ **V65.3** Unspecified occupant of heavy transport vehicle injured in collision with railway train or railway vehicle in nontraffic accident

✓x7ᵗʰ **V65.4** Person boarding or alighting a heavy transport vehicle injured in collision with railway train or railway vehicle

✓x7ᵗʰ **V65.5** Driver of heavy transport vehicle injured in collision with railway train or railway vehicle in traffic accident

✓x7ᵗʰ **V65.6** Passenger in heavy transport vehicle injured in collision with railway train or railway vehicle in traffic accident

✓x7ᵗʰ **V65.7** Person on outside of heavy transport vehicle injured in collision with railway train or railway vehicle in traffic accident

✓x7ᵗʰ **V65.9** Unspecified occupant of heavy transport vehicle injured in collision with railway train or railway vehicle in traffic accident

✓4ᵗʰ **V66** Occupant of heavy transport vehicle injured in collision with other nonmotor vehicle

INCLUDES collision with animal-drawn vehicle, animal being ridden, streetcar

✓x7ᵗʰ **V66.Ø** Driver of heavy transport vehicle injured in collision with other nonmotor vehicle in nontraffic accident

✓x7ᵗʰ **V66.1** Passenger in heavy transport vehicle injured in collision with other nonmotor vehicle in nontraffic accident

✓x7ᵗʰ **V66.2** Person on outside of heavy transport vehicle injured in collision with other nonmotor vehicle in nontraffic accident

✓x7ᵗʰ **V66.3** Unspecified occupant of heavy transport vehicle injured in collision with other nonmotor vehicle in nontraffic accident

✓x7ᵗʰ **V66.4** Person boarding or alighting a heavy transport vehicle injured in collision with other nonmotor vehicle

✓x7ᵗʰ **V66.5** Driver of heavy transport vehicle injured in collision with other nonmotor vehicle in traffic accident

✓x7ᵗʰ **V66.6** Passenger in heavy transport vehicle injured in collision with other nonmotor vehicle in traffic accident

✓x7ᵗʰ **V66.7** Person on outside of heavy transport vehicle injured in collision with other nonmotor vehicle in traffic accident

✓x7ᵗʰ **V66.9** Unspecified occupant of heavy transport vehicle injured in collision with other nonmotor vehicle in traffic accident

✓4ᵗʰ **V67** Occupant of heavy transport vehicle injured in collision with fixed or stationary object

✓x7ᵗʰ **V67.Ø** Driver of heavy transport vehicle injured in collision with fixed or stationary object in nontraffic accident

✓x7ᵗʰ **V67.1** Passenger in heavy transport vehicle injured in collision with fixed or stationary object in nontraffic accident

✓x7ᵗʰ **V67.2** Person on outside of heavy transport vehicle injured in collision with fixed or stationary object in nontraffic accident

✓x7ᵗʰ **V67.3** Unspecified occupant of heavy transport vehicle injured in collision with fixed or stationary object in nontraffic accident

✓x7ᵗʰ **V67.4** Person boarding or alighting a heavy transport vehicle injured in collision with fixed or stationary object

✓x7ᵗʰ **V67.5** Driver of heavy transport vehicle injured in collision with fixed or stationary object in traffic accident

✓x7ᵗʰ **V67.6** Passenger in heavy transport vehicle injured in collision with fixed or stationary object in traffic accident

✓x7ᵗʰ **V67.7** Person on outside of heavy transport vehicle injured in collision with fixed or stationary object in traffic accident

✓x7ᵗʰ **V67.9** Unspecified occupant of heavy transport vehicle injured in collision with fixed or stationary object in traffic accident

✓4ᵗʰ **V68** Occupant of heavy transport vehicle injured in noncollision transport accident

INCLUDES overturning heavy transport vehicle NOS
overturning heavy transport vehicle without collision

✓x7ᵗʰ **V68.Ø** Driver of heavy transport vehicle injured in noncollision transport accident in nontraffic accident

✓x7ᵗʰ **V68.1** Passenger in heavy transport vehicle injured in noncollision transport accident in nontraffic accident

✓x7ᵗʰ **V68.2** Person on outside of heavy transport vehicle injured in noncollision transport accident in nontraffic accident

✓x7ᵗʰ **V68.3** Unspecified occupant of heavy transport vehicle injured in noncollision transport accident in nontraffic accident

✓x7ᵗʰ **V68.4** Person boarding or alighting a heavy transport vehicle injured in noncollision transport accident

✓x7ᵗʰ **V68.5** Driver of heavy transport vehicle injured in noncollision transport accident in traffic accident

✓x7ᵗʰ **V68.6** Passenger in heavy transport vehicle injured in noncollision transport accident in traffic accident

✓x7ᵗʰ **V68.7** Person on outside of heavy transport vehicle injured in noncollision transport accident in traffic accident

✓x7ᵗʰ **V68.9** Unspecified occupant of heavy transport vehicle injured in noncollision transport accident in traffic accident

✓4ᵗʰ **V69** Occupant of heavy transport vehicle injured in other and unspecified transport accidents

✓5ᵗʰ **V69.Ø** Driver of heavy transport vehicle injured in collision with other and unspecified motor vehicles in nontraffic accident

✓x7ᵗʰ **V69.ØØ** Driver of heavy transport vehicle injured in collision with unspecified motor vehicles in nontraffic accident

✓x7ᵗʰ **V69.Ø9** Driver of heavy transport vehicle injured in collision with other motor vehicles in nontraffic accident

✓5ᵗʰ **V69.1** Passenger in heavy transport vehicle injured in collision with other and unspecified motor vehicles in nontraffic accident

✓x7ᵗʰ **V69.1Ø** Passenger in heavy transport vehicle injured in collision with unspecified motor vehicles in nontraffic accident

✓x7ᵗʰ **V69.19** Passenger in heavy transport vehicle injured in collision with other motor vehicles in nontraffic accident

✓5ᵗʰ **V69.2** Unspecified occupant of heavy transport vehicle injured in collision with other and unspecified motor vehicles in nontraffic accident

✓x7ᵗʰ **V69.2Ø** Unspecified occupant of heavy transport vehicle injured in collision with unspecified motor vehicles in nontraffic accident

Collision NOS involving heavy transport vehicle, nontraffic

✓x7ᵗʰ **V69.29** Unspecified occupant of heavy transport vehicle injured in collision with other motor vehicles in nontraffic accident

✓x7ᵗʰ **V69.3** Occupant (driver) (passenger) of heavy transport vehicle injured in unspecified nontraffic accident

     Accident NOS involving heavy transport vehicle, nontraffic

     Occupant of heavy transport vehicle injured in nontraffic accident NOS

✓5ᵗʰ **V69.4** Driver of heavy transport vehicle injured in collision with other and unspecified motor vehicles in traffic accident

   ✓x7ᵗʰ **V69.40** Driver of heavy transport vehicle injured in collision with unspecified motor vehicles in traffic accident

   ✓x7ᵗʰ **V69.49** Driver of heavy transport vehicle injured in collision with other motor vehicles in traffic accident

✓5ᵗʰ **V69.5** Passenger in heavy transport vehicle injured in collision with other and unspecified motor vehicles in traffic accident

   ✓x7ᵗʰ **V69.50** Passenger in heavy transport vehicle injured in collision with unspecified motor vehicles in traffic accident

   ✓x7ᵗʰ **V69.59** Passenger in heavy transport vehicle injured in collision with other motor vehicles in traffic accident

✓5ᵗʰ **V69.6** Unspecified occupant of heavy transport vehicle injured in collision with other and unspecified motor vehicles in traffic accident

   ✓x7ᵗʰ **V69.60** Unspecified occupant of heavy transport vehicle injured in collision with unspecified motor vehicles in traffic accident

     Collision NOS involving heavy transport vehicle (traffic)

   ✓x7ᵗʰ **V69.69** Unspecified occupant of heavy transport vehicle injured in collision with other motor vehicles in traffic accident

✓5ᵗʰ **V69.8** Occupant (driver) (passenger) of heavy transport vehicle injured in other specified transport accidents

   ✓x7ᵗʰ **V69.81** Occupant (driver) (passenger) of heavy transport vehicle injured in transport accidents with military vehicle

   ✓x7ᵗʰ **V69.88** Occupant (driver) (passenger) of heavy transport vehicle injured in other specified transport accidents

✓x7ᵗʰ **V69.9** Occupant (driver) (passenger) of heavy transport vehicle injured in unspecified traffic accident

     Accident NOS involving heavy transport vehicle

Bus occupant injured in transport accident (V70-V79)

INCLUDES motorcoach
EXCLUDES 1 minibus (V50-V59)

The appropriate 7th character is to be added to each code from categories V70-V79.
A   initial encounter
D   subsequent encounter
S   sequela

✓4ᵗʰ **V70** Bus occupant injured in collision with pedestrian or animal

   EXCLUDES 1 *bus collision with animal-drawn vehicle or animal being ridden (V76.-)*

   ✓x7ᵗʰ **V70.0** Driver of bus injured in collision with pedestrian or animal in nontraffic accident

   ✓x7ᵗʰ **V70.1** Passenger on bus injured in collision with pedestrian or animal in nontraffic accident

   ✓x7ᵗʰ **V70.2** Person on outside of bus injured in collision with pedestrian or animal in nontraffic accident

   ✓x7ᵗʰ **V70.3** Unspecified occupant of bus injured in collision with pedestrian or animal in nontraffic accident

   ✓x7ᵗʰ **V70.4** Person boarding or alighting from bus injured in collision with pedestrian or animal

   ✓x7ᵗʰ **V70.5** Driver of bus injured in collision with pedestrian or animal in traffic accident

   ✓x7ᵗʰ **V70.6** Passenger on bus injured in collision with pedestrian or animal in traffic accident

   ✓x7ᵗʰ **V70.7** Person on outside of bus injured in collision with pedestrian or animal in traffic accident

   ✓x7ᵗʰ **V70.9** Unspecified occupant of bus injured in collision with pedestrian or animal in traffic accident

✓4ᵗʰ **V71** Bus occupant injured in collision with pedal cycle

   ✓x7ᵗʰ **V71.0** Driver of bus injured in collision with pedal cycle in nontraffic accident

   ✓x7ᵗʰ **V71.1** Passenger on bus injured in collision with pedal cycle in nontraffic accident

   ✓x7ᵗʰ **V71.2** Person on outside of bus injured in collision with pedal cycle in nontraffic accident

   ✓x7ᵗʰ **V71.3** Unspecified occupant of bus injured in collision with pedal cycle in nontraffic accident

   ✓x7ᵗʰ **V71.4** Person boarding or alighting from bus injured in collision with pedal cycle

   ✓x7ᵗʰ **V71.5** Driver of bus injured in collision with pedal cycle in traffic accident

   ✓x7ᵗʰ **V71.6** Passenger on bus injured in collision with pedal cycle in traffic accident

   ✓x7ᵗʰ **V71.7** Person on outside of bus injured in collision with pedal cycle in traffic accident

   ✓x7ᵗʰ **V71.9** Unspecified occupant of bus injured in collision with pedal cycle in traffic accident

✓4ᵗʰ **V72** Bus occupant injured in collision with two- or three-wheeled motor vehicle

   ✓x7ᵗʰ **V72.0** Driver of bus injured in collision with two- or three-wheeled motor vehicle in nontraffic accident

   ✓x7ᵗʰ **V72.1** Passenger on bus injured in collision with two- or three-wheeled motor vehicle in nontraffic accident

   ✓x7ᵗʰ **V72.2** Person on outside of bus injured in collision with two- or three-wheeled motor vehicle in nontraffic accident

   ✓x7ᵗʰ **V72.3** Unspecified occupant of bus injured in collision with two- or three-wheeled motor vehicle in nontraffic accident

   ✓x7ᵗʰ **V72.4** Person boarding or alighting from bus injured in collision with two- or three-wheeled motor vehicle

   ✓x7ᵗʰ **V72.5** Driver of bus injured in collision with two- or three-wheeled motor vehicle in traffic accident

   ✓x7ᵗʰ **V72.6** Passenger on bus injured in collision with two- or three-wheeled motor vehicle in traffic accident

   ✓x7ᵗʰ **V72.7** Person on outside of bus injured in collision with two- or three-wheeled motor vehicle in traffic accident

   ✓x7ᵗʰ **V72.9** Unspecified occupant of bus injured in collision with two- or three-wheeled motor vehicle in traffic accident

✓4ᵗʰ **V73** Bus occupant injured in collision with car, pick-up truck or van

   ✓x7ᵗʰ **V73.0** Driver of bus injured in collision with car, pick-up truck or van in nontraffic accident

   ✓x7ᵗʰ **V73.1** Passenger on bus injured in collision with car, pick-up truck or van in nontraffic accident

   ✓x7ᵗʰ **V73.2** Person on outside of bus injured in collision with car, pick-up truck or van in nontraffic accident

   ✓x7ᵗʰ **V73.3** Unspecified occupant of bus injured in collision with car, pick-up truck or van in nontraffic accident

   ✓x7ᵗʰ **V73.4** Person boarding or alighting from bus injured in collision with car, pick-up truck or van

   ✓x7ᵗʰ **V73.5** Driver of bus injured in collision with car, pick-up truck or van in traffic accident

   ✓x7ᵗʰ **V73.6** Passenger on bus injured in collision with car, pick-up truck or van in traffic accident

   ✓x7ᵗʰ **V73.7** Person on outside of bus injured in collision with car, pick-up truck or van in traffic accident

   ✓x7ᵗʰ **V73.9** Unspecified occupant of bus injured in collision with car, pick-up truck or van in traffic accident

✓4ᵗʰ **V74** Bus occupant injured in collision with heavy transport vehicle or bus

   EXCLUDES 1 *bus occupant injured in collision with military vehicle (V79.81)*

   ✓x7ᵗʰ **V74.0** Driver of bus injured in collision with heavy transport vehicle or bus in nontraffic accident

   ✓x7ᵗʰ **V74.1** Passenger on bus injured in collision with heavy transport vehicle or bus in nontraffic accident

   ✓x7ᵗʰ **V74.2** Person on outside of bus injured in collision with heavy transport vehicle or bus in nontraffic accident

   ✓x7ᵗʰ **V74.3** Unspecified occupant of bus injured in collision with heavy transport vehicle or bus in nontraffic accident

   ✓x7ᵗʰ **V74.4** Person boarding or alighting from bus injured in collision with heavy transport vehicle or bus

   ✓x7ᵗʰ **V74.5** Driver of bus injured in collision with heavy transport vehicle or bus in traffic accident

   ✓x7ᵗʰ **V74.6** Passenger on bus injured in collision with heavy transport vehicle or bus in traffic accident

   ✓x7ᵗʰ **V74.7** Person on outside of bus injured in collision with heavy transport vehicle or bus in traffic accident

   ✓x7ᵗʰ **V74.9** Unspecified occupant of bus injured in collision with heavy transport vehicle or bus in traffic accident

✓4ᵗʰ **V75** Bus occupant injured in collision with railway train or railway vehicle

   ✓x7ᵗʰ **V75.0** Driver of bus injured in collision with railway train or railway vehicle in nontraffic accident

   ✓x7ᵗʰ **V75.1** Passenger on bus injured in collision with railway train or railway vehicle in nontraffic accident

   ✓x7ᵗʰ **V75.2** Person on outside of bus injured in collision with railway train or railway vehicle in nontraffic accident

Chapter 20. External Causes of Morbidity

V69.29–V75.2

√x7ᵗʰ **V75.3** Unspecified occupant of bus injured in collision with railway train or railway vehicle **in nontraffic accident**

√x7ᵗʰ **V75.4** Person boarding or alighting **from bus injured in collision with railway train or railway vehicle**

√x7ᵗʰ **V75.5** Driver of bus injured in collision with railway train or railway vehicle **in traffic accident**

√x7ᵗʰ **V75.6** Passenger **on bus injured in collision with railway train or railway vehicle** in traffic accident

√x7ᵗʰ **V75.7** Person on outside **of bus injured in collision with railway train or railway vehicle** in traffic accident

√x7ᵗʰ **V75.9** Unspecified occupant of bus injured in collision with railway train or railway vehicle **in traffic accident**

√4ᵗʰ **V76** **Bus occupant injured in collision with other nonmotor vehicle**

     INCLUDES   collision with animal-drawn vehicle, animal being ridden, streetcar

√x7ᵗʰ **V76.0** Driver **of bus injured in collision with other nonmotor vehicle in nontraffic accident**

√x7ᵗʰ **V76.1** Passenger **on bus injured in collision with other nonmotor vehicle** in nontraffic accident

√x7ᵗʰ **V76.2** Person on outside **of bus injured in collision with other nonmotor vehicle** in nontraffic accident

√x7ᵗʰ **V76.3** Unspecified occupant of bus injured in collision with other nonmotor vehicle **in nontraffic accident**

√x7ᵗʰ **V76.4** Person boarding or alighting **from bus injured in collision with other nonmotor vehicle**

√x7ᵗʰ **V76.5** Driver **of bus injured in collision with other nonmotor vehicle in traffic accident**

√x7ᵗʰ **V76.6** Passenger **on bus injured in collision with other nonmotor vehicle** in traffic accident

√x7ᵗʰ **V76.7** Person on outside **of bus injured in collision with other nonmotor vehicle** in traffic accident

√x7ᵗʰ **V76.9** Unspecified occupant of bus injured in collision with other nonmotor vehicle **in traffic accident**

√4ᵗʰ **V77** **Bus occupant injured in collision with fixed or stationary object**

√x7ᵗʰ **V77.0** Driver **of bus injured in collision with fixed or stationary object** in nontraffic accident

√x7ᵗʰ **V77.1** Passenger **on bus injured in collision with fixed or stationary object** in nontraffic accident

√x7ᵗʰ **V77.2** Person on outside **of bus injured in collision with fixed or stationary object** in nontraffic accident

√x7ᵗʰ **V77.3** Unspecified occupant of bus injured in collision with fixed or stationary object **in nontraffic accident**

√x7ᵗʰ **V77.4** Person boarding or alighting **from bus injured in collision with fixed or stationary object**

√x7ᵗʰ **V77.5** Driver **of bus injured in collision with fixed or stationary object** in traffic accident

√x7ᵗʰ **V77.6** Passenger **on bus injured in collision with fixed or stationary object** in traffic accident

√x7ᵗʰ **V77.7** Person on outside **of bus injured in collision with fixed or stationary object** in traffic accident

√x7ᵗʰ **V77.9** Unspecified occupant of bus injured in collision with fixed or stationary object **in traffic accident**

√4ᵗʰ **V78** **Bus occupant injured in noncollision transport accident**

     INCLUDES   overturning bus NOS

                 overturning bus without collision

√x7ᵗʰ **V78.0** Driver **of bus injured in noncollision transport accident** in nontraffic accident

√x7ᵗʰ **V78.1** Passenger **on bus injured in noncollision transport accident** in nontraffic accident

√x7ᵗʰ **V78.2** Person on outside **of bus injured in noncollision transport accident** in nontraffic accident

√x7ᵗʰ **V78.3** Unspecified occupant of bus injured in noncollision transport accident **in nontraffic accident**

√x7ᵗʰ **V78.4** Person boarding or alighting **from bus injured in noncollision transport accident**

√x7ᵗʰ **V78.5** Driver **of bus injured in noncollision transport accident** in traffic accident

√x7ᵗʰ **V78.6** Passenger **on bus injured in noncollision transport accident** in traffic accident

√x7ᵗʰ **V78.7** Person on outside **of bus injured in noncollision transport accident** in traffic accident

√x7ᵗʰ **V78.9** Unspecified occupant of bus injured in noncollision transport accident **in traffic accident**

√4ᵗʰ **V79** **Bus occupant injured in other and unspecified transport accidents**

√5ᵗʰ **V79.0** Driver **of bus injured in collision with other and unspecified motor vehicles** in nontraffic accident

√x7ᵗʰ **V79.00** Driver of bus injured in collision with unspecified motor vehicles in nontraffic accident

√x7ᵗʰ **V79.09** Driver of bus injured in collision with other motor vehicles in nontraffic accident

√5ᵗʰ **V79.1** Passenger **on bus injured in collision with other and unspecified motor vehicles** in nontraffic accident

√x7ᵗʰ **V79.10** Passenger on bus injured in collision with unspecified motor vehicles in nontraffic accident

√x7ᵗʰ **V79.19** Passenger on bus injured in collision with other motor vehicles in nontraffic accident

√5ᵗʰ **V79.2** Unspecified bus occupant injured in collision with other and unspecified motor vehicles **in nontraffic accident**

√x7ᵗʰ **V79.20** Unspecified bus occupant injured in collision with unspecified motor vehicles in nontraffic accident

         Bus collision NOS, nontraffic

√x7ᵗʰ **V79.29** Unspecified bus occupant injured in collision with other motor vehicles in nontraffic accident

√x7ᵗʰ **V79.3** **Bus occupant (driver) (passenger) injured in unspecified nontraffic accident**

         Bus accident NOS, nontraffic

         Bus occupant injured in nontraffic accident NOS

√5ᵗʰ **V79.4** Driver **of bus injured in collision with other and unspecified motor vehicles** in traffic accident

√x7ᵗʰ **V79.40** Driver of bus injured in collision with unspecified motor vehicles in traffic accident

√x7ᵗʰ **V79.49** Driver of bus injured in collision with other motor vehicles in traffic accident

√5ᵗʰ **V79.5** Passenger **on bus injured in collision with other and unspecified motor vehicles** in traffic accident

√x7ᵗʰ **V79.50** Passenger on bus injured in collision with unspecified motor vehicles in traffic accident

√x7ᵗʰ **V79.59** Passenger on bus injured in collision with other motor vehicles in traffic accident

√5ᵗʰ **V79.6** Unspecified bus occupant injured in collision with other and unspecified motor vehicles **in traffic accident**

√x7ᵗʰ **V79.60** Unspecified bus occupant injured in collision with unspecified motor vehicles in traffic accident

         Bus collision NOS (traffic)

√x7ᵗʰ **V79.69** Unspecified bus occupant injured in collision with other motor vehicles in traffic accident

√5ᵗʰ **V79.8** **Bus occupant (driver) (passenger) injured in other specified transport accidents**

√x7ᵗʰ **V79.81** Bus occupant (driver) (passenger) injured in transport accidents with military vehicle

√x7ᵗʰ **V79.88** Bus occupant (driver) (passenger) injured in other specified transport accidents

√x7ᵗʰ **V79.9** **Bus occupant (driver) (passenger) injured in unspecified traffic accident**

         Bus accident NOS

Other land transport accidents (V80–V89)

The appropriate 7th character is to be added to each code from categories V80-V89.

A   initial encounter
D   subsequent encounter
S   sequela

√4ᵗʰ **V80** **Animal-rider or occupant of animal-drawn vehicle injured in transport accident**

√5ᵗʰ **V80.0** **Animal-rider or occupant of animal drawn vehicle injured by fall from or being thrown from animal or animal-drawn vehicle** in noncollision accident

√6ᵗʰ **V80.01** Animal-rider injured by fall from or being thrown from animal in noncollision accident

√7ᵗʰ **V80.010** Animal-rider injured by fall from or being thrown from horse in noncollision accident

√7ᵗʰ **V80.018** Animal-rider injured by fall from or being thrown from other animal in noncollision accident

√x7ᵗʰ **V80.02** Occupant of animal-drawn vehicle injured by fall from or being thrown from animal-drawn vehicle in noncollision accident

         Overturning animal-drawn vehicle NOS

         Overturning animal-drawn vehicle without collision

√5ᵗʰ **V80.1** **Animal-rider or occupant of animal-drawn vehicle injured in collision with pedestrian or animal**

     EXCLUDES 1   *animal-rider or animal-drawn vehicle collision with animal-drawn vehicle or animal being ridden (V80.7)*

√x7ᵗʰ **V80.11** Animal-rider injured in collision with pedestrian or animal

√x7ᵗʰ **V80.12** Occupant of animal-drawn vehicle injured in collision with pedestrian or animal

HCC CMS-HCC   **Rx** Rx HCC   **ESR** ESRD HCC   **COM** Commercial HCC   **N** Newborn: 0   **P** Pediatric: 0-17   **M** Maternity: 9-64   **A** Adult: 15-124

1216   ICD-10-CM 2023

√5ᵗʰ **V80.2** **Animal-rider or occupant of animal-drawn vehicle injured in collision with** pedal cycle

  √x7ᵗʰ **V80.21** Animal-rider **injured in collision with pedal cycle**

  √x7ᵗʰ **V80.22** Occupant **of animal-drawn vehicle injured in collision with pedal cycle**

√5ᵗʰ **V80.3** **Animal-rider or occupant of animal-drawn vehicle injured in collision with** two- or three-wheeled motor vehicle

  √x7ᵗʰ **V80.31** Animal-rider **injured in collision with two- or three-wheeled motor vehicle**

  √x7ᵗʰ **V80.32** Occupant **of animal-drawn vehicle injured in collision with two- or three-wheeled motor vehicle**

√5ᵗʰ **V80.4** **Animal-rider or occupant of animal-drawn vehicle injured in collision with** car, pick-up truck, van, heavy transport vehicle or bus

    EXCLUDES 1   *animal-rider injured in collision with military vehicle (V80.910)*

              occupant of animal-drawn vehicle injured in collision with military vehicle (V80.920)

  √x7ᵗʰ **V80.41** Animal-rider **injured in collision with car, pick-up truck, van, heavy transport vehicle or bus**

  √x7ᵗʰ **V80.42** Occupant **of animal-drawn vehicle injured in collision with car, pick-up truck, van, heavy transport vehicle or bus**

√5ᵗʰ **V80.5** **Animal-rider or occupant of animal-drawn vehicle injured in collision with other specified motor vehicle**

  √x7ᵗʰ **V80.51** Animal-rider **injured in collision with other specified motor vehicle**

  √x7ᵗʰ **V80.52** Occupant **of animal-drawn vehicle injured in collision with other specified motor vehicle**

√5ᵗʰ **V80.6** **Animal-rider or occupant of animal-drawn vehicle injured in collision with** railway train or railway vehicle

  √x7ᵗʰ **V80.61** Animal-rider **injured in collision with railway train or railway vehicle**

  √x7ᵗʰ **V80.62** Occupant **of animal-drawn vehicle injured in collision with railway train or railway vehicle**

√5ᵗʰ **V80.7** **Animal-rider or occupant of animal-drawn vehicle injured in collision with other nonmotor vehicles**

  √6ᵗʰ **V80.71** **Animal-rider or occupant of animal-drawn vehicle injured in collision with** animal being ridden

    √7ᵗʰ **V80.710** Animal-rider **injured in collision with other animal being ridden**

    √7ᵗʰ **V80.711** Occupant **of animal-drawn vehicle injured in collision with animal being ridden**

  √6ᵗʰ **V80.72** **Animal-rider or occupant of animal-drawn vehicle injured in collision with** other animal-drawn vehicle

    √7ᵗʰ **V80.720** Animal-rider **injured in collision with animal-drawn vehicle**

    √7ᵗʰ **V80.721** Occupant **of animal-drawn vehicle injured in collision with other animal-drawn vehicle**

  √6ᵗʰ **V80.73** **Animal-rider or occupant of animal-drawn vehicle injured in collision with** streetcar

    √7ᵗʰ **V80.730** Animal-rider **injured in collision with streetcar**

    √7ᵗʰ **V80.731** Occupant **of animal-drawn vehicle injured in collision with streetcar**

  √6ᵗʰ **V80.79** **Animal-rider or occupant of animal-drawn vehicle injured in collision with** other nonmotor vehicles

    √7ᵗʰ **V80.790** Animal-rider **injured in collision with other nonmotor vehicles**

    √7ᵗʰ **V80.791** Occupant **of animal-drawn vehicle injured in collision with other nonmotor vehicles**

√5ᵗʰ **V80.8** **Animal-rider or occupant of animal-drawn vehicle injured in collision with** fixed or stationary object

  √x7ᵗʰ **V80.81** Animal-rider **injured in collision with fixed or stationary object**

  √x7ᵗʰ **V80.82** Occupant **of animal-drawn vehicle injured in collision with fixed or stationary object**

√5ᵗʰ **V80.9** **Animal-rider or occupant of animal-drawn vehicle injured in other and unspecified transport accidents**

  √6ᵗʰ **V80.91** Animal-rider **injured in other and unspecified transport accidents**

    √7ᵗʰ **V80.910** **Animal-rider injured in transport accident with** military vehicle

    √7ᵗʰ **V80.918** **Animal-rider injured in other transport accident**

    √7ᵗʰ **V80.919** **Animal-rider injured in unspecified transport accident**

        Animal rider accident NOS

  √6ᵗʰ **V80.92** Occupant **of animal-drawn vehicle injured in other and unspecified transport accidents**

    √7ᵗʰ **V80.920** **Occupant of animal-drawn vehicle injured in transport accident with** military vehicle

    √7ᵗʰ **V80.928** **Occupant of animal-drawn vehicle injured in other transport accident**

    √7ᵗʰ **V80.929** **Occupant of animal-drawn vehicle injured in unspecified transport accident**

        Animal-drawn vehicle accident NOS

√4ᵗʰ **V81** **Occupant of railway train or railway vehicle injured in transport accident**

  INCLUDES   derailment of railway train or railway vehicle

              person on outside of train

  EXCLUDES 1   *streetcar (V82.-)*

√x7ᵗʰ **V81.0** **Occupant of railway train or railway vehicle injured in collision with motor vehicle** in nontraffic accident

    EXCLUDES 1   *occupant of railway train or railway vehicle injured due to collision with military vehicle (V81.83)*

√x7ᵗʰ **V81.1** **Occupant of railway train or railway vehicle injured in collision with motor vehicle** in traffic accident

    EXCLUDES 1   *occupant of railway train or railway vehicle injured due to collision with military vehicle (V81.83)*

√x7ᵗʰ **V81.2** **Occupant of railway train or railway vehicle injured in collision with or** hit by rolling stock

√x7ᵗʰ **V81.3** **Occupant of railway train or railway vehicle injured in collision with other object**

    Railway collision NOS

√x7ᵗʰ **V81.4** **Person injured** while boarding or alighting **from railway train or railway vehicle**

√x7ᵗʰ **V81.5** **Occupant of railway train or railway vehicle injured by fall** in railway train **or railway vehicle**

√x7ᵗʰ **V81.6** **Occupant of railway train or railway vehicle injured by fall** from railway train **or railway vehicle**

√x7ᵗʰ **V81.7** **Occupant of railway train or railway vehicle injured in** derailment without antecedent collision

√5ᵗʰ **V81.8** **Occupant of railway train or railway vehicle injured in other specified railway accidents**

  √x7ᵗʰ **V81.81** **Occupant of railway train or railway vehicle injured due to** explosion or fire **on train**

  √x7ᵗʰ **V81.82** **Occupant of railway train or railway vehicle injured due to** object falling onto **train**

    Occupant of railway train or railway vehicle injured due to falling earth onto train

    Occupant of railway train or railway vehicle injured due to falling rocks onto train

    Occupant of railway train or railway vehicle injured due to falling snow onto train

    Occupant of railway train or railway vehicle injured due to falling trees onto train

  √x7ᵗʰ **V81.83** **Occupant of railway train or railway vehicle injured due to** collision with military vehicle

  √x7ᵗʰ **V81.89** **Occupant of railway train or railway vehicle injured due to other specified railway accident**

√x7ᵗʰ **V81.9** **Occupant of railway train or railway vehicle injured in unspecified railway accident**

    Railway accident NOS

√4ᵗʰ **V82** **Occupant of powered streetcar injured in transport accident**

  INCLUDES   interurban electric car

              person on outside of streetcar

              tram (car)

              trolley (car)

  EXCLUDES 1   *bus (V70-V79)*

              motorcoach (V70-V79)

              nonpowered streetcar (V76.-)

              train (V81.-)

√x7ᵗʰ **V82.0** **Occupant of streetcar injured in collision with motor vehicle** in nontraffic accident

√x7ᵗʰ **V82.1** **Occupant of streetcar injured in collision with motor vehicle** in traffic accident

√x7ᵗʰ **V82.2** **Occupant of streetcar injured in collision with or** hit by rolling stock

√x7ᵗʰ **V82.3** **Occupant of streetcar injured in collision with other object**

    EXCLUDES 1   *collision with animal-drawn vehicle or animal being ridden (V82.8)*

√x7ᵗʰ **V82.4** **Person injured** while boarding or alighting **from streetcar**

✅ Additional Character Required   √x7ᵗʰ Placeholder Alert   Manifestation   Unspecified Dx   Q QPP   UPD Unacceptable PDx

√x7ᵗʰ **V82.5 Occupant of streetcar injured by fall in streetcar**
> EXCLUDES 1   *fall in streetcar:*
>> *while boarding or alighting (V82.4)*
>> *with antecedent collision (V82.0-V82.3)*

√x7ᵗʰ **V82.6 Occupant of streetcar injured by fall from streetcar**
> EXCLUDES 1   *fall from streetcar:*
>> *while boarding or alighting (V82.4)*
>> *with antecedent collision (V82.0-V82.3)*

√x7ᵗʰ **V82.7 Occupant of streetcar injured in derailment without antecedent collision**
> EXCLUDES 1   *occupant of streetcar injured in derailment with antecedent collision (V82.0-V82.3)*

√x7ᵗʰ **V82.8 Occupant of streetcar injured in other specified transport accidents**
> Streetcar collision with military vehicle
> Streetcar collision with train or nonmotor vehicles

√x7ᵗʰ **V82.9 Occupant of streetcar injured in unspecified traffic accident**
> Streetcar accident NOS

√4ᵗʰ **V83 Occupant of special vehicle mainly used on industrial premises injured in transport accident**
> INCLUDES   battery-powered airport passenger vehicle
> battery-powered truck (baggage) (mail)
> coal-car in mine
> forklift (truck)
> logging car
> self-propelled industrial truck
> station baggage truck (powered)
> tram, truck, or tub (powered) in mine or quarry
> EXCLUDES 1   *special construction vehicles (V85.-)*
>> *special industrial vehicle in stationary use or maintenance (W31.-)*

√x7ᵗʰ **V83.0 Driver of special industrial vehicle injured in traffic accident**

√x7ᵗʰ **V83.1 Passenger of special industrial vehicle injured in traffic accident**

√x7ᵗʰ **V83.2 Person on outside of special industrial vehicle injured in traffic accident**

√x7ᵗʰ **V83.3 Unspecified occupant of special industrial vehicle injured in traffic accident**

√x7ᵗʰ **V83.4 Person injured while boarding or alighting from special industrial vehicle**

√x7ᵗʰ **V83.5 Driver of special industrial vehicle injured in nontraffic accident**

√x7ᵗʰ **V83.6 Passenger of special industrial vehicle injured in nontraffic accident**

√x7ᵗʰ **V83.7 Person on outside of special industrial vehicle injured in nontraffic accident**

√x7ᵗʰ **V83.9 Unspecified occupant of special industrial vehicle injured in nontraffic accident**
> Special-industrial-vehicle accident NOS

√4ᵗʰ **V84 Occupant of special vehicle mainly used in agriculture injured in transport accident**
> INCLUDES   self-propelled farm machinery
> tractor (and trailer)
> EXCLUDES 1   *animal-powered farm machinery accident (W30.8-)*
>> *contact with combine harvester (W30.0)*
>> *special agricultural vehicle in stationary use or maintenance (W30.-)*

√x7ᵗʰ **V84.0 Driver of special agricultural vehicle injured in traffic accident**

√x7ᵗʰ **V84.1 Passenger of special agricultural vehicle injured in traffic accident**

√x7ᵗʰ **V84.2 Person on outside of special agricultural vehicle injured in traffic accident**

√x7ᵗʰ **V84.3 Unspecified occupant of special agricultural vehicle injured in traffic accident**

√x7ᵗʰ **V84.4 Person injured while boarding or alighting from special agricultural vehicle**

√x7ᵗʰ **V84.5 Driver of special agricultural vehicle injured in nontraffic accident**

√x7ᵗʰ **V84.6 Passenger of special agricultural vehicle injured in nontraffic accident**

√x7ᵗʰ **V84.7 Person on outside of special agricultural vehicle injured in nontraffic accident**

√x7ᵗʰ **V84.9 Unspecified occupant of special agricultural vehicle injured in nontraffic accident**
> Special-agricultural vehicle accident NOS

√4ᵗʰ **V85 Occupant of special construction vehicle injured in transport accident**
> INCLUDES   bulldozer
> digger
> dump truck
> earth-leveller
> mechanical shovel
> road-roller
> EXCLUDES 1   *special industrial vehicle (V83.-)*
>> *special construction vehicle in stationary use or maintenance (W31.-)*

√x7ᵗʰ **V85.0 Driver of special construction vehicle injured in traffic accident**

√x7ᵗʰ **V85.1 Passenger of special construction vehicle injured in traffic accident**

√x7ᵗʰ **V85.2 Person on outside of special construction vehicle injured in traffic accident**

√x7ᵗʰ **V85.3 Unspecified occupant of special construction vehicle injured in traffic accident**

√x7ᵗʰ **V85.4 Person injured while boarding or alighting from special construction vehicle**

√x7ᵗʰ **V85.5 Driver of special construction vehicle injured in nontraffic accident**

√x7ᵗʰ **V85.6 Passenger of special construction vehicle injured in nontraffic accident**

√x7ᵗʰ **V85.7 Person on outside of special construction vehicle injured in nontraffic accident**

√x7ᵗʰ **V85.9 Unspecified occupant of special construction vehicle injured in nontraffic accident**
> Special-construction-vehicle accident NOS

√4ᵗʰ **V86 Occupant of special all-terrain or other off-road motor vehicle, injured in transport accident**
> EXCLUDES 1   *special all-terrain vehicle in stationary use or maintenance (W31.-)*
>> *sport-utility vehicle (V50-V59)*
>> *three-wheeled motor vehicle designed for on-road use (V30-V39)*
> **AHA:** 2017,4Q,26

√5ᵗʰ **V86.0 Driver of special all-terrain or other off-road motor vehicle injured in traffic accident**

√x7ᵗʰ **V86.01 Driver of ambulance or fire engine injured in traffic accident**

√x7ᵗʰ **V86.02 Driver of snowmobile injured in traffic accident**

√x7ᵗʰ **V86.03 Driver of dune buggy injured in traffic accident**

√x7ᵗʰ **V86.04 Driver of military vehicle injured in traffic accident**

√x7ᵗʰ **V86.05 Driver of 3- or 4- wheeled all-terrain vehicle (ATV) injured in traffic accident**

√x7ᵗʰ **V86.06 Driver of dirt bike or motor/cross bike injured in traffic accident**

√x7ᵗʰ **V86.09 Driver of other special all-terrain or other off-road motor vehicle injured in traffic accident**
> Driver of go cart injured in traffic accident
> Driver of golf cart injured in traffic accident

√5ᵗʰ **V86.1 Passenger of special all-terrain or other off-road motor vehicle injured in traffic accident**

√x7ᵗʰ **V86.11 Passenger of ambulance or fire engine injured in traffic accident**

√x7ᵗʰ **V86.12 Passenger of snowmobile injured in traffic accident**

√x7ᵗʰ **V86.13 Passenger of dune buggy injured in traffic accident**

√x7ᵗʰ **V86.14 Passenger of military vehicle injured in traffic accident**

√x7ᵗʰ **V86.15 Passenger of 3- or 4- wheeled all-terrain vehicle (ATV) injured in traffic accident**

√x7ᵗʰ **V86.16 Passenger of dirt bike or motor/cross bike injured in traffic accident**

√x7ᵗʰ **V86.19 Passenger of other special all-terrain or other off-road motor vehicle injured in traffic accident**
> Passenger of go cart injured in traffic accident
> Passenger of golf cart injured in traffic accident

√5ᵗʰ **V86.2 Person on outside of special all-terrain or other off-road motor vehicle injured in traffic accident**

√x7ᵗʰ **V86.21 Person on outside of ambulance or fire engine injured in traffic accident**

√x7ᵗʰ **V86.22 Person on outside of snowmobile injured in traffic accident**

√x7ᵗʰ **V86.23 Person on outside of dune buggy injured in traffic accident**

√x7ᵗʰ **V86.24 Person on outside of military vehicle injured in traffic accident**

√x7ᵗʰ **V86.25** Person on outside of 3- or 4- wheeled all-terrain vehicle (ATV) injured in traffic accident

√x7ᵗʰ **V86.26** Person on outside of dirt bike or motor/cross bike injured in traffic accident

√x7ᵗʰ **V86.29** Person on outside of other special all-terrain or other off-road motor vehicle injured in traffic accident

     Person on outside of go cart in traffic accident

     Person on outside of golf cart injured in traffic accident

√5ᵗʰ **V86.3** Unspecified occupant of special all-terrain or other off-road motor vehicle injured in traffic accident

√x7ᵗʰ **V86.31** Unspecified occupant of ambulance or fire engine injured in traffic accident

√x7ᵗʰ **V86.32** Unspecified occupant of snowmobile injured in traffic accident

√x7ᵗʰ **V86.33** Unspecified occupant of dune buggy injured in traffic accident

√x7ᵗʰ **V86.34** Unspecified occupant of military vehicle injured in traffic accident

√x7ᵗʰ **V86.35** Unspecified occupant of 3- or 4- wheeled all-terrain vehicle (ATV) injured in traffic accident

√x7ᵗʰ **V86.36** Unspecified occupant of dirt bike or motor/cross bike injured in traffic accident

√x7ᵗʰ **V86.39** Unspecified occupant of other special all-terrain or other off-road motor vehicle injured in traffic accident

     Unspecified occupant of go cart injured in traffic accident

     Unspecified occupant of golf cart injured in traffic accident

√5ᵗʰ **V86.4** Person injured while boarding or alighting from special all-terrain or other off-road motor vehicle

√x7ᵗʰ **V86.41** Person injured while boarding or alighting from ambulance or fire engine

√x7ᵗʰ **V86.42** Person injured while boarding or alighting from snowmobile

√x7ᵗʰ **V86.43** Person injured while boarding or alighting from dune buggy

√x7ᵗʰ **V86.44** Person injured while boarding or alighting from military vehicle

√x7ᵗʰ **V86.45** Person injured while boarding or alighting from a 3- or 4- wheeled all-terrain vehicle (ATV)

√x7ᵗʰ **V86.46** Person injured while boarding or alighting from a dirt bike or motor/cross bike

√x7ᵗʰ **V86.49** Person injured while boarding or alighting from other special all-terrain or other off-road motor vehicle

     Person injured while boarding or alighting from go cart

     Person injured while boarding or alighting from golf cart

√5ᵗʰ **V86.5** Driver of special all-terrain or other off-road motor vehicle injured in nontraffic accident

√x7ᵗʰ **V86.51** Driver of ambulance or fire engine injured in nontraffic accident

√x7ᵗʰ **V86.52** Driver of snowmobile injured in nontraffic accident

√x7ᵗʰ **V86.53** Driver of dune buggy injured in nontraffic accident

√x7ᵗʰ **V86.54** Driver of military vehicle injured in nontraffic accident

√x7ᵗʰ **V86.55** Driver of 3- or 4- wheeled all-terrain vehicle (ATV) injured in nontraffic accident

√x7ᵗʰ **V86.56** Driver of dirt bike or motor/cross bike injured in nontraffic accident

√x7ᵗʰ **V86.59** Driver of other special all-terrain or other off-road motor vehicle injured in nontraffic accident

     Driver of go cart injured in nontraffic accident

     Driver of golf cart injured in nontraffic accident

√5ᵗʰ **V86.6** Passenger of special all-terrain or other off-road motor vehicle injured in nontraffic accident

√x7ᵗʰ **V86.61** Passenger of ambulance or fire engine injured in nontraffic accident

√x7ᵗʰ **V86.62** Passenger of snowmobile injured in nontraffic accident

√x7ᵗʰ **V86.63** Passenger of dune buggy injured in nontraffic accident

√x7ᵗʰ **V86.64** Passenger of military vehicle injured in nontraffic accident

√x7ᵗʰ **V86.65** Passenger of 3- or 4- wheeled all-terrain vehicle (ATV) injured in nontraffic accident

√x7ᵗʰ **V86.66** Passenger of dirt bike or motor/cross bike injured in nontraffic accident

√x7ᵗʰ **V86.69** Passenger of other special all-terrain or other off-road motor vehicle injured in nontraffic accident

     Passenger of go cart injured in nontraffic accident

     Passenger of golf cart injured in nontraffic accident

√5ᵗʰ **V86.7** Person on outside of special all-terrain or other off-road motor vehicle injured in nontraffic accident

√x7ᵗʰ **V86.71** Person on outside of ambulance or fire engine injured in nontraffic accident

√x7ᵗʰ **V86.72** Person on outside of snowmobile injured in nontraffic accident

√x7ᵗʰ **V86.73** Person on outside of dune buggy injured in nontraffic accident

√x7ᵗʰ **V86.74** Person on outside of military vehicle injured in nontraffic accident

√x7ᵗʰ **V86.75** Person on outside of 3- or 4- wheeled all-terrain vehicle (ATV) injured in nontraffic accident

√x7ᵗʰ **V86.76** Person on outside of dirt bike or motor/cross bike injured in nontraffic accident

√x7ᵗʰ **V86.79** Person on outside of other special all-terrain or other off-road motor vehicles injured in nontraffic accident

     Person on outside of go cart injured in nontraffic accident

     Person on outside of golf cart injured in nontraffic accident

√5ᵗʰ **V86.9** Unspecified occupant of special all-terrain or other off-road motor vehicle injured in nontraffic accident

√x7ᵗʰ **V86.91** Unspecified occupant of ambulance or fire engine injured in nontraffic accident

√x7ᵗʰ **V86.92** Unspecified occupant of snowmobile injured in nontraffic accident

√x7ᵗʰ **V86.93** Unspecified occupant of dune buggy injured in nontraffic accident

√x7ᵗʰ **V86.94** Unspecified occupant of military vehicle injured in nontraffic accident

√x7ᵗʰ **V86.95** Unspecified occupant of 3- or 4- wheeled all-terrain vehicle (ATV) injured in nontraffic accident

√x7ᵗʰ **V86.96** Unspecified occupant of dirt bike or motor/cross bike injured in nontraffic accident

√x7ᵗʰ **V86.99** Unspecified occupant of other special all-terrain or other off-road motor vehicle injured in nontraffic accident

     Off-road motor-vehicle accident NOS

     Other motor-vehicle accident NOS

     Unspecified occupant of go cart injured in nontraffic accident

     Unspecified occupant of golf cart injured in nontraffic accident

√4ᵗʰ **V87** Traffic accident of specified type but victim's mode of transport unknown

     EXCLUDES 1   collision involving:

         pedal cycle (V10-V19)

         pedestrian (V01-V09)

√x7ᵗʰ **V87.0** Person injured in collision between car and two- or three-wheeled powered vehicle (traffic)

√x7ᵗʰ **V87.1** Person injured in collision between other motor vehicle and two- or three-wheeled motor vehicle (traffic)

√x7ᵗʰ **V87.2** Person injured in collision between car and pick-up truck or van (traffic)

√x7ᵗʰ **V87.3** Person injured in collision between car and bus (traffic)

√x7ᵗʰ **V87.4** Person injured in collision between car and heavy transport vehicle (traffic)

√x7ᵗʰ **V87.5** Person injured in collision between heavy transport vehicle and bus (traffic)

√x7ᵗʰ **V87.6** Person injured in collision between railway train or railway vehicle and car (traffic)

√x7ᵗʰ **V87.7** Person injured in collision between other specified motor vehicles (traffic)

√x7ᵗʰ **V87.8** Person injured in other specified noncollision transport accidents involving motor vehicle (traffic)

√x7ᵗʰ **V87.9** Person injured in other specified (collision)(noncollision) transport accidents involving nonmotor vehicle (traffic)

☑ Additional Character Required   √x7ᵗʰ Placeholder Alert   Manifestation   Unspecified Dx   ℚ QPP   UPD Unacceptable PDx

√4ᵗʰ **V88 Nontraffic accident of specified type but victim's mode of transport unknown**

> EXCLUDES 1 collision involving:
> pedal cycle (V10-V19)
> pedestrian (V01-V09)

√x7ᵗʰ **V88.0 Person injured in collision between** car and two- or three-wheeled motor vehicle, **nontraffic**

√x7ᵗʰ **V88.1 Person injured in collision between other** motor vehicle and two- or three-wheeled motor vehicle, **nontraffic**

√x7ᵗʰ **V88.2 Person injured in collision between** car and pick-up truck or van, **nontraffic**

√x7ᵗʰ **V88.3 Person injured in collision between** car and bus, **nontraffic**

√x7ᵗʰ **V88.4 Person injured in collision between** car and heavy transport vehicle, **nontraffic**

√x7ᵗʰ **V88.5 Person injured in collision between** heavy transport vehicle and bus, **nontraffic**

√x7ᵗʰ **V88.6 Person injured in collision between** railway train or railway vehicle and car, **nontraffic**

√x7ᵗʰ **V88.7 Person injured in collision between other specified motor vehicle, nontraffic**

√x7ᵗʰ **V88.8 Person injured in other specified** noncollision **transport accidents** involving motor vehicle, **nontraffic**

√x7ᵗʰ **V88.9 Person injured in other specified (collision)(noncollision) transport accidents** involving nonmotor vehicle, **nontraffic**

√4ᵗʰ **V89 Motor- or nonmotor-vehicle accident, type of vehicle unspecified**

√x7ᵗʰ **V89.0 Person injured in unspecified** motor-vehicle **accident, nontraffic**

> Motor-vehicle accident NOS, nontraffic

√x7ᵗʰ **V89.1 Person injured in unspecified** nonmotor-vehicle **accident, nontraffic**

> Nonmotor-vehicle accident NOS (nontraffic)

√x7ᵗʰ **V89.2 Person injured in unspecified** motor-vehicle **accident,** traffic

> Motor-vehicle accident [MVA] NOS
> Road (traffic) accident [RTA] NOS

√x7ᵗʰ **V89.3 Person injured in unspecified** nonmotor-vehicle **accident, traffic**

> Nonmotor-vehicle traffic accident NOS

√x7ᵗʰ **V89.9 Person injured in unspecified vehicle accident**

> Collision NOS

Water transport accidents (V90-V94)

The appropriate 7th character is to be added to each code from categories V90-V94.
A   initial encounter
D   subsequent encounter
S   sequela

√4ᵗʰ **V90 Drowning and submersion due to accident to watercraft**

> EXCLUDES 1 civilian water transport accident involving military watercraft (V94.81-)
> fall into water not from watercraft (W16.-)
> military watercraft accident in military or war operations (Y36.0-, Y37.0-)
> water-transport-related drowning or submersion without accident to watercraft (V92.-)

√5ᵗʰ **V90.0 Drowning and submersion due to** watercraft overturning

√x7ᵗʰ **V90.00 Drowning and submersion due to** merchant ship **overturning**

√x7ᵗʰ **V90.01 Drowning and submersion due to** passenger ship **overturning**

> Drowning and submersion due to Ferry-boat overturning
> Drowning and submersion due to Liner overturning

√x7ᵗʰ **V90.02 Drowning and submersion due to** fishing boat **overturning**

√x7ᵗʰ **V90.03 Drowning and submersion due to other** powered watercraft **overturning**

> Drowning and submersion due to Hovercraft (on open water) overturning
> Drowning and submersion due to Jet ski overturning

√x7ᵗʰ **V90.04 Drowning and submersion due to** sailboat **overturning**

√x7ᵗʰ **V90.05 Drowning and submersion due to** canoe or kayak **overturning**

√x7ᵗʰ **V90.06 Drowning and submersion due to (nonpowered)** inflatable craft **overturning**

√x7ᵗʰ **V90.08 Drowning and submersion due to other** unpowered watercraft **overturning**

> Drowning and submersion due to windsurfer overturning

√x7ᵗʰ **V90.09 Drowning and submersion due to unspecified watercraft overturning**

> Drowning and submersion due to boat NOS overturning
> Drowning and submersion due to ship NOS overturning
> Drowning and submersion due to watercraft NOS overturning

√5ᵗʰ **V90.1 Drowning and submersion due to** watercraft sinking

√x7ᵗʰ **V90.10 Drowning and submersion due to** merchant ship **sinking**

√x7ᵗʰ **V90.11 Drowning and submersion due to** passenger ship **sinking**

> Drowning and submersion due to Ferry-boat sinking
> Drowning and submersion due to Liner sinking

√x7ᵗʰ **V90.12 Drowning and submersion due to** fishing boat **sinking**

√x7ᵗʰ **V90.13 Drowning and submersion due to other** powered watercraft **sinking**

> Drowning and submersion due to Hovercraft (on open water) sinking
> Drowning and submersion due to Jet ski sinking

√x7ᵗʰ **V90.14 Drowning and submersion due to** sailboat **sinking**

√x7ᵗʰ **V90.15 Drowning and submersion due to** canoe or kayak **sinking**

√x7ᵗʰ **V90.16 Drowning and submersion due to (nonpowered)** inflatable craft **sinking**

√x7ᵗʰ **V90.18 Drowning and submersion due to other** unpowered watercraft **sinking**

√x7ᵗʰ **V90.19 Drowning and submersion due to unspecified watercraft sinking**

> Drowning and submersion due to boat NOS sinking
> Drowning and submersion due to ship NOS sinking
> Drowning and submersion due to watercraft NOS sinking

√5ᵗʰ **V90.2 Drowning and submersion due to** falling or jumping from burning watercraft

√x7ᵗʰ **V90.20 Drowning and submersion due to falling or jumping from burning** merchant ship

√x7ᵗʰ **V90.21 Drowning and submersion due to falling or jumping from burning** passenger ship

> Drowning and submersion due to falling or jumping from burning Ferry-boat
> Drowning and submersion due to falling or jumping from burning Liner

√x7ᵗʰ **V90.22 Drowning and submersion due to falling or jumping from burning** fishing boat

√x7ᵗʰ **V90.23 Drowning and submersion due to falling or jumping from other burning** powered **watercraft**

> Drowning and submersion due to falling and jumping from burning Hovercraft (on open water)
> Drowning and submersion due to falling and jumping from burning Jet ski

√x7ᵗʰ **V90.24 Drowning and submersion due to falling or jumping from burning** sailboat

√x7ᵗʰ **V90.25 Drowning and submersion due to falling or jumping from burning** canoe or kayak

√x7ᵗʰ **V90.26 Drowning and submersion due to falling or jumping from burning (nonpowered)** inflatable craft

√x7ᵗʰ **V90.27 Drowning and submersion due to falling or jumping from burning** water-skis

√x7ᵗʰ **V90.28 Drowning and submersion due to falling or jumping from other burning** unpowered **watercraft**

> Drowning and submersion due to falling and jumping from burning surf-board
> Drowning and submersion due to falling and jumping from burning windsurfer

√x7ᵗʰ **V90.29 Drowning and submersion due to falling or jumping from unspecified burning watercraft**

> Drowning and submersion due to falling or jumping from burning boat NOS
> Drowning and submersion due to falling or jumping from burning ship NOS
> Drowning and submersion due to falling or jumping from burning watercraft NOS

✓5ᵗʰ **V90.3** **Drowning and submersion due to** falling or jumping from crushed watercraft

✓x7ᵗʰ **V90.30** **Drowning and submersion due to falling or jumping from crushed** merchant ship

✓x7ᵗʰ **V90.31** **Drowning and submersion due to falling or jumping from crushed** passenger ship
Drowning and submersion due to falling and jumping from crushed Ferry boat
Drowning and submersion due to falling and jumping from crushed Liner

✓x7ᵗʰ **V90.32** **Drowning and submersion due to falling or jumping from crushed** fishing boat

✓x7ᵗʰ **V90.33** **Drowning and submersion due to falling or jumping from other crushed** powered **watercraft**
Drowning and submersion due to falling and jumping from crushed Hovercraft
Drowning and submersion due to falling and jumping from crushed Jet ski

✓x7ᵗʰ **V90.34** **Drowning and submersion due to falling or jumping from crushed** sailboat

✓x7ᵗʰ **V90.35** **Drowning and submersion due to falling or jumping from crushed** canoe or kayak

✓x7ᵗʰ **V90.36** **Drowning and submersion due to falling or jumping from crushed (nonpowered)** inflatable craft

✓x7ᵗʰ **V90.37** **Drowning and submersion due to falling or jumping from crushed** water-skis

✓x7ᵗʰ **V90.38** **Drowning and submersion due to falling or jumping from other crushed** unpowered **watercraft**
Drowning and submersion due to falling and jumping from crushed surf-board
Drowning and submersion due to falling and jumping from crushed windsurfer

✓x7ᵗʰ **V90.39** **Drowning and submersion due to falling or jumping from crushed unspecified watercraft**
Drowning and submersion due to falling and jumping from crushed boat NOS
Drowning and submersion due to falling and jumping from crushed ship NOS
Drowning and submersion due to falling and jumping from crushed watercraft NOS

✓5ᵗʰ **V90.8** **Drowning and submersion due to other accident to watercraft**

✓x7ᵗʰ **V90.80** **Drowning and submersion due to other accident to** merchant ship

✓x7ᵗʰ **V90.81** **Drowning and submersion due to other accident to** passenger ship
Drowning and submersion due to other accident to Ferry-boat
Drowning and submersion due to other accident to Liner

✓x7ᵗʰ **V90.82** **Drowning and submersion due to other accident to** fishing boat

✓x7ᵗʰ **V90.83** **Drowning and submersion due to other** powered **watercraft**
Drowning and submersion due to other accident to Hovercraft (on open water)
Drowning and submersion due to other accident to Jet ski

✓x7ᵗʰ **V90.84** **Drowning and submersion due to other accident to** sailboat

✓x7ᵗʰ **V90.85** **Drowning and submersion due to other accident to** canoe or kayak

✓x7ᵗʰ **V90.86** **Drowning and submersion due to other accident to (nonpowered)** inflatable craft

✓x7ᵗʰ **V90.87** **Drowning and submersion due to other accident to** water-skis

✓x7ᵗʰ **V90.88** **Drowning and submersion due to other accident to other** unpowered **watercraft**
Drowning and submersion due to other accident to surf-board
Drowning and submersion due to other accident to windsurfer

✓x7ᵗʰ **V90.89** **Drowning and submersion due to other accident to unspecified watercraft**
Drowning and submersion due to other accident to boat NOS
Drowning and submersion due to other accident to ship NOS
Drowning and submersion due to other accident to watercraft NOS

✓4ᵗʰ **V91** **Other injury due to accident to watercraft**

INCLUDES   any injury except drowning and submersion as a result of an accident to watercraft

EXCLUDES 1   civilian water transport accident involving military watercraft (V94.81-)
military watercraft accident in military or war operations (Y36, Y37.-)

EXCLUDES 2   drowning and submersion due to accident to watercraft (V90.-)

✓5ᵗʰ **V91.0** **Burn due to watercraft on fire**

EXCLUDES 1   burn from localized fire or explosion on board ship without accident to watercraft (V93.-)

✓x7ᵗʰ **V91.00** **Burn due to** merchant ship **on fire**

✓x7ᵗʰ **V91.01** **Burn due to** passenger ship **on fire**
Burn due to Ferry-boat on fire
Burn due to Liner on fire

✓x7ᵗʰ **V91.02** **Burn due to** fishing boat **on fire**

✓x7ᵗʰ **V91.03** **Burn due to other** powered **watercraft on fire**
Burn due to Hovercraft (on open water) on fire
Burn due to Jet ski on fire

✓x7ᵗʰ **V91.04** **Burn due to** sailboat **on fire**

✓x7ᵗʰ **V91.05** **Burn due to** canoe or kayak **on fire**

✓x7ᵗʰ **V91.06** **Burn due to (nonpowered)** inflatable craft **on fire**

✓x7ᵗʰ **V91.07** **Burn due to** water-skis **on fire**

✓x7ᵗʰ **V91.08** **Burn due to other** unpowered **watercraft on fire**

✓x7ᵗʰ **V91.09** **Burn due to unspecified watercraft on fire**
Burn due to boat NOS on fire
Burn due to ship NOS on fire
Burn due to watercraft NOS on fire

✓5ᵗʰ **V91.1** **Crushed between watercraft and other watercraft or other object due to collision**
Crushed by lifeboat after abandoning ship in a collision

NOTE   Select the specified type of watercraft that the victim was on at the time of the collision

✓x7ᵗʰ **V91.10** **Crushed between** merchant ship **and other watercraft or other object due to collision**

✓x7ᵗʰ **V91.11** **Crushed between** passenger ship **and other watercraft or other object due to collision**
Crushed between Ferry-boat and other watercraft or other object due to collision
Crushed between Liner and other watercraft or other object due to collision

✓x7ᵗʰ **V91.12** **Crushed between** fishing boat **and other watercraft or other object due to collision**

✓x7ᵗʰ **V91.13** **Crushed between other** powered **watercraft and other watercraft or other object due to collision**
Crushed between Hovercraft (on open water) and other watercraft or other object due to collision
Crushed between Jet ski and other watercraft or other object due to collision

✓x7ᵗʰ **V91.14** **Crushed between** sailboat **and other watercraft or other object due to collision**

✓x7ᵗʰ **V91.15** **Crushed between** canoe or kayak **and other watercraft or other object due to collision**

✓x7ᵗʰ **V91.16** **Crushed between (nonpowered)** inflatable craft **and other watercraft or other object due to collision**

✓x7ᵗʰ **V91.18** **Crushed between other** unpowered **watercraft and other watercraft or other object due to collision**
Crushed between surfboard and other watercraft or other object due to collision
Crushed between windsurfer and other watercraft or other object due to collision

√x7ᵗʰ **V91.19 Crushed between unspecified watercraft and other watercraft or other object due to collision**
Crushed between boat NOS and other watercraft or other object due to collision
Crushed between ship NOS and other watercraft or other object due to collision
Crushed between watercraft NOS and other watercraft or other object due to collision

√5ᵗʰ **V91.2 Fall due to collision between watercraft and other watercraft or other object**
Fall while remaining on watercraft after collision

NOTE Select the specified type of watercraft that the victim was on at the time of the collision

EXCLUDES 1 *crushed between watercraft and other watercraft and other object due to collision (V91.1-)*
drowning and submersion due to falling from crushed watercraft (V90.3-)

√x7ᵗʰ **V91.20 Fall due to collision between merchant ship and other watercraft or other object**

√x7ᵗʰ **V91.21 Fall due to collision between passenger ship and other watercraft or other object**
Fall due to collision between Ferry-boat and other watercraft or other object
Fall due to collision between Liner and other watercraft or other object

√x7ᵗʰ **V91.22 Fall due to collision between fishing boat and other watercraft or other object**

√x7ᵗʰ **V91.23 Fall due to collision between other powered watercraft and other watercraft or other object**
Fall due to collision between Hovercraft (on open water) and other watercraft or other object
Fall due to collision between Jet ski and other watercraft or other object

√x7ᵗʰ **V91.24 Fall due to collision between sailboat and other watercraft or other object**

√x7ᵗʰ **V91.25 Fall due to collision between canoe or kayak and other watercraft or other object**

√x7ᵗʰ **V91.26 Fall due to collision between (nonpowered) inflatable craft and other watercraft or other object**

√x7ᵗʰ **V91.29 Fall due to collision between unspecified watercraft and other watercraft or other object**
Fall due to collision between boat NOS and other watercraft or other object
Fall due to collision between ship NOS and other watercraft or other object
Fall due to collision between watercraft NOS and other watercraft or other object

√5ᵗʰ **V91.3 Hit or struck by falling object due to accident to watercraft**
Hit or struck by falling object (part of damaged watercraft or other object) after falling or jumping from damaged watercraft

EXCLUDES 2 *drowning or submersion due to fall or jumping from damaged watercraft (V90.2-, V90.3-)*

√x7ᵗʰ **V91.30 Hit or struck by falling object due to accident to merchant ship**

√x7ᵗʰ **V91.31 Hit or struck by falling object due to accident to passenger ship**
Hit or struck by falling object due to accident to Ferry-boat
Hit or struck by falling object due to accident to Liner

√x7ᵗʰ **V91.32 Hit or struck by falling object due to accident to fishing boat**

√x7ᵗʰ **V91.33 Hit or struck by falling object due to accident to other powered watercraft**
Hit or struck by falling object due to accident to Hovercraft (on open water)
Hit or struck by falling object due to accident to Jet ski

√x7ᵗʰ **V91.34 Hit or struck by falling object due to accident to sailboat**

√x7ᵗʰ **V91.35 Hit or struck by falling object due to accident to canoe or kayak**

√x7ᵗʰ **V91.36 Hit or struck by falling object due to accident to (nonpowered) inflatable craft**

√x7ᵗʰ **V91.37 Hit or struck by falling object due to accident to water-skis**
Hit by water-skis after jumping off of waterskis

√x7ᵗʰ **V91.38 Hit or struck by falling object due to accident to other unpowered watercraft**
Hit or struck by surf-board after falling off damaged surf-board
Hit or struck by windsurfer after falling off damaged windsurfer

√x7ᵗʰ **V91.39 Hit or struck by falling object due to accident to unspecified watercraft**
Hit or struck by falling object due to accident to boat NOS
Hit or struck by falling object due to accident to ship NOS
Hit or struck by falling object due to accident to watercraft NOS

√5ᵗʰ **V91.8 Other injury due to other accident to watercraft**

√x7ᵗʰ **V91.80 Other injury due to other accident to merchant ship**

√x7ᵗʰ **V91.81 Other injury due to other accident to passenger ship**
Other injury due to other accident to Ferry-boat
Other injury due to other accident to Liner

√x7ᵗʰ **V91.82 Other injury due to other accident to fishing boat**

√x7ᵗʰ **V91.83 Other injury due to other accident to other powered watercraft**
Other injury due to other accident to Hovercraft (on open water)
Other injury due to other accident to Jet ski

√x7ᵗʰ **V91.84 Other injury due to other accident to sailboat**

√x7ᵗʰ **V91.85 Other injury due to other accident to canoe or kayak**

√x7ᵗʰ **V91.86 Other injury due to other accident to (nonpowered) inflatable craft**

√x7ᵗʰ **V91.87 Other injury due to other accident to water-skis**

√x7ᵗʰ **V91.88 Other injury due to other accident to other unpowered watercraft**
Other injury due to other accident to surf-board
Other injury due to other accident to windsurfer

√x7ᵗʰ **V91.89 Other injury due to other accident to unspecified watercraft**
Other injury due to other accident to boat NOS
Other injury due to other accident to ship NOS
Other injury due to other accident to watercraft NOS

√4ᵗʰ **V92 Drowning and submersion due to accident on board watercraft, without accident to watercraft**

EXCLUDES 1 *civilian water transport accident involving military watercraft (V94.81-)*
drowning or submersion due to accident to watercraft (V90-V91)
drowning or submersion of diver who voluntarily jumps from boat not involved in an accident (W16.711, W16.721)
fall into water without watercraft (W16.-)
military watercraft accident in military or war operations (Y36, Y37)

√5ᵗʰ **V92.0 Drowning and submersion due to fall off watercraft**
Drowning and submersion due to fall from gangplank of watercraft
Drowning and submersion due to fall overboard watercraft

EXCLUDES 2 *hitting head on object or bottom of body of water due to fall from watercraft (V94.0-)*

√x7ᵗʰ **V92.00 Drowning and submersion due to fall off merchant ship**

√x7ᵗʰ **V92.01 Drowning and submersion due to fall off passenger ship**
Drowning and submersion due to fall off Ferry-boat
Drowning and submersion due to fall off Liner

√x7ᵗʰ **V92.02 Drowning and submersion due to fall off fishing boat**

√x7ᵗʰ **V92.03 Drowning and submersion due to fall off other powered watercraft**
Drowning and submersion due to fall off Hovercraft (on open water)
Drowning and submersion due to fall off Jet ski

√x7ᵗʰ **V92.04 Drowning and submersion due to fall off sailboat**

√x7ᵗʰ **V92.05 Drowning and submersion due to fall off canoe or kayak**

√x7ᵗʰ **V92.06 Drowning and submersion due to fall off (nonpowered) inflatable craft**

✓x7th **V92.07 Drowning and submersion due to fall off** water-skis

    EXCLUDES 1   *drowning and submersion due to falling off burning water-skis (V90.27)*

            drowning and submersion due to falling off crushed water-skis (V90.37)

            hit by boat while water-skiing NOS (V94.X)

✓x7th **V92.08 Drowning and submersion due to fall off other** unpowered **watercraft**

     Drowning and submersion due to fall off surf-board

     Drowning and submersion due to fall off windsurfer

    EXCLUDES 1   *drowning and submersion due to fall off burning unpowered watercraft (V90.28)*

            drowning and submersion due to fall off crushed unpowered watercraft (V90.38)

            drowning and submersion due to fall off damaged unpowered watercraft (V90.88)

            drowning and submersion due to rider of nonpowered watercraft being hit by other watercraft (V94.-)

            other injury due to rider of nonpowered watercraft being hit by other watercraft (V94.-)

✓x7th **V92.09 Drowning and submersion due to fall off unspecified watercraft**

     Drowning and submersion due to fall off boat NOS

     Drowning and submersion due to fall off ship

     Drowning and submersion due to fall off watercraft NOS

✓5th **V92.1 Drowning and submersion due to being** thrown overboard **by motion of watercraft**

    EXCLUDES 1   *drowning and submersion due to fall off surf-board (V92.08)*

            drowning and submersion due to fall off water-skis (V92.07)

            drowning and submersion due to fall off windsurfer (V92.08)

✓x7th **V92.10 Drowning and submersion due to being thrown overboard by motion of** merchant ship

✓x7th **V92.11 Drowning and submersion due to being thrown overboard by motion of** passenger ship

     Drowning and submersion due to being thrown overboard by motion of Ferry-boat

     Drowning and submersion due to being thrown overboard by motion of Liner

✓x7th **V92.12 Drowning and submersion due to being thrown overboard by motion of** fishing boat

✓x7th **V92.13 Drowning and submersion due to being thrown overboard by motion of other** powered **watercraft**

     Drowning and submersion due to being thrown overboard by motion of Hovercraft

✓x7th **V92.14 Drowning and submersion due to being thrown overboard by motion of** sailboat

✓x7th **V92.15 Drowning and submersion due to being thrown overboard by motion of** canoe or kayak

✓x7th **V92.16 Drowning and submersion due to being thrown overboard by motion of** (nonpowered) inflatable craft

✓x7th **V92.19 Drowning and submersion due to being thrown overboard by motion of unspecified watercraft**

     Drowning and submersion due to being thrown overboard by motion of boat NOS

     Drowning and submersion due to being thrown overboard by motion of ship NOS

     Drowning and submersion due to being thrown overboard by motion of watercraft NOS

✓5th **V92.2 Drowning and submersion due to being** washed overboard **from watercraft**

     Code first any associated cataclysm (X37.0-)

✓x7th **V92.20 Drowning and submersion due to being washed overboard from** merchant ship

✓x7th **V92.21 Drowning and submersion due to being washed overboard from** passenger ship

     Drowning and submersion due to being washed overboard from Ferry-boat

     Drowning and submersion due to being washed overboard from Liner

✓x7th **V92.22 Drowning and submersion due to being washed overboard from** fishing boat

✓x7th **V92.23 Drowning and submersion due to being washed overboard from other** powered **watercraft**

     Drowning and submersion due to being washed overboard from Hovercraft (on open water)

     Drowning and submersion due to being washed overboard from Jet ski

✓x7th **V92.24 Drowning and submersion due to being washed overboard from** sailboat

✓x7th **V92.25 Drowning and submersion due to being washed overboard from** canoe or kayak

✓x7th **V92.26 Drowning and submersion due to being washed overboard from** (nonpowered) inflatable craft

✓x7th **V92.27 Drowning and submersion due to being washed overboard from** water-skis

    EXCLUDES 1   *drowning and submersion due to fall off water-skis (V92.07)*

✓x7th **V92.28 Drowning and submersion due to being washed overboard from other** unpowered **watercraft**

     Drowning and submersion due to being washed overboard from surf-board

     Drowning and submersion due to being washed overboard from windsurfer

✓x7th **V92.29 Drowning and submersion due to being washed overboard from unspecified watercraft**

     Drowning and submersion due to being washed overboard from boat NOS

     Drowning and submersion due to being washed overboard from ship NOS

     Drowning and submersion due to being washed overboard from watercraft NOS

✓4th **V93 Other injury due to accident on board watercraft, without accident to watercraft**

    EXCLUDES 1   *civilian water transport accident involving military watercraft (V94.81-)*

            other injury due to accident to watercraft (V91.-)

            military watercraft accident in military or war operations (Y36, Y37.-)

    EXCLUDES 2   *drowning and submersion due to accident on board watercraft, without accident to watercraft (V92.-)*

✓5th **V93.0 Burn due to localized fire on board watercraft**

    EXCLUDES 1   *burn due to watercraft on fire (V91.0-)*

✓x7th **V93.00 Burn due to localized fire on board** merchant vessel

✓x7th **V93.01 Burn due to localized fire on board** passenger vessel

     Burn due to localized fire on board Ferry-boat

     Burn due to localized fire on board Liner

✓x7th **V93.02 Burn due to localized fire on board** fishing boat

✓x7th **V93.03 Burn due to localized fire on board other** powered **watercraft**

     Burn due to localized fire on board Hovercraft

     Burn due to localized fire on board Jet ski

✓x7th **V93.04 Burn due to localized fire on board** sailboat

✓x7th **V93.09 Burn due to localized fire on board unspecified watercraft**

     Burn due to localized fire on board boat NOS

     Burn due to localized fire on board ship NOS

     Burn due to localized fire on board watercraft NOS

✓5th **V93.1 Other burn on board watercraft**

     Burn due to source other than fire on board watercraft

    EXCLUDES 1   *burn due to watercraft on fire (V91.0-)*

✓x7th **V93.10 Other burn on board** merchant vessel

✓x7th **V93.11 Other burn on board** passenger vessel

     Other burn on board Ferry-boat

     Other burn on board Liner

✓x7th **V93.12 Other burn on board** fishing boat

✓x7th **V93.13 Other burn on board other** powered **watercraft**

     Other burn on board Hovercraft

     Other burn on board Jet ski

✓x7th **V93.14 Other burn on board** sailboat

☑ Additional Character Required   ✓x7th Placeholder Alert   Manifestation   Unspecified Dx   Q QPP   UPD Unacceptable PDx

√x7ᵗʰ **V93.19 Other burn on board unspecified watercraft**
  Other burn on board boat NOS
  Other burn on board ship NOS
  Other burn on board watercraft NOS

√5ᵗʰ **V93.2 Heat exposure on board watercraft**
  EXCLUDES 1   exposure to man-made heat not aboard watercraft (W92)
  exposure to natural heat while on board watercraft (X30)
  exposure to sunlight while on board watercraft (X32)
  EXCLUDES 2   burn due to fire on board watercraft (V93.0-)

√x7ᵗʰ **V93.20 Heat exposure on board merchant ship**

√x7ᵗʰ **V93.21 Heat exposure on board passenger ship**
  Heat exposure on board Ferry-boat
  Heat exposure on board Liner

√x7ᵗʰ **V93.22 Heat exposure on board fishing boat**

√x7ᵗʰ **V93.23 Heat exposure on board other powered watercraft**
  Heat exposure on board hovercraft

√x7ᵗʰ **V93.24 Heat exposure on board sailboat**

√x7ᵗʰ **V93.29 Heat exposure on board unspecified watercraft**
  Heat exposure on board boat NOS
  Heat exposure on board ship NOS
  Heat exposure on board watercraft NOS

√5ᵗʰ **V93.3 Fall on board watercraft**
  EXCLUDES 1   fall due to collision of watercraft (V91.2-)

√x7ᵗʰ **V93.30 Fall on board merchant ship**

√x7ᵗʰ **V93.31 Fall on board passenger ship**
  Fall on board Ferry-boat
  Fall on board Liner

√x7ᵗʰ **V93.32 Fall on board fishing boat**

√x7ᵗʰ **V93.33 Fall on board other powered watercraft**
  Fall on board Hovercraft (on open water)
  Fall on board Jet ski

√x7ᵗʰ **V93.34 Fall on board sailboat**

√x7ᵗʰ **V93.35 Fall on board canoe or kayak**

√x7ᵗʰ **V93.36 Fall on board (nonpowered) inflatable craft**

√x7ᵗʰ **V93.38 Fall on board other unpowered watercraft**

√x7ᵗʰ **V93.39 Fall on board unspecified watercraft**
  Fall on board boat NOS
  Fall on board ship NOS
  Fall on board watercraft NOS

√5ᵗʰ **V93.4 Struck by falling object on board watercraft**
  Hit by falling object on board watercraft
  EXCLUDES 1   struck by falling object due to accident to watercraft (V91.3)

√x7ᵗʰ **V93.40 Struck by falling object on merchant ship**

√x7ᵗʰ **V93.41 Struck by falling object on passenger ship**
  Struck by falling object on Ferry-boat
  Struck by falling object on Liner

√x7ᵗʰ **V93.42 Struck by falling object on fishing boat**

√x7ᵗʰ **V93.43 Struck by falling object on other powered watercraft**
  Struck by falling object on Hovercraft

√x7ᵗʰ **V93.44 Struck by falling object on sailboat**

√x7ᵗʰ **V93.48 Struck by falling object on other unpowered watercraft**

√x7ᵗʰ **V93.49 Struck by falling object on unspecified watercraft**

√5ᵗʰ **V93.5 Explosion on board watercraft**
  Boiler explosion on steamship
  EXCLUDES 2   fire on board watercraft (V93.0-)

√x7ᵗʰ **V93.50 Explosion on board merchant ship**

√x7ᵗʰ **V93.51 Explosion on board passenger ship**
  Explosion on board Ferry-boat
  Explosion on board Liner

√x7ᵗʰ **V93.52 Explosion on board fishing boat**

√x7ᵗʰ **V93.53 Explosion on board other powered watercraft**
  Explosion on board Hovercraft
  Explosion on board Jet ski

√x7ᵗʰ **V93.54 Explosion on board sailboat**

√x7ᵗʰ **V93.59 Explosion on board unspecified watercraft**
  Explosion on board boat NOS
  Explosion on board ship NOS
  Explosion on board watercraft NOS

√5ᵗʰ **V93.6 Machinery accident on board watercraft**
  EXCLUDES 1   machinery explosion on board watercraft (V93.4-)
  machinery fire on board watercraft (V93.0-)

√x7ᵗʰ **V93.60 Machinery accident on board merchant ship**

√x7ᵗʰ **V93.61 Machinery accident on board passenger ship**
  Machinery accident on board Ferry-boat
  Machinery accident on board Liner

√x7ᵗʰ **V93.62 Machinery accident on board fishing boat**

√x7ᵗʰ **V93.63 Machinery accident on board other powered watercraft**
  Machinery accident on board Hovercraft

√x7ᵗʰ **V93.64 Machinery accident on board sailboat**

√x7ᵗʰ **V93.69 Machinery accident on board unspecified watercraft**
  Machinery accident on board boat NOS
  Machinery accident on board ship NOS
  Machinery accident on board watercraft NOS

√5ᵗʰ **V93.8 Other injury due to other accident on board watercraft**
  Accidental poisoning by gases or fumes on watercraft

√x7ᵗʰ **V93.80 Other injury due to other accident on board merchant ship**

√x7ᵗʰ **V93.81 Other injury due to other accident on board passenger ship**
  Other injury due to other accident on board Ferry-boat
  Other injury due to other accident on board Liner

√x7ᵗʰ **V93.82 Other injury due to other accident on board fishing boat**

√x7ᵗʰ **V93.83 Other injury due to other accident on board other powered watercraft**
  Other injury due to other accident on board Hovercraft
  Other injury due to other accident on board Jet ski

√x7ᵗʰ **V93.84 Other injury due to other accident on board sailboat**

√x7ᵗʰ **V93.85 Other injury due to other accident on board canoe or kayak**

√x7ᵗʰ **V93.86 Other injury due to other accident on board (nonpowered) inflatable craft**

√x7ᵗʰ **V93.87 Other injury due to other accident on board water-skis**
  Hit or struck by object while waterskiing

√x7ᵗʰ **V93.88 Other injury due to other accident on board other unpowered watercraft**
  Hit or struck by object while surfing
  Hit or struck by object while on board windsurfer

√x7ᵗʰ **V93.89 Other injury due to other accident on board unspecified watercraft**
  Other injury due to other accident on board boat NOS
  Other injury due to other accident on board ship NOS
  Other injury due to other accident on board watercraft NOS

√4ᵗʰ **V94 Other and unspecified water transport accidents**
  EXCLUDES 1   military watercraft accidents in military or war operations (Y36, Y37)

√x7ᵗʰ **V94.0 Hitting object or bottom of body of water due to fall from watercraft**
  EXCLUDES 2   drowning and submersion due to fall from watercraft (V92.0-)

√5ᵗʰ **V94.1 Bather struck by watercraft**
  Swimmer hit by watercraft

√x7ᵗʰ **V94.11 Bather struck by powered watercraft**

√x7ᵗʰ **V94.12 Bather struck by nonpowered watercraft**

√5ᵗʰ **V94.2 Rider of nonpowered watercraft struck by other watercraft**

√x7ᵗʰ **V94.21 Rider of nonpowered watercraft struck by other nonpowered watercraft**
  Canoer hit by other nonpowered watercraft
  Surfer hit by other nonpowered watercraft
  Windsurfer hit by other nonpowered watercraft

√x7ᵗʰ V94.22 Rider of nonpowered watercraft struck by powered **watercraft**
     Canoer hit by motorboat
     Surfer hit by motorboat
     Windsurfer hit by motorboat

√5ᵗʰ V94.3 Injury to rider of (inflatable) watercraft being pulled behind other watercraft

  √x7ᵗʰ V94.31 Injury to rider of (inflatable) recreational **watercraft being pulled behind other watercraft**
     Injury to rider of inner-tube pulled behind motor boat

  √x7ᵗʰ V94.32 Injury to rider of non-recreational **watercraft being pulled behind other watercraft**
     Injury to occupant of dingy being pulled behind boat or ship
     Injury to occupant of life-raft being pulled behind boat or ship

√x7ᵗʰ V94.4 Injury to barefoot water-skier
     Injury to person being pulled behind boat or ship

√5ᵗʰ V94.8 Other water transport accident

  √6ᵗʰ V94.81 Water transport accident involving military watercraft

    √7ᵗʰ V94.810 Civilian watercraft involved in water transport accident with military watercraft
       Passenger on civilian watercraft injured due to accident with military watercraft

    √7ᵗʰ V94.811 Civilian in water injured by military watercraft

    √7ᵗʰ V94.818 Other water transport accident involving military watercraft

  √x7ᵗʰ V94.89 Other water transport accident

√x7ᵗʰ V94.9 Unspecified water transport accident
     Water transport accident NOS

Air and space transport accidents (V95-V97)

EXCLUDES 1   *military aircraft accidents in military or war operations (Y36, Y37)*

The appropriate 7th character is to be added to each code from categories V95-V97.
A   initial encounter
D   subsequent encounter
S   sequela

√4ᵗʰ V95 Accident to powered aircraft causing injury to occupant

 √5ᵗʰ V95.0 Helicopter **accident injuring occupant**

  √x7ᵗʰ V95.00 Unspecified helicopter accident injuring occupant

  √x7ᵗʰ V95.01 Helicopter crash **injuring occupant**

  √x7ᵗʰ V95.02 Forced landing **of helicopter injuring occupant**

  √x7ᵗʰ V95.03 Helicopter collision **injuring occupant**
     Helicopter collision with any object, fixed, movable or moving

  √x7ᵗʰ V95.04 Helicopter fire **injuring occupant**

  √x7ᵗʰ V95.05 Helicopter explosion **injuring occupant**

  √x7ᵗʰ V95.09 Other helicopter accident injuring occupant

 √5ᵗʰ V95.1 Ultralight, microlight or powered-glider **accident injuring occupant**

  √x7ᵗʰ V95.10 Unspecified ultralight, microlight or powered-glider accident injuring occupant

  √x7ᵗʰ V95.11 Ultralight, microlight or powered-glider crash **injuring occupant**

  √x7ᵗʰ V95.12 Forced landing **of ultralight, microlight or powered-glider injuring occupant**

  √x7ᵗʰ V95.13 Ultralight, microlight or powered-glider collision **injuring occupant**
     Ultralight, microlight or powered-glider collision with any object, fixed, movable or moving

  √x7ᵗʰ V95.14 Ultralight, microlight or powered-glider fire **injuring occupant**

  √x7ᵗʰ V95.15 Ultralight, microlight or powered-glider explosion **injuring occupant**

  √x7ᵗʰ V95.19 Other ultralight, microlight or powered-glider accident injuring occupant

 √5ᵗʰ V95.2 Other private fixed-wing aircraft accident injuring occupant

  √x7ᵗʰ V95.20 Unspecified accident to other private fixed-wing aircraft, injuring occupant

  √x7ᵗʰ V95.21 Other private fixed-wing aircraft crash injuring occupant

  √x7ᵗʰ V95.22 Forced landing **of other private fixed-wing aircraft injuring occupant**

  √x7ᵗʰ V95.23 Other private fixed-wing aircraft collision **injuring occupant**
     Other private fixed-wing aircraft collision with any object, fixed, movable or moving

  √x7ᵗʰ V95.24 Other private fixed-wing aircraft fire **injuring occupant**

  √x7ᵗʰ V95.25 Other private fixed-wing aircraft explosion **injuring occupant**

  √x7ᵗʰ V95.29 Other accident to other private fixed-wing aircraft injuring occupant

 √6ᵗʰ V95.3 Commercial fixed-wing **aircraft accident injuring occupant**

  √x7ᵗʰ V95.30 Unspecified accident to commercial fixed-wing aircraft injuring occupant

  √x7ᵗʰ V95.31 Commercial fixed-wing aircraft crash injuring occupant

  √x7ᵗʰ V95.32 Forced landing **of commercial fixed-wing aircraft injuring occupant**

  √x7ᵗʰ V95.33 Commercial fixed-wing aircraft collision **injuring occupant**
     Commercial fixed-wing aircraft collision with any object, fixed, movable or moving

  √x7ᵗʰ V95.34 Commercial fixed-wing aircraft fire **injuring occupant**

  √x7ᵗʰ V95.35 Commercial fixed-wing aircraft explosion **injuring occupant**

  √x7ᵗʰ V95.39 Other accident to commercial fixed-wing aircraft injuring occupant

 √5ᵗʰ V95.4 Spacecraft **accident injuring occupant**

  √x7ᵗʰ V95.40 Unspecified spacecraft accident injuring occupant

  √x7ᵗʰ V95.41 Spacecraft crash **injuring occupant**

  √x7ᵗʰ V95.42 Forced landing **of spacecraft injuring occupant**

  √x7ᵗʰ V95.43 Spacecraft collision **injuring occupant**
     Spacecraft collision with any object, fixed, moveable or moving

  √x7ᵗʰ V95.44 Spacecraft fire **injuring occupant**

  √x7ᵗʰ V95.45 Spacecraft explosion **injuring occupant**

  √x7ᵗʰ V95.49 Other spacecraft accident injuring occupant

 √x7ᵗʰ V95.8 Other powered aircraft accidents injuring occupant

 √x7ᵗʰ V95.9 Unspecified aircraft accident injuring occupant
     Aircraft accident NOS
     Air transport accident NOS

√4ᵗʰ V96 Accident to nonpowered aircraft causing injury to occupant

 √5ᵗʰ V96.0 Balloon **accident injuring occupant**

  √x7ᵗʰ V96.00 Unspecified balloon accident injuring occupant

  √x7ᵗʰ V96.01 Balloon crash **injuring occupant**

  √x7ᵗʰ V96.02 Forced landing **of balloon injuring occupant**

  √x7ᵗʰ V96.03 Balloon collision **injuring occupant**
     Balloon collision with any object, fixed, moveable or moving

  √x7ᵗʰ V96.04 Balloon fire **injuring occupant**

  √x7ᵗʰ V96.05 Balloon explosion **injuring occupant**

  √x7ᵗʰ V96.09 Other balloon accident injuring occupant

 √5ᵗʰ V96.1 Hang-glider **accident injuring occupant**

  √x7ᵗʰ V96.10 Unspecified hang-glider accident injuring occupant

  √x7ᵗʰ V96.11 Hang-glider crash **injuring occupant**

  √x7ᵗʰ V96.12 Forced landing **of hang-glider injuring occupant**

  √x7ᵗʰ V96.13 Hang-glider collision **injuring occupant**
     Hang-glider collision with any object, fixed, moveable or moving

  √x7ᵗʰ V96.14 Hang-glider fire **injuring occupant**

  √x7ᵗʰ V96.15 Hang-glider explosion **injuring occupant**

  √x7ᵗʰ V96.19 Other hang-glider accident injuring occupant

 √6ᵗʰ V96.2 Glider (nonpowered) **accident injuring occupant**

  √x7ᵗʰ V96.20 Unspecified glider (nonpowered) accident injuring occupant

  √x7ᵗʰ V96.21 Glider (nonpowered) crash injuring occupant

  √x7ᵗʰ V96.22 Forced landing **of glider (nonpowered) injuring occupant**

√x7ᵗʰ **V96.23 Glider (nonpowered) collision injuring occupant**
　　　Glider (nonpowered) collision with any object, fixed, moveable or moving

√x7ᵗʰ **V96.24 Glider (nonpowered) fire injuring occupant**

√x7ᵗʰ **V96.25 Glider (nonpowered) explosion injuring occupant**

√x7ᵗʰ **V96.29 Other glider (nonpowered) accident injuring occupant**

√x7ᵗʰ **V96.8 Other nonpowered-aircraft accidents injuring occupant**
　　　Kite carrying a person accident injuring occupant

√x7ᵗʰ **V96.9 Unspecified nonpowered-aircraft accident injuring occupant**
　　　Nonpowered-aircraft accident NOS

√4ᵗʰ **V97 Other specified air transport accidents**

√x7ᵗʰ **V97.0 Occupant of aircraft injured in other specified air transport accidents**
　　　Fall in, on or from aircraft in air transport accident
　　　EXCLUDES 1　*accident while boarding or alighting aircraft (V97.1)*

√x7ᵗʰ **V97.1 Person injured while boarding or alighting from aircraft**

√5ᵗʰ **V97.2 Parachutist accident**

　　√x7ᵗʰ **V97.21 Parachutist entangled in object**
　　　　Parachutist landing in tree

　　√x7ᵗʰ **V97.22 Parachutist injured on landing**

　　√x7ᵗʰ **V97.29 Other parachutist accident**

√5ᵗʰ **V97.3 Person on ground injured in air transport accident**

　　√x7ᵗʰ **V97.31 Hit by object falling from aircraft**
　　　　Hit by crashing aircraft
　　　　Injured by aircraft hitting house
　　　　Injured by aircraft hitting car

　　√x7ᵗʰ **V97.32 Injured by rotating propeller**

　　√x7ᵗʰ **V97.33 Sucked into jet engine**

　　√x7ᵗʰ **V97.39 Other injury to person on ground due to air transport accident**

√5ᵗʰ **V97.8 Other air transport accidents, not elsewhere classified**
　　EXCLUDES 1　*aircraft accident NOS (V95.9)*
　　　　exposure to changes in air pressure during ascent or descent (V94.-)

　　√6ᵗʰ **V97.81 Air transport accident involving military aircraft**

　　　√7ᵗʰ **V97.810 Civilian aircraft involved in air transport accident with military aircraft**
　　　　　Passenger in civilian aircraft injured due to accident with military aircraft

　　　√7ᵗʰ **V97.811 Civilian injured by military aircraft**

　　　√7ᵗʰ **V97.818 Other air transport accident involving military aircraft**

　　√x7ᵗʰ **V97.89 Other air transport accidents, not elsewhere classified**
　　　　Injury from machinery on aircraft

Other and unspecified transport accidents (V98-V99)

EXCLUDES 1　*vehicle accident, type of vehicle unspecified (V89.-)*

The appropriate 7th character is to be added to each code from categories V98-V99.
A　initial encounter
D　subsequent encounter
S　sequela

√4ᵗʰ **V98 Other specified transport accidents**

√x7ᵗʰ **V98.0 Accident to, on or involving cable-car, not on rails**
　　　Caught or dragged by cable-car, not on rails
　　　Fall or jump from cable-car, not on rails
　　　Object thrown from or in cable-car, not on rails

√x7ᵗʰ **V98.1 Accident to, on or involving land-yacht**

√x7ᵗʰ **V98.2 Accident to, on or involving ice yacht**

√x7ᵗʰ **V98.3 Accident to, on or involving ski lift**
　　　Accident to, on or involving ski chair-lift
　　　Accident to, on or involving ski-lift with gondola

√x7ᵗʰ **V98.8 Other specified transport accidents**

√x7ᵗʰ **V99 Unspecified transport accident**

OTHER EXTERNAL CAUSES OF ACCIDENTAL INJURY (W00-X58)

Slipping, tripping, stumbling and falls (W00-W19)

EXCLUDES 1　*assault involving a fall (Y01-Y02)*
　　　fall from animal (V80.-)
　　　fall (in) (from) machinery (in operation) (W28-W31)
　　　fall (in) (from) transport vehicle (V01-V99)
　　　intentional self-harm involving a fall (X80-X81)

EXCLUDES 2　*at risk for fall (history of fall) Z91.81*
　　　fall (in) (from) burning building (X00.-)
　　　fall into fire (X00-X04, X08)

The appropriate 7th character is to be added to each code from categories W00-W19.
A　initial encounter
D　subsequent encounter
S　sequela

√4ᵗʰ **W00 Fall due to ice and snow**
　　INCLUDES　pedestrian on foot falling (slipping) on ice and snow
　　EXCLUDES 1　*fall on (from) ice and snow involving pedestrian conveyance (V00.-)*
　　　fall from stairs and steps not due to ice and snow (W10.-)
　　AHA: 2016,2Q,4

√x7ᵗʰ **W00.0 Fall on same level due to ice and snow**

√x7ᵗʰ **W00.1 Fall from stairs and steps due to ice and snow**

√x7ᵗʰ **W00.2 Other fall from one level to another due to ice and snow**

√x7ᵗʰ **W00.9 Unspecified fall due to ice and snow**

√4ᵗʰ **W01 Fall on same level from slipping, tripping and stumbling**
　　INCLUDES　fall on moving sidewalk
　　EXCLUDES 1　*fall due to bumping (striking) against object (W18.0-)*
　　　fall in shower or bathtub (W18.2-)
　　　fall on same level NOS (W18.30)
　　　fall on same level from slipping, tripping and stumbling due to ice or snow (W00.0)
　　　fall off or from toilet (W18.1-)
　　　slipping, tripping and stumbling NOS (W18.40)
　　　slipping, tripping and stumbling without falling (W18.4-)

√x7ᵗʰ **W01.0 Fall on same level from slipping, tripping and stumbling without subsequent striking against object**
　　　Falling over animal

√5ᵗʰ **W01.1 Fall on same level from slipping, tripping and stumbling with subsequent striking against object**

　　√x7ᵗʰ **W01.10 Fall on same level from slipping, tripping and stumbling with subsequent striking against unspecified object**

　　√6ᵗʰ **W01.11 Fall on same level from slipping, tripping and stumbling with subsequent striking against sharp object**

　　　√7ᵗʰ **W01.110 Fall on same level from slipping, tripping and stumbling with subsequent striking against sharp glass**

　　　√7ᵗʰ **W01.111 Fall on same level from slipping, tripping and stumbling with subsequent striking against power tool or machine**

　　　√7ᵗʰ **W01.118 Fall on same level from slipping, tripping and stumbling with subsequent striking against other sharp object**

　　　√7ᵗʰ **W01.119 Fall on same level from slipping, tripping and stumbling with subsequent striking against unspecified sharp object**

　　√6ᵗʰ **W01.19 Fall on same level from slipping, tripping and stumbling with subsequent striking against other object**

　　　√7ᵗʰ **W01.190 Fall on same level from slipping, tripping and stumbling with subsequent striking against furniture**

　　　√7ᵗʰ **W01.198 Fall on same level from slipping, tripping and stumbling with subsequent striking against other object**

☑x7ᵗʰ **W03** **Other fall on same level due to collision with another person**
- Fall due to non-transport collision with other person
  - EXCLUDES 1   *collision with another person without fall (W51)*
  - *crushed or pushed by a crowd or human stampede (W52)*
  - *fall involving pedestrian conveyance (V00-V09)*
  - *fall due to ice or snow (W00)*
  - *fall on same level NOS (W18.30)*
  - AHA: 2012,4Q,108

☑x7ᵗʰ **W04** **Fall while being carried or supported by other persons**
- Accidentally dropped while being carried

☑4ᵗʰ **W05** **Fall from non-moving wheelchair, nonmotorized scooter and motorized mobility scooter**
- EXCLUDES 1   *fall from moving wheelchair (powered) (V00.811)*
- *fall from moving motorized mobility scooter (V00.831)*
- *fall from nonmotorized scooter (V00.141)*

☑x7ᵗʰ **W05.0** **Fall from non-moving wheelchair**
- AHA: 2019,2Q,27

☑x7ᵗʰ **W05.1** **Fall from non-moving nonmotorized scooter**

☑x7ᵗʰ **W05.2** **Fall from non-moving motorized mobility scooter**

☑x7ᵗʰ **W06** **Fall from bed**

☑x7ᵗʰ **W07** **Fall from chair**

☑x7ᵗʰ **W08** **Fall from other furniture**
- ▶Fall from stool◀

☑4ᵗʰ **W09** **Fall on and from playground equipment**
- EXCLUDES 1   *fall involving recreational machinery (W31)*

☑x7ᵗʰ **W09.0** **Fall on or from playground slide**

☑x7ᵗʰ **W09.1** **Fall from playground swing**

☑x7ᵗʰ **W09.2** **Fall on or from jungle gym**

☑x7ᵗʰ **W09.8** **Fall on or from other playground equipment**

☑4ᵗʰ **W10** **Fall on and from stairs and steps**
- EXCLUDES 1   *Fall from stairs and steps due to ice and snow (W00.1)*

☑x7ᵗʰ **W10.0** **Fall (on)(from) escalator**

☑x7ᵗʰ **W10.1** **Fall (on)(from) sidewalk curb**

☑x7ᵗʰ **W10.2** **Fall (on)(from) incline**
- Fall (on) (from) ramp

☑x7ᵗʰ **W10.8** **Fall (on) (from) other stairs and steps**

☑x7ᵗʰ **W10.9** **Fall (on) (from) unspecified stairs and steps**

☑x7ᵗʰ **W11** **Fall on and from ladder**

☑x7ᵗʰ **W12** **Fall on and from scaffolding**

☑4ᵗʰ **W13** **Fall from, out of or through building or structure**

☑x7ᵗʰ **W13.0** **Fall from, out of or through balcony**
- Fall from, out of or through railing

☑x7ᵗʰ **W13.1** **Fall from, out of or through bridge**

☑x7ᵗʰ **W13.2** **Fall from, out of or through roof**

☑x7ᵗʰ **W13.3** **Fall through floor**

☑x7ᵗʰ **W13.4** **Fall from, out of or through window**
- EXCLUDES 2   *fall with subsequent striking against sharp glass (W01.110-)*

☑x7ᵗʰ **W13.8** **Fall from, out of or through other building or structure**
- Fall from, out of or through viaduct
- Fall from, out of or through wall
- Fall from, out of or through flag-pole

☑x7ᵗʰ **W13.9** **Fall from, out of or through building, not otherwise specified**
- EXCLUDES 1   *collapse of a building or structure (W20.-)*
- *fall or jump from burning building or structure (X00.-)*

☑x7ᵗʰ **W14** **Fall from tree**

☑x7ᵗʰ **W15** **Fall from cliff**

☑4ᵗʰ **W16** **Fall, jump or diving into water**
- EXCLUDES 1   *accidental non-watercraft drowning and submersion not involving fall (W65-W74)*
- *effects of air pressure from diving (W94.-)*
- *fall into water from watercraft (V90-V94)*
- *hitting an object or against bottom when falling from watercraft (V94.0)*
- EXCLUDES 2   *striking or hitting diving board (W21.4)*

☑5ᵗʰ **W16.0** **Fall into swimming pool**
- Fall into swimming pool NOS
  - EXCLUDES 1   *fall into empty swimming pool (W17.3)*

☑6ᵗʰ **W16.01** **Fall into swimming pool striking water surface**

☑7ᵗʰ **W16.011** **Fall into swimming pool striking water surface causing drowning and submersion**
- EXCLUDES 1   *drowning and submersion while in swimming pool without fall (W67)*

☑7ᵗʰ **W16.012** **Fall into swimming pool striking water surface causing other injury**

☑6ᵗʰ **W16.02** **Fall into swimming pool striking bottom**

☑7ᵗʰ **W16.021** **Fall into swimming pool striking bottom causing drowning and submersion**
- EXCLUDES 1   *drowning and submersion while in swimming pool without fall (W67)*

☑7ᵗʰ **W16.022** **Fall into swimming pool striking bottom causing other injury**

☑6ᵗʰ **W16.03** **Fall into swimming pool striking wall**

☑7ᵗʰ **W16.031** **Fall into swimming pool striking wall causing drowning and submersion**
- EXCLUDES 1   *drowning and submersion while in swimming pool without fall (W67)*

☑7ᵗʰ **W16.032** **Fall into swimming pool striking wall causing other injury**

☑5ᵗʰ **W16.1** **Fall into natural body of water**
- Fall into lake
- Fall into open sea
- Fall into river
- Fall into stream

☑6ᵗʰ **W16.11** **Fall into natural body of water striking water surface**

☑7ᵗʰ **W16.111** **Fall into natural body of water striking water surface causing drowning and submersion**
- EXCLUDES 1   *drowning and submersion while in natural body of water without fall (W69)*

☑7ᵗʰ **W16.112** **Fall into natural body of water striking water surface causing other injury**

☑6ᵗʰ **W16.12** **Fall into natural body of water striking bottom**

☑7ᵗʰ **W16.121** **Fall into natural body of water striking bottom causing drowning and submersion**
- EXCLUDES 1   *drowning and submersion while in natural body of water without fall (W69)*

☑7ᵗʰ **W16.122** **Fall into natural body of water striking bottom causing other injury**

☑6ᵗʰ **W16.13** **Fall into natural body of water striking side**

☑7ᵗʰ **W16.131** **Fall into natural body of water striking side causing drowning and submersion**
- EXCLUDES 1   *drowning and submersion while in natural body of water without fall (W69)*

☑7ᵗʰ **W16.132** **Fall into natural body of water striking side causing other injury**

☑5ᵗʰ **W16.2** **Fall in (into) filled bathtub or bucket of water**

☑6ᵗʰ **W16.21** **Fall in (into) filled bathtub**
- EXCLUDES 1   *fall into empty bathtub (W18.2)*

☑7ᵗʰ **W16.211** **Fall in (into) filled bathtub causing drowning and submersion**
- EXCLUDES 1   *drowning and submersion while in filled bathtub without fall (W65)*

☑7ᵗʰ **W16.212** **Fall in (into) filled bathtub causing other injury**

√6ᵗʰ **W16.22**   **Fall in (into)** bucket of water
- √7ᵗʰ **W16.221**   **Fall in (into) bucket of water causing** drowning and submersion
- √7ᵗʰ **W16.222**   **Fall in (into) bucket of water causing** other injury

√5ᵗʰ **W16.3**   **Fall into other water**
- Fall into fountain
- Fall into reservoir
- √6ᵗʰ **W16.31**   **Fall into other water** striking water surface
  - √7ᵗʰ **W16.311**   **Fall into other water striking water surface causing** drowning and submersion
    - *EXCLUDES 1*   *drowning and submersion while in other water without fall (W73)*
  - √7ᵗʰ **W16.312**   **Fall into other water striking water surface causing other injury**
- √6ᵗʰ **W16.32**   **Fall into other water** striking bottom
  - √7ᵗʰ **W16.321**   **Fall into other water striking bottom causing** drowning and submersion
    - *EXCLUDES 1*   *drowning and submersion while in other water without fall (W73)*
  - √7ᵗʰ **W16.322**   **Fall into other water striking bottom causing other injury**
- √6ᵗʰ **W16.33**   **Fall into other water** striking wall
  - √7ᵗʰ **W16.331**   **Fall into other water striking wall causing** drowning and submersion
    - *EXCLUDES 1*   *drowning and submersion while in other water without fall (W73)*
  - √7ᵗʰ **W16.332**   **Fall into other water striking wall causing other injury**

√5ᵗʰ **W16.4**   **Fall into unspecified water**
- √x7ᵗʰ **W16.41**   **Fall into unspecified water causing** drowning and submersion
- √x7ᵗʰ **W16.42**   **Fall into unspecified water causing other injury**

√5ᵗʰ **W16.5**   **Jumping or diving into** swimming pool
- √6ᵗʰ **W16.51**   **Jumping or diving into swimming pool** striking water surface
  - √7ᵗʰ **W16.511**   **Jumping or diving into swimming pool striking water surface causing** drowning and submersion
    - *EXCLUDES 1*   *drowning and submersion while in swimming pool without jumping or diving (W67)*
  - √7ᵗʰ **W16.512**   **Jumping or diving into swimming pool striking water surface causing other injury**
- √6ᵗʰ **W16.52**   **Jumping or diving into swimming pool** striking bottom
  - √7ᵗʰ **W16.521**   **Jumping or diving into swimming pool striking bottom causing** drowning and submersion
    - *EXCLUDES 1*   *drowning and submersion while in swimming pool without jumping or diving (W67)*
  - √7ᵗʰ **W16.522**   **Jumping or diving into swimming pool striking bottom causing other injury**
- √6ᵗʰ **W16.53**   **Jumping or diving into swimming pool** striking wall
  - √7ᵗʰ **W16.531**   **Jumping or diving into swimming pool striking wall causing** drowning and submersion
    - *EXCLUDES 1*   *drowning and submersion while in swimming pool without jumping or diving (W67)*
  - √7ᵗʰ **W16.532**   **Jumping or diving into swimming pool striking wall causing other injury**

√5ᵗʰ **W16.6**   **Jumping or diving into** natural body of water
- Jumping or diving into lake
- Jumping or diving into open sea
- Jumping or diving into river
- Jumping or diving into stream
- √6ᵗʰ **W16.61**   **Jumping or diving into natural body of water** striking water surface
  - √7ᵗʰ **W16.611**   **Jumping or diving into natural body of water striking water surface causing** drowning and submersion
    - *EXCLUDES 1*   *drowning and submersion while in natural body of water without jumping or diving (W69)*
  - √7ᵗʰ **W16.612**   **Jumping or diving into natural body of water striking water surface causing other injury**
- √6ᵗʰ **W16.62**   **Jumping or diving into natural body of water** striking bottom
  - √7ᵗʰ **W16.621**   **Jumping or diving into natural body of water striking bottom causing** drowning and submersion
    - *EXCLUDES 1*   *drowning and submersion while in natural body of water without jumping or diving (W69)*
  - √7ᵗʰ **W16.622**   **Jumping or diving into natural body of water striking bottom causing other injury**

√5ᵗʰ **W16.7**   **Jumping or diving** from boat
- *EXCLUDES 1*   *fall from boat into water - see watercraft accident (V90-V94)*
- √6ᵗʰ **W16.71**   **Jumping or diving from boat** striking water surface
  - √7ᵗʰ **W16.711**   **Jumping or diving from boat striking water surface causing** drowning and submersion
  - √7ᵗʰ **W16.712**   **Jumping or diving from boat striking water surface causing other injury**
- √6ᵗʰ **W16.72**   **Jumping or diving from boat** striking bottom
  - √7ᵗʰ **W16.721**   **Jumping or diving from boat striking bottom causing** drowning and submersion
  - √7ᵗʰ **W16.722**   **Jumping or diving from boat striking bottom causing other injury**

√5ᵗʰ **W16.8**   **Jumping or diving into** other water
- Jumping or diving into fountain
- Jumping or diving into reservoir
- √6ᵗʰ **W16.81**   **Jumping or diving into other water** striking water surface
  - √7ᵗʰ **W16.811**   **Jumping or diving into other water striking water surface causing** drowning and submersion
    - *EXCLUDES 1*   *drowning and submersion while in other water without jumping or diving (W73)*
  - √7ᵗʰ **W16.812**   **Jumping or diving into other water striking water surface causing other injury**
- √6ᵗʰ **W16.82**   **Jumping or diving into other water** striking bottom
  - √7ᵗʰ **W16.821**   **Jumping or diving into other water striking bottom causing** drowning and submersion
    - *EXCLUDES 1*   *drowning and submersion while in other water without jumping or diving (W73)*
  - √7ᵗʰ **W16.822**   **Jumping or diving into other water striking bottom causing other injury**
- √6ᵗʰ **W16.83**   **Jumping or diving into other water** striking wall
  - √7ᵗʰ **W16.831**   **Jumping or diving into other water striking wall causing** drowning and submersion
    - *EXCLUDES 1*   *drowning and submersion while in other water without jumping or diving (W73)*
  - √7ᵗʰ **W16.832**   **Jumping or diving into other water striking wall causing other injury**

HCC CMS-HCC   **Rx** Rx HCC   **ESR** ESRD HCC   **COM** Commercial HCC   **N** Newborn: 0   **P** Pediatric: 0-17   **M** Maternity: 9-64   **A** Adult: 15-124

1228   ICD-10-CM 2023

✓5ᵗʰ **W16.9 Jumping or diving into unspecified water**
- ✓x7ᵗʰ **W16.91 Jumping or diving into unspecified water causing drowning and submersion**
- ✓x7ᵗʰ **W16.92 Jumping or diving into unspecified water causing other injury**

✓4ᵗʰ **W17 Other fall from one level to another**
- ✓x7ᵗʰ **W17.0 Fall into well**
- ✓x7ᵗʰ **W17.1 Fall into storm drain or manhole**
- ✓x7ᵗʰ **W17.2 Fall into hole**
  - Fall into pit
- ✓x7ᵗʰ **W17.3 Fall into empty swimming pool**
  - EXCLUDES 1 *fall into filled swimming pool (W16.0-)*
- ✓x7ᵗʰ **W17.4 Fall from dock**
- ✓5ᵗʰ **W17.8 Other fall from one level to another**
  - ✓x7ᵗʰ **W17.81 Fall down embankment (hill)**
  - ✓x7ᵗʰ **W17.82 Fall from (out of) grocery cart**
    - Fall due to grocery cart tipping over
  - ✓x7ᵗʰ **W17.89 Other fall from one level to another**
    - Fall from cherry picker
    - Fall from lifting device
    - Fall from mobile elevated work platform [MEWP]
    - Fall from sky lift
    - AHA: 2015,2Q,6

✓4ᵗʰ **W18 Other slipping, tripping and stumbling and falls**
- ✓5ᵗʰ **W18.0 Fall due to bumping against object**
  - Striking against object with subsequent fall
  - EXCLUDES 1 *fall on same level due to slipping, tripping, or stumbling with subsequent striking against object (W01.1-)*
  - ✓x7ᵗʰ **W18.00 Striking against unspecified object with subsequent fall**
  - ✓x7ᵗʰ **W18.01 Striking against sports equipment with subsequent fall**
  - ✓x7ᵗʰ **W18.02 Striking against glass with subsequent fall**
  - ✓x7ᵗʰ **W18.09 Striking against other object with subsequent fall**
- ✓5ᵗʰ **W18.1 Fall from or off toilet**
  - ✓x7ᵗʰ **W18.11 Fall from or off toilet without subsequent striking against object**
    - Fall from (off) toilet NOS
  - ✓x7ᵗʰ **W18.12 Fall from or off toilet with subsequent striking against object**
- ✓x7ᵗʰ **W18.2 Fall in (into) shower or empty bathtub**
  - EXCLUDES 1 *fall in full bathtub causing drowning or submersion (W16.21-)*
- ✓5ᵗʰ **W18.3 Other and unspecified fall on same level**
  - ✓x7ᵗʰ **W18.30 Fall on same level, unspecified**
  - ✓x7ᵗʰ **W18.31 Fall on same level due to stepping on an object**
    - Fall on same level due to stepping on an animal
    - EXCLUDES 1 *slipping, tripping and stumbling without fall due to stepping on animal (W18.41)*
  - ✓x7ᵗʰ **W18.39 Other fall on same level**
- ✓5ᵗʰ **W18.4 Slipping, tripping and stumbling without falling**
  - EXCLUDES 1 *collision with another person without fall (W51)*
  - ✓x7ᵗʰ **W18.40 Slipping, tripping and stumbling without falling, unspecified**
  - ✓x7ᵗʰ **W18.41 Slipping, tripping and stumbling without falling due to stepping on object**
    - Slipping, tripping and stumbling without falling due to stepping on animal
    - EXCLUDES 1 *slipping, tripping and stumbling with fall due to stepping on animal (W18.31)*
  - ✓x7ᵗʰ **W18.42 Slipping, tripping and stumbling without falling due to stepping into hole or opening**
  - ✓x7ᵗʰ **W18.43 Slipping, tripping and stumbling without falling due to stepping from one level to another**
  - ✓x7ᵗʰ **W18.49 Other slipping, tripping and stumbling without falling**

✓x7ᵗʰ **W19 Unspecified fall**
- Accidental fall NOS
- AHA: 2012,4Q,95

Exposure to inanimate mechanical forces (W20-W49)

EXCLUDES 1 *assault (X92-Y09)*
contact or collision with animals or persons (W50-W64)
exposure to inanimate mechanical forces involving military or war operations (Y36.-, Y37.-)
intentional self-harm (X71-X83)

The appropriate 7th character is to be added to each code from categories W20-W49.
A   initial encounter
D   subsequent encounter
S   sequela

✓4ᵗʰ **W20 Struck by thrown, projected or falling object**
- Code first any associated:
- cataclysm (X34-X39)
- lightning strike (T75.00)
- EXCLUDES 1 *falling object in machinery accident (W24, W28-W31)*
  falling object in transport accident (V01-V99)
  object set in motion by explosion (W35-W40)
  object set in motion by firearm (W32-W34)
  struck by thrown sports equipment (W21.-)
- ✓x7ᵗʰ **W20.0 Struck by falling object in cave-in**
  - EXCLUDES 2 *asphyxiation due to cave-in (T71.21)*
- ✓x7ᵗʰ **W20.1 Struck by object due to collapse of building**
  - EXCLUDES 1 *struck by object due to collapse of burning building (X00.2, X02.2)*
- ✓x7ᵗʰ **W20.8 Other cause of strike by thrown, projected or falling object**
  - EXCLUDES 1 *struck by thrown sports equipment (W21.-)*

✓4ᵗʰ **W21 Striking against or struck by sports equipment**
- EXCLUDES 1 *assault with sports equipment (Y08.0-)*
  striking against or struck by sports equipment with subsequent fall (W18.01)
- ✓5ᵗʰ **W21.0 Struck by hit or thrown ball**
  - ✓x7ᵗʰ **W21.00 Struck by hit or thrown ball, unspecified type**
  - ✓x7ᵗʰ **W21.01 Struck by football**
  - ✓x7ᵗʰ **W21.02 Struck by soccer ball**
  - ✓x7ᵗʰ **W21.03 Struck by baseball**
  - ✓x7ᵗʰ **W21.04 Struck by golf ball**
  - ✓x7ᵗʰ **W21.05 Struck by basketball**
  - ✓x7ᵗʰ **W21.06 Struck by volleyball**
  - ✓x7ᵗʰ **W21.07 Struck by softball**
  - ✓x7ᵗʰ **W21.09 Struck by other hit or thrown ball**
- ✓5ᵗʰ **W21.1 Struck by bat, racquet or club**
  - ✓x7ᵗʰ **W21.11 Struck by baseball bat**
  - ✓x7ᵗʰ **W21.12 Struck by tennis racquet**
  - ✓x7ᵗʰ **W21.13 Struck by golf club**
  - ✓x7ᵗʰ **W21.19 Struck by other bat, racquet or club**
- ✓5ᵗʰ **W21.2 Struck by hockey stick or puck**
  - ✓6ᵗʰ **W21.21 Struck by hockey stick**
    - ✓7ᵗʰ **W21.210 Struck by ice hockey stick**
    - ✓7ᵗʰ **W21.211 Struck by field hockey stick**
  - ✓6ᵗʰ **W21.22 Struck by hockey puck**
    - ✓7ᵗʰ **W21.220 Struck by ice hockey puck**
    - ✓7ᵗʰ **W21.221 Struck by field hockey puck**
- ✓5ᵗʰ **W21.3 Struck by sports foot wear**
  - ✓x7ᵗʰ **W21.31 Struck by shoe cleats**
    - Stepped on by shoe cleats
  - ✓x7ᵗʰ **W21.32 Struck by skate blades**
    - Skated over by skate blades
  - ✓x7ᵗʰ **W21.39 Struck by other sports foot wear**
- ✓x7ᵗʰ **W21.4 Striking against diving board**
  - Use additional code for subsequent falling into water, if applicable (W16.-)
- ✓5ᵗʰ **W21.8 Striking against or struck by other sports equipment**
  - ✓x7ᵗʰ **W21.81 Striking against or struck by football helmet**
  - ✓x7ᵗʰ **W21.89 Striking against or struck by other sports equipment**
- ✓x7ᵗʰ **W21.9 Striking against or struck by unspecified sports equipment**

Chapter 20. External Causes of Morbidity

✓4ᵗʰ **W22 Striking against or struck by other objects**
> EXCLUDES 1   striking against or struck by object with subsequent fall (W18.09)

✓5ᵗʰ **W22.0 Striking against stationary object**
> EXCLUDES 1   striking against stationary sports equipment (W21.8)

✓7ᵗʰ **W22.01 Walked into wall**

✓7ᵗʰ **W22.02 Walked into lamppost**

✓7ᵗʰ **W22.03 Walked into furniture**

✓6ᵗʰ **W22.04 Striking against wall of swimming pool**

    7ᵗʰ **W22.041 Striking against wall of swimming pool causing drowning and submersion**
> EXCLUDES 1   drowning and submersion while swimming without striking against wall (W67)

    7ᵗʰ **W22.042 Striking against wall of swimming pool causing other injury**

✓7ᵗʰ **W22.09 Striking against other stationary object**

✓5ᵗʰ **W22.1 Striking against or struck by automobile airbag**

✓7ᵗʰ **W22.10 Striking against or struck by unspecified automobile airbag**

✓7ᵗʰ **W22.11 Striking against or struck by driver side automobile airbag**

✓7ᵗʰ **W22.12 Striking against or struck by front passenger side automobile airbag**

✓7ᵗʰ **W22.19 Striking against or struck by other automobile airbag**

✓7ᵗʰ **W22.8 Striking against or struck by other objects**
> Striking against or struck by object NOS
> EXCLUDES 1   struck by thrown, projected or falling object (W20.-)

✓4ᵗʰ **W23 Caught, crushed, jammed or pinched in or between objects**
> EXCLUDES 1   injury caused by cutting or piercing instruments (W25-W27)
> injury caused by firearms malfunction (W32.1, W33.1-, W34.1-)
> injury caused by lifting and transmission devices (W24.-)
> injury caused by machinery (W28-W31)
> injury caused by nonpowered hand tools (W27.-)
> injury caused by transport vehicle being used as a means of transportation (V01-V99)
> injury caused by struck by thrown, projected or falling object (W20.-)

✓7ᵗʰ **W23.0 Caught, crushed, jammed, or pinched between moving objects**

✓7ᵗʰ **W23.1 Caught, crushed, jammed, or pinched between stationary objects**

● ✓7ᵗʰ **W23.2 Caught, crushed, jammed or pinched between a moving and stationary object**

✓4ᵗʰ **W24 Contact with lifting and transmission devices, not elsewhere classified**
> EXCLUDES 1   transport accidents (V01-V99)

✓7ᵗʰ **W24.0 Contact with lifting devices, not elsewhere classified**
> Contact with chain hoist
> Contact with drive belt
> Contact with pulley (block)

✓7ᵗʰ **W24.1 Contact with transmission devices, not elsewhere classified**
> Contact with transmission belt or cable

✓7ᵗʰ **W25 Contact with sharp glass**
> Code first any associated:
> injury due to flying glass from explosion or firearm discharge (W32-W40)
> transport accident (V00-V99)
> EXCLUDES 1   fall on same level due to slipping, tripping and stumbling with subsequent striking against sharp glass (W01.110-)
> striking against sharp glass with subsequent fall (W18.02-)
> EXCLUDES 2   glass embedded in skin (W45.-)

✓4ᵗʰ **W26 Contact with other sharp objects**
> EXCLUDES 2   sharp object(s) embedded in skin (W45.-)
> AHA: 2016,4Q,73

✓7ᵗʰ **W26.0 Contact with knife**
> EXCLUDES 1   contact with electric knife (W29.1)

✓7ᵗʰ **W26.1 Contact with sword or dagger**

✓7ᵗʰ **W26.2 Contact with edge of stiff paper**
> Paper cut

✓7ᵗʰ **W26.8 Contact with other sharp object(s), not elsewhere classified**
> Contact with tin can lid

✓7ᵗʰ **W26.9 Contact with unspecified sharp object(s)**

✓4ᵗʰ **W27 Contact with nonpowered hand tool**

✓7ᵗʰ **W27.0 Contact with workbench tool**
> Contact with auger
> Contact with axe
> Contact with chisel
> Contact with handsaw
> Contact with screwdriver

✓7ᵗʰ **W27.1 Contact with garden tool**
> Contact with hoe
> Contact with nonpowered lawn mower
> Contact with pitchfork
> Contact with rake

✓7ᵗʰ **W27.2 Contact with scissors**

✓7ᵗʰ **W27.3 Contact with needle (sewing)**
> EXCLUDES 1   contact with hypodermic needle (W46.-)

✓7ᵗʰ **W27.4 Contact with kitchen utensil**
> Contact with fork
> Contact with ice-pick
> Contact with can-opener NOS

✓7ᵗʰ **W27.5 Contact with paper-cutter**

✓7ᵗʰ **W27.8 Contact with other nonpowered hand tool**
> Contact with nonpowered sewing machine
> Contact with shovel

✓7ᵗʰ **W28 Contact with powered lawn mower**
> Powered lawn mower (commercial) (residential)
> EXCLUDES 1   contact with nonpowered lawn mower (W27.1)
> EXCLUDES 2   exposure to electric current (W86.-)

✓4ᵗʰ **W29 Contact with other powered hand tools and household machinery**
> EXCLUDES 1   contact with commercial machinery (W31.82)
> contact with hot household appliance (X15)
> contact with nonpowered hand tool (W27.-)
> exposure to electric current (W86)

✓7ᵗʰ **W29.0 Contact with powered kitchen appliance**
> Contact with blender
> Contact with can-opener
> Contact with garbage disposal
> Contact with mixer

✓7ᵗʰ **W29.1 Contact with electric knife**

✓7ᵗʰ **W29.2 Contact with other powered household machinery**
> Contact with electric fan
> Contact with powered dryer (clothes) (powered) (spin)
> Contact with washing-machine
> Contact with sewing machine

✓7ᵗʰ **W29.3 Contact with powered garden and outdoor hand tools and machinery**
> Contact with chainsaw
> Contact with edger
> Contact with garden cultivator (tiller)
> Contact with hedge trimmer
> Contact with other powered garden tool
> EXCLUDES 1   contact with powered lawn mower (W28)

✓7ᵗʰ **W29.4 Contact with nail gun**

✓7ᵗʰ **W29.8 Contact with other powered hand tools and household machinery**
> Contact with do-it-yourself tool NOS

✓4ᵗʰ **W30 Contact with agricultural machinery**
> INCLUDES   animal-powered farm machine
> EXCLUDES 1   agricultural transport vehicle accident (V01-V99)
> explosion of grain store (W40.8)
> exposure to electric current (W86.-)

✓7ᵗʰ **W30.0 Contact with combine harvester**
> Contact with reaper
> Contact with thresher

✓7ᵗʰ **W30.1 Contact with power take-off devices (PTO)**

✓7ᵗʰ **W30.2 Contact with hay derrick**

√x7ᵗʰ **W30.3** **Contact with grain storage elevator**
　　　　EXCLUDES 1　*explosion of grain store (W40.8)*

√5ᵗʰ **W30.8** **Contact with other specified agricultural machinery**

　　√x7ᵗʰ **W30.81** **Contact with agricultural transport vehicle in stationary use**
　　　　　Contact with agricultural transport vehicle under repair, not on public roadway
　　　　　EXCLUDES 1　*agricultural transport vehicle accident (V01-V99)*

　　√x7ᵗʰ **W30.89** **Contact with other specified agricultural machinery**

√x7ᵗʰ **W30.9** **Contact with unspecified agricultural machinery**
　　　　Contact with farm machinery NOS

√4ᵗʰ **W31** **Contact with other and unspecified machinery**
　　　　EXCLUDES 1　*contact with agricultural machinery (W30.-)*
　　　　　contact with machinery in transport under own power or being towed by a vehicle (V01-V99)
　　　　　exposure to electric current (W86)

√x7ᵗʰ **W31.0** **Contact with mining and earth-drilling machinery**
　　　　Contact with bore or drill (land) (seabed)
　　　　Contact with shaft hoist
　　　　Contact with shaft lift
　　　　Contact with undercutter

√x7ᵗʰ **W31.1** **Contact with metalworking machines**
　　　　Contact with abrasive wheel
　　　　Contact with forging machine
　　　　Contact with lathe
　　　　Contact with mechanical shears
　　　　Contact with metal drilling machine
　　　　Contact with milling machine
　　　　Contact with power press
　　　　Contact with rolling-mill
　　　　Contact with metal sawing machine

√x7ᵗʰ **W31.2** **Contact with powered woodworking and forming machines**
　　　　Contact with band saw
　　　　Contact with bench saw
　　　　Contact with circular saw
　　　　Contact with molding machine
　　　　Contact with overhead plane
　　　　Contact with powered saw
　　　　Contact with radial saw
　　　　Contact with sander
　　　　EXCLUDES 1　*nonpowered woodworking tools (W27.0)*

√x7ᵗʰ **W31.3** **Contact with prime movers**
　　　　Contact with gas turbine
　　　　Contact with internal combustion engine
　　　　Contact with steam engine
　　　　Contact with water driven turbine

√5ᵗʰ **W31.8** **Contact with other specified machinery**

　　√x7ᵗʰ **W31.81** **Contact with recreational machinery**
　　　　　Contact with roller coaster

　　√x7ᵗʰ **W31.82** **Contact with other commercial machinery**
　　　　　Contact with commercial electric fan
　　　　　Contact with commercial kitchen appliances
　　　　　Contact with commercial powered dryer (clothes) (powered) (spin)
　　　　　Contact with commercial washing-machine
　　　　　Contact with commercial sewing machine
　　　　　EXCLUDES 1　*contact with household machinery (W29.-)*
　　　　　　contact with powered lawn mower (W28)

　　√x7ᵗʰ **W31.83** **Contact with special construction vehicle in stationary use**
　　　　　Contact with special construction vehicle under repair, not on public roadway
　　　　　EXCLUDES 1　*special construction vehicle accident (V01-V99)*

　　√x7ᵗʰ **W31.89** **Contact with other specified machinery**

√x7ᵗʰ **W31.9** **Contact with unspecified machinery**
　　　　Contact with machinery NOS

√4ᵗʰ **W32** **Accidental handgun discharge and malfunction**
　　　　INCLUDES　accidental discharge and malfunction of gun for single hand use
　　　　　accidental discharge and malfunction of pistol
　　　　　accidental discharge and malfunction of revolver
　　　　　handgun discharge and malfunction NOS
　　　　EXCLUDES 1　*accidental airgun discharge and malfunction (W34.010, W34.110)*
　　　　　accidental BB gun discharge and malfunction (W34.010, W34.110)
　　　　　accidental pellet gun discharge and malfunction (W34.010, W34.110)
　　　　　accidental shotgun discharge and malfunction (W33.01, W33.11)
　　　　　assault by handgun discharge (X93)
　　　　　handgun discharge involving legal intervention (Y35.0-)
　　　　　handgun discharge involving military or war operations (Y36.4-)
　　　　　intentional self-harm by handgun discharge (X72)
　　　　　Very pistol discharge and malfunction (W34.09, W34.19)

√x7ᵗʰ **W32.0** **Accidental handgun discharge**

√x7ᵗʰ **W32.1** **Accidental handgun malfunction**
　　　　Injury due to explosion of handgun (parts)
　　　　Injury due to malfunction of mechanism or component of handgun
　　　　Injury due to recoil of handgun
　　　　Powder burn from handgun

√4ᵗʰ **W33** **Accidental rifle, shotgun and larger firearm discharge and malfunction**
　　　　INCLUDES　rifle, shotgun and larger firearm discharge and malfunction NOS
　　　　EXCLUDES 1　*accidental airgun discharge and malfunction (W34.010, W34.110)*
　　　　　accidental BB gun discharge and malfunction (W34.010, W34.110)
　　　　　accidental handgun discharge and malfunction (W32.-)
　　　　　accidental pellet gun discharge and malfunction (W34.010, W34.110)
　　　　　assault by rifle, shotgun and larger firearm discharge (X94)
　　　　　firearm discharge involving legal intervention (Y35.0-)
　　　　　firearm discharge involving military or war operations (Y36.4-)
　　　　　intentional self-harm by rifle, shotgun and larger firearm discharge (X73)

√5ᵗʰ **W33.0** **Accidental rifle, shotgun and larger firearm discharge**

　　√x7ᵗʰ **W33.00** **Accidental discharge of unspecified larger firearm**
　　　　　Discharge of unspecified larger firearm NOS

　　√x7ᵗʰ **W33.01** **Accidental discharge of shotgun**
　　　　　Discharge of shotgun NOS

　　√x7ᵗʰ **W33.02** **Accidental discharge of hunting rifle**
　　　　　Discharge of hunting rifle NOS

　　√x7ᵗʰ **W33.03** **Accidental discharge of machine gun**
　　　　　Discharge of machine gun NOS

　　√x7ᵗʰ **W33.09** **Accidental discharge of other larger firearm**
　　　　　Discharge of other larger firearm NOS

√5ᵗʰ **W33.1** **Accidental rifle, shotgun and larger firearm malfunction**
　　　　Injury due to explosion of rifle, shotgun and larger firearm (parts)
　　　　Injury due to malfunction of mechanism or component of rifle, shotgun and larger firearm
　　　　Injury due to piercing, cutting, crushing or pinching due to (by) slide trigger mechanism, scope or other gun part
　　　　Injury due to recoil of rifle, shotgun and larger firearm
　　　　Powder burn from rifle, shotgun and larger firearm

　　√x7ᵗʰ **W33.10** **Accidental malfunction of unspecified larger firearm**
　　　　　Malfunction of unspecified larger firearm NOS

　　√x7ᵗʰ **W33.11** **Accidental malfunction of shotgun**
　　　　　Malfunction of shotgun NOS

　　√x7ᵗʰ **W33.12** **Accidental malfunction of hunting rifle**
　　　　　Malfunction of hunting rifle NOS

　　√x7ᵗʰ **W33.13** **Accidental malfunction of machine gun**
　　　　　Malfunction of machine gun NOS

✓x7ᵗʰ **W33.19** **Accidental malfunction of other larger firearm**

Malfunction of other larger firearm NOS

✓4ᵗʰ **W34** **Accidental discharge and malfunction from other and unspecified firearms and guns**

✓5ᵗʰ **W34.0** **Accidental discharge from other and unspecified firearms and guns**

✓x7ᵗʰ **W34.00** **Accidental discharge from unspecified firearms or gun**

Discharge from firearm NOS
Gunshot wound NOS
Shot NOS

✓6ᵗʰ **W34.01** **Accidental discharge of gas, air or spring-operated guns**

✓7ᵗʰ **W34.010** **Accidental discharge of airgun**

Accidental discharge of BB gun
Accidental discharge of pellet gun

✓7ᵗʰ **W34.011** **Accidental discharge of paintball gun**

Accidental injury due to paintball discharge

✓7ᵗʰ **W34.018** **Accidental discharge of other gas, air or spring-operated gun**

✓x7ᵗʰ **W34.09** **Accidental discharge from other specified firearms**

Accidental discharge from Very pistol [flare]

✓5ᵗʰ **W34.1** **Accidental malfunction from other and unspecified firearms and guns**

✓x7ᵗʰ **W34.10** **Accidental malfunction from unspecified firearms or gun**

Firearm malfunction NOS

✓6ᵗʰ **W34.11** **Accidental malfunction of gas, air or spring-operated guns**

✓7ᵗʰ **W34.110** **Accidental malfunction of airgun**

Accidental malfunction of BB gun
Accidental malfunction of pellet gun

✓7ᵗʰ **W34.111** **Accidental malfunction of paintball gun**

Accidental injury due to paintball gun malfunction

✓7ᵗʰ **W34.118** **Accidental malfunction of other gas, air or spring-operated gun**

✓x7ᵗʰ **W34.19** **Accidental malfunction from other specified firearms**

Accidental malfunction from Very pistol [flare]

✓x7ᵗʰ **W35** **Explosion and rupture of boiler**

EXCLUDES 1   *explosion and rupture of boiler on watercraft (V93.4)*

✓4ᵗʰ **W36** **Explosion and rupture of gas cylinder**

✓x7ᵗʰ **W36.1** **Explosion and rupture of aerosol can**

✓x7ᵗʰ **W36.2** **Explosion and rupture of air tank**

✓x7ᵗʰ **W36.3** **Explosion and rupture of pressurized-gas tank**

✓x7ᵗʰ **W36.8** **Explosion and rupture of other gas cylinder**

✓x7ᵗʰ **W36.9** **Explosion and rupture of unspecified gas cylinder**

✓4ᵗʰ **W37** **Explosion and rupture of pressurized tire, pipe or hose**

✓x7ᵗʰ **W37.0** **Explosion of bicycle tire**

✓x7ᵗʰ **W37.8** **Explosion and rupture of other pressurized tire, pipe or hose**

✓x7ᵗʰ **W38** **Explosion and rupture of other specified pressurized devices**

✓x7ᵗʰ **W39** **Discharge of firework**

✓4ᵗʰ **W40** **Explosion of other materials**

EXCLUDES 1   *assault by explosive material (X96)*
explosion involving legal intervention (Y35.1-)
explosion involving military or war operations (Y36.0-, Y36.2-)
intentional self-harm by explosive material (X75)

✓x7ᵗʰ **W40.0** **Explosion of blasting material**

Explosion of blasting cap
Explosion of detonator
Explosion of dynamite
Explosion of explosive (any) used in blasting operations

✓x7ᵗʰ **W40.1** **Explosion of explosive gases**

Explosion of acetylene
Explosion of butane
Explosion of coal gas
Explosion in mine NOS
Explosion of explosive gas
Explosion of fire damp
Explosion of gasoline fumes
Explosion of methane
Explosion of propane

✓x7ᵗʰ **W40.8** **Explosion of other specified explosive materials**

Explosion in dump NOS
Explosion in factory NOS
Explosion in grain store
Explosion in munitions

EXCLUDES 1   *explosion involving legal intervention (Y35.1-)*
explosion involving military or war operations (Y36.0-, Y36.2-)

✓x7ᵗʰ **W40.9** **Explosion of unspecified explosive materials**

Explosion NOS

✓4ᵗʰ **W42** **Exposure to noise**

✓x7ᵗʰ **W42.0** **Exposure to supersonic waves**

✓x7ᵗʰ **W42.9** **Exposure to other noise**

Exposure to sound waves NOS

✓4ᵗʰ **W45** **Foreign body or object entering through skin**

INCLUDES   foreign body or object embedded in skin
nail embedded in skin

EXCLUDES 2   *contact with hand tools (nonpowered) (powered) (W27-W29)*
contact with other sharp objects (W26.-)
contact with sharp glass (W25.-)
struck by objects (W20-W22)

✓x7ᵗʰ **W45.0** **Nail entering through skin**

✓x7ᵗʰ **W45.8** **Other foreign body or object entering through skin**

Splinter in skin NOS

✓4ᵗʰ **W46** **Contact with hypodermic needle**

✓x7ᵗʰ **W46.0** **Contact with hypodermic needle**

Hypodermic needle stick NOS

✓x7ᵗʰ **W46.1** **Contact with contaminated hypodermic needle**

✓4ᵗʰ **W49** **Exposure to other inanimate mechanical forces**

INCLUDES   exposure to abnormal gravitational [G] forces
exposure to inanimate mechanical forces NEC

EXCLUDES 1   *exposure to inanimate mechanical forces involving military or war operations (Y36.-, Y37.-)*

✓5ᵗʰ **W49.0** **Item causing external constriction**

✓x7ᵗʰ **W49.01** **Hair causing external constriction**

✓x7ᵗʰ **W49.02** **String or thread causing external constriction**

✓x7ᵗʰ **W49.03** **Rubber band causing external constriction**

✓x7ᵗʰ **W49.04** **Ring or other jewelry causing external constriction**

✓x7ᵗʰ **W49.09** **Other specified item causing external constriction**

✓x7ᵗʰ **W49.9** **Exposure to other inanimate mechanical forces**

Exposure to animate mechanical forces (W50-W64)

EXCLUDES 1   *toxic effect of contact with venomous animals and plants (T63.-)*

The appropriate 7th character is to be added to each code from categories W50-W64.
A   initial encounter
D   subsequent encounter
S   sequela

✓4ᵗʰ **W50** **Accidental hit, strike, kick, twist, bite or scratch by another person**

INCLUDES   hit, strike, kick, twist, bite, or scratch by another person NOS

EXCLUDES 1   *assault by bodily force (Y04)*
struck by objects (W20-W22)

✓x7ᵗʰ **W50.0** **Accidental hit or strike by another person**

Hit or strike by another person NOS

✓x7ᵗʰ **W50.1** **Accidental kick by another person**

Kick by another person NOS

✓x7ᵗʰ **W50.2** **Accidental twist by another person**

Twist by another person NOS

√x7ᵗʰ **W50.3 Accidental bite by another person**
Human bite
Bite by another person NOS

√x7ᵗʰ **W50.4 Accidental scratch by another person**
Scratch by another person NOS

√x7ᵗʰ **W51 Accidental striking against or bumped into by another person**
EXCLUDES 1   *assault by striking against or bumping into by another person (Y04.2)*
fall due to collision with another person (W03)

√x7ᵗʰ **W52 Crushed, pushed or stepped on by crowd or human stampede**
Crushed, pushed or stepped on by crowd or human stampede with or without fall

√4ᵗʰ **W53 Contact with rodent**
INCLUDES   contact with saliva, feces or urine of rodent

√5ᵗʰ **W53.0 Contact with mouse**
√x7ᵗʰ **W53.01   Bitten by mouse**
√x7ᵗʰ **W53.09   Other contact with mouse**

√5ᵗʰ **W53.1 Contact with rat**
√x7ᵗʰ **W53.11   Bitten by rat**
√x7ᵗʰ **W53.19   Other contact with rat**

√5ᵗʰ **W53.2 Contact with squirrel**
√x7ᵗʰ **W53.21   Bitten by squirrel**
√x7ᵗʰ **W53.29   Other contact with squirrel**

√5ᵗʰ **W53.8 Contact with other rodent**
√x7ᵗʰ **W53.81   Bitten by other rodent**
√x7ᵗʰ **W53.89   Other contact with other rodent**

√4ᵗʰ **W54 Contact with dog**
INCLUDES   contact with saliva, feces or urine of dog

√x7ᵗʰ **W54.0   Bitten by dog**
√x7ᵗʰ **W54.1   Struck by dog**
Knocked over by dog
√x7ᵗʰ **W54.8   Other contact with dog**

√4ᵗʰ **W55 Contact with other mammals**
INCLUDES   contact with saliva, feces or urine of mammal
EXCLUDES 1   *animal being ridden - see transport accidents*
bitten or struck by dog (W54)
bitten or struck by rodent (W53.-)
contact with marine mammals (W56.-)

√5ᵗʰ **W55.0 Contact with cat**
√x7ᵗʰ **W55.01   Bitten by cat**
√x7ᵗʰ **W55.03   Scratched by cat**
√x7ᵗʰ **W55.09   Other contact with cat**

√5ᵗʰ **W55.1 Contact with horse**
√x7ᵗʰ **W55.11   Bitten by horse**
√x7ᵗʰ **W55.12   Struck by horse**
√x7ᵗʰ **W55.19   Other contact with horse**

√5ᵗʰ **W55.2 Contact with cow**
Contact with bull
√x7ᵗʰ **W55.21   Bitten by cow**
√x7ᵗʰ **W55.22   Struck by cow**
Gored by bull
√x7ᵗʰ **W55.29   Other contact with cow**

√5ᵗʰ **W55.3 Contact with other hoof stock**
Contact with goats
Contact with sheep
√x7ᵗʰ **W55.31   Bitten by other hoof stock**
√x7ᵗʰ **W55.32   Struck by other hoof stock**
Gored by goat
Gored by ram
√x7ᵗʰ **W55.39   Other contact with other hoof stock**

√5ᵗʰ **W55.4 Contact with pig**
√x7ᵗʰ **W55.41   Bitten by pig**
√x7ᵗʰ **W55.42   Struck by pig**
√x7ᵗʰ **W55.49   Other contact with pig**

√5ᵗʰ **W55.5 Contact with raccoon**
√x7ᵗʰ **W55.51   Bitten by raccoon**

√x7ᵗʰ **W55.52   Struck by raccoon**
√x7ᵗʰ **W55.59   Other contact with raccoon**

√5ᵗʰ **W55.8 Contact with other mammals**
√x7ᵗʰ **W55.81   Bitten by other mammals**
√x7ᵗʰ **W55.82   Struck by other mammals**
√x7ᵗʰ **W55.89   Other contact with other mammals**

√4ᵗʰ **W56 Contact with nonvenomous marine animal**
EXCLUDES 1   *contact with venomous marine animal (T63.-)*

√5ᵗʰ **W56.0 Contact with dolphin**
√x7ᵗʰ **W56.01   Bitten by dolphin**
√x7ᵗʰ **W56.02   Struck by dolphin**
√x7ᵗʰ **W56.09   Other contact with dolphin**

√5ᵗʰ **W56.1 Contact with sea lion**
√x7ᵗʰ **W56.11   Bitten by sea lion**
√x7ᵗʰ **W56.12   Struck by sea lion**
√x7ᵗʰ **W56.19   Other contact with sea lion**

√5ᵗʰ **W56.2 Contact with orca**
Contact with killer whale
√x7ᵗʰ **W56.21   Bitten by orca**
√x7ᵗʰ **W56.22   Struck by orca**
√x7ᵗʰ **W56.29   Other contact with orca**

√5ᵗʰ **W56.3 Contact with other marine mammals**
√x7ᵗʰ **W56.31   Bitten by other marine mammals**
√x7ᵗʰ **W56.32   Struck by other marine mammals**
√x7ᵗʰ **W56.39   Other contact with other marine mammals**

√5ᵗʰ **W56.4 Contact with shark**
√x7ᵗʰ **W56.41   Bitten by shark**
√x7ᵗʰ **W56.42   Struck by shark**
√x7ᵗʰ **W56.49   Other contact with shark**

√5ᵗʰ **W56.5 Contact with other fish**
√x7ᵗʰ **W56.51   Bitten by other fish**
√x7ᵗʰ **W56.52   Struck by other fish**
√x7ᵗʰ **W56.59   Other contact with other fish**

√5ᵗʰ **W56.8 Contact with other nonvenomous marine animals**
√x7ᵗʰ **W56.81   Bitten by other nonvenomous marine animals**
√x7ᵗʰ **W56.82   Struck by other nonvenomous marine animals**
√x7ᵗʰ **W56.89   Other contact with other nonvenomous marine animals**

√x7ᵗʰ **W57 Bitten or stung by nonvenomous insect and other nonvenomous arthropods**
EXCLUDES 1   *contact with venomous insects and arthropods (T63.2-, T63.3-, T63.4-)*

√4ᵗʰ **W58 Contact with crocodile or alligator**
√5ᵗʰ **W58.0 Contact with alligator**
√x7ᵗʰ **W58.01   Bitten by alligator**
√x7ᵗʰ **W58.02   Struck by alligator**
√x7ᵗʰ **W58.03   Crushed by alligator**
√x7ᵗʰ **W58.09   Other contact with alligator**

√5ᵗʰ **W58.1 Contact with crocodile**
√x7ᵗʰ **W58.11   Bitten by crocodile**
√x7ᵗʰ **W58.12   Struck by crocodile**
√x7ᵗʰ **W58.13   Crushed by crocodile**
√x7ᵗʰ **W58.19   Other contact with crocodile**

√4ᵗʰ **W59 Contact with other nonvenomous reptiles**
EXCLUDES 1   *contact with venomous reptile (T63.0-, T63.1-)*

√5ᵗʰ **W59.0 Contact with nonvenomous lizards**
√x7ᵗʰ **W59.01   Bitten by nonvenomous lizards**
√x7ᵗʰ **W59.02   Struck by nonvenomous lizards**
√x7ᵗʰ **W59.09   Other contact with nonvenomous lizards**
Exposure to nonvenomous lizards

√5ᵗʰ **W59.1 Contact with nonvenomous snakes**
√x7ᵗʰ **W59.11   Bitten by nonvenomous snake**
√x7ᵗʰ **W59.12   Struck by nonvenomous snake**
√x7ᵗʰ **W59.13   Crushed by nonvenomous snake**
√x7ᵗʰ **W59.19   Other contact with nonvenomous snake**

Chapter 20. External Causes of Morbidity

W59.2–W88.1

√5ᵗʰ **W59.2** **Contact with** turtles

    EXCLUDES 1   contact with tortoises (W59.8-)

  √x7ᵗʰ **W59.21** **Bitten by turtle**

  √x7ᵗʰ **W59.22** **Struck by turtle**

  √x7ᵗʰ **W59.29** **Other contact with turtle**

    Exposure to turtles

√5ᵗʰ **W59.8** **Contact with other nonvenomous reptiles**

  √x7ᵗʰ **W59.81** **Bitten by other nonvenomous reptiles**

  √x7ᵗʰ **W59.82** **Struck by other nonvenomous reptiles**

  √x7ᵗʰ **W59.83** **Crushed by other nonvenomous reptiles**

  √x7ᵗʰ **W59.89** **Other contact with other nonvenomous reptiles**

√x7ᵗʰ **W60** **Contact with nonvenomous plant thorns and spines and sharp leaves**

    EXCLUDES 1   contact with venomous plants (T63.7-)

√4ᵗʰ **W61** **Contact with birds (domestic) (wild)**

    INCLUDES   contact with excreta of birds

√5ᵗʰ **W61.0** **Contact with** parrot

  √x7ᵗʰ **W61.01** **Bitten by parrot**

  √x7ᵗʰ **W61.02** **Struck by parrot**

  √x7ᵗʰ **W61.09** **Other contact with parrot**

    Exposure to parrots

√5ᵗʰ **W61.1** **Contact with** macaw

  √x7ᵗʰ **W61.11** **Bitten by macaw**

  √x7ᵗʰ **W61.12** **Struck by macaw**

  √x7ᵗʰ **W61.19** **Other contact with macaw**

    Exposure to macaws

√5ᵗʰ **W61.2** **Contact with other** psittacines

  √x7ᵗʰ **W61.21** **Bitten by other psittacines**

  √x7ᵗʰ **W61.22** **Struck by other psittacines**

  √x7ᵗʰ **W61.29** **Other contact with other psittacines**

    Exposure to other psittacines

√5ᵗʰ **W61.3** **Contact with** chicken

  √x7ᵗʰ **W61.32** **Struck by chicken**

  √x7ᵗʰ **W61.33** **Pecked by chicken**

  √x7ᵗʰ **W61.39** **Other contact with chicken**

    Exposure to chickens

√5ᵗʰ **W61.4** **Contact with** turkey

  √x7ᵗʰ **W61.42** **Struck by turkey**

  √x7ᵗʰ **W61.43** **Pecked by turkey**

  √x7ᵗʰ **W61.49** **Other contact with turkey**

√5ᵗʰ **W61.5** **Contact with** goose

  √x7ᵗʰ **W61.51** **Bitten by goose**

  √x7ᵗʰ **W61.52** **Struck by goose**

  √x7ᵗʰ **W61.59** **Other contact with goose**

√5ᵗʰ **W61.6** **Contact with** duck

  √x7ᵗʰ **W61.61** **Bitten by duck**

  √x7ᵗʰ **W61.62** **Struck by duck**

  √x7ᵗʰ **W61.69** **Other contact with duck**

√5ᵗʰ **W61.9** **Contact with other birds**

  √x7ᵗʰ **W61.91** **Bitten by other birds**

  √x7ᵗʰ **W61.92** **Struck by other birds**

  √x7ᵗʰ **W61.99** **Other contact with other birds**

    Contact with bird NOS

√4ᵗʰ **W62** **Contact with nonvenomous amphibians**

    EXCLUDES 1   contact with venomous amphibians (T63.81-R63.83)

√x7ᵗʰ **W62.0** **Contact with nonvenomous** frogs

√x7ᵗʰ **W62.1** **Contact with nonvenomous** toads

√x7ᵗʰ **W62.9** **Contact with other nonvenomous amphibians**

√x7ᵗʰ **W64** **Exposure to other animate mechanical forces**

    INCLUDES   exposure to nonvenomous animal NOS

    EXCLUDES 1   contact with venomous animal (T63.-)

Accidental non-transport drowning and submersion (W65-W74)

  EXCLUDES 1   accidental drowning and submersion due to fall into water (W16.-)

            accidental drowning and submersion due to water transport accident (V90.-, V92.-)

  EXCLUDES 2   accidental drowning and submersion due to cataclysm (X34-X39)

The appropriate 7th character is to be added to each code from categories W65-W74.

A   initial encounter
D   subsequent encounter
S   sequela

√x7ᵗʰ **W65** **Accidental drowning and submersion while in** bath-tub

    EXCLUDES 1   accidental drowning and submersion due to fall in (into) bathtub (W16.211)

√x7ᵗʰ **W67** **Accidental drowning and submersion while in** swimming-pool

    EXCLUDES 1   accidental drowning and submersion due to fall into swimming pool (W16.011, W16.021, W16.031)

            accidental drowning and submersion due to striking into wall of swimming pool (W22.041)

√x7ᵗʰ **W69** **Accidental drowning and submersion while in** natural water

    Accidental drowning and submersion while in lake

    Accidental drowning and submersion while in open sea

    Accidental drowning and submersion while in river

    Accidental drowning and submersion while in stream

    EXCLUDES 1   accidental drowning and submersion due to fall into natural body of water (W16.111, W16.121, W16.131)

√x7ᵗʰ **W73** **Other specified cause of accidental non-transport drowning and submersion**

    Accidental drowning and submersion while in quenching tank

    Accidental drowning and submersion while in reservoir

    EXCLUDES 1   accidental drowning and submersion due to fall into other water (W16.311, W16.321, W16.331)

√x7ᵗʰ **W74** **Unspecified cause of accidental drowning and submersion**

    Drowning NOS

Exposure to electric current, radiation and extreme ambient air temperature and pressure (W85-W99)

  EXCLUDES 1   exposure to:

      failure in dosage of radiation or temperature during surgical and medical care (Y63.2-Y63.5)

      lightning (T75.0-)

      natural cold (X31)

      natural heat (X30)

      natural radiation NOS (X39)

      radiological procedure and radiotherapy (Y84.2)

      sunlight (X32)

AHA: 2018,2Q,7-8

The appropriate 7th character is to be added to each code from categories W85-W99.

A   initial encounter
D   subsequent encounter
S   sequela

√x7ᵗʰ **W85** **Exposure to electric transmission lines**

    Broken power line

√4ᵗʰ **W86** **Exposure to other specified electric current**

√x7ᵗʰ **W86.0** **Exposure to domestic wiring and appliances**

√x7ᵗʰ **W86.1** **Exposure to industrial wiring, appliances and electrical machinery**

    Exposure to conductors

    Exposure to control apparatus

    Exposure to electrical equipment and machinery

    Exposure to transformers

√x7ᵗʰ **W86.8** **Exposure to other electric current**

    Exposure to wiring and appliances in or on farm (not farmhouse)

    Exposure to wiring and appliances outdoors

    Exposure to wiring and appliances in or on public building

    Exposure to wiring and appliances in or on residential institutions

    Exposure to wiring and appliances in or on schools

√4ᵗʰ **W88** **Exposure to ionizing radiation**

    EXCLUDES 1   exposure to sunlight (X32)

√x7ᵗʰ **W88.0** **Exposure to** X-rays

√x7ᵗʰ **W88.1** **Exposure to** radioactive isotopes

√x7ᵗʰ **W88.8**   **Exposure to other ionizing radiation**

✅4ᵗʰ **W89**   **Exposure to man-made visible and ultraviolet light**
> INCLUDES   exposure to welding light (arc)
> EXCLUDES 2   *exposure to sunlight (X32)*

  √x7ᵗʰ **W89.0**   **Exposure to welding light (arc)**

  √x7ᵗʰ **W89.1**   **Exposure to tanning bed**

  √x7ᵗʰ **W89.8**   **Exposure to other man-made visible and ultraviolet light**

  √x7ᵗʰ **W89.9**   **Exposure to unspecified man-made visible and ultraviolet light**

✅4ᵗʰ **W90**   **Exposure to other nonionizing radiation**
> EXCLUDES 2   *exposure to sunlight (X32)*
> AHA: 2019,1Q,21

  √x7ᵗʰ **W90.0**   **Exposure to radiofrequency**

  √x7ᵗʰ **W90.1**   **Exposure to infrared radiation**

  √x7ᵗʰ **W90.2**   **Exposure to laser radiation**

  √x7ᵗʰ **W90.8**   **Exposure to other nonionizing radiation**

√x7ᵗʰ **W92**   **Exposure to excessive heat of man-made origin**

✅4ᵗʰ **W93**   **Exposure to excessive cold of man-made origin**

  ✅5ᵗʰ **W93.0**   **Contact with or inhalation of dry ice**

    √x7ᵗʰ **W93.01**   **Contact with dry ice**

    √x7ᵗʰ **W93.02**   **Inhalation of dry ice**

  ✅5ᵗʰ **W93.1**   **Contact with or inhalation of liquid air**

    √x7ᵗʰ **W93.11**   **Contact with liquid air**
       Contact with liquid hydrogen
       Contact with liquid nitrogen

    √x7ᵗʰ **W93.12**   **Inhalation of liquid air**
       Inhalation of liquid hydrogen
       Inhalation of liquid nitrogen

  √x7ᵗʰ **W93.2**   **Prolonged exposure in deep freeze unit or refrigerator**

  √x7ᵗʰ **W93.8**   **Exposure to other excessive cold of man-made origin**

✅4ᵗʰ **W94**   **Exposure to high and low air pressure and changes in air pressure**

  √x7ᵗʰ **W94.0**   **Exposure to prolonged high air pressure**

  ✅5ᵗʰ **W94.1**   **Exposure to prolonged low air pressure**

    √x7ᵗʰ **W94.11**   **Exposure to residence or prolonged visit at high altitude**

    √x7ᵗʰ **W94.12**   **Exposure to other prolonged low air pressure**

  ✅5ᵗʰ **W94.2**   **Exposure to rapid changes in air pressure during ascent**

    √x7ᵗʰ **W94.21**   **Exposure to reduction in atmospheric pressure while surfacing from deep-water diving**

    √x7ᵗʰ **W94.22**   **Exposure to reduction in atmospheric pressure while surfacing from underground**

    √x7ᵗʰ **W94.23**   **Exposure to sudden change in air pressure in aircraft during ascent**

    √x7ᵗʰ **W94.29**   **Exposure to other rapid changes in air pressure during ascent**

  ✅5ᵗʰ **W94.3**   **Exposure to rapid changes in air pressure during descent**

    √x7ᵗʰ **W94.31**   **Exposure to sudden change in air pressure in aircraft during descent**

    √x7ᵗʰ **W94.32**   **Exposure to high air pressure from rapid descent in water**

    √x7ᵗʰ **W94.39**   **Exposure to other rapid changes in air pressure during descent**

√x7ᵗʰ **W99**   **Exposure to other man-made environmental factors**

Exposure to smoke, fire and flames (X00-X08)

> EXCLUDES 1   *arson (X97)*
> EXCLUDES 2   *explosions (W35-W40)*
>   *lightning (T75.0-)*
>   *transport accident (V01-V99)*

AHA: 2018,2Q,7-8

The appropriate 7th character is to be added to each code from categories X00-X08.
A   initial encounter
D   subsequent encounter
S   sequela

✅4ᵗʰ **X00**   **Exposure to uncontrolled fire in building or structure**
> INCLUDES   conflagration in building or structure
> Code first any associated cataclysm
> EXCLUDES 2   *exposure to ignition or melting of nightwear (X05)*
>   *exposure to ignition or melting of other clothing and apparel (X06.-)*
>   *exposure to other specified smoke, fire and flames (X08.-)*
> AHA: 2016,2Q,5

  √x7ᵗʰ **X00.0**   **Exposure to flames in uncontrolled fire in building or structure**

  √x7ᵗʰ **X00.1**   **Exposure to smoke in uncontrolled fire in building or structure**

  √x7ᵗʰ **X00.2**   **Injury due to collapse of burning building or structure in uncontrolled fire**
> EXCLUDES 1   *injury due to collapse of building not on fire (W20.1)*

  √x7ᵗʰ **X00.3**   **Fall from burning building or structure in uncontrolled fire**

  √x7ᵗʰ **X00.4**   **Hit by object from burning building or structure in uncontrolled fire**
> AHA: 2016,2Q,4

  √x7ᵗʰ **X00.5**   **Jump from burning building or structure in uncontrolled fire**

  √x7ᵗʰ **X00.8**   **Other exposure to uncontrolled fire in building or structure**

✅4ᵗʰ **X01**   **Exposure to uncontrolled fire, not in building or structure**
> INCLUDES   exposure to forest fire

  √x7ᵗʰ **X01.0**   **Exposure to flames in uncontrolled fire, not in building or structure**

  √x7ᵗʰ **X01.1**   **Exposure to smoke in uncontrolled fire, not in building or structure**

  √x7ᵗʰ **X01.3**   **Fall due to uncontrolled fire, not in building or structure**

  √x7ᵗʰ **X01.4**   **Hit by object due to uncontrolled fire, not in building or structure**

  √x7ᵗʰ **X01.8**   **Other exposure to uncontrolled fire, not in building or structure**

✅4ᵗʰ **X02**   **Exposure to controlled fire in building or structure**
> INCLUDES   exposure to fire in fireplace
>   exposure to fire in stove

  √x7ᵗʰ **X02.0**   **Exposure to flames in controlled fire in building or structure**

  √x7ᵗʰ **X02.1**   **Exposure to smoke in controlled fire in building or structure**

  √x7ᵗʰ **X02.2**   **Injury due to collapse of burning building or structure in controlled fire**
> EXCLUDES 1   *injury due to collapse of building not on fire (W20.1)*

  √x7ᵗʰ **X02.3**   **Fall from burning building or structure in controlled fire**

  √x7ᵗʰ **X02.4**   **Hit by object from burning building or structure in controlled fire**

  √x7ᵗʰ **X02.5**   **Jump from burning building or structure in controlled fire**

  √x7ᵗʰ **X02.8**   **Other exposure to controlled fire in building or structure**

✅4ᵗʰ **X03**   **Exposure to controlled fire, not in building or structure**
> INCLUDES   exposure to bon fire
>   exposure to camp-fire
>   exposure to trash fire

  √x7ᵗʰ **X03.0**   **Exposure to flames in controlled fire, not in building or structure**

  √x7ᵗʰ **X03.1**   **Exposure to smoke in controlled fire, not in building or structure**

  √x7ᵗʰ **X03.3**   **Fall due to controlled fire, not in building or structure**

  √x7ᵗʰ **X03.4**   **Hit by object due to controlled fire, not in building or structure**

  √x7ᵗʰ **X03.8**   **Other exposure to controlled fire, not in building or structure**

√x7ᵗʰ **X04** **Exposure to ignition of highly flammable material**
    Exposure to ignition of gasoline
    Exposure to ignition of kerosene
    Exposure to ignition of petrol
    EXCLUDES 2   *exposure to ignition or melting of nightwear (X05)*
      exposure to ignition or melting of other clothing and apparel (X06)
    AHA: 2016,2Q,4

√x7ᵗʰ **X05** **Exposure to ignition or melting of nightwear**
    EXCLUDES 2   *exposure to uncontrolled fire in building or structure (X00.-)*
      exposure to uncontrolled fire, not in building or structure (X01.-)
      exposure to controlled fire in building or structure (X02.-)
      exposure to controlled fire, not in building or structure (X03.-)
      exposure to ignition of highly flammable materials (X04.-)

√4ᵗʰ **X06** **Exposure to ignition or melting of other clothing and apparel**
    EXCLUDES 2   *exposure to uncontrolled fire in building or structure (X00.-)*
      exposure to uncontrolled fire, not in building or structure (X01.-)
      exposure to controlled fire in building or structure (X02.-)
      exposure to controlled fire, not in building or structure (X03.-)
      exposure to ignition of highly flammable materials (X04.-)

    √x7ᵗʰ **X06.0** **Exposure to ignition of plastic jewelry**
    √x7ᵗʰ **X06.1** **Exposure to melting of plastic jewelry**
    √x7ᵗʰ **X06.2** **Exposure to ignition of other clothing and apparel**
    √x7ᵗʰ **X06.3** **Exposure to melting of other clothing and apparel**

√4ᵗʰ **X08** **Exposure to other specified smoke, fire and flames**
    √5ᵗʰ **X08.0** **Exposure to bed fire**
      Exposure to mattress fire
      √x7ᵗʰ **X08.00** **Exposure to bed fire due to unspecified burning material**
      √x7ᵗʰ **X08.01** **Exposure to bed fire due to burning cigarette**
      √x7ᵗʰ **X08.09** **Exposure to bed fire due to other burning material**
    √5ᵗʰ **X08.1** **Exposure to sofa fire**
      √x7ᵗʰ **X08.10** **Exposure to sofa fire due to unspecified burning material**
      √x7ᵗʰ **X08.11** **Exposure to sofa fire due to burning cigarette**
      √x7ᵗʰ **X08.19** **Exposure to sofa fire due to other burning material**
    √5ᵗʰ **X08.2** **Exposure to other furniture fire**
      √x7ᵗʰ **X08.20** **Exposure to other furniture fire due to unspecified burning material**
      √x7ᵗʰ **X08.21** **Exposure to other furniture fire due to burning cigarette**
      √x7ᵗʰ **X08.29** **Exposure to other furniture fire due to other burning material**
    √x7ᵗʰ **X08.8** **Exposure to other specified smoke, fire and flames**

Contact with heat and hot substances (X10-X19)

EXCLUDES 1   *exposure to excessive natural heat (X30)*
     exposure to fire and flames (X00-X08)
AHA: 2018,2Q,7-8

The appropriate 7th character is to be added to each code from categories X10-X19.
A   initial encounter
D   subsequent encounter
S   sequela

√4ᵗʰ **X10** **Contact with hot drinks, food, fats and cooking oils**
    √x7ᵗʰ **X10.0** **Contact with hot drinks**
    √x7ᵗʰ **X10.1** **Contact with hot food**
    √x7ᵗʰ **X10.2** **Contact with fats and cooking oils**

√4ᵗʰ **X11** **Contact with hot tap-water**
    INCLUDES   contact with boiling tap-water
      contact with boiling water NOS
    EXCLUDES 1   *contact with water heated on stove (X12)*
    √x7ᵗʰ **X11.0** **Contact with hot water in bath or tub**
      EXCLUDES 1   *contact with running hot water in bath or tub (X11.1)*
    √x7ᵗʰ **X11.1** **Contact with running hot water**
      Contact with hot water running out of hose
      Contact with hot water running out of tap

√x7ᵗʰ **X11.8** **Contact with other hot tap-water**
      Contact with hot water in bucket
      Contact with hot tap-water NOS

√x7ᵗʰ **X12** **Contact with other hot fluids**
    Contact with water heated on stove
    EXCLUDES 1   *hot (liquid) metals (X18)*

√4ᵗʰ **X13** **Contact with steam and other hot vapors**
    √x7ᵗʰ **X13.0** **Inhalation of steam and other hot vapors**
    √x7ᵗʰ **X13.1** **Other contact with steam and other hot vapors**

√4ᵗʰ **X14** **Contact with hot air and other hot gases**
    √x7ᵗʰ **X14.0** **Inhalation of hot air and gases**
    √x7ᵗʰ **X14.1** **Other contact with hot air and other hot gases**

√4ᵗʰ **X15** **Contact with hot household appliances**
    EXCLUDES 1   *contact with heating appliances (X16)*
      contact with powered household appliances (W29.-)
      exposure to controlled fire in building or structure due to household appliance (X02.8)
      exposure to household appliances electrical current (W86.0)
    √x7ᵗʰ **X15.0** **Contact with hot stove (kitchen)**
    √x7ᵗʰ **X15.1** **Contact with hot toaster**
    √x7ᵗʰ **X15.2** **Contact with hotplate**
    √x7ᵗʰ **X15.3** **Contact with hot saucepan or skillet**
      ▶Contact with hot cooking pan◄
      ▶Contact with hot cooking pot◄
    √x7ᵗʰ **X15.8** **Contact with other hot household appliances**
      Contact with cooker
      Contact with kettle
      Contact with light bulbs

√x7ᵗʰ **X16** **Contact with hot heating appliances, radiators and pipes**
    EXCLUDES 1   *contact with powered appliances (W29.-)*
      exposure to controlled fire in building or structure due to appliance (X02.8)
      exposure to industrial appliances electrical current (W86.1)

√x7ᵗʰ **X17** **Contact with hot engines, machinery and tools**
    EXCLUDES 1   *contact with hot heating appliances, radiators and pipes (X16)*
      contact with hot household appliances (X15)

√x7ᵗʰ **X18** **Contact with other hot metals**
    Contact with liquid metal

√x7ᵗʰ **X19** **Contact with other heat and hot substances**
    EXCLUDES 1   *objects that are not normally hot, e.g., an object made hot by a house fire (X00-X08)*

Exposure to forces of nature (X30-X39)

AHA: 2018,2Q,7-8

The appropriate 7th character is to be added to each code from categories X30-X39.
A   initial encounter
D   subsequent encounter
S   sequela

√x7ᵗʰ **X30** **Exposure to excessive natural heat**
    Exposure to excessive heat as the cause of sunstroke
    Exposure to heat NOS
    EXCLUDES 1   *excessive heat of man-made origin (W92)*
      exposure to man-made radiation (W89)
      exposure to sunlight (X32)
      exposure to tanning bed (W89)

√x7ᵗʰ **X31** **Exposure to excessive natural cold**
    Excessive cold as the cause of chilblains NOS
    Excessive cold as the cause of immersion foot or hand
    Exposure to cold NOS
    Exposure to weather conditions
    EXCLUDES 1   *cold of man-made origin (W93.-)*
      contact with or inhalation of dry ice (W93.-)
      contact with or inhalation of liquefied gas (W93.-)

√x7ᵗʰ **X32** **Exposure to sunlight**
    EXCLUDES 1   *man-made radiation (tanning bed) (W89)*
    EXCLUDES 2   *radiation-related disorders of the skin and subcutaneous tissue (L55-L59)*

Chapter 20. External Causes of Morbidity

✓x7ᵗʰ X34 Earthquake
     EXCLUDES 2   *tidal wave (tsunami) due to earthquake (X37.41)*

✓x7ᵗʰ X35 Volcanic eruption
     EXCLUDES 2   *tidal wave (tsunami) due to volcanic eruption (X37.41)*

✓4ᵗʰ X36 Avalanche, landslide and other earth movements
     INCLUDES   victim of mudslide of cataclysmic nature
     EXCLUDES 1   *earthquake (X34)*
     EXCLUDES 2   *transport accident involving collision with avalanche or landslide not in motion (V01-V99)*

   ✓x7ᵗʰ X36.0 Collapse of dam or man-made structure causing earth movement
   ✓x7ᵗʰ X36.1 Avalanche, landslide, or mudslide

✓4ᵗʰ X37 Cataclysmic storm
   ✓x7ᵗʰ X37.0 Hurricane
     Storm surge
     Typhoon
   ✓x7ᵗʰ X37.1 Tornado
     Cyclone
     Twister
   ✓x7ᵗʰ X37.2 Blizzard (snow)(ice)
   ✓x7ᵗʰ X37.3 Dust storm
   ✓5ᵗʰ X37.4 Tidalwave
     ✓x7ᵗʰ X37.41 Tidal wave due to earthquake or volcanic eruption
       Tidal wave NOS
       Tsunami
     ✓x7ᵗʰ X37.42 Tidal wave due to storm
     ✓x7ᵗʰ X37.43 Tidal wave due to landslide
   ✓x7ᵗʰ X37.8 Other cataclysmic storms
     Cloudburst
     Torrential rain
     EXCLUDES 2   *flood (X38)*
   ✓x7ᵗʰ X37.9 Unspecified cataclysmic storm
     Storm NOS
     EXCLUDES 1   *collapse of dam or man-made structure causing earth movement (X36.0)*

✓x7ᵗʰ X38 Flood
     Flood arising from remote storm
     Flood of cataclysmic nature arising from melting snow
     Flood resulting directly from storm
     EXCLUDES 1   *collapse of dam or man-made structure causing earth movement (X36.0)*
                tidal wave NOS (X37.41)
                tidal wave caused by storm (X37.42)

✓4ᵗʰ X39 Exposure to other forces of nature
   ✓5ᵗʰ X39.0 Exposure to natural radiation
     EXCLUDES 1   *contact with and (suspected) exposure to radon and other naturally occurring radiation (Z77.123)*
                exposure to man-made radiation (W88-W90)
                exposure to sunlight (X32)
     ✓x7ᵗʰ X39.01 Exposure to radon
     ✓x7ᵗʰ X39.08 Exposure to other natural radiation
   ✓x7ᵗʰ X39.8 Other exposure to forces of nature

Overexertion and strenuous or repetitive movements (X50)

✓4ᵗʰ X50 Overexertion and strenuous or repetitive movements
     AHA: 2018,2Q,7-8; 2016,4Q,73-74

     The appropriate 7th character is to be added to each code from category X50.
     A   initial encounter
     D   subsequent encounter
     S   sequela

   ✓x7ᵗʰ X50.0 Overexertion from strenuous movement or load
     Lifting heavy objects
     Lifting weights

   ✓x7ᵗʰ X50.1 Overexertion from prolonged static or awkward postures
     Prolonged bending
     Prolonged kneeling
     Prolonged reaching
     Prolonged sitting
     Prolonged standing
     Prolonged twisting
     Static bending
     Static kneeling
     Static reaching
     Static sitting
     Static standing
     Static twisting

   ✓x7ᵗʰ X50.3 Overexertion from repetitive movements
     Use of hand as hammer
     EXCLUDES 2   *overuse from prolonged static or awkward postures (X50.1)*

   ✓x7ᵗʰ X50.9 Other and unspecified overexertion or strenuous movements or postures
     Contact pressure
     Contact stress

Accidental exposure to other specified factors (X52-X58)

AHA: 2018,2Q,7-8

The appropriate 7th character is to be added to each code from categories X52-X58.
A   initial encounter
D   subsequent encounter
S   sequela

✓x7ᵗʰ X52 Prolonged stay in weightless environment
     Weightlessness in spacecraft (simulator)

✓x7ᵗʰ X58 Exposure to other specified factors
     Accident NOS
     Exposure NOS

Intentional self-harm (X71-X83)

Purposely self-inflicted injury
Suicide (attempted)

The appropriate 7th character is to be added to each code from categories X71-X83.
A   initial encounter
D   subsequent encounter
S   sequela

✓4ᵗʰ X71 Intentional self-harm by drowning and submersion
   ✓x7ᵗʰ X71.0 Intentional self-harm by drowning and submersion while in bathtub HCC Rx ESR COM
   ✓x7ᵗʰ X71.1 Intentional self-harm by drowning and submersion while in swimming pool HCC Rx ESR COM
   ✓x7ᵗʰ X71.2 Intentional self-harm by drowning and submersion after jump into swimming pool HCC Rx ESR COM
   ✓x7ᵗʰ X71.3 Intentional self-harm by drowning and submersion in natural water HCC Rx ESR COM
   ✓x7ᵗʰ X71.8 Other intentional self-harm by drowning and submersion HCC Rx ESR COM
   ✓x7ᵗʰ X71.9 Intentional self-harm by drowning and submersion, unspecified HCC Rx ESR COM

✓x7ᵗʰ X72 Intentional self-harm by handgun discharge HCC Rx ESR COM
     Intentional self-harm by gun for single hand use
     Intentional self-harm by pistol
     Intentional self-harm by revolver
     EXCLUDES 1   *Very pistol (X74.8)*

✓4ᵗʰ X73 Intentional self-harm by rifle, shotgun and larger firearm discharge
     EXCLUDES 1   *airgun (X74.01)*
   ✓x7ᵗʰ X73.0 Intentional self-harm by shotgun discharge HCC Rx ESR COM
   ✓x7ᵗʰ X73.1 Intentional self-harm by hunting rifle discharge HCC Rx ESR COM
   ✓x7ᵗʰ X73.2 Intentional self-harm by machine gun HCC Rx ESR COM
   ✓x7ᵗʰ X73.8 Intentional self-harm by other larger firearm discharge HCC Rx ESR COM
   ✓x7ᵗʰ X73.9 Intentional self-harm by unspecified larger firearm discharge HCC Rx ESR COM

Chapter 20. External Causes of Morbidity

√4th **X74 Intentional self-harm by other and unspecified firearm and gun discharge**

√5th **X74.0 Intentional self-harm by gas, air or spring-operated guns**

√x7th **X74.01 Intentional self-harm by airgun** HCC Rx ESR COM
Intentional self-harm by BB gun discharge
Intentional self-harm by pellet gun discharge

√x7th **X74.02 Intentional self-harm by paintball gun** HCC Rx ESR COM

√x7th **X74.09 Intentional self-harm by other gas, air or spring-operated gun** HCC Rx ESR COM

√x7th **X74.8 Intentional self-harm by other firearm discharge** HCC Rx ESR COM
Intentional self-harm by Very pistol [flare] discharge

√x7th **X74.9 Intentional self-harm by unspecified firearm discharge** HCC Rx ESR COM

√x7th **X75 Intentional self-harm by explosive material** HCC Rx ESR COM

√x7th **X76 Intentional self-harm by smoke, fire and flames** HCC Rx ESR COM

√4th **X77 Intentional self-harm by steam, hot vapors and hot objects**

√x7th **X77.0 Intentional self-harm by steam or hot vapors** HCC Rx ESR COM

√x7th **X77.1 Intentional self-harm by hot tap water** HCC Rx ESR COM

√x7th **X77.2 Intentional self-harm by other hot fluids** HCC Rx ESR COM

√x7th **X77.3 Intentional self-harm by hot household appliances** HCC Rx ESR COM

√x7th **X77.8 Intentional self-harm by other hot objects** HCC Rx ESR COM

√x7th **X77.9 Intentional self-harm by unspecified hot objects** HCC Rx ESR COM

√4th **X78 Intentional self-harm by sharp object**

√x7th **X78.0 Intentional self-harm by sharp glass** HCC Rx ESR COM

√x7th **X78.1 Intentional self-harm by knife** HCC Rx ESR COM

√x7th **X78.2 Intentional self-harm by sword or dagger** HCC Rx ESR COM

√x7th **X78.8 Intentional self-harm by other sharp object** HCC Rx ESR COM
AHA: 2022,1Q,27

√x7th **X78.9 Intentional self-harm by unspecified sharp object** HCC Rx ESR COM

√x7th **X79 Intentional self-harm by blunt object** HCC Rx ESR COM

√x7th **X80 Intentional self-harm by jumping from a high place** HCC Rx ESR COM
Intentional fall from one level to another

√4th **X81 Intentional self-harm by jumping or lying in front of moving object**

√x7th **X81.0 Intentional self-harm by jumping or lying in front of motor vehicle** HCC Rx ESR COM

√x7th **X81.1 Intentional self-harm by jumping or lying in front of (subway) train** HCC Rx ESR COM

√x7th **X81.8 Intentional self-harm by jumping or lying in front of other moving object** HCC Rx ESR COM

√4th **X82 Intentional self-harm by crashing of motor vehicle**

√x7th **X82.0 Intentional collision of motor vehicle with other motor vehicle** HCC Rx ESR COM

√x7th **X82.1 Intentional collision of motor vehicle with train** HCC Rx ESR COM

√x7th **X82.2 Intentional collision of motor vehicle with tree** HCC Rx ESR COM

√x7th **X82.8 Other intentional self-harm by crashing of motor vehicle** HCC Rx ESR COM

√4th **X83 Intentional self-harm by other specified means**

EXCLUDES 1 *intentional self-harm by poisoning or contact with toxic substance - see Table of Drugs and Chemicals*

√x7th **X83.0 Intentional self-harm by crashing of aircraft** HCC Rx ESR COM

√x7th **X83.1 Intentional self-harm by electrocution** HCC Rx ESR COM

√x7th **X83.2 Intentional self-harm by exposure to extremes of cold** HCC Rx ESR COM

√x7th **X83.8 Intentional self-harm by other specified means** HCC Rx ESR COM

Assault (X92-Y09)

INCLUDES   homicide
injuries inflicted by another person with intent to injure or kill, by any means

EXCLUDES 1 *injuries due to legal intervention (Y35.-)*
injuries due to operations of war (Y36.-)
injuries due to terrorism (Y38.-)

The appropriate 7th character is to be added to each code from categories X92-Y04 and Y08.
A   initial encounter
D   subsequent encounter
S   sequela

√4th **X92 Assault by drowning and submersion**

√x7th **X92.0 Assault by drowning and submersion while in bathtub**

√x7th **X92.1 Assault by drowning and submersion while in swimming pool**

√x7th **X92.2 Assault by drowning and submersion after push into swimming pool**

√x7th **X92.3 Assault by drowning and submersion in natural water**

√x7th **X92.8 Other assault by drowning and submersion**

√x7th **X92.9 Assault by drowning and submersion, unspecified**

√x7th **X93 Assault by handgun discharge**
Assault by discharge of gun for single hand use
Assault by discharge of pistol
Assault by discharge of revolver
EXCLUDES 1 *Very pistol (X95.8)*

√4th **X94 Assault by rifle, shotgun and larger firearm discharge**
EXCLUDES 1 *airgun (X95.01)*

√x7th **X94.0 Assault by shotgun**

√x7th **X94.1 Assault by hunting rifle**

√x7th **X94.2 Assault by machine gun**

√x7th **X94.8 Assault by other larger firearm discharge**

√x7th **X94.9 Assault by unspecified larger firearm discharge**

√4th **X95 Assault by other and unspecified firearm and gun discharge**

√5th **X95.0 Assault by gas, air or spring-operated guns**

√x7th **X95.01 Assault by airgun discharge**
Assault by BB gun discharge
Assault by pellet gun discharge

√x7th **X95.02 Assault by paintball gun discharge**

√x7th **X95.09 Assault by other gas, air or spring-operated gun**

√x7th **X95.8 Assault by other firearm discharge**
Assault by Very pistol [flare] discharge

√x7th **X95.9 Assault by unspecified firearm discharge**

√4th **X96 Assault by explosive material**
EXCLUDES 1 *incendiary device (X97)*
terrorism involving explosive material (Y38.2-)

√x7th **X96.0 Assault by antipersonnel bomb**
EXCLUDES 1 *antipersonnel bomb use in military or war (Y36.2-)*

√x7th **X96.1 Assault by gasoline bomb**

√x7th **X96.2 Assault by letter bomb**

√x7th **X96.3 Assault by fertilizer bomb**

√x7th **X96.4 Assault by pipe bomb**

√x7th **X96.8 Assault by other specified explosive**

√x7th **X96.9 Assault by unspecified explosive**

√x7th **X97 Assault by smoke, fire and flames**
Assault by arson
Assault by cigarettes
Assault by incendiary device

√4th **X98 Assault by steam, hot vapors and hot objects**

√x7th **X98.0 Assault by steam or hot vapors**

√x7th **X98.1 Assault by hot tap water**

√x7th **X98.2 Assault by hot fluids**

√x7th **X98.3 Assault by hot household appliances**

√x7th **X98.8 Assault by other hot objects**

√x7th **X98.9 Assault by unspecified hot objects**

☑️4ᵗʰ **X99 Assault by sharp object**

> EXCLUDES 1   *assault by strike by sports equipment (Y08.0-)*

✓x7ᵗʰ **X99.0 Assault by sharp glass**

✓x7ᵗʰ **X99.1 Assault by knife**

✓x7ᵗʰ **X99.2 Assault by sword or dagger**

✓x7ᵗʰ **X99.8 Assault by other sharp object**

✓x7ᵗʰ **X99.9 Assault by unspecified sharp object**

> Assault by stabbing NOS

✓x7ᵗʰ **Y00 Assault by blunt object**

> EXCLUDES 1   *assault by strike by sports equipment (Y08.0-)*

✓x7ᵗʰ **Y01 Assault by pushing from high place**

☑️4ᵗʰ **Y02 Assault by pushing or placing victim in front of moving object**

✓x7ᵗʰ **Y02.0 Assault by pushing or placing victim in front of motor vehicle**

✓x7ᵗʰ **Y02.1 Assault by pushing or placing victim in front of (subway) train**

✓x7ᵗʰ **Y02.8 Assault by pushing or placing victim in front of other moving object**

☑️4ᵗʰ **Y03 Assault by crashing of motor vehicle**

✓x7ᵗʰ **Y03.0 Assault by being hit or run over by motor vehicle**

✓x7ᵗʰ **Y03.8 Other assault by crashing of motor vehicle**

☑️4ᵗʰ **Y04 Assault by bodily force**

> EXCLUDES 1   *assault by:*
> *submersion (X92.-)*
> *use of weapon (X93-X95, X99, Y00)*

✓x7ᵗʰ **Y04.0 Assault by unarmed brawl or fight**

✓x7ᵗʰ **Y04.1 Assault by human bite**

✓x7ᵗʰ **Y04.2 Assault by strike against or bumped into by another person**

✓x7ᵗʰ **Y04.8 Assault by other bodily force**

> Assault by bodily force NOS

☑️4ᵗʰ **Y07 Perpetrator of assault, maltreatment and neglect**

> **NOTE**   Codes from this category are for use only in cases of confirmed abuse (T74.-)
>
> Selection of the correct perpetrator code is based on the relationship between the perpetrator and the victim
>
> **INCLUDES**   perpetrator of abandonment
> perpetrator of emotional neglect
> perpetrator of mental cruelty
> perpetrator of physical abuse
> perpetrator of physical neglect
> perpetrator of sexual abuse
> perpetrator of torture

☑️5ᵗʰ **Y07.0 Spouse or partner, perpetrator of maltreatment and neglect**

> Spouse or partner, perpetrator of maltreatment and neglect against spouse or partner

Y07.01 Husband, perpetrator of maltreatment and neglect

Y07.02 Wife, perpetrator of maltreatment and neglect

Y07.03 Male partner, perpetrator of maltreatment and neglect

Y07.04 Female partner, perpetrator of maltreatment and neglect

☑️5ᵗʰ **Y07.1 Parent (adoptive) (biological), perpetrator of maltreatment and neglect**

Y07.11 Biological father, perpetrator of maltreatment and neglect

Y07.12 Biological mother, perpetrator of maltreatment and neglect

Y07.13 Adoptive father, perpetrator of maltreatment and neglect

Y07.14 Adoptive mother, perpetrator of maltreatment and neglect

☑️5ᵗʰ **Y07.4 Other family member, perpetrator of maltreatment and neglect**

☑️6ᵗʰ **Y07.41 Sibling, perpetrator of maltreatment and neglect**

> EXCLUDES 1   *stepsibling, perpetrator of maltreatment and neglect (Y07.435, Y07.436)*

Y07.410 Brother, perpetrator of maltreatment and neglect

Y07.411 Sister, perpetrator of maltreatment and neglect

☑️6ᵗʰ **Y07.42 Foster parent, perpetrator of maltreatment and neglect**

Y07.420 Foster father, perpetrator of maltreatment and neglect

Y07.421 Foster mother, perpetrator of maltreatment and neglect

☑️6ᵗʰ **Y07.43 Stepparent or stepsibling, perpetrator of maltreatment and neglect**

Y07.430 Stepfather, perpetrator of maltreatment and neglect

Y07.432 Male friend of parent (co-residing in household), perpetrator of maltreatment and neglect

Y07.433 Stepmother, perpetrator of maltreatment and neglect

Y07.434 Female friend of parent (co-residing in household), perpetrator of maltreatment and neglect

Y07.435 Stepbrother, perpetrator or maltreatment and neglect

Y07.436 Stepsister, perpetrator of maltreatment and neglect

☑️6ᵗʰ **Y07.49 Other family member, perpetrator of maltreatment and neglect**

Y07.490 Male cousin, perpetrator of maltreatment and neglect

Y07.491 Female cousin, perpetrator of maltreatment and neglect

Y07.499 Other family member, perpetrator of maltreatment and neglect

☑️5ᵗʰ **Y07.5 Non-family member, perpetrator of maltreatment and neglect**

Y07.50 Unspecified non-family member, perpetrator of maltreatment and neglect

☑️6ᵗʰ **Y07.51 Daycare provider, perpetrator of maltreatment and neglect**

Y07.510 At-home childcare provider, perpetrator of maltreatment and neglect

Y07.511 Daycare center childcare provider, perpetrator of maltreatment and neglect

Y07.512 At-home adultcare provider, perpetrator of maltreatment and neglect

Y07.513 Adultcare center provider, perpetrator of maltreatment and neglect

Y07.519 Unspecified daycare provider, perpetrator of maltreatment and neglect

☑️6ᵗʰ **Y07.52 Healthcare provider, perpetrator of maltreatment and neglect**

Y07.521 Mental health provider, perpetrator of maltreatment and neglect

Y07.528 Other therapist or healthcare provider, perpetrator of maltreatment and neglect

> Nurse perpetrator of maltreatment and neglect
> Occupational therapist perpetrator of maltreatment and neglect
> Physical therapist perpetrator of maltreatment and neglect
> Speech therapist perpetrator of maltreatment and neglect

Y07.529 Unspecified healthcare provider, perpetrator of maltreatment and neglect

Y07.53 Teacher or instructor, perpetrator of maltreatment and neglect

> Coach, perpetrator of maltreatment and neglect

Y07.59 Other non-family member, perpetrator of maltreatment and neglect

Y07.6 Multiple perpetrators of maltreatment and neglect

> AHA: 2018,4Q,32

Y07.9 Unspecified perpetrator of maltreatment and neglect

☑️4ᵗʰ **Y08 Assault by other specified means**

☑️5ᵗʰ **Y08.0 Assault by strike by sport equipment**

✓x7ᵗʰ **Y08.01 Assault by strike by hockey stick**

✓x7ᵗʰ **Y08.02 Assault by strike by baseball bat**

✓x7ᵗʰ **Y08.09 Assault by strike by other specified type of sport equipment**

☑️5ᵗʰ **Y08.8 Assault by other specified means**

✓x7ᵗʰ **Y08.81 Assault by crashing of aircraft**

✓x7ᵗʰ **Y08.89 Assault by other specified means**

Y09 Assault by unspecified means
Assassination (attempted) NOS
Homicide (attempted) NOS
Manslaughter (attempted) NOS
Murder (attempted) NOS

Event of undetermined intent (Y21-Y33)

Undetermined intent is only for use when there is specific documentation in the record that the intent of the injury cannot be determined. If no such documentation is present, code to accidental (unintentional).

The appropriate 7th character is to be added to each code from categories Y21-Y33.
A   initial encounter
D   subsequent encounter
S   sequela

√4th **Y21 Drowning and submersion, undetermined intent**

√x7th **Y21.0 Drowning and submersion** while in bathtub, **undetermined intent**

√x7th **Y21.1 Drowning and submersion** after fall into bathtub, **undetermined intent**

√x7th **Y21.2 Drowning and submersion** while in swimming pool, **undetermined intent**

√x7th **Y21.3 Drowning and submersion** after fall into swimming pool, **undetermined intent**

√x7th **Y21.4 Drowning and submersion** in natural water, **undetermined intent**

√x7th **Y21.8 Other drowning and submersion, undetermined intent**

√x7th **Y21.9 Unspecified drowning and submersion, undetermined intent**

√x7th **Y22 Handgun discharge, undetermined intent**
Discharge of gun for single hand use, undetermined intent
Discharge of pistol, undetermined intent
Discharge of revolver, undetermined intent
EXCLUDES 2   Very pistol (Y24.8)

√4th **Y23 Rifle, shotgun and larger firearm discharge, undetermined intent**
EXCLUDES 2   airgun (Y24.0)

√x7th **Y23.0 Shotgun discharge, undetermined intent**

√x7th **Y23.1 Hunting rifle discharge, undetermined intent**

√x7th **Y23.2 Military firearm discharge, undetermined intent**

√x7th **Y23.3 Machine gun discharge, undetermined intent**

√x7th **Y23.8 Other larger firearm discharge, undetermined intent**

√x7th **Y23.9 Unspecified larger firearm discharge, undetermined intent**

√4th **Y24 Other and unspecified firearm discharge, undetermined intent**

√x7th **Y24.0 Airgun discharge, undetermined intent**
BB gun discharge, undetermined intent
Pellet gun discharge, undetermined intent

√x7th **Y24.8 Other firearm discharge, undetermined intent**
Paintball gun discharge, undetermined intent
Very pistol [flare] discharge, undetermined intent

√x7th **Y24.9 Unspecified firearm discharge, undetermined intent**

√x7th **Y25 Contact with explosive material, undetermined intent**

√x7th **Y26 Exposure to smoke, fire and flames, undetermined intent**

√4th **Y27 Contact with steam, hot vapors and hot objects, undetermined intent**

√x7th **Y27.0 Contact with steam and hot vapors, undetermined intent**

√x7th **Y27.1 Contact with hot tap water, undetermined intent**

√x7th **Y27.2 Contact with hot fluids, undetermined intent**

√x7th **Y27.3 Contact with hot household appliance, undetermined intent**

√x7th **Y27.8 Contact with other hot objects, undetermined intent**

√x7th **Y27.9 Contact with unspecified hot objects, undetermined intent**

√4th **Y28 Contact with sharp object, undetermined intent**

√x7th **Y28.0 Contact with sharp glass, undetermined intent**

√x7th **Y28.1 Contact with knife, undetermined intent**

√x7th **Y28.2 Contact with sword or dagger, undetermined intent**

√x7th **Y28.8 Contact with other sharp object, undetermined intent**

√x7th **Y28.9 Contact with unspecified sharp object, undetermined intent**

√x7th **Y29 Contact with blunt object, undetermined intent**

√x7th **Y30 Falling, jumping or pushed from a high place, undetermined intent**
Victim falling from one level to another, undetermined intent

√x7th **Y31 Falling, lying or running before or into moving object, undetermined intent**

√x7th **Y32 Crashing of motor vehicle, undetermined intent**

√x7th **Y33 Other specified events, undetermined Intent**

Legal intervention, operations of war, military operations, and terrorism (Y35-Y38)

The appropriate 7th character is to be added to each code from categories Y35-Y38.
A   initial encounter
D   subsequent encounter
S   sequela

√4th **Y35 Legal intervention**
INCLUDES   any injury sustained as a result of an encounter with any law enforcement official, serving in any capacity at the time of the encounter, whether on-duty or off-duty. Includes injury to law enforcement official, suspect and bystander
AHA: 2019,4Q,18-19

√5th **Y35.0 Legal intervention involving firearm discharge**

√6th **Y35.00 Legal intervention involving unspecified firearm discharge**
Legal intervention involving gunshot wound
Legal intervention involving shot NOS

√7th **Y35.001 Legal intervention involving unspecified firearm discharge, law enforcement official injured**

√7th **Y35.002 Legal intervention involving unspecified firearm discharge, bystander injured**

√7th **Y35.003 Legal intervention involving unspecified firearm discharge, suspect injured**

√7th **Y35.009 Legal intervention involving unspecified firearm discharge, unspecified person injured**

√6th **Y35.01 Legal intervention involving injury by machine gun**

√7th **Y35.011 Legal intervention involving injury by machine gun, law enforcement official injured**

√7th **Y35.012 Legal intervention involving injury by machine gun, bystander injured**

√7th **Y35.013 Legal intervention involving injury by machine gun, suspect injured**

√7th **Y35.019 Legal intervention involving injury by machine gun, unspecified person injured**

√6th **Y35.02 Legal intervention involving injury by handgun**

√7th **Y35.021 Legal intervention involving injury by handgun, law enforcement official injured**

√7th **Y35.022 Legal intervention involving injury by handgun, bystander injured**

√7th **Y35.023 Legal intervention involving injury by handgun, suspect injured**

√7th **Y35.029 Legal intervention involving injury by handgun, unspecified person injured**

√6th **Y35.03 Legal intervention involving injury by rifle pellet**

√7th **Y35.031 Legal intervention involving injury by rifle pellet, law enforcement official injured**

√7th **Y35.032 Legal intervention involving injury by rifle pellet, bystander injured**

√7th **Y35.033 Legal intervention involving injury by rifle pellet, suspect injured**

√7th **Y35.039 Legal intervention involving injury by rifle pellet, unspecified person injured**

√6th **Y35.04 Legal intervention involving injury by rubber bullet**

√7th **Y35.041 Legal intervention involving injury by rubber bullet, law enforcement official injured**

√7th **Y35.042 Legal intervention involving injury by rubber bullet, bystander injured**

√7th **Y35.043 Legal intervention involving injury by rubber bullet, suspect injured**

√7th **Y35.049 Legal intervention involving injury by rubber bullet, unspecified person injured**

√6th **Y35.09 Legal intervention involving other firearm discharge**

√7th **Y35.091 Legal intervention involving other firearm discharge, law enforcement official injured**

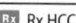

√7ᵗʰ **Y35.092** Legal intervention involving other firearm discharge, **bystander** injured

√7ᵗʰ **Y35.093** Legal intervention involving other firearm discharge, **suspect** injured

√7ᵗʰ **Y35.099** Legal intervention involving other firearm discharge, unspecified person injured

√5ᵗʰ **Y35.1** Legal intervention involving **explosives**

√6ᵗʰ **Y35.10** Legal intervention involving unspecified explosives

√7ᵗʰ **Y35.101** Legal intervention involving unspecified explosives, **law enforcement official** injured

√7ᵗʰ **Y35.102** Legal intervention involving unspecified explosives, **bystander** injured

√7ᵗʰ **Y35.103** Legal intervention involving unspecified explosives, **suspect** injured

√7ᵗʰ **Y35.109** Legal intervention involving unspecified explosives, unspecified person injured

√6ᵗʰ **Y35.11** Legal intervention involving injury by **dynamite**

√7ᵗʰ **Y35.111** Legal intervention involving injury by dynamite, **law enforcement official** injured

√7ᵗʰ **Y35.112** Legal intervention involving injury by dynamite, **bystander** injured

√7ᵗʰ **Y35.113** Legal intervention involving injury by dynamite, **suspect** injured

√7ᵗʰ **Y35.119** Legal intervention involving injury by dynamite, unspecified person injured

√6ᵗʰ **Y35.12** Legal intervention involving injury by **explosive shell**

√7ᵗʰ **Y35.121** Legal intervention involving injury by explosive shell, **law enforcement official** injured

√7ᵗʰ **Y35.122** Legal intervention involving injury by explosive shell, **bystander** injured

√7ᵗʰ **Y35.123** Legal intervention involving injury by explosive shell, **suspect** injured

√7ᵗʰ **Y35.129** Legal intervention involving injury by explosive shell, unspecified person injured

√6ᵗʰ **Y35.19** Legal intervention involving other explosives

Legal intervention involving injury by grenade

Legal intervention involving injury by mortar bomb

√7ᵗʰ **Y35.191** Legal intervention involving other explosives, **law enforcement official** injured

√7ᵗʰ **Y35.192** Legal intervention involving other explosives, **bystander** injured

√7ᵗʰ **Y35.193** Legal intervention involving other explosives, **suspect** injured

√7ᵗʰ **Y35.199** Legal intervention involving other explosives, unspecified person injured

√5ᵗʰ **Y35.2** Legal intervention involving **gas**

Legal intervention involving asphyxiation by gas

Legal intervention involving poisoning by gas

√6ᵗʰ **Y35.20** Legal intervention involving unspecified gas

√7ᵗʰ **Y35.201** Legal intervention involving unspecified gas, **law enforcement official** injured

√7ᵗʰ **Y35.202** Legal intervention involving unspecified gas, **bystander** injured

√7ᵗʰ **Y35.203** Legal intervention involving unspecified gas, **suspect** injured

√7ᵗʰ **Y35.209** Legal intervention involving unspecified gas, unspecified person injured

√6ᵗʰ **Y35.21** Legal intervention involving injury by **tear gas**

√7ᵗʰ **Y35.211** Legal intervention involving injury by tear gas, **law enforcement official** injured

√7ᵗʰ **Y35.212** Legal intervention involving injury by tear gas, **bystander** injured

√7ᵗʰ **Y35.213** Legal intervention involving injury by tear gas, **suspect** injured

√7ᵗʰ **Y35.219** Legal intervention involving injury by tear gas, unspecified person injured

√6ᵗʰ **Y35.29** Legal intervention involving other gas

√7ᵗʰ **Y35.291** Legal intervention involving other gas, **law enforcement official** injured

√7ᵗʰ **Y35.292** Legal intervention involving other gas, **bystander** injured

√7ᵗʰ **Y35.293** Legal intervention involving other gas, **suspect** injured

√7ᵗʰ **Y35.299** Legal intervention involving other gas, unspecified person injured

√5ᵗʰ **Y35.3** Legal intervention involving **blunt objects**

Legal intervention involving being hit or struck by blunt object

√6ᵗʰ **Y35.30** Legal intervention involving unspecified blunt objects

√7ᵗʰ **Y35.301** Legal intervention involving unspecified blunt objects, **law enforcement official** injured

√7ᵗʰ **Y35.302** Legal intervention involving unspecified blunt objects, **bystander** injured

√7ᵗʰ **Y35.303** Legal intervention involving unspecified blunt objects, **suspect** injured

√7ᵗʰ **Y35.309** Legal intervention involving unspecified blunt objects, unspecified person injured

√6ᵗʰ **Y35.31** Legal intervention involving **baton**

√7ᵗʰ **Y35.311** Legal intervention involving baton, **law enforcement official** injured

√7ᵗʰ **Y35.312** Legal intervention involving baton, **bystander** injured

√7ᵗʰ **Y35.313** Legal intervention involving baton, **suspect** injured

√7ᵗʰ **Y35.319** Legal intervention involving baton, unspecified person injured

√6ᵗʰ **Y35.39** Legal intervention involving other blunt objects

√7ᵗʰ **Y35.391** Legal intervention involving other blunt objects, **law enforcement official** injured

√7ᵗʰ **Y35.392** Legal intervention involving other blunt objects, **bystander** injured

√7ᵗʰ **Y35.393** Legal intervention involving other blunt objects, **suspect** injured

√7ᵗʰ **Y35.399** Legal intervention involving other blunt objects, unspecified person injured

√5ᵗʰ **Y35.4** Legal intervention involving **sharp objects**

Legal intervention involving being cut by sharp objects

Legal intervention involving being stabbed by sharp objects

√6ᵗʰ **Y35.40** Legal intervention involving unspecified sharp objects

√7ᵗʰ **Y35.401** Legal intervention involving unspecified sharp objects, **law enforcement official** injured

√7ᵗʰ **Y35.402** Legal intervention involving unspecified sharp objects, **bystander** injured

√7ᵗʰ **Y35.403** Legal intervention involving unspecified sharp objects, **suspect** injured

√7ᵗʰ **Y35.409** Legal intervention involving unspecified sharp objects, unspecified person injured

√6ᵗʰ **Y35.41** Legal intervention involving **bayonet**

√7ᵗʰ **Y35.411** Legal intervention involving bayonet, **law enforcement official** injured

√7ᵗʰ **Y35.412** Legal intervention involving bayonet, **bystander** injured

√7ᵗʰ **Y35.413** Legal intervention involving bayonet, **suspect** injured

√7ᵗʰ **Y35.419** Legal intervention involving bayonet, unspecified person injured

√6ᵗʰ **Y35.49** Legal intervention involving other sharp objects

√7ᵗʰ **Y35.491** Legal intervention involving other sharp objects, **law enforcement official** injured

√7ᵗʰ **Y35.492** Legal intervention involving other sharp objects, **bystander** injured

√7ᵗʰ **Y35.493** Legal intervention involving other sharp objects, **suspect** injured

√7ᵗʰ **Y35.499** Legal intervention involving other sharp objects, unspecified person injured

√6ᵗʰ **Y35.8** Legal intervention involving other specified means

AHA: 2019,4Q,19

√6ᵗʰ **Y35.81** Legal intervention involving **manhandling**

√7ᵗʰ **Y35.811** Legal intervention involving manhandling, **law enforcement official** injured

√7ᵗʰ **Y35.812** Legal intervention involving manhandling, **bystander** injured

√7ᵗʰ **Y35.813** Legal intervention involving manhandling, **suspect** injured

√7ᵗʰ **Y35.819** Legal intervention involving manhandling, unspecified person injured

---

☑ Additional Character Required   √x7ᵗʰ Placeholder Alert   Manifestation   Unspecified Dx   ◘ QPP   UPD Unacceptable PDx

Chapter 20. External Causes of Morbidity

✓6ᵗʰ **Y35.83 Legal intervention involving a** conducted energy device
Electroshock device (taser)
Stun gun

✓7ᵗʰ **Y35.831 Legal intervention involving a conducted energy device,** law enforcement official injured

✓7ᵗʰ **Y35.832 Legal intervention involving a conducted energy device,** bystander injured

✓7ᵗʰ **Y35.833 Legal intervention involving a conducted energy device,** suspect injured

✓7ᵗʰ **Y35.839 Legal intervention involving a conducted energy device,** unspecified person injured

✓6ᵗʰ **Y35.89 Legal intervention involving other specified means**

✓7ᵗʰ **Y35.891 Legal intervention involving other specified means,** law enforcement official injured

✓7ᵗʰ **Y35.892 Legal intervention involving other specified means,** bystander injured

✓7ᵗʰ **Y35.893 Legal intervention involving other specified means,** suspect injured
AHA: 2018,1Q,5

✓7ᵗʰ **Y35.899 Legal intervention involving other specified means, unspecified person injured**

✓5ᵗʰ **Y35.9 Legal intervention, means unspecified**

✓x7ᵗʰ **Y35.91 Legal intervention, means unspecified,** law enforcement official injured

✓x7ᵗʰ **Y35.92 Legal intervention, means unspecified,** bystander injured

✓x7ᵗʰ **Y35.93 Legal intervention, means unspecified,** suspect injured

✓x7ᵗʰ **Y35.99 Legal intervention, means unspecified, unspecified person injured**

✓4ᵗʰ **Y36 Operations of war**

INCLUDES   injuries to military personnel and civilians caused by war, civil insurrection, and peacekeeping missions

EXCLUDES 1   injury to military personnel occurring during peacetime military operations (Y37.-)
military vehicles involved in transport accidents with non-military vehicle during peacetime ▶(V09.01, V09.21, V19.81, V29.818, V39.81, V49.81, V59.81, V69.81, V79.81)◀

AHA: 2014,3Q,4

✓5ᵗʰ **Y36.0 War operations involving** explosion of marine weapons

✓6ᵗʰ **Y36.00 War operations involving explosion of unspecified marine weapon**
War operations involving underwater blast NOS

✓7ᵗʰ **Y36.000 War operations involving explosion of unspecified marine weapon,** military personnel

✓7ᵗʰ **Y36.001 War operations involving explosion of unspecified marine weapon,** civilian

✓6ᵗʰ **Y36.01 War operations involving explosion of** depth-charge

✓7ᵗʰ **Y36.010 War operations involving explosion of depth-charge,** military personnel

✓7ᵗʰ **Y36.011 War operations involving explosion of depth-charge,** civilian

✓6ᵗʰ **Y36.02 War operations involving explosion of** marine mine
War operations involving explosion of marine mine, at sea or in harbor

✓7ᵗʰ **Y36.020 War operations involving explosion of marine mine,** military personnel

✓7ᵗʰ **Y36.021 War operations involving explosion of marine mine,** civilian

✓6ᵗʰ **Y36.03 War operations involving explosion of** sea-based artillery shell

✓7ᵗʰ **Y36.030 War operations involving explosion of sea-based artillery shell,** military personnel

✓7ᵗʰ **Y36.031 War operations involving explosion of sea-based artillery shell,** civilian

✓6ᵗʰ **Y36.04 War operations involving explosion of** torpedo

✓7ᵗʰ **Y36.040 War operations involving explosion of torpedo,** military personnel

✓7ᵗʰ **Y36.041 War operations involving explosion of torpedo,** civilian

✓6ᵗʰ **Y36.05 War operations involving** accidental detonation of onboard marine weapons

✓7ᵗʰ **Y36.050 War operations involving accidental detonation of onboard marine weapons,** military personnel

✓7ᵗʰ **Y36.051 War operations involving accidental detonation of onboard marine weapons,** civilian

✓6ᵗʰ **Y36.09 War operations involving explosion of other marine weapons**

✓7ᵗʰ **Y36.090 War operations involving explosion of other marine weapons,** military personnel

✓7ᵗʰ **Y36.091 War operations involving explosion of other marine weapons,** civilian

✓5ᵗʰ **Y36.1 War operations involving** destruction of aircraft

✓6ᵗʰ **Y36.10 War operations involving unspecified destruction of aircraft**

✓7ᵗʰ **Y36.100 War operations involving unspecified destruction of aircraft,** military personnel

✓7ᵗʰ **Y36.101 War operations involving unspecified destruction of aircraft,** civilian

✓6ᵗʰ **Y36.11 War operations involving destruction of aircraft due to** enemy fire or explosives
War operations involving destruction of aircraft due to air to air missile
War operations involving destruction of aircraft due to explosive placed on aircraft
War operations involving destruction of aircraft due to rocket propelled grenade [RPG]
War operations involving destruction of aircraft due to small arms fire
War operations involving destruction of aircraft due to surface to air missile

✓7ᵗʰ **Y36.110 War operations involving destruction of aircraft due to enemy fire or explosives,** military personnel

✓7ᵗʰ **Y36.111 War operations involving destruction of aircraft due to enemy fire or explosives,** civilian

✓6ᵗʰ **Y36.12 War operations involving destruction of aircraft due to** collision with other aircraft

✓7ᵗʰ **Y36.120 War operations involving destruction of aircraft due to collision with other aircraft,** military personnel

✓7ᵗʰ **Y36.121 War operations involving destruction of aircraft due to collision with other aircraft,** civilian

✓6ᵗʰ **Y36.13 War operations involving destruction of aircraft due to** onboard fire

✓7ᵗʰ **Y36.130 War operations involving destruction of aircraft due to onboard fire,** military personnel

✓7ᵗʰ **Y36.131 War operations involving destruction of aircraft due to onboard fire,** civilian

✓6ᵗʰ **Y36.14 War operations involving destruction of aircraft due to** accidental detonation of onboard munitions and explosives

✓7ᵗʰ **Y36.140 War operations involving destruction of aircraft due to accidental detonation of onboard munitions and explosives,** military personnel

✓7ᵗʰ **Y36.141 War operations involving destruction of aircraft due to accidental detonation of onboard munitions and explosives,** civilian

✓6ᵗʰ **Y36.19 War operations involving other destruction of aircraft**

✓7ᵗʰ **Y36.190 War operations involving other destruction of aircraft,** military personnel

✓7ᵗʰ **Y36.191 War operations involving other destruction of aircraft,** civilian

✓5th **Y36.2 War operations involving other explosions and fragments**

EXCLUDES 1 *war operations involving explosion of aircraft (Y36.1-)*
war operations involving explosion of marine weapons (Y36.0-)
war operations involving explosion of nuclear weapons (Y36.5-)
war operations involving explosion occurring after cessation of hostilities (Y36.8-)

✓6th **Y36.20 War operations involving unspecified explosion and fragments**
War operations involving air blast NOS
War operations involving blast NOS
War operations involving blast fragments NOS
War operations involving blast wave NOS
War operations involving blast wind NOS
War operations involving explosion NOS
War operations involving explosion of bomb NOS

✓7th **Y36.200 War operations involving unspecified explosion and fragments, military personnel**

✓7th **Y36.201 War operations involving unspecified explosion and fragments, civilian**

✓6th **Y36.21 War operations involving explosion of aerial bomb**

✓7th **Y36.210 War operations involving explosion of aerial bomb, military personnel**

✓7th **Y36.211 War operations involving explosion of aerial bomb, civilian**

✓6th **Y36.22 War operations involving explosion of guided missile**

✓7th **Y36.220 War operations involving explosion of guided missile, military personnel**

✓7th **Y36.221 War operations involving explosion of guided missile, civilian**

✓6th **Y36.23 War operations involving explosion of improvised explosive device [IED]**
War operations involving explosion of person-borne improvised explosive device [IED]
War operations involving explosion of vehicle-borne improvised explosive device [IED]
War operations involving explosion of roadside improvised explosive device [IED]

✓7th **Y36.230 War operations involving explosion of improvised explosive device [IED], military personnel**

✓7th **Y36.231 War operations involving explosion of improvised explosive device [IED], civilian**

✓6th **Y36.24 War operations involving explosion due to accidental detonation and discharge of own munitions or munitions launch device**

✓7th **Y36.240 War operations involving explosion due to accidental detonation and discharge of own munitions or munitions launch device, military personnel**

✓7th **Y36.241 War operations involving explosion due to accidental detonation and discharge of own munitions or munitions launch device, civilian**

✓6th **Y36.25 War operations involving fragments from munitions**

✓7th **Y36.250 War operations involving fragments from munitions, military personnel**

✓7th **Y36.251 War operations involving fragments from munitions, civilian**

✓6th **Y36.26 War operations involving fragments of improvised explosive device [IED]**
War operations involving fragments of person-borne improvised explosive device [IED]
War operations involving fragments of vehicle-borne improvised explosive device [IED]
War operations involving fragments of roadside improvised explosive device [IED]

✓7th **Y36.260 War operations involving fragments of improvised explosive device [IED], military personnel**

✓7th **Y36.261 War operations involving fragments of improvised explosive device [IED], civilian**

✓6th **Y36.27 War operations involving fragments from weapons**

✓7th **Y36.270 War operations involving fragments from weapons, military personnel**

✓7th **Y36.271 War operations involving fragments from weapons, civilian**

✓6th **Y36.29 War operations involving other explosions and fragments**
War operations involving explosion of grenade
War operations involving explosions of land mine
War operations involving shrapnel NOS

✓7th **Y36.290 War operations involving other explosions and fragments, military personnel**

✓7th **Y36.291 War operations involving other explosions and fragments, civilian**

✓5th **Y36.3 War operations involving fires, conflagrations and hot substances**
War operations involving smoke, fumes, and heat from fires, conflagrations and hot substances

EXCLUDES 1 *war operations involving fires and conflagrations aboard military aircraft (Y36.1-)*
war operations involving fires and conflagrations aboard military watercraft (Y36.0-)
war operations involving fires and conflagrations caused indirectly by conventional weapons (Y36.2-)
war operations involving fires and thermal effects of nuclear weapons (Y36.53-)

✓6th **Y36.30 War operations involving unspecified fire, conflagration and hot substance**

✓7th **Y36.300 War operations involving unspecified fire, conflagration and hot substance, military personnel**

✓7th **Y36.301 War operations involving unspecified fire, conflagration and hot substance, civilian**

✓6th **Y36.31 War operations involving gasoline bomb**
War operations involving incendiary bomb
War operations involving petrol bomb

✓7th **Y36.310 War operations involving gasoline bomb, military personnel**

✓7th **Y36.311 War operations involving gasoline bomb, civilian**

✓6th **Y36.32 War operations involving incendiary bullet**

✓7th **Y36.320 War operations involving incendiary bullet, military personnel**

✓7th **Y36.321 War operations involving incendiary bullet, civilian**

✓6th **Y36.33 War operations involving flamethrower**

✓7th **Y36.330 War operations involving flamethrower, military personnel**

✓7th **Y36.331 War operations involving flamethrower, civilian**

✓6th **Y36.39 War operations involving other fires, conflagrations and hot substances**

✓7th **Y36.390 War operations involving other fires, conflagrations and hot substances, military personnel**

✓7th **Y36.391 War operations involving other fires, conflagrations and hot substances, civilian**

✓5th **Y36.4 War operations involving firearm discharge and other forms of conventional warfare**

✓6th **Y36.41 War operations involving rubber bullets**

✓7th **Y36.410 War operations involving rubber bullets, military personnel**

✓7th **Y36.411 War operations involving rubber bullets, civilian**

✓6th **Y36.42 War operations involving firearms pellets**

✓7th **Y36.420 War operations involving firearms pellets, military personnel**

✓7th **Y36.421 War operations involving firearms pellets, civilian**

✓6th **Y36.43 War operations involving other firearms discharge**
War operations involving bullets NOS

EXCLUDES 1 *war operations involving munitions fragments (Y36.25-)*
war operations involving incendiary bullets (Y36.32-)

✓7th **Y36.430 War operations involving other firearms discharge, military personnel**

✓7th **Y36.431 War operations involving other firearms discharge, civilian**

Chapter 20. External Causes of Morbidity

Y36.44 War operations involving unarmed hand to hand combat

EXCLUDES 1
war operations involving combat using blunt or piercing object (Y36.45-)
war operations involving intentional restriction of air and airway (Y36.46-)
war operations involving unintentional restriction of air and airway (Y36.47-)

Y36.440 War operations involving unarmed hand to hand combat, military personnel
Y36.441 War operations involving unarmed hand to hand combat, civilian

Y36.45 War operations involving combat using blunt or piercing object
Y36.450 War operations involving combat using blunt or piercing object, military personnel
Y36.451 War operations involving combat using blunt or piercing object, civilian

Y36.46 War operations involving intentional restriction of air and airway
Y36.460 War operations involving intentional restriction of air and airway, military personnel
Y36.461 War operations involving intentional restriction of air and airway, civilian

Y36.47 War operations involving unintentional restriction of air and airway
Y36.470 War operations involving unintentional restriction of air and airway, military personnel
Y36.471 War operations involving unintentional restriction of air and airway, civilian

Y36.49 War operations involving other forms of conventional warfare
Y36.490 War operations involving other forms of conventional warfare, military personnel
Y36.491 War operations involving other forms of conventional warfare, civilian

Y36.5 War operations involving nuclear weapons
War operations involving dirty bomb NOS

Y36.50 War operations involving unspecified effect of nuclear weapon
Y36.500 War operations involving unspecified effect of nuclear weapon, military personnel
Y36.501 War operations involving unspecified effect of nuclear weapon, civilian

Y36.51 War operations involving direct blast effect of nuclear weapon
War operations involving blast pressure of nuclear weapon
Y36.510 War operations involving direct blast effect of nuclear weapon, military personnel
Y36.511 War operations involving direct blast effect of nuclear weapon, civilian

Y36.52 War operations involving indirect blast effect of nuclear weapon
War operations involving being thrown by blast of nuclear weapon
War operations involving being struck or crushed by blast debris of nuclear weapon
Y36.520 War operations involving indirect blast effect of nuclear weapon, military personnel
Y36.521 War operations involving indirect blast effect of nuclear weapon, civilian

Y36.53 War operations involving thermal radiation effect of nuclear weapon
War operations involving direct heat from nuclear weapon
War operation involving fireball effects from nuclear weapon
Y36.530 War operations involving thermal radiation effect of nuclear weapon, military personnel
Y36.531 War operations involving thermal radiation effect of nuclear weapon, civilian

Y36.54 War operation involving nuclear radiation effects of nuclear weapon
War operation involving acute radiation exposure from nuclear weapon
War operation involving exposure to immediate ionizing radiation from nuclear weapon
War operation involving fallout exposure from nuclear weapon
War operation involving secondary effects of nuclear weapons
Y36.540 War operation involving nuclear radiation effects of nuclear weapon, military personnel
Y36.541 War operation involving nuclear radiation effects of nuclear weapon, civilian

Y36.59 War operation involving other effects of nuclear weapons
Y36.590 War operation involving other effects of nuclear weapons, military personnel
Y36.591 War operation involving other effects of nuclear weapons, civilian

Y36.6 War operations involving biological weapons
Y36.6X War operations involving biological weapons
Y36.6X0 War operations involving biological weapons, military personnel
Y36.6X1 War operations involving biological weapons, civilian

Y36.7 War operations involving chemical weapons and other forms of unconventional warfare
EXCLUDES 1 war operations involving incendiary devices (Y36.3-, Y36.5-)
Y36.7X War operations involving chemical weapons and other forms of unconventional warfare
Y36.7X0 War operations involving chemical weapons and other forms of unconventional warfare, military personnel
Y36.7X1 War operations involving chemical weapons and other forms of unconventional warfare, civilian

Y36.8 War operations occurring after cessation of hostilities
War operations classifiable to categories Y36.0-Y36.8 but occurring after cessation of hostilities
Y36.81 Explosion of mine placed during war operations but exploding after cessation of hostilities
Y36.810 Explosion of mine placed during war operations but exploding after cessation of hostilities, military personnel
Y36.811 Explosion of mine placed during war operations but exploding after cessation of hostilities, civilian
Y36.82 Explosion of bomb placed during war operations but exploding after cessation of hostilities
Y36.820 Explosion of bomb placed during war operations but exploding after cessation of hostilities, military personnel
Y36.821 Explosion of bomb placed during war operations but exploding after cessation of hostilities, civilian
Y36.88 Other war operations occurring after cessation of hostilities
Y36.880 Other war operations occurring after cessation of hostilities, military personnel
Y36.881 Other war operations occurring after cessation of hostilities, civilian
Y36.89 Unspecified war operations occurring after cessation of hostilities
Y36.890 Unspecified war operations occurring after cessation of hostilities, military personnel
Y36.891 Unspecified war operations occurring after cessation of hostilities, civilian

Y36.9 Other and unspecified war operations
Y36.90 War operations, unspecified
Y36.91 War operations involving unspecified weapon of mass destruction [WMD]
Y36.92 War operations involving friendly fire

☑4ᵗʰ **Y37 Military operations**

> INCLUDES   injuries to military personnel and civilians occurring during peacetime on military property and during routine military exercises and operations
>
> EXCLUDES 1   *military aircraft involved in aircraft accident with civilian aircraft (V97.81-)*
> *military vehicles involved in transport accident with civilian vehicle ▶(V09.01, V09.21, V19.81, V29.818, V39.81, V49.81, V59.81, V69.81, V79.81)◀*
> *military watercraft involved in water transport accident with civilian watercraft (V94.81-)*
> *war operations (Y36.-)*

☑5ᵗʰ **Y37.0 Military operations involving** explosion of marine weapons

    ☑6ᵗʰ **Y37.00 Military operations involving explosion of unspecified marine weapon**

         Military operations involving underwater blast NOS

        ☑7ᵗʰ **Y37.000 Military operations involving explosion of unspecified marine weapon, military personnel**

        ☑7ᵗʰ **Y37.001 Military operations involving explosion of unspecified marine weapon, civilian**

    ☑6ᵗʰ **Y37.01 Military operations involving explosion of depth-charge**

        ☑7ᵗʰ **Y37.010 Military operations involving explosion of depth-charge, military personnel**

        ☑7ᵗʰ **Y37.011 Military operations involving explosion of depth-charge, civilian**

    ☑6ᵗʰ **Y37.02 Military operations involving explosion of** marine mine

         Military operations involving explosion of marine mine, at sea or in harbor

        ☑7ᵗʰ **Y37.020 Military operations involving explosion of marine mine, military personnel**

        ☑7ᵗʰ **Y37.021 Military operations involving explosion of marine mine, civilian**

    ☑6ᵗʰ **Y37.03 Military operations involving explosion of** sea-based artillery shell

        ☑7ᵗʰ **Y37.030 Military operations involving explosion of sea-based artillery shell, military personnel**

        ☑7ᵗʰ **Y37.031 Military operations involving explosion of sea-based artillery shell, civilian**

    ☑6ᵗʰ **Y37.04 Military operations involving explosion of** torpedo

        ☑7ᵗʰ **Y37.040 Military operations involving explosion of torpedo, military personnel**

        ☑7ᵗʰ **Y37.041 Military operations involving explosion of torpedo, civilian**

    ☑6ᵗʰ **Y37.05 Military operations involving accidental detonation of** onboard marine weapons

        ☑7ᵗʰ **Y37.050 Military operations involving accidental detonation of onboard marine weapons, military personnel**

        ☑7ᵗʰ **Y37.051 Military operations involving accidental detonation of onboard marine weapons, civilian**

    ☑6ᵗʰ **Y37.09 Military operations involving explosion of other marine weapons**

        ☑7ᵗʰ **Y37.090 Military operations involving explosion of other marine weapons, military personnel**

        ☑7ᵗʰ **Y37.091 Military operations involving explosion of other marine weapons, civilian**

☑5ᵗʰ **Y37.1 Military operations involving** destruction of aircraft

    ☑6ᵗʰ **Y37.10 Military operations involving unspecified destruction of aircraft**

        ☑7ᵗʰ **Y37.100 Military operations involving unspecified destruction of aircraft, military personnel**

        ☑7ᵗʰ **Y37.101 Military operations involving unspecified destruction of aircraft, civilian**

☑6ᵗʰ **Y37.11 Military operations involving destruction of aircraft due to enemy fire or explosives**

     Military operations involving destruction of aircraft due to air to air missile

     Military operations involving destruction of aircraft due to explosive placed on aircraft

     Military operations involving destruction of aircraft due to rocket propelled grenade [RPG]

     Military operations involving destruction of aircraft due to small arms fire

     Military operations involving destruction of aircraft due to surface to air missile

    ☑7ᵗʰ **Y37.110 Military operations involving destruction of aircraft due to enemy fire or explosives, military personnel**

    ☑7ᵗʰ **Y37.111 Military operations involving destruction of aircraft due to enemy fire or explosives, civilian**

☑6ᵗʰ **Y37.12 Military operations involving destruction of aircraft due to collision with other aircraft**

    ☑7ᵗʰ **Y37.120 Military operations involving destruction of aircraft due to collision with other aircraft, military personnel**

    ☑7ᵗʰ **Y37.121 Military operations involving destruction of aircraft due to collision with other aircraft, civilian**

☑6ᵗʰ **Y37.13 Military operations involving destruction of aircraft due to onboard fire**

    ☑7ᵗʰ **Y37.130 Military operations involving destruction of aircraft due to onboard fire, military personnel**

    ☑7ᵗʰ **Y37.131 Military operations involving destruction of aircraft due to onboard fire, civilian**

☑6ᵗʰ **Y37.14 Military operations involving destruction of aircraft due to** accidental detonation of onboard munitions and explosives

    ☑7ᵗʰ **Y37.140 Military operations involving destruction of aircraft due to accidental detonation of onboard munitions and explosives, military personnel**

    ☑7ᵗʰ **Y37.141 Military operations involving destruction of aircraft due to accidental detonation of onboard munitions and explosives, civilian**

☑6ᵗʰ **Y37.19 Military operations involving other destruction of aircraft**

    ☑7ᵗʰ **Y37.190 Military operations involving other destruction of aircraft, military personnel**

    ☑7ᵗʰ **Y37.191 Military operations involving other destruction of aircraft, civilian**

☑5ᵗʰ **Y37.2 Military operations involving** other explosions and fragments

> EXCLUDES 1   *military operations involving explosion of aircraft (Y37.1-)*
> *military operations involving explosion of marine weapons (Y37.0-)*
> *military operations involving explosion of nuclear weapons (Y37.5-)*

    ☑6ᵗʰ **Y37.20 Military operations involving unspecified explosion and fragments**

     Military operations involving air blast NOS

     Military operations involving blast NOS

     Military operations involving blast fragments NOS

     Military operations involving blast wave NOS

     Military operations involving blast wind NOS

     Military operations involving explosion NOS

     Military operations involving explosion of bomb NOS

    ☑7ᵗʰ **Y37.200 Military operations involving unspecified explosion and fragments, military personnel**

    ☑7ᵗʰ **Y37.201 Military operations involving unspecified explosion and fragments, civilian**

    ☑6ᵗʰ **Y37.21 Military operations involving explosion of** aerial bomb

        ☑7ᵗʰ **Y37.210 Military operations involving explosion of aerial bomb, military personnel**

        ☑7ᵗʰ **Y37.211 Military operations involving explosion of aerial bomb, civilian**

    ☑6ᵗʰ **Y37.22 Military operations involving explosion of** guided missile

        ☑7ᵗʰ **Y37.220 Military operations involving explosion of guided missile, military personnel**

√7ᵗʰ **Y37.221 Military operations involving explosion of guided missile,** civilian

√6ᵗʰ **Y37.23 Military operations involving explosion of** improvised explosive device [IED]

Military operations involving explosion of person-borne improvised explosive device [IED]

Military operations involving explosion of vehicle-borne improvised explosive device [IED]

Military operations involving explosion of roadside improvised explosive device [IED]

√7ᵗʰ **Y37.230 Military operations involving explosion of improvised explosive device [IED], military personnel**

√7ᵗʰ **Y37.231 Military operations involving explosion of improvised explosive device [IED], civilian**

√6ᵗʰ **Y37.24 Military operations involving explosion** due to accidental detonation and discharge of own munitions or munitions launch device

√7ᵗʰ **Y37.240 Military operations involving explosion due to accidental detonation and discharge of own munitions or munitions launch device, military personnel**

√7ᵗʰ **Y37.241 Military operations involving explosion due to accidental detonation and discharge of own munitions or munitions launch device, civilian**

√6ᵗʰ **Y37.25 Military operations involving** fragments from munitions

√7ᵗʰ **Y37.250 Military operations involving fragments from munitions, military personnel**

√7ᵗʰ **Y37.251 Military operations involving fragments from munitions, civilian**

√6ᵗʰ **Y37.26 Military operations involving** fragments of improvised explosive device [IED]

Military operations involving fragments of person-borne improvised explosive device [IED]

Military operations involving fragments of vehicle-borne improvised explosive device [IED]

Military operations involving fragments of roadside improvised explosive device [IED]

√7ᵗʰ **Y37.260 Military operations involving fragments of improvised explosive device [IED], military personnel**

√7ᵗʰ **Y37.261 Military operations involving fragments of improvised explosive device [IED], civilian**

√6ᵗʰ **Y37.27 Military operations involving** fragments from weapons

√7ᵗʰ **Y37.270 Military operations involving fragments from weapons, military personnel**

√7ᵗʰ **Y37.271 Military operations involving fragments from weapons, civilian**

√6ᵗʰ **Y37.29 Military operations involving other explosions and fragments**

Military operations involving explosion of grenade

Military operations involving explosions of land mine

Military operations involving shrapnel NOS

√7ᵗʰ **Y37.290 Military operations involving other explosions and fragments, military personnel**

√7ᵗʰ **Y37.291 Military operations involving other explosions and fragments, civilian**

√5ᵗʰ **Y37.3 Military operations involving** fires, conflagrations and hot substances

Military operations involving smoke, fumes, and heat from fires, conflagrations and hot substances

EXCLUDES 1 *military operations involving fires and conflagrations aboard military aircraft (Y37.1-)*

military operations involving fires and conflagrations aboard military watercraft (Y37.0-)

military operations involving fires and conflagrations caused indirectly by conventional weapons (Y37.2-)

military operations involving fires and thermal effects of nuclear weapons (Y36.53-)

√6ᵗʰ **Y37.30 Military operations involving unspecified fire, conflagration and hot substance**

√7ᵗʰ **Y37.300 Military operations involving unspecified fire, conflagration and hot substance, military personnel**

√7ᵗʰ **Y37.301 Military operations involving unspecified fire, conflagration and hot substance, civilian**

√6ᵗʰ **Y37.31 Military operations involving** gasoline bomb

Military operations involving incendiary bomb

Military operations involving petrol bomb

√7ᵗʰ **Y37.310 Military operations involving gasoline bomb, military personnel**

√7ᵗʰ **Y37.311 Military operations involving gasoline bomb, civilian**

√6ᵗʰ **Y37.32 Military operations involving** incendiary bullet

√7ᵗʰ **Y37.320 Military operations involving incendiary bullet, military personnel**

√7ᵗʰ **Y37.321 Military operations involving incendiary bullet, civilian**

√6ᵗʰ **Y37.33 Military operations involving** flamethrower

√7ᵗʰ **Y37.330 Military operations involving flamethrower, military personnel**

√7ᵗʰ **Y37.331 Military operations involving flamethrower, civilian**

√6ᵗʰ **Y37.39 Military operations involving other fires, conflagrations and hot substances**

√7ᵗʰ **Y37.390 Military operations involving other fires, conflagrations and hot substances, military personnel**

√7ᵗʰ **Y37.391 Military operations involving other fires, conflagrations and hot substances, civilian**

√5ᵗʰ **Y37.4 Military operations involving firearm discharge and other forms of conventional warfare**

√6ᵗʰ **Y37.41 Military operations involving** rubber bullets

√7ᵗʰ **Y37.410 Military operations involving rubber bullets, military personnel**

√7ᵗʰ **Y37.411 Military operations involving rubber bullets, civilian**

√6ᵗʰ **Y37.42 Military operations involving** firearms pellets

√7ᵗʰ **Y37.420 Military operations involving firearms pellets, military personnel**

√7ᵗʰ **Y37.421 Military operations involving firearms pellets, civilian**

√6ᵗʰ **Y37.43 Military operations involving other firearms discharge**

Military operations involving bullets NOS

EXCLUDES 1 *military operations involving munitions fragments (Y37.25-)*

military operations involving incendiary bullets (Y37.32-)

√7ᵗʰ **Y37.430 Military operations involving other firearms discharge, military personnel**

√7ᵗʰ **Y37.431 Military operations involving other firearms discharge, civilian**

√6ᵗʰ **Y37.44 Military operations involving** unarmed hand to hand combat

EXCLUDES 1 *military operations involving combat using blunt or piercing object (Y37.45-)*

military operations involving intentional restriction of air and airway (Y37.46-)

military operations involving unintentional restriction of air and airway (Y37.47-)

√7ᵗʰ **Y37.440 Military operations involving unarmed hand to hand combat, military personnel**

√7ᵗʰ **Y37.441 Military operations involving unarmed hand to hand combat, civilian**

√6ᵗʰ **Y37.45 Military operations involving** combat using blunt or piercing object

√7ᵗʰ **Y37.450 Military operations involving combat using blunt or piercing object, military personnel**

√7ᵗʰ **Y37.451 Military operations involving combat using blunt or piercing object, civilian**

√6ᵗʰ **Y37.46 Military operations involving** intentional restriction of air and airway

√7ᵗʰ **Y37.460 Military operations involving intentional restriction of air and airway, military personnel**

√7ᵗʰ **Y37.461 Military operations involving intentional restriction of air and airway, civilian**

HCC CMS-HCC   **Rx** Rx HCC   **ESR** ESRD HCC   **COM** Commercial HCC   **N** Newborn: 0   **P** Pediatric: 0-17   **M** Maternity: 9-64   **A** Adult: 15-124

1246   ICD-10-CM 2023

√6ᵗʰ **Y37.47** **Military operations involving** unintentional restriction of air and airway

    √7ᵗʰ **Y37.470** **Military operations involving unintentional restriction of air and airway,** military personnel

    √7ᵗʰ **Y37.471** **Military operations involving unintentional restriction of air and airway,** civilian

√6ᵗʰ **Y37.49** **Military operations involving other forms of conventional warfare**

    √7ᵗʰ **Y37.490** **Military operations involving other forms of conventional warfare,** military personnel

    √7ᵗʰ **Y37.491** **Military operations involving other forms of conventional warfare,** civilian

√5ᵗʰ **Y37.5** **Military operations involving** nuclear weapons

    Military operation involving dirty bomb NOS

√6ᵗʰ **Y37.50** **Military operations involving unspecified effect of nuclear weapon**

    √7ᵗʰ **Y37.500** **Military operations involving unspecified effect of nuclear weapon,** military personnel

    √7ᵗʰ **Y37.501** **Military operations involving unspecified effect of nuclear weapon,** civilian

√6ᵗʰ **Y37.51** **Military operations involving** direct blast effect **of nuclear weapon**

    Military operations involving blast pressure of nuclear weapon

    √7ᵗʰ **Y37.510** **Military operations involving direct blast effect of nuclear weapon,** military personnel

    √7ᵗʰ **Y37.511** **Military operations involving direct blast effect of nuclear weapon,** civilian

√6ᵗʰ **Y37.52** **Military operations involving** indirect blast effect **of nuclear weapon**

    Military operations involving being thrown by blast of nuclear weapon

    Military operations involving being struck or crushed by blast debris of nuclear weapon

    √7ᵗʰ **Y37.520** **Military operations involving indirect blast effect of nuclear weapon,** military personnel

    √7ᵗʰ **Y37.521** **Military operations involving indirect blast effect of nuclear weapon,** civilian

√6ᵗʰ **Y37.53** **Military operations involving** thermal radiation effect **of nuclear weapon**

    Military operations involving direct heat from nuclear weapon

    Military operation involving fireball effects from nuclear weapon

    √7ᵗʰ **Y37.530** **Military operations involving thermal radiation effect of nuclear weapon,** military personnel

    √7ᵗʰ **Y37.531** **Military operations involving thermal radiation effect of nuclear weapon,** civilian

√6ᵗʰ **Y37.54** **Military operation involving** nuclear radiation effects **of nuclear weapon**

    Military operation involving acute radiation exposure from nuclear weapon

    Military operation involving exposure to immediate ionizing radiation from nuclear weapon

    Military operation involving fallout exposure from nuclear weapon

    Military operation involving secondary effects of nuclear weapons

    √7ᵗʰ **Y37.540** **Military operation involving nuclear radiation effects of nuclear weapon,** military personnel

    √7ᵗʰ **Y37.541** **Military operation involving nuclear radiation effects of nuclear weapon,** civilian

√6ᵗʰ **Y37.59** **Military operation involving other effects of nuclear weapons**

    √7ᵗʰ **Y37.590** **Military operation involving other effects of nuclear weapons,** military personnel

    √7ᵗʰ **Y37.591** **Military operation involving other effects of nuclear weapons,** civilian

√5ᵗʰ **Y37.6** **Military operations involving** biological weapons

√6ᵗʰ **Y37.6X** **Military operations involving biological weapons**

    √7ᵗʰ **Y37.6X0** **Military operations involving biological weapons,** military personnel

    √7ᵗʰ **Y37.6X1** **Military operations involving biological weapons,** civilian

√5ᵗʰ **Y37.7** **Military operations involving chemical weapons and other forms of unconventional warfare**

    EXCLUDES 1 *military operations involving incendiary devices (Y36.3-, Y36.5-)*

√6ᵗʰ **Y37.7X** **Military operations involving** chemical weapons and other forms of unconventional warfare

    √7ᵗʰ **Y37.7X0** **Military operations involving chemical weapons and other forms of unconventional warfare,** military personnel

    √7ᵗʰ **Y37.7X1** **Military operations involving chemical weapons and other forms of unconventional warfare,** civilian

√6ᵗʰ **Y37.9** **Other and unspecified military operations**

    √×7ᵗʰ **Y37.90** **Military operations, unspecified**

    √×7ᵗʰ **Y37.91** **Military operations involving unspecified** weapon of mass destruction [WMD]

    √×7ᵗʰ **Y37.92** **Military operations involving** friendly fire

√4ᵗʰ **Y38** **Terrorism**

    NOTE These codes are for use to identify injuries resulting from the unlawful use of force or violence against persons or property to intimidate or coerce a Government, the civilian population, or any segment thereof, in furtherance of political or social objective

    Use additional code for place of occurrence (Y92.-)

√5ᵗʰ **Y38.0** **Terrorism involving explosion of marine weapons**

    Terrorism involving depth-charge
    Terrorism involving marine mine
    Terrorism involving mine NOS, at sea or in harbor
    Terrorism involving sea-based artillery shell
    Terrorism involving torpedo
    Terrorism involving underwater blast

√6ᵗʰ **Y38.0X** **Terrorism involving explosion of** marine weapons

    √7ᵗʰ **Y38.0X1** **Terrorism involving explosion of marine weapons,** public safety official **injured**

    √7ᵗʰ **Y38.0X2** **Terrorism involving explosion of marine weapons,** civilian **injured**

    √7ᵗʰ **Y38.0X3** **Terrorism involving explosion of marine weapons,** terrorist **injured**

√5ᵗʰ **Y38.1** **Terrorism involving destruction of aircraft**

    Terrorism involving aircraft burned
    Terrorism involving aircraft exploded
    Terrorism involving aircraft being shot down
    Terrorism involving aircraft used as a weapon

√6ᵗʰ **Y38.1X** **Terrorism involving** destruction of aircraft

    √7ᵗʰ **Y38.1X1** **Terrorism involving destruction of aircraft,** public safety official **injured**

    √7ᵗʰ **Y38.1X2** **Terrorism involving destruction of aircraft,** civilian **injured**

    √7ᵗʰ **Y38.1X3** **Terrorism involving destruction of aircraft,** terrorist **injured**

√5ᵗʰ **Y38.2** **Terrorism involving other explosions and fragments**

    Terrorism involving antipersonnel (fragments) bomb
    Terrorism involving blast NOS
    Terrorism involving explosion NOS
    Terrorism involving explosion of breech block
    Terrorism involving explosion of cannon block
    Terrorism involving explosion (fragments) of artillery shell
    Terrorism involving explosion (fragments) of bomb
    Terrorism involving explosion (fragments) of grenade
    Terrorism involving explosion (fragments) of guided missile
    Terrorism involving explosion (fragments) of land mine
    Terrorism involving explosion of mortar bomb
    Terrorism involving explosion of munitions
    Terrorism involving explosion (fragments) of rocket
    Terrorism involving explosion (fragments) of shell
    Terrorism involving shrapnel
    Terrorism involving mine NOS, on land

    EXCLUDES 1 *terrorism involving explosion of nuclear weapon (Y38.5)*
    terrorism involving suicide bomber (Y38.81)

√6ᵗʰ **Y38.2X** **Terrorism involving other explosions and fragments**

    √7ᵗʰ **Y38.2X1** **Terrorism involving other explosions and fragments,** public safety official **injured**

✓7th **Y38.2X2 Terrorism involving other explosions and fragments, civilian injured**

✓7th **Y38.2X3 Terrorism involving other explosions and fragments, terrorist injured**

✓5th **Y38.3 Terrorism involving fires, conflagration and hot substances**

Terrorism involving conflagration NOS
Terrorism involving fire NOS
Terrorism involving petrol bomb

EXCLUDES 1   *terrorism involving fire or heat of nuclear weapon (Y38.5)*

✓6th **Y38.3X Terrorism involving fires, conflagration and hot substances**

✓7th **Y38.3X1 Terrorism involving fires, conflagration and hot substances, public safety official injured**

✓7th **Y38.3X2 Terrorism involving fires, conflagration and hot substances, civilian injured**

✓7th **Y38.3X3 Terrorism involving fires, conflagration and hot substances, terrorist injured**

✓5th **Y38.4 Terrorism involving firearms**

Terrorism involving carbine bullet
Terrorism involving machine gun bullet
Terrorism involving pellets (shotgun)
Terrorism involving pistol bullet
Terrorism involving rifle bullet
Terrorism involving rubber (rifle) bullet

✓6th **Y38.4X Terrorism involving firearms**

✓7th **Y38.4X1 Terrorism involving firearms, public safety official injured**

✓7th **Y38.4X2 Terrorism involving firearms, civilian injured**

✓7th **Y38.4X3 Terrorism involving firearms, terrorist injured**

✓5th **Y38.5 Terrorism involving nuclear weapons**

Terrorism involving blast effects of nuclear weapon
Terrorism involving exposure to ionizing radiation from nuclear weapon
Terrorism involving fireball effect of nuclear weapon
Terrorism involving heat from nuclear weapon

✓6th **Y38.5X Terrorism involving nuclear weapons**

✓7th **Y38.5X1 Terrorism involving nuclear weapons, public safety official injured**

✓7th **Y38.5X2 Terrorism involving nuclear weapons, civilian injured**

✓7th **Y38.5X3 Terrorism involving nuclear weapons, terrorist injured**

✓6th **Y38.6 Terrorism involving biological weapons**

Terrorism involving anthrax
Terrorism involving cholera
Terrorism involving smallpox

✓6th **Y38.6X Terrorism involving biological weapons**

✓7th **Y38.6X1 Terrorism involving biological weapons, public safety official injured**

✓7th **Y38.6X2 Terrorism involving biological weapons, civilian injured**

✓7th **Y38.6X3 Terrorism involving biological weapons, terrorist injured**

✓5th **Y38.7 Terrorism involving chemical weapons**

Terrorism involving gases, fumes, chemicals
Terrorism involving hydrogen cyanide
Terrorism involving phosgene
Terrorism involving sarin

✓6th **Y38.7X Terrorism involving chemical weapons**

✓7th **Y38.7X1 Terrorism involving chemical weapons, public safety official injured**

✓7th **Y38.7X2 Terrorism involving chemical weapons, civilian injured**

✓7th **Y38.7X3 Terrorism involving chemical weapons, terrorist injured**

✓5th **Y38.8 Terrorism involving other and unspecified means**

✓x7th **Y38.80 Terrorism involving unspecified means**

Terrorism NOS

✓6th **Y38.81 Terrorism involving suicide bomber**

✓7th **Y38.811 Terrorism involving suicide bomber, public safety official injured**

✓7th **Y38.812 Terrorism involving suicide bomber, civilian injured**

✓6th **Y38.89 Terrorism involving other means**

Terrorism involving drowning and submersion
Terrorism involving lasers
Terrorism involving piercing or stabbing instruments

✓7th **Y38.891 Terrorism involving other means, public safety official injured**

✓7th **Y38.892 Terrorism involving other means, civilian injured**

✓7th **Y38.893 Terrorism involving other means, terrorist injured**

✓5th **Y38.9 Terrorism, secondary effects**

NOTE   This code is for use to identify conditions occurring subsequent to a terrorist attack not those that are due to the initial terrorist attack

✓6th **Y38.9X Terrorism, secondary effects**

✓7th **Y38.9X1 Terrorism, secondary effects, public safety official injured**

✓7th **Y38.9X2 Terrorism, secondary effects, civilian injured**

COMPLICATIONS OF MEDICAL AND SURGICAL CARE (Y62-Y84)

INCLUDES   complications of medical devices
surgical and medical procedures as the cause of abnormal reaction of the patient, or of later complication, without mention of misadventure at the time of the procedure

Misadventures to patients during surgical and medical care (Y62-Y69)

EXCLUDES 1   *surgical and medical procedures as the cause of abnormal reaction of the patient, without mention of misadventure at the time of the procedure (Y83-Y84)*

EXCLUDES 2   *breakdown or malfunctioning of medical device (during procedure) (after implantation) (ongoing use) (Y70-Y82)*

✓4th **Y62 Failure of sterile precautions during surgical and medical care**

Y62.0 Failure of sterile precautions during surgical operation

Y62.1 Failure of sterile precautions during infusion or transfusion

Y62.2 Failure of sterile precautions during kidney dialysis and other perfusion   HCC Rx ESR

Y62.3 Failure of sterile precautions during injection or immunization

Y62.4 Failure of sterile precautions during endoscopic examination

Y62.5 Failure of sterile precautions during heart catheterization

Y62.6 Failure of sterile precautions during aspiration, puncture and other catheterization

Y62.8 Failure of sterile precautions during other surgical and medical care

Y62.9 Failure of sterile precautions during unspecified surgical and medical care

✓4th **Y63 Failure in dosage during surgical and medical care**

EXCLUDES 2   *accidental overdose of drug or wrong drug given in error (T36-T50)*

Y63.0 Excessive amount of blood or other fluid given during transfusion or infusion

Y63.1 Incorrect dilution of fluid used during infusion

Y63.2 Overdose of radiation given during therapy

Y63.3 Inadvertent exposure of patient to radiation during medical care

Y63.4 Failure in dosage in electroshock or insulin-shock therapy

Y63.5 Inappropriate temperature in local application and packing

Y63.6 Underdosing and nonadministration of necessary drug, medicament or biological substance
AHA: 2018,4Q,72

Y63.8 Failure in dosage during other surgical and medical care
AHA: 2018,4Q,72

Y63.9 Failure in dosage during unspecified surgical and medical care
AHA: 2018,4Q,72

✓4th **Y64 Contaminated medical or biological substances**

Y64.0 Contaminated medical or biological substance, transfused or infused

Y64.1 Contaminated medical or biological substance, injected or used for immunization

Y64.8 Contaminated medical or biological substance administered by other means

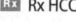

Y64.9 Contaminated medical or biological substance administered by unspecified means
Administered contaminated medical or biological substance NOS

☑4ᵗʰ **Y65 Other misadventures during surgical and medical care**

Y65.0 Mismatched blood in transfusion

Y65.1 Wrong fluid used in infusion

Y65.2 Failure in suture or ligature during surgical operation

Y65.3 Endotracheal tube wrongly placed during anesthetic procedure

Y65.4 Failure to introduce or to remove other tube or instrument

☑5ᵗʰ **Y65.5 Performance of wrong procedure (operation)**

Y65.51 Performance of wrong procedure (operation) on correct patient
Wrong device implanted into correct surgical site
EXCLUDES 1 *performance of correct procedure (operation) on wrong side or body part (Y65.53)*

Y65.52 Performance of procedure (operation) on patient not scheduled for surgery
Performance of procedure (operation) intended for another patient
Performance of procedure (operation) on wrong patient

Y65.53 Performance of correct procedure (operation) on wrong side or body part
Performance of correct procedure (operation) on wrong side
Performance of correct procedure (operation) on wrong site

Y65.8 Other specified misadventures during surgical and medical care
AHA: 2022,1Q,22; 2019,2Q,23-24

Y66 Nonadministration of surgical and medical care
Premature cessation of surgical and medical care
EXCLUDES 1 *DNR status (Z66)*
palliative care (Z51.5)

Y69 Unspecified misadventure during surgical and medical care

Medical devices associated with adverse incidents in diagnostic and therapeutic use (Y70-Y82)

INCLUDES breakdown or malfunction of medical devices (during use) (after implantation) (ongoing use)

EXCLUDES 2 *later complications following use of medical devices without breakdown or malfunctioning of device (Y83-Y84)*
misadventure to patients during surgical and medical care, classifiable to (Y62-Y69)
surgical and other medical procedures as the cause of abnormal reaction of the patient, or of later complication, without mention of misadventure at the time of the procedure (Y83-Y84)

☑4ᵗʰ **Y70 Anesthesiology devices associated with adverse incidents**

Y70.0 Diagnostic and monitoring anesthesiology devices associated with adverse incidents

Y70.1 Therapeutic (nonsurgical) and rehabilitative anesthesiology devices associated with adverse incidents

Y70.2 Prosthetic and other implants, materials and accessory anesthesiology devices associated with adverse incidents

Y70.3 Surgical instruments, materials and anesthesiology devices (including sutures) associated with adverse incidents

Y70.8 Miscellaneous anesthesiology devices associated with adverse incidents, not elsewhere classified

☑4ᵗʰ **Y71 Cardiovascular devices associated with adverse incidents**

Y71.0 Diagnostic and monitoring cardiovascular devices associated with adverse incidents

Y71.1 Therapeutic (nonsurgical) and rehabilitative cardiovascular devices associated with adverse incidents

Y71.2 Prosthetic and other implants, materials and accessory cardiovascular devices associated with adverse incidents

Y71.3 Surgical instruments, materials and cardiovascular devices (including sutures) associated with adverse incidents

Y71.8 Miscellaneous cardiovascular devices associated with adverse incidents, not elsewhere classified

☑4ᵗʰ **Y72 Otorhinolaryngological devices associated with adverse incidents**

Y72.0 Diagnostic and monitoring otorhinolaryngological devices associated with adverse incidents

Y72.1 Therapeutic (nonsurgical) and rehabilitative otorhinolaryngological devices associated with adverse incidents

Y72.2 Prosthetic and other implants, materials and accessory otorhinolaryngological devices associated with adverse incidents

Y72.3 Surgical instruments, materials and otorhinolaryngological devices (including sutures) associated with adverse incidents

Y72.8 Miscellaneous otorhinolaryngological devices associated with adverse incidents, not elsewhere classified

☑4ᵗʰ **Y73 Gastroenterology and urology devices associated with adverse incidents**

Y73.0 Diagnostic and monitoring gastroenterology and urology devices associated with adverse incidents

Y73.1 Therapeutic (nonsurgical) and rehabilitative gastroenterology and urology devices associated with adverse incidents

Y73.2 Prosthetic and other implants, materials and accessory gastroenterology and urology devices associated with adverse incidents

Y73.3 Surgical instruments, materials and gastroenterology and urology devices (including sutures) associated with adverse incidents

Y73.8 Miscellaneous gastroenterology and urology devices associated with adverse incidents, not elsewhere classified

☑4ᵗʰ **Y74 General hospital and personal-use devices associated with adverse incidents**

Y74.0 Diagnostic and monitoring general hospital and personal-use devices associated with adverse incidents

Y74.1 Therapeutic (nonsurgical) and rehabilitative general hospital and personal-use devices associated with adverse incidents

Y74.2 Prosthetic and other implants, materials and accessory general hospital and personal-use devices associated with adverse incidents

Y74.3 Surgical instruments, materials and general hospital and personal-use devices (including sutures) associated with adverse incidents

Y74.8 Miscellaneous general hospital and personal-use devices associated with adverse incidents, not elsewhere classified

☑4ᵗʰ **Y75 Neurological devices associated with adverse incidents**

Y75.0 Diagnostic and monitoring neurological devices associated with adverse incidents

Y75.1 Therapeutic (nonsurgical) and rehabilitative neurological devices associated with adverse incidents

Y75.2 Prosthetic and other implants, materials and neurological devices associated with adverse incidents

Y75.3 Surgical instruments, materials and neurological devices (including sutures) associated with adverse incidents

Y75.8 Miscellaneous neurological devices associated with adverse incidents, not elsewhere classified

☑4ᵗʰ **Y76 Obstetric and gynecological devices associated with adverse incidents**

Y76.0 Diagnostic and monitoring obstetric and gynecological devices associated with adverse incidents ♀

Y76.1 Therapeutic (nonsurgical) and rehabilitative obstetric and gynecological devices associated with adverse incidents ♀

Y76.2 Prosthetic and other implants, materials and accessory obstetric and gynecological devices associated with adverse incidents ♀

Y76.3 Surgical instruments, materials and obstetric and gynecological devices (including sutures) associated with adverse incidents ♀

Y76.8 Miscellaneous obstetric and gynecological devices associated with adverse incidents, not elsewhere classified ♀

☑4ᵗʰ **Y77 Ophthalmic devices associated with adverse incidents**

Y77.0 Diagnostic and monitoring ophthalmic devices associated with adverse incidents

☑5ᵗʰ **Y77.1 Therapeutic (nonsurgical) and rehabilitative ophthalmic devices associated with adverse incidents**
AHA: 2020,4Q,41

Y77.11 Contact lens associated with adverse incidents
Rigid gas permeable contact lens associated with adverse incidents
Soft (hydrophilic) contact lens associated with adverse incidents

Y77.19 Other therapeutic (nonsurgical) and rehabilitative ophthalmic devices associated with adverse incidents

Y77.2 Prosthetic and other implants, materials and accessory ophthalmic devices associated with adverse incidents

Y77.3 Surgical instruments, materials and ophthalmic devices (including sutures) associated with adverse incidents

Y77.8 Miscellaneous ophthalmic devices associated with adverse incidents, not elsewhere classified

☑4ᵗʰ **Y78** Radiological devices associated with adverse incidents

Y78.0 Diagnostic and monitoring radiological devices associated with adverse incidents

Y78.1 Therapeutic (nonsurgical) and rehabilitative radiological devices associated with adverse incidents

Y78.2 Prosthetic and other implants, materials and accessory radiological devices associated with adverse incidents

Y78.3 Surgical instruments, materials and radiological devices (including sutures) associated with adverse incidents

Y78.8 Miscellaneous radiological devices associated with adverse incidents, not elsewhere classified

☑4ᵗʰ **Y79** Orthopedic devices associated with adverse incidents

Y79.0 Diagnostic and monitoring orthopedic devices associated with adverse incidents

Y79.1 Therapeutic (nonsurgical) and rehabilitative orthopedic devices associated with adverse incidents

Y79.2 Prosthetic and other implants, materials and accessory orthopedic devices associated with adverse incidents

Y79.3 Surgical instruments, materials and orthopedic devices (including sutures) associated with adverse incidents

Y79.8 Miscellaneous orthopedic devices associated with adverse incidents, not elsewhere classified

☑4ᵗʰ **Y80** Physical medicine devices associated with adverse incidents

Y80.0 Diagnostic and monitoring physical medicine devices associated with adverse incidents

Y80.1 Therapeutic (nonsurgical) and rehabilitative physical medicine devices associated with adverse incidents

Y80.2 Prosthetic and other implants, materials and accessory physical medicine devices associated with adverse incidents

Y80.3 Surgical instruments, materials and physical medicine devices (including sutures) associated with adverse incidents

Y80.8 Miscellaneous physical medicine devices associated with adverse incidents, not elsewhere classified

☑4ᵗʰ **Y81** General- and plastic-surgery devices associated with adverse incidents

Y81.0 Diagnostic and monitoring general- and plastic-surgery devices associated with adverse incidents

Y81.1 Therapeutic (nonsurgical) and rehabilitative general- and plastic-surgery devices associated with adverse incidents

Y81.2 Prosthetic and other implants, materials and accessory general- and plastic-surgery devices associated with adverse incidents

Y81.3 Surgical instruments, materials and general- and plastic-surgery devices (including sutures) associated with adverse incidents

Y81.8 Miscellaneous general- and plastic-surgery devices associated with adverse incidents, not elsewhere classified

☑4ᵗʰ **Y82** Other and unspecified medical devices associated with adverse incidents

Y82.8 Other medical devices associated with adverse incidents

Y82.9 Unspecified medical devices associated with adverse incidents

Surgical and other medical procedures as the cause of abnormal reaction of the patient, or of later complication, without mention of misadventure at the time of the procedure (Y83-Y84)

EXCLUDES 1   misadventures to patients during surgical and medical care, classifiable to (Y62-Y69)

EXCLUDES 2   breakdown or malfunctioning of medical device (during procedure) (after implantation) (ongoing use) (Y70-Y82)

☑4ᵗʰ **Y83** Surgical operation and other surgical procedures as the cause of abnormal reaction of the patient, or of later complication, without mention of misadventure at the time of the procedure

Y83.0 Surgical operation with transplant of whole organ as the cause of abnormal reaction of the patient, or of later complication, without mention of misadventure at the time of the procedure

Y83.1 Surgical operation with implant of artificial internal device as the cause of abnormal reaction of the patient, or of later complication, without mention of misadventure at the time of the procedure

Y83.2 Surgical operation with anastomosis, bypass or graft as the cause of abnormal reaction of the patient, or of later complication, without mention of misadventure at the time of the procedure

Y83.3 Surgical operation with formation of external stoma as the cause of abnormal reaction of the patient, or of later complication, without mention of misadventure at the time of the procedure

Y83.4 Other reconstructive surgery as the cause of abnormal reaction of the patient, or of later complication, without mention of misadventure at the time of the procedure

Y83.5 Amputation of limb(s) as the cause of abnormal reaction of the patient, or of later complication, without mention of misadventure at the time of the procedure

Y83.6 Removal of other organ (partial) (total) as the cause of abnormal reaction of the patient, or of later complication, without mention of misadventure at the time of the procedure

Y83.8 Other surgical procedures as the cause of abnormal reaction of the patient, or of later complication, without mention of misadventure at the time of the procedure

Y83.9 Surgical procedure, unspecified as the cause of abnormal reaction of the patient, or of later complication, without mention of misadventure at the time of the procedure

☑4ᵗʰ **Y84** Other medical procedures as the cause of abnormal reaction of the patient, or of later complication, without mention of misadventure at the time of the procedure

Y84.0 Cardiac catheterization as the cause of abnormal reaction of the patient, or of later complication, without mention of misadventure at the time of the procedure

Y84.1 Kidney dialysis as the cause of abnormal reaction of the patient, or of later complication, without mention of misadventure at the time of the procedure

Y84.2 Radiological procedure and radiotherapy as the cause of abnormal reaction of the patient, or of later complication, without mention of misadventure at the time of the procedure
AHA: 2019,1Q,21; 2017,1Q,33

Y84.3 Shock therapy as the cause of abnormal reaction of the patient, or of later complication, without mention of misadventure at the time of the procedure

Y84.4 Aspiration of fluid as the cause of abnormal reaction of the patient, or of later complication, without mention of misadventure at the time of the procedure

Y84.5 Insertion of gastric or duodenal sound as the cause of abnormal reaction of the patient, or of later complication, without mention of misadventure at the time of the procedure

Y84.6 Urinary catheterization as the cause of abnormal reaction of the patient, or of later complication, without mention of misadventure at the time of the procedure

Y84.7 Blood-sampling as the cause of abnormal reaction of the patient, or of later complication, without mention of misadventure at the time of the procedure

Y84.8 Other medical procedures as the cause of abnormal reaction of the patient, or of later complication, without mention of misadventure at the time of the procedure
AHA: 2021,1Q,5; 2014,4Q,24

Y84.9 Medical procedure, unspecified as the cause of abnormal reaction of the patient, or of later complication, without mention of misadventure at the time of the procedure

Supplementary factors related to causes of morbidity classified elsewhere (Y90-Y99)

NOTE   These categories may be used to provide supplementary information concerning causes of morbidity. They are not to be used for single-condition coding.

☑4ᵗʰ **Y90** Evidence of alcohol involvement determined by blood alcohol level
Code first any associated alcohol related disorders (F10)

Y90.0 Blood alcohol level of less than 20 mg/100 ml

Y90.1 Blood alcohol level of 20-39 mg/100 ml

Y90.2 Blood alcohol level of 40-59 mg/100 ml

Y90.3 Blood alcohol level of 60-79 mg/100 ml

Y90.4 Blood alcohol level of 80-99 mg/100 ml

Y90.5 Blood alcohol level of 100-119 mg/100 ml

Y90.6 Blood alcohol level of 120-199 mg/100 ml

Y90.7 Blood alcohol level of 200-239 mg/100 ml

Y90.8 Blood alcohol level of 240 mg/100 ml or more

Y90.9 Presence of alcohol in blood, level not specified

☑4ᵗʰ Y92 Place of occurrence of the external cause

The following category is for use, when relevant, to identify the place of occurrence of the external cause. Use in conjunction with an activity code.

Place of occurrence should be recorded only at the initial encounter for treatment

☑5ᵗʰ Y92.0 Non-institutional (private) residence as the place of occurrence of the external cause

> EXCLUDES 1   abandoned or derelict house (Y92.89)
> home under construction but not yet occupied (Y92.6-)
> institutional place of residence (Y92.1-)

☑6ᵗʰ Y92.00 Unspecified non-institutional (private) residence as the place of occurrence of the external cause

Y92.000   **Kitchen of unspecified non-institutional (private) residence as the place of occurrence of the external cause**

Y92.001   **Dining room of unspecified non-institutional (private) residence as the place of occurrence of the external cause**

Y92.002   **Bathroom of unspecified non-institutional (private) residence as the place of occurrence of the external cause**

Y92.003   **Bedroom of unspecified non-institutional (private) residence as the place of occurrence of the external cause**

Y92.007   **Garden or yard of unspecified non-institutional (private) residence as the place of occurrence of the external cause**

Y92.008   **Other place in unspecified non-institutional (private) residence as the place of occurrence of the external cause**

Y92.009   **Unspecified place in unspecified non-institutional (private) residence as the place of occurrence of the external cause**

> Home (NOS) as the place of occurrence of the external cause

☑6ᵗʰ Y92.01 Single-family non-institutional (private) house as the place of occurrence of the external cause

> Farmhouse as the place of occurrence of the external cause

> EXCLUDES 1   barn (Y92.71)
> chicken coop or hen house (Y92.72)
> farm field (Y92.73)
> orchard (Y92.74)
> single family mobile home or trailer (Y92.02-)
> slaughter house (Y92.86)

Y92.010   **Kitchen of single-family (private) house as the place of occurrence of the external cause**

Y92.011   **Dining room of single-family (private) house as the place of occurrence of the external cause**

Y92.012   **Bathroom of single-family (private) house as the place of occurrence of the external cause**

Y92.013   **Bedroom of single-family (private) house as the place of occurrence of the external cause**

Y92.014   **Private driveway to single-family (private) house as the place of occurrence of the external cause**

Y92.015   **Private garage of single-family (private) house as the place of occurrence of the external cause**

Y92.016   **Swimming-pool in single-family (private) house or garden as the place of occurrence of the external cause**

Y92.017   **Garden or yard in single-family (private) house as the place of occurrence of the external cause**

Y92.018   **Other place in single-family (private) house as the place of occurrence of the external cause**

Y92.019   **Unspecified place in single-family (private) house as the place of occurrence of the external cause**

☑6ᵗʰ Y92.02 Mobile home as the place of occurrence of the external cause

Y92.020   **Kitchen in mobile home as the place of occurrence of the external cause**

Y92.021   **Dining room in mobile home as the place of occurrence of the external cause**

Y92.022   **Bathroom in mobile home as the place of occurrence of the external cause**

Y92.023   **Bedroom in mobile home as the place of occurrence of the external cause**

Y92.024   **Driveway of mobile home as the place of occurrence of the external cause**

Y92.025   **Garage of mobile home as the place of occurrence of the external cause**

Y92.026   **Swimming-pool of mobile home as the place of occurrence of the external cause**

Y92.027   **Garden or yard of mobile home as the place of occurrence of the external cause**

Y92.028   **Other place in mobile home as the place of occurrence of the external cause**

Y92.029   **Unspecified place in mobile home as the place of occurrence of the external cause**

☑6ᵗʰ Y92.03 Apartment as the place of occurrence of the external cause

> Condominium as the place of occurrence of the external cause
> Co-op apartment as the place of occurrence of the external cause

Y92.030   **Kitchen in apartment as the place of occurrence of the external cause**

Y92.031   **Bathroom in apartment as the place of occurrence of the external cause**

Y92.032   **Bedroom in apartment as the place of occurrence of the external cause**

Y92.038   **Other place in apartment as the place of occurrence of the external cause**

Y92.039   **Unspecified place in apartment as the place of occurrence of the external cause**

☑6ᵗʰ Y92.04 Boarding-house as the place of occurrence of the external cause

Y92.040   **Kitchen in boarding-house as the place of occurrence of the external cause**

Y92.041   **Bathroom in boarding-house as the place of occurrence of the external cause**

Y92.042   **Bedroom in boarding-house as the place of occurrence of the external cause**

Y92.043   **Driveway of boarding-house as the place of occurrence of the external cause**

Y92.044   **Garage of boarding-house as the place of occurrence of the external cause**

Y92.045   **Swimming-pool of boarding-house as the place of occurrence of the external cause**

Y92.046   **Garden or yard of boarding-house as the place of occurrence of the external cause**

Y92.048   **Other place in boarding-house as the place of occurrence of the external cause**

Y92.049   **Unspecified place in boarding-house as the place of occurrence of the external cause**

☑6ᵗʰ Y92.09 Other non-institutional residence as the place of occurrence of the external cause

> AHA: 2017,2Q,10

Y92.090   **Kitchen in other non-institutional residence as the place of occurrence of the external cause**

Y92.091   **Bathroom in other non-institutional residence as the place of occurrence of the external cause**

Y92.092   **Bedroom in other non-institutional residence as the place of occurrence of the external cause**

Y92.093   **Driveway of other non-institutional residence as the place of occurrence of the external cause**

Y92.094   **Garage of other non-institutional residence as the place of occurrence of the external cause**

Y92.095   **Swimming-pool of other non-institutional residence as the place of occurrence of the external cause**

Y92.096   **Garden or yard of other non-institutional residence as the place of occurrence of the external cause**

Y92.Ø98   **Other place in other non-institutional residence as the place of occurrence of the external cause**

Y92.Ø99   **Unspecified place in other non-institutional residence as the place of occurrence of the external cause**

✓5ᵗʰ   **Y92.1**   **Institutional (nonprivate) residence as the place of occurrence of the external cause**

Y92.1Ø   **Unspecified residential institution as the place of occurrence of the external cause**

✓6ᵗʰ   **Y92.11**   **Children's home and orphanage as the place of occurrence of the external cause**

Y92.11Ø   **Kitchen in children's home and orphanage as the place of occurrence of the external cause**

Y92.111   **Bathroom in children's home and orphanage as the place of occurrence of the external cause**

Y92.112   **Bedroom in children's home and orphanage as the place of occurrence of the external cause**

Y92.113   **Driveway of children's home and orphanage as the place of occurrence of the external cause**

Y92.114   **Garage of children's home and orphanage as the place of occurrence of the external cause**

Y92.115   **Swimming-pool of children's home and orphanage as the place of occurrence of the external cause**

Y92.116   **Garden or yard of children's home and orphanage as the place of occurrence of the external cause**

Y92.118   **Other place in children's home and orphanage as the place of occurrence of the external cause**

Y92.119   **Unspecified place in children's home and orphanage as the place of occurrence of the external cause**

✓6ᵗʰ   **Y92.12**   **Nursing home as the place of occurrence of the external cause**

Home for the sick as the place of occurrence of the external cause

Hospice as the place of occurrence of the external cause

AHA: 2017,2Q,10

Y92.12Ø   **Kitchen in nursing home as the place of occurrence of the external cause**

Y92.121   **Bathroom in nursing home as the place of occurrence of the external cause**

Y92.122   **Bedroom in nursing home as the place of occurrence of the external cause**

Y92.123   **Driveway of nursing home as the place of occurrence of the external cause**

Y92.124   **Garage of nursing home as the place of occurrence of the external cause**

Y92.125   **Swimming-pool of nursing home as the place of occurrence of the external cause**

Y92.126   **Garden or yard of nursing home as the place of occurrence of the external cause**

Y92.128   **Other place in nursing home as the place of occurrence of the external cause**

Y92.129   **Unspecified place in nursing home as the place of occurrence of the external cause**

✓6ᵗʰ   **Y92.13**   **Military base as the place of occurrence of the external cause**

EXCLUDES 1   *military training grounds (Y92.84)*

Y92.13Ø   **Kitchen on military base as the place of occurrence of the external cause**

Y92.131   **Mess hall on military base as the place of occurrence of the external cause**

Y92.133   **Barracks on military base as the place of occurrence of the external cause**

Y92.135   **Garage on military base as the place of occurrence of the external cause**

Y92.136   **Swimming-pool on military base as the place of occurrence of the external cause**

Y92.137   **Garden or yard on military base as the place of occurrence of the external cause**

Y92.138   **Other place on military base as the place of occurrence of the external cause**

Y92.139   **Unspecified place military base as the place of occurrence of the external cause**

✓6ᵗʰ   **Y92.14**   **Prison as the place of occurrence of the external cause**

Y92.14Ø   **Kitchen in prison as the place of occurrence of the external cause**

Y92.141   **Dining room in prison as the place of occurrence of the external cause**

Y92.142   **Bathroom in prison as the place of occurrence of the external cause**

Y92.143   **Cell of prison as the place of occurrence of the external cause**

Y92.146   **Swimming-pool of prison as the place of occurrence of the external cause**

Y92.147   **Courtyard of prison as the place of occurrence of the external cause**

Y92.148   **Other place in prison as the place of occurrence of the external cause**

Y92.149   **Unspecified place in prison as the place of occurrence of the external cause**

✓6ᵗʰ   **Y92.15**   **Reform school as the place of occurrence of the external cause**

Y92.15Ø   **Kitchen in reform school as the place of occurrence of the external cause**

Y92.151   **Dining room in reform school as the place of occurrence of the external cause**

Y92.152   **Bathroom in reform school as the place of occurrence of the external cause**

Y92.153   **Bedroom in reform school as the place of occurrence of the external cause**

Y92.154   **Driveway of reform school as the place of occurrence of the external cause**

Y92.155   **Garage of reform school as the place of occurrence of the external cause**

Y92.156   **Swimming-pool of reform school as the place of occurrence of the external cause**

Y92.157   **Garden or yard of reform school as the place of occurrence of the external cause**

Y92.158   **Other place in reform school as the place of occurrence of the external cause**

Y92.159   **Unspecified place in reform school as the place of occurrence of the external cause**

✓6ᵗʰ   **Y92.16**   **School dormitory as the place of occurrence of the external cause**

EXCLUDES 1   *reform school as the place of occurrence of the external cause (Y92.15-)*

school buildings and grounds as the place of occurrence of the external cause (Y92.2-)

school sports and athletic areas as the place of occurrence of the external cause (Y92.3-)

Y92.16Ø   **Kitchen in school dormitory as the place of occurrence of the external cause**

Y92.161   **Dining room in school dormitory as the place of occurrence of the external cause**

Y92.162   **Bathroom in school dormitory as the place of occurrence of the external cause**

Y92.163   **Bedroom in school dormitory as the place of occurrence of the external cause**

Y92.168   **Other place in school dormitory as the place of occurrence of the external cause**

Y92.169   **Unspecified place in school dormitory as the place of occurrence of the external cause**

✓6ᵗʰ   **Y92.19**   **Other specified residential institution as the place of occurrence of the external cause**

AHA: 2017,2Q,10

Y92.19Ø   **Kitchen in other specified residential institution as the place of occurrence of the external cause**

Y92.191   **Dining room in other specified residential institution as the place of occurrence of the external cause**

Y92.192   **Bathroom in other specified residential institution as the place of occurrence of the external cause**

Y92.193   **Bedroom in other specified residential institution as the place of occurrence of the external cause**

Y92.194   **Driveway of other specified residential institution as the place of occurrence of the external cause**

Y92.195   **Garage** of other specified residential institution as the place of occurrence of the external cause

Y92.196   **Pool** of other specified residential institution as the place of occurrence of the external cause

Y92.197   **Garden or yard** of other specified residential institution as the place of occurrence of the external cause

Y92.198   **Other place** in other specified residential institution as the place of occurrence of the external cause

Y92.199   **Unspecified place** in other specified residential institution as the place of occurrence of the external cause

✓5ᵗʰ **Y92.2**   **School, other institution and public administrative area** as the place of occurrence of the external cause

Building and adjacent grounds used by the general public or by a particular group of the public

> EXCLUDES 1   *building under construction as the place of occurrence of the external cause (Y92.6)*
> *residential institution as the place of occurrence of the external cause (Y92.1)*
> *school dormitory as the place of occurrence of the external cause (Y92.16-)*
> *sports and athletics area of schools as the place of occurrence of the external cause (Y92.3-)*

✓6ᵗʰ **Y92.21**   **School (private) (public) (state)** as the place of occurrence of the external cause

Y92.210   **Daycare center** as the place of occurrence of the external cause

Y92.211   **Elementary school** as the place of occurrence of the external cause

> Kindergarten as the place of occurrence of the external cause

Y92.212   **Middle school** as the place of occurrence of the external cause

Y92.213   **High school** as the place of occurrence of the external cause

> **AHA:** 2012,4Q,108

Y92.214   **College** as the place of occurrence of the external cause

> University as the place of occurrence of the external cause

Y92.215   **Trade school** as the place of occurrence of the external cause

Y92.218   **Other school** as the place of occurrence of the external cause

Y92.219   **Unspecified school** as the place of occurrence of the external cause

Y92.22   **Religious institution** as the place of occurrence of the external cause

> Church as the place of occurrence of the external cause
> Mosque as the place of occurrence of the external cause
> Synagogue as the place of occurrence of the external cause

✓6ᵗʰ **Y92.23**   **Hospital** as the place of occurrence of the external cause

> EXCLUDES 1   *ambulatory (outpatient) health services establishments (Y92.53-)*
> *home for the sick as the place of occurrence of the external cause (Y92.12-)*
> *hospice as the place of occurrence of the external cause (Y92.12-)*
> *nursing home as the place of occurrence of the external cause (Y92.12-)*

Y92.230   **Patient room** in hospital as the place of occurrence of the external cause

Y92.231   **Patient bathroom** in hospital as the place of occurrence of the external cause

Y92.232   **Corridor** of hospital as the place of occurrence of the external cause

Y92.233   **Cafeteria** of hospital as the place of occurrence of the external cause

Y92.234   **Operating room** of hospital as the place of occurrence of the external cause

Y92.238   **Other place** in hospital as the place of occurrence of the external cause

Y92.239   **Unspecified place** in hospital as the place of occurrence of the external cause

✓6ᵗʰ **Y92.24**   **Public administrative building** as the place of occurrence of the external cause

Y92.240   **Courthouse** as the place of occurrence of the external cause

Y92.241   **Library** as the place of occurrence of the external cause

Y92.242   **Post office** as the place of occurrence of the external cause

Y92.243   **City hall** as the place of occurrence of the external cause

Y92.248   **Other public administrative building** as the place of occurrence of the external cause

✓6ᵗʰ **Y92.25**   **Cultural building** as the place of occurrence of the external cause

Y92.250   **Art Gallery** as the place of occurrence of the external cause

Y92.251   **Museum** as the place of occurrence of the external cause

Y92.252   **Music hall** as the place of occurrence of the external cause

Y92.253   **Opera house** as the place of occurrence of the external cause

Y92.254   **Theater (live)** as the place of occurrence of the external cause

Y92.258   **Other cultural public building** as the place of occurrence of the external cause

Y92.26   **Movie house or cinema** as the place of occurrence of the external cause

Y92.29   **Other specified public building** as the place of occurrence of the external cause

> Assembly hall as the place of occurrence of the external cause
> Clubhouse as the place of occurrence of the external cause

✓5ᵗʰ **Y92.3**   **Sports and athletics area** as the place of occurrence of the external cause

✓6ᵗʰ **Y92.31**   **Athletic court** as the place of occurrence of the external cause

> EXCLUDES 1   *tennis court in private home or garden (Y92.09)*

Y92.310   **Basketball court** as the place of occurrence of the external cause

Y92.311   **Squash court** as the place of occurrence of the external cause

Y92.312   **Tennis court** as the place of occurrence of the external cause

Y92.318   **Other athletic court** as the place of occurrence of the external cause

✓6ᵗʰ **Y92.32**   **Athletic field** as the place of occurrence of the external cause

Y92.320   **Baseball field** as the place of occurrence of the external cause

Y92.321   **Football field** as the place of occurrence of the external cause

Y92.322   **Soccer field** as the place of occurrence of the external cause

Y92.328   **Other athletic field** as the place of occurrence of the external cause

> Cricket field as the place of occurrence of the external cause
> Hockey field as the place of occurrence of the external cause

✓6ᵗʰ **Y92.33**   **Skating rink** as the place of occurrence of the external cause

Y92.330   **Ice skating rink (indoor) (outdoor)** as the place of occurrence of the external cause

Y92.331   **Roller skating rink** as the place of occurrence of the external cause

Y92.34   **Swimming pool (public)** as the place of occurrence of the external cause

> EXCLUDES 1   *swimming pool in private home or garden (Y92.016)*

Y92.39 Other specified sports and athletic area as the place of occurrence of the external cause
Golf-course as the place of occurrence of the external cause
Gymnasium as the place of occurrence of the external cause
Riding-school as the place of occurrence of the external cause
Stadium as the place of occurrence of the external cause

✓5ᵗʰ **Y92.4 Street, highway and other paved roadways as the place of occurrence of the external cause**
EXCLUDES 1 *private driveway of residence (Y92.014, Y92.024, Y92.043, Y92.093, Y92.113, Y92.123, Y92.154, Y92.194)*

✓6ᵗʰ **Y92.41 Street and highway as the place of occurrence of the external cause**
Y92.410 Unspecified street and highway as the place of occurrence of the external cause
Road NOS as the place of occurrence of the external cause
Y92.411 Interstate highway as the place of occurrence of the external cause
Freeway as the place of occurrence of the external cause
Motorway as the place of occurrence of the external cause
Y92.412 Parkway as the place of occurrence of the external cause
Y92.413 State road as the place of occurrence of the external cause
Y92.414 Local residential or business street as the place of occurrence of the external cause
Y92.415 Exit ramp or entrance ramp of street or highway as the place of occurrence of the external cause

✓6ᵗʰ **Y92.48 Other paved roadways as the place of occurrence of the external cause**
Y92.480 Sidewalk as the place of occurrence of the external cause
Y92.481 Parking lot as the place of occurrence of the external cause
Y92.482 Bike path as the place of occurrence of the external cause
Y92.488 Other paved roadways as the place of occurrence of the external cause

✓5ᵗʰ **Y92.5 Trade and service area as the place of occurrence of the external cause**
EXCLUDES 1 *garage in private home (Y92.015)*
schools and other public administration buildings (Y92.2-)

✓6ᵗʰ **Y92.51 Private commercial establishments as the place of occurrence of the external cause**
Y92.510 Bank as the place of occurrence of the external cause
Y92.511 Restaurant or café as the place of occurrence of the external cause
Y92.512 Supermarket, store or market as the place of occurrence of the external cause
Y92.513 Shop (commercial) as the place of occurrence of the external cause

✓6ᵗʰ **Y92.52 Service areas as the place of occurrence of the external cause**
Y92.520 Airport as the place of occurrence of the external cause
Y92.521 Bus station as the place of occurrence of the external cause
Y92.522 Railway station as the place of occurrence of the external cause
Y92.523 Highway rest stop as the place of occurrence of the external cause
Y92.524 Gas station as the place of occurrence of the external cause
Petroleum station as the place of occurrence of the external cause
Service station as the place of occurrence of the external cause

✓6ᵗʰ **Y92.53 Ambulatory health services establishments as the place of occurrence of the external cause**
Y92.530 Ambulatory surgery center as the place of occurrence of the external cause
Outpatient surgery center, including that connected with a hospital as the place of occurrence of the external cause
Same day surgery center, including that connected with a hospital as the place of occurrence of the external cause
Y92.531 Health care provider office as the place of occurrence of the external cause
Physician office as the place of occurrence of the external cause
Y92.532 Urgent care center as the place of occurrence of the external cause
Y92.538 Other ambulatory health services establishments as the place of occurrence of the external cause
AHA: 2019,1Q,21

Y92.59 Other trade areas as the place of occurrence of the external cause
Office building as the place of occurrence of the external cause
Casino as the place of occurrence of the external cause
Garage (commercial) as the place of occurrence of the external cause
Hotel as the place of occurrence of the external cause
Radio or television station as the place of occurrence of the external cause
Shopping mall as the place of occurrence of the external cause
Warehouse as the place of occurrence of the external cause

✓5ᵗʰ **Y92.6 Industrial and construction area as the place of occurrence of the external cause**
Y92.61 Building [any] under construction as the place of occurrence of the external cause
Y92.62 Dock or shipyard as the place of occurrence of the external cause
Dockyard as the place of occurrence of the external cause
Dry dock as the place of occurrence of the external cause
Shipyard as the place of occurrence of the external cause
Y92.63 Factory as the place of occurrence of the external cause
Factory building as the place of occurrence of the external cause
Factory premises as the place of occurrence of the external cause
Industrial yard as the place of occurrence of the external cause
Y92.64 Mine or pit as the place of occurrence of the external cause
Mine as the place of occurrence of the external cause
Y92.65 Oil rig as the place of occurrence of the external cause
Pit (coal) (gravel) (sand) as the place of occurrence of the external cause
Y92.69 Other specified industrial and construction area as the place of occurrence of the external cause
Gasworks as the place of occurrence of the external cause
Power-station (coal) (nuclear) (oil) as the place of occurrence of the external cause
Tunnel under construction as the place of occurrence of the external cause
Workshop as the place of occurrence of the external cause

✓5ᵗʰ **Y92.7 Farm as the place of occurrence of the external cause**
Ranch as the place of occurrence of the external cause
EXCLUDES 1 *farmhouse and home premises of farm (Y92.01-)*
Y92.71 Barn as the place of occurrence of the external cause

Y92.72   **Chicken coop** as the place of occurrence of the external cause

     Hen house as the place of occurrence of the external cause

Y92.73   **Farm field** as the place of occurrence of the external cause

Y92.74   **Orchard** as the place of occurrence of the external cause

Y92.79   **Other farm location** as the place of occurrence of the external cause

✓5ᵗʰ **Y92.8**   **Other places as the place of occurrence of the external cause**

   ✓6ᵗʰ **Y92.81**   **Transport vehicle** as the place of occurrence of the external cause

     EXCLUDES 1   *transport accidents (V00-V99)*

     Y92.810   **Car** as the place of occurrence of the external cause

     Y92.811   **Bus** as the place of occurrence of the external cause

     Y92.812   **Truck** as the place of occurrence of the external cause

     Y92.813   **Airplane** as the place of occurrence of the external cause

     Y92.814   **Boat** as the place of occurrence of the external cause

     Y92.815   **Train** as the place of occurrence of the external cause

     Y92.816   **Subway car** as the place of occurrence of the external cause

     Y92.818   **Other transport vehicle** as the place of occurrence of the external cause

   ✓6ᵗʰ **Y92.82**   **Wilderness area**

     Y92.820   **Desert** as the place of occurrence of the external cause

     Y92.821   **Forest** as the place of occurrence of the external cause

     Y92.828   **Other wilderness area** as the place of occurrence of the external cause

       Swamp as the place of occurrence of the external cause

       Mountain as the place of occurrence of the external cause

       Marsh as the place of occurrence of the external cause

       Prairie as the place of occurrence of the external cause

   ✓6ᵗʰ **Y92.83**   **Recreation area** as the place of occurrence of the external cause

     Y92.830   **Public park** as the place of occurrence of the external cause

     Y92.831   **Amusement park** as the place of occurrence of the external cause

     Y92.832   **Beach** as the place of occurrence of the external cause

       Seashore as the place of occurrence of the external cause

     Y92.833   **Campsite** as the place of occurrence of the external cause

     Y92.834   **Zoological garden (Zoo)** as the place of occurrence of the external cause

     Y92.838   **Other recreation area** as the place of occurrence of the external cause

   Y92.84   **Military training ground** as the place of occurrence of the external cause

   Y92.85   **Railroad track** as the place of occurrence of the external cause

   Y92.86   **Slaughter house** as the place of occurrence of the external cause

   Y92.89   **Other specified places** as the place of occurrence of the external cause

       Derelict house as the place of occurrence of the external cause

Y92.9   **Unspecified place or not applicable**

✓4ᵗʰ **Y93**   **Activity codes**

   NOTE   Category Y93 is provided for use to indicate the activity of the person seeking healthcare for an injury or health condition, such as a heart attack while shoveling snow, which resulted from, or was contributed to, by the activity. These codes are appropriate for use for both acute injuries, such as those from chapter 19, and conditions that are due to the long-term, cumulative effects of an activity, such as those from chapter 13. They are also appropriate for use with external cause codes for cause and intent if identifying the activity provides additional information on the event. These codes should be used in conjunction with codes for external cause status (Y99) and place of occurrence (Y92).

This section contains the following broad activity categories:

Y93.0	Activities involving walking and running
Y93.1	Activities involving water and water craft
Y93.2	Activities involving ice and snow
Y93.3	Activities involving climbing, rappelling, and jumping off
Y93.4	Activities involving dancing and other rhythmic movement
Y93.5	Activities involving other sports and athletics played individually
Y93.6	Activities involving other sports and athletics played as a team or group
Y93.7	Activities involving other specified sports and athletics
Y93.A	Activities involving other cardiorespiratory exercise
Y93.B	Activities involving other muscle strengthening exercises
Y93.C	Activities involving computer technology and electronic devices
Y93.D	Activities involving arts and handcrafts
Y93.E	Activities involving personal hygiene and interior property and clothing maintenance
Y93.F	Activities involving caregiving
Y93.G	Activities involving food preparation, cooking and grilling
Y93.H	Activities involving exterior property and land maintenance, building and construction
Y93.I	Activities involving roller coasters and other types of external motion
Y93.J	Activities involving playing musical instrument
Y93.K	Activities involving animal care
Y93.8	Activities, other specified
Y93.9	Activity, unspecified

✓5ᵗʰ **Y93.0**   **Activities involving walking and running**

     EXCLUDES 1   *activity, walking an animal (Y93.K1)*

                activity, walking or running on a treadmill (Y93.A1)

   Y93.01   **Activity, walking, marching and hiking**

     Activity, walking, marching and hiking on level or elevated terrain

     EXCLUDES 1   *activity, mountain climbing (Y93.31)*

   Y93.02   **Activity, running**

✓5ᵗʰ **Y93.1**   **Activities involving water and water craft**

     EXCLUDES 1   *activities involving ice (Y93.2-)*

   Y93.11   **Activity, swimming**

   Y93.12   **Activity, springboard and platform diving**

   Y93.13   **Activity, water polo**

   Y93.14   **Activity, water aerobics and water exercise**

   Y93.15   **Activity, underwater diving and snorkeling**

     Activity, SCUBA diving

   Y93.16   **Activity, rowing, canoeing, kayaking, rafting and tubing**

     Activity, canoeing, kayaking, rafting and tubing in calm and turbulent water

   Y93.17   **Activity, water skiing and wake boarding**

   Y93.18   **Activity, surfing, windsurfing and boogie boarding**

     Activity, water sliding

   Y93.19   **Activity, other involving water and watercraft**

     Activity involving water NOS

     Activity, parasailing

     Activity, water survival training and testing

☑5ᵗʰ **Y93.2 Activities involving ice and snow**
> **EXCLUDES 1** activity, shoveling ice and snow (Y93.H1)

Y93.21 Activity, ice skating
Activity, figure skating (singles) (pairs)
Activity, ice dancing
> **EXCLUDES 1** activity, ice hockey (Y93.22)

Y93.22 Activity, ice hockey

Y93.23 Activity, snow (alpine) (downhill) skiing, snowboarding, sledding, tobogganing and snow tubing
> **EXCLUDES 1** activity, cross country skiing (Y93.24)

Y93.24 Activity, cross country skiing
Activity, nordic skiing

Y93.29 Activity, other involving ice and snow
Activity involving ice and snow NOS

☑5ᵗʰ **Y93.3 Activities involving climbing, rappelling and jumping off**
> **EXCLUDES 1** activity, hiking on level or elevated terrain (Y93.Ø1)
> activity, jumping rope (Y93.56)
> activity, trampoline jumping (Y93.44)

Y93.31 Activity, mountain climbing, rock climbing and wall climbing

Y93.32 Activity, rappelling

Y93.33 Activity, BASE jumping
Activity, Building, Antenna, Span, Earth jumping

Y93.34 Activity, bungee jumping

Y93.35 Activity, hang gliding

Y93.39 Activity, other involving climbing, rappelling and jumping off

☑5ᵗʰ **Y93.4 Activities involving dancing and other rhythmic movement**
> **EXCLUDES 1** activity, martial arts (Y93.75)

Y93.41 Activity, dancing
AHA: 2012,4Q,108

Y93.42 Activity, yoga

Y93.43 Activity, gymnastics
Activity, rhythmic gymnastics
> **EXCLUDES 1** activity, trampolining (Y93.44)

Y93.44 Activity, trampolining

Y93.45 Activity, cheerleading

Y93.49 Activity, other involving dancing and other rhythmic movements

☑5ᵗʰ **Y93.5 Activities involving other sports and athletics played individually**
> **EXCLUDES 1** activity, dancing (Y93.41)
> activity, gymnastic (Y93.43)
> activity, trampolining (Y93.44)
> activity, yoga (Y93.42)

Y93.51 Activity, roller skating (inline) and skateboarding

Y93.52 Activity, horseback riding

Y93.53 Activity, golf

Y93.54 Activity, bowling

Y93.55 Activity, bike riding

Y93.56 Activity, jumping rope

Y93.57 Activity, non-running track and field events
> **EXCLUDES 1** activity, running (any form) (Y93.Ø2)

Y93.59 Activity, other involving other sports and athletics played individually
> **EXCLUDES 1** activities involving climbing, rappelling, and jumping (Y93.3-)
> activities involving ice and snow (Y93.2-)
> activities involving walking and running (Y93.Ø-)
> activities involving water and watercraft (Y93.1-)

☑5ᵗʰ **Y93.6 Activities involving other sports and athletics played as a team or group**
> **EXCLUDES 1** activity, ice hockey (Y93.22)
> activity, water polo (Y93.13)

Y93.61 Activity, American tackle football
Activity, football NOS

Y93.62 Activity, American flag or touch football

Y93.63 Activity, rugby

Y93.64 Activity, baseball
Activity, softball

Y93.65 Activity, lacrosse and field hockey

Y93.66 Activity, soccer

Y93.67 Activity, basketball

Y93.68 Activity, volleyball (beach) (court)

Y93.6A Activity, physical games generally associated with school recess, summer camp and children
Activity, capture the flag
Activity, dodge ball
Activity, four square
Activity, kickball

Y93.69 Activity, other involving other sports and athletics played as a team or group
Activity, cricket

☑5ᵗʰ **Y93.7 Activities involving other specified sports and athletics**

Y93.71 Activity, boxing

Y93.72 Activity, wrestling

Y93.73 Activity, racquet and hand sports
Activity, handball
Activity, racquetball
Activity, squash
Activity, tennis

Y93.74 Activity, frisbee
Activity, ultimate frisbee

Y93.75 Activity, martial arts
Activity, combatives

Y93.79 Activity, other specified sports and athletics
> **EXCLUDES 1** sports and athletics activities specified in categories Y93.Ø-Y93.6

☑5ᵗʰ **Y93.A Activities involving other cardiorespiratory exercise**
Activities involving physical training

Y93.A1 Activity, exercise machines primarily for cardiorespiratory conditioning
Activity, elliptical and stepper machines
Activity, stationary bike
Activity, treadmill

Y93.A2 Activity, calisthenics
Activity, jumping jacks
Activity, warm up and cool down

Y93.A3 Activity, aerobic and step exercise

Y93.A4 Activity, circuit training

Y93.A5 Activity, obstacle course
Activity, challenge course
Activity, confidence course

Y93.A6 Activity, grass drills
Activity, guerilla drills

Y93.A9 Activity, other involving cardiorespiratory exercise
> **EXCLUDES 1** activities involving cardiorespiratory exercise specified in categories Y93.Ø-Y93.7

☑5ᵗʰ **Y93.B Activities involving other muscle strengthening exercises**

Y93.B1 Activity, exercise machines primarily for muscle strengthening

Y93.B2 Activity, push-ups, pull-ups, sit-ups

Y93.B3 Activity, free weights
Activity, barbells
Activity, dumbbells

Y93.B4 Activity, pilates

Y93.B9 Activity, other involving muscle strengthening exercises
> **EXCLUDES 1** activities involving muscle strengthening specified in categories Y93.Ø-Y93.A

☑5ᵗʰ **Y93.C Activities involving computer technology and electronic devices**
> **EXCLUDES 1** activity, electronic musical keyboard or instruments (Y93.J-)

Y93.C1 Activity, computer keyboarding
Activity, electronic game playing using keyboard or other stationary device

Y93.C2 Activity, hand held interactive electronic device
Activity, cellular telephone and communication device
Activity, electronic game playing using interactive device
> **EXCLUDES 1** activity, electronic game playing using keyboard or other stationary device (Y93.C1)

Y93.C9 Activity, other involving computer technology and electronic devices

☑5ᵗʰ **Y93.D Activities involving arts and handcrafts**
> **EXCLUDES 1** activities involving playing musical instrument (Y93.J-)

Y93.D1 Activity, knitting and crocheting

Y93.D2 **Activity,** sewing

Y93.D3 **Activity,** furniture building and finishing

Activity, furniture repair

Y93.D9 **Activity, other involving arts and handcrafts**

✓5ᵗʰ **Y93.E** **Activities involving personal hygiene and interior property and clothing maintenance**

EXCLUDES 1 *activities involving cooking and grilling (Y93.G-)*

activities involving exterior property and land maintenance, building and construction (Y93.H-)

activities involving caregiving (Y93.F-)

activity, dishwashing (Y93.G1)

activity, food preparation (Y93.G1)

activity, gardening (Y93.H2)

Y93.E1 **Activity,** personal bathing and showering

Y93.E2 **Activity,** laundry

Y93.E3 **Activity,** vacuuming

Y93.E4 **Activity,** ironing

Y93.E5 **Activity,** floor mopping and cleaning

Y93.E6 **Activity,** residential relocation

Activity, packing up and unpacking involved in moving to a new residence

Y93.E8 **Activity, other personal hygiene**

Y93.E9 **Activity, other interior property and clothing maintenance**

✓5ᵗʰ **Y93.F** **Activities involving** caregiving

Activity involving the provider of caregiving

Y93.F1 **Activity, caregiving,** bathing

Y93.F2 **Activity, caregiving,** lifting

Y93.F9 **Activity, other caregiving**

✓5ᵗʰ **Y93.G** **Activities involving food preparation, cooking and grilling**

Y93.G1 **Activity,** food preparation and clean up

Activity, dishwashing

Y93.G2 **Activity,** grilling and smoking food

Y93.G3 **Activity,** cooking and baking

Activity, use of stove, oven and microwave oven

Y93.G9 **Activity, other involving cooking and grilling**

✓5ᵗʰ **Y93.H** **Activities involving exterior property and land maintenance, building and construction**

Y93.H1 **Activity,** digging, shoveling and raking

Activity, dirt digging

Activity, raking leaves

Activity, snow shoveling

Y93.H2 **Activity,** gardening and landscaping

Activity, pruning, trimming shrubs, weeding

Y93.H3 **Activity,** building and construction

Y93.H9 **Activity, other involving exterior property and land maintenance, building and construction**

✓5ᵗʰ **Y93.I** **Activities involving roller coasters and other types of external motion**

Y93.I1 **Activity,** rollercoaster riding

Y93.I9 **Activity, other involving external motion**

✓5ᵗʰ **Y93.J** **Activities involving playing musical instrument**

Activity involving playing electric musical instrument

Y93.J1 **Activity,** piano playing

Activity, musical keyboard (electronic) playing

Y93.J2 **Activity,** drum and other percussion instrument playing

Y93.J3 **Activity,** string instrument playing

Y93.J4 **Activity,** winds and brass instrument playing

✓5ᵗʰ **Y93.K** **Activities involving animal care**

EXCLUDES 1 *activity, horseback riding (Y93.52)*

Y93.K1 **Activity,** walking an animal

Y93.K2 **Activity,** milking an animal

Y93.K3 **Activity,** grooming and shearing an animal

Y93.K9 **Activity, other involving animal care**

✓5ᵗʰ **Y93.8** **Activities, other specified**

Y93.81 **Activity,** refereeing a sports activity

Y93.82 **Activity,** spectator at an event

Y93.83 **Activity,** rough housing and horseplay

Y93.84 **Activity,** sleeping

Y93.85 **Activity,** choking game

Activity, blackout game

Activity, fainting game

Activity, pass out game

AHA: 2016,4Q,74-76

Y93.89 **Activity, other specified**

Y93.9 **Activity, unspecified**

Y95 **Nosocomial condition**

AHA: 2013,4Q,119

✓4ᵗʰ **Y99** **External cause status**

NOTE A single code from category Y99 should be used in conjunction with the external cause code(s) assigned to a record to indicate the status of the person at the time the event occurred.

Y99.0 **Civilian** activity done for income or pay

Civilian activity done for financial or other compensation

EXCLUDES 1 *military activity (Y99.1)*

volunteer activity (Y99.2)

Y99.1 **Military** activity

EXCLUDES 1 *activity of off duty military personnel (Y99.8)*

Y99.2 **Volunteer** activity

EXCLUDES 1 *activity of child or other family member assisting in compensated work of other family member (Y99.8)*

Y99.8 **Other external cause status**

Activity NEC

Activity of child or other family member assisting in compensated work of other family member

Hobby not done for income

Leisure activity

Off-duty activity of military personnel

Recreation or sport not for income or while a student

Student activity

EXCLUDES 1 *civilian activity done for income or compensation (Y99.0)*

military activity (Y99.1)

AHA: 2012,4Q,108

Y99.9 **Unspecified external cause status**

Chapter 21. Factors Influencing Health Status and Contact with Health Services (Z00–Z99)

Chapter-specific Guidelines with Coding Examples

The chapter-specific guidelines from the ICD-10-CM Official Guidelines for Coding and Reporting have been provided below. Along with these guidelines are coding examples, contained in the shaded boxes, that have been developed to help illustrate the coding and/or sequencing guidance found in these guidelines.

Note: The chapter-specific guidelines provide additional information about the use of Z codes for specified encounters.

a. Use of Z Codes in any healthcare setting

Z codes are for use in any healthcare setting. Z codes may be used as either a first-listed (principal diagnosis code in the inpatient setting) or secondary code, depending on the circumstances of the encounter. Certain Z codes may only be used as first-listed or principal diagnosis.

> Patient with middle lobe lung cancer presents for initiation of chemotherapy
>
> **Z51.11**   **Encounter for antineoplastic chemotherapy**
>
> **C34.2**   **Malignant neoplasm of middle lobe, bronchus or lung**
>
> *Explanation:* A Z code can be used as first-listed in this situation based on guidelines in this chapter as well as chapter 2, "Neoplasms."

> Patient has chronic lymphocytic leukemia for which the patient had previous chemotherapy and is now in remission
>
> **C91.11**   **Chronic lymphocytic leukemia of B-cell type in remission**
>
> **Z92.21**   **Personal history of antineoplastic chemotherapy**
>
> *Explanation:* The personal history Z code is used to describe a secondary (supplementary) diagnosis to identify that this patient has had chemotherapy in the past.

b. Z Codes indicate a reason for an encounter or provide additional information about a patient encounter

Z codes are not procedure codes. A corresponding procedure code must accompany a Z code to describe any procedure performed.

c. Categories of Z Codes

1) Contact/exposure

Category Z20 indicates contact with, and suspected exposure to, communicable diseases. These codes are for patients who are suspected to have been exposed to a disease by close personal contact with an infected individual or are in an area where a disease is epidemic.

Category Z77, Other contact with and (suspected) exposures hazardous to health, indicates contact with and suspected exposures hazardous to health.

Contact/exposure codes may be used as a first-listed code to explain an encounter for testing, or, more commonly, as a secondary code to identify a potential risk.

2) Inoculations and vaccinations

Code Z23 is for encounters for inoculations and vaccinations. It indicates that a patient is being seen to receive a prophylactic inoculation against a disease. Procedure codes are required to identify the actual administration of the injection and the type(s) of immunizations given. Code Z23 may be used as a secondary code if the inoculation is given as a routine part of preventive health care, such as a well-baby visit.

3) Status

Status codes indicate that a patient is either a carrier of a disease or has the sequelae or residual of a past disease or condition. This includes such things as the presence of prosthetic or mechanical devices resulting from past treatment. A status code is informative, because the status may affect the course of treatment and its outcome. A status code is distinct from a history code. The history code indicates that the patient no longer has the condition.

A status code should not be used with a diagnosis code from one of the body system chapters, if the diagnosis code includes the information provided by the status code. For example, code Z94.1, Heart transplant status, should not be used with a code from subcategory T86.2, Complications of heart transplant. The status code does not provide additional information. The complication code indicates that the patient is a heart transplant patient.

For encounters for weaning from a mechanical ventilator, assign a code from subcategory J96.1, Chronic respiratory failure, followed by code Z99.11, Dependence on respirator [ventilator] status.

The status Z codes/categories are:

Z14   Genetic carrier

Genetic carrier status indicates that a person carries a gene, associated with a particular disease, which may be passed to offspring who may develop that disease. The person does not have the disease and is not at risk of developing the disease.

Z15   Genetic susceptibility to disease

Genetic susceptibility indicates that a person has a gene that increases the risk of that person developing the disease.

Codes from category Z15 should not be used as principal or first-listed codes. If the patient has the condition to which he/she is susceptible, and that condition is the reason for the encounter, the code for the current condition should be sequenced first. If the patient is being seen for follow-up after completed treatment for this condition, and the condition no longer exists, a follow-up code should be sequenced first, followed by the appropriate personal history and genetic susceptibility codes. If the purpose of the encounter is genetic counseling associated with procreative management, code Z31.5, Encounter for genetic counseling, should be assigned as the first-listed code, followed by a code from category Z15. Additional codes should be assigned for any applicable family or personal history.

Z16   Resistance to antimicrobial drugs

This code indicates that a patient has a condition that is resistant to antimicrobial drug treatment. Sequence the infection code first.

Z17   Estrogen receptor status

Z18   Retained foreign body fragments

Z19   Hormone sensitivity malignancy status

Z21   Asymptomatic HIV infection status

This code indicates that a patient has tested positive for HIV but has manifested no signs or symptoms of the disease.

Z22   Carrier of infectious disease

Carrier status indicates that a person harbors the specific organisms of a disease without manifest symptoms and is capable of transmitting the infection.

Z28.3   Underimmunization status

See Section I.B.14. for underimmunization documentation by clinicians other than the patient's provider.

Z33.1   Pregnant state, incidental

This code is a secondary code only for use when the pregnancy is in no way complicating the reason for visit. Otherwise, a code from the obstetric chapter is required.

Z66   Do not resuscitate

This code may be used when it is documented by the provider that a patient is on do not resuscitate status at any time during the stay.

Z67   Blood type

Z68   Body mass index (BMI)

BMI codes should only be assigned when there is an associated, reportable diagnosis (such as obesity). Do not assign BMI codes during pregnancy.

See Section I.B.14. for BMI documentation by clinicians other than the patient's provider.

> Patient seen today for chest pain, noncardiac in nature. Nurses notes identify a BMI of 20.5.
>
> **R07.89**   **Other chest pain**
>
> *Explanation:* Section I.B.14 stipulates that the BMI can be assigned from documentation of someone other than the patient's provider, such as nursing notes, only when the provider has documented that the diagnosis is associated with the BMI. As there is no supporting documentation from the provider linking the BMI to an associated condition, no code is assigned for the BMI.

Chapter 21. Factors Influencing Health Status and Contact with Health Services

Z74.Ø1   Bed confinement status

Z76.82   Awaiting organ transplant status

Z78   Other specified health status

Code Z78.1, Physical restraint status, may be used when it is documented by the provider that a patient has been put in restraints during the current encounter. Please note that this code should not be reported when it is documented by the provider that a patient is temporarily restrained during a procedure.

Z79   Long-term (current) drug therapy

Codes from this category indicate a patient's continuous use of a prescribed drug (including such things as aspirin therapy) for the long-term treatment of a condition or for prophylactic use. It is not for use for patients who have addictions to drugs. This subcategory is not for use of medications for detoxification or maintenance programs to prevent withdrawal symptoms (e.g., methadone maintenance for opiate dependence). Assign the appropriate code for the drug use, abuse, or dependence instead.

Assign a code from Z79 if the patient is receiving a medication for an extended period as a prophylactic measure (such as for the prevention of deep vein thrombosis) or as treatment of a chronic condition (such as arthritis) or a disease requiring a lengthy course of treatment (such as cancer). Do not assign a code from category Z79 for medication being administered for a brief period of time to treat an acute illness or injury (such as a course of antibiotics to treat acute bronchitis).

Z88   Allergy status to drugs, medicaments and biological substances

Except: Z88.9, Allergy status to unspecified drugs, medicaments and biological substances status

Z89   Acquired absence of limb

Z9Ø   Acquired absence of organs, not elsewhere classified

Z91.Ø-   Allergy status, other than to drugs and biological substances

Z92.82   Status post administration of tPA (rtPA) in a different facility within the last 24 hours prior to admission to a current facility

Assign code Z92.82, Status post administration of tPA (rtPA) in a different facility within the last 24 hours prior to admission to current facility, as a secondary diagnosis when a patient is received by transfer into a facility and documentation indicates they were administered tissue plasminogen activator (tPA) within the last 24 hours prior to admission to the current facility.

This guideline applies even if the patient is still receiving the tPA at the time they are received into the current facility.

The appropriate code for the condition for which the tPA was administered (such as cerebrovascular disease or myocardial infarction) should be assigned first.

Code Z92.82 is only applicable to the receiving facility record and not to the transferring facility record.

Z93   Artificial opening status

Z94   Transplanted organ and tissue status

Z95   Presence of cardiac and vascular implants and grafts

Z96   Presence of other functional implants

Z97   Presence of other devices

Z98   Other postprocedural states

Assign code Z98.85, Transplanted organ removal status, to indicate that a transplanted organ has been previously removed. This code should not be assigned for the encounter in which the transplanted organ is removed. The complication necessitating removal of the transplant organ should be assigned for that encounter.

See section I.C.19. for information on the coding of organ transplant complications.

Z99   Dependence on enabling machines and devices, not elsewhere classified

Note: Categories Z89-Z9Ø and Z93-Z99 are for use only if there are no complications or malfunctions of the organ or tissue replaced, the amputation site or the equipment on which the patient is dependent.

4) History (of)

There are two types of history Z codes, personal and family. Personal history codes explain a patient's past medical condition that no longer exists and is not receiving any treatment, but that has the potential for recurrence, and therefore may require continued monitoring.

Family history codes are for use when a patient has a family member(s) who has had a particular disease that causes the patient to be at higher risk of also contracting the disease.

Personal history codes may be used in conjunction with follow-up codes and family history codes may be used in conjunction with screening codes to explain the need for a test or procedure. History codes are also acceptable on any medical record regardless of the reason for visit. A history of an illness, even if no longer present, is important information that may alter the type of treatment ordered.

The reason for the encounter (for example, screening or counseling) should be sequenced first and the appropriate personal and/or family history code(s) should be assigned as additional diagnos(es).

The history Z code categories are:

Z80   Family history of primary malignant neoplasm

Z81   Family history of mental and behavioral disorders

Z82   Family history of certain disabilities and chronic diseases (leading to disablement)

Z83   Family history of other specific disorders

Z84   Family history of other conditions

Z85   Personal history of malignant neoplasm

Z86   Personal history of certain other diseases

Z87   Personal history of other diseases and conditions

Z91.4-   Personal history of psychological trauma, not elsewhere classified

Z91.5-   Personal history of self-harm

Z91.81   History of falling

Z91.82   Personal history of military deployment

Z92   Personal history of medical treatment

Except: Z92.Ø, Personal history of contraception

Except: Z92.82, Status post administration of tPA (rtPA) in a different facility within the last 24 hours prior to admission to a current facility

5) Screening

Screening is the testing for disease or disease precursors in seemingly well individuals so that early detection and treatment can be provided for those who test positive for the disease (e.g., screening mammogram).

The testing of a person to rule out or confirm a suspected diagnosis because the patient has some sign or symptom is a diagnostic examination, not a screening. In these cases, the sign or symptom is used to explain the reason for the test.

A screening code may be a first-listed code if the reason for the visit is specifically the screening exam. It may also be used as an additional code if the screening is done during an office visit for other health problems. A screening code is not necessary if the screening is inherent to a routine examination, such as a pap smear done during a routine pelvic examination.

Should a condition be discovered during the screening then the code for the condition may be assigned as an additional diagnosis.

Prostate screening of healthy 50-year-old male patient; PSA noted to be elevated but normal digital rectal exam

Z12.5   **Encounter for screening for malignant neoplasm of prostate**

R97.2Ø   **Elevated prostate specific antigen [PSA]**

Explanation: The patient had no signs or symptoms of any prostate-related illness prior to coming in for the screening. The screening code is appropriately used as the first-listed code to signify that this was for routine screening. The elevated PSA is reported as a secondary diagnosis to reflect that an abnormal lab value was found as a result of the screening procedure(s).

The Z code indicates that a screening exam is planned. A procedure code is required to confirm that the screening was performed.

The screening Z codes/categories:

Z11   Encounter for screening for infectious and parasitic diseases

Z12   Encounter for screening for malignant neoplasms

Z13   Encounter for screening for other diseases and disorders

Except: Z13.9, Encounter for screening, unspecified

Z36   Encounter for antenatal screening for mother

6) Observation

There are three observation Z code categories. They are for use in very limited circumstances when a person is being observed for a suspected condition that is ruled out. The observation codes are not for use if an injury or illness or any signs or symptoms related to the suspected condition are present. In such cases the diagnosis/symptom code is used with the corresponding external cause code.

The observation codes are primarily to be used as a principal/first-listed diagnosis. An observation code may be assigned as a secondary diagnosis code when the patient is being observed for a condition that is ruled out and is unrelated to the principal/first-listed diagnosis. Also, when the principal diagnosis is required to be a code from category Z38, Liveborn infants according to place of birth and type of delivery. Then a code from category Z05, Encounter for observation and evaluation of newborn for suspected diseases and conditions ruled out, is sequenced after the Z38 code. Additional codes may be used in addition to the observation code but only if they are unrelated to the suspected condition being observed.

Codes from subcategory Z03.7, Encounter for suspected maternal and fetal conditions ruled out, may either be used as a first-listed or as an additional code assignment depending on the case. They are for use in very limited circumstances on a maternal record when an encounter is for a suspected maternal or fetal condition that is ruled out during that encounter (for example, a maternal or fetal condition may be suspected due to an abnormal test result). These codes should not be used when the condition is confirmed. In those cases, the confirmed condition should be coded. In addition, these codes are not for use if an illness or any signs or symptoms related to the suspected condition or problem are present. In such cases the diagnosis/symptom code is used.

Additional codes may be used in addition to the code from subcategory Z03.7, but only if they are unrelated to the suspected condition being evaluated.

Codes from subcategory Z03.7 may not be used for encounters for antenatal screening of mother. *See Section I.C.21. Screening.*

For encounters for suspected fetal condition that are inconclusive following testing and evaluation, assign the appropriate code from category O35, O36, O40 or O41.

The observation Z code categories:

Z03   Encounter for medical observation for suspected diseases and conditions ruled out

Z04   Encounter for examination and observation for other reasons
        Except: Z04.9, Encounter for examination and observation for unspecified reason

Z05   Encounter for observation and evaluation of newborn for suspected diseases and conditions ruled out

7) Aftercare

Aftercare visit codes cover situations when the initial treatment of a disease has been performed and the patient requires continued care during the healing or recovery phase, or for the long-term consequences of the disease. The aftercare Z code should not be used if treatment is directed at a current, acute disease. The diagnosis code is to be used in these cases. Exceptions to this rule are codes Z51.0, Encounter for antineoplastic radiation therapy, and codes from subcategory Z51.1, Encounter for antineoplastic chemotherapy and immunotherapy. These codes are to be first listed, followed by the diagnosis code when a patient's encounter is solely to receive radiation therapy, chemotherapy, or immunotherapy for the treatment of a neoplasm. If the reason for the encounter is more than one type of antineoplastic therapy, code Z51.0 and a code from subcategory Z51.1 may be assigned together, in which case one of these codes would be reported as a secondary diagnosis.

The aftercare Z codes should also not be used for aftercare for injuries. For aftercare of an injury, assign the acute injury code with the appropriate 7th character (for subsequent encounter).

The aftercare codes are generally first listed to explain the specific reason for the encounter. An aftercare code may be used as an additional code when some type of aftercare is provided in addition to the reason for admission and no diagnosis code is applicable. An example of this would be the closure of a colostomy during an encounter for treatment of another condition.

Aftercare codes should be used in conjunction with other aftercare codes or diagnosis codes to provide better detail on the specifics of an aftercare encounter visit, unless otherwise directed by the classification. The sequencing of multiple aftercare codes depends on the circumstances of the encounter.

Patient presents for third round of gemcitabine and first dose of antineoplastic radiation therapy for advanced pancreatic carcinoma

Z51.11	**Encounter for antineoplastic chemotherapy**
Z51.0	**Encounter for antineoplastic radiation therapy**
C25.9	**Malignant neoplasm of pancreas, unspecified**

Explanation: Gemcitabine is an antineoplastic chemotherapy. Since the encounter was solely to administer antineoplastic treatment, both forms of treatment are reported and either code can be the first-listed diagnosis, followed by the neoplastic condition code. Aftercare codes are typically not assigned for current treatment of disease; however, Z51.0 and subcategory Z51.1 are an exception to this standard.

Certain aftercare Z code categories need a secondary diagnosis code to describe the resolving condition or sequelae. For others, the condition is included in the code title.

Additional Z code aftercare category terms include fitting and adjustment, and attention to artificial openings.

Status Z codes may be used with aftercare Z codes to indicate the nature of the aftercare. For example code Z95.1, Presence of aortocoronary bypass graft, may be used with code Z48.812, Encounter for surgical aftercare following surgery on the circulatory system, to indicate the surgery for which the aftercare is being performed. A status code should not be used when the aftercare code indicates the type of status, such as using Z43.0, Encounter for attention to tracheostomy, with Z93.0, Tracheostomy status.

The aftercare Z category/codes:

Z42   Encounter for plastic and reconstructive surgery following medical procedure or healed injury

Z43   Encounter for attention to artificial openings

Z44   Encounter for fitting and adjustment of external prosthetic device

Z45   Encounter for adjustment and management of implanted device

Z46   Encounter for fitting and adjustment of other devices

Z47   Orthopedic aftercare

Z48   Encounter for other postprocedural aftercare

Z49   Encounter for care involving renal dialysis

Z51   Encounter for other aftercare and medical care

8) Follow-up

The follow-up codes are used to explain continuing surveillance following completed treatment of a disease, condition, or injury. They imply that the condition has been fully treated and no longer exists. They should not be confused with aftercare codes, or injury codes with a 7th character for subsequent encounter, that explain ongoing care of a healing condition or its sequelae. Follow-up codes may be used in conjunction with history codes to provide the full picture of the healed condition and its treatment. The follow-up code is sequenced first, followed by the history code.

A follow-up code may be used to explain multiple visits. Should a condition be found to have recurred on the follow-up visit, then the diagnosis code for the condition should be assigned in place of the follow-up code.

The follow-up Z code categories:

Z08   Encounter for follow-up examination after completed treatment for malignant neoplasm

Z09   Encounter for follow-up examination after completed treatment for conditions other than malignant neoplasm

Z39   Encounter for maternal postpartum care and examination

Follow-up for patient several months after completing a regime of IV antibiotics for recurrent pneumonia; lungs are clear and pneumonia is resolved

| Z09 | **Encounter for follow-up examination after completed treatment for conditions other than malignant neoplasm** |
| Z87.01 | **Personal history of pneumonia (recurrent)** |

Explanation: Code Z09 identifies the follow-up visit as being unrelated to a malignant neoplasm, and code Z87 describes the condition that has now resolved.

Follow-up for patient several months after completing a regime of IV antibiotics for recurrent pneumonia; pneumonia has recurred, and a new antibiotic regimen has been prescribed

> **J18.9　　　Pneumonia, unspecified organism**
>
> *Explanation:* Since the follow-up exam for pneumonia determined that the pneumonia was not resolved or recurred, code Z09 Encounter for follow-up examination after completed treatment for conditions other than malignant neoplasm, no longer applies. Instead the first-listed code describes the pneumonia.

9) Donor

Codes in category Z52, Donors of organs and tissues, are used for living individuals who are donating blood or other body tissue. These codes are for individuals donating for others, as well as for self-donations. They are not used to identify cadaveric donations.

10) Counseling

Counseling Z codes are used when a patient or family member receives assistance in the aftermath of an illness or injury, or when support is required in coping with family or social problems.

The counseling Z codes/categories:

Z30.0-	Encounter for general counseling and advice on contraception
Z31.5	Encounter for procreative genetic counseling
Z31.6-	Encounter for general counseling and advice on procreation
Z32.2	Encounter for childbirth instruction
Z32.3	Encounter for childcare instruction
Z69	Encounter for mental health services for victim and perpetrator of abuse
Z70	Counseling related to sexual attitude, behavior and orientation
Z71	Persons encountering health services for other counseling and medical advice, not elsewhere classified

Note: Code Z71.84, Encounter for health counseling related to travel, is to be used for health risk and safety counseling for future travel purposes.

Code Z71.85, Encounter for immunization safety counseling, is to be used for counseling of the patient or caregiver regarding the safety of a vaccine. This code should not be used for the provision of general information regarding risks and potential side effects during routine encounters for the administration of vaccines.

Code Z71.87, Encounter for pediatric-to-adult transition counseling, should be assigned when pediatric-to-adult transition counseling is the sole reason for the encounter or when this counseling is provided in addition to other services, such as treatment of a chronic condition. If both transition counseling and treatment of a medical condition are provided during the same encounter, the code(s) for the medical condition(s) treated and code Z71.87 should be assigned, with sequencing depending on the circumstances of the encounter.

Z76.81	Expectant mother prebirth pediatrician visit

11) Encounters for obstetrical and reproductive services

See Section I.C.15. Pregnancy, Childbirth, and the Puerperium, for further instruction on the use of these codes.

Z codes for pregnancy are for use in those circumstances when none of the problems or complications included in the codes from the Obstetrics chapter exist (a routine prenatal visit or postpartum care). Codes in category Z34, Encounter for supervision of normal pregnancy, are always first-listed and are not to be used with any other code from the OB chapter.

Codes in category Z3A, Weeks of gestation, may be assigned to provide additional information about the pregnancy. Category Z3A codes should not be assigned for pregnancies with abortive outcomes (categories O00-O08), elective termination of pregnancy (code Z33.2), nor for postpartum conditions, as category Z3A is not applicable to these conditions. The date of the admission should be used to determine weeks of gestation for inpatient admissions that encompass more than one gestational week.

The outcome of delivery, category Z37, should be included on all maternal delivery records. It is always a secondary code.

Codes in category Z37 should not be used on the newborn record.

Z codes for family planning (contraceptive) or procreative management and counseling should be included on an obstetric record either during the pregnancy or the postpartum stage, if applicable.

Z codes/categories for obstetrical and reproductive services:

Z30	Encounter for contraceptive management
Z31	Encounter for procreative management
Z32.2	Encounter for childbirth instruction
Z32.3	Encounter for childcare instruction
Z33	Pregnant state
Z34	Encounter for supervision of normal pregnancy
Z36	Encounter for antenatal screening of mother
Z3A	Weeks of gestation
Z37	Outcome of delivery
Z39	Encounter for maternal postpartum care and examination
Z76.81	Expectant mother prebirth pediatrician visit

12) Newborns and infants

See Section I.C.16. Newborn (Perinatal) Guidelines, for further instruction on the use of these codes.

Newborn Z codes/categories:

Z76.1	Encounter for health supervision and care of foundling
Z00.1-	Encounter for routine child health examination
Z38	Liveborn infants according to place of birth and type of delivery

13) Routine and administrative examinations

The Z codes allow for the description of encounters for routine examinations, such as, a general check-up, or, examinations for administrative purposes, such as, a pre-employment physical. The codes are not to be used if the examination is for diagnosis of a suspected condition or for treatment purposes. In such cases the diagnosis code is used. During a routine exam, should a diagnosis or condition be discovered, it should be coded as an additional code. Pre-existing and chronic conditions and history codes may also be included as additional codes as long as the examination is for administrative purposes and not focused on any particular condition.

Some of the codes for routine health examinations distinguish between "with" and "without" abnormal findings. Code assignment depends on the information that is known at the time the encounter is being coded. For example, if no abnormal findings were found during the examination, but the encounter is being coded before test results are back, it is acceptable to assign the code for "without abnormal findings." When assigning a code for "with abnormal findings," additional code(s) should be assigned to identify the specific abnormal finding(s).

> 12-month-old boy presented for well-child visit; pediatrician notices some eczema on the child's scalp and back of the knees
>
> **Z00.121　　Encounter for routine child health examination with abnormal findings**
>
> **L30.9　　　Dermatitis, unspecified**
>
> *Explanation:* The Z code identifying that this is a routine well-child visit is reported first. Because an abnormal finding (eczema) was documented, a code for this condition may also be appended.

Pre-operative examination and pre-procedural laboratory examination Z codes are for use only in those situations when a patient is being cleared for a procedure or surgery and no treatment is given.

The Z codes/categories for routine and administrative examinations:

Z00	Encounter for general examination without complaint, suspected or reported diagnosis
Z01	Encounter for other special examination without complaint, suspected or reported diagnosis
Z02	Encounter for administrative examination
	Except: Z02.9, Encounter for administrative examinations, unspecified
Z32.0-	Encounter for pregnancy test

14) Miscellaneous Z codes

The miscellaneous Z codes capture a number of other health care encounters that do not fall into one of the other categories. Some of these codes identify the reason for the encounter; others are for use as additional codes that provide useful information on circumstances that may affect a patient's care and treatment.

Prophylactic organ removal

For encounters specifically for prophylactic removal of an organ (such as prophylactic removal of breasts due to a genetic susceptibility to cancer or a family history of cancer), the principal or first-listed code should be a code from category Z40, Encounter for prophylactic surgery, followed by the appropriate codes to identify the associated risk factor (such as genetic susceptibility or family history).

If the patient has a malignancy of one site and is having prophylactic removal at another site to prevent either a new primary malignancy or metastatic disease, a code for the malignancy should also be assigned in addition to a code from subcategory Z40.0, Encounter for prophylactic surgery for risk factors related to malignant neoplasms. A Z40.0 code should not be assigned if the patient is having organ removal for treatment of a malignancy, such as the removal of the testes for the treatment of prostate cancer.

Miscellaneous Z codes/categories:

Z28	Immunization not carried out
	Except: Z28.3-, Underimmunization status
Z29	Encounter for other prophylactic measures
Z40	Encounter for prophylactic surgery
Z41	Encounter for procedures for purposes other than remedying health state
	Except: Z41.9, Encounter for procedure for purposes other than remedying health state, unspecified
Z53	Persons encountering health services for specific procedures and treatment, not carried out
Z72	Problems related to lifestyle
	Note: These codes should be assigned only when the documentation specifies that the patient has an associated problem
Z73	Problems related to life management difficulty
	Note: These codes should be assigned only when the documentation specifies that the patient has an associated problem.
Z74	Problems related to care provider dependency
	Except: Z74.01, Bed confinement status
Z75	Problems related to medical facilities and other health care
Z76.0	Encounter for issue of repeat prescription
Z76.3	Healthy person accompanying sick person
Z76.4	Other boarder to healthcare facility
Z76.5	Malingerer [conscious simulation]
Z91.1-	Patient's noncompliance with medical treatment and regimen
Z91.83	Wandering in diseases classified elsewhere
Z91.84-	Oral health risk factors
Z91.89	Other specified personal risk factors, not elsewhere classified

See Section I.B.14. for Z55-Z65 Persons with potential health hazards related to socioeconomic and psychosocial circumstances, documentation by clinicians other than the patient's provider

15) Nonspecific Z codes

Certain Z codes are so non-specific, or potentially redundant with other codes in the classification, that there can be little justification for their use in the inpatient setting. Their use in the outpatient setting should be limited to those instances when there is no further documentation to permit more precise coding. Otherwise, any sign or symptom or any other reason for visit that is captured in another code should be used.

Nonspecific Z codes/categories:

Z02.9	Encounter for administrative examinations, unspecified
Z04.9	Encounter for examination and observation for unspecified reason
Z13.9	Encounter for screening, unspecified
Z41.9	Encounter for procedure for purposes other than remedying health state, unspecified
Z52.9	Donor of unspecified organ or tissue
Z86.59	Personal history of other mental and behavioral disorders
Z88.9	Allergy status to unspecified drugs, medicaments and biological substances status
Z92.0	Personal history of contraception

16) Z codes that may only be principal/first-listed diagnosis

The following Z codes/categories may only be reported as the principal/first-listed diagnosis, except when there are multiple encounters on the same day and the medical records for the encounters are combined:

Z00	Encounter for general examination without complaint, suspected or reported diagnosis
	Except: Z00.6
Z01	Encounter for other special examination without complaint, suspected or reported diagnosis
Z02	Encounter for administrative examination
Z04	Encounter for examination and observation for other reasons
Z33.2	Encounter for elective termination of pregnancy
Z31.81	Encounter for male factor infertility in female patient
Z31.83	Encounter for assisted reproductive fertility procedure cycle
Z31.84	Encounter for fertility preservation procedure

Z34	Encounter for supervision of normal pregnancy
Z39	Encounter for maternal postpartum care and examination
Z38	Liveborn infants according to place of birth and type of delivery
Z40	Encounter for prophylactic surgery
Z42	Encounter for plastic and reconstructive surgery following medical procedure or healed injury
Z51.0	Encounter for antineoplastic radiation therapy
Z51.1-	Encounter for antineoplastic chemotherapy and immunotherapy
Z52	Donors of organs and tissues
	Except: Z52.9, Donor of unspecified organ or tissue
Z76.1	Encounter for health supervision and care of foundling
Z76.2	Encounter for health supervision and care of other healthy infant and child
Z99.12	Encounter for respirator [ventilator] dependence during power failure

Female patient seen at 32 weeks' gestation to check the progress of her first pregnancy

Z34.03 **Encounter for supervision of normal first pregnancy, third trimester**

Z3A.32 **32 weeks gestation of pregnancy**

Explanation: Category Z34 is appropriate as a first-listed diagnosis. Category Z3A helps to clarify at which point in the pregnancy the patient was provided supervision.

17) Social determinants of health

Codes describing **problems or risk factors related to** social determinants of health (SDOH) should be assigned when this information is documented. **Assign as many SDOH codes as are necessary to describe all of the problems or risk factors. These codes should be assigned only when the documentation specifies that the patient has an associated problem or risk factor. For example, not every individual living alone would be assigned code Z60.2, Problems related to living alone.**

For social determinants of health, such as information found in categories Z55-Z65, Persons with potential health hazards related to socioeconomic and psychosocial circumstances, code assignment may be based on medical record documentation from clinicians involved in the care of the patient who are not the patient's provider since this information represents social information, rather than medical diagnoses.

For example, coding professionals may utilize documentation of social information from social workers, community health workers, case managers, or nurses, if their documentation is included in the official medical record.

Patient self-reported documentation may be used to assign codes for social determinants of health, as long as the patient self-reported information is signed-off by and incorporated into the medical record by either a clinician or provider.

Social determinants of health codes are located primarily in these Z code categories:

Z55	Problems related to education and literacy
Z56	Problems related to employment and unemployment
Z57	Occupational exposure to risk factors
Z58	Problems related to physical environment
Z59	Problems related to housing and economic circumstances
Z60	Problems related to social environment
Z62	Problems related to upbringing
Z63	Other problems related to primary support group, including family circumstances
Z64	Problems related to certain psychosocial circumstances
Z65	Problems related to other psychosocial circumstances

See Section I.B.14. Documentation by Clinicians Other than the Patient's Provider.

Chapter 21. Factors Influencing Health Status and Contact With Health Services

Z00–Z01.01

Chapter 21. Factors Influencing Health Status and Contact With Health Services (Z00-Z99)

> **NOTE** Z codes represent reasons for encounters. A corresponding procedure code must accompany a Z code if a procedure is performed. Categories Z00-Z99 are provided for occasions when circumstances other than a disease, injury or external cause classifiable to categories A00-Y89 are recorded as "diagnoses" or "problems." This can arise in two main ways:
>
> (a) When a person who may or may not be sick encounters the health services for some specific purpose, such as to receive limited care or service for a current condition, to donate an organ or tissue, to receive prophylactic vaccination (immunization), or to discuss a problem which is in itself not a disease or injury.
>
> (b) When some circumstance or problem is present which influences the person's health status but is not in itself a current illness or injury.

AHA: 2018,4Q,60-61

This chapter contains the following blocks:

Z00-Z13	Persons encountering health services for examinations
Z14-Z15	Genetic carrier and genetic susceptibility to disease
Z16	Resistance to antimicrobial drugs
Z17	Estrogen receptor status
Z18	Retained foreign body fragments
Z19	Hormone sensitivity malignancy status
Z20-Z29	Persons with potential health hazards related to communicable diseases
Z30-Z39	Persons encountering health services in circumstances related to reproduction
Z40-Z53	Encounters for other specific health care
Z55-Z65	Persons with potential health hazards related to socioeconomic and psychosocial circumstances
Z66	Do not resuscitate status
Z67	Blood type
Z68	Body mass index (BMI)
Z69-Z76	Persons encountering health services in other circumstances
Z77-Z99	Persons with potential health hazards related to family and personal history and certain conditions influencing health status

Persons encountering health services for examinations (Z00-Z13)

> **NOTE** Nonspecific abnormal findings disclosed at the time of these examinations are classified to categories R70-R94.

> **EXCLUDES 1** examinations related to pregnancy and reproduction (Z30-Z36, Z39.-)

✓4ᵗʰ Z00 Encounter for general examination without complaint, suspected or reported diagnosis

> **EXCLUDES 1** encounter for examination for administrative purposes (Z02.-)
> **EXCLUDES 2** encounter for pre-procedural examinations (Z01.81-)
> special screening examinations (Z11-Z13)

AHA: 2017,4Q,95

✓5ᵗʰ Z00.0 Encounter for general adult medical examination

Encounter for adult periodic examination (annual) (physical) and any associated laboratory and radiologic examinations

> **EXCLUDES 1** encounter for examination of sign or symptom - code to sign or symptom
> general health check-up of infant or child (Z00.12.-)

Z00.00 Encounter for general adult medical examination without abnormal findings `PDx` `A`

Encounter for adult health check-up NOS

AHA: 2016,1Q,36

Z00.01 Encounter for general adult medical examination with abnormal findings `PDx` `A`

Use additional code to identify abnormal findings

AHA: 2016,1Q,35-36

✓5ᵗʰ Z00.1 Encounter for newborn, infant and child health examinations

✓6ᵗʰ Z00.11 Newborn health examination

Health check for child under 29 days old

Use additional code to identify any abnormal findings

> **EXCLUDES 1** health check for child over 28 days old (Z00.12-)

Z00.110 Health examination for newborn under 8 days old `PDx` `N`

Health check for newborn under 8 days old

Z00.111 Health examination for newborn 8 to 28 days old `PDx` `N`

Health check for newborn 8 to 28 days old

Newborn weight check

✓6ᵗʰ Z00.12 Encounter for routine child health examination

Health check (routine) for child over 28 days old

Immunizations appropriate for age

Routine developmental screening of infant or child

Routine vison and hearing testing

> **EXCLUDES 1** health check for child under 29 days old (Z00.11-)
> health supervision of foundling or other healthy infant or child (Z76.1-Z76.2)
> newborn health examination (Z00.11-)

AHA: 2018,4Q,36

Z00.121 Encounter for routine child health examination with abnormal findings `PDx` `P`

Use additional code to identify abnormal findings

AHA: 2016,1Q,34-35

Z00.129 Encounter for routine child health examination without abnormal findings `PDx` `P`

Encounter for routine child health examination NOS

AHA: 2016,1Q,34

Z00.2 Encounter for examination for period of rapid growth in childhood `PDx` `P`

Z00.3 Encounter for examination for adolescent development state `PDx` `P`

Encounter for puberty development state

Z00.5 Encounter for examination of potential donor of organ and tissue `PDx`

Z00.6 Encounter for examination for normal comparison and control in clinical research program

Examination of participant or control in clinical research program

✓5ᵗʰ Z00.7 Encounter for examination for period of delayed growth in childhood

Z00.70 Encounter for examination for period of delayed growth in childhood without abnormal findings `PDx` `P`

Z00.71 Encounter for examination for period of delayed growth in childhood with abnormal findings `PDx` `P`

Use additional code to identify abnormal findings

Z00.8 Encounter for other general examination `PDx`

Encounter for health examination in population surveys

✓4ᵗʰ Z01 Encounter for other special examination without complaint, suspected or reported diagnosis

> **INCLUDES** routine examination of specific system

> **NOTE** Codes from category Z01 represent the reason for the encounter. A separate procedure code is required to identify any examinations or procedures performed

> **EXCLUDES 1** encounter for examination for administrative purposes (Z02.-)
> encounter for examination for suspected conditions, proven not to exist (Z03.-)
> encounter for laboratory and radiologic examinations as a component of general medical examinations (Z00.0-)
> encounter for laboratory, radiologic and imaging examinations for sign(s) and symptom(s) - code to the sign(s) or symptom(s)

> **EXCLUDES 2** screening examinations (Z11-Z13)

✓5ᵗʰ Z01.0 Encounter for examination of eyes and vision

> **EXCLUDES 1** examination for driving license (Z02.4)

Z01.00 Encounter for examination of eyes and vision without abnormal findings `PDx`

Encounter for examination of eyes and vision NOS

Z01.01 Encounter for examination of eyes and vision with abnormal findings `PDx`

Use additional code to identify abnormal findings

AHA: 2016,4Q,21

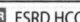 **HCC** CMS-HCC   **Rx** Rx HCC   **ESR** ESRD HCC   **COM** Commercial HCC   **PDx** Primary Dx Only   **N** Newborn: 0   **P** Pediatric: 0-17   **M** Maternity: 9-64   **A** Adult: 15-124

1264   ICD-10-CM 2023

☑6ᵗʰ **Z01.02** **Encounter for examination of eyes and vision following failed vision screening**

EXCLUDES 1   *encounter for examination of eyes and vision with abnormal findings (Z01.01)*

encounter for examination of eyes and vision without abnormal findings (Z01.00)

AHA: 2019,4Q,20

Z01.020 **Encounter for examination of eyes and vision following failed vision screening without abnormal findings** PDx

Z01.021 **Encounter for examination of eyes and vision following failed vision screening with abnormal findings** PDx

Use additional code to identify abnormal findings

☑5ᵗʰ **Z01.1** **Encounter for examination of ears and hearing**

Z01.10 **Encounter for examination of ears and hearing without abnormal findings** PDx

Encounter for examination of ears and hearing NOS

AHA: 2016,4Q,24

☑6ᵗʰ **Z01.11** **Encounter for examination of ears and hearing with abnormal findings**

AHA: 2016,3Q,17-18

Z01.110 **Encounter for hearing examination following failed hearing screening** PDx

Z01.118 **Encounter for examination of ears and hearing with other abnormal findings** PDx

Use additional code to identify abnormal findings

Z01.12 **Encounter for hearing conservation and treatment** PDx

☑5ᵗʰ **Z01.2** **Encounter for dental examination and cleaning**

Z01.20 **Encounter for dental examination and cleaning without abnormal findings** PDx

Encounter for dental examination and cleaning NOS

Z01.21 **Encounter for dental examination and cleaning with abnormal findings** PDx

Use additional code to identify abnormal findings

☑5ᵗʰ **Z01.3** **Encounter for examination of blood pressure**

Z01.30 **Encounter for examination of blood pressure without abnormal findings** PDx

Encounter for examination of blood pressure NOS

Z01.31 **Encounter for examination of blood pressure with abnormal findings** PDx

Use additional code to identify abnormal findings

☑5ᵗʰ **Z01.4** **Encounter for gynecological examination**

EXCLUDES 2   *pregnancy examination or test (Z32.0-)*

routine examination for contraceptive maintenance (Z30.4-)

☑6ᵗʰ **Z01.41** **Encounter for routine gynecological examination**

Encounter for general gynecological examination with or without cervical smear

Encounter for gynecological examination (general) (routine) NOS

Encounter for pelvic examination (annual) (periodic)

Use additional code:

for screening for human papillomavirus, if applicable, (Z11.51)

for screening vaginal pap smear, if applicable (Z12.72)

to identify acquired absence of uterus, if applicable (Z90.71-)

EXCLUDES 1   *gynecologic examination status-post hysterectomy for malignant condition (Z08)*

screening cervical pap smear not a part of a routine gynecological examination (Z12.4)

Z01.411 **Encounter for gynecological examination (general) (routine) with abnormal findings** PDx ♀

Use additional code to identify abnormal findings

Z01.419 **Encounter for gynecological examination (general) (routine) without abnormal findings** PDx ♀

Z01.42 **Encounter for cervical smear to confirm findings of recent normal smear following initial abnormal smear** PDx ♀

☑5ᵗʰ **Z01.8** **Encounter for other specified special examinations**

☑6ᵗʰ **Z01.81** **Encounter for preprocedural examinations**

Encounter for preoperative examinations

Encounter for radiological and imaging examinations as part of preprocedural examination

TIP: Assign a code for the condition necessitating surgery and any findings as additional diagnoses.

Z01.810 **Encounter for preprocedural cardiovascular examination** PDx

Z01.811 **Encounter for preprocedural respiratory examination** PDx

Z01.812 **Encounter for preprocedural laboratory examination** PDx

Blood and urine tests prior to treatment or procedure

AHA: 2020,3Q,14

TIP: During the COVID-19 pandemic, assign this code followed by code Z20.822 Contact with and (suspected) exposure to COVID-19, when COVID-19 testing is being performed as part of preoperative testing.

Z01.818 **Encounter for other preprocedural examination** PDx

Encounter for preprocedural examination NOS

Encounter for examinations prior to antineoplastic chemotherapy

Z01.82 **Encounter for allergy testing** PDx

EXCLUDES 1   *encounter for antibody response examination (Z01.84)*

Z01.83 **Encounter for blood typing** PDx

Encounter for Rh typing

Z01.84 **Encounter for antibody response examination** PDx

Encounter for immunity status testing

EXCLUDES 1   *encounter for allergy testing (Z01.82)*

AHA: 2020,2Q,11

Z01.89 **Encounter for other specified special examinations** PDx

☑4ᵗʰ **Z02** **Encounter for administrative examination**

Z02.0 **Encounter for examination for admission to educational institution** PDx

Encounter for examination for admission to preschool (education)

Encounter for examination for re-admission to school following illness or medical treatment

Z02.1 **Encounter for pre-employment examination** PDx

Z02.2 **Encounter for examination for admission to residential institution** PDx

EXCLUDES 1   *examination for admission to prison (Z02.89)*

Z02.3 **Encounter for examination for recruitment to armed forces** PDx

Z02.4 **Encounter for examination for driving license** PDx

Z02.5 **Encounter for examination for participation in sport** PDx

EXCLUDES 1   *blood-alcohol and blood-drug test (Z02.83)*

Z02.6 **Encounter for examination for insurance purposes** PDx

☑5ᵗʰ **Z02.7** **Encounter for issue of medical certificate**

EXCLUDES 1   *encounter for general medical examination (Z00-Z01, Z02.0-Z02.6, Z02.8-Z02.9)*

Z02.71 **Encounter for disability determination** PDx

Encounter for issue of medical certificate of incapacity

Encounter for issue of medical certificate of invalidity

Z02.79 **Encounter for issue of other medical certificate** PDx

☑5ᵗʰ **Z02.8** **Encounter for other administrative examinations**

Z02.81 **Encounter for paternity testing** PDx

Z02.82 **Encounter for adoption services** PDx

Z02.83 **Encounter for** blood-alcohol and blood-drug test ◻PDx◻
　　Use additional code for findings of alcohol or drugs in blood (R78.-)

Z02.89 **Encounter for other administrative examinations** ◻PDx◻
　　Encounter for examination for admission to prison
　　Encounter for examination for admission to summer camp
　　Encounter for immigration examination
　　Encounter for naturalization examination
　　Encounter for premarital examination
　　EXCLUDES 1　health supervision of foundling or other healthy infant or child (Z76.1-Z76.2)

Z02.9 **Encounter for administrative examinations, unspecified** ◻PDx◻

✔4ᵗʰ Z03 **Encounter for** medical observation **for suspected diseases and conditions ruled out**
　　This category is to be used when a person without a diagnosis is suspected of having an abnormal condition, without signs or symptoms, which requires study, but after examination and observation, is ruled out. This category is also for use for administrative and legal observation status.
　　EXCLUDES 1　contact with and (suspected) exposures hazardous to health (Z77.-)
　　　　encounter for observation and evaluation of newborn for suspected diseases and conditions ruled out (Z05.-)
　　　　person with feared complaint in whom no diagnosis is made (Z71.1)
　　　　signs or symptoms under study - code to signs or symptoms
　　AHA: 2020,2Q,8; 2018,2Q,7-8; 2017,4Q,27

Z03.6 **Encounter for observation for suspected** toxic effect from ingested substance **ruled out**
　　Encounter for observation for suspected adverse effect from drug
　　Encounter for observation for suspected poisoning

✔5ᵗʰ Z03.7 **Encounter for suspected** maternal and fetal conditions **ruled out**
　　Encounter for suspected maternal and fetal conditions not found
　　EXCLUDES 1　known or suspected fetal anomalies affecting management of mother, not ruled out (O26.-, O35.-, O36.-, O40.-, O41.-)

Z03.71 **Encounter for suspected problem with** amniotic cavity and membrane **ruled out** Ⓜ♀
　　Encounter for suspected oligohydramnios ruled out
　　Encounter for suspected polyhydramnios ruled out

Z03.72 **Encounter for suspected** placental problem **ruled out** Ⓜ♀

Z03.73 **Encounter for suspected** fetal anomaly **ruled out** Ⓜ♀

Z03.74 **Encounter for suspected** problem with fetal growth **ruled out** Ⓜ♀

Z03.75 **Encounter for suspected** cervical shortening **ruled out** Ⓜ♀

Z03.79 **Encounter for other suspected maternal and fetal conditions ruled out** Ⓜ♀

✔5ᵗʰ Z03.8 **Encounter for** observation **for other suspected diseases and conditions ruled out**

✔6ᵗʰ Z03.81 **Encounter for observation for suspected** exposure to biological agents **ruled out**
　　Z03.810 **Encounter for observation for suspected exposure to** anthrax **ruled out**
　　Z03.818 **Encounter for observation for suspected exposure to other biological agents ruled out**
　　　　AHA: 2020,2Q,8; 2020,1Q,34-36
　　　　TIP: During the COVID-19 pandemic, possible exposure to COVID-19 should be coded using Z20.822 Contact with and (suspected) exposure to COVID-19, even when the COVID-19 infection has been ruled out.

✔6ᵗʰ Z03.82 **Encounter for observation for suspected** foreign body **ruled out**
　　EXCLUDES 1　retained foreign body (Z18.-)
　　　　retained foreign body in eyelid (H02.81)
　　　　residual foreign body in soft tissue (M79.5)
　　EXCLUDES 2　confirmed foreign body ingestion or aspiration including:
　　　　foreign body in alimentary tract (T18)
　　　　foreign body in ear (T16)
　　　　foreign body on external eye (T15)
　　　　foreign body in respiratory tract (T17)
　　AHA: 2020,4Q,42

Z03.821 **Encounter for observation for suspected** ingested **foreign body ruled out**

Z03.822 **Encounter for observation for suspected** aspirated (inhaled) **foreign body ruled out**

Z03.823 **Encounter for observation for suspected** inserted (injected) **foreign body ruled out**
　　Encounter for observation for suspected inserted (injected) foreign body in eye ruled out
　　Encounter for observation for suspected inserted (injected) foreign body in orifice ruled out
　　Encounter for observation for suspected inserted (injected) foreign body in skin ruled out

● **Z03.83** **Encounter for observation for suspected conditions related to** home physiologic monitoring device **ruled out**
　　Encounter for observation for apnea alarm without findings
　　Encounter for observation for bradycardia alarm without findings
　　Encounter for observation for malfunction of home cardiorespiratory monitor
　　Encounter for observation for non-specific findings home physiologic monitoring device
　　Encounter for observation for pulse oximeter alarm without findings
　　EXCLUDES 1　apnea NOS (R06.81)
　　　　neonatal bradycardia (P29.12)
　　　　newborn apnea (P28.4-)
　　　　primary sleep apnea of newborn (P28.3-)
　　　　sleep apnea (G47.3-)

Z03.89 **Encounter for observation for other suspected diseases and conditions ruled out**

✔4ᵗʰ Z04 **Encounter for examination and observation for other reasons**
　　INCLUDES　encounter for examination for medicolegal reasons
　　This category is to be used when a person without a diagnosis is suspected of having an abnormal condition, without signs or symptoms, which requires study, but after examination and observation, is ruled-out. This category is also for use for administrative and legal observation status.
　　AHA: 2018,2Q,7-8

Z04.1 **Encounter for examination and observation following** transport accident ◻PDx◻
　　EXCLUDES 1　encounter for examination and observation following work accident (Z04.2)
　　AHA: 2019,2Q,11; 2018,2Q,8

Z04.2 **Encounter for examination and observation following** work accident ◻PDx◻

Z04.3 **Encounter for examination and observation following other** accident ◻PDx◻

✔5ᵗʰ Z04.4 **Encounter for examination and observation following** alleged rape
　　Encounter for examination and observation of victim following alleged rape
　　Encounter for examination and observation of victim following alleged sexual abuse

Z04.41 **Encounter for examination and observation following alleged** adult **rape** ◻PDx◻ Ⓐ
　　Suspected adult rape, ruled out
　　Suspected adult sexual abuse, ruled out

Z04.42 **Encounter for examination and observation following alleged** child rape   PDx P
    Suspected child rape, ruled out
    Suspected child sexual abuse, ruled out

Z04.6 **Encounter for** general psychiatric examination, requested by authority   PDx

☑5ᵗʰ **Z04.7** **Encounter for examination and observation following** alleged physical abuse

    Z04.71 **Encounter for examination and observation following alleged** adult physical abuse   PDx A
       Suspected adult physical abuse, ruled out
       EXCLUDES 1   *confirmed case of adult physical abuse (T74.-)*
          encounter for examination and observation following alleged adult sexual abuse (Z04.41)
          suspected case of adult physical abuse, not ruled out (T76.-)

    Z04.72 **Encounter for examination and observation following alleged** child physical abuse   PDx P
       Suspected child physical abuse, ruled out
       EXCLUDES 1   *confirmed case of child physical abuse (T74.-)*
          encounter for examination and observation following alleged child sexual abuse (Z04.42)
          suspected case of child physical abuse, not ruled out (T76.-)

☑5ᵗʰ **Z04.8** **Encounter for examination and observation for** other specified reasons
    Encounter for examination and observation for request for expert evidence
    AHA: 2018,4Q,32,35,72

    Z04.81 **Encounter for examination and observation of** victim following forced sexual exploitation   PDx
    Z04.82 **Encounter for examination and observation of** victim following forced labor exploitation   PDx
    Z04.89 **Encounter for examination and observation for** other specified reasons   PDx

Z04.9 **Encounter for examination and observation for unspecified** reason   PDx
    Encounter for observation NOS

☑4ᵗʰ **Z05** **Encounter for observation and evaluation of newborn for** suspected diseases and conditions ruled out
    This category is to be used for newborns, within the neonatal period (the first 28 days of life), who are suspected of having an abnormal condition, but without signs or symptoms, and which, after examination and observation, is ruled out.
    AHA: 2022,1Q,17-18; 2017,4Q,27; 2016,4Q,77

    Z05.0 **Observation and evaluation of newborn for suspected** cardiac condition ruled out   N
    Z05.1 **Observation and evaluation of newborn for suspected** infectious condition ruled out   N
       AHA: 2019,2Q,10
    Z05.2 **Observation and evaluation of newborn for suspected** neurological condition ruled out   N
    Z05.3 **Observation and evaluation of newborn for suspected** respiratory condition ruled out   N

☑5ᵗʰ **Z05.4** **Observation and evaluation of newborn for suspected** genetic, metabolic or immunologic condition ruled out
    Z05.41 **Observation and evaluation of newborn for suspected** genetic condition ruled out
       AHA: 2016,4Q,55
    Z05.42 **Observation and evaluation of newborn for suspected** metabolic condition ruled out   N
    Z05.43 **Observation and evaluation of newborn for suspected** immunologic condition ruled out   N

    Z05.5 **Observation and evaluation of newborn for suspected** gastrointestinal condition ruled out   N
    Z05.6 **Observation and evaluation of newborn for suspected** genitourinary condition ruled out   N

☑5ᵗʰ **Z05.7** **Observation and evaluation of newborn for suspected** skin, subcutaneous, musculoskeletal and connective tissue condition ruled out
    Z05.71 **Observation and evaluation of newborn for suspected** skin and subcutaneous tissue condition ruled out   N

    Z05.72 **Observation and evaluation of newborn for suspected** musculoskeletal condition ruled out   N
    Z05.73 **Observation and evaluation of newborn for suspected** connective tissue condition ruled out   N

    Z05.8 **Observation and evaluation of newborn for other specified suspected condition ruled out**   N
       AHA: 2022,1Q,17-18
    Z05.9 **Observation and evaluation of newborn for unspecified suspected condition ruled out**   N

Z08 **Encounter for** follow-up examination after completed treatment for malignant neoplasm
    Medical surveillance following completed treatment
    Use additional code to identify any acquired absence of organs (Z90.-)
    Use additional code to identify the personal history of malignant neoplasm (Z85.-)
    EXCLUDES 1   *aftercare following medical care (Z43-Z49, Z51)*
    AHA: 2020,3Q,30

Z09 **Encounter for** follow-up examination after completed treatment for conditions other than malignant neoplasm
    Medical surveillance following completed treatment
    Use additional code to identify any applicable history of disease code (Z86.-, Z87.-)
    EXCLUDES 1   *aftercare following medical care (Z43-Z49, Z51)*
          surveillance of contraception (Z30.4-)
          surveillance of prosthetic and other medical devices (Z44-Z46)
    AHA: 2021,1Q,33; 2020,2Q,10; 2017,1Q,9; 2015,1Q,8

☑4ᵗʰ **Z11** **Encounter for** screening for infectious and parasitic diseases
    Screening is the testing for disease or disease precursors in asymptomatic individuals so that early detection and treatment can be provided for those who test positive for the disease.
    EXCLUDES 1   *encounter for diagnostic examination - code to sign or symptom*

    Z11.0 **Encounter for screening for** intestinal infectious diseases
    Z11.1 **Encounter for screening for** respiratory tuberculosis
       Encounter for screening for active tuberculosis disease
    Z11.2 **Encounter for screening for** other bacterial diseases
    Z11.3 **Encounter for screening for infections with a** predominantly sexual mode of transmission
       EXCLUDES 2   *encounter for screening for human immunodeficiency virus [HIV] (Z11.4)*
          encounter for screening for human papillomavirus (Z11.51)
    Z11.4 **Encounter for screening for** human immunodeficiency virus [HIV]

☑5ᵗʰ **Z11.5** **Encounter for screening for other viral diseases**
       EXCLUDES 2   *encounter for screening for viral intestinal disease (Z11.0)*
    Z11.51 **Encounter for screening for** human papillomavirus (HPV)
    Z11.52 **Encounter for screening for** COVID-19
       AHA: 2021,1Q,27,37,41
       TIP: This code is not appropriate for use during the pandemic phase of COVID-19. Use Z20.822 Contact with or (suspected) exposure to COVID-19, instead.
    Z11.59 **Encounter for screening for other viral diseases**
       AHA: 2020,3Q,14

    Z11.6 **Encounter for screening for other protozoal diseases and helminthiases**
       EXCLUDES 2   *encounter for screening for protozoal intestinal disease (Z11.0)*
    Z11.7 **Encounter for testing for** latent tuberculosis infection
       AHA: 2019,4Q,20
    Z11.8 **Encounter for screening for other infectious and parasitic diseases**
       Encounter for screening for chlamydia
       Encounter for screening for rickettsial
       Encounter for screening for spirochetal
       Encounter for screening for mycoses
    Z11.9 **Encounter for screening for infectious and parasitic diseases, unspecified**

☑4ᵗʰ Z12 Encounter for screening for malignant neoplasms

Screening is the testing for disease or disease precursors in asymptomatic individuals so that early detection and treatment can be provided for those who test positive for the disease.

Use additional code to identify any family history of malignant neoplasm (Z80.-)

EXCLUDES 1 *encounter for diagnostic examination - code to sign or symptom*

Z12.Ø Encounter for screening for malignant neoplasm of stomach

☑5ᵗʰ Z12.1 Encounter for screening for malignant neoplasm of intestinal tract

AHA: 2017,1Q,8,9

Z12.1Ø Encounter for screening for malignant neoplasm of intestinal tract, unspecified

Z12.11 Encounter for screening for malignant neoplasm of colon Q

Encounter for screening colonoscopy NOS

AHA: 2019,1Q,32-33; 2018,1Q,6

TIP: Surveillance colonoscopies are a type of screening exam used to screen for malignancies in those patients with history of polyps and/or cancer (previously removed). If polyps or cancer are removed during the colonoscopy, code the appropriate neoplasm code instead of Z12.11.

Z12.12 Encounter for screening for malignant neoplasm of rectum

AHA: 2018,1Q,6

Z12.13 Encounter for screening for malignant neoplasm of small intestine

Z12.2 Encounter for screening for malignant neoplasm of respiratory organs

☑5ᵗʰ Z12.3 Encounter for screening for malignant neoplasm of breast

Z12.31 Encounter for screening mammogram for malignant neoplasm of breast

EXCLUDES 1 *inconclusive mammogram (R92.2)*

AHA: 2015,1Q,24

Z12.39 Encounter for other screening for malignant neoplasm of breast

Z12.4 Encounter for screening for malignant neoplasm of cervix ♀

Encounter for screening pap smear for malignant neoplasm of cervix

EXCLUDES 1 *when screening is part of general gynecological examination (Z01.4-)*

EXCLUDES 2 *encounter for screening for human papillomavirus (Z11.51)*

Z12.5 Encounter for screening for malignant neoplasm of prostate ♂

Z12.6 Encounter for screening for malignant neoplasm of bladder

☑5ᵗʰ Z12.7 Encounter for screening for malignant neoplasm of other genitourinary organs

Z12.71 Encounter for screening for malignant neoplasm of testis ♂

Z12.72 Encounter for screening for malignant neoplasm of vagina ♀

Vaginal pap smear status-post hysterectomy for non-malignant condition

Use additional code to identify acquired absence of uterus (Z90.71-)

EXCLUDES 1 *vaginal pap smear status-post hysterectomy for malignant conditions (Z08)*

Z12.73 Encounter for screening for malignant neoplasm of ovary ♀

Z12.79 Encounter for screening for malignant neoplasm of other genitourinary organs

☑5ᵗʰ Z12.8 Encounter for screening for malignant neoplasm of other sites

Z12.81 Encounter for screening for malignant neoplasm of oral cavity

Z12.82 Encounter for screening for malignant neoplasm of nervous system

Z12.83 Encounter for screening for malignant neoplasm of skin

Z12.89 Encounter for screening for malignant neoplasm of other sites

AHA: 2021,1Q,14

Z12.9 Encounter for screening for malignant neoplasm, site unspecified

☑4ᵗʰ Z13 Encounter for screening for other diseases and disorders

Screening is the testing for disease or disease precursors in asymptomatic individuals so that early detection and treatment can be provided for those who test positive for the disease.

EXCLUDES 1 *encounter for diagnostic examination - code to sign or symptom*

Z13.Ø Encounter for screening for diseases of the blood and blood-forming organs and certain disorders involving the immune mechanism

Z13.1 Encounter for screening for diabetes mellitus

☑5ᵗʰ Z13.2 Encounter for screening for nutritional, metabolic and other endocrine disorders

Z13.21 Encounter for screening for nutritional disorder

☑6ᵗʰ Z13.22 Encounter for screening for metabolic disorder

Z13.22Ø Encounter for screening for lipoid disorders

Encounter for screening for cholesterol level

Encounter for screening for hypercholesterolemia

Encounter for screening for hyperlipidemia

Z13.228 Encounter for screening for other metabolic disorders

Z13.29 Encounter for screening for other suspected endocrine disorder

EXCLUDES 2 *encounter for screening for diabetes mellitus (Z13.1)*

☑5ᵗʰ Z13.3 Encounter for screening examination for mental health and behavioral disorders

AHA: 2018,4Q,35-36

Z13.3Ø Encounter for screening examination for mental health and behavioral disorders, unspecified

Z13.31 Encounter for screening for depression

Encounter for screening for depression, adult

Encounter for screening for depression for child or adolescent

Z13.32 Encounter for screening for maternal depression ♀

Encounter for screening for perinatal depression

Z13.39 Encounter for screening examination for other mental health and behavioral disorders

Encounter for screening for alcoholism

Encounter for screening for intellectual disabilities

☑5ᵗʰ Z13.4 Encounter for screening for certain developmental disorders in childhood

Encounter for development testing of infant or child

Encounter for screening for developmental handicaps in early childhood

EXCLUDES 2 *encounter for routine child health examination (Z00.12-)*

AHA: 2018,4Q,36

Z13.4Ø Encounter for screening for unspecified developmental delays

Z13.41 Encounter for autism screening

Z13.42 Encounter for screening for global developmental delays (milestones)

Encounter for screening for developmental handicaps in early childhood

Z13.49 Encounter for screening for other developmental delays

Z13.5 Encounter for screening for eye and ear disorders

EXCLUDES 2 *encounter for general hearing examination (Z01.1-)*
encounter for general vision examination (Z01.0-)

AHA: 2016,3Q,17

Z13.6 Encounter for screening for cardiovascular disorders

☑5ᵗʰ Z13.7 Encounter for screening for genetic and chromosomal anomalies

EXCLUDES 1 *genetic testing for procreative management (Z31.4-)*

Z13.71 Encounter for nonprocreative screening for genetic disease carrier status

Z13.79 Encounter for other screening for genetic and chromosomal anomalies

☑5ᵗʰ Z13.8 Encounter for screening for other specified diseases and disorders

EXCLUDES 2 *screening for malignant neoplasms (Z12.-)*

☑6ᵗʰ Z13.81 Encounter for screening for digestive system disorders

Z13.81Ø Encounter for screening for upper gastrointestinal disorder

HCC CMS-HCC Rx Rx HCC ESR ESRD HCC COM Commercial HCC PDx Primary Dx Only N Newborn: 0 P Pediatric: 0-17 M Maternity: 9-64 A Adult: 15-124

1268 ICD-10-CM 2023

Z13.811 Encounter for screening for lower gastrointestinal disorder
> EXCLUDES 1 *encounter for screening for intestinal infectious disease (Z11.0)*

Z13.818 Encounter for screening for other digestive system disorders

√6ᵗʰ **Z13.82 Encounter for screening for musculoskeletal disorder**

Z13.820 Encounter for screening for osteoporosis

Z13.828 Encounter for screening for other musculoskeletal disorder

Z13.83 Encounter for screening for respiratory disorder NEC
> EXCLUDES 1 *encounter for screening for respiratory tuberculosis (Z11.1)*

Z13.84 Encounter for screening for dental disorders

√6ᵗʰ **Z13.85 Encounter for screening for nervous system disorders**

Z13.850 Encounter for screening for traumatic brain injury

Z13.858 Encounter for screening for other nervous system disorders

Z13.88 Encounter for screening for disorder due to exposure to contaminants
> EXCLUDES 1 *those exposed to contaminants without suspected disorders (Z57.-, Z77.-)*

Z13.89 Encounter for screening for other disorder
Encounter for screening for genitourinary disorders

Z13.9 Encounter for screening, unspecified

Genetic carrier and genetic susceptibility to disease (Z14-Z15)

√4ᵗʰ **Z14 Genetic carrier**
> **DEF:** Individuals carrying a gene mutation associated with a certain disease that typically do not develop the disease but are able to pass the mutated genes to offspring.

√5ᵗʰ **Z14.0 Hemophilia A carrier**

Z14.01 Asymptomatic hemophilia A carrier

Z14.02 Symptomatic hemophilia A carrier

Z14.1 Cystic fibrosis carrier

Z14.8 Genetic carrier of other disease

√4ᵗʰ **Z15 Genetic susceptibility to disease**
> INCLUDES confirmed abnormal gene
> Use additional code, if applicable, for any associated family history of the disease (Z80-Z84)
> EXCLUDES 1 *chromosomal anomalies (Q90-Q99)*

√5ᵗʰ **Z15.0 Genetic susceptibility to malignant neoplasm**
> Code first, if applicable, any current malignant neoplasm (C00-C75, C81-C96)
> Use additional code, if applicable, for any personal history of malignant neoplasm (Z85.-)

Z15.01 Genetic susceptibility to malignant neoplasm of breast

Z15.02 Genetic susceptibility to malignant neoplasm of ovary ♀

Z15.03 Genetic susceptibility to malignant neoplasm of prostate ♂

Z15.04 Genetic susceptibility to malignant neoplasm of endometrium ♀

Z15.09 Genetic susceptibility to other malignant neoplasm
> **AHA:** 2021,1Q,14

√5ᵗʰ **Z15.8 Genetic susceptibility to other disease**

Z15.81 Genetic susceptibility to multiple endocrine neoplasia [MEN]
> EXCLUDES 1 *multiple endocrine neoplasia [MEN] syndromes (E31.2-)*
> **DEF:** Group of conditions in which several endocrine glands grow excessively (such as in adenomatous hyperplasia) and/or develop benign or malignant tumors. Tumors and hyperplasia associated with MEN often produce excess hormones, which impede normal physiology. There is no comprehensive cure known for MEN syndrome. Treatment is directed at the hyperplasia or tumors in each individual gland. Tumors are usually surgically removed and oral medications or hormonal injections are used to correct hormone imbalances.

Z15.89 Genetic susceptibility to other disease

Resistance to antimicrobial drugs (Z16)

√4ᵗʰ **Z16 Resistance to antimicrobial drugs**
> NOTE The codes in this category are provided for use as additional codes to identify the resistance and non-responsiveness of a condition to antimicrobial drugs.
> Code first the infection
> EXCLUDES 1 *Methicillin resistant Staphylococcus aureus infection (A49.02)*
> *Methicillin resistant Staphylococcus aureus pneumonia (J15.212)*
> *sepsis due to Methicillin resistant Staphylococcus aureus (A41.02)*

√5ᵗʰ **Z16.1 Resistance to beta lactam antibiotics**

Z16.10 Resistance to unspecified beta lactam antibiotics UPD

Z16.11 Resistance to penicillins UPD
Resistance to amoxicillin
Resistance to ampicillin

Z16.12 Extended spectrum beta lactamase (ESBL) resistance UPD
> EXCLUDES 2 *Methicillin resistant Staphylococcus aureus infection in diseases classified elsewhere (B95.62)*

Z16.19 Resistance to other specified beta lactam antibiotics UPD
Resistance to cephalosporins

√5ᵗʰ **Z16.2 Resistance to other antibiotics**

Z16.20 Resistance to unspecified antibiotic UPD
Resistance to antibiotics NOS

Z16.21 Resistance to vancomycin UPD

Z16.22 Resistance to vancomycin related antibiotics UPD

Z16.23 Resistance to quinolones and fluoroquinolones UPD

Z16.24 Resistance to multiple antibiotics UPD

Z16.29 Resistance to other single specified antibiotic UPD
Resistance to aminoglycosides
Resistance to macrolides
Resistance to sulfonamides
Resistance to tetracyclines

√5ᵗʰ **Z16.3 Resistance to other antimicrobial drugs**
> EXCLUDES 1 *resistance to antibiotics (Z16.1-, Z16.2-)*

Z16.30 Resistance to unspecified antimicrobial drugs UPD
Drug resistance NOS

Z16.31 Resistance to antiparasitic drug(s) UPD
Resistance to quinine and related compounds

Z16.32 Resistance to antifungal drug(s) UPD

Z16.33 Resistance to antiviral drug(s) UPD

√6ᵗʰ **Z16.34 Resistance to antimycobacterial drug(s)**
Resistance to tuberculostatics

Z16.341 Resistance to single antimycobacterial drug UPD
Resistance to antimycobacterial drug NOS

Z16.342 Resistance to multiple antimycobacterial drugs UPD

Z16.35 Resistance to multiple antimicrobial drugs UPD
> EXCLUDES 1 *resistance to multiple antibiotics only (Z16.24)*

Z16.39 Resistance to other specified antimicrobial drug UPD

Estrogen receptor status (Z17)

√4ᵗʰ **Z17 Estrogen receptor status**
> Code first malignant neoplasm of breast (C50.-)
> **DEF:** Receptor status of breast cancer cells for the hormone estrogen that is used to help determine treatment and evaluate prognosis. ER+ breast cancer responds to hormone therapies while ER- breast cancer does not.

Z17.0 Estrogen receptor positive status [ER+] UPD

Z17.1 Estrogen receptor negative status [ER-] UPD

Chapter 21. Factors Influencing Health Status and Contact With Health Services

Retained foreign body fragments (Z18)

✓4th Z18 Retained foreign body fragments

INCLUDES   embedded fragment (status)
embedded splinter (status)
retained foreign body status

EXCLUDES 1   artificial joint prosthesis status (Z96.6-)
foreign body accidentally left during a procedure (T81.5-)
foreign body entering through orifice (T15-T19)
in situ cardiac device (Z95.-)
organ or tissue replaced by means other than transplant (Z96.-, Z97.-)
organ or tissue replaced by transplant (Z94.-)
personal history of retained foreign body fully removed Z87.821
superficial foreign body (non-embedded splinter) - code to superficial foreign body, by site

DEF: Embedded or retained fragment, splinter, or foreign body, natural or synthetic that can cause infection.

✓5th Z18.0 Retained radioactive fragments

    Z18.01 Retained depleted uranium fragments

    Z18.09 Other retained radioactive fragments
       Other retained depleted isotope fragments
       Retained nontherapeutic radioactive fragments

✓5th Z18.1 Retained metal fragments

    EXCLUDES 1   retained radioactive metal fragments (Z18.01-Z18.09)

    Z18.10 Retained metal fragments, unspecified
       Retained metal fragment NOS

    Z18.11 Retained magnetic metal fragments

    Z18.12 Retained nonmagnetic metal fragments

Z18.2 Retained plastic fragments
    Acrylics fragments
    Diethylhexyl phthalates fragments
    Isocyanate fragments

✓5th Z18.3 Retained organic fragments

    Z18.31 Retained animal quills or spines

    Z18.32 Retained tooth

    Z18.33 Retained wood fragments

    Z18.39 Other retained organic fragments

✓5th Z18.8 Other specified retained foreign body

    Z18.81 Retained glass fragments

    Z18.83 Retained stone or crystalline fragments
       Retained concrete or cement fragments

    Z18.89 Other specified retained foreign body fragments

Z18.9 Retained foreign body fragments, unspecified material

Hormone sensitivity malignancy status (Z19)

✓4th Z19 Hormone sensitivity malignancy status

    Code first malignant neoplasm — see Table of Neoplasms, by site, malignant

    AHA: 2016,4Q,76

    Z19.1 Hormone sensitive malignancy status   UPD

    Z19.2 Hormone resistant malignancy status   UPD
       Castrate resistant prostate malignancy status

Persons with potential health hazards related to communicable diseases (Z20-Z29)

✓4th Z20 Contact with and (suspected) exposure to communicable diseases

    EXCLUDES 1   carrier of infectious disease (Z22.-)
       diagnosed current infectious or parasitic disease - see Alphabetic Index

    EXCLUDES 2   personal history of infectious and parasitic diseases (Z86.1-)

    ✓5th Z20.0 Contact with and (suspected) exposure to intestinal infectious diseases

       Z20.01 Contact with and (suspected) exposure to intestinal infectious diseases due to Escherichia coli (E. coli)

       Z20.09 Contact with and (suspected) exposure to other intestinal infectious diseases

    Z20.1 Contact with and (suspected) exposure to tuberculosis

    Z20.2 Contact with and (suspected) exposure to infections with a predominantly sexual mode of transmission

    Z20.3 Contact with and (suspected) exposure to rabies

    Z20.4 Contact with and (suspected) exposure to rubella

    Z20.5 Contact with and (suspected) exposure to viral hepatitis

    Z20.6 Contact with and (suspected) exposure to human immunodeficiency virus [HIV]

       EXCLUDES 1   asymptomatic human immunodeficiency virus [HIV] HIV infection status (Z21)

    Z20.7 Contact with and (suspected) exposure to pediculosis, acariasis and other infestations

    ✓5th Z20.8 Contact with and (suspected) exposure to other communicable diseases

       ✓6th Z20.81 Contact with and (suspected) exposure to other bacterial communicable diseases

         Z20.810 Contact with and (suspected) exposure to anthrax

         Z20.811 Contact with and (suspected) exposure to meningococcus

         Z20.818 Contact with and (suspected) exposure to other bacterial communicable diseases
           AHA: 2019,2Q,10

       ✓6th Z20.82 Contact with and (suspected) exposure to other viral communicable diseases

         Z20.820 Contact with and (suspected) exposure to varicella

         Z20.821 Contact with and (suspected) exposure to Zika virus
           AHA: 2018,4Q,35,64

         Z20.822 Contact with and (suspected) exposure to COVID-19
           Contact with and (suspected) exposure to SARS-CoV-2
           AHA: 2022,2Q,28-29; 2021,4Q,109; 2021,1Q,27-29,37-38,41

         Z20.828 Contact with and (suspected) exposure to other viral communicable diseases
           AHA: 2021,1Q,37-38; 2020,4Q,99; 2020,3Q,14-15; 2020,2Q,4,8; 2020,1Q,34-36

       Z20.89 Contact with and (suspected) exposure to other communicable diseases

    Z20.9 Contact with and (suspected) exposure to unspecified communicable disease

Z21 Asymptomatic human immunodeficiency virus [HIV] infection status   HCC Rx ESR COM

    HIV positive NOS
    Code first human immunodeficiency virus [HIV] disease complicating pregnancy, childbirth and the puerperium, if applicable (O98.7-)

    EXCLUDES 1   acquired immunodeficiency syndrome (B20)
       contact with human immunodeficiency virus [HIV] (Z20.6)
       exposure to human immunodeficiency virus [HIV] (Z20.6)
       human immunodeficiency virus [HIV] disease (B20)
       inconclusive laboratory evidence of human immunodeficiency virus [HIV] (R75)

    AHA: 2022,1Q,36; 2019,1Q,8-11
    DEF: Phase of human immunodeficiency virus (HIV) infection with no clinical symptoms. This phase may last for 10 years or more.

✓4th Z22 Carrier of infectious disease

    INCLUDES   colonization status
       suspected carrier

    EXCLUDES 2   carrier of viral hepatitis (B18.-)

    Z22.0 Carrier of typhoid

    Z22.1 Carrier of other intestinal infectious diseases

    Z22.2 Carrier of diphtheria

    ✓5th Z22.3 Carrier of other specified bacterial diseases

       Z22.31 Carrier of bacterial disease due to meningococci

       ✓6th Z22.32 Carrier of bacterial disease due to staphylococci

         Z22.321 Carrier or suspected carrier of Methicillin susceptible Staphylococcus aureus
           MSSA colonization

         Z22.322 Carrier or suspected carrier of Methicillin resistant Staphylococcus aureus
           MRSA colonization
           DEF: Carriers (colonization) of methicillin resistant *Staphylococcus aureus* (MRSA) have MRSA on their skin or in their body but do not exhibit signs of infection. These individuals are able to pass MRSA on to others who may develop an infection.

HCC CMS-HCC   Rx Rx HCC   ESR ESRD HCC   COM Commercial HCC   PDx Primary Dx Only   N Newborn: 0   P Pediatric: 0-17   M Maternity: 9-64   A Adult: 15-124

1270   ICD-10-CM 2023

✓6ᵗʰ **Z22.33 Carrier of bacterial disease due to** streptococci

Z22.330 Carrier of Group B **streptococcus**
> EXCLUDES 1   *carrier of streptococcus group B (GBS) complicating pregnancy, childbirth and the puerperium (O99.82-)*

Z22.338 Carrier of other streptococcus

Z22.39 Carrier of other specified bacterial diseases

Z22.4 Carrier of infections with a predominantly sexual mode of transmission

Z22.6 Carrier of human T-lymphotropic virus type-1 **[HTLV-1] infection**

Z22.7 Latent tuberculosis
Latent tuberculosis infection (LTBI)
> EXCLUDES 1   *nonspecific reaction to cell mediated immunity measurement of gamma interferon antigen response without active tuberculosis (R76.12) nonspecific reaction to tuberculin skin test without active tuberculosis (R76.11)*

AHA: 2019,4Q,19

Z22.8 Carrier of other infectious diseases

Z22.9 Carrier of infectious disease, unspecified

Z23 Encounter for immunization
> NOTE   Procedure codes are required to identify the types of immunizations given

Code first any routine childhood examination
Code also, if applicable, encounter for immunization safety counseling (Z71.85)

✓4ᵗʰ **Z28 Immunization not carried out and underimmunization status**
> INCLUDES   vaccination not carried out

Code also, if applicable, encounter for immunization safety counseling (Z71.85)

✓5ᵗʰ **Z28.0 Immunization not carried out because of** contraindication
> DEF: Contraindication: Situation where a drug, surgery, or other procedure may negatively affect or cause harm to a patient.

Z28.01 Immunization not carried out because of acute illness **of patient**

Z28.02 Immunization not carried out because of chronic illness **or condition of patient**

Z28.03 Immunization not carried out because of immune compromised state **of patient**

Z28.04 Immunization not carried out because of patient allergy to vaccine or component

Z28.09 Immunization not carried out because of other contraindication

Z28.1 Immunization not carried out because of patient decision for reasons of belief or group pressure
Immunization not carried out because of religious belief

✓5ᵗʰ **Z28.2 Immunization not carried out because of patient decision for** other and unspecified **reason**

Z28.20 Immunization not carried out because of patient decision for unspecified reason

Z28.21 Immunization not carried out because of patient refusal

Z28.29 Immunization not carried out because of patient decision for other reason

▲ ✓5ᵗʰ **Z28.3 Underimmunization status**
~~Delinquent immunization status~~
~~Lapsed immunization schedule status~~
▶Use additional code, if applicable, to identify:◀
▶immunization not carried out because of contraindication (Z28.0-)◀
▶immunization not carried out because of patient decision for other and unspecified reason (Z28.2-)◀
▶immunization not carried out because of patient decision for reasons of belief or group pressure (Z28.1)◀
▶immunization not carried out for other reason (Z28.8-)◀
AHA: 2022,1Q,4-5

● ✓6ᵗʰ **Z28.31 Underimmunization for COVID-19 status**
> NOTE   These codes should not be used for individuals who are not eligible for the COVID-19 vaccines, as determined by the healthcare provider.

● **Z28.310 Unvaccinated for COVID-19** UPD
● **Z28.311 Partially vaccinated for COVID-19** UPD

● **Z28.39 Other underimmunization status** UPD
Delinquent immunization status
Lapsed immunization schedule status

✓5ᵗʰ **Z28.8 Immunization not carried out for other reason**

Z28.81 Immunization not carried out due to patient having had the disease

Z28.82 Immunization not carried out because of caregiver refusal
Immunization not carried out because of guardian refusal
Immunization not carried out because of parent refusal
> EXCLUDES 1   *immunization not carried out because of caregiver refusal because of religious belief (Z28.1)*

Z28.83 Immunization not carried out due to unavailability of vaccine
Delay in delivery of vaccine
Lack of availability of vaccine
Manufacturer delay of vaccine
AHA: 2018,4Q,36

Z28.89 Immunization not carried out for other reason

Z28.9 Immunization not carried out for unspecified reason

✓4ᵗʰ **Z29 Encounter for other prophylactic measures**
> EXCLUDES 1   *desensitization to allergens (Z51.6) prophylactic surgery (Z40.-)*

AHA: 2016,4Q,78-79

✓5ᵗʰ **Z29.1 Encounter for prophylactic immunotherapy**
Encounter for administration of immunoglobulin

Z29.11 Encounter for prophylactic immunotherapy for respiratory syncytial virus (RSV)

Z29.12 Encounter for prophylactic antivenin

Z29.13 Encounter for prophylactic Rho(D) immune globulin
AHA: 2019,3Q,5

Z29.14 Encounter for prophylactic rabies immune globin

Z29.3 Encounter for prophylactic fluoride administration

Z29.8 Encounter for other specified prophylactic measures
AHA: 2022,2Q,27

Z29.9 Encounter for prophylactic measures, unspecified

Persons encountering health services in circumstances related to reproduction (Z30-Z39)

✓4ᵗʰ **Z30 Encounter for contraceptive management**
AHA: 2016,4Q,78
> DEF: Contraceptive management to prevent pregnancy. Methods include oral medications, intrauterine devices, and surgical procedures for males and females (sterilization).

✓5ᵗʰ **Z30.0 Encounter for general counseling and advice on** contraception

✓6ᵗʰ **Z30.01 Encounter for** initial prescription **of contraceptives**
> EXCLUDES 1   *encounter for surveillance of contraceptives (Z30.4-)*

Z30.011 Encounter for initial prescription of **contraceptive pills** ♀

Z30.012 Encounter for prescription of emergency **contraception** ♀
Encounter for postcoital contraception

Z30.013 Encounter for initial prescription of injectable **contraceptive** ♀

Z30.014 Encounter for initial prescription of intrauterine **contraceptive device** ♀
> EXCLUDES 1   *encounter for insertion of intrauterine contraceptive device (Z30.430, Z30.432)*

Z30.015 Encounter for initial prescription of vaginal ring hormonal **contraceptive** ♀

Z30.016 Encounter for initial prescription of transdermal patch hormonal **contraceptive device**

Z30.017 Encounter for initial prescription of implantable subdermal **contraceptive**

Z30.018   **Encounter for initial prescription of other contraceptives** ♀

Encounter for initial prescription of barrier contraception

Encounter for initial prescription of diaphragm

Z30.019   **Encounter for initial prescription of contraceptives, unspecified** ♀

Z30.02   **Counseling and instruction in** natural family planning **to avoid pregnancy**

Z30.09   **Encounter for other general counseling and advice on contraception**

Encounter for family planning advice NOS

Z30.2   **Encounter for** sterilization

AHA: 2021,3Q,13

✓5ᵗʰ **Z30.4**   **Encounter for** surveillance **of contraceptives**

Z30.40   **Encounter for surveillance of contraceptives, unspecified**

Z30.41   **Encounter for surveillance of contraceptive** pills ♀

Encounter for repeat prescription for contraceptive pill

Z30.42   **Encounter for surveillance of** injectable **contraceptive** ♀

✓6ᵗʰ **Z30.43**   **Encounter for surveillance of** intrauterine **contraceptive device**

Z30.430   **Encounter for** insertion **of intrauterine contraceptive device** ♀

Z30.431   **Encounter for** routine checking **of intrauterine contraceptive device** ♀

Z30.432   **Encounter for** removal **of intrauterine contraceptive device** ♀

Z30.433   **Encounter for** removal and reinsertion **of intrauterine contraceptive device** ♀

Encounter for replacement of intrauterine contraceptive device

Z30.44   **Encounter for surveillance of** vaginal ring hormonal **contraceptive device** ♀

Z30.45   **Encounter for surveillance of** transdermal patch hormonal **contraceptive device** ♀

Z30.46   **Encounter for surveillance of** implantable subdermal **contraceptive** ♀

Encounter for checking, reinsertion or removal of implantable subdermal contraceptive

Z30.49   **Encounter for surveillance of other contraceptives** ♀

Encounter for surveillance of barrier contraception

Encounter for surveillance of diaphragm

Z30.8   **Encounter for other contraceptive management**

Encounter for postvasectomy sperm count

Encounter for routine examination for contraceptive maintenance

EXCLUDES 1   *sperm count following sterilization reversal (Z31.42)*

sperm count for fertility testing (Z31.41)

Z30.9   **Encounter for contraceptive management, unspecified**

✓4ᵗʰ **Z31**   **Encounter for procreative management**

EXCLUDES 2   *complications associated with artificial fertilization (N98.-)*

female infertility (N97.-)

male infertility (N46.-)

Z31.0   **Encounter for reversal of previous sterilization**

✓5ᵗʰ **Z31.4**   **Encounter for** procreative investigation and testing

EXCLUDES 1   *postvasectomy sperm count (Z30.8)*

Z31.41   **Encounter for** fertility testing

Encounter for fallopian tube patency testing

Encounter for sperm count for fertility testing

Z31.42   Aftercare **following** sterilization reversal

Sperm count following sterilization reversal

✓6ᵗʰ **Z31.43**   **Encounter for genetic testing of** female **for procreative management**

Use additional code for recurrent pregnancy loss, if applicable (N96, O26.2-)

EXCLUDES 1   *nonprocreative genetic testing (Z13.7-)*

Z31.430   **Encounter of female for testing for genetic** disease carrier status **for procreative management** ♀

Z31.438   **Encounter for other genetic testing of female for procreative management** ♀

✓6ᵗʰ **Z31.44**   **Encounter for genetic testing of** male **for procreative management**

EXCLUDES 1   *nonprocreative genetic testing (Z13.7-)*

Z31.440   **Encounter of male for testing for genetic disease carrier status for procreative management** ♂

Z31.441   **Encounter for testing of male partner of patient with** recurrent pregnancy loss 🅰♂

Z31.448   **Encounter for other genetic testing of male for procreative management** 🅰♂

Z31.49   **Encounter for other procreative investigation and testing**

Z31.5   **Encounter for procreative genetic counseling**

AHA: 2017,4Q,27

✓5ᵗʰ **Z31.6**   **Encounter for general counseling and advice on procreation**

Z31.61   **Procreative counseling and advice using** natural family planning

Z31.62   **Encounter for** fertility preservation **counseling**

Encounter for fertility preservation counseling prior to cancer therapy

Encounter for fertility preservation counseling prior to surgical removal of gonads

Z31.69   **Encounter for other general counseling and advice on procreation**

Z31.7   **Encounter for procreative management and counseling for gestational carrier** ♀

EXCLUDES 1   *pregnant state, gestational carrier (Z33.3)*

AHA: 2016,4Q,78

✓5ᵗʰ **Z31.8**   **Encounter for other procreative management**

Z31.81   **Encounter for** male factor **infertility in female patient** PDx ♀

Z31.82   **Encounter for** Rh incompatibility status

AHA: 2015,3Q,40; 2014,4Q,17

Z31.83   **Encounter for** assisted reproductive fertility procedure cycle PDx ♀

Patient undergoing in vitro fertilization cycle

Use additional code to identify the type of infertility

EXCLUDES 1   *pre-cycle diagnosis and testing - code to reason for encounter*

AHA: 2022,2Q,15-16

Z31.84   **Encounter for** fertility preservation procedure PDx

Encounter for fertility preservation procedure prior to cancer therapy

Encounter for fertility preservation procedure prior to surgical removal of gonads

Z31.89   **Encounter for other procreative management**

Z31.9   **Encounter for procreative management, unspecified**

✓4ᵗʰ **Z32**   **Encounter for pregnancy test and childbirth and childcare instruction**

✓5ᵗʰ **Z32.0**   **Encounter for** pregnancy test

Z32.00   **Encounter for pregnancy test,** result unknown ♀

Encounter for pregnancy test NOS

Z32.01   **Encounter for pregnancy test,** result positive COM Ⓜ ♀

Z32.02   **Encounter for pregnancy test,** result negative ♀

Z32.2   **Encounter for** childbirth instruction

Z32.3   **Encounter for** childcare instruction

Encounter for prenatal or postpartum childcare instruction

✓4ᵗʰ **Z33**   **Pregnant state**

Z33.1   **Pregnant state,** incidental COM Ⓜ ♀

Pregnancy NOS

Pregnant state NOS

EXCLUDES 1   *complications of pregnancy (O00-O9A)*

pregnant state, gestational carrier (Z33.3)

Z33.2   **Encounter for** elective termination of pregnancy PDx Ⓜ ♀

EXCLUDES 1   *early fetal death with retention of dead fetus (O02.1)*

late fetal death (O36.4)

spontaneous abortion (O03)

AHA: 2022,1Q,20

TIP: Do not assign a code from category Z3A with this code.

HCC CMS-HCC   Rx Rx HCC   ESR ESRD HCC   COM Commercial HCC   PDx Primary Dx Only   Ⓝ Newborn: 0   Ⓟ Pediatric: 0-17   Ⓜ Maternity: 9-64   🅰 Adult: 15-124

1272

ICD-10-CM 2023

Z33.3 Pregnant state, gestational carrier COM M ♀
> EXCLUDES 1   encounter for procreative management and counseling for gestational carrier (Z31.7)
> AHA: 2016,4Q,78

Z34 Encounter for supervision of normal pregnancy
> EXCLUDES 1   any complication of pregnancy (O00-O9A)
> encounter for pregnancy test (Z32.0-)
> encounter for supervision of high risk pregnancy (O09.-)
> AHA: 2019,3Q,5; 2014,4Q,17

Z34.0 Encounter for supervision of normal first pregnancy
- **Z34.00** Encounter for supervision of normal first pregnancy, unspecified trimester COM PDx M ♀
- **Z34.01** Encounter for supervision of normal first pregnancy, first trimester COM PDx M ♀
- **Z34.02** Encounter for supervision of normal first pregnancy, second trimester COM PDx M ♀
- **Z34.03** Encounter for supervision of normal first pregnancy, third trimester COM PDx M ♀

Z34.8 Encounter for supervision of other normal pregnancy
- **Z34.80** Encounter for supervision of other normal pregnancy, unspecified trimester COM PDx M ♀
- **Z34.81** Encounter for supervision of other normal pregnancy, first trimester COM PDx M ♀
- **Z34.82** Encounter for supervision of other normal pregnancy, second trimester COM PDx M ♀
- **Z34.83** Encounter for supervision of other normal pregnancy, third trimester COM PDx M ♀

Z34.9 Encounter for supervision of normal pregnancy, unspecified
- **Z34.90** Encounter for supervision of normal pregnancy, unspecified, unspecified trimester COM PDx M ♀
- **Z34.91** Encounter for supervision of normal pregnancy, unspecified, first trimester COM PDx M ♀
- **Z34.92** Encounter for supervision of normal pregnancy, unspecified, second trimester COM PDx M ♀
- **Z34.93** Encounter for supervision of normal pregnancy, unspecified, third trimester COM PDx M ♀

Z36 Encounter for antenatal screening of mother
> INCLUDES   encounter for placental sample (taken vaginally)
> screening is the testing for disease or disease precursors in asymptomatic individuals so that early detection and treatment can be provided for those who test positive for the disease.
> EXCLUDES 1   diagnostic examination - code to sign or symptom
> encounter for suspected maternal and fetal conditions ruled out (Z03.7-)
> suspected fetal condition affecting management of pregnancy - code to condition in Chapter 15
> EXCLUDES 2   abnormal findings on antenatal screening of mother (O28.-)
> genetic counseling and testing (Z31.43-, Z31.5)
> routine prenatal care (Z34)
> AHA: 2017,4Q,28

Z36.0 Encounter for antenatal screening for chromosomal anomalies COM M ♀

Z36.1 Encounter for antenatal screening for raised alphafetoprotein level COM M ♀
> Encounter for antenatal screening for elevated maternal serum alphafetoprotein level
> DEF: High levels of alpha-fetoprotein (AFP) that may indicate a possibility of spina bifida and other neural tube defects, anencephaly, or omphalocele in the fetus.

Z36.2 Encounter for other antenatal screening follow-up COM M ♀
> Non-visualized anatomy on a previous scan

Z36.3 Encounter for antenatal screening for malformations COM M ♀
> Screening for a suspected anomaly

Z36.4 Encounter for antenatal screening for fetal growth retardation COM M ♀
> Intrauterine growth restriction (IUGR)/small-for-dates

Z36.5 Encounter for antenatal screening for isoimmunization COM M ♀

Z36.8 Encounter for other antenatal screening
- **Z36.81** Encounter for antenatal screening for hydrops fetalis COM M ♀
  > DEF: Hydrops fetalis: Abnormal accumulation of fluid in two or more parts of the fetus, such as ascites, effusion of the pleural or pericardial tissues, or edema.
- **Z36.82** Encounter for antenatal screening for nuchal translucency COM M ♀
- **Z36.83** Encounter for fetal screening for congenital cardiac abnormalities COM M ♀
- **Z36.84** Encounter for antenatal screening for fetal lung maturity COM M ♀
- **Z36.85** Encounter for antenatal screening for Streptococcus B COM M ♀
- **Z36.86** Encounter for antenatal screening for cervical length COM M ♀
  > Screening for risk of pre-term labor
- **Z36.87** Encounter for antenatal screening for uncertain dates COM M ♀
- **Z36.88** Encounter for antenatal screening for fetal macrosomia COM M ♀
  > Screening for large-for-dates
- **Z36.89** Encounter for other specified antenatal screening COM M ♀
- **Z36.8A** Encounter for antenatal screening for other genetic defects COM M ♀

Z36.9 Encounter for antenatal screening, unspecified COM M ♀

Z3A Weeks of gestation
> NOTE   Codes from category Z3A are for use, only on the maternal record, to indicate the weeks of gestation of the pregnancy, if known.
> Code first obstetric condition or encounter for delivery (O09-O60, O80-O82)
> AHA: 2022,2Q,3; 2019,2Q,11; 2016,2Q,34; 2014,3Q,17; 2014,2Q,9; 2013,2Q,33
> TIP: Do not assign a code from this category with codes from categories O00-O08 or code Z33.2.

Z3A.0 Weeks of gestation of pregnancy, unspecified or less than 10 weeks
- **Z3A.00** Weeks of gestation of pregnancy not specified COM UPD M ♀
- **Z3A.01** Less than 8 weeks gestation of pregnancy COM UPD M ♀
- **Z3A.08** 8 weeks gestation of pregnancy COM UPD M ♀
- **Z3A.09** 9 weeks gestation of pregnancy COM UPD M ♀

Z3A.1 Weeks of gestation of pregnancy, weeks 10-19
- **Z3A.10** 10 weeks gestation of pregnancy COM UPD M ♀
- **Z3A.11** 11 weeks gestation of pregnancy COM UPD M ♀
- **Z3A.12** 12 weeks gestation of pregnancy COM UPD M ♀
- **Z3A.13** 13 weeks gestation of pregnancy COM UPD M ♀
- **Z3A.14** 14 weeks gestation of pregnancy COM UPD M ♀
- **Z3A.15** 15 weeks gestation of pregnancy COM UPD M ♀
- **Z3A.16** 16 weeks gestation of pregnancy COM UPD M ♀
- **Z3A.17** 17 weeks gestation of pregnancy COM UPD M ♀
- **Z3A.18** 18 weeks gestation of pregnancy COM UPD M ♀
- **Z3A.19** 19 weeks gestation of pregnancy COM UPD M ♀

Z3A.2 Weeks of gestation of pregnancy, weeks 20-29
- **Z3A.20** 20 weeks gestation of pregnancy COM UPD M ♀
- **Z3A.21** 21 weeks gestation of pregnancy COM UPD M ♀
- **Z3A.22** 22 weeks gestation of pregnancy COM UPD M ♀
- **Z3A.23** 23 weeks gestation of pregnancy COM UPD M ♀
- **Z3A.24** 24 weeks gestation of pregnancy COM UPD M ♀
- **Z3A.25** 25 weeks gestation of pregnancy COM UPD M ♀
- **Z3A.26** 26 weeks gestation of pregnancy COM UPD M ♀
- **Z3A.27** 27 weeks gestation of pregnancy COM UPD M ♀
- **Z3A.28** 28 weeks gestation of pregnancy COM UPD M ♀
- **Z3A.29** 29 weeks gestation of pregnancy COM UPD M ♀

Z3A.3 Weeks of gestation of pregnancy, weeks 30-39
- **Z3A.30** 30 weeks gestation of pregnancy COM UPD M ♀
- **Z3A.31** 31 weeks gestation of pregnancy COM UPD M ♀
- **Z3A.32** 32 weeks gestation of pregnancy COM UPD M ♀
- **Z3A.33** 33 weeks gestation of pregnancy COM UPD M ♀
- **Z3A.34** 34 weeks gestation of pregnancy COM UPD M ♀
- **Z3A.35** 35 weeks gestation of pregnancy COM UPD M ♀

Z3A.36   36 weeks **gestation of pregnancy** `COM` `UPD` `M` ♀
Z3A.37   37 weeks **gestation of pregnancy** `COM` `UPD` `M` ♀
Z3A.38   38 weeks **gestation of pregnancy** `COM` `UPD` `M` ♀
Z3A.39   39 weeks **gestation of pregnancy** `COM` `UPD` `M` ♀

√5ᵗʰ **Z3A.4**   **Weeks of gestation of pregnancy, weeks 40 or greater**
     AHA: 2014,4Q,23

Z3A.40   40 weeks **gestation of pregnancy** `COM` `UPD` `M` ♀
Z3A.41   41 weeks **gestation of pregnancy** `COM` `UPD` `M` ♀
Z3A.42   42 weeks **gestation of pregnancy** `COM` `UPD` `M` ♀
Z3A.49   **Greater than 42 weeks gestation of pregnancy** `COM` `UPD` `M` ♀

√4ᵗʰ **Z37**   **Outcome of delivery**

This category is intended for use as an additional code to identify the outcome of delivery on the mother's record. It is not for use on the newborn record.

   EXCLUDES 1   stillbirth (P95)

Z37.0   **Single live birth** `COM` `UPD` `M` ♀
     AHA: 2016,2Q,34; 2014,2Q,9

Z37.1   **Single stillbirth** `COM` `UPD` `M` ♀
Z37.2   **Twins, both liveborn** `COM` `UPD` `M` ♀
Z37.3   **Twins, one liveborn and one stillborn** `COM` `UPD` `M` ♀
Z37.4   **Twins, both stillborn** `COM` `UPD` `M` ♀

√5ᵗʰ **Z37.5**   **Other multiple births, all liveborn**

Z37.50   **Multiple births, unspecified, all liveborn** `COM` `UPD` `M` ♀
Z37.51   **Triplets, all liveborn** `COM` `UPD` `M` ♀
Z37.52   **Quadruplets, all liveborn** `COM` `UPD` `M` ♀
Z37.53   **Quintuplets, all liveborn** `COM` `UPD` `M` ♀
Z37.54   **Sextuplets, all liveborn** `COM` `UPD` `M` ♀
Z37.59   **Other multiple births, all liveborn** `COM` `UPD` `M` ♀

√5ᵗʰ **Z37.6**   **Other multiple births, some liveborn**

Z37.60   **Multiple births, unspecified, some liveborn** `COM` `UPD` `M` ♀
Z37.61   **Triplets, some liveborn** `COM` `UPD` `M` ♀
Z37.62   **Quadruplets, some liveborn** `COM` `UPD` `M` ♀
Z37.63   **Quintuplets, some liveborn** `COM` `UPD` `M` ♀
Z37.64   **Sextuplets, some liveborn** `COM` `UPD` `M` ♀
Z37.69   **Other multiple births, some liveborn** `COM` `UPD` `M` ♀

Z37.7   **Other multiple births, all stillborn** `COM` `UPD` `M` ♀
Z37.9   **Outcome of delivery, unspecified** `COM` `UPD` `M` ♀
     Multiple birth NOS
     Single birth NOS

√4ᵗʰ **Z38**   **Liveborn infants according to place of birth and type of delivery**

This category is for use as the principal code on the initial record of a newborn baby. It is to be used for the initial birth record only. It is not to be used on the mother's record.

AHA: 2020,2Q,13; 2017,2Q,5-7; 2016,3Q,18; 2015,2Q,15

TIP: For attending physician services, a code from this category can be reported as first listed every time the physician visits the newborn during the birth admission.

√5ᵗʰ **Z38.0**   **Single liveborn infant, born in hospital**

     Single liveborn infant, born in birthing center or other health care facility

Z38.00   **Single liveborn infant, delivered vaginally** `COM` `PDx` `N`
Z38.01   **Single liveborn infant, delivered by cesarean** `COM` `PDx` `N`

Z38.1   **Single liveborn infant, born outside hospital** `COM` `PDx` `N`
Z38.2   **Single liveborn infant, unspecified as to place of birth** `COM` `PDx` `N`
     Single liveborn infant NOS

√5ᵗʰ **Z38.3**   **Twin liveborn infant, born in hospital**

Z38.30   **Twin liveborn infant, delivered vaginally** `COM` `PDx` `N`
Z38.31   **Twin liveborn infant, delivered by cesarean** `COM` `PDx` `N`

Z38.4   **Twin liveborn infant, born outside hospital** `COM` `PDx` `N`
Z38.5   **Twin liveborn infant, unspecified as to place of birth** `COM` `PDx` `N`

√5ᵗʰ **Z38.6**   **Other multiple liveborn infant, born in hospital**

Z38.61   **Triplet liveborn infant, delivered vaginally** `COM` `PDx` `N`

Z38.62   **Triplet liveborn infant, delivered by cesarean** `COM` `PDx` `N`
Z38.63   **Quadruplet liveborn infant, delivered vaginally** `COM` `PDx` `N`
Z38.64   **Quadruplet liveborn infant, delivered by cesarean** `COM` `PDx` `N`
Z38.65   **Quintuplet liveborn infant, delivered vaginally** `COM` `PDx` `N`
Z38.66   **Quintuplet liveborn infant, delivered by cesarean** `COM` `PDx` `N`
Z38.68   **Other multiple liveborn infant, delivered vaginally** `COM` `PDx` `N`
Z38.69   **Other multiple liveborn infant, delivered by cesarean** `COM` `PDx` `N`

Z38.7   **Other multiple liveborn infant, born outside hospital** `COM` `PDx` `N`
Z38.8   **Other multiple liveborn infant, unspecified as to place of birth** `COM` `PDx` `N`

√4ᵗʰ **Z39**   **Encounter for maternal postpartum care and examination**

Z39.0   **Encounter for care and examination of mother immediately after delivery** `COM` `PDx` `M` ♀
     Care and observation in uncomplicated cases when the delivery occurs outside a healthcare facility
   EXCLUDES 1   care for postpartum complication - see Alphabetic Index
     AHA: 2021,3Q,13

Z39.1   **Encounter for care and examination of lactating mother** `PDx` `M` ♀
     Encounter for supervision of lactation
   EXCLUDES 1   disorders of lactation (O92.-)

Z39.2   **Encounter for routine postpartum follow-up** `COM` `PDx` `M` ♀

Encounters for other specific health care (Z40-Z53)

Categories Z40-Z53 are intended for use to indicate a reason for care. They may be used for patients who have already been treated for a disease or injury, but who are receiving aftercare or prophylactic care, or care to consolidate the treatment, or to deal with a residual state

   EXCLUDES 2   follow-up examination for medical surveillance after treatment (Z08-Z09)

√4ᵗʰ **Z40**   **Encounter for prophylactic surgery**

   EXCLUDES 1   organ donations (Z52.-)
         therapeutic organ removal - code to condition

DEF: Treatment measure intended to prevent or ward off a disease or condition.

√5ᵗʰ **Z40.0**   **Encounter for prophylactic surgery for risk factors related to malignant neoplasms**
     Admission for prophylactic organ removal
     Use additional code to identify risk factor
     AHA: 2017,4Q,28-29

Z40.00   **Encounter for prophylactic removal of unspecified organ** `PDx`
Z40.01   **Encounter for prophylactic removal of breast** `PDx`
Z40.02   **Encounter for prophylactic removal of ovary(s)** `PDx` ♀
     Encounter for prophylactic removal of ovary(s) and fallopian tube(s)
Z40.03   **Encounter for prophylactic removal of fallopian tube(s)** `PDx` ♀
Z40.09   **Encounter for prophylactic removal of other organ** `PDx`

Z40.8   **Encounter for other prophylactic surgery** `PDx`
Z40.9   **Encounter for prophylactic surgery, unspecified** `PDx`

√4ᵗʰ **Z41**   **Encounter for procedures for purposes other than remedying health state**

Z41.1   **Encounter for cosmetic surgery**
     Encounter for cosmetic breast implant
     Encounter for cosmetic procedure
   EXCLUDES 1   encounter for plastic and reconstructive surgery following medical procedure or healed injury (Z42.-)
         encounter for post-mastectomy breast implantation (Z42.1)

`HCC` CMS-HCC   `Rx` Rx HCC   `ESR` ESRD HCC   `COM` Commercial HCC   `PDx` Primary Dx Only   `N` Newborn: 0   `P` Pediatric: 0-17   `M` Maternity: 9-64   `A` Adult: 15-124

1274   ICD-10-CM 2023

Z41.2 Encounter for routine and ritual male circumcision ♂
  AHA: 2018,3Q,15
  TIP: This code should only be reported when the circumcision is elective (unrelated to a specific diagnosis) and was not performed during the birth admission.

Z41.3 Encounter for ear piercing

Z41.8 Encounter for other procedures for purposes other than remedying health state

Z41.9 Encounter for procedure for purposes other than remedying health state, unspecified

✓4ᵗʰ **Z42** Encounter for plastic and reconstructive surgery following medical procedure or healed injury
  EXCLUDES 1 encounter for cosmetic plastic surgery (Z41.1)
              encounter for plastic surgery for treatment of current injury - code to relevent injury

Z42.1 Encounter for breast reconstruction following mastectomy PDx A
  EXCLUDES 1 deformity and disproportion of reconstructed breast (N65.1-)

Z42.8 Encounter for other plastic and reconstructive surgery following medical procedure or healed injury PDx
  AHA: 2017,1Q,42

✓4ᵗʰ **Z43** Encounter for attention to artificial openings
  INCLUDES closure of artificial openings
            passage of sounds or bougies through artificial openings
            reforming artificial openings
            removal of catheter from artificial openings
            toilet or cleansing of artificial openings
  EXCLUDES 1 complications of external stoma (J95.0-, K94.-, N99.5-)
  EXCLUDES 2 fitting and adjustment of prosthetic and other devices (Z44-Z46)
  AHA: 2019,2Q,33

Z43.0 Encounter for attention to tracheostomy HCC ESR COM

Z43.1 Encounter for attention to gastrostomy HCC ESR COM
  EXCLUDES 2 artificial opening status only, without need for care (Z93.-)

Z43.2 Encounter for attention to ileostomy HCC ESR COM

Z43.3 Encounter for attention to colostomy HCC ESR COM

Z43.4 Encounter for attention to other artificial openings of digestive tract HCC ESR COM

Z43.5 Encounter for attention to cystostomy HCC ESR COM

Z43.6 Encounter for attention to other artificial openings of urinary tract HCC ESR COM
  Encounter for attention to nephrostomy
  Encounter for attention to ureterostomy
  Encounter for attention to urethrostomy

Z43.7 Encounter for attention to artificial vagina

Z43.8 Encounter for attention to other artificial openings HCC ESR COM

Z43.9 Encounter for attention to unspecified artificial opening HCC ESR COM

✓4ᵗʰ **Z44** Encounter for fitting and adjustment of external prosthetic device
  INCLUDES removal or replacement of external prosthetic device
  EXCLUDES 1 malfunction or other complications of device - see Alphabetical Index
              presence of prosthetic device (Z97.-)

✓5ᵗʰ **Z44.0** Encounter for fitting and adjustment of artificial arm

  ✓6ᵗʰ **Z44.00** Encounter for fitting and adjustment of unspecified artificial arm
    Z44.001 Encounter for fitting and adjustment of unspecified right artificial arm COM
    Z44.002 Encounter for fitting and adjustment of unspecified left artificial arm COM
    Z44.009 Encounter for fitting and adjustment of unspecified artificial arm, unspecified arm COM

  ✓6ᵗʰ **Z44.01** Encounter for fitting and adjustment of complete artificial arm
    Z44.011 Encounter for fitting and adjustment of complete right artificial arm COM
    Z44.012 Encounter for fitting and adjustment of complete left artificial arm COM
    Z44.019 Encounter for fitting and adjustment of complete artificial arm, unspecified arm COM

  ✓6ᵗʰ **Z44.02** Encounter for fitting and adjustment of partial artificial arm
    Z44.021 Encounter for fitting and adjustment of partial artificial right arm COM
    Z44.022 Encounter for fitting and adjustment of partial artificial left arm COM
    Z44.029 Encounter for fitting and adjustment of partial artificial arm, unspecified arm COM

✓5ᵗʰ **Z44.1** Encounter for fitting and adjustment of artificial leg

  ✓6ᵗʰ **Z44.10** Encounter for fitting and adjustment of unspecified artificial leg
    Z44.101 Encounter for fitting and adjustment of unspecified right artificial leg HCC ESR COM
    Z44.102 Encounter for fitting and adjustment of unspecified left artificial leg HCC ESR COM
    Z44.109 Encounter for fitting and adjustment of unspecified artificial leg, unspecified leg HCC ESR COM

  ✓6ᵗʰ **Z44.11** Encounter for fitting and adjustment of complete artificial leg
    Z44.111 Encounter for fitting and adjustment of complete right artificial leg HCC ESR COM
    Z44.112 Encounter for fitting and adjustment of complete left artificial leg HCC ESR COM
    Z44.119 Encounter for fitting and adjustment of complete artificial leg, unspecified leg HCC ESR COM

  ✓6ᵗʰ **Z44.12** Encounter for fitting and adjustment of partial artificial leg
    Z44.121 Encounter for fitting and adjustment of partial artificial right leg HCC ESR COM
    Z44.122 Encounter for fitting and adjustment of partial artificial left leg HCC ESR COM
    Z44.129 Encounter for fitting and adjustment of partial artificial leg, unspecified leg HCC ESR COM

✓5ᵗʰ **Z44.2** Encounter for fitting and adjustment of artificial eye
  EXCLUDES 1 mechanical complication of ocular prosthesis (T85.3)

  Z44.20 Encounter for fitting and adjustment of artificial eye, unspecified

  Z44.21 Encounter for fitting and adjustment of artificial right eye

  Z44.22 Encounter for fitting and adjustment of artificial left eye

✓5ᵗʰ **Z44.3** Encounter for fitting and adjustment of external breast prosthesis
  EXCLUDES 1 complications of breast implant (T85.4-)
              encounter for adjustment or removal of breast implant (Z45.81-)
              encounter for initial breast implant insertion for cosmetic breast augmentation (Z41.1)
              encounter for breast reconstruction following mastectomy (Z42.1)

  Z44.30 Encounter for fitting and adjustment of external breast prosthesis, unspecified breast

  Z44.31 Encounter for fitting and adjustment of external right breast prosthesis

  Z44.32 Encounter for fitting and adjustment of external left breast prosthesis

Z44.8 Encounter for fitting and adjustment of other external prosthetic devices

Z44.9 Encounter for fitting and adjustment of unspecified external prosthetic device

Chapter 21. Factors Influencing Health Status and Contact With Health Services

Z45–Z46.59

√4ᵗʰ **Z45** **Encounter for adjustment and management of implanted device**

     INCLUDES   removal or replacement of implanted device

     EXCLUDES 1   *malfunction or other complications of device - see Alphabetical Index*

     EXCLUDES 2   *encounter for fitting and adjustment of non-implanted device (Z46.-)*

√5ᵗʰ **Z45.0** **Encounter for adjustment and management of** cardiac device

     TIP: Assign an additional code for the associated condition if that condition requires constant intervention from the device, as in cases of sick sinus syndrome. For conditions that do not require constant intervention from the device, as in cases of ventricular fibrillation, an additional code for the associated condition should be assigned only if the patient is experiencing the condition and the device is firing during the current admission.

     √6ᵗʰ **Z45.01** **Encounter for adjustment and management of** cardiac pacemaker

         Encounter for adjustment and management of cardiac resynchronization therapy pacemaker (CRT-P)

         EXCLUDES 1   *encounter for adjustment and management of automatic implantable cardiac defibrillator with synchronous cardiac pacemaker (Z45.02)*

         Z45.010 **Encounter for checking and testing of cardiac pacemaker** pulse generator **[battery]**

             Encounter for replacing cardiac pacemaker pulse generator [battery]

         Z45.018 **Encounter for adjustment and management of other part of cardiac pacemaker**

             EXCLUDES 1   *presence of other part of cardiac pacemaker (Z95.0)*

             EXCLUDES 2   *presence of prosthetic and other devices (Z95.1-Z95.5, Z95.811-Z97)*

     Z45.02 **Encounter for adjustment and management of** automatic implantable cardiac defibrillator

         Encounter for adjustment and management of automatic implantable cardiac defibrillator with synchronous cardiac pacemaker

         Encounter for adjustment and management of cardiac resynchronization therapy defibrillator (CRT-D)

     Z45.09 **Encounter for adjustment and management of other cardiac device**

Z45.1 **Encounter for adjustment and management of** infusion pump

Z45.2 **Encounter for adjustment and management of** vascular access device

     Encounter for adjustment and management of vascular catheters

     EXCLUDES 1   *encounter for adjustment and management of renal dialysis catheter (Z49.01)*

     AHA: 2020,2Q,21; 2018,3Q,20

√5ᵗʰ **Z45.3** **Encounter for adjustment and management of implanted devices of the special senses**

     Z45.31 **Encounter for adjustment and management of implanted** visual substitution device

     √6ᵗʰ **Z45.32** **Encounter for adjustment and management of implanted** hearing device

         EXCLUDES 1   *encounter for fitting and adjustment of hearing aide (Z46.1)*

         Z45.320 **Encounter for adjustment and management of** bone conduction **device**

         Z45.321 **Encounter for adjustment and management of** cochlear **device**

         Z45.328 **Encounter for adjustment and management of other implanted hearing device**

√5ᵗʰ **Z45.4** **Encounter for adjustment and management of implanted nervous system device**

     Z45.41 **Encounter for adjustment and management of** cerebrospinal fluid drainage **device**

         Encounter for adjustment and management of cerebral ventricular (communicating) shunt

Z45.42 **Encounter for adjustment and management of** neurostimulator

     Encounter for adjustment and management of brain neurostimulator

     Encounter for adjustment and management of gastric neurostimulator

     Encounter for adjustment and management of peripheral nerve neurostimulator

     Encounter for adjustment and management of sacral nerve neurostimulator

     Encounter for adjustment and management of spinal cord neurostimulator

     Encounter for adjustment and management of vagus nerve neurostimulator

Z45.49 **Encounter for adjustment and management of other implanted nervous system device**

     AHA: 2014,3Q,19

√5ᵗʰ **Z45.8** **Encounter for adjustment and management of other implanted devices**

     √6ᵗʰ **Z45.81** **Encounter for adjustment or** removal of breast implant

         Encounter for elective implant exchange (different material) (different size)

         Encounter for removal of tissue expander with or without synchronous insertion of permanent implant

         EXCLUDES 1   *complications of breast implant (T85.4-)*

              encounter for initial breast implant insertion for cosmetic breast augmentation (Z41.1)

              encounter for breast reconstruction following mastectomy (Z42.1)

         Z45.811 **Encounter for adjustment or removal of** right breast implant

         Z45.812 **Encounter for adjustment or removal of** left breast implant

         Z45.819 **Encounter for adjustment or removal of unspecified breast implant**

     Z45.82 **Encounter for** adjustment or removal of myringotomy device **(stent) (tube)**

     Z45.89 **Encounter for adjustment and management of other implanted devices**

         AHA: 2014,4Q,26-28

Z45.9 **Encounter for adjustment and management of unspecified implanted device**

√4ᵗʰ **Z46** **Encounter for fitting and adjustment of other devices**

     INCLUDES   removal or replacement of other device

     EXCLUDES 1   *malfunction or other complications of device - see Alphabetical Index*

     EXCLUDES 2   *encounter for fitting and management of implanted devices (Z45.-)*

         issue of repeat prescription only (Z76.0)

         presence of prosthetic and other devices (Z95-Z97)

Z46.0 **Encounter for fitting and adjustment of** spectacles and contact lenses

Z46.1 **Encounter for fitting and adjustment of** hearing aid

     EXCLUDES 1   *encounter for adjustment and management of implanted hearing device (Z45.32-)*

Z46.2 **Encounter for fitting and adjustment of other devices related to nervous system and special senses**

     EXCLUDES 2   *encounter for adjustment and management of implanted nervous system device (Z45.4-)*

         encounter for adjustment and management of implanted visual substitution device (Z45.31)

Z46.3 **Encounter for fitting and adjustment of** dental prosthetic device

     Encounter for fitting and adjustment of dentures

Z46.4 **Encounter for fitting and adjustment of** orthodontic device

√5ᵗʰ **Z46.5** **Encounter for fitting and adjustment of other** gastrointestinal appliance and device

     EXCLUDES 1   *encounter for attention to artificial openings of digestive tract (Z43.1-Z43.4)*

     Z46.51 **Encounter for fitting and adjustment of** gastric lap band

     Z46.59 **Encounter for fitting and adjustment of other gastrointestinal appliance and device**

HCC CMS-HCC   Rx Rx HCC   ESR ESRD HCC   COM Commercial HCC   PDx Primary Dx Only   N Newborn: 0   P Pediatric: 0-17   M Maternity: 9-64   A Adult: 15-124

1276   ICD-10-CM 2023

Z46.6 Encounter for fitting and adjustment of urinary device
  EXCLUDES 2 *attention to artificial openings of urinary tract (Z43.5, Z43.6)*

☑5ᵗʰ Z46.8 Encounter for fitting and adjustment of other specified devices
  Z46.81 Encounter for fitting and adjustment of insulin pump
    Encounter for insulin pump instruction and training
    Encounter for insulin pump titration
  Z46.82 Encounter for fitting and adjustment of non-vascular catheter
  Z46.89 Encounter for fitting and adjustment of other specified devices
    Encounter for fitting and adjustment of wheelchair

Z46.9 Encounter for fitting and adjustment of unspecified device

☑4ᵗʰ Z47 Orthopedic aftercare
  EXCLUDES 1 *aftercare for healing fracture - code to fracture with 7th character D*

  Z47.1 Aftercare following joint replacement surgery
    Use additional code to identify the joint (Z96.6-)
    AHA: 2020,1Q,23

  Z47.2 Encounter for removal of internal fixation device
    EXCLUDES 1 *encounter for adjustment of internal fixation device for fracture treatment - code to fracture with appropriate 7th character*
    encounter for removal of external fixation device - code to fracture with 7th character D
    infection or inflammatory reaction to internal fixation device (T84.6-)
    mechanical complication of internal fixation device (T84.1-)

  ☑5ᵗʰ Z47.3 Aftercare following explantation of joint prosthesis
    Aftercare following explantation of joint prosthesis, staged procedure
    Encounter for joint prosthesis insertion following prior explantation of joint prosthesis
    AHA: 2020,1Q,23; 2015,1Q,16
    TIP: For staged removal of elbow joint prosthesis, assign code Z47.1.
    Z47.31 Aftercare following explantation of shoulder joint prosthesis
      EXCLUDES 1 *acquired absence of shoulder joint following prior explantation of shoulder joint prosthesis (Z89.23-)*
      shoulder joint prosthesis explantation status (Z89.23-)
    Z47.32 Aftercare following explantation of hip joint prosthesis
      EXCLUDES 1 *acquired absence of hip joint following prior explantation of hip joint prosthesis (Z89.62-)*
      hip joint prosthesis explantation status (Z89.62-)
    Z47.33 Aftercare following explantation of knee joint prosthesis
      EXCLUDES 1 *acquired absence of knee joint following prior explantation of knee prosthesis (Z89.52-)*
      knee joint prosthesis explantation status (Z89.52-)

  ☑5ᵗʰ Z47.8 Encounter for other orthopedic aftercare
    Z47.81 Encounter for orthopedic aftercare following surgical amputation
      Use additional code to identify the limb amputated (Z89.-)
    Z47.82 Encounter for orthopedic aftercare following scoliosis surgery
    Z47.89 Encounter for other orthopedic aftercare
      AHA: 2015,1Q,8

☑4ᵗʰ Z48 Encounter for other postprocedural aftercare
  EXCLUDES 1 *encounter for aftercare following injury - code to Injury, by site, with appropriate 7th character for subsequent encounter*
  encounter for follow-up examination after completed treatment (Z08-Z09)
  EXCLUDES 2 *encounter for attention to artificial openings (Z43.-)*
  encounter for fitting and adjustment of prosthetic and other devices (Z44-Z46)
  AHA: 2015,4Q,38; 2015,1Q,6-7

  ☑5ᵗʰ Z48.0 Encounter for attention to dressings, sutures and drains
    EXCLUDES 1 *encounter for planned postprocedural wound closure (Z48.1)*
    Z48.00 Encounter for change or removal of nonsurgical wound dressing
      Encounter for change or removal of wound dressing NOS
    Z48.01 Encounter for change or removal of surgical wound dressing
      AHA: 2019,2Q,33
    Z48.02 Encounter for removal of sutures
      Encounter for removal of staples
    Z48.03 Encounter for change or removal of drains
      AHA: 2019,2Q,33

  Z48.1 Encounter for planned postprocedural wound closure
    EXCLUDES 1 *encounter for attention to dressings and sutures (Z48.0-)*

  ☑5ᵗʰ Z48.2 Encounter for aftercare following organ transplant
    Z48.21 Encounter for aftercare following heart transplant HCC Rx ESR COM
    Z48.22 Encounter for aftercare following kidney transplant Rx COM
    Z48.23 Encounter for aftercare following liver transplant HCC Rx ESR COM
    Z48.24 Encounter for aftercare following lung transplant HCC Rx ESR COM
    ☑6ᵗʰ Z48.28 Encounter for aftercare following multiple organ transplant
      Z48.280 Encounter for aftercare following heart-lung transplant HCC Rx ESR COM
      Z48.288 Encounter for aftercare following multiple organ transplant
    ☑6ᵗʰ Z48.29 Encounter for aftercare following other organ transplant
      Z48.290 Encounter for aftercare following bone marrow transplant HCC Rx ESR COM
      Z48.298 Encounter for aftercare following other organ transplant

  Z48.3 Aftercare following surgery for neoplasm
    Use additional code to identify the neoplasm

  ☑5ᵗʰ Z48.8 Encounter for other specified postprocedural aftercare
    ☑6ᵗʰ Z48.81 Encounter for surgical aftercare following surgery on specified body systems
      These codes identify the body system requiring aftercare. They are for use in conjunction with other aftercare codes to fully explain the aftercare encounter. The condition treated should also be coded if still present.
      EXCLUDES 1 *aftercare for injury - code the injury with 7th character D*
      aftercare following surgery for neoplasm (Z48.3)
      EXCLUDES 2 *aftercare following organ transplant (Z48.2-)*
      orthopedic aftercare (Z47.-)
      AHA: 2015,4Q,38
      Z48.810 Encounter for surgical aftercare following surgery on the sense organs
      Z48.811 Encounter for surgical aftercare following surgery on the nervous system
        EXCLUDES 2 *encounter for surgical aftercare following surgery on the sense organs (Z48.810)*
      Z48.812 Encounter for surgical aftercare following surgery on the circulatory system
        AHA: 2012,4Q,96

Z48.813 Encounter for surgical aftercare following surgery on the respiratory system
AHA: 2019,2Q,33

Z48.814 Encounter for surgical aftercare following surgery on the teeth or oral cavity

Z48.815 Encounter for surgical aftercare following surgery on the digestive system

Z48.816 Encounter for surgical aftercare following surgery on the genitourinary system
EXCLUDES 1 encounter for aftercare following sterilization reversal (Z31.42)

Z48.817 Encounter for surgical aftercare following surgery on the skin and subcutaneous tissue

Z48.89 Encounter for other specified surgical aftercare

✓4ᵗʰ **Z49** Encounter for care involving renal dialysis
Code also associated end stage renal disease (N18.6)

✓5ᵗʰ **Z49.0** Preparatory care for renal dialysis
Encounter for dialysis instruction and training

Z49.01 Encounter for fitting and adjustment of extracorporeal dialysis catheter HCC Rx ESR
Removal or replacement of renal dialysis catheter
Toilet or cleansing of renal dialysis catheter

Z49.02 Encounter for fitting and adjustment of peritoneal dialysis catheter HCC Rx ESR

✓5ᵗʰ **Z49.3** Encounter for adequacy testing for dialysis

Z49.31 Encounter for adequacy testing for hemodialysis HCC Rx ESR

Z49.32 Encounter for adequacy testing for peritoneal dialysis HCC Rx ESR
Encounter for peritoneal equilibration test

✓4ᵗʰ **Z51** Encounter for other aftercare and medical care
Code also condition requiring care
EXCLUDES 1 follow-up examination after treatment (Z08-Z09)

Z51.0 Encounter for antineoplastic radiation therapy PDx
AHA: 2017,4Q,103
TIP: Do not assign when admission is for insertion/implantation of radioactive elements. Assign a code for the malignancy instead. Any complications related to the radioactive elements should be assigned as secondary diagnoses.

✓5ᵗʰ **Z51.1** Encounter for antineoplastic chemotherapy and immunotherapy
EXCLUDES 2 encounter for chemotherapy and immunotherapy for nonneoplastic condition - code to condition

Z51.11 Encounter for antineoplastic chemotherapy PDx
AHA: 2022,1Q,16; 2015,3Q,19

Z51.12 Encounter for antineoplastic immunotherapy PDx

Z51.5 Encounter for palliative care
AHA: 2022,1Q,18; 2020,4Q,98; 2017,1Q,48

Z51.6 Encounter for desensitization to allergens
AHA: 2016,4Q,77

✓5ᵗʰ **Z51.8** Encounter for other specified aftercare
EXCLUDES 1 holiday relief care (Z75.5)

Z51.81 Encounter for therapeutic drug level monitoring
Code also any long-term (current) drug therapy (Z79.-)
EXCLUDES 1 encounter for blood-drug test for administrative or medicolegal reasons (Z02.83)
DEF: Drug monitoring: Measurement of the level of a specific drug in the body or measurement of a specific function to assess effectiveness of a drug.

Z51.89 Encounter for other specified aftercare
AHA: 2012,4Q,95-97

✓4ᵗʰ **Z52** Donors of organs and tissues
INCLUDES autologous and other living donors
EXCLUDES 1 cadaveric donor - omit code
examination of potential donor (Z00.5)
AHA: 2012,4Q,99

✓5ᵗʰ **Z52.0** Blood donor

✓6ᵗʰ **Z52.00** Unspecified blood donor

Z52.000 Unspecified donor, whole blood PDx

Z52.001 Unspecified donor, stem cells PDx

Z52.008 Unspecified donor, other blood PDx

✓6ᵗʰ **Z52.01** Autologous blood donor

Z52.010 Autologous donor, whole blood PDx

Z52.011 Autologous donor, stem cells PDx

Z52.018 Autologous donor, other blood PDx

✓6ᵗʰ **Z52.09** Other blood donor
Volunteer donor

Z52.090 Other blood donor, whole blood PDx

Z52.091 Other blood donor, stem cells PDx

Z52.098 Other blood donor, other blood PDx

✓5ᵗʰ **Z52.1** Skin donor

Z52.10 Skin donor, unspecified PDx

Z52.11 Skin donor, autologous PDx

Z52.19 Skin donor, other PDx

✓5ᵗʰ **Z52.2** Bone donor

Z52.20 Bone donor, unspecified PDx

Z52.21 Bone donor, autologous PDx

Z52.29 Bone donor, other PDx

Z52.3 Bone marrow donor PDx

Z52.4 Kidney donor PDx

Z52.5 Cornea donor PDx

Z52.6 Liver donor PDx

✓5ᵗʰ **Z52.8** Donor of other specified organs or tissues

✓6ᵗʰ **Z52.81** Egg (Oocyte) donor

Z52.810 Egg (Oocyte) donor under age 35, anonymous recipient PDx ♀
Egg donor under age 35 NOS

Z52.811 Egg (Oocyte) donor under age 35, designated recipient PDx ♀

Z52.812 Egg (Oocyte) donor age 35 and over, anonymous recipient PDx ♀
Egg donor age 35 and over NOS

Z52.813 Egg (Oocyte) donor age 35 and over, designated recipient PDx ♀

Z52.819 Egg (Oocyte) donor, unspecified PDx ♀

Z52.89 Donor of other specified organs or tissues PDx

Z52.9 Donor of unspecified organ or tissue
Donor NOS

✓4ᵗʰ **Z53** Persons encountering health services for specific procedures and treatment, not carried out

✓5ᵗʰ **Z53.0** Procedure and treatment not carried out because of contraindication

Z53.01 Procedure and treatment not carried out due to patient smoking

Z53.09 Procedure and treatment not carried out because of other contraindication

Z53.1 Procedure and treatment not carried out because of patient's decision for reasons of belief and group pressure

✓5ᵗʰ **Z53.2** Procedure and treatment not carried out because of patient's decision for other and unspecified reasons

Z53.20 Procedure and treatment not carried out because of patient's decision for unspecified reasons

Z53.21 Procedure and treatment not carried out due to patient leaving prior to being seen by health care provider

Z53.29 Procedure and treatment not carried out because of patient's decision for other reasons

✓5ᵗʰ **Z53.3** Procedure converted to open procedure
AHA: 2016,4Q,79

Z53.31 Laparoscopic surgical procedure converted to open procedure UPD

Z53.32 Thoracoscopic surgical procedure converted to open procedure UPD

Z53.33 Arthroscopic surgical procedure converted to open procedure UPD

Z53.39 Other specified procedure converted to open procedure UPD

Z53.8 Procedure and treatment not carried out for other reasons

Z53.9 Procedure and treatment not carried out, unspecified reason

Persons with potential health hazards related to socioeconomic and psychosocial circumstances (Z55-Z65)

AHA: 2021,4Q,34-37; 2019,4Q,66; 2018,4Q,58,73; 2018,1Q,18
DEF: Social determinants of health: Socioeconomic factors that can affect a person's health, including both environmental and societal conditions such as education and literacy, employment, health behaviors, housing, lack of adequate food or water, occupational exposure to risk factors, social support, transportation, and violence. Tracking social needs that impact patients allows providers to identify population health trends and to promote the personalized care that addresses the medical and social needs of individual patients. *Synonym(s): SDOH.*
TIP: Because codes in these categories represent social information rather than medical diagnoses, they can be assigned based on documentation by nonphysician clinicians involved in the care of these patients as well as self-reported documentation from the patient, as long as the information is approved and incorporated into the medical record by a clinician or provider.

✓4ᵗʰ Z55 Problems related to education and literacy
> EXCLUDES 1   *disorders of psychological development (F80-F89)*

    Z55.0 Illiteracy and low-level literacy
    Z55.1 Schooling unavailable and unattainable
    Z55.2 Failed school examinations
    Z55.3 Underachievement in school
    Z55.4 Educational maladjustment and discord with teachers and classmates
    Z55.5 Less than a high school diploma   UPD
        No general equivalence degree (GED)
    Z55.8 Other problems related to education and literacy
        Problems related to inadequate teaching
    Z55.9 Problems related to education and literacy, unspecified
        Academic problems NOS

✓4ᵗʰ Z56 Problems related to employment and unemployment
> EXCLUDES 2   *occupational exposure to risk factors (Z57.-)*
>   *problems related to housing and economic circumstances (Z59.-)*

    Z56.0 Unemployment, unspecified
    Z56.1 Change of job   A
    Z56.2 Threat of job loss
    Z56.3 Stressful work schedule
    Z56.4 Discord with boss and workmates
    Z56.5 Uncongenial work environment
        Difficult conditions at work
    Z56.6 Other physical and mental strain related to work
    ✓5ᵗʰ Z56.8 Other problems related to employment
        Z56.81 Sexual harassment on the job
        Z56.82 Military deployment status
            Individual (civilian or military) currently deployed in theater or in support of military war, peacekeeping and humanitarian operations
        Z56.89 Other problems related to employment
    Z56.9 Unspecified problems related to employment
        Occupational problems NOS

✓4ᵗʰ Z57 Occupational exposure to risk factors

    Z57.0 Occupational exposure to noise
    Z57.1 Occupational exposure to radiation
    Z57.2 Occupational exposure to dust
    ✓5ᵗʰ Z57.3 Occupational exposure to other air contaminants
        Z57.31 Occupational exposure to environmental tobacco smoke
        > EXCLUDES 2   *exposure to environmental tobacco smoke (Z77.22)*
        Z57.39 Occupational exposure to other air contaminants
    Z57.4 Occupational exposure to toxic agents in agriculture
        Occupational exposure to solids, liquids, gases or vapors in agriculture
    Z57.5 Occupational exposure to toxic agents in other industries
        Occupational exposure to solids, liquids, gases or vapors in other industries
    Z57.6 Occupational exposure to extreme temperature
    Z57.7 Occupational exposure to vibration
    Z57.8 Occupational exposure to other risk factors
    Z57.9 Occupational exposure to unspecified risk factor

✓4ᵗʰ Z58 Problems related to physical environment
> EXCLUDES 2   *occupational exposure (Z57.-)*

    Z58.6 Inadequate drinking-water supply
        Lack of safe drinking water
        > EXCLUDES 2   *deprivation of water (T73.1)*

✓4ᵗʰ Z59 Problems related to housing and economic circumstances
> EXCLUDES 2   *problems related to upbringing (Z62.-)*

    ✓5ᵗʰ Z59.0 Homelessness
        Z59.00 Homelessness unspecified   UPD
        Z59.01 Sheltered homelessness   UPD
            Doubled up
            Living in a shelter such as: motel, scattered site housing, temporary or transitional living situation
        Z59.02 Unsheltered homelessness   UPD
            Residing in place not meant for human habitation such as: abandoned buildings, cars, parks, sidewalk
            Residing on the street
    Z59.1 Inadequate housing
        Lack of heating
        Restriction of space
        Technical defects in home preventing adequate care
        Unsatisfactory surroundings
        > EXCLUDES 1   *problems related to the natural and physical environment (Z77.1-)*
    Z59.2 Discord with neighbors, lodgers and landlord
    Z59.3 Problems related to living in residential institution
        Boarding-school resident
        > EXCLUDES 1   *institutional upbringing (Z62.2)*
    ✓5ᵗʰ Z59.4 Lack of adequate food
        > EXCLUDES 2   *deprivation of food (T73.0)*
             effects of hunger (T73.0)
             inappropriate diet or eating habits (Z72.4)
             malnutrition (E40-E46)
        Z59.41 Food insecurity   UPD
        Z59.48 Other specified lack of adequate food   UPD
            Inadequate food
            Lack of food
    Z59.5 Extreme poverty
    Z59.6 Low income
    Z59.7 Insufficient social insurance and welfare support
    ✓5ᵗʰ Z59.8 Other problems related to housing and economic circumstances
        ✓6ᵗʰ Z59.81 Housing instability, housed
            Foreclosure on home loan
            Past due on rent or mortgage
            Unwanted multiple moves in the last 12 months
            Z59.811 Housing instability, housed, with risk of homelessness   UPD
                Imminent risk of homelessness
            Z59.812 Housing instability, housed, homelessness in past 12 months   UPD
            Z59.819 Housing instability, housed unspecified   UPD
        ● **Z59.82 Transportation insecurity**
            Excessive transportation time
            Inaccessible transportation
            Inadequate transportation
            Lack of transportation
            Unaffordable transportation
            Unreliable transportation
            Unsafe transportation

●   **Z59.86**   **Financial insecurity**
         Bankruptcy
         Burdensome debt
         Economic strain
         Financial strain
         Money problems
         Running out of money
         Unable to make ends meet
         EXCLUDES 2   *extreme poverty (Z59.5)*
                low income (Z59.6)
                material hardship, not elsewhere classified (Z59.87)

●   **Z59.87**   **Material hardship**
         Material deprivation
         Unable to obtain adequate childcare
         Unable to obtain adequate clothing
         Unable to obtain adequate utilities
         Unable to obtain basic needs
         EXCLUDES 2   *extreme poverty (Z59.5)*
                financial insecurity, not elsewhere classified (Z59.86)
                low income (Z59.6)

     Z59.89   **Other problems related to housing and economic circumstances**   UPD
         Foreclosure on loan
         Isolated dwelling
         Problems with creditors

     Z59.9   **Problem related to housing and economic circumstances, unspecified**

✓4ᵗʰ **Z60**   **Problems related to social environment**

     Z60.0   **Problems of adjustment to life-cycle transitions**
         Empty nest syndrome
         Phase of life problem
         Problem with adjustment to retirement [pension]

     Z60.2   **Problems related to living alone**

     Z60.3   **Acculturation difficulty**
         Problem with migration
         Problem with social transplantation
         DEF: Problem adapting to a different culture or environment not based on any coexisting mental disorder.

     Z60.4   **Social exclusion and rejection**
         Exclusion and rejection on the basis of personal characteristics, such as unusual physical appearance, illness or behavior.
         EXCLUDES 1   *target of adverse discrimination such as for racial or religious reasons (Z60.5)*

     Z60.5   **Target of (perceived) adverse discrimination and persecution**
         EXCLUDES 1   *social exclusion and rejection (Z60.4)*

     Z60.8   **Other problems related to social environment**

     Z60.9   **Problem related to social environment, unspecified**

✓4ᵗʰ **Z62**   **Problems related to upbringing**
     INCLUDES   current and past negative life events in childhood
              current and past problems of a child related to upbringing
     EXCLUDES 2   *maltreatment syndrome (T74.-)*
              problems related to housing and economic circumstances (Z59.-)

     Z62.0   **Inadequate parental supervision and control**

     Z62.1   **Parental overprotection**

✓5ᵗʰ   **Z62.2**   **Upbringing away from parents**
         EXCLUDES 1   *problems with boarding school (Z59.3)*

         Z62.21   **Child in welfare custody**   P
              Child in care of non-parental family member
              Child in foster care
              EXCLUDES 2   *problem for parent due to child in welfare custody (Z63.5)*

         Z62.22   **Institutional upbringing**
              Child living in orphanage or group home

         Z62.29   **Other upbringing away from parents**

     Z62.3   **Hostility towards and scapegoating of child**   P

     Z62.6   **Inappropriate (excessive) parental pressure**

✓5ᵗʰ   **Z62.8**   **Other specified problems related to upbringing**

      ✓6ᵗʰ   **Z62.81**   **Personal history of abuse in childhood**

         Z62.810   **Personal history of physical and sexual abuse in childhood**
              EXCLUDES 1   *current child physical abuse (T74.12, T76.12)*
                   current child sexual abuse (T74.22, T76.22)

         Z62.811   **Personal history of psychological abuse in childhood**
              EXCLUDES 1   *current child psychological abuse (T74.32, T76.32)*

         Z62.812   **Personal history of neglect in childhood**
              EXCLUDES 1   *current child neglect (T74.02, T76.02)*

         Z62.813   **Personal history of forced labor or sexual exploitation in childhood**
              AHA: 2018,4Q,32,35

         Z62.819   **Personal history of unspecified abuse in childhood**
              EXCLUDES 1   *current child abuse NOS (T74.92, T76.92)*

      ✓6ᵗʰ   **Z62.82**   **Parent-child conflict**

         Z62.820   **Parent-biological child conflict**
              Parent-child problem NOS

         Z62.821   **Parent-adopted child conflict**

         Z62.822   **Parent-foster child conflict**

      ✓6ᵗʰ   **Z62.89**   **Other specified problems related to upbringing**

         Z62.890   **Parent-child estrangement NEC**

         Z62.891   **Sibling rivalry**

         Z62.898   **Other specified problems related to upbringing**

     Z62.9   **Problem related to upbringing, unspecified**

✓4ᵗʰ **Z63**   **Other problems related to primary support group, including family circumstances**
     EXCLUDES 2   *maltreatment syndrome (T74.-, T76)*
              parent-child problems (Z62.-)
              problems related to negative life events in childhood (Z62.-)
              problems related to upbringing (Z62.-)

     Z63.0   **Problems in relationship with spouse or partner**
         Relationship distress with spouse or intimate partner
         EXCLUDES 1   *counseling for spousal or partner abuse problems (Z69.1)*
                counseling related to sexual attitude, behavior, and orientation (Z70.-)

     Z63.1   **Problems in relationship with in-laws**

✓5ᵗʰ   **Z63.3**   **Absence of family member**
         EXCLUDES 1   *absence of family member due to disappearance and death (Z63.4)*
                absence of family member due to separation and divorce (Z63.5)

         Z63.31   **Absence of family member due to military deployment**
              Individual or family affected by other family member being on military deployment
              EXCLUDES 1   *family disruption due to return of family member from military deployment (Z63.71)*

         Z63.32   **Other absence of family member**

     Z63.4   **Disappearance and death of family member**
         Assumed death of family member
         Bereavement
         AHA: 2014,1Q,25

     Z63.5   **Disruption of family by separation and divorce**
         Marital estrangement

     Z63.6   **Dependent relative needing care at home**

✓5ᵗʰ   **Z63.7**   **Other stressful life events affecting family and household**

         Z63.71   **Stress on family due to return of family member from military deployment**
              Individual or family affected by family member having returned from military deployment (current or past conflict)

         Z63.72   **Alcoholism and drug addiction in family**

Z63.79   **Other stressful life events affecting family and household**
Anxiety (normal) about sick person in family
Health problems within family
Ill or disturbed family member
Isolated family

Z63.8   **Other specified problems related to primary support group**
Family discord NOS
Family estrangement NOS
High expressed emotional level within family
Inadequate family support NOS
Inadequate or distorted communication within family

Z63.9   **Problem related to primary support group, unspecified**
Relationship disorder NOS

✓4ᵗʰ **Z64**   **Problems related to certain psychosocial circumstances**

Z64.0   **Problems related to unwanted pregnancy** ♀

Z64.1   **Problems related to multiparity** ♀

Z64.4   **Discord with counselors**
Discord with probation officer
Discord with social worker

✓4ᵗʰ **Z65**   **Problems related to other psychosocial circumstances**

Z65.0   **Conviction in civil and criminal proceedings without imprisonment**

Z65.1   **Imprisonment and other incarceration**

Z65.2   **Problems related to release from prison**

Z65.3   **Problems related to other legal circumstances**
Arrest
Child custody or support proceedings
Litigation
Prosecution

Z65.4   **Victim of crime and terrorism**
Victim of torture

Z65.5   **Exposure to disaster, war and other hostilities**
EXCLUDES 1   target of perceived discrimination or persecution (Z60.5)

Z65.8   **Other specified problems related to psychosocial circumstances**
Religious or spiritual problem

Z65.9   **Problem related to unspecified psychosocial circumstances**

Do not resuscitate status (Z66)

Z66   **Do not resuscitate**
DNR status
DEF: Medical order written by a physician that instructs others not to perform cardiopulmonary resuscitation (CPR), intubation, or advanced cardiac life support (ACLS). It prevents unnecessary invasive treatment to prolong life should breathing stop or cardiac arrest occur.

Blood type (Z67)

✓4ᵗʰ **Z67**   **Blood type**
AHA: 2015,3Q,40

✓5ᵗʰ **Z67.1**   **Type A blood**
     Z67.10   **Type A blood, Rh positive**
     Z67.11   **Type A blood, Rh negative**

✓5ᵗʰ **Z67.2**   **Type B blood**
     Z67.20   **Type B blood, Rh positive**
     Z67.21   **Type B blood, Rh negative**

✓5ᵗʰ **Z67.3**   **Type AB blood**
     Z67.30   **Type AB blood, Rh positive**
     Z67.31   **Type AB blood, Rh negative**

✓5ᵗʰ **Z67.4**   **Type O blood**
     Z67.40   **Type O blood, Rh positive**
     Z67.41   **Type O blood, Rh negative**

✓5ᵗʰ **Z67.9**   **Unspecified blood type**
     Z67.90   **Unspecified blood type, Rh positive**
     Z67.91   **Unspecified blood type, Rh negative**

Body mass index [BMI] (Z68)

✓4ᵗʰ **Z68**   **Body mass index [BMI]**
Kilograms per meters squared

NOTE   BMI adult codes are for use for persons 20 years of age or older
BMI pediatric codes are for use for persons 2-19 years of age.
These percentiles are based on the growth charts published by the Centers for Disease Control and Prevention (CDC)

AHA: 2019,4Q,19,57; 2018,4Q,73,77-83; 2017,1Q,39
DEF: Index used to help determine whether an individual is underweight, a healthy weight, overweight, or obese.
TIP: A BMI code may be assigned to support an associated condition based on medical record documentation from clinicians who are not the patient's provider.
TIP: In order to assign a BMI code, the associated condition must meet the definition of a reportable diagnosis for outpatient encounters, per section IV.J of the *ICD-10-CM Official Guidelines for Coding and Reporting*.

Z68.1   **Body mass index [BMI] 19.9 or less, adult**   UPD A

✓5ᵗʰ **Z68.2**   **Body mass index [BMI] 20-29, adult**
     Z68.20   **Body mass index [BMI] 20.0-20.9, adult**   UPD A
     Z68.21   **Body mass index [BMI] 21.0-21.9, adult**   UPD A
     Z68.22   **Body mass index [BMI] 22.0-22.9, adult**   UPD A
     Z68.23   **Body mass index [BMI] 23.0-23.9, adult**   UPD A
     Z68.24   **Body mass index [BMI] 24.0-24.9, adult**   UPD A
     Z68.25   **Body mass index [BMI] 25.0-25.9, adult**   UPD A
     Z68.26   **Body mass index [BMI] 26.0-26.9, adult**   UPD A
     Z68.27   **Body mass index [BMI] 27.0-27.9, adult**   UPD A
     Z68.28   **Body mass index [BMI] 28.0-28.9, adult**   UPD A
     Z68.29   **Body mass index [BMI] 29.0-29.9, adult**   UPD A

✓5ᵗʰ **Z68.3**   **Body mass index [BMI] 30-39, adult**
     Z68.30   **Body mass index [BMI] 30.0-30.9, adult**   UPD A
     Z68.31   **Body mass index [BMI] 31.0-31.9, adult**   UPD A
     Z68.32   **Body mass index [BMI] 32.0-32.9, adult**   UPD A
     Z68.33   **Body mass index [BMI] 33.0-33.9, adult**   UPD A
     Z68.34   **Body mass index [BMI] 34.0-34.9, adult**   UPD A
     Z68.35   **Body mass index [BMI] 35.0-35.9, adult**   UPD A
     Z68.36   **Body mass index [BMI] 36.0-36.9, adult**   UPD A
     Z68.37   **Body mass index [BMI] 37.0-37.9, adult**   UPD A
     Z68.38   **Body mass index [BMI] 38.0-38.9, adult**   UPD A
     Z68.39   **Body mass index [BMI] 39.0-39.9, adult**   UPD A

✓5ᵗʰ **Z68.4**   **Body mass index [BMI] 40 or greater, adult**
     Z68.41   **Body mass index [BMI] 40.0-44.9, adult**   HCC ESR UPD A
     Z68.42   **Body mass index [BMI] 45.0-49.9, adult**   HCC ESR UPD A
     Z68.43   **Body mass index [BMI] 50.0-59.9, adult**   HCC ESR UPD A
     Z68.44   **Body mass index [BMI] 60.0-69.9, adult**   HCC ESR UPD A
     Z68.45   **Body mass index [BMI] 70 or greater, adult**   HCC ESR UPD A

✓5ᵗʰ **Z68.5**   **Body mass index [BMI] pediatric**
AHA: 2018,4Q,81-82
     Z68.51   **Body mass index [BMI] pediatric, less than 5th percentile for age**   UPD
     Z68.52   **Body mass index [BMI] pediatric, 5th percentile to less than 85th percentile for age**   UPD
     Z68.53   **Body mass index [BMI] pediatric, 85th percentile to less than 95th percentile for age**   UPD
     Z68.54   **Body mass index [BMI] pediatric, greater than or equal to 95th percentile for age**   UPD

☑ Additional Character Required   ✓x7ᵗʰ Placeholder Alert   **Manifestation**   Unspecified Dx   Q QPP   UPD Unacceptable PDx

Chapter 21. Factors Influencing Health Status and Contact With Health Services

Z69–Z71.51

Persons encountering health services in other circumstances (Z69-Z76)

√4ᵗʰ Z69 Encounter for mental health services for victim and perpetrator of abuse

> INCLUDES   counseling for victims and perpetrators of abuse

√5ᵗʰ Z69.0 Encounter for mental health services for child abuse problems

√6ᵗʰ Z69.01 Encounter for mental health services for parental child abuse

Z69.010 Encounter for mental health services for victim of parental child abuse P

> Encounter for mental health services for victim of child abuse by parent
> Encounter for mental health services for victim of child neglect by parent
> Encounter for mental health services for victim of child psychological abuse by parent
> Encounter for mental health services for victim of child sexual abuse by parent

Z69.011 Encounter for mental health services for perpetrator of parental child abuse

> Encounter for mental health services for perpetrator of parental child neglect
> Encounter for mental health services for perpetrator of parental child psychological abuse
> Encounter for mental health services for perpetrator of parental child sexual abuse

> EXCLUDES 1   encounter for mental health services for non-parental child abuse (Z69.02-)

√6ᵗʰ Z69.02 Encounter for mental health services for non-parental child abuse

Z69.020 Encounter for mental health services for victim of non-parental child abuse P

> Encounter for mental health services for victim of non-parental child neglect
> Encounter for mental health services for victim of non-parental child psychological abuse
> Encounter for mental health services for victim of non-parental child sexual abuse

Z69.021 Encounter for mental health services for perpetrator of non-parental child abuse

> Encounter for mental health services for perpetrator of non-parental child neglect
> Encounter for mental health services for perpetrator of non-parental child psychological abuse
> Encounter for mental health services for perpetrator of non-parental child sexual abuse

√5ᵗʰ Z69.1 Encounter for mental health services for spousal or partner abuse problems

Z69.11 Encounter for mental health services for victim of spousal or partner abuse

> Encounter for mental health services for victim of spouse or partner neglect
> Encounter for mental health services for victim of spouse or partner psychological abuse
> Encounter for mental health services for victim of spouse or partner violence, physical

Z69.12 Encounter for mental health services for perpetrator of spousal or partner abuse

> Encounter for mental health services for perpetrator of spouse or partner neglect
> Encounter for mental health services for perpetrator of spouse or partner psychological abuse
> Encounter for mental health services for perpetrator of spouse or partner violence, physical
> Encounter for mental health services for perpetrator of spouse or partner violence, sexual

√5ᵗʰ Z69.8 Encounter for mental health services for victim or perpetrator of other abuse

Z69.81 Encounter for mental health services for victim of other abuse

> Encounter for mental health services for victim of non-spousal adult abuse
> Encounter for mental health services for victim of spouse or partner violence, sexual
> Encounter for rape victim counseling

Z69.82 Encounter for mental health services for perpetrator of other abuse

> Encounter for mental health services for perpetrator of non-spousal adult abuse

√4ᵗʰ Z70 Counseling related to sexual attitude, behavior and orientation

> INCLUDES   encounter for mental health services for sexual attitude, behavior and orientation

> EXCLUDES 2   contraceptive or procreative counseling (Z30-Z31)

Z70.0 Counseling related to sexual attitude

Z70.1 Counseling related to patient's sexual behavior and orientation

> Patient concerned regarding impotence
> Patient concerned regarding non-responsiveness
> Patient concerned regarding promiscuity
> Patient concerned regarding sexual orientation

Z70.2 Counseling related to sexual behavior and orientation of third party

> Advice sought regarding sexual behavior and orientation of child
> Advice sought regarding sexual behavior and orientation of partner
> Advice sought regarding sexual behavior and orientation of spouse

Z70.3 Counseling related to combined concerns regarding sexual attitude, behavior and orientation

Z70.8 Other sex counseling

> Encounter for sex education

Z70.9 Sex counseling, unspecified

√4ᵗʰ Z71 Persons encountering health services for other counseling and medical advice, not elsewhere classified

> EXCLUDES 2   contraceptive or procreation counseling (Z30-Z31)
> sex counseling (Z70.-)

Z71.0 Person encountering health services to consult on behalf of another person

> Person encountering health services to seek advice or treatment for non-attending third party

> EXCLUDES 2   anxiety (normal) about sick person in family (Z63.7)
> expectant (adoptive) parent(s) pre-birth pediatrician visit (Z76.81)

Z71.1 Person with feared health complaint in whom no diagnosis is made

> Person encountering health services with feared condition which was not demonstrated
> Person encountering health services in which problem was normal state
> "Worried well"

> EXCLUDES 1   medical observation for suspected diseases and conditions proven not to exist (Z03.-)

Z71.2 Person consulting for explanation of examination or test findings

Z71.3 Dietary counseling and surveillance

> Use additional code for any associated underlying medical condition
> Use additional code to identify body mass index (BMI), if known (Z68.-)

√5ᵗʰ Z71.4 Alcohol abuse counseling and surveillance

> Use additional code for alcohol abuse or dependence (F10.-)

Z71.41 Alcohol abuse counseling and surveillance of alcoholic

Z71.42 Counseling for family member of alcoholic

> Counseling for significant other, partner, or friend of alcoholic

√5ᵗʰ Z71.5 Drug abuse counseling and surveillance

> Use additional code for drug abuse or dependence (F11-F16, F18-F19)

Z71.51 Drug abuse counseling and surveillance of drug abuser

HCC CMS-HCC   Rx Rx HCC   ESR ESRD HCC   COM Commercial HCC   PDx Primary Dx Only   N Newborn: 0   P Pediatric: 0-17   M Maternity: 9-64   A Adult: 15-124

1282   ICD-10-CM 2023

Z71.52   Counseling for family member of drug abuser
Counseling for significant other, partner, or friend of drug abuser

Z71.6   Tobacco abuse counseling
Use additional code for nicotine dependence (F17.-)

Z71.7   Human immunodeficiency virus [HIV] counseling

✓5ᵗʰ **Z71.8   Other specified counseling**
EXCLUDES 2   *counseling for contraception (Z30.0-)*
AHA: 2017,4Q,27

Z71.81   Spiritual or religious counseling

Z71.82   Exercise counseling

Z71.83   Encounter for nonprocreative genetic counseling
EXCLUDES 1   *counseling for procreative genetics (Z31.5)*
counseling for procreative management (Z31.6)

Z71.84   Encounter for health counseling related to travel
Encounter for health risk and safety counseling for (international) travel
Code also, if applicable, encounter for immunization (Z23)
EXCLUDES 2   *encounter for administrative examination (Z02.-)*
encounter for other special examination without complaint, suspected or reported diagnosis (Z01.-)
AHA: 2019,4Q,20,57

Z71.85   Encounter for immunization safety counseling
Encounter for vaccine product safety counseling
Code also, if applicable, encounter for immunization (Z23)
Code also, if applicable, immunization not carried out (Z28.-)
EXCLUDES 1   *encounter for health counseling related to travel (Z71.84)*
AHA: 2021,4Q,34

● **Z71.87   Encounter for pediatric-to-adult transition counseling**
Code also chronic condition, if applicable, such as:
autism spectrum disorder (F84.0)
congenital malformations of the circulatory system (Q20-Q28)
cystic fibrosis (E84-)
sickle-cell disorder (D57-)

● **Z71.88   Encounter for counseling for socioeconomic factors**

Z71.89   Other specified counseling

Z71.9   Counseling, unspecified
Encounter for medical advice NOS

✓4ᵗʰ **Z72   Problems related to lifestyle**
EXCLUDES 2   *problems related to life-management difficulty (Z73.-)*
problems related to socioeconomic and psychosocial circumstances (Z55-Z65)

Z72.0   Tobacco use
Tobacco use NOS
EXCLUDES 1   *history of tobacco dependence (Z87.891)*
nicotine dependence (F17.2-)
tobacco dependence (F17.2-)
tobacco use during pregnancy (O99.33-)

Z72.3   Lack of physical exercise

Z72.4   Inappropriate diet and eating habits
EXCLUDES 1   *behavioral eating disorders of infancy or childhood (F98.2-F98.3)*
eating disorders (F50.-)
lack of adequate food (Z59.48)
malnutrition and other nutritional deficiencies (E40-E64)

✓5ᵗʰ **Z72.5   High risk sexual behavior**
Promiscuity
EXCLUDES 1   *paraphilias (F65)*

Z72.51   High risk heterosexual behavior

Z72.52   High risk homosexual behavior

Z72.53   High risk bisexual behavior

Z72.6   Gambling and betting
EXCLUDES 1   *compulsive or pathological gambling (F63.0)*

✓5ᵗʰ **Z72.8   Other problems related to lifestyle**

✓6ᵗʰ **Z72.81   Antisocial behavior**
EXCLUDES 1   *conduct disorders (F91.-)*

Z72.810   Child and adolescent antisocial behavior   P
Antisocial behavior (child) (adolescent) without manifest psychiatric disorder
Delinquency NOS
Group delinquency
Offenses in the context of gang membership
Stealing in company with others
Truancy from school

Z72.811   Adult antisocial behavior   A
Adult antisocial behavior without manifest psychiatric disorder

✓6ᵗʰ **Z72.82   Problems related to sleep**

Z72.820   Sleep deprivation
Lack of adequate sleep
EXCLUDES 1   *insomnia (G47.0-)*

Z72.821   Inadequate sleep hygiene
Bad sleep habits
Irregular sleep habits
Unhealthy sleep wake schedule
EXCLUDES 1   *insomnia (F51.0-, G47.0-)*

Z72.823   Risk of suffocation (smothering) under another while sleeping
Child-caregiver co-sleeping
Infant bed-sharing

Z72.89   Other problems related to lifestyle
Self-damaging behavior

Z72.9   Problem related to lifestyle, unspecified

✓4ᵗʰ **Z73   Problems related to life management difficulty**
EXCLUDES 2   *problems related to socioeconomic and psychosocial circumstances (Z55-Z65)*
DEF: State of emotional, mental, and physical exhaustion causing difficulties in managing personal, school, or work circumstances. It is usually due to prolonged stress or poor interpersonal relationship skills or parenting skills.

Z73.0   Burn-out

Z73.1   Type A behavior pattern

Z73.2   Lack of relaxation and leisure

Z73.3   Stress, not elsewhere classified
Physical and mental strain NOS
EXCLUDES 1   *stress related to employment or unemployment (Z56.-)*

Z73.4   Inadequate social skills, not elsewhere classified

Z73.5   Social role conflict, not elsewhere classified

Z73.6   Limitation of activities due to disability
EXCLUDES 1   *care-provider dependency (Z74.-)*

✓5ᵗʰ **Z73.8   Other problems related to life management difficulty**

✓6ᵗʰ **Z73.81   Behavioral insomnia of childhood**
DEF: Behaviors on the part of the child or caregivers that cause negative compliance with a child's sleep schedule resulting in lack of adequate sleep.

Z73.810   Behavioral insomnia of childhood, sleep-onset association type   P

Z73.811   Behavioral insomnia of childhood, limit setting type   P

Z73.812   Behavioral insomnia of childhood, combined type   P

Z73.819   Behavioral insomnia of childhood, unspecified type   P

Z73.82   Dual sensory impairment

Z73.89   Other problems related to life management difficulty

Z73.9   Problem related to life management difficulty, unspecified

✓4ᵗʰ **Z74   Problems related to care provider dependency**
EXCLUDES 2   *dependence on enabling machines or devices NEC (Z99.-)*

✓5ᵗʰ **Z74.0   Reduced mobility**

Z74.01   Bed confinement status
Bedridden

☑ Additional Character Required   ✓7ᵗʰ Placeholder Alert   Manifestation   Unspecified Dx   Q QPP   UPD Unacceptable PDx

Z74.09 Other reduced mobility
   Chair ridden
   Reduced mobility NOS
   EXCLUDES 2 *wheelchair dependence (Z99.3)*

Z74.1 Need for assistance with personal care

Z74.2 Need for assistance at home and no other household member able to render care

Z74.3 Need for continuous supervision

Z74.8 Other problems related to care provider dependency

Z74.9 Problem related to care provider dependency, unspecified

☑4ᵗʰ **Z75 Problems related to medical facilities and other health care**

Z75.0 Medical services not available in home
   EXCLUDES 1 *no other household member able to render care (Z74.2)*

Z75.1 Person awaiting admission **to adequate facility elsewhere**

Z75.2 Other waiting period for investigation and treatment

Z75.3 Unavailability and inaccessibility of health-care facilities
   EXCLUDES 1 *bed unavailable (Z75.1)*

Z75.4 Unavailability and inaccessibility of other helping agencies

Z75.5 Holiday relief care

Z75.8 Other problems related to medical facilities and other health care

Z75.9 Unspecified problem related to medical facilities and other health care

☑4ᵗʰ **Z76 Persons encountering health services in other circumstances**

Z76.0 Encounter for issue of repeat prescription
   Encounter for issue of repeat prescription for appliance
   Encounter for issue of repeat prescription for medicaments
   Encounter for issue of repeat prescription for spectacles
   EXCLUDES 2 *issue of medical certificate (Z02.7)*
          repeat prescription for contraceptive (Z30.4-)

Z76.1 Encounter for health supervision and care of foundling PDx

Z76.2 Encounter for health supervision and care of other healthy infant and child PDx P
   Encounter for medical or nursing care or supervision of healthy infant under circumstances such as adverse socioeconomic conditions at home
   Encounter for medical or nursing care or supervision of healthy infant under circumstances such as awaiting foster or adoptive placement
   Encounter for medical or nursing care or supervision of healthy infant under circumstances such as maternal illness
   Encounter for medical or nursing care or supervision of healthy infant under circumstances such as number of children at home preventing or interfering with normal care

Z76.3 Healthy person accompanying sick person

Z76.4 Other boarder to healthcare facility
   EXCLUDES 1 *homelessness (Z59.0-)*

Z76.5 Malingerer [conscious simulation]
   Person feigning illness (with obvious motivation)
   EXCLUDES 1 *factitious disorder (F68.1-, F68.A)*
          peregrinating patient (F68.1-)
   DEF: Act of intentionally exaggerating an illness or disability in order to receive personal gain or to avoid punishment or responsibility.

☑5ᵗʰ **Z76.8 Persons encountering health services in other specified circumstances**

Z76.81 Expectant parent(s) prebirth pediatrician visit
   Pre-adoption pediatrician visit for adoptive parent(s)

Z76.82 Awaiting organ transplant status
   Patient waiting for organ availability

Z76.89 Persons encountering health services in other specified circumstances
   Persons encountering health services NOS
   AHA: 2014,2Q,10

Persons with potential health hazards related to family and personal history and certain conditions influencing health status (Z77-Z99)

Code also any follow-up examination (Z08-Z09)

☑4ᵗʰ **Z77 Other contact with and (suspected) exposures hazardous to health**
   INCLUDES contact with and (suspected) exposures to potential hazards to health
   EXCLUDES 2 *contact with and (suspected) exposure to communicable diseases (Z20.-)*
          exposure to (parental) (environmental) tobacco smoke in the perinatal period (P96.81)
          newborn affected by noxious substances transmitted via placenta or breast milk (P04.-)
          occupational exposure to risk factors (Z57.-)
          retained foreign body (Z18.-)
          retained foreign body fully removed (Z87.821)
          toxic effects of substances chiefly nonmedicinal as to source (T51-T65)

☑5ᵗʰ **Z77.0 Contact with and (suspected) exposure to** hazardous, chiefly nonmedicinal, **chemicals**

☑6ᵗʰ **Z77.01 Contact with and (suspected) exposure to hazardous** metals

Z77.010 Contact with and (suspected) exposure to arsenic

Z77.011 Contact with and (suspected) exposure to lead

Z77.012 Contact with and (suspected) exposure to uranium
   EXCLUDES 1 *retained depleted uranium fragments (Z18.01)*

Z77.018 Contact with and (suspected) exposure to other hazardous metals
   Contact with and (suspected) exposure to chromium compounds
   Contact with and (suspected) exposure to nickel dust

☑6ᵗʰ **Z77.02 Contact with and (suspected) exposure to hazardous** aromatic compounds

Z77.020 Contact with and (suspected) exposure to aromatic amines

Z77.021 Contact with and (suspected) exposure to benzene

Z77.028 Contact with and (suspected) exposure to other hazardous aromatic compounds
   Aromatic dyes NOS
   Polycyclic aromatic hydrocarbons

☑6ᵗʰ **Z77.09 Contact with and (suspected) exposure to other hazardous, chiefly** nonmedicinal, **chemicals**

Z77.090 Contact with and (suspected) exposure to asbestos

Z77.098 Contact with and (suspected) exposure to other hazardous, chiefly nonmedicinal, chemicals
   Dyes NOS

☑5ᵗʰ **Z77.1 Contact with and (suspected) exposure to** environmental pollution and hazards in the physical environment

☑6ᵗʰ **Z77.11 Contact with and (suspected) exposure to** environmental pollution

Z77.110 Contact with and (suspected) exposure to air **pollution**

Z77.111 Contact with and (suspected) exposure to water **pollution**

Z77.112 Contact with and (suspected) exposure to soil **pollution**

Z77.118 Contact with and (suspected) exposure to other environmental pollution

☑6ᵗʰ **Z77.12 Contact with and (suspected) exposure to** hazards in the physical environment

Z77.120 Contact with and (suspected) exposure to mold **(toxic)**

Z77.121 **Contact with and (suspected) exposure to** harmful algae and algae toxins
Contact with and (suspected) exposure to (harmful) algae bloom NOS
Contact with and (suspected) exposure to blue-green algae bloom
Contact with and (suspected) exposure to brown tide
Contact with and (suspected) exposure to cyanobacteria bloom
Contact with and (suspected) exposure to Florida red tide
Contact with and (suspected) exposure to pfiesteria piscicida
Contact with and (suspected) exposure to red tide

Z77.122 **Contact with and (suspected) exposure to** noise

Z77.123 **Contact with and (suspected) exposure to** radon and other naturally occurring radiation
EXCLUDES 2   *radiation exposure as the cause of a confirmed condition (W88-W90, X39.0-)*
radiation sickness NOS (T66)

Z77.128 **Contact with and (suspected) exposure to other hazards in the physical environment**

✓5ᵗʰ **Z77.2** **Contact with and (suspected) exposure to other hazardous substances**

Z77.21 **Contact with and (suspected) exposure to potentially hazardous** body fluids

Z77.22 **Contact with and (suspected) exposure to** environmental tobacco smoke **(acute) (chronic)**
Exposure to second hand tobacco smoke (acute) (chronic)
Passive smoking (acute) (chronic)
EXCLUDES 1   *nicotine dependence (F17.-)*
tobacco use (Z72.0)
EXCLUDES 2   *occupational exposure to environmental tobacco smoke (Z57.31)*

Z77.29 **Contact with and (suspected) exposure to other hazardous substances**
AHA: 2016,2Q,33

Z77.9 **Other contact with and (suspected) exposures hazardous to health**

✓4ᵗʰ **Z78** **Other specified health status**
EXCLUDES 2   *asymptomatic human immunodeficiency virus [HIV] infection status (Z21)*
postprocedural status (Z93-Z99)
sex reassignment status (Z87.890)

Z78.0 **Asymptomatic menopausal state**   A ♀
Menopausal state NOS
Postmenopausal status NOS
EXCLUDES 2   *symptomatic menopausal state (N95.1)*

Z78.1 **Physical restraint status**
EXCLUDES 1   *physical restraint due to a procedure - omit code*
DEF: Application of mechanical restraining devices or manual restraints to limit physical mobility of a patient.

Z78.9 **Other specified health status**

✓4ᵗʰ **Z79** **Long term (current) drug therapy**
INCLUDES   long term (current) drug use for prophylactic purposes
Code also any therapeutic drug level monitoring (Z51.81)
EXCLUDES 2   *drug abuse and dependence (F11-F19)*
drug use complicating pregnancy, childbirth, and the puerperium (O99.32-)
AHA: 2021,1Q,12

✓5ᵗʰ **Z79.0** **Long term (current) use of anticoagulants and antithrombotics/antiplatelets**
EXCLUDES 2   *long term (current) use of aspirin (Z79.82)*

Z79.01 **Long term (current) use of** anticoagulants
AHA: 2022,2Q,17; 2021,1Q,4; 2020,2Q,20

Z79.02 **Long term (current) use of** antithrombotics/antiplatelets   UPD

Z79.1 **Long term (current) use of** non-steroidal anti-inflammatories (NSAID)   UPD
EXCLUDES 2   *long term (current) use of aspirin (Z79.82)*

Z79.2 **Long term (current) use of** antibiotics   UPD

Z79.3 **Long term (current) use of** hormonal contraceptives
Long term (current) use of birth control pill or patch

Z79.4 **Long term (current) use of** insulin   HCC Rx ESR COM
EXCLUDES 2   ▶*long-term (current) use of injectable non-insulin antidiabetic drugs (Z79.85)*◀
long term (current) use of oral antidiabetic drugs (Z79.84)
long term (current) use of oral hypoglycemic drugs (Z79.84)
AHA: 2020,3Q,31

✓5ᵗʰ **Z79.5** **Long term (current) use of steroids**

Z79.51 **Long term (current) use of** inhaled steroids   UPD

Z79.52 **Long term (current) use of** systemic steroids   UPD

✓5ᵗʰ **Z79.6** **Long term (current) use of immunomodulators and immunosuppressants**
EXCLUDES 2   *long term (current) use of steroids (Z79.5-)*
long term (current) use of agents affecting estrogen receptors and estrogen levels (Z79.81-)

Z79.60 **Long term (current) use of unspecified immunomodulators and immunosuppressants**

Z79.61 **Long term (current) use of** immunomodulator
Long term (current) use of apremilast
Long term (current) use of immunomodulatory imide drug
Long term (current) use of lenalidomide
Long term (current) use of pomalidomide

✓6ᵗʰ **Z79.62** **Long term (current) use of** immunosuppressant

Z79.620 **Long term (current) use of immunosuppressive biologic**
Long term (current) use of adalimumab
Long term (current) use of etanercept
Long term (current) use of infliximab
Long term (current) use of monoclonal antibodies

Z79.621 **Long term (current) use of** calcineurin inhibitor
Long term (current) use of cyclosporine
Long term (current) use of tacrolimus

Z79.622 **Long term (current) use of** Janus kinase inhibitor
Long term (current) use of tofacitinib

Z79.623 **Long term (current) use of** mammalian target of rapamycin (mTOR) inhibitor
Long term (current) use of sirolimus

Z79.624 **Long term (current) use of** inhibitors of nucleotide synthesis
Long term (current) use of azathioprine
Long term (current) use omycophenolate
Long term (current) use of purine synthesis (IMDH) inhibitors

✓6ᵗʰ **Z79.63** **Long term (current) use of chemotherapeutic agent**

Z79.630 **Long term (current) use of** alkylating agent
Long term (current) use of chlorambucil
Long term (current) use of cisplatin
Long term (current) use of cyclophosphamide

Z79.631 **Long term (current) use of** antimetabolite agent
Long term (current) use of 5-fluorouracil
Long term (current) use of 6-mercaptopurine
Long term (current) use of cytarabine
Long term (current) use of methotrexate

Z79.632 **Long term (current) use of** antitumor antibiotic
Long term (current) use of bleomycin
Long term (current) use of doxorubicin
Long term (current) use of mitomycin C

Z79.633 **Long term (current) use of** mitotic inhibitor
Long term (current) use of paclitaxel
Long term (current) use of plant alkaloids
Long term (current) use of vinblastine
Long term (current) use of vincristine

✅ Additional Character Required   ✓x7ᵗʰ Placeholder Alert   Manifestation   Unspecified Dx   Q QPP   UPD Unacceptable PDx

- **Z79.634** **Long term (current) use of** topoisomerase inhibitor
  - Long term (current) use of etoposide
  - Long term (current) use of irinotecan
  - Long term (current) use of topotecan
- **Z79.64** **Long term (current) use of** myelosuppressive agent
  - Long term (current) use of hydroxyurea
- **Z79.69** **Long term (current) use of other immunomodulators and immunosuppressants**
- √5ᵗʰ **Z79.8** **Other long term (current) drug therapy**
  - √6ᵗʰ **Z79.81** **Long term (current) use of agents affecting estrogen receptors and estrogen levels**
    - Code first, if applicable:
      - malignant neoplasm of breast (C50.-)
      - malignant neoplasm of prostate (C61)
    - Use additional code, if applicable, to identify:
      - estrogen receptor positive status (Z17.0)
      - family history of breast cancer (Z80.3)
      - genetic susceptibility to malignant neoplasm (cancer) (Z15.0-)
      - personal history of breast cancer (Z85.3)
      - personal history of prostate cancer (Z85.46)
      - postmenopausal status (Z78.0)
    - *EXCLUDES 1* hormone replacement therapy (Z79.890)
    - **Z79.810** **Long term (current) use of selective estrogen receptor modulators (SERMs)** UPD
      - Long term (current) use of raloxifene (Evista)
      - Long term (current) use of tamoxifen (Nolvadex)
      - Long term (current) use of toremifene (Fareston)
    - **Z79.811** **Long term (current) use of** aromatase inhibitors UPD
      - Long term (current) use of anastrozole (Arimidex)
      - Long term (current) use of exemestane (Aromasin)
      - Long term (current) use of letrozole (Femara)
    - **Z79.818** **Long term (current) use of other agents affecting estrogen receptors and estrogen levels** UPD
      - Long term (current) use of estrogen receptor downregulators
      - Long term (current) use of fulvestrant (Faslodex)
      - Long term (current) use of gonadotropin-releasing hormone (GnRH) agonist
      - Long term (current) use of goserelin acetate (Zoladex)
      - Long term (current) use of leuprolide acetate (leuprorelin) (Lupron)
      - Long term (current) use of megestrol acetate (Megace)
  - **Z79.82** **Long term (current) use of** aspirin
  - **Z79.83** **Long term (current) use of** bisphosphonates UPD
    - **AHA:** 2016,4Q,42
  - **Z79.84** **Long term (current) use of** oral hypoglycemic drugs UPD
    - Long term (current) use of oral antidiabetic drugs
    - *EXCLUDES 2* ▶long-term (current) use of injectable non-insulin antidiabetic drugs (Z79.85)◄
      - long term (current) use of insulin (Z79.4)
    - **AHA:** 2020,3Q,31; 2016,4Q,76
- **Z79.85** **Long-term (current) use of** injectable non-insulin antidiabetic drugs
  - *EXCLUDES 2* long term (current) use of insulin (Z79.4)
    - long term (current) use of oral hypoglycemic drugs (Z79.84)
  - √6ᵗʰ **Z79.89** **Other long term (current) drug therapy**
    - **Z79.890** Hormone replacement therapy UPD

- **Z79.891** **Long term (current) use of** opiate analgesic
  - Long term (current) use of methadone for pain management
  - *EXCLUDES 1* methadone use NOS (F11.9-)
    - use of methadone for treatment of heroin addiction (F11.2-)
- **Z79.899** **Other long term (current) drug therapy**
  - **AHA:** 2020,4Q,11; 2020,3Q,31; 2020,2Q,14; 2015,4Q,34; 2015,3Q,21

√4ᵗʰ **Z80** **Family history of primary malignant neoplasm**
- **Z80.0** **Family history of malignant neoplasm of** digestive organs UPD
  - Conditions classifiable to C15-C26
  - **AHA:** 2018,1Q,6
- **Z80.1** **Family history of malignant neoplasm of** trachea, bronchus and lung UPD
  - Conditions classifiable to C33-C34
- **Z80.2** **Family history of malignant neoplasm of other respiratory and intrathoracic organs** UPD
  - Conditions classifiable to C30-C32, C37-C39
- **Z80.3** **Family history of malignant neoplasm of** breast UPD
  - Conditions classifiable to C50.-
- √5ᵗʰ **Z80.4** **Family history of malignant neoplasm of genital organs**
  - Conditions classifiable to C51-C63
  - **Z80.41** **Family history of malignant neoplasm of** ovary UPD
  - **Z80.42** **Family history of malignant neoplasm of** prostate UPD
  - **Z80.43** **Family history of malignant neoplasm of** testis UPD
  - **Z80.49** **Family history of malignant neoplasm of other** genital organs UPD
- √5ᵗʰ **Z80.5** **Family history of malignant neoplasm of urinary tract**
  - Conditions classifiable to C64-C68
  - **Z80.51** **Family history of malignant neoplasm of** kidney UPD
  - **Z80.52** **Family history of malignant neoplasm of** bladder UPD
  - **Z80.59** **Family history of malignant neoplasm of other** urinary tract organ UPD
- **Z80.6** **Family history of** leukemia UPD
  - Conditions classifiable to C91-C95
- **Z80.7** **Family history of other malignant neoplasms of** lymphoid, hematopoietic and related tissues UPD
  - Conditions classifiable to C81-C90, C96.-
- **Z80.8** **Family history of malignant neoplasm of other organs or systems** UPD
  - Conditions classifiable to C00-C14, C40-C49, C69-C79
- **Z80.9** **Family history of malignant neoplasm, unspecified** UPD
  - Conditions classifiable to C80.1

√4ᵗʰ **Z81** **Family history of mental and behavioral disorders**
- **Z81.0** **Family history of** intellectual disabilities
  - Conditions classifiable to F70-F79
- **Z81.1** **Family history of** alcohol abuse and dependence
  - Conditions classifiable to F10.-
- **Z81.2** **Family history of** tobacco abuse and dependence
  - Conditions classifiable to F17.-
- **Z81.3** **Family history of other psychoactive substance abuse and dependence**
  - Conditions classifiable to F11-F16, F18-F19
- **Z81.4** **Family history of other substance abuse and dependence**
  - Conditions classifiable to F55
- **Z81.8** **Family history of other mental and behavioral disorders**
  - Conditions classifiable elsewhere in F01-F99

√4ᵗʰ **Z82** **Family history of certain disabilities and chronic diseases (leading to disablement)**
- **Z82.0** **Family history of** epilepsy and other diseases of the nervous system UPD
  - Conditions classifiable to G00-G99
- **Z82.1** **Family history of** blindness and visual loss UPD
  - Conditions classifiable to H54.-
- **Z82.2** **Family history of** deafness and hearing loss UPD
  - Conditions classifiable to H90-H91

Z82.3   **Family history of** stroke   `UPD`
Conditions classifiable to I60-I64

√5ᵗʰ   **Z82.4**   **Family history of ischemic heart disease and other diseases of the circulatory system**
Conditions classifiable to I00-I5A, I65-I99

   Z82.41   **Family history of** sudden cardiac death   `UPD`
   Z82.49   **Family history of** ischemic heart disease **and other diseases of the circulatory system**   `UPD`

Z82.5   **Family history of** asthma **and other chronic lower respiratory diseases**   `UPD`
Conditions classifiable to J40-J47
EXCLUDES 2   family history of other diseases of the respiratory system (Z83.6)

√5ᵗʰ   **Z82.6**   **Family history of arthritis and other diseases of the musculoskeletal system and connective tissue**
Conditions classifiable to M00-M99

   Z82.61   **Family history of** arthritis   `UPD`
   Z82.62   **Family history of** osteoporosis   `UPD`
   Z82.69   **Family history of other diseases of the musculoskeletal system and connective tissue**   `UPD`

√5ᵗʰ   **Z82.7**   **Family history of congenital malformations, deformations and chromosomal abnormalities**
Conditions classifiable to Q00-Q99

   Z82.71   **Family history of** polycystic kidney   `UPD`
   Z82.79   **Family history of other congenital malformations, deformations and chromosomal abnormalities**   `UPD`

Z82.8   **Family history of other disabilities and chronic diseases leading to disablement, not elsewhere classified**   `UPD`

√4ᵗʰ   **Z83**   **Family history of other specific disorders**
EXCLUDES 2   contact with and (suspected) exposure to communicable disease in the family (Z20.-)

Z83.0   **Family history of** human immunodeficiency virus **[HIV] disease**   `UPD`
Conditions classifiable to B20

Z83.1   **Family history of other infectious and parasitic diseases**   `UPD`
Conditions classifiable to A00-B19, B25-B94, B99

Z83.2   **Family history of diseases of the** blood and blood-forming organs **and certain disorders involving the immune mechanism**   `UPD`
Conditions classifiable to D50-D89

Z83.3   **Family history of** diabetes mellitus   `UPD`
Conditions classifiable to E08-E13

√5ᵗʰ   **Z83.4**   **Family history of other endocrine, nutritional and metabolic diseases**
Conditions classifiable to E00-E07, E15-E88

   Z83.41   **Family history of** multiple endocrine neoplasia **[MEN] syndrome**   `UPD`
   Z83.42   **Family history of** familial hypercholesterolemia   `UPD`
AHA: 2016,4Q,77

√6ᵗʰ   **Z83.43**   **Family history of other disorder of lipoprotein metabolism and other lipidemias**
AHA: 2018,4Q,6,35

      Z83.430   **Family history of** elevated lipoprotein(a)   `UPD`
Family history of elevated Lp(a)

      Z83.438   **Family history of other disorder of lipoprotein metabolism and other lipidemia**   `UPD`
Family history of familial combined hyperlipidemia

   Z83.49   **Family history of other endocrine, nutritional and metabolic diseases**   `UPD`

√5ᵗʰ   **Z83.5**   **Family history of eye and ear disorders**

√6ᵗʰ   **Z83.51**   **Family history of** eye **disorders**
Conditions classifiable to H00-H53, H55-H59
EXCLUDES 2   family history of blindness and visual loss (Z82.1)

      Z83.511   **Family history of** glaucoma   `UPD`
      Z83.518   **Family history of other specified eye disorder**   `UPD`

Z83.52   **Family history of** ear **disorders**   `UPD`
Conditions classifiable to H60-H83, H92-H95
EXCLUDES 2   family history of deafness and hearing loss (Z82.2)

Z83.6   **Family history of other diseases of the** respiratory system   `UPD`
Conditions classifiable to J00-J39, J60-J99
EXCLUDES 2   family history of asthma and other chronic lower respiratory diseases (Z82.5)

√5ᵗʰ   **Z83.7**   **Family history of diseases of the digestive system**
Conditions classifiable to K00-K93

   Z83.71   **Family history of** colonic polyps   `UPD`
EXCLUDES 2   family history of malignant neoplasm of digestive organs (Z80.0)
AHA: 2021,1Q,14

   Z83.79   **Family history of other diseases of the digestive system**   `UPD`

√4ᵗʰ   **Z84**   **Family history of other conditions**

Z84.0   **Family history of diseases of the** skin and subcutaneous tissue   `UPD`
Conditions classifiable to L00-L99

Z84.1   **Family history of disorders of** kidney and ureter   `UPD`
Conditions classifiable to N00-N29

Z84.2   **Family history of other diseases of the** genitourinary system   `UPD`
Conditions classifiable to N30-N99

Z84.3   **Family history of** consanguinity   `UPD`

√5ᵗʰ   **Z84.8**   **Family history of other specified conditions**

   Z84.81   **Family history of carrier of** genetic disease   `UPD`
AHA: 2021,1Q,14

   Z84.82   **Family history of** sudden infant death syndrome   `UPD`
Family history of SIDS
AHA: 2016,4Q,77

   Z84.89   **Family history of other specified conditions**   `UPD`

√4ᵗʰ   **Z85**   **Personal history of malignant neoplasm**
Code first any follow-up examination after treatment of malignant neoplasm (Z08)
Use additional code to identify:
   alcohol use and dependence (F10.-)
   exposure to environmental tobacco smoke (Z77.22)
   history of tobacco dependence (Z87.891)
   occupational exposure to environmental tobacco smoke (Z57.31)
   tobacco dependence (F17.-)
   tobacco use (Z72.0)
EXCLUDES 2   personal history of benign neoplasm (Z86.01-)
            personal history of carcinoma-in-situ (Z86.00-)
AHA: 2020,3Q,30; 2018,4Q,64

√5ᵗʰ   **Z85.0**   **Personal history of malignant neoplasm of** digestive organs
AHA: 2017,1Q,9

   Z85.00   **Personal history of malignant neoplasm of unspecified digestive organ**

   Z85.01   **Personal history of malignant neoplasm of** esophagus
Conditions classifiable to C15

√6ᵗʰ   **Z85.02**   **Personal history of malignant neoplasm of** stomach

      Z85.020   **Personal history of malignant** carcinoid tumor **of stomach**
Conditions classifiable to C7A.092

      Z85.028   **Personal history of other malignant neoplasm of stomach**
Conditions classifiable to C16

√6ᵗʰ   **Z85.03**   **Personal history of malignant neoplasm of** large intestine

      Z85.030   **Personal history of malignant** carcinoid tumor **of large intestine**
Conditions classifiable to C7A.022-C7A.025, C7A.029

      Z85.038   **Personal history of other malignant neoplasm of large intestine**
Conditions classifiable to C18

√6ᵗʰ   **Z85.04**   **Personal history of malignant neoplasm of** rectum, rectosigmoid junction, and anus

      Z85.040   **Personal history of malignant** carcinoid tumor **of rectum**
Conditions classifiable to C7A.026

Z85.Ø48 **Personal history of other malignant neoplasm of rectum, rectosigmoid junction, and anus**
Conditions classifiable to C19-C21

Z85.Ø5 **Personal history of malignant neoplasm of** liver
Conditions classifiable to C22

✓6ᵗʰ Z85.Ø6 **Personal history of malignant neoplasm of** small intestine

Z85.Ø6Ø **Personal history of malignant** carcinoid tumor of small intestine
Conditions classifiable to C7A.Ø1-

Z85.Ø68 **Personal history of other malignant neoplasm of small intestine**
Conditions classifiable to C17

Z85.Ø7 **Personal history of malignant neoplasm of** pancreas
Conditions classifiable to C25

Z85.Ø9 **Personal history of malignant neoplasm of other digestive organs**

✓5ᵗʰ Z85.1 **Personal history of malignant neoplasm of** trachea, bronchus and lung

✓6ᵗʰ Z85.11 **Personal history of malignant neoplasm of** bronchus and lung

Z85.11Ø **Personal history of malignant** carcinoid tumor of bronchus and lung
Conditions classifiable to C7A.Ø9Ø

Z85.118 **Personal history of other malignant neoplasm of bronchus and lung**
Conditions classifiable to C34

Z85.12 **Personal history of malignant neoplasm of** trachea
Conditions classifiable to C33

✓5ᵗʰ Z85.2 **Personal history of malignant neoplasm of other** respiratory and intrathoracic organs

Z85.2Ø **Personal history of malignant neoplasm of unspecified respiratory organ**

Z85.21 **Personal history of malignant neoplasm of** larynx
Conditions classifiable to C32

Z85.22 **Personal history of malignant neoplasm of** nasal cavities, middle ear, and accessory sinuses
Conditions classifiable to C3Ø-C31

✓6ᵗʰ Z85.23 **Personal history of malignant neoplasm of** thymus

Z85.23Ø **Personal history of malignant** carcinoid tumor of thymus
Conditions classifiable to C7A.Ø91

Z85.238 **Personal history of other malignant neoplasm of thymus**
Conditions classifiable to C37

Z85.29 **Personal history of malignant neoplasm of other respiratory and intrathoracic organs**

Z85.3 **Personal history of malignant neoplasm of** breast
Conditions classifiable to C5Ø.-

✓5ᵗʰ Z85.4 **Personal history of malignant neoplasm of** genital organs
Conditions classifiable to C51-C63

Z85.4Ø **Personal history of malignant neoplasm of unspecified** female **genital organ** ♀

Z85.41 **Personal history of malignant neoplasm of** cervix uteri ♀

Z85.42 **Personal history of malignant neoplasm of other parts of uterus** ♀

Z85.43 **Personal history of malignant neoplasm of** ovary ♀

Z85.44 **Personal history of malignant neoplasm of other** female **genital organs** ♀

Z85.45 **Personal history of malignant neoplasm of unspecified** male **genital organ** ♂

Z85.46 **Personal history of malignant neoplasm of** prostate ♂

Z85.47 **Personal history of malignant neoplasm of** testis ♂

Z85.48 **Personal history of malignant neoplasm of** epididymis ♂

Z85.49 **Personal history of malignant neoplasm of other** male **genital organs** ♂

✓5ᵗʰ Z85.5 **Personal history of malignant neoplasm of** urinary tract
Conditions classifiable to C64-C68

Z85.5Ø **Personal history of malignant neoplasm of unspecified urinary tract organ**

Z85.51 **Personal history of malignant neoplasm of** bladder

✓6ᵗʰ Z85.52 **Personal history of malignant neoplasm of** kidney
EXCLUDES 1   personal history of malignant neoplasm of renal pelvis (Z85.53)

Z85.52Ø **Personal history of malignant** carcinoid tumor **of kidney**
Conditions classifiable to C7A.Ø93

Z85.528 **Personal history of other malignant neoplasm of kidney**
Conditions classifiable to C64

Z85.53 **Personal history of malignant neoplasm of** renal pelvis

Z85.54 **Personal history of malignant neoplasm of** ureter

Z85.59 **Personal history of malignant neoplasm of other urinary tract organ**

Z85.6 **Personal history of** leukemia
Conditions classifiable to C91-C95
EXCLUDES 1   leukemia in remission C91.Ø-C95.9 with 5th character 1

✓5ᵗʰ Z85.7 **Personal history of other malignant neoplasms of lymphoid, hematopoietic and related tissues**

Z85.71 **Personal history of** Hodgkin lymphoma
Conditions classifiable to C81

Z85.72 **Personal history of** non-Hodgkin lymphomas
Conditions classifiable to C82-C85

Z85.79 **Personal history of other malignant neoplasms of lymphoid, hematopoietic and related tissues**
Conditions classifiable to C88-C9Ø, C96
EXCLUDES 1   multiple myeloma in remission (C9Ø.Ø1)
plasma cell leukemia in remission (C9Ø.11)
plasmacytoma in remission (C9Ø.21)

✓5ᵗʰ Z85.8 **Personal history of malignant neoplasms of other organs and systems**
Conditions classifiable to CØØ-C14, C4Ø-C49, C69-C75, C7A.Ø98, C76-C79

✓6ᵗʰ Z85.81 **Personal history of malignant neoplasm of** lip, oral cavity, and pharynx
Conditions classifiable to CØØ-C14

Z85.81Ø **Personal history of malignant neoplasm of tongue**

Z85.818 **Personal history of malignant neoplasm of other sites of lip, oral cavity, and pharynx**

Z85.819 **Personal history of malignant neoplasm of unspecified site of lip, oral cavity, and pharynx**

✓6ᵗʰ Z85.82 **Personal history of malignant neoplasm of** skin

Z85.82Ø **Personal history of malignant** melanoma of skin
Conditions classifiable to C43

Z85.821 **Personal history of** Merkel cell carcinoma
Conditions classifiable to C4A

Z85.828 **Personal history of other malignant neoplasm of skin**
Conditions classifiable to C44

✓6ᵗʰ Z85.83 **Personal history of malignant neoplasm of** bone and soft tissue
Conditions classifiable to C4Ø-C41; C45-C49

Z85.83Ø **Personal history of malignant neoplasm of bone**

Z85.831 **Personal history of malignant neoplasm of soft tissue**
EXCLUDES 2   personal history of malignant neoplasm of skin (Z85.82-)

✓6ᵗʰ Z85.84 **Personal history of malignant neoplasm of** eye and nervous tissue
Conditions classifiable to C69-C72

Z85.84Ø **Personal history of malignant neoplasm of eye**

Z85.841 **Personal history of malignant neoplasm of brain**

Z85.848 **Personal history of malignant neoplasm of other parts of nervous tissue**

✓6ᵗʰ Z85.85 **Personal history of malignant neoplasm of** endocrine glands
Conditions classifiable to C73-C75

Z85.85Ø **Personal history of malignant neoplasm of thyroid**

Z85.858 **Personal history of malignant neoplasm of other endocrine glands**

Z85.89   **Personal history of malignant neoplasm of other organs and systems**
Conditions classifiable to C7A.098, C76, C77-C79

Z85.9   **Personal history of malignant neoplasm, unspecified**
Conditions classifiable to C7A.00, C80.1

✓4th **Z86**   **Personal history of certain other diseases**
Code first any follow-up examination after treatment (Z09)

✓5th **Z86.0**   **Personal history of in-situ and benign neoplasms and neoplasms of uncertain behavior**
EXCLUDES 2   personal history of malignant neoplasms (Z85.-)
AHA: 2017,1Q,9

✓6th **Z86.00**   **Personal history of in-situ neoplasm**
Conditions classifiable to D00-D09
AHA: 2019,4Q,20

Z86.000   **Personal history of in-situ neoplasm of breast**
Conditions classifiable to D05

Z86.001   **Personal history of in-situ neoplasm of cervix uteri**   ♀
Conditions classifiable to D06
Personal history of cervical intraepithelial neoplasia III [CIN III]

Z86.002   **Personal history of in-situ neoplasm of other and unspecified genital organs**
Conditions classifiable to D07
Personal history of high-grade prostatic intraepithelial neoplasia III [HGPIN III]
Personal history of vaginal intraepithelial neoplasia III [VAIN III]
Personal history of vulvar intraepithelial neoplasia III [VIN III]

Z86.003   **Personal history of in-situ neoplasm of oral cavity, esophagus and stomach**
Conditions classifiable to D00

Z86.004   **Personal history of in-situ neoplasm of other and unspecified digestive organs**
Conditions classifiable to D01
Personal history of anal intraepithelial neoplasia (AIN III)

Z86.005   **Personal history of in-situ neoplasm of middle ear and respiratory system**
Conditions classifiable to D02

Z86.006   **Personal history of melanoma in-situ**
Conditions classifiable to D03
EXCLUDES 2   sites other than skin - code to personal history of in-situ neoplasm of the site

Z86.007   **Personal history of in-situ neoplasm of skin**
Conditions classifiable to D04
Personal history of carcinoma in situ of skin

Z86.008   **Personal history of in-situ neoplasm of other site**
Conditions classifiable to D09

✓6th **Z86.01**   **Personal history of benign neoplasm**

Z86.010   **Personal history of colonic polyps**
AHA: 2021,1Q,14; 2017,1Q,14

Z86.011   **Personal history of benign neoplasm of the brain**

Z86.012   **Personal history of benign carcinoid tumor**

Z86.018   **Personal history of other benign neoplasm**
AHA: 2017,1Q,14

Z86.03   **Personal history of neoplasm of uncertain behavior**

✓5th **Z86.1**   **Personal history of infectious and parasitic diseases**
Conditions classifiable to A00-B89, B99
EXCLUDES 1   personal history of infectious diseases specific to a body system
sequelae of infectious and parasitic diseases (B90-B94)

Z86.11   **Personal history of tuberculosis**

Z86.12   **Personal history of poliomyelitis**

Z86.13   **Personal history of malaria**

Z86.14   **Personal history of Methicillin resistant Staphylococcus aureus infection**
Personal history of MRSA infection

Z86.15   **Personal history of latent tuberculosis infection**

Z86.16   **Personal history of COVID-19**   UPD
EXCLUDES 1   post COVID-19 condition (U09.9)
AHA: 2021,4Q,107-108; 2021,1Q,28-29,33-35,40-41,44-45

Z86.19   **Personal history of other infectious and parasitic diseases**
AHA: 2021,1Q,33-34,40; 2020,3Q,13; 2020,2Q,10,12

Z86.2   **Personal history of diseases of the blood and blood-forming organs and certain disorders involving the immune mechanism**
Conditions classifiable to D50-D89

✓5th **Z86.3**   **Personal history of endocrine, nutritional and metabolic diseases**
Conditions classifiable to E00-E88

Z86.31   **Personal history of diabetic foot ulcer**
EXCLUDES 2   current diabetic foot ulcer (E08.621, E09.621, E10.621, E11.621, E13.621)

Z86.32   **Personal history of gestational diabetes**   ♀
Personal history of conditions classifiable to O24.4-
EXCLUDES 1   gestational diabetes mellitus in current pregnancy (O24.4-)

Z86.39   **Personal history of other endocrine, nutritional and metabolic disease**
AHA: 2020,1Q,12

✓5th **Z86.5**   **Personal history of mental and behavioral disorders**
Conditions classifiable to F40-F59

Z86.51   **Personal history of combat and operational stress reaction**   A

Z86.59   **Personal history of other mental and behavioral disorders**

✓5th **Z86.6**   **Personal history of diseases of the nervous system and sense organs**
Conditions classifiable to G00-G99, H00-H95

Z86.61   **Personal history of infections of the central nervous system**
Personal history of encephalitis
Personal history of meningitis

Z86.69   **Personal history of other diseases of the nervous system and sense organs**
AHA: 2016,4Q,24

✓5th **Z86.7**   **Personal history of diseases of the circulatory system**
Conditions classifiable to I00-I99
EXCLUDES 2   old myocardial infarction (I25.2)
personal history of anaphylactic shock (Z87.892)
postmyocardial infarction syndrome (I24.1)

✓6th **Z86.71**   **Personal history of venous thrombosis and embolism**

Z86.711   **Personal history of pulmonary embolism**

Z86.718   **Personal history of other venous thrombosis and embolism**
AHA: 2020,2Q,20

Z86.72   **Personal history of thrombophlebitis**

Z86.73   **Personal history of transient ischemic attack (TIA), and cerebral infarction without residual deficits**
Personal history of prolonged reversible ischemic neurological deficit (PRIND)
Personal history of stroke NOS without residual deficits
EXCLUDES 1   personal history of traumatic brain injury (Z87.820)
sequelae of cerebrovascular disease (I69.-)
AHA: 2012,4Q,92

Z86.74   **Personal history of sudden cardiac arrest**
Personal history of sudden cardiac death successfully resuscitated

Z86.79   **Personal history of other diseases of the circulatory system**
AHA: 2022,2Q,14; 2020,1Q,12

✓4th **Z87**   **Personal history of other diseases and conditions**
Code first any follow-up examination after treatment (Z09)

✓5th **Z87.0**   **Personal history of diseases of the respiratory system**
Conditions classifiable to J00-J99

Z87.01   **Personal history of pneumonia (recurrent)**

Z87.09   **Personal history of other diseases of the respiratory system**

✓5th **Z87.1**   **Personal history of diseases of the digestive system**
Conditions classifiable to K00-K93

Z87.11   **Personal history of peptic ulcer disease**

Z87.19 Personal history of other diseases of the digestive system
AHA: 2017,1Q,14

Z87.2 Personal history of diseases of the skin and subcutaneous tissue
Conditions classifiable to L00-L99
EXCLUDES 2 personal history of diabetic foot ulcer (Z86.31)

√5ᵗʰ **Z87.3 Personal history of diseases of the musculoskeletal system and connective tissue**
Conditions classifiable to M00-M99
EXCLUDES 2 personal history of (healed) traumatic fracture (Z87.81)

√6ᵗʰ **Z87.31 Personal history of (healed) nontraumatic fracture**

Z87.310 Personal history of (healed) osteoporosis fracture
Personal history of (healed) fragility fracture
Personal history of (healed) collapsed vertebra due to osteoporosis
TIP: Assign for history of osteoporosis fractures that have resolved, even when a code from category M80 indicating current osteoporosis fracture is also reported.

Z87.311 Personal history of (healed) other pathological fracture
Personal history of (healed) collapsed vertebra NOS
EXCLUDES 2 personal history of osteoporosis fracture (Z87.310)

Z87.312 Personal history of (healed) stress fracture
Personal history of (healed) fatigue fracture

Z87.39 Personal history of other diseases of the musculoskeletal system and connective tissue

√5ᵗʰ **Z87.4 Personal history of diseases of the genitourinary system**
Conditions classifiable to N00-N99

√6ᵗʰ **Z87.41 Personal history of dysplasia of the female genital tract**
EXCLUDES 1 personal history of intraepithelial neoplasia III of female genital tract (Z86.001, Z86.008)
personal history of malignant neoplasm of female genital tract (Z85.40-Z85.44)

Z87.410 Personal history of cervical dysplasia ♀

Z87.411 Personal history of vaginal dysplasia ♀

Z87.412 Personal history of vulvar dysplasia ♀

Z87.42 Personal history of other diseases of the female genital tract ♀

√6ᵗʰ **Z87.43 Personal history of diseases of the male genital organs**

Z87.430 Personal history of prostatic dysplasia ♂
EXCLUDES 1 personal history of malignant neoplasm of prostate (Z85.46)

Z87.438 Personal history of other diseases of male genital organs ♂

√6ᵗʰ **Z87.44 Personal history of diseases of the urinary system**
EXCLUDES 1 personal history of malignant neoplasm of cervix uteri (Z85.41)

Z87.440 Personal history of urinary (tract) infections

Z87.441 Personal history of nephrotic syndrome

Z87.442 Personal history of urinary calculi
Personal history of kidney stones

Z87.448 Personal history of other diseases of urinary system

√5ᵗʰ **Z87.5 Personal history of complications of pregnancy, childbirth and the puerperium**
Conditions classifiable to O00-O9A
EXCLUDES 2 recurrent pregnancy loss (N96)

Z87.51 Personal history of pre-term labor ♀
EXCLUDES 1 current pregnancy with history of pre-term labor (O09.21-)

Z87.59 Personal history of other complications of pregnancy, childbirth and the puerperium ♀
Personal history of trophoblastic disease

√5ᵗʰ **Z87.6 Personal history of certain (corrected) conditions arising in the perinatal period**
Conditions classifiable to P00-P96
EXCLUDES 1 personal history of (corrected) congenital malformations (Z87.7-)

Z87.61 Personal history of (corrected) necrotizing enterocolitis of newborn

Z87.68 Personal history of other (corrected) conditions arising in the perinatal period

√5ᵗʰ **Z87.7 Personal history of (corrected) congenital malformations**
Conditions classifiable to Q00-Q89 that have been repaired or corrected
AHA: 2013,1Q,
EXCLUDES 1 congenital malformations that have been partially corrected or repair but which still require medical treatment – code to condition
EXCLUDES 2 ▶congenital malformations that have been partially corrected or repaired but which still require medical treatment - code to condition◀
other postprocedural states (Z98.-)
personal history of medical treatment (Z92.-)
presence of cardiac and vascular implants and grafts (Z95.-)
presence of other devices (Z97.-)
presence of other functional implants (Z96.-)
transplanted organ and tissue status (Z94.-)

√6ᵗʰ **Z87.71 Personal history of (corrected) congenital malformations of genitourinary system**

Z87.710 Personal history of (corrected) hypospadias ♂

Z87.718 Personal history of other specified (corrected) congenital malformations of genitourinary system

√6ᵗʰ **Z87.72 Personal history of (corrected) congenital malformations of nervous system and sense organs**

Z87.720 Personal history of (corrected) congenital malformations of eye

Z87.721 Personal history of (corrected) congenital malformations of ear

Z87.728 Personal history of other specified (corrected) congenital malformations of nervous system and sense organs

√6ᵗʰ **Z87.73 Personal history of (corrected) congenital malformations of digestive system**

Z87.730 Personal history of (corrected) cleft lip and palate

Z87.731 Personal history of (corrected) tracheoesophageal fistula or atresia

Z87.732 Personal history of (corrected) persistent cloaca or cloacal malformations

Z87.738 Personal history of other specified (corrected) congenital malformations of digestive system

Z87.74 Personal history of (corrected) congenital malformations of heart and circulatory system

Z87.75 Personal history of (corrected) congenital malformations of respiratory system

√6ᵗʰ **Z87.76 Personal history of (corrected) congenital malformations of integument, limbs and musculoskeletal system**

Z87.760 Personal history of (corrected) congenital diaphragmatic hernia or other congenital diaphragm malformations

Z87.761 Personal history of (corrected) gastroschisis

Z87.762 Personal history of (corrected) prune belly malformation

Z87.763 Personal history of other (corrected) congenital abdominal wall malformations

Z87.768 Personal history of other specified (corrected) congenital malformations of integument, limbs and musculoskeletal system

√6ᵗʰ **Z87.79 Personal history of other (corrected) congenital malformations**

Z87.790 Personal history of (corrected) congenital malformations of face and neck

Z87.798 Personal history of other (corrected) congenital malformations

√5ᵗʰ **Z87.8**   **Personal history of other specified conditions**
- EXCLUDES 2   *personal history of self harm (Z91.5-)*

Z87.81   **Personal history of (healed)** traumatic fracture
- EXCLUDES 2   *personal history of (healed) nontraumatic fracture (Z87.31-)*

√6ᵗʰ **Z87.82**   **Personal history of other (healed)** physical injury and trauma
- Conditions classifiable to S00–T88, except traumatic fractures

Z87.820   **Personal history of** traumatic brain injury
- EXCLUDES 1   *personal history of transient ischemic attack (TIA), and cerebral infarction without residual deficits (Z86.73)*

Z87.821   **Personal history of** retained foreign body fully removed

Z87.828   **Personal history of other (healed) physical injury and trauma**

√6ᵗʰ **Z87.89**   **Personal history of other specified conditions**

Z87.890   **Personal history of** sex reassignment

Z87.891   **Personal history of** nicotine dependence
- EXCLUDES 1   *current nicotine dependence (F17.2-)*
- AHA: 2017,2Q,27

Z87.892   **Personal history of** anaphylaxis
- Code also allergy status such as:
  - allergy status to drugs, medicaments and biological substances (Z88.-)
  - allergy status, other than to drugs and biological substances (Z91.0-)

Z87.898   **Personal history of other specified conditions**
- AHA: 2013,1Q,21

√4ᵗʰ **Z88**   **Allergy status to drugs, medicaments and biological substances**
- EXCLUDES 2   *allergy status, other than to drugs and biological substances (Z91.0-)*
- AHA: 2015,3Q,23

Z88.0   **Allergy status to** penicillin

Z88.1   **Allergy status to other antibiotic agents**

Z88.2   **Allergy status to** sulfonamides

Z88.3   **Allergy status to other anti-infective agents**

Z88.4   **Allergy status to** anesthetic **agent**

Z88.5   **Allergy status to** narcotic **agent**

Z88.6   **Allergy status to** analgesic **agent**

Z88.7   **Allergy status to** serum and vaccine

Z88.8   **Allergy status to other drugs, medicaments and biological substances**

Z88.9   **Allergy status to unspecified drugs, medicaments and biological substances**

√4ᵗʰ **Z89**   **Acquired absence of limb**
- INCLUDES   amputation status
  - postprocedural loss of limb
  - post-traumatic loss of limb
- EXCLUDES 1   *acquired deformities of limbs (M20-M21)*
  - *congenital absence of limbs (Q71-Q73)*

√5ᵗʰ **Z89.0**   **Acquired absence of** thumb and other finger(s)

√6ᵗʰ **Z89.01**   **Acquired absence of** thumb

Z89.011   **Acquired absence of** right **thumb**

Z89.012   **Acquired absence of** left **thumb**

Z89.019   **Acquired absence of unspecified thumb**

√6ᵗʰ **Z89.02**   **Acquired absence of other** finger(s)
- EXCLUDES 2   *acquired absence of thumb (Z89.01-)*

Z89.021   **Acquired absence of** right **finger(s)**

Z89.022   **Acquired absence of** left **finger(s)**

Z89.029   **Acquired absence of unspecified finger(s)**

√5ᵗʰ **Z89.1**   **Acquired absence of** hand and wrist

√6ᵗʰ **Z89.11**   **Acquired absence of** hand

Z89.111   **Acquired absence of** right **hand**   COM

Z89.112   **Acquired absence of** left **hand**   COM

Z89.119   **Acquired absence of unspecified hand**   COM

√6ᵗʰ **Z89.12**   **Acquired absence of** wrist
- Disarticulation at wrist

Z89.121   **Acquired absence of** right **wrist**   COM

Z89.122   **Acquired absence of** left **wrist**   COM

Z89.129   **Acquired absence of unspecified wrist**   COM

√5ᵗʰ **Z89.2**   **Acquired absence of** upper limb above wrist

√6ᵗʰ **Z89.20**   **Acquired absence of upper limb, unspecified level**

Z89.201   **Acquired absence of** right **upper limb, unspecified level**   COM

Z89.202   **Acquired absence of** left **upper limb, unspecified level**   COM

Z89.209   **Acquired absence of unspecified upper limb, unspecified level**   COM
- Acquired absence of arm NOS

√6ᵗʰ **Z89.21**   **Acquired absence of** upper limb below elbow

Z89.211   **Acquired absence of** right **upper limb below elbow**   COM

Z89.212   **Acquired absence of** left **upper limb below elbow**   COM

Z89.219   **Acquired absence of unspecified upper limb below elbow**   COM

√6ᵗʰ **Z89.22**   **Acquired absence of** upper limb above elbow
- Disarticulation at elbow

Z89.221   **Acquired absence of** right **upper limb above elbow**   COM

Z89.222   **Acquired absence of** left **upper limb above elbow**   COM

Z89.229   **Acquired absence of unspecified upper limb above elbow**   COM

√6ᵗʰ **Z89.23**   **Acquired absence of** shoulder
- Acquired absence of shoulder joint following explantation of shoulder joint prosthesis, with or without presence of antibiotic-impregnated cement spacer

Z89.231   **Acquired absence of** right **shoulder**

Z89.232   **Acquired absence of** left **shoulder**

Z89.239   **Acquired absence of unspecified shoulder**

√5ᵗʰ **Z89.4**   **Acquired absence of** toe(s), foot, and ankle

√6ᵗʰ **Z89.41**   **Acquired absence of** great toe

Z89.411   **Acquired absence of** right **great toe**   HCC ESR

Z89.412   **Acquired absence of** left **great toe**   HCC ESR

Z89.419   **Acquired absence of unspecified great toe**   HCC ESR

√6ᵗʰ **Z89.42**   **Acquired absence of other** toe(s)
- EXCLUDES 2   *acquired absence of great toe (Z89.41-)*

Z89.421   **Acquired absence of other** right **toe(s)**   HCC ESR

Z89.422   **Acquired absence of other** left **toe(s)**   HCC ESR

Z89.429   **Acquired absence of other toe(s), unspecified side**   HCC ESR

√6ᵗʰ **Z89.43**   **Acquired absence of** foot

Z89.431   **Acquired absence of** right **foot**   HCC ESR COM

Z89.432   **Acquired absence of** left **foot**   HCC ESR COM

Z89.439   **Acquired absence of unspecified foot**   HCC ESR COM

√6ᵗʰ **Z89.44**   **Acquired absence of** ankle
- Disarticulation of ankle

Z89.441   **Acquired absence of** right **ankle**   HCC ESR COM

Z89.442   **Acquired absence of** left **ankle**   HCC ESR COM

Z89.449   **Acquired absence of unspecified ankle**   HCC ESR COM

√5ᵗʰ **Z89.5**   **Acquired absence of leg below knee**

√6ᵗʰ **Z89.51**   **Acquired absence of** leg below knee

Z89.511   **Acquired absence of** right **leg below knee**   HCC ESR COM

Z89.512   **Acquired absence of** left **leg below knee**   HCC ESR COM

Z89.519   **Acquired absence of unspecified leg below knee**   HCC ESR COM

☑ Additional Character Required   √x7ᵗʰ Placeholder Alert   **Manifestation**   Unspecified Dx   ⑩ QPP   UPD Unacceptable PDx

✓6ᵗʰ **Z89.52 Acquired absence of** knee

Acquired absence of knee joint following explantation of knee joint prosthesis, with or without presence of antibiotic-impregnated cement spacer

Z89.521 Acquired absence of right **knee**

Z89.522 Acquired absence of left **knee**

Z89.529 Acquired absence of unspecified knee

✓5ᵗʰ **Z89.6 Acquired absence of leg above knee**

✓6ᵗʰ **Z89.61 Acquired absence of** leg above knee

Acquired absence of leg NOS
Disarticulation at knee

Z89.611 Acquired absence of right **leg above knee**   HCC ESR COM

Z89.612 Acquired absence of left **leg above knee**   HCC ESR COM

Z89.619 Acquired absence of unspecified leg above knee   HCC ESR COM

✓6ᵗʰ **Z89.62 Acquired absence of** hip

Acquired absence of hip joint following explantation of hip joint prosthesis, with or without presence of antibiotic-impregnated cement spacer
Disarticulation at hip

Z89.621 Acquired absence of right **hip joint**

Z89.622 Acquired absence of left **hip joint**

Z89.629 Acquired absence of unspecified hip joint

Z89.9 Acquired absence of limb, unspecified   COM

✓4ᵗʰ **Z90 Acquired absence of organs, not elsewhere classified**

INCLUDES   postprocedural or post-traumatic loss of body part NEC

EXCLUDES 1   congenital absence - see Alphabetical Index

EXCLUDES 2   postprocedural absence of endocrine glands (E89.-)

✓5ᵗʰ **Z90.0 Acquired absence of part of** head and neck

Z90.01 Acquired absence of eye

Z90.02 Acquired absence of larynx

Z90.09 Acquired absence of other part of head and neck

Acquired absence of nose

EXCLUDES 2   teeth (K08.1)

✓5ᵗʰ **Z90.1 Acquired absence of** breast and nipple

Z90.10 Acquired absence of unspecified breast and nipple

Z90.11 Acquired absence of right **breast and nipple**

Z90.12 Acquired absence of left **breast and nipple**

Z90.13 Acquired absence of bilateral **breasts and nipples**

Z90.2 Acquired absence of lung **[part of]**

Z90.3 Acquired absence of stomach **[part of]**

✓5ᵗʰ **Z90.4 Acquired absence of other specified parts of digestive tract**

✓6ᵗʰ **Z90.41 Acquired absence of** pancreas

Code also exocrine pancreatic insufficiency (K86.81)
Use additional code to identify any associated:
diabetes mellitus, postpancreatectomy (E13.-)
insulin use (Z79.4)

Z90.410 Acquired total absence **of pancreas**

Acquired absence of pancreas NOS

Z90.411 Acquired partial absence **of pancreas**

Z90.49 Acquired absence of other specified parts of digestive tract

Z90.5 Acquired absence of kidney

Z90.6 Acquired absence of other parts of urinary tract

Acquired absence of bladder

✓5ᵗʰ **Z90.7 Acquired absence of** genital organ(s)

EXCLUDES 1   personal history of sex reassignment (Z87.890)

EXCLUDES 2   female genital mutilation status (N90.81-)

✓6ᵗʰ **Z90.71 Acquired absence of** cervix and uterus

Z90.710 Acquired absence of both cervix and uterus   ♀

Acquired absence of uterus NOS
Status post total hysterectomy

Z90.711 Acquired absence of uterus with remaining cervical stump   ♀

Status post partial hysterectomy with remaining cervical stump

Z90.712 Acquired absence of cervix with remaining uterus   ♀

✓6ᵗʰ **Z90.72 Acquired absence of** ovaries

Z90.721 Acquired absence of ovaries, unilateral   ♀

Z90.722 Acquired absence of ovaries, bilateral   ♀

Z90.79 Acquired absence of other genital organ(s)

✓5ᵗʰ **Z90.8 Acquired absence of other organs**

Z90.81 Acquired absence of spleen

Z90.89 Acquired absence of other organs

✓4ᵗʰ **Z91 Personal risk factors, not elsewhere classified**

EXCLUDES 2   contact with and (suspected) exposures hazardous to health (Z77.-)

exposure to pollution and other problems related to physical environment (Z77.1-)

female genital mutilation status (N90.81-)

personal history of physical injury and trauma (Z87.81, Z87.82-)

occupational exposure to risk factors (Z57.-)

✓5ᵗʰ **Z91.0 Allergy status, other than to drugs and biological substances**

EXCLUDES 2   allergy status to drugs, medicaments, and biological substances (Z88.-)

✓6ᵗʰ **Z91.01 Food allergy status**

EXCLUDES 2   food additives allergy status (Z91.02)

Z91.010 Allergy to peanuts

Z91.011 Allergy to milk products

EXCLUDES 1   lactose intolerance (E73.-)

Z91.012 Allergy to eggs

Z91.013 Allergy to seafood

Allergy to shellfish
Allergy to octopus or squid ink

Z91.014 Allergy to mammalian meats

Allergy to beef
Allergy to lamb
Allergy to pork
Allergy to red meats
AHA: 2021,4Q,33

Z91.018 Allergy to other foods

Allergy to nuts other than peanuts

Z91.02 Food additives allergy status

✓6ᵗʰ **Z91.03 Insect allergy status**

Z91.030 Bee allergy status

Z91.038 Other insect allergy status

✓6ᵗʰ **Z91.04 Nonmedicinal substance allergy status**

Z91.040 Latex allergy status

Latex sensitivity status

Z91.041 Radiographic dye allergy status

Allergy status to contrast media used for diagnostic X-ray procedure

Z91.048 Other nonmedicinal substance allergy status

Z91.09 Other allergy status, other than to drugs and biological substances

✓5ᵗʰ **Z91.1 Patient's noncompliance with medical treatment and regimen**

EXCLUDES 2   ▶caregiver noncompliance with patient's medical treatment and regimen (Z91.A-)◄

✓6ᵗʰ ▲ **Z91.11 Patient's noncompliance with** dietary regimen

▶Code also, if applicable, food insecurity (Z59.4-)◄

● **Z91.110 Patient's noncompliance with dietary regimen due to** financial hardship

● **Z91.118 Patient's noncompliance with dietary regimen for other reason**

Inability to comply with dietary regimen

● **Z91.119 Patient's noncompliance with dietary regimen due to unspecified reason**

✓6ᵗʰ **Z91.12 Patient's** intentional underdosing **of medication regimen**

Code first underdosing of medication (T36-T50) with fifth or sixth character 6

EXCLUDES 1   adverse effect of prescribed drug taken as directed - code to adverse effect
poisoning (overdose) - code to poisoning

AHA: 2018,4Q,72

Z91.120 Patient's intentional underdosing of medication regimen due to financial hardship

Z91.128 Patient's intentional underdosing of medication regimen for other reason

HCC CMS-HCC   Rx Rx HCC   ESR ESRD HCC   COM Commercial HCC   PDx Primary Dx Only   N Newborn: 0   P Pediatric: 0-17   M Maternity: 9-64   A Adult: 15-124

1292   ICD-10-CM 2023

√6th **Z91.13** **Patient's unintentional underdosing of medication regimen**

Code first underdosing of medication (T36-T50) with fifth or sixth character 6

EXCLUDES 1   *adverse effect of prescribed drug taken as directed - code to adverse effect*
poisoning (overdose) - code to poisoning

AHA: 2018,4Q,72

Z91.130 **Patient's unintentional underdosing of medication regimen due to age-related debility**

Z91.138 **Patient's unintentional underdosing of medication regimen for other reason**

Z91.14 **Patient's other noncompliance with medication regimen**

Patient's underdosing of medication NOS

AHA: 2022,1Q,36; 2018,4Q,72

Z91.15 **Patient's noncompliance with renal dialysis**   HCC Rx ESR

▲ √6th **Z91.19** **Patient's noncompliance with other medical treatment and regimen**

▶Patient's nonadherence to medical treatment◀

● **Z91.190** **Patient's noncompliance with other medical treatment and regimen due to financial hardship**

● **Z91.198** **Patient's noncompliance with other medical treatment and regimen for other reason**

● **Z91.199** **Patient's noncompliance with other medical treatment and regimen due to unspecified reason**

● √5th **Z91.A** **Caregiver's noncompliance with patient's medical treatment and regimen**

● √6th **Z91.A1** **Caregiver's noncompliance with patient's dietary regimen**

Caregiver's inability to comply with patient's dietary regimen

Code also, if applicable, food insecurity (Z59.4-)

● **Z91.A10** **Caregiver's noncompliance with patient's dietary regimen due to financial hardship**

● **Z91.A18** **Caregiver's noncompliance with patient's dietary regimen for other reason**

● √6th **Z91.A2** **Caregiver's intentional underdosing of patient's medication regimen**

Code first underdosing of medication (T36-T50) with fifth or sixth character 6

● **Z91.A20** **Caregiver's intentional underdosing of patient's medication regimen due to financial hardship**

● **Z91.A28** **Caregiver's intentional underdosing of medication regimen for other reason**

● **Z91.A3** **Caregiver's unintentional underdosing of patient's medication regimen**

Code first underdosing of medication (T36-T50) with fifth or sixth character 6

● **Z91.A4** **Caregiver's other noncompliance with patient's medication regimen**

Caregiver's underdosing of patient's medication NOS

● **Z91.A5** **Caregiver's noncompliance with patient's renal dialysis**

● **Z91.A9** **Caregiver's noncompliance with patient's other medical treatment and regimen**

Caregiver's nonadherence to patient's medical treatment

√5th **Z91.4** **Personal history of psychological trauma, not elsewhere classified**

√6th **Z91.41** **Personal history of adult abuse**

EXCLUDES 2   *personal history of abuse in childhood (Z62.81-)*

Z91.410 **Personal history of adult physical and sexual abuse**   A

EXCLUDES 1   *current adult physical abuse (T74.11, T76.11)*
current adult sexual abuse (T74.21, T76.11)

Z91.411 **Personal history of adult psychological abuse**   A

Z91.412 **Personal history of adult neglect**   A

EXCLUDES 1   *current adult neglect (T74.01, T76.01)*

Z91.419 **Personal history of unspecified adult abuse**   A

Z91.42 **Personal history of forced labor or sexual exploitation**

AHA: 2018,4Q,32,35

Z91.49 **Other personal history of psychological trauma, not elsewhere classified**

√5th **Z91.5** **Personal history of self-harm**

Code also mental health disorder, if known

AHA: 2021,4Q,33

Z91.51 **Personal history of suicidal behavior**   UPD

Personal history of parasuicide
Personal history of self-poisoning
Personal history of suicide attempt

Z91.52 **Personal history of nonsuicidal self-harm**   UPD

Personal history of nonsuicidal self-injury
Personal history of self-inflicted injury without suicidal intent
Personal history of self-mutilation

√5th **Z91.8** **Other specified personal risk factors, not elsewhere classified**

Z91.81 **History of falling**

At risk for falling

Z91.82 **Personal history of military deployment**   A

Individual (civilian or military) with past history of military war, peacekeeping and humanitarian deployment (current or past conflict)
Returned from military deployment

Z91.83 *Wandering in diseases classified elsewhere*

Code first underlying disorder such as:
Alzheimer's disease (G30.-)
autism or pervasive developmental disorder (F84.-)
intellectual disabilities (F70-F79)
unspecified dementia with behavioral disturbance ▶(F03.9-, F03.A-, F03.B-, F03.C-)◀

√6th **Z91.84** **Oral health risk factors**

AHA: 2017,4Q,29

Z91.841 **Risk for dental caries, low**

Z91.842 **Risk for dental caries, moderate**

Z91.843 **Risk for dental caries, high**

Z91.849 **Unspecified risk for dental caries**

Z91.89 **Other specified personal risk factors, not elsewhere classified**

AHA: 2017,1Q,45

√4th **Z92** **Personal history of medical treatment**

EXCLUDES 2   *postprocedural states (Z98.-)*

Z92.0 **Personal history of contraception**

EXCLUDES 1   *counseling or management of current contraceptive practices (Z30.-)*
long term (current) use of contraception (Z79.3)
presence of (intrauterine) contraceptive device (Z97.5)

√5th **Z92.2** **Personal history of drug therapy**

EXCLUDES 2   *long term (current) drug therapy (Z79.-)*

Z92.21 **Personal history of antineoplastic chemotherapy**

Z92.22 **Personal history of monoclonal drug therapy**

Z92.23 **Personal history of estrogen therapy**

√6th **Z92.24** **Personal history of steroid therapy**

Z92.240 **Personal history of inhaled steroid therapy**

Z92.241 **Personal history of systemic steroid therapy**

Personal history of steroid therapy NOS

Z92.25 **Personal history of immunosuppression therapy**

EXCLUDES 2   *personal history of steroid therapy (Z92.24)*

Z92.29 **Personal history of other drug therapy**

Z92.3 **Personal history of irradiation**

Personal history of exposure to therapeutic radiation

EXCLUDES 1   *exposure to radiation in the physical environment (Z77.12)*
occupational exposure to radiation (Z57.1)

√5th **Z92.8** **Personal history of other medical treatment**

Z92.81 **Personal history of extracorporeal membrane oxygenation (ECMO)**

Z92.82   **Status post administration of tPA (rtPA) in a different facility within the last 24 hours prior to admission to current facility**   UPD
     Code first condition requiring tPA administration, such as:
     acute cerebral infarction (I63.-)
     acute myocardial infarction (I21.-, I22.-)
     AHA: 2013,4Q,124

Z92.83   **Personal history of** failed moderate sedation
     Personal history of failed conscious sedation
     EXCLUDES 2   failed moderate sedation during procedure (T88.52)

Z92.84   **Personal history of** unintended awareness under general anesthesia
     EXCLUDES 2   unintended awareness under general anesthesia during procedure (T88.53)
     AHA: 2016,4Q,72-73,77

✓6ᵗʰ **Z92.85**   **Personal history of cellular therapy**
     AHA: 2021,4Q,33-34

     Z92.850   **Personal history of** Chimeric Antigen Receptor T-cell therapy   UPD
         Personal history of CAR T-cell therapy

     Z92.858   **Personal history of other cellular therapy**   UPD

     Z92.859   **Personal history of cellular therapy, unspecified**   UPD

Z92.86   **Personal history of** gene therapy   UPD
     AHA: 2021,4Q,33-34

Z92.89   **Personal history of other medical treatment**
     AHA: 2020,1Q,18

✓4ᵗʰ **Z93**   **Artificial opening status**
     EXCLUDES 1   artificial openings requiring attention or management (Z43.-)
         complications of external stoma (J95.0-, K94.-, N99.5-)

Z93.0   **Tracheostomy status**   HCC ESR COM
     AHA: 2013,4Q,129

Z93.1   **Gastrostomy status**   HCC ESR COM

Z93.2   **Ileostomy status**   HCC ESR COM

Z93.3   **Colostomy status**   HCC ESR COM

Z93.4   **Other artificial openings of gastrointestinal tract status**   HCC ESR COM

✓5ᵗʰ **Z93.5**   **Cystostomy status**

     Z93.50   **Unspecified cystostomy status**   HCC ESR COM

     Z93.51   **Cutaneous-vesicostomy status**   HCC ESR COM

     Z93.52   **Appendico-vesicostomy status**   HCC ESR COM

     Z93.59   **Other cystostomy status**   HCC ESR COM

Z93.6   **Other artificial openings of** urinary tract **status**   HCC ESR COM
     Nephrostomy status
     Ureterostomy status
     Urethrostomy status

Z93.8   **Other artificial opening status**   HCC ESR COM

Z93.9   **Artificial opening status, unspecified**   HCC ESR COM

✓4ᵗʰ **Z94**   **Transplanted organ and tissue status**
     INCLUDES   organ or tissue replaced by heterogenous or homogenous transplant
     EXCLUDES 1   complications of transplanted organ or tissue - see Alphabetical Index
     EXCLUDES 2   presence of vascular grafts (Z95.-)

Z94.0   **Kidney transplant status**   Rx COM

Z94.1   **Heart transplant status**   HCC Rx ESR COM
     EXCLUDES 1   artificial heart status (Z95.812)
         heart-valve replacement status (Z95.2-Z95.4)

Z94.2   **Lung transplant status**   HCC Rx ESR COM

Z94.3   **Heart and lungs transplant status**   HCC Rx ESR COM

Z94.4   **Liver transplant status**   HCC Rx ESR COM

Z94.5   **Skin transplant status**
     Autogenous skin transplant status

Z94.6   **Bone transplant status**

Z94.7   **Corneal transplant status**

✓5ᵗʰ **Z94.8**   **Other transplanted organ and tissue status**

     Z94.81   **Bone marrow transplant status**   HCC Rx ESR COM

     Z94.82   **Intestine transplant status**   HCC Rx ESR COM

     Z94.83   **Pancreas transplant status**   HCC Rx ESR COM

     Z94.84   **Stem cells transplant status**   HCC Rx ESR COM

Z94.89   **Other transplanted organ and tissue status**

Z94.9   **Transplanted organ and tissue status, unspecified**

✓4ᵗʰ **Z95**   **Presence of cardiac and vascular implants and grafts**
     EXCLUDES 2   complications of cardiac and vascular devices, implants and grafts (T82.-)

Z95.0   **Presence of** cardiac pacemaker
     Presence of cardiac resynchronization therapy (CRT-P) pacemaker
     EXCLUDES 1   adjustment or management of cardiac device (Z45.0-)
         adjustment or management of cardiac pacemaker (Z45.0)
         presence of automatic (implantable) cardiac defibrillator with synchronous cardiac pacemaker (Z95.810)
     AHA: 2022,2Q,14; 2019,1Q,33
     TIP: Assign an additional code for the associated condition if that condition requires constant intervention from the device, as in cases of sick sinus syndrome. For conditions that do not require constant intervention from the device, as in cases of ventricular fibrillation, an additional code for the associated condition should be assigned only if the patient is experiencing the condition and the device is firing during the current admission.

Z95.1   **Presence of** aortocoronary bypass graft
     Presence of coronary artery bypass graft

Z95.2   **Presence of** prosthetic heart valve
     Presence of heart valve NOS

Z95.3   **Presence of** xenogenic heart valve

Z95.4   **Presence of other heart-valve replacement**

Z95.5   **Presence of** coronary angioplasty **implant and graft**
     EXCLUDES 1   coronary angioplasty status without implant and graft (Z98.61)

✓5ᵗʰ **Z95.8**   **Presence of other cardiac and vascular implants and grafts**

✓6ᵗʰ **Z95.81**   **Presence of other cardiac implants and grafts**

     Z95.810   **Presence of** automatic (implantable) cardiac defibrillator
         Presence of automatic (implantable) cardiac defibrillator with synchronous cardiac pacemaker
         Presence of cardiac resynchronization therapy defibrillator (CRT-D)
         Presence of cardioverter-defibrillator (ICD)
         AHA: 2022,2Q,14; 2019,1Q,33
         TIP: Assign an additional code for the associated condition if that condition requires constant intervention from the device, as in cases of sick sinus syndrome. For conditions that do not require constant intervention from the device, as in cases of ventricular fibrillation, an additional code for the associated condition should be assigned only if the patient is experiencing the condition and the device is firing during the current admission.

     Z95.811   **Presence of** heart assist device   HCC ESR COM

     Z95.812   **Presence of** fully implantable artificial heart   HCC ESR COM

     Z95.818   **Presence of other cardiac implants and grafts**

✓6ᵗʰ **Z95.82**   **Presence of other vascular implants and grafts**

     Z95.820   **Peripheral** vascular angioplasty status **with implants and grafts**
         EXCLUDES 1   peripheral vascular angioplasty without implant and graft (Z98.62)

     Z95.828   **Presence of other vascular implants and grafts**
         Presence of intravascular prosthesis NEC

Z95.9   **Presence of cardiac and vascular implant and graft, unspecified**

✓4ᵗʰ **Z96**   **Presence of other functional implants**
     EXCLUDES 2   complications of internal prosthetic devices, implants and grafts (T82-T85)
         fitting and adjustment of prosthetic and other devices (Z44-Z46)

Z96.0   **Presence of** urogenital **implants**

Z96.1   **Presence of** intraocular lens
     Presence of pseudophakia

√5ᵗʰ   **Z96.2**   **Presence of** otological and audiological **implants**

     Z96.20   **Presence of otological and audiological implant, unspecified**

     Z96.21   **Cochlear implant status**

     Z96.22   **Myringotomy tube(s) status**

     Z96.29   **Presence of other otological and audiological implants**
        Presence of bone-conduction hearing device
        Presence of eustachian tube stent
        Stapes replacement

Z96.3   **Presence of** artificial larynx

√5ᵗʰ   **Z96.4**   **Presence of** endocrine **implants**

     Z96.41   **Presence of** insulin pump **(external) (internal)**

     Z96.49   **Presence of other endocrine implants**

Z96.5   **Presence of** tooth-root and mandibular **implants**

√5ᵗʰ   **Z96.6**   **Presence of** orthopedic joint **implants**
     AHA: 2019,3Q,16

     Z96.60   **Presence of unspecified orthopedic joint implant**

    √6ᵗʰ   **Z96.61**   **Presence of** artificial shoulder joint

        Z96.611   **Presence of** right **artificial shoulder joint**
        Z96.612   **Presence of** left **artificial shoulder joint**
        Z96.619   **Presence of unspecified artificial shoulder joint**

    √6ᵗʰ   **Z96.62**   **Presence of** artificial elbow joint

        Z96.621   **Presence of** right **artificial elbow joint**
        Z96.622   **Presence of** left **artificial elbow joint**
        Z96.629   **Presence of unspecified artificial elbow joint**

    √6ᵗʰ   **Z96.63**   **Presence of** artificial wrist joint

        Z96.631   **Presence of** right **artificial wrist joint**
        Z96.632   **Presence of** left **artificial wrist joint**
        Z96.639   **Presence of unspecified artificial wrist joint**

    √6ᵗʰ   **Z96.64**   **Presence of** artificial hip joint
        Hip-joint replacement (partial) (total)
        Z96.641   **Presence of** right **artificial hip joint**
        Z96.642   **Presence of** left **artificial hip joint**
        Z96.643   **Presence of artificial hip joint, bilateral**
        Z96.649   **Presence of unspecified artificial hip joint**

    √6ᵗʰ   **Z96.65**   **Presence of** artificial knee joint

        Z96.651   **Presence of** right **artificial knee joint**
        Z96.652   **Presence of** left **artificial knee joint**
        Z96.653   **Presence of artificial knee joint, bilateral**
        Z96.659   **Presence of unspecified artificial knee joint**

    √6ᵗʰ   **Z96.66**   **Presence of** artificial ankle joint

        Z96.661   **Presence of** right **artificial ankle joint**
        Z96.662   **Presence of** left **artificial ankle joint**
        Z96.669   **Presence of unspecified artificial ankle joint**

    √6ᵗʰ   **Z96.69**   **Presence of** other orthopedic joint implants

        Z96.691   **Finger-joint replacement of** right **hand**
        Z96.692   **Finger-joint replacement of** left **hand**
        Z96.693   **Finger-joint replacement, bilateral**
        Z96.698   **Presence of other orthopedic joint implants**

Z96.7   **Presence of other bone and tendon implants**
     Presence of skull plate

√5ᵗʰ   **Z96.8**   **Presence of other specified functional implants**

     Z96.81   **Presence of** artificial skin

     Z96.82   **Presence of** neurostimulator
        Presence of brain neurostimulator
        Presence of gastric neurostimulator
        Presence of peripheral nerve neurostimulator
        Presence of sacral nerve neurostimulator
        Presence of spinal cord neurostimulator
        Presence of vagus nerve neurostimulator
        AHA: 2019,4Q,19

     Z96.89   **Presence of other specified functional implants**

     Z96.9   **Presence of functional implant, unspecified**

√4ᵗʰ   **Z97**   **Presence of other devices**

     EXCLUDES 1   complications of internal prosthetic devices, implants and grafts (T82-T85)

     EXCLUDES 2   fitting and adjustment of prosthetic and other devices (Z44-Z46)
        presence of cerebrospinal fluid drainage device (Z98.2)

     Z97.0   **Presence of** artificial eye

√5ᵗʰ   **Z97.1**   **Presence of** artificial limb (complete) (partial)

     Z97.10   **Presence of artificial limb (complete) (partial), unspecified**   COM

     Z97.11   **Presence of artificial** right **arm (complete) (partial)**   COM

     Z97.12   **Presence of artificial** left **arm (complete) (partial)**   COM

     Z97.13   **Presence of artificial** right **leg (complete) (partial)**   COM

     Z97.14   **Presence of artificial** left **leg (complete) (partial)**   COM

     Z97.15   **Presence of artificial arms, bilateral (complete) (partial)**   COM

     Z97.16   **Presence of artificial legs, bilateral (complete) (partial)**   COM

     Z97.2   **Presence of** dental prosthetic device **(complete) (partial)**
        Presence of dentures (complete) (partial)

     Z97.3   **Presence of** spectacles and contact lenses

     Z97.4   **Presence of** external hearing-aid

     Z97.5   **Presence of (intrauterine)** contraceptive device   ♀
        EXCLUDES 1   checking, reinsertion or removal of implantable subdermal contraceptive (Z30.46)
            checking, reinsertion or removal of intrauterine contraceptive device (Z30.43-)

     Z97.8   **Presence of other specified devices**

√4ᵗʰ   **Z98**   **Other postprocedural states**

     EXCLUDES 2   aftercare (Z43-Z49, Z51)
        follow-up medical care (Z08-Z09)
        postprocedural complication - see Alphabetical Index

     Z98.0   **Intestinal bypass and anastomosis status**
        EXCLUDES 2   bariatric surgery status (Z98.84)
            gastric bypass status (Z98.84)
            obesity surgery status (Z98.84)

     Z98.1   **Arthrodesis status**

     Z98.2   **Presence of cerebrospinal fluid drainage device**
        Presence of CSF shunt

     Z98.3   **Post therapeutic collapse of lung status**   UPD
        Code first underlying disease

√5ᵗʰ   **Z98.4**   **Cataract extraction status**
        Use additional code to identify intraocular lens implant status (Z96.1)
        EXCLUDES 1   aphakia (H27.0)

     Z98.41   **Cataract extraction status,** right **eye**
     Z98.42   **Cataract extraction status,** left **eye**
     Z98.49   **Cataract extraction status, unspecified eye**

√5ᵗʰ   **Z98.5**   **Sterilization status**
        EXCLUDES 1   female infertility (N97.-)
            male infertility (N46.-)

     Z98.51   **Tubal ligation status**   ♀
     Z98.52   **Vasectomy status**   A ♂

√5ᵗʰ   **Z98.6**   **Angioplasty status**

     Z98.61   **Coronary angioplasty status**
        EXCLUDES 1   coronary angioplasty status with implant and graft (Z95.5)

     Z98.62   **Peripheral vascular angioplasty status**
        EXCLUDES 1   peripheral vascular angioplasty status with implant and graft (Z95.820)

√5ᵗʰ   **Z98.8**   **Other specified postprocedural states**

    √6ᵗʰ   **Z98.81**   **Dental procedure status**

        Z98.810   **Dental sealant status**
        Z98.811   **Dental restoration status**
            Dental crown status
            Dental fillings status
        Z98.818   **Other dental procedure status**

     Z98.82   **Breast implant status**
        EXCLUDES 1   breast implant removal status (Z98.86)

Z98.83 Filtering (vitreous) bleb after glaucoma surgery status
> EXCLUDES 1   inflammation (infection) of postprocedural bleb (H59.4-)

AHA: 2020,3Q,29

Z98.84 Bariatric surgery status
Gastric banding status
Gastric bypass status for obesity
Obesity surgery status
> EXCLUDES 1   bariatric surgery status complicating pregnancy, childbirth, or the puerperium (O99.84)
> EXCLUDES 2   intestinal bypass and anastomosis status (Z98.0)

AHA: 2020,1Q,12

Z98.85 Transplanted organ removal status
Transplanted organ previously removed due to complication, failure, rejection or infection
> EXCLUDES 1   encounter for removal of transplanted organ - code to complication of transplanted organ (T86.-)

Z98.86 Personal history of breast implant removal

√6ᵗʰ **Z98.87 Personal history of in utero procedure**

Z98.870 Personal history of in utero procedure during pregnancy ♀
> EXCLUDES 2   complications from in utero procedure for current pregnancy (O35.7)
> supervision of current pregnancy with history of in utero procedure during previous pregnancy (O09.82-)

Z98.871 Personal history of in utero procedure while a fetus

√6ᵗʰ **Z98.89 Other specified postprocedural states**

Z98.890 Other specified postprocedural states
Personal history of surgery, not elsewhere classified

Z98.891 History of uterine scar from previous surgery ♀
> EXCLUDES 1   maternal care due to uterine scar from previous surgery (O34.2-)

AHA: 2016,4Q,51-52,76

√4ᵗʰ **Z99 Dependence on enabling machines and devices, not elsewhere classified**
AHA: 2020,1Q,11

Z99.0 Dependence on aspirator

√5ᵗʰ **Z99.1 Dependence on respirator**
Dependence on ventilator

Z99.11 Dependence on respirator [ventilator] status HCC ESR COM
AHA: 2015,1Q,21

Z99.12 Encounter for respirator [ventilator] dependence during power failure HCC ESR COM PDx
> EXCLUDES 1   mechanical complication of respirator [ventilator] (J95.850)

Z99.2 Dependence on renal dialysis HCC Rx ESR
Hemodialysis status
Peritoneal dialysis status
Presence of arteriovenous shunt for dialysis
Renal dialysis status NOS
> EXCLUDES 1   encounter for fitting and adjustment of dialysis catheter (Z49.0-)
> EXCLUDES 2   noncompliance with renal dialysis (Z91.15)

AHA: 2016,1Q,12; 2013,4Q,125

Z99.3 Dependence on wheelchair
Wheelchair confinement status
Code first cause of dependence, such as:
muscular dystrophy (G71.0-)
obesity (E66.-)

√5ᵗʰ **Z99.8 Dependence on other enabling machines and devices**

Z99.81 Dependence on supplemental oxygen
Dependence on long-term oxygen
AHA: 2013,4Q,129

Z99.89 Dependence on other enabling machines and devices
Dependence on machine or device NOS
AHA: 2020,1Q,11

HCC CMS-HCC   Rx Rx HCC   ESR ESRD HCC   COM Commercial HCC   PDx Primary Dx Only   N Newborn: 0   P Pediatric: 0-17   M Maternity: 9-64   A Adult: 15-124

1296   ICD-10-CM 2023

Chapter 22. Codes for Special Purposes (U00–U85)

Chapter-specific Guidelines

U07.0	Vaping-related disorder (see Section I.C.10.e., Vaping-related disorders)
U07.1	COVID-19 (see Section I.C.1.g.1., COVID-19 infection)
U09.9	Post COVID-19 condition, unspecified (see Section I.C.1.g.1.m.)

Chapter 22. Codes for Special Purposes (U00-U85)

This chapter contains the following blocks:

U00-U49   Provisional assignment of new diseases of uncertain etiology or emergency use

Provisional assignment of new diseases of uncertain etiology or emergency use (U00-U49)

✓4ᵗʰ **U07** **Emergency use of U07**

    U07.0 **Vaping-related disorder**

         Dabbing related lung damage

         Dabbing related lung injury

         E-cigarette, or vaping, product use associated lung injury [EVALI]

         Electronic cigarette related lung damage

         Electronic cigarette related lung injury

         Use additional code, to identify manifestations, such as:

            abdominal pain (R10.84)

            acute respiratory distress syndrome (J80)

            diarrhea (R19.7)

            drug-induced interstitial lung disorder (J70.4)

            lipoid pneumonia (J69.1)

            weight loss (R63.4)

         DEF: Respiratory illness or injury caused by harmful aerosolized substances and chemicals produced by electronic cigarettes, vapes, e-pipes, and other battery-powered vaping devices. Symptoms may include shortness of breath and fever, while some patients experience severe, sometimes fatal, lung damage. ***Synonym(s):*** *e-cigarette and vaping product use-associated lung injury, EVALI.*

    U07.1 **COVID-19**

         Use additional code to identify pneumonia or other manifestations, such as:

         pneumonia due to COVID-19 (J12.82)

         EXCLUDES 2   *coronavirus as the cause of diseases classified elsewhere (B97.2-)*

                 coronavirus infection, unspecified (B34.2)

                 pneumonia due to SARS-associated coronavirus (J12.81)

         AHA: 2022,2Q,28; 2021,4Q,101,107-108; 2021,1Q,25-30,31-49; 2020,4Q,14,99; 2020,3Q,9-16; 2020,2Q,3-13

         DEF: First diagnosed in December 2019 in China, coronavirus disease 2019 (COVID-19) is a respiratory infection caused by a newly identified (novel) virus not previously seen in humans, known as severe acute respiratory syndrome coronavirus 2 (SARS-CoV-2). Symptoms of this lower respiratory illness include fever, dry cough, and tiredness that may progress to include difficulty breathing. Older patients and those with high blood pressure, heart problems, and diabetes are more likely to develop serious symptoms of the illness. ***Synonym(s):*** *SARS-CoV-2, coronavirus disease 2019.*

         TIP: Only a confirmed diagnosis of COVID-19 can be coded to U07.1; a positive COVID-19 test result or documentation by the provider that the disease is confirmed is sufficient.

         TIP: Assign for asymptomatic individuals who test positive for COVID-19. Even though asymptomatic, the individual is considered to have the COVID-19 infection due to the positive test result.

         TIP: Assign appropriate codes for presenting signs/symptoms associated with COVID-19 (cough, fever, shortness of breath), instead of U07.1, if a definitive diagnosis has not been established.

✓4ᵗʰ **U09** **Post COVID-19 condition**

    U09.9 **Post COVID-19 condition, unspecified**

         NOTE   This code enables establishment of a link with COVID-19.

                 This code is not to be used in cases that are still presenting with active COVID-19. However, an exception is made in cases of re-infection with COVID-19, occurring with a condition related to prior COVID-19.

         ~~Post-acute sequela of COVID-19~~

         ▶Post-acute sequela of COVID-19◀

         Code first the specific condition related to COVID-19 if known, such as:

         chronic respiratory failure (J96.1-)

         loss of smell (R43.8)

         loss of taste (R43.8)

         multisystem inflammatory syndrome (M35.81)

         pulmonary embolism (I26.-)

         pulmonary fibrosis (J84.10)

         AHA: 2021,4Q,31-32,102-106

Notes

Notes

Notes

Notes

A09	Infectious gastroenteritis and colitis, unspecified
A33	Tetanus neonatorum
A34	Obstetrical tetanus
A35	Other tetanus
A46	Erysipelas
A55	Chlamydial lymphogranuloma (venereum)
A57	Chancroid
A58	Granuloma inguinale
A64	Unspecified sexually transmitted disease
A65	Nonvenereal syphilis
A70	Chlamydia psittaci infections
A78	Q fever
A86	Unspecified viral encephalitis
A89	Unspecified viral infection of central nervous system
A90	Dengue fever [classical dengue]
A91	Dengue hemorrhagic fever
A94	Unspecified arthropod-borne viral fever
A99	Unspecified viral hemorrhagic fever
B03	Smallpox
B04	Monkeypox
B09	Unspecified viral infection characterized by skin and mucous membrane lesions
B20	Human immunodeficiency virus [HIV] disease
B49	Unspecified mycosis
B54	Unspecified malaria
B59	Pneumocystosis
B64	Unspecified protozoal disease
B72	Dracunculiasis
B75	Trichinellosis
B79	Trichuriasis
B80	Enterobiasis
B86	Scabies
B89	Unspecified parasitic disease
B91	Sequelae of poliomyelitis
B92	Sequelae of leprosy
C01	Malignant neoplasm of base of tongue
C07	Malignant neoplasm of parotid gland
C12	Malignant neoplasm of pyriform sinus
C19	Malignant neoplasm of rectosigmoid junction
C20	Malignant neoplasm of rectum
C23	Malignant neoplasm of gallbladder
C33	Malignant neoplasm of trachea
C37	Malignant neoplasm of thymus
C52	Malignant neoplasm of vagina
C55	Malignant neoplasm of uterus, part unspecified
C58	Malignant neoplasm of placenta
C61	Malignant neoplasm of prostate
C73	Malignant neoplasm of thyroid gland
D34	Benign neoplasm of thyroid gland
D45	Polycythemia vera
D62	Acute posthemorrhagic anemia
D65	Disseminated intravascular coagulation [defibrination syndrome]
D66	Hereditary factor VIII deficiency
D67	Hereditary factor IX deficiency
D71	Functional disorders of polymorphonuclear neutrophils
D77	Other disorders of blood and blood-forming organs in diseases classified elsewhere
E02	Subclinical iodine-deficiency hypothyroidism
E15	Nondiabetic hypoglycemic coma
E35	Disorders of endocrine glands in diseases classified elsewhere
E40	Kwashiorkor
E41	Nutritional marasmus
E42	Marasmic kwashiorkor
E43	Unspecified severe protein-calorie malnutrition
E45	Retarded development following protein-calorie malnutrition

E46	Unspecified protein-calorie malnutrition
E52	Niacin deficiency [pellagra]
E54	Ascorbic acid deficiency
E58	Dietary calcium deficiency
E59	Dietary selenium deficiency
E60	Dietary zinc deficiency
E65	Localized adiposity
E68	Sequelae of hyperalimentation
F04	Amnestic disorder due to known physiological condition
F05	Delirium due to known physiological condition
F09	Unspecified mental disorder due to known physiological condition
F21	Schizotypal disorder
F22	Delusional disorders
F23	Brief psychotic disorder
F24	Shared psychotic disorder
F28	Other psychotic disorder not due to a substance or known physiological condition
F29	Unspecified psychosis not due to a substance or known physiological condition
F39	Unspecified mood [affective] disorder
F54	Psychological and behavioral factors associated with disorders or diseases classified elsewhere
F59	Unspecified behavioral syndromes associated with physiological disturbances and physical factors
F66	Other sexual disorders
F69	Unspecified disorder of adult personality and behavior
F70	Mild intellectual disabilities
F71	Moderate intellectual disabilities
F72	Severe intellectual disabilities
F73	Profound intellectual disabilities
F79	Unspecified intellectual disabilities
F82	Specific developmental disorder of motor function
F88	Other disorders of psychological development
F89	Unspecified disorder of psychological development
F99	Mental disorder, not otherwise specified
G01	Meningitis in bacterial diseases classified elsewhere
G02	Meningitis in other infectious and parasitic diseases classified elsewhere
G07	Intracranial and intraspinal abscess and granuloma in diseases classified elsewhere
G08	Intracranial and intraspinal phlebitis and thrombophlebitis
G09	Sequelae of inflammatory diseases of central nervous system
G10	Huntington's disease
G14	Postpolio syndrome
G20	Parkinson's disease
G26	Extrapyramidal and movement disorders in diseases classified elsewhere
G35	Multiple sclerosis
G53	Cranial nerve disorders in diseases classified elsewhere
G55	Nerve root and plexus compressions in diseases classified elsewhere
G59	Mononeuropathy in diseases classified elsewhere
G63	Polyneuropathy in diseases classified elsewhere
G64	Other disorders of peripheral nervous system
G94	Other disorders of brain in diseases classified elsewhere
H22	Disorders of iris and ciliary body in diseases classified elsewhere
H28	Cataract in diseases classified elsewhere
H32	Chorioretinal disorders in diseases classified elsewhere
H36	Retinal disorders in diseases classified elsewhere
H42	Glaucoma in diseases classified elsewhere
I00	Rheumatic fever without heart involvement
I10	Essential (primary) hypertension
I32	Pericarditis in diseases classified elsewhere
I38	Endocarditis, valve unspecified
I39	Endocarditis and heart valve disorders in diseases classified elsewhere

Appendix A: Valid 3-character ICD-10-CM Codes

I41	Myocarditis in diseases classified elsewhere
I43	Cardiomyopathy in diseases classified elsewhere
I52	Other heart disorders in diseases classified elsewhere
I5A	Non-ischemic myocardial injury (non-traumatic)
I76	Septic arterial embolism
I81	Portal vein thrombosis
I96	Gangrene, not elsewhere classified
J00	Acute nasopharyngitis (common cold)
J13	Pneumonia due to Streptococcus pneumoniae
J14	Pneumonia due to Hemophilus influenzae
J17	Pneumonia in diseases classified elsewhere
J22	Unspecified acute lower respiratory infection
J36	Peritonsillar abscess
J40	Bronchitis, not specified as acute or chronic
J42	Unspecified chronic bronchitis
J60	Coalworker's pneumoconiosis
J61	Pneumoconiosis due to asbestos and other mineral fibers
J64	Unspecified pneumoconiosis
J65	Pneumoconiosis associated with tuberculosis
J80	Acute respiratory distress syndrome
J90	Pleural effusion, not elsewhere classified
J99	Respiratory disorders in diseases classified elsewhere
K23	Disorders of esophagus in diseases classified elsewhere
K30	Functional dyspepsia
K36	Other appendicitis
K37	Unspecified appendicitis
K67	Disorders of peritoneum in infectious diseases classified elsewhere
K77	Liver disorders in diseases classified elsewhere
K87	Disorders of gallbladder, biliary tract and pancreas in diseases classified elsewhere
L00	Staphylococcal scalded skin syndrome
L14	Bullous disorders in diseases classified elsewhere
L22	Diaper dermatitis
L26	Exfoliative dermatitis
L42	Pityriasis rosea
L45	Papulosquamous disorders in diseases classified elsewhere
L52	Erythema nodosum
L54	Erythema in diseases classified elsewhere
L62	Nail disorders in diseases classified elsewhere
L80	Vitiligo
L83	Acanthosis nigricans
L84	Corns and callosities
L86	Keratoderma in diseases classified elsewhere
L88	Pyoderma gangrenosum
L99	Other disorders of skin and subcutaneous tissue in diseases classified elsewhere
N08	Glomerular disorders in diseases classified elsewhere
N10	Acute tubulo-interstitial nephritis
N12	Tubulo-interstitial nephritis, not specified as acute or chronic
N16	Renal tubulo-interstitial disorders in diseases classified elsewhere
N19	Unspecified kidney failure
N22	Calculus of urinary tract in diseases classified elsewhere
N23	Unspecified renal colic
N29	Other disorders of kidney and ureter in diseases classified elsewhere
N33	Bladder disorders in diseases classified elsewhere
N37	Urethral disorders in diseases classified elsewhere
N51	Disorders of male genital organs in diseases classified elsewhere
N62	Hypertrophy of breast
N72	Inflammatory disease of cervix uteri
N74	Female pelvic inflammatory disorders in diseases classified elsewhere
N86	Erosion and ectropion of cervix uteri
N96	Recurrent pregnancy loss
O68	Labor and delivery complicated by abnormality of fetal acid-base balance

O76	Abnormality in fetal heart rate and rhythm complicating labor and delivery
O80	Encounter for full-term uncomplicated delivery
O82	Encounter for cesarean delivery without indication
O85	Puerperal sepsis
O94	Sequelae of complication of pregnancy, childbirth, and the puerperium
P53	Hemorrhagic disease of newborn
P60	Disseminated intravascular coagulation of newborn
P84	Other problems with newborn
P90	Convulsions of newborn
P95	Stillbirth
Q02	Microcephaly
R12	Heartburn
R17	Unspecified jaundice
R21	Rash and other nonspecific skin eruption
R32	Unspecified urinary incontinence
R34	Anuria and oliguria
R37	Sexual dysfunction, unspecified
R42	Dizziness and giddiness
R52	Pain, unspecified
R54	Age-related physical debility
R55	Syncope and collapse
R58	Hemorrhage, not elsewhere classified
R61	Generalized hyperhidrosis
R64	Cachexia
R69	Illness, unspecified
R75	Inconclusive laboratory evidence of human immunodeficiency virus [HIV]
R81	Glycosuria
R99	Ill-defined and unknown cause of mortality
Y09	Assault by unspecified means
Y66	Nonadministration of surgical and medical care
Y69	Unspecified misadventure during surgical and medical care
Y95	Nosocomial condition
Z08	Encounter for follow-up examination after completed treatment for malignant neoplasm
Z09	Encounter for follow-up examination after completed treatment for conditions other than malignant neoplasm
Z21	Asymptomatic human immunodeficiency virus [HIV] infection status
Z23	Encounter for immunization
Z66	Do not resuscitate

Appendix B: Pharmacology List 2023

This section enables the coder to quickly review drugs, drug actions, and indications that are often associated with overlooked or undocumented diagnoses. The coder should review the patient's medication record and know what condition the physician is treating with the prescribed medication based on documentation in the medical record. When documentation is lacking, the coder can reference this section to locate the drug, determine the drug action, confirm drug indications, and when necessary query the physician. When applicable, some of the drugs provided in this resource have also been mapped to their appropriate Z code for long-term drug use.

Drug	Z Code	Drug Action/Classification	Indications
5-fluorouracil (5-FU) [fluorouracil]	Z79.631	Antimetabolite agent	Skin, colorectal, breast, stomach, and pancreas cancer
6-mercaptopurine (6-MP) [mercaptopurine]	Z79.631	Antimetabolite agent	Acute lymphoblastic leukemia
Abilify [aripiprazole]		Antipsychotic	Depression; bipolar disorder; schizophrenia; autism symptoms
Acarbose [acarbose]	Z79.84	Oral hypoglycemic	Diabetes mellitus
Accupril [quinapril hydrochloride]		ACE inhibitor	Congestive heart failure; hypertension
Acetaminophen with codeine [acetaminophen/codeine phosphate]	Z79.891	Analgesic, narcotic	Pain, moderate to severe
Aclasta [zoledronic acid]	Z79.83	Bisphosphonate	Paget's disease; bone loss prevention in postmenopausal women
Actemra [tocilizumab]	Z79.620	Immunosuppressive biologic; monoclonal antibody	Rheumatoid arthritis; systemic sclerosis-associated interstitial lung disease; giant cell arteritis; polyarticular or systemic juvenile idiopathic arthritis; cytokine release syndrome
Actimmune [interferon gamma-1b]	Z79.69	Other immunosuppressant/immunomodulator	Chronic granulomatous disease; malignant osteopetrosis
Activella [estradiol/norethindrone acetate]	Z79.890	Estrogen therapy	Menopause symptoms; vaginal and vulvar atrophy; osteoporosis prevention
Actonel [risedronate sodium]	Z79.83	Bisphosphonate	Decrease in bone loss in multiple myeloma patients; Paget's disease; hyperparathyroidism; osteoporosis
Actoplus Met [metformin hydrochloride/pioglitazone hydrochloride]	Z79.84	Oral hypoglycemic	Diabetes mellitus
Actos [pioglitazone hydrochloride]	Z79.84	Oral hypoglycemic	Diabetes mellitus
Aczone [dapsone]		Acne agent, topical	Acne vulgaris
Adalat CC [nifedipine]		Calcium channel blocker	Vasospastic angina; chronic stable angina; hypertension
Adderall XR [amphetamine aspartate and sulfate/dextroamphetamine saccharate and sulfate]		CNS stimulant	Attention deficit hyperactivity disorder (ADHD)
Adlarity [donepezil hydrochloride]		Acetylcholinesterase/cholinesterase inhibitors	Dementia due to Alzheimer's
Adlyxin [lixisenatide]	Z79.85	Antidiabetic – non-insulin injectable	Diabetes mellitus
Admelog [insulin lispro]	Z79.4	Insulin	Diabetes mellitus
Advair [fluticasone propionate/salmeterol xinafoate]	Z79.51	Corticosteroid – inhaled; antiasthmatic	Prophylaxis and treatment of asthma and COPD
Advil [ibuprofen]	Z79.1	Nonsteroidal anti-inflammatory drug (NSAID)	Pain or fever relief
Afrezza [human insulin recombinant]	Z79.899	Insulin – inhaled	Diabetes mellitus
Aggrastat [tirofiban hydrochloride]	Z79.02	Antiplatelet	Unstable angina; heart attacks
Aggrenox [aspirin/dipyridamole]	Z79.02	Antiplatelet	Lessening of the chance of heart attack or stroke
Aimovig [erenumab-aooe]	Z79.620	Immunosuppressive biologic; monoclonal antibody	Migraine headache prevention
AirDuo RespiClick [fluticasone propionate/salmeterol xinafoate]	Z79.51	Corticosteroid – inhaled; antiasthmatic	Asthma
Aklief [trifarotene]		Acne agent, topical	Acne vulgaris
Aldactone [spironolactone]		Cardiovascular agent; antihypertensive agent; diuretic; electrolytic and renal agent	Severe heart failure; ascites associated with cirrhosis; hypokalemia
Aleve [naproxen sodium]	Z79.1	Nonsteroidal anti-inflammatory drug (NSAID)	Reduction of temporary aches and pains
Allegra allergy [fexofenadine hydrochloride]		Antihistamine	Seasonal allergic rhinitis
Allopurinol [allopurinol]		Antigout	Gouty arthritis; renal calculus; hyperuricemia; hyperuricemia secondary to leukemia; hyperuricemia secondary to lymphoma

Drug	Z Code	Drug Action/Classification	Indications
Alora [estradiol]	Z79.890	Estrogen therapy	Menopause symptoms
Alphagan P [brimonidine tartrate]		Antiglaucoma agent (ophthalmic); antihypertensive, ocular	Open angle glaucoma or another condition in which pressure in the eye is too high (ocular hypertension)
Alprazolam [alprazolam]		Antianxiety; sedative/hypnotic	Anxiety and panic disorders
Altabax [retapamulin]	Z79.2	Antibiotic, topical	Skin infections
Altace [ramipril]		ACE inhibitor	Congestive heart failure; hypertension
Altavera [ethinyl estradiol/levonorgestrel]	Z79.3	Contraceptive	Prevention of pregnancy
Alvesco [ciclesonide]	Z79.51	Corticosteroid – inhaled; antiasthmatic	Prophylaxis and treatment of asthma
Alyacen [ethinyl estradiol/norethindrone]	Z79.3	Contraceptive	Prevention of pregnancy
Amaryl [glimepiride]	Z79.84	Oral hypoglycemic	Diabetes mellitus
Ambien [zolpidem tartrate]		CNS depressant; anxiolytic/sedative/hypnotic	Insomnia
Amikacin [amikacin sulfate]	Z79.2	Antibiotic	Gram-negative bacterial infections such as Pseudomonas, Escherichia coli (E. coli), Proteus, Klebsiella-Enterobacter-Serratia
Amitriptyline HCl [amitriptyline hydrochloride]		Antidepressant	Depression
Amoxicillin [amoxicillin]	Z79.2	Antibiotic	Treatment of infections with a broad spectrum of bactericidal activity against many gram-positive and gram-negative microorganisms; otitis media, gonorrhea, skin, respiratory, gastrointestinal, and genitourinary infections
Ampicillin [ampicillin sodium]	Z79.2	Antibiotic	Bacterial infections
Ampyra [dalfampridine]		Potassium channel blocker	Improvement in walking in patients with multiple sclerosis
Amrix [cyclobenzaprine hydrochloride]		Muscle relaxant	Adjunct to rest and physical therapy for muscle spasms
Anaprox DS [naproxen sodium]	Z79.1	Nonsteroidal anti-inflammatory drug (NSAID)	Pain, inflammation or fever relief
Anastrozole [anastrozole]	Z79.811	Aromatase inhibitor	Postmenopausal breast cancer
Androderm [testosterone]	Z79.890	Testosterone therapy – topical	Primary hypogonadism; hypogonadotropic hypogonadism
AndroGel [testosterone]	Z79.890	Testosterone therapy – topical	Primary hypogonadism; hypogonadotropic hypogonadism
Angeliq [drospirenone/estradiol]	Z79.890	Estrogen therapy	Menopause symptoms
Angiomax [bivalirudin]	Z79.01	Anticoagulant	Prevention of blood clots
Antabuse [disulfiram]		Alcohol treatment	Alcoholism
Antineoplastic/chemotherapy	Z79.899	Antineoplastic	Cancer
Apidra [insulin glulisine recombinant]	Z79.4	Insulin	Diabetes mellitus
Aranelle [ethinyl estradiol/norethindrone]	Z79.3	Contraceptive	Prevention of pregnancy; acne
Aranesp [darbepoetin alfa]		Erythropoiesis-stimulating agent (ESA)	Treatment of lower than normal blood cells (anemia) from disorders such as CKD and neoplasms
Aredia [pamidronate disodium]	Z79.83	Bisphosphonate	Prevention of thinning of the bones (osteoporosis)
Argatroban [argatroban]	Z79.01	Anticoagulant	Prophylaxis and treatment of venous thrombosis in thrombocytopenia patients
Aricept [donepezil hydrochloride]		Acetylcholinesterase/cholinesterase inhibitors	Dementia due to Alzheimer's
Arimidex [anastrozole]	Z79.811	Aromatase inhibitor	Postmenopausal breast cancer
Aristospan [triamcinolone hexacetonide]	Z79.52	Corticosteroid	Severe inflammation
Arixtra [fondaparinux sodium]	Z79.01	Anticoagulant	Venous thrombosis and pulmonary embolism
Arnuity Ellipta [fluticasone furoate]	Z79.51	Corticosteroid – inhaled; antiasthmatic	Prophylaxis and treatment of asthma
Aromasin [exemestane]	Z79.811	Aromatase inhibitor	Postmenopausal breast cancer
Arthrotec [diclofenac sodium/misoprostol]	Z79.1	Nonsteroidal anti-inflammatory drug (NSAID)-prostaglandin combo	Treatment of patients with arthritis who may develop stomach ulcers from taking nonsteroidal anti-inflammatory drugs (NSAIDs) alone; used to help relieve some symptoms of arthritis, such as inflammation, swelling, stiffness, and joint pain
Asacol HD [mesalamine]		Anti-inflammatory	Ulcerative colitis
Ashlyna [ethinyl estradiol/levonorgestrel]	Z79.3	Contraceptive	Prevention of pregnancy

Drug	Z Code	Drug Action/Classification	Indications
Asmanex [mometasone furoate]	Z79.51	Corticosteroid – inhaled; antiasthmatic	Prophylaxis and treatment of asthma
Astagraf XL [tacrolimus]	Z79.621	Calcineurin inhibitor	Prophylaxis of organ transplant rejection
Atelvia [risedronate sodium]	Z79.83	Bisphosphonate	Prevention of thinning of the bones (osteoporosis)
Atenolol [atenolol]		Beta blocker	Angina pectoris; hypertension; acute myocardial infarction
Ativan [lorazepam]		Antianxiety; sedative/hypnotic	Anxiety disorder associated with depressive symptoms; controls tension, agitation, irritability, and insomnia
Atripla [efavirenz/emtricitabine/tenofovir disoproxil fumarate]	Z79.899	Antiretroviral	HIV
Atrovent HFA [ipratropium bromide]		Antiasthmatic/bronchodilator	Chronic bronchitis, emphysema; bronchial asthma
Augmentin [amoxicillin/clavulanate potassium]	Z79.2	Antibiotic	Middle ear, lower respiratory, sinus, skin and skin structures, and urinary tract infections
Avandia [rosiglitazone maleate]	Z79.84	Oral hypoglycemic	Diabetes mellitus
Avapro [irbesartan]		Antihypertensive	Hypertension
Avelox [moxifloxacin hydrochloride]	Z79.2	Antibiotic	Bacterial infections of the skin, sinuses, lungs, or stomach; plague
Aviane-28 [ethinyl estradiol/levonorgestrel]	Z79.3	Contraceptive	Prevention of pregnancy
Avonex [interferon beta-1a]	Z79.69	Other immunosuppressant/immunomodulator	Treatment of relapsing multiple sclerosis
Axid AR [nizatidine]		Histamine H2-receptor antagonist	Acid/peptic disorder; gastroesophageal reflux; duodenal, gastric, and peptic ulcers
Ayvakit [avapritinib]		Multikinase inhibitor	Unresectable or metastatic gastrointestinal stromal tumor (GIST); advanced systemic mastocytosis
Azactam [aztreonam]	Z79.2	Antibiotic	Severe bacterial infections
Azithromycin [azithromycin]	Z79.2	Antibiotic	Bacterial infections
Azstarys [serdexmethylphenidate and dexmethylphenidate]		CNS stimulant	Attention deficit hyperactivity disorder (ADHD)
Bactrim [sulfamethoxazole/trimethoprim]	Z79.2	Antibiotic	Treatment of urinary tract infections, acute otitis media, acute exacerbation of chronic bronchitis, shigellosis, and pneumocystis carinii
Bactroban [mupirocin topical]	Z79.2	Antibiotic, topical	Bacterial skin infections
Balziva-28 [ethinyl estradiol/norethindrone]	Z79.3	Contraceptive	Prevention of pregnancy
Basaglar [insulin glargine]	Z79.4	Insulin	Diabetes mellitus
Bayer [acetylsalicylic acid]	Z79.82	Aspirin	Prophylaxis and treatment of heart attacks, angina or strokes; reduction of fever, pain and inflammation
Beconase AQ [beclomethasone dipropionate monohydrate]	Z79.899	Corticosteroid – intranasal	Perennial and seasonal allergies; vasomotor rhinitis
Bekyree [desogestrel/ethinyl estradiol]	Z79.3	Contraceptive	Prevention of pregnancy
Betaseron [interferon beta-1b]	Z79.69	Other immunosuppressant/immunomodulator	Treatment of relapsing multiple sclerosis
Betoptic [betaxolol hydrochloride]		Beta blocker; ophthalmic glaucoma agent	Lowering of intraocular pressure; also used for treatment of ocular hypertension and chronic open-angle glaucoma
Bevyxxa [betrixaban]	Z79.01	Anticoagulant	Prophylaxis of venous thromboembolism
Beyaz [drospirenone/ethinyl estradiol/levomefolate calcium]	Z79.3	Contraceptive	Prevention of pregnancy; acne
Biaxin XL [clarithromycin]	Z79.2	Antibiotic	Acid/peptic disorder or ulcer; acute exacerbation chronic bronchitis; human immunodeficiency virus; lower and upper respiratory tract infection; sinus infection; prophylaxis mycobacterium avium complex; pharyngitis; pneumonia; tonsillitis
Bijuva [estradiol/progesterone]	Z79.890	Estrogen/progesterone therapy	Menopausal symptoms
Biktarvy [bictegravir sodium/emtricitabine/ tenofovir alafenamide fumarate]	Z79.899	Antiretroviral	HIV
Biltricide [praziquantel]		Antiparasitic	Infections from Schistosoma species and liver flukes
Binosto [alendronate sodium]	Z79.83	Bisphosphonate	Prevention of thinning of the bones (osteoporosis)
Bleomycin [bleomycin]	Z79.632	Antitumor antibiotic	Squamous cell carcinoma; Hodgkin's disease; non-Hodgkin's lymphoma; malignant pleural effusion; testicular cancer

Drug	Z Code	Drug Action/Classification	Indications
Boniva [ibandronate sodium]	Z79.83	Bisphosphonate	Prevention of thinning of the bones (osteoporosis)
Breo Ellipta [fluticasone furoate/vilanterol trifenatate]	Z79.51	Corticosteroid – inhaled; antiasthmatic	Maintenance treatment of asthma and COPD
Brevicon 28-day [ethinyl estradiol/norethindrone]	Z79.3	Contraceptive	Prevention of pregnancy; acne
Brexafemme [ibrexafungerp]		Antifungal	Vulvovaginal candidiasis
Briellyn [ethinyl estradiol/norethindrone]	Z79.3	Contraceptive	Prevention of pregnancy
Brilinta [ticagrelor]	Z79.02	Antiplatelet	Unstable angina; heart attacks; prevention of blood clots
Brisdelle [paroxetine]		Selective serotonin reuptake inhibitor (SSRI)	Vasomotor symptoms related to menopause
Bufferin [aspirin]	Z79.82	Aspirin	Pain, reduce fever or inflammation; prophylaxis and treatment of heart attack, stroke, angina
Buprenex [buprenorphine hydrochloride]	Z79.891	Analgesic, narcotic	Moderate to severe pain
Buprenorphine HCl and Naloxone HCl [buprenorphine hydrochloride/naloxone hydrochloride]	Z79.891	Analgesic, narcotic	Moderate to severe pain
Buspirone HCl [buspirone hydrochloride]		Antianxiety	Generalized anxiety disorder
Busulfex [busulfan]	Z79.630	Chemotherapeutic alkylating agent	Chronic myelogenous leukemia
Butrans [buprenorphine]	Z79.891	Analgesic, narcotic	Chronic pain
Bydureon [exenatide]	Z79.85	Antidiabetic – non-insulin injectable	Diabetes mellitus
Byetta [exenatide]	Z79.85	Antidiabetic – non-insulin injectable	Diabetes mellitus
Calan [verapamil hydrochloride]		Calcium channel blocker	Angina pectoris at rest and chronic stable, arrhythmia, atrial fibrillation, atrial flutter, paroxysmal supraventricular tachycardia, ventricular arrhythmia, hypertension
Caldolor [ibuprofen]	Z79.1	Nonsteroidal anti-inflammatory drug (NSAID)	Pain or fever relief
Cambia [diclofenac potassium]	Z79.1	Nonsteroidal anti-inflammatory drug (NSAID)	Migraine headache
Camila [norethindrone]	Z79.3	Contraceptive	Prevention of pregnancy; menstrual disorders
Camptosar [irinotecan]	Z79.634	Topoisomerase inhibitor	Metastatic colon or rectal cancer
Caplyta [lumateperone]		Antipsychotic	Schizophrenia
Cardizem CD [diltiazem hydrochloride]		Calcium channel blocker	Chronic stable angina, atrial fibrillation, atrial flutter, hypertension, paroxysmal supraventricular tachycardia
Cardura [doxazosin mesylate]		Antihypertensive	Benign prostatic hyperplasia; hypertension
Carmustine [carmustine]	Z79.630	Chemotherapeutic alkylating agent	Brain tumors; Hodgkin's disease; multiple myeloma; non-Hodgkin's lymphoma
Cefazolin sodium [cefazolin sodium]	Z79.2	Antibiotic	Respiratory tract infections due to Streptococcus pneumoniae, Klebsiella species, Haemophilus influenzae (H. influenzae), Staphylococcus aureus, and group A beta-hemolytic streptococci; urinary tract infections due to E. coli, Proteus mirabilis, Klebsiella species, and some strains of Enterobacter and enterococci; skin and skin structure infections, biliary tract infections, bone and joint infections, genital infections, septicemia, and endocarditis
Ceftriaxone [ceftriaxone sodium]	Z79.2	Antibiotic	Bacterial infections
Cefzil [cefprozil]	Z79.2	Antibiotic	Acute exacerbation and chronic bronchitis, lower respiratory tract infection, upper respiratory tract infection, pharyngitis, tonsillitis
Celebrex [celecoxib]	Z79.1	Nonsteroidal anti-inflammatory drug (NSAID)	Relief of symptoms caused by arthritis, such as inflammation, swelling, stiffness, and joint pain
Celestone Soluspan [betamethasone acetate/betamethasone sodium phosphate]	Z79.52	Corticosteroid; antiasthmatic	Asthma; severe inflammation
Celexa [citalopram hydrobromide]		Antidepressant	Depression
CellCept [mycophenolate mofetil]	Z79.624	Inhibitors of nucleotide synthesis	Prophylaxis of organ transplant rejection
Centany [mupirocin]	Z79.2	Antibiotic, topical	Bacterial skin infections
Cephalexin [cephalexin]	Z79.2	Antibiotic	Bacterial infections
Cerubidine [daunorubicin hydrochloride]	Z79.632	Antitumor antibiotic	Leukemia
Chantix [varenicline tartrate]		Smoking cessation aid	Nicotine addiction, smoking

Drug	Z Code	Drug Action/Classification	Indications
Chlorambucil [chlorambucil]	Z79.630	Chemotherapeutic alkylating agent	Chronic lymphocytic leukemia; malignant lymphoma
Cibinqo [abrocitinib]	Z79.622	Janus kinase (JAK) inhibitor	Atopic dermatitis
Cimduo [lamivudine/tenofovir disoproxil fumarate]	Z79.899	Antiretroviral	HIV; chronic hepatitis B
Cipro [ciprofloxacin hydrochloride]	Z79.2	Antibiotic	Cystitis; infectious diarrhea; gonorrhea; bone and joint infection; gastrointestinal tract infection; lower and upper respiratory tract infection; sinus infection; urinary tract infection; nosocomial pneumonia; chronic prostatitis
Ciprofloxacin [ciprofloxacin]	Z79.2	Antibiotic	Bacterial infections
Cisplatin [cisplatin]	Z79.630	Chemotherapeutic alkylating agent	Cancer
Clarithromycin [clarithromycin]	Z79.2	Antibiotic	Skin and respiratory bacterial infections
Claritin [loratadine]		Antihistamine	Seasonal allergic rhinitis; chronic idiopathic urticaria
Cleocin [clindamycin phosphate]	Z79.2	Antibiotic	Bacterial infections
Climara [estradiol]	Z79.890	Estrogen therapy	Osteoporosis prevention and to treat menopausal symptoms; vaginal and vulvar atrophy; hypoestrogenism; ovarian failure
Clindamycin [clindamycin phosphate]	Z79.2	Antibiotic	Bacterial infections
Clonazepam [clonazepam]		Anticonvulsant	Absence, akinetic, and myoclonic epilepsy; Lennox-Gastaut syndrome
Clonidine HCl [clonidine hydrochloride]		Antihypertensive	Hypertension
Clopidogrel bisulfate [clopidogrel bisulfate]	Z79.02	Antiplatelet	Unstable angina; heart attacks; prevention of blood clots
Codeine [codeine sulfate]	Z79.891	Analgesic, narcotic	Mild to moderate pain
Cogentin [benztropine mesylate]		Antiparkinsonism	Parkinson's disease
Colace [docusate sodium]		Gastrointestinal agent; laxative, stool softener	Constipation
Colazal [balsalazide]		Anti-inflammatory	Ulcerative colitis
Colocort [hydrocortisone]	Z79.52	Corticosteroid	Inflammation of the colon
CombiPatch [ethinyl estradiol/norethindrone acetate]	Z79.890	Estrogen therapy	Menopause symptoms; vaginal and vulvar atrophy; osteoporosis prevention
Combivent Respimat [ipratropium bromide/albuterol sulfate]		Antiasthmatic/bronchodilator	Chronic bronchitis, emphysema; bronchial asthma
Compro [prochlorperazine]		Antiemetic; antipsychotic	Nausea, vomiting, and manic phase of bipolar syndrome or schizophrenia
Conjupri [levamlodipine maleate]		Antihypertensive	Hypertension
Copaxone [glatiramer acetate]	Z79.69	Other immunosuppressant/immunomodulator	Treatment of relapsing multiple sclerosis
Coreg [carvedilol]		Beta blocker	Hypertension; chronic heart failure; left ventricular dysfunction following myocardial infarction
Coreg CR [carvedilol phosphate]		Beta blocker	Hypertension; chronic heart failure; left ventricular dysfunction following myocardial infarction
Cortef [hydrocortisone]	Z79.52	Corticosteroid	Severe inflammation
Cortenema [hydrocortisone]	Z79.52	Corticosteroid	Inflammation of the colon
Cortifoam [hydrocortisone acetate]	Z79.52	Corticosteroid	Colon and rectum inflammation
Cortisone acetate [cortisone acetate]	Z79.52	Corticosteroid	Inflammation
Cortisporin [hydrocortisone acetate/neomycin sulfate/polymyxin B sulfate]		Topical anti-infective, topical steroid	Dermatosis
Cosentyx [secukinumab]	Z79.620	Immunosuppressive biologic; monoclonal antibody	Plaque psoriasis; psoriatic arthritis; ankylosing spondylitis
Coumadin [warfarin sodium]	Z79.01	Anticoagulant	Prophylaxis and treatment of venous thrombosis; treatment of atrial fibrillation with embolization (pulmonary embolism), arrhythmias, myocardial infarction, and stroke prevention
Cozaar [losartan potassium]		Antihypertensive	Hypertension
Crestor [rosuvastatin calcium]		HMG-CoA reductase inhibitor (statin)	Hypercholesterolemia; hyperlipidemia; hyperproteinemia
Cryselle [ethinyl estradiol/norgestrel]	Z79.3	Contraceptive	Prevention of pregnancy
Cubicin [daptomycin]	Z79.2	Antibiotic	Bacterial skin infections; Staphylococcus aureus bloodstream infections

Appendix B: Pharmacology List 2023

Drug	Z Code	Drug Action/Classification	Indications
Cyclafem [ethinyl estradiol/norethindrone]	Z79.3	Contraceptive	Prevention of pregnancy
Cyclessa [desogestrel/ethinyl estradiol]	Z79.3	Contraceptive	Prevention of pregnancy
Cyclosporine [cyclosporine]	Z79.621	Calcineurin inhibitor	Prophylaxis of organ transplant rejection
Cyltezo [adalimumab-abdm]	Z79.620	Immunosuppressive biologic; monoclonal antibody	Rheumatoid arthritis; juvenile idiopathic arthritis; psoriatic arthritis; Crohn's disease; ulcerative colitis; plaque psoriasis
Cymbalta [duloxetine hydrochloride]		Antidepressant, serotonin and norepinephrine reuptake inhibitor (SNRI)	Major depressive disorder; general anxiety disorder; fibromyalgia; diabetic peripheral neuropathy; chronic musculoskeletal pain
Cytarabine [cytarabine]	Z79.631	Antimetabolite agent	Leukemia
Cytomel [liothyronine sodium]		Thyroid hormone	Hypothyroidism or prevention of euthyroid goiters
Cytoxan [cyclophosphamide]	Z79.630	Chemotherapeutic alkylating agent	Cancer
Daptomycin [daptomycin]	Z79.2	Antibiotic	Skin and underlying tissue bacterial infections
Dasetta [ethinyl estradiol/norethindrone]	Z79.3	Contraceptive	Prevention of pregnancy
Daypro [oxaprozin]	Z79.1	Nonsteroidal anti-inflammatory drug (NSAID)	Osteoarthritis and rheumatoid arthritis
Daysee [ethinyl estradiol/levonorgestrel]	Z79.3	Contraceptive	Prevention of pregnancy
Delestrogen [estradiol valerate]	Z79.890	Estrogen therapy	Menopause symptoms
Demerol [meperidine hydrochloride]	Z79.891	Analgesic, narcotic	Moderate to severe pain
Depakote [divalproex sodium]		Anticonvulsant	Bipolar affective disorder; complex absence, complex partial and mixed pattern epilepsy; migraine headache
Depo-Medrol [methylprednisolone acetate]	Z79.52	Corticosteroid	Arthritis; joint disorders
Depo-Provera [medroxyprogesterone acetate]	Z79.3, Z79.890	Antineoplastic; contraceptive; progestin	Amenorrhea; carcinoma, endometrium, adjunct; carcinoma, renal; prevention of pregnancy; hemorrhage
Depo-SubQ Provera [medroxyprogesterone acetate]	Z79.3	Contraceptive	Prevention of pregnancy; menstrual disorder pain
Descovy [emtricitabine/tenofovir alafenamide]	Z79.899	Antiretroviral	HIV
Desogen [desogestrel/ethinyl estradiol]	Z79.3	Contraceptive	Prevention of pregnancy
Detrol [tolterodine tartrate]		Muscarinic receptor antagonist	Overactive bladders in patients with urinary frequency, urgency, or urge incontinence
Dexamethasone Intensol [dexamethasone]	Z79.52	Corticosteroid	Arthritis; allergic disorders; breathing disorders; lupus
Dexilant [dexlansoprazole]		Proton pump inhibitor	Healing of erosive esophagitis; relieve of heartburn; treatment of nonerosive gastroesophageal reflux disease
DiaBeta [glyburide]	Z79.84	Oral hypoglycemic	Diabetes mellitus
Diclegis [doxylamine succinate/pyridoxine hydrochloride]		Antiemetic	Nausea/vomiting in pregnancy
Dificid [fidaxomicin]	Z79.2	Antibiotic	Clostridium difficile
Diflucan [fluconazole]		Antifungal	Oropharyngeal and esophageal candidiasis and cryptococcal meningitis in AIDS patients
Digoxin [digoxin]		Cardiotonic glycoside	Heart failure, atrial flutter, atrial fibrillation, and supraventricular tachycardia
Dilantin [phenytoin sodium]		Anticonvulsant	Grand mal and psychomotor seizures
Dilaudid [hydromorphone hydrochloride]	Z79.891	Analgesic, narcotic	Moderate to severe pain
Diovan [valsartan]		Antihypertensive	Hypertension
Diskets [methadone hydrochloride]		Opioid agonist	Treatment of opioid addiction
Divigel [estradiol]	Z79.890	Estrogen therapy – topical	Menopause symptoms
Dolophine HCl [methadone hydrochloride]	Z79.891	Analgesic, narcotic; opioid agonist	Pain; treatment of opioid addiction
Dovato [dolutegravir sodium/lamivudine]	Z79.899	Antiretroviral	HIV; chronic hepatitis B
Doxorubicin [doxorubicin]	Z79.632	Antitumor antibiotic	Hodgkin lymphoma; non-Hodgkin lymphoma; specific types of cancers and leukemias
Doxycycline [doxycycline]	Z79.2	Antibiotic	Bacterial infections; acne

Drug	Z Code	Drug Action/Classification	Indications
Duavee [bazedoxifene acetate/conjugated estrogens]	Z79.890	Estrogen therapy	Menopause symptoms; osteoporosis prevention
Duetact [glimepiride/pioglitazone hydrochloride]	Z79.84	Oral hypoglycemic	Diabetes mellitus
Duexis [famotidine/ibuprofen]	Z79.1	Nonsteroidal anti-inflammatory drug (NSAID)	Symptomatic treatment of osteoarthritis and rheumatoid arthritis; reduce risk of ulcers
Dulera [formoterol fumarate/mometasone furoate]	Z79.51	Corticosteroid – inhaled; antiasthmatic	Prophylaxis and treatment of asthma
Dupixent [dupilumab]	Z79.620	Immunosuppressive biologic; monoclonal antibody	Atopic dermatitis; asthma
Duragesic [fentanyl]	Z79.891	Analgesic, narcotic	Chronic pain
Duramorph PF [morphine sulfate]	Z79.891	Analgesic, narcotic	Moderate to severe pain
Durlaza [aspirin]	Z79.82	Aspirin	Prevention of heart attack, stroke, angina
Dymista [azelastine/fluticasone]	Z79.899	Corticosteroid – intranasal	Seasonal allergies
Dynacin [minocycline hydrochloride]	Z79.2	Antibiotic	Severe acne treatment
E.E.S. [erythromycin ethylsuccinate]	Z79.2	Antibiotic	Bacterial infections
Effexor XR [venlafaxine hydrochloride]		Antidepressant, serotonin and norepinephrine reuptake inhibitors (SNRIs)	Major depressive disorder; social anxiety disorder; panic disorder
Effient [prasugrel hydrochloride]	Z79.02	Antiplatelet	Lessening of the chance of heart attack or stroke
Elestrin [estradiol]	Z79.890	Estrogen therapy	Menopause symptoms
Eligard [leuprolide acetate]	Z79.818	Agents affecting estrogen receptors and estrogen levels	Palliative treatment of prostate cancer symptoms
Elinest [norgestrel/ethinyl estradiol]	Z79.3	Contraceptive	Prevention of pregnancy
Eliquis [apixaban]	Z79.01	Anticoagulant	Venous thrombosis
Elyxyb [celecoxib]	Z79.1	Nonsteroidal anti-inflammatory drug (NSAID)	Migraine headache
Emoquette [ethinyl estradiol/desogestrel]	Z79.3	Contraceptive	Prevention of pregnancy
Emtriva [emtricitabine]	Z79.899	Antiretroviral	HIV
Enbrel [etanercept]	Z79.620	Immunosuppressive biologic	Rheumatoid arthritis; polyarticular juvenile idiopathic arthritis; psoriatic arthritis; ankylosing spondylitis; plaque psoriasis
Enpresse-28 [ethinyl estradiol/levonorgestrel]	Z79.3	Contraceptive	Prevention of pregnancy
Enskyce [desogestrel/ethinyl estradiol]	Z79.3	Contraceptive	Prevention of pregnancy
Entocort EC [budesonide]	Z79.52	Corticosteroid	Crohn's disease; ulcerative colitis
Entresto [sacubitril/valsartan]		Angiotensin II receptor blocker; neprilysin inhibitor	Chronic heart failure
Entyvio [vedolizumab]	Z79.620	Immunosuppressive biologic; monoclonal antibody	Ulcerative colitis; Crohn's disease
Envarsus XR [tacrolimus]	Z79.621	Calcineurin inhibitor	Prophylaxis of organ transplant rejection
Epinephrine [epinephrine]		Bronchodilator, cardiotonic	Most commonly, relief of distress due to bronchospasm and restoration of cardiac rhythm in cardiac arrest
Epivir, Epivir-HBV [lamivudine]	Z79.899	Antiretroviral	HIV; chronic hepatitis B
Erelzi [etanercept-szzs]	Z79.899	Antirheumatic	Rheumatoid arthritis; polyarticular juvenile idiopathic arthritis; psoriatic arthritis; ankylosing spondylitis; plaque psoriasis
Errin [norethindrone]	Z79.3	Contraceptive	Prevention of pregnancy
Ertapenem [ertapenem sodium]	Z79.2	Antibiotic	Stomach, urinary tract, pelvis, skin and lung infections
ERYC [erythromycin]	Z79.2	Antibiotic	Respiratory tract infections
Erygel [erythromycin]	Z79.2	Antibiotic, topical	Bacterial skin infections
EryPed [erythromycin ethylsuccinate]	Z79.2	Antibiotic	Bacterial infections; rheumatic fever attacks
Ery-Tab [erythromycin]	Z79.2	Antibiotic	Bacterial infections
Erythrocin [erythromycin lactobionate]	Z79.2	Antibiotic	Bacterial infections
Erythromycin [erythromycin]	Z79.2	Antibiotic	Respiratory tract infections
Estarylla [ethinyl estradiol/norgestimate]	Z79.3	Contraceptive	Prevention of pregnancy
Estrace [estradiol]	Z79.890	Estrogen therapy	Vaginal cream for treatment of vaginal and vulvar atrophy

Drug	Z Code	Drug Action/Classification	Indications
EstroGel [estradiol]	Z79.890	Estrogen therapy – topical	Menopause symptoms
Estrostep Fe [ethinyl estradiol/norethindrone acetate]	Z79.3	Contraceptive	Prevention of pregnancy
Etoposide [etoposide]	Z79.634	Topoisomerase inhibitor	Small cell lung cancer
Evista [raloxifene hydrochloride]	Z79.810	Selective estrogen receptor modulator (SERM)	Prevention of thinning of the bones (osteoporosis) only in postmenopausal women
Exemestane [exemestane]	Z79.811	Aromatase inhibitor	Postmenopausal breast cancer
Factive [gemifloxacin mesylate]	Z79.2	Antibiotic	Bacterial lung infections
Falmina [ethinyl estradiol/levonorgestrel]	Z79.3	Contraceptive	Prevention of pregnancy
Fareston [toremifene citrate]	Z79.810	Selective estrogen receptor modulator (SERM)	Treatment of metastatic breast cancer in postmenopausal women
Farxiga [dapagliflozin propanediol]	Z79.84	Oral hypoglycemic	Diabetes mellitus
Faslodex [fulvestrant]	Z79.818	Agents affecting estrogen receptors and estrogen levels	Hormone-related breast cancer; metastatic breast cancer
Feldene [piroxicam]	Z79.1	Nonsteroidal anti-inflammatory drug (NSAID)	Treatment of pain and inflammation due to arthritis
Femara [letrozole]	Z79.811	Aromatase inhibitor	Postmenopausal breast cancer
Femhrt [ethinyl estradiol/norethindrone acetate]	Z79.3, Z79.890	Contraceptive; estrogen therapy	Prevention of pregnancy; menopause symptoms; osteoporosis prevention
Femring [estradiol acetate]	Z79.890	Estrogen therapy	Osteoporosis prevention and to treat menopausal symptoms; hypoestrogenism; ovarian failure
Fentanyl citrate [fentanyl citrate]	Z79.891	Analgesic, narcotic	Postprocedural or chronic pain
Fentora [fentanyl citrate]	Z79.891	Analgesic, narcotic	Breakthrough cancer pain
Fetroja [cefiderocol]	Z79.2	Antibiotic	Complicated urinary tract infections; pyelonephritis
Fiasp [insulin aspart]	Z79.4	Insulin	Diabetes mellitus
Fioricet with codeine [acetaminophen/butalbital/caffeine/codeine phosphate]	Z79.891	Analgesic, narcotic	Tension headaches
Firmagon [degarelix]	Z79.890	Hormone therapy	Prostate cancer
Flagyl [metronidazole]	Z79.2	Antibiotic	Bacterial infections
Flavoxate HCl [flavoxate hydrochloride]		Urinary tract spasmolytic	Relief of dysuria, urgency, nocturia, suprapubic pain, frequency, and incontinence associated with cystitis, prostatitis, urethritis, and urethrocystitis/urethrotrigonitis
Flomax [tamsulosin hydrochloride]		Antiadrenergic	Benign prostatic hyperplasia
Flonase allergy relief [fluticasone propionate]	Z79.899	Corticosteroid – intranasal	Perennial and seasonal allergic rhinitis
Flovent HFA [fluticasone propionate]	Z79.51	Corticosteroid – inhaled; antiasthmatic	Asthma
Fortaz [ceftazidime]	Z79.2	Antibiotic	Pneumonia and lower respiratory infections
Fosamax [alendronate sodium]	Z79.83	Bisphosphonate	Osteoporosis; Paget's disease
Fosinopril sodium [fosinopril sodium]		ACE inhibitor	Hypertension
Fosrenol [lanthanum carbonate]		Phosphate binder	End-stage renal disease (ESRD)
Fragmin [dalteparin sodium]	Z79.01	Anticoagulant	Prophylaxis and treatment of blood clots
Garamycin [gentamicin sulfate]	Z79.2	Antibiotic	Severe bacterial infections
Gengraf [cyclosporine]	Z79.621	Calcineurin inhibitor	Prophylaxis of organ transplant rejection
Gentamicin sulfate [gentamicin sulfate]	Z79.2	Antibiotic	Severe bacterial infections
Gildagia [ethinyl estradiol/norethindrone]	Z79.3	Contraceptive	Prevention of pregnancy
Gildess [ethinyl estradiol/norethindrone acetate]	Z79.3	Contraceptive	Prevention of pregnancy
Glimepiride [glimepiride]	Z79.84	Oral hypoglycemic	Diabetes mellitus
Glucotrol [glipizide]	Z79.84	Oral hypoglycemic	Diabetes mellitus
Glumetza [metformin hydrochloride]	Z79.84	Oral hypoglycemic	Diabetes mellitus
Glyburide (micronized) [glyburide]	Z79.84	Oral hypoglycemic	Diabetes mellitus
Glynase [glyburide]	Z79.84	Oral hypoglycemic	Diabetes mellitus
Glyset [miglitol]	Z79.84	Oral hypoglycemic	Diabetes mellitus

Drug	Z Code	Drug Action/Classification	Indications
Harvoni [ledipasvir/sofosbuvir]	Z79.899	Antiviral	Chronic hepatitis C
Heparin sodium [heparin sodium]	Z79.01	Anticoagulant	Prophylaxis and treatment of venous thrombosis, pulmonary embolism; prevention of cerebral thrombosis, and treatment of consumptive coagulopathies
Hiprex [methenamine]	Z79.2	Antibiotic	Recurring bladder infection
Humalog [insulin lispro recombinant]	Z79.4	Insulin	Diabetes mellitus
Humira [adalimumab]	Z79.620	Immunosuppressive biologic; monoclonal antibody	Rheumatoid arthritis; juvenile idiopathic arthritis; psoriatic arthritis; Crohn's disease; ulcerative colitis; plaque psoriasis; hidradenitis suppurativa; uveitis
Humulin R [insulin recombinant]	Z79.4	Insulin	Diabetes mellitus
Hycamtin [topotecan]	Z79.634	Topoisomerase inhibitor	Cancer
Hydrocodone [acetaminophen/hydrocodone bitartrate]	Z79.891	Analgesic, narcotic	Moderate to severe pain
Hydrocodone bitartrate and acetaminophen [acetaminophen/ hydrocodone bitartrate]	Z79.891	Analgesic, narcotic	Pain, moderate to severe
Hydrocortisone [hydrocortisone]	Z79.52	Corticosteroid	Addison's disease; arthritis; immune disorders; allergies; breathing problems
Hydromorphone HCl [hydromorphone hydrochloride]	Z79.891	Analgesic, narcotic	Moderate to severe pain
Hydroxyurea [hydroxyurea]	Z79.64	Myelosuppressive agent	Pain related to sickle cell disease; chronic myeloid leukemia; ovarian cancer
Hyrimoz [adalimumab-adaz]	Z79.620	Immunosuppressive biologic; monoclonal antibody	Rheumatoid arthritis; juvenile idiopathic arthritis; psoriatic arthritis; Crohn's disease; ulcerative colitis; plaque psoriasis
Hyzaar [hydrochlorothiazide/ losartan potassium]		Antihypertensive	Hypertension
Ibsrela [tenapanor hydrochloride]		NHE-3 inhibitor	Irritable bowel syndrome with constipation (IBS-C)
Ibuprofen [ibuprofen]	Z79.1	Nonsteroidal anti-inflammatory drug (NSAID)	Pain or fever relief
Imitrex [sumatriptan succinate]		Antimigraine	Migraine headache
Imuran [azathioprine]	Z79.624	Inhibitors of nucleotide synthesis	Rheumatoid arthritis; prophylaxis of organ transplant rejection
Inderal XL [propranolol hydrochloride]		Beta blocker	Angina pectoris; hypertension; cardiac arrhythmias
Indocin [indomethacin]	Z79.1	Nonsteroidal anti-inflammatory drug (NSAID)	Treatment of pain and inflammation
Integrilin [eptifibatide]	Z79.02	Antiplatelet	Unstable angina; heart attacks; prevention of blood clots
Intron A [interferon alfa 2-b]	Z79.69	Other immunosuppressant/ immunomodulator	Cancer; hepatitis
Introvale [levonorgestrel/ethinyl estradiol]	Z79.3	Contraceptive	Prevention of pregnancy
Invanz [ertapenem sodium]	Z79.2	Antibiotic	Stomach, urinary tract, pelvis, skin, and lung infections
Invokamet [canagliflozin/metformin hydrochloride]	Z79.84	Oral hypoglycemic	Diabetes mellitus
Invokana [canagliflozin]	Z79.84	Oral hypoglycemic	Diabetes mellitus
Isoniazid [isoniazid]	Z79.2	Antibiotic	Tuberculosis
Isopto Carpine [pilocarpine hydrochloride]		Cholinergic parasympathomimetic agent	Reduction of intraocular pressure in open-angle glaucoma or ocular hypertension; management of acute angle-closure glaucoma
Isordil Titradose [isosorbide dinitrate]		Smooth muscle relaxant	Acute anginal attacks
Isturisa [osilodrostat]		Cortisol synthesis inhibitor	Cushing's disease in adults
Isuprel [isoproterenol hydrochloride]		Adrenergic agent	Bronchodilator for asthma, chronic pulmonary emphysema, bronchitis, and other conditions accompanied by bronchospasm; can be used in cardiogenic shock cases
Ixempra [ixabepilone]	Z79.633	Mitotic inhibitor	Advanced breast cancer
Jantoven [warfarin sodium]	Z79.01	Anticoagulant	Prophylaxis and treatment of venous thrombosis, pulmonary embolism; prevention of cerebral thrombosis, and treatment of consumptive coagulopathies
Janumet [metformin hydrochloride/sitagliptin phosphate]	Z79.84	Oral hypoglycemic	Diabetes mellitus

Drug	Z Code	Drug Action/Classification	Indications
Januvia [sitagliptin phosphate]	Z79.84	Oral hypoglycemic	Diabetes mellitus
Jencycla [norethindrone]	Z79.3	Contraceptive	Prevention of pregnancy
Jentadueto [linagliptin/metformin hydrochloride]]	Z79.84	Oral hypoglycemic	Diabetes mellitus
Junel [ethinyl estradiol/norethindrone acetate]	Z79.3	Contraceptive	Prevention of pregnancy
Kadian [morphine sulfate]	Z79.891	Analgesic, narcotic	Moderate to severe pain
Kariva [desogestrel/ethinyl estradiol]	Z79.3	Contraceptive	Prevention of pregnancy
Katerzia [amlodipine benzoate]		Antihypertensive	Hypertension; coronary artery disease (CAD); chronic stable angina; prinzmetal's angina; variant angina
Kazano [alogliptin benzoate/metformin hydrochloride]	Z79.84	Oral hypoglycemic	Diabetes mellitus
Keflex [cephalexin]	Z79.2	Antibiotic	Bone, middle ear, skin and skin structures, upper respiratory tract and urinary tract infections; acute prostatitis
Kelnor [ethynodiol diacetate/ethinyl estradiol]	Z79.3	Contraceptive	Prevention of pregnancy
Kenalog-10; Kenalog-40 [triamcinolone acetonide]	Z79.52	Corticosteroid	Gouty arthritis; bursitis; tenosynovitis; epicondylitis; rheumatoid arthritis; synovitis; osteoarthritis
Keytruda [pembrolizumab]	Z79.620	Immunosuppressive biologic; monoclonal antibody	Cancer
Kimidess [ethinyl estradiol/desogestrel]	Z79.3	Contraceptive	Prevention of pregnancy
Klaron [sulfacetamide sodium]	Z79.2	Antibiotic, topical	Acne vulgaris
Klonopin [clonazepam]		Anticonvulsant; CNS depressant	Epilepsy; seizures; panic disorder
Klor-Con [potassium chloride]		Replaces potassium and maintains potassium level	Hypokalemia
Kombiglyze [metformin hydrochloride/saxagliptin hydrochloride]	Z79.84	Oral hypoglycemic	Diabetes mellitus
K-Tab [potassium chloride]		Replaces potassium and maintains potassium level	Hypokalemia
Kurvelo [ethinyl estradiol/levonorgestrel]	Z79.3	Contraceptive	Prevention of pregnancy; menstrual disorders
Kyleena [levonorgestrel]	Z79.3	Contraceptive	Prevention of pregnancy
Lamisil [terbinafine hydrochloride]		Antifungal	Tinea cruris (jock itch); T. pedis (athlete's foot); T. corporis (ringworm)
Lanoxin [digoxin]		Cardiotonic glycoside	Congestive heart failure
Lantus [insulin glargine recombinant]	Z79.4	Insulin	Diabetes mellitus
Larin [ethinyl estradiol/norethindrone acetate]	Z79.3	Contraceptive	Prevention of pregnancy
Lasix [furosemide]		Antihypertensive; diuretic	Management of edema associated with congestive heart failure, renal disease, including nephrotic syndrome and hypertension
Lazanda [fentanyl citrate]	Z79.891	Analgesics, narcotic	Breakthrough cancer pain
Lescol XL [fluvastatin sodium]		HMG-CoA reductase inhibitor (statin)	Hypercholesterolemia; hyperlipidemia; hyperlipoproteinemia
Lessina-28 [ethinyl estradiol/levonorgestrel]	Z79.3	Contraceptive	Prevention of pregnancy
Letrozole [letrozole]	Z79.811	Aromatase inhibitor	Postmenopausal breast cancer
Leukeran [chlorambucil]	Z79.630	Chemotherapeutic alkylating agent	Cancer
Levemir [insulin detemir recombinant]	Z79.4	Insulin	Diabetes mellitus
Levonest [levonorgestrel/ethinyl estradiol]	Z79.3	Contraceptive	Prevention of pregnancy; menstrual disorders; acne
Levora [levonorgestrel/ethinyl estradiol]	Z79.3	Contraceptive	Prevention of pregnancy
Levoxyl [levothyroxine sodium]		Thyroid hormone	Euthyroid goiter; hypothyroidism
Lexapro [escitalopram oxalate]		Antidepressant, selective serotonin reuptake inhibitor (SSRI)	Depression; anxiety
Lialda [mesalamine]		Anti-inflammatory	Ulcerative colitis
Lidocaine HCl [lidocaine hydrochloride]		Antiarrhythmic	Management of ventricular arrhythmias or during cardiac manipulation, such as cardiac surgery

Drug	Z Code	Drug Action/Classification	Indications
Liletta [levonorgestrel]	Z79.3	Contraceptive	Intrauterine device to prevent pregnancy
Lincocin [lincocin hydrochloride]	Z79.2	Antibiotic	Severe bacterial infections
Lipitor [atorvastatin calcium]		HMG-CoA reductase inhibitor (statin)	Hypercholesterolemia; hyperlipidemia; hyperproteinemia
Lithium carbonate [lithium carbonate]		Antimanic	Control of manic episodes in bipolar disorders
Livtencity [maribavir]	Z79.899	Antiviral	Post-transplant CMV infection/disease
Lo Loestrin Fe [ethinyl estradiol/norethindrone acetate]	Z79.3	Contraceptive	Prevention of pregnancy
Locoid [hydrocortisone butyrate]	Z79.52	Corticosteroid – topical	Atopic dermatitis; other dermatoses
Loestrin [ethinyl estradiol/norethindrone acetate]	Z79.3	Contraceptive	Prevention of pregnancy
Lomotil [diphenoxylate hydrochloride/atropine sulfate]		Antidiarrheal	Symptoms of chronic and functional diarrhea
Lopid [gemfibrozil]		Lipid regulating agent	Hypercholesterolemia; hyperlipidemia; hyperlipoproteinemia; hypertriglyceridemia
Lopressor [metoprolol tartrate]		Beta blocker	Angina pectoris; hypertension; acute myocardial infarction
Lorazepam [lorazepam]		Antianxiety; sedative/hypnotic	Anxiety disorder associated with depressive symptoms; controls tension, agitation, irritability, and insomnia
Loryna [drospirenone/ethinyl estradiol]	Z79.3	Contraceptive	Prevention of pregnancy
LoSeasonique [ethinyl estradiol/levonorgestrel]	Z79.3	Contraceptive	Prevention of pregnancy
Lotensin [benazepril hydrochloride]		ACE inhibitor	Hypertension
Lotrel [amlodipine besylate/benazepril hydrochloride]		Antihypertensive	Hypertension
Lotrisone [clotrimazole/ betamethasone dipropionate]		Antifungal-corticosteroid	Relief of redness, swelling, itching, and other discomfort of fungus infections
Lovastatin [lovastatin]		HMG-CoA reductase inhibitor (statin)	Hypercholesterolemia; hyperlipidemia; hyperlipoproteinemia
Lovenox [enoxaparin sodium]	Z79.01	Anticoagulant	Prophylaxis and treatment of venous thrombosis and pulmonary embolism
Low-Ogestrel-28 [norgestrel/ethinyl estradiol]	Z79.3	Contraceptive	Prevention of pregnancy
Lupkynis [voclosporin]	Z79.621	Calcineurin inhibitor	Lupus nephritis
Lupron Depot [leuprolide acetate]	Z79.818	Agents affecting estrogen receptors and estrogen levels	Endometriosis symptoms; uterine fibroids
Macrobid [nitrofurantoin]	Z79.2	Antibiotic	Urinary tract infections
Macrodantin [nitrofurantoin]	Z79.2	Antibiotic	Urinary tract infections
Marlissa [ethinyl estradiol/levonorgestrel]	Z79.3	Contraceptive	Prevention of pregnancy
Maxipime [cefepime hydrochloride]	Z79.2	Antibiotic	Bacterial infections
Meclizine hydrochloride [meclizine hydrochloride]		Antihistamine	Nausea and vomiting, and dizziness associated with motion sickness
Medrol [methylprednisolone]	Z79.52	Corticosteroid	Endocrine, rheumatic, hematologic disorders; collagen, dermatological, ophthalmic, respiratory, neoplastic, gastrointestinal, nervous system disorders; allergic and edematous states
Megace ES [megestrol acetate]	Z79.818	Agents affecting estrogen receptors and estrogen levels	Endometrial or advanced breast cancers; weight loss due to AIDS
Menest [esterified estrogens]	Z79.890	Estrogen therapy	Menopause symptoms; ovarian failure
Menostar [estradiol]	Z79.890	Estrogen therapy	Menopause symptoms; osteoporosis prevention
Mepron [atovaquone]	Z79.2	Antibiotic	Pneumonia due to pneumocystis jirovecii
Merrem [meropenem]	Z79.2	Antibiotic	Bacterial infections of skin or stomach; bacterial meningitis
Metformin [metformin hydrochloride]	Z79.84	Oral hypoglycemic	Diabetes mellitus
Methadone HCl [methadone hydrochloride]	Z79.891	Analgesic, narcotic; opioid agonist	Pain; treatment of opioid addiction
Methadose [methadone hydrochloride]	Z79.891	Analgesic, narcotic	Acute and chronic pain
Methergine [methylergonovine maleate]		Oxytocic agent	Routine management of postpartum hemorrhage after delivery of placenta
Methotrexate [methotrexate]	Z79.631	Antimetabolite agent	Cancer

Drug	Z Code	Drug Action/Classification	Indications
Methylprednisolone [methylprednisolone]	Z79.52	Corticosteroid	Inflammatory disorders
Metronidazole [metronidazole]	Z79.2	Antibiotic	Bacterial infections
Miacalcin [calcitonin salmon]		Calcitonin; a peptide hormone	Hypercalcemia; osteoporosis; postmenopausal symptoms; Paget's disease
Microgestin [ethinyl estradiol/norethindrone acetate]	Z79.3	Contraceptive	Prevention of pregnancy
Minastrin [ethinyl estradiol/norethindrone acetate]	Z79.3	Contraceptive	Prevention of pregnancy
Minivelle [estradiol]	Z79.890	Estrogen therapy	Menopause symptoms; osteoporosis prevention
Minocin [minocycline hydrochloride]	Z79.2	Antibiotic	Bacterial infections; acne
Mirena [levonorgestrel]	Z79.3	Contraceptive	Intrauterine device for prevention of pregnancy; menstrual disorders
Mitomycin [mitomycin]	Z79.632	Antitumor antibiotic	Stomach and pancreas cancer
Mobic [meloxicam]	Z79.1	Nonsteroidal anti-inflammatory drug (NSAID)	Treatment of pain and inflammation due to osteoarthritis and rheumatoid arthritis
Monoclonal antibodies	Z79.620	Immunosuppressive biologic	Cancer; prophylaxis of organ transplant rejection
Monodox [doxycycline]	Z79.2	Antibiotic	Bacterial infections; acne
Mono-Linyah [norgestimate/ethinyl estradiol]	Z79.3	Contraceptive	Prevention of pregnancy; menstrual disorders; acne
Monurol [fosfomycin tromethamine]	Z79.2	Antibiotic	Bacterial bladder infections
Morphine sulfate [morphine sulfate]	Z79.891	Analgesic, narcotic	Moderate to severe pain
Motrin IB [ibuprofen]	Z79.1	Nonsteroidal anti-inflammatory drug (NSAID)	Pain or fever relief
MS Contin [morphine sulfate]	Z79.891	Analgesic, narcotic	Moderate to severe pain
Multaq [dronedarone hydrochloride]		Cardiac rhythm regulator	Treatment of patients with recent episodes of atrial fibrillation or atrial flutter
Mycobutin [rifabutin]	Z79.2	Antibiotic	Mycobacterium avium complex (MAC) prophylactic in HIV patients
Mytesi [crofelemer]		Antidiarrheal	Diarrhea occurring in HIV/AIDs patient's on anti-retroviral therapy
Myzilra [ethinyl estradiol/levonorgestrel]	Z79.3	Contraceptive	Prevention of pregnancy
Nabumetone [nabumetone]	Z79.1	Nonsteroidal anti-inflammatory drug (NSAID)	Osteoarthritis and rheumatoid arthritis
Nalfon [fenoprofen calcium]	Z79.1	Nonsteroidal anti-inflammatory drug (NSAID)	Pain or inflammation relief
Namzaric [memantine/donepezil hydrochlorides]		Acetylcholinesterase/cholinesterase inhibitors	Dementia due to Alzheimer's
Naprelan [naproxen sodium]	Z79.1	Nonsteroidal anti-inflammatory drug (NSAID)	Pain or inflammation relief
Naprosyn [naproxen]	Z79.1	Nonsteroidal anti-inflammatory drug (NSAID)	Rheumatoid, gouty arthritis and osteoarthritis; ankylosing spondylitis; bursitis; dysmenorrhea; pain, mild to moderate; tendonitis
Natazia [estradiol valerate/dienogest]	Z79.3	Contraceptive	Prevention of pregnancy; menstrual disorders
Nebupent [pentamidine isethionate]	Z79.2	Antibiotic	Severe bacterial lung infection in high risk patients with HIV
Nefazodone HCl [nefazodone hydrochloride]		Antidepressant	Depression
Nembutal sodium [pentobarbital sodium]		Sedative/hypnotic	Adjunct medication in diagnostic procedures or for emergency use with convulsive disorders
NeoProfen [ibuprofen lysine]	Z79.1	Nonsteroidal anti-inflammatory drug (NSAID)	Pain or fever relief
Neoral [cyclosporine]	Z79.621	Calcineurin inhibitor	Prophylaxis of organ transplant rejection
Neosporin [bacitracin, neomycin]	Z79.2	Antibiotic, topical	Bacterial skin infections
Neurontin [gabapentin]		Anticonvulsant	Epilepsy, partial
Nexium [esomeprazole magnesium]		Proton pump inhibitor	Gastroesophageal reflux disease (GERD), erosive esophagitis
Nexletol [bempedoic acid]	Z79.899	Antihyperlipidemic	Heterozygous familial hypercholesterolemia; established atherosclerotic cardiovascular disease requiring additional lowering of LDL-C
Nexplanon [etonogestrel]	Z79.3	Contraceptive	Implantable device used for prevention of pregnancy

Appendix B: Pharmacology List 2023

Drug	Z Code	Drug Action/Classification	Indications
Nextstellis [drospirenone and estetrol]	Z79.3	Contraceptive	Prevention of pregnancy
Nitrofurantoin [nitrofurantoin]	Z79.2	Antibiotic	Bacterial urinary tract infections
Nitropress [sodium nitroprusside]		Vasodilator	Potent, rapid action in reducing blood pressure in hypertensive crisis or for controlling bleeding during anesthesia by producing controlled hypotension
Nitrostat [nitroglycerin]		Muscle relaxant; antianginal; antihypertensive; coronary vasodilator	Prophylaxis and treatment of angina pectoris; heart failure associated with myocardial infarction; hypertension, perioperative; surgery, adjunct
Norco [acetaminophen/hydrocodone bitartrate]	Z79.891	Analgesic, narcotic	Moderate to severe pain
Norinyl [mestranol/norethisterone]	Z79.3	Contraceptive	Prevention of pregnancy
Norpace [disopyramide phosphate]		Antiarrhythmic	Coronary artery disease, for prevention, recurrence, and control of unifocal, multifocal, and paired PVCs
Nortrel [ethinyl estradiol/norethindrone]	Z79.3	Contraceptive	Prevention of pregnancy
Norvasc [amlodipine besylate]		Antihypertensive	Hypertension; coronary artery disease (CAD); chronic stable angina; prinzmetal's angina; variant angina
Novolin [insulin recombinant]	Z79.4	Insulin	Diabetes mellitus
Novolog [insulin aspart recombinant]	Z79.4	Insulin	Diabetes mellitus
Nucynta [tapentadol hydrochloride]	Z79.891	Analgesic, narcotic	Moderate to severe pain
NuvaRing [etonogestrel/ethinyl estradiol]	Z79.3	Contraceptive	Vaginal ring to prevent pregnancy
Ogestrel [norgestrel/ethinyl estradiol]	Z79.3	Contraceptive	Prevention of pregnancy
Olumiant [baricitinib]	Z79.622	Janus kinase (JAK) inhibitor	Rheumatoid arthritis
Onglyza [saxagliptin hydrochloride]	Z79.84	Oral hypoglycemic	Diabetes mellitus
Oracea [doxycycline]	Z79.2	Antibiotic	Rosacea
Orapred ODT [prednisolone sodium phosphate]	Z79.52	Corticosteroid	Inflammatory disorders
Orbactiv [oritavancin diphosphate]	Z79.2	Antibiotic	Bacterial skin infections
Orencia [abatacept]	Z79.69	Other immunosuppressant/immunomodulator	Rheumatoid arthritis; polyarticular juvenile idiopathic arthritis; psoriatic arthritis
Orilissa [elagolix]	Z79.890	Hormone therapy	Pain associated with endometriosis
Orphenadrine citrate [orphenadrine citrate]		Muscle relaxant	Acute spasms, tension, and post-trauma cases
Orsythia [ethinyl estradiol/levonorgestrel]	Z79.3	Contraceptive	Prevention of pregnancy
Ortho-Novum [norethindrone/ethinyl estradiol]	Z79.3	Contraceptive	Prevention of pregnancy
Oseni [alogliptin benzoate/pioglitazone hydrochloride]	Z79.84	Oral hypoglycemic	Diabetes mellitus
Osphena [ospemifene]	Z79.810, Z79.890	Selective estrogen receptor modulator (SERM)	Postmenopausal dyspareunia due to vaginal atrophy; osteoporosis prevention and treatment of menopausal symptoms
Otezla [apremilast]	Z79.61	Antirheumatic; immunomodulator	Psoriatic arthritis; plaque psoriasis
Oxazepam [oxazepam]		Antianxiety	Anxiety, tension, and alcohol withdrawal
Oxbryta [voxelotor]		Hemoglobin S polymerization inhibitor	Sickle cell disease
Oxycodone HCl [oxycodone hydrochloride]	Z79.891	Analgesic, narcotic	Moderate to severe pain
OxyContin [oxycodone hydrochloride]	Z79.891	Analgesic, narcotic	Moderate to severe pain
Ozempic [semaglutide]	Z79.85	Antidiabetic – non-insulin injectable	Diabetes mellitus
Paclitaxel [paclitaxel]	Z79.633	Mitotic inhibitor	Cancer
Paxil [paroxetine hydrochloride]		Antidepressant	Anxiety with panic disorder and depression; obsessive-compulsive disorder
PediaPred [prednisolone sodium phosphate]	Z79.52	Corticosteroid	Inflammatory disorders
PegIntron [peginterferon alfa-2b]	Z79.69	Other immunosuppressant/immunomodulator	Hepatitis C

Drug	Z Code	Drug Action/Classification	Indications
Penicillin-VK [penicillin V potassium]	Z79.2	Antibiotic	Chorea, prevention; endocarditis, prevention, secondary to tooth extraction; erysipelas; infections of the skin and skin structures, upper respiratory tract; rheumatic fever, prophylaxis; scarlet fever; Vincent's gingivitis; Vincent's pharyngitis
Pentam [pentamidine isethionate]	Z79.2	Antibiotic	Severe bacterial lung infections
Pentasa [mesalamine]		Anti-inflammatory	Ulcerative colitis and Crohn's disease
Pepcid [famotidine]		Histamine H2-receptor inhibitor	Acid/peptic disorder; adenoma, secretory; gastroesophageal reflux; duodenal and gastric ulcer; Zollinger-Ellison syndrome
Percocet [oxycodone hydrochloride/acetaminophen]	Z79.891	Analgesic, narcotic	Pain, moderate to severe
Persantine [dipyridamole]	Z79.02	Antiplatelet	Therapy for chronic angina pectoris, preventing clots post heart valve surgery
Pfizerpen [penicillin g potassium]	Z79.2	Antibiotic	Severe bacterial infections
Phenobarbital [phenobarbital sodium]		Anticonvulsant	Grand mal epilepsy
Philith [ethinyl estradiol/norethindrone]	Z79.3	Contraceptive	Prevention of pregnancy
Pimtrea [desogestrel/ethinyl estradiol]	Z79.3	Contraceptive	Prevention of pregnancy
Piqray [alpelisib]		Kinase inhibitor	Postmenopausal advanced or metastatic breast cancer that is HR positive, HER2 negative
Pirmella [ethinyl estradiol/norethindrone]	Z79.3	Contraceptive	Prevention of pregnancy
Pitocin [oxytocin]		Uterotonic	Induction or stimulation of labor at term
Plan B One-Step [levonorgestrel]	Z79.3	Contraceptive	Prevention of pregnancy
Plavix [clopidogrel bisulfate]	Z79.02	Antiplatelet	Lessening of the chance of heart attack or stroke
Pluvicto [lutetium Lu 177 vipivotide tetraxetan]		Radioligand therapeutic agent	Metastatic castration-resistant prostate cancer (mCRPC)
Pomalyst [pomalidomide]	Z79.61	Immunomodulator	Multiple myeloma; Kaposi sarcoma
Ponstel [mefenamic acid]	Z79.1	Nonsteroidal anti-inflammatory drug (NSAID)	Treatment of pain
Ponvory [ponesimod]	Z79.69	Other immunosuppressant/immunomodulator	Relapsing forms of multiple sclerosis (MS)
Portia-28 [ethinyl estradiol/levonorgestrel]	Z79.3	Contraceptive	Prevention of pregnancy
Pradaxa [dabigatran etexilate mesylate]	Z79.01	Anticoagulant	Prophylaxis and treatment of blood clots in patients with atrial fibrillation
Prasugrel [prasugrel hydrochloride]	Z79.02	Antiplatelet	Lessening the chance of heart attack or stroke
Pravachol [pravastatin sodium]		HMG-CoA reductase inhibitor (statin)	Hypercholesterolemia; hyperlipidemia; hyperlipoproteinemia
Prednisolone [prednisolone]	Z79.52	Corticosteroid	Inflammatory disorders
Prednisone [prednisone]	Z79.52	Corticosteroid	Used for its immunosuppressant effects and for relief of inflammation; used in arthritis, polymyositis and other systemic diseases
Pregnyl [chorionic gonadotropin]		Gonadotropic hormone	Prepubertal cryptorchidism; hypogonadism; corpus luteum insufficiency and infertility
Prempro [conjugated estrogens/medroxyprogesterone acetate]	Z79.890	Estrogen/progesterone therapy	Menopause; osteoporosis; atrophic vaginitis
Prevacid [lansoprazole]		Proton pump inhibitor	Acid/peptic disorder; erosive esophagitis; duodenal ulcer; Zollinger-Ellison syndrome
Previfem [ethinyl estradiol/norgestimate]	Z79.3	Contraceptive	Prevention of pregnancy
Prezcobix [darunavir/cobicistat]	Z79.899	Antiretroviral	HIV
Prezista [darunavir]	Z79.899	Antiretroviral	HIV
Priftin [rifapentine]	Z79.2	Antibiotic	Tuberculosis
Prilosec [omeprazole magnesium]		Proton pump inhibitor	Acid/peptic disorder; endocrine adenoma; erosive esophagitis; systemic mastocytosis; gastroesophageal reflux; duodenal, peptic and gastric ulcer; Zollinger-Ellison syndrome
Primaxin [cilastatin sodium/imipenem]	Z79.2	Antibiotic	Skin, stomach, bone, joint, endocarditis, UTI, female reproductive organs or lower respiratory tract infections
Prinivil [lisinopril]		ACE inhibitor	Congestive heart failure; hypertension

Drug	Z Code	Drug Action/Classification	Indications
Pristiq [desvenlafaxine]		Antidepressant; serotonin and norepinephrine reuptake inhibitor (SNRI)	Major depressive disorder
Procardia [nifedipine]		Calcium channel blocker	Management of vasospastic angina and chronic stable angina, hypertension
Prograf [tacrolimus]	Z79.621	Calcineurin inhibitor	Prophylaxis of organ transplant rejection
Prolia [denosumab]	Z79.620	Immunosuppressive biologic; monoclonal antibody	Treatment and prevention of bone resorption and prevention of bone fracture
Promethazine hydrochloride [promethazine hydrochloride]		Anesthesia, adjunct to; antiemetic; antihistamine; antitussive/expectorant; sedative/hypnotic; vertigo/motion sickness/vomiting	Anesthesia; adjunct; angioedema; conjunctivitis; dermographism; hypersensitivity, motion sickness; pain; perennial, seasonal, and allergic rhinitis; sedation, obstetrical; urticaria
Protonix [pantoprazole]		Proton pump inhibitor	Short-term treatment and maintenance therapy of erosive esophagitis associated with gastroesophageal reflux disease (GERD)
Protopic [tacrolimus]	Z79.621	Calcineurin inhibitor	Atomic dermatitis (eczema)
Proventil-HFA [albuterol sulfate]		Antiasthmatic/bronchodilator	Asthma
Provera [medroxyprogesterone acetate]	Z79.3, Z79.890	Antineoplastic; contraceptive; progestin	Amenorrhea; carcinoma, endometrium, adjunct; carcinoma, renal; prevention of pregnancy; hemorrhage
Prozac [fluoxetine hydrochloride]		Selective serotonin reuptake inhibitor (SSRI)	Bulimia nervosa; depression; obsessive-compulsive disorder
Pulmicort [budesonide]	Z79.51	Corticosteroid – inhaled; antiasthmatic	Prophylaxis and treatment of asthma
Qelbree [viloxazine hydrochloride]		Selective norepinephrine reuptake inhibitor	Attention deficit hyperactivity disorder (ADHD)
Qnasl [beclomethasone dipropionate]	Z79.899	Corticosteroid – intranasal	Perennial and seasonal allergies; vasomotor rhinitis
Qtern [dapagliflozin/saxagliptin]	Z79.84	Oral hypoglycemic	Diabetes mellitus
Quartette [levonorgestrel/ethinyl estradiol]	Z79.3	Contraceptive	Prevention of pregnancy
Qulipta [atogepant]		Calcitonin gene-related peptide inhibitor	Migraine headache prevention
Quviviq [daridorexant hydrochloride]		CNS depressant	Insomnia
Qvar Redihaler [beclomethasone dipropionate]	Z79.51	Corticosteroid – inhaled; antiasthmatic	Prophylaxis and treatment of asthma
Raloxifene HCl [raloxifene hydrochloride]	Z79.810	Selective estrogen receptor modulator (SERM)	Prevention of thinning of the bones (osteoporosis) only in postmenopausal women
Rapaflo [silodosin]		Antiadrenergic	Benign prostatic hyperplasia
Rapamune [sirolimus]	Z79.623	Mammalian target of rapamycin (mTOR) inhibitor	Prophylaxis of organ transplant rejection
Rayos [prednisone]	Z79.52	Corticosteroid; antiasthmatic	Arthritis; blood disorders; allergies; asthma
Rebetol [ribavirin]	Z79.899	Antiviral	Chronic hepatitis C
Rebif [interferon beta-1a]	Z79.69	Other immunosuppressant/ immunomodulator	Treatment of relapsing multiple sclerosis
Reclast [zoledronic acid]	Z79.83	Bisphosphonate	Prevention of thinning of the bones (osteoporosis); Paget's disease; bone cancer
Relenza [zanamivir]		Antiviral	Treat and prevent influenza A and B
Remicade [infliximab]	Z79.620	Immunosuppressive biologic; monoclonal antibody	Ankylosing spondylitis; psoriatic arthritis; rheumatoid arthritis; Crohn's disease; ulcerative colitis
Renvela [sevelamer carbonate]		Phosphate binder	Chronic kidney disease (CKD) on dialysis
Repaglinide [repaglinide]	Z79.84	Oral hypoglycemic	Diabetes mellitus
Restasis [cyclosporine ophthalmic emulsion]		Anti-inflammatory, ophthalmic	Ocular inflammation due to keratoconjunctivitis sicca
Restoril [temazepam]		Sedative/hypnotic	Insomnia
Retrovir [zidovudine]	Z79.899	Antiretroviral	HIV
Revlimid [lenalidomide]	Z79.61	Immunomodulator	Multiple myeloma following autologous stem cell transplant; myelodysplastic syndromes; mantle cell lymphoma
Reyvow [lasmiditan]		Antimigraine	Migraine headache
Rifadin [rifampin]	Z79.2	Antibiotic	Tuberculosis
Rimactane [rifampin]	Z79.2	Antibiotic	Tuberculosis
Rinvoq [upadacitinib]	Z79.622	Janus kinase (JAK) inhibitor	Rheumatoid arthritis; psoriatic arthritis; ankylosing spondylitis; ulcerative colitis
Riomet [metformin hydrochloride]	Z79.84	Oral hypoglycemic	Diabetes mellitus

Drug	Z Code	Drug Action/Classification	Indications
Risperdal [risperidone]		Antipsychotic/antimanic	Schizophrenia; bipolar I disorder
Ritalin [methylphenidate hydrochloride]		CNS stimulant	Attention deficit hyperactivity disorder (ADHD); narcolepsy
Rituxan [rituximab]	Z79.620	Immunosuppressive biologic; monoclonal antibody	Non-Hodgkin's lymphoma; chronic lymphocytic leukemia; rheumatoid arthritis; granulomatosis with polyangiitis; pemphigus vulgaris
Roxicet [oxycodone hydrochloride/acetaminophen]	Z79.891	Analgesic, narcotic	Pain, moderate to severe
Roxicodone [oxycodone hydrochloride]	Z79.891	Analgesic, narcotic	Pain relief
Rukobia [fostemsavir tromethamine]	Z79.899	Antiretroviral	HIV
Rybelsus [semaglutide]	Z79.84	Oral hypoglycemic	Diabetes mellitus
Sabril [vigabatrin]		Anticonvulsant	Refractory complex partial seizures
Safyral [drospirenone/ethinyl estradiol/levomefolate calcium]	Z79.3	Contraceptive	Prevention of pregnancy
Sandimmune [cyclosporine]	Z79.621	Calcineurin inhibitor	Prophylaxis of organ transplant rejection
Sarafem [fluoxetine hydrochloride]		Selective serotonin reuptake inhibitor (SSRI)	Premenstrual dysphoric disorder (PMDD)
Savaysa [edoxaban tosylate]	Z79.01	Anticoagulant	Prophylaxis and treatment of venous thrombosis, pulmonary embolism; prevention of blood clots due to atrial fibrillation
Scemblix [asciminib hydrochloride]		Kinase inhibitor	Philadelphia chromosome-positive chronic myeloid leukemia
Seasonale [levonorgestrel/ethinyl estradiol]	Z79.3	Contraceptive	Prevention of pregnancy
Seasonique [ethinyl estradiol/levonorgestrel]	Z79.3	Contraceptive	Prevention of pregnancy
Septra [sulfamethoxazole trimethoprim]	Z79.2	Antibiotic	Urinary tract infections; acute otitis media; acute exacerbations of chronic bronchitis; shigellosis
Serevent [salmeterol xinafoate]		Bronchodilator	Asthma
Seromycin [cycloserine]	Z79.2	Antibiotic	Tuberculosis; urinary tract infections
Seroquel XR [quetiapine fumarate]		Antipsychotic	Schizophrenia; bipolar disorder; major depressive disorder
Setlakin [ethinyl estradiol/levonorgestrel]	Z79.3	Contraceptive	Prevention of pregnancy
Silvadene [silver sulfadiazine]	Z79.2	Antibiotic, topical	Wound sepsis due to second/third degree burns
Simulect [basiliximab]	Z79.620	Immunosuppressive biologic; monoclonal antibody	Prophylaxis of organ transplant rejection
Sinemet [carbidopa/levodopa]		Antiparkinsonism	Parkinson's disease
Singulair [montelukast sodium]		Antiasthmatic	Asthma; exercise-induced bronchoconstriction; perennial and seasonal allergic rhinitis
Sirolimus [sirolimus]	Z79.623	Mammalian target of rapamycin (mTOR) inhibitor	Prophylaxis of organ transplant rejection
Sitagliptin [sitagliptin/metformin hydrochloride]	Z79.84	Oral hypoglycemic	Diabetes mellitus
Sivextro [tedizolid phosphate]	Z79.2	Antibiotic	Skin infections including MRSA
Skyla [levonorgestrel]	Z79.3	Contraceptive	Intrauterine device to prevent pregnancy
Skyrizi [risankizumab]	Z79.620	Immunosuppressive biologic; monoclonal antibody	Plaque psoriasis
Soliqua [insulin glargine/lixisenatide]	Z79.4	Insulin	Diabetes mellitus
Solodyn [minocycline hydrochloride]	Z79.2	Antibiotic	Bacterial infections
Solosec [secnidazole]	Z79.2	Antibiotic	Bacterial vaginal inflammation; trichomoniasis
Soltamox [tamoxifen citrate]	Z79.810	Selective estrogen receptor modulator (SERM)	Breast cancer
Solu-Cortef [hydrocortisone sodium succinate]	Z79.52	Corticosteroid; antiasthmatic	Asthma; severe inflammation; allergic reactions
Solu-Medrol [methylprednisolone sodium succinate]	Z79.52	Corticosteroid	Anti-inflammatory and antiallergenic for shock and ulcerative colitis
Spiriva [tiotropium bromide]		Antiasthmatic/bronchodilator	Chronic obstructive pulmonary disease (COPD); asthma
Sprintec [norgestimate/ethinyl estradiol]	Z79.3	Contraceptive	Prevention of pregnancy
Stelara [ustekinumab]	Z79.620	Immunosuppressive biologic; monoclonal antibody	Plaque psoriasis; psoriatic arthritis; Crohn's disease; ulcerative colitis

Drug	Z Code	Drug Action/Classification	Indications
Strattera [atomoxetine hydrochloride]		CNS stimulant	Severe bacterial infections
Streptomycin sulfate [streptomycin sulfate]	Z79.2	Antibiotic	Treatment of opioid addiction
Suboxone [buprenorphine/naloxone]		Opioid agonist	Precocious puberty
Supprelin LA [histrelin acetate]	Z79.818	Agents affecting estrogen receptors and estrogen levels	Bacterial infections
Suprax [cefixime]	Z79.2	Antibiotic	Various bacterial infections
Sustiva [efavirenz]	Z79.899	Antiretroviral	HIV
Syeda [drospirenone/ethinyl estradiol]	Z79.3	Contraceptive	Prevention of pregnancy
Sylatron [peginterferon alfa-2b]	Z79.69	Other immunosuppressant/immunomodulator	Prevention of recurrent malignant melanoma
Symbicort [budesonide/formoterol fumarate dihydrate]	Z79.51	Corticosteroid – inhaled; antiasthmatic	Prophylaxis and treatment of asthma and COPD
Symbyax [olanzapine/fluoxetine]		Antidepressant	Acute depressive episodes associated with bipolar I disorder; treatment resistant depression
Symlin [pramlintide]	Z79.85	Antidiabetic – non-insulin injectable	Diabetes mellitus
Symtuza [darunavir/cobicistat/emtricitabine/tenofovir alafenamide]	Z79.899	Antiretroviral	HIV
Synarel [nafarelin acetate]	Z79.818	Agents affecting estrogen receptors and estrogen levels	Endometriosis symptoms; precocious puberty
Synercid [dalfopristin/quinupristin]	Z79.2	Antibiotic	Severe blood infections
Synjardy [empagliflozin/metformin hydrochloride]	Z79.84	Oral hypoglycemic	Diabetes mellitus
Synthroid [levothyroxine sodium]		Thyroid hormone	Hypothyroidism
Tacrolimus [tacrolimus]	Z79.621	Calcineurin inhibitor	Prophylaxis of organ transplant rejection
Talicia [omeprazole magnesium/amoxicillin/rifabutin]	Z79.2	Combination antibiotic	Helicobacter pylori infection
Taltz [ixekizumab]	Z79.620	Immunosuppressive biologic; monoclonal antibody	Plaque psoriasis; psoriatic arthritis; ankylosing spondylitis; axial spondyloarthritis
Tamiflu [oseltamivir phosphate]		Antiviral	Treatment and prevention of influenza A and B
Tamoxifen citrate [tamoxifen citrate]	Z79.810	Selective estrogen receptor modulator (SERM)	Metastatic breast cancer in postmenopausal women
Tavneos [avacopan]	Z79.69	Other immunosuppressant/immunomodulator	ANCA-associated vasculitis
Taxotere [docetaxel]	Z79.633	Mitotic inhibitor	Cancer
Tazicef [ceftazidime]	Z79.2	Antibiotic	Confirmed or suspected bacterial infections
Teflaro [ceftaroline fosamil]	Z79.2	Antibiotic	Bacterial skin infections; pneumonia
Tegretol [carbamazepine]		Anticonvulsant; analgesic	Epilepsy, especially with complex symptomatology; specific analgesic for trigeminal neuralgia
Temozolomide [temozolomide]	Z79.630	Chemotherapeutic alkylating agent	Chronic myelogenous leukemia
Tenormin [atenolol]		Beta blocker	Angina pectoris; hypertension; acute myocardial infarction
Terazosin HCl [terazosin hydrochloride]		Antiadrenergic	Benign prostatic hypertrophy; hypertension
Testim [testosterone]	Z79.890	Testosterone therapy – topical	Primary hypogonadism
Tetracycline [tetracycline]	Z79.2	Antibiotic	Bacterial infections
Thalidomide [thalidomide]	Z79.61	Immunomodulator	Multiple myeloma; erythema nodosum leprosum
Tiazac [diltiazem hydrochloride]		Calcium channel blocker	Chronic stable angina; atrial fibrillation; atrial flutter; hypertension; paroxysmal supraventricular tachycardia
Tivorbex [indomethacin]	Z79.1	Nonsteroidal anti-inflammatory drug (NSAID)	Treatment of pain, inflammation, and joint stiffness
Tobradex [tobramycin/dexamethasone]		Aminoglycoside ocular anti-infective; anti-inflammatory	Infectious conjunctivitis; dermatosis, corticosteroid-responsive with secondary infection; foreign body in eye; corneal inflammation; uveitis
Tobramycin [dexamethasone/tobramycin]	Z79.2	Antibiotic	Bacterial eye infections
Topamax [topiramate]		Anticonvulsant	Epilepsy; primary generalized tonic-clonic seizures; seizures associated with Lennox-Gastaut syndrome; migraine headache

Appendix B: Pharmacology List 2023

Drug	Z Code	Drug Action/Classification	Indications
Toprol-XL [metoprolol succinate]		Beta blocker	Angina pectoris; hypertension
Toremifene citrate [toremifene citrate]	Z79.810	Selective estrogen receptor modulator (SERM)	Metastatic breast cancer in postmenopausal women
Torisel [temsirolimus]	Z79.623	Mammalian target of rapamycin (mTOR) inhibitor	Renal cell carcinoma
Toujeo Solostar [insulin glargine recombinant]	Z79.4	Insulin	Diabetes mellitus
Tradjenta [linagliptin]	Z79.84	Oral hypoglycemic	Diabetes mellitus
Trazodone HCl [trazodone hydrochloride]		Antidepressant	Depression
Trelegy Ellipta [fluticasone furoate/umeclidinium bromide/vilanterol trifenatate]	Z79.51	Corticosteroid -- inhaled; antiasthmatic	COPD
Trelstar [triptorelin pamoate]	Z79.818	Agents affecting estrogen receptors and estrogen levels	Palliative treatment of prostate cancer symptoms
Tremfya [guselkumab]	Z79.620	Immunosuppressive biologic; monoclonal antibody	Plaque psoriasis
Tresiba [insulin degludec]	Z79.4	Insulin	Diabetes mellitus
Triamterene and hydrochlorothiazide [triamterene/ hydrochlorothiazide]		Antihypertensive; diuretic	Edema; hypertension
Tri-Estarylla [ethinyl estradiol/norgestimate]	Z79.3	Contraceptive	Prevention of pregnancy; acne
Trijardy XR [empagliflozin/linagliptin/metformin hydrochloride]	Z79.84	Oral hypoglycemic	Diabetes mellitus
Tri-Legest [ethinyl estradiol/norethindrone acetate]	Z79.3	Contraceptive	Prevention of pregnancy
Tri-Linyah [ethinyl estradiol/norgestimate]	Z79.3	Contraceptive	Prevention of pregnancy
Tri-Lo-Estarylla [ethinyl estradiol/norgestimate]	Z79.3	Contraceptive	Prevention of pregnancy
Tri-Lo-Sprintec [ethinyl estradiol/norgestimate]	Z79.3	Contraceptive	Prevention of pregnancy
Trimethoprim [trimethoprim]	Z79.2	Antibiotic	Acute exacerbation chronic bronchitis; travelers' diarrhea; infections of the middle, lower respiratory tract, and urinary tract; pneumonia, pneumocystis; shigellosis
Tri-Previfem [ethinyl estradiol/norgestimate]	Z79.3	Contraceptive	Prevention of pregnancy
Triptodur [triptorelin]	Z79.818	Agents affecting estrogen receptors and estrogen levels	Precocious puberty
Tri-Sprintec [ethinyl estradiol/norgestimate]	Z79.3	Contraceptive	Prevention of pregnancy; acne
Trivora-28 [ethinyl estradiol/ levonorgestrel]	Z79.3	Contraceptive	Prevention of pregnancy
Trokendi XR [topiramate]		Anticonvulsant	Epilepsy; primary generalized tonic-clonic seizures; seizures associated with Lennox-Gastaut syndrome; migraine headache
Trulicity [dulaglutide]	Z79.85	Antidiabetic – non-insulin injectable	Diabetes mellitus
Truvada [emtricitabine/tenofovir disoproxil fumarate]	Z79.899	Antiretroviral	HIV
Turalio [pexidartinib]		Kinase inhibitor	Symptomatic tenosynovial giant cell tumor
Tygacil [tigecycline]	Z79.2	Antibiotic	Bacterial skin or digestive system infections; pneumonia
Tylenol with codeine [acetaminophen/codeine phosphate]	Z79.891	Analgesic, narcotic	Pain and cough
Ubrelvy [ubrogepant]		Calcitonin gene-related peptide inhibitor	Migraine headache
Ultram [tramadol hydrochloride]	Z79.891	Analgesic, non-narcotic (opiate, narcotic-like)	Moderate to severe pain
Unasyn [ampicillin sodium/sulbactam sodium]	Z79.2	Antibiotic	Bacterial infections
Vabomere [meropenem; vaborbactam]	Z79.2	Antibiotic	Complicated urinary tract infections; pyelonephritis
Vagifem [estradiol]	Z79.890	Estrogen therapy	Menopause symptoms

Drug	Z Code	Drug Action/Classification	Indications
Valium [diazepam]		Antianxiety; muscle relaxant; anticonvulsant	Anxiety, tension, withdrawal from alcohol, muscle spasms and anticonvulsant therapy; epilepsy, generalized tonic-clonic; status epilepticus; stiff-man syndrome; tetanus
Vancocin HCl [vancomycin hydrochloride]	Z79.2	Antibiotic	Severe bacterial infections
Vancomycin HCl [vancomycin hydrochloride]	Z79.2	Antibiotic	Severe bacterial infections
Vantas [histrelin acetate]	Z79.818	Agents affecting estrogen receptors and estrogen levels	Palliative treatment of prostate cancer symptoms
Vasotec [enalaprilat maleate]		ACE inhibitor	Congestive heart failure; hypertension
Velivet [desogestrel/ethinyl estradiol]	Z79.3	Contraceptive	Prevention of pregnancy
Venlafaxine HCl [venlafaxine hydrochloride]		Antidepressant, serotonin and norepinephrine reuptake inhibitor (SNRI)	Major depressive disorder; social anxiety disorder; panic disorder
Ventolin HFA [albuterol sulfate]		Antiasthmatic/bronchodilator	Asthma
Verapamil HCL [verapamil hydrochloride]		Calcium channel blocker	Angina pectoris; chronic stable angina; atrial fibrillation; atrial flutter; paroxysmal supraventricular tachycardia; ventricular arrhythmia; hypertension
Viagra [sildenafil citrate]		Phosphodiesterase-5 (PDE5) inhibitor	Erectile dysfunction
Vibativ [telavancin hydrochloride]	Z79.2	Antibiotic	Pneumonia; severe bacterial skin infections
Vibramycin [doxycycline calcium]	Z79.2	Antibiotic	Bacterial infections
Victoza [liraglutide]	Z79.85	Antidiabetic – non-insulin injectable	Diabetes mellitus
Vienva [ethinyl estradiol/levonorgestrel]	Z79.3	Contraceptive	Prevention of pregnancy
Vinblastine [vinblastine]	Z79.633	Mitotic inhibitor	Cancer
Vincristine [vincristine]	Z79.633	Mitotic inhibitor	Cancer
Viorele [desogestrel/ethinyl estradiol]	Z79.3	Contraceptive	Prevention of pregnancy
Virazole [ribavirin]	Z79.899	Antiviral	Respiratory syncytial virus (RSV)
Viread [tenofovir disoproxil fumarate]	Z79.899	Antiretroviral	HIV; chronic hepatitis B
Voltaren [diclofenac sodium]	Z79.1	Nonsteroidal anti-inflammatory drug (NSAID)	Treatment of pain, inflammation, and joint stiffness due to arthritis
Vumerity [diroximel fumarate]	Z79.69	Other immunosuppressant/immunomodulator	Relapsing forms of multiple sclerosis (MS)
Vytorin [ezetimibe/simvastatin]		HMG-CoA reductase inhibitor (statin); cholesterol absorption inhibitor	Hyperlipidemia; hypercholesterolemia
Wakix [pitolisant hydrochloride]		CNS stimulant	Narcolepsy
Warfarin [warfarin sodium]	Z79.01	Anticoagulant	Prophylaxis and treatment of venous thrombosis; treatment of atrial fibrillation with embolization (pulmonary embolism), arrhythmias, myocardial infarction, and stroke prevention
Wellbutrin SR, Wellbutrin XL [bupropion hydrochloride]		Antidepressant	Depression
Wera [ethinyl estradiol/norethindrone]	Z79.3	Contraceptive	Prevention of pregnancy
Xalatan [latanoprost]		Prostaglandin F2α analogue	Glaucoma, open-angle; ocular hypertension
Xanax, Xanax XR [alprazolam]		Antianxiety; sedative/hypnotic	Anxiety disorders with panic disorder and depression
Xarelto [rivaroxaban]	Z79.01	Anticoagulant	Prophylaxis and treatment of venous thrombosis, pulmonary embolism; prevention of blood clots due to atrial fibrillation
Xeljanz, Xeljanz XR [tofacitinib]	Z79.622	Janus kinase (JAK) inhibitor	Rheumatoid arthritis; psoriatic arthritis
Xeloda [capecitabine]	Z79.631	Antimetabolite agent	Breast cancer, colon/colorectal cancer
Xelstrym [dextroamphetamine]		CNS stimulant	Attention deficit hyperactivity disorder (ADHD)
Xenleta [lefamulin acetate]	Z79.2	Antibiotic	Community-acquired bacterial pneumonia
Xgeva [denosumab]	Z79.620	Immunosuppressive biologic; monoclonal antibody	Treatment and prevention of bone resorption and prevention of bone fracture
Xifaxan [rifaximin]	Z79.2	Antibiotic	E. coli diarrhea
Xigduo [dapagliflozin propanediol/metformin hydrochloride]	Z79.84	Oral hypoglycemic	Diabetes mellitus
Xpovio [selinexor]	Z79.899	Antineoplastic	Multiple myeloma in adults
Xultophy [insulin degludec/liraglutide]	Z79.4	Insulin	Diabetes mellitus

Appendix B: Pharmacology List 2023

Drug	Z Code	Drug Action/Classification	Indications
Xyrem [sodium oxybate]		CNS depressant; anxiolytic/sedative/hypnotic	Cataplexy and/or excessive daytime sleepiness in narcolepsy
Xyzal [levocetirizine dihydrochloride]		Antihistamine	Perennial allergic rhinitis; chronic idiopathic urticaria
Yasmin [drospirenone/ethinyl estradiol]	Z79.3	Contraceptive	Prevention of pregnancy
Yaz [drospirenone/ethinyl estradiol]	Z79.3	Contraceptive	Prevention of pregnancy; menstrual disorders
Zerbaxa [ceftolozane sulfate/tazobactam sodium]	Z79.2	Antibiotic	Complicated urinary tract and intra-abdominal infections
Zestoretic [lisinopril/hydrochlorothiazide]		ACE inhibitor	Congestive heart failure; hypertension
Zestril [lisinopril]		ACE inhibitor	Congestive heart failure; hypertension
Zetia [ezetimibe]		Antihyperlipidemic	Hypercholesterolemia; sitosterolemia
Ziac [bisoprolol fumarate/hydrochlorothiazide]		Antihypertensive	Hypertension
Zinacef [cefuroxime sodium]	Z79.2	Antibiotic	Bacterial infections
Zipsor [diclofenac potassium]	Z79.1	Nonsteroidal anti-inflammatory drug (NSAID)	Pain and inflammation relief
Zithromax [azithromycin]	Z79.2	Antibiotic	Infections of the cervix, lower respiratory tract, skin and skin structures, urethra, nongonococcal; mycobacterium avium complex; pharyngitis, streptococcal pneumonia; tonsillitis
Zocor [simvastatin]		HMG-CoA reductase inhibitor (statin)	Hypercholesterolemia; hyperlipidemia; hyperlipoproteinemia; hypertriglyceridemia
Zoladex [goserelin acetate]	Z79.818	Agents affecting estrogen receptors and estrogen levels	Palliative treatment of prostate cancer and breast cancer symptoms; endometriosis
Zoloft [sertraline hydrochloride]		Antidepressant	Anxiety with panic disorder and depression; obsessive-compulsive disorder
Zometa [zoledronic acid]	Z79.83	Bisphosphonate	Multiple myeloma; Paget's disease
Zortress [everolimus]	Z79.623	Mammalian target of rapamycin (mTOR) inhibitor	Prophylaxis of organ transplant rejection
Zorvolex [diclofenac]	Z79.1	Nonsteroidal anti-inflammatory drug (NSAID)	Pain, inflammation or fever relief
Zosyn [piperacillin sodium/tazobactam sodium]	Z79.2	Antibiotic	Bacterial infections
Zovia [ethynodiol diacetate/ethinyl estradiol]	Z79.3	Contraceptive	Prevention of pregnancy
Zovirax [acyclovir]	Z79.899	Antiviral	Genital herpes and herpes zoster infections
Zubsolv [buprenorphine/naloxone]		Opioid agonist	Treatment of opioid addiction
Zyloprim [allopurinol]		Antigout	Gouty arthritis; renal calculus; hyperuricemia; hyperuricemia secondary to leukemia; hyperuricemia secondary to lymphoma
Zyprexa [olanzapine]		Antipsychotic/antimanic	Psychotic disorders; schizophrenia
Zyrtec allergy [cetirizine hydrochloride]		Antihistamine	Perennial and seasonal allergic rhinitis; chronic urticaria
Zyvox [linezolid]	Z79.2	Antibiotic	Severe bacterial infections

Appendix C: Z Codes for Long-Term Drug Use with Associated Drugs

This resource correlates the Z codes that are used to identify current long-term drug use with a list of drugs that are typically categorized to that class of drug. These lists are not all-inclusive, providing only the more commonly used drugs.

Z79.01 Long term (current) use of anticoagulants
- Angiomax
- Argatroban
- Arixtra
- Bevyxxa
- Coumadin
- Eliquis
- Fragmin
- Heparin
- Jantoven
- Lovenox
- Pradaxa
- Savaysa
- Warfarin
- Xarelto

Z79.02 Long term (current) use of antithrombotics/antiplatelets
- Aggrastat
- Aggrenox
- Brilinta
- Clopidogrel bisulfate
- Effient
- Integrilin
- Persantine
- Plavix
- Prasugrel

Z79.1 Long term (current) use of non-steroidal anti-inflammatories (NSAID)
- Advil
- Aleve
- Anaprox DS
- Arthrotec
- Caldolor
- Cambia
- Celebrex
- Daypro
- Duexis
- Elyxyb
- Feldene
- Ibuprofen
- Indocin
- Mobic
- Motrin IB
- Nabumetone
- Nalfon
- Naprelan
- Naprosyn
- NeoProfen
- Ponstel
- Tivorbex
- Voltaren
- Zipsor
- Zorvolex

Z79.2 Long term (current) use of antibiotics
- Altabax
- Amikacin
- Amoxicillin
- Ampicillin
- Augmentin
- Avelox
- Azactam
- Azithromycin

- Bactrim
- Bactroban
- Biaxin XL
- Cefazolin sodium
- Ceftriaxone
- Cefzil
- Centany
- Cephalexin
- Cipro
- Ciprofloxacin
- Clarithromycin
- Cleocin
- Clindamycin
- Cubicin
- Daptomycin
- Dificid
- Doxycycline
- Dynacin
- E.E.S.
- Ertapenem
- ERYC
- Erygel
- EryPed
- Ery-Tab
- Erythrocin
- Erythromycin
- Factive
- Fetroja
- Flagyl
- Fortaz
- Garamycin
- Gentamicin sulfate
- Hiprex
- Invanz
- Isoniazid
- Keflex
- Klaron
- Lincocin
- Macrobid
- Macrodantin
- Maxipime
- Mepron
- Merrem
- Metronidazole
- Minocin
- Monodox
- Monurol
- Mycobutin
- Nebupent
- Neosporin
- Nitrofurantoin
- Oracea
- Orbactiv
- Penicillin-VK
- Pentam
- Pfizerpen
- Priftin
- Primaxin
- Rifadin
- Rimactane
- Septra
- Seromycin
- Silvadene
- Sivextro

- Solodyn
- Solosec
- Streptomycin sulfate
- Suprax
- Synercid
- Talicia
- Tazicef
- Teflaro
- Tetracycline
- Tobramycin
- Trimethoprim
- Tygacil
- Unasyn
- Vabomere
- Vancocin HCl
- Vancomycin HCl
- Vibativ
- Vibramycin
- Xenleta
- Xifaxan
- Zerbaxa
- Zinacef
- Zithromax
- Zosyn
- Zyvox

Z79.3 Long term (current) use of hormonal contraceptives
- Altavera
- Alyacen
- Aranelle
- Ashlyna
- Aviane-28
- Balziva-28
- Bekyree
- Beyaz
- Brevicon 28-day
- Briellyn
- Camila
- Cryselle
- Cyclafem
- Cyclessa
- Dasetta
- Daysee
- Depo-Provera
- Depo-SubQ Provera
- Desogen
- Elinest
- Emoquette
- Enpresse-28
- Enskyce
- Errin
- Estarylla
- Estrostep Fe
- Falmina
- Femhrt
- Gildagia
- Gildess
- Introvale
- Jencycla
- Junel
- Kariva
- Kelnor
- Kimidess
- Kurvelo

Kyleena
Larin
Lessina-28
Levonest
Levora
Liletta
Lo Loestrin Fe
Loestrin
Loryna
LoSeasonique
Low-Ogestrel-28
Marlissa
Microgestin
Minastrin
Mirena
Mono-Linyah
Myzilra
Natazia
Nexplanon
Nextstellis
Norinyl
Nortrel
NuvaRing
Ogestrel
Orsythia
Ortho-Novum
Philith
Pimtrea
Pirmella
Plan B One-Step
Portia-28
Previfem
Provera
Quartette
Safyral
Seasonale
Seasonique
Setlakin
Skyla
Sprintec
Syeda
Tri-Estarylla
Tri-Legest
Tri-Linyah
Tri-Lo-Estarylla
Tri-Lo-Sprintec
Tri-Previfem
Tri-Sprintec
Trivora-28
Velivet
Vienva
Viorele
Wera
Yasmin
Yaz
Zovia

Z79.4 Long term (current) use of insulin
Admelog
Apidra
Basaglar
Fiasp
Humalog
Humulin R
Lantus
Levemir
Novolin
Novolog
Soliqua
Toujeo Solostar

Tresiba
Xultophy

Z79.51 Long term (current) use of inhaled steroids
Advair
AirDuo RespiClick
Alvesco
Arnuity Ellipta
Asmanex
Breo Ellipta
Dulera
Flovent HFA
Pulmicort
Qvar Redihaler
Symbicort
Trelegy Ellipta

Z79.52 Long term (current) use of systemic steroids
Aristospan
Celestone Soluspan
Colocort
Cortef
Cortenema
Cortifoam
Cortisone acetate
Depo-Medrol
Dexamethasone Intensol
Entocort EC
Hydrocortisone
Kenalog-10
Kenalog-40
Locoid
Medrol
Methylprednisolone
Orapred ODT
PediaPred
Prednisolone
Prednisone
Rayos
Solu-Cortef
Solu-Medrol

Z79.61 Long term (current) use of immunomodulator
Apremilast
Otezla
Pomalyst
Revlimid
Thalidomide

Z79.620 Long term (current) use of immunosuppressive biologic
Actemra
Aimovig
Cosentyx
Cyltezo
Dupixent
Enbrel
Entyvio
Humira
Hyrimoz
Keytruda
Monoclonal antibodies
Prolia
Remicade
Rituxan
Simulect
Skyrizi
Stelara
Taltz
Tremfya

Xgeva

Z79.621 Long term (current) use of calcineurin inhibitor
Astagraf XL
Cyclosporin
Envarsus XR
Gengraf
Lupkynis
Neoral
Prograf
Protopic
Sandimmune
Tacrolimus

Z79.622 Long term (current) use of Janus kinase inhibitor
Cibinqo
Olumiant
Rinvoq
Xeljanz XR

Z79.623 Long term (current) use of mammalian target of rapamycin (mTOR) inhibitor
Rapamune
Sirolimus
Torisel
Zortress

Z79.624 Long term (current) use of inhibitors of nucleotide synthesis
CellCept
Imuran

Z79.630 Long term (current) use of alkylating agent
Busulfex
Carmustine
Chlorambucil
Cisplatin
Cytoxan
Leukeran
Temozolomide

Z79.631 Long term (current) use of antimetabolite agent
5-fluorouracil (5-FU)
6-mercaptopurine (6-MP)
Cytarabine
Methotrexate
Xeloda

Z79.632 Long term (current) use of antitumor antibiotic
Bleomycin
Cerubidine
Doxorubicin
Mitomycin

Z79.633 Long term (current) use of mitotic inhibitor
Ixempra
Paclitaxel
Taxotere
Vinblastine
Vincristine

Z79.634 Long term (current) use of topoisomerase inhibitor
Camptosar
Etoposide
Hycamtin

Z79.64 Long term (current) use of myelosuppressive agent
Hydroxyurea

Z79.69   **Long term (current) use of other immunomodulators and immunosuppressants**
Actimmune
Avonex
Betaseron
Copaxone
Intron A
Orencia
PegIntron
Ponvory
Rebif
Sylatron
Tavneos
Vumerity

Z79.810   **Long term (current) use of selective estrogen receptor modulators (SERMs)**
Evista
Fareston
Osphena
Raloxifene HCl
Soltamox
Tamoxifen citrate
Toremifene citrate

Z79.811   **Long term (current) use of aromatase inhibitors**
Anastrozole
Arimidex
Aromasin
Exemestane
Femara
Letrozole

Z79.818   **Long term (current) use of other agents affecting estrogen receptors and estrogen levels**
Eligard
Faslodex
Lupron Depot
Megace ES
Supprelin LA
Synarel
Trelstar
Triptodur
Vantas
Zoladex

Z79.82   **Long term (current) use of aspirin**
Bayer
Bufferin
Durlaza

Z79.83   **Long term (current) use of bisphosphonates**
Aclasta
Actonel
Aredia
Atelvia
Binosto
Boniva
Fosamax
Reclast
Zometa

Z79.84   **Long term (current) use of oral hypoglycemic drugs**
Acarbose
Actoplus Met
Actos

Amaryl
Avandia
DiaBeta
Duetact
Farxiga
Glimepiride
Glucotrol
Glumetza
Glyburide
Glynase
Glyset
Invokamet
Invokana
Janumet
Januvia
Jentadueto
Kazano
Kombiglyze
Metformin
Onglyza
Oseni
Qtern
Repaglinide
Riomet
Rybelsus
Sitagliptin
Synjardy
Tradjenta
Trijardy XR
Xigduo

Z79.85   **Long-term (current) use of injectable non-insulin antidiabetic drugs**
Adlyxin
Bydureon
Byetta
Ozempic
Symlin
Trulicity
Victoza

Z79.890   **Hormone replacement therapy**
Activella
Alora
Androderm
AndroGel
Angeliq
Bijuva
Climara
CombiPatch
Delestrogen
Depo-Provera
Divigel
Duavee
Elestrin
Estrace
EstroGel
Femhrt
Femring
Firmagon
Menest
Menostar
Minivelle
Orilissa
Osphena
Prempro
Provera
Testim
Vagifem

Z79.891   **Long term (current) use of opiate analgesic**
Acetaminophen with codeine
Buprenex
Buprenorphine HCl and Naloxone HCl
Butrans
Codeine
Demerol
Dilaudid
Dolophine HCl
Duragesic
Duramorph PF
Fentanyl citrate
Fentora
Fioricet with codeine
Hydrocodone
Hydrocodone bitartrate and acetaminophen
Hydromorphone HCl
Kadian
Lazanda
Methadone HCl
Methadose
Morphine sulfate
MS Contin
Norco
Nucynta
Oxycodone HCl
OxyContin
Percocet
Roxicet
Roxicodone
Tylenol with codeine
Ultram

Z79.899   **Other long term (current) drug therapy**
Afrezza
Antineoplastic/chemotherapy
Atripla
Beconase AQ
Biktarvy
Cimduo
Descovy
Dovato
Dymista
Emtriva
Epivir
Epivir-HBV
Erelzi
Flonase
Harvoni
Livtencity
Nexletol
Prezcobix
Prezista
Qnasl
Rebetol
Retrovir
Rukobia
Sustiva
Symtuza
Truvada
Virazole
Viread
Xpovio
Zovirax

Appendix D: Z Codes Only as Principal/First-Listed Diagnosis

Z00.00	Z01.118	Z02.1	Z04.6	Z34.83	Z38.66	Z51.11	Z52.4
Z00.01	Z01.12	Z02.2	Z04.71	Z34.90	Z38.68	Z51.12	Z52.5
Z00.110	Z01.20	Z02.3	Z04.72	Z34.91	Z38.69	Z52.000	Z52.6
Z00.111	Z01.21	Z02.4	Z04.81	Z34.92	Z38.7	Z52.001	Z52.810
Z00.121	Z01.30	Z02.5	Z04.82	Z34.93	Z38.8	Z52.008	Z52.811
Z00.129	Z01.31	Z02.6	Z04.89	Z38.00	Z39.0	Z52.010	Z52.812
Z00.2	Z01.411	Z02.71	Z04.9	Z38.01	Z39.1	Z52.011	Z52.813
Z00.3	Z01.419	Z02.79	Z31.81	Z38.1	Z39.2	Z52.018	Z52.819
Z00.5	Z01.42	Z02.81	Z31.83	Z38.2	Z40.00	Z52.090	Z52.89
Z00.70	Z01.810	Z02.82	Z31.84	Z38.30	Z40.01	Z52.091	Z76.1
Z00.71	Z01.811	Z02.83	Z33.2	Z38.31	Z40.02	Z52.098	Z76.2
Z00.8	Z01.812	Z02.89	Z34.00	Z38.4	Z40.03	Z52.10	Z99.12
Z01.00	Z01.818	Z02.9	Z34.01	Z38.5	Z40.09	Z52.11	
Z01.01	Z01.82	Z04.1	Z34.02	Z38.61	Z40.8	Z52.19	
Z01.020	Z01.83	Z04.2	Z34.03	Z38.62	Z40.9	Z52.20	
Z01.021	Z01.84	Z04.3	Z34.80	Z38.63	Z42.1	Z52.21	
Z01.10	Z01.89	Z04.41	Z34.81	Z38.64	Z42.8	Z52.29	
Z01.110	Z02.0	Z04.42	Z34.82	Z38.65	Z51.0	Z52.3	

Appendix E: Centers for Medicare & Medicaid Services Hierarchical Condition Categories (CMS-HCC)

In the 1970s, Medicare began demonstration projects that contracted with health maintenance organizations (HMOs) to provide care for Medicare beneficiaries in exchange for prospective payments. In 1985, this project changed from demonstration status to a regular part of the Medicare program, Medicare Part C. The Balanced Budget Act (BBA) of 1997 named Medicare's Part C managed care program Medicare+Choice, and the Medicare Modernization Act (MMA) of 2003 again renamed it to Medicare Advantage (MA).

Medicare is one of the world's largest health insurance programs, and about one-third of the beneficiaries on Medicare are enrolled in a MA private health care plan. Due to the great variance in the health status of Medicare beneficiaries, risk adjustment provides a means of adequately compensating those plans with large numbers of seriously ill patients while not overburdening other plans that have healthier individuals. Medicare Advantage (MA) plans have been using the Hierarchical Condition Category (HCC) risk adjustment model since 2004.

The Risk Adjustment Model

The primary purpose of a risk adjustment model is to predict (on average) the future health care costs for specific consortiums enrolled in Medicare Advantage (MA) health plans. CMS is then able to provide capitation payments to these private health plans. Capitation payments are an incentive for health plans to enroll not only healthier individuals but those with chronic conditions or who are more seriously ill by removing some of the financial burden.

The MA risk adjustment model uses HCCs to assess the disease burden of its enrollees. HCC diagnostic groupings were created after examining claims data so that enrollees with similar disease processes, and consequently similar health care expenditures, could be pooled into a larger data set in which an average expenditure rate could be determined. The medical conditions included in HCC categories are those that were determined to most predictably affect the health status and health care costs of any individual. Several important principles to the risk adjustment model and the development of the HCC categories include but are not limited to:

1. The HCC diagnostic categories should be clinically meaningful.
   - Diagnostic categories are well-defined.
   - Clinically specific diseases or medical conditions are grouped to each category.
2. The HCC diagnostic categories should predict medical expenditures.
   - The diagnoses grouped to a specific category should have as close to the same cost burden not only in the current year but also in the future.
3. The HCC diagnostic categories should have adequate sample sizes and discretionary categories excluded to be as accurate and stable in their estimate of costs as possible.
   - A diagnostic category that groups extremely rare diseases or conditions would not be reliably effective in determining current or future costs.
   - Codes that are not credible as cost predictors or may be subject to coding variation should be excluded, when possible.
4. The HCC diagnostic categories should be both hierarchical and additive.
   - Hierarchical measurement is used within a specific disease process.
   - Disease processes that are unrelated to each other are measured additively.
5. The diagnostic classification should encourage specificity and should not reward coding proliferation.
   - More diagnosis codes and vague diagnosis codes do not equal greater disease burden.

More than 10,000 ICD-10-CM diagnosis codes map to 86 HCCs in the current risk adjustment model. Diagnoses are excluded from mapping when they do not predict future cost or are vague or variable in diagnosis, coding, or treatment, such as symptoms or osteoarthritis. Also excluded are diagnosis codes from laboratories, radiology, and home health claims.

Risk Adjustment Factors

The CMS-HCC risk adjustment model uses "risk adjustment factors" to calculate a risk score for each member. This score summarizes that particular patient's expected cost of care relative to other members'. Each member's risk score is based on demographic and health status information and is calculated as the sum of these demographic and health factors weighted by their estimated marginal contributions to total risk. The model also takes into account where the patient resides (community or institutional), Medicaid eligibility (full or partial benefits), the patient's Medicare enrollment status (new or established), age, disability status, whether the patient is frail or has end-stage renal disease (ESRD), and even prescription drug use.

No procedure codes, ICD-10-PCS or CPT, are included in the MA risk adjustment model. The model relies solely on diagnostic and demographic data. Not all ICD-10-CM diagnoses map to an HCC, and there is no specific code sequencing involved. The CMS-HCC model is additive as well as hierarchical. The additive functionality allows a patient to have more than one HCC category assigned, providing a more complete clinical picture and prediction of resource consumption. The hierarchical aspect of the model provides a means of ranking diagnoses that are similar in disease process, by severity. The hierarchy of the condition categories ensures the patient's conditions are classified to the most severe condition within the related group. Less severe conditions within a particular hierarchy are superseded by more severe diagnoses within the same group. The hierarchy and additive relationship permits this model to characterize the person's illness level within each disease process, while still allowing the effects of unrelated disease processes to be counted in the patient's overall score.

Certain combinations of coexisting diagnoses for an individual can increase medical costs. The CMS-HCC model adjusts for these higher costs by the addition of "disease interaction" factors. For each patient, multiple HCCs assigned, along with demographic and disease interaction factors, are used to calculate a single, combined risk adjustment factor (RAF). The RAF score for an individual member represents all of the HCCs that have been submitted from all sources for that member to CMS during the course of an entire calendar year.

There are separate CMS-HCC models for new enrollees and continuing enrollees. The new enrollee model uses demographic factors only, such as age, sex, and disability status, and is used when the enrollee has less than 12 months of medical history. The community model accounts for age, sex, original reason for Medicare entitlement (age or disability), Medicaid eligibility, and clinical conditions as measured by HCCs. In the second step, expected costs are adjusted for outliers based on the member's risk score and whether the patient has ESRD.

Demographic data (age, sex, eligibility) as well as health status (diagnoses codes submitted on claims to CMS) of an MA population are used to determine the reimbursement to the health plan to care for their members.

CMS considers a RAF score of 1.0 as the benchmark to indicate the score of the average healthy patient with the same demographic and diagnostic factors. These patients are expected to use average or lower-than-average resources. When the RAF score is higher than 1.0, CMS considers the patient to be sicker than the average patient with the same criteria and expects greater-than-average resource utilization.

A low RAF score may accurately indicate a healthier patient, but it may also falsely indicate a healthier patient due to incomplete or inaccurate coding, incomplete or insufficient record documentation, or patients who fail to complete an annual assessment.

A high RAF score may accurately indicate a sicker patient, or it may be falsely inflated from overcoding due to diagnoses that are reported but not documented, or from copying and pasting from previous encounters or problem lists of resolved conditions.

Documentation Requirements

Payment is made per HCC category (not per diagnosis code). No matter how many times in the year the diagnosis codes are reported, a single payment is made to the MA plan each year. Each year the list of HCCs and the RAF for each patient is "reset." This means the annual health assessment is extremely important, and adequate documentation is critical. Accurate risk adjustment payment relies on complete medical record documentation and diagnosis coding. CMS requires that all applicable diagnosis codes be reported and that all diagnoses be reported to the highest level of specificity and that these be substantiated by the medical record.

CMS's Guiding Principle:

The risk adjustment diagnosis must be based on clinical medical record documentation from a face-to-face encounter, coded according to the *ICD-10-CM Guidelines for Coding and Reporting*; assigned based on dates of service within the data collection period, submitted to the MA organization from an appropriate risk adjustment provider type and an appropriate risk adjustment physician data source.

A "face-to-face" health service encounter between a patient and healthcare provider describes an encounter between the patient and the provider (MD, DO), including qualified nonphysician practitioners (NPP) (e.g. nurse practitioner or physician's assistant), which is face-to-face with the patient. CMS provides a current listing of acceptable physician specialty types for risk adjustment data submission within the 2012 Regional Technical Assistance Participant Guide. The only exception to the face-to-face encounter requirement is pathology services (professional component only). Due to the 2019 coronavirus disease (COVID-19) pandemic, CMS is allowing MA organizations to submit diagnoses from telehealth services that meet the risk adjustment face-to-face requirement when the services are provided using interactive audio and video telecommunications systems that permit real-time interactive communication. Currently, CMS does not provide a listing of all services that are considered face-to-face visits for risk adjustment data, but does provide guidance on what types of services are not acceptable for risk adjustment in the Participant Guide. For example, diagnostic radiology does not qualify because diagnostic radiologists typically do not document confirmed diagnoses. Other examples of services that are not acceptable include diagnostic reports that have not been interpreted, such as laboratory reports.

It is essential that the medical record documentation show evidence by provider authentication that the direct face-to-face service was personally furnished by the physician or qualified NPP. Examples of these services include office visits, hospital visits, preoperative anesthesia assessment, and surgical and invasive procedures.

Risk adjustment relies on annual health information. Each enrollee is assigned an individual risk score based on the health status information obtained from the diagnosis codes on the claims. The CMS-HCC model relies on ICD-10-CM coding specificity for accurate risk adjustment by using the most specific code available that is substantiated by the documentation in the medical record. Providers should fully document and accurately code the evaluation and management of all severe and chronic conditions to ensure a full, complete, and accurate clinical record of the patient's condition and reflect the work involved in caring for the patient, particularly those with complex and challenging health issues. All conditions affecting the treatment or management of the patient's health should be documented at least once a year, as applicable to care provided, to accurately describe the true complexity and severity of the patient's health. If the diagnosis coding on the claim is not accurate or complete, the claim may indicate that the provider did much less medical decision-making, evaluation, and management than was actually performed.

Documentation to support or validate risk adjustment conditions may be found anywhere in the note for the face-to-face encounter. It is important to ensure that the note accurately reflects all chronic conditions that affect the health and care of the patient. Each encounter must be unique and reflect only that visit as it occurred. Insufficient documentation influences the assignment of diagnosis codes and directly affects the patient's risk score.

Documentation should properly validate all reported conditions. Each page of progress notes should be properly authenticated and include the patient's name and the date.

Providers should document each clinical diagnosis to the highest degree of specificity per encounter, including all complications and/or manifestations, including clear links to causal conditions. Only confirmed conditions should be documented—no rule-out conditions or abnormal findings without clinical significance. All known conditions, including chronic conditions, that affect the care and treatment of the patient at least once per year should be noted.

Providers should specifically document the condition and clinical significance, and pertinent changes using terminology such as decreased, increased, worsening, improving, or unchanged, or abnormal findings.

Documentation Tips
- Document all cause-and-effect relationships.
- Report the most specific diagnosis code available that is supported by the documentation.
- Include all current diagnoses as part of the current medical decision-making, and document for every visit.
- Identify diagnoses that are current or chronic problems rather than a past medical history or previous resolved condition.
- Document history of heart attack, status codes, etc., that affect the patient's care as "history of" or "PMH" when they no longer exist or are not current conditions.
- Ensure each progress note has the date, signature, and credentials/specialty.
- Document the thought processes used to assess each condition.

- Know high revenue HCCs that are often undiagnosed or undercoded.
- Avoid "unspecified" codes.
- Ensure the codes reported are accurate.
- Ensure each encounter is billed.
- Review rejection reports, and audit reports to assess risks.

Audits
Because reimbursement is by patient, rather than based on an average of the entire population, and is based upon documentation, there is the potential for upcoding. Audits are conducted by the MA plan and CMS recovery auditors.

Initial Validation Audit (IVA)
CMS requires that the MA plan validate HCCs. This is usually performed by an independent auditor working with the plan or a contracted vendor to validate the MA plan's data submitted to CMS.

The MA plan submits the one best medical record that supports each HCC identified for the beneficiary.

Risk Adjustment Data Validation Audit
Risk adjustment data validation (RADV) audits were introduced in 2011 and updated for 2015. They are performed by CMS to validate the integrity and accuracy of risk-adjusted payments by verifying that the diagnosis codes the MA plans submit are supported by the medical record documentation for a member. On March 30, 2020, CMS announced it was suspending RADV activities related to the payment year 2015 audit and will not initiate any additional contract-level audits until after the 2019 coronavirus public health emergency (PHE) has ended, at which time CMS will make an announcement when normal audit activities will resume.

MA plans can be selected by CMS for RADV audits annually and if chosen are required to submit their members' medical records to CMS. Providers are required to assist the MA plan by providing the medical record documentation included in the audit. Even though each diagnosis needs to be reported only once in a calendar year, during a RADV audit up to five dates of service may be submitted to support any one HCC.

To be validated, medical record documentation must meet certain criteria and standards. Even if the diagnosis is documented and coded correctly, any deficiency in the documentation can make the encounter and the HCC invalid. Diagnoses that cannot be validated are considered payment errors. The results of the audit are communicated to the MA plan, which then communicates these results to the provider. Under- and overpayments are subject to payment adjustment. The results of RADV audits can be extrapolated over the MA plan population to calculate potential payment errors and overpayments/recoupments. Regulations include a RADV appeal process, a document dispute process, and a procedure for obtaining physician-signature attestations.

The following items are reviewed during the validation process:
- The record is for the correct enrollee.
- The record is from the correct calendar year for the payment year being audited.
- The record is legible.
- The date of service is present on the records and is for a face-to-face visit.
- The record is from a valid provider type.
- Valid credentials and/or a valid physician specialty are documented on the record.
- The record contains a signature from an acceptable type of physician.
- There is a diagnosis on the record.
- The diagnosis supports an HCC.
- The diagnosis supports the submitted HCC.

Mitigate audit risk by coding each reportable diagnosis each time it meets reporting guidelines. Audit regularly to assess areas of risk and in need of improvement and to capture conditions documented but not coded. Check for additional qualifying HCCs. Ensure claims are submitted and that corrected claims are submitted when indicated. There are three claims submission deadlines: January, March, and September. CMS adjusts each member's risk score twice a year, with the final reconciliation in August of the year after the plan year.

If providers emphasize correct coding and documentation and perform internal audits to determine where the risks are and prepare for audits, incorrect payment is less likely. For additional information on risk adjustment coding, see Optum's *Risk Adjustment Coding and HCC Guide*.

Appendix F: Centers for Medicare & Medicaid Services Quality Payment Program

In 2015, in an effort to repeal the faulty Medicare sustainable growth rate (SGR), focus on quality of patient outcomes, and control Medicare spending, Congress passed the Medicare Access and CHIP Reauthorization Act (MACRA), which included sweeping changes for practitioners who provide services reimbursed under the Medicare physician fee schedule (MPFS). MACRA repealed the Medicare SGR methodology used for updating the MPFS and replaced it with the Quality Payment Program (QPP).

Under the QPP, providers who demonstrate success at controlling costs while providing high-quality care to their patients are eligible to earn increased payments. Clinicians who successfully report on determined criteria receive a larger payment. Those who do not participate at all or do not fulfill the defined requirements receive a negative payment adjustment of 9 percent of Medicare Part B reimbursements based on 2020 performance to be applied in 2022, negative payment adjustment of up to 9 percent of Medicare Part B reimbursements based on 2021 performance to be applied in 2023.

Passage of the Medicare Access and CHIP Reauthorization Act of 2015

The final rule for implementing MACRA was published November 4, 2016. The final rule primarily provided details on how the QPP was to be implemented, including requiring the secretary of Health and Human Services (HHS) to sunset the value-based (VM) modifier incentive program, the Medicare electronic health record (EHR) incentive program, and the Physician Quality Reporting System (PQRS), and incorporated these incentive programs into the QPP.

Replacement of the Sustainable Growth Rate

Under the SGR, if overall physician costs were higher than a targeted Medicare expenditure, payments were reduced across the board. With the SGR method, payments to clinicians would have resulted in substantial cuts.

Because the QPP replaces the SGR methodology, the following revisions were detailed in MACRA:

- Established conversion factor updates:
  - a Medicare physician fee schedule conversion factor adjustment of 0.5 percent in 2016–2019 and a conversion factor adjustment of 0.00 percent for 2020–2025
  - the qualifying participant (QP) alternative payment models (APM) conversion factor of 0.75 percent and a nonqualifying provider APM conversion factor of 0.25 percent for 2026 and each subsequent year

Under the QPP, the Centers for Medicare and Medicaid Services (CMS) aims to:

- Support quality of patient care improvement by focusing on better outcomes for patients, decreasing provider burden, and preserving the independent clinical practice
- Promote the adoption of APMs, which align incentives across healthcare stakeholders
- Advance existing efforts of delivery system reform, including ensuring a smooth transition to a new system that promotes high-quality, efficient care through unification of CMS legacy programs such as the EHR incentive program

Quality Payment Program Established

The MACRA final rule established the Quality Payment Program (QPP) effective January 1, 2017. Within the QPP there are two interrelated pathways: Advanced Alternative Payment Models (APM) and the Merit-based Incentive Payment System (MIPS).

Eligible clinicians (EC) select the track/pathway—MIPS or advanced APMs—they wish to participate in based on the practice size, specialty, location, and patient population. Unlike previous quality initiatives, a provider does not have to enroll in the QPP. However, groups wishing to participate in the MIPS program via the Consumer Assessment of Healthcare Providers and Systems (CAHPS) for MIPS survey measures or CMS Web Interface (WI) must register by June 30 each year. Note that beginning with the 2022 performance period, the CMS WI will no longer be available as a submission or collection type. The CAHPS for MIPS survey is an optional quality measure that groups participating in MIPS can elect to administer.

In the 2020 Physician Fee Schedule Final Rule, CMS finalized a new participation framework to begin in 2021 known as MIPS Value Pathways (MVPs). The MVPs allow for a more cohesive participation experience by connecting activities and measures that are relevant to a specialty, medical condition, or a particular population. Due to the 2019 Coronavirus public health emergency (PHE), CMS postponed the implementation of MVPs as a reporting option for MIPS measures and activities through at least 2021. CMS finalized proposed updates for the criteria, process and MVP implementation, and anticipate the first MVP candidates to be proposed in the CY2022 notice of proposed rule making (NPRM). For additional and updated information on MVPs, see https://qpp.cms.gov/mips/mips-value-pathways.

Merit-based Incentive Payment System

MIPS is the track for clinicians who opt to participate in traditional Medicare as opposed to participating through an advanced APM. In doing so, clinicians may earn a payment adjustment related to evidence-based and practice-specific quality data. As a result, depending on the degree and success of performance in all four categories for CY 2021, clinicians receive one of the following:

- Positive payment adjustment in which additional compensation is received; bonuses are also available for meeting the exceptional performance threshold
- Neutral payment adjustment that neither increases nor reduces Medicare payments
- Negative payment adjustment of up to 9 percent of Medicare payment furnished in calendar year (CY) 2023

Participation in the MIPS track is determined based on the amount billed to Medicare and the number of beneficiaries seen per year. The following provider types are eligible for participation if they meet or exceed at least one of the following criteria:

- Medicare billings are greater than $90,000
- Care is provided for more than 200 covered services
- Care is provided to 200 or more Medicare patients each year

For 2021, the following clinician types are considered ECs:

- Physicians (MD, DO, DDS, DMD, DPM, OD)
- Physician assistants (PA)
- Nurse practitioners (NP)
- Clinical nurse specialists (CNS)
- Certified registered nurse anesthetists (CRNA)
- Physical therapists (PT)
- Occupational therapists (OT)
- Qualified speech-language pathologists
- Qualified audiologists
- Clinical psychologists
- Osteopathic practitioners
- Chiropractor
- Registered dieticians or nutrition professionals
- Any clinician group that includes one of the professionals listed above

Anatomy of MIPS

A measurement-based regime creates a single reporting framework for physicians that comprise four performance categories:

- Quality
- Improvement Activities (IA)—implemented in 2017
- Promoting Interoperability
- Cost

MIPS eligible clinicians may participate in the program as an individual clinician, group, virtual group, or APM entity (applicable for 2021). Each of the four performance categories has been weighted, with greatest emphasis placed on the Quality category. Performance category weights for individuals, groups, and virtual groups placed the Quality category at 40 percent, Promoting Interoperability is second at 25 percent, IA at 15 percent, and Cost at 20 percent. Performance category weights for APM entities reporting traditional MIPS for the 2021 performance period are weighted differently than these participation levels. The emphasis is still on the Quality category at 50 percent, Promoting Interoperability is second at 30 percent, Improvement Activities is third at 20 percent, and Cost is at 0 percent. Beginning with the 2022 performance period regardless of participation level (e.g., individual, group, etc.) the quality and cost performance categories will be equally weighted at 30%.

The 2021 MIPS performance threshold equates to 60 points out of a possible 100 points. Simply put, eligible clinicians are required to score 60 points to avoid the negative 9 percent payment adjustment.

Quality Performance
Under the MIPS Quality performance category, ECs and groups must select six measures from a listing of more than 200 measures, with at least one of the six measures being an outcome measure, high-priority measure (in absences of outcome measure), or complete specialty measure set. Patient outcomes such as mortality, whether a patient is readmitted to the hospital, and the patient's experience are areas that CMS and the healthcare industry seek to improve. An outcome measure is the way CMS can quantify changes in the health of an individual, groups of individuals, and even certain populations that they can attribute back to a specific intervention or series of interventions.

Quality measures are tools for quantifying, or measuring, healthcare processes and patient outcomes and perceptions, as well as organizational structure and/or systems linked to the ability to provide high-quality healthcare. These measures play an important role under the MIPS. Reporting should be done on a minimum of half of the EC's or group practice's Medicare Part B patients. Performance data is reported for 70 percent of the patients who qualify for each measure. Each measure is worth up to 10 points and is compared to a national benchmark.

Improvement Activities
The IA category assesses to what degree a clinician participates in activities designed to improve clinical practices. ECs are required to attest that they have participated in two high-weighted activities, one high-weighted activity and two medium-weighted activities, or four medium-weighted activities. The activities may be selected from an expanded inventory of more than 100 activities across eight subcategories for 90 consecutive days. These eight subcategories include:

- Expanded practice access
- Population management
- Care coordination
- Beneficiary engagement
- Patient safety and practice assessment
- Achieving health equity
- Integrating behavioral and mental health
- Emergency preparedness and response

This category was created with some inherent flexibility; for example, for groups with 15 or fewer participants, nonpatient-facing clinicians (e.g., pathologists), or those ECs in a rural or health professional shortage area (HPSA) receive two times the points when they report activities for at least 90 consecutive days.

Promoting Interoperability
CMS wants to encourage and promote the use of certified EHR technology (CEHRT) among providers and, in particular, the use of interoperability and sharing of information among clinicians and between providers and patients. In response to the 21st Century Cures Act Final Rule, CMS updated the CEHRT requirements to include technology certified to the 2015 Edition Cures Update certification criteria, the current 2015 Edition certification criteria, or a combination of both criteria to collect and report PI data.

Successful reporting of measures in this category require the EC to report measures from the four objectives and measures based exclusively on the 2015 edition of CEHRT and, as applicable, claim an exclusion. Exclusions are reported by submitting a "0" in addition to the exclusion type that applies to the EC because some measures may be associated with more than one exclusion.

The PI performance category contains four objectives:

- E-Prescribing
- Health Information Exchange
- Provider to Patient Exchange
- Public Health and Clinical Data Exchange

Data collected for each of the four objectives must be submitted for the same minimum continuous 90 days (unless an exclusion is applicable).

Cost
In this performance category, CMS determines an EC or group practice's cost score by calculating data from two measures previously included in the value-based payment modifier that involves the total cost of care for attributed beneficiaries and what Medicare spends per beneficiary. This amount is the total of both Medicare Part A and B payments from three days before through 30 days after a beneficiary has had an inpatient hospitalization episode. CMS then determines which ECs and practices have an adequate number of beneficiaries and hospitalizations associated with them. This number is compared to national benchmarks established for the performance period.

There are a total of 20 cost measures:
- Total Per Capita Cost (TPCC)
- Medicare Spending Per Beneficiary Clinician (MSPB Clinician)
- 13 Procedural episode-based measures and 5 acute inpatient medical condition episode-based measures (18 measures)

For procedure episodes, the case minimum established is 10 with credit for the episodes going to the clinician who performs the procedure. For acute inpatient medical condition episodes, the case minimum is set at 20, and credit is assigned to each clinician who bills the inpatient evaluation and management (E/M) claim lines during a triggered inpatient hospitalization under a TIN that furnishes at least 30 percent of the inpatient E/M claim lines during that particular hospitalization.

Clinicians have no additional submission responsibilities associated with this category as the score is determined from Medicare administrative claims data.

The category also has separate benchmarks. The Cost score is determined and compared with those benchmarks with points assigned based on the decile system in a similar manner to the Quality performance category with some differences such as:

- Benchmarks for performance are for the *same* year versus prior year performance.
- Scores are determined once case minimum requirements for each of the two measures in this category have been met.

MIPS Scoring
CMS uses scoring to determine an EC's successful participation in the QPP and thereby determine if the clinician's reimbursement will be negative, neutral, or positive.

The scoring methodology is a unified approach across all performance categories, allowing eligible clinicians to understand what is expected so they can perform successfully in the MIPS. For more information and details on QPP, see https:/qpp.cms.gov.

Illustrations

Chapter 3. Diseases of the Blood and Blood-forming Organs and Certain Disorders Involving the Immune Mechanism (D50–D89)

Red Blood Cells

White Blood Cell

Platelet

Coagulation

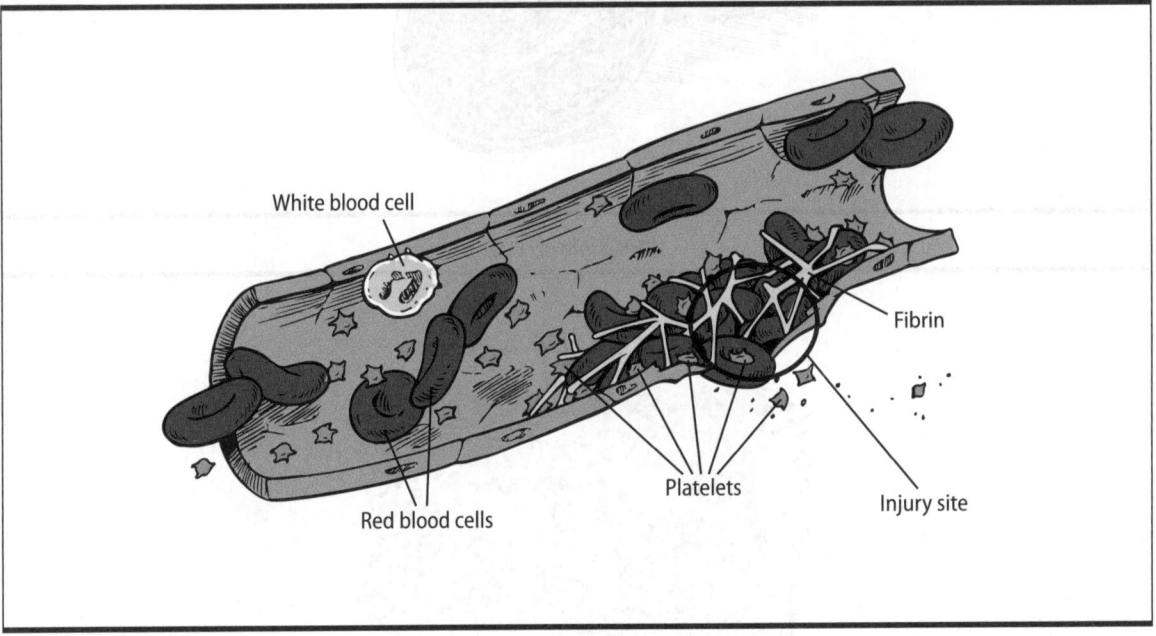

White blood cell

Fibrin

Platelets

Injury site

Red blood cells

Heart Valves

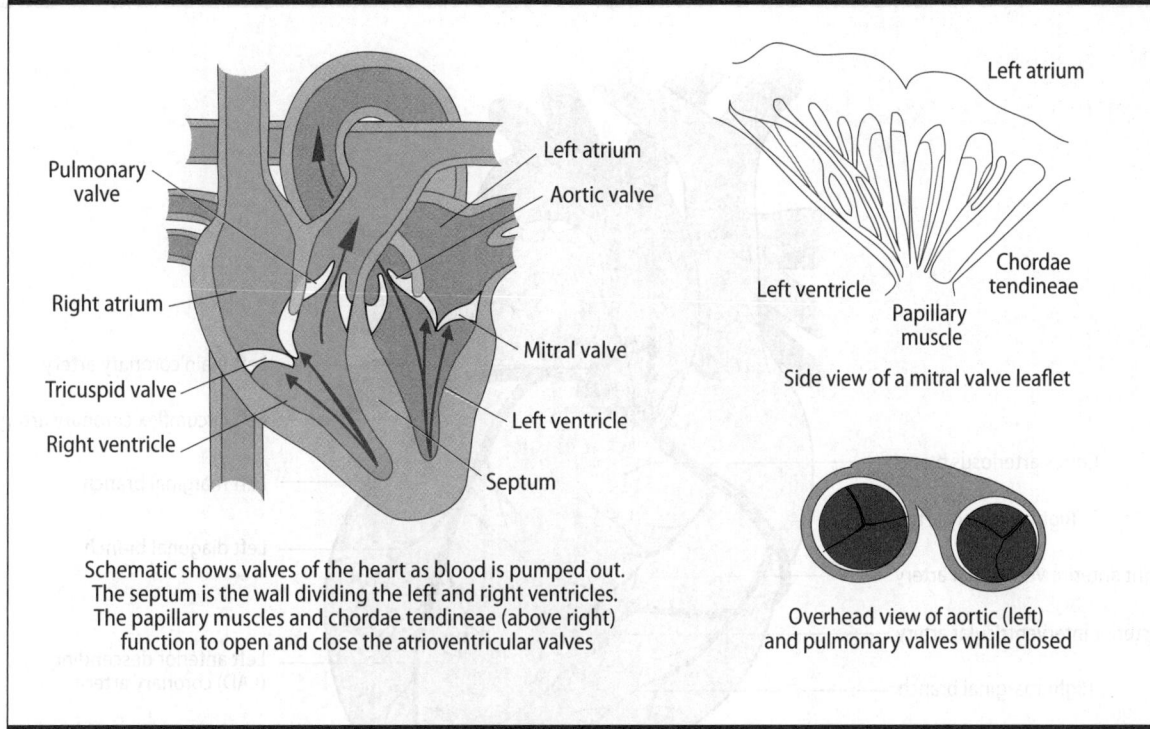

Schematic shows valves of the heart as blood is pumped out.
The septum is the wall dividing the left and right ventricles.
The papillary muscles and chordae tendineae (above right)
function to open and close the atrioventricular valves

Side view of a mitral valve leaflet

Overhead view of aortic (left)
and pulmonary valves while closed

Heart Conduction System

Coronary Arteries

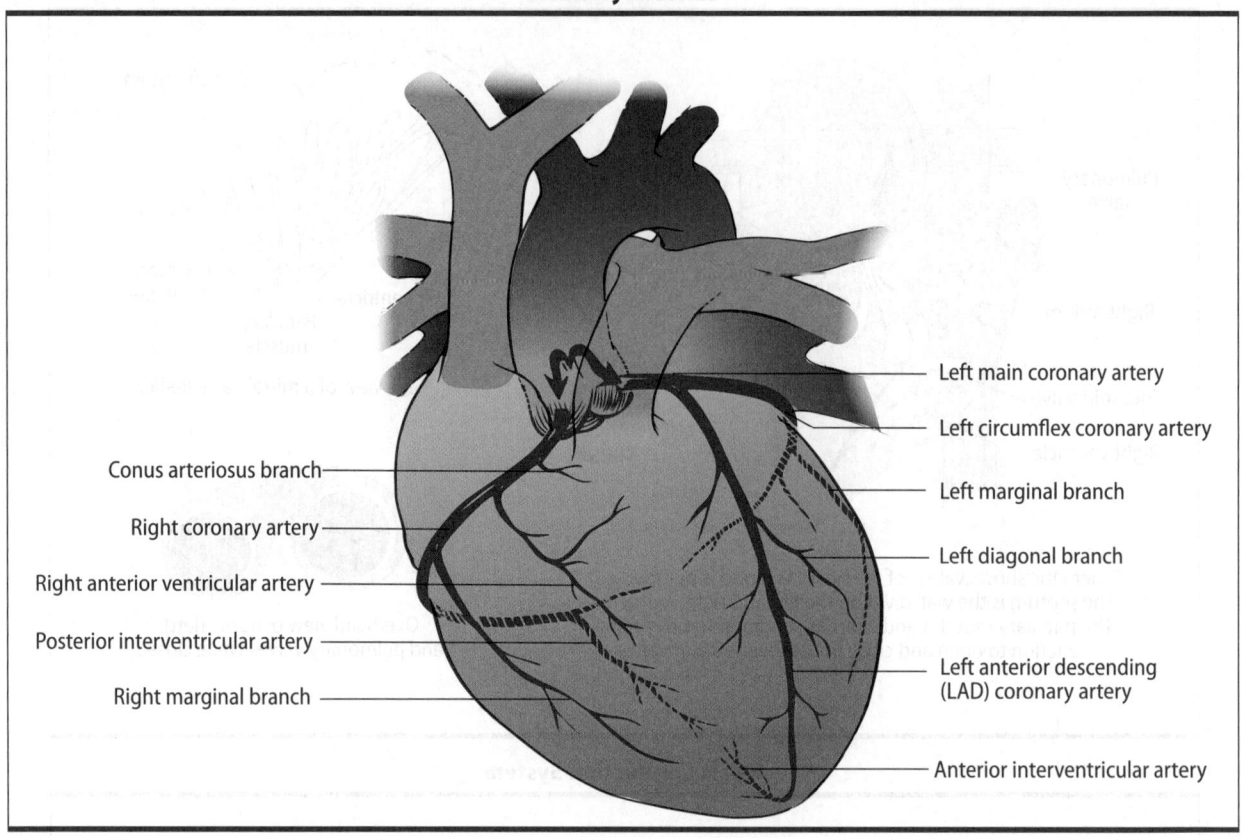

Conus arteriosus branch —

Right coronary artery —

Right anterior ventricular artery —

Posterior interventricular artery —

Right marginal branch —

Left main coronary artery

Left circumflex coronary artery

Left marginal branch

Left diagonal branch

Left anterior descending (LAD) coronary artery

Anterior interventricular artery

Arteries

Veins

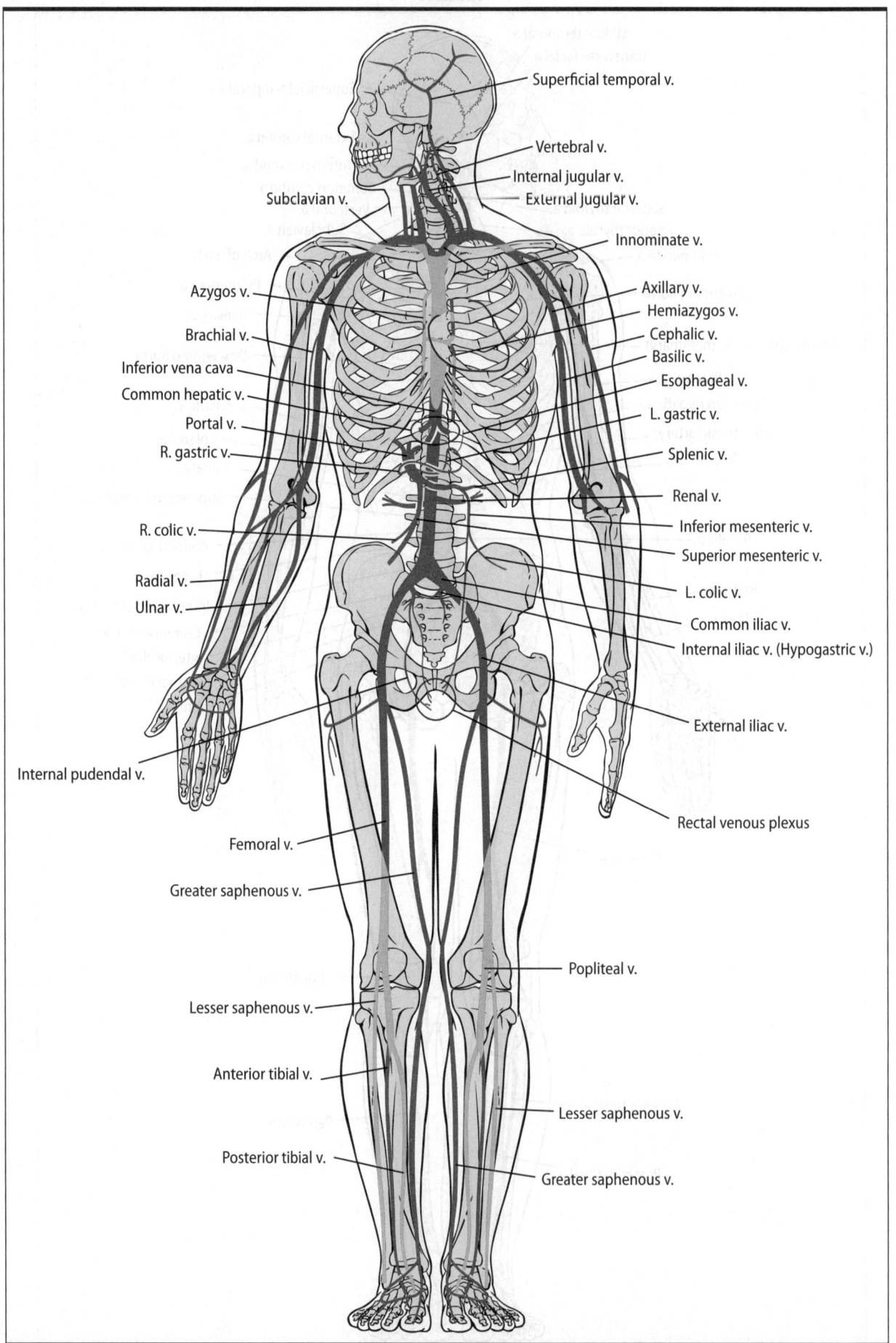

Superficial temporal v.

Vertebral v.

Internal jugular v.

External Jugular v.

Subclavian v.

Innominate v.

Azygos v.

Axillary v.

Hemiazygos v.

Brachial v.

Cephalic v.

Basilic v.

Inferior vena cava

Esophageal v.

Common hepatic v.

L. gastric v.

Portal v.

R. gastric v.

Splenic v.

Renal v.

R. colic v.

Inferior mesenteric v.

Superior mesenteric v.

Radial v.

L. colic v.

Ulnar v.

Common iliac v.

Internal iliac v. (Hypogastric v.)

External iliac v.

Internal pudendal v.

Rectal venous plexus

Femoral v.

Greater saphenous v.

Popliteal v.

Lesser saphenous v.

Anterior tibial v.

Lesser saphenous v.

Posterior tibial v.

Greater saphenous v.

Internal Carotid and Vertebral Arteries and Branches

Side View

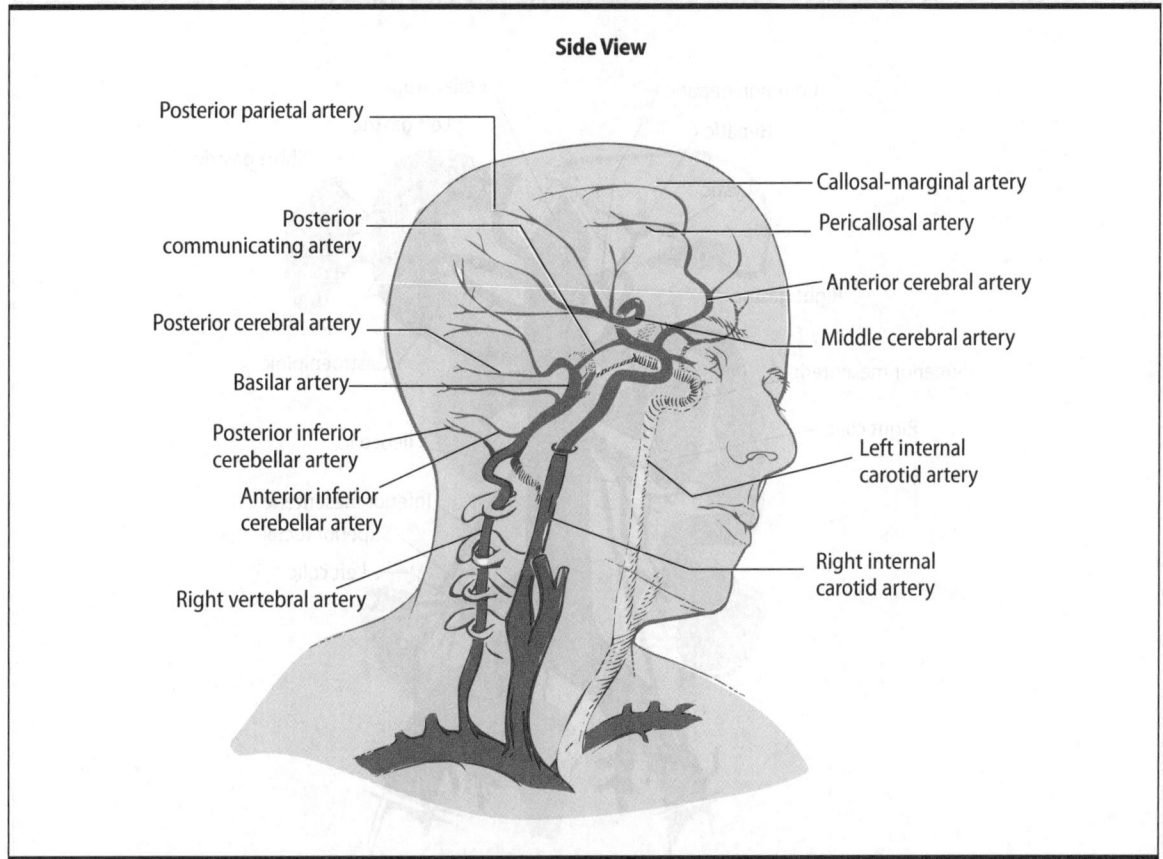

External Carotid Artery and Branches

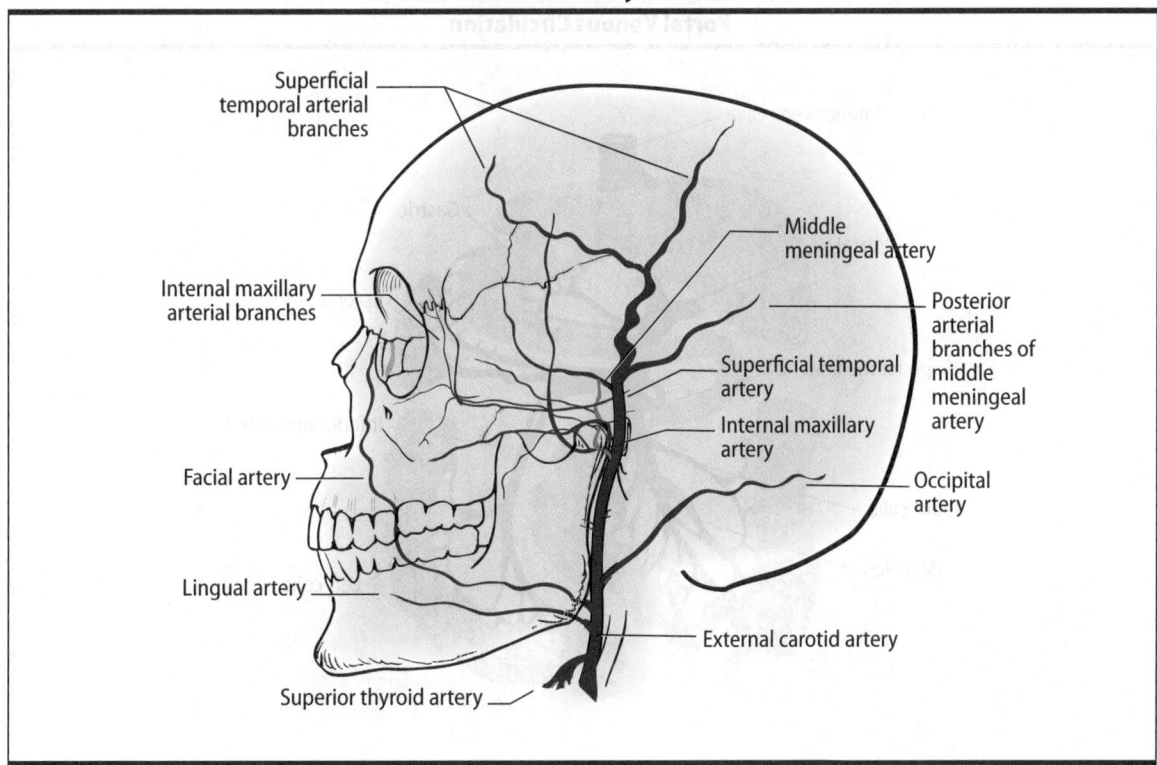

Branches of Abdominal Aorta

Portal Venous Circulation

Lymphatic System

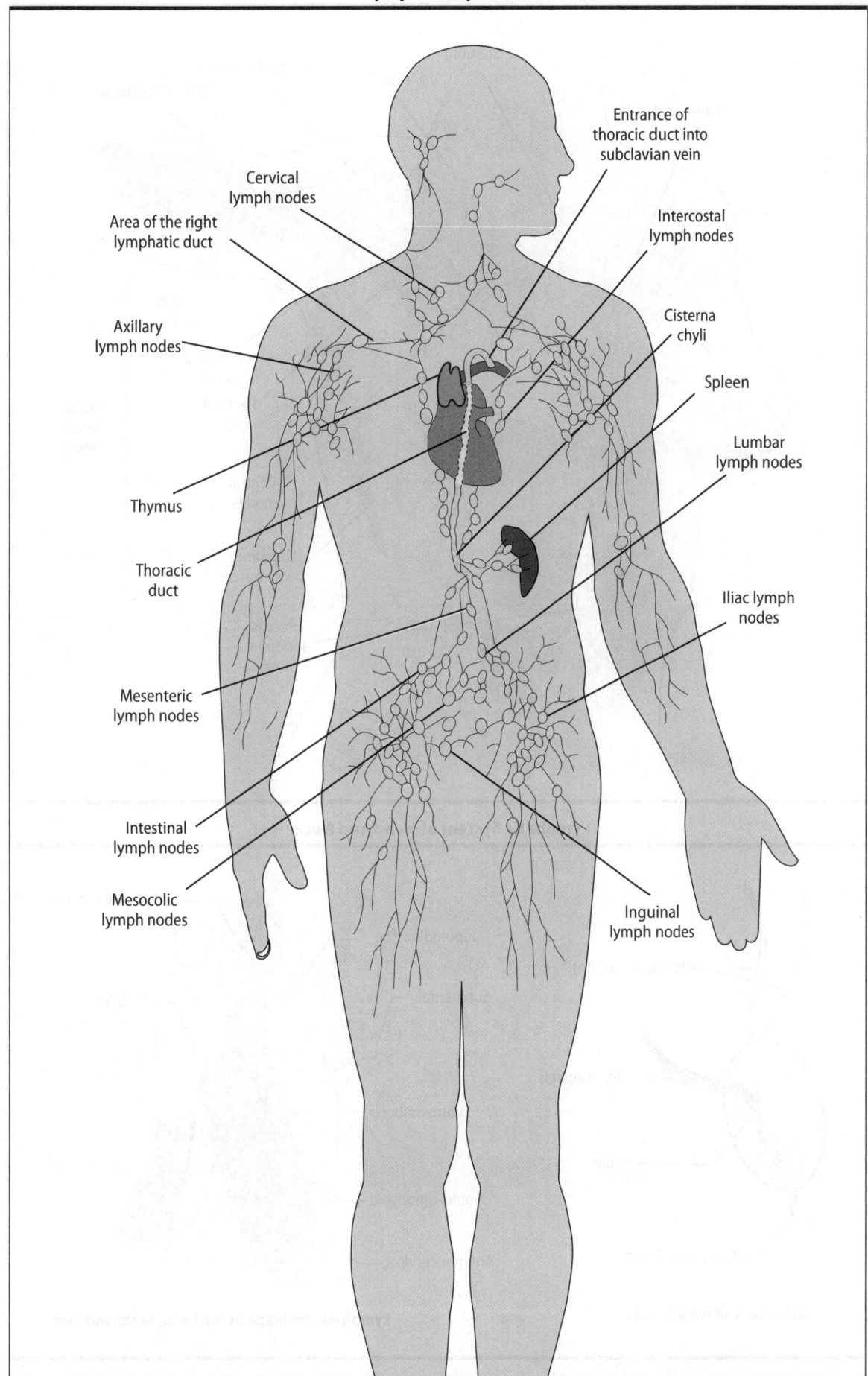

Axillary Lymph Nodes

Sternum

Clavicle

Deltoid muscle

Brachialis muscle

Parasternal nodes

Lateral nodes

Subscapular nodes

Pectoral nodes

Axillary lymph nodes

Central nodes

Latissimus dorsi muscle

Rectus abdominis muscle

Lymphatic System of Head and Neck

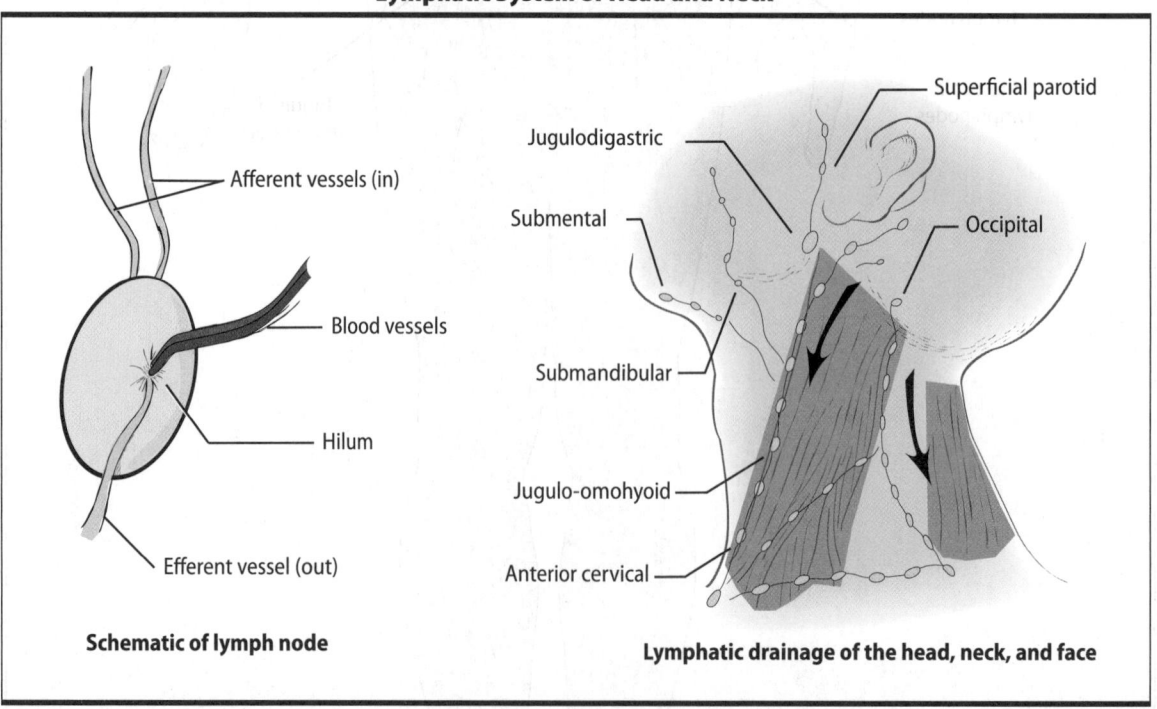

Afferent vessels (in)

Blood vessels

Hilum

Efferent vessel (out)

Schematic of lymph node

Jugulodigastric

Superficial parotid

Submental

Occipital

Submandibular

Jugulo-omohyoid

Anterior cervical

Lymphatic drainage of the head, neck, and face

Lymphatic Capillaries

Schematic of lymphatic capillaries

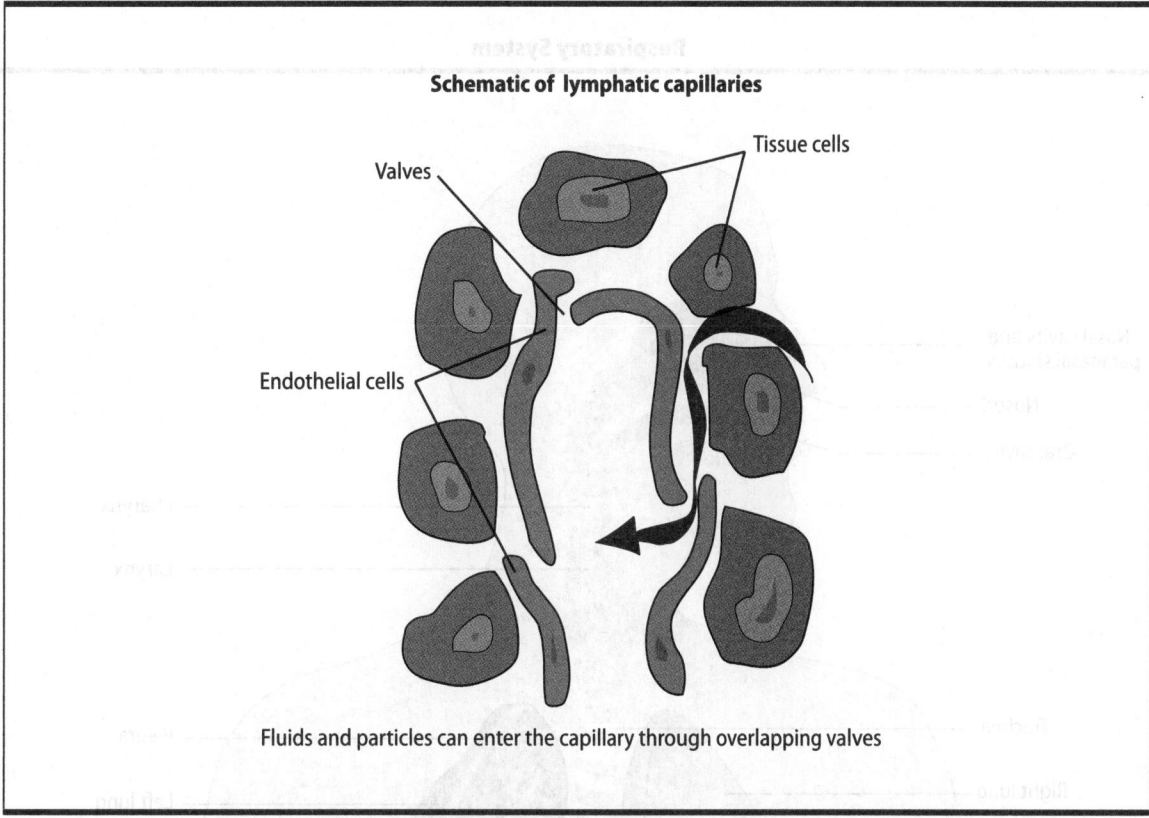

Tissue cells

Valves

Endothelial cells

Fluids and particles can enter the capillary through overlapping valves

Lymphatic Drainage

Lymphatic drainage of the colon follows blood supply

Middle colic nodes

Paracolic nodes

Left colic nodes

Ascending colon

Cecum

Rectum

Chapter 10. Diseases of the Respiratory System (J00–J99)

Respiratory System

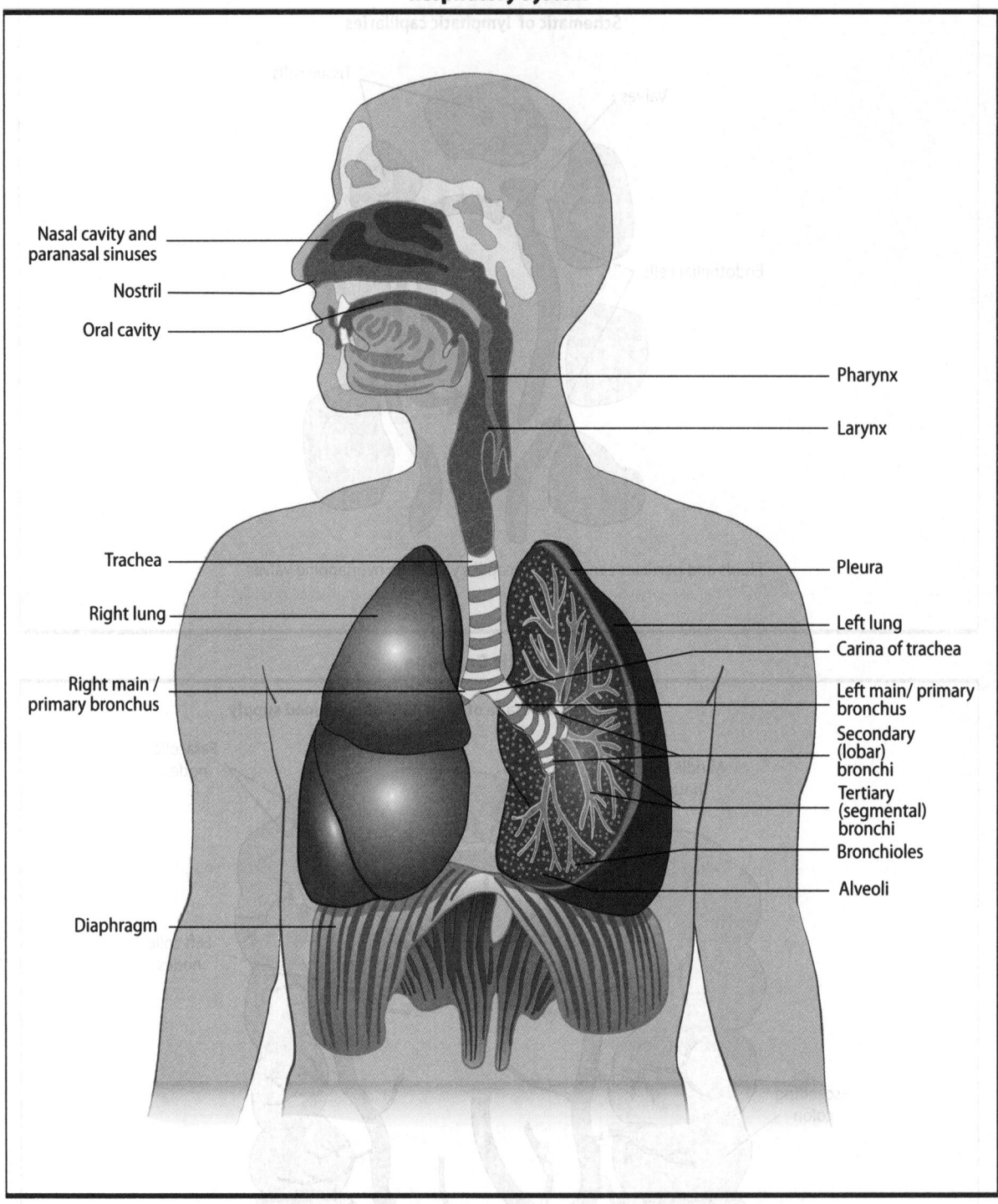

Nasal cavity and paranasal sinuses

Nostril

Oral cavity

Pharynx

Larynx

Trachea

Right lung

Pleura

Left lung

Carina of trachea

Right main / primary bronchus

Left main/ primary bronchus

Secondary (lobar) bronchi

Tertiary (segmental) bronchi

Bronchioles

Alveoli

Diaphragm

Upper Respiratory System

Lower Respiratory System

Paranasal Sinuses

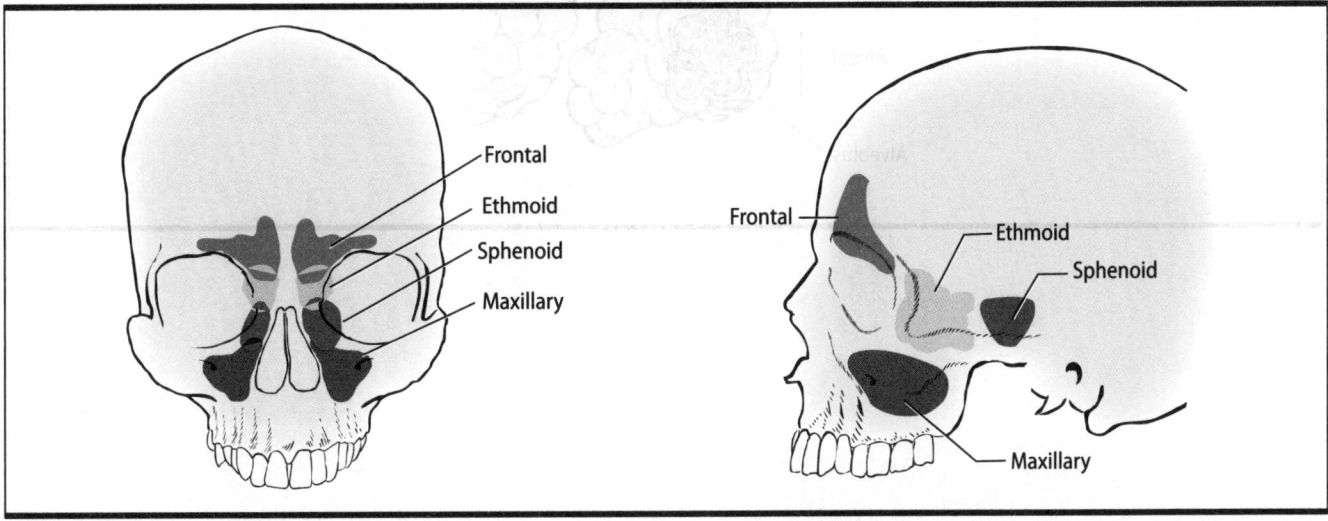

Lung Segments

Right lung   Left lung

Apical
segment

Apical-posterior
segment

Anterior segment

Superior
lobe

Superior
lobe

Posterior
segment

Superior lingular
segment

Inferior lingular
segment

Anterior
segment

Medial
basal
segment

Superior
basal
segment

Lateral
segment

Middle
lobe

Superior
segment

Lateral
basal
segment

Inferior
lobe

Posterior
basal
segment

Inferior
lobe

Anterior
medial
segment

Anterior
basal segment

Horizontal fissure

Oblique fissures

Alveoli

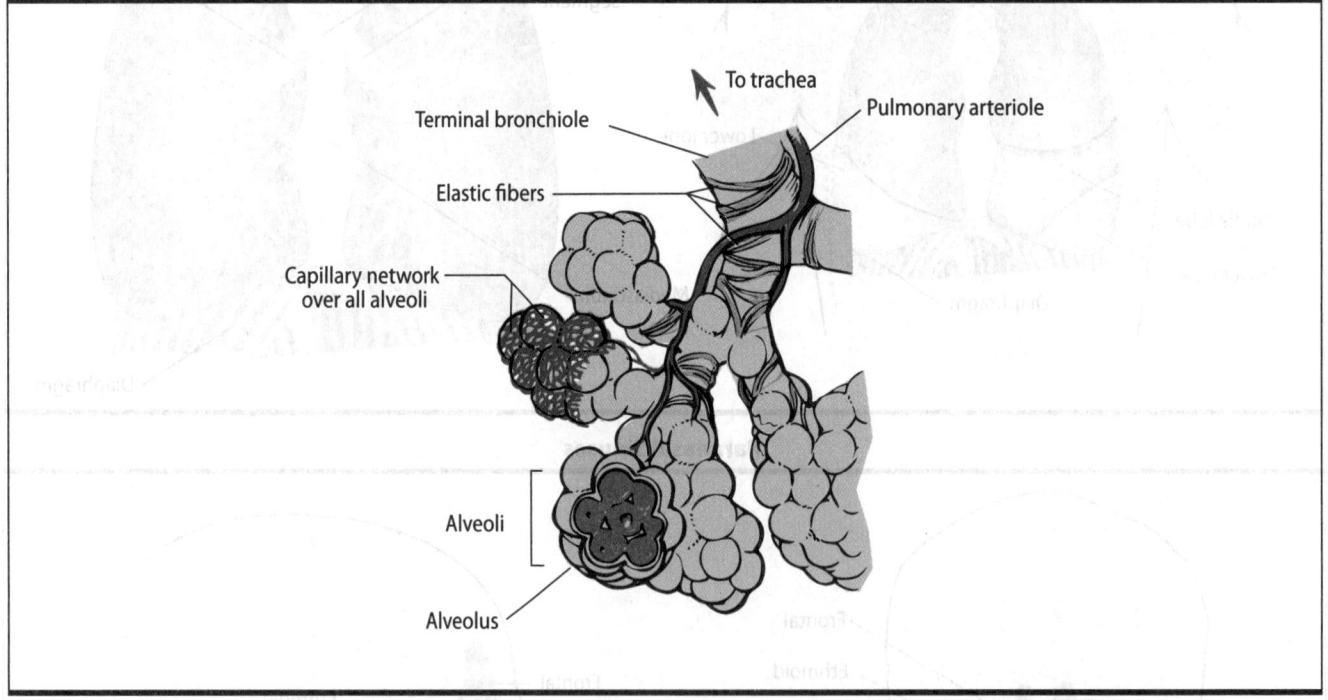

To trachea

Terminal bronchiole

Pulmonary arteriole

Elastic fibers

Capillary network
over all alveoli

Alveoli

Alveolus

Chapter 11. Diseases of the Digestive System (KØØ–K95)

Digestive System

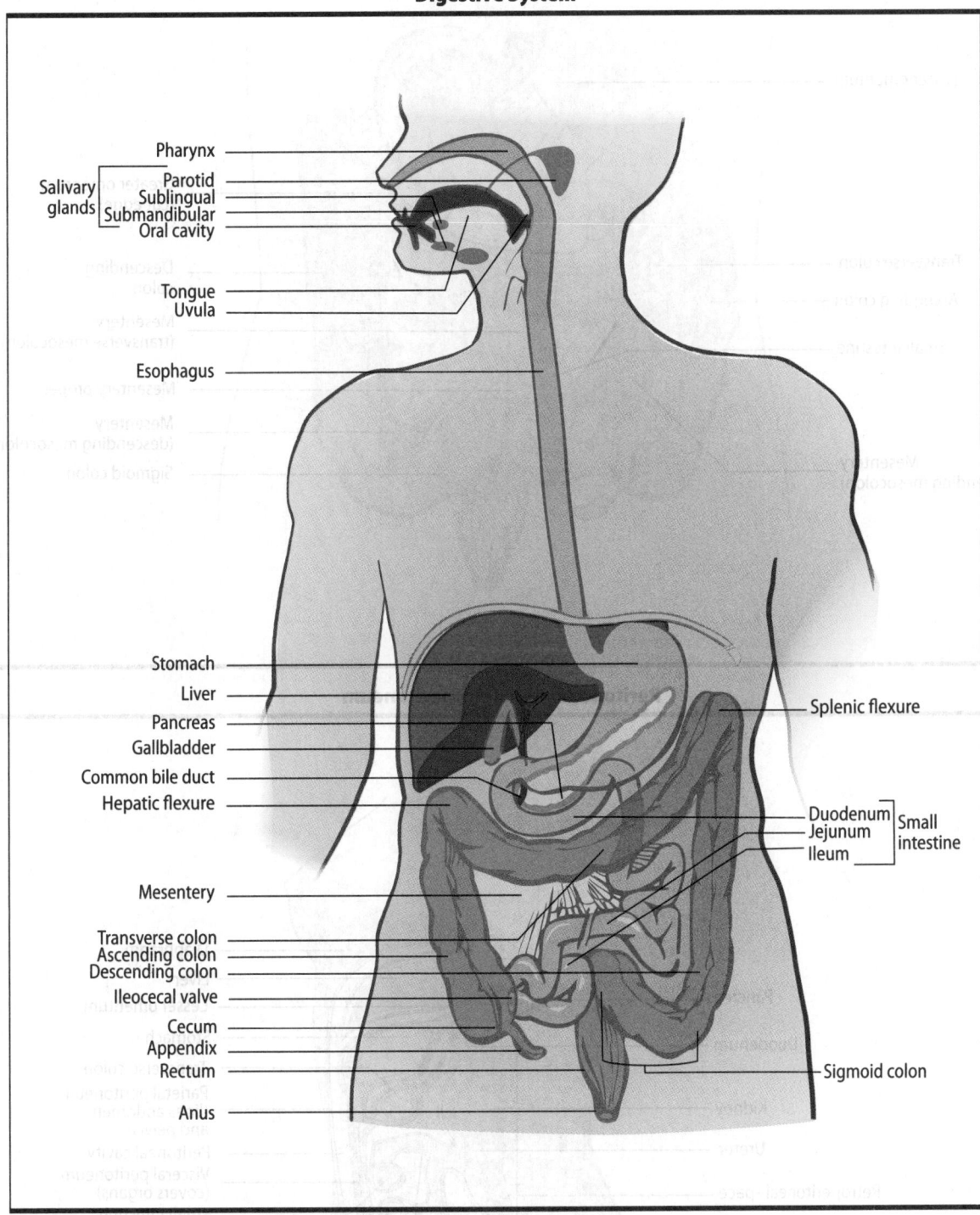

Omentum and Mesentery

Lesser omentum

Transverse colon

Ascending colon

Small intestine

Mesentery
(ascending mesocolon)

Greater omentum
(cut edge)

Descending
colon

Mesentery
(transverse mesocolon)

Mesentery proper

Mesentery
(descending mesocolon)

Sigmoid colon

Peritoneum and Retroperitoneum

Pancreas

Duodenum

Kidney

Ureter

Retroperitoneal space

Sigmoid colon

Bladder

Rectum

Diaphragm

Liver

Lesser omentum

Stomach

Transverse colon

Parietal peritoneum
(lines abdomen
and pelvis)

Peritoneal cavity

Visceral peritoneum
(covers organs)

Small intestine

Mesentery

Greater omentum

Chapter 12. Diseases of the Skin and Subcutaneous Tissue (L00–L99)

Nail Anatomy

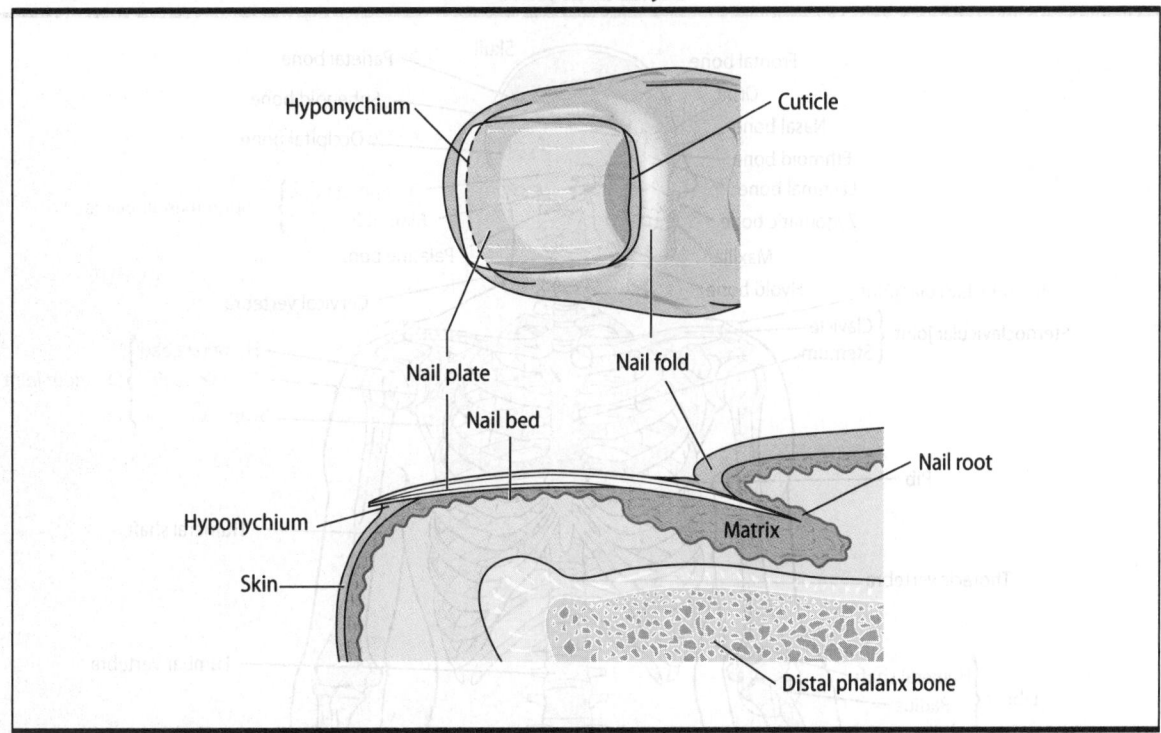

Hyponychium
Cuticle
Nail plate
Nail fold
Nail bed
Nail root
Hyponychium
Matrix
Skin
Distal phalanx bone

Skin and Subcutaneous Tissue

Hair
Basal layer
Corneal layer (corneum)
Epidermis
Hair shaft
Dermis
Sebaceous gland
Bulb
Hypodermis (subcutaneous layer)
Hair follicles
Sweat (eccrine gland)
Sensory nerve
Adipose tissue
Blood vessels

Chapter 13. Diseases of the Musculoskeletal System and Connective Tissue (M00–M99)

Bones and Joints

Shoulder Anterior View

Shoulder Posterior View

Elbow Anterior View

Elbow Posterior View

Hand

Hip Anterior View

Hip Posterior View

Knee Anterior View

Knee Posterior View

Foot

Muscles

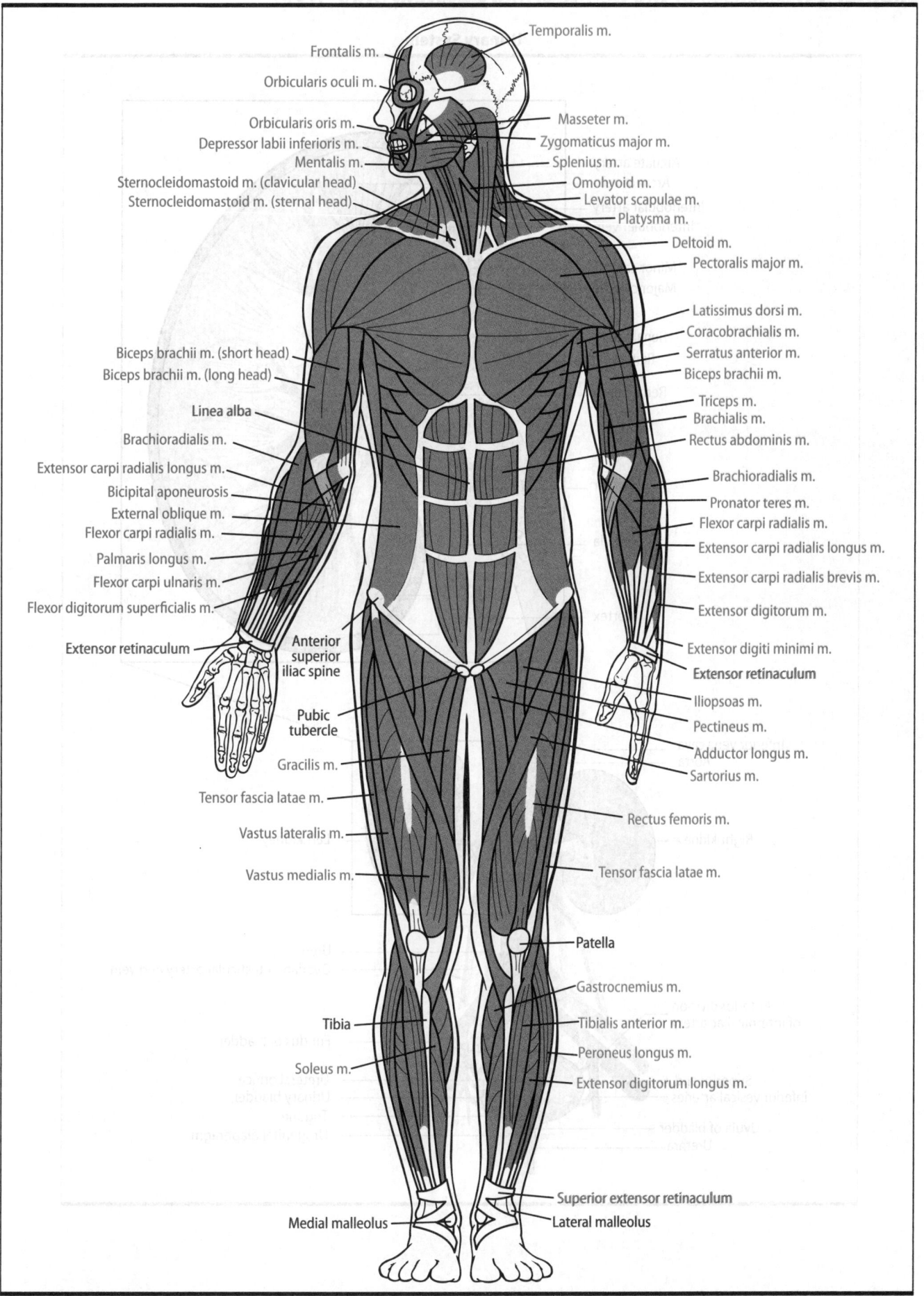

Chapter 14. Diseases of the Genitourinary System (NØØ–N99)

Urinary System

Male Genitourinary System

Female Internal Genitalia

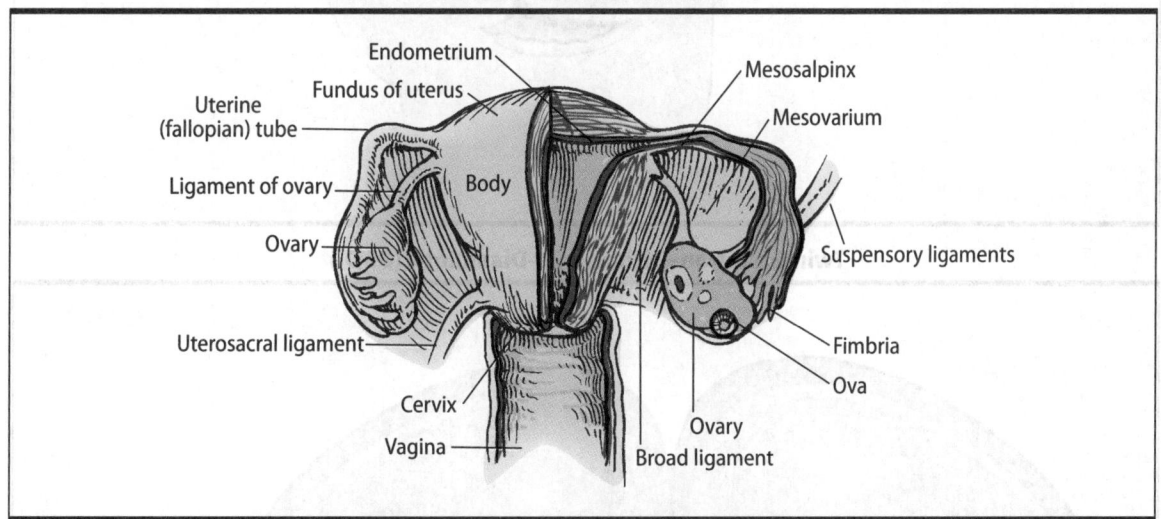

Female Genitourinary Tract Lateral View

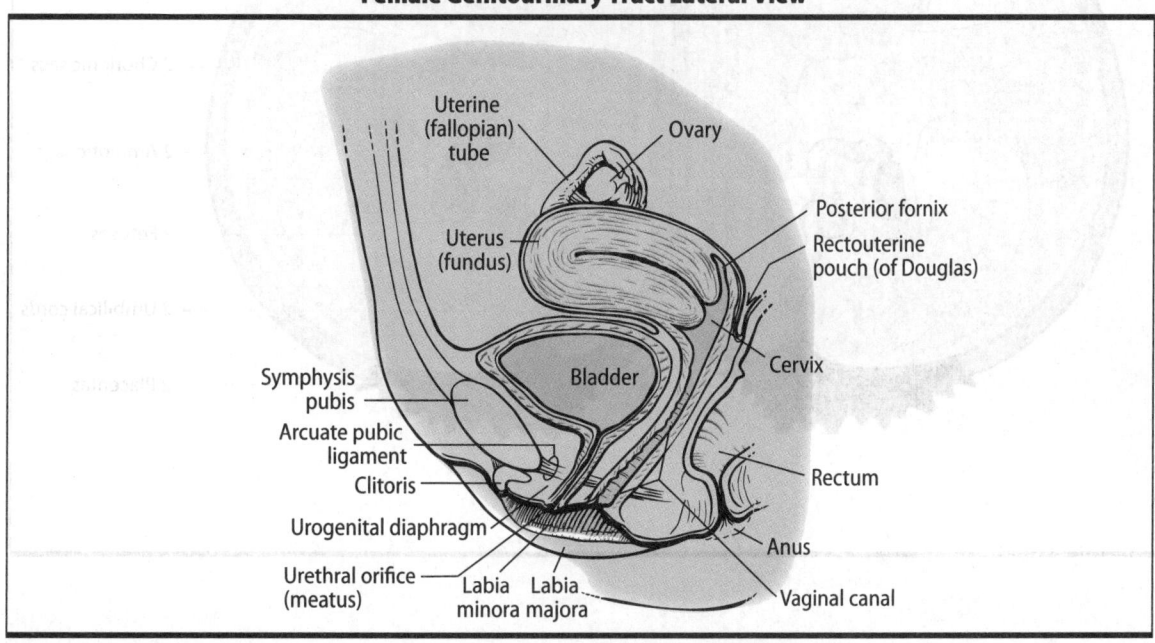

Chapter 15. Pregnancy, Childbirth and the Puerperium (O00–O9A)

Term Pregnancy – Single Gestation

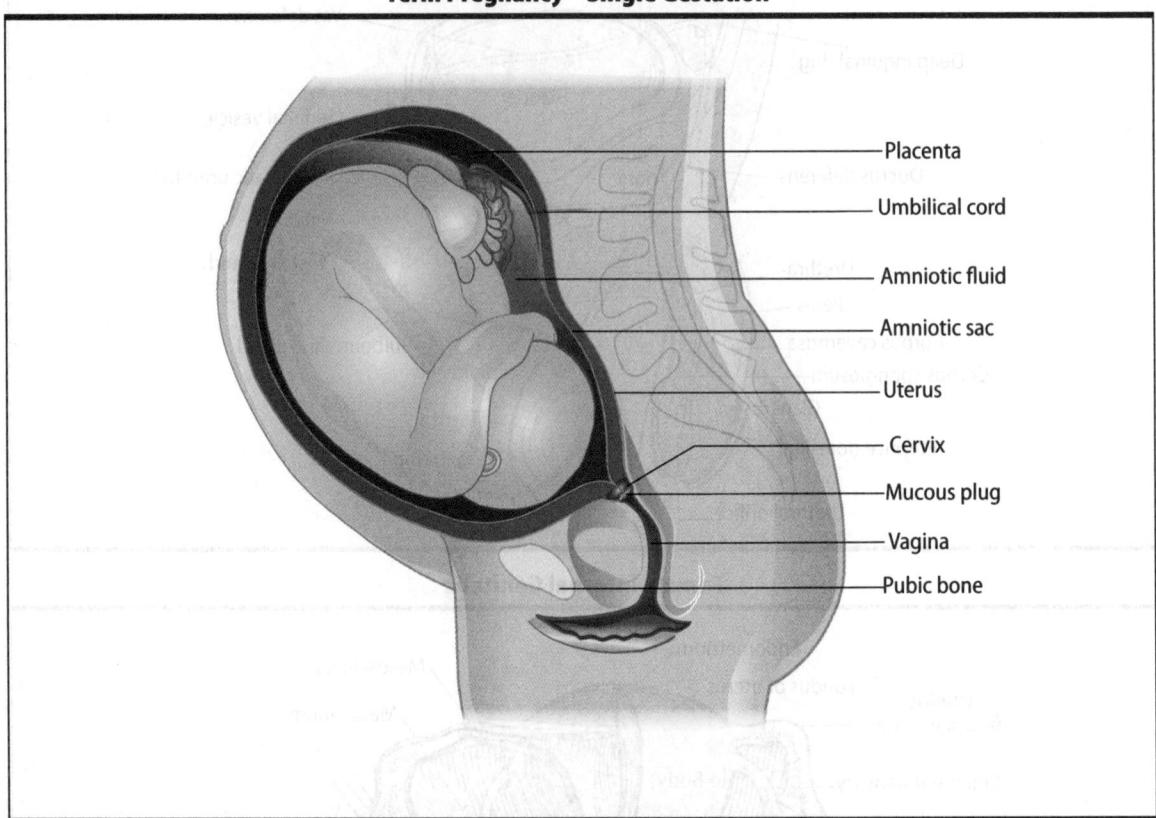

Placenta

Umbilical cord

Amniotic fluid

Amniotic sac

Uterus

Cervix

Mucous plug

Vagina

Pubic bone

Twin Gestation–Dichorionic–Diamniotic (DI-DI)

2 Chorionic sacs

2 Amniotic sacs

2 Fetuses

2 Umbilical cords

2 Placentas

Twin Gestation–Monochorionic–Diamniotic (MO-DI)

1 Chorionic sac

2 Amniotic sacs

2 Fetuses

2 Umbilical cords

1 Placenta

Twin Gestation–Monochorionic–Monoamniotic (MO-MO)

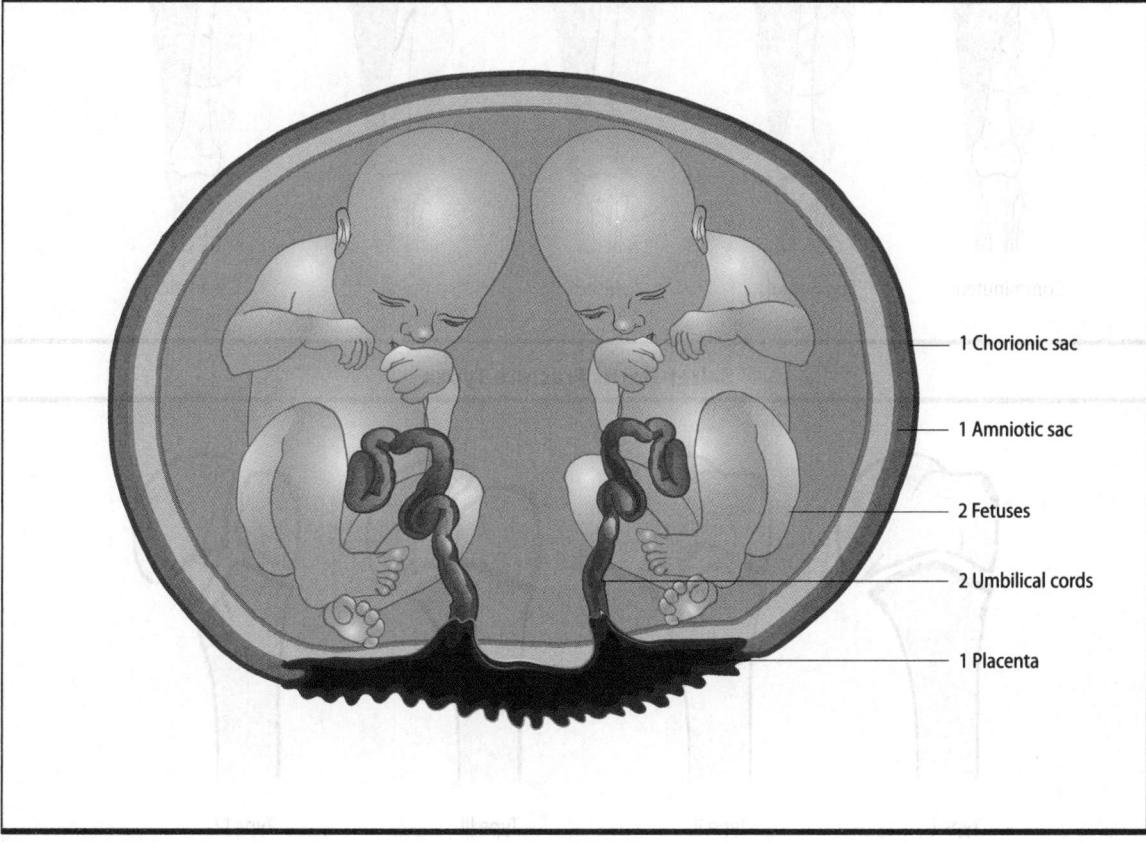

1 Chorionic sac

1 Amniotic sac

2 Fetuses

2 Umbilical cords

1 Placenta

Chapter 19. Injury, Poisoning and Certain Other Consequences of External Causes (SØØ–T88)

Types of Fractures

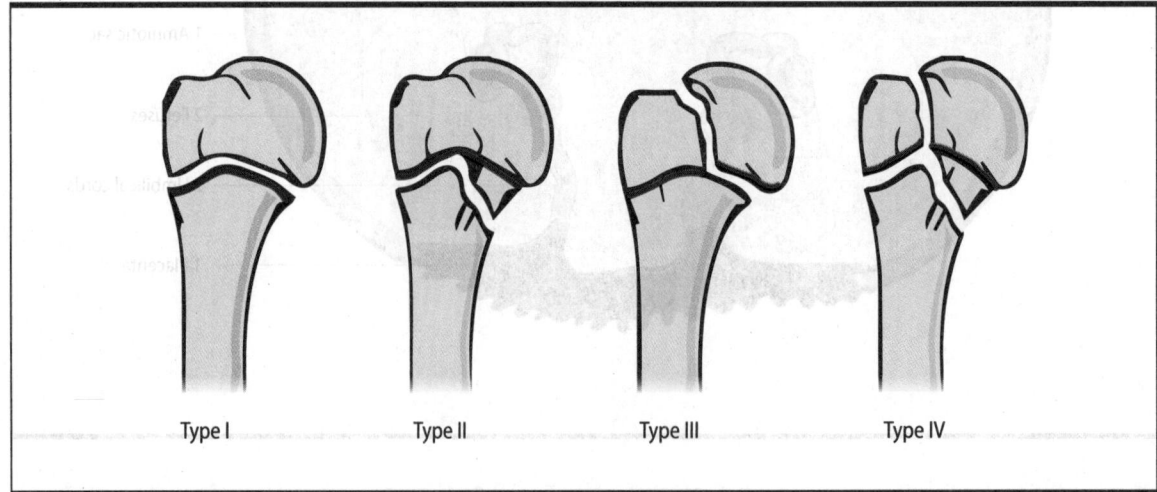

Normal	Transverse	Open/Compound	Oblique	Oblique displaced
Comminuted	Segmental	Avulsed	Spiral	Greenstick

Salter-Harris Fracture Types

Type I	Type II	Type III	Type IV